KEYED TO PDR®

63 EDITION

2009

PDR®

Guide to Drug Interactions, Side Effects, and Indications

ISBN: 978-1-56363-711-7

FOREWORD

Welcome to one of the most useful drug references in current clinical practice, the 2009 edition of the *PDR® Guide to Drug Interactions, Side Effects, and Indications*. Cross-referenced with key facts from the 2009 *Physicians' Desk Reference®*, this unique handbook can help you to provide safe drug management. From its Indications Index, which permits you to instantly identify pharmaceutical alternatives for any given illness, to its Contraindications Index, which just as swiftly singles out alternatives to avoid, this *PDR* guide is designed to make safe, effective prescribing as fast, easy, and accurate as possible. Whether the challenge is identification of an unknown tablet or capsule, detecting the source of an adverse reaction, or avoiding a negative interaction, the *PDR Guide to Drug Interactions, Side Effects, and Indications* provides the tools you need to quickly find the answer. Here's a brief overview of the many features offered in the 2009 edition:

Interactions Index. In this section you'll find an entry for each product described in *PDR* and its companion volumes. Listed are generic compounds and dietary items that may interact with the product, as well as the specific brands containing each generic ingredient. A brief description of the interaction also appears. (Because product labeling varies in the scope of its interaction reporting, be sure to check the listing for each product in the patient's regimen.)

Food Interactions Cross-Reference. If you suspect an interaction with a specific dietary item, turn to this section. There you'll find potential drug/food and drug/alcohol interactions cross-referenced alphabetically by the name or type of food. Each entry includes a list of implicated drugs and a brief description of each interaction.

Side Effects Index. When a multidrug regimen masks the source of a side effect, this section provides the solution. It contains an alphabetical list of more than 4,000 distinct reactions cited throughout *PDR* and its companion volumes. Each entry includes an alphabetical list of the brands that have been associated with the problem. To help target the most likely offenders, incidence data are included whenever found in the official labeling.

Indications Index. If you need to locate an alternative to a problem medication—or simply want to review the full range of options for a particular diagnosis—turn to this part of the book. Here each indication cited in *PDR* and its companions is listed alphabetically, with a cross-reference to all brands approved for that purpose. For easy comparison, the listings include the generic name and manufacturer of each product. (Only FDA-approved indications are referenced.)

Contraindications Index. When therapy is complicated by other medical conditions, this convenient index will enable you to eliminate quickly contraindicated drugs from consideration. Here each contraindication cited in *PDR* is listed alphabetically, together with the drugs to avoid when the problem occurs.

International Drug Name Index. This section enables you to determine quickly a U.S. equivalent when you're confronted with a medication from another country. The index describes the product's country of origin, the closest domestic generic equivalent, all associated *PDR* brand-name entries and their *PDR* page number. Included are more than 33,000 entries covering products from more than 35 nations.

Generic Availability Guide. If you've ever had trouble remembering whether there's a generic alternative for a particular brand, you're sure to appreciate this handy guide. It alerts you to the existence of alternatives, form by form, and strength by strength. Included are all prescription drugs described in *PDR* and *PDR® for Ophthalmic Medicines*.

Imprint Identification Guide. This table permits you to establish quickly the identity of virtually any unknown tablet or capsule. Organized alphabetically by imprint, it supplies the brand or generic name of the drug, its strength and manufacturer, and, to confirm its identity, the color, form, and shape.

Based on the FDA-approved labeling in the 2009 editions of *Physicians' Desk Reference, PDR for Ophthalmic Medicines,* and *PDR® for Nonprescription Drugs, Dietary Supplements, and Herbs*—and augmented with a wealth of authoritative data from such *PDR* affiliates as *Red Book®* and Micromedex—the entries in the *PDR Guide to Drug Interactions, Side Effects, and Indications* cover some 2,400 domestic drug products. Please note, however, that because the entries in the Indications, Contraindications, Interactions, and Side Effects indices are derived directly from the FDA-approved prescribing information published by *PDR*, only products described in *Physicians' Desk Reference* and its main companion volumes are cited in these sections. Please note, also, that the publisher cannot guarantee that all entries are totally accurate or complete, nor is the publisher responsible for misuse of a product due to typographical error. Remember that important qualifications of the information listed in these indices may reside in the underlying text. Use this Guide as a convenient cross-reference, but consult the *PDR* text, as well as the medical literature, when more detailed information is needed.

Web-Based Clinical Resources

PDR.net, a web portal designed specifically for healthcare professionals, provides a wealth of clinical information, including full drug and disease monographs, specialty-specific resource centers, patient education, clinical news, and conference information. PDR.net gives prescribers online access to evidence-based information they need to support or confirm diagnosis and treatment decisions, including:

- Daily feeds of specialty news, conference coverage, and monthly summaries
- FDA-approved and other manufacturer-supplied product labeling for more than 2,400 brand-name drugs
- Multidrug interaction checker and other tools
- Extensive disease diagnosis and treatment information
- Customizable patient education
- Professional resources

PDR.net is also home to our **Clinical Resource Centers**, giving you the latest medical news and disease information all in one easy place. Log on to *www.PDR.net* to visit one of these clinical specialties:

- Allergy and Immunology
- Breast Cancer
- Cardiovascular
- Dermatology
- Diabetes and Endocrinology
- Nephrology
- Neurology
- Pediatrics
- Psychiatry
- Pulmonology
- Rheumatology
- Urology
- Women's Health
- And more

Online access is **free** for U.S.-based MDs, DOs, dentists, NPs, and PAs in full-time patient practice, as well as for medical students, residents, and other select prescribing allied health professionals. Register today at *www.PDR.net.*

Other Clinical Information Products from PDR
For those times when all you need is quick confirmation of a particular dosage, consult the 2009 **PDR® Pharmacopoeia Pocket Dosing Guide**. Only slightly larger than an index card and a half inch thick, it fits easily into any pocket, and provides you with FDA-approved dosing recommendations for more than 1,500 drugs. Unlike other condensed drug references, the information is drawn almost exclusively from the FDA-approved drug labeling published in *Physicians' Desk Reference*. Plus, its tabular presentation makes lookups quick and easy.

PDR® for Nutritional Supplements, 2nd Edition
The **PDR® for Nutritional Supplements, 2nd Edition** is acknowledged as one of the leading, most reliable and comprehensive reference sources on supplements. You'll find in-depth, up-to-date science-based information on these key categories:

- Vitamins
- Metabolites and cofactors
- Proteins
- Lipids
- Probiotics and Prebiotics
- Phytosupplements
- Nucleic Acids
- Amino Acids and Oligopeptides
- Mycosupplements
- Glycosupplements
- Hormonal products

Plus you'll find new additions such as hyaluronic acid, lactotripeptides, and food peptides, and major updates on supplements such as beta-carotene, brewer's yeast, calcium, flaxseed oil, and copper.

Since supplements are not regulated by the FDA, healthcare providers need a trusted, research-based resource to help guide them in learning how supplements work, including the presence of any adverse reactions or interactions. The **PDR® for Nutritional Supplements, 2nd Edition** helps separate fact from fiction.

For counseling patients who favor herbal remedies, the newly updated **PDR® for Herbal Medicines, Fourth Edition** provides you with a recent science-based assessment of more than 700 botanicals. Indexed by scientific and common names (as well as Western, Asian, and homeopathic indications), this volume also includes a Side Effects Index, a Drug/Herb Interactions Guide, an Herb Identification Guide with nearly 400 color photos, and a Safety Guide that lists herbs to be avoided during pregnancy and herbs to be used only under professional supervision. Although botanical products are not officially regulated or monitored in the United States, *PDR for Herbal Medicines* provides you with authoritative information—the findings of the German Regulatory Authority's expert committee on herbal medicines, Commission E.

PDR and its major companion volumes are also found in the **PDR® Electronic Library** on CD-ROM. This Windows-compatible disc provides users with a complete database of *PDR* prescribing information, electronically searchable for instant retrieval. A standard subscription includes *PDR's* sophisticated search software and an extensive file of chemical structures, illustrations, and full-color product photographs. Optional enhancements include the complete contents of *The Merck Manual Seventeenth Edition, Stedman's Medical Dictionary*, and *Stedman's Spellchecker*. For anyone who wants to run a fast double check on a proposed prescription, there's also the *PDR® Drug Interactions and Side Effects System*—sophisticated software capable of automatically screening a 20-drug regimen for conflicts, then proposing alternatives for any problematic medication. This unique decision-making tool comes free with the *PDR Electronic Library*. For more information on these or any other members of the growing family of *PDR* products, please call, toll-free, 800-232-7379 or fax 201-722-2680.

CONTENTS

Section 1
Interactions Index ... 1

Section 2
Food Interactions Cross-Reference ... 1703

Section 3
Side Effects Index ... 1715

Section 4
Indications Index ... 1957

Section 5
Contraindications Index ... 2005

Section 6
International Drug Name Index ... 2019

Section 7
Generic Availability Guide ... 2117

Section 8
Imprint Identification Guide ... 2127

Key to Controlled Substances Categories ... 2237
Gives the definition of each category and the prescribing limitations that apply.

Key to FDA Use-In-Pregnancy Ratings ... 2237
Provides at-a-glance description of each risk/benefit rating.

U.S. Food and Drug Administration Telephone Directory ... 2239
Gives numbers of key reporting programs and information services.

Poison Control Centers ... 2241
A national directory arranged alphabetically by state and city.

Drug Information Centers ... 2245
A national directory arranged alphabetically by state and city.

SECTION 1

INTERACTIONS INDEX

Cataloged in this section are all interactions found during a review of the labeling published in *PDR®*, *PDR® For Nonprescription Drugs, Dietary Supplements and Herbs,* and *PDR® For Ophthalmic Medicines.* The list is arranged alphabetically by brand or, when applicable, generic name.

Whenever appropriate, each brand-name heading is followed by a summary of the major pharmaceutical categories with which the product is said to interact. Beneath this summary is an alphabetical list of the compounds in these categories, each followed by a brief notation regarding the results of concurrent administration with the brand in question. After each notation is an alphabetical list of the brands of the compound found in *PDR®* and its companion volumes.

Page numbers refer to the 2009 editions of *PDR®*, *PDR® For Ophthalmic Medicines* and *PDR® For Nonprescription Drugs, Dietary Supplements and Herbs.* A key to the symbols denoting the companion volumes appears in the bottom margin of every other page.

Following the list of interactive drugs is a similar list of foods. Note that interactions with alcohol are listed here as well.

This index lists only interactions cited in official prescribing information as published by *PDR®*. Because product labeling varies in the scope of its interaction reporting, the most prudent course is to check each product in the patient's regimen. Note also that cross-sensitivity reactions and effects on laboratory results are not included in the listings.

ABELCET INJECTION
(Amphotericin B Lipid Complex) 1134
May interact with aminoglycosides, antineoplastics, corticosteroids, curariform skeletal muscle relaxants, cardiac glycosides, imidazoles, and certain other agents. Compounds in these categories include:

ACTH (Concurrent use may potentiate hypokalemia which could predispose the patient to cardiac dysfunction).
No products indexed under this heading.

Altretamine (Concurrent use may enhance the potential for renal toxicity, bronchospasm and hypotension). Products include:
Hexalen Capsules 1078

Amikacin Sulfate (Concurrent use may enhance the potential for drug-induced renal toxicity).
No products indexed under this heading.

Anastrozole (Concurrent use may enhance the potential for renal toxicity, bronchospasm and hypotension). Products include:
Arimidex Tablets 672

Asparaginase (Concurrent use may enhance the potential for renal toxicity, bronchospasm and hypotension). Products include:
Elspar for Injection 1990
Elspar for Injection 2488

Atracurium Besylate (Amphotericin B-induced hypokalemia may enhance the curariform effect of skeletal relaxants).
No products indexed under this heading.

Betamethasone Acetate (Concurrent use may potentiate hypokalemia which could predispose the patient to cardiac dysfunction).
No products indexed under this heading.

Betamethasone Sodium Phosphate (Concurrent use may potentiate hypokalemia which could predispose the patient to cardiac dysfunction).
No products indexed under this heading.

Bicalutamide (Concurrent use may enhance the potential for renal toxicity, bronchospasm and hypotension). Products include:
No products indexed under this heading.

Bleomycin Sulfate (Concurrent use may enhance the potential for renal toxicity, bronchospasm and hypotension).
No products indexed under this heading.

Budesonide (Concurrent use may potentiate hypokalemia which could predispose the patient to cardiac dysfunction). Products include:
Pulmicort Flexhaler 654
Symbicort 80/4.5 Inhalation Aerosol 659
Symbicort 160/4.5 Inhalation Aerosol 659

Busulfan (Concurrent use may enhance the potential for renal toxicity, bronchospasm and hypotension). Products include:
Busulfex Injection 2477
Myleran Tablets 1530

Carboplatin (Concurrent use may enhance the potential for renal toxicity, bronchospasm and hypotension).
No products indexed under this heading.

Carmustine (BCNU) (Concurrent use may enhance the potential for renal toxicity, bronchospasm and hypotension).
No products indexed under this heading.

Chlorambucil (Concurrent use may enhance the potential for renal toxicity, bronchospasm and hypotension). Products include:
Leukeran Tablets 1508

Ciclesonide (Concurrent use may potentiate hypokalemia which could predispose the patient to cardiac dysfunction). Products include:
Alvesco Inhalation Aerosol 2985
Omnaris Nasal Spray 2998

Cisatracurium Besylate (Amphotericin B-induced hypokalemia may enhance the curariform effect of skeletal relaxants). Products include:
Nimbex Injection 484

Cisplatin (Concurrent use may enhance the potential for renal toxicity, bronchospasm and hypotension).
No products indexed under this heading.

Clotrimazole (Antagonism between amphotericin B and imidazole derivatives, which inhibit ergosterol synthesis, has been reported; clinical significance of this finding has not been determined). Products include:
Lotrisone 2881

Cortisone Acetate (Concurrent use may potentiate hypokalemia which could predispose the patient to cardiac dysfunction).
No products indexed under this heading.

Cyclophosphamide (Concurrent use may enhance the potential for renal toxicity, bronchospasm and hypotension).
No products indexed under this heading.

Cyclosporine (Concurrent initiation of cyclosporine and Abelcet within several days of bone marrow ablation may be associated with increased nephrotoxicity). Products include:
Gengraf Capsules 435
Neoral Oral Solution 2280
Neoral Soft Gelatin Capsules 2280
Restasis Ophthalmic Emulsion 557
Sandimmune 2296

Dacarbazine (Concurrent use may enhance the potential for renal toxicity, bronchospasm and hypotension).
No products indexed under this heading.

IMPORTANT NOTE: Always consult each drug listing in the patient's regimen for possible interactions.

Daunorubicin Citrate (Concurrent use may enhance the potential for renal toxicity, bronchospasm and hypotension).
No products indexed under this heading.

Daunorubicin Hydrochloride (Concurrent use may enhance the potential for renal toxicity, bronchospasm and hypotension).
No products indexed under this heading.

Denileukin Diftitox (Concurrent use may enhance the potential for renal toxicity, bronchospasm and hypotension). Products include:
Ontak Vials **1079**

Deslanoside (Concurrent use may induce hypokalemia and may potentiate digitalis toxicity).
No products indexed under this heading.

Dexamethasone (Concurrent use may potentiate hypokalemia which could predispose the patient to cardiac dysfunction). Products include:
Ciprodex Otic Suspension **541**

Dexamethasone Acetate (Concurrent use may potentiate hypokalemia which could predispose the patient to cardiac dysfunction).
No products indexed under this heading.

Dexamethasone Sodium Phosphate (Concurrent use may potentiate hypokalemia which could predispose the patient to cardiac dysfunction).
No products indexed under this heading.

Digitalis Glycoside Preparations (Concurrent use may induce hypokalemia and may potentiate digitalis toxicity).
No products indexed under this heading.

Digitoxin (Concurrent use may induce hypokalemia and may potentiate digitalis toxicity).
No products indexed under this heading.

Digoxin (Concurrent use may induce hypokalemia and may potentiate digitalis toxicity). Products include:
Lanoxin Injection **1498**
Lanoxin Injection Pediatric **1502**
Lanoxin Tablets **1505**

Docetaxel (Concurrent use may enhance the potential for renal toxicity, bronchospasm and hypotension). Products include:
Taxotere Injection Concentrate **2773**

Doxacurium Chloride (Amphotericin B-induced hypokalemia may enhance the curariform effect of skeletal relaxants).
No products indexed under this heading.

Doxorubicin Hydrochloride (Concurrent use may enhance the potential for renal toxicity, bronchospasm and hypotension).
No products indexed under this heading.

Epirubicin Hydrochloride (Concurrent use may enhance the potential for renal toxicity, bronchospasm and hypotension).
No products indexed under this heading.

Estramustine Phosphate Sodium (Concurrent use may enhance the potential for renal toxicity, bronchospasm and hypotension).
No products indexed under this heading.

Etoposide (Concurrent use may enhance the potential for renal toxicity, bronchospasm and hypotension).
No products indexed under this heading.

Exemestane (Concurrent use may enhance the potential for renal toxicity, bronchospasm and hypotension).
No products indexed under this heading.

Floxuridine (Concurrent use may enhance the potential for renal toxicity, bronchospasm and hypotension).
No products indexed under this heading.

Fluconazole (Antagonism between amphotericin B and imidazole derivatives, which inhibit ergosterol synthesis, has been reported; clinical significance of this finding has not been determined).
No products indexed under this heading.

Flucytosine (Concurrent use may increase the toxicity of flucytosine by possibly increasing its cellular uptake and/or impairing its renal excretion).
No products indexed under this heading.

Fludrocortisone Acetate (Concurrent use may potentiate hypokalemia which could predispose the patient to cardiac dysfunction).
No products indexed under this heading.

Flunisolide (Concurrent use may potentiate hypokalemia which could predispose the patient to cardiac dysfunction). Products include:
Aerobid/Aerobid-M **1153**

Fluorouracil (Concurrent use may enhance the potential for renal toxicity, bronchospasm and hypotension). Products include:
Carac Cream 0.5% **2722**

Flutamide (Concurrent use may enhance the potential for renal toxicity, bronchospasm and hypotension).
No products indexed under this heading.

Fluticasone Propionate (Concurrent use may potentiate hypokalemia which could predispose the patient to cardiac dysfunction). Products include:
Advair Diskus 100/50 .... **1276**
Advair Diskus 250/50 .... **1276**
Advair Diskus 500/50 .... **1276**
Advair HFA 45/21 Inhalation Aerosol...................................... **1288**
Advair HFA 115/21 Inhalation Aerosol...................................... **1288**
Advair HFA 230/21 Inhalation Aerosol...................................... **1288**
Flonase Nasal Spray **1431**
Flovent Diskus 50 mcg **1435**

Fluticasone Propionate HFA (Concurrent use may potentiate hypokalemia which could predispose the patient to cardiac dysfunction). Products include:
Flovent HFA **1440**

Gemcitabine Hydrochloride (Concurrent use may enhance the potential for renal toxicity, bronchospasm and hypotension). Products include:
Gemzar for Injection **1820**

Gentamicin Sulfate (Concurrent use may enhance the potential for drug-induced renal toxicity). Products include:
Pred-G Ophthalmic Ointment .... ⊙**229**
Pred-G Ophthalmic Suspension ...... ⊙**228**

Hydrocortisone (Concurrent use may potentiate hypokalemia which could predispose the patient to cardiac dysfunction).
No products indexed under this heading.

Hydrocortisone Acetate (Concurrent use may potentiate hypokalemia which could predispose the patient to cardiac dysfunction). Products include:
Analpram-HC **1140**
Pramosone **1141**

Hydrocortisone Sodium Phosphate (Concurrent use may potentiate hypokalemia which could predispose the patient to cardiac dysfunction).
No products indexed under this heading.

Hydrocortisone Sodium Succinate (Concurrent use may potentiate hypokalemia which could predispose the patient to cardiac dysfunction).
No products indexed under this heading.

Hydroxyurea (Concurrent use may enhance the potential for renal toxicity, bronchospasm and hypotension).
No products indexed under this heading.

Idarubicin Hydrochloride (Concurrent use may enhance the potential for renal toxicity, bronchospasm and hypotension).
No products indexed under this heading.

Ifosfamide (Concurrent use may enhance the potential for renal toxicity, bronchospasm and hypotension).
No products indexed under this heading.

Interferon alfa-2a, Recombinant (Concurrent use may enhance the potential for renal toxicity, bronchospasm and hypotension).
No products indexed under this heading.

Interferon alfa-2b, Recombinant (Concurrent use may enhance the potential for renal toxicity, bronchospasm and hypotension). Products include:
Intron A for Injection **2859**

Irinotecan Hydrochloride (Concurrent use may enhance the potential for renal toxicity, bronchospasm and hypotension).
No products indexed under this heading.

Kanamycin Sulfate (Concurrent use may enhance the potential for drug-induced renal toxicity).
No products indexed under this heading.

Ketoconazole (Antagonism between amphotericin B and imidazole derivatives, which inhibit ergosterol synthesis, has been reported; clinical significance of this finding has not been determined). Products include:
Extina Foam, 2% **3057**
Nizoral A-D Shampoo **1901**

Leukocyte Transfusions (Concurrent use has resulted in acute pulmonary toxicity; concurrent use should be avoided).
No products indexed under this heading.

Levamisole Hydrochloride (Concurrent use may enhance the potential for renal toxicity, bronchospasm and hypotension).
No products indexed under this heading.

Lomustine (CCNU) (Concurrent use may enhance the potential for renal toxicity, bronchospasm and hypotension).
No products indexed under this heading.

Mechlorethamine Hydrochloride (Concurrent use may enhance the potential for renal toxicity, bronchospasm and hypotension). Products include:
Mustargen for Injection **2492**

Megestrol Acetate (Concurrent use may enhance the potential for renal toxicity, bronchospasm and hypotension). Products include:
Megace ES Oral Suspension **2499**

Melphalan (Concurrent use may enhance the potential for renal toxicity, bronchospasm and hypotension).
No products indexed under this heading.

Mercaptopurine (Concurrent use may enhance the potential for renal toxicity, bronchospasm and hypotension).
No products indexed under this heading.

Methotrexate Sodium (Concurrent use may enhance the potential for renal toxicity, bronchospasm and hypotension).
No products indexed under this heading.

Methylprednisolone Acetate (Concurrent use may potentiate hypokalemia which could predispose the patient to cardiac dysfunction).
No products indexed under this heading.

Methylprednisolone Sodium Succinate (Concurrent use may potentiate hypokalemia which could predispose the patient to cardiac dysfunction).
No products indexed under this heading.

Metocurine Iodide (Amphotericin B-induced hypokalemia may enhance the curariform effect of skeletal relaxants).
No products indexed under this heading.

Miconazole (Antagonism between amphotericin B and imidazole derivatives, which inhibit ergosterol synthesis, has been reported; clinical significance of this finding has not been determined).
No products indexed under this heading.

Miconazole Nitrate (Antagonism between amphotericin B and imidazole derivatives, which inhibit ergosterol synthesis, has been reported; clinical significance of this finding has not been determined).
No products indexed under this heading.

Mitomycin (Mitomycin-C) (Concurrent use may enhance the potential for renal toxicity, bronchospasm and hypotension).
No products indexed under this heading.

Mitotane (Concurrent use may enhance the potential for renal toxicity, bronchospasm and hypotension).
No products indexed under this heading.

Mitoxantrone Hydrochloride (Concurrent use may enhance the potential for renal toxicity, bronchospasm and hypotension). Products include:

Novantrone for Injection Concentrate 1100

Mivacurium Chloride (Amphotericin B-induced hypokalemia may enhance the curariform effect of skeletal relaxants).
No products indexed under this heading.

Mometasone Furoate (Concurrent use may potentiate hypokalemia which could predispose the patient to cardiac dysfunction). Products include:
Asmanex Twisthaler 2797
Elocon Cream 0.1% 2840
Elocon Lotion 0.1% 2841
Elocon Ointment 0.1% 2842

Mometasone Furoate Monohydrate (Concurrent use may potentiate hypokalemia which could predispose the patient to cardiac dysfunction). Products include:
Nasonex Nasal Spray 2883

Oxaliplatin (Concurrent use may enhance the potential for renal toxicity, bronchospasm and hypotension). Products include:
Eloxatin for Injection 2731

Paclitaxel (Concurrent use may enhance the potential for renal toxicity, bronchospasm and hypotension).
No products indexed under this heading.

Pancuronium Bromide (Amphotericin B-induced hypokalemia may enhance the curariform effect of skeletal relaxants).
No products indexed under this heading.

Pentamidine Isethionate (Concurrent use may enhance the potential for drug-induced renal toxicity).
No products indexed under this heading.

Pipecuronium Bromide (Amphotericin B-induced hypokalemia may enhance the curariform effect of skeletal relaxants).
No products indexed under this heading.

Prednisolone Acetate (Concurrent use may potentiate hypokalemia which could predispose the patient to cardiac dysfunction). Products include:
Pred Forte Ophthalmic Suspension .... ⊙227
Pred Mild Ophthalmic Suspension .... ⊙230
Pred-G Ophthalmic Ointment .... ⊙229
Pred-G Ophthalmic Suspension .... ⊙228

Prednisolone Sodium Phosphate (Concurrent use may potentiate hypokalemia which could predispose the patient to cardiac dysfunction).
No products indexed under this heading.

Prednisolone Tebutate (Concurrent use may potentiate hypokalemia which could predispose the patient to cardiac dysfunction).
No products indexed under this heading.

Prednisone (Concurrent use may potentiate hypokalemia which could predispose the patient to cardiac dysfunction).
No products indexed under this heading.

Procarbazine Hydrochloride (Concurrent use may enhance the potential for renal toxicity, bronchospasm and hypotension).
No products indexed under this heading.

Rapacuronium Bromide (Amphotericin B-induced hypokalemia may enhance the curariform effect of skeletal relaxants).
No products indexed under this heading.

Rocuronium Bromide (Amphotericin B-induced hypokalemia may enhance the curariform effect of skeletal relaxants). Products include:
Zemuron Injection 2947

Streptomycin Sulfate (Concurrent use may enhance the potential for drug-induced renal toxicity).
No products indexed under this heading.

Streptozocin (Concurrent use may enhance the potential for renal toxicity, bronchospasm and hypotension).
No products indexed under this heading.

Tamoxifen Citrate (Concurrent use may enhance the potential for renal toxicity, bronchospasm and hypotension).
No products indexed under this heading.

Teniposide (Concurrent use may enhance the potential for renal toxicity, bronchospasm and hypotension).
No products indexed under this heading.

Thioguanine (Concurrent use may enhance the potential for renal toxicity, bronchospasm and hypotension). Products include:
Tabloid Tablets 1601

Thiotepa (Concurrent use may enhance the potential for renal toxicity, bronchospasm and hypotension).
No products indexed under this heading.

Tobramycin (Concurrent use may enhance the potential for drug-induced renal toxicity). Products include:
Zylet Ophthalmic Suspension .... ⊙247

Tobramycin Sulfate (Concurrent use may enhance the potential for drug-induced renal toxicity).
No products indexed under this heading.

Topotecan Hydrochloride (Concurrent use may enhance the potential for renal toxicity, bronchospasm and hypotension). Products include:
Hycamtin for Injection 1459
Hycamtin Capsules 1456

Toremifene Citrate (Concurrent use may enhance the potential for renal toxicity, bronchospasm and hypotension).
No products indexed under this heading.

Triamcinolone (Concurrent use may potentiate hypokalemia which could predispose the patient to cardiac dysfunction).
No products indexed under this heading.

Triamcinolone Acetonide (Concurrent use may potentiate hypokalemia which could predispose the patient to cardiac dysfunction). Products include:
Azmacort Inhalation Aerosol 407
Nasacort AQ Nasal Spray 2765
Triesence Injectable Suspension .... ⊙209

Triamcinolone Diacetate (Concurrent use may potentiate hypokalemia which could predispose the patient to cardiac dysfunction).
No products indexed under this heading.

Triamcinolone Hexacetonide (Concurrent use may potentiate hypokalemia which could predispose the patient to cardiac dysfunction).
No products indexed under this heading.

Tubocurarine Chloride (Amphotericin B-induced hypokalemia may enhance the curariform effect of skeletal muscle relaxants).
No products indexed under this heading.

Valrubicin (Concurrent use may enhance the potential for renal toxicity, bronchospasm and hypotension). Products include:
Valstar Sterile Solution for Intravesical Instillation 1735

Vecuronium Bromide (Amphotericin B-induced hypokalemia may enhance the curariform effect of skeletal relaxants).
No products indexed under this heading.

Vincristine Sulfate (Concurrent use may enhance the potential for renal toxicity, bronchospasm and hypotension).
No products indexed under this heading.

Vinorelbine Tartrate (Concurrent use may enhance the potential for renal toxicity, bronchospasm and hypotension).
No products indexed under this heading.

Zidovudine (Potential for increased myelotoxicity and nephrotoxicity). Products include:
Combivir Tablets 1384
Retrovir 1574
Retrovir IV Infusion 1579
Trizivir Tablets 1622

ABILIFY INJECTION

(Aripiprazole) 881
See Abilify Tablets

ABILIFY INJECTION

(Aripiprazole) 2466
See Abilify Tablets

ABILIFY ORAL SOLUTION

(Aripiprazole) 881
See Abilify Tablets

ABILIFY ORAL SOLUTION

(Aripiprazole) 2466
See Abilify Tablets

ABILIFY DISCMELT ORALLY DISINTEGRATING TABLETS

(Aripiprazole) 881
See Abilify Tablets

ABILIFY DISCMELT ORALLY DISINTEGRATING TABLETS

(Aripiprazole) 2466
See Abilify Tablets

ABILIFY TABLETS

(Aripiprazole) 881

May interact with antihypertensives, central nervous system depressants, central nervous system stimulants, cytochrome p450 2d6 inhibitors (selected), cytochrome p450 3a4 inducers (selected), cytochrome p450 3a4 inhibitors (selected), cytochrome p450 3a4 inhibitors, potent, quinidine, and certain other agents. Compounds in these categories include:

Acebutolol Hydrochloride (Due to its alpha-1-adrenergic receptor antagonism, aripiprazole has the potential to enhance the effect of certain antihypertensive agents).
No products indexed under this heading.

Acetazolamide (Inhibitors of CYP3A4 can inhibit aripiprazole elimination and cause increased blood levels).
No products indexed under this heading.

Alfentanil Hydrochloride (Given the primary CNS effects of aripiprazole, caution should be used when co-administered with other centrally acting drugs).
No products indexed under this heading.

Aliskiren (Due to its alpha-1-adrenergic receptor antagonism, aripiprazole has the potential to enhance the effect of certain antihypertensive agents). Products include:
Tekturna Tablets 2321
Tekturna HCT Tablets 2324

Allium sativum (Agents that induce CYP3A4 could cause an increase in aripiprazole clearance and lower blood levels).
No products indexed under this heading.

Alprazolam (Given the primary CNS effects of aripiprazole, caution should be used when co-administered with other centrally acting drugs).
No products indexed under this heading.

Amiodarone Hydrochloride (Inhibitors of CYP3A4 can inhibit aripiprazole elimination and cause increased blood levels).
No products indexed under this heading.

Amitriptyline Hydrochloride (Inhibitors of CYP2D6 can inhibit aripiprazole elimination and cause increased blood levels).
No products indexed under this heading.

Amlodipine Besylate (Due to its alpha-1-adrenergic receptor antagonism, aripiprazole has the potential to enhance the effect of certain antihypertensive agents). Products include:
Azor Tablets 1005
Exforge Tablets 2238

Amoxapine (Inhibitors of CYP2D6 can inhibit aripiprazole elimination and cause increased blood levels).
No products indexed under this heading.

Amphetamine Resins (Given the primary CNS effects of aripiprazole, caution should be used when co-administered with other centrally acting drugs).
No products indexed under this heading.

Amprenavir (Strong inhibitors of CYP3A4 may increase levels of aripiprazole and its active metabolite; dose reduction of aripiprazole should be considered).
No products indexed under this heading.

Anastrozole (Inhibitors of CYP3A4 can inhibit aripiprazole elimination and cause increased blood levels). Products include:
Arimidex Tablets 672

Aprepitant (Agents that induce CYP3A4 could cause an increase in aripiprazole clearance and lower blood levels). Products include:
Emend Capsules 1992

Aprobarbital (Given the primary CNS effects of aripiprazole, caution should be used when co-administered with other centrally acting drugs).
No products indexed under this heading.

Atazanavir (Strong inhibitors of CYP3A4 may increase levels of aripiprazole and its active metabolite; dose reduction of aripiprazole should be considered).
No products indexed under this heading.

Atazanavir Sulfate (Strong inhibitors of CYP3A4 may increase levels of aripiprazole and its active metabolite; dose reduction of aripiprazole should be considered). Products include:
Reyataz Capsules 3299

Atenolol (Due to its alpha-1-adrenergic receptor antagonism, aripiprazole has the potential to enhance the effect of certain antihypertensive agents).
No products indexed under this heading.

Benazepril Hydrochloride (Due to its alpha-1-adrenergic receptor antagonism, aripiprazole has the potential to enhance the effect of certain antihypertensive agents).
No products indexed under this heading.

Bendroflumethiazide (Due to its alpha-1-adrenergic receptor antagonism, aripiprazole has the potential to enhance the effect of certain antihypertensive agents).
No products indexed under this heading.

Betamethasone Acetate (Agents that induce CYP3A4 could cause an increase in aripiprazole clearance and lower blood levels).
No products indexed under this heading.

Betamethasone Sodium Phosphate (Agents that induce CYP3A4 could cause an increase in aripiprazole clearance and lower blood levels).
No products indexed under this heading.

Betaxolol Hydrochloride (Due to its alpha-1-adrenergic receptor antagonism, aripiprazole has the potential to enhance the effect of certain antihypertensive agents).
No products indexed under this heading.

Bisoprolol Fumarate (Due to its alpha-1-adrenergic receptor antagonism, aripiprazole has the potential to enhance the effect of certain antihypertensive agents).
No products indexed under this heading.

Buprenorphine Hydrochloride (Given the primary CNS effects of aripiprazole, caution should be used when co-administered with other centrally acting drugs). Products include:
Suboxone Tablets 2601
Subutex Tablets 2601

Bupropion Hydrochloride (Inhibitors of CYP2D6 can inhibit aripiprazole elimination and cause increased blood levels). Products include:
Wellbutrin Tablets 1648
Wellbutrin SR Sustained-Release Tablets 1653
Wellbutrin XL Extended-Release Tablets 1659
Zyban Sustained-Release Tablets 1692

Buspirone Hydrochloride (Given the primary CNS effects of aripiprazole, caution should be used when co-administered with other centrally acting drugs).
No products indexed under this heading.

Butabarbital (Given the primary CNS effects of aripiprazole, caution should be used when co-administered with other centrally acting drugs).
No products indexed under this heading.

Butalbital (Given the primary CNS effects of aripiprazole, caution should be used when co-administered with other centrally acting drugs).
No products indexed under this heading.

Candesartan Cilexetil (Due to its alpha-1-adrenergic receptor antagonism, aripiprazole has the potential to enhance the effect of certain antihypertensive agents). Products include:
Atacand Tablets 639
Atacand HCT 642

Captopril (Due to its alpha-1-adrenergic receptor antagonism, aripiprazole has the potential to enhance the effect of certain antihypertensive agents). Products include:
Captopril Tablets 2182

Carbamazepine (Co-administration of carbamazepine, a potent CYP3A4 inducer, with aripiprazole resulted in an approximate 70% decrease in Cmax and AUC values of both aripiprazole and its active metabolite, dehydro-aripiprazole. When carbamazepine is added to aripiprazole therapy, aripiprazole dose should be doubled. When carbamazepine is withdrawn from combination therapy, aripiprazole dose should then be reduced). Products include:
Carbatrol Capsules 3019
Equetro Extended-Release Capsules 3174

Carteolol Hydrochloride (Due to its alpha-1-adrenergic receptor antagonism, aripiprazole has the potential to enhance the effect of certain antihypertensive agents).
No products indexed under this heading.

Celecoxib (Inhibitors of CYP2D6 can inhibit aripiprazole elimination and cause increased blood levels). Products include:
Celebrex Capsules 2979

Chlordiazepoxide (Given the primary CNS effects of aripiprazole, caution should be used when co-administered with other centrally acting drugs).
No products indexed under this heading.

Chlordiazepoxide Hydrochloride (Given the primary CNS effects of aripiprazole, caution should be used when co-administered with other centrally acting drugs).
No products indexed under this heading.

Chloroquine Hydrochloride (Inhibitors of CYP2D6 can inhibit aripiprazole elimination and cause increased blood levels).
No products indexed under this heading.

Chloroquine Phosphate (Inhibitors of CYP2D6 can inhibit aripiprazole elimination and cause increased blood levels).
No products indexed under this heading.

Chlorothiazide (Due to its alpha-1-adrenergic receptor antagonism, aripiprazole has the potential to enhance the effect of certain antihypertensive agents).
No products indexed under this heading.

Chlorothiazide Sodium (Due to its alpha-1-adrenergic receptor antagonism, aripiprazole has the potential to enhance the effect of certain antihypertensive agents). Products include:
Intravenous Sodium Diuril 2490

Chlorpheniramine (Inhibitors of CYP2D6 can inhibit aripiprazole elimination and cause increased blood levels).
No products indexed under this heading.

Chlorpheniramine Maleate (Inhibitors of CYP2D6 can inhibit aripiprazole elimination and cause increased blood levels). Products include:
Actifed Cold & Allergy Tablets 1895
Sudafed PE Sinus & Allergy Tablets 1908
Tylenol Allergy Multi-Symptom Caplets with Cool Burst and Rapid Release Gelcaps 1916
Children's Tylenol Plus Cold Suspension Liquid 1912
Children's Tylenol Plus Cough & Runny Nose Suspension Liquid 1912
Children's Tylenol Plus Flu Suspension Liquid 1914
Children's Tylenol Plus Multi-Symptom Cold Suspension Liquid 1912
Tylenol Cold Head Congestion Nighttime Caplets with Cool Burst 1910
Tylenol Cold Multi-Symptom Nighttime Caplets with Cool Burst 1913
Tylenol Sinus Congestion & Pain Nighttime Caplets with Cool Burst 1917

Chlorpheniramine Polistirex (Inhibitors of CYP2D6 can inhibit aripiprazole elimination and cause increased blood levels). Products include:
Tussionex Pennkinetic Extended-Release Suspension 3154

Chlorpheniramine Tannate (Inhibitors of CYP2D6 can inhibit aripiprazole elimination and cause increased blood levels).
No products indexed under this heading.

Chlorpromazine (Given the primary CNS effects of aripiprazole, caution should be used when co-administered with other centrally acting drugs).
No products indexed under this heading.

Chlorpromazine Hydrochloride (Given the primary CNS effects of aripiprazole, caution should be used when co-administered with other centrally acting drugs).
No products indexed under this heading.

Chlorprothixene (Given the primary CNS effects of aripiprazole, caution should be used when co-administered with other centrally acting drugs).
No products indexed under this heading.

Chlorprothixene Hydrochloride (Given the primary CNS effects of aripiprazole, caution should be used when co-administered with other centrally acting drugs).
No products indexed under this heading.

Chlorprothixene Lactate (Given the primary CNS effects of aripiprazole, caution should be used when co-administered with other centrally acting drugs).
No products indexed under this heading.

Chlorthalidone (Due to its alpha-1-adrenergic receptor antagonism, aripiprazole has the potential to enhance the effect of certain antihypertensive agents). Products include:
Clorpres Tablets 2185

Cimetidine (Inhibitors of CYP3A4 can inhibit aripiprazole elimination and cause increased blood levels).
No products indexed under this heading.

Cimetidine Hydrochloride (Inhibitors of CYP3A4 can inhibit aripiprazole elimination and cause increased blood levels).
No products indexed under this heading.

Ciprofloxacin (Inhibitors of CYP3A4 can inhibit aripiprazole elimination and cause increased blood levels). Products include:
Cipro I.V. 2817
Cipro Oral Suspension 2810
Cipro XR Tablets 2823
Ciprodex Otic Suspension 541

Ciprofloxacin Hydrochloride (Agents that induce CYP3A4 could cause an increase in aripiprazole clearance and lower blood levels). Products include:
Cipro Tablets 2810

Cisplatin (Agents that induce CYP3A4 could cause an increase in aripiprazole clearance and lower blood levels).
No products indexed under this heading.

Citalopram Hydrobromide (Inhibitors of CYP2D6 can inhibit aripiprazole elimination and cause increased blood levels). Products include:
Celexa 1160

Clarithromycin (Strong inhibitors of CYP3A4 may increase levels of aripiprazole and its active metabolite; dose reduction of aripiprazole should be considered). Products include:
Biaxin/Biaxin XL 411

Clomipramine Hydrochloride (Inhibitors of CYP2D6 can inhibit aripiprazole elimination and cause increased blood levels).
No products indexed under this heading.

Clonidine (Due to its alpha-1-adrenergic receptor antagonism, aripiprazole has the potential to enhance the effect of certain antihypertensive agents). Products include:
Catapres-TTS 842

Clonidine Hydrochloride (Due to its alpha-1-adrenergic receptor antagonism, aripiprazole has the potential to enhance the effect of certain antihypertensive agents). Products include:
Catapres Tablets 841
Clorpres Tablets 2185

Clorazepate Dipotassium (Given the primary CNS effects of aripiprazole, caution should be used when co-administered with other centrally acting drugs).
No products indexed under this heading.

Clotrimazole (Inhibitors of CYP3A4 can inhibit aripiprazole elimination and cause increased blood levels). Products include:
Lotrisone 2881

Clozapine (Given the primary CNS effects of aripiprazole, caution should be used when co-administered with other centrally acting drugs).
No products indexed under this heading.

Cocaine Hydrochloride (Inhibitors of CYP2D6 can inhibit aripiprazole elimination and cause increased blood levels).
No products indexed under this heading.

Codeine Phosphate (Given the primary CNS effects of aripiprazole, caution should be used when co-administered with other centrally acting drugs). Products include:
Tylenol with Codeine Tablets 2427

Cortisone Acetate (Agents that induce CYP3A4 could cause an increase in aripiprazole clearance and lower blood levels).
No products indexed under this heading.

Cyclosporine (Inhibitors of CYP3A4 can inhibit aripiprazole elimination and cause increased blood levels). Products include:
Gengraf Capsules 435
Neoral Oral Solution 2280
Neoral Soft Gelatin Capsules 2280
Restasis Ophthalmic Emulsion 557
Sandimmune 2296

Dalfopristin (Inhibitors of CYP3A4 can inhibit aripiprazole elimination and cause increased blood levels).
No products indexed under this heading.

Danazol (Inhibitors of CYP3A4 can inhibit aripiprazole elimination and cause increased blood levels).
No products indexed under this heading.

Delavirdine Mesylate (Strong inhibitors of CYP3A4 may increase levels of aripiprazole and its active metabolite; dose reduction of aripiprazole should be considered).
No products indexed under this heading.

Delavirine (Strong inhibitors of CYP3A4 may increase levels of aripiprazole and its active metabolite; dose reduction of aripiprazole should be considered).
No products indexed under this heading.

Deserpidine (Due to its alpha-1-adrenergic receptor antagonism, aripiprazole has the potential to enhance the effect of certain antihypertensive agents).
No products indexed under this heading.

Desflurane (Given the primary CNS effects of aripiprazole, caution should be used when co-administered with other centrally acting drugs).
No products indexed under this heading.

Desipramine Hydrochloride (Inhibitors of CYP2D6 can inhibit aripiprazole elimination and cause increased blood levels).
No products indexed under this heading.

Dexamethasone (Agents that induce CYP3A4 could cause an increase in aripiprazole clearance and lower blood levels). Products include:
Ciprodex Otic Suspension 541

Dexamethasone Acetate (Agents that induce CYP3A4 could cause an increase in aripiprazole clearance and lower blood levels).
No products indexed under this heading.

Dexamethasone Sodium Phosphate (Agents that induce CYP3A4 could cause an increase in aripiprazole clearance and lower blood levels).
No products indexed under this heading.

Dextroamphetamine Sulfate (Given the primary CNS effects of aripiprazole, caution should be used when co-administered with other centrally acting drugs). Products include:
Adderall XR Capsules 3012
Dexedrine 1401

Dezocine (Given the primary CNS effects of aripiprazole, caution should be used when co-administered with other centrally acting drugs).
No products indexed under this heading.

Diazepam (Given the primary CNS effects of aripiprazole, caution should be used when co-administered with other centrally acting drugs). Products include:
Valium Tablets 2658

Diazoxide (Due to its alpha-1-adrenergic receptor antagonism, aripiprazole has the potential to enhance the effect of certain antihypertensive agents). Products include:
Proglycem Capsules 1185
Proglycem Suspension 1185

Diltiazem Hydrochloride (Due to its alpha-1-adrenergic receptor antagonism, aripiprazole has the potential to enhance the effect of certain antihypertensive agents). Products include:
Cardizem LA Extended Release Tablets 421

Diltiazem Maleate (Inhibitors of CYP3A4 can inhibit aripiprazole elimination and cause increased blood levels).
No products indexed under this heading.

Diphenhydramine (Inhibitors of CYP2D6 can inhibit aripiprazole elimination and cause increased blood levels).
No products indexed under this heading.

Diphenhydramine Hydrochloride (Inhibitors of CYP2D6 can inhibit aripiprazole elimination and cause increased blood levels). Products include:
Benadryl Allergy & Cold Kapgels 1895
Benadryl Allergy & Sinus Headache Kapgels 1895
Benadryl Severe Allergy & Sinus Headache Caplets 1897
Benadryl Dye-Free Allergy Liqui-gels Softgels 1897
Benadryl Allergy Kapgels 1895
Benadryl Allergy Quick Dissolve Strips 1896
Benadryl Allergy Ultratab Tablets 1896
Children's Benadryl Dye-Free Allergy Liquid 1897
Children's Benadryl Allergy Fastmelts 1897
Children's Benadryl Allergy Liquid 1898
Children's Benadryl Allergy Perfect Measure 1896
Children's Benadryl-D Allergy & Sinus Liquid 1896
Benadryl-D Allergy & Sinus Tablet 1896
PediaCare Children's Allergy & Cold Liquid 1902
PediaCare Children's Allergy Liquid 1902
Simply Sleep Caplets 1905
Sudafed PE Nighttime Cold Caplets 1907
Sudafed PE Severe Cold Caplets 1908
Extra Strength Tylenol PM Caplets, Geltabs, Liquid, and Rapid Release Gels 1915
Tylenol Allergy Multi-Symptom Nighttime Caplets with Cool Burst 1916
Tylenol Severe Allergy Caplets 1916
Children's Tylenol Plus Cold & Allergy Suspension Liquid 1914
Tylenol Sore Throat Nighttime Liquid with Cool Burst 1918

Doxazosin Mesylate (Due to its alpha-1-adrenergic receptor antagonism, aripiprazole has the potential to enhance the effect of certain antihypertensive agents).
No products indexed under this heading.

Doxepin Hydrochloride (Inhibitors of CYP2D6 can inhibit aripiprazole elimination and cause increased blood levels).
No products indexed under this heading.

Doxorubicin Hydrochloride (Agents that induce CYP3A4 could cause an increase in aripiprazole clearance and lower blood levels).
No products indexed under this heading.

Droperidol (Given the primary CNS effects of aripiprazole, caution should be used when co-administered with other centrally acting drugs).
No products indexed under this heading.

Efavirenz (Agents that induce CYP3A4 could cause an increase in aripiprazole clearance and lower blood levels). Products include:
Atripla Tablets 938
Sustiva Capsules 930
Sustiva Tablets 930

Enalapril Maleate (Due to its alpha-1-adrenergic receptor antagonism, aripiprazole has the potential to enhance the effect of certain antihypertensive agents).
No products indexed under this heading.

Enalaprilat (Due to its alpha-1-adrenergic receptor antagonism, aripiprazole has the potential to enhance the effect of certain antihypertensive agents).
No products indexed under this heading.

Enflurane (Given the primary CNS effects of aripiprazole, caution should be used when co-administered with other centrally acting drugs).
No products indexed under this heading.

Eprosartan Mesylate (Due to its alpha-1-adrenergic receptor antagonism, aripiprazole has the potential to enhance the effect of certain antihypertensive agents). Products include:
Teveten Tablets 515
Teveten HCT Tablets 517

Erythromycin (Inhibitors of CYP3A4 can inhibit aripiprazole elimination and cause increased blood levels).
No products indexed under this heading.

Erythromycin Estolate (Inhibitors of CYP3A4 can inhibit aripiprazole elimination and cause increased blood levels).
No products indexed under this heading.

Erythromycin Ethylsuccinate (Inhibitors of CYP3A4 can inhibit aripiprazole elimination and cause increased blood levels). Products include:
E.E.S. 433
EryPed 431

Erythromycin Gluceptate (Inhibitors of CYP3A4 can inhibit aripiprazole elimination and cause increased blood levels).
No products indexed under this heading.

Erythromycin Lactobionate (Inhibitors of CYP3A4 can inhibit aripiprazole elimination and cause increased blood levels).
No products indexed under this heading.

Erythromycin Stearate (Inhibitors of CYP3A4 can inhibit aripiprazole elimination and cause increased blood levels).
No products indexed under this heading.

Escitalopram Oxalate (Inhibitors of CYP2D6 can inhibit aripiprazole elimination and cause increased blood levels). Products include:
Lexapro Oral Suspension 1174
Lexapro Tablets 1174

Esmolol Hydrochloride (Due to its alpha-1-adrenergic receptor antagonism, aripiprazole has the potential to enhance the effect of certain antihypertensive agents).
No products indexed under this heading.

Esomeprazole Magnesium (Inhibitors of CYP3A4 can inhibit aripiprazole elimination and cause increased blood levels). Products include:
Nexium Delayed-Release Capsules 645

IMPORTANT NOTE: Always consult each drug listing in the patient's regimen for possible interactions.

Nexium Delayed-Release Oral Suspension 645

Estazolam (Given the primary CNS effects of aripiprazole, caution should be used when co-administered with other centrally acting drugs).
No products indexed under this heading.

Ethanol (Given the primary CNS effects of aripiprazole, caution should be used when co-administered with other centrally acting drugs).
No products indexed under this heading.

Ethchlorvynol (Given the primary CNS effects of aripiprazole, caution should be used when co-administered with other centrally acting drugs).
No products indexed under this heading.

Ethinamate (Given the primary CNS effects of aripiprazole, caution should be used when co-administered with other centrally acting drugs).
No products indexed under this heading.

Ethosuximide (Agents that induce CYP3A4 could cause an increase in aripiprazole clearance and lower blood levels).
No products indexed under this heading.

Ethyl Alcohol (Given the primary CNS effects of aripiprazole, caution should be used when co-administered with other centrally acting drugs).
No products indexed under this heading.

Famotidine (Co-administration will decrease the solubility of aripiprazole and hence its rate of absorption. No dosage adjustment is required). Products include:
Pepcid Tablets 2075
Original Strength Pepcid AC Gelcaps 1771
Original Strength Pepcid AC Tablets 1771
Maximum Strength Pepcid AC Tablets 1771
Pepcid Complete Chewable Tablets 1771

Felbamate (Agents that induce CYP3A4 could cause an increase in aripiprazole clearance and lower blood levels).
No products indexed under this heading.

Felodipine (Due to its alpha-1-adrenergic receptor antagonism, aripiprazole has the potential to enhance the effect of certain antihypertensive agents).
No products indexed under this heading.

Fentanyl (Given the primary CNS effects of aripiprazole, caution should be used when co-administered with other centrally acting drugs). Products include:
Duragesic Transdermal System 2405
Ionsys Transdermal System 2410

Fentanyl Citrate (Given the primary CNS effects of aripiprazole, caution should be used when co-administered with other centrally acting drugs). Products include:
Actiq 959
Fentora Tablets 968

Fluconazole (Inhibitors of CYP3A4 can inhibit aripiprazole elimination and cause increased blood levels).
No products indexed under this heading.

Fludrocortisone Acetate (Agents that induce CYP3A4 could cause an increase in aripiprazole clearance and lower blood levels).
No products indexed under this heading.

Fluoxetine (When concomitant administration of potential CYP2D6 inhibitors such as quinidine, fluoxetine, or paroxetine with aripiprazole occurs, aripiprazole dose should be reduced at least to one-half of its normal dose. When the CYP2D6 inhibitor is withdrawn from the combination therapy, the aripiprazole dose should then be increased. When adjunctive aripiprazole is administered to patients with major depressive disorder, aripiprazole should be administered without dosage adjustment as specified).
No products indexed under this heading.

Fluoxetine Hydrochloride (When concomitant administration of potential CYP2D6 inhibitors such as quinidine, fluoxetine, or paroxetine with aripiprazole occurs, aripiprazole dose should be reduced at least to one-half of its normal dose. When the CYP2D6 inhibitor is withdrawn from the combination therapy, the aripiprazole dose should then be increased. When adjunctive aripiprazole is administered to patients with major depressive disorder, aripiprazole should be administered without dosage adjustment as specified). Products include:
Prozac Weekly Capsules 1852
Prozac Pulvules and Liquid 1852
Symbyax Capsules 1871

Fluphenazine Decanoate (Inhibitors of CYP2D6 can inhibit aripiprazole elimination and cause increased blood levels).
No products indexed under this heading.

Fluphenazine Enanthate (Inhibitors of CYP2D6 can inhibit aripiprazole elimination and cause increased blood levels).
No products indexed under this heading.

Fluphenazine Hydrochloride (Inhibitors of CYP2D6 can inhibit aripiprazole elimination and cause increased blood levels).
No products indexed under this heading.

Flurazepam Hydrochloride (Given the primary CNS effects of aripiprazole, caution should be used when co-administered with other centrally acting drugs).
No products indexed under this heading.

Fluvoxamine Maleate (Inhibitors of CYP3A4 can inhibit aripiprazole elimination and cause increased blood levels). Products include:
Luvox CR Extended-Release Capsules 1759

Fosamprenavir Calcium (Strong inhibitors of CYP3A4 may increase levels of aripiprazole and its active metabolite; dose reduction of aripiprazole should be considered). Products include:
Lexiva Oral Suspension 1510
Lexiva Tablets 1510

Fosinopril Sodium (Due to its alpha-1-adrenergic receptor antagonism, aripiprazole has the potential to enhance the effect of certain antihypertensive agents).
No products indexed under this heading.

Fosphenytoin Sodium (Agents that induce CYP3A4 could cause an increase in aripiprazole clearance and lower blood levels).
No products indexed under this heading.

Furosemide (Due to its alpha-1-adrenergic receptor antagonism, aripiprazole has the potential to enhance the effect of certain antihypertensive agents). Products include:
Furosemide Tablets 2186

Garlic Extract (Agents that induce CYP3A4 could cause an increase in aripiprazole clearance and lower blood levels).
No products indexed under this heading.

Garlic Oil (Agents that induce CYP3A4 could cause an increase in aripiprazole clearance and lower blood levels).
No products indexed under this heading.

Glutethimide (Given the primary CNS effects of aripiprazole, caution should be used when co-administered with other centrally acting drugs).
No products indexed under this heading.

Guanabenz Acetate (Due to its alpha-1-adrenergic receptor antagonism, aripiprazole has the potential to enhance the effect of certain antihypertensive agents).
No products indexed under this heading.

Guanethidine Monosulfate (Due to its alpha-1-adrenergic receptor antagonism, aripiprazole has the potential to enhance the effect of certain antihypertensive agents).
No products indexed under this heading.

Halofantrine Hydrochloride (Inhibitors of CYP2D6 can inhibit aripiprazole elimination and cause increased blood levels).
No products indexed under this heading.

Haloperidol (Inhibitors of CYP2D6 can inhibit aripiprazole elimination and cause increased blood levels).
No products indexed under this heading.

Haloperidol Decanoate (Inhibitors of CYP2D6 can inhibit aripiprazole elimination and cause increased blood levels).
No products indexed under this heading.

Hydralazine Hydrochloride (Due to its alpha-1-adrenergic receptor antagonism, aripiprazole has the potential to enhance the effect of certain antihypertensive agents).
No products indexed under this heading.

Hydrochlorothiazide (Due to its alpha-1-adrenergic receptor antagonism, aripiprazole has the potential to enhance the effect of certain antihypertensive agents). Products include:
Atacand HCT 642
Avalide Tablets 892
Avalide Tablets 2713
Benicar HCT Tablets 1010
Diovan HCT Tablets 2216
Dyazide Capsules 1405
Micardis HCT Tablets 854
Prinzide Tablets 2092
Tekturna HCT Tablets 2324
Teveten HCT Tablets 517

Hydrocodone Bitartrate (Given the primary CNS effects of aripiprazole, caution should be used when co-administered with other centrally acting drugs). Products include:
Lortab 5/500 Tablets 3143
Lortab 7.5/500 Tablets 3144
Lortab 10/500 Tablets 3144
Vicodin Tablets 529
Vicodin ES Tablets 530
Vicodin HP Tablets 531
Vicoprofen Tablets 533
Zydone Tablets 1132

Hydrocodone Polistirex (Given the primary CNS effects of aripiprazole, caution should be used when co-administered with other centrally acting drugs). Products include:
Tussionex Pennkinetic Extended-Release Suspension 3154

Hydrocortisone (Agents that induce CYP3A4 could cause an increase in aripiprazole clearance and lower blood levels).
No products indexed under this heading.

Hydrocortisone Acetate (Agents that induce CYP3A4 could cause an increase in aripiprazole clearance and lower blood levels). Products include:
Analpram-HC 1140
Pramosone 1141

Hydrocortisone Butyrate (Agents that induce CYP3A4 could cause an increase in aripiprazole clearance and lower blood levels).
No products indexed under this heading.

Hydrocortisone Cypionate (Agents that induce CYP3A4 could cause an increase in aripiprazole clearance and lower blood levels).
No products indexed under this heading.

Hydrocortisone Hemisuccinate (Agents that induce CYP3A4 could cause an increase in aripiprazole clearance and lower blood levels).
No products indexed under this heading.

Hydrocortisone Probutate (Agents that induce CYP3A4 could cause an increase in aripiprazole clearance and lower blood levels).
No products indexed under this heading.

Hydrocortisone Sodium Phosphate (Agents that induce CYP3A4 could cause an increase in aripiprazole clearance and lower blood levels).
No products indexed under this heading.

Hydrocortisone Sodium Succinate (Agents that induce CYP3A4 could cause an increase in aripiprazole clearance and lower blood levels).
No products indexed under this heading.

Hydrocortisone Valerate (Agents that induce CYP3A4 could cause an increase in aripiprazole clearance and lower blood levels).
No products indexed under this heading.

Hydroflumethiazide (Due to its alpha-1-adrenergic receptor antagonism, aripiprazole has the potential to enhance the effect of certain antihypertensive agents).
No products indexed under this heading.

Hydromorphone Hydrochloride (Given the primary CNS effects of aripiprazole, caution should be used when co-administered with other centrally acting drugs).
No products indexed under this heading.

Hydroxychloroquine Sulfate (Inhibitors of CYP2D6 can inhibit aripiprazole elimination and cause increased blood levels).
No products indexed under this heading.

Hydroxyzine Hydrochloride (Given the primary CNS effects of aripiprazole, caution should be used when co-administered with other centrally acting drugs).
No products indexed under this heading.

Hypericum (Agents that induce CYP3A4 could cause an increase in aripiprazole clearance and lower blood levels). Products include:
Satieté Tablets 640

Hypericum Perforatum (Agents that induce CYP3A4 could cause an increase in aripiprazole clearance and lower blood levels).
No products indexed under this heading.

Imatinib Mesylate (Inhibitors of CYP2D6 can inhibit aripiprazole elimination and cause increased blood levels). Products include:
Gleevec Tablets 2255

Imipramine Hydrochloride (Inhibitors of CYP2D6 can inhibit aripiprazole elimination and cause increased blood levels).
No products indexed under this heading.

Imipramine Pamoate (Inhibitors of CYP2D6 can inhibit aripiprazole elimination and cause increased blood levels).
No products indexed under this heading.

Indapamide (Due to its alpha-1-adrenergic receptor antagonism, aripiprazole has the potential to enhance the effect of certain antihypertensive agents). Products include:
Indapamide Tablets 2188

Indinavir Sulfate (Strong inhibitors of CYP3A4 may increase levels of aripiprazole and its active metabolite; dose reduction of aripiprazole should be considered). Products include:
Crixivan Capsules 1979

Irbesartan (Due to its alpha-1-adrenergic receptor antagonism, aripiprazole has the potential to enhance the effect of certain antihypertensive agents). Products include:
Avalide Tablets 892
Avalide Tablets 2713
Avapro Tablets 897
Avapro Tablets 2718

Isoflurane (Given the primary CNS effects of aripiprazole, caution should be used when co-administered with other centrally acting drugs).
No products indexed under this heading.

Isoniazid (Inhibitors of CYP3A4 can inhibit aripiprazole elimination and cause increased blood levels).
No products indexed under this heading.

Isradipine (Due to its alpha-1-adrenergic receptor antagonism, aripiprazole has the potential to enhance the effect of certain antihypertensive agents). Products include:
DynaCirc CR Controlled Release Tablets 1407

Itraconazole (Co-administration with ketoconazole increased the AUC of aripiprazole and its active metabolite by 63% and 77%, respectively. When concomitant administration of ketoconazole with aripiprazole occurs, aripiprazole dose should be reduced to one-half of its normal dose. Other strong inhibitors of CYP3A4 (itraconazole) would be expected to have similar effects and need similar dose reductions. When the CYP3A4 inhibitor is withdrawn from the combination therapy, aripiprazole dose should then be increased).
No products indexed under this heading.

Ketamine Hydrochloride (Given the primary CNS effects of aripiprazole, caution should be used when co-administered with other centrally acting drugs).
No products indexed under this heading.

Ketoconazole (Co-administration with ketoconazole increased the AUC of aripiprazole and its active metabolite by 63% and 77%, respectively. When concomitant administration of ketoconazole with aripiprazole occurs, aripiprazole dose should be reduced to one-half of its normal dose. When the CYP3A4 inhibitor is withdrawn from the combination therapy, aripiprazole dose should then be increased). Products include:
Extina Foam, 2% 3057
Nizoral A-D Shampoo 1901

Labetalol Hydrochloride (Due to its alpha-1-adrenergic receptor antagonism, aripiprazole has the potential to enhance the effect of certain antihypertensive agents).
No products indexed under this heading.

Levomethadyl Acetate Hydrochloride (Given the primary CNS effects of aripiprazole, caution should be used when co-administered with other centrally acting drugs).
No products indexed under this heading.

Levorphanol Tartrate (Given the primary CNS effects of aripiprazole, caution should be used when co-administered with other centrally acting drugs).
No products indexed under this heading.

Lisinopril (Due to its alpha-1-adrenergic receptor antagonism, aripiprazole has the potential to enhance the effect of certain antihypertensive agents). Products include:
Prinivil Tablets 2087
Prinzide Tablets 2092

Lopinavir (Strong inhibitors of CYP3A4 may increase levels of aripiprazole and its active metabolite; dose reduction of aripiprazole should be considered). Products include:
Kaletra 452

Loratadine (Inhibitors of CYP3A4 can inhibit aripiprazole elimination and cause increased blood levels).
No products indexed under this heading.

Lorazepam (Given the primary CNS effects of aripiprazole, caution should be used when co-administered with other centrally acting drugs).
No products indexed under this heading.

Losartan Potassium (Due to its alpha-1-adrenergic receptor antagonism, aripiprazole has the potential to enhance the effect of certain antihypertensive agents). Products include:
Cozaar Tablets 1973

Loxapine Hydrochloride (Given the primary CNS effects of aripiprazole, caution should be used when co-administered with other centrally acting drugs).
No products indexed under this heading.

Loxapine Succinate (Given the primary CNS effects of aripiprazole, caution should be used when co-administered with other centrally acting drugs).
No products indexed under this heading.

Maprotiline Hydrochloride (Inhibitors of CYP2D6 can inhibit aripiprazole elimination and cause increased blood levels).
No products indexed under this heading.

Mecamylamine Hydrochloride (Due to its alpha-1-adrenergic receptor antagonism, aripiprazole has the potential to enhance the effect of certain antihypertensive agents).
No products indexed under this heading.

Meperidine Hydrochloride (Given the primary CNS effects of aripiprazole, caution should be used when co-administered with other centrally acting drugs).
No products indexed under this heading.

Mephenytoin (Agents that induce CYP3A4 could cause an increase in aripiprazole clearance and lower blood levels).
No products indexed under this heading.

Mephobarbital (Given the primary CNS effects of aripiprazole, caution should be used when co-administered with other centrally acting drugs).
No products indexed under this heading.

Meprobamate (Given the primary CNS effects of aripiprazole, caution should be used when co-administered with other centrally acting drugs).
No products indexed under this heading.

Mesoridazine Besylate (Given the primary CNS effects of aripiprazole, caution should be used when co-administered with other centrally acting drugs).
No products indexed under this heading.

Methadone Hydrochloride (Inhibitors of CYP2D6 can inhibit aripiprazole elimination and cause increased blood levels).
No products indexed under this heading.

Methamphetamine Hydrochloride (Given the primary CNS effects of aripiprazole, caution should be used when co-administered with other centrally acting drugs).
No products indexed under this heading.

Methohexital Sodium (Given the primary CNS effects of aripiprazole, caution should be used when co-administered with other centrally acting drugs).
No products indexed under this heading.

Methotrimeprazine (Given the primary CNS effects of aripiprazole, caution should be used when co-administered with other centrally acting drugs).
No products indexed under this heading.

Methoxyflurane (Given the primary CNS effects of aripiprazole, caution should be used when co-administered with other centrally acting drugs).
No products indexed under this heading.

Methsuximide (Agents that induce CYP3A4 could cause an increase in aripiprazole clearance and lower blood levels).
No products indexed under this heading.

Methyclothiazide (Due to its alpha-1-adrenergic receptor antagonism, aripiprazole has the potential to enhance the effect of certain antihypertensive agents).
No products indexed under this heading.

Methyldopa (Due to its alpha-1-adrenergic receptor antagonism, aripiprazole has the potential to enhance the effect of certain antihypertensive agents).
No products indexed under this heading.

Methyldopate Hydrochloride (Due to its alpha-1-adrenergic receptor antagonism, aripiprazole has the potential to enhance the effect of certain antihypertensive agents).
No products indexed under this heading.

Methylphenidate (Given the primary CNS effects of aripiprazole, caution should be used when co-administered with other centrally acting drugs). Products include:
Daytrana Transdermal Patch 3022

Methylphenidate Hydrochloride (Given the primary CNS effects of aripiprazole, caution should be used when co-administered with other centrally acting drugs). Products include:
Concerta Extended-Release Tablets 1925
Metadate CD Capsules 3146

Methylprednisolone (Agents that induce CYP3A4 could cause an increase in aripiprazole clearance and lower blood levels).
No products indexed under this heading.

IMPORTANT NOTE: Always consult each drug listing in the patient's regimen for possible interactions.

Methylprednisolone Acetate (Agents that induce CYP3A4 could cause an increase in aripiprazole clearance and lower blood levels).
No products indexed under this heading.

Methylprednisolone Sodium Succinate (Agents that induce CYP3A4 could cause an increase in aripiprazole clearance and lower blood levels).
No products indexed under this heading.

Metolazone (Due to its alpha-1-adrenergic receptor antagonism, aripiprazole has the potential to enhance the effect of certain antihypertensive agents).
No products indexed under this heading.

Metoprolol Succinate (Due to its alpha-1-adrenergic receptor antagonism, aripiprazole has the potential to enhance the effect of certain antihypertensive agents). Products include:
Toprol-XL Tablets 666

Metoprolol Tartrate (Due to its alpha-1-adrenergic receptor antagonism, aripiprazole has the potential to enhance the effect of certain antihypertensive agents).
No products indexed under this heading.

Metronidazole (Inhibitors of CYP3A4 can inhibit aripiprazole elimination and cause increased blood levels). Products include:
Pylera Capsules 714

Metronidazole Benzoate (Inhibitors of CYP3A4 can inhibit aripiprazole elimination and cause increased blood levels).
No products indexed under this heading.

Metronidazole Hydrochloride (Inhibitors of CYP3A4 can inhibit aripiprazole elimination and cause increased blood levels).
No products indexed under this heading.

Metronidazole Sodium (Inhibitors of CYP3A4 can inhibit aripiprazole elimination and cause increased blood levels).
No products indexed under this heading.

Metyrosine (Due to its alpha-1-adrenergic receptor antagonism, aripiprazole has the potential to enhance the effect of certain antihypertensive agents). Products include:
Demser Capsules 1989

Mibefradil Dihydrochloride (Due to its alpha-1-adrenergic receptor antagonism, aripiprazole has the potential to enhance the effect of certain antihypertensive agents).
No products indexed under this heading.

Miconazole (Inhibitors of CYP3A4 can inhibit aripiprazole elimination and cause increased blood levels).
No products indexed under this heading.

Miconazole Nitrate (Inhibitors of CYP3A4 can inhibit aripiprazole elimination and cause increased blood levels).
No products indexed under this heading.

Midazolam Hydrochloride (Given the primary CNS effects of aripiprazole, caution should be used when co-administered with other centrally acting drugs).
No products indexed under this heading.

Minoxidil (Due to its alpha-1-adrenergic receptor antagonism, aripiprazole has the potential to enhance the effect of certain antihypertensive agents).
No products indexed under this heading.

Moclobemide (Inhibitors of CYP2D6 can inhibit aripiprazole elimination and cause increased blood levels).
No products indexed under this heading.

Modafinil (Agents that induce CYP3A4 could cause an increase in aripiprazole clearance and lower blood levels). Products include:
Provigil Tablets 977

Moexipril Hydrochloride (Due to its alpha-1-adrenergic receptor antagonism, aripiprazole has the potential to enhance the effect of certain antihypertensive agents).
No products indexed under this heading.

Molindone Hydrochloride (Given the primary CNS effects of aripiprazole, caution should be used when co-administered with other centrally acting drugs). Products include:
Moban Tablets 1116

Morphine Sulfate (Given the primary CNS effects of aripiprazole, caution should be used when co-administered with other centrally acting drugs). Products include:
Avinza Capsules 1772
DepoDur Injection 1095
MS Contin Tablets 2585

Nadolol (Due to its alpha-1-adrenergic receptor antagonism, aripiprazole has the potential to enhance the effect of certain antihypertensive agents). Products include:
Nadolol Tablets 2191

Nebivolol (Due to its alpha-1-adrenergic receptor antagonism, aripiprazole has the potential to enhance the effect of certain antihypertensive agents). Products include:
Bystolic Tablets 1155

Nefazodone Hydrochloride (Strong inhibitors of CYP3A4 may increase levels of aripiprazole and its active metabolite; dose reduction of aripiprazole should be considered).
No products indexed under this heading.

Nelfinavir Mesylate (Strong inhibitors of CYP3A4 may increase levels of aripiprazole and its active metabolite; dose reduction of aripiprazole should be considered).
No products indexed under this heading.

Nevirapine (Agents that induce CYP3A4 could cause an increase in aripiprazole clearance and lower blood levels). Products include:
Viramune Oral Suspension 873
Viramune Tablets 873

Niacinamide (Inhibitors of CYP3A4 can inhibit aripiprazole elimination and cause increased blood levels). Products include:
BioLean Free Tablets .... ▣635

Nicardipine Hydrochloride (Due to its alpha-1-adrenergic receptor antagonism, aripiprazole has the potential to enhance the effect of certain antihypertensive agents). Products include:
Cardene I.V. 1093

Nicotinamide (Inhibitors of CYP3A4 can inhibit aripiprazole elimination and cause increased blood levels).
No products indexed under this heading.

Nifedipine (Due to its alpha-1-adrenergic receptor antagonism, aripiprazole has the potential to enhance the effect of certain antihypertensive agents).
No products indexed under this heading.

Nisoldipine (Due to its alpha-1-adrenergic receptor antagonism, aripiprazole has the potential to enhance the effect of certain antihypertensive agents). Products include:
Sular Extended Release Tablets 2975

Nitroglycerin (Due to its alpha-1-adrenergic receptor antagonism, aripiprazole has the potential to enhance the effect of certain antihypertensive agents). Products include:
Nitro-Dur Transdermal Infusion System 2887
Nitrolingual Pumpspray 2965

Norfloxacin (Inhibitors of CYP3A4 can inhibit aripiprazole elimination and cause increased blood levels). Products include:
Noroxin Tablets 2069

Nortriptyline Hydrochloride (Inhibitors of CYP2D6 can inhibit aripiprazole elimination and cause increased blood levels).
No products indexed under this heading.

Olanzapine (Given the primary CNS effects of aripiprazole, caution should be used when co-administered with other centrally acting drugs). Products include:
Symbyax Capsules 1871
Zyprexa Tablets 1883
Zyprexa IntraMuscular 1883
Zyprexa ZYDIS Orally Disintegrating Tablets 1883

Omeprazole (Inhibitors of CYP3A4 can inhibit aripiprazole elimination and cause increased blood levels).
No products indexed under this heading.

Oxazepam (Given the primary CNS effects of aripiprazole, caution should be used when co-administered with other centrally acting drugs).
No products indexed under this heading.

Oxcarbazepine (Agents that induce CYP3A4 could cause an increase in aripiprazole clearance and lower blood levels).
No products indexed under this heading.

Oxycodone Hydrochloride (Given the primary CNS effects of aripiprazole, caution should be used when co-administered with other centrally acting drugs). Products include:
OxyContin Tablets 2589
OxyIR Capsules 2593
Percocet Tablets 1127
Percodan Tablets 1130

Paroxetine Hydrochloride (When concomitant administration of potential CYP2D6 inhibitors such as quinidine, fluoxetine, or paroxetine with aripiprazole occurs, aripiprazole dose should be reduced at least to one-half of its normal dose. When the CYP2D6 inhibitor is withdrawn from the combination therapy, the aripiprazole dose should then be increased. When adjunctive aripiprazole is administered to patients with major depressive disorder, aripiprazole should be administered without dosage adjustment as specified). Products include:
Paxil 1535
Paxil CR Controlled-Release Tablets 1544

Paroxetine Mesylate (When concomitant administration of potential CYP2D6 inhibitors such as quinidine, fluoxetine, or paroxetine with aripiprazole occurs, aripiprazole dose should be reduced at least to one-half of its normal dose. When the CYP2D6 inhibitor is withdrawn from the combination therapy, the aripiprazole dose should then be increased. When adjunctive aripiprazole is administered to patients with major depressive disorder, aripiprazole should be administered without dosage adjustment as specified).
No products indexed under this heading.

Pemoline (Given the primary CNS effects of aripiprazole, caution should be used when co-administered with other centrally acting drugs).
No products indexed under this heading.

Penbutolol Sulfate (Due to its alpha-1-adrenergic receptor antagonism, aripiprazole has the potential to enhance the effect of certain antihypertensive agents).
No products indexed under this heading.

Pentobarbital Sodium (Given the primary CNS effects of aripiprazole, caution should be used when co-administered with other centrally acting drugs). Products include:
Nembutal Sodium Solution, USP 2494

Perindopril Erbumine (Due to its alpha-1-adrenergic receptor antagonism, aripiprazole has the potential to enhance the effect of certain antihypertensive agents). Products include:
Aceon Tablets (2 mg, 4 mg, 8 mg) 3038

Perphenazine (Inhibitors of CYP2D6 can inhibit aripiprazole elimination and cause increased blood levels).
No products indexed under this heading.

Phenobarbital (Agents that induce CYP3A4 could cause an increase in aripiprazole clearance and lower blood levels). Products include:
Donnatal Extentabs 2507

Phenobarbital Sodium (Agents that induce CYP3A4 could cause an increase in aripiprazole clearance and lower blood levels).
No products indexed under this heading.

Phenoxybenzamine Hydrochloride (Due to its alpha-1-adrenergic receptor antagonism, aripiprazole has the potential to enhance the effect of certain antihypertensive agents). Products include:
Dibenzyline Capsules 3188

Phentolamine Mesylate (Due to its alpha-1-adrenergic receptor antagonism, aripiprazole has the potential to enhance the effect of certain antihypertensive agents).
No products indexed under this heading.

Phenytoin (Agents that induce CYP3A4 could cause an increase in aripiprazole clearance and lower blood levels).
No products indexed under this heading.

Phenytoin Sodium (Agents that induce CYP3A4 could cause an increase in aripiprazole clearance and lower blood levels). Products include:
Phenytek Capsules **2192**

Pindolol (Due to its alpha-1-adrenergic receptor antagonism, aripiprazole has the potential to enhance the effect of certain antihypertensive agents).
No products indexed under this heading.

Polythiazide (Due to its alpha-1-adrenergic receptor antagonism, aripiprazole has the potential to enhance the effect of certain antihypertensive agents).
No products indexed under this heading.

Prazepam (Given the primary CNS effects of aripiprazole, caution should be used when co-administered with other centrally acting drugs).
No products indexed under this heading.

Prazosin Hydrochloride (Due to its alpha-1-adrenergic receptor antagonism, aripiprazole has the potential to enhance the effect of certain antihypertensive agents).
No products indexed under this heading.

Prednisolone Acetate (Agents that induce CYP3A4 could cause an increase in aripiprazole clearance and lower blood levels). Products include:
Pred Forte Ophthalmic Suspension .... ⊙**227**
Pred Mild Ophthalmic Suspension .... ⊙**230**
Pred-G Ophthalmic Ointment .... ⊙**229**
Pred-G Ophthalmic Suspension ...... ⊙**228**

Prednisolone Sodium Phosphate (Agents that induce CYP3A4 could cause an increase in aripiprazole clearance and lower blood levels).
No products indexed under this heading.

Prednisolone Tebutate (Agents that induce CYP3A4 could cause an increase in aripiprazole clearance and lower blood levels).
No products indexed under this heading.

Prednisone (Agents that induce CYP3A4 could cause an increase in aripiprazole clearance and lower blood levels).
No products indexed under this heading.

Primidone (Agents that induce CYP3A4 could cause an increase in aripiprazole clearance and lower blood levels).
No products indexed under this heading.

Prochlorperazine (Given the primary CNS effects of aripiprazole, caution should be used when co-administered with other centrally acting drugs).
No products indexed under this heading.

Promethazine Hydrochloride (Given the primary CNS effects of aripiprazole, caution should be used when co-administered with other centrally acting drugs).
No products indexed under this heading.

Propafenone Hydrochloride (Inhibitors of CYP2D6 can inhibit aripiprazole elimination and cause increased blood levels). Products include:
Rythmol Tablets **1586**
Rythmol SR Capsules **1590**

Propofol (Given the primary CNS effects of aripiprazole, caution should be used when co-administered with other centrally acting drugs).
No products indexed under this heading.

Propoxyphene Hydrochloride (Inhibitors of CYP3A4 can inhibit aripiprazole elimination and cause increased blood levels).
No products indexed under this heading.

Propoxyphene Napsylate (Inhibitors of CYP3A4 can inhibit aripiprazole elimination and cause increased blood levels).
No products indexed under this heading.

Propranolol Hydrochloride (Due to its alpha-1-adrenergic receptor antagonism, aripiprazole has the potential to enhance the effect of certain antihypertensive agents). Products include:
InnoPran XL Extended Release Capsules **1484**

Protriptyline Hydrochloride (Inhibitors of CYP2D6 can inhibit aripiprazole elimination and cause increased blood levels).
No products indexed under this heading.

Quazepam (Given the primary CNS effects of aripiprazole, caution should be used when co-administered with other centrally acting drugs).
No products indexed under this heading.

Quetiapine Fumarate (Given the primary CNS effects of aripiprazole, caution should be used when co-administered with other centrally acting drugs).
No products indexed under this heading.

Quinacrine Hydrochloride (Inhibitors of CYP2D6 can inhibit aripiprazole elimination and cause increased blood levels).
No products indexed under this heading.

Quinapril Hydrochloride (Due to its alpha-1-adrenergic receptor antagonism, aripiprazole has the potential to enhance the effect of certain antihypertensive agents).
No products indexed under this heading.

Quinidine (When concomitant administration of potential CYP2D6 inhibitors such as quinidine, fluoxetine, or paroxetine with aripiprazole occurs, aripiprazole dose should be reduce at least to one-half of its normal dose. When the CYP2D6 inhibitor is withdrawn from the combination therapy, the aripiprazole dose should then be increased. When adjunctive aripiprazole is administered to patients with major depressive disorder, aripiprazole should be administered without dosage adjustment as specified).
No products indexed under this heading.

Quinidine Gluconate (When concomitant administration of potential CYP2D6 inhibitors such as quinidine, fluoxetine, or paroxetine with aripiprazole occurs, aripiprazole dose should be reduce at least to one-half of its normal dose. When the CYP2D6 inhibitor is withdrawn from the combination therapy, the aripiprazole dose should then be increased. When adjunctive aripiprazole is administered to patients with major depressive disorder, aripiprazole should be administered without dosage adjustment as specified).
No products indexed under this heading.

Quinidine Hydrochloride (When concomitant administration of potential CYP2D6 inhibitors such as quinidine, fluoxetine, or paroxetine with aripiprazole occurs, aripiprazole dose should be reduce at least to one-half of its normal dose. When the CYP2D6 inhibitor is withdrawn from the combination therapy, the aripiprazole dose should then be increased. When adjunctive aripiprazole is administered to patients with major depressive disorder, aripiprazole should be administered without dosage adjustment as specified).
No products indexed under this heading.

Quinidine Polygalacturonate (When concomitant administration of potential CYP2D6 inhibitors such as quinidine, fluoxetine, or paroxetine with aripiprazole occurs, aripiprazole dose should be reduce at least to one-half of its normal dose. When the CYP2D6 inhibitor is withdrawn from the combination therapy, the aripiprazole dose should then be increased. When adjunctive aripiprazole is administered to patients with major depressive disorder, aripiprazole should be administered without dosage adjustment as specified).
No products indexed under this heading.

Quinidine Sulfate (When concomitant administration of potential CYP2D6 inhibitors such as quinidine, fluoxetine, or paroxetine with aripiprazole occurs, aripiprazole dose should be reduce at least to one-half of its normal dose. When the CYP2D6 inhibitor is withdrawn from the combination therapy, the aripiprazole dose should then be increased. When adjunctive aripiprazole is administered to patients with major depressive disorder, aripiprazole should be administered without dosage adjustment as specified).
No products indexed under this heading.

Quinine (Inhibitors of CYP3A4 can inhibit aripiprazole elimination and cause increased blood levels).
No products indexed under this heading.

Quinine Sulfate (Inhibitors of CYP3A4 can inhibit aripiprazole elimination and cause increased blood levels).
No products indexed under this heading.

Quinupristin (Inhibitors of CYP3A4 can inhibit aripiprazole elimination and cause increased blood levels).
No products indexed under this heading.

Ramipril (Due to its alpha-1-adrenergic receptor antagonism, aripiprazole has the potential to enhance the effect of certain antihypertensive agents).
No products indexed under this heading.

Ranitidine Bismuth Citrate (Inhibitors of CYP3A4 can inhibit aripiprazole elimination and cause increased blood levels).
No products indexed under this heading.

Ranitidine Hydrochloride (Inhibitors of CYP3A4 can inhibit aripiprazole elimination and cause increased blood levels). Products include:
Zantac 75 Tablets .... ▣**603**
Zantac **1670**
Zantac Injection **1666**
Zantac Injection Pharmacy Bulk Package **1668**
Maximum Strength Zantac 150 Tablets .... ▣**603**
Maximum Strength Zantac 150 Cool Mint Tablets .... ▣**603**

Rauwolfia Serpentina (Due to its alpha-1-adrenergic receptor antagonism, aripiprazole has the potential to enhance the effect of certain antihypertensive agents).
No products indexed under this heading.

Remifentanil Hydrochloride (Given the primary CNS effects of aripiprazole, caution should be used when co-administered with other centrally acting drugs).
No products indexed under this heading.

Rescinnamine (Due to its alpha-1-adrenergic receptor antagonism, aripiprazole has the potential to enhance the effect of certain antihypertensive agents).
No products indexed under this heading.

Reserpine (Due to its alpha-1-adrenergic receptor antagonism, aripiprazole has the potential to enhance the effect of certain antihypertensive agents).
No products indexed under this heading.

Rifabutin (Agents that induce CYP3A4 could cause an increase in aripiprazole clearance and lower blood levels).
No products indexed under this heading.

Rifampicin (Agents that induce CYP3A4 could cause an increase in aripiprazole clearance and lower blood levels).
No products indexed under this heading.

Rifampin (Agents that induce CYP3A4 could cause an increase in aripiprazole clearance and lower blood levels).
No products indexed under this heading.

IMPORTANT NOTE: Always consult each drug listing in the patient's regimen for possible interactions.

Rifapentine (Agents that induce CYP3A4 could cause an increase in aripiprazole clearance and lower blood levels).
No products indexed under this heading.

Risperidone (Given the primary CNS effects of aripiprazole, caution should be used when co-administered with other centrally acting drugs). Products include:
Risperdal Consta Long-Acting Injection 1753

Ritonavir (Strong inhibitors of CYP3A4 may increase levels of aripiprazole and its active metabolite; dose reduction of aripiprazole should be considered). Products include:
Kaletra 452
Norvir 489

Saquinavir (Strong inhibitors of CYP3A4 may increase levels of aripiprazole and its active metabolite; dose reduction of aripiprazole should be considered).
No products indexed under this heading.

Saquinavir Mesylate (Strong inhibitors of CYP3A4 may increase levels of aripiprazole and its active metabolite; dose reduction of aripiprazole should be considered).
No products indexed under this heading.

Secobarbital Sodium (Given the primary CNS effects of aripiprazole, caution should be used when co-administered with other centrally acting drugs).
No products indexed under this heading.

Sertraline Hydrochloride (Inhibitors of CYP3A4 can inhibit aripiprazole elimination and cause increased blood levels).
No products indexed under this heading.

Sevoflurane (Given the primary CNS effects of aripiprazole, caution should be used when co-administered with other centrally acting drugs). Products include:
Ultane Liquid for Inhalation 524

Sildenafil Citrate (Inhibitors of CYP3A4 can inhibit aripiprazole elimination and cause increased blood levels).
No products indexed under this heading.

Sodium Nitroprusside (Due to its alpha-1-adrenergic receptor antagonism, aripiprazole has the potential to enhance the effect of certain antihypertensive agents).
No products indexed under this heading.

Sodium Oxybate (Given the primary CNS effects of aripiprazole, caution should be used when co-administered with other centrally acting drugs). Products include:
Xyrem Oral Solution 1766

Sotalol Hydrochloride (Due to its alpha-1-adrenergic receptor antagonism, aripiprazole has the potential to enhance the effect of certain antihypertensive agents).
No products indexed under this heading.

Spirapril Hydrochloride (Due to its alpha-1-adrenergic receptor antagonism, aripiprazole has the potential to enhance the effect of certain antihypertensive agents).
No products indexed under this heading.

Sufentanil Citrate (Given the primary CNS effects of aripiprazole, caution should be used when co-administered with other centrally acting drugs).
No products indexed under this heading.

Sulfinpyrazone (Agents that induce CYP3A4 could cause an increase in aripiprazole clearance and lower blood levels).
No products indexed under this heading.

Telithromycin (Strong inhibitors of CYP3A4 may increase levels of aripiprazole and its active metabolite; dose reduction of aripiprazole should be considered). Products include:
Ketek Tablets 2744

Telmisartan (Due to its alpha-1-adrenergic receptor antagonism, aripiprazole has the potential to enhance the effect of certain antihypertensive agents). Products include:
Micardis Tablets 852
Micardis HCT Tablets 854

Temazepam (Given the primary CNS effects of aripiprazole, caution should be used when co-administered with other centrally acting drugs).
No products indexed under this heading.

Terazosin Hydrochloride (Due to its alpha-1-adrenergic receptor antagonism, aripiprazole has the potential to enhance the effect of certain antihypertensive agents).
No products indexed under this heading.

Terbinafine Hydrochloride (Inhibitors of CYP2D6 can inhibit aripiprazole elimination and cause increased blood levels). Products include:
Lamisil Oral Granules 2264
Lamisil Tablets 2266

Theophylline (Agents that induce CYP3A4 could cause an increase in aripiprazole clearance and lower blood levels).
No products indexed under this heading.

Theophylline Anhydrous (Agents that induce CYP3A4 could cause an increase in aripiprazole clearance and lower blood levels). Products include:
Uniphyl Tablets 2595

Theophylline Calcium Salicylate (Agents that induce CYP3A4 could cause an increase in aripiprazole clearance and lower blood levels).
No products indexed under this heading.

Theophylline Dihydroxypropyl (Glyceryl) (Agents that induce CYP3A4 could cause an increase in aripiprazole clearance and lower blood levels).
No products indexed under this heading.

Theophylline Ethylenediamine (Agents that induce CYP3A4 could cause an increase in aripiprazole clearance and lower blood levels).
No products indexed under this heading.

Thiamylal Sodium (Given the primary CNS effects of aripiprazole, caution should be used when co-administered with other centrally acting drugs).
No products indexed under this heading.

Thioridazine Hydrochloride (Inhibitors of CYP2D6 can inhibit aripiprazole elimination and cause increased blood levels). Products include:
Thioridazine Hydrochloride Tablets 2195

Thiothixene (Given the primary CNS effects of aripiprazole, caution should be used when co-administered with other centrally acting drugs). Products include:
Thiothixene Capsules 2197

Timolol Maleate (Due to its alpha-1-adrenergic receptor antagonism, aripiprazole has the potential to enhance the effect of certain antihypertensive agents). Products include:
Combigan Ophthalmic Solution 553
Cosopt Sterile Ophthalmic Solution 1969
Timoptic Sterile Ophthalmic Solution 2121
Timoptic in Ocudose 2124
Timoptic-XE Sterile Ophthalmic Gel Forming Solution 2125

Torsemide (Due to its alpha-1-adrenergic receptor antagonism, aripiprazole has the potential to enhance the effect of certain antihypertensive agents). Products include:
Demadex Injection 2630
Demadex Tablets 2630

Trandolapril (Due to its alpha-1-adrenergic receptor antagonism, aripiprazole has the potential to enhance the effect of certain antihypertensive agents). Products include:
Mavik Tablets 472
Tarka Tablets 511

Triamcinolone (Agents that induce CYP3A4 could cause an increase in aripiprazole clearance and lower blood levels).
No products indexed under this heading.

Triamcinolone Acetonide (Agents that induce CYP3A4 could cause an increase in aripiprazole clearance and lower blood levels). Products include:
Azmacort Inhalation Aerosol 407
Nasacort AQ Nasal Spray 2765
Triesence Injectable Suspension .... ⊙ 209

Triamcinolone Diacetate (Agents that induce CYP3A4 could cause an increase in aripiprazole clearance and lower blood levels).
No products indexed under this heading.

Triamcinolone Hexacetonide (Agents that induce CYP3A4 could cause an increase in aripiprazole clearance and lower blood levels).
No products indexed under this heading.

Triazolam (Given the primary CNS effects of aripiprazole, caution should be used when co-administered with other centrally acting drugs).
No products indexed under this heading.

Trifluoperazine Hydrochloride (Given the primary CNS effects of aripiprazole, caution should be used when co-administered with other centrally acting drugs).
No products indexed under this heading.

Trimethaphan Camsylate (Due to its alpha-1-adrenergic receptor antagonism, aripiprazole has the potential to enhance the effect of certain antihypertensive agents).
No products indexed under this heading.

Trimipramine Maleate (Inhibitors of CYP2D6 can inhibit aripiprazole elimination and cause increased blood levels).
No products indexed under this heading.

Troglitazone (Agents that induce CYP3A4 could cause an increase in aripiprazole clearance and lower blood levels).
No products indexed under this heading.

Troleandomycin (Strong inhibitors of CYP3A4 may increase levels of aripiprazole and its active metabolite; dose reduction of aripiprazole should be considered).
No products indexed under this heading.

Valproate Sodium (Inhibitors of CYP3A4 can inhibit aripiprazole elimination and cause increased blood levels).
No products indexed under this heading.

Valsartan (Due to its alpha-1-adrenergic receptor antagonism, aripiprazole has the potential to enhance the effect of certain antihypertensive agents). Products include:
Diovan Tablets 2212
Diovan HCT Tablets 2216
Exforge Tablets 2238

Vardenafil Hydrochloride (Inhibitors of CYP3A4 can inhibit aripiprazole elimination and cause increased blood levels). Products include:
Levitra Tablets 2876

Verapamil Hydrochloride (Due to its alpha-1-adrenergic receptor antagonism, aripiprazole has the potential to enhance the effect of certain antihypertensive agents). Products include:
Tarka Tablets 511

Voriconazole (Strong inhibitors of CYP3A4 may increase levels of aripiprazole and its active metabolite; dose reduction of aripiprazole should be considered).
No products indexed under this heading.

Zafirlukast (Inhibitors of CYP3A4 can inhibit aripiprazole elimination and cause increased blood levels). Products include:
Accolate Tablets 669

Zaleplon (Given the primary CNS effects of aripiprazole, caution should be used when co-administered with other centrally acting drugs).
No products indexed under this heading.

Zileuton (Inhibitors of CYP3A4 can inhibit aripiprazole elimination and cause increased blood levels).
No products indexed under this heading.

Ziprasidone Hydrochloride (Given the primary CNS effects of aripiprazole, caution should be used when co-administered with other centrally acting drugs). Products include:
Geodon Capsules 2520

Zolpidem Tartrate (Given the primary CNS effects of aripiprazole,

caution should be used when co-administered with other centrally acting drugs). Products include:
Ambien Tablets ... 2692
Ambien CR Tablets ... 2696

Food Interactions

Alcohol (Given the primary CNS effects of aripiprazole, caution should be used when co-administered with alcohol; patients should be advised to avoid alcohol while taking aripiprazole).

Grapefruit (Inhibitors of CYP3A4 can inhibit aripiprazole elimination and cause increased blood levels).

Grapefruit Juice (Inhibitors of CYP3A4 can inhibit aripiprazole elimination and cause increased blood levels).

ABILIFY TABLETS

(Aripiprazole) ... 2466
May interact with antihypertensives, central nervous system depressants, central nervous system stimulants, cytochrome p450 2d6 inhibitors (selected), cytochrome p450 3a4 inducers (selected), cytochrome p450 3a4 inhibitors (selected), cytochrome p450 3a4 inhibitors, potent, quinidine, and certain other agents. Compounds in these categories include:

Acebutolol Hydrochloride (Due to its alpha-1-adrenergic receptor antagonism, aripiprazole has the potential to enhance the effect of certain antihypertensive agents).
No products indexed under this heading.

Acetazolamide (Inhibitors of CYP3A4 can inhibit aripiprazole elimination and cause increased blood levels).
No products indexed under this heading.

Alfentanil Hydrochloride (Given the primary CNS effects of aripiprazole, caution should be used when co-administered with other centrally acting drugs).
No products indexed under this heading.

Aliskiren (Due to its alpha-1-adrenergic receptor antagonism, aripiprazole has the potential to enhance the effect of certain antihypertensive agents). Products include:
Tekturna Tablets ... 2321
Tekturna HCT Tablets ... 2324

Allium sativum (Agents that induce CYP3A4 could cause an increase in aripiprazole clearance and lower blood levels).
No products indexed under this heading.

Alprazolam (Given the primary CNS effects of aripiprazole, caution should be used when co-administered with other centrally acting drugs).
No products indexed under this heading.

Amiodarone Hydrochloride (Inhibitors of CYP3A4 can inhibit aripiprazole elimination and cause increased blood levels).
No products indexed under this heading.

Amitriptyline Hydrochloride (Inhibitors of CYP2D6 can inhibit aripiprazole elimination and cause increased blood levels).
No products indexed under this heading.

Amlodipine Besylate (Due to its alpha-1-adrenergic receptor antagonism, aripiprazole has the potential to enhance the effect of certain antihypertensive agents). Products include:
Azor Tablets ... 1005
Exforge Tablets ... 2238

Amoxapine (Inhibitors of CYP2D6 can inhibit aripiprazole elimination and cause increased blood levels).
No products indexed under this heading.

Amphetamine Resins (Given the primary CNS effects of aripiprazole, caution should be used when co-administered with other centrally acting drugs).
No products indexed under this heading.

Amprenavir (Strong inhibitors of CYP3A4 may increase levels of aripiprazole and its active metabolite; dose reduction of aripiprazole should be considered).
No products indexed under this heading.

Anastrozole (Inhibitors of CYP3A4 can inhibit aripiprazole elimination and cause increased blood levels). Products include:
Arimidex Tablets ... 672

Aprepitant (Agents that induce CYP3A4 could cause an increase in aripiprazole clearance and lower blood levels). Products include:
Emend Capsules ... 1992

Aprobarbital (Given the primary CNS effects of aripiprazole, caution should be used when co-administered with other centrally acting drugs).
No products indexed under this heading.

Atazanavir (Strong inhibitors of CYP3A4 may increase levels of aripiprazole and its active metabolite; dose reduction of aripiprazole should be considered).
No products indexed under this heading.

Atazanavir Sulfate (Strong inhibitors of CYP3A4 may increase levels of aripiprazole and its active metabolite; dose reduction of aripiprazole should be considered). Products include:
Reyataz Capsules ... 3299

Atenolol (Due to its alpha-1-adrenergic receptor antagonism, aripiprazole has the potential to enhance the effect of certain antihypertensive agents).
No products indexed under this heading.

Benazepril Hydrochloride (Due to its alpha-1-adrenergic receptor antagonism, aripiprazole has the potential to enhance the effect of certain antihypertensive agents).
No products indexed under this heading.

Bendroflumethiazide (Due to its alpha-1-adrenergic receptor antagonism, aripiprazole has the potential to enhance the effect of certain antihypertensive agents).
No products indexed under this heading.

Betamethasone Acetate (Agents that induce CYP3A4 could cause an increase in aripiprazole clearance and lower blood levels).
No products indexed under this heading.

Betamethasone Sodium Phosphate (Agents that induce CYP3A4 could cause an increase in aripiprazole clearance and lower blood levels).
No products indexed under this heading.

Betaxolol Hydrochloride (Due to its alpha-1-adrenergic receptor antagonism, aripiprazole has the potential to enhance the effect of certain antihypertensive agents).
No products indexed under this heading.

Bisoprolol Fumarate (Due to its alpha-1-adrenergic receptor antagonism, aripiprazole has the potential to enhance the effect of certain antihypertensive agents).
No products indexed under this heading.

Buprenorphine Hydrochloride (Given the primary CNS effects of aripiprazole, caution should be used when co-administered with other centrally acting drugs). Products include:
Suboxone Tablets ... 2601
Subutex Tablets ... 2601

Bupropion Hydrochloride (Inhibitors of CYP2D6 can inhibit aripiprazole elimination and cause increased blood levels). Products include:
Wellbutrin Tablets ... 1648
Wellbutrin SR Sustained-Release Tablets ... 1653
Wellbutrin XL Extended-Release Tablets ... 1659
Zyban Sustained-Release Tablets ... 1692

Buspirone Hydrochloride (Given the primary CNS effects of aripiprazole, caution should be used when co-administered with other centrally acting drugs).
No products indexed under this heading.

Butabarbital (Given the primary CNS effects of aripiprazole, caution should be used when co-administered with other centrally acting drugs).
No products indexed under this heading.

Butalbital (Given the primary CNS effects of aripiprazole, caution should be used when co-administered with other centrally acting drugs).
No products indexed under this heading.

Candesartan Cilexetil (Due to its alpha-1-adrenergic receptor antagonism, aripiprazole has the potential to enhance the effect of certain antihypertensive agents). Products include:
Atacand Tablets ... 639
Atacand HCT ... 642

Captopril (Due to its alpha-1-adrenergic receptor antagonism, aripiprazole has the potential to enhance the effect of certain antihypertensive agents). Products include:
Captopril Tablets ... 2182

Carbamazepine (Co-administration of carbamazepine, a potent CYP3A4 inducer, with aripiprazole resulted in an approximate 70% decrease in Cmax and AUC values of both aripiprazole and its active metabolite, dehydro-aripiprazole. When carbamazepine is added to aripiprazole therapy, aripiprazole dose should be doubled. When carbamazepine is withdrawn from combination therapy, aripiprazole dose should then be reduced). Products include:
Carbatrol Capsules ... 3019
Equetro Extended-Release Capsules ... 3174

Carteolol Hydrochloride (Due to its alpha-1-adrenergic receptor antagonism, aripiprazole has the potential to enhance the effect of certain antihypertensive agents).
No products indexed under this heading.

Celecoxib (Inhibitors of CYP2D6 can inhibit aripiprazole elimination and cause increased blood levels). Products include:
Celebrex Capsules ... 2979

Chlordiazepoxide (Given the primary CNS effects of aripiprazole, caution should be used when co-administered with other centrally acting drugs).
No products indexed under this heading.

Chlordiazepoxide Hydrochloride (Given the primary CNS effects of aripiprazole, caution should be used when co-administered with other centrally acting drugs).
No products indexed under this heading.

Chloroquine Hydrochloride (Inhibitors of CYP2D6 can inhibit aripiprazole elimination and cause increased blood levels).
No products indexed under this heading.

Chloroquine Phosphate (Inhibitors of CYP2D6 can inhibit aripiprazole elimination and cause increased blood levels).
No products indexed under this heading.

Chlorothiazide (Due to its alpha-1-adrenergic receptor antagonism, aripiprazole has the potential to enhance the effect of certain antihypertensive agents).
No products indexed under this heading.

Chlorothiazide Sodium (Due to its alpha-1-adrenergic receptor antagonism, aripiprazole has the potential to enhance the effect of certain antihypertensive agents). Products include:
Intravenous Sodium Diuril ... 2490

Chlorpheniramine (Inhibitors of CYP2D6 can inhibit aripiprazole elimination and cause increased blood levels).
No products indexed under this heading.

Chlorpheniramine Maleate (Inhibitors of CYP2D6 can inhibit aripiprazole elimination and cause increased blood levels). Products include:
Actifed Cold & Allergy Tablets ... 1895
Sudafed PE Sinus & Allergy Tablets ... 1908
Tylenol Allergy Multi-Symptom Caplets with Cool Burst and Rapid Release Gelcaps ... 1916
Children's Tylenol Plus Cold Suspension Liquid ... 1912
Children's Tylenol Plus Cough & Runny Nose Suspension Liquid ... 1912
Children's Tylenol Plus Flu Suspension Liquid ... 1914
Children's Tylenol Plus Multi-Symptom Cold Suspension Liquid ... 1912
Tylenol Cold Head Congestion Nighttime Caplets with Cool Burst ... 1910

IMPORTANT NOTE: Always consult each drug listing in the patient's regimen for possible interactions.

Tylenol Cold Multi-Symptom Nighttime Caplets with Cool Burst ... 1913
Tylenol Sinus Congestion & Pain Nighttime Caplets with Cool Burst ... 1917

Chlorpheniramine Polistirex (Inhibitors of CYP2D6 can inhibit aripiprazole elimination and cause increased blood levels). Products include:
Tussionex Pennkinetic Extended-Release Suspension ... 3154

Chlorpheniramine Tannate (Inhibitors of CYP2D6 can inhibit aripiprazole elimination and cause increased blood levels).
No products indexed under this heading.

Chlorpromazine (Given the primary CNS effects of aripiprazole, caution should be used when co-administered with other centrally acting drugs).
No products indexed under this heading.

Chlorpromazine Hydrochloride (Given the primary CNS effects of aripiprazole, caution should be used when co-administered with other centrally acting drugs).
No products indexed under this heading.

Chlorprothixene (Given the primary CNS effects of aripiprazole, caution should be used when co-administered with other centrally acting drugs).
No products indexed under this heading.

Chlorprothixene Hydrochloride (Given the primary CNS effects of aripiprazole, caution should be used when co-administered with other centrally acting drugs).
No products indexed under this heading.

Chlorprothixene Lactate (Given the primary CNS effects of aripiprazole, caution should be used when co-administered with other centrally acting drugs).
No products indexed under this heading.

Chlorthalidone (Due to its alpha-1-adrenergic receptor antagonism, aripiprazole has the potential to enhance the effect of certain antihypertensive agents). Products include:
Clorpres Tablets ... 2185

Cimetidine (Inhibitors of CYP3A4 can inhibit aripiprazole elimination and cause increased blood levels).
No products indexed under this heading.

Cimetidine Hydrochloride (Inhibitors of CYP3A4 can inhibit aripiprazole elimination and cause increased blood levels).
No products indexed under this heading.

Ciprofloxacin (Inhibitors of CYP3A4 can inhibit aripiprazole elimination and cause increased blood levels). Products include:
Cipro I.V. ... 2817
Cipro Oral Suspension ... 2810
Cipro XR Tablets ... 2823
Ciprodex Otic Suspension ... 541

Ciprofloxacin Hydrochloride (Agents that induce CYP3A4 could cause an increase in aripiprazole clearance and lower blood levels). Products include:
Cipro Tablets ... 2810

Cisplatin (Agents that induce CYP3A4 could cause an increase in aripiprazole clearance and lower blood levels).
No products indexed under this heading.

Citalopram Hydrobromide (Inhibitors of CYP2D6 can inhibit aripiprazole elimination and cause increased blood levels). Products include:
Celexa ... 1160

Clarithromycin (Strong inhibitors of CYP3A4 may increase levels of aripiprazole and its active metabolite; dose reduction of aripiprazole should be considered). Products include:
Biaxin/Biaxin XL ... 411

Clomipramine Hydrochloride (Inhibitors of CYP2D6 can inhibit aripiprazole elimination and cause increased blood levels).
No products indexed under this heading.

Clonidine (Due to its alpha-1-adrenergic receptor antagonism, aripiprazole has the potential to enhance the effect of certain antihypertensive agents). Products include:
Catapres-TTS ... 842

Clonidine Hydrochloride (Due to its alpha-1-adrenergic receptor antagonism, aripiprazole has the potential to enhance the effect of certain antihypertensive agents). Products include:
Catapres Tablets ... 841
Clorpres Tablets ... 2185

Clorazepate Dipotassium (Given the primary CNS effects of aripiprazole, caution should be used when co-administered with other centrally acting drugs).
No products indexed under this heading.

Clotrimazole (Inhibitors of CYP3A4 can inhibit aripiprazole elimination and cause increased blood levels). Products include:
Lotrisone ... 2881

Clozapine (Given the primary CNS effects of aripiprazole, caution should be used when co-administered with other centrally acting drugs).
No products indexed under this heading.

Cocaine Hydrochloride (Inhibitors of CYP2D6 can inhibit aripiprazole elimination and cause increased blood levels).
No products indexed under this heading.

Codeine Phosphate (Given the primary CNS effects of aripiprazole, caution should be used when co-administered with other centrally acting drugs). Products include:
Tylenol with Codeine Tablets ... 2427

Cortisone Acetate (Agents that induce CYP3A4 could cause an increase in aripiprazole clearance and lower blood levels).
No products indexed under this heading.

Cyclosporine (Inhibitors of CYP3A4 can inhibit aripiprazole elimination and cause increased blood levels). Products include:
Gengraf Capsules ... 435
Neoral Oral Solution ... 2280
Neoral Soft Gelatin Capsules ... 2280
Restasis Ophthalmic Emulsion ... 557
Sandimmune ... 2296

Dalfopristin (Inhibitors of CYP3A4 can inhibit aripiprazole elimination and cause increased blood levels).
No products indexed under this heading.

Danazol (Inhibitors of CYP3A4 can inhibit aripiprazole elimination and cause increased blood levels).
No products indexed under this heading.

Delavirdine Mesylate (Strong inhibitors of CYP3A4 may increase levels of aripiprazole and its active metabolite; dose reduction of aripiprazole should be considered).
No products indexed under this heading.

Delavirine (Strong inhibitors of CYP3A4 may increase levels of aripiprazole and its active metabolite; dose reduction of aripiprazole should be considered).
No products indexed under this heading.

Deserpidine (Due to its alpha-1-adrenergic receptor antagonism, aripiprazole has the potential to enhance the effect of certain antihypertensive agents).
No products indexed under this heading.

Desflurane (Given the primary CNS effects of aripiprazole, caution should be used when co-administered with other centrally acting drugs).
No products indexed under this heading.

Desipramine Hydrochloride (Inhibitors of CYP2D6 can inhibit aripiprazole elimination and cause increased blood levels).
No products indexed under this heading.

Dexamethasone (Agents that induce CYP3A4 could cause an increase in aripiprazole clearance and lower blood levels). Products include:
Ciprodex Otic Suspension ... 541

Dexamethasone Acetate (Agents that induce CYP3A4 could cause an increase in aripiprazole clearance and lower blood levels).
No products indexed under this heading.

Dexamethasone Sodium Phosphate (Agents that induce CYP3A4 could cause an increase in aripiprazole clearance and lower blood levels).
No products indexed under this heading.

Dextroamphetamine Sulfate (Given the primary CNS effects of aripiprazole, caution should be used when co-administered with other centrally acting drugs). Products include:
Adderall XR Capsules ... 3012
Dexedrine ... 1401

Dezocine (Given the primary CNS effects of aripiprazole, caution should be used when co-administered with other centrally acting drugs).
No products indexed under this heading.

Diazepam (Given the primary CNS effects of aripiprazole, caution should be used when co-administered with other centrally acting drugs). Products include:
Valium Tablets ... 2658

Diazoxide (Due to its alpha-1-adrenergic receptor antagonism, aripiprazole has the potential to enhance the effect of certain antihypertensive agents). Products include:
Proglycem Capsules ... 1185
Proglycem Suspension ... 1185

Diltiazem Hydrochloride (Due to its alpha-1-adrenergic receptor antagonism, aripiprazole has the potential to enhance the effect of certain antihypertensive agents). Products include:
Cardizem LA Extended Release Tablets ... 421

Diltiazem Maleate (Inhibitors of CYP3A4 can inhibit aripiprazole elimination and cause increased blood levels).
No products indexed under this heading.

Diphenhydramine (Inhibitors of CYP2D6 can inhibit aripiprazole elimination and cause increased blood levels).
No products indexed under this heading.

Diphenhydramine Hydrochloride (Inhibitors of CYP2D6 can inhibit aripiprazole elimination and cause increased blood levels). Products include:
Benadryl Allergy & Cold Kapgels ... 1895
Benadryl Allergy & Sinus Headache Kapgels ... 1895
Benadryl Severe Allergy & Sinus Headache Caplets ... 1897
Benadryl Dye-Free Allergy Liqui-gels Softgels ... 1897
Benadryl Allergy Kapgels ... 1895
Benadryl Allergy Quick Dissolve Strips ... 1896
Benadryl Allergy Ultratab Tablets ... 1896
Children's Benadryl Dye-Free Allergy Liquid ... 1897
Children's Benadryl Allergy Fastmelts ... 1897
Children's Benadryl Allergy Liquid ... 1898
Children's Benadryl Allergy Perfect Measure ... 1896
Children's Benadryl-D Allergy & Sinus Liquid ... 1896
Benadryl-D Allergy & Sinus Tablet ... 1896
PediaCare Children's Allergy & Cold Liquid ... 1902
PediaCare Children's Allergy Liquid ... 1902
Simply Sleep Caplets ... 1905
Sudafed PE Nighttime Cold Caplets ... 1907
Sudafed PE Severe Cold Caplets ... 1908
Extra Strength Tylenol PM Caplets, Geltabs, Liquid, and Rapid Release Gels ... 1915
Tylenol Allergy Multi-Symptom Nighttime Caplets with Cool Burst ... 1916
Tylenol Severe Allergy Caplets ... 1916
Children's Tylenol Plus Cold & Allergy Suspension Liquid ... 1914
Tylenol Sore Throat Nighttime Liquid with Cool Burst ... 1918

Doxazosin Mesylate (Due to its alpha-1-adrenergic receptor antagonism, aripiprazole has the potential to enhance the effect of certain antihypertensive agents).
No products indexed under this heading.

Doxepin Hydrochloride (Inhibitors of CYP2D6 can inhibit aripiprazole elimination and cause increased blood levels).
No products indexed under this heading.

Doxorubicin Hydrochloride (Agents that induce CYP3A4 could cause an increase in aripiprazole clearance and lower blood levels).
No products indexed under this heading.

Droperidol (Given the primary CNS effects of aripiprazole, caution should be used when co-administered with other centrally acting drugs).
No products indexed under this heading.

Efavirenz (Agents that induce CYP3A4 could cause an increase in aripiprazole clearance and lower blood levels). Products include:
Atripla Tablets 938
Sustiva Capsules 930
Sustiva Tablets 930

Enalapril Maleate (Due to its alpha-1-adrenergic receptor antagonism, aripiprazole has the potential to enhance the effect of certain antihypertensive agents).
No products indexed under this heading.

Enalaprilat (Due to its alpha-1-adrenergic receptor antagonism, aripiprazole has the potential to enhance the effect of certain antihypertensive agents).
No products indexed under this heading.

Enflurane (Given the primary CNS effects of aripiprazole, caution should be used when co-administered with other centrally acting drugs).
No products indexed under this heading.

Eprosartan Mesylate (Due to its alpha-1-adrenergic receptor antagonism, aripiprazole has the potential to enhance the effect of certain antihypertensive agents). Products include:
Teveten Tablets 515
Teveten HCT Tablets 517

Erythromycin (Inhibitors of CYP3A4 can inhibit aripiprazole elimination and cause increased blood levels).
No products indexed under this heading.

Erythromycin Estolate (Inhibitors of CYP3A4 can inhibit aripiprazole elimination and cause increased blood levels).
No products indexed under this heading.

Erythromycin Ethylsuccinate (Inhibitors of CYP3A4 can inhibit aripiprazole elimination and cause increased blood levels). Products include:
E.E.S. 433
EryPed 431

Erythromycin Gluceptate (Inhibitors of CYP3A4 can inhibit aripiprazole elimination and cause increased blood levels).
No products indexed under this heading.

Erythromycin Lactobionate (Inhibitors of CYP3A4 can inhibit aripiprazole elimination and cause increased blood levels).
No products indexed under this heading.

Erythromycin Stearate (Inhibitors of CYP3A4 can inhibit aripiprazole elimination and cause increased blood levels).
No products indexed under this heading.

Escitalopram Oxalate (Inhibitors of CYP2D6 can inhibit aripiprazole elimination and cause increased blood levels). Products include:
Lexapro Oral Suspension 1174
Lexapro Tablets 1174

Esmolol Hydrochloride (Due to its alpha-1-adrenergic receptor antagonism, aripiprazole has the potential to enhance the effect of certain antihypertensive agents).
No products indexed under this heading.

Esomeprazole Magnesium (Inhibitors of CYP3A4 can inhibit aripiprazole elimination and cause increased blood levels). Products include:
Nexium Delayed-Release Capsules 645
Nexium Delayed-Release Oral Suspension 645

Estazolam (Given the primary CNS effects of aripiprazole, caution should be used when co-administered with other centrally acting drugs).
No products indexed under this heading.

Ethanol (Given the primary CNS effects of aripiprazole, caution should be used when co-administered with other centrally acting drugs).
No products indexed under this heading.

Ethchlorvynol (Given the primary CNS effects of aripiprazole, caution should be used when co-administered with other centrally acting drugs).
No products indexed under this heading.

Ethinamate (Given the primary CNS effects of aripiprazole, caution should be used when co-administered with other centrally acting drugs).
No products indexed under this heading.

Ethosuximide (Agents that induce CYP3A4 could cause an increase in aripiprazole clearance and lower blood levels).
No products indexed under this heading.

Ethyl Alcohol (Given the primary CNS effects of aripiprazole, caution should be used when co-administered with other centrally acting drugs).
No products indexed under this heading.

Famotidine (Co-administration will decrease the solubility of aripiprazole and hence its rate of absorption. No dosage adjustment is required). Products include:
Pepcid Tablets 2075
Original Strength Pepcid AC Gelcaps 1771
Original Strength Pepcid AC Tablets 1771
Maximum Strength Pepcid AC Tablets 1771
Pepcid Complete Chewable Tablets 1771

Felbamate (Agents that induce CYP3A4 could cause an increase in aripiprazole clearance and lower blood levels).
No products indexed under this heading.

Felodipine (Due to its alpha-1-adrenergic receptor antagonism, aripiprazole has the potential to enhance the effect of certain antihypertensive agents).
No products indexed under this heading.

Fentanyl (Given the primary CNS effects of aripiprazole, caution should be used when co-administered with other centrally acting drugs). Products include:
Duragesic Transdermal System 2405
Ionsys Transdermal System 2410

Fentanyl Citrate (Given the primary CNS effects of aripiprazole, caution should be used when co-administered with other centrally acting drugs). Products include:
Actiq 959
Fentora Tablets 968

Fluconazole (Inhibitors of CYP3A4 can inhibit aripiprazole elimination and cause increased blood levels).
No products indexed under this heading.

Fludrocortisone Acetate (Agents that induce CYP3A4 could cause an increase in aripiprazole clearance and lower blood levels).
No products indexed under this heading.

Fluoxetine (When concomitant administration of potential CYP2D6 inhibitors such as quinidine, fluoxetine, or paroxetine with aripiprazole occurs, aripiprazole dose should be reduced at least to one-half of its normal dose. When the CYP2D6 inhibitor is withdrawn from the combination therapy, the aripiprazole dose should then be increased. When adjunctive aripiprazole is administered to patients with major depressive disorder, aripiprazole should be administered without dosage adjustment as specified).
No products indexed under this heading.

Fluoxetine Hydrochloride (When concomitant administration of potential CYP2D6 inhibitors such as quinidine, fluoxetine, or paroxetine with aripiprazole occurs, aripiprazole dose should be reduced at least to one-half of its normal dose. When the CYP2D6 inhibitor is withdrawn from the combination therapy, the aripiprazole dose should then be increased. When adjunctive aripiprazole is administered to patients with major depressive disorder, aripiprazole should be administered without dosage adjustment as specified). Products include:
Prozac Weekly Capsules 1852
Prozac Pulvules and Liquid 1852
Symbyax Capsules 1871

Fluphenazine Decanoate (Inhibitors of CYP2D6 can inhibit aripiprazole elimination and cause increased blood levels).
No products indexed under this heading.

Fluphenazine Enanthate (Inhibitors of CYP2D6 can inhibit aripiprazole elimination and cause increased blood levels).
No products indexed under this heading.

Fluphenazine Hydrochloride (Inhibitors of CYP2D6 can inhibit aripiprazole elimination and cause increased blood levels).
No products indexed under this heading.

Flurazepam Hydrochloride (Given the primary CNS effects of aripiprazole, caution should be used when co-administered with other centrally acting drugs).
No products indexed under this heading.

Fluvoxamine Maleate (Inhibitors of CYP3A4 can inhibit aripiprazole elimination and cause increased blood levels). Products include:
Luvox CR Extended-Release Capsules 1759

Fosamprenavir Calcium (Strong inhibitors of CYP3A4 may increase levels of aripiprazole and its active metabolite; dose reduction of aripiprazole should be considered). Products include:
Lexiva Oral Suspension 1510
Lexiva Tablets 1510

Fosinopril Sodium (Due to its alpha-1-adrenergic receptor antagonism, aripiprazole has the potential to enhance the effect of certain antihypertensive agents).
No products indexed under this heading.

Fosphenytoin Sodium (Agents that induce CYP3A4 could cause an increase in aripiprazole clearance and lower blood levels).
No products indexed under this heading.

Furosemide (Due to its alpha-1-adrenergic receptor antagonism, aripiprazole has the potential to enhance the effect of certain antihypertensive agents). Products include:
Furosemide Tablets 2186

Garlic Extract (Agents that induce CYP3A4 could cause an increase in aripiprazole clearance and lower blood levels).
No products indexed under this heading.

Garlic Oil (Agents that induce CYP3A4 could cause an increase in aripiprazole clearance and lower blood levels).
No products indexed under this heading.

Glutethimide (Given the primary CNS effects of aripiprazole, caution should be used when co-administered with other centrally acting drugs).
No products indexed under this heading.

Guanabenz Acetate (Due to its alpha-1-adrenergic receptor antagonism, aripiprazole has the potential to enhance the effect of certain antihypertensive agents).
No products indexed under this heading.

Guanethidine Monosulfate (Due to its alpha-1-adrenergic receptor antagonism, aripiprazole has the potential to enhance the effect of certain antihypertensive agents).
No products indexed under this heading.

Halofantrine Hydrochloride (Inhibitors of CYP2D6 can inhibit aripiprazole elimination and cause increased blood levels).
No products indexed under this heading.

Haloperidol (Inhibitors of CYP2D6 can inhibit aripiprazole elimination and cause increased blood levels).
No products indexed under this heading.

Haloperidol Decanoate (Inhibitors of CYP2D6 can inhibit aripiprazole elimination and cause increased blood levels).
No products indexed under this heading.

IMPORTANT NOTE: Always consult each drug listing in the patient's regimen for possible interactions.

Hydralazine Hydrochloride (Due to its alpha-1-adrenergic receptor antagonism, aripiprazole has the potential to enhance the effect of certain antihypertensive agents).
No products indexed under this heading.

Hydrochlorothiazide (Due to its alpha-1-adrenergic receptor antagonism, aripiprazole has the potential to enhance the effect of certain antihypertensive agents). Products include:
Atacand HCT 642
Avalide Tablets 892
Avalide Tablets 2713
Benicar HCT Tablets 1010
Diovan HCT Tablets 2216
Dyazide Capsules 1405
Micardis HCT Tablets 854
Prinzide Tablets 2092
Tekturna HCT Tablets 2324
Teveten HCT Tablets 517

Hydrocodone Bitartrate (Given the primary CNS effects of aripiprazole, caution should be used when co-administered with other centrally acting drugs). Products include:
Lortab 5/500 Tablets 3143
Lortab 7.5/500 Tablets 3144
Lortab 10/500 Tablets 3144
Vicodin Tablets 529
Vicodin ES Tablets 530
Vicodin HP Tablets 531
Vicoprofen Tablets 533
Zydone Tablets 1132

Hydrocodone Polistirex (Given the primary CNS effects of aripiprazole, caution should be used when co-administered with other centrally acting drugs). Products include:
Tussionex Pennkinetic Extended-Release Suspension 3154

Hydrocortisone (Agents that induce CYP3A4 could cause an increase in aripiprazole clearance and lower blood levels).
No products indexed under this heading.

Hydrocortisone Acetate (Agents that induce CYP3A4 could cause an increase in aripiprazole clearance and lower blood levels). Products include:
Analpram-HC 1140
Pramosone 1141

Hydrocortisone Butyrate (Agents that induce CYP3A4 could cause an increase in aripiprazole clearance and lower blood levels).
No products indexed under this heading.

Hydrocortisone Cypionate (Agents that induce CYP3A4 could cause an increase in aripiprazole clearance and lower blood levels).
No products indexed under this heading.

Hydrocortisone Hemisuccinate (Agents that induce CYP3A4 could cause an increase in aripiprazole clearance and lower blood levels).
No products indexed under this heading.

Hydrocortisone Probutate (Agents that induce CYP3A4 could cause an increase in aripiprazole clearance and lower blood levels).
No products indexed under this heading.

Hydrocortisone Sodium Phosphate (Agents that induce CYP3A4 could cause an increase in aripiprazole clearance and lower blood levels).
No products indexed under this heading.

Hydrocortisone Sodium Succinate (Agents that induce CYP3A4 could cause an increase in aripiprazole clearance and lower blood levels).
No products indexed under this heading.

Hydrocortisone Valerate (Agents that induce CYP3A4 could cause an increase in aripiprazole clearance and lower blood levels).
No products indexed under this heading.

Hydroflumethiazide (Due to its alpha-1-adrenergic receptor antagonism, aripiprazole has the potential to enhance the effect of certain antihypertensive agents).
No products indexed under this heading.

Hydromorphone Hydrochloride (Given the primary CNS effects of aripiprazole, caution should be used when co-administered with other centrally acting drugs).
No products indexed under this heading.

Hydroxychloroquine Sulfate (Inhibitors of CYP2D6 can inhibit aripiprazole elimination and cause increased blood levels).
No products indexed under this heading.

Hydroxyzine Hydrochloride (Given the primary CNS effects of aripiprazole, caution should be used when co-administered with other centrally acting drugs).
No products indexed under this heading.

Hypericum (Agents that induce CYP3A4 could cause an increase in aripiprazole clearance and lower blood levels). Products include:
Satieté Tablets .... ▣ 640

Hypericum Perforatum (Agents that induce CYP3A4 could cause an increase in aripiprazole clearance and lower blood levels).
No products indexed under this heading.

Imatinib Mesylate (Inhibitors of CYP2D6 can inhibit aripiprazole elimination and cause increased blood levels). Products include:
Gleevec Tablets 2255

Imipramine Hydrochloride (Inhibitors of CYP2D6 can inhibit aripiprazole elimination and cause increased blood levels).
No products indexed under this heading.

Imipramine Pamoate (Inhibitors of CYP2D6 can inhibit aripiprazole elimination and cause increased blood levels).
No products indexed under this heading.

Indapamide (Due to its alpha-1-adrenergic receptor antagonism, aripiprazole has the potential to enhance the effect of certain antihypertensive agents). Products include:
Indapamide Tablets 2188

Indinavir Sulfate (Strong inhibitors of CYP3A4 may increase levels of aripiprazole and its active metabolite; dose reduction of aripiprazole should be considered). Products include:
Crixivan Capsules 1979

Irbesartan (Due to its alpha-1-adrenergic receptor antagonism, aripiprazole has the potential to enhance the effect of certain antihypertensive agents). Products include:
Avalide Tablets 892
Avalide Tablets 2713
Avapro Tablets 897
Avapro Tablets 2718

Isoflurane (Given the primary CNS effects of aripiprazole, caution should be used when co-administered with other centrally acting drugs).
No products indexed under this heading.

Isoniazid (Inhibitors of CYP3A4 can inhibit aripiprazole elimination and cause increased blood levels).
No products indexed under this heading.

Isradipine (Due to its alpha-1-adrenergic receptor antagonism, aripiprazole has the potential to enhance the effect of certain antihypertensive agents). Products include:
DynaCirc CR Controlled Release Tablets 1407

Itraconazole (Co-administration with ketoconazole increased the AUC of aripiprazole and its active metabolite by 63% and 77%, respectively. When concomitant administration of ketoconazole with aripiprazole occurs, aripiprazole dose should be reduced to one-half of its normal dose. Other strong inhibitors of CYP3A4 (itraconazole) would be expected to have similar effects and need similar dose reductions. When the CYP3A4 inhibitor is withdrawn from the combination therapy, aripiprazole dose should then be increased).
No products indexed under this heading.

Ketamine Hydrochloride (Given the primary CNS effects of aripiprazole, caution should be used when co-administered with other centrally acting drugs).
No products indexed under this heading.

Ketoconazole (Co-administration with ketoconazole increased the AUC of aripiprazole and its active metabolite by 63% and 77%, respectively. When concomitant administration of ketoconazole with aripiprazole occurs, aripiprazole dose should be reduced to one-half of its normal dose. When the CYP3A4 inhibitor is withdrawn from the combination therapy, aripiprazole dose should then be increased). Products include:
Extina Foam, 2% 3057
Nizoral A-D Shampoo 1901

Labetalol Hydrochloride (Due to its alpha-1-adrenergic receptor antagonism, aripiprazole has the potential to enhance the effect of certain antihypertensive agents).
No products indexed under this heading.

Levomethadyl Acetate Hydrochloride (Given the primary CNS effects of aripiprazole, caution should be used when co-administered with other centrally acting drugs).
No products indexed under this heading.

Levorphanol Tartrate (Given the primary CNS effects of aripiprazole, caution should be used when co-administered with other centrally acting drugs).
No products indexed under this heading.

Lisinopril (Due to its alpha-1-adrenergic receptor antagonism, aripiprazole has the potential to enhance the effect of certain antihypertensive agents). Products include:
Prinivil Tablets 2087
Prinzide Tablets 2092

Lopinavir (Strong inhibitors of CYP3A4 may increase levels of aripiprazole and its active metabolite; dose reduction of aripiprazole should be considered). Products include:
Kaletra 452

Loratadine (Inhibitors of CYP3A4 can inhibit aripiprazole elimination and cause increased blood levels).
No products indexed under this heading.

Lorazepam (Given the primary CNS effects of aripiprazole, caution should be used when co-administered with other centrally acting drugs).
No products indexed under this heading.

Losartan Potassium (Due to its alpha-1-adrenergic receptor antagonism, aripiprazole has the potential to enhance the effect of certain antihypertensive agents). Products include:
Cozaar Tablets 1973

Loxapine Hydrochloride (Given the primary CNS effects of aripiprazole, caution should be used when co-administered with other centrally acting drugs).
No products indexed under this heading.

Loxapine Succinate (Given the primary CNS effects of aripiprazole, caution should be used when co-administered with other centrally acting drugs).
No products indexed under this heading.

Maprotiline Hydrochloride (Inhibitors of CYP2D6 can inhibit aripiprazole elimination and cause increased blood levels).
No products indexed under this heading.

Mecamylamine Hydrochloride (Due to its alpha-1-adrenergic receptor antagonism, aripiprazole has the potential to enhance the effect of certain antihypertensive agents).
No products indexed under this heading.

Meperidine Hydrochloride (Given the primary CNS effects of aripiprazole, caution should be used when co-administered with other centrally acting drugs).
No products indexed under this heading.

Mephenytoin (Agents that induce CYP3A4 could cause an increase in aripiprazole clearance and lower blood levels).
No products indexed under this heading.

Mephobarbital (Given the primary CNS effects of aripiprazole, caution should be used when co-administered with other centrally acting drugs).
No products indexed under this heading.

Meprobamate (Given the primary CNS effects of aripiprazole, caution should be used when co-administered with other centrally acting drugs).
No products indexed under this heading.

Mesoridazine Besylate (Given the primary CNS effects of aripiprazole, caution should be used when co-administered with other centrally acting drugs).
No products indexed under this heading.

Methadone Hydrochloride (Inhibitors of CYP2D6 can inhibit aripiprazole elimination and cause increased blood levels).
No products indexed under this heading.

Methamphetamine Hydrochloride (Given the primary CNS effects of aripiprazole, caution should be used when co-administered with other centrally acting drugs).
No products indexed under this heading.

Methohexital Sodium (Given the primary CNS effects of aripiprazole, caution should be used when co-administered with other centrally acting drugs).
No products indexed under this heading.

Methotrimeprazine (Given the primary CNS effects of aripiprazole, caution should be used when co-administered with other centrally acting drugs).
No products indexed under this heading.

Methoxyflurane (Given the primary CNS effects of aripiprazole, caution should be used when co-administered with other centrally acting drugs).
No products indexed under this heading.

Methsuximide (Agents that induce CYP3A4 could cause an increase in aripiprazole clearance and lower blood levels).
No products indexed under this heading.

Methyclothiazide (Due to its alpha-1-adrenergic receptor antagonism, aripiprazole has the potential to enhance the effect of certain antihypertensive agents).
No products indexed under this heading.

Methyldopa (Due to its alpha-1-adrenergic receptor antagonism, aripiprazole has the potential to enhance the effect of certain antihypertensive agents).
No products indexed under this heading.

Methyldopate Hydrochloride (Due to its alpha-1-adrenergic receptor antagonism, aripiprazole has the potential to enhance the effect of certain antihypertensive agents).
No products indexed under this heading.

Methylphenidate (Given the primary CNS effects of aripiprazole, caution should be used when co-administered with other centrally acting drugs). Products include:
Daytrana Transdermal Patch 3022

Methylphenidate Hydrochloride (Given the primary CNS effects of aripiprazole, caution should be used when co-administered with other centrally acting drugs). Products include:
Concerta Extended-Release Tablets 1925
Metadate CD Capsules 3146

Methylprednisolone (Agents that induce CYP3A4 could cause an increase in aripiprazole clearance and lower blood levels).
No products indexed under this heading.

Methylprednisolone Acetate (Agents that induce CYP3A4 could cause an increase in aripiprazole clearance and lower blood levels).
No products indexed under this heading.

Methylprednisolone Sodium Succinate (Agents that induce CYP3A4 could cause an increase in aripiprazole clearance and lower blood levels).
No products indexed under this heading.

Metolazone (Due to its alpha-1-adrenergic receptor antagonism, aripiprazole has the potential to enhance the effect of certain antihypertensive agents).
No products indexed under this heading.

Metoprolol Succinate (Due to its alpha-1-adrenergic receptor antagonism, aripiprazole has the potential to enhance the effect of certain antihypertensive agents). Products include:
Toprol-XL Tablets 666

Metoprolol Tartrate (Due to its alpha-1-adrenergic receptor antagonism, aripiprazole has the potential to enhance the effect of certain antihypertensive agents).
No products indexed under this heading.

Metronidazole (Inhibitors of CYP3A4 can inhibit aripiprazole elimination and cause increased blood levels). Products include:
Pylera Capsules 714

Metronidazole Benzoate (Inhibitors of CYP3A4 can inhibit aripiprazole elimination and cause increased blood levels).
No products indexed under this heading.

Metronidazole Hydrochloride (Inhibitors of CYP3A4 can inhibit aripiprazole elimination and cause increased blood levels).
No products indexed under this heading.

Metronidazole Sodium (Inhibitors of CYP3A4 can inhibit aripiprazole elimination and cause increased blood levels).
No products indexed under this heading.

Metyrosine (Due to its alpha-1-adrenergic receptor antagonism, aripiprazole has the potential to enhance the effect of certain antihypertensive agents). Products include:
Demser Capsules 1989

Mibefradil Dihydrochloride (Due to its alpha-1-adrenergic receptor antagonism, aripiprazole has the potential to enhance the effect of certain antihypertensive agents).
No products indexed under this heading.

Miconazole (Inhibitors of CYP3A4 can inhibit aripiprazole elimination and cause increased blood levels).
No products indexed under this heading.

Miconazole Nitrate (Inhibitors of CYP3A4 can inhibit aripiprazole elimination and cause increased blood levels).
No products indexed under this heading.

Midazolam Hydrochloride (Given the primary CNS effects of aripiprazole, caution should be used when co-administered with other centrally acting drugs).
No products indexed under this heading.

Minoxidil (Due to its alpha-1-adrenergic receptor antagonism, aripiprazole has the potential to enhance the effect of certain antihypertensive agents).
No products indexed under this heading.

Moclobemide (Inhibitors of CYP2D6 can inhibit aripiprazole elimination and cause increased blood levels).
No products indexed under this heading.

Modafinil (Agents that induce CYP3A4 could cause an increase in aripiprazole clearance and lower blood levels). Products include:
Provigil Tablets 977

Moexipril Hydrochloride (Due to its alpha-1-adrenergic receptor antagonism, aripiprazole has the potential to enhance the effect of certain antihypertensive agents).
No products indexed under this heading.

Molindone Hydrochloride (Given the primary CNS effects of aripiprazole, caution should be used when co-administered with other centrally acting drugs). Products include:
Moban Tablets 1116

Morphine Sulfate (Given the primary CNS effects of aripiprazole, caution should be used when co-administered with other centrally acting drugs). Products include:
Avinza Capsules 1772
DepoDur Injection 1095
MS Contin Tablets 2585

Nadolol (Due to its alpha-1-adrenergic receptor antagonism, aripiprazole has the potential to enhance the effect of certain antihypertensive agents). Products include:
Nadolol Tablets 2191

Nebivolol (Due to its alpha-1-adrenergic receptor antagonism, aripiprazole has the potential to enhance the effect of certain antihypertensive agents). Products include:
Bystolic Tablets 1155

Nefazodone Hydrochloride (Strong inhibitors of CYP3A4 may increase levels of aripiprazole and its active metabolite; dose reduction of aripiprazole should be considered).
No products indexed under this heading.

Nelfinavir Mesylate (Strong inhibitors of CYP3A4 may increase levels of aripiprazole and its active metabolite; dose reduction of aripiprazole should be considered).
No products indexed under this heading.

Nevirapine (Agents that induce CYP3A4 could cause an increase in aripiprazole clearance and lower blood levels). Products include:
Viramune Oral Suspension 873
Viramune Tablets 873

Niacinamide (Inhibitors of CYP3A4 can inhibit aripiprazole elimination and cause increased blood levels). Products include:
BioLean Free Tablets .... ◙635

Nicardipine Hydrochloride (Due to its alpha-1-adrenergic receptor antagonism, aripiprazole has the potential to enhance the effect of certain antihypertensive agents). Products include:
Cardene I.V. 1093

Nicotinamide (Inhibitors of CYP3A4 can inhibit aripiprazole elimination and cause increased blood levels).
No products indexed under this heading.

Nifedipine (Due to its alpha-1-adrenergic receptor antagonism, aripiprazole has the potential to enhance the effect of certain antihypertensive agents).
No products indexed under this heading.

Nisoldipine (Due to its alpha-1-adrenergic receptor antagonism, aripiprazole has the potential to enhance the effect of certain antihypertensive agents). Products include:
Sular Extended Release Tablets 2975

Nitroglycerin (Due to its alpha-1-adrenergic receptor antagonism, aripiprazole has the potential to enhance the effect of certain antihypertensive agents). Products include:
Nitro-Dur Transdermal Infusion System 2887
Nitrolingual Pumpspray 2965

Norfloxacin (Inhibitors of CYP3A4 can inhibit aripiprazole elimination and cause increased blood levels). Products include:
Noroxin Tablets 2069

Nortriptyline Hydrochloride (Inhibitors of CYP2D6 can inhibit aripiprazole elimination and cause increased blood levels).
No products indexed under this heading.

Olanzapine (Given the primary CNS effects of aripiprazole, caution should be used when co-administered with other centrally acting drugs). Products include:
Symbyax Capsules 1871
Zyprexa Tablets 1883
Zyprexa IntraMuscular 1883
Zyprexa ZYDIS Orally Disintegrating Tablets 1883

Omeprazole (Inhibitors of CYP3A4 can inhibit aripiprazole elimination and cause increased blood levels).
No products indexed under this heading.

Oxazepam (Given the primary CNS effects of aripiprazole, caution should be used when co-administered with other centrally acting drugs).
No products indexed under this heading.

Oxcarbazepine (Agents that induce CYP3A4 could cause an increase in aripiprazole clearance and lower blood levels).
No products indexed under this heading.

Oxycodone Hydrochloride (Given the primary CNS effects of aripipra-

zole, caution should be used when co-administered with other centrally acting drugs). Products include:

- OxyContin Tablets 2589
- OxyIR Capsules 2593
- Percocet Tablets 1127
- Percodan Tablets 1130

Paroxetine Hydrochloride (When concomitant administration of potential CYP2D6 inhibitors such as quinidine, fluoxetine, or paroxetine with aripiprazole occurs, aripiprazole dose should be reduced at least to one-half of its normal dose. When the CYP2D6 inhibitor is withdrawn from the combination therapy, the aripiprazole dose should then be increased. When adjunctive aripiprazole is administered to patients with major depressive disorder, aripiprazole should be administered without dosage adjustment as specified). Products include:

- Paxil 1535
- Paxil CR Controlled-Release Tablets 1544

Paroxetine Mesylate (When concomitant administration of potential CYP2D6 inhibitors such as quinidine, fluoxetine, or paroxetine with aripiprazole occurs, aripiprazole dose should be reduced at least to one-half of its normal dose. When the CYP2D6 inhibitor is withdrawn from the combination therapy, the aripiprazole dose should then be increased. When adjunctive aripiprazole is administered to patients with major depressive disorder, aripiprazole should be administered without dosage adjustment as specified).

No products indexed under this heading.

Pemoline (Given the primary CNS effects of aripiprazole, caution should be used when co-administered with other centrally acting drugs).

No products indexed under this heading.

Penbutolol Sulfate (Due to its alpha-1-adrenergic receptor antagonism, aripiprazole has the potential to enhance the effect of certain antihypertensive agents).

No products indexed under this heading.

Pentobarbital Sodium (Given the primary CNS effects of aripiprazole, caution should be used when co-administered with other centrally acting drugs). Products include:

- Nembutal Sodium Solution, USP 2494

Perindopril Erbumine (Due to its alpha-1-adrenergic receptor antagonism, aripiprazole has the potential to enhance the effect of certain antihypertensive agents). Products include:

- Aceon Tablets (2 mg, 4 mg, 8 mg) 3038

Perphenazine (Inhibitors of CYP2D6 can inhibit aripiprazole elimination and cause increased blood levels).

No products indexed under this heading.

Phenobarbital (Agents that induce CYP3A4 could cause an increase in aripiprazole clearance and lower blood levels). Products include:

- Donnatal Extentabs 2507

Phenobarbital Sodium (Agents that induce CYP3A4 could cause an increase in aripiprazole clearance and lower blood levels).

No products indexed under this heading.

Phenoxybenzamine Hydrochloride (Due to its alpha-1-adrenergic receptor antagonism, aripiprazole has the potential to enhance the effect of certain antihypertensive agents). Products include:

- Dibenzyline Capsules 3188

Phentolamine Mesylate (Due to its alpha-1-adrenergic receptor antagonism, aripiprazole has the potential to enhance the effect of certain antihypertensive agents).

No products indexed under this heading.

Phenytoin (Agents that induce CYP3A4 could cause an increase in aripiprazole clearance and lower blood levels).

No products indexed under this heading.

Phenytoin Sodium (Agents that induce CYP3A4 could cause an increase in aripiprazole clearance and lower blood levels). Products include:

- Phenytek Capsules 2192

Pindolol (Due to its alpha-1-adrenergic receptor antagonism, aripiprazole has the potential to enhance the effect of certain antihypertensive agents).

No products indexed under this heading.

Polythiazide (Due to its alpha-1-adrenergic receptor antagonism, aripiprazole has the potential to enhance the effect of certain antihypertensive agents).

No products indexed under this heading.

Prazepam (Given the primary CNS effects of aripiprazole, caution should be used when co-administered with other centrally acting drugs).

No products indexed under this heading.

Prazosin Hydrochloride (Due to its alpha-1-adrenergic receptor antagonism, aripiprazole has the potential to enhance the effect of certain antihypertensive agents).

No products indexed under this heading.

Prednisolone Acetate (Agents that induce CYP3A4 could cause an increase in aripiprazole clearance and lower blood levels). Products include:

- Pred Forte Ophthalmic Suspension .... ⊙ 227
- Pred Mild Ophthalmic Suspension .... ⊙ 230
- Pred-G Ophthalmic Ointment .... ⊙ 229
- Pred-G Ophthalmic Suspension ...... ⊙ 228

Prednisolone Sodium Phosphate (Agents that induce CYP3A4 could cause an increase in aripiprazole clearance and lower blood levels).

No products indexed under this heading.

Prednisolone Tebutate (Agents that induce CYP3A4 could cause an increase in aripiprazole clearance and lower blood levels).

No products indexed under this heading.

Prednisone (Agents that induce CYP3A4 could cause an increase in aripiprazole clearance and lower blood levels).

No products indexed under this heading.

Primidone (Agents that induce CYP3A4 could cause an increase in aripiprazole clearance and lower blood levels).

No products indexed under this heading.

Prochlorperazine (Given the primary CNS effects of aripiprazole, caution should be used when co-administered with other centrally acting drugs).

No products indexed under this heading.

Promethazine Hydrochloride (Given the primary CNS effects of aripiprazole, caution should be used when co-administered with other centrally acting drugs).

No products indexed under this heading.

Propafenone Hydrochloride (Inhibitors of CYP2D6 can inhibit aripiprazole elimination and cause increased blood levels). Products include:

- Rythmol Tablets 1586
- Rythmol SR Capsules 1590

Propofol (Given the primary CNS effects of aripiprazole, caution should be used when co-administered with other centrally acting drugs).

No products indexed under this heading.

Propoxyphene Hydrochloride (Inhibitors of CYP3A4 can inhibit aripiprazole elimination and cause increased blood levels).

No products indexed under this heading.

Propoxyphene Napsylate (Inhibitors of CYP3A4 can inhibit aripiprazole elimination and cause increased blood levels).

No products indexed under this heading.

Propranolol Hydrochloride (Due to its alpha-1-adrenergic receptor antagonism, aripiprazole has the potential to enhance the effect of certain antihypertensive agents). Products include:

- InnoPran XL Extended Release Capsules 1484

Protriptyline Hydrochloride (Inhibitors of CYP2D6 can inhibit aripiprazole elimination and cause increased blood levels).

No products indexed under this heading.

Quazepam (Given the primary CNS effects of aripiprazole, caution should be used when co-administered with other centrally acting drugs).

No products indexed under this heading.

Quetiapine Fumarate (Given the primary CNS effects of aripiprazole, caution should be used when co-administered with other centrally acting drugs).

No products indexed under this heading.

Quinacrine Hydrochloride (Inhibitors of CYP2D6 can inhibit aripiprazole elimination and cause increased blood levels).

No products indexed under this heading.

Quinapril Hydrochloride (Due to its alpha-1-adrenergic receptor antagonism, aripiprazole has the potential to enhance the effect of certain antihypertensive agents).

No products indexed under this heading.

Quinidine (When concomitant administration of potential CYP2D6 inhibitors such as quinidine, fluoxetine, or paroxetine with aripiprazole occurs, aripiprazole dose should be reduced at least to one-half of its normal dose. When the CYP2D6 inhibitor is withdrawn fromthe combination therapy, the aripiprazole dose should then be increased. When adjunctive aripiprazole is administered to patients with major depressive disorder, aripiprazole should be administered without dosage adjustment as specified).

No products indexed under this heading.

Quinidine Gluconate (When concomitant administration of potential CYP2D6 inhibitors such as quinidine, fluoxetine, or paroxetine with aripiprazole occurs, aripiprazole dose should be reduced at least to one-half of its normal dose. When the CYP2D6 inhibitor is withdrawn fromthe combination therapy, the aripiprazole dose should then be increased. When adjunctive aripiprazole is administered to patients with major depressive disorder, aripiprazole should be administered without dosage adjustment as specified).

No products indexed under this heading.

Quinidine Hydrochloride (When concomitant administration of potential CYP2D6 inhibitors such as quinidine, fluoxetine, or paroxetine with aripiprazole occurs, aripiprazole dose should be reduced at least to one-half of its normal dose. When the CYP2D6 inhibitor is withdrawn fromthe combination therapy, the aripiprazole dose should then be increased. When adjunctive aripiprazole is administered to patients with major depressive disorder, aripiprazole should be administered without dosage adjustment as specified).

No products indexed under this heading.

Quinidine Polygalacturonate (When concomitant administration of potential CYP2D6 inhibitors such as quinidine, fluoxetine, or paroxetine with aripiprazole occurs, aripiprazole dose should be reduced at least to one-half of its normal dose. When the CYP2D6 inhibitor is withdrawn fromthe combination therapy, the aripiprazole dose should then be increased. When adjunctive aripiprazole is administered to patients with major depressive disorder, aripiprazole should be administered without dosage adjustment as specified).

No products indexed under this heading.

Quinidine Sulfate (When concomitant administration of potential CYP2D6 inhibitors such as quinidine, fluoxetine, or paroxetine with aripiprazole occurs, aripiprazole dose should be reduced at least to one-half of its normal dose. When the CYP2D6 inhibitor is withdrawn fromthe combination therapy, the aripiprazole dose should then be increased. When adjunctive aripiprazole is administered to patients with major depressive disorder, aripiprazole should be administered without dosage adjustment as specified).

No products indexed under this heading.

Quinine (Inhibitors of CYP3A4 can inhibit aripiprazole elimination and cause increased blood levels).
No products indexed under this heading.

Quinine Sulfate (Inhibitors of CYP3A4 can inhibit aripiprazole elimination and cause increased blood levels).
No products indexed under this heading.

Quinupristin (Inhibitors of CYP3A4 can inhibit aripiprazole elimination and cause increased blood levels).
No products indexed under this heading.

Ramipril (Due to its alpha-1-adrenergic receptor antagonism, aripiprazole has the potential to enhance the effect of certain antihypertensive agents).
No products indexed under this heading.

Ranitidine Bismuth Citrate (Inhibitors of CYP3A4 can inhibit aripiprazole elimination and cause increased blood levels).
No products indexed under this heading.

Ranitidine Hydrochloride (Inhibitors of CYP3A4 can inhibit aripiprazole elimination and cause increased blood levels). Products include:
Zantac 75 Tablets .... ⊡603
Zantac 1670
Zantac Injection 1666
Zantac Injection Pharmacy Bulk Package 1668
Maximum Strength Zantac 150 Tablets .... ⊡603
Maximum Strength Zantac 150 Cool Mint Tablets .... ⊡603

Rauwolfia Serpentina (Due to its alpha-1-adrenergic receptor antagonism, aripiprazole has the potential to enhance the effect of certain antihypertensive agents).
No products indexed under this heading.

Remifentanil Hydrochloride (Given the primary CNS effects of aripiprazole, caution should be used when co-administered with other centrally acting drugs).
No products indexed under this heading.

Rescinnamine (Due to its alpha-1-adrenergic receptor antagonism, aripiprazole has the potential to enhance the effect of certain antihypertensive agents).
No products indexed under this heading.

Reserpine (Due to its alpha-1-adrenergic receptor antagonism, aripiprazole has the potential to enhance the effect of certain antihypertensive agents).
No products indexed under this heading.

Rifabutin (Agents that induce CYP3A4 could cause an increase in aripiprazole clearance and lower blood levels).
No products indexed under this heading.

Rifampicin (Agents that induce CYP3A4 could cause an increase in aripiprazole clearance and lower blood levels).
No products indexed under this heading.

Rifampin (Agents that induce CYP3A4 could cause an increase in aripiprazole clearance and lower blood levels).
No products indexed under this heading.

Rifapentine (Agents that induce CYP3A4 could cause an increase in aripiprazole clearance and lower blood levels).
No products indexed under this heading.

Risperidone (Given the primary CNS effects of aripiprazole, caution should be used when co-administered with other centrally acting drugs). Products include:
Risperdal Consta Long-Acting Injection 1753

Ritonavir (Strong inhibitors of CYP3A4 may increase levels of aripiprazole and its active metabolite; dose reduction of aripiprazole should be considered). Products include:
Kaletra 452
Norvir 489

Saquinavir (Strong inhibitors of CYP3A4 may increase levels of aripiprazole and its active metabolite; dose reduction of aripiprazole should be considered).
No products indexed under this heading.

Saquinavir Mesylate (Strong inhibitors of CYP3A4 may increase levels of aripiprazole and its active metabolite; dose reduction of aripiprazole should be considered).
No products indexed under this heading.

Secobarbital Sodium (Given the primary CNS effects of aripiprazole, caution should be used when co-administered with other centrally acting drugs).
No products indexed under this heading.

Sertraline Hydrochloride (Inhibitors of CYP3A4 can inhibit aripiprazole elimination and cause increased blood levels).
No products indexed under this heading.

Sevoflurane (Given the primary CNS effects of aripiprazole, caution should be used when co-administered with other centrally acting drugs). Products include:
Ultane Liquid for Inhalation 524

Sildenafil Citrate (Inhibitors of CYP3A4 can inhibit aripiprazole elimination and cause increased blood levels).
No products indexed under this heading.

Sodium Nitroprusside (Due to its alpha-1-adrenergic receptor antagonism, aripiprazole has the potential to enhance the effect of certain antihypertensive agents).
No products indexed under this heading.

Sodium Oxybate (Given the primary CNS effects of aripiprazole, caution should be used when co-administered with other centrally acting drugs). Products include:
Xyrem Oral Solution 1766

Sotalol Hydrochloride (Due to its alpha-1-adrenergic receptor antagonism, aripiprazole has the potential to enhance the effect of certain antihypertensive agents).
No products indexed under this heading.

Spirapril Hydrochloride (Due to its alpha-1-adrenergic receptor antagonism, aripiprazole has the potential to enhance the effect of certain antihypertensive agents).
No products indexed under this heading.

Sufentanil Citrate (Given the primary CNS effects of aripiprazole, caution should be used when co-administered with other centrally acting drugs).
No products indexed under this heading.

Sulfinpyrazone (Agents that induce CYP3A4 could cause an increase in aripiprazole clearance and lower blood levels).
No products indexed under this heading.

Telithromycin (Strong inhibitors of CYP3A4 may increase levels of aripiprazole and its active metabolite; dose reduction of aripiprazole should be considered). Products include:
Ketek Tablets 2744

Telmisartan (Due to its alpha-1-adrenergic receptor antagonism, aripiprazole has the potential to enhance the effect of certain antihypertensive agents). Products include:
Micardis Tablets 852
Micardis HCT Tablets 854

Temazepam (Given the primary CNS effects of aripiprazole, caution should be used when co-administered with other centrally acting drugs).
No products indexed under this heading.

Terazosin Hydrochloride (Due to its alpha-1-adrenergic receptor antagonism, aripiprazole has the potential to enhance the effect of certain antihypertensive agents).
No products indexed under this heading.

Terbinafine Hydrochloride (Inhibitors of CYP2D6 can inhibit aripiprazole elimination and cause increased blood levels). Products include:
Lamisil Oral Granules 2264
Lamisil Tablets 2266

Theophylline (Agents that induce CYP3A4 could cause an increase in aripiprazole clearance and lower blood levels).
No products indexed under this heading.

Theophylline Anhydrous (Agents that induce CYP3A4 could cause an increase in aripiprazole clearance and lower blood levels). Products include:
Uniphyl Tablets 2595

Theophylline Calcium Salicylate (Agents that induce CYP3A4 could cause an increase in aripiprazole clearance and lower blood levels).
No products indexed under this heading.

Theophylline Dihydroxypropyl (Glyceryl) (Agents that induce CYP3A4 could cause an increase in aripiprazole clearance and lower blood levels).
No products indexed under this heading.

Theophylline Ethylenediamine (Agents that induce CYP3A4 could cause an increase in aripiprazole clearance and lower blood levels).
No products indexed under this heading.

Thiamylal Sodium (Given the primary CNS effects of aripiprazole, caution should be used when co-administered with other centrally acting drugs).
No products indexed under this heading.

Thioridazine Hydrochloride (Inhibitors of CYP2D6 can inhibit aripiprazole elimination and cause increased blood levels). Products include:
Thioridazine Hydrochloride Tablets 2195

Thiothixene (Given the primary CNS effects of aripiprazole, caution should be used when co-administered with other centrally acting drugs). Products include:
Thiothixene Capsules 2197

Timolol Maleate (Due to its alpha-1-adrenergic receptor antagonism, aripiprazole has the potential to enhance the effect of certain antihypertensive agents). Products include:
Combigan Ophthalmic Solution 553
Cosopt Sterile Ophthalmic Solution 1969
Timoptic Sterile Ophthalmic Solution 2121
Timoptic in Ocudose 2124
Timoptic-XE Sterile Ophthalmic Gel Forming Solution 2125

Torsemide (Due to its alpha-1-adrenergic receptor antagonism, aripiprazole has the potential to enhance the effect of certain antihypertensive agents). Products include:
Demadex Injection 2630
Demadex Tablets 2630

Trandolapril (Due to its alpha-1-adrenergic receptor antagonism, aripiprazole has the potential to enhance the effect of certain antihypertensive agents). Products include:
Mavik Tablets 472
Tarka Tablets 511

Triamcinolone (Agents that induce CYP3A4 could cause an increase in aripiprazole clearance and lower blood levels).
No products indexed under this heading.

Triamcinolone Acetonide (Agents that induce CYP3A4 could cause an increase in aripiprazole clearance and lower blood levels). Products include:
Azmacort Inhalation Aerosol 407
Nasacort AQ Nasal Spray 2765
Triesence Injectable Suspension .... ⊙209

Triamcinolone Diacetate (Agents that induce CYP3A4 could cause an increase in aripiprazole clearance and lower blood levels).
No products indexed under this heading.

Triamcinolone Hexacetonide (Agents that induce CYP3A4 could cause an increase in aripiprazole clearance and lower blood levels).
No products indexed under this heading.

Triazolam (Given the primary CNS effects of aripiprazole, caution should be used when co-administered with other centrally acting drugs).
No products indexed under this heading.

IMPORTANT NOTE: Always consult each drug listing in the patient's regimen for possible interactions.

Trifluoperazine Hydrochloride (Given the primary CNS effects of aripiprazole, caution should be used when co-administered with other centrally acting drugs).
No products indexed under this heading.

Trimethaphan Camsylate (Due to its alpha-1-adrenergic receptor antagonism, aripiprazole has the potential to enhance the effect of certain antihypertensive agents).
No products indexed under this heading.

Trimipramine Maleate (Inhibitors of CYP2D6 can inhibit aripiprazole elimination and cause increased blood levels).
No products indexed under this heading.

Troglitazone (Agents that induce CYP3A4 could cause an increase in aripiprazole clearance and lower blood levels).
No products indexed under this heading.

Troleandomycin (Strong inhibitors of CYP3A4 may increase levels of aripiprazole and its active metabolite; dose reduction of aripiprazole should be considered).
No products indexed under this heading.

Valproate Sodium (Inhibitors of CYP3A4 can inhibit aripiprazole elimination and cause increased blood levels).
No products indexed under this heading.

Valsartan (Due to its alpha-1-adrenergic receptor antagonism, aripiprazole has the potential to enhance the effect of certain antihypertensive agents). Products include:
Diovan Tablets 2212
Diovan HCT Tablets 2216
Exforge Tablets 2238

Vardenafil Hydrochloride (Inhibitors of CYP3A4 can inhibit aripiprazole elimination and cause increased blood levels). Products include:
Levitra Tablets 2876

Verapamil Hydrochloride (Due to its alpha-1-adrenergic receptor antagonism, aripiprazole has the potential to enhance the effect of certain antihypertensive agents). Products include:
Tarka Tablets 511

Voriconazole (Strong inhibitors of CYP3A4 may increase levels of aripiprazole and its active metabolite; dose reduction of aripiprazole should be considered).
No products indexed under this heading.

Zafirlukast (Inhibitors of CYP3A4 can inhibit aripiprazole elimination and cause increased blood levels). Products include:
Accolate Tablets 669

Zaleplon (Given the primary CNS effects of aripiprazole, caution should be used when co-administered with other centrally acting drugs).
No products indexed under this heading.

Zileuton (Inhibitors of CYP3A4 can inhibit aripiprazole elimination and cause increased blood levels).
No products indexed under this heading.

Ziprasidone Hydrochloride (Given the primary CNS effects of aripiprazole, caution should be used when co-administered with other centrally acting drugs). Products include:
Geodon Capsules 2520

Zolpidem Tartrate (Given the primary CNS effects of aripiprazole, caution should be used when co-administered with other centrally acting drugs). Products include:
Ambien Tablets 2692
Ambien CR Tablets 2696

Food Interactions

Alcohol (Given the primary CNS effects of aripiprazole, caution should be used when co-administered with alcohol; patients should be advised to avoid alcohol while taking aripiprazole).

Grapefruit (Inhibitors of CYP3A4 can inhibit aripiprazole elimination and cause increased blood levels).

Grapefruit Juice (Inhibitors of CYP3A4 can inhibit aripiprazole elimination and cause increased blood levels).

ACCELERATOR TABLETS

(Amino Acid Preparations, Calcium Carbonate, Calcium Phosphate, Dibasic, Herbals, Multiple) .... ▣634
None cited in PDR database.

ACCOLATE TABLETS

(Zafirlukast) 669
May interact with xanthines and certain other agents. Compounds in these categories include:

Acarbose (No formal drug-drug interaction studies with zafirlukast and other drugs known to be metabolized by the cytochrome P450 2C9 isoenzyme (e.g., tolbutamide, phenytoin, carbamazepine) have been conducted; however, care should be exercised when zafirlukast is co-administered with these drugs). Products include:
Precose Tablets 792

Alfentanil Hydrochloride (No formal drug-drug interaction studies between zafirlukast and marketed drugs known to be metabolized by the P450 3A4 (CYP3A4) isoenzyme (e.g., dihydropyridine calcium-channel blockers, cyclosporin, cisapride) have been conducted. As zafirlukast is known to be an inhibitor of CYP3A4 in vitro, it is reasonable to employ appropriate clinical monitoring when these drugs are co-administered with zafirlukast).
No products indexed under this heading.

Alprazolam (No formal drug-drug interaction studies between zafirlukast and marketed drugs known to be metabolized by the P450 3A4 (CYP3A4) isoenzyme (e.g., dihydropyridine calcium-channel blockers, cyclosporin, cisapride) have been conducted. As zafirlukast is known to be an inhibitor of CYP3A4 in vitro, it is reasonable to employ appropriate clinical monitoring when these drugs are co-administered with zafirlukast).
No products indexed under this heading.

Aminophylline (Rare cases of patients experiencing increased theophylline levels with or without clinical signs or symptoms of theophylline toxicity after the addition of zafirlukast to an existing theophylline regimen have been reported).
No products indexed under this heading.

Amiodarone Hydrochloride (No formal drug-drug interaction studies between zafirlukast and marketed drugs known to be metabolized by the P450 3A4 (CYP3A4) isoenzyme (e.g., dihydropyridine calcium-channel blockers, cyclosporin, cisapride) have been conducted. As zafirlukast is known to be an inhibitor of CYP3A4 in vitro, it is reasonable to employ appropriate clinical monitoring when these drugs are co-administered with zafirlukast).
No products indexed under this heading.

Amitriptyline Hydrochloride (No formal drug-drug interaction studies with zafirlukast and other drugs known to be metabolized by the cytochrome P450 2C9 isoenzyme (e.g., tolbutamide, phenytoin, carbamazepine) have been conducted; however, care should be exercised when zafirlukast is co-administered with these drugs).
No products indexed under this heading.

Amlodipine Besylate (No formal drug-drug interaction studies between zafirlukast and marketed drugs known to be metabolized by the P450 3A4 (CYP3A4) isoenzyme (e.g., dihydropyridine calcium-channel blockers, cyclosporin, cisapride) have been conducted. As zafirlukast is known to be an inhibitor of CYP3A4 in vitro, it is reasonable to employ appropriate clinical monitoring when these drugs are co-administered with zafirlukast). Products include:
Azor Tablets 1005
Exforge Tablets 2238

Anisindione (In a drug interaction study in 16 healthy male volunteers, co-administration of multiple doses of zafirlukast (160 mg/day) to steady-state with a single 25 mg dose of warfarin resulted in a significant increase in the mean AUC (+63%) and half-life (+36%) of S-warfarin. The mean prothrombin time (PT) increased by approximately 35%. This interaction is probably due to an inhibition by zafirlukast of the cytochrome P450 2C9 isoenzyme system. Patients on oral warfarin anticoagulant therapy and zafirlukast should have their prothrombin times monitored closely and anticoagulant dose adjusted accordingly).
No products indexed under this heading.

Aprepitant (No formal drug-drug interaction studies between zafirlukast and marketed drugs known to be metabolized by the P450 3A4 (CYP3A4) isoenzyme (e.g., dihydropyridine calcium-channel blockers, cyclosporin, cisapride) have been conducted. As zafirlukast is known to be an inhibitor of CYP3A4 in vitro, it is reasonable to employ appropriate clinical monitoring when these drugs are co-administered with zafirlukast). Products include:
Emend Capsules 1992

Aspirin (Co-administration of zafirlukast (40 mg/day) with aspirin (650 mg four times daily) resulted in mean increased plasma levels of zafirlukast by approximately 45%). Products include:
Aggrenox Capsules 819
Bayer Aspirin 750
Percodan Tablets 1130
St. Joseph 81 mg Aspirin Chewable and Enteric Coated Tablets 1903

Aspirin, Enteric Coated (Co-administration of zafirlukast (40 mg/day) with aspirin (650 mg four times daily) resulted in mean increased plasma levels of zafirlukast by approximately 45%).
No products indexed under this heading.

Aspirin Buffered (Co-administration of zafirlukast (40 mg/day) with aspirin (650 mg four times daily) resulted in mean increased plasma levels of zafirlukast by approximately 45%).
No products indexed under this heading.

Astemizole (No formal drug-drug interaction studies between zafirlukast and marketed drugs known to be metabolized by the P450 3A4 (CYP3A4) isoenzyme (e.g., dihydropyridine calcium-channel blockers, cyclosporin, cisapride) have been conducted. As zafirlukast is known to be an inhibitor of CYP3A4 in vitro, it is reasonable to employ appropriate clinical monitoring when these drugs are co-administered with zafirlukast).
No products indexed under this heading.

Atorvastatin Calcium (No formal drug-drug interaction studies between zafirlukast and marketed drugs known to be metabolized by the P450 3A4 (CYP3A4) isoenzyme (e.g., dihydropyridine calcium-channel blockers, cyclosporin, cisapride) have been conducted. As zafirlukast is known to be an inhibitor of CYP3A4 in vitro, it is reasonable to employ appropriate clinical monitoring when these drugs are co-administered with zafirlukast). Products include:
Lipitor Tablets 2501

Belladonna Ergotamine (No formal drug-drug interaction studies between zafirlukast and marketed drugs known to be metabolized by the P450 3A4 (CYP3A4) isoenzyme (e.g., dihydropyridine calcium-channel blockers, cyclosporin, cisapride) have been conducted. As zafirlukast is known to be an inhibitor of CYP3A4 in vitro, it is reasonable to employ appropriate clinical monitoring when these drugs are co-administered with zafirlukast).
No products indexed under this heading.

Buspirone Hydrochloride (No formal drug-drug interaction studies between zafirlukast and marketed drugs known to be metabolized by the P450 3A4 (CYP3A4) isoenzyme (e.g., dihydropyridine calcium-channel blockers, cyclosporin, cisapride) have been conducted. As zafirlukast is known to be an inhibitor of CYP3A4 in vitro, it is reasonable to employ appropriate clinical monitoring when these drugs are co-administered with zafirlukast).
No products indexed under this heading.

Busulfan (No formal drug-drug interaction studies between zafirlukast and marketed drugs known to be metabolized by the P450 3A4 (CYP3A4) isoenzyme (e.g., dihydropyridine calcium-channel blockers, cyclosporin, cisapride) have been conducted. As zafirlukast is known to be an inhibitor of CYP3A4 in vitro, it is reasonable to employ appropriate clinical monitoring when these drugs are co-administered with zafirlukast). Products include:

- Busulfex Injection 2477
- Myleran Tablets 1530

Candesartan Cilexetil (No formal drug-drug interaction studies with zafirlukast and other drugs known to be metabolized by the cytochrome P450 2C9 isoenzyme (e.g., tolbutamide, phenytoin, carbamazepine) have been conducted; however, care should be exercised when zafirlukast is co-administered with these drugs). Products include:

- Atacand Tablets 639
- Atacand HCT 642

Carbamazepine (No formal drug-drug interaction studies with zafirlukast and other drugs known to be metabolized by the cytochrome P450 2C9 isoenzyme (e.g., tolbutamide, phenytoin, carbamazepine) have been conducted; however, care should be exercised when zafirlukast is co-administered with these drugs). Products include:

- Carbatrol Capsules 3019
- Equetro Extended-Release Capsules 3174

Carvedilol (No formal drug-drug interaction studies with zafirlukast and other drugs known to be metabolized by the cytochrome P450 2C9 isoenzyme (e.g., tolbutamide, phenytoin, carbamazepine) have been conducted; however, care should be exercised when zafirlukast is co-administered with these drugs). Products include:

- Coreg Tablets 1387

Celecoxib (No formal drug-drug interaction studies with zafirlukast and other drugs known to be metabolized by the cytochrome P450 2C9 isoenzyme (e.g., tolbutamide, phenytoin, carbamazepine) have been conducted; however, care should be exercised when zafirlukast is co-administered with these drugs). Products include:

- Celebrex Capsules 2979

Cerivastatin Sodium (No formal drug-drug interaction studies between zafirlukast and marketed drugs known to be metabolized by the P450 3A4 (CYP3A4) isoenzyme (e.g., dihydropyridine calcium-channel blockers, cyclosporin, cisapride) have been conducted. As zafirlukast is known to be an inhibitor of CYP3A4 in vitro, it is reasonable to employ appropriate clinical monitoring when these drugs are co-administered with zafirlukast).

No products indexed under this heading.

Chlorpheniramine (No formal drug-drug interaction studies between zafirlukast and marketed drugs known to be metabolized by the P450 3A4 (CYP3A4) isoenzyme (e.g., dihydropyridine calcium-channel blockers, cyclosporin, cisapride) have been conducted. As zafirlukast is known to be an inhibitor of CYP3A4 in vitro, it is reasonable to employ appropriate clinical monitoring when these drugs are co-administered with zafirlukast).

No products indexed under this heading.

Chlorpheniramine Maleate (No formal drug-drug interaction studies between zafirlukast and marketed drugs known to be metabolized by the P450 3A4 (CYP3A4) isoenzyme (e.g., dihydropyridine calcium-channel blockers, cyclosporin, cisapride) have been conducted. As zafirlukast is known to be an inhibitor of CYP3A4 in vitro, it is reasonable to employ appropriate clinical monitoring when these drugs are co-administered with zafirlukast). Products include:

- Actifed Cold & Allergy Tablets 1895
- Sudafed PE Sinus & Allergy Tablets 1908
- Tylenol Allergy Multi-Symptom Caplets with Cool Burst and Rapid Release Gelcaps 1916
- Children's Tylenol Plus Cold Suspension Liquid 1912
- Children's Tylenol Plus Cough & Runny Nose Suspension Liquid 1912
- Children's Tylenol Plus Flu Suspension Liquid 1914
- Children's Tylenol Plus Multi-Symptom Cold Suspension Liquid 1912
- Tylenol Cold Head Congestion Nighttime Caplets with Cool Burst 1910
- Tylenol Cold Multi-Symptom Nighttime Caplets with Cool Burst 1913
- Tylenol Sinus Congestion & Pain Nighttime Caplets with Cool Burst 1917

Chlorpheniramine Polistirex (No formal drug-drug interaction studies between zafirlukast and marketed drugs known to be metabolized by the P450 3A4 (CYP3A4) isoenzyme (e.g., dihydropyridine calcium-channel blockers, cyclosporin, cisapride) have been conducted. As zafirlukast is known to be an inhibitor of CYP3A4 in vitro, it is reasonable to employ appropriate clinical monitoring when these drugs are co-administered with zafirlukast). Products include:

- Tussionex Pennkinetic Extended-Release Suspension 3154

Chlorpheniramine Tannate (No formal drug-drug interaction studies between zafirlukast and marketed drugs known to be metabolized by the P450 3A4 (CYP3A4) isoenzyme (e.g., dihydropyridine calcium-channel blockers, cyclosporin, cisapride) have been conducted. As zafirlukast is known to be an inhibitor of CYP3A4 in vitro, it is reasonable to employ appropriate clinical monitoring when these drugs are co-administered with zafirlukast).

No products indexed under this heading.

Chlorpropamide (No formal drug-drug interaction studies with zafirlukast and other drugs known to be metabolized by the cytochrome P450 2C9 isoenzyme (e.g., tolbutamide, phenytoin, carbamazepine) have been conducted; however, care should be exercised when zafirlukast is co-administered with these drugs).

No products indexed under this heading.

Cisapride (No formal drug-drug interaction studies between zafirlukast and marketed drugs known to be metabolized by the P450 3A4 (CYP3A4) isoenzyme (e.g., dihydropyridine calcium-channel blockers, cyclosporin, cisapride) have been conducted. As zafirlukast is known to be an inhibitor of CYP3A4 in vitro, it is reasonable to employ appropriate clinical monitoring when these drugs are co-administered with zafirlukast).

No products indexed under this heading.

Clarithromycin (No formal drug-drug interaction studies between zafirlukast and marketed drugs known to be metabolized by the P450 3A4 (CYP3A4) isoenzyme (e.g., dihydropyridine calcium-channel blockers, cyclosporin, cisapride) have been conducted. As zafirlukast is known to be an inhibitor of CYP3A4 in vitro, it is reasonable to employ appropriate clinical monitoring when these drugs are co-administered with zafirlukast). Products include:

- Biaxin/Biaxin XL 411

Clomipramine Hydrochloride (No formal drug-drug interaction studies with zafirlukast and other drugs known to be metabolized by the cytochrome P450 2C9 isoenzyme (e.g., tolbutamide, phenytoin, carbamazepine) have been conducted; however, care should be exercised when zafirlukast is co-administered with these drugs).

No products indexed under this heading.

Cyclosporine (No formal drug-drug interaction studies between zafirlukast and marketed drugs known to be metabolized by the P450 3A4 (CYP3A4) isoenzyme (e.g., dihydropyridine calcium-channel blockers, cyclosporin, cisapride) have been conducted. As zafirlukast is known to be an inhibitor of CYP3A4 in vitro, it is reasonable to employ appropriate clinical monitoring when these drugs are co-administered with zafirlukast). Products include:

- Gengraf Capsules 435
- Neoral Oral Solution 2280
- Neoral Soft Gelatin Capsules 2280
- Restasis Ophthalmic Emulsion 557
- Sandimmune 2296

Desogestrel (No formal drug-drug interaction studies with zafirlukast and other drugs known to be metabolized by the cytochrome P450 2C9 isoenzyme (e.g., tolbutamide, phenytoin, carbamazepine) have been conducted; however, care should be exercised when zafirlukast is co-administered with these drugs). Products include:

- Mircette Tablets 1034

Dextromethorphan (No formal drug-drug interaction studies with zafirlukast and other drugs known to be metabolized by the cytochrome P450 2C9 isoenzyme (e.g., tolbutamide, phenytoin, carbamazepine) have been conducted; however, care should be exercised when zafirlukast is co-administered with these drugs).

No products indexed under this heading.

Diazepam (No formal drug-drug interaction studies with zafirlukast and other drugs known to be metabolized by the cytochrome P450 2C9 isoenzyme (e.g., tolbutamide, phenytoin, carbamazepine) have been conducted; however, care should be exercised when zafirlukast is co-administered with these drugs). Products include:

- Valium Tablets 2658

Diclofenac Potassium (No formal drug-drug interaction studies with zafirlukast and other drugs known to be metabolized by the cytochrome P450 2C9 isoenzyme (e.g., tolbutamide, phenytoin, carbamazepine) have been conducted; however, care should be exercised when zafirlukast is co-administered with these drugs).

No products indexed under this heading.

Diclofenac Sodium (No formal drug-drug interaction studies with zafirlukast and other drugs known to be metabolized by the cytochrome P450 2C9 isoenzyme (e.g., tolbutamide, phenytoin, carbamazepine) have been conducted; however, care should be exercised when zafirlukast is co-administered with these drugs). Products include:

- Diclofenac Sodium Ophthalmic Solution .... ⊙240
- Voltaren Ophthalmic Solution 2336
- Voltaren Tablets 2334
- Voltaren-XR Tablets 2337

Dicumarol (In a drug interaction study in 16 healthy male volunteers, co-administration of multiple doses of zafirlukast (160 mg/day) to steady-state with a single 25 mg dose of warfarin resulted in a significant increase in the mean AUC (+63%) and half-life (+36%) of S-warfarin. The mean prothrombin time (PT) increased by approximately 35%. This interaction is probably due to an inhibition by zafirlukast of the cytochrome P450 2C9 isoenzyme system. Patients on oral warfarin anticoagulant therapy and zafirlukast should have their prothrombin times monitored closely and anticoagulant dose adjusted accordingly).

No products indexed under this heading.

Dihydroergotamine Mesylate (No formal drug-drug interaction studies between zafirlukast and marketed drugs known to be metabolized by the P450 3A4 (CYP3A4) isoenzyme (e.g., dihydropyridine calcium-channel blockers, cyclosporin, cisapride) have been conducted. As zafirlukast is known to be an inhibitor of CYP3A4 in vitro, it is reasonable to employ appropriate clinical monitoring when these drugs are co-administered with zafirlukast).

No products indexed under this heading.

Diltiazem Hydrochloride (No formal drug-drug interaction studies between zafirlukast and marketed drugs known to be metabolized by the P450 3A4 (CYP3A4) isoenzyme (e.g., dihydropyridine calcium-channel blockers, cyclosporin, cisapride) have been conducted. As zafirlukast is known to be an inhibitor of CYP3A4 in vitro, it is reasonable to employ appropriate clinical monitoring when these drugs are co-administered with zafirlukast). Products include:

- Cardizem LA Extended Release Tablets 421

Diltiazem Maleate (No formal drug-drug interaction studies between zafirlukast and marketed drugs known to be metabolized by the P450 3A4 (CYP3A4) isoenzyme (e.g., dihydropyridine calcium-channel blockers, cyclosporin, cisapride) have been conducted. As zafirlukast is known to be an inhibitor of CYP3A4 in vitro, it is reasonable to employ appropriate clinical monitoring when these drugs are co-administered with zafirlukast).

No products indexed under this heading.

Disopyramide (No formal drug-drug interaction studies between zafirlukast and marketed drugs known to be metabolized by the P450 3A4 (CYP3A4) isoenzyme (e.g., dihydropyridine calcium-channel blockers, cyclosporin, cisapride) have been conducted. As zafirlukast is known to be an inhibitor of CYP3A4 in vitro, it is reasonable to employ appropriate clinical monitoring when these drugs are co-administered with zafirlukast).

No products indexed under this heading.

Disopyramide Phosphate (No formal drug-drug interaction studies between zafirlukast and marketed drugs known to be metabolized by the P450 3A4 (CYP3A4) isoenzyme (e.g., dihydropyridine calcium-channel blockers, cyclosporin, cisapride) have been conducted. As zafirlukast is known to be an inhibitor of CYP3A4 in vitro, it is reasonable to employ appropriate clinical monitoring when these drugs are co-administered with zafirlukast).

No products indexed under this heading.

Disulfiram (No formal drug-drug interaction studies between zafirlukast and marketed drugs known to be metabolized by the P450 3A4 (CYP3A4) isoenzyme (e.g., dihydropyridine calcium-channel blockers, cyclosporin, cisapride) have been conducted. As zafirlukast is known to be an inhibitor of CYP3A4 in vitro, it is reasonable to employ appropriate clinical monitoring when these drugs are co-administered with zafirlukast).

No products indexed under this heading.

Doxorubicin Hydrochloride (No formal drug-drug interaction studies between zafirlukast and marketed drugs known to be metabolized by the P450 3A4 (CYP3A4) isoenzyme (e.g., dihydropyridine calcium-channel blockers, cyclosporin, cisapride) have been conducted. As zafirlukast is known to be an inhibitor of CYP3A4 in vitro, it is reasonable to employ appropriate clinical monitoring when these drugs are co-administered with zafirlukast).

No products indexed under this heading.

Dronabinol (No formal drug-drug interaction studies with zafirlukast and other drugs known to be metabolized by the cytochrome P450 2C9 isoenzyme (e.g., tolbutamide, phenytoin, carbamazepine) have been conducted; however, care should be exercised when zafirlukast is co-administered with these drugs).
Products include:

Marinol Capsules **3163**

Dyphylline (Rare cases of patients experiencing increased theophylline levels with or without clinical signs or symptoms of theophylline toxicity after the addition of zafirlukast to an existing theophylline regimen have been reported).

No products indexed under this heading.

Eprosartan Mesylate (No formal drug-drug interaction studies with zafirlukast and other drugs known to be metabolized by the cytochrome P450 2C9 isoenzyme (e.g., tolbutamide, phenytoin, carbamazepine) have been conducted; however, care should be exercised when zafirlukast is co-administered with these drugs).
Products include:

Teveten Tablets **515**
Teveten HCT Tablets **517**

Ergotamine Tartrate (No formal drug-drug interaction studies between zafirlukast and marketed drugs known to be metabolized by the P450 3A4 (CYP3A4) isoenzyme (e.g., dihydropyridine calcium-channel blockers, cyclosporin, cisapride) have been conducted. As zafirlukast is known to be an inhibitor of CYP3A4 in vitro, it is reasonable to employ appropriate clinical monitoring when these drugs are co-administered with zafirlukast).

No products indexed under this heading.

Erythromycin (In a drug interaction study in 11 asthmatic patients, co-administration of a single dose of zafirlukast (40 mg) with erythromycin (500 mg three times daily for 5 days) to steady-state resulted in decreased mean plasma levels of zafirlukast by approximately 40% due to a decrease in zafirlukast bioavailability).

No products indexed under this heading.

Erythromycin Estolate (In a drug interaction study in 11 asthmatic patients, co-administration of a single dose of zafirlukast (40 mg) with erythromycin (500 mg three times daily for 5 days) to steady-state resulted in decreased mean plasma levels of zafirlukast by approximately 40% due to a decrease in zafirlukast bioavailability).

No products indexed under this heading.

Erythromycin Ethylsuccinate (In a drug interaction study in 11 asthmatic patients, co-administration of a single dose of zafirlukast (40 mg) with erythromycin (500 mg three times daily for 5 days) to steady-state resulted in decreased mean plasma levels of zafirlukast by approximately 40% due to a decrease in zafirlukast bioavailability). Products include:

E.E.S. **433**
EryPed **431**

Erythromycin Gluceptate (In a drug interaction study in 11 asthmatic patients, co-administration of a single dose of zafirlukast (40 mg) with erythromycin (500 mg three times daily for 5 days) to steady-state resulted in decreased mean plasma levels of zafirlukast by approximately 40% due to a decrease in zafirlukast bioavailability).

No products indexed under this heading.

Erythromycin Lactobionate (In a drug interaction study in 11 asthmatic patients, co-administration of a single dose of zafirlukast (40 mg) with erythromycin (500 mg three times daily for 5 days) to steady-state resulted in decreased mean plasma levels of zafirlukast by approximately 40% due to a decrease in zafirlukast bioavailability).

No products indexed under this heading.

Erythromycin Stearate (In a drug interaction study in 11 asthmatic patients, co-administration of a single dose of zafirlukast (40 mg) with erythromycin (500 mg three times daily for 5 days) to steady-state resulted in decreased mean plasma levels of zafirlukast by approximately 40% due to a decrease in zafirlukast bioavailability).

No products indexed under this heading.

Estradiol (No formal drug-drug interaction studies between zafirlukast and marketed drugs known to be metabolized by the P450 3A4 (CYP3A4) isoenzyme (e.g., dihydropyridine calcium-channel blockers, cyclosporin, cisapride) have been conducted. As zafirlukast is known to be an inhibitor of CYP3A4 in vitro, it is reasonable to employ appropriate clinical monitoring when these drugs are co-administered with zafirlukast).
Products include:

Activella Tablets **2347**
Angeliq Tablets **751**
Climara Transdermal System **763**
Climara Pro Transdermal System **768**
Divigel **3167**
Vagifem Tablets **2375**

Estradiol Benzoate (No formal drug-drug interaction studies between zafirlukast and marketed drugs known to be metabolized by the P450 3A4 (CYP3A4) isoenzyme (e.g., dihydropyridine calcium-channel blockers, cyclosporin, cisapride) have been conducted. As zafirlukast is known to be an inhibitor of CYP3A4 in vitro, it is reasonable to employ appropriate clinical monitoring when these drugs are co-administered with zafirlukast).

No products indexed under this heading.

Estradiol Cypionate (No formal drug-drug interaction studies between zafirlukast and marketed drugs known to be metabolized by the P450 3A4 (CYP3A4) isoenzyme (e.g., dihydropyridine calcium-channel blockers, cyclosporin, cisapride) have been conducted. As zafirlukast is known to be an inhibitor of CYP3A4 in vitro, it is reasonable to employ appropriate clinical monitoring when these drugs are co-administered with zafirlukast).

No products indexed under this heading.

Estradiol Valerate (No formal drug-drug interaction studies between zafirlukast and marketed drugs known to be metabolized by the P450 3A4 (CYP3A4) isoenzyme (e.g., dihydropyridine calcium-channel blockers, cyclosporin, cisapride) have been conducted. As zafirlukast is known to be an inhibitor of CYP3A4 in vitro, it is reasonable to employ appropriate clinical monitoring when these drugs are co-administered with zafirlukast).

No products indexed under this heading.

Ethinyl Estradiol (No formal drug-drug interaction studies between zafirlukast and marketed drugs known to be metabolized by the P450 3A4 (CYP3A4) isoenzyme (e.g., dihydropyridine calcium-channel blockers, cyclosporin, cisapride) have been conducted. As zafirlukast is known to be an inhibitor of CYP3A4 in vitro, it is reasonable to employ appropriate clinical monitoring when these drugs are co-administered with zafirlukast).
Products include:

Lybrel Tablets **3204**
Mircette Tablets **1034**
NuvaRing **2897**
Ortho-Cyclen/Ortho Tri-Cyclen **2449**
Ortho Evra Transdermal System **2437**
Ortho Tri-Cyclen Lo Tablets **2458**
Seasonique Tablets **1046**
Yaz Tablets **805**

Ethosuximide (No formal drug-drug interaction studies between zafirlukast and marketed drugs known to be metabolized by the P450 3A4 (CYP3A4) isoenzyme (e.g., dihydropyridine calcium-channel blockers, cyclosporin, cisapride) have been conducted. As zafirlukast is known to be an inhibitor of CYP3A4 in vitro, it is reasonable to employ appropriate clinical monitoring when these drugs are co-administered with zafirlukast).

No products indexed under this heading.

Ethynodiol Diacetate (No formal drug-drug interaction studies between zafirlukast and marketed drugs known to be metabolized by the P450 3A4 (CYP3A4) isoenzyme (e.g., dihydropyridine calcium-channel blockers, cyclosporin, cisapride) have been conducted. As zafirlukast is known to be an inhibitor of CYP3A4 in vitro, it is reasonable to employ appropriate clinical monitoring when these drugs are co-administered with zafirlukast).

No products indexed under this heading.

Etodolac (No formal drug-drug interaction studies with zafirlukast and other drugs known to be metabolized by the cytochrome P450 2C9 isoenzyme (e.g., tolbutamide, phenytoin, carbamazepine) have been conducted; however, care should be exercised when zafirlukast is co-administered with these drugs).

No products indexed under this heading.

Etoposide (No formal drug-drug interaction studies between zafirlukast and marketed drugs known to be metabolized by the P450 3A4 (CYP3A4) isoenzyme (e.g., dihydropyridine calcium-channel blockers, cyclosporin, cisapride) have been conducted. As zafirlukast is known to be an inhibitor of CYP3A4 in vitro, it is reasonable to employ appropriate clinical monitoring when these drugs are co-administered with zafirlukast).

No products indexed under this heading.

Etoposide Phosphate (No formal drug-drug interaction studies between zafirlukast and marketed drugs known to be metabolized by the P450 3A4 (CYP3A4) isoenzyme (e.g., dihydropyridine calcium-channel blockers, cyclosporin, cisapride) have been conducted. As zafirlukast is known to be an inhibitor of CYP3A4 in vitro, it is reasonable to employ appropriate clinical monitoring when these drugs are co-administered with zafirlukast).

No products indexed under this heading.

Felodipine (No formal drug-drug interaction studies between zafirlukast and marketed drugs known to be metabolized by the P450 3A4 (CYP3A4) isoenzyme (e.g., dihydropyridine calcium-channel blockers, cyclosporin, cisapride) have been conducted. As zafirlukast is known to be an inhibitor of CYP3A4 in vitro, it is reasonable to employ appropriate clinical monitoring when these drugs are co-administered with zafirlukast).

No products indexed under this heading.

Fenoprofen Calcium (No formal drug-drug interaction studies with

zafirlukast and other drugs known to be metabolized by the cytochrome P450 2C9 isoenzyme (e.g., tolbutamide, phenytoin, carbamazepine) have been conducted; however, care should be exercised when zafirlukast is co-administered with these drugs). Products include:
Nalfon Capsules 2508

Fentanyl (No formal drug-drug interaction studies between zafirlukast and marketed drugs known to be metabolized by the P450 3A4 (CYP3A4) isoenzyme (e.g., dihydropyridine calcium-channel blockers, cyclosporin, cisapride) have been conducted. As zafirlukast is known to be an inhibitor of CYP3A4 in vitro, it is reasonable to employ appropriate clinical monitoring when these drugs are co-administered with zafirlukast). Products include:
Duragesic Transdermal System 2405
Ionsys Transdermal System 2410

Fentanyl Citrate (No formal drug-drug interaction studies between zafirlukast and marketed drugs known to be metabolized by the P450 3A4 (CYP3A4) isoenzyme (e.g., dihydropyridine calcium-channel blockers, cyclosporin, cisapride) have been conducted. As zafirlukast is known to be an inhibitor of CYP3A4 in vitro, it is reasonable to employ appropriate clinical monitoring when these drugs are co-administered with zafirlukast). Products include:
Actiq 959
Fentora Tablets 968

Fluoxetine Hydrochloride (No formal drug-drug interaction studies with zafirlukast and other drugs known to be metabolized by the cytochrome P450 2C9 isoenzyme (e.g., tolbutamide, phenytoin, carbamazepine) have been conducted; however, care should be exercised when zafirlukast is co-administered with these drugs). Products include:
Prozac Weekly Capsules 1852
Prozac Pulvules and Liquid 1852
Symbyax Capsules 1871

Flurbiprofen (No formal drug-drug interaction studies with zafirlukast and other drugs known to be metabolized by the cytochrome P450 2C9 isoenzyme (e.g., tolbutamide, phenytoin, carbamazepine) have been conducted; however, care should be exercised when zafirlukast is co-administered with these drugs).
No products indexed under this heading.

Flurbiprofen Sodium (No formal drug-drug interaction studies with zafirlukast and other drugs known to be metabolized by the cytochrome P450 2C9 isoenzyme (e.g., tolbutamide, phenytoin, carbamazepine) have been conducted; however, care should be exercised when zafirlukast is co-administered with these drugs).
No products indexed under this heading.

Fluvastatin Sodium (No formal drug-drug interaction studies with zafirlukast and other drugs known to be metabolized by the cytochrome P450 2C9 isoenzyme (e.g., tolbutamide, phenytoin, carbamazepine) have been conducted; however, care should be exercised when zafirlukast is co-administered with these drugs). Products include:
Lescol Capsules 2268
Lescol XL Tablets 2268

Glimepiride (No formal drug-drug interaction studies with zafirlukast and other drugs known to be metabolized by the cytochrome P450 2C9 isoenzyme (e.g., tolbutamide, phenytoin, carbamazepine) have been conducted; however, care should be exercised when zafirlukast is co-administered with these drugs). Products include:
Avandaryl Tablets 1344
Duetact Tablets 3085

Glipizide (No formal drug-drug interaction studies with zafirlukast and other drugs known to be metabolized by the cytochrome P450 2C9 isoenzyme (e.g., tolbutamide, phenytoin, carbamazepine) have been conducted; however, care should be exercised when zafirlukast is co-administered with these drugs).
No products indexed under this heading.

Haloperidol (No formal drug-drug interaction studies between zafirlukast and marketed drugs known to be metabolized by the P450 3A4 (CYP3A4) isoenzyme (e.g., dihydropyridine calcium-channel blockers, cyclosporin, cisapride) have been conducted. As zafirlukast is known to be an inhibitor of CYP3A4 in vitro, it is reasonable to employ appropriate clinical monitoring when these drugs are co-administered with zafirlukast).
No products indexed under this heading.

Haloperidol Decanoate (No formal drug-drug interaction studies between zafirlukast and marketed drugs known to be metabolized by the P450 3A4 (CYP3A4) isoenzyme (e.g., dihydropyridine calcium-channel blockers, cyclosporin, cisapride) have been conducted. As zafirlukast is known to be an inhibitor of CYP3A4 in vitro, it is reasonable to employ appropriate clinical monitoring when these drugs are co-administered with zafirlukast).
No products indexed under this heading.

Haloperidol Lactate (No formal drug-drug interaction studies between zafirlukast and marketed drugs known to be metabolized by the P450 3A4 (CYP3A4) isoenzyme (e.g., dihydropyridine calcium-channel blockers, cyclosporin, cisapride) have been conducted. As zafirlukast is known to be an inhibitor of CYP3A4 in vitro, it is reasonable to employ appropriate clinical monitoring when these drugs are co-administered with zafirlukast).
No products indexed under this heading.

Ibuprofen (No formal drug-drug interaction studies with zafirlukast and other drugs known to be metabolized by the cytochrome P450 2C9 isoenzyme (e.g., tolbutamide, phenytoin, carbamazepine) have been conducted; however, care should be exercised when zafirlukast is co-administered with these drugs). Products include:
Motrin IB Tablets and Caplets 1900
Children's Motrin Oral Suspension ... 1901
Children's Motrin Non-Staining Dye-Free Oral Suspension 1901
Children's Motrin Cold Oral Suspension 1899
Infants' Motrin Concentrated Drops 1901
Infants' Motrin Non-Staining Dye-Free Concentrated Drops 1901
Junior Strength Motrin Caplets and Chewable Tablets 1901
Vicoprofen Tablets 533

Imipramine Hydrochloride (No formal drug-drug interaction studies with zafirlukast and other drugs known to be metabolized by the cytochrome P450 2C9 isoenzyme (e.g., tolbutamide, phenytoin, carbamazepine) have been conducted; however, care should be exercised when zafirlukast is co-administered with these drugs).
No products indexed under this heading.

Indinavir Sulfate (No formal drug-drug interaction studies between zafirlukast and marketed drugs known to be metabolized by the P450 3A4 (CYP3A4) isoenzyme (e.g., dihydropyridine calcium-channel blockers, cyclosporin, cisapride) have been conducted. As zafirlukast is known to be an inhibitor of CYP3A4 in vitro, it is reasonable to employ appropriate clinical monitoring when these drugs are co-administered with zafirlukast). Products include:
Crixivan Capsules 1979

Indomethacin (No formal drug-drug interaction studies with zafirlukast and other drugs known to be metabolized by the cytochrome P450 2C9 isoenzyme (e.g., tolbutamide, phenytoin, carbamazepine) have been conducted; however, care should be exercised when zafirlukast is co-administered with these drugs). Products include:
Indocin 2024

Indomethacin Sodium Trihydrate (No formal drug-drug interaction studies with zafirlukast and other drugs known to be metabolized by the cytochrome P450 2C9 isoenzyme (e.g., tolbutamide, phenytoin, carbamazepine) have been conducted; however, care should be exercised when zafirlukast is co-administered with these drugs). Products include:
Indocin I.V. 2489

Irbesartan (No formal drug-drug interaction studies with zafirlukast and other drugs known to be metabolized by the cytochrome P450 2C9 isoenzyme (e.g., tolbutamide, phenytoin, carbamazepine) have been conducted; however, care should be exercised when zafirlukast is co-administered with these drugs). Products include:
Avalide Tablets 892
Avalide Tablets 2713
Avapro Tablets 897
Avapro Tablets 2718

Isradipine (No formal drug-drug interaction studies between zafirlukast and marketed drugs known to be metabolized by the P450 3A4 (CYP3A4) isoenzyme (e.g., dihydropyridine calcium-channel blockers, cyclosporin, cisapride) have been conducted. As zafirlukast is known to be an inhibitor of CYP3A4 in vitro, it is reasonable to employ appropriate clinical monitoring when these drugs are co-administered with zafirlukast). Products include:
DynaCirc CR Controlled Release Tablets 1407

Itraconazole (No formal drug-drug interaction studies between zafirlukast and marketed drugs known to be metabolized by the P450 3A4 (CYP3A4) isoenzyme (e.g., dihydropyridine calcium-channel blockers, cyclosporin, cisapride) have been conducted. As zafirlukast is known to be an inhibitor of CYP3A4 in vitro, it is reasonable to employ appropriate clinical monitoring when these drugs are co-administered with zafirlukast).
No products indexed under this heading.

Ixabepilone (No formal drug-drug interaction studies between zafirlukast and marketed drugs known to be metabolized by the P450 3A4 (CYP3A4) isoenzyme (e.g., dihydropyridine calcium-channel blockers, cyclosporin, cisapride) have been conducted. As zafirlukast is known to be an inhibitor of CYP3A4 in vitro, it is reasonable to employ appropriate clinical monitoring when these drugs are co-administered with zafirlukast). Products include:
Ixempra Kit for Injection 915

Ketoconazole (No formal drug-drug interaction studies between zafirlukast and marketed drugs known to be metabolized by the P450 3A4 (CYP3A4) isoenzyme (e.g., dihydropyridine calcium-channel blockers, cyclosporin, cisapride) have been conducted. As zafirlukast is known to be an inhibitor of CYP3A4 in vitro, it is reasonable to employ appropriate clinical monitoring when these drugs are co-administered with zafirlukast). Products include:
Extina Foam, 2% 3057
Nizoral A-D Shampoo 1901

Ketoprofen (No formal drug-drug interaction studies with zafirlukast and other drugs known to be metabolized by the cytochrome P450 2C9 isoenzyme (e.g., tolbutamide, phenytoin, carbamazepine) have been conducted; however, care should be exercised when zafirlukast is co-administered with these drugs).
No products indexed under this heading.

Ketorolac Tromethamine (No formal drug-drug interaction studies with zafirlukast and other drugs known to be metabolized by the cytochrome P450 2C9 isoenzyme (e.g., tolbutamide, phenytoin, carbamazepine) have been conducted; however, care should be exercised when zafirlukast is co-administered with these drugs).
No products indexed under this heading.

Lansoprazole (No formal drug-drug interaction studies with zafirlukast and other drugs known to be metabolized by the cytochrome P450 2C9 isoenzyme (e.g., tolbutamide, phenytoin, carbamazepine) have been conducted; however, care should be exercised when zafirlukast is co-administered with these drugs).
No products indexed under this heading.

Levonorgestrel (No formal drug-drug interaction studies between zafirlukast and marketed drugs known to be metabolized by the P450 3A4 (CYP3A4) isoenzyme (e.g., dihydropyridine calcium-channel blockers, cyclosporin, cisapride) have been conducted. As zafirlukast is known to be an inhibitor of CYP3A4 in vitro, it is reasonable to employ appropriate clinical moni-

toring when these drugs are co-administered with zafirlukast).
Products include:
Climara Pro Transdermal System **768**
Lybrel Tablets **3204**
Mirena Intrauterine System **779**
Plan B Tablets **1044**
Seasonique Tablets **1046**

Lidocaine (No formal drug-drug interaction studies between zafirlukast and marketed drugs known to be metabolized by the P450 3A4 (CYP3A4) isoenzyme (e.g., dihydropyridine calcium-channel blockers, cyclosporin, cisapride) have been conducted. As zafirlukast is known to be an inhibitor of CYP3A4 in vitro, it is reasonable to employ appropriate clinical monitoring when these drugs are co-administered with zafirlukast).
Products include:
Lidoderm Patch **1114**

Lidocaine Hydrochloride (No formal drug-drug interaction studies between zafirlukast and marketed drugs known to be metabolized by the P450 3A4 (CYP3A4) isoenzyme (e.g., dihydropyridine calcium-channel blockers, cyclosporin, cisapride) have been conducted. As zafirlukast is known to be an inhibitor of CYP3A4 in vitro, it is reasonable to employ appropriate clinical monitoring when these drugs are co-administered with zafirlukast).
No products indexed under this heading.

Losartan Potassium (No formal drug-drug interaction studies with zafirlukast and other drugs known to be metabolized by the cytochrome P450 2C9 isoenzyme (e.g., tolbutamide, phenytoin, carbamazepine) have been conducted; however, care should be exercised when zafirlukast is co-administered with these drugs).
Products include:
Cozaar Tablets **1973**

Lovastatin (No formal drug-drug interaction studies between zafirlukast and marketed drugs known to be metabolized by the P450 3A4 (CYP3A4) isoenzyme (e.g., dihydropyridine calcium-channel blockers, cyclosporin, cisapride) have been conducted. As zafirlukast is known to be an inhibitor of CYP3A4 in vitro, it is reasonable to employ appropriate clinical monitoring when these drugs are co-administered with zafirlukast).
Products include:
Advicor Tablets **402**
Mevacor Tablets **2063**

Meclofenamate Sodium (No formal drug-drug interaction studies with zafirlukast and other drugs known to be metabolized by the cytochrome P450 2C9 isoenzyme (e.g., tolbutamide, phenytoin, carbamazepine) have been conducted; however, care should be exercised when zafirlukast is co-administered with these drugs).
No products indexed under this heading.

Mefenamic Acid (No formal drug-drug interaction studies with zafirlukast and other drugs known to be metabolized by the cytochrome P450 2C9 isoenzyme (e.g., tolbutamide, phenytoin, carbamazepine) have been conducted; however, care should be exercised when zafirlukast is co-administered with these drugs).
No products indexed under this heading.

Meloxicam (No formal drug-drug interaction studies with zafirlukast and other drugs known to be metabolized by the cytochrome P450 2C9 isoenzyme (e.g., tolbutamide, phenytoin, carbamazepine) have been conducted; however, care should be exercised when zafirlukast is co-administered with these drugs).
Products include:
Mobic Oral Suspension **863**
Mobic Tablets **863**

Mestranol (No formal drug-drug interaction studies between zafirlukast and marketed drugs known to be metabolized by the P450 3A4 (CYP3A4) isoenzyme (e.g., dihydropyridine calcium-channel blockers, cyclosporin, cisapride) have been conducted. As zafirlukast is known to be an inhibitor of CYP3A4 in vitro, it is reasonable to employ appropriate clinical monitoring when these drugs are co-administered with zafirlukast).
No products indexed under this heading.

Metformin Hydrochloride (No formal drug-drug interaction studies with zafirlukast and other drugs known to be metabolized by the cytochrome P450 2C9 isoenzyme (e.g., tolbutamide, phenytoin, carbamazepine) have been conducted; however, care should be exercised when zafirlukast is co-administered with these drugs). Products include:
ActoPlus Met Tablets **3071**
Avandamet Tablets **1336**
Janumet Tablets **2041**
PrandiMet Tablets **2967**

Methadone Hydrochloride (No formal drug-drug interaction studies between zafirlukast and marketed drugs known to be metabolized by the P450 3A4 (CYP3A4) isoenzyme (e.g., dihydropyridine calcium-channel blockers, cyclosporin, cisapride) have been conducted. As zafirlukast is known to be an inhibitor of CYP3A4 in vitro, it is reasonable to employ appropriate clinical monitoring when these drugs are co-administered with zafirlukast).
No products indexed under this heading.

Midazolam Hydrochloride (No formal drug-drug interaction studies between zafirlukast and marketed drugs known to be metabolized by the P450 3A4 (CYP3A4) isoenzyme (e.g., dihydropyridine calcium-channel blockers, cyclosporin, cisapride) have been conducted. As zafirlukast is known to be an inhibitor of CYP3A4 in vitro, it is reasonable to employ appropriate clinical monitoring when these drugs are co-administered with zafirlukast).
No products indexed under this heading.

Miglitol (No formal drug-drug interaction studies with zafirlukast and other drugs known to be metabolized by the cytochrome P450 2C9 isoenzyme (e.g., tolbutamide, phenytoin, carbamazepine) have been conducted; however, care should be exercised when zafirlukast is co-administered with these drugs).
No products indexed under this heading.

Mirtazapine (No formal drug-drug interaction studies with zafirlukast and other drugs known to be metabolized by the cytochrome P450 2C9 isoenzyme (e.g., tolbutamide, phenytoin, carbamazepine) have been conducted; however, care should be exercised when zafirlukast is co-administered with these drugs).
Products include:
Remeron Tablets **2924**
RemeronSolTab Tablets **2927**

Montelukast Sodium (No formal drug-drug interaction studies with zafirlukast and other drugs known to be metabolized by the cytochrome P450 2C9 isoenzyme (e.g., tolbutamide, phenytoin, carbamazepine) have been conducted; however, care should be exercised when zafirlukast is co-administered with these drugs).
Products include:
Singulair **2114**

Nabumetone (No formal drug-drug interaction studies with zafirlukast and other drugs known to be metabolized by the cytochrome P450 2C9 isoenzyme (e.g., tolbutamide, phenytoin, carbamazepine) have been conducted; however, care should be exercised when zafirlukast is co-administered with these drugs).
No products indexed under this heading.

Naproxen (No formal drug-drug interaction studies with zafirlukast and other drugs known to be metabolized by the cytochrome P450 2C9 isoenzyme (e.g., tolbutamide, phenytoin, carbamazepine) have been conducted; however, care should be exercised when zafirlukast is co-administered with these drugs).
Products include:
EC-Naprosyn Delayed-Release Tablets **2632**
Naprosyn Suspension **2632**
Naprosyn Tablets **2632**

Naproxen Sodium (No formal drug-drug interaction studies with zafirlukast and other drugs known to be metabolized by the cytochrome P450 2C9 isoenzyme (e.g., tolbutamide, phenytoin, carbamazepine) have been conducted; however, care should be exercised when zafirlukast is co-administered with these drugs).
Products include:
Anaprox Tablets **2632**
Anaprox DS Tablets **2632**
Treximet Tablets **1616**

Nateglinide (No formal drug-drug interaction studies with zafirlukast and other drugs known to be metabolized by the cytochrome P450 2C9 isoenzyme (e.g., tolbutamide, phenytoin, carbamazepine) have been conducted; however, care should be exercised when zafirlukast is co-administered with these drugs).
Products include:
Starlix Tablets **2314**

Nefazodone Hydrochloride (No formal drug-drug interaction studies between zafirlukast and marketed drugs known to be metabolized by the P450 3A4 (CYP3A4) isoenzyme (e.g., dihydropyridine calcium-channel blockers, cyclosporin, cisapride) have been conducted. As zafirlukast is known to be an inhibitor of CYP3A4 in vitro, it is reasonable to employ appropriate clinical monitoring when these drugs are co-administered with zafirlukast).
No products indexed under this heading.

Nelfinavir Mesylate (No formal drug-drug interaction studies between zafirlukast and marketed drugs known to be metabolized by the P450 3A4 (CYP3A4) isoenzyme (e.g., dihydropyridine calcium-channel blockers, cyclosporin, cisapride) have been conducted. As zafirlukast is known to be an inhibitor of CYP3A4 in vitro, it is reasonable to employ appropriate clinical monitoring when these drugs are co-administered with zafirlukast).
No products indexed under this heading.

Nicardipine Hydrochloride (No formal drug-drug interaction studies between zafirlukast and marketed drugs known to be metabolized by the P450 3A4 (CYP3A4) isoenzyme (e.g., dihydropyridine calcium-channel blockers, cyclosporin, cisapride) have been conducted. As zafirlukast is known to be an inhibitor of CYP3A4 in vitro, it is reasonable to employ appropriate clinical monitoring when these drugs are co-administered with zafirlukast).
Products include:
Cardene I.V. **1093**

Nifedipine (No formal drug-drug interaction studies with zafirlukast and other drugs known to be metabolized by the cytochrome P450 2C9 isoenzyme (e.g., tolbutamide, phenytoin, carbamazepine) have been conducted; however, care should be exercised when zafirlukast is co-administered with these drugs).
No products indexed under this heading.

Nimodipine (No formal drug-drug interaction studies between zafirlukast and marketed drugs known to be metabolized by the P450 3A4 (CYP3A4) isoenzyme (e.g., dihydropyridine calcium-channel blockers, cyclosporin, cisapride) have been conducted. As zafirlukast is known to be an inhibitor of CYP3A4 in vitro, it is reasonable to employ appropriate clinical monitoring when these drugs are co-administered with zafirlukast).
Products include:
Nimotop Capsules **790**

Nisoldipine (No formal drug-drug interaction studies between zafirlukast and marketed drugs known to be metabolized by the P450 3A4 (CYP3A4) isoenzyme (e.g., dihydropyridine calcium-channel blockers, cyclosporin, cisapride) have been conducted. As zafirlukast is known to be an inhibitor of CYP3A4 in vitro, it is reasonable to employ appropriate clinical monitoring when these drugs are co-administered with zafirlukast).
Products include:
Sular Extended Release Tablets **2975**

Nitrendipine (No formal drug-drug interaction studies between zafirlukast and marketed drugs known to be metabolized by the P450 3A4 (CYP3A4) isoenzyme (e.g., dihydropyridine calcium-channel blockers, cyclosporin, cisapride) have been conducted. As zafirlukast is known to be an inhibitor of CYP3A4 in vitro, it is reasonable to employ appropriate clinical monitoring when these drugs are co-administered with zafirlukast).
No products indexed under this heading.

Norethindrone (No formal drug-drug interaction studies between zafirlukast and marketed drugs known to be metabolized by the P450 3A4 (CYP3A4) isoenzyme (e.g., dihydropyridine calcium-channel blockers, cyclosporin, cisapride) have been conducted. As zafirlukast is known to be an inhibitor

of CYP3A4 in vitro, it is reasonable to employ appropriate clinical monitoring when these drugs are co-administered with zafirlukast).
Products include:
Ortho Micronor Tablets **2446**

Norethindrone Acetate (No formal drug-drug interaction studies between zafirlukast and marketed drugs known to be metabolized by the P450 3A4 (CYP3A4) isoenzyme (e.g., dihydropyridine calcium-channel blockers, cyclosporin, cisapride) have been conducted. As zafirlukast is known to be an inhibitor of CYP3A4 in vitro, it is reasonable to employ appropriate clinical monitoring when these drugs are co-administered with zafirlukast).
Products include:
Activella Tablets **2347**

Norgestrel (No formal drug-drug interaction studies between zafirlukast and marketed drugs known to be metabolized by the P450 3A4 (CYP3A4) isoenzyme (e.g., dihydropyridine calcium-channel blockers, cyclosporin, cisapride) have been conducted. As zafirlukast is known to be an inhibitor of CYP3A4 in vitro, it is reasonable to employ appropriate clinical monitoring when these drugs are co-administered with zafirlukast).
No products indexed under this heading.

Omeprazole (No formal drug-drug interaction studies with zafirlukast and other drugs known to be metabolized by the cytochrome P450 2C9 isoenzyme (e.g., tolbutamide, phenytoin, carbamazepine) have been conducted; however, care should be exercised when zafirlukast is co-administered with these drugs).
No products indexed under this heading.

Ondansetron (No formal drug-drug interaction studies between zafirlukast and marketed drugs known to be metabolized by the P450 3A4 (CYP3A4) isoenzyme (e.g., dihydropyridine calcium-channel blockers, cyclosporin, cisapride) have been conducted. As zafirlukast is known to be an inhibitor of CYP3A4 in vitro, it is reasonable to employ appropriate clinical monitoring when these drugs are co-administered with zafirlukast).
Products include:
Zofran ODT Orally Disintegrating Tablets **1687**

Ondansetron Hydrochloride (No formal drug-drug interaction studies between zafirlukast and marketed drugs known to be metabolized by the P450 3A4 (CYP3A4) isoenzyme (e.g., dihydropyridine calcium-channel blockers, cyclosporin, cisapride) have been conducted. As zafirlukast is known to be an inhibitor of CYP3A4 in vitro, it is reasonable to employ appropriate clinical monitoring when these drugs are co-administered with zafirlukast).
Products include:
Zofran Injection **1682**
Zofran **1687**

Oxaprozin (No formal drug-drug interaction studies with zafirlukast and other drugs known to be metabolized by the cytochrome P450 2C9 isoenzyme (e.g., tolbutamide, phenytoin, carbamazepine) have been conducted; however, care should be exercised when zafirlukast is co-administered with these drugs).
No products indexed under this heading.

Paclitaxel (No formal drug-drug interaction studies between zafirlukast and marketed drugs known to be metabolized by the P450 3A4 (CYP3A4) isoenzyme (e.g., dihydropyridine calcium-channel blockers, cyclosporin, cisapride) have been conducted. As zafirlukast is known to be an inhibitor of CYP3A4 in vitro, it is reasonable to employ appropriate clinical monitoring when these drugs are co-administered with zafirlukast).
No products indexed under this heading.

Phenylbutazone (No formal drug-drug interaction studies with zafirlukast and other drugs known to be metabolized by the cytochrome P450 2C9 isoenzyme (e.g., tolbutamide, phenytoin, carbamazepine) have been conducted; however, care should be exercised when zafirlukast is co-administered with these drugs).
No products indexed under this heading.

Phenytoin (No formal drug-drug interaction studies with zafirlukast and other drugs known to be metabolized by the cytochrome P450 2C9 isoenzyme (e.g., tolbutamide, phenytoin, carbamazepine) have been conducted; however, care should be exercised when zafirlukast is co-administered with these drugs).
No products indexed under this heading.

Phenytoin Sodium (No formal drug-drug interaction studies with zafirlukast and other drugs known to be metabolized by the cytochrome P450 2C9 isoenzyme (e.g., tolbutamide, phenytoin, carbamazepine) have been conducted; however, care should be exercised when zafirlukast is co-administered with these drugs).
Products include:
Phenytek Capsules **2192**

Pimozide (No formal drug-drug interaction studies between zafirlukast and marketed drugs known to be metabolized by the P450 3A4 (CYP3A4) isoenzyme (e.g., dihydropyridine calcium-channel blockers, cyclosporin, cisapride) have been conducted. As zafirlukast is known to be an inhibitor of CYP3A4 in vitro, it is reasonable to employ appropriate clinical monitoring when these drugs are co-administered with zafirlukast).
No products indexed under this heading.

Pioglitazone Hydrochloride (No formal drug-drug interaction studies with zafirlukast and other drugs known to be metabolized by the cytochrome P450 2C9 isoenzyme (e.g., tolbutamide, phenytoin, carbamazepine) have been conducted; however, care should be exercised when zafirlukast is co-administered with these drugs). Products include:
ActoPlus Met Tablets **3071**
Actos Tablets **3077**
Duetact Tablets **3085**

Piroxicam (No formal drug-drug interaction studies with zafirlukast and other drugs known to be metabolized by the cytochrome P450 2C9 isoenzyme (e.g., tolbutamide, phenytoin, carbamazepine) have been conducted; however, care should be exercised when zafirlukast is co-administered with these drugs).
No products indexed under this heading.

Polyestradiol Phosphate (No formal drug-drug interaction studies between zafirlukast and marketed drugs known to be metabolized by the P450 3A4 (CYP3A4) isoenzyme (e.g., dihydropyridine calcium-channel blockers, cyclosporin, cisapride) have been conducted. As zafirlukast is known to be an inhibitor of CYP3A4 in vitro, it is reasonable to employ appropriate clinical monitoring when these drugs are co-administered with zafirlukast).
No products indexed under this heading.

Quinidine Gluconate (No formal drug-drug interaction studies between zafirlukast and marketed drugs known to be metabolized by the P450 3A4 (CYP3A4) isoenzyme (e.g., dihydropyridine calcium-channel blockers, cyclosporin, cisapride) have been conducted. As zafirlukast is known to be an inhibitor of CYP3A4 in vitro, it is reasonable to employ appropriate clinical monitoring when these drugs are co-administered with zafirlukast).
No products indexed under this heading.

Quinidine Polygalacturonate (No formal drug-drug interaction studies between zafirlukast and marketed drugs known to be metabolized by the P450 3A4 (CYP3A4) isoenzyme (e.g., dihydropyridine calcium-channel blockers, cyclosporin, cisapride) have been conducted. As zafirlukast is known to be an inhibitor of CYP3A4 in vitro, it is reasonable to employ appropriate clinical monitoring when these drugs are co-administered with zafirlukast).
No products indexed under this heading.

Quinidine Sulfate (No formal drug-drug interaction studies between zafirlukast and marketed drugs known to be metabolized by the P450 3A4 (CYP3A4) isoenzyme (e.g., dihydropyridine calcium-channel blockers, cyclosporin, cisapride) have been conducted. As zafirlukast is known to be an inhibitor of CYP3A4 in vitro, it is reasonable to employ appropriate clinical monitoring when these drugs are co-administered with zafirlukast).
No products indexed under this heading.

Repaglinide (No formal drug-drug interaction studies with zafirlukast and other drugs known to be metabolized by the cytochrome P450 2C9 isoenzyme (e.g., tolbutamide, phenytoin, carbamazepine) have been conducted; however, care should be exercised when zafirlukast is co-administered with these drugs).
Products include:
PrandiMet Tablets **2967**
Prandin Tablets **2971**

Rifabutin (No formal drug-drug interaction studies between zafirlukast and marketed drugs known to be metabolized by the P450 3A4 (CYP3A4) isoenzyme (e.g., dihydropyridine calcium-channel blockers, cyclosporin, cisapride) have been conducted. As zafirlukast is known to be an inhibitor of CYP3A4 in vitro, it is reasonable to employ appropriate clinical monitoring when these drugs are co-administered with zafirlukast).
No products indexed under this heading.

Ritonavir (No formal drug-drug interaction studies between zafirlukast and marketed drugs known to be metabolized by the P450 3A4 (CYP3A4) isoenzyme (e.g., dihydropyridine calcium-channel blockers, cyclosporin, cisapride) have been conducted. As zafirlukast is known to be an inhibitor of CYP3A4 in vitro, it is reasonable to employ appropriate clinical monitoring when these drugs are co-administered with zafirlukast).
Products include:
Kaletra **452**
Norvir **489**

Rofecoxib (No formal drug-drug interaction studies with zafirlukast and other drugs known to be metabolized by the cytochrome P450 2C9 isoenzyme (e.g., tolbutamide, phenytoin, carbamazepine) have been conducted; however, care should be exercised when zafirlukast is co-administered with these drugs).
No products indexed under this heading.

Rosiglitazone Maleate (No formal drug-drug interaction studies with zafirlukast and other drugs known to be metabolized by the cytochrome P450 2C9 isoenzyme (e.g., tolbutamide, phenytoin, carbamazepine) have been conducted; however, care should be exercised when zafirlukast is co-administered with these drugs).
Products include:
Avandamet Tablets **1336**
Avandaryl Tablets **1344**
Avandia Tablets **1351**

Saquinavir (No formal drug-drug interaction studies between zafirlukast and marketed drugs known to be metabolized by the P450 3A4 (CYP3A4) isoenzyme (e.g., dihydropyridine calcium-channel blockers, cyclosporin, cisapride) have been conducted. As zafirlukast is known to be an inhibitor of CYP3A4 in vitro, it is reasonable to employ appropriate clinical monitoring when these drugs are co-administered with zafirlukast).
No products indexed under this heading.

Saquinavir Mesylate (No formal drug-drug interaction studies between zafirlukast and marketed drugs known to be metabolized by the P450 3A4 (CYP3A4) isoenzyme (e.g., dihydropyridine calcium-channel blockers, cyclosporin, cisapride) have been conducted. As zafirlukast is known to be an inhibitor of CYP3A4 in vitro, it is reasonable to employ appropriate clinical monitoring when these drugs are co-administered with zafirlukast).
No products indexed under this heading.

Sertraline Hydrochloride (No formal drug-drug interaction studies between zafirlukast and marketed drugs known to be metabolized by the P450 3A4 (CYP3A4) isoenzyme (e.g., dihydropyridine calcium-channel blockers, cyclosporin, cisapride) have been conducted. As zafirlukast is known to be an inhibitor of CYP3A4 in vitro, it is reasonable to employ appropriate clinical monitoring when these drugs are co-administered with zafirlukast).

No products indexed under this heading.

Sildenafil Citrate (No formal drug-drug interaction studies with zafirlukast and other drugs known to be metabolized by the cytochrome P450 2C9 isoenzyme (e.g., tolbutamide, phenytoin, carbamazepine) have been conducted; however, care should be exercised when zafirlukast is co-administered with these drugs).

No products indexed under this heading.

Simvastatin (No formal drug-drug interaction studies between zafirlukast and marketed drugs known to be metabolized by the P450 3A4 (CYP3A4) isoenzyme (e.g., dihydropyridine calcium-channel blockers, cyclosporin, cisapride) have been conducted. As zafirlukast is known to be an inhibitor of CYP3A4 in vitro, it is reasonable to employ appropriate clinical monitoring when these drugs are co-administered with zafirlukast).

Products include:

Simcor Tablets 502
Vytorin 10/10 Tablets 2149
Vytorin 10/10 Tablets 2939
Vytorin 10/20 Tablets 2149
Vytorin 10/20 Tablets 2939
Vytorin 10/40 Tablets 2149
Vytorin 10/40 Tablets 2939
Vytorin 10/80 Tablets 2149
Vytorin 10/80 Tablets 2939
Zocor Tablets 2136

Sirolimus (No formal drug-drug interaction studies between zafirlukast and marketed drugs known to be metabolized by the P450 3A4 (CYP3A4) isoenzyme (e.g., dihydropyridine calcium-channel blockers, cyclosporin, cisapride) have been conducted. As zafirlukast is known to be an inhibitor of CYP3A4 in vitro, it is reasonable to employ appropriate clinical monitoring when these drugs are co-administered with zafirlukast).

Products include:

Rapamune 3260

Sulfamethoxazole (No formal drug-drug interaction studies with zafirlukast and other drugs known to be metabolized by the cytochrome P450 2C9 isoenzyme (e.g., tolbutamide, phenytoin, carbamazepine) have been conducted; however, care should be exercised when zafirlukast is co-administered with these drugs).

No products indexed under this heading.

Sulindac (No formal drug-drug interaction studies with zafirlukast and other drugs known to be metabolized by the cytochrome P450 2C9 isoenzyme (e.g., tolbutamide, phenytoin, carbamazepine) have been conducted; however, care should be exercised when zafirlukast is co-administered with these drugs).

Products include:

Clinoril Tablets 1962

Suprofen (No formal drug-drug interaction studies with zafirlukast and other drugs known to be metabolized by the cytochrome P450 2C9 isoenzyme (e.g., tolbutamide, phenytoin, carbamazepine) have been conducted; however, care should be exercised when zafirlukast is co-administered with these drugs).

No products indexed under this heading.

Tacrolimus (No formal drug-drug interaction studies between zafirlukast and marketed drugs known to be metabolized by the P450 3A4 (CYP3A4) isoenzyme (e.g., dihydropyridine calcium-channel blockers, cyclosporin, cisapride) have been conducted. As zafirlukast is known to be an inhibitor of CYP3A4 in vitro, it is reasonable to employ appropriate clinical monitoring when these drugs are co-administered with zafirlukast).

Products include:

Prograf Capsules and Injection 622
Protopic Ointment 628

Tadalafil (No formal drug-drug interaction studies between zafirlukast and marketed drugs known to be metabolized by the P450 3A4 (CYP3A4) isoenzyme (e.g., dihydropyridine calcium-channel blockers, cyclosporin, cisapride) have been conducted. As zafirlukast is known to be an inhibitor of CYP3A4 in vitro, it is reasonable to employ appropriate clinical monitoring when these drugs are co-administered with zafirlukast). Products include:

Cialis Tablets 1792

Tamoxifen Citrate (No formal drug-drug interaction studies with zafirlukast and other drugs known to be metabolized by the cytochrome P450 2C9 isoenzyme (e.g., tolbutamide, phenytoin, carbamazepine) have been conducted; however, care should be exercised when zafirlukast is co-administered with these drugs).

No products indexed under this heading.

Telmisartan (No formal drug-drug interaction studies with zafirlukast and other drugs known to be metabolized by the cytochrome P450 2C9 isoenzyme (e.g., tolbutamide, phenytoin, carbamazepine) have been conducted; however, care should be exercised when zafirlukast is co-administered with these drugs).

Products include:

Micardis Tablets 852
Micardis HCT Tablets 854

Theophylline (Rare cases of patients experiencing increased theophylline levels with or without clinical signs or symptoms of theophylline toxicity after the addition of zafirlukast to an existing theophylline regimen have been reported).

No products indexed under this heading.

Theophylline Anhydrous (Rare cases of patients experiencing increased theophylline levels with or without clinical signs or symptoms of theophylline toxicity after the addition of zafirlukast to an existing theophylline regimen have been reported). Products include:

Uniphyl Tablets 2595

Theophylline Calcium Salicylate (Rare cases of patients experiencing increased theophylline levels with or without clinical signs or symptoms of theophylline toxicity after the addition of zafirlukast to an existing theophylline regimen have been reported).

No products indexed under this heading.

Theophylline Dihydroxypropyl (Glyceryl) (Rare cases of patients experiencing increased theophylline levels with or without clinical signs or symptoms of theophylline toxicity after the addition of zafirlukast to an existing theophylline regimen have been reported).

No products indexed under this heading.

Theophylline Ethylenediamine (Rare cases of patients experiencing increased theophylline levels with or without clinical signs or symptoms of theophylline toxicity after the addition of zafirlukast to an existing theophylline regimen have been reported).

No products indexed under this heading.

Theophylline Sodium Glycinate (Rare cases of patients experiencing increased theophylline levels with or without clinical signs or symptoms of theophylline toxicity after the addition of zafirlukast to an existing theophylline regimen have been reported).

No products indexed under this heading.

Tiagabine Hydrochloride (No formal drug-drug interaction studies between zafirlukast and marketed drugs known to be metabolized by the P450 3A4 (CYP3A4) isoenzyme (e.g., dihydropyridine calcium-channel blockers, cyclosporin, cisapride) have been conducted. As zafirlukast is known to be an inhibitor of CYP3A4 in vitro, it is reasonable to employ appropriate clinical monitoring when these drugs are co-administered with zafirlukast).

Products include:

Gabitril Tablets 973

Tolazamide (No formal drug-drug interaction studies with zafirlukast and other drugs known to be metabolized by the cytochrome P450 2C9 isoenzyme (e.g., tolbutamide, phenytoin, carbamazepine) have been conducted; however, care should be exercised when zafirlukast is co-administered with these drugs).

No products indexed under this heading.

Tolbutamide (No formal drug-drug interaction studies with zafirlukast and other drugs known to be metabolized by the cytochrome P450 2C9 isoenzyme (e.g., tolbutamide, phenytoin, carbamazepine) have been conducted; however, care should be exercised when zafirlukast is co-administered with these drugs).

No products indexed under this heading.

Tolbutamide Sodium (No formal drug-drug interaction studies with zafirlukast and other drugs known to be metabolized by the cytochrome P450 2C9 isoenzyme (e.g., tolbutamide, phenytoin, carbamazepine) have been conducted; however, care should be exercised when zafirlukast is co-administered with these drugs).

No products indexed under this heading.

Tolmetin Sodium (No formal drug-drug interaction studies with zafirlukast and other drugs known to be metabolized by the cytochrome P450 2C9 isoenzyme (e.g., tolbutamide, phenytoin, carbamazepine) have been conducted; however, care should be exercised when zafirlukast is co-administered with these drugs).

No products indexed under this heading.

Tolterodine Tartrate (No formal drug-drug interaction studies between zafirlukast and marketed drugs known to be metabolized by the P450 3A4 (CYP3A4) isoenzyme (e.g., dihydropyridine calcium-channel blockers, cyclosporin, cisapride) have been conducted. As zafirlukast is known to be an inhibitor of CYP3A4 in vitro, it is reasonable to employ appropriate clinical monitoring when these drugs are co-administered with zafirlukast).

No products indexed under this heading.

Torsemide (No formal drug-drug interaction studies with zafirlukast and other drugs known to be metabolized by the cytochrome P450 2C9 isoenzyme (e.g., tolbutamide, phenytoin, carbamazepine) have been conducted; however, care should be exercised when zafirlukast is co-administered with these drugs).

Products include:

Demadex Injection 2630
Demadex Tablets 2630

Trazodone Hydrochloride (No formal drug-drug interaction studies between zafirlukast and marketed drugs known to be metabolized by the P450 3A4 (CYP3A4) isoenzyme (e.g., dihydropyridine calcium-channel blockers, cyclosporin, cisapride) have been conducted. As zafirlukast is known to be an inhibitor of CYP3A4 in vitro, it is reasonable to employ appropriate clinical monitoring when these drugs are co-administered with zafirlukast).

No products indexed under this heading.

Triazolam (No formal drug-drug interaction studies between zafirlukast and marketed drugs known to be metabolized by the P450 3A4 (CYP3A4) isoenzyme (e.g., dihydropyridine calcium-channel blockers, cyclosporin, cisapride) have been conducted. As zafirlukast is known to be an inhibitor of CYP3A4 in vitro, it is reasonable to employ appropriate clinical monitoring when these drugs are co-administered with zafirlukast).

No products indexed under this heading.

Troglitazone (No formal drug-drug interaction studies with zafirlukast and other drugs known to be metabolized by the cytochrome P450 2C9 isoenzyme (e.g., tolbutamide, phenytoin, carbamazepine) have been conducted; however, care should be exercised when zafirlukast is co-administered with these drugs).

No products indexed under this heading.

Valdecoxib (No formal drug-drug interaction studies with zafirlukast and other drugs known to be metabolized by the cytochrome P450 2C9 isoenzyme (e.g., tolbutamide, phenytoin, carbamazepine) have been conducted; however, care should be exercised when zafirlukast is co-administered with these drugs).
No products indexed under this heading.

Valsartan (No formal drug-drug interaction studies with zafirlukast and other drugs known to be metabolized by the cytochrome P450 2C9 isoenzyme (e.g., tolbutamide, phenytoin, carbamazepine) have been conducted; however, care should be exercised when zafirlukast is co-administered with these drugs). Products include:
Diovan Tablets 2212
Diovan HCT Tablets 2216
Exforge Tablets 2238

Vardenafil Hydrochloride (No formal drug-drug interaction studies with zafirlukast and other drugs known to be metabolized by the cytochrome P450 2C9 isoenzyme (e.g., tolbutamide, phenytoin, carbamazepine) have been conducted; however, care should be exercised when zafirlukast is co-administered with these drugs). Products include:
Levitra Tablets 2876

Verapamil Hydrochloride (No formal drug-drug interaction studies with zafirlukast and other drugs known to be metabolized by the cytochrome P450 2C9 isoenzyme (e.g., tolbutamide, phenytoin, carbamazepine) have been conducted; however, care should be exercised when zafirlukast is co-administered with these drugs). Products include:
Tarka Tablets 511

Vinblastine Sulfate (No formal drug-drug interaction studies between zafirlukast and marketed drugs known to be metabolized by the P450 3A4 (CYP3A4) isoenzyme (e.g., dihydropyridine calcium-channel blockers, cyclosporin, cisapride) have been conducted. As zafirlukast is known to be an inhibitor of CYP3A4 in vitro, it is reasonable to employ appropriate clinical monitoring when these drugs are co-administered with zafirlukast).
No products indexed under this heading.

Vincristine Sulfate (No formal drug-drug interaction studies between zafirlukast and marketed drugs known to be metabolized by the P450 3A4 (CYP3A4) isoenzyme (e.g., dihydropyridine calcium-channel blockers, cyclosporin, cisapride) have been conducted. As zafirlukast is known to be an inhibitor of CYP3A4 in vitro, it is reasonable to employ appropriate clinical monitoring when these drugs are co-administered with zafirlukast).
No products indexed under this heading.

Voriconazole (No formal drug-drug interaction studies with zafirlukast and other drugs known to be metabolized by the cytochrome P450 2C9 isoenzyme (e.g., tolbutamide, phenytoin, carbamazepine) have been conducted; however, care should be exercised when zafirlukast is co-administered with these drugs).
No products indexed under this heading.

Warfarin Sodium (In a drug interaction study in 16 healthy male volunteers, co-administration of multiple doses of zafirlukast (160 mg/day) to steady-state with a single 25 mg dose of warfarin resulted in a significant increase in the mean AUC (+63%) and half-life (+36%) of S-warfarin. The mean prothrombin time (PT) increased by approximately 35%. This interaction is probably due to an inhibition by zafirlukast of the cytochrome P450 2C9 isoenzyme system. Patients on oral warfarin anticoagulant therapy and zafirlukast should have their prothrombin times monitored closely and anticoagulant dose adjusted accordingly).
No products indexed under this heading.

Zileuton (No formal drug-drug interaction studies with zafirlukast and other drugs known to be metabolized by the cytochrome P450 2C9 isoenzyme (e.g., tolbutamide, phenytoin, carbamazepine) have been conducted; however, care should be exercised when zafirlukast is co-administered with these drugs).
No products indexed under this heading.

Food Interactions

Food, unspecified (The bioavailability of zafirlukast may be decreased when taken with food. Patients should be instructed to take zafirlukast at least 1 hour before or 2 hours after meals).

ACCUTANE CAPSULES

(Isotretinoin) 2607
May interact with corticosteroids, phenytoin, tetracyclines, and certain other agents. Compounds in these categories include:

Betamethasone Acetate (Systemic corticosteroids are known to cause osteoporosis; caution is advised if used concurrently because of potential interactive effect on bone loss between systemic corticosteroids and Accutane).
No products indexed under this heading.

Betamethasone Sodium Phosphate (Systemic corticosteroids are known to cause osteoporosis; caution is advised if used concurrently because of potential interactive effect on bone loss between systemic corticosteroids and Accutane).
No products indexed under this heading.

Budesonide (Systemic corticosteroids are known to cause osteoporosis; caution is advised if used concurrently because of potential interactive effect on bone loss between systemic corticosteroids and Accutane). Products include:
Pulmicort Flexhaler 654
Symbicort 80/4.5 Inhalation Aerosol 659
Symbicort 160/4.5 Inhalation Aerosol 659

Ciclesonide (Systemic corticosteroids are known to cause osteoporosis; caution is advised if used concurrently because of potential interactive effect on bone loss between systemic corticosteroids and Accutane). Products include:
Alvesco Inhalation Aerosol 2985
Omnaris Nasal Spray 2998

Cortisone Acetate (Systemic corticosteroids are known to cause osteoporosis; caution is advised if used concurrently because of potential interactive effect on bone loss between systemic corticosteroids and Accutane).
No products indexed under this heading.

Demeclocycline Hydrochloride (Concomitant treatment with Accutane and tetracyclines should be avoided because Accutane is associated with a number of cases of pseudotumor cerebri, some of which involved concomitant use of tetracyclines).
No products indexed under this heading.

Dexamethasone (Systemic corticosteroids are known to cause osteoporosis; caution is advised if used concurrently because of potential interactive effect on bone loss between systemic corticosteroids and Accutane). Products include:
Ciprodex Otic Suspension 541

Dexamethasone Acetate (Systemic corticosteroids are known to cause osteoporosis; caution is advised if used concurrently because of potential interactive effect on bone loss between systemic corticosteroids and Accutane).
No products indexed under this heading.

Dexamethasone Sodium Phosphate (Systemic corticosteroids are known to cause osteoporosis; caution is advised if used concurrently because of potential interactive effect on bone loss between systemic corticosteroids and Accutane).
No products indexed under this heading.

Doxycycline Calcium (Concomitant treatment with Accutane and tetracyclines should be avoided because Accutane is associated with a number of cases of pseudotumor cerebri, some of which involved concomitant use of tetracyclines).
No products indexed under this heading.

Doxycycline Hyclate (Concomitant treatment with Accutane and tetracyclines should be avoided because Accutane is associated with a number of cases of pseudotumor cerebri, some of which involved concomitant use of tetracyclines).
No products indexed under this heading.

Doxycycline Monohydrate (Concomitant treatment with Accutane and tetracyclines should be avoided because Accutane is associated with a number of cases of pseudotumor cerebri, some of which involved concomitant use of tetracyclines).
No products indexed under this heading.

Fludrocortisone Acetate (Systemic corticosteroids are known to cause osteoporosis; caution is advised if used concurrently because of potential interactive effect on bone loss between systemic corticosteroids and Accutane).
No products indexed under this heading.

Flunisolide (Systemic corticosteroids are known to cause osteoporosis; caution is advised if used concurrently because of potential interactive effect on bone loss between systemic corticosteroids and Accutane). Products include:
Aerobid/Aerobid-M 1153

Fluticasone Propionate (Systemic corticosteroids are known to cause osteoporosis; caution is advised if used concurrently because of potential interactive effect on bone loss between systemic corticosteroids and Accutane). Products include:
Advair Diskus 100/50 1276
Advair Diskus 250/50 1276
Advair Diskus 500/50 1276
Advair HFA 45/21 Inhalation Aerosol 1288
Advair HFA 115/21 Inhalation Aerosol 1288
Advair HFA 230/21 Inhalation Aerosol 1288
Flonase Nasal Spray 1431
Flovent Diskus 50 mcg 1435

Fluticasone Propionate HFA (Systemic corticosteroids are known to cause osteoporosis; caution is advised if used concurrently because of potential interactive effect on bone loss between systemic corticosteroids and Accutane). Products include:
Flovent HFA 1440

Fosphenytoin Sodium (Phenytoin is known to cause osteomalacia; caution is advised if used concurrently because of potential interactive effect on bone loss between phenytoin and Accutane).
No products indexed under this heading.

Hydrocortisone (Systemic corticosteroids are known to cause osteoporosis; caution is advised if used concurrently because of potential interactive effect on bone loss between systemic corticosteroids and Accutane).
No products indexed under this heading.

Hydrocortisone Acetate (Systemic corticosteroids are known to cause osteoporosis; caution is advised if used concurrently because of potential interactive effect on bone loss between systemic corticosteroids and Accutane). Products include:
Analpram-HC 1140
Pramosone 1141

Hydrocortisone Sodium Phosphate (Systemic corticosteroids are known to cause osteoporosis; caution is advised if used concurrently because of potential interactive effect on bone loss between systemic corticosteroids and Accutane).
No products indexed under this heading.

Hydrocortisone Sodium Succinate (Systemic corticosteroids are known to cause osteoporosis; caution is advised if used concurrently because of potential interactive effect on bone loss between systemic corticosteroids and Accutane).
No products indexed under this heading.

Hypericum (Avoid St. John's Wort due to a possible interaction based on reports of breakthrough bleeding being reported on oral contraceptives shortly after starting St. John's Wort. Pregnancies have been reported by users of combined hormonal contraceptives who also used some form of St. John's Wort). Products include:
Satieté Tablets 640

Methacycline Hydrochloride (Concomitant treatment with Accutane and tetracyclines should be avoided because Accutane is associated with a number of cases of pseudotumor cerebri, some of which involved concomitant use of tetracyclines).
No products indexed under this heading.

Methylprednisolone Acetate (Systemic corticosteroids are known to cause osteoporosis; caution is advised if used concurrently because of potential interactive effect on bone loss between systemic corticosteroids and Accutane).
No products indexed under this heading.

Methylprednisolone Sodium Succinate (Systemic corticosteroids are known to cause osteoporosis; caution is advised if used concurrently because of potential interactive effect on bone loss between systemic corticosteroids and Accutane).
No products indexed under this heading.

Minocycline Hydrochloride (Concomitant treatment with Accutane and tetracyclines should be avoided because Accutane is associated with a number of cases of pseudotumor cerebri, some of which involved concomitant use of tetracyclines). Products include:
Solodyn Extended Release Tablets ... 1938

Mometasone Furoate (Systemic corticosteroids are known to cause osteoporosis; caution is advised if used concurrently because of potential interactive effect on bone loss between systemic corticosteroids and Accutane). Products include:
Asmanex Twisthaler ... 2797
Elocon Cream 0.1% ... 2840
Elocon Lotion 0.1% ... 2841
Elocon Ointment 0.1% ... 2842

Mometasone Furoate Monohydrate (Systemic corticosteroids are known to cause osteoporosis; caution is advised if used concurrently because of potential interactive effect on bone loss between systemic corticosteroids and Accutane). Products include:
Nasonex Nasal Spray ... 2883

Norethindrone (Microdosed progesterone preparations (minipills) may be an inadequate method of contraception during Accutane therapy). Products include:
Ortho Micronor Tablets ... 2446

Oxytetracycline Hydrochloride (Concomitant treatment with Accutane and tetracyclines should be avoided because Accutane is associated with a number of cases of pseudotumor cerebri, some of which involved concomitant use of tetracyclines).
No products indexed under this heading.

Phenytoin (Phenytoin is known to cause osteomalacia; caution is advised if used concurrently because of potential interactive effect on bone loss between phenytoin and Accutane).
No products indexed under this heading.

Phenytoin Sodium (Phenytoin is known to cause osteomalacia; caution is advised if used concurrently because of potential interactive effect on bone loss between phenytoin and Accutane). Products include:
Phenytek Capsules ... 2192

Prednisolone Acetate (Systemic corticosteroids are known to cause osteoporosis; caution is advised if used concurrently because of potential interactive effect on bone loss between systemic corticosteroids and Accutane). Products include:
Pred Forte Ophthalmic Suspension ... ⊙227
Pred Mild Ophthalmic Suspension ... ⊙230
Pred-G Ophthalmic Ointment ... ⊙229
Pred-G Ophthalmic Suspension ... ⊙228

Prednisolone Sodium Phosphate (Systemic corticosteroids are known to cause osteoporosis; caution is advised if used concurrently because of potential interactive effect on bone loss between systemic corticosteroids and Accutane).
No products indexed under this heading.

Prednisolone Tebutate (Systemic corticosteroids are known to cause osteoporosis; caution is advised if used concurrently because of potential interactive effect on bone loss between systemic corticosteroids and Accutane).
No products indexed under this heading.

Prednisone (Systemic corticosteroids are known to cause osteoporosis; caution is advised if used concurrently because of potential interactive effect on bone loss between systemic corticosteroids and Accutane).
No products indexed under this heading.

Tetracycline Hydrochloride (Concomitant treatment with Accutane and tetracyclines should be avoided because Accutane is associated with a number of cases of pseudotumor cerebri, some of which involved concomitant use of tetracyclines). Products include:
Pylera Capsules ... 714

Triamcinolone (Systemic corticosteroids are known to cause osteoporosis; caution is advised if used concurrently because of potential interactive effect on bone loss between systemic corticosteroids and Accutane).
No products indexed under this heading.

Triamcinolone Acetonide (Systemic corticosteroids are known to cause osteoporosis; caution is advised if used concurrently because of potential interactive effect on bone loss between systemic corticosteroids and Accutane). Products include:
Azmacort Inhalation Aerosol ... 407
Nasacort AQ Nasal Spray ... 2765
Triesence Injectable Suspension ... ⊙209

Triamcinolone Diacetate (Systemic corticosteroids are known to cause osteoporosis; caution is advised if used concurrently because of potential interactive effect on bone loss between systemic corticosteroids and Accutane).
No products indexed under this heading.

Triamcinolone Hexacetonide (Systemic corticosteroids are known to cause osteoporosis; caution is advised if used concurrently because of potential interactive effect on bone loss between systemic corticosteroids and Accutane).
No products indexed under this heading.

Vitamin A (Additive Vitamin A toxicity). Products include:
Norwegian Cod Liver Oil ... 949

ACCUZYME DEBRIDING OINTMENT

(Papain, Urea) ... 1723
None cited in PDR database.

ACCUZYME SE SPRAY EMULSION

(Papain, Urea) ... 1723
May interact with:

Heavy metal salts, unspecified (Papain may be inactivated by the salts of heavy metals).
No products indexed under this heading.

Hydrogen Peroxide (May inactivate papain).
No products indexed under this heading.

ACEON TABLETS (2 MG, 4 MG, 8 MG)

(Perindopril Erbumine) ... 3038
May interact with diuretics, lithium preparations, potassium preparations, potassium sparing diuretics, and certain other agents. Compounds in these categories include:

Amiloride Hydrochloride (Co-administration of perindopril with potassium-sparing diuretics may increase the risk of hyperkalemia).
No products indexed under this heading.

Bendroflumethiazide (Patients on diuretics, and especially those started recently, may occasionally experience an excessive reduction in blood pressure after initiation of perindopril therapy; co-administration has resulted in reduced bioavailability of perindopril).
No products indexed under this heading.

Bumetanide (Patients on diuretics, and especially those started recently, may occasionally experience an excessive reduction in blood pressure after initiation of perindopril therapy; co-administration has resulted in reduced bioavailability of perindopril).
No products indexed under this heading.

Chlorothiazide (Patients on diuretics, and especially those started recently, may occasionally experience an excessive reduction in blood pressure after initiation of perindopril therapy; co-administration has resulted in reduced bioavailability of perindopril).
No products indexed under this heading.

Chlorothiazide Sodium (Patients on diuretics, and especially those started recently, may occasionally experience an excessive reduction in blood pressure after initiation of perindopril therapy; co-administration has resulted in reduced bioavailability of perindopril). Products include:
Intravenous Sodium Diuril ... 2490

Chlorthalidone (Patients on diuretics, and especially those started recently, may occasionally experience an excessive reduction in blood pressure after initiation of perindopril therapy; co-administration has resulted in reduced bioavailability of perindopril). Products include:
Clorpres Tablets ... 2185

Cyclosporine (Co-administration of perindopril with other drugs capable of increasing serum potassium, such as cyclosporine, may increase the risk of hyperkalemia). Products include:
Gengraf Capsules ... 435
Neoral Oral Solution ... 2280
Neoral Soft Gelatin Capsules ... 2280
Restasis Ophthalmic Emulsion ... 557
Sandimmune ... 2296

Ethacrynic Acid (Patients on diuretics, and especially those started recently, may occasionally experience an excessive reduction in blood pressure after initiation of perindopril therapy; co-administration has resulted in reduced bioavailability of perindopril). Products include:
Edecrin Tablets ... 698

Furosemide (Patients on diuretics, and especially those started recently, may occasionally experience an excessive reduction in blood pressure after initiation of perindopril therapy; co-administration has resulted in reduced bioavailability of perindopril). Products include:
Furosemide Tablets ... 2186

Gentamicin Sulfate (Animal data has suggested the possibility of an interaction between gentamicin and perindopril; co-administration should proceed with caution). Products include:
Pred-G Ophthalmic Ointment ... ⊙229
Pred-G Ophthalmic Suspension ... ⊙228

Gold Sodium Thiomalate (Nitritoid reactions (symptoms include facial flushing, nausea, vomiting, and hypotension) have been reported rarely in patients on therapy with injectible gold (sodium aurothimalate) and concomitant ACE inhibitor therapy).
No products indexed under this heading.

Heparin Sodium (Co-administration of perindopril with other drugs capable of increasing serum potassium, such as heparin, may increase the risk of hyperkalemia).
No products indexed under this heading.

Hydrochlorothiazide (Patients on diuretics, and especially those started recently, may occasionally experience an excessive reduction in blood pressure after initiation of perindopril therapy; co-administration has resulted in reduced bioavailability of perindopril). Products include:
Atacand HCT ... 642
Avalide Tablets ... 892
Avalide Tablets ... 2713
Benicar HCT Tablets ... 1010
Diovan HCT Tablets ... 2216
Dyazide Capsules ... 1405
Micardis HCT Tablets ... 854
Prinzide Tablets ... 2092
Tekturna HCT Tablets ... 2324
Teveten HCT Tablets ... 517

Hydroflumethiazide (Patients on diuretics, and especially those started recently, may occasionally experience an excessive reduction in blood pressure after initiation of perindopril therapy; co-administration has resulted in reduced bioavailability of perindopril).
No products indexed under this heading.

Indapamide (Patients on diuretics, and especially those started recently, may occasionally experience an excessive reduction in blood pressure after initiation of perindopril therapy; co-administration has resulted in reduced bioavailability of perindopril). Products include:
Indapamide Tablets 2188

Indomethacin (Co-administration of perindopril with other drugs capable of increasing serum potassium, such as indomethacin, may increase the risk of hyperkalemia). Products include:
Indocin 2024

Lithium (Co-administration of ACE inhibitors and lithium has resulted in increased serum lithium levels and symptoms of lithium toxicity).
No products indexed under this heading.

Lithium Carbonate (Co-administration of ACE inhibitors and lithium has resulted in increased serum lithium levels and symptoms of lithium toxicity).
No products indexed under this heading.

Lithium Citrate (Co-administration of ACE inhibitors and lithium has resulted in increased serum lithium levels and symptoms of lithium toxicity).
No products indexed under this heading.

Methyclothiazide (Patients on diuretics, and especially those started recently, may occasionally experience an excessive reduction in blood pressure after initiation of perindopril therapy; co-administration has resulted in reduced bioavailability of perindopril).
No products indexed under this heading.

Metolazone (Patients on diuretics, and especially those started recently, may occasionally experience an excessive reduction in blood pressure after initiation of perindopril therapy; co-administration has resulted in reduced bioavailability of perindopril).
No products indexed under this heading.

Polythiazide (Patients on diuretics, and especially those started recently, may occasionally experience an excessive reduction in blood pressure after initiation of perindopril therapy; co-administration has resulted in reduced bioavailability of perindopril).
No products indexed under this heading.

Potassium Acid Phosphate (Co-administration of perindopril with potassium supplements may increase the risk of hyperkalemia). Products include:
K-Phos Original (Sodium Free) Tablets 814

Potassium Bicarbonate (Co-administration of perindopril with potassium supplements may increase the risk of hyperkalemia).
No products indexed under this heading.

Potassium Chloride (Co-administration of perindopril with potassium supplements may increase the risk of hyperkalemia). Products include:
MoviPrep Oral Solution 2679

Potassium Citrate (Co-administration of perindopril with potassium supplements may increase the risk of hyperkalemia). Products include:
BioLean Free Tablets .... ▣635
Urocit-K Tablets 2176

Potassium Gluconate (Co-administration of perindopril with potassium supplements may increase the risk of hyperkalemia).
No products indexed under this heading.

Potassium Phosphate (Co-administration of perindopril with potassium supplements may increase the risk of hyperkalemia). Products include:
K-Phos Neutral Tablets 813

Spironolactone (Co-administration of perindopril with potassium-sparing diuretics may increase the risk of hyperkalemia).
No products indexed under this heading.

Torsemide (Patients on diuretics, and especially those started recently, may occasionally experience an excessive reduction in blood pressure after initiation of perindopril therapy; co-administration has resulted in reduced bioavailability of perindopril). Products include:
Demadex Injection 2630
Demadex Tablets 2630

Triamterene (Co-administration of perindopril with potassium-sparing diuretics may increase the risk of hyperkalemia). Products include:
Dyazide Capsules 1405
Dyrenium Capsules 3189

Food Interactions

Food, unspecified (The presence of food in the GI tract does not affect the rate or extent of absorption of perindopril but reduces bioavailability of perindoprilat by about 35%; in clinical trials, perindopril was generally administered in a non-fasting state).

ACETADOTE INJECTION

(Acetylcysteine) 1001
None cited in PDR database.

ACIPHEX TABLETS

(Rabeprazole Sodium) 1053
May interact with drugs whose absorption can be affected by the level of gastric acidity (selected) and certain other agents. Compounds in these categories include:

Amoxicillin (Combined administration consisting of rabeprazole, amoxicillin, and clarithromycin resulted in increases in plasma concentrations of rabeprazole and 14-hydroxyclarithromycin). Products include:
Amoxil Capsules 1305
Amoxil Chewable Tablets 1305
Amoxil Pediatric Drops for Oral Suspension 1305
Amoxil Powder for Oral Suspension 1305
Amoxil Tablets 1305
Augmentin 1323
Augmentin Tablets 1327
Augmentin XR Extended Release Tablets 1333
Augmentin ES-600 Powder for Oral Suspension 1329
Moxatag Tablets 2165

Amoxicillin Trihydrate (Combined administration consisting of rabeprazole, amoxicillin, and clarithromycin resulted in increases in plasma concentrations of rabeprazole and 14-hydroxyclarithromycin).
No products indexed under this heading.

Atazanavir (Co-administration of atazanavir with proton pump inhibitors is expected to substantially decrease atazanavir plasma concentrations and thereby reduce its therapeutic effect. Concomitant use of atazanavir and proton pump inhibitors is not recommended).
No products indexed under this heading.

Atazanavir Sulfate (Co-administration of atazanavir with proton pump inhibitors is expected to substantially decrease atazanavir plasma concentrations and thereby reduce its therapeutic effect. Concomitant use of atazanavir and proton pump inhibitors is not recommended). Products include:
Reyataz Capsules 3299

Clarithromycin (Combined administration consisting of rabeprazole, amoxicillin, and clarithromycin resulted in increases in plasma concentrations of rabeprazole and 14-hydroxyclarithromycin). Products include:
Biaxin/Biaxin XL 411

Cyclosporine (In vitro incubations employing human liver microsomes indicated that rabeprazole inhibited cyclosporine metabolism with an IC50 of 62 micromolar, a concentration that is over 50 times higher than the Cmax in healthy volunteers following 14 days of dosing with 20 mg of rabeprazole). Products include:
Gengraf Capsules 435
Neoral Oral Solution 2280
Neoral Soft Gelatin-Capsules 2280
Restasis Ophthalmic Emulsion 557
Sandimmune 2296

Dapsone (Rabeprazole produces sustained inhibition of gastric acid secretion. An interaction with compounds which are dependent on gastric pH for absorption may occur due to the magnitude of acid suppression observed with rabeprazole. Patients may need to be monitored when such drugs are taken concomitantly with rabeprazole). Products include:
Aczone Gel 5% 3296
Dapsone Tablets USP 1746

Digoxin (Rabeprazole produces sustained inhibition of gastric acid secretion. An interaction with compounds which are dependent on gastric pH for absorption may occur due to the magnitude of acid suppression observed with rabeprazole. For example, in normal subjects, co-administration of rabeprazole 20 mg q.d. resulted in the AUC and Cmax for digoxin of 19% and 29%, respectively. Therefore, patients may need to be monitored when digoxin is taken concomitantly with rabeprazole). Products include:
Lanoxin Injection 1498
Lanoxin Injection Pediatric 1502
Lanoxin Tablets 1505

Ketoconazole (Rabeprazole produces sustained inhibition of gastric acid secretion. An interaction with compounds which are dependent on gastric pH for absorption may occur due to the magnitude of acid suppression observed with rabeprazole. For example, in normal subjects, co-administration of rabeprazole 20 mg q.d. resulted in an approximately 30% decrease in the bioavailability of ketoconazole. Therefore, patients may need to be monitored when ketoconazole is taken concomitantly with rabeprazole). Products include:
Extina Foam, 2% 3057
Nizoral A-D Shampoo 1901

Warfarin Sodium (There have been reports of increased INR and prothrombin time in patients receiving proton pump inhibitors, including rabeprazole, and warfarin concomitantly. Increases in INR and prothrombin time may lead to abnormal bleeding and even death).
No products indexed under this heading.

ACTIFED COLD & ALLERGY TABLETS

(Chlorpheniramine Maleate, Phenylephrine Hydrochloride) 1895
May interact with hypnotics and sedatives, monoamine oxidase inhibitors, tranquilizers, and certain other agents. Compounds in these categories include:

Alprazolam (Concomitant use may cause increased drowsiness).
No products indexed under this heading.

Buspirone Hydrochloride (Concomitant use may cause increased drowsiness).
No products indexed under this heading.

Butabarbital (Concomitant use may cause increased drowsiness).
No products indexed under this heading.

Butabarbital Sodium (Concomitant use may cause increased drowsiness).
No products indexed under this heading.

Chloral Hydrate (Concomitant use may cause increased drowsiness).
No products indexed under this heading.

Chlordiazepoxide (Concomitant use may cause increased drowsiness).
No products indexed under this heading.

Chlordiazepoxide Hydrochloride (Concomitant use may cause increased drowsiness).
No products indexed under this heading.

Chlorpromazine (Concomitant use may cause increased drowsiness).
No products indexed under this heading.

Chlorpromazine Hydrochloride (Concomitant use may cause increased drowsiness).
No products indexed under this heading.

Chlorprothixene (Concomitant use may cause increased drowsiness).
No products indexed under this heading.

Chlorprothixene Hydrochloride (Concomitant use may cause increased drowsiness).
No products indexed under this heading.

Clorazepate Dipotassium (Concomitant use may cause increased drowsiness).
No products indexed under this heading.

Diazepam (Concomitant use may cause increased drowsiness). Products include:
Valium Tablets 2658

Droperidol (Concomitant use may cause increased drowsiness).
No products indexed under this heading.

Estazolam (Concomitant use may cause increased drowsiness).
No products indexed under this heading.

Ethchlorvynol (Concomitant use may cause increased drowsiness).
No products indexed under this heading.

Ethinamate (Concomitant use may cause increased drowsiness).
No products indexed under this heading.

Fluphenazine Decanoate (Concomitant use may cause increased drowsiness).
No products indexed under this heading.

Fluphenazine Enanthate (Concomitant use may cause increased drowsiness).
No products indexed under this heading.

Fluphenazine Hydrochloride (Concomitant use may cause increased drowsiness).
No products indexed under this heading.

Flurazepam Hydrochloride (Concomitant use may cause increased drowsiness).
No products indexed under this heading.

Glutethimide (Concomitant use may cause increased drowsiness).
No products indexed under this heading.

Haloperidol (Concomitant use may cause increased drowsiness).
No products indexed under this heading.

Haloperidol Decanoate (Concomitant use may cause increased drowsiness).
No products indexed under this heading.

Hydroxyzine Hydrochloride (Concomitant use may cause increased drowsiness).
No products indexed under this heading.

Isocarboxazid (Avoid with MAO inhibitors, or for two weeks after stopping MAO inhibitor). Products include:
Marplan Tablets 3177

Lorazepam (Concomitant use may cause increased drowsiness).
No products indexed under this heading.

Loxapine Hydrochloride (Concomitant use may cause increased drowsiness).
No products indexed under this heading.

Loxapine Succinate (Concomitant use may cause increased drowsiness).
No products indexed under this heading.

Meprobamate (Concomitant use may cause increased drowsiness).
No products indexed under this heading.

Mesoridazine Besylate (Concomitant use may cause increased drowsiness).
No products indexed under this heading.

Midazolam Hydrochloride (Concomitant use may cause increased drowsiness).
No products indexed under this heading.

Moclobemide (Avoid with MAO inhibitors, or for two weeks after stopping MAO inhibitor).
No products indexed under this heading.

Molindone Hydrochloride (Concomitant use may cause increased drowsiness). Products include:
Moban Tablets 1116

Oxazepam (Concomitant use may cause increased drowsiness).
No products indexed under this heading.

Pargyline Hydrochloride (Avoid with MAO inhibitors, or for two weeks after stopping MAO inhibitor).
No products indexed under this heading.

Perphenazine (Concomitant use may cause increased drowsiness).
No products indexed under this heading.

Phenelzine Sulfate (Avoid with MAO inhibitors, or for two weeks after stopping MAO inhibitor).
No products indexed under this heading.

Prazepam (Concomitant use may cause increased drowsiness).
No products indexed under this heading.

Procarbazine Hydrochloride (Avoid with MAO inhibitors, or for two weeks after stopping MAO inhibitor).
No products indexed under this heading.

Prochlorperazine (Concomitant use may cause increased drowsiness).
No products indexed under this heading.

Promethazine Hydrochloride (Concomitant use may cause increased drowsiness).
No products indexed under this heading.

Propofol (Concomitant use may cause increased drowsiness).
No products indexed under this heading.

Quazepam (Concomitant use may cause increased drowsiness).
No products indexed under this heading.

Ramelteon (Concomitant use may cause increased drowsiness). Products include:
Rozerem Tablets 3091

Rasagiline Mesylate (Avoid with MAO inhibitors, or for two weeks after stopping MAO inhibitor). Products include:
Azilect Tablets 3106

Secobarbital Sodium (Concomitant use may cause increased drowsiness).
No products indexed under this heading.

Selegiline (Avoid with MAO inhibitors, or for two weeks after stopping MAO inhibitor). Products include:
Emsam Transdermal System 905

Selegiline Hydrochloride (Avoid with MAO inhibitors, or for two weeks after stopping MAO inhibitor). Products include:
Eldepryl Capsules 3052

Sodium Butabarbital (Concomitant use may cause increased drowsiness).
No products indexed under this heading.

Temazepam (Concomitant use may cause increased drowsiness).
No products indexed under this heading.

Thioridazine Hydrochloride (Concomitant use may cause increased drowsiness). Products include:
Thioridazine Hydrochloride Tablets 2195

Thiothixene (Concomitant use may cause increased drowsiness). Products include:
Thiothixene Capsules 2197

Tranylcypromine Sulfate (Avoid with MAO inhibitors, or for two weeks after stopping MAO inhibitor). Products include:
Parnate Tablets 1532

Triazolam (Concomitant use may cause increased drowsiness).
No products indexed under this heading.

Trifluoperazine Hydrochloride (Concomitant use may cause increased drowsiness).
No products indexed under this heading.

Zaleplon (Concomitant use may cause increased drowsiness).
No products indexed under this heading.

Zolpidem Tartrate (Concomitant use may cause increased drowsiness). Products include:
Ambien Tablets 2692
Ambien CR Tablets 2696

Food Interactions

Alcohol (Concomitant use may cause increased drowsiness).

ACTIMMUNE

(Interferon Gamma-1B) 1743
May interact with:

Bone Marrow Depressants, unspecified (Caution should be exercised when administering with other potentially myelosuppressive agents).
No products indexed under this heading.

ACTIQ

(Fentanyl Citrate) 959
May interact with central nervous system depressants, cytochrome p450 3a4 inducers (selected), cytochrome p450 3a4 inhibitors (selected), cytochrome p450 3a inhibitors (selected), erythromycin, general anesthetics, hypnotics and sedatives, monoamine oxidase inhibitors, narcotic analgesics, phenothiazines, sedating antihistamines, tranquilizers, and certain other agents. Compounds in these categories include:

Acetazolamide (Concomitant use of fentanyl with strong CYP3A4 inhibitors (eg, ritonavir, ketoconazole, itraconazole, troleandomycin, clarthromycin, nelfinavir, and nefazodone) or moderate CYP3A4 inhibitors (eg, amprenavir, aprepitant, diltiazem, erythromycin, fluconazole, fosamprenavir, and verapamil) may result in increased fentanyl plasma concentrations, potentially causing serious adverse drug effects including fatal respiratory depression. Concurrent use with moderate or strong CYP3A4 inhibitors should be carefullymonitored for an extended period of time. Dosage increase should be done conservatively).
No products indexed under this heading.

Acrivastine (Co-administration with sedating antihistamines may result in increased depressant effects).
No products indexed under this heading.

Alfentanil Hydrochloride (Co-administration may result in increased depressant effects; hypoventilation, hypotension, and profound sedation may occur. Monitor for change in opioid effects and consider adjusting dose of fentanyl if warranted).
No products indexed under this heading.

Allium sativum (Concomitant use of fentanyl with drugs that induce cytochrome P450 3A4 activity may result in decreased fentanyl plasma concentrations).
No products indexed under this heading.

Alprazolam (Co-administration may result in increased depressant effects; hypoventilation, hypotension, and profound sedation may occur. Monitor for change in opioid effects and consider adjusting dose of fentanyl if warranted).
No products indexed under this heading.

Amiodarone Hydrochloride (Concomitant use of fentanyl with strong CYP3A4 inhibitors (eg, ritonavir, ketoconazole, itraconazole, troleandomycin, clarthromycin, nelfinavir, and nefazodone) or moderate CYP3A4 inhibitors (eg, amprenavir, aprepitant, diltiazem, erythromycin, fluconazole, fosamprenavir, and verapamil) may result in increased fentanyl plasma concentrations, potentially causing serious adverse drug effects including fatal respiratory depression. Concurrent use with moderate or strong CYP3A4 inhibitors should be carefullymonitored for an extended period of time. Dosage increase should be done conservatively).
No products indexed under this heading.

Amprenavir (Concomitant use of fentanyl with strong CYP3A4 inhibitors (eg, ritonavir, ketoconazole, itraconazole, troleandomycin, clarthromycin, nelfinavir, and nefazodone) or moderate CYP3A4 inhibitors (eg, amprenavir, aprepitant, diltiazem, erythromycin, fluconazole, fosamprenavir, and verapamil) may result in increased fentanyl plasma concentrations, potentially causing serious adverse drug effects including fatal respiratory depression. Concurrent use with moderate or strong CYP3A4 inhibitors should be carefullymonitored for an extended period of time. Dosage increase should be

done conservatively).

No products indexed under this heading.

Anastrozole (Concomitant use of fentanyl with strong CYP3A4 inhibitors (eg, ritonavir, ketoconazole, itraconazole, troleandomycin, clarthromycin, nelfinavir, and nefazodone) or moderate CYP3A4 inhibitors (eg, amprenavir, aprepitant, diltiazem, erythromycin, fluconazole, fosamprenavir, and verapamil) may result in increased fentanyl plasma concentrations, potentially causing serious adverse drug effects including fatal respiratory depression. Concurrent use with moderate or strong CYP3A4 inhibitors should be carefullymonitored for an extended period of time. Dosage increase should be done conservatively). Products include:

Arimidex Tablets 672

Aprepitant (Concomitant use of fentanyl with strong CYP3A4 inhibitors (eg, ritonavir, ketoconazole, itraconazole, troleandomycin, clarthromycin, nelfinavir, and nefazodone) or moderate CYP3A4 inhibitors (eg, amprenavir, aprepitant, diltiazem, erythromycin, fluconazole, fosamprenavir, and verapamil) may result in increased fentanyl plasma concentrations, potentially causing serious adverse drug effects including fatal respiratory depression. Concurrent use with moderate or strong CYP3A4 inhibitors should be carefullymonitored for an extended period of time. Dosage increase should be done conservatively). Products include:

Emend Capsules 1992

Aprobarbital (Co-administration may result in increased depressant effects; hypoventilation, hypotension, and profound sedation may occur. Monitor for change in opiod effects and consider adjusting dose of fentanyl if warranted).

No products indexed under this heading.

Atazanavir (Concomitant use of fentanyl with strong CYP3A4 inhibitors (eg, ritonavir, ketoconazole, itraconazole, troleandomycin, clarthromycin, nelfinavir, and nefazodone) or moderate CYP3A4 inhibitors (eg, amprenavir, aprepitant, diltiazem, erythromycin, fluconazole, fosamprenavir, and verapamil) may result in increased fentanyl plasma concentrations, potentially causing serious adverse drug effects including fatal respiratory depression. Concurrent use with moderate or strong CYP3A4 inhibitors should be carefullymonitored for an extended period of time. Dosage increase should be done conservatively).

No products indexed under this heading.

Atazanavir Sulfate (Concomitant use of fentanyl with strong CYP3A4 inhibitors (eg, ritonavir, ketoconazole, itraconazole, troleandomycin, clarthromycin, nelfinavir, and nefazodone) or moderate CYP3A4 inhibitors (eg, amprenavir, aprepitant, diltiazem, erythromycin, fluconazole, fosamprenavir, and verapamil) may result in increased fentanyl plasma concentrations, potentially causing serious adverse drug effects including fatal respiratory depression. Concurrent use with moderate or strong CYP3A4 inhibitors should be carefullymonitored for an extended period of time. Dosage increase should be done conservatively). Products include:

Reyataz Capsules 3299

Azatadine Maleate (Co-administration with sedating antihistamines may result in increased depressant effects).

No products indexed under this heading.

Betamethasone Acetate (Concomitant use of fentanyl with drugs that induce cytochrome P450 3A4 activity may result in decreased fentanyl plasma concentrations).

No products indexed under this heading.

Betamethasone Sodium Phosphate (Concomitant use of fentanyl with drugs that induce cytochrome P450 3A4 activity may result in decreased fentanyl plasma concentrations).

No products indexed under this heading.

Bromodiphenhydramine Hydrochloride (Co-administration with sedating antihistamines may result in increased depressant effects).

No products indexed under this heading.

Brompheniramine Maleate (Co-administration with sedating antihistamines may result in increased depressant effects).

No products indexed under this heading.

Buprenorphine Hydrochloride (Co-administration may result in increased depressant effects; hypoventilation, hypotension, and profound sedation may occur. Monitor for change in opiod effects and consider adjusting dose of fentanyl if warranted). Products include:

Suboxone Tablets 2601
Subutex Tablets 2601

Buspirone Hydrochloride (Co-administration may result in increased depressant effects; hypoventilation, hypotension, and profound sedation may occur. Monitor for change in opiod effects and consider adjusting dose of fentanyl if warranted).

No products indexed under this heading.

Butabarbital (Co-administration may result in increased depressant effects; hypoventilation, hypotension, and profound sedation may occur).

No products indexed under this heading.

Butabarbital Sodium (Co-administration may result in increased depressant effects; hypoventilation, hypotension, and profound sedation may occur).

No products indexed under this heading.

Butalbital (Co-administration may result in increased depressant effects; hypoventilation, hypotension, and profound sedation may occur. Monitor for change in opiod effects and consider adjusting dose of fentanyl if warranted).

No products indexed under this heading.

Carbamazepine (Concomitant use of fentanyl with drugs that induce cytochrome P450 3A4 activity may result in decreased fentanyl plasma concentrations). Products include:

Carbatrol Capsules 3019
Equetro Extended-Release Capsules 3174

Chloral Hydrate (Co-administration may result in increased depressant effects; hypoventilation, hypotension, and profound sedation may occur).

No products indexed under this heading.

Chlordiazepoxide (Co-administration may result in increased depressant effects; hypoventilation, hypotension, and profound sedation may occur. Monitor for change in opiod effects and consider adjusting dose of fentanyl if warranted).

No products indexed under this heading.

Chlordiazepoxide Hydrochloride (Co-administration may result in increased depressant effects; hypoventilation, hypotension, and profound sedation may occur. Monitor for change in opiod effects and consider adjusting dose of fentanyl if warranted).

No products indexed under this heading.

Chlorpheniramine Maleate (Co-administration with sedating antihistamines may result in increased depressant effects). Products include:

Actifed Cold & Allergy Tablets 1895
Sudafed PE Sinus & Allergy Tablets 1908
Tylenol Allergy Multi-Symptom Caplets with Cool Burst and Rapid Release Gelcaps 1916
Children's Tylenol Plus Cold Suspension Liquid 1912
Children's Tylenol Plus Cough & Runny Nose Suspension Liquid 1912
Children's Tylenol Plus Flu Suspension Liquid 1914
Children's Tylenol Plus Multi-Symptom Cold Suspension Liquid 1912
Tylenol Cold Head Congestion Nighttime Caplets with Cool Burst 1910
Tylenol Cold Multi-Symptom Nighttime Caplets with Cool Burst 1913
Tylenol Sinus Congestion & Pain Nighttime Caplets with Cool Burst 1917

Chlorpheniramine Polistirex (Co-administration with sedating antihistamines may result in increased depressant effects). Products include:

Tussionex Pennkinetic Extended-Release Suspension 3154

Chlorpheniramine Tannate (Co-administration with sedating antihistamines may result in increased depressant effects).

No products indexed under this heading.

Chlorpromazine (Co-administration may result in increased depressant effects; hypoventilation, hypotension, and profound sedation may occur. Monitor for change in opiod effects and consider adjusting dose of fentanyl if warranted).

No products indexed under this heading.

Chlorpromazine Hydrochloride (Co-administration may result in increased depressant effects; hypoventilation, hypotension, and profound sedation may occur. Monitor for change in opiod effects and consider adjusting dose of fentanyl if warranted).

No products indexed under this heading.

Chlorprothixene (Co-administration may result in increased depressant effects; hypoventilation, hypotension, and profound sedation may occur. Monitor for change in opiod effects and consider adjusting dose of fentanyl if warranted).

No products indexed under this heading.

Chlorprothixene Hydrochloride (Co-administration may result in increased depressant effects; hypoventilation, hypotension, and profound sedation may occur. Monitor for change in opiod effects and consider adjusting dose of fentanyl if warranted).

No products indexed under this heading.

Chlorprothixene Lactate (Co-administration may result in increased depressant effects; hypoventilation, hypotension, and profound sedation may occur. Monitor for change in opiod effects and consider adjusting dose of fentanyl if warranted).

No products indexed under this heading.

Cimetidine (Concomitant use of fentanyl with strong CYP3A4 inhibitors (eg, ritonavir, ketoconazole, itraconazole, troleandomycin, clarthromycin, nelfinavir, and nefazodone) or moderate CYP3A4 inhibitors (eg, amprenavir, aprepitant, diltiazem, erythromycin, fluconazole, fosamprenavir, and verapamil) may result in increased fentanyl plasma concentrations, potentially causing serious adverse drug effects including fatal respiratory depression. Concurrent use with moderate or strong CYP3A4 inhibitors should be carefullymonitored for an extended period of time. Dosage increase should be done conservatively).

No products indexed under this heading.

Cimetidine Hydrochloride (Concomitant use of fentanyl with strong CYP3A4 inhibitors (eg, ritonavir, ketoconazole, itraconazole, troleandomycin, clarthromycin, nelfinavir, and nefazodone) or moderate CYP3A4 inhibitors (eg, amprenavir, aprepitant, diltiazem, erythromycin, fluconazole, fosamprenavir, and verapamil) may result in increased fentanyl plasma concentrations, potentially causing serious adverse drug effects including fatal respiratory depression. Concurrent use with moderate or strong CYP3A4 inhibitors should be carefullymonitored for an extended period of time. Dosage increase should be done conservatively).

No products indexed under this heading.

Ciprofloxacin (Concomitant use of fentanyl with strong CYP3A4 inhibitors (eg, ritonavir, ketoconazole, itraconazole, troleandomycin, clarthromycin, nelfinavir, and nefazodone) or moderate CYP3A4 inhibitors (eg, amprenavir, aprepitant, diltiazem, erythromycin, fluconazole, fosamprenavir, and verapamil) may result in increased fentanyl plasma concentrations, potentially causing serious adverse drug effects including fatal respiratory depression. Concurrent use with moderate or strong CYP3A4 inhibitors should be carefullymonitored for an extended period of time. Dosage increase should be done conservatively). Products include:

Cipro I.V. 2817
Cipro Oral Suspension 2810
Cipro XR Tablets 2823
Ciprodex Otic Suspension 541

Ciprofloxacin Hydrochloride (Concomitant use of fentanyl with strong CYP3A4 inhibitors (eg, ritonavir, ketoconazole, itraconazole, troleandomycin, clarthromycin, nelfinavir, and nefazodone) or moderate CYP3A4 inhibitors (eg, amprenavir, aprepitant, diltiazem, erythromycin, fluconazole, fosamprenavir, and verapamil) may result in increased fentanyl plasma concentrations, potentially causing serious adverse drug effects including fatal respiratory depression. Concurrent use with moderate or strong CYP3A4 inhibitors should be carefullymonitored for an extended period of time. Dosage increase should be done conservatively). Products include:

Cipro Tablets 2810

Cisplatin (Concomitant use of fentanyl with drugs that induce cytochrome P450 3A4 activity may result in decreased fentanyl plasma concentrations).

No products indexed under this heading.

Clarithromycin (Concomitant use of fentanyl with strong CYP3A4 inhibitors (eg, ritonavir, ketoconazole, itraconazole, troleandomycin, clarthromycin, nelfinavir, and nefazodone) or moderate CYP3A4 inhibitors (eg, amprenavir, aprepitant, diltiazem, erythromycin, fluconazole, fosamprenavir, and verapamil) may result in increased fentanyl plasma concentrations, potentially causing serious adverse drug effects including fatal respiratory depression. Concurrent use with moderate or strong CYP3A4 inhibitors should be carefullymonitored for an extended period of time. Dosage increase should be done conservatively). Products include:

Biaxin/Biaxin XL 411

Clemastine Fumarate (Co-administration with sedating antihistamines may result in increased depressant effects).

No products indexed under this heading.

Clorazepate Dipotassium (Co-administration may result in increased depressant effects; hypoventilation, hypotension, and profound sedation may occur. Monitor for change in opioid effects and consider adjusting dose of fentanyl if warranted).

No products indexed under this heading.

Clotrimazole (Concomitant use of fentanyl with strong CYP3A4 inhibitors (eg, ritonavir, ketoconazole, itraconazole, troleandomycin, clarthromycin, nelfinavir, and nefazodone) or moderate CYP3A4 inhibitors (eg, amprenavir, aprepitant, diltiazem, erythromycin, fluconazole, fosamprenavir, and verapamil) may result in increased fentanyl plasma concentrations, potentially causing serious adverse drug effects including fatal respiratory depression. Concurrent use with moderate or strong CYP3A4 inhibitors should be carefullymonitored for an extended period of time. Dosage increase should be done conservatively). Products include:

Lotrisone 2881

Clozapine (Co-administration may result in increased depressant effects; hypoventilation, hypotension, and profound sedation may occur. Monitor for change in opioid effects and consider adjusting dose of fentanyl if warranted).

No products indexed under this heading.

Codeine Phosphate (Co-administration may result in increased depressant effects; hypoventilation, hypotension, and profound sedation may occur. Monitor for change in opioid effects and consider adjusting dose of fentanyl if warranted). Products include:

Tylenol with Codeine Tablets 2427

Cortisone Acetate (Concomitant use of fentanyl with drugs that induce cytochrome P450 3A4 activity may result in decreased fentanyl plasma concentrations).

No products indexed under this heading.

Cyclosporine (Concomitant use of fentanyl with strong CYP3A4 inhibitors (eg, ritonavir, ketoconazole, itraconazole, troleandomycin, clarthromycin, nelfinavir, and nefazodone) or moderate CYP3A4 inhibitors (eg, amprenavir, aprepitant, diltiazem, erythromycin, fluconazole, fosamprenavir, and verapamil) may result in increased fentanyl plasma concentrations, potentially causing serious adverse drug effects including fatal respiratory depression. Concurrent use with moderate or strong CYP3A4 inhibitors should be carefullymonitored for an extended period of time. Dosage increase should be done conservatively). Products include:

Gengraf Capsules 435
Neoral Oral Solution 2280
Neoral Soft Gelatin Capsules 2280
Restasis Ophthalmic Emulsion 557
Sandimmune 2296

Cyproheptadine Hydrochloride (Co-administration with sedating antihistamines may result in increased depressant effects).

No products indexed under this heading.

Dalfopristin (Concomitant use of fentanyl with strong CYP3A4 inhibitors (eg, ritonavir, ketoconazole, itraconazole, troleandomycin, clarthromycin, nelfinavir, and nefazodone) or moderate CYP3A4 inhibitors (eg, amprenavir, aprepitant, diltiazem, erythromycin, fluconazole, fosamprenavir, and verapamil) may result in increased fentanyl plasma concentrations, potentially causing serious adverse drug effects including fatal respiratory depression. Concurrent use with moderate or strong CYP3A4 inhibitors should be carefullymonitored for an extended period of time. Dosage increase should be done conservatively).

No products indexed under this heading.

Danazol (Concomitant use of fentanyl with strong CYP3A4 inhibitors (eg, ritonavir, ketoconazole, itraconazole, troleandomycin, clarthromycin, nelfinavir, and nefazodone) or moderate CYP3A4 inhibitors (eg, amprenavir, aprepitant, diltiazem, erythromycin, fluconazole, fosamprenavir, and verapamil) may result in increased fentanyl plasma concentrations, potentially causing serious adverse drug effects including fatal respiratory depression. Concurrent use with moderate or strong CYP3A4 inhibitors should be carefullymonitored for an extended period of time. Dosage increase should be done conservatively).

No products indexed under this heading.

Delavirdine Mesylate (Concomitant use of fentanyl with strong CYP3A4 inhibitors (eg, ritonavir, ketoconazole, itraconazole, troleandomycin, clarthromycin, nelfinavir, and nefazodone) or moderate CYP3A4 inhibitors (eg, amprenavir, aprepitant, diltiazem, erythromycin, fluconazole, fosamprenavir, and verapamil) may result in increased fentanyl plasma concentrations, potentially causing serious adverse drug effects including fatal respiratory depression. Concurrent use with moderate or strong CYP3A4 inhibitors should be carefullymonitored for an extended period of time. Dosage increase should be done conservatively).

No products indexed under this heading.

Desflurane (Co-administration may result in increased depressant effects; hypoventilation, hypotension, and profound sedation may occur. Monitor for change in opioid effects and consider adjusting dose of fentanyl if warranted).

No products indexed under this heading.

Dexamethasone (Concomitant use of fentanyl with drugs that induce cytochrome P450 3A4 activity may result in decreased fentanyl plasma concentrations). Products include:

Ciprodex Otic Suspension 541

Dexamethasone Acetate (Concomitant use of fentanyl with drugs that induce cytochrome P450 3A4 activity may result in decreased fentanyl plasma concentrations).

No products indexed under this heading.

Dexamethasone Sodium Phosphate (Concomitant use of fentanyl with drugs that induce cytochrome P450 3A4 activity may result in decreased fentanyl plasma concentrations).

No products indexed under this heading.

Dexchlorpheniramine Maleate (Co-administration with sedating antihistamines may result in increased depressant effects).

No products indexed under this heading.

Dezocine (Co-administration may result in increased depressant effects; hypoventilation, hypotension, and profound sedation may occur. Monitor for change in opioid effects and consider adjusting dose of fentanyl if warranted).

No products indexed under this heading.

Diazepam (Co-administration may result in increased depressant effects; hypoventilation, hypotension, and profound sedation may occur. Monitor for change in opioid effects and consider adjusting dose of fentanyl if warranted). Products include:

Valium Tablets 2658

Diltiazem Hydrochloride (Concomitant use of fentanyl with strong CYP3A4 inhibitors (eg, ritonavir, ketoconazole, itraconazole, troleandomycin, clarthromycin, nelfinavir, and nefazodone) or moderate CYP3A4 inhibitors (eg, amprenavir, aprepitant, diltiazem, erythromycin, fluconazole, fosamprenavir, and verapamil) may result in increased fentanyl plasma concentrations, potentially causing serious adverse drug effects including fatal respiratory depression. Concurrent use with moderate or strong CYP3A4 inhibitors should be carefullymonitored for an extended period of time. Dosage increase should be done conservatively). Products include:

Cardizem LA Extended Release Tablets 421

Diltiazem Maleate (Concomitant use of fentanyl with strong CYP3A4 inhibitors (eg, ritonavir, ketoconazole, itraconazole, troleandomycin, clarthromycin, nelfinavir, and nefazodone) or moderate CYP3A4 inhibitors (eg, amprenavir, aprepitant, diltiazem, erythromycin, fluconazole, fosamprenavir, and verapamil) may result in increased fentanyl plasma concentrations, potentially causing serious adverse drug effects including fatal respiratory depression. Concurrent use with moderate or strong CYP3A4 inhibitors should be carefullymonitored for an extended period of time. Dosage increase should be done conservatively).

No products indexed under this heading.

Diphenhydramine Citrate (Co-administration with sedating antihistamines may result in increased depressant effects).

No products indexed under this heading.

Diphenhydramine Hydrochloride (Co-administration with sedating antihistamines may result in increased depressant effects). Products include:

Benadryl Allergy & Cold Kapgels 1895
Benadryl Allergy & Sinus Headache Kapgels 1895
Benadryl Severe Allergy & Sinus Headache Caplets 1897
Benadryl Dye-Free Allergy Liqui-gels Softgels 1897
Benadryl Allergy Kapgels 1895
Benadryl Allergy Quick Dissolve Strips 1896
Benadryl Allergy Ultratab Tablets 1896
Children's Benadryl Dye-Free Allergy Liquid 1897
Children's Benadryl Allergy Fastmelts 1897
Children's Benadryl Allergy Liquid 1898
Children's Benadryl Allergy Perfect Measure 1896
Children's Benadryl-D Allergy & Sinus Liquid 1896
Benadryl-D Allergy & Sinus Tablet 1896
PediaCare Children's Allergy & Cold Liquid 1902
PediaCare Children's Allergy Liquid 1902
Simply Sleep Caplets 1905
Sudafed PE Nighttime Cold Caplets 1907
Sudafed PE Severe Cold Caplets 1908
Extra Strength Tylenol PM Caplets, Geltabs, Liquid, and Rapid Release Gels 1915
Tylenol Allergy Multi-Symptom Nighttime Caplets with Cool Burst 1916
Tylenol Severe Allergy Caplets 1916
Children's Tylenol Plus Cold & Allergy Suspension Liquid 1914
Tylenol Sore Throat Nighttime Liquid with Cool Burst 1918

Diphenylpyraline Hydrochloride (Co-administration with sedating antihistamines may result in increased depressant effects).

No products indexed under this heading.

Doxorubicin Hydrochloride (Concomitant use of fentanyl with drugs that induce cytochrome P450 3A4 activity may result in decreased fentanyl plasma concentrations).

No products indexed under this heading.

Droperidol (Co-administration may result in increased depressant effects; hypoventilation, hypotension, and profound sedation may occur. Monitor for change in opiod effects and consider adjusting dose of fentanyl if warranted).

No products indexed under this heading.

Efavirenz (Concomitant use of fentanyl with strong CYP3A4 inhibitors (eg, ritonavir, ketoconazole, itraconazole, troleandomycin, clarthromycin, nelfinavir, and nefazodone) or moderate CYP3A4 inhibitors (eg, amprenavir, aprepitant, diltiazem, erythromycin, fluconazole, fosamprenavir, and verapamil) may result in increased fentanyl plasma concentrations, potentially causing serious adverse drug effects including fatal respiratory depression. Concurrent use with moderate or strong CYP3A4 inhibitors should be carefullymonitored for an extended period of time. Dosage increase should be done conservatively). Products include:

Atripla Tablets 938
Sustiva Capsules 930
Sustiva Tablets 930

Enflurane (Co-administration may result in increased depressant effects; hypoventilation, hypotension, and profound sedation may occur).

No products indexed under this heading.

Erythromycin (Co-administration with potent inhibitors of CYP450 3A4 isoform, such as erythromycin, may increase the bioavailability of swallowed fentanyl by decreasing intestinal and hepatic first pass metabolism and may decrease the systemic clearance resulting in increased or prolonged opioid effects).

No products indexed under this heading.

Erythromycin Estolate (Co-administration with potent inhibitors of CYP450 3A4 isoform, such as erythromycin, may increase the bioavailability of swallowed fentanyl by decreasing intestinal and hepatic first pass metabolism and may decrease the systemic clearance resulting in increased or prolonged opioid effects).

No products indexed under this heading.

Erythromycin Ethylsuccinate (Co-administration with potent inhibitors of CYP450 3A4 isoform, such as erythromycin, may increase the bioavailability of swallowed fentanyl by decreasing intestinal and hepatic first pass metabolism and may decrease the systemic clearance resulting in increased or prolonged opioid effects). Products include:

E.E.S. 433
EryPed 431

Erythromycin Gluceptate (Co-administration with potent inhibitors of CYP450 3A4 isoform, such as erythromycin, may increase the bioavailability of swallowed fentanyl by decreasing intestinal and hepatic first pass metabolism and may decrease the systemic clearance resulting in increased or prolonged opioid effects).

No products indexed under this heading.

Erythromycin Lactobionate (Co-administration with potent inhibitors of CYP450 3A4 isoform, such as erythromycin, may increase the bioavailability of swallowed fentanyl by decreasing intestinal and hepatic first pass metabolism and may decrease the systemic clearance resulting in increased or prolonged opioid effects).

No products indexed under this heading.

Erythromycin Stearate (Co-administration with potent inhibitors of CYP450 3A4 isoform, such as erythromycin, may increase the bioavailability of swallowed fentanyl by decreasing intestinal and hepatic first pass metabolism and may decrease the systemic clearance resulting in increased or prolonged opioid effects).

No products indexed under this heading.

Esomeprazole Magnesium (Concomitant use of fentanyl with strong CYP3A4 inhibitors (eg, ritonavir, ketoconazole, itraconazole, troleandomycin, clarthromycin, nelfinavir, and nefazodone) or moderate CYP3A4 inhibitors (eg, amprenavir, aprepitant, diltiazem, erythromycin, fluconazole, fosamprenavir, and verapamil) may result in increased fentanyl plasma concentrations, potentially causing serious adverse drug effects including fatal respiratory depression. Concurrent use with moderate or strong CYP3A4 inhibitors should be carefullymonitored for an extended period of time. Dosage increase should be done conservatively). Products include:

Nexium Delayed-Release Capsules 645
Nexium Delayed-Release Oral Suspension 645

Estazolam (Co-administration may result in increased depressant effects; hypoventilation, hypotension, and profound sedation may occur).

No products indexed under this heading.

Ethanol (Co-administration may result in increased depressant effects; hypoventilation, hypotension, and profound sedation may occur. Monitor for change in opiod effects and consider adjusting dose of fentanyl if warranted).

No products indexed under this heading.

Ethchlorvynol (Co-administration may result in increased depressant effects; hypoventilation, hypotension, and profound sedation may occur).

No products indexed under this heading.

Ethinamate (Co-administration may result in increased depressant effects; hypoventilation, hypotension, and profound sedation may occur).

No products indexed under this heading.

Ethosuximide (Concomitant use of fentanyl with drugs that induce cytochrome P450 3A4 activity may result in decreased fentanyl plasma concentrations).

No products indexed under this heading.

Ethyl Alcohol (Co-administration may result in increased depressant effects; hypoventilation, hypotension, and profound sedation may occur. Monitor for change in opiod effects and consider adjusting dose of fentanyl if warranted).

No products indexed under this heading.

Felbamate (Concomitant use of fentanyl with drugs that induce cytochrome P450 3A4 activity may result in decreased fentanyl plasma concentrations).

No products indexed under this heading.

Fentanyl (Co-administration may result in increased depressant effects; hypoventilation, hypotension, and profound sedation may occur. Monitor for change in opiod effects and consider adjusting dose of fentanyl if warranted). Products include:

Duragesic Transdermal System 2405
Ionsys Transdermal System 2410

Fluconazole (Concomitant use of fentanyl with strong CYP3A4 inhibitors (eg, ritonavir, ketoconazole, itraconazole, troleandomycin, clarthromycin, nelfinavir, and nefazodone) or moderate CYP3A4 inhibitors (eg, amprenavir, aprepitant, diltiazem, erythromycin, fluconazole, fosamprenavir, and verapamil) may result in increased fentanyl plasma concentrations, potentially causing serious adverse drug effects including fatal respiratory depression. Concurrent use with moderate or strong CYP3A4 inhibitors should be carefullymonitored for an extended period of time. Dosage increase should be done conservatively).

No products indexed under this heading.

Fludrocortisone Acetate (Concomitant use of fentanyl with drugs that induce cytochrome P450 3A4 activity may result in decreased fentanyl plasma concentrations).

No products indexed under this heading.

Fluoxetine (Concomitant use of fentanyl with strong CYP3A4 inhibitors (eg, ritonavir, ketoconazole, itraconazole, troleandomycin, clarthromycin, nelfinavir, and nefazodone) or moderate CYP3A4 inhibitors (eg, amprenavir, aprepitant, diltiazem, erythromycin, fluconazole, fosamprenavir, and verapamil) may result in increased fentanyl plasma concentrations, potentially causing serious adverse drug effects including fatal respiratory depression. Concurrent use with moderate or strong CYP3A4 inhibitors should be carefullymonitored for an extended period of time. Dosage increase should be done conservatively).

No products indexed under this heading.

Fluoxetine Hydrochloride (Concomitant use of fentanyl with strong CYP3A4 inhibitors (eg, ritonavir, ketoconazole, itraconazole, troleandomycin, clarthromycin, nelfinavir, and nefazodone) or moderate CYP3A4 inhibitors (eg, amprenavir, aprepitant, diltiazem, erythromycin, fluconazole, fosamprenavir, and verapamil) may result in increased fentanyl plasma concentrations, potentially causing serious adverse drug effects including fatal respiratory depression. Concurrent use with moderate or strong CYP3A4 inhibitors should be carefullymonitored for an extended period of time. Dosage increase should be done conservatively). Products include:

Prozac Weekly Capsules 1852
Prozac Pulvules and Liquid 1852
Symbyax Capsules 1871

Fluphenazine Decanoate (Co-administration may result in increased depressant effects; hypoventilation, hypotension, and profound sedation may occur. Monitor for change in opiod effects and consider adjusting dose of fentanyl if warranted).

No products indexed under this heading.

Fluphenazine Enanthate (Co-administration may result in increased depressant effects; hypoventilation, hypotension, and profound sedation may occur. Monitor for change in opiod effects and consider adjusting dose of fentanyl if warranted).

No products indexed under this heading.

Fluphenazine Hydrochloride (Co-administration may result in increased depressant effects; hypoventilation, hypotension, and profound sedation may occur. Monitor for change in opiod effects and consider adjusting dose of fentanyl if warranted).

No products indexed under this heading.

Flurazepam Hydrochloride (Co-administration may result in increased depressant effects; hypoventilation, hypotension, and profound sedation may occur).

No products indexed under this heading.

Fluvoxamine Maleate (Concomitant use of fentanyl with strong CYP3A4 inhibitors (eg, ritonavir, ketoconazole, itraconazole, troleandomycin, clarthromycin, nelfinavir, and nefazodone) or moderate CYP3A4 inhibitors (eg, amprenavir, aprepitant, diltiazem, erythromycin, fluconazole, fosamprenavir, and verapamil) may result in increased fentanyl plasma concentrations, potentially causing serious adverse drug effects including fatal respiratory depression. Concurrent use with moderate or strong CYP3A4 inhibitors should be carefullymonitored for an extended period of time. Dosage increase should be done conservatively). Products include:

Luvox CR Extended-Release Capsules 1759

Fosamprenavir Calcium (Concomitant use of fentanyl with strong CYP3A4 inhibitors (eg, ritonavir, ketoconazole, itraconazole, troleandomycin, clarthromycin, nelfinavir, and nefazodone) or moderate CYP3A4 inhibitors (eg, amprenavir, aprepitant, diltiazem, erythromycin,

fluconazole, fosamprenavir, and verapamil) may result in increased fentanyl plasma concentrations, potentially causing serious adverse drug effects including fatal respiratory depression. Concurrent use with moderate or strong CYP3A4 inhibitors should be carefullymonitored for an extended period of time. Dosage increase should be done conservatively). Products include:

Lexiva Oral Suspension 1510
Lexiva Tablets 1510

Fosphenytoin Sodium (Concomitant use of fentanyl with drugs that induce cytochrome P450 3A4 activity may result in decreased fentanyl plasma concentrations).

No products indexed under this heading.

Garlic Extract (Concomitant use of fentanyl with drugs that induce cytochrome P450 3A4 activity may result in decreased fentanyl plasma concentrations).

No products indexed under this heading.

Garlic Oil (Concomitant use of fentanyl with drugs that induce cytochrome P450 3A4 activity may result in decreased fentanyl plasma concentrations).

No products indexed under this heading.

Glutethimide (Co-administration may result in increased depressant effects; hypoventilation, hypotension, and profound sedation may occur).

No products indexed under this heading.

Haloperidol (Co-administration may result in increased depressant effects; hypoventilation, hypotension, and profound sedation may occur. Monitor for change in opiod effects and consider adjusting dose of fentanyl if warranted).

No products indexed under this heading.

Haloperidol Decanoate (Co-administration may result in increased depressant effects; hypoventilation, hypotension, and profound sedation may occur. Monitor for change in opiod effects and consider adjusting dose of fentanyl if warranted).

No products indexed under this heading.

Hydrocodone Bitartrate (Co-administration may result in increased depressant effects; hypoventilation, hypotension, and profound sedation may occur. Monitor for change in opiod effects and consider adjusting dose of fentanyl if warranted). Products include:

Lortab 5/500 Tablets 3143
Lortab 7.5/500 Tablets 3144
Lortab 10/500 Tablets 3144
Vicodin Tablets 529
Vicodin ES Tablets 530
Vicodin HP Tablets 531
Vicoprofen Tablets 533
Zydone Tablets 1132

Hydrocodone Polistirex (Co-administration may result in increased depressant effects; hypoventilation, hypotension, and profound sedation may occur. Monitor for change in opiod effects and consider adjusting dose of fentanyl if warranted). Products include:

Tussionex Pennkinetic
Extended-Release Suspension...... 3154

Hydrocortisone (Concomitant use of fentanyl with drugs that induce cytochrome P450 3A4 activity may result in decreased fentanyl plasma concentrations).

No products indexed under this heading.

Hydrocortisone Acetate (Concomitant use of fentanyl with drugs that induce cytochrome P450 3A4 activity may result in decreased fentanyl plasma concentrations). Products include:

Analpram-HC 1140
Pramosone 1141

Hydrocortisone Butyrate (Concomitant use of fentanyl with drugs that induce cytochrome P450 3A4 activity may result in decreased fentanyl plasma concentrations).

No products indexed under this heading.

Hydrocortisone Cypionate (Concomitant use of fentanyl with drugs that induce cytochrome P450 3A4 activity may result in decreased fentanyl plasma concentrations).

No products indexed under this heading.

Hydrocortisone Hemisuccinate (Concomitant use of fentanyl with drugs that induce cytochrome P450 3A4 activity may result in decreased fentanyl plasma concentrations).

No products indexed under this heading.

Hydrocortisone Probutate (Concomitant use of fentanyl with drugs that induce cytochrome P450 3A4 activity may result in decreased fentanyl plasma concentrations).

No products indexed under this heading.

Hydrocortisone Sodium Phosphate (Concomitant use of fentanyl with drugs that induce cytochrome P450 3A4 activity may result in decreased fentanyl plasma concentrations).

No products indexed under this heading.

Hydrocortisone Sodium Succinate (Concomitant use of fentanyl with drugs that induce cytochrome P450 3A4 activity may result in decreased fentanyl plasma concentrations).

No products indexed under this heading.

Hydrocortisone Valerate (Concomitant use of fentanyl with drugs that induce cytochrome P450 3A4 activity may result in decreased fentanyl plasma concentrations).

No products indexed under this heading.

Hydromorphone Hydrochloride (Co-administration may result in increased depressant effects; hypoventilation, hypotension, and profound sedation may occur. Monitor for change in opiod effects and consider adjusting dose of fentanyl if warranted).

No products indexed under this heading.

Hydroxyzine Hydrochloride (Co-administration may result in increased depressant effects; hypoventilation, hypotension, and profound sedation may occur. Monitor for change in opiod effects and consider adjusting dose of fentanyl if warranted).

No products indexed under this heading.

Hypericum (Concomitant use of fentanyl with drugs that induce cytochrome P450 3A4 activity may result in decreased fentanyl plasma concentrations). Products include:

Satieté Tablets .... ▣ 640

Hypericum Perforatum (Concomitant use of fentanyl with drugs that induce cytochrome P450 3A4 activity may result in decreased fentanyl plasma concentrations).

No products indexed under this heading.

Indinavir Sulfate (Concomitant use of fentanyl with strong CYP3A4 inhibitors (eg, ritonavir, ketoconazole, itraconazole, troleandomycin, clarthromycin, nelfinavir, and nefazodone) or moderate CYP3A4 inhibitors (eg, amprenavir, aprepitant, diltiazem, erythromycin, fluconazole, fosamprenavir, and verapamil) may result in increased fentanyl plasma concentrations, potentially causing serious adverse drug effects including fatal respiratory depression. Concurrent use with moderate or strong CYP3A4 inhibitors should be carefullymonitored for an extended period of time. Dosage increase should be done conservatively). Products include:

Crixivan Capsules 1979

Isocarboxazid (Concurrent and/or sequential use with MAO inhibitors is not recommended; potential for severe and unpredictable potentiation of MAO inhibitors has been reported with opioid analgesics). Products include:

Marplan Tablets 3177

Isoflurane (Co-administration may result in increased depressant effects; hypoventilation, hypotension, and profound sedation may occur).

No products indexed under this heading.

Isoniazid (Concomitant use of fentanyl with strong CYP3A4 inhibitors (eg, ritonavir, ketoconazole, itraconazole, troleandomycin, clarthromycin, nelfinavir, and nefazodone) or moderate CYP3A4 inhibitors (eg, amprenavir, aprepitant, diltiazem, erythromycin, fluconazole, fosamprenavir, and verapamil) may result in increased fentanyl plasma concentrations, potentially causing serious adverse drug effects including fatal respiratory depression. Concurrent use with moderate or strong CYP3A4 inhibitors should be carefullymonitored for an extended period of time. Dosage increase should be done conservatively).

No products indexed under this heading.

Itraconazole (Co-administration with potent inhibitors of CYP450 3A4 isoform, such as azole antifungal itraconazole, may increase the bioavailability of swallowed fentanyl by decreasing intestinal and hepatic first pass metabolism and may decrease the systemic clearance resulting in increased or prolonged opioid effects).

No products indexed under this heading.

Ketamine Hydrochloride (Co-administration may result in increased depressant effects; hypoventilation, hypotension, and profound sedation may occur).

No products indexed under this heading.

Ketoconazole (Co-administration with potent inhibitors of CYP450 3A4 isoform, such as azole antifungal ketoconazole, may increase the bioavailability of swallowed fentanyl by decreasing intestinal and hepatic first pass metabolism and may decrease the systemic clearance resulting in increased or prolonged opioid effects). Products include:

Extina Foam, 2% 3057
Nizoral A-D Shampoo 1901

Levomethadyl Acetate Hydrochloride (Co-administration may result in increased depressant effects; hypoventilation, hypotension, and profound sedation may occur. Monitor for change in opiod effects and consider adjusting dose of fentanyl if warranted).

No products indexed under this heading.

Levorphanol Tartrate (Co-administration may result in increased depressant effects; hypoventilation, hypotension, and profound sedation may occur. Monitor for change in opiod effects and consider adjusting dose of fentanyl if warranted).

No products indexed under this heading.

Lopinavir (Concomitant use of fentanyl with strong CYP3A4 inhibitors (eg, ritonavir, ketoconazole, itraconazole, troleandomycin, clarthromycin, nelfinavir, and nefazodone) or moderate CYP3A4 inhibitors (eg, amprenavir, aprepitant, diltiazem, erythromycin, fluconazole, fosamprenavir, and verapamil) may result in increased fentanyl plasma concentrations, potentially causing serious adverse drug effects including fatal respiratory depression. Concurrent use with moderate or strong CYP3A4 inhibitors should be carefullymonitored for an extended period of time. Dosage increase should be done conservatively). Products include:

Kaletra 452

Loratadine (Concomitant use of fentanyl with strong CYP3A4 inhibitors (eg, ritonavir, ketoconazole, itraconazole, troleandomycin, clarthromycin, nelfinavir, and nefazodone) or moderate CYP3A4 inhibitors (eg, amprenavir, aprepitant, diltiazem, erythromycin, fluconazole, fosamprenavir, and verapamil) may result in increased fentanyl plasma concentrations, potentially causing serious adverse drug effects including fatal respiratory depression. Concurrent use with moderate or strong CYP3A4 inhibitors should be carefullymonitored for an extended period of time. Dosage increase should be done conservatively).

No products indexed under this heading.

Lorazepam (Co-administration may result in increased depressant effects; hypoventilation, hypotension, and profound sedation may occur).

No products indexed under this heading.

Loxapine Hydrochloride (Co-administration may result in increased depressant effects; hypoventilation, hypotension, and profound sedation may occur. Monitor for change in opiod effects and consider adjusting dose of fentanyl if warranted).

No products indexed under this heading.

Loxapine Succinate (Co-administration may result in increased depressant effects; hypoventilation, hypotension, and profound sedation may occur. Monitor for change in opiod effects and consider adjusting dose of fentanyl if warranted).
No products indexed under this heading.

Meperidine Hydrochloride (Co-administration may result in increased depressant effects; hypoventilation, hypotension, and profound sedation may occur. Monitor for change in opiod effects and consider adjusting dose of fentanyl if warranted).
No products indexed under this heading.

Mephenytoin (Concomitant use of fentanyl with drugs that induce cytochrome P450 3A4 activity may result in decreased fentanyl plasma concentrations).
No products indexed under this heading.

Mephobarbital (Co-administration may result in increased depressant effects; hypoventilation, hypotension, and profound sedation may occur. Monitor for change in opiod effects and consider adjusting dose of fentanyl if warranted).
No products indexed under this heading.

Meprobamate (Co-administration may result in increased depressant effects; hypoventilation, hypotension, and profound sedation may occur. Monitor for change in opiod effects and consider adjusting dose of fentanyl if warranted).
No products indexed under this heading.

Mesoridazine Besylate (Co-administration may result in increased depressant effects; hypoventilation, hypotension, and profound sedation may occur. Monitor for change in opiod effects and consider adjusting dose of fentanyl if warranted).
No products indexed under this heading.

Methadone Hydrochloride (Co-administration may result in increased depressant effects; hypoventilation, hypotension, and profound sedation may occur. Monitor for change in opiod effects and consider adjusting dose of fentanyl if warranted).
No products indexed under this heading.

Methdilazine Hydrochloride (Co-administration with sedating antihistamines may result in increased depressant effects).
No products indexed under this heading.

Methohexital Sodium (Co-administration may result in increased depressant effects; hypoventilation, hypotension, and profound sedation may occur).
No products indexed under this heading.

Methotrimeprazine (Co-administration may result in increased depressant effects; hypoventilation, hypotension, and profound sedation may occur. Monitor for change in opiod effects and consider adjusting dose of fentanyl if warranted).
No products indexed under this heading.

Methoxyflurane (Co-administration may result in increased depressant effects; hypoventilation, hypotension, and profound sedation may occur).
No products indexed under this heading.

Methsuximide (Concomitant use of fentanyl with drugs that induce cytochrome P450 3A4 activity may result in decreased fentanyl plasma concentrations).
No products indexed under this heading.

Methylprednisolone (Concomitant use of fentanyl with drugs that induce cytochrome P450 3A4 activity may result in decreased fentanyl plasma concentrations).
No products indexed under this heading.

Methylprednisolone Acetate (Concomitant use of fentanyl with drugs that induce cytochrome P450 3A4 activity may result in decreased fentanyl plasma concentrations).
No products indexed under this heading.

Methylprednisolone Sodium Succinate (Concomitant use of fentanyl with drugs that induce cytochrome P450 3A4 activity may result in decreased fentanyl plasma concentrations).
No products indexed under this heading.

Metronidazole (Concomitant use of fentanyl with strong CYP3A4 inhibitors (eg, ritonavir, ketoconazole, itraconazole, troleandomycin, clarthromycin, nelfinavir, and nefazodone) or moderate CYP3A4 inhibitors (eg, amprenavir, aprepitant, diltiazem, erythromycin, fluconazole, fosamprenavir, and verapamil) may result in increased fentanyl plasma concentrations, potentially causing serious adverse drug effects including fatal respiratory depression. Concurrent use with moderate or strong CYP3A4 inhibitors should be carefullymonitored for an extended period of time. Dosage increase should be done conservatively). Products include:
Pylera Capsules 714

Metronidazole Benzoate (Concomitant use of fentanyl with strong CYP3A4 inhibitors (eg, ritonavir, ketoconazole, itraconazole, troleandomycin, clarthromycin, nelfinavir, and nefazodone) or moderate CYP3A4 inhibitors (eg, amprenavir, aprepitant, diltiazem, erythromycin, fluconazole, fosamprenavir, and verapamil) may result in increased fentanyl plasma concentrations, potentially causing serious adverse drug effects including fatal respiratory depression. Concurrent use with moderate or strong CYP3A4 inhibitors should be carefullymonitored for an extended period of time. Dosage increase should be done conservatively).
No products indexed under this heading.

Metronidazole Hydrochloride (Concomitant use of fentanyl with strong CYP3A4 inhibitors (eg, ritonavir, ketoconazole, itraconazole, troleandomycin, clarthromycin, nelfinavir, and nefazodone) or moderate CYP3A4 inhibitors (eg, amprenavir, aprepitant, diltiazem, erythromycin, fluconazole, fosamprenavir, and verapamil) may result in increased fentanyl plasma concentrations, potentially causing serious adverse drug effects including fatal respiratory depression. Concurrent use with moderate or strong CYP3A4 inhibitors should be carefullymonitored for an extended period of time. Dosage increase should be done conservatively).
No products indexed under this heading.

Miconazole (Concomitant use of fentanyl with strong CYP3A4 inhibitors (eg, ritonavir, ketoconazole, itraconazole, troleandomycin, clarthromycin, nelfinavir, and nefazodone) or moderate CYP3A4 inhibitors (eg, amprenavir, aprepitant, diltiazem, erythromycin, fluconazole, fosamprenavir, and verapamil) may result in increased fentanyl plasma concentrations, potentially causing serious adverse drug effects including fatal respiratory depression. Concurrent use with moderate or strong CYP3A4 inhibitors should be carefullymonitored for an extended period of time. Dosage increase should be done conservatively).
No products indexed under this heading.

Miconazole Nitrate (Concomitant use of fentanyl with strong CYP3A4 inhibitors (eg, ritonavir, ketoconazole, itraconazole, troleandomycin, clarthromycin, nelfinavir, and nefazodone) or moderate CYP3A4 inhibitors (eg, amprenavir, aprepitant, diltiazem, erythromycin, fluconazole, fosamprenavir, and verapamil) may result in increased fentanyl plasma concentrations, potentially causing serious adverse drug effects including fatal respiratory depression. Concurrent use with moderate or strong CYP3A4 inhibitors should be carefullymonitored for an extended period of time. Dosage increase should be done conservatively).
No products indexed under this heading.

Midazolam Hydrochloride (Co-administration may result in increased depressant effects; hypoventilation, hypotension, and profound sedation may occur).
No products indexed under this heading.

Moclobemide (Concurrent and/or sequential use with MAO inhibitors is not recommended; potential for severe and unpredictable potentiation of MAO inhibitors has been reported with opioid analgesics).
No products indexed under this heading.

Modafinil (Concomitant use of fentanyl with drugs that induce cytochrome P450 3A4 activity may result in decreased fentanyl plasma concentrations). Products include:
Provigil Tablets 977

Molindone Hydrochloride (Co-administration may result in increased depressant effects; hypoventilation, hypotension, and profound sedation may occur. Monitor for change in opiod effects and consider adjusting dose of fentanyl if warranted). Products include:
Moban Tablets 1116

Morphine Sulfate (Co-administration may result in increased depressant effects; hypoventilation, hypotension, and profound sedation may occur. Monitor for change in opiod effects and consider adjusting dose of fentanyl if warranted). Products include:
Avinza Capsules 1772
DepoDur Injection 1095
MS Contin Tablets 2585

Nefazodone Hydrochloride (Concomitant use of fentanyl with strong CYP3A4 inhibitors (eg, ritonavir, ketoconazole, itraconazole, troleandomycin, clarthromycin, nelfinavir, and nefazodone) or moderate CYP3A4 inhibitors (eg, amprenavir, aprepitant, diltiazem, erythromycin, fluconazole, fosamprenavir, and verapamil) may result in increased fentanyl plasma concentrations, potentially causing serious adverse drug effects including fatal respiratory depression. Concurrent use with moderate or strong CYP3A4 inhibitors should be carefullymonitored for an extended period of time. Dosage increase should be done conservatively).
No products indexed under this heading.

Nelfinavir Mesylate (Concomitant use of fentanyl with strong CYP3A4 inhibitors (eg, ritonavir, ketoconazole, itraconazole, troleandomycin, clarthromycin, nelfinavir, and nefazodone) or moderate CYP3A4 inhibitors (eg, amprenavir, aprepitant, diltiazem, erythromycin, fluconazole, fosamprenavir, and verapamil) may result in increased fentanyl plasma concentrations, potentially causing serious adverse drug effects including fatal respiratory depression. Concurrent use with moderate or strong CYP3A4 inhibitors should be carefullymonitored for an extended period of time. Dosage increase should be done conservatively).
No products indexed under this heading.

Nevirapine (Concomitant use of fentanyl with strong CYP3A4 inhibitors (eg, ritonavir, ketoconazole, itraconazole, troleandomycin, clarthromycin, nelfinavir, and nefazodone) or moderate CYP3A4 inhibitors (eg, amprenavir, aprepitant, diltiazem, erythromycin, fluconazole, fosamprenavir, and verapamil) may result in increased fentanyl plasma concentrations, potentially causing serious adverse drug effects including fatal respiratory depression. Concurrent use with moderate or strong CYP3A4 inhibitors should be carefullymonitored for an extended period of time. Dosage increase should be done conservatively). Products include:
Viramune Oral Suspension 873
Viramune Tablets 873

Niacinamide (Concomitant use of fentanyl with strong CYP3A4 inhibitors (eg, ritonavir, ketoconazole, itraconazole, troleandomycin, clarthromycin, nelfinavir, and nefazodone) or moderate CYP3A4 inhibitors (eg, amprenavir, aprepitant, diltiazem, erythromycin, fluconazole, fosamprenavir, and verapamil) may result in increased fentanyl plasma concentrations, potentially causing serious adverse drug effects including fatal respiratory depression. Concurrent use with moderate or strong CYP3A4 inhibitors should be carefullymonitored for an extended period of time. Dosage increase should be done conservatively). Products include:
BioLean Free Tablets 635

Nicotinamide (Concomitant use of fentanyl with strong CYP3A4 inhibitors (eg, ritonavir, ketoconazole, itraconazole, troleandomycin, clarthromycin, nelfinavir, and nefazodone) or moderate CYP3A4 inhibitors (eg, amprenavir, aprepitant, diltiazem, erythromycin, fluconazole, fosamprenavir, and verapamil) may result in increased fentanyl plasma concentrations, potentially causing serious adverse drug effects including fatal respiratory depression. Concurrent use with moderate or strong CYP3A4 inhibitors should be carefullymonitored for an extended period of time. Dosage increase should be done conservatively).
No products indexed under this heading.

Nifedipine (Concomitant use of fentanyl with strong CYP3A4 inhibitors (eg, ritonavir, ketoconazole, itraconazole, troleandomycin, clarthromycin, nelfinavir, and nefazodone) or moderate CYP3A4 inhibitors (eg, amprenavir, aprepitant, diltiazem, erythromycin, fluconazole, fosamprenavir, and verapamil) may result in increased fentanyl plasma concentrations, potentially causing serious adverse drug effects including fatal respiratory depression. Concurrent use with moderate or strong CYP3A4 inhibitors should be carefullymonitored for an extended period of time. Dosage increase should be done conservatively).
No products indexed under this heading.

Norfloxacin (Concomitant use of fentanyl with strong CYP3A4 inhibitors (eg, ritonavir, ketoconazole, itraconazole, troleandomycin, clarthromycin, nelfinavir, and nefazodone) or moderate CYP3A4 inhibitors (eg, amprenavir, aprepitant, diltiazem, erythromycin, fluconazole, fosamprenavir, and verapamil) may result in increased fentanyl plasma concentrations, potentially causing serious adverse drug effects including fatal respiratory depression. Concurrent use with moderate or strong CYP3A4 inhibitors should be carefullymonitored for an extended period of time. Dosage increase should be done conservatively). Products include:
Noroxin Tablets 2069

Olanzapine (Co-administration may result in increased depressant effects; hypoventilation, hypotension, and profound sedation may occur. Monitor for change in opiod effects and consider adjusting dose of fentanyl if warranted). Products include:
Symbyax Capsules 1871
Zyprexa Tablets 1883
Zyprexa IntraMuscular 1883
Zyprexa ZYDIS Orally Disintegrating Tablets.................. 1883

Omeprazole (Concomitant use of fentanyl with strong CYP3A4 inhibitors (eg, ritonavir, ketoconazole, itraconazole, troleandomycin, clarthromycin, nelfinavir, and nefazodone) or moderate CYP3A4 inhibitors (eg, amprenavir, aprepitant, diltiazem, erythromycin, fluconazole, fosamprenavir, and verapamil) may result in increased fentanyl plasma concentrations, potentially causing serious adverse drug effects including fatal respiratory depression. Concurrent use with moderate or strong CYP3A4 inhibitors should be carefullymonitored for an extended period of time. Dosage increase should be done conservatively).
No products indexed under this heading.

Oxazepam (Co-administration may result in increased depressant effects; hypoventilation, hypotension, and profound sedation may occur. Monitor for change in opiod effects and consider adjusting dose of fentanyl if warranted).
No products indexed under this heading.

Oxcarbazepine (Concomitant use of fentanyl with drugs that induce cytochrome P450 3A4 activity may result in decreased fentanyl plasma concentrations).
No products indexed under this heading.

Oxycodone Hydrochloride (Co-administration may result in increased depressant effects; hypoventilation, hypotension, and profound sedation may occur. Monitor for change in opiod effects and consider adjusting dose of fentanyl if warranted). Products include:
OxyContin Tablets 2589
OxyIR Capsules 2593
Percocet Tablets 1127
Percodan Tablets 1130

Pargyline Hydrochloride (Concurrent and/or sequential use with MAO inhibitors is not recommended; potential for severe and unpredictable potentiation of MAO inhibitors has been reported with opioid analgesics).
No products indexed under this heading.

Paroxetine Hydrochloride (Concomitant use of fentanyl with strong CYP3A4 inhibitors (eg, ritonavir, ketoconazole, itraconazole, troleandomycin, clarthromycin, nelfinavir, and nefazodone) or moderate CYP3A4 inhibitors (eg, amprenavir, aprepitant, diltiazem, erythromycin, fluconazole, fosamprenavir, and verapamil) may result in increased fentanyl plasma concentrations, potentially causing serious adverse drug effects including fatal respiratory depression. Concurrent use with moderate or strong CYP3A4 inhibitors should be carefullymonitored for an extended period of time. Dosage increase should be done conservatively). Products include:
Paxil 1535
Paxil CR Controlled-Release Tablets 1544

Pentobarbital Sodium (Co-administration may result in increased depressant effects; hypoventilation, hypotension, and profound sedation may occur. Monitor for change in opiod effects and consider adjusting dose of fentanyl if warranted). Products include:
Nembutal Sodium Solution, USP 2494

Perphenazine (Co-administration may result in increased depressant effects; hypoventilation, hypotension, and profound sedation may occur. Monitor for change in opiod effects and consider adjusting dose of fentanyl if warranted).
No products indexed under this heading.

Phenelzine Sulfate (Concurrent and/or sequential use with MAO inhibitors is not recommended; potential for severe and unpredictable potentiation of MAO inhibitors has been reported with opioid analgesics).
No products indexed under this heading.

Phenobarbital (Co-administration may result in increased depressant effects; hypoventilation, hypotension, and profound sedation may occur. Monitor for change in opiod effects and consider adjusting dose of fentanyl if warranted). Products include:
Donnatal Extentabs 2507

Phenobarbital Sodium (Concomitant use of fentanyl with drugs that induce cytochrome P450 3A4 activity may result in decreased fentanyl plasma concentrations).
No products indexed under this heading.

Phenytoin (Concomitant use of fentanyl with drugs that induce cytochrome P450 3A4 activity may result in decreased fentanyl plasma concentrations).
No products indexed under this heading.

Phenytoin Sodium (Concomitant use of fentanyl with drugs that induce cytochrome P450 3A4 activity may result in decreased fentanyl plasma concentrations). Products include:
Phenytek Capsules 2192

Prazepam (Co-administration may result in increased depressant effects; hypoventilation, hypotension, and profound sedation may occur. Monitor for change in opiod effects and consider adjusting dose of fentanyl if warranted).
No products indexed under this heading.

Prednisolone Acetate (Concomitant use of fentanyl with drugs that induce cytochrome P450 3A4 activity may result in decreased fentanyl plasma concentrations). Products include:
Pred Forte Ophthalmic Suspension .... ⊙ 227
Pred Mild Ophthalmic Suspension .... ⊙ 230
Pred-G Ophthalmic Ointment .... ⊙ 229
Pred-G Ophthalmic Suspension ..... ⊙ 228

Prednisolone Sodium Phosphate (Concomitant use of fentanyl with drugs that induce cytochrome P450 3A4 activity may result in decreased fentanyl plasma concentrations).
No products indexed under this heading.

Prednisolone Tebutate (Concomitant use of fentanyl with drugs that induce cytochrome P450 3A4 activity may result in decreased fentanyl plasma concentrations).
No products indexed under this heading.

Prednisone (Concomitant use of fentanyl with drugs that induce cytochrome P450 3A4 activity may result in decreased fentanyl plasma concentrations).
No products indexed under this heading.

Primidone (Concomitant use of fentanyl with drugs that induce cytochrome P450 3A4 activity may result in decreased fentanyl plasma concentrations).
No products indexed under this heading.

Procarbazine Hydrochloride (Concurrent and/or sequential use with MAO inhibitors is not recommended; potential for severe and unpredictable potentiation of MAO inhibitors has been reported with opioid analgesics).
No products indexed under this heading.

Prochlorperazine (Co-administration may result in increased depressant effects; hypoventilation, hypotension, and profound sedation may occur. Monitor for change in opiod effects and consider adjusting dose of fentanyl if warranted).
No products indexed under this heading.

Promethazine Hydrochloride (Co-administration with sedating antihistamines may result in increased depressant effects).
No products indexed under this heading.

Propofol (Co-administration may result in increased depressant effects; hypoventilation, hypotension, and profound sedation may occur).
No products indexed under this heading.

Propoxyphene Hydrochloride (Co-administration may result in increased depressant effects; hypoventilation, hypotension, and profound sedation may occur. Monitor for change in opiod effects and consider adjusting dose of fentanyl if warranted).
No products indexed under this heading.

Propoxyphene Napsylate (Co-administration may result in increased depressant effects; hypoventilation, hypotension, and profound sedation may occur. Monitor for change in opiod effects and consider adjusting dose of fentanyl if warranted).
No products indexed under this heading.

Pyrilamine Maleate (Co-administration with sedating antihistamines may result in increased depressant effects).
No products indexed under this heading.

Pyrilamine Tannate (Co-administration with sedating antihistamines may result in increased depressant effects).
No products indexed under this heading.

Quazepam (Co-administration may result in increased depressant effects; hypoventilation, hypotension, and profound sedation may occur).
No products indexed under this heading.

Quetiapine Fumarate (Co-administration may result in increased depressant effects; hypoventilation, hypotension, and profound sedation may occur. Monitor for change in opiod effects and consider adjusting dose of fentanyl if warranted).
No products indexed under this heading.

Quinidine (Concomitant use of fentanyl with strong CYP3A4 inhibitors (eg, ritonavir, ketoconazole, itraconazole, troleandomycin, clarthromycin, nelfinavir, and nefazodone) or moderate CYP3A4 inhibitors (eg, amprenavir, aprepitant, diltiazem, erythromycin, fluconazole, fosamprenavir, and verapamil) may result in increased fentanyl plasma concentrations, potentially causing serious adverse drug effects including fatal respiratory depression. Concurrent use with moderate or strong CYP3A4 inhibitors should be carefullymonitored for an extended period of time. Dosage increase should be done conservatively).

No products indexed under this heading.

Quinidine Hydrochloride (Concomitant use of fentanyl with strong CYP3A4 inhibitors (eg, ritonavir, ketoconazole, itraconazole, troleandomycin, clarthromycin, nelfinavir, and nefazodone) or moderate CYP3A4 inhibitors (eg, amprenavir, aprepitant, diltiazem, erythromycin, fluconazole, fosamprenavir, and verapamil) may result in increased fentanyl plasma concentrations, potentially causing serious adverse drug effects including fatal respiratory depression. Concurrent use with moderate or strong CYP3A4 inhibitors should be carefullymonitored for an extended period of time. Dosage increase should be done conservatively).

No products indexed under this heading.

Quinidine Polygalacturonate (Concomitant use of fentanyl with strong CYP3A4 inhibitors (eg, ritonavir, ketoconazole, itraconazole, troleandomycin, clarthromycin, nelfinavir, and nefazodone) or moderate CYP3A4 inhibitors (eg, amprenavir, aprepitant, diltiazem, erythromycin, fluconazole, fosamprenavir, and verapamil) may result in increased fentanyl plasma concentrations, potentially causing serious adverse drug effects including fatal respiratory depression. Concurrent use with moderate or strong CYP3A4 inhibitors should be carefullymonitored for an extended period of time. Dosage increase should be done conservatively).

No products indexed under this heading.

Quinidine Sulfate (Concomitant use of fentanyl with strong CYP3A4 inhibitors (eg, ritonavir, ketoconazole, itraconazole, troleandomycin, clarthromycin, nelfinavir, and nefazodone) or moderate CYP3A4 inhibitors (eg, amprenavir, aprepitant, diltiazem, erythromycin, fluconazole, fosamprenavir, and verapamil) may result in increased fentanyl plasma concentrations, potentially causing serious adverse drug effects including fatal respiratory depression. Concurrent use with moderate or strong CYP3A4 inhibitors should be carefullymonitored for an extended period of time. Dosage increase should be done conservatively).

No products indexed under this heading.

Quinine (Concomitant use of fentanyl with strong CYP3A4 inhibitors (eg, ritonavir, ketoconazole, itraconazole, troleandomycin, clarthromycin, nelfinavir, and nefazodone) or moderate CYP3A4 inhibitors (eg, amprenavir, aprepitant, diltiazem, erythromycin, fluconazole, fosamprenavir, and verapamil) may result in increased fentanyl plasma concentrations, potentially causing serious adverse drug effects including fatal respiratory depression. Concurrent use with moderate or strong CYP3A4 inhibitors should be carefullymonitored for an extended period of time. Dosage increase should be done conservatively).

No products indexed under this heading.

Quinine Sulfate (Concomitant use of fentanyl with strong CYP3A4 inhibitors (eg, ritonavir, ketoconazole, itraconazole, troleandomycin, clarthromycin, nelfinavir, and nefazodone) or moderate CYP3A4 inhibitors (eg, amprenavir, aprepitant, diltiazem, erythromycin, fluconazole, fosamprenavir, and verapamil) may result in increased fentanyl plasma concentrations, potentially causing serious adverse drug effects including fatal respiratory depression. Concurrent use with moderate or strong CYP3A4 inhibitors should be carefullymonitored for an extended period of time. Dosage increase should be done conservatively).

No products indexed under this heading.

Quinupristin (Concomitant use of fentanyl with strong CYP3A4 inhibitors (eg, ritonavir, ketoconazole, itraconazole, troleandomycin, clarthromycin, nelfinavir, and nefazodone) or moderate CYP3A4 inhibitors (eg, amprenavir, aprepitant, diltiazem, erythromycin, fluconazole, fosamprenavir, and verapamil) may result in increased fentanyl plasma concentrations, potentially causing serious adverse drug effects including fatal respiratory depression. Concurrent use with moderate or strong CYP3A4 inhibitors should be carefullymonitored for an extended period of time. Dosage increase should be done conservatively).

No products indexed under this heading.

Ramelteon (Co-administration may result in increased depressant effects; hypoventilation, hypotension, and profound sedation may occur). Products include:

Rozerem Tablets **3091**

Ranitidine Bismuth Citrate (Concomitant use of fentanyl with strong CYP3A4 inhibitors (eg, ritonavir, ketoconazole, itraconazole, troleandomycin, clarthromycin, nelfinavir, and nefazodone) or moderate CYP3A4 inhibitors (eg, amprenavir, aprepitant, diltiazem, erythromycin, fluconazole, fosamprenavir, and verapamil) may result in increased fentanyl plasma concentrations, potentially causing serious adverse drug effects including fatal respiratory depression. Concurrent use with moderate or strong CYP3A4 inhibitors should be carefullymonitored for an extended period of time. Dosage increase should be done conservatively).

No products indexed under this heading.

Ranitidine Hydrochloride (Concomitant use of fentanyl with strong CYP3A4 inhibitors (eg, ritonavir, ketoconazole, itraconazole, troleandomycin, clarthromycin, nelfinavir, and nefazodone) or moderate CYP3A4 inhibitors (eg, amprenavir, aprepitant, diltiazem, erythromycin, fluconazole, fosamprenavir, and verapamil) may result in increased fentanyl plasma concentrations, potentially causing serious adverse drug effects including fatal respiratory depression. Concurrent use with moderate or strong CYP3A4 inhibitors should be carefullymonitored for an extended period of time. Dosage increase should be done conservatively). Products include:

Zantac 75 Tablets **603**
Zantac **1670**
Zantac Injection **1666**
Zantac Injection Pharmacy Bulk Package **1668**
Maximum Strength Zantac 150 Tablets **603**
Maximum Strength Zantac 150 Cool Mint Tablets **603**

Rasagiline Mesylate (Concurrent and/or sequential use with MAO inhibitors is not recommended; potential for severe and unpredictable potentiation of MAO inhibitors has been reported with opioid analgesics). Products include:

Azilect Tablets **3106**

Remifentanil Hydrochloride (Co-administration may result in increased depressant effects; hypoventilation, hypotension, and profound sedation may occur. Monitor for change in opioid effects and consider adjusting dose of fentanyl if warranted).

No products indexed under this heading.

Rifabutin (Concomitant use of fentanyl with drugs that induce cytochrome P450 3A4 activity may result in decreased fentanyl plasma concentrations).

No products indexed under this heading.

Rifampicin (Concomitant use of fentanyl with drugs that induce cytochrome P450 3A4 activity may result in decreased fentanyl plasma concentrations).

No products indexed under this heading.

Rifampin (Concomitant use of fentanyl with drugs that induce cytochrome P450 3A4 activity may result in decreased fentanyl plasma concentrations).

No products indexed under this heading.

Rifapentine (Concomitant use of fentanyl with drugs that induce cytochrome P450 3A4 activity may result in decreased fentanyl plasma concentrations).

No products indexed under this heading.

Risperidone (Co-administration may result in increased depressant effects; hypoventilation, hypotension, and profound sedation may occur. Monitor for change in opioid effects and consider adjusting dose of fentanyl if warranted). Products include:

Risperdal Consta Long-Acting Injection **1753**

Ritonavir (Co-administration with potent inhibitors of CYP450 3A4 isoform, such as protease inhibitor ritonavir, may increase the bioavailability of swallowed fentanyl by decreasing intestinal and hepatic first pass metabolism and may decrease the systemic clearance resulting in increased or prolonged opioid effects). Products include:

Kaletra **452**
Norvir **489**

Saquinavir (Concomitant use of fentanyl with strong CYP3A4 inhibitors (eg, ritonavir, ketoconazole, itraconazole, troleandomycin, clarthromycin, nelfinavir, and nefazodone) or moderate CYP3A4 inhibitors (eg, amprenavir, aprepitant, diltiazem, erythromycin, fluconazole, fosamprenavir, and verapamil) may result in increased fentanyl plasma concentrations, potentially causing serious adverse drug effects including fatal respiratory depression. Concurrent use with moderate or strong CYP3A4 inhibitors should be carefullymonitored for an extended period of time. Dosage increase should be done conservatively).

No products indexed under this heading.

Saquinavir Mesylate (Concomitant use of fentanyl with strong CYP3A4 inhibitors (eg, ritonavir, ketoconazole, itraconazole, troleandomycin, clarthromycin, nelfinavir, and nefazodone) or moderate CYP3A4 inhibitors (eg, amprenavir, aprepitant, diltiazem, erythromycin, fluconazole, fosamprenavir, and verapamil) may result in increased fentanyl plasma concentrations, potentially causing serious adverse drug effects including fatal respiratory depression. Concurrent use with moderate or strong CYP3A4 inhibitors should be carefullymonitored for an extended period of time. Dosage increase should be done conservatively).

No products indexed under this heading.

Secobarbital Sodium (Co-administration may result in increased depressant effects; hypoventilation, hypotension, and profound sedation may occur).

No products indexed under this heading.

Selegiline (Concurrent and/or sequential use with MAO inhibitors is not recommended; potential for severe and unpredictable potentiation of MAO inhibitors has been reported with opioid analgesics). Products include:

Emsam Transdermal System **905**

Selegiline Hydrochloride (Concurrent and/or sequential use with MAO inhibitors is not recommended; potential for severe and unpredictable potentiation of MAO inhibitors has been reported with opioid analgesics). Products include:

Eldepryl Capsules **3052**

Sertraline Hydrochloride (Concomitant use of fentanyl with strong CYP3A4 inhibitors (eg, ritonavir, ketoconazole, itraconazole, troleandomycin, clarthromycin, nelfinavir, and nefazodone) or moderate CYP3A4 inhibitors (eg, amprenavir, aprepitant, diltiazem, erythromycin, fluconazole, fosamprenavir, and verapamil) may result in increased fentanyl plasma concentrations, potentially causing serious adverse drug effects including fatal respiratory depression. Concurrent use with moderate or strong CYP3A4 inhibitors should be carefullymonitored for an extended period of time. Dosage increase should be done conservatively).

No products indexed under this heading.

Sevoflurane (Co-administration may result in increased depressant effects; hypoventilation, hypotension, and profound sedation may occur). Products include:

Ultane Liquid for Inhalation **524**

Sildenafil Citrate (Concomitant use of fentanyl with strong CYP3A4 inhibitors (eg, ritonavir, ketoconazole, itraconazole, troleandomycin, clarthromycin, nelfinavir, and nefazodone) or moderate CYP3A4 inhibitors (eg, amprenavir, aprepitant, diltiazem, erythromycin, fluconazole, fosamprenavir, and verapamil) may result in increased fentanyl plasma concentrations, potentially causing serious adverse drug effects including fatal respiratory depression. Concurrent use with moderate or strong CYP3A4 inhibitors should be carefullymonitored for an extended period of time. Dosage increase should be done conservatively).
No products indexed under this heading.

Sodium Butabarbital (Co-administration may result in increased depressant effects; hypoventilation, hypotension, and profound sedation may occur).
No products indexed under this heading.

Sodium Oxybate (Co-administration may result in increased depressant effects; hypoventilation, hypotension, and profound sedation may occur. Monitor for change in opiod effects and consider adjusting dose of fentanyl if warranted). Products include:
Xyrem Oral Solution 1766

Sufentanil Citrate (Co-administration may result in increased depressant effects; hypoventilation, hypotension, and profound sedation may occur. Monitor for change in opiod effects and consider adjusting dose of fentanyl if warranted).
No products indexed under this heading.

Sulfinpyrazone (Concomitant use of fentanyl with drugs that induce cytochrome P450 3A4 activity may result in decreased fentanyl plasma concentrations).
No products indexed under this heading.

Telithromycin (Concomitant use of fentanyl with strong CYP3A4 inhibitors (eg, ritonavir, ketoconazole, itraconazole, troleandomycin, clarthromycin, nelfinavir, and nefazodone) or moderate CYP3A4 inhibitors (eg, amprenavir, aprepitant, diltiazem, erythromycin, fluconazole, fosamprenavir, and verapamil) may result in increased fentanyl plasma concentrations, potentially causing serious adverse drug effects including fatal respiratory depression. Concurrent use with moderate or strong CYP3A4 inhibitors should be carefullymonitored for an extended period of time. Dosage increase should be done conservatively). Products include:
Ketek Tablets 2744

Temazepam (Co-administration may result in increased depressant effects; hypoventilation, hypotension, and profound sedation may occur).
No products indexed under this heading.

Theophylline (Concomitant use of fentanyl with drugs that induce cytochrome P450 3A4 activity may result in decreased fentanyl plasma concentrations).
No products indexed under this heading.

Theophylline Anhydrous (Concomitant use of fentanyl with drugs that induce cytochrome P450 3A4 activity may result in decreased fentanyl plasma concentrations). Products include:
Uniphyl Tablets 2595

Theophylline Calcium Salicylate (Concomitant use of fentanyl with drugs that induce cytochrome P450 3A4 activity may result in decreased fentanyl plasma concentrations).
No products indexed under this heading.

Theophylline Dihydroxypropyl (Glyceryl) (Concomitant use of fentanyl with drugs that induce cytochrome P450 3A4 activity may result in decreased fentanyl plasma concentrations).
No products indexed under this heading.

Theophylline Ethylenediamine (Concomitant use of fentanyl with drugs that induce cytochrome P450 3A4 activity may result in decreased fentanyl plasma concentrations).
No products indexed under this heading.

Thiamylal Sodium (Co-administration may result in increased depressant effects; hypoventilation, hypotension, and profound sedation may occur. Monitor for change in opiod effects and consider adjusting dose of fentanyl if warranted).
No products indexed under this heading.

Thioridazine Hydrochloride (Co-administration may result in increased depressant effects; hypoventilation, hypotension, and profound sedation may occur. Monitor for change in opiod effects and consider adjusting dose of fentanyl if warranted). Products include:
Thioridazine Hydrochloride Tablets 2195

Thiothixene (Co-administration may result in increased depressant effects; hypoventilation, hypotension, and profound sedation may occur. Monitor for change in opiod effects and consider adjusting dose of fentanyl if warranted). Products include:
Thiothixene Capsules 2197

Tranylcypromine Sulfate (Concurrent and/or sequential use with MAO inhibitors is not recommended; potential for severe and unpredictable potentiation of MAO inhibitors has been reported with opioid analgesics). Products include:
Parnate Tablets 1532

Triamcinolone (Concomitant use of fentanyl with drugs that induce cytochrome P450 3A4 activity may result in decreased fentanyl plasma concentrations).
No products indexed under this heading.

Triamcinolone Acetonide (Concomitant use of fentanyl with drugs that induce cytochrome P450 3A4 activity may result in decreased fentanyl plasma concentrations). Products include:
Azmacort Inhalation Aerosol 407
Nasacort AQ Nasal Spray 2765
Triesence Injectable Suspension .... ⊙209

Triamcinolone Diacetate (Concomitant use of fentanyl with drugs that induce cytochrome P450 3A4 activity may result in decreased fentanyl plasma concentrations).
No products indexed under this heading.

Triamcinolone Hexacetonide (Concomitant use of fentanyl with drugs that induce cytochrome P450 3A4 activity may result in decreased fentanyl plasma concentrations).
No products indexed under this heading.

Triazolam (Co-administration may result in increased depressant effects; hypoventilation, hypotension, and profound sedation may occur).
No products indexed under this heading.

Trifluoperazine Hydrochloride (Co-administration may result in increased depressant effects; hypoventilation, hypotension, and profound sedation may occur. Monitor for change in opiod effects and consider adjusting dose of fentanyl if warranted).
No products indexed under this heading.

Trimeprazine Tartrate (Co-administration with sedating antihistamines may result in increased depressant effects).
No products indexed under this heading.

Tripelennamine Hydrochloride (Co-administration with sedating antihistamines may result in increased depressant effects).
No products indexed under this heading.

Triprolidine Hydrochloride (Co-administration with sedating antihistamines may result in increased depressant effects).
No products indexed under this heading.

Troglitazone (Concomitant use of fentanyl with strong CYP3A4 inhibitors (eg, ritonavir, ketoconazole, itraconazole, troleandomycin, clarthromycin, nelfinavir, and nefazodone) or moderate CYP3A4 inhibitors (eg, amprenavir, aprepitant, diltiazem, erythromycin, fluconazole, fosamprenavir, and verapamil) may result in increased fentanyl plasma concentrations, potentially causing serious adverse drug effects including fatal respiratory depression. Concurrent use with moderate or strong CYP3A4 inhibitors should be carefullymonitored for an extended period of time. Dosage increase should be done conservatively).
No products indexed under this heading.

Troleandomycin (Concomitant use of fentanyl with strong CYP3A4 inhibitors (eg, ritonavir, ketoconazole, itraconazole, troleandomycin, clarthromycin, nelfinavir, and nefazodone) or moderate CYP3A4 inhibitors (eg, amprenavir, aprepitant, diltiazem, erythromycin, fluconazole, fosamprenavir, and verapamil) may result in increased fentanyl plasma concentrations, potentially causing serious adverse drug effects including fatal respiratory depression. Concurrent use with moderate or strong CYP3A4 inhibitors should be carefullymonitored for an extended period of time. Dosage increase should be done conservatively).
No products indexed under this heading.

Valproate Sodium (Concomitant use of fentanyl with strong CYP3A4 inhibitors (eg, ritonavir, ketoconazole, itraconazole, troleandomycin, clarthromycin, nelfinavir, and nefazodone) or moderate CYP3A4 inhibitors (eg, amprenavir, aprepitant, diltiazem, erythromycin, fluconazole, fosamprenavir, and verapamil) may result in increased fentanyl plasma concentrations, potentially causing serious adverse drug effects including fatal respiratory depression. Concurrent use with moderate or strong CYP3A4 inhibitors should be carefullymonitored for an extended period of time. Dosage increase should be done conservatively).
No products indexed under this heading.

Vardenafil Hydrochloride (Concomitant use of fentanyl with strong CYP3A4 inhibitors (eg, ritonavir, ketoconazole, itraconazole, troleandomycin, clarthromycin, nelfinavir, and nefazodone) or moderate CYP3A4 inhibitors (eg, amprenavir, aprepitant, diltiazem, erythromycin, fluconazole, fosamprenavir, and verapamil) may result in increased fentanyl plasma concentrations, potentially causing serious adverse drug effects including fatal respiratory depression. Concurrent use with moderate or strong CYP3A4 inhibitors should be carefullymonitored for an extended period of time. Dosage increase should be done conservatively). Products include:
Levitra Tablets 2876

Venlafaxine Hydrochloride (Concomitant use of fentanyl with strong CYP3A4 inhibitors (eg, ritonavir, ketoconazole, itraconazole, troleandomycin, clarthromycin, nelfinavir, and nefazodone) or moderate CYP3A4 inhibitors (eg, amprenavir, aprepitant, diltiazem, erythromycin, fluconazole, fosamprenavir, and verapamil) may result in increased fentanyl plasma concentrations, potentially causing serious adverse drug effects including fatal respiratory depression. Concurrent use with moderate or strong CYP3A4 inhibitors should be carefullymonitored for an extended period of time. Dosage increase should be done conservatively). Products include:
Effexor XR Extended-Release Capsules 3195
Venlafaxine Hydrochloride Tablets ... 2199

Verapamil Hydrochloride (Concomitant use of fentanyl with strong CYP3A4 inhibitors (eg, ritonavir, ketoconazole, itraconazole, troleandomycin, clarthromycin, nelfinavir, and nefazodone) or moderate CYP3A4 inhibitors (eg, amprenavir, aprepitant, diltiazem, erythromycin, fluconazole, fosamprenavir, and verapamil) may result in increased fentanyl plasma concentrations, potentially causing serious adverse drug effects including fatal respiratory depression. Concurrent use with moderate or strong CYP3A4 inhibitors should be carefullymonitored for an extended period of time. Dosage increase should be done conservatively). Products include:
Tarka Tablets 511

Voriconazole (Concomitant use of fentanyl with strong CYP3A4 inhibitors (eg, ritonavir, ketoconazole,

itraconazole, troleandomycin, clarthromycin, nelfinavir, and nefazodone) or moderate CYP3A4 inhibitors (eg, amprenavir, aprepitant, diltiazem, erythromycin, fluconazole, fosamprenavir, and verapamil) may result in increased fentanyl plasma concentrations, potentially causing serious adverse drug effects including fatal respiratory depression. Concurrent use with moderate or strong CYP3A4 inhibitors should be carefullymonitored for an extended period of time. Dosage increase should be done conservatively).

No products indexed under this heading.

Zafirlukast (Concomitant use of fentanyl with strong CYP3A4 inhibitors (eg, ritonavir, ketoconazole, itraconazole, troleandomycin, clarthromycin, nelfinavir, and nefazodone) or moderate CYP3A4 inhibitors (eg, amprenavir, aprepitant, diltiazem, erythromycin, fluconazole, fosamprenavir, and verapamil) may result in increased fentanyl plasma concentrations, potentially causing serious adverse drug effects including fatal respiratory depression. Concurrent use with moderate or strong CYP3A4 inhibitors should be carefullymonitored for an extended period of time. Dosage increase should be done conservatively). Products include:

Accolate Tablets 669

Zaleplon (Co-administration may result in increased depressant effects; hypoventilation, hypotension, and profound sedation may occur).

No products indexed under this heading.

Zileuton (Concomitant use of fentanyl with strong CYP3A4 inhibitors (eg, ritonavir, ketoconazole, itraconazole, troleandomycin, clarthromycin, nelfinavir, and nefazodone) or moderate CYP3A4 inhibitors (eg, amprenavir, aprepitant, diltiazem, erythromycin, fluconazole, fosamprenavir, and verapamil) may result in increased fentanyl plasma concentrations, potentially causing serious adverse drug effects including fatal respiratory depression. Concurrent use with moderate or strong CYP3A4 inhibitors should be carefullymonitored for an extended period of time. Dosage increase should be done conservatively).

No products indexed under this heading.

Ziprasidone Hydrochloride (Co-administration may result in increased depressant effects; hypoventilation, hypotension, and profound sedation may occur. Monitor for change in opioid effects and consider adjusting dose of fentanyl if warranted). Products include:

Geodon Capsules 2520

Zolpidem Tartrate (Co-administration may result in increased depressant effects; hypoventilation, hypotension, and profound sedation may occur). Products include:

Ambien Tablets 2692
Ambien CR Tablets 2696

Food Interactions

Alcohol (Concurrent use with alcoholic beverages may result in increased depressant effects; hypoventilation, hypotension, and profound sedation may occur).

Grapefruit (Grapefruit and grapefruit juice decrease CYP3A4 activity, increasing blood concentrations of fentanyl; concurrent use should be avoided).

Grapefruit Juice (Grapefruit and grapefruit juice decrease CYP3A4 activity, increasing blood concentrations of fentanyl; concurrent use should be avoided).

ACTIVASE I.V.

(Alteplase) 1188

May interact with ACE inhibitors, vitamin K antagonists, and certain other agents. Compounds in these categories include:

Abciximab (Drugs that alter platelet function, such as abciximab, may increase the risk of bleeding if administered prior to or after alteplase therapy). Products include:

ReoPro Vials 1860

Aspirin (Drugs that alter platelet function, such as aspirin, may increase the risk of bleeding if administered prior to or after alteplase therapy). Products include:

Aggrenox Capsules 819
Bayer Aspirin 750
Percodan Tablets 1130
St. Joseph 81 mg Aspirin Chewable and Enteric Coated Tablets 1903

Benazepril Hydrochloride (Post-marketing reports of orolingual angioedema associated with alteplase have primarily been in acute ischemic stroke patients receiving concomitant ACE inhibitors).

No products indexed under this heading.

Captopril (Post-marketing reports of orolingual angioedema associated with alteplase have primarily been in acute ischemic stroke patients receiving concomitant ACE inhibitors). Products include:

Captopril Tablets 2182

Clopidogrel Bisulfate (Drugs that alter platelet function, such as clopidogrel, may increase the risk of bleeding if administered prior to or after alteplase therapy). Products include:

Plavix Tablets 926
Plavix Tablets 2767

Dicumarol (Co-administration increases the risk of bleeding).

No products indexed under this heading.

Dipyridamole (Drugs that alter platelet function, such as dipyridamole, may increase the risk of bleeding if administered prior to or after alteplase therapy). Products include:

Aggrenox Capsules 819
Persantine Tablets 869

Enalapril Maleate (Post-marketing reports of orolingual angioedema associated with alteplase have primarily been in acute ischemic stroke patients receiving concomitant ACE inhibitors).

No products indexed under this heading.

Enalaprilat (Post-marketing reports of orolingual angioedema associated with alteplase have primarily been in acute ischemic stroke patients receiving concomitant ACE inhibitors).

No products indexed under this heading.

Eptifibatide (Drugs that alter platelet function, such as eptifibatide, may increase the risk of bleeding if administered prior to or after alteplase therapy). Products include:

Integrilin Injection 2855

Fosinopril Sodium (Post-marketing reports of orolingual angioedema associated with alteplase have primarily been in acute ischemic stroke patients receiving concomitant ACE inhibitors).

No products indexed under this heading.

Heparin Sodium (Co-administration increases the risk of bleeding).

No products indexed under this heading.

Lisinopril (Post-marketing reports of orolingual angioedema associated with alteplase have primarily been in acute ischemic stroke patients receiving concomitant ACE inhibitors). Products include:

Prinivil Tablets 2087
Prinzide Tablets 2092

Moexipril Hydrochloride (Post-marketing reports of orolingual angioedema associated with alteplase have primarily been in acute ischemic stroke patients receiving concomitant ACE inhibitors).

No products indexed under this heading.

Perindopril Erbumine (Post-marketing reports of orolingual angioedema associated with alteplase have primarily been in acute ischemic stroke patients receiving concomitant ACE inhibitors). Products include:

Aceon Tablets (2 mg, 4 mg, 8 mg) 3038

Quinapril Hydrochloride (Post-marketing reports of orolingual angioedema associated with alteplase have primarily been in acute ischemic stroke patients receiving concomitant ACE inhibitors).

No products indexed under this heading.

Ramipril (Post-marketing reports of orolingual angioedema associated with alteplase have primarily been in acute ischemic stroke patients receiving concomitant ACE inhibitors).

No products indexed under this heading.

Spirapril Hydrochloride (Post-marketing reports of orolingual angioedema associated with alteplase have primarily been in acute ischemic stroke patients receiving concomitant ACE inhibitors).

No products indexed under this heading.

Ticlopidine Hydrochloride (Drugs that alter platelet function, such as ticlopidine, may increase the risk of bleeding if administered prior to or after alteplase therapy).

No products indexed under this heading.

Tirofiban Hydrochloride (Drugs that alter platelet function, such as tirofiban, may increase the risk of bleeding if administered prior to or after alteplase therapy).

No products indexed under this heading.

Trandolapril (Post-marketing reports of orolingual angioedema associated with alteplase have primarily been in acute ischemic stroke patients receiving concomitant ACE inhibitors). Products include:

Mavik Tablets 472
Tarka Tablets 511

Warfarin Sodium (Co-administration increases the risk of bleeding).

No products indexed under this heading.

ACTIVE CALCIUM TABLETS

(Calcium Citrate, Vitamin D) 3173

None cited in PDR database.

ACTIVELLA TABLETS

(Estradiol, Norethindrone Acetate) 2347

May interact with thyroid preparations. Compounds in these categories include:

Levothyroxine Sodium (Estrogen administration leads to increased thyroid-binding globulin (TBG) levels. Patients with normal thyroid function can compensate for the increased TBG by making more thyroid hormone, thus maintaining free T4 and T3 serum concentrations in the normal range. Patients dependent on thyroid hormone replacement therapy who are also receiving estrogen may require increased doses of their thyroid replacement therapy. These patients should have their thyroid function monitored to maintain their free throid hormone levels in an acceptable range). Products include:

Levothroid Tablets 1170
Levoxyl Tablets 1780
Synthroid Tablets 507

Liothyronine Sodium (Estrogen administration leads to increased thyroid-binding globulin (TBG) levels. Patients with normal thyroid function can compensate for the increased TBG by making more thyroid hormone, thus maintaining free T4 and T3 serum concentrations in the normal range. Patients dependent on thyroid hormone replacement therapy who are also receiving estrogen may require increased doses of their thyroid replacement therapy. These patients should have their thyroid function monitored to maintain their free throid hormone levels in an acceptable range). Products include:

Cytomel Tablets 1778

Liotrix (Estrogen administration leads to increased thyroid-binding globulin (TBG) levels. Patients with normal thyroid function can compensate for the increased TBG by making more thyroid hormone, thus maintaining free T4 and T3 serum concentrations in the normal range. Patients dependent on thyroid hormone replacement therapy who are also receiving estrogen may require increased doses of their thyroid replacement therapy. These patients should have their thyroid function monitored to maintain their free throid hormone levels in an acceptable range).

No products indexed under this heading.

Thyroglobulin (Estrogen administration leads to increased thyroid-binding globulin (TBG) levels. Patients with normal thyroid function can compensate for the increased TBG by making more thyroid hormone, thus maintaining free T4 and T3 serum concentrations in the normal range. Patients dependent on thyroid hormone replacement therapy who are also receiving estrogen may require increased doses of their thyroid replacement therapy. These patients should have their thyroid function monitored to maintain their free throid hormone levels in an acceptable range).

No products indexed under this heading.

Thyroid (Estrogen administration leads to increased thyroid-binding globulin (TBG) levels. Patients with normal thyroid function can compensate for the increased TBG by making more thyroid hormone, thus maintaining free T4 and T3 serum concentrations in the normal range. Patients dependent on thyroid hormone replacement therapy who are also receiving estrogen may require increased doses of their thyroid replacement therapy. These patients should have their thyroid function monitored to maintain their free throid hormone levels in an acceptable range). Products include:

Naturethroid Tablets 2605

Thyroxine (Estrogen administration leads to increased thyroid-binding globulin (TBG) levels. Patients with normal thyroid function can compensate for the increased TBG by making more thyroid hormone, thus maintaining free T4 and T3 serum concentrations in the normal range. Patients dependent on thyroid hormone replacement therapy who are also receiving estrogen may require increased doses of their thyroid replacement therapy. These patients should have their thyroid function monitored to maintain their free throid hormone levels in an acceptable range).

No products indexed under this heading.

Thyroxine Sodium (Estrogen administration leads to increased thyroid-binding globulin (TBG) levels. Patients with normal thyroid function can compensate for the increased TBG by making more thyroid hormone, thus maintaining free T4 and T3 serum concentrations in the normal range. Patients dependent on thyroid hormone replacement therapy who are also receiving estrogen may require increased doses of their thyroid replacement therapy. These patients should have their thyroid function monitored to maintain their free throid hormone levels in an acceptable range).

No products indexed under this heading.

ACTONEL TABLETS

(Risedronate Sodium) 2568

May interact with antacids containing aluminum, calcium and magnesium, calcium preparations, cations, and certain other agents. Compounds in these categories include:

Aluminum Carbonate (Antacids may interfere with the absorption of risedronate sodium; antacids should be taken at a different time of the day).

No products indexed under this heading.

Aluminum-containing Compounds, unspecified (Medications containing divalent cations may interfere with the absorption of risedronate sodium: these medications should be taken at a different time of the day).

No products indexed under this heading.

Aluminum Hydroxide (Antacids may interfere with the absorption of risedronate sodium; antacids should be taken at a different time of the day).

No products indexed under this heading.

Aspirin (The incidence of gastrointestinal adverse events is, in general, higher with co-administration; caution should be used). Products include:

Aggrenox Capsules 819
Bayer Aspirin 750
Percodan Tablets 1130
St. Joseph 81 mg Aspirin Chewable and Enteric Coated Tablets 1903

Calcium (Medications containing divalent cations may interfere with the absorption of risedronate sodium: these medications should be taken at a different time of the day). Products include:

Phyto-Vite Tablets .... ■ 639
Vibe Liquid Multi-Nutrient Supplement .... ■ 626

Calcium Carbonate (Calcium-containing preparations may interfere with the absorption of risedronate sodium; calcium preparations should be taken at a different time of the day). Products include:

Accelerator Tablets .... ■ 634
Actonel with Calcium Tablets 2574
BioLean II Tablets .... ■ 635
Calcet Triple Calcium + Vitamin D Tablets .... ■ 629
D-Cal Chewable Caplets .... ■ 624
Elixir Capsules .... ■ 636
Pepcid Complete Chewable Tablets 1771
Extra Strength Rolaids Plus Gas Relief Tropical Fruit Softchews 1903
Extra Strength Rolaids Softchews Vanilla Creme 1903
Extra Strength Rolaids Freshmint Tablets 1903
Rolaids Multi-Symptom Berry Tablets 1903
Rolaids Original Peppermint Tablets 1903

Calcium Chloride (Calcium-containing preparations may interfere with the absorption of risedronate sodium; calcium preparations should be taken at a different time of the day).

No products indexed under this heading.

Calcium Citrate (Calcium-containing preparations may interfere with the absorption of risedronate sodium; calcium preparations should be taken at a different time of the day). Products include:

Active Calcium Tablets 3173
CitraNatal DHA Tablets 2175
CitraNatal 90 DHA Tablets 2175

Calcium Glubionate (Calcium-containing preparations may interfere with the absorption of risedronate sodium; calcium preparations should be taken at a different time of the day).

No products indexed under this heading.

Iron (Medications containing divalent cations may interfere with the absorption of risedronate sodium: these medications should be taken at a different time of the day). Products include:

Phyto-Vite Tablets .... ■ 639

Magaldrate (Antacids may interfere with the absorption of risedronate sodium; antacids should be taken at a different time of the day).

No products indexed under this heading.

Magnesium (Medications containing divalent cations may interfere with the absorption of risedronate sodium: these medications should be taken at a different time of the day). Products include:

Protector Capsules .... ■ 639
Vibe Liquid Multi-Nutrient Supplement .... ■ 626

Magnesium Hydroxide (Antacids may interfere with the absorption of risedronate sodium; antacids should be taken at a different time of the day). Products include:

Fleet Pedia-Lax Chewable Tablets 1145
Pepcid Complete Chewable Tablets 1771
Extra Strength Rolaids Freshmint Tablets 1903
Rolaids Multi-Symptom Berry Tablets 1903
Rolaids Original Peppermint Tablets 1903

Magnesium Oxide (Antacids may interfere with the absorption of risedronate sodium; antacids should be taken at a different time of the day). Products include:

Beelith Tablets 813

Zinc (Medications containing divalent cations may interfere with the absorption of risedronate sodium: these medications should be taken at a different time of the day). Products include:

Comax Dietary Supplement 995
Glaucofit Dietary Supplement 995
Glauma Dietary Supplement 995
Tonox Dietary Supplement 995
Vibe Liquid Multi-Nutrient Supplement .... ■ 626
Visutein Capsules 3159

Food Interactions

Food, unspecified (Mean oral bioavailability is decreased when risedronate is administered with food; risedronate sodium is effective when administered at least 30 minutes before breakfast).

ACTONEL WITH CALCIUM TABLETS

(Calcium Carbonate, Risedronate Sodium) 2574

May interact with antacids, antacids containing aluminum, calcium and magnesium, bisphosphonates, calcium preparations, cations, fluoroquinolone antibiotics, glucocorticoids, iron containing oral preparations, tetracyclines, thiazides, and certain other agents. Compounds in these categories include:

Alatrofloxacin Mesylate (Concomitant administration of a fluoroquinolone and calcium carbonate may decrease the absorption of the flouroquinolone).

No products indexed under this heading.

Alendronate Sodium (Co-administration with calcium may lead to a decrease in biphosphonate absorption). Products include:

Fosamax 2005
Fosamax Plus D Tablets 2013

Aluminum Carbonate (Antacids may interfere with the absorption of risedronate sodium; antacids should be taken at a different time of the day).

No products indexed under this heading.

Aluminum-containing Compounds, unspecified (Co-administration of risedronate sodium and calcium, antacids, or oral medications containing divalent cations will interfere with the absorption of risedronate sodium).

No products indexed under this heading.

Aluminum Hydroxide (Antacids may interfere with the absorption of risedronate sodium; antacids should be taken at a different time of the day).

No products indexed under this heading.

Aspirin (The incidence of gastrointestinal adverse events is, in general, higher with co-administration; caution should be used). Products include:

Aggrenox Capsules 819
Bayer Aspirin 750
Percodan Tablets 1130
St. Joseph 81 mg Aspirin Chewable and Enteric Coated Tablets 1903

Bendroflumethiazide (Reduced urinary excretion of calcium has been reported during concomitant use of calcium carbonate and thiazide diuretics).

No products indexed under this heading.

Betamethasone Acetate (Calcium absorption is reduced when calcium carbonate is taken concomitantly with systemic glucocorticoids).

No products indexed under this heading.

Betamethasone Sodium Phosphate (Calcium absorption is reduced when calcium carbonate is taken concomitantly with systemic glucocorticoids).

No products indexed under this heading.

Calcitriol (Absorption of calcium may be increased when calcium carbonate is given concomitantly with vitamin D analogues). Products include:

Calcijex Injection 419
Rocaltrol Capsules 1150
Rocaltrol Oral Solution 1150

Calcium (Co-administration of risedronate sodium and calcium, antacids, or oral medications containing divalent cations will interfere with the absorption of risedronate sodium). Products include:

Phyto-Vite Tablets .... ■ 639
Vibe Liquid Multi-Nutrient Supplement .... ■ 626

Calcium Chloride (Co-administration of risedronate sodium and calcium, antacids, or oral medications containing divalent cations will interfere with the absorption of risedronate sodium).

No products indexed under this heading.

Calcium Citrate (Co-administration of risedronate sodium and calcium, antacids, or oral medications containing divalent cations will interfere with the absorption of risedronate sodium). Products include:

Active Calcium Tablets 3173
CitraNatal DHA Tablets 2175
CitraNatal 90 DHA Tablets 2175

Calcium Glubionate (Co-administration of risedronate sodium and calcium, antacids, or oral medications containing divalent cations will interfere with the absorption of risedronate sodium).
No products indexed under this heading.

Chlorothiazide (Reduced urinary excretion of calcium has been reported during concomitant use of calcium carbonate and thiazide diuretics).
No products indexed under this heading.

Chlorothiazide Sodium (Reduced urinary excretion of calcium has been reported during concomitant use of calcium carbonate and thiazide diuretics). Products include:
Intravenous Sodium Diuril 2490

Ciprofloxacin (Concomitant administration of a fluoroquinolone and calcium carbonate may decrease the absorption of the flouroquinolone). Products include:
Cipro I.V. 2817
Cipro Oral Suspension 2810
Cipro XR Tablets 2823
Ciprodex Otic Suspension 541

Ciprofloxacin Hydrochloride (Concomitant administration of a fluoroquinolone and calcium carbonate may decrease the absorption of the flouroquinolone). Products include:
Cipro Tablets 2810

Cortisone Acetate (Calcium absorption is reduced when calcium carbonate is taken concomitantly with systemic glucocorticoids).
No products indexed under this heading.

Demeclocycline Hydrochloride (Concomitant administration of a tetracycline and a calcium carbonate may decrease the absorption of the tetracycline).
No products indexed under this heading.

Dexamethasone (Calcium absorption is reduced when calcium carbonate is taken concomitantly with systemic glucocorticoids). Products include:
Ciprodex Otic Suspension 541

Dexamethasone Acetate (Calcium absorption is reduced when calcium carbonate is taken concomitantly with systemic glucocorticoids).
No products indexed under this heading.

Dexamethasone Sodium Phosphate (Calcium absorption is reduced when calcium carbonate is taken concomitantly with systemic glucocorticoids).
No products indexed under this heading.

Doxercalciferol (Absorption of calcium may be increased when calcium carbonate is given concomitantly with vitamin D analogues).
No products indexed under this heading.

Doxycycline Calcium (Concomitant administration of a tetracycline and a calcium carbonate may decrease the absorption of the tetracycline).
No products indexed under this heading.

Doxycycline Hyclate (Concomitant administration of a tetracycline and a calcium carbonate may decrease the absorption of the tetracycline).
No products indexed under this heading.

Doxycycline Monohydrate (Concomitant administration of a tetracycline and a calcium carbonate may decrease the absorption of the tetracycline).
No products indexed under this heading.

Enoxacin (Concomitant administration of a fluoroquinolone and calcium carbonate may decrease the absorption of the flouroquinolone).
No products indexed under this heading.

Etidronate Disodium (Co-administration with calcium may lead to a decrease in biphosphonate absorption). Products include:
Didronel Tablets 2583

Ferrous Fumarate (Calcium may interfere with the absorption of iron. Patients being treated for iron-deficiency should take iron and calcium at different times of the day).
No products indexed under this heading.

Ferrous Gluconate (Calcium may interfere with the absorption of iron. Patients being treated for iron-deficiency should take iron and calcium at different times of the day). Products include:
CitraNatal DHA Tablets 2175

Ferrous Sulfate (Calcium may interfere with the absorption of iron. Patients being treated for iron-deficiency should take iron and calcium at different times of the day).
No products indexed under this heading.

Fludrocortisone Acetate (Calcium absorption is reduced when calcium carbonate is taken concomitantly with systemic glucocorticoids).
No products indexed under this heading.

Gatifloxacin (Concomitant administration of a fluoroquinolone and calcium carbonate may decrease the absorption of the flouroquinolone).
No products indexed under this heading.

Grepafloxacin Hydrochloride (Concomitant administration of a fluoroquinolone and calcium carbonate may decrease the absorption of the flouroquinolone).
No products indexed under this heading.

Hydrochlorothiazide (Reduced urinary excretion of calcium has been reported during concomitant use of calcium carbonate and thiazide diuretics). Products include:
Atacand HCT 642
Avalide Tablets 892
Avalide Tablets 2713
Benicar HCT Tablets 1010
Diovan HCT Tablets 2216
Dyazide Capsules 1405
Micardis HCT Tablets 854
Prinzide Tablets 2092
Tekturna HCT Tablets 2324
Teveten HCT Tablets 517

Hydrocortisone (Calcium absorption is reduced when calcium carbonate is taken concomitantly with systemic glucocorticoids).
No products indexed under this heading.

Hydrocortisone Acetate (Calcium absorption is reduced when calcium carbonate is taken concomitantly with systemic glucocorticoids). Products include:
Analpram-HC 1140
Pramosone 1141

Hydrocortisone Sodium Phosphate (Calcium absorption is reduced when calcium carbonate is taken concomitantly with systemic glucocorticoids).
No products indexed under this heading.

Hydrocortisone Sodium Succinate (Calcium absorption is reduced when calcium carbonate is taken concomitantly with systemic glucocorticoids).
No products indexed under this heading.

Hydroflumethiazide (Reduced urinary excretion of calcium has been reported during concomitant use of calcium carbonate and thiazide diuretics).
No products indexed under this heading.

Iron (Calcium may interfere with the absorption of iron. Patients being treated for iron-deficiency should take iron and calcium at different times of the day). Products include:
Phyto-Vite Tablets .... ▣ 639

Levofloxacin (Concomitant administration of a fluoroquinolone and calcium carbonate may decrease the absorption of the flouroquinolone). Products include:
Iquix Ophthalmic Solution 3183
Levaquin 2416
Levaquin in 5% Dextrose Injection 2416
Quixin Ophthalmic Solution 3184

Levothyroxine Sodium (Concomitant intake of levothyroxine and calcium carbonate was found to reduce levothyroxine absorption and increase serum thyrotropin levels). Products include:
Levothroid Tablets 1170
Levoxyl Tablets 1780
Synthroid Tablets 507

Lomefloxacin Hydrochloride (Concomitant administration of a fluoroquinolone and calcium carbonate may decrease the absorption of the flouroquinolone).
No products indexed under this heading.

Magaldrate (Antacids may interfere with the absorption of risedronate sodium; antacids should be taken at a different time of the day).
No products indexed under this heading.

Magnesium (Co-administration of risedronate sodium and calcium, antacids, or oral medications containing divalent cations will interfere with the absorption of risedronate sodium). Products include:
Protector Capsules .... ▣ 639
Vibe Liquid Multi-Nutrient Supplement .... ▣ 626

Magnesium Hydroxide (Antacids may interfere with the absorption of risedronate sodium; antacids should be taken at a different time of the day). Products include:
Fleet Pedia-Lax Chewable Tablets 1145
Pepcid Complete Chewable Tablets 1771
Extra Strength Rolaids Freshmint Tablets 1903
Rolaids Multi-Symptom Berry Tablets 1903
Rolaids Original Peppermint Tablets 1903

Magnesium Oxide (Antacids may interfere with the absorption of risedronate sodium; antacids should be taken at a different time of the day). Products include:
Beelith Tablets 813

Methacycline Hydrochloride (Concomitant administration of a tetracycline and a calcium carbonate may decrease the absorption of the tetracycline).
No products indexed under this heading.

Methyclothiazide (Reduced urinary excretion of calcium has been reported during concomitant use of calcium carbonate and thiazide diuretics).
No products indexed under this heading.

Methylprednisolone Acetate (Calcium absorption is reduced when calcium carbonate is taken concomitantly with systemic glucocorticoids).
No products indexed under this heading.

Methylprednisolone Sodium Succinate (Calcium absorption is reduced when calcium carbonate is taken concomitantly with systemic glucocorticoids).
No products indexed under this heading.

Minocycline Hydrochloride (Concomitant administration of a tetracycline and a calcium carbonate may decrease the absorption of the tetracycline). Products include:
Solodyn Extended Release Tablets 1938

Moxifloxacin Hydrochloride (Concomitant administration of a fluoroquinolone and calcium carbonate may decrease the absorption of the flouroquinolone). Products include:
Avelox 2803
Vigamox Ophthalmic Solution 548

Norfloxacin (Concomitant administration of a fluoroquinolone and calcium carbonate may decrease the absorption of the flouroquinolone). Products include:
Noroxin Tablets 2069

Ofloxacin (Concomitant administration of a fluoroquinolone and calcium carbonate may decrease the absorption of the flouroquinolone). Products include:
Ofloxacin Ophthalmic Solution 0.3% .... ⊙ 243

Oxytetracycline Hydrochloride (Concomitant administration of a tetracycline and a calcium carbonate may decrease the absorption of the tetracycline).
No products indexed under this heading.

Paricalcitol (Absorption of calcium may be increased when calcium carbonate is given concomitantly with vitamin D analogues). Products include:
Zemplar Capsules 536
Zemplar Injection 538

Polysaccharide Iron Complex (Calcium may interfere with the absorption of iron. Patients being treated for iron-deficiency should take iron and calcium at different times of the day). Products include:
Nu-Iron 150 Capsules 2165

IMPORTANT NOTE: Always consult each drug listing in the patient's regimen for possible interactions.

Polythiazide (Reduced urinary excretion of calcium has been reported during concomitant use of calcium carbonate and thiazide diuretics).
No products indexed under this heading.

Prednisolone Acetate (Calcium absorption is reduced when calcium carbonate is taken concomitantly with systemic glucocorticoids).
Products include:
- Pred Forte Ophthalmic Suspension .... ⊙ 227
- Pred Mild Ophthalmic Suspension .... ⊙ 230
- Pred-G Ophthalmic Ointment .... ⊙ 229
- Pred-G Ophthalmic Suspension .... ⊙ 228

Prednisolone Sodium Phosphate (Calcium absorption is reduced when calcium carbonate is taken concomitantly with systemic glucocorticoids).
No products indexed under this heading.

Prednisolone Tebutate (Calcium absorption is reduced when calcium carbonate is taken concomitantly with systemic glucocorticoids).
No products indexed under this heading.

Prednisone (Calcium absorption is reduced when calcium carbonate is taken concomitantly with systemic glucocorticoids).
No products indexed under this heading.

Sodium Bicarbonate (Co-administration of risedronate sodium and calcium, antacids, or oral medications containing divalent cations will interfere with the absorption of risedronate sodium). Products include:
- Ceo-Two Laxative Suppository 815

Tetracycline Hydrochloride (Concomitant administration of a tetracycline and a calcium carbonate may decrease the absorption of the tetracycline). Products include:
- Pylera Capsules 714

Tiludronate Disodium (Co-administration with calcium may lead to a decrease in biphosphonate absorption).
No products indexed under this heading.

Triamcinolone (Calcium absorption is reduced when calcium carbonate is taken concomitantly with systemic glucocorticoids).
No products indexed under this heading.

Triamcinolone Acetonide (Calcium absorption is reduced when calcium carbonate is taken concomitantly with systemic glucocorticoids). Products include:
- Azmacort Inhalation Aerosol 407
- Nasacort AQ Nasal Spray 2765
- Triesence Injectable Suspension .... ⊙ 209

Triamcinolone Diacetate (Calcium absorption is reduced when calcium carbonate is taken concomitantly with systemic glucocorticoids).
No products indexed under this heading.

Triamcinolone Hexacetonide (Calcium absorption is reduced when calcium carbonate is taken concomitantly with systemic glucocorticoids).
No products indexed under this heading.

Trovafloxacin Mesylate (Concomitant administration of a fluoroquinolone and calcium carbonate may decrease the absorption of the flouroquinolone).
No products indexed under this heading.

Vitamin D (Absorption of calcium may be increased when calcium carbonate is given concomitantly with vitamin D analogues). Products include:
- Active Calcium Tablets 3173
- D-Cal Chewable Caplets .... ▣ 624
- Norwegian Cod Liver Oil 949

Zinc (Co-administration of risedronate sodium and calcium, antacids, or oral medications containing divalent cations will interfere with the absorption of risedronate sodium).
Products include:
- Comax Dietary Supplement 995
- Glaucofit Dietary Supplement 995
- Glauma Dietary Supplement 995
- Tonox Dietary Supplement 995
- Vibe Liquid Multi-Nutrient Supplement .... ▣ 626
- Visutein Capsules 3159

Food Interactions

Food, unspecified (Mean oral bioavailability is decreased when risedronate is administered with food; risedronate sodium is effective when administered at least 30 minutes before breakfast).

ACTOPLUS MET TABLETS

(Metformin Hydrochloride, Pioglitazone Hydrochloride) 3071

May interact with cationic drugs that are eliminated by renal tubular, calcium channel blockers, corticosteroids, cytochrome p450 3a4 substrates (selected), diuretics, estrogens, oral hypoglycemic agents, insulin, oral contraceptives, phenothiazines, phenytoin, sympathomimetics, thiazides, thyroid preparations, and certain other agents. Compounds in these categories include:

Acarbose (Pioglitazone, like other thiazolidinediones, can cause fluid retention when used alone or in combination with other antihyperglycemic agents, including insulin). Products include:
- Precose Tablets 792

Albuterol (Certain drugs, including sympathomimetics, tend to produce hyperglycemia and may lead to loss of glycemic control. When such drugs are administered to a patient receiving Actoplus Met, the patient should be closely observed to maintain adequate glycemic control).
No products indexed under this heading.

Albuterol Sulfate (Certain drugs, including sympathomimetics, tend to produce hyperglycemia and may lead to loss of glycemic control. When such drugs are administered to a patient receiving Actoplus Met, the patient should be closely observed to maintain adequate glycemic control). Products include:
- Combivent Inhalation Aerosol 845
- ProAir HFA Inhalation Aerosol 3113
- Proventil HFA Inhalation Aerosol 2914
- Ventolin HFA Inhalation Aerosol 1638

Alfentanil Hydrochloride (Studies have suggested that pioglitazone may be a weak inducer of CYP450 isoform 3A4 substrate).
No products indexed under this heading.

Alprazolam (Studies have suggested that pioglitazone may be a weak inducer of CYP450 isoform 3A4 substrate).
No products indexed under this heading.

Amiloride Hydrochloride (Cationic drugs that are eliminated by renal tubular secretion theoretically have the potential for interaction with metformin by competing for common renal tubular transport systems. Although such interactions remain theoretical, careful patient monitoring and dose adjustment of Actoplus Met and/or the interfering drug is recommended in patients who are taking cationic medications that are excreted via the proximal renal tubular secretory system).
No products indexed under this heading.

Amiodarone Hydrochloride (Studies have suggested that pioglitazone may be a weak inducer of CYP450 isoform 3A4 substrate).
No products indexed under this heading.

Amitriptyline Hydrochloride (Studies have suggested that pioglitazone may be a weak inducer of CYP450 isoform 3A4 substrate).
No products indexed under this heading.

Amlodipine Besylate (Certain drugs, including calcium channel blockers, tend to produce hyperglycemia and may lead to loss of glycemic control. When such drugs are administered to a patient receiving Actoplus Met, the patient should be closely observed to maintain adequate glycemic control). Products include:
- Azor Tablets 1005
- Exforge Tablets 2238

Aprepitant (Studies have suggested that pioglitazone may be a weak inducer of CYP450 isoform 3A4 substrate). Products include:
- Emend Capsules 1992

Astemizole (Studies have suggested that pioglitazone may be a weak inducer of CYP450 isoform 3A4 substrate).
No products indexed under this heading.

Atorvastatin Calcium (Studies have suggested that pioglitazone may be a weak inducer of CYP450 isoform 3A4 substrate). Products include:
- Lipitor Tablets 2501

Belladonna Ergotamine (Studies have suggested that pioglitazone may be a weak inducer of CYP450 isoform 3A4 substrate).
No products indexed under this heading.

Bendroflumethiazide (Certain drugs, including thiazide diuretics, tend to produce hyperglycemia and may lead to loss of glycemic control. When such drugs are administered to a patient receiving Actoplus Met, the patient should be closely observed to maintain adequate glycemic control).
No products indexed under this heading.

Bepridil Hydrochloride (Certain drugs, including calcium channel blockers, tend to produce hyperglycemia and may lead to loss of glycemic control. When such drugs are administered to a patient receiving Actoplus Met, the patient should be closely observed to maintain adequate glycemic control).
No products indexed under this heading.

Betamethasone Acetate (Certain drugs, including corticosteroids, tend to produce hyperglycemia and may lead to loss of glycemic control. When such drugs are administered to a patient receiving Actoplus Met, the patient should be closely observed to maintain adequate glycemic control).
No products indexed under this heading.

Betamethasone Sodium Phosphate (Certain drugs, including corticosteroids, tend to produce hyperglycemia and may lead to loss of glycemic control. When such drugs are administered to a patient receiving Actoplus Met, the patient should be closely observed to maintain adequate glycemic control).
No products indexed under this heading.

Budesonide (Certain drugs, including corticosteroids, tend to produce hyperglycemia and may lead to loss of glycemic control. When such drugs are administered to a patient receiving Actoplus Met, the patient should be closely observed to maintain adequate glycemic control). Products include:
- Pulmicort Flexhaler 654
- Symbicort 80/4.5 Inhalation Aerosol 659
- Symbicort 160/4.5 Inhalation Aerosol 659

Bumetanide (Certain drugs, including diuretics, tend to produce hyperglycemia and may lead to loss of glycemic control. When such drugs are administered to a patient receiving Actoplus Met, the patient should be closely observed to maintain adequate glycemic control).
No products indexed under this heading.

Buspirone Hydrochloride (Studies have suggested that pioglitazone may be a weak inducer of CYP450 isoform 3A4 substrate).
No products indexed under this heading.

Busulfan (Studies have suggested that pioglitazone may be a weak inducer of CYP450 isoform 3A4 substrate). Products include:
- Busulfex Injection 2477
- Myleran Tablets 1530

Carbamazepine (Studies have suggested that pioglitazone may be a weak inducer of CYP450 isoform 3A4 substrate). Products include:
- Carbatrol Capsules 3019
- Equetro Extended-Release Capsules 3174

Cerivastatin Sodium (Studies have suggested that pioglitazone may be a weak inducer of CYP450 isoform 3A4 substrate).
No products indexed under this heading.

Chlorothiazide (Certain drugs, including thiazide diuretics, tend to produce hyperglycemia and may lead to loss of glycemic control. When such drugs are administered to a patient receiving Actoplus Met, the patient should be closely observed to maintain adequate glycemic control).
No products indexed under this heading.

Chlorothiazide Sodium (Certain drugs, including thiazide diuretics, tend to produce hyperglycemia and may lead to loss of glycemic control. When such drugs are administered to a patient receiving Actoplus Met, the patient should be closely observed to maintain adequate glycemic control). Products include:
Intravenous Sodium Diuril 2490

Chlorotrianisene (Certain drugs, including estrogens, tend to produce hyperglycemia and may lead to loss of glycemic control. When such drugs are administered to a patient receiving Actoplus Met, the patient should be closely observed to maintain adequate glycemic control).
No products indexed under this heading.

Chlorpheniramine (Studies have suggested that pioglitazone may be a weak inducer of CYP450 isoform 3A4 substrate).
No products indexed under this heading.

Chlorpheniramine Maleate (Studies have suggested that pioglitazone may be a weak inducer of CYP450 isoform 3A4 substrate). Products include:
Actifed Cold & Allergy Tablets 1895
Sudafed PE Sinus & Allergy Tablets 1908
Tylenol Allergy Multi-Symptom Caplets with Cool Burst and Rapid Release Gelcaps 1916
Children's Tylenol Plus Cold Suspension Liquid 1912
Children's Tylenol Plus Cough & Runny Nose Suspension Liquid 1912
Children's Tylenol Plus Flu Suspension Liquid 1914
Children's Tylenol Plus Multi-Symptom Cold Suspension Liquid 1912
Tylenol Cold Head Congestion Nighttime Caplets with Cool Burst 1910
Tylenol Cold Multi-Symptom Nighttime Caplets with Cool Burst 1913
Tylenol Sinus Congestion & Pain Nighttime Caplets with Cool Burst 1917

Chlorpheniramine Polistirex (Studies have suggested that pioglitazone may be a weak inducer of CYP450 isoform 3A4 substrate). Products include:
Tussionex Pennkinetic Extended-Release Suspension 3154

Chlorpheniramine Tannate (Studies have suggested that pioglitazone may be a weak inducer of CYP450 isoform 3A4 substrate).
No products indexed under this heading.

Chlorpromazine (Certain drugs, including phenothiazines, tend to produce hyperglycemia and may lead to loss of glycemic control. When such drugs are administered to a patient receiving Actoplus Met, the patient should be closely observed to maintain adequate glycemic control).
No products indexed under this heading.

Chlorpromazine Hydrochloride (Certain drugs, including phenothiazines, tend to produce hyperglycemia and may lead to loss of glycemic control. When such drugs are administered to a patient receiving Actoplus Met, the patient should be closely observed to maintain adequate glycemic control).
No products indexed under this heading.

Chlorpropamide (Pioglitazone, like other thiazolidinediones, can cause fluid retention when used alone or in combination with other antihyperglycemic agents, including insulin).
No products indexed under this heading.

Chlorthalidone (Certain drugs, including diuretics, tend to produce hyperglycemia and may lead to loss of glycemic control. When such drugs are administered to a patient receiving Actoplus Met, the patient should be closely observed to maintain adequate glycemic control). Products include:
Clorpres Tablets 2185

Ciclesonide (Certain drugs, including corticosteroids, tend to produce hyperglycemia and may lead to loss of glycemic control. When such drugs are administered to a patient receiving Actoplus Met, the patient should be closely observed to maintain adequate glycemic control). Products include:
Alvesco Inhalation Aerosol 2985
Omnaris Nasal Spray 2998

Cimetidine (Cationic drugs that are eliminated by renal tubular secretion and theoretically have the potential for interaction with metformin by competing for common renal tubular transport systems. Although such interactions remain theoretical (except for cimetidine), careful patient monitoring and dose adjustment of Actolus Met and/or the interfering drug is recommended in patients who are taking cationic medications that are excreted via the proximal renal tubular secretory system).
No products indexed under this heading.

Cimetidine Hydrochloride (Cationic drugs that are eliminated by renal tubular secretion and theoretically have the potential for interaction with metformin by competing for common renal tubular transport systems. Although such interactions remain theoretical (except for cimetidine), careful patient monitoring and dose adjustment of Actolus Met and/or the interfering drug is recommended in patients who are taking cationic medications that are excreted via the proximal renal tubular secretory system).
No products indexed under this heading.

Cisapride (Studies have suggested that pioglitazone may be a weak inducer of CYP450 isoform 3A4 substrate).
No products indexed under this heading.

Clarithromycin (Studies have suggested that pioglitazone may be a weak inducer of CYP450 isoform 3A4 substrate). Products include:
Biaxin/Biaxin XL 411

Cortisone Acetate (Certain drugs, including corticosteroids, tend to produce hyperglycemia and may lead to loss of glycemic control. When such drugs are administered to a patient receiving Actoplus Met, the patient should be closely observed to maintain adequate glycemic control).
No products indexed under this heading.

Cyclosporine (Studies have suggested that pioglitazone may be a weak inducer of CYP450 isoform 3A4 substrate). Products include:
Gengraf Capsules 435
Neoral Oral Solution 2280
Neoral Soft Gelatin Capsules 2280
Restasis Ophthalmic Emulsion 557
Sandimmune 2296

Desogestrel (Certain drugs, including oral contraceptives, tend to produce hyperglycemia and may lead to loss of glycemic control. When such drugs are administered to a patient receiving Actoplus Met, the patient should be closely observed to maintain adequate glycemic control). Products include:
Mircette Tablets 1034

Dexamethasone (Certain drugs, including corticosteroids, tend to produce hyperglycemia and may lead to loss of glycemic control. When such drugs are administered to a patient receiving Actoplus Met, the patient should be closely observed to maintain adequate glycemic control). Products include:
Ciprodex Otic Suspension 541

Dexamethasone Acetate (Certain drugs, including corticosteroids, tend to produce hyperglycemia and may lead to loss of glycemic control. When such drugs are administered to a patient receiving Actoplus Met, the patient should be closely observed to maintain adequate glycemic control).
No products indexed under this heading.

Dexamethasone Sodium Phosphate (Certain drugs, including corticosteroids, tend to produce hyperglycemia and may lead to loss of glycemic control. When such drugs are administered to a patient receiving Actoplus Met, the patient should be closely observed to maintain adequate glycemic control).
No products indexed under this heading.

Diazepam (Studies have suggested that pioglitazone may be a weak inducer of CYP450 isoform 3A4 substrate). Products include:
Valium Tablets 2658

Dienestrol (Certain drugs, including estrogens, tend to produce hyperglycemia and may lead to loss of glycemic control. When such drugs are administered to a patient receiving Actoplus Met, the patient should be closely observed to maintain adequate glycemic control).
No products indexed under this heading.

Diethylstilbestrol (Certain drugs, including estrogens, tend to produce hyperglycemia and may lead to loss of glycemic control. When such drugs are administered to a patient receiving Actoplus Met, the patient should be closely observed to maintain adequate glycemic control).
No products indexed under this heading.

Digoxin (Cationic drugs that are eliminated by renal tubular secretion theoretically have the potential for interaction with metformin by competing for common renal tubular transport systems. Although such interactions remain theoretical, careful patient monitoring and dose adjustment of Actoplus Met and/or the interfering drug is recommended in patients who are taking cationic medications that are excreted via the proximal renal tubular secretory system). Products include:
Lanoxin Injection 1498
Lanoxin Injection Pediatric 1502
Lanoxin Tablets 1505

Dihydroergotamine Mesylate (Studies have suggested that pioglitazone may be a weak inducer of CYP450 isoform 3A4 substrate).
No products indexed under this heading.

Diltiazem Hydrochloride (Certain drugs, including calcium channel blockers, tend to produce hyperglycemia and may lead to loss of glycemic control. When such drugs are administered to a patient receiving Actoplus Met, the patient should be closely observed to maintain adequate glycemic control). Products include:
Cardizem LA Extended Release Tablets 421

Diltiazem Maleate (Studies have suggested that pioglitazone may be a weak inducer of CYP450 isoform 3A4 substrate).
No products indexed under this heading.

Disopyramide (Studies have suggested that pioglitazone may be a weak inducer of CYP450 isoform 3A4 substrate).
No products indexed under this heading.

Disopyramide Phosphate (Studies have suggested that pioglitazone may be a weak inducer of CYP450 isoform 3A4 substrate).
No products indexed under this heading.

Disulfiram (Studies have suggested that pioglitazone may be a weak inducer of CYP450 isoform 3A4 substrate).
No products indexed under this heading.

Dobutamine Hydrochloride (Certain drugs, including sympathomimetics, tend to produce hyperglycemia and may lead to loss of glycemic control. When such drugs are administered to a patient receiving Actoplus Met, the patient should be closely observed to maintain adequate glycemic control).
No products indexed under this heading.

Dopamine Hydrochloride (Certain drugs, including sympathomimetics, tend to produce hyperglycemia and may lead to loss of glycemic control. When such drugs are administered to a patient receiving Actoplus Met, the patient should be closely observed to maintain adequate glycemic control)..
No products indexed under this heading.

Doxorubicin Hydrochloride (Studies have suggested that pioglitazone may be a weak inducer of CYP450 isoform 3A4 substrate).
No products indexed under this heading.

IMPORTANT NOTE: Always consult each drug listing in the patient's regimen for possible interactions.

Dronabinol (Studies have suggested that pioglitazone may be a weak inducer of CYP450 isoform 3A4 substrate). Products include:
Marinol Capsules 3163

Ephedrine Hydrochloride (Certain drugs, including sympathomimetics, tend to produce hyperglycemia and may lead to loss of glycemic control. When such drugs are administered to a patient receiving Actoplus Met, the patient should be closely observed to maintain adequate glycemic control).
No products indexed under this heading.

Ephedrine Sulfate (Certain drugs, including sympathomimetics, tend to produce hyperglycemia and may lead to loss of glycemic control. When such drugs are administered to a patient receiving Actoplus Met, the patient should be closely observed to maintain adequate glycemic control).
No products indexed under this heading.

Ephedrine Tannate (Certain drugs, including sympathomimetics, tend to produce hyperglycemia and may lead to loss of glycemic control. When such drugs are administered to a patient receiving Actoplus Met, the patient should be closely observed to maintain adequate glycemic control).
No products indexed under this heading.

Epinephrine (Certain drugs, including sympathomimetics, tend to produce hyperglycemia and may lead to loss of glycemic control. When such drugs are administered to a patient receiving Actoplus Met, the patient should be closely observed to maintain adequate glycemic control). Products include:
EpiPen 1024

Epinephrine Bitartrate (Certain drugs, including sympathomimetics, tend to produce hyperglycemia and may lead to loss of glycemic control. When such drugs are administered to a patient receiving Actoplus Met, the patient should be closely observed to maintain adequate glycemic control).
No products indexed under this heading.

Epinephrine Hydrochloride (Certain drugs, including sympathomimetics, tend to produce hyperglycemia and may lead to loss of glycemic control. When such drugs are administered to a patient receiving Actoplus Met, the patient should be closely observed to maintain adequate glycemic control).
No products indexed under this heading.

Ergotamine Tartrate (Studies have suggested that pioglitazone may be a weak inducer of CYP450 isoform 3A4 substrate).
No products indexed under this heading.

Erythromycin (Studies have suggested that pioglitazone may be a weak inducer of CYP450 isoform 3A4 substrate).
No products indexed under this heading.

Erythromycin Estolate (Studies have suggested that pioglitazone may be a weak inducer of CYP450 isoform 3A4 substrate).
No products indexed under this heading.

Erythromycin Ethylsuccinate (Studies have suggested that pioglitazone may be a weak inducer of CYP450 isoform 3A4 substrate). Products include:
E.E.S. 433
EryPed 431

Erythromycin Gluceptate (Studies have suggested that pioglitazone may be a weak inducer of CYP450 isoform 3A4 substrate).
No products indexed under this heading.

Erythromycin Lactobionate (Studies have suggested that pioglitazone may be a weak inducer of CYP450 isoform 3A4 substrate).
No products indexed under this heading.

Erythromycin Stearate (Studies have suggested that pioglitazone may be a weak inducer of CYP450 isoform 3A4 substrate).
No products indexed under this heading.

Estradiol (Certain drugs, including estrogens, tend to produce hyperglycemia and may lead to loss of glycemic control. When such drugs are administered to a patient receiving Actoplus Met, the patient should be closely observed to maintain adequate glycemic control). Products include:
Activella Tablets 2347
Angeliq Tablets 751
Climara Transdermal System 763
Climara Pro Transdermal System 768
Divigel 3167
Vagifem Tablets 2375

Estradiol Benzoate (Studies have suggested that pioglitazone may be a weak inducer of CYP450 isoform 3A4 substrate).
No products indexed under this heading.

Estradiol Cypionate (Studies have suggested that pioglitazone may be a weak inducer of CYP450 isoform 3A4 substrate).
No products indexed under this heading.

Estradiol Valerate (Studies have suggested that pioglitazone may be a weak inducer of CYP450 isoform 3A4 substrate).
No products indexed under this heading.

Estrogens, Conjugated (Certain drugs, including estrogens, tend to produce hyperglycemia and may lead to loss of glycemic control. When such drugs are administered to a patient receiving Actoplus Met, the patient should be closely observed to maintain adequate glycemic control). Products include:
Premarin Intravenous 3217
Premarin Tablets 3221
Premarin Vaginal Cream 3228
Premphase Tablets 3232
Prempro Tablets 3232

Estrogens, Esterified (Certain drugs, including estrogens, tend to produce hyperglycemia and may lead to loss of glycemic control. When such drugs are administered to a patient receiving Actoplus Met, the patient should be closely observed to maintain adequate glycemic control). Products include:
Estratest Tablets 3043
Estratest H.S. Tablets 3043

Estropipate (Certain drugs, including estrogens, tend to produce hyperglycemia and may lead to loss of glycemic control. When such drugs are administered to a patient receiving Actoplus Met, the patient should be closely observed to maintain adequate glycemic control).
No products indexed under this heading.

Ethacrynic Acid (Certain drugs, including diuretics, tend to produce hyperglycemia and may lead to loss of glycemic control. When such drugs are administered to a patient receiving Actoplus Met, the patient should be closely observed to maintain adequate glycemic control). Products include:
Edecrin Tablets 698

Ethinyl Estradiol (Certain drugs, including oral contraceptives, tend to produce hyperglycemia and may lead to loss of glycemic control. When such drugs are administered to a patient receiving Actoplus Met, the patient should be closely observed to maintain adequate glycemic control). Products include:
Lybrel Tablets 3204
Mircette Tablets 1034
NuvaRing 2897
Ortho-Cyclen/Ortho Tri-Cyclen 2449
Ortho Evra Transdermal System 2437
Ortho Tri-Cyclen Lo Tablets 2458
Seasonique Tablets 1046
Yaz Tablets 805

Ethosuximide (Studies have suggested that pioglitazone may be a weak inducer of CYP450 isoform 3A4 substrate).
No products indexed under this heading.

Ethyl Alcohol (Alcohol is known to potentiate the effect of metformin on lactate metabolism. Patients, therefore, should be warned against excessive alcohol intake, acute or chronic, while receiving Actoplus Met).
No products indexed under this heading.

Ethynodiol Diacetate (Certain drugs, including oral contraceptives, tend to produce hyperglycemia and may lead to loss of glycemic control. When such drugs are administered to a patient receiving Actoplus Met, the patient should be closely observed to maintain adequate glycemic control).
No products indexed under this heading.

Etoposide (Studies have suggested that pioglitazone may be a weak inducer of CYP450 isoform 3A4 substrate).
No products indexed under this heading.

Etoposide Phosphate (Studies have suggested that pioglitazone may be a weak inducer of CYP450 isoform 3A4 substrate).
No products indexed under this heading.

Felodipine (Certain drugs, including calcium channel blockers, tend to produce hyperglycemia and may lead to loss of glycemic control. When such drugs are administered to a patient receiving Actoplus Met, the patient should be closely observed to maintain adequate glycemic control).
No products indexed under this heading.

Fentanyl (Studies have suggested that pioglitazone may be a weak inducer of CYP450 isoform 3A4 substrate). Products include:
Duragesic Transdermal System 2405
Ionsys Transdermal System 2410

Fentanyl Citrate (Studies have suggested that pioglitazone may be a weak inducer of CYP450 isoform 3A4 substrate). Products include:
Actiq 959
Fentora Tablets 968

Fludrocortisone Acetate (Certain drugs, including corticosteroids, tend to produce hyperglycemia and may lead to loss of glycemic control. When such drugs are administered to a patient receiving Actoplus Met, the patient should be closely observed to maintain adequate glycemic control).
No products indexed under this heading.

Flunisolide (Certain drugs, including corticosteroids, tend to produce hyperglycemia and may lead to loss of glycemic control. When such drugs are administered to a patient receiving Actoplus Met, the patient should be closely observed to maintain adequate glycemic control). Products include:
Aerobid/Aerobid-M 1153

Fluphenazine Decanoate (Certain drugs, including phenothiazines, tend to produce hyperglycemia and may lead to loss of glycemic control. When such drugs are administered to a patient receiving Actoplus Met, the patient should be closely observed to maintain adequate glycemic control).
No products indexed under this heading.

Fluphenazine Enanthate (Certain drugs, including phenothiazines, tend to produce hyperglycemia and may lead to loss of glycemic control. When such drugs are administered to a patient receiving Actoplus Met, the patient should be closely observed to maintain adequate glycemic control).
No products indexed under this heading.

Fluphenazine Hydrochloride (Certain drugs, including phenothiazines, tend to produce hyperglycemia and may lead to loss of glycemic control. When such drugs are administered to a patient receiving Actoplus Met, the patient should be closely observed to maintain adequate glycemic control).
No products indexed under this heading.

Fluticasone Propionate (Certain drugs, including corticosteroids, tend to produce hyperglycemia and may lead to loss of glycemic control. When such drugs are administered to a patient receiving Actoplus Met, the patient should be closely observed to maintain adequate glycemic control). Products include:
Advair Diskus 100/50 1276
Advair Diskus 250/50 1276
Advair Diskus 500/50 1276
Advair HFA 45/21 Inhalation Aerosol 1288
Advair HFA 115/21 Inhalation Aerosol 1288
Advair HFA 230/21 Inhalation Aerosol 1288
Flonase Nasal Spray 1431
Flovent Diskus 50 mcg 1435

Fluticasone Propionate HFA (Certain drugs, including corticosteroids,

tend to produce hyperglycemia and may lead to loss of glycemic control. When such drugs are administered to a patient receiving Actoplus Met, the patient should be closely observed to maintain adequate glycemic control). Products include:

Flovent HFA 1440

Fosphenytoin Sodium (Certain drugs, including phenytoin, tend to produce hyperglycemia and may lead to loss of glycemic control. When such drugs are administered to a patient receiving Actoplus Met, the patient should be closely observed to maintain adequate glycemic control).

No products indexed under this heading.

Furosemide (A single-dose, metformin-furosemide drug interaction study in healthy subjects demonstrated that pharmacokinetic parameters of both compounds were affected by co-administration. Furosemide increased the metformin plasma and blood Cmax by 22% and blood AUC by 15%, without any significant change in metformin renal clearance. When administered with metformin, the Cmax and AUC of furosemide were 31% and 12% smaller, respectively, than when administered alone and the terminal half-life was decreased by 31%,without any significant change in furosemide renal clearance. No information is available about the interaction of metformin and furosemide when co-administered chronically). Products include:

Furosemide Tablets 2186

Gemfibrozil (Concomitant administration of gemfibrozil (oral 600 mg twice daily), an inhibitor of CYP2C8, with pioglitazone (oral 30 mg) in 10 healthy volunteers pre-treated for 2 days prior with gemfibrozil (oral 600 mg twice daily) resulted in pioglitazone exposure (AUC 0-24) being 226% of the pioglitazone exposure in the absence of gemfibrozil).

No products indexed under this heading.

Glimepiride (Pioglitazone, like other thiazolidinediones, can cause fluid retention when used alone or in combination with other antihyperglycemic agents, including insulin). Products include:

Avandaryl Tablets 1344
Duetact Tablets 3085

Glipizide (Pioglitazone, like other thiazolidinediones, can cause fluid retention when used alone or in combination with other antihyperglycemic agents, including insulin).

No products indexed under this heading.

Glyburide (Pioglitazone, like other thiazolidinediones, can cause fluid retention when used alone or in combination with other antihyperglycemic agents, including insulin).

No products indexed under this heading.

Haloperidol (Studies have suggested that pioglitazone may be a weak inducer of CYP450 isoform 3A4 substrate).

No products indexed under this heading.

Haloperidol Decanoate (Studies have suggested that pioglitazone may be a weak inducer of CYP450 isoform 3A4 substrate).

No products indexed under this heading.

Haloperidol Lactate (Studies have suggested that pioglitazone may be a weak inducer of CYP450 isoform 3A4 substrate).

No products indexed under this heading.

Hydrochlorothiazide (Certain drugs, including thiazide diuretics, tend to produce hyperglycemia and may lead to loss of glycemic control. When such drugs are administered to a patient receiving Actoplus Met, the patient should be closely observed to maintain adequate glycemic control). Products include:

Atacand HCT 642
Avalide Tablets 892
Avalide Tablets 2713
Benicar HCT Tablets 1010
Diovan HCT Tablets 2216
Dyazide Capsules 1405
Micardis HCT Tablets 854
Prinzide Tablets 2092
Tekturna HCT Tablets 2324
Teveten HCT Tablets 517

Hydrocortisone (Certain drugs, including corticosteroids, tend to produce hyperglycemia and may lead to loss of glycemic control. When such drugs are administered to a patient receiving Actoplus Met, the patient should be closely observed to maintain adequate glycemic control).

No products indexed under this heading.

Hydrocortisone Acetate (Certain drugs, including corticosteroids, tend to produce hyperglycemia and may lead to loss of glycemic control. When such drugs are administered to a patient receiving Actoplus Met, the patient should be closely observed to maintain adequate glycemic control). Products include:

Analpram-HC 1140
Pramosone 1141

Hydrocortisone Sodium Phosphate (Certain drugs, including corticosteroids, tend to produce hyperglycemia and may lead to loss of glycemic control. When such drugs are administered to a patient receiving Actoplus Met, the patient should be closely observed to maintain adequate glycemic control).

No products indexed under this heading.

Hydrocortisone Sodium Succinate (Certain drugs, including corticosteroids, tend to produce hyperglycemia and may lead to loss of glycemic control. When such drugs are administered to a patient receiving Actoplus Met, the patient should be closely observed to maintain adequate glycemic control).

No products indexed under this heading.

Hydroflumethiazide (Certain drugs, including thiazide diuretics, tend to produce hyperglycemia and may lead to loss of glycemic control. When such drugs are administered to a patient receiving Actoplus Met, the patient should be closely observed to maintain adequate glycemic control).

No products indexed under this heading.

Indapamide (Certain drugs, including diuretics, tend to produce hyperglycemia and may lead to loss of glycemic control. When such drugs are administered to a patient receiving Actoplus Met, the patient should be closely observed to maintain adequate glycemic control). Products include:

Indapamide Tablets 2188

Indinavir Sulfate (Studies have suggested that pioglitazone may be a weak inducer of CYP450 isoform 3A4 substrate). Products include:

Crixivan Capsules 1979

Insulin (Pioglitazone, like other thiazolidinediones, can cause fluid retention when used alone or in combination with other antihyperglycemic agents, including insulin).

No products indexed under this heading.

Insulin, Human, Zinc Suspension (Pioglitazone, like other thiazolidinediones, can cause fluid retention when used alone or in combination with other antihyperglycemic agents, including insulin).

No products indexed under this heading.

Insulin, Human (rDNA origin) (Pioglitazone, like other thiazolidinediones, can cause fluid retention when used alone or in combination with other antihyperglycemic agents, including insulin). Products include:

Exubera Inhalation Powder 2515

Insulin, Human NPH (Pioglitazone, like other thiazolidinediones, can cause fluid retention when used alone or in combination with other antihyperglycemic agents, including insulin). Products include:

Humulin N Vial 1846

Insulin, Human Regular (Pioglitazone, like other thiazolidinediones, can cause fluid retention when used alone or in combination with other antihyperglycemic agents, including insulin). Products include:

Humulin R 1849
Humulin R (U-500) 1850

Insulin, Human Regular and Human NPH Mixture (Pioglitazone, like other thiazolidinediones, can cause fluid retention when used alone or in combination with other antihyperglycemic agents, including insulin). Products include:

Humulin 50/50, 100 Units 1843
Humulin 70/30 Vial 1844

Insulin, NPH (Pioglitazone, like other thiazolidinediones, can cause fluid retention when used alone or in combination with other antihyperglycemic agents, including insulin).

No products indexed under this heading.

Insulin, Regular (Pioglitazone, like other thiazolidinediones, can cause fluid retention when used alone or in combination with other antihyperglycemic agents, including insulin).

No products indexed under this heading.

Insulin, Regular and NPH mixture (Pioglitazone, like other thiazolidinediones, can cause fluid retention when used alone or in combination with other antihyperglycemic agents, including insulin).

No products indexed under this heading.

Insulin, Zinc Crystals (Pioglitazone, like other thiazolidinediones, can cause fluid retention when used alone or in combination with other antihyperglycemic agents, including insulin).

No products indexed under this heading.

Insulin, Zinc Suspension (Pioglitazone, like other thiazolidinediones, can cause fluid retention when used alone or in combination with other antihyperglycemic agents, including insulin).

No products indexed under this heading.

Insulin Aspart (Pioglitazone, like other thiazolidinediones, can cause fluid retention when used alone or in combination with other antihyperglycemic agents, including insulin).

No products indexed under this heading.

Insulin Aspart, Human (Pioglitazone, like other thiazolidinediones, can cause fluid retention when used alone or in combination with other antihyperglycemic agents, including insulin). Products include:

NovoLog Mix 70/30 2364

Insulin Aspart, Human Regular (Pioglitazone, like other thiazolidinediones, can cause fluid retention when used alone or in combination with other antihyperglycemic agents, including insulin). Products include:

NovoLog Injection 2359

Insulin Aspart Protamine, Human (Pioglitazone, like other thiazolidinediones, can cause fluid retention when used alone or in combination with other antihyperglycemic agents, including insulin). Products include:

NovoLog Mix 70/30 2364

Insulin Detemir (rDNA Origin) (Pioglitazone, like other thiazolidinediones, can cause fluid retention when used alone or in combination with other antihyperglycemic agents, including insulin). Products include:

Levemir Injection 2352

Insulin glargine (Pioglitazone, like other thiazolidinediones, can cause fluid retention when used alone or in combination with other antihyperglycemic agents, including insulin). Products include:

Lantus Injection 2749

Insulin Glulisine (Pioglitazone, like other thiazolidinediones, can cause fluid retention when used alone or in combination with other antihyperglycemic agents, including insulin). Products include:

Apidra Injection 2706

Insulin Lispro, Human (Pioglitazone, like other thiazolidinediones, can cause fluid retention when used alone or in combination with other antihyperglycemic agents, including insulin). Products include:

Humalog-Pen and KwikPen 1829
Humalog Mix 50/50-Pen and KwikPen 1833
Humalog Mix 75/25-Pen and KwikPen 1835

Insulin Lispro Protamine, Human (Pioglitazone, like other thiazolidinediones, can cause fluid retention when used alone or in combination with other antihyperglycemic agents, including insulin). Products include:

Humalog Mix 50/50-Pen and KwikPen 1833
Humalog Mix 75/25-Pen and KwikPen 1835

Isoniazid (Certain drugs, including isoniazid, tend to produce hyperglycemia and may lead to loss of glycemic control. When such drugs are administered to a patient receiving Actoplus Met, the patient should be closely observed to maintain adequate glycemic control).
No products indexed under this heading.

Isoproterenol Hydrochloride (Certain drugs, including sympathomimetics, tend to produce hyperglycemia and may lead to loss of glycemic control. When such drugs are administered to a patient receiving Actoplus Met, the patient should be closely observed to maintain adequate glycemic control).
No products indexed under this heading.

Isoproterenol Sulfate (Certain drugs, including sympathomimetics, tend to produce hyperglycemia and may lead to loss of glycemic control. When such drugs are administered to a patient receiving Actoplus Met, the patient should be closely observed to maintain adequate glycemic control).
No products indexed under this heading.

Isradipine (Certain drugs, including calcium channel blockers, tend to produce hyperglycemia and may lead to loss of glycemic control. When such drugs are administered to a patient receiving Actoplus Met, the patient should be closely observed to maintain adequate glycemic control). Products include:
DynaCirc CR Controlled Release Tablets 1407

Itraconazole (Studies have suggested that pioglitazone may be a weak inducer of CYP450 isoform 3A4 substrate).
No products indexed under this heading.

Ixabepilone (Studies have suggested that pioglitazone may be a weak inducer of CYP450 isoform 3A4 substrate). Products include:
Ixempra Kit for Injection 915

Ketoconazole (Studies have suggested that pioglitazone may be a weak inducer of CYP450 isoform 3A4 substrate). Products include:
Extina Foam, 2% 3057
Nizoral A-D Shampoo 1901

Levalbuterol Hydrochloride (Certain drugs, including sympathomimetics, tend to produce hyperglycemia and may lead to loss of glycemic control. When such drugs are administered to a patient receiving Actoplus Met, the patient should be closely observed to maintain adequate glycemic control). Products include:
Xopenex Inhalation Solution 3001
Xopenex Inhalation Solution Concentrate 3005

Levonorgestrel (Certain drugs, including oral contraceptives, tend to produce hyperglycemia and may lead to loss of glycemic control. When such drugs are administered to a patient receiving Actoplus Met, the patient should be closely observed to maintain adequate glycemic control). Products include:
Climara Pro Transdermal System 768
Lybrel Tablets 3204
Mirena Intrauterine System 779
Plan B Tablets 1044
Seasonique Tablets 1046

Levothyroxine Sodium (Certain drugs, including thyroid products, tend to produce hyperglycemia and may lead to loss of glycemic control. When such drugs are administered to a patient receiving Actoplus Met, the patient should be closely observed to maintain adequate glycemic control). Products include:
Levothroid Tablets 1170
Levoxyl Tablets 1780
Synthroid Tablets 507

Lidocaine (Studies have suggested that pioglitazone may be a weak inducer of CYP450 isoform 3A4 substrate). Products include:
Lidoderm Patch 1114

Lidocaine Hydrochloride (Studies have suggested that pioglitazone may be a weak inducer of CYP450 isoform 3A4 substrate).
No products indexed under this heading.

Liothyronine Sodium (Certain drugs, including thyroid products, tend to produce hyperglycemia and may lead to loss of glycemic control. When such drugs are administered to a patient receiving Actoplus Met, the patient should be closely observed to maintain adequate glycemic control). Products include:
Cytomel Tablets 1778

Liotrix (Certain drugs, including thyroid products, tend to produce hyperglycemia and may lead to loss of glycemic control. When such drugs are administered to a patient receiving Actoplus Met, the patient should be closely observed to maintain adequate glycemic control).
No products indexed under this heading.

Lovastatin (Studies have suggested that pioglitazone may be a weak inducer of CYP450 isoform 3A4 substrate). Products include:
Advicor Tablets 402
Mevacor Tablets 2063

Mesoridazine Besylate (Certain drugs, including phenothiazines, tend to produce hyperglycemia and may lead to loss of glycemic control. When such drugs are administered to a patient receiving Actoplus Met, the patient should be closely observed to maintain adequate glycemic control).
No products indexed under this heading.

Mestranol (Certain drugs, including oral contraceptives, tend to produce hyperglycemia and may lead to loss of glycemic control. When such drugs are administered to a patient receiving Actoplus Met, the patient should be closely observed to maintain adequate glycemic control).
No products indexed under this heading.

Metaproterenol Sulfate (Certain drugs, including sympathomimetics, tend to produce hyperglycemia and may lead to loss of glycemic control. When such drugs are administered to a patient receiving Actoplus Met, the patient should be closely observed to maintain adequate glycemic control).
No products indexed under this heading.

Metaraminol Bitartrate (Certain drugs, including sympathomimetics, tend to produce hyperglycemia and may lead to loss of glycemic control. When such drugs are administered to a patient receiving Actoplus Met, the patient should be closely observed to maintain adequate glycemic control).
No products indexed under this heading.

Methadone Hydrochloride (Studies have suggested that pioglitazone may be a weak inducer of CYP450 isoform 3A4 substrate).
No products indexed under this heading.

Methotrimeprazine (Certain drugs, including phenothiazines, tend to produce hyperglycemia and may lead to loss of glycemic control. When such drugs are administered to a patient receiving Actoplus Met, the patient should be closely observed to maintain adequate glycemic control).
No products indexed under this heading.

Methoxamine Hydrochloride (Certain drugs, including sympathomimetics, tend to produce hyperglycemia and may lead to loss of glycemic control. When such drugs are administered to a patient receiving Actoplus Met, the patient should be closely observed to maintain adequate glycemic control).
No products indexed under this heading.

Methyclothiazide (Certain drugs, including thiazide diuretics, tend to produce hyperglycemia and may lead to loss of glycemic control. When such drugs are administered to a patient receiving Actoplus Met, the patient should be closely observed to maintain adequate glycemic control).
No products indexed under this heading.

Methylprednisolone Acetate (Certain drugs, including corticosteroids, tend to produce hyperglycemia and may lead to loss of glycemic control. When such drugs are administered to a patient receiving Actoplus Met, the patient should be closely observed to maintain adequate glycemic control).
No products indexed under this heading.

Methylprednisolone Sodium Succinate (Certain drugs, including corticosteroids, tend to produce hyperglycemia and may lead to loss of glycemic control. When such drugs are administered to a patient receiving Actoplus Met, the patient should be closely observed to maintain adequate glycemic control).
No products indexed under this heading.

Metolazone (Certain drugs, including diuretics, tend to produce hyperglycemia and may lead to loss of glycemic control. When such drugs are administered to a patient receiving Actoplus Met, the patient should be closely observed to maintain adequate glycemic control).
No products indexed under this heading.

Mibefradil Dihydrochloride (Certain drugs, including calcium channel blockers, tend to produce hyperglycemia and may lead to loss of glycemic control. When such drugs are administered to a patient receiving Actoplus Met, the patient should be closely observed to maintain adequate glycemic control).
No products indexed under this heading.

Midazolam Hydrochloride (Studies have suggested that pioglitazone may be a weak inducer of CYP450 isoform 3A4 substrate).
No products indexed under this heading.

Miglitol (Pioglitazone, like other thiazolidinediones, can cause fluid retention when used alone or in combination with other antihyperglycemic agents, including insulin).
No products indexed under this heading.

Mometasone Furoate (Certain drugs, including corticosteroids, tend to produce hyperglycemia and may lead to loss of glycemic control. When such drugs are administered to a patient receiving Actoplus Met, the patient should be closely observed to maintain adequate glycemic control). Products include:
Asmanex Twisthaler 2797
Elocon Cream 0.1% 2840
Elocon Lotion 0.1% 2841
Elocon Ointment 0.1% 2842

Mometasone Furoate Monohydrate (Certain drugs, including corticosteroids, tend to produce hyperglycemia and may lead to loss of glycemic control. When such drugs are administered to a patient receiving Actoplus Met, the patient should be closely observed to maintain adequate glycemic control). Products include:
Nasonex Nasal Spray 2883

Morphine Sulfate (Cationic drugs that are eliminated by renal tubular secretion theoretically have the potential for interaction with metformin by competing for common renal tubular transport systems. Although such interactions remain theoretical, careful patient monitoring and dose adjustment of Actoplus Met and/or the interfering drug is recommended in patients who are taking cationic medications that are excreted via the proximal renal tubular secretory system). Products include:
Avinza Capsules 1772
DepoDur Injection 1095
MS Contin Tablets 2585

Nateglinide (Pioglitazone, like other thiazolidinediones, can cause fluid retention when used alone or in combination with other antihyperglycemic agents, including insulin). Products include:
Starlix Tablets 2314

Nefazodone Hydrochloride (Studies have suggested that pioglitazone may be a weak inducer of CYP450 isoform 3A4 substrate).
No products indexed under this heading.

Nelfinavir Mesylate (Studies have suggested that pioglitazone may be a weak inducer of CYP450 isoform 3A4 substrate).
No products indexed under this heading.

Nicardipine Hydrochloride (Certain drugs, including calcium channel blockers, tend to produce hypergly-

cemia and may lead to loss of glycemic control. When such drugs are administered to a patient receiving Actoplus Met, the patient should be closely observed to maintain adequate glycemic control). Products include:

Cardene I.V. 1093

Nicotinic Acid (Certain drugs, including nicotinic acid, tend to produce hyperglycemia and may lead to loss of glycemic control. When such drugs are administered to a patient receiving Actoplus Met, the patient should be closely observed to maintain adequate glycemic control).

No products indexed under this heading.

Nifedipine (A single-dose, metformin-nifedipine drug interaction study in normal healthy volunteers demonstrated that co-administration of nifedipine increased plasma metformin Cmax and AUC by 20% and 9%, respectively, and increased the amount excreted in the urine. Tmax and half-life were unaffected. Nifedipine appears to enhance the absorption of metformin. Metformin had minimal effects on nifedipine).

No products indexed under this heading.

Nimodipine (Certain drugs, including calcium channel blockers, tend to produce hyperglycemia and may lead to loss of glycemic control. When such drugs are administered to a patient receiving Actoplus Met, the patient should be closely observed to maintain adequate glycemic control). Products include:

Nimotop Capsules 790

Nisoldipine (Certain drugs, including calcium channel blockers, tend to produce hyperglycemia and may lead to loss of glycemic control. When such drugs are administered to a patient receiving Actoplus Met, the patient should be closely observed to maintain adequate glycemic control). Products include:

Sular Extended Release Tablets 2975

Nitrendipine (Studies have suggested that pioglitazone may be a weak inducer of CYP450 isoform 3A4 substrate).

No products indexed under this heading.

Norepinephrine Bitartrate (Certain drugs, including sympathomimetics, tend to produce hyperglycemia and may lead to loss of glycemic control. When such drugs are administered to a patient receiving Actoplus Met, the patient should be closely observed to maintain adequate glycemic control).

No products indexed under this heading.

Norethindrone (Certain drugs, including oral contraceptives, tend to produce hyperglycemia and may lead to loss of glycemic control. When such drugs are administered to a patient receiving Actoplus Met, the patient should be closely observed to maintain adequate glycemic control). Products include:

Ortho Micronor Tablets 2446

Norethindrone Acetate (Studies have suggested that pioglitazone may be a weak inducer of CYP450 isoform 3A4 substrate). Products include:

Activella Tablets 2347

Norethynodrel (Certain drugs, including oral contraceptives, tend to produce hyperglycemia and may lead to loss of glycemic control. When such drugs are administered to a patient receiving Actoplus Met, the patient should be closely observed to maintain adequate glycemic control).

No products indexed under this heading.

Norgestimate (Certain drugs, including oral contraceptives, tend to produce hyperglycemia and may lead to loss of glycemic control. When such drugs are administered to a patient receiving Actoplus Met, the patient should be closely observed to maintain adequate glycemic control). Products include:

Ortho-Cyclen/Ortho Tri-Cyclen 2449
Ortho Tri-Cyclen Lo Tablets 2458

Norgestrel (Certain drugs, including oral contraceptives, tend to produce hyperglycemia and may lead to loss of glycemic control. When such drugs are administered to a patient receiving Actoplus Met, the patient should be closely observed to maintain adequate glycemic control).

No products indexed under this heading.

Ondansetron (Studies have suggested that pioglitazone may be a weak inducer of CYP450 isoform 3A4 substrate). Products include:

Zofran ODT Orally Disintegrating Tablets 1687

Ondansetron Hydrochloride (Studies have suggested that pioglitazone may be a weak inducer of CYP450 isoform 3A4 substrate). Products include:

Zofran Injection 1682
Zofran 1687

Paclitaxel (Studies have suggested that pioglitazone may be a weak inducer of CYP450 isoform 3A4 substrate).

No products indexed under this heading.

Perphenazine (Certain drugs, including phenothiazines, tend to produce hyperglycemia and may lead to loss of glycemic control. When such drugs are administered to a patient receiving Actoplus Met, the patient should be closely observed to maintain adequate glycemic control).

No products indexed under this heading.

Phenylephrine Bitartrate (Certain drugs, including sympathomimetics, tend to produce hyperglycemia and may lead to loss of glycemic control. When such drugs are administered to a patient receiving Actoplus Met, the patient should be closely observed to maintain adequate glycemic control).

No products indexed under this heading.

Phenylephrine Hydrochloride (Certain drugs, including sympathomimetics, tend to produce hyperglycemia and may lead to loss of glycemic control. When such drugs are administered to a patient receiving Actoplus Met, the patient should be closely observed to maintain adequate glycemic control). Products include:

Actifed Cold & Allergy Tablets 1895
Benadryl Allergy & Cold Kapgels 1895
Benadryl Allergy & Sinus Headache Kapgels 1895
Benadryl Severe Allergy & Sinus Headache Caplets 1897
Children's Benadryl-D Allergy & Sinus Liquid 1896
Benadryl-D Allergy & Sinus Tablet 1896
PediaCare Children's Allergy & Cold Liquid 1902
PediaCare Children's Decongestant Liquid 1902
PediaCare Children's Liquid Multi-Symptom Cold 1902
Sinutab Non-Drying Caplets 1905
Sinutab Sinus Caplets 1905
Children's Sudafed PE Cold & Cough Liquid 1907
Children's Sudafed PE Nasal Decongestant Liquid 1906
Sudafed PE Cold & Cough Caplets 1907
Sudafed PE Nasal Decongestant Tablets 1907
Sudafed PE Nighttime Cold Caplets 1907
Sudafed PE Non-Drying Sinus Caplets 1908
Sudafed PE Severe Cold Caplets 1908
Sudafed PE Sinus & Allergy Tablets 1908
Sudafed PE Sinus Headache Caplets 1908
Tylenol Allergy Multi-Symptom Caplets with Cool Burst and Rapid Release Gelcaps 1916
Tylenol Allergy Multi-Symptom Nighttime Caplets with Cool Burst 1916
Children's Tylenol Plus Cold Suspension Liquid 1912
Children's Tylenol Plus Cold & Allergy Suspension Liquid 1914
Children's Tylenol Plus Flu Suspension Liquid 1914
Children's Tylenol Plus Multi-Symptom Cold Suspension Liquid 1912
Tylenol Cold Head Congestion Daytime Caplets with Cool Burst 1910
Tylenol Cold Head Congestion Nighttime Caplets with Cool Burst 1910
Tylenol Cold Head Congestion Severe Daytime Caplets with Cool Burst 1910
Tylenol Cold Multi-Symptom Daytime Caplets with Cool Burst and Rapid Release Gels 1913
Tylenol Cold Multi-Symptom Daytime Liquid with Citrus Burst ... 1913
Tylenol Cold Multi-Symptom Nighttime Caplets with Cool Burst 1913
Tylenol Cold Multi-Symptom Nighttime Liquid with Cool Burst ... 1913
Tylenol Cold Multi-Symptom Severe Caplets with Cool Burst..... 1913
Tylenol Cold Multi-Symptom Severe Daytime Liquid with Citrus Burst 1913
Tylenol Sinus Congestion & Pain Daytime Caplets with Cool Burst and Gelcaps 1917
Tylenol Sinus Congestion & Pain Nighttime Caplets with Cool Burst 1917
Tylenol Sinus Congestion & Pain Severe Caplets with Cool Burst..... 1917
Vicks DayQuil Cold & Flu Multi-Symptom Relief .... ▪616
Vicks DayQuil LiquiCaps 2567
Vicks DayQuil Liquid 2567
Vicks DayQuil Multi-Symptom Cold/Flu Relief 2567

Phenylephrine Tannate (Certain drugs, including sympathomimetics, tend to produce hyperglycemia and may lead to loss of glycemic control. When such drugs are administered to a patient receiving Actoplus Met, the patient should be closely observed to maintain adequate glycemic control).

No products indexed under this heading.

Phenylpropanolamine Hydrochloride (Certain drugs, including sympathomimetics, tend to produce hyperglycemia and may lead to loss of glycemic control. When such drugs are administered to a patient receiving Actoplus Met, the patient should be closely observed to maintain adequate glycemic control).

No products indexed under this heading.

Phenytoin (Certain drugs, including phenytoin, tend to produce hyperglycemia and may lead to loss of glycemic control. When such drugs are administered to a patient receiving Actoplus Met, the patient should be closely observed to maintain adequate glycemic control).

No products indexed under this heading.

Phenytoin Sodium (Certain drugs, including phenytoin, tend to produce hyperglycemia and may lead to loss of glycemic control. When such drugs are administered to a patient receiving Actoplus Met, the patient should be closely observed to maintain adequate glycemic control). Products include:

Phenytek Capsules 2192

Pimozide (Studies have suggested that pioglitazone may be a weak inducer of CYP450 isoform 3A4 substrate).

No products indexed under this heading.

Pirbuterol Acetate (Certain drugs, including sympathomimetics, tend to produce hyperglycemia and may lead to loss of glycemic control. When such drugs are administered to a patient receiving Actoplus Met, the patient should be closely observed to maintain adequate glycemic control). Products include:

Maxair Autohaler 1705

Polyestradiol Phosphate (Certain drugs, including estrogens, tend to produce hyperglycemia and may lead to loss of glycemic control. When such drugs are administered to a patient receiving Actoplus Met, the patient should be closely observed to maintain adequate glycemic control).

No products indexed under this heading.

Polythiazide (Certain drugs, including thiazide diuretics, tend to produce hyperglycemia and may lead to loss of glycemic control. When such drugs are administered to a patient receiving Actoplus Met, the patient should be closely observed to maintain adequate glycemic control).

No products indexed under this heading.

Prednisolone Acetate (Certain drugs, including corticosteroids, tend to produce hyperglycemia and may lead to loss of glycemic control. When such drugs are administered to a patient receiving Actoplus Met, the patient should be closely observed to maintain adequate glycemic control). Products include:

Pred Forte Ophthalmic Suspension .... ⊙227
Pred Mild Ophthalmic Suspension .... ⊙230
Pred-G Ophthalmic Ointment .... ⊙229
Pred-G Ophthalmic Suspension ...... ⊙228

Prednisolone Sodium Phosphate (Certain drugs, including corticosteroids, tend to produce hyperglycemia and may lead to loss of glycemic control. When such drugs are administered to a patient receiving Actoplus Met, the patient should be closely observed to maintain adequate glycemic control).
No products indexed under this heading.

Prednisolone Tebutate (Certain drugs, including corticosteroids, tend to produce hyperglycemia and may lead to loss of glycemic control. When such drugs are administered to a patient receiving Actoplus Met, the patient should be closely observed to maintain adequate glycemic control).
No products indexed under this heading.

Prednisone (Certain drugs, including corticosteroids, tend to produce hyperglycemia and may lead to loss of glycemic control. When such drugs are administered to a patient receiving Actoplus Met, the patient should be closely observed to maintain adequate glycemic control).
No products indexed under this heading.

Procainamide Hydrochloride (Cationic drugs that are eliminated by renal tubular secretion theoretically have the potential for interaction with metformin by competing for common renal tubular transport systems. Although such interactions remain theoretical, careful patient monitoring and dose adjustment of Actoplus Met and/or the interfering drug is recommended in patients who are taking cationic medications that are excreted via the proximal renal tubular secretory system).
No products indexed under this heading.

Prochlorperazine (Certain drugs, including phenothiazines, tend to produce hyperglycemia and may lead to loss of glycemic control. When such drugs are administered to a patient receiving Actoplus Met, the patient should be closely observed to maintain adequate glycemic control).
No products indexed under this heading.

Promethazine Hydrochloride (Certain drugs, including phenothiazines, tend to produce hyperglycemia and may lead to loss of glycemic control. When such drugs are administered to a patient receiving Actoplus Met, the patient should be closely observed to maintain adequate glycemic control).
No products indexed under this heading.

Pseudoephedrine Hydrochloride (Certain drugs, including sympathomimetics, tend to produce hyperglycemia and may lead to loss of glycemic control. When such drugs are administered to a patient receiving Actoplus Met, the patient should be closely observed to maintain adequate glycemic control). Products include:

- Allegra-D 12 Hour Extended-Release Tablets **2687**
- Allegra-D 24 Hour Extended-Release Tablets **2690**
- Children's Motrin Cold Oral Suspension **1899**
- Sudafed 12 Hour Nasal Decongestant Non-Drowsy Caplets **1909**
- Sudafed 24 Hour Non-Drowsy Nasal Decongestant Tablets **1906**
- Children's Sudafed Nasal Decongestant Liquid **1906**
- Sudafed Nasal Decongestant Tablets **1906**
- Tylenol Cold Severe Congestion Daytime Caplets with Cool Burst **1912**
- Tylenol Sinus Severe Congestion Caplets with Cool Burst **1917**
- Vicks NyQuil LiquiCaps **2567**
- Vicks NyQuil Liquid **2567**
- Vicks NyQuil Multi-Symptom Cold/Flu Relief **2567**
- Zyrtec-D 12 Hour Extended Release Tablets **1923**
- Zyrtec-D Allergy & Congestion Extended-Release Tablets **1923**

Pseudoephedrine Sulfate (Certain drugs, including sympathomimetics, tend to produce hyperglycemia and may lead to loss of glycemic control. When such drugs are administered to a patient receiving Actoplus Met, the patient should be closely observed to maintain adequate glycemic control). Products include:

- Clarinex-D 12-Hour Extended-Release Tablets **2831**
- Clarinex-D 24-Hour Extended-Release Tablets **2834**

Quinestrol (Certain drugs, including estrogens, tend to produce hyperglycemia and may lead to loss of glycemic control. When such drugs are administered to a patient receiving Actoplus Met, the patient should be closely observed to maintain adequate glycemic control).
No products indexed under this heading.

Quinidine Gluconate (Cationic drugs that are eliminated by renal tubular secretion theoretically have the potential for interaction with metformin by competing for common renal tubular transport systems. Although such interactions remain theoretical, careful patient monitoring and dose adjustment of Actoplus Met and/or the interfering drug is recommended in patients who are taking cationic medications that are excreted via the proximal renal tubular secretory system).
No products indexed under this heading.

Quinidine Polygalacturonate (Cationic drugs that are eliminated by renal tubular secretion theoretically have the potential for interaction with metformin by competing for common renal tubular transport systems. Although such interactions remain theoretical, careful patient monitoring and dose adjustment of Actoplus Met and/or the interfering drug is recommended in patients who are taking cationic medications that are excreted via the proximal renal tubular secretory system).
No products indexed under this heading.

Quinidine Sulfate (Cationic drugs that are eliminated by renal tubular secretion theoretically have the potential for interaction with metformin by competing for common renal tubular transport systems. Although such interactions remain theoretical, careful patient monitoring and dose adjustment of Actoplus Met and/or the interfering drug is recommended in patients who are taking cationic medications that are excreted via the proximal renal tubular secretory system).
No products indexed under this heading.

Quinine Sulfate (Cationic drugs that are eliminated by renal tubular secretion theoretically have the potential for interaction with metformin by competing for common renal tubular transport systems. Although such interactions remain theoretical, careful patient monitoring and dose adjustment of Actoplus Met and/or the interfering drug is recommended in patients who are taking cationic medications that are excreted via the proximal renal tubular secretory system).
No products indexed under this heading.

Ranitidine Hydrochloride (Cationic drugs that are eliminated by renal tubular secretion theoretically have the potential for interaction with metformin by competing for common renal tubular transport systems. Although such interactions remain theoretical, careful patient monitoring and dose adjustment of Actoplus Met and/or the interfering drug is recommended in patients who are taking cationic medications that are excreted via the proximal renal tubular secretory system). Products include:

- Zantac 75 Tablets .... ■**603**
- Zantac **1670**
- Zantac Injection **1666**
- Zantac Injection Pharmacy Bulk Package **1668**
- Maximum Strength Zantac 150 Tablets .... ■**603**
- Maximum Strength Zantac 150 Cool Mint Tablets .... ■**603**

Repaglinide (Pioglitazone, like other thiazolidinediones, can cause fluid retention when used alone or in combination with other antihyperglycemic agents, including insulin). Products include:

- PrandiMet Tablets **2967**
- Prandin Tablets **2971**

Rifabutin (Studies have suggested that pioglitazone may be a weak inducer of CYP450 isoform 3A4 substrate).
No products indexed under this heading.

Rifampin (Concomitant administration of rifampin (oral 600 mg once daily), an inducer of CYP2C8 with pioglitazone (oral 30 mg) in 10 healthy volunteers pre-treated for 5 days prior with rifampin (oral 600 mg once daily) resulted in a decrease in the AUC of pioglitazone by 54%).
No products indexed under this heading.

Ritonavir (Studies have suggested that pioglitazone may be a weak inducer of CYP450 isoform 3A4 substrate). Products include:

- Kaletra **452**
- Norvir **489**

Rosiglitazone Maleate (Pioglitazone, like other thiazolidinediones, can cause fluid retention when used alone or in combination with other antihyperglycemic agents, including insulin). Products include:

- Avandamet Tablets **1336**
- Avandaryl Tablets **1344**
- Avandia Tablets **1351**

Salmeterol Xinafoate (Certain drugs, including sympathomimetics, tend to produce hyperglycemia and may lead to loss of glycemic control. When such drugs are administered to a patient receiving Actoplus Met, the patient should be closely observed to maintain adequate glycemic control). Products include:

- Advair Diskus 100/50 .... **1276**
- Advair Diskus 250/50 .... **1276**
- Advair Diskus 500/50 .... **1276**
- Advair HFA 45/21 Inhalation Aerosol **1288**
- Advair HFA 115/21 Inhalation Aerosol **1288**
- Advair HFA 230/21 Inhalation Aerosol **1288**
- Serevent Diskus **1594**

Saquinavir (Studies have suggested that pioglitazone may be a weak inducer of CYP450 isoform 3A4 substrate).
No products indexed under this heading.

Saquinavir Mesylate (Studies have suggested that pioglitazone may be a weak inducer of CYP450 isoform 3A4 substrate).
No products indexed under this heading.

Sertraline Hydrochloride (Studies have suggested that pioglitazone may be a weak inducer of CYP450 isoform 3A4 substrate).
No products indexed under this heading.

Sildenafil Citrate (Studies have suggested that pioglitazone may be a weak inducer of CYP450 isoform 3A4 substrate).
No products indexed under this heading.

Simvastatin (Studies have suggested that pioglitazone may be a weak inducer of CYP450 isoform 3A4 substrate). Products include:

- Simcor Tablets **502**
- Vytorin 10/10 Tablets **2149**
- Vytorin 10/10 Tablets **2939**
- Vytorin 10/20 Tablets **2149**
- Vytorin 10/20 Tablets **2939**
- Vytorin 10/40 Tablets **2149**
- Vytorin 10/40 Tablets **2939**
- Vytorin 10/80 Tablets **2149**
- Vytorin 10/80 Tablets **2939**
- Zocor Tablets **2136**

Sirolimus (Studies have suggested that pioglitazone may be a weak inducer of CYP450 isoform 3A4 substrate). Products include:

- Rapamune **3260**

Sitagliptin Phosphate (Pioglitazone, like other thiazolidinediones, can cause fluid retention when used alone or in combination with other antihyperglycemic agents, including insulin). Products include:

- Janumet Tablets **2041**
- Januvia Tablets **2048**

Spironolactone (Certain drugs, including diuretics, tend to produce hyperglycemia and may lead to loss of glycemic control. When such drugs are administered to a patient receiving Actoplus Met, the patient should be closely observed to maintain adequate glycemic control).
No products indexed under this heading.

Tacrolimus (Studies have suggested that pioglitazone may be a weak inducer of CYP450 isoform 3A4 substrate). Products include:

- Prograf Capsules and Injection **622**
- Protopic Ointment **628**

Tadalafil (Studies have suggested that pioglitazone may be a weak inducer of CYP450 isoform 3A4 substrate). Products include:

- Cialis Tablets **1792**

Tamoxifen Citrate (Studies have suggested that pioglitazone may be a weak inducer of CYP450 isoform 3A4 substrate).
No products indexed under this heading.

Terbutaline Sulfate (Certain drugs, including sympathomimetics, tend to produce hyperglycemia and may lead to loss of glycemic control. When such drugs are administered to a patient receiving Actoplus Met, the patient should be closely observed to maintain adequate glycemic control).
No products indexed under this heading.

Thioridazine Hydrochloride (Certain drugs, including phenothiazines, tend to produce hyperglycemia and may lead to loss of glycemic control. When such drugs are administered to a patient receiving Actoplus Met, the patient should be closely observed to maintain adequate glycemic control). Products include:
Thioridazine Hydrochloride Tablets 2195

Thyroglobulin (Certain drugs, including thyroid products, tend to produce hyperglycemia and may lead to loss of glycemic control. When such drugs are administered to a patient receiving Actoplus Met, the patient should be closely observed to maintain adequate glycemic control).
No products indexed under this heading.

Thyroid (Certain drugs, including thyroid products, tend to produce hyperglycemia and may lead to loss of glycemic control. When such drugs are administered to a patient receiving Actoplus Met, the patient should be closely observed to maintain adequate glycemic control). Products include:
Naturethroid Tablets 2605

Thyroxine (Certain drugs, including thyroid products, tend to produce hyperglycemia and may lead to loss of glycemic control. When such drugs are administered to a patient receiving Actoplus Met, the patient should be closely observed to maintain adequate glycemic control).
No products indexed under this heading.

Thyroxine Sodium (Certain drugs, including thyroid products, tend to produce hyperglycemia and may lead to loss of glycemic control. When such drugs are administered to a patient receiving Actoplus Met, the patient should be closely observed to maintain adequate glycemic control).
No products indexed under this heading.

Tiagabine Hydrochloride (Studies have suggested that pioglitazone may be a weak inducer of CYP450 isoform 3A4 substrate). Products include:
Gabitril Tablets 973

Tolazamide (Pioglitazone, like other thiazolidinediones, can cause fluid retention when used alone or in combination with other antihyperglycemic agents, including insulin).
No products indexed under this heading.

Tolbutamide (Pioglitazone, like other thiazolidinediones, can cause fluid retention when used alone or in combination with other antihyperglycemic agents, including insulin).
No products indexed under this heading.

Tolterodine Tartrate (Studies have suggested that pioglitazone may be a weak inducer of CYP450 isoform 3A4 substrate).
No products indexed under this heading.

Torsemide (Certain drugs, including diuretics, tend to produce hyperglycemia and may lead to loss of glycemic control. When such drugs are administered to a patient receiving Actoplus Met, the patient should be closely observed to maintain adequate glycemic control). Products include:
Demadex Injection 2630
Demadex Tablets 2630

Trazodone Hydrochloride (Studies have suggested that pioglitazone may be a weak inducer of CYP450 isoform 3A4 substrate).
No products indexed under this heading.

Triamcinolone (Certain drugs, including corticosteroids, tend to produce hyperglycemia and may lead to loss of glycemic control. When such drugs are administered to a patient receiving Actoplus Met, the patient should be closely observed to maintain adequate glycemic control).
No products indexed under this heading.

Triamcinolone Acetonide (Certain drugs, including corticosteroids, tend to produce hyperglycemia and may lead to loss of glycemic control. When such drugs are administered to a patient receiving Actoplus Met, the patient should be closely observed to maintain adequate glycemic control). Products include:
Azmacort Inhalation Aerosol 407
Nasacort AQ Nasal Spray 2765
Triesence Injectable Suspension .... ⊙209

Triamcinolone Diacetate (Certain drugs, including corticosteroids, tend to produce hyperglycemia and may lead to loss of glycemic control. When such drugs are administered to a patient receiving Actoplus Met, the patient should be closely observed to maintain adequate glycemic control).
No products indexed under this heading.

Triamcinolone Hexacetonide (Certain drugs, including corticosteroids, tend to produce hyperglycemia and may lead to loss of glycemic control. When such drugs are administered to a patient receiving Actoplus Met, the patient should be closely observed to maintain adequate glycemic control).
No products indexed under this heading.

Triamterene (Cationic drugs that are eliminated by renal tubular secretion theoretically have the potential for interaction with metformin by competing for common renal tubular transport systems. Although such interactions remain theoretical, careful patient monitoring and dose adjustment of Actoplus Met and/or the interfering drug is recommended in patients who are taking cationic medications that are excreted via the proximal renal tubular secretory system). Products include:
Dyazide Capsules 1405
Dyrenium Capsules 3189

Triazolam (Studies have suggested that pioglitazone may be a weak inducer of CYP450 isoform 3A4 substrate).
No products indexed under this heading.

Trifluoperazine Hydrochloride (Certain drugs, including phenothiazines, tend to produce hyperglycemia and may lead to loss of glycemic control. When such drugs are administered to a patient receiving Actoplus Met, the patient should be closely observed to maintain adequate glycemic control).
No products indexed under this heading.

Trimethoprim (Cationic drugs that are eliminated by renal tubular secretion theoretically have the potential for interaction with metformin by competing for common renal tubular transport systems. Although such interactions remain theoretical, careful patient monitoring and dose adjustment of Actoplus Met and/or the interfering drug is recommended in patients who are taking cationic medications that are excreted via the proximal renal tubular secretory system).
No products indexed under this heading.

Trimethoprim Sulfate (Cationic drugs that are eliminated by renal tubular secretion theoretically have the potential for interaction with metformin by competing for common renal tubular transport systems. Although such interactions remain theoretical, careful patient monitoring and dose adjustment of Actoplus Met and/or the interfering drug is recommended in patients who are taking cationic medications that are excreted via the proximal renal tubular secretory system).
No products indexed under this heading.

Troglitazone (Pioglitazone, like other thiazolidinediones, can cause fluid retention when used alone or in combination with other antihyperglycemic agents, including insulin).
No products indexed under this heading.

Vancomycin Hydrochloride (Cationic drugs that are eliminated by renal tubular secretion theoretically have the potential for interaction with metformin by competing for common renal tubular transport systems. Although such interactions remain theoretical, careful patient monitoring and dose adjustment of Actoplus Met and/or the interfering drug is recommended in patients who are taking cationic medications that are excreted via the proximal renal tubular secretory system).
No products indexed under this heading.

Vardenafil Hydrochloride (Studies have suggested that pioglitazone may be a weak inducer of CYP450 isoform 3A4 substrate). Products include:
Levitra Tablets 2876

Verapamil Hydrochloride (Certain drugs, including calcium channel blockers, tend to produce hyperglycemia and may lead to loss of glycemic control. When such drugs are administered to a patient receiving Actoplus Met, the patient should be closely observed to maintain adequate glycemic control). Products include:
Tarka Tablets 511

Vinblastine Sulfate (Studies have suggested that pioglitazone may be a weak inducer of CYP450 isoform 3A4 substrate).
No products indexed under this heading.

Vincristine Sulfate (Studies have suggested that pioglitazone may be a weak inducer of CYP450 isoform 3A4 substrate).
No products indexed under this heading.

Warfarin Sodium (Studies have suggested that pioglitazone may be a weak inducer of CYP450 isoform 3A4 substrate).
No products indexed under this heading.

Food Interactions

Alcohol (Alcohol is known to potentiate the effect of metformin on lactate metabolism. Patients, therefore, should be warned against excessive alcohol intake, acute or chronic, while receiving Actoplus Met).

ACTOS TABLETS

(Pioglitazone Hydrochloride) 3077
May interact with cytochrome p450 2c8 inducers (selected), cytochrome p450 2c8 inhibitors (selected), cytochrome p450 3a4 substrates (selected), oral hypoglycemic agents, insulin, oral contraceptives, sulfonylureas, and certain other agents. Compounds in these categories include:

Acarbose (Patients receiving pioglitazone in combination with oral hypoglycemic agents may be at risk for hypoglycemia. Pioglitazone can cause fluid retention when used alone or in combination with other antidiabetic agents). Products include:
Precose Tablets 792

Alfentanil Hydrochloride (Pioglitazone may be a weak inducer of CYP450 isoform 3A4 substrate).
No products indexed under this heading.

Alprazolam (Pioglitazone may be a weak inducer of CYP450 isoform 3A4 substrate).
No products indexed under this heading.

Amiodarone Hydrochloride (Pioglitazone may be a weak inducer of CYP450 isoform 3A4 substrate).
No products indexed under this heading.

Amitriptyline Hydrochloride (Pioglitazone may be a weak inducer of CYP450 isoform 3A4 substrate).
No products indexed under this heading.

Amlodipine Besylate (Pioglitazone may be a weak inducer of CYP450 isoform 3A4 substrate). Products include:
Azor Tablets 1005
Exforge Tablets 2238

Anastrozole (An enzyme inhibitor of CYP2C8 may significantly increase the AUC of pioglitazone; therefore, if an enzyme inhibitor of CYP2C8 is started or stopped during treatment with pioglitazone, changes in diabetes treatment may be needed). Products include:

Arimidex Tablets 672

Aprepitant (Pioglitazone may be a weak inducer of CYP450 isoform 3A4 substrate). Products include:

Emend Capsules 1992

Astemizole (Pioglitazone may be a weak inducer of CYP450 isoform 3A4 substrate).

No products indexed under this heading.

Atorvastatin Calcium (Atorvastatin appears to induce the metabolism of pioglitazone; pioglitazone appears to induce the metabolism of atorvastatin). Products include:

Lipitor Tablets 2501

Belladonna Ergotamine (Pioglitazone may be a weak inducer of CYP450 isoform 3A4 substrate).

No products indexed under this heading.

Buspirone Hydrochloride (Pioglitazone may be a weak inducer of CYP450 isoform 3A4 substrate).

No products indexed under this heading.

Busulfan (Pioglitazone may be a weak inducer of CYP450 isoform 3A4 substrate). Products include:

Busulfex Injection 2477
Myleran Tablets 1530

Carbamazepine (An enzyme inducer of CYP2C8 may significantly decrease the AUC of pioglitazone; therefore, if an enzyme inducer of CYP2C8 is started or stopped during treatment with pioglitazone, changes in diabetes treatment may be needed). Products include:

Carbatrol Capsules 3019
Equetro Extended-Release Capsules 3174

Cerivastatin Sodium (Pioglitazone may be a weak inducer of CYP450 isoform 3A4 substrate).

No products indexed under this heading.

Chlorpheniramine (Pioglitazone may be a weak inducer of CYP450 isoform 3A4 substrate).

No products indexed under this heading.

Chlorpheniramine Maleate (Pioglitazone may be a weak inducer of CYP450 isoform 3A4 substrate). Products include:

Actifed Cold & Allergy Tablets 1895
Sudafed PE Sinus & Allergy Tablets 1908
Tylenol Allergy Multi-Symptom Caplets with Cool Burst and Rapid Release Gelcaps 1916
Children's Tylenol Plus Cold Suspension Liquid 1912
Children's Tylenol Plus Cough & Runny Nose Suspension Liquid 1912
Children's Tylenol Plus Flu Suspension Liquid 1914
Children's Tylenol Plus Multi-Symptom Cold Suspension Liquid 1912
Tylenol Cold Head Congestion Nighttime Caplets with Cool Burst 1910
Tylenol Cold Multi-Symptom Nighttime Caplets with Cool Burst 1913
Tylenol Sinus Congestion & Pain Nighttime Caplets with Cool Burst 1917

Chlorpheniramine Polistirex (Pioglitazone may be a weak inducer of CYP450 isoform 3A4 substrate). Products include:

Tussionex Pennkinetic Extended-Release Suspension 3154

Chlorpheniramine Tannate (Pioglitazone may be a weak inducer of CYP450 isoform 3A4 substrate).

No products indexed under this heading.

Chlorpropamide (Patients receiving pioglitazone in combination with oral hypoglycemic agents may be at risk for hypoglycemia. Pioglitazone can cause fluid retention when used alone or in combination with other antidiabetic agents).

No products indexed under this heading.

Cimetidine (An enzyme inhibitor of CYP2C8 may significantly increase the AUC of pioglitazone; therefore, if an enzyme inhibitor of CYP2C8 is started or stopped during treatment with pioglitazone, changes in diabetes treatment may be needed).

No products indexed under this heading.

Cimetidine Hydrochloride (An enzyme inhibitor of CYP2C8 may significantly increase the AUC of pioglitazone; therefore, if an enzyme inhibitor of CYP2C8 is started or stopped during treatment with pioglitazone, changes in diabetes treatment may be needed).

No products indexed under this heading.

Cisapride (Pioglitazone may be a weak inducer of CYP450 isoform 3A4 substrate).

No products indexed under this heading.

Clarithromycin (Pioglitazone may be a weak inducer of CYP450 isoform 3A4 substrate). Products include:

Biaxin/Biaxin XL 411

Cyclosporine (Pioglitazone may be a weak inducer of CYP450 isoform 3A4 substrate). Products include:

Gengraf Capsules 435
Neoral Oral Solution 2280
Neoral Soft Gelatin Capsules 2280
Restasis Ophthalmic Emulsion 557
Sandimmune 2296

Desogestrel (Co-administration of pioglitazone hydrochloride (45mg once daily) and an oral contraceptive (1mg norethindrone plus 0.035mg ethinyl estradiol once daily) for 21 days, resulted in an 11% decrease in ethinyl estradiol AUC (0-24h) and an 11% to 14% decrease in C_{max}. There were no significant changes in norethindrone AUC (0-24h) and C_{max}). Products include:

Mircette Tablets 1034

Diazepam (Pioglitazone may be a weak inducer of CYP450 isoform 3A4 substrate). Products include:

Valium Tablets 2658

Dihydroergotamine Mesylate (Pioglitazone may be a weak inducer of CYP450 isoform 3A4 substrate).

No products indexed under this heading.

Diltiazem Hydrochloride (Pioglitazone may be a weak inducer of CYP450 isoform 3A4 substrate). Products include:

Cardizem LA Extended Release Tablets 421

Diltiazem Maleate (Pioglitazone may be a weak inducer of CYP450 isoform 3A4 substrate).

No products indexed under this heading.

Disopyramide (Pioglitazone may be a weak inducer of CYP450 isoform 3A4 substrate).

No products indexed under this heading.

Disopyramide Phosphate (Pioglitazone may be a weak inducer of CYP450 isoform 3A4 substrate).

No products indexed under this heading.

Disulfiram (Pioglitazone may be a weak inducer of CYP450 isoform 3A4 substrate).

No products indexed under this heading.

Doxorubicin Hydrochloride (Pioglitazone may be a weak inducer of CYP450 isoform 3A4 substrate).

No products indexed under this heading.

Dronabinol (Pioglitazone may be a weak inducer of CYP450 isoform 3A4 substrate). Products include:

Marinol Capsules 3163

Ergotamine Tartrate (Pioglitazone may be a weak inducer of CYP450 isoform 3A4 substrate).

No products indexed under this heading.

Erythromycin (Pioglitazone may be a weak inducer of CYP450 isoform 3A4 substrate).

No products indexed under this heading.

Erythromycin Estolate (Pioglitazone may be a weak inducer of CYP450 isoform 3A4 substrate).

No products indexed under this heading.

Erythromycin Ethylsuccinate (Pioglitazone may be a weak inducer of CYP450 isoform 3A4 substrate). Products include:

E.E.S. 433
EryPed 431

Erythromycin Gluceptate (Pioglitazone may be a weak inducer of CYP450 isoform 3A4 substrate).

No products indexed under this heading.

Erythromycin Lactobionate (Pioglitazone may be a weak inducer of CYP450 isoform 3A4 substrate).

No products indexed under this heading.

Erythromycin Stearate (Pioglitazone may be a weak inducer of CYP450 isoform 3A4 substrate).

No products indexed under this heading.

Estradiol (Pioglitazone may be a weak inducer of CYP450 isoform 3A4 substrate). Products include:

Activella Tablets 2347
Angeliq Tablets 751
Climara Transdermal System 763
Climara Pro Transdermal System 768
Divigel 3167
Vagifem Tablets 2375

Estradiol Benzoate (Pioglitazone may be a weak inducer of CYP450 isoform 3A4 substrate).

No products indexed under this heading.

Estradiol Cypionate (Pioglitazone may be a weak inducer of CYP450 isoform 3A4 substrate).

No products indexed under this heading.

Estradiol Valerate (Pioglitazone may be a weak inducer of CYP450 isoform 3A4 substrate).

No products indexed under this heading.

Ethinyl Estradiol (Co-administration of pioglitazone hydrochloride (45mg once daily) and an oral contraceptive (1mg norethindrone plus 0.035mg ethinyl estradiol once daily) for 21 days, resulted in an 11% decrease in ethinyl estradiol AUC (0-24h) and an 11% to 14% decrease in C_{max}. There were no significant changes in norethindrone AUC (0-24h) and C_{max}). Products include:

Lybrel Tablets 3204
Mircette Tablets 1034
NuvaRing 2897
Ortho-Cyclen/Ortho Tri-Cyclen 2449
Ortho Evra Transdermal System 2437
Ortho Tri-Cyclen Lo Tablets 2458
Seasonique Tablets 1046
Yaz Tablets 805

Ethosuximide (Pioglitazone may be a weak inducer of CYP450 isoform 3A4 substrate).

No products indexed under this heading.

Ethynodiol Diacetate (Co-administration of pioglitazone hydrochloride (45mg once daily) and an oral contraceptive (1mg norethindrone plus 0.035mg ethinyl estradiol once daily) for 21 days, resulted in an 11% decrease in ethinyl estradiol AUC (0-24h) and an 11% to 14% decrease in C_{max}. There were no significant changes in norethindrone AUC (0-24h) and C_{max}).

No products indexed under this heading.

Etoposide (Pioglitazone may be a weak inducer of CYP450 isoform 3A4 substrate).

No products indexed under this heading.

Etoposide Phosphate (Pioglitazone may be a weak inducer of CYP450 isoform 3A4 substrate).

No products indexed under this heading.

Felodipine (Pioglitazone may be a weak inducer of CYP450 isoform 3A4 substrate).

No products indexed under this heading.

Fentanyl (Pioglitazone may be a weak inducer of CYP450 isoform 3A4 substrate). Products include:

Duragesic Transdermal System 2405
Ionsys Transdermal System 2410

Fentanyl Citrate (Pioglitazone may be a weak inducer of CYP450 isoform 3A4 substrate). Products include:

Actiq 959
Fentora Tablets 968

Gemfibrozil (Concomitant administration of gemfibrozil (oral 600 mg twice daily), an inhibitor of CYP2C8, with pioglitazone (oral 30 mg) in 10 healthy volunteers pre-treated for 2 days prior with gemfibrozil (oral 600 mg twice daily) resulted in pioglitazone exposure (AUC 0-24) being 226% of the pioglitazone exposure in the absence of gemfibrozil).

No products indexed under this heading.

Glimepiride (Patients receiving pioglitazone in combination with oral hypoglycemic agents may be at risk for hypoglycemia. Pioglitazone can cause fluid retention when used alone or in combination with other antidiabetic agents). Products include:

Avandaryl Tablets 1344
Duetact Tablets 3085

Glipizide (Patients receiving pioglitazone in combination with oral hypoglycemic agents may be at risk for hypoglycemia. Pioglitazone can cause fluid retention when used alone or in combination with other antidiabetic agents).
No products indexed under this heading.

Glyburide (Patients receiving pioglitazone in combination with oral hypoglycemic agents may be at risk for hypoglycemia. Pioglitazone can cause fluid retention when used alone or in combination with other antidiabetic agents).
No products indexed under this heading.

Haloperidol (Pioglitazone may be a weak inducer of CYP450 isoform 3A4 substrate).
No products indexed under this heading.

Haloperidol Decanoate (Pioglitazone may be a weak inducer of CYP450 isoform 3A4 substrate).
No products indexed under this heading.

Haloperidol Lactate (Pioglitazone may be a weak inducer of CYP450 isoform 3A4 substrate).
No products indexed under this heading.

Indinavir Sulfate (Pioglitazone may be a weak inducer of CYP450 isoform 3A4 substrate). Products include:
Crixivan Capsules 1979

Insulin (Patients receiving pioglitazone in combination with insulin may be at risk for hypoglycemia; pioglitazone can cause fluid retention when used alone or in combination with insulin; anemia was reported in less than or equal 2% of patients treated with pioglitazone and metformin).
No products indexed under this heading.

Insulin, Human, Zinc Suspension (Patients receiving pioglitazone in combination with insulin may be at risk for hypoglycemia; pioglitazone can cause fluid retention when used alone or in combination with insulin; anemia was reported in less than or equal 2% of patients treated with pioglitazone and metformin).
No products indexed under this heading.

Insulin, Human (rDNA origin) (Patients receiving pioglitazone in combination with insulin may be at risk for hypoglycemia; pioglitazone can cause fluid retention when used alone or in combination with insulin; anemia was reported in less than or equal 2% of patients treated with pioglitazone and metformin). Products include:
Exubera Inhalation Powder 2515

Insulin, Human NPH (Patients receiving pioglitazone in combination with insulin may be at risk for hypoglycemia; pioglitazone can cause fluid retention when used alone or in combination with insulin; anemia was reported in less than or equal 2% of patients treated with pioglitazone and metformin). Products include:
Humulin N Vial 1846

Insulin, Human Regular (Patients receiving pioglitazone in combination with insulin may be at risk for hypoglycemia; pioglitazone can cause fluid retention when used alone or in combination with insulin; anemia was reported in less than or equal 2% of patients treated with pioglitazone and metformin). Products include:
Humulin R 1849
Humulin R (U-500) 1850

Insulin, Human Regular and Human NPH Mixture (Patients receiving pioglitazone in combination with insulin may be at risk for hypoglycemia; pioglitazone can cause fluid retention when used alone or in combination with insulin; anemia was reported in less than or equal 2% of patients treated with pioglitazone and metformin). Products include:
Humulin 50/50, 100 Units 1843
Humulin 70/30 Vial 1844

Insulin, NPH (Patients receiving pioglitazone in combination with insulin may be at risk for hypoglycemia; pioglitazone can cause fluid retention when used alone or in combination with insulin; anemia was reported in less than or equal 2% of patients treated with pioglitazone and metformin).
No products indexed under this heading.

Insulin, Regular (Patients receiving pioglitazone in combination with insulin may be at risk for hypoglycemia; pioglitazone can cause fluid retention when used alone or in combination with insulin; anemia was reported in less than or equal 2% of patients treated with pioglitazone and metformin).
No products indexed under this heading.

Insulin, Regular and NPH mixture (Patients receiving pioglitazone in combination with insulin may be at risk for hypoglycemia; pioglitazone can cause fluid retention when used alone or in combination with insulin; anemia was reported in less than or equal 2% of patients treated with pioglitazone and metformin).
No products indexed under this heading.

Insulin, Zinc Crystals (Patients receiving pioglitazone in combination with insulin may be at risk for hypoglycemia; pioglitazone can cause fluid retention when used alone or in combination with insulin; anemia was reported in less than or equal 2% of patients treated with pioglitazone and metformin).
No products indexed under this heading.

Insulin, Zinc Suspension (Patients receiving pioglitazone in combination with insulin may be at risk for hypoglycemia; pioglitazone can cause fluid retention when used alone or in combination with insulin; anemia was reported in less than or equal 2% of patients treated with pioglitazone and metformin).
No products indexed under this heading.

Insulin Aspart (Patients receiving pioglitazone in combination with insulin may be at risk for hypoglycemia; pioglitazone can cause fluid retention when used alone or in combination with insulin; anemia was reported in less than or equal 2% of patients treated with pioglitazone and metformin).
No products indexed under this heading.

Insulin Aspart, Human (Patients receiving pioglitazone in combination with insulin may be at risk for hypoglycemia; pioglitazone can cause fluid retention when used alone or in combination with insulin; anemia was reported in less than or equal 2% of patients treated with pioglitazone and metformin). Products include:
NovoLog Mix 70/30 2364

Insulin Aspart, Human Regular (Patients receiving pioglitazone in combination with insulin may be at risk for hypoglycemia; pioglitazone can cause fluid retention when used alone or in combination with insulin; anemia was reported in less than or equal 2% of patients treated with pioglitazone and metformin). Products include:
NovoLog Injection 2359

Insulin Aspart Protamine, Human (Patients receiving pioglitazone in combination with insulin may be at risk for hypoglycemia; pioglitazone can cause fluid retention when used alone or in combination with insulin; anemia was reported in less than or equal 2% of patients treated with pioglitazone and metformin). Products include:
NovoLog Mix 70/30 2364

Insulin Detemir (rDNA Origin) (Patients receiving pioglitazone in combination with insulin may be at risk for hypoglycemia; pioglitazone can cause fluid retention when used alone or in combination with insulin; anemia was reported in less than or equal 2% of patients treated with pioglitazone and metformin). Products include:
Levemir Injection 2352

Insulin glargine (Patients receiving pioglitazone in combination with insulin may be at risk for hypoglycemia; pioglitazone can cause fluid retention when used alone or in combination with insulin; anemia was reported in less than or equal 2% of patients treated with pioglitazone and metformin). Products include:
Lantus Injection 2749

Insulin Glulisine (Patients receiving pioglitazone in combination with insulin may be at risk for hypoglycemia; pioglitazone can cause fluid retention when used alone or in combination with insulin; anemia was reported in less than or equal 2% of patients treated with pioglitazone and metformin). Products include:
Apidra Injection 2706

Insulin Lispro, Human (Patients receiving pioglitazone in combination with insulin may be at risk for hypoglycemia; pioglitazone can cause fluid retention when used alone or in combination with insulin; anemia was reported in less than or equal 2% of patients treated with pioglitazone and metformin). Products include:
Humalog-Pen and KwikPen 1829
Humalog Mix 50/50-Pen and KwikPen 1833
Humalog Mix 75/25-Pen and KwikPen 1835

Insulin Lispro Protamine, Human (Patients receiving pioglitazone in combination with insulin may be at risk for hypoglycemia; pioglitazone can cause fluid retention when used alone or in combination with insulin; anemia was reported in less than or equal 2% of patients treated with pioglitazone and metformin). Products include:
Humalog Mix 50/50-Pen and KwikPen 1833
Humalog Mix 75/25-Pen and KwikPen 1835

Isradipine (Pioglitazone may be a weak inducer of CYP450 isoform 3A4 substrate). Products include:
DynaCirc CR Controlled Release Tablets 1407

Itraconazole (Pioglitazone may be a weak inducer of CYP450 isoform 3A4 substrate).
No products indexed under this heading.

Ixabepilone (Pioglitazone may be a weak inducer of CYP450 isoform 3A4 substrate). Products include:
Ixempra Kit for Injection 915

Ketoconazole (Pioglitazone may be a weak inducer of CYP450 isoform 3A4 substrate). Products include:
Extina Foam, 2% 3057
Nizoral A-D Shampoo 1901

Levonorgestrel (Co-administration of pioglitazone hydrochloride (45mg once daily) and an oral contraceptive (1mg norethindrone plus 0.035mg ethinyl estradiol once daily) for 21 days, resulted in an 11% decrease in ethinyl estradiol AUC (0-24h) and an 11% to 14% decrease in C_{max}. There were no significant changes in norethindrone AUC (0-24h) and C_{max}). Products include:
Climara Pro Transdermal System 768
Lybrel Tablets 3204
Mirena Intrauterine System 779
Plan B Tablets 1044
Seasonique Tablets 1046

Lidocaine (Pioglitazone may be a weak inducer of CYP450 isoform 3A4 substrate). Products include:
Lidoderm Patch 1114

Lidocaine Hydrochloride (Pioglitazone may be a weak inducer of CYP450 isoform 3A4 substrate).
No products indexed under this heading.

Lovastatin (Pioglitazone may be a weak inducer of CYP450 isoform 3A4 substrate). Products include:
Advicor Tablets 402
Mevacor Tablets 2063

Mestranol (Co-administration of pioglitazone hydrochloride (45mg once daily) and an oral contraceptive (1mg norethindrone plus 0.035mg ethinyl estradiol once daily) for 21 days, resulted in an 11% decrease in ethinyl estradiol AUC (0-24h) and an 11% to 14% decrease in C_{max}. There were no significant changes in norethindrone AUC (0-24h) and C_{max}).
No products indexed under this heading.

Metformin (Anemia was reported in less than or equal to 2% of patients with pioglitazone and metformin).
No products indexed under this heading.

Metformin Hydrochloride (Anemia was reported in less than or equal to 2% of patients with pioglitazone and metformin). Products include:
ActoPlus Met Tablets 3071
Avandamet Tablets 1336
Janumet Tablets 2041
PrandiMet Tablets 2967

Methadone Hydrochloride (Pioglitazone may be a weak inducer of CYP450 isoform 3A4 substrate).
No products indexed under this heading.

Midazolam Hydrochloride (Pioglitazone appears to induce the metabolism of midazolam with a 26% reduction of midazolam Cmax and AUC).
No products indexed under this heading.

Miglitol (Patients receiving pioglitazone in combination with oral hypoglycemic agents may be at risk for hypoglycemia. Pioglitazone can cause fluid retention when used alone or in combination with other antidiabetic agents).
No products indexed under this heading.

Nateglinide (Patients receiving pioglitazone in combination with oral hypoglycemic agents may be at risk for hypoglycemia. Pioglitazone can cause fluid retention when used alone or in combination with other antidiabetic agents). Products include:
Starlix Tablets ... 2314

Nefazodone Hydrochloride (Pioglitazone may be a weak inducer of CYP450 isoform 3A4 substrate).
No products indexed under this heading.

Nelfinavir Mesylate (Pioglitazone may be a weak inducer of CYP450 isoform 3A4 substrate).
No products indexed under this heading.

Nicardipine Hydrochloride (An enzyme inhibitor of CYP2C8 may significantly increase the AUC of pioglitazone; therefore, if an enzyme inhibitor of CYP2C8 is started or stopped during treatment with pioglitazone, changes in diabetes treatment may be needed). Products include:
Cardene I.V. ... 1093

Nifedipine (Pioglitazone may be a weak inducer of CYP450 isoform 3A4 substrate).
No products indexed under this heading.

Nimodipine (Pioglitazone may be a weak inducer of CYP450 isoform 3A4 substrate). Products include:
Nimotop Capsules ... 790

Nisoldipine (Pioglitazone may be a weak inducer of CYP450 isoform 3A4 substrate). Products include:
Sular Extended Release Tablets ... 2975

Nitrendipine (Pioglitazone may be a weak inducer of CYP450 isoform 3A4 substrate).
No products indexed under this heading.

Norethindrone (Co-administration of pioglitazone hydrochloride (45mg once daily) and an oral contraceptive (1mg norethindrone plus 0.035mg ethinyl estradiol once daily) for 21 days, resulted in an 11% decrease in ethinyl estradiol AUC (0-24h) and an 11% to 14% decrease in C_{max}. There were no significant changes in norethindrone AUC (0-24h) and C_{max}). Products include:
Ortho Micronor Tablets ... 2446

Norethindrone Acetate (Pioglitazone may be a weak inducer of CYP450 isoform 3A4 substrate). Products include:
Activella Tablets ... 2347

Norethynodrel (Co-administration of pioglitazone hydrochloride (45mg once daily) and an oral contraceptive (1mg norethindrone plus 0.035mg ethinyl estradiol once daily) for 21 days, resulted in an 11% decrease in ethinyl estradiol AUC (0-24h) and an 11% to 14% decrease in C_{max}. There were no significant changes in norethindrone AUC (0-24h) and C_{max}).
No products indexed under this heading.

Norgestimate (Co-administration of pioglitazone hydrochloride (45mg once daily) and an oral contraceptive (1mg norethindrone plus 0.035mg ethinyl estradiol once daily) for 21 days, resulted in an 11% decrease in ethinyl estradiol AUC (0-24h) and an 11% to 14% decrease in C_{max}. There were no significant changes in norethindrone AUC (0-24h) and C_{max}). Products include:
Ortho-Cyclen/Ortho Tri-Cyclen ... 2449
Ortho Tri-Cyclen Lo Tablets ... 2458

Norgestrel (Co-administration of pioglitazone hydrochloride (45mg once daily) and an oral contraceptive (1mg norethindrone plus 0.035mg ethinyl estradiol once daily) for 21 days, resulted in an 11% decrease in ethinyl estradiol AUC (0-24h) and an 11% to 14% decrease in C_{max}. There were no significant changes in norethindrone AUC (0-24h) and C_{max}).
No products indexed under this heading.

Omeprazole (An enzyme inhibitor of CYP2C8 may significantly increase the AUC of pioglitazone; therefore, if an enzyme inhibitor of CYP2C8 is started or stopped during treatment with pioglitazone, changes in diabetes treatment may be needed).
No products indexed under this heading.

Ondansetron (Pioglitazone may be a weak inducer of CYP450 isoform 3A4 substrate). Products include:
Zofran ODT Orally Disintegrating Tablets ... 1687

Ondansetron Hydrochloride (Pioglitazone may be a weak inducer of CYP450 isoform 3A4 substrate). Products include:
Zofran Injection ... 1682
Zofran ... 1687

Paclitaxel (Pioglitazone may be a weak inducer of CYP450 isoform 3A4 substrate).
No products indexed under this heading.

Phenobarbital (An enzyme inducer of CYP2C8 may significantly decrease the AUC of pioglitazone; therefore, if an enzyme inducer of CYP2C8 is started or stopped during treatment with pioglitazone, changes in diabetes treatment may be needed). Products include:
Donnatal Extentabs ... 2507

Pimozide (Pioglitazone may be a weak inducer of CYP450 isoform 3A4 substrate).
No products indexed under this heading.

Polyestradiol Phosphate (Pioglitazone may be a weak inducer of CYP450 isoform 3A4 substrate).
No products indexed under this heading.

Primidone (An enzyme inducer of CYP2C8 may significantly decrease the AUC of pioglitazone; therefore, if an enzyme inducer of CYP2C8 is started or stopped during treatment with pioglitazone, changes in diabetes treatment may be needed).
No products indexed under this heading.

Quercetin (An enzyme inhibitor of CYP2C8 may significantly increase the AUC of pioglitazone; therefore, if an enzyme inhibitor of CYP2C8 is started or stopped during treatment with pioglitazone, changes in diabetes treatment may be needed).
No products indexed under this heading.

Quinidine Gluconate (Pioglitazone may be a weak inducer of CYP450 isoform 3A4 substrate).
No products indexed under this heading.

Quinidine Polygalacturonate (Pioglitazone may be a weak inducer of CYP450 isoform 3A4 substrate).
No products indexed under this heading.

Quinidine Sulfate (Pioglitazone may be a weak inducer of CYP450 isoform 3A4 substrate).
No products indexed under this heading.

Repaglinide (Patients receiving pioglitazone in combination with oral hypoglycemic agents may be at risk for hypoglycemia. Pioglitazone can cause fluid retention when used alone or in combination with other antidiabetic agents). Products include:
PrandiMet Tablets ... 2967
Prandin Tablets ... 2971

Rifabutin (An enzyme inducer of CYP2C8 may significantly decrease the AUC of pioglitazone; therefore, if an enzyme inducer of CYP2C8 is started or stopped during treatment with pioglitazone, changes in diabetes treatment may be needed).
No products indexed under this heading.

Rifampin (Concomitant administration of rifampin (oral 600 mg twice daily), an inducer of CYP2C8 with pioglitazone (oral 30 mg) in 10 healthy volunteers pre-treated for 5 days prior with rifampin (oral 600 mg twice daily) resulted in a decrease in the AUC of pioglitazone by 54%).
No products indexed under this heading.

Ritonavir (Pioglitazone may be a weak inducer of CYP450 isoform 3A4 substrate). Products include:
Kaletra ... 452
Norvir ... 489

Rosiglitazone Maleate (Patients receiving pioglitazone in combination with oral hypoglycemic agents may be at risk for hypoglycemia. Pioglitazone can cause fluid retention when used alone or in combination with other antidiabetic agents). Products include:
Avandamet Tablets ... 1336
Avandaryl Tablets ... 1344
Avandia Tablets ... 1351

Rosiglitazone/Metformin (Anemia was reported in less than or equal to 2% of patients with pioglitazone and metformin).
No products indexed under this heading.

Saquinavir (Pioglitazone may be a weak inducer of CYP450 isoform 3A4 substrate).
No products indexed under this heading.

Saquinavir Mesylate (Pioglitazone may be a weak inducer of CYP450 isoform 3A4 substrate).
No products indexed under this heading.

Sertraline Hydrochloride (Pioglitazone may be a weak inducer of CYP450 isoform 3A4 substrate).
No products indexed under this heading.

Sildenafil Citrate (Pioglitazone may be a weak inducer of CYP450 isoform 3A4 substrate).
No products indexed under this heading.

Simvastatin (Pioglitazone may be a weak inducer of CYP450 isoform 3A4 substrate). Products include:
Simcor Tablets ... 502
Vytorin 10/10 Tablets ... 2149
Vytorin 10/10 Tablets ... 2939
Vytorin 10/20 Tablets ... 2149
Vytorin 10/20 Tablets ... 2939
Vytorin 10/40 Tablets ... 2149
Vytorin 10/40 Tablets ... 2939
Vytorin 10/80 Tablets ... 2149
Vytorin 10/80 Tablets ... 2939
Zocor Tablets ... 2136

Sirolimus (Pioglitazone may be a weak inducer of CYP450 isoform 3A4 substrate). Products include:
Rapamune ... 3260

Sitagliptin Phosphate (Patients receiving pioglitazone in combination with oral hypoglycemic agents may be at risk for hypoglycemia. Pioglitazone can cause fluid retention when used alone or in combination with other antidiabetic agents). Products include:
Janumet Tablets ... 2041
Januvia Tablets ... 2048

Sulfaphenazole (An enzyme inhibitor of CYP2C8 may significantly increase the AUC of pioglitazone; therefore, if an enzyme inhibitor of CYP2C8 is started or stopped during treatment with pioglitazone, changes in diabetes treatment may be needed).
No products indexed under this heading.

Sulfinpyrazone (An enzyme inhibitor of CYP2C8 may significantly increase the AUC of pioglitazone; therefore, if an enzyme inhibitor of CYP2C8 is started or stopped during treatment with pioglitazone, changes in diabetes treatment may be needed).
No products indexed under this heading.

Tacrolimus (Pioglitazone may be a weak inducer of CYP450 isoform 3A4 substrate). Products include:
Prograf Capsules and Injection ... 622
Protopic Ointment ... 628

Tadalafil (Pioglitazone may be a weak inducer of CYP450 isoform 3A4 substrate). Products include:
Cialis Tablets ... 1792

Tamoxifen Citrate (Pioglitazone may be a weak inducer of CYP450 isoform 3A4 substrate).
No products indexed under this heading.

Tiagabine Hydrochloride (Pioglitazone may be a weak inducer of CYP450 isoform 3A4 substrate). Products include:
Gabitril Tablets ... 973

Tolazamide (Patients receiving pioglitazone in combination with oral hypoglycemic agents may be at risk for hypoglycemia. Pioglitazone can cause fluid retention when used alone or in combination with other antidiabetic agents).
No products indexed under this heading.

Tolbutamide (Patients receiving pioglitazone in combination with oral hypoglycemic agents may be at risk for hypoglycemia. Pioglitazone can cause fluid retention when used alone or in combination with other antidiabetic agents).
No products indexed under this heading.

Tolterodine Tartrate (Pioglitazone may be a weak inducer of CYP450 isoform 3A4 substrate).
No products indexed under this heading.

Trazodone Hydrochloride (Pioglitazone may be a weak inducer of CYP450 isoform 3A4 substrate).
No products indexed under this heading.

Triazolam (Pioglitazone may be a weak inducer of CYP450 isoform 3A4 substrate).
No products indexed under this heading.

Trimethoprim (An enzyme inhibitor of CYP2C8 may significantly increase the AUC of pioglitazone; therefore, if an enzyme inhibitor of CYP2C8 is started or stopped during treatment with pioglitazone, changes in diabetes treatment may be needed).
No products indexed under this heading.

Trimethoprim Hydrochloride (An enzyme inhibitor of CYP2C8 may significantly increase the AUC of pioglitazone; therefore, if an enzyme inhibitor of CYP2C8 is started or stopped during treatment with pioglitazone, changes in diabetes treatment may be needed).
No products indexed under this heading.

Troglitazone (Patients receiving pioglitazone in combination with oral hypoglycemic agents may be at risk for hypoglycemia. Pioglitazone can cause fluid retention when used alone or in combination with other antidiabetic agents).
No products indexed under this heading.

Vardenafil Hydrochloride (Pioglitazone may be a weak inducer of CYP450 isoform 3A4 substrate). Products include:
Levitra Tablets 2876

Verapamil Hydrochloride (Pioglitazone may be a weak inducer of CYP450 isoform 3A4 substrate). Products include:
Tarka Tablets 511

Vinblastine Sulfate (Pioglitazone may be a weak inducer of CYP450 isoform 3A4 substrate).
No products indexed under this heading.

Vincristine Sulfate (Pioglitazone may be a weak inducer of CYP450 isoform 3A4 substrate).
No products indexed under this heading.

Warfarin Sodium (Pioglitazone may be a weak inducer of CYP450 isoform 3A4 substrate).
No products indexed under this heading.

ACZONE GEL 5%

(Dapsone) 3296

May interact with antimalarials, anticonvulsants, and certain other agents. Compounds in these categories include:

Benzoyl Peroxide (Topical application of dapsone gel dapsone gel followed by benzoyl peroxide in subjects with acne vulgaris resulted in a temporary local yellow or orange discoloration of the skin and facial hair (reported 7 out of 95 subjects) with resolution in 4 to 57 days). Products include:
Benzaclin Topical Gel 2721
Brevoxyl 3054
Brevoxyl 3054
Duac Topical Gel 3054

Carbamazepine (Concomitant administration may increase the formation of dapsone hydroxylamine, a metabolite of dapsone associated with hemolysis). Products include:
Carbatrol Capsules 3019
Equetro Extended-Release Capsules 3174

Chloroquine Hydrochloride (Dapsone gel, 5% should not be used in patients who are taking antimalarial medications because of the potential for hemolytic reactions).
No products indexed under this heading.

Chloroquine Phosphate (Dapsone gel, 5% should not be used in patients who are taking antimalarial medications because of the potential for hemolytic reactions).
No products indexed under this heading.

Divalproex Sodium (Concomitant administration may increase the formation of dapsone hydroxylamine, a metabolite of dapsone associated with hemolysis). Products include:
Depakote ER Tablets 423

Ethosuximide (Concomitant administration may increase the formation of dapsone hydroxylamine, a metabolite of dapsone associated with hemolysis).
No products indexed under this heading.

Ethotoin (Concomitant administration may increase the formation of dapsone hydroxylamine, a metabolite of dapsone associated with hemolysis).
No products indexed under this heading.

Felbamate (Concomitant administration may increase the formation of dapsone hydroxylamine, a metabolite of dapsone associated with hemolysis).
No products indexed under this heading.

Fosphenytoin (Concomitant administration may increase the formation of dapsone hydroxylamine, a metabolite of dapsone associated with hemolysis).
No products indexed under this heading.

Fosphenytoin Sodium (Concomitant administration may increase the formation of dapsone hydroxylamine, a metabolite of dapsone associated with hemolysis).
No products indexed under this heading.

Gabapentin (Concomitant administration may increase the formation of dapsone hydroxylamine, a metabolite of dapsone associated with hemolysis).
No products indexed under this heading.

Hypericum (Certain concomitant medications such as St. John's wort, may increase the formation of dapsone hydroxylamine, a metabolite of dapsone associated with hemolysis). Products include:
Satieté Tablets 640

Lamotrigine (Concomitant administration may increase the formation of dapsone hydroxylamine, a metabolite of dapsone associated with hemolysis). Products include:
Lamictal 1488

Levetiracetam (Concomitant administration may increase the formation of dapsone hydroxylamine, a metabolite of dapsone associated with hemolysis). Products include:
Keppra Injection 3137
Keppra Oral Solution 3131
Keppra Tablets 3131

Mefloquine Hydrochloride (Dapsone gel, 5% should not be used in patients who are taking antimalarial medications because of the potential for hemolytic reactions).
No products indexed under this heading.

Mephenytoin (Concomitant administration may increase the formation of dapsone hydroxylamine, a metabolite of dapsone associated with hemolysis).
No products indexed under this heading.

Methsuximide (Concomitant administration may increase the formation of dapsone hydroxylamine, a metabolite of dapsone associated with hemolysis).
No products indexed under this heading.

Oxcarbazepine (Concomitant administration may increase the formation of dapsone hydroxylamine, a metabolite of dapsone associated with hemolysis).
No products indexed under this heading.

Paramethadione (Concomitant administration may increase the formation of dapsone hydroxylamine, a metabolite of dapsone associated with hemolysis).
No products indexed under this heading.

Phenacemide (Concomitant administration may increase the formation of dapsone hydroxylamine, a metabolite of dapsone associated with hemolysis).
No products indexed under this heading.

Phenobarbital (Concomitant administration may increase the formation of dapsone hydroxylamine, a metabolite of dapsone associated with hemolysis). Products include:
Donnatal Extentabs 2507

Phensuximide (Concomitant administration may increase the formation of dapsone hydroxylamine, a metabolite of dapsone associated with hemolysis).
No products indexed under this heading.

Phenytoin (Concomitant administration may increase the formation of dapsone hydroxylamine, a metabolite of dapsone associated with hemolysis).
No products indexed under this heading.

Phenytoin Sodium (Concomitant administration may increase the formation of dapsone hydroxylamine, a metabolite of dapsone associated with hemolysis). Products include:
Phenytek Capsules 2192

Primidone (Concomitant administration may increase the formation of dapsone hydroxylamine, a metabolite of dapsone associated with hemolysis).
No products indexed under this heading.

Pyrimethamine (With oral dapsone treatment, folic acid antagonists such as pyrimethamine have been noted to possibly increase the likelihood of hematologic reactions). Products include:
Daraprim Tablets 1400
Fansidar Tablets 2636

Rifampin (Certain concomitant medications such as rifampin may increase the formation of dapson hydroxylamine, a metabolite of dapsone associated with hemolysis).
No products indexed under this heading.

Sulfamethoxazole (A study evaluated the effect of the use of dapsone gel in combination with trimethoprim-sulfamethoxazole (TMP/SMX). During co-administration, system levels of TMP and SMX were essentially unchanged. However, levels of dapsone and its metabolites increased in the presence of TMP/SMX. Systemic exposure (AUC 0-24) of dapsone and N-acetyl-dapsone were increased by about 40% and 20%, respectively, in the presence of TMP/SMX. Systemic exposure (AUC 0-24) of dapsone hydroxylamine was more than doubled in the presence of TMP/SMX. Exposure from the proposed topical dose is about 1% of that from the 100 mg oral dose, even when co-administered with TMP/SMX. Use of dapsone gel with TMP/SMX may increase the likelihood of hemolysis in patients with G6PD deficiency).
No products indexed under this heading.

Tiagabine Hydrochloride (Concomitant administration may increase the formation of dapsone hydroxylamine, a metabolite of dapsone associated with hemolysis). Products include:
Gabitril Tablets 973

Topiramate (Concomitant administration may increase the formation of dapsone hydroxylamine, a metabolite of dapsone associated with hemolysis).
No products indexed under this heading.

Trimethadione (Concomitant administration may increase the formation of dapsone hydroxylamine, a metabolite of dapsone associated with hemolysis).
No products indexed under this heading.

Trimethoprim (A study evaluated the effect of the use of dapsone gel in combination with trimethoprim-sulfamethoxazole (TMP/SMX). During co-administration, system levels of TMP and SMX were essentially unchanged. However, levels of dapsone and its metabolites increased in the presence of TMP/SMX. Systemic exposure (AUC 0-24) of dapsone and N-acetyl-dapsone were increased by about 40% and 20%, respectively, in the presence of TMP/SMX. Systemic exposure (AUC 0-24) of dapsone hydroxylamine was more than doubled in the presence of TMP/SMX. Exposure from the proposed topical dose is about 1% of that from the 100 mg oral dose, even when co-administered with TMP/SMX. Use of dapsone gel with TMP/SMX may increase the likelihood of hemolysis in patients with G6PD deficiency).
No products indexed under this heading.

Trimethoprim Hydrochloride (A study evaluated the effect of the use of dapsone gel in combination with trimethoprim-sulfamethoxazole (TMP/SMX). During co-administration, system levels of TMP and SMX were essentially unchanged. However, levels of dapsone and its metabolites increased in the presence of TMP/SMX. Systemic exposure (AUC 0-24) of dapsone and N-acetyl-dapsone were increased by about 40% and 20%, respectively, in the presence of TMP/SMX. Systemic exposure (AUC 0-24) of dapsone hydroxylamine was more than doubled in the presence of TMP/SMX. Exposure from the proposed topical dose is about 1% of that from the 100 mg oral dose, even when co-administered with TMP/SMX. Use of dapsone gel with TMP/SMX may increase the likelihood of hemolysis in patients with G6PD deficiency).
No products indexed under this heading.

Trimethoprim Sulfate (A study evaluated the effect of the use of dapsone gel in combination with trimethoprim-sulfamethoxazole (TMP/SMX). During co-administration, system levels of TMP and SMX were essentially unchanged. However, levels of dapsone and its metabolites increased in the presence of TMP/SMX. Systemic exposure (AUC 0-24) of dapsone and N-acetyl-dapsone were increased by about 40% and 20%, respectively, in the presence of TMP/SMX. Systemic exposure (AUC 0-24) of dapsone hydroxylamine was more than doubled in the presence of TMP/SMX. Exposure from the proposed topical dose is about 1% of that from the 100 mg oral dose, even when co-administered with TMP/SMX. Use of dapsone gel with TMP/SMX may increase the likelihood of hemolysis in patients with G6PD deficiency).
No products indexed under this heading.

Valproate Sodium (Concomitant administration may increase the formation of dapsone hydroxylamine, a metabolite of dapsone associated with hemolysis).
No products indexed under this heading.

Valproic Acid (Concomitant administration may increase the formation of dapsone hydroxylamine, a metabolite of dapsone associated with hemolysis).
No products indexed under this heading.

Zonisamide (Concomitant administration may increase the formation of dapsone hydroxylamine, a metabolite of dapsone associated with hemolysis). Products include:
Zonegran Capsules 1089

ADDERALL XR CAPSULES

(Amphetamine Aspartate, Amphetamine Sulfate, Dextroamphetamine Saccharate, Dextroamphetamine Sulfate).............. 3012
May interact with antacids, antihistamines, antihypertensives, beta blockers, monoamine oxidase inhibitors, methenamine, phenytoin, thiazides, tricyclic antidepressants, urinary alkalinizing agents, veratrum alkaloids, and certain other agents. Compounds in these categories include:

Acebutolol Hydrochloride (Adrenergic blockers are inhibited by amphetamines; amphetamines may antagonize the hypotensive effects of antihypertensives).
No products indexed under this heading.

Acetazolamide (Co-administration with urinary alkalinizing agents, such as acetazolamide, increase the concentration of the non-ionized species of the amphetamine molecule, thereby decreasing urinary excretion resulting in increased blood levels and potentiate the actions of amphetamines).
No products indexed under this heading.

Acetazolamide Sodium (Co-administration with urinary alkalinizing agents, such as acetazolamide, increase the concentration of the non-ionized species of the amphetamine molecule, thereby decreasing urinary excretion resulting in increased blood levels and potentiate the actions of amphetamines).
No products indexed under this heading.

Acrivastine (Amphetamines may counteract the sedative effect of antihistamines).
No products indexed under this heading.

Aliskiren (Amphetamines may antagonize the hypotensive effects of antihypertensives). Products include:
Tekturna Tablets 2321
Tekturna HCT Tablets 2324

Aluminum Carbonate (Co-administration with gastrointestinal alkalinizing agents, such as antacids, may increase the absorption of amphetamines; concurrent use should be avoided).
No products indexed under this heading.

Aluminum Hydroxide (Co-administration with gastrointestinal alkalinizing agents, such as antacids, may increase the absorption of amphetamines; concurrent use should be avoided).
No products indexed under this heading.

Amitriptyline Hydrochloride (Enhanced activity of tricyclic antidepressants or sympathomimetics; possible increases in d-amphetamine resulting in potentiation of cardiovascular effects).
No products indexed under this heading.

Amlodipine Besylate (Amphetamines may antagonize the hypotensive effects of antihypertensives). Products include:
Azor Tablets 1005
Exforge Tablets 2238

Ammonium Chloride (Co-administration with urinary acidifying agents increases the concentration of the ionized species of the amphetamine molecule, thereby increasing urinary excretion resulting in reduced blood levels and efficacy of amphetamines).
No products indexed under this heading.

Amoxapine (Enhanced activity of tricyclic antidepressants or sympathomimetics; possible increases in d-amphetamine resulting in potentiation of cardiovascular effects).
No products indexed under this heading.

Astemizole (Amphetamines may counteract the sedative effect of antihistamines).
No products indexed under this heading.

Atenolol (Adrenergic blockers are inhibited by amphetamines; amphetamines may antagonize the hypotensive effects of antihypertensives).
No products indexed under this heading.

Azatadine Maleate (Amphetamines may counteract the sedative effect of antihistamines).
No products indexed under this heading.

Benazepril Hydrochloride (Amphetamines may antagonize the hypotensive effects of antihypertensives).
No products indexed under this heading.

Bendroflumethiazide (Co-administration with urinary alkalinizing agents, such as certain thiazides, increase the concentration of the non-ionized species of the amphetamine molecule, thereby decreasing urinary excretion resulting in increased blood levels and potentiation ofactions of amphetamines; amphetamines may antagonize the hypotensive effects of antihypertensives).
No products indexed under this heading.

Betaxolol Hydrochloride (Adrenergic blockers are inhibited by amphetamines; amphetamines may antagonize the hypotensive effects of antihypertensives).
No products indexed under this heading.

Bisoprolol Fumarate (Adrenergic blockers are inhibited by amphetamines; amphetamines may antagonize the hypotensive effects of antihypertensives).
No products indexed under this heading.

Bromodiphenhydramine Hydrochloride (Amphetamines may counteract the sedative effect of antihistamines).
No products indexed under this heading.

Brompheniramine Maleate (Amphetamines may counteract the sedative effect of antihistamines).
No products indexed under this heading.

Candesartan Cilexetil (Amphetamines may antagonize the hypotensive effects of antihypertensives). Products include:
Atacand Tablets 639
Atacand HCT 642

Captopril (Amphetamines may antagonize the hypotensive effects of antihypertensives). Products include:
Captopril Tablets 2182

Carteolol Hydrochloride (Adrenergic blockers are inhibited by amphetamines; amphetamines may antagonize the hypotensive effects of antihypertensives).
No products indexed under this heading.

Cetirizine Hydrochloride (Amphetamines may counteract the sedative effect of antihistamines). Products include:
Zyrtec Allergy Tablets 1919
Zyrtec Chewable Tablets 1920
Children's Zyrtec Allergy Chewable Tablets 1922
Children's Zyrtec Allergy Syrup 1920
Children's Zyrtec Hives Relief Syrup 1920
Zyrtec Syrup 1920
Zyrtec Tablets 1920
Zyrtec-D 12 Hour Extended Release Tablets 1923
Zyrtec-D Allergy & Congestion Extended-Release Tablets 1923

Chlorothiazide (Co-administration with urinary alkalinizing agents, such as certain thiazides, increase the concentration of the non-ionized species of the amphetamine molecule, thereby decreasing urinary excretion resulting in increased blood levels and potentiation ofactions of amphetamines; amphetamines may antagonize the hypotensive effects of antihypertensives).
No products indexed under this heading.

Chlorothiazide Sodium (Co-administration with urinary alkalinizing agents, such as certain thiazides, increase the concentration of the non-ionized species of the amphetamine molecule, thereby decreasing urinary excretion resulting in increased blood levels and potentiation ofactions of ampheta-

mines; amphetamines may antagonize the hypotensive effects of antihypertensives). Products include:
- Intravenous Sodium Diuril 2490

Chlorpheniramine Maleate (Amphetamines may counteract the sedative effect of antihistamines). Products include:
- Actifed Cold & Allergy Tablets 1895
- Sudafed PE Sinus & Allergy Tablets 1908
- Tylenol Allergy Multi-Symptom Caplets with Cool Burst and Rapid Release Gelcaps 1916
- Children's Tylenol Plus Cold Suspension Liquid 1912
- Children's Tylenol Plus Cough & Runny Nose Suspension Liquid 1912
- Children's Tylenol Plus Flu Suspension Liquid 1914
- Children's Tylenol Plus Multi-Symptom Cold Suspension Liquid 1912
- Tylenol Cold Head Congestion Nighttime Caplets with Cool Burst 1910
- Tylenol Cold Multi-Symptom Nighttime Caplets with Cool Burst 1913
- Tylenol Sinus Congestion & Pain Nighttime Caplets with Cool Burst 1917

Chlorpheniramine Polistirex (Amphetamines may counteract the sedative effect of antihistamines). Products include:
- Tussionex Pennkinetic Extended-Release Suspension 3154

Chlorpheniramine Tannate (Amphetamines may counteract the sedative effect of antihistamines).
No products indexed under this heading.

Chlorpromazine (Blocks the dopamine and norepinephrine receptors, thus inhibiting the central stimulant effects of amphetamines).
No products indexed under this heading.

Chlorpromazine Hydrochloride (Blocks the dopamine and norepinephrine receptors, thus inhibiting the central stimulant effects of amphetamines).
No products indexed under this heading.

Chlorthalidone (Amphetamines may antagonize the hypotensive effects of antihypertensives). Products include:
- Clorpres Tablets 2185

Clemastine Fumarate (Amphetamines may counteract the sedative effect of antihistamines).
No products indexed under this heading.

Clomipramine Hydrochloride (Enhanced activity of tricyclic antidepressants or sympathomimetics; possible increases in d-amphetamine resulting in potentiation of cardiovascular effects).
No products indexed under this heading.

Clonidine (Amphetamines may antagonize the hypotensive effects of antihypertensives). Products include:
- Catapres-TTS 842

Clonidine Hydrochloride (Amphetamines may antagonize the hypotensive effects of antihypertensives). Products include:
- Catapres Tablets 841
- Clorpres Tablets 2185

Cryptenamine Preparations (Amphetamines inhibit the hypotensive effect of veratrum alkaloids).
No products indexed under this heading.

Cyproheptadine Hydrochloride (Amphetamines may counteract the sedative effect of antihistamines).
No products indexed under this heading.

Deserpidine (Amphetamines may antagonize the hypotensive effects of antihypertensives).
No products indexed under this heading.

Desipramine Hydrochloride (Enhanced activity of tricyclic antidepressants or sympathomimetics; possible increases in d-amphetamine resulting in potentiation of cardiovascular effects).
No products indexed under this heading.

Dexchlorpheniramine Maleate (Amphetamines may counteract the sedative effect of antihistamines).
No products indexed under this heading.

Diazoxide (Amphetamines may antagonize the hypotensive effects of antihypertensives). Products include:
- Proglycem Capsules 1185
- Proglycem Suspension 1185

Diltiazem Hydrochloride (Amphetamines may antagonize the hypotensive effects of antihypertensives). Products include:
- Cardizem LA Extended Release Tablets 421

Diphenhydramine Citrate (Amphetamines may counteract the sedative effect of antihistamines).
No products indexed under this heading.

Diphenhydramine Hydrochloride (Amphetamines may counteract the sedative effect of antihistamines). Products include:
- Benadryl Allergy & Cold Kapgels 1895
- Benadryl Allergy & Sinus Headache Kapgels 1895
- Benadryl Severe Allergy & Sinus Headache Caplets 1897
- Benadryl Dye-Free Allergy Liqui-gels Softgels 1897
- Benadryl Allergy Kapgels 1895
- Benadryl Allergy Quick Dissolve Strips 1896
- Benadryl Allergy Ultratab Tablets 1896
- Children's Benadryl Dye-Free Allergy Liquid 1897
- Children's Benadryl Allergy Fastmelts 1897
- Children's Benadryl Allergy Liquid 1898
- Children's Benadryl Allergy Perfect Measure 1896
- Children's Benadryl-D Allergy & Sinus Liquid 1896
- Benadryl-D Allergy & Sinus Tablet 1896
- PediaCare Children's Allergy & Cold Liquid 1902
- PediaCare Children's Allergy Liquid 1902
- Simply Sleep Caplets 1905
- Sudafed PE Nighttime Cold Caplets 1907
- Sudafed PE Severe Cold Caplets 1908
- Extra Strength Tylenol PM Caplets, Geltabs, Liquid, and Rapid Release Gels 1915
- Tylenol Allergy Multi-Symptom Nighttime Caplets with Cool Burst 1916
- Tylenol Severe Allergy Caplets 1916
- Children's Tylenol Plus Cold & Allergy Suspension Liquid 1914
- Tylenol Sore Throat Nighttime Liquid with Cool Burst 1918

Diphenylpyraline Hydrochloride (Amphetamines may counteract the sedative effect of antihistamines).
No products indexed under this heading.

Doxazosin Mesylate (Amphetamines may antagonize the hypotensive effects of antihypertensives).
No products indexed under this heading.

Doxepin Hydrochloride (Enhanced activity of tricyclic antidepressants or sympathomimetics; possible increases in d-amphetamine resulting in potentiation of cardiovascular effects).
No products indexed under this heading.

Enalapril Maleate (Amphetamines may antagonize the hypotensive effects of antihypertensives).
No products indexed under this heading.

Enalaprilat (Amphetamines may antagonize the hypotensive effects of antihypertensives).
No products indexed under this heading.

Eprosartan Mesylate (Amphetamines may antagonize the hypotensive effects of antihypertensives). Products include:
- Teveten Tablets 515
- Teveten HCT Tablets 517

Esmolol Hydrochloride (Adrenergic blockers are inhibited by amphetamines; amphetamines may antagonize the hypotensive effects of antihypertensives).
No products indexed under this heading.

Ethosuximide (Amphetamines may delay intestinal absorption of ethosuximide).
No products indexed under this heading.

Felodipine (Amphetamines may antagonize the hypotensive effects of antihypertensives).
No products indexed under this heading.

Fexofenadine Hydrochloride (Amphetamines may counteract the sedative effect of antihistamines). Products include:
- Allegra Oral Solution 2684
- Allegra Tablets 2684
- Allegra-D 12 Hour Extended-Release Tablets 2687
- Allegra-D 24 Hour Extended-Release Tablets 2690

Fosinopril Sodium (Amphetamines may antagonize the hypotensive effects of antihypertensives).
No products indexed under this heading.

Fosphenytoin Sodium (Amphetamines may delay intestinal absorption of phenytoin; co-administration may produce a synergistic anticonvulsant action).
No products indexed under this heading.

Furazolidone (Concurrent use with metabolite of furazolidone may result in hypertensive crises; may slow the metabolism of amphetamines with resultant increase in their effect on release of norepinephrine and other monoamines from adrenergic nerve ending; this can cause headaches and other signs of hypertensice crises).
No products indexed under this heading.

Furosemide (Amphetamines may antagonize the hypotensive effects of antihypertensives). Products include:
- Furosemide Tablets 2186

Glutamic Acid Hydrochloride (Co-administration with gastrointestinal acidifying agents, such as glutamic acid, lowers absorption of amphetamines resulting in reduced blood levels and efficacy of amphetamines).
No products indexed under this heading.

Guanabenz Acetate (Amphetamines may antagonize the hypotensive effects of antihypertensives).
No products indexed under this heading.

Guanethidine Monosulfate (Co-administration with gastrointestinal acidifying agents, such as guanethidine, lowers absorption of amphetamines resulting in reduced blood levels and efficacy of amphetamines; amphetamines may antagonize the hypotensive effects of antihypertensives).
No products indexed under this heading.

Haloperidol (Blocks the dopamine receptors, thus inhibiting the central stimulant effects of amphetamines).
No products indexed under this heading.

Haloperidol Decanoate (Blocks the dopamine receptors, thus inhibiting the central stimulant effects of amphetamines).
No products indexed under this heading.

Hydralazine Hydrochloride (Amphetamines may antagonize the hypotensive effects of antihypertensives).
No products indexed under this heading.

Hydrochlorothiazide (Co-administration with urinary alkalinizing agents, such as certain thiazides, increase the concentration of the non-ionized species of the amphetamine molecule, thereby decreasing urinary excretion resulting in increased blood levels and potentiation ofactions of amphetamines; amphetamines may antagonize the hypotensive effects of antihypertensives). Products include:
- Atacand HCT 642
- Avalide Tablets 892
- Avalide Tablets 2713
- Benicar HCT Tablets 1010
- Diovan HCT Tablets 2216
- Dyazide Capsules 1405
- Micardis HCT Tablets 854
- Prinzide Tablets 2092
- Tekturna HCT Tablets 2324
- Teveten HCT Tablets 517

Hydroflumethiazide (Co-administration with urinary alkalinizing agents, such as certain thiazides, increase the concentration of the non-ionized species of the amphetamine molecule, thereby decreasing urinary excretion resulting in increased blood levels and potentiation ofactions of amphetamines; amphetamines may antagonize the hypotensive effects of antihypertensives).
No products indexed under this heading.

IMPORTANT NOTE: Always consult each drug listing in the patient's regimen for possible interactions.

Imipramine Hydrochloride (Enhanced activity of tricyclic antidepressants or sympathomimetics; possible increases in d-amphetamine resulting in potentiation of cardiovascular effects).
No products indexed under this heading.

Imipramine Pamoate (Enhanced activity of tricyclic antidepressants or sympathomimetics; possible increases in d-amphetamine resulting in potentiation of cardiovascular effects).
No products indexed under this heading.

Indapamide (Amphetamines may antagonize the hypotensive effects of antihypertensives). Products include:
Indapamide Tablets 2188

Irbesartan (Amphetamines may antagonize the hypotensive effects of antihypertensives). Products include:
Avalide Tablets 892
Avalide Tablets 2713
Avapro Tablets 897
Avapro Tablets 2718

Isocarboxazid (Concurrent and/or sequential use may result in hypertensive crises; MAOI may slow the metabolism of amphetamines with resultant increase in their effect on release of norepinephrine and other monoamines from adrenergic nerve ending; this can cause headaches and other signs of hypertensive crises; concurrent and/or sequential use is contraindicated). Products include:
Marplan Tablets 3177

Isradipine (Amphetamines may antagonize the hypotensive effects of antihypertensives). Products include:
DynaCirc CR Controlled Release Tablets 1407

Labetalol Hydrochloride (Adrenergic blockers are inhibited by amphetamines; amphetamines may antagonize the hypotensive effects of antihypertensives).
No products indexed under this heading.

Levobunolol Hydrochloride (Adrenergic blockers are inhibited by amphetamines; amphetamines may antagonize the hypotensive effects of antihypertensives).
No products indexed under this heading.

Lisinopril (Amphetamines may antagonize the hypotensive effects of antihypertensives). Products include:
Prinivil Tablets 2087
Prinzide Tablets 2092

Lithium Carbonate (Anorectic and stimulatory effects of amphetamines may be inhibited by lithium carbonate).
No products indexed under this heading.

Loratadine (Amphetamines may counteract the sedative effect of antihistamines).
No products indexed under this heading.

Losartan Potassium (Amphetamines may antagonize the hypotensive effects of antihypertensives). Products include:
Cozaar Tablets 1973

Magaldrate (Co-administration with gastrointestinal alkalinizing agents, such as antacids, may increase the absorption of amphetamines; concurrent use should be avoided).
No products indexed under this heading.

Magnesium Hydroxide (Co-administration with gastrointestinal alkalinizing agents, such as antacids, may increase the absorption of amphetamines; concurrent use should be avoided). Products include:
Fleet Pedia-Lax Chewable Tablets 1145
Pepcid Complete Chewable Tablets 1771
Extra Strength Rolaids Freshmint Tablets 1903
Rolaids Multi-Symptom Berry Tablets 1903
Rolaids Original Peppermint Tablets 1903

Magnesium Oxide (Co-administration with gastrointestinal alkalinizing agents, such as antacids, may increase the absorption of amphetamines; concurrent use should be avoided). Products include:
Beelith Tablets 813

Maprotiline Hydrochloride (Enhanced activity of tricyclic antidepressants or sympathomimetics; possible increases in d-amphetamine resulting in potentiation of cardiovascular effects).
No products indexed under this heading.

Mecamylamine Hydrochloride (Amphetamines may antagonize the hypotensive effects of antihypertensives).
No products indexed under this heading.

Meperidine Hydrochloride (Amphetamines potentiate the analgesic effect of meperidine).
No products indexed under this heading.

Methdilazine Hydrochloride (Amphetamines may counteract the sedative effect of antihistamines).
No products indexed under this heading.

Methenamine (Urinary excretion of amphetamines is increased, and efficacy is reduced by acidifying agents used in methenamine therapy).
No products indexed under this heading.

Methenamine Hippurate (Urinary excretion of amphetamines is increased, and efficacy is reduced by acidifying agents used in methenamine therapy).
No products indexed under this heading.

Methenamine Mandelate (Urinary excretion of amphetamines is increased, and efficacy is reduced by acidifying agents used in methenamine therapy). Products include:
Uroqid-Acid No. 2 Tablets 814

Methyclothiazide (Co-administration with urinary alkalinizing agents, such as certain thiazides, increase the concentration of the non-ionized species of the amphetamine molecule, thereby decreasing urinary excretion resulting in increased blood levels and potentiation ofactions of amphetamines; amphetamines may antagonize the hypotensive effects of antihypertensives).
No products indexed under this heading.

Methyldopa (Amphetamines may antagonize the hypotensive effects of antihypertensives).
No products indexed under this heading.

Methyldopate Hydrochloride (Amphetamines may antagonize the hypotensive effects of antihypertensives).
No products indexed under this heading.

Metipranolol Hydrochloride (Adrenergic blockers are inhibited by amphetamines; amphetamines may antagonize the hypotensive effects of antihypertensives).
No products indexed under this heading.

Metolazone (Amphetamines may antagonize the hypotensive effects of antihypertensives).
No products indexed under this heading.

Metoprolol Succinate (Adrenergic blockers are inhibited by amphetamines; amphetamines may antagonize the hypotensive effects of antihypertensives). Products include:
Toprol-XL Tablets 666

Metoprolol Tartrate (Adrenergic blockers are inhibited by amphetamines; amphetamines may antagonize the hypotensive effects of antihypertensives).
No products indexed under this heading.

Metyrosine (Amphetamines may antagonize the hypotensive effects of antihypertensives). Products include:
Demser Capsules 1989

Mibefradil Dihydrochloride (Amphetamines may antagonize the hypotensive effects of antihypertensives).
No products indexed under this heading.

Minoxidil (Amphetamines may antagonize the hypotensive effects of antihypertensives).
No products indexed under this heading.

Moclobemide (Concurrent and/or sequential use may result in hypertensive crises; MAOI may slow the metabolism of amphetamines with resultant increase in their effect on release of norepinephrine and other monoamines from adrenergic nerve ending; this can cause headaches and other signs of hypertensive crises; concurrent and/or sequential use is contraindicated).
No products indexed under this heading.

Moexipril Hydrochloride (Amphetamines may antagonize the hypotensive effects of antihypertensives).
No products indexed under this heading.

Nadolol (Adrenergic blockers are inhibited by amphetamines; amphetamines may antagonize the hypotensive effects of antihypertensives). Products include:
Nadolol Tablets 2191

Nebivolol (Adrenergic blockers are inhibited by amphetamines; amphetamines may antagonize the hypotensive effects of antihypertensives). Products include:
Bystolic Tablets 1155

Nicardipine Hydrochloride (Amphetamines may antagonize the hypotensive effects of antihypertensives). Products include:
Cardene I.V. 1093

Nifedipine (Amphetamines may antagonize the hypotensive effects of antihypertensives).
No products indexed under this heading.

Nisoldipine (Amphetamines may antagonize the hypotensive effects of antihypertensives). Products include:
Sular Extended Release Tablets 2975

Nitroglycerin (Amphetamines may antagonize the hypotensive effects of antihypertensives). Products include:
Nitro-Dur Transdermal Infusion System 2887
Nitrolingual Pumpspray 2965

Norepinephrine Bitartrate (Amphetamines enhance the adrenergic effect of norepinephrine).
No products indexed under this heading.

Nortriptyline Hydrochloride (Enhanced activity of tricyclic antidepressants or sympathomimetics; possible increases in d-amphetamine resulting in potentiation of cardiovascular effects).
No products indexed under this heading.

Pargyline Hydrochloride (Concurrent and/or sequential use may result in hypertensive crises; MAOI may slow the metabolism of amphetamines with resultant increase in their effect on release of norepinephrine and other monoamines from adrenergic nerve ending; this can cause headaches and other signs of hypertensive crises; concurrent and/or sequential use is contraindicated).
No products indexed under this heading.

Penbutolol Sulfate (Adrenergic blockers are inhibited by amphetamines; amphetamines may antagonize the hypotensive effects of antihypertensives).
No products indexed under this heading.

Perindopril Erbumine (Amphetamines may antagonize the hypotensive effects of antihypertensives). Products include:
Aceon Tablets (2 mg, 4 mg, 8 mg) 3038

Phenelzine Sulfate (Concurrent and/or sequential use may result in hypertensive crises; MAOI may slow the metabolism of amphetamines with resultant increase in their effect on release of norepinephrine and other monoamines from adrenergic nerve ending; this can cause headaches and other signs of hypertensive crises; concurrent and/or sequential use is contraindicated).
No products indexed under this heading.

Phenobarbital (Amphetamines may delay intestinal absorption of phenobarbital; co-administration may produce a synergistic anticonvulsant action). Products include:
Donnatal Extentabs 2507

Phenoxybenzamine Hydrochloride (Amphetamines may antagonize the hypotensive effects of antihypertensives). Products include:
Dibenzyline Capsules 3188

Phentolamine Mesylate (Amphetamines may antagonize the hypotensive effects of antihypertensives).
No products indexed under this heading.

Phenytoin (Amphetamines may delay intestinal absorption of phenytoin; co-administration may produce a synergistic anticonvulsant action).
No products indexed under this heading.

Phenytoin Sodium (Amphetamines may delay intestinal absorption of phenytoin; co-administration may produce a synergistic anticonvulsant action). Products include:
Phenytek Capsules **2192**

Pindolol (Adrenergic blockers are inhibited by amphetamines; amphetamines may antagonize the hypotensive effects of antihypertensives).
No products indexed under this heading.

Polythiazide (Co-administration with urinary alkalinizing agents, such as certain thiazides, increase the concentration of the non-ionized species of the amphetamine molecule, thereby decreasing urinary excretion resulting in increased blood levels and potentiation ofactions of amphetamines; amphetamines may antagonize the hypotensive effects of antihypertensives).
No products indexed under this heading.

Potassium Citrate (Co-administration with urinary acidifying agents increases the concentration of the ionized species of the amphetamine molecule, thereby increasing urinary excretion resulting in reduced blood levels and efficacy of amphetamines). Products include:
BioLean Free Tablets **635**
Urocit-K Tablets **2176**

Prazosin Hydrochloride (Amphetamines may antagonize the hypotensive effects of antihypertensives).
No products indexed under this heading.

Procarbazine Hydrochloride (Concurrent and/or sequential use may result in hypertensive crises; MAOI may slow the metabolism of amphetamines with resultant increase in their effect on release of norepinephrine and other monoamines from adrenergic nerve ending; this can cause headaches and other signs of hypertensive crises; concurrent and/or sequential use is contraindicated).
No products indexed under this heading.

Promethazine Hydrochloride (Amphetamines may counteract the sedative effect of antihistamines).
No products indexed under this heading.

Propoxyphene Hydrochloride (In cases of propoxyphene overdosage, amphetamine CNS stimulation is potentiated and fatal convulstions can occur).
No products indexed under this heading.

Propoxyphene Napsylate (In cases of propoxyphene overdosage, amphetamine CNS stimulation is potentiated and fatal convulstions can occur).
No products indexed under this heading.

Propranolol Hydrochloride (Adrenergic blockers are inhibited by amphetamines; amphetamines may antagonize the hypotensive effects of antihypertensives). Products include:
InnoPran XL Extended Release Capsules **1484**

Protriptyline Hydrochloride (Enhanced activity of tricyclic antidepressants or sympathomimetics; possible increases in d-amphetamine resulting in potentiation of cardiovascular effects).
No products indexed under this heading.

Pyrilamine Maleate (Amphetamines may counteract the sedative effect of antihistamines).
No products indexed under this heading.

Pyrilamine Tannate (Amphetamines may counteract the sedative effect of antihistamines).
No products indexed under this heading.

Quinapril Hydrochloride (Amphetamines may antagonize the hypotensive effects of antihypertensives).
No products indexed under this heading.

Ramipril (Amphetamines may antagonize the hypotensive effects of antihypertensives).
No products indexed under this heading.

Rasagiline Mesylate (Concurrent and/or sequential use may result in hypertensive crises; MAOI may slow the metabolism of amphetamines with resultant increase in their effect on release of norepinephrine and other monoamines from adrenergic nerve ending; this can cause headaches and other signs of hypertensive crises; concurrent and/or sequential use is contraindicated). Products include:
Azilect Tablets **3106**

Rauwolfia Serpentina (Amphetamines may antagonize the hypotensive effects of antihypertensives).
No products indexed under this heading.

Rescinnamine (Amphetamines may antagonize the hypotensive effects of antihypertensives).
No products indexed under this heading.

Reserpine (Co-administration with gastrointestinal acidifying agents, such as reserpine, lowers absorption of amphetamines resulting in reduced blood levels and efficacy of amphetamines; amphetamines may antagonize the hypotensive effects of antihypertensives).
No products indexed under this heading.

Selegiline (Concurrent and/or sequential use may result in hypertensive crises; MAOI may slow the metabolism of amphetamines with resultant increase in their effect on release of norepinephrine and other monoamines from adrenergic nerve ending; this can cause headaches and other signs of hypertensive crises; concurrent and/or sequential use is contraindicated). Products include:
Emsam Transdermal System **905**

Selegiline Hydrochloride (Concurrent and/or sequential use may result in hypertensive crises; MAOI may slow the metabolism of amphetamines with resultant increase in their effect on release of norepinephrine and other monoamines from adrenergic nerve ending; this can cause headaches and other signs of hypertensive crises; concurrent and/or sequential use is contraindicated). Products include:
Eldepryl Capsules **3052**

Sodium Bicarbonate (Co-administration with gastrointestinal alkalinizing agents, such as systemic disodium bicarbonate, increases the absorption of amphetamines). Products include:
Ceo-Two Laxative Suppository **815**

Sodium Citrate (Co-administration with urinary acidifying agents increases the concentration of the ionized species of the amphetamine molecule, thereby increasing urinary excretion resulting in reduced blood levels and efficacy of amphetamines).
No products indexed under this heading.

Sodium Nitroprusside (Amphetamines may antagonize the hypotensive effects of antihypertensives).
No products indexed under this heading.

Sotalol Hydrochloride (Adrenergic blockers are inhibited by amphetamines; amphetamines may antagonize the hypotensive effects of antihypertensives).
No products indexed under this heading.

Spirapril Hydrochloride (Amphetamines may antagonize the hypotensive effects of antihypertensives).
No products indexed under this heading.

Telmisartan (Amphetamines may antagonize the hypotensive effects of antihypertensives). Products include:
Micardis Tablets **852**
Micardis HCT Tablets **854**

Terazosin Hydrochloride (Amphetamines may antagonize the hypotensive effects of antihypertensives).
No products indexed under this heading.

Terfenadine (Amphetamines may counteract the sedative effect of antihistamines).
No products indexed under this heading.

Timolol Hemihydrate (Adrenergic blockers are inhibited by amphetamines; amphetamines may antagonize the hypotensive effects of antihypertensives). Products include:
Betimol Ophthalmic Solution **3181**

Timolol Maleate (Adrenergic blockers are inhibited by amphetamines; amphetamines may antagonize the hypotensive effects of antihypertensives). Products include:
Combigan Ophthalmic Solution **553**
Cosopt Sterile Ophthalmic Solution.. **1969**
Timoptic Sterile Ophthalmic Solution.. **2121**
Timoptic in Ocudose **2124**
Timoptic-XE Sterile Ophthalmic Gel Forming Solution..................... **2125**

Torsemide (Amphetamines may antagonize the hypotensive effects of antihypertensives). Products include:
Demadex Injection **2630**
Demadex Tablets **2630**

Trandolapril (Amphetamines may antagonize the hypotensive effects of antihypertensives). Products include:
Mavik Tablets **472**
Tarka Tablets **511**

Tranylcypromine Sulfate (Concurrent and/or sequential use may result in hypertensive crises; MAOI may slow the metabolism of amphetamines with resultant increase in their effect on release of norepinephrine and other monoamines from adrenergic nerve ending; this can cause headaches and other signs of hypertensive crises; concurrent and/or sequential use is contraindicated). Products include:
Parnate Tablets **1532**

Trimeprazine Tartrate (Amphetamines may counteract the sedative effect of antihistamines).
No products indexed under this heading.

Trimethaphan Camsylate (Amphetamines may antagonize the hypotensive effects of antihypertensives).
No products indexed under this heading.

Trimipramine Maleate (Enhanced activity of tricyclic antidepressants or sympathomimetics; possible increases in d-amphetamine resulting in potentiation of cardiovascular effects).
No products indexed under this heading.

Tripelennamine Hydrochloride (Amphetamines may counteract the sedative effect of antihistamines).
No products indexed under this heading.

Triprolidine Hydrochloride (Amphetamines may counteract the sedative effect of antihistamines).
No products indexed under this heading.

Valsartan (Amphetamines may antagonize the hypotensive effects of antihypertensives). Products include:
Diovan Tablets **2212**
Diovan HCT Tablets **2216**
Exforge Tablets **2238**

Verapamil Hydrochloride (Amphetamines may antagonize the hypotensive effects of antihypertensives). Products include:
Tarka Tablets **511**

Vitamin C (Co-administration with gastrointestinal acidifying agents, such as vitamin C, lowers absorption of amphetamines resulting in reduced blood levels and efficacy of amphetamines). Products include:
Bausch & Lomb Ocuvite Adult 50+ Vitamin and Mineral Supplement.................................. ⊙**237**
Comax Dietary Supplement **995**
Ferralet 90 Tablets **2175**
Glaucofit Dietary Supplement **995**
Glauma Dietary Supplement **995**
MoviPrep Oral Solution **2679**
Procosa II Tablets **3174**
Proflavanol 90 Tablets **3174**
Tonox Dietary Supplement **995**
Vibe Liquid Multi-Nutrient Supplement.................................. **626**

Food Interactions

Food, unspecified (Concurrent use with food prolongs T_{max} by 2.5 hours, however, food does not affect the extent of absorption).

IMPORTANT NOTE: Always consult each drug listing in the patient's regimen for possible interactions.

ADENOCARD IV INJECTION

(Adenosine) 603

May interact with cardiac glycosides, xanthines, and certain other agents. Compounds in these categories include:

Aminophylline (The effects of adenosine are antagonized by co-administration with methylxanthines, such as theophylline; larger doses of adenosine may be required or adenosine may not be effective).

No products indexed under this heading.

Caffeine (The effects of adenosine are antagonized by co-administration with methylxanthines, such as caffeine; larger doses of adenosine may be required or adenosine may not be effective). Products include:

BioLean Free Tablets .... ▣635
BioLean II Tablets .... ▣635
Winrgy Dietary Supplement .... ▣642

Carbamazepine (Adenosine decreases the conduction through AV node, higher degrees of heart block may be produced in the presence of carbamazepine). Products include:

Carbatrol Capsules 3019
Equetro Extended-Release Capsules 3174

Deslanoside (The use of adenosine in patients receiving digitalis may be rarely associated with ventricular fibrillation).

No products indexed under this heading.

Digitalis Glycoside Preparations (The use of adenosine in patients receiving digitalis may be rarely associated with ventricular fibrillation).

No products indexed under this heading.

Digitoxin (The use of adenosine in patients receiving digitalis may be rarely associated with ventricular fibrillation).

No products indexed under this heading.

Digoxin (The use of adenosine in patients receiving digitalis may be rarely associated with ventricular fibrillation). Products include:

Lanoxin Injection 1498
Lanoxin Injection Pediatric 1502
Lanoxin Tablets 1505

Dipyridamole (Adenosine effects are potentiated by dipyridamole; smaller doses of adenosine may be effective with concurrent use). Products include:

Aggrenox Capsules 819
Persantine Tablets 869

Dyphylline (The effects of adenosine are antagonized by co-administration with methylxanthines, such as theophylline; larger doses of adenosine may be required or adenosine may not be effective).

No products indexed under this heading.

Theophylline (The effects of adenosine are antagonized by co-administration with methylxanthines, such as theophylline; larger doses of adenosine may be required or adenosine may not be effective).

No products indexed under this heading.

Theophylline Anhydrous (The effects of adenosine are antagonized by co-administration with methylxanthines, such as theophylline; larger doses of adenosine may be required or adenosine may not be effective). Products include:

Uniphyl Tablets 2595

Theophylline Calcium Salicylate (The effects of adenosine are antagonized by co-administration with methylxanthines, such as theophylline; larger doses of adenosine may be required or adenosine may not be effective).

No products indexed under this heading.

Theophylline Dihydroxypropyl (Glyceryl) (The effects of adenosine are antagonized by co-administration with methylxanthines, such as theophylline; larger doses of adenosine may be required or adenosine may not be effective).

No products indexed under this heading.

Theophylline Ethylenediamine (The effects of adenosine are antagonized by co-administration with methylxanthines, such as theophylline; larger doses of adenosine may be required or adenosine may not be effective).

No products indexed under this heading.

Theophylline Sodium Glycinate (The effects of adenosine are antagonized by co-administration with methylxanthines, such as theophylline; larger doses of adenosine may be required or adenosine may not be effective).

No products indexed under this heading.

Verapamil Hydrochloride (Digoxin and verapamil use may be rarely associated with ventricular fibrillation when combined with adenosine; potential for additive or synergistic depressant effects on the SA and AV nodes). Products include:

Tarka Tablets 511

ADENOSCAN

(Adenosine) 605

May interact with adenosine receptor antagonists, beta blockers, calcium channel blockers, cardiac glycosides, and nucleoside transport inhibitors. Compounds in these categories include:

Acebutolol Hydrochloride (Potential for additive or synergistic depressant effects on the SA or AV nodes; adenosine should be used with caution in the presence of these agents; no adverse interactions have been reported when co-administered).

No products indexed under this heading.

Aminophylline (The vasoactive effects of adenosine are inhibited by adenosine receptor antagonists such as methylxanthines).

No products indexed under this heading.

Amlodipine Besylate (Potential for additive or synergistic depressant effects on the SA or AV nodes; adenosine should be used with caution in the presence of these agents; no adverse interactions have been reported when co-administered). Products include:

Azor Tablets 1005
Exforge Tablets 2238

Atenolol (Potential for additive or synergistic depressant effects on the SA or AV nodes; adenosine should be used with caution in the presence of these agents; no adverse interactions have been reported when co-administered).

No products indexed under this heading.

Bepridil Hydrochloride (Potential for additive or synergistic depressant effects on the SA or AV nodes; adenosine should be used with caution in the presence of these agents; no adverse interactions have been reported when co-administered).

No products indexed under this heading.

Betaxolol Hydrochloride (Potential for additive or synergistic depressant effects on the SA or AV nodes; adenosine should be used with caution in the presence of these agents; no adverse interactions have been reported when co-administered).

No products indexed under this heading.

Bisoprolol Fumarate (Potential for additive or synergistic depressant effects on the SA or AV nodes; adenosine should be used with caution in the presence of these agents; no adverse interactions have been reported when co-administered).

No products indexed under this heading.

Caffeine (The vasoactive effects of adenosine are inhibited by adenosine receptor antagonists such as methylxanthines). Products include:

BioLean Free Tablets .... ▣635
BioLean II Tablets .... ▣635
Winrgy Dietary Supplement .... ▣642

Carteolol Hydrochloride (Potential for additive or synergistic depressant effects on the SA or AV nodes; adenosine should be used with caution in the presence of these agents; no adverse interactions have been reported when co-administered).

No products indexed under this heading.

Deslanoside (Potential for additive or synergistic depressant effects on the SA or AV nodes; adenosine should be used with caution in the presence of these agents; no adverse interactions have been reported when co-administered).

No products indexed under this heading.

Digitalis Glycoside Preparations (Potential for additive or synergistic depressant effects on the SA or AV nodes; adenosine should be used with caution in the presence of these agents; no adverse interactions have been reported when co-administered).

No products indexed under this heading.

Digitoxin (Potential for additive or synergistic depressant effects on the SA or AV nodes; adenosine should be used with caution in the presence of these agents; no adverse interactions have been reported when co-administered).

No products indexed under this heading.

Digoxin (Potential for additive or synergistic depressant effects on the SA or AV nodes; adenosine should be used with caution in the presence of these agents; no adverse interactions have been reported when co-administered). Products include:

Lanoxin Injection 1498
Lanoxin Injection Pediatric 1502
Lanoxin Tablets 1505

Diltiazem Hydrochloride (Potential for additive or synergistic depressant effects on the SA or AV nodes; adenosine should be used with caution in the presence of these agents; no adverse interactions have been reported when co-administered). Products include:

Cardizem LA Extended Release Tablets 421

Dipyridamole (Vasoactive effects of adenosine are potentiated by nucleoside transport inhibitors). Products include:

Aggrenox Capsules 819
Persantine Tablets 869

Dyphylline (The vasoactive effects of adenosine are inhibited by adenosine receptor antagonists such as methylxanthines).

No products indexed under this heading.

Esmolol Hydrochloride (Potential for additive or synergistic depressant effects on the SA or AV nodes; adenosine should be used with caution in the presence of these agents; no adverse interactions have been reported when co-administered).

No products indexed under this heading.

Felodipine (Potential for additive or synergistic depressant effects on the SA or AV nodes; adenosine should be used with caution in the presence of these agents; no adverse interactions have been reported when co-administered).

No products indexed under this heading.

Isradipine (Potential for additive or synergistic depressant effects on the SA or AV nodes; adenosine should be used with caution in the presence of these agents; no adverse interactions have been reported when co-administered). Products include:

DynaCirc CR Controlled Release Tablets 1407

Labetalol Hydrochloride (Potential for additive or synergistic depressant effects on the SA or AV nodes; adenosine should be used with caution in the presence of these agents; no adverse interactions have been reported when co-administered).

No products indexed under this heading.

Levobunolol Hydrochloride (Potential for additive or synergistic depressant effects on the SA or AV nodes; adenosine should be used with caution in the presence of these agents; no adverse interactions have been reported when co-administered).

No products indexed under this heading.

Metipranolol Hydrochloride (Potential for additive or synergistic depressant effects on the SA or AV nodes; adenosine should be used with caution in the presence of these agents; no adverse interactions have been reported when co-administered).

No products indexed under this heading.

Metoprolol Succinate (Potential for additive or synergistic depressant effects on the SA or AV nodes; adenosine should be used with caution in the presence of these agents; no adverse interactions have been reported when co-administered). Products include:

Toprol-XL Tablets 666

Metoprolol Tartrate (Potential for additive or synergistic depressant effects on the SA or AV nodes; adenosine should be used with caution in the presence of these agents; no adverse interactions have been reported when co-administered).

No products indexed under this heading.

Mibefradil Dihydrochloride (Potential for additive or synergistic depressant effects on the SA or AV nodes; adenosine should be used with caution in the presence of these agents; no adverse interactions have been reported when co-administered).

No products indexed under this heading.

Nadolol (Potential for additive or synergistic depressant effects on the SA or AV nodes; adenosine should be used with caution in the presence of these agents; no adverse interactions have been reported when co-administered). Products include:

Nadolol Tablets 2191

Nebivolol (Potential for additive or synergistic depressant effects on the SA or AV nodes; adenosine should be used with caution in the presence of these agents; no adverse interactions have been reported when co-administered). Products include:

Bystolic Tablets 1155

Nicardipine Hydrochloride (Potential for additive or synergistic depressant effects on the SA or AV nodes; adenosine should be used with caution in the presence of these agents; no adverse interactions have been reported when co-administered). Products include:

Cardene I.V. 1093

Nifedipine (Potential for additive or synergistic depressant effects on the SA or AV nodes; adenosine should be used with caution in the presence of these agents; no adverse interactions have been reported when co-administered).

No products indexed under this heading.

Nimodipine (Potential for additive or synergistic depressant effects on the SA or AV nodes; adenosine should be used with caution in the presence of these agents; no adverse interactions have been reported when co-administered). Products include:

Nimotop Capsules 790

Nisoldipine (Potential for additive or synergistic depressant effects on the SA or AV nodes; adenosine should be used with caution in the presence of these agents; no adverse interactions have been reported when co-administered). Products include:

Sular Extended Release Tablets 2975

Penbutolol Sulfate (Potential for additive or synergistic depressant effects on the SA or AV nodes; adenosine should be used with caution in the presence of these agents; no adverse interactions have been reported when co-administered).

No products indexed under this heading.

Pindolol (Potential for additive or synergistic depressant effects on the SA or AV nodes; adenosine should be used with caution in the presence of these agents; no adverse interactions have been reported when co-administered).

No products indexed under this heading.

Propranolol Hydrochloride (Potential for additive or synergistic depressant effects on the SA or AV nodes; adenosine should be used with caution in the presence of these agents; no adverse interactions have been reported when co-administered). Products include:

InnoPran XL Extended Release Capsules 1484

Sotalol Hydrochloride (Potential for additive or synergistic depressant effects on the SA or AV nodes; adenosine should be used with caution in the presence of these agents; no adverse interactions have been reported when co-administered).

No products indexed under this heading.

Theophylline (The vasoactive effects of adenosine are inhibited by adenosine receptor antagonists such as methylxanthines).

No products indexed under this heading.

Theophylline Calcium Salicylate (The vasoactive effects of adenosine are inhibited by adenosine receptor antagonists such as methylxanthines).

No products indexed under this heading.

Theophylline Sodium Glycinate (The vasoactive effects of adenosine are inhibited by adenosine receptor antagonists such as methylxanthines).

No products indexed under this heading.

Timolol Hemihydrate (Potential for additive or synergistic depressant effects on the SA or AV nodes; adenosine should be used with caution in the presence of these agents; no adverse interactions have been reported when co-administered). Products include:

Betimol Ophthalmic Solution 3181

Timolol Maleate (Potential for additive or synergistic depressant effects on the SA or AV nodes; adenosine should be used with caution in the presence of these agents; no adverse interactions have been reported when co-administered). Products include:

Combigan Ophthalmic Solution 553
Cosopt Sterile Ophthalmic Solution 1969
Timoptic Sterile Ophthalmic Solution 2121
Timoptic in Ocudose 2124
Timoptic-XE Sterile Ophthalmic Gel Forming Solution 2125

Verapamil Hydrochloride (Potential for additive or synergistic depressant effects on the SA or AV nodes; adenosine should be used with caution in the presence of these agents; no adverse interactions have been reported when co-administered). Products include:

Tarka Tablets 511

ADIPEX-P CAPSULES

(Phentermine Hydrochloride) 1185

See Adipex-P Tablets

ADIPEX-P TABLETS

(Phentermine Hydrochloride) 1185

May interact with insulin, monoamine oxidase inhibitors, selective serotonin reuptake inhibitors, and certain other agents. Compounds in these categories include:

Citalopram Hydrobromide (The safety and efficacy of combination therapy with phentermine and any other drug products for weight loss, including selective serotonin reuptake inhibitors, have not been established; co-administration of these products for weight loss is not recommended). Products include:

Celexa 1160

Dexfenfluramine Hydrochloride (Co-administration has resulted in primary pulmonary hypertension, a rare, frequently fatal disease of the lungs and serious regurgitant cardiac valvular disease).

No products indexed under this heading.

Escitalopram Oxalate (The safety and efficacy of combination therapy with phentermine and any other drug products for weight loss, including selective serotonin reuptake inhibitors, have not been established; co-administration of these products for weight loss is not recommended). Products include:

Lexapro Oral Suspension 1174
Lexapro Tablets 1174

Fenfluramine Hydrochloride (Co-administration has resulted in primary pulmonary hypertension, a rare, frequently fatal disease of the lungs and serious regurgitant cardiac valvular disease).

No products indexed under this heading.

Fluoxetine (The safety and efficacy of combination therapy with phentermine and any other drug products for weight loss, including selective serotonin reuptake inhibitors, have not been established; co-administration of these products for weight loss is not recommended).

No products indexed under this heading.

Fluoxetine Hydrochloride (The safety and efficacy of combination therapy with phentermine and any other drug products for weight loss, including selective serotonin reuptake inhibitors, have not been established; co-administration of these products for weight loss is not recommended). Products include:

Prozac Weekly Capsules 1852
Prozac Pulvules and Liquid 1852
Symbyax Capsules 1871

Fluvoxamine Maleate (The safety and efficacy of combination therapy with phentermine and any other drug products for weight loss, including selective serotonin reuptake inhibitors, have not been established; co-administration of these products for weight loss is not recommended). Products include:

Luvox CR Extended-Release Capsules 1759

Guanethidine Monosulfate (Decreased hypotensive effect of guanethidine).

No products indexed under this heading.

Insulin (Insulin requirement may be altered).

No products indexed under this heading.

Insulin, Human, Zinc Suspension (Insulin requirement may be altered).

No products indexed under this heading.

Insulin, Human (rDNA origin) (Insulin requirement may be altered). Products include:

Exubera Inhalation Powder 2515

Insulin, Human NPH (Insulin requirement may be altered). Products include:

Humulin N Vial 1846

Insulin, Human Regular (Insulin requirement may be altered). Products include:

Humulin R 1849
Humulin R (U-500) 1850

Insulin, Human Regular and Human NPH Mixture (Insulin requirement may be altered). Products include:

Humulin 50/50, 100 Units 1843
Humulin 70/30 Vial 1844

Insulin, NPH (Insulin requirement may be altered).

No products indexed under this heading.

Insulin, Regular (Insulin requirement may be altered).

No products indexed under this heading.

Insulin, Regular and NPH mixture (Insulin requirement may be altered).

No products indexed under this heading.

Insulin, Zinc Crystals (Insulin requirement may be altered).

No products indexed under this heading.

Insulin, Zinc Suspension (Insulin requirement may be altered).

No products indexed under this heading.

Insulin Aspart (Insulin requirement may be altered).

No products indexed under this heading.

Insulin Aspart, Human (Insulin requirement may be altered). Products include:

NovoLog Mix 70/30 2364

Insulin Aspart, Human Regular (Insulin requirement may be altered). Products include:

NovoLog Injection 2359

Insulin Aspart Protamine, Human (Insulin requirement may be altered). Products include:

NovoLog Mix 70/30 2364

Insulin Detemir (rDNA Origin) (Insulin requirement may be altered). Products include:

Levemir Injection 2352

Insulin glargine (Insulin requirement may be altered). Products include:

Lantus Injection 2749

Insulin Glulisine (Insulin requirement may be altered). Products include:

Apidra Injection 2706

Insulin Lispro, Human (Insulin requirement may be altered). Products include:

Humalog-Pen and KwikPen 1829

IMPORTANT NOTE: Always consult each drug listing in the patient's regimen for possible interactions.

Humalog Mix 50/50-Pen and KwikPen 1833
Humalog Mix 75/25-Pen and KwikPen 1835

Insulin Lispro Protamine, Human (Insulin requirement may be altered). Products include:
Humalog Mix 50/50-Pen and KwikPen 1833
Humalog Mix 75/25-Pen and KwikPen 1835

Isocarboxazid (Concurrent and/or sequential administration with MAO inhibitors may result in hypertensive crises; co-administration is contraindicated). Products include:
Marplan Tablets 3177

Moclobemide (Concurrent and/or sequential administration with MAO inhibitors may result in hypertensive crises; co-administration is contraindicated).
No products indexed under this heading.

Pargyline Hydrochloride (Concurrent and/or sequential administration with MAO inhibitors may result in hypertensive crises; co-administration is contraindicated).
No products indexed under this heading.

Paroxetine Hydrochloride (The safety and efficacy of combination therapy with phentermine and any other drug products for weight loss, including selective serotonin reuptake inhibitors, have not been established; co-administration of these products for weight loss is not recommended). Products include:
Paxil 1535
Paxil CR Controlled-Release Tablets 1544

Phenelzine Sulfate (Concurrent and/or sequential administration with MAO inhibitors may result in hypertensive crises; co-administration is contraindicated).
No products indexed under this heading.

Procarbazine Hydrochloride (Concurrent and/or sequential administration with MAO inhibitors may result in hypertensive crises; co-administration is contraindicated).
No products indexed under this heading.

Rasagiline Mesylate (Concurrent and/or sequential administration with MAO inhibitors may result in hypertensive crises; co-administration is contraindicated). Products include:
Azilect Tablets 3106

Selegiline (Concurrent and/or sequential administration with MAO inhibitors may result in hypertensive crises; co-administration is contraindicated). Products include:
Emsam Transdermal System 905

Selegiline Hydrochloride (Concurrent and/or sequential administration with MAO inhibitors may result in hypertensive crises; co-administration is contraindicated). Products include:
Eldepryl Capsules 3052

Sertraline Hydrochloride (The safety and efficacy of combination therapy with phentermine and any other drug products for weight loss, including selective serotonin reuptake inhibitors, have not been established; co-administration of these products for weight loss is not recommended).
No products indexed under this heading.

Tranylcypromine Sulfate (Concurrent and/or sequential administration with MAO inhibitors may result in hypertensive crises; co-administration is contraindicated). Products include:
Parnate Tablets 1532

Food Interactions

Alcohol (May result in adverse drug interaction).

ADVAIR DISKUS 100/50

(Fluticasone Propionate, Salmeterol Xinafoate) 1276
May interact with beta blockers, cytochrome p450 3a4 inhibitors (selected), monoamine oxidase inhibitors, potassium-depleting diuretics, tricyclic antidepressants, and certain other agents. Compounds in these categories include:

Acebutolol Hydrochloride (Co-administration with beta-blockers not only blocks the pulmonary effect of beta-agonists, such as salmeterol, but may produce severe bronchospasm in patients with asthma).
No products indexed under this heading.

Acetazolamide (Fluticasone propionate and salmeterol, the individual components of Advair Diskus, are substrates of CYP3A4. The use of strong CYP3A4 inhibitors (e.g., ritonavir, atazanavir, clarithromycin, indinavir, itraconazole, nefazodone, nelfinavir, saquinavir, ketoconazole, telithromycin) with Advair Diskus is not recommended because increased corticosteroid and increased cardiovascular adverse effects may occur).
No products indexed under this heading.

Amiodarone Hydrochloride (Fluticasone propionate and salmeterol, the individual components of Advair Diskus, are substrates of CYP3A4. The use of strong CYP3A4 inhibitors (e.g., ritonavir, atazanavir, clarithromycin, indinavir, itraconazole, nefazodone, nelfinavir, saquinavir, ketoconazole, telithromycin) with Advair Diskus is not recommended because increased corticosteroid and increased cardiovascular adverse effects may occur).
No products indexed under this heading.

Amitriptyline Hydrochloride (Concurrent and/or sequential administration with tricyclic antidepressants may potentiate the action of salmeterol on the vascular system).
No products indexed under this heading.

Amoxapine (Concurrent and/or sequential administration with tricyclic antidepressants may potentiate the action of salmeterol on the vascular system).
No products indexed under this heading.

Amprenavir (Fluticasone propionate and salmeterol, the individual components of Advair Diskus, are substrates of CYP3A4. The use of strong CYP3A4 inhibitors (e.g., ritonavir, atazanavir, clarithromycin, indinavir, itraconazole, nefazodone, nelfinavir, saquinavir, ketoconazole, telithromycin) with Advair Diskus is not recommended because increased corticosteroid and increased cardiovascular adverse effects may occur).
No products indexed under this heading.

Anastrozole (Fluticasone propionate and salmeterol, the individual components of Advair Diskus, are substrates of CYP3A4. The use of strong CYP3A4 inhibitors (e.g., ritonavir, atazanavir, clarithromycin, indinavir, itraconazole, nefazodone, nelfinavir, saquinavir, ketoconazole, telithromycin) with Advair Diskus is not recommended because increased corticosteroid and increased cardiovascular adverse effects may occur). Products include:
Arimidex Tablets 672

Aprepitant (Fluticasone propionate and salmeterol, the individual components of Advair Diskus, are substrates of CYP3A4. The use of strong CYP3A4 inhibitors (e.g., ritonavir, atazanavir, clarithromycin, indinavir, itraconazole, nefazodone, nelfinavir, saquinavir, ketoconazole, telithromycin) with Advair Diskus is not recommended because increased corticosteroid and increased cardiovascular adverse effects may occur). Products include:
Emend Capsules 1992

Atazanavir (Fluticasone propionate and salmeterol, the individual components of Advair Diskus, are substrates of CYP3A4. The use of strong CYP3A4 inhibitors (e.g., ritonavir, atazanavir, clarithromycin, indinavir, itraconazole, nefazodone, nelfinavir, saquinavir, ketoconazole, telithromycin) with Advair Diskus is not recommended because increased corticosteroid and increased cardiovascular adverse effects may occur).
No products indexed under this heading.

Atazanavir Sulfate (Fluticasone propionate and salmeterol, the individual components of Advair Diskus, are substrates of CYP3A4. The use of strong CYP3A4 inhibitors (e.g., ritonavir, atazanavir, clarithromycin, indinavir, itraconazole, nefazodone, nelfinavir, saquinavir, ketoconazole, telithromycin) with Advair Diskus is not recommended because increased corticosteroid and increased cardiovascular adverse effects may occur). Products include:
Reyataz Capsules 3299

Atenolol (Co-administration with beta-blockers not only blocks the pulmonary effect of beta-agonists, such as salmeterol, but may produce severe bronchospasm in patients with asthma).
No products indexed under this heading.

Bendroflumethiazide (The ECG changes and/or hypokalemia that may result from the administration of non-potassium sparing diuretics can be acutely worsened by beta-agonists, especially when the recommended dose of beta-agonist is exceeded).
No products indexed under this heading.

Betaxolol Hydrochloride (Co-administration with beta-blockers not only blocks the pulmonary effect of beta-agonists, such as salmeterol, but may produce severe bronchospasm in patients with asthma).
No products indexed under this heading.

Bisoprolol Fumarate (Co-administration with beta-blockers not only blocks the pulmonary effect of beta-agonists, such as salmeterol, but may produce severe bronchospasm in patients with asthma).
No products indexed under this heading.

Bumetanide (The ECG changes and/or hypokalemia that may result from the administration of non-potassium sparing diuretics can be acutely worsened by beta-agonists, especially when the recommended dose of beta-agonist is exceeded).
No products indexed under this heading.

Carteolol Hydrochloride (Co-administration with beta-blockers not only blocks the pulmonary effect of beta-agonists, such as salmeterol, but may produce severe bronchospasm in patients with asthma).
No products indexed under this heading.

Chlorothiazide (The ECG changes and/or hypokalemia that may result from the administration of non-potassium sparing diuretics can be acutely worsened by beta-agonists, especially when the recommended dose of beta-agonist is exceeded).
No products indexed under this heading.

Chlorothiazide Sodium (The ECG changes and/or hypokalemia that may result from the administration of non-potassium sparing diuretics can be acutely worsened by beta-agonists, especially when the recommended dose of beta-agonist is exceeded). Products include:
Intravenous Sodium Diuril 2490

Cimetidine (Fluticasone propionate and salmeterol, the individual components of Advair Diskus, are substrates of CYP3A4. The use of strong CYP3A4 inhibitors (e.g., ritonavir, atazanavir, clarithromycin, indinavir, itraconazole, nefazodone, nelfinavir, saquinavir, ketoconazole, telithromycin) with Advair Diskus is not recommended because increased corticosteroid and increased cardiovascular adverse effects may occur).
No products indexed under this heading.

Cimetidine Hydrochloride (Fluticasone propionate and salmeterol, the individual components of Advair Diskus, are substrates of CYP3A4. The use of strong CYP3A4 inhibitors (e.g., ritonavir, atazanavir, clarithromycin, indinavir, itraconazole, nefazodone, nelfinavir, saquinavir, ketoconazole, telithromycin) with Advair Diskus is not recommended because increased corticosteroid and increased cardiovascular adverse effects may occur).
No products indexed under this heading.

Ciprofloxacin (Fluticasone propionate and salmeterol, the individual components of Advair Diskus, are substrates of CYP3A4. The use of strong CYP3A4 inhibitors (e.g., ritonavir, atazanavir, clarithromycin, indinavir, itraconazole, nefazodone, nelfinavir, saquinavir, ketoconazole, telithromycin) with Advair Diskus is not recommended because increased corticosteroid and increased cardiovascular adverse effects may occur). Products include:

Cipro I.V. 2817
Cipro Oral Suspension 2810
Cipro XR Tablets 2823
Ciprodex Otic Suspension 541

Clarithromycin (Fluticasone propionate and salmeterol, the individual components of Advair Diskus, are substrates of CYP3A4. The use of strong CYP3A4 inhibitors (e.g., ritonavir, atazanavir, clarithromycin, indinavir, itraconazole, nefazodone, nelfinavir, saquinavir, ketoconazole, telithromycin) with Advair Diskus is not recommended because increased corticosteroid and increased cardiovascular adverse effects may occur). Products include:

Biaxin/Biaxin XL 411

Clomipramine Hydrochloride (Concurrent and/or sequential administration with tricyclic antidepressants may potentiate the action of salmeterol on the vascular system).

No products indexed under this heading.

Clotrimazole (Fluticasone propionate and salmeterol, the individual components of Advair Diskus, are substrates of CYP3A4. The use of strong CYP3A4 inhibitors (e.g., ritonavir, atazanavir, clarithromycin, indinavir, itraconazole, nefazodone, nelfinavir, saquinavir, ketoconazole, telithromycin) with Advair Diskus is not recommended because increased corticosteroid and increased cardiovascular adverse effects may occur). Products include:

Lotrisone 2881

Cyclosporine (Fluticasone propionate and salmeterol, the individual components of Advair Diskus, are substrates of CYP3A4. The use of strong CYP3A4 inhibitors (e.g., ritonavir, atazanavir, clarithromycin, indinavir, itraconazole, nefazodone, nelfinavir, saquinavir, ketoconazole, telithromycin) with Advair Diskus is not recommended because increased corticosteroid and increased cardiovascular adverse effects may occur). Products include:

Gengraf Capsules 435
Neoral Oral Solution 2280
Neoral Soft Gelatin Capsules 2280
Restasis Ophthalmic Emulsion 557
Sandimmune 2296

Dalfopristin (Fluticasone propionate and salmeterol, the individual components of Advair Diskus, are substrates of CYP3A4. The use of strong CYP3A4 inhibitors (e.g., ritonavir, atazanavir, clarithromycin, indinavir, itraconazole, nefazodone, nelfinavir, saquinavir, ketoconazole, telithromycin) with Advair Diskus is not recommended because increased corticosteroid and increased cardiovascular adverse effects may occur).

No products indexed under this heading.

Danazol (Fluticasone propionate and salmeterol, the individual components of Advair Diskus, are substrates of CYP3A4. The use of strong CYP3A4 inhibitors (e.g., ritonavir, atazanavir, clarithromycin, indinavir, itraconazole, nefazodone, nelfinavir, saquinavir, ketoconazole, telithromycin) with Advair Diskus is not recommended because increased corticosteroid and increased cardiovascular adverse effects may occur).

No products indexed under this heading.

Delavirdine Mesylate (Fluticasone propionate and salmeterol, the individual components of Advair Diskus, are substrates of CYP3A4. The use of strong CYP3A4 inhibitors (e.g., ritonavir, atazanavir, clarithromycin, indinavir, itraconazole, nefazodone, nelfinavir, saquinavir, ketoconazole, telithromycin) with Advair Diskus is not recommended because increased corticosteroid and increased cardiovascular adverse effects may occur).

No products indexed under this heading.

Desipramine Hydrochloride (Concurrent and/or sequential administration with tricyclic antidepressants may potentiate the action of salmeterol on the vascular system).

No products indexed under this heading.

Diltiazem Hydrochloride (Fluticasone propionate and salmeterol, the individual components of Advair Diskus, are substrates of CYP3A4. The use of strong CYP3A4 inhibitors (e.g., ritonavir, atazanavir, clarithromycin, indinavir, itraconazole, nefazodone, nelfinavir, saquinavir, ketoconazole, telithromycin) with Advair Diskus is not recommended because increased corticosteroid and increased cardiovascular adverse effects may occur). Products include:

Cardizem LA Extended Release Tablets 421

Diltiazem Maleate (Fluticasone propionate and salmeterol, the individual components of Advair Diskus, are substrates of CYP3A4. The use of strong CYP3A4 inhibitors (e.g., ritonavir, atazanavir, clarithromycin, indinavir, itraconazole, nefazodone, nelfinavir, saquinavir, ketoconazole, telithromycin) with Advair Diskus is not recommended because increased corticosteroid and increased cardiovascular adverse effects may occur).

No products indexed under this heading.

Doxepin Hydrochloride (Concurrent and/or sequential administration with tricyclic antidepressants may potentiate the action of salmeterol on the vascular system).

No products indexed under this heading.

Efavirenz (Fluticasone propionate and salmeterol, the individual components of Advair Diskus, are substrates of CYP3A4. The use of strong CYP3A4 inhibitors (e.g., ritonavir, atazanavir, clarithromycin, indinavir, itraconazole, nefazodone, nelfinavir, saquinavir, ketoconazole, telithromycin) with Advair Diskus is not recommended because increased corticosteroid and increased cardiovascular adverse effects may occur). Products include:

Atripla Tablets 938
Sustiva Capsules 930
Sustiva Tablets 930

Erythromycin (Fluticasone propionate and salmeterol, the individual components of Advair Diskus, are substrates of CYP3A4. The use of strong CYP3A4 inhibitors (e.g., ritonavir, atazanavir, clarithromycin, indinavir, itraconazole, nefazodone, nelfinavir, saquinavir, ketoconazole, telithromycin) with Advair Diskus is not recommended because increased corticosteroid and increased cardiovascular adverse effects may occur).

No products indexed under this heading.

Erythromycin Estolate (Fluticasone propionate and salmeterol, the individual components of Advair Diskus, are substrates of CYP3A4. The use of strong CYP3A4 inhibitors (e.g., ritonavir, atazanavir, clarithromycin, indinavir, itraconazole, nefazodone, nelfinavir, saquinavir, ketoconazole, telithromycin) with Advair Diskus is not recommended because increased corticosteroid and increased cardiovascular adverse effects may occur).

No products indexed under this heading.

Erythromycin Ethylsuccinate (Fluticasone propionate and salmeterol, the individual components of Advair Diskus, are substrates of CYP3A4. The use of strong CYP3A4 inhibitors (e.g., ritonavir, atazanavir, clarithromycin, indinavir, itraconazole, nefazodone, nelfinavir, saquinavir, ketoconazole, telithromycin) with Advair Diskus is not recommended because increased corticosteroid and increased cardiovascular adverse effects may occur). Products include:

E.E.S. 433
EryPed 431

Erythromycin Gluceptate (Fluticasone propionate and salmeterol, the individual components of Advair Diskus, are substrates of CYP3A4. The use of strong CYP3A4 inhibitors (e.g., ritonavir, atazanavir, clarithromycin, indinavir, itraconazole, nefazodone, nelfinavir, saquinavir, ketoconazole, telithromycin) with Advair Diskus is not recommended because increased corticosteroid and increased cardiovascular adverse effects may occur).

No products indexed under this heading.

Erythromycin Lactobionate (Fluticasone propionate and salmeterol, the individual components of Advair Diskus, are substrates of CYP3A4. The use of strong CYP3A4 inhibitors (e.g., ritonavir, atazanavir, clarithromycin, indinavir, itraconazole, nefazodone, nelfinavir, saquinavir, ketoconazole, telithromycin) with Advair Diskus is not recommended because increased corticosteroid and increased cardiovascular adverse effects may occur).

No products indexed under this heading.

Erythromycin Stearate (Fluticasone propionate and salmeterol, the individual components of Advair Diskus, are substrates of CYP3A4. The use of strong CYP3A4 inhibitors (e.g., ritonavir, atazanavir, clarithromycin, indinavir, itraconazole, nefazodone, nelfinavir, saquinavir, ketoconazole, telithromycin) with Advair Diskus is not recommended because increased corticosteroid and increased cardiovascular adverse effects may occur).

No products indexed under this heading.

Esmolol Hydrochloride (Co-administration with beta-blockers not only blocks the pulmonary effect of beta-agonists, such as salmeterol, but may produce severe bronchospasm in patients with asthma).

No products indexed under this heading.

Esomeprazole Magnesium (Fluticasone propionate and salmeterol, the individual components of Advair Diskus, are substrates of CYP3A4. The use of strong CYP3A4 inhibitors (e.g., ritonavir, atazanavir, clarithromycin, indinavir, itraconazole, nefazodone, nelfinavir, saquinavir, ketoconazole, telithromycin) with Advair Diskus is not recommended because increased corticosteroid and increased cardiovascular adverse effects may occur). Products include:

Nexium Delayed-Release Capsules 645
Nexium Delayed-Release Oral Suspension 645

Ethacrynic Acid (The ECG changes and/or hypokalemia that may result from the administration of non-potassium sparing diuretics can be acutely worsened by beta-agonists, especially when the recommended dose of beta-agonist is exceeded). Products include:

Edecrin Tablets 698

Fluconazole (Fluticasone propionate and salmeterol, the individual components of Advair Diskus, are substrates of CYP3A4. The use of strong CYP3A4 inhibitors (e.g., ritonavir, atazanavir, clarithromycin, indinavir, itraconazole, nefazodone, nelfinavir, saquinavir, ketoconazole, telithromycin) with Advair Diskus is not recommended because increased corticosteroid and increased cardiovascular adverse effects may occur).

No products indexed under this heading.

Fluoxetine (Fluticasone propionate and salmeterol, the individual components of Advair Diskus, are substrates of CYP3A4. The use of strong CYP3A4 inhibitors (e.g., ritonavir, atazanavir, clarithromycin, indinavir, itraconazole, nefazodone, nelfinavir, saquinavir, ketoconazole, telithromycin) with Advair Diskus is not recommended because increased corticosteroid and increased cardiovascular adverse effects may occur).

No products indexed under this heading.

Fluoxetine Hydrochloride (Fluticasone propionate and salmeterol, the individual components of Advair Diskus, are substrates of CYP3A4. The use of strong CYP3A4 inhibitors (e.g., ritonavir, atazanavir, clarithromycin, indinavir, itraconazole, nefazodone, nelfinavir, saquinavir, ketoconazole, telithromycin) with Advair Diskus is not recommended because increased corticosteroid and increased cardiovascular adverse effects may occur). Products include:

Prozac Weekly Capsules 1852
Prozac Pulvules and Liquid 1852
Symbyax Capsules 1871

Fluvoxamine Maleate (Fluticasone propionate and salmeterol, the individual components of Advair Diskus, are substrates of CYP3A4. The use of strong CYP3A4 inhibitors (e.g., ritonavir, atazanavir, clarithromycin,

indinavir, itraconazole, nefazodone, nelfinavir, saquinavir, ketoconazole, telithromycin) with Advair Diskus is not recommended because increased corticosteroid and increased cardiovascular adverse effects may occur). Products include:

Luvox CR Extended-Release Capsules 1759

Fosamprenavir Calcium (Fluticasone propionate and salmeterol, the individual components of Advair Diskus, are substrates of CYP3A4. The use of strong CYP3A4 inhibitors (e.g., ritonavir, atazanavir, clarithromycin, indinavir, itraconazole, nefazodone, nelfinavir, saquinavir, ketoconazole, telithromycin) with Advair Diskus is not recommended because increased corticosteroid and increased cardiovascular adverse effects may occur). Products include:

Lexiva Oral Suspension 1510
Lexiva Tablets 1510

Furosemide (The ECG changes and/or hypokalemia that may result from the administration of non-potassium sparing diuretics can be acutely worsened by beta-agonists, especially when the recommended dose of beta-agonist is exceeded). Products include:

Furosemide Tablets 2186

Hydrochlorothiazide (The ECG changes and/or hypokalemia that may result from the administration of non-potassium sparing diuretics can be acutely worsened by beta-agonists, especially when the recommended dose of beta-agonist is exceeded). Products include:

Atacand HCT 642
Avalide Tablets 892
Avalide Tablets 2713
Benicar HCT Tablets 1010
Diovan HCT Tablets 2216
Dyazide Capsules 1405
Micardis HCT Tablets 854
Prinzide Tablets 2092
Tekturna HCT Tablets 2324
Teveten HCT Tablets 517

Hydroflumethiazide (The ECG changes and/or hypokalemia that may result from the administration of non-potassium sparing diuretics can be acutely worsened by beta-agonists, especially when the recommended dose of beta-agonist is exceeded).

No products indexed under this heading.

Imipramine Hydrochloride (Concurrent and/or sequential administration with tricyclic antidepressants may potentiate the action of salmeterol on the vascular system).

No products indexed under this heading.

Imipramine Pamoate (Concurrent and/or sequential administration with tricyclic antidepressants may potentiate the action of salmeterol on the vascular system).

No products indexed under this heading.

Indinavir Sulfate (Fluticasone propionate and salmeterol, the individual components of Advair Diskus, are substrates of CYP3A4. The use of strong CYP3A4 inhibitors (e.g., ritonavir, atazanavir, clarithromycin, indinavir, itraconazole, nefazodone, nelfinavir, saquinavir, ketoconazole, telithromycin) with Advair Diskus is not recommended because increased corticosteroid and increased cardiovascular adverse effects may occur). Products include:

Crixivan Capsules 1979

Isocarboxazid (Concurrent and/or sequential administration with MAO inhibitors may potentiate the action of salmeterol on the vascular system. Advair Diskus should be administered with extreme caution to patients being treated with monoamine oxidase inhibitors, or within 2 weeks of discontinuation of such agents). Products include:

Marplan Tablets 3177

Isoniazid (Fluticasone propionate and salmeterol, the individual components of Advair Diskus, are substrates of CYP3A4. The use of strong CYP3A4 inhibitors (e.g., ritonavir, atazanavir, clarithromycin, indinavir, itraconazole, nefazodone, nelfinavir, saquinavir, ketoconazole, telithromycin) with Advair Diskus is not recommended because increased corticosteroid and increased cardiovascular adverse effects may occur).

No products indexed under this heading.

Itraconazole (Fluticasone propionate and salmeterol, the individual components of Advair Diskus, are substrates of CYP3A4. The use of strong CYP3A4 inhibitors (e.g., ritonavir, atazanavir, clarithromycin, indinavir, itraconazole, nefazodone, nelfinavir, saquinavir, ketoconazole, telithromycin) with Advair Diskus is not recommended because increased corticosteroid and increased cardiovascular adverse effects may occur).

No products indexed under this heading.

Ketoconazole (Co-administration of salmeterol and ketoconazole was associated with more frequent increase in QTc duration compared with salmeterol and placebo administration. Co-administration of orally inhaled fluticasone propionate and ketoconazole resulted in increased plasma fluticasone propionate exposure and reduced plasma cortisol area under the curve, but had no effect on urinary excretion of cortisol). Products include:

Extina Foam, 2% 3057
Nizoral A-D Shampoo 1901

Labetalol Hydrochloride (Co-administration with beta-blockers not only blocks the pulmonary effect of beta-agonists, such as salmeterol, but may produce severe bronchospasm in patients with asthma).

No products indexed under this heading.

Levobunolol Hydrochloride (Co-administration with beta-blockers not only blocks the pulmonary effect of beta-agonists, such as salmeterol, but may produce severe bronchospasm in patients with asthma).

No products indexed under this heading.

Lopinavir (Fluticasone propionate and salmeterol, the individual components of Advair Diskus, are substrates of CYP3A4. The use of strong CYP3A4 inhibitors (e.g., ritonavir, atazanavir, clarithromycin, indinavir, itraconazole, nefazodone, nelfinavir, saquinavir, ketoconazole, telithromycin) with Advair Diskus is not recommended because increased corticosteroid and increased cardiovascular adverse effects may occur). Products include:

Kaletra 452

Loratadine (Fluticasone propionate and salmeterol, the individual components of Advair Diskus, are substrates of CYP3A4. The use of strong CYP3A4 inhibitors (e.g., ritonavir, atazanavir, clarithromycin, indinavir, itraconazole, nefazodone, nelfinavir, saquinavir, ketoconazole, telithromycin) with Advair Diskus is not recommended because increased corticosteroid and increased cardiovascular adverse effects may occur).

No products indexed under this heading.

Maprotiline Hydrochloride (Concurrent and/or sequential administration with tricyclic antidepressants may potentiate the action of salmeterol on the vascular system).

No products indexed under this heading.

Methyclothiazide (The ECG changes and/or hypokalemia that may result from the administration of non-potassium sparing diuretics can be acutely worsened by beta-agonists, especially when the recommended dose of beta-agonist is exceeded).

No products indexed under this heading.

Metipranolol Hydrochloride (Co-administration with beta-blockers not only blocks the pulmonary effect of beta-agonists, such as salmeterol, but may produce severe bronchospasm in patients with asthma).

No products indexed under this heading.

Metoprolol Succinate (Co-administration with beta-blockers not only blocks the pulmonary effect of beta-agonists, such as salmeterol, but may produce severe bronchospasm in patients with asthma). Products include:

Toprol-XL Tablets 666

Metoprolol Tartrate (Co-administration with beta-blockers not only blocks the pulmonary effect of beta-agonists, such as salmeterol, but may produce severe bronchospasm in patients with asthma).

No products indexed under this heading.

Metronidazole (Fluticasone propionate and salmeterol, the individual components of Advair Diskus, are substrates of CYP3A4. The use of strong CYP3A4 inhibitors (e.g., ritonavir, atazanavir, clarithromycin, indinavir, itraconazole, nefazodone, nelfinavir, saquinavir, ketoconazole, telithromycin) with Advair Diskus is not recommended because increased corticosteroid and increased cardiovascular adverse effects may occur). Products include:

Pylera Capsules 714

Metronidazole Benzoate (Fluticasone propionate and salmeterol, the individual components of Advair Diskus, are substrates of CYP3A4. The use of strong CYP3A4 inhibitors (e.g., ritonavir, atazanavir, clarithromycin, indinavir, itraconazole, nefazodone, nelfinavir, saquinavir, ketoconazole, telithromycin) with Advair Diskus is not recommended because increased corticosteroid and increased cardiovascular adverse effects may occur).

No products indexed under this heading.

Metronidazole Hydrochloride (Fluticasone propionate and salmeterol, the individual components of Advair Diskus, are substrates of CYP3A4. The use of strong CYP3A4 inhibitors (e.g., ritonavir, atazanavir, clarithromycin, indinavir, itraconazole, nefazodone, nelfinavir, saquinavir, ketoconazole, telithromycin) with Advair Diskus is not recommended because increased corticosteroid and increased cardiovascular adverse effects may occur).

No products indexed under this heading.

Metronidazole Sodium (Fluticasone propionate and salmeterol, the individual components of Advair Diskus, are substrates of CYP3A4. The use of strong CYP3A4 inhibitors (e.g., ritonavir, atazanavir, clarithromycin, indinavir, itraconazole, nefazodone, nelfinavir, saquinavir, ketoconazole, telithromycin) with Advair Diskus is not recommended because increased corticosteroid and increased cardiovascular adverse effects may occur).

No products indexed under this heading.

Miconazole (Fluticasone propionate and salmeterol, the individual components of Advair Diskus, are substrates of CYP3A4. The use of strong CYP3A4 inhibitors (e.g., ritonavir, atazanavir, clarithromycin, indinavir, itraconazole, nefazodone, nelfinavir, saquinavir, ketoconazole, telithromycin) with Advair Diskus is not recommended because increased corticosteroid and increased cardiovascular adverse effects may occur).

No products indexed under this heading.

Miconazole Nitrate (Fluticasone propionate and salmeterol, the individual components of Advair Diskus, are substrates of CYP3A4. The use of strong CYP3A4 inhibitors (e.g., ritonavir, atazanavir, clarithromycin, indinavir, itraconazole, nefazodone, nelfinavir, saquinavir, ketoconazole, telithromycin) with Advair Diskus is not recommended because increased corticosteroid and increased cardiovascular adverse effects may occur).

No products indexed under this heading.

Moclobemide (Concurrent and/or sequential administration with MAO inhibitors may potentiate the action of salmeterol on the vascular system. Advair Diskus should be administered with extreme caution to patients being treated with monoamine oxidase inhibitors, or within 2 weeks of discontinuation of such agents).

No products indexed under this heading.

Nadolol (Co-administration with beta-blockers not only blocks the pulmonary effect of beta-agonists, such as salmeterol, but may produce severe bronchospasm in patients with asthma). Products include:

Nadolol Tablets 2191

Nebivolol (Co-administration with beta-blockers not only blocks the pulmonary effect of beta-agonists, such as salmeterol, but may pro-

duce severe bronchospasm in patients with asthma). Products include:

Bystolic Tablets 1155

Nefazodone Hydrochloride (Fluticasone propionate and salmeterol, the individual components of Advair Diskus, are substrates of CYP3A4. The use of strong CYP3A4 inhibitors (e.g., ritonavir, atazanavir, clarithromycin, indinavir, itraconazole, nefazodone, nelfinavir, saquinavir, ketoconazole, telithromycin) with Advair Diskus is not recommended because increased corticosteroid and increased cardiovascular adverse effects may occur).

No products indexed under this heading.

Nelfinavir Mesylate (Fluticasone propionate and salmeterol, the individual components of Advair Diskus, are substrates of CYP3A4. The use of strong CYP3A4 inhibitors (e.g., ritonavir, atazanavir, clarithromycin, indinavir, itraconazole, nefazodone, nelfinavir, saquinavir, ketoconazole, telithromycin) with Advair Diskus is not recommended because increased corticosteroid and increased cardiovascular adverse effects may occur).

No products indexed under this heading.

Nevirapine (Fluticasone propionate and salmeterol, the individual components of Advair Diskus, are substrates of CYP3A4. The use of strong CYP3A4 inhibitors (e.g., ritonavir, atazanavir, clarithromycin, indinavir, itraconazole, nefazodone, nelfinavir, saquinavir, ketoconazole, telithromycin) with Advair Diskus is not recommended because increased corticosteroid and increased cardiovascular adverse effects may occur). Products include:

Viramune Oral Suspension 873
Viramune Tablets 873

Niacinamide (Fluticasone propionate and salmeterol, the individual components of Advair Diskus, are substrates of CYP3A4. The use of strong CYP3A4 inhibitors (e.g., ritonavir, atazanavir, clarithromycin, indinavir, itraconazole, nefazodone, nelfinavir, saquinavir, ketoconazole, telithromycin) with Advair Diskus is not recommended because increased corticosteroid and increased cardiovascular adverse effects may occur). Products include:

BioLean Free Tablets 635

Nicotinamide (Fluticasone propionate and salmeterol, the individual components of Advair Diskus, are substrates of CYP3A4. The use of strong CYP3A4 inhibitors (e.g., ritonavir, atazanavir, clarithromycin, indinavir, itraconazole, nefazodone, nelfinavir, saquinavir, ketoconazole, telithromycin) with Advair Diskus is not recommended because increased corticosteroid and increased cardiovascular adverse effects may occur).

No products indexed under this heading.

Nifedipine (Fluticasone propionate and salmeterol, the individual components of Advair Diskus, are substrates of CYP3A4. The use of strong CYP3A4 inhibitors (e.g., ritonavir, atazanavir, clarithromycin, indinavir, itraconazole, nefazodone, nelfinavir, saquinavir, ketoconazole, telithromycin) with Advair Diskus is not recommended because increased corticosteroid and increased cardiovascular adverse effects may occur).

No products indexed under this heading.

Norfloxacin (Fluticasone propionate and salmeterol, the individual components of Advair Diskus, are substrates of CYP3A4. The use of strong CYP3A4 inhibitors (e.g., ritonavir, atazanavir, clarithromycin, indinavir, itraconazole, nefazodone, nelfinavir, saquinavir, ketoconazole, telithromycin) with Advair Diskus is not recommended because increased corticosteroid and increased cardiovascular adverse effects may occur). Products include:

Noroxin Tablets 2069

Nortriptyline Hydrochloride (Concurrent and/or sequential administration with tricyclic antidepressants may potentiate the action of salmeterol on the vascular system).

No products indexed under this heading.

Omeprazole (Fluticasone propionate and salmeterol, the individual components of Advair Diskus, are substrates of CYP3A4. The use of strong CYP3A4 inhibitors (e.g., ritonavir, atazanavir, clarithromycin, indinavir, itraconazole, nefazodone, nelfinavir, saquinavir, ketoconazole, telithromycin) with Advair Diskus is not recommended because increased corticosteroid and increased cardiovascular adverse effects may occur).

No products indexed under this heading.

Pargyline Hydrochloride (Concurrent and/or sequential administration with MAO inhibitors may potentiate the action of salmeterol on the vascular system. Advair Diskus should be administered with extreme caution to patients being treated with monoamine oxidase inhibitors, or within 2 weeks of discontinuation of such agents).

No products indexed under this heading.

Paroxetine Hydrochloride (Fluticasone propionate and salmeterol, the individual components of Advair Diskus, are substrates of CYP3A4. The use of strong CYP3A4 inhibitors (e.g., ritonavir, atazanavir, clarithromycin, indinavir, itraconazole, nefazodone, nelfinavir, saquinavir, ketoconazole, telithromycin) with Advair Diskus is not recommended because increased corticosteroid and increased cardiovascular adverse effects may occur). Products include:

Paxil 1535
Paxil CR Controlled-Release Tablets 1544

Penbutolol Sulfate (Co-administration with beta-blockers not only blocks the pulmonary effect of beta-agonists, such as salmeterol, but may produce severe bronchospasm in patients with asthma).

No products indexed under this heading.

Phenelzine Sulfate (Concurrent and/or sequential administration with MAO inhibitors may potentiate the action of salmeterol on the vascular system. Advair Diskus should be administered with extreme caution to patients being treated with monoamine oxidase inhibitors, or within 2 weeks of discontinuation of such agents).

No products indexed under this heading.

Pindolol (Co-administration with beta-blockers not only blocks the pulmonary effect of beta-agonists, such as salmeterol, but may produce severe bronchospasm in patients with asthma).

No products indexed under this heading.

Polythiazide (The ECG changes and/or hypokalemia that may result from the administration of non-potassium sparing diuretics can be acutely worsened by beta-agonists, especially when the recommended dose of beta-agonist is exceeded).

No products indexed under this heading.

Procarbazine Hydrochloride (Concurrent and/or sequential administration with MAO inhibitors may potentiate the action of salmeterol on the vascular system. Advair Diskus should be administered with extreme caution to patients being treated with monoamine oxidase inhibitors, or within 2 weeks of discontinuation of such agents).

No products indexed under this heading.

Propoxyphene Hydrochloride (Fluticasone propionate and salmeterol, the individual components of Advair Diskus, are substrates of CYP3A4. The use of strong CYP3A4 inhibitors (e.g., ritonavir, atazanavir, clarithromycin, indinavir, itraconazole, nefazodone, nelfinavir, saquinavir, ketoconazole, telithromycin) with Advair Diskus is not recommended because increased corticosteroid and increased cardiovascular adverse effects may occur).

No products indexed under this heading.

Propoxyphene Napsylate (Fluticasone propionate and salmeterol, the individual components of Advair Diskus, are substrates of CYP3A4. The use of strong CYP3A4 inhibitors (e.g., ritonavir, atazanavir, clarithromycin, indinavir, itraconazole, nefazodone, nelfinavir, saquinavir, ketoconazole, telithromycin) with Advair Diskus is not recommended because increased corticosteroid and increased cardiovascular adverse effects may occur).

No products indexed under this heading.

Propranolol Hydrochloride (Co-administration with beta-blockers not only blocks the pulmonary effect of beta-agonists, such as salmeterol, but may produce severe bronchospasm in patients with asthma). Products include:

InnoPran XL Extended Release Capsules 1484

Protriptyline Hydrochloride (Concurrent and/or sequential administration with tricyclic antidepressants may potentiate the action of salmeterol on the vascular system).

No products indexed under this heading.

Quinidine (Fluticasone propionate and salmeterol, the individual components of Advair Diskus, are substrates of CYP3A4. The use of strong CYP3A4 inhibitors (e.g., ritonavir, atazanavir, clarithromycin, indinavir, itraconazole, nefazodone, nelfinavir, saquinavir, ketoconazole, telithromycin) with Advair Diskus is not recommended because increased corticosteroid and increased cardiovascular adverse effects may occur).

No products indexed under this heading.

Quinidine Hydrochloride (Fluticasone propionate and salmeterol, the individual components of Advair Diskus, are substrates of CYP3A4. The use of strong CYP3A4 inhibitors (e.g., ritonavir, atazanavir, clarithromycin, indinavir, itraconazole, nefazodone, nelfinavir, saquinavir, ketoconazole, telithromycin) with Advair Diskus is not recommended because increased corticosteroid and increased cardiovascular adverse effects may occur).

No products indexed under this heading.

Quinidine Polygalacturonate (Fluticasone propionate and salmeterol, the individual components of Advair Diskus, are substrates of CYP3A4. The use of strong CYP3A4 inhibitors (e.g., ritonavir, atazanavir, clarithromycin, indinavir, itraconazole, nefazodone, nelfinavir, saquinavir, ketoconazole, telithromycin) with Advair Diskus is not recommended because increased corticosteroid and increased cardiovascular adverse effects may occur).

No products indexed under this heading.

Quinidine Sulfate (Fluticasone propionate and salmeterol, the individual components of Advair Diskus, are substrates of CYP3A4. The use of strong CYP3A4 inhibitors (e.g., ritonavir, atazanavir, clarithromycin, indinavir, itraconazole, nefazodone, nelfinavir, saquinavir, ketoconazole, telithromycin) with Advair Diskus is not recommended because increased corticosteroid and increased cardiovascular adverse effects may occur).

No products indexed under this heading.

Quinine (Fluticasone propionate and salmeterol, the individual components of Advair Diskus, are substrates of CYP3A4. The use of strong CYP3A4 inhibitors (e.g., ritonavir, atazanavir, clarithromycin, indinavir, itraconazole, nefazodone, nelfinavir, saquinavir, ketoconazole, telithromycin) with Advair Diskus is not recommended because increased corticosteroid and increased cardiovascular adverse effects may occur).

No products indexed under this heading.

Quinine Sulfate (Fluticasone propionate and salmeterol, the individual components of Advair Diskus, are substrates of CYP3A4. The use of strong CYP3A4 inhibitors (e.g., ritonavir, atazanavir, clarithromycin, indinavir, itraconazole, nefazodone, nelfinavir, saquinavir, ketoconazole, telithromycin) with Advair Diskus is not recommended because increased corticosteroid and increased cardiovascular adverse

effects may occur).
No products indexed under this heading.

Quinupristin (Fluticasone propionate and salmeterol, the individual components of Advair Diskus, are substrates of CYP3A4. The use of strong CYP3A4 inhibitors (e.g., ritonavir, atazanavir, clarithromycin, indinavir, itraconazole, nefazodone, nelfinavir, saquinavir, ketoconazole, telithromycin) with Advair Diskus is not recommended because increased corticosteroid and increased cardiovascular adverse effects may occur).
No products indexed under this heading.

Ranitidine Bismuth Citrate (Fluticasone propionate and salmeterol, the individual components of Advair Diskus, are substrates of CYP3A4. The use of strong CYP3A4 inhibitors (e.g., ritonavir, atazanavir, clarithromycin, indinavir, itraconazole, nefazodone, nelfinavir, saquinavir, ketoconazole, telithromycin) with Advair Diskus is not recommended because increased corticosteroid and increased cardiovascular adverse effects may occur).
No products indexed under this heading.

Ranitidine Hydrochloride (Fluticasone propionate and salmeterol, the individual components of Advair Diskus, are substrates of CYP3A4. The use of strong CYP3A4 inhibitors (e.g., ritonavir, atazanavir, clarithromycin, indinavir, itraconazole, nefazodone, nelfinavir, saquinavir, ketoconazole, telithromycin) with Advair Diskus is not recommended because increased corticosteroid and increased cardiovascular adverse effects may occur). Products include:
- Zantac 75 Tablets .... ▣603
- Zantac 1670
- Zantac Injection 1666
- Zantac Injection Pharmacy Bulk Package 1668
- Maximum Strength Zantac 150 Tablets .... ▣603
- Maximum Strength Zantac 150 Cool Mint Tablets .... ▣603

Rasagiline Mesylate (Concurrent and/or sequential administration with MAO inhibitors may potentiate the action of salmeterol on the vascular system. Advair Diskus should be administered with extreme caution to patients being treated with monoamine oxidase inhibitors, or within 2 weeks of discontinuation of such agents). Products include:
- Azilect Tablets 3106

Ritonavir (Ritonavir, a potent CYP3A4 inhibitor, can significantly increase plasma fluticasone exposure, resulting in reduced serum cortisol concentrations. Cushing syndrome and adrenal suppression have been reported; therefore, co-administration is not recommended unless the potential benefit outweighs the risks). Products include:
- Kaletra 452
- Norvir 489

Saquinavir (Fluticasone propionate and salmeterol, the individual components of Advair Diskus, are substrates of CYP3A4. The use of strong CYP3A4 inhibitors (e.g., ritonavir, atazanavir, clarithromycin, indinavir, itraconazole, nefazodone, nelfinavir, saquinavir, ketoconazole, telithromycin) with Advair Diskus is not recommended because increased corticosteroid and increased cardiovascular adverse effects may occur).
No products indexed under this heading.

Saquinavir Mesylate (Fluticasone propionate and salmeterol, the individual components of Advair Diskus, are substrates of CYP3A4. The use of strong CYP3A4 inhibitors (e.g., ritonavir, atazanavir, clarithromycin, indinavir, itraconazole, nefazodone, nelfinavir, saquinavir, ketoconazole, telithromycin) with Advair Diskus is not recommended because increased corticosteroid and increased cardiovascular adverse effects may occur).
No products indexed under this heading.

Selegiline (Concurrent and/or sequential administration with MAO inhibitors may potentiate the action of salmeterol on the vascular system. Advair Diskus should be administered with extreme caution to patients being treated with monoamine oxidase inhibitors, or within 2 weeks of discontinuation of such agents). Products include:
- Emsam Transdermal System 905

Selegiline Hydrochloride (Concurrent and/or sequential administration with MAO inhibitors may potentiate the action of salmeterol on the vascular system. Advair Diskus should be administered with extreme caution to patients being treated with monoamine oxidase inhibitors, or within 2 weeks of discontinuation of such agents). Products include:
- Eldepryl Capsules 3052

Sertraline Hydrochloride (Fluticasone propionate and salmeterol, the individual components of Advair Diskus, are substrates of CYP3A4. The use of strong CYP3A4 inhibitors (e.g., ritonavir, atazanavir, clarithromycin, indinavir, itraconazole, nefazodone, nelfinavir, saquinavir, ketoconazole, telithromycin) with Advair Diskus is not recommended because increased corticosteroid and increased cardiovascular adverse effects may occur).
No products indexed under this heading.

Sildenafil Citrate (Fluticasone propionate and salmeterol, the individual components of Advair Diskus, are substrates of CYP3A4. The use of strong CYP3A4 inhibitors (e.g., ritonavir, atazanavir, clarithromycin, indinavir, itraconazole, nefazodone, nelfinavir, saquinavir, ketoconazole, telithromycin) with Advair Diskus is not recommended because increased corticosteroid and increased cardiovascular adverse effects may occur).
No products indexed under this heading.

Sotalol Hydrochloride (Co-administration with beta-blockers not only blocks the pulmonary effect of beta-agonists, such as salmeterol, but may produce severe bronchospasm in patients with asthma).
No products indexed under this heading.

Telithromycin (Fluticasone propionate and salmeterol, the individual components of Advair Diskus, are substrates of CYP3A4. The use of strong CYP3A4 inhibitors (e.g., ritonavir, atazanavir, clarithromycin, indinavir, itraconazole, nefazodone, nelfinavir, saquinavir, ketoconazole, telithromycin) with Advair Diskus is not recommended because increased corticosteroid and increased cardiovascular adverse effects may occur). Products include:
- Ketek Tablets 2744

Timolol Hemihydrate (Co-administration with beta-blockers not only blocks the pulmonary effect of beta-agonists, such as salmeterol, but may produce severe bronchospasm in patients with asthma). Products include:
- Betimol Ophthalmic Solution 3181

Timolol Maleate (Co-administration with beta-blockers not only blocks the pulmonary effect of beta-agonists, such as salmeterol, but may produce severe bronchospasm in patients with asthma). Products include:
- Combigan Ophthalmic Solution 553
- Cosopt Sterile Ophthalmic Solution 1969
- Timoptic Sterile Ophthalmic Solution 2121
- Timoptic in Ocudose 2124
- Timoptic-XE Sterile Ophthalmic Gel Forming Solution 2125

Torsemide (The ECG changes and/or hypokalemia that may result from the administration of non-potassium sparing diuretics can be acutely worsened by beta-agonists, especially when the recommended dose of beta-agonist is exceeded). Products include:
- Demadex Injection 2630
- Demadex Tablets 2630

Tranylcypromine Sulfate (Concurrent and/or sequential administration with MAO inhibitors may potentiate the action of salmeterol on the vascular system. Advair Diskus should be administered with extreme caution to patients being treated with monoamine oxidase inhibitors, or within 2 weeks of discontinuation of such agents). Products include:
- Parnate Tablets 1532

Trimipramine Maleate (Concurrent and/or sequential administration with tricyclic antidepressants may potentiate the action of salmeterol on the vascular system).
No products indexed under this heading.

Troglitazone (Fluticasone propionate and salmeterol, the individual components of Advair Diskus, are substrates of CYP3A4. The use of strong CYP3A4 inhibitors (e.g., ritonavir, atazanavir, clarithromycin, indinavir, itraconazole, nefazodone, nelfinavir, saquinavir, ketoconazole, telithromycin) with Advair Diskus is not recommended because increased corticosteroid and increased cardiovascular adverse effects may occur).
No products indexed under this heading.

Troleandomycin (Fluticasone propionate and salmeterol, the individual components of Advair Diskus, are substrates of CYP3A4. The use of strong CYP3A4 inhibitors (e.g., ritonavir, atazanavir, clarithromycin, indinavir, itraconazole, nefazodone, nelfinavir, saquinavir, ketoconazole, telithromycin) with Advair Diskus is not recommended because increased corticosteroid and increased cardiovascular adverse effects may occur).
No products indexed under this heading.

Valproate Sodium (Fluticasone propionate and salmeterol, the individual components of Advair Diskus, are substrates of CYP3A4. The use of strong CYP3A4 inhibitors (e.g., ritonavir, atazanavir, clarithromycin, indinavir, itraconazole, nefazodone, nelfinavir, saquinavir, ketoconazole, telithromycin) with Advair Diskus is not recommended because increased corticosteroid and increased cardiovascular adverse effects may occur).
No products indexed under this heading.

Vardenafil Hydrochloride (Fluticasone propionate and salmeterol, the individual components of Advair Diskus, are substrates of CYP3A4. The use of strong CYP3A4 inhibitors (e.g., ritonavir, atazanavir, clarithromycin, indinavir, itraconazole, nefazodone, nelfinavir, saquinavir, ketoconazole, telithromycin) with Advair Diskus is not recommended because increased corticosteroid and increased cardiovascular adverse effects may occur). Products include:
- Levitra Tablets 2876

Verapamil Hydrochloride (Fluticasone propionate and salmeterol, the individual components of Advair Diskus, are substrates of CYP3A4. The use of strong CYP3A4 inhibitors (e.g., ritonavir, atazanavir, clarithromycin, indinavir, itraconazole, nefazodone, nelfinavir, saquinavir, ketoconazole, telithromycin) with Advair Diskus is not recommended because increased corticosteroid and increased cardiovascular adverse effects may occur). Products include:
- Tarka Tablets 511

Voriconazole (Fluticasone propionate and salmeterol, the individual components of Advair Diskus, are substrates of CYP3A4. The use of strong CYP3A4 inhibitors (e.g., ritonavir, atazanavir, clarithromycin, indinavir, itraconazole, nefazodone, nelfinavir, saquinavir, ketoconazole, telithromycin) with Advair Diskus is not recommended because increased corticosteroid and increased cardiovascular adverse effects may occur).
No products indexed under this heading.

Zafirlukast (Fluticasone propionate and salmeterol, the individual components of Advair Diskus, are substrates of CYP3A4. The use of strong CYP3A4 inhibitors (e.g., ritonavir, atazanavir, clarithromycin, indinavir, itraconazole, nefazodone, nelfinavir, saquinavir, ketoconazole, telithromycin) with Advair Diskus is not recommended because increased corticosteroid and increased cardiovascular adverse effects may occur). Products include:
- Accolate Tablets 669

Zileuton (Fluticasone propionate and salmeterol, the individual components of Advair Diskus, are substrates of CYP3A4. The use of strong CYP3A4 inhibitors (e.g., ritonavir, atazanavir, clarithromycin, indinavir, itraconazole, nefazodone, nelfinavir, saquinavir, ketoconazole, telithromycin) with Advair Diskus is not recommended because

increased corticosteroid and increased cardiovascular adverse effects may occur).
No products indexed under this heading.

Food Interactions

Grapefruit (Fluticasone propionate and salmeterol, the individual components of Advair Diskus, are substrates of CYP3A4. The use of strong CYP3A4 inhibitors (e.g., ritonavir, atazanavir, clarithromycin, indinavir, itraconazole, nefazodone, nelfinavir, saquinavir, ketoconazole, telithromycin) with Advair Diskus is not recommended because increased corticosteroid and increased cardiovascular adverse effects may occur).

Grapefruit Juice (Fluticasone propionate and salmeterol, the individual components of Advair Diskus, are substrates of CYP3A4. The use of strong CYP3A4 inhibitors (e.g., ritonavir, atazanavir, clarithromycin, indinavir, itraconazole, nefazodone, nelfinavir, saquinavir, ketoconazole, telithromycin) with Advair Diskus is not recommended because increased corticosteroid and increased cardiovascular adverse effects may occur).

ADVAIR DISKUS 250/50
(Fluticasone Propionate, Salmeterol Xinafoate) 1276
See Advair Diskus 100/50

ADVAIR DISKUS 500/50
(Fluticasone Propionate, Salmeterol Xinafoate) 1276
See Advair Diskus 100/50

ADVAIR HFA 45/21 INHALATION AEROSOL
(Fluticasone Propionate, Salmeterol Xinafoate) 1288
May interact with beta blockers, cytochrome p450 3a4 inhibitors (selected), monoamine oxidase inhibitors, potassium-depleting diuretics, tricyclic antidepressants, and certain other agents. Compounds in these categories include:

Acebutolol Hydrochloride (Co-administration with beta-blockers not only blocks the pulmonary effect of beta-agonists, such as salmeterol, but may produce severe bronchospasm in patients with asthma).
No products indexed under this heading.

Acetazolamide (Concomitant administration of erythromycin (a moderate CYP3A4 inhibitor) and salmeterol inhalation aerosol resulted in a 40% increase in salmeterol Cmax at steady state, a 3.6-beat/min. increase in heart rate, a 5.8-msec increase in QTc interval, and no change in plasma potassium. Due to the potential increased risk of cardiovascular events, the concomitant use of salmeterol with strong CYP3A4 inhibitors (e.g., ketoconazole, ritonavir, atazanavir, clarithromycin, indinavir, itraconazole, nefazodone, nelfinavir, saquinavir, telithromycin) is not recommended).
No products indexed under this heading.

Amiodarone Hydrochloride (Concomitant administration of erythromycin (a moderate CYP3A4 inhibitor) and salmeterol inhalation aerosol resulted in a 40% increase in salmeterol Cmax at steady state, a 3.6-beat/min. increase in heart rate, a 5.8-msec increase in QTc interval, and no change in plasma potassium. Due to the potential increased risk of cardiovascular events, the concomitant use of salmeterol with strong CYP3A4 inhibitors (e.g., ketoconazole, ritonavir, atazanavir, clarithromycin, indinavir, itraconazole, nefazodone, nelfinavir, saquinavir, telithromycin) is not recommended).
No products indexed under this heading.

Amitriptyline Hydrochloride (Concurrent and/or sequential administration with tricyclic antidepressants may potentiate the action of salmeterol on the vascular system).
No products indexed under this heading.

Amoxapine (Concurrent and/or sequential administration with tricyclic antidepressants may potentiate the action of salmeterol on the vascular system).
No products indexed under this heading.

Amprenavir (Concomitant administration of erythromycin (a moderate CYP3A4 inhibitor) and salmeterol inhalation aerosol resulted in a 40% increase in salmeterol Cmax at steady state, a 3.6-beat/min. increase in heart rate, a 5.8-msec increase in QTc interval, and no change in plasma potassium. Due to the potential increased risk of cardiovascular events, the concomitant use of salmeterol with strong CYP3A4 inhibitors (e.g., ketoconazole, ritonavir, atazanavir, clarithromycin, indinavir, itraconazole, nefazodone, nelfinavir, saquinavir, telithromycin) is not recommended).
No products indexed under this heading.

Anastrozole (Concomitant administration of erythromycin (a moderate CYP3A4 inhibitor) and salmeterol inhalation aerosol resulted in a 40% increase in salmeterol Cmax at steady state, a 3.6-beat/min. increase in heart rate, a 5.8-msec increase in QTc interval, and no change in plasma potassium. Due to the potential increased risk of cardiovascular events, the concomitant use of salmeterol with strong CYP3A4 inhibitors (e.g., ketoconazole, ritonavir, atazanavir, clarithromycin, indinavir, itraconazole, nefazodone, nelfinavir, saquinavir, telithromycin) is not recommended). Products include:
Arimidex Tablets 672

Aprepitant (Concomitant administration of erythromycin (a moderate CYP3A4 inhibitor) and salmeterol inhalation aerosol resulted in a 40% increase in salmeterol Cmax at steady state, a 3.6-beat/min. increase in heart rate, a 5.8-msec increase in QTc interval, and no change in plasma potassium. Due to the potential increased risk of cardiovascular events, the concomitant use of salmeterol with strong CYP3A4 inhibitors (e.g., ketoconazole, ritonavir, atazanavir, clarithromycin, indinavir, itraconazole, nefazodone, nelfinavir, saquinavir, telithromycin) is not recommended). Products include:
Emend Capsules 1992

Atazanavir (Concomitant administration of erythromycin (a moderate CYP3A4 inhibitor) and salmeterol inhalation aerosol resulted in a 40% increase in salmeterol Cmax at steady state, a 3.6-beat/min. increase in heart rate, a 5.8-msec increase in QTc interval, and no change in plasma potassium. Due to the potential increased risk of cardiovascular events, the concomitant use of salmeterol with strong CYP3A4 inhibitors (e.g., ketoconazole, ritonavir, atazanavir, clarithromycin, indinavir, itraconazole, nefazodone, nelfinavir, saquinavir, telithromycin) is not recommended).
No products indexed under this heading.

Atazanavir Sulfate (Concomitant administration of erythromycin (a moderate CYP3A4 inhibitor) and salmeterol inhalation aerosol resulted in a 40% increase in salmeterol Cmax at steady state, a 3.6-beat/min. increase in heart rate, a 5.8-msec increase in QTc interval, and no change in plasma potassium. Due to the potential increased risk of cardiovascular events, the concomitant use of salmeterol with strong CYP3A4 inhibitors (e.g., ketoconazole, ritonavir, atazanavir, clarithromycin, indinavir, itraconazole, nefazodone, nelfinavir, saquinavir, telithromycin) is not recommended). Products include:
Reyataz Capsules 3299

Atenolol (Co-administration with beta-blockers not only blocks the pulmonary effect of beta-agonists, such as salmeterol, but may produce severe bronchospasm in patients with asthma).
No products indexed under this heading.

Bendroflumethiazide (The ECG changes and/or hypokalemia that may result from the administration of non-potassium sparing diuretics can be acutely worsened by beta-agonists, especially when the recommended dose of beta-agonist is exceeded).
No products indexed under this heading.

Betaxolol Hydrochloride (Co-administration with beta-blockers not only blocks the pulmonary effect of beta-agonists, such as salmeterol, but may produce severe bronchospasm in patients with asthma).
No products indexed under this heading.

Bisoprolol Fumarate (Co-administration with beta-blockers not only blocks the pulmonary effect of beta-agonists, such as salmeterol, but may produce severe bronchospasm in patients with asthma).
No products indexed under this heading.

Bumetanide (The ECG changes and/or hypokalemia that may result from the administration of non-potassium sparing diuretics can be acutely worsened by beta-agonists, especially when the recommended dose of beta-agonist is exceeded).
No products indexed under this heading.

Carteolol Hydrochloride (Co-administration with beta-blockers not only blocks the pulmonary effect of beta-agonists, such as salmeterol, but may produce severe bronchospasm in patients with asthma).
No products indexed under this heading.

Chlorothiazide (The ECG changes and/or hypokalemia that may result from the administration of non-potassium sparing diuretics can be acutely worsened by beta-agonists, especially when the recommended dose of beta-agonist is exceeded).
No products indexed under this heading.

Chlorothiazide Sodium (The ECG changes and/or hypokalemia that may result from the administration of non-potassium sparing diuretics can be acutely worsened by beta-agonists, especially when the recommended dose of beta-agonist is exceeded). Products include:
Intravenous Sodium Diuril 2490

Cimetidine (Concomitant administration of erythromycin (a moderate CYP3A4 inhibitor) and salmeterol inhalation aerosol resulted in a 40% increase in salmeterol Cmax at steady state, a 3.6-beat/min. increase in heart rate, a 5.8-msec increase in QTc interval, and no change in plasma potassium. Due to the potential increased risk of cardiovascular events, the concomitant use of salmeterol with strong CYP3A4 inhibitors (e.g., ketoconazole, ritonavir, atazanavir, clarithromycin, indinavir, itraconazole, nefazodone, nelfinavir, saquinavir, telithromycin) is not recommended).
No products indexed under this heading.

Cimetidine Hydrochloride (Concomitant administration of erythromycin (a moderate CYP3A4 inhibitor) and salmeterol inhalation aerosol resulted in a 40% increase in salmeterol Cmax at steady state, a 3.6-beat/min. increase in heart rate, a 5.8-msec increase in QTc interval, and no change in plasma potassium. Due to the potential increased risk of cardiovascular events, the concomitant use of salmeterol with strong CYP3A4 inhibitors (e.g., ketoconazole, ritonavir, atazanavir, clarithromycin, indinavir, itraconazole, nefazodone, nelfinavir, saquinavir, telithromycin) is not recommended).
No products indexed under this heading.

Ciprofloxacin (Concomitant administration of erythromycin (a moderate CYP3A4 inhibitor) and salmeterol inhalation aerosol resulted in a 40% increase in salmeterol Cmax at steady state, a 3.6-beat/min. increase in heart rate, a 5.8-msec increase in QTc interval, and no change in plasma potassium. Due to the potential increased risk of cardiovascular events, the concomitant use of salmeterol with strong CYP3A4 inhibitors (e.g., ketoconazole, ritonavir, atazanavir, clarithromycin, indinavir, itraconazole, nefazodone, nelfinavir, saquinavir, telithromycin) is not recommended). Products include:
Cipro I.V. 2817
Cipro Oral Suspension 2810
Cipro XR Tablets 2823
Ciprodex Otic Suspension 541

Clarithromycin (Concomitant administration of erythromycin (a moderate CYP3A4 inhibitor) and salmeterol inhalation aerosol resulted in a 40% increase in salmeterol Cmax at steady state, a 3.6-beat/min. increase in heart rate, a 5.8-msec increase in QTc interval, and no change in plasma potassium. Due to the potential increased risk of cardio-

vascular events, the concomitant use of salmeterol with strong CYP3A4 inhibitors (e.g., ketoconazole, ritonavir, atazanavir, clarithromycin, indinavir, itraconazone, nefazodone, nelfinavir, saquinavir, telithromycin) is not recommended). Products include:

Biaxin/Biaxin XL 411

Clomipramine Hydrochloride (Concurrent and/or sequential administration with tricyclic antidepressants may potentiate the action of salmeterol on the vascular system).

No products indexed under this heading.

Clotrimazole (Concomitant administration of erythromycin (a moderate CYP3A4 inhibitor) and salmeterol inhalation aerosol resulted in a 40% increase in salmeterol Cmax at steady state, a 3.6-beat/min. increase in heart rate, a 5.8-msec increase in QTc interval, and no change in plasma potassium. Due to the potential increased risk of cardiovascular events, the concomitant use of salmeterol with strong CYP3A4 inhibitors (e.g., ketoconazole, ritonavir, atazanavir, clarithromycin, indinavir, itraconazone, nefazodone, nelfinavir, saquinavir, telithromycin) is not recommended). Products include:

Lotrisone 2881

Cyclosporine (Concomitant administration of erythromycin (a moderate CYP3A4 inhibitor) and salmeterol inhalation aerosol resulted in a 40% increase in salmeterol Cmax at steady state, a 3.6-beat/min. increase in heart rate, a 5.8-msec increase in QTc interval, and no change in plasma potassium. Due to the potential increased risk of cardiovascular events, the concomitant use of salmeterol with strong CYP3A4 inhibitors (e.g., ketoconazole, ritonavir, atazanavir, clarithromycin, indinavir, itraconazone, nefazodone, nelfinavir, saquinavir, telithromycin) is not recommended). Products include:

Gengraf Capsules 435
Neoral Oral Solution 2280
Neoral Soft Gelatin Capsules 2280
Restasis Ophthalmic Emulsion 557
Sandimmune 2296

Dalfopristin (Concomitant administration of erythromycin (a moderate CYP3A4 inhibitor) and salmeterol inhalation aerosol resulted in a 40% increase in salmeterol Cmax at steady state, a 3.6-beat/min. increase in heart rate, a 5.8-msec increase in QTc interval, and no change in plasma potassium. Due to the potential increased risk of cardiovascular events, the concomitant use of salmeterol with strong CYP3A4 inhibitors (e.g., ketoconazole, ritonavir, atazanavir, clarithromycin, indinavir, itraconazone, nefazodone, nelfinavir, saquinavir, telithromycin) is not recommended).

No products indexed under this heading.

Danazol (Concomitant administration of erythromycin (a moderate CYP3A4 inhibitor) and salmeterol inhalation aerosol resulted in a 40% increase in salmeterol Cmax at steady state, a 3.6-beat/min. increase in heart rate, a 5.8-msec increase in QTc interval, and no change in plasma potassium. Due to the potential increased risk of cardiovascular events, the concomitant use of salmeterol with strong CYP3A4 inhibitors (e.g., ketoconazole, ritonavir, atazanavir, clarithromycin, indinavir, itraconazone, nefazodone, nelfinavir, saquinavir, telithromycin) is not recommended).

No products indexed under this heading.

Delavirdine Mesylate (Concomitant administration of erythromycin (a moderate CYP3A4 inhibitor) and salmeterol inhalation aerosol resulted in a 40% increase in salmeterol Cmax at steady state, a 3.6-beat/min. increase in heart rate, a 5.8-msec increase in QTc interval, and no change in plasma potassium. Due to the potential increased risk of cardiovascular events, the concomitant use of salmeterol with strong CYP3A4 inhibitors (e.g., ketoconazole, ritonavir, atazanavir, clarithromycin, indinavir, itraconazone, nefazodone, nelfinavir, saquinavir, telithromycin) is not recommended).

No products indexed under this heading.

Desipramine Hydrochloride (Concurrent and/or sequential administration with tricyclic antidepressants may potentiate the action of salmeterol on the vascular system).

No products indexed under this heading.

Diltiazem Hydrochloride (Concomitant administration of erythromycin (a moderate CYP3A4 inhibitor) and salmeterol inhalation aerosol resulted in a 40% increase in salmeterol Cmax at steady state, a 3.6-beat/min. increase in heart rate, a 5.8-msec increase in QTc interval, and no change in plasma potassium. Due to the potential increased risk of cardiovascular events, the concomitant use of salmeterol with strong CYP3A4 inhibitors (e.g., ketoconazole, ritonavir, atazanavir, clarithromycin, indinavir, itraconazone, nefazodone, nelfinavir, saquinavir, telithromycin) is not recommended). Products include:

Cardizem LA Extended Release Tablets 421

Diltiazem Maleate (Concomitant administration of erythromycin (a moderate CYP3A4 inhibitor) and salmeterol inhalation aerosol resulted in a 40% increase in salmeterol Cmax at steady state, a 3.6-beat/min. increase in heart rate, a 5.8-msec increase in QTc interval, and no change in plasma potassium. Due to the potential increased risk of cardiovascular events, the concomitant use of salmeterol with strong CYP3A4 inhibitors (e.g., ketoconazole, ritonavir, atazanavir, clarithromycin, indinavir, itraconazone, nefazodone, nelfinavir, saquinavir, telithromycin) is not recommended).

No products indexed under this heading.

Doxepin Hydrochloride (Concurrent and/or sequential administration with tricyclic antidepressants may potentiate the action of salmeterol on the vascular system).

No products indexed under this heading.

Efavirenz (Concomitant administration of erythromycin (a moderate CYP3A4 inhibitor) and salmeterol inhalation aerosol resulted in a 40% increase in salmeterol Cmax at steady state, a 3.6-beat/min. increase in heart rate, a 5.8-msec increase in QTc interval, and no change in plasma potassium. Due to the potential increased risk of cardiovascular events, the concomitant use of salmeterol with strong CYP3A4 inhibitors (e.g., ketoconazole, ritonavir, atazanavir, clarithromycin, indinavir, itraconazone, nefazodone, nelfinavir, saquinavir, telithromycin) is not recommended). Products include:

Atripla Tablets 938
Sustiva Capsules 930
Sustiva Tablets 930

Erythromycin (Concomitant administration of erythromycin (a moderate CYP3A4 inhibitor) and salmeterol inhalation aerosol resulted in a 40% increase in salmeterol Cmax at steady state, a 3.6-beat/min. increase in heart rate, a 5.8-msec increase in QTc interval, and no change in plasma potassium. Due to the potential increased risk of cardiovascular events, the concomitant use of salmeterol with strong CYP3A4 inhibitors (e.g., ketoconazole, ritonavir, atazanavir, clarithromycin, indinavir, itraconazone, nefazodone, nelfinavir, saquinavir, telithromycin) is not recommended).

No products indexed under this heading.

Erythromycin Estolate (Concomitant administration of erythromycin (a moderate CYP3A4 inhibitor) and salmeterol inhalation aerosol resulted in a 40% increase in salmeterol Cmax at steady state, a 3.6-beat/min. increase in heart rate, a 5.8-msec increase in QTc interval, and no change in plasma potassium. Due to the potential increased risk of cardiovascular events, the concomitant use of salmeterol with strong CYP3A4 inhibitors (e.g., ketoconazole, ritonavir, atazanavir, clarithromycin, indinavir, itraconazone, nefazodone, nelfinavir, saquinavir, telithromycin) is not recommended).

No products indexed under this heading.

Erythromycin Ethylsuccinate (Concomitant administration of erythromycin (a moderate CYP3A4 inhibitor) and salmeterol inhalation aerosol resulted in a 40% increase in salmeterol Cmax at steady state, a 3.6-beat/min. increase in heart rate, a 5.8-msec increase in QTc interval, and no change in plasma potassium. Due to the potential increased risk of cardiovascular events, the concomitant use of salmeterol with strong CYP3A4 inhibitors (e.g., ketoconazole, ritonavir, atazanavir, clarithromycin, indinavir, itraconazone, nefazodone, nelfinavir, saquinavir, telithromycin) is not recommended). Products include:

E.E.S. 433
EryPed 431

Erythromycin Gluceptate (Concomitant administration of erythromycin (a moderate CYP3A4 inhibitor) and salmeterol inhalation aerosol resulted in a 40% increase in salmeterol Cmax at steady state, a 3.6-beat/min. increase in heart rate, a 5.8-msec increase in QTc interval, and no change in plasma potassium. Due to the potential increased risk of cardiovascular events, the concomitant use of salmeterol with strong CYP3A4 inhibitors (e.g., ketoconazole, ritonavir, atazanavir, clarithromycin, indinavir, itraconazone, nefazodone, nelfinavir, saquinavir, telithromycin) is not recommended).

No products indexed under this heading.

Erythromycin Lactobionate (Concomitant administration of erythromycin (a moderate CYP3A4 inhibitor) and salmeterol inhalation aerosol resulted in a 40% increase in salmeterol Cmax at steady state, a 3.6-beat/min. increase in heart rate, a 5.8-msec increase in QTc interval, and no change in plasma potassium. Due to the potential increased risk of cardiovascular events, the concomitant use of salmeterol with strong CYP3A4 inhibitors (e.g., ketoconazole, ritonavir, atazanavir, clarithromycin, indinavir, itraconazone, nefazodone, nelfinavir, saquinavir, telithromycin) is not recommended).

No products indexed under this heading.

Erythromycin Stearate (Concomitant administration of erythromycin (a moderate CYP3A4 inhibitor) and salmeterol inhalation aerosol resulted in a 40% increase in salmeterol Cmax at steady state, a 3.6-beat/min. increase in heart rate, a 5.8-msec increase in QTc interval, and no change in plasma potassium. Due to the potential increased risk of cardiovascular events, the concomitant use of salmeterol with strong CYP3A4 inhibitors (e.g., ketoconazole, ritonavir, atazanavir, clarithromycin, indinavir, itraconazone, nefazodone, nelfinavir, saquinavir, telithromycin) is not recommended).

No products indexed under this heading.

Esmolol Hydrochloride (Co-administration with beta-blockers not only blocks the pulmonary effect of beta-agonists, such as salmeterol, but may produce severe bronchospasm in patients with asthma).

No products indexed under this heading.

Esomeprazole Magnesium (Concomitant administration of erythromycin (a moderate CYP3A4 inhibitor) and salmeterol inhalation aerosol resulted in a 40% increase in salmeterol Cmax at steady state, a 3.6-beat/min. increase in heart rate, a 5.8-msec increase in QTc interval, and no change in plasma potassium. Due to the potential increased risk of cardiovascular events, the concomitant use of salmeterol with strong CYP3A4 inhibitors (e.g., ketoconazole, ritonavir, atazanavir, clarithromycin, indinavir, itraconazone, nefazodone, nelfinavir, saquinavir, telithromycin) is not recommended). Products include:

Nexium Delayed-Release Capsules 645
Nexium Delayed-Release Oral Suspension 645

Ethacrynic Acid (The ECG changes and/or hypokalemia that may result from the administration of non-potassium sparing diuretics can be acutely worsened by beta-agonists, especially when the recommended dose of beta-agonist is exceeded). Products include:

Edecrin Tablets 698

Fluconazole (Concomitant administration of erythromycin (a moderate CYP3A4 inhibitor) and salmeterol inhalation aerosol resulted in a 40% increase in salmeterol Cmax at steady state, a 3.6-beat/min. increase in heart rate, a 5.8-msec increase in QTc interval, and no change in plasma potassium. Due to the potential increased risk of cardiovascular events, the concomitant use of salmeterol with strong CYP3A4 inhibitors (e.g., ketoconazole, ritonavir, atazanavir, clarithromycin, indinavir, itraconazole, nefazodone, nelfinavir, saquinavir, telithromycin) is not recommended).

No products indexed under this heading.

Fluoxetine (Concomitant administration of erythromycin (a moderate CYP3A4 inhibitor) and salmeterol inhalation aerosol resulted in a 40% increase in salmeterol Cmax at steady state, a 3.6-beat/min. increase in heart rate, a 5.8-msec increase in QTc interval, and no change in plasma potassium. Due to the potential increased risk of cardiovascular events, the concomitant use of salmeterol with strong CYP3A4 inhibitors (e.g., ketoconazole, ritonavir, atazanavir, clarithromycin, indinavir, itraconazole, nefazodone, nelfinavir, saquinavir, telithromycin) is not recommended).

No products indexed under this heading.

Fluoxetine Hydrochloride (Concomitant administration of erythromycin (a moderate CYP3A4 inhibitor) and salmeterol inhalation aerosol resulted in a 40% increase in salmeterol Cmax at steady state, a 3.6-beat/min. increase in heart rate, a 5.8-msec increase in QTc interval, and no change in plasma potassium. Due to the potential increased risk of cardiovascular events, the concomitant use of salmeterol with strong CYP3A4 inhibitors (e.g., ketoconazole, ritonavir, atazanavir, clarithromycin, indinavir, itraconazole, nefazodone, nelfinavir, saquinavir, telithromycin) is not recommended). Products include:

Prozac Weekly Capsules 1852
Prozac Pulvules and Liquid 1852
Symbyax Capsules 1871

Fluvoxamine Maleate (Concomitant administration of erythromycin (a moderate CYP3A4 inhibitor) and salmeterol inhalation aerosol resulted in a 40% increase in salmeterol Cmax at steady state, a 3.6-beat/min. increase in heart rate, a 5.8-msec increase in QTc interval, and no change in plasma potassium. Due to the potential increased risk of cardiovascular events, the concomitant use of salmeterol with strong CYP3A4 inhibitors (e.g., ketoconazole, ritonavir, atazanavir, clarithromycin, indinavir, itraconazole, nefazodone, nelfinavir, saquinavir, telithromycin) is not recommended). Products include:

Luvox CR Extended-Release Capsules.................................... 1759

Fosamprenavir Calcium (Concomitant administration of erythromycin (a moderate CYP3A4 inhibitor) and salmeterol inhalation aerosol resulted in a 40% increase in salmeterol Cmax at steady state, a 3.6-beat/min. increase in heart rate, a 5.8-msec increase in QTc interval, and no change in plasma potassium. Due to the potential increased risk of cardiovascular events, the concomitant use of salmeterol with strong CYP3A4 inhibitors (e.g., ketoconazole, ritonavir, atazanavir, clarithromycin, indinavir, itraconazole, nefazodone, nelfinavir, saquinavir, telithromycin) is not recommended). Products include:

Lexiva Oral Suspension 1510
Lexiva Tablets 1510

Furosemide (The ECG changes and/or hypokalemia that may result from the administration of non-potassium sparing diuretics can be acutely worsened by beta-agonists, especially when the recommended dose of beta-agonist is exceeded). Products include:

Furosemide Tablets 2186

Hydrochlorothiazide (The ECG changes and/or hypokalemia that may result from the administration of non-potassium sparing diuretics can be acutely worsened by beta-agonists, especially when the recommended dose of beta-agonist is exceeded). Products include:

Atacand HCT 642
Avalide Tablets 892
Avalide Tablets 2713
Benicar HCT Tablets 1010
Diovan HCT Tablets 2216
Dyazide Capsules 1405
Micardis HCT Tablets 854
Prinzide Tablets 2092
Tekturna HCT Tablets 2324
Teveten HCT Tablets 517

Hydroflumethiazide (The ECG changes and/or hypokalemia that may result from the administration of non-potassium sparing diuretics can be acutely worsened by beta-agonists, especially when the recommended dose of beta-agonist is exceeded).

No products indexed under this heading.

Imipramine Hydrochloride (Concurrent and/or sequential administration with tricyclic antidepressants may potentiate the action of salmeterol on the vascular system).

No products indexed under this heading.

Imipramine Pamoate (Concurrent and/or sequential administration with tricyclic antidepressants may potentiate the action of salmeterol on the vascular system).

No products indexed under this heading.

Indinavir Sulfate (Concomitant administration of erythromycin (a moderate CYP3A4 inhibitor) and salmeterol inhalation aerosol resulted in a 40% increase in salmeterol Cmax at steady state, a 3.6-beat/min. increase in heart rate, a 5.8-msec increase in QTc interval, and no change in plasma potassium. Due to the potential increased risk of cardiovascular events, the concomitant use of salmeterol with strong CYP3A4 inhibitors (e.g., ketoconazole, ritonavir, atazanavir, clarithromycin, indinavir, itraconazole, nefazodone, nelfinavir, saquinavir, telithromycin) is not recommended). Products include:

Crixivan Capsules 1979

Isocarboxazid (Concurrent and/or sequential administration with MAO inhibitors may potentiate the action of salmeterol on the vascular system. Advair Diskus should be administered with extreme caution to patients being treated with monoamine oxidase inhibitors, or within 2 weeks of discontinuation of such agents). Products include:

Marplan Tablets 3177

Isoniazid (Concomitant administration of erythromycin (a moderate CYP3A4 inhibitor) and salmeterol inhalation aerosol resulted in a 40% increase in salmeterol Cmax at steady state, a 3.6-beat/min. increase in heart rate, a 5.8-msec increase in QTc interval, and no change in plasma potassium. Due to the potential increased risk of cardiovascular events, the concomitant use of salmeterol with strong CYP3A4 inhibitors (e.g., ketoconazole, ritonavir, atazanavir, clarithromycin, indinavir, itraconazole, nefazodone, nelfinavir, saquinavir, telithromycin) is not recommended).

No products indexed under this heading.

Itraconazole (Concomitant administration of erythromycin (a moderate CYP3A4 inhibitor) and salmeterol inhalation aerosol resulted in a 40% increase in salmeterol Cmax at steady state, a 3.6-beat/min. increase in heart rate, a 5.8-msec increase in QTc interval, and no change in plasma potassium. Due to the potential increased risk of cardiovascular events, the concomitant use of salmeterol with strong CYP3A4 inhibitors (e.g., ketoconazole, ritonavir, atazanavir, clarithromycin, indinavir, itraconazole, nefazodone, nelfinavir, saquinavir, telithromycin) is not recommended).

No products indexed under this heading.

Ketoconazole (Co-administration of salmeterol and the strong CYP3A4 inhibitor ketoconazole resulted in a significant increase in plasma salmeterol exposure mainly due to increased bioavailability of the swallowed portion of the dose. Peak plasma salmeterol concentrations were increased by 1.4-fold. Due to the potential increased risk of cardiovascular events, the concomitant use of salmeterol with strong CYP3A4 inhibitors (eg, ketoconazole) is not recommended). Products include:

Extina Foam, 2% 3057
Nizoral A-D Shampoo 1901

Labetalol Hydrochloride (Co-administration with beta-blockers not only blocks the pulmonary effect of beta-agonists, such as salmeterol, but may produce severe bronchospasm in patients with asthma).

No products indexed under this heading.

Levobunolol Hydrochloride (Co-administration with beta-blockers not only blocks the pulmonary effect of beta-agonists, such as salmeterol, but may produce severe bronchospasm in patients with asthma).

No products indexed under this heading.

Lopinavir (Concomitant administration of erythromycin (a moderate CYP3A4 inhibitor) and salmeterol inhalation aerosol resulted in a 40% increase in salmeterol Cmax at steady state, a 3.6-beat/min. increase in heart rate, a 5.8-msec increase in QTc interval, and no change in plasma potassium. Due to the potential increased risk of cardiovascular events, the concomitant use of salmeterol with strong CYP3A4 inhibitors (e.g., ketoconazole, ritonavir, atazanavir, clarithromycin, indinavir, itraconazole, nefazodone, nelfinavir, saquinavir, telithromycin) is not recommended). Products include:

Kaletra 452

Loratadine (Concomitant administration of erythromycin (a moderate CYP3A4 inhibitor) and salmeterol inhalation aerosol resulted in a 40% increase in salmeterol Cmax at steady state, a 3.6-beat/min. increase in heart rate, a 5.8-msec increase in QTc interval, and no change in plasma potassium. Due to the potential increased risk of cardiovascular events, the concomitant use of salmeterol with strong CYP3A4 inhibitors (e.g., ketoconazole, ritonavir, atazanavir, clarithromycin, indinavir, itraconazole, nefazodone, nelfinavir, saquinavir, telithromycin) is not recommended).

No products indexed under this heading.

Maprotiline Hydrochloride (Concurrent and/or sequential administration with tricyclic antidepressants may potentiate the action of salmeterol on the vascular system).

No products indexed under this heading.

Methyclothiazide (The ECG changes and/or hypokalemia that may result from the administration of non-potassium sparing diuretics can be acutely worsened by beta-agonists, especially when the recommended dose of beta-agonist is exceeded).

No products indexed under this heading.

Metipranolol Hydrochloride (Co-administration with beta-blockers not only blocks the pulmonary effect of beta-agonists, such as salmeterol, but may produce severe bronchospasm in patients with asthma).

No products indexed under this heading.

Metoprolol Succinate (Co-administration with beta-blockers not only blocks the pulmonary effect of beta-agonists, such as salmeterol, but may produce severe bronchospasm in patients with asthma). Products include:

Toprol-XL Tablets 666

Metoprolol Tartrate (Co-administration with beta-blockers not only blocks the pulmonary effect of beta-agonists, such as salmeterol, but may produce severe bronchospasm in patients with asthma).

No products indexed under this heading.

Metronidazole (Concomitant administration of erythromycin (a moderate CYP3A4 inhibitor) and salmeterol inhalation aerosol resulted in a 40% increase in salmeterol Cmax at steady state, a 3.6-beat/min. increase in heart rate, a 5.8-msec increase in QTc interval, and no change in plasma potassium. Due to the potential increased risk of cardiovascular events, the concomitant use of salmeterol with strong CYP3A4 inhibitors (e.g., ketoconazole, ritonavir, atazanavir, clarithromycin, indinavir, itraconazole, nefazodone, nelfinavir, saquinavir, telithromycin) is not recommended). Products include:

Pylera Capsules 714

Metronidazole Benzoate (Concomitant administration of erythromycin (a moderate CYP3A4 inhibitor) and salmeterol inhalation aerosol resulted in a 40% increase in salmeterol Cmax at steady state, a 3.6-beat/min. increase in heart rate, a 5.8-msec increase in QTc interval, and no change in plasma potassium. Due to the potential increased risk of cardiovascular events, the concomitant use of salmeterol with strong CYP3A4 inhibitors (e.g., ketoconazole, ritonavir, atazanavir, clarithromycin, indinavir, itraconazone, nefazodone, nelfinavir, saquinavir, telithromycin) is not recommended).

No products indexed under this heading.

Metronidazole Hydrochloride (Concomitant administration of erythromycin (a moderate CYP3A4 inhibitor) and salmeterol inhalation aerosol resulted in a 40% increase in salmeterol Cmax at steady state, a 3.6-beat/min. increase in heart rate, a 5.8-msec increase in QTc interval, and no change in plasma potassium. Due to the potential increased risk of cardiovascular events, the concomitant use of salmeterol with strong CYP3A4 inhibitors (e.g., ketoconazole, ritonavir, atazanavir, clarithromycin, indinavir, itraconazone, nefazodone, nelfinavir, saquinavir, telithromycin) is not recommended).

No products indexed under this heading.

Metronidazole Sodium (Concomitant administration of erythromycin (a moderate CYP3A4 inhibitor) and salmeterol inhalation aerosol resulted in a 40% increase in salmeterol Cmax at steady state, a 3.6-beat/min. increase in heart rate, a 5.8-msec increase in QTc interval, and no change in plasma potassium. Due to the potential increased risk of cardiovascular events, the concomitant use of salmeterol with strong CYP3A4 inhibitors (e.g., ketoconazole, ritonavir, atazanavir, clarithromycin, indinavir, itraconazone, nefazodone, nelfinavir, saquinavir, telithromycin) is not recommended).

No products indexed under this heading.

Miconazole (Concomitant administration of erythromycin (a moderate CYP3A4 inhibitor) and salmeterol inhalation aerosol resulted in a 40% increase in salmeterol Cmax at steady state, a 3.6-beat/min. increase in heart rate, a 5.8-msec increase in QTc interval, and no change in plasma potassium. Due to the potential increased risk of cardiovascular events, the concomitant use of salmeterol with strong CYP3A4 inhibitors (e.g., ketoconazole, ritonavir, atazanavir, clarithromycin, indinavir, itraconazone, nefazodone, nelfinavir, saquinavir, telithromycin) is not recommended).

No products indexed under this heading.

Miconazole Nitrate (Concomitant administration of erythromycin (a moderate CYP3A4 inhibitor) and salmeterol inhalation aerosol resulted in a 40% increase in salmeterol Cmax at steady state, a 3.6-beat/min. increase in heart rate, a 5.8-msec increase in QTc interval, and no change in plasma potassium. Due to the potential increased risk of cardiovascular events, the concomitant use of salmeterol with strong CYP3A4 inhibitors (e.g., ketoconazole, ritonavir, atazanavir, clarithromycin, indinavir, itraconazone, nefazodone, nelfinavir, saquinavir, telithromycin) is not recommended).

No products indexed under this heading.

Moclobemide (Concurrent and/or sequential administration with MAO inhibitors may potentiate the action of salmeterol on the vascular system. Advair Diskus should be administered with extreme caution to patients being treated with monoamine oxidase inhibitors, or within 2 weeks of discontinuation of such agents).

No products indexed under this heading.

Nadolol (Co-administration with beta-blockers not only blocks the pulmonary effect of beta-agonists, such as salmeterol, but may produce severe bronchospasm in patients with asthma). Products include:

Nadolol Tablets **2191**

Nebivolol (Co-administration with beta-blockers not only blocks the pulmonary effect of beta-agonists, such as salmeterol, but may produce severe bronchospasm in patients with asthma). Products include:

Bystolic Tablets **1155**

Nefazodone Hydrochloride (Concomitant administration of erythromycin (a moderate CYP3A4 inhibitor) and salmeterol inhalation aerosol resulted in a 40% increase in salmeterol Cmax at steady state, a 3.6-beat/min. increase in heart rate, a 5.8-msec increase in QTc interval, and no change in plasma potassium. Due to the potential increased risk of cardiovascular events, the concomitant use of salmeterol with strong CYP3A4 inhibitors (e.g., ketoconazole, ritonavir, atazanavir, clarithromycin, indinavir, itraconazone, nefazodone, nelfinavir, saquinavir, telithromycin) is not recommended).

No products indexed under this heading.

Nelfinavir Mesylate (Concomitant administration of erythromycin (a moderate CYP3A4 inhibitor) and salmeterol inhalation aerosol resulted in a 40% increase in salmeterol Cmax at steady state, a 3.6-beat/min. increase in heart rate, a 5.8-msec increase in QTc interval, and no change in plasma potassium. Due to the potential increased risk of cardiovascular events, the concomitant use of salmeterol with strong CYP3A4 inhibitors (e.g., ketoconazole, ritonavir, atazanavir, clarithromycin, indinavir, itraconazone, nefazodone, nelfinavir, saquinavir, telithromycin) is not recommended).

No products indexed under this heading.

Nevirapine (Concomitant administration of erythromycin (a moderate CYP3A4 inhibitor) and salmeterol inhalation aerosol resulted in a 40% increase in salmeterol Cmax at steady state, a 3.6-beat/min. increase in heart rate, a 5.8-msec increase in QTc interval, and no change in plasma potassium. Due to the potential increased risk of cardiovascular events, the concomitant use of salmeterol with strong CYP3A4 inhibitors (e.g., ketoconazole, ritonavir, atazanavir, clarithromycin, indinavir, itraconazone, nefazodone, nelfinavir, saquinavir, telithromycin) is not recommended). Products include:

Viramune Oral Suspension **873**
Viramune Tablets **873**

Niacinamide (Concomitant administration of erythromycin (a moderate CYP3A4 inhibitor) and salmeterol inhalation aerosol resulted in a 40% increase in salmeterol Cmax at steady state, a 3.6-beat/min. increase in heart rate, a 5.8-msec increase in QTc interval, and no change in plasma potassium. Due to the potential increased risk of cardiovascular events, the concomitant use of salmeterol with strong CYP3A4 inhibitors (e.g., ketoconazole, ritonavir, atazanavir, clarithromycin, indinavir, itraconazone, nefazodone, nelfinavir, saquinavir, telithromycin) is not recommended). Products include:

BioLean Free Tablets .... ■□ **635**

Nicotinamide (Concomitant administration of erythromycin (a moderate CYP3A4 inhibitor) and salmeterol inhalation aerosol resulted in a 40% increase in salmeterol Cmax at steady state, a 3.6-beat/min. increase in heart rate, a 5.8-msec increase in QTc interval, and no change in plasma potassium. Due to the potential increased risk of cardiovascular events, the concomitant use of salmeterol with strong CYP3A4 inhibitors (e.g., ketoconazole, ritonavir, atazanavir, clarithromycin, indinavir, itraconazone, nefazodone, nelfinavir, saquinavir, telithromycin) is not recommended).

No products indexed under this heading.

Nifedipine (Concomitant administration of erythromycin (a moderate CYP3A4 inhibitor) and salmeterol inhalation aerosol resulted in a 40% increase in salmeterol Cmax at steady state, a 3.6-beat/min. increase in heart rate, a 5.8-msec increase in QTc interval, and no change in plasma potassium. Due to the potential increased risk of cardiovascular events, the concomitant use of salmeterol with strong CYP3A4 inhibitors (e.g., ketoconazole, ritonavir, atazanavir, clarithromycin, indinavir, itraconazone, nefazodone, nelfinavir, saquinavir, telithromycin) is not recommended).

No products indexed under this heading.

Norfloxacin (Concomitant administration of erythromycin (a moderate CYP3A4 inhibitor) and salmeterol inhalation aerosol resulted in a 40% increase in salmeterol Cmax at steady state, a 3.6-beat/min. increase in heart rate, a 5.8-msec increase in QTc interval, and no change in plasma potassium. Due to the potential increased risk of cardiovascular events, the concomitant use of salmeterol with strong CYP3A4 inhibitors (e.g., ketoconazole, ritonavir, atazanavir, clarithromycin, indinavir, itraconazone, nefazodone, nelfinavir, saquinavir, telithromycin) is not recommended). Products include:

Noroxin Tablets **2069**

Nortriptyline Hydrochloride (Concurrent and/or sequential administration with tricyclic antidepressants may potentiate the action of salmeterol on the vascular system).

No products indexed under this heading.

Omeprazole (Concomitant administration of erythromycin (a moderate CYP3A4 inhibitor) and salmeterol inhalation aerosol resulted in a 40% increase in salmeterol Cmax at steady state, a 3.6-beat/min. increase in heart rate, a 5.8-msec increase in QTc interval, and no change in plasma potassium. Due to the potential increased risk of cardiovascular events, the concomitant use of salmeterol with strong CYP3A4 inhibitors (e.g., ketoconazole, ritonavir, atazanavir, clarithromycin, indinavir, itraconazone, nefazodone, nelfinavir, saquinavir, telithromycin) is not recommended).

No products indexed under this heading.

Pargyline Hydrochloride (Concurrent and/or sequential administration with MAO inhibitors may potentiate the action of salmeterol on the vascular system. Advair Diskus should be administered with extreme caution to patients being treated with monoamine oxidase inhibitors, or within 2 weeks of discontinuation of such agents).

No products indexed under this heading.

Paroxetine Hydrochloride (Concomitant administration of erythromycin (a moderate CYP3A4 inhibitor) and salmeterol inhalation aerosol resulted in a 40% increase in salmeterol Cmax at steady state, a 3.6-beat/min. increase in heart rate, a 5.8-msec increase in QTc interval, and no change in plasma potassium. Due to the potential increased risk of cardiovascular events, the concomitant use of salmeterol with strong CYP3A4 inhibitors (e.g., ketoconazole, ritonavir, atazanavir, clarithromycin, indinavir, itraconazone, nefazodone, nelfinavir, saquinavir, telithromycin) is not recommended). Products include:

Paxil **1535**
Paxil CR Controlled-Release Tablets **1544**

Penbutolol Sulfate (Co-administration with beta-blockers not only blocks the pulmonary effect of beta-agonists, such as salmeterol, but may produce severe bronchospasm in patients with asthma).

No products indexed under this heading.

Phenelzine Sulfate (Concurrent and/or sequential administration with MAO inhibitors may potentiate the action of salmeterol on the vascular system. Advair Diskus should be administered with extreme caution to patients being treated with monoamine oxidase inhibitors, or within 2 weeks of discontinuation of such agents).

No products indexed under this heading.

Pindolol (Co-administration with beta-blockers not only blocks the pulmonary effect of beta-agonists, such as salmeterol, but may produce severe bronchospasm in patients with asthma).

No products indexed under this heading.

Polythiazide (The ECG changes and/or hypokalemia that may result from the administration of non-potassium sparing diuretics can be acutely worsened by beta-agonists, especially when the recommended dose of beta-agonist is exceeded).

No products indexed under this heading.

Procarbazine Hydrochloride (Concurrent and/or sequential administration with MAO inhibitors may potentiate the action of salmeterol on the vascular system. Advair Diskus should be administered with extreme caution to patients being treated with monoamine oxidase inhibitors, or within 2 weeks of discontinuation of such agents).
No products indexed under this heading.

Propoxyphene Hydrochloride (Concomitant administration of erythromycin (a moderate CYP3A4 inhibitor) and salmeterol inhalation aerosol resulted in a 40% increase in salmeterol Cmax at steady state, a 3.6-beat/min. increase in heart rate, a 5.8-msec increase in QTc interval, and no change in plasma potassium. Due to the potential increased risk of cardiovascular events, the concomitant use of salmeterol with strong CYP3A4 inhibitors (e.g., ketoconazole, ritonavir, atazanavir, clarithromycin, indinavir, itraconazone, nefazodone, nelfinavir, saquinavir, telithromycin) is not recommended).
No products indexed under this heading.

Propoxyphene Napsylate (Concomitant administration of erythromycin (a moderate CYP3A4 inhibitor) and salmeterol inhalation aerosol resulted in a 40% increase in salmeterol Cmax at steady state, a 3.6-beat/min. increase in heart rate, a 5.8-msec increase in QTc interval, and no change in plasma potassium. Due to the potential increased risk of cardiovascular events, the concomitant use of salmeterol with strong CYP3A4 inhibitors (e.g., ketoconazole, ritonavir, atazanavir, clarithromycin, indinavir, itraconazone, nefazodone, nelfinavir, saquinavir, telithromycin) is not recommended).
No products indexed under this heading.

Propranolol Hydrochloride (Coadministration with beta-blockers not only blocks the pulmonary effect of beta-agonists, such as salmeterol, but may produce severe bronchospasm in patients with asthma). Products include:
InnoPran XL Extended Release Capsules 1484

Protriptyline Hydrochloride (Concurrent and/or sequential administration with tricyclic antidepressants may potentiate the action of salmeterol on the vascular system).
No products indexed under this heading.

Quinidine (Concomitant administration of erythromycin (a moderate CYP3A4 inhibitor) and salmeterol inhalation aerosol resulted in a 40% increase in salmeterol Cmax at steady state, a 3.6-beat/min. increase in heart rate, a 5.8-msec increase in QTc interval, and no change in plasma potassium. Due to the potential increased risk of cardiovascular events, the concomitant use of salmeterol with strong CYP3A4 inhibitors (e.g., ketoconazole, ritonavir, atazanavir, clarithromycin, indinavir, itraconazone, nefazodone, nelfinavir, saquinavir, telithromycin) is not recommended).
No products indexed under this heading.

Quinidine Hydrochloride (Concomitant administration of erythromycin (a moderate CYP3A4 inhibitor) and salmeterol inhalation aerosol resulted in a 40% increase in salmeterol Cmax at steady state, a 3.6-beat/min. increase in heart rate, a 5.8-msec increase in QTc interval, and no change in plasma potassium. Due to the potential increased risk of cardiovascular events, the concomitant use of salmeterol with strong CYP3A4 inhibitors (e.g., ketoconazole, ritonavir, atazanavir, clarithromycin, indinavir, itraconazone, nefazodone, nelfinavir, saquinavir, telithromycin) is not recommended).
No products indexed under this heading.

Quinidine Polygalacturonate (Concomitant administration of erythromycin (a moderate CYP3A4 inhibitor) and salmeterol inhalation aerosol resulted in a 40% increase in salmeterol Cmax at steady state, a 3.6-beat/min. increase in heart rate, a 5.8-msec increase in QTc interval, and no change in plasma potassium. Due to the potential increased risk of cardiovascular events, the concomitant use of salmeterol with strong CYP3A4 inhibitors (e.g., ketoconazole, ritonavir, atazanavir, clarithromycin, indinavir, itraconazone, nefazodone, nelfinavir, saquinavir, telithromycin) is not recommended).
No products indexed under this heading.

Quinidine Sulfate (Concomitant administration of erythromycin (a moderate CYP3A4 inhibitor) and salmeterol inhalation aerosol resulted in a 40% increase in salmeterol Cmax at steady state, a 3.6-beat/min. increase in heart rate, a 5.8-msec increase in QTc interval, and no change in plasma potassium. Due to the potential increased risk of cardiovascular events, the concomitant use of salmeterol with strong CYP3A4 inhibitors (e.g., ketoconazole, ritonavir, atazanavir, clarithromycin, indinavir, itraconazone, nefazodone, nelfinavir, saquinavir, telithromycin) is not recommended).
No products indexed under this heading.

Quinine (Concomitant administration of erythromycin (a moderate CYP3A4 inhibitor) and salmeterol inhalation aerosol resulted in a 40% increase in salmeterol Cmax at steady state, a 3.6-beat/min. increase in heart rate, a 5.8-msec increase in QTc interval, and no change in plasma potassium. Due to the potential increased risk of cardiovascular events, the concomitant use of salmeterol with strong CYP3A4 inhibitors (e.g., ketoconazole, ritonavir, atazanavir, clarithromycin, indinavir, itraconazone, nefazodone, nelfinavir, saquinavir, telithromycin) is not recommended).
No products indexed under this heading.

Quinine Sulfate (Concomitant administration of erythromycin (a moderate CYP3A4 inhibitor) and salmeterol inhalation aerosol resulted in a 40% increase in salmeterol Cmax at steady state, a 3.6-beat/min. increase in heart rate, a 5.8-msec increase in QTc interval, and no change in plasma potassium. Due to the potential increased risk of cardiovascular events, the concomitant use of salmeterol with strong CYP3A4 inhibitors (e.g., ketoconazole, ritonavir, atazanavir, clarithromycin, indinavir, itraconazone, nefazodone, nelfinavir, saquinavir, telithromycin) is not recommended).
No products indexed under this heading.

Quinupristin (Concomitant administration of erythromycin (a moderate CYP3A4 inhibitor) and salmeterol inhalation aerosol resulted in a 40% increase in salmeterol Cmax at steady state, a 3.6-beat/min. increase in heart rate, a 5.8-msec increase in QTc interval, and no change in plasma potassium. Due to the potential increased risk of cardiovascular events, the concomitant use of salmeterol with strong CYP3A4 inhibitors (e.g., ketoconazole, ritonavir, atazanavir, clarithromycin, indinavir, itraconazone, nefazodone, nelfinavir, saquinavir, telithromycin) is not recommended).
No products indexed under this heading.

Ranitidine Bismuth Citrate (Concomitant administration of erythromycin (a moderate CYP3A4 inhibitor) and salmeterol inhalation aerosol resulted in a 40% increase in salmeterol Cmax at steady state, a 3.6-beat/min. increase in heart rate, a 5.8-msec increase in QTc interval, and no change in plasma potassium. Due to the potential increased risk of cardiovascular events, the concomitant use of salmeterol with strong CYP3A4 inhibitors (e.g., ketoconazole, ritonavir, atazanavir, clarithromycin, indinavir, itraconazone, nefazodone, nelfinavir, saquinavir, telithromycin) is not recommended).
No products indexed under this heading.

Ranitidine Hydrochloride (Concomitant administration of erythromycin (a moderate CYP3A4 inhibitor) and salmeterol inhalation aerosol resulted in a 40% increase in salmeterol Cmax at steady state, a 3.6-beat/min. increase in heart rate, a 5.8-msec increase in QTc interval, and no change in plasma potassium. Due to the potential increased risk of cardiovascular events, the concomitant use of salmeterol with strong CYP3A4 inhibitors (e.g., ketoconazole, ritonavir, atazanavir, clarithromycin, indinavir, itraconazone, nefazodone, nelfinavir, saquinavir, telithromycin) is not recommended). Products include:
Zantac 75 Tablets 603
Zantac 1670
Zantac Injection 1666
Zantac Injection Pharmacy Bulk Package.................................... 1668
Maximum Strength Zantac 150 Tablets.. 603
Maximum Strength Zantac 150 Cool Mint Tablets 603

Rasagiline Mesylate (Concurrent and/or sequential administration with MAO inhibitors may potentiate the action of salmeterol on the vascular system. Advair Diskus should be administered with extreme caution to patients being treated with monoamine oxidase inhibitors, or within 2 weeks of discontinuation of such agents). Products include:
Azilect Tablets 3106

Ritonavir (Ritonavir, a potent CYP3A4 inhibitor, can significantly increase plasma fluticasone exposure, resulting in reduced serum cortisol concentrations. Cushing syndrome and adrenal suppression have been reported; therefore, coadministration is not recommended unless the potential benefit outweighs the risks). Products include:
Kaletra 452
Norvir 489

Saquinavir (Concomitant administration of erythromycin (a moderate CYP3A4 inhibitor) and salmeterol inhalation aerosol resulted in a 40% increase in salmeterol Cmax at steady state, a 3.6-beat/min. increase in heart rate, a 5.8-msec increase in QTc interval, and no change in plasma potassium. Due to the potential increased risk of cardiovascular events, the concomitant use of salmeterol with strong CYP3A4 inhibitors (e.g., ketoconazole, ritonavir, atazanavir, clarithromycin, indinavir, itraconazone, nefazodone, nelfinavir, saquinavir, telithromycin) is not recommended).
No products indexed under this heading.

Saquinavir Mesylate (Concomitant administration of erythromycin (a moderate CYP3A4 inhibitor) and salmeterol inhalation aerosol resulted in a 40% increase in salmeterol Cmax at steady state, a 3.6-beat/min. increase in heart rate, a 5.8-msec increase in QTc interval, and no change in plasma potassium. Due to the potential increased risk of cardiovascular events, the concomitant use of salmeterol with strong CYP3A4 inhibitors (e.g., ketoconazole, ritonavir, atazanavir, clarithromycin, indinavir, itraconazone, nefazodone, nelfinavir, saquinavir, telithromycin) is not recommended).
No products indexed under this heading.

Selegiline (Concurrent and/or sequential administration with MAO inhibitors may potentiate the action of salmeterol on the vascular system. Advair Diskus should be administered with extreme caution to patients being treated with monoamine oxidase inhibitors, or within 2 weeks of discontinuation of such agents). Products include:
Emsam Transdermal System 905

Selegiline Hydrochloride (Concurrent and/or sequential administration with MAO inhibitors may potentiate the action of salmeterol on the vascular system. Advair Diskus should be administered with extreme caution to patients being treated with monoamine oxidase inhibitors, or within 2 weeks of discontinuation of such agents). Products include:
Eldepryl Capsules 3052

Sertraline Hydrochloride (Concomitant administration of erythromycin (a moderate CYP3A4 inhibitor) and salmeterol inhalation aerosol resulted in a 40% increase in salmeterol Cmax at steady state, a 3.6-beat/min. increase in heart rate, a 5.8-msec increase in QTc interval, and no change in plasma potassium. Due to the potential increased risk of cardiovascular events, the concomitant use of salmeterol with strong CYP3A4 inhibitors (e.g., ketoconazole, ritonavir, atazanavir, clarithromycin, indinavir, itraconazone, nefazodone, nelfinavir, saquinavir, telithromycin) is not recommended).
No products indexed under this heading.

Sildenafil Citrate (Concomitant administration of erythromycin (a moderate CYP3A4 inhibitor) and salmeterol inhalation aerosol resulted in a 40% increase in salmeterol Cmax

at steady state, a 3.6-beat/min. increase in heart rate, a 5.8-msec increase in QTc interval, and no change in plasma potassium. Due to the potential increased risk of cardiovascular events, the concomitant use of salmeterol with strong CYP3A4 inhibitors (e.g., ketoconazole, ritonavir, atazanavir, clarithromycin, indinavir, itraconazone, nefazodone, nelfinavir, saquinavir, telithromycin) is not recommended).
No products indexed under this heading.

Sotalol Hydrochloride (Co-administration with beta-blockers not only blocks the pulmonary effect of beta-agonists, such as salmeterol, but may produce severe bronchospasm in patients with asthma).
No products indexed under this heading.

Telithromycin (Concomitant administration of erythromycin (a moderate CYP3A4 inhibitor) and salmeterol inhalation aerosol resulted in a 40% increase in salmeterol Cmax at steady state, a 3.6-beat/min. increase in heart rate, a 5.8-msec increase in QTc interval, and no change in plasma potassium. Due to the potential increased risk of cardiovascular events, the concomitant use of salmeterol with strong CYP3A4 inhibitors (e.g., ketoconazole, ritonavir, atazanavir, clarithromycin, indinavir, itraconazone, nefazodone, nelfinavir, saquinavir, telithromycin) is not recommended). Products include:
Ketek Tablets 2744

Timolol Hemihydrate (Co-administration with beta-blockers not only blocks the pulmonary effect of beta-agonists, such as salmeterol, but may produce severe bronchospasm in patients with asthma). Products include:
Betimol Ophthalmic Solution 3181

Timolol Maleate (Co-administration with beta-blockers not only blocks the pulmonary effect of beta-agonists, such as salmeterol, but may produce severe bronchospasm in patients with asthma). Products include:
Combigan Ophthalmic Solution 553
Cosopt Sterile Ophthalmic Solution.. 1969
Timoptic Sterile Ophthalmic Solution.. 2121
Timoptic in Ocudose 2124
Timoptic-XE Sterile Ophthalmic Gel Forming Solution.................... 2125

Torsemide (The ECG changes and/or hypokalemia that may result from the administration of non-potassium sparing diuretics can be acutely worsened by beta-agonists, especially when the recommended dose of beta-agonist is exceeded). Products include:
Demadex Injection 2630
Demadex Tablets 2630

Tranylcypromine Sulfate (Concurrent and/or sequential administration with MAO inhibitors may potentiate the action of salmeterol on the vascular system. Advair Diskus should be administered with extreme caution to patients being treated with monoamine oxidase inhibitors, or within 2 weeks of discontinuation of such agents). Products include:
Parnate Tablets 1532

Trimipramine Maleate (Concurrent and/or sequential administration with tricyclic antidepressants may potentiate the action of salmeterol on the vascular system).
No products indexed under this heading.

Troglitazone (Concomitant administration of erythromycin (a moderate CYP3A4 inhibitor) and salmeterol inhalation aerosol resulted in a 40% increase in salmeterol Cmax at steady state, a 3.6-beat/min. increase in heart rate, a 5.8-msec increase in QTc interval, and no change in plasma potassium. Due to the potential increased risk of cardiovascular events, the concomitant use of salmeterol with strong CYP3A4 inhibitors (e.g., ketoconazole, ritonavir, atazanavir, clarithromycin, indinavir, itraconazone, nefazodone, nelfinavir, saquinavir, telithromycin) is not recommended).
No products indexed under this heading.

Troleandomycin (Concomitant administration of erythromycin (a moderate CYP3A4 inhibitor) and salmeterol inhalation aerosol resulted in a 40% increase in salmeterol Cmax at steady state, a 3.6-beat/min. increase in heart rate, a 5.8-msec increase in QTc interval, and no change in plasma potassium. Due to the potential increased risk of cardiovascular events, the concomitant use of salmeterol with strong CYP3A4 inhibitors (e.g., ketoconazole, ritonavir, atazanavir, clarithromycin, indinavir, itraconazone, nefazodone, nelfinavir, saquinavir, telithromycin) is not recommended).
No products indexed under this heading.

Valproate Sodium (Concomitant administration of erythromycin (a moderate CYP3A4 inhibitor) and salmeterol inhalation aerosol resulted in a 40% increase in salmeterol Cmax at steady state, a 3.6-beat/min. increase in heart rate, a 5.8-msec increase in QTc interval, and no change in plasma potassium. Due to the potential increased risk of cardiovascular events, the concomitant use of salmeterol with strong CYP3A4 inhibitors (e.g., ketoconazole, ritonavir, atazanavir, clarithromycin, indinavir, itraconazone, nefazodone, nelfinavir, saquinavir, telithromycin) is not recommended).
No products indexed under this heading.

Vardenafil Hydrochloride (Concomitant administration of erythromycin (a moderate CYP3A4 inhibitor) and salmeterol inhalation aerosol resulted in a 40% increase in salmeterol Cmax at steady state, a 3.6-beat/min. increase in heart rate, a 5.8-msec increase in QTc interval, and no change in plasma potassium. Due to the potential increased risk of cardiovascular events, the concomitant use of salmeterol with strong CYP3A4 inhibitors (e.g., ketoconazole, ritonavir, atazanavir, clarithromycin, indinavir, itraconazone, nefazodone, nelfinavir, saquinavir, telithromycin) is not recommended). Products include:
Levitra Tablets 2876

Verapamil Hydrochloride (Concomitant administration of erythromycin (a moderate CYP3A4 inhibitor) and salmeterol inhalation aerosol resulted in a 40% increase in salmeterol Cmax at steady state, a 3.6-beat/min. increase in heart rate, a 5.8-msec increase in QTc interval, and no change in plasma potassium. Due to the potential increased risk of cardiovascular events, the concomitant use of salmeterol with strong CYP3A4 inhibitors (e.g., ketoconazole, ritonavir, atazanavir, clarithromycin, indinavir, itraconazone, nefazodone, nelfinavir, saquinavir, telithromycin) is not recommended). Products include:
Tarka Tablets 511

Voriconazole (Concomitant administration of erythromycin (a moderate CYP3A4 inhibitor) and salmeterol inhalation aerosol resulted in a 40% increase in salmeterol Cmax at steady state, a 3.6-beat/min. increase in heart rate, a 5.8-msec increase in QTc interval, and no change in plasma potassium. Due to the potential increased risk of cardiovascular events, the concomitant use of salmeterol with strong CYP3A4 inhibitors (e.g., ketoconazole, ritonavir, atazanavir, clarithromycin, indinavir, itraconazone, nefazodone, nelfinavir, saquinavir, telithromycin) is not recommended).
No products indexed under this heading.

Zafirlukast (Concomitant administration of erythromycin (a moderate CYP3A4 inhibitor) and salmeterol inhalation aerosol resulted in a 40% increase in salmeterol Cmax at steady state, a 3.6-beat/min. increase in heart rate, a 5.8-msec increase in QTc interval, and no change in plasma potassium. Due to the potential increased risk of cardiovascular events, the concomitant use of salmeterol with strong CYP3A4 inhibitors (e.g., ketoconazole, ritonavir, atazanavir, clarithromycin, indinavir, itraconazone, nefazodone, nelfinavir, saquinavir, telithromycin) is not recommended). Products include:
Accolate Tablets 669

Zileuton (Concomitant administration of erythromycin (a moderate CYP3A4 inhibitor) and salmeterol inhalation aerosol resulted in a 40% increase in salmeterol Cmax at steady state, a 3.6-beat/min. increase in heart rate, a 5.8-msec increase in QTc interval, and no change in plasma potassium. Due to the potential increased risk of cardiovascular events, the concomitant use of salmeterol with strong CYP3A4 inhibitors (e.g., ketoconazole, ritonavir, atazanavir, clarithromycin, indinavir, itraconazone, nefazodone, nelfinavir, saquinavir, telithromycin) is not recommended).
No products indexed under this heading.

Food Interactions

Grapefruit (Concomitant administration of erythromycin (a moderate CYP3A4 inhibitor) and salmeterol inhalation aerosol resulted in a 40% increase in salmeterol Cmax at steady state, a 3.6-beat/min. increase in heart rate, a 5.8-msec increase in QTc interval, and no change in plasma potassium. Due to the potential increased risk of cardiovascular events, the concomitant use of salmeterol with strong CYP3A4 inhibitors (e.g., ketoconazole, ritonavir, atazanavir, clarithromycin, indinavir, itraconazone, nefazodone, nelfinavir, saquinavir, telithromycin) is not recommended).

Grapefruit Juice (Concomitant administration of erythromycin (a moderate CYP3A4 inhibitor) and salmeterol inhalation aerosol resulted in a 40% increase in salmeterol Cmax at steady state, a 3.6-beat/min. increase in heart rate, a 5.8-msec increase in QTc interval, and no change in plasma potassium. Due to the potential increased risk of cardiovascular events, the concomitant use of salmeterol with strong CYP3A4 inhibitors (e.g., ketoconazole, ritonavir, atazanavir, clarithromycin, indinavir, itraconazone, nefazodone, nelfinavir, saquinavir, telithromycin) is not recommended).

ADVAIR HFA 115/21 INHALATION AEROSOL

(Fluticasone Propionate, Salmeterol Xinafoate)...................... 1288
See Advair HFA 45/21 Inhalation Aerosol

ADVAIR HFA 230/21 INHALATION AEROSOL

(Fluticasone Propionate, Salmeterol Xinafoate)...................... 1288
See Advair HFA 45/21 Inhalation Aerosol

ADVATE

(Antihemophilic Factor (Recombinant)).............................. 721
None cited in PDR database.

ADVICOR TABLETS

(Lovastatin, Niacin) 402
May interact with azole antifungals, beta blockers, calcium channel blockers, oral anticoagulants, cytochrome p450 3a4 inhibitors (selected), erythromycin, fibrates, nitrates and nitrites, protease inhibitors, and certain other agents. Compounds in these categories include:

Acebutolol Hydrochloride (Co-administration of niacin with vasoactive drugs, such as adrenergic blocking agents, may result in postural hypotension, particularly in patients with unstable angina or acute phase of myocardial infarction).
No products indexed under this heading.

Acetazolamide (The risk of myopathy appears to be increased by high levels of HMG-CoA reductase inhibitory activity in plasma. Lovastatin is metabolized by the cytochrome P450 isoform 3A4. Certain drugs which share this metabolic pathway can raise the plasma levels of lovastatin and may increase the risk of myopathy).
No products indexed under this heading.

Amiodarone Hydrochloride (The risk of myopathy appears to be increased by high levels of HMG-CoA reductase inhibitory activity in plasma. Lovastatin is metabolized by the cytochrome P450 isoform 3A4. Certain drugs which share this metabolic pathway can raise the plasma levels of lovastatin and may increase the risk of myopathy).
No products indexed under this heading.

Amlodipine Besylate (Co-administration of niacin with vasoactive drugs, such as calcium channel blockers, may result in postural hypotension, particularly in patients with unstable angina or acute phase of myocardial infarction). Products include:
Azor Tablets 1005
Exforge Tablets 2238

Amprenavir (Co-administration results in serious skeletal muscle disorders, such as rhabdomyolysis and myopathy).
No products indexed under this heading.

Amyl Nitrite (Co-administration of niacin with vasoactive drugs, such as nitrates, may result in postural hypotension, particularly in patients with unstable angina or acute phase of myocardial infarction).
No products indexed under this heading.

Anastrozole (The risk of myopathy appears to be increased by high levels of HMG-CoA reductase inhibitory activity in plasma. Lovastatin is metabolized by the cytochrome P450 isoform 3A4. Certain drugs which share this metabolic pathway can raise the plasma levels of lovastatin and may increase the risk of myopathy). Products include:
Arimidex Tablets 672

Anisindione (Co-administration has resulted in increased bleeding and/or prothrombin time).
No products indexed under this heading.

Aprepitant (The risk of myopathy appears to be increased by high levels of HMG-CoA reductase inhibitory activity in plasma. Lovastatin is metabolized by the cytochrome P450 isoform 3A4. Certain drugs which share this metabolic pathway can raise the plasma levels of lovastatin and may increase the risk of myopathy). Products include:
Emend Capsules 1992

Aspirin (May decrease the metabolic clearance of niacin; the clinical relevance of this finding is unclear). Products include:
Aggrenox Capsules 819
Bayer Aspirin 750
Percodan Tablets 1130
St. Joseph 81 mg Aspirin Chewable and Enteric Coated Tablets 1903

Atazanavir (The risk of myopathy appears to be increased by high levels of HMG-CoA reductase inhibitory activity in plasma. Lovastatin is metabolized by the cytochrome P450 isoform 3A4. Certain drugs which share this metabolic pathway can raise the plasma levels of lovastatin and may increase the risk of myopathy).
No products indexed under this heading.

Atazanavir Sulfate (The risk of myopathy appears to be increased by high levels of HMG-CoA reductase inhibitory activity in plasma. Lovastatin is metabolized by the cytochrome P450 isoform 3A4. Certain drugs which share this metabolic pathway can raise the plasma levels of lovastatin and may increase the risk of myopathy). Products include:
Reyataz Capsules 3299

Atenolol (Co-administration of niacin with vasoactive drugs, such as adrenergic blocking agents, may result in postural hypotension, particularly in patients with unstable angina or acute phase of myocardial infarction).
No products indexed under this heading.

Bepridil Hydrochloride (Co-administration of niacin with vasoactive drugs, such as calcium channel blockers, may result in postural hypotension, particularly in patients with unstable angina or acute phase of myocardial infarction).
No products indexed under this heading.

Betaxolol Hydrochloride (Co-administration of niacin with vasoactive drugs, such as adrenergic blocking agents, may result in postural hypotension, particularly in patients with unstable angina or acute phase of myocardial infarction).
No products indexed under this heading.

Bisoprolol Fumarate (Co-administration of niacin with vasoactive drugs, such as adrenergic blocking agents, may result in postural hypotension, particularly in patients with unstable angina or acute phase of myocardial infarction).
No products indexed under this heading.

Carteolol Hydrochloride (Co-administration of niacin with vasoactive drugs, such as adrenergic blocking agents, may result in postural hypotension, particularly in patients with unstable angina or acute phase of myocardial infarction).
No products indexed under this heading.

Cholestyramine (In-vitro study resulted in approximately 10% to 30% of available niacin bound to cholestyramine; 4 to 6 hours should elapse between ingestion of bile acid-binding resins and the administration of Advicor).
No products indexed under this heading.

Cimetidine (The risk of myopathy appears to be increased by high levels of HMG-CoA reductase inhibitory activity in plasma. Lovastatin is metabolized by the cytochrome P450 isoform 3A4. Certain drugs which share this metabolic pathway can raise the plasma levels of lovastatin and may increase the risk of myopathy).
No products indexed under this heading.

Cimetidine Hydrochloride (The risk of myopathy appears to be increased by high levels of HMG-CoA reductase inhibitory activity in plasma. Lovastatin is metabolized by the cytochrome P450 isoform 3A4. Certain drugs which share this metabolic pathway can raise the plasma levels of lovastatin and may increase the risk of myopathy).
No products indexed under this heading.

Ciprofloxacin (The risk of myopathy appears to be increased by high levels of HMG-CoA reductase inhibitory activity in plasma. Lovastatin is metabolized by the cytochrome P450 isoform 3A4. Certain drugs which share this metabolic pathway can raise the plasma levels of lovastatin and may increase the risk of myopathy). Products include:
Cipro I.V. 2817
Cipro Oral Suspension 2810
Cipro XR Tablets 2823
Ciprodex Otic Suspension 541

Clarithromycin (Co-administration results in serious skeletal muscle disorders, such as rhabdomyolysis and myopathy). Products include:
Biaxin/Biaxin XL 411

Clofibrate (The incidence and severity of myopathy are increased by co-administration of Advicor with drugs that cause myopathy when given alone, such as fibrates; combined use should be avoided).
No products indexed under this heading.

Clotrimazole (Co-administration results in serious skeletal muscle disorders, such as rhabdomyolysis and myopathy). Products include:
Lotrisone 2881

Colestipol Hydrochloride (In-vitro study resulted in approximately 90% of available niacin bound to colestipol; 4 to 6 hours should elapse between ingestion of bile acid-binding resins and the administration of Advicor).
No products indexed under this heading.

Cyclosporine (Co-administration results in serious skeletal muscle disorders, such as rhabdomyolysis and myopathy. Cyclosporine has been shown to increase the AUC of HMG-CoA reductase inhibitors). Products include:
Gengraf Capsules 435
Neoral Oral Solution 2280
Neoral Soft Gelatin Capsules 2280
Restasis Ophthalmic Emulsion 557
Sandimmune 2296

Dalfopristin (The risk of myopathy appears to be increased by high levels of HMG-CoA reductase inhibitory activity in plasma. Lovastatin is metabolized by the cytochrome P450 isoform 3A4. Certain drugs which share this metabolic pathway can raise the plasma levels of lovastatin and may increase the risk of myopathy).
No products indexed under this heading.

Danazol (Co-administration results in serious skeletal muscle disorders, such as rhabdomyolysis and myopathy).
No products indexed under this heading.

Darunavir (Co-administration results in serious skeletal muscle disorders, such as rhabdomyolysis and myopathy).
No products indexed under this heading.

Delavirdine Mesylate (The risk of myopathy appears to be increased by high levels of HMG-CoA reductase inhibitory activity in plasma. Lovastatin is metabolized by the cytochrome P450 isoform 3A4. Certain drugs which share this metabolic pathway can raise the plasma levels of lovastatin and may increase the risk of myopathy).
No products indexed under this heading.

Dicumarol (Co-administration has resulted in increased bleeding and/or prothrombin time).
No products indexed under this heading.

Diltiazem Hydrochloride (Co-administration of niacin with vasoactive drugs, such as calcium channel blockers, may result in postural hypotension, particularly in patients with unstable angina or acute phase of myocardial infarction). Products include:
Cardizem LA Extended Release Tablets 421

Diltiazem Maleate (The risk of myopathy appears to be increased by high levels of HMG-CoA reductase inhibitory activity in plasma. Lovastatin is metabolized by the cytochrome P450 isoform 3A4. Certain drugs which share this metabolic pathway can raise the plasma levels of lovastatin and may increase the risk of myopathy).
No products indexed under this heading.

Efavirenz (The risk of myopathy appears to be increased by high levels of HMG-CoA reductase inhibitory activity in plasma. Lovastatin is metabolized by the cytochrome P450 isoform 3A4. Certain drugs which share this metabolic pathway can raise the plasma levels of lovastatin and may increase the risk of myopathy). Products include:
Atripla Tablets 938
Sustiva Capsules 930
Sustiva Tablets 930

Erythrityl Tetranitrate (Co-administration of niacin with vasoactive drugs, such as nitrates, may result in postural hypotension, particularly in patients with unstable angina or acute phase of myocardial infarction).
No products indexed under this heading.

Erythromycin (Co-administration results in serious skeletal muscle disorders, such as rhabdomyolysis and myopathy).
No products indexed under this heading.

Erythromycin Estolate (Co-administration results in serious skeletal muscle disorders, such as rhabdomyolysis and myopathy).
No products indexed under this heading.

Erythromycin Ethylsuccinate (Co-administration results in serious skeletal muscle disorders, such as rhabdomyolysis and myopathy). Products include:
E.E.S. 433
EryPed 431

Erythromycin Gluceptate (Co-administration results in serious skeletal muscle disorders, such as rhabdomyolysis and myopathy).
No products indexed under this heading.

Erythromycin Lactobionate (Co-administration results in serious skeletal muscle disorders, such as rhabdomyolysis and myopathy).
No products indexed under this heading.

Erythromycin Stearate (Co-administration results in serious skeletal muscle disorders, such as rhabdomyolysis and myopathy).
No products indexed under this heading.

Esmolol Hydrochloride (Co-administration of niacin with vasoactive drugs, such as adrenergic blocking agents, may result in postural hypotension, particularly in patients with unstable angina or acute phase of myocardial infarction).
No products indexed under this heading.

Esomeprazole Magnesium (The risk of myopathy appears to be increased by high levels of HMG-CoA reductase inhibitory activity in plasma. Lovastatin is metabolized by the cytochrome P450 isoform 3A4. Certain drugs which share this metabolic pathway can raise the plasma levels of lovastatin and may increase the risk of myopathy). Products include:

Nexium Delayed-Release Capsules 645
Nexium Delayed-Release Oral Suspension 645

Felodipine (Co-administration of niacin with vasoactive drugs, such as calcium channel blockers, may result in postural hypotension, particularly in patients with unstable angina or acute phase of myocardial infarction).

No products indexed under this heading.

Fenofibrate (The incidence and severity of myopathy are increased by co-administration of Advicor with drugs that cause myopathy when given alone, such as fibrates; combined use should be avoided). Products include:

Fenoglide Tablets 2960
Tricor Tablets 520

Fluconazole (Co-administration results in serious skeletal muscle disorders, such as rhabdomyolysis and myopathy).

No products indexed under this heading.

Fluoxetine (The risk of myopathy appears to be increased by high levels of HMG-CoA reductase inhibitory activity in plasma. Lovastatin is metabolized by the cytochrome P450 isoform 3A4. Certain drugs which share this metabolic pathway can raise the plasma levels of lovastatin and may increase the risk of myopathy).

No products indexed under this heading.

Fluoxetine Hydrochloride (The risk of myopathy appears to be increased by high levels of HMG-CoA reductase inhibitory activity in plasma. Lovastatin is metabolized by the cytochrome P450 isoform 3A4. Certain drugs which share this metabolic pathway can raise the plasma levels of lovastatin and may increase the risk of myopathy). Products include:

Prozac Weekly Capsules 1852
Prozac Pulvules and Liquid 1852
Symbyax Capsules 1871

Fluvoxamine Maleate (The risk of myopathy appears to be increased by high levels of HMG-CoA reductase inhibitory activity in plasma. Lovastatin is metabolized by the cytochrome P450 isoform 3A4. Certain drugs which share this metabolic pathway can raise the plasma levels of lovastatin and may increase the risk of myopathy). Products include:

Luvox CR Extended-Release Capsules 1759

Fosamprenavir Calcium (Co-administration results in serious skeletal muscle disorders, such as rhabdomyolysis and myopathy). Products include:

Lexiva Oral Suspension 1510
Lexiva Tablets 1510

Gemfibrozil (The incidence and severity of myopathy are increased by co-administration of Advicor with drugs that cause myopathy when given alone, such as fibrates; combined use should be avoided).

No products indexed under this heading.

Indinavir Sulfate (Co-administration results in serious skeletal muscle disorders, such as rhabdomyolysis and myopathy). Products include:

Crixivan Capsules 1979

Isoniazid (The risk of myopathy appears to be increased by high levels of HMG-CoA reductase inhibitory activity in plasma. Lovastatin is metabolized by the cytochrome P450 isoform 3A4. Certain drugs which share this metabolic pathway can raise the plasma levels of lovastatin and may increase the risk of myopathy).

No products indexed under this heading.

Isosorbide Dinitrate (Co-administration of niacin with vasoactive drugs, such as nitrates, may result in postural hypotension, particularly in patients with unstable angina or acute phase of myocardial infarction).

No products indexed under this heading.

Isosorbide Mononitrate (Co-administration of niacin with vasoactive drugs, such as nitrates, may result in postural hypotension, particularly in patients with unstable angina or acute phase of myocardial infarction).

No products indexed under this heading.

Isradipine (Co-administration of niacin with vasoactive drugs, such as calcium channel blockers, may result in postural hypotension, particularly in patients with unstable angina or acute phase of myocardial infarction). Products include:

DynaCirc CR Controlled Release Tablets 1407

Itraconazole (Co-administration results in serious skeletal muscle disorders, such as rhabdomyolysis and myopathy).

No products indexed under this heading.

Ketoconazole (Co-administration results in serious skeletal muscle disorders, such as rhabdomyolysis and myopathy). Products include:

Extina Foam, 2% 3057
Nizoral A-D Shampoo 1901

Labetalol Hydrochloride (Co-administration of niacin with vasoactive drugs, such as adrenergic blocking agents, may result in postural hypotension, particularly in patients with unstable angina or acute phase of myocardial infarction).

No products indexed under this heading.

Levobunolol Hydrochloride (Co-administration of niacin with vasoactive drugs, such as adrenergic blocking agents, may result in postural hypotension, particularly in patients with unstable angina or acute phase of myocardial infarction).

No products indexed under this heading.

Lopinavir (Co-administration results in serious skeletal muscle disorders, such as rhabdomyolysis and myopathy). Products include:

Kaletra 452

Loratadine (The risk of myopathy appears to be increased by high levels of HMG-CoA reductase inhibitory activity in plasma. Lovastatin is metabolized by the cytochrome P450 isoform 3A4. Certain drugs which share this metabolic pathway can raise the plasma levels of lovastatin and may increase the risk of myopathy).

No products indexed under this heading.

Metipranolol Hydrochloride (Co-administration of niacin with vasoactive drugs, such as adrenergic blocking agents, may result in postural hypotension, particularly in patients with unstable angina or acute phase of myocardial infarction).

No products indexed under this heading.

Metoprolol Succinate (Co-administration of niacin with vasoactive drugs, such as adrenergic blocking agents, may result in postural hypotension, particularly in patients with unstable angina or acute phase of myocardial infarction). Products include:

Toprol-XL Tablets 666

Metoprolol Tartrate (Co-administration of niacin with vasoactive drugs, such as adrenergic blocking agents, may result in postural hypotension, particularly in patients with unstable angina or acute phase of myocardial infarction).

No products indexed under this heading.

Metronidazole (The risk of myopathy appears to be increased by high levels of HMG-CoA reductase inhibitory activity in plasma. Lovastatin is metabolized by the cytochrome P450 isoform 3A4. Certain drugs which share this metabolic pathway can raise the plasma levels of lovastatin and may increase the risk of myopathy). Products include:

Pylera Capsules 714

Metronidazole Benzoate (The risk of myopathy appears to be increased by high levels of HMG-CoA reductase inhibitory activity in plasma. Lovastatin is metabolized by the cytochrome P450 isoform 3A4. Certain drugs which share this metabolic pathway can raise the plasma levels of lovastatin and may increase the risk of myopathy).

No products indexed under this heading.

Metronidazole Hydrochloride (The risk of myopathy appears to be increased by high levels of HMG-CoA reductase inhibitory activity in plasma. Lovastatin is metabolized by the cytochrome P450 isoform 3A4. Certain drugs which share this metabolic pathway can raise the plasma levels of lovastatin and may increase the risk of myopathy).

No products indexed under this heading.

Mibefradil Dihydrochloride (Co-administration of niacin with vasoactive drugs, such as calcium channel blockers, may result in postural hypotension, particularly in patients with unstable angina or acute phase of myocardial infarction).

No products indexed under this heading.

Miconazole (Co-administration results in serious skeletal muscle disorders, such as rhabdomyolysis and myopathy).

No products indexed under this heading.

Miconazole Nitrate (The risk of myopathy appears to be increased by high levels of HMG-CoA reductase inhibitory activity in plasma. Lovastatin is metabolized by the cytochrome P450 isoform 3A4. Certain drugs which share this metabolic pathway can raise the plasma levels of lovastatin and may increase the risk of myopathy).

No products indexed under this heading.

Nadolol (Co-administration of niacin with vasoactive drugs, such as adrenergic blocking agents, may result in postural hypotension, particularly in patients with unstable angina or acute phase of myocardial infarction). Products include:

Nadolol Tablets 2191

Nebivolol (Co-administration of niacin with vasoactive drugs, such as adrenergic blocking agents, may result in postural hypotension, particularly in patients with unstable angina or acute phase of myocardial infarction). Products include:

Bystolic Tablets 1155

Nefazodone Hydrochloride (Co-administration results in serious skeletal muscle disorders, such as rhabdomyolysis and myopathy).

No products indexed under this heading.

Nelfinavir Mesylate (Co-administration results in serious skeletal muscle disorders, such as rhabdomyolysis and myopathy).

No products indexed under this heading.

Nevirapine (The risk of myopathy appears to be increased by high levels of HMG-CoA reductase inhibitory activity in plasma. Lovastatin is metabolized by the cytochrome P450 isoform 3A4. Certain drugs which share this metabolic pathway can raise the plasma levels of lovastatin and may increase the risk of myopathy). Products include:

Viramune Oral Suspension 873
Viramune Tablets 873

Niacinamide (The risk of myopathy appears to be increased by high levels of HMG-CoA reductase inhibitory activity in plasma. Lovastatin is metabolized by the cytochrome P450 isoform 3A4. Certain drugs which share this metabolic pathway can raise the plasma levels of lovastatin and may increase the risk of myopathy). Products include:

BioLean Free Tablets .... ■■635

Nicardipine Hydrochloride (Co-administration of niacin with vasoactive drugs, such as calcium channel blockers, may result in postural hypotension, particularly in patients with unstable angina or acute phase of myocardial infarction). Products include:

Cardene I.V. 1093

Nicotinamide (May potentiate the adverse effects of Advicor).

No products indexed under this heading.

Nifedipine (Co-administration of niacin with vasoactive drugs, such as calcium channel blockers, may result in postural hypotension, particularly in patients with unstable angina or acute phase of myocardial infarction).
No products indexed under this heading.

Nimodipine (Co-administration of niacin with vasoactive drugs, such as calcium channel blockers, may result in postural hypotension, particularly in patients with unstable angina or acute phase of myocardial infarction). Products include:
Nimotop Capsules 790

Nisoldipine (Co-administration of niacin with vasoactive drugs, such as calcium channel blockers, may result in postural hypotension, particularly in patients with unstable angina or acute phase of myocardial infarction). Products include:
Sular Extended Release Tablets 2975

Nitroglycerin (Co-administration of niacin with vasoactive drugs, such as nitrates, may result in postural hypotension, particularly in patients with unstable angina or acute phase of myocardial infarction). Products include:
Nitro-Dur Transdermal Infusion System 2887
Nitrolingual Pumpspray 2965

Norfloxacin (The risk of myopathy appears to be increased by high levels of HMG-CoA reductase inhibitory activity in plasma. Lovastatin is metabolized by the cytochrome P450 isoform 3A4. Certain drugs which share this metabolic pathway can raise the plasma levels of lovastatin and may increase the risk of myopathy). Products include:
Noroxin Tablets 2069

Omeprazole (The risk of myopathy appears to be increased by high levels of HMG-CoA reductase inhibitory activity in plasma. Lovastatin is metabolized by the cytochrome P450 isoform 3A4. Certain drugs which share this metabolic pathway can raise the plasma levels of lovastatin and may increase the risk of myopathy).
No products indexed under this heading.

Oxiconazole Nitrate (Co-administration results in serious skeletal muscle disorders, such as rhabdomyolysis and myopathy).
No products indexed under this heading.

Paroxetine Hydrochloride (The risk of myopathy appears to be increased by high levels of HMG-CoA reductase inhibitory activity in plasma. Lovastatin is metabolized by the cytochrome P450 isoform 3A4. Certain drugs which share this metabolic pathway can raise the plasma levels of lovastatin and may increase the risk of myopathy). Products include:
Paxil 1535
Paxil CR Controlled-Release Tablets 1544

Penbutolol Sulfate (Co-administration of niacin with vasoactive drugs, such as adrenergic blocking agents, may result in postural hypotension, particularly in patients with unstable angina or acute phase of myocardial infarction).
No products indexed under this heading.

Pentaerythritol Tetranitrate (Co-administration of niacin with vasoactive drugs, such as nitrates, may result in postural hypotension, particularly in patients with unstable angina or acute phase of myocardial infarction).
No products indexed under this heading.

Pindolol (Co-administration of niacin with vasoactive drugs, such as adrenergic blocking agents, may result in postural hypotension, particularly in patients with unstable angina or acute phase of myocardial infarction).
No products indexed under this heading.

Posaconazole (Co-administration results in serious skeletal muscle disorders, such as rhabdomyolysis and myopathy). Products include:
Noxafil Oral Suspension 2889

Propoxyphene Hydrochloride (The risk of myopathy appears to be increased by high levels of HMG-CoA reductase inhibitory activity in plasma. Lovastatin is metabolized by the cytochrome P450 isoform 3A4. Certain drugs which share this metabolic pathway can raise the plasma levels of lovastatin and may increase the risk of myopathy).
No products indexed under this heading.

Propoxyphene Napsylate (The risk of myopathy appears to be increased by high levels of HMG-CoA reductase inhibitory activity in plasma. Lovastatin is metabolized by the cytochrome P450 isoform 3A4. Certain drugs which share this metabolic pathway can raise the plasma levels of lovastatin and may increase the risk of myopathy).
No products indexed under this heading.

Propranolol Hydrochloride (Co-administration of niacin with vasoactive drugs, such as adrenergic blocking agents, may result in postural hypotension, particularly in patients with unstable angina or acute phase of myocardial infarction). Products include:
InnoPran XL Extended Release Capsules 1484

Quinidine (The risk of myopathy appears to be increased by high levels of HMG-CoA reductase inhibitory activity in plasma. Lovastatin is metabolized by the cytochrome P450 isoform 3A4. Certain drugs which share this metabolic pathway can raise the plasma levels of lovastatin and may increase the risk of myopathy).
No products indexed under this heading.

Quinidine Hydrochloride (The risk of myopathy appears to be increased by high levels of HMG-CoA reductase inhibitory activity in plasma. Lovastatin is metabolized by the cytochrome P450 isoform 3A4. Certain drugs which share this metabolic pathway can raise the plasma levels of lovastatin and may increase the risk of myopathy).
No products indexed under this heading.

Quinidine Polygalacturonate (The risk of myopathy appears to be increased by high levels of HMG-CoA reductase inhibitory activity in plasma. Lovastatin is metabolized by the cytochrome P450 isoform 3A4. Certain drugs which share this metabolic pathway can raise the plasma levels of lovastatin and may increase the risk of myopathy).
No products indexed under this heading.

Quinidine Sulfate (The risk of myopathy appears to be increased by high levels of HMG-CoA reductase inhibitory activity in plasma. Lovastatin is metabolized by the cytochrome P450 isoform 3A4. Certain drugs which share this metabolic pathway can raise the plasma levels of lovastatin and may increase the risk of myopathy).
No products indexed under this heading.

Quinine (The risk of myopathy appears to be increased by high levels of HMG-CoA reductase inhibitory activity in plasma. Lovastatin is metabolized by the cytochrome P450 isoform 3A4. Certain drugs which share this metabolic pathway can raise the plasma levels of lovastatin and may increase the risk of myopathy).
No products indexed under this heading.

Quinine Sulfate (The risk of myopathy appears to be increased by high levels of HMG-CoA reductase inhibitory activity in plasma. Lovastatin is metabolized by the cytochrome P450 isoform 3A4. Certain drugs which share this metabolic pathway can raise the plasma levels of lovastatin and may increase the risk of myopathy).
No products indexed under this heading.

Quinupristin (The risk of myopathy appears to be increased by high levels of HMG-CoA reductase inhibitory activity in plasma. Lovastatin is metabolized by the cytochrome P450 isoform 3A4. Certain drugs which share this metabolic pathway can raise the plasma levels of lovastatin and may increase the risk of myopathy).
No products indexed under this heading.

Ranitidine Bismuth Citrate (The risk of myopathy appears to be increased by high levels of HMG-CoA reductase inhibitory activity in plasma. Lovastatin is metabolized by the cytochrome P450 isoform 3A4. Certain drugs which share this metabolic pathway can raise the plasma levels of lovastatin and may increase the risk of myopathy).
No products indexed under this heading.

Ranitidine Hydrochloride (The risk of myopathy appears to be increased by high levels of HMG-CoA reductase inhibitory activity in plasma. Lovastatin is metabolized by the cytochrome P450 isoform 3A4. Certain drugs which share this metabolic pathway can raise the plasma levels of lovastatin and may increase the risk of myopathy). Products include:
Zantac 75 Tablets 603
Zantac 1670
Zantac Injection 1666
Zantac Injection Pharmacy Bulk Package 1668
Maximum Strength Zantac 150 Tablets 603
Maximum Strength Zantac 150 Cool Mint Tablets 603

Ritonavir (Co-administration results in serious skeletal muscle disorders, such as rhabdomyolysis and myopathy). Products include:
Kaletra 452
Norvir 489

Saquinavir (Co-administration results in serious skeletal muscle disorders, such as rhabdomyolysis and myopathy).
No products indexed under this heading.

Saquinavir Mesylate (Co-administration results in serious skeletal muscle disorders, such as rhabdomyolysis and myopathy).
No products indexed under this heading.

Sertraline Hydrochloride (The risk of myopathy appears to be increased by high levels of HMG-CoA reductase inhibitory activity in plasma. Lovastatin is metabolized by the cytochrome P450 isoform 3A4. Certain drugs which share this metabolic pathway can raise the plasma levels of lovastatin and may increase the risk of myopathy).
No products indexed under this heading.

Sildenafil Citrate (The risk of myopathy appears to be increased by high levels of HMG-CoA reductase inhibitory activity in plasma. Lovastatin is metabolized by the cytochrome P450 isoform 3A4. Certain drugs which share this metabolic pathway can raise the plasma levels of lovastatin and may increase the risk of myopathy).
No products indexed under this heading.

Sotalol Hydrochloride (Co-administration of niacin with vasoactive drugs, such as adrenergic blocking agents, may result in postural hypotension, particularly in patients with unstable angina or acute phase of myocardial infarction).
No products indexed under this heading.

Telithromycin (Co-administration results in serious skeletal muscle disorders, such as rhabdomyolysis and myopathy). Products include:
Ketek Tablets 2744

Terconazole (Co-administration results in serious skeletal muscle disorders, such as rhabdomyolysis and myopathy).
No products indexed under this heading.

Timolol Hemihydrate (Co-administration of niacin with vasoactive drugs, such as adrenergic blocking agents, may result in postural hypotension, particularly in patients with unstable angina or acute phase of myocardial infarction). Products include:
Betimol Ophthalmic Solution 3181

Timolol Maleate (Co-administration of niacin with vasoactive drugs, such as adrenergic blocking agents, may result in postural hypotension, particularly in patients with unstable angina or acute phase of myocardial infarction). Products include:
Combigan Ophthalmic Solution 553
Cosopt Sterile Ophthalmic Solution 1969

Timoptic Sterile Ophthalmic Solution 2121
Timoptic in Ocudose 2124
Timoptic-XE Sterile Ophthalmic Gel Forming Solution 2125

Tipranavir (Co-administration results in serious skeletal muscle disorders, such as rhabdomyolysis and myopathy). Products include:
Aptivus Capsules 823
Aptivus Oral Solution 823

Troglitazone (The risk of myopathy appears to be increased by high levels of HMG-CoA reductase inhibitory activity in plasma. Lovastatin is metabolized by the cytochrome P450 isoform 3A4. Certain drugs which share this metabolic pathway can raise the plasma levels of lovastatin and may increase the risk of myopathy).
No products indexed under this heading.

Troleandomycin (The risk of myopathy appears to be increased by high levels of HMG-CoA reductase inhibitory activity in plasma. Lovastatin is metabolized by the cytochrome P450 isoform 3A4. Certain drugs which share this metabolic pathway can raise the plasma levels of lovastatin and may increase the risk of myopathy).
No products indexed under this heading.

Valproate Sodium (The risk of myopathy appears to be increased by high levels of HMG-CoA reductase inhibitory activity in plasma. Lovastatin is metabolized by the cytochrome P450 isoform 3A4. Certain drugs which share this metabolic pathway can raise the plasma levels of lovastatin and may increase the risk of myopathy).
No products indexed under this heading.

Vardenafil Hydrochloride (The risk of myopathy appears to be increased by high levels of HMG-CoA reductase inhibitory activity in plasma. Lovastatin is metabolized by the cytochrome P450 isoform 3A4. Certain drugs which share this metabolic pathway can raise the plasma levels of lovastatin and may increase the risk of myopathy). Products include:
Levitra Tablets 2876

Verapamil Hydrochloride (Co-administration of niacin with vasoactive drugs, such as calcium channel blockers, may result in postural hypotension, particularly in patients with unstable angina or acute phase of myocardial infarction). Products include:
Tarka Tablets 511

Voriconazole (Co-administration results in serious skeletal muscle disorders, such as rhabdomyolysis and myopathy).
No products indexed under this heading.

Warfarin Sodium (Co-administration has resulted in increased bleeding and/or prothrombin time).
No products indexed under this heading.

Zafirlukast (The risk of myopathy appears to be increased by high levels of HMG-CoA reductase inhibitory activity in plasma. Lovastatin is metabolized by the cytochrome P450 isoform 3A4. Certain drugs which share this metabolic pathway can raise the plasma levels of lovastatin and may increase the risk of myopathy). Products include:
Accolate Tablets 669

Zileuton (The risk of myopathy appears to be increased by high levels of HMG-CoA reductase inhibitory activity in plasma. Lovastatin is metabolized by the cytochrome P450 isoform 3A4. Certain drugs which share this metabolic pathway can raise the plasma levels of lovastatin and may increase the risk of myopathy).
No products indexed under this heading.

Food Interactions

Alcohol (Concomitant alcohol may increase the flushing and its use should be avoided around the time of Advicor administration).

Drinks, hot, unspecified (Concomitant hot drinks may increase the flushing and its use should be avoided around the time of Advicor administration).

Grapefruit (The risk of myopathy appears to be increased by high levels of HMG-CoA reductase inhibitory activity in plasma. Lovastatin is metabolized by the cytochrome P450 isoform 3A4. Certain drugs which share this metabolic pathway can raise the plasma levels of lovastatin and may increase the risk of myopathy).

Grapefruit Juice (Inhibits CYP3A4 and can increase the plasma concentration of lovastatin; concurrent use should be avoided).

AEROBID INHALER SYSTEM

(Flunisolide) 1153
None cited in PDR database.

AEROBID-M INHALER SYSTEM

(Flunisolide) 1153
None cited in PDR database.

AEROCHAMBER PLUS AND AEROCHAMBER PLUS WITH MASK

(Spacer, Inhalation) 1154
None cited in PDR database.

AGGRENOX CAPSULES

(Aspirin, Dipyridamole) 819
May interact with ACE inhibitors, anticholinesterase drugs, beta blockers, anticoagulants, diuretics, oral hypoglycemic agents, non-steroidal anti-inflammatory agents, phenytoin, valproate, and certain other agents. Compounds in these categories include:

Acarbose (Moderate doses of aspirin may increase the effectiveness of renal hypoglycemic drugs, leading to hypoglycemia). Products include:
Precose Tablets 792

Acebutolol Hydrochloride (The hypertensive effects of beta-blockers may be diminished by the concomitant administration of aspirin due to inhibition of renal prostaglandins, leading to decreased renal blood flow and salt and fluid retention).
No products indexed under this heading.

Acetazolamide (Co-administration can lead to high serum concentrations of acetazolamide (and toxicity) due to competition at the renal tube for secretion).
No products indexed under this heading.

Acetazolamide Sodium (Co-administration can lead to high serum concentrations of acetazolamide (and toxicity) due to competition at the renal tube for secretion).
No products indexed under this heading.

Adenosine (Dipyridamole has been reported to increase the plasma levels and cardiovascular effects of adenosine). Products include:
Adenocard IV Injection 603
Adenoscan 605

Amiloride Hydrochloride (The effectiveness of diuretics in patients with underlying renal or cardiovascular disease may be diminished by co-administration of aspirin due to inhibition of renal prostaglandins, leading to decreased renal blood flow and salt and fluid retention).
No products indexed under this heading.

Anisindione (Patients on anticoagulation therapy are at risk for bleeding).
No products indexed under this heading.

Ardeparin Sodium (Patients on anticoagulation therapy are at risk for bleeding).
No products indexed under this heading.

Atenolol (The hypertensive effects of beta-blockers may be diminished by the concomitant administration of aspirin due to inhibition of renal prostaglandins, leading to decreased renal blood flow and salt and fluid retention).
No products indexed under this heading.

Benazepril Hydrochloride (Co-administration can result in diminished hypotensive and hyponatremic effects of ACE inhibitors due to the effect of aspirin on the renin-angiotensin conversion pathway).
No products indexed under this heading.

Bendroflumethiazide (The effectiveness of diuretics in patients with underlying renal or cardiovascular disease may be diminished by co-administration of aspirin due to inhibition of renal prostaglandins, leading to decreased renal blood flow and salt and fluid retention).
No products indexed under this heading.

Betaxolol Hydrochloride (The hypertensive effects of beta-blockers may be diminished by the concomitant administration of aspirin due to inhibition of renal prostaglandins, leading to decreased renal blood flow and salt and fluid retention).
No products indexed under this heading.

Bisoprolol Fumarate (The hypertensive effects of beta-blockers may be diminished by the concomitant administration of aspirin due to inhibition of renal prostaglandins, leading to decreased renal blood flow and salt and fluid retention).
No products indexed under this heading.

Bumetanide (The effectiveness of diuretics in patients with underlying renal or cardiovascular disease may be diminished by co-administration of aspirin due to inhibition of renal prostaglandins, leading to decreased renal blood flow and salt and fluid retention).
No products indexed under this heading.

Captopril (Co-administration can result in diminished hypotensive and hyponatremic effects of ACE inhibitors due to the effect of aspirin on the renin-angiotensin conversion pathway). Products include:
Captopril Tablets 2182

Carteolol Hydrochloride (The hypertensive effects of beta-blockers may be diminished by the concomitant administration of aspirin due to inhibition of renal prostaglandins, leading to decreased renal blood flow and salt and fluid retention).
No products indexed under this heading.

Celecoxib (Co-administration of non-steroidal anti-inflammatory drugs with aspirin may increase bleeding or lead to decreased renal function). Products include:
Celebrex Capsules 2979

Chlorothiazide (The effectiveness of diuretics in patients with underlying renal or cardiovascular disease may be diminished by co-administration of aspirin due to inhibition of renal prostaglandins, leading to decreased renal blood flow and salt and fluid retention).
No products indexed under this heading.

Chlorothiazide Sodium (The effectiveness of diuretics in patients with underlying renal or cardiovascular disease may be diminished by co-administration of aspirin due to inhibition of renal prostaglandins, leading to decreased renal blood flow and salt and fluid retention). Products include:
Intravenous Sodium Diuril 2490

Chlorpropamide (Moderate doses of aspirin may increase the effectiveness of renal hypoglycemic drugs, leading to hypoglycemia).
No products indexed under this heading.

Chlorthalidone (The effectiveness of diuretics in patients with underlying renal or cardiovascular disease may be diminished by co-administration of aspirin due to inhibition of renal prostaglandins, leading to decreased renal blood flow and salt and fluid retention). Products include:
Clorpres Tablets 2185

Dalteparin Sodium (Patients on anticoagulation therapy are at risk for bleeding). Products include:
Fragmin Injection 1070

Danaparoid Sodium (Patients on anticoagulation therapy are at risk for bleeding).
No products indexed under this heading.

Diclofenac Epolamine (Co-administration of non-steroidal anti-inflammatory drugs with aspirin may increase bleeding or lead to decreased renal function). Products include:
Flector Patch 561

Diclofenac Potassium (Co-administration of non-steroidal anti-inflammatory drugs with aspirin may increase bleeding or lead to decreased renal function).
No products indexed under this heading.

Diclofenac Sodium (Co-administration of non-steroidal anti-inflammatory drugs with aspirin may increase bleeding or lead to decreased renal function). Products include:
Diclofenac Sodium Ophthalmic Solution ⊙ 240
Voltaren Ophthalmic Solution 2336
Voltaren Tablets 2334
Voltaren-XR Tablets 2337

Dicumarol (Patients on anticoagulation therapy are at risk for bleeding).
No products indexed under this heading.

Divalproex Sodium (Salicylic acid can displace protein-bound valproic acid leading to an increase in serum valproic acid levels). Products include:
Depakote ER Tablets 423

Donepezil Hydrochloride (Dipyridamole may counteract the anticholinesterase effect of cholinesterase inhibitors, thereby potentially aggravating myasthenia gravis). Products include:
Aricept Tablets 1062
Aricept ODT Tablets 1062

Enalapril Maleate (Co-administration can result in diminished hypotensive and hyponatremic effects of ACE inhibitors due to the effect of aspirin on the renin-angiotensin conversion pathway).
No products indexed under this heading.

Enalaprilat (Co-administration can result in diminished hypotensive and hyponatremic effects of ACE inhibitors due to the effect of aspirin on the renin-angiotensin conversion pathway).
No products indexed under this heading.

Enoxaparin Sodium (Patients on anticoagulation therapy are at risk for bleeding). Products include:
Lovenox Injection 2756

Esmolol Hydrochloride (The hypertensive effects of beta-blockers may be diminished by the concomitant administration of aspirin due to inhibition of renal prostaglandins, leading to decreased renal blood flow and salt and fluid retention).
No products indexed under this heading.

Ethacrynic Acid (The effectiveness of diuretics in patients with underlying renal or cardiovascular disease may be diminished by co-administration of aspirin due to inhibition of renal prostaglandins, leading to decreased renal blood flow and salt and fluid retention). Products include:
Edecrin Tablets 698

Etodolac (Co-administration of non-steroidal anti-inflammatory drugs with aspirin may increase bleeding or lead to decreased renal function).
No products indexed under this heading.

Fenoprofen Calcium (Co-administration of non-steroidal anti-inflammatory drugs with aspirin may increase bleeding or lead to decreased renal function). Products include:
Nalfon Capsules 2508

Flurbiprofen (Co-administration of non-steroidal anti-inflammatory drugs with aspirin may increase bleeding or lead to decreased renal function).
No products indexed under this heading.

Fondaparinux Sodium (Patients on anticoagulation therapy are at risk for bleeding). Products include:
Arixtra Injection 1313

Fosinopril Sodium (Co-administration can result in diminished hypotensive and hyponatremic effects of ACE inhibitors due to the effect of aspirin on the renin-angiotensin conversion pathway).
No products indexed under this heading.

Fosphenytoin Sodium (Salicylic acid can displace protein-bound phenytoin leading to a decrease in the total concentration of phenytoin).
No products indexed under this heading.

Furosemide (The effectiveness of diuretics in patients with underlying renal or cardiovascular disease may be diminished by co-administration of aspirin due to inhibition of renal prostaglandins, leading to decreased renal blood flow and salt and fluid retention). Products include:
Furosemide Tablets 2186

Galantamine Hydrobromide (Dipyridamole may counteract the anticholinesterase effect of cholinesterase inhibitors, thereby potentially aggravating myasthenia gravis).
No products indexed under this heading.

Glimepiride (Moderate doses of aspirin may increase the effectiveness of renal hypoglycemic drugs, leading to hypoglycemia). Products include:
Avandaryl Tablets 1344
Duetact Tablets 3085

Glipizide (Moderate doses of aspirin may increase the effectiveness of renal hypoglycemic drugs, leading to hypoglycemia).
No products indexed under this heading.

Glyburide (Moderate doses of aspirin may increase the effectiveness of renal hypoglycemic drugs, leading to hypoglycemia).
No products indexed under this heading.

Heparin Calcium (Patients on anticoagulation therapy are at risk for bleeding).
No products indexed under this heading.

Heparin Sodium (Aspirin can increase the anticoagulant activity of heparin, increasing bleeding risk).
No products indexed under this heading.

Hydrochlorothiazide (The effectiveness of diuretics in patients with underlying renal or cardiovascular disease may be diminished by co-administration of aspirin due to inhibition of renal prostaglandins, leading to decreased renal blood flow and salt and fluid retention). Products include:
Atacand HCT 642
Avalide Tablets 892
Avalide Tablets 2713
Benicar HCT Tablets 1010
Diovan HCT Tablets 2216
Dyazide Capsules 1405
Micardis HCT Tablets 854
Prinzide Tablets 2092
Tekturna HCT Tablets 2324
Teveten HCT Tablets 517

Hydroflumethiazide (The effectiveness of diuretics in patients with underlying renal or cardiovascular disease may be diminished by co-administration of aspirin due to inhibition of renal prostaglandins, leading to decreased renal blood flow and salt and fluid retention).
No products indexed under this heading.

Ibuprofen (Co-administration of non-steroidal anti-inflammatory drugs with aspirin may increase bleeding or lead to decreased renal function). Products include:
Motrin IB Tablets and Caplets 1900
Children's Motrin Oral Suspension 1901
Children's Motrin Non-Staining Dye-Free Oral Suspension 1901
Children's Motrin Cold Oral Suspension 1899
Infants' Motrin Concentrated Drops 1901
Infants' Motrin Non-Staining Dye-Free Concentrated Drops 1901
Junior Strength Motrin Caplets and Chewable Tablets 1901
Vicoprofen Tablets 533

Indapamide (The effectiveness of diuretics in patients with underlying renal or cardiovascular disease may be diminished by co-administration of aspirin due to inhibition of renal prostaglandins, leading to decreased renal blood flow and salt and fluid retention). Products include:
Indapamide Tablets 2188

Indomethacin (Co-administration of non-steroidal anti-inflammatory drugs with aspirin may increase bleeding or lead to decreased renal function). Products include:
Indocin 2024

Indomethacin Sodium Trihydrate (Co-administration of non-steroidal anti-inflammatory drugs with aspirin may increase bleeding or lead to decreased renal function). Products include:
Indocin I.V. 2489

Ketoprofen (Co-administration of non-steroidal anti-inflammatory drugs with aspirin may increase bleeding or lead to decreased renal function).
No products indexed under this heading.

Ketorolac Tromethamine (Co-administration of non-steroidal anti-inflammatory drugs with aspirin may increase bleeding or lead to decreased renal function).
No products indexed under this heading.

Labetalol Hydrochloride (The hypertensive effects of beta-blockers may be diminished by the concomitant administration of aspirin due to inhibition of renal prostaglandins, leading to decreased renal blood flow and salt and fluid retention).
No products indexed under this heading.

Levobunolol Hydrochloride (The hypertensive effects of beta-blockers may be diminished by the concomitant administration of aspirin due to inhibition of renal prostaglandins, leading to decreased renal blood flow and salt and fluid retention).
No products indexed under this heading.

Lisinopril (Co-administration can result in diminished hypotensive and hyponatremic effects of ACE inhibitors due to the effect of aspirin on the renin-angiotensin conversion pathway). Products include:
Prinivil Tablets 2087
Prinzide Tablets 2092

Low Molecular Weight Heparins (Patients on anticoagulation therapy are at risk for bleeding).
No products indexed under this heading.

Meclofenamate Sodium (Co-administration of non-steroidal anti-inflammatory drugs with aspirin may increase bleeding or lead to decreased renal function).
No products indexed under this heading.

Mefenamic Acid (Co-administration of non-steroidal anti-inflammatory drugs with aspirin may increase bleeding or lead to decreased renal function).
No products indexed under this heading.

Meloxicam (Co-administration of non-steroidal anti-inflammatory drugs with aspirin may increase bleeding or lead to decreased renal function). Products include:
Mobic Oral Suspension 863
Mobic Tablets 863

Metformin Hydrochloride (Moderate doses of aspirin may increase the effectiveness of renal hypoglycemic drugs, leading to hypoglycemia). Products include:
ActoPlus Met Tablets 3071
Avandamet Tablets 1336
Janumet Tablets 2041
PrandiMet Tablets 2967

Methotrexate Sodium (Salicylic acid can inhibit renal clearance of methotrexate, leading to bone marrow toxicity, especially in the elderly or renal impaired).
No products indexed under this heading.

Methyclothiazide (The effectiveness of diuretics in patients with underlying renal or cardiovascular disease may be diminished by co-administration of aspirin due to inhibition of renal prostaglandins, leading to decreased renal blood flow and salt and fluid retention).
No products indexed under this heading.

Metipranolol Hydrochloride (The hypertensive effects of beta-blockers may be diminished by the concomitant administration of aspirin due to inhibition of renal prostaglandins, leading to decreased renal blood flow and salt and fluid retention).
No products indexed under this heading.

Metolazone (The effectiveness of diuretics in patients with underlying renal or cardiovascular disease may be diminished by co-administration of aspirin due to inhibition of renal prostaglandins, leading to decreased renal blood flow and salt and fluid retention).
No products indexed under this heading.

Metoprolol Succinate (The hypertensive effects of beta-blockers may be diminished by the concomitant administration of aspirin due to inhibition of renal prostaglandins, leading to decreased renal blood flow and salt and fluid retention). Products include:
Toprol-XL Tablets 666

Metoprolol Tartrate (The hypertensive effects of beta-blockers may be diminished by the concomitant administration of aspirin due to inhibition of renal prostaglandins, leading to decreased renal blood flow and salt and fluid retention).
No products indexed under this heading.

Miglitol (Moderate doses of aspirin may increase the effectiveness of renal hypoglycemic drugs, leading to hypoglycemia).
No products indexed under this heading.

Moexipril Hydrochloride (Co-administration can result in diminished hypotensive and hyponatremic effects of ACE inhibitors due to the effect of aspirin on the renin-angiotensin conversion pathway).
No products indexed under this heading.

Nabumetone (Co-administration of non-steroidal anti-inflammatory drugs with aspirin may increase bleeding or lead to decreased renal function).
No products indexed under this heading.

Nadolol (The hypertensive effects of beta-blockers may be diminished by the concomitant administration of aspirin due to inhibition of renal prostaglandins, leading to decreased renal blood flow and salt and fluid retention). Products include:
Nadolol Tablets 2191

Naproxen (Co-administration of non-steroidal anti-inflammatory drugs with aspirin may increase bleeding or lead to decreased renal function). Products include:
EC-Naprosyn Delayed-Release Tablets 2632
Naprosyn Suspension 2632
Naprosyn Tablets 2632

Naproxen Sodium (Co-administration of non-steroidal anti-inflammatory drugs with aspirin may increase bleeding or lead to decreased renal function). Products include:
Anaprox Tablets 2632
Anaprox DS Tablets 2632
Treximet Tablets 1616

Nateglinide (Moderate doses of aspirin may increase the effectiveness of renal hypoglycemic drugs, leading to hypoglycemia). Products include:
Starlix Tablets 2314

Nebivolol (The hypertensive effects of beta-blockers may be diminished by the concomitant administration of aspirin due to inhibition of renal prostaglandins, leading to decreased renal blood flow and salt and fluid retention). Products include:
Bystolic Tablets 1155

Neostigmine Bromide (Dipyridamole may counteract the anticholinesterase effect of cholinesterase inhibitors, thereby potentially aggravating myasthenia gravis).
No products indexed under this heading.

Neostigmine Methylsulfate (Dipyridamole may counteract the anticholinesterase effect of cholinesterase inhibitors, thereby potentially aggravating myasthenia gravis).
No products indexed under this heading.

Oxaprozin (Co-administration of non-steroidal anti-inflammatory drugs with aspirin may increase bleeding or lead to decreased renal function).
No products indexed under this heading.

Penbutolol Sulfate (The hypertensive effects of beta-blockers may be diminished by the concomitant administration of aspirin due to inhibition of renal prostaglandins, leading to decreased renal blood flow and salt and fluid retention).
No products indexed under this heading.

Perindopril Erbumine (Co-administration can result in diminished hypotensive and hyponatremic effects of ACE inhibitors due to the effect of aspirin on the renin-angiotensin conversion pathway). Products include:
Aceon Tablets (2 mg, 4 mg, 8 mg) 3038

Phenylbutazone (Co-administration of non-steroidal anti-inflammatory drugs with aspirin may increase bleeding or lead to decreased renal function).
No products indexed under this heading.

Phenytoin (Salicylic acid can displace protein-bound phenytoin leading to a decrease in the total concentration of phenytoin).
No products indexed under this heading.

Phenytoin Sodium (Salicylic acid can displace protein-bound phenytoin leading to a decrease in the total concentration of phenytoin). Products include:
Phenytek Capsules 2192

Pindolol (The hypertensive effects of beta-blockers may be diminished by the concomitant administration of aspirin due to inhibition of renal prostaglandins, leading to decreased renal blood flow and salt and fluid retention).
No products indexed under this heading.

Pioglitazone Hydrochloride (Moderate doses of aspirin may increase the effectiveness of renal hypoglycemic drugs, leading to hypoglycemia). Products include:
ActoPlus Met Tablets 3071
Actos Tablets 3077
Duetact Tablets 3085

Piroxicam (Co-administration of non-steroidal anti-inflammatory drugs with aspirin may increase bleeding or lead to decreased renal function).
No products indexed under this heading.

Polythiazide (The effectiveness of diuretics in patients with underlying renal or cardiovascular disease may be diminished by co-administration of aspirin due to inhibition of renal prostaglandins, leading to decreased renal blood flow and salt and fluid retention).
No products indexed under this heading.

Probenecid (Salicylates antagonize the uricosuric action of uricosuric agents, such as probenecid).
No products indexed under this heading.

Propranolol Hydrochloride (The hypertensive effects of beta-blockers may be diminished by the concomitant administration of aspirin due to inhibition of renal prostaglandins, leading to decreased renal blood flow and salt and fluid retention). Products include:
InnoPran XL Extended Release Capsules 1484

Pyridostigmine Bromide (Dipyridamole may counteract the anticholinesterase effect of cholinesterase inhibitors, thereby potentially aggravating myasthenia gravis).
No products indexed under this heading.

Quinapril Hydrochloride (Co-administration can result in diminished hypotensive and hyponatremic effects of ACE inhibitors due to the effect of aspirin on the renin-angiotensin conversion pathway).
No products indexed under this heading.

Ramipril (Co-administration can result in diminished hypotensive and hyponatremic effects of ACE inhibitors due to the effect of aspirin on the renin-angiotensin conversion pathway).
No products indexed under this heading.

Repaglinide (Moderate doses of aspirin may increase the effectiveness of renal hypoglycemic drugs, leading to hypoglycemia). Products include:
PrandiMet Tablets 2967
Prandin Tablets 2971

Rivastigmine Tartrate (Dipyridamole may counteract the anticholinesterase effect of cholinesterase inhibitors, thereby potentially aggravating myasthenia gravis). Products include:
Exelon Capsules 2229
Exelon Oral Solution 2229
Exelon Patch 2233

Rofecoxib (Co-administration of non-steroidal anti-inflammatory drugs with aspirin may increase bleeding or lead to decreased renal function).
No products indexed under this heading.

Rosiglitazone Maleate (Moderate doses of aspirin may increase the effectiveness of renal hypoglycemic drugs, leading to hypoglycemia). Products include:
Avandamet Tablets 1336
Avandaryl Tablets 1344
Avandia Tablets 1351

Sitagliptin Phosphate (Moderate doses of aspirin may increase the effectiveness of renal hypoglycemic drugs, leading to hypoglycemia). Products include:
Janumet Tablets 2041
Januvia Tablets 2048

Sotalol Hydrochloride (The hypertensive effects of beta-blockers may be diminished by the concomitant administration of aspirin due to inhibition of renal prostaglandins, leading to decreased renal blood flow and salt and fluid retention).
No products indexed under this heading.

Spirapril Hydrochloride (Co-administration can result in diminished hypotensive and hyponatremic effects of ACE inhibitors due to the effect of aspirin on the renin-angiotensin conversion pathway).
No products indexed under this heading.

Spironolactone (The effectiveness of diuretics in patients with underlying renal or cardiovascular disease may be diminished by co-administration of aspirin due to inhibition of renal prostaglandins, leading to decreased renal blood flow and salt and fluid retention).
No products indexed under this heading.

Sulfinpyrazone (Salicylates antagonize the uricosuric action of uricosuric agents, such as sulfinpyrazone).
No products indexed under this heading.

Sulindac (Co-administration of non-steroidal anti-inflammatory drugs with aspirin may increase bleeding or lead to decreased renal function). Products include:
Clinoril Tablets 1962

Tacrine Hydrochloride (Dipyridamole may counteract the anticholinesterase effect of cholinesterase inhibitors, thereby potentially aggravating myasthenia gravis).
No products indexed under this heading.

Timolol Hemihydrate (The hypertensive effects of beta-blockers may be diminished by the concomitant administration of aspirin due to inhibition of renal prostaglandins, leading to decreased renal blood flow and salt and fluid retention). Products include:
Betimol Ophthalmic Solution 3181

Timolol Maleate (The hypertensive effects of beta-blockers may be diminished by the concomitant administration of aspirin due to inhibition of renal prostaglandins, leading to decreased renal blood flow and salt and fluid retention). Products include:
Combigan Ophthalmic Solution 553
Cosopt Sterile Ophthalmic Solution 1969
Timoptic Sterile Ophthalmic Solution 2121
Timoptic in Ocudose 2124
Timoptic-XE Sterile Ophthalmic Gel Forming Solution 2125

Tinzaparin Sodium (Patients on anticoagulation therapy are at risk for bleeding).
No products indexed under this heading.

Tolazamide (Moderate doses of aspirin may increase the effectiveness of renal hypoglycemic drugs, leading to hypoglycemia).
No products indexed under this heading.

Tolbutamide (Moderate doses of aspirin may increase the effectiveness of renal hypoglycemic drugs, leading to hypoglycemia).
No products indexed under this heading.

Tolmetin Sodium (Co-administration of non-steroidal anti-inflammatory drugs with aspirin may increase bleeding or lead to decreased renal function).

No products indexed under this heading.

Torsemide (The effectiveness of diuretics in patients with underlying renal or cardiovascular disease may be diminished by co-administration of aspirin due to inhibition of renal prostaglandins, leading to decreased renal blood flow and salt and fluid retention). Products include:

Demadex Injection **2630**
Demadex Tablets **2630**

Trandolapril (Co-administration can result in diminished hypotensive and hyponatremic effects of ACE inhibitors due to the effect of aspirin on the renin-angiotensin conversion pathway). Products include:

Mavik Tablets **472**
Tarka Tablets **511**

Triamterene (The effectiveness of diuretics in patients with underlying renal or cardiovascular disease may be diminished by co-administration of aspirin due to inhibition of renal prostaglandins, leading to decreased renal blood flow and salt and fluid retention). Products include:

Dyazide Capsules **1405**
Dyrenium Capsules **3189**

Troglitazone (Moderate doses of aspirin may increase the effectiveness of renal hypoglycemic drugs, leading to hypoglycemia).

No products indexed under this heading.

Valdecoxib (Co-administration of non-steroidal anti-inflammatory drugs with aspirin may increase bleeding or lead to decreased renal function).

No products indexed under this heading.

Valproate Sodium (Salicylic acid can displace protein-bound valproic acid leading to an increase in serum valproic acid levels).

No products indexed under this heading.

Valproic Acid (Salicylic acid can displace protein-bound valproic acid leading to an increase in serum valproic acid levels).

No products indexed under this heading.

Warfarin Sodium (Aspirin can displace warfarin from protein binding sites, leading to a prolongation of both the prothrombin time and the bleeding time).

No products indexed under this heading.

Food Interactions

Alcohol (Patients who consume three or more alcoholic drinks every day should be counseled about the bleeding risks involved with chronic, heavy alcohol use while taking aspirin).

AGRYLIN CAPSULES

(Anagrelide Hydrochloride) **3017**

May interact with aspirin-acetylsalicylic acid, cytochrome p450 1a2 inhibitors (selected), cytochrome p450 1a2 substrates (selected), and certain other agents. Compounds in these categories include:

Acetaminophen (Anagrelide demonstrates some limited inhibitory activity towards CYP1A2 which may present a theoretical potential for interaction with other co-administered medicinal products sharing that clearance mechanism). Products include:

Benadryl Allergy & Cold Kapgels **1895**
Benadryl Allergy & Sinus Headache Kapgels **1895**
Benadryl Severe Allergy & Sinus Headache Caplets **1897**
Lortab 5/500 Tablets **3143**
Lortab 7.5/500 Tablets **3144**
Lortab 10/500 Tablets **3144**
Percocet Tablets **1127**
Sinutab Sinus Caplets **1905**
Sudafed PE Cold & Cough Caplets **1907**
Sudafed PE Nighttime Cold Caplets **1907**
Sudafed PE Severe Cold Caplets **1908**
Sudafed PE Sinus Headache Caplets **1908**
Regular Strength Tylenol Tablets **1915**
Tylenol 8 Hour Extended Release Caplets **1915**
Extra Strength Tylenol Caplets, Cool Caplets, and EZ Tabs **1915**
Extra Strength Tylenol Adult Rapid Blast Liquid **1915**
Extra Strength Tylenol PM Caplets, Geltabs, Liquid, and Rapid Release Gels **1915**
Extra Strength Tylenol Rapid Release Gels **1915**
Tylenol with Codeine Tablets **2427**
Tylenol Allergy Multi-Symptom Caplets with Cool Burst and Rapid Release Gelcaps **1916**
Tylenol Allergy Multi-Symptom Nighttime Caplets with Cool Burst **1916**
Tylenol Severe Allergy Caplets **1916**
Tylenol Arthritis Pain Extended Release Geltabs/Caplets **1915**
Tylenol Chest Congestion Caplets with Cool Burst **1910**
Tylenol Chest Congestion Liquid with Cool Burst **1910**
Children's Tylenol Plus Cold Suspension Liquid **1912**
Children's Tylenol Plus Cold & Allergy Suspension Liquid **1914**
Children's Tylenol Plus Cough & Runny Nose Suspension Liquid **1912**
Children's Tylenol Plus Cough & Sore Throat Suspension Liquid **1912**
Children's Tylenol Plus Flu Suspension Liquid **1914**
Children's Tylenol Suspension Liquid **1909**
Children's Tylenol Meltaways **1909**
Children's Tylenol Plus Multi-Symptom Cold Suspension Liquid **1912**
Tylenol Cold Severe Congestion Daytime Caplets with Cool Burst **1912**
Tylenol Cold Head Congestion Daytime Caplets with Cool Burst **1910**
Tylenol Cold Head Congestion Nighttime Caplets with Cool Burst **1910**
Tylenol Cold Head Congestion Severe Daytime Caplets with Cool Burst **1910**
Tylenol Cold Multi-Symptom Daytime Caplets with Cool Burst and Rapid Release Gels **1913**
Tylenol Cold Multi-Symptom Daytime Liquid with Citrus Burst **1913**
Tylenol Cold Multi-Symptom Nighttime Caplets with Cool Burst **1913**
Tylenol Cold Multi-Symptom Nighttime Liquid with Cool Burst **1913**
Tylenol Cold Multi-Symptom Severe Caplets with Cool Burst **1913**
Tylenol Cold Multi-Symptom Severe Daytime Liquid with Citrus Burst **1913**
Tylenol Cough & Sore Throat Daytime Liquid with Cool Burst **1918**
Tylenol Cough & Sore Throat Nighttime Liquid with Cool Burst **1918**
Concentrated Tylenol Infants' Drops **1909**
Jr. Tylenol Meltaways **1909**
Tylenol Sinus Congestion & Pain Daytime Caplets with Cool Burst and Gelcaps **1917**
Tylenol Sinus Congestion & Pain Nighttime Caplets with Cool Burst **1917**
Tylenol Sinus Congestion & Pain Severe Caplets with Cool Burst **1917**
Tylenol Sinus Severe Congestion Caplets with Cool Burst **1917**
Tylenol Sore Throat Daytime Liquid with Cool Burst **1918**
Tylenol Sore Throat Nighttime Liquid with Cool Burst **1918**
Women's Tylenol Menstrual Relief Caplets **1919**
Vicks DayQuil Cold & Flu Multi-Symptom Relief **616**
Vicks DayQuil LiquiCaps **2567**
Vicks DayQuil Liquid **2567**
Vicks DayQuil Multi-Symptom Cold/Flu Relief **2567**
Vicks NyQuil Cold & Flu Multi-Symptom Relief **617**
Vicks NyQuil LiquiCaps **2567**
Vicks NyQuil Liquid **2567**
Vicks NyQuil Multi-Symptom Cold/Flu Relief **2567**
Vicodin Tablets **529**
Vicodin ES Tablets **530**
Vicodin HP Tablets **531**
Zydone Tablets **1132**

Alatrofloxacin Mesylate (Anagrelide is metabolized at least in part by CYP1A2. Therefore, CYP1A2 inhibitors could theoretically adversely influence the clearance of anagrelide).

No products indexed under this heading.

Amiodarone Hydrochloride (Anagrelide is metabolized at least in part by CYP1A2. Therefore, CYP1A2 inhibitors could theoretically adversely influence the clearance of anagrelide).

No products indexed under this heading.

Amitriptyline Hydrochloride (Anagrelide demonstrates some limited inhibitory activity towards CYP1A2 which may present a theoretical potential for interaction with other co-administered medicinal products sharing that clearance mechanism).

No products indexed under this heading.

Amoxapine (Anagrelide demonstrates some limited inhibitory activity towards CYP1A2 which may present a theoretical potential for interaction with other co-administered medicinal products sharing that clearance mechanism).

No products indexed under this heading.

Amrinone Lactate (Anagrelide is an inhibitor of AMP PDE III. The effects of medicinal products with similar properties, such as amrinone, may be exacerbated by anagrelide).

No products indexed under this heading.

Anastrozole (Anagrelide is metabolized at least in part by CYP1A2. Therefore, CYP1A2 inhibitors could theoretically adversely influence the clearance of anagrelide). Products include:

Arimidex Tablets **672**

Aspirin (Anagrelide may slightly enhance the inhibition of platelet aggregation by aspirin). Products include:

Aggrenox Capsules **819**
Bayer Aspirin **750**
Percodan Tablets **1130**
St. Joseph 81 mg Aspirin Chewable and Enteric Coated Tablets **1903**

Aspirin, Enteric Coated (Anagrelide may slightly enhance the inhibition of platelet aggregation by aspirin).

No products indexed under this heading.

Aspirin Buffered (Anagrelide may slightly enhance the inhibition of platelet aggregation by aspirin).

No products indexed under this heading.

Caffeine (Anagrelide demonstrates some limited inhibitory activity towards CYP1A2 which may present a theoretical potential for interaction with other co-administered medicinal products sharing that clearance mechanism). Products include:

BioLean Free Tablets **635**
BioLean II Tablets **635**
Winrgy Dietary Supplement **642**

Caffeine Anhydrous (Anagrelide demonstrates some limited inhibitory activity towards CYP1A2 which may present a theoretical potential for interaction with other co-administered medicinal products sharing that clearance mechanism).

No products indexed under this heading.

Chlordiazepoxide (Anagrelide demonstrates some limited inhibitory activity towards CYP1A2 which may present a theoretical potential for interaction with other co-administered medicinal products sharing that clearance mechanism).

No products indexed under this heading.

Chlordiazepoxide Hydrochloride (Anagrelide demonstrates some limited inhibitory activity towards CYP1A2 which may present a theoretical potential for interaction with other co-administered medicinal products sharing that clearance mechanism).

No products indexed under this heading.

Cilostazol (Anagrelide is an inhibitor of AMP PDE III. The effects of medicinal products with similar properties, such as cilostazol, may be exacerbated by anagrelide). Products include:

Pletal Tablets **2481**

Cimetidine (Anagrelide is metabolized at least in part by CYP1A2. Therefore, CYP1A2 inhibitors could theoretically adversely influence the clearance of anagrelide).

No products indexed under this heading.

Cimetidine Hydrochloride (Anagrelide is metabolized at least in part by CYP1A2. Therefore, CYP1A2 inhibitors could theoretically adversely influence the clearance of anagrelide).

No products indexed under this heading.

Ciprofloxacin (Anagrelide is metabolized at least in part by CYP1A2. Therefore, CYP1A2 inhibitors could theoretically adversely influence the clearance of anagrelide). Products include:

Cipro I.V. **2817**
Cipro Oral Suspension **2810**
Cipro XR Tablets **2823**
Ciprodex Otic Suspension **541**

Ciprofloxacin Hydrochloride (Anagrelide is metabolized at least in part by CYP1A2. Therefore, CYP1A2

inhibitors could theoretically adversely influence the clearance of anagrelide). Products include:
Cipro Tablets 2810

Clarithromycin (Anagrelide is metabolized at least in part by CYP1A2. Therefore, CYP1A2 inhibitors could theoretically adversely influence the clearance of anagrelide). Products include:
Biaxin/Biaxin XL 411

Clomipramine Hydrochloride (Anagrelide demonstrates some limited inhibitory activity towards CYP1A2 which may present a theoretical potential for interaction with other co-administered medicinal products sharing that clearance mechanism).
No products indexed under this heading.

Clopidogrel Bisulfate (Anagrelide demonstrates some limited inhibitory activity towards CYP1A2 which may present a theoretical potential for interaction with other co-administered medicinal products sharing that clearance mechanism). Products include:
Plavix Tablets 926
Plavix Tablets 2767

Clozapine (Anagrelide demonstrates some limited inhibitory activity towards CYP1A2 which may present a theoretical potential for interaction with other co-administered medicinal products sharing that clearance mechanism).
No products indexed under this heading.

Cyclobenzaprine (Anagrelide demonstrates some limited inhibitory activity towards CYP1A2 which may present a theoretical potential for interaction with other co-administered medicinal products sharing that clearance mechanism).
No products indexed under this heading.

Cyclobenzaprine Hydrochloride (Anagrelide demonstrates some limited inhibitory activity towards CYP1A2 which may present a theoretical potential for interaction with other co-administered medicinal products sharing that clearance mechanism). Products include:
Amrix Capsules 966

Desipramine Hydrochloride (Anagrelide demonstrates some limited inhibitory activity towards CYP1A2 which may present a theoretical potential for interaction with other co-administered medicinal products sharing that clearance mechanism).
No products indexed under this heading.

Desogestrel (Anagrelide is metabolized at least in part by CYP1A2. Therefore, CYP1A2 inhibitors could theoretically adversely influence the clearance of anagrelide). Products include:
Mircette Tablets 1034

Diazepam (Anagrelide demonstrates some limited inhibitory activity towards CYP1A2 which may present a theoretical potential for interaction with other co-administered medicinal products sharing that clearance mechanism). Products include:
Valium Tablets 2658

Diltiazem Hydrochloride (Anagrelide demonstrates some limited inhibitory activity towards CYP1A2 which may present a theoretical potential for interaction with other co-administered medicinal products sharing that clearance mechanism). Products include:
Cardizem LA Extended Release Tablets 421

Diltiazem Maleate (Anagrelide demonstrates some limited inhibitory activity towards CYP1A2 which may present a theoretical potential for interaction with other co-administered medicinal products sharing that clearance mechanism).
No products indexed under this heading.

Doxepin Hydrochloride (Anagrelide demonstrates some limited inhibitory activity towards CYP1A2 which may present a theoretical potential for interaction with other co-administered medicinal products sharing that clearance mechanism).
No products indexed under this heading.

Enoxacin (Anagrelide is metabolized at least in part by CYP1A2. Therefore, CYP1A2 inhibitors could theoretically adversely influence the clearance of anagrelide).
No products indexed under this heading.

Enoximone (Anagrelide is an inhibitor of AMP PDE III. The effects of medicinal products with similar properties, such as enoximone, may be exacerbated by anagrelide).
No products indexed under this heading.

Erythromycin (Anagrelide demonstrates some limited inhibitory activity towards CYP1A2 which may present a theoretical potential for interaction with other co-administered medicinal products sharing that clearance mechanism).
No products indexed under this heading.

Erythromycin Estolate (Anagrelide demonstrates some limited inhibitory activity towards CYP1A2 which may present a theoretical potential for interaction with other co-administered medicinal products sharing that clearance mechanism).
No products indexed under this heading.

Erythromycin Ethylsuccinate (Anagrelide demonstrates some limited inhibitory activity towards CYP1A2 which may present a theoretical potential for interaction with other co-administered medicinal products sharing that clearance mechanism). Products include:
E.E.S. 433
EryPed 431

Erythromycin Gluceptate (Anagrelide demonstrates some limited inhibitory activity towards CYP1A2 which may present a theoretical potential for interaction with other co-administered medicinal products sharing that clearance mechanism).
No products indexed under this heading.

Erythromycin Lactobionate (Anagrelide demonstrates some limited inhibitory activity towards CYP1A2 which may present a theoretical potential for interaction with other co-administered medicinal products sharing that clearance mechanism).
No products indexed under this heading.

Erythromycin Stearate (Anagrelide demonstrates some limited inhibitory activity towards CYP1A2 which may present a theoretical potential for interaction with other co-administered medicinal products sharing that clearance mechanism).
No products indexed under this heading.

Estradiol (Anagrelide demonstrates some limited inhibitory activity towards CYP1A2 which may present a theoretical potential for interaction with other co-administered medicinal products sharing that clearance mechanism). Products include:
Activella Tablets 2347
Angeliq Tablets 751
Climara Transdermal System 763
Climara Pro Transdermal System 768
Divigel 3167
Vagifem Tablets 2375

Estradiol Benzoate (Anagrelide demonstrates some limited inhibitory activity towards CYP1A2 which may present a theoretical potential for interaction with other co-administered medicinal products sharing that clearance mechanism).
No products indexed under this heading.

Estradiol Cypionate (Anagrelide demonstrates some limited inhibitory activity towards CYP1A2 which may present a theoretical potential for interaction with other co-administered medicinal products sharing that clearance mechanism).
No products indexed under this heading.

Ethinyl Estradiol (Anagrelide is metabolized at least in part by CYP1A2. Therefore, CYP1A2 inhibitors could theoretically adversely influence the clearance of anagrelide). Products include:
Lybrel Tablets 3204
Mircette Tablets 1034
NuvaRing 2897
Ortho-Cyclen/Ortho Tri-Cyclen 2449
Ortho Evra Transdermal System 2437
Ortho Tri-Cyclen Lo Tablets 2458
Seasonique Tablets 1046
Yaz Tablets 805

Flutamide (Anagrelide demonstrates some limited inhibitory activity towards CYP1A2 which may present a theoretical potential for interaction with other co-administered medicinal products sharing that clearance mechanism).
No products indexed under this heading.

Fluticasone Propionate (Anagrelide demonstrates some limited inhibitory activity towards CYP1A2 which may present a theoretical potential for interaction with other co-administered medicinal products sharing that clearance mechanism). Products include:
Advair Diskus 100/50 1276
Advair Diskus 250/50 1276
Advair Diskus 500/50 1276
Advair HFA 45/21 Inhalation Aerosol 1288
Advair HFA 115/21 Inhalation Aerosol 1288
Advair HFA 230/21 Inhalation Aerosol 1288
Flonase Nasal Spray 1431
Flovent Diskus 50 mcg 1435

Fluvoxamine (Anagrelide is metabolized at least in part by CYP1A2. Therefore, CYP1A2 inhibitors could theoretically adversely influence the clearance of anagrelide).
No products indexed under this heading.

Fluvoxamine Maleate (Anagrelide is metabolized at least in part by CYP1A2. Therefore, CYP1A2 inhibitors could theoretically adversely influence the clearance of anagrelide). Products include:
Luvox CR Extended-Release Capsules 1759

Gatifloxacin (Anagrelide is metabolized at least in part by CYP1A2. Therefore, CYP1A2 inhibitors could theoretically adversely influence the clearance of anagrelide).
No products indexed under this heading.

Gemifloxacin Mesylate (Anagrelide is metabolized at least in part by CYP1A2. Therefore, CYP1A2 inhibitors could theoretically adversely influence the clearance of anagrelide).
No products indexed under this heading.

Grepafloxacin Hydrochloride (Anagrelide is metabolized at least in part by CYP1A2. Therefore, CYP1A2 inhibitors could theoretically adversely influence the clearance of anagrelide).
No products indexed under this heading.

Haloperidol (Anagrelide demonstrates some limited inhibitory activity towards CYP1A2 which may present a theoretical potential for interaction with other co-administered medicinal products sharing that clearance mechanism).
No products indexed under this heading.

Haloperidol Decanoate (Anagrelide demonstrates some limited inhibitory activity towards CYP1A2 which may present a theoretical potential for interaction with other co-administered medicinal products sharing that clearance mechanism).
No products indexed under this heading.

Haloperidol Lactate (Anagrelide demonstrates some limited inhibitory activity towards CYP1A2 which may present a theoretical potential for interaction with other co-administered medicinal products sharing that clearance mechanism).
No products indexed under this heading.

Imipramine Hydrochloride (Anagrelide demonstrates some limited inhibitory activity towards CYP1A2 which may present a theoretical potential for interaction with other co-administered medicinal products sharing that clearance mechanism).
No products indexed under this heading.

Imipramine Pamoate (Anagrelide demonstrates some limited inhibitory activity towards CYP1A2 which may present a theoretical potential for interaction with other co-administered medicinal products sharing that clearance mechanism).
No products indexed under this heading.

Isoniazid (Anagrelide is metabolized at least in part by CYP1A2. Therefore, CYP1A2 inhibitors could theoretically adversely influence the clearance of anagrelide).
No products indexed under this heading.

Ketoconazole (Anagrelide is metabolized at least in part by CYP1A2. Therefore, CYP1A2 inhibitors could theoretically adversely influence the clearance of anagrelide). Products include:
Extina Foam, 2% 3057
Nizoral A-D Shampoo 1901

Levobupivacaine Hydrochloride (Anagrelide demonstrates some limited inhibitory activity towards CYP1A2 which may present a theoretical potential for interaction with other co-administered medicinal products sharing that clearance mechanism).
No products indexed under this heading.

Levofloxacin (Anagrelide is metabolized at least in part by CYP1A2. Therefore, CYP1A2 inhibitors could theoretically adversely influence the clearance of anagrelide). Products include:
Iquix Ophthalmic Solution 3183
Levaquin 2416
Levaquin in 5% Dextrose Injection 2416
Quixin Ophthalmic Solution 3184

Levonorgestrel (Anagrelide is metabolized at least in part by CYP1A2. Therefore, CYP1A2 inhibitors could theoretically adversely influence the clearance of anagrelide). Products include:
Climara Pro Transdermal System 768
Lybrel Tablets 3204
Mirena Intrauterine System 779
Plan B Tablets 1044
Seasonique Tablets 1046

Lomefloxacin Hydrochloride (Anagrelide is metabolized at least in part by CYP1A2. Therefore, CYP1A2 inhibitors could theoretically adversely influence the clearance of anagrelide).
No products indexed under this heading.

Maprotiline Hydrochloride (Anagrelide demonstrates some limited inhibitory activity towards CYP1A2 which may present a theoretical potential for interaction with other co-administered medicinal products sharing that clearance mechanism).
No products indexed under this heading.

Mestranol (Anagrelide is metabolized at least in part by CYP1A2. Therefore, CYP1A2 inhibitors could theoretically adversely influence the clearance of anagrelide).
No products indexed under this heading.

Methadone Hydrochloride (Anagrelide demonstrates some limited inhibitory activity towards CYP1A2 which may present a theoretical potential for interaction with other co-administered medicinal products sharing that clearance mechanism).
No products indexed under this heading.

Methoxsalen (Anagrelide is metabolized at least in part by CYP1A2. Therefore, CYP1A2 inhibitors could theoretically adversely influence the clearance of anagrelide).
No products indexed under this heading.

Mexiletine Hydrochloride (Anagrelide is metabolized at least in part by CYP1A2. Therefore, CYP1A2 inhibitors could theoretically adversely influence the clearance of anagrelide).
No products indexed under this heading.

Mibefradil Dihydrochloride (Anagrelide is metabolized at least in part by CYP1A2. Therefore, CYP1A2 inhibitors could theoretically adversely influence the clearance of anagrelide).
No products indexed under this heading.

Milrinone Lactate (Anagrelide is an inhibitor of cyclic AMP PDE III. The effects of medicinal products with similar properties, such as milrinone, may be exacerbated by anagrelide).
No products indexed under this heading.

Mirtazapine (Anagrelide demonstrates some limited inhibitory activity towards CYP1A2 which may present a theoretical potential for interaction with other co-administered medicinal products sharing that clearance mechanism). Products include:
Remeron Tablets 2924
RemeronSolTab Tablets 2927

Moxifloxacin Hydrochloride (Anagrelide is metabolized at least in part by CYP1A2. Therefore, CYP1A2 inhibitors could theoretically adversely influence the clearance of anagrelide). Products include:
Avelox 2803
Vigamox Ophthalmic Solution 548

Nafcillin Sodium (Anagrelide demonstrates some limited inhibitory activity towards CYP1A2 which may present a theoretical potential for interaction with other co-administered medicinal products sharing that clearance mechanism).
No products indexed under this heading.

Nalidixic Acid (Anagrelide is metabolized at least in part by CYP1A2. Therefore, CYP1A2 inhibitors could theoretically adversely influence the clearance of anagrelide).
No products indexed under this heading.

Naproxen (Anagrelide demonstrates some limited inhibitory activity towards CYP1A2 which may present a theoretical potential for interaction with other co-administered medicinal products sharing that clearance mechanism). Products include:
EC-Naprosyn Delayed-Release Tablets 2632
Naprosyn Suspension 2632
Naprosyn Tablets 2632

Naproxen Sodium (Anagrelide demonstrates some limited inhibitory activity towards CYP1A2 which may present a theoretical potential for interaction with other co-administered medicinal products sharing that clearance mechanism). Products include:
Anaprox Tablets 2632
Anaprox DS Tablets 2632
Treximet Tablets 1616

Nicotine Polacrilex (Anagrelide demonstrates some limited inhibitory activity towards CYP1A2 which may present a theoretical potential for interaction with other co-administered medicinal products sharing that clearance mechanism).
No products indexed under this heading.

Nicotine Salicylate (Anagrelide demonstrates some limited inhibitory activity towards CYP1A2 which may present a theoretical potential for interaction with other co-administered medicinal products sharing that clearance mechanism).
No products indexed under this heading.

Nicotine Sulfate (Anagrelide demonstrates some limited inhibitory activity towards CYP1A2 which may present a theoretical potential for interaction with other co-administered medicinal products sharing that clearance mechanism).
No products indexed under this heading.

Norethindrone (Anagrelide is metabolized at least in part by CYP1A2. Therefore, CYP1A2 inhibitors could theoretically adversely influence the clearance of anagrelide). Products include:
Ortho Micronor Tablets 2446

Norethindrone Acetate (Anagrelide demonstrates some limited inhibitory activity towards CYP1A2 which may present a theoretical potential for interaction with other co-administered medicinal products sharing that clearance mechanism). Products include:
Activella Tablets 2347

Norfloxacin (Anagrelide is metabolized at least in part by CYP1A2. Therefore, CYP1A2 inhibitors could theoretically adversely influence the clearance of anagrelide). Products include:
Noroxin Tablets 2069

Norgestrel (Anagrelide is metabolized at least in part by CYP1A2. Therefore, CYP1A2 inhibitors could theoretically adversely influence the clearance of anagrelide).
No products indexed under this heading.

Nortriptyline Hydrochloride (Anagrelide demonstrates some limited inhibitory activity towards CYP1A2 which may present a theoretical potential for interaction with other co-administered medicinal products sharing that clearance mechanism).
No products indexed under this heading.

Ofloxacin (Anagrelide is metabolized at least in part by CYP1A2. Therefore, CYP1A2 inhibitors could theoretically adversely influence the clearance of anagrelide). Products include:
Ofloxacin Ophthalmic Solution 0.3% .... ⊙243

Olanzapine (Anagrelide demonstrates some limited inhibitory activity towards CYP1A2 which may present a theoretical potential for interaction with other co-administered medicinal products sharing that clearance mechanism). Products include:
Symbyax Capsules 1871
Zyprexa Tablets 1883
Zyprexa IntraMuscular 1883
Zyprexa ZYDIS Orally Disintegrating Tablets 1883

Olprinone (Anagrelide is an inhibitor of AMP PDE III. The effects of medicinal products with similar properties, such as olprinone, may be exacerbated by anagrelide).
No products indexed under this heading.

Omeprazole (Anagrelide is metabolized at least in part by CYP1A2. Therefore, CYP1A2 inhibitors could theoretically adversely influence the clearance of anagrelide).
No products indexed under this heading.

Ondansetron (Anagrelide demonstrates some limited inhibitory activity towards CYP1A2 which may present a theoretical potential for interaction with other co-administered medicinal products sharing that clearance mechanism). Products include:
Zofran ODT Orally Disintegrating Tablets 1687

Ondansetron Hydrochloride (Anagrelide demonstrates some limited inhibitory activity towards CYP1A2 which may present a theoretical potential for interaction with other co-administered medicinal products sharing that clearance mechanism). Products include:
Zofran Injection 1682
Zofran 1687

Paroxetine Hydrochloride (Anagrelide is metabolized at least in part by CYP1A2. Therefore, CYP1A2 inhibitors could theoretically adversely influence the clearance of anagrelide). Products include:
Paxil 1535
Paxil CR Controlled-Release Tablets 1544

Phenobarbital Sodium (Anagrelide demonstrates some limited inhibitory activity towards CYP1A2 which may present a theoretical potential for interaction with other co-administered medicinal products sharing that clearance mechanism).
No products indexed under this heading.

Phenytoin Sodium (Anagrelide demonstrates some limited inhibitory activity towards CYP1A2 which may present a theoretical potential for interaction with other co-administered medicinal products sharing that clearance mechanism). Products include:
Phenytek Capsules 2192

Propafenone Hydrochloride (Anagrelide demonstrates some limited inhibitory activity towards CYP1A2 which may present a theoretical potential for interaction with other co-administered medicinal products sharing that clearance mechanism). Products include:
Rythmol Tablets 1586
Rythmol SR Capsules 1590

Propranolol Hydrochloride (Anagrelide demonstrates some limited inhibitory activity towards CYP1A2 which may present a theoretical potential for interaction with other co-administered medicinal products sharing that clearance mechanism). Products include:
InnoPran XL Extended Release Capsules 1484

Protriptyline Hydrochloride (Anagrelide demonstrates some limited inhibitory activity towards CYP1A2 which may present a theoretical potential for interaction with other co-administered medicinal products sharing that clearance mechanism).
No products indexed under this heading.

Ranitidine Hydrochloride (Anagrelide is metabolized at least in part by CYP1A2. Therefore, CYP1A2 inhibitors could theoretically adversely influence the clearance of anagrelide). Products include:
Zantac 75 Tablets .... ▣ 603
Zantac 1670
Zantac Injection 1666
Zantac Injection Pharmacy Bulk Package 1668
Maximum Strength Zantac 150 Tablets .... ▣ 603
Maximum Strength Zantac 150 Cool Mint Tablets .... ▣ 603

Riluzole (Anagrelide demonstrates some limited inhibitory activity towards CYP1A2 which may present a theoretical potential for interaction with other co-administered medicinal products sharing that clearance mechanism). Products include:
Rilutek Tablets 2771

Ritonavir (Anagrelide is metabolized at least in part by CYP1A2. Therefore, CYP1A2 inhibitors could theoretically adversely influence the clearance of anagrelide). Products include:
Kaletra 452
Norvir 489

Ropinirole Hydrochloride (Anagrelide demonstrates some limited inhibitory activity towards CYP1A2 which may present a theoretical potential for interaction with other co-administered medicinal products sharing that clearance mechanism). Products include:
Requip Tablets 1561
Requip XL Tablets 1568

Ropivacaine Hydrochloride (Anagrelide demonstrates some limited inhibitory activity towards CYP1A2 which may present a theoretical potential for interaction with other co-administered medicinal products sharing that clearance mechanism).
No products indexed under this heading.

Sildenafil Citrate (Anagrelide is metabolized at least in part by CYP1A2. Therefore, CYP1A2 inhibitors could theoretically adversely influence the clearance of anagrelide).
No products indexed under this heading.

Sparfloxacin (Anagrelide is metabolized at least in part by CYP1A2. Therefore, CYP1A2 inhibitors could theoretically adversely influence the clearance of anagrelide).
No products indexed under this heading.

Sucralfate (There is a single case report which suggests that sucralfate may interfere with anagrelide absorption). Products include:
Carafate Suspension 706
Carafate Tablets 707

Tacrine Hydrochloride (Anagrelide is metabolized at least in part by CYP1A2. Therefore, CYP1A2 inhibitors could theoretically adversely influence the clearance of anagrelide).
No products indexed under this heading.

Tamoxifen Citrate (Anagrelide demonstrates some limited inhibitory activity towards CYP1A2 which may present a theoretical potential for interaction with other co-administered medicinal products sharing that clearance mechanism).
No products indexed under this heading.

Theophylline (Anagrelide demonstrates some limited inhibitory activity towards CYP1A2 which may present a theoretical potential for interaction with other co-administered medicinal products sharing that clearance mechanism).
No products indexed under this heading.

Theophylline Anhydrous (Anagrelide demonstrates some limited inhibitory activity towards CYP1A2 which may present a theoretical potential for interaction with other co-administered medicinal products sharing that clearance mechanism). Products include:
Uniphyl Tablets 2595

Theophylline Calcium Salicylate (Anagrelide demonstrates some limited inhibitory activity towards CYP1A2 which may present a theoretical potential for interaction with other co-administered medicinal products sharing that clearance mechanism).
No products indexed under this heading.

Theophylline Dihydroxypropyl (Glyceryl) (Anagrelide demonstrates some limited inhibitory activity towards CYP1A2 which may present a theoretical potential for interaction with other co-administered medicinal products sharing that clearance mechanism).
No products indexed under this heading.

Theophylline Ethylenediamine (Anagrelide demonstrates some limited inhibitory activity towards CYP1A2 which may present a theoretical potential for interaction with other co-administered medicinal products sharing that clearance mechanism).
No products indexed under this heading.

Ticlopidine Hydrochloride (Anagrelide is metabolized at least in part by CYP1A2. Therefore, CYP1A2 inhibitors could theoretically adversely influence the clearance of anagrelide).
No products indexed under this heading.

Trimethaphan Camsylate (Anagrelide demonstrates some limited inhibitory activity towards CYP1A2 which may present a theoretical potential for interaction with other co-administered medicinal products sharing that clearance mechanism).
No products indexed under this heading.

Trimipramine Maleate (Anagrelide demonstrates some limited inhibitory activity towards CYP1A2 which may present a theoretical potential for interaction with other co-administered medicinal products sharing that clearance mechanism).
No products indexed under this heading.

Troleandomycin (Anagrelide is metabolized at least in part by CYP1A2. Therefore, CYP1A2 inhibitors could theoretically adversely influence the clearance of anagrelide).
No products indexed under this heading.

Trovafloxacin Mesylate (Anagrelide is metabolized at least in part by CYP1A2. Therefore, CYP1A2 inhibitors could theoretically adversely influence the clearance of anagrelide).
No products indexed under this heading.

Vardenafil Hydrochloride (Anagrelide is metabolized at least in part by CYP1A2. Therefore, CYP1A2 inhibitors could theoretically adversely influence the clearance of anagrelide). Products include:
Levitra Tablets 2876

Verapamil Hydrochloride (Anagrelide demonstrates some limited inhibitory activity towards CYP1A2 which may present a theoretical potential for interaction with other co-administered medicinal products sharing that clearance mechanism). Products include:
Tarka Tablets 511

Warfarin Sodium (Anagrelide demonstrates some limited inhibitory activity towards CYP1A2 which may present a theoretical potential for interaction with other co-administered medicinal products sharing that clearance mechanism).
No products indexed under this heading.

Zileuton (Anagrelide is metabolized at least in part by CYP1A2. Therefore, CYP1A2 inhibitors could theoretically adversely influence the clearance of anagrelide).
No products indexed under this heading.

Zolmitriptan (Anagrelide demonstrates some limited inhibitory activity towards CYP1A2 which may present a theoretical potential for interaction with other co-administered medicinal products sharing that clearance mechanism). Products include:
Zomig Tablets 694
Zomig Nasal Spray 689
Zomig-ZMT Tablets 694

Food Interactions

Grapefruit Juice (Anagrelide is metabolized at least in part by CYP1A2. Therefore, CYP1A2 inhibitors could theoretically adversely influence the clearance of anagrelide).

ALAMAST OPHTHALMIC SOLUTION

(Pemirolast Potassium) 3181
None cited in PDR database.

ALBENZA TABLETS

(Albendazole) 1297
May interact with theophyllines and certain other agents. Compounds in these categories include:

Cimetidine (Co-administration has resulted in increased albendazole sulfoxide concentrations in bile and cystic fluid in hydatid cyst).
No products indexed under this heading.

Cimetidine Hydrochloride (Co-administration has resulted in increased albendazole sulfoxide concentrations in bile and cystic fluid in hydatid cyst).
No products indexed under this heading.

Dexamethasone (Co-administration has resulted in higher steady-state trough concentrations of albendazole sulfoxide). Products include:
Ciprodex Otic Suspension 541

Dexamethasone Acetate (Co-administration has resulted in higher steady-state trough concentrations of albendazole sulfoxide).
No products indexed under this heading.

Dexamethasone Sodium Phosphate (Co-administration has resulted in higher steady-state trough concentrations of albendazole sulfoxide).
No products indexed under this heading.

Praziquantel (Co-administration has resulted in increased mean maximum plasma concentration and area under the curve of albendazole sulfoxide).
No products indexed under this heading.

Theophylline (Monitoring theophylline plasma concentrations during and after treatment with albendazole is recommended).
No products indexed under this heading.

Theophylline Anhydrous (Monitoring theophylline plasma concentrations during and after treatment with albendazole is recommended). Products include:
Uniphyl Tablets 2595

Theophylline Calcium Salicylate (Monitoring theophylline plasma concentrations during and after treatment with albendazole is recommended).
No products indexed under this heading.

Theophylline Dihydroxypropyl (Glyceryl) (Monitoring theophylline plasma concentrations during and after treatment with albendazole is recommended).
No products indexed under this heading.

Theophylline Ethylenediamine (Monitoring theophylline plasma concentrations during and after treatment with albendazole is recommended).
No products indexed under this heading.

Theophylline Sodium Glycinate (Monitoring theophylline plasma concentrations during and after treatment with albendazole is recommended).
No products indexed under this heading.

Food Interactions

Diet, high-lipid (Oral bioavailability appears to be enhanced when albendazole is co-administered with a fatty meal).

ALBUTEIN 5%

(Albumin (human)) 1707
None cited in PDR database.

ALBUTEIN 25%

(Albumin (human)) 1708
None cited in PDR database.

ALDARA CREAM, 5%

(Imiquimod) 1699
None cited in PDR database.

ALFERON N INJECTION

(Interferon alfa-N3 (Human Leukocyte Derived)).......................... 1726
None cited in PDR database.

ALIGN DAILY PROBIOTIC SUPPLEMENT

(Bifidobacteria) 2563
None cited in PDR database.

ALIMTA FOR INJECTION

(Pemetrexed) 1786
May interact with nephrotoxic agents, non-steroidal anti-inflammatory agents, and certain other agents. Compounds in these categories include:

Abacavir Sulfate (Concomitant administration of nephrotoxic drugs could result in delayed clearance of pemetrexed). Products include:
Epzicom Tablets 1422
Trizivir Tablets 1622
Ziagen 1673

Acyclovir (Concomitant administration of nephrotoxic drugs could result in delayed clearance of pemetrexed). Products include:
Zovirax 1690
Zovirax Cream 817
Zovirax Ointment 819

Acyclovir Sodium (Concomitant administration of nephrotoxic drugs could result in delayed clearance of pemetrexed).
No products indexed under this heading.

Alatrofloxacin Mesylate (Concomitant administration of nephrotoxic drugs could result in delayed clearance of pemetrexed).
No products indexed under this heading.

Aldesleukin (Concomitant administration of nephrotoxic drugs could result in delayed clearance of pemetrexed). Products include:
Proleukin for Injection 2287

Amikacin Sulfate (Concomitant administration of nephrotoxic drugs could result in delayed clearance of pemetrexed).
No products indexed under this heading.

Amoxicillin (Concomitant administration of nephrotoxic drugs could result in delayed clearance of pemetrexed). Products include:
Amoxil Capsules 1305
Amoxil Chewable Tablets 1305
Amoxil Pediatric Drops for Oral Suspension 1305
Amoxil Powder for Oral Suspension 1305
Amoxil Tablets 1305
Augmentin 1323
Augmentin Tablets 1327
Augmentin XR Extended Release Tablets 1333
Augmentin ES-600 Powder for Oral Suspension 1329
Moxatag Tablets 2165

Amoxicillin Trihydrate (Concomitant administration of nephrotoxic drugs could result in delayed clearance of pemetrexed).
No products indexed under this heading.

Amphotericin B (Concomitant administration of nephrotoxic drugs could result in delayed clearance of pemetrexed).
No products indexed under this heading.

Amphotericin B, liposomal (Concomitant administration of nephrotoxic drugs could result in delayed clearance of pemetrexed). Products include:
AmBisome for Injection 606

Amphotericin B Cholesteryl Sulfate (Concomitant administration of nephrotoxic drugs could result in delayed clearance of pemetrexed).
No products indexed under this heading.

Amphotericin B Lipid Complex (Concomitant administration of nephrotoxic drugs could result in delayed clearance of pemetrexed). Products include:
Abelcet Injection 1134

Ampicillin (Concomitant administration of nephrotoxic drugs could result in delayed clearance of pemetrexed).
No products indexed under this heading.

Ampicillin Sodium (Concomitant administration of nephrotoxic drugs could result in delayed clearance of pemetrexed).
No products indexed under this heading.

Ampicillin Trihydrate (Concomitant administration of nephrotoxic drugs could result in delayed clearance of pemetrexed).
No products indexed under this heading.

Amprenavir (Concomitant administration of nephrotoxic drugs could result in delayed clearance of pemetrexed).
No products indexed under this heading.

Aspirin (Concomitant administration of nephrotoxic drugs could result in delayed clearance of pemetrexed). Products include:
Aggrenox Capsules 819
Bayer Aspirin 750
Percodan Tablets 1130
St. Joseph 81 mg Aspirin Chewable and Enteric Coated Tablets 1903

Atazanavir (Concomitant administration of nephrotoxic drugs could result in delayed clearance of pemetrexed).
No products indexed under this heading.

Atorvastatin Calcium (Concomitant administration of nephrotoxic drugs could result in delayed clearance of pemetrexed). Products include:
Lipitor Tablets 2501

Azithromycin Dihydrate (Concomitant administration of nephrotoxic drugs could result in delayed clearance of pemetrexed).
No products indexed under this heading.

Azlocillin Sodium (Concomitant administration of nephrotoxic drugs could result in delayed clearance of pemetrexed).
No products indexed under this heading.

Aztreonam (Concomitant administration of nephrotoxic drugs could result in delayed clearance of pemetrexed).
No products indexed under this heading.

Bacampicillin Hydrochloride (Concomitant administration of nephrotoxic drugs could result in delayed clearance of pemetrexed).
No products indexed under this heading.

Balsalazide Disodium (Concomitant administration of nephrotoxic drugs could result in delayed clearance of pemetrexed).
No products indexed under this heading.

Benazepril Hydrochloride (Concomitant administration of nephrotoxic drugs could result in delayed clearance of pemetrexed).
No products indexed under this heading.

Bendroflumethiazide (Concomitant administration of nephrotoxic drugs could result in delayed clearance of pemetrexed).
No products indexed under this heading.

Caffeine (Concomitant administration of nephrotoxic drugs could result in delayed clearance of pemetrexed). Products include:
BioLean Free Tablets 635
BioLean II Tablets 635
Winrgy Dietary Supplement 642

Captopril (Concomitant administration of nephrotoxic drugs could result in delayed clearance of pemetrexed). Products include:
Captopril Tablets 2182

Carbenicillin Disodium (Concomitant administration of nephrotoxic drugs could result in delayed clearance of pemetrexed).
No products indexed under this heading.

Carbenicillin Indanyl Sodium (Concomitant administration of nephrotoxic drugs could result in delayed clearance of pemetrexed).
No products indexed under this heading.

Carboplatin (Concomitant administration of nephrotoxic drugs could result in delayed clearance of pemetrexed).
No products indexed under this heading.

Carmustine (BCNU) (Concomitant administration of nephrotoxic drugs could result in delayed clearance of pemetrexed).
No products indexed under this heading.

Cefaclor (Concomitant administration of nephrotoxic drugs could result in delayed clearance of pemetrexed).
No products indexed under this heading.

Cefadroxil (Concomitant administration of nephrotoxic drugs could result in delayed clearance of pemetrexed).
No products indexed under this heading.

Cefamandole Nafate (Concomitant administration of nephrotoxic drugs could result in delayed clearance of pemetrexed).
No products indexed under this heading.

Cefazolin Sodium (Concomitant administration of nephrotoxic drugs could result in delayed clearance of pemetrexed).
No products indexed under this heading.

Cefdinir (Concomitant administration of nephrotoxic drugs could result in delayed clearance of pemetrexed). Products include:
Omnicef Capsules 497
Omnicef for Oral Suspension 497

Cefepime Hydrochloride (Concomitant administration of nephrotoxic drugs could result in delayed clearance of pemetrexed).
No products indexed under this heading.

Cefixime (Concomitant administration of nephrotoxic drugs could result in delayed clearance of pemetrexed). Products include:
Suprax for Oral Suspension 1891
Suprax Tablets 1891

Cefmetazole Sodium (Concomitant administration of nephrotoxic drugs could result in delayed clearance of pemetrexed).
No products indexed under this heading.

Cefonicid Sodium (Concomitant administration of nephrotoxic drugs could result in delayed clearance of pemetrexed).
No products indexed under this heading.

Cefoperazone Sodium (Concomitant administration of nephrotoxic drugs could result in delayed clearance of pemetrexed).
No products indexed under this heading.

Ceforanide (Concomitant administration of nephrotoxic drugs could result in delayed clearance of pemetrexed).
No products indexed under this heading.

Cefotaxime Sodium (Concomitant administration of nephrotoxic drugs could result in delayed clearance of pemetrexed).
No products indexed under this heading.

Cefotetan (Concomitant administration of nephrotoxic drugs could result in delayed clearance of pemetrexed).
No products indexed under this heading.

Cefoxitin Sodium (Concomitant administration of nephrotoxic drugs could result in delayed clearance of pemetrexed).
No products indexed under this heading.

Cefpodoxime Proxetil (Concomitant administration of nephrotoxic drugs could result in delayed clearance of pemetrexed).
No products indexed under this heading.

Cefprozil (Concomitant administration of nephrotoxic drugs could result in delayed clearance of pemetrexed).
No products indexed under this heading.

Ceftazidime (Concomitant administration of nephrotoxic drugs could result in delayed clearance of pemetrexed). Products include:
Fortaz 1450

Ceftizoxime Sodium (Concomitant administration of nephrotoxic drugs could result in delayed clearance of pemetrexed).
No products indexed under this heading.

Ceftriaxone Sodium (Concomitant administration of nephrotoxic drugs could result in delayed clearance of pemetrexed). Products include:
Rocephin Injectable Vials, ADD-Vantage, Galaxy, Bulk 2642

Cefuroxime Axetil (Concomitant administration of nephrotoxic drugs could result in delayed clearance of pemetrexed). Products include:
Ceftin 1380

Cefuroxime Sodium (Concomitant administration of nephrotoxic drugs could result in delayed clearance of pemetrexed).
No products indexed under this heading.

Celecoxib (Patients with mild to moderate renal insufficiency should avoid NSAIDs with short elimination half-lives two days before, the day of, and two days following administration of pemetrexed. All patients should avoid NSAIDs with longer half-lives at least five days before, the day of, and two days following pemetrexed administration. If concomitant administration of an NSAID is necessary, patients should be monitored closely for toxicity, especially myelosuppression, renal and gastrointestinal toxicity). Products include:
Celebrex Capsules 2979

Cephalexin (Concomitant administration of nephrotoxic drugs could result in delayed clearance of pemetrexed).
No products indexed under this heading.

Cephalothin Sodium (Concomitant administration of nephrotoxic drugs could result in delayed clearance of pemetrexed).
No products indexed under this heading.

Cephapirin Sodium (Concomitant administration of nephrotoxic drugs could result in delayed clearance of pemetrexed).
No products indexed under this heading.

Cephradine (Concomitant administration of nephrotoxic drugs could result in delayed clearance of pemetrexed).
No products indexed under this heading.

Cerivastatin Sodium (Concomitant administration of nephrotoxic drugs could result in delayed clearance of pemetrexed).
No products indexed under this heading.

Chlorothiazide (Concomitant administration of nephrotoxic drugs could result in delayed clearance of pemetrexed).
No products indexed under this heading.

Chlorothiazide Sodium (Concomitant administration of nephrotoxic drugs could result in delayed clearance of pemetrexed). Products include:
Intravenous Sodium Diuril 2490

Chlorpropamide (Concomitant administration of nephrotoxic drugs could result in delayed clearance of pemetrexed).
No products indexed under this heading.

Cidofovir (Concomitant administration of nephrotoxic drugs could result in delayed clearance of pemetrexed).
No products indexed under this heading.

Cilastatin Sodium (Concomitant administration of nephrotoxic drugs could result in delayed clearance of pemetrexed). Products include:
Primaxin I.M. 2080
Primaxin I.V. 2083

Cimetidine (Concomitant administration of nephrotoxic drugs could result in delayed clearance of pemetrexed).
No products indexed under this heading.

Cimetidine Hydrochloride (Concomitant administration of nephrotoxic drugs could result in delayed clearance of pemetrexed).
No products indexed under this heading.

Cisplatin (Concomitant administration of nephrotoxic drugs could result in delayed clearance of pemetrexed).
No products indexed under this heading.

Cladribine (Concomitant administration of nephrotoxic drugs could result in delayed clearance of pemetrexed). Products include:
Leustatin Injection 2384

Clozapine (Concomitant administration of nephrotoxic drugs could result in delayed clearance of pemetrexed).
No products indexed under this heading.

Colistimethate Sodium (Concomitant administration of nephrotoxic drugs could result in delayed clearance of pemetrexed).
No products indexed under this heading.

Colistin Sulfate (Concomitant administration of nephrotoxic drugs could result in delayed clearance of pemetrexed).
No products indexed under this heading.

Cyclophosphamide (Concomitant administration of nephrotoxic drugs could result in delayed clearance of pemetrexed).
No products indexed under this heading.

Cyclosporine (Concomitant administration of nephrotoxic drugs could result in delayed clearance of pemetrexed). Products include:
Gengraf Capsules 435
Neoral Oral Solution 2280
Neoral Soft Gelatin Capsules 2280
Restasis Ophthalmic Emulsion 557
Sandimmune 2296

Cytarabine (Concomitant administration of nephrotoxic drugs could result in delayed clearance of pemetrexed).
No products indexed under this heading.

Cytarabine Liposome (Concomitant administration of nephrotoxic drugs could result in delayed clearance of pemetrexed). Products include:
DepoCyt Injection 1136

Delavirdine Mesylate (Concomitant administration of nephrotoxic drugs could result in delayed clearance of pemetrexed).
No products indexed under this heading.

Diatrizoate Meglumine (Concomitant administration of nephrotoxic drugs could result in delayed clearance of pemetrexed).
No products indexed under this heading.

Diatrizoate Sodium (Concomitant administration of nephrotoxic drugs could result in delayed clearance of pemetrexed).
No products indexed under this heading.

Diclofenac Epolamine (Patients with mild to moderate renal insufficiency should avoid NSAIDs with short elimination half-lives two days before, the day of, and two days following administration of pemetrexed. All patients should avoid NSAIDs with longer half-lives at least five days before, the day of, and two days following pemetrexed administration. If concomitant administration of an NSAID is necessary, patients should be monitored closely for toxicity, especially myelosuppression, renal and gastrointestinal toxicity). Products include:
Flector Patch 561

Diclofenac Potassium (Patients with mild to moderate renal insufficiency should avoid NSAIDs with short elimination half-lives two days before, the day of, and two days following administration of pemetrexed. All patients should avoid NSAIDs with longer half-lives at least five days before, the day of, and two days following pemetrexed administration. If concomitant administration of an NSAID is necessary, patients should be monitored closely for toxicity, especially myelosuppression, renal and gastrointestinal toxicity).
No products indexed under this heading.

Diclofenac Sodium (Patients with mild to moderate renal insufficiency should avoid NSAIDs with short elimination half-lives two days before, the day of, and two days following administration of pemetrexed. All patients should avoid NSAIDs with longer half-lives at least five days before, the day of, and two days following pemetrexed administration. If concomitant administration of an NSAID is necessary, patients should be monitored closely for toxicity, especially myelosuppression, renal and gastrointestinal toxicity). Products include:
Diclofenac Sodium Ophthalmic Solution .... ⊙ 240
Voltaren Ophthalmic Solution 2336
Voltaren Tablets 2334
Voltaren-XR Tablets 2337

Dicloxacillin Sodium (Concomitant administration of nephrotoxic drugs could result in delayed clearance of pemetrexed).
No products indexed under this heading.

Didanosine (Concomitant administration of nephrotoxic drugs could result in delayed clearance of pemetrexed).
No products indexed under this heading.

Efavirenz (Concomitant administration of nephrotoxic drugs could result in delayed clearance of pemetrexed). Products include:
Atripla Tablets 938
Sustiva Capsules 930
Sustiva Tablets 930

Emtricitabine (Concomitant administration of nephrotoxic drugs could result in delayed clearance of pemetrexed). Products include:
Atripla Tablets 938
Emtriva Capsules 1246
Emtriva Oral Solution 1246
Truvada Tablets 1262

Enalapril Maleate (Concomitant administration of nephrotoxic drugs could result in delayed clearance of pemetrexed).
No products indexed under this heading.

Enalaprilat (Concomitant administration of nephrotoxic drugs could result in delayed clearance of pemetrexed).
No products indexed under this heading.

Enfuvirtide (Concomitant administration of nephrotoxic drugs could result in delayed clearance of pemetrexed).
No products indexed under this heading.

Ethiodized Oil (Concomitant administration of nephrotoxic drugs could result in delayed clearance of pemetrexed).
No products indexed under this heading.

Etodolac (Patients with mild to moderate renal insufficiency should avoid NSAIDs with short elimination half-lives two days before, the day of, and two days following administration of pemetrexed. All patients should avoid NSAIDs with longer half-lives at least five days before, the day of, and two days following pemetrexed administration. If concomitant administration of an NSAID is necessary, patients should be monitored closely for toxicity, especially myelosuppression, renal and gastrointestinal toxicity).
No products indexed under this heading.

Fenoprofen Calcium (Patients with mild to moderate renal insufficiency should avoid NSAIDs with short elimination half-lives two days before, the day of, and two days following administration of pemetrexed. All patients should avoid NSAIDs with longer half-lives at least five days before, the day of, and two days following pemetrexed administration. If concomitant administration of an NSAID is necessary, patients should be monitored closely for toxicity, especially myelosuppression, renal and gastrointestinal toxicity). Products include:
Nalfon Capsules 2508

Filgrastim (Concomitant administration of nephrotoxic drugs could result in delayed clearance of pemetrexed). Products include:
Neupogen for Injection 589

Fluorouracil (Concomitant administration of nephrotoxic drugs could result in delayed clearance of pemetrexed). Products include:
Carac Cream 0.5% 2722

Flurbiprofen (Patients with mild to moderate renal insufficiency should avoid NSAIDs with short elimination half-lives two days before, the day

of, and two days following administration of pemetrexed. All patients should avoid NSAIDs with longer half-lives at least five days before, the day of, and two days following pemetrexed administration. If concomitant administration of an NSAID is necessary, patients should be monitored closely for toxicity, especially myelosuppression, renal and gastrointestinal toxicity).
No products indexed under this heading.

Fluvastatin Sodium (Concomitant administration of nephrotoxic drugs could result in delayed clearance of pemetrexed). Products include:
Lescol Capsules ... **2268**
Lescol XL Tablets ... **2268**

Foscarnet Sodium (Concomitant administration of nephrotoxic drugs could result in delayed clearance of pemetrexed).
No products indexed under this heading.

Fosinopril Sodium (Concomitant administration of nephrotoxic drugs could result in delayed clearance of pemetrexed).
No products indexed under this heading.

Furosemide (Concomitant administration of nephrotoxic drugs could result in delayed clearance of pemetrexed). Products include:
Furosemide Tablets ... **2186**

Gadopentetate Dimeglumine (Concomitant administration of nephrotoxic drugs could result in delayed clearance of pemetrexed).
No products indexed under this heading.

Gentamicin (Concomitant administration of nephrotoxic drugs could result in delayed clearance of pemetrexed).
No products indexed under this heading.

Gentamicin Sulfate (Concomitant administration of nephrotoxic drugs could result in delayed clearance of pemetrexed). Products include:
Pred-G Ophthalmic Ointment ... ⊙ **229**
Pred-G Ophthalmic Suspension ... ⊙ **228**

Glipizide (Concomitant administration of nephrotoxic drugs could result in delayed clearance of pemetrexed).
No products indexed under this heading.

Globulin, Immune (Human) (Concomitant administration of nephrotoxic drugs could result in delayed clearance of pemetrexed). Products include:
Flebogamma 5% ... **1715**

Glyburide (Concomitant administration of nephrotoxic drugs could result in delayed clearance of pemetrexed).
No products indexed under this heading.

Gold Therapy (Concomitant administration of nephrotoxic drugs could result in delayed clearance of pemetrexed).
No products indexed under this heading.

HMG-CoA Reductase Inhibitors (Concomitant administration of nephrotoxic drugs could result in delayed clearance of pemetrexed).
No products indexed under this heading.

Hydrochlorothiazide (Concomitant administration of nephrotoxic drugs could result in delayed clearance of pemetrexed). Products include:
Atacand HCT ... **642**
Avalide Tablets ... **892**
Avalide Tablets ... **2713**
Benicar HCT Tablets ... **1010**
Diovan HCT Tablets ... **2216**
Dyazide Capsules ... **1405**
Micardis HCT Tablets ... **854**
Prinzide Tablets ... **2092**
Tekturna HCT Tablets ... **2324**
Teveten HCT Tablets ... **517**

Hydroflumethiazide (Concomitant administration of nephrotoxic drugs could result in delayed clearance of pemetrexed).
No products indexed under this heading.

Ibuprofen (Caution should be used when administering ibuprofen concurrently with pemetrexed to patients with mild to moderate renal insufficiency (CrCl 45-79 mL/min)). Products include:
Motrin IB Tablets and Caplets ... **1900**
Children's Motrin Oral Suspension ... **1901**
Children's Motrin Non-Staining Dye-Free Oral Suspension ... **1901**
Children's Motrin Cold Oral Suspension ... **1899**
Infants' Motrin Concentrated Drops ... **1901**
Infants' Motrin Non-Staining Dye-Free Concentrated Drops ... **1901**
Junior Strength Motrin Caplets and Chewable Tablets ... **1901**
Vicoprofen Tablets ... **533**

Idarubicin Hydrochloride (Concomitant administration of nephrotoxic drugs could result in delayed clearance of pemetrexed).
No products indexed under this heading.

Ifosfamide (Concomitant administration of nephrotoxic drugs could result in delayed clearance of pemetrexed).
No products indexed under this heading.

Imipenem (Concomitant administration of nephrotoxic drugs could result in delayed clearance of pemetrexed). Products include:
Primaxin I.M. ... **2080**
Primaxin I.V. ... **2083**

Immune Globulin Intravenous (Human) (Concomitant administration of nephrotoxic drugs could result in delayed clearance of pemetrexed). Products include:
Flebogamma 5% DIF ... **1718**
Gammagard Liquid ... **730**
Gammagard S/D ... **734**
Gamunex ... **3094**

Indinavir Sulfate (Concomitant administration of nephrotoxic drugs could result in delayed clearance of pemetrexed). Products include:
Crixivan Capsules ... **1979**

Indomethacin (Patients with mild to moderate renal insufficiency should avoid NSAIDs with short elimination half-lives two days before, the day of, and two days following administration of pemetrexed. All patients should avoid NSAIDs with longer half-lives at least five days before, the day of, and two days following pemetrexed administration. If concomitant administration of an NSAID is necessary, patients should be monitored closely for toxicity, especially myelosuppression, renal and gastrointestinal toxicity). Products include:
Indocin ... **2024**

Indomethacin Sodium Trihydrate (Patients with mild to moderate renal insufficiency should avoid NSAIDs with short elimination half-lives two days before, the day of, and two days following administration of pemetrexed. All patients should avoid NSAIDs with longer half-lives at least five days before, the day of, and two days following pemetrexed administration. If concomitant administration of an NSAID is necessary, patients should be monitored closely for toxicity, especially myelosuppression, renal and gastrointestinal toxicity). Products include:
Indocin I.V. ... **2489**

Interferon Beta-1b (Concomitant administration of nephrotoxic drugs could result in delayed clearance of pemetrexed). Products include:
Betaseron for SC Injection ... **756**

Interleukin-2 (Concomitant administration of nephrotoxic drugs could result in delayed clearance of pemetrexed).
No products indexed under this heading.

Iodamide Meglumine (Concomitant administration of nephrotoxic drugs could result in delayed clearance of pemetrexed).
No products indexed under this heading.

Iohexol (Concomitant administration of nephrotoxic drugs could result in delayed clearance of pemetrexed).
No products indexed under this heading.

Iopamidol (Concomitant administration of nephrotoxic drugs could result in delayed clearance of pemetrexed).
No products indexed under this heading.

Iopanoic Acid (Concomitant administration of nephrotoxic drugs could result in delayed clearance of pemetrexed).
No products indexed under this heading.

Iothalamate Meglumine (Concomitant administration of nephrotoxic drugs could result in delayed clearance of pemetrexed).
No products indexed under this heading.

Ioxaglate Meglumine (Concomitant administration of nephrotoxic drugs could result in delayed clearance of pemetrexed).
No products indexed under this heading.

Ioxaglate Sodium (Concomitant administration of nephrotoxic drugs could result in delayed clearance of pemetrexed).
No products indexed under this heading.

Kanamycin Sulfate (Concomitant administration of nephrotoxic drugs could result in delayed clearance of pemetrexed).
No products indexed under this heading.

Ketoprofen (Patients with mild to moderate renal insufficiency should avoid NSAIDs with short elimination half-lives two days before, the day of, and two days following administration of pemetrexed. All patients should avoid NSAIDs with longer half-lives at least five days before, the day of, and two days following pemetrexed administration. If concomitant administration of an NSAID is necessary, patients should be monitored closely for toxicity, especially myelosuppression, renal and gastrointestinal toxicity).
No products indexed under this heading.

Ketorolac Tromethamine (Patients with mild to moderate renal insufficiency should avoid NSAIDs with short elimination half-lives two days before, the day of, and two days following administration of pemetrexed. All patients should avoid NSAIDs with longer half-lives at least five days before, the day of, and two days following pemetrexed administration. If concomitant administration of an NSAID is necessary, patients should be monitored closely for toxicity, especially myelosuppression, renal and gastrointestinal toxicity).
No products indexed under this heading.

Lamium album (Concomitant administration of nephrotoxic drugs could result in delayed clearance of pemetrexed).
No products indexed under this heading.

Lisinopril (Concomitant administration of nephrotoxic drugs could result in delayed clearance of pemetrexed). Products include:
Prinivil Tablets ... **2087**
Prinzide Tablets ... **2092**

Lithium (Concomitant administration of nephrotoxic drugs could result in delayed clearance of pemetrexed).
No products indexed under this heading.

Lithium Carbonate (Concomitant administration of nephrotoxic drugs could result in delayed clearance of pemetrexed).
No products indexed under this heading.

Lithium Citrate (Concomitant administration of nephrotoxic drugs could result in delayed clearance of pemetrexed).
No products indexed under this heading.

Lopinavir (Concomitant administration of nephrotoxic drugs could result in delayed clearance of pemetrexed). Products include:
Kaletra ... **452**

Loracarbef (Concomitant administration of nephrotoxic drugs could result in delayed clearance of pemetrexed).
No products indexed under this heading.

Lovastatin (Concomitant administration of nephrotoxic drugs could result in delayed clearance of pemetrexed). Products include:
Advicor Tablets ... **402**
Mevacor Tablets ... **2063**

Meclofenamate Sodium (Patients with mild to moderate renal insufficiency should avoid NSAIDs with short elimination half-lives two days before, the day of, and two days following administration of pemetrexed. All patients should avoid NSAIDs with longer half-lives at least five days before, the day of, and two days following pemetrexed administration. If concomitant administration of an NSAID is necessary, patients should be monitored closely for toxicity, especially myelosuppression,

renal and gastrointestinal toxicity).
No products indexed under this heading.

Mefenamic Acid (Patients with mild to moderate renal insufficiency should avoid NSAIDs with short elimination half-lives two days before, the day of, and two days following administration of pemetrexed. All patients should avoid NSAIDs with longer half-lives at least five days before, the day of, and two days following pemetrexed administration. If concomitant administration of an NSAID is necessary, patients should be monitored closely for toxicity, especially myelosuppression, renal and gastrointestinal toxicity).
No products indexed under this heading.

Meloxicam (Patients with mild to moderate renal insufficiency should avoid NSAIDs with short elimination half-lives two days before, the day of, and two days following administration of pemetrexed. All patients should avoid NSAIDs with longer half-lives at least five days before, the day of, and two days following pemetrexed administration. If concomitant administration of an NSAID is necessary, patients should be monitored closely for toxicity, especially myelosuppression, renal and gastrointestinal toxicity). Products include:
Mobic Oral Suspension 863
Mobic Tablets 863

Melphalan Hydrochloride (Concomitant administration of nephrotoxic drugs could result in delayed clearance of pemetrexed).
No products indexed under this heading.

Mesalamine (Concomitant administration of nephrotoxic drugs could result in delayed clearance of pemetrexed). Products include:
Asacol Delayed-Release Tablets 2579
Canasa Rectal Suppositories 705
Lialda Tablets 3029
Pentasa Capsules 3030

Methimazole (Concomitant administration of nephrotoxic drugs could result in delayed clearance of pemetrexed).
No products indexed under this heading.

Methotrexate (Concomitant administration of nephrotoxic drugs could result in delayed clearance of pemetrexed).
No products indexed under this heading.

Methotrexate Sodium (Concomitant administration of nephrotoxic drugs could result in delayed clearance of pemetrexed).
No products indexed under this heading.

Methyclothiazide (Concomitant administration of nephrotoxic drugs could result in delayed clearance of pemetrexed).
No products indexed under this heading.

Mezlocillin Sodium (Concomitant administration of nephrotoxic drugs could result in delayed clearance of pemetrexed).
No products indexed under this heading.

Minocycline Hydrochloride (Concomitant administration of nephrotoxic drugs could result in delayed clearance of pemetrexed). Products include:
Solodyn Extended Release Tablets 1938

Mitomycin (Mitomycin-C) (Concomitant administration of nephrotoxic drugs could result in delayed clearance of pemetrexed).
No products indexed under this heading.

Moexipril Hydrochloride (Concomitant administration of nephrotoxic drugs could result in delayed clearance of pemetrexed).
No products indexed under this heading.

Muromonab-CD3 (Concomitant administration of nephrotoxic drugs could result in delayed clearance of pemetrexed). Products include:
Orthoclone OKT3 Sterile Solution 2387

Nabumetone (Patients with mild to moderate renal insufficiency should avoid NSAIDs with short elimination half-lives two days before, the day of, and two days following administration of pemetrexed. All patients should avoid NSAIDs with longer half-lives at least five days before, the day of, and two days following pemetrexed administration. If concomitant administration of an NSAID is necessary, patients should be monitored closely for toxicity, especially myelosuppression, renal and gastrointestinal toxicity).
No products indexed under this heading.

Nafcillin Sodium (Concomitant administration of nephrotoxic drugs could result in delayed clearance of pemetrexed).
No products indexed under this heading.

Naproxen (Patients with mild to moderate renal insufficiency should avoid NSAIDs with short elimination half-lives two days before, the day of, and two days following administration of pemetrexed. All patients should avoid NSAIDs with longer half-lives at least five days before, the day of, and two days following pemetrexed administration. If concomitant administration of an NSAID is necessary, patients should be monitored closely for toxicity, especially myelosuppression, renal and gastrointestinal toxicity). Products include:
EC-Naprosyn Delayed-Release Tablets 2632
Naprosyn Suspension 2632
Naprosyn Tablets 2632

Naproxen Sodium (Patients with mild to moderate renal insufficiency should avoid NSAIDs with short elimination half-lives two days before, the day of, and two days following administration of pemetrexed. All patients should avoid NSAIDs with longer half-lives at least five days before, the day of, and two days following pemetrexed administration. If concomitant administration of an NSAID is necessary, patients should be monitored closely for toxicity, especially myelosuppression, renal and gastrointestinal toxicity). Products include:
Anaprox Tablets 2632
Anaprox DS Tablets 2632
Treximet Tablets 1616

Nelfinavir Mesylate (Concomitant administration of nephrotoxic drugs could result in delayed clearance of pemetrexed).
No products indexed under this heading.

Neomycin (Concomitant administration of nephrotoxic drugs could result in delayed clearance of pemetrexed).
No products indexed under this heading.

Neomycin, oral (Concomitant administration of nephrotoxic drugs could result in delayed clearance of pemetrexed).
No products indexed under this heading.

Neomycin Sulfate (Concomitant administration of nephrotoxic drugs could result in delayed clearance of pemetrexed). Products include:
Neosporin Ophthalmic Solution Sterile .... ⊙252

Nevirapine (Concomitant administration of nephrotoxic drugs could result in delayed clearance of pemetrexed). Products include:
Viramune Oral Suspension 873
Viramune Tablets 873

Norfloxacin (Concomitant administration of nephrotoxic drugs could result in delayed clearance of pemetrexed). Products include:
Noroxin Tablets 2069

Olsalazine Sodium (Concomitant administration of nephrotoxic drugs could result in delayed clearance of pemetrexed).
No products indexed under this heading.

Omeprazole (Concomitant administration of nephrotoxic drugs could result in delayed clearance of pemetrexed).
No products indexed under this heading.

Oxaprozin (Patients with mild to moderate renal insufficiency should avoid NSAIDs with short elimination half-lives two days before, the day of, and two days following administration of pemetrexed. All patients should avoid NSAIDs with longer half-lives at least five days before, the day of, and two days following pemetrexed administration. If concomitant administration of an NSAID is necessary, patients should be monitored closely for toxicity, especially myelosuppression, renal and gastrointestinal toxicity).
No products indexed under this heading.

Pamidronate Disodium (Concomitant administration of nephrotoxic drugs could result in delayed clearance of pemetrexed).
No products indexed under this heading.

Paroxetine Hydrochloride (Concomitant administration of nephrotoxic drugs could result in delayed clearance of pemetrexed). Products include:
Paxil 1535
Paxil CR Controlled-Release Tablets 1544

Penicillamine (Concomitant administration of nephrotoxic drugs could result in delayed clearance of pemetrexed). Products include:
Cuprimine Capsules 1986

Penicillin G Benzathine (Concomitant administration of nephrotoxic drugs could result in delayed clearance of pemetrexed). Products include:
Bicillin C-R Injectable Suspension 1775
Bicillin L-A Injection 1777

Penicillin G Potassium (Concomitant administration of nephrotoxic drugs could result in delayed clearance of pemetrexed).
No products indexed under this heading.

Penicillin G Procaine (Concomitant administration of nephrotoxic drugs could result in delayed clearance of pemetrexed). Products include:
Bicillin C-R Injectable Suspension 1775
Bicillin L-A Injection 1777

Penicillin G Sodium (Concomitant administration of nephrotoxic drugs could result in delayed clearance of pemetrexed).
No products indexed under this heading.

Penicillin V Potassium (Concomitant administration of nephrotoxic drugs could result in delayed clearance of pemetrexed).
No products indexed under this heading.

Pentamidine Isethionate (Concomitant administration of nephrotoxic drugs could result in delayed clearance of pemetrexed).
No products indexed under this heading.

Perindopril Erbumine (Concomitant administration of nephrotoxic drugs could result in delayed clearance of pemetrexed). Products include:
Aceon Tablets (2 mg, 4 mg, 8 mg) 3038

Phenylbutazone (Patients with mild to moderate renal insufficiency should avoid NSAIDs with short elimination half-lives two days before, the day of, and two days following administration of pemetrexed. All patients should avoid NSAIDs with longer half-lives at least five days before, the day of, and two days following pemetrexed administration. If concomitant administration of an NSAID is necessary, patients should be monitored closely for toxicity, especially myelosuppression, renal and gastrointestinal toxicity).
No products indexed under this heading.

Piroxicam (Patients with mild to moderate renal insufficiency should avoid NSAIDs with short elimination half-lives two days before, the day of, and two days following administration of pemetrexed. All patients should avoid NSAIDs with longer half-lives at least five days before, the day of, and two days following pemetrexed administration. If concomitant administration of an NSAID is necessary, patients should be monitored closely for toxicity, especially myelosuppression, renal and gastrointestinal toxicity).
No products indexed under this heading.

Plicamycin (Concomitant administration of nephrotoxic drugs could result in delayed clearance of pemetrexed).
No products indexed under this heading.

Polymyxin (Concomitant administration of nephrotoxic drugs could result in delayed clearance of pemetrexed).
No products indexed under this heading.

Polymyxin B Sulfate (Concomitant administration of nephrotoxic drugs could result in delayed clearance of pemetrexed). Products include:
- Neosporin Ophthalmic Solution Sterile ⊙252

Polythiazide (Concomitant administration of nephrotoxic drugs could result in delayed clearance of pemetrexed).
- No products indexed under this heading.

Pravastatin Sodium (Concomitant administration of nephrotoxic drugs could result in delayed clearance of pemetrexed).
- No products indexed under this heading.

Probenecid (Concomitant administration of substances that are also tubularly secreted (e.g., probenecid) could potentially result in delayed clearance of pemetrexed).
- No products indexed under this heading.

Quinapril Hydrochloride (Concomitant administration of nephrotoxic drugs could result in delayed clearance of pemetrexed).
- No products indexed under this heading.

Rabeprazole Sodium (Concomitant administration of nephrotoxic drugs could result in delayed clearance of pemetrexed). Products include:
- Aciphex Tablets 1053

Ramipril (Concomitant administration of nephrotoxic drugs could result in delayed clearance of pemetrexed).
- No products indexed under this heading.

Rifampin (Concomitant administration of nephrotoxic drugs could result in delayed clearance of pemetrexed).
- No products indexed under this heading.

Riluzole (Concomitant administration of nephrotoxic drugs could result in delayed clearance of pemetrexed). Products include:
- Rilutek Tablets 2771

Ritonavir (Concomitant administration of nephrotoxic drugs could result in delayed clearance of pemetrexed). Products include:
- Kaletra 452
- Norvir 489

Rofecoxib (Patients with mild to moderate renal insufficiency should avoid NSAIDs with short elimination half-lives two days before, the day of, and two days following administration of pemetrexed. All patients should avoid NSAIDs with longer half-lives at least five days before, the day of, and two days following pemetrexed administration. If concomitant administration of an NSAID is necessary, patients should be monitored closely for toxicity, especially myelosuppression, renal and gastrointestinal toxicity).
- No products indexed under this heading.

Saquinavir (Concomitant administration of nephrotoxic drugs could result in delayed clearance of pemetrexed).
- No products indexed under this heading.

Sibutramine Hydrochloride Monohydrate (Concomitant administration of nephrotoxic drugs could result in delayed clearance of pemetrexed). Products include:
- Meridia Capsules 475

Simvastatin (Concomitant administration of nephrotoxic drugs could result in delayed clearance of pemetrexed). Products include:
- Simcor Tablets 502
- Vytorin 10/10 Tablets 2149
- Vytorin 10/10 Tablets 2939
- Vytorin 10/20 Tablets 2149
- Vytorin 10/20 Tablets 2939
- Vytorin 10/40 Tablets 2149
- Vytorin 10/40 Tablets 2939
- Vytorin 10/80 Tablets 2149
- Vytorin 10/80 Tablets 2939
- Zocor Tablets 2136

Spirapril Hydrochloride (Concomitant administration of nephrotoxic drugs could result in delayed clearance of pemetrexed).
- No products indexed under this heading.

Stavudine (Concomitant administration of nephrotoxic drugs could result in delayed clearance of pemetrexed).
- No products indexed under this heading.

Streptomycin Sulfate (Concomitant administration of nephrotoxic drugs could result in delayed clearance of pemetrexed).
- No products indexed under this heading.

Streptozocin (Concomitant administration of nephrotoxic drugs could result in delayed clearance of pemetrexed).
- No products indexed under this heading.

Sulfacytine (Concomitant administration of nephrotoxic drugs could result in delayed clearance of pemetrexed).
- No products indexed under this heading.

Sulfamethizole (Concomitant administration of nephrotoxic drugs could result in delayed clearance of pemetrexed).
- No products indexed under this heading.

Sulfamethoxazole (Concomitant administration of nephrotoxic drugs could result in delayed clearance of pemetrexed).
- No products indexed under this heading.

Sulfasalazine (Concomitant administration of nephrotoxic drugs could result in delayed clearance of pemetrexed).
- No products indexed under this heading.

Sulfinpyrazone (Concomitant administration of nephrotoxic drugs could result in delayed clearance of pemetrexed).
- No products indexed under this heading.

Sulfisoxazole Acetyl (Concomitant administration of nephrotoxic drugs could result in delayed clearance of pemetrexed).
- No products indexed under this heading.

Sulfisoxazole Diolamine (Concomitant administration of nephrotoxic drugs could result in delayed clearance of pemetrexed).
- No products indexed under this heading.

Sulindac (Patients with mild to moderate renal insufficiency should avoid NSAIDs with short elimination half-lives two days before, the day of, and two days following administration of pemetrexed. All patients should avoid NSAIDs with longer half-lives at least five days before, the day of, and two days following pemetrexed administration. If concomitant administration of an NSAID is necessary, patients should be monitored closely for toxicity, especially myelosuppression, renal and gastrointestinal toxicity). Products include:
- Clinoril Tablets 1962

Tacrolimus (Concomitant administration of nephrotoxic drugs could result in delayed clearance of pemetrexed). Products include:
- Prograf Capsules and Injection 622
- Protopic Ointment 628

Tenofovir Disoproxil Fumarate (Concomitant administration of nephrotoxic drugs could result in delayed clearance of pemetrexed). Products include:
- Atripla Tablets 938
- Truvada Tablets 1262
- Viread Tablets 1268

Thioguanine (Concomitant administration of nephrotoxic drugs could result in delayed clearance of pemetrexed). Products include:
- Tabloid Tablets 1601

Ticarcillin Disodium (Concomitant administration of nephrotoxic drugs could result in delayed clearance of pemetrexed). Products include:
- Timentin ADD-Vantage 1606
- Timentin Injection Galaxy Container 1609
- Timentin IV Infusion 1603
- Timentin Pharmacy Bulk Package 1613

Tobramycin (Concomitant administration of nephrotoxic drugs could result in delayed clearance of pemetrexed). Products include:
- Zylet Ophthalmic Suspension ⊙247

Tobramycin Sulfate (Concomitant administration of nephrotoxic drugs could result in delayed clearance of pemetrexed).
- No products indexed under this heading.

Tolazamide (Concomitant administration of nephrotoxic drugs could result in delayed clearance of pemetrexed).
- No products indexed under this heading.

Tolbutamide (Concomitant administration of nephrotoxic drugs could result in delayed clearance of pemetrexed).
- No products indexed under this heading.

Tolmetin Sodium (Patients with mild to moderate renal insufficiency should avoid NSAIDs with short elimination half-lives two days before, the day of, and two days following administration of pemetrexed. All patients should avoid NSAIDs with longer half-lives at least five days before, the day of, and two days following pemetrexed administration. If concomitant administration of an NSAID is necessary, patients should be monitored closely for toxicity, especially myelosuppression, renal and gastrointestinal toxicity).
- No products indexed under this heading.

Trandolapril (Concomitant administration of nephrotoxic drugs could result in delayed clearance of pemetrexed). Products include:
- Mavik Tablets 472
- Tarka Tablets 511

Triamterene (Concomitant administration of nephrotoxic drugs could result in delayed clearance of pemetrexed). Products include:
- Dyazide Capsules 1405
- Dyrenium Capsules 3189

Trimethadione (Concomitant administration of nephrotoxic drugs could result in delayed clearance of pemetrexed).
- No products indexed under this heading.

Trovafloxacin Mesylate (Concomitant administration of nephrotoxic drugs could result in delayed clearance of pemetrexed).
- No products indexed under this heading.

Tyropanoate Sodium (Concomitant administration of nephrotoxic drugs could result in delayed clearance of pemetrexed).
- No products indexed under this heading.

Valacyclovir Hydrochloride (Concomitant administration of nephrotoxic drugs could result in delayed clearance of pemetrexed). Products include:
- Valtrex Caplets 1635

Valdecoxib (Patients with mild to moderate renal insufficiency should avoid NSAIDs with short elimination half-lives two days before, the day of, and two days following administration of pemetrexed. All patients should avoid NSAIDs with longer half-lives at least five days before, the day of, and two days following pemetrexed administration. If concomitant administration of an NSAID is necessary, patients should be monitored closely for toxicity, especially myelosuppression, renal and gastrointestinal toxicity).
- No products indexed under this heading.

Vancomycin Hydrochloride (Concomitant administration of nephrotoxic drugs could result in delayed clearance of pemetrexed).
- No products indexed under this heading.

Voriconazole (Concomitant administration of nephrotoxic drugs could result in delayed clearance of pemetrexed).
- No products indexed under this heading.

Zalcitabine (Concomitant administration of nephrotoxic drugs could result in delayed clearance of pemetrexed).
- No products indexed under this heading.

Zidovudine (Concomitant administration of nephrotoxic drugs could result in delayed clearance of pemetrexed). Products include:
- Combivir Tablets 1384
- Retrovir 1574
- Retrovir IV Infusion 1579
- Trizivir Tablets 1622

Zoledronic acid (Concomitant administration of nephrotoxic drugs could result in delayed clearance of pemetrexed). Products include:
- Reclast Injection 2291
- Zometa for Intravenous Infusion 2341

IMPORTANT NOTE: Always consult each drug listing in the patient's regimen for possible interactions.

ALINIA FOR ORAL SUSPENSION

(Nitazoxanide) 2677
May interact with highly protein bound drugs (selected). Compounds in these categories include:

Amiodarone Hydrochloride (Metabolite is highly bound to plasma protein. Use caution when administering nitazoxanide concurrently with other highly plasma protein-bound drugs with narrow therapeutic indices).
No products indexed under this heading.

Amitriptyline Hydrochloride (Metabolite is highly bound to plasma protein. Use caution when administering nitazoxanide concurrently with other highly plasma protein-bound drugs with narrow therapeutic indices).
No products indexed under this heading.

Atovaquone (Metabolite is highly bound to plasma protein. Use caution when administering nitazoxanide concurrently with other highly plasma protein-bound drugs with narrow therapeutic indices). Products include:
Malarone Pediatric Tablets 1521
Malarone Tablets 1521
Mepron Suspension 1526

Cefonicid Sodium (Metabolite is highly bound to plasma protein. Use caution when administering nitazoxanide concurrently with other highly plasma protein-bound drugs with narrow therapeutic indices).
No products indexed under this heading.

Celecoxib (Metabolite is highly bound to plasma protein. Use caution when administering nitazoxanide concurrently with other highly plasma protein-bound drugs with narrow therapeutic indices). Products include:
Celebrex Capsules 2979

Chlordiazepoxide (Metabolite is highly bound to plasma protein. Use caution when administering nitazoxanide concurrently with other highly plasma protein-bound drugs with narrow therapeutic indices).
No products indexed under this heading.

Chlordiazepoxide Hydrochloride (Metabolite is highly bound to plasma protein. Use caution when administering nitazoxanide concurrently with other highly plasma protein-bound drugs with narrow therapeutic indices).
No products indexed under this heading.

Chlorpromazine (Metabolite is highly bound to plasma protein. Use caution when administering nitazoxanide concurrently with other highly plasma protein-bound drugs with narrow therapeutic indices).
No products indexed under this heading.

Chlorpromazine Hydrochloride (Metabolite is highly bound to plasma protein. Use caution when administering nitazoxanide concurrently with other highly plasma protein-bound drugs with narrow therapeutic indices).
No products indexed under this heading.

Clomipramine Hydrochloride (Metabolite is highly bound to plasma protein. Use caution when administering nitazoxanide concurrently with other highly plasma protein-bound drugs with narrow therapeutic indices).
No products indexed under this heading.

Clozapine (Metabolite is highly bound to plasma protein. Use caution when administering nitazoxanide concurrently with other highly plasma protein-bound drugs with narrow therapeutic indices).
No products indexed under this heading.

Cyclosporine (Metabolite is highly bound to plasma protein. Use caution when administering nitazoxanide concurrently with other highly plasma protein-bound drugs with narrow therapeutic indices). Products include:
Gengraf Capsules 435
Neoral Oral Solution 2280
Neoral Soft Gelatin Capsules 2280
Restasis Ophthalmic Emulsion 557
Sandimmune 2296

Diazepam (Metabolite is highly bound to plasma protein. Use caution when administering nitazoxanide concurrently with other highly plasma protein-bound drugs with narrow therapeutic indices). Products include:
Valium Tablets 2658

Diclofenac Potassium (Metabolite is highly bound to plasma protein. Use caution when administering nitazoxanide concurrently with other highly plasma protein-bound drugs with narrow therapeutic indices).
No products indexed under this heading.

Diclofenac Sodium (Metabolite is highly bound to plasma protein. Use caution when administering nitazoxanide concurrently with other highly plasma protein-bound drugs with narrow therapeutic indices).
Products include:
Diclofenac Sodium Ophthalmic Solution.. ⊙240
Voltaren Ophthalmic Solution 2336
Voltaren Tablets 2334
Voltaren-XR Tablets 2337

Dipyridamole (Metabolite is highly bound to plasma protein. Use caution when administering nitazoxanide concurrently with other highly plasma protein-bound drugs with narrow therapeutic indices). Products include:
Aggrenox Capsules 819
Persantine Tablets 869

Fenoprofen Calcium (Metabolite is highly bound to plasma protein. Use caution when administering nitazoxanide concurrently with other highly plasma protein-bound drugs with narrow therapeutic indices).
Products include:
Nalfon Capsules 2508

Flurazepam Hydrochloride (Metabolite is highly bound to plasma protein. Use caution when administering nitazoxanide concurrently with other highly plasma protein-bound drugs with narrow therapeutic indices).
No products indexed under this heading.

Flurbiprofen (Metabolite is highly bound to plasma protein. Use caution when administering nitazoxanide concurrently with other highly plasma protein-bound drugs with narrow therapeutic indices).
No products indexed under this heading.

Glipizide (Metabolite is highly bound to plasma protein. Use caution when administering nitazoxanide concurrently with other highly plasma protein-bound drugs with narrow therapeutic indices).
No products indexed under this heading.

Ibuprofen (Metabolite is highly bound to plasma protein. Use caution when administering nitazoxanide concurrently with other highly plasma protein-bound drugs with narrow therapeutic indices). Products include:
Motrin IB Tablets and Caplets 1900
Children's Motrin Oral Suspension ... 1901
Children's Motrin Non-Staining Dye-Free Oral Suspension............ 1901
Children's Motrin Cold Oral Suspension 1899
Infants' Motrin Concentrated Drops.. 1901
Infants' Motrin Non-Staining Dye-Free Concentrated Drops....... 1901
Junior Strength Motrin Caplets and Chewable Tablets.................. 1901
Vicoprofen Tablets 533

Imipramine Hydrochloride (Metabolite is highly bound to plasma protein. Use caution when administering nitazoxanide concurrently with other highly plasma protein-bound drugs with narrow therapeutic indices).
No products indexed under this heading.

Imipramine Pamoate (Metabolite is highly bound to plasma protein. Use caution when administering nitazoxanide concurrently with other highly plasma protein-bound drugs with narrow therapeutic indices).
No products indexed under this heading.

Indomethacin (Metabolite is highly bound to plasma protein. Use caution when administering nitazoxanide concurrently with other highly plasma protein-bound drugs with narrow therapeutic indices). Products include:
Indocin 2024

Indomethacin Sodium Trihydrate (Metabolite is highly bound to plasma protein. Use caution when administering nitazoxanide concurrently with other highly plasma protein-bound drugs with narrow therapeutic indices). Products include:
Indocin I.V. 2489

Ketoprofen (Metabolite is highly bound to plasma protein. Use caution when administering nitazoxanide concurrently with other highly plasma protein-bound drugs with narrow therapeutic indices).
No products indexed under this heading.

Ketorolac Tromethamine (Metabolite is highly bound to plasma protein. Use caution when administering nitazoxanide concurrently with other highly plasma protein-bound drugs with narrow therapeutic indices).
No products indexed under this heading.

Meclofenamate Sodium (Metabolite is highly bound to plasma protein. Use caution when administering nitazoxanide concurrently with other highly plasma protein-bound drugs with narrow therapeutic indices).
No products indexed under this heading.

Mefenamic Acid (Metabolite is highly bound to plasma protein. Use caution when administering nitazoxanide concurrently with other highly plasma protein-bound drugs with narrow therapeutic indices).
No products indexed under this heading.

Midazolam Hydrochloride (Metabolite is highly bound to plasma protein. Use caution when administering nitazoxanide concurrently with other highly plasma protein-bound drugs with narrow therapeutic indices).
No products indexed under this heading.

Naproxen (Metabolite is highly bound to plasma protein. Use caution when administering nitazoxanide concurrently with other highly plasma protein-bound drugs with narrow therapeutic indices). Products include:
EC-Naprosyn Delayed-Release Tablets 2632
Naprosyn Suspension 2632
Naprosyn Tablets 2632

Naproxen Sodium (Metabolite is highly bound to plasma protein. Use caution when administering nitazoxanide concurrently with other highly plasma protein-bound drugs with narrow therapeutic indices).
Products include:
Anaprox Tablets 2632
Anaprox DS Tablets 2632
Treximet Tablets 1616

Nortriptyline Hydrochloride (Metabolite is highly bound to plasma protein. Use caution when administering nitazoxanide concurrently with other highly plasma protein-bound drugs with narrow therapeutic indices).
No products indexed under this heading.

Oxaprozin (Metabolite is highly bound to plasma protein. Use caution when administering nitazoxanide concurrently with other highly plasma protein-bound drugs with narrow therapeutic indices).
No products indexed under this heading.

Oxazepam (Metabolite is highly bound to plasma protein. Use caution when administering nitazoxanide concurrently with other highly plasma protein-bound drugs with narrow therapeutic indices).
No products indexed under this heading.

Phenylbutazone (Metabolite is highly bound to plasma protein. Use caution when administering nitazoxanide concurrently with other highly plasma protein-bound drugs with narrow therapeutic indices).
No products indexed under this heading.

Piroxicam (Metabolite is highly bound to plasma protein. Use caution when administering nitazoxanide concurrently with other highly plasma protein-bound drugs with narrow therapeutic indices).
No products indexed under this heading.

Propranolol Hydrochloride (Metabolite is highly bound to plasma protein. Use caution when administering nitazoxanide concurrently with other highly plasma protein-bound drugs with narrow therapeutic indices). Products include:

InnoPran XL Extended Release Capsules 1484

Sulindac (Metabolite is highly bound to plasma protein. Use caution when administering nitazoxanide concurrently with other highly plasma protein-bound drugs with narrow therapeutic indices). Products include:

Clinoril Tablets 1962

Temazepam (Metabolite is highly bound to plasma protein. Use caution when administering nitazoxanide concurrently with other highly plasma protein-bound drugs with narrow therapeutic indices).

No products indexed under this heading.

Tolbutamide (Metabolite is highly bound to plasma protein. Use caution when administering nitazoxanide concurrently with other highly plasma protein-bound drugs with narrow therapeutic indices).

No products indexed under this heading.

Tolmetin Sodium (Metabolite is highly bound to plasma protein. Use caution when administering nitazoxanide concurrently with other highly plasma protein-bound drugs with narrow therapeutic indices).

No products indexed under this heading.

Trimipramine Maleate (Metabolite is highly bound to plasma protein. Use caution when administering nitazoxanide concurrently with other highly plasma protein-bound drugs with narrow therapeutic indices).

No products indexed under this heading.

Warfarin Sodium (Metabolite is highly bound to plasma protein. Use caution when administering nitazoxanide concurrently with other highly plasma protein-bound drugs with narrow therapeutic indices).

No products indexed under this heading.

ALINIA TABLETS

(Nitazoxanide) 2677

See Alinia for Oral Suspension

ALLEGRA ORAL SOLUTION

(Fexofenadine Hydrochloride) 2684

See Allegra Tablets

ALLEGRA TABLETS

(Fexofenadine Hydrochloride) 2684

May interact with erythromycin and certain other agents. Compounds in these categories include:

Aluminum Hydroxide (Administration of fexofenadine within 15 minutes of an aluminum and magnesium containing antacid decreased fexofenadine AUC by 41% and Cmax by 43%; Allegra should not be taken closely in time with aluminum and magnesium containing antacids).

No products indexed under this heading.

Erythromycin (Co-administration with erythromycin has led to increased plasma levels of fexofenadine).

No products indexed under this heading.

Erythromycin Estolate (Co-administration with erythromycin has led to increased plasma levels of fexofenadine).

No products indexed under this heading.

Erythromycin Ethylsuccinate (Co-administration with erythromycin has led to increased plasma levels of fexofenadine). Products include:

E.E.S. 433
EryPed 431

Erythromycin Gluceptate (Co-administration with erythromycin has led to increased plasma levels of fexofenadine).

No products indexed under this heading.

Erythromycin Lactobionate (Co-administration with erythromycin has led to increased plasma levels of fexofenadine).

No products indexed under this heading.

Erythromycin Stearate (Co-administration with erythromycin has led to increased plasma levels of fexofenadine).

No products indexed under this heading.

Ketoconazole (Co-administration with ketoconazole as led to increased plasma levels of fexofenadine). Products include:

Extina Foam, 2% 3057
Nizoral A-D Shampoo 1901

Magnesium Hydroxide (Administration of fexofenadine within 15 minutes of an aluminum and magnesium containing antacid decreased fexofenadine AUC by 41% and Cmax by 43%; Allegra should not be taken closely in time with aluminum and magnesium containing antacids). Products include:

Fleet Pedia-Lax Chewable Tablets 1145
Pepcid Complete Chewable Tablets 1771
Extra Strength Rolaids Freshmint Tablets 1903
Rolaids Multi-Symptom Berry Tablets 1903
Rolaids Original Peppermint Tablets 1903

Food Interactions

Fruit juices, unspecified (Grapefruit, orange and apple may reduce the bioavailability and exposure of fexofenadine; it is recommended that fexofenadine should be taken with water).

ALLEGRA-D 12 HOUR EXTENDED-RELEASE TABLETS

(Fexofenadine Hydrochloride, Pseudoephedrine Hydrochloride) 2687

May interact with antacids, erythromycin, cardiac glycosides, monoamine oxidase inhibitors, sympathomimetics, and certain other agents. Compounds in these categories include:

Albuterol (Combined effects of pseudoephedrine with other sympathomimetics on cardiovascular system may be harmful to the patient).

No products indexed under this heading.

Albuterol Sulfate (Combined effects of pseudoephedrine with other sympathomimetics on cardiovascular system may be harmful to the patient). Products include:

Combivent Inhalation Aerosol 845
ProAir HFA Inhalation Aerosol 3113
Proventil HFA Inhalation Aerosol 2914
Ventolin HFA Inhalation Aerosol 1638

Aluminum Carbonate (Co-administration with fexofenadine HCL may decrease fexofenadine AUC by 41% and Cmax by 43%).

No products indexed under this heading.

Aluminum Hydroxide (Co-administration with fexofenadine HCL may decrease fexofenadine AUC by 41% and Cmax by 43%).

No products indexed under this heading.

Deslanoside (Increased ectopic pacemaker activity can occur when pseudoephedrine is used concomitantly with digitalis).

No products indexed under this heading.

Digitalis Glycoside Preparations (Increased ectopic pacemaker activity can occur when pseudoephedrine is used concomitantly with digitalis).

No products indexed under this heading.

Digitoxin (Increased ectopic pacemaker activity can occur when pseudoephedrine is used concomitantly with digitalis).

No products indexed under this heading.

Digoxin (Increased ectopic pacemaker activity can occur when pseudoephedrine is used concomitantly with digitalis). Products include:

Lanoxin Injection 1498
Lanoxin Injection Pediatric 1502
Lanoxin Tablets 1505

Dobutamine Hydrochloride (Combined effects of pseudoephedrine with other sympathomimetics on cardiovascular system may be harmful to the patient).

No products indexed under this heading.

Dopamine Hydrochloride (Combined effects of pseudoephedrine with other sympathomimetics on cardiovascular system may be harmful to the patient).

No products indexed under this heading.

Ephedrine Hydrochloride (Combined effects of pseudoephedrine with other sympathomimetics on cardiovascular system may be harmful to the patient).

No products indexed under this heading.

Ephedrine Sulfate (Combined effects of pseudoephedrine with other sympathomimetics on cardiovascular system may be harmful to the patient).

No products indexed under this heading.

Ephedrine Tannate (Combined effects of pseudoephedrine with other sympathomimetics on cardiovascular system may be harmful to the patient).

No products indexed under this heading.

Epinephrine (Combined effects of pseudoephedrine with other sympathomimetics on cardiovascular system may be harmful to the patient). Products include:

EpiPen 1024

Epinephrine Bitartrate (Combined effects of pseudoephedrine with other sympathomimetics on cardiovascular system may be harmful to the patient).

No products indexed under this heading.

Epinephrine Hydrochloride (Combined effects of pseudoephedrine with other sympathomimetics on cardiovascular system may be harmful to the patient).

No products indexed under this heading.

Erythromycin (Co-administration with erythromycin enhances fexofenadine gastrointestinal absorption thereby increasing plasma levels of fexofenadine; in vivo animal studies suggest that erythromycin may also decrease biliary excretion).

No products indexed under this heading.

Erythromycin Estolate (Co-administration with erythromycin enhances fexofenadine gastrointestinal absorption thereby increasing plasma levels of fexofenadine; in vivo animal studies suggest that erythromycin may also decrease biliary excretion).

No products indexed under this heading.

Erythromycin Ethylsuccinate (Co-administration with erythromycin enhances fexofenadine gastrointestinal absorption thereby increasing plasma levels of fexofenadine; in vivo animal studies suggest that erythromycin may also decrease biliary excretion). Products include:

E.E.S. 433
EryPed 431

Erythromycin Gluceptate (Co-administration with erythromycin enhances fexofenadine gastrointestinal absorption thereby increasing plasma levels of fexofenadine; in vivo animal studies suggest that erythromycin may also decrease biliary excretion).

No products indexed under this heading.

Erythromycin Lactobionate (Co-administration with erythromycin enhances fexofenadine gastrointestinal absorption thereby increasing plasma levels of fexofenadine; in vivo animal studies suggest that erythromycin may also decrease biliary excretion).

No products indexed under this heading.

Erythromycin Stearate (Co-administration with erythromycin enhances fexofenadine gastrointestinal absorption thereby increasing plasma levels of fexofenadine; in vivo animal studies suggest that erythromycin may also decrease biliary excretion).

No products indexed under this heading.

Isocarboxazid (Concurrent and/or sequential use with MAO inhibitors is contraindicated). Products include:

Marplan Tablets 3177

Isoproterenol Hydrochloride (Combined effects of pseudoephedrine with other sympathomimetics on cardiovascular system may be harmful to the patient).

No products indexed under this heading.

Isoproterenol Sulfate (Combined effects of pseudoephedrine with other sympathomimetics on cardiovascular system may be harmful to the patient).

No products indexed under this heading.

Ketoconazole (Co-administration with ketoconazole enhances fexofenadine gastrointestinal absorption thereby increasing plasma levels of fexofenadine; in vivo animal studies suggest that ketoconazole may also decrease fexofenadine gastrointestinal secretion). Products include:

Extina Foam, 2% 3057
Nizoral A-D Shampoo 1901

Levalbuterol Hydrochloride (Combined effects of pseudoephedrine with other sympathomimetics on cardiovascular system may be harmful to the patient). Products include:

Xopenex Inhalation Solution 3001
Xopenex Inhalation Solution Concentrate 3005

Magaldrate (Co-administration with fexofenadine HCL may decrease fexofenadine AUC by 41% and Cmax by 43%).

No products indexed under this heading.

Magnesium Hydroxide (Co-administration with fexofenadine HCL may decrease fexofenadine AUC by 41% and Cmax by 43%). Products include:

Fleet Pedia-Lax Chewable Tablets 1145
Pepcid Complete Chewable Tablets 1771
Extra Strength Rolaids Freshmint Tablets 1903
Rolaids Multi-Symptom Berry Tablets 1903
Rolaids Original Peppermint Tablets 1903

Magnesium Oxide (Co-administration with fexofenadine HCL may decrease fexofenadine AUC by 41% and Cmax by 43%). Products include:

Beelith Tablets 813

Mecamylamine Hydrochloride (Reduced antihypertensive effects).

No products indexed under this heading.

Metaproterenol Sulfate (Combined effects of pseudoephedrine with other sympathomimetics on cardiovascular system may be harmful to the patient).

No products indexed under this heading.

Metaraminol Bitartrate (Combined effects of pseudoephedrine with other sympathomimetics on cardiovascular system may be harmful to the patient).

No products indexed under this heading.

Methoxamine Hydrochloride (Combined effects of pseudoephedrine with other sympathomimetics on cardiovascular system may be harmful to the patient).

No products indexed under this heading.

Methyldopa (Reduced antihypertensive effects).

No products indexed under this heading.

Methyldopate Hydrochloride (Reduced antihypertensive effects).

No products indexed under this heading.

Moclobemide (Concurrent and/or sequential use with MAO inhibitors is contraindicated).

No products indexed under this heading.

Norepinephrine Bitartrate (Combined effects of pseudoephedrine with other sympathomimetics on cardiovascular system may be harmful to the patient).

No products indexed under this heading.

Pargyline Hydrochloride (Concurrent and/or sequential use with MAO inhibitors is contraindicated).

No products indexed under this heading.

Phenelzine Sulfate (Concurrent and/or sequential use with MAO inhibitors is contraindicated).

No products indexed under this heading.

Phenylephrine Bitartrate (Combined effects of pseudoephedrine with other sympathomimetics on cardiovascular system may be harmful to the patient).

No products indexed under this heading.

Phenylephrine Hydrochloride (Combined effects of pseudoephedrine with other sympathomimetics on cardiovascular system may be harmful to the patient). Products include:

Actifed Cold & Allergy Tablets 1895
Benadryl Allergy & Cold Kapgels 1895
Benadryl Allergy & Sinus Headache Kapgels 1895
Benadryl Severe Allergy & Sinus Headache Caplets 1897
Children's Benadryl-D Allergy & Sinus Liquid 1896
Benadryl-D Allergy & Sinus Tablet 1896
PediaCare Children's Allergy & Cold Liquid 1902
PediaCare Children's Decongestant Liquid 1902
PediaCare Children's Liquid Multi-Symptom Cold 1902
Sinutab Non-Drying Caplets 1905
Sinutab Sinus Caplets 1905
Children's Sudafed PE Cold & Cough Liquid 1907
Children's Sudafed PE Nasal Decongestant Liquid 1906
Sudafed PE Cold & Cough Caplets 1907
Sudafed PE Nasal Decongestant Tablets 1907
Sudafed PE Nighttime Cold Caplets 1907
Sudafed PE Non-Drying Sinus Caplets 1908
Sudafed PE Severe Cold Caplets 1908
Sudafed PE Sinus & Allergy Tablets 1908
Sudafed PE Sinus Headache Caplets 1908
Tylenol Allergy Multi-Symptom Caplets with Cool Burst and Rapid Release Gelcaps 1916
Tylenol Allergy Multi-Symptom Nighttime Caplets with Cool Burst 1916
Children's Tylenol Plus Cold Suspension Liquid 1912
Children's Tylenol Plus Cold & Allergy Suspension Liquid 1914
Children's Tylenol Plus Flu Suspension Liquid 1914
Children's Tylenol Plus Multi-Symptom Cold Suspension Liquid 1912
Tylenol Cold Head Congestion Daytime Caplets with Cool Burst 1910
Tylenol Cold Head Congestion Nighttime Caplets with Cool Burst 1910
Tylenol Cold Head Congestion Severe Daytime Caplets with Cool Burst 1910
Tylenol Cold Multi-Symptom Daytime Caplets with Cool Burst and Rapid Release Gels 1913
Tylenol Cold Multi-Symptom Daytime Liquid with Citrus Burst 1913
Tylenol Cold Multi-Symptom Nighttime Caplets with Cool Burst 1913
Tylenol Cold Multi-Symptom Nighttime Liquid with Cool Burst 1913
Tylenol Cold Multi-Symptom Severe Caplets with Cool Burst 1913
Tylenol Cold Multi-Symptom Severe Daytime Liquid with Citrus Burst 1913
Tylenol Sinus Congestion & Pain Daytime Caplets with Cool Burst and Gelcaps 1917
Tylenol Sinus Congestion & Pain Nighttime Caplets with Cool Burst 1917
Tylenol Sinus Congestion & Pain Severe Caplets with Cool Burst 1917
Vicks DayQuil Cold & Flu Multi-Symptom Relief .... ■ 616
Vicks DayQuil LiquiCaps 2567
Vicks DayQuil Liquid 2567
Vicks DayQuil Multi-Symptom Cold/Flu Relief 2567

Phenylephrine Tannate (Combined effects of pseudoephedrine with other sympathomimetics on cardiovascular system may be harmful to the patient).

No products indexed under this heading.

Phenylpropanolamine Hydrochloride (Combined effects of pseudoephedrine with other sympathomimetics on cardiovascular system may be harmful to the patient).

No products indexed under this heading.

Pirbuterol Acetate (Combined effects of pseudoephedrine with other sympathomimetics on cardiovascular system may be harmful to the patient). Products include:

Maxair Autohaler 1705

Procarbazine Hydrochloride (Concurrent and/or sequential use with MAO inhibitors is contraindicated).

No products indexed under this heading.

Pseudoephedrine Sulfate (Combined effects of pseudoephedrine with other sympathomimetics on cardiovascular system may be harmful to the patient). Products include:

Clarinex-D 12-Hour Extended-Release Tablets 2831
Clarinex-D 24-Hour Extended-Release Tablets 2834

Rasagiline Mesylate (Concurrent and/or sequential use with MAO inhibitors is contraindicated). Products include:

Azilect Tablets 3106

Reserpine (Reduced antihypertensive effects).

No products indexed under this heading.

Salmeterol Xinafoate (Combined effects of pseudoephedrine with other sympathomimetics on cardiovascular system may be harmful to the patient). Products include:

Advair Diskus 100/50 1276
Advair Diskus 250/50 1276
Advair Diskus 500/50 1276
Advair HFA 45/21 Inhalation Aerosol 1288
Advair HFA 115/21 Inhalation Aerosol 1288
Advair HFA 230/21 Inhalation Aerosol 1288
Serevent Diskus 1594

Selegiline (Concurrent and/or sequential use with MAO inhibitors is contraindicated). Products include:

Emsam Transdermal System 905

Selegiline Hydrochloride (Concurrent and/or sequential use with MAO inhibitors is contraindicated). Products include:

Eldepryl Capsules 3052

Sodium Bicarbonate (Co-administration with fexofenadine HCL may decrease fexofenadine AUC by 41% and Cmax by 43%). Products include:

Ceo-Two Laxative Suppository 815

Terbutaline Sulfate (Combined effects of pseudoephedrine with other sympathomimetics on cardiovascular system may be harmful to the patient).

No products indexed under this heading.

Tranylcypromine Sulfate (Concurrent and/or sequential use with MAO inhibitors is contraindicated). Products include:

Parnate Tablets 1532

Food Interactions

Apple Juice (Co-administration with grapefruit, orange or apple juice will reduce the bioavailability and exposure or fexofenadine).

Diet, high-lipid (Co-administration with a high-fat meal decreased fexofenadine plasma concentrations Cmax and AUC, and Tmax was delayed by 50%; the rate of extent of pseudoephedrine absorption was not affected by food; administration of Allegra-D with food should be avoided).

Grapefruit Juice (Co-administration with grapefruit, orange or apple juice will reduce the bioavailability and exposure or fexofenadine).

Orange Juice (Co-administration with grapefruit, orange or apple juice will reduce the bioavailability and exposure or fexofenadine).

ALLEGRA-D 24 HOUR EXTENDED-RELEASE TABLETS

(Fexofenadine Hydrochloride, Pseudoephedrine Hydrochloride) 2690

See Allegra-D 12 Hour Extended-Release Tablets

ALOXI INJECTION

(Palonosetron Hydrochloride) 1059

None cited in PDR database.

ALPHAGAN P OPHTHALMIC SOLUTION

(Brimonidine Tartrate) 549

May interact with anesthetics, antihypertensives, barbiturates, beta blockers, central nervous system depressants, cardiac glycosides, hypnotics and sedatives, monoamine oxidase inhibitors, narcotic analgesics, tricyclic antidepressants, and certain other agents. Compounds in these categories include:

Acebutolol Hydrochloride (Concurrent use of brimonidine, an alpha adrenergic agonist, with beta blockers (ophthalmic and systemic) may reduce pulse and blood pressure, however, in clinical trials brimonidine did not have any significant effects on pulse and blood pressure).

No products indexed under this heading.

Alfentanil Hydrochloride (Possible additive or potentiating effect with CNS depressants).

No products indexed under this heading.

Aliskiren (Concurrent use of brimonidine, an alpha adrenergic agonist, with antihypertensives may reduce pulse and blood pressure, however, in clinical trials brimonidine did not have any significant effects on pulse and blood pressure). Products include:

Tekturna Tablets 2321
Tekturna HCT Tablets 2324

Alprazolam (Possible additive or potentiating effect with CNS depressants).
No products indexed under this heading.

Amitriptyline Hydrochloride (Tricyclic antidepressants have been reported to blunt the hypotensive effect of systemic clonidine, an alpha adrenergic agonist; it is not known whether the concurrent use of these agents with brimonidine can lead to interference in IOP-lowering effect; caution is advised).
No products indexed under this heading.

Amlodipine Besylate (Concurrent use of brimonidine, an alpha adrenergic agonist, with antihypertensives may reduce pulse and blood pressure, however, in clinical trials brimonidine did not have any significant effects on pulse and blood pressure). Products include:
Azor Tablets **1005**
Exforge Tablets **2238**

Amoxapine (Tricyclic antidepressants have been reported to blunt the hypotensive effect of systemic clonidine, an alpha adrenergic agonist; it is not known whether the concurrent use of these agents with brimonidine can lead to interference in IOP-lowering effect; caution is advised).
No products indexed under this heading.

Aprobarbital (Possible additive or potentiating effect with CNS depressants).
No products indexed under this heading.

Atenolol (Concurrent use of brimonidine, an alpha adrenergic agonist, with beta blockers (ophthalmic and systemic) may reduce pulse and blood pressure, however, in clinical trials brimonidine did not have any significant effects on pulse and blood pressure).
No products indexed under this heading.

Benazepril Hydrochloride (Concurrent use of brimonidine, an alpha adrenergic agonist, with antihypertensives may reduce pulse and blood pressure, however, in clinical trials brimonidine did not have any significant effects on pulse and blood pressure).
No products indexed under this heading.

Bendroflumethiazide (Concurrent use of brimonidine, an alpha adrenergic agonist, with antihypertensives may reduce pulse and blood pressure, however, in clinical trials brimonidine did not have any significant effects on pulse and blood pressure).
No products indexed under this heading.

Betaxolol Hydrochloride (Concurrent use of brimonidine, an alpha adrenergic agonist, with beta blockers (ophthalmic and systemic) may reduce pulse and blood pressure, however, in clinical trials brimonidine did not have any significant effects on pulse and blood pressure).
No products indexed under this heading.

Bisoprolol Fumarate (Concurrent use of brimonidine, an alpha adrenergic agonist, with beta blockers (ophthalmic and systemic) may reduce pulse and blood pressure, however, in clinical trials brimonidine did not have any significant effects on pulse and blood pressure).
No products indexed under this heading.

Buprenorphine Hydrochloride (Possible additive or potentiating effect with CNS depressants). Products include:
Suboxone Tablets **2601**
Subutex Tablets **2601**

Buspirone Hydrochloride (Possible additive or potentiating effect with CNS depressants).
No products indexed under this heading.

Butabarbital (Possible additive or potentiating effect with CNS depressants).
No products indexed under this heading.

Butabarbital Sodium (Possible additive or potentiating effect with CNS depressants).
No products indexed under this heading.

Butalbital (Possible additive or potentiating effect with CNS depressants).
No products indexed under this heading.

Candesartan Cilexetil (Concurrent use of brimonidine, an alpha adrenergic agonist, with antihypertensives may reduce pulse and blood pressure, however, in clinical trials brimonidine did not have any significant effects on pulse and blood pressure). Products include:
Atacand Tablets **639**
Atacand HCT **642**

Captopril (Concurrent use of brimonidine, an alpha adrenergic agonist, with antihypertensives may reduce pulse and blood pressure, however, in clinical trials brimonidine did not have any significant effects on pulse and blood pressure). Products include:
Captopril Tablets **2182**

Carteolol Hydrochloride (Concurrent use of brimonidine, an alpha adrenergic agonist, with beta blockers (ophthalmic and systemic) may reduce pulse and blood pressure, however, in clinical trials brimonidine did not have any significant effects on pulse and blood pressure).
No products indexed under this heading.

Chloral Hydrate (Possible additive or potentiating effect with CNS depressants).
No products indexed under this heading.

Chlordiazepoxide (Possible additive or potentiating effect with CNS depressants).
No products indexed under this heading.

Chlordiazepoxide Hydrochloride (Possible additive or potentiating effect with CNS depressants).
No products indexed under this heading.

Chlorothiazide (Concurrent use of brimonidine, an alpha adrenergic agonist, with antihypertensives may reduce pulse and blood pressure, however, in clinical trials brimonidine did not have any significant effects on pulse and blood pressure).
No products indexed under this heading.

Chlorothiazide Sodium (Concurrent use of brimonidine, an alpha adrenergic agonist, with antihypertensives may reduce pulse and blood pressure, however, in clinical trials brimonidine did not have any significant effects on pulse and blood pressure). Products include:
Intravenous Sodium Diuril **2490**

Chlorpromazine (Possible additive or potentiating effect with CNS depressants).
No products indexed under this heading.

Chlorpromazine Hydrochloride (Possible additive or potentiating effect with CNS depressants).
No products indexed under this heading.

Chlorprothixene (Possible additive or potentiating effect with CNS depressants).
No products indexed under this heading.

Chlorprothixene Hydrochloride (Possible additive or potentiating effect with CNS depressants).
No products indexed under this heading.

Chlorprothixene Lactate (Possible additive or potentiating effect with CNS depressants).
No products indexed under this heading.

Chlorthalidone (Concurrent use of brimonidine, an alpha adrenergic agonist, with antihypertensives may reduce pulse and blood pressure, however, in clinical trials brimonidine did not have any significant effects on pulse and blood pressure). Products include:
Clorpres Tablets **2185**

Clomipramine Hydrochloride (Tricyclic antidepressants have been reported to blunt the hypotensive effect of systemic clonidine, an alpha adrenergic agonist; it is not known whether the concurrent use of these agents with brimonidine can lead to interference in IOP-lowering effect; caution is advised).
No products indexed under this heading.

Clonidine (Concurrent use of brimonidine, an alpha adrenergic agonist, with antihypertensives may reduce pulse and blood pressure, however, in clinical trials brimonidine did not have any significant effects on pulse and blood pressure). Products include:
Catapres-TTS **842**

Clonidine Hydrochloride (Concurrent use of brimonidine, an alpha adrenergic agonist, with antihypertensives may reduce pulse and blood pressure, however, in clinical trials brimonidine did not have any significant effects on pulse and blood pressure). Products include:
Catapres Tablets **841**
Clorpres Tablets **2185**

Clorazepate Dipotassium (Possible additive or potentiating effect with CNS depressants).
No products indexed under this heading.

Clozapine (Possible additive or potentiating effect with CNS depressants).
No products indexed under this heading.

Codeine Phosphate (Possible additive or potentiating effect with CNS depressants). Products include:
Tylenol with Codeine Tablets **2427**

Deserpidine (Concurrent use of brimonidine, an alpha adrenergic agonist, with antihypertensives may reduce pulse and blood pressure, however, in clinical trials brimonidine did not have any significant effects on pulse and blood pressure).
No products indexed under this heading.

Desflurane (Possible additive or potentiating effect with CNS depressants).
No products indexed under this heading.

Desipramine Hydrochloride (Tricyclic antidepressants have been reported to blunt the hypotensive effect of systemic clonidine, an alpha adrenergic agonist; it is not known whether the concurrent use of these agents with brimonidine can lead to interference in IOP-lowering effect; caution is advised).
No products indexed under this heading.

Deslanoside (Concurrent use of brimonidine, an alpha adrenergic agonist, with cardiac glycosides may reduce pulse and blood pressure, however, in clinical trials brimonidine did not have any significant effects on pulse and blood pressure).
No products indexed under this heading.

Dezocine (Possible additive or potentiating effect with CNS depressants).
No products indexed under this heading.

Diazepam (Possible additive or potentiating effect with CNS depressants). Products include:
Valium Tablets **2658**

Diazoxide (Concurrent use of brimonidine, an alpha adrenergic agonist, with antihypertensives may reduce pulse and blood pressure, however, in clinical trials brimonidine did not have any significant effects on pulse and blood pressure). Products include:
Proglycem Capsules **1185**
Proglycem Suspension **1185**

Digitalis Glycoside Preparations (Concurrent use of brimonidine, an alpha adrenergic agonist, with cardiac glycosides may reduce pulse and blood pressure, however, in clinical trials brimonidine did not have any significant effects on pulse and blood pressure).
No products indexed under this heading.

Digitoxin (Concurrent use of brimonidine, an alpha adrenergic agonist, with cardiac glycosides may reduce pulse and blood pressure, however, in clinical trials brimonidine did not have any significant effects on pulse and blood pressure).
No products indexed under this heading.

Digoxin (Concurrent use of brimonidine, an alpha adrenergic agonist, with cardiac glycosides may reduce pulse and blood pressure, however, in clinical trials brimonidine did not have any significant effects on pulse and blood pressure). Products include:

Lanoxin Injection 1498
Lanoxin Injection Pediatric 1502
Lanoxin Tablets 1505

Diltiazem Hydrochloride (Concurrent use of brimonidine, an alpha adrenergic agonist, with antihypertensives may reduce pulse and blood pressure, however, in clinical trials brimonidine did not have any significant effects on pulse and blood pressure). Products include:

Cardizem LA Extended Release Tablets 421

Doxazosin Mesylate (Concurrent use of brimonidine, an alpha adrenergic agonist, with antihypertensives may reduce pulse and blood pressure, however, in clinical trials brimonidine did not have any significant effects on pulse and blood pressure).

No products indexed under this heading.

Doxepin Hydrochloride (Tricyclic antidepressants have been reported to blunt the hypotensive effect of systemic clonidine, an alpha adrenergic agonist; it is not known whether the concurrent use of these agents with brimonidine can lead to interference in IOP-lowering effect; caution is advised).

No products indexed under this heading.

Droperidol (Possible additive or potentiating effect with CNS depressants).

No products indexed under this heading.

Enalapril Maleate (Concurrent use of brimonidine, an alpha adrenergic agonist, with antihypertensives may reduce pulse and blood pressure, however, in clinical trials brimonidine did not have any significant effects on pulse and blood pressure).

No products indexed under this heading.

Enalaprilat (Concurrent use of brimonidine, an alpha adrenergic agonist, with antihypertensives may reduce pulse and blood pressure, however, in clinical trials brimonidine did not have any significant effects on pulse and blood pressure).

No products indexed under this heading.

Enflurane (Possible additive or potentiating effect with CNS depressants).

No products indexed under this heading.

Eprosartan Mesylate (Concurrent use of brimonidine, an alpha adrenergic agonist, with antihypertensives may reduce pulse and blood pressure, however, in clinical trials brimonidine did not have any significant effects on pulse and blood pressure). Products include:

Teveten Tablets 515
Teveten HCT Tablets 517

Esmolol Hydrochloride (Concurrent use of brimonidine, an alpha adrenergic agonist, with beta blockers (ophthalmic and systemic) may reduce pulse and blood pressure, however, in clinical trials brimonidine did not have any significant effects on pulse and blood pressure).

No products indexed under this heading.

Estazolam (Possible additive or potentiating effect with CNS depressants).

No products indexed under this heading.

Ethanol (Possible additive or potentiating effect with CNS depressants).

No products indexed under this heading.

Ethchlorvynol (Possible additive or potentiating effect with CNS depressants).

No products indexed under this heading.

Ethinamate (Possible additive or potentiating effect with CNS depressants).

No products indexed under this heading.

Ethyl Alcohol (Possible additive or potentiating effect with CNS depressants).

No products indexed under this heading.

Felodipine (Concurrent use of brimonidine, an alpha adrenergic agonist, with antihypertensives may reduce pulse and blood pressure, however, in clinical trials brimonidine did not have any significant effects on pulse and blood pressure).

No products indexed under this heading.

Fentanyl (Possible additive or potentiating effect with CNS depressants). Products include:

Duragesic Transdermal System 2405
Ionsys Transdermal System 2410

Fentanyl Citrate (Possible additive or potentiating effect with CNS depressants). Products include:

Actiq 959
Fentora Tablets 968

Fluphenazine Decanoate (Possible additive or potentiating effect with CNS depressants).

No products indexed under this heading.

Fluphenazine Enanthate (Possible additive or potentiating effect with CNS depressants).

No products indexed under this heading.

Fluphenazine Hydrochloride (Possible additive or potentiating effect with CNS depressants).

No products indexed under this heading.

Flurazepam Hydrochloride (Possible additive or potentiating effect with CNS depressants).

No products indexed under this heading.

Fosinopril Sodium (Concurrent use of brimonidine, an alpha adrenergic agonist, with antihypertensives may reduce pulse and blood pressure, however, in clinical trials brimonidine did not have any significant effects on pulse and blood pressure).

No products indexed under this heading.

Furosemide (Concurrent use of brimonidine, an alpha adrenergic agonist, with antihypertensives may reduce pulse and blood pressure, however, in clinical trials brimonidine did not have any significant effects on pulse and blood pressure). Products include:

Furosemide Tablets 2186

Glutethimide (Possible additive or potentiating effect with CNS depressants).

No products indexed under this heading.

Guanabenz Acetate (Concurrent use of brimonidine, an alpha adrenergic agonist, with antihypertensives may reduce pulse and blood pressure, however, in clinical trials brimonidine did not have any significant effects on pulse and blood pressure).

No products indexed under this heading.

Guanethidine Monosulfate (Concurrent use of brimonidine, an alpha adrenergic agonist, with antihypertensives may reduce pulse and blood pressure, however, in clinical trials brimonidine did not have any significant effects on pulse and blood pressure).

No products indexed under this heading.

Haloperidol (Possible additive or potentiating effect with CNS depressants).

No products indexed under this heading.

Haloperidol Decanoate (Possible additive or potentiating effect with CNS depressants).

No products indexed under this heading.

Halothane (Possible additive or potentiating effect with CNS depressants).

No products indexed under this heading.

Hydralazine Hydrochloride (Concurrent use of brimonidine, an alpha adrenergic agonist, with antihypertensives may reduce pulse and blood pressure, however, in clinical trials brimonidine did not have any significant effects on pulse and blood pressure).

No products indexed under this heading.

Hydrochlorothiazide (Concurrent use of brimonidine, an alpha adrenergic agonist, with antihypertensives may reduce pulse and blood pressure, however, in clinical trials brimonidine did not have any significant effects on pulse and blood pressure). Products include:

Atacand HCT 642
Avalide Tablets 892
Avalide Tablets 2713
Benicar HCT Tablets 1010
Diovan HCT Tablets 2216
Dyazide Capsules 1405
Micardis HCT Tablets 854
Prinzide Tablets 2092
Tekturna HCT Tablets 2324
Teveten HCT Tablets 517

Hydrocodone Bitartrate (Possible additive or potentiating effect with CNS depressants). Products include:

Lortab 5/500 Tablets 3143
Lortab 7.5/500 Tablets 3144
Lortab 10/500 Tablets 3144
Vicodin Tablets 529
Vicodin ES Tablets 530
Vicodin HP Tablets 531
Vicoprofen Tablets 533
Zydone Tablets 1132

Hydrocodone Polistirex (Possible additive or potentiating effect with CNS depressants). Products include:

Tussionex Pennkinetic Extended-Release Suspension 3154

Hydroflumethiazide (Concurrent use of brimonidine, an alpha adrenergic agonist, with antihypertensives may reduce pulse and blood pressure, however, in clinical trials brimonidine did not have any significant effects on pulse and blood pressure).

No products indexed under this heading.

Hydromorphone Hydrochloride (Possible additive or potentiating effect with CNS depressants).

No products indexed under this heading.

Hydroxyzine Hydrochloride (Possible additive or potentiating effect with CNS depressants).

No products indexed under this heading.

Imipramine Hydrochloride (Tricyclic antidepressants have been reported to blunt the hypotensive effect of systemic clonidine, an alpha adrenergic agonist; it is not known whether the concurrent use of these agents with brimonidine can lead to interference in IOP-lowering effect; caution is advised).

No products indexed under this heading.

Imipramine Pamoate (Tricyclic antidepressants have been reported to blunt the hypotensive effect of systemic clonidine, an alpha adrenergic agonist; it is not known whether the concurrent use of these agents with brimonidine can lead to interference in IOP-lowering effect; caution is advised).

No products indexed under this heading.

Indapamide (Concurrent use of brimonidine, an alpha adrenergic agonist, with antihypertensives may reduce pulse and blood pressure, however, in clinical trials brimonidine did not have any significant effects on pulse and blood pressure). Products include:

Indapamide Tablets 2188

Irbesartan (Concurrent use of brimonidine, an alpha adrenergic agonist, with antihypertensives may reduce pulse and blood pressure, however, in clinical trials brimonidine did not have any significant effects on pulse and blood pressure). Products include:

Avalide Tablets 892
Avalide Tablets 2713
Avapro Tablets 897
Avapro Tablets 2718

Isocarboxazid (Concurrent use of brimonidine, an alpha adrenergic agonist, and MAO inhibitor is contraindicated). Products include:

Marplan Tablets 3177

Isoflurane (Possible additive or potentiating effect with CNS depressants).

No products indexed under this heading.

Isradipine (Concurrent use of brimonidine, an alpha adrenergic agonist, with antihypertensives may reduce pulse and blood pressure, however, in clinical trials brimonidine did not have any significant effects on pulse and blood pressure). Products include:

DynaCirc CR Controlled Release Tablets 1407

Ketamine Hydrochloride (Possible additive or potentiating effect with CNS depressants).
No products indexed under this heading.

Labetalol Hydrochloride (Concurrent use of brimonidine, an alpha adrenergic agonist, with beta blockers (ophthalmic and systemic) may reduce pulse and blood pressure, however, in clinical trials brimonidine did not have any significant effects on pulse and blood pressure).
No products indexed under this heading.

Levobunolol Hydrochloride (Concurrent use of brimonidine, an alpha adrenergic agonist, with beta blockers (ophthalmic and systemic) may reduce pulse and blood pressure, however, in clinical trials brimonidine did not have any significant effects on pulse and blood pressure).
No products indexed under this heading.

Levomethadyl Acetate Hydrochloride (Possible additive or potentiating effect with CNS depressants).
No products indexed under this heading.

Levorphanol Tartrate (Possible additive or potentiating effect with CNS depressants).
No products indexed under this heading.

Lisinopril (Concurrent use of brimonidine, an alpha adrenergic agonist, with antihypertensives may reduce pulse and blood pressure, however, in clinical trials brimonidine did not have any significant effects on pulse and blood pressure). Products include:
Prinivil Tablets 2087
Prinzide Tablets 2092

Lorazepam (Possible additive or potentiating effect with CNS depressants).
No products indexed under this heading.

Losartan Potassium (Concurrent use of brimonidine, an alpha adrenergic agonist, with antihypertensives may reduce pulse and blood pressure, however, in clinical trials brimonidine did not have any significant effects on pulse and blood pressure). Products include:
Cozaar Tablets 1973

Loxapine Hydrochloride (Possible additive or potentiating effect with CNS depressants).
No products indexed under this heading.

Loxapine Succinate (Possible additive or potentiating effect with CNS depressants).
No products indexed under this heading.

Maprotiline Hydrochloride (Tricyclic antidepressants have been reported to blunt the hypotensive effect of systemic clonidine, an alpha adrenergic agonist; it is not known whether the concurrent use of these agents with brimonidine can lead to interference in IOP-lowering effect; caution is advised).
No products indexed under this heading.

Mecamylamine Hydrochloride (Concurrent use of brimonidine, an alpha adrenergic agonist, with antihypertensives may reduce pulse and blood pressure, however, in clinical trials brimonidine did not have any significant effects on pulse and blood pressure).
No products indexed under this heading.

Meperidine Hydrochloride (Possible additive or potentiating effect with CNS depressants).
No products indexed under this heading.

Mephobarbital (Possible additive or potentiating effect with CNS depressants).
No products indexed under this heading.

Meprobamate (Possible additive or potentiating effect with CNS depressants).
No products indexed under this heading.

Mesoridazine Besylate (Possible additive or potentiating effect with CNS depressants).
No products indexed under this heading.

Methadone Hydrochloride (Possible additive or potentiating effect with CNS depressants).
No products indexed under this heading.

Methohexital Sodium (Possible additive or potentiating effect with CNS depressants).
No products indexed under this heading.

Methotrimeprazine (Possible additive or potentiating effect with CNS depressants).
No products indexed under this heading.

Methoxyflurane (Possible additive or potentiating effect with CNS depressants).
No products indexed under this heading.

Methyclothiazide (Concurrent use of brimonidine, an alpha adrenergic agonist, with antihypertensives may reduce pulse and blood pressure, however, in clinical trials brimonidine did not have any significant effects on pulse and blood pressure).
No products indexed under this heading.

Methyldopa (Concurrent use of brimonidine, an alpha adrenergic agonist, with antihypertensives may reduce pulse and blood pressure, however, in clinical trials brimonidine did not have any significant effects on pulse and blood pressure).
No products indexed under this heading.

Methyldopate Hydrochloride (Concurrent use of brimonidine, an alpha adrenergic agonist, with antihypertensives may reduce pulse and blood pressure, however, in clinical trials brimonidine did not have any significant effects on pulse and blood pressure).
No products indexed under this heading.

Metipranolol Hydrochloride (Concurrent use of brimonidine, an alpha adrenergic agonist, with beta blockers (ophthalmic and systemic) may reduce pulse and blood pressure, however, in clinical trials brimonidine did not have any significant effects on pulse and blood pressure).
No products indexed under this heading.

Metolazone (Concurrent use of brimonidine, an alpha adrenergic agonist, with antihypertensives may reduce pulse and blood pressure, however, in clinical trials brimonidine did not have any significant effects on pulse and blood pressure).
No products indexed under this heading.

Metoprolol Succinate (Concurrent use of brimonidine, an alpha adrenergic agonist, with beta blockers (ophthalmic and systemic) may reduce pulse and blood pressure, however, in clinical trials brimonidine did not have any significant effects on pulse and blood pressure). Products include:
Toprol-XL Tablets 666

Metoprolol Tartrate (Concurrent use of brimonidine, an alpha adrenergic agonist, with beta blockers (ophthalmic and systemic) may reduce pulse and blood pressure, however, in clinical trials brimonidine did not have any significant effects on pulse and blood pressure).
No products indexed under this heading.

Metyrosine (Concurrent use of brimonidine, an alpha adrenergic agonist, with antihypertensives may reduce pulse and blood pressure, however, in clinical trials brimonidine did not have any significant effects on pulse and blood pressure). Products include:
Demser Capsules 1989

Mibefradil Dihydrochloride (Concurrent use of brimonidine, an alpha adrenergic agonist, with antihypertensives may reduce pulse and blood pressure, however, in clinical trials brimonidine did not have any significant effects on pulse and blood pressure).
No products indexed under this heading.

Midazolam Hydrochloride (Possible additive or potentiating effect with CNS depressants).
No products indexed under this heading.

Minoxidil (Concurrent use of brimonidine, an alpha adrenergic agonist, with antihypertensives may reduce pulse and blood pressure, however, in clinical trials brimonidine did not have any significant effects on pulse and blood pressure).
No products indexed under this heading.

Moclobemide (Concurrent use of brimonidine, an alpha adrenergic agonist, and MAO inhibitor is contraindicated).
No products indexed under this heading.

Moexipril Hydrochloride (Concurrent use of brimonidine, an alpha adrenergic agonist, with antihypertensives may reduce pulse and blood pressure, however, in clinical trials brimonidine did not have any significant effects on pulse and blood pressure).
No products indexed under this heading.

Molindone Hydrochloride (Possible additive or potentiating effect with CNS depressants). Products include:
Moban Tablets 1116

Morphine Sulfate (Possible additive or potentiating effect with CNS depressants). Products include:
Avinza Capsules 1772
DepoDur Injection 1095
MS Contin Tablets 2585

Nadolol (Concurrent use of brimonidine, an alpha adrenergic agonist, with beta blockers (ophthalmic and systemic) may reduce pulse and blood pressure, however, in clinical trials brimonidine did not have any significant effects on pulse and blood pressure). Products include:
Nadolol Tablets 2191

Nebivolol (Concurrent use of brimonidine, an alpha adrenergic agonist, with beta blockers (ophthalmic and systemic) may reduce pulse and blood pressure, however, in clinical trials brimonidine did not have any significant effects on pulse and blood pressure). Products include:
Bystolic Tablets 1155

Nicardipine Hydrochloride (Concurrent use of brimonidine, an alpha adrenergic agonist, with antihypertensives may reduce pulse and blood pressure, however, in clinical trials brimonidine did not have any significant effects on pulse and blood pressure). Products include:
Cardene I.V. 1093

Nifedipine (Concurrent use of brimonidine, an alpha adrenergic agonist, with antihypertensives may reduce pulse and blood pressure, however, in clinical trials brimonidine did not have any significant effects on pulse and blood pressure).
No products indexed under this heading.

Nisoldipine (Concurrent use of brimonidine, an alpha adrenergic agonist, with antihypertensives may reduce pulse and blood pressure, however, in clinical trials brimonidine did not have any significant effects on pulse and blood pressure). Products include:
Sular Extended Release Tablets 2975

Nitroglycerin (Concurrent use of brimonidine, an alpha adrenergic agonist, with antihypertensives may reduce pulse and blood pressure, however, in clinical trials brimonidine did not have any significant effects on pulse and blood pressure). Products include:
Nitro-Dur Transdermal Infusion System 2887
Nitrolingual Pumpspray 2965

Nortriptyline Hydrochloride (Tricyclic antidepressants have been reported to blunt the hypotensive effect of systemic clonidine, an alpha adrenergic agonist; it is not known whether the concurrent use of these agents with brimonidine can lead to interference in IOP-lowering effect; caution is advised).
No products indexed under this heading.

Olanzapine (Possible additive or potentiating effect with CNS depressants). Products include:
Symbyax Capsules 1871
Zyprexa Tablets 1883
Zyprexa IntraMuscular 1883
Zyprexa ZYDIS Orally Disintegrating Tablets 1883

Oxazepam (Possible additive or potentiating effect with CNS depressants).
No products indexed under this heading.

Oxycodone Hydrochloride (Possible additive or potentiating effect with CNS depressants). Products include:
OxyContin Tablets 2589
OxyIR Capsules 2593
Percocet Tablets 1127
Percodan Tablets 1130

Pargyline Hydrochloride (Concurrent use of brimonidine, an alpha adrenergic agonist, and MAO inhibitor is contraindicated).
No products indexed under this heading.

Penbutolol Sulfate (Concurrent use of brimonidine, an alpha adrenergic agonist, with beta blockers (ophthalmic and systemic) may reduce pulse and blood pressure, however, in clinical trials brimonidine did not have any significant effects on pulse and blood pressure).
No products indexed under this heading.

Pentobarbital Sodium (Possible additive or potentiating effect with CNS depressants). Products include:
Nembutal Sodium Solution, USP 2494

Perindopril Erbumine (Concurrent use of brimonidine, an alpha adrenergic agonist, with antihypertensives may reduce pulse and blood pressure, however, in clinical trials brimonidine did not have any significant effects on pulse and blood pressure). Products include:
Aceon Tablets (2 mg, 4 mg, 8 mg) 3038

Perphenazine (Possible additive or potentiating effect with CNS depressants).
No products indexed under this heading.

Phenelzine Sulfate (Concurrent use of brimonidine, an alpha adrenergic agonist, and MAO inhibitor is contraindicated).
No products indexed under this heading.

Phenobarbital (Possible additive or potentiating effect with CNS depressants). Products include:
Donnatal Extentabs 2507

Phenoxybenzamine Hydrochloride (Concurrent use of brimonidine, an alpha adrenergic agonist, with antihypertensives may reduce pulse and blood pressure, however, in clinical trials brimonidine did not have any significant effects on pulse and blood pressure). Products include:
Dibenzyline Capsules 3188

Phentolamine Mesylate (Concurrent use of brimonidine, an alpha adrenergic agonist, with antihypertensives may reduce pulse and blood pressure, however, in clinical trials brimonidine did not have any significant effects on pulse and blood pressure).
No products indexed under this heading.

Pindolol (Concurrent use of brimonidine, an alpha adrenergic agonist, with beta blockers (ophthalmic and systemic) may reduce pulse and blood pressure, however, in clinical trials brimonidine did not have any significant effects on pulse and blood pressure).
No products indexed under this heading.

Polythiazide (Concurrent use of brimonidine, an alpha adrenergic agonist, with antihypertensives may reduce pulse and blood pressure, however, in clinical trials brimonidine did not have any significant effects on pulse and blood pressure).
No products indexed under this heading.

Prazepam (Possible additive or potentiating effect with CNS depressants).
No products indexed under this heading.

Prazosin Hydrochloride (Concurrent use of brimonidine, an alpha adrenergic agonist, with antihypertensives may reduce pulse and blood pressure, however, in clinical trials brimonidine did not have any significant effects on pulse and blood pressure).
No products indexed under this heading.

Procarbazine Hydrochloride (Concurrent use of brimonidine, an alpha adrenergic agonist, and MAO inhibitor is contraindicated).
No products indexed under this heading.

Prochlorperazine (Possible additive or potentiating effect with CNS depressants).
No products indexed under this heading.

Promethazine Hydrochloride (Possible additive or potentiating effect with CNS depressants).
No products indexed under this heading.

Propofol (Possible additive or potentiating effect with CNS depressants).
No products indexed under this heading.

Propoxyphene Hydrochloride (Possible additive or potentiating effect with CNS depressants).
No products indexed under this heading.

Propoxyphene Napsylate (Possible additive or potentiating effect with CNS depressants).
No products indexed under this heading.

Propranolol Hydrochloride (Concurrent use of brimonidine, an alpha adrenergic agonist, with beta blockers (ophthalmic and systemic) may reduce pulse and blood pressure, however, in clinical trials brimonidine did not have any significant effects on pulse and blood pressure). Products include:
InnoPran XL Extended Release Capsules 1484

Protriptyline Hydrochloride (Tricyclic antidepressants have been reported to blunt the hypotensive effect of systemic clonidine, an alpha adrenergic agonist; it is not known whether the concurrent use of these agents with brimonidine can lead to interference in IOP-lowering effect; caution is advised).
No products indexed under this heading.

Quazepam (Possible additive or potentiating effect with CNS depressants).
No products indexed under this heading.

Quetiapine Fumarate (Possible additive or potentiating effect with CNS depressants).
No products indexed under this heading.

Quinapril Hydrochloride (Concurrent use of brimonidine, an alpha adrenergic agonist, with antihypertensives may reduce pulse and blood pressure, however, in clinical trials brimonidine did not have any significant effects on pulse and blood pressure).
No products indexed under this heading.

Ramelteon (Possible additive or potentiating effect with CNS depressants). Products include:
Rozerem Tablets 3091

Ramipril (Concurrent use of brimonidine, an alpha adrenergic agonist, with antihypertensives may reduce pulse and blood pressure, however, in clinical trials brimonidine did not have any significant effects on pulse and blood pressure).
No products indexed under this heading.

Rasagiline Mesylate (Concurrent use of brimonidine, an alpha adrenergic agonist, and MAO inhibitor is contraindicated). Products include:
Azilect Tablets 3106

Rauwolfia Serpentina (Concurrent use of brimonidine, an alpha adrenergic agonist, with antihypertensives may reduce pulse and blood pressure, however, in clinical trials brimonidine did not have any significant effects on pulse and blood pressure).
No products indexed under this heading.

Remifentanil Hydrochloride (Possible additive or potentiating effect with CNS depressants).
No products indexed under this heading.

Rescinnamine (Concurrent use of brimonidine, an alpha adrenergic agonist, with antihypertensives may reduce pulse and blood pressure, however, in clinical trials brimonidine did not have any significant effects on pulse and blood pressure).
No products indexed under this heading.

Reserpine (Concurrent use of brimonidine, an alpha adrenergic agonist, with antihypertensives may reduce pulse and blood pressure, however, in clinical trials brimonidine did not have any significant effects on pulse and blood pressure).
No products indexed under this heading.

Risperidone (Possible additive or potentiating effect with CNS depressants). Products include:
Risperdal Consta Long-Acting Injection 1753

Secobarbital Sodium (Possible additive or potentiating effect with CNS depressants).
No products indexed under this heading.

Selegiline (Concurrent use of brimonidine, an alpha adrenergic agonist, and MAO inhibitor is contraindicated). Products include:
Emsam Transdermal System 905

Selegiline Hydrochloride (Concurrent use of brimonidine, an alpha adrenergic agonist, and MAO inhibitor is contraindicated). Products include:
Eldepryl Capsules 3052

Sevoflurane (Possible additive or potentiating effect with CNS depressants). Products include:
Ultane Liquid for Inhalation 524

Sodium Butabarbital (Possible additive or potentiating effect with CNS depressants).
No products indexed under this heading.

Sodium Nitroprusside (Concurrent use of brimonidine, an alpha adrenergic agonist, with antihypertensives may reduce pulse and blood pressure, however, in clinical trials brimonidine did not have any significant effects on pulse and blood pressure).
No products indexed under this heading.

Sodium Oxybate (Possible additive or potentiating effect with CNS depressants). Products include:
Xyrem Oral Solution 1766

Sotalol Hydrochloride (Concurrent use of brimonidine, an alpha adrenergic agonist, with beta blockers (ophthalmic and systemic) may reduce pulse and blood pressure, however, in clinical trials brimonidine did not have any significant effects on pulse and blood pressure).
No products indexed under this heading.

Spirapril Hydrochloride (Concurrent use of brimonidine, an alpha adrenergic agonist, with antihypertensives may reduce pulse and blood pressure, however, in clinical trials brimonidine did not have any significant effects on pulse and blood pressure).
No products indexed under this heading.

Sufentanil Citrate (Possible additive or potentiating effect with CNS depressants).
No products indexed under this heading.

Telmisartan (Concurrent use of brimonidine, an alpha adrenergic agonist, with antihypertensives may reduce pulse and blood pressure, however, in clinical trials brimonidine did not have any significant effects on pulse and blood pressure). Products include:
Micardis Tablets 852
Micardis HCT Tablets 854

Temazepam (Possible additive or potentiating effect with CNS depressants).
No products indexed under this heading.

Terazosin Hydrochloride (Concurrent use of brimonidine, an alpha adrenergic agonist, with antihypertensives may reduce pulse and blood pressure, however, in clinical trials brimonidine did not have any significant effects on pulse and blood pressure).
No products indexed under this heading.

Thiamylal Sodium (Possible additive or potentiating effect with CNS depressants).
No products indexed under this heading.

Thioridazine Hydrochloride (Possible additive or potentiating effect with CNS depressants). Products include:
Thioridazine Hydrochloride Tablets 2195

Thiothixene (Possible additive or potentiating effect with CNS depressants). Products include:
Thiothixene Capsules 2197

Timolol Hemihydrate (Concurrent use of brimonidine, an alpha adrenergic agonist, with beta blockers (oph-

thalmic and systemic) may reduce pulse and blood pressure, however, in clinical trials brimonidine did not have any significant effects on pulse and blood pressure). Products include:

Betimol Ophthalmic Solution 3181

Timolol Maleate (Concurrent use of brimonidine, an alpha adrenergic agonist, with beta blockers (ophthalmic and systemic) may reduce pulse and blood pressure, however, in clinical trials brimonidine did not have any significant effects on pulse and blood pressure). Products include:

Combigan Ophthalmic Solution 553
Cosopt Sterile Ophthalmic Solution 1969
Timoptic Sterile Ophthalmic Solution 2121
Timoptic in Ocudose 2124
Timoptic-XE Sterile Ophthalmic Gel Forming Solution 2125

Torsemide (Concurrent use of brimonidine, an alpha adrenergic agonist, with antihypertensives may reduce pulse and blood pressure, however, in clinical trials brimonidine did not have any significant effects on pulse and blood pressure). Products include:

Demadex Injection 2630
Demadex Tablets 2630

Trandolapril (Concurrent use of brimonidine, an alpha adrenergic agonist, with antihypertensives may reduce pulse and blood pressure, however, in clinical trials brimonidine did not have any significant effects on pulse and blood pressure). Products include:

Mavik Tablets 472
Tarka Tablets 511

Tranylcypromine Sulfate (Concurrent use of brimonidine, an alpha adrenergic agonist, and MAO inhibitor is contraindicated). Products include:

Parnate Tablets 1532

Triazolam (Possible additive or potentiating effect with CNS depressants).

No products indexed under this heading.

Trifluoperazine Hydrochloride (Possible additive or potentiating effect with CNS depressants).

No products indexed under this heading.

Trimethaphan Camsylate (Concurrent use of brimonidine, an alpha adrenergic agonist, with antihypertensives may reduce pulse and blood pressure, however, in clinical trials brimonidine did not have any significant effects on pulse and blood pressure).

No products indexed under this heading.

Trimipramine Maleate (Tricyclic antidepressants have been reported to blunt the hypotensive effect of systemic clonidine, an alpha adrenergic agonist; it is not known whether the concurrent use of these agents with brimonidine can lead to interference in IOP-lowering effect; caution is advised).

No products indexed under this heading.

Valsartan (Concurrent use of brimonidine, an alpha adrenergic agonist, with antihypertensives may reduce pulse and blood pressure, however, in clinical trials brimonidine did not have any significant effects on pulse and blood pressure). Products include:

Diovan Tablets 2212
Diovan HCT Tablets 2216
Exforge Tablets 2238

Verapamil Hydrochloride (Concurrent use of brimonidine, an alpha adrenergic agonist, with antihypertensives may reduce pulse and blood pressure, however, in clinical trials brimonidine did not have any significant effects on pulse and blood pressure). Products include:

Tarka Tablets 511

Zaleplon (Possible additive or potentiating effect with CNS depressants).

No products indexed under this heading.

Ziprasidone Hydrochloride (Possible additive or potentiating effect with CNS depressants). Products include:

Geodon Capsules 2520

Zolpidem Tartrate (Possible additive or potentiating effect with CNS depressants). Products include:

Ambien Tablets 2692
Ambien CR Tablets 2696

Food Interactions

Alcohol (Possible additive or potentiating effect with CNS depressants).

ALPHANATE

(Antihemophilic Factor (Human), von Willebrand Factor (Human))........... 1709
None cited in PDR database.

ALPHANINE SD

(Factor IX (Human)) 1713
None cited in PDR database.

ALREX OPHTHALMIC SUSPENSION 0.2%

(Loteprednol Etabonate) .... ⊙236
None cited in PDR database.

ALTABAX OINTMENT

(Retapamulin) 1299
May interact with:

Ketoconazole (Co-administration of oral ketoconazole 200 mg twice daily increased retapamulin geometric mean AUC and Cmax by 81% after topical application of retapamulin ointment, 1% on the abraded skin of healthy adult males. Due to low systemic exposure to retapamulin following topical application in patients, dosage adjustments for retapamulin are unnecessary when co-administered with CYP3A4 inhibitors, such as ketoconazole). Products include:

Extina Foam, 2% 3057
Nizoral A-D Shampoo 1901

ALVESCO INHALATION AEROSOL

(Ciclesonide) 2985
May interact with:

Ketoconazole (In clinical studies, co-administration of orally inhaled ciclesonide and oral ketoconazole, a potent inhibitor of cytochrome P450 3A4, increased the exposure (AUC) of ciclesonide active metabolite, des-ciclesonide, by approximately 3.6-fold at steady state, while levels of ciclesonide remained unchanged). Products include:

Extina Foam, 2% 3057
Nizoral A-D Shampoo 1901

AMBIEN TABLETS

(Zolpidem Tartrate) 2692
May interact with central nervous system depressants, cytochrome p450 3a inhibitors (selected), and certain other agents. Compounds in these categories include:

Alfentanil Hydrochloride (Since the systematic evaluations of zolpidem in combination with other CNS-active drugs have been limited, careful consideration should be given to the pharmacology of any CNS-active drug to be used with zolpidem. Any drug with CNS-depressant effects could potentially enhance the CNS depressant effects of zolpidem. Dosage adjustments may be necessary when zolpidem is combined with other CNS depressant drugs).

No products indexed under this heading.

Alprazolam (Since the systematic evaluations of zolpidem in combination with other CNS-active drugs have been limited, careful consideration should be given to the pharmacology of any CNS-active drug to be used with zolpidem. Any drug with CNS-depressant effects could potentially enhance the CNS depressant effects of zolpidem. Dosage adjustments may be necessary when zolpidem is combined with other CNS depressant drugs).

No products indexed under this heading.

Amiodarone Hydrochloride (Some compounds known to inhibit CYP3A may increase exposure to zolpidem).

No products indexed under this heading.

Amprenavir (Some compounds known to inhibit CYP3A may increase exposure to zolpidem).

No products indexed under this heading.

Aprepitant (Some compounds known to inhibit CYP3A may increase exposure to zolpidem). Products include:

Emend Capsules 1992

Aprobarbital (Since the systematic evaluations of zolpidem in combination with other CNS-active drugs have been limited, careful consideration should be given to the pharmacology of any CNS-active drug to be used with zolpidem. Any drug with CNS-depressant effects could potentially enhance the CNS depressant effects of zolpidem. Dosage adjustments may be necessary when zolpidem is combined with other CNS depressant drugs).

No products indexed under this heading.

Buprenorphine Hydrochloride (Since the systematic evaluations of zolpidem in combination with other CNS-active drugs have been limited, careful consideration should be given to the pharmacology of any CNS-active drug to be used with zolpidem. Any drug with CNS-depressant effects could potentially enhance the CNS depressant effects of zolpidem. Dosage adjustments may be necessary when zolpidem is combined with other CNS depressant drugs). Products include:

Suboxone Tablets 2601
Subutex Tablets 2601

Buspirone Hydrochloride (Since the systematic evaluations of zolpidem in combination with other CNS-active drugs have been limited, careful consideration should be given to the pharmacology of any CNS-active drug to be used with zolpidem. Any drug with CNS-depressant effects could potentially enhance the CNS depressant effects of zolpidem. Dosage adjustments may be necessary when zolpidem is combined with other CNS depressant drugs).

No products indexed under this heading.

Butabarbital (Since the systematic evaluations of zolpidem in combination with other CNS-active drugs have been limited, careful consideration should be given to the pharmacology of any CNS-active drug to be used with zolpidem. Any drug with CNS-depressant effects could potentially enhance the CNS depressant effects of zolpidem. Dosage adjustments may be necessary when zolpidem is combined with other CNS depressant drugs).

No products indexed under this heading.

Butalbital (Since the systematic evaluations of zolpidem in combination with other CNS-active drugs have been limited, careful consideration should be given to the pharmacology of any CNS-active drug to be used with zolpidem. Any drug with CNS-depressant effects could potentially enhance the CNS depressant effects of zolpidem. Dosage adjustments may be necessary when zolpidem is combined with other CNS depressant drugs).

No products indexed under this heading.

Chlordiazepoxide (Since the systematic evaluations of zolpidem in combination with other CNS-active drugs have been limited, careful consideration should be given to the pharmacology of any CNS-active drug to be used with zolpidem. Any drug with CNS-depressant effects could potentially enhance the CNS depressant effects of zolpidem. Dosage adjustments may be necessary when zolpidem is combined with other CNS depressant drugs).

No products indexed under this heading.

Chlordiazepoxide Hydrochloride (Since the systematic evaluations of zolpidem in combination with other CNS-active drugs have been limited, careful consideration should be given to the pharmacology of any CNS-active drug to be used with zolpidem. Any drug with CNS-depressant effects could potentially enhance the CNS depressant effects of zolpidem. Dosage adjustments may be necessary when zolpidem is combined with other CNS depressant drugs).

No products indexed under this heading.

Chlorpromazine (The systematic evaluations of zolpidem in combination with other CNS-active drugs has been limited. Zolpidem was evaluated in healthy subjects in a single dose interaction study. Chlorpromazine in combination with zolpidem produced no pharmacokinetic interaction, but there was an additive effect of decreased alertness and psychomotor performance).

No products indexed under this heading.

Chlorpromazine Hydrochloride (The systematic evaluations of zolpidem in combination with other CNS-active drugs has been limited. Zolpidem was evaluated in healthy subjects in a single dose interaction study. Chlorpromazine in combination with zolpidem produced no pharmacokinetic interaction, but there was an additive effect of decreased alertness and psychomotor performance).
No products indexed under this heading.

Chlorprothixene (Since the systematic evaluations of zolpidem in combination with other CNS-active drugs have been limited, careful consideration should be given to the pharmacology of any CNS-active drug to be used with zolpidem. Any drug with CNS-depressant effects could potentially enhance the CNS depressant effects of zolpidem. Dosage adjustments may be necessary when zolpidem is combined with other CNS depressant drugs).
No products indexed under this heading.

Chlorprothixene Hydrochloride (Since the systematic evaluations of zolpidem in combination with other CNS-active drugs have been limited, careful consideration should be given to the pharmacology of any CNS-active drug to be used with zolpidem. Any drug with CNS-depressant effects could potentially enhance the CNS depressant effects of zolpidem. Dosage adjustments may be necessary when zolpidem is combined with other CNS depressant drugs).
No products indexed under this heading.

Chlorprothixene Lactate (Since the systematic evaluations of zolpidem in combination with other CNS-active drugs have been limited, careful consideration should be given to the pharmacology of any CNS-active drug to be used with zolpidem. Any drug with CNS-depressant effects could potentially enhance the CNS depressant effects of zolpidem. Dosage adjustments may be necessary when zolpidem is combined with other CNS depressant drugs).
No products indexed under this heading.

Cimetidine (Some compounds known to inhibit CYP3A may increase exposure to zolpidem).
No products indexed under this heading.

Cimetidine Hydrochloride (Some compounds known to inhibit CYP3A may increase exposure to zolpidem).
No products indexed under this heading.

Ciprofloxacin (Some compounds known to inhibit CYP3A may increase exposure to zolpidem). Products include:
Cipro I.V. **2817**
Cipro Oral Suspension **2810**
Cipro XR Tablets **2823**
Ciprodex Otic Suspension **541**

Ciprofloxacin Hydrochloride (Some compounds known to inhibit CYP3A may increase exposure to zolpidem). Products include:
Cipro Tablets **2810**

Clarithromycin (Some compounds known to inhibit CYP3A may increase exposure to zolpidem). Products include:
Biaxin/Biaxin XL **411**

Clorazepate Dipotassium (Since the systematic evaluations of zolpidem in combination with other CNS-active drugs have been limited, careful consideration should be given to the pharmacology of any CNS-active drug to be used with zolpidem. Any drug with CNS-depressant effects could potentially enhance the CNS depressant effects of zolpidem. Dosage adjustments may be necessary when zolpidem is combined with other CNS depressant drugs).
No products indexed under this heading.

Clozapine (Since the systematic evaluations of zolpidem in combination with other CNS-active drugs have been limited, careful consideration should be given to the pharmacology of any CNS-active drug to be used with zolpidem. Any drug with CNS-depressant effects could potentially enhance the CNS depressant effects of zolpidem. Dosage adjustments may be necessary when zolpidem is combined with other CNS depressant drugs).
No products indexed under this heading.

Codeine Phosphate (Since the systematic evaluations of zolpidem in combination with other CNS-active drugs have been limited, careful consideration should be given to the pharmacology of any CNS-active drug to be used with zolpidem. Any drug with CNS-depressant effects could potentially enhance the CNS depressant effects of zolpidem. Dosage adjustments may be necessary when zolpidem is combined with other CNS depressant drugs). Products include:
Tylenol with Codeine Tablets **2427**

Cyclosporine (Some compounds known to inhibit CYP3A may increase exposure to zolpidem). Products include:
Gengraf Capsules **435**
Neoral Oral Solution **2280**
Neoral Soft Gelatin Capsules **2280**
Restasis Ophthalmic Emulsion **557**
Sandimmune **2296**

Delavirdine Mesylate (Some compounds known to inhibit CYP3A may increase exposure to zolpidem).
No products indexed under this heading.

Desflurane (Since the systematic evaluations of zolpidem in combination with other CNS-active drugs have been limited, careful consideration should be given to the pharmacology of any CNS-active drug to be used with zolpidem. Any drug with CNS-depressant effects could potentially enhance the CNS depressant effects of zolpidem. Dosage adjustments may be necessary when zolpidem is combined with other CNS depressant drugs).
No products indexed under this heading.

Dezocine (Since the systematic evaluations of zolpidem in combination with other CNS-active drugs have been limited, careful consideration should be given to the pharmacology of any CNS-active drug to be used with zolpidem. Any drug with CNS-depressant effects could potentially enhance the CNS depressant effects of zolpidem. Dosage adjustments may be necessary when zolpidem is combined with other CNS depressant drugs).
No products indexed under this heading.

Diazepam (Since the systematic evaluations of zolpidem in combination with other CNS-active drugs have been limited, careful consideration should be given to the pharmacology of any CNS-active drug to be used with zolpidem. Any drug with CNS-depressant effects could potentially enhance the CNS depressant effects of zolpidem. Dosage adjustments may be necessary when zolpidem is combined with other CNS depressant drugs). Products include:
Valium Tablets **2658**

Diltiazem Hydrochloride (Some compounds known to inhibit CYP3A may increase exposure to zolpidem). Products include:
Cardizem LA Extended Release Tablets **421**

Diltiazem Maleate (Some compounds known to inhibit CYP3A may increase exposure to zolpidem).
No products indexed under this heading.

Droperidol (Since the systematic evaluations of zolpidem in combination with other CNS-active drugs have been limited, careful consideration should be given to the pharmacology of any CNS-active drug to be used with zolpidem. Any drug with CNS-depressant effects could potentially enhance the CNS depressant effects of zolpidem. Dosage adjustments may be necessary when zolpidem is combined with other CNS depressant drugs).
No products indexed under this heading.

Efavirenz (Some compounds known to inhibit CYP3A may increase exposure to zolpidem). Products include:
Atripla Tablets **938**
Sustiva Capsules **930**
Sustiva Tablets **930**

Enflurane (Since the systematic evaluations of zolpidem in combination with other CNS-active drugs have been limited, careful consideration should be given to the pharmacology of any CNS-active drug to be used with zolpidem. Any drug with CNS-depressant effects could potentially enhance the CNS depressant effects of zolpidem. Dosage adjustments may be necessary when zolpidem is combined with other CNS depressant drugs).
No products indexed under this heading.

Erythromycin (Some compounds known to inhibit CYP3A may increase exposure to zolpidem).
No products indexed under this heading.

Estazolam (Since the systematic evaluations of zolpidem in combination with other CNS-active drugs have been limited, careful consideration should be given to the pharmacology of any CNS-active drug to be used with zolpidem. Any drug with CNS-depressant effects could potentially enhance the CNS depressant effects of zolpidem. Dosage adjustments may be necessary when zolpidem is combined with other CNS depressant drugs).
No products indexed under this heading.

Ethanol (An additive effect on psychomotor performance between alcohol and zolpidem was demonstrated. Zolpidem should not be taken with alcohol).
No products indexed under this heading.

Ethchlorvynol (Since the systematic evaluations of zolpidem in combination with other CNS-active drugs have been limited, careful consideration should be given to the pharmacology of any CNS-active drug to be used with zolpidem. Any drug with CNS-depressant effects could potentially enhance the CNS depressant effects of zolpidem. Dosage adjustments may be necessary when zolpidem is combined with other CNS depressant drugs).
No products indexed under this heading.

Ethinamate (Since the systematic evaluations of zolpidem in combination with other CNS-active drugs have been limited, careful consideration should be given to the pharmacology of any CNS-active drug to be used with zolpidem. Any drug with CNS-depressant effects could potentially enhance the CNS depressant effects of zolpidem. Dosage adjustments may be necessary when zolpidem is combined with other CNS depressant drugs).
No products indexed under this heading.

Ethyl Alcohol (An additive effect on psychomotor performance between alcohol and zolpidem was demonstrated. Zolpidem should not be taken with alcohol).
No products indexed under this heading.

Fentanyl (Since the systematic evaluations of zolpidem in combination with other CNS-active drugs have been limited, careful consideration should be given to the pharmacology of any CNS-active drug to be used with zolpidem. Any drug with CNS-depressant effects could potentially enhance the CNS depressant effects of zolpidem. Dosage adjustments may be necessary when zolpidem is combined with other CNS depressant drugs). Products include:
Duragesic Transdermal System **2405**
Ionsys Transdermal System **2410**

Fentanyl Citrate (Since the systematic evaluations of zolpidem in combination with other CNS-active drugs have been limited, careful consideration should be given to the pharmacology of any CNS-active drug to be used with zolpidem. Any drug with CNS-depressant effects could potentially enhance the CNS depressant effects of zolpidem. Dosage adjustments may be necessary when zolpidem is combined with other CNS depressant drugs). Products include:
Actiq **959**
Fentora Tablets **968**

Fluconazole (Some compounds known to inhibit CYP3A may increase exposure to zolpidem).
No products indexed under this heading.

Fluoxetine (A single dose interaction study with zolpidem 10 mg and fluoxetine 20 mg at steady-state levels in male volunteers did not demonstrate any clinically significant pharmacokinetic or pharmacodynamic interactions. When multiple doses of zolpidem and fluoxetine at

steady-state concentrations were evaluated in healthy females, the only significant change was a 17% increase in zolpidem half-life. There was no evidence of an additive effect in psychomotor performance).

No products indexed under this heading.

Fluoxetine Hydrochloride (A single dose interaction study with zolpidem 10 mg and fluoxetine 20 mg at steady-state levels in male volunteers did not demonstrate any clinically significant pharmacokinetic or pharmacodynamic interactions. When multiple doses of zolpidem and fluoxetine at steady-state concentrations were evaluated in healthy females, the only significant change was a 17% increase in zolpidem half-life. There was no evidence of an additive effect in psychomotor performance). Products include:

Prozac Weekly Capsules **1852**
Prozac Pulvules and Liquid **1852**
Symbyax Capsules **1871**

Fluphenazine Decanoate (Since the systematic evaluations of zolpidem in combination with other CNS-active drugs have been limited, careful consideration should be given to the pharmacology of any CNS-active drug to be used with zolpidem. Any drug with CNS-depressant effects could potentially enhance the CNS depressant effects of zolpidem. Dosage adjustments may be necessary when zolpidem is combined with other CNS depressant drugs).

No products indexed under this heading.

Fluphenazine Enanthate (Since the systematic evaluations of zolpidem in combination with other CNS-active drugs have been limited, careful consideration should be given to the pharmacology of any CNS-active drug to be used with zolpidem. Any drug with CNS-depressant effects could potentially enhance the CNS depressant effects of zolpidem. Dosage adjustments may be necessary when zolpidem is combined with other CNS depressant drugs).

No products indexed under this heading.

Fluphenazine Hydrochloride (Since the systematic evaluations of zolpidem in combination with other CNS-active drugs have been limited, careful consideration should be given to the pharmacology of any CNS-active drug to be used with zolpidem. Any drug with CNS-depressant effects could potentially enhance the CNS depressant effects of zolpidem. Dosage adjustments may be necessary when zolpidem is combined with other CNS depressant drugs).

No products indexed under this heading.

Flurazepam Hydrochloride (Since the systematic evaluations of zolpidem in combination with other CNS-active drugs have been limited, careful consideration should be given to the pharmacology of any CNS-active drug to be used with zolpidem. Any drug with CNS-depressant effects could potentially enhance the CNS depressant effects of zolpidem. Dosage adjustments may be necessary when zolpidem is combined with other CNS depressant drugs).

No products indexed under this heading.

Fluvoxamine Maleate (Some compounds known to inhibit CYP3A may increase exposure to zolpidem). Products include:

Luvox CR Extended-Release Capsules **1759**

Glutethimide (Since the systematic evaluations of zolpidem in combination with other CNS-active drugs have been limited, careful consideration should be given to the pharmacology of any CNS-active drug to be used with zolpidem. Any drug with CNS-depressant effects could potentially enhance the CNS depressant effects of zolpidem. Dosage adjustments may be necessary when zolpidem is combined with other CNS depressant drugs).

No products indexed under this heading.

Haloperidol (The systematic evaluations of zolpidem in combination with other CNS-active drugs has been limited. Zolpidem was evaluated in healthy subjects in a single dose interaction study. A study involving haloperidol and zolpidem revealed no effect of haloperidol on the pharmacokinetics or pharmacodynamics of zolpidem. The lack of drug interaction following single dose administration does not predict a lack of a drug interaction following chronic administration).

No products indexed under this heading.

Haloperidol Decanoate (The systematic evaluations of zolpidem in combination with other CNS-active drugs has been limited. Zolpidem was evaluated in healthy subjects in a single dose interaction study. A study involving haloperidol and zolpidem revealed no effect of haloperidol on the pharmacokinetics or pharmacodynamics of zolpidem. The lack of drug interaction following single dose administration does not predict a lack of a drug interaction following chronic administration).

No products indexed under this heading.

Haloperidol Lactate (The systematic evaluations of zolpidem in combination with other CNS-active drugs has been limited. Zolpidem was evaluated in healthy subjects in a single dose interaction study. A study involving haloperidol and zolpidem revealed no effect of haloperidol on the pharmacokinetics or pharmacodynamics of zolpidem. The lack of drug interaction following single dose administration does not predict a lack of a drug interaction following chronic administration).

No products indexed under this heading.

Hydrocodone Bitartrate (Since the systematic evaluations of zolpidem in combination with other CNS-active drugs have been limited, careful consideration should be given to the pharmacology of any CNS-active drug to be used with zolpidem. Any drug with CNS-depressant effects could potentially enhance the CNS depressant effects of zolpidem. Dosage adjustments may be necessary when zolpidem is combined with other CNS depressant drugs). Products include:

Lortab 5/500 Tablets **3143**
Lortab 7.5/500 Tablets **3144**
Lortab 10/500 Tablets **3144**
Vicodin Tablets **529**
Vicodin ES Tablets **530**
Vicodin HP Tablets **531**
Vicoprofen Tablets **533**
Zydone Tablets **1132**

Hydrocodone Polistirex (Since the systematic evaluations of zolpidem in combination with other CNS-active drugs have been limited, careful consideration should be given to the pharmacology of any CNS-active drug to be used with zolpidem. Any drug with CNS-depressant effects could potentially enhance the CNS depressant effects of zolpidem. Dosage adjustments may be necessary when zolpidem is combined with other CNS depressant drugs). Products include:

Tussionex Pennkinetic Extended-Release Suspension...... **3154**

Hydromorphone Hydrochloride (Since the systematic evaluations of zolpidem in combination with other CNS-active drugs have been limited, careful consideration should be given to the pharmacology of any CNS-active drug to be used with zolpidem. Any drug with CNS-depressant effects could potentially enhance the CNS depressant effects of zolpidem. Dosage adjustments may be necessary when zolpidem is combined with other CNS depressant drugs).

No products indexed under this heading.

Hydroxyzine Hydrochloride (Since the systematic evaluations of zolpidem in combination with other CNS-active drugs have been limited, careful consideration should be given to the pharmacology of any CNS-active drug to be used with zolpidem. Any drug with CNS-depressant effects could potentially enhance the CNS depressant effects of zolpidem. Dosage adjustments may be necessary when zolpidem is combined with other CNS depressant drugs).

No products indexed under this heading.

Imipramine Hydrochloride (The systematic evaluations of zolpidem in combination with other CNS-active drugs has been limited. Zolpidem was evaluated in healthy subjects in a single dose interaction study. Imipramine in combination with zolpidem produced no pharmacokinetic interaction other than a 20% decrease in peak levels of imipramine, but there was an additive effect of decreased alertness).

No products indexed under this heading.

Imipramine Pamoate (The systematic evaluations of zolpidem in combination with other CNS-active drugs has been limited. Zolpidem was evaluated in healthy subjects in a single dose interaction study. Imipramine in combination with zolpidem produced no pharmacokinetic interaction other than a 20% decrease in peak levels of imipramine, but there was an additive effect of decreased alertness).

No products indexed under this heading.

Indinavir Sulfate (Some compounds known to inhibit CYP3A may increase exposure to zolpidem). Products include:

Crixivan Capsules **1979**

Isoflurane (Since the systematic evaluations of zolpidem in combination with other CNS-active drugs have been limited, careful consideration should be given to the pharmacology of any CNS-active drug to be used with zolpidem. Any drug with CNS-depressant effects could potentially enhance the CNS depressant effects of zolpidem. Dosage adjustments may be necessary when zolpidem is combined with other CNS depressant drugs).

No products indexed under this heading.

Isoniazid (Some compounds known to inhibit CYP3A may increase exposure to zolpidem).

No products indexed under this heading.

Itraconazole (A randomized, double-blind, crossover interaction study in ten healthy volunteers between itraconazole (200 mg QD for 4 days) and a single dose of zolpidem (10 mg) given 5 hours after the last dose of itraconazole resulted in a 34% increase in AUC of zolpidem. There were no significant pharmacodynamic effects of zolpidem on subjective drowsiness, postural sway, or psychomotor performance).

No products indexed under this heading.

Ketamine Hydrochloride (Since the systematic evaluations of zolpidem in combination with other CNS-active drugs have been limited, careful consideration should be given to the pharmacology of any CNS-active drug to be used with zolpidem. Any drug with CNS-depressant effects could potentially enhance the CNS depressant effects of zolpidem. Dosage adjustments may be necessary when zolpidem is combined with other CNS depressant drugs).

No products indexed under this heading.

Ketoconazole (A randomized, double-blind, crossover interaction study in 12 healthy subjects showed that co-administration of a single 5 mg dose of zolpidem with ketoconazole, a potent CYP3A4 inhibitor, given as 200 mg bid for two days increased Cmax of zolpidem by a factor of 1.3 and increased the total AUC of zolpidem by a factor of 1.7 compared to zolpidem alone and prolonged the elimination half-life by approximately 30% along with an increase in the pharmacodynamic effects of zolpidem. Caution should be used when ketoconazole is given with zolpidem and consideration should be given to using a lower dose of zolpidem when ketoconazole and zolpidem are given together. Patients should be advised that the use of zolpidem with ketoconazole may enhance sedative effects). Products include:

Extina Foam, 2% **3057**
Nizoral A-D Shampoo **1901**

Levomethadyl Acetate Hydrochloride (Since the systematic evaluations of zolpidem in combination with other CNS-active drugs have been limited, careful consideration should be given to the pharmacology of any CNS-active drug to be used with zolpidem. Any drug with CNS-depressant effects could potentially enhance the CNS depressant effects of zolpidem. Dosage adjustments may be necessary when zolpidem is combined with other CNS depressant drugs).

No products indexed under this heading.

Levorphanol Tartrate (Since the systematic evaluations of zolpidem

in combination with other CNS-active drugs have been limited, careful consideration should be given to the pharmacology of any CNS-active drug to be used with zolpidem. Any drug with CNS-depressant effects could potentially enhance the CNS depressant effects of zolpidem. Dosage adjustments may be necessary when zolpidem is combined with other CNS depressant drugs).
No products indexed under this heading.

Lopinavir (Some compounds known to inhibit CYP3A may increase exposure to zolpidem). Products include:
Kaletra 452

Lorazepam (Since the systematic evaluations of zolpidem in combination with other CNS-active drugs have been limited, careful consideration should be given to the pharmacology of any CNS-active drug to be used with zolpidem. Any drug with CNS-depressant effects could potentially enhance the CNS depressant effects of zolpidem. Dosage adjustments may be necessary when zolpidem is combined with other CNS depressant drugs).
No products indexed under this heading.

Loxapine Hydrochloride (Since the systematic evaluations of zolpidem in combination with other CNS-active drugs have been limited, careful consideration should be given to the pharmacology of any CNS-active drug to be used with zolpidem. Any drug with CNS-depressant effects could potentially enhance the CNS depressant effects of zolpidem. Dosage adjustments may be necessary when zolpidem is combined with other CNS depressant drugs).
No products indexed under this heading.

Loxapine Succinate (Since the systematic evaluations of zolpidem in combination with other CNS-active drugs have been limited, careful consideration should be given to the pharmacology of any CNS-active drug to be used with zolpidem. Any drug with CNS-depressant effects could potentially enhance the CNS depressant effects of zolpidem. Dosage adjustments may be necessary when zolpidem is combined with other CNS depressant drugs).
No products indexed under this heading.

Meperidine Hydrochloride (Since the systematic evaluations of zolpidem in combination with other CNS-active drugs have been limited, careful consideration should be given to the pharmacology of any CNS-active drug to be used with zolpidem. Any drug with CNS-depressant effects could potentially enhance the CNS depressant effects of zolpidem. Dosage adjustments may be necessary when zolpidem is combined with other CNS depressant drugs).
No products indexed under this heading.

Mephobarbital (Since the systematic evaluations of zolpidem in combination with other CNS-active drugs have been limited, careful consideration should be given to the pharmacology of any CNS-active drug to be used with zolpidem. Any drug with CNS-depressant effects could potentially enhance the CNS depressant effects of zolpidem. Dosage adjustments may be necessary when zolpidem is combined with other CNS depressant drugs).
No products indexed under this heading.

Meprobamate (Since the systematic evaluations of zolpidem in combination with other CNS-active drugs have been limited, careful consideration should be given to the pharmacology of any CNS-active drug to be used with zolpidem. Any drug with CNS-depressant effects could potentially enhance the CNS depressant effects of zolpidem. Dosage adjustments may be necessary when zolpidem is combined with other CNS depressant drugs).
No products indexed under this heading.

Mesoridazine Besylate (Since the systematic evaluations of zolpidem in combination with other CNS-active drugs have been limited, careful consideration should be given to the pharmacology of any CNS-active drug to be used with zolpidem. Any drug with CNS-depressant effects could potentially enhance the CNS depressant effects of zolpidem. Dosage adjustments may be necessary when zolpidem is combined with other CNS depressant drugs).
No products indexed under this heading.

Methadone Hydrochloride (Since the systematic evaluations of zolpidem in combination with other CNS-active drugs have been limited, careful consideration should be given to the pharmacology of any CNS-active drug to be used with zolpidem. Any drug with CNS-depressant effects could potentially enhance the CNS depressant effects of zolpidem. Dosage adjustments may be necessary when zolpidem is combined with other CNS depressant drugs).
No products indexed under this heading.

Methohexital Sodium (Since the systematic evaluations of zolpidem in combination with other CNS-active drugs have been limited, careful consideration should be given to the pharmacology of any CNS-active drug to be used with zolpidem. Any drug with CNS-depressant effects could potentially enhance the CNS depressant effects of zolpidem. Dosage adjustments may be necessary when zolpidem is combined with other CNS depressant drugs).
No products indexed under this heading.

Methotrimeprazine (Since the systematic evaluations of zolpidem in combination with other CNS-active drugs have been limited, careful consideration should be given to the pharmacology of any CNS-active drug to be used with zolpidem. Any drug with CNS-depressant effects could potentially enhance the CNS depressant effects of zolpidem. Dosage adjustments may be necessary when zolpidem is combined with other CNS depressant drugs).
No products indexed under this heading.

Methoxyflurane (Since the systematic evaluations of zolpidem in combination with other CNS-active drugs have been limited, careful consideration should be given to the pharmacology of any CNS-active drug to be used with zolpidem. Any drug with CNS-depressant effects could potentially enhance the CNS depressant effects of zolpidem. Dosage adjustments may be necessary when zolpidem is combined with other CNS depressant drugs).
No products indexed under this heading.

Metronidazole (Some compounds known to inhibit CYP3A may increase exposure to zolpidem). Products include:
Pylera Capsules 714

Metronidazole Benzoate (Some compounds known to inhibit CYP3A may increase exposure to zolpidem).
No products indexed under this heading.

Metronidazole Hydrochloride (Some compounds known to inhibit CYP3A may increase exposure to zolpidem).
No products indexed under this heading.

Miconazole (Some compounds known to inhibit CYP3A may increase exposure to zolpidem).
No products indexed under this heading.

Midazolam Hydrochloride (Since the systematic evaluations of zolpidem in combination with other CNS-active drugs have been limited, careful consideration should be given to the pharmacology of any CNS-active drug to be used with zolpidem. Any drug with CNS-depressant effects could potentially enhance the CNS depressant effects of zolpidem. Dosage adjustments may be necessary when zolpidem is combined with other CNS depressant drugs).
No products indexed under this heading.

Molindone Hydrochloride (Since the systematic evaluations of zolpidem in combination with other CNS-active drugs have been limited, careful consideration should be given to the pharmacology of any CNS-active drug to be used with zolpidem. Any drug with CNS-depressant effects could potentially enhance the CNS depressant effects of zolpidem. Dosage adjustments may be necessary when zolpidem is combined with other CNS depressant drugs). Products include:
Moban Tablets 1116

Morphine Sulfate (Since the systematic evaluations of zolpidem in combination with other CNS-active drugs have been limited, careful consideration should be given to the pharmacology of any CNS-active drug to be used with zolpidem. Any drug with CNS-depressant effects could potentially enhance the CNS depressant effects of zolpidem. Dosage adjustments may be necessary when zolpidem is combined with other CNS depressant drugs). Products include:
Avinza Capsules 1772
DepoDur Injection 1095
MS Contin Tablets 2585

Nefazodone Hydrochloride (Some compounds known to inhibit CYP3A may increase exposure to zolpidem).
No products indexed under this heading.

Nelfinavir Mesylate (Some compounds known to inhibit CYP3A may increase exposure to zolpidem).
No products indexed under this heading.

Nifedipine (Some compounds known to inhibit CYP3A may increase exposure to zolpidem).
No products indexed under this heading.

Norfloxacin (Some compounds known to inhibit CYP3A may increase exposure to zolpidem). Products include:
Noroxin Tablets 2069

Olanzapine (Since the systematic evaluations of zolpidem in combination with other CNS-active drugs have been limited, careful consideration should be given to the pharmacology of any CNS-active drug to be used with zolpidem. Any drug with CNS-depressant effects could potentially enhance the CNS depressant effects of zolpidem. Dosage adjustments may be necessary when zolpidem is combined with other CNS depressant drugs). Products include:
Symbyax Capsules 1871
Zyprexa Tablets 1883
Zyprexa IntraMuscular 1883
Zyprexa ZYDIS Orally Disintegrating Tablets 1883

Oxazepam (Since the systematic evaluations of zolpidem in combination with other CNS-active drugs have been limited, careful consideration should be given to the pharmacology of any CNS-active drug to be used with zolpidem. Any drug with CNS-depressant effects could potentially enhance the CNS depressant effects of zolpidem. Dosage adjustments may be necessary when zolpidem is combined with other CNS depressant drugs).
No products indexed under this heading.

Oxycodone Hydrochloride (Since the systematic evaluations of zolpidem in combination with other CNS-active drugs have been limited, careful consideration should be given to the pharmacology of any CNS-active drug to be used with zolpidem. Any drug with CNS-depressant effects could potentially enhance the CNS depressant effects of zolpidem. Dosage adjustments may be necessary when zolpidem is combined with other CNS depressant drugs). Products include:
OxyContin Tablets 2589
OxyIR Capsules 2593
Percocet Tablets 1127
Percodan Tablets 1130

Paroxetine Hydrochloride (Some compounds known to inhibit CYP3A may increase exposure to zolpidem). Products include:
Paxil 1535
Paxil CR Controlled-Release Tablets 1544

Pentobarbital Sodium (Since the systematic evaluations of zolpidem in combination with other CNS-active drugs have been limited, careful consideration should be given to the pharmacology of any CNS-active drug to be used with zolpidem. Any drug with CNS-depressant effects could potentially enhance the CNS depressant effects of zolpidem. Dosage adjustments may be necessary when zolpidem is combined with other CNS depressant drugs). Products include:
Nembutal Sodium Solution, USP 2494

Perphenazine (Since the systematic evaluations of zolpidem in combination with other CNS-active drugs have been limited, careful consideration should be given to the pharmacology of any CNS-active drug to be used with zolpidem. Any drug with CNS-depressant effects could potentially enhance the CNS depressant effects of zolpidem. Dosage adjustments may be necessary when zolpidem is combined with other CNS depressant drugs).

No products indexed under this heading.

Phenobarbital (Since the systematic evaluations of zolpidem in combination with other CNS-active drugs have been limited, careful consideration should be given to the pharmacology of any CNS-active drug to be used with zolpidem. Any drug with CNS-depressant effects could potentially enhance the CNS depressant effects of zolpidem. Dosage adjustments may be necessary when zolpidem is combined with other CNS depressant drugs). Products include:

Donnatal Extentabs **2507**

Prazepam (Since the systematic evaluations of zolpidem in combination with other CNS-active drugs have been limited, careful consideration should be given to the pharmacology of any CNS-active drug to be used with zolpidem. Any drug with CNS-depressant effects could potentially enhance the CNS depressant effects of zolpidem. Dosage adjustments may be necessary when zolpidem is combined with other CNS depressant drugs).

No products indexed under this heading.

Prochlorperazine (Since the systematic evaluations of zolpidem in combination with other CNS-active drugs have been limited, careful consideration should be given to the pharmacology of any CNS-active drug to be used with zolpidem. Any drug with CNS-depressant effects could potentially enhance the CNS depressant effects of zolpidem. Dosage adjustments may be necessary when zolpidem is combined with other CNS depressant drugs).

No products indexed under this heading.

Promethazine Hydrochloride (Since the systematic evaluations of zolpidem in combination with other CNS-active drugs have been limited, careful consideration should be given to the pharmacology of any CNS-active drug to be used with zolpidem. Any drug with CNS-depressant effects could potentially enhance the CNS depressant effects of zolpidem. Dosage adjustments may be necessary when zolpidem is combined with other CNS depressant drugs).

No products indexed under this heading.

Propofol (Since the systematic evaluations of zolpidem in combination with other CNS-active drugs have been limited, careful consideration should be given to the pharmacology of any CNS-active drug to be used with zolpidem. Any drug with CNS-depressant effects could potentially enhance the CNS depressant effects of zolpidem. Dosage adjustments may be necessary when zolpidem is combined with other CNS depressant drugs).

No products indexed under this heading.

Propoxyphene Hydrochloride (Since the systematic evaluations of zolpidem in combination with other CNS-active drugs have been limited, careful consideration should be given to the pharmacology of any CNS-active drug to be used with zolpidem. Any drug with CNS-depressant effects could potentially enhance the CNS depressant effects of zolpidem. Dosage adjustments may be necessary when zolpidem is combined with other CNS depressant drugs).

No products indexed under this heading.

Propoxyphene Napsylate (Since the systematic evaluations of zolpidem in combination with other CNS-active drugs have been limited, careful consideration should be given to the pharmacology of any CNS-active drug to be used with zolpidem. Any drug with CNS-depressant effects could potentially enhance the CNS depressant effects of zolpidem. Dosage adjustments may be necessary when zolpidem is combined with other CNS depressant drugs).

No products indexed under this heading.

Quazepam (Since the systematic evaluations of zolpidem in combination with other CNS-active drugs have been limited, careful consideration should be given to the pharmacology of any CNS-active drug to be used with zolpidem. Any drug with CNS-depressant effects could potentially enhance the CNS depressant effects of zolpidem. Dosage adjustments may be necessary when zolpidem is combined with other CNS depressant drugs).

No products indexed under this heading.

Quetiapine Fumarate (Since the systematic evaluations of zolpidem in combination with other CNS-active drugs have been limited, careful consideration should be given to the pharmacology of any CNS-active drug to be used with zolpidem. Any drug with CNS-depressant effects could potentially enhance the CNS depressant effects of zolpidem. Dosage adjustments may be necessary when zolpidem is combined with other CNS depressant drugs).

No products indexed under this heading.

Quinine (Some compounds known to inhibit CYP3A may increase exposure to zolpidem).

No products indexed under this heading.

Quinine Sulfate (Some compounds known to inhibit CYP3A may increase exposure to zolpidem).

No products indexed under this heading.

Remifentanil Hydrochloride (Since the systematic evaluations of zolpidem in combination with other CNS-active drugs have been limited, careful consideration should be given to the pharmacology of any CNS-active drug to be used with zolpidem. Any drug with CNS-depressant effects could potentially enhance the CNS depressant effects of zolpidem. Dosage adjustments may be necessary when zolpidem is combined with other CNS depressant drugs).

No products indexed under this heading.

Rifampin (A randomized, placebo-controlled, crossover interaction study in eight healthy female subjects between five consecutive daily doses of rifampin (600 mg) and a single dose of zolpidem (20 mg) given 17 hours after the last dose of rifampin showed significant reductions of the AUC (-73%), Cmax (-58) and T1/2 (-36) of zolpidem together with significant reductions in the pharmacodynamics of zolpidem).

No products indexed under this heading.

Risperidone (Since the systematic evaluations of zolpidem in combination with other CNS-active drugs have been limited, careful consideration should be given to the pharmacology of any CNS-active drug to be used with zolpidem. Any drug with CNS-depressant effects could potentially enhance the CNS depressant effects of zolpidem. Dosage adjustments may be necessary when zolpidem is combined with other CNS depressant drugs). Products include:

Risperdal Consta Long-Acting Injection **1753**

Ritonavir (Some compounds known to inhibit CYP3A may increase exposure to zolpidem). Products include:

Kaletra **452**
Norvir **489**

Saquinavir (Some compounds known to inhibit CYP3A may increase exposure to zolpidem).

No products indexed under this heading.

Saquinavir Mesylate (Some compounds known to inhibit CYP3A may increase exposure to zolpidem).

No products indexed under this heading.

Secobarbital Sodium (Since the systematic evaluations of zolpidem in combination with other CNS-active drugs have been limited, careful consideration should be given to the pharmacology of any CNS-active drug to be used with zolpidem. Any drug with CNS-depressant effects could potentially enhance the CNS depressant effects of zolpidem. Dosage adjustments may be necessary when zolpidem is combined with other CNS depressant drugs).

No products indexed under this heading.

Sertraline Hydrochloride (Following five consecutive nightly doses of zolpidem 10 mg in the presence of sertaline 50 mg (17 consecutive daily doses, at 7:00 am, in healthy female volunteers), zolpidem Cmax was significantly higher (43%) and Tmax was significantly decreased (53%).Pharmacokinetics of sertraline and N-desmethylsertraline were unaffected by zolpidem).

No products indexed under this heading.

Sevoflurane (Since the systematic evaluations of zolpidem in combination with other CNS-active drugs have been limited, careful consideration should be given to the pharmacology of any CNS-active drug to be used with zolpidem. Any drug with CNS-depressant effects could potentially enhance the CNS depressant effects of zolpidem. Dosage adjustments may be necessary when zolpidem is combined with other CNS depressant drugs). Products include:

Ultane Liquid for Inhalation **524**

Sodium Oxybate (Since the systematic evaluations of zolpidem in combination with other CNS-active drugs have been limited, careful consideration should be given to the pharmacology of any CNS-active drug to be used with zolpidem. Any drug with CNS-depressant effects could potentially enhance the CNS depressant effects of zolpidem. Dosage adjustments may be necessary when zolpidem is combined with other CNS depressant drugs). Products include:

Xyrem Oral Solution **1766**

Sufentanil Citrate (Since the systematic evaluations of zolpidem in combination with other CNS-active drugs have been limited, careful consideration should be given to the pharmacology of any CNS-active drug to be used with zolpidem. Any drug with CNS-depressant effects could potentially enhance the CNS depressant effects of zolpidem. Dosage adjustments may be necessary when zolpidem is combined with other CNS depressant drugs).

No products indexed under this heading.

Temazepam (Since the systematic evaluations of zolpidem in combination with other CNS-active drugs have been limited, careful consideration should be given to the pharmacology of any CNS-active drug to be used with zolpidem. Any drug with CNS-depressant effects could potentially enhance the CNS depressant effects of zolpidem. Dosage adjustments may be necessary when zolpidem is combined with other CNS depressant drugs).

No products indexed under this heading.

Thiamylal Sodium (Since the systematic evaluations of zolpidem in combination with other CNS-active drugs have been limited, careful consideration should be given to the pharmacology of any CNS-active drug to be used with zolpidem. Any drug with CNS-depressant effects could potentially enhance the CNS depressant effects of zolpidem. Dosage adjustments may be necessary when zolpidem is combined with other CNS depressant drugs).

No products indexed under this heading.

Thioridazine Hydrochloride (Since the systematic evaluations of zolpidem in combination with other CNS-active drugs have been limited, careful consideration should be given to the pharmacology of any CNS-active drug to be used with zolpidem. Any drug with CNS-depressant effects could potentially enhance the CNS depressant effects of zolpidem. Dosage adjustments may be necessary when zolpidem is combined with other CNS depressant drugs). Products include:

Thioridazine Hydrochloride Tablets **2195**

Thiothixene (Since the systematic evaluations of zolpidem in combination with other CNS-active drugs have been limited, careful consideration should be given to the pharmacology of any CNS-active drug to be used with zolpidem. Any drug with CNS-depressant effects could potentially enhance the CNS depressant effects of zolpidem. Dosage adjustments may be necessary when zolpidem is combined with other CNS depressant drugs). Products include:

Thiothixene Capsules **2197**

Triazolam (Since the systematic evaluations of zolpidem in combination with other CNS-active drugs have been limited, careful consideration should be given to the pharma-

cology of any CNS-active drug to be used with zolpidem. Any drug with CNS-depressant effects could potentially enhance the CNS depressant effects of zolpidem. Dosage adjustments may be necessary when zolpidem is combined with other CNS depressant drugs).

No products indexed under this heading.

Trifluoperazine Hydrochloride (Since the systematic evaluations of zolpidem in combination with other CNS-active drugs have been limited, careful consideration should be given to the pharmacology of any CNS-active drug to be used with zolpidem. Any drug with CNS-depressant effects could potentially enhance the CNS depressant effects of zolpidem. Dosage adjustments may be necessary when zolpidem is combined with other CNS depressant drugs).

No products indexed under this heading.

Troleandomycin (Some compounds known to inhibit CYP3A may increase exposure to zolpidem).

No products indexed under this heading.

Venlafaxine Hydrochloride (Some compounds known to inhibit CYP3A may increase exposure to zolpidem). Products include:

Effexor XR Extended-Release Capsules **3195**
Venlafaxine Hydrochloride Tablets ... **2199**

Verapamil Hydrochloride (Some compounds known to inhibit CYP3A may increase exposure to zolpidem). Products include:

Tarka Tablets **511**

Voriconazole (Some compounds known to inhibit CYP3A may increase exposure to zolpidem).

No products indexed under this heading.

Zafirlukast (Some compounds known to inhibit CYP3A may increase exposure to zolpidem). Products include:

Accolate Tablets **669**

Zaleplon (Since the systematic evaluations of zolpidem in combination with other CNS-active drugs have been limited, careful consideration should be given to the pharmacology of any CNS-active drug to be used with zolpidem. Any drug with CNS-depressant effects could potentially enhance the CNS depressant effects of zolpidem. Dosage adjustments may be necessary when zolpidem is combined with other CNS depressant drugs).

No products indexed under this heading.

Zileuton (Some compounds known to inhibit CYP3A may increase exposure to zolpidem).

No products indexed under this heading.

Ziprasidone Hydrochloride (Since the systematic evaluations of zolpidem in combination with other CNS-active drugs have been limited, careful consideration should be given to the pharmacology of any CNS-active drug to be used with zolpidem. Any drug with CNS-depressant effects could potentially enhance the CNS depressant effects of zolpidem. Dosage adjustments may be necessary when zolpidem is combined with other CNS depressant drugs). Products include:

Geodon Capsules **2520**

Food Interactions

Alcohol (An additive effect on psychomotor performance between alcohol and zolpidem was demonstrated. Zolpidem should not be taken with alcohol).

Grapefruit (Some compounds known to inhibit CYP3A may increase exposure to zolpidem).

Meal, unspecified (The effect of zolpidem may be slowed by ingestion with or immediately after a meal).

AMBIEN CR TABLETS

(Zolpidem Tartrate) **2696**

May interact with central nervous system depressants, central nervous system stimulants, cytochrome p450 3a inhibitors (selected), and certain other agents. Compounds in these categories include:

Alfentanil Hydrochloride (Any drug with CNS-depressant effects could potentially enhance the CNS-depressant effects of zolpidem tartrate. Dosage adjustments may be necessary when zolpidem tartrate is combined with other CNS depressant drugs).

No products indexed under this heading.

Alprazolam (Any drug with CNS-depressant effects could potentially enhance the CNS-depressant effects of zolpidem tartrate. Dosage adjustments may be necessary when zolpidem tartrate is combined with other CNS depressant drugs).

No products indexed under this heading.

Amiodarone Hydrochloride (Some compounds known to inhibit CYP3A4 may increase exposure to zolpidem tartrate).

No products indexed under this heading.

Amphetamine Resins (The systematic evaluation of zolpidem tartrate in combination with other CNS-active drugs has been very limited. Therefore, careful consideration should be given to the pharmacology of any CNS-active drug to be used with zolpidem tartrate).

No products indexed under this heading.

Amprenavir (Some compounds known to inhibit CYP3A4 may increase exposure to zolpidem tartrate).

No products indexed under this heading.

Aprepitant (Some compounds known to inhibit CYP3A4 may increase exposure to zolpidem tartrate). Products include:

Emend Capsules **1992**

Aprobarbital (Any drug with CNS-depressant effects could potentially enhance the CNS-depressant effects of zolpidem tartrate. Dosage adjustments may be necessary when zolpidem tartrate is combined with other CNS depressant drugs).

No products indexed under this heading.

Buprenorphine Hydrochloride (Any drug with CNS-depressant effects could potentially enhance the CNS-depressant effects of zolpidem tartrate. Dosage adjustments may be necessary when zolpidem tartrate is combined with other CNS depressant drugs). Products include:

Suboxone Tablets **2601**
Subutex Tablets **2601**

Buspirone Hydrochloride (Any drug with CNS-depressant effects could potentially enhance the CNS-depressant effects of zolpidem tartrate. Dosage adjustments may be necessary when zolpidem tartrate is combined with other CNS depressant drugs).

No products indexed under this heading.

Butabarbital (Any drug with CNS-depressant effects could potentially enhance the CNS-depressant effects of zolpidem tartrate. Dosage adjustments may be necessary when zolpidem tartrate is combined with other CNS depressant drugs).

No products indexed under this heading.

Butalbital (Any drug with CNS-depressant effects could potentially enhance the CNS-depressant effects of zolpidem tartrate. Dosage adjustments may be necessary when zolpidem tartrate is combined with other CNS depressant drugs).

No products indexed under this heading.

Chlordiazepoxide (Any drug with CNS-depressant effects could potentially enhance the CNS-depressant effects of zolpidem tartrate. Dosage adjustments may be necessary when zolpidem tartrate is combined with other CNS depressant drugs).

No products indexed under this heading.

Chlordiazepoxide Hydrochloride (Any drug with CNS-depressant effects could potentially enhance the CNS-depressant effects of zolpidem tartrate. Dosage adjustments may be necessary when zolpidem tartrate is combined with other CNS depressant drugs).

No products indexed under this heading.

Chlorpromazine (Chlorpromazine in combination with zolpidem tartrate produced no pharmacokinetic interaction, but there was an additive effect of decreased alertness and psychomotor performance).

No products indexed under this heading.

Chlorpromazine Hydrochloride (Chlorpromazine in combination with zolpidem tartrate produced no pharmacokinetic interaction, but there was an additive effect of decreased alertness and psychomotor performance).

No products indexed under this heading.

Chlorprothixene (Any drug with CNS-depressant effects could potentially enhance the CNS-depressant effects of zolpidem tartrate. Dosage adjustments may be necessary when zolpidem tartrate is combined with other CNS depressant drugs).

No products indexed under this heading.

Chlorprothixene Hydrochloride (Any drug with CNS-depressant effects could potentially enhance the CNS-depressant effects of zolpidem tartrate. Dosage adjustments may be necessary when zolpidem tartrate is combined with other CNS depressant drugs).

No products indexed under this heading.

Chlorprothixene Lactate (Any drug with CNS-depressant effects could potentially enhance the CNS-depressant effects of zolpidem tartrate. Dosage adjustments may be necessary when zolpidem tartrate is combined with other CNS depressant drugs).

No products indexed under this heading.

Cimetidine (Some compounds known to inhibit CYP3A4 may increase exposure to zolpidem tartrate).

No products indexed under this heading.

Cimetidine Hydrochloride (Some compounds known to inhibit CYP3A4 may increase exposure to zolpidem tartrate).

No products indexed under this heading.

Ciprofloxacin (Some compounds known to inhibit CYP3A4 may increase exposure to zolpidem tartrate). Products include:

Cipro I.V. **2817**
Cipro Oral Suspension **2810**
Cipro XR Tablets **2823**
Ciprodex Otic Suspension **541**

Ciprofloxacin Hydrochloride (Some compounds known to inhibit CYP3A4 may increase exposure to zolpidem tartrate). Products include:

Cipro Tablets **2810**

Clarithromycin (Some compounds known to inhibit CYP3A4 may increase exposure to zolpidem tartrate). Products include:

Biaxin/Biaxin XL **411**

Clorazepate Dipotassium (Any drug with CNS-depressant effects could potentially enhance the CNS-depressant effects of zolpidem tartrate. Dosage adjustments may be necessary when zolpidem tartrate is combined with other CNS depressant drugs).

No products indexed under this heading.

Clozapine (Any drug with CNS-depressant effects could potentially enhance the CNS-depressant effects of zolpidem tartrate. Dosage adjustments may be necessary when zolpidem tartrate is combined with other CNS depressant drugs).

No products indexed under this heading.

Codeine Phosphate (Any drug with CNS-depressant effects could potentially enhance the CNS-depressant effects of zolpidem tartrate. Dosage adjustments may be necessary when zolpidem tartrate is combined with other CNS depressant drugs). Products include:

Tylenol with Codeine Tablets **2427**

Cyclosporine (Some compounds known to inhibit CYP3A4 may increase exposure to zolpidem tartrate). Products include:

Gengraf Capsules **435**
Neoral Oral Solution **2280**
Neoral Soft Gelatin Capsules **2280**
Restasis Ophthalmic Emulsion **557**
Sandimmune **2296**

Delavirdine Mesylate (Some compounds known to inhibit CYP3A4 may increase exposure to zolpidem tartrate).

No products indexed under this heading.

Desflurane (Any drug with CNS-depressant effects could potentially enhance the CNS-depressant effects of zolpidem tartrate. Dosage adjustments may be necessary when zolpidem tartrate is combined with other CNS depressant drugs).
No products indexed under this heading.

Dextroamphetamine Sulfate (The systematic evaluation of zolpidem tartrate in combination with other CNS-active drugs has been very limited. Therefore, careful consideration should be given to the pharmacology of any CNS-active drug to be used with zolpidem tartrate). Products include:
Adderall XR Capsules 3012
Dexedrine 1401

Dezocine (Any drug with CNS-depressant effects could potentially enhance the CNS-depressant effects of zolpidem tartrate. Dosage adjustments may be necessary when zolpidem tartrate is combined with other CNS depressant drugs).
No products indexed under this heading.

Diazepam (Any drug with CNS-depressant effects could potentially enhance the CNS-depressant effects of zolpidem tartrate. Dosage adjustments may be necessary when zolpidem tartrate is combined with other CNS depressant drugs). Products include:
Valium Tablets 2658

Diltiazem Hydrochloride (Some compounds known to inhibit CYP3A4 may increase exposure to zolpidem tartrate). Products include:
Cardizem LA Extended Release Tablets 421

Diltiazem Maleate (Some compounds known to inhibit CYP3A4 may increase exposure to zolpidem tartrate).
No products indexed under this heading.

Droperidol (Any drug with CNS-depressant effects could potentially enhance the CNS-depressant effects of zolpidem tartrate. Dosage adjustments may be necessary when zolpidem tartrate is combined with other CNS depressant drugs).
No products indexed under this heading.

Efavirenz (Some compounds known to inhibit CYP3A4 may increase exposure to zolpidem tartrate). Products include:
Atripla Tablets 938
Sustiva Capsules 930
Sustiva Tablets 930

Enflurane (Any drug with CNS-depressant effects could potentially enhance the CNS-depressant effects of zolpidem tartrate. Dosage adjustments may be necessary when zolpidem tartrate is combined with other CNS depressant drugs).
No products indexed under this heading.

Erythromycin (Some compounds known to inhibit CYP3A4 may increase exposure to zolpidem tartrate).
No products indexed under this heading.

Estazolam (Any drug with CNS-depressant effects could potentially enhance the CNS-depressant effects of zolpidem tartrate. Dosage adjustments may be necessary when zolpidem tartrate is combined with other CNS depressant drugs).
No products indexed under this heading.

Ethanol (Zolpidem tartrate has shown additive effects when combined with alcohol and should not be taken with alcohol).
No products indexed under this heading.

Ethchlorvynol (Any drug with CNS-depressant effects could potentially enhance the CNS-depressant effects of zolpidem tartrate. Dosage adjustments may be necessary when zolpidem tartrate is combined with other CNS depressant drugs).
No products indexed under this heading.

Ethinamate (Any drug with CNS-depressant effects could potentially enhance the CNS-depressant effects of zolpidem tartrate. Dosage adjustments may be necessary when zolpidem tartrate is combined with other CNS depressant drugs).
No products indexed under this heading.

Ethyl Alcohol (Zolpidem tartrate has shown additive effects when combined with alcohol and should not be taken with alcohol).
No products indexed under this heading.

Fentanyl (Any drug with CNS-depressant effects could potentially enhance the CNS-depressant effects of zolpidem tartrate. Dosage adjustments may be necessary when zolpidem tartrate is combined with other CNS depressant drugs). Products include:
Duragesic Transdermal System 2405
Ionsys Transdermal System 2410

Fentanyl Citrate (Any drug with CNS-depressant effects could potentially enhance the CNS-depressant effects of zolpidem tartrate. Dosage adjustments may be necessary when zolpidem tartrate is combined with other CNS depressant drugs). Products include:
Actiq 959
Fentora Tablets 968

Fluconazole (Some compounds known to inhibit CYP3A4 may increase exposure to zolpidem tartrate).
No products indexed under this heading.

Fluoxetine (A single-dose interaction study with zolpidem tartrate 10 mg and fluoxetine 20 mg at steady-state levels in male volunteers did not demonstrate any clinically significant pharmacokinetic or pharmacodynamic interactions. When multiple doses of zolpidem tartrate and fluoxetine at steady-state concentrations were evaluated in healthy females, the only significant change was a 17% increase in the zolpidem tartrate half-life. There was no evidence of an additive effect in psychomotor performance).
No products indexed under this heading.

Fluoxetine Hydrochloride (A single-dose interaction study with zolpidem tartrate 10 mg and fluoxetine 20 mg at steady-state levels in male volunteers did not demonstrate any clinically significant pharmacokinetic or pharmacodynamic interactions. When multiple doses of zolpidem tartrate and fluoxetine at steady-state concentrations were evaluated in healthy females, the only significant change was a 17% increase in the zolpidem tartrate half-life. There was no evidence of an additive effect in psychomotor performance). Products include:
Prozac Weekly Capsules 1852
Prozac Pulvules and Liquid 1852
Symbyax Capsules 1871

Fluphenazine Decanoate (Any drug with CNS-depressant effects could potentially enhance the CNS-depressant effects of zolpidem tartrate. Dosage adjustments may be necessary when zolpidem tartrate is combined with other CNS depressant drugs).
No products indexed under this heading.

Fluphenazine Enanthate (Any drug with CNS-depressant effects could potentially enhance the CNS-depressant effects of zolpidem tartrate. Dosage adjustments may be necessary when zolpidem tartrate is combined with other CNS depressant drugs).
No products indexed under this heading.

Fluphenazine Hydrochloride (Any drug with CNS-depressant effects could potentially enhance the CNS-depressant effects of zolpidem tartrate. Dosage adjustments may be necessary when zolpidem tartrate is combined with other CNS depressant drugs).
No products indexed under this heading.

Flurazepam Hydrochloride (Any drug with CNS-depressant effects could potentially enhance the CNS-depressant effects of zolpidem tartrate. Dosage adjustments may be necessary when zolpidem tartrate is combined with other CNS depressant drugs).
No products indexed under this heading.

Fluvoxamine Maleate (Some compounds known to inhibit CYP3A4 may increase exposure to zolpidem tartrate). Products include:
Luvox CR Extended-Release Capsules 1759

Glutethimide (Any drug with CNS-depressant effects could potentially enhance the CNS-depressant effects of zolpidem tartrate. Dosage adjustments may be necessary when zolpidem tartrate is combined with other CNS depressant drugs).
No products indexed under this heading.

Haloperidol (A study involving haloperidol and zolpidem tartrate revealed no effect of haloperidol on the pharmacokinetics or pharmacodynamics of zolpidem tartrate. The lack of a drug interaction following a single-dose administration does not predict a lack following chronic administration).
No products indexed under this heading.

Haloperidol Decanoate (A study involving haloperidol and zolpidem tartrate revealed no effect of haloperidol on the pharmacokinetics or pharmacodynamics of zolpidem tartrate. The lack of a drug interaction following a single-dose administration does not predict a lack following chronic administration).
No products indexed under this heading.

Haloperidol Lactate (A study involving haloperidol and zolpidem tartrate revealed no effect of haloperidol on the pharmacokinetics or pharmacodynamics of zolpidem tartrate. The lack of a drug interaction following a single-dose administration does not predict a lack following chronic administration).
No products indexed under this heading.

Hydrocodone Bitartrate (Any drug with CNS-depressant effects could potentially enhance the CNS-depressant effects of zolpidem tartrate. Dosage adjustments may be necessary when zolpidem tartrate is combined with other CNS depressant drugs). Products include:
Lortab 5/500 Tablets 3143
Lortab 7.5/500 Tablets 3144
Lortab 10/500 Tablets 3144
Vicodin Tablets 529
Vicodin ES Tablets 530
Vicodin HP Tablets 531
Vicoprofen Tablets 533
Zydone Tablets 1132

Hydrocodone Polistirex (Any drug with CNS-depressant effects could potentially enhance the CNS-depressant effects of zolpidem tartrate. Dosage adjustments may be necessary when zolpidem tartrate is combined with other CNS depressant drugs). Products include:
Tussionex Pennkinetic Extended-Release Suspension 3154

Hydromorphone Hydrochloride (Any drug with CNS-depressant effects could potentially enhance the CNS-depressant effects of zolpidem tartrate. Dosage adjustments may be necessary when zolpidem tartrate is combined with other CNS depressant drugs).
No products indexed under this heading.

Hydroxyzine Hydrochloride (Any drug with CNS-depressant effects could potentially enhance the CNS-depressant effects of zolpidem tartrate. Dosage adjustments may be necessary when zolpidem tartrate is combined with other CNS depressant drugs).
No products indexed under this heading.

Imipramine Hydrochloride (Imipramine in combination with zolpidem tartrate produced no pharmacokinetic interaction other than a 20% decrease in peak levels of imipramine, but there was an additive effect of decreased alertness).
No products indexed under this heading.

Imipramine Pamoate (Imipramine in combination with zolpidem tartrate produced no pharmacokinetic interaction other than a 20% decrease in peak levels of imipramine, but there was an additive effect of decreased alertness).
No products indexed under this heading.

Indinavir Sulfate (Some compounds known to inhibit CYP3A4 may increase exposure to zolpidem tartrate). Products include:

Crixivan Capsules 1979

Isoflurane (Any drug with CNS-depressant effects could potentially enhance the CNS-depressant effects of zolpidem tartrate. Dosage adjustments may be necessary when zolpidem tartrate is combined with other CNS depressant drugs).

No products indexed under this heading.

Isoniazid (Some compounds known to inhibit CYP3A4 may increase exposure to zolpidem tartrate).

No products indexed under this heading.

Itraconazole (A randomized, double-blind, crossover interaction study in 10 healthy volunteers between itraconazole (200 mg once daily for 4 days) and a single dose of zolpidem tartrate (10 mg) given 5 hours after the last dose of itraconazole resulted in a 34% increase in AUC of zolpidem tartrate. There were no significant pharmacodynamic effects of zolpidem tartrate on subjective drowsiness, postural sway, or psychomotor performance).

No products indexed under this heading.

Ketamine Hydrochloride (Any drug with CNS-depressant effects could potentially enhance the CNS-depressant effects of zolpidem tartrate. Dosage adjustments may be necessary when zolpidem tartrate is combined with other CNS depressant drugs).

No products indexed under this heading.

Ketoconazole (A study in 12 healthy subjects showed that co-administration of a single 5 mg dose of immediate-release zolpidem tartrate with ketoconazole, a potent CYP3A4 inhibitor, given as 200 mg b.i.d. for 2 days increased Cmax of zolpidem by a factor of 1.3 and increased the total AUC of zolpidem by a factor of 1.7 compared to zolpidem alone and prolonged the elimination T1/2 by approximately 30% along with an increase in the pharmacodynamic effects of zolpidem. Caution should be used when ketoconazole is given with zolpidem and consideration should be given to using a lower dose of zolpidem when ketoconazole and zolpidem are given together. Advise patients that the use of zolpidem tartrate extended release tablets with ketoconazole may enhance the sedative effects). Products include:

Extina Foam, 2% 3057
Nizoral A-D Shampoo 1901

Levomethadyl Acetate Hydrochloride (Any drug with CNS-depressant effects could potentially enhance the CNS-depressant effects of zolpidem tartrate. Dosage adjustments may be necessary when zolpidem tartrate is combined with other CNS depressant drugs).

No products indexed under this heading.

Levorphanol Tartrate (Any drug with CNS-depressant effects could potentially enhance the CNS-depressant effects of zolpidem tartrate. Dosage adjustments may be necessary when zolpidem tartrate is combined with other CNS depressant drugs).

No products indexed under this heading.

Lopinavir (Some compounds known to inhibit CYP3A4 may increase exposure to zolpidem tartrate). Products include:

Kaletra 452

Lorazepam (Any drug with CNS-depressant effects could potentially enhance the CNS-depressant effects of zolpidem tartrate. Dosage adjustments may be necessary when zolpidem tartrate is combined with other CNS depressant drugs).

No products indexed under this heading.

Loxapine Hydrochloride (Any drug with CNS-depressant effects could potentially enhance the CNS-depressant effects of zolpidem tartrate. Dosage adjustments may be necessary when zolpidem tartrate is combined with other CNS depressant drugs).

No products indexed under this heading.

Loxapine Succinate (Any drug with CNS-depressant effects could potentially enhance the CNS-depressant effects of zolpidem tartrate. Dosage adjustments may be necessary when zolpidem tartrate is combined with other CNS depressant drugs).

No products indexed under this heading.

Meperidine Hydrochloride (Any drug with CNS-depressant effects could potentially enhance the CNS-depressant effects of zolpidem tartrate. Dosage adjustments may be necessary when zolpidem tartrate is combined with other CNS depressant drugs).

No products indexed under this heading.

Mephobarbital (Any drug with CNS-depressant effects could potentially enhance the CNS-depressant effects of zolpidem tartrate. Dosage adjustments may be necessary when zolpidem tartrate is combined with other CNS depressant drugs).

No products indexed under this heading.

Meprobamate (Any drug with CNS-depressant effects could potentially enhance the CNS-depressant effects of zolpidem tartrate. Dosage adjustments may be necessary when zolpidem tartrate is combined with other CNS depressant drugs).

No products indexed under this heading.

Mesoridazine Besylate (Any drug with CNS-depressant effects could potentially enhance the CNS-depressant effects of zolpidem tartrate. Dosage adjustments may be necessary when zolpidem tartrate is combined with other CNS depressant drugs).

No products indexed under this heading.

Methadone Hydrochloride (Any drug with CNS-depressant effects could potentially enhance the CNS-depressant effects of zolpidem tartrate. Dosage adjustments may be necessary when zolpidem tartrate is combined with other CNS depressant drugs).

No products indexed under this heading.

Methamphetamine Hydrochloride (The systematic evaluation of zolpidem tartrate in combination with other CNS-active drugs has been very limited. Therefore, careful consideration should be given to the pharmacology of any CNS-active drug to be used with zolpidem tartrate).

No products indexed under this heading.

Methohexital Sodium (Any drug with CNS-depressant effects could potentially enhance the CNS-depressant effects of zolpidem tartrate. Dosage adjustments may be necessary when zolpidem tartrate is combined with other CNS depressant drugs).

No products indexed under this heading.

Methotrimeprazine (Any drug with CNS-depressant effects could potentially enhance the CNS-depressant effects of zolpidem tartrate. Dosage adjustments may be necessary when zolpidem tartrate is combined with other CNS depressant drugs).

No products indexed under this heading.

Methoxyflurane (Any drug with CNS-depressant effects could potentially enhance the CNS-depressant effects of zolpidem tartrate. Dosage adjustments may be necessary when zolpidem tartrate is combined with other CNS depressant drugs).

No products indexed under this heading.

Methylphenidate (The systematic evaluation of zolpidem tartrate in combination with other CNS-active drugs has been very limited. Therefore, careful consideration should be given to the pharmacology of any CNS-active drug to be used with zolpidem tartrate). Products include:

Daytrana Transdermal Patch 3022

Methylphenidate Hydrochloride (The systematic evaluation of zolpidem tartrate in combination with other CNS-active drugs has been very limited. Therefore, careful consideration should be given to the pharmacology of any CNS-active drug to be used with zolpidem tartrate). Products include:

Concerta Extended-Release Tablets 1925
Metadate CD Capsules 3146

Metronidazole (Some compounds known to inhibit CYP3A4 may increase exposure to zolpidem tartrate). Products include:

Pylera Capsules 714

Metronidazole Benzoate (Some compounds known to inhibit CYP3A4 may increase exposure to zolpidem tartrate).

No products indexed under this heading.

Metronidazole Hydrochloride (Some compounds known to inhibit CYP3A4 may increase exposure to zolpidem tartrate).

No products indexed under this heading.

Miconazole (Some compounds known to inhibit CYP3A4 may increase exposure to zolpidem tartrate).

No products indexed under this heading.

Midazolam Hydrochloride (Any drug with CNS-depressant effects could potentially enhance the CNS-depressant effects of zolpidem tartrate. Dosage adjustments may be necessary when zolpidem tartrate is combined with other CNS depressant drugs).

No products indexed under this heading.

Molindone Hydrochloride (Any drug with CNS-depressant effects could potentially enhance the CNS-depressant effects of zolpidem tartrate. Dosage adjustments may be necessary when zolpidem tartrate is combined with other CNS depressant drugs). Products include:

Moban Tablets 1116

Morphine Sulfate (Any drug with CNS-depressant effects could potentially enhance the CNS-depressant effects of zolpidem tartrate. Dosage adjustments may be necessary when zolpidem tartrate is combined with other CNS depressant drugs). Products include:

Avinza Capsules 1772
DepoDur Injection 1095
MS Contin Tablets 2585

Nefazodone Hydrochloride (Some compounds known to inhibit CYP3A4 may increase exposure to zolpidem tartrate).

No products indexed under this heading.

Nelfinavir Mesylate (Some compounds known to inhibit CYP3A4 may increase exposure to zolpidem tartrate).

No products indexed under this heading.

Nifedipine (Some compounds known to inhibit CYP3A4 may increase exposure to zolpidem tartrate).

No products indexed under this heading.

Norfloxacin (Some compounds known to inhibit CYP3A4 may increase exposure to zolpidem tartrate). Products include:

Noroxin Tablets 2069

Olanzapine (Any drug with CNS-depressant effects could potentially enhance the CNS-depressant effects of zolpidem tartrate. Dosage adjustments may be necessary when zolpidem tartrate is combined with other CNS depressant drugs). Products include:

Symbyax Capsules 1871
Zyprexa Tablets 1883
Zyprexa IntraMuscular 1883
Zyprexa ZYDIS Orally Disintegrating Tablets 1883

Oxazepam (Any drug with CNS-depressant effects could potentially enhance the CNS-depressant effects of zolpidem tartrate. Dosage adjustments may be necessary when zolpidem tartrate is combined with other CNS depressant drugs).

No products indexed under this heading.

Oxycodone Hydrochloride (Any drug with CNS-depressant effects could potentially enhance the CNS-depressant effects of zolpidem tartrate. Dosage adjustments may be

necessary when zolpidem tartrate is combined with other CNS depressant drugs). Products include:
OxyContin Tablets 2589
OxyIR Capsules 2593
Percocet Tablets 1127
Percodan Tablets 1130

Paroxetine Hydrochloride (Some compounds known to inhibit CYP3A4 may increase exposure to zolpidem tartrate). Products include:
Paxil 1535
Paxil CR Controlled-Release Tablets 1544

Pemoline (The systematic evaluation of zolpidem tartrate in combination with other CNS-active drugs has been very limited. Therefore, careful consideration should be given to the pharmacology of any CNS-active drug to be used with zolpidem tartrate).
No products indexed under this heading.

Pentobarbital Sodium (Any drug with CNS-depressant effects could potentially enhance the CNS-depressant effects of zolpidem tartrate. Dosage adjustments may be necessary when zolpidem tartrate is combined with other CNS depressant drugs). Products include:
Nembutal Sodium Solution, USP 2494

Perphenazine (Any drug with CNS-depressant effects could potentially enhance the CNS-depressant effects of zolpidem tartrate. Dosage adjustments may be necessary when zolpidem tartrate is combined with other CNS depressant drugs).
No products indexed under this heading.

Phenobarbital (Any drug with CNS-depressant effects could potentially enhance the CNS-depressant effects of zolpidem tartrate. Dosage adjustments may be necessary when zolpidem tartrate is combined with other CNS depressant drugs). Products include:
Donnatal Extentabs 2507

Prazepam (Any drug with CNS-depressant effects could potentially enhance the CNS-depressant effects of zolpidem tartrate. Dosage adjustments may be necessary when zolpidem tartrate is combined with other CNS depressant drugs).
No products indexed under this heading.

Prochlorperazine (Any drug with CNS-depressant effects could potentially enhance the CNS-depressant effects of zolpidem tartrate. Dosage adjustments may be necessary when zolpidem tartrate is combined with other CNS depressant drugs).
No products indexed under this heading.

Promethazine Hydrochloride (Any drug with CNS-depressant effects could potentially enhance the CNS-depressant effects of zolpidem tartrate. Dosage adjustments may be necessary when zolpidem tartrate is combined with other CNS depressant drugs).
No products indexed under this heading.

Propofol (Any drug with CNS-depressant effects could potentially enhance the CNS-depressant effects of zolpidem tartrate. Dosage adjustments may be necessary when zolpidem tartrate is combined with other CNS depressant drugs).
No products indexed under this heading.

Propoxyphene Hydrochloride (Any drug with CNS-depressant effects could potentially enhance the CNS-depressant effects of zolpidem tartrate. Dosage adjustments may be necessary when zolpidem tartrate is combined with other CNS depressant drugs).
No products indexed under this heading.

Propoxyphene Napsylate (Any drug with CNS-depressant effects could potentially enhance the CNS-depressant effects of zolpidem tartrate. Dosage adjustments may be necessary when zolpidem tartrate is combined with other CNS depressant drugs).
No products indexed under this heading.

Quazepam (Any drug with CNS-depressant effects could potentially enhance the CNS-depressant effects of zolpidem tartrate. Dosage adjustments may be necessary when zolpidem tartrate is combined with other CNS depressant drugs).
No products indexed under this heading.

Quetiapine Fumarate (Any drug with CNS-depressant effects could potentially enhance the CNS-depressant effects of zolpidem tartrate. Dosage adjustments may be necessary when zolpidem tartrate is combined with other CNS depressant drugs).
No products indexed under this heading.

Quinine (Some compounds known to inhibit CYP3A4 may increase exposure to zolpidem tartrate).
No products indexed under this heading.

Quinine Sulfate (Some compounds known to inhibit CYP3A4 may increase exposure to zolpidem tartrate).
No products indexed under this heading.

Remifentanil Hydrochloride (Any drug with CNS-depressant effects could potentially enhance the CNS-depressant effects of zolpidem tartrate. Dosage adjustments may be necessary when zolpidem tartrate is combined with other CNS depressant drugs).
No products indexed under this heading.

Rifampin (A randomized, placebo-controlled, crossover interaction study in 8 healthy female subjects between 5 consecutive daily doses of rifampin (600 mg) and a single dose of an immediate-release formulation of zolpidem tartrate (20 mg) given 17 hours after the last dose of rifampin showed significant reductions of the AUC (-73%), Cmax (-58%), and T1/2 (-36%) of zolpidem tartrate together with significant reductions in the pharmacodynamic effects of zolpidem tartrate).
No products indexed under this heading.

Risperidone (Any drug with CNS-depressant effects could potentially enhance the CNS-depressant effects of zolpidem tartrate. Dosage adjustments may be necessary when zolpidem tartrate is combined with other CNS depressant drugs). Products include:
Risperdal Consta Long-Acting Injection 1753

Ritonavir (Some compounds known to inhibit CYP3A4 may increase exposure to zolpidem tartrate). Products include:
Kaletra 452
Norvir 489

Saquinavir (Some compounds known to inhibit CYP3A4 may increase exposure to zolpidem tartrate).
No products indexed under this heading.

Saquinavir Mesylate (Some compounds known to inhibit CYP3A4 may increase exposure to zolpidem tartrate).
No products indexed under this heading.

Secobarbital Sodium (Any drug with CNS-depressant effects could potentially enhance the CNS-depressant effects of zolpidem tartrate. Dosage adjustments may be necessary when zolpidem tartrate is combined with other CNS depressant drugs).
No products indexed under this heading.

Sertraline Hydrochloride (Following five consecutive nightly doses of zolpidem tartrate 10 mg in the presence of sertraline 50 mg (17 consecutive daily doses, at 7:00 AM, in healthy female volunteers), zolpidem tartrate Cmax was significantly higher (43%) and Tmax was significantly decreased (53%). Pharmacokinetics of sertraline and N-desmethylsertraline were unaffected by zolpidem tartrate).
No products indexed under this heading.

Sevoflurane (Any drug with CNS-depressant effects could potentially enhance the CNS-depressant effects of zolpidem tartrate. Dosage adjustments may be necessary when zolpidem tartrate is combined with other CNS depressant drugs). Products include:
Ultane Liquid for Inhalation 524

Sodium Oxybate (Any drug with CNS-depressant effects could potentially enhance the CNS-depressant effects of zolpidem tartrate. Dosage adjustments may be necessary when zolpidem tartrate is combined with other CNS depressant drugs). Products include:
Xyrem Oral Solution 1766

Sufentanil Citrate (Any drug with CNS-depressant effects could potentially enhance the CNS-depressant effects of zolpidem tartrate. Dosage adjustments may be necessary when zolpidem tartrate is combined with other CNS depressant drugs).
No products indexed under this heading.

Temazepam (Any drug with CNS-depressant effects could potentially enhance the CNS-depressant effects of zolpidem tartrate. Dosage adjustments may be necessary when zolpidem tartrate is combined with other CNS depressant drugs).
No products indexed under this heading.

Thiamylal Sodium (Any drug with CNS-depressant effects could potentially enhance the CNS-depressant effects of zolpidem tartrate. Dosage adjustments may be necessary when zolpidem tartrate is combined with other CNS depressant drugs).
No products indexed under this heading.

Thioridazine Hydrochloride (Any drug with CNS-depressant effects could potentially enhance the CNS-depressant effects of zolpidem tartrate. Dosage adjustments may be necessary when zolpidem tartrate is combined with other CNS depressant drugs). Products include:
Thioridazine Hydrochloride Tablets 2195

Thiothixene (Any drug with CNS-depressant effects could potentially enhance the CNS-depressant effects of zolpidem tartrate. Dosage adjustments may be necessary when zolpidem tartrate is combined with other CNS depressant drugs). Products include:
Thiothixene Capsules 2197

Triazolam (Any drug with CNS-depressant effects could potentially enhance the CNS-depressant effects of zolpidem tartrate. Dosage adjustments may be necessary when zolpidem tartrate is combined with other CNS depressant drugs).
No products indexed under this heading.

Trifluoperazine Hydrochloride (Any drug with CNS-depressant effects could potentially enhance the CNS-depressant effects of zolpidem tartrate. Dosage adjustments may be necessary when zolpidem tartrate is combined with other CNS depressant drugs).
No products indexed under this heading.

Troleandomycin (Some compounds known to inhibit CYP3A4 may increase exposure to zolpidem tartrate).
No products indexed under this heading.

Venlafaxine Hydrochloride (Some compounds known to inhibit CYP3A4 may increase exposure to zolpidem tartrate). Products include:
Effexor XR Extended-Release Capsules 3195
Venlafaxine Hydrochloride Tablets 2199

Verapamil Hydrochloride (Some compounds known to inhibit CYP3A4 may increase exposure to zolpidem tartrate). Products include:
Tarka Tablets 511

Voriconazole (Some compounds known to inhibit CYP3A4 may increase exposure to zolpidem tartrate).
No products indexed under this heading.

Zafirlukast (Some compounds known to inhibit CYP3A4 may increase exposure to zolpidem tartrate). Products include:
Accolate Tablets 669

Zaleplon (Any drug with CNS-depressant effects could potentially enhance the CNS-depressant effects of zolpidem tartrate. Dosage adjustments may be necessary when zolpidem tartrate is combined with other CNS depressant drugs).
No products indexed under this heading.

Zileuton (Some compounds known to inhibit CYP3A4 may increase exposure to zolpidem tartrate).
No products indexed under this heading.

Ziprasidone Hydrochloride (Any drug with CNS-depressant effects could potentially enhance the CNS-depressant effects of zolpidem tartrate. Dosage adjustments may be

necessary when zolpidem tartrate is combined with other CNS depressant drugs). Products include:

Geodon Capsules 2520

Food Interactions

Alcohol (Zolpidem tartrate has shown additive effects when combined with alcohol and should not be taken with alcohol).

Grapefruit (Some compounds known to inhibit CYP3A4 may increase exposure to zolpidem tartrate).

AMBISOME FOR INJECTION

(Amphotericin B, liposomal) 606

May interact with aminoglycosides, antineoplastics, corticosteroids, curariform skeletal muscle relaxants, cardiac glycosides, imidazoles, and certain other agents. Compounds in these categories include:

ACTH (Concurrent use of ACTH and amphotericin B may potentiate hypokalemia which could predispose the patient to cardiac dysfunction).

No products indexed under this heading.

Altretamine (Concurrent use of antineoplastic agents and amphotericin B may enhance the potential for renal toxicity, bronchospasm, and hypotension). Products include:

Hexalen Capsules 1078

Amikacin Sulfate (Concurrent use of amphotericin B and other nephrotoxic agents, such as aminoglycosides, may enhance the potential for drug-induced renal toxicity).

No products indexed under this heading.

Anastrozole (Concurrent use of antineoplastic agents and amphotericin B may enhance the potential for renal toxicity, bronchospasm, and hypotension). Products include:

Arimidex Tablets 672

Asparaginase (Concurrent use of antineoplastic agents and amphotericin B may enhance the potential for renal toxicity, bronchospasm, and hypotension). Products include:

Elspar for Injection 1990

Elspar for Injection 2488

Atracurium Besylate (Amphotericin B-induced hypokalemia may enhance the curariform effect of skeletal relaxants).

No products indexed under this heading.

Betamethasone Acetate (Concurrent use of corticosteroids and amphotericin B may potentiate hypokalemia which could predispose the patient to cardiac dysfunction).

No products indexed under this heading.

Betamethasone Sodium Phosphate (Concurrent use of corticosteroids and amphotericin B may potentiate hypokalemia which could predispose the patient to cardiac dysfunction).

No products indexed under this heading.

Bicalutamide (Concurrent use of antineoplastic agents and amphotericin B may enhance the potential for renal toxicity, bronchospasm, and hypotension). Products include:

No products indexed under this heading.

Bleomycin Sulfate (Concurrent use of antineoplastic agents and amphotericin B may enhance the potential for renal toxicity, bronchospasm, and hypotension).

No products indexed under this heading.

Budesonide (Concurrent use of corticosteroids and amphotericin B may potentiate hypokalemia which could predispose the patient to cardiac dysfunction). Products include:

Pulmicort Flexhaler 654

Symbicort 80/4.5 Inhalation Aerosol 659

Symbicort 160/4.5 Inhalation Aerosol 659

Busulfan (Concurrent use of antineoplastic agents and amphotericin B may enhance the potential for renal toxicity, bronchospasm, and hypotension). Products include:

Busulfex Injection 2477

Myleran Tablets 1530

Carboplatin (Concurrent use of antineoplastic agents and amphotericin B may enhance the potential for renal toxicity, bronchospasm, and hypotension).

No products indexed under this heading.

Carmustine (BCNU) (Concurrent use of antineoplastic agents and amphotericin B may enhance the potential for renal toxicity, bronchospasm, and hypotension).

No products indexed under this heading.

Chlorambucil (Concurrent use of antineoplastic agents and amphotericin B may enhance the potential for renal toxicity, bronchospasm, and hypotension). Products include:

Leukeran Tablets 1508

Ciclesonide (Concurrent use of corticosteroids and amphotericin B may potentiate hypokalemia which could predispose the patient to cardiac dysfunction). Products include:

Alvesco Inhalation Aerosol 2985

Omnaris Nasal Spray 2998

Cisatracurium Besylate (Amphotericin B-induced hypokalemia may enhance the curariform effect of skeletal relaxants). Products include:

Nimbex Injection 484

Cisplatin (Concurrent use of antineoplastic agents and amphotericin B may enhance the potential for renal toxicity, bronchospasm, and hypotension).

No products indexed under this heading.

Clotrimazole (Imidazoles may induce fungal resistance to amphotericin B; combination therapy should be administered with caution, especially in immunocompromised patients). Products include:

Lotrisone 2881

Cortisone Acetate (Concurrent use of corticosteroids and amphotericin B may potentiate hypokalemia which could predispose the patient to cardiac dysfunction).

No products indexed under this heading.

Cyclophosphamide (Concurrent use of antineoplastic agents and amphotericin B may enhance the potential for renal toxicity, bronchospasm, and hypotension).

No products indexed under this heading.

Cyclosporine (Concurrent use of amphotericin B and other nephrotoxic agents, such as cyclosporine, may enhance the potential for drug-induced renal toxicity). Products include:

Gengraf Capsules 435

Neoral Oral Solution 2280

Neoral Soft Gelatin Capsules 2280

Restasis Ophthalmic Emulsion 557

Sandimmune 2296

Dacarbazine (Concurrent use of antineoplastic agents and amphotericin B may enhance the potential for renal toxicity, bronchospasm, and hypotension).

No products indexed under this heading.

Daunorubicin Citrate (Concurrent use of antineoplastic agents and amphotericin B may enhance the potential for renal toxicity, bronchospasm, and hypotension).

No products indexed under this heading.

Daunorubicin Hydrochloride (Concurrent use of antineoplastic agents and amphotericin B may enhance the potential for renal toxicity, bronchospasm, and hypotension).

No products indexed under this heading.

Denileukin Diftitox (Concurrent use of antineoplastic agents and amphotericin B may enhance the potential for renal toxicity, bronchospasm, and hypotension). Products include:

Ontak Vials 1079

Deslanoside (Concurrent use of digitalis and amphotericin B may induce hypokalemia and may potentiate digitalis toxicity).

No products indexed under this heading.

Dexamethasone (Concurrent use of corticosteroids and amphotericin B may potentiate hypokalemia which could predispose the patient to cardiac dysfunction). Products include:

Ciprodex Otic Suspension 541

Dexamethasone Acetate (Concurrent use of corticosteroids and amphotericin B may potentiate hypokalemia which could predispose the patient to cardiac dysfunction).

No products indexed under this heading.

Dexamethasone Sodium Phosphate (Concurrent use of corticosteroids and amphotericin B may potentiate hypokalemia which could predispose the patient to cardiac dysfunction).

No products indexed under this heading.

Digitalis Glycoside Preparations (Concurrent use of digitalis and amphotericin B may induce hypokalemia and may potentiate digitalis toxicity).

No products indexed under this heading.

Digitoxin (Concurrent use of digitalis and amphotericin B may induce hypokalemia and may potentiate digitalis toxicity).

No products indexed under this heading.

Digoxin (Concurrent use of digitalis and amphotericin B may induce hypokalemia and may potentiate digitalis toxicity). Products include:

Lanoxin Injection 1498

Lanoxin Injection Pediatric 1502

Lanoxin Tablets 1505

Docetaxel (Concurrent use of antineoplastic agents and amphotericin B may enhance the potential for renal toxicity, bronchospasm, and hypotension). Products include:

Taxotere Injection Concentrate 2773

Doxacurium Chloride (Amphotericin B-induced hypokalemia may enhance the curariform effect of skeletal relaxants).

No products indexed under this heading.

Doxorubicin Hydrochloride (Concurrent use of antineoplastic agents and amphotericin B may enhance the potential for renal toxicity, bronchospasm, and hypotension).

No products indexed under this heading.

Epirubicin Hydrochloride (Concurrent use of antineoplastic agents and amphotericin B may enhance the potential for renal toxicity, bronchospasm, and hypotension).

No products indexed under this heading.

Estramustine Phosphate Sodium (Concurrent use of antineoplastic agents and amphotericin B may enhance the potential for renal toxicity, bronchospasm, and hypotension).

No products indexed under this heading.

Etoposide (Concurrent use of antineoplastic agents and amphotericin B may enhance the potential for renal toxicity, bronchospasm, and hypotension).

No products indexed under this heading.

Exemestane (Concurrent use of antineoplastic agents and amphotericin B may enhance the potential for renal toxicity, bronchospasm, and hypotension).

No products indexed under this heading.

Floxuridine (Concurrent use of antineoplastic agents and amphotericin B may enhance the potential for renal toxicity, bronchospasm, and hypotension).

No products indexed under this heading.

Fluconazole (Imidazoles may induce fungal resistance to amphotericin B; combination therapy should be administered with caution, especially in immunocompromised patients).

No products indexed under this heading.

Flucytosine (Concurrent use may increase the toxicity of flucytosine by possibly increasing its cellular uptake and/or impairing its renal excretion).

No products indexed under this heading.

Fludrocortisone Acetate (Concurrent use of corticosteroids and amphotericin B may potentiate hypokalemia which could predispose the patient to cardiac dysfunction).

No products indexed under this heading.

Flunisolide (Concurrent use of corticosteroids and amphotericin B may potentiate hypokalemia which could predispose the patient to cardiac dysfunction). Products include:

Aerobid/Aerobid-M 1153

Fluorouracil (Concurrent use of antineoplastic agents and amphotericin B may enhance the potential for renal toxicity, bronchospasm, and hypotension). Products include:

Carac Cream 0.5% 2722

Flutamide (Concurrent use of antineoplastic agents and amphotericin B may enhance the potential for renal toxicity, bronchospasm, and hypotension).
No products indexed under this heading.

Fluticasone Propionate (Concurrent use of corticosteroids and amphotericin B may potentiate hypokalemia which could predispose the patient to cardiac dysfunction). Products include:
Advair Diskus 100/50 1276
Advair Diskus 250/50 1276
Advair Diskus 500/50 1276
Advair HFA 45/21 Inhalation Aerosol.................................... 1288
Advair HFA 115/21 Inhalation Aerosol.................................... 1288
Advair HFA 230/21 Inhalation Aerosol.................................... 1288
Flonase Nasal Spray 1431
Flovent Diskus 50 mcg 1435

Fluticasone Propionate HFA (Concurrent use of corticosteroids and amphotericin B may potentiate hypokalemia which could predispose the patient to cardiac dysfunction). Products include:
Flovent HFA 1440

Gemcitabine Hydrochloride (Concurrent use of antineoplastic agents and amphotericin B may enhance the potential for renal toxicity, bronchospasm, and hypotension). Products include:
Gemzar for Injection 1820

Gentamicin Sulfate (Concurrent use of amphotericin B and other nephrotoxic agents, such as aminoglycosides, may enhance the potential for drug-induced renal toxicity). Products include:
Pred-G Ophthalmic Ointment .... ⊙ 229
Pred-G Ophthalmic Suspension ...... ⊙ 228

Hydrocortisone (Concurrent use of corticosteroids and amphotericin B may potentiate hypokalemia which could predispose the patient to cardiac dysfunction).
No products indexed under this heading.

Hydrocortisone Acetate (Concurrent use of corticosteroids and amphotericin B may potentiate hypokalemia which could predispose the patient to cardiac dysfunction). Products include:
Analpram-HC 1140
Pramosone 1141

Hydrocortisone Sodium Phosphate (Concurrent use of corticosteroids and amphotericin B may potentiate hypokalemia which could predispose the patient to cardiac dysfunction).
No products indexed under this heading.

Hydrocortisone Sodium Succinate (Concurrent use of corticosteroids and amphotericin B may potentiate hypokalemia which could predispose the patient to cardiac dysfunction).
No products indexed under this heading.

Hydroxyurea (Concurrent use of antineoplastic agents and amphotericin B may enhance the potential for renal toxicity, bronchospasm, and hypotension).
No products indexed under this heading.

Idarubicin Hydrochloride (Concurrent use of antineoplastic agents and amphotericin B may enhance the potential for renal toxicity, bronchospasm, and hypotension).
No products indexed under this heading.

Ifosfamide (Concurrent use of antineoplastic agents and amphotericin B may enhance the potential for renal toxicity, bronchospasm, and hypotension).
No products indexed under this heading.

Interferon alfa-2a, Recombinant (Concurrent use of antineoplastic agents and amphotericin B may enhance the potential for renal toxicity, bronchospasm, and hypotension).
No products indexed under this heading.

Interferon alfa-2b, Recombinant (Concurrent use of antineoplastic agents and amphotericin B may enhance the potential for renal toxicity, bronchospasm, and hypotension). Products include:
Intron A for Injection 2859

Irinotecan Hydrochloride (Concurrent use of antineoplastic agents and amphotericin B may enhance the potential for renal toxicity, bronchospasm, and hypotension).
No products indexed under this heading.

Kanamycin Sulfate (Concurrent use of amphotericin B and other nephrotoxic agents, such as aminoglycosides, may enhance the potential for drug-induced renal toxicity).
No products indexed under this heading.

Ketoconazole (Imidazoles may induce fungal resistance to amphotericin B; combination therapy should be administered with caution, especially in immunocompromised patients). Products include:
Extina Foam, 2% 3057
Nizoral A-D Shampoo 1901

Levamisole Hydrochloride (Concurrent use of antineoplastic agents and amphotericin B may enhance the potential for renal toxicity, bronchospasm, and hypotension).
No products indexed under this heading.

Lomustine (CCNU) (Concurrent use of antineoplastic agents and amphotericin B may enhance the potential for renal toxicity, bronchospasm, and hypotension).
No products indexed under this heading.

Mechlorethamine Hydrochloride (Concurrent use of antineoplastic agents and amphotericin B may enhance the potential for renal toxicity, bronchospasm, and hypotension). Products include:
Mustargen for Injection 2492

Megestrol Acetate (Concurrent use of antineoplastic agents and amphotericin B may enhance the potential for renal toxicity, bronchospasm, and hypotension). Products include:
Megace ES Oral Suspension 2499

Melphalan (Concurrent use of antineoplastic agents and amphotericin B may enhance the potential for renal toxicity, bronchospasm, and hypotension).
No products indexed under this heading.

Mercaptopurine (Concurrent use of antineoplastic agents and amphotericin B may enhance the potential for renal toxicity, bronchospasm, and hypotension).
No products indexed under this heading.

Methotrexate Sodium (Concurrent use of antineoplastic agents and amphotericin B may enhance the potential for renal toxicity, bronchospasm, and hypotension).
No products indexed under this heading.

Methylprednisolone Acetate (Concurrent use of corticosteroids and amphotericin B may potentiate hypokalemia which could predispose the patient to cardiac dysfunction).
No products indexed under this heading.

Methylprednisolone Sodium Succinate (Concurrent use of corticosteroids and amphotericin B may potentiate hypokalemia which could predispose the patient to cardiac dysfunction).
No products indexed under this heading.

Metocurine Iodide (Amphotericin B-induced hypokalemia may enhance the curariform effect of skeletal relaxants).
No products indexed under this heading.

Miconazole (Imidazoles may induce fungal resistance to amphotericin B; combination therapy should be administered with caution, especially in immunocompromised patients).
No products indexed under this heading.

Miconazole Nitrate (Imidazoles may induce fungal resistance to amphotericin B; combination therapy should be administered with caution, especially in immunocompromised patients).
No products indexed under this heading.

Mitomycin (Mitomycin-C) (Concurrent use of antineoplastic agents and amphotericin B may enhance the potential for renal toxicity, bronchospasm, and hypotension).
No products indexed under this heading.

Mitotane (Concurrent use of antineoplastic agents and amphotericin B may enhance the potential for renal toxicity, bronchospasm, and hypotension).
No products indexed under this heading.

Mitoxantrone Hydrochloride (Concurrent use of antineoplastic agents and amphotericin B may enhance the potential for renal toxicity, bronchospasm, and hypotension). Products include:
Novantrone for Injection Concentrate.............................. 1100

Mivacurium Chloride (Amphotericin B-induced hypokalemia may enhance the curariform effect of skeletal relaxants).
No products indexed under this heading.

Mometasone Furoate (Concurrent use of corticosteroids and amphotericin B may potentiate hypokalemia which could predispose the patient to cardiac dysfunction). Products include:
Asmanex Twisthaler 2797
Elocon Cream 0.1% 2840
Elocon Lotion 0.1% 2841
Elocon Ointment 0.1% 2842

Mometasone Furoate Monohydrate (Concurrent use of corticosteroids and amphotericin B may potentiate hypokalemia which could predispose the patient to cardiac dysfunction). Products include:
Nasonex Nasal Spray 2883

Oxaliplatin (Concurrent use of antineoplastic agents and amphotericin B may enhance the potential for renal toxicity, bronchospasm, and hypotension). Products include:
Eloxatin for Injection 2731

Paclitaxel (Concurrent use of antineoplastic agents and amphotericin B may enhance the potential for renal toxicity, bronchospasm, and hypotension).
No products indexed under this heading.

Pancuronium Bromide (Amphotericin B-induced hypokalemia may enhance the curariform effect of skeletal relaxants).
No products indexed under this heading.

Pentamidine Isethionate (Concurrent use of amphotericin B and other nephrotoxic agents, such as pentamidine, may enhance the potential for drug-induced renal toxicity).
No products indexed under this heading.

Pipecuronium Bromide (Amphotericin B-induced hypokalemia may enhance the curariform effect of skeletal relaxants).
No products indexed under this heading.

Prednisolone Acetate (Concurrent use of corticosteroids and amphotericin B may potentiate hypokalemia which could predispose the patient to cardiac dysfunction). Products include:
Pred Forte Ophthalmic Suspension............................... ⊙ 227
Pred Mild Ophthalmic Suspension............................... ⊙ 230
Pred-G Ophthalmic Ointment .... ⊙ 229
Pred-G Ophthalmic Suspension ...... ⊙ 228

Prednisolone Sodium Phosphate (Concurrent use of corticosteroids and amphotericin B may potentiate hypokalemia which could predispose the patient to cardiac dysfunction).
No products indexed under this heading.

Prednisolone Tebutate (Concurrent use of corticosteroids and amphotericin B may potentiate hypokalemia which could predispose the patient to cardiac dysfunction).
No products indexed under this heading.

Prednisone (Concurrent use of corticosteroids and amphotericin B may potentiate hypokalemia which could predispose the patient to cardiac dysfunction).
No products indexed under this heading.

Procarbazine Hydrochloride (Concurrent use of antineoplastic agents and amphotericin B may enhance the potential for renal toxicity, bronchospasm, and hypotension).
No products indexed under this heading.

Rapacuronium Bromide (Amphotericin B-induced hypokalemia may enhance the curariform effect of skeletal relaxants).
No products indexed under this heading.

Rocuronium Bromide (Amphotericin B-induced hypokalemia may enhance the curariform effect of skeletal relaxants). Products include:
Zemuron Injection 2947

Streptomycin Sulfate (Concurrent use of amphotericin B and other nephrotoxic agents, such as aminoglycosides, may enhance the potential for drug-induced renal toxicity).
No products indexed under this heading.

Streptozocin (Concurrent use of antineoplastic agents and amphotericin B may enhance the potential for renal toxicity, bronchospasm, and hypotension).
No products indexed under this heading.

Tamoxifen Citrate (Concurrent use of antineoplastic agents and amphotericin B may enhance the potential for renal toxicity, bronchospasm, and hypotension).
No products indexed under this heading.

Teniposide (Concurrent use of antineoplastic agents and amphotericin B may enhance the potential for renal toxicity, bronchospasm, and hypotension).
No products indexed under this heading.

Thioguanine (Concurrent use of antineoplastic agents and amphotericin B may enhance the potential for renal toxicity, bronchospasm, and hypotension). Products include:
Tabloid Tablets 1601

Thiotepa (Concurrent use of antineoplastic agents and amphotericin B may enhance the potential for renal toxicity, bronchospasm, and hypotension).
No products indexed under this heading.

Tobramycin (Concurrent use of amphotericin B and other nephrotoxic agents, such as aminoglycosides, may enhance the potential for drug-induced renal toxicity). Products include:
Zylet Ophthalmic Suspension .... ⊙247

Tobramycin Sulfate (Concurrent use of amphotericin B and other nephrotoxic agents, such as aminoglycosides, may enhance the potential for drug-induced renal toxicity).
No products indexed under this heading.

Topotecan Hydrochloride (Concurrent use of antineoplastic agents and amphotericin B may enhance the potential for renal toxicity, bronchospasm, and hypotension). Products include:
Hycamtin for Injection 1459
Hycamtin Capsules 1456

Toremifene Citrate (Concurrent use of antineoplastic agents and amphotericin B may enhance the potential for renal toxicity, bronchospasm, and hypotension).
No products indexed under this heading.

Triamcinolone (Concurrent use of corticosteroids and amphotericin B may potentiate hypokalemia which could predispose the patient to cardiac dysfunction).
No products indexed under this heading.

Triamcinolone Acetonide (Concurrent use of corticosteroids and amphotericin B may potentiate hypokalemia which could predispose the patient to cardiac dysfunction). Products include:
Azmacort Inhalation Aerosol 407
Nasacort AQ Nasal Spray 2765
Triesence Injectable Suspension .... ⊙209

Triamcinolone Diacetate (Concurrent use of corticosteroids and amphotericin B may potentiate hypokalemia which could predispose the patient to cardiac dysfunction).
No products indexed under this heading.

Triamcinolone Hexacetonide (Concurrent use of corticosteroids and amphotericin B may potentiate hypokalemia which could predispose the patient to cardiac dysfunction).
No products indexed under this heading.

Tubocurarine Chloride (Amphotericin B-induced hypokalemia may enhance the curariform effect of skeletal relaxants).
No products indexed under this heading.

Valrubicin (Concurrent use of antineoplastic agents and amphotericin B may enhance the potential for renal toxicity, bronchospasm, and hypotension). Products include:
Valstar Sterile Solution for Intravesical Instillation.................. 1735

Vecuronium Bromide (Amphotericin B-induced hypokalemia may enhance the curariform effect of skeletal relaxants).
No products indexed under this heading.

Vincristine Sulfate (Concurrent use of antineoplastic agents and amphotericin B may enhance the potential for renal toxicity, bronchospasm, and hypotension).
No products indexed under this heading.

Vinorelbine Tartrate (Concurrent use of antineoplastic agents and amphotericin B may enhance the potential for renal toxicity, bronchospasm, and hypotension).
No products indexed under this heading.

AMERGE TABLETS

(Naratriptan Hydrochloride) 1301
May interact with 5HT1-receptor agonists, ergot-containing drugs, oral contraceptives, Serotonin and Norepinephrine Reuptake Inhibitors, and selective serotonin reuptake inhibitors. Compounds in these categories include:

Almotriptan Malate (Co-administration with other 5-HT$_1$ agonists within 24 hours of each other is contraindicated because of the vasospastic effects may be additive). Products include:
Axert Tablets 2431

Citalopram Hydrobromide (Cases of life-threatening serotonin syndrome, including mental status changes, autonomic instability, neuromuscular aberrations, and/or GI symptoms, have been reported during combination use of selective serotonin reuptake inhibitors and triptans. If concomitant treatment with naratriptan and an SSRI is clinically warranted, careful observation of the patient is advised, particularly during treatment initiation and dose increases). Products include:
Celexa 1160

Desogestrel (Co-administration with oral contraceptives has resulted in reduced clearance by 32% and volume of distribution by 22%, producing slightly higher concentrations of naratriptan). Products include:
Mircette Tablets 1034

Desvenlafaxine Succinate (Cases of life-threatening serotonin syndrome, including mental status changes, autonomic instability, neuromuscular aberrations, and/or GI symptoms, have been reported during combination use of selective serotonin reuptake inhibitors and triptans. If concomitant treatment with naratriptan and an SSRI is clinically waranted, careful observation of the patient is advised, particularly during treatment initiation and dose increases). Products include:
Pristiq Extended-Release Tablets 3247

Dihydroergotamine Mesylate (Ergot-containing drugs have been reported to cause prolonged vasospastic reactions; because there is a theoretical basis that these effects may be additive, use of ergot-type agents and naratriptan within 24 hours is contraindicated).
No products indexed under this heading.

Duloxetine Hydrochloride (Cases of life-threatening serotonin syndrome, including mental status changes, autonomic instability, neuromuscular aberrations, and/or GI symptoms, have been reported during combination use of serotonin and norepinephrine reuptake inhibitors and triptans. If concomitant treatment with naratriptan and an SNRI is clinically warranted, careful observation of the patient is advised, particularly during treatment initiation and dose increases). Products include:
Cymbalta Delayed-Release Capsules..................................... 1801

Eletriptan Hydrobromide (Co-administration with other 5-HT$_1$ agonists within 24 hours of each other is contraindicated because of the vasospastic effects may be additive).
No products indexed under this heading.

Ergonovine Maleate (Ergot-containing drugs have been reported to cause prolonged vasospastic reactions; because there is a theoretical basis that these effects may be additive, use of ergot-type agents and naratriptan within 24 hours is contraindicated).
No products indexed under this heading.

Ergotamine Tartrate (Ergot-containing drugs have been reported to cause prolonged vasospastic reactions; because there is a theoretical basis that these effects may be additive, use of ergot-type agents and naratriptan within 24 hours is contraindicated).
No products indexed under this heading.

Escitalopram Oxalate (Cases of life-threatening serotonin syndrome, including mental status changes, autonomic instability, neuromuscular aberrations, and/or GI symptoms, have been reported during combination use of selective serotonin reuptake inhibitors and triptans. If concomitant treatment with naratriptan and an SSRI is clinically warranted, careful observation of the patient is advised, particularly during treatment initiation and dose increases). Products include:
Lexapro Oral Suspension 1174
Lexapro Tablets 1174

Ethinyl Estradiol (Co-administration with oral contraceptives has resulted in reduced clearance by 32% and volume of distribution by 22%, producing slightly higher concentrations of naratriptan). Products include:
Lybrel Tablets 3204
Mircette Tablets 1034
NuvaRing 2897
Ortho-Cyclen/Ortho Tri-Cyclen 2449
Ortho Evra Transdermal System 2437
Ortho Tri-Cyclen Lo Tablets 2458
Seasonique Tablets 1046
Yaz Tablets 805

Ethynodiol Diacetate (Co-administration with oral contraceptives has resulted in reduced clearance by 32% and volume of distribution by 22%, producing slightly higher concentrations of naratriptan).
No products indexed under this heading.

Fluoxetine (Cases of life-threatening serotonin syndrome, including mental status changes, autonomic instability, neuromuscular aberrations, and/or GI symptoms, have been reported during combination use of selective serotonin reuptake inhibitors and triptans. If concomitant treatment with naratriptan and an SSRI is clinically warranted, careful observation of the patient is advised, particularly during treatment initiation and dose increases).
No products indexed under this heading.

Fluoxetine Hydrochloride (Cases of life-threatening serotonin syndrome, including mental status changes, autonomic instability, neuromuscular aberrations, and/or GI symptoms, have been reported during combination use of selective serotonin reuptake inhibitors and triptans. If concomitant treatment with naratriptan and an SSRI is clinically warranted, careful observation of the patient is advised, particularly during treatment initiation and dose increases). Products include:
Prozac Weekly Capsules 1852
Prozac Pulvules and Liquid 1852
Symbyax Capsules 1871

Fluvoxamine Maleate (Cases of life-threatening serotonin syndrome, including mental status changes, autonomic instability, neuromuscular aberrations, and/or GI symptoms, have been reported during combination use of selective serotonin reuptake inhibitors and triptans. If concomitant treatment with naratriptan and an SSRI is clinically warranted, careful observation of the patient is advised, particularly during treatment initiation and dose increases). Products include:
Luvox CR Extended-Release Capsules.................................... 1759

Frovatriptan Succinate (Co-administration with other 5-HT$_1$ agonists within 24 hours of each other is contraindicated because of the vasospastic effects may be additive). Products include:
Frova Tablets 1111

Levonorgestrel (Co-administration with oral contraceptives has resulted in reduced clearance by 32% and volume of distribution by 22%, producing slightly higher concentrations of naratriptan). Products include:

Climara Pro Transdermal System 768
Lybrel Tablets 3204
Mirena Intrauterine System 779
Plan B Tablets 1044
Seasonique Tablets 1046

Mestranol (Co-administration with oral contraceptives has resulted in reduced clearance by 32% and volume of distribution by 22%, producing slightly higher concentrations of naratriptan).
No products indexed under this heading.

Methylergonovine Maleate (Ergot-containing drugs have been reported to cause prolonged vasospastic reactions; because there is a theoretical basis that these effects may be additive, use of ergot-type agents and naratriptan within 24 hours is contraindicated).
No products indexed under this heading.

Methysergide Maleate (Ergot-containing drugs have been reported to cause prolonged vasospastic reactions; because there is a theoretical basis that these effects may be additive, use of ergot-type agents and naratriptan within 24 hours is contraindicated).
No products indexed under this heading.

Nefazodone Hydrochloride (Cases of life-threatening serotonin syndrome, including mental status changes, autonomic instability, neuromuscular aberrations, and/or GI symptoms, have been reported during combination use of serotonin and norepinephrine reuptake inhibitors and triptans. If concomitant treatment with naratriptan and an SNRI is clinically warranted, careful observation of the patient is advised, particularly during treatment initiation and dose increases).
No products indexed under this heading.

Norethindrone (Co-administration with oral contraceptives has resulted in reduced clearance by 32% and volume of distribution by 22%, producing slightly higher concentrations of naratriptan). Products include:
Ortho Micronor Tablets 2446

Norethynodrel (Co-administration with oral contraceptives has resulted in reduced clearance by 32% and volume of distribution by 22%, producing slightly higher concentrations of naratriptan).
No products indexed under this heading.

Norgestimate (Co-administration with oral contraceptives has resulted in reduced clearance by 32% and volume of distribution by 22%, producing slightly higher concentrations of naratriptan). Products include:
Ortho-Cyclen/Ortho Tri-Cyclen 2449
Ortho Tri-Cyclen Lo Tablets 2458

Norgestrel (Co-administration with oral contraceptives has resulted in reduced clearance by 32% and volume of distribution by 22%, producing slightly higher concentrations of naratriptan).
No products indexed under this heading.

Paroxetine Hydrochloride (Cases of life-threatening serotonin syndrome, including mental status changes, autonomic instability, neuromuscular aberrations, and/or GI symptoms, have been reported during combination use of selective serotonin reuptake inhibitors and triptans. If concomitant treatment with naratriptan and an SSRI is clinically warranted, careful observation of the patient is advised, particularly during treatment initiation and dose increases). Products include:
Paxil 1535
Paxil CR Controlled-Release Tablets 1544

Rizatriptan Benzoate (Co-administration with other 5-HT_1 agonists within 24 hours of each other is contraindicated because of the vasospastic effects may be additive). Products include:
Maxalt Tablets 2056
Maxalt-MLT Orally Disintegrating Tablets 2056

Sertraline Hydrochloride (Cases of life-threatening serotonin syndrome, including mental status changes, autonomic instability, neuromuscular aberrations, and/or GI symptoms, have been reported during combination use of selective serotonin reuptake inhibitors and triptans. If concomitant treatment with naratriptan and an SSRI is clinically warranted, careful observation of the patient is advised, particularly during treatment initiation and dose increases).
No products indexed under this heading.

Sumatriptan (Co-administration with other 5-HT_1 agonists within 24 hours of each other is contraindicated because of the vasospastic effects may be additive). Products include:
Imitrex Nasal Spray 1470

Sumatriptan Succinate (Co-administration with other 5-HT_1 agonists within 24 hours of each other is contraindicated because of the vasospastic effects may be additive). Products include:
Imitrex Injection 1465
Imitrex Tablets 1474
Treximet Tablets 1616

Venlafaxine Hydrochloride (Cases of life-threatening serotonin syndrome, including mental status changes, autonomic instability, neuromuscular aberrations, and/or GI symptoms, have been reported during combination use of serotonin and norepinephrine reuptake inhibitors and triptans. If concomitant treatment with naratriptan and an SNRI is clinically warranted, careful observation of the patient is advised, particularly during treatment initiation and dose increases). Products include:
Effexor XR Extended-Release Capsules 3195
Venlafaxine Hydrochloride Tablets ... 2199

Zolmitriptan (Co-administration with other 5-HT_1 agonists within 24 hours of each other is contraindicated because of the vasospastic effects may be additive). Products include:
Zomig Tablets 694
Zomig Nasal Spray 689
Zomig-ZMT Tablets 694

AMEVIVE

(Alefacept) 611
None cited in PDR database.

AMINOHIPPURATE SODIUM "PAH" INJECTION

(Aminohippurate Sodium) 1950
May interact with sulfonamides and certain other agents. Compounds in these categories include:

Bendroflumethiazide (Co-administration with sulfonamides interfere with chemical color development essential to the analytical procedures).
No products indexed under this heading.

Chlorothiazide (Co-administration with sulfonamides interfere with chemical color development essential to the analytical procedures).
No products indexed under this heading.

Chlorothiazide Sodium (Co-administration with sulfonamides interfere with chemical color development essential to the analytical procedures). Products include:
Intravenous Sodium Diuril 2490

Chlorpropamide (Co-administration with sulfonamides interfere with chemical color development essential to the analytical procedures).
No products indexed under this heading.

Glipizide (Co-administration with sulfonamides interfere with chemical color development essential to the analytical procedures).
No products indexed under this heading.

Glyburide (Co-administration with sulfonamides interfere with chemical color development essential to the analytical procedures).
No products indexed under this heading.

Hydrochlorothiazide (Co-administration with sulfonamides interfere with chemical color development essential to the analytical procedures). Products include:
Atacand HCT 642
Avalide Tablets 892
Avalide Tablets 2713
Benicar HCT Tablets 1010
Diovan HCT Tablets 2216
Dyazide Capsules 1405
Micardis HCT Tablets 854
Prinzide Tablets 2092
Tekturna HCT Tablets 2324
Teveten HCT Tablets 517

Hydroflumethiazide (Co-administration with sulfonamides interfere with chemical color development essential to the analytical procedures).
No products indexed under this heading.

Methyclothiazide (Co-administration with sulfonamides interfere with chemical color development essential to the analytical procedures).
No products indexed under this heading.

Polythiazide (Co-administration with sulfonamides interfere with chemical color development essential to the analytical procedures).
No products indexed under this heading.

Probenecid (Tubular secretion of PAH depressed).
No products indexed under this heading.

Procaine Hydrochloride (Renal clearance measurements impaired).
No products indexed under this heading.

Sulfacytine (Co-administration with sulfonamides interfere with chemical color development essential to the analytical procedures).
No products indexed under this heading.

Sulfamethizole (Co-administration with sulfonamides interfere with chemical color development essential to the analytical procedures).
No products indexed under this heading.

Sulfamethoxazole (Co-administration with sulfonamides interfere with chemical color development essential to the analytical procedures).
No products indexed under this heading.

Sulfasalazine (Co-administration with sulfonamides interfere with chemical color development essential to the analytical procedures).
No products indexed under this heading.

Sulfinpyrazone (Co-administration with sulfonamides interfere with chemical color development essential to the analytical procedures).
No products indexed under this heading.

Sulfisoxazole Acetyl (Co-administration with sulfonamides interfere with chemical color development essential to the analytical procedures).
No products indexed under this heading.

Sulfisoxazole Diolamine (Co-administration with sulfonamides interfere with chemical color development essential to the analytical procedures).
No products indexed under this heading.

Tolazamide (Co-administration with sulfonamides interfere with chemical color development essential to the analytical procedures).
No products indexed under this heading.

Tolbutamide (Co-administration with sulfonamides interfere with chemical color development essential to the analytical procedures).
No products indexed under this heading.

AMITIZA CAPSULES

(Lubiprostone) 3082
None cited in PDR database.

AMOXIL CAPSULES

(Amoxicillin) 1305
See Amoxil Tablets

AMOXIL CHEWABLE TABLETS

(Amoxicillin) 1305
See Amoxil Tablets

AMOXIL PEDIATRIC DROPS FOR ORAL SUSPENSION

(Amoxicillin) 1305
See Amoxil Tablets

AMOXIL POWDER FOR ORAL SUSPENSION

(Amoxicillin) 1305
See Amoxil Tablets

AMOXIL TABLETS
(Amoxicillin) 1305
May interact with certain other agents. Compounds in these categories include:

Azithromycin Dihydrate (May interfere with bactericidal effects of penicillin. This has been demonstrated in vitro; however, the clinical significance of the interaction is not well documented).
No products indexed under this heading.

Bendroflumethiazide (May interfere with bactericidal effects of penicillin. This has been demonstrated in vitro; however, the clinical significance of the interaction is not well documented).
No products indexed under this heading.

Chloramphenicol Sodium Succinate (May interfere with bactericidal effects of penicillin. This has been demonstrated in vitro; however, the clinical significance of the interaction is not well documented).
No products indexed under this heading.

Chlorothiazide (May interfere with bactericidal effects of penicillin. This has been demonstrated in vitro; however, the clinical significance of the interaction is not well documented).
No products indexed under this heading.

Chlorothiazide Sodium (May interfere with bactericidal effects of penicillin. This has been demonstrated in vitro; however, the clinical significance of the interaction is not well documented). Products include:
Intravenous Sodium Diuril 2490

Chlorpropamide (May interfere with bactericidal effects of penicillin. This has been demonstrated in vitro; however, the clinical significance of the interaction is not well documented).
No products indexed under this heading.

Clarithromycin (May interfere with bactericidal effects of penicillin. This has been demonstrated in vitro; however, the clinical significance of the interaction is not well documented). Products include:
Biaxin/Biaxin XL 411

Demeclocycline Hydrochloride (May interfere with bactericidal effects of penicillin. This has been demonstrated in vitro; however, the clinical significance of the interaction is not well documented).
No products indexed under this heading.

Desogestrel (In common with other antibiotics, amoxicillin may affect the gut flora, leading to lower estrogen reabsorption and reduce efficacy of combined oral estrogen/progesterone contraceptives). Products include:
Mircette Tablets 1034

Dirithromycin (May interfere with bactericidal effects of penicillin. This has been demonstrated in vitro; however, the clinical significance of the interaction is not well documented).
No products indexed under this heading.

Doxycycline Calcium (May interfere with bactericidal effects of penicillin. This has been demonstrated in vitro; however, the clinical significance of the interaction is not well documented).
No products indexed under this heading.

Doxycycline Hyclate (May interfere with bactericidal effects of penicillin. This has been demonstrated in vitro; however, the clinical significance of the interaction is not well documented).
No products indexed under this heading.

Doxycycline Monohydrate (May interfere with bactericidal effects of penicillin. This has been demonstrated in vitro; however, the clinical significance of the interaction is not well documented).
No products indexed under this heading.

Erythromycin (May interfere with bactericidal effects of penicillin. This has been demonstrated in vitro; however, the clinical significance of the interaction is not well documented).
No products indexed under this heading.

Erythromycin Estolate (May interfere with bactericidal effects of penicillin. This has been demonstrated in vitro; however, the clinical significance of the interaction is not well documented).
No products indexed under this heading.

Erythromycin Ethylsuccinate (May interfere with bactericidal effects of penicillin. This has been demonstrated in vitro; however, the clinical significance of the interaction is not well documented). Products include:
E.E.S. 433
EryPed 431

Erythromycin Gluceptate (May interfere with bactericidal effects of penicillin. This has been demonstrated in vitro; however, the clinical significance of the interaction is not well documented).
No products indexed under this heading.

Erythromycin Stearate (May interfere with bactericidal effects of penicillin. This has been demonstrated in vitro; however, the clinical significance of the interaction is not well documented).
No products indexed under this heading.

Ethinyl Estradiol (In common with other antibiotics, amoxicillin may affect the gut flora, leading to lower estrogen reabsorption and reduce efficacy of combined oral estrogen/progesterone contraceptives). Products include:
Lybrel Tablets 3204
Mircette Tablets 1034
NuvaRing 2897
Ortho-Cyclen/Ortho Tri-Cyclen 2449
Ortho Evra Transdermal System 2437
Ortho Tri-Cyclen Lo Tablets 2458
Seasonique Tablets 1046
Yaz Tablets 805

Ethynodiol Diacetate (In common with other antibiotics, amoxicillin may affect the gut flora, leading to lower estrogen reabsorption and reduce efficacy of combined oral estrogen/progesterone contraceptives).
No products indexed under this heading.

Glipizide (May interfere with bactericidal effects of penicillin. This has been demonstrated in vitro; however, the clinical significance of the interaction is not well documented).
No products indexed under this heading.

Glyburide (May interfere with bactericidal effects of penicillin. This has been demonstrated in vitro; however, the clinical significance of the interaction is not well documented).
No products indexed under this heading.

Hydrochlorothiazide (May interfere with bactericidal effects of penicillin. This has been demonstrated in vitro; however, the clinical significance of the interaction is not well documented). Products include:
Atacand HCT 642
Avalide Tablets 892
Avalide Tablets 2713
Benicar HCT Tablets 1010
Diovan HCT Tablets 2216
Dyazide Capsules 1405
Micardis HCT Tablets 854
Prinzide Tablets 2092
Tekturna HCT Tablets 2324
Teveten HCT Tablets 517

Hydroflumethiazide (May interfere with bactericidal effects of penicillin. This has been demonstrated in vitro; however, the clinical significance of the interaction is not well documented).
No products indexed under this heading.

Levonorgestrel (In common with other antibiotics, amoxicillin may affect the gut flora, leading to lower estrogen reabsorption and reduce efficacy of combined oral estrogen/progesterone contraceptives). Products include:
Climara Pro Transdermal System 768
Lybrel Tablets 3204
Mirena Intrauterine System 779
Plan B Tablets 1044
Seasonique Tablets 1046

Mestranol (In common with other antibiotics, amoxicillin may affect the gut flora, leading to lower estrogen reabsorption and reduce efficacy of combined oral estrogen/progesterone contraceptives).
No products indexed under this heading.

Methacycline Hydrochloride (May interfere with bactericidal effects of penicillin. This has been demonstrated in vitro; however, the clinical significance of the interaction is not well documented).
No products indexed under this heading.

Methyclothiazide (May interfere with bactericidal effects of penicillin. This has been demonstrated in vitro; however, the clinical significance of the interaction is not well documented).
No products indexed under this heading.

Minocycline Hydrochloride (May interfere with bactericidal effects of penicillin. This has been demonstrated in vitro; however, the clinical significance of the interaction is not well documented). Products include:
Solodyn Extended Release Tablets 1938

Norethindrone (In common with other antibiotics, amoxicillin may affect the gut flora, leading to lower estrogen reabsorption and reduce efficacy of combined oral estrogen/progesterone contraceptives). Products include:
Ortho Micronor Tablets 2446

Norethynodrel (In common with other antibiotics, amoxicillin may affect the gut flora, leading to lower estrogen reabsorption and reduce efficacy of combined oral estrogen/progesterone contraceptives).
No products indexed under this heading.

Norgestimate (In common with other antibiotics, amoxicillin may affect the gut flora, leading to lower estrogen reabsorption and reduce efficacy of combined oral estrogen/progesterone contraceptives). Products include:
Ortho-Cyclen/Ortho Tri-Cyclen 2449
Ortho Tri-Cyclen Lo Tablets 2458

Norgestrel (In common with other antibiotics, amoxicillin may affect the gut flora, leading to lower estrogen reabsorption and reduce efficacy of combined oral estrogen/progesterone contraceptives).
No products indexed under this heading.

Oxytetracycline Hydrochloride (May interfere with bactericidal effects of penicillin. This has been demonstrated in vitro; however, the clinical significance of the interaction is not well documented).
No products indexed under this heading.

Polythiazide (May interfere with bactericidal effects of penicillin. This has been demonstrated in vitro; however, the clinical significance of the interaction is not well documented).
No products indexed under this heading.

Probenecid (Decreases the renal tubular secretion of amoxicillin; concurrent use may result in increased and prolonged blood levels).
No products indexed under this heading.

Sulfacytine (May interfere with bactericidal effects of penicillin. This has been demonstrated in vitro; however, the clinical significance of the interaction is not well documented).
No products indexed under this heading.

Sulfamethizole (May interfere with bactericidal effects of penicillin. This has been demonstrated in vitro; however, the clinical significance of the interaction is not well documented).
No products indexed under this heading.

Sulfamethoxazole (May interfere with bactericidal effects of penicillin. This has been demonstrated in vitro; however, the clinical significance of the interaction is not well documented).
No products indexed under this heading.

Sulfisoxazole Acetyl (May interfere with bactericidal effects of penicillin. This has been demonstrated in vitro; however, the clinical significance of the interaction is not well documented).
No products indexed under this heading.

Tetracycline Hydrochloride (May interfere with bactericidal effects of penicillin. This has been demonstrated in vitro; however, the clinical significance of the interaction is not well documented). Products include:
Pylera Capsules 714

Troleandomycin (May interfere with bactericidal effects of penicillin. This has been demonstrated in vitro; however, the clinical significance of the interaction is not well documented).
No products indexed under this heading.

AMRIX CAPSULES
(Cyclobenzaprine Hydrochloride) 966
May interact with barbiturates, central nervous system depressants, monoamine oxidase inhibitors, and certain other agents. Compounds in these categories include:

Alfentanil Hydrochloride (Concomitant use with cyclobenzaprine HCl may enhance the effects of CNS depressants).
No products indexed under this heading.

Alprazolam (Concomitant use with cyclobenzaprine HCl may enhance the effects of CNS depressants).
No products indexed under this heading.

Aprobarbital (Concomitant use with cyclobenzaprine HCl may enhance the effects of barbiturates).
No products indexed under this heading.

Buprenorphine Hydrochloride (Concomitant use with cyclobenzaprine HCl may enhance the effects of CNS depressants). Products include:
Suboxone Tablets 2601
Subutex Tablets 2601

Buspirone Hydrochloride (Concomitant use with cyclobenzaprine HCl may enhance the effects of CNS depressants).
No products indexed under this heading.

Butabarbital (Concomitant use with cyclobenzaprine HCl may enhance the effects of barbiturates).
No products indexed under this heading.

Butalbital (Concomitant use with cyclobenzaprine HCl may enhance the effects of barbiturates).
No products indexed under this heading.

Chlordiazepoxide (Concomitant use with cyclobenzaprine HCl may enhance the effects of CNS depressants).
No products indexed under this heading.

Chlordiazepoxide Hydrochloride (Concomitant use with cyclobenzaprine HCl may enhance the effects of CNS depressants).
No products indexed under this heading.

Chlorpromazine (Concomitant use with cyclobenzaprine HCl may enhance the effects of CNS depressants).
No products indexed under this heading.

Chlorpromazine Hydrochloride (Concomitant use with cyclobenzaprine HCl may enhance the effects of CNS depressants).
No products indexed under this heading.

Chlorprothixene (Concomitant use with cyclobenzaprine HCl may enhance the effects of CNS depressants).
No products indexed under this heading.

Chlorprothixene Hydrochloride (Concomitant use with cyclobenzaprine HCl may enhance the effects of CNS depressants).
No products indexed under this heading.

Chlorprothixene Lactate (Concomitant use with cyclobenzaprine HCl may enhance the effects of CNS depressants).
No products indexed under this heading.

Clorazepate Dipotassium (Concomitant use with cyclobenzaprine HCl may enhance the effects of CNS depressants).
No products indexed under this heading.

Clozapine (Concomitant use with cyclobenzaprine HCl may enhance the effects of CNS depressants).
No products indexed under this heading.

Codeine Phosphate (Concomitant use with cyclobenzaprine HCl may enhance the effects of CNS depressants). Products include:
Tylenol with Codeine Tablets 2427

Desflurane (Concomitant use with cyclobenzaprine HCl may enhance the effects of CNS depressants).
No products indexed under this heading.

Dezocine (Concomitant use with cyclobenzaprine HCl may enhance the effects of CNS depressants).
No products indexed under this heading.

Diazepam (Concomitant use with cyclobenzaprine HCl may enhance the effects of CNS depressants). Products include:
Valium Tablets 2658

Droperidol (Concomitant use with cyclobenzaprine HCl may enhance the effects of CNS depressants).
No products indexed under this heading.

Enflurane (Concomitant use with cyclobenzaprine HCl may enhance the effects of CNS depressants).
No products indexed under this heading.

Estazolam (Concomitant use with cyclobenzaprine HCl may enhance the effects of CNS depressants).
No products indexed under this heading.

Ethanol (Concomitant use with cyclobenzaprine HCl may enhance the effects of CNS depressants).
No products indexed under this heading.

Ethchlorvynol (Concomitant use with cyclobenzaprine HCl may enhance the effects of CNS depressants).
No products indexed under this heading.

Ethinamate (Concomitant use with cyclobenzaprine HCl may enhance the effects of CNS depressants).
No products indexed under this heading.

Ethyl Alcohol (Concomitant use with cyclobenzaprine HCl may enhance the effects of CNS depressants).
No products indexed under this heading.

Fentanyl (Concomitant use with cyclobenzaprine HCl may enhance the effects of CNS depressants). Products include:
Duragesic Transdermal System 2405
Ionsys Transdermal System 2410

Fentanyl Citrate (Concomitant use with cyclobenzaprine HCl may enhance the effects of CNS depressants). Products include:
Actiq 959
Fentora Tablets 968

Fluphenazine Decanoate (Concomitant use with cyclobenzaprine HCl may enhance the effects of CNS depressants).
No products indexed under this heading.

Fluphenazine Enanthate (Concomitant use with cyclobenzaprine HCl may enhance the effects of CNS depressants).
No products indexed under this heading.

Fluphenazine Hydrochloride (Concomitant use with cyclobenzaprine HCl may enhance the effects of CNS depressants).
No products indexed under this heading.

Flurazepam Hydrochloride (Concomitant use with cyclobenzaprine HCl may enhance the effects of CNS depressants).
No products indexed under this heading.

Glutethimide (Concomitant use with cyclobenzaprine HCl may enhance the effects of CNS depressants).
No products indexed under this heading.

Guanethidine (Tricyclic antidepressants may block the antihypertensive action of guanethidine and similarly acting compounds).
No products indexed under this heading.

Haloperidol (Concomitant use with cyclobenzaprine HCl may enhance the effects of CNS depressants).
No products indexed under this heading.

Haloperidol Decanoate (Concomitant use with cyclobenzaprine HCl may enhance the effects of CNS depressants).
No products indexed under this heading.

Hydrocodone Bitartrate (Concomitant use with cyclobenzaprine HCl may enhance the effects of CNS depressants). Products include:
Lortab 5/500 Tablets 3143
Lortab 7.5/500 Tablets 3144
Lortab 10/500 Tablets 3144
Vicodin Tablets 529
Vicodin ES Tablets 530
Vicodin HP Tablets 531
Vicoprofen Tablets 533
Zydone Tablets 1132

Hydrocodone Polistirex (Concomitant use with cyclobenzaprine HCl may enhance the effects of CNS depressants). Products include:
Tussionex Pennkinetic Extended-Release Suspension 3154

Hydromorphone Hydrochloride (Concomitant use with cyclobenzaprine HCl may enhance the effects of CNS depressants).
No products indexed under this heading.

Hydroxyzine Hydrochloride (Concomitant use with cyclobenzaprine HCl may enhance the effects of CNS depressants).
No products indexed under this heading.

Isocarboxazid (Cyclobenzaprine HCl may have life-threatening interactions with MAO inhibitors. Concomitant use of monoamine oxidase (MAO) inhibitors or within 14 days after their discontinuation is contraindicated). Products include:
Marplan Tablets 3177

Isoflurane (Concomitant use with cyclobenzaprine HCl may enhance the effects of CNS depressants).
No products indexed under this heading.

Ketamine Hydrochloride (Concomitant use with cyclobenzaprine HCl may enhance the effects of CNS depressants).
No products indexed under this heading.

Levomethadyl Acetate Hydrochloride (Concomitant use with cyclobenzaprine HCl may enhance the effects of CNS depressants).
No products indexed under this heading.

Levorphanol Tartrate (Concomitant use with cyclobenzaprine HCl may enhance the effects of CNS depressants).
No products indexed under this heading.

Lorazepam (Concomitant use with cyclobenzaprine HCl may enhance the effects of CNS depressants).
No products indexed under this heading.

Loxapine Hydrochloride (Concomitant use with cyclobenzaprine HCl may enhance the effects of CNS depressants).
No products indexed under this heading.

Loxapine Succinate (Concomitant use with cyclobenzaprine HCl may enhance the effects of CNS depressants).
No products indexed under this heading.

Meperidine Hydrochloride (Concomitant use with cyclobenzaprine HCl may enhance the effects of CNS depressants).
No products indexed under this heading.

Mephobarbital (Concomitant use with cyclobenzaprine HCl may enhance the effects of barbiturates).
No products indexed under this heading.

Meprobamate (Concomitant use with cyclobenzaprine HCl may enhance the effects of CNS depressants).
No products indexed under this heading.

Mesoridazine Besylate (Concomitant use with cyclobenzaprine HCl may enhance the effects of CNS depressants).
No products indexed under this heading.

Methadone Hydrochloride (Concomitant use with cyclobenzaprine HCl may enhance the effects of CNS depressants).
No products indexed under this heading.

Methohexital Sodium (Concomitant use with cyclobenzaprine HCl may enhance the effects of CNS depressants).
No products indexed under this heading.

Methotrimeprazine (Concomitant use with cyclobenzaprine HCl may enhance the effects of CNS depressants).
No products indexed under this heading.

Methoxyflurane (Concomitant use with cyclobenzaprine HCl may enhance the effects of CNS depressants).
No products indexed under this heading.

Midazolam Hydrochloride (Concomitant use with cyclobenzaprine HCl may enhance the effects of CNS depressants).
No products indexed under this heading.

Moclobemide (Cyclobenzaprine HCl may have life-threatening interactions with MAO inhibitors. Concomitant use of monoamine oxidase (MAO) inhibitors or within 14 days after their discontinuation is contraindicated).
No products indexed under this heading.

Molindone Hydrochloride (Concomitant use with cyclobenzaprine HCl may enhance the effects of CNS depressants). Products include:
Moban Tablets 1116

Morphine Sulfate (Concomitant use with cyclobenzaprine HCl may enhance the effects of CNS depressants). Products include:
Avinza Capsules 1772
DepoDur Injection 1095
MS Contin Tablets 2585

Olanzapine (Concomitant use with cyclobenzaprine HCl may enhance the effects of CNS depressants).
Products include:
Symbyax Capsules 1871
Zyprexa Tablets 1883
Zyprexa IntraMuscular 1883
Zyprexa ZYDIS Orally Disintegrating Tablets 1883

Oxazepam (Concomitant use with cyclobenzaprine HCl may enhance the effects of CNS depressants).
No products indexed under this heading.

Oxycodone Hydrochloride (Concomitant use with cyclobenzaprine HCl may enhance the effects of CNS depressants). Products include:
OxyContin Tablets 2589
OxyIR Capsules 2593
Percocet Tablets 1127
Percodan Tablets 1130

Pargyline Hydrochloride (Cyclobenzaprine HCl may have life-threatening interactions with MAO inhibitors. Concomitant use of monoamine oxidase (MAO) inhibitors or within 14 days after their discontinuation is contraindicated).
No products indexed under this heading.

Pentobarbital Sodium (Concomitant use with cyclobenzaprine HCl may enhance the effects of barbiturates). Products include:
Nembutal Sodium Solution, USP 2494

Perphenazine (Concomitant use with cyclobenzaprine HCl may enhance the effects of CNS depressants).
No products indexed under this heading.

Phenelzine Sulfate (Cyclobenzaprine HCl may have life-threatening interactions with MAO inhibitors. Concomitant use of monoamine oxidase (MAO) inhibitors or within 14 days after their discontinuation is contraindicated).
No products indexed under this heading.

Phenobarbital (Concomitant use with cyclobenzaprine HCl may enhance the effects of barbiturates). Products include:
Donnatal Extentabs 2507

Prazepam (Concomitant use with cyclobenzaprine HCl may enhance the effects of CNS depressants).
No products indexed under this heading.

Procarbazine Hydrochloride (Cyclobenzaprine HCl may have life-threatening interactions with MAO inhibitors. Concomitant use of monoamine oxidase (MAO) inhibitors or within 14 days after their discontinuation is contraindicated).
No products indexed under this heading.

Prochlorperazine (Concomitant use with cyclobenzaprine HCl may enhance the effects of CNS depressants).
No products indexed under this heading.

Promethazine Hydrochloride (Concomitant use with cyclobenzaprine HCl may enhance the effects of CNS depressants).
No products indexed under this heading.

Propofol (Concomitant use with cyclobenzaprine HCl may enhance the effects of CNS depressants).
No products indexed under this heading.

Propoxyphene Hydrochloride (Concomitant use with cyclobenzaprine HCl may enhance the effects of CNS depressants).
No products indexed under this heading.

Propoxyphene Napsylate (Concomitant use with cyclobenzaprine HCl may enhance the effects of CNS depressants).
No products indexed under this heading.

Quazepam (Concomitant use with cyclobenzaprine HCl may enhance the effects of CNS depressants).
No products indexed under this heading.

Quetiapine Fumarate (Concomitant use with cyclobenzaprine HCl may enhance the effects of CNS depressants).
No products indexed under this heading.

Rasagiline Mesylate (Cyclobenzaprine HCl may have life-threatening interactions with MAO inhibitors. Concomitant use of monoamine oxidase (MAO) inhibitors or within 14 days after their discontinuation is contraindicated). Products include:
Azilect Tablets 3106

Remifentanil Hydrochloride (Concomitant use with cyclobenzaprine HCl may enhance the effects of CNS depressants).
No products indexed under this heading.

Risperidone (Concomitant use with cyclobenzaprine HCl may enhance the effects of CNS depressants).
Products include:
Risperdal Consta Long-Acting Injection 1753

Secobarbital Sodium (Concomitant use with cyclobenzaprine HCl may enhance the effects of barbiturates).
No products indexed under this heading.

Selegiline (Cyclobenzaprine HCl may have life-threatening interactions with MAO inhibitors. Concomitant use of monoamine oxidase (MAO) inhibitors or within 14 days after their discontinuation is contraindicated). Products include:
Emsam Transdermal System 905

Selegiline Hydrochloride (Cyclobenzaprine HCl may have life-threatening interactions with MAO inhibitors. Concomitant use of monoamine oxidase (MAO) inhibitors or within 14 days after their discontinuation is contraindicated). Products include:
Eldepryl Capsules 3052

Sevoflurane (Concomitant use with cyclobenzaprine HCl may enhance the effects of CNS depressants).
Products include:
Ultane Liquid for Inhalation 524

Sodium Oxybate (Concomitant use with cyclobenzaprine HCl may enhance the effects of CNS depressants). Products include:
Xyrem Oral Solution 1766

Sufentanil Citrate (Concomitant use with cyclobenzaprine HCl may enhance the effects of CNS depressants).
No products indexed under this heading.

Temazepam (Concomitant use with cyclobenzaprine HCl may enhance the effects of CNS depressants).
No products indexed under this heading.

Thiamylal Sodium (Concomitant use with cyclobenzaprine HCl may enhance the effects of barbiturates).
No products indexed under this heading.

Thioridazine Hydrochloride (Concomitant use with cyclobenzaprine HCl may enhance the effects of CNS depressants). Products include:
Thioridazine Hydrochloride Tablets 2195

Thiothixene (Concomitant use with cyclobenzaprine HCl may enhance the effects of CNS depressants).
Products include:
Thiothixene Capsules 2197

Tramadol Hydrochloride (Tricyclic antidepressants may enhance the seizure risk in patients taking tramadol). Products include:
Ultram ER Extended-Release Tablets 2428

Tranylcypromine Sulfate (Cyclobenzaprine HCl may have life-threatening interactions with MAO inhibitors. Concomitant use of monoamine oxidase (MAO) inhibitors or within 14 days after their discontinuation is contraindicated). Products include:
Parnate Tablets 1532

Triazolam (Concomitant use with cyclobenzaprine HCl may enhance the effects of CNS depressants).
No products indexed under this heading.

Trifluoperazine Hydrochloride (Concomitant use with cyclobenzaprine HCl may enhance the effects of CNS depressants).
No products indexed under this heading.

Zaleplon (Concomitant use with cyclobenzaprine HCl may enhance the effects of CNS depressants).
No products indexed under this heading.

Ziprasidone Hydrochloride (Concomitant use with cyclobenzaprine HCl may enhance the effects of CNS depressants). Products include:
Geodon Capsules 2520

Zolpidem Tartrate (Concomitant use with cyclobenzaprine HCl may enhance the effects of CNS depressants). Products include:
Ambien Tablets 2692
Ambien CR Tablets 2696

Food Interactions

Alcohol (Concomitant use with cyclobenzaprine HCl may enhance the effects of alcohol).

ANALPRAM HC CREAM, 1% AND 2.5%

(Hydrocortisone Acetate, Pramoxine Hydrochloride) 1140
None cited in PDR database.

ANALPRAM HC LOTION, 2.5%

(Hydrocortisone Acetate, Pramoxine Hydrochloride) 1140
None cited in PDR database.

ANAPROX TABLETS

(Naproxen Sodium) 2632
See EC-Naprosyn Delayed-Release Tablets

ANAPROX DS TABLETS

(Naproxen Sodium) 2632
See EC-Naprosyn Delayed-Release Tablets

ANDROGEL

(Testosterone) 3159
May interact with corticosteroids, oral anticoagulants, insulin, and certain other agents. Compounds in these categories include:

ACTH (The concurrent use of testosterone with ACTH or corticosteroids may result in increased fluid retention and should be monitored cautiously, particularly in patients with cardiac, renal, or hepatic disease).
No products indexed under this heading.

Anisindione (Changes in anticoagulant activity may be seen with androgens. More frequent monitoring of INR and prothrombin time are recommended in patients taking anticoagulants, especially at the initiation and termination of androgen therapy).
No products indexed under this heading.

Betamethasone Acetate (The concurrent use of testosterone with ACTH or corticosteroids may result in increased fluid retention and should be monitored cautiously, particularly in patients with cardiac, renal, or hepatic disease).
No products indexed under this heading.

Betamethasone Sodium Phosphate (The concurrent use of testosterone with ACTH or corticosteroids may result in increased fluid retention and should be monitored cautiously, particularly in patients with cardiac, renal, or hepatic disease).
No products indexed under this heading.

Budesonide (The concurrent use of testosterone with ACTH or corticosteroids may result in increased fluid retention and should be monitored cautiously, particularly in patients with cardiac, renal, or hepatic disease). Products include:
Pulmicort Flexhaler 654
Symbicort 80/4.5 Inhalation Aerosol.. 659
Symbicort 160/4.5 Inhalation Aerosol.. 659

Ciclesonide (The concurrent use of testosterone with ACTH or corticosteroids may result in increased fluid retention and should be monitored cautiously, particularly in patients with cardiac, renal, or hepatic disease). Products include:
Alvesco Inhalation Aerosol 2985
Omnaris Nasal Spray 2998

Cortisone Acetate (The concurrent use of testosterone with ACTH or corticosteroids may result in increased fluid retention and should be monitored cautiously, particularly in patients with cardiac, renal, or hepatic disease).
No products indexed under this heading.

Dexamethasone (The concurrent use of testosterone with ACTH or corticosteroids may result in increased fluid retention and should be monitored cautiously, particularly in patients with cardiac, renal, or hepatic disease). Products include:
Ciprodex Otic Suspension 541

Dexamethasone Acetate (The concurrent use of testosterone with ACTH or corticosteroids may result in increased fluid retention and should be monitored cautiously, particularly in patients with cardiac, renal, or hepatic disease).
No products indexed under this heading.

Dexamethasone Sodium Phosphate (The concurrent use of testosterone with ACTH or corticosteroids may result in increased fluid retention and should be monitored cautiously, particularly in patients with cardiac, renal, or hepatic disease).
No products indexed under this heading.

Dicumarol (Changes in anticoagulant activity may be seen with androgens. More frequent monitoring of INR and prothrombin time are recommended in patients taking anticoagulants, especially at the initiation and termination of androgen therapy).
No products indexed under this heading.

Fludrocortisone Acetate (The concurrent use of testosterone with ACTH or corticosteroids may result in increased fluid retention and should be monitored cautiously, particularly in patients with cardiac, renal, or hepatic disease).
No products indexed under this heading.

Flunisolide (The concurrent use of testosterone with ACTH or corticosteroids may result in increased fluid retention and should be monitored cautiously, particularly in patients with cardiac, renal, or hepatic disease). Products include:
Aerobid/Aerobid-M 1153

Fluticasone Propionate (The concurrent use of testosterone with ACTH or corticosteroids may result in increased fluid retention and should be monitored cautiously, particularly in patients with cardiac, renal, or hepatic disease). Products include:
Advair Diskus 100/50 1276
Advair Diskus 250/50 1276
Advair Diskus 500/50 1276
Advair HFA 45/21 Inhalation Aerosol.. 1288
Advair HFA 115/21 Inhalation Aerosol.. 1288
Advair HFA 230/21 Inhalation Aerosol.. 1288
Flonase Nasal Spray 1431
Flovent Diskus 50 mcg 1435

Fluticasone Propionate HFA (The concurrent use of testosterone with ACTH or corticosteroids may result in increased fluid retention and should be monitored cautiously, particularly in patients with cardiac, renal, or hepatic disease). Products include:
Flovent HFA.................................... 1440

Hydrocortisone (The concurrent use of testosterone with ACTH or corticosteroids may result in increased fluid retention and should be monitored cautiously, particularly in patients with cardiac, renal, or hepatic disease).
No products indexed under this heading.

Hydrocortisone Acetate (The concurrent use of testosterone with ACTH or corticosteroids may result in increased fluid retention and should be monitored cautiously, particularly in patients with cardiac, renal, or hepatic disease). Products include:
Analpram-HC 1140
Pramosone 1141

Hydrocortisone Sodium Phosphate (The concurrent use of testosterone with ACTH or corticosteroids may result in increased fluid retention and should be monitored cautiously, particularly in patients with cardiac, renal, or hepatic disease).
No products indexed under this heading.

Hydrocortisone Sodium Succinate (The concurrent use of testosterone with ACTH or corticosteroids may result in increased fluid retention and should be monitored cautiously, particularly in patients with cardiac, renal, or hepatic disease).
No products indexed under this heading.

Insulin (Changes in insulin sensitivity or glycemic control may occur in patients treated with androgens. In diabetic patients, the metabolic effects of androgens may decrease blood glucose and, therefore, insulin requirements).
No products indexed under this heading.

Insulin, Human, Zinc Suspension (Changes in insulin sensitivity or glycemic control may occur in patients treated with androgens. In diabetic patients, the metabolic effects of androgens may decrease blood glucose and, therefore, insulin requirements).
No products indexed under this heading.

Insulin, Human (rDNA origin) (Changes in insulin sensitivity or glycemic control may occur in patients treated with androgens. In diabetic patients, the metabolic effects of androgens may decrease blood glucose and, therefore, insulin requirements). Products include:
Exubera Inhalation Powder 2515

Insulin, Human NPH (Changes in insulin sensitivity or glycemic control may occur in patients treated with androgens. In diabetic patients, the metabolic effects of androgens may decrease blood glucose and, therefore, insulin requirements). Products include:
Humulin N Vial 1846

Insulin, Human Regular (Changes in insulin sensitivity or glycemic control may occur in patients treated with androgens. In diabetic patients, the metabolic effects of androgens may decrease blood glucose and, therefore, insulin requirements). Products include:
Humulin R 1849
Humulin R (U-500) 1850

Insulin, Human Regular and Human NPH Mixture (Changes in insulin sensitivity or glycemic control may occur in patients treated with androgens. In diabetic patients, the metabolic effects of androgens may decrease blood glucose and, therefore, insulin requirements). Products include:
Humulin 50/50, 100 Units 1843
Humulin 70/30 Vial 1844

Insulin, NPH (Changes in insulin sensitivity or glycemic control may occur in patients treated with androgens. In diabetic patients, the metabolic effects of androgens may decrease blood glucose and, therefore, insulin requirements).
No products indexed under this heading.

Insulin, Regular (Changes in insulin sensitivity or glycemic control may occur in patients treated with androgens. In diabetic patients, the metabolic effects of androgens may decrease blood glucose and, therefore, insulin requirements).
No products indexed under this heading.

Insulin, Regular and NPH mixture (Changes in insulin sensitivity or glycemic control may occur in patients treated with androgens. In diabetic patients, the metabolic effects of androgens may decrease blood glucose and, therefore, insulin requirements).
No products indexed under this heading.

Insulin, Zinc Crystals (Changes in insulin sensitivity or glycemic control may occur in patients treated with androgens. In diabetic patients, the metabolic effects of androgens may decrease blood glucose and, therefore, insulin requirements).
No products indexed under this heading.

Insulin, Zinc Suspension (Changes in insulin sensitivity or glycemic control may occur in patients treated with androgens. In diabetic patients, the metabolic effects of androgens may decrease blood glucose and, therefore, insulin requirements).
No products indexed under this heading.

Insulin Aspart (Changes in insulin sensitivity or glycemic control may occur in patients treated with androgens. In diabetic patients, the metabolic effects of androgens may decrease blood glucose and, therefore, insulin requirements).
No products indexed under this heading.

Insulin Aspart, Human (Changes in insulin sensitivity or glycemic control may occur in patients treated with androgens. In diabetic patients, the metabolic effects of androgens may decrease blood glucose and, therefore, insulin requirements). Products include:
NovoLog Mix 70/30 2364

Insulin Aspart, Human Regular (Changes in insulin sensitivity or glycemic control may occur in patients treated with androgens. In diabetic patients, the metabolic effects of androgens may decrease blood glucose and, therefore, insulin requirements). Products include:
NovoLog Injection 2359

Insulin Aspart Protamine, Human (Changes in insulin sensitivity or glycemic control may occur in patients treated with androgens. In diabetic patients, the metabolic effects of androgens may decrease blood glucose and, therefore, insulin requirements). Products include:
NovoLog Mix 70/30 2364

Insulin Detemir (rDNA Origin) (Changes in insulin sensitivity or glycemic control may occur in patients treated with androgens. In diabetic patients, the metabolic effects of androgens may decrease blood glucose and, therefore, insulin requirements). Products include:
Levemir Injection 2352

Insulin glargine (Changes in insulin sensitivity or glycemic control may occur in patients treated with androgens. In diabetic patients, the metabolic effects of androgens may decrease blood glucose and, therefore, insulin requirements). Products include:
Lantus Injection 2749

Insulin Glulisine (Changes in insulin sensitivity or glycemic control may occur in patients treated with androgens. In diabetic patients, the metabolic effects of androgens may decrease blood glucose and, therefore, insulin requirements). Products include:
Apidra Injection 2706

Insulin Lispro, Human (Changes in insulin sensitivity or glycemic control may occur in patients treated with androgens. In diabetic patients, the metabolic effects of androgens may decrease blood glucose and, therefore, insulin requirements). Products include:
Humalog-Pen and KwikPen 1829
Humalog Mix 50/50-Pen and KwikPen.. 1833
Humalog Mix 75/25-Pen and KwikPen.. 1835

Insulin Lispro Protamine, Human (Changes in insulin sensitivity or gly-

cemic control may occur in patients treated with androgens. In diabetic patients, the metabolic effects of androgens may decrease blood glucose and, therefore, insulin requirements). Products include:
Humalog Mix 50/50-Pen and KwikPen 1833
Humalog Mix 75/25-Pen and KwikPen 1835

Methylprednisolone Acetate (The concurrent use of testosterone with ACTH or corticosteroids may result in increased fluid retention and should be monitored cautiously, particularly in patients with cardiac, renal, or hepatic disease).
No products indexed under this heading.

Methylprednisolone Sodium Succinate (The concurrent use of testosterone with ACTH or corticosteroids may result in increased fluid retention and should be monitored cautiously, particularly in patients with cardiac, renal, or hepatic disease).
No products indexed under this heading.

Mometasone Furoate (The concurrent use of testosterone with ACTH or corticosteroids may result in increased fluid retention and should be monitored cautiously, particularly in patients with cardiac, renal, or hepatic disease). Products include:
Asmanex Twisthaler 2797
Elocon Cream 0.1% 2840
Elocon Lotion 0.1% 2841
Elocon Ointment 0.1% 2842

Mometasone Furoate Monohydrate (The concurrent use of testosterone with ACTH or corticosteroids may result in increased fluid retention and should be monitored cautiously, particularly in patients with cardiac, renal, or hepatic disease). Products include:
Nasonex Nasal Spray 2883

Oxyphenbutazone (Co-administration of androgens and oxyphenbutazone may result in elevated serum levels of oxyphenbutazone).
No products indexed under this heading.

Prednisolone Acetate (The concurrent use of testosterone with ACTH or corticosteroids may result in increased fluid retention and should be monitored cautiously, particularly in patients with cardiac, renal, or hepatic disease). Products include:
Pred Forte Ophthalmic Suspension .... ⊙227
Pred Mild Ophthalmic Suspension .... ⊙230
Pred-G Ophthalmic Ointment .... ⊙229
Pred-G Ophthalmic Suspension .... ⊙228

Prednisolone Sodium Phosphate (The concurrent use of testosterone with ACTH or corticosteroids may result in increased fluid retention and should be monitored cautiously, particularly in patients with cardiac, renal, or hepatic disease).
No products indexed under this heading.

Prednisolone Tebutate (The concurrent use of testosterone with ACTH or corticosteroids may result in increased fluid retention and should be monitored cautiously, particularly in patients with cardiac, renal, or hepatic disease).
No products indexed under this heading.

Prednisone (The concurrent use of testosterone with ACTH or corticosteroids may result in increased fluid retention and should be monitored cautiously, particularly in patients with cardiac, renal, or hepatic disease).
No products indexed under this heading.

Propranolol Hydrochloride (Co-administration of injectable testosterone cypionate has resulted in an increased clearance of propranolol). Products include:
InnoPran XL Extended Release Capsules 1484

Triamcinolone (The concurrent use of testosterone with ACTH or corticosteroids may result in increased fluid retention and should be monitored cautiously, particularly in patients with cardiac, renal, or hepatic disease).
No products indexed under this heading.

Triamcinolone Acetonide (The concurrent use of testosterone with ACTH or corticosteroids may result in increased fluid retention and should be monitored cautiously, particularly in patients with cardiac, renal, or hepatic disease). Products include:
Azmacort Inhalation Aerosol 407
Nasacort AQ Nasal Spray 2765
Triesence Injectable Suspension .... ⊙209

Triamcinolone Diacetate (The concurrent use of testosterone with ACTH or corticosteroids may result in increased fluid retention and should be monitored cautiously, particularly in patients with cardiac, renal, or hepatic disease).
No products indexed under this heading.

Triamcinolone Hexacetonide (The concurrent use of testosterone with ACTH or corticosteroids may result in increased fluid retention and should be monitored cautiously, particularly in patients with cardiac, renal, or hepatic disease).
No products indexed under this heading.

Warfarin Sodium (Changes in anticoagulant activity may be seen with androgens. More frequent monitoring of INR and prothrombin time are recommended in patients taking anticoagulants, especially at the initiation and termination of androgen therapy).
No products indexed under this heading.

ANDROMON DIETARY SUPPLEMENT
(Dehydroepiandrosterone, Herbal Medicines, unspecified, Vitex agnus-castus) 995
None cited in PDR database.

ANGELIQ TABLETS
(Drospirenone, Estradiol) 751
May interact with ACE inhibitors, angiotensin-II receptor antagonists, cytochrome p450 3a4 inducers (selected), cytochrome p450 3a4 inhibitors (selected), and non-steroidal anti-inflammatory agents. Compounds in these categories include:

Acetazolamide (Inhibitors of CYP3A4 such as erythromycin, clarithromycin, ketoconazole, itraconazole, ritonavir and grapefruit juice may increase plasma concentrations of estrogens and may result in side effects).
No products indexed under this heading.

Allium sativum (Inducers of CYP3A4, such as St. John's Wort preparations (Hypericum perforatum), phenobarbital, carbamazepine, and rifampin, may reduce plasma concentrations of estrogens, possibly resulting in a decrease in therapeutic effects and/or changes in the uterine bleeding profile).
No products indexed under this heading.

Amiodarone Hydrochloride (Inhibitors of CYP3A4 such as erythromycin, clarithromycin, ketoconazole, itraconazole, ritonavir and grapefruit juice may increase plasma concentrations of estrogens and may result in side effects).
No products indexed under this heading.

Amprenavir (Inhibitors of CYP3A4 such as erythromycin, clarithromycin, ketoconazole, itraconazole, ritonavir and grapefruit juice may increase plasma concentrations of estrogens and may result in side effects).
No products indexed under this heading.

Anastrozole (Inhibitors of CYP3A4 such as erythromycin, clarithromycin, ketoconazole, itraconazole, ritonavir and grapefruit juice may increase plasma concentrations of estrogens and may result in side effects). Products include:
Arimidex Tablets 672

Aprepitant (Inhibitors of CYP3A4 such as erythromycin, clarithromycin, ketoconazole, itraconazole, ritonavir and grapefruit juice may increase plasma concentrations of estrogens and may result in side effects). Products include:
Emend Capsules 1992

Atazanavir (Inhibitors of CYP3A4 such as erythromycin, clarithromycin, ketoconazole, itraconazole, ritonavir and grapefruit juice may increase plasma concentrations of estrogens and may result in side effects).
No products indexed under this heading.

Atazanavir Sulfate (Inhibitors of CYP3A4 such as erythromycin, clarithromycin, ketoconazole, itraconazole, ritonavir and grapefruit juice may increase plasma concentrations of estrogens and may result in side effects). Products include:
Reyataz Capsules 3299

Benazepril Hydrochloride (There is potential for an increase in serum potassium in women taking drospirenone with other drugs that may affect electrolytes).
No products indexed under this heading.

Betamethasone Acetate (Inducers of CYP3A4, such as St. John's Wort preparations (Hypericum perforatum), phenobarbital, carbamazepine, and rifampin, may reduce plasma concentrations of estrogens, possibly resulting in a decrease in therapeutic effects and/or changes in the uterine bleeding profile).
No products indexed under this heading.

Betamethasone Sodium Phosphate (Inducers of CYP3A4, such as St. John's Wort preparations (Hypericum perforatum), phenobarbital, carbamazepine, and rifampin, may reduce plasma concentrations of estrogens, possibly resulting in a decrease in therapeutic effects and/or changes in the uterine bleeding profile).
No products indexed under this heading.

Candesartan Cilexetil (There is potential for an increase in serum potassium in women taking drospirenone with other drugs that may affect electrolytes). Products include:
Atacand Tablets 639
Atacand HCT 642

Captopril (There is potential for an increase in serum potassium in women taking drospirenone with other drugs that may affect electrolytes). Products include:
Captopril Tablets 2182

Carbamazepine (Inducers of CYP3A4, such as St. John's Wort preparations (Hypericum perforatum), phenobarbital, carbamazepine, and rifampin, may reduce plasma concentrations of estrogens, possibly resulting in a decrease in therapeutic effects and/or changes in the uterine bleeding profile). Products include:
Carbatrol Capsules 3019
Equetro Extended-Release Capsules 3174

Celecoxib (There is potential for an increase in serum potassium in women taking drospirenone with other drugs that may affect electrolytes). Products include:
Celebrex Capsules 2979

Cimetidine (Inhibitors of CYP3A4 such as erythromycin, clarithromycin, ketoconazole, itraconazole, ritonavir and grapefruit juice may increase plasma concentrations of estrogens and may result in side effects).
No products indexed under this heading.

Cimetidine Hydrochloride (Inhibitors of CYP3A4 such as erythromycin, clarithromycin, ketoconazole, itraconazole, ritonavir and grapefruit juice may increase plasma concentrations of estrogens and may result in side effects).
No products indexed under this heading.

Ciprofloxacin (Inhibitors of CYP3A4 such as erythromycin, clarithromycin, ketoconazole, itraconazole, ritonavir and grapefruit juice may increase plasma concentrations of estrogens and may result in side effects). Products include:
Cipro I.V. 2817
Cipro Oral Suspension 2810
Cipro XR Tablets 2823
Ciprodex Otic Suspension 541

Ciprofloxacin Hydrochloride (Inducers of CYP3A4, such as St. John's Wort preparations (Hypericum perforatum), phenobarbital, carbamazepine, and rifampin, may reduce plasma concentrations of estrogens, possibly resulting in a decrease in therapeutic effects and/or changes in the uterine bleeding profile). Products include:
- Cipro Tablets ... 2810

Cisplatin (Inducers of CYP3A4, such as St. John's Wort preparations (Hypericum perforatum), phenobarbital, carbamazepine, and rifampin, may reduce plasma concentrations of estrogens, possibly resulting in a decrease in therapeutic effects and/or changes in the uterine bleeding profile).
No products indexed under this heading.

Clarithromycin (Inhibitors of CYP3A4 such as erythromycin, clarithromycin, ketoconazole, itraconazole, ritonavir and grapefruit juice may increase plasma concentrations of estrogens and may result in side effects). Products include:
- Biaxin/Biaxin XL ... 411

Clotrimazole (Inhibitors of CYP3A4 such as erythromycin, clarithromycin, ketoconazole, itraconazole, ritonavir and grapefruit juice may increase plasma concentrations of estrogens and may result in side effects). Products include:
- Lotrisone ... 2881

Cortisone Acetate (Inducers of CYP3A4, such as St. John's Wort preparations (Hypericum perforatum), phenobarbital, carbamazepine, and rifampin, may reduce plasma concentrations of estrogens, possibly resulting in a decrease in therapeutic effects and/or changes in the uterine bleeding profile).
No products indexed under this heading.

Cyclosporine (Inhibitors of CYP3A4 such as erythromycin, clarithromycin, ketoconazole, itraconazole, ritonavir and grapefruit juice may increase plasma concentrations of estrogens and may result in side effects). Products include:
- Gengraf Capsules ... 435
- Neoral Oral Solution ... 2280
- Neoral Soft Gelatin Capsules ... 2280
- Restasis Ophthalmic Emulsion ... 557
- Sandimmune ... 2296

Dalfopristin (Inhibitors of CYP3A4 such as erythromycin, clarithromycin, ketoconazole, itraconazole, ritonavir and grapefruit juice may increase plasma concentrations of estrogens and may result in side effects).
No products indexed under this heading.

Danazol (Inhibitors of CYP3A4 such as erythromycin, clarithromycin, ketoconazole, itraconazole, ritonavir and grapefruit juice may increase plasma concentrations of estrogens and may result in side effects).
No products indexed under this heading.

Delavirdine Mesylate (Inhibitors of CYP3A4 such as erythromycin, clarithromycin, ketoconazole, itraconazole, ritonavir and grapefruit juice may increase plasma concentrations of estrogens and may result in side effects).
No products indexed under this heading.

Dexamethasone (Inducers of CYP3A4, such as St. John's Wort preparations (Hypericum perforatum), phenobarbital, carbamazepine, and rifampin, may reduce plasma concentrations of estrogens, possibly resulting in a decrease in therapeutic effects and/or changes in the uterine bleeding profile). Products include:
- Ciprodex Otic Suspension ... 541

Dexamethasone Acetate (Inducers of CYP3A4, such as St. John's Wort preparations (Hypericum perforatum), phenobarbital, carbamazepine, and rifampin, may reduce plasma concentrations of estrogens, possibly resulting in a decrease in therapeutic effects and/or changes in the uterine bleeding profile).
No products indexed under this heading.

Dexamethasone Sodium Phosphate (Inducers of CYP3A4, such as St. John's Wort preparations (Hypericum perforatum), phenobarbital, carbamazepine, and rifampin, may reduce plasma concentrations of estrogens, possibly resulting in a decrease in therapeutic effects and/or changes in the uterine bleeding profile).
No products indexed under this heading.

Diclofenac Epolamine (There is potential for an increase in serum potassium in women taking drospirenone with other drugs that may affect electrolytes). Products include:
- Flector Patch ... 561

Diclofenac Potassium (There is potential for an increase in serum potassium in women taking drospirenone with other drugs that may affect electrolytes).
No products indexed under this heading.

Diclofenac Sodium (There is potential for an increase in serum potassium in women taking drospirenone with other drugs that may affect electrolytes). Products include:
- Diclofenac Sodium Ophthalmic Solution ... ⊙ 240
- Voltaren Ophthalmic Solution ... 2336
- Voltaren Tablets ... 2334
- Voltaren-XR Tablets ... 2337

Diltiazem Hydrochloride (Inhibitors of CYP3A4 such as erythromycin, clarithromycin, ketoconazole, itraconazole, ritonavir and grapefruit juice may increase plasma concentrations of estrogens and may result in side effects). Products include:
- Cardizem LA Extended Release Tablets ... 421

Diltiazem Maleate (Inhibitors of CYP3A4 such as erythromycin, clarithromycin, ketoconazole, itraconazole, ritonavir and grapefruit juice may increase plasma concentrations of estrogens and may result in side effects).
No products indexed under this heading.

Doxorubicin Hydrochloride (Inducers of CYP3A4, such as St. John's Wort preparations (Hypericum perforatum), phenobarbital, carbamazepine, and rifampin, may reduce plasma concentrations of estrogens, possibly resulting in a decrease in therapeutic effects and/or changes in the uterine bleeding profile).
No products indexed under this heading.

Efavirenz (Inhibitors of CYP3A4 such as erythromycin, clarithromycin, ketoconazole, itraconazole, ritonavir and grapefruit juice may increase plasma concentrations of estrogens and may result in side effects). Products include:
- Atripla Tablets ... 938
- Sustiva Capsules ... 930
- Sustiva Tablets ... 930

Enalapril Maleate (There is potential for an increase in serum potassium in women taking drospirenone with other drugs that may affect electrolytes).
No products indexed under this heading.

Enalaprilat (There is potential for an increase in serum potassium in women taking drospirenone with other drugs that may affect electrolytes).
No products indexed under this heading.

Eprosartan Mesylate (There is potential for an increase in serum potassium in women taking drospirenone with other drugs that may affect electrolytes). Products include:
- Teveten Tablets ... 515
- Teveten HCT Tablets ... 517

Erythromycin (Inhibitors of CYP3A4 such as erythromycin, clarithromycin, ketoconazole, itraconazole, ritonavir and grapefruit juice may increase plasma concentrations of estrogens and may result in side effects).
No products indexed under this heading.

Erythromycin Estolate (Inhibitors of CYP3A4 such as erythromycin, clarithromycin, ketoconazole, itraconazole, ritonavir and grapefruit juice may increase plasma concentrations of estrogens and may result in side effects).
No products indexed under this heading.

Erythromycin Ethylsuccinate (Inhibitors of CYP3A4 such as erythromycin, clarithromycin, ketoconazole, itraconazole, ritonavir and grapefruit juice may increase plasma concentrations of estrogens and may result in side effects). Products include:
- E.E.S. ... 433
- EryPed ... 431

Erythromycin Gluceptate (Inhibitors of CYP3A4 such as erythromycin, clarithromycin, ketoconazole, itraconazole, ritonavir and grapefruit juice may increase plasma concentrations of estrogens and may result in side effects).
No products indexed under this heading.

Erythromycin Lactobionate (Inhibitors of CYP3A4 such as erythromycin, clarithromycin, ketoconazole, itraconazole, ritonavir and grapefruit juice may increase plasma concentrations of estrogens and may result in side effects).
No products indexed under this heading.

Erythromycin Stearate (Inhibitors of CYP3A4 such as erythromycin, clarithromycin, ketoconazole, itraconazole, ritonavir and grapefruit juice may increase plasma concentrations of estrogens and may result in side effects).
No products indexed under this heading.

Esomeprazole Magnesium (Inhibitors of CYP3A4 such as erythromycin, clarithromycin, ketoconazole, itraconazole, ritonavir and grapefruit juice may increase plasma concentrations of estrogens and may result in side effects). Products include:
- Nexium Delayed-Release Capsules ... 645
- Nexium Delayed-Release Oral Suspension ... 645

Ethosuximide (Inducers of CYP3A4, such as St. John's Wort preparations (Hypericum perforatum), phenobarbital, carbamazepine, and rifampin, may reduce plasma concentrations of estrogens, possibly resulting in a decrease in therapeutic effects and/or changes in the uterine bleeding profile).
No products indexed under this heading.

Etodolac (There is potential for an increase in serum potassium in women taking drospirenone with other drugs that may affect electrolytes).
No products indexed under this heading.

Felbamate (Inducers of CYP3A4, such as St. John's Wort preparations (Hypericum perforatum), phenobarbital, carbamazepine, and rifampin, may reduce plasma concentrations of estrogens, possibly resulting in a decrease in therapeutic effects and/or changes in the uterine bleeding profile).
No products indexed under this heading.

Fenoprofen Calcium (There is potential for an increase in serum potassium in women taking drospirenone with other drugs that may affect electrolytes). Products include:
- Nalfon Capsules ... 2508

Fluconazole (Inhibitors of CYP3A4 such as erythromycin, clarithromycin, ketoconazole, itraconazole, ritonavir and grapefruit juice may increase plasma concentrations of estrogens and may result in side effects).
No products indexed under this heading.

Fludrocortisone Acetate (Inducers of CYP3A4, such as St. John's Wort preparations (Hypericum perforatum), phenobarbital, carbamazepine, and rifampin, may reduce plasma concentrations of estrogens, possibly resulting in a decrease in therapeutic effects and/or changes in the uterine bleeding profile).
No products indexed under this heading.

Fluoxetine (Inhibitors of CYP3A4 such as erythromycin, clarithromycin, ketoconazole, itraconazole, ritonavir and grapefruit juice may increase plasma concentrations of estrogens and may result in side effects).
No products indexed under this heading.

Fluoxetine Hydrochloride (Inhibitors of CYP3A4 such as erythromycin, clarithromycin, ketoconazole, itraconazole, ritonavir and grapefruit juice may increase plasma concentrations of estrogens and may result in side effects). Products include:
- Prozac Weekly Capsules ... 1852
- Prozac Pulvules and Liquid ... 1852
- Symbyax Capsules ... 1871

IMPORTANT NOTE: Always consult each drug listing in the patient's regimen for possible interactions.

Flurbiprofen (There is potential for an increase in serum potassium in women taking drospirenone with other drugs that may affect electrolytes).
No products indexed under this heading.

Fluvoxamine Maleate (Inhibitors of CYP3A4 such as erythromycin, clarithromycin, ketoconazole, itraconazole, ritonavir and grapefruit juice may increase plasma concentrations of estrogens and may result in side effects). Products include:
Luvox CR Extended-Release Capsules 1759

Fosamprenavir Calcium (Inhibitors of CYP3A4 such as erythromycin, clarithromycin, ketoconazole, itraconazole, ritonavir and grapefruit juice may increase plasma concentrations of estrogens and may result in side effects). Products include:
Lexiva Oral Suspension 1510
Lexiva Tablets 1510

Fosinopril Sodium (There is potential for an increase in serum potassium in women taking drospirenone with other drugs that may affect electrolytes).
No products indexed under this heading.

Fosphenytoin Sodium (Inducers of CYP3A4, such as St. John's Wort preparations (Hypericum perforatum), phenobarbital, carbamazepine, and rifampin, may reduce plasma concentrations of estrogens, possibly resulting in a decrease in therapeutic effects and/or changes in the uterine bleeding profile).
No products indexed under this heading.

Garlic Extract (Inducers of CYP3A4, such as St. John's Wort preparations (Hypericum perforatum), phenobarbital, carbamazepine, and rifampin, may reduce plasma concentrations of estrogens, possibly resulting in a decrease in therapeutic effects and/or changes in the uterine bleeding profile).
No products indexed under this heading.

Garlic Oil (Inducers of CYP3A4, such as St. John's Wort preparations (Hypericum perforatum), phenobarbital, carbamazepine, and rifampin, may reduce plasma concentrations of estrogens, possibly resulting in a decrease in therapeutic effects and/or changes in the uterine bleeding profile).
No products indexed under this heading.

Hydrocortisone (Inducers of CYP3A4, such as St. John's Wort preparations (Hypericum perforatum), phenobarbital, carbamazepine, and rifampin, may reduce plasma concentrations of estrogens, possibly resulting in a decrease in therapeutic effects and/or changes in the uterine bleeding profile).
No products indexed under this heading.

Hydrocortisone Acetate (Inducers of CYP3A4, such as St. John's Wort preparations (Hypericum perforatum), phenobarbital, carbamazepine, and rifampin, may reduce plasma concentrations of estrogens, possibly resulting in a decrease in therapeutic effects and/or changes in the uterine bleeding profile). Products include:
Analpram-HC 1140
Pramosone 1141

Hydrocortisone Butyrate (Inducers of CYP3A4, such as St. John's Wort preparations (Hypericum perforatum), phenobarbital, carbamazepine, and rifampin, may reduce plasma concentrations of estrogens, possibly resulting in a decrease in therapeutic effects and/or changes in the uterine bleeding profile).
No products indexed under this heading.

Hydrocortisone Cypionate (Inducers of CYP3A4, such as St. John's Wort preparations (Hypericum perforatum), phenobarbital, carbamazepine, and rifampin, may reduce plasma concentrations of estrogens, possibly resulting in a decrease in therapeutic effects and/or changes in the uterine bleeding profile).
No products indexed under this heading.

Hydrocortisone Hemisuccinate (Inducers of CYP3A4, such as St. John's Wort preparations (Hypericum perforatum), phenobarbital, carbamazepine, and rifampin, may reduce plasma concentrations of estrogens, possibly resulting in a decrease in therapeutic effects and/or changes in the uterine bleeding profile).
No products indexed under this heading.

Hydrocortisone Probutate (Inducers of CYP3A4, such as St. John's Wort preparations (Hypericum perforatum), phenobarbital, carbamazepine, and rifampin, may reduce plasma concentrations of estrogens, possibly resulting in a decrease in therapeutic effects and/or changes in the uterine bleeding profile).
No products indexed under this heading.

Hydrocortisone Sodium Phosphate (Inducers of CYP3A4, such as St. John's Wort preparations (Hypericum perforatum), phenobarbital, carbamazepine, and rifampin, may reduce plasma concentrations of estrogens, possibly resulting in a decrease in therapeutic effects and/or changes in the uterine bleeding profile).
No products indexed under this heading.

Hydrocortisone Sodium Succinate (Inducers of CYP3A4, such as St. John's Wort preparations (Hypericum perforatum), phenobarbital, carbamazepine, and rifampin, may reduce plasma concentrations of estrogens, possibly resulting in a decrease in therapeutic effects and/or changes in the uterine bleeding profile).
No products indexed under this heading.

Hydrocortisone Valerate (Inducers of CYP3A4, such as St. John's Wort preparations (Hypericum perforatum), phenobarbital, carbamazepine, and rifampin, may reduce plasma concentrations of estrogens, possibly resulting in a decrease in therapeutic effects and/or changes in the uterine bleeding profile).
No products indexed under this heading.

Hypericum (Inducers of CYP3A4, such as St. John's Wort preparations (Hypericum perforatum), phenobarbital, carbamazepine, and rifampin, may reduce plasma concentrations of estrogens, possibly resulting in a decrease in therapeutic effects and/or changes in the uterine bleeding profile). Products include:
Satieté Tablets .... ▣640

Hypericum Perforatum (Inducers of CYP3A4, such as St. John's Wort preparations (Hypericum perforatum), phenobarbital, carbamazepine, and rifampin, may reduce plasma concentrations of estrogens, possibly resulting in a decrease in therapeutic effects and/or changes in the uterine bleeding profile).
No products indexed under this heading.

Ibuprofen (There is potential for an increase in serum potassium in women taking drospirenone with other drugs that may affect electrolytes). Products include:
Motrin IB Tablets and Caplets 1900
Children's Motrin Oral Suspension ... 1901
Children's Motrin Non-Staining Dye-Free Oral Suspension 1901
Children's Motrin Cold Oral Suspension 1899
Infants' Motrin Concentrated Drops 1901
Infants' Motrin Non-Staining Dye-Free Concentrated Drops 1901
Junior Strength Motrin Caplets and Chewable Tablets 1901
Vicoprofen Tablets 533

Indinavir Sulfate (Inhibitors of CYP3A4 such as erythromycin, clarithromycin, ketoconazole, itraconazole, ritonavir and grapefruit juice may increase plasma concentrations of estrogens and may result in side effects). Products include:
Crixivan Capsules 1979

Indomethacin (There is potential for an increase in serum potassium in women taking drospirenone with other drugs that may affect electrolytes). Products include:
Indocin 2024

Indomethacin Sodium Trihydrate (There is potential for an increase in serum potassium in women taking drospirenone with other drugs that may affect electrolytes). Products include:
Indocin I.V. 2489

Irbesartan (There is potential for an increase in serum potassium in women taking drospirenone with other drugs that may affect electrolytes). Products include:
Avalide Tablets 892
Avalide Tablets 2713
Avapro Tablets 897
Avapro Tablets 2718

Isoniazid (Inhibitors of CYP3A4 such as erythromycin, clarithromycin, ketoconazole, itraconazole, ritonavir and grapefruit juice may increase plasma concentrations of estrogens and may result in side effects).
No products indexed under this heading.

Itraconazole (Inhibitors of CYP3A4 such as erythromycin, clarithromycin, ketoconazole, itraconazole, ritonavir and grapefruit juice may increase plasma concentrations of estrogens and may result in side effects).
No products indexed under this heading.

Ketoconazole (Inhibitors of CYP3A4 such as erythromycin, clarithromycin, ketoconazole, itraconazole, ritonavir and grapefruit juice may increase plasma concentrations of estrogens and may result in side effects). Products include:
Extina Foam, 2% 3057
Nizoral A-D Shampoo 1901

Ketoprofen (There is potential for an increase in serum potassium in women taking drospirenone with other drugs that may affect electrolytes).
No products indexed under this heading.

Ketorolac Tromethamine (There is potential for an increase in serum potassium in women taking drospirenone with other drugs that may affect electrolytes).
No products indexed under this heading.

Lisinopril (There is potential for an increase in serum potassium in women taking drospirenone with other drugs that may affect electrolytes). Products include:
Prinivil Tablets 2087
Prinzide Tablets 2092

Lopinavir (Inhibitors of CYP3A4 such as erythromycin, clarithromycin, ketoconazole, itraconazole, ritonavir and grapefruit juice may increase plasma concentrations of estrogens and may result in side effects). Products include:
Kaletra 452

Loratadine (Inhibitors of CYP3A4 such as erythromycin, clarithromycin, ketoconazole, itraconazole, ritonavir and grapefruit juice may increase plasma concentrations of estrogens and may result in side effects).
No products indexed under this heading.

Losartan Potassium (There is potential for an increase in serum potassium in women taking drospirenone with other drugs that may affect electrolytes). Products include:
Cozaar Tablets 1973

Meclofenamate Sodium (There is potential for an increase in serum potassium in women taking drospirenone with other drugs that may affect electrolytes).
No products indexed under this heading.

Mefenamic Acid (There is potential for an increase in serum potassium in women taking drospirenone with other drugs that may affect electrolytes).
No products indexed under this heading.

Meloxicam (There is potential for an increase in serum potassium in women taking drospirenone with other drugs that may affect electrolytes). Products include:
Mobic Oral Suspension 863
Mobic Tablets 863

Mephenytoin (Inducers of CYP3A4, such as St. John's Wort preparations (Hypericum perforatum), phenobarbital, carbamazepine, and rifampin, may reduce plasma concentrations of estrogens, possibly resulting in a decrease in therapeutic effects and/or changes in the uterine bleeding profile).
No products indexed under this heading.

Methsuximide (Inducers of CYP3A4, such as St. John's Wort preparations (Hypericum perforatum), phenobarbital, carbamazepine, and rifampin, may reduce plasma concentrations of estrogens, possibly resulting in a decrease in therapeutic effects and/or changes in the uterine bleeding profile).
No products indexed under this heading.

Methylprednisolone (Inducers of CYP3A4, such as St. John's Wort preparations (Hypericum perforatum), phenobarbital, carbamazepine, and rifampin, may reduce plasma concentrations of estrogens, possibly resulting in a decrease in therapeutic effects and/or changes in the uterine bleeding profile).
No products indexed under this heading.

Methylprednisolone Acetate (Inducers of CYP3A4, such as St. John's Wort preparations (Hypericum perforatum), phenobarbital, carbamazepine, and rifampin, may reduce plasma concentrations of estrogens, possibly resulting in a decrease in therapeutic effects and/or changes in the uterine bleeding profile).
No products indexed under this heading.

Methylprednisolone Sodium Succinate (Inducers of CYP3A4, such as St. John's Wort preparations (Hypericum perforatum), phenobarbital, carbamazepine, and rifampin, may reduce plasma concentrations of estrogens, possibly resulting in a decrease in therapeutic effects and/or changes in the uterine bleeding profile).
No products indexed under this heading.

Metronidazole (Inhibitors of CYP3A4 such as erythromycin, clarithromycin, ketoconazole, itraconazole, ritonavir and grapefruit juice may increase plasma concentrations of estrogens and may result in side effects). Products include:
Pylera Capsules 714

Metronidazole Benzoate (Inhibitors of CYP3A4 such as erythromycin, clarithromycin, ketoconazole, itraconazole, ritonavir and grapefruit juice may increase plasma concentrations of estrogens and may result in side effects).
No products indexed under this heading.

Metronidazole Hydrochloride (Inhibitors of CYP3A4 such as erythromycin, clarithromycin, ketoconazole, itraconazole, ritonavir and grapefruit juice may increase plasma concentrations of estrogens and may result in side effects).
No products indexed under this heading.

Miconazole (Inhibitors of CYP3A4 such as erythromycin, clarithromycin, ketoconazole, itraconazole, ritonavir and grapefruit juice may increase plasma concentrations of estrogens and may result in side effects).
No products indexed under this heading.

Miconazole Nitrate (Inhibitors of CYP3A4 such as erythromycin, clarithromycin, ketoconazole, itraconazole, ritonavir and grapefruit juice may increase plasma concentrations of estrogens and may result in side effects).
No products indexed under this heading.

Modafinil (Inducers of CYP3A4, such as St. John's Wort preparations (Hypericum perforatum), phenobarbital, carbamazepine, and rifampin, may reduce plasma concentrations of estrogens, possibly resulting in a decrease in therapeutic effects and/or changes in the uterine bleeding profile). Products include:
Provigil Tablets 977

Moexipril Hydrochloride (There is potential for an increase in serum potassium in women taking drospirenone with other drugs that may affect electrolytes).
No products indexed under this heading.

Nabumetone (There is potential for an increase in serum potassium in women taking drospirenone with other drugs that may affect electrolytes).
No products indexed under this heading.

Naproxen (There is potential for an increase in serum potassium in women taking drospirenone with other drugs that may affect electrolytes). Products include:
EC-Naprosyn Delayed-Release Tablets 2632
Naprosyn Suspension 2632
Naprosyn Tablets 2632

Naproxen Sodium (There is potential for an increase in serum potassium in women taking drospirenone with other drugs that may affect electrolytes). Products include:
Anaprox Tablets 2632
Anaprox DS Tablets 2632
Treximet Tablets 1616

Nefazodone Hydrochloride (Inhibitors of CYP3A4 such as erythromycin, clarithromycin, ketoconazole, itraconazole, ritonavir and grapefruit juice may increase plasma concentrations of estrogens and may result in side effects).
No products indexed under this heading.

Nelfinavir Mesylate (Inhibitors of CYP3A4 such as erythromycin, clarithromycin, ketoconazole, itraconazole, ritonavir and grapefruit juice may increase plasma concentrations of estrogens and may result in side effects).
No products indexed under this heading.

Nevirapine (Inhibitors of CYP3A4 such as erythromycin, clarithromycin, ketoconazole, itraconazole, ritonavir and grapefruit juice may increase plasma concentrations of estrogens and may result in side effects). Products include:
Viramune Oral Suspension 873
Viramune Tablets 873

Niacinamide (Inhibitors of CYP3A4 such as erythromycin, clarithromycin, ketoconazole, itraconazole, ritonavir and grapefruit juice may increase plasma concentrations of estrogens and may result in side effects). Products include:
BioLean Free Tablets 635

Nicotinamide (Inhibitors of CYP3A4 such as erythromycin, clarithromycin, ketoconazole, itraconazole, ritonavir and grapefruit juice may increase plasma concentrations of estrogens and may result in side effects).
No products indexed under this heading.

Nifedipine (Inhibitors of CYP3A4 such as erythromycin, clarithromycin, ketoconazole, itraconazole, ritonavir and grapefruit juice may increase plasma concentrations of estrogens and may result in side effects).
No products indexed under this heading.

Norfloxacin (Inhibitors of CYP3A4 such as erythromycin, clarithromycin, ketoconazole, itraconazole, ritonavir and grapefruit juice may increase plasma concentrations of estrogens and may result in side effects). Products include:
Noroxin Tablets 2069

Omeprazole (Inhibitors of CYP3A4 such as erythromycin, clarithromycin, ketoconazole, itraconazole, ritonavir and grapefruit juice may increase plasma concentrations of estrogens and may result in side effects).
No products indexed under this heading.

Oxaprozin (There is potential for an increase in serum potassium in women taking drospirenone with other drugs that may affect electrolytes).
No products indexed under this heading.

Oxcarbazepine (Inducers of CYP3A4, such as St. John's Wort preparations (Hypericum perforatum), phenobarbital, carbamazepine, and rifampin, may reduce plasma concentrations of estrogens, possibly resulting in a decrease in therapeutic effects and/or changes in the uterine bleeding profile).
No products indexed under this heading.

Paroxetine Hydrochloride (Inhibitors of CYP3A4 such as erythromycin, clarithromycin, ketoconazole, itraconazole, ritonavir and grapefruit juice may increase plasma concentrations of estrogens and may result in side effects). Products include:
Paxil 1535
Paxil CR Controlled-Release Tablets 1544

Perindopril Erbumine (There is potential for an increase in serum potassium in women taking drospirenone with other drugs that may affect electrolytes). Products include:
Aceon Tablets (2 mg, 4 mg, 8 mg) 3038

Phenobarbital (Inducers of CYP3A4, such as St. John's Wort preparations (Hypericum perforatum), phenobarbital, carbamazepine, and rifampin, may reduce plasma concentrations of estrogens, possibly resulting in a decrease in therapeutic effects and/or changes in the uterine bleeding profile). Products include:
Donnatal Extentabs 2507

Phenobarbital Sodium (Inducers of CYP3A4, such as St. John's Wort preparations (Hypericum perforatum), phenobarbital, carbamazepine, and rifampin, may reduce plasma concentrations of estrogens, possibly resulting in a decrease in therapeutic effects and/or changes in the uterine bleeding profile).
No products indexed under this heading.

Phenylbutazone (There is potential for an increase in serum potassium in women taking drospirenone with other drugs that may affect electrolytes).
No products indexed under this heading.

Phenytoin (Inducers of CYP3A4, such as St. John's Wort preparations (Hypericum perforatum), phenobarbital, carbamazepine, and rifampin, may reduce plasma concentrations of estrogens, possibly resulting in a decrease in therapeutic effects and/or changes in the uterine bleeding profile).
No products indexed under this heading.

Phenytoin Sodium (Inducers of CYP3A4, such as St. John's Wort preparations (Hypericum perforatum), phenobarbital, carbamazepine, and rifampin, may reduce plasma concentrations of estrogens, possibly resulting in a decrease in therapeutic effects and/or changes in the uterine bleeding profile). Products include:
Phenytek Capsules 2192

Piroxicam (There is potential for an increase in serum potassium in women taking drospirenone with other drugs that may affect electrolytes).
No products indexed under this heading.

Prednisolone Acetate (Inducers of CYP3A4, such as St. John's Wort preparations (Hypericum perforatum), phenobarbital, carbamazepine, and rifampin, may reduce plasma concentrations of estrogens, possibly resulting in a decrease in therapeutic effects and/or changes in the uterine bleeding profile). Products include:
Pred Forte Ophthalmic Suspension .... ⊙227
Pred Mild Ophthalmic Suspension .... ⊙230
Pred-G Ophthalmic Ointment .... ⊙229
Pred-G Ophthalmic Suspension .... ⊙228

Prednisolone Sodium Phosphate (Inducers of CYP3A4, such as St. John's Wort preparations (Hypericum perforatum), phenobarbital, carbamazepine, and rifampin, may reduce plasma concentrations of estrogens, possibly resulting in a decrease in therapeutic effects and/or changes in the uterine bleeding profile).
No products indexed under this heading.

Prednisolone Tebutate (Inducers of CYP3A4, such as St. John's Wort preparations (Hypericum perforatum), phenobarbital, carbamazepine, and rifampin, may reduce plasma concentrations of estrogens, possibly resulting in a decrease in therapeutic effects and/or changes in the uterine bleeding profile).
No products indexed under this heading.

Prednisone (Inducers of CYP3A4, such as St. John's Wort preparations (Hypericum perforatum), phenobarbital, carbamazepine, and rifampin, may reduce plasma concentrations of estrogens, possibly resulting in a decrease in therapeutic effects and/or changes in the uterine bleeding profile).
No products indexed under this heading.

Primidone (Inducers of CYP3A4, such as St. John's Wort preparations (Hypericum perforatum), phenobarbital, carbamazepine, and rifampin, may reduce plasma concentrations of estrogens, possibly resulting in a decrease in therapeutic effects and/or changes in the uterine bleeding profile).
No products indexed under this heading.

Propoxyphene Hydrochloride (Inhibitors of CYP3A4 such as erythromycin, clarithromycin, ketoconazole, itraconazole, ritonavir and grapefruit juice may increase plasma concentrations of estrogens and may result in side effects).
No products indexed under this heading.

Propoxyphene Napsylate (Inhibitors of CYP3A4 such as erythromycin, clarithromycin, ketoconazole, itraconazole, ritonavir and grapefruit juice may increase plasma concentrations of estrogens and may result in side effects).
No products indexed under this heading.

Quinapril Hydrochloride (There is potential for an increase in serum potassium in women taking drospirenone with other drugs that may affect electrolytes).
No products indexed under this heading.

Quinidine (Inhibitors of CYP3A4 such as erythromycin, clarithromycin, ketoconazole, itraconazole, ritonavir and grapefruit juice may increase plasma concentrations of estrogens and may result in side effects).
No products indexed under this heading.

Quinidine Hydrochloride (Inhibitors of CYP3A4 such as erythromycin, clarithromycin, ketoconazole, itraconazole, ritonavir and grapefruit juice may increase plasma concentrations of estrogens and may result in side effects).
No products indexed under this heading.

Quinidine Polygalacturonate (Inhibitors of CYP3A4 such as erythromycin, clarithromycin, ketoconazole, itraconazole, ritonavir and grapefruit juice may increase plasma concentrations of estrogens and may result in side effects).
No products indexed under this heading.

Quinidine Sulfate (Inhibitors of CYP3A4 such as erythromycin, clarithromycin, ketoconazole, itraconazole, ritonavir and grapefruit juice may increase plasma concentrations of estrogens and may result in side effects).
No products indexed under this heading.

Quinine (Inhibitors of CYP3A4 such as erythromycin, clarithromycin, ketoconazole, itraconazole, ritonavir and grapefruit juice may increase plasma concentrations of estrogens and may result in side effects).
No products indexed under this heading.

Quinine Sulfate (Inhibitors of CYP3A4 such as erythromycin, clarithromycin, ketoconazole, itraconazole, ritonavir and grapefruit juice may increase plasma concentrations of estrogens and may result in side effects).
No products indexed under this heading.

Quinupristin (Inhibitors of CYP3A4 such as erythromycin, clarithromycin, ketoconazole, itraconazole, ritonavir and grapefruit juice may increase plasma concentrations of estrogens and may result in side effects).
No products indexed under this heading.

Ramipril (There is potential for an increase in serum potassium in women taking drospirenone with other drugs that may affect electrolytes).
No products indexed under this heading.

Ranitidine Bismuth Citrate (Inhibitors of CYP3A4 such as erythromycin, clarithromycin, ketoconazole, itraconazole, ritonavir and grapefruit juice may increase plasma concentrations of estrogens and may result in side effects).
No products indexed under this heading.

Ranitidine Hydrochloride (Inhibitors of CYP3A4 such as erythromycin, clarithromycin, ketoconazole, itraconazole, ritonavir and grapefruit juice may increase plasma concentrations of estrogens and may result in side effects). Products include:
Zantac 75 Tablets .... ▣ 603
Zantac 1670
Zantac Injection 1666
Zantac Injection Pharmacy Bulk Package 1668
Maximum Strength Zantac 150 Tablets .... ▣ 603
Maximum Strength Zantac 150 Cool Mint Tablets .... ▣ 603

Rifabutin (Inducers of CYP3A4, such as St. John's Wort preparations (Hypericum perforatum), phenobarbital, carbamazepine, and rifampin, may reduce plasma concentrations of estrogens, possibly resulting in a decrease in therapeutic effects and/or changes in the uterine bleeding profile).
No products indexed under this heading.

Rifampicin (Inducers of CYP3A4, such as St. John's Wort preparations (Hypericum perforatum), phenobarbital, carbamazepine, and rifampin, may reduce plasma concentrations of estrogens, possibly resulting in a decrease in therapeutic effects and/or changes in the uterine bleeding profile).
No products indexed under this heading.

Rifampin (Inducers of CYP3A4, such as St. John's Wort preparations (Hypericum perforatum), phenobarbital, carbamazepine, and rifampin, may reduce plasma concentrations of estrogens, possibly resulting in a decrease in therapeutic effects and/or changes in the uterine bleeding profile).
No products indexed under this heading.

Rifapentine (Inducers of CYP3A4, such as St. John's Wort preparations (Hypericum perforatum), phenobarbital, carbamazepine, and rifampin, may reduce plasma concentrations of estrogens, possibly resulting in a decrease in therapeutic effects and/or changes in the uterine bleeding profile).
No products indexed under this heading.

Ritonavir (Inhibitors of CYP3A4 such as erythromycin, clarithromycin, ketoconazole, itraconazole, ritonavir and grapefruit juice may increase plasma concentrations of estrogens and may result in side effects). Products include:
Kaletra 452
Norvir 489

Rofecoxib (There is potential for an increase in serum potassium in women taking drospirenone with other drugs that may affect electrolytes).
No products indexed under this heading.

Saquinavir (Inhibitors of CYP3A4 such as erythromycin, clarithromycin, ketoconazole, itraconazole, ritonavir and grapefruit juice may increase plasma concentrations of estrogens and may result in side effects).
No products indexed under this heading.

Saquinavir Mesylate (Inhibitors of CYP3A4 such as erythromycin, clarithromycin, ketoconazole, itraconazole, ritonavir and grapefruit juice may increase plasma concentrations of estrogens and may result in side effects).
No products indexed under this heading.

Sertraline Hydrochloride (Inhibitors of CYP3A4 such as erythromycin, clarithromycin, ketoconazole, itraconazole, ritonavir and grapefruit juice may increase plasma concentrations of estrogens and may result in side effects).
No products indexed under this heading.

Sildenafil Citrate (Inhibitors of CYP3A4 such as erythromycin, clarithromycin, ketoconazole, itraconazole, ritonavir and grapefruit juice may increase plasma concentrations of estrogens and may result in side effects).
No products indexed under this heading.

Spirapril Hydrochloride (There is potential for an increase in serum potassium in women taking drospirenone with other drugs that may affect electrolytes).
No products indexed under this heading.

Sulfinpyrazone (Inducers of CYP3A4, such as St. John's Wort preparations (Hypericum perforatum), phenobarbital, carbamazepine, and rifampin, may reduce plasma concentrations of estrogens, possibly resulting in a decrease in therapeutic effects and/or changes in the uterine bleeding profile).
No products indexed under this heading.

Sulindac (There is potential for an increase in serum potassium in women taking drospirenone with other drugs that may affect electrolytes). Products include:
Clinoril Tablets 1962

Telithromycin (Inhibitors of CYP3A4 such as erythromycin, clarithromycin, ketoconazole, itraconazole, ritonavir and grapefruit juice may increase plasma concentrations of estrogens and may result in side effects). Products include:
Ketek Tablets 2744

Telmisartan (There is potential for an increase in serum potassium in women taking drospirenone with other drugs that may affect electrolytes). Products include:
Micardis Tablets 852
Micardis HCT Tablets 854

Theophylline (Inducers of CYP3A4, such as St. John's Wort preparations (Hypericum perforatum), phenobarbital, carbamazepine, and rifampin, may reduce plasma concentrations of estrogens, possibly resulting in a decrease in therapeutic effects and/or changes in the uterine bleeding profile).
No products indexed under this heading.

Theophylline Anhydrous (Inducers of CYP3A4, such as St. John's Wort preparations (Hypericum perforatum), phenobarbital, carbamazepine, and rifampin, may reduce plasma concentrations of estrogens, possibly resulting in a decrease in therapeutic effects and/or changes in the uterine bleeding profile). Products include:
Uniphyl Tablets 2595

Theophylline Calcium Salicylate (Inducers of CYP3A4, such as St. John's Wort preparations (Hypericum perforatum), phenobarbital, carbamazepine, and rifampin, may reduce plasma concentrations of estrogens, possibly resulting in a decrease in therapeutic effects and/or changes in the uterine bleeding profile).
No products indexed under this heading.

Theophylline Dihydroxypropyl (Glyceryl) (Inducers of CYP3A4, such as St. John's Wort preparations (Hypericum perforatum), phenobarbital, carbamazepine, and rifampin, may reduce plasma concentrations of estrogens, possibly resulting in a decrease in therapeutic effects and/or changes in the uterine bleeding profile).
No products indexed under this heading.

Theophylline Ethylenediamine (Inducers of CYP3A4, such as St. John's Wort preparations (Hypericum perforatum), phenobarbital, carbamazepine, and rifampin, may reduce plasma concentrations of estrogens, possibly resulting in a decrease in therapeutic effects and/or changes in the uterine bleeding profile).
No products indexed under this heading.

Tolmetin Sodium (There is potential for an increase in serum potassium in women taking drospirenone with other drugs that may affect electrolytes).
No products indexed under this heading.

Trandolapril (There is potential for an increase in serum potassium in women taking drospirenone with other drugs that may affect electrolytes). Products include:
Mavik Tablets 472
Tarka Tablets 511

Triamcinolone (Inducers of CYP3A4, such as St. John's Wort preparations (Hypericum perforatum), phenobarbital, carbamazepine, and rifampin, may reduce plasma concentrations of estrogens, possibly resulting in a decrease in therapeutic effects and/or changes in the uterine bleeding profile).
No products indexed under this heading.

Triamcinolone Acetonide (Inducers of CYP3A4, such as St. John's Wort preparations (Hypericum perforatum), phenobarbital, carbamazepine, and rifampin, may reduce plasma concentrations of estrogens, possibly resulting in a decrease in therapeutic effects and/or changes in the uterine bleeding profile). Products include:
Azmacort Inhalation Aerosol 407
Nasacort AQ Nasal Spray 2765
Triesence Injectable Suspension .... ⊙ 209

Triamcinolone Diacetate (Inducers of CYP3A4, such as St. John's Wort preparations (Hypericum perforatum), phenobarbital, carbamazepine, and rifampin, may reduce plasma concentrations of estrogens, possibly resulting in a decrease in therapeutic effects and/or changes in the uterine bleeding profile).
No products indexed under this heading.

Triamcinolone Hexacetonide (Inducers of CYP3A4, such as St. John's Wort preparations (Hypericum perforatum), phenobarbital, carbamazepine, and rifampin, may reduce plasma concentrations of estrogens, possibly resulting in a decrease in therapeutic effects and/or changes in the uterine bleeding profile).
No products indexed under this heading.

Troglitazone (Inhibitors of CYP3A4 such as erythromycin, clarithromycin, ketoconazole, itraconazole, ritonavir and grapefruit juice may increase plasma concentrations of estrogens and may result in side effects).
No products indexed under this heading.

Troleandomycin (Inhibitors of CYP3A4 such as erythromycin, clarithromycin, ketoconazole, itraconazole, ritonavir and grapefruit juice may increase plasma concentrations of estrogens and may result in side effects).
No products indexed under this heading.

Valdecoxib (There is potential for an increase in serum potassium in women taking drospirenone with other drugs that may affect electrolytes).
No products indexed under this heading.

Valproate Sodium (Inhibitors of CYP3A4 such as erythromycin, clarithromycin, ketoconazole, itraconazole, ritonavir and grapefruit juice may increase plasma concentrations of estrogens and may result in side effects).
No products indexed under this heading.

Valsartan (There is potential for an increase in serum potassium in women taking drospirenone with other drugs that may affect electrolytes). Products include:
Diovan Tablets 2212
Diovan HCT Tablets 2216
Exforge Tablets 2238

Vardenafil Hydrochloride (Inhibitors of CYP3A4 such as erythromycin, clarithromycin, ketoconazole, itraconazole, ritonavir and grapefruit juice may increase plasma concentrations of estrogens and may result in side effects). Products include:
Levitra Tablets 2876

Verapamil Hydrochloride (Inhibitors of CYP3A4 such as erythromycin, clarithromycin, ketoconazole, itraconazole, ritonavir and grapefruit juice may increase plasma concentrations of estrogens and may result in side effects). Products include:
Tarka Tablets 511

Voriconazole (Inhibitors of CYP3A4 such as erythromycin, clarithromycin, ketoconazole, itraconazole, ritonavir and grapefruit juice may increase plasma concentrations of estrogens and may result in side effects).
No products indexed under this heading.

Zafirlukast (Inhibitors of CYP3A4 such as erythromycin, clarithromycin, ketoconazole, itraconazole, ritonavir and grapefruit juice may increase plasma concentrations of estrogens and may result in side effects). Products include:
Accolate Tablets 669

Zileuton (Inhibitors of CYP3A4 such as erythromycin, clarithromycin, ketoconazole, itraconazole, ritonavir and grapefruit juice may increase plasma concentrations of estrogens and may result in side effects).
No products indexed under this heading.

Food Interactions

Grapefruit (Inhibitors of CYP3A4 such as erythromycin, clarithromycin, ketoconazole, itraconazole, ritonavir and grapefruit juice may increase plasma concentrations of estrogens and may result in side effects).

Grapefruit Juice (Inhibitors of CYP3A4 such as erythromycin, clarithromycin, ketoconazole, itraconazole, ritonavir and grapefruit juice may increase plasma concentrations of estrogens and may result in side effects).

ANGIOMAX FOR INJECTION

(Bivalirudin) 1933
May interact with glycoprotein (GP) IIb/IIIa inhibitors, thrombolytics, and certain other agents. Compounds in these categories include:

Abciximab (Co-administration was associated with increased risks of major bleeding events). Products include:
ReoPro Vials 1860

Alteplase (Co-administration was associated with increased risks of major bleeding events). Products include:
Activase I.V. 1188
Cathflo Activase 1198

Anistreplase (Co-administration was associated with increased risks of major bleeding events).
No products indexed under this heading.

Eptifibatide (Co-administration was associated with increased risks of major bleeding events). Products include:
Integrilin Injection 2855

Heparin Sodium (Co-administration was associated with increased risks of major bleeding events).
No products indexed under this heading.

Reteplase (Co-administration was associated with increased risks of major bleeding events).
No products indexed under this heading.

Streptokinase (Co-administration was associated with increased risks of major bleeding events).
No products indexed under this heading.

Tirofiban Hydrochloride (Co-administration was associated with increased risks of major bleeding events).
No products indexed under this heading.

Urokinase (Co-administration was associated with increased risks of major bleeding events).
No products indexed under this heading.

Warfarin Sodium (Co-administration was associated with increased risks of major bleeding events).
No products indexed under this heading.

ANIMI-3 CAPSULES

(Docosahexaenoic Acid (DHA), Eicosapentaenoic Acid (EPA), Folic Acid, Omega-3 Acids, Phytosterols, Vitamin B_{12}, Vitamin B_6) 2506
None cited in PDR database.

ANTIVENIN (BLACK WIDOW SPIDER ANTIVENIN)

(Black Widow Spider Antivenin (Equine)) 1951
None cited in PDR database.

ANZEMET INJECTION

(Dolasetron Mesylate) 2701
See Anzemet Tablets

ANZEMET TABLETS

(Dolasetron Mesylate) 2704
May interact with antiarrhythmics, anthracyclines, diuretics, drugs that prolong the QT interval, and certain other agents. Compounds in these categories include:

Acebutolol Hydrochloride (Dolasetron should be administered with caution in patients who have or may develop prolongation of cardiac conduction intervals, particularly QTc. This includes patients taking anti-arrhythmic drugs).
No products indexed under this heading.

Adenosine (Dolasetron should be administered with caution in patients who have or may develop prolongation of cardiac conduction intervals, particularly QTc. This includes patients taking anti-arrhythmic drugs). Products include:
Adenocard IV Injection 603
Adenoscan 605

Alprazolam (Dolasetron should be administered with caution in patients who have or may develop prolongation of cardiac conduction intervals, particularly QTc. This includes patients taking drugs which lead to QT prolongation).
No products indexed under this heading.

Amiloride Hydrochloride (Dolasetron should be administered with caution in patients who have or may develop prolongation of cardiac conduction intervals, particularly QTc. This includes patients taking diuretics with potential for inducing electrolyte abnormalities).
No products indexed under this heading.

Amiodarone Hydrochloride (Dolasetron should be administered with caution in patients who have or may develop prolongation of cardiac conduction intervals, particularly QTc. This includes patients taking drugs which lead to QT prolongation).
No products indexed under this heading.

Amitriptyline Hydrochloride (Dolasetron should be administered with caution in patients who have or may develop prolongation of cardiac conduction intervals, particularly QTc. This includes patients taking drugs which lead to QT prolongation).
No products indexed under this heading.

Amoxapine (Dolasetron should be administered with caution in patients who have or may develop prolongation of cardiac conduction intervals, particularly QTc. This includes patients taking drugs which lead to QT prolongation).
No products indexed under this heading.

Astemizole (Dolasetron should be administered with caution in patients who have or may develop prolongation of cardiac conduction intervals, particularly QTc. This includes patients taking drugs which lead to QT prolongation).
No products indexed under this heading.

Atenolol (Clearance of hydrodolasetron, the active metabolite of dolasetron, decreased by about 27% when dolasetron was administered intravenously concomitantly with atenolol).
No products indexed under this heading.

Bendroflumethiazide (Dolasetron should be administered with caution in patients who have or may develop prolongation of cardiac conduction intervals, particularly QTc. This includes patients taking diuretics with potential for inducing electrolyte abnormalities).
No products indexed under this heading.

Bretylium Tosylate (Dolasetron should be administered with caution in patients who have or may develop prolongation of cardiac conduction intervals, particularly QTc. This includes patients taking drugs which lead to QT prolongation).
No products indexed under this heading.

Bumetanide (Dolasetron should be administered with caution in patients who have or may develop prolongation of cardiac conduction intervals, particularly QTc. This includes patients taking diuretics with potential for inducing electrolyte abnormalities).
No products indexed under this heading.

Buspirone Hydrochloride (Dolasetron should be administered with caution in patients who have or may develop prolongation of cardiac conduction intervals, particularly QTc. This includes patients taking drugs which lead to QT prolongation).
No products indexed under this heading.

Chlordiazepoxide (Dolasetron should be administered with caution in patients who have or may develop prolongation of cardiac conduction intervals, particularly QTc. This includes patients taking drugs which lead to QT prolongation).
No products indexed under this heading.

Chlordiazepoxide Hydrochloride (Dolasetron should be administered with caution in patients who have or may develop prolongation of cardiac conduction intervals, particularly QTc. This includes patients taking drugs which lead to QT prolongation).
No products indexed under this heading.

Chlorothiazide (Dolasetron should be administered with caution in patients who have or may develop prolongation of cardiac conduction intervals, particularly QTc. This includes patients taking diuretics with potential for inducing electrolyte abnormalities).
No products indexed under this heading.

Chlorothiazide Sodium (Dolasetron should be administered with caution in patients who have or may develop prolongation of cardiac conduction intervals, particularly QTc. This includes patients taking diuretics with potential for inducing electrolyte abnormalities). Products include:
Intravenous Sodium Diuril 2490

Chlorpromazine (Dolasetron should be administered with caution in patients who have or may develop prolongation of cardiac conduction intervals, particularly QTc. This includes patients taking drugs which lead to QT prolongation).
No products indexed under this heading.

Chlorpromazine Hydrochloride (Dolasetron should be administered with caution in patients who have or may develop prolongation of cardiac conduction intervals, particularly QTc. This includes patients taking drugs which lead to QT prolongation).
No products indexed under this heading.

Chlorprothixene (Dolasetron should be administered with caution in patients who have or may develop prolongation of cardiac conduction intervals, particularly QTc. This includes patients taking drugs which lead to QT prolongation).
No products indexed under this heading.

Chlorprothixene Hydrochloride (Dolasetron should be administered with caution in patients who have or may develop prolongation of cardiac conduction intervals, particularly QTc. This includes patients taking drugs which lead to QT prolongation).
No products indexed under this heading.

Chlorthalidone (Dolasetron should be administered with caution in patients who have or may develop prolongation of cardiac conduction intervals, particularly QTc. This includes patients taking diuretics with potential for inducing electrolyte abnormalities). Products include:
Clorpres Tablets 2185

Cimetidine (Blood levels of hydrodolasetron, the active metabolite of dolasetron, increased 24% when dolasetron was co-administered for seven days with cimetidine, a nonselective inhibitor of cytochrome P-450).
No products indexed under this heading.

Cimetidine Hydrochloride (Blood levels of hydrodolasetron, the active metabolite of dolasetron, increased 24% when dolasetron was co-administered for seven days with cimetidine, a nonselective inhibitor of cytochrome P-450).
No products indexed under this heading.

Clomipramine Hydrochloride (Dolasetron should be administered with caution in patients who have or may develop prolongation of cardiac conduction intervals, particularly QTc. This includes patients taking drugs which lead to QT prolongation).
No products indexed under this heading.

Clorazepate Dipotassium (Dolasetron should be administered with caution in patients who have or may develop prolongation of cardiac conduction intervals, particularly QTc. This includes patients taking drugs which lead to QT prolongation).
No products indexed under this heading.

Clozapine (Dolasetron should be administered with caution in patients who have or may develop prolongation of cardiac conduction intervals, particularly QTc. This includes patients taking drugs which lead to QT prolongation).
No products indexed under this heading.

Daunorubicin Hydrochloride (Dolasetron should be administered with caution in patients who have or may develop prolongation of cardiac conduction intervals, particularly QTc. This includes patients receiving cumulative high dose anthracycline therapy).
No products indexed under this heading.

Desipramine Hydrochloride (Dolasetron should be administered with caution in patients who have or may develop prolongation of cardiac conduction intervals, particularly QTc. This includes patients taking drugs which lead to QT prolongation).
No products indexed under this heading.

Diazepam (Dolasetron should be administered with caution in patients who have or may develop prolongation of cardiac conduction intervals, particularly QTc. This includes patients taking drugs which lead to QT prolongation). Products include:
Valium Tablets 2658

Disopyramide Phosphate (Dolasetron should be administered with caution in patients who have or may develop prolongation of cardiac conduction intervals, particularly QTc. This includes patients taking drugs which lead to QT prolongation).
No products indexed under this heading.

Dofetilide (Dolasetron should be administered with caution in patients who have or may develop prolongation of cardiac conduction intervals, particularly QTc. This includes patients taking drugs which lead to QT prolongation).
No products indexed under this heading.

Doxepin Hydrochloride (Dolasetron should be administered with caution in patients who have or may develop prolongation of cardiac conduction intervals, particularly QTc. This includes patients taking drugs which lead to QT prolongation).
No products indexed under this heading.

Doxorubicin Hydrochloride (Dolasetron should be administered with caution in patients who have or may develop prolongation of cardiac conduction intervals, particularly QTc. This includes patients receiving cumulative high dose anthracycline therapy).
No products indexed under this heading.

Droperidol (Dolasetron should be administered with caution in patients who have or may develop prolongation of cardiac conduction intervals, particularly QTc. This includes patients taking drugs which lead to QT prolongation).
No products indexed under this heading.

Epirubicin Hydrochloride (Dolasetron should be administered with caution in patients who have or may develop prolongation of cardiac conduction intervals, particularly QTc. This includes patients receiving cumulative high dose anthracycline therapy).
No products indexed under this heading.

Erythromycin (Dolasetron should be administered with caution in patients who have or may develop prolongation of cardiac conduction intervals, particularly QTc. This includes patients taking drugs which lead to QT prolongation).
No products indexed under this heading.

Erythromycin Estolate (Dolasetron should be administered with caution in patients who have or may develop prolongation of cardiac conduction intervals, particularly QTc. This includes patients taking drugs which lead to QT prolongation).
No products indexed under this heading.

Erythromycin Ethylsuccinate (Dolasetron should be administered with caution in patients who have or may develop prolongation of cardiac conduction intervals, particularly QTc. This includes patients taking drugs which lead to QT prolongation). Products include:
E.E.S. 433
EryPed 431

Erythromycin Gluceptate (Dolasetron should be administered with caution in patients who have or may develop prolongation of cardiac conduction intervals, particularly QTc. This includes patients taking drugs which lead to QT prolongation).
No products indexed under this heading.

Erythromycin Lactobionate (Dolasetron should be administered with caution in patients who have or may develop prolongation of cardiac conduction intervals, particularly QTc. This includes patients taking drugs which lead to QT prolongation).
No products indexed under this heading.

Erythromycin Stearate (Dolasetron should be administered with caution in patients who have or may develop prolongation of cardiac conduction intervals, particularly QTc. This includes patients taking drugs which lead to QT prolongation).
No products indexed under this heading.

Ethacrynic Acid (Dolasetron should be administered with caution in patients who have or may develop prolongation of cardiac conduction intervals, particularly QTc. This includes patients taking diuretics with potential for inducing electrolyte abnormalities). Products include:
Edecrin Tablets 698

Flecainide Acetate (Dolasetron should be administered with caution in patients who have or may develop prolongation of cardiac conduction intervals, particularly QTc. This includes patients taking drugs which lead to QT prolongation).
No products indexed under this heading.

Fluphenazine Decanoate (Dolasetron should be administered with caution in patients who have or may develop prolongation of cardiac conduction intervals, particularly QTc. This includes patients taking drugs which lead to QT prolongation).
No products indexed under this heading.

Fluphenazine Enanthate (Dolasetron should be administered with caution in patients who have or may develop prolongation of cardiac conduction intervals, particularly QTc. This includes patients taking drugs which lead to QT prolongation).
No products indexed under this heading.

Fluphenazine Hydrochloride (Dolasetron should be administered with caution in patients who have or may develop prolongation of cardiac conduction intervals, particularly QTc. This includes patients taking drugs which lead to QT prolongation).
No products indexed under this heading.

Furosemide (Dolasetron should be administered with caution in patients who have or may develop prolongation of cardiac conduction intervals, particularly QTc. This includes patients taking diuretics with potential for inducing electrolyte abnormalities). Products include:
Furosemide Tablets 2186

Haloperidol (Dolasetron should be administered with caution in patients who have or may develop prolongation of cardiac conduction intervals, particularly QTc. This includes patients taking drugs which lead to QT prolongation).
No products indexed under this heading.

Haloperidol Decanoate (Dolasetron should be administered with caution in patients who have or may develop prolongation of cardiac conduction intervals, particularly QTc. This includes patients taking drugs which lead to QT prolongation).
No products indexed under this heading.

Hydrochlorothiazide (Dolasetron should be administered with caution in patients who have or may develop prolongation of cardiac conduction intervals, particularly QTc. This includes patients taking diuretics with potential for inducing electrolyte abnormalities). Products include:
Atacand HCT 642
Avalide Tablets 892
Avalide Tablets 2713
Benicar HCT Tablets 1010
Diovan HCT Tablets 2216
Dyazide Capsules 1405
Micardis HCT Tablets 854
Prinzide Tablets 2092
Tekturna HCT Tablets 2324
Teveten HCT Tablets 517

Hydroflumethiazide (Dolasetron should be administered with caution in patients who have or may develop prolongation of cardiac conduction intervals, particularly QTc. This includes patients taking diuretics with potential for inducing electrolyte abnormalities).
No products indexed under this heading.

Hydroxyzine Hydrochloride (Dolasetron should be administered with caution in patients who have or may develop prolongation of cardiac conduction intervals, particularly QTc. This includes patients taking drugs which lead to QT prolongation).
No products indexed under this heading.

Idarubicin Hydrochloride (Dolasetron should be administered with caution in patients who have or may develop prolongation of cardiac conduction intervals, particularly QTc. This includes patients receiving cumulative high dose anthracycline therapy).
No products indexed under this heading.

Imipramine Hydrochloride (Dolasetron should be administered with caution in patients who have or may develop prolongation of cardiac conduction intervals, particularly QTc. This includes patients taking drugs which lead to QT prolongation).
No products indexed under this heading.

Imipramine Pamoate (Dolasetron should be administered with caution in patients who have or may develop prolongation of cardiac conduction intervals, particularly QTc. This includes patients taking drugs which lead to QT prolongation).
No products indexed under this heading.

Indapamide (Dolasetron should be administered with caution in patients who have or may develop prolongation of cardiac conduction intervals, particularly QTc. This includes patients taking diuretics with potential for inducing electrolyte abnormalities). Products include:
Indapamide Tablets 2188

Isocarboxazid (Dolasetron should be administered with caution in patients who have or may develop prolongation of cardiac conduction intervals, particularly QTc. This includes patients taking drugs which lead to QT prolongation). Products include:
Marplan Tablets 3177

Lidocaine Hydrochloride (Dolasetron should be administered with caution in patients who have or may develop prolongation of cardiac conduction intervals, particularly QTc. This includes patients taking drugs which lead to QT prolongation).
No products indexed under this heading.

Lithium Carbonate (Dolasetron should be administered with caution in patients who have or may develop prolongation of cardiac conduction intervals, particularly QTc. This includes patients taking drugs which lead to QT prolongation).
No products indexed under this heading.

Lithium Citrate (Dolasetron should be administered with caution in patients who have or may develop prolongation of cardiac conduction intervals, particularly QTc. This includes patients taking drugs which lead to QT prolongation).
No products indexed under this heading.

Lorazepam (Dolasetron should be administered with caution in patients who have or may develop prolongation of cardiac conduction intervals, particularly QTc. This includes patients taking drugs which lead to QT prolongation).
No products indexed under this heading.

Loxapine Hydrochloride (Dolasetron should be administered with caution in patients who have or may develop prolongation of cardiac conduction intervals, particularly QTc. This includes patients taking drugs which lead to QT prolongation).
No products indexed under this heading.

Loxapine Succinate (Dolasetron should be administered with caution in patients who have or may develop prolongation of cardiac conduction intervals, particularly QTc. This includes patients taking drugs which lead to QT prolongation).
No products indexed under this heading.

Maprotiline Hydrochloride (Dolasetron should be administered with caution in patients who have or may develop prolongation of cardiac conduction intervals, particularly QTc. This includes patients taking drugs which lead to QT prolongation).
No products indexed under this heading.

Meprobamate (Dolasetron should be administered with caution in patients who have or may develop prolongation of cardiac conduction intervals, particularly QTc. This includes patients taking drugs which lead to QT prolongation).
No products indexed under this heading.

Mesoridazine Besylate (Dolasetron should be administered with caution in patients who have or may develop prolongation of cardiac conduction intervals, particularly QTc. This includes patients taking drugs which lead to QT prolongation).
No products indexed under this heading.

Methyclothiazide (Dolasetron should be administered with caution in patients who have or may develop prolongation of cardiac conduction intervals, particularly QTc. This includes patients taking diuretics with potential for inducing electrolyte abnormalities).
No products indexed under this heading.

Metolazone (Dolasetron should be administered with caution in patients who have or may develop prolongation of cardiac conduction intervals, particularly QTc. This includes patients taking diuretics with potential for inducing electrolyte abnormalities).
No products indexed under this heading.

Mexiletine Hydrochloride (Dolasetron should be administered with caution in patients who have or may develop prolongation of cardiac conduction intervals, particularly QTc. This includes patients taking drugs which lead to QT prolongation).
No products indexed under this heading.

Midazolam Hydrochloride (Dolasetron should be administered with caution in patients who have or may develop prolongation of cardiac conduction intervals, particularly QTc. This includes patients taking drugs which lead to QT prolongation).
No products indexed under this heading.

Molindone Hydrochloride (Dolasetron should be administered with caution in patients who have or may develop prolongation of cardiac conduction intervals, particularly QTc. This includes patients taking drugs which lead to QT prolongation). Products include:
Moban Tablets 1116

Moricizine Hydrochloride (Dolasetron should be administered with caution in patients who have or may develop prolongation of cardiac conduction intervals, particularly QTc. This includes patients taking antiarrhythmic drugs).
No products indexed under this heading.

Nortriptyline Hydrochloride (Dolasetron should be administered with caution in patients who have or may develop prolongation of cardiac conduction intervals, particularly QTc. This includes patients taking drugs which lead to QT prolongation).
No products indexed under this heading.

Olanzapine (Dolasetron should be administered with caution in patients who have or may develop prolongation of cardiac conduction intervals, particularly QTc. This includes patients taking drugs which lead to QT prolongation). Products include:
Symbyax Capsules 1871
Zyprexa Tablets 1883
Zyprexa IntraMuscular 1883
Zyprexa ZYDIS Orally Disintegrating Tablets 1883

Oxazepam (Dolasetron should be administered with caution in patients who have or may develop prolongation of cardiac conduction intervals, particularly QTc. This includes patients taking drugs which lead to QT prolongation).
No products indexed under this heading.

Perphenazine (Dolasetron should be administered with caution in patients who have or may develop prolongation of cardiac conduction intervals, particularly QTc. This includes patients taking drugs which lead to QT prolongation).
No products indexed under this heading.

Phenelzine Sulfate (Dolasetron should be administered with caution in patients who have or may develop prolongation of cardiac conduction intervals, particularly QTc. This includes patients taking drugs which lead to QT prolongation).
No products indexed under this heading.

Polythiazide (Dolasetron should be administered with caution in patients who have or may develop prolongation of cardiac conduction intervals, particularly QTc. This includes patients taking diuretics with potential for inducing electrolyte abnormalities).
No products indexed under this heading.

Prazepam (Dolasetron should be administered with caution in patients who have or may develop prolongation of cardiac conduction intervals, particularly QTc. This includes patients taking drugs which lead to QT prolongation).
No products indexed under this heading.

Procainamide Hydrochloride (Dolasetron should be administered with caution in patients who have or may develop prolongation of cardiac conduction intervals, particularly QTc. This includes patients taking drugs which lead to QT prolongation).
No products indexed under this heading.

Prochlorperazine (Dolasetron should be administered with caution in patients who have or may develop prolongation of cardiac conduction intervals, particularly QTc. This includes patients taking drugs which lead to QT prolongation).
No products indexed under this heading.

Promethazine Hydrochloride (Dolasetron should be administered with caution in patients who have or may develop prolongation of cardiac conduction intervals, particularly QTc. This includes patients taking drugs which lead to QT prolongation).
No products indexed under this heading.

Propafenone Hydrochloride (Dolasetron should be administered with caution in patients who have or may develop prolongation of cardiac conduction intervals, particularly QTc. This includes patients taking drugs which lead to QT prolongation). Products include:
Rythmol Tablets 1586
Rythmol SR Capsules 1590

Propranolol Hydrochloride (Dolasetron should be administered with

caution in patients who have or may develop prolongation of cardiac conduction intervals, particularly QTc. This includes patients taking anti-arrhythmic drugs). Products include:
- InnoPran XL Extended Release Capsules 1484

Protriptyline Hydrochloride (Dolasetron should be administered with caution in patients who have or may develop prolongation of cardiac conduction intervals, particularly QTc. This includes patients taking drugs which lead to QT prolongation).
No products indexed under this heading.

Quetiapine Fumarate (Dolasetron should be administered with caution in patients who have or may develop prolongation of cardiac conduction intervals, particularly QTc. This includes patients taking drugs which lead to QT prolongation).
No products indexed under this heading.

Quinidine Gluconate (Dolasetron should be administered with caution in patients who have or may develop prolongation of cardiac conduction intervals, particularly QTc. This includes patients taking drugs which lead to QT prolongation).
No products indexed under this heading.

Quinidine Polygalacturonate (Dolasetron should be administered with caution in patients who have or may develop prolongation of cardiac conduction intervals, particularly QTc. This includes patients taking drugs which lead to QT prolongation).
No products indexed under this heading.

Quinidine Sulfate (Dolasetron should be administered with caution in patients who have or may develop prolongation of cardiac conduction intervals, particularly QTc. This includes patients taking drugs which lead to QT prolongation).
No products indexed under this heading.

Rifampin (Blood levels of hydrodolasetron, the active metabolite of dolasetron, decreased 28% with co-administration for seven days with rifampin, a potent inducer of cytochrome P-450).
No products indexed under this heading.

Risperidone (Dolasetron should be administered with caution in patients who have or may develop prolongation of cardiac conduction intervals, particularly QTc. This includes patients taking drugs which lead to QT prolongation). Products include:
- Risperdal Consta Long-Acting Injection 1753

Sotalol Hydrochloride (Dolasetron should be administered with caution in patients who have or may develop prolongation of cardiac conduction intervals, particularly QTc. This includes patients taking anti-arrhythmic drugs).
No products indexed under this heading.

Spironolactone (Dolasetron should be administered with caution in patients who have or may develop prolongation of cardiac conduction intervals, particularly QTc. This includes patients taking diuretics with potential for inducing electrolyte abnormalities).
No products indexed under this heading.

Thioridazine Hydrochloride (Dolasetron should be administered with caution in patients who have or may develop prolongation of cardiac conduction intervals, particularly QTc. This includes patients taking drugs which lead to QT prolongation). Products include:
- Thioridazine Hydrochloride Tablets 2195

Thiothixene (Dolasetron should be administered with caution in patients who have or may develop prolongation of cardiac conduction intervals, particularly QTc. This includes patients taking drugs which lead to QT prolongation). Products include:
- Thiothixene Capsules 2197

Tocainide Hydrochloride (Dolasetron should be administered with caution in patients who have or may develop prolongation of cardiac conduction intervals, particularly QTc. This includes patients taking drugs which lead to QT prolongation).
No products indexed under this heading.

Torsemide (Dolasetron should be administered with caution in patients who have or may develop prolongation of cardiac conduction intervals, particularly QTc. This includes patients taking diuretics with potential for inducing electrolyte abnormalities). Products include:
- Demadex Injection 2630
- Demadex Tablets 2630

Tranylcypromine Sulfate (Dolasetron should be administered with caution in patients who have or may develop prolongation of cardiac conduction intervals, particularly QTc. This includes patients taking drugs which lead to QT prolongation). Products include:
- Parnate Tablets 1532

Triamterene (Dolasetron should be administered with caution in patients who have or may develop prolongation of cardiac conduction intervals, particularly QTc. This includes patients taking diuretics with potential for inducing electrolyte abnormalities). Products include:
- Dyazide Capsules 1405
- Dyrenium Capsules 3189

Trifluoperazine Hydrochloride (Dolasetron should be administered with caution in patients who have or may develop prolongation of cardiac conduction intervals, particularly QTc. This includes patients taking drugs which lead to QT prolongation).
No products indexed under this heading.

Trimipramine Maleate (Dolasetron should be administered with caution in patients who have or may develop prolongation of cardiac conduction intervals, particularly QTc. This includes patients taking drugs which lead to QT prolongation).
No products indexed under this heading.

Valrubicin (Dolasetron should be administered with caution in patients who have or may develop prolongation of cardiac conduction intervals, particularly QTc. This includes patients receiving cumulative high dose anthracycline therapy). Products include:
- Valstar Sterile Solution for Intravesical Instillation 1735

Verapamil Hydrochloride (Dolasetron should be administered with caution in patients who have or may develop prolongation of cardiac conduction intervals, particularly QTc. This includes patients taking anti-arrhythmic drugs). Products include:
- Tarka Tablets 511

Ziprasidone Hydrochloride (Dolasetron should be administered with caution in patients who have or may develop prolongation of cardiac conduction intervals, particularly QTc. This includes patients taking drugs which lead to QT prolongation). Products include:
- Geodon Capsules 2520

APIDRA INJECTION

(Insulin Glulisine) 2706

May interact with ACE inhibitors, atypical antipsychotics, beta blockers, corticosteroids, diuretics, estrogens, fibrates, oral hypoglycemic agents, lithium preparations, monoamine oxidase inhibitors, phenothiazines, progestins, protease inhibitors, salicylates, sulfonamides, sympathomimetics, thyroid preparations, tions, and certain other agents. Compounds in these categories include:

Acarbose (Oral antidiabetic products may increase the blood glucose-lowering effect and susceptibility to hypoglycemia of insulin). Products include:
- Precose Tablets 792

Acebutolol Hydrochloride (Beta-blockers may either potentiate or weaken the blood glucose-lowering effect of insulin and reduce or hide the signs of hypoglycemia).
No products indexed under this heading.

Albuterol (Sympathomimetic agents may reduce the blood glucose-lowering effect of insulin).
No products indexed under this heading.

Albuterol Sulfate (Sympathomimetic agents may reduce the blood glucose-lowering effect of insulin). Products include:
- Combivent Inhalation Aerosol 845
- ProAir HFA Inhalation Aerosol 3113
- Proventil HFA Inhalation Aerosol 2914
- Ventolin HFA Inhalation Aerosol 1638

Amiloride Hydrochloride (Diuretics may reduce the blood glucose-lowering effect of insulin).
No products indexed under this heading.

Amprenavir (Protease inhibitors may reduce the blood glucose-lowering effect of insulin).
No products indexed under this heading.

Aripiprazole (Atypical antipsychotics may reduce the blood glucose-lowering effect of insulin). Products include:
- Abilify Injection 881
- Abilify Injection 2466
- Abilify Oral Solution 881
- Abilify Oral Solution 2466
- Abilify Discmelt Orally Disintegrating Tablets 881
- Abilify Discmelt Orally Disintegrating Tablets 2466
- Abilify Tablets 881
- Abilify Tablets 2466

Aspirin (Salicylates may increase the blood glucose-lowering effect and susceptibility to hypoglycemia of insulin). Products include:
- Aggrenox Capsules 819
- Bayer Aspirin 750
- Percodan Tablets 1130
- St. Joseph 81 mg Aspirin Chewable and Enteric Coated Tablets 1903

Aspirin, Enteric Coated (Salicylates may increase the blood glucose-lowering effect and susceptibility to hypoglycemia of insulin).
No products indexed under this heading.

Aspirin Buffered (Salicylates may increase the blood glucose-lowering effect and susceptibility to hypoglycemia of insulin).
No products indexed under this heading.

Atenolol (Beta-blockers may either potentiate or weaken the blood glucose-lowering effect of insulin and reduce or hide the signs of hypoglycemia).
No products indexed under this heading.

Benazepril Hydrochloride (ACE inhibitors may increase the blood glucose-lowering effect and susceptibility to hypoglycemia of insulin).
No products indexed under this heading.

Bendroflumethiazide (Diuretics may reduce the blood glucose-lowering effect of insulin).
No products indexed under this heading.

Betamethasone Acetate (Corticosteroids may reduce the blood glucose-lowering effect of insulin).
No products indexed under this heading.

Betamethasone Sodium Phosphate (Corticosteroids may reduce the blood glucose-lowering effect of insulin).
No products indexed under this heading.

Betaxolol Hydrochloride (Beta-blockers may either potentiate or weaken the blood glucose-lowering effect of insulin and reduce or hide the signs of hypoglycemia).
No products indexed under this heading.

Bisoprolol Fumarate (Beta-blockers may either potentiate or weaken the blood glucose-lowering effect of insulin and reduce or hide the signs of hypoglycemia).
No products indexed under this heading.

Budesonide (Corticosteroids may reduce the blood glucose-lowering effect of insulin). Products include:
- Pulmicort Flexhaler 654
- Symbicort 80/4.5 Inhalation Aerosol 659
- Symbicort 160/4.5 Inhalation Aerosol 659

Bumetanide (Diuretics may reduce the blood glucose-lowering effect of insulin).
No products indexed under this heading.

Captopril (ACE inhibitors may increase the blood glucose-lowering effect and susceptibility to hypoglycemia of insulin). Products include:
- Captopril Tablets 2182

Carteolol Hydrochloride (Beta-blockers may either potentiate or weaken the blood glucose-lowering effect of insulin and reduce or hide the signs of hypoglycemia).
No products indexed under this heading.

Chlorothiazide (Diuretics may reduce the blood glucose-lowering effect of insulin).
No products indexed under this heading.

Chlorothiazide Sodium (Diuretics may reduce the blood glucose-lowering effect of insulin). Products include:
Intravenous Sodium Diuril ... 2490

Chlorotrianisene (Estrogens may reduce the blood glucose-lowering effect of insulin).
No products indexed under this heading.

Chlorpromazine (Phenothiazine derivatives may reduce the blood glucose-lowering effect of insulin).
No products indexed under this heading.

Chlorpromazine Hydrochloride (Phenothiazine derivatives may reduce the blood glucose-lowering effect of insulin).
No products indexed under this heading.

Chlorpropamide (Oral antidiabetic products may increase the blood glucose-lowering effect and susceptibility to hypoglycemia of insulin).
No products indexed under this heading.

Chlorthalidone (Diuretics may reduce the blood glucose-lowering effect of insulin). Products include:
Clorpres Tablets ... 2185

Choline Magnesium Trisalicylate (Salicylates may increase the blood glucose-lowering effect and susceptibility to hypoglycemia of insulin).
No products indexed under this heading.

Ciclesonide (Corticosteroids may reduce the blood glucose-lowering effect of insulin). Products include:
Alvesco Inhalation Aerosol ... 2985
Omnaris Nasal Spray ... 2998

Clofibrate (Fibrates may increase the blood glucose-lowering effect and susceptibility to hypoglycemia of insulin).
No products indexed under this heading.

Clonidine (Clonidine may either potentiate or weaken the blood glucose-lowering effect of insulin and reduce or hide the signs of hypoglycemia). Products include:
Catapres-TTS ... 842

Clonidine Hydrochloride (Clonidine may either potentiate or weaken the blood glucose-lowering effect of insulin and reduce or hide the signs of hypoglycemia). Products include:
Catapres Tablets ... 841
Clorpres Tablets ... 2185

Clozapine (Atypical antipsychotics may reduce the blood glucose-lowering effect of insulin).
No products indexed under this heading

Cortisone Acetate (Corticosteroids may reduce the blood glucose-lowering effect of insulin).
No products indexed under this heading.

Danazol (Danazol may reduce the blood glucose-lowering effect of insulin).
No products indexed under this heading.

Darunavir (Protease inhibitors may reduce the blood glucose-lowering effect of insulin).
No products indexed under this heading.

Desogestrel (Progestogens may reduce the blood glucose-lowering effect of insulin). Products include:
Mircette Tablets ... 1034

Dexamethasone (Corticosteroids may reduce the blood glucose-lowering effect of insulin). Products include:
Ciprodex Otic Suspension ... 541

Dexamethasone Acetate (Corticosteroids may reduce the blood glucose-lowering effect of insulin).
No products indexed under this heading.

Dexamethasone Sodium Phosphate (Corticosteroids may reduce the blood glucose-lowering effect of insulin).
No products indexed under this heading.

Diazoxide (Diazoxide may reduce the blood glucose-lowering effect of insulin). Products include:
Proglycem Capsules ... 1185
Proglycem Suspension ... 1185

Dienestrol (Estrogens may reduce the blood glucose-lowering effect of insulin).
No products indexed under this heading.

Diethylstilbestrol (Estrogens may reduce the blood glucose-lowering effect of insulin).
No products indexed under this heading.

Diflunisal (Salicylates may increase the blood glucose-lowering effect and susceptibility to hypoglycemia of insulin).
No products indexed under this heading.

Disopyramide (Disopyramide may increase the blood glucose-lowering effect and susceptibility to hypoglycemia of insulin).
No products indexed under this heading.

Disopyramide Phosphate (Disopyramide may increase the blood glucose-lowering effect and susceptibility to hypoglycemia of insulin).
No products indexed under this heading.

Dobutamine Hydrochloride (Sympathomimetic agents may reduce the blood glucose-lowering effect of insulin).
No products indexed under this heading.

Dopamine Hydrochloride (Sympathomimetic agents may reduce the blood glucose-lowering effect of insulin).
No products indexed under this heading.

Enalapril Maleate (ACE inhibitors may increase the blood glucose-lowering effect and susceptibility to hypoglycemia of insulin).
No products indexed under this heading.

Enalaprilat (ACE inhibitors may increase the blood glucose-lowering effect and susceptibility to hypoglycemia of insulin).
No products indexed under this heading.

Ephedrine Hydrochloride (Sympathomimetic agents may reduce the blood glucose-lowering effect of insulin).
No products indexed under this heading.

Ephedrine Sulfate (Sympathomimetic agents may reduce the blood glucose-lowering effect of insulin).
No products indexed under this heading.

Ephedrine Tannate (Sympathomimetic agents may reduce the blood glucose-lowering effect of insulin).
No products indexed under this heading.

Epinephrine (Sympathomimetic agents may reduce the blood glucose-lowering effect of insulin). Products include:
EpiPen ... 1024

Epinephrine Bitartrate (Sympathomimetic agents may reduce the blood glucose-lowering effect of insulin).
No products indexed under this heading.

Epinephrine Hydrochloride (Sympathomimetic agents may reduce the blood glucose-lowering effect of insulin).
No products indexed under this heading.

Esmolol Hydrochloride (Beta-blockers may either potentiate or weaken the blood glucose-lowering effect of insulin and reduce or hide the signs of hypoglycemia).
No products indexed under this heading.

Estradiol (Estrogens may reduce the blood glucose-lowering effect of insulin). Products include:
Activella Tablets ... 2347
Angeliq Tablets ... 751
Climara Transdermal System ... 763
Climara Pro Transdermal System ... 768
Divigel ... 3167
Vagifem Tablets ... 2375

Estrogens, Conjugated (Estrogens may reduce the blood glucose-lowering effect of insulin). Products include:
Premarin Intravenous ... 3217
Premarin Tablets ... 3221
Premarin Vaginal Cream ... 3228
Premphase Tablets ... 3232
Prempro Tablets ... 3232

Estrogens, Esterified (Estrogens may reduce the blood glucose-lowering effect of insulin). Products include:
Estratest Tablets ... 3043
Estratest H.S. Tablets ... 3043

Estropipate (Estrogens may reduce the blood glucose-lowering effect of insulin).
No products indexed under this heading.

Ethacrynic Acid (Diuretics may reduce the blood glucose-lowering effect of insulin). Products include:
Edecrin Tablets ... 698

Ethinyl Estradiol (Estrogens may reduce the blood glucose-lowering effect of insulin). Products include:
Lybrel Tablets ... 3204
Mircette Tablets ... 1034
NuvaRing ... 2897
Ortho-Cyclen/Ortho Tri-Cyclen ... 2449
Ortho Evra Transdermal System ... 2437
Ortho Tri-Cyclen Lo Tablets ... 2458
Seasonique Tablets ... 1046
Yaz Tablets ... 805

Fenofibrate (Fibrates may increase the blood glucose-lowering effect and susceptibility to hypoglycemia of insulin). Products include:
Fenoglide Tablets ... 2960
Tricor Tablets ... 520

Fludrocortisone Acetate (Corticosteroids may reduce the blood glucose-lowering effect of insulin).
No products indexed under this heading.

Flunisolide (Corticosteroids may reduce the blood glucose-lowering effect of insulin). Products include:
Aerobid/Aerobid-M ... 1153

Fluoxetine (Fluoxetine may increase the blood glucose-lowering effect and susceptibility to hypoglycemia of insulin).
No products indexed under this heading.

Fluoxetine Hydrochloride (Fluoxetine may increase the blood glucose-lowering effect and susceptibility to hypoglycemia of insulin). Products include:
Prozac Weekly Capsules ... 1852
Prozac Pulvules and Liquid ... 1852
Symbyax Capsules ... 1871

Fluphenazine Decanoate (Phenothiazine derivatives may reduce the blood glucose-lowering effect of insulin).
No products indexed under this heading.

Fluphenazine Enanthate (Phenothiazine derivatives may reduce the blood glucose-lowering effect of insulin).
No products indexed under this heading.

Fluphenazine Hydrochloride (Phenothiazine derivatives may reduce the blood glucose-lowering effect of insulin).
No products indexed under this heading.

Fluticasone Propionate (Corticosteroids may reduce the blood glucose-lowering effect of insulin). Products include:
Advair Diskus 100/50 ... 1276
Advair Diskus 250/50 ... 1276
Advair Diskus 500/50 ... 1276
Advair HFA 45/21 Inhalation Aerosol ... 1288
Advair HFA 115/21 Inhalation Aerosol ... 1288
Advair HFA 230/21 Inhalation Aerosol ... 1288
Flonase Nasal Spray ... 1431
Flovent Diskus 50 mcg ... 1435

Fluticasone Propionate HFA (Corticosteroids may reduce the blood glucose-lowering effect of insulin). Products include:
Flovent HFA ... 1440

Fosamprenavir Calcium (Protease inhibitors may reduce the blood glucose-lowering effect of insulin). Products include:
Lexiva Oral Suspension ... 1510
Lexiva Tablets ... 1510

Fosinopril Sodium (ACE inhibitors may increase the blood glucose-lowering effect and susceptibility to hypoglycemia of insulin).
No products indexed under this heading.

Furosemide (Diuretics may reduce the blood glucose-lowering effect of insulin). Products include:
Furosemide Tablets ... 2186

IMPORTANT NOTE: Always consult each drug listing in the patient's regimen for possible interactions.

Gemfibrozil (Fibrates may increase the blood glucose-lowering effect and susceptibility to hypoglycemia of insulin).
No products indexed under this heading.

Glimepiride (Oral antidiabetic products may increase the blood glucose-lowering effect and susceptibility to hypoglycemia of insulin). Products include:
Avandaryl Tablets 1344
Duetact Tablets 3085

Glipizide (Oral antidiabetic products may increase the blood glucose-lowering effect and susceptibility to hypoglycemia of insulin).
No products indexed under this heading.

Glucagon (Glucagon may reduce the blood glucose-lowering effect of insulin). Products include:
Glucagon for Injection Vials and Emergency Kit 1827

Glyburide (Oral antidiabetic products may increase the blood glucose-lowering effect and susceptibility to hypoglycemia of insulin).
No products indexed under this heading.

Guanethidine (Under the influence of sympatholytic medicinal products, such as guanethidine, the signs of hypoglycemia may be reduced or absent).
No products indexed under this heading.

Guanethidine Monosulfate (Under the influence of sympatholytic medicinal products, such as guanethidine, the signs of hypoglycemia may be reduced or absent).
No products indexed under this heading.

Guanethidine Sulfate (Under the influence of sympatholytic medicinal products, such as guanethidine, the signs of hypoglycemia may be reduced or absent).
No products indexed under this heading.

Hydrochlorothiazide (Diuretics may reduce the blood glucose-lowering effect of insulin). Products include:
Atacand HCT 642
Avalide Tablets 892
Avalide Tablets 2713
Benicar HCT Tablets 1010
Diovan HCT Tablets 2216
Dyazide Capsules 1405
Micardis HCT Tablets 854
Prinzide Tablets 2092
Tekturna HCT Tablets 2324
Teveten HCT Tablets 517

Hydrocortisone (Corticosteroids may reduce the blood glucose-lowering effect of insulin).
No products indexed under this heading.

Hydrocortisone Acetate (Corticosteroids may reduce the blood glucose-lowering effect of insulin). Products include:
Analpram-HC 1140
Pramosone 1141

Hydrocortisone Sodium Phosphate (Corticosteroids may reduce the blood glucose-lowering effect of insulin).
No products indexed under this heading.

Hydrocortisone Sodium Succinate (Corticosteroids may reduce the blood glucose-lowering effect of insulin).
No products indexed under this heading.

Hydroflumethiazide (Diuretics may reduce the blood glucose-lowering effect of insulin).
No products indexed under this heading.

Indapamide (Diuretics may reduce the blood glucose-lowering effect of insulin). Products include:
Indapamide Tablets 2188

Indinavir Sulfate (Protease inhibitors may reduce the blood glucose-lowering effect of insulin). Products include:
Crixivan Capsules 1979

Isocarboxazid (MAO inhibitors may increase the blood glucose-lowering effect and susceptibility to hypoglycemia of insulin). Products include:
Marplan Tablets 3177

Isoniazid (Isoniazid may reduce the blood glucose-lowering effect of insulin).
No products indexed under this heading.

Isoproterenol Hydrochloride (Sympathomimetic agents may reduce the blood glucose-lowering effect of insulin).
No products indexed under this heading.

Isoproterenol Sulfate (Sympathomimetic agents may reduce the blood glucose-lowering effect of insulin).
No products indexed under this heading.

Labetalol Hydrochloride (Beta-blockers may either potentiate or weaken the blood glucose-lowering effect of insulin and reduce or hide the signs of hypoglycemia).
No products indexed under this heading.

Levalbuterol Hydrochloride (Sympathomimetic agents may reduce the blood glucose-lowering effect of insulin). Products include:
Xopenex Inhalation Solution 3001
Xopenex Inhalation Solution Concentrate 3005

Levobunolol Hydrochloride (Beta-blockers may either potentiate or weaken the blood glucose-lowering effect of insulin and reduce or hide the signs of hypoglycemia).
No products indexed under this heading.

Levothyroxine Sodium (Thyroid hormones may reduce the blood glucose-lowering effect of insulin). Products include:
Levothroid Tablets 1170
Levoxyl Tablets 1780
Synthroid Tablets 507

Liothyronine Sodium (Thyroid hormones may reduce the blood glucose-lowering effect of insulin). Products include:
Cytomel Tablets 1778

Liotrix (Thyroid hormones may reduce the blood glucose-lowering effect of insulin).
No products indexed under this heading.

Lisinopril (ACE inhibitors may increase the blood glucose-lowering effect and susceptibility to hypoglycemia of insulin). Products include:
Prinivil Tablets 2087
Prinzide Tablets 2092

Lithium (Lithium salts may either potentiate or weaken the blood-glucose-lowering effect of insulin).
No products indexed under this heading.

Lithium Carbonate (Lithium salts may either potentiate or weaken the blood-glucose-lowering effect of insulin).
No products indexed under this heading.

Lithium Citrate (Lithium salts may either potentiate or weaken the blood-glucose-lowering effect of insulin).
No products indexed under this heading.

Lopinavir (Protease inhibitors may reduce the blood glucose-lowering effect of insulin). Products include:
Kaletra 452

Magnesium Salicylate (Salicylates may increase the blood glucose-lowering effect and susceptibility to hypoglycemia of insulin).
No products indexed under this heading.

Medroxyprogesterone Acetate (Progestogens may reduce the blood glucose-lowering effect of insulin). Products include:
Premphase Tablets 3232
Prempro Tablets 3232

Megestrol Acetate (Progestogens may reduce the blood glucose-lowering effect of insulin). Products include:
Megace ES Oral Suspension 2499

Mesoridazine Besylate (Phenothiazine derivatives may reduce the blood glucose-lowering effect of insulin).
No products indexed under this heading.

Metaproterenol Sulfate (Sympathomimetic agents may reduce the blood glucose-lowering effect of insulin).
No products indexed under this heading.

Metaraminol Bitartrate (Sympathomimetic agents may reduce the blood glucose-lowering effect of insulin).
No products indexed under this heading.

Metformin Hydrochloride (Oral antidiabetic products may increase the blood glucose-lowering effect and susceptibility to hypoglycemia of insulin). Products include:
ActoPlus Met Tablets 3071
Avandamet Tablets 1336
Janumet Tablets 2041
PrandiMet Tablets 2967

Methotrimeprazine (Phenothiazine derivatives may reduce the blood glucose-lowering effect of insulin).
No products indexed under this heading.

Methoxamine Hydrochloride (Sympathomimetic agents may reduce the blood glucose-lowering effect of insulin).
No products indexed under this heading.

Methyclothiazide (Diuretics may reduce the blood glucose-lowering effect of insulin).
No products indexed under this heading.

Methylprednisolone Acetate (Corticosteroids may reduce the blood glucose-lowering effect of insulin).
No products indexed under this heading.

Methylprednisolone Sodium Succinate (Corticosteroids may reduce the blood glucose-lowering effect of insulin).
No products indexed under this heading.

Metipranolol Hydrochloride (Beta-blockers may either potentiate or weaken the blood glucose-lowering effect of insulin and reduce or hide the signs of hypoglycemia).
No products indexed under this heading.

Metolazone (Diuretics may reduce the blood glucose-lowering effect of insulin).
No products indexed under this heading.

Metoprolol Succinate (Beta-blockers may either potentiate or weaken the blood glucose-lowering effect of insulin and reduce or hide the signs of hypoglycemia). Products include:
Toprol-XL Tablets 666

Metoprolol Tartrate (Beta-blockers may either potentiate or weaken the blood glucose-lowering effect of insulin and reduce or hide the signs of hypoglycemia).
No products indexed under this heading.

Miglitol (Oral antidiabetic products may increase the blood glucose-lowering effect and susceptibility to hypoglycemia of insulin).
No products indexed under this heading.

Moclobemide (MAO inhibitors may increase the blood glucose-lowering effect and susceptibility to hypoglycemia of insulin).
No products indexed under this heading.

Moexipril Hydrochloride (ACE inhibitors may increase the blood glucose-lowering effect and susceptibility to hypoglycemia of insulin).
No products indexed under this heading.

Mometasone Furoate (Corticosteroids may reduce the blood glucose-lowering effect of insulin). Products include:
Asmanex Twisthaler 2797
Elocon Cream 0.1% 2840
Elocon Lotion 0.1% 2841
Elocon Ointment 0.1% 2842

Mometasone Furoate Monohydrate (Corticosteroids may reduce the blood glucose-lowering effect of insulin). Products include:
Nasonex Nasal Spray 2883

Nadolol (Beta-blockers may either potentiate or weaken the blood glucose-lowering effect of insulin and reduce or hide the signs of hypoglycemia). Products include:
Nadolol Tablets 2191

Nateglinide (Oral antidiabetic products may increase the blood glucose-lowering effect and susceptibility to hypoglycemia of insulin). Products include:
Starlix Tablets 2314

Nebivolol (Beta-blockers may either potentiate or weaken the blood glucose-lowering effect of insulin and reduce or hide the signs of hypoglycemia). Products include:
Bystolic Tablets 1155

Nelfinavir Mesylate (Protease inhibitors may reduce the blood glucose-lowering effect of insulin).
No products indexed under this heading.

Norepinephrine Bitartrate (Sympathomimetic agents may reduce the blood glucose-lowering effect of insulin).
No products indexed under this heading.

Norgestimate (Progestogens may reduce the blood glucose-lowering effect of insulin). Products include:
Ortho-Cyclen/Ortho Tri-Cyclen **2449**
Ortho Tri-Cyclen Lo Tablets **2458**

Olanzapine (Atypical antipsychotics may reduce the blood glucose-lowering effect of insulin). Products include:
Symbyax Capsules **1871**
Zyprexa Tablets **1883**
Zyprexa IntraMuscular **1883**
Zyprexa ZYDIS Orally Disintegrating Tablets **1883**

Pargyline Hydrochloride (MAO inhibitors may increase the blood glucose-lowering effect and susceptibility to hypoglycemia of insulin).
No products indexed under this heading.

Penbutolol Sulfate (Beta-blockers may either potentiate or weaken the blood glucose-lowering effect of insulin and reduce or hide the signs of hypoglycemia).
No products indexed under this heading.

Pentamidine Isethionate (Pentamidine may cause hypoglycemia, which may sometimes be followed by hyperglycemia).
No products indexed under this heading.

Pentoxifylline (Pentoxifylline may increase the blood glucose-lowering effect and susceptibility to hypoglycemia of insulin).
No products indexed under this heading.

Perindopril Erbumine (ACE inhibitors may increase the blood glucose-lowering effect and susceptibility to hypoglycemia of insulin). Products include:
Aceon Tablets (2 mg, 4 mg, 8 mg) **3038**

Perphenazine (Phenothiazine derivatives may reduce the blood glucose-lowering effect of insulin).
No products indexed under this heading.

Phenelzine Sulfate (MAO inhibitors may increase the blood glucose-lowering effect and susceptibility to hypoglycemia of insulin).
No products indexed under this heading.

Phenylephrine Bitartrate (Sympathomimetic agents may reduce the blood glucose-lowering effect of insulin).
No products indexed under this heading.

Phenylephrine Hydrochloride (Sympathomimetic agents may reduce the blood glucose-lowering effect of insulin). Products include:
Actifed Cold & Allergy Tablets **1895**
Benadryl Allergy & Cold Kapgels **1895**
Benadryl Allergy & Sinus Headache Kapgels **1895**
Benadryl Severe Allergy & Sinus Headache Caplets **1897**
Children's Benadryl-D Allergy & Sinus Liquid **1896**
Benadryl-D Allergy & Sinus Tablet **1896**
PediaCare Children's Allergy & Cold Liquid **1902**
PediaCare Children's Decongestant Liquid.................... **1902**
PediaCare Children's Liquid Multi-Symptom Cold..................... **1902**
Sinutab Non-Drying Caplets **1905**
Sinutab Sinus Caplets **1905**
Children's Sudafed PE Cold & Cough Liquid **1907**
Children's Sudafed PE Nasal Decongestant Liquid.................... **1906**
Sudafed PE Cold & Cough Caplets....................................... **1907**
Sudafed PE Nasal Decongestant Tablets **1907**
Sudafed PE Nighttime Cold Caplets.. **1907**
Sudafed PE Non-Drying Sinus Caplets.. **1908**
Sudafed PE Severe Cold Caplets **1908**
Sudafed PE Sinus & Allergy Tablets **1908**
Sudafed PE Sinus Headache Caplets.. **1908**
Tylenol Allergy Multi-Symptom Caplets with Cool Burst and Rapid Release Gelcaps **1916**
Tylenol Allergy Multi-Symptom Nighttime Caplets with Cool Burst **1916**
Children's Tylenol Plus Cold Suspension Liquid **1912**
Children's Tylenol Plus Cold & Allergy Suspension Liquid **1914**
Children's Tylenol Plus Flu Suspension Liquid **1914**
Children's Tylenol Plus Multi-Symptom Cold Suspension Liquid **1912**
Tylenol Cold Head Congestion Daytime Caplets with Cool Burst **1910**
Tylenol Cold Head Congestion Nighttime Caplets with Cool Burst **1910**
Tylenol Cold Head Congestion Severe Daytime Caplets with Cool Burst **1910**
Tylenol Cold Multi-Symptom Daytime Caplets with Cool Burst and Rapid Release Gels **1913**
Tylenol Cold Multi-Symptom Daytime Liquid with Citrus Burst ... **1913**
Tylenol Cold Multi-Symptom Nighttime Caplets with Cool Burst **1913**
Tylenol Cold Multi-Symptom Nighttime Liquid with Cool Burst ... **1913**
Tylenol Cold Multi-Symptom Severe Caplets with Cool Burst..... **1913**
Tylenol Cold Multi-Symptom Severe Daytime Liquid with Citrus Burst **1913**
Tylenol Sinus Congestion & Pain Daytime Caplets with Cool Burst and Gelcaps...................... **1917**
Tylenol Sinus Congestion & Pain Nighttime Caplets with Cool Burst **1917**
Tylenol Sinus Congestion & Pain Severe Caplets with Cool Burst..... **1917**
Vicks DayQuil Cold & Flu Multi-Symptom Relief **616**
Vicks DayQuil LiquiCaps **2567**
Vicks DayQuil Liquid **2567**
Vicks DayQuil Multi-Symptom Cold/Flu Relief............................ **2567**

Phenylephrine Tannate (Sympathomimetic agents may reduce the blood glucose-lowering effect of insulin).
No products indexed under this heading.

Phenylpropanolamine Hydrochloride (Sympathomimetic agents may reduce the blood glucose-lowering effect of insulin).
No products indexed under this heading.

Pindolol (Beta-blockers may either potentiate or weaken the blood glucose-lowering effect of insulin and reduce or hide the signs of hypoglycemia).
No products indexed under this heading.

Pioglitazone Hydrochloride (Oral antidiabetic products may increase the blood glucose-lowering effect and susceptibility to hypoglycemia of insulin). Products include:
ActoPlus Met Tablets **3071**
Actos Tablets **3077**
Duetact Tablets **3085**

Pirbuterol Acetate (Sympathomimetic agents may reduce the blood glucose-lowering effect of insulin). Products include:
Maxair Autohaler **1705**

Polyestradiol Phosphate (Estrogens may reduce the blood glucose-lowering effect of insulin).
No products indexed under this heading.

Polythiazide (Diuretics may reduce the blood glucose-lowering effect of insulin).
No products indexed under this heading.

Prednisolone Acetate (Corticosteroids may reduce the blood glucose-lowering effect of insulin). Products include:
Pred Forte Ophthalmic Suspension .... ⊙ **227**
Pred Mild Ophthalmic Suspension .... ⊙ **230**
Pred-G Ophthalmic Ointment .... ⊙ **229**
Pred-G Ophthalmic Suspension ...... ⊙ **228**

Prednisolone Sodium Phosphate (Corticosteroids may reduce the blood glucose-lowering effect of insulin).
No products indexed under this heading.

Prednisolone Tebutate (Corticosteroids may reduce the blood glucose-lowering effect of insulin).
No products indexed under this heading.

Prednisone (Corticosteroids may reduce the blood glucose-lowering effect of insulin).
No products indexed under this heading.

Procarbazine Hydrochloride (MAO inhibitors may increase the blood glucose-lowering effect and susceptibility to hypoglycemia of insulin).
No products indexed under this heading.

Prochlorperazine (Phenothiazine derivatives may reduce the blood glucose-lowering effect of insulin).
No products indexed under this heading.

Promethazine Hydrochloride (Phenothiazine derivatives may reduce the blood glucose-lowering effect of insulin).
No products indexed under this heading.

Propoxyphene Hydrochloride (Propoxyphene may increase the blood glucose-lowering effect and susceptibility to hypoglycemia of insulin).
No products indexed under this heading.

Propoxyphene Napsylate (Propoxyphene may increase the blood glucose-lowering effect and susceptibility to hypoglycemia of insulin).
No products indexed under this heading.

Propranolol Hydrochloride (Beta-blockers may either potentiate or weaken the blood glucose-lowering effect of insulin and reduce or hide the signs of hypoglycemia). Products include:
InnoPran XL Extended Release Capsules....................................... **1484**

Pseudoephedrine Hydrochloride (Sympathomimetic agents may reduce the blood glucose-lowering effect of insulin). Products include:
Allegra-D 12 Hour Extended-Release Tablets............ **2687**
Allegra-D 24 Hour Extended-Release Tablets............ **2690**
Children's Motrin Cold Oral Suspension **1899**
Sudafed 12 Hour Nasal Decongestant Non-Drowsy Caplets.. **1909**
Sudafed 24 Hour Non-Drowsy Nasal Decongestant Tablets......... **1906**
Children's Sudafed Nasal Decongestant Liquid.................... **1906**
Sudafed Nasal Decongestant Tablets **1906**
Tylenol Cold Severe Congestion Daytime Caplets with Cool Burst **1912**
Tylenol Sinus Severe Congestion Caplets with Cool Burst **1917**
Vicks NyQuil LiquiCaps **2567**
Vicks NyQuil Liquid **2567**
Vicks NyQuil Multi-Symptom Cold/Flu Relief............................ **2567**
Zyrtec-D 12 Hour Extended Release Tablets **1923**
Zyrtec-D Allergy & Congestion Extended-Release Tablets............ **1923**

Pseudoephedrine Sulfate (Sympathomimetic agents may reduce the blood glucose-lowering effect of insulin). Products include:
Clarinex-D 12-Hour Extended-Release Tablets............ **2831**
Clarinex-D 24-Hour Extended-Release Tablets............ **2834**

Quetiapine Fumarate (Atypical antipsychotics may reduce the blood glucose-lowering effect of insulin).
No products indexed under this heading.

Quinapril Hydrochloride (ACE inhibitors may increase the blood glucose-lowering effect and susceptibility to hypoglycemia of insulin).
No products indexed under this heading.

Quinestrol (Estrogens may reduce the blood glucose-lowering effect of insulin).
No products indexed under this heading.

Ramipril (ACE inhibitors may increase the blood glucose-lowering effect and susceptibility to hypoglycemia of insulin).
No products indexed under this heading.

Rasagiline Mesylate (MAO inhibitors may increase the blood glucose-lowering effect and susceptibility to hypoglycemia of insulin). Products include:
Azilect Tablets **3106**

Repaglinide (Oral antidiabetic products may increase the blood glucose-lowering effect and susceptibility to hypoglycemia of insulin). Products include:
PrandiMet Tablets **2967**
Prandin Tablets **2971**

Reserpine (Under the influence of sympatholytic medicinal products, such as reserpine, the signs of hypoglycemia may be reduced or absent).
No products indexed under this heading.

Risperidone (Atypical antipsychotics may reduce the blood glucose-lowering effect of insulin). Products include:
Risperdal Consta Long-Acting Injection **1753**

Ritonavir (Protease inhibitors may reduce the blood glucose-lowering effect of insulin). Products include:
Kaletra 452
Norvir 489

Rosiglitazone Maleate (Oral antidiabetic products may increase the blood glucose-lowering effect and susceptibility to hypoglycemia of insulin). Products include:
Avandamet Tablets 1336
Avandaryl Tablets 1344
Avandia Tablets 1351

Salmeterol Xinafoate (Sympathomimetic agents may reduce the blood glucose-lowering effect of insulin). Products include:
Advair Diskus 100/50 1276
Advair Diskus 250/50 1276
Advair Diskus 500/50 1276
Advair HFA 45/21 Inhalation Aerosol........ 1288
Advair HFA 115/21 Inhalation Aerosol........ 1288
Advair HFA 230/21 Inhalation Aerosol........ 1288
Serevent Diskus 1594

Salsalate (Salicylates may increase the blood glucose-lowering effect and susceptibility to hypoglycemia of insulin).
No products indexed under this heading.

Saquinavir (Protease inhibitors may reduce the blood glucose-lowering effect of insulin).
No products indexed under this heading.

Saquinavir Mesylate (Protease inhibitors may reduce the blood glucose-lowering effect of insulin).
No products indexed under this heading.

Selegiline (MAO inhibitors may increase the blood glucose-lowering effect and susceptibility to hypoglycemia of insulin). Products include:
Emsam Transdermal System 905

Selegiline Hydrochloride (MAO inhibitors may increase the blood glucose-lowering effect and susceptibility to hypoglycemia of insulin). Products include:
Eldepryl Capsules 3052

Sitagliptin Phosphate (Oral antidiabetic products may increase the blood glucose-lowering effect and susceptibility to hypoglycemia of insulin). Products include:
Janumet Tablets 2041
Januvia Tablets 2048

Somatropin (Somatropin may reduce the blood glucose-lowering effect of insulin). Products include:
Genotropin Lyophilized Powder 2547
Humatrope Vials and Cartridges 1838
Nutropin for Injection 1208
Nutropin AQ Injection 1212
Nutropin AQ NuSpin Injection 1212
Nutropin AQ Pen 1212
Nutropin AQ Pen Cartridge 1212

Sotalol Hydrochloride (Beta-blockers may either potentiate or weaken the blood glucose-lowering effect of insulin and reduce or hide the signs of hypoglycemia).
No products indexed under this heading.

Spirapril Hydrochloride (ACE inhibitors may increase the blood glucose-lowering effect and susceptibility to hypoglycemia of insulin).
No products indexed under this heading.

Spironolactone (Diuretics may reduce the blood glucose-lowering effect of insulin).
No products indexed under this heading.

Sulfacytine (Sulfonamide antibiotics may increase the blood glucose-lowering effect and susceptibility to hypoglycemia of insulin).
No products indexed under this heading.

Sulfamethizole (Sulfonamide antibiotics may increase the blood glucose-lowering effect and susceptibility to hypoglycemia of insulin).
No products indexed under this heading.

Sulfamethoxazole (Sulfonamide antibiotics may increase the blood glucose-lowering effect and susceptibility to hypoglycemia of insulin).
No products indexed under this heading.

Sulfasalazine (Sulfonamide antibiotics may increase the blood glucose-lowering effect and susceptibility to hypoglycemia of insulin).
No products indexed under this heading.

Sulfinpyrazone (Sulfonamide antibiotics may increase the blood glucose-lowering effect and susceptibility to hypoglycemia of insulin).
No products indexed under this heading.

Sulfisoxazole Acetyl (Sulfonamide antibiotics may increase the blood glucose-lowering effect and susceptibility to hypoglycemia of insulin).
No products indexed under this heading.

Sulfisoxazole Diolamine (Sulfonamide antibiotics may increase the blood glucose-lowering effect and susceptibility to hypoglycemia of insulin).
No products indexed under this heading.

Terbutaline Sulfate (Sympathomimetic agents may reduce the blood glucose-lowering effect of insulin).
No products indexed under this heading.

Thioridazine Hydrochloride (Phenothiazine derivatives may reduce the blood glucose-lowering effect of insulin). Products include:
Thioridazine Hydrochloride Tablets 2195

Thyroglobulin (Thyroid hormones may reduce the blood glucose-lowering effect of insulin).
No products indexed under this heading.

Thyroid (Thyroid hormones may reduce the blood glucose-lowering effect of insulin). Products include:
Naturethroid Tablets 2605

Thyroxine (Thyroid hormones may reduce the blood glucose-lowering effect of insulin).
No products indexed under this heading.

Thyroxine Sodium (Thyroid hormones may reduce the blood glucose-lowering effect of insulin).
No products indexed under this heading.

Timolol Hemihydrate (Beta-blockers may either potentiate or weaken the blood glucose-lowering effect of insulin and reduce or hide the signs of hypoglycemia). Products include:
Betimol Ophthalmic Solution 3181

Timolol Maleate (Beta-blockers may either potentiate or weaken the blood glucose-lowering effect of insulin and reduce or hide the signs of hypoglycemia). Products include:
Combigan Ophthalmic Solution 553
Cosopt Sterile Ophthalmic Solution 1969
Timoptic Sterile Ophthalmic Solution 2121
Timoptic in Ocudose 2124
Timoptic-XE Sterile Ophthalmic Gel Forming Solution 2125

Tipranavir (Protease inhibitors may reduce the blood glucose-lowering effect of insulin). Products include:
Aptivus Capsules 823
Aptivus Oral Solution 823

Tolazamide (Oral antidiabetic products may increase the blood glucose-lowering effect and susceptibility to hypoglycemia of insulin).
No products indexed under this heading.

Tolbutamide (Oral antidiabetic products may increase the blood glucose-lowering effect and susceptibility to hypoglycemia of insulin).
No products indexed under this heading.

Torsemide (Diuretics may reduce the blood glucose-lowering effect of insulin). Products include:
Demadex Injection 2630
Demadex Tablets 2630

Trandolapril (ACE inhibitors may increase the blood glucose-lowering effect and susceptibility to hypoglycemia of insulin). Products include:
Mavik Tablets 472
Tarka Tablets 511

Tranylcypromine Sulfate (MAO inhibitors may increase the blood glucose-lowering effect and susceptibility to hypoglycemia of insulin). Products include:
Parnate Tablets 1532

Triamcinolone (Corticosteroids may reduce the blood glucose-lowering effect of insulin).
No products indexed under this heading.

Triamcinolone Acetonide (Corticosteroids may reduce the blood glucose-lowering effect of insulin). Products include:
Azmacort Inhalation Aerosol 407
Nasacort AQ Nasal Spray 2765
Triesence Injectable Suspension .... ⊙209

Triamcinolone Diacetate (Corticosteroids may reduce the blood glucose-lowering effect of insulin).
No products indexed under this heading.

Triamcinolone Hexacetonide (Corticosteroids may reduce the blood glucose-lowering effect of insulin).
No products indexed under this heading.

Triamterene (Diuretics may reduce the blood glucose-lowering effect of insulin). Products include:
Dyazide Capsules 1405
Dyrenium Capsules 3189

Trifluoperazine Hydrochloride (Phenothiazine derivatives may reduce the blood glucose-lowering effect of insulin).
No products indexed under this heading.

Troglitazone (Oral antidiabetic products may increase the blood glucose-lowering effect and susceptibility to hypoglycemia of insulin).
No products indexed under this heading.

Ziprasidone Hydrochloride (Atypical antipsychotics may reduce the blood glucose-lowering effect of insulin). Products include:
Geodon Capsules 2520

Ziprasidone Mesylate (Atypical antipsychotics may reduce the blood glucose-lowering effect of insulin). Products include:
Geodon for Injection 2520

Food Interactions

Alcohol (Alcohol may either potentiate or weaken the blood glucose-lowering effect of insulin).

APPEAREX TABLETS

(Biotin) 2163

May interact with phenytoin and certain other agents. Compounds in these categories include:

Antibiotics, unspecified (The use of antibiotics may reduce the contribution of biotin made by bacteria within the large intestine).
No products indexed under this heading.

Carbamazepine (May accelerate biotin metabolism, leading to a reduction in available biotin). Products include:
Carbatrol Capsules 3019
Equetro Extended-Release Capsules 3174

Fosphenytoin Sodium (May accelerate biotin metabolism, leading to a reduction in available biotin).
No products indexed under this heading.

Phenobarbital (May accelerate biotin metabolism, leading to a reduction in available biotin). Products include:
Donnatal Extentabs 2507

Phenytoin (May accelerate biotin metabolism, leading to a reduction in available biotin).
No products indexed under this heading.

Phenytoin Sodium (May accelerate biotin metabolism, leading to a reduction in available biotin). Products include:
Phenytek Capsules 2192

Primidone (May accelerate biotin metabolism, leading to a reduction in available biotin).
No products indexed under this heading.

APTIVUS CAPSULES

(Tipranavir) 823

May interact with oral anticoagulants, cytochrome p450 3a inducers (selected), cytochrome p450 3a substrates (selected), estrogens, oral hypoglycemic agents, insulin, oral contraceptives, P-glycoprotein inhibitors, phenytoin, platelet inhibitors, quinidine, valproate, and certain other agents. Compounds in these categories include:

Abacavir Sulfate (Concomitant use with abacavir led to a decrease in AUC of abacavir by 40%. The clinical relevance of reduction in abacavir levels has not been established. Dose adjustment of abacavir cannot be recommended at this time). Products include:
Epzicom Tablets 1422
Trizivir Tablets 1622
Ziagen 1673

Acarbose (New onset diabetes mellitus, exacerbation of pre-existing diabetes mellitus, and hyperglycemia have been reported during post-

marketing surveillance in HIV-1 infected patients receiving protease inhibitor therapy. Some patients require either dose initiation or dose adjustments of oral hypoglycemic agents for treatment of these events). Products include:
Precose Tablets 792

Alfentanil Hydrochloride (Tipranavir co-administered with ritonavir at the recommended dose is a net inhibitor of CYP3A and may increase plasma concentrations of agents that are primarily metabolized by CYP3A. Thus, co-administration of tipranavir/ritonavir with drugs highly dependent on CYP3A for clearance and for which elevated plasma concentrations are associated with serious and/or life-threatening events is contraindicated. Co-administration with other CYP3A substrates may require a dose adjustment or additional monitoring).
No products indexed under this heading.

Allium sativum (Co-administration of tipranavir with ritonavir with drugs that are potent CYP3A inducers is contraindicated).
No products indexed under this heading.

Alprazolam (Tipranavir co-administered with ritonavir at the recommended dose is a net inhibitor of CYP3A and may increase plasma concentrations of agents that are primarily metabolized by CYP3A. Thus, co-administration of tipranavir/ritonavir with drugs highly dependent on CYP3A for clearance and for which elevated plasma concentrations are associated with serious and/or life-threatening events is contraindicated. Co-administration with other CYP3A substrates may require a dose adjustment or additional monitoring).
No products indexed under this heading.

Aminophylline (Tipranavir co-administered with ritonavir at the recommended dose is a net inhibitor of CYP3A and may increase plasma concentrations of agents that are primarily metabolized by CYP3A. Thus, co-administration of tipranavir/ritonavir with drugs highly dependent on CYP3A for clearance and for which elevated plasma concentrations are associated with serious and/or life-threatening events is contraindicated. Co-administration with other CYP3A substrates may require a dose adjustment or additional monitoring).
No products indexed under this heading.

Amiodarone Hydrochloride (Co-administration of tipranavir/ritonavir and amiodarone may lead to potential for serious and/or life-threatening reactions such as cardiac arrhythmias secondary to increases in plasma concentrations of antiarrhythmics. Concomitant use of tipranavir/ritonavir and amiodarone is contraindicated).
No products indexed under this heading.

Amitriptyline Hydrochloride (Tipranavir co-administered with ritonavir at the recommended dose is a net inhibitor of CYP3A and may increase plasma concentrations of agents that are primarily metabolized by CYP3A. Thus, co-administration of tipranavir/ritonavir with drugs highly dependent on CYP3A for clearance and for which elevated plasma concentrations are associated with serious and/or life-threatening events is contraindicated. Co-administration with other CYP3A substrates may require a dose adjustment or additional monitoring).
No products indexed under this heading.

Amlodipine Besylate (Tipranavir co-administered with ritonavir at the recommended dose is a net inhibitor of CYP3A and may increase plasma concentrations of agents that are primarily metabolized by CYP3A. Thus, co-administration of tipranavir/ritonavir with drugs highly dependent on CYP3A for clearance and for which elevated plasma concentrations are associated with serious and/or life-threatening events is contraindicated. Co-administration with other CYP3A substrates may require a dose adjustment or additional monitoring). Products include:
Azor Tablets 1005
Exforge Tablets 2238

Anisindione (Tipranavir/ritonavir should be used with caution in patients who are receiving medications known to increase the risk of bleeding, such as anticoagulants).
No products indexed under this heading.

Aprepitant (Tipranavir co-administered with ritonavir at the recommended dose is a net inhibitor of CYP3A and may increase plasma concentrations of agents that are primarily metabolized by CYP3A. Thus, co-administration of tipranavir/ritonavir with drugs highly dependent on CYP3A for clearance and for which elevated plasma concentrations are associated with serious and/or life-threatening events is contraindicated. Co-administration with other CYP3A substrates may require a dose adjustment or additional monitoring). Products include:
Emend Capsules 1992

Aspirin (Tipranavir/ritonavir should be used with caution in patients who are receiving medications known to increase the risk of bleeding, such as antiplatelet agents). Products include:
Aggrenox Capsules 819
Bayer Aspirin 750
Percodan Tablets 1130
St. Joseph 81 mg Aspirin Chewable and Enteric Coated Tablets 1903

Aspirin, Enteric Coated (Tipranavir/ritonavir should be used with caution in patients who are receiving medications known to increase the risk of bleeding, such as antiplatelet agents).
No products indexed under this heading.

Aspirin Buffered (Tipranavir/ritonavir should be used with caution in patients who are receiving medications known to increase the risk of bleeding, such as antiplatelet agents).
No products indexed under this heading.

Astemizole (Tipranavir co-administered with ritonavir at the recommended dose is a net inhibitor of CYP3A and may increase plasma concentrations of agents that are primarily metabolized by CYP3A. Thus, co-administration of tipranavir/ritonavir with drugs highly dependent on CYP3A for clearance and for which elevated plasma concentrations are associated with serious and/or life-threatening events is contraindicated. Co-administration with other CYP3A substrates may require a dose adjustment or additional monitoring).
No products indexed under this heading.

Atazanavir (Concomitant use of atazanavir with tipranavir and 100 mg of ritonavir led to a decrease in concentrations of atazanavir and an increase in concentrations of tipranavir. Combining a protease inhibitor with tipranavir/ritonavir is not recommended).
No products indexed under this heading.

Atazanavir Sulfate (Concomitant use of atazanavir with tipranavir and 100 mg of ritonavir led to a decrease in concentrations of atazanavir and an increase in concentrations of tipranavir. Combining a protease inhibitor with tipranavir/ritonavir is not recommended). Products include:
Reyataz Capsules 3299

Atenolol (Co-administration with drugs that inhibit P-gp may increase tipranavir plasma concentrations).
No products indexed under this heading.

Atorvastatin Calcium (Concomitant use may increase concentrations of atorvastatin and/or tipranavir and decrease concentrations of hydroxy-atorvastatin metabolites. Start with the lowest possible dose of atorvastatin with careful monitoring, or consider other HMG-CoA reductase inhibitors such as pravastatin or fluvastatin when in concomitant use of tipranavir, co-administered with 200 mg of ritonavir). Products include:
Lipitor Tablets 2501

Azithromycin Dihydrate (Co-administration with drugs that inhibit P-gp may increase tipranavir plasma concentrations).
No products indexed under this heading.

Azlocillin Sodium (Tipranavir/ritonavir should be used with caution in patients who are receiving medications known to increase the risk of bleeding, such as antiplatelet agents).
No products indexed under this heading.

Bepridil Hydrochloride (Co-administration of tipranavir/ritonavir and bepridil may lead to potential for serious and/or life-threatening reactions such as cardiac arrhythmias secondary to increases in plasma concentrations of antiarrhythmics. Concomitant use of tipranavir/ritonavir and bepridil is contraindicated).
No products indexed under this heading.

Buspirone Hydrochloride (Tipranavir co-administered with ritonavir at the recommended dose is a net inhibitor of CYP3A and may increase plasma concentrations of agents that are primarily metabolized by CYP3A. Thus, co-administration of tipranavir/ritonavir with drugs highly dependent on CYP3A for clearance and for which elevated plasma concentrations are associated with serious and/or life-threatening events is contraindicated. Co-administration with other CYP3A substrates may require a dose adjustment or additional monitoring).
No products indexed under this heading.

Busulfan (Tipranavir co-administered with ritonavir at the recommended dose is a net inhibitor of CYP3A and may increase plasma concentrations of agents that are primarily metabolized by CYP3A. Thus, co-administration of tipranavir/ritonavir with drugs highly dependent on CYP3A for clearance and for which elevated plasma concentrations are associated with serious and/or life-threatening events is contraindicated. Co-administration with other CYP3A substrates may require a dose adjustment or additional monitoring). Products include:
Busulfex Injection 2477
Myleran Tablets 1530

Carbamazepine (Concomitant use may lead to a decrease in tipranavir concentrations. Caution should be used when prescribing carbamazepine, phenobarbital, and or phenytoin. Tipranavir may be less effective due to decreased tipranavir plasma concentrations in patients taking these agents concomitantly). Products include:
Carbatrol Capsules 3019
Equetro Extended-Release Capsules 3174

Carbenicillin Indanyl Sodium (Tipranavir/ritonavir should be used with caution in patients who are receiving medications known to increase the risk of bleeding, such as antiplatelet agents).
No products indexed under this heading.

Cerivastatin Sodium (Tipranavir co-administered with ritonavir at the recommended dose is a net inhibitor of CYP3A and may increase plasma concentrations of agents that are primarily metabolized by CYP3A. Thus, co-administration of tipranavir/ritonavir with drugs highly dependent on CYP3A for clearance and for which elevated plasma concentrations are associated with serious and/or life-threatening events is contraindicated. Co-administration with other CYP3A substrates may require a dose adjustment or additional monitoring).
No products indexed under this heading.

Chlorotrianisene (Concomitant use may decrease ethinyl estradiol concentrations by 50%. Alternative methods of non-hormonal contraception should be used when estrogen-based oral contraceptives are co-administered with tipranavir and 200 mg or ritonavir. Patients using estrogens as hormone replacement therapy should be clinically monitored for signs of estrogen deficiency. Women using estrogens may have an increased risk of non-serious rash).
No products indexed under this heading.

Chlorpheniramine (Tipranavir co-administered with ritonavir at the recommended dose is a net inhibitor of CYP3A and may increase plasma concentrations of agents that are primarily metabolized by CYP3A.

Thus, co-administration of tipranavir/ritonavir with drugs highly dependent on CYP3A for clearance and for which elevated plasma concentrations are associated with serious and/or life-threatening events is contraindicated. Co-administration with other CYP3A substrates may require a dose adjustment or additional monitoring).

No products indexed under this heading.

Chlorpheniramine Maleate (Tipranavir co-administered with ritonavir at the recommended dose is a net inhibitor of CYP3A and may increase plasma concentrations of agents that are primarily metabolized by CYP3A. Thus, co-administration of tipranavir/ritonavir with drugs highly dependent on CYP3A for clearance and for which elevated plasma concentrations are associated with serious and/or life-threatening events is contraindicated. Co-administration with other CYP3A substrates may require a dose adjustment or additional monitoring). Products include:

Actifed Cold & Allergy Tablets 1895
Sudafed PE Sinus & Allergy Tablets 1908
Tylenol Allergy Multi-Symptom Caplets with Cool Burst and Rapid Release Gelcaps 1916
Children's Tylenol Plus Cold Suspension Liquid 1912
Children's Tylenol Plus Cough & Runny Nose Suspension Liquid 1912
Children's Tylenol Plus Flu Suspension Liquid 1914
Children's Tylenol Plus Multi-Symptom Cold Suspension Liquid 1912
Tylenol Cold Head Congestion Nighttime Caplets with Cool Burst 1910
Tylenol Cold Multi-Symptom Nighttime Caplets with Cool Burst 1913
Tylenol Sinus Congestion & Pain Nighttime Caplets with Cool Burst 1917

Chlorpheniramine Polistirex (Tipranavir co-administered with ritonavir at the recommended dose is a net inhibitor of CYP3A and may increase plasma concentrations of agents that are primarily metabolized by CYP3A. Thus, co-administration of tipranavir/ritonavir with drugs highly dependent on CYP3A for clearance and for which elevated plasma concentrations are associated with serious and/or life-threatening events is contraindicated. Co-administration with other CYP3A substrates may require a dose adjustment or additional monitoring). Products include:

Tussionex Pennkinetic Extended-Release Suspension 3154

Chlorpheniramine Tannate (Tipranavir co-administered with ritonavir at the recommended dose is a net inhibitor of CYP3A and may increase plasma concentrations of agents that are primarily metabolized by CYP3A. Thus, co-administration of tipranavir/ritonavir with drugs highly dependent on CYP3A for clearance and for which elevated plasma concentrations are associated with serious and/or life-threatening events is contraindicated. Co-administration with other CYP3A substrates may require a dose adjustment or additional monitoring).

No products indexed under this heading.

Chlorpropamide (New onset diabetes mellitus, exacerbation of pre-existing diabetes mellitus, and hyperglycemia have been reported during post-marketing surveillance in HIV-1 infected patients receiving protease inhibitor therapy. Some patients require either dose initiation or dose adjustments of oral hypoglycemic agents for treatment of these events).

No products indexed under this heading.

Choline Magnesium Trisalicylate (Tipranavir/ritonavir should be used with caution in patients who are receiving medications known to increase the risk of bleeding, such as antiplatelet agents).

No products indexed under this heading.

Cisapride (Co-administration of tipranavir/ritonavir and cisapride may lead to the potential for cardiac arrhythmias. Concomitant use of tipranavir/ritonavir and cisapride is contraindicated).

No products indexed under this heading.

Clarithromycin (Concomitant use may lead to an increase in concentrations of tipranavir and/or clarithromycin and a decrease in the 14-hydroxy-clarithromycin metabolite. No dose adjustment of tipranavir or clarithromycin for patients with normal renal function is necessary. For patients with a CrCl of 30 to 60 mL/min., the dose of clarithromycin should be reduced by 50%. For patients with a CrCl of less than 30 mL/min., the dose of clarithromycin should be decreased by 75%). Products include:

Biaxin/Biaxin XL 411

Clopidogrel Bisulfate (Tipranavir/ritonavir should be used with caution in patients who are receiving medications known to increase the risk of bleeding, such as antiplatelet agents). Products include:

Plavix Tablets 926
Plavix Tablets 2767

Cyclosporine (Concomitant use may increase or decrease concentrations of cyclosporine. Increased frequency of monitoring plasma levels of immunosuppressant drugs is recommended). Products include:

Gengraf Capsules 435
Neoral Oral Solution 2280
Neoral Soft Gelatin Capsules 2280
Restasis Ophthalmic Emulsion 557
Sandimmune 2296

Desipramine Hydrochloride (Concomitant use may lead to an increase in concentrations of desipramine. Dosage reduction and concentration monitoring of desipramine is recommended).

No products indexed under this heading.

Desogestrel (Alternative methods of non-hormonal contraception should be used when estrogen-based oral contraceptives are co-administered with tipranavir and 200 mg of ritonavir). Products include:

Mircette Tablets 1034

Dexamethasone (Tipranavir co-administered with ritonavir at the recommended dose is a net inhibitor of CYP3A and may increase plasma concentrations of agents that are primarily metabolized by CYP3A. Thus, co-administration of tipranavir/ritonavir with drugs highly dependent on CYP3A for clearance and for which elevated plasma concentrations are associated with serious and/or life-threatening events is contraindicated. Co-administration with other CYP3A substrates may require a dose adjustment or additional monitoring). Products include:

Ciprodex Otic Suspension 541

Dexamethasone Acetate (Tipranavir co-administered with ritonavir at the recommended dose is a net inhibitor of CYP3A and may increase plasma concentrations of agents that are primarily metabolized by CYP3A. Thus, co-administration of tipranavir/ritonavir with drugs highly dependent on CYP3A for clearance and for which elevated plasma concentrations are associated with serious and/or life-threatening events is contraindicated. Co-administration with other CYP3A substrates may require a dose adjustment or additional monitoring).

No products indexed under this heading.

Dexamethasone Phosphate (Tipranavir co-administered with ritonavir at the recommended dose is a net inhibitor of CYP3A and may increase plasma concentrations of agents that are primarily metabolized by CYP3A. Thus, co-administration of tipranavir/ritonavir with drugs highly dependent on CYP3A for clearance and for which elevated plasma concentrations are associated with serious and/or life-threatening events is contraindicated. Co-administration with other CYP3A substrates may require a dose adjustment or additional monitoring).

No products indexed under this heading.

Dexamethasone Sodium (Tipranavir co-administered with ritonavir at the recommended dose is a net inhibitor of CYP3A and may increase plasma concentrations of agents that are primarily metabolized by CYP3A. Thus, co-administration of tipranavir/ritonavir with drugs highly dependent on CYP3A for clearance and for which elevated plasma concentrations are associated with serious and/or life-threatening events is contraindicated. Co-administration with other CYP3A substrates may require a dose adjustment or additional monitoring).

No products indexed under this heading.

Dexamethasone Sodium Phosphate (Tipranavir co-administered with ritonavir at the recommended dose is a net inhibitor of CYP3A and may increase plasma concentrations of agents that are primarily metabolized by CYP3A. Thus, co-administration of tipranavir/ritonavir with drugs highly dependent on CYP3A for clearance and for which elevated plasma concentrations are associated with serious and/or life-threatening events is contraindicated. Co-administration with other CYP3A substrates may require a dose adjustment or additional monitoring).

No products indexed under this heading.

Diazepam (Tipranavir co-administered with ritonavir at the recommended dose is a net inhibitor of CYP3A and may increase plasma concentrations of agents that are primarily metabolized by CYP3A. Thus, co-administration of tipranavir/ritonavir with drugs highly dependent on CYP3A for clearance and for which elevated plasma concentrations are associated with serious and/or life-threatening events is contraindicated. Co-administration with other CYP3A substrates may require a dose adjustment or additional monitoring). Products include:

Valium Tablets 2658

Diclofenac Potassium (Tipranavir/ritonavir should be used with caution in patients who are receiving medications known to increase the risk of bleeding, such as antiplatelet agents).

No products indexed under this heading.

Diclofenac Sodium (Tipranavir/ritonavir should be used with caution in patients who are receiving medications known to increase the risk of bleeding, such as antiplatelet agents). Products include:

Diclofenac Sodium Ophthalmic Solution .... ⊙ 240
Voltaren Ophthalmic Solution 2336
Voltaren Tablets 2334
Voltaren-XR Tablets 2337

Dicumarol (Tipranavir/ritonavir should be used with caution in patients who are receiving medications known to increase the risk of bleeding, such as anticoagulants).

No products indexed under this heading.

Didanosine (Concomitant use with didanosine decreased concentration levels of didanosine. The clinical relevance of reduction in didanosine levels has not been established. For optimal absorption, didanosine should be separated from tipranavir/ritonavir dosing by at least 2 hours).

No products indexed under this heading.

Dienestrol (Concomitant use may decrease ethinyl estradiol concentrations by 50%. Alternative methods of non-hormonal contraception should be used when estrogen-based oral contraceptives are co-administered with tipranavir and 200 mg or ritonavir. Patients using estrogens as hormone replacement therapy should be clinically monitored for signs of estrogen deficiency. Women using estrogens may have an increased risk of non-serious rash).

No products indexed under this heading.

Diethylstilbestrol (Concomitant use may decrease ethinyl estradiol concentrations by 50%. Alternative methods of non-hormonal contraception should be used when estrogen-based oral contraceptives are co-administered with tipranavir and 200 mg or ritonavir. Patients using estrogens as hormone replacement therapy should be clinically monitored for signs of estrogen deficiency. Women using estrogens may have an increased risk of non-serious rash).

No products indexed under this heading.

monitoring).
No products indexed under this heading.

Estrogens, Conjugated (Concomitant use may decrease ethinyl estradiol concentrations by 50%. Alternative methods of non-hormonal contraception should be used when estrogen-based oral contraceptives are co-administered with tipranavir and 200 mg or ritonavir. Patients using estrogens as hormone replacement therapy should be clinically monitored for signs of estrogen deficiency. Women using estrogens may have an increased risk of non-serious rash). Products include:
Premarin Intravenous **3217**
Premarin Tablets **3221**
Premarin Vaginal Cream **3228**
Premphase Tablets **3232**
Prempro Tablets **3232**

Estrogens, Conjugated, Synthetic A (Tipranavir co-administered with ritonavir at the recommended dose is a net inhibitor of CYP3A and may increase plasma concentrations of agents that are primarily metabolized by CYP3A. Thus, co-administration of tipranavir/ritonavir with drugs highly dependent on CYP3A for clearance and for which elevated plasma concentrations are associated with serious and/or life-threatening events is contraindicated. Co-administration with other CYP3A substrates may require a dose adjustment or additional monitoring).
No products indexed under this heading.

Estrogens, Esterified (Concomitant use may decrease ethinyl estradiol concentrations by 50%. Alternative methods of non-hormonal contraception should be used when estrogen-based oral contraceptives are co-administered with tipranavir and 200 mg or ritonavir. Patients using estrogens as hormone replacement therapy should be clinically monitored for signs of estrogen deficiency. Women using estrogens may have an increased risk of non-serious rash). Products include:
Estratest Tablets **3043**
Estratest H.S. Tablets **3043**

Estropipate (Concomitant use may decrease ethinyl estradiol concentrations by 50%. Alternative methods of non-hormonal contraception should be used when estrogen-based oral contraceptives are co-administered with tipranavir and 200 mg or ritonavir. Patients using estrogens as hormone replacement therapy should be clinically monitored for signs of estrogen deficiency. Women using estrogens may have an increased risk of non-serious rash).
No products indexed under this heading.

Ethinyl Estradiol (Concomitant use may decrease ethinyl estradiol concentrations by 50%. Alternative methods of non-hormonal contraception should be used when estrogen-based oral contraceptives are co-administered with tipranavir and 200 mg or ritonavir. Patients using estrogens as hormone replacement therapy should be clinically monitored for signs of estrogen deficiency. Women using estrogens may have an increased risk of non-serious rash). Products include:
Lybrel Tablets **3204**
Mircette Tablets **1034**
NuvaRing **2897**
Ortho-Cyclen/Ortho Tri-Cyclen **2449**
Ortho Evra Transdermal System **2437**
Ortho Tri-Cyclen Lo Tablets **2458**
Seasonique Tablets **1046**
Yaz Tablets **805**

Ethosuximide (Tipranavir co-administered with ritonavir at the recommended dose is a net inhibitor of CYP3A and may increase plasma concentrations of agents that are primarily metabolized by CYP3A. Thus, co-administration of tipranavir/ritonavir with drugs highly dependent on CYP3A for clearance and for which elevated plasma concentrations are associated with serious and/or life-threatening events is contraindicated. Co-administration with other CYP3A substrates may require a dose adjustment or additional monitoring).
No products indexed under this heading.

Ethynodiol Diacetate (Alternative methods of non-hormonal contraception should be used when estrogen-based oral contraceptives are co-administered with tipranavir and 200 mg of ritonavir).
No products indexed under this heading.

Etoposide (Tipranavir co-administered with ritonavir at the recommended dose is a net inhibitor of CYP3A and may increase plasma concentrations of agents that are primarily metabolized by CYP3A. Thus, co-administration of tipranavir/ritonavir with drugs highly dependent on CYP3A for clearance and for which elevated plasma concentrations are associated with serious and/or life-threatening events is contraindicated. Co-administration with other CYP3A substrates may require a dose adjustment or additional monitoring).
No products indexed under this heading.

Etoposide Phosphate (Tipranavir co-administered with ritonavir at the recommended dose is a net inhibitor of CYP3A and may increase plasma concentrations of agents that are primarily metabolized by CYP3A. Thus, co-administration of tipranavir/ritonavir with drugs highly dependent on CYP3A for clearance and for which elevated plasma concentrations are associated with serious and/or life-threatening events is contraindicated. Co-administration with other CYP3A substrates may require a dose adjustment or additional monitoring).
No products indexed under this heading.

Felodipine (Concomitant use may increase felodipine concentrations. Caution is warranted and clinical monitoring of patients is recommended).
No products indexed under this heading.

Fenoprofen Calcium (Tipranavir/ritonavir should be used with caution in patients who are receiving medications known to increase the risk of bleeding, such as antiplatelet agents). Products include:
Nalfon Capsules **2508**

Fentanyl (Tipranavir co-administered with ritonavir at the recommended dose is a net inhibitor of CYP3A and may increase plasma concentrations of agents that are primarily metabolized by CYP3A. Thus, co-administration of tipranavir/ritonavir with drugs highly dependent on CYP3A for clearance and for which elevated plasma concentrations are associated with serious and/or life-threatening events is contraindicated. Co-administration with other CYP3A substrates may require a dose adjustment or additional monitoring). Products include:
Duragesic Transdermal System **2405**
Ionsys Transdermal System **2410**

Fentanyl Citrate (Tipranavir co-administered with ritonavir at the recommended dose is a net inhibitor of CYP3A and may increase plasma concentrations of agents that are primarily metabolized by CYP3A. Thus, co-administration of tipranavir/ritonavir with drugs highly dependent on CYP3A for clearance and for which elevated plasma concentrations are associated with serious and/or life-threatening events is contraindicated. Co-administration with other CYP3A substrates may require a dose adjustment or additional monitoring). Products include:
Actiq **959**
Fentora Tablets **968**

Flecainide Acetate (Co-administration of tipranavir/ritonavir and flecainide may lead to potential for serious and/or life-threatening reactions such as cardiac arrhythmias secondary to increases in plasma concentrations of antiarrhythmics. Concomitant use of tipranavir/ritonavir and flecainide is contraindicated).
No products indexed under this heading.

Fluconazole (Concomitant use with fluconazole may increase tipranavir concentrations but dose adjustments are not needed. Fluconazole doses greater than 200 mg/day are not recommended).
No products indexed under this heading.

Fluoxetine (Concomitant use may increase concentrations of fluoxetine. Fluoxetine doses may need to be adjusted upon initiation of tipranavir/ritonavir therapy).
No products indexed under this heading.

Fluoxetine Hydrochloride (Concomitant use may increase concentrations of fluoxetine. Fluoxetine doses may need to be adjusted upon initiation of tipranavir/ritonavir therapy). Products include:
Prozac Weekly Capsules **1852**
Prozac Pulvules and Liquid **1852**
Symbyax Capsules **1871**

Flurbiprofen (Tipranavir/ritonavir should be used with caution in patients who are receiving medications known to increase the risk of bleeding, such as antiplatelet agents).
No products indexed under this heading.

Fluticasone Propionate (Concomitant use of fluticasone propionate and tipranavir/ritonavir may increase plasma concentrations of fluticasone propionate, resulting in significantly reduced serum cortisol concentrations. Co-administration of fluticasone propionate and tipranavir/ritonavir is not recommended unless the potential benefit to the patient outweighs the risk of systemic corticosteroid side effects). Products include:
Advair Diskus 100/50 .... **1276**
Advair Diskus 250/50 .... **1276**
Advair Diskus 500/50 .... **1276**
Advair HFA 45/21 Inhalation Aerosol **1288**
Advair HFA 115/21 Inhalation Aerosol **1288**
Advair HFA 230/21 Inhalation Aerosol **1288**
Flonase Nasal Spray **1431**
Flovent Diskus 50 mcg **1435**

Fluticasone Propionate HFA (Concomitant use of fluticasone propionate and tipranavir/ritonavir may increase plasma concentrations of fluticasone propionate, resulting in significantly reduced serum cortisol concentrations. Co-administration of fluticasone propionate and tipranavir/ritonavir is not recommended unless the potential benefit to the patient outweighs the risk of systemic corticosteroid side effects). Products include:
Flovent HFA **1440**

Fosamprenavir Calcium (Concomitant use of fosamprenavir with tipranavir and 200 mg of ritonavir led to a decrease in concentrations of amprenavir. Combining a protease inhibitor with tipranavir/ritonavir is not recommended). Products include:
Lexiva Oral Suspension **1510**
Lexiva Tablets **1510**

Fosphenytoin Sodium (Concomitant use may lead to a decrease in tipranavir concentrations. Caution should be used when prescribing carbamazepine, phenobarbital, and or phenytoin. Tipranavir may be less effective due to decreased tipranavir plasma concentrations in patients taking these agents concomitantly).
No products indexed under this heading.

Glimepiride (Concomitant use led to no changes in concentrations of glimepiride. However careful glucose monitoring is warranted). Products include:
Avandaryl Tablets **1344**
Duetact Tablets **3085**

Glipizide (Concomitant use led to no changes in concentrations of glipizide. However careful glucose monitoring is warranted).
No products indexed under this heading.

Glyburide (Concomitant use led to no changes in concentrations of glyburide. However careful glucose monitoring is warranted).
No products indexed under this heading.

Haloperidol (Tipranavir co-administered with ritonavir at the recommended dose is a net inhibitor of CYP3A and may increase plasma concentrations of agents that are primarily metabolized by CYP3A. Thus, co-administration of tipranavir/ritonavir with drugs highly dependent on CYP3A for clearance and for which elevated plasma concentrations are associated with serious and/or life-threatening events is contraindicated. Co-administration with other CYP3A substrates may require a dose adjustment or additional monitoring).
No products indexed under this heading.

Haloperidol Decanoate (Tipranavir co-administered with ritonavir at the recommended dose is a net inhibitor of CYP3A and may increase plasma concentrations of

agents that are primarily metabolized by CYP3A. Thus, co-administration of tipranavir/ritonavir with drugs highly dependent on CYP3A for clearance and for which elevated plasma concentrations are associated with serious and/or life-threatening events is contraindicated. Co-administration with other CYP3A substrates may require a dose adjustment or additional monitoring).
No products indexed under this heading.

Hypericum (Co-administration of tipranavir/ritonavir and St. John's Wort may lead to loss of virologic response and possible resistance to tipranavir or the class of protease inhibitors. Concomitant use of tipranavir/ritonavir and St. John's Wort is contraindicated). Products include:
Satieté Tablets .... ▣640

Ibuprofen (Tipranavir/ritonavir should be used with caution in patients who are receiving medications known to increase the risk of bleeding, such as antiplatelet agents). Products include:
Motrin IB Tablets and Caplets 1900
Children's Motrin Oral Suspension ... 1901
Children's Motrin Non-Staining Dye-Free Oral Suspension............ 1901
Children's Motrin Cold Oral Suspension 1899
Infants' Motrin Concentrated Drops.. 1901
Infants' Motrin Non-Staining Dye-Free Concentrated Drops....... 1901
Junior Strength Motrin Caplets and Chewable Tablets.................. 1901
Vicoprofen Tablets 533

Imipramine Hydrochloride (Tipranavir co-administered with ritonavir at the recommended dose is a net inhibitor of CYP3A and may increase plasma concentrations of agents that are primarily metabolized by CYP3A. Thus, co-administration of tipranavir/ritonavir with drugs highly dependent on CYP3A for clearance and for which elevated plasma concentrations are associated with serious and/or life-threatening events is contraindicated. Co-administration with other CYP3A substrates may require a dose adjustment or additional monitoring).
No products indexed under this heading.

Imipramine Pamoate (Tipranavir co-administered with ritonavir at the recommended dose is a net inhibitor of CYP3A and may increase plasma concentrations of agents that are primarily metabolized by CYP3A. Thus, co-administration of tipranavir/ritonavir with drugs highly dependent on CYP3A for clearance and for which elevated plasma concentrations are associated with serious and/or life-threatening events is contraindicated. Co-administration with other CYP3A substrates may require a dose adjustment or additional monitoring).
No products indexed under this heading.

Indinavir Sulfate (Tipranavir co-administered with ritonavir at the recommended dose is a net inhibitor of CYP3A and may increase plasma concentrations of agents that are primarily metabolized by CYP3A. Thus, co-administration of tipranavir/ritonavir with drugs highly dependent on CYP3A for clearance and for which elevated plasma concentrations are associated with serious and/or life-threatening events is contraindicated. Co-administration with other CYP3A substrates may require a dose adjustment or additional monitoring). Products include:
Crixivan Capsules 1979

Indomethacin (Tipranavir/ritonavir should be used with caution in patients who are receiving medications known to increase the risk of bleeding, such as antiplatelet agents). Products include:
Indocin 2024

Indomethacin Sodium Trihydrate (Tipranavir/ritonavir should be used with caution in patients who are receiving medications known to increase the risk of bleeding, such as antiplatelet agents). Products include:
Indocin I.V. 2489

Insulin (New onset diabetes mellitus, exacerbation of pre-existing diabetes mellitus, and hyperglycemia have been reported during post-marketing surveillance in HIV-1 infected patients receiving protease inhibitor therapy. Some patients require either dose initiation or dose adjustments of insulin for treatment of these events).
No products indexed under this heading.

Insulin, Human, Zinc Suspension (New onset diabetes mellitus, exacerbation of pre-existing diabetes mellitus, and hyperglycemia have been reported during post-marketing surveillance in HIV-1 infected patients receiving protease inhibitor therapy. Some patients require either dose initiation or dose adjustments of insulin for treatment of these events).
No products indexed under this heading.

Insulin, Human (rDNA origin) (New onset diabetes mellitus, exacerbation of pre-existing diabetes mellitus, and hyperglycemia have been reported during post-marketing surveillance in HIV-1 infected patients receiving protease inhibitor therapy. Some patients require either dose initiation or dose adjustments of insulin for treatment of these events). Products include:
Exubera Inhalation Powder 2515

Insulin, Human NPH (New onset diabetes mellitus, exacerbation of pre-existing diabetes mellitus, and hyperglycemia have been reported during post-marketing surveillance in HIV-1 infected patients receiving protease inhibitor therapy. Some patients require either dose initiation or dose adjustments of insulin for treatment of these events). Products include:
Humulin N Vial 1846

Insulin, Human Regular (New onset diabetes mellitus, exacerbation of pre-existing diabetes mellitus, and hyperglycemia have been reported during post-marketing surveillance in HIV-1 infected patients receiving protease inhibitor therapy. Some patients require either dose initiation or dose adjustments of insulin for treatment of these events). Products include:
Humulin R.. 1849
Humulin R (U-500) 1850

Insulin, Human Regular and Human NPH Mixture (New onset diabetes mellitus, exacerbation of pre-existing diabetes mellitus, and hyperglycemia have been reported during post-marketing surveillance in HIV-1 infected patients receiving protease inhibitor therapy. Some patients require either dose initiation or dose adjustments of insulin for treatment of these events). Products include:
Humulin 50/50, 100 Units 1843
Humulin 70/30 Vial 1844

Insulin, NPH (New onset diabetes mellitus, exacerbation of pre-existing diabetes mellitus, and hyperglycemia have been reported during post-marketing surveillance in HIV-1 infected patients receiving protease inhibitor therapy. Some patients require either dose initiation or dose adjustments of insulin for treatment of these events).
No products indexed under this heading.

Insulin, Regular (New onset diabetes mellitus, exacerbation of pre-existing diabetes mellitus, and hyperglycemia have been reported during post-marketing surveillance in HIV-1 infected patients receiving protease inhibitor therapy. Some patients require either dose initiation or dose adjustments of insulin for treatment of these events).
No products indexed under this heading.

Insulin, Regular and NPH mixture (New onset diabetes mellitus, exacerbation of pre-existing diabetes mellitus, and hyperglycemia have been reported during post-marketing surveillance in HIV-1 infected patients receiving protease inhibitor therapy. Some patients require either dose initiation or dose adjustments of insulin for treatment of these events).
No products indexed under this heading.

Insulin, Zinc Crystals (New onset diabetes mellitus, exacerbation of pre-existing diabetes mellitus, and hyperglycemia have been reported during post-marketing surveillance in HIV-1 infected patients receiving protease inhibitor therapy. Some patients require either dose initiation or dose adjustments of insulin for treatment of these events).
No products indexed under this heading.

Insulin, Zinc Suspension (New onset diabetes mellitus, exacerbation of pre-existing diabetes mellitus, and hyperglycemia have been reported during post-marketing surveillance in HIV-1 infected patients receiving protease inhibitor therapy. Some patients require either dose initiation or dose adjustments of insulin for treatment of these events).
No products indexed under this heading.

Insulin Aspart (New onset diabetes mellitus, exacerbation of pre-existing diabetes mellitus, and hyperglycemia have been reported during post-marketing surveillance in HIV-1 infected patients receiving protease inhibitor therapy. Some patients require either dose initiation or dose adjustments of insulin for treatment of these events).
No products indexed under this heading.

Insulin Aspart, Human (New onset diabetes mellitus, exacerbation of pre-existing diabetes mellitus, and hyperglycemia have been reported during post-marketing surveillance in HIV-1 infected patients receiving protease inhibitor therapy. Some patients require either dose initiation or dose adjustments of insulin for treatment of these events). Products include:
NovoLog Mix 70/30 2364

Insulin Aspart, Human Regular (New onset diabetes mellitus, exacerbation of pre-existing diabetes mellitus, and hyperglycemia have been reported during post-marketing surveillance in HIV-1 infected patients receiving protease inhibitor therapy. Some patients require either dose initiation or dose adjustments of insulin for treatment of these events). Products include:
NovoLog Injection 2359

Insulin Aspart Protamine, Human (New onset diabetes mellitus, exacerbation of pre-existing diabetes mellitus, and hyperglycemia have been reported during post-marketing surveillance in HIV-1 infected patients receiving protease inhibitor therapy. Some patients require either dose initiation or dose adjustments of insulin for treatment of these events). Products include:
NovoLog Mix 70/30 2364

Insulin Detemir (rDNA Origin) (New onset diabetes mellitus, exacerbation of pre-existing diabetes mellitus, and hyperglycemia have been reported during post-marketing surveillance in HIV-1 infected patients receiving protease inhibitor therapy. Some patients require either dose initiation or dose adjustments of insulin for treatment of these events). Products include:
Levemir Injection 2352

Insulin glargine (New onset diabetes mellitus, exacerbation of pre-existing diabetes mellitus, and hyperglycemia have been reported during post-marketing surveillance in HIV-1 infected patients receiving protease inhibitor therapy. Some patients require either dose initiation or dose adjustments of insulin for treatment of these events). Products include:
Lantus Injection 2749

Insulin Glulisine (New onset diabetes mellitus, exacerbation of pre-existing diabetes mellitus, and hyperglycemia have been reported during post-marketing surveillance in HIV-1 infected patients receiving protease inhibitor therapy. Some patients require either dose initiation or dose adjustments of insulin for treatment of these events). Products include:
Apidra Injection 2706

Insulin Lispro, Human (New onset diabetes mellitus, exacerbation of pre-existing diabetes mellitus, and hyperglycemia have been reported during post-marketing surveillance in HIV-1 infected patients receiving protease inhibitor therapy. Some patients require either dose initiation or dose adjustments of insulin for treatment of these events). Products include:
Humalog-Pen and KwikPen 1829
Humalog Mix 50/50-Pen and KwikPen.. 1833
Humalog Mix 75/25-Pen and KwikPen.. 1835

Insulin Lispro Protamine, Human (New onset diabetes mellitus, exacerbation of pre-existing diabetes mellitus, and hyperglycemia have been reported during post-marketing surveillance in HIV-1 infected patients receiving protease inhibitor therapy. Some patients require either dose initiation or dose adjustments of insulin for treatment of these events). Products include:

Humalog Mix 50/50-Pen and KwikPen 1833
Humalog Mix 75/25-Pen and KwikPen 1835

Isradipine (Tipranavir co-administered with ritonavir at the recommended dose is a net inhibitor of CYP3A and may increase plasma concentrations of agents that are primarily metabolized by CYP3A. Thus, co-administration of tipranavir/ritonavir with drugs highly dependent on CYP3A for clearance and for which elevated plasma concentrations are associated with serious and/or life-threatening events is contraindicated. Co-administration with other CYP3A substrates may require a dose adjustment or additional monitoring). Products include:

DynaCirc CR Controlled Release Tablets 1407

Itraconazole (Concomitant use with itraconazole may increase itraconazole concentrations. Based on theoretical considerations, itraconazole should be used with caution with tipranavir/ritonavir. High doses (greater than 200 mg/day) are not recommended).

No products indexed under this heading.

Ketoconazole (Concomitant use may increase ketoconazole concentrations. Based on theoretical considerations, ketoconazole should be used with caution with tipranavir/ritonavir. High doses (greater than 200 mg/day) are not recommended). Products include:

Extina Foam, 2% 3057
Nizoral A-D Shampoo 1901

Ketoprofen (Tipranavir/ritonavir should be used with caution in patients who are receiving medications known to increase the risk of bleeding, such as antiplatelet agents).

No products indexed under this heading.

Levonorgestrel (Alternative methods of non-hormonal contraception should be used when estrogen-based oral contraceptives are co-administered with tipranavir and 200 mg of ritonavir). Products include:

Climara Pro Transdermal System 768
Lybrel Tablets 3204
Mirena Intrauterine System 779
Plan B Tablets 1044
Seasonique Tablets 1046

Lidocaine (Tipranavir co-administered with ritonavir at the recommended dose is a net inhibitor of CYP3A and may increase plasma concentrations of agents that are primarily metabolized by CYP3A. Thus, co-administration of tipranavir/ritonavir with drugs highly dependent on CYP3A for clearance and for which elevated plasma concentrations are associated with serious and/or life-threatening events is contraindicated. Co-administration with other CYP3A substrates may require a dose adjustment or additional monitoring). Products include:

Lidoderm Patch 1114

Lidocaine Hydrochloride (Tipranavir co-administered with ritonavir at the recommended dose is a net inhibitor of CYP3A and may increase plasma concentrations of agents that are primarily metabolized by CYP3A. Thus, co-administration of tipranavir/ritonavir with drugs highly dependent on CYP3A for clearance and for which elevated plasma concentrations are associated with serious and/or life-threatening events is contraindicated. Co-administration with other CYP3A substrates may require a dose adjustment or additional monitoring).

No products indexed under this heading.

Lopinavir (Concomitant use of lopinavir with tipranavir and 200 mg of ritonavir led to a decrease in concentrations of lopinavir. Combining a protease inhibitor with tipranavir/ritonavir is not recommended). Products include:

Kaletra 452

Lovastatin (Co-administration of tipranavir/ritonavir and lovastatin may lead to the potential for myopathy including rhabdomyolysis. Concomitant use of tipranavir/ritonavir and lovastatin is contraindicated). Products include:

Advicor Tablets 402
Mevacor Tablets 2063

Magnesium Salicylate (Tipranavir/ritonavir should be used with caution in patients who are receiving medications known to increase the risk of bleeding, such as antiplatelet agents).

No products indexed under this heading.

Meclofenamate Sodium (Tipranavir/ritonavir should be used with caution in patients who are receiving medications known to increase the risk of bleeding, such as antiplatelet agents).

No products indexed under this heading.

Mefenamic Acid (Tipranavir/ritonavir should be used with caution in patients who are receiving medications known to increase the risk of bleeding, such as antiplatelet agents).

No products indexed under this heading.

Meperidine Hydrochloride (Concomitant use may decrease concentrations of meperidine and increase concentrations of normeperidine. Dosage increase and long-term use of meperidine are not recommended due to increased concentrations of the metabolite normeperidine which has both analgesic activity and CNS stimulant activity (eg, seizures)).

No products indexed under this heading.

Mestranol (Alternative methods of non-hormonal contraception should be used when estrogen-based oral contraceptives are co-administered with tipranavir and 200 mg of ritonavir).

No products indexed under this heading.

Metformin Hydrochloride (New onset diabetes mellitus, exacerbation of pre-existing diabetes mellitus, and hyperglycemia have been reported during post-marketing surveillance in HIV-1 infected patients receiving protease inhibitor therapy. Some patients require either dose initiation or dose adjustments of oral hypoglycemic agents for treatment of these events). Products include:

ActoPlus Met Tablets 3071
Avandamet Tablets 1336
Janumet Tablets 2041
PrandiMet Tablets 2967

Methadone Hydrochloride (Concomitant use may decrease concentrations of methadone. Dosage of methadone may need to be increased when co-administered with tipranavir and 200 mg of ritonavir).

No products indexed under this heading.

Methylergonovine Maleate (Co-administration of tipranavir/ritonavir with methylergonovine may lead to the potential for acute ergot toxicity characterized by peripheral vasospasm and ischemia of the extremities and other tissues. Concomitant use of tipranavir/ritonavir with methylergonovine is contraindicated).

No products indexed under this heading.

Metronidazole (Tipranavir capsules contain alcohol that can produce disulfiram-like reactions when co-administered with metronidazole or other drugs which produce this reaction). Products include:

Pylera Capsules 714

Metronidazole Benzoate (Tipranavir capsules contain alcohol that can produce disulfiram-like reactions when co-administered with metronidazole or other drugs which produce this reaction).

No products indexed under this heading.

Metronidazole Hydrochloride (Tipranavir capsules contain alcohol that can produce disulfiram-like reactions when co-administered with metronidazole or other drugs which produce this reaction).

No products indexed under this heading.

Metronidazole Sodium (Tipranavir capsules contain alcohol that can produce disulfiram-like reactions when co-administered with metronidazole or other drugs which produce this reaction).

No products indexed under this heading.

Mezlocillin Sodium (Tipranavir/ritonavir should be used with caution in patients who are receiving medications known to increase the risk of bleeding, such as antiplatelet agents).

No products indexed under this heading.

Mibefradil Dihydrochloride (Co-administration with drugs that inhibit P-gp may increase tipranavir plasma concentrations).

No products indexed under this heading.

Midazolam Hydrochloride (Co-administration of tipranavir/ritonavir and oral midazolam may lead to prolonged or increased sedation or respiratory depression. Concomitant use of tipranavir/ritonavir and oral midazolam is contraindicated. If tipranavir is co-administered with parenteral midazolam, close clinical monitoring for respiratory depression and/or prolonged sedation should be exercised and dosage adjustments should be considered).

No products indexed under this heading.

Miglitol (New onset diabetes mellitus, exacerbation of pre-existing diabetes mellitus, and hyperglycemia have been reported during post-marketing surveillance in HIV-1 infected patients receiving protease inhibitor therapy. Some patients require either dose initiation or dose adjustments of oral hypoglycemic agents for treatment of these events).

No products indexed under this heading.

Modafinil (Co-administration of tipranavir with ritonavir with drugs that are potent CYP3A inducers is contraindicated). Products include:

Provigil Tablets 977

Nafcillin Sodium (Tipranavir/ritonavir should be used with caution in patients who are receiving medications known to increase the risk of bleeding, such as antiplatelet agents).

No products indexed under this heading.

Naproxen (Tipranavir/ritonavir should be used with caution in patients who are receiving medications known to increase the risk of bleeding, such as antiplatelet agents). Products include:

EC-Naprosyn Delayed-Release Tablets 2632
Naprosyn Suspension 2632
Naprosyn Tablets 2632

Naproxen Sodium (Tipranavir/ritonavir should be used with caution in patients who are receiving medications known to increase the risk of bleeding, such as antiplatelet agents). Products include:

Anaprox Tablets 2632
Anaprox DS Tablets 2632
Treximet Tablets 1616

Nateglinide (New onset diabetes mellitus, exacerbation of pre-existing diabetes mellitus, and hyperglycemia have been reported during post-marketing surveillance in HIV-1 infected patients receiving protease inhibitor therapy. Some patients require either dose initiation or dose adjustments of oral hypoglycemic agents for treatment of these events). Products include:

Starlix Tablets 2314

Nefazodone Hydrochloride (Tipranavir co-administered with ritonavir at the recommended dose is a net inhibitor of CYP3A and may increase plasma concentrations of agents that are primarily metabolized by CYP3A. Thus, co-administration of tipranavir/ritonavir with drugs highly dependent on CYP3A for clearance and for which elevated plasma concentrations are associated with serious and/or life-threatening events is contraindicated. Co-administration with other CYP3A substrates may require a dose adjustment or additional monitoring).

No products indexed under this heading.

Nelfinavir Mesylate (Tipranavir co-administered with ritonavir at the recommended dose is a net inhibitor of CYP3A and may increase plasma concentrations of agents that are primarily metabolized by CYP3A. Thus, co-administration of tipranavir/ritonavir with drugs highly dependent on CYP3A for clearance and for which elevated plasma concentrations are associated with serious and/or life-threatening events is contraindicated. Co-administration with other CYP3A substrates may require a dose adjustment or additional monitoring).

No products indexed under this heading.

Nevirapine (Co-administration of tipranavir with ritonavir with drugs that are potent CYP3A inducers is contraindicated). Products include:

Viramune Oral Suspension 873
Viramune Tablets 873

Nicardipine (Concomitant use may increase or decrease nicardipine concentrations. Caution is warranted and clinical monitoring of patients is recommended).

No products indexed under this heading.

Nicardipine Hydrochloride (Concomitant use may increase or decrease nicardipine concentrations. Caution is warranted and clinical monitoring of patients is recommended). Products include:

Cardene I.V. 1093

Nifedipine (Tipranavir co-administered with ritonavir at the recommended dose is a net inhibitor of CYP3A and may increase plasma concentrations of agents that are primarily metabolized by CYP3A. Thus, co-administration of tipranavir/ritonavir with drugs highly dependent on CYP3A for clearance and for which elevated plasma concentrations are associated with serious and/or life-threatening events is contraindicated. Co-administration with other CYP3A substrates may require a dose adjustment or additional monitoring).

No products indexed under this heading.

Nimodipine (Tipranavir co-administered with ritonavir at the recommended dose is a net inhibitor of CYP3A and may increase plasma concentrations of agents that are primarily metabolized by CYP3A. Thus, co-administration of tipranavir/ritonavir with drugs highly dependent on CYP3A for clearance and for which elevated plasma concentrations are associated with serious and/or life-threatening events is contraindicated. Co-administration with other CYP3A substrates may require a dose adjustment or additional monitoring). Products include:

Nimotop Capsules 790

Nisoldipine (Concomitant use may increase or decrease nisoldipine concentrations. Caution is warranted and clinical monitoring of patients is recommended). Products include:

Sular Extended Release Tablets 2975

Norethindrone (Alternative methods of non-hormonal contraception should be used when estrogen-based oral contraceptives are co-administered with tipranavir and 200 mg of ritonavir). Products include:

Ortho Micronor Tablets 2446

Norethynodrel (Alternative methods of non-hormonal contraception should be used when estrogen-based oral contraceptives are co-administered with tipranavir and 200 mg of ritonavir).

No products indexed under this heading.

Norgestimate (Alternative methods of non-hormonal contraception should be used when estrogen-based oral contraceptives are co-administered with tipranavir and 200 mg of ritonavir). Products include:

Ortho-Cyclen/Ortho Tri-Cyclen 2449
Ortho Tri-Cyclen Lo Tablets 2458

Norgestrel (Alternative methods of non-hormonal contraception should be used when estrogen-based oral contraceptives are co-administered with tipranavir and 200 mg of ritonavir).

No products indexed under this heading.

Omeprazole (Concomitant use may decrease concentrations of omeprazole. Dosage of omeprazole may need to be increased when co-administered with tipranavir and ritonavir).

No products indexed under this heading.

Omeprazole Magnesium (Concomitant use may decrease concentrations of omeprazole. Dosage of omeprazole may need to be increased when co-administered with tipranavir and ritonavir). Products include:

Prilosec OTC Tablets 2565

Ondansetron Hydrochloride (Tipranavir co-administered with ritonavir at the recommended dose is a net inhibitor of CYP3A and may increase plasma concentrations of agents that are primarily metabolized by CYP3A. Thus, co-administration of tipranavir/ritonavir with drugs highly dependent on CYP3A for clearance and for which elevated plasma concentrations are associated with serious and/or life-threatening events is contraindicated. Co-administration with other CYP3A substrates may require a dose adjustment or additional monitoring). Products include:

Zofran Injection 1682
Zofran 1687

Paclitaxel (Tipranavir co-administered with ritonavir at the recommended dose is a net inhibitor of CYP3A and may increase plasma concentrations of agents that are primarily metabolized by CYP3A. Thus, co-administration of tipranavir/ritonavir with drugs highly dependent on CYP3A for clearance and for which elevated plasma concentrations are associated with serious and/or life-threatening events is contraindicated. Co-administration with other CYP3A substrates may require a dose adjustment or additional monitoring).

No products indexed under this heading.

Paroxetine (Concomitant use may increase concentrations of paroxetine. Paroxetine doses may need to be adjusted upon initiation of tipranavir/ritonavir therapy).

No products indexed under this heading.

Paroxetine Hydrochloride (Concomitant use may increase concentrations of paroxetine. Paroxetine doses may need to be adjusted upon initiation of tipranavir/ritonavir therapy). Products include:

Paxil 1535
Paxil CR Controlled-Release Tablets 1544

Paroxetine Mesylate (Concomitant use may increase concentrations of paroxetine. Paroxetine doses may need to be adjusted upon initiation of tipranavir/ritonavir therapy).

No products indexed under this heading.

Penicillin G Benzathine (Tipranavir/ritonavir should be used with caution in patients who are receiving medications known to increase the risk of bleeding, such as antiplatelet agents). Products include:

Bicillin C-R Injectable Suspension 1775
Bicillin L-A Injection 1777

Penicillin G Procaine (Tipranavir/ritonavir should be used with caution in patients who are receiving medications known to increase the risk of bleeding, such as antiplatelet agents). Products include:

Bicillin C-R Injectable Suspension 1775
Bicillin L-A Injection 1777

Phenobarbital (Concomitant use may lead to a decrease in tipranavir concentrations. Caution should be used when prescribing carbamazepine, phenobarbital, and or phenytoin. Tipranavir may be less effective due to decreased tipranavir plasma concentrations in patients taking these agents concomitantly). Products include:

Donnatal Extentabs 2507

Phenobarbital Sodium (Concomitant use may lead to a decrease in tipranavir concentrations. Caution should be used when prescribing carbamazepine, phenobarbital, and or phenytoin. Tipranavir may be less effective due to decreased tipranavir plasma concentrations in patients taking these agents concomitantly).

No products indexed under this heading.

Phenylbutazone (Tipranavir/ritonavir should be used with caution in patients who are receiving medications known to increase the risk of bleeding, such as antiplatelet agents).

No products indexed under this heading.

Phenytoin (Concomitant use may lead to a decrease in tipranavir concentrations. Caution should be used when prescribing carbamazepine, phenobarbital, and or phenytoin. Tipranavir may be less effective due to decreased tipranavir plasma concentrations in patients taking these agents concomitantly).

No products indexed under this heading.

Phenytoin Sodium (Concomitant use may lead to a decrease in tipranavir concentrations. Caution should be used when prescribing carbamazepine, phenobarbital, and or phenytoin. Tipranavir may be less effective due to decreased tipranavir plasma concentrations in patients taking these agents concomitantly). Products include:

Phenytek Capsules 2192

Pimozide (Co-administration of tipranavir/ritonavir and pimozide may lead to the potential for cardiac arrhythmias. Concomitant use of tipranavir/ritonavir and pimozide is contraindicated).

No products indexed under this heading.

Pioglitazone Hydrochloride (Concomitant use may increase or decrease concentrations of pioglitazone. Careful glucose monitoring is warranted). Products include:

ActoPlus Met Tablets 3071
Actos Tablets 3077
Duetact Tablets 3085

Piroxicam (Tipranavir/ritonavir should be used with caution in patients who are receiving medications known to increase the risk of bleeding, such as antiplatelet agents).

No products indexed under this heading.

Polyestradiol Phosphate (Concomitant use may decrease ethinyl estradiol concentrations by 50%. Alternative methods of non-hormonal contraception should be used when estrogen-based oral contraceptives are co-administered with tipranavir and 200 mg or ritonavir. Patients using estrogens as hormone replacement therapy should be clinically monitored for signs of estrogen deficiency. Women using estrogens may have an increased risk of non-serious rash).

No products indexed under this heading.

Propafenone Hydrochloride (Co-administration of tipranavir/ritonavir and propafenone may lead to potential for serious and/or life-threatening reactions such as cardiac arrhythmias secondary to increases in plasma concentrations of antiarrhythmics. Concomitant use of tipranavir/ritonavir and propafenone is contraindicated). Products include:

Rythmol Tablets 1586
Rythmol SR Capsules 1590

Quinestrol (Concomitant use may decrease ethinyl estradiol concentrations by 50%. Alternative methods of non-hormonal contraception should be used when estrogen-based oral contraceptives are co-administered with tipranavir and 200 mg or ritonavir. Patients using estrogens as hormone replacement therapy should be clinically monitored for signs of estrogen deficiency. Women using estrogens may have an increased risk of non-serious rash).

No products indexed under this heading.

Quinidine (Co-administration of tipranavir/ritonavir with quinidine may lead to potential for serious and/or life-threatening reactions such as cardiac arrhythmias secondary to increases in plasma concentrations of antiarrhythmics. Concomitant use of tipranavir/ritonavir and quinidine is contraindicated).

No products indexed under this heading.

Quinidine Gluconate (Co-administration of tipranavir/ritonavir with quinidine may lead to potential for serious and/or life-threatening reactions such as cardiac arrhythmias secondary to increases in plasma concentrations of antiarrhythmics. Concomitant use of tipranavir/ritonavir and quinidine is contraindicated).

No products indexed under this heading.

Testosterone Enanthate (Tipranavir co-administered with ritonavir at the recommended dose is a net inhibitor of CYP3A and may increase plasma concentrations of agents that are primarily metabolized by CYP3A. Thus, co-administration of tipranavir/ritonavir with drugs highly dependent on CYP3A for clearance and for which elevated plasma concentrations are associated with serious and/or life-threatening events is contraindicated. Co-administration with other CYP3A substrates may require a dose adjustment or additional monitoring). Products include:

Testosterone Propionate (Tipranavir co-administered with ritonavir at the recommended dose is a net inhibitor of CYP3A and may increase plasma concentrations of agents that are primarily metabolized by CYP3A. Thus, co-administration of tipranavir/ritonavir with drugs highly dependent on CYP3A for clearance and for which elevated plasma concentrations are associated with serious and/or life-threatening events is contraindicated. Co-administration with other CYP3A substrates may require a dose adjustment or additional monitoring).

No products indexed under this heading.

Theophylline (Tipranavir co-administered with ritonavir at the recommended dose is a net inhibitor of CYP3A and may increase plasma concentrations of agents that are primarily metabolized by CYP3A. Thus, co-administration of tipranavir/ritonavir with drugs highly dependent on CYP3A for clearance and for which elevated plasma concentrations are associated with serious and/or life-threatening events is contraindicated. Co-administration with other CYP3A substrates may require a dose adjustment or additional monitoring).

No products indexed under this heading.

Theophylline Anhydrous (Tipranavir co-administered with ritonavir at the recommended dose is a net inhibitor of CYP3A and may increase plasma concentrations of agents that are primarily metabolized by CYP3A. Thus, co-administration of tipranavir/ritonavir with drugs highly dependent on CYP3A for clearance and for which elevated plasma concentrations are associated with serious and/or life-threatening events is contraindicated. Co-administration with other CYP3A substrates may require a dose adjustment or additional monitoring). Products include:

Theophylline Calcium Salicylate (Tipranavir co-administered with ritonavir at the recommended dose is a net inhibitor of CYP3A and may increase plasma concentrations of agents that are primarily metabolized by CYP3A. Thus, co-administration of tipranavir/ritonavir with drugs highly dependent on CYP3A for clearance and for which elevated plasma concentrations are associated with serious and/or life-threatening events is contraindicated. Co-administration with other CYP3A substrates may require a dose adjustment or additional monitoring).

No products indexed under this heading.

Theophylline Sodium Glycinate (Tipranavir co-administered with ritonavir at the recommended dose is a net inhibitor of CYP3A and may increase plasma concentrations of agents that are primarily metabolized by CYP3A. Thus, co-administration of tipranavir/ritonavir with drugs highly dependent on CYP3A for clearance and for which elevated plasma concentrations are associated with serious and/or life-threatening events is contraindicated. Co-administration with other CYP3A substrates may require a dose adjustment or additional monitoring).

No products indexed under this heading.

Tiagabine Hydrochloride (Tipranavir co-administered with ritonavir at the recommended dose is a net inhibitor of CYP3A and may increase plasma concentrations of agents that are primarily metabolized by CYP3A. Thus, co-administration of tipranavir/ritonavir with drugs highly dependent on CYP3A for clearance and for which elevated plasma concentrations are associated with serious and/or life-threatening events is contraindicated. Co-administration with other CYP3A substrates may require a dose adjustment or additional monitoring). Products include:

Ticarcillin Disodium (Tipranavir/ritonavir should be used with caution in patients who are receiving medications known to increase the risk of bleeding, such as antiplatelet agents). Products include:

Ticlopidine Hydrochloride (Tipranavir/ritonavir should be used with caution in patients who are receiving medications known to increase the risk of bleeding, such as antiplatelet agents).

No products indexed under this heading.

Tolazamide (New onset diabetes mellitus, exacerbation of pre-existing diabetes mellitus, and hyperglycemia have been reported during post-marketing surveillance in HIV-1 infected patients receiving protease inhibitor therapy. Some patients require either dose initiation or dose adjustments of oral hypoglycemic agents for treatment of these events).

No products indexed under this heading.

Tolbutamide (Concomitant use led to no changes in concentrations of tolbutamide. However careful glucose monitoring is warranted).

No products indexed under this heading.

Tolbutamide Sodium (Concomitant use led to no changes in concentrations of tolbutamide. However careful glucose monitoring is warranted).

No products indexed under this heading.

Tolmetin Sodium (Tipranavir/ritonavir should be used with caution in patients who are receiving medications known to increase the risk of bleeding, such as antiplatelet agents).

No products indexed under this heading.

Tolterodine Tartrate (Tipranavir co-administered with ritonavir at the recommended dose is a net inhibitor of CYP3A and may increase plasma concentrations of agents that are primarily metabolized by CYP3A. Thus, co-administration of tipranavir/ritonavir with drugs highly dependent on CYP3A for clearance and for which elevated plasma concentrations are associated with serious and/or life-threatening events is contraindicated. Co-administration with other CYP3A substrates may require a dose adjustment or additional monitoring).

No products indexed under this heading.

Trazodone Hydrochloride (Concomitant use of trazodone and tipranavir/ritonavir may increase plasma concentrations of trazodone. Adverse events of nausea, dizziness, hypotension, and syncope have been observed following co-administration of trazodone and ritonavir. If trazodone is used with a CYP3A4 inhibitor such as tipranavir/ritonavir, the combination should be used with caution and a lower dose of trazodone should be considered).

No products indexed under this heading.

Triazolam (Co-administration of tipranavir/ritonavir and triazolam may lead to prolonged or increased sedation or respiratory depression. Concomitant use with triazolam is contraindicated).

No products indexed under this heading.

Troglitazone (New onset diabetes mellitus, exacerbation of pre-existing diabetes mellitus, and hyperglycemia have been reported during post-marketing surveillance in HIV-1 infected patients receiving protease inhibitor therapy. Some patients require either dose initiation or dose adjustments of oral hypoglycemic agents for treatment of these events).

No products indexed under this heading.

Troleandomycin (Co-administration with drugs that inhibit P-gp may increase tipranavir plasma concentrations).

No products indexed under this heading.

Valproate Sodium (Concomitant use may decrease concentrations of valproic acid. Caution should be used when prescribing valproic acid. Valproic acid may be less effective due to decreased valproic acid concentrations in patients taking tipranavir concomitantly).

No products indexed under this heading.

Valproic Acid (Concomitant use may decrease concentrations of valproic acid. Caution should be used when prescribing valproic acid. Valproic acid may be less effective due to decreased valproic acid concentrations in patients taking tipranavir concomitantly).

No products indexed under this heading.

Vardenafil Hydrochloride (Concomitant use may increase levels of vardenafil. Concurrent use of PDE-5 inhibitors with tipranavir and ritonavir should be used with caution and in no case should the starting dose of vardenafil exceed 2.5 mg every 72 hours). Products include:

Venlafaxine Hydrochloride (Tipranavir co-administered with ritonavir at the recommended dose is a net inhibitor of CYP3A and may increase plasma concentrations of agents that are primarily metabolized by CYP3A. Thus, co-administration of tipranavir/ritonavir with drugs highly dependent on CYP3A for clearance and for which elevated plasma concentrations are associated with serious and/or life-threatening events is contraindicated. Co-administration with other CYP3A substrates may require a dose adjustment or additional monitoring). Products include:

Verapamil Hydrochloride (Concomitant use may increase or decrease verapamil concentrations. Caution is warranted and clinical monitoring of patients is recommended). Products include:

Vinblastine Sulfate (Tipranavir co-administered with ritonavir at the recommended dose is a net inhibitor of CYP3A and may increase plasma concentrations of agents that are primarily metabolized by CYP3A. Thus, co-administration of tipranavir/ritonavir with drugs highly dependent on CYP3A for clearance and for which elevated plasma concentrations are associated with serious and/or life-threatening events is contraindicated. Co-administration with other CYP3A substrates may require a dose adjustment or additional monitoring).

No products indexed under this heading.

Vincristine Sulfate (Tipranavir co-administered with ritonavir at the recommended dose is a net inhibitor of CYP3A and may increase plasma concentrations of agents that are primarily metabolized by CYP3A. Thus, co-administration of tipranavir/ritonavir with drugs highly dependent on CYP3A for clearance and for which elevated plasma concentrations are associated with serious and/or life-threatening events is contraindicated. Co-administration with other CYP3A substrates may require a dose adjustment or additional monitoring).

No products indexed under this heading.

Voriconazole (Due to multiple enzymes involved with voriconazole metabolism, it is difficult to predict the interaction).

No products indexed under this heading.

Warfarin Sodium (Frequent INF (international normalized ratio) monitoring upon initiation of tipranavir/ritonavir therapy is recommended).

No products indexed under this heading.

Zidovudine (Concomitant use with zidovudine decreased zidovudine AUC by approximately 35%. The clinical relevance of reduction in zidovudine levels has not been established. Dose adjustment of zidovudine cannot be recommended at this time). Products include:

Combivir Tablets 1384
Retrovir 1574
Retrovir IV Infusion 1579
Trizivir Tablets 1622

APTIVUS ORAL SOLUTION

(Tipranavir) 823

May interact with oral anticoagulants, cytochrome p450 3a inducers (selected), cytochrome p450 3a substrates (selected), estrogens, oral hypoglycemic agents, insulin, oral contraceptives, P-glycoprotein inhibitors, phenytoin, platelet inhibitors, quinidine, valproate, and certain other agents. Compounds in these categories include:

Abacavir Sulfate (Concomitant use with abacavir led to a decrease in AUC of abacavir by 40%. The clinical relevance of reduction in abacavir levels has not been established. Dose adjustment of abacavir cannot be recommended at this time). Products include:

Epzicom Tablets 1422
Trizivir Tablets 1622
Ziagen 1673

Acarbose (New onset diabetes mellitus, exacerbation of pre-existing diabetes mellitus, and hyperglycemia have been reported during post-marketing surveillance in HIV-1 infected patients receiving protease inhibitor therapy. Some patients require either dose initiation or dose adjustments of oral hypoglycemic agents for treatment of these events). Products include:

Precose Tablets 792

Alfentanil Hydrochloride (Tipranavir co-administered with ritonavir at the recommended dose is a net inhibitor of CYP3A and may increase plasma concentrations of agents that are primarily metabolized by CYP3A. Thus, co-administration of tipranavir/ritonavir with drugs highly dependent on CYP3A for clearance and for which elevated plasma concentrations are associated with serious and/or life-threatening events is contraindicated. Co-administration with other CYP3A substrates may require a dose adjustment or additional monitoring).

No products indexed under this heading.

Allium sativum (Co-administration of tipranavir with ritonavir with other drugs that are potent CYP3A inducers is contraindicated).

No products indexed under this heading.

Alprazolam (Tipranavir co-administered with ritonavir at the recommended dose is a net inhibitor of CYP3A and may increase plasma concentrations of agents that are primarily metabolized by CYP3A. Thus, co-administration of tipranavir/ritonavir with drugs highly dependent on CYP3A for clearance and for which elevated plasma concentrations are associated with serious and/or life-threatening events is contraindicated. Co-administration with other CYP3A substrates may require a dose adjustment or additional monitoring).

No products indexed under this heading.

Aminophylline (Tipranavir co-administered with ritonavir at the recommended dose is a net inhibitor of CYP3A and may increase plasma concentrations of agents that are primarily metabolized by CYP3A. Thus, co-administration of tipranavir/ritonavir with drugs highly dependent on CYP3A for clearance and for which elevated plasma concentrations are associated with serious and/or life-threatening events is contraindicated. Co-administration with other CYP3A substrates may require a dose adjustment or additional monitoring).

No products indexed under this heading.

Amiodarone Hydrochloride (Co-administration of tipranavir/ritonavir and amiodarone may lead to potential for serious and/or life-threatening reactions such as cardiac arrhythmias secondary to increases in plasma concentrations of antiarrhythmics. Concomitant use of tipranavir/ritonavir and amiodarone is contraindicated).

No products indexed under this heading.

Amitriptyline Hydrochloride (Tipranavir co-administered with ritonavir at the recommended dose is a net inhibitor of CYP3A and may increase plasma concentrations of agents that are primarily metabolized by CYP3A. Thus, co-administration of tipranavir/ritonavir with drugs highly dependent on CYP3A for clearance and for which elevated plasma concentrations are associated with serious and/or life-threatening events is contraindicated. Co-administration with other CYP3A substrates may require a dose adjustment or additional monitoring).

No products indexed under this heading.

Amlodipine Besylate (Tipranavir co-administered with ritonavir at the recommended dose is a net inhibitor of CYP3A and may increase plasma concentrations of agents that are primarily metabolized by CYP3A. Thus, co-administration of tipranavir/ritonavir with drugs highly dependent on CYP3A for clearance and for which elevated plasma concentrations are associated with serious and/or life-threatening events is contraindicated. Co-administration with other CYP3A substrates may require a dose adjustment or additional monitoring). Products include:

Azor Tablets 1005
Exforge Tablets 2238

Anisindione (Tipranavir/ritonavir should be used with caution in patients who are receiving medications known to increase the risk of bleeding, such as anticoagulants).

No products indexed under this heading.

Aprepitant (Tipranavir co-administered with ritonavir at the recommended dose is a net inhibitor of CYP3A and may increase plasma concentrations of agents that are primarily metabolized by CYP3A. Thus, co-administration of tipranavir/ritonavir with drugs highly dependent on CYP3A for clearance and for which elevated plasma concentrations are associated with serious and/or life-threatening events is contraindicated. Co-administration with other CYP3A substrates may require a dose adjustment or additional monitoring). Products include:

Emend Capsules 1992

Aspirin (Tipranavir/ritonavir should be used with caution in patients who are receiving medications known to increase the risk of bleeding, such as antiplatelet agents). Products include:

Aggrenox Capsules 819
Bayer Aspirin 750
Percodan Tablets 1130
St. Joseph 81 mg Aspirin Chewable and Enteric Coated Tablets 1903

Aspirin, Enteric Coated (Tipranavir/ritonavir should be used with caution in patients who are receiving medications known to increase the risk of bleeding, such as antiplatelet agents).

No products indexed under this heading.

Aspirin Buffered (Tipranavir/ritonavir should be used with caution in patients who are receiving medications known to increase the risk of bleeding, such as antiplatelet agents).

No products indexed under this heading.

Astemizole (Tipranavir co-administered with ritonavir at the recommended dose is a net inhibitor of CYP3A and may increase plasma concentrations of agents that are primarily metabolized by CYP3A. Thus, co-administration of tipranavir/ritonavir with drugs highly dependent on CYP3A for clearance and for which elevated plasma concentrations are associated with serious and/or life-threatening events is contraindicated. Co-administration with other CYP3A substrates may require a dose adjustment or additional monitoring).

No products indexed under this heading.

Atazanavir (Concomitant use of atazanavir with tipranavir and 100 mg of ritonavir led to a decrease in concentrations of atazanavir and an increase in concentrations of tipranavir. Combining a protease inhibitor with tipranavir/ritonavir is not recommended).

No products indexed under this heading.

Atazanavir Sulfate (Concomitant use of atazanavir with tipranavir and 100 mg of ritonavir led to a decrease in concentrations of atazanavir and an increase in concentrations of tipranavir. Combining a protease inhibitor with tipranavir/ritonavir is not recommended). Products include:

Reyataz Capsules 3299

Atenolol (Co-administration with drugs that inhibit P-gp may increase tipranavir plasma concentrations).

No products indexed under this heading.

Atorvastatin Calcium (Concomitant use may increase concentrations of atorvastatin and/or tipranavir and decrease concentrations of hydroxy-atorvastatin metabolites. Start with the lowest possible dose of atorvastatin with careful monitoring, or consider other HMG-CoA reductase inhibitors such as pravastatin or fluvastatin when in concomitant use of tipranavir, co-administered with 200 mg of ritonavir). Products include:

Lipitor Tablets 2501

Azithromycin Dihydrate (Co-administration with drugs that inhibit P-gp may increase tipranavir plasma concentrations).

No products indexed under this heading.

Azlocillin Sodium (Tipranavir/ritonavir should be used with caution in patients who are receiving medications known to increase the risk of bleeding, such as antiplatelet agents).

No products indexed under this heading.

Bepridil Hydrochloride (Co-administration of tipranavir/ritonavir and bepridil may lead to potential for serious and/or life-threatening reactions such as cardiac arrhythmias secondary to increases in plasma concentrations of antiarrhythmics. Concomitant use of tipranavir/ritonavir and bepridil is contraindicated).

No products indexed under this heading.

Buspirone Hydrochloride (Tipranavir co-administered with ritonavir at the recommended dose is a net inhibitor of CYP3A and may increase plasma concentrations of agents that are primarily metabolized by CYP3A. Thus, co-administration of tipranavir/ritonavir with drugs highly dependent on CYP3A for clearance and for which elevated plasma concentrations are associated with serious and/or life-threatening events is contraindicated. Co-administration with other CYP3A substrates may require a dose adjustment or additional monitoring).

No products indexed under this heading.

Busulfan (Tipranavir co-administered with ritonavir at the recommended dose is a net inhibitor of CYP3A and may increase plasma concentrations of agents that are primarily metabolized by CYP3A. Thus, co-administration of tipranavir/ritonavir with drugs highly dependent on CYP3A for clearance and for which elevated plasma concentrations are associated with serious and/or life-threatening events is contraindicated. Co-administration with other CYP3A substrates may require a dose adjustment or additional monitoring). Products include:

Busulfex Injection 2477
Myleran Tablets 1530

Carbamazepine (Concomitant use may lead to a decrease in tipranavir concentrations. Caution should be used when prescribing carbamazepine, phenobarbital, and or phenytoin. Tipranavir may be less effective due to decreased tipranavir plasma concentrations in patients taking these agents concomitantly). Products include:

Carbatrol Capsules 3019
Equetro Extended-Release Capsules 3174

Carbenicillin Indanyl Sodium (Tipranavir/ritonavir should be used with caution in patients who are receiving medications known to increase the risk of bleeding, such as antiplatelet agents).

No products indexed under this heading.

Cerivastatin Sodium (Tipranavir co-administered with ritonavir at the recommended dose is a net inhibitor of CYP3A and may increase plasma concentrations of agents that are primarily metabolized by CYP3A. Thus, co-administration of tipranavir/ritonavir with drugs highly dependent on CYP3A for clearance and for which elevated plasma concentrations are associated with serious and/or life-threatening events is contraindicated. Co-administration with other CYP3A substrates may require a dose adjustment or additional monitoring).

No products indexed under this heading.

Chlorotrianisene (Concomitant use may decrease ethinyl estradiol concentrations by 50%. Alternative methods of non-hormonal contraception should be used when estrogen-based oral contraceptives are co-administered with tipranavir and 200 mg or ritonavir. Patients using estrogens as hormone replacement therapy should be clinically monitored for signs of estrogen deficiency. Women using estrogens may have an increased risk of non-serious rash).

No products indexed under this heading.

Chlorpheniramine (Tipranavir co-administered with ritonavir at the recommended dose is a net inhibitor of CYP3A and may increase plasma concentrations of agents that are primarily metabolized by CYP3A. Thus, co-administration of tipranavir/ritonavir with drugs highly dependent on CYP3A for clearance and for which elevated plasma concentrations are associated with serious and/or life-threatening events is contraindicated. Co-administration with other CYP3A substrates may require a dose adjustment or additional monitoring).

No products indexed under this heading.

Chlorpheniramine Maleate (Tipranavir co-administered with ritonavir at the recommended dose is a net inhibitor of CYP3A and may increase plasma concentrations of agents that are primarily metabolized by CYP3A. Thus, co-administration of tipranavir/ritonavir with drugs highly dependent on CYP3A for clearance and for which elevated plasma concentrations are associated with serious and/or life-threatening events is contraindicated. Co-administration with other CYP3A substrates may require a dose adjustment or additional monitoring). Products include:

Actifed Cold & Allergy Tablets 1895
Sudafed PE Sinus & Allergy Tablets 1908
Tylenol Allergy Multi-Symptom Caplets with Cool Burst and Rapid Release Gelcaps 1916
Children's Tylenol Plus Cold Suspension Liquid 1912
Children's Tylenol Plus Cough & Runny Nose Suspension Liquid 1912
Children's Tylenol Plus Flu Suspension Liquid 1914
Children's Tylenol Plus Multi-Symptom Cold Suspension Liquid 1912
Tylenol Cold Head Congestion Nighttime Caplets with Cool Burst 1910
Tylenol Cold Multi-Symptom Nighttime Caplets with Cool Burst 1913
Tylenol Sinus Congestion & Pain Nighttime Caplets with Cool Burst 1917

Chlorpheniramine Polistirex (Tipranavir co-administered with ritonavir at the recommended dose is a net inhibitor of CYP3A and may increase plasma concentrations of agents that are primarily metabolized by CYP3A. Thus, co-administration of tipranavir/ritonavir with drugs highly dependent on CYP3A for clearance and for which elevated plasma concentrations are associated with serious and/or life-threatening events is contraindicated. Co-administration with other CYP3A substrates may require a dose adjustment or additional monitoring). Products include:

Tussionex Pennkinetic Extended-Release Suspension 3154

Chlorpheniramine Tannate (Tipranavir co-administered with ritonavir at the recommended dose is a net inhibitor of CYP3A and may increase plasma concentrations of agents that are primarily metabolized by CYP3A. Thus, co-administration of tipranavir/ritonavir with drugs highly dependent on CYP3A for clearance and for which elevated plasma concentrations are associated with serious and/or life-threatening events is contraindicated. Co-administration with other CYP3A substrates may require a dose adjustment or additional monitoring).

No products indexed under this heading.

Chlorpropamide (New onset diabetes mellitus, exacerbation of pre-existing diabetes mellitus, and hyperglycemia have been reported during post-marketing surveillance in HIV-1 infected patients receiving protease inhibitor therapy. Some patients require either dose initiation or dose adjustments of oral hypoglycemic agents for treatment of these events).

No products indexed under this heading.

Choline Magnesium Trisalicylate (Tipranavir/ritonavir should be used with caution in patients who are receiving medications known to increase the risk of bleeding, such as antiplatelet agents).

No products indexed under this heading.

Cisapride (Co-administration of tipranavir/ritonavir and cisapride may lead to the potential for cardiac arrhythmias. Concomitant use of tipranavir/ritonavir and cisapride is contraindicated).

No products indexed under this heading.

Clarithromycin (Concomitant use may lead to an increase in concentrations of tipranavir and/or clarithromycin and a decrease in the 14-hydroxy-clarithromycin metabolite. No dose adjustment of tipranavir or clarithromycin for patients with normal renal function is necessary. For patients with a CrCl of 30 to 60 mL/min., the dose of clarithromycin should be reduced by 50%. For patients with a CrCl of less than 30 mL/min., the dose of clarithromycin should be decreased by 75%). Products include:

Biaxin/Biaxin XL 411

Clopidogrel Bisulfate (Tipranavir/ritonavir should be used with caution in patients who are receiving medications known to increase the risk of bleeding, such as antiplatelet agents). Products include:

Plavix Tablets 926
Plavix Tablets 2767

Cyclosporine (Concomitant use may increase or decrease concentrations of cyclosporine. Increased frequency of monitoring plasma levels of immunosuppressant drugs is recommended). Products include:

Gengraf Capsules 435
Neoral Oral Solution 2280
Neoral Soft Gelatin Capsules 2280
Restasis Ophthalmic Emulsion 557
Sandimmune 2296

Desipramine Hydrochloride (Concomitant use may lead to an increase in concentrations of desipramine. Dosage reduction and concentration monitoring of desipramine is recommended).

No products indexed under this heading.

Desogestrel (Alternative methods of non-hormonal contraception should be used when estrogen-based oral contraceptives are co-administered with tipranavir and 200 mg or ritonavir). Products include:

Mircette Tablets 1034

Dexamethasone (Tipranavir co-administered with ritonavir at the recommended dose is a net inhibitor of CYP3A and may increase plasma concentrations of agents that are primarily metabolized by CYP3A. Thus, co-administration of tipranavir/ritonavir with drugs highly dependent on CYP3A for clearance and for which elevated plasma concentrations are associated with serious and/or life-threatening events is contraindicated. Co-administration with other CYP3A substrates may require a dose adjustment or additional monitoring). Products include:

Ciprodex Otic Suspension 541

Dexamethasone Acetate (Tipranavir co-administered with ritonavir at the recommended dose is a net inhibitor of CYP3A and may increase plasma concentrations of agents that are primarily metabolized by CYP3A. Thus, co-administration of tipranavir/ritonavir with drugs highly dependent on CYP3A for clearance and for which elevated plasma concentrations are associated with serious and/or life-threatening events is contraindicated. Co-administration with other CYP3A substrates may require a dose adjustment or additional monitoring).

No products indexed under this heading.

Dexamethasone Phosphate (Tipranavir co-administered with ritonavir at the recommended dose is a net inhibitor of CYP3A and may increase plasma concentrations of agents that are primarily metabolized by CYP3A. Thus, co-administration of tipranavir/ritonavir with drugs highly dependent on CYP3A for clearance and for which elevated plasma concentrations are associated with serious and/or life-threatening events is contraindicated. Co-administration with other CYP3A substrates may require a dose adjustment or additional monitoring).

No products indexed under this heading.

Dexamethasone Sodium (Tipranavir co-administered with ritonavir at the recommended dose is a net inhibitor of CYP3A and may increase plasma concentrations of agents that are primarily metabolized by CYP3A. Thus, co-administration of tipranavir/ritonavir with drugs highly dependent on CYP3A for clearance and for which elevated plasma concentrations are associated with serious and/or life-threatening events is contraindicated. Co-administration with other CYP3A substrates may require a dose adjustment or additional monitoring).

No products indexed under this heading.

Dexamethasone Sodium Phosphate (Tipranavir co-administered with ritonavir at the recommended dose is a net inhibitor of CYP3A and may increase plasma concentrations of agents that are primarily metabolized by CYP3A. Thus, co-administration of tipranavir/ritonavir with drugs highly dependent on CYP3A for clearance and for which elevated plasma concentrations are associated with serious and/or life-threatening events is contraindicated. Co-administration with other CYP3A substrates may require a dose adjustment or additional monitoring).

No products indexed under this heading.

Diazepam (Tipranavir co-administered with ritonavir at the recommended dose is a net inhibitor of CYP3A and may increase plasma concentrations of agents that are primarily metabolized by CYP3A. Thus, co-administration of tipranavir/ritonavir with drugs highly dependent on CYP3A for clearance and for which elevated plasma concentrations are associated with serious and/or life-threatening events is contraindicated. Co-administration with other CYP3A substrates may require a dose adjustment or additional monitoring). Products include:

Valium Tablets 2658

Diclofenac Potassium (Tipranavir/ritonavir should be used with caution in patients who are receiving medications known to increase the risk of bleeding, such as antiplatelet agents).

No products indexed under this heading.

Diclofenac Sodium (Tipranavir/ritonavir should be used with caution in patients who are receiving medications known to increase the risk of bleeding, such as antiplatelet agents). Products include:

Diclofenac Sodium Ophthalmic Solution .... ⊙ 240
Voltaren Ophthalmic Solution 2336
Voltaren Tablets 2334
Voltaren-XR Tablets 2337

Dicumarol (Tipranavir/ritonavir should be used with caution in patients who are receiving medications known to increase the risk of bleeding, such as anticoagulants).

No products indexed under this heading.

Didanosine (Concomitant use with didanosine decreased concentration levels of didanosine. The clinical relevance of reduction in didanosine levels has not been established. For optimal absorption, didanosine should be separated from tipranavir/ritonavir dosing by at least 2 hours).
No products indexed under this heading.

Dienestrol (Concomitant use may decrease ethinyl estradiol concentrations by 50%. Alternative methods of non-hormonal contraception should be used when estrogen-based oral contraceptives are co-administered with tipranavir and 200 mg or ritonavir. Patients using estrogens as hormone replacement therapy should be clinically monitored for signs of estrogen deficiency. Women using estrogens may have an increased risk of non-serious rash).
No products indexed under this heading.

Diethylstilbestrol (Concomitant use may decrease ethinyl estradiol concentrations by 50%. Alternative methods of non-hormonal contraception should be used when estrogen-based oral contraceptives are co-administered with tipranavir and 200 mg or ritonavir. Patients using estrogens as hormone replacement therapy should be clinically monitored for signs of estrogen deficiency. Women using estrogens may have an increased risk of non-serious rash).
No products indexed under this heading.

Diflunisal (Tipranavir/ritonavir should be used with caution in patients who are receiving medications known to increase the risk of bleeding, such as antiplatelet agents).
No products indexed under this heading.

Digoxin (Co-administration with drugs that inhibit P-gp may increase tipranavir plasma concentrations). Products include:
Lanoxin Injection **1498**
Lanoxin Injection Pediatric **1502**
Lanoxin Tablets **1505**

Dihydroergotamine Mesylate (Co-administration of tipranavir/ritonavir with dihydroergotamine may lead to the potential for acute ergot toxicity characterized by peripheral vasospasm and ischemia of the extremities and other tissues. Concomitant use of tipranavir/ritonavir with dihydroergotamine is contraindicated).
No products indexed under this heading.

Diltiazem Hydrochloride (Concomitant use may increase or decrease diltiazem concentrations. Caution is warranted and clinical monitoring of patients is recommended). Products include:
Cardizem LA Extended Release Tablets **421**

Diltiazem Maleate (Concomitant use may increase or decrease diltiazem concentrations. Caution is warranted and clinical monitoring of patients is recommended).
No products indexed under this heading.

Dipyridamole (Tipranavir/ritonavir should be used with caution in patients who are receiving medications known to increase the risk of bleeding, such as antiplatelet agents). Products include:
Aggrenox Capsules **819**
Persantine Tablets **869**

Dirithromycin (Co-administration with drugs that inhibit P-gp may increase tipranavir plasma concentrations).
No products indexed under this heading.

Disopyramide Phosphate (Tipranavir co-administered with ritonavir at the recommended dose is a net inhibitor of CYP3A and may increase plasma concentrations of agents that are primarily metabolized by CYP3A. Thus, co-administration of tipranavir/ritonavir with drugs highly dependent on CYP3A for clearance and for which elevated plasma concentrations are associated with serious and/or life-threatening events is contraindicated. Co-administration with other CYP3A substrates may require a dose adjustment or additional monitoring).
No products indexed under this heading.

Divalproex Sodium (Concomitant use may decrease concentrations of valproic acid. Caution should be used when prescribing valproic acid. Valproic acid may be less effective due to decreased valproic acid concentrations in patients taking tipranavir concomitantly). Products include:
Depakote ER Tablets **423**

Doxorubicin Hydrochloride (Tipranavir co-administered with ritonavir at the recommended dose is a net inhibitor of CYP3A and may increase plasma concentrations of agents that are primarily metabolized by CYP3A. Thus, co-administration of tipranavir/ritonavir with drugs highly dependent on CYP3A for clearance and for which elevated plasma concentrations are associated with serious and/or life-threatening events is contraindicated. Co-administration with other CYP3A substrates may require a dose adjustment or additional monitoring).
No products indexed under this heading.

Dronabinol (Tipranavir co-administered with ritonavir at the recommended dose is a net inhibitor of CYP3A and may increase plasma concentrations of agents that are primarily metabolized by CYP3A. Thus, co-administration of tipranavir/ritonavir with drugs highly dependent on CYP3A for clearance and for which elevated plasma concentrations are associated with serious and/or life-threatening events is contraindicated. Co-administration with other CYP3A substrates may require a dose adjustment or additional monitoring). Products include:
Marinol Capsules **3163**

Dyphylline (Tipranavir co-administered with ritonavir at the recommended dose is a net inhibitor of CYP3A and may increase plasma concentrations of agents that are primarily metabolized by CYP3A. Thus, co-administration of tipranavir/ritonavir with drugs highly dependent on CYP3A for clearance and for which elevated plasma concentrations are associated with serious and/or life-threatening events is contraindicated. Co-administration with other CYP3A substrates may require a dose adjustment or additional monitoring).
No products indexed under this heading.

Efavirenz (Co-administration of tipranavir with ritonavir with other drugs that are potent CYP3A inducers is contraindicated). Products include:
Atripla Tablets **938**
Sustiva Capsules **930**
Sustiva Tablets **930**

Elacridar (Co-administration with drugs that inhibit P-gp may increase tipranavir plasma concentrations).
No products indexed under this heading.

Ergonovine Maleate (Co-administration of tipranavir/ritonavir with ergotamine may lead to the potential for acute ergot toxicity characterized by peripheral vasospasm and ischemia of the extremities and other tissues. Concomitant use of tipranavir/ritonavir with ergotamineis contraindicated).
No products indexed under this heading.

Ergotamine Tartrate (Co-administration of tipranavir/ritonavir with ergotamine may lead to the potential for acute ergot toxicity characterized by peripheral vasospasm and ischemia of the extremities and other tissues. Concomitant use of tipranavir/ritonavir with ergotamine is contraindicated).
No products indexed under this heading.

Erythromycin (Tipranavir co-administered with ritonavir at the recommended dose is a net inhibitor of CYP3A and may increase plasma concentrations of agents that are primarily metabolized by CYP3A. Thus, co-administration of tipranavir/ritonavir with drugs highly dependent on CYP3A for clearance and for which elevated plasma concentrations are associated with serious and/or life-threatening events is contraindicated. Co-administration with other CYP3A substrates may require a dose adjustment or additional monitoring).
No products indexed under this heading.

Erythromycin Estolate (Tipranavir co-administered with ritonavir at the recommended dose is a net inhibitor of CYP3A and may increase plasma concentrations of agents that are primarily metabolized by CYP3A. Thus, co-administration of tipranavir/ritonavir with drugs highly dependent on CYP3A for clearance and for which elevated plasma concentrations are associated with serious and/or life-threatening events is contraindicated. Co-administration with other CYP3A substrates may require a dose adjustment or additional monitoring).
No products indexed under this heading.

Erythromycin Ethylsuccinate (Tipranavir co-administered with ritonavir at the recommended dose is a net inhibitor of CYP3A and may increase plasma concentrations of agents that are primarily metabolized by CYP3A. Thus, co-administration of tipranavir/ritonavir with drugs highly dependent on CYP3A for clearance and for which elevated plasma concentrations are associated with serious and/or life-threatening events is contraindicated. Co-administration with other CYP3A substrates may require a dose adjustment or additional monitoring). Products include:
E.E.S. **433**
EryPed **431**

Erythromycin Gluceptate (Tipranavir co-administered with ritonavir at the recommended dose is a net inhibitor of CYP3A and may increase plasma concentrations of agents that are primarily metabolized by CYP3A. Thus, co-administration of tipranavir/ritonavir with drugs highly dependent on CYP3A for clearance and for which elevated plasma concentrations are associated with serious and/or life-threatening events is contraindicated. Co-administration with other CYP3A substrates may require a dose adjustment or additional monitoring).
No products indexed under this heading.

Erythromycin Lactobionate (Tipranavir co-administered with ritonavir at the recommended dose is a net inhibitor of CYP3A and may increase plasma concentrations of agents that are primarily metabolized by CYP3A. Thus, co-administration of tipranavir/ritonavir with drugs highly dependent on CYP3A for clearance and for which elevated plasma concentrations are associated with serious and/or life-threatening events is contraindicated. Co-administration with other CYP3A substrates may require a dose adjustment or additional monitoring).
No products indexed under this heading.

Erythromycin Stearate (Tipranavir co-administered with ritonavir at the recommended dose is a net inhibitor of CYP3A and may increase plasma concentrations of agents that are primarily metabolized by CYP3A. Thus, co-administration of tipranavir/ritonavir with drugs highly dependent on CYP3A for clearance and for which elevated plasma concentrations are associated with serious and/or life-threatening events is contraindicated. Co-administration with other CYP3A substrates may require a dose adjustment or additional monitoring).
No products indexed under this heading.

Esomeprazole Magnesium (Concomitant use may decrease concentrations of omeprazole. Dosage of omeprazole may need to be increased when co-administered with tipranavir and ritonavir). Products include:
Nexium Delayed-Release Capsules **645**
Nexium Delayed-Release Oral Suspension **645**

Esomeprazole Sodium (Concomitant use may decrease concentrations of omeprazole. Dosage of omeprazole may need to be increased when co-administered with tipranavir and ritonavir). Products include:
Nexium I.V. **652**

Estradiol (Concomitant use may decrease ethinyl estradiol concentrations by 50%. Alternative methods of non-hormonal contraception should be used when estrogen-based oral

Glipizide (Concomitant use led to no changes in concentrations of glipizide. However careful glucose monitoring is warranted).
No products indexed under this heading.

Glyburide (Concomitant use led to no changes in concentrations of glyburide. However careful glucose monitoring is warranted).
No products indexed under this heading.

Haloperidol (Tipranavir co-administered with ritonavir at the recommended dose is a net inhibitor of CYP3A and may increase plasma concentrations of agents that are primarily metabolized by CYP3A. Thus, co-administration of tipranavir/ritonavir with drugs highly dependent on CYP3A for clearance and for which elevated plasma concentrations are associated with serious and/or life-threatening events is contraindicated. Co-administration with other CYP3A substrates may require a dose adjustment or additional monitoring).
No products indexed under this heading.

Haloperidol Decanoate (Tipranavir co-administered with ritonavir at the recommended dose is a net inhibitor of CYP3A and may increase plasma concentrations of agents that are primarily metabolized by CYP3A. Thus, co-administration of tipranavir/ritonavir with drugs highly dependent on CYP3A for clearance and for which elevated plasma concentrations are associated with serious and/or life-threatening events is contraindicated. Co-administration with other CYP3A substrates may require a dose adjustment or additional monitoring).
No products indexed under this heading.

Hypericum (Co-administration of tipranavir/ritonavir and St. John's Wort may lead to loss of virologic response and possible resistance to tipranavir or to the class of protease inhibitors. Concomitant use of tipranavir/ritonavir and St. John's Wort is contraindicated). Products include:
Satieté Tablets .... ▣ 640

Ibuprofen (Tipranavir/ritonavir should be used with caution in patients who are receiving medications known to increase the risk of bleeding, such as antiplatelet agents). Products include:
Motrin IB Tablets and Caplets 1900
Children's Motrin Oral Suspension ... 1901
Children's Motrin Non-Staining Dye-Free Oral Suspension............ 1901
Children's Motrin Cold Oral Suspension.................................. 1899
Infants' Motrin Concentrated Drops... 1901
Infants' Motrin Non-Staining Dye-Free Concentrated Drops....... 1901
Junior Strength Motrin Caplets and Chewable Tablets.................. 1901
Vicoprofen Tablets 533

Imipramine Hydrochloride (Tipranavir co-administered with ritonavir at the recommended dose is a net inhibitor of CYP3A and may increase plasma concentrations of agents that are primarily metabolized by CYP3A. Thus, co-administration of tipranavir/ritonavir with drugs highly dependent on CYP3A for clearance and for which elevated plasma concentrations are associated with serious and/or life-threatening events is contraindicated. Co-administration with other CYP3A substrates may require a dose adjustment or additional monitoring).
No products indexed under this heading.

Imipramine Pamoate (Tipranavir co-administered with ritonavir at the recommended dose is a net inhibitor of CYP3A and may increase plasma concentrations of agents that are primarily metabolized by CYP3A. Thus, co-administration of tipranavir/ritonavir with drugs highly dependent on CYP3A for clearance and for which elevated plasma concentrations are associated with serious and/or life-threatening events is contraindicated. Co-administration with other CYP3A substrates may require a dose adjustment or additional monitoring).
No products indexed under this heading.

Indinavir Sulfate (Tipranavir co-administered with ritonavir at the recommended dose is a net inhibitor of CYP3A and may increase plasma concentrations of agents that are primarily metabolized by CYP3A. Thus, co-administration of tipranavir/ritonavir with drugs highly dependent on CYP3A for clearance and for which elevated plasma concentrations are associated with serious and/or life-threatening events is contraindicated. Co-administration with other CYP3A substrates may require a dose adjustment or additional monitoring). Products include:
Crixivan Capsules 1979

Indomethacin (Tipranavir/ritonavir should be used with caution in patients who are receiving medications known to increase the risk of bleeding, such as antiplatelet agents). Products include:
Indocin 2024

Indomethacin Sodium Trihydrate (Tipranavir/ritonavir should be used with caution in patients who are receiving medications known to increase the risk of bleeding, such as antiplatelet agents). Products include:
Indocin I.V. 2489

Insulin (New onset diabetes mellitus, exacerbation of pre-existing diabetes mellitus, and hyperglycemia have been reported during post-marketing surveillance in HIV-1 infected patients receiving protease inhibitor therapy. Some patients require either dose initiation or dose adjustments of insulin for treatment of these events).
No products indexed under this heading.

Insulin, Human, Zinc Suspension (New onset diabetes mellitus, exacerbation of pre-existing diabetes mellitus, and hyperglycemia have been reported during post-marketing surveillance in HIV-1 infected patients receiving protease inhibitor therapy. Some patients require either dose initiation or dose adjustments of insulin for treatment of these events).
No products indexed under this heading.

Insulin, Human (rDNA origin) (New onset diabetes mellitus, exacerbation of pre-existing diabetes mellitus, and hyperglycemia have been reported during post-marketing surveillance in HIV-1 infected patients receiving protease inhibitor therapy. Some patients require either dose initiation or dose adjustments of insulin for treatment of these events). Products include:
Exubera Inhalation Powder 2515

Insulin, Human NPH (New onset diabetes mellitus, exacerbation of pre-existing diabetes mellitus, and hyperglycemia have been reported during post-marketing surveillance in HIV-1 infected patients receiving protease inhibitor therapy. Some patients require either dose initiation or dose adjustments of insulin for treatment of these events). Products include:
Humulin N Vial 1846

Insulin, Human Regular (New onset diabetes mellitus, exacerbation of pre-existing diabetes mellitus, and hyperglycemia have been reported during post-marketing surveillance in HIV-1 infected patients receiving protease inhibitor therapy. Some patients require either dose initiation or dose adjustments of insulin for treatment of these events). Products include:
Humulin R 1849
Humulin R (U-500) 1850

Insulin, Human Regular and Human NPH Mixture (New onset diabetes mellitus, exacerbation of pre-existing diabetes mellitus, and hyperglycemia have been reported during post-marketing surveillance in HIV-1 infected patients receiving protease inhibitor therapy. Some patients require either dose initiation or dose adjustments of insulin for treatment of these events). Products include:
Humulin 50/50, 100 Units 1843
Humulin 70/30 Vial 1844

Insulin, NPH (New onset diabetes mellitus, exacerbation of pre-existing diabetes mellitus, and hyperglycemia have been reported during post-marketing surveillance in HIV-1 infected patients receiving protease inhibitor therapy. Some patients require either dose initiation or dose adjustments of insulin for treatment of these events).
No products indexed under this heading.

Insulin, Regular (New onset diabetes mellitus, exacerbation of pre-existing diabetes mellitus, and hyperglycemia have been reported during post-marketing surveillance in HIV-1 infected patients receiving protease inhibitor therapy. Some patients require either dose initiation or dose adjustments of insulin for treatment of these events).
No products indexed under this heading.

Insulin, Regular and NPH mixture (New onset diabetes mellitus, exacerbation of pre-existing diabetes mellitus, and hyperglycemia have been reported during post-marketing surveillance in HIV-1 infected patients receiving protease inhibitor therapy. Some patients require either dose initiation or dose adjustments of insulin for treatment of these events).
No products indexed under this heading.

Insulin, Zinc Crystals (New onset diabetes mellitus, exacerbation of pre-existing diabetes mellitus, and hyperglycemia have been reported during post-marketing surveillance in HIV-1 infected patients receiving protease inhibitor therapy. Some patients require either dose initiation or dose adjustments of insulin for treatment of these events).
No products indexed under this heading.

Insulin, Zinc Suspension (New onset diabetes mellitus, exacerbation of pre-existing diabetes mellitus, and hyperglycemia have been reported during post-marketing surveillance in HIV-1 infected patients receiving protease inhibitor therapy. Some patients require either dose initiation or dose adjustments of insulin for treatment of these events).
No products indexed under this heading.

Insulin Aspart (New onset diabetes mellitus, exacerbation of pre-existing diabetes mellitus, and hyperglycemia have been reported during post-marketing surveillance in HIV-1 infected patients receiving protease inhibitor therapy. Some patients require either dose initiation or dose adjustments of insulin for treatment of these events).
No products indexed under this heading.

Insulin Aspart, Human (New onset diabetes mellitus, exacerbation of pre-existing diabetes mellitus, and hyperglycemia have been reported during post-marketing surveillance in HIV-1 infected patients receiving protease inhibitor therapy. Some patients require either dose initiation or dose adjustments of insulin for treatment of these events). Products include:
NovoLog Mix 70/30 2364

Insulin Aspart, Human Regular (New onset diabetes mellitus, exacerbation of pre-existing diabetes mellitus, and hyperglycemia have been reported during post-marketing surveillance in HIV-1 infected patients receiving protease inhibitor therapy. Some patients require either dose initiation or dose adjustments of insulin for treatment of these events). Products include:
NovoLog Injection 2359

Insulin Aspart Protamine, Human (New onset diabetes mellitus, exacerbation of pre-existing diabetes mellitus, and hyperglycemia have been reported during post-marketing surveillance in HIV-1 infected patients receiving protease inhibitor therapy. Some patients require either dose initiation or dose adjustments of insulin for treatment of these events). Products include:
NovoLog Mix 70/30 2364

Insulin Detemir (rDNA Origin) (New onset diabetes mellitus, exacerbation of pre-existing diabetes mellitus, and hyperglycemia have been reported during post-marketing surveillance in HIV-1 infected patients receiving protease inhibitor therapy. Some patients require either dose initiation or dose adjustments of insulin for treatment of these events). Products include:
Levemir Injection 2352

Insulin glargine (New onset diabetes mellitus, exacerbation of pre-existing diabetes mellitus, and hyperglycemia have been reported during post-marketing surveillance in HIV-1 infected patients receiving protease inhibitor therapy. Some patients require either dose initiation or dose adjustments of insulin for treatment of these events). Products include:

Lantus Injection 2749

Insulin Glulisine (New onset diabetes mellitus, exacerbation of pre-existing diabetes mellitus, and hyperglycemia have been reported during post-marketing surveillance in HIV-1 infected patients receiving protease inhibitor therapy. Some patients require either dose initiation or dose adjustments of insulin for treatment of these events). Products include:

Apidra Injection 2706

Insulin Lispro, Human (New onset diabetes mellitus, exacerbation of pre-existing diabetes mellitus, and hyperglycemia have been reported during post-marketing surveillance in HIV-1 infected patients receiving protease inhibitor therapy. Some patients require either dose initiation or dose adjustments of insulin for treatment of these events). Products include:

Humalog-Pen and KwikPen 1829
Humalog Mix 50/50-Pen and KwikPen 1833
Humalog Mix 75/25-Pen and KwikPen 1835

Insulin Lispro Protamine, Human (New onset diabetes mellitus, exacerbation of pre-existing diabetes mellitus, and hyperglycemia have been reported during post-marketing surveillance in HIV-1 infected patients receiving protease inhibitor therapy. Some patients require either dose initiation or dose adjustments of insulin for treatment of these events). Products include:

Humalog Mix 50/50-Pen and KwikPen 1833
Humalog Mix 75/25-Pen and KwikPen 1835

Isradipine (Tipranavir co-administered with ritonavir at the recommended dose is a net inhibitor of CYP3A and may increase plasma concentrations of agents that are primarily metabolized by CYP3A. Thus, co-administration of tipranavir/ritonavir with drugs highly dependent on CYP3A for clearance and for which elevated plasma concentrations are associated with serious and/or life-threatening events is contraindicated. Co-administration with other CYP3A substrates may require a dose adjustment or additional monitoring). Products include:

DynaCirc CR Controlled Release Tablets 1407

Itraconazole (Concomitant use with itraconazole may increase itraconazole concentrations. Based on theoretical considerations, itraconazole should be used with caution with tipranavir/ritonavir. High doses (greater than 200 mg/day) are not recommended).

No products indexed under this heading.

Ketoconazole (Concomitant use may increase ketoconazole concentrations. Based on theoretical considerations, ketoconazole should be used with caution with tipranavir/ritonavir. High doses (greater than 200 mg/day) are not recommended). Products include:

Extina Foam, 2% 3057
Nizoral A-D Shampoo 1901

Ketoprofen (Tipranavir/ritonavir should be used with caution in patients who are receiving medications known to increase the risk of bleeding, such as antiplatelet agents).

No products indexed under this heading.

Levonorgestrel (Alternative methods of non-hormonal contraception should be used when estrogen-based oral contraceptives are co-administered with tipranavir and 200 mg or ritonavir). Products include:

Climara Pro Transdermal System 768
Lybrel Tablets 3204
Mirena Intrauterine System 779
Plan B Tablets 1044
Seasonique Tablets 1046

Lidocaine (Tipranavir co-administered with ritonavir at the recommended dose is a net inhibitor of CYP3A and may increase plasma concentrations of agents that are primarily metabolized by CYP3A. Thus, co-administration of tipranavir/ritonavir with drugs highly dependent on CYP3A for clearance and for which elevated plasma concentrations are associated with serious and/or life-threatening events is contraindicated. Co-administration with other CYP3A substrates may require a dose adjustment or additional monitoring). Products include:

Lidoderm Patch 1114

Lidocaine Hydrochloride (Tipranavir co-administered with ritonavir at the recommended dose is a net inhibitor of CYP3A and may increase plasma concentrations of agents that are primarily metabolized by CYP3A. Thus, co-administration of tipranavir/ritonavir with drugs highly dependent on CYP3A for clearance and for which elevated plasma concentrations are associated with serious and/or life-threatening events is contraindicated. Co-administration with other CYP3A substrates may require a dose adjustment or additional monitoring).

No products indexed under this heading.

Lopinavir (Concomitant use of lopinavir with tipranavir and 200 mg of ritonavir led to a decrease in concentrations of lopinavir. Combining a protease inhibitor with tipranavir/ritonavir is not recommended). Products include:

Kaletra 452

Lovastatin (Co-administration of tipranavir/ritonavir and lovastatin may lead to the potential for myopathy including rhabdomyolysis. Concomitant use of tipranavir/ritonavir and lovastatin is contraindicated). Products include:

Advicor Tablets 402
Mevacor Tablets 2063

Magnesium Salicylate (Tipranavir/ritonavir should be used with caution in patients who are receiving medications known to increase the risk of bleeding, such as antiplatelet agents).

No products indexed under this heading.

Meclofenamate Sodium (Tipranavir/ritonavir should be used with caution in patients who are receiving medications known to increase the risk of bleeding, such as antiplatelet agents).

No products indexed under this heading.

Mefenamic Acid (Tipranavir/ritonavir should be used with caution in patients who are receiving medications known to increase the risk of bleeding, such as antiplatelet agents).

No products indexed under this heading.

Meperidine Hydrochloride (Concomitant use may decrease concentrations of meperidine and increase concentrations of normeperidine. Dosage increase and long-term use of meperidine are not recommended due to increased concentrations of the metabolite normeperidine which has both analgesic activity and CNS stimulant activity (eg, seizures)).

No products indexed under this heading.

Mestranol (Alternative methods of non-hormonal contraception should be used when estrogen-based oral contraceptives are co-administered with tipranavir and 200 mg or ritonavir).

No products indexed under this heading.

Metformin Hydrochloride (New onset diabetes mellitus, exacerbation of pre-existing diabetes mellitus, and hyperglycemia have been reported during post-marketing surveillance in HIV-1 infected patients receiving protease inhibitor therapy. Some patients require either dose initiation or dose adjustments of oral hypoglycemic agents for treatment of these events). Products include:

ActoPlus Met Tablets 3071
Avandamet Tablets 1336
Janumet Tablets 2041
PrandiMet Tablets 2967

Methadone Hydrochloride (Concomitant use may decrease concentrations of methadone. Dosage of methadone may need to be increased when co-administered with tipranavir and 200 mg of ritonavir).

No products indexed under this heading.

Methylergonovine Maleate (Co-administration of tipranavir/ritonavir with methylergonovine may lead to the potential for acute ergot toxicity characterized by peripheral vasospasm and ischemia of the extremities and other tissues. Concomitant use of tipranavir/ritonavir with methylergonovine is contraindicated).

No products indexed under this heading.

Mezlocillin Sodium (Tipranavir/ritonavir should be used with caution in patients who are receiving medications known to increase the risk of bleeding, such as antiplatelet agents).

No products indexed under this heading.

Mibefradil Dihydrochloride (Co-administration with drugs that inhibit P-gp may increase tipranavir plasma concentrations).

No products indexed under this heading.

Midazolam Hydrochloride (Co-administration of tipranavir/ritonavir and oral midazolam may lead to prolonged or increased sedation or respiratory depression. Concomitant use of tipranavir/ritonavir and oral midazolam is contraindicated. If tipranavir is co-administered with parenteral midazolam, close clinical monitoring for respiratory depression and/or prolonged sedation should be exercised and dosage adjustments should be considered).

No products indexed under this heading.

Miglitol (New onset diabetes mellitus, exacerbation of pre-existing diabetes mellitus, and hyperglycemia have been reported during post-marketing surveillance in HIV-1 infected patients receiving protease inhibitor therapy. Some patients require either dose initiation or dose adjustments of oral hypoglycemic agents for treatment of these events).

No products indexed under this heading.

Modafinil (Co-administration of tipranavir with ritonavir with other drugs that are potent CYP3A inducers is contraindicated). Products include:

Provigil Tablets 977

Nafcillin Sodium (Tipranavir/ritonavir should be used with caution in patients who are receiving medications known to increase the risk of bleeding, such as antiplatelet agents).

No products indexed under this heading.

Naproxen (Tipranavir/ritonavir should be used with caution in patients who are receiving medications known to increase the risk of bleeding, such as antiplatelet agents). Products include:

EC-Naprosyn Delayed-Release Tablets 2632
Naprosyn Suspension 2632
Naprosyn Tablets 2632

Naproxen Sodium (Tipranavir/ritonavir should be used with caution in patients who are receiving medications known to increase the risk of bleeding, such as antiplatelet agents). Products include:

Anaprox Tablets 2632
Anaprox DS Tablets 2632
Treximet Tablets 1616

Nateglinide (New onset diabetes mellitus, exacerbation of pre-existing diabetes mellitus, and hyperglycemia have been reported during post-marketing surveillance in HIV-1 infected patients receiving protease inhibitor therapy. Some patients require either dose initiation or dose adjustments of oral hypoglycemic agents for treatment of these events). Products include:

Starlix Tablets 2314

Nefazodone Hydrochloride (Tipranavir co-administered with ritonavir at the recommended dose is a net inhibitor of CYP3A and may increase plasma concentrations of agents that are primarily metabolized by CYP3A. Thus, co-administration of tipranavir/ritonavir with drugs highly dependent on CYP3A for clearance and for which elevated plasma concentrations are associated with serious and/or life-threatening events is contraindicated. Co-administration with other CYP3A substrates may require a dose adjustment or additional

Quinidine Gluconate (Co-administration of tipranavir/ritonavir with quinidine may lead to potential for serious and/or life-threatening reactions such as cardiac arrhythmias secondary to increases in plasma concentrations of antiarrhythmics. Concomitant use of tipranavir/ritonavir and quinidine is contraindicated).
No products indexed under this heading.

Quinidine Hydrochloride (Co-administration of tipranavir/ritonavir with quinidine may lead to potential for serious and/or life-threatening reactions such as cardiac arrhythmias secondary to increases in plasma concentrations of antiarrhythmics. Concomitant use of tipranavir/ritonavir and quinidine is contraindicated).
No products indexed under this heading.

Quinidine Polygalacturonate (Co-administration of tipranavir/ritonavir with quinidine may lead to potential for serious and/or life-threatening reactions such as cardiac arrhythmias secondary to increases in plasma concentrations of antiarrhythmics. Concomitant use of tipranavir/ritonavir and quinidine is contraindicated).
No products indexed under this heading.

Quinidine Sulfate (Co-administration of tipranavir/ritonavir with quinidine may lead to potential for serious and/or life-threatening reactions such as cardiac arrhythmias secondary to increases in plasma concentrations of antiarrhythmics. Concomitant use of tipranavir/ritonavir and quinidine is contraindicated).
No products indexed under this heading.

Quinine (Tipranavir co-administered with ritonavir at the recommended dose is a net inhibitor of CYP3A and may increase plasma concentrations of agents that are primarily metabolized by CYP3A. Thus, co-administration of tipranavir/ritonavir with drugs highly dependent on CYP3A for clearance and for which elevated plasma concentrations are associated with serious and/or life-threatening events is contraindicated. Co-administration with other CYP3A substrates may require a dose adjustment or additional monitoring).
No products indexed under this heading.

Quinine Sulfate (Tipranavir co-administered with ritonavir at the recommended dose is a net inhibitor of CYP3A and may increase plasma concentrations of agents that are primarily metabolized by CYP3A. Thus, co-administration of tipranavir/ritonavir with drugs highly dependent on CYP3A for clearance and for which elevated plasma concentrations are associated with serious and/or life-threatening events is contraindicated. Co-administration with other CYP3A substrates may require a dose adjustment or additional monitoring).
No products indexed under this heading.

Repaglinide (Concomitant use may increase or decrease concentrations of repaglinide. Careful glucose monitoring is warranted). Products include:
PrandiMet Tablets 2967
Prandin Tablets 2971

Rifabutin (Concomitant use may lead to increased concentrations of rifabutin and desacetyl-rifabutin. Dosage reductions of rifabutin by 75% are recommended (eg, 150 mg every other day). Increased monitoring for adverse events in patients receiving the combination is warranted. Further dosage reduction may be required).
No products indexed under this heading.

Rifampicin (Co-administration of tipranavir with ritonavir with other drugs that are potent CYP3A inducers is contraindicated).
No products indexed under this heading.

Rifampin (Co-administration of tipranavir/ritonavir with rifampin may lead to loss of virologic response and possible resistance to tipranavir or to the class of protease inhibitors or other co-administered antiretroviral agents. Concomitant use of tipranavir/ritonavir with rifampin is contraindicated).
No products indexed under this heading.

Rifapentine (Co-administration of tipranavir with ritonavir with other drugs that are potent CYP3A inducers is contraindicated).
No products indexed under this heading.

Ritonavir (Tipranavir co-administered with ritonavir at the recommended dose is a net inhibitor of CYP3A and may increase plasma concentrations of agents that are primarily metabolized by CYP3A. Thus, co-administration of tipranavir/ritonavir with drugs highly dependent on CYP3A for clearance and for which elevated plasma concentrations are associated with serious and/or life-threatening events is contraindicated. Co-administration with other CYP3A substrates may require a dose adjustment or additional monitoring). Products include:
Kaletra 452
Norvir 489

Rosiglitazone Maleate (New onset diabetes mellitus, exacerbation of pre-existing diabetes mellitus, and hyperglycemia have been reported during post-marketing surveillance in HIV-1 infected patients receiving protease inhibitor therapy. Some patients require either dose initiation or dose adjustments of oral hypoglycemic agents for treatment of these events). Products include:
Avandamet Tablets 1336
Avandaryl Tablets 1344
Avandia Tablets 1351

Rosuvastatin Calcium (Concomitant use may increase concentrations of rosuvastatin and/or tipranavir. Start with the lowest possible dose of rosuvastatin with careful monitoring, or consider other HMG-CoA reductase inhibitors such as pravastatin or fluvastatin when in concomitant use of tipranavir, co-administered with 200 mg of ritonavir). Products include:
Crestor Tablets 677

Salsalate (Tipranavir/ritonavir should be used with caution in patients who are receiving medications known to increase the risk of bleeding, such as antiplatelet agents).
No products indexed under this heading.

Saquinavir (Concomitant use of saquinavir with tipranavir and 200 mg of ritonavir led to a decrease in the concentrations of saquinavir. Combining a protease inhibitor with tipranavir/ritonavir is not recommended).
No products indexed under this heading.

Saquinavir Mesylate (Concomitant use of saquinavir with tipranavir and 200 mg of ritonavir led to a decrease in the concentrations of saquinavir. Combining a protease inhibitor with tipranavir/ritonavir is not recommended).
No products indexed under this heading.

Sertraline Hydrochloride (Concomitant use may increase concentrations of sertraline. Sertraline doses may need to be adjusted upon initiation of tipranavir/ritonavir therapy).
No products indexed under this heading.

Sildenafil Citrate (Concomitant use may increase concentrations of sildenafil. Concurrent use of PDE-5 inhibitors with tipranavir and ritonavir should be used with caution and in no case should the starting dose of sildenafil exceed 25 mg within 48 hours).
No products indexed under this heading.

Simvastatin (Co-administration of tipranavir/ritonavir and simvastatin may lead to the potential for myopathy including rhabdomyolysis. Concomitant use of tipranavir/ritonavir and simvastatin is contraindicated). Products include:
Simcor Tablets 502
Vytorin 10/10 Tablets 2149
Vytorin 10/10 Tablets 2939
Vytorin 10/20 Tablets 2149
Vytorin 10/20 Tablets 2939
Vytorin 10/40 Tablets 2149
Vytorin 10/40 Tablets 2939
Vytorin 10/80 Tablets 2149
Vytorin 10/80 Tablets 2939
Zocor Tablets 2136

Sirolimus (Concomitant use may increase or decrease concentrations of sirolimus. Increased frequency of monitoring plasma levels of immunosuppressant drugs is recommended). Products include:
Rapamune 3260

Sitagliptin Phosphate (New onset diabetes mellitus, exacerbation of pre-existing diabetes mellitus, and hyperglycemia have been reported during post-marketing surveillance in HIV-1 infected patients receiving protease inhibitor therapy. Some patients require either dose initiation or dose adjustments of oral hypoglycemic agents for treatment of these events). Products include:
Janumet Tablets 2041
Januvia Tablets 2048

Sulindac (Tipranavir/ritonavir should be used with caution in patients who are receiving medications known to increase the risk of bleeding, such as antiplatelet agents). Products include:
Clinoril Tablets 1962

Tacrolimus (Concomitant use may increase or decrease concentrations of tacrolimus. Increased frequency of monitoring plasma levels of immunosuppressant drugs is recommended). Products include:
Prograf Capsules and Injection 622
Protopic Ointment 628

Tadalafil (Following the first dose of tipranavir/ritonavir, concentrations of tadalafil were shown to increase. At steady state of tipranavir/ritonavir, no changes in tadalafil concentration were seen. Concurrent use of PDE-5 inhibitors with tipranavir and ritonavir should be used with caution and in no case should the starting dose of tadalafil exceed 10 mg every 72 hours). Products include:
Cialis Tablets 1792

Tamoxifen Citrate (Tipranavir co-administered with ritonavir at the recommended dose is a net inhibitor of CYP3A and may increase plasma concentrations of agents that are primarily metabolized by CYP3A. Thus, co-administration of tipranavir/ritonavir with drugs highly dependent on CYP3A for clearance and for which elevated plasma concentrations are associated with serious and/or life-threatening events is contraindicated. Co-administration with other CYP3A substrates may require a dose adjustment or additional monitoring).
No products indexed under this heading.

Terfenadine (Tipranavir co-administered with ritonavir at the recommended dose is a net inhibitor of CYP3A and may increase plasma concentrations of agents that are primarily metabolized by CYP3A. Thus, co-administration of tipranavir/ritonavir with drugs highly dependent on CYP3A for clearance and for which elevated plasma concentrations are associated with serious and/or life-threatening events is contraindicated. Co-administration with other CYP3A substrates may require a dose adjustment or additional monitoring).
No products indexed under this heading.

Testosterone (Tipranavir co-administered with ritonavir at the recommended dose is a net inhibitor of CYP3A and may increase plasma concentrations of agents that are primarily metabolized by CYP3A. Thus, co-administration of tipranavir/ritonavir with drugs highly dependent on CYP3A for clearance and for which elevated plasma concentrations are associated with serious and/or life-threatening events is contraindicated. Co-administration with other CYP3A substrates may require a dose adjustment or additional monitoring). Products include:
AndroGel 3159
Testim 1% Gel 701

Testosterone Cypionate (Tipranavir co-administered with ritonavir at the recommended dose is a net inhibitor of CYP3A and may increase plasma concentrations of agents that are primarily metabolized by CYP3A. Thus, co-administration of tipranavir/ritonavir with drugs highly dependent on CYP3A for clearance and for which elevated plasma concentrations are associated with serious and/or life-

threatening events is contraindicated. Co-administration with other CYP3A substrates may require a dose adjustment or additional monitoring).
No products indexed under this heading.

Testosterone Enanthate (Tipranavir co-administered with ritonavir at the recommended dose is a net inhibitor of CYP3A and may increase plasma concentrations of agents that are primarily metabolized by CYP3A. Thus, co-administration of tipranavir/ritonavir with drugs highly dependent on CYP3A for clearance and for which elevated plasma concentrations are associated with serious and/or life-threatening events is contraindicated. Co-administration with other CYP3A substrates may require a dose adjustment or additional monitoring). Products include:
Delatestryl Injection 1730

Testosterone Propionate (Tipranavir co-administered with ritonavir at the recommended dose is a net inhibitor of CYP3A and may increase plasma concentrations of agents that are primarily metabolized by CYP3A. Thus, co-administration of tipranavir/ritonavir with drugs highly dependent on CYP3A for clearance and for which elevated plasma concentrations are associated with serious and/or life-threatening events is contraindicated. Co-administration with other CYP3A substrates may require a dose adjustment or additional monitoring).
No products indexed under this heading.

Theophylline (Tipranavir co-administered with ritonavir at the recommended dose is a net inhibitor of CYP3A and may increase plasma concentrations of agents that are primarily metabolized by CYP3A. Thus, co-administration of tipranavir/ritonavir with drugs highly dependent on CYP3A for clearance and for which elevated plasma concentrations are associated with serious and/or life-threatening events is contraindicated. Co-administration with other CYP3A substrates may require a dose adjustment or additional monitoring).
No products indexed under this heading.

Theophylline Anhydrous (Tipranavir co-administered with ritonavir at the recommended dose is a net inhibitor of CYP3A and may increase plasma concentrations of agents that are primarily metabolized by CYP3A. Thus, co-administration of tipranavir/ritonavir with drugs highly dependent on CYP3A for clearance and for which elevated plasma concentrations are associated with serious and/or life-threatening events is contraindicated. Co-administration with other CYP3A substrates may require a dose adjustment or additional monitoring). Products include:
Uniphyl Tablets 2595

Theophylline Calcium Salicylate (Tipranavir co-administered with ritonavir at the recommended dose is a net inhibitor of CYP3A and may increase plasma concentrations of agents that are primarily metabolized by CYP3A. Thus, co-administration of tipranavir/ritonavir with drugs highly dependent on CYP3A for clearance and for which elevated plasma concentrations are associated with serious and/or life-threatening events is contraindicated. Co-administration with other CYP3A substrates may require a dose adjustment or additional monitoring).
No products indexed under this heading.

Theophylline Sodium Glycinate (Tipranavir co-administered with ritonavir at the recommended dose is a net inhibitor of CYP3A and may increase plasma concentrations of agents that are primarily metabolized by CYP3A. Thus, co-administration of tipranavir/ritonavir with drugs highly dependent on CYP3A for clearance and for which elevated plasma concentrations are associated with serious and/or life-threatening events is contraindicated. Co-administration with other CYP3A substrates may require a dose adjustment or additional monitoring).
No products indexed under this heading.

Tiagabine Hydrochloride (Tipranavir co-administered with ritonavir at the recommended dose is a net inhibitor of CYP3A and may increase plasma concentrations of agents that are primarily metabolized by CYP3A. Thus, co-administration of tipranavir/ritonavir with drugs highly dependent on CYP3A for clearance and for which elevated plasma concentrations are associated with serious and/or life-threatening events is contraindicated. Co-administration with other CYP3A substrates may require a dose adjustment or additional monitoring). Products include:
Gabitril Tablets 973

Ticarcillin Disodium (Tipranavir/ritonavir should be used with caution in patients who are receiving medications known to increase the risk of bleeding, such as antiplatelet agents). Products include:
Timentin ADD-Vantage 1606
Timentin Injection Galaxy Container 1609
Timentin IV Infusion 1603
Timentin Pharmacy Bulk Package 1613

Ticlopidine Hydrochloride (Tipranavir/ritonavir should be used with caution in patients who are receiving medications known to increase the risk of bleeding, such as antiplatelet agents).
No products indexed under this heading.

Tolazamide (New onset diabetes mellitus, exacerbation of pre-existing diabetes mellitus, and hyperglycemia have been reported during post-marketing surveillance in HIV-1 infected patients receiving protease inhibitor therapy. Some patients require either dose initiation or dose adjustments of oral hypoglycemic agents for treatment of these events).
No products indexed under this heading.

Tolbutamide (Concomitant use led to no changes in concentrations of tolbutamide. However careful glucose monitoring is warranted).
No products indexed under this heading.

Tolbutamide Sodium (Concomitant use led to no changes in concentrations of tolbutamide. However careful glucose monitoring is warranted).
No products indexed under this heading.

Tolmetin Sodium (Tipranavir/ritonavir should be used with caution in patients who are receiving medications known to increase the risk of bleeding, such as antiplatelet agents).
No products indexed under this heading.

Tolterodine Tartrate (Tipranavir co-administered with ritonavir at the recommended dose is a net inhibitor of CYP3A and may increase plasma concentrations of agents that are primarily metabolized by CYP3A. Thus, co-administration of tipranavir/ritonavir with drugs highly dependent on CYP3A for clearance and for which elevated plasma concentrations are associated with serious and/or life-threatening events is contraindicated. Co-administration with other CYP3A substrates may require a dose adjustment or additional monitoring).
No products indexed under this heading.

Trazodone Hydrochloride (Concomitant use of trazodone and tipranavir/ritonavir may increase plasma concentrations of trazodone. Adverse events of nausea, dizziness, hypotension, and syncope have been observed following co-administration of trazodone and ritonavir. If trazodoneis used with a CYP3A4 inhibitor such as tipranavir/ritonavir, the combination should be used with caution and a lower dose of trazodone should be considered).
No products indexed under this heading.

Triazolam (Co-administration of tipranavir/ritonavir and triazolam may lead to prolonged or increased sedation or respiratory depression. Concomitant use with triazolam is contraindicated).
No products indexed under this heading.

Troglitazone (New onset diabetes mellitus, exacerbation of pre-existing diabetes mellitus, and hyperglycemia have been reported during post-marketing surveillance in HIV-1 infected patients receiving protease inhibitor therapy. Some patients require either dose initiation or dose adjustments of oral hypoglycemic agents for treatment of these events).
No products indexed under this heading.

Troleandomycin (Co-administration with drugs that inhibit P-gp may increase tipranavir plasma concentrations).
No products indexed under this heading.

Valproate Sodium (Concomitant use may decrease concentrations of valproic acid. Caution should be used when prescribing valproic acid. Valproic acid may be less effective due to decreased valproic acid concentrations in patients taking tipranavir concomitantly).
No products indexed under this heading.

Valproic Acid (Concomitant use may decrease concentrations of valproic acid. Caution should be used when prescribing valproic acid. Valproic acid may be less effective due to decreased valproic acid concentrations in patients taking tipranavir concomitantly).
No products indexed under this heading.

Vardenafil Hydrochloride (Concomitant use may increase levels of vardenafil. Concurrent use of PDE-5 inhibitors with tipranavir and ritonavir should be used with caution and in no case should the starting dose of vardenafil exceed 2.5 mg every 72 hours). Products include:
Levitra Tablets 2876

Venlafaxine Hydrochloride (Tipranavir co-administered with ritonavir at the recommended dose is a net inhibitor of CYP3A and may increase plasma concentrations of agents that are primarily metabolized by CYP3A. Thus, co-administration of tipranavir/ritonavir with drugs highly dependent on CYP3A for clearance and for which elevated plasma concentrations are associated with serious and/or life-threatening events is contraindicated. Co-administration with other CYP3A substrates may require a dose adjustment or additional monitoring). Products include:
Effexor XR Extended-Release Capsules 3195
Venlafaxine Hydrochloride Tablets ... 2199

Verapamil Hydrochloride (Concomitant use may increase or decrease verapamil concentrations. Caution is warranted and clinical monitoring of patients is recommended). Products include:
Tarka Tablets 511

Vinblastine Sulfate (Tipranavir co-administered with ritonavir at the recommended dose is a net inhibitor of CYP3A and may increase plasma concentrations of agents that are primarily metabolized by CYP3A. Thus, co-administration of tipranavir/ritonavir with drugs highly dependent on CYP3A for clearance and for which elevated plasma concentrations are associated with serious and/or life-threatening events is contraindicated. Co-administration with other CYP3A substrates may require a dose adjustment or additional monitoring).
No products indexed under this heading.

Vincristine Sulfate (Tipranavir co-administered with ritonavir at the recommended dose is a net inhibitor of CYP3A and may increase plasma concentrations of agents that are primarily metabolized by CYP3A. Thus, co-administration of tipranavir/ritonavir with drugs highly dependent on CYP3A for clearance and for which elevated plasma concentrations are associated with serious and/or life-threatening events is contraindicated. Co-administration with other CYP3A substrates may require a dose adjustment or additional monitoring).
No products indexed under this heading.

Vitamin E (Patients taking tipranavir oral solution should be advised not to take supplemental vitamin E greater than a standard multivitamin as tipranavir oral solution contains 116 IU/mL of vitamin E and when taken at the recommended dose of 500 mg/200 mg tipranavir/ritonavir b.i.d., results in a daily dose of 1160 IU. This intake is higher than the Reference Daily Intake (adults 30 IU, pediatrics approximately 10 IU)). Products include:

Bausch & Lomb Ocuvite Adult 50+ Vitamin and Mineral Supplement .... ⊙ 237
Comax Dietary Supplement 995
Glaucofit Dietary Supplement 995
Glauma Dietary Supplement 995
MarineOmega Softgel Capsules 2560
Norwegian Cod Liver Oil 949
Tonox Dietary Supplement 995
Vibe Liquid Multi-Nutrient Supplement .... ▣ 626

Voriconazole (Due to multiple enzymes involved with voriconazole metabolism, it is difficult to predict the interaction).
No products indexed under this heading.

Warfarin Sodium (Frequent INR (international normalized ratio) monitoring upon initiation of tipranavir/ritonavir therapy is recommended).
No products indexed under this heading.

Zidovudine (Concomitant use with zidovudine decreased zidovudine AUC by approximately 35%. The clinical relevance of reduction in zidovudine levels has not been established. Dose adjustment of zidovudine cannot be recommended at this time). Products include:

Combivir Tablets 1384
Retrovir 1574
Retrovir IV Infusion 1579
Trizivir Tablets 1622

ARALAST

(Alpha$_1$-Proteinase Inhibitor (Human)) 726
None cited in PDR database.

ARANESP FOR INJECTION

(Darbepoetin alfa) 564
None cited in PDR database.

ARGATROBAN INJECTION

(Argatroban) 1308
May interact with anticoagulants, thrombolytics, and certain other agents. Compounds in these categories include:

Alteplase (Co-administration with thrombolytic agents may increase the risk of bleeding). Products include:

Activase I.V. 1188
Cathflo Activase 1198

Anisindione (Co-administration with other anticoagulants may increase the risk of bleeding).
No products indexed under this heading.

Anistreplase (Co-administration with thrombolytic agents may increase the risk of bleeding).
No products indexed under this heading.

Ardeparin Sodium (Co-administration with other anticoagulants may increase the risk of bleeding).
No products indexed under this heading.

Aspirin (Co-administration with antiplatelet agents, such as aspirin, may increase the risk of bleeding). Products include:

Aggrenox Capsules 819
Bayer Aspirin 750
Percodan Tablets 1130
St. Joseph 81 mg Aspirin Chewable and Enteric Coated Tablets 1903

Bivalirudin (Co-administration with thrombolytic agents may increase the risk of bleeding). Products include:

Angiomax for Injection 1933

Clopidogrel Bisulfate (Co-administration with antiplatelet agents may increase the risk of bleeding). Products include:

Plavix Tablets 926
Plavix Tablets 2767

Dalteparin Sodium (Co-administration with other anticoagulants may increase the risk of bleeding). Products include:

Fragmin Injection 1070

Danaparoid Sodium (Co-administration with other anticoagulants may increase the risk of bleeding).
No products indexed under this heading.

Dicumarol (Co-administration with other anticoagulants may increase the risk of bleeding).
No products indexed under this heading.

Dipyridamole (Co-administration with antiplatelet agents may increase the risk of bleeding). Products include:

Aggrenox Capsules 819
Persantine Tablets 869

Enoxaparin Sodium (Co-administration with other anticoagulants may increase the risk of bleeding). Products include:

Lovenox Injection 2756

Fondaparinux Sodium (Co-administration with other anticoagulants may increase the risk of bleeding). Products include:

Arixtra Injection 1313

Heparin Calcium (Co-administration with other anticoagulants may increase the risk of bleeding).
No products indexed under this heading.

Heparin Sodium (Co-administration with other anticoagulants may increase the risk of bleeding).
No products indexed under this heading.

Low Molecular Weight Heparins (Co-administration with other anticoagulants may increase the risk of bleeding).
No products indexed under this heading.

Reteplase (Co-administration with thrombolytic agents may increase the risk of bleeding).
No products indexed under this heading.

Streptokinase (Co-administration with thrombolytic agents may increase the risk of bleeding).
No products indexed under this heading.

Tinzaparin Sodium (Co-administration with other anticoagulants may increase the risk of bleeding).
No products indexed under this heading.

Urokinase (Co-administration with thrombolytic agents may increase the risk of bleeding).
No products indexed under this heading.

Warfarin Sodium (Co-administration with other anticoagulants may increase the risk of bleeding).
No products indexed under this heading.

ARICEPT TABLETS

(Donepezil Hydrochloride) 1062
May interact with anticholinergics, cytochrome p450 2d6 inducers (selected), cytochrome p450 3a4 inducers (selected), dexamethasone, non-steroidal anti-inflammatory agents, phenytoin, quinidine, and certain other agents. Compounds in these categories include:

Allium sativum (Inducers of CYP3A4 could increase the rate of elimination of donepezil).
No products indexed under this heading.

Aprepitant (Inducers of CYP3A4 could increase the rate of elimination of donepezil). Products include:

Emend Capsules 1992

Atropine Sulfate (Donepezil, a cholinesterase inhibitor, has the potential to interfere with the activity of anticholinergic medications). Products include:

Donnatal Extentabs 2507

Belladonna Alkaloids (Donepezil, a cholinesterase inhibitor, has the potential to interfere with the activity of anticholinergic medications). Products include:

Hyland's Teething Tablets .... ▣ 621

Benztropine Mesylate (Donepezil, a cholinesterase inhibitor, has the potential to interfere with the activity of anticholinergic medications).
No products indexed under this heading.

Betamethasone Acetate (Inducers of CYP3A4 could increase the rate of elimination of donepezil).
No products indexed under this heading.

Betamethasone Sodium Phosphate (Inducers of CYP3A4 could increase the rate of elimination of donepezil).
No products indexed under this heading.

Bethanechol Chloride (Potential for synergistic effect).
No products indexed under this heading.

Biperiden Hydrochloride (Donepezil, a cholinesterase inhibitor, has the potential to interfere with the activity of anticholinergic medications).
No products indexed under this heading.

Carbamazepine (Inducers of CYP2D6 and CYP3A4, such as carbamazepine, could increase the rate of elimination of donepezil). Products include:

Carbatrol Capsules 3019
Equetro Extended-Release Capsules 3174

Celecoxib (Cholinesterase inhibitors, such as donepezil, may be expected to increase gastric acid secretion due to increased cholinergic activity, therefore, patients on concurrent NSAID therapy should be monitored closely for increased risk of developing ulcers or symptoms of active or occult gastrointestinal bleeding). Products include:

Celebrex Capsules 2979

Ciprofloxacin Hydrochloride (Inducers of CYP3A4 could increase the rate of elimination of donepezil). Products include:

Cipro Tablets 2810

Cisplatin (Inducers of CYP3A4 could increase the rate of elimination of donepezil).
No products indexed under this heading.

Clidinium Bromide (Donepezil, a cholinesterase inhibitor, has the potential to interfere with the activity of anticholinergic medications).
No products indexed under this heading.

Cortisone Acetate (Inducers of CYP3A4 could increase the rate of elimination of donepezil).
No products indexed under this heading.

Dexamethasone (Inducers of CYP2D6 and CYP3A4, such as dexamethasone, could increase the rate of elimination of donepezil). Products include:

Ciprodex Otic Suspension 541

Dexamethasone Acetate (Inducers of CYP2D6 and CYP3A4, such as dexamethasone, could increase the rate of elimination of donepezil).
No products indexed under this heading.

Dexamethasone Sodium Phosphate (Inducers of CYP2D6 and CYP3A4, such as dexamethasone, could increase the rate of elimination of donepezil).
No products indexed under this heading.

Diclofenac Epolamine (Cholinesterase inhibitors, such as donepezil, may be expected to increase gastric acid secretion due to increased cholinergic activity, therefore, patients on concurrent NSAID therapy should be monitored closely for increased risk of developing ulcers or symptoms of active or occult gastrointestinal bleeding). Products include:

Flector Patch 561

Diclofenac Potassium (Cholinesterase inhibitors, such as donepezil, may be expected to increase gastric acid secretion due to increased cholinergic activity, therefore, patients on concurrent NSAID therapy should be monitored closely for increased risk of developing ulcers or symptoms of active or occult gastrointestinal bleeding).
No products indexed under this heading.

Diclofenac Sodium (Cholinesterase inhibitors, such as donepezil, may be expected to increase gastric acid secretion due to increased cholinergic activity, therefore, patients on concurrent NSAID therapy should be monitored closely for increased risk of developing ulcers or symptoms of active or occult gastrointestinal bleeding). Products include:

Diclofenac Sodium Ophthalmic Solution .... ⊙ 240
Voltaren Ophthalmic Solution 2336
Voltaren Tablets 2334
Voltaren-XR Tablets 2337

Dicyclomine Hydrochloride (Donepezil, a cholinesterase inhibitor, has the potential to interfere with the activity of anticholinergic medications). Products include:

Bentyl Capsules 703
Bentyl Injection 703
Bentyl Syrup 703
Bentyl Tablets 703

Doxorubicin Hydrochloride (Inducers of CYP3A4 could increase the rate of elimination of donepezil).
No products indexed under this heading.

Efavirenz (Inducers of CYP3A4 could increase the rate of elimination of donepezil). Products include:
Atripla Tablets **938**
Sustiva Capsules **930**
Sustiva Tablets **930**

Ethanol (Inducers of CYP2D6 could increase the rate of elimination of donepezil).
No products indexed under this heading.

Ethosuximide (Inducers of CYP3A4 could increase the rate of elimination of donepezil).
No products indexed under this heading.

Etodolac (Cholinesterase inhibitors, such as donepezil, may be expected to increase gastric acid secretion due to increased cholinergic activity, therefore, patients on concurrent NSAID therapy should be monitored closely for increased risk of developing ulcers or symptoms of active or occult gastrointestinal bleeding).
No products indexed under this heading.

Felbamate (Inducers of CYP3A4 could increase the rate of elimination of donepezil).
No products indexed under this heading.

Fenoprofen Calcium (Cholinesterase inhibitors, such as donepezil, may be expected to increase gastric acid secretion due to increased cholinergic activity, therefore, patients on concurrent NSAID therapy should be monitored closely for increased risk of developing ulcers or symptoms of active or occult gastrointestinal bleeding). Products include:
Nalfon Capsules **2508**

Fludrocortisone Acetate (Inducers of CYP3A4 could increase the rate of elimination of donepezil).
No products indexed under this heading.

Flurbiprofen (Cholinesterase inhibitors, such as donepezil, may be expected to increase gastric acid secretion due to increased cholinergic activity, therefore, patients on concurrent NSAID therapy should be monitored closely for increased risk of developing ulcers or symptoms of active or occult gastrointestinal bleeding).
No products indexed under this heading.

Fosphenytoin Sodium (Inducers of CYP2D6 and CYP3A4, such as phenytoin, could increase the rate of elimination of donepezil).
No products indexed under this heading.

Garlic Extract (Inducers of CYP3A4 could increase the rate of elimination of donepezil).
No products indexed under this heading.

Garlic Oil (Inducers of CYP3A4 could increase the rate of elimination of donepezil).
No products indexed under this heading.

Glycopyrrolate (Donepezil, a cholinesterase inhibitor, has the potential to interfere with the activity of anticholinergic medications).
No products indexed under this heading.

Hydrocortisone (Inducers of CYP3A4 could increase the rate of elimination of donepezil).
No products indexed under this heading.

Hydrocortisone Acetate (Inducers of CYP3A4 could increase the rate of elimination of donepezil). Products include:
Analpram-HC **1140**
Pramosone **1141**

Hydrocortisone Butyrate (Inducers of CYP3A4 could increase the rate of elimination of donepezil).
No products indexed under this heading.

Hydrocortisone Cypionate (Inducers of CYP3A4 could increase the rate of elimination of donepezil).
No products indexed under this heading.

Hydrocortisone Hemisuccinate (Inducers of CYP3A4 could increase the rate of elimination of donepezil).
No products indexed under this heading.

Hydrocortisone Probutate (Inducers of CYP3A4 could increase the rate of elimination of donepezil).
No products indexed under this heading.

Hydrocortisone Sodium Phosphate (Inducers of CYP3A4 could increase the rate of elimination of donepezil).
No products indexed under this heading.

Hydrocortisone Sodium Succinate (Inducers of CYP3A4 could increase the rate of elimination of donepezil).
No products indexed under this heading.

Hydrocortisone Valerate (Inducers of CYP3A4 could increase the rate of elimination of donepezil).
No products indexed under this heading.

Hyoscyamine (Donepezil, a cholinesterase inhibitor, has the potential to interfere with the activity of anticholinergic medications).
No products indexed under this heading.

Hyoscyamine Sulfate (Donepezil, a cholinesterase inhibitor, has the potential to interfere with the activity of anticholinergic medications). Products include:
Donnatal Extentabs **2507**

Hypericum (Inducers of CYP3A4 could increase the rate of elimination of donepezil). Products include:
Satieté Tablets .... ▣ **640**

Hypericum Perforatum (Inducers of CYP3A4 could increase the rate of elimination of donepezil).
No products indexed under this heading.

Ibuprofen (Cholinesterase inhibitors, such as donepezil, may be expected to increase gastric acid secretion due to increased cholinergic activity, therefore, patients on concurrent NSAID therapy should be monitored closely for increased risk of developing ulcers or symptoms of active or occult gastrointestinal bleeding). Products include:
Motrin IB Tablets and Caplets **1900**
Children's Motrin Oral Suspension ... **1901**
Children's Motrin Non-Staining Dye-Free Oral Suspension **1901**
Children's Motrin Cold Oral Suspension **1899**
Infants' Motrin Concentrated Drops **1901**
Infants' Motrin Non-Staining Dye-Free Concentrated Drops **1901**
Junior Strength Motrin Caplets and Chewable Tablets **1901**
Vicoprofen Tablets **533**

Indomethacin (Cholinesterase inhibitors, such as donepezil, may be expected to increase gastric acid secretion due to increased cholinergic activity, therefore, patients on concurrent NSAID therapy should be monitored closely for increased risk of developing ulcers or symptoms of active or occult gastrointestinal bleeding). Products include:
Indocin **2024**

Indomethacin Sodium Trihydrate (Cholinesterase inhibitors, such as donepezil, may be expected to increase gastric acid secretion due to increased cholinergic activity, therefore, patients on concurrent NSAID therapy should be monitored closely for increased risk of developing ulcers or symptoms of active or occult gastrointestinal bleeding). Products include:
Indocin I.V. **2489**

Ipratropium Bromide (Donepezil, a cholinesterase inhibitor, has the potential to interfere with the activity of anticholinergic medications). Products include:
Atrovent HFA Inhalation Aerosol **839**
Atrovent Nasal Spray 0.03% **834**
Atrovent Nasal Spray 0.06% **836**
Combivent Inhalation Aerosol **845**

Ketoconazole (Inhibitors of CYP450, 2D6 and 3A4, such as ketoconazole, inhibit donepezil metabolism in vitro. In a crossover study, ketoconazole increased mean donepezil concentrations by 36%; the clinical relevance is unknown). Products include:
Extina Foam, 2% **3057**
Nizoral A-D Shampoo **1901**

Ketoprofen (Cholinesterase inhibitors, such as donepezil, may be expected to increase gastric acid secretion due to increased cholinergic activity, therefore, patients on concurrent NSAID therapy should be monitored closely for increased risk of developing ulcers or symptoms of active or occult gastrointestinal bleeding).
No products indexed under this heading.

Ketorolac Tromethamine (Cholinesterase inhibitors, such as donepezil, may be expected to increase gastric acid secretion due to increased cholinergic activity, therefore, patients on concurrent NSAID therapy should be monitored closely for increased risk of developing ulcers or symptoms of active or occult gastrointestinal bleeding).
No products indexed under this heading.

Meclofenamate Sodium (Cholinesterase inhibitors, such as donepezil, may be expected to increase gastric acid secretion due to increased cholinergic activity, therefore, patients on concurrent NSAID therapy should be monitored closely for increased risk of developing ulcers or symptoms of active or occult gastrointestinal bleeding).
No products indexed under this heading.

Mefenamic Acid (Cholinesterase inhibitors, such as donepezil, may be expected to increase gastric acid secretion due to increased cholinergic activity, therefore, patients on concurrent NSAID therapy should be monitored closely for increased risk of developing ulcers or symptoms of active or occult gastrointestinal bleeding).
No products indexed under this heading.

Meloxicam (Cholinesterase inhibitors, such as donepezil, may be expected to increase gastric acid secretion due to increased cholinergic activity, therefore, patients on concurrent NSAID therapy should be monitored closely for increased risk of developing ulcers or symptoms of active or occult gastrointestinal bleeding). Products include:
Mobic Oral Suspension **863**
Mobic Tablets **863**

Mepenzolate Bromide (Donepezil, a cholinesterase inhibitor, has the potential to interfere with the activity of anticholinergic medications).
No products indexed under this heading.

Mephenytoin (Inducers of CYP3A4 could increase the rate of elimination of donepezil).
No products indexed under this heading.

Methsuximide (Inducers of CYP3A4 could increase the rate of elimination of donepezil).
No products indexed under this heading.

Methylprednisolone (Inducers of CYP3A4 could increase the rate of elimination of donepezil).
No products indexed under this heading.

Methylprednisolone Acetate (Inducers of CYP3A4 could increase the rate of elimination of donepezil).
No products indexed under this heading.

Methylprednisolone Sodium Succinate (Inducers of CYP3A4 could increase the rate of elimination of donepezil).
No products indexed under this heading.

Modafinil (Inducers of CYP3A4 could increase the rate of elimination of donepezil). Products include:
Provigil Tablets **977**

Nabumetone (Cholinesterase inhibitors, such as donepezil, may be expected to increase gastric acid secretion due to increased cholinergic activity, therefore, patients on concurrent NSAID therapy should be monitored closely for increased risk of developing ulcers or symptoms of active or occult gastrointestinal bleeding).
No products indexed under this heading.

Naproxen (Cholinesterase inhibitors, such as donepezil, may be expected to increase gastric acid secretion due to increased cholinergic activity, therefore, patients on concurrent NSAID therapy should be monitored closely for increased risk of developing ulcers or symptoms of active or occult gastrointestinal bleeding). Products include:
EC-Naprosyn Delayed-Release Tablets **2632**
Naprosyn Suspension **2632**
Naprosyn Tablets **2632**

Naproxen Sodium (Cholinesterase inhibitors, such as donepezil, may be expected to increase gastric acid secretion due to increased cholinergic activity, therefore, patients on concurrent NSAID therapy should be monitored closely for increased risk of developing ulcers or symptoms of active or occult gastrointestinal bleeding). Products include:
- Anaprox Tablets 2632
- Anaprox DS Tablets 2632
- Treximet Tablets 1616

Nevirapine (Inducers of CYP3A4 could increase the rate of elimination of donepezil). Products include:
- Viramune Oral Suspension 873
- Viramune Tablets 873

Oxaprozin (Cholinesterase inhibitors, such as donepezil, may be expected to increase gastric acid secretion due to increased cholinergic activity, therefore, patients on concurrent NSAID therapy should be monitored closely for increased risk of developing ulcers or symptoms of active or occult gastrointestinal bleeding).
No products indexed under this heading.

Oxcarbazepine (Inducers of CYP3A4 could increase the rate of elimination of donepezil).
No products indexed under this heading.

Oxybutynin Chloride (Donepezil, a cholinesterase inhibitor, has the potential to interfere with the activity of anticholinergic medications).
No products indexed under this heading.

Phenobarbital (Inducers of CYP2D6 and CYP3A4, such as phenobarbital, could increase the rate of elimination of donepezil). Products include:
- Donnatal Extentabs 2507

Phenobarbital Sodium (Inducers of CYP3A4 could increase the rate of elimination of donepezil).
No products indexed under this heading.

Phenylbutazone (Cholinesterase inhibitors, such as donepezil, may be expected to increase gastric acid secretion due to increased cholinergic activity, therefore, patients on concurrent NSAID therapy should be monitored closely for increased risk of developing ulcers or symptoms of active or occult gastrointestinal bleeding).
No products indexed under this heading.

Phenytoin (Inducers of CYP2D6 and CYP3A4, such as phenytoin, could increase the rate of elimination of donepezil).
No products indexed under this heading.

Phenytoin Sodium (Inducers of CYP2D6 and CYP3A4, such as phenytoin, could increase the rate of elimination of donepezil). Products include:
- Phenytek Capsules 2192

Piroxicam (Cholinesterase inhibitors, such as donepezil, may be expected to increase gastric acid secretion due to increased cholinergic activity, therefore, patients on concurrent NSAID therapy should be monitored closely for increased risk of developing ulcers or symptoms of active or occult gastrointestinal bleeding).
No products indexed under this heading.

Prednisolone Acetate (Inducers of CYP3A4 could increase the rate of elimination of donepezil). Products include:
- Pred Forte Ophthalmic Suspension .... ⊙227
- Pred Mild Ophthalmic Suspension .... ⊙230
- Pred-G Ophthalmic Ointment .... ⊙229
- Pred-G Ophthalmic Suspension .... ⊙228

Prednisolone Sodium Phosphate (Inducers of CYP3A4 could increase the rate of elimination of donepezil).
No products indexed under this heading.

Prednisolone Tebutate (Inducers of CYP3A4 could increase the rate of elimination of donepezil).
No products indexed under this heading.

Prednisone (Inducers of CYP3A4 could increase the rate of elimination of donepezil).
No products indexed under this heading.

Primidone (Inducers of CYP3A4 could increase the rate of elimination of donepezil).
No products indexed under this heading.

Procyclidine Hydrochloride (Donepezil, a cholinesterase inhibitor, has the potential to interfere with the activity of anticholinergic medications).
No products indexed under this heading.

Propantheline Bromide (Donepezil, a cholinesterase inhibitor, has the potential to interfere with the activity of anticholinergic medications).
No products indexed under this heading.

Quinidine (Inhibitors of CYP450, 2D6 and 3A4, such as quinidine, inhibit donepezil metabolism in vitro).
No products indexed under this heading.

Quinidine Gluconate (Inhibitors of CYP450, 2D6 and 3A4, such as quinidine, inhibit donepezil metabolism in vitro).
No products indexed under this heading.

Quinidine Hydrochloride (Inhibitors of CYP450, 2D6 and 3A4, such as quinidine, inhibit donepezil metabolism in vitro).
No products indexed under this heading.

Quinidine Polygalacturonate (Inhibitors of CYP450, 2D6 and 3A4, such as quinidine, inhibit donepezil metabolism in vitro).
No products indexed under this heading.

Quinidine Sulfate (Inhibitors of CYP450, 2D6 and 3A4, such as quinidine, inhibit donepezil metabolism in vitro).
No products indexed under this heading.

Rifabutin (Inducers of CYP3A4 could increase the rate of elimination of donepezil).
No products indexed under this heading.

Rifampicin (Inducers of CYP3A4 could increase the rate of elimination of donepezil).
No products indexed under this heading.

Rifampin (Inducers of CYP2D6 and CYP3A4, such as rifampin, could increase the rate of elimination of donepezil).
No products indexed under this heading.

Rifapentine (Inducers of CYP3A4 could increase the rate of elimination of donepezil).
No products indexed under this heading.

Ritonavir (Inducers of CYP2D6 could increase the rate of elimination of donepezil). Products include:
- Kaletra 452
- Norvir 489

Rofecoxib (Cholinesterase inhibitors, such as donepezil, may be expected to increase gastric acid secretion due to increased cholinergic activity, therefore, patients on concurrent NSAID therapy should be monitored closely for increased risk of developing ulcers or symptoms of active or occult gastrointestinal bleeding).
No products indexed under this heading.

Scopolamine (Donepezil, a cholinesterase inhibitor, has the potential to interfere with the activity of anticholinergic medications). Products include:
- Transderm Scōp Transdermal Therapeutic System 2206

Scopolamine Hydrobromide (Donepezil, a cholinesterase inhibitor, has the potential to interfere with the activity of anticholinergic medications). Products include:
- Donnatal Extentabs 2507

Succinylcholine Chloride (Potential for synergistic effect).
No products indexed under this heading.

Sulfinpyrazone (Inducers of CYP3A4 could increase the rate of elimination of donepezil).
No products indexed under this heading.

Sulindac (Cholinesterase inhibitors, such as donepezil, may be expected to increase gastric acid secretion due to increased cholinergic activity, therefore, patients on concurrent NSAID therapy should be monitored closely for increased risk of developing ulcers or symptoms of active or occult gastrointestinal bleeding). Products include:
- Clinoril Tablets 1962

Theophylline (Inducers of CYP3A4 could increase the rate of elimination of donepezil).
No products indexed under this heading.

Theophylline Anhydrous (Inducers of CYP3A4 could increase the rate of elimination of donepezil). Products include:
- Uniphyl Tablets 2595

Theophylline Calcium Salicylate (Inducers of CYP3A4 could increase the rate of elimination of donepezil).
No products indexed under this heading.

Theophylline Dihydroxypropyl (Glyceryl) (Inducers of CYP3A4 could increase the rate of elimination of donepezil).
No products indexed under this heading.

Theophylline Ethylenediamine (Inducers of CYP3A4 could increase the rate of elimination of donepezil).
No products indexed under this heading.

Tolmetin Sodium (Cholinesterase inhibitors, such as donepezil, may be expected to increase gastric acid secretion due to increased cholinergic activity, therefore, patients on concurrent NSAID therapy should be monitored closely for increased risk of developing ulcers or symptoms of active or occult gastrointestinal bleeding).
No products indexed under this heading.

Tolterodine Tartrate (Donepezil, a cholinesterase inhibitor, has the potential to interfere with the activity of anticholinergic medications).
No products indexed under this heading.

Triamcinolone (Inducers of CYP3A4 could increase the rate of elimination of donepezil).
No products indexed under this heading.

Triamcinolone Acetonide (Inducers of CYP3A4 could increase the rate of elimination of donepezil). Products include:
- Azmacort Inhalation Aerosol 407
- Nasacort AQ Nasal Spray 2765
- Triesence Injectable Suspension .... ⊙209

Triamcinolone Diacetate (Inducers of CYP3A4 could increase the rate of elimination of donepezil).
No products indexed under this heading.

Triamcinolone Hexacetonide (Inducers of CYP3A4 could increase the rate of elimination of donepezil).
No products indexed under this heading.

Tridihexethyl Chloride (Donepezil, a cholinesterase inhibitor, has the potential to interfere with the activity of anticholinergic medications).
No products indexed under this heading.

Trihexyphenidyl Hydrochloride (Donepezil, a cholinesterase inhibitor, has the potential to interfere with the activity of anticholinergic medications).
No products indexed under this heading.

Troglitazone (Inducers of CYP3A4 could increase the rate of elimination of donepezil).
No products indexed under this heading.

Valdecoxib (Cholinesterase inhibitors, such as donepezil, may be expected to increase gastric acid secretion due to increased cholinergic activity, therefore, patients on concurrent NSAID therapy should be monitored closely for increased risk of developing ulcers or symptoms of active or occult gastrointestinal bleeding).
No products indexed under this heading.

ARICEPT ODT TABLETS

(Donepezil Hydrochloride) 1062
See Aricept Tablets

ARIMIDEX TABLETS

(Anastrozole) 672
May interact with estrogens and certain other agents. Compounds in these categories include:

Chlorotrianisene (Estrogen-containing therapies should not be used with anastrozole as they may diminish its pharmacologic action).
No products indexed under this heading.

Dienestrol (Estrogen-containing therapies should not be used with anastrozole as they may diminish its pharmacologic action).
No products indexed under this heading.

Diethylstilbestrol (Estrogen-containing therapies should not be used with anastrozole as they may diminish its pharmacologic action).
No products indexed under this heading.

Estradiol (Estrogen-containing therapies should not be used with anastrozole as they may diminish its pharmacologic action). Products include:
Activella Tablets 2347
Angeliq Tablets 751
Climara Transdermal System 763
Climara Pro Transdermal System 768
Divigel 3167
Vagifem Tablets 2375

Estrogens, Conjugated (Estrogen-containing therapies should not be used with anastrozole as they may diminish its pharmacologic action).
Products include:
Premarin Intravenous 3217
Premarin Tablets 3221
Premarin Vaginal Cream 3228
Premphase Tablets 3232
Prempro Tablets 3232

Estrogens, Esterified (Estrogen-containing therapies should not be used with anastrozole as they may diminish its pharmacologic action).
Products include:
Estratest Tablets 3043
Estratest H.S. Tablets 3043

Estropipate (Estrogen-containing therapies should not be used with anastrozole as they may diminish its pharmacologic action).
No products indexed under this heading.

Ethinyl Estradiol (Estrogen-containing therapies should not be used with anastrozole as they may diminish its pharmacologic action).
Products include:
Lybrel Tablets 3204
Mircette Tablets 1034
NuvaRing 2897
Ortho-Cyclen/Ortho Tri-Cyclen 2449
Ortho Evra Transdermal System 2437
Ortho Tri-Cyclen Lo Tablets 2458
Seasonique Tablets 1046
Yaz Tablets 805

Polyestradiol Phosphate (Estrogen-containing therapies should not be used with anastrozole as they may diminish its pharmacologic action).
No products indexed under this heading.

Quinestrol (Estrogen-containing therapies should not be used with anastrozole as they may diminish its pharmacologic action).
No products indexed under this heading.

Tamoxifen Citrate (Co-administration of tamoxifen and anastrozole may reduce anastrozole plasma concentration; avoid co-administration).
No products indexed under this heading.

ARIXTRA INJECTION

(Fondaparinux Sodium) 1313
May interact with anticoagulants, non-steroidal anti-inflammatory agents, and certain other agents. Compounds in these categories include:

Abciximab (Agents that may enhance the risk of hemorrhage, such as abciximab, should be discontinued prior to initiation of fondaparinux sodium therapy. If co-administration is essential, close monitoring may be appropriate). Products include:
ReoPro Vials 1860

Anisindione (Agents that may enhance the risk of hemorrhage, such as anticoagulants, should be discontinued prior to initiation of fondaparinux sodium therapy. If co-administration is essential, close monitoring may be appropriate).
No products indexed under this heading.

Ardeparin Sodium (Agents that may enhance the risk of hemorrhage, such as anticoagulants, should be discontinued prior to initiation of fondaparinux sodium therapy. If co-administration is essential, close monitoring may be appropriate).
No products indexed under this heading.

Aspirin (Agents that may enhance the risk of hemorrhage, such as aspirin, should be discontinued prior to initiation of fondaparinux sodium therapy. If co-administration is essential, close monitoring may be appropriate). Products include:
Aggrenox Capsules 819
Bayer Aspirin 750
Percodan Tablets 1130
St. Joseph 81 mg Aspirin Chewable and Enteric Coated Tablets 1903

Celecoxib (Agents that may enhance the risk of hemorrhage, such as non-steroidal anti-inflammatory agents, should be discontinued prior to initiation of fondaparinux sodium therapy. If co-administration is essential, close monitoring may be appropriate). Products include:
Celebrex Capsules 2979

Clopidogrel Bisulfate (Agents that may enhance the risk of hemorrhage, such as clopidogrel bisulfate, should be discontinued prior to initiation of fondaparinux sodium therapy. If co-administration is essential, close monitoring may be appropriate). Products include:
Plavix Tablets 926
Plavix Tablets 2767

Dalteparin Sodium (Agents that may enhance the risk of hemorrhage, such as anticoagulants, should be discontinued prior to initiation of fondaparinux sodium therapy. If co-administration is essential, close monitoring may be appropriate). Products include:
Fragmin Injection 1070

Danaparoid Sodium (Agents that may enhance the risk of hemorrhage, such as anticoagulants, should be discontinued prior to initiation of fondaparinux sodium therapy. If co-administration is essential, close monitoring may be appropriate).
No products indexed under this heading.

Diclofenac Epolamine (Agents that may enhance the risk of hemorrhage, such as non-steroidal anti-inflammatory agents, should be discontinued prior to initiation of fondaparinux sodium therapy. If co-administration is essential, close monitoring may be appropriate).
Products include:
Flector Patch 561

Diclofenac Potassium (Agents that may enhance the risk of hemorrhage, such as non-steroidal anti-inflammatory agents, should be discontinued prior to initiation of fondaparinux sodium therapy. If co-administration is essential, close monitoring may be appropriate).
No products indexed under this heading.

Diclofenac Sodium (Agents that may enhance the risk of hemorrhage, such as non-steroidal anti-inflammatory agents, should be discontinued prior to initiation of fondaparinux sodium therapy. If co-administration is essential, close monitoring may be appropriate).
Products include:
Diclofenac Sodium Ophthalmic Solution .... ⊙ 240
Voltaren Ophthalmic Solution 2336
Voltaren Tablets 2334
Voltaren-XR Tablets 2337

Dicumarol (Agents that may enhance the risk of hemorrhage, such as anticoagulants, should be discontinued prior to initiation of fondaparinux sodium therapy. If co-administration is essential, close monitoring may be appropriate).
No products indexed under this heading.

Dipyridamole (Agents that may enhance the risk of hemorrhage, such as dipyridamole, should be discontinued prior to initiation of fondaparinux sodium therapy. If co-administration is essential, close monitoring may be appropriate).
Products include:
Aggrenox Capsules 819
Persantine Tablets 869

Enoxaparin Sodium (Agents that may enhance the risk of hemorrhage, such as anticoagulants, should be discontinued prior to initiation of fondaparinux sodium therapy. If co-administration is essential, close monitoring may be appropriate). Products include:
Lovenox Injection 2756

Eptifibatide (Agents that may enhance the risk of hemorrhage, such as eptifibatide, should be discontinued prior to initiation of fondaparinux sodium therapy. If co-administration is essential, close monitoring may be appropriate).
Products include:
Integrilin Injection 2855

Etodolac (Agents that may enhance the risk of hemorrhage, such as non-steroidal anti-inflammatory agents, should be discontinued prior to initiation of fondaparinux sodium therapy. If co-administration is essential, close monitoring may be appropriate).
No products indexed under this heading.

Fenoprofen Calcium (Agents that may enhance the risk of hemorrhage, such as non-steroidal anti-inflammatory agents, should be discontinued prior to initiation of fondaparinux sodium therapy. If co-administration is essential, close monitoring may be appropriate).
Products include:
Nalfon Capsules 2508

Flurbiprofen (Agents that may enhance the risk of hemorrhage, such as non-steroidal anti-inflammatory agents, should be discontinued prior to initiation of fondaparinux sodium therapy. If co-administration is essential, close monitoring may be appropriate).
No products indexed under this heading.

Heparin Calcium (Agents that may enhance the risk of hemorrhage, such as anticoagulants, should be discontinued prior to initiation of fondaparinux sodium therapy. If co-administration is essential, close monitoring may be appropriate).
No products indexed under this heading.

Heparin Sodium (Agents that may enhance the risk of hemorrhage, such as anticoagulants, should be discontinued prior to initiation of fondaparinux sodium therapy. If co-administration is essential, close monitoring may be appropriate).
No products indexed under this heading.

Ibuprofen (Agents that may enhance the risk of hemorrhage, such as non-steroidal anti-inflammatory agents, should be discontinued prior to initiation of fondaparinux sodium therapy. If co-administration is essential, close monitoring may be appropriate). Products include:
Motrin IB Tablets and Caplets 1900
Children's Motrin Oral Suspension 1901
Children's Motrin Non-Staining Dye-Free Oral Suspension 1901
Children's Motrin Cold Oral Suspension 1899
Infants' Motrin Concentrated Drops 1901
Infants' Motrin Non-Staining Dye-Free Concentrated Drops 1901
Junior Strength Motrin Caplets and Chewable Tablets 1901
Vicoprofen Tablets 533

Indomethacin (Agents that may enhance the risk of hemorrhage, such as non-steroidal anti-inflammatory agents, should be discontinued prior to initiation of fondaparinux sodium therapy. If co-administration is essential, close monitoring may be appropriate). Products include:
Indocin 2024

Indomethacin Sodium Trihydrate (Agents that may enhance the risk of hemorrhage, such as non-steroidal anti-inflammatory agents, should be discontinued prior to initiation of fondaparinux sodium therapy. If co-administration is essential, close monitoring may be appropriate). Products include:
Indocin I.V. 2489

Ketoprofen (Agents that may enhance the risk of hemorrhage, such as non-steroidal anti-inflammatory agents, should be discontinued prior to initiation of fondaparinux sodium therapy. If co-administration is essential, close monitoring may be appropriate).
No products indexed under this heading.

Ketorolac Tromethamine (Agents that may enhance the risk of hemorrhage, such as non-steroidal anti-inflammatory agents, should be discontinued prior to initiation of fondaparinux sodium therapy. If co-administration is essential, close monitoring may be appropriate).
No products indexed under this heading.

Low Molecular Weight Heparins (Agents that may enhance the risk of hemorrhage, such as anticoagulants, should be discontinued prior to initiation of fondaparinux sodium therapy. If co-administration is essential, close monitoring may be appropriate).
No products indexed under this heading.

Meclofenamate Sodium (Agents that may enhance the risk of hemorrhage, such as non-steroidal anti-inflammatory agents, should be discontinued prior to initiation of fondaparinux sodium therapy. If co-administration is essential, close monitoring may be appropriate).
No products indexed under this heading.

Mefenamic Acid (Agents that may enhance the risk of hemorrhage, such as non-steroidal anti-inflammatory agents, should be discontinued prior to initiation of fondaparinux sodium therapy. If co-administration is essential, close monitoring may be appropriate).
No products indexed under this heading.

Meloxicam (Agents that may enhance the risk of hemorrhage, such as non-steroidal anti-inflammatory agents, should be discontinued prior to initiation of fondaparinux sodium therapy. If co-administration is essential, close monitoring may be appropriate). Products include:
Mobic Oral Suspension 863
Mobic Tablets 863

Nabumetone (Agents that may enhance the risk of hemorrhage, such as non-steroidal anti-inflammatory agents, should be discontinued prior to initiation of fondaparinux sodium therapy. If co-administration is essential, close monitoring may be appropriate).
No products indexed under this heading.

Naproxen (Agents that may enhance the risk of hemorrhage, such as non-steroidal anti-inflammatory agents, should be discontinued prior to initiation of fondaparinux sodium therapy. If co-administration is essential, close monitoring may be appropriate). Products include:
EC-Naprosyn Delayed-Release Tablets 2632
Naprosyn Suspension 2632
Naprosyn Tablets 2632

Naproxen Sodium (Agents that may enhance the risk of hemorrhage, such as non-steroidal anti-inflammatory agents, should be discontinued prior to initiation of fondaparinux sodium therapy. If co-administration is essential, close monitoring may be appropriate). Products include:
Anaprox Tablets 2632
Anaprox DS Tablets 2632
Treximet Tablets 1616

Oxaprozin (Agents that may enhance the risk of hemorrhage, such as non-steroidal anti-inflammatory agents, should be discontinued prior to initiation of fondaparinux sodium therapy. If co-administration is essential, close monitoring may be appropriate).
No products indexed under this heading.

Phenylbutazone (Agents that may enhance the risk of hemorrhage, such as non-steroidal anti-inflammatory agents, should be discontinued prior to initiation of fondaparinux sodium therapy. If co-administration is essential, close monitoring may be appropriate).
No products indexed under this heading.

Piroxicam (Agents that may enhance the risk of hemorrhage, such as non-steroidal anti-inflammatory agents, should be discontinued prior to initiation of fondaparinux sodium therapy. If co-administration is essential, close monitoring may be appropriate).
No products indexed under this heading.

Rofecoxib (Agents that may enhance the risk of hemorrhage, such as non-steroidal anti-inflammatory agents, should be discontinued prior to initiation of fondaparinux sodium therapy. If co-administration is essential, close monitoring may be appropriate).
No products indexed under this heading.

Sulindac (Agents that may enhance the risk of hemorrhage, such as non-steroidal anti-inflammatory agents, should be discontinued prior to initiation of fondaparinux sodium therapy. If co-administration is essential, close monitoring may be appropriate). Products include:
Clinoril Tablets 1962

Tinzaparin Sodium (Agents that may enhance the risk of hemorrhage, such as anticoagulants, should be discontinued prior to initiation of fondaparinux sodium therapy. If co-administration is essential, close monitoring may be appropriate).
No products indexed under this heading.

Tirofiban Hydrochloride (Agents that may enhance the risk of hemorrhage, such as tirofiban hydrochloride, should be discontinued prior to initiation of fondaparinux sodium therapy. If co-administration is essential, close monitoring may be appropriate).
No products indexed under this heading.

Tolmetin Sodium (Agents that may enhance the risk of hemorrhage, such as non-steroidal anti-inflammatory agents, should be discontinued prior to initiation of fondaparinux sodium therapy. If co-administration is essential, close monitoring may be appropriate).
No products indexed under this heading.

Valdecoxib (Agents that may enhance the risk of hemorrhage, such as non-steroidal anti-inflammatory agents, should be discontinued prior to initiation of fondaparinux sodium therapy. If co-administration is essential, close monitoring may be appropriate).
No products indexed under this heading.

Warfarin Sodium (Agents that may enhance the risk of hemorrhage, such as anticoagulants, should be discontinued prior to initiation of fondaparinux sodium therapy. If co-administration is essential, close monitoring may be appropriate).
No products indexed under this heading.

ARRANON INJECTION

(Nelarabine) 1319
May interact with:

Pentostatin (Co-administration of nelarabine with adenosine deaminase inhibitors, such as pentostatin, is not recommended).
No products indexed under this heading.

ASACOL DELAYED-RELEASE TABLETS

(Mesalamine) 2579
None cited in PDR database.

ASMANEX TWISTHALER

(Mometasone Furoate) 2797
May interact with:

Ketoconazole (Ketoconazone, a strong inhibitor of cytochrome P4503A4, may increase plasma levels of mometasone furoate during concomitant dosing). Products include:
Extina Foam, 2% 3057
Nizoral A-D Shampoo 1901

ATACAND TABLETS

(Candesartan Cilexetil) 639
May interact with lithium preparations. Compounds in these categories include:

Lithium (An increase in serum lithium concentration has been reported during concomitant administration of lithium with candesartan cilexetil, so careful monitoring of serum lithium levels is recommended during concomitant use).
No products indexed under this heading.

Lithium Carbonate (An increase in serum lithium concentration has been reported during concomitant administration of lithium with candesartan cilexetil, so careful monitoring of serum lithium levels is recommended during concomitant use).
No products indexed under this heading.

Lithium Citrate (An increase in serum lithium concentration has been reported during concomitant administration of lithium with candesartan cilexetil, so careful monitoring of serum lithium levels is recommended during concomitant use).
No products indexed under this heading.

ATACAND HCT 16-12.5 TABLETS

(Candesartan Cilexetil, Hydrochlorothiazide).......................... 642
May interact with antihypertensives, barbiturates, corticosteroids, oral hypoglycemic agents, insulin, lithium preparations, narcotic analgesics, nondepolarizing neuromuscular blocking agents, non-steroidal anti-inflammatory agents, and certain other agents. Compounds in these categories include:

Acarbose (Hyperglycemia may occur with thiazide diuretics; dosage adjustment of the antidiabetic drugs may be required). Products include:
Precose Tablets 792

Acebutolol Hydrochloride (Co-administration with other antihypertensive drugs may result in additive effect or potentiation of the antihypertensive effects with a potential for aggravation of orthostatic hypotension).
No products indexed under this heading.

ACTH (Co-administration with ACTH intensifies the electrolyte depletion, particularly hypokalemia).
No products indexed under this heading.

Alfentanil Hydrochloride (Narcotics may aggravate orthostatic hypotension produced by hydrochlorothiazide).
No products indexed under this heading.

Aliskiren (Co-administration with other antihypertensive drugs may result in additive effect or potentiation of the antihypertensive effects with a potential for aggravation of orthostatic hypotension). Products include:
Tekturna Tablets 2321
Tekturna HCT Tablets 2324

Amlodipine Besylate (Co-administration with other antihypertensive drugs may result in additive effect or potentiation of the antihypertensive effects with a potential for aggravation of orthostatic hypotension). Products include:
Azor Tablets 1005
Exforge Tablets 2238

Aprobarbital (Barbiturates may aggravate orthostatic hypotension produced by hydrochlorothiazide).
No products indexed under this heading.

Atenolol (Co-administration with other antihypertensive drugs may result in additive effect or potentiation of the antihypertensive effects with a potential for aggravation of orthostatic hypotension).
No products indexed under this heading.

Atracurium Besylate (Possible increased responsiveness to the muscle relaxant).
No products indexed under this heading.

Benazepril Hydrochloride (Co-administration with other antihypertensive drugs may result in additive effect or potentiation of the antihypertensive effects with a potential for aggravation of orthostatic hypotension).
No products indexed under this heading.

Bendroflumethiazide (Co-administration with other antihypertensive drugs may result in additive effect or potentiation of the antihypertensive effects with a potential for aggravation of orthostatic hypotension).
No products indexed under this heading.

Betamethasone Acetate (Co-administration with corticosteroids intensifies the electrolyte depletion, particularly hypokalemia).
No products indexed under this heading.

Betamethasone Sodium Phosphate (Co-administration with corticosteroids intensifies the electrolyte depletion, particularly hypokalemia).
No products indexed under this heading.

Betaxolol Hydrochloride (Co-administration with other antihypertensive drugs may result in additive effect or potentiation of the antihypertensive effects with a potential for aggravation of orthostatic hypotension).
No products indexed under this heading.

Bisoprolol Fumarate (Co-administration with other antihypertensive drugs may result in additive effect or potentiation of the antihypertensive effects with a potential for aggravation of orthostatic hypotension).
No products indexed under this heading.

Budesonide (Co-administration with corticosteroids intensifies the electrolyte depletion, particularly hypokalemia). Products include:
Pulmicort Flexhaler 654
Symbicort 80/4.5 Inhalation Aerosol 659
Symbicort 160/4.5 Inhalation Aerosol 659

Buprenorphine Hydrochloride (Narcotics may aggravate orthostatic hypotension produced by hydrochlorothiazide). Products include:
Suboxone Tablets 2601
Subutex Tablets 2601

Butabarbital (Barbiturates may aggravate orthostatic hypotension produced by hydrochlorothiazide).
No products indexed under this heading.

Butalbital (Barbiturates may aggravate orthostatic hypotension produced by hydrochlorothiazide).
No products indexed under this heading.

Captopril (Co-administration with other antihypertensive drugs may result in additive effect or potentiation of the antihypertensive effects with a potential for aggravation of orthostatic hypotension). Products include:
Captopril Tablets 2182

Carteolol Hydrochloride (Co-administration with other antihypertensive drugs may result in additive effect or potentiation of the antihypertensive effects with a potential for aggravation of orthostatic hypotension).
No products indexed under this heading.

Celecoxib (Co-administration of non-steroidal anti-inflammatory agents can reduce the diuretic, natriuretic, and antihypertensive effects of thiazide diuretics). Products include:
Celebrex Capsules 2979

Chlorothiazide (Co-administration with other antihypertensive drugs may result in additive effect or potentiation of the antihypertensive effects with a potential for aggravation of orthostatic hypotension).
No products indexed under this heading.

Chlorothiazide Sodium (Co-administration with other antihypertensive drugs may result in additive effect or potentiation of the antihypertensive effects with a potential for aggravation of orthostatic hypotension). Products include:
Intravenous Sodium Diuril 2490

Chlorpropamide (Hyperglycemia may occur with thiazide diuretics; dosage adjustment of the antidiabetic drugs may be required).
No products indexed under this heading.

Chlorthalidone (Co-administration with other antihypertensive drugs may result in additive effect or potentiation of the antihypertensive effects with a potential for aggravation of orthostatic hypotension). Products include:
Clorpres Tablets 2185

Cholestyramine (Co-administration with anionic exchange resins, such as cholestyramine, binds the hydrochlorothiazide and reduces its absorption by up to 85 percent).
No products indexed under this heading.

Ciclesonide (Co-administration with corticosteroids intensifies the electrolyte depletion, particularly hypokalemia). Products include:
Alvesco Inhalation Aerosol 2985
Omnaris Nasal Spray 2998

Cisatracurium Besylate (Possible increased responsiveness to the muscle relaxant). Products include:
Nimbex Injection 484

Clonidine (Co-administration with other antihypertensive drugs may result in additive effect or potentiation of the antihypertensive effects with a potential for aggravation of orthostatic hypotension). Products include:
Catapres-TTS 842

Clonidine Hydrochloride (Co-administration with other antihypertensive drugs may result in additive effect or potentiation of the antihypertensive effects with a potential for aggravation of orthostatic hypotension). Products include:
Catapres Tablets 841
Clorpres Tablets 2185

Codeine Phosphate (Narcotics may aggravate orthostatic hypotension produced by hydrochlorothiazide). Products include:
Tylenol with Codeine Tablets 2427

Colestipol Hydrochloride (Co-administration with anionic exchange resins, such as colestipol, binds the hydrochlorothiazide and reduces its absorption by up to 43 percent).
No products indexed under this heading.

Cortisone Acetate (Co-administration with corticosteroids intensifies the electrolyte depletion, particularly hypokalemia).
No products indexed under this heading.

Deserpidine (Co-administration with other antihypertensive drugs may result in additive effect or potentiation of the antihypertensive effects with a potential for aggravation of orthostatic hypotension).
No products indexed under this heading.

Dexamethasone (Co-administration with corticosteroids intensifies the electrolyte depletion, particularly hypokalemia). Products include:
Ciprodex Otic Suspension 541

Dexamethasone Acetate (Co-administration with corticosteroids intensifies the electrolyte depletion, particularly hypokalemia).
No products indexed under this heading.

Dexamethasone Sodium Phosphate (Co-administration with corticosteroids intensifies the electrolyte depletion, particularly hypokalemia).
No products indexed under this heading.

Dezocine (Narcotics may aggravate orthostatic hypotension produced by hydrochlorothiazide).
No products indexed under this heading.

Diazoxide (Co-administration with other antihypertensive drugs may result in additive effect or potentiation of the antihypertensive effects with a potential for aggravation of orthostatic hypotension). Products include:
Proglycem Capsules 1185
Proglycem Suspension 1185

Diclofenac Epolamine (Co-administration of non-steroidal anti-inflammatory agents can reduce the diuretic, natriuretic, and antihypertensive effects of thiazide diuretics). Products include:
Flector Patch 561

Diclofenac Potassium (Co-administration of non-steroidal anti-inflammatory agents can reduce the diuretic, natriuretic, and antihypertensive effects of thiazide diuretics).
No products indexed under this heading.

Diclofenac Sodium (Co-administration of non-steroidal anti-inflammatory agents can reduce the diuretic, natriuretic, and antihypertensive effects of thiazide diuretics). Products include:
Diclofenac Sodium Ophthalmic Solution .... ⊙240
Voltaren Ophthalmic Solution 2336
Voltaren Tablets 2334
Voltaren-XR Tablets 2337

Diltiazem Hydrochloride (Co-administration with other antihypertensive drugs may result in additive effect or potentiation of the antihypertensive effects with a potential for aggravation of orthostatic hypotension). Products include:
Cardizem LA Extended Release Tablets 421

Doxazosin Mesylate (Co-administration with other antihypertensive drugs may result in additive effect or potentiation of the antihypertensive effects with a potential for aggravation of orthostatic hypotension).
No products indexed under this heading.

Enalapril Maleate (Co-administration with other antihypertensive drugs may result in additive effect or potentiation of the antihypertensive effects with a potential for aggravation of orthostatic hypotension).
No products indexed under this heading.

Enalaprilat (Co-administration with other antihypertensive drugs may result in additive effect or potentiation of the antihypertensive effects with a potential for aggravation of orthostatic hypotension).
No products indexed under this heading.

Eprosartan Mesylate (Co-administration with other antihypertensive drugs may result in additive effect or potentiation of the antihypertensive effects with a potential for aggravation of orthostatic hypotension). Products include:
Teveten Tablets 515
Teveten HCT Tablets 517

Esmolol Hydrochloride (Co-administration with other antihypertensive drugs may result in additive effect or potentiation of the antihypertensive effects with a potential for aggravation of orthostatic hypotension).
No products indexed under this heading.

Etodolac (Co-administration of non-steroidal anti-inflammatory agents can reduce the diuretic, natriuretic, and antihypertensive effects of thiazide diuretics).
No products indexed under this heading.

Felodipine (Co-administration with other antihypertensive drugs may result in additive effect or potentiation of the antihypertensive effects with a potential for aggravation of orthostatic hypotension).
No products indexed under this heading.

Fenoprofen Calcium (Co-administration of non-steroidal anti-inflammatory agents can reduce the diuretic, natriuretic, and antihypertensive effects of thiazide diuretics). Products include:
Nalfon Capsules 2508

Fentanyl (Narcotics may aggravate orthostatic hypotension produced by hydrochlorothiazide). Products include:
Duragesic Transdermal System 2405
Ionsys Transdermal System 2410

Fentanyl Citrate (Narcotics may aggravate orthostatic hypotension produced by hydrochlorothiazide). Products include:
Actiq 959
Fentora Tablets 968

Fludrocortisone Acetate (Co-administration with corticosteroids intensifies the electrolyte depletion, particularly hypokalemia).
No products indexed under this heading.

Flunisolide (Co-administration with corticosteroids intensifies the electrolyte depletion, particularly hypokalemia). Products include:
Aerobid/Aerobid-M 1153

Flurbiprofen (Co-administration of non-steroidal anti-inflammatory agents can reduce the diuretic, natriuretic, and antihypertensive effects of thiazide diuretics).
No products indexed under this heading.

Fluticasone Propionate (Co-administration with corticosteroids intensifies the electrolyte depletion, particularly hypokalemia). Products include:
Advair Diskus 100/50 1276
Advair Diskus 250/50 1276
Advair Diskus 500/50 1276
Advair HFA 45/21 Inhalation Aerosol 1288
Advair HFA 115/21 Inhalation Aerosol 1288
Advair HFA 230/21 Inhalation Aerosol 1288
Flonase Nasal Spray 1431
Flovent Diskus 50 mcg 1435

Fluticasone Propionate HFA (Co-administration with corticosteroids intensifies the electrolyte depletion, particularly hypokalemia). Products include:
Flovent HFA 1440

Fosinopril Sodium (Co-administration with other antihypertensive drugs may result in additive effect or potentiation of the antihypertensive effects with a potential for aggravation of orthostatic hypotension).
No products indexed under this heading.

Furosemide (Co-administration with other antihypertensive drugs may result in additive effect or potentiation of the antihypertensive effects with a potential for aggravation of orthostatic hypotension). Products include:
Furosemide Tablets 2186

Glimepiride (Hyperglycemia may occur with thiazide diuretics; dosage adjustment of the antidiabetic drugs may be required). Products include:
Avandaryl Tablets 1344
Duetact Tablets 3085

Glipizide (Hyperglycemia may occur with thiazide diuretics; dosage adjustment of the antidiabetic drugs may be required).
No products indexed under this heading.

Glyburide (Hyperglycemia may occur with thiazide diuretics; dosage adjustment of the antidiabetic drugs may be required).
No products indexed under this heading.

Guanabenz Acetate (Co-administration with other antihypertensive drugs may result in additive effect or potentiation of the antihypertensive effects with a potential for aggravation of orthostatic hypotension).
No products indexed under this heading.

Guanethidine Monosulfate (Co-administration with other antihypertensive drugs may result in additive effect or potentiation of the antihypertensive effects with a potential for aggravation of orthostatic hypotension).
No products indexed under this heading.

Hydralazine Hydrochloride (Co-administration with other antihypertensive drugs may result in additive effect or potentiation of the antihypertensive effects with a potential for aggravation of orthostatic hypotension).
No products indexed under this heading.

Hydrocodone Bitartrate (Narcotics may aggravate orthostatic hypotension produced by hydrochlorothiazide). Products include:
Lortab 5/500 Tablets 3143
Lortab 7.5/500 Tablets 3144
Lortab 10/500 Tablets 3144
Vicodin Tablets 529
Vicodin ES Tablets 530
Vicodin HP Tablets 531
Vicoprofen Tablets 533
Zydone Tablets 1132

Hydrocodone Polistirex (Narcotics may aggravate orthostatic hypotension produced by hydrochlorothiazide). Products include:
Tussionex Pennkinetic Extended-Release Suspension 3154

Hydrocortisone (Co-administration with corticosteroids intensifies the electrolyte depletion, particularly hypokalemia).
No products indexed under this heading.

Hydrocortisone Acetate (Co-administration with corticosteroids intensifies the electrolyte depletion, particularly hypokalemia). Products include:
Analpram-HC 1140
Pramosone 1141

Hydrocortisone Sodium Phosphate (Co-administration with corticosteroids intensifies the electrolyte depletion, particularly hypokalemia).
No products indexed under this heading.

Hydrocortisone Sodium Succinate (Co-administration with corticosteroids intensifies the electrolyte depletion, particularly hypokalemia).
No products indexed under this heading.

Hydroflumethiazide (Co-administration with other antihypertensive drugs may result in additive effect or potentiation of the antihypertensive effects with a potential for aggravation of orthostatic hypotension).
No products indexed under this heading.

Hydromorphone Hydrochloride (Narcotics may aggravate orthostatic hypotension produced by hydrochlorothiazide).
No products indexed under this heading.

Ibuprofen (Co-administration of non-steroidal anti-inflammatory agents can reduce the diuretic, natriuretic, and antihypertensive effects of thiazide diuretics). Products include:
Motrin IB Tablets and Caplets 1900
Children's Motrin Oral Suspension ... 1901
Children's Motrin Non-Staining Dye-Free Oral Suspension 1901
Children's Motrin Cold Oral Suspension 1899
Infants' Motrin Concentrated Drops 1901
Infants' Motrin Non-Staining Dye-Free Concentrated Drops 1901
Junior Strength Motrin Caplets and Chewable Tablets 1901
Vicoprofen Tablets 533

Indapamide (Co-administration with other antihypertensive drugs may result in additive effect or potentiation of the antihypertensive effects with a potential for aggravation of orthostatic hypotension). Products include:
Indapamide Tablets 2188

Indomethacin (Co-administration of non-steroidal anti-inflammatory agents can reduce the diuretic, natriuretic, and antihypertensive effects of thiazide diuretics). Products include:
Indocin 2024

Indomethacin Sodium Trihydrate (Co-administration of non-steroidal anti-inflammatory agents can reduce the diuretic, natriuretic, and antihypertensive effects of thiazide diuretics). Products include:
Indocin I.V. 2489

Insulin (Hyperglycemia may occur with thiazide diuretics; dosage adjustment of the insulin may be required).
No products indexed under this heading.

Insulin, Human, Zinc Suspension (Hyperglycemia may occur with thiazide diuretics; dosage adjustment of the insulin may be required).
No products indexed under this heading.

Insulin, Human (rDNA origin) (Hyperglycemia may occur with thiazide diuretics; dosage adjustment of the insulin may be required). Products include:
Exubera Inhalation Powder 2515

Insulin, Human NPH (Hyperglycemia may occur with thiazide diuretics; dosage adjustment of the insulin may be required). Products include:
Humulin N Vial 1846

Insulin, Human Regular (Hyperglycemia may occur with thiazide diuretics; dosage adjustment of the insulin may be required). Products include:
Humulin R 1849
Humulin R (U-500) 1850

Insulin, Human Regular and Human NPH Mixture (Hyperglycemia may occur with thiazide diuretics; dosage adjustment of the insulin may be required). Products include:
Humulin 50/50, 100 Units 1843
Humulin 70/30 Vial 1844

Insulin, NPH (Hyperglycemia may occur with thiazide diuretics; dosage adjustment of the insulin may be required).
No products indexed under this heading.

Insulin, Regular (Hyperglycemia may occur with thiazide diuretics; dosage adjustment of the insulin may be required).
No products indexed under this heading.

Insulin, Regular and NPH mixture (Hyperglycemia may occur with thiazide diuretics; dosage adjustment of the insulin may be required).
No products indexed under this heading.

Insulin, Zinc Crystals (Hyperglycemia may occur with thiazide diuretics; dosage adjustment of the insulin may be required).
No products indexed under this heading.

Insulin, Zinc Suspension (Hyperglycemia may occur with thiazide diuretics; dosage adjustment of the insulin may be required).
No products indexed under this heading.

Insulin Aspart (Hyperglycemia may occur with thiazide diuretics; dosage adjustment of the insulin may be required).
No products indexed under this heading.

Insulin Aspart, Human (Hyperglycemia may occur with thiazide diuretics; dosage adjustment of the insulin may be required). Products include:
NovoLog Mix 70/30 2364

Insulin Aspart, Human Regular (Hyperglycemia may occur with thiazide diuretics; dosage adjustment of the insulin may be required). Products include:
NovoLog Injection 2359

Insulin Aspart Protamine, Human (Hyperglycemia may occur with thiazide diuretics; dosage adjustment of the insulin may be required). Products include:
NovoLog Mix 70/30 2364

Insulin Detemir (rDNA Origin) (Hyperglycemia may occur with thiazide diuretics; dosage adjustment of the insulin may be required). Products include:
Levemir Injection 2352

Insulin glargine (Hyperglycemia may occur with thiazide diuretics; dosage adjustment of the insulin may be required). Products include:
Lantus Injection 2749

Insulin Glulisine (Hyperglycemia may occur with thiazide diuretics; dosage adjustment of the insulin may be required). Products include:
Apidra Injection 2706

Insulin Lispro, Human (Hyperglycemia may occur with thiazide diuretics; dosage adjustment of the insulin may be required). Products include:
Humalog-Pen and KwikPen 1829
Humalog Mix 50/50-Pen and KwikPen 1833
Humalog Mix 75/25-Pen and KwikPen 1835

Insulin Lispro Protamine, Human (Hyperglycemia may occur with thiazide diuretics; dosage adjustment of the insulin may be required). Products include:
Humalog Mix 50/50-Pen and KwikPen 1833
Humalog Mix 75/25-Pen and KwikPen 1835

Irbesartan (Co-administration with other antihypertensive drugs may result in additive effect or potentiation of the antihypertensive effects with a potential for aggravation of orthostatic hypotension). Products include:
Avalide Tablets 892
Avalide Tablets 2713
Avapro Tablets 897
Avapro Tablets 2718

Isradipine (Co-administration with other antihypertensive drugs may result in additive effect or potentiation of the antihypertensive effects with a potential for aggravation of orthostatic hypotension). Products include:
DynaCirc CR Controlled Release Tablets 1407

Ketoprofen (Co-administration of non-steroidal anti-inflammatory agents can reduce the diuretic, natriuretic, and antihypertensive effects of thiazide diuretics).
No products indexed under this heading.

Ketorolac Tromethamine (Co-administration of non-steroidal anti-inflammatory agents can reduce the diuretic, natriuretic, and antihypertensive effects of thiazide diuretics).
No products indexed under this heading.

Labetalol Hydrochloride (Co-administration with other antihypertensive drugs may result in additive effect or potentiation of the antihypertensive effects with a potential for aggravation of orthostatic hypotension).
No products indexed under this heading.

Levorphanol Tartrate (Narcotics may aggravate orthostatic hypotension produced by hydrochlorothiazide).
No products indexed under this heading.

Lisinopril (Co-administration with other antihypertensive drugs may result in additive effect or potentiation of the antihypertensive effects with a potential for aggravation of orthostatic hypotension). Products include:
Prinivil Tablets 2087
Prinzide Tablets 2092

Lithium (Hydrochlorothiazide reduces the renal clearance of lithium and can cause a high risk of lithium toxicity; in general, lithium should not be given with diuretics. An increase in serum lithium concentration has been reported during concomitant administration of lithium with candesartan cilexetil; careful monitoring of serum lithium levels is recommended during concomitant use).
No products indexed under this heading.

Lithium Carbonate (Hydrochlorothiazide reduces the renal clearance of lithium and can cause a high risk of lithium toxicity; in general, lithium should not be given with diuretics. An increase in serum lithium concentration has been reported during concomitant administration of lithium with candesartan cilexetil; careful monitoring of serum lithium levels is recommended during concomitant use).
No products indexed under this heading.

Lithium Citrate (Hydrochlorothiazide reduces the renal clearance of lithium and can cause a high risk of lithium toxicity; in general, lithium should not be given with diuretics. An increase in serum lithium concentration has been reported during concomitant administration of lithium with candesartan cilexetil; careful monitoring of serum lithium levels is recommended during concomitant use).
No products indexed under this heading.

Losartan Potassium (Co-administration with other antihypertensive drugs may result in additive effect or potentiation of the antihypertensive effects with a potential for aggravation of orthostatic hypotension). Products include:
Cozaar Tablets 1973

Mecamylamine Hydrochloride (Co-administration with other antihypertensive drugs may result in additive effect or potentiation of the antihypertensive effects with a potential for aggravation of orthostatic hypotension).
No products indexed under this heading.

Meclofenamate Sodium (Co-administration of non-steroidal anti-inflammatory agents can reduce the diuretic, natriuretic, and antihypertensive effects of thiazide diuretics).
No products indexed under this heading.

Mefenamic Acid (Co-administration of non-steroidal anti-inflammatory agents can reduce the diuretic, natriuretic, and antihypertensive effects of thiazide diuretics).
No products indexed under this heading.

Meloxicam (Co-administration of non-steroidal anti-inflammatory agents can reduce the diuretic, natriuretic, and antihypertensive effects of thiazide diuretics). Products include:
Mobic Oral Suspension 863
Mobic Tablets 863

Meperidine Hydrochloride (Narcotics may aggravate orthostatic hypotension produced by hydrochlorothiazide).
No products indexed under this heading.

Mephobarbital (Barbiturates may aggravate orthostatic hypotension produced by hydrochlorothiazide).
No products indexed under this heading.

Metformin Hydrochloride (Hyperglycemia may occur with thiazide diuretics; dosage adjustment of the antidiabetic drugs may be required). Products include:
ActoPlus Met Tablets 3071
Avandamet Tablets 1336
Janumet Tablets 2041
PrandiMet Tablets 2967

Methadone Hydrochloride (Narcotics may aggravate orthostatic hypotension produced by hydrochlorothiazide).
No products indexed under this heading.

Methyclothiazide (Co-administration with other antihypertensive drugs may result in additive effect or potentiation of the antihypertensive effects with a potential for aggravation of orthostatic hypotension).
No products indexed under this heading.

Methyldopa (Co-administration with other antihypertensive drugs may result in additive effect or potentiation of the antihypertensive effects with a potential for aggravation of orthostatic hypotension).
No products indexed under this heading.

Methyldopate Hydrochloride (Co-administration with other antihypertensive drugs may result in additive effect or potentiation of the antihypertensive effects with a potential for aggravation of orthostatic hypotension).
No products indexed under this heading.

Methylprednisolone Acetate (Co-administration with corticosteroids intensifies the electrolyte depletion, particularly hypokalemia).
No products indexed under this heading.

Methylprednisolone Sodium Succinate (Co-administration with corticosteroids intensifies the electrolyte depletion, particularly hypokalemia).
No products indexed under this heading.

Metocurine Iodide (Possible increased responsiveness to the muscle relaxant).
No products indexed under this heading.

Metolazone (Co-administration with other antihypertensive drugs may result in additive effect or potentiation of the antihypertensive effects with a potential for aggravation of orthostatic hypotension).
No products indexed under this heading.

Metoprolol Succinate (Co-administration with other antihypertensive drugs may result in additive effect or potentiation of the antihypertensive effects with a potential for aggravation of orthostatic hypotension). Products include:
Toprol-XL Tablets 666

Metoprolol Tartrate (Co-administration with other antihypertensive drugs may result in additive effect or potentiation of the antihypertensive effects with a potential for aggravation of orthostatic hypotension).
No products indexed under this heading.

Metyrosine (Co-administration with other antihypertensive drugs may result in additive effect or potentiation of the antihypertensive effects with a potential for aggravation of orthostatic hypotension). Products include:
Demser Capsules 1989

Mibefradil Dihydrochloride (Co-administration with other antihypertensive drugs may result in additive effect or potentiation of the antihypertensive effects with a potential for aggravation of orthostatic hypotension).
No products indexed under this heading.

Miglitol (Hyperglycemia may occur with thiazide diuretics; dosage adjustment of the antidiabetic drugs may be required).
No products indexed under this heading.

Minoxidil (Co-administration with other antihypertensive drugs may result in additive effect or potentiation of the antihypertensive effects with a potential for aggravation of orthostatic hypotension).
No products indexed under this heading.

Mivacurium Chloride (Possible increased responsiveness to the muscle relaxant).
No products indexed under this heading.

Moexipril Hydrochloride (Co-administration with other antihypertensive drugs may result in additive effect or potentiation of the antihypertensive effects with a potential for aggravation of orthostatic hypotension).
No products indexed under this heading.

Mometasone Furoate (Co-administration with corticosteroids intensifies the electrolyte depletion, particularly hypokalemia). Products include:
Asmanex Twisthaler 2797
Elocon Cream 0.1% 2840
Elocon Lotion 0.1% 2841
Elocon Ointment 0.1% 2842

Mometasone Furoate Monohydrate (Co-administration with corticosteroids intensifies the electrolyte depletion, particularly hypokalemia). Products include:
Nasonex Nasal Spray 2883

Morphine Sulfate (Narcotics may aggravate orthostatic hypotension produced by hydrochlorothiazide). Products include:
Avinza Capsules 1772
DepoDur Injection 1095
MS Contin Tablets 2585

Nabumetone (Co-administration of non-steroidal anti-inflammatory agents can reduce the diuretic, natriuretic, and antihypertensive effects of thiazide diuretics).
No products indexed under this heading.

Nadolol (Co-administration with other antihypertensive drugs may result in additive effect or potentiation of the antihypertensive effects with a potential for aggravation of orthostatic hypotension). Products include:
Nadolol Tablets 2191

Naproxen (Co-administration of non-steroidal anti-inflammatory agents can reduce the diuretic, natriuretic, and antihypertensive effects of thiazide diuretics). Products include:
EC-Naprosyn Delayed-Release Tablets 2632
Naprosyn Suspension 2632
Naprosyn Tablets 2632

Naproxen Sodium (Co-administration of non-steroidal anti-inflammatory agents can reduce the diuretic, natriuretic, and antihypertensive effects of thiazide diuretics). Products include:
Anaprox Tablets 2632
Anaprox DS Tablets 2632
Treximet Tablets 1616

Nateglinide (Hyperglycemia may occur with thiazide diuretics; dosage adjustment of the antidiabetic drugs may be required). Products include:
Starlix Tablets 2314

Nebivolol (Co-administration with other antihypertensive drugs may result in additive effect or potentiation of the antihypertensive effects with a potential for aggravation of orthostatic hypotension). Products include:
Bystolic Tablets 1155

Nicardipine Hydrochloride (Co-administration with other antihypertensive drugs may result in additive effect or potentiation of the antihypertensive effects with a potential for aggravation of orthostatic hypotension). Products include:
Cardene I.V. 1093

Nifedipine (Co-administration with other antihypertensive drugs may result in additive effect or potentiation of the antihypertensive effects with a potential for aggravation of orthostatic hypotension).
No products indexed under this heading.

Nisoldipine (Co-administration with other antihypertensive drugs may result in additive effect or potentiation of the antihypertensive effects with a potential for aggravation of orthostatic hypotension). Products include:
Sular Extended Release Tablets 2975

Nitroglycerin (Co-administration with other antihypertensive drugs may result in additive effect or potentiation of the antihypertensive effects with a potential for aggravation of orthostatic hypotension). Products include:
Nitro-Dur Transdermal Infusion System 2887
Nitrolingual Pumpspray 2965

Norepinephrine Bitartrate (Possible decreased response to pressor amines).
No products indexed under this heading.

Oxaprozin (Co-administration of non-steroidal anti-inflammatory agents can reduce the diuretic, natriuretic, and antihypertensive effects of thiazide diuretics).
No products indexed under this heading.

Oxycodone Hydrochloride (Narcotics may aggravate orthostatic hypotension produced by hydrochlorothiazide). Products include:
OxyContin Tablets 2589

OxyIR Capsules 2593
Percocet Tablets 1127
Percodan Tablets 1130

Pancuronium Bromide (Possible increased responsiveness to the muscle relaxant).
No products indexed under this heading.

Penbutolol Sulfate (Co-administration with other antihypertensive drugs may result in additive effect or potentiation of the antihypertensive effects with a potential for aggravation of orthostatic hypotension).
No products indexed under this heading.

Pentobarbital Sodium (Barbiturates may aggravate orthostatic hypotension produced by hydrochlorothiazide). Products include:
Nembutal Sodium Solution, USP 2494

Perindopril Erbumine (Co-administration with other antihypertensive drugs may result in additive effect or potentiation of the antihypertensive effects with a potential for aggravation of orthostatic hypotension). Products include:
Aceon Tablets (2 mg, 4 mg, 8 mg) 3038

Phenobarbital (Barbiturates may aggravate orthostatic hypotension produced by hydrochlorothiazide). Products include:
Donnatal Extentabs 2507

Phenoxybenzamine Hydrochloride (Co-administration with other antihypertensive drugs may result in additive effect or potentiation of the antihypertensive effects with a potential for aggravation of orthostatic hypotension). Products include:
Dibenzyline Capsules 3188

Phentolamine Mesylate (Co-administration with other antihypertensive drugs may result in additive effect or potentiation of the antihypertensive effects with a potential for aggravation of orthostatic hypotension).
No products indexed under this heading.

Phenylbutazone (Co-administration of non-steroidal anti-inflammatory agents can reduce the diuretic, natriuretic, and antihypertensive effects of thiazide diuretics).
No products indexed under this heading.

Pindolol (Co-administration with other antihypertensive drugs may result in additive effect or potentiation of the antihypertensive effects with a potential for aggravation of orthostatic hypotension).
No products indexed under this heading.

Pioglitazone Hydrochloride (Hyperglycemia may occur with thiazide diuretics; dosage adjustment of the antidiabetic drugs may be required). Products include:
ActoPlus Met Tablets 3071
Actos Tablets 3077
Duetact Tablets 3085

Piroxicam (Co-administration of non-steroidal anti-inflammatory agents can reduce the diuretic, natriuretic, and antihypertensive effects of thiazide diuretics).
No products indexed under this heading.

Polythiazide (Co-administration with other antihypertensive drugs may result in additive effect or potentiation of the antihypertensive effects with a potential for aggravation of orthostatic hypotension).
No products indexed under this heading.

Prazosin Hydrochloride (Co-administration with other antihypertensive drugs may result in additive effect or potentiation of the antihypertensive effects with a potential for aggravation of orthostatic hypotension).
No products indexed under this heading.

Prednisolone Acetate (Co-administration with corticosteroids intensifies the electrolyte depletion, particularly hypokalemia). Products include:
Pred Forte Ophthalmic Suspension .... ⊙ 227
Pred Mild Ophthalmic Suspension .... ⊙ 230
Pred-G Ophthalmic Ointment .... ⊙ 229
Pred-G Ophthalmic Suspension ...... ⊙ 228

Prednisolone Sodium Phosphate (Co-administration with corticosteroids intensifies the electrolyte depletion, particularly hypokalemia).
No products indexed under this heading.

Prednisolone Tebutate (Co-administration with corticosteroids intensifies the electrolyte depletion, particularly hypokalemia).
No products indexed under this heading.

Prednisone (Co-administration with corticosteroids intensifies the electrolyte depletion, particularly hypokalemia).
No products indexed under this heading.

Propoxyphene Hydrochloride (Narcotics may aggravate orthostatic hypotension produced by hydrochlorothiazide).
No products indexed under this heading.

Propoxyphene Napsylate (Narcotics may aggravate orthostatic hypotension produced by hydrochlorothiazide).
No products indexed under this heading.

Propranolol Hydrochloride (Co-administration with other antihypertensive drugs may result in additive effect or potentiation of the antihypertensive effects with a potential for aggravation of orthostatic hypotension). Products include:
InnoPran XL Extended Release Capsules 1484

Quinapril Hydrochloride (Co-administration with other antihypertensive drugs may result in additive effect or potentiation of the antihypertensive effects with a potential for aggravation of orthostatic hypotension).
No products indexed under this heading.

Ramipril (Co-administration with other antihypertensive drugs may result in additive effect or potentiation of the antihypertensive effects with a potential for aggravation of orthostatic hypotension).
No products indexed under this heading.

Rapacuronium Bromide (Possible increased responsiveness to the muscle relaxant).
No products indexed under this heading.

Rauwolfia Serpentina (Co-administration with other antihypertensive drugs may result in additive effect or potentiation of the antihypertensive effects with a potential for aggravation of orthostatic hypotension).
No products indexed under this heading.

Remifentanil Hydrochloride (Narcotics may aggravate orthostatic hypotension produced by hydrochlorothiazide).
No products indexed under this heading.

Repaglinide (Hyperglycemia may occur with thiazide diuretics; dosage adjustment of the antidiabetic drugs may be required). Products include:
PrandiMet Tablets 2967
Prandin Tablets 2971

Rescinnamine (Co-administration with other antihypertensive drugs may result in additive effect or potentiation of the antihypertensive effects with a potential for aggravation of orthostatic hypotension).
No products indexed under this heading.

Reserpine (Co-administration with other antihypertensive drugs may result in additive effect or potentiation of the antihypertensive effects with a potential for aggravation of orthostatic hypotension).
No products indexed under this heading.

Rocuronium Bromide (Possible increased responsiveness to the muscle relaxant). Products include:
Zemuron Injection 2947

Rofecoxib (Co-administration of non-steroidal anti-inflammatory agents can reduce the diuretic, natriuretic, and antihypertensive effects of thiazide diuretics).
No products indexed under this heading.

Rosiglitazone Maleate (Hyperglycemia may occur with thiazide diuretics; dosage adjustment of the antidiabetic drugs may be required). Products include:
Avandamet Tablets 1336
Avandaryl Tablets 1344
Avandia Tablets 1351

Secobarbital Sodium (Barbiturates may aggravate orthostatic hypotension produced by hydrochlorothiazide).
No products indexed under this heading.

Sitagliptin Phosphate (Hyperglycemia may occur with thiazide diuretics; dosage adjustment of the antidiabetic drugs may be required). Products include:
Janumet Tablets 2041
Januvia Tablets 2048

Sodium Nitroprusside (Co-administration with other antihypertensive drugs may result in additive effect or potentiation of the antihypertensive effects with a potential for aggravation of orthostatic hypotension).
No products indexed under this heading.

Sotalol Hydrochloride (Co-administration with other antihypertensive drugs may result in additive effect or potentiation of the antihypertensive effects with a potential for aggravation of orthostatic hypotension).
No products indexed under this heading.

Spirapril Hydrochloride (Co-administration with other antihypertensive drugs may result in additive effect or potentiation of the antihypertensive effects with a potential for aggravation of orthostatic hypotension).
No products indexed under this heading.

Sufentanil Citrate (Narcotics may aggravate orthostatic hypotension produced by hydrochlorothiazide).
No products indexed under this heading.

Sulindac (Co-administration of non-steroidal anti-inflammatory agents can reduce the diuretic, natriuretic, and antihypertensive effects of thiazide diuretics). Products include:
Clinoril Tablets 1962

Telmisartan (Co-administration with other antihypertensive drugs may result in additive effect or potentiation of the antihypertensive effects with a potential for aggravation of orthostatic hypotension). Products include:
Micardis Tablets 852
Micardis HCT Tablets 854

Terazosin Hydrochloride (Co-administration with other antihypertensive drugs may result in additive effect or potentiation of the antihypertensive effects with a potential for aggravation of orthostatic hypotension).
No products indexed under this heading.

Thiamylal Sodium (Barbiturates may aggravate orthostatic hypotension produced by hydrochlorothiazide).
No products indexed under this heading.

Timolol Maleate (Co-administration with other antihypertensive drugs may result in additive effect or potentiation of the antihypertensive effects with a potential for aggravation of orthostatic hypotension). Products include:
Combigan Ophthalmic Solution 553
Cosopt Sterile Ophthalmic Solution 1969
Timoptic Sterile Ophthalmic Solution 2121
Timoptic in Ocudose 2124
Timoptic-XE Sterile Ophthalmic Gel Forming Solution 2125

Tolazamide (Hyperglycemia may occur with thiazide diuretics; dosage adjustment of the antidiabetic drugs may be required).
No products indexed under this heading.

Tolbutamide (Hyperglycemia may occur with thiazide diuretics; dosage adjustment of the antidiabetic drugs may be required).
No products indexed under this heading.

Tolmetin Sodium (Co-administration of non-steroidal anti-inflammatory agents can reduce the diuretic, natriuretic, and antihypertensive effects of thiazide diuretics).
No products indexed under this heading.

IMPORTANT NOTE: Always consult each drug listing in the patient's regimen for possible interactions.

Torsemide (Co-administration with other antihypertensive drugs may result in additive effect or potentiation of the antihypertensive effects with a potential for aggravation of orthostatic hypotension). Products include:
Demadex Injection 2630
Demadex Tablets 2630

Trandolapril (Co-administration with other antihypertensive drugs may result in additive effect or potentiation of the antihypertensive effects with a potential for aggravation of orthostatic hypotension). Products include:
Mavik Tablets 472
Tarka Tablets 511

Triamcinolone (Co-administration with corticosteroids intensifies the electrolyte depletion, particularly hypokalemia).
No products indexed under this heading.

Triamcinolone Acetonide (Co-administration with corticosteroids intensifies the electrolyte depletion, particularly hypokalemia). Products include:
Azmacort Inhalation Aerosol 407
Nasacort AQ Nasal Spray 2765
Triesence Injectable Suspension .... ⊙209

Triamcinolone Diacetate (Co-administration with corticosteroids intensifies the electrolyte depletion, particularly hypokalemia).
No products indexed under this heading.

Triamcinolone Hexacetonide (Co-administration with corticosteroids intensifies the electrolyte depletion, particularly hypokalemia).
No products indexed under this heading.

Trimethaphan Camsylate (Co-administration with other antihypertensive drugs may result in additive effect or potentiation of the antihypertensive effects with a potential for aggravation of orthostatic hypotension).
No products indexed under this heading.

Troglitazone (Hyperglycemia may occur with thiazide diuretics; dosage adjustment of the antidiabetic drugs may be required).
No products indexed under this heading.

Tubocurarine Chloride (Possible increased responsiveness to the muscle relaxant).
No products indexed under this heading.

Valdecoxib (Co-administration of non-steroidal anti-inflammatory agents can reduce the diuretic, natriuretic, and antihypertensive effects of thiazide diuretics).
No products indexed under this heading.

Valsartan (Co-administration with other antihypertensive drugs may result in additive effect or potentiation of the antihypertensive effects with a potential for aggravation of orthostatic hypotension). Products include:
Diovan Tablets 2212
Diovan HCT Tablets 2216
Exforge Tablets 2238

Vecuronium Bromide (Possible increased responsiveness to the muscle relaxant).
No products indexed under this heading.

Verapamil Hydrochloride (Co-administration with other antihypertensive drugs may result in additive effect or potentiation of the antihypertensive effects with a potential for aggravation of orthostatic hypotension). Products include:
Tarka Tablets 511

Food Interactions

Alcohol (May aggravate orthostatic hypotension produced by hydrochlorothiazide).

ATACAND HCT 32-12.5 TABLETS

(Candesartan Cilexetil, Hydrochlorothiazide).......... 642
See Atacand HCT 16-12.5 Tablets

ATRIPLA TABLETS

(Efavirenz, Emtricitabine, Tenofovir Disoproxil Fumarate).......... 938
May interact with cytochrome p450 2c19 substrates (selected), cytochrome p450 2c9 substrates (selected), cytochrome p450 3a4 inducers (selected), cytochrome p450 3a4 substrates (selected), nephrotoxic agents, and certain other agents. Compounds in these categories include:

Abacavir Sulfate (Renal impairment, including cases of acute renal failure and Fanconi syndrome (renal tubular injury with severe hypophosphatemia), has been reported in association with the use of tenofovir DF. The majority of these cases occurred in patients with underlying systemic or renal disease, or in patients taking nephrotoxic agents; however, some cases occured in patients without identified risk factors. Atripla should be avoided with concurrent or recent use of a nephrotoxic agent). Products include:
Epzicom Tablets 1422
Trizivir Tablets 1622
Ziagen 1673

Acarbose (In vitro studies have demonstrated that efavirenz inhibits CYP2C9 in the range of observed efavirenz plasma concentrations. Co-administration of efavirenz with drugs primarily metabolized by CYP2C9 may result in altered plasma concentrations of the co-administered drug. Therefore, appropriate dose adjustments may be necessary for these drugs). Products include:
Precose Tablets 792

Acyclovir (Since emtricitabine and tenofovir are primarily eliminated by the kidneys, co-administration of ATRIPLA with drugs that reduce renal fuction or compete for active tubular secretion may increase serum concentrations of emtricitabine, tenofovir, and/or other renally eliminated drugs). Products include:
Zovirax 1690
Zovirax Cream 817
Zovirax Ointment 819

Acyclovir Sodium (Since emtricitabine and tenofovir are primarily eliminated by the kidneys, co-administration of ATRIPLA with drugs that reduce renal fuction or compete for active tubular secretion may increase serum concentrations of emtricitabine, tenofovir, and/or other renally eliminated drugs).
No products indexed under this heading.

Adefovir dipivoxil (Since emtricitabine and tenofovir are primarily eliminated by the kidneys, co-administration of ATRIPLA with drugs that reduce renal fuction or compete for active tubular secretion may increase serum concentrations of emtricitabine, tenofovir, and/or other renally eliminated drugs). Products include:
Hepsera Tablets 1253

Alatrofloxacin Mesylate (Renal impairment, including cases of acute renal failure and Fanconi syndrome (renal tubular injury with severe hypophosphatemia), has been reported in association with the use of tenofovir DF. The majority of these cases occurred in patients with underlying systemic or renal disease, or in patients taking nephrotoxic agents; however, some cases occured in patients without identified risk factors. Atripla should be avoided with concurrent or recent use of a nephrotoxic agent).
No products indexed under this heading.

Aldesleukin (Renal impairment, including cases of acute renal failure and Fanconi syndrome (renal tubular injury with severe hypophosphatemia), has been reported in association with the use of tenofovir DF. The majority of these cases occurred in patients with underlying systemic or renal disease, or in patients taking nephrotoxic agents; however, some cases occured in patients without identified risk factors. Atripla should be avoided with concurrent or recent use of a nephrotoxic agent). Products include:
Proleukin for Injection 2287

Alfentanil Hydrochloride (Efavirenz has been shown in vivo to induce CYP3A4. Other compounds that are substrates of CYP3A4 may have decreased plasma concentrations when co-administered with efavirenz).
No products indexed under this heading.

Allium sativum (Drugs which induce CYP3A4 activity would be expected to increase the clearance of efavirenz resulting in lower plasma concentrations).
No products indexed under this heading.

Alprazolam (Efavirenz has been shown in vivo to induce CYP3A4. Other compounds that are substrates of CYP3A4 may have decreased plasma concentrations when co-administered with efavirenz).
No products indexed under this heading.

Amikacin Sulfate (Renal impairment, including cases of acute renal failure and Fanconi syndrome (renal tubular injury with severe hypophosphatemia), has been reported in association with the use of tenofovir DF. The majority of these cases occurred in patients with underlying systemic or renal disease, or in patients taking nephrotoxic agents; however, some cases occured in patients without identified risk factors. Atripla should be avoided with concurrent or recent use of a nephrotoxic agent).
No products indexed under this heading.

Amiodarone Hydrochloride (Efavirenz has been shown in vivo to induce CYP3A4. Other compounds that are substrates of CYP3A4 may have decreased plasma concentrations when co-administered with efavirenz).
No products indexed under this heading.

Amitriptyline Hydrochloride (Efavirenz has been shown in vivo to induce CYP3A4. Other compounds that are substrates of CYP3A4 may have decreased plasma concentrations when co-administered with efavirenz).
No products indexed under this heading.

Amlodipine Besylate (Efavirenz has been shown in vivo to induce CYP3A4. Other compounds that are substrates of CYP3A4 may have decreased plasma concentrations when co-administered with efavirenz). Products include:
Azor Tablets 1005
Exforge Tablets 2238

Amoxapine (In vitro studies have demonstrated that efavirenz inhibits CYP2C19 in the range of observed efavirenz plasma concentrations. Co-administration of efavirenz with drugs primarily metabolized by CYP2C19 may result in altered plasma concentrations of the co-administered drug. Therefore, appropriate dose adjustments may be necessary for these drugs).
No products indexed under this heading.

Amoxicillin (Renal impairment, including cases of acute renal failure and Fanconi syndrome (renal tubular injury with severe hypophosphatemia), has been reported in association with the use of tenofovir DF. The majority of these cases occurred in patients with underlying systemic or renal disease, or in patients taking nephrotoxic agents; however, some cases occured in patients without identified risk factors. Atripla should be avoided with concurrent or recent use of a nephrotoxic agent). Products include:
Amoxil Capsules 1305
Amoxil Chewable Tablets 1305
Amoxil Pediatric Drops for Oral Suspension 1305
Amoxil Powder for Oral Suspension 1305
Amoxil Tablets 1305
Augmentin 1323
Augmentin Tablets 1327
Augmentin XR Extended Release Tablets 1333
Augmentin ES-600 Powder for Oral Suspension 1329
Moxatag Tablets 2165

Amoxicillin Trihydrate (Renal impairment, including cases of acute renal failure and Fanconi syndrome (renal tubular injury with severe hypophosphatemia), has been reported in association with the use of tenofovir DF. The majority of these cases occurred in patients with underlying systemic or renal disease, or in patients taking nephrotoxic agents; however, some cases occured in patients without identified risk factors. Atripla should be avoided with concurrent or recent use of a nephrotoxic agent).
No products indexed under this heading.

Amphotericin B (Renal impairment, including cases of acute renal failure and Fanconi syndrome (renal tubular

injury with severe hypophosphatemia), has been reported in association with the use of tenofovir DF. The majority of these cases occurred in patients with underlying systemic or renal disease, or in patients taking nephrotoxic agents; however, some cases occured in patients without identified risk factors. Atripla should be avoided with concurrent or recent use of a nephrotoxic agent).
No products indexed under this heading.

Amphotericin B, liposomal (Renal impairment, including cases of acute renal failure and Fanconi syndrome (renal tubular injury with severe hypophosphatemia), has been reported in association with the use of tenofovir DF. The majority of these cases occurred in patients with underlying systemic or renal disease, or in patients taking nephrotoxic agents; however, some cases occured in patients without identified risk factors. Atripla should be avoided with concurrent or recent use of a nephrotoxic agent). Products include:
AmBisome for Injection **606**

Amphotericin B Cholesteryl Sulfate (Renal impairment, including cases of acute renal failure and Fanconi syndrome (renal tubular injury with severe hypophosphatemia), has been reported in association with the use of tenofovir DF. The majority of these cases occurred in patients with underlying systemic or renal disease, or in patients taking nephrotoxic agents; however, some cases occured in patients without identified risk factors. Atripla should be avoided with concurrent or recent use of a nephrotoxic agent).
No products indexed under this heading.

Amphotericin B Lipid Complex (Renal impairment, including cases of acute renal failure and Fanconi syndrome (renal tubular injury with severe hypophosphatemia), has been reported in association with the use of tenofovir DF. The majority of these cases occurred in patients with underlying systemic or renal disease, or in patients taking nephrotoxic agents; however, some cases occured in patients without identified risk factors. Atripla should be avoided with concurrent or recent use of a nephrotoxic agent). Products include:
Abelcet Injection **1134**

Ampicillin (Renal impairment, including cases of acute renal failure and Fanconi syndrome (renal tubular injury with severe hypophosphatemia), has been reported in association with the use of tenofovir DF. The majority of these cases occurred in patients with underlying systemic or renal disease, or in patients taking nephrotoxic agents; however, some cases occured in patients without identified risk factors. Atripla should be avoided with concurrent or recent use of a nephrotoxic agent).
No products indexed under this heading.

Ampicillin Sodium (Renal impairment, including cases of acute renal failure and Fanconi syndrome (renal tubular injury with severe hypophosphatemia), has been reported in association with the use of tenofovir DF. The majority of these cases occurred in patients with underlying systemic or renal disease, or in patients taking nephrotoxic agents; however, some cases occured in patients without identified risk factors. Atripla should be avoided with concurrent or recent use of a nephrotoxic agent).
No products indexed under this heading.

Ampicillin Trihydrate (Renal impairment, including cases of acute renal failure and Fanconi syndrome (renal tubular injury with severe hypophosphatemia), has been reported in association with the use of tenofovir DF. The majority of these cases occurred in patients with underlying systemic or renal disease, or in patients taking nephrotoxic agents; however, some cases occured in patients without identified risk factors. Atripla should be avoided with concurrent or recent use of a nephrotoxic agent).
No products indexed under this heading.

Amprenavir (Efavirenz has the potential to decrease serum concentrations of amprenavir).
No products indexed under this heading.

Aprepitant (Efavirenz has been shown in vivo to induce CYP3A4. Other compounds that are substrates of CYP3A4 may have decreased plasma concentrations when co-administered with efavirenz). Products include:
Emend Capsules **1992**

Aspirin (Renal impairment, including cases of acute renal failure and Fanconi syndrome (renal tubular injury with severe hypophosphatemia), has been reported in association with the use of tenofovir DF. The majority of these cases occurred in patients with underlying systemic or renal disease, or in patients taking nephrotoxic agents; however, some cases occured in patients without identified risk factors. Atripla should be avoided with concurrent or recent use of a nephrotoxic agent). Products include:
Aggrenox Capsules **819**
Bayer Aspirin **750**
Percodan Tablets **1130**
St. Joseph 81 mg Aspirin Chewable and Enteric Coated Tablets **1903**

Astemizole (Due to the potential for serious and/or life-threatening reactions, such as cardiac arrhythmias with astemizole, concomitant use is contraindicated).
No products indexed under this heading.

Atazanavir (Atazanavir has been shown to increase tenofovir concentrations. The mechanism of this interaction is unknown. Higher tenofovir concentrations could potentiate tenofovir-associated adverse events, including renal disorders. Patients receiving either atazanavir with tenofovir DF should be monitored for tenofovir-associated adverse events. Atripla should be discontinued in patients who develop tenofovir-assocatied adverse events).
No products indexed under this heading.

Atorvastatin Calcium (Plasma concentrations of atorvastatin, pravastatin, and simvastatin decreased with efavirenz. Consult the complete prescribing information for the HMG-CoA reductase inhibitor for guidance on individualizing the dose). Products include:
Lipitor Tablets **2501**

Azithromycin Dihydrate (Renal impairment, including cases of acute renal failure and Fanconi syndrome (renal tubular injury with severe hypophosphatemia), has been reported in association with the use of tenofovir DF. The majority of these cases occurred in patients with underlying systemic or renal disease, or in patients taking nephrotoxic agents; however, some cases occured in patients without identified risk factors. Atripla should be avoided with concurrent or recent use of a nephrotoxic agent).
No products indexed under this heading.

Azlocillin Sodium (Renal impairment, including cases of acute renal failure and Fanconi syndrome (renal tubular injury with severe hypophosphatemia), has been reported in association with the use of tenofovir DF. The majority of these cases occurred in patients with underlying systemic or renal disease, or in patients taking nephrotoxic agents; however, some cases occured in patients without identified risk factors. Atripla should be avoided with concurrent or recent use of a nephrotoxic agent).
No products indexed under this heading.

Aztreonam (Renal impairment, including cases of acute renal failure and Fanconi syndrome (renal tubular injury with severe hypophosphatemia), has been reported in association with the use of tenofovir DF. The majority of these cases occurred in patients with underlying systemic or renal disease, or in patients taking nephrotoxic agents; however, some cases occured in patients without identified risk factors. Atripla should be avoided with concurrent or recent use of a nephrotoxic agent).
No products indexed under this heading.

Bacampicillin Hydrochloride (Renal impairment, including cases of acute renal failure and Fanconi syndrome (renal tubular injury with severe hypophosphatemia), has been reported in association with the use of tenofovir DF. The majority of these cases occurred in patients with underlying systemic or renal disease, or in patients taking nephrotoxic agents; however, some cases occured in patients without identified risk factors. Atripla should be avoided with concurrent or recent use of a nephrotoxic agent).
No products indexed under this heading.

Balsalazide Disodium (Renal impairment, including cases of acute renal failure and Fanconi syndrome (renal tubular injury with severe hypophosphatemia), has been reported in association with the use of tenofovir DF. The majority of these cases occurred in patients with underlying systemic or renal disease, or in patients taking nephrotoxic agents; however, some cases occured in patients without identified risk factors. Atripla should be avoided with concurrent or recent use of a nephrotoxic agent).
No products indexed under this heading.

Belladonna Ergotamine (Efavirenz has been shown in vivo to induce CYP3A4. Other compounds that are substrates of CYP3A4 may have decreased plasma concentrations when co-administered with efavirenz).
No products indexed under this heading.

Benazepril Hydrochloride (Renal impairment, including cases of acute renal failure and Fanconi syndrome (renal tubular injury with severe hypophosphatemia), has been reported in association with the use of tenofovir DF. The majority of these cases occurred in patients with underlying systemic or renal disease, or in patients taking nephrotoxic agents; however, some cases occured in patients without identified risk factors. Atripla should be avoided with concurrent or recent use of a nephrotoxic agent).
No products indexed under this heading.

Bendroflumethiazide (Renal impairment, including cases of acute renal failure and Fanconi syndrome (renal tubular injury with severe hypophosphatemia), has been reported in association with the use of tenofovir DF. The majority of these cases occurred in patients with underlying systemic or renal disease, or in patients taking nephrotoxic agents; however, some cases occured in patients without identified risk factors. Atripla should be avoided with concurrent or recent use of a nephrotoxic agent).
No products indexed under this heading.

Bepridil Hydrochloride (Due to the potential for serious and/or life threatening reactions, such as cardiac arrhythmias, concomitant use with bepridil is contraindicated).
No products indexed under this heading.

Betamethasone Acetate (Drugs which induce CYP3A4 activity would be expected to increase the clearance of efavirenz resulting in lower plasma concentrations).
No products indexed under this heading.

Betamethasone Sodium Phosphate (Drugs which induce CYP3A4 activity would be expected to increase the clearance of efavirenz resulting in lower plasma concentrations).
No products indexed under this heading.

Buspirone Hydrochloride (Efavirenz has been shown in vivo to induce CYP3A4. Other compounds that are substrates of CYP3A4 may have decreased plasma concentrations when co-administered with efavirenz).
No products indexed under this heading.

Busulfan (Efavirenz has been shown in vivo to induce CYP3A4. Other compounds that are substrates of CYP3A4 may have decreased plasma concentrations when co-administered with efavirenz). Products include:
Busulfex Injection **2477**
Myleran Tablets **1530**

Caffeine (Renal impairment, including cases of acute renal failure and Fanconi syndrome (renal tubular injury with severe hypophosphatemia),

has been reported in association with the use of tenofovir DF. The majority of these cases occurred in patients with underlying systemic or renal disease, or in patients taking nephrotoxic agents; however, some cases occured in patients without identified risk factors. Atripla should be avoided with concurrent or recent use of a nephrotoxic agent).
Products include:
BioLean Free Tablets .... ▣635
BioLean II Tablets .... ▣635
Winrgy Dietary Supplement .... ▣642

Candesartan Cilexetil (In vitro studies have demonstrated that efavirenz inhibits CYP2C9 in the range of observed efavirenz plasma concentrations. Co-administration of efavirenz with drugs primarily metabolized by CYP2C9 may result in altered plasma concentrations of the co-administered drug. Therefore, appropriate dose adjustments may be necessary for these drugs).
Products include:
Atacand Tablets 639
Atacand HCT 642

Captopril (Renal impairment, including cases of acute renal failure and Fanconi syndrome (renal tubular injury with severe hypophosphatemia), has been reported in association with the use of tenofovir DF. The majority of these cases occurred in patients with underlying systemic or renal disease, or in patients taking nephrotoxic agents; however, some cases occured in patients without identified risk factors. Atripla should be avoided with concurrent or recent use of a nephrotoxic agent).
Products include:
Captopril Tablets 2182

Carbamazepine (Alternative anticonvulsant treatments should be used due to decreases in both carbamazepine and efavirenz concentrations). Products include:
Carbatrol Capsules 3019
Equetro Extended-Release Capsules 3174

Carbenicillin Disodium (Renal impairment, including cases of acute renal failure and Fanconi syndrome (renal tubular injury with severe hypophosphatemia), has been reported in association with the use of tenofovir DF. The majority of these cases occurred in patients with underlying systemic or renal disease, or in patients taking nephrotoxic agents; however, some cases occured in patients without identified risk factors. Atripla should be avoided with concurrent or recent use of a nephrotoxic agent).
No products indexed under this heading.

Carbenicillin Indanyl Sodium (Renal impairment, including cases of acute renal failure and Fanconi syndrome (renal tubular injury with severe hypophosphatemia), has been reported in association with the use of tenofovir DF. The majority of these cases occurred in patients with underlying systemic or renal disease, or in patients taking nephrotoxic agents; however, some cases occured in patients without identified risk factors. Atripla should be avoided with concurrent or recent use of a nephrotoxic agent).
No products indexed under this heading.

Carboplatin (Renal impairment, including cases of acute renal failure and Fanconi syndrome (renal tubular injury with severe hypophosphatemia), has been reported in association with the use of tenofovir DF. The majority of these cases occurred in patients with underlying systemic or renal disease, or in patients taking nephrotoxic agents; however, some cases occured in patients without identified risk factors. Atripla should be avoided with concurrent or recent use of a nephrotoxic agent).
No products indexed under this heading.

Carisoprodol (In vitro studies have demonstrated that efavirenz inhibits CYP2C19 in the range of observed efavirenz plasma concentrations. Co-administration of efavirenz with drugs primarily metabolized by CYP2C19 may result in altered plasma concentrations of the co-administered drug. Therefore, appropriate dose adjustments may be necessary for these drugs).
Products include:
Soma Tablets 1931

Carmustine (BCNU) (Renal impairment, including cases of acute renal failure and Fanconi syndrome (renal tubular injury with severe hypophosphatemia), has been reported in association with the use of tenofovir DF. The majority of these cases occurred in patients with underlying systemic or renal disease, or in patients taking nephrotoxic agents; however, some cases occured in patients without identified risk factors. Atripla should be avoided with concurrent or recent use of a nephrotoxic agent).
No products indexed under this heading.

Carvedilol (In vitro studies have demonstrated that efavirenz inhibits CYP2C9 in the range of observed efavirenz plasma concentrations. Co-administration of efavirenz with drugs primarily metabolized by CYP2C9 may result in altered plasma concentrations of the co-administered drug. Therefore, appropriate dose adjustments may be necessary for these drugs).
Products include:
Coreg Tablets 1387

Cefaclor (Renal impairment, including cases of acute renal failure and Fanconi syndrome (renal tubular injury with severe hypophosphatemia), has been reported in association with the use of tenofovir DF. The majority of these cases occurred in patients with underlying systemic or renal disease, or in patients taking nephrotoxic agents; however, some cases occured in patients without identified risk factors. Atripla should be avoided with concurrent or recent use of a nephrotoxic agent).
No products indexed under this heading.

Cefadroxil (Renal impairment, including cases of acute renal failure and Fanconi syndrome (renal tubular injury with severe hypophosphatemia), has been reported in association with the use of tenofovir DF. The majority of these cases occurred in patients with underlying systemic or renal disease, or in patients taking nephrotoxic agents; however, some cases occured in patients without identified risk factors. Atripla should be avoided with concurrent or recent use of a nephrotoxic agent).
No products indexed under this heading.

Cefamandole Nafate (Renal impairment, including cases of acute renal failure and Fanconi syndrome (renal tubular injury with severe hypophosphatemia), has been reported in association with the use of tenofovir DF. The majority of these cases occurred in patients with underlying systemic or renal disease, or in patients taking nephrotoxic agents; however, some cases occured in patients without identified risk factors. Atripla should be avoided with concurrent or recent use of a nephrotoxic agent).
No products indexed under this heading.

Cefazolin Sodium (Renal impairment, including cases of acute renal failure and Fanconi syndrome (renal tubular injury with severe hypophosphatemia), has been reported in association with the use of tenofovir DF. The majority of these cases occurred in patients with underlying systemic or renal disease, or in patients taking nephrotoxic agents; however, some cases occured in patients without identified risk factors. Atripla should be avoided with concurrent or recent use of a nephrotoxic agent).
No products indexed under this heading.

Cefdinir (Renal impairment, including cases of acute renal failure and Fanconi syndrome (renal tubular injury with severe hypophosphatemia), has been reported in association with the use of tenofovir DF. The majority of these cases occurred in patients with underlying systemic or renal disease, or in patients taking nephrotoxic agents; however, some cases occured in patients without identified risk factors. Atripla should be avoided with concurrent or recent use of a nephrotoxic agent).
Products include:
Omnicef Capsules 497
Omnicef for Oral Suspension 497

Cefepime Hydrochloride (Renal impairment, including cases of acute renal failure and Fanconi syndrome (renal tubular injury with severe hypophosphatemia), has been reported in association with the use of tenofovir DF. The majority of these cases occurred in patients with underlying systemic or renal disease, or in patients taking nephrotoxic agents; however, some cases occured in patients without identified risk factors. Atripla should be avoided with concurrent or recent use of a nephrotoxic agent).
No products indexed under this heading.

Cefixime (Renal impairment, including cases of acute renal failure and Fanconi syndrome (renal tubular injury with severe hypophosphatemia), has been reported in association with the use of tenofovir DF. The majority of these cases occurred in patients with underlying systemic or renal disease, or in patients taking nephrotoxic agents; however, some cases occured in patients without identified risk factors. Atripla should be avoided with concurrent or recent use of a nephrotoxic agent).
Products include:
Suprax for Oral Suspension 1891
Suprax Tablets 1891

Cefmetazole Sodium (Renal impairment, including cases of acute renal failure and Fanconi syndrome (renal tubular injury with severe hypophosphatemia), has been reported in association with the use of tenofovir DF. The majority of these cases occurred in patients with underlying systemic or renal disease, or in patients taking nephrotoxic agents; however, some cases occured in patients without identified risk factors. Atripla should be avoided with concurrent or recent use of a nephrotoxic agent).
No products indexed under this heading.

Cefonicid Sodium (Renal impairment, including cases of acute renal failure and Fanconi syndrome (renal tubular injury with severe hypophosphatemia), has been reported in association with the use of tenofovir DF. The majority of these cases occurred in patients with underlying systemic or renal disease, or in patients taking nephrotoxic agents; however, some cases occured in patients without identified risk factors. Atripla should be avoided with concurrent or recent use of a nephrotoxic agent).
No products indexed under this heading.

Cefoperazone Sodium (Renal impairment, including cases of acute renal failure and Fanconi syndrome (renal tubular injury with severe hypophosphatemia), has been reported in association with the use of tenofovir DF. The majority of these cases occurred in patients with underlying systemic or renal disease, or in patients taking nephrotoxic agents; however, some cases occured in patients without identified risk factors. Atripla should be avoided with concurrent or recent use of a nephrotoxic agent).
No products indexed under this heading.

Ceforanide (Renal impairment, including cases of acute renal failure and Fanconi syndrome (renal tubular injury with severe hypophosphatemia), has been reported in association with the use of tenofovir DF. The majority of these cases occurred in patients with underlying systemic or renal disease, or in patients taking nephrotoxic agents; however, some cases occured in patients without identified risk factors. Atripla should be avoided with concurrent or recent use of a nephrotoxic agent).
No products indexed under this heading.

Cefotaxime Sodium (Renal impairment, including cases of acute renal failure and Fanconi syndrome (renal tubular injury with severe hypophosphatemia), has been reported in association with the use of tenofovir DF. The majority of these cases occurred in patients with underlying systemic or renal disease, or in patients taking nephrotoxic agents; however, some cases occured in patients without identified risk factors. Atripla should be avoided with concurrent or recent use of a nephrotoxic agent).
No products indexed under this heading.

Cefotetan (Renal impairment, including cases of acute renal failure and Fanconi syndrome (renal tubular injury with severe hypophosphatemia), has been reported in association with the use of tenofovir DF. The majority of these cases occurred in patients with underlying systemic or renal disease, or in patients taking nephrotoxic agents; however, some cases occured in patients without identified risk factors. Atripla should be avoided with concurrent or recent use of a nephrotoxic agent).

No products indexed under this heading.

Cefoxitin Sodium (Renal impairment, including cases of acute renal failure and Fanconi syndrome (renal tubular injury with severe hypophosphatemia), has been reported in association with the use of tenofovir DF. The majority of these cases occurred in patients with underlying systemic or renal disease, or in patients taking nephrotoxic agents; however, some cases occured in patients without identified risk factors. Atripla should be avoided with concurrent or recent use of a nephrotoxic agent).

No products indexed under this heading.

Cefpodoxime Proxetil (Renal impairment, including cases of acute renal failure and Fanconi syndrome (renal tubular injury with severe hypophosphatemia), has been reported in association with the use of tenofovir DF. The majority of these cases occurred in patients with underlying systemic or renal disease, or in patients taking nephrotoxic agents; however, some cases occured in patients without identified risk factors. Atripla should be avoided with concurrent or recent use of a nephrotoxic agent).

No products indexed under this heading.

Cefprozil (Renal impairment, including cases of acute renal failure and Fanconi syndrome (renal tubular injury with severe hypophosphatemia), has been reported in association with the use of tenofovir DF. The majority of these cases occurred in patients with underlying systemic or renal disease, or in patients taking nephrotoxic agents; however, some cases occured in patients without identified risk factors. Atripla should be avoided with concurrent or recent use of a nephrotoxic agent).

No products indexed under this heading.

Ceftazidime (Renal impairment, including cases of acute renal failure and Fanconi syndrome (renal tubular injury with severe hypophosphatemia), has been reported in association with the use of tenofovir DF. The majority of these cases occurred in patients with underlying systemic or renal disease, or in patients taking nephrotoxic agents; however, some cases occured in patients without identified risk factors. Atripla should be avoided with concurrent or recent use of a nephrotoxic agent). Products include:

Fortaz **1450**

Ceftizoxime Sodium (Renal impairment, including cases of acute renal failure and Fanconi syndrome (renal tubular injury with severe hypophosphatemia), has been reported in association with the use of tenofovir DF. The majority of these cases occurred in patients with underlying systemic or renal disease, or in patients taking nephrotoxic agents; however, some cases occured in patients without identified risk factors. Atripla should be avoided with concurrent or recent use of a nephrotoxic agent).

No products indexed under this heading.

Ceftriaxone Sodium (Renal impairment, including cases of acute renal failure and Fanconi syndrome (renal tubular injury with severe hypophosphatemia), has been reported in association with the use of tenofovir DF. The majority of these cases occurred in patients with underlying systemic or renal disease, or in patients taking nephrotoxic agents; however, some cases occured in patients without identified risk factors. Atripla should be avoided with concurrent or recent use of a nephrotoxic agent). Products include:

Rocephin Injectable Vials, ADD-Vantage, Galaxy, Bulk **2642**

Cefuroxime Axetil (Renal impairment, including cases of acute renal failure and Fanconi syndrome (renal tubular injury with severe hypophosphatemia), has been reported in association with the use of tenofovir DF. The majority of these cases occurred in patients with underlying systemic or renal disease, or in patients taking nephrotoxic agents; however, some cases occured in patients without identified risk factors. Atripla should be avoided with concurrent or recent use of a nephrotoxic agent). Products include:

Ceftin **1380**

Cefuroxime Sodium (Renal impairment, including cases of acute renal failure and Fanconi syndrome (renal tubular injury with severe hypophosphatemia), has been reported in association with the use of tenofovir DF. The majority of these cases occurred in patients with underlying systemic or renal disease, or in patients taking nephrotoxic agents; however, some cases occured in patients without identified risk factors. Atripla should be avoided with concurrent or recent use of a nephrotoxic agent).

No products indexed under this heading.

Celecoxib (Renal impairment, including cases of acute renal failure and Fanconi syndrome (renal tubular injury with severe hypophosphatemia), has been reported in association with the use of tenofovir DF. The majority of these cases occurred in patients with underlying systemic or renal disease, or in patients taking nephrotoxic agents; however, some cases occured in patients without identified risk factors. Atripla should be avoided with concurrent or recent use of a nephrotoxic agent). Products include:

Celebrex Capsules **2979**

Cephalexin (Renal impairment, including cases of acute renal failure and Fanconi syndrome (renal tubular injury with severe hypophosphatemia), has been reported in association with the use of tenofovir DF. The majority of these cases occurred in patients with underlying systemic or renal disease, or in patients taking nephrotoxic agents; however, some cases occured in patients without identified risk factors. Atripla should be avoided with concurrent or recent use of a nephrotoxic agent).

No products indexed under this heading.

Cephalothin Sodium (Renal impairment, including cases of acute renal failure and Fanconi syndrome (renal tubular injury with severe hypophosphatemia), has been reported in association with the use of tenofovir DF. The majority of these cases occurred in patients with underlying systemic or renal disease, or in patients taking nephrotoxic agents; however, some cases occured in patients without identified risk factors. Atripla should be avoided with concurrent or recent use of a nephrotoxic agent).

No products indexed under this heading.

Cephapirin Sodium (Renal impairment, including cases of acute renal failure and Fanconi syndrome (renal tubular injury with severe hypophosphatemia), has been reported in association with the use of tenofovir DF. The majority of these cases occurred in patients with underlying systemic or renal disease, or in patients taking nephrotoxic agents; however, some cases occured in patients without identified risk factors. Atripla should be avoided with concurrent or recent use of a nephrotoxic agent).

No products indexed under this heading.

Cephradine (Renal impairment, including cases of acute renal failure and Fanconi syndrome (renal tubular injury with severe hypophosphatemia), has been reported in association with the use of tenofovir DF. The majority of these cases occurred in patients with underlying systemic or renal disease, or in patients taking nephrotoxic agents; however, some cases occured in patients without identified risk factors. Atripla should be avoided with concurrent or recent use of a nephrotoxic agent).

No products indexed under this heading.

Cerivastatin Sodium (Renal impairment, including cases of acute renal failure and Fanconi syndrome (renal tubular injury with severe hypophosphatemia), has been reported in association with the use of tenofovir DF. The majority of these cases occurred in patients with underlying systemic or renal disease, or in patients taking nephrotoxic agents; however, some cases occured in patients without identified risk factors. Atripla should be avoided with concurrent or recent use of a nephrotoxic agent).

No products indexed under this heading.

Chlorothiazide (Renal impairment, including cases of acute renal failure and Fanconi syndrome (renal tubular injury with severe hypophosphatemia), has been reported in association with the use of tenofovir DF. The majority of these cases occurred in patients with underlying systemic or renal disease, or in patients taking nephrotoxic agents; however, some cases occured in patients without identified risk factors. Atripla should be avoided with concurrent or recent use of a nephrotoxic agent).

No products indexed under this heading.

Chlorothiazide Sodium (Renal impairment, including cases of acute renal failure and Fanconi syndrome (renal tubular injury with severe hypophosphatemia), has been reported in association with the use of tenofovir DF. The majority of these cases occurred in patients with underlying systemic or renal disease, or in patients taking nephrotoxic agents; however, some cases occured in patients without identified risk factors. Atripla should be avoided with concurrent or recent use of a nephrotoxic agent). Products include:

Intravenous Sodium Diuril **2490**

Chlorpheniramine (Efavirenz has been shown in vivo to induce CYP3A4. Other compounds that are substrates of CYP3A4 may have decreased plasma concentrations when co-administered with efavirenz).

No products indexed under this heading.

Chlorpheniramine Maleate (Efavirenz has been shown in vivo to induce CYP3A4. Other compounds that are substrates of CYP3A4 may have decreased plasma concentrations when co-administered with efavirenz). Products include:

Actifed Cold & Allergy Tablets **1895**
Sudafed PE Sinus & Allergy Tablets **1908**
Tylenol Allergy Multi-Symptom Caplets with Cool Burst and Rapid Release Gelcaps **1916**
Children's Tylenol Plus Cold Suspension Liquid **1912**
Children's Tylenol Plus Cough & Runny Nose Suspension Liquid **1912**
Children's Tylenol Plus Flu Suspension Liquid **1914**
Children's Tylenol Plus Multi-Symptom Cold Suspension Liquid **1912**
Tylenol Cold Head Congestion Nighttime Caplets with Cool Burst **1910**
Tylenol Cold Multi-Symptom Nighttime Caplets with Cool Burst **1913**
Tylenol Sinus Congestion & Pain Nighttime Caplets with Cool Burst **1917**

Chlorpheniramine Polistirex (Efavirenz has been shown in vivo to induce CYP3A4. Other compounds that are substrates of CYP3A4 may have decreased plasma concentrations when co-administered with efavirenz). Products include:

Tussionex Pennkinetic Extended-Release Suspension **3154**

Chlorpheniramine Tannate (Efavirenz has been shown in vivo to induce CYP3A4. Other compounds that are substrates of CYP3A4 may have decreased plasma concentrations when co-administered with efavirenz).

No products indexed under this heading.

Chlorpropamide (Renal impairment, including cases of acute renal failure and Fanconi syndrome (renal tubular injury with severe hypophosphatemia), has been reported in association with the use of tenofovir DF. The majority of these cases occurred in patients with underlying systemic or renal disease, or in patients taking nephrotoxic agents; however, some cases occured in patients without identified risk factors. Atripla should be avoided with concurrent or recent use of a nephrotoxic agent).

No products indexed under this heading.

Cidofovir (Since emtricitabine and tenofovir are primarily eliminated by the kidneys, co-administration of Atripla with drugs that reduce renal fuction or compete for active tubular secretion may increase serum concentrations of emtricitabine, tenofovir, and/or other renally eliminated drugs).
No products indexed under this heading.

Cilastatin Sodium (Renal impairment, including cases of acute renal failure and Fanconi syndrome (renal tubular injury with severe hypophosphatemia), has been reported in association with the use of tenofovir DF. The majority of these cases occurred in patients with underlying systemic or renal disease, or in patients taking nephrotoxic agents; however, some cases occured in patients without identified risk factors. Atripla should be avoided with concurrent or recent use of a nephrotoxic agent). Products include:
Primaxin I.M. 2080
Primaxin I.V. 2083

Cilostazol (In vitro studies have demonstrated that efavirenz inhibits CYP2C19 in the range of observed efavirenz plasma concentrations. Co-administration of efavirenz with drugs primarily metabolized by CYP2C19 may result in altered plasma concentrations of the co-administered drug. Therefore, appropriate dose adjustments may be necessary for these drugs).
Products include:
Pletal Tablets 2481

Cimetidine (Renal impairment, including cases of acute renal failure and Fanconi syndrome (renal tubular injury with severe hypophosphatemia), has been reported in association with the use of tenofovir DF. The majority of these cases occurred in patients with underlying systemic or renal disease, or in patients taking nephrotoxic agents; however, some cases occured in patients without identified risk factors. Atripla should be avoided with concurrent or recent use of a nephrotoxic agent).
No products indexed under this heading.

Cimetidine Hydrochloride (Renal impairment, including cases of acute renal failure and Fanconi syndrome (renal tubular injury with severe hypophosphatemia), has been reported in association with the use of tenofovir DF. The majority of these cases occurred in patients with underlying systemic or renal disease, or in patients taking nephrotoxic agents; however, some cases occured in patients without identified risk factors. Atripla should be avoided with concurrent or recent use of a nephrotoxic agent).
No products indexed under this heading.

Ciprofloxacin Hydrochloride (Drugs which induce CYP3A4 activity would be expected to increase the clearance of efavirenz resulting in lower plasma concentrations).
Products include:
Cipro Tablets 2810

Cisapride (Due to the potential for serious and/or life-threatening reactions, such as cardiac arrhythmias, concomitant use with cisapride is contraindicated).
No products indexed under this heading.

Cisplatin (Renal impairment, including cases of acute renal failure and Fanconi syndrome (renal tubular injury with severe hypophosphatemia), has been reported in association with the use of tenofovir DF. The majority of these cases occurred in patients with underlying systemic or renal disease, or in patients taking nephrotoxic agents; however, some cases occured in patients without identified risk factors. Atripla should be avoided with concurrent or recent use of a nephrotoxic agent).
No products indexed under this heading.

Citalopram Hydrobromide (In vitro studies have demonstrated that efavirenz inhibits CYP2C19 in the range of observed efavirenz plasma concentrations. Co-administration of efavirenz with drugs primarily metabolized by CYP2C19 may result in altered plasma concentrations of the co-administered drug. Therefore, appropriate dose adjustments may be necessary for these drugs).
Products include:
Celexa 1160

Cladribine (Renal impairment, including cases of acute renal failure and Fanconi syndrome (renal tubular injury with severe hypophosphatemia), has been reported in association with the use of tenofovir DF. The majority of these cases occurred in patients with underlying systemic or renal disease, or in patients taking nephrotoxic agents; however, some cases occured in patients without identified risk factors. Atripla should be avoided with concurrent or recent use of a nephrotoxic agent).
Products include:
Leustatin Injection 2384

Clarithromycin (In uninfected volunteers, 46% developed a rash while receiving efavirenz and clarithromycin. No dose adjustment of Atripla is recommended when given with clarithromycin. Alternatives to clarithromycin, such as azithromycin, should be considered. Other macrolide antibiotics, such as erythromycin, have not been studied in combination with Atripla). Products include:
Biaxin/Biaxin XL 411

Clomipramine Hydrochloride (In vitro studies have demonstrated that efavirenz inhibits CYP2C9 in the range of observed efavirenz plasma concentrations. Co-administration of efavirenz with drugs primarily metabolized by CYP2C9 may result in altered plasma concentrations of the co-administered drug. Therefore, appropriate dose adjustments may be necessary for these drugs).
No products indexed under this heading.

Clozapine (Renal impairment, including cases of acute renal failure and Fanconi syndrome (renal tubular injury with severe hypophosphatemia), has been reported in association with the use of tenofovir DF. The majority of these cases occurred in patients with underlying systemic or renal disease, or in patients taking nephrotoxic agents; however, some cases occured in patients without identified risk factors. Atripla should be avoided with concurrent or recent use of a nephrotoxic agent).
No products indexed under this heading.

Colistimethate Sodium (Renal impairment, including cases of acute renal failure and Fanconi syndrome (renal tubular injury with severe hypophosphatemia), has been reported in association with the use of tenofovir DF. The majority of these cases occurred in patients with underlying systemic or renal disease, or in patients taking nephrotoxic agents; however, some cases occured in patients without identified risk factors. Atripla should be avoided with concurrent or recent use of a nephrotoxic agent).
No products indexed under this heading.

Colistin Sulfate (Renal impairment, including cases of acute renal failure and Fanconi syndrome (renal tubular injury with severe hypophosphatemia), has been reported in association with the use of tenofovir DF. The majority of these cases occurred in patients with underlying systemic or renal disease, or in patients taking nephrotoxic agents; however, some cases occured in patients without identified risk factors. Atripla should be avoided with concurrent or recent use of a nephrotoxic agent).
No products indexed under this heading.

Cortisone Acetate (Drugs which induce CYP3A4 activity would be expected to increase the clearance of efavirenz resulting in lower plasma concentrations).
No products indexed under this heading.

Cyclophosphamide (Renal impairment, including cases of acute renal failure and Fanconi syndrome (renal tubular injury with severe hypophosphatemia), has been reported in association with the use of tenofovir DF. The majority of these cases occurred in patients with underlying systemic or renal disease, or in patients taking nephrotoxic agents; however, some cases occured in patients without identified risk factors. Atripla should be avoided with concurrent or recent use of a nephrotoxic agent).
No products indexed under this heading.

Cyclosporine (Renal impairment, including cases of acute renal failure and Fanconi syndrome (renal tubular injury with severe hypophosphatemia), has been reported in association with the use of tenofovir DF. The majority of these cases occurred in patients with underlying systemic or renal disease, or in patients taking nephrotoxic agents; however, some cases occured in patients without identified risk factors. Atripla should be avoided with concurrent or recent use of a nephrotoxic agent).
Products include:
Gengraf Capsules 435
Neoral Oral Solution 2280
Neoral Soft Gelatin Capsules 2280
Restasis Ophthalmic Emulsion 557
Sandimmune 2296

Cytarabine (Renal impairment, including cases of acute renal failure and Fanconi syndrome (renal tubular injury with severe hypophosphatemia), has been reported in association with the use of tenofovir DF. The majority of these cases occurred in patients with underlying systemic or renal disease, or in patients taking nephrotoxic agents; however, some cases occured in patients without identified risk factors. Atripla should be avoided with concurrent or recent use of a nephrotoxic agent).
No products indexed under this heading.

Cytarabine Liposome (Renal impairment, including cases of acute renal failure and Fanconi syndrome (renal tubular injury with severe hypophosphatemia), has been reported in association with the use of tenofovir DF. The majority of these cases occurred in patients with underlying systemic or renal disease, or in patients taking nephrotoxic agents; however, some cases occured in patients without identified risk factors. Atripla should be avoided with concurrent or recent use of a nephrotoxic agent). Products include:
DepoCyt Injection 1136

Delavirdine Mesylate (Renal impairment, including cases of acute renal failure and Fanconi syndrome (renal tubular injury with severe hypophosphatemia), has been reported in association with the use of tenofovir DF. The majority of these cases occurred in patients with underlying systemic or renal disease, or in patients taking nephrotoxic agents; however, some cases occured in patients without identified risk factors. Atripla should be avoided with concurrent or recent use of a nephrotoxic agent).
No products indexed under this heading.

Desipramine Hydrochloride (In vitro studies have demonstrated that efavirenz inhibits CYP2C19 in the range of observed efavirenz plasma concentrations. Co-administration of efavirenz with drugs primarily metabolized by CYP2C19 may result in altered plasma concentrations of the co-administered drug. Therefore, appropriate dose adjustments may be necessary for these drugs).
No products indexed under this heading.

Desogestrel (Efavirenz has been shown in vivo to induce CYP3A4. Other compounds that are substrates of CYP3A4 may have decreased plasma concentrations when co-administered with efavirenz). Products include:
Mircette Tablets 1034

Dexamethasone (Drugs which induce CYP3A4 activity would be expected to increase the clearance of efavirenz resulting in lower plasma concentrations). Products include:
Ciprodex Otic Suspension 541

Dexamethasone Acetate (Drugs which induce CYP3A4 activity would be expected to increase the clearance of efavirenz resulting in lower plasma concentrations).
No products indexed under this heading.

Dexamethasone Sodium Phosphate (Drugs which induce CYP3A4 activity would be expected to increase the clearance of efavirenz resulting in lower plasma concentrations).
No products indexed under this heading.

Dextromethorphan (In vitro studies have demonstrated that efavirenz inhibits CYP2C9 in the range of observed efavirenz plasma concentrations. Co-administration of efavirenz with drugs primarily metabolized by CYP2C9 may result in altered plasma concentrations of the co-administered drug. Therefore, appropriate dose adjustments may be necessary for these drugs).
No products indexed under this heading.

Dextromethorphan Hydrobromide (In vitro studies have demonstrated that efavirenz inhibits CYP2C19 in the range of observed efavirenz plasma concentrations. Co-administration of efavirenz with drugs primarily metabolized by CYP2C19 may result in altered plasma concentrations of the co-administered drug. Therefore, appropriate dose adjustments may be necessary for these drugs).
Products include:
PediaCare Children's Liquid Multi-Symptom Cold **1902**
PediaCare Children's Long-Acting Cough **1902**
Children's Sudafed PE Cold & Cough Liquid **1907**
Sudafed PE Cold & Cough Caplets **1907**
Children's Tylenol Plus Cough & Runny Nose Suspension Liquid **1912**
Children's Tylenol Plus Cough & Sore Throat Suspension Liquid **1912**
Children's Tylenol Plus Flu Suspension Liquid **1914**
Children's Tylenol Plus Multi-Symptom Cold Suspension Liquid **1912**
Tylenol Cold Severe Congestion Daytime Caplets with Cool Burst **1912**
Tylenol Cold Head Congestion Daytime Caplets with Cool Burst **1910**
Tylenol Cold Head Congestion Nighttime Caplets with Cool Burst **1910**
Tylenol Cold Head Congestion Severe Daytime Caplets with Cool Burst **1910**
Tylenol Cold Multi-Symptom Daytime Caplets with Cool Burst and Rapid Release Gels **1913**
Tylenol Cold Multi-Symptom Daytime Liquid with Citrus Burst **1913**
Tylenol Cold Multi-Symptom Nighttime Caplets with Cool Burst **1913**
Tylenol Cold Multi-Symptom Nighttime Liquid with Cool Burst **1913**
Tylenol Cold Multi-Symptom Severe Caplets with Cool Burst **1913**
Tylenol Cold Multi-Symptom Severe Daytime Liquid with Citrus Burst **1913**
Tylenol Cough & Sore Throat Daytime Liquid with Cool Burst **1918**
Tylenol Cough & Sore Throat Nighttime Liquid with Cool Burst **1918**
Vicks DayQuil Cold & Flu Multi-Symptom Relief **616**
Vicks DayQuil LiquiCaps **2567**
Vicks DayQuil Liquid **2567**
Vicks DayQuil Multi-Symptom Cold/Flu Relief **2567**
Vicks NyQuil Cold & Flu Multi-Symptom Relief **617**
Vicks NyQuil LiquiCaps **2567**
Vicks NyQuil Liquid **2567**
Vicks NyQuil Multi-Symptom Cold/Flu Relief **2567**

Diatrizoate Meglumine (Renal impairment, including cases of acute renal failure and Fanconi syndrome (renal tubular injury with severe hypophosphatemia), has been reported in association with the use of tenofovir DF. The majority of these cases occurred in patients with underlying systemic or renal disease, or in patients taking nephrotoxic agents; however, some cases occured in patients without identified risk factors. Atripla should be avoided with concurrent or recent use of a nephrotoxic agent).
No products indexed under this heading.

Diatrizoate Sodium (Renal impairment, including cases of acute renal failure and Fanconi syndrome (renal tubular injury with severe hypophosphatemia), has been reported in association with the use of tenofovir DF. The majority of these cases occurred in patients with underlying systemic or renal disease, or in patients taking nephrotoxic agents; however, some cases occured in patients without identified risk factors. Atripla should be avoided with concurrent or recent use of a nephrotoxic agent).
No products indexed under this heading.

Diazepam (Efavirenz has been shown in vivo to induce CYP3A4. Other compounds that are substrates of CYP3A4 may have decreased plasma concentrations when co-administered with efavirenz). Products include:
Valium Tablets **2658**

Diclofenac Potassium (Renal impairment, including cases of acute renal failure and Fanconi syndrome (renal tubular injury with severe hypophosphatemia), has been reported in association with the use of tenofovir DF. The majority of these cases occurred in patients with underlying systemic or renal disease, or in patients taking nephrotoxic agents; however, some cases occured in patients without identified risk factors. Atripla should be avoided with concurrent or recent use of a nephrotoxic agent).
No products indexed under this heading.

Diclofenac Sodium (Renal impairment, including cases of acute renal failure and Fanconi syndrome (renal tubular injury with severe hypophosphatemia), has been reported in association with the use of tenofovir DF. The majority of these cases occurred in patients with underlying systemic or renal disease, or in patients taking nephrotoxic agents; however, some cases occured in patients without identified risk factors. Atripla should be avoided with concurrent or recent use of a nephrotoxic agent). Products include:
Diclofenac Sodium Ophthalmic Solution .... ⊙ **240**
Voltaren Ophthalmic Solution **2336**
Voltaren Tablets **2334**
Voltaren-XR Tablets **2337**

Dicloxacillin Sodium (Renal impairment, including cases of acute renal failure and Fanconi syndrome (renal tubular injury with severe hypophosphatemia), has been reported in association with the use of tenofovir DF. The majority of these cases occurred in patients with underlying systemic or renal disease, or in patients taking nephrotoxic agents; however, some cases occured in patients without identified risk factors. Atripla should be avoided with concurrent or recent use of a nephrotoxic agent).
No products indexed under this heading.

Didanosine (Co-administration of tenofovir DF and didanosine should be undertaken with caution and patients receiving this combination should be monitored closely for didanosine-associated adverse events. Didanosine should be discontinued in patients who develop didanosine-associated adverse events).
No products indexed under this heading.

Dihydroergotamine Mesylate (Due to the potential for serious and/or life-threatening reactions, such as acute ergot toxicity characterized by peripheral vasospasm and ischemia of the extremities and other tissues, concomitant use with ergot derivatives is contraindicated).
No products indexed under this heading.

Diltiazem Hydrochloride (Efavirenz has been shown in vivo to induce CYP3A4. Other compounds that are substrates of CYP3A4 may have decreased plasma concentrations when co-administered with efavirenz). Products include:
Cardizem LA Extended Release Tablets **421**

Diltiazem Maleate (Efavirenz has been shown in vivo to induce CYP3A4. Other compounds that are substrates of CYP3A4 may have decreased plasma concentrations when co-administered with efavirenz).
No products indexed under this heading.

Disopyramide (Efavirenz has been shown in vivo to induce CYP3A4. Other compounds that are substrates of CYP3A4 may have decreased plasma concentrations when co-administered with efavirenz).
No products indexed under this heading.

Disopyramide Phosphate (Efavirenz has been shown in vivo to induce CYP3A4. Other compounds that are substrates of CYP3A4 may have decreased plasma concentrations when co-administered with efavirenz).
No products indexed under this heading.

Disulfiram (Efavirenz has been shown in vivo to induce CYP3A4. Other compounds that are substrates of CYP3A4 may have decreased plasma concentrations when co-administered with efavirenz).
No products indexed under this heading.

Divalproex Sodium (In vitro studies have demonstrated that efavirenz inhibits CYP2C19 in the range of observed efavirenz plasma concentrations. Co-administration of efavirenz with drugs primarily metabolized by CYP2C19 may result in altered plasma concentrations of the co-administered drug. Therefore, appropriate dose adjustments may be necessary for these drugs). Products include:
Depakote ER Tablets **423**

Doxepin Hydrochloride (In vitro studies have demonstrated that efavirenz inhibits CYP2C19 in the range of observed efavirenz plasma concentrations. Co-administration of efavirenz with drugs primarily metabolized by CYP2C19 may result in altered plasma concentrations of the co-administered drug. Therefore, appropriate dose adjustments may be necessary for these drugs).
No products indexed under this heading.

Doxorubicin Hydrochloride (Efavirenz has been shown in vivo to induce CYP3A4. Other compounds that are substrates of CYP3A4 may have decreased plasma concentrations when co-administered with efavirenz).
No products indexed under this heading.

Dronabinol (Efavirenz has been shown in vivo to induce CYP3A4. Other compounds that are substrates of CYP3A4 may have decreased plasma concentrations when co-administered with efavirenz). Products include:
Marinol Capsules **3163**

Enalapril Maleate (Renal impairment, including cases of acute renal failure and Fanconi syndrome (renal tubular injury with severe hypophosphatemia), has been reported in association with the use of tenofovir DF. The majority of these cases occurred in patients with underlying systemic or renal disease, or in patients taking nephrotoxic agents; however, some cases occured in patients without identified risk factors. Atripla should be avoided with concurrent or recent use of a nephrotoxic agent).
No products indexed under this heading.

Enalaprilat (Renal impairment, including cases of acute renal failure and Fanconi syndrome (renal tubular injury with severe hypophosphatemia), has been reported in association with the use of tenofovir DF. The majority of these cases occurred in patients with underlying systemic or renal disease, or in patients taking nephrotoxic agents; however, some cases occured in patients without identified risk factors. Atripla should be avoided with concurrent or recent use of a nephrotoxic agent).
No products indexed under this heading.

Enfuvirtide (Renal impairment, including cases of acute renal failure and Fanconi syndrome (renal tubular injury with severe hypophosphatemia), has been reported in association with the use of tenofovir DF. The majority of these cases occurred in patients with underlying systemic or renal disease, or in patients taking nephrotoxic agents; however, some cases occured in patients without identified risk factors. Atripla should be avoided with concurrent or recent use of a nephrotoxic agent).
No products indexed under this heading.

Eprosartan Mesylate (In vitro studies have demonstrated that efavirenz inhibits CYP2C9 in the range of observed efavirenz plasma concentrations. Co-administration of efavirenz with drugs primarily metabolized by CYP2C9 may result in altered plasma concentrations of the co-administered drug. Therefore,

appropriate dose adjustments may be necessary for these drugs). Products include:
- Teveten Tablets 515
- Teveten HCT Tablets 517

Ergonovine Maleate (Due to the potential for serious and/or life-threatening reactions, such as acute ergot toxicity characterized by peripheral vasospasm and ischemia of the extremities and other tissues, concomitant use with ergot derivatives is contraindicated).
No products indexed under this heading.

Ergotamine Tartrate (Due to the potential for serious and/or life-threatening reactions, such as acute ergot toxicity characterized by peripheral vasospasm and ischemia of the extremities and other tissues, concomitant use with ergot derivatives is contraindicated).
No products indexed under this heading.

Erythromycin (Efavirenz has been shown in vivo to induce CYP3A4. Other compounds that are substrates of CYP3A4 may have decreased plasma concentrations when co-administered with efavirenz).
No products indexed under this heading.

Erythromycin Estolate (Efavirenz has been shown in vivo to induce CYP3A4. Other compounds that are substrates of CYP3A4 may have decreased plasma concentrations when co-administered with efavirenz).
No products indexed under this heading.

Erythromycin Ethylsuccinate (Efavirenz has been shown in vivo to induce CYP3A4. Other compounds that are substrates of CYP3A4 may have decreased plasma concentrations when co-administered with efavirenz). Products include:
- E.E.S. 433
- EryPed 431

Erythromycin Gluceptate (Efavirenz has been shown in vivo to induce CYP3A4. Other compounds that are substrates of CYP3A4 may have decreased plasma concentrations when co-administered with efavirenz).
No products indexed under this heading.

Erythromycin Lactobionate (Efavirenz has been shown in vivo to induce CYP3A4. Other compounds that are substrates of CYP3A4 may have decreased plasma concentrations when co-administered with efavirenz).
No products indexed under this heading.

Erythromycin Stearate (Efavirenz has been shown in vivo to induce CYP3A4. Other compounds that are substrates of CYP3A4 may have decreased plasma concentrations when co-administered with efavirenz).
No products indexed under this heading.

Esomeprazole Magnesium (In vitro studies have demonstrated that efavirenz inhibits CYP2C19 in the range of observed efavirenz plasma concentrations. Co-administration of efavirenz with drugs primarily metabolized by CYP2C19 may result in altered plasma concentrations of the co-administered drug. Therefore, appropriate dose adjustments may be necessary for these drugs). Products include:
- Nexium Delayed-Release Capsules 645
- Nexium Delayed-Release Oral Suspension 645

Estradiol (Efavirenz has been shown in vivo to induce CYP3A4. Other compounds that are substrates of CYP3A4 may have decreased plasma concentrations when co-administered with efavirenz). Products include:
- Activella Tablets 2347
- Angeliq Tablets 751
- Climara Transdermal System 763
- Climara Pro Transdermal System 768
- Divigel 3167
- Vagifem Tablets 2375

Estradiol Benzoate (Efavirenz has been shown in vivo to induce CYP3A4. Other compounds that are substrates of CYP3A4 may have decreased plasma concentrations when co-administered with efavirenz).
No products indexed under this heading.

Estradiol Cypionate (Efavirenz has been shown in vivo to induce CYP3A4. Other compounds that are substrates of CYP3A4 may have decreased plasma concentrations when co-administered with efavirenz).
No products indexed under this heading.

Estradiol Valerate (Efavirenz has been shown in vivo to induce CYP3A4. Other compounds that are substrates of CYP3A4 may have decreased plasma concentrations when co-administered with efavirenz).
No products indexed under this heading.

Ethinyl Estradiol (Because the potential interaction of efavirenz with oral contraceptives has not been fully characterized, a reliable method of barrier contraception should be used in addition to oral contraceptives). Products include:
- Lybrel Tablets 3204
- Mircette Tablets 1034
- NuvaRing 2897
- Ortho-Cyclen/Ortho Tri-Cyclen 2449
- Ortho Evra Transdermal System 2437
- Ortho Tri-Cyclen Lo Tablets 2458
- Seasonique Tablets 1046
- Yaz Tablets 805

Ethiodized Oil (Renal impairment, including cases of acute renal failure and Fanconi syndrome (renal tubular injury with severe hypophosphatemia), has been reported in association with the use of tenofovir DF. The majority of these cases occurred in patients with underlying systemic or renal disease, or in patients taking nephrotoxic agents; however, some cases occured in patients without identified risk factors. Atripla should be avoided with concurrent or recent use of a nephrotoxic agent).
No products indexed under this heading.

Ethosuximide (Efavirenz has been shown in vivo to induce CYP3A4. Other compounds that are substrates of CYP3A4 may have decreased plasma concentrations when co-administered with efavirenz).
No products indexed under this heading.

Ethotoin (In vitro studies have demonstrated that efavirenz inhibits CYP2C19 in the range of observed efavirenz plasma concentrations. Co-administration of efavirenz with drugs primarily metabolized by CYP2C19 may result in altered plasma concentrations of the co-administered drug. Therefore, appropriate dose adjustments may be necessary for these drugs).
No products indexed under this heading.

Ethynodiol Diacetate (Efavirenz has been shown in vivo to induce CYP3A4. Other compounds that are substrates of CYP3A4 may have decreased plasma concentrations when co-administered with efavirenz).
No products indexed under this heading.

Etodolac (Renal impairment, including cases of acute renal failure and Fanconi syndrome (renal tubular injury with severe hypophosphatemia), has been reported in association with the use of tenofovir DF. The majority of these cases occurred in patients with underlying systemic or renal disease, or in patients taking nephrotoxic agents; however, some cases occured in patients without identified risk factors. Atripla should be avoided with concurrent or recent use of a nephrotoxic agent).
No products indexed under this heading.

Etoposide (Efavirenz has been shown in vivo to induce CYP3A4. Other compounds that are substrates of CYP3A4 may have decreased plasma concentrations when co-administered with efavirenz).
No products indexed under this heading.

Etoposide Phosphate (Efavirenz has been shown in vivo to induce CYP3A4. Other compounds that are substrates of CYP3A4 may have decreased plasma concentrations when co-administered with efavirenz).
No products indexed under this heading.

Felbamate (Drugs which induce CYP3A4 activity would be expected to increase the clearance of efavirenz resulting in lower plasma concentrations).
No products indexed under this heading.

Felodipine (Efavirenz has been shown in vivo to induce CYP3A4. Other compounds that are substrates of CYP3A4 may have decreased plasma concentrations when co-administered with efavirenz).
No products indexed under this heading.

Fenoprofen Calcium (Renal impairment, including cases of acute renal failure and Fanconi syndrome (renal tubular injury with severe hypophosphatemia), has been reported in association with the use of tenofovir DF. The majority of these cases occurred in patients with underlying systemic or renal disease, or in patients taking nephrotoxic agents; however, some cases occured in patients without identified risk factors. Atripla should be avoided with concurrent or recent use of a nephrotoxic agent). Products include:
- Nalfon Capsules 2508

Fentanyl (Efavirenz has been shown in vivo to induce CYP3A4. Other compounds that are substrates of CYP3A4 may have decreased plasma concentrations when co-administered with efavirenz). Products include:
- Duragesic Transdermal System 2405
- Ionsys Transdermal System 2410

Fentanyl Citrate (Efavirenz has been shown in vivo to induce CYP3A4. Other compounds that are substrates of CYP3A4 may have decreased plasma concentrations when co-administered with efavirenz). Products include:
- Actiq 959
- Fentora Tablets 968

Filgrastim (Renal impairment, including cases of acute renal failure and Fanconi syndrome (renal tubular injury with severe hypophosphatemia), has been reported in association with the use of tenofovir DF. The majority of these cases occurred in patients with underlying systemic or renal disease, or in patients taking nephrotoxic agents; however, some cases occured in patients without identified risk factors. Atripla should be avoided with concurrent or recent use of a nephrotoxic agent). Products include:
- Neupogen for Injection 589

Fludrocortisone Acetate (Drugs which induce CYP3A4 activity would be expected to increase the clearance of efavirenz resulting in lower plasma concentrations).
No products indexed under this heading.

Fluorouracil (Renal impairment, including cases of acute renal failure and Fanconi syndrome (renal tubular injury with severe hypophosphatemia), has been reported in association with the use of tenofovir DF. The majority of these cases occurred in patients with underlying systemic or renal disease, or in patients taking nephrotoxic agents; however, some cases occured in patients without identified risk factors. Atripla should be avoided with concurrent or recent use of a nephrotoxic agent). Products include:
- Carac Cream 0.5% 2722

Fluoxetine Hydrochloride (In vitro studies have demonstrated that efavirenz inhibits CYP2C9 in the range of observed efavirenz plasma concentrations. Co-administration of efavirenz with drugs primarily metabolized by CYP2C9 may result in altered plasma concentrations of the co-administered drug. Therefore, appropriate dose adjustments may be necessary for these drugs). Products include:
- Prozac Weekly Capsules 1852
- Prozac Pulvules and Liquid 1852
- Symbyax Capsules 1871

Flurbiprofen (Renal impairment, including cases of acute renal failure and Fanconi syndrome (renal tubular injury with severe hypophosphatemia), has been reported in association with the use of tenofovir DF. The majority of these cases occurred in patients with underlying systemic or renal disease, or in patients taking nephrotoxic agents; however, some cases occured in patients without identified risk factors. Atripla should be avoided with concurrent or recent

use of a nephrotoxic agent).
No products indexed under this heading.

Flurbiprofen Sodium (In vitro studies have demonstrated that efavirenz inhibits CYP2C9 in the range of observed efavirenz plasma concentrations. Co-administration of efavirenz with drugs primarily metabolized by CYP2C9 may result in altered plasma concentrations of the co-administered drug. Therefore, appropriate dose adjustments may be necessary for these drugs).
No products indexed under this heading.

Fluvastatin Sodium (Renal impairment, including cases of acute renal failure and Fanconi syndrome (renal tubular injury with severe hypophosphatemia), has been reported in association with the use of tenofovir DF. The majority of these cases occurred in patients with underlying systemic or renal disease, or in patients taking nephrotoxic agents; however, some cases occured in patients without identified risk factors. Atripla should be avoided with concurrent or recent use of a nephrotoxic agent). Products include:
Lescol Capsules **2268**
Lescol XL Tablets **2268**

Formoterol Fumarate (In vitro studies have demonstrated that efavirenz inhibits CYP2C19 in the range of observed efavirenz plasma concentrations. Co-administration of efavirenz with drugs primarily metabolized by CYP2C19 may result in altered plasma concentrations of the co-administered drug. Therefore, appropriate dose adjustments may be necessary for these drugs).
Products include:
Foradil Aerolizer **2849**
Perforomist Inhalation Solution **1025**

Fosamprenavir Calcium (An additional 100 mg/day (300 mg total) of ritonavir is recommended when Atripla is administered with fosamprenavir/ritonavir once daily. No change in the ritonavir dose is required when Atripla is administered with fosamprenavir plus ritonavir twice daily). Products include:
Lexiva Oral Suspension **1510**
Lexiva Tablets **1510**

Foscarnet Sodium (Renal impairment, including cases of acute renal failure and Fanconi syndrome (renal tubular injury with severe hypophosphatemia), has been reported in association with the use of tenofovir DF. The majority of these cases occurred in patients with underlying systemic or renal disease, or in patients taking nephrotoxic agents; however, some cases occured in patients without identified risk factors. Atripla should be avoided with concurrent or recent use of a nephrotoxic agent).
No products indexed under this heading.

Fosinopril Sodium (Renal impairment, including cases of acute renal failure and Fanconi syndrome (renal tubular injury with severe hypophosphatemia), has been reported in association with the use of tenofovir DF. The majority of these cases occurred in patients with underlying systemic or renal disease, or in patients taking nephrotoxic agents; however, some cases occured in patients without identified risk factors. Atripla should be avoided with concurrent or recent use of a nephrotoxic agent).
No products indexed under this heading.

Fosphenytoin (In vitro studies have demonstrated that efavirenz inhibits CYP2C19 in the range of observed efavirenz plasma concentrations. Co-administration of efavirenz with drugs primarily metabolized by CYP2C19 may result in altered plasma concentrations of the co-administered drug. Therefore, appropriate dose adjustments may be necessary for these drugs).
No products indexed under this heading.

Fosphenytoin Sodium (Drugs which induce CYP3A4 activity would be expected to increase the clearance of efavirenz resulting in lower plasma concentrations).
No products indexed under this heading.

Furosemide (Renal impairment, including cases of acute renal failure and Fanconi syndrome (renal tubular injury with severe hypophosphatemia), has been reported in association with the use of tenofovir DF. The majority of these cases occurred in patients with underlying systemic or renal disease, or in patients taking nephrotoxic agents; however, some cases occured in patients without identified risk factors. Atripla should be avoided with concurrent or recent use of a nephrotoxic agent).
Products include:
Furosemide Tablets **2186**

Gabapentin (In vitro studies have demonstrated that efavirenz inhibits CYP2C19 in the range of observed efavirenz plasma concentrations. Co-administration of efavirenz with drugs primarily metabolized by CYP2C19 may result in altered plasma concentrations of the co-administered drug. Therefore, appropriate dose adjustments may be necessary for these drugs).
No products indexed under this heading.

Gadopentetate Dimeglumine (Renal impairment, including cases of acute renal failure and Fanconi syndrome (renal tubular injury with severe hypophosphatemia), has been reported in association with the use of tenofovir DF. The majority of these cases occurred in patients with underlying systemic or renal disease, or in patients taking nephrotoxic agents; however, some cases occured in patients without identified risk factors. Atripla should be avoided with concurrent or recent use of a nephrotoxic agent).
No products indexed under this heading.

Ganciclovir (Since emtricitabine and tenofovir are primarily eliminated by the kidneys, co-administration of Atripla with drugs that reduce renal fuction or compete for active tubular secretion may increase serum concentrations of emtricitabine, tenofovir, and/or other renally eliminated drugs).
No products indexed under this heading.

Ganciclovir Sodium (Since emtricitabine and tenofovir are primarily eliminated by the kidneys, co-administration of Atripla with drugs that reduce renal fuction or compete for active tubular secretion may increase serum concentrations of emtricitabine, tenofovir, and/or other renally eliminated drugs).
No products indexed under this heading.

Garlic Extract (Drugs which induce CYP3A4 activity would be expected to increase the clearance of efavirenz resulting in lower plasma concentrations).
No products indexed under this heading.

Garlic Oil (Drugs which induce CYP3A4 activity would be expected to increase the clearance of efavirenz resulting in lower plasma concentrations).
No products indexed under this heading.

Gentamicin (Renal impairment, including cases of acute renal failure and Fanconi syndrome (renal tubular injury with severe hypophosphatemia), has been reported in association with the use of tenofovir DF. The majority of these cases occurred in patients with underlying systemic or renal disease, or in patients taking nephrotoxic agents; however, some cases occured in patients without identified risk factors. Atripla should be avoided with concurrent or recent use of a nephrotoxic agent).
No products indexed under this heading.

Gentamicin Sulfate (Renal impairment, including cases of acute renal failure and Fanconi syndrome (renal tubular injury with severe hypophosphatemia), has been reported in association with the use of tenofovir DF. The majority of these cases occurred in patients with underlying systemic or renal disease, or in patients taking nephrotoxic agents; however, some cases occured in patients without identified risk factors. Atripla should be avoided with concurrent or recent use of a nephrotoxic agent). Products include:
Pred-G Ophthalmic Ointment .... ⊙**229**
Pred-G Ophthalmic Suspension ...... ⊙**228**

Glimepiride (In vitro studies have demonstrated that efavirenz inhibits CYP2C9 in the range of observed efavirenz plasma concentrations. Co-administration of efavirenz with drugs primarily metabolized by CYP2C9 may result in altered plasma concentrations of the co-administered drug. Therefore, appropriate dose adjustments may be necessary for these drugs).
Products include:
Avandaryl Tablets **1344**
Duetact Tablets **3085**

Glipizide (Renal impairment, including cases of acute renal failure and Fanconi syndrome (renal tubular injury with severe hypophosphatemia), has been reported in association with the use of tenofovir DF. The majority of these cases occurred in patients with underlying systemic or renal disease, or in patients taking nephrotoxic agents; however, some cases occured in patients without identified risk factors. Atripla should be avoided with concurrent or recent use of a nephrotoxic agent).
No products indexed under this heading.

Globulin, Immune (Human) (Renal impairment, including cases of acute renal failure and Fanconi syndrome (renal tubular injury with severe hypophosphatemia), has been reported in association with the use of tenofovir DF. The majority of these cases occurred in patients with underlying systemic or renal disease, or in patients taking nephrotoxic agents; however, some cases occured in patients without identified risk factors. Atripla should be avoided with concurrent or recent use of a nephrotoxic agent).
Products include:
Flebogamma 5% **1715**

Glyburide (Renal impairment, including cases of acute renal failure and Fanconi syndrome (renal tubular injury with severe hypophosphatemia), has been reported in association with the use of tenofovir DF. The majority of these cases occurred in patients with underlying systemic or renal disease, or in patients taking nephrotoxic agents; however, some cases occured in patients without identified risk factors. Atripla should be avoided with concurrent or recent use of a nephrotoxic agent).
No products indexed under this heading.

Gold Therapy (Renal impairment, including cases of acute renal failure and Fanconi syndrome (renal tubular injury with severe hypophosphatemia), has been reported in association with the use of tenofovir DF. The majority of these cases occurred in patients with underlying systemic or renal disease, or in patients taking nephrotoxic agents; however, some cases occured in patients without identified risk factors. Atripla should be avoided with concurrent or recent use of a nephrotoxic agent).
No products indexed under this heading.

Haloperidol (Efavirenz has been shown in vivo to induce CYP3A4. Other compounds that are substrates of CYP3A4 may have decreased plasma concentrations when co-administered with efavirenz).
No products indexed under this heading.

Haloperidol Decanoate (Efavirenz has been shown in vivo to induce CYP3A4. Other compounds that are substrates of CYP3A4 may have decreased plasma concentrations when co-administered with efavirenz).
No products indexed under this heading.

Haloperidol Lactate (Efavirenz has been shown in vivo to induce CYP3A4. Other compounds that are substrates of CYP3A4 may have decreased plasma concentrations when co-administered with efavirenz).
No products indexed under this heading.

HMG-CoA Reductase Inhibitors (Renal impairment, including cases of acute renal failure and Fanconi syndrome (renal tubular injury with severe hypophosphatemia), has been reported in association with the use of tenofovir DF. The majority of these cases occurred in patients with underlying systemic or renal disease, or in patients taking nephrotoxic agents; however, some cases occured in patients without identified risk factors. Atripla should be avoided with concurrent or recent use of a nephrotoxic agent).

No products indexed under this heading.

Hydrochlorothiazide (Renal impairment, including cases of acute renal failure and Fanconi syndrome (renal tubular injury with severe hypophosphatemia), has been reported in association with the use of tenofovir DF. The majority of these cases occurred in patients with underlying systemic or renal disease, or in patients taking nephrotoxic agents; however, some cases occured in patients without identified risk factors. Atripla should be avoided with concurrent or recent use of a nephrotoxic agent). Products include:

Atacand HCT 642
Avalide Tablets 892
Avalide Tablets 2713
Benicar HCT Tablets 1010
Diovan HCT Tablets 2216
Dyazide Capsules 1405
Micardis HCT Tablets 854
Prinzide Tablets 2092
Tekturna HCT Tablets 2324
Teveten HCT Tablets 517

Hydrocortisone (Drugs which induce CYP3A4 activity would be expected to increase the clearance of efavirenz resulting in lower plasma concentrations).

No products indexed under this heading.

Hydrocortisone Acetate (Drugs which induce CYP3A4 activity would be expected to increase the clearance of efavirenz resulting in lower plasma concentrations). Products include:

Analpram-HC 1140
Pramosone 1141

Hydrocortisone Butyrate (Drugs which induce CYP3A4 activity would be expected to increase the clearance of efavirenz resulting in lower plasma concentrations).

No products indexed under this heading.

Hydrocortisone Cypionate (Drugs which induce CYP3A4 activity would be expected to increase the clearance of efavirenz resulting in lower plasma concentrations).

No products indexed under this heading.

Hydrocortisone Hemisuccinate (Drugs which induce CYP3A4 activity would be expected to increase the clearance of efavirenz resulting in lower plasma concentrations).

No products indexed under this heading.

Hydrocortisone Probutate (Drugs which induce CYP3A4 activity would be expected to increase the clearance of efavirenz resulting in lower plasma concentrations).

No products indexed under this heading.

Hydrocortisone Sodium Phosphate (Drugs which induce CYP3A4 activity would be expected to increase the clearance of efavirenz resulting in lower plasma concentrations).

No products indexed under this heading.

Hydrocortisone Sodium Succinate (Drugs which induce CYP3A4 activity would be expected to increase the clearance of efavirenz resulting in lower plasma concentrations).

No products indexed under this heading.

Hydrocortisone Valerate (Drugs which induce CYP3A4 activity would be expected to increase the clearance of efavirenz resulting in lower plasma concentrations).

No products indexed under this heading.

Hydroflumethiazide (Renal impairment, including cases of acute renal failure and Fanconi syndrome (renal tubular injury with severe hypophosphatemia), has been reported in association with the use of tenofovir DF. The majority of these cases occurred in patients with underlying systemic or renal disease, or in patients taking nephrotoxic agents; however, some cases occured in patients without identified risk factors. Atripla should be avoided with concurrent or recent use of a nephrotoxic agent).

No products indexed under this heading.

Hypericum (Drugs which induce CYP3A4 activity would be expected to increase the clearance of efavirenz resulting in lower plasma concentrations). Products include:

Satieté Tablets .... ▣ 640

Hypericum Perforatum (Hypericum perforatum is expected to substantially decrease plasma levels of efavirenz. It has not been studied in combination with efavirenz, but concomitant use is not recommended).

No products indexed under this heading.

Ibuprofen (Renal impairment, including cases of acute renal failure and Fanconi syndrome (renal tubular injury with severe hypophosphatemia), has been reported in association with the use of tenofovir DF. The majority of these cases occurred in patients with underlying systemic or renal disease, or in patients taking nephrotoxic agents; however, some cases occured in patients without identified risk factors. Atripla should be avoided with concurrent or recent use of a nephrotoxic agent). Products include:

Motrin IB Tablets and Caplets 1900
Children's Motrin Oral Suspension ... 1901
Children's Motrin Non-Staining Dye-Free Oral Suspension 1901
Children's Motrin Cold Oral Suspension 1899
Infants' Motrin Concentrated Drops 1901
Infants' Motrin Non-Staining Dye-Free Concentrated Drops 1901
Junior Strength Motrin Caplets and Chewable Tablets 1901
Vicoprofen Tablets 533

Idarubicin Hydrochloride (Renal impairment, including cases of acute renal failure and Fanconi syndrome (renal tubular injury with severe hypophosphatemia), has been reported in association with the use of tenofovir DF. The majority of these cases occurred in patients with underlying systemic or renal disease, or in patients taking nephrotoxic agents; however, some cases occured in patients without identified risk factors. Atripla should be avoided with concurrent or recent use of a nephrotoxic agent).

No products indexed under this heading.

Ifosfamide (Renal impairment, including cases of acute renal failure and Fanconi syndrome (renal tubular injury with severe hypophosphatemia), has been reported in association with the use of tenofovir DF. The majority of these cases occurred in patients with underlying systemic or renal disease, or in patients taking nephrotoxic agents; however, some cases occured in patients without identified risk factors. Atripla should be avoided with concurrent or recent use of a nephrotoxic agent).

No products indexed under this heading.

Imipenem (Renal impairment, including cases of acute renal failure and Fanconi syndrome (renal tubular injury with severe hypophosphatemia), has been reported in association with the use of tenofovir DF. The majority of these cases occurred in patients with underlying systemic or renal disease, or in patients taking nephrotoxic agents; however, some cases occured in patients without identified risk factors. Atripla should be avoided with concurrent or recent use of a nephrotoxic agent). Products include:

Primaxin I.M. 2080
Primaxin I.V. 2083

Imipramine Hydrochloride (In vitro studies have demonstrated that efavirenz inhibits CYP2C9 in the range of observed efavirenz plasma concentrations. Co-administration of efavirenz with drugs primarily metabolized by CYP2C9 may result in altered plasma concentrations of the co-administered drug. Therefore, appropriate dose adjustments may be necessary for these drugs).

No products indexed under this heading.

Imipramine Pamoate (In vitro studies have demonstrated that efavirenz inhibits CYP2C19 in the range of observed efavirenz plasma concentrations. Co-administration of efavirenz with drugs primarily metabolized by CYP2C19 may result in altered plasma concentrations of the co-administered drug. Therefore, appropriate dose adjustments may be necessary for these drugs).

No products indexed under this heading.

Immune Globulin Intravenous (Human) (Renal impairment, including cases of acute renal failure and Fanconi syndrome (renal tubular injury with severe hypophosphatemia), has been reported in association with the use of tenofovir DF. The majority of these cases occurred in patients with underlying systemic or renal disease, or in patients taking nephrotoxic agents; however, some cases occured in patients without identified risk factors. Atripla should be avoided with concurrent or recent use of a nephrotoxic agent). Products include:

Flebogamma 5% DIF 1718
Gammagard Liquid 730
Gammagard S/D 734
Gamunex 3094

Indinavir Sulfate (The optimal dose of indinavir, when given in combination with efavirenz, is not known. Increasing the indinavir dose to 1000 mg every 8 hours does not compensate for the increased indinavir metabolism due to efavirenz). Products include:

Crixivan Capsules 1979

Indomethacin (Renal impairment, including cases of acute renal failure and Fanconi syndrome (renal tubular injury with severe hypophosphatemia), has been reported in association with the use of tenofovir DF. The majority of these cases occurred in patients with underlying systemic or renal disease, or in patients taking nephrotoxic agents; however, some cases occured in patients without identified risk factors. Atripla should be avoided with concurrent or recent use of a nephrotoxic agent). Products include:

Indocin 2024

Indomethacin Sodium Trihydrate (Renal impairment, including cases of acute renal failure and Fanconi syndrome (renal tubular injury with severe hypophosphatemia), has been reported in association with the use of tenofovir DF. The majority of these cases occurred in patients with underlying systemic or renal disease, or in patients taking nephrotoxic agents; however, some cases occured in patients without identified risk factors. Atripla should be avoided with concurrent or recent use of a nephrotoxic agent). Products include:

Indocin I.V. 2489

Interferon Beta-1b (Renal impairment, including cases of acute renal failure and Fanconi syndrome (renal tubular injury with severe hypophosphatemia), has been reported in association with the use of tenofovir DF. The majority of these cases occurred in patients with underlying systemic or renal disease, or in patients taking nephrotoxic agents; however, some cases occured in patients without identified risk factors. Atripla should be avoided with concurrent or recent use of a nephrotoxic agent). Products include:

Betaseron for SC Injection 756

Interleuken-2 (Renal impairment, including cases of acute renal failure and Fanconi syndrome (renal tubular injury with severe hypophosphatemia), has been reported in association with the use of tenofovir DF. The majority of these cases occurred in patients with underlying systemic or renal disease, or in patients taking nephrotoxic agents; however, some cases occured in patients without identified risk factors. Atripla should be avoided with concurrent or recent use of a nephrotoxic agent).

No products indexed under this heading.

Iodamide Meglumine (Renal impairment, including cases of acute renal failure and Fanconi syndrome (renal tubular injury with severe hypophosphatemia), has been reported in association with the use of tenofovir DF. The majority of these cases occurred in patients with underlying systemic or renal disease, or in patients taking nephrotoxic agents; however, some cases occured in patients without identified risk factors. Atripla should be avoided with concurrent or recent use of a nephrotoxic agent).

No products indexed under this heading.

Iohexol (Renal impairment, including cases of acute renal failure and Fanconi syndrome (renal tubular injury with severe hypophosphatemia), has been reported in association with the use of tenofovir DF. The majority of these cases occurred in patients with underlying systemic or renal disease, or in patients taking nephrotoxic agents; however, some cases occured in patients without identified risk factors. Atripla should be avoided with concurrent or recent use of a nephrotoxic agent).

No products indexed under this heading.

Iopamidol (Renal impairment, including cases of acute renal failure and Fanconi syndrome (renal tubular injury with severe hypophosphatemia), has been reported in association with the use of tenofovir DF. The majority of these cases occurred in patients with underlying systemic or renal disease, or in patients taking nephrotoxic agents; however, some cases occured in patients without identified risk factors. Atripla should be avoided with concurrent or recent use of a nephrotoxic agent).

No products indexed under this heading.

Iopanoic Acid (Renal impairment, including cases of acute renal failure and Fanconi syndrome (renal tubular injury with severe hypophosphatemia), has been reported in association with the use of tenofovir DF. The majority of these cases occurred in patients with underlying systemic or renal disease, or in patients taking nephrotoxic agents; however, some cases occured in patients without identified risk factors. Atripla should be avoided with concurrent or recent use of a nephrotoxic agent).

No products indexed under this heading.

Iothalamate Meglumine (Renal impairment, including cases of acute renal failure and Fanconi syndrome (renal tubular injury with severe hypophosphatemia), has been reported in association with the use of tenofovir DF. The majority of these cases occurred in patients with underlying systemic or renal disease, or in patients taking nephrotoxic agents; however, some cases occured in patients without identified risk factors. Atripla should be avoided with concurrent or recent use of a nephrotoxic agent).

No products indexed under this heading.

Ioxaglate Meglumine (Renal impairment, including cases of acute renal failure and Fanconi syndrome (renal tubular injury with severe hypophosphatemia), has been reported in association with the use of tenofovir DF. The majority of these cases occurred in patients with underlying systemic or renal disease, or in patients taking nephrotoxic agents; however, some cases occured in patients without identified risk factors. Atripla should be avoided with concurrent or recent use of a nephrotoxic agent).

No products indexed under this heading.

Ioxaglate Sodium (Renal impairment, including cases of acute renal failure and Fanconi syndrome (renal tubular injury with severe hypophosphatemia), has been reported in association with the use of tenofovir DF. The majority of these cases occurred in patients with underlying systemic or renal disease, or in patients taking nephrotoxic agents; however, some cases occured in patients without identified risk factors. Atripla should be avoided with concurrent or recent use of a nephrotoxic agent).

No products indexed under this heading.

Irbesartan (In vitro studies have demonstrated that efavirenz inhibits CYP2C9 in the range of observed efavirenz plasma concentrations. Co-administration of efavirenz with drugs primarily metabolized by CYP2C9 may result in altered plasma concentrations of the co-administered drug. Therefore, appropriate dose adjustments may be necessary for these drugs). Products include:

Avalide Tablets ... 892
Avalide Tablets ... 2713
Avapro Tablets ... 897
Avapro Tablets ... 2718

Isradipine (Efavirenz has been shown in vivo to induce CYP3A4. Other compounds that are substrates of CYP3A4 may have decreased plasma concentrations when co-administered with efavirenz). Products include:

DynaCirc CR Controlled Release Tablets ... 1407

Itraconazole (Drug interaction studies with Atripla and these imidazole and triazole antifungals have not been conducted. Efavirenz has the potential to decrease plasma concentrations of itraconazole and ketoconazole).

No products indexed under this heading.

Ixabepilone (Efavirenz has been shown in vivo to induce CYP3A4. Other compounds that are substrates of CYP3A4 may have decreased plasma concentrations when co-administered with efavirenz). Products include:

Ixempra Kit for Injection ... 915

Kanamycin Sulfate (Renal impairment, including cases of acute renal failure and Fanconi syndrome (renal tubular injury with severe hypophosphatemia), has been reported in association with the use of tenofovir DF. The majority of these cases occurred in patients with underlying systemic or renal disease, or in patients taking nephrotoxic agents; however, some cases occured in patients without identified risk factors. Atripla should be avoided with concurrent or recent use of a nephrotoxic agent).

No products indexed under this heading.

Ketoconazole (Drug interaction studies with Atripla and these imidazole and triazole antifungals have not been conducted. Efavirenz has the potential to decrease plasma concentrations of itraconazole and ketoconazole). Products include:

Extina Foam, 2% ... 3057
Nizoral A-D Shampoo ... 1901

Ketoprofen (Renal impairment, including cases of acute renal failure and Fanconi syndrome (renal tubular injury with severe hypophosphatemia), has been reported in association with the use of tenofovir DF. The majority of these cases occurred in patients with underlying systemic or renal disease, or in patients taking nephrotoxic agents; however, some cases occured in patients without identified risk factors. Atripla should be avoided with concurrent or recent use of a nephrotoxic agent).

No products indexed under this heading.

Ketorolac Tromethamine (Renal impairment, including cases of acute renal failure and Fanconi syndrome (renal tubular injury with severe hypophosphatemia), has been reported in association with the use of tenofovir DF. The majority of these cases occurred in patients with underlying systemic or renal disease, or in patients taking nephrotoxic agents; however, some cases occured in patients without identified risk factors. Atripla should be avoided with concurrent or recent use of a nephrotoxic agent).

No products indexed under this heading.

Lamium album (Renal impairment, including cases of acute renal failure and Fanconi syndrome (renal tubular injury with severe hypophosphatemia), has been reported in association with the use of tenofovir DF. The majority of these cases occurred in patients with underlying systemic or renal disease, or in patients taking nephrotoxic agents; however, some cases occured in patients without identified risk factors. Atripla should be avoided with concurrent or recent use of a nephrotoxic agent).

No products indexed under this heading.

Lamotrigine (In vitro studies have demonstrated that efavirenz inhibits CYP2C19 in the range of observed efavirenz plasma concentrations. Co-administration of efavirenz with drugs primarily metabolized by CYP2C19 may result in altered plasma concentrations of the co-administered drug. Therefore, appropriate dose adjustments may be necessary for these drugs). Products include:

Lamictal ... 1488

Lansoprazole (In vitro studies have demonstrated that efavirenz inhibits CYP2C9 in the range of observed efavirenz plasma concentrations. Co-administration of efavirenz with drugs primarily metabolized by CYP2C9 may result in altered plasma concentrations of the co-administered drug. Therefore, appropriate dose adjustments may be necessary for these drugs).

No products indexed under this heading.

Levetiracetam (In vitro studies have demonstrated that efavirenz inhibits CYP2C19 in the range of observed efavirenz plasma concentrations. Co-administration of efavirenz with drugs primarily metabolized by CYP2C19 may result in altered plasma concentrations of the co-administered drug. Therefore, appropriate dose adjustments may be necessary for these drugs). Products include:

Keppra Injection ... 3137
Keppra Oral Solution ... 3131
Keppra Tablets ... 3131

Levonorgestrel (Efavirenz has been shown in vivo to induce CYP3A4. Other compounds that are substrates of CYP3A4 may have decreased plasma concentrations when co-administered with efavirenz). Products include:

Climara Pro Transdermal System ... 768
Lybrel Tablets ... 3204
Mirena Intrauterine System ... 779
Plan B Tablets ... 1044
Seasonique Tablets ... 1046

Lidocaine (Efavirenz has been shown in vivo to induce CYP3A4. Other compounds that are substrates of CYP3A4 may have decreased plasma concentrations when co-administered with efavirenz). Products include:

Lidoderm Patch ... 1114

Lidocaine Hydrochloride (Efavirenz has been shown in vivo to induce CYP3A4. Other compounds that are substrates of CYP3A4 may have decreased plasma concentrations when co-administered with efavirenz).

No products indexed under this heading.

Lisinopril (Renal impairment, including cases of acute renal failure and Fanconi syndrome (renal tubular injury with severe hypophosphatemia), has been reported in association with the use of tenofovir DF. The majority of these cases occurred in patients with underlying systemic or renal disease, or in patients taking nephrotoxic agents; however, some cases occured in patients without identified risk factors. Atripla should be avoided with concurrent or recent use of a nephrotoxic agent). Products include:

Prinivil Tablets ... 2087
Prinzide Tablets ... 2092

Lithium (Renal impairment, including cases of acute renal failure and Fanconi syndrome (renal tubular injury with severe hypophosphatemia), has been reported in association with the use of tenofovir DF. The majority of these cases occurred in patients with underlying systemic or renal disease, or in patients taking nephrotoxic agents; however, some cases occured in patients without identified risk factors. Atripla should be avoided with concurrent or recent use of a nephrotoxic agent).

No products indexed under this heading.

Lithium Carbonate (Renal impairment, including cases of acute renal failure and Fanconi syndrome (renal tubular injury with severe hypophosphatemia), has been reported in association with the use of tenofovir DF. The majority of these cases occurred in patients with underlying systemic or renal disease, or in patients taking nephrotoxic agents; however, some cases occured in patients without identified risk factors. Atripla should be avoided with concurrent or recent use of a nephrotoxic agent).

No products indexed under this heading.

Lithium Citrate (Renal impairment, including cases of acute renal failure and Fanconi syndrome (renal tubular injury with severe hypophosphatemia), has been reported in association with the use of tenofovir DF. The majority of these cases occurred in patients with underlying systemic or renal disease, or in patients taking nephrotoxic agents; however, some cases occured in patients without identified risk factors. Atripla should be avoided with concurrent or recent use of a nephrotoxic agent).

No products indexed under this heading.

Lopinavir (Kaletra has been shown to increase tenofovir concentrations. The mechanism of this interaction is unknown. Higher tenofovir concentrations could potentiate tenofovir-associated adverse events, including renal disorders. Patients receiving Kaletra with tenofovir DF should be monitored for tenofovir-associated adverse events. Atripla should be discontinued in patients who develop tenofovir-associated adverse events). Products include:

Kaletra 452

Loracarbef (Renal impairment, including cases of acute renal failure and Fanconi syndrome (renal tubular injury with severe hypophosphatemia), has been reported in association with the use of tenofovir DF. The majority of these cases occurred in patients with underlying systemic or renal disease, or in patients taking nephrotoxic agents; however, some cases occured in patients without identified risk factors. Atripla should be avoided with concurrent or recent use of a nephrotoxic agent).

No products indexed under this heading.

Losartan Potassium (In vitro studies have demonstrated that efavirenz inhibits CYP2C9 in the range of observed efavirenz plasma concentrations. Co-administration of efavirenz with drugs primarily metabolized by CYP2C9 may result in altered plasma concentrations of the co-administered drug. Therefore, appropriate dose adjustments may be necessary for these drugs). Products include:

Cozaar Tablets 1973

Lovastatin (Renal impairment, including cases of acute renal failure and Fanconi syndrome (renal tubular injury with severe hypophosphatemia), has been reported in association with the use of tenofovir DF. The majority of these cases occurred in patients with underlying systemic or renal disease, or in patients taking nephrotoxic agents; however, some cases occured in patients without identified risk factors. Atripla should be avoided with concurrent or recent use of a nephrotoxic agent). Products include:

Advicor Tablets 402
Mevacor Tablets 2063

Maprotiline Hydrochloride (In vitro studies have demonstrated that efavirenz inhibits CYP2C19 in the range of observed efavirenz plasma concentrations. Co-administration of efavirenz with drugs primarily metabolized by CYP2C19 may result in altered plasma concentrations of the co-administered drug. Therefore, appropriate dose adjustments may be necessary for these drugs).

No products indexed under this heading.

Meclofenamate Sodium (Renal impairment, including cases of acute renal failure and Fanconi syndrome (renal tubular injury with severe hypophosphatemia), has been reported in association with the use of tenofovir DF. The majority of these cases occurred in patients with underlying systemic or renal disease, or in patients taking nephrotoxic agents; however, some cases occured in patients without identified risk factors. Atripla should be avoided with concurrent or recent use of a nephrotoxic agent).

No products indexed under this heading.

Mefenamic Acid (Renal impairment, including cases of acute renal failure and Fanconi syndrome (renal tubular injury with severe hypophosphatemia), has been reported in association with the use of tenofovir DF. The majority of these cases occurred in patients with underlying systemic or renal disease, or in patients taking nephrotoxic agents; however, some cases occured in patients without identified risk factors. Atripla should be avoided with concurrent or recent use of a nephrotoxic agent).

No products indexed under this heading.

Meloxicam (Renal impairment, including cases of acute renal failure and Fanconi syndrome (renal tubular injury with severe hypophosphatemia), has been reported in association with the use of tenofovir DF. The majority of these cases occurred in patients with underlying systemic or renal disease, or in patients taking nephrotoxic agents; however, some cases occured in patients without identified risk factors. Atripla should be avoided with concurrent or recent use of a nephrotoxic agent). Products include:

Mobic Oral Suspension 863
Mobic Tablets 863

Melphalan Hydrochloride (Renal impairment, including cases of acute renal failure and Fanconi syndrome (renal tubular injury with severe hypophosphatemia), has been reported in association with the use of tenofovir DF. The majority of these cases occurred in patients with underlying systemic or renal disease, or in patients taking nephrotoxic agents; however, some cases occured in patients without identified risk factors. Atripla should be avoided with concurrent or recent use of a nephrotoxic agent).

No products indexed under this heading.

Mephenytoin (Drugs which induce CYP3A4 activity would be expected to increase the clearance of efavirenz resulting in lower plasma concentrations).

No products indexed under this heading.

Mephobarbital (In vitro studies have demonstrated that efavirenz inhibits CYP2C19 in the range of observed efavirenz plasma concentrations. Co-administration of efavirenz with drugs primarily metabolized by CYP2C19 may result in altered plasma concentrations of the co-administered drug. Therefore, appropriate dose adjustments may be necessary for these drugs).

No products indexed under this heading.

Meprobamate (In vitro studies have demonstrated that efavirenz inhibits CYP2C19 in the range of observed efavirenz plasma concentrations. Co-administration of efavirenz with drugs primarily metabolized by CYP2C19 may result in altered plasma concentrations of the co-administered drug. Therefore, appropriate dose adjustments may be necessary for these drugs).

No products indexed under this heading.

Mesalamine (Renal impairment, including cases of acute renal failure and Fanconi syndrome (renal tubular injury with severe hypophosphatemia), has been reported in association with the use of tenofovir DF. The majority of these cases occurred in patients with underlying systemic or renal disease, or in patients taking nephrotoxic agents; however, some cases occured in patients without identified risk factors. Atripla should be avoided with concurrent or recent use of a nephrotoxic agent). Products include:

Asacol Delayed-Release Tablets 2579
Canasa Rectal Suppositories 705
Lialda Tablets 3029
Pentasa Capsules 3030

Mestranol (Efavirenz has been shown in vivo to induce CYP3A4. Other compounds that are substrates of CYP3A4 may have decreased plasma concentrations when co-administered with efavirenz).

No products indexed under this heading.

Metformin Hydrochloride (In vitro studies have demonstrated that efavirenz inhibits CYP2C9 in the range of observed efavirenz plasma concentrations. Co-administration of efavirenz with drugs primarily metabolized by CYP2C9 may result in altered plasma concentrations of the co-administered drug. Therefore, appropriate dose adjustments may be necessary for these drugs). Products include:

ActoPlus Met Tablets 3071
Avandamet Tablets 1336
Janumet Tablets 2041
PrandiMet Tablets 2967

Methadone Hydrochloride (Co-administration of efavirenz in HIV-infected individuals with a history of injection drug use resulted in decreased plasma levels of methadone and signs of opiate withdrawal. Methadone dose was increased by a mean of 22% to alleviate withdrawal symptoms. Patients should be monitored for signs of withdrawal and their methadone dose increased as required to alleviate withdrawal symptoms).

No products indexed under this heading.

Methimazole (Renal impairment, including cases of acute renal failure and Fanconi syndrome (renal tubular injury with severe hypophosphatemia), has been reported in association with the use of tenofovir DF. The majority of these cases occurred in patients with underlying systemic or renal disease, or in patients taking nephrotoxic agents; however, some cases occured in patients without identified risk factors. Atripla should be avoided with concurrent or recent use of a nephrotoxic agent).

No products indexed under this heading.

Methotrexate (Renal impairment, including cases of acute renal failure and Fanconi syndrome (renal tubular injury with severe hypophosphatemia), has been reported in association with the use of tenofovir DF. The majority of these cases occurred in patients with underlying systemic or renal disease, or in patients taking nephrotoxic agents; however, some cases occured in patients without identified risk factors. Atripla should be avoided with concurrent or recent use of a nephrotoxic agent).

No products indexed under this heading.

Methotrexate Sodium (Renal impairment, including cases of acute renal failure and Fanconi syndrome (renal tubular injury with severe hypophosphatemia), has been reported in association with the use of tenofovir DF. The majority of these cases occurred in patients with underlying systemic or renal disease, or in patients taking nephrotoxic agents; however, some cases occured in patients without identified risk factors. Atripla should be avoided with concurrent or recent use of a nephrotoxic agent).

No products indexed under this heading.

Methsuximide (Drugs which induce CYP3A4 activity would be expected to increase the clearance of efavirenz resulting in lower plasma concentrations).

No products indexed under this heading.

Methyclothiazide (Renal impairment, including cases of acute renal failure and Fanconi syndrome (renal tubular injury with severe hypophosphatemia), has been reported in association with the use of tenofovir DF. The majority of these cases occurred in patients with underlying systemic or renal disease, or in patients taking nephrotoxic agents; however, some cases occured in patients without identified risk factors. Atripla should be avoided with concurrent or recent use of a nephrotoxic agent).

No products indexed under this heading.

Methylergonovine Maleate (Due to the potential for serious and/or life-threatening reactions, such as acute ergot toxicity characterized by peripheral vasospasm and ischemia of the extremities and other tissues, concomitant use with ergot derivatives is contraindicated).

No products indexed under this heading.

Methylprednisolone (Drugs which induce CYP3A4 activity would be expected to increase the clearance of efavirenz resulting in lower plasma concentrations).

No products indexed under this heading.

Methylprednisolone Acetate (Drugs which induce CYP3A4 activity would be expected to increase the clearance of efavirenz resulting in lower plasma concentrations).

No products indexed under this heading.

Methylprednisolone Sodium Succinate (Drugs which induce CYP3A4 activity would be expected to increase the clearance of efavirenz resulting in lower plasma concentrations).

No products indexed under this heading.

Mezlocillin Sodium (Renal impairment, including cases of acute renal failure and Fanconi syndrome (renal tubular injury with severe hypophosphatemia), has been reported in association with the use of tenofovir DF. The majority of these cases occurred in patients with underlying systemic or renal disease, or in patients taking nephrotoxic agents; however, some cases occured in

patients without identified risk factors. Atripla should be avoided with concurrent or recent use of a nephrotoxic agent).
No products indexed under this heading.

Midazolam Hydrochloride (Due to the potential for serious and/or life-threatening reactions, such as prolonged or increased sedation or respiratory depression, concomitant use with midazolam hydrochloride is contraindicated).
No products indexed under this heading.

Miglitol (In vitro studies have demonstrated that efavirenz inhibits CYP2C9 in the range of observed efavirenz plasma concentrations. Co-administration of efavirenz with drugs primarily metabolized by CYP2C9 may result in altered plasma concentrations of the co-administered drug. Therefore, appropriate dose adjustments may be necessary for these drugs).
No products indexed under this heading.

Minocycline Hydrochloride (Renal impairment, including cases of acute renal failure and Fanconi syndrome (renal tubular injury with severe hypophosphatemia), has been reported in association with the use of tenofovir DF. The majority of these cases occurred in patients with underlying systemic or renal disease, or in patients taking nephrotoxic agents; however, some cases occured in patients without identified risk factors. Atripla should be avoided with concurrent or recent use of a nephrotoxic agent).
Products include:
Solodyn Extended Release Tablets 1938

Mirtazapine (In vitro studies have demonstrated that efavirenz inhibits CYP2C9 in the range of observed efavirenz plasma concentrations. Co-administration of efavirenz with drugs primarily metabolized by CYP2C9 may result in altered plasma concentrations of the co-administered drug. Therefore, appropriate dose adjustments may be necessary for these drugs).
Products include:
Remeron Tablets 2924
RemeronSolTab Tablets 2927

Mitomycin (Mitomycin-C) (Renal impairment, including cases of acute renal failure and Fanconi syndrome (renal tubular injury with severe hypophosphatemia), has been reported in association with the use of tenofovir DF. The majority of these cases occurred in patients with underlying systemic or renal disease, or in patients taking nephrotoxic agents; however, some cases occured in patients without identified risk factors. Atripla should be avoided with concurrent or recent use of a nephrotoxic agent).
No products indexed under this heading.

Modafinil (Drugs which induce CYP3A4 activity would be expected to increase the clearance of efavirenz resulting in lower plasma concentrations). Products include:
Provigil Tablets 977

Moexipril Hydrochloride (Renal impairment, including cases of acute renal failure and Fanconi syndrome (renal tubular injury with severe hypophosphatemia), has been reported in association with the use of tenofovir DF. The majority of these cases occurred in patients with underlying systemic or renal disease, or in patients taking nephrotoxic agents; however, some cases occured in patients without identified risk factors. Atripla should be avoided with concurrent or recent use of a nephrotoxic agent).
No products indexed under this heading.

Montelukast Sodium (In vitro studies have demonstrated that efavirenz inhibits CYP2C9 in the range of observed efavirenz plasma concentrations. Co-administration of efavirenz with drugs primarily metabolized by CYP2C9 may result in altered plasma concentrations of the co-administered drug. Therefore, appropriate dose adjustments may be necessary for these drugs).
Products include:
Singulair 2114

Muromonab-CD3 (Renal impairment, including cases of acute renal failure and Fanconi syndrome (renal tubular injury with severe hypophosphatemia), has been reported in association with the use of tenofovir DF. The majority of these cases occurred in patients with underlying systemic or renal disease, or in patients taking nephrotoxic agents; however, some cases occured in patients without identified risk factors. Atripla should be avoided with concurrent or recent use of a nephrotoxic agent). Products include:
Orthoclone OKT3 Sterile Solution 2387

Nabumetone (Renal impairment, including cases of acute renal failure and Fanconi syndrome (renal tubular injury with severe hypophosphatemia), has been reported in association with the use of tenofovir DF. The majority of these cases occurred in patients with underlying systemic or renal disease, or in patients taking nephrotoxic agents; however, some cases occured in patients without identified risk factors. Atripla should be avoided with concurrent or recent use of a nephrotoxic agent).
No products indexed under this heading.

Nafcillin Sodium (Renal impairment, including cases of acute renal failure and Fanconi syndrome (renal tubular injury with severe hypophosphatemia), has been reported in association with the use of tenofovir DF. The majority of these cases occurred in patients with underlying systemic or renal disease, or in patients taking nephrotoxic agents; however, some cases occured in patients without identified risk factors. Atripla should be avoided with concurrent or recent use of a nephrotoxic agent).
No products indexed under this heading.

Naproxen (Renal impairment, including cases of acute renal failure and Fanconi syndrome (renal tubular injury with severe hypophosphatemia), has been reported in association with the use of tenofovir DF. The majority of these cases occurred in patients with underlying systemic or renal disease, or in patients taking nephrotoxic agents; however, some cases occured in patients without identified risk factors. Atripla should be avoided with concurrent or recent use of a nephrotoxic agent).
Products include:
EC-Naprosyn Delayed-Release Tablets 2632
Naprosyn Suspension 2632
Naprosyn Tablets 2632

Naproxen Sodium (Renal impairment, including cases of acute renal failure and Fanconi syndrome (renal tubular injury with severe hypophosphatemia), has been reported in association with the use of tenofovir DF. The majority of these cases occurred in patients with underlying systemic or renal disease, or in patients taking nephrotoxic agents; however, some cases occured in patients without identified risk factors. Atripla should be avoided with concurrent or recent use of a nephrotoxic agent). Products include:
Anaprox Tablets 2632
Anaprox DS Tablets 2632
Treximet Tablets 1616

Nateglinide (In vitro studies have demonstrated that efavirenz inhibits CYP2C9 in the range of observed efavirenz plasma concentrations. Co-administration of efavirenz with drugs primarily metabolized by CYP2C9 may result in altered plasma concentrations of the co-administered drug. Therefore, appropriate dose adjustments may be necessary for these drugs).
Products include:
Starlix Tablets 2314

Nefazodone Hydrochloride (Efavirenz has been shown in vivo to induce CYP3A4. Other compounds that are substrates of CYP3A4 may have decreased plasma concentrations when co-administered with efavirenz).
No products indexed under this heading.

Nelfinavir Mesylate (Renal impairment, including cases of acute renal failure and Fanconi syndrome (renal tubular injury with severe hypophosphatemia), has been reported in association with the use of tenofovir DF. The majority of these cases occurred in patients with underlying systemic or renal disease, or in patients taking nephrotoxic agents; however, some cases occured in patients without identified risk factors. Atripla should be avoided with concurrent or recent use of a nephrotoxic agent).
No products indexed under this heading.

Neomycin (Renal impairment, including cases of acute renal failure and Fanconi syndrome (renal tubular injury with severe hypophosphatemia), has been reported in association with the use of tenofovir DF. The majority of these cases occurred in patients with underlying systemic or renal disease, or in patients taking nephrotoxic agents; however, some cases occured in patients without identified risk factors. Atripla should be avoided with concurrent or recent use of a nephrotoxic agent).
No products indexed under this heading.

Neomycin, oral (Renal impairment, including cases of acute renal failure and Fanconi syndrome (renal tubular injury with severe hypophosphatemia), has been reported in association with the use of tenofovir DF. The majority of these cases occurred in patients with underlying systemic or renal disease, or in patients taking nephrotoxic agents; however, some cases occured in patients without identified risk factors. Atripla should be avoided with concurrent or recent use of a nephrotoxic agent).
No products indexed under this heading.

Neomycin Sulfate (Renal impairment, including cases of acute renal failure and Fanconi syndrome (renal tubular injury with severe hypophosphatemia), has been reported in association with the use of tenofovir DF. The majority of these cases occurred in patients with underlying systemic or renal disease, or in patients taking nephrotoxic agents; however, some cases occured in patients without identified risk factors. Atripla should be avoided with concurrent or recent use of a nephrotoxic agent). Products include:
Neosporin Ophthalmic Solution Sterile .... ⊙252

Nevirapine (Renal impairment, including cases of acute renal failure and Fanconi syndrome (renal tubular injury with severe hypophosphatemia), has been reported in association with the use of tenofovir DF. The majority of these cases occurred in patients with underlying systemic or renal disease, or in patients taking nephrotoxic agents; however, some cases occured in patients without identified risk factors. Atripla should be avoided with concurrent or recent use of a nephrotoxic agent).
Products include:
Viramune Oral Suspension 873
Viramune Tablets 873

Nicardipine Hydrochloride (Efavirenz has been shown in vivo to induce CYP3A4. Other compounds that are substrates of CYP3A4 may have decreased plasma concentrations when co-administered with efavirenz). Products include:
Cardene I.V. 1093

Nifedipine (Efavirenz has been shown in vivo to induce CYP3A4. Other compounds that are substrates of CYP3A4 may have decreased plasma concentrations when co-administered with efavirenz).
No products indexed under this heading.

Nilutamide (In vitro studies have demonstrated that efavirenz inhibits CYP2C19 in the range of observed efavirenz plasma concentrations. Co-administration of efavirenz with drugs primarily metabolized by CYP2C19 may result in altered plasma concentrations of the co-administered drug. Therefore, appropriate dose adjustments may be necessary for these drugs).
No products indexed under this heading.

Nimodipine (Efavirenz has been shown in vivo to induce CYP3A4. Other compounds that are substrates of CYP3A4 may have decreased plasma concentrations when co-administered with efavirenz). Products include:
Nimotop Capsules 790

Nisoldipine (Efavirenz has been shown in vivo to induce CYP3A4. Other compounds that are substrates of CYP3A4 may have decreased plasma concentrations when co-administered with efavirenz). Products include:

Sular Extended Release Tablets 2975

Nitrendipine (Efavirenz has been shown in vivo to induce CYP3A4. Other compounds that are substrates of CYP3A4 may have decreased plasma concentrations when co-administered with efavirenz).
No products indexed under this heading.

Norethindrone (Efavirenz has been shown in vivo to induce CYP3A4. Other compounds that are substrates of CYP3A4 may have decreased plasma concentrations when co-administered with efavirenz). Products include:
Ortho Micronor Tablets 2446

Norethindrone Acetate (Efavirenz has been shown in vivo to induce CYP3A4. Other compounds that are substrates of CYP3A4 may have decreased plasma concentrations when co-administered with efavirenz). Products include:
Activella Tablets 2347

Norfloxacin (Renal impairment, including cases of acute renal failure and Fanconi syndrome (renal tubular injury with severe hypophosphatemia), has been reported in association with the use of tenofovir DF. The majority of these cases occurred in patients with underlying systemic or renal disease, or in patients taking nephrotoxic agents; however, some cases occured in patients without identified risk factors. Atripla should be avoided with concurrent or recent use of a nephrotoxic agent). Products include:
Noroxin Tablets 2069

Norgestrel (Efavirenz has been shown in vivo to induce CYP3A4. Other compounds that are substrates of CYP3A4 may have decreased plasma concentrations when co-administered with efavirenz).
No products indexed under this heading.

Nortriptyline Hydrochloride (In vitro studies have demonstrated that efavirenz inhibits CYP2C19 in the range of observed efavirenz plasma concentrations. Co-administration of efavirenz with drugs primarily metabolized by CYP2C19 may result in altered plasma concentrations of the co-administered drug. Therefore, appropriate dose adjustments may be necessary for these drugs).
No products indexed under this heading.

Olsalazine Sodium (Renal impairment, including cases of acute renal failure and Fanconi syndrome (renal tubular injury with severe hypophosphatemia), has been reported in association with the use of tenofovir DF. The majority of these cases occurred in patients with underlying systemic or renal disease, or in patients taking nephrotoxic agents; however, some cases occured in patients without identified risk factors. Atripla should be avoided with concurrent or recent use of a nephrotoxic agent).
No products indexed under this heading.

Omeprazole (Renal impairment, including cases of acute renal failure and Fanconi syndrome (renal tubular injury with severe hypophosphatemia), has been reported in association with the use of tenofovir DF. The majority of these cases occurred in patients with underlying systemic or renal disease, or in patients taking nephrotoxic agents; however, some cases occured in patients without identified risk factors. Atripla should be avoided with concurrent or recent use of a nephrotoxic agent).
No products indexed under this heading.

Ondansetron (Efavirenz has been shown in vivo to induce CYP3A4. Other compounds that are substrates of CYP3A4 may have decreased plasma concentrations when co-administered with efavirenz). Products include:
Zofran ODT Orally Disintegrating Tablets 1687

Ondansetron Hydrochloride (Efavirenz has been shown in vivo to induce CYP3A4. Other compounds that are substrates of CYP3A4 may have decreased plasma concentrations when co-administered with efavirenz). Products include:
Zofran Injection 1682
Zofran 1687

Oxaprozin (Renal impairment, including cases of acute renal failure and Fanconi syndrome (renal tubular injury with severe hypophosphatemia), has been reported in association with the use of tenofovir DF. The majority of these cases occurred in patients with underlying systemic or renal disease, or in patients taking nephrotoxic agents; however, some cases occured in patients without identified risk factors. Atripla should be avoided with concurrent or recent use of a nephrotoxic agent).
No products indexed under this heading.

Oxcarbazepine (Drugs which induce CYP3A4 activity would be expected to increase the clearance of efavirenz resulting in lower plasma concentrations).
No products indexed under this heading.

Paclitaxel (Efavirenz has been shown in vivo to induce CYP3A4. Other compounds that are substrates of CYP3A4 may have decreased plasma concentrations when co-administered with efavirenz).
No products indexed under this heading.

Pamidronate Disodium (Renal impairment, including cases of acute renal failure and Fanconi syndrome (renal tubular injury with severe hypophosphatemia), has been reported in association with the use of tenofovir DF. The majority of these cases occurred in patients with underlying systemic or renal disease, or in patients taking nephrotoxic agents; however, some cases occured in patients without identified risk factors. Atripla should be avoided with concurrent or recent use of a nephrotoxic agent).
No products indexed under this heading.

Pantoprazole Sodium (In vitro studies have demonstrated that efavirenz inhibits CYP2C19 in the range of observed efavirenz plasma concentrations. Co-administration of efavirenz with drugs primarily metabolized by CYP2C19 may result in altered plasma concentrations of the co-administered drug. Therefore, appropriate dose adjustments may be necessary for these drugs). Products include:
Protonix for Delayed-Release Oral Suspension 3254
Protonix Delayed-Release Tablets 3254
Protonix I.V. 3257

Paramethadione (In vitro studies have demonstrated that efavirenz inhibits CYP2C19 in the range of observed efavirenz plasma concentrations. Co-administration of efavirenz with drugs primarily metabolized by CYP2C19 may result in altered plasma concentrations of the co-administered drug. Therefore, appropriate dose adjustments may be necessary for these drugs).
No products indexed under this heading.

Paroxetine Hydrochloride (Renal impairment, including cases of acute renal failure and Fanconi syndrome (renal tubular injury with severe hypophosphatemia), has been reported in association with the use of tenofovir DF. The majority of these cases occurred in patients with underlying systemic or renal disease, or in patients taking nephrotoxic agents; however, some cases occured in patients without identified risk factors. Atripla should be avoided with concurrent or recent use of a nephrotoxic agent). Products include:
Paxil 1535
Paxil CR Controlled-Release Tablets 1544

Penicillamine (Renal impairment, including cases of acute renal failure and Fanconi syndrome (renal tubular injury with severe hypophosphatemia), has been reported in association with the use of tenofovir DF. The majority of these cases occurred in patients with underlying systemic or renal disease, or in patients taking nephrotoxic agents; however, some cases occured in patients without identified risk factors. Atripla should be avoided with concurrent or recent use of a nephrotoxic agent). Products include:
Cuprimine Capsules 1986

Penicillin G Benzathine (Renal impairment, including cases of acute renal failure and Fanconi syndrome (renal tubular injury with severe hypophosphatemia), has been reported in association with the use of tenofovir DF. The majority of these cases occurred in patients with underlying systemic or renal disease, or in patients taking nephrotoxic agents; however, some cases occured in patients without identified risk factors. Atripla should be avoided with concurrent or recent use of a nephrotoxic agent). Products include:
Bicillin C-R Injectable Suspension 1775
Bicillin L-A Injection 1777

Penicillin G Potassium (Renal impairment, including cases of acute renal failure and Fanconi syndrome (renal tubular injury with severe hypophosphatemia), has been reported in association with the use of tenofovir DF. The majority of these cases occurred in patients with underlying systemic or renal disease, or in patients taking nephrotoxic agents; however, some cases occured in patients without identified risk factors. Atripla should be avoided with concurrent or recent use of a nephrotoxic agent).
No products indexed under this heading.

Penicillin G Procaine (Renal impairment, including cases of acute renal failure and Fanconi syndrome (renal tubular injury with severe hypophosphatemia), has been reported in association with the use of tenofovir DF. The majority of these cases occurred in patients with underlying systemic or renal disease, or in patients taking nephrotoxic agents; however, some cases occured in patients without identified risk factors. Atripla should be avoided with concurrent or recent use of a nephrotoxic agent). Products include:
Bicillin C-R Injectable Suspension 1775
Bicillin L-A Injection 1777

Penicillin G Sodium (Renal impairment, including cases of acute renal failure and Fanconi syndrome (renal tubular injury with severe hypophosphatemia), has been reported in association with the use of tenofovir DF. The majority of these cases occurred in patients with underlying systemic or renal disease, or in patients taking nephrotoxic agents; however, some cases occured in patients without identified risk factors. Atripla should be avoided with concurrent or recent use of a nephrotoxic agent).
No products indexed under this heading.

Penicillin V Potassium (Renal impairment, including cases of acute renal failure and Fanconi syndrome (renal tubular injury with severe hypophosphatemia), has been reported in association with the use of tenofovir DF. The majority of these cases occurred in patients with underlying systemic or renal disease, or in patients taking nephrotoxic agents; however, some cases occured in patients without identified risk factors. Atripla should be avoided with concurrent or recent use of a nephrotoxic agent).
No products indexed under this heading.

Pentamidine Isethionate (Renal impairment, including cases of acute renal failure and Fanconi syndrome (renal tubular injury with severe hypophosphatemia), has been reported in association with the use of tenofovir DF. The majority of these cases occurred in patients with underlying systemic or renal disease, or in patients taking nephrotoxic agents; however, some cases occured in patients without identified risk factors. Atripla should be avoided with concurrent or recent use of a nephrotoxic agent).
No products indexed under this heading.

Perindopril Erbumine (Renal impairment, including cases of acute renal failure and Fanconi syndrome (renal tubular injury with severe hypophosphatemia), has been reported in association with the use of tenofovir DF. The majority of these cases occurred in patients with underlying systemic or renal disease, or in patients taking nephrotoxic agents; however, some cases occured in patients without identified risk factors. Atripla should be avoided with concurrent or recent use of a nephrotoxic agent). Products include:
Aceon Tablets (2 mg, 4 mg, 8 mg) 3038

Phenacemide (In vitro studies have demonstrated that efavirenz inhibits CYP2C19 in the range of observed efavirenz plasma concentrations. Co-administration of efavirenz with drugs primarily metabolized by CYP2C19 may result in altered plasma concentrations of the co-administered drug. Therefore, appropriate dose adjustments may be necessary for these drugs).
No products indexed under this heading.

Phenobarbital (Potential for reduction in anticonvulsant and/or efavirenz plasma levels; periodic monitoring of anticonvulsant plasma levels should be conducted).
Products include:
Donnatal Extentabs 2507

Phenobarbital Sodium (Potential for reduction in anticonvulsant and/or efavirenz plasma levels; periodic monitoring of anticonvulsant plasma levels should be conducted).
No products indexed under this heading.

Phensuximide (In vitro studies have demonstrated that efavirenz inhibits CYP2C19 in the range of observed efavirenz plasma concentrations. Co-administration of efavirenz with drugs primarily metabolized by CYP2C19 may result in altered plasma concentrations of the co-administered drug. Therefore, appropriate dose adjustments may be necessary for these drugs).
No products indexed under this heading.

Phenylbutazone (Renal impairment, including cases of acute renal failure and Fanconi syndrome (renal tubular injury with severe hypophosphatemia), has been reported in association with the use of tenofovir DF. The majority of these cases occurred in patients with underlying systemic or renal disease, or in patients taking nephrotoxic agents; however, some cases occured in patients without identified risk factors. Atripla should be avoided with concurrent or recent use of a nephrotoxic agent).
No products indexed under this heading.

Phenytoin (Potential for reduction in anticonvulsant and/or efavirenz plasma levels; periodic monitoring of anticonvulsant plasma levels should be conducted).
No products indexed under this heading.

Phenytoin Sodium (Potential for reduction in anticonvulsant and/or efavirenz plasma levels; periodic monitoring of anticonvulsant plasma levels should be conducted).
Products include:
Phenytek Capsules 2192

Pimozide (Due to the potential for serious and/or life threatening reactions, such as cardiac arrhythmias, concomitant use with pimozide is contraindicated).
No products indexed under this heading.

Pioglitazone Hydrochloride (In vitro studies have demonstrated that efavirenz inhibits CYP2C9 in the range of observed efavirenz plasma concentrations. Co-administration of efavirenz with drugs primarily metabolized by CYP2C9 may result in altered plasma concentrations of the co-administered drug. Therefore, appropriate dose adjustments may be necessary for these drugs).
Products include:
ActoPlus Met Tablets 3071
Actos Tablets 3077
Duetact Tablets 3085

Piroxicam (Renal impairment, including cases of acute renal failure and Fanconi syndrome (renal tubular injury with severe hypophosphatemia), has been reported in association with the use of tenofovir DF. The majority of these cases occurred in patients with underlying systemic or renal disease, or in patients taking nephrotoxic agents; however, some cases occured in patients without identified risk factors. Atripla should be avoided with concurrent or recent use of a nephrotoxic agent).
No products indexed under this heading.

Plicamycin (Renal impairment, including cases of acute renal failure and Fanconi syndrome (renal tubular injury with severe hypophosphatemia), has been reported in association with the use of tenofovir DF. The majority of these cases occurred in patients with underlying systemic or renal disease, or in patients taking nephrotoxic agents; however, some cases occured in patients without identified risk factors. Atripla should be avoided with concurrent or recent use of a nephrotoxic agent).
No products indexed under this heading.

Polyestradiol Phosphate (Efavirenz has been shown in vivo to induce CYP3A4. Other compounds that are substrates of CYP3A4 may have decreased plasma concentrations when co-administered with efavirenz).
No products indexed under this heading.

Polymyxin (Renal impairment, including cases of acute renal failure and Fanconi syndrome (renal tubular injury with severe hypophosphatemia), has been reported in association with the use of tenofovir DF. The majority of these cases occurred in patients with underlying systemic or renal disease, or in patients taking nephrotoxic agents; however, some cases occured in patients without identified risk factors. Atripla should be avoided with concurrent or recent use of a nephrotoxic agent).
No products indexed under this heading.

Polymyxin B Sulfate (Renal impairment, including cases of acute renal failure and Fanconi syndrome (renal tubular injury with severe hypophosphatemia), has been reported in association with the use of tenofovir DF. The majority of these cases occurred in patients with underlying systemic or renal disease, or in patients taking nephrotoxic agents; however, some cases occured in patients without identified risk factors. Atripla should be avoided with concurrent or recent use of a nephrotoxic agent). Products include:
Neosporin Ophthalmic Solution Sterile .... ⊙252

Polythiazide (Renal impairment, including cases of acute renal failure and Fanconi syndrome (renal tubular injury with severe hypophosphatemia), has been reported in association with the use of tenofovir DF. The majority of these cases occurred in patients with underlying systemic or renal disease, or in patients taking nephrotoxic agents; however, some cases occured in patients without identified risk factors. Atripla should be avoided with concurrent or recent use of a nephrotoxic agent).
No products indexed under this heading.

Pravastatin Sodium (Plasma concentrations of atorvastatin, pravastatin, and simvastatin decreased with efavirenz. Consult the complete prescribing information for the HMGCoA reductase inhibitor for guidance on individualizing the dose).
No products indexed under this heading.

Prednisolone Acetate (Drugs which induce CYP3A4 activity would be expected to increase the clearance of efavirenz resulting in lower plasma concentrations). Products include:
Pred Forte Ophthalmic Suspension .... ⊙227
Pred Mild Ophthalmic Suspension .... ⊙230
Pred-G Ophthalmic Ointment .... ⊙229
Pred-G Ophthalmic Suspension ...... ⊙228

Prednisolone Sodium Phosphate (Drugs which induce CYP3A4 activity would be expected to increase the clearance of efavirenz resulting in lower plasma concentrations).
No products indexed under this heading.

Prednisolone Tebutate (Drugs which induce CYP3A4 activity would be expected to increase the clearance of efavirenz resulting in lower plasma concentrations).
No products indexed under this heading.

Prednisone (Drugs which induce CYP3A4 activity would be expected to increase the clearance of efavirenz resulting in lower plasma concentrations).
No products indexed under this heading.

Primidone (Drugs which induce CYP3A4 activity would be expected to increase the clearance of efavirenz resulting in lower plasma concentrations).
No products indexed under this heading.

Probenecid (Renal impairment, including cases of acute renal failure and Fanconi syndrome (renal tubular injury with severe hypophosphatemia), has been reported in association with the use of tenofovir DF. The majority of these cases occurred in patients with underlying systemic or renal disease, or in patients taking nephrotoxic agents; however, some cases occured in patients without identified risk factors. Atripla should be avoided with concurrent or recent use of a nephrotoxic agent).
No products indexed under this heading.

Progesterone (In vitro studies have demonstrated that efavirenz inhibits CYP2C19 in the range of observed efavirenz plasma concentrations. Co-administration of efavirenz with drugs primarily metabolized by CYP2C19 may result in altered plasma concentrations of the co-administered drug. Therefore, appropriate dose adjustments may be necessary for these drugs).
Products include:
Crinone 4% Gel 992
Crinone 8% Gel 992
Prometrium Capsules (100 mg, 200 mg) 3047

Proguanil Hydrochloride (In vitro studies have demonstrated that efavirenz inhibits CYP2C19 in the range of observed efavirenz plasma concentrations. Co-administration of efavirenz with drugs primarily metabolized by CYP2C19 may result in altered plasma concentrations of the co-administered drug. Therefore, appropriate dose adjustments may be necessary for these drugs).
Products include:
Malarone Pediatric Tablets 1521
Malarone Tablets 1521

Propranolol Hydrochloride (In vitro studies have demonstrated that efavirenz inhibits CYP2C19 in the range of observed efavirenz plasma concentrations. Co-administration of efavirenz with drugs primarily metabolized by CYP2C19 may result in altered plasma concentrations of the co-administered drug. Therefore, appropriate dose adjustments may be necessary for these drugs).
Products include:
InnoPran XL Extended Release Capsules 1484

Protriptyline Hydrochloride (In vitro studies have demonstrated that efavirenz inhibits CYP2C19 in the range of observed efavirenz plasma concentrations. Co-administration of efavirenz with drugs primarily metabolized by CYP2C19 may result in altered plasma concentrations of the co-administered drug. Therefore, appropriate dose adjustments may be necessary for these drugs).
No products indexed under this heading.

Quinapril Hydrochloride (Renal impairment, including cases of acute renal failure and Fanconi syndrome (renal tubular injury with severe hypophosphatemia), has been reported in association with the use of tenofovir DF. The majority of these cases occurred in patients with underlying systemic or renal disease, or in patients taking nephrotoxic agents; however, some cases occured in patients without identified risk factors. Atripla should be avoided with concurrent or recent use of a nephrotoxic agent).
No products indexed under this heading.

Quinidine Gluconate (Efavirenz has been shown in vivo to induce CYP3A4. Other compounds that are substrates of CYP3A4 may have decreased plasma concentrations when co-administered with efavirenz).
No products indexed under this heading.

Quinidine Polygalacturonate (Efavirenz has been shown in vivo to induce CYP3A4. Other compounds that are substrates of CYP3A4 may have decreased plasma concentrations when co-administered with efavirenz).
No products indexed under this heading.

Quinidine Sulfate (Efavirenz has been shown in vivo to induce CYP3A4. Other compounds that are substrates of CYP3A4 may have decreased plasma concentrations when co-administered with efavirenz).
No products indexed under this heading.

Rabeprazole Sodium (Renal impairment, including cases of acute renal failure and Fanconi syndrome (renal tubular injury with severe hypophosphatemia), has been reported in association with the use of tenofovir DF. The majority of these cases occurred in patients with underlying systemic or renal disease, or in patients taking nephrotoxic agents; however, some cases occured in patients without identified risk factors. Atripla should be avoided with concurrent or recent use of a nephrotoxic agent). Products include:

Aciphex Tablets 1053

Ramipril (Renal impairment, including cases of acute renal failure and Fanconi syndrome (renal tubular injury with severe hypophosphatemia), has been reported in association with the use of tenofovir DF. The majority of these cases occurred in patients with underlying systemic or renal disease, or in patients taking nephrotoxic agents; however, some cases occured in patients without identified risk factors. Atripla should be avoided with concurrent or recent use of a nephrotoxic agent).

No products indexed under this heading.

Repaglinide (In vitro studies have demonstrated that efavirenz inhibits CYP2C9 in the range of observed efavirenz plasma concentrations. Co-administration of efavirenz with drugs primarily metabolized by CYP2C9 may result in altered plasma concentrations of the co-administered drug. Therefore, appropriate dose adjustments may be necessary for these drugs). Products include:

PrandiMet Tablets 2967
Prandin Tablets 2971

Rifabutin (Increase daily dose of rifabutin by 50%. Consider doubling the rifabutin dose regimens where rifabutin is given 2 or 3 times a week).

No products indexed under this heading.

Rifampicin (Drugs which induce CYP3A4 activity would be expected to increase the clearance of efavirenz resulting in lower plasma concentrations).

No products indexed under this heading.

Rifampin (Rifampin reduced plasma concentrations of efavirenz).

No products indexed under this heading.

Rifapentine (Drugs which induce CYP3A4 activity would be expected to increase the clearance of efavirenz resulting in lower plasma concentrations).

No products indexed under this heading.

Riluzole (Renal impairment, including cases of acute renal failure and Fanconi syndrome (renal tubular injury with severe hypophosphatemia), has been reported in association with the use of tenofovir DF. The majority of these cases occurred in patients with underlying systemic or renal disease, or in patients taking nephrotoxic agents; however, some cases occured in patients without identified risk factors. Atripla should be avoided with concurrent or recent use of a nephrotoxic agent). Products include:

Rilutek Tablets 2771

Ritonavir (Kaletra may increase tenofovir concentrations. The mechanism of this interaction is unknown. Higher tenofovir concentrations could potentiate tenofovir-associated adverse events. Patients receiving Kaletra with tenofovir DF should be monitored for tenofovir-associated adverse events. Atripla should be discontinued in patients who develop tenofovir-assocatied adverse events. When ritonavir 500 mg every 12 hours was co-administered with efavirenz 600 mg once daily, the combination was associated with a higher frequency of adverse clinical experiences (e.g., dizziness, nausea, paresthesia) and lab abnormalities (elevated liver enzymes). Monitoring of liver enzymes is recommended when Atripla is used with ritonavir). Products include:

Kaletra 452
Norvir 489

Rofecoxib (Renal impairment, including cases of acute renal failure and Fanconi syndrome (renal tubular injury with severe hypophosphatemia), has been reported in association with the use of tenofovir DF. The majority of these cases occurred in patients with underlying systemic or renal disease, or in patients taking nephrotoxic agents; however, some cases occured in patients without identified risk factors. Atripla should be avoided with concurrent or recent use of a nephrotoxic agent).

No products indexed under this heading.

Rosiglitazone Maleate (In vitro studies have demonstrated that efavirenz inhibits CYP2C9 in the range of observed efavirenz plasma concentrations. Co-administration of efavirenz with drugs primarily metabolized by CYP2C9 may result in altered plasma concentrations of the co-administered drug. Therefore, appropriate dose adjustments may be necessary for these drugs). Products include:

Avandamet Tablets 1336
Avandaryl Tablets 1344
Avandia Tablets 1351

Saquinavir (Due to a decrease in its concentration, saquinavir should not be used as sole protease inhibitor in combination with Atripla).

No products indexed under this heading.

Saquinavir Mesylate (Due to a decrease in its concentration, saquinavir should not be used as sole protease inhibitor in combination with Atripla).

No products indexed under this heading.

Sertraline Hydrochloride (Increases in sertraline dose should be guided by clinical response).

No products indexed under this heading.

Sibutramine Hydrochloride Monohydrate (Renal impairment, including cases of acute renal failure and Fanconi syndrome (renal tubular injury with severe hypophosphatemia), has been reported in association with the use of tenofovir DF. The majority of these cases occurred in patients with underlying systemic or renal disease, or in patients taking nephrotoxic agents; however, some cases occured in patients without identified risk factors. Atripla should be avoided with concurrent or recent use of a nephrotoxic agent). Products include:

Meridia Capsules 475

Sildenafil Citrate (Efavirenz has been shown in vivo to induce CYP3A4. Other compounds that are substrates of CYP3A4 may have decreased plasma concentrations when co-administered with efavirenz).

No products indexed under this heading.

Simvastatin (Plasma concentrations of atorvastatin, pravastatin, and simvastatin decreased with efavirenz. Consult the complete prescribing information for the HMGCoA reductase inhibitor for guidance on individualizing the dose). Products include:

Simcor Tablets 502
Vytorin 10/10 Tablets 2149
Vytorin 10/10 Tablets 2939
Vytorin 10/20 Tablets 2149
Vytorin 10/20 Tablets 2939
Vytorin 10/40 Tablets 2149
Vytorin 10/40 Tablets 2939
Vytorin 10/80 Tablets 2149
Vytorin 10/80 Tablets 2939
Zocor Tablets 2136

Sirolimus (Efavirenz has been shown in vivo to induce CYP3A4. Other compounds that are substrates of CYP3A4 may have decreased plasma concentrations when co-administered with efavirenz). Products include:

Rapamune 3260

Spirapril Hydrochloride (Renal impairment, including cases of acute renal failure and Fanconi syndrome (renal tubular injury with severe hypophosphatemia), has been reported in association with the use of tenofovir DF. The majority of these cases occurred in patients with underlying systemic or renal disease, or in patients taking nephrotoxic agents; however, some cases occured in patients without identified risk factors. Atripla should be avoided with concurrent or recent use of a nephrotoxic agent).

No products indexed under this heading.

Stavudine (Renal impairment, including cases of acute renal failure and Fanconi syndrome (renal tubular injury with severe hypophosphatemia), has been reported in association with the use of tenofovir DF. The majority of these cases occurred in patients with underlying systemic or renal disease, or in patients taking nephrotoxic agents; however, some cases occured in patients without identified risk factors. Atripla should be avoided with concurrent or recent use of a nephrotoxic agent).

No products indexed under this heading.

Streptomycin Sulfate (Renal impairment, including cases of acute renal failure and Fanconi syndrome (renal tubular injury with severe hypophosphatemia), has been reported in association with the use of tenofovir DF. The majority of these cases occurred in patients with underlying systemic or renal disease, or in patients taking nephrotoxic agents; however, some cases occured in patients without identified risk factors. Atripla should be avoided with concurrent or recent use of a nephrotoxic agent).

No products indexed under this heading.

Streptozocin (Renal impairment, including cases of acute renal failure and Fanconi syndrome (renal tubular injury with severe hypophosphatemia), has been reported in association with the use of tenofovir DF. The majority of these cases occurred in patients with underlying systemic or renal disease, or in patients taking nephrotoxic agents; however, some cases occured in patients without identified risk factors. Atripla should be avoided with concurrent or recent use of a nephrotoxic agent).

No products indexed under this heading.

Sulfacytine (Renal impairment, including cases of acute renal failure and Fanconi syndrome (renal tubular injury with severe hypophosphatemia), has been reported in association with the use of tenofovir DF. The majority of these cases occurred in patients with underlying systemic or renal disease, or in patients taking nephrotoxic agents; however, some cases occured in patients without identified risk factors. Atripla should be avoided with concurrent or recent use of a nephrotoxic agent).

No products indexed under this heading.

Sulfamethizole (Renal impairment, including cases of acute renal failure and Fanconi syndrome (renal tubular injury with severe hypophosphatemia), has been reported in association with the use of tenofovir DF. The majority of these cases occurred in patients with underlying systemic or renal disease, or in patients taking nephrotoxic agents; however, some cases occured in patients without identified risk factors. Atripla should be avoided with concurrent or recent use of a nephrotoxic agent).

No products indexed under this heading.

Sulfamethoxazole (Renal impairment, including cases of acute renal failure and Fanconi syndrome (renal tubular injury with severe hypophosphatemia), has been reported in association with the use of tenofovir DF. The majority of these cases occurred in patients with underlying systemic or renal disease, or in patients taking nephrotoxic agents; however, some cases occured in patients without identified risk factors. Atripla should be avoided with concurrent or recent use of a nephrotoxic agent).

No products indexed under this heading.

Sulfasalazine (Renal impairment, including cases of acute renal failure and Fanconi syndrome (renal tubular injury with severe hypophosphatemia), has been reported in association with the use of tenofovir DF. The majority of these cases occurred in patients with underlying systemic or renal disease, or in patients taking nephrotoxic agents; however, some cases occured in patients without identified risk factors. Atripla should be avoided with concurrent or recent use of a nephrotoxic agent).

No products indexed under this heading.

Sulfinpyrazone (Renal impairment, including cases of acute renal failure and Fanconi syndrome (renal tubular injury with severe hypophosphatemia), has been reported in association with the use of tenofovir DF. The majority of these cases occurred in patients with underlying systemic or renal disease, or in patients taking nephrotoxic agents; however, some cases occured in patients without identified risk factors. Atripla should be avoided with concurrent or recent use of a nephrotoxic agent).

No products indexed under this heading.

Sulfisoxazole Acetyl (Renal impairment, including cases of acute renal failure and Fanconi syndrome (renal tubular injury with severe hypophosphatemia), has been reported in association with the use of tenofovir DF. The majority of these cases occurred in patients with underlying systemic or renal disease, or in patients taking nephrotoxic agents; however, some cases occured in patients without identified risk factors. Atripla should be avoided with concurrent or recent use of a nephrotoxic agent).

No products indexed under this heading.

Sulfisoxazole Diolamine (Renal impairment, including cases of acute renal failure and Fanconi syndrome (renal tubular injury with severe hypophosphatemia), has been reported in association with the use of tenofovir DF. The majority of these cases occurred in patients with underlying systemic or renal disease, or in patients taking nephrotoxic agents; however, some cases occured in patients without identified risk factors. Atripla should be avoided with concurrent or recent use of a nephrotoxic agent).

No products indexed under this heading.

Sulindac (Renal impairment, including cases of acute renal failure and Fanconi syndrome (renal tubular injury with severe hypophosphatemia), has been reported in association with the use of tenofovir DF. The majority of these cases occurred in patients with underlying systemic or renal disease, or in patients taking nephrotoxic agents; however, some cases occured in patients without identified risk factors. Atripla should be avoided with concurrent or recent use of a nephrotoxic agent).

Products include:

Clinoril Tablets 1962

Suprofen (In vitro studies have demonstrated that efavirenz inhibits CYP2C9 in the range of observed efavirenz plasma concentrations. Co-administration of efavirenz with drugs primarily metabolized by CYP2C9 may result in altered plasma concentrations of the co-administered drug. Therefore, appropriate dose adjustments may be necessary for these drugs).

No products indexed under this heading.

Tacrolimus (Renal impairment, including cases of acute renal failure and Fanconi syndrome (renal tubular injury with severe hypophosphatemia), has been reported in association with the use of tenofovir DF. The majority of these cases occurred in patients with underlying systemic or renal disease, or in patients taking nephrotoxic agents; however, some cases occured in patients without identified risk factors. Atripla should be avoided with concurrent or recent use of a nephrotoxic agent).

Products include:

Prograf Capsules and Injection 622

Protopic Ointment 628

Tadalafil (Efavirenz has been shown in vivo to induce CYP3A4. Other compounds that are substrates of CYP3A4 may have decreased plasma concentrations when co-administered with efavirenz).

Products include:

Cialis Tablets 1792

Tamoxifen Citrate (Efavirenz has been shown in vivo to induce CYP3A4. Other compounds that are substrates of CYP3A4 may have decreased plasma concentrations when co-administered with efavirenz).

No products indexed under this heading.

Telmisartan (In vitro studies have demonstrated that efavirenz inhibits CYP2C9 in the range of observed efavirenz plasma concentrations. Co-administration of efavirenz with drugs primarily metabolized by CYP2C9 may result in altered plasma concentrations of the co-administered drug. Therefore, appropriate dose adjustments may be necessary for these drugs).

Products include:

Micardis Tablets 852

Micardis HCT Tablets 854

Teniposide (In vitro studies have demonstrated that efavirenz inhibits CYP2C19 in the range of observed efavirenz plasma concentrations. Co-administration of efavirenz with drugs primarily metabolized by CYP2C19 may result in altered plasma concentrations of the co-administered drug. Therefore, appropriate dose adjustments may be necessary for these drugs).

No products indexed under this heading.

Theophylline (Drugs which induce CYP3A4 activity would be expected to increase the clearance of efavirenz resulting in lower plasma concentrations).

No products indexed under this heading.

Theophylline Anhydrous (Drugs which induce CYP3A4 activity would be expected to increase the clearance of efavirenz resulting in lower plasma concentrations). Products include:

Uniphyl Tablets 2595

Theophylline Calcium Salicylate (Drugs which induce CYP3A4 activity would be expected to increase the clearance of efavirenz resulting in lower plasma concentrations).

No products indexed under this heading.

Theophylline Dihydroxypropyl (Glyceryl) (Drugs which induce CYP3A4 activity would be expected to increase the clearance of efavirenz resulting in lower plasma concentrations).

No products indexed under this heading.

Theophylline Ethylenediamine (Drugs which induce CYP3A4 activity would be expected to increase the clearance of efavirenz resulting in lower plasma concentrations).

No products indexed under this heading.

Thioguanine (Renal impairment, including cases of acute renal failure and Fanconi syndrome (renal tubular injury with severe hypophosphatemia), has been reported in association with the use of tenofovir DF. The majority of these cases occurred in patients with underlying systemic or renal disease, or in patients taking nephrotoxic agents; however, some cases occured in patients without identified risk factors. Atripla should be avoided with concurrent or recent use of a nephrotoxic agent).

Products include:

Tabloid Tablets 1601

Thioridazine (In vitro studies have demonstrated that efavirenz inhibits CYP2C19 in the range of observed efavirenz plasma concentrations. Co-administration of efavirenz with drugs primarily metabolized by CYP2C19 may result in altered plasma concentrations of the co-administered drug. Therefore, appropriate dose adjustments may be necessary for these drugs).

No products indexed under this heading.

Thioridazine Hydrochloride (In vitro studies have demonstrated that efavirenz inhibits CYP2C19 in the range of observed efavirenz plasma concentrations. Co-administration of efavirenz with drugs primarily metabolized by CYP2C19 may result in altered plasma concentrations of the co-administered drug. Therefore, appropriate dose adjustments may be necessary for these drugs).

Products include:

Thioridazine Hydrochloride Tablets 2195

Tiagabine Hydrochloride (Efavirenz has been shown in vivo to induce CYP3A4. Other compounds that are substrates of CYP3A4 may have decreased plasma concentrations when co-administered with efavirenz). Products include:

Gabitril Tablets 973

Ticarcillin Disodium (Renal impairment, including cases of acute renal failure and Fanconi syndrome (renal tubular injury with severe hypophosphatemia), has been reported in association with the use of tenofovir DF. The majority of these cases occurred in patients with underlying systemic or renal disease, or in patients taking nephrotoxic agents; however, some cases occured in patients without identified risk factors. Atripla should be avoided with concurrent or recent use of a nephrotoxic agent). Products include:

Timentin ADD-Vantage 1606

Timentin Injection Galaxy Container 1609

Timentin IV Infusion 1603

Timentin Pharmacy Bulk Package 1613

Tobramycin (Renal impairment, including cases of acute renal failure and Fanconi syndrome (renal tubular injury with severe hypophosphatemia), has been reported in association with the use of tenofovir DF. The majority of these cases occurred in patients with underlying systemic or renal disease, or in patients taking nephrotoxic agents; however, some cases occured in patients without identified risk factors. Atripla should be avoided with concurrent or recent use of a nephrotoxic agent).

Products include:

Zylet Ophthalmic Suspension .... ⊙ 247

Tobramycin Sulfate (Renal impairment, including cases of acute renal failure and Fanconi syndrome (renal tubular injury with severe hypophosphatemia), has been reported in association with the use of tenofovir DF. The majority of these cases occurred in patients with underlying systemic or renal disease, or in patients taking nephrotoxic agents; however, some cases occured in patients without identified risk factors. Atripla should be avoided with concurrent or recent use of a nephrotoxic agent).

No products indexed under this heading.

Tolazamide (Renal impairment, including cases of acute renal failure and Fanconi syndrome (renal tubular injury with severe hypophosphatemia), has been reported in association with the use of tenofovir DF. The majority of these cases occurred in patients with underlying systemic or renal disease, or in patients taking nephrotoxic agents; however, some cases occured in patients without identified risk factors. Atripla should be avoided with concurrent or recent use of a nephrotoxic agent).

No products indexed under this heading.

Tolbutamide (Renal impairment, including cases of acute renal failure and Fanconi syndrome (renal tubular injury with severe hypophosphatemia), has been reported in association with the use of tenofovir DF. The majority of these cases occurred in patients with underlying systemic or renal disease, or in patients taking nephrotoxic agents; however, some cases occured in patients without identified risk factors. Atripla should be avoided with concurrent or recent use of a nephrotoxic agent).

No products indexed under this heading.

Tolbutamide Sodium (In vitro studies have demonstrated that efavirenz inhibits CYP2C9 in the range of observed efavirenz plasma concentrations. Co-administration of efavirenz with drugs primarily metabolized by CYP2C9 may result in altered plasma concentrations of the co-administered drug. Therefore, appropriate dose adjustments may be necessary for these drugs).

No products indexed under this heading.

Tolmetin Sodium (Renal impairment, including cases of acute renal failure and Fanconi syndrome (renal tubular injury with severe hypophosphatemia), has been reported in association with the use of tenofovir DF. The majority of these cases occurred in patients with underlying systemic or renal disease, or in patients taking nephrotoxic agents; however, some cases occured in patients without identified risk factors. Atripla should be avoided with concurrent or recent use of a nephrotoxic agent).

No products indexed under this heading.

Tolterodine Tartrate (Efavirenz has been shown in vivo to induce CYP3A4. Other compounds that are substrates of CYP3A4 may have decreased plasma concentrations when co-administered with efavirenz).

No products indexed under this heading.

Topiramate (In vitro studies have demonstrated that efavirenz inhibits CYP2C19 in the range of observed efavirenz plasma concentrations. Co-administration of efavirenz with drugs primarily metabolized by CYP2C19 may result in altered plasma concentrations of the co-administered drug. Therefore, appropriate dose adjustments may be necessary for these drugs).

No products indexed under this heading.

Torsemide (In vitro studies have demonstrated that efavirenz inhibits CYP2C9 in the range of observed efavirenz plasma concentrations. Co-administration of efavirenz with drugs primarily metabolized by CYP2C9 may result in altered plasma concentrations of the co-administered drug. Therefore, appropriate dose adjustments may be necessary for these drugs). Products include:

Demadex Injection 2630
Demadex Tablets 2630

Trandolapril (Renal impairment, including cases of acute renal failure and Fanconi syndrome (renal tubular injury with severe hypophosphatemia), has been reported in association with the use of tenofovir DF. The majority of these cases occurred in patients with underlying systemic or renal disease, or in patients taking nephrotoxic agents; however, some cases occured in patients without identified risk factors. Atripla should be avoided with concurrent or recent use of a nephrotoxic agent). Products include:

Mavik Tablets 472
Tarka Tablets 511

Trazodone Hydrochloride (Efavirenz has been shown in vivo to induce CYP3A4. Other compounds that are substrates of CYP3A4 may have decreased plasma concentrations when co-administered with efavirenz).

No products indexed under this heading.

Triamcinolone (Drugs which induce CYP3A4 activity would be expected to increase the clearance of efavirenz resulting in lower plasma concentrations).

No products indexed under this heading.

Triamcinolone Acetonide (Drugs which induce CYP3A4 activity would be expected to increase the clearance of efavirenz resulting in lower plasma concentrations). Products include:

Azmacort Inhalation Aerosol 407
Nasacort AQ Nasal Spray 2765
Triesence Injectable Suspension .... ⊙209

Triamcinolone Diacetate (Drugs which induce CYP3A4 activity would be expected to increase the clearance of efavirenz resulting in lower plasma concentrations).

No products indexed under this heading.

Triamcinolone Hexacetonide (Drugs which induce CYP3A4 activity would be expected to increase the clearance of efavirenz resulting in lower plasma concentrations).

No products indexed under this heading.

Triamterene (Renal impairment, including cases of acute renal failure and Fanconi syndrome (renal tubular injury with severe hypophosphatemia), has been reported in association with the use of tenofovir DF. The majority of these cases occurred in patients with underlying systemic or renal disease, or in patients taking nephrotoxic agents; however, some cases occured in patients without identified risk factors. Atripla should be avoided with concurrent or recent use of a nephrotoxic agent). Products include:

Dyazide Capsules 1405
Dyrenium Capsules 3189

Triazolam (Due to the potential for serious and/or life-threatening reactions, such as prolonged or increased sedation or respiratory depression, concomitant use with triazolam is contraindicated).

No products indexed under this heading.

Trimethadione (Renal impairment, including cases of acute renal failure and Fanconi syndrome (renal tubular injury with severe hypophosphatemia), has been reported in association with the use of tenofovir DF. The majority of these cases occurred in patients with underlying systemic or renal disease, or in patients taking nephrotoxic agents; however, some cases occured in patients without identified risk factors. Atripla should be avoided with concurrent or recent use of a nephrotoxic agent).

No products indexed under this heading.

Trimipramine Maleate (In vitro studies have demonstrated that efavirenz inhibits CYP2C19 in the range of observed efavirenz plasma concentrations. Co-administration of efavirenz with drugs primarily metabolized by CYP2C19 may result in altered plasma concentrations of the co-administered drug. Therefore, appropriate dose adjustments may be necessary for these drugs).

No products indexed under this heading.

Troglitazone (Drugs which induce CYP3A4 activity would be expected to increase the clearance of efavirenz resulting in lower plasma concentrations).

No products indexed under this heading.

Trovafloxacin Mesylate (Renal impairment, including cases of acute renal failure and Fanconi syndrome (renal tubular injury with severe hypophosphatemia), has been reported in association with the use of tenofovir DF. The majority of these cases occurred in patients with underlying systemic or renal disease, or in patients taking nephrotoxic agents; however, some cases occured in patients without identified risk factors. Atripla should be avoided with concurrent or recent use of a nephrotoxic agent).

No products indexed under this heading.

Tyropanoate Sodium (Renal impairment, including cases of acute renal failure and Fanconi syndrome (renal tubular injury with severe hypophosphatemia), has been reported in association with the use of tenofovir DF. The majority of these cases occurred in patients with underlying systemic or renal disease, or in patients taking nephrotoxic agents; however, some cases occured in patients without identified risk factors. Atripla should be avoided with concurrent or recent use of a nephrotoxic agent).

No products indexed under this heading.

Valacyclovir Hydrochloride (Since emtricitabine and tenofovir are primarily eliminated by the kidneys, co-administration of Atripla with drugs that reduce renal fuction or compete for active tubular secretion may increase serum concentrations of emtricitabine, tenofovir, and/or other renally eliminated drugs). Products include:

Valtrex Caplets 1635

Valdecoxib (Renal impairment, including cases of acute renal failure and Fanconi syndrome (renal tubular injury with severe hypophosphatemia), has been reported in association with the use of tenofovir DF. The majority of these cases occurred in patients with underlying systemic or renal disease, or in patients taking nephrotoxic agents; however, some cases occured in patients without identified risk factors. Atripla should be avoided with concurrent or recent use of a nephrotoxic agent).

No products indexed under this heading.

Valganciclovir Hydrochloride (Since emtricitabine and tenofovir are primarily eliminated by the kidneys, co-administration of Atripla with drugs that reduce renal fuction or compete for active tubular secretion may increase serum concentrations of emtricitabine, tenofovir, and/or other renally eliminated drugs). Products include:

Valcyte Tablets 2654

Valproate Sodium (In vitro studies have demonstrated that efavirenz inhibits CYP2C19 in the range of observed efavirenz plasma concentrations. Co-administration of efavirenz with drugs primarily metabolized by CYP2C19 may result in altered plasma concentrations of the co-administered drug. Therefore, appropriate dose adjustments may be necessary for these drugs).

No products indexed under this heading.

Valproic Acid (In vitro studies have demonstrated that efavirenz inhibits CYP2C19 in the range of observed efavirenz plasma concentrations. Co-administration of efavirenz with drugs primarily metabolized by CYP2C19 may result in altered plasma concentrations of the co-administered drug. Therefore, appropriate dose adjustments may be necessary for these drugs).

No products indexed under this heading.

Valsartan (In vitro studies have demonstrated that efavirenz inhibits CYP2C9 in the range of observed efavirenz plasma concentrations. Co-administration of efavirenz with drugs primarily metabolized by CYP2C9 may result in altered plasma concentrations of the co-administered drug. Therefore, appropriate dose adjustments may be necessary for these drugs). Products include:

Diovan Tablets 2212
Diovan HCT Tablets 2216
Exforge Tablets 2238

Vancomycin Hydrochloride (Renal impairment, including cases of acute renal failure and Fanconi syndrome (renal tubular injury with severe hypophosphatemia), has been reported in association with the use of tenofovir DF. The majority of these cases occurred in patients with underlying systemic or renal disease, or in patients taking nephrotoxic agents; however, some cases occured in patients without identified risk factors. Atripla should be avoided with concurrent or recent use of a nephrotoxic agent).

No products indexed under this heading.

Vardenafil Hydrochloride (Efavirenz has been shown in vivo to induce CYP3A4. Other compounds that are substrates of CYP3A4 may have decreased plasma concentrations when co-administered with efavirenz). Products include:

Levitra Tablets 2876

Verapamil Hydrochloride (Efavirenz has been shown in vivo to induce CYP3A4. Other compounds that are substrates of CYP3A4 may have decreased plasma concentrations when co-administered with efavirenz). Products include:

Tarka Tablets 511

Vinblastine Sulfate (Efavirenz has been shown in vivo to induce CYP3A4. Other compounds that are substrates of CYP3A4 may have decreased plasma concentrations when co-administered with efavirenz).

No products indexed under this heading.

Vincristine Sulfate (Efavirenz has been shown in vivo to induce CYP3A4. Other compounds that are substrates of CYP3A4 may have decreased plasma concentrations when co-administered with efavirenz).

No products indexed under this heading.

Voriconazole (Efavirenz significantly decreases voriconazole plasma concentrations, and co-administration may decrease the therapeutic effectiveness of voriconazole. Also, voriconazole significantly increases efavirenz plasma concentrations, which may increase the risk of efavirenz-associated side effects. Concomitant use is contraindicated).

No products indexed under this heading.

Warfarin Sodium (Plasma concentrations and effects to warfarin sodium potentially increased or decreased by efavirenz).

No products indexed under this heading.

Zafirlukast (In vitro studies have demonstrated that efavirenz inhibits CYP2C9 in the range of observed efavirenz plasma concentrations. Co-administration of efavirenz with drugs primarily metabolized by CYP2C9 may result in altered plasma concentrations of the co-administered drug. Therefore, appropriate dose adjustments may be necessary for these drugs). Products include:

Accolate Tablets 669

Zalcitabine (Renal impairment, including cases of acute renal failure and Fanconi syndrome (renal tubular injury with severe hypophosphatemia), has been reported in association with the use of tenofovir DF. The majority of these cases occurred in patients with underlying systemic or renal disease, or in patients taking nephrotoxic agents; however, some cases occured in patients without identified risk factors. Atripla should be avoided with concurrent or recent use of a nephrotoxic agent).

No products indexed under this heading.

Zidovudine (Renal impairment, including cases of acute renal failure and Fanconi syndrome (renal tubular injury with severe hypophosphatemia), has been reported in association with the use of tenofovir DF. The majority of these cases occurred in patients with underlying systemic or renal disease, or in patients taking nephrotoxic agents; however, some cases occured in patients without identified risk factors. Atripla should be avoided with concurrent or recent use of a nephrotoxic agent). Products include:

Combivir Tablets 1384
Retrovir 1574
Retrovir IV Infusion 1579
Trizivir Tablets 1622

Zileuton (In vitro studies have demonstrated that efavirenz inhibits CYP2C9 in the range of observed efavirenz plasma concentrations. Co-administration of efavirenz with drugs primarily metabolized by CYP2C9 may result in altered plasma concentrations of the co-administered drug. Therefore, appropriate dose adjustments may be necessary for these drugs).

No products indexed under this heading.

Zoledronic acid (Renal impairment, including cases of acute renal failure and Fanconi syndrome (renal tubular injury with severe hypophosphatemia), has been reported in association with the use of tenofovir DF. The majority of these cases occurred in patients with underlying systemic or renal disease, or in patients taking nephrotoxic agents; however, some cases occured in patients without identified risk factors. Atripla should be avoided with concurrent or recent use of a nephrotoxic agent). Products include:

Reclast Injection 2291
Zometa for Intravenous Infusion 2341

Zonisamide (In vitro studies have demonstrated that efavirenz inhibits CYP2C19 in the range of observed efavirenz plasma concentrations. Co-administration of efavirenz with drugs primarily metabolized by CYP2C19 may result in altered plasma concentrations of the co-administered drug. Therefore, appropriate dose adjustments may be necessary for these drugs). Products include:

Zonegran Capsules 1089

ATROVENT HFA INHALATION AEROSOL

(Ipratropium Bromide) 839

May interact with anticholinergics. Compounds in these categories include:

Atropine Sulfate (Although ipratropium bromide is minimally absorbed into the systemic circulation, there is some potential for an additive interaction with concomitantly used anticholinergic medications. Caution is therefore advised in the co-administration of ipratropium bromide HFA Inhalation Aerosol with other anticholinergic-containing drugs). Products include:

Donnatal Extentabs 2507

Belladonna Alkaloids (Although ipratropium bromide is minimally absorbed into the systemic circulation, there is some potential for an additive interaction with concomitantly used anticholinergic medications. Caution is therefore advised in the co-administration of ipratropium bromide HFA Inhalation Aerosol with other anticholinergic-containing drugs). Products include:

Hyland's Teething Tablets 621

Benztropine Mesylate (Although ipratropium bromide is minimally absorbed into the systemic circulation, there is some potential for an additive interaction with concomitantly used anticholinergic medications. Caution is therefore advised in the co-administration of ipratropium bromide HFA Inhalation Aerosol with other anticholinergic-containing drugs).

No products indexed under this heading.

Biperiden Hydrochloride (Although ipratropium bromide is minimally absorbed into the systemic circulation, there is some potential for an additive interaction with concomitantly used anticholinergic medications. Caution is therefore advised in the co-administration of ipratropium bromide HFA Inhalation Aerosol with other anticholinergic-containing drugs).

No products indexed under this heading.

Clidinium Bromide (Although ipratropium bromide is minimally absorbed into the systemic circulation, there is some potential for an additive interaction with concomitantly used anticholinergic medications. Caution is therefore advised in the co-administration of ipratropium bromide HFA Inhalation Aerosol with other anticholinergic-containing drugs).

No products indexed under this heading.

Dicyclomine Hydrochloride (Although ipratropium bromide is minimally absorbed into the systemic circulation, there is some potential for an additive interaction with concomitantly used anticholinergic medications. Caution is therefore advised in the co-administration of ipratropium bromide HFA Inhalation Aerosol with other anticholinergic-containing drugs). Products include:

Bentyl Capsules 703
Bentyl Injection 703
Bentyl Syrup 703
Bentyl Tablets 703

Glycopyrrolate (Although ipratropium bromide is minimally absorbed into the systemic circulation, there is some potential for an additive interaction with concomitantly used anticholinergic medications. Caution is therefore advised in the co-administration of ipratropium bromide HFA Inhalation Aerosol with other anticholinergic-containing drugs).

No products indexed under this heading.

Hyoscyamine (Although ipratropium bromide is minimally absorbed into the systemic circulation, there is some potential for an additive interaction with concomitantly used anticholinergic medications. Caution is therefore advised in the co-administration of ipratropium bromide HFA Inhalation Aerosol with other anticholinergic-containing drugs).

No products indexed under this heading.

Hyoscyamine Sulfate (Although ipratropium bromide is minimally absorbed into the systemic circulation, there is some potential for an additive interaction with concomitantly used anticholinergic medications. Caution is therefore advised in the co-administration of ipratropium bromide HFA Inhalation Aerosol with other anticholinergic-containing drugs). Products include:

Donnatal Extentabs 2507

Mepenzolate Bromide (Although ipratropium bromide is minimally absorbed into the systemic circulation, there is some potential for an additive interaction with concomitantly used anticholinergic medications. Caution is therefore advised in the co-administration of ipratropium bromide HFA Inhalation Aerosol with other anticholinergic-containing drugs).

No products indexed under this heading.

Oxybutynin Chloride (Although ipratropium bromide is minimally absorbed into the systemic circulation, there is some potential for an additive interaction with concomitantly used anticholinergic medications. Caution is therefore advised in the co-administration of ipratropium bromide HFA Inhalation Aerosol with other anticholinergic-containing drugs).

No products indexed under this heading.

Procyclidine Hydrochloride (Although ipratropium bromide is minimally absorbed into the systemic circulation, there is some potential for an additive interaction with concomitantly used anticholinergic medications. Caution is therefore advised in the co-administration of ipratropium bromide HFA Inhalation Aerosol with other anticholinergic-containing drugs).

No products indexed under this heading.

Propantheline Bromide (Although ipratropium bromide is minimally absorbed into the systemic circulation, there is some potential for an additive interaction with concomitantly used anticholinergic medications. Caution is therefore advised in the co-administration of ipratropium bromide HFA Inhalation Aerosol with other anticholinergic-containing drugs).

No products indexed under this heading.

Scopolamine (Although ipratropium bromide is minimally absorbed into the systemic circulation, there is some potential for an additive interaction with concomitantly used anticholinergic medications. Caution is therefore advised in the co-administration of ipratropium bromide HFA Inhalation Aerosol with other anticholinergic-containing drugs). Products include:

Transderm Scōp Transdermal Therapeutic System 2206

Scopolamine Hydrobromide (Although ipratropium bromide is minimally absorbed into the systemic circulation, there is some potential for an additive interaction with concomitantly used anticholinergic medications. Caution is therefore advised in the co-administration of ipratropium bromide HFA Inhalation Aerosol with other anticholinergic-containing drugs). Products include:

Donnatal Extentabs 2507

Tolterodine Tartrate (Although ipratropium bromide is minimally absorbed into the systemic circulation, there is some potential for an additive interaction with concomitantly used anticholinergic medications. Caution is therefore advised in the co-administration of ipratropium bromide HFA Inhalation Aerosol with other anticholinergic-containing drugs).

No products indexed under this heading.

Tridihexethyl Chloride (Although ipratropium bromide is minimally absorbed into the systemic circulation, there is some potential for an additive interaction with concomitantly used anticholinergic medications. Caution is therefore advised in the co-administration of ipratropium bromide HFA Inhalation Aerosol with other anticholinergic-containing drugs).

No products indexed under this heading.

Trihexyphenidyl Hydrochloride (Although ipratropium bromide is minimally absorbed into the systemic circulation, there is some potential for an additive interaction with concomitantly used anticholinergic medications. Caution is therefore advised in the co-administration of ipratropium bromide HFA Inhalation Aerosol with other anticholinergic-containing drugs).

No products indexed under this heading.

ATROVENT NASAL SPRAY 0.03%

(Ipratropium Bromide) 834

May interact with anticholinergics. Compounds in these categories include:

Atropine Sulfate (No controlled clinical trials were conducted to investigate potential drug-drug interactions. Ipratropium bromide 0.03% nasal spray is minimally absorbed into the systemic circulation. Nonetheless, there is some potential for an additive interaction with other concomitantly-administered medications with anticholinergic properties). Products include:

Donnatal Extentabs 2507

Belladonna Alkaloids (No controlled clinical trials were conducted to investigate potential drug-drug interactions. Ipratropium bromide 0.03% nasal spray is minimally absorbed into the systemic circulation. Nonetheless, there is some potential for an additive interaction with other concomitantly-administered medications with anticholinergic properties). Products include:

Hyland's Teething Tablets 621

Benztropine Mesylate (No controlled clinical trials were conducted to investigate potential drug-drug interactions. Ipratropium bromide 0.03% nasal spray is minimally absorbed into the systemic circulation. Nonetheless, there is some potential for an additive interaction with other concomitantly-administered medications with anticholinergic properties).
No products indexed under this heading.

Biperiden Hydrochloride (No controlled clinical trials were conducted to investigate potential drug-drug interactions. Ipratropium bromide 0.03% nasal spray is minimally absorbed into the systemic circulation. Nonetheless, there is some potential for an additive interaction with other concomitantly-administered medications with anticholinergic properties).
No products indexed under this heading.

Clidinium Bromide (No controlled clinical trials were conducted to investigate potential drug-drug interactions. Ipratropium bromide 0.03% nasal spray is minimally absorbed into the systemic circulation. Nonetheless, there is some potential for an additive interaction with other concomitantly-administered medications with anticholinergic properties).
No products indexed under this heading.

Dicyclomine Hydrochloride (No controlled clinical trials were conducted to investigate potential drug-drug interactions. Ipratropium bromide 0.03% nasal spray is minimally absorbed into the systemic circulation. Nonetheless, there is some potential for an additive interaction with other concomitantly-administered medications with anticholinergic properties). Products include:
Bentyl Capsules **703**
Bentyl Injection **703**
Bentyl Syrup **703**
Bentyl Tablets **703**

Glycopyrrolate (No controlled clinical trials were conducted to investigate potential drug-drug interactions. Ipratropium bromide 0.03% nasal spray is minimally absorbed into the systemic circulation. Nonetheless, there is some potential for an additive interaction with other concomitantly-administered medications with anticholinergic properties).
No products indexed under this heading.

Hyoscyamine (No controlled clinical trials were conducted to investigate potential drug-drug interactions. Ipratropium bromide 0.03% nasal spray is minimally absorbed into the systemic circulation. Nonetheless, there is some potential for an additive interaction with other concomitantly-administered medications with anticholinergic properties).
No products indexed under this heading.

Hyoscyamine Sulfate (No controlled clinical trials were conducted to investigate potential drug-drug interactions. Ipratropium bromide 0.03% nasal spray is minimally absorbed into the systemic circulation. Nonetheless, there is some potential for an additive interaction with other concomitantly-administered medications with anticholinergic properties). Products include:
Donnatal Extentabs **2507**

Mepenzolate Bromide (No controlled clinical trials were conducted to investigate potential drug-drug interactions. Ipratropium bromide 0.03% nasal spray is minimally absorbed into the systemic circulation. Nonetheless, there is some potential for an additive interaction with other concomitantly-administered medications with anticholinergic properties).
No products indexed under this heading.

Oxybutynin Chloride (No controlled clinical trials were conducted to investigate potential drug-drug interactions. Ipratropium bromide 0.03% nasal spray is minimally absorbed into the systemic circulation. Nonetheless, there is some potential for an additive interaction with other concomitantly-administered medications with anticholinergic properties).
No products indexed under this heading.

Procyclidine Hydrochloride (No controlled clinical trials were conducted to investigate potential drug-drug interactions. Ipratropium bromide 0.03% nasal spray is minimally absorbed into the systemic circulation. Nonetheless, there is some potential for an additive interaction with other concomitantly-administered medications with anticholinergic properties).
No products indexed under this heading.

Propantheline Bromide (No controlled clinical trials were conducted to investigate potential drug-drug interactions. Ipratropium bromide 0.03% nasal spray is minimally absorbed into the systemic circulation. Nonetheless, there is some potential for an additive interaction with other concomitantly-administered medications with anticholinergic properties).
No products indexed under this heading.

Scopolamine (No controlled clinical trials were conducted to investigate potential drug-drug interactions. Ipratropium bromide 0.03% nasal spray is minimally absorbed into the systemic circulation. Nonetheless, there is some potential for an additive interaction with other concomitantly-administered medications with anticholinergic properties). Products include:
Transderm Scōp Transdermal Therapeutic System **2206**

Scopolamine Hydrobromide (No controlled clinical trials were conducted to investigate potential drug-drug interactions. Ipratropium bromide 0.03% nasal spray is minimally absorbed into the systemic circulation. Nonetheless, there is some potential for an additive interaction with other concomitantly-administered medications with anticholinergic properties). Products include:
Donnatal Extentabs **2507**

Tolterodine Tartrate (No controlled clinical trials were conducted to investigate potential drug-drug interactions. Ipratropium bromide 0.03% nasal spray is minimally absorbed into the systemic circulation. Nonetheless, there is some potential for an additive interaction with other concomitantly-administered medications with anticholinergic properties).
No products indexed under this heading.

Tridihexethyl Chloride (No controlled clinical trials were conducted to investigate potential drug-drug interactions. Ipratropium bromide 0.03% nasal spray is minimally absorbed into the systemic circulation. Nonetheless, there is some potential for an additive interaction with other concomitantly-administered medications with anticholinergic properties).
No products indexed under this heading.

Trihexyphenidyl Hydrochloride (No controlled clinical trials were conducted to investigate potential drug-drug interactions. Ipratropium bromide 0.03% nasal spray is minimally absorbed into the systemic circulation. Nonetheless, there is some potential for an additive interaction with other concomitantly-administered medications with anticholinergic properties).
No products indexed under this heading.

ATROVENT NASAL SPRAY 0.06%

(Ipratropium Bromide) **836**
May interact with anticholinergics. Compounds in these categories include:

Atropine Sulfate (Some potential for an additive interaction with other concomitantly administered anticholinergic drugs). Products include:
Donnatal Extentabs **2507**

Belladonna Alkaloids (Some potential for an additive interaction with other concomitantly administered anticholinergic drugs). Products include:
Hyland's Teething Tablets .... ▣**621**

Benztropine Mesylate (Some potential for an additive interaction with other concomitantly administered anticholinergic drugs).
No products indexed under this heading.

Biperiden Hydrochloride (Some potential for an additive interaction with other concomitantly administered anticholinergic drugs).
No products indexed under this heading.

Clidinium Bromide (Some potential for an additive interaction with other concomitantly administered anticholinergic drugs).
No products indexed under this heading.

Dicyclomine Hydrochloride (Some potential for an additive interaction with other concomitantly administered anticholinergic drugs). Products include:
Bentyl Capsules **703**
Bentyl Injection **703**
Bentyl Syrup **703**
Bentyl Tablets **703**

Glycopyrrolate (Some potential for an additive interaction with other concomitantly administered anticholinergic drugs).
No products indexed under this heading.

Hyoscyamine (Some potential for an additive interaction with other concomitantly administered anticholinergic drugs).
No products indexed under this heading.

Hyoscyamine Sulfate (Some potential for an additive interaction with other concomitantly administered anticholinergic drugs). Products include:
Donnatal Extentabs **2507**

Mepenzolate Bromide (Some potential for an additive interaction with other concomitantly administered anticholinergic drugs).
No products indexed under this heading.

Oxybutynin Chloride (Some potential for an additive interaction with other concomitantly administered anticholinergic drugs).
No products indexed under this heading.

Procyclidine Hydrochloride (Some potential for an additive interaction with other concomitantly administered anticholinergic drugs).
No products indexed under this heading.

Propantheline Bromide (Some potential for an additive interaction with other concomitantly administered anticholinergic drugs).
No products indexed under this heading.

Scopolamine (Some potential for an additive interaction with other concomitantly administered anticholinergic drugs). Products include:
Transderm Scōp Transdermal Therapeutic System **2206**

Scopolamine Hydrobromide (Some potential for an additive interaction with other concomitantly administered anticholinergic drugs). Products include:
Donnatal Extentabs **2507**

Tolterodine Tartrate (Some potential for an additive interaction with other concomitantly administered anticholinergic drugs).
No products indexed under this heading.

Tridihexethyl Chloride (Some potential for an additive interaction with other concomitantly administered anticholinergic drugs).
No products indexed under this heading.

Trihexyphenidyl Hydrochloride (Some potential for an additive interaction with other concomitantly administered anticholinergic drugs).
No products indexed under this heading.

ATTENUVAX

(Measles Virus Vaccine Live) **1951**
May interact with immunosuppressive agents. Compounds in these categories include:

Azathioprine (Concurrent use in individuals on immunosuppressive therapy is contraindicated).
No products indexed under this heading.

Basiliximab (Concurrent use in individuals on immunosuppressive therapy is contraindicated). Products include:

Simulect for Injection 2306

Cyclosporine (Concurrent use in individuals on immunosuppressive therapy is contraindicated). Products include:

Gengraf Capsules 435
Neoral Oral Solution 2280
Neoral Soft Gelatin Capsules 2280
Restasis Ophthalmic Emulsion 557
Sandimmune 2296

Muromonab-CD3 (Concurrent use in individuals on immunosuppressive therapy is contraindicated). Products include:

Orthoclone OKT3 Sterile Solution 2387

Mycophenolate Mofetil (Concurrent use in individuals on immunosuppressive therapy is contraindicated). Products include:

CellCept Capsules 2622
CellCept Oral Suspension 2622
CellCept Tablets 2622

Sirolimus (Concurrent use in individuals on immunosuppressive therapy is contraindicated). Products include:

Rapamune 3260

Tacrolimus (Concurrent use in individuals on immunosuppressive therapy is contraindicated). Products include:

Prograf Capsules and Injection 622
Protopic Ointment 628

AUGMENTIN CHEWABLE TABLETS

(Amoxicillin, Clavulanate Potassium) 1323

See Augmentin ES-600 Powder for Oral Suspension

AUGMENTIN POWDER FOR ORAL SUSPENSION

(Amoxicillin, Clavulanate Potassium) 1323

See Augmentin ES-600 Powder for Oral Suspension

AUGMENTIN TABLETS

(Amoxicillin, Clavulanate Potassium) 1327

See Augmentin ES-600 Powder for Oral Suspension

AUGMENTIN XR EXTENDED RELEASE TABLETS

(Amoxicillin, Clavulanate Potassium) 1333

See Augmentin ES-600 Powder for Oral Suspension

AUGMENTIN ES-600 POWDER FOR ORAL SUSPENSION

(Amoxicillin, Clavulanate Potassium) 1329

May interact with anticoagulants, oral contraceptives, and certain other agents. Compounds in these categories include:

Allopurinol (Co-administration of ampicillin with allopurinol substantially increases the incidence of rashes; there are no data with Augmentin and allopurinol administered concurrently).

No products indexed under this heading.

Anisindione (There have been reports of increased prothrombin time in patients receiving Augmentin and anticoagulant therapy concomitantly).

No products indexed under this heading.

Ardeparin Sodium (There have been reports of increased prothrombin time in patients receiving Augmentin and anticoagulant therapy concomitantly).

No products indexed under this heading.

Dalteparin Sodium (There have been reports of increased prothrombin time in patients receiving Augmentin and anticoagulant therapy concomitantly). Products include:

Fragmin Injection 1070

Danaparoid Sodium (There have been reports of increased prothrombin time in patients receiving Augmentin and anticoagulant therapy concomitantly).

No products indexed under this heading.

Desogestrel (Potential for reduced efficacy of oral contraceptives). Products include:

Mircette Tablets 1034

Dicumarol (There have been reports of increased prothrombin time in patients receiving Augmentin and anticoagulant therapy concomitantly).

No products indexed under this heading.

Enoxaparin Sodium (There have been reports of increased prothrombin time in patients receiving Augmentin and anticoagulant therapy concomitantly). Products include:

Lovenox Injection 2756

Ethinyl Estradiol (Potential for reduced efficacy of oral contraceptives). Products include:

Lybrel Tablets 3204
Mircette Tablets 1034
NuvaRing 2897
Ortho-Cyclen/Ortho Tri-Cyclen 2449
Ortho Evra Transdermal System 2437
Ortho Tri-Cyclen Lo Tablets 2458
Seasonique Tablets 1046
Yaz Tablets 805

Ethynodiol Diacetate (Potential for reduced efficacy of oral contraceptives).

No products indexed under this heading.

Fondaparinux Sodium (There have been reports of increased prothrombin time in patients receiving Augmentin and anticoagulant therapy concomitantly). Products include:

Arixtra Injection 1313

Heparin Calcium (There have been reports of increased prothrombin time in patients receiving Augmentin and anticoagulant therapy concomitantly).

No products indexed under this heading.

Heparin Sodium (There have been reports of increased prothrombin time in patients receiving Augmentin and anticoagulant therapy concomitantly).

No products indexed under this heading.

Levonorgestrel (Potential for reduced efficacy of oral contraceptives). Products include:

Climara Pro Transdermal System 768
Lybrel Tablets 3204
Mirena Intrauterine System 779
Plan B Tablets 1044
Seasonique Tablets 1046

Low Molecular Weight Heparins (There have been reports of increased prothrombin time in patients receiving Augmentin and anticoagulant therapy concomitantly).

No products indexed under this heading.

Mestranol (Potential for reduced efficacy of oral contraceptives).

No products indexed under this heading.

Norethindrone (Potential for reduced efficacy of oral contraceptives). Products include:

Ortho Micronor Tablets 2446

Norethynodrel (Potential for reduced efficacy of oral contraceptives).

No products indexed under this heading.

Norgestimate (Potential for reduced efficacy of oral contraceptives). Products include:

Ortho-Cyclen/Ortho Tri-Cyclen 2449
Ortho Tri-Cyclen Lo Tablets 2458

Norgestrel (Potential for reduced efficacy of oral contraceptives).

No products indexed under this heading.

Probenecid (Decreases the renal tubular secretion of amoxicillin; concurrent use may result in increased and prolonged blood levels of amoxicillin; therefore, concomitant use is not recommended).

No products indexed under this heading.

Tinzaparin Sodium (There have been reports of increased prothrombin time in patients receiving Augmentin and anticoagulant therapy concomitantly).

No products indexed under this heading.

Warfarin Sodium (There have been reports of increased prothrombin time in patients receiving Augmentin and anticoagulant therapy concomitantly).

No products indexed under this heading.

AUTHIA CREAM

(Thiamine Disulfide, Vitamin B_{12}) 3190

None cited in PDR database.

AVALIDE TABLETS

(Hydrochlorothiazide, Irbesartan) 892

May interact with antihypertensives, barbiturates, corticosteroids, cardiac glycosides, oral hypoglycemic agents, insulin, lithium preparations, narcotic analgesics, nondepolarizing neuromuscular blocking agents, nonsteroidal anti-inflammatory agents, and certain other agents. Compounds in these categories include:

Acarbose (Hydrochlorothiazide may cause hyperglycemia, therefore, dosage adjustment of oral hypoglycemic agent may be required). Products include:

Precose Tablets 792

Acebutolol Hydrochloride (Hydrochlorothiazide may add to or potentiate the therapeutic effect of other antihypertensive drugs).

No products indexed under this heading.

ACTH (Co-administration with ACTH intensifies electrolyte depletion particularly hypokalemia).

No products indexed under this heading.

Alfentanil Hydrochloride (Potentiation of orthostatic hypotension may occur).

No products indexed under this heading.

Aliskiren (Hydrochlorothiazide may add to or potentiate the therapeutic effect of other antihypertensive drugs). Products include:

Tekturna Tablets 2321
Tekturna HCT Tablets 2324

Amlodipine Besylate (Hydrochlorothiazide may add to or potentiate the therapeutic effect of other antihypertensive drugs). Products include:

Azor Tablets 1005
Exforge Tablets 2238

Aprobarbital (Potentiation of orthostatic hypotension may occur).

No products indexed under this heading.

Atenolol (Hydrochlorothiazide may add to or potentiate the therapeutic effect of other antihypertensive drugs).

No products indexed under this heading.

Atracurium Besylate (Possible increased responsiveness to the muscle relaxants).

No products indexed under this heading.

Benazepril Hydrochloride (Hydrochlorothiazide may add to or potentiate the therapeutic effect of other antihypertensive drugs).

No products indexed under this heading.

Bendroflumethiazide (Hydrochlorothiazide may add to or potentiate the therapeutic effect of other antihypertensive drugs).

No products indexed under this heading.

Betamethasone Acetate (Co-administration with corticosteroids intensifies electrolyte depletion particularly hypokalemia).

No products indexed under this heading.

Betamethasone Sodium Phosphate (Co-administration with corticosteroids intensifies electrolyte depletion particularly hypokalemia).

No products indexed under this heading.

Betaxolol Hydrochloride (Hydrochlorothiazide may add to or potentiate the therapeutic effect of other antihypertensive drugs).

No products indexed under this heading.

Bisoprolol Fumarate (Hydrochlorothiazide may add to or potentiate the therapeutic effect of other antihypertensive drugs).

No products indexed under this heading.

Budesonide (Co-administration with corticosteroids intensifies electrolyte depletion particularly hypokalemia). Products include:

Pulmicort Flexhaler 654
Symbicort 80/4.5 Inhalation Aerosol 659
Symbicort 160/4.5 Inhalation Aerosol 659

Buprenorphine Hydrochloride (Potentiation of orthostatic hypotension may occur). Products include:

Suboxone Tablets 2601
Subutex Tablets 2601

Butabarbital (Potentiation of orthostatic hypotension may occur).

No products indexed under this heading.

Butalbital (Potentiation of orthostatic hypotension may occur).
No products indexed under this heading.

Candesartan Cilexetil (Hydrochlorothiazide may add to or potentiate the therapeutic effect of other antihypertensive drugs). Products include:
Atacand Tablets ... 639
Atacand HCT ... 642

Captopril (Hydrochlorothiazide may add to or potentiate the therapeutic effect of other antihypertensive drugs). Products include:
Captopril Tablets ... 2182

Carteolol Hydrochloride (Hydrochlorothiazide may add to or potentiate the therapeutic effect of other antihypertensive drugs).
No products indexed under this heading.

Celecoxib (Co-administration with non-steroidal anti-inflammatory agents may reduce the natriuretic and antihypertensive effects of thiazides). Products include:
Celebrex Capsules ... 2979

Chlorothiazide (Hydrochlorothiazide may add to or potentiate the therapeutic effect of other antihypertensive drugs).
No products indexed under this heading.

Chlorothiazide Sodium (Hydrochlorothiazide may add to or potentiate the therapeutic effect of other antihypertensive drugs). Products include:
Intravenous Sodium Diuril ... 2490

Chlorpropamide (Hydrochlorothiazide may cause hyperglycemia, therefore, dosage adjustment of oral hypoglycemic agent may be required).
No products indexed under this heading.

Chlorthalidone (Hydrochlorothiazide may add to or potentiate the therapeutic effect of other antihypertensive drugs). Products include:
Clorpres Tablets ... 2185

Cholestyramine (Absorption of hydrochlorothiazide is impaired in the presence of anionic exchange resins; single dose of cholestyramine binds the hydrochlorothiazide and reduces its absorption from GI tract by 85%).
No products indexed under this heading.

Ciclesonide (Co-administration with corticosteroids intensifies electrolyte depletion particularly hypokalemia). Products include:
Alvesco Inhalation Aerosol ... 2985
Omnaris Nasal Spray ... 2998

Cisatracurium Besylate (Possible increased responsiveness to the muscle relaxants). Products include:
Nimbex Injection ... 484

Clonidine (Hydrochlorothiazide may add to or potentiate the therapeutic effect of other antihypertensive drugs). Products include:
Catapres-TTS ... 842

Clonidine Hydrochloride (Hydrochlorothiazide may add to or potentiate the therapeutic effect of other antihypertensive drugs). Products include:
Catapres Tablets ... 841
Clorpres Tablets ... 2185

Codeine Phosphate (Potentiation of orthostatic hypotension may occur). Products include:
Tylenol with Codeine Tablets ... 2427

Colestipol Hydrochloride (Absorption of hydrochlorothiazide is impaired in the presence of anionic exchange resins; single dose of colestipol binds the hydrochlorothiazide and reduces its absorption from GI tract by 43%).
No products indexed under this heading.

Cortisone Acetate (Co-administration with corticosteroids intensifies electrolyte depletion particularly hypokalemia).
No products indexed under this heading.

Deserpidine (Hydrochlorothiazide may add to or potentiate the therapeutic effect of other antihypertensive drugs).
No products indexed under this heading.

Deslanoside (Concurrent digitalis therapy may exaggerate metabolic effects of hypokalemia, especially myocardial effects, e.g., increased ventricular irritability).
No products indexed under this heading.

Dexamethasone (Co-administration with corticosteroids intensifies electrolyte depletion particularly hypokalemia). Products include:
Ciprodex Otic Suspension ... 541

Dexamethasone Acetate (Co-administration with corticosteroids intensifies electrolyte depletion particularly hypokalemia).
No products indexed under this heading.

Dexamethasone Sodium Phosphate (Co-administration with corticosteroids intensifies electrolyte depletion particularly hypokalemia).
No products indexed under this heading.

Dezocine (Potentiation of orthostatic hypotension may occur).
No products indexed under this heading.

Diazoxide (Hydrochlorothiazide may add to or potentiate the therapeutic effect of other antihypertensive drugs). Products include:
Proglycem Capsules ... 1185
Proglycem Suspension ... 1185

Diclofenac Epolamine (Co-administration with non-steroidal anti-inflammatory agents may reduce the natriuretic and antihypertensive effects of thiazides). Products include:
Flector Patch ... 561

Diclofenac Potassium (Co-administration with non-steroidal anti-inflammatory agents may reduce the natriuretic and antihypertensive effects of thiazides).
No products indexed under this heading.

Diclofenac Sodium (Co-administration with non-steroidal anti-inflammatory agents may reduce the natriuretic and antihypertensive effects of thiazides). Products include:
Diclofenac Sodium Ophthalmic Solution ... ⊙ 240
Voltaren Ophthalmic Solution ... 2336
Voltaren Tablets ... 2334
Voltaren-XR Tablets ... 2337

Digitalis Glycoside Preparations (Concurrent digitalis therapy may exaggerate metabolic effects of hypokalemia, especially myocardial effects, e.g., increased ventricular irritability).
No products indexed under this heading.

Digitoxin (Concurrent digitalis therapy may exaggerate metabolic effects of hypokalemia, especially myocardial effects, e.g., increased ventricular irritability).
No products indexed under this heading.

Digoxin (Concurrent digitalis therapy may exaggerate metabolic effects of hypokalemia, especially myocardial effects, e.g., increased ventricular irritability). Products include:
Lanoxin Injection ... 1498
Lanoxin Injection Pediatric ... 1502
Lanoxin Tablets ... 1505

Diltiazem Hydrochloride (Hydrochlorothiazide may add to or potentiate the therapeutic effect of other antihypertensive drugs). Products include:
Cardizem LA Extended Release Tablets ... 421

Doxazosin Mesylate (Hydrochlorothiazide may add to or potentiate the therapeutic effect of other antihypertensive drugs).
No products indexed under this heading.

Enalapril Maleate (Hydrochlorothiazide may add to or potentiate the therapeutic effect of other antihypertensive drugs).
No products indexed under this heading.

Enalaprilat (Hydrochlorothiazide may add to or potentiate the therapeutic effect of other antihypertensive drugs).
No products indexed under this heading.

Eprosartan Mesylate (Hydrochlorothiazide may add to or potentiate the therapeutic effect of other antihypertensive drugs). Products include:
Teveten Tablets ... 515
Teveten HCT Tablets ... 517

Esmolol Hydrochloride (Hydrochlorothiazide may add to or potentiate the therapeutic effect of other antihypertensive drugs).
No products indexed under this heading.

Etodolac (Co-administration with non-steroidal anti-inflammatory agents may reduce the natriuretic and antihypertensive effects of thiazides).
No products indexed under this heading.

Felodipine (Hydrochlorothiazide may add to or potentiate the therapeutic effect of other antihypertensive drugs).
No products indexed under this heading.

Fenoprofen Calcium (Co-administration with non-steroidal anti-inflammatory agents may reduce the natriuretic and antihypertensive effects of thiazides). Products include:
Nalfon Capsules ... 2508

Fentanyl (Potentiation of orthostatic hypotension may occur). Products include:
Duragesic Transdermal System ... 2405
Ionsys Transdermal System ... 2410

Fentanyl Citrate (Potentiation of orthostatic hypotension may occur). Products include:
Actiq ... 959
Fentora Tablets ... 968

Fludrocortisone Acetate (Co-administration with corticosteroids intensifies electrolyte depletion particularly hypokalemia).
No products indexed under this heading.

Flunisolide (Co-administration with corticosteroids intensifies electrolyte depletion particularly hypokalemia). Products include:
Aerobid/Aerobid-M ... 1153

Flurbiprofen (Co-administration with non-steroidal anti-inflammatory agents may reduce the natriuretic and antihypertensive effects of thiazides).
No products indexed under this heading.

Fluticasone Propionate (Co-administration with corticosteroids intensifies electrolyte depletion particularly hypokalemia). Products include:
Advair Diskus 100/50 ... 1276
Advair Diskus 250/50 ... 1276
Advair Diskus 500/50 ... 1276
Advair HFA 45/21 Inhalation Aerosol ... 1288
Advair HFA 115/21 Inhalation Aerosol ... 1288
Advair HFA 230/21 Inhalation Aerosol ... 1288
Flonase Nasal Spray ... 1431
Flovent Diskus 50 mcg ... 1435

Fluticasone Propionate HFA (Co-administration with corticosteroids intensifies electrolyte depletion particularly hypokalemia). Products include:
Flovent HFA ... 1440

Fosinopril Sodium (Hydrochlorothiazide may add to or potentiate the therapeutic effect of other antihypertensive drugs).
No products indexed under this heading.

Furosemide (Hydrochlorothiazide may add to or potentiate the therapeutic effect of other antihypertensive drugs). Products include:
Furosemide Tablets ... 2186

Glimepiride (Hydrochlorothiazide may cause hyperglycemia, therefore, dosage adjustment of oral hypoglycemic agent may be required). Products include:
Avandaryl Tablets ... 1344
Duetact Tablets ... 3085

Glipizide (Hydrochlorothiazide may cause hyperglycemia, therefore, dosage adjustment of oral hypoglycemic agent may be required).
No products indexed under this heading.

Glyburide (Hydrochlorothiazide may cause hyperglycemia, therefore, dosage adjustment of oral hypoglycemic agent may be required).
No products indexed under this heading.

Guanabenz Acetate (Hydrochlorothiazide may add to or potentiate the therapeutic effect of other antihypertensive drugs).
No products indexed under this heading.

Guanethidine Monosulfate (Hydrochlorothiazide may add to or potentiate the therapeutic effect of other antihypertensive drugs).
No products indexed under this heading.

Hydralazine Hydrochloride (Hydrochlorothiazide may add to or potentiate the therapeutic effect of other antihypertensive drugs).
No products indexed under this heading.

Hydrocodone Bitartrate (Potentiation of orthostatic hypotension may occur). Products include:
Lortab 5/500 Tablets 3143
Lortab 7.5/500 Tablets 3144
Lortab 10/500 Tablets 3144
Vicodin Tablets 529
Vicodin ES Tablets 530
Vicodin HP Tablets 531
Vicoprofen Tablets 533
Zydone Tablets 1132

Hydrocodone Polistirex (Potentiation of orthostatic hypotension may occur). Products include:
Tussionex Pennkinetic Extended-Release Suspension 3154

Hydrocortisone (Co-administration with corticosteroids intensifies electrolyte depletion particularly hypokalemia).
No products indexed under this heading.

Hydrocortisone Acetate (Co-administration with corticosteroids intensifies electrolyte depletion particularly hypokalemia). Products include:
Analpram-HC 1140
Pramosone 1141

Hydrocortisone Sodium Phosphate (Co-administration with corticosteroids intensifies electrolyte depletion particularly hypokalemia).
No products indexed under this heading.

Hydrocortisone Sodium Succinate (Co-administration with corticosteroids intensifies electrolyte depletion particularly hypokalemia).
No products indexed under this heading.

Hydroflumethiazide (Hydrochlorothiazide may add to or potentiate the therapeutic effect of other antihypertensive drugs).
No products indexed under this heading.

Hydromorphone Hydrochloride (Potentiation of orthostatic hypotension may occur).
No products indexed under this heading.

Ibuprofen (Co-administration with non-steroidal anti-inflammatory agents may reduce the natriuretic and antihypertensive effects of thiazides). Products include:
Motrin IB Tablets and Caplets 1900
Children's Motrin Oral Suspension ... 1901
Children's Motrin Non-Staining Dye-Free Oral Suspension 1901
Children's Motrin Cold Oral Suspension 1899
Infants' Motrin Concentrated Drops 1901
Infants' Motrin Non-Staining Dye-Free Concentrated Drops 1901
Junior Strength Motrin Caplets and Chewable Tablets 1901
Vicoprofen Tablets 533

Indapamide (Hydrochlorothiazide may add to or potentiate the therapeutic effect of other antihypertensive drugs). Products include:
Indapamide Tablets 2188

Indomethacin (Co-administration with non-steroidal anti-inflammatory agents may reduce the natriuretic and antihypertensive effects of thiazides). Products include:
Indocin 2024

Indomethacin Sodium Trihydrate (Co-administration with non-steroidal anti-inflammatory agents may reduce the natriuretic and antihypertensive effects of thiazides). Products include:
Indocin I.V. 2489

Insulin (Hydrochlorothiazide may cause hyperglycemia, therefore, dosage adjustment of insulin may be required).
No products indexed under this heading.

Insulin, Human, Zinc Suspension (Hydrochlorothiazide may cause hyperglycemia, therefore, dosage adjustment of insulin may be required).
No products indexed under this heading.

Insulin, Human (rDNA origin) (Hydrochlorothiazide may cause hyperglycemia, therefore, dosage adjustment of insulin may be required). Products include:
Exubera Inhalation Powder 2515

Insulin, Human NPH (Hydrochlorothiazide may cause hyperglycemia, therefore, dosage adjustment of insulin may be required). Products include:
Humulin N Vial 1846

Insulin, Human Regular (Hydrochlorothiazide may cause hyperglycemia, therefore, dosage adjustment of insulin may be required). Products include:
Humulin R 1849
Humulin R (U-500) 1850

Insulin, Human Regular and Human NPH Mixture (Hydrochlorothiazide may cause hyperglycemia, therefore, dosage adjustment of insulin may be required). Products include:
Humulin 50/50, 100 Units 1843
Humulin 70/30 Vial 1844

Insulin, NPH (Hydrochlorothiazide may cause hyperglycemia, therefore, dosage adjustment of insulin may be required).
No products indexed under this heading.

Insulin, Regular (Hydrochlorothiazide may cause hyperglycemia, therefore, dosage adjustment of insulin may be required).
No products indexed under this heading.

Insulin, Regular and NPH mixture (Hydrochlorothiazide may cause hyperglycemia, therefore, dosage adjustment of insulin may be required).
No products indexed under this heading.

Insulin, Zinc Crystals (Hydrochlorothiazide may cause hyperglycemia, therefore, dosage adjustment of insulin may be required).
No products indexed under this heading.

Insulin, Zinc Suspension (Hydrochlorothiazide may cause hyperglycemia, therefore, dosage adjustment of insulin may be required).
No products indexed under this heading.

Insulin Aspart (Hydrochlorothiazide may cause hyperglycemia, therefore, dosage adjustment of insulin may be required).
No products indexed under this heading.

Insulin Aspart, Human (Hydrochlorothiazide may cause hyperglycemia, therefore, dosage adjustment of insulin may be required). Products include:
NovoLog Mix 70/30 2364

Insulin Aspart, Human Regular (Hydrochlorothiazide may cause hyperglycemia, therefore, dosage adjustment of insulin may be required). Products include:
NovoLog Injection 2359

Insulin Aspart Protamine, Human (Hydrochlorothiazide may cause hyperglycemia, therefore, dosage adjustment of insulin may be required). Products include:
NovoLog Mix 70/30 2364

Insulin Detemir (rDNA Origin) (Hydrochlorothiazide may cause hyperglycemia, therefore, dosage adjustment of insulin may be required). Products include:
Levemir Injection 2352

Insulin glargine (Hydrochlorothiazide may cause hyperglycemia, therefore, dosage adjustment of insulin may be required). Products include:
Lantus Injection 2749

Insulin Glulisine (Hydrochlorothiazide may cause hyperglycemia, therefore, dosage adjustment of insulin may be required). Products include:
Apidra Injection 2706

Insulin Lispro, Human (Hydrochlorothiazide may cause hyperglycemia, therefore, dosage adjustment of insulin may be required). Products include:
Humalog-Pen and KwikPen 1829
Humalog Mix 50/50-Pen and KwikPen 1833
Humalog Mix 75/25-Pen and KwikPen 1835

Insulin Lispro Protamine, Human (Hydrochlorothiazide may cause hyperglycemia, therefore, dosage adjustment of insulin may be required). Products include:
Humalog Mix 50/50-Pen and KwikPen 1833
Humalog Mix 75/25-Pen and KwikPen 1835

Isradipine (Hydrochlorothiazide may add to or potentiate the therapeutic effect of other antihypertensive drugs). Products include:
DynaCirc CR Controlled Release Tablets 1407

Ketoprofen (Co-administration with non-steroidal anti-inflammatory agents may reduce the natriuretic and antihypertensive effects of thiazides).
No products indexed under this heading.

Ketorolac Tromethamine (Co-administration with non-steroidal anti-inflammatory agents may reduce the natriuretic and antihypertensive effects of thiazides).
No products indexed under this heading.

Labetalol Hydrochloride (Hydrochlorothiazide may add to or potentiate the therapeutic effect of other antihypertensive drugs).
No products indexed under this heading.

Levorphanol Tartrate (Potentiation of orthostatic hypotension may occur).
No products indexed under this heading.

Lisinopril (Hydrochlorothiazide may add to or potentiate the therapeutic effect of other antihypertensive drugs). Products include:
Prinivil Tablets 2087
Prinzide Tablets 2092

Lithium (Diuretics reduce lithium's renal clearance and add a high risk of lithium toxicity).
No products indexed under this heading.

Lithium Carbonate (Diuretics reduce lithium's renal clearance and add a high risk of lithium toxicity).
No products indexed under this heading.

Lithium Citrate (Diuretics reduce lithium's renal clearance and add a high risk of lithium toxicity).
No products indexed under this heading.

Losartan Potassium (Hydrochlorothiazide may add to or potentiate the therapeutic effect of other antihypertensive drugs). Products include:
Cozaar Tablets 1973

Mecamylamine Hydrochloride (Hydrochlorothiazide may add to or potentiate the therapeutic effect of other antihypertensive drugs).
No products indexed under this heading.

Meclofenamate Sodium (Co-administration with non-steroidal anti-inflammatory agents may reduce the natriuretic and antihypertensive effects of thiazides).
No products indexed under this heading.

Mefenamic Acid (Co-administration with non-steroidal anti-inflammatory agents may reduce the natriuretic and antihypertensive effects of thiazides).
No products indexed under this heading.

Meloxicam (Co-administration with non-steroidal anti-inflammatory agents may reduce the natriuretic and antihypertensive effects of thiazides). Products include:
Mobic Oral Suspension 863
Mobic Tablets 863

Meperidine Hydrochloride (Potentiation of orthostatic hypotension may occur).
No products indexed under this heading.

Mephobarbital (Potentiation of orthostatic hypotension may occur).
No products indexed under this heading.

Metformin Hydrochloride (Hydrochlorothiazide may cause hyperglycemia, therefore, dosage adjustment of oral hypoglycemic agent may be required). Products include:
ActoPlus Met Tablets 3071
Avandamet Tablets 1336
Janumet Tablets 2041
PrandiMet Tablets 2967

Methadone Hydrochloride (Potentiation of orthostatic hypotension may occur).
No products indexed under this heading.

Methyclothiazide (Hydrochlorothiazide may add to or potentiate the therapeutic effect of other antihypertensive drugs).
No products indexed under this heading.

Methyldopa (Hydrochlorothiazide may add to or potentiate the therapeutic effect of other antihypertensive drugs).
No products indexed under this heading.

Methyldopate Hydrochloride (Hydrochlorothiazide may add to or potentiate the therapeutic effect of other antihypertensive drugs).
No products indexed under this heading.

Methylprednisolone Acetate (Co-administration with corticosteroids intensifies electrolyte depletion particularly hypokalemia).
No products indexed under this heading.

Methylprednisolone Sodium Succinate (Co-administration with corticosteroids intensifies electrolyte depletion particularly hypokalemia).
No products indexed under this heading.

Metocurine Iodide (Possible increased responsiveness to the muscle relaxants).
No products indexed under this heading.

Metolazone (Hydrochlorothiazide may add to or potentiate the therapeutic effect of other antihypertensive drugs).
No products indexed under this heading.

Metoprolol Succinate (Hydrochlorothiazide may add to or potentiate the therapeutic effect of other antihypertensive drugs). Products include:
Toprol-XL Tablets ... 666

Metoprolol Tartrate (Hydrochlorothiazide may add to or potentiate the therapeutic effect of other antihypertensive drugs).
No products indexed under this heading.

Metyrosine (Hydrochlorothiazide may add to or potentiate the therapeutic effect of other antihypertensive drugs). Products include:
Demser Capsules ... 1989

Mibefradil Dihydrochloride (Hydrochlorothiazide may add to or potentiate the therapeutic effect of other antihypertensive drugs).
No products indexed under this heading.

Miglitol (Hydrochlorothiazide may cause hyperglycemia, therefore, dosage adjustment of oral hypoglycemic agent may be required).
No products indexed under this heading.

Minoxidil (Hydrochlorothiazide may add to or potentiate the therapeutic effect of other antihypertensive drugs).
No products indexed under this heading.

Mivacurium Chloride (Possible increased responsiveness to the muscle relaxants).
No products indexed under this heading.

Moexipril Hydrochloride (Hydrochlorothiazide may add to or potentiate the therapeutic effect of other antihypertensive drugs).
No products indexed under this heading.

Mometasone Furoate (Co-administration with corticosteroids intensifies electrolyte depletion particularly hypokalemia). Products include:
Asmanex Twisthaler ... 2797
Elocon Cream 0.1% ... 2840
Elocon Lotion 0.1% ... 2841
Elocon Ointment 0.1% ... 2842

Mometasone Furoate Monohydrate (Co-administration with corticosteroids intensifies electrolyte depletion particularly hypokalemia). Products include:
Nasonex Nasal Spray ... 2883

Morphine Sulfate (Potentiation of orthostatic hypotension may occur). Products include:
Avinza Capsules ... 1772
DepoDur Injection ... 1095
MS Contin Tablets ... 2585

Nabumetone (Co-administration with non-steroidal anti-inflammatory agents may reduce the natriuretic and antihypertensive effects of thiazides).
No products indexed under this heading.

Nadolol (Hydrochlorothiazide may add to or potentiate the therapeutic effect of other antihypertensive drugs). Products include:
Nadolol Tablets ... 2191

Naproxen (Co-administration with non-steroidal anti-inflammatory agents may reduce the natriuretic and antihypertensive effects of thiazides). Products include:
EC-Naprosyn Delayed-Release Tablets ... 2632
Naprosyn Suspension ... 2632
Naprosyn Tablets ... 2632

Naproxen Sodium (Co-administration with non-steroidal anti-inflammatory agents may reduce the natriuretic and antihypertensive effects of thiazides). Products include:
Anaprox Tablets ... 2632
Anaprox DS Tablets ... 2632
Treximet Tablets ... 1616

Nateglinide (Hydrochlorothiazide may cause hyperglycemia, therefore, dosage adjustment of oral hypoglycemic agent may be required). Products include:
Starlix Tablets ... 2314

Nebivolol (Hydrochlorothiazide may add to or potentiate the therapeutic effect of other antihypertensive drugs). Products include:
Bystolic Tablets ... 1155

Nicardipine Hydrochloride (Hydrochlorothiazide may add to or potentiate the therapeutic effect of other antihypertensive drugs). Products include:
Cardene I.V. ... 1093

Nifedipine (In vitro studies show significant inhibition of the formation of oxidized irbesartan metabolites with the known cytochrome CYP 2C9 substrate/inhibitor, nifedipine; the pharmacokinetics of irbesartan were not affected by co-administration of nifedipine; hydrochlorothiazide may add to or potentiate the therapeutic effect of other antihypertensive drugs).
No products indexed under this heading.

Nisoldipine (Hydrochlorothiazide may add to or potentiate the therapeutic effect of other antihypertensive drugs). Products include:
Sular Extended Release Tablets ... 2975

Nitroglycerin (Hydrochlorothiazide may add to or potentiate the therapeutic effect of other antihypertensive drugs). Products include:
Nitro-Dur Transdermal Infusion System ... 2887
Nitrolingual Pumpspray ... 2965

Norepinephrine Bitartrate (Thiazides may decrease arterial responsiveness to norepinephrine).
No products indexed under this heading.

Oxaprozin (Co-administration with non-steroidal anti-inflammatory agents may reduce the natriuretic and antihypertensive effects of thiazides).
No products indexed under this heading.

Oxycodone Hydrochloride (Potentiation of orthostatic hypotension may occur). Products include:
OxyContin Tablets ... 2589
OxyIR Capsules ... 2593
Percocet Tablets ... 1127
Percodan Tablets ... 1130

Pancuronium Bromide (Possible increased responsiveness to the muscle relaxants).
No products indexed under this heading.

Penbutolol Sulfate (Hydrochlorothiazide may add to or potentiate the therapeutic effect of other antihypertensive drugs).
No products indexed under this heading.

Pentobarbital Sodium (Potentiation of orthostatic hypotension may occur). Products include:
Nembutal Sodium Solution, USP ... 2494

Perindopril Erbumine (Hydrochlorothiazide may add to or potentiate the therapeutic effect of other antihypertensive drugs). Products include:
Aceon Tablets (2 mg, 4 mg, 8 mg) ... 3038

Phenobarbital (Potentiation of orthostatic hypotension may occur). Products include:
Donnatal Extentabs ... 2507

Phenoxybenzamine Hydrochloride (Hydrochlorothiazide may add to or potentiate the therapeutic effect of other antihypertensive drugs). Products include:
Dibenzyline Capsules ... 3188

Phentolamine Mesylate (Hydrochlorothiazide may add to or potentiate the therapeutic effect of other antihypertensive drugs).
No products indexed under this heading.

Phenylbutazone (Co-administration with non-steroidal anti-inflammatory agents may reduce the natriuretic and antihypertensive effects of thiazides).
No products indexed under this heading.

Pindolol (Hydrochlorothiazide may add to or potentiate the therapeutic effect of other antihypertensive drugs).
No products indexed under this heading.

Pioglitazone Hydrochloride (Hydrochlorothiazide may cause hyperglycemia, therefore, dosage adjustment of oral hypoglycemic agent may be required). Products include:
ActoPlus Met Tablets ... 3071
Actos Tablets ... 3077
Duetact Tablets ... 3085

Piroxicam (Co-administration with non-steroidal anti-inflammatory agents may reduce the natriuretic and antihypertensive effects of thiazides).
No products indexed under this heading.

Polythiazide (Hydrochlorothiazide may add to or potentiate the therapeutic effect of other antihypertensive drugs).
No products indexed under this heading.

Prazosin Hydrochloride (Hydrochlorothiazide may add to or potentiate the therapeutic effect of other antihypertensive drugs).
No products indexed under this heading.

Prednisolone Acetate (Co-administration with corticosteroids intensifies electrolyte depletion particularly hypokalemia). Products include:
Pred Forte Ophthalmic Suspension ... ⊙ 227
Pred Mild Ophthalmic Suspension ... ⊙ 230
Pred-G Ophthalmic Ointment ... ⊙ 229
Pred-G Ophthalmic Suspension ... ⊙ 228

Prednisolone Sodium Phosphate (Co-administration with corticosteroids intensifies electrolyte depletion particularly hypokalemia).
No products indexed under this heading.

Prednisolone Tebutate (Co-administration with corticosteroids intensifies electrolyte depletion particularly hypokalemia).
No products indexed under this heading.

Prednisone (Co-administration with corticosteroids intensifies electrolyte depletion particularly hypokalemia).
No products indexed under this heading.

Propoxyphene Hydrochloride (Potentiation of orthostatic hypotension may occur).
No products indexed under this heading.

Propoxyphene Napsylate (Potentiation of orthostatic hypotension may occur).
No products indexed under this heading.

Propranolol Hydrochloride (Hydrochlorothiazide may add to or potentiate the therapeutic effect of other antihypertensive drugs). Products include:
InnoPran XL Extended Release Capsules ... 1484

Quinapril Hydrochloride (Hydrochlorothiazide may add to or potentiate the therapeutic effect of other antihypertensive drugs).
No products indexed under this heading.

Ramipril (Hydrochlorothiazide may add to or potentiate the therapeutic effect of other antihypertensive drugs).
No products indexed under this heading.

Rapacuronium Bromide (Possible increased responsiveness to the muscle relaxants).
No products indexed under this heading.

Rauwolfia Serpentina (Hydrochlorothiazide may add to or potentiate the therapeutic effect of other antihypertensive drugs).
No products indexed under this heading.

Remifentanil Hydrochloride (Potentiation of orthostatic hypotension may occur).
No products indexed under this heading.

Repaglinide (Hydrochlorothiazide may cause hyperglycemia, therefore, dosage adjustment of oral hypoglycemic agent may be required). Products include:
PrandiMet Tablets ... 2967
Prandin Tablets ... 2971

Rescinnamine (Hydrochlorothiazide may add to or potentiate the therapeutic effect of other antihypertensive drugs).
No products indexed under this heading.

Reserpine (Hydrochlorothiazide may add to or potentiate the therapeutic effect of other antihypertensive drugs).
No products indexed under this heading.

Rocuronium Bromide (Possible increased responsiveness to the muscle relaxants). Products include:
Zemuron Injection **2947**

Rofecoxib (Co-administration with non-steroidal anti-inflammatory agents may reduce the natriuretic and antihypertensive effects of thiazides).
No products indexed under this heading.

Rosiglitazone Maleate (Hydrochlorothiazide may cause hyperglycemia, therefore, dosage adjustment of oral hypoglycemic agent may be required). Products include:
Avandamet Tablets **1336**
Avandaryl Tablets **1344**
Avandia Tablets **1351**

Secobarbital Sodium (Potentiation of orthostatic hypotension may occur).
No products indexed under this heading.

Sitagliptin Phosphate (Hydrochlorothiazide may cause hyperglycemia, therefore, dosage adjustment of oral hypoglycemic agent may be required). Products include:
Janumet Tablets **2041**
Januvia Tablets **2048**

Sodium Nitroprusside (Hydrochlorothiazide may add to or potentiate the therapeutic effect of other antihypertensive drugs).
No products indexed under this heading.

Sotalol Hydrochloride (Hydrochlorothiazide may add to or potentiate the therapeutic effect of other antihypertensive drugs).
No products indexed under this heading.

Spirapril Hydrochloride (Hydrochlorothiazide may add to or potentiate the therapeutic effect of other antihypertensive drugs).
No products indexed under this heading.

Sufentanil Citrate (Potentiation of orthostatic hypotension may occur).
No products indexed under this heading.

Sulindac (Co-administration with non-steroidal anti-inflammatory agents may reduce the natriuretic and antihypertensive effects of thiazides). Products include:
Clinoril Tablets **1962**

Telmisartan (Hydrochlorothiazide may add to or potentiate the therapeutic effect of other antihypertensive drugs). Products include:
Micardis Tablets **852**
Micardis HCT Tablets **854**

Terazosin Hydrochloride (Hydrochlorothiazide may add to or potentiate the therapeutic effect of other antihypertensive drugs).
No products indexed under this heading.

Thiamylal Sodium (Potentiation of orthostatic hypotension may occur).
No products indexed under this heading.

Timolol Maleate (Hydrochlorothiazide may add to or potentiate the therapeutic effect of other antihypertensive drugs). Products include:
Combigan Ophthalmic Solution **553**
Cosopt Sterile Ophthalmic Solution **1969**
Timoptic Sterile Ophthalmic Solution **2121**
Timoptic in Ocudose **2124**
Timoptic-XE Sterile Ophthalmic Gel Forming Solution **2125**

Tolazamide (Hydrochlorothiazide may cause hyperglycemia, therefore, dosage adjustment of oral hypoglycemic agent may be required).
No products indexed under this heading.

Tolbutamide (In vitro studies show significant inhibition of the formation of oxidized irbesartan metabolites with the known cytochrome CYP 2C9 substrate/inhibitor, tolbutamide; hydrochlorothiazide may cause hyperglycemia, therefore dosage adjustment of oral hypoglycemic agent may be required).
No products indexed under this heading.

Tolmetin Sodium (Co-administration with non-steroidal anti-inflammatory agents may reduce the natriuretic and antihypertensive effects of thiazides).
No products indexed under this heading.

Torsemide (Hydrochlorothiazide may add to or potentiate the therapeutic effect of other antihypertensive drugs). Products include:
Demadex Injection **2630**
Demadex Tablets **2630**

Trandolapril (Hydrochlorothiazide may add to or potentiate the therapeutic effect of other antihypertensive drugs). Products include:
Mavik Tablets **472**
Tarka Tablets **511**

Triamcinolone (Co-administration with corticosteroids intensifies electrolyte depletion particularly hypokalemia).
No products indexed under this heading.

Triamcinolone Acetonide (Co-administration with corticosteroids intensifies electrolyte depletion particularly hypokalemia). Products include:
Azmacort Inhalation Aerosol **407**
Nasacort AQ Nasal Spray **2765**
Triesence Injectable Suspension .... ⊙**209**

Triamcinolone Diacetate (Co-administration with corticosteroids intensifies electrolyte depletion particularly hypokalemia).
No products indexed under this heading.

Triamcinolone Hexacetonide (Co-administration with corticosteroids intensifies electrolyte depletion particularly hypokalemia).
No products indexed under this heading.

Trimethaphan Camsylate (Hydrochlorothiazide may add to or potentiate the therapeutic effect of other antihypertensive drugs).
No products indexed under this heading.

Troglitazone (Hydrochlorothiazide may cause hyperglycemia, therefore, dosage adjustment of oral hypoglycemic agent may be required).
No products indexed under this heading.

Tubocurarine Chloride (Possible increased responsiveness to the muscle relaxants).
No products indexed under this heading.

Valdecoxib (Co-administration with non-steroidal anti-inflammatory agents may reduce the natriuretic and antihypertensive effects of thiazides).
No products indexed under this heading.

Valsartan (Hydrochlorothiazide may add to or potentiate the therapeutic effect of other antihypertensive drugs). Products include:
Diovan Tablets **2212**
Diovan HCT Tablets **2216**
Exforge Tablets **2238**

Vecuronium Bromide (Possible increased responsiveness to the muscle relaxants).
No products indexed under this heading.

Verapamil Hydrochloride (Hydrochlorothiazide may add to or potentiate the therapeutic effect of other antihypertensive drugs). Products include:
Tarka Tablets **511**

Food Interactions

Alcohol (Potentiation of orthostatic hypotension may occur).

AVALIDE TABLETS

(Hydrochlorothiazide, Irbesartan) **2713**
May interact with antihypertensives, barbiturates, corticosteroids, oral hypoglycemic agents, insulin, lithium preparations, narcotic analgesics, nondepolarizing neuromuscular blocking agents, non-steroidal anti-inflammatory agents, and certain other agents. Compounds in these categories include:

Acarbose (Hyperglycemia may occur with thiazide diuretics, therefore dosage adjustment of the oral hypoglycemic agent may be required). Products include:
Precose Tablets **792**

Acebutolol Hydrochloride (Hydrochlorothiazide may produce an additive or potentiated effect).
No products indexed under this heading.

ACTH (Concurrent use with ACTH may cause intensified electrolyte depletion, particularly hypokalemia).
No products indexed under this heading.

Alfentanil Hydrochloride (Potentiation of orthostatic hypertension may occur).
No products indexed under this heading.

Aliskiren (Hydrochlorothiazide may produce an additive or potentiated effect). Products include:
Tekturna Tablets **2321**
Tekturna HCT Tablets **2324**

Amlodipine Besylate (Hydrochlorothiazide may produce an additive or potentiated effect). Products include:
Azor Tablets **1005**
Exforge Tablets **2238**

Aprobarbital (Potentiation of orthostatic hypertension may occur).
No products indexed under this heading.

Atenolol (Hydrochlorothiazide may produce an additive or potentiated effect).
No products indexed under this heading.

Atracurium Besylate (May cause a possible increased responsiveness to the muscle relaxant).
No products indexed under this heading.

Benazepril Hydrochloride (Hydrochlorothiazide may produce an additive or potentiated effect).
No products indexed under this heading.

Bendroflumethiazide (Hydrochlorothiazide may produce an additive or potentiated effect).
No products indexed under this heading.

Betamethasone Acetate (Concurrent use with corticosteroids may cause intensified electrolyte depletion, particularly hypokalemia).
No products indexed under this heading.

Betamethasone Sodium Phosphate (Concurrent use with corticosteroids may cause intensified electrolyte depletion, particularly hypokalemia).
No products indexed under this heading.

Betaxolol Hydrochloride (Hydrochlorothiazide may produce an additive or potentiated effect).
No products indexed under this heading.

Bisoprolol Fumarate (Hydrochlorothiazide may produce an additive or potentiated effect).
No products indexed under this heading.

Budesonide (Concurrent use with corticosteroids may cause intensified electrolyte depletion, particularly hypokalemia). Products include:
Pulmicort Flexhaler **654**
Symbicort 80/4.5 Inhalation Aerosol **659**
Symbicort 160/4.5 Inhalation Aerosol **659**

Buprenorphine Hydrochloride (Potentiation of orthostatic hypertension may occur). Products include:
Suboxone Tablets **2601**
Subutex Tablets **2601**

Butabarbital (Potentiation of orthostatic hypertension may occur).
No products indexed under this heading.

Butalbital (Potentiation of orthostatic hypertension may occur).
No products indexed under this heading.

Candesartan Cilexetil (Hydrochlorothiazide may produce an additive or potentiated effect). Products include:
Atacand Tablets **639**
Atacand HCT **642**

Captopril (Hydrochlorothiazide may produce an additive or potentiated effect). Products include:
Captopril Tablets **2182**

Carteolol Hydrochloride (Hydrochlorothiazide may produce an additive or potentiated effect).
No products indexed under this heading.

Celecoxib (In some patients, the administration of a non-steroidal

anti-inflammatory agent can reduce the diuretic, natriuretic, and antihypertensive effects of loop, potassium-sparing and thiazide diuretics. Therefore, when Avalide tablets and non-steroidal anti-inflammatory agents are used concomitantly, the patient should be observed closely to determine if the desired effect on the diuretic is obtained). Products include:
Celebrex Capsules 2979

Chlorothiazide (Hydrochlorothiazide may produce an additive or potentiated effect).
No products indexed under this heading.

Chlorothiazide Sodium (Hydrochlorothiazide may produce an additive or potentiated effect). Products include:
Intravenous Sodium Diuril 2490

Chlorpropamide (Hyperglycemia may occur with thiazide diuretics, therefore dosage adjustment of the oral hypoglycemic agent may be required).
No products indexed under this heading.

Chlorthalidone (Hydrochlorothiazide may produce an additive or potentiated effect). Products include:
Clorpres Tablets 2185

Cholestyramine (Absorption of hydrochlorothiazide is impaired in the presence of anionic exchange resins. Single doses of cholestyramine bind the hydrochlorothiazide and reduce its absorption from the gastrointestinal tract by up to 85%).
No products indexed under this heading.

Ciclesonide (Concurrent use with corticosteroids may cause intensified electrolyte depletion, particularly hypokalemia). Products include:
Alvesco Inhalation Aerosol 2985
Omnaris Nasal Spray 2998

Cisatracurium Besylate (May cause a possible increased responsiveness to the muscle relaxant). Products include:
Nimbex Injection 484

Clonidine (Hydrochlorothiazide may produce an additive or potentiated effect). Products include:
Catapres-TTS 842

Clonidine Hydrochloride (Hydrochlorothiazide may produce an additive or potentiated effect). Products include:
Catapres Tablets 841
Clorpres Tablets 2185

Codeine Phosphate (Potentiation of orthostatic hypertension may occur). Products include:
Tylenol with Codeine Tablets 2427

Colestipol (Absorption of hydrochlorothiazide is impaired in the presence of anionic exchange resins. Single doses of colestipol resins bind the hydrochlorothiazide and reduce its absorption from the gastrointestinal tract by up to 43%).
No products indexed under this heading.

Colestipol Hydrochloride (Absorption of hydrochlorothiazide is impaired in the presence of anionic exchange resins. Single doses of colestipol resins bind the hydrochlorothiazide and reduce its absorption from the gastrointestinal tract by up to 43%).
No products indexed under this heading.

Cortisone Acetate (Concurrent use with corticosteroids may cause intensified electrolyte depletion, particularly hypokalemia).
No products indexed under this heading.

Deserpidine (Hydrochlorothiazide may produce an additive or potentiated effect).
No products indexed under this heading.

Dexamethasone (Concurrent use with corticosteroids may cause intensified electrolyte depletion, particularly hypokalemia). Products include:
Ciprodex Otic Suspension 541

Dexamethasone Acetate (Concurrent use with corticosteroids may cause intensified electrolyte depletion, particularly hypokalemia).
No products indexed under this heading.

Dexamethasone Sodium Phosphate (Concurrent use with corticosteroids may cause intensified electrolyte depletion, particularly hypokalemia).
No products indexed under this heading.

Dezocine (Potentiation of orthostatic hypertension may occur).
No products indexed under this heading.

Diazoxide (Hydrochlorothiazide may produce an additive or potentiated effect). Products include:
Proglycem Capsules 1185
Proglycem Suspension 1185

Diclofenac Epolamine (In some patients, the administration of a non-steroidal anti-inflammatory agent can reduce the diuretic, natriuretic, and antihypertensive effects of loop, potassium-sparing and thiazide diuretics. Therefore, when Avalide tablets and non-steroidal anti-inflammatory agents are used concomitantly, the patient should be observed closely to determine if the desired effect on the diuretic is obtained). Products include:
Flector Patch 561

Diclofenac Potassium (In some patients, the administration of a non-steroidal anti-inflammatory agent can reduce the diuretic, natriuretic, and antihypertensive effects of loop, potassium-sparing and thiazide diuretics. Therefore, when Avalide tablets and non-steroidal anti-inflammatory agents are used concomitantly, the patient should be observed closely to determine if the desired effect on the diuretic is obtained).
No products indexed under this heading.

Diclofenac Sodium (In some patients, the administration of a non-steroidal anti-inflammatory agent can reduce the diuretic, natriuretic, and antihypertensive effects of loop, potassium-sparing and thiazide diuretics. Therefore, when Avalide tablets and non-steroidal anti-inflammatory agents are used concomitantly, the patient should be observed closely to determine if the desired effect on the diuretic is obtained). Products include:
Diclofenac Sodium Ophthalmic Solution .... ⊙ 240
Voltaren Ophthalmic Solution 2336
Voltaren Tablets 2334
Voltaren-XR Tablets 2337

Diltiazem Hydrochloride (Hydrochlorothiazide may produce an additive or potentiated effect). Products include:
Cardizem LA Extended Release Tablets 421

Doxazosin Mesylate (Hydrochlorothiazide may produce an additive or potentiated effect).
No products indexed under this heading.

Enalapril Maleate (Hydrochlorothiazide may produce an additive or potentiated effect).
No products indexed under this heading.

Enalaprilat (Hydrochlorothiazide may produce an additive or potentiated effect).
No products indexed under this heading.

Eprosartan Mesylate (Hydrochlorothiazide may produce an additive or potentiated effect). Products include:
Teveten Tablets 515
Teveten HCT Tablets 517

Esmolol Hydrochloride (Hydrochlorothiazide may produce an additive or potentiated effect).
No products indexed under this heading.

Ethanol (Potentiation of orthostatic hypertension may occur).
No products indexed under this heading.

Ethyl Alcohol (Potentiation of orthostatic hypertension may occur).
No products indexed under this heading.

Etodolac (In some patients, the administration of a non-steroidal anti-inflammatory agent can reduce the diuretic, natriuretic, and antihypertensive effects of loop, potassium-sparing and thiazide diuretics. Therefore, when Avalide tablets and non-steroidal anti-inflammatory agents are used concomitantly, the patient should be observed closely to determine if the desired effect on the diuretic is obtained).
No products indexed under this heading.

Felodipine (Hydrochlorothiazide may produce an additive or potentiated effect).
No products indexed under this heading.

Fenoprofen Calcium (In some patients, the administration of a non-steroidal anti-inflammatory agent can reduce the diuretic, natriuretic, and antihypertensive effects of loop, potassium-sparing and thiazide diuretics. Therefore, when Avalide tablets and non-steroidal anti-inflammatory agents are used concomitantly, the patient should be observed closely to determine if the desired effect on the diuretic is obtained). Products include:
Nalfon Capsules 2508

Fentanyl (Potentiation of orthostatic hypertension may occur). Products include:
Duragesic Transdermal System 2405
Ionsys Transdermal System 2410

Fentanyl Citrate (Potentiation of orthostatic hypertension may occur). Products include:
Actiq 959
Fentora Tablets 968

Fludrocortisone Acetate (Concurrent use with corticosteroids may cause intensified electrolyte depletion, particularly hypokalemia).
No products indexed under this heading.

Flunisolide (Concurrent use with corticosteroids may cause intensified electrolyte depletion, particularly hypokalemia). Products include:
Aerobid/Aerobid-M 1153

Flurbiprofen (In some patients, the administration of a non-steroidal anti-inflammatory agent can reduce the diuretic, natriuretic, and antihypertensive effects of loop, potassium-sparing and thiazide diuretics. Therefore, when Avalide tablets and non-steroidal anti-inflammatory agents are used concomitantly, the patient should be observed closely to determine if the desired effect on the diuretic is obtained).
No products indexed under this heading.

Fluticasone Propionate (Concurrent use with corticosteroids may cause intensified electrolyte depletion, particularly hypokalemia). Products include:
Advair Diskus 100/50 1276
Advair Diskus 250/50 1276
Advair Diskus 500/50 1276
Advair HFA 45/21 Inhalation Aerosol 1288
Advair HFA 115/21 Inhalation Aerosol 1288
Advair HFA 230/21 Inhalation Aerosol 1288
Flonase Nasal Spray 1431
Flovent Diskus 50 mcg 1435

Fluticasone Propionate HFA (Concurrent use with corticosteroids may cause intensified electrolyte depletion, particularly hypokalemia). Products include:
Flovent HFA 1440

Fosinopril Sodium (Hydrochlorothiazide may produce an additive or potentiated effect).
No products indexed under this heading.

Furosemide (Hydrochlorothiazide may produce an additive or potentiated effect). Products include:
Furosemide Tablets 2186

Glimepiride (Hyperglycemia may occur with thiazide diuretics, therefore dosage adjustment of the oral hypoglycemic agent may be required). Products include:
Avandaryl Tablets 1344
Duetact Tablets 3085

Glipizide (Hyperglycemia may occur with thiazide diuretics, therefore dosage adjustment of the oral hypoglycemic agent may be required).
No products indexed under this heading.

Glyburide (Hyperglycemia may occur with thiazide diuretics, therefore dosage adjustment of the oral hypoglycemic agent may be required).
No products indexed under this heading.

Guanabenz Acetate (Hydrochlorothiazide may produce an additive or potentiated effect).
No products indexed under this heading.

Guanethidine Monosulfate (Hydrochlorothiazide may produce an additive or potentiated effect).
No products indexed under this heading.

Hydralazine Hydrochloride (Hydrochlorothiazide may produce an additive or potentiated effect).
No products indexed under this heading.

Hydrocodone Bitartrate (Potentiation of orthostatic hypertension may occur). Products include:
Lortab 5/500 Tablets **3143**
Lortab 7.5/500 Tablets **3144**
Lortab 10/500 Tablets **3144**
Vicodin Tablets **529**
Vicodin ES Tablets **530**
Vicodin HP Tablets **531**
Vicoprofen Tablets **533**
Zydone Tablets **1132**

Hydrocodone Polistirex (Potentiation of orthostatic hypertension may occur). Products include:
Tussionex Pennkinetic Extended-Release Suspension **3154**

Hydrocortisone (Concurrent use with corticosteroids may cause intensified electrolyte depletion, particularly hypokalemia).
No products indexed under this heading.

Hydrocortisone Acetate (Concurrent use with corticosteroids may cause intensified electrolyte depletion, particularly hypokalemia). Products include:
Analpram-HC **1140**
Pramosone **1141**

Hydrocortisone Sodium Phosphate (Concurrent use with corticosteroids may cause intensified electrolyte depletion, particularly hypokalemia).
No products indexed under this heading.

Hydrocortisone Sodium Succinate (Concurrent use with corticosteroids may cause intensified electrolyte depletion, particularly hypokalemia).
No products indexed under this heading.

Hydroflumethiazide (Hydrochlorothiazide may produce an additive or potentiated effect).
No products indexed under this heading.

Hydromorphone Hydrochloride (Potentiation of orthostatic hypertension may occur).
No products indexed under this heading.

Ibuprofen (In some patients, the administration of a non-steroidal anti-inflammatory agent can reduce the diuretic, natriuretic, and antihypertensive effects of loop, potassium-sparing and thiazide diuretics. Therefore, when Avalide tablets and non-steroidal anti-inflammatory agents are used concomitantly, the patient should be observed closely to determine if the desired effect on the diuretic is obtained). Products include:
Motrin IB Tablets and Caplets **1900**
Children's Motrin Oral Suspension ... **1901**
Children's Motrin Non-Staining Dye-Free Oral Suspension **1901**
Children's Motrin Cold Oral Suspension **1899**
Infants' Motrin Concentrated Drops **1901**
Infants' Motrin Non-Staining Dye-Free Concentrated Drops **1901**
Junior Strength Motrin Caplets and Chewable Tablets **1901**
Vicoprofen Tablets **533**

Indapamide (Hydrochlorothiazide may produce an additive or potentiated effect). Products include:
Indapamide Tablets **2188**

Indomethacin (In some patients, the administration of a non-steroidal anti-inflammatory agent can reduce the diuretic, natriuretic, and antihypertensive effects of loop, potassium-sparing and thiazide diuretics. Therefore, when Avalide tablets and non-steroidal anti-inflammatory agents are used concomitantly, the patient should be observed closely to determine if the desired effect on the diuretic is obtained). Products include:
Indocin **2024**

Indomethacin Sodium Trihydrate (In some patients, the administration of a non-steroidal anti-inflammatory agent can reduce the diuretic, natriuretic, and antihypertensive effects of loop, potassium-sparing and thiazide diuretics. Therefore, when Avalide tablets and non-steroidal anti-inflammatory agents are used concomitantly, the patient should be observed closely to determine if the desired effect on the diuretic is obtained). Products include:
Indocin I.V. **2489**

Insulin (Hyperglycemia may occur with thiazide diuretics, therefore dosage adjustment of insulin may be required).
No products indexed under this heading.

Insulin, Human, Zinc Suspension (Hyperglycemia may occur with thiazide diuretics, therefore dosage adjustment of insulin may be required).
No products indexed under this heading.

Insulin, Human (rDNA origin) (Hyperglycemia may occur with thiazide diuretics, therefore dosage adjustment of insulin may be required). Products include:
Exubera Inhalation Powder **2515**

Insulin, Human NPH (Hyperglycemia may occur with thiazide diuretics, therefore dosage adjustment of insulin may be required). Products include:
Humulin N Vial **1846**

Insulin, Human Regular (Hyperglycemia may occur with thiazide diuretics, therefore dosage adjustment of insulin may be required). Products include:
Humulin R **1849**
Humulin R (U-500) **1850**

Insulin, Human Regular and Human NPH Mixture (Hyperglycemia may occur with thiazide diuretics, therefore dosage adjustment of insulin may be required). Products include:
Humulin 50/50, 100 Units **1843**
Humulin 70/30 Vial **1844**

Insulin, NPH (Hyperglycemia may occur with thiazide diuretics, therefore dosage adjustment of insulin may be required).
No products indexed under this heading.

Insulin, Regular (Hyperglycemia may occur with thiazide diuretics, therefore dosage adjustment of insulin may be required).
No products indexed under this heading.

Insulin, Regular and NPH mixture (Hyperglycemia may occur with thiazide diuretics, therefore dosage adjustment of insulin may be required).
No products indexed under this heading.

Insulin, Zinc Crystals (Hyperglycemia may occur with thiazide diuretics, therefore dosage adjustment of insulin may be required).
No products indexed under this heading.

Insulin, Zinc Suspension (Hyperglycemia may occur with thiazide diuretics, therefore dosage adjustment of insulin may be required).
No products indexed under this heading.

Insulin Aspart (Hyperglycemia may occur with thiazide diuretics, therefore dosage adjustment of insulin may be required).
No products indexed under this heading.

Insulin Aspart, Human (Hyperglycemia may occur with thiazide diuretics, therefore dosage adjustment of insulin may be required). Products include:
NovoLog Mix 70/30 .... **2364**

Insulin Aspart, Human Regular (Hyperglycemia may occur with thiazide diuretics, therefore dosage adjustment of insulin may be required). Products include:
NovoLog Injection **2359**

Insulin Aspart Protamine, Human (Hyperglycemia may occur with thiazide diuretics, therefore dosage adjustment of insulin may be required). Products include:
NovoLog Mix 70/30 .... **2364**

Insulin Detemir (rDNA Origin) (Hyperglycemia may occur with thiazide diuretics, therefore dosage adjustment of insulin may be required). Products include:
Levemir Injection **2352**

Insulin glargine (Hyperglycemia may occur with thiazide diuretics, therefore dosage adjustment of insulin may be required). Products include:
Lantus Injection **2749**

Insulin Glulisine (Hyperglycemia may occur with thiazide diuretics, therefore dosage adjustment of insulin may be required). Products include:
Apidra Injection **2706**

Insulin Lispro, Human (Hyperglycemia may occur with thiazide diuretics, therefore dosage adjustment of insulin may be required). Products include:
Humalog-Pen and KwikPen **1829**
Humalog Mix 50/50-Pen and KwikPen **1833**
Humalog Mix 75/25-Pen and KwikPen **1835**

Insulin Lispro Protamine, Human (Hyperglycemia may occur with thiazide diuretics, therefore dosage adjustment of insulin may be required). Products include:
Humalog Mix 50/50-Pen and KwikPen **1833**
Humalog Mix 75/25-Pen and KwikPen **1835**

Isradipine (Hydrochlorothiazide may produce an additive or potentiated effect). Products include:
DynaCirc CR Controlled Release Tablets **1407**

Ketoprofen (In some patients, the administration of a non-steroidal anti-inflammatory agent can reduce the diuretic, natriuretic, and antihypertensive effects of loop, potassium-sparing and thiazide diuretics. Therefore, when Avalide tablets and non-steroidal anti-inflammatory agents are used concomitantly, the patient should be observed closely to determine if the desired effect on the diuretic is obtained).
No products indexed under this heading.

Ketorolac Tromethamine (In some patients, the administration of a non-steroidal anti-inflammatory agent can reduce the diuretic, natriuretic, and antihypertensive effects of loop, potassium-sparing and thiazide diuretics. Therefore, when Avalide tablets and non-steroidal anti-inflammatory agents are used concomitantly, the patient should be observed closely to determine if the desired effect on the diuretic is obtained).
No products indexed under this heading.

Labetalol Hydrochloride (Hydrochlorothiazide may produce an additive or potentiated effect).
No products indexed under this heading.

Levorphanol Tartrate (Potentiation of orthostatic hypertension may occur).
No products indexed under this heading.

Lisinopril (Hydrochlorothiazide may produce an additive or potentiated effect). Products include:
Prinivil Tablets **2087**
Prinzide Tablets **2092**

Lithium (Should not generally be given with diuretics. Diuretic agents reduce the renal clearance of lithium and add a high risk of lithium toxicity).
No products indexed under this heading.

Lithium Carbonate (Should not generally be given with diuretics. Diuretic agents reduce the renal clearance of lithium and add a high risk of lithium toxicity).
No products indexed under this heading.

Lithium Citrate (Should not generally be given with diuretics. Diuretic agents reduce the renal clearance of lithium and add a high risk of lithium toxicity).
No products indexed under this heading.

Losartan Potassium (Hydrochlorothiazide may produce an additive or potentiated effect). Products include:
Cozaar Tablets **1973**

Mecamylamine Hydrochloride (Hydrochlorothiazide may produce an additive or potentiated effect).
No products indexed under this heading.

Meclofenamate Sodium (In some patients, the administration of a non-steroidal anti-inflammatory agent can reduce the diuretic, natriuretic, and antihypertensive effects of loop, potassium-sparing and thiazide

IMPORTANT NOTE: Always consult each drug listing in the patient's regimen for possible interactions.

diuretics. Therefore, when Avalide tablets and non-steroidal anti-inflammatory agents are used concomitantly, the patient should be observed closely to determine if the desired effect on the diuretic is obtained).

No products indexed under this heading.

Mefenamic Acid (In some patients, the administration of a non-steroidal anti-inflammatory agent can reduce the diuretic, natriuretic, and antihypertensive effects of loop, potassium-sparing and thiazide diuretics. Therefore, when Avalide tablets and non-steroidal anti-inflammatory agents are used concomitantly, the patient should be observed closely to determine if the desired effect on the diuretic is obtained).

No products indexed under this heading.

Meloxicam (In some patients, the administration of a non-steroidal anti-inflammatory agent can reduce the diuretic, natriuretic, and antihypertensive effects of loop, potassium-sparing and thiazide diuretics. Therefore, when Avalide tablets and non-steroidal anti-inflammatory agents are used concomitantly, the patient should be observed closely to determine if the desired effect on the diuretic is obtained). Products include:

Mobic Oral Suspension **863**
Mobic Tablets **863**

Meperidine Hydrochloride (Potentiation of orthostatic hypertension may occur).

No products indexed under this heading.

Mephobarbital (Potentiation of orthostatic hypertension may occur).

No products indexed under this heading.

Metformin Hydrochloride (Hyperglycemia may occur with thiazide diuretics, therefore dosage adjustment of the oral hypoglycemic agent may be required). Products include:

ActoPlus Met Tablets **3071**
Avandamet Tablets **1336**
Janumet Tablets **2041**
PrandiMet Tablets **2967**

Methadone Hydrochloride (Potentiation of orthostatic hypertension may occur).

No products indexed under this heading.

Methyclothiazide (Hydrochlorothiazide may produce an additive or potentiated effect).

No products indexed under this heading.

Methyldopa (Hydrochlorothiazide may produce an additive or potentiated effect).

No products indexed under this heading.

Methyldopate Hydrochloride (Hydrochlorothiazide may produce an additive or potentiated effect).

No products indexed under this heading.

Methylprednisolone Acetate (Concurrent use with corticosteroids may cause intensified electrolyte depletion, particularly hypokalemia).

No products indexed under this heading.

Methylprednisolone Sodium Succinate (Concurrent use with corticosteroids may cause intensified electrolyte depletion, particularly hypokalemia).

No products indexed under this heading.

Metocurine Iodide (May cause a possible increased responsiveness to the muscle relaxant).

No products indexed under this heading.

Metolazone (Hydrochlorothiazide may produce an additive or potentiated effect).

No products indexed under this heading.

Metoprolol Succinate (Hydrochlorothiazide may produce an additive or potentiated effect). Products include:

Toprol-XL Tablets **666**

Metoprolol Tartrate (Hydrochlorothiazide may produce an additive or potentiated effect).

No products indexed under this heading.

Metyrosine (Hydrochlorothiazide may produce an additive or potentiated effect). Products include:

Demser Capsules **1989**

Mibefradil Dihydrochloride (Hydrochlorothiazide may produce an additive or potentiated effect).

No products indexed under this heading.

Miglitol (Hyperglycemia may occur with thiazide diuretics, therefore dosage adjustment of the oral hypoglycemic agent may be required).

No products indexed under this heading.

Minoxidil (Hydrochlorothiazide may produce an additive or potentiated effect).

No products indexed under this heading.

Mivacurium Chloride (May cause a possible increased responsiveness to the muscle relaxant).

No products indexed under this heading.

Moexipril Hydrochloride (Hydrochlorothiazide may produce an additive or potentiated effect).

No products indexed under this heading.

Mometasone Furoate (Concurrent use with corticosteroids may cause intensified electrolyte depletion, particularly hypokalemia). Products include:

Asmanex Twisthaler **2797**
Elocon Cream 0.1% **2840**
Elocon Lotion 0.1% **2841**
Elocon Ointment 0.1% **2842**

Mometasone Furoate Monohydrate (Concurrent use with corticosteroids may cause intensified electrolyte depletion, particularly hypokalemia). Products include:

Nasonex Nasal Spray **2883**

Morphine Sulfate (Potentiation of orthostatic hypertension may occur). Products include:

Avinza Capsules **1772**
DepoDur Injection **1095**
MS Contin Tablets **2585**

Nabumetone (In some patients, the administration of a non-steroidal anti-inflammatory agent can reduce the diuretic, natriuretic, and antihypertensive effects of loop, potassium-sparing and thiazide diuretics. Therefore, when Avalide tablets and non-steroidal anti-inflammatory agents are used concomitantly, the patient should be observed closely to determine if the desired effect on the diuretic is obtained).

No products indexed under this heading.

Nadolol (Hydrochlorothiazide may produce an additive or potentiated effect). Products include:

Nadolol Tablets **2191**

Naproxen (In some patients, the administration of a non-steroidal anti-inflammatory agent can reduce the diuretic, natriuretic, and antihypertensive effects of loop, potassium-sparing and thiazide diuretics. Therefore, when Avalide tablets and non-steroidal anti-inflammatory agents are used concomitantly, the patient should be observed closely to determine if the desired effect on the diuretic is obtained). Products include:

EC-Naprosyn Delayed-Release Tablets **2632**
Naprosyn Suspension **2632**
Naprosyn Tablets **2632**

Naproxen Sodium (In some patients, the administration of a non-steroidal anti-inflammatory agent can reduce the diuretic, natriuretic, and antihypertensive effects of loop, potassium-sparing and thiazide diuretics. Therefore, when Avalide tablets and non-steroidal anti-inflammatory agents are used concomitantly, the patient should be observed closely to determine if the desired effect on the diuretic is obtained). Products include:

Anaprox Tablets **2632**
Anaprox DS Tablets **2632**
Treximet Tablets **1616**

Nateglinide (Hyperglycemia may occur with thiazide diuretics, therefore dosage adjustment of the oral hypoglycemic agent may be required). Products include:

Starlix Tablets **2314**

Nebivolol (Hydrochlorothiazide may produce an additive or potentiated effect). Products include:

Bystolic Tablets **1155**

Nicardipine Hydrochloride (Hydrochlorothiazide may produce an additive or potentiated effect). Products include:

Cardene I.V. **1093**

Nifedipine (Hydrochlorothiazide may produce an additive or potentiated effect).

No products indexed under this heading.

Nisoldipine (Hydrochlorothiazide may produce an additive or potentiated effect). Products include:

Sular Extended Release Tablets **2975**

Nitroglycerin (Hydrochlorothiazide may produce an additive or potentiated effect). Products include:

Nitro-Dur Transdermal Infusion System **2887**
Nitrolingual Pumpspray **2965**

Norepinephrine Bitartrate (Possible decreased response to pressor amines (e.g., norepinephrine) but not sufficient to preclude their use).

No products indexed under this heading.

Norepinephrine Hydrochloride (Possible decreased response to pressor amines (e.g., norepinephrine) but not sufficient to preclude their use).

No products indexed under this heading.

Oxaprozin (In some patients, the administration of a non-steroidal anti-inflammatory agent can reduce the diuretic, natriuretic, and antihypertensive effects of loop, potassium-sparing and thiazide diuretics. Therefore, when Avalide tablets and non-steroidal anti-inflammatory agents are used concomitantly, the patient should be observed closely to determine if the desired effect on the diuretic is obtained).

No products indexed under this heading.

Oxycodone Hydrochloride (Potentiation of orthostatic hypertension may occur). Products include:

OxyContin Tablets **2589**
OxyIR Capsules **2593**
Percocet Tablets **1127**
Percodan Tablets **1130**

Pancuronium Bromide (May cause a possible increased responsiveness to the muscle relaxant).

No products indexed under this heading.

Penbutolol Sulfate (Hydrochlorothiazide may produce an additive or potentiated effect).

No products indexed under this heading.

Pentobarbital Sodium (Potentiation of orthostatic hypertension may occur). Products include:

Nembutal Sodium Solution, USP **2494**

Perindopril Erbumine (Hydrochlorothiazide may produce an additive or potentiated effect). Products include:

Aceon Tablets (2 mg, 4 mg, 8 mg) **3038**

Phenobarbital (Potentiation of orthostatic hypertension may occur). Products include:

Donnatal Extentabs **2507**

Phenoxybenzamine Hydrochloride (Hydrochlorothiazide may produce an additive or potentiated effect). Products include:

Dibenzyline Capsules **3188**

Phentolamine Mesylate (Hydrochlorothiazide may produce an additive or potentiated effect).

No products indexed under this heading.

Phenylbutazone (In some patients, the administration of a non-steroidal anti-inflammatory agent can reduce the diuretic, natriuretic, and antihypertensive effects of loop, potassium-sparing and thiazide diuretics. Therefore, when Avalide tablets and non-steroidal anti-inflammatory agents are used concomitantly, the patient should be observed closely to determine if the desired effect on the diuretic is obtained).

No products indexed under this heading.

Pindolol (Hydrochlorothiazide may produce an additive or potentiated effect).

No products indexed under this heading.

Pioglitazone Hydrochloride (Hyperglycemia may occur with thiazide diuretics, therefore dosage adjustment of the oral hypoglycemic agent may be required). Products include:

ActoPlus Met Tablets **3071**
Actos Tablets **3077**
Duetact Tablets **3085**

Piroxicam (In some patients, the administration of a non-steroidal

anti-inflammatory agent can reduce the diuretic, natriuretic, and antihypertensive effects of loop, potassium-sparing and thiazide diuretics. Therefore, when Avalide tablets and non-steroidal anti-inflammatory agents are used concomitantly, the patient should be observed closely to determine if the desired effect on the diuretic is obtained).
No products indexed under this heading.

Polythiazide (Hydrochlorothiazide may produce an additive or potentiated effect).
No products indexed under this heading.

Prazosin Hydrochloride (Hydrochlorothiazide may produce an additive or potentiated effect).
No products indexed under this heading.

Prednisolone Acetate (Concurrent use with corticosteroids may cause intensified electrolyte depletion, particularly hypokalemia). Products include:
Pred Forte Ophthalmic Suspension ⊙ 227
Pred Mild Ophthalmic Suspension ⊙ 230
Pred-G Ophthalmic Ointment ⊙ 229
Pred-G Ophthalmic Suspension ⊙ 228

Prednisolone Sodium Phosphate (Concurrent use with corticosteroids may cause intensified electrolyte depletion, particularly hypokalemia).
No products indexed under this heading.

Prednisolone Tebutate (Concurrent use with corticosteroids may cause intensified electrolyte depletion, particularly hypokalemia).
No products indexed under this heading.

Prednisone (Concurrent use with corticosteroids may cause intensified electrolyte depletion, particularly hypokalemia).
No products indexed under this heading.

Propoxyphene Hydrochloride (Potentiation of orthostatic hypertension may occur).
No products indexed under this heading.

Propoxyphene Napsylate (Potentiation of orthostatic hypertension may occur).
No products indexed under this heading.

Propranolol Hydrochloride (Hydrochlorothiazide may produce an additive or potentiated effect). Products include:
InnoPran XL Extended Release Capsules 1484

Quinapril Hydrochloride (Hydrochlorothiazide may produce an additive or potentiated effect).
No products indexed under this heading.

Ramipril (Hydrochlorothiazide may produce an additive or potentiated effect).
No products indexed under this heading.

Rapacuronium Bromide (May cause a possible increased responsiveness to the muscle relaxant).
No products indexed under this heading.

Rauwolfia Serpentina (Hydrochlorothiazide may produce an additive or potentiated effect).
No products indexed under this heading.

Remifentanil Hydrochloride (Potentiation of orthostatic hypertension may occur).
No products indexed under this heading.

Repaglinide (Hyperglycemia may occur with thiazide diuretics, therefore dosage adjustment of the oral hypoglycemic agent may be required). Products include:
PrandiMet Tablets 2967
Prandin Tablets 2971

Rescinnamine (Hydrochlorothiazide may produce an additive or potentiated effect).
No products indexed under this heading.

Reserpine (Hydrochlorothiazide may produce an additive or potentiated effect).
No products indexed under this heading.

Rocuronium Bromide (May cause a possible increased responsiveness to the muscle relaxant). Products include:
Zemuron Injection 2947

Rofecoxib (In some patients, the administration of a non-steroidal anti-inflammatory agent can reduce the diuretic, natriuretic, and antihypertensive effects of loop, potassium-sparing and thiazide diuretics. Therefore, when Avalide tablets and non-steroidal anti-inflammatory agents are used concomitantly, the patient should be observed closely to determine if the desired effect on the diuretic is obtained).
No products indexed under this heading.

Rosiglitazone Maleate (Hyperglycemia may occur with thiazide diuretics, therefore dosage adjustment of the oral hypoglycemic agent may be required). Products include:
Avandamet Tablets 1336
Avandaryl Tablets 1344
Avandia Tablets 1351

Secobarbital Sodium (Potentiation of orthostatic hypertension may occur).
No products indexed under this heading.

Sitagliptin Phosphate (Hyperglycemia may occur with thiazide diuretics, therefore dosage adjustment of the oral hypoglycemic agent may be required). Products include:
Janumet Tablets 2041
Januvia Tablets 2048

Sodium Nitroprusside (Hydrochlorothiazide may produce an additive or potentiated effect).
No products indexed under this heading.

Sotalol Hydrochloride (Hydrochlorothiazide may produce an additive or potentiated effect).
No products indexed under this heading.

Spirapril Hydrochloride (Hydrochlorothiazide may produce an additive or potentiated effect).
No products indexed under this heading.

Sufentanil Citrate (Potentiation of orthostatic hypertension may occur).
No products indexed under this heading.

Sulindac (In some patients, the administration of a non-steroidal anti-inflammatory agent can reduce the diuretic, natriuretic, and antihypertensive effects of loop, potassium-sparing and thiazide diuretics. Therefore, when Avalide tablets and non-steroidal anti-inflammatory agents are used concomitantly, the patient should be observed closely to determine if the desired effect on the diuretic is obtained). Products include:
Clinoril Tablets 1962

Telmisartan (Hydrochlorothiazide may produce an additive or potentiated effect). Products include:
Micardis Tablets 852
Micardis HCT Tablets 854

Terazosin Hydrochloride (Hydrochlorothiazide may produce an additive or potentiated effect).
No products indexed under this heading.

Thiamylal Sodium (Potentiation of orthostatic hypertension may occur).
No products indexed under this heading.

Timolol Maleate (Hydrochlorothiazide may produce an additive or potentiated effect). Products include:
Combigan Ophthalmic Solution 553
Cosopt Sterile Ophthalmic Solution 1969
Timoptic Sterile Ophthalmic Solution 2121
Timoptic in Ocudose 2124
Timoptic-XE Sterile Ophthalmic Gel Forming Solution 2125

Tolazamide (Hyperglycemia may occur with thiazide diuretics, therefore dosage adjustment of the oral hypoglycemic agent may be required).
No products indexed under this heading.

Tolbutamide (Hyperglycemia may occur with thiazide diuretics, therefore dosage adjustment of the oral hypoglycemic agent may be required).
No products indexed under this heading.

Tolmetin Sodium (In some patients, the administration of a non-steroidal anti-inflammatory agent can reduce the diuretic, natriuretic, and antihypertensive effects of loop, potassium-sparing and thiazide diuretics. Therefore, when Avalide tablets and non-steroidal anti-inflammatory agents are used concomitantly, the patient should be observed closely to determine if the desired effect on the diuretic is obtained).
No products indexed under this heading.

Torsemide (Hydrochlorothiazide may produce an additive or potentiated effect). Products include:
Demadex Injection 2630
Demadex Tablets 2630

Trandolapril (Hydrochlorothiazide may produce an additive or potentiated effect). Products include:
Mavik Tablets 472
Tarka Tablets 511

Triamcinolone (Concurrent use with corticosteroids may cause intensified electrolyte depletion, particularly hypokalemia).
No products indexed under this heading.

Triamcinolone Acetonide (Concurrent use with corticosteroids may cause intensified electrolyte depletion, particularly hypokalemia). Products include:
Azmacort Inhalation Aerosol 407
Nasacort AQ Nasal Spray 2765
Triesence Injectable Suspension ⊙ 209

Triamcinolone Diacetate (Concurrent use with corticosteroids may cause intensified electrolyte depletion, particularly hypokalemia).
No products indexed under this heading.

Triamcinolone Hexacetonide (Concurrent use with corticosteroids may cause intensified electrolyte depletion, particularly hypokalemia).
No products indexed under this heading.

Trimethaphan Camsylate (Hydrochlorothiazide may produce an additive or potentiated effect).
No products indexed under this heading.

Troglitazone (Hyperglycemia may occur with thiazide diuretics, therefore dosage adjustment of the oral hypoglycemic agent may be required).
No products indexed under this heading.

Tubocurarine Chloride (May cause a possible increased responsiveness to tubocurarine).
No products indexed under this heading.

Valdecoxib (In some patients, the administration of a non-steroidal anti-inflammatory agent can reduce the diuretic, natriuretic, and antihypertensive effects of loop, potassium-sparing and thiazide diuretics. Therefore, when Avalide tablets and non-steroidal anti-inflammatory agents are used concomitantly, the patient should be observed closely to determine if the desired effect on the diuretic is obtained).
No products indexed under this heading.

Valsartan (Hydrochlorothiazide may produce an additive or potentiated effect). Products include:
Diovan Tablets 2212
Diovan HCT Tablets 2216
Exforge Tablets 2238

Vecuronium Bromide (May cause a possible increased responsiveness to the muscle relaxant).
No products indexed under this heading.

Verapamil Hydrochloride (Hydrochlorothiazide may produce an additive or potentiated effect). Products include:
Tarka Tablets 511

Food Interactions

Alcohol (Potentiation of orthostatic hypertension may occur).

AVANDAMET TABLETS

(Metformin Hydrochloride, Rosiglitazone Maleate) 1336
May interact with cationic drugs that are eliminated by renal tubular, calcium channel blockers, corticosteroids, cytochrome p450 2c8 inducers (selected), cytochrome p450 2c8 inhibitors (selected), diuretics, estrogens, oral hypoglycemic agents, insulin, oral contraceptives, phenothiazines, phenytoin, quinidine, radiographic iodinated contrast media, sulfonylureas, sympathomimetics, thiazides, thyroid preparations, and certain other agents. Compounds in these categories include:

Acarbose (Patients receiving rosiglitazone in combination with other hypoglycemic agents may be at risk for hypoglycemia and a reduction in the dose of the concomitant agent may be necessary). Products include:

Precose Tablets 792

Albuterol (Certain drugs, such as sympathomimetics, tend to produce hyperglycemia and may lead to loss of glycemic control).

No products indexed under this heading.

Albuterol Sulfate (Certain drugs, such as sympathomimetics, tend to produce hyperglycemia and may lead to loss of glycemic control). Products include:

Combivent Inhalation Aerosol 845
ProAir HFA Inhalation Aerosol 3113
Proventil HFA Inhalation Aerosol 2914
Ventolin HFA Inhalation Aerosol 1638

Amiloride Hydrochloride (Potential for loss of glycemic control; theoretical potential for interaction with metformin by competing for common renal tubular transport system).

No products indexed under this heading.

Amlodipine Besylate (Certain drugs, such as calcium channel blockers, tend to produce hyperglycemia and may lead to loss of glycemic control). Products include:

Azor Tablets 1005
Exforge Tablets 2238

Anastrozole (An inhibitor of CYP2C8 may increase the AUC of rosiglitazone). Products include:

Arimidex Tablets 672

Bendroflumethiazide (Certain drugs, such as thiazides and other diuretics, tend to produce hyperglycemia and may lead to loss of glycemic control).

No products indexed under this heading.

Bepridil Hydrochloride (Certain drugs, such as calcium channel blockers, tend to produce hyperglycemia and may lead to loss of glycemic control).

No products indexed under this heading.

Betamethasone Acetate (Certain drugs, such as corticosteroids, tend to produce hyperglycemia and may lead to loss of glycemic control).

No products indexed under this heading.

Betamethasone Sodium Phosphate (Certain drugs, such as corticosteroids, tend to produce hyperglycemia and may lead to loss of glycemic control).

No products indexed under this heading.

Budesonide (Certain drugs, such as corticosteroids, tend to produce hyperglycemia and may lead to loss of glycemic control). Products include:

Pulmicort Flexhaler 654
Symbicort 80/4.5 Inhalation Aerosol.. 659
Symbicort 160/4.5 Inhalation Aerosol.. 659

Bumetanide (Certain drugs, such as diuretics, tend to produce hyperglycemia and may lead to loss of glycemic control).

No products indexed under this heading.

Carbamazepine (An inducer of CYP2C8 may decrease the AUC of rosiglitazone). Products include:

Carbatrol Capsules 3019
Equetro Extended-Release Capsules 3174

Chlorothiazide (Certain drugs, such as thiazides and other diuretics, tend to produce hyperglycemia and may lead to loss of glycemic control).

No products indexed under this heading.

Chlorothiazide Sodium (Certain drugs, such as thiazides and other diuretics, tend to produce hyperglycemia and may lead to loss of glycemic control). Products include:

Intravenous Sodium Diuril 2490

Chlorotrianisene (Certain drugs, such as estrogens, tend to produce hyperglycemia and may lead to loss of glycemic control).

No products indexed under this heading.

Chlorpromazine (Certain drugs, such as phenothiazines, tend to produce hyperglycemia and may lead to loss of glycemic control).

No products indexed under this heading.

Chlorpromazine Hydrochloride (Certain drugs, such as phenothiazines, tend to produce hyperglycemia and may lead to loss of glycemic control).

No products indexed under this heading.

Chlorpropamide (An increased incidence of heart failure has been observed when rosiglitazone was added to a sulfonylurea or to a sulfonylurea plus metformin).

No products indexed under this heading.

Chlorthalidone (Certain drugs, such as diuretics, tend to produce hyperglycemia and may lead to loss of glycemic control). Products include:

Clorpres Tablets 2185

Ciclesonide (Certain drugs, such as corticosteroids, tend to produce hyperglycemia and may lead to loss of glycemic control). Products include:

Alvesco Inhalation Aerosol 2985
Omnaris Nasal Spray 2998

Cimetidine (Co-administered with oral cimetidine may increase peak metformin plasma and whole blood concentrations by 60% and a 40% increase in plasma and whole blood metformin AUC).

No products indexed under this heading.

Cimetidine Hydrochloride (An inhibitor of CYP2C8 may increase the AUC of rosiglitazone).

No products indexed under this heading.

Cortisone Acetate (Certain drugs, such as corticosteroids, tend to produce hyperglycemia and may lead to loss of glycemic control).

No products indexed under this heading.

Desogestrel (Certain drugs, such as oral contraceptives, tend to produce hyperglycemia and may lead to loss of glycemic control). Products include:

Mircette Tablets 1034

Dexamethasone (Certain drugs, such as corticosteroids, tend to produce hyperglycemia and may lead to loss of glycemic control). Products include:

Ciprodex Otic Suspension 541

Dexamethasone Acetate (Certain drugs, such as corticosteroids, tend to produce hyperglycemia and may lead to loss of glycemic control).

No products indexed under this heading.

Dexamethasone Sodium Phosphate (Certain drugs, such as corticosteroids, tend to produce hyperglycemia and may lead to loss of glycemic control).

No products indexed under this heading.

Diatrizoate Meglumine (Potential for acute alteration of renal function; metformin should be temporarily withheld in patients undergoing radiologic studies involving parenteral iodinated contrast material).

No products indexed under this heading.

Diatrizoate Sodium (Potential for acute alteration of renal function; metformin should be temporarily withheld in patients undergoing radiologic studies involving parenteral iodinated contrast material).

No products indexed under this heading.

Dienestrol (Certain drugs, such as estrogens, tend to produce hyperglycemia and may lead to loss of glycemic control).

No products indexed under this heading.

Diethylstilbestrol (Certain drugs, such as estrogens, tend to produce hyperglycemia and may lead to loss of glycemic control).

No products indexed under this heading.

Digoxin (Theoretical potential for interaction with metformin by competing for common renal tubular transport system). Products include:

Lanoxin Injection 1498
Lanoxin Injection Pediatric 1502
Lanoxin Tablets 1505

Diltiazem Hydrochloride (Certain drugs, such as calcium channel blockers, tend to produce hyperglycemia and may lead to loss of glycemic control). Products include:

Cardizem LA Extended Release Tablets 421

Dobutamine Hydrochloride (Certain drugs, such as sympathomimetics, tend to produce hyperglycemia and may lead to loss of glycemic control).

No products indexed under this heading.

Dopamine Hydrochloride (Certain drugs, such as sympathomimetics, tend to produce hyperglycemia and may lead to loss of glycemic control).

No products indexed under this heading.

Ephedrine Hydrochloride (Certain drugs, such as sympathomimetics, tend to produce hyperglycemia and may lead to loss of glycemic control).

No products indexed under this heading.

Ephedrine Sulfate (Certain drugs, such as sympathomimetics, tend to produce hyperglycemia and may lead to loss of glycemic control).

No products indexed under this heading.

Ephedrine Tannate (Certain drugs, such as sympathomimetics, tend to produce hyperglycemia and may lead to loss of glycemic control).

No products indexed under this heading.

Epinephrine (Certain drugs, such as sympathomimetics, tend to produce hyperglycemia and may lead to loss of glycemic control). Products include:

EpiPen 1024

Epinephrine Bitartrate (Certain drugs, such as sympathomimetics, tend to produce hyperglycemia and may lead to loss of glycemic control).

No products indexed under this heading.

Epinephrine Hydrochloride (Certain drugs, such as sympathomimetics, tend to produce hyperglycemia and may lead to loss of glycemic control).

No products indexed under this heading.

Estradiol (Certain drugs, such as estrogens, tend to produce hyperglycemia and may lead to loss of glycemic control). Products include:

Activella Tablets 2347
Angeliq Tablets 751
Climara Transdermal System 763
Climara Pro Transdermal System 768
Divigel 3167
Vagifem Tablets 2375

Estrogens, Conjugated (Certain drugs, such as estrogens, tend to produce hyperglycemia and may lead to loss of glycemic control). Products include:

Premarin Intravenous 3217
Premarin Tablets 3221
Premarin Vaginal Cream 3228
Premphase Tablets 3232
Prempro Tablets 3232

Estrogens, Esterified (Certain drugs, such as estrogens, tend to produce hyperglycemia and may lead to loss of glycemic control). Products include:

Estratest Tablets 3043
Estratest H.S. Tablets 3043

Estropipate (Certain drugs, such as estrogens, tend to produce hyperglycemia and may lead to loss of glycemic control).

No products indexed under this heading.

Ethacrynic Acid (Certain drugs, such as diuretics, tend to produce hyperglycemia and may lead to loss of glycemic control). Products include:

Edecrin Tablets 698

Ethinyl Estradiol (Certain drugs, such as estrogens, tend to produce hyperglycemia and may lead to loss of glycemic control). Products include:

Lybrel Tablets 3204
Mircette Tablets 1034
NuvaRing 2897
Ortho-Cyclen/Ortho Tri-Cyclen 2449
Ortho Evra Transdermal System 2437
Ortho Tri-Cyclen Lo Tablets 2458
Seasonique Tablets 1046
Yaz Tablets 805

Ethiodized Oil (Potential for acute alteration of renal function; metformin should be temporarily withheld in patients undergoing radiologic studies involving parenteral iodinated contrast material).

No products indexed under this heading.

Ethynodiol Diacetate (Certain drugs, such as oral contraceptives, tend to produce hyperglycemia and may lead to loss of glycemic control).
No products indexed under this heading.

Felodipine (Certain drugs, such as calcium channel blockers, tend to produce hyperglycemia and may lead to loss of glycemic control).
No products indexed under this heading.

Fludrocortisone Acetate (Certain drugs, such as corticosteroids, tend to produce hyperglycemia and may lead to loss of glycemic control).
No products indexed under this heading.

Flunisolide (Certain drugs, such as corticosteroids, tend to produce hyperglycemia and may lead to loss of glycemic control). Products include:
Aerobid/Aerobid-M 1153

Fluphenazine Decanoate (Certain drugs, such as phenothiazines, tend to produce hyperglycemia and may lead to loss of glycemic control).
No products indexed under this heading.

Fluphenazine Enanthate (Certain drugs, such as phenothiazines, tend to produce hyperglycemia and may lead to loss of glycemic control).
No products indexed under this heading.

Fluphenazine Hydrochloride (Certain drugs, such as phenothiazines, tend to produce hyperglycemia and may lead to loss of glycemic control).
No products indexed under this heading.

Fluticasone Propionate (Certain drugs, such as corticosteroids, tend to produce hyperglycemia and may lead to loss of glycemic control). Products include:
Advair Diskus 100/50 1276
Advair Diskus 250/50 1276
Advair Diskus 500/50 1276
Advair HFA 45/21 Inhalation Aerosol 1288
Advair HFA 115/21 Inhalation Aerosol 1288
Advair HFA 230/21 Inhalation Aerosol 1288
Flonase Nasal Spray 1431
Flovent Diskus 50 mcg 1435

Fluticasone Propionate HFA (Certain drugs, such as corticosteroids, tend to produce hyperglycemia and may lead to loss of glycemic control). Products include:
Flovent HFA 1440

Fosphenytoin Sodium (Certain drugs, such as phenytoin, tend to produce hyperglycemia and may lead to loss of glycemic control).
No products indexed under this heading.

Furosemide (Increases metformin plasma and blood Cmax by 22% and blood AUC by 15%; the Cmax and AUC of furosemide were 31% and 12% smaller when co-administered; potential for loss of glycemic control). Products include:
Furosemide Tablets 2186

Gadopentetate Dimeglumine (Potential for acute alteration of renal function; metformin should be temporarily withheld in patients undergoing radiologic studies involving parenteral iodinated contrast material).
No products indexed under this heading.

Gemfibrozil (Concomitant administration of gemfibrozil (600 mg bid), an inhibitor of CYP2C8, and rosiglitazone (4 mg qd) for 7 days increased rosiglitazone AUC by 127%, compared to administration of rosiglitazone (4 mg qd) alone).
No products indexed under this heading.

Glimepiride (An increased incidence of heart failure has been observed when rosiglitazone was added to a sulfonylurea or to a sulfonylurea plus metformin). Products include:
Avandaryl Tablets 1344
Duetact Tablets 3085

Glipizide (An increased incidence of heart failure has been observed when rosiglitazone was added to a sulfonylurea or to a sulfonylurea plus metformin).
No products indexed under this heading.

Glyburide (Decrease in glyburide AUC and Cmax have been observed, but were highly variable).
No products indexed under this heading.

Hydrochlorothiazide (Certain drugs, such as thiazides and other diuretics, tend to produce hyperglycemia and may lead to loss of glycemic control). Products include:
Atacand HCT 642
Avalide Tablets 892
Avalide Tablets 2713
Benicar HCT Tablets 1010
Diovan HCT Tablets 2216
Dyazide Capsules 1405
Micardis HCT Tablets 854
Prinzide Tablets 2092
Tekturna HCT Tablets 2324
Teveten HCT Tablets 517

Hydrocortisone (Certain drugs, such as corticosteroids, tend to produce hyperglycemia and may lead to loss of glycemic control).
No products indexed under this heading.

Hydrocortisone Acetate (Certain drugs, such as corticosteroids, tend to produce hyperglycemia and may lead to loss of glycemic control). Products include:
Analpram-HC 1140
Pramosone 1141

Hydrocortisone Sodium Phosphate (Certain drugs, such as corticosteroids, tend to produce hyperglycemia and may lead to loss of glycemic control).
No products indexed under this heading.

Hydrocortisone Sodium Succinate (Certain drugs, such as corticosteroids, tend to produce hyperglycemia and may lead to loss of glycemic control).
No products indexed under this heading.

Hydroflumethiazide (Certain drugs, such as thiazides and other diuretics, tend to produce hyperglycemia and may lead to loss of glycemic control).
No products indexed under this heading.

Indapamide (Certain drugs, such as diuretics, tend to produce hyperglycemia and may lead to loss of glycemic control). Products include:
Indapamide Tablets 2188

Insulin (Co-administration of rosiglitazone with insulin has resulted in increased incidence of cardiac failure and other cardiovascular adverse events).
No products indexed under this heading.

Insulin, Human, Zinc Suspension (Co-administration of rosiglitazone with insulin has resulted in increased incidence of cardiac failure and other cardiovascular adverse events).
No products indexed under this heading.

Insulin, Human (rDNA origin) (Co-administration of rosiglitazone with insulin has resulted in increased incidence of cardiac failure and other cardiovascular adverse events). Products include:
Exubera Inhalation Powder 2515

Insulin, Human NPH (Co-administration of rosiglitazone with insulin has resulted in increased incidence of cardiac failure and other cardiovascular adverse events). Products include:
Humulin N Vial 1846

Insulin, Human Regular (Co-administration of rosiglitazone with insulin has resulted in increased incidence of cardiac failure and other cardiovascular adverse events). Products include:
Humulin R 1849
Humulin R (U-500) 1850

Insulin, Human Regular and Human NPH Mixture (Co-administration of rosiglitazone with insulin has resulted in increased incidence of cardiac failure and other cardiovascular adverse events). Products include:
Humulin 50/50, 100 Units 1843
Humulin 70/30 Vial 1844

Insulin, NPH (Co-administration of rosiglitazone with insulin has resulted in increased incidence of cardiac failure and other cardiovascular adverse events).
No products indexed under this heading.

Insulin, Regular (Co-administration of rosiglitazone with insulin has resulted in increased incidence of cardiac failure and other cardiovascular adverse events).
No products indexed under this heading.

Insulin, Regular and NPH mixture (Co-administration of rosiglitazone with insulin has resulted in increased incidence of cardiac failure and other cardiovascular adverse events).
No products indexed under this heading.

Insulin, Zinc Crystals (Co-administration of rosiglitazone with insulin has resulted in increased incidence of cardiac failure and other cardiovascular adverse events).
No products indexed under this heading.

Insulin, Zinc Suspension (Co-administration of rosiglitazone with insulin has resulted in increased incidence of cardiac failure and other cardiovascular adverse events).
No products indexed under this heading.

Insulin Aspart (Co-administration of rosiglitazone with insulin has resulted in increased incidence of cardiac failure and other cardiovascular adverse events).
No products indexed under this heading.

Insulin Aspart, Human (Co-administration of rosiglitazone with insulin has resulted in increased incidence of cardiac failure and other cardiovascular adverse events). Products include:
NovoLog Mix 70/30 2364

Insulin Aspart, Human Regular (Co-administration of rosiglitazone with insulin has resulted in increased incidence of cardiac failure and other cardiovascular adverse events). Products include:
NovoLog Injection 2359

Insulin Aspart Protamine, Human (Co-administration of rosiglitazone with insulin has resulted in increased incidence of cardiac failure and other cardiovascular adverse events). Products include:
NovoLog Mix 70/30 2364

Insulin Detemir (rDNA Origin) (Co-administration of rosiglitazone with insulin has resulted in increased incidence of cardiac failure and other cardiovascular adverse events). Products include:
Levemir Injection 2352

Insulin glargine (Co-administration of rosiglitazone with insulin has resulted in increased incidence of cardiac failure and other cardiovascular adverse events). Products include:
Lantus Injection 2749

Insulin Glulisine (Co-administration of rosiglitazone with insulin has resulted in increased incidence of cardiac failure and other cardiovascular adverse events). Products include:
Apidra Injection 2706

Insulin Lispro, Human (Co-administration of rosiglitazone with insulin has resulted in increased incidence of cardiac failure and other cardiovascular adverse events). Products include:
Humalog-Pen and KwikPen 1829
Humalog Mix 50/50-Pen and KwikPen 1833
Humalog Mix 75/25-Pen and KwikPen 1835

Insulin Lispro Protamine, Human (Co-administration of rosiglitazone with insulin has resulted in increased incidence of cardiac failure and other cardiovascular adverse events). Products include:
Humalog Mix 50/50-Pen and KwikPen 1833
Humalog Mix 75/25-Pen and KwikPen 1835

Iodamide Meglumine (Potential for acute alteration of renal function; metformin should be temporarily withheld in patients undergoing radiologic studies involving parenteral iodinated contrast material).
No products indexed under this heading.

Iohexol (Potential for acute alteration of renal function; metformin should be temporarily withheld in patients undergoing radiologic studies involving parenteral iodinated contrast material).
No products indexed under this heading.

IMPORTANT NOTE: Always consult each drug listing in the patient's regimen for possible interactions.

Iopamidol (Potential for acute alteration of renal function; metformin should be temporarily withheld in patients undergoing radiologic studies involving parenteral iodinated contrast material).
No products indexed under this heading.

Iopanoic Acid (Potential for acute alteration of renal function; metformin should be temporarily withheld in patients undergoing radiologic studies involving parenteral iodinated contrast material).
No products indexed under this heading.

Iothalamate Meglumine (Potential for acute alteration of renal function; metformin should be temporarily withheld in patients undergoing radiologic studies involving parenteral iodinated contrast material).
No products indexed under this heading.

Ioxaglate Meglumine (Potential for acute alteration of renal function; metformin should be temporarily withheld in patients undergoing radiologic studies involving parenteral iodinated contrast material).
No products indexed under this heading.

Ioxaglate Sodium (Potential for acute alteration of renal function; metformin should be temporarily withheld in patients undergoing radiologic studies involving parenteral iodinated contrast material).
No products indexed under this heading.

Isoniazid (Certain drugs, such as isoniazid, tend to produce hyperglycemia and may lead to loss of glycemic control).
No products indexed under this heading.

Isoproterenol Hydrochloride (Certain drugs, such as sympathomimetics, tend to produce hyperglycemia and may lead to loss of glycemic control).
No products indexed under this heading.

Isoproterenol Sulfate (Certain drugs, such as sympathomimetics, tend to produce hyperglycemia and may lead to loss of glycemic control).
No products indexed under this heading.

Isradipine (Certain drugs, such as calcium channel blockers, tend to produce hyperglycemia and may lead to loss of glycemic control). Products include:
DynaCirc CR Controlled Release Tablets 1407

Levalbuterol Hydrochloride (Certain drugs, such as sympathomimetics, tend to produce hyperglycemia and may lead to loss of glycemic control). Products include:
Xopenex Inhalation Solution 3001
Xopenex Inhalation Solution Concentrate 3005

Levonorgestrel (Certain drugs, such as oral contraceptives, tend to produce hyperglycemia and may lead to loss of glycemic control). Products include:
Climara Pro Transdermal System 768
Lybrel Tablets 3204
Mirena Intrauterine System 779
Plan B Tablets 1044
Seasonique Tablets 1046

Levothyroxine Sodium (Certain drugs, such as thyroid products, tend to produce hyperglycemia and may lead to loss of glycemic control). Products include:
Levothroid Tablets 1170
Levoxyl Tablets 1780
Synthroid Tablets 507

Liothyronine Sodium (Certain drugs, such as thyroid products, tend to produce hyperglycemia and may lead to loss of glycemic control). Products include:
Cytomel Tablets 1778

Liotrix (Certain drugs, such as thyroid products, tend to produce hyperglycemia and may lead to loss of glycemic control).
No products indexed under this heading.

Mesoridazine Besylate (Certain drugs, such as phenothiazines, tend to produce hyperglycemia and may lead to loss of glycemic control).
No products indexed under this heading.

Mestranol (Certain drugs, such as oral contraceptives, tend to produce hyperglycemia and may lead to loss of glycemic control).
No products indexed under this heading.

Metaproterenol Sulfate (Certain drugs, such as sympathomimetics, tend to produce hyperglycemia and may lead to loss of glycemic control).
No products indexed under this heading.

Metaraminol Bitartrate (Certain drugs, such as sympathomimetics, tend to produce hyperglycemia and may lead to loss of glycemic control).
No products indexed under this heading.

Methotrimeprazine (Certain drugs, such as phenothiazines, tend to produce hyperglycemia and may lead to loss of glycemic control).
No products indexed under this heading.

Methoxamine Hydrochloride (Certain drugs, such as sympathomimetics, tend to produce hyperglycemia and may lead to loss of glycemic control).
No products indexed under this heading.

Methyclothiazide (Certain drugs, such as thiazides and other diuretics, tend to produce hyperglycemia and may lead to loss of glycemic control).
No products indexed under this heading.

Methylprednisolone Acetate (Certain drugs, such as corticosteroids, tend to produce hyperglycemia and may lead to loss of glycemic control).
No products indexed under this heading.

Methylprednisolone Sodium Succinate (Certain drugs, such as corticosteroids, tend to produce hyperglycemia and may lead to loss of glycemic control).
No products indexed under this heading.

Metolazone (Certain drugs, such as diuretics, tend to produce hyperglycemia and may lead to loss of glycemic control).
No products indexed under this heading.

Mibefradil Dihydrochloride (Certain drugs, such as calcium channel blockers, tend to produce hyperglycemia and may lead to loss of glycemic control).
No products indexed under this heading.

Miglitol (Patients receiving rosiglitazone in combination with other hypoglycemic agents may be at risk for hypoglycemia and a reduction in the dose of the concomitant agent may be necessary).
No products indexed under this heading.

Mometasone Furoate (Certain drugs, such as corticosteroids, tend to produce hyperglycemia and may lead to loss of glycemic control). Products include:
Asmanex Twisthaler 2797
Elocon Cream 0.1% 2840
Elocon Lotion 0.1% 2841
Elocon Ointment 0.1% 2842

Mometasone Furoate Monohydrate (Certain drugs, such as corticosteroids, tend to produce hyperglycemia and may lead to loss of glycemic control). Products include:
Nasonex Nasal Spray 2883

Morphine Sulfate (Theoretical potential for interaction with metformin by competing for common renal tubular transport system). Products include:
Avinza Capsules 1772
DepoDur Injection 1095
MS Contin Tablets 2585

Nateglinide (Patients receiving rosiglitazone in combination with other hypoglycemic agents may be at risk for hypoglycemia and a reduction in the dose of the concomitant agent may be necessary). Products include:
Starlix Tablets 2314

Niacin (Certain drugs, such as niacin, tend to produce hyperglycemia and may lead to loss of glycemic control). Products include:
Advicor Tablets 402
Bausch & Lomb Ocuvite DF Vitamin Supplement .... ⊙ 238
Dismutax Dietary Supplement 995
Niaspan Extended-Release Tablets 480
NT-Kinase Dietary Supplement 995
Simcor Tablets 502

Nicardipine Hydrochloride (Certain drugs, such as calcium channel blockers, tend to produce hyperglycemia and may lead to loss of glycemic control). Products include:
Cardene I.V. 1093

Nicotinic Acid (Potential for loss of glycemic control).
No products indexed under this heading.

Nifedipine (Enhances the absorption of metformin by increasing plasma metformin Cmax and AUC; potential for loss of glycemic control).
No products indexed under this heading.

Nimodipine (Certain drugs, such as calcium channel blockers, tend to produce hyperglycemia and may lead to loss of glycemic control). Products include:
Nimotop Capsules 790

Nisoldipine (Certain drugs, such as calcium channel blockers, tend to produce hyperglycemia and may lead to loss of glycemic control). Products include:
Sular Extended Release Tablets 2975

Norepinephrine Bitartrate (Certain drugs, such as sympathomimetics, tend to produce hyperglycemia and may lead to loss of glycemic control).
No products indexed under this heading.

Norethindrone (Certain drugs, such as oral contraceptives, tend to produce hyperglycemia and may lead to loss of glycemic control). Products include:
Ortho Micronor Tablets 2446

Norethynodrel (Certain drugs, such as oral contraceptives, tend to produce hyperglycemia and may lead to loss of glycemic control).
No products indexed under this heading.

Norgestimate (Certain drugs, such as oral contraceptives, tend to produce hyperglycemia and may lead to loss of glycemic control). Products include:
Ortho-Cyclen/Ortho Tri-Cyclen 2449
Ortho Tri-Cyclen Lo Tablets 2458

Norgestrel (Certain drugs, such as oral contraceptives, tend to produce hyperglycemia and may lead to loss of glycemic control).
No products indexed under this heading.

Omeprazole (An inhibitor of CYP2C8 may increase the AUC of rosiglitazone).
No products indexed under this heading.

Perphenazine (Certain drugs, such as phenothiazines, tend to produce hyperglycemia and may lead to loss of glycemic control).
No products indexed under this heading.

Phenobarbital (An inducer of CYP2C8 may decrease the AUC of rosiglitazone). Products include:
Donnatal Extentabs 2507

Phenylephrine Bitartrate (Certain drugs, such as sympathomimetics, tend to produce hyperglycemia and may lead to loss of glycemic control).
No products indexed under this heading.

Phenylephrine Hydrochloride (Certain drugs, such as sympathomimetics, tend to produce hyperglycemia and may lead to loss of glycemic control). Products include:
Actifed Cold & Allergy Tablets 1895
Benadryl Allergy & Cold Kapgels 1895
Benadryl Allergy & Sinus Headache Kapgels 1895
Benadryl Severe Allergy & Sinus Headache Caplets 1897
Children's Benadryl-D Allergy & Sinus Liquid 1896
Benadryl-D Allergy & Sinus Tablet 1896
PediaCare Children's Allergy & Cold Liquid 1902
PediaCare Children's Decongestant Liquid 1902
PediaCare Children's Liquid Multi-Symptom Cold 1902
Sinutab Non-Drying Caplets 1905
Sinutab Sinus Caplets 1905
Children's Sudafed PE Cold & Cough Liquid 1907
Children's Sudafed PE Nasal Decongestant Liquid 1906
Sudafed PE Cold & Cough Caplets 1907
Sudafed PE Nasal Decongestant Tablets 1907
Sudafed PE Nighttime Cold Caplets 1907
Sudafed PE Non-Drying Sinus Caplets 1908
Sudafed PE Severe Cold Caplets 1908

Sudafed PE Sinus & Allergy Tablets 1908
Sudafed PE Sinus Headache Caplets 1908
Tylenol Allergy Multi-Symptom Caplets with Cool Burst and Rapid Release Gelcaps 1916
Tylenol Allergy Multi-Symptom Nighttime Caplets with Cool Burst 1916
Children's Tylenol Plus Cold Suspension Liquid 1912
Children's Tylenol Plus Cold & Allergy Suspension Liquid 1914
Children's Tylenol Plus Flu Suspension Liquid 1914
Children's Tylenol Plus Multi-Symptom Cold Suspension Liquid 1912
Tylenol Cold Head Congestion Daytime Caplets with Cool Burst 1910
Tylenol Cold Head Congestion Nighttime Caplets with Cool Burst 1910
Tylenol Cold Head Congestion Severe Daytime Caplets with Cool Burst 1910
Tylenol Cold Multi-Symptom Daytime Caplets with Cool Burst and Rapid Release Gels 1913
Tylenol Cold Multi-Symptom Daytime Liquid with Citrus Burst 1913
Tylenol Cold Multi-Symptom Nighttime Caplets with Cool Burst 1913
Tylenol Cold Multi-Symptom Nighttime Liquid with Cool Burst 1913
Tylenol Cold Multi-Symptom Severe Caplets with Cool Burst 1913
Tylenol Cold Multi-Symptom Severe Daytime Liquid with Citrus Burst 1913
Tylenol Sinus Congestion & Pain Daytime Caplets with Cool Burst and Gelcaps 1917
Tylenol Sinus Congestion & Pain Nighttime Caplets with Cool Burst 1917
Tylenol Sinus Congestion & Pain Severe Caplets with Cool Burst 1917
Vicks DayQuil Cold & Flu Multi-Symptom Relief 616
Vicks DayQuil LiquiCaps 2567
Vicks DayQuil Liquid 2567
Vicks DayQuil Multi-Symptom Cold/Flu Relief 2567

Phenylephrine Tannate (Certain drugs, such as sympathomimetics, tend to produce hyperglycemia and may lead to loss of glycemic control).
No products indexed under this heading.

Phenylpropanolamine Hydrochloride (Certain drugs, such as sympathomimetics, tend to produce hyperglycemia and may lead to loss of glycemic control).
No products indexed under this heading.

Phenytoin (Certain drugs, such as phenytoin, tend to produce hyperglycemia and may lead to loss of glycemic control).
No products indexed under this heading.

Phenytoin Sodium (Certain drugs, such as phenytoin, tend to produce hyperglycemia and may lead to loss of glycemic control). Products include:
Phenytek Capsules 2192

Pioglitazone Hydrochloride (Patients receiving rosiglitazone in combination with other hypoglycemic agents may be at risk for hypoglycemia and a reduction in the dose of the concomitant agent may be necessary). Products include:
ActoPlus Met Tablets 3071
Actos Tablets 3077
Duetact Tablets 3085

Pirbuterol Acetate (Certain drugs, such as sympathomimetics, tend to produce hyperglycemia and may lead to loss of glycemic control). Products include:
Maxair Autohaler 1705

Polyestradiol Phosphate (Certain drugs, such as estrogens, tend to produce hyperglycemia and may lead to loss of glycemic control).
No products indexed under this heading.

Polythiazide (Certain drugs, such as thiazides and other diuretics, tend to produce hyperglycemia and may lead to loss of glycemic control).
No products indexed under this heading.

Prednisolone Acetate (Certain drugs, such as corticosteroids, tend to produce hyperglycemia and may lead to loss of glycemic control). Products include:
Pred Forte Ophthalmic Suspension .... ⊙ 227
Pred Mild Ophthalmic Suspension .... ⊙ 230
Pred-G Ophthalmic Ointment .... ⊙ 229
Pred-G Ophthalmic Suspension .... ⊙ 228

Prednisolone Sodium Phosphate (Certain drugs, such as corticosteroids, tend to produce hyperglycemia and may lead to loss of glycemic control).
No products indexed under this heading.

Prednisolone Tebutate (Certain drugs, such as corticosteroids, tend to produce hyperglycemia and may lead to loss of glycemic control).
No products indexed under this heading.

Prednisone (Certain drugs, such as corticosteroids, tend to produce hyperglycemia and may lead to loss of glycemic control).
No products indexed under this heading.

Primidone (An inducer of CYP2C8 may decrease the AUC of rosiglitazone).
No products indexed under this heading.

Procainamide Hydrochloride (Theoretical potential for interaction with metformin by competing for common renal tubular transport system).
No products indexed under this heading.

Prochlorperazine (Certain drugs, such as phenothiazines, tend to produce hyperglycemia and may lead to loss of glycemic control).
No products indexed under this heading.

Promethazine Hydrochloride (Certain drugs, such as phenothiazines, tend to produce hyperglycemia and may lead to loss of glycemic control).
No products indexed under this heading.

Pseudoephedrine Hydrochloride (Certain drugs, such as sympathomimetics, tend to produce hyperglycemia and may lead to loss of glycemic control). Products include:
Allegra-D 12 Hour Extended-Release Tablets 2687
Allegra-D 24 Hour Extended-Release Tablets 2690
Children's Motrin Cold Oral Suspension 1899
Sudafed 12 Hour Nasal Decongestant Non-Drowsy Caplets 1909
Sudafed 24 Hour Non-Drowsy Nasal Decongestant Tablets 1906
Children's Sudafed Nasal Decongestant Liquid 1906
Sudafed Nasal Decongestant Tablets 1906
Tylenol Cold Severe Congestion Daytime Caplets with Cool Burst 1912
Tylenol Sinus Severe Congestion Caplets with Cool Burst 1917
Vicks NyQuil LiquiCaps 2567
Vicks NyQuil Liquid 2567
Vicks NyQuil Multi-Symptom Cold/Flu Relief 2567
Zyrtec-D 12 Hour Extended Release Tablets 1923
Zyrtec-D Allergy & Congestion Extended-Release Tablets 1923

Pseudoephedrine Sulfate (Certain drugs, such as sympathomimetics, tend to produce hyperglycemia and may lead to loss of glycemic control). Products include:
Clarinex-D 12-Hour Extended-Release Tablets 2831
Clarinex-D 24-Hour Extended-Release Tablets 2834

Quercetin (An inhibitor of CYP2C8 may increase the AUC of rosiglitazone).
No products indexed under this heading.

Quinestrol (Certain drugs, such as estrogens, tend to produce hyperglycemia and may lead to loss of glycemic control).
No products indexed under this heading.

Quinidine (Theoretical potential for interaction with metformin by competing for common renal tubular transport system).
No products indexed under this heading.

Quinidine Gluconate (Theoretical potential for interaction with metformin by competing for common renal tubular transport system).
No products indexed under this heading.

Quinidine Hydrochloride (Theoretical potential for interaction with metformin by competing for common renal tubular transport system).
No products indexed under this heading.

Quinidine Polygalacturonate (Theoretical potential for interaction with metformin by competing for common renal tubular transport system).
No products indexed under this heading.

Quinidine Sulfate (Theoretical potential for interaction with metformin by competing for common renal tubular transport system).
No products indexed under this heading.

Quinine Sulfate (Theoretical potential for interaction with metformin by competing for common renal tubular transport system).
No products indexed under this heading.

Ranitidine Hydrochloride (Theoretical potential for interaction with metformin by competing for common renal tubular transport system). Products include:
Zantac 75 Tablets 603
Zantac 1670
Zantac Injection 1666
Zantac Injection Pharmacy Bulk Package 1668
Maximum Strength Zantac 150 Tablets 603
Maximum Strength Zantac 150 Cool Mint Tablets 603

Repaglinide (Patients receiving rosiglitazone in combination with other hypoglycemic agents may be at risk for hypoglycemia and a reduction in the dose of the concomitant agent may be necessary). Products include:
PrandiMet Tablets 2967
Prandin Tablets 2971

Rifabutin (An inducer of CYP2C8 may decrease the AUC of rosiglitazone).
No products indexed under this heading.

Rifampin (Rifampin administration (600 mg qd) an inducer of CYP2C8, for 6 days is reported to decrease rosiglitazone AUC by 66%, compared to administration of rosiglitazone (8 mg) alone).
No products indexed under this heading.

Salmeterol Xinafoate (Certain drugs, such as sympathomimetics, tend to produce hyperglycemia and may lead to loss of glycemic control). Products include:
Advair Diskus 100/50 1276
Advair Diskus 250/50 1276
Advair Diskus 500/50 1276
Advair HFA 45/21 Inhalation Aerosol 1288
Advair HFA 115/21 Inhalation Aerosol 1288
Advair HFA 230/21 Inhalation Aerosol 1288
Serevent Diskus 1594

Sitagliptin Phosphate (Patients receiving rosiglitazone in combination with other hypoglycemic agents may be at risk for hypoglycemia and a reduction in the dose of the concomitant agent may be necessary). Products include:
Janumet Tablets 2041
Januvia Tablets 2048

Spironolactone (Certain drugs, such as diuretics, tend to produce hyperglycemia and may lead to loss of glycemic control).
No products indexed under this heading.

Sulfaphenazole (An inhibitor of CYP2C8 may increase the AUC of rosiglitazone).
No products indexed under this heading.

Sulfinpyrazone (An inhibitor of CYP2C8 may increase the AUC of rosiglitazone).
No products indexed under this heading.

Terbutaline Sulfate (Certain drugs, such as sympathomimetics, tend to produce hyperglycemia and may lead to loss of glycemic control).
No products indexed under this heading.

Thioridazine Hydrochloride (Certain drugs, such as phenothiazines, tend to produce hyperglycemia and may lead to loss of glycemic control). Products include:
Thioridazine Hydrochloride Tablets 2195

Thyroglobulin (Certain drugs, such as thyroid products, tend to produce hyperglycemia and may lead to loss of glycemic control).
No products indexed under this heading.

Thyroid (Certain drugs, such as thyroid products, tend to produce hyperglycemia and may lead to loss of glycemic control). Products include:

IMPORTANT NOTE: Always consult each drug listing in the patient's regimen for possible interactions.

Naturethroid Tablets 2605

Thyroxine (Certain drugs, such as thyroid products, tend to produce hyperglycemia and may lead to loss of glycemic control).
No products indexed under this heading.

Thyroxine Sodium (Certain drugs, such as thyroid products, tend to produce hyperglycemia and may lead to loss of glycemic control).
No products indexed under this heading.

Tolazamide (An increased incidence of heart failure has been observed when rosiglitazone was added to a sulfonylurea or to a sulfonylurea plus metformin).
No products indexed under this heading.

Tolbutamide (An increased incidence of heart failure has been observed when rosiglitazone was added to a sulfonylurea or to a sulfonylurea plus metformin).
No products indexed under this heading.

Torsemide (Certain drugs, such as diuretics, tend to produce hyperglycemia and may lead to loss of glycemic control). Products include:
Demadex Injection 2630
Demadex Tablets 2630

Triamcinolone (Certain drugs, such as corticosteroids, tend to produce hyperglycemia and may lead to loss of glycemic control).
No products indexed under this heading.

Triamcinolone Acetonide (Certain drugs, such as corticosteroids, tend to produce hyperglycemia and may lead to loss of glycemic control). Products include:
Azmacort Inhalation Aerosol 407
Nasacort AQ Nasal Spray 2765
Triesence Injectable Suspension .... ⊙209

Triamcinolone Diacetate (Certain drugs, such as corticosteroids, tend to produce hyperglycemia and may lead to loss of glycemic control).
No products indexed under this heading.

Triamcinolone Hexacetonide (Certain drugs, such as corticosteroids, tend to produce hyperglycemia and may lead to loss of glycemic control).
No products indexed under this heading.

Triamterene (Potential for loss of glycemic control; theoretical potential for interaction with metformin by competing for common renal tubular transport system). Products include:
Dyazide Capsules 1405
Dyrenium Capsules 3189

Trifluoperazine Hydrochloride (Certain drugs, such as phenothiazines, tend to produce hyperglycemia and may lead to loss of glycemic control).
No products indexed under this heading.

Trimethoprim (Theoretical potential for interaction with metformin by competing for common renal tubular transport system).
No products indexed under this heading.

Trimethoprim Hydrochloride (An inhibitor of CYP2C8 may increase the AUC of rosiglitazone).
No products indexed under this heading.

Trimethoprim Sulfate (Theoretical potential for interaction with metformin by competing for common renal tubular transport system).
No products indexed under this heading.

Troglitazone (Patients receiving rosiglitazone in combination with other hypoglycemic agents may be at risk for hypoglycemia and a reduction in the dose of the concomitant agent may be necessary).
No products indexed under this heading.

Tyropanoate Sodium (Potential for acute alteration of renal function; metformin should be temporarily withheld in patients undergoing radiologic studies involving parenteral iodinated contrast material).
No products indexed under this heading.

Vancomycin Hydrochloride (Theoretical potential for interaction with metformin by competing for common renal tubular transport system).
No products indexed under this heading.

Verapamil Hydrochloride (Certain drugs, such as calcium channel blockers, tend to produce hyperglycemia and may lead to loss of glycemic control). Products include:
Tarka Tablets 511

Food Interactions

Alcohol (Alcohol potentiates the effect of metformin on lactate metabolism; patients should be warned against excessive alcohol intake, acute or chronic).

Food, unspecified (Food decreases the extent and slightly delays the absorption of metformin).

AVANDARYL TABLETS

(Glimepiride, Rosiglitazone Maleate) 1344

May interact with non-steroidal anti-inflammatory agents, oral contraceptives, phenothiazines, salicylates, sulfonamides, sympathomimetics, thiazides, thyroid preparations, and certain other agents. Compounds in these categories include:

Acebutolol Hydrochloride (May potentiate hypoglycemic action).
No products indexed under this heading.

Albuterol (Sympathomimetics tend to produce hyperglycemia and concurrent use may lead to loss of control).
No products indexed under this heading.

Albuterol Sulfate (Sympathomimetics tend to produce hyperglycemia and concurrent use may lead to loss of control). Products include:
Combivent Inhalation Aerosol 845
ProAir HFA Inhalation Aerosol 3113
Proventil HFA Inhalation Aerosol 2914
Ventolin HFA Inhalation Aerosol 1638

Amiloride Hydrochloride (Diuretics tend to produce hyperglycemia and concurrent use may lead to loss of control).
No products indexed under this heading.

Anastrozole (An inhibitor of CYP2C8 may decrease the AUC of rosiglitazone. Therefore, if an inducer of CYP2C8 is started or stopped during treatment with rosiglitazone, changes in diabetes treatment may be needed upon clinical response). Products include:
Arimidex Tablets 672

Anisindione (May potentiate hypoglycemic action).
No products indexed under this heading.

Aspirin (Co-administration of aspirin (1 g tid) led to a 34% decrease in the mean glimepiride AUC and, therefore, a 34% increase in the mean CL/f; no hypoglycemic symptoms were reported). Products include:
Aggrenox Capsules 819
Bayer Aspirin 750
Percodan Tablets 1130
St. Joseph 81 mg Aspirin Chewable and Enteric Coated Tablets 1903

Aspirin, Enteric Coated (May potentiate hypoglycemic action; clinical trials data indicate no evidence of significant adverse interaction with concurrent use).
No products indexed under this heading.

Aspirin Buffered (May potentiate hypoglycemic action; clinical trials data indicate no evidence of significant adverse interaction with concurrent use).
No products indexed under this heading.

Atenolol (May potentiate hypoglycemic action).
No products indexed under this heading.

Bendroflumethiazide (Diuretics tend to produce hyperglycemia and concurrent use may lead to loss of control).
No products indexed under this heading.

Betamethasone Acetate (Corticosteroids tend to produce hyperglycemia and concurrent use may lead to loss of control).
No products indexed under this heading.

Betamethasone Sodium Phosphate (Corticosteroids tend to produce hyperglycemia and concurrent use may lead to loss of control).
No products indexed under this heading.

Betaxolol Hydrochloride (May potentiate hypoglycemic action).
No products indexed under this heading.

Bisoprolol Fumarate (May potentiate hypoglycemic action).
No products indexed under this heading.

Budesonide (Corticosteroids tend to produce hyperglycemia and concurrent use may lead to loss of control). Products include:
Pulmicort Flexhaler 654
Symbicort 80/4.5 Inhalation Aerosol 659
Symbicort 160/4.5 Inhalation Aerosol 659

Bumetanide (Diuretics tend to produce hyperglycemia and concurrent use may lead to loss of control).
No products indexed under this heading.

Carbamazepine (An inhibitor of CYP2C8 may decrease the AUC of rosiglitazone. Therefore, if an inducer of CYP2C8 is started or stopped during treatment with rosiglitazone, changes in diabetes treatment may be needed upon clinical response). Products include:
Carbatrol Capsules 3019
Equetro Extended-Release Capsules 3174

Carteolol Hydrochloride (May potentiate hypoglycemic action).
No products indexed under this heading.

Celecoxib (May potentiate hypoglycemic action). Products include:
Celebrex Capsules 2979

Chloramphenicol (May potentiate hypoglycemic action).
No products indexed under this heading.

Chloramphenicol Palmitate (May potentiate hypoglycemic action).
No products indexed under this heading.

Chloramphenicol Sodium Succinate (May potentiate hypoglycemic action).
No products indexed under this heading.

Chlorothiazide (Diuretics tend to produce hyperglycemia and concurrent use may lead to loss of control).
No products indexed under this heading.

Chlorothiazide Sodium (Diuretics tend to produce hyperglycemia and concurrent use may lead to loss of control). Products include:
Intravenous Sodium Diuril 2490

Chlorotrianisene (Estrogens tend to produce hyperglycemia and concurrent use may lead to loss of control).
No products indexed under this heading.

Chlorpromazine (Phenothiazines tend to produce hyperglycemia and concurrent use may lead to loss of control).
No products indexed under this heading.

Chlorpromazine Hydrochloride (Phenothiazines tend to produce hyperglycemia and concurrent use may lead to loss of control).
No products indexed under this heading.

Chlorpropamide (May potentiate hypoglycemic action).
No products indexed under this heading.

Chlorthalidone (Diuretics tend to produce hyperglycemia and concurrent use may lead to loss of control). Products include:
Clorpres Tablets 2185

Choline Magnesium Trisalicylate (May potentiate hypoglycemic action; clinical trials data indicate no evidence of significant adverse interaction with concurrent use).
No products indexed under this heading.

Ciclesonide (Corticosteroids tend to produce hyperglycemia and concurrent use may lead to loss of control). Products include:
Alvesco Inhalation Aerosol 2985
Omnaris Nasal Spray 2998

Cimetidine (An inhibitor of CYP2C8 may decrease the AUC of rosiglitazone. Therefore, if an inducer of CYP2C8 is started or stopped during treatment with rosiglitazone, changes in diabetes treatment may be needed upon clinical response).
No products indexed under this heading.

Cimetidine Hydrochloride (An inhibitor of CYP2C8 may decrease the AUC of rosiglitazone. Therefore, if an inducer of CYP2C8 is started or stopped during treatment with rosiglitazone, changes in diabetes treatment may be needed upon clinical response).
No products indexed under this heading.

Cortisone Acetate (Corticosteroids tend to produce hyperglycemia and concurrent use may lead to loss of control).
No products indexed under this heading.

Desogestrel (Oral contraceptives tend to produce hyperglycemia and concurrent use may lead to loss of control). Products include:
Mircette Tablets 1034

Dexamethasone (Corticosteroids tend to produce hyperglycemia and concurrent use may lead to loss of control). Products include:
Ciprodex Otic Suspension 541

Dexamethasone Acetate (Corticosteroids tend to produce hyperglycemia and concurrent use may lead to loss of control).
No products indexed under this heading.

Dexamethasone Sodium Phosphate (Corticosteroids tend to produce hyperglycemia and concurrent use may lead to loss of control).
No products indexed under this heading.

Diclofenac Epolamine (May potentiate hypoglycemic action). Products include:
Flector Patch 561

Diclofenac Potassium (May potentiate hypoglycemic action).
No products indexed under this heading.

Diclofenac Sodium (May potentiate hypoglycemic action). Products include:
Diclofenac Sodium Ophthalmic Solution .... ⊙ 240
Voltaren Ophthalmic Solution 2336
Voltaren Tablets 2334
Voltaren-XR Tablets 2337

Dicumarol (May potentiate hypoglycemic action).
No products indexed under this heading.

Dienestrol (Estrogens tend to produce hyperglycemia and concurrent use may lead to loss of control).
No products indexed under this heading.

Diethylstilbestrol (Estrogens tend to produce hyperglycemia and concurrent use may lead to loss of control).
No products indexed under this heading.

Diflunisal (May potentiate hypoglycemic action; clinical trials data indicate no evidence of significant adverse interaction with concurrent use).
No products indexed under this heading.

Dobutamine Hydrochloride (Sympathomimetics tend to produce hyperglycemia and concurrent use may lead to loss of control).
No products indexed under this heading.

Dopamine Hydrochloride (Sympathomimetics tend to produce hyperglycemia and concurrent use may lead to loss of control).
No products indexed under this heading.

Ephedrine Hydrochloride (Sympathomimetics tend to produce hyperglycemia and concurrent use may lead to loss of control).
No products indexed under this heading.

Ephedrine Sulfate (Sympathomimetics tend to produce hyperglycemia and concurrent use may lead to loss of control).
No products indexed under this heading.

Ephedrine Tannate (Sympathomimetics tend to produce hyperglycemia and concurrent use may lead to loss of control).
No products indexed under this heading.

Epinephrine (Sympathomimetics tend to produce hyperglycemia and concurrent use may lead to loss of control). Products include:
EpiPen 1024

Epinephrine Bitartrate (Sympathomimetics tend to produce hyperglycemia and concurrent use may lead to loss of control).
No products indexed under this heading.

Epinephrine Hydrochloride (Sympathomimetics tend to produce hyperglycemia and concurrent use may lead to loss of control).
No products indexed under this heading.

Esmolol Hydrochloride (May potentiate hypoglycemic action).
No products indexed under this heading.

Estradiol (Estrogens tend to produce hyperglycemia and concurrent use may lead to loss of control). Products include:
Activella Tablets 2347
Angeliq Tablets 751
Climara Transdermal System 763
Climara Pro Transdermal System 768
Divigel 3167
Vagifem Tablets 2375

Estrogens, Conjugated (Estrogens tend to produce hyperglycemia and concurrent use may lead to loss of control). Products include:
Premarin Intravenous 3217
Premarin Tablets 3221
Premarin Vaginal Cream 3228
Premphase Tablets 3232
Prempro Tablets 3232

Estrogens, Esterified (Estrogens tend to produce hyperglycemia and concurrent use may lead to loss of control). Products include:
Estratest Tablets 3043
Estratest H.S. Tablets 3043

Estropipate (Estrogens tend to produce hyperglycemia and concurrent use may lead to loss of control).
No products indexed under this heading.

Ethacrynic Acid (Diuretics tend to produce hyperglycemia and concurrent use may lead to loss of control). Products include:
Edecrin Tablets 698

Ethinyl Estradiol (Estrogens tend to produce hyperglycemia and concurrent use may lead to loss of control). Products include:
Lybrel Tablets 3204
Mircette Tablets 1034
NuvaRing 2897
Ortho-Cyclen/Ortho Tri-Cyclen 2449
Ortho Evra Transdermal System 2437
Ortho Tri-Cyclen Lo Tablets 2458
Seasonique Tablets 1046
Yaz Tablets 805

Ethynodiol Diacetate (Oral contraceptives tend to produce hyperglycemia and concurrent use may lead to loss of control).
No products indexed under this heading.

Etodolac (May potentiate hypoglycemic action).
No products indexed under this heading.

Fenoprofen Calcium (May potentiate hypoglycemic action). Products include:
Nalfon Capsules 2508

Fludrocortisone Acetate (Corticosteroids tend to produce hyperglycemia and concurrent use may lead to loss of control).
No products indexed under this heading.

Flunisolide (Corticosteroids tend to produce hyperglycemia and concurrent use may lead to loss of control). Products include:
Aerobid/Aerobid-M 1153

Fluphenazine Decanoate (Phenothiazines tend to produce hyperglycemia and concurrent use may lead to loss of control).
No products indexed under this heading.

Fluphenazine Enanthate (Phenothiazines tend to produce hyperglycemia and concurrent use may lead to loss of control).
No products indexed under this heading.

Fluphenazine Hydrochloride (Phenothiazines tend to produce hyperglycemia and concurrent use may lead to loss of control).
No products indexed under this heading.

Flurbiprofen (May potentiate hypoglycemic action).
No products indexed under this heading.

Fluticasone Propionate (Corticosteroids tend to produce hyperglycemia and concurrent use may lead to loss of control). Products include:
Advair Diskus 100/50 1276
Advair Diskus 250/50 1276
Advair Diskus 500/50 1276
Advair HFA 45/21 Inhalation Aerosol 1288
Advair HFA 115/21 Inhalation Aerosol 1288
Advair HFA 230/21 Inhalation Aerosol 1288
Flonase Nasal Spray 1431
Flovent Diskus 50 mcg 1435

Fluticasone Propionate HFA (Corticosteroids tend to produce hyperglycemia and concurrent use may lead to loss of control). Products include:
Flovent HFA 1440

Furosemide (Diuretics tend to produce hyperglycemia and concurrent use may lead to loss of control). Products include:
Furosemide Tablets 2186

Gemfibrozil (Concomitant administration of gemfibrozil (600 mg twice daily), an inhibitor of CYP2C8 and rosiglitazone (4 mg once daily) for 7 days increased rosiglitazone AUC by 127% compared to the administration of rosiglitazone (4 mg once daily) alone. Given the potential for dose-related adverse events with rosiglitazone, a decrease in the dose of rosiglitazone may be needed when gemfibrozil is introduced).
No products indexed under this heading.

Glipizide (May potentiate hypoglycemic action).
No products indexed under this heading.

Glyburide (Rosiglitazone (2 mg twice daily) taken concomitantly with glyburide (3.75 to 10 mg/day) for 7 days did not alter the mean steady-state 24-hour plasma glucose concentrations in diabetic patients stabilized on glyburide therapy. Repeat doses of rosiglitazone (8 mg once daily) for 8 days in healthy adult Caucasian subjects caused a decrease in glyburide AUC (32%) and Cmax (35%). In Japanese subjects, glyburide AUC (14%) and Cmax (31%) slightly increased following co-administration of rosiglitazone).
No products indexed under this heading.

Hydrochlorothiazide (Diuretics tend to produce hyperglycemia and concurrent use may lead to loss of control). Products include:
Atacand HCT 642
Avalide Tablets 892
Avalide Tablets 2713
Benicar HCT Tablets 1010
Diovan HCT Tablets 2216
Dyazide Capsules 1405
Micardis HCT Tablets 854
Prinzide Tablets 2092
Tekturna HCT Tablets 2324
Teveten HCT Tablets 517

Hydrocortisone (Corticosteroids tend to produce hyperglycemia and concurrent use may lead to loss of control).
No products indexed under this heading.

Hydrocortisone Acetate (Corticosteroids tend to produce hyperglycemia and concurrent use may lead to loss of control). Products include:
Analpram-HC 1140
Pramosone 1141

Hydrocortisone Sodium Phosphate (Corticosteroids tend to produce hyperglycemia and concurrent use may lead to loss of control).
No products indexed under this heading.

Hydrocortisone Sodium Succinate (Corticosteroids tend to produce hyperglycemia and concurrent use may lead to loss of control).
No products indexed under this heading.

Hydroflumethiazide (Diuretics tend to produce hyperglycemia and concurrent use may lead to loss of control).
No products indexed under this heading.

Ibuprofen (May potentiate hypoglycemic action). Products include:
Motrin IB Tablets and Caplets 1900
Children's Motrin Oral Suspension 1901
Children's Motrin Non-Staining Dye-Free Oral Suspension 1901
Children's Motrin Cold Oral Suspension 1899
Infants' Motrin Concentrated Drops 1901
Infants' Motrin Non-Staining Dye-Free Concentrated Drops 1901
Junior Strength Motrin Caplets and Chewable Tablets 1901
Vicoprofen Tablets 533

Indapamide (Diuretics tend to produce hyperglycemia and concurrent use may lead to loss of control). Products include:
Indapamide Tablets 2188

Indomethacin (May potentiate hypoglycemic action). Products include:
Indocin 2024

Indomethacin Sodium Trihydrate (May potentiate hypoglycemic action). Products include:
Indocin I.V. 2489

Insulin (Co-administration of glimepiride with insulin may increase the potential for hypoglycemia. Co-administration of rosiglitazone with insulin has resulted in increased incidence of cardiac failure and other cardiovascular adverse events).
No products indexed under this heading.

Insulin, Human, Zinc Suspension (Co-administration of glimepiride with insulin may increase the potential for hypoglycemia. Co-administration of rosiglitazone with insulin has resulted in increased incidence of cardiac failure and other cardiovascular adverse events).
No products indexed under this heading.

Insulin, Human (rDNA origin) (Co-administration of glimepiride with insulin may increase the potential for hypoglycemia. Co-administration of rosiglitazone with insulin has resulted in increased incidence of cardiac failure and other cardiovascular adverse events). Products include:
Exubera Inhalation Powder 2515

Insulin, Human NPH (Co-administration of glimepiride with insulin may increase the potential for hypoglycemia. Co-administration of rosiglitazone with insulin has resulted in increased incidence of cardiac failure and other cardiovascular adverse events). Products include:
Humulin N Vial 1846

Insulin, Human Regular (Co-administration of glimepiride with insulin may increase the potential for hypoglycemia. Co-administration of rosiglitazone with insulin has resulted in increased incidence of cardiac failure and other cardiovascular adverse events). Products include:
Humulin R 1849
Humulin R (U-500) 1850

Insulin, Human Regular and Human NPH Mixture (Co-administration of glimepiride with insulin may increase the potential for hypoglycemia. Co-administration of rosiglitazone with insulin has resulted in increased incidence of cardiac failure and other cardiovascular adverse events). Products include:
Humulin 50/50, 100 Units 1843
Humulin 70/30 Vial 1844

Insulin, NPH (Co-administration of glimepiride with insulin may increase the potential for hypoglycemia. Co-administration of rosiglitazone with insulin has resulted in increased incidence of cardiac failure and other cardiovascular adverse events).
No products indexed under this heading.

Insulin, Regular (Co-administration of glimepiride with insulin may increase the potential for hypoglycemia. Co-administration of rosiglitazone with insulin has resulted in increased incidence of cardiac failure and other cardiovascular adverse events).
No products indexed under this heading.

Insulin, Regular and NPH mixture (Co-administration of glimepiride with insulin may increase the potential for hypoglycemia. Co-administration of rosiglitazone with insulin has resulted in increased incidence of cardiac failure and other cardiovascular adverse events).
No products indexed under this heading.

Insulin, Zinc Crystals (Co-administration of glimepiride with insulin may increase the potential for hypoglycemia. Co-administration of rosiglitazone with insulin has resulted in increased incidence of cardiac failure and other cardiovascular adverse events).
No products indexed under this heading.

Insulin, Zinc Suspension (Co-administration of glimepiride with insulin may increase the potential for hypoglycemia. Co-administration of rosiglitazone with insulin has resulted in increased incidence of cardiac failure and other cardiovascular adverse events).
No products indexed under this heading.

Insulin Aspart (Co-administration of glimepiride with insulin may increase the potential for hypoglycemia. Co-administration of rosiglitazone with insulin has resulted in increased incidence of cardiac failure and other cardiovascular adverse events).
No products indexed under this heading.

Insulin Aspart, Human (Co-administration of glimepiride with insulin may increase the potential for hypoglycemia. Co-administration of rosiglitazone with insulin has resulted in increased incidence of cardiac failure and other cardiovascular adverse events). Products include:
NovoLog Mix 70/30 2364

Insulin Aspart, Human Regular (Co-administration of glimepiride with insulin may increase the potential for hypoglycemia. Co-administration of rosiglitazone with insulin has resulted in increased incidence of cardiac failure and other cardiovascular adverse events). Products include:
NovoLog Injection 2359

Insulin Aspart Protamine, Human (Co-administration of glimepiride with insulin may increase the potential for hypoglycemia. Co-administration of rosiglitazone with insulin has resulted in increased incidence of cardiac failure and other cardiovascular adverse events). Products include:
NovoLog Mix 70/30 2364

Insulin Detemir (rDNA Origin) (Co-administration of glimepiride with insulin may increase the potential for hypoglycemia. Co-administration of rosiglitazone with insulin has resulted in increased incidence of cardiac failure and other cardiovascular adverse events). Products include:
Levemir Injection 2352

Insulin glargine (Co-administration of glimepiride with insulin may increase the potential for hypoglycemia. Co-administration of rosiglitazone with insulin has resulted in increased incidence of cardiac failure and other cardiovascular adverse events). Products include:
Lantus Injection 2749

Insulin Glulisine (Co-administration of glimepiride with insulin may increase the potential for hypoglycemia. Co-administration of rosiglitazone with insulin has resulted in increased incidence of cardiac failure and other cardiovascular adverse events). Products include:
Apidra Injection 2706

Insulin Lispro, Human (Co-administration of glimepiride with insulin may increase the potential for hypoglycemia. Co-administration of rosiglitazone with insulin has resulted in increased incidence of cardiac failure and other cardiovascular adverse events). Products include:
Humalog-Pen and KwikPen 1829
Humalog Mix 50/50-Pen and KwikPen 1833
Humalog Mix 75/25-Pen and KwikPen 1835

Insulin Lispro Protamine, Human (Co-administration of glimepiride with insulin may increase the potential for hypoglycemia. Co-administration of rosiglitazone with insulin has resulted in increased incidence of cardiac failure and other cardiovascular adverse events). Products include:
Humalog Mix 50/50-Pen and KwikPen 1833
Humalog Mix 75/25-Pen and KwikPen 1835

Isocarboxazid (May potentiate hypoglycemic action). Products include:
Marplan Tablets 3177

Isoniazid (Isoniazid tends to produce hyperglycemia and concurrent use may lead to loss of control).
No products indexed under this heading.

Isoproterenol Hydrochloride (Sympathomimetics tend to produce hyperglycemia and concurrent use may lead to loss of control).
No products indexed under this heading.

Isoproterenol Sulfate (Sympathomimetics tend to produce hyperglycemia and concurrent use may lead to loss of control).
No products indexed under this heading.

Ketoprofen (May potentiate hypoglycemic action).
No products indexed under this heading.

Ketorolac Tromethamine (May potentiate hypoglycemic action).
No products indexed under this heading.

Labetalol Hydrochloride (May potentiate hypoglycemic action).
No products indexed under this heading.

Levalbuterol Hydrochloride (Sympathomimetics tend to produce hyperglycemia and concurrent use may lead to loss of control).
Products include:
Xopenex Inhalation Solution 3001
Xopenex Inhalation Solution Concentrate 3005

Levobunolol Hydrochloride (May potentiate hypoglycemic action).
No products indexed under this heading.

Levonorgestrel (Oral contraceptives tend to produce hyperglycemia and concurrent use may lead to loss of control). Products include:
Climara Pro Transdermal System 768
Lybrel Tablets 3204
Mirena Intrauterine System 779
Plan B Tablets 1044
Seasonique Tablets 1046

Levothyroxine Sodium (Thyroid products tend to produce hyperglycemia and concurrent use may lead to loss of control). Products include:
Levothroid Tablets 1170
Levoxyl Tablets 1780
Synthroid Tablets 507

Liothyronine Sodium (Thyroid products tend to produce hyperglycemia and concurrent use may lead to loss of control). Products include:
Cytomel Tablets 1778

Liotrix (Thyroid products tend to produce hyperglycemia and concurrent use may lead to loss of control).
No products indexed under this heading.

Magnesium Salicylate (May potentiate hypoglycemic action; clinical trials data indicate no evidence of significant adverse interaction with concurrent use).
No products indexed under this heading.

Meclofenamate Sodium (May potentiate hypoglycemic action).
No products indexed under this heading.

Mefenamic Acid (May potentiate hypoglycemic action).
No products indexed under this heading.

Meloxicam (May potentiate hypoglycemic action). Products include:
Mobic Oral Suspension 863
Mobic Tablets 863

Mesoridazine Besylate (Phenothiazines tend to produce hyperglycemia and concurrent use may lead to loss of control).
No products indexed under this heading.

Mestranol (Oral contraceptives tend to produce hyperglycemia and concurrent use may lead to loss of control).
No products indexed under this heading.

Metaproterenol Sulfate (Sympathomimetics tend to produce hyperglycemia and concurrent use may lead to loss of control).
No products indexed under this heading.

Metaraminol Bitartrate (Sympathomimetics tend to produce hyperglycemia and concurrent use may lead to loss of control).
No products indexed under this heading.

Metformin Hydrochloride (Co-administration of glimepiride with metformin may increase the potential for hypoglycemia). Products include:
ActoPlus Met Tablets 3071
Avandamet Tablets 1336
Janumet Tablets 2041
PrandiMet Tablets 2967

Methotrimeprazine (Phenothiazines tend to produce hyperglycemia and concurrent use may lead to loss of control).
No products indexed under this heading.

Methoxamine Hydrochloride (Sympathomimetics tend to produce hyperglycemia and concurrent use may lead to loss of control).
No products indexed under this heading.

Methyclothiazide (Diuretics tend to produce hyperglycemia and concurrent use may lead to loss of control).
No products indexed under this heading.

Methylprednisolone Acetate (Corticosteroids tend to produce hyperglycemia and concurrent use may lead to loss of control).
No products indexed under this heading.

Methylprednisolone Sodium Succinate (Corticosteroids tend to produce hyperglycemia and concurrent use may lead to loss of control).
No products indexed under this heading.

Metipranolol Hydrochloride (May potentiate hypoglycemic action).
No products indexed under this heading.

Metolazone (Diuretics tend to produce hyperglycemia and concurrent use may lead to loss of control).
No products indexed under this heading.

Metoprolol Succinate (May potentiate hypoglycemic action). Products include:
Toprol-XL Tablets **666**

Metoprolol Tartrate (May potentiate hypoglycemic action).
No products indexed under this heading.

Miconazole (A potential interaction between oral miconazole and oral hypoglycemic agents leading to severe hypoglycemia has been reported).
No products indexed under this heading.

Moclobemide (May potentiate hypoglycemic action).
No products indexed under this heading.

Mometasone Furoate (Corticosteroids tend to produce hyperglycemia and concurrent use may lead to loss of control). Products include:
Asmanex Twisthaler **2797**
Elocon Cream 0.1% **2840**
Elocon Lotion 0.1% **2841**
Elocon Ointment 0.1% **2842**

Mometasone Furoate Monohydrate (Corticosteroids tend to produce hyperglycemia and concurrent use may lead to loss of control). Products include:
Nasonex Nasal Spray **2883**

Nabumetone (May potentiate hypoglycemic action).
No products indexed under this heading.

Nadolol (May potentiate hypoglycemic action). Products include:
Nadolol Tablets **2191**

Naproxen (May potentiate hypoglycemic action). Products include:
EC-Naprosyn Delayed-Release Tablets **2632**
Naprosyn Suspension **2632**
Naprosyn Tablets **2632**

Naproxen Sodium (May potentiate hypoglycemic action). Products include:
Anaprox Tablets **2632**
Anaprox DS Tablets **2632**
Treximet Tablets **1616**

Nebivolol (May potentiate hypoglycemic action). Products include:
Bystolic Tablets **1155**

Nicardipine Hydrochloride (An inhibitor of CYP2C8 may decrease the AUC of rosiglitazone. Therefore, if an inducer of CYP2C8 is started or stopped during treatment with rosiglitazone, changes in diabetes treatment may be needed upon clinical response). Products include:
Cardene I.V. **1093**

Nicotinic Acid (Nicotinic acid tends to produce hyperglycemia and concurrent use may lead to loss of control).
No products indexed under this heading.

Norepinephrine Bitartrate (Sympathomimetics tend to produce hyperglycemia and concurrent use may lead to loss of control).
No products indexed under this heading.

Norethindrone (Oral contraceptives tend to produce hyperglycemia and concurrent use may lead to loss of control). Products include:
Ortho Micronor Tablets **2446**

Norethynodrel (Oral contraceptives tend to produce hyperglycemia and concurrent use may lead to loss of control).
No products indexed under this heading.

Norgestimate (Oral contraceptives tend to produce hyperglycemia and concurrent use may lead to loss of control). Products include:
Ortho-Cyclen/Ortho Tri-Cyclen **2449**
Ortho Tri-Cyclen Lo Tablets **2458**

Norgestrel (Oral contraceptives tend to produce hyperglycemia and concurrent use may lead to loss of control).
No products indexed under this heading.

Omeprazole (An inhibitor of CYP2C8 may decrease the AUC of rosiglitazone. Therefore, if an inducer of CYP2C8 is started or stopped during treatment with rosiglitazone, changes in diabetes treatment may be needed upon clinical response).
No products indexed under this heading.

Oxaprozin (May potentiate hypoglycemic action).
No products indexed under this heading.

Pargyline Hydrochloride (May potentiate hypoglycemic action).
No products indexed under this heading.

Penbutolol Sulfate (May potentiate hypoglycemic action).
No products indexed under this heading.

Perphenazine (Phenothiazines tend to produce hyperglycemia and concurrent use may lead to loss of control).
No products indexed under this heading.

Phenelzine Sulfate (May potentiate hypoglycemic action).
No products indexed under this heading.

Phenobarbital (An inhibitor of CYP2C8 may decrease the AUC of rosiglitazone. Therefore, if an inducer of CYP2C8 is started or stopped during treatment with rosiglitazone, changes in diabetes treatment may be needed upon clinical response). Products include:
Donnatal Extentabs **2507**

Phenylbutazone (May potentiate hypoglycemic action).
No products indexed under this heading.

Phenylephrine Bitartrate (Sympathomimetics tend to produce hyperglycemia and concurrent use may lead to loss of control).
No products indexed under this heading.

Phenylephrine Hydrochloride (Sympathomimetics tend to produce hyperglycemia and concurrent use may lead to loss of control). Products include:
Actifed Cold & Allergy Tablets **1895**
Benadryl Allergy & Cold Kapgels **1895**
Benadryl Allergy & Sinus Headache Kapgels **1895**
Benadryl Severe Allergy & Sinus Headache Caplets **1897**
Children's Benadryl-D Allergy & Sinus Liquid **1896**
Benadryl-D Allergy & Sinus Tablet **1896**
PediaCare Children's Allergy & Cold Liquid **1902**
PediaCare Children's Decongestant Liquid **1902**
PediaCare Children's Liquid Multi-Symptom Cold **1902**
Sinutab Non-Drying Caplets **1905**
Sinutab Sinus Caplets **1905**
Children's Sudafed PE Cold & Cough Liquid **1907**
Children's Sudafed PE Nasal Decongestant Liquid **1906**
Sudafed PE Cold & Cough Caplets **1907**
Sudafed PE Nasal Decongestant Tablets **1907**
Sudafed PE Nighttime Cold Caplets **1907**
Sudafed PE Non-Drying Sinus Caplets **1908**
Sudafed PE Severe Cold Caplets **1908**
Sudafed PE Sinus & Allergy Tablets **1908**
Sudafed PE Sinus Headache Caplets **1908**
Tylenol Allergy Multi-Symptom Caplets with Cool Burst and Rapid Release Gelcaps **1916**
Tylenol Allergy Multi-Symptom Nighttime Caplets with Cool Burst **1916**
Children's Tylenol Plus Cold Suspension Liquid **1912**
Children's Tylenol Plus Cold & Allergy Suspension Liquid **1914**
Children's Tylenol Plus Flu Suspension Liquid **1914**
Children's Tylenol Plus Multi-Symptom Cold Suspension Liquid **1912**
Tylenol Cold Head Congestion Daytime Caplets with Cool Burst **1910**
Tylenol Cold Head Congestion Nighttime Caplets with Cool Burst **1910**
Tylenol Cold Head Congestion Severe Daytime Caplets with Cool Burst **1910**
Tylenol Cold Multi-Symptom Daytime Caplets with Cool Burst and Rapid Release Gels **1913**
Tylenol Cold Multi-Symptom Daytime Liquid with Citrus Burst **1913**
Tylenol Cold Multi-Symptom Nighttime Caplets with Cool Burst **1913**
Tylenol Cold Multi-Symptom Nighttime Liquid with Cool Burst **1913**
Tylenol Cold Multi-Symptom Severe Caplets with Cool Burst **1913**
Tylenol Cold Multi-Symptom Severe Daytime Liquid with Citrus Burst **1913**
Tylenol Sinus Congestion & Pain Daytime Caplets with Cool Burst and Gelcaps **1917**
Tylenol Sinus Congestion & Pain Nighttime Caplets with Cool Burst **1917**
Tylenol Sinus Congestion & Pain Severe Caplets with Cool Burst **1917**
Vicks DayQuil Cold & Flu Multi-Symptom Relief .... ■**616**
Vicks DayQuil LiquiCaps **2567**
Vicks DayQuil Liquid **2567**
Vicks DayQuil Multi-Symptom Cold/Flu Relief **2567**

Phenylephrine Tannate (Sympathomimetics tend to produce hyperglycemia and concurrent use may lead to loss of control).
No products indexed under this heading.

Phenylpropanolamine Hydrochloride (Sympathomimetics tend to produce hyperglycemia and concurrent use may lead to loss of control).
No products indexed under this heading.

Phenytoin (Phenytoin tends to produce hyperglycemia and concurrent use may lead to loss of control).
No products indexed under this heading.

Phenytoin Sodium (Phenytoin tends to produce hyperglycemia and concurrent use may lead to loss of control). Products include:
Phenytek Capsules **2192**

Pindolol (May potentiate hypoglycemic action).
No products indexed under this heading.

Pirbuterol Acetate (Sympathomimetics tend to produce hyperglycemia and concurrent use may lead to loss of control). Products include:
Maxair Autohaler **1705**

Piroxicam (May potentiate hypoglycemic action).
No products indexed under this heading.

Polyestradiol Phosphate (Estrogens tend to produce hyperglycemia and concurrent use may lead to loss of control).
No products indexed under this heading.

Polythiazide (Diuretics tend to produce hyperglycemia and concurrent use may lead to loss of control).
No products indexed under this heading.

Prednisolone Acetate (Corticosteroids tend to produce hyperglycemia and concurrent use may lead to loss of control). Products include:
Pred Forte Ophthalmic Suspension .... ⊙**227**
Pred Mild Ophthalmic Suspension .... ⊙**230**
Pred-G Ophthalmic Ointment .... ⊙**229**
Pred-G Ophthalmic Suspension .... ⊙**228**

Prednisolone Sodium Phosphate (Corticosteroids tend to produce hyperglycemia and concurrent use may lead to loss of control).
No products indexed under this heading.

Prednisolone Tebutate (Corticosteroids tend to produce hyperglycemia and concurrent use may lead to loss of control).
No products indexed under this heading.

Prednisone (Corticosteroids tend to produce hyperglycemia and concurrent use may lead to loss of control).
No products indexed under this heading.

Primidone (An inhibitor of CYP2C8 may decrease the AUC of rosiglitazone. Therefore, if an inducer of CYP2C8 is started or stopped during treatment with rosiglitazone, changes in diabetes treatment may be needed upon clinical response).
No products indexed under this heading.

Probenecid (May potentiate hypoglycemic action).
No products indexed under this heading.

Procarbazine Hydrochloride (May potentiate hypoglycemic action).
No products indexed under this heading.

Prochlorperazine (Phenothiazines tend to produce hyperglycemia and concurrent use may lead to loss of control).
No products indexed under this heading.

Promethazine Hydrochloride (Phenothiazines tend to produce hyperglycemia and concurrent use may lead to loss of control).
No products indexed under this heading.

Propranolol Hydrochloride (Coadministration increases Cmax AUC, and T1/2 of glimepiride by 23%, 22% and 15% respectively and it decreased CL/f by 18%; no evidence of clinically significant adverse interactions). Products include:
InnoPran XL Extended Release Capsules 1484

Pseudoephedrine Hydrochloride (Sympathomimetics tend to produce hyperglycemia and concurrent use may lead to loss of control).
Products include:
Allegra-D 12 Hour Extended-Release Tablets 2687
Allegra-D 24 Hour Extended-Release Tablets 2690
Children's Motrin Cold Oral Suspension 1899
Sudafed 12 Hour Nasal Decongestant Non-Drowsy Caplets 1909
Sudafed 24 Hour Non-Drowsy Nasal Decongestant Tablets 1906
Children's Sudafed Nasal Decongestant Liquid 1906
Sudafed Nasal Decongestant Tablets 1906
Tylenol Cold Severe Congestion Daytime Caplets with Cool Burst 1912
Tylenol Sinus Severe Congestion Caplets with Cool Burst 1917
Vicks NyQuil LiquiCaps 2567
Vicks NyQuil Liquid 2567
Vicks NyQuil Multi-Symptom Cold/Flu Relief 2567
Zyrtec-D 12 Hour Extended Release Tablets 1923
Zyrtec-D Allergy & Congestion Extended-Release Tablets 1923

Pseudoephedrine Sulfate (Sympathomimetics tend to produce hyperglycemia and concurrent use may lead to loss of control).
Products include:
Clarinex-D 12-Hour Extended-Release Tablets 2831
Clarinex-D 24-Hour Extended-Release Tablets 2834

Quercetin (An inhibitor of CYP2C8 may decrease the AUC of rosiglitazone. Therefore, if an inducer of CYP2C8 is started or stopped during treatment with rosiglitazone, changes in diabetes treatment may be needed upon clinical response).
No products indexed under this heading.

Quinestrol (Estrogens tend to produce hyperglycemia and concurrent use may lead to loss of control).
No products indexed under this heading.

Rasagiline Mesylate (May potentiate hypoglycemic action). Products include:
Azilect Tablets 3106

Rifabutin (An inhibitor of CYP2C8 may decrease the AUC of rosiglitazone. Therefore, if an inducer of CYP2C8 is started or stopped during treatment with rosiglitazone, changes in diabetes treatment may be needed upon clinical response).
No products indexed under this heading.

Rifampin (Rifampin administration (600 mg twice daily), an inducer of CYP2C8, for 6 days is reported to decrease rosiglitazone AUC by 66%, compared to the administration of rosiglitazone (8 mg) alone).
No products indexed under this heading.

Rofecoxib (May potentiate hypoglycemic action).
No products indexed under this heading.

Salmeterol Xinafoate (Sympathomimetics tend to produce hyperglycemia and concurrent use may lead to loss of control). Products include:
Advair Diskus 100/50 1276
Advair Diskus 250/50 1276
Advair Diskus 500/50 1276
Advair HFA 45/21 Inhalation Aerosol 1288
Advair HFA 115/21 Inhalation Aerosol 1288
Advair HFA 230/21 Inhalation Aerosol 1288
Serevent Diskus 1594

Salsalate (May potentiate hypoglycemic action; clinical trials data indicate no evidence of significant adverse interaction with concurrent use).
No products indexed under this heading.

Selegiline (May potentiate hypoglycemic action). Products include:
Emsam Transdermal System 905

Selegiline Hydrochloride (May potentiate hypoglycemic action).
Products include:
Eldepryl Capsules 3052

Sotalol Hydrochloride (May potentiate hypoglycemic action).
No products indexed under this heading.

Spironolactone (Diuretics tend to produce hyperglycemia and concurrent use may lead to loss of control).
No products indexed under this heading.

Sulfacytine (May potentiate hypoglycemic action).
No products indexed under this heading.

Sulfamethizole (May potentiate hypoglycemic action).
No products indexed under this heading.

Sulfamethoxazole (May potentiate hypoglycemic action).
No products indexed under this heading.

Sulfaphenazole (An inhibitor of CYP2C8 may decrease the AUC of rosiglitazone. Therefore, if an inducer of CYP2C8 is started or stopped during treatment with rosiglitazone, changes in diabetes treatment may be needed upon clinical response).
No products indexed under this heading.

Sulfasalazine (May potentiate hypoglycemic action).
No products indexed under this heading.

Sulfinpyrazone (May potentiate hypoglycemic action).
No products indexed under this heading.

Sulfisoxazole Acetyl (May potentiate hypoglycemic action).
No products indexed under this heading.

Sulfisoxazole Diolamine (May potentiate hypoglycemic action).
No products indexed under this heading.

Sulindac (May potentiate hypoglycemic action). Products include:
Clinoril Tablets 1962

Terbutaline Sulfate (Sympathomimetics tend to produce hyperglycemia and concurrent use may lead to loss of control).
No products indexed under this heading.

Thioridazine Hydrochloride (Phenothiazines tend to produce hyperglycemia and concurrent use may lead to loss of control). Products include:
Thioridazine Hydrochloride Tablets 2195

Thyroglobulin (Thyroid products tend to produce hyperglycemia and concurrent use may lead to loss of control).
No products indexed under this heading.

Thyroid (Thyroid products tend to produce hyperglycemia and concurrent use may lead to loss of control).
Products include:
Naturethroid Tablets 2605

Thyroxine (Thyroid products tend to produce hyperglycemia and concurrent use may lead to loss of control).
No products indexed under this heading.

Thyroxine Sodium (Thyroid products tend to produce hyperglycemia and concurrent use may lead to loss of control).
No products indexed under this heading.

Timolol Hemihydrate (May potentiate hypoglycemic action). Products include:
Betimol Ophthalmic Solution 3181

Timolol Maleate (May potentiate hypoglycemic action). Products include:
Combigan Ophthalmic Solution 553
Cosopt Sterile Ophthalmic Solution 1969
Timoptic Sterile Ophthalmic Solution 2121
Timoptic in Ocudose 2124
Timoptic-XE Sterile Ophthalmic Gel Forming Solution 2125

Tolazamide (May potentiate hypoglycemic action).
No products indexed under this heading.

Tolbutamide (May potentiate hypoglycemic action).
No products indexed under this heading.

Tolmetin Sodium (May potentiate hypoglycemic action).
No products indexed under this heading.

Torsemide (Diuretics tend to produce hyperglycemia and concurrent use may lead to loss of control).
Products include:
Demadex Injection 2630
Demadex Tablets 2630

Tranylcypromine Sulfate (May potentiate hypoglycemic action).
Products include:
Parnate Tablets 1532

Triamcinolone (Corticosteroids tend to produce hyperglycemia and concurrent use may lead to loss of control).
No products indexed under this heading.

Triamcinolone Acetonide (Corticosteroids tend to produce hyperglycemia and concurrent use may lead to loss of control). Products include:
Azmacort Inhalation Aerosol 407
Nasacort AQ Nasal Spray 2765
Triesence Injectable Suspension .... ⊙209

Triamcinolone Diacetate (Corticosteroids tend to produce hyperglycemia and concurrent use may lead to loss of control).
No products indexed under this heading.

Triamcinolone Hexacetonide (Corticosteroids tend to produce hyperglycemia and concurrent use may lead to loss of control).
No products indexed under this heading.

Triamterene (Diuretics tend to produce hyperglycemia and concurrent use may lead to loss of control).
Products include:
Dyazide Capsules 1405
Dyrenium Capsules 3189

Trifluoperazine Hydrochloride (Phenothiazines tend to produce hyperglycemia and concurrent use may lead to loss of control).
No products indexed under this heading.

Trimethoprim (An inhibitor of CYP2C8 may decrease the AUC of rosiglitazone. Therefore, if an inducer of CYP2C8 is started or stopped during treatment with rosiglitazone, changes in diabetes treatment may be needed upon clinical response).
No products indexed under this heading.

Trimethoprim Hydrochloride (An inhibitor of CYP2C8 may decrease the AUC of rosiglitazone. Therefore, if an inducer of CYP2C8 is started or stopped during treatment with rosiglitazone, changes in diabetes treatment may be needed upon clinical response).
No products indexed under this heading.

Valdecoxib (May potentiate hypoglycemic action).
No products indexed under this heading.

Warfarin Sodium (May potentiate hypoglycemic action).
No products indexed under this heading.

Food Interactions

Meal, unspecified (When glimepiride is given with meals the mean Tmax is slightly increased (12%) and mean Cmax and AUC are slightly decreased).

AVANDIA TABLETS

(Rosiglitazone Maleate) 1351

May interact with cytochrome p450 2c8 inducers (selected), cytochrome p450 2c8 inhibitors (selected), insulin, sulfonylureas, and certain other agents. Compounds in these categories include:

Anastrozole (An inhibitor of CYP2C8 may increase the AUC of rosiglitazone. Therefore, if an inhibitor of CYP2C8 is started or stopped during treatment with rosiglitazone, changes in diabetes treatment may be needed upon clinical response). Products include:

Arimidex Tablets 672

Carbamazepine (An inducer of CYP2C8 may decrease the AUC of rosiglitazone. Therefore, if an inducer of CYP2C8 is started or stopped during treatment with rosiglitazone, changes in diabetes treatment may be needed upon clinical response). Products include:

Carbatrol Capsules 3019

Equetro Extended-Release Capsules 3174

Chlorpropamide (An increased incidence of heart failure has been observed when rosiglitazone was added to a sulfonylurea or to a sulfonylurea plus metformin).

No products indexed under this heading.

Cimetidine (An inhibitor of CYP2C8 may increase the AUC of rosiglitazone. Therefore, if an inhibitor of CYP2C8 is started or stopped during treatment with rosiglitazone, changes in diabetes treatment may be needed upon clinical response).

No products indexed under this heading.

Cimetidine Hydrochloride (An inhibitor of CYP2C8 may increase the AUC of rosiglitazone. Therefore, if an inhibitor of CYP2C8 is started or stopped during treatment with rosiglitazone, changes in diabetes treatment may be needed upon clinical response).

No products indexed under this heading.

Gemfibrozil (Concomitant administration of gemfibrozil (600 mg twice daily), an inhibitor of CYP2C8, and rosiglitazone (4 mg once daily) for 7 days increased rosiglitazone AUC by 127% compared to the administration of rosiglitazone (4 mg once daily) alone. Given the potential for dose-related adverse events with rosiglitazone, a decrease in the dose of rosiglitazone may be needed when gemfibrozil is introduced).

No products indexed under this heading.

Glimepiride (An increased incidence of heart failure has been observed when rosiglitazone was added to a sulfonylurea or to a sulfonylurea plus metformin). Products include:

Avandaryl Tablets 1344

Duetact Tablets 3085

Glipizide (An increased incidence of heart failure has been observed when rosiglitazone was added to a sulfonylurea or to a sulfonylurea plus metformin).

No products indexed under this heading.

Glyburide (Rosiglitazone (2 mg twice daily) taken concomitantly with glyburide (3.75 to 10 mg/day) for 7 days did not alter the mean steady-state 24-hour plasma glucose concentrations in diabetic patients stabilized on glyburide therapy. Repeat doses of rosiglitazone (8 mg once daily) for 8 days in healthy adult Caucasian subjects caused a decrease in glyburide AUC and Cmax of approximately 30%. In Japanese subjects, glyburide AUC (14%) and Cmax (31%) slightly increased following co-administration of rosiglitazone).

No products indexed under this heading.

Insulin (Co-administration of rosiglitazone with insulin has resulted in increased incidence of cardiac failure and other cardiovascular adverse events. Co-administration of rosiglitazone and insulin is not recommended).

No products indexed under this heading.

Insulin, Human, Zinc Suspension (Co-administration of rosiglitazone with insulin has resulted in increased incidence of cardiac failure and other cardiovascular adverse events. Co-administration of rosiglitazone and insulin is not recommended).

No products indexed under this heading.

Insulin, Human (rDNA origin) (Co-administration of rosiglitazone with insulin has resulted in increased incidence of cardiac failure and other cardiovascular adverse events. Co-administration of rosiglitazone and insulin is not recommended). Products include:

Exubera Inhalation Powder 2515

Insulin, Human NPH (Co-administration of rosiglitazone with insulin has resulted in increased incidence of cardiac failure and other cardiovascular adverse events. Co-administration of rosiglitazone and insulin is not recommended). Products include:

Humulin N Vial 1846

Insulin, Human Regular (Co-administration of rosiglitazone with insulin has resulted in increased incidence of cardiac failure and other cardiovascular adverse events. Co-administration of rosiglitazone and insulin is not recommended). Products include:

Humulin R 1849

Humulin R (U-500) 1850

Insulin, Human Regular and Human NPH Mixture (Co-administration of rosiglitazone with insulin has resulted in increased incidence of cardiac failure and other cardiovascular adverse events. Co-administration of rosiglitazone and insulin is not recommended). Products include:

Humulin 50/50, 100 Units 1843

Humulin 70/30 Vial 1844

Insulin, NPH (Co-administration of rosiglitazone with insulin has resulted in increased incidence of cardiac failure and other cardiovascular adverse events. Co-administration of rosiglitazone and insulin is not recommended).

No products indexed under this heading.

Insulin, Regular (Co-administration of rosiglitazone with insulin has resulted in increased incidence of cardiac failure and other cardiovascular adverse events. Co-administration of rosiglitazone and insulin is not recommended).

No products indexed under this heading.

Insulin, Regular and NPH mixture (Co-administration of rosiglitazone with insulin has resulted in increased incidence of cardiac failure and other cardiovascular adverse events. Co-administration of rosiglitazone and insulin is not recommended).

No products indexed under this heading.

Insulin, Zinc Crystals (Co-administration of rosiglitazone with insulin has resulted in increased incidence of cardiac failure and other cardiovascular adverse events. Co-administration of rosiglitazone and insulin is not recommended).

No products indexed under this heading.

Insulin, Zinc Suspension (Co-administration of rosiglitazone with insulin has resulted in increased incidence of cardiac failure and other cardiovascular adverse events. Co-administration of rosiglitazone and insulin is not recommended).

No products indexed under this heading.

Insulin Aspart (Co-administration of rosiglitazone with insulin has resulted in increased incidence of cardiac failure and other cardiovascular adverse events. Co-administration of rosiglitazone and insulin is not recommended).

No products indexed under this heading.

Insulin Aspart, Human (Co-administration of rosiglitazone with insulin has resulted in increased incidence of cardiac failure and other cardiovascular adverse events. Co-administration of rosiglitazone and insulin is not recommended). Products include:

NovoLog Mix 70/30 2364

Insulin Aspart, Human Regular (Co-administration of rosiglitazone with insulin has resulted in increased incidence of cardiac failure and other cardiovascular adverse events. Co-administration of rosiglitazone and insulin is not recommended). Products include:

NovoLog Injection 2359

Insulin Aspart Protamine, Human (Co-administration of rosiglitazone with insulin has resulted in increased incidence of cardiac failure and other cardiovascular adverse events. Co-administration of rosiglitazone and insulin is not recommended). Products include:

NovoLog Mix 70/30 2364

Insulin Detemir (rDNA Origin) (Co-administration of rosiglitazone with insulin has resulted in increased incidence of cardiac failure and other cardiovascular adverse events. Co-administration of rosiglitazone and insulin is not recommended). Products include:

Levemir Injection 2352

Insulin glargine (Co-administration of rosiglitazone with insulin has resulted in increased incidence of cardiac failure and other cardiovascular adverse events. Co-administration of rosiglitazone and insulin is not recommended). Products include:

Lantus Injection 2749

Insulin Glulisine (Co-administration of rosiglitazone with insulin has resulted in increased incidence of cardiac failure and other cardiovascular adverse events. Co-administration of rosiglitazone and insulin is not recommended). Products include:

Apidra Injection 2706

Insulin Lispro, Human (Co-administration of rosiglitazone with insulin has resulted in increased incidence of cardiac failure and other cardiovascular adverse events. Co-administration of rosiglitazone and insulin is not recommended). Products include:

Humalog-Pen and KwikPen 1829

Humalog Mix 50/50-Pen and KwikPen 1833

Humalog Mix 75/25-Pen and KwikPen 1835

Insulin Lispro Protamine, Human (Co-administration of rosiglitazone with insulin has resulted in increased incidence of cardiac failure and other cardiovascular adverse events. Co-administration of rosiglitazone and insulin is not recommended). Products include:

Humalog Mix 50/50-Pen and KwikPen 1833

Humalog Mix 75/25-Pen and KwikPen 1835

Nicardipine Hydrochloride (An inhibitor of CYP2C8 may increase the AUC of rosiglitazone. Therefore, if an inhibitor of CYP2C8 is started or stopped during treatment with rosiglitazone, changes in diabetes treatment may be needed upon clinical response). Products include:

Cardene I.V. 1093

Omeprazole (An inhibitor of CYP2C8 may increase the AUC of rosiglitazone. Therefore, if an inhibitor of CYP2C8 is started or stopped during treatment with rosiglitazone, changes in diabetes treatment may be needed upon clinical response).

No products indexed under this heading.

Phenobarbital (An inducer of CYP2C8 may decrease the AUC of rosiglitazone. Therefore, if an inducer of CYP2C8 is started or stopped during treatment with rosiglitazone, changes in diabetes treatment may be needed upon clinical response). Products include:

Donnatal Extentabs 2507

Primidone (An inducer of CYP2C8 may decrease the AUC of rosiglitazone. Therefore, if an inducer of CYP2C8 is started or stopped during treatment with rosiglitazone, changes in diabetes treatment may be needed upon clinical response).

No products indexed under this heading.

Quercetin (An inhibitor of CYP2C8 may increase the AUC of rosiglitazone. Therefore, if an inhibitor of CYP2C8 is started or stopped during treatment with rosiglitazone, changes in diabetes treatment may be needed upon clinical response).
No products indexed under this heading.

Rifabutin (An inducer of CYP2C8 may decrease the AUC of rosiglitazone. Therefore, if an inducer of CYP2C8 is started or stopped during treatment with rosiglitazone, changes in diabetes treatment may be needed upon clinical response).
No products indexed under this heading.

Rifampin (Rifampin administration (600 mg twice daily), an inducer of CYP2C8, for 6 days is reported to decrease rosiglitazone AUC by 66%, compared to the administration of rosiglitazone (8 mg) alone).
No products indexed under this heading.

Sulfaphenazole (An inhibitor of CYP2C8 may increase the AUC of rosiglitazone. Therefore, if an inhibitor of CYP2C8 is started or stopped during treatment with rosiglitazone, changes in diabetes treatment may be needed upon clinical response).
No products indexed under this heading.

Sulfinpyrazone (An inhibitor of CYP2C8 may increase the AUC of rosiglitazone. Therefore, if an inhibitor of CYP2C8 is started or stopped during treatment with rosiglitazone, changes in diabetes treatment may be needed upon clinical response).
No products indexed under this heading.

Tolazamide (An increased incidence of heart failure has been observed when rosiglitazone was added to a sulfonylurea or to a sulfonylurea plus metformin).
No products indexed under this heading.

Tolbutamide (An increased incidence of heart failure has been observed when rosiglitazone was added to a sulfonylurea or to a sulfonylurea plus metformin).
No products indexed under this heading.

Trimethoprim (An inhibitor of CYP2C8 may increase the AUC of rosiglitazone. Therefore, if an inhibitor of CYP2C8 is started or stopped during treatment with rosiglitazone, changes in diabetes treatment may be needed upon clinical response).
No products indexed under this heading.

Trimethoprim Hydrochloride (An inhibitor of CYP2C8 may increase the AUC of rosiglitazone. Therefore, if an inhibitor of CYP2C8 is started or stopped during treatment with rosiglitazone, changes in diabetes treatment may be needed upon clinical response).
No products indexed under this heading.

AVAPRO TABLETS

(Irbesartan) 897
None cited in PDR database.

AVAPRO TABLETS

(Irbesartan) 2718
None cited in PDR database.

AVASTIN IV

(Bevacizumab) 1192
None cited in PDR database.

AVELOX I.V.

(Moxifloxacin Hydrochloride) 2803
See Avelox Tablets

AVELOX TABLETS

(Moxifloxacin Hydrochloride) 2803
May interact with antacids containing aluminum, calcium and magnesium, class 1A antiarrhythmics, class III antiarrhythmics, calcium preparations, corticosteroids, oral anticoagulants, erythromycin, iron containing oral preparations, nonsteroidal anti-inflammatory agents, phenothiazines, quinidine, tricyclic antidepressants, and certain other agents. Compounds in these categories include:

Aluminum Carbonate (Quinolones form chelates with alkaline earth and transition metal cations. When moxifloxacin (single 400 mg tablet dose) was administered two hours before, concomitantly, or 4 hours after an aluminum/magnesium-containing antacid (900 mg aluminum hydroxide and 600 mg magnesium hydroxide as a single oral dose) to 12 healthy volunteers there was a 26%, 60%, and 23% reduction in the mean AUC of moxifloxacin, respectively. Moxifloxacin should be taken at least 4 hours before or 8 hours after antacids containing magnesium or aluminum).
No products indexed under this heading.

Aluminum Hydroxide (Quinolones form chelates with alkaline earth and transition metal cations. When moxifloxacin (single 400 mg tablet dose) was administered two hours before, concomitantly, or 4 hours after an aluminum/magnesium-containing antacid (900 mg aluminum hydroxide and 600 mg magnesium hydroxide as a single oral dose) to 12 healthy volunteers there was a 26%, 60%, and 23% reduction in the mean AUC of moxifloxacin, respectively. Moxifloxacin should be taken at least 4 hours before or 8 hours after antacids containing magnesium or aluminum).
No products indexed under this heading.

Amiodarone Hydrochloride (Moxifloxacin has been shown to prolong the QT interval of the electrocardiogram in some patients. The drug should be avoided in patients receiving Class III antiarrhythmic agents such as amiodarone, due to the lack of clinical experience with the drug in this patient population).
No products indexed under this heading.

Amitriptyline Hydrochloride (Moxifloxacin has been shown to prolong the QT interval of the electrocardiogram in some patients. Pharmacokinetic studies between moxifloxacin and other drugs that prolong the QT interval such as tricyclic antidepressants have not been performed. An additive effect of moxifloxacin and tricyclic antidepressants cannot be excluded, therefore, caution should be exercised when moxifloxacin is given concurrently with tricyclic antidepressants).
No products indexed under this heading.

Amoxapine (Moxifloxacin has been shown to prolong the QT interval of the electrocardiogram in some patients. Pharmacokinetic studies between moxifloxacin and other drugs that prolong the QT interval such as tricyclic antidepressants have not been performed. An additive effect of moxifloxacin and tricyclic antidepressants cannot be excluded, therefore, caution should be exercised when moxifloxacin is given concurrently with tricyclic antidepressants).
No products indexed under this heading.

Anisindione (No significant effect of moxifloxacin on R- and S-warfarin was detected in a clinical study involving 24 healthy volunteers. No significant changes in prothrombin time were noted in the presence of moxifloxacin. Quinolones, including moxifloxacin, have been reported to enhance the anticoagulant effects of warfarin or its derivatives in the patient population. In addition, infectious disease and its accompanying inflammatory process, age, and general status of the patient are risk factors for increased anticoagulant activity. Therefore, the prothrombin time, International Normalized Ratio (INR), or other suitable anticoagulation tests should be closely monitored if a quinolone is administered concomitantly with warfarin or its derivatives).
No products indexed under this heading.

Atenolol (In a crossover study involving 24 healthy volunteers (12 male; 12 female), the mean atenolol AUC following a single oral dose of 50 mg atenolol with placebo was similar to that observed when atenolol was given concomitantly with a single 400 mg oral dose of moxifloxacin. The mean Cmax of single dose atenolol decreased by about 10% following co-administration with a single dose of moxifloxacin).
No products indexed under this heading.

Betamethasone Acetate (Ruptures of the shoulder, hand, Achilles tendon or other tendons that required surgical repair or resulted in prolonged disability have been reported in patients receiving quinolones, including moxifloxacin, Post-marketing surveillance reports indicate that this risk may be increased in patients receiving concomitant corticosteroids, especially the elderly).
No products indexed under this heading.

Betamethasone Sodium Phosphate (Ruptures of the shoulder, hand, Achilles tendon or other tendons that required surgical repair or resulted in prolonged disability have been reported in patients receiving quinolones, including moxifloxacin, Post-marketing surveillance reports indicate that this risk may be increased in patients receiving concomitant corticosteroids, especially the elderly).
No products indexed under this heading.

Bretylium Tosylate (Moxifloxacin has been shown to prolong QT interval of the electrocardiogram in some patients. The drug should be avoided in patients receiving Class III antiarrhythmic agents, due to lack of clinical experience with the drug in these populations).
No products indexed under this heading.

Budesonide (Ruptures of the shoulder, hand, Achilles tendon or other tendons that required surgical repair or resulted in prolonged disability have been reported in patients receiving quinolones, including moxifloxacin, Post-marketing surveillance reports indicate that this risk may be increased in patients receiving concomitant corticosteroids, especially the elderly). Products include:

Pulmicort Flexhaler 654
Symbicort 80/4.5 Inhalation Aerosol.. 659
Symbicort 160/4.5 Inhalation Aerosol.. 659

Calcium Carbonate (Twelve healthy volunteers were administered concomitant moxifloxacin (single 400 mg dose) and calcium (single dose of 500 mg Ca++ dietary supplement) followed by an additional two doses of calcium 12 and 24 hours after moxifloxacin administration. Calcium had no significant effect on the mean AUC of moxifloxacin. The mean Cmax was slightly reduced and the time to maximum plasma concentration was prolonged when moxifloxacin was given with calcium compared to when moxifloxacin was given alone (2.5 hours versus 0.9 hours). These differences are not considered to be clinically significant). Products include:

Accelerator Tablets .... ▣634
Actonel with Calcium Tablets 2574
BioLean II Tablets .... ▣635
Calcet Triple Calcium + Vitamin D Tablets.. ▣629
D-Cal Chewable Caplets .... ▣624
Elixir Capsules .... ▣636
Pepcid Complete Chewable Tablets.. 1771
Extra Strength Rolaids Plus Gas Relief Tropical Fruit Softchews...... 1903
Extra Strength Rolaids Softchews Vanilla Creme 1903
Extra Strength Rolaids Freshmint Tablets.. 1903
Rolaids Multi-Symptom Berry Tablets.. 1903
Rolaids Original Peppermint Tablets.. 1903

Calcium Chloride (Twelve healthy volunteers were administered concomitant moxifloxacin (single 400 mg dose) and calcium (single dose of 500 mg Ca++ dietary supplement) followed by an additional two doses of calcium 12 and 24 hours after moxifloxacin administration. Calcium had no significant effect on the mean AUC of moxifloxacin. The mean Cmax was slightly reduced and the time to maximum plasma concentration was prolonged when moxifloxacin was given with calcium compared to when moxifloxacin was given alone (2.5 hours versus 0.9 hours). These differences are not considered to be clinically significant).
No products indexed under this heading.

Calcium Citrate (Twelve healthy volunteers were administered concomitant moxifloxacin (single 400 mg dose) and calcium (single dose of 500 mg Ca++ dietary supplement) followed by an additional two doses of calcium 12 and 24 hours after moxifloxacin administration. Calcium had no significant effect on the mean AUC of moxifloxacin. The mean Cmax was slightly reduced and the time to maximum plasma concentration was prolonged when moxifloxacin was given with calcium compared to when moxifloxacin was given alone (2.5 hours versus 0.9 hours). These differences are not considered to be clinically significant). Products include:

- Active Calcium Tablets 3173
- CitraNatal DHA Tablets 2175
- CitraNatal 90 DHA Tablets 2175

Calcium Glubionate (Twelve healthy volunteers were administered concomitant moxifloxacin (single 400 mg dose) and calcium (single dose of 500 mg Ca++ dietary supplement) followed by an additional two doses of calcium 12 and 24 hours after moxifloxacin administration. Calcium had no significant effect on the mean AUC of moxifloxacin. The mean Cmax was slightly reduced and the time to maximum plasma concentration was prolonged when moxifloxacin was given with calcium compared to when moxifloxacin was given alone (2.5 hours versus 0.9 hours). These differences are not considered to be clinically significant).

No products indexed under this heading.

Celecoxib (Although not observed with moxifloxacin in preclinical and clinical trials, the concomitant administration of a nonsteriodal anti-inflammatory drug with a quinolone may increase the risks of CNS stimulation and convulsions). Products include:

- Celebrex Capsules 2979

Chlorpromazine (Moxifloxacin has been shown to prolong the QT interval of the electrocardiogram in some patients. Pharmacokinetic studies between moxifloxacin and other drugs that prolong the QT interval such as antipsychotic phenthiazines has not been performed. An additive effect of moxifloxacin and antipsychotic phenthiazines cannot be excluded, therefore, caution should be exercised when moxifloxacin is given concurrently with antipsychotic phenthiazines).

No products indexed under this heading.

Chlorpromazine Hydrochloride (Moxifloxacin has been shown to prolong the QT interval of the electrocardiogram in some patients. Pharmacokinetic studies between moxifloxacin and other drugs that prolong the QT interval such as antipsychotic phenthiazines has not been performed. An additive effect of moxifloxacin and antipsychotic phenthiazines cannot be excluded, therefore, caution should be exercised when moxifloxacin is given concurrently with antipsychotic phenthiazines).

No products indexed under this heading.

Ciclesonide (Ruptures of the shoulder, hand, Achilles tendon or other tendons that required surgical repair or resulted in prolonged disability have been reported in patients receiving quinolones, including moxifloxacin, Post-marketing surveillance reports indicate that this risk may be increased in patients receiving concomitant corticosteroids, especially the elderly). Products include:

- Alvesco Inhalation Aerosol 2985
- Omnaris Nasal Spray 2998

Cisapride (Moxifloxacin has been shown to prolong the QT interval of the electrocardiogram in some patients. Pharmacokinetic studies between moxifloxacin and other drugs that prolong the QT interval such as cisapride has not been performed. An additive effect of moxifloxacin and cisapride cannot be excluded, therefore, caution should be exercised when moxifloxacin is given concurrently with cisapride).

No products indexed under this heading.

Clomipramine Hydrochloride (Moxifloxacin has been shown to prolong the QT interval of the electrocardiogram in some patients. Pharmacokinetic studies between moxifloxacin and other drugs that prolong the QT interval such as tricyclic antidepressants have not been performed. An additive effect of moxifloxacin and tricyclic antidepressants cannot be excluded, therefore, caution should be exercised when moxifloxacin is given concurrently with tricyclic antidepressants).

No products indexed under this heading.

Cortisone Acetate (Ruptures of the shoulder, hand, Achilles tendon or other tendons that required surgical repair or resulted in prolonged disability have been reported in patients receiving quinolones, including moxifloxacin, Post-marketing surveillance reports indicate that this risk may be increased in patients receiving concomitant corticosteroids, especially the elderly).

No products indexed under this heading.

Desipramine Hydrochloride (Moxifloxacin has been shown to prolong the QT interval of the electrocardiogram in some patients. Pharmacokinetic studies between moxifloxacin and other drugs that prolong the QT interval such as tricyclic antidepressants have not been performed. An additive effect of moxifloxacin and tricyclic antidepressants cannot be excluded, therefore, caution should be exercised when moxifloxacin is given concurrently with tricyclic antidepressants).

No products indexed under this heading.

Dexamethasone (Ruptures of the shoulder, hand, Achilles tendon or other tendons that required surgical repair or resulted in prolonged disability have been reported in patients receiving quinolones, including moxifloxacin, Post-marketing surveillance reports indicate that this risk may be increased in patients receiving concomitant corticosteroids, especially the elderly). Products include:

- Ciprodex Otic Suspension 541

Dexamethasone Acetate (Ruptures of the shoulder, hand, Achilles tendon or other tendons that required surgical repair or resulted in prolonged disability have been reported in patients receiving quinolones, including moxifloxacin, Post-marketing surveillance reports indicate that this risk may be increased in patients receiving concomitant corticosteroids, especially the elderly).

No products indexed under this heading.

Dexamethasone Sodium Phosphate (Ruptures of the shoulder, hand, Achilles tendon or other tendons that required surgical repair or resulted in prolonged disability have been reported in patients receiving quinolones, including moxifloxacin, Post-marketing surveillance reports indicate that this risk may be increased in patients receiving concomitant corticosteroids, especially the elderly).

No products indexed under this heading.

Diclofenac Epolamine (Although not observed with moxifloxacin in preclinical and clinical trials, the concomitant administration of a nonsteriodal anti-inflammatory drug with a quinolone may increase the risks of CNS stimulation and convulsions). Products include:

- Flector Patch 561

Diclofenac Potassium (Although not observed with moxifloxacin in preclinical and clinical trials, the concomitant administration of a nonsteriodal anti-inflammatory drug with a quinolone may increase the risks of CNS stimulation and convulsions).

No products indexed under this heading.

Diclofenac Sodium (Although not observed with moxifloxacin in preclinical and clinical trials, the concomitant administration of a nonsteriodal anti-inflammatory drug with a quinolone may increase the risks of CNS stimulation and convulsions). Products include:

- Diclofenac Sodium Ophthalmic Solution.................................... ⊙240
- Voltaren Ophthalmic Solution 2336
- Voltaren Tablets 2334
- Voltaren-XR Tablets 2337

Dicumarol (No significant effect of moxifloxacin on R- and S-warfarin was detected in a clinical study involving 24 healthy volunteers. No significant changes in prothrombin time were noted in the presence of moxifloxacin. Quinolones, including moxifloxacin, have been reported to enhance the anticoagulant effects of warfarin or its derivatives in the patient population. In addition, infectious disease and its accompanying inflammatory process, age, and general status of the patient are risk factors for increased anticoagulant activity. Therefore, the prothrombin time, International Normalized Ratio (INR), or other suitable anticoagulation tests should be closely monitored if a quinolone is administered concomitantly with warfarin or its derivatives).

No products indexed under this heading.

Didanosine (Quinolones form chelates with alkaline earth and transition metal cations. Oral administration of quinolones with formulations containing divalent and trivalent cations such as didanosine chewable/buffered tablets or the pediatric powder for oral solution, may substantially interfere with the absorption of quinolones, resulting in systemic concentrations considerably lower than desired. Therefore, moxifloxacin should be taken at least 4 hours before or 8 hours after didanosine).

No products indexed under this heading.

Digoxin (No significant effect of moxifloxacin (400 mg once daily for 2 days) on digoxin (0.6 mg as a single dose) AUC was detected in a study involving 12 healthy volunteers. The mean digoxin Cmax increased by about 50% during the distrubution phase of digoxin. This transient increase in digoxin Cmax is not viewed to be clinically significant. Moxifloxacin pharmacokinetics were similar in the presence or absence of digoxin. No dosage adjustment for moxifloxacin or digoxin is required when these drugs are administered concomitantly). Products include:

- Lanoxin Injection 1498
- Lanoxin Injection Pediatric 1502
- Lanoxin Tablets 1505

Disopyramide (Moxifloxacin has been shown to prolong the QT interval of the electrocardiogram in some patients. The drug should be avoided in patients receiving Class IA antiarrhythmic agents, due to the lack of clinical experience with the drug in these patient populations).

No products indexed under this heading.

Doxepin Hydrochloride (Moxifloxacin has been shown to prolong the QT interval of the electrocardiogram in some patients. Pharmacokinetic studies between moxifloxacin and other drugs that prolong the QT interval such as tricyclic antidepressants have not been performed. An additive effect of moxifloxacin and tricyclic antidepressants cannot be excluded, therefore, caution should be exercised when moxifloxacin is given concurrently with tricyclic antidepressants).

No products indexed under this heading.

Erythromycin (Moxifloxacine has been shown to prolong the QT interval of the electrocardiogram in some patients. Pharmacokinetic studies between moxifloxacin and other drugs that prolong the QT interval such as erythromycin has not been performed. An additive effect of moxifloxacin and erythromycin cannot be excluded, therefore, caution should be exercised when moxifloxacin is given concurrently with erythromycin).

No products indexed under this heading.

Erythromycin Estolate (Moxifloxacine has been shown to prolong the QT interval of the electrocardiogram in some patients. Pharmacokinetic studies between moxifloxacin and other drugs that prolong the QT interval such as erythromycin has not been performed. An additive effect of moxifloxacin and erythromycin cannot be excluded, therefore, caution should be exercised when moxifloxacin is given concurrently with erythromycin).

No products indexed under this heading.

Erythromycin Ethylsuccinate (Moxifloxacine has been shown to prolong the QT interval of the electrocardiogram in some patients. Pharmacokinetic studies between moxifloxacin and other drugs that prolong the QT interval such as erythromycin has not been performed. An additive effect of moxifloxacin and erythromycin cannot be excluded, therefore, caution should be exercised when moxifloxacin is given concurrently with erythromycin). Products include:

- E.E.S. 433
- EryPed 431

Erythromycin Gluceptate (Moxifloxacine has been shown to prolong the QT interval of the electrocardiogram in some patients. Pharmacokinetic studies between moxifloxacin and other drugs that prolong the QT interval such as erythromycin has

not been performed. An additive effect of moxifloxacin and erythromycin cannot be excluded, therefore, caution should be exercised when moxifloxacin is given concurrently with erythromycin).
No products indexed under this heading.

Erythromycin Lactobionate (Moxifloxacine has been shown to prolong the QT interval of the electrocardiogram in some patients. Pharmacokinetic studies between moxifloxacin and other drugs that prolong the QT interval such as erythromycin has not been performed. An additive effect of moxifloxacin and erythromycin cannot be excluded, therefore, caution should be exercised when moxifloxacin is given concurrently with erythromycin).
No products indexed under this heading.

Erythromycin Stearate (Moxifloxacine has been shown to prolong the QT interval of the electrocardiogram in some patients. Pharmacokinetic studies between moxifloxacin and other drugs that prolong the QT interval such as erythromycin has not been performed. An additive effect of moxifloxacin and erythromycin cannot be excluded, therefore, caution should be exercised when moxifloxacin is given concurrently with erythromycin).
No products indexed under this heading.

Etodolac (Although not observed with moxifloxacin in preclinical and clinical trials, the concomitant administration of a nonsteriodal anti-inflammatory drug with a quinolone may increase the risks of CNS stimulation and convulsions).
No products indexed under this heading.

Fenoprofen Calcium (Although not observed with moxifloxacin in preclinical and clinical trials, the concomitant administration of a nonsteriodal anti-inflammatory drug with a quinolone may increase the risks of CNS stimulation and convulsions). Products include:

Nalfon Capsules 2508

Ferrous Fumarate (Quinolones form chelates with alkaline earth and transition metal cations. When moxifloxacin tablets were administered concomitantly with iron (ferrous sulfate 100 mg once daily for two days), the mean AUC and Cmax of moxifloxacin was reduced by 39% and59%, respectively. Moxifloxacin should only be taken more than 4 hours before or 8 hours after iron products).
No products indexed under this heading.

Ferrous Gluconate (Quinolones form chelates with alkaline earth and transition metal cations. When moxifloxacin tablets were administered concomitantly with iron (ferrous sulfate 100 mg once daily for two days), the mean AUC and Cmax of moxifloxacin was reduced by 39% and59%, respectively. Moxifloxacin should only be taken more than 4 hours before or 8 hours after iron products). Products include:

CitraNatal DHA Tablets 2175

Ferrous Sulfate (Quinolones form chelates with alkaline earth and transition metal cations. When moxifloxacin tablets were administered concomitantly with iron (ferrous sulfate 100 mg once daily for two days), the mean AUC and Cmax of moxifloxacin was reduced by 39% and59%, respectively. Moxifloxacin should only be taken more than 4 hours before or 8 hours after iron products).
No products indexed under this heading.

Fludrocortisone Acetate (Ruptures of the shoulder, hand, Achilles tendon or other tendons that required surgical repair or resulted in prolonged disability have been reported in patients receiving quinolones, including moxifloxacin, Post-marketing surveillance reports indicate that this risk may be increased in patients receiving concomitant corticosteroids, especially the elderly).
No products indexed under this heading.

Flunisolide (Ruptures of the shoulder, hand, Achilles tendon or other tendons that required surgical repair or resulted in prolonged disability have been reported in patients receiving quinolones, including moxifloxacin, Post-marketing surveillance reports indicate that this risk may be increased in patients receiving concomitant corticosteroids, especially the elderly). Products include:

Aerobid/Aerobid-M 1153

Fluphenazine Decanoate (Moxifloxacin has been shown to prolong the QT interval of the electrocardiogram in some patients. Pharmacokinetic studies between moxifloxacin and other drugs that prolong the QT interval such as antipsychotic phenthiazines has not been performed. An additive effect of moxifloxacin and antipsychotic phenthiazines cannot be excluded, therefore, caution should be exercised when moxifloxacin is given concurrently with antipsychotic phenthiazines).
No products indexed under this heading.

Fluphenazine Enanthate (Moxifloxacin has been shown to prolong the QT interval of the electrocardiogram in some patients. Pharmacokinetic studies between moxifloxacin and other drugs that prolong the QT interval such as antipsychotic phenthiazines has not been performed. An additive effect of moxifloxacin and antipsychotic phenthiazines cannot be excluded, therefore, caution should be exercised when moxifloxacin is given concurrently with antipsychotic phenthiazines).
No products indexed under this heading.

Fluphenazine Hydrochloride (Moxifloxacin has been shown to prolong the QT interval of the electrocardiogram in some patients. Pharmacokinetic studies between moxifloxacin and other drugs that prolong the QT interval such as antipsychotic phenthiazines has not been performed. An additive effect of moxifloxacin and antipsychotic phenthiazines cannot be excluded, therefore, caution should be exercised when moxifloxacin is given concurrently with antipsychotic phenthiazines).
No products indexed under this heading.

Flurbiprofen (Although not observed with moxifloxacin in preclinical and clinical trials, the concomitant administration of a nonsteriodal anti-inflammatory drug with a quinolone may increase the risks of CNS stimulation and convulsions).
No products indexed under this heading.

Fluticasone Propionate (Ruptures of the shoulder, hand, Achilles tendon or other tendons that required surgical repair or resulted in prolonged disability have been reported in patients receiving quinolones, including moxifloxacin, Post-marketing surveillance reports indicate that this risk may be increased in patients receiving concomitant corticosteroids, especially the elderly). Products include:

Advair Diskus 100/50 1276
Advair Diskus 250/50 1276
Advair Diskus 500/50 1276
Advair HFA 45/21 Inhalation Aerosol.. 1288
Advair HFA 115/21 Inhalation Aerosol.. 1288
Advair HFA 230/21 Inhalation Aerosol.. 1288
Flonase Nasal Spray 1431
Flovent Diskus 50 mcg 1435

Fluticasone Propionate HFA (Ruptures of the shoulder, hand, Achilles tendon or other tendons that required surgical repair or resulted in prolonged disability have been reported in patients receiving quinolones, including moxifloxacin, Post-marketing surveillance reports indicate that this risk may be increased in patients receiving concomitant corticosteroids, especially the elderly). Products include:

Flovent HFA 1440

Glyburide (In diabetics, glyburide (2.5 mg once daily for two weeks pretreatment and for five days concurrently) mean AUC and Cmax were 12% and 21% lower, respectively, when taken with moxifloxacin (400 mg once daily for five days) in comparison to placebo. Nonetheless, blood glucose levels were decreased slightly in patients taking glyburide and moxifloxacin in comparison to those taking glyburide alone, suggesting no interference by moxifloxacin on the activity of glyburide. These interaction results are not viewed as clinically significant).
No products indexed under this heading.

Hydrocortisone (Ruptures of the shoulder, hand, Achilles tendon or other tendons that required surgical repair or resulted in prolonged disability have been reported in patients receiving quinolones, including moxifloxacin, Post-marketing surveillance reports indicate that this risk may be increased in patients receiving concomitant corticosteroids, especially the elderly).
No products indexed under this heading.

Hydrocortisone Acetate (Ruptures of the shoulder, hand, Achilles tendon or other tendons that required surgical repair or resulted in prolonged disability have been reported in patients receiving quinolones, including moxifloxacin, Post-marketing surveillance reports indicate that this risk may be increased in patients receiving concomitant corticosteroids, especially the elderly). Products include:

Analpram-HC 1140
Pramosone 1141

Hydrocortisone Sodium Phosphate (Ruptures of the shoulder, hand, Achilles tendon or other tendons that required surgical repair or resulted in prolonged disability have been reported in patients receiving quinolones, including moxifloxacin, Post-marketing surveillance reports indicate that this risk may be increased in patients receiving concomitant corticosteroids, especially the elderly).
No products indexed under this heading.

Hydrocortisone Sodium Succinate (Ruptures of the shoulder, hand, Achilles tendon or other tendons that required surgical repair or resulted in prolonged disability have been reported in patients receiving quinolones, including moxifloxacin, Post-marketing surveillance reports indicate that this risk may be increased in patients receiving concomitant corticosteroids, especially the elderly).
No products indexed under this heading.

Ibuprofen (Although not observed with moxifloxacin in preclinical and clinical trials, the concomitant administration of a nonsteriodal anti-inflammatory drug with a quinolone may increase the risks of CNS stimulation and convulsions). Products include:

Motrin IB Tablets and Caplets 1900
Children's Motrin Oral Suspension ... 1901
Children's Motrin Non-Staining Dye-Free Oral Suspension............ 1901
Children's Motrin Cold Oral Suspension 1899
Infants' Motrin Concentrated Drops.. 1901
Infants' Motrin Non-Staining Dye-Free Concentrated Drops....... 1901
Junior Strength Motrin Caplets and Chewable Tablets.................. 1901
Vicoprofen Tablets 533

Imipramine Hydrochloride (Moxifloxacin has been shown to prolong the QT interval of the electrocardiogram in some patients. Pharmacokinetic studies between moxifloxacin and other drugs that prolong the QT interval such as tricyclic antidepressants have not been performed. An additive effect of moxifloxacin and tricyclic antidepressants cannot be excluded, therefore, caution should be exercised when moxifloxacin is given concurrently with tricyclic antidepressants).
No products indexed under this heading.

Imipramine Pamoate (Moxifloxacin has been shown to prolong the QT interval of the electrocardiogram in some patients. Pharmacokinetic studies between moxifloxacin and other drugs that prolong the QT interval such as tricyclic antidepressants have not been performed. An additive effect of moxifloxacin and tricyclic antidepressants cannot be excluded, therefore, caution should be exercised when moxifloxacin is given concurrently with tricyclic antidepressants).
No products indexed under this heading.

Indomethacin (Although not observed with moxifloxacin in preclinical and clinical trials, the concomitant administration of a nonsteriodal anti-inflammatory drug with a quinolone may increase the risks of CNS stimulation and convulsions). Products include:

Indocin 2024

Indomethacin Sodium Trihydrate (Although not observed with moxifloxacin in preclinical and clinical trials, the concomitant administration of a nonsteriodal anti-inflammatory drug with a quinolone may increase the risks of CNS stimulation and convulsions). Products include:

Indocin I.V. 2489

Iron (Quinolones form chelates with alkaline earth and transition metal cations. When moxifloxacin tablets were administered concomitantly with iron (ferrous sulfate 100 mg once daily for two days), the mean AUC and Cmax of moxifloxacin was reduced by 39% and59%, respectively. Moxifloxacin should only be taken more than 4 hours before or 8 hours after iron products). Products include:

Phyto-Vite Tablets 639

Ketoprofen (Although not observed with moxifloxacin in preclinical and clinical trials, the concomitant administration of a nonsteriodal anti-inflammatory drug with a quinolone may increase the risks of CNS stimulation and convulsions).

No products indexed under this heading.

Ketorolac Tromethamine (Although not observed with moxifloxacin in preclinical and clinical trials, the concomitant administration of a nonsteriodal anti-inflammatory drug with a quinolone may increase the risks of CNS stimulation and convulsions).

No products indexed under this heading.

Magaldrate (Quinolones form chelates with alkaline earth and transition metal cations. When moxifloxacin (single 400 mg tablet dose) was administered two hours before, concomitantly, or 4 hours after an aluminum/magnesium-containing antacid (900 mg aluminum hydroxide and 600 mg magnesium hydroxide as a single oral dose) to 12 healthy volunteers there was a 26%, 60%, and 23% reduction in the mean AUC of moxifloxacin, respectively. Moxifloxacin should be taken at least 4 hours before or 8 hours after antacids containing magnesium or aluminum).

No products indexed under this heading.

Magnesium Hydroxide (Quinolones form chelates with alkaline earth and transition metal cations. When moxifloxacin (single 400 mg tablet dose) was administered two hours before, concomitantly, or 4 hours after an aluminum/magnesium-containing antacid (900 mg aluminum hydroxide and 600 mg magnesium hydroxide as a single oral dose) to 12 healthy volunteers there was a 26%, 60%, and 23% reduction in the mean AUC of moxifloxacin, respectively. Moxifloxacin should be taken at least 4 hours before or 8 hours after antacids containing magnesium or aluminum). Products include:

Fleet Pedia-Lax Chewable Tablets 1145
Pepcid Complete Chewable Tablets 1771
Extra Strength Rolaids Freshmint Tablets 1903
Rolaids Multi-Symptom Berry Tablets 1903
Rolaids Original Peppermint Tablets 1903

Magnesium Oxide (Quinolones form chelates with alkaline earth and transition metal cations. When moxifloxacin (single 400 mg tablet dose) was administered two hours before, concomitantly, or 4 hours after an aluminum/magnesium-containing antacid (900 mg aluminum hydroxide and 600 mg magnesium hydroxide as a single oral dose) to 12 healthy volunteers there was a 26%, 60%, and 23% reduction in the mean AUC of moxifloxacin, respectively. Moxifloxacin should be taken at least 4 hours before or 8 hours after antacids containing magnesium or aluminum). Products include:

Beelith Tablets 813

Maprotiline Hydrochloride (Moxifloxacin has been shown to prolong the QT interval of the electrocardiogram in some patients. Pharmacokinetic studies between moxifloxacin and other drugs that prolong the QT interval such as tricyclic antidepressants have not been performed. An additive effect of moxifloxacin and tricyclic antidepressants cannot be excluded, therefore, caution should be exercised when moxifloxacin is given concurrently with tricyclic antidepressants).

No products indexed under this heading.

Meclofenamate Sodium (Although not observed with moxifloxacin in preclinical and clinical trials, the concomitant administration of a nonsteriodal anti-inflammatory drug with a quinolone may increase the risks of CNS stimulation and convulsions).

No products indexed under this heading.

Mefenamic Acid (Although not observed with moxifloxacin in preclinical and clinical trials, the concomitant administration of a nonsteriodal anti-inflammatory drug with a quinolone may increase the risks of CNS stimulation and convulsions).

No products indexed under this heading.

Meloxicam (Although not observed with moxifloxacin in preclinical and clinical trials, the concomitant administration of a nonsteriodal anti-inflammatory drug with a quinolone may increase the risks of CNS stimulation and convulsions). Products include:

Mobic Oral Suspension 863
Mobic Tablets 863

Mesoridazine Besylate (Moxifloxacin has been shown to prolong the QT interval of the electrocardiogram in some patients. Pharmacokinetic studies between moxifloxacin and other drugs that prolong the QT interval such as antipsychotic phenthiazines has not been performed. An additive effect of moxifloxacin and antipsychotic phenthiazines cannot be excluded, therefore, caution should be exercised when moxifloxacin is given concurrently with antipsychotic phenthiazines).

No products indexed under this heading.

Methotrimeprazine (Moxifloxacin has been shown to prolong the QT interval of the electrocardiogram in some patients. Pharmacokinetic studies between moxifloxacin and other drugs that prolong the QT interval such as antipsychotic phenthiazines has not been performed. An additive effect of moxifloxacin and antipsychotic phenthiazines cannot be excluded, therefore, caution should be exercised when moxifloxacin is given concurrently with antipsychotic phenthiazines).

No products indexed under this heading.

Methylprednisolone Acetate (Ruptures of the shoulder, hand, Achilles tendon or other tendons that required surgical repair or resulted in prolonged disability have been reported in patients receiving quinolones, including moxifloxacin, Post-marketing surveillance reports indicate that this risk may be increased in patients receiving concomitant corticosteroids, especially the elderly).

No products indexed under this heading.

Methylprednisolone Sodium Succinate (Ruptures of the shoulder, hand, Achilles tendon or other tendons that required surgical repair or resulted in prolonged disability have been reported in patients receiving quinolones, including moxifloxacin, Post-marketing surveillance reports indicate that this risk may be increased in patients receiving concomitant corticosteroids, especially the elderly).

No products indexed under this heading.

Mometasone Furoate (Ruptures of the shoulder, hand, Achilles tendon or other tendons that required surgical repair or resulted in prolonged disability have been reported in patients receiving quinolones, including moxifloxacin, Post-marketing surveillance reports indicate that this risk may be increased in patients receiving concomitant corticosteroids, especially the elderly). Products include:

Asmanex Twisthaler 2797
Elocon Cream 0.1% 2840
Elocon Lotion 0.1% 2841
Elocon Ointment 0.1% 2842

Mometasone Furoate Monohydrate (Ruptures of the shoulder, hand, Achilles tendon or other tendons that required surgical repair or resulted in prolonged disability have been reported in patients receiving quinolones, including moxifloxacin, Post-marketing surveillance reports indicate that this risk may be increased in patients receiving concomitant corticosteroids, especially the elderly). Products include:

Nasonex Nasal Spray 2883

Moricizine Hydrochloride (Moxifloxacin has been shown to prolong the QT interval of the electrocardiogram in some patients. The drug should be avoided in patients receiving Class IA antiarrhythmic agents, due to the lack of clinical experience with the drug in these patient populations).

No products indexed under this heading.

Nabumetone (Although not observed with moxifloxacin in preclinical and clinical trials, the concomitant administration of a nonsteriodal anti-inflammatory drug with a quinolone may increase the risks of CNS stimulation and convulsions).

No products indexed under this heading.

Naproxen (Although not observed with moxifloxacin in preclinical and clinical trials, the concomitant administration of a nonsteriodal anti-inflammatory drug with a quinolone may increase the risks of CNS stimulation and convulsions). Products include:

EC-Naprosyn Delayed-Release Tablets 2632
Naprosyn Suspension 2632
Naprosyn Tablets 2632

Naproxen Sodium (Although not observed with moxifloxacin in preclinical and clinical trials, the concomitant administration of a nonsteriodal anti-inflammatory drug with a quinolone may increase the risks of CNS stimulation and convulsions). Products include:

Anaprox Tablets 2632
Anaprox DS Tablets 2632
Treximet Tablets 1616

Nortriptyline Hydrochloride (Moxifloxacin has been shown to prolong the QT interval of the electrocardiogram in some patients. Pharmacokinetic studies between moxifloxacin and other drugs that prolong the QT interval such as tricyclic antidepressants have not been performed. An additive effect of moxifloxacin and tricyclic antidepressants cannot be excluded, therefore, caution should be exercised when moxifloxacin is given concurrently with tricyclic antidepressants).

No products indexed under this heading.

Oxaprozin (Although not observed with moxifloxacin in preclinical and clinical trials, the concomitant administration of a nonsteriodal anti-inflammatory drug with a quinolone may increase the risks of CNS stimulation and convulsions).

No products indexed under this heading.

Perphenazine (Moxifloxacin has been shown to prolong the QT interval of the electrocardiogram in some patients. Pharmacokinetic studies between moxifloxacin and other drugs that prolong the QT interval such as antipsychotic phenthiazines has not been performed. An additive effect of moxifloxacin and antipsychotic phenthiazines cannot be excluded, therefore, caution should be exercised when moxifloxacin is given concurrently with antipsychotic phenthiazines).

No products indexed under this heading.

Phenylbutazone (Although not observed with moxifloxacin in preclinical and clinical trials, the concomitant administration of a nonsteriodal anti-inflammatory drug with a quinolone may increase the risks of CNS stimulation and convulsions).

No products indexed under this heading.

Piroxicam (Although not observed with moxifloxacin in preclinical and clinical trials, the concomitant administration of a nonsteriodal anti-inflammatory drug with a quinolone may increase the risks of CNS stimulation and convulsions).

No products indexed under this heading.

Polysaccharide Iron Complex (Quinolones form chelates with alkaline earth and transition metal cations. When moxifloxacin tablets were administered concomitantly with iron (ferrous sulfate 100 mg once daily for two days), the mean AUC and

Cmax of moxifloxacin was reduced by 39% and59%, respectively. Moxifloxacin should only be taken more than 4 hours before or 8 hours after iron products). Products include:

Nu-Iron 150 Capsules 2165

Prednisolone Acetate (Ruptures of the shoulder, hand, Achilles tendon or other tendons that required surgical repair or resulted in prolonged disability have been reported in patients receiving quinolones, including moxifloxacin, Post-marketing surveillance reports indicate that this risk may be increased in patients receiving concomitant corticosteroids, especially the elderly). Products include:

Pred Forte Ophthalmic Suspension .... ⊙ 227
Pred Mild Ophthalmic Suspension .... ⊙ 230
Pred-G Ophthalmic Ointment .... ⊙ 229
Pred-G Ophthalmic Suspension ...... ⊙ 228

Prednisolone Sodium Phosphate (Ruptures of the shoulder, hand, Achilles tendon or other tendons that required surgical repair or resulted in prolonged disability have been reported in patients receiving quinolones, including moxifloxacin, Post-marketing surveillance reports indicate that this risk may be increased in patients receiving concomitant corticosteroids, especially the elderly).

No products indexed under this heading.

Prednisolone Tebutate (Ruptures of the shoulder, hand, Achilles tendon or other tendons that required surgical repair or resulted in prolonged disability have been reported in patients receiving quinolones, including moxifloxacin, Post-marketing surveillance reports indicate that this risk may be increased in patients receiving concomitant corticosteroids, especially the elderly).

No products indexed under this heading.

Prednisone (Ruptures of the shoulder, hand, Achilles tendon or other tendons that required surgical repair or resulted in prolonged disability have been reported in patients receiving quinolones, including moxifloxacin, Post-marketing surveillance reports indicate that this risk may be increased in patients receiving concomitant corticosteroids, especially the elderly).

No products indexed under this heading.

Procainamide (Moxifloxacin has been shown to prolong the QT interval of the electrocardiogram in some patients. The drug should be avoided in patients receiving Class IA antiarrhythmic agents such as procainamide, due to the lack of clinical experience with the drug in this patient population).

No products indexed under this heading.

Procainamide Hydrochloride (Moxifloxacin has been shown to prolong the QT interval of the electrocardiogram in some patients. The drug should be avoided in patients receiving Class IA antiarrhythmic agents such as procainamide, due to the lack of clinical experience with the drug in this patient population).

No products indexed under this heading.

Prochlorperazine (Moxifloxacin has been shown to prolong the QT interval of the electrocardiogram in some patients. Pharmacokinetic studies between moxifloxacin and other drugs that prolong the QT interval such as antipsychotic phenthiazines has not been performed. An additive effect of moxifloxacin and antipsychotic phenthiazines cannot be excluded, therefore, caution should be exercised when moxifloxacin is given concurrently with antipsychotic phenthiazines).

No products indexed under this heading.

Promethazine Hydrochloride (Moxifloxacin has been shown to prolong the QT interval of the electrocardiogram in some patients. Pharmacokinetic studies between moxifloxacin and other drugs that prolong the QT interval such as antipsychotic phenthiazines has not been performed. An additive effect of moxifloxacin and antipsychotic phenthiazines cannot be excluded, therefore, caution should be exercised when moxifloxacin is given concurrently with antipsychotic phenthiazines).

No products indexed under this heading.

Protriptyline Hydrochloride (Moxifloxacin has been shown to prolong the QT interval of the electrocardiogram in some patients. Pharmacokinetic studies between moxifloxacin and other drugs that prolong the QT interval such as tricyclic antidepressants have not been performed. An additive effect of moxifloxacin and tricyclic antidepressants cannot be excluded, therefore, caution should be exercised when moxifloxacin is given concurrently with tricyclic antidepressants).

No products indexed under this heading.

Quinidine (Moxifloxacin has been shown to prolong the QT interval of the electrocardiogram in some patients. The drug should be avoided in patients receiving Class IA antiarrhythmic agents, due to the lack of clinical experience with the drug in these patient populations).

No products indexed under this heading.

Quinidine Gluconate (Moxifloxacin has been shown to prolong the QT interval of the electrocardiogram in some patients. The drug should be avoided in patients receiving Class IA antiarrhythmic agents, due to the lack of clinical experience with the drug in these patient populations).

No products indexed under this heading.

Quinidine Hydrochloride (Moxifloxacin has been shown to prolong the QT interval of the electrocardiogram in some patients. The drug should be avoided in patients receiving Class IA antiarrhythmic agents, due to the lack of clinical experience with the drug in these patient populations).

No products indexed under this heading.

Quinidine Polygalacturonate (Moxifloxacin has been shown to prolong the QT interval of the electrocardiogram in some patients. The drug should be avoided in patients receiving Class IA antiarrhythmic agents, due to the lack of clinical experience with the drug in these patient populations).

No products indexed under this heading.

Quinidine Sulfate (Moxifloxacin has been shown to prolong the QT interval of the electrocardiogram in some patients. The drug should be avoided in patients receiving Class IA antiarrhythmic agents, due to the lack of clinical experience with the drug in these patient populations).

No products indexed under this heading.

Rofecoxib (Although not observed with moxifloxacin in preclinical and clinical trials, the concomitant administration of a nonsteriodal anti-inflammatory drug with a quinolone may increase the risks of CNS stimulation and convulsions).

No products indexed under this heading.

Sotalol Hydrochloride (Moxifloxacin has been shown to prolong the QT interval of the electrocardiogram in some patients. The drug should be avoided in patients receiving Class III antiarrhythmic agents such as sotalol, due to the lack of clinical experience with the drug in this patient population).

No products indexed under this heading.

Sucralfate (Quinolones form chelates with alkaline earth and transition metal cations. Oral administration of quinolones with sucralfate, may substantially interfere with the absorption of quinolones, resulting in systemic concentrations considerably lower than desired. Therefore, moxifloxacin should be taken at least 4 hours before or 8 hours after these agents). Products include:

Carafate Suspension 706
Carafate Tablets 707

Sulindac (Although not observed with moxifloxacin in preclinical and clinical trials, the concomitant administration of a nonsteriodal anti-inflammatory drug with a quinolone may increase the risks of CNS stimulation and convulsions). Products include:

Clinoril Tablets 1962

Thioridazine Hydrochloride (Moxifloxacin has been shown to prolong the QT interval of the electrocardiogram in some patients. Pharmacokinetic studies between moxifloxacin and other drugs that prolong the QT interval such as antipsychotic phenthiazines has not been performed. An additive effect of moxifloxacin and antipsychotic phenthiazines cannot be excluded, therefore, caution should be exercised when moxifloxacin is given concurrently with antipsychotic phenthiazines). Products include:

Thioridazine Hydrochloride Tablets 2195

Tolmetin Sodium (Although not observed with moxifloxacin in preclinical and clinical trials, the concomitant administration of a nonsteriodal anti-inflammatory drug with a quinolone may increase the risks of CNS stimulation and convulsions).

No products indexed under this heading.

Triamcinolone (Ruptures of the shoulder, hand, Achilles tendon or other tendons that required surgical repair or resulted in prolonged disability have been reported in patients receiving quinolones, including moxifloxacin, Post-marketing surveillance reports indicate that this risk may be increased in patients receiving concomitant corticosteroids, especially the elderly).

No products indexed under this heading.

Triamcinolone Acetonide (Ruptures of the shoulder, hand, Achilles tendon or other tendons that required surgical repair or resulted in prolonged disability have been reported in patients receiving quinolones, including moxifloxacin, Post-marketing surveillance reports indicate that this risk may be increased in patients receiving concomitant corticosteroids, especially the elderly). Products include:

Azmacort Inhalation Aerosol 407
Nasacort AQ Nasal Spray 2765
Triesence Injectable Suspension .... ⊙ 209

Triamcinolone Diacetate (Ruptures of the shoulder, hand, Achilles tendon or other tendons that required surgical repair or resulted in prolonged disability have been reported in patients receiving quinolones, including moxifloxacin, Post-marketing surveillance reports indicate that this risk may be increased in patients receiving concomitant corticosteroids, especially the elderly).

No products indexed under this heading.

Triamcinolone Hexacetonide (Ruptures of the shoulder, hand, Achilles tendon or other tendons that required surgical repair or resulted in prolonged disability have been reported in patients receiving quinolones, including moxifloxacin, Post-marketing surveillance reports indicate that this risk may be increased in patients receiving concomitant corticosteroids, especially the elderly).

No products indexed under this heading.

Trifluoperazine Hydrochloride (Moxifloxacin has been shown to prolong the QT interval of the electrocardiogram in some patients. Pharmacokinetic studies between moxifloxacin and other drugs that prolong the QT interval such as antipsychotic phenthiazines has not been performed. An additive effect of moxifloxacin and antipsychotic phenthiazines cannot be excluded, therefore, caution should be exercised when moxifloxacin is given concurrently with antipsychotic phenthiazines).

No products indexed under this heading.

Trimipramine Maleate (Moxifloxacin has been shown to prolong the QT interval of the electrocardiogram in some patients. Pharmacokinetic studies between moxifloxacin and other drugs that prolong the QT interval such as tricyclic antidepressants have not been performed. An additive effect of moxifloxacin and tricyclic antidepressants cannot be excluded, therefore, caution should be exercised when moxifloxacin is given concurrently with tricyclic

antidepressants).
No products indexed under this heading.

Valdecoxib (Although not observed with moxifloxacin in preclinical and clinical trials, the concomitant administration of a nonsteriodal anti-inflammatory drug with a quinolone may increase the risks of CNS stimulation and convulsions).
No products indexed under this heading.

Vitamins with Iron (Quinolones form chelates with alkaline earth and transition metal cations. Oral administration of quinolones with multivitamins containing iron or zinc, may substantially interfere with the absorption of quinolones, resulting in systemic concentrations considerably lower than desired. Therefore, moxifloxacin should be taken at least 4 hours before or 8 hours after these agents).
No products indexed under this heading.

Warfarin Sodium (No significant effect of moxifloxacin on R- and S-warfarin was detected in a clinical study involving 24 healthy volunteers. No significant changes in prothrombin time were noted in the presence of moxifloxacin. Quinolones, including moxifloxacin, have been reported to enhance the anticoagulant effects of warfarin or its derivatives in the patient population. In addition, infectious disease and its accompanying inflammatory process, age, and general status of the patient are risk factors for increased anticoagulant activity. Therefore, the prothrombin time, International Normalized Ratio (INR), or other suitable anticoagulation tests should be closely monitored if a quinolone is administered concomitantly with warfarin or its derivatives).
No products indexed under this heading.

Zinc (Quinolones form chelates with alkaline earth and transition metal cations. Oral administration of quinolones with metal cations may substantially interfere with the absorption of quinolones, resulting in systemic concentrations considerably lower than desired. Therefore, moxifloxacin should be taken at least 4 hours before or 8 hours after metal cations such as zinc). Products include:
Comax Dietary Supplement 995
Glaucofit Dietary Supplement 995
Glauma Dietary Supplement 995
Tonox Dietary Supplement 995
Vibe Liquid Multi-Nutrient Supplement 626
Visutein Capsules 3159

Zinc-Containing Multivitamins (Quinolones form chelates with alkaline earth and transition metal cations. Oral administration of quinolones with multivitamins containing iron or zinc, may substantially interfere with the absorption of quinolones, resulting in systemic concentrations considerably lower than desired. Therefore, moxifloxacin should be taken at least 4 hours before or 8 hours after these agents).
No products indexed under this heading.

AVINZA CAPSULES

(Morphine Sulfate) 1772
May interact with central nervous system depressants, monoamine oxidase inhibitors, mixed agonist/antagonist opioid analgesics, muscle relaxants, and certain other agents. Compounds in these categories include:

Alfentanil Hydrochloride (Co-administration increases the risk of respiratory depression, hypotension, profound sedation, or coma).
No products indexed under this heading.

Alprazolam (Co-administration increases the risk of respiratory depression, hypotension, profound sedation, or coma).
No products indexed under this heading.

Aprobarbital (Co-administration increases the risk of respiratory depression, hypotension, profound sedation, or coma).
No products indexed under this heading.

Atracurium Besylate (Morphine may enhance the neuromuscular blocking action of skeletal muscle relaxants and produce an increased degree of respiratory depression).
No products indexed under this heading.

Baclofen (Morphine may enhance the neuromuscular blocking action of skeletal muscle relaxants and produce an increased degree of respiratory depression).
No products indexed under this heading.

Buprenorphine Hydrochloride (Mixed agonist/antagonist analgesics may reduce the analgesic effect and/or may precipitate withdrawal symptoms; mixed agonist/antagonist analgesics should NOT be administered to patients who have received or are receiving a course of therapy with pure opioid agonist analgesic). Products include:
Suboxone Tablets 2601
Subutex Tablets 2601

Buspirone Hydrochloride (Co-administration increases the risk of respiratory depression, hypotension, profound sedation, or coma).
No products indexed under this heading.

Butabarbital (Co-administration increases the risk of respiratory depression, hypotension, profound sedation, or coma).
No products indexed under this heading.

Butalbital (Co-administration increases the risk of respiratory depression, hypotension, profound sedation, or coma).
No products indexed under this heading.

Butorphanol Tartrate (Mixed agonist/antagonist analgesics may reduce the analgesic effect and/or may precipitate withdrawal symptoms; mixed agonist/antagonist analgesics should NOT be administered to patients who have received or are receiving a course of therapy with pure opioid agonist analgesic).
No products indexed under this heading.

Carisoprodol (Morphine may enhance the neuromuscular blocking action of skeletal muscle relaxants and produce an increased degree of respiratory depression). Products include:
Soma Tablets 1931

Chlordiazepoxide (Co-administration increases the risk of respiratory depression, hypotension, profound sedation, or coma).
No products indexed under this heading.

Chlordiazepoxide Hydrochloride (Co-administration increases the risk of respiratory depression, hypotension, profound sedation, or coma).
No products indexed under this heading.

Chlorpromazine (Co-administration increases the risk of respiratory depression, hypotension, profound sedation, or coma).
No products indexed under this heading.

Chlorpromazine Hydrochloride (Co-administration increases the risk of respiratory depression, hypotension, profound sedation, or coma).
No products indexed under this heading.

Chlorprothixene (Co-administration increases the risk of respiratory depression, hypotension, profound sedation, or coma).
No products indexed under this heading.

Chlorprothixene Hydrochloride (Co-administration increases the risk of respiratory depression, hypotension, profound sedation, or coma).
No products indexed under this heading.

Chlorprothixene Lactate (Co-administration increases the risk of respiratory depression, hypotension, profound sedation, or coma).
No products indexed under this heading.

Chlorzoxazone (Morphine may enhance the neuromuscular blocking action of skeletal muscle relaxants and produce an increased degree of respiratory depression).
No products indexed under this heading.

Cimetidine (Co-administration has been reported to precipitate apnea, confusion and muscle twitching in an isolated report).
No products indexed under this heading.

Cisatracurium Besylate (Morphine may enhance the neuromuscular blocking action of skeletal muscle relaxants and produce an increased degree of respiratory depression). Products include:
Nimbex Injection 484

Clorazepate Dipotassium (Co-administration increases the risk of respiratory depression, hypotension, profound sedation, or coma).
No products indexed under this heading.

Clozapine (Co-administration increases the risk of respiratory depression, hypotension, profound sedation, or coma).
No products indexed under this heading.

Codeine Phosphate (Co-administration increases the risk of respiratory depression, hypotension, profound sedation, or coma). Products include:
Tylenol with Codeine Tablets 2427

Cyclobenzaprine Hydrochloride (Morphine may enhance the neuromuscular blocking action of skeletal muscle relaxants and produce an increased degree of respiratory depression). Products include:
Amrix Capsules 966

Dantrolene Sodium (Morphine may enhance the neuromuscular blocking action of skeletal muscle relaxants and produce an increased degree of respiratory depression). Products include:
Dantrium Capsules 2580
Dantrium Intravenous 2582

Desflurane (Co-administration increases the risk of respiratory depression, hypotension, profound sedation, or coma).
No products indexed under this heading.

Dezocine (Co-administration increases the risk of respiratory depression, hypotension, profound sedation, or coma).
No products indexed under this heading.

Diazepam (Co-administration increases the risk of respiratory depression, hypotension, profound sedation, or coma). Products include:
Valium Tablets 2658

Doxacurium Chloride (Morphine may enhance the neuromuscular blocking action of skeletal muscle relaxants and produce an increased degree of respiratory depression).
No products indexed under this heading.

Droperidol (Co-administration increases the risk of respiratory depression, hypotension, profound sedation, or coma).
No products indexed under this heading.

Enflurane (Co-administration increases the risk of respiratory depression, hypotension, profound sedation, or coma).
No products indexed under this heading.

Estazolam (Co-administration increases the risk of respiratory depression, hypotension, profound sedation, or coma).
No products indexed under this heading.

Ethanol (Co-administration increases the risk of respiratory depression, hypotension, profound sedation, or coma).
No products indexed under this heading.

Ethchlorvynol (Co-administration increases the risk of respiratory depression, hypotension, profound sedation, or coma).
No products indexed under this heading.

Ethinamate (Co-administration increases the risk of respiratory depression, hypotension, profound sedation, or coma).
No products indexed under this heading.

Ethyl Alcohol (Co-administration increases the risk of respiratory depression, hypotension, profound sedation, or coma).
No products indexed under this heading.

Fentanyl (Co-administration increases the risk of respiratory depression, hypotension, profound sedation, or coma). Products include:
Duragesic Transdermal System 2405

Ionsys Transdermal System 2410

Fentanyl Citrate (Co-administration increases the risk of respiratory depression, hypotension, profound sedation, or coma). Products include:
Actiq 959
Fentora Tablets 968

Fluphenazine Decanoate (Co-administration increases the risk of respiratory depression, hypotension, profound sedation, or coma).
No products indexed under this heading.

Fluphenazine Enanthate (Co-administration increases the risk of respiratory depression, hypotension, profound sedation, or coma).
No products indexed under this heading.

Fluphenazine Hydrochloride (Co-administration increases the risk of respiratory depression, hypotension, profound sedation, or coma).
No products indexed under this heading.

Flurazepam Hydrochloride (Co-administration increases the risk of respiratory depression, hypotension, profound sedation, or coma).
No products indexed under this heading.

Glutethimide (Co-administration increases the risk of respiratory depression, hypotension, profound sedation, or coma).
No products indexed under this heading.

Haloperidol (Co-administration increases the risk of respiratory depression, hypotension, profound sedation, or coma).
No products indexed under this heading.

Haloperidol Decanoate (Co-administration increases the risk of respiratory depression, hypotension, profound sedation, or coma).
No products indexed under this heading.

Hydrocodone Bitartrate (Co-administration increases the risk of respiratory depression, hypotension, profound sedation, or coma). Products include:
Lortab 5/500 Tablets 3143
Lortab 7.5/500 Tablets 3144
Lortab 10/500 Tablets 3144
Vicodin Tablets 529
Vicodin ES Tablets 530
Vicodin HP Tablets 531
Vicoprofen Tablets 533
Zydone Tablets 1132

Hydrocodone Polistirex (Co-administration increases the risk of respiratory depression, hypotension, profound sedation, or coma). Products include:
Tussionex Pennkinetic Extended-Release Suspension 3154

Hydromorphone Hydrochloride (Co-administration increases the risk of respiratory depression, hypotension, profound sedation, or coma).
No products indexed under this heading.

Hydroxyzine Hydrochloride (Co-administration increases the risk of respiratory depression, hypotension, profound sedation, or coma).
No products indexed under this heading.

Isocarboxazid (MAO inhibitors markedly potentiate the action of morphine; concurrent and/or sequential use should be avoided). Products include:
Marplan Tablets 3177

Isoflurane (Co-administration increases the risk of respiratory depression, hypotension, profound sedation, or coma).
No products indexed under this heading.

Ketamine Hydrochloride (Co-administration increases the risk of respiratory depression, hypotension, profound sedation, or coma).
No products indexed under this heading.

Levomethadyl Acetate Hydrochloride (Co-administration increases the risk of respiratory depression, hypotension, profound sedation, or coma).
No products indexed under this heading.

Levorphanol Tartrate (Co-administration increases the risk of respiratory depression, hypotension, profound sedation, or coma).
No products indexed under this heading.

Lorazepam (Co-administration increases the risk of respiratory depression, hypotension, profound sedation, or coma).
No products indexed under this heading.

Loxapine Hydrochloride (Co-administration increases the risk of respiratory depression, hypotension, profound sedation, or coma).
No products indexed under this heading.

Loxapine Succinate (Co-administration increases the risk of respiratory depression, hypotension, profound sedation, or coma).
No products indexed under this heading.

Meperidine Hydrochloride (Co-administration increases the risk of respiratory depression, hypotension, profound sedation, or coma).
No products indexed under this heading.

Mephobarbital (Co-administration increases the risk of respiratory depression, hypotension, profound sedation, or coma).
No products indexed under this heading.

Meprobamate (Co-administration increases the risk of respiratory depression, hypotension, profound sedation, or coma).
No products indexed under this heading.

Mesoridazine Besylate (Co-administration increases the risk of respiratory depression, hypotension, profound sedation, or coma).
No products indexed under this heading.

Metaxalone (Morphine may enhance the neuromuscular blocking action of skeletal muscle relaxants and produce an increased degree of respiratory depression). Products include:
Skelaxin Tablets 1784

Methadone Hydrochloride (Co-administration increases the risk of respiratory depression, hypotension, profound sedation, or coma).
No products indexed under this heading.

Methocarbamol (Morphine may enhance the neuromuscular blocking action of skeletal muscle relaxants and produce an increased degree of respiratory depression).
No products indexed under this heading.

Methohexital Sodium (Co-administration increases the risk of respiratory depression, hypotension, profound sedation, or coma).
No products indexed under this heading.

Methotrimeprazine (Co-administration increases the risk of respiratory depression, hypotension, profound sedation, or coma).
No products indexed under this heading.

Methoxyflurane (Co-administration increases the risk of respiratory depression, hypotension, profound sedation, or coma).
No products indexed under this heading.

Metocurine Iodide (Morphine may enhance the neuromuscular blocking action of skeletal muscle relaxants and produce an increased degree of respiratory depression).
No products indexed under this heading.

Midazolam Hydrochloride (Co-administration increases the risk of respiratory depression, hypotension, profound sedation, or coma).
No products indexed under this heading.

Mivacurium Chloride (Morphine may enhance the neuromuscular blocking action of skeletal muscle relaxants and produce an increased degree of respiratory depression).
No products indexed under this heading.

Moclobemide (MAO inhibitors markedly potentiate the action of morphine; concurrent and/or sequential use should be avoided).
No products indexed under this heading.

Molindone Hydrochloride (Co-administration increases the risk of respiratory depression, hypotension, profound sedation, or coma). Products include:
Moban Tablets 1116

Nalbuphine Hydrochloride (Mixed agonist/antagonist analgesics may reduce the analgesic effect and/or may precipitate withdrawal symptoms; mixed agonist/antagonist analgesics should NOT be administered to patients who have received or are receiving a course of therapy with pure opioid agonist analgesic).
No products indexed under this heading.

Olanzapine (Co-administration increases the risk of respiratory depression, hypotension, profound sedation, or coma). Products include:
Symbyax Capsules 1871
Zyprexa Tablets 1883
Zyprexa IntraMuscular 1883
Zyprexa ZYDIS Orally Disintegrating Tablets 1883

Orphenadrine Citrate (Morphine may enhance the neuromuscular blocking action of skeletal muscle relaxants and produce an increased degree of respiratory depression).
No products indexed under this heading.

Oxazepam (Co-administration increases the risk of respiratory depression, hypotension, profound sedation, or coma).
No products indexed under this heading.

Oxycodone Hydrochloride (Co-administration increases the risk of respiratory depression, hypotension, profound sedation, or coma). Products include:
OxyContin Tablets 2589
OxyIR Capsules 2593
Percocet Tablets 1127
Percodan Tablets 1130

Pancuronium Bromide (Morphine may enhance the neuromuscular blocking action of skeletal muscle relaxants and produce an increased degree of respiratory depression).
No products indexed under this heading.

Pargyline Hydrochloride (MAO inhibitors markedly potentiate the action of morphine; concurrent and/or sequential use should be avoided).
No products indexed under this heading.

Pentazocine Hydrochloride (Mixed agonist/antagonist analgesics may reduce the analgesic effect and/or may precipitate withdrawal symptoms; mixed agonist/antagonist analgesics should NOT be administered to patients who have received or are receiving a course of therapy with pure opioid agonist analgesic).
No products indexed under this heading.

Pentazocine Lactate (Mixed agonist/antagonist analgesics may reduce the analgesic effect and/or may precipitate withdrawal symptoms; mixed agonist/antagonist analgesics should NOT be administered to patients who have received or are receiving a course of therapy with pure opioid agonist analgesic).
No products indexed under this heading.

Pentobarbital Sodium (Co-administration increases the risk of respiratory depression, hypotension, profound sedation, or coma). Products include:
Nembutal Sodium Solution, USP 2494

Perphenazine (Co-administration increases the risk of respiratory depression, hypotension, profound sedation, or coma).
No products indexed under this heading.

Phenelzine Sulfate (MAO inhibitors markedly potentiate the action of morphine; concurrent and/or sequential use should be avoided).
No products indexed under this heading.

Phenobarbital (Co-administration increases the risk of respiratory depression, hypotension, profound sedation, or coma). Products include:
Donnatal Extentabs 2507

Prazepam (Co-administration increases the risk of respiratory depression, hypotension, profound sedation, or coma).
No products indexed under this heading.

Procarbazine Hydrochloride (MAO inhibitors markedly potentiate the action of morphine; concurrent and/or sequential use should be avoided).
No products indexed under this heading.

Prochlorperazine (Co-administration increases the risk of respiratory depression, hypotension, profound sedation, or coma).
No products indexed under this heading.

Promethazine Hydrochloride (Co-administration increases the risk of respiratory depression, hypotension, profound sedation, or coma).
No products indexed under this heading.

Propofol (Co-administration increases the risk of respiratory depression, hypotension, profound sedation, or coma).
No products indexed under this heading.

Propoxyphene Hydrochloride (Co-administration increases the risk of respiratory depression, hypotension, profound sedation, or coma).
No products indexed under this heading.

Propoxyphene Napsylate (Co-administration increases the risk of respiratory depression, hypotension, profound sedation, or coma).
No products indexed under this heading.

Quazepam (Co-administration increases the risk of respiratory depression, hypotension, profound sedation, or coma).
No products indexed under this heading.

Quetiapine Fumarate (Co-administration increases the risk of respiratory depression, hypotension, profound sedation, or coma).
No products indexed under this heading.

Rapacuronium Bromide (Morphine may enhance the neuromuscular blocking action of skeletal muscle relaxants and produce an increased degree of respiratory depression).
No products indexed under this heading.

Rasagiline Mesylate (MAO inhibitors markedly potentiate the action of morphine; concurrent and/or sequential use should be avoided). Products include:
Azilect Tablets 3106

Remifentanil Hydrochloride (Co-administration increases the risk of respiratory depression, hypotension, profound sedation, or coma).
No products indexed under this heading.

Risperidone (Co-administration increases the risk of respiratory depression, hypotension, profound sedation, or coma). Products include:
Risperdal Consta Long-Acting Injection 1753

Rocuronium Bromide (Morphine may enhance the neuromuscular blocking action of skeletal muscle relaxants and produce an increased degree of respiratory depression). Products include:
Zemuron Injection 2947

Secobarbital Sodium (Co-administration increases the risk of respiratory depression, hypotension, profound sedation, or coma).
No products indexed under this heading.

Selegiline (MAO inhibitors markedly potentiate the action of morphine; concurrent and/or sequential use should be avoided). Products include:
Emsam Transdermal System 905

Selegiline Hydrochloride (MAO inhibitors markedly potentiate the action of morphine; concurrent and/or sequential use should be avoided). Products include:
Eldepryl Capsules 3052

Sevoflurane (Co-administration increases the risk of respiratory depression, hypotension, profound sedation, or coma). Products include:
Ultane Liquid for Inhalation 524

Sodium Oxybate (Co-administration increases the risk of respiratory depression, hypotension, profound sedation, or coma). Products include:
Xyrem Oral Solution 1766

Succinylcholine Chloride (Morphine may enhance the neuromuscular blocking action of skeletal muscle relaxants and produce an increased degree of respiratory depression).
No products indexed under this heading.

Sufentanil Citrate (Co-administration increases the risk of respiratory depression, hypotension, profound sedation, or coma).
No products indexed under this heading.

Temazepam (Co-administration increases the risk of respiratory depression, hypotension, profound sedation, or coma).
No products indexed under this heading.

Thiamylal Sodium (Co-administration increases the risk of respiratory depression, hypotension, profound sedation, or coma).
No products indexed under this heading.

Thioridazine Hydrochloride (Co-administration increases the risk of respiratory depression, hypotension, profound sedation, or coma). Products include:
Thioridazine Hydrochloride Tablets 2195

Thiothixene (Co-administration increases the risk of respiratory depression, hypotension, profound sedation, or coma). Products include:
Thiothixene Capsules 2197

Tranylcypromine Sulfate (MAO inhibitors markedly potentiate the action of morphine; concurrent and/or sequential use should be avoided). Products include:
Parnate Tablets 1532

Triazolam (Co-administration increases the risk of respiratory depression, hypotension, profound sedation, or coma).
No products indexed under this heading.

Trifluoperazine Hydrochloride (Co-administration increases the risk of respiratory depression, hypotension, profound sedation, or coma).
No products indexed under this heading.

Vecuronium Bromide (Morphine may enhance the neuromuscular blocking action of skeletal muscle relaxants and produce an increased degree of respiratory depression).
No products indexed under this heading.

Zaleplon (Co-administration increases the risk of respiratory depression, hypotension, profound sedation, or coma).
No products indexed under this heading.

Ziprasidone Hydrochloride (Co-administration increases the risk of respiratory depression, hypotension, profound sedation, or coma). Products include:
Geodon Capsules 2520

Zolpidem Tartrate (Co-administration increases the risk of respiratory depression, hypotension, profound sedation, or coma). Products include:
Ambien Tablets 2692
Ambien CR Tablets 2696

Food Interactions

Alcohol (Patients must not consume alcoholic beverages, prescription or non-prescription medications containing alcohol while on morphine sulfate therapy. Consumption of alcohol while taking morphine sulfate may result in the rapid release and absoption of a potentially fatal dose of morphine).

AVODART SOFT GELATIN CAPSULES

(Dutasteride) 1359
May interact with cytochrome p450 3a4 inhibitors (selected) and certain other agents. Compounds in these categories include:

Acetazolamide (Blood concentrations of dutasteride may increase in the presence of CYP3A4 inhibitors).
No products indexed under this heading.

Amiodarone Hydrochloride (Blood concentrations of dutasteride may increase in the presence of CYP3A4 inhibitors).
No products indexed under this heading.

Amprenavir (Blood concentrations of dutasteride may increase in the presence of CYP3A4 inhibitors).
No products indexed under this heading.

Anastrozole (Blood concentrations of dutasteride may increase in the presence of CYP3A4 inhibitors). Products include:
Arimidex Tablets 672

Aprepitant (Blood concentrations of dutasteride may increase in the presence of CYP3A4 inhibitors). Products include:
Emend Capsules 1992

Atazanavir (Blood concentrations of dutasteride may increase in the presence of CYP3A4 inhibitors).
No products indexed under this heading.

Atazanavir Sulfate (Blood concentrations of dutasteride may increase in the presence of CYP3A4 inhibitors). Products include:
Reyataz Capsules 3299

Cimetidine (Blood concentrations of dutasteride may increase in the presence of CYP3A4 inhibitors).
No products indexed under this heading.

Cimetidine Hydrochloride (Blood concentrations of dutasteride may increase in the presence of CYP3A4 inhibitors).
No products indexed under this heading.

Ciprofloxacin (Blood concentrations of dutasteride may increase in the presence of CYP3A4 inhibitors). Products include:
Cipro I.V. 2817
Cipro Oral Suspension 2810
Cipro XR Tablets 2823
Ciprodex Otic Suspension 541

Clarithromycin (Blood concentrations of dutasteride may increase in the presence of CYP3A4 inhibitors). Products include:
Biaxin/Biaxin XL 411

Clotrimazole (Blood concentrations of dutasteride may increase in the presence of CYP3A4 inhibitors). Products include:
Lotrisone 2881

Cyclosporine (Blood concentrations of dutasteride may increase in the presence of CYP3A4 inhibitors). Products include:
Gengraf Capsules 435
Neoral Oral Solution 2280
Neoral Soft Gelatin Capsules 2280
Restasis Ophthalmic Emulsion 557
Sandimmune 2296

Dalfopristin (Blood concentrations of dutasteride may increase in the presence of CYP3A4 inhibitors).
No products indexed under this heading.

Danazol (Blood concentrations of dutasteride may increase in the presence of CYP3A4 inhibitors).
No products indexed under this heading.

Delavirdine Mesylate (Blood concentrations of dutasteride may increase in the presence of CYP3A4 inhibitors).
No products indexed under this heading.

Diltiazem Hydrochloride (Co-administration of diltiazem decreases dutasteride clearance and leads to increased exposure to dutasteride. The change in dutasteride exposure is not considered to be clinically significant. No dose adjustment is recommended). Products include:
Cardizem LA Extended Release Tablets 421

Diltiazem Maleate (Blood concentrations of dutasteride may increase in the presence of CYP3A4 inhibitors).
No products indexed under this heading.

Efavirenz (Blood concentrations of dutasteride may increase in the presence of CYP3A4 inhibitors). Products include:
Atripla Tablets 938
Sustiva Capsules 930
Sustiva Tablets 930

Erythromycin (Blood concentrations of dutasteride may increase in the presence of CYP3A4 inhibitors).
No products indexed under this heading.

Erythromycin Estolate (Blood concentrations of dutasteride may increase in the presence of CYP3A4 inhibitors).
No products indexed under this heading.

Erythromycin Ethylsuccinate (Blood concentrations of dutasteride

may increase in the presence of CYP3A4 inhibitors). Products include:
- E.E.S. 433
- EryPed 431

Erythromycin Gluceptate (Blood concentrations of dutasteride may increase in the presence of CYP3A4 inhibitors).
No products indexed under this heading.

Erythromycin Lactobionate (Blood concentrations of dutasteride may increase in the presence of CYP3A4 inhibitors).
No products indexed under this heading.

Erythromycin Stearate (Blood concentrations of dutasteride may increase in the presence of CYP3A4 inhibitors).
No products indexed under this heading.

Esomeprazole Magnesium (Blood concentrations of dutasteride may increase in the presence of CYP3A4 inhibitors). Products include:
- Nexium Delayed-Release Capsules 645
- Nexium Delayed-Release Oral Suspension 645

Fluconazole (Blood concentrations of dutasteride may increase in the presence of CYP3A4 inhibitors).
No products indexed under this heading.

Fluoxetine (Blood concentrations of dutasteride may increase in the presence of CYP3A4 inhibitors).
No products indexed under this heading.

Fluoxetine Hydrochloride (Blood concentrations of dutasteride may increase in the presence of CYP3A4 inhibitors). Products include:
- Prozac Weekly Capsules 1852
- Prozac Pulvules and Liquid 1852
- Symbyax Capsules 1871

Fluvoxamine Maleate (Blood concentrations of dutasteride may increase in the presence of CYP3A4 inhibitors). Products include:
- Luvox CR Extended-Release Capsules 1759

Fosamprenavir Calcium (Blood concentrations of dutasteride may increase in the presence of CYP3A4 inhibitors). Products include:
- Lexiva Oral Suspension 1510
- Lexiva Tablets 1510

Indinavir Sulfate (Blood concentrations of dutasteride may increase in the presence of CYP3A4 inhibitors). Products include:
- Crixivan Capsules 1979

Isoniazid (Blood concentrations of dutasteride may increase in the presence of CYP3A4 inhibitors).
No products indexed under this heading.

Itraconazole (Blood concentrations of dutasteride may increase in the presence of CYP3A4 inhibitors).
No products indexed under this heading.

Ketoconazole (Blood concentrations of dutasteride may increase in the presence of CYP3A4 inhibitors). Products include:
- Extina Foam, 2% 3057
- Nizoral A-D Shampoo 1901

Lopinavir (Blood concentrations of dutasteride may increase in the presence of CYP3A4 inhibitors). Products include:
- Kaletra 452

Loratadine (Blood concentrations of dutasteride may increase in the presence of CYP3A4 inhibitors).
No products indexed under this heading.

Metronidazole (Blood concentrations of dutasteride may increase in the presence of CYP3A4 inhibitors). Products include:
- Pylera Capsules 714

Metronidazole Benzoate (Blood concentrations of dutasteride may increase in the presence of CYP3A4 inhibitors).
No products indexed under this heading.

Metronidazole Hydrochloride (Blood concentrations of dutasteride may increase in the presence of CYP3A4 inhibitors).
No products indexed under this heading.

Metronidazole Sodium (Blood concentrations of dutasteride may increase in the presence of CYP3A4 inhibitors).
No products indexed under this heading.

Miconazole (Blood concentrations of dutasteride may increase in the presence of CYP3A4 inhibitors).
No products indexed under this heading.

Miconazole Nitrate (Blood concentrations of dutasteride may increase in the presence of CYP3A4 inhibitors).
No products indexed under this heading.

Nefazodone Hydrochloride (Blood concentrations of dutasteride may increase in the presence of CYP3A4 inhibitors).
No products indexed under this heading.

Nelfinavir Mesylate (Blood concentrations of dutasteride may increase in the presence of CYP3A4 inhibitors).
No products indexed under this heading.

Nevirapine (Blood concentrations of dutasteride may increase in the presence of CYP3A4 inhibitors). Products include:
- Viramune Oral Suspension 873
- Viramune Tablets 873

Niacinamide (Blood concentrations of dutasteride may increase in the presence of CYP3A4 inhibitors). Products include:
- BioLean Free Tablets .... ■ 635

Nicotinamide (Blood concentrations of dutasteride may increase in the presence of CYP3A4 inhibitors).
No products indexed under this heading.

Nifedipine (Blood concentrations of dutasteride may increase in the presence of CYP3A4 inhibitors).
No products indexed under this heading.

Norfloxacin (Blood concentrations of dutasteride may increase in the presence of CYP3A4 inhibitors). Products include:
- Noroxin Tablets 2069

Omeprazole (Blood concentrations of dutasteride may increase in the presence of CYP3A4 inhibitors).
No products indexed under this heading.

Paroxetine Hydrochloride (Blood concentrations of dutasteride may increase in the presence of CYP3A4 inhibitors). Products include:
- Paxil 1535
- Paxil CR Controlled-Release Tablets 1544

Propoxyphene Hydrochloride (Blood concentrations of dutasteride may increase in the presence of CYP3A4 inhibitors).
No products indexed under this heading.

Propoxyphene Napsylate (Blood concentrations of dutasteride may increase in the presence of CYP3A4 inhibitors).
No products indexed under this heading.

Quinidine (Blood concentrations of dutasteride may increase in the presence of CYP3A4 inhibitors).
No products indexed under this heading.

Quinidine Hydrochloride (Blood concentrations of dutasteride may increase in the presence of CYP3A4 inhibitors).
No products indexed under this heading.

Quinidine Polygalacturonate (Blood concentrations of dutasteride may increase in the presence of CYP3A4 inhibitors).
No products indexed under this heading.

Quinidine Sulfate (Blood concentrations of dutasteride may increase in the presence of CYP3A4 inhibitors).
No products indexed under this heading.

Quinine (Blood concentrations of dutasteride may increase in the presence of CYP3A4 inhibitors).
No products indexed under this heading.

Quinine Sulfate (Blood concentrations of dutasteride may increase in the presence of CYP3A4 inhibitors).
No products indexed under this heading.

Quinupristin (Blood concentrations of dutasteride may increase in the presence of CYP3A4 inhibitors).
No products indexed under this heading.

Ranitidine Bismuth Citrate (Blood concentrations of dutasteride may increase in the presence of CYP3A4 inhibitors).
No products indexed under this heading.

Ranitidine Hydrochloride (Blood concentrations of dutasteride may increase in the presence of CYP3A4 inhibitors). Products include:
- Zantac 75 Tablets .... ■ 603
- Zantac 1670
- Zantac Injection 1666
- Zantac Injection Pharmacy Bulk Package 1668
- Maximum Strength Zantac 150 Tablets .... ■ 603
- Maximum Strength Zantac 150 Cool Mint Tablets .... ■ 603

Ritonavir (Blood concentrations of dutasteride may increase in the presence of CYP3A4 inhibitors). Products include:
- Kaletra 452
- Norvir 489

Saquinavir (Blood concentrations of dutasteride may increase in the presence of CYP3A4 inhibitors).
No products indexed under this heading.

Saquinavir Mesylate (Blood concentrations of dutasteride may increase in the presence of CYP3A4 inhibitors).
No products indexed under this heading.

Sertraline Hydrochloride (Blood concentrations of dutasteride may increase in the presence of CYP3A4 inhibitors).
No products indexed under this heading.

Sildenafil Citrate (Blood concentrations of dutasteride may increase in the presence of CYP3A4 inhibitors).
No products indexed under this heading.

Telithromycin (Blood concentrations of dutasteride may increase in the presence of CYP3A4 inhibitors). Products include:
- Ketek Tablets 2744

Troglitazone (Blood concentrations of dutasteride may increase in the presence of CYP3A4 inhibitors).
No products indexed under this heading.

Troleandomycin (Blood concentrations of dutasteride may increase in the presence of CYP3A4 inhibitors).
No products indexed under this heading.

Valproate Sodium (Blood concentrations of dutasteride may increase in the presence of CYP3A4 inhibitors).
No products indexed under this heading.

Vardenafil Hydrochloride (Blood concentrations of dutasteride may increase in the presence of CYP3A4 inhibitors). Products include:
- Levitra Tablets 2876

Verapamil Hydrochloride (Co-administration of verapamil decreases dutasteride clearance and leads to increased exposure to dutasteride. The change in dutasteride exposure is not considered to be clinically significant. No dose adjustment is recommended). Products include:
- Tarka Tablets 511

Voriconazole (Blood concentrations of dutasteride may increase in the presence of CYP3A4 inhibitors).
No products indexed under this heading.

Zafirlukast (Blood concentrations of dutasteride may increase in the presence of CYP3A4 inhibitors). Products include:
- Accolate Tablets 669

Zileuton (Blood concentrations of dutasteride may increase in the presence of CYP3A4 inhibitors).
No products indexed under this heading.

Food Interactions

Grapefruit (Blood concentrations of dutasteride may increase in the presence of CYP3A4 inhibitors).

Grapefruit Juice (Blood concentrations of dutasteride may increase in the presence of CYP3A4 inhibitors).

AWARENESS CLEAR CAPSULES

(Herbals, Multiple) .... ■ 624
None cited in PDR database.

AWARENESS FEMALE BALANCE

(Herbals, Multiple) .... ■ 624
None cited in PDR database.

AXERT TABLETS
(Almotriptan Malate) 2431
May interact with 5HT1-receptor agonists, ergot-containing drugs, erythromycin, Serotonin and Norepinephrine Reuptake Inhibitors, selective serotonin reuptake inhibitors, and certain other agents. Compounds in these categories include:

Citalopram Hydrobromide (Cases of life-threatening serotonin syndrome have been reported during combined use of selective serotonin reuptake inhibitors and triptans). Products include:
Celexa 1160

Desvenlafaxine Succinate (Cases of life-threatening serotonin syndrome have been reported during combined use of selective serotonin norepinephrine reuptake inhibitors and triptans). Products include:
Pristiq Extended-Release Tablets 3247

Dihydroergotamine Mesylate (Ergot-containing drugs have been reported to cause prolonged vasospastic reactions; because there is a theoretical basis that these effects may be additive, use of ergot-type agents and almotriptan within 24 hours is contraindicated).
No products indexed under this heading.

Duloxetine Hydrochloride (Cases of life-threatening serotonin syndrome have been reported during combined use of selective serotonin norepinephrine reuptake inhibitors and triptans). Products include:
Cymbalta Delayed-Release Capsules 1801

Eletriptan Hydrobromide (Co-administration with other 5HT1 agonists within 24 hours of treatment with almotriptan is contraindicated).
No products indexed under this heading.

Ergonovine Maleate (Ergot-containing drugs have been reported to cause prolonged vasospastic reactions; because there is a theoretical basis that these effects may be additive, use of ergot-type agents and almotriptan within 24 hours is contraindicated).
No products indexed under this heading.

Ergotamine Tartrate (Ergot-containing drugs have been reported to cause prolonged vasospastic reactions; because there is a theoretical basis that these effects may be additive, use of ergot-type agents and almotriptan within 24 hours is contraindicated).
No products indexed under this heading.

Erythromycin (Co-administration with other potent inhibitors of CYP3A4 inhibitors, such as erythromycin, may result in increased exposures to almotriptan).
No products indexed under this heading.

Erythromycin Estolate (Co-administration with other potent inhibitors of CYP3A4 inhibitors, such as erythromycin, may result in increased exposures to almotriptan).
No products indexed under this heading.

Erythromycin Ethylsuccinate (Co-administration with other potent inhibitors of CYP3A4 inhibitors, such as erythromycin, may result in increased exposures to almotriptan). Products include:
E.E.S. 433
EryPed 431

Erythromycin Gluceptate (Co-administration with other potent inhibitors of CYP3A4 inhibitors, such as erythromycin, may result in increased exposures to almotriptan).
No products indexed under this heading.

Erythromycin Lactobionate (Co-administration with other potent inhibitors of CYP3A4 inhibitors, such as erythromycin, may result in increased exposures to almotriptan).
No products indexed under this heading.

Erythromycin Stearate (Co-administration with other potent inhibitors of CYP3A4 inhibitors, such as erythromycin, may result in increased exposures to almotriptan).
No products indexed under this heading.

Escitalopram Oxalate (Cases of life-threatening serotonin syndrome have been reported during combined use of selective serotonin reuptake inhibitors and triptans). Products include:
Lexapro Oral Suspension 1174
Lexapro Tablets 1174

Fluoxetine (Cases of life-threatening serotonin syndrome have been reported during combined use of selective serotonin reuptake inhibitors and triptans).
No products indexed under this heading.

Fluoxetine Hydrochloride (Co-administration has resulted in an increase in maximal concentrations of almotriptan by 18%; this difference is not clinically significant; co-administration of SSRI and 5HT1 agonist have been rarely reported to cause weakness, hyperreflexia, and incoordination). Products include:
Prozac Weekly Capsules 1852
Prozac Pulvules and Liquid 1852
Symbyax Capsules 1871

Fluvoxamine Maleate (Cases of life-threatening serotonin syndrome have been reported during combined use of selective serotonin reuptake inhibitors and triptans). Products include:
Luvox CR Extended-Release Capsules 1759

Frovatriptan Succinate (Co-administration with other 5HT1 agonists within 24 hours of treatment with almotriptan is contraindicated). Products include:
Frova Tablets 1111

Itraconazole (Co-administration with other potent inhibitors of CYP3A4 inhibitors, such as itraconazole, may result in increased exposures to almotriptan).
No products indexed under this heading.

Ketoconazole (Co-administration has resulted in an approximately 60% increase in the AUC and maximal plasma concentrations of almotriptan). Products include:
Extina Foam, 2% 3057
Nizoral A-D Shampoo 1901

Methylergonovine Maleate (Ergot-containing drugs have been reported to cause prolonged vasospastic reactions; because there is a theoretical basis that these effects may be additive, use of ergot-type agents and almotriptan within 24 hours is contraindicated).
No products indexed under this heading.

Methysergide Maleate (Ergot-containing drugs have been reported to cause prolonged vasospastic reactions; because there is a theoretical basis that these effects may be additive, use of ergot-type agents and almotriptan within 24 hours is contraindicated).
No products indexed under this heading.

Moclobemide (Co-administration has resulted in a 27% decrease in almotriptan clearance).
No products indexed under this heading.

Naratriptan Hydrochloride (Co-administration with other 5HT1 agonists within 24 hours of treatment with almotriptan is contraindicated). Products include:
Amerge Tablets 1301

Nefazodone Hydrochloride (Cases of life-threatening serotonin syndrome have been reported during combined use of selective serotonin norepinephrine reuptake inhibitors and triptans).
No products indexed under this heading.

Paroxetine Hydrochloride (Cases of life-threatening serotonin syndrome have been reported during combined use of selective serotonin reuptake inhibitors and triptans). Products include:
Paxil 1535
Paxil CR Controlled-Release Tablets 1544

Ritonavir (Co-administration with other potent inhibitors of CYP3A4 inhibitors, such as ritonavir, may result in increased exposures to almotriptan). Products include:
Kaletra 452
Norvir 489

Rizatriptan Benzoate (Co-administration with other 5HT1 agonists within 24 hours of treatment with almotriptan is contraindicated). Products include:
Maxalt Tablets 2056
Maxalt-MLT Orally Disintegrating Tablets 2056

Sertraline Hydrochloride (Cases of life-threatening serotonin syndrome have been reported during combined use of selective serotonin reuptake inhibitors and triptans).
No products indexed under this heading.

Sumatriptan (Co-administration with other 5HT1 agonists within 24 hours of treatment with almotriptan is contraindicated). Products include:
Imitrex Nasal Spray 1470

Sumatriptan Succinate (Co-administration with other 5HT1 agonists within 24 hours of treatment with almotriptan is contraindicated). Products include:
Imitrex Injection 1465
Imitrex Tablets 1474
Treximet Tablets 1616

Venlafaxine Hydrochloride (Cases of life-threatening serotonin syndrome have been reported during combined use of selective serotonin norepinephrine reuptake inhibitors and triptans). Products include:
Effexor XR Extended-Release Capsules 3195
Venlafaxine Hydrochloride Tablets 2199

Verapamil Hydrochloride (Co-administration has resulted in a 20% increase in AUC and a 24% increase in maximal plasma concentrations of almotriptan; neither of these changes is clinically significant). Products include:
Tarka Tablets 511

Zolmitriptan (Co-administration with other 5HT1 agonists within 24 hours of treatment with almotriptan is contraindicated). Products include:
Zomig Tablets 694
Zomig Nasal Spray 689
Zomig-ZMT Tablets 694

AXID CAPSULES
(Nizatidine) 1364
May interact with aspirin-acetylsalicylic acid. Compounds in these categories include:

Aspirin (In patients given very high doses (3,900 mg) of aspirin daily, increases in serum salicylate levels were seen when nizatidine, 150 mg b.i.d., were administered concurrently). Products include:
Aggrenox Capsules 819
Bayer Aspirin 750
Percodan Tablets 1130
St. Joseph 81 mg Aspirin Chewable and Enteric Coated Tablets 1903

Aspirin, Enteric Coated (In patients given very high doses (3,900 mg) of aspirin daily, increases in serum salicylate levels were seen when nizatidine, 150 mg b.i.d., were administered concurrently).
No products indexed under this heading.

Aspirin Buffered (In patients given very high doses (3,900 mg) of aspirin daily, increases in serum salicylate levels were seen when nizatidine, 150 mg b.i.d., were administered concurrently).
No products indexed under this heading.

AZASITE OPHTHALMIC DROPS
(Azithromycin) 1740
None cited in PDR database.

AZILECT TABLETS
(Rasagiline Mesylate) 3106
May interact with cytochrome p450 1a2 inhibitors (selected), monoamine oxidase inhibitors, nonselective MAO inhibitors, Serotonin and Norepinephrine Reuptake Inhibitors, selective serotonin reuptake inhibitors, sympathomimetics, tricyclic antidepressants, and certain other agents. Compounds in these categories include:

Alatrofloxacin Mesylate (Rasagiline plasma concentrations may increase up to 2 fold in patients using concomitant CYP1A2 inhibitors).
No products indexed under this heading.

Albuterol (Severe hypertensive reactions have followed the administration of sympathomimetics and non-selective MAO inhibitors and concomitant use is contraindicated).
No products indexed under this heading.

Albuterol Sulfate (Severe hypertensive reactions have followed the administration of sympathomimetics and non-selective MAO inhibitors and concomitant use is contraindicated). Products include:
- Combivent Inhalation Aerosol 845
- ProAir HFA Inhalation Aerosol 3113
- Proventil HFA Inhalation Aerosol 2914
- Ventolin HFA Inhalation Aerosol 1638

Amiodarone Hydrochloride (Rasagiline plasma concentrations may increase up to 2 fold in patients using concomitant CYP1A2 inhibitors).
No products indexed under this heading.

Amitriptyline Hydrochloride (Severe CNS toxicity associated with hyperpyrexia and death has been reported with the combination of tricyclic antidepressants (TCAs) and non-selective MAOIs or selective MAO-B inhibitors. Because the mechanisms of these reactions are not fully understood, the combination of rasagiline with TCAs should be avoided. At least 14 days should elapse between discontinuation of rasagiline and initiation of treatment with a TCA).
No products indexed under this heading.

Amoxapine (Severe CNS toxicity associated with hyperpyrexia and death has been reported with the combination of tricyclic antidepressants (TCAs) and non-selective MAOIs or selective MAO-B inhibitors. Because the mechanisms of these reactions are not fully understood, the combination of rasagiline with TCAs should be avoided. At least 14 days should elapse between discontinuation of rasagiline and initiation of treatment with a TCA).
No products indexed under this heading.

Anastrozole (Rasagiline plasma concentrations may increase up to 2 fold in patients using concomitant CYP1A2 inhibitors). Products include:
- Arimidex Tablets 672

Cimetidine (Rasagiline plasma concentrations may increase up to 2 fold in patients using concomitant CYP1A2 inhibitors).
No products indexed under this heading.

Cimetidine Hydrochloride (Rasagiline plasma concentrations may increase up to 2 fold in patients using concomitant CYP1A2 inhibitors).
No products indexed under this heading.

Ciprofloxacin (Rasagiline plasma concentrations may increase up to 2 fold in patients using concomitant ciprofloxacin). Products include:
- Cipro I.V. 2817
- Cipro Oral Suspension 2810
- Cipro XR Tablets 2823
- Ciprodex Otic Suspension 541

Ciprofloxacin Hydrochloride (Rasagiline plasma concentrations may increase up to 2 fold in patients using concomitant ciprofloxacin). Products include:
- Cipro Tablets 2810

Citalopram Hydrobromide (Severe CNS toxicity associated with hyperpyrexia and death has been reported with the combination of selective serotonin reuptake inhibitors (SSRIs) and non-selective MAOIs or selective MAO-B inhibitors. Because the mechanisms of these reactions are not fully understood, the combination of rasagiline with SSRI antidepressants should be avoided. At least 14 days should elapse between discontinuation of rasagiline and initiation of treatment with a SSRI antidepressant. Because of the long half lives offluoxetine and its active metabolite, at least five weeks (perhaps longer, especially if fluoxetine has been prescribed chronically and/or at higher doses) should elapse between discontinuation of fluoxetine and inititation of rasagiline). Products include:
- Celexa 1160

Clarithromycin (Rasagiline plasma concentrations may increase up to 2 fold in patients using concomitant CYP1A2 inhibitors). Products include:
- Biaxin/Biaxin XL 411

Clomipramine Hydrochloride (Severe CNS toxicity associated with hyperpyrexia and death has been reported with the combination of tricyclic antidepressants (TCAs) and non-selective MAOIs or selective MAO-B inhibitors. Because the mechanisms of these reactions are not fully understood, the combination of rasagiline with TCAs should be avoided. At least 14 days should elapse between discontinuation of rasagiline and initiation of treatment with a TCA).
No products indexed under this heading.

Cyclobenzaprine (Rasagiline is contraindicated for use with cyclobenzaprine).
No products indexed under this heading.

Cyclobenzaprine Hydrochloride (Rasagiline is contraindicated for use with cyclobenzaprine). Products include:
- Amrix Capsules 966

Desipramine Hydrochloride (Severe CNS toxicity associated with hyperpyrexia and death has been reported with the combination of tricyclic antidepressants (TCAs) and non-selective MAOIs or selective MAO-B inhibitors. Because the mechanisms of these reactions are not fully understood, the combination of rasagiline with TCAs should be avoided. At least 14 days should elapse between discontinuation of rasagiline and initiation of treatment with a TCA).
No products indexed under this heading.

Desogestrel (Rasagiline plasma concentrations may increase up to 2 fold in patients using concomitant CYP1A2 inhibitors). Products include:
- Mircette Tablets 1034

Desvenlafaxine Succinate (Severe CNS toxicity associated with hyperpyrexia and death has been reported with the combination of serotonin-norepinephrine reuptake inhibitors (SNRIs) and non-selective MAOIs or selective MAO-B inhibitors. Furthermore, because the mechanisms of these reactions are not fully understood, it seems prudent, in general, to avoid the combination of rasagiline with SNRI antidepressants. At least 14 days should elapse between discontinuation of rasagiline and initiation of treatment with a SNRI antidepressant). Products include:
- Pristiq Extended-Release Tablets 3247

Dextromethorphan (The combination of MAO inhibitors and dextromethorphan has been reported to cause brief episodes of psychosis or bizarre behavior and concomitant use is contraindicated).
No products indexed under this heading.

Dextromethorphan Hydrobromide (The combination of MAO inhibitors and dextromethorphan has been reported to cause brief episodes of psychosis or bizarre behavior and concomitant use is contraindicated). Products include:
- PediaCare Children's Liquid Multi-Symptom Cold 1902
- PediaCare Children's Long-Acting Cough 1902
- Children's Sudafed PE Cold & Cough Liquid 1907
- Sudafed PE Cold & Cough Caplets 1907
- Children's Tylenol Plus Cough & Runny Nose Suspension Liquid 1912
- Children's Tylenol Plus Cough & Sore Throat Suspension Liquid 1912
- Children's Tylenol Plus Flu Suspension Liquid 1914
- Children's Tylenol Plus Multi-Symptom Cold Suspension Liquid 1912
- Tylenol Cold Severe Congestion Daytime Caplets with Cool Burst 1912
- Tylenol Cold Head Congestion Daytime Caplets with Cool Burst 1910
- Tylenol Cold Head Congestion Nighttime Caplets with Cool Burst 1910
- Tylenol Cold Head Congestion Severe Daytime Caplets with Cool Burst 1910
- Tylenol Cold Multi-Symptom Daytime Caplets with Cool Burst and Rapid Release Gels 1913
- Tylenol Cold Multi-Symptom Daytime Liquid with Citrus Burst 1913
- Tylenol Cold Multi-Symptom Nighttime Caplets with Cool Burst 1913
- Tylenol Cold Multi-Symptom Nighttime Liquid with Cool Burst 1913
- Tylenol Cold Multi-Symptom Severe Caplets with Cool Burst 1913
- Tylenol Cold Multi-Symptom Severe Daytime Liquid with Citrus Burst 1913
- Tylenol Cough & Sore Throat Daytime Liquid with Cool Burst 1918
- Tylenol Cough & Sore Throat Nighttime Liquid with Cool Burst 1918
- Vicks DayQuil Cold & Flu Multi-Symptom Relief .... ▣616
- Vicks DayQuil LiquiCaps 2567
- Vicks DayQuil Liquid 2567
- Vicks DayQuil Multi-Symptom Cold/Flu Relief 2567
- Vicks NyQuil Cold & Flu Multi-Symptom Relief .... ▣617
- Vicks NyQuil LiquiCaps 2567
- Vicks NyQuil Liquid 2567
- Vicks NyQuil Multi-Symptom Cold/Flu Relief 2567

Dextromethorphan Polistirex (The combination of MAO inhibitors and dextromethorphan has been reported to cause brief episodes of psychosis or bizarre behavior and concomitant use is contraindicated).
No products indexed under this heading.

Dobutamine Hydrochloride (Severe hypertensive reactions have followed the administration of sympathomimetics and non-selective MAO inhibitors and concomitant use is contraindicated).
No products indexed under this heading.

Dopamine Hydrochloride (Severe hypertensive reactions have followed the administration of sympathomimetics and non-selective MAO inhibitors and concomitant use is contraindicated).
No products indexed under this heading.

Doxepin Hydrochloride (Severe CNS toxicity associated with hyperpyrexia and death has been reported with the combination of tricyclic antidepressants (TCAs) and non-selective MAOIs or selective MAO-B inhibitors. Because the mechanisms of these reactions are not fully understood, the combination of rasagiline with TCAs should be avoided. At least 14 days should elapse between discontinuation of rasagiline and initiation of treatment with a TCA).
No products indexed under this heading.

Duloxetine Hydrochloride (Severe CNS toxicity associated with hyperpyrexia and death has been reported with the combination of serotonin-norepinephrine reuptake inhibitors (SNRIs) and non-selective MAOIs or selective MAO-B inhibitors. Furthermore, because the mechanisms of these reactions are not fully understood, it seems prudent, in general, to avoid the combination of rasagiline with SNRI antidepressants. At least 14 days should elapse between discontinuation of rasagiline and initiation of treatment with a SNRI antidepressant). Products include:
- Cymbalta Delayed-Release Capsules 1801

Enoxacin (Rasagiline plasma concentrations may increase up to 2 fold in patients using concomitant CYP1A2 inhibitors).
No products indexed under this heading.

Ephedrine Hydrochloride (Severe hypertensive reactions have followed the administration of sympathomimetics and non-selective MAO inhibitors and concomitant use is contraindicated).
No products indexed under this heading.

Ephedrine Sulfate (Severe hypertensive reactions have followed the administration of sympathomimetics and non-selective MAO inhibitors and concomitant use is contraindicated).
No products indexed under this heading.

Ephedrine Tannate (Severe hypertensive reactions have followed the administration of sympathomimetics and non-selective MAO inhibitors and concomitant use is contraindicated).
No products indexed under this heading.

Epinephrine (Severe hypertensive reactions have followed the administration of sympathomimetics and non-selective MAO inhibitors and concomitant use is contraindicated). Products include:
- EpiPen 1024

Epinephrine Bitartrate (Severe hypertensive reactions have followed the administration of sympathomimetics and non-selective MAO inhibitors and concomitant use is contraindicated).
No products indexed under this heading.

Epinephrine Hydrochloride
(Severe hypertensive reactions have followed the administration of sympathomimetics and non-selective MAO inhibitors and concomitant use is contraindicated).
No products indexed under this heading.

Escitalopram Oxalate (Severe CNS toxicity associated with hyperpyrexia and death has been reported with the combination of selective serotonin reuptake inhibitors (SSRIs) and non-selective MAOIs or selective MAO-B inhibitors. Because the mechanisms of these reactions are not fully understood, the combination of rasagiline with SSRI antidepressants should be avoided. At least 14 days should elapse between discontinuation of rasagiline and initiation of treatment with a SSRI antidepressant. Because of the long half lives offluxetine and its active metabolite, at least five weeks (perhaps longer, especially if fluoxetine has been prescribed chronically and/or at higher doses) should elapse between discontinuation of fluoxetine and inititation of rasagiline). Products include:
Lexapro Oral Suspension 1174
Lexapro Tablets 1174

Ethinyl Estradiol (Rasagiline plasma concentrations may increase up to 2 fold in patients using concomitant CYP1A2 inhibitors). Products include:
Lybrel Tablets 3204
Mircette Tablets 1034
NuvaRing 2897
Ortho-Cyclen/Ortho Tri-Cyclen 2449
Ortho Evra Transdermal System 2437
Ortho Tri-Cyclen Lo Tablets 2458
Seasonique Tablets 1046
Yaz Tablets 805

Fluoxetine (Severe CNS toxicity associated with hyperpyrexia and death has been reported with the combination of selective serotonin reuptake inhibitors (SSRIs) and non-selective MAOIs or selective MAO-B inhibitors. Because the mechanisms of these reactions are not fully understood, the combination of rasagiline with SSRI antidepressants should be avoided. At least 14 days should elapse between discontinuation of rasagiline and initiation of treatment with a SSRI antidepressant. Because of the long half lives offluxetine and its active metabolite, at least five weeks (perhaps longer, especially if fluoxetine has been prescribed chronically and/or at higher doses) should elapse between discontinuation of fluoxetine and inititation of rasagiline).
No products indexed under this heading.

Fluoxetine Hydrochloride (Severe CNS toxicity associated with hyperpyrexia and death has been reported with the combination of selective serotonin reuptake inhibitors (SSRIs) and non-selective MAOIs or selective MAO-B inhibitors. Because the mechanisms of these reactions are not fully understood, the combination of rasagiline with SSRI antidepressants should be avoided. At least 14 days should elapse between discontinuation of rasagiline and initiation of treatment with a SSRI antidepressant. Because of the long half lives offluxetine and its active metabolite, at least five weeks (perhaps longer, especially if fluoxetine has been prescribed chronically and/or at higher doses) should elapse between discontinuation of fluoxetine and inititation of rasagiline). Products include:
Prozac Weekly Capsules 1852
Prozac Pulvules and Liquid 1852
Symbyax Capsules 1871

Fluvoxamine (Rasagiline plasma concentrations may increase up to 2 fold in patients using concomitant CYP1A2 inhibitors).
No products indexed under this heading.

Fluvoxamine Maleate (Severe CNS toxicity associated with hyperpyrexia and death has been reported with the combination of selective serotonin reuptake inhibitors (SSRIs) and non-selective MAOIs or selective MAO-B inhibitors. Because the mechanisms of these reactions are not fully understood, the combination of rasagiline with SSRI antidepressants should be avoided. At least 14 days should elapse between discontinuation of rasagiline and initiation of treatment with a SSRI antidepressant. Because of the long half lives offluxetine and its active metabolite, at least five weeks (perhaps longer, especially if fluoxetine has been prescribed chronically and/or at higher doses) should elapse between discontinuation of fluoxetine and inititation of rasagiline). Products include:
Luvox CR Extended-Release Capsules 1759

Gatifloxacin (Rasagiline plasma concentrations may increase up to 2 fold in patients using concomitant CYP1A2 inhibitors).
No products indexed under this heading.

Gemifloxacin Mesylate (Rasagiline plasma concentrations may increase up to 2 fold in patients using concomitant CYP1A2 inhibitors).
No products indexed under this heading.

Grepafloxacin Hydrochloride
(Rasagiline plasma concentrations may increase up to 2 fold in patients using concomitant CYP1A2 inhibitors).
No products indexed under this heading.

Hypericum (Rasagiline is contraindicated for use with St. John's wort). Products include:
Satieté Tablets 640

Hypericum Perforatum (Rasagiline is contraindicated for use with St. John's wort).
No products indexed under this heading.

Imipramine Hydrochloride
(Severe CNS toxicity associated with hyperpyrexia and death has been reported with the combination of tricyclic antidepressants (TCAs) and non-selective MAOIs or selective MAO-B inhibitors. Because the mechanisms of these reactions are not fully understood, the combination of rasagiline with TCAs should be avoided. At least 14 days should elapse between discontinuation of rasagiline and initiation of treatment with a TCA).
No products indexed under this heading.

Imipramine Pamoate (Severe CNS toxicity associated with hyperpyrexia and death has been reported with the combination of tricyclic antidepressants (TCAs) and non-selective MAOIs or selective MAO-B inhibitors. Because the mechanisms of these reactions are not fully understood, the combination of rasagiline with TCAs should be avoided. At least 14 days should elapse between discontinuation of rasagiline and initiation of treatment with a TCA).
No products indexed under this heading.

Isocarboxazid (Rasagiline should not be administered along with other MAO inhibitors because of the increased risk of non-selective MAO inhibition that may lead to a hypertensive crisis. At least 14 days should elapse between discontinuation of rasagiline and initiation of treatment with MAO inhibitors). Products include:
Marplan Tablets 3177

Isoniazid (Rasagiline plasma concentrations may increase up to 2 fold in patients using concomitant CYP1A2 inhibitors).
No products indexed under this heading.

Isoproterenol Hydrochloride
(Severe hypertensive reactions have followed the administration of sympathomimetics and non-selective MAO inhibitors and concomitant use is contraindicated).
No products indexed under this heading.

Isoproterenol Sulfate (Severe hypertensive reactions have followed the administration of sympathomimetics and non-selective MAO inhibitors and concomitant use is contraindicated).
No products indexed under this heading.

Ketoconazole (Rasagiline plasma concentrations may increase up to 2 fold in patients using concomitant CYP1A2 inhibitors). Products include:
Extina Foam, 2% 3057
Nizoral A-D Shampoo 1901

Levalbuterol Hydrochloride
(Severe hypertensive reactions have followed the administration of sympathomimetics and non-selective MAO inhibitors and concomitant use is contraindicated). Products include:
Xopenex Inhalation Solution 3001
Xopenex Inhalation Solution Concentrate 3005

Levofloxacin (Rasagiline plasma concentrations may increase up to 2 fold in patients using concomitant CYP1A2 inhibitors). Products include:
Iquix Ophthalmic Solution 3183
Levaquin 2416
Levaquin in 5% Dextrose Injection 2416
Quixin Ophthalmic Solution 3184

Levonorgestrel (Rasagiline plasma concentrations may increase up to 2 fold in patients using concomitant CYP1A2 inhibitors). Products include:
Climara Pro Transdermal System 768
Lybrel Tablets 3204
Mirena Intrauterine System 779
Plan B Tablets 1044
Seasonique Tablets 1046

Lomefloxacin Hydrochloride
(Rasagiline plasma concentrations may increase up to 2 fold in patients using concomitant CYP1A2 inhibitors).
No products indexed under this heading.

Maprotiline Hydrochloride
(Severe CNS toxicity associated with hyperpyrexia and death has been reported with the combination of tricyclic antidepressants (TCAs) and non-selective MAOIs or selective MAO-B inhibitors. Because the mechanisms of these reactions are not fully understood, the combination of rasagiline with TCAs should be avoided. At least 14 days should elapse between discontinuation of rasagiline and initiation of treatment with a TCA).
No products indexed under this heading.

Meperidine Hydrochloride (Serious, sometimes fatal reactions have been precipitated with concomitant use of meperidine and MAO inhibitors and concomitant use is contraindicated).
No products indexed under this heading.

Mestranol (Rasagiline plasma concentrations may increase up to 2 fold in patients using concomitant CYP1A2 inhibitors).
No products indexed under this heading.

Metaproterenol Sulfate (Severe hypertensive reactions have followed the administration of sympathomimetics and non-selective MAO inhibitors and concomitant use is contraindicated).
No products indexed under this heading.

Metaraminol Bitartrate (Severe hypertensive reactions have followed the administration of sympathomimetics and non-selective MAO inhibitors and concomitant use is contraindicated).
No products indexed under this heading.

Methadone Hydrochloride (Serious, sometimes fatal reactions have been precipitated with concomitant use of methadone and MAO inhibitors and concomitant use is contraindicated).
No products indexed under this heading.

Methoxamine Hydrochloride
(Severe hypertensive reactions have followed the administration of sympathomimetics and non-selective MAO inhibitors and concomitant use is contraindicated).
No products indexed under this heading.

Methoxsalen (Rasagiline plasma concentrations may increase up to 2 fold in patients using concomitant CYP1A2 inhibitors).
No products indexed under this heading.

Mexiletine Hydrochloride (Rasagiline plasma concentrations may increase up to 2 fold in patients using concomitant CYP1A2 inhibitors).
No products indexed under this heading.

Mibefradil Dihydrochloride (Rasagiline plasma concentrations may increase up to 2 fold in patients using concomitant CYP1A2 inhibitors).
No products indexed under this heading.

Mirtazapine (Rasagiline is contraindicated for use with mirtazapine). Products include:
Remeron Tablets 2924
RemeronSolTab Tablets 2927

Moclobemide (Rasagiline should not be administered along with other MAO inhibitors because of the increased risk of non-selective MAO inhibition that may lead to a hypertensive crisis. At least 14 days should elapse between discontinuation of rasagiline and initiation of treatment with MAO inhibitors).
No products indexed under this heading.

Moxifloxacin Hydrochloride (Rasagiline plasma concentrations may increase up to 2 fold in patients using concomitant CYP1A2 inhibitors). Products include:
Avelox 2803
Vigamox Ophthalmic Solution 548

Nalidixic Acid (Rasagiline plasma concentrations may increase up to 2 fold in patients using concomitant CYP1A2 inhibitors).
No products indexed under this heading.

Nefazodone Hydrochloride (Severe CNS toxicity associated with hyperpyrexia and death has been reported with the combination of serotonin-norepinephrine reuptake inhibitors (SNRIs) and non-selective MAOIs or selective MAO-B inhibitors. Furthermore, because the mechanisms of these reactions are not fully understood, it seems prudent, in general, to avoid the combination of rasagiline with SNRI antidepressants. At least 14 days should elapse between discontinuation of rasagiline and initiation of treatment with a SNRI antidepressant).
No products indexed under this heading.

Norepinephrine Bitartrate (Severe hypertensive reactions have followed the administration of sympathomimetics and non-selective MAO inhibitors and concomitant use is contraindicated).
No products indexed under this heading.

Norethindrone (Rasagiline plasma concentrations may increase up to 2 fold in patients using concomitant CYP1A2 inhibitors). Products include:
Ortho Micronor Tablets 2446

Norfloxacin (Rasagiline plasma concentrations may increase up to 2 fold in patients using concomitant CYP1A2 inhibitors). Products include:
Noroxin Tablets 2069

Norgestrel (Rasagiline plasma concentrations may increase up to 2 fold in patients using concomitant CYP1A2 inhibitors).
No products indexed under this heading.

Nortriptyline Hydrochloride (Severe CNS toxicity associated with hyperpyrexia and death has been reported with the combination of tricyclic antidepressants (TCAs) and non-selective MAOIs or selective MAO-B inhibitors. Because the mechanisms of these reactions are not fully understood, the combination of rasagiline with TCAs should be avoided. At least 14 days should elapse between discontinuation of rasagiline and initiation of treatment with a TCA).
No products indexed under this heading.

Ofloxacin (Rasagiline plasma concentrations may increase up to 2 fold in patients using concomitant CYP1A2 inhibitors). Products include:
Ofloxacin Ophthalmic Solution 0.3% .... ⊙243

Omeprazole (Rasagiline plasma concentrations may increase up to 2 fold in patients using concomitant CYP1A2 inhibitors).
No products indexed under this heading.

Pargyline Hydrochloride (Rasagiline should not be administered along with other MAO inhibitors because of the increased risk of non-selective MAO inhibition that may lead to a hypertensive crisis. At least 14 days should elapse between discontinuation of rasagiline and initiation of treatment with MAO inhibitors).
No products indexed under this heading.

Paroxetine Hydrochloride (Severe CNS toxicity associated with hyperpyrexia and death has been reported with the combination of selective serotonin reuptake inhibitors (SSRIs) and non-selective MAOIs or selective MAO-B inhibitors. Because the mechanisms of these reactions are not fully understood, the combination of rasagiline with SSRI antidepressants should be avoided. At least 14 days should elapse between discontinuation of rasagiline and initiation of treatment with a SSRI antidepressant. Because of the long half lives offluoxetine and its active metabolite, at least five weeks (perhaps longer, especially if fluoxetine has been prescribed chronically and/or at higher doses) should elapse between discontinuation of fluoxetine and inititation of rasagiline). Products include:
Paxil 1535
Paxil CR Controlled-Release Tablets 1544

Phenelzine Sulfate (Rasagiline should not be administered along with other MAO inhibitors because of the increased risk of non-selective MAO inhibition that may lead to a hypertensive crisis. At least 14 days should elapse between discontinuation of rasagiline and initiation of treatment with MAO inhibitors).
No products indexed under this heading.

Phenylephrine Bitartrate (Severe hypertensive reactions have followed the administration of sympathomimetics and non-selective MAO inhibitors and concomitant use is contraindicated).
No products indexed under this heading.

Phenylephrine Hydrochloride (Severe hypertensive reactions have followed the administration of sympathomimetics and non-selective MAO inhibitors and concomitant use is contraindicated). Products include:
Actifed Cold & Allergy Tablets 1895
Benadryl Allergy & Cold Kapgels 1895
Benadryl Allergy & Sinus Headache Kapgels 1895
Benadryl Severe Allergy & Sinus Headache Caplets 1897
Children's Benadryl-D Allergy & Sinus Liquid................................ 1896
Benadryl-D Allergy & Sinus Tablet 1896
PediaCare Children's Allergy & Cold Liquid 1902
PediaCare Children's Decongestant Liquid...................... 1902
PediaCare Children's Liquid Multi-Symptom Cold..................... 1902
Sinutab Non-Drying Caplets 1905
Sinutab Sinus Caplets 1905
Children's Sudafed PE Cold & Cough Liquid 1907
Children's Sudafed PE Nasal Decongestant Liquid...................... 1906
Sudafed PE Cold & Cough Caplets.. 1907
Sudafed PE Nasal Decongestant Tablets 1907
Sudafed PE Nighttime Cold Caplets.. 1907
Sudafed PE Non-Drying Sinus Caplets.. 1908
Sudafed PE Severe Cold Caplets 1908
Sudafed PE Sinus & Allergy Tablets 1908
Sudafed PE Sinus Headache Caplets.. 1908
Tylenol Allergy Multi-Symptom Caplets with Cool Burst and Rapid Release Gelcaps................ 1916
Tylenol Allergy Multi-Symptom Nighttime Caplets with Cool Burst 1916
Children's Tylenol Plus Cold Suspension Liquid 1912
Children's Tylenol Plus Cold & Allergy Suspension Liquid............ 1914
Children's Tylenol Plus Flu Suspension Liquid 1914
Children's Tylenol Plus Multi-Symptom Cold Suspension Liquid 1912
Tylenol Cold Head Congestion Daytime Caplets with Cool Burst 1910
Tylenol Cold Head Congestion Nighttime Caplets with Cool Burst 1910
Tylenol Cold Head Congestion Severe Daytime Caplets with Cool Burst.................................... 1910
Tylenol Cold Multi-Symptom Daytime Caplets with Cool Burst and Rapid Release Gels....... 1913
Tylenol Cold Multi-Symptom Daytime Liquid with Citrus Burst... 1913
Tylenol Cold Multi-Symptom Nighttime Caplets with Cool Burst 1913
Tylenol Cold Multi-Symptom Nighttime Liquid with Cool Burst... 1913
Tylenol Cold Multi-Symptom Severe Caplets with Cool Burst..... 1913
Tylenol Cold Multi-Symptom Severe Daytime Liquid with Citrus Burst 1913
Tylenol Sinus Congestion & Pain Daytime Caplets with Cool Burst and Gelcaps....................... 1917
Tylenol Sinus Congestion & Pain Nighttime Caplets with Cool Burst.. 1917
Tylenol Sinus Congestion & Pain Severe Caplets with Cool Burst..... 1917
Vicks DayQuil Cold & Flu Multi-Symptom Relief .... ▣616
Vicks DayQuil LiquiCaps 2567
Vicks DayQuil Liquid 2567
Vicks DayQuil Multi-Symptom Cold/Flu Relief............................ 2567

Phenylephrine Tannate (Severe hypertensive reactions have followed the administration of sympathomimetics and non-selective MAO inhibitors and concomitant use is contraindicated).
No products indexed under this heading.

Phenylpropanolamine Hydrochloride (Severe hypertensive reactions have followed the administration of sympathomimetics and non-selective MAO inhibitors and concomitant use is contraindicated).
No products indexed under this heading.

Pirbuterol Acetate (Severe hypertensive reactions have followed the administration of sympathomimetics and non-selective MAO inhibitors and concomitant use is contraindicated). Products include:
Maxair Autohaler 1705

Procarbazine Hydrochloride (Rasagiline should not be administered along with other MAO inhibitors because of the increased risk of non-selective MAO inhibition that may lead to a hypertensive crisis. At least 14 days should elapse between discontinuation of rasagiline and initiation of treatment with MAO inhibitors).
No products indexed under this heading.

Protriptyline Hydrochloride (Severe CNS toxicity associated with hyperpyrexia and death has been reported with the combination of tricyclic antidepressants (TCAs) and non-selective MAOIs or selective MAO-B inhibitors. Because the mechanisms of these reactions are not fully understood, the combination of rasagiline with TCAs should be avoided. At least 14 days should elapse between discontinuation of rasagiline and initiation of treatment with a TCA).
No products indexed under this heading.

Pseudoephedrine Hydrochloride (Severe hypertensive reactions have followed the administration of sympathomimetics and non-selective MAO inhibitors and concomitant use is contraindicated). Products include:
Allegra-D 12 Hour Extended-Release Tablets............ 2687
Allegra-D 24 Hour Extended-Release Tablets............ 2690
Children's Motrin Cold Oral Suspension 1899
Sudafed 12 Hour Nasal Decongestant Non-Drowsy Caplets.. 1909
Sudafed 24 Hour Non-Drowsy Nasal Decongestant Tablets......... 1906
Children's Sudafed Nasal Decongestant Liquid...................... 1906
Sudafed Nasal Decongestant Tablets 1906
Tylenol Cold Severe Congestion Daytime Caplets with Cool Burst.. 1912
Tylenol Sinus Severe Congestion Caplets with Cool Burst.............. 1917
Vicks NyQuil LiquiCaps 2567
Vicks NyQuil Liquid 2567
Vicks NyQuil Multi-Symptom Cold/Flu Relief............................ 2567
Zyrtec-D 12 Hour Extended Release Tablets 1923
Zyrtec-D Allergy & Congestion Extended-Release Tablets........... 1923

Pseudoephedrine Sulfate (Severe hypertensive reactions have followed the administration of sympathomimetics and non-selective MAO inhibitors and concomitant use is contraindicated). Products include:
Clarinex-D 12-Hour Extended-Release Tablets............ 2831
Clarinex-D 24-Hour Extended-Release Tablets............ 2834

Ranitidine Hydrochloride (Rasagiline plasma concentrations may increase up to 2 fold in patients using concomitant CYP1A2 inhibitors). Products include:

Zantac 75 Tablets 603
Zantac 1670
Zantac Injection 1666
Zantac Injection Pharmacy Bulk Package 1668
Maximum Strength Zantac 150 Tablets 603
Maximum Strength Zantac 150 Cool Mint Tablets 603

Ritonavir (Rasagiline plasma concentrations may increase up to 2 fold in patients using concomitant CYP1A2 inhibitors). Products include:

Kaletra 452
Norvir 489

Salmeterol Xinafoate (Severe hypertensive reactions have followed the administration of sympathomimetics and non-selective MAO inhibitors and concomitant use is contraindicated). Products include:

Advair Diskus 100/50 1276
Advair Diskus 250/50 1276
Advair Diskus 500/50 1276
Advair HFA 45/21 Inhalation Aerosol 1288
Advair HFA 115/21 Inhalation Aerosol 1288
Advair HFA 230/21 Inhalation Aerosol 1288
Serevent Diskus 1594

Selegiline (Rasagiline should not be administered along with other MAO inhibitors because of the increased risk of non-selective MAO inhibition that may lead to a hypertensive crisis. At least 14 days should elapse between discontinuation of rasagiline and initiation of treatment with MAO inhibitors). Products include:

Emsam Transdermal System 905

Selegiline Hydrochloride (Rasagiline should not be administered along with other MAO inhibitors because of the increased risk of non-selective MAO inhibition that may lead to a hypertensive crisis. At least 14 days should elapse between discontinuation of rasagiline and initiation of treatment with MAO inhibitors). Products include:

Eldepryl Capsules 3052

Sertraline Hydrochloride (Severe CNS toxicity associated with hyperpyrexia and death has been reported with the combination of selective serotonin reuptake inhibitors (SSRIs) and non-selective MAOIs or selective MAO-B inhibitors. Because the mechanisms of these reactions are not fully understood, the combination of rasagiline with SSRI antidepressants should be avoided. At least 14 days should elapse between discontinuation of rasagiline and initiation of treatment with a SSRI antidepressant. Because of the long half lives offluoxetine and its active metabolite, at least five weeks (perhaps longer, especially if fluoxetine has been prescribed chronically and/or at higher doses) should elapse between discontinuation of fluoxetine and initiation of rasagiline).

No products indexed under this heading.

Sildenafil Citrate (Rasagiline plasma concentrations may increase up to 2 fold in patients using concomitant CYP1A2 inhibitors).

No products indexed under this heading.

Sparfloxacin (Rasagiline plasma concentrations may increase up to 2 fold in patients using concomitant CYP1A2 inhibitors).

No products indexed under this heading.

Tacrine Hydrochloride (Rasagiline plasma concentrations may increase up to 2 fold in patients using concomitant CYP1A2 inhibitors).

No products indexed under this heading.

Terbutaline Sulfate (Severe hypertensive reactions have followed the administration of sympathomimetics and non-selective MAO inhibitors and concomitant use is contraindicated).

No products indexed under this heading.

Ticlopidine Hydrochloride (Rasagiline plasma concentrations may increase up to 2 fold in patients using concomitant CYP1A2 inhibitors).

No products indexed under this heading.

Tramadol Hydrochloride (Serious, sometimes fatal reactions have been precipitated with concomitant use of tramadol and MAO inhibitors and concomitant use is contraindicated). Products include:

Ultram ER Extended-Release Tablets 2428

Tranylcypromine Sulfate (Rasagiline should not be administered along with other MAO inhibitors because of the increased risk of non-selective MAO inhibition that may lead to a hypertensive crisis. At least 14 days should elapse between discontinuation of rasagiline and initiation of treatment with MAO inhibitors). Products include:

Parnate Tablets 1532

Trimipramine Maleate (Severe CNS toxicity associated with hyperpyrexia and death has been reported with the combination of tricyclic antidepressants (TCAs) and non-selective MAOIs or selective MAO-B inhibitors. Because the mechanisms of these reactions are not fully understood, the combination of rasagiline with TCAs should be avoided. At least 14 days should elapse between discontinuation of rasagiline and initiation of treatment with a TCA).

No products indexed under this heading.

Troleandomycin (Rasagiline plasma concentrations may increase up to 2 fold in patients using concomitant CYP1A2 inhibitors).

No products indexed under this heading.

Trovafloxacin Mesylate (Rasagiline plasma concentrations may increase up to 2 fold in patients using concomitant CYP1A2 inhibitors).

No products indexed under this heading.

Vardenafil Hydrochloride (Rasagiline plasma concentrations may increase up to 2 fold in patients using concomitant CYP1A2 inhibitors). Products include:

Levitra Tablets 2876

Venlafaxine Hydrochloride (Severe CNS toxicity associated with hyperpyrexia and death has been reported with the combination of serotonin-norepinephrine reuptake inhibitors (SNRIs) and non-selective MAOIs or selective MAO-B inhibitors. Furthermore, because the mechanisms of these reactions are not fully understood, it seems prudent, in general, to avoid the combination of rasagiline with SNRI antidepressants. At least 14 days should elapse between discontinuation of rasagiline and initiation of treatment with a SNRI antidepressant). Products include:

Effexor XR Extended-Release Capsules 3195
Venlafaxine Hydrochloride Tablets ... 2199

Zileuton (Rasagiline plasma concentrations may increase up to 2 fold in patients using concomitant CYP1A2 inhibitors).

No products indexed under this heading.

Food Interactions

Beverages with high tyramine (Severe hypertensive reactions have followed the administration of tyramine rich beverages and non-selective MAO inhibitors).

Food high in tyramine (Severe hypertensive reactions have followed the administration of tyramine rich foods and non-selective MAO inhibitors).

Grapefruit Juice (Rasagiline plasma concentrations may increase up to 2 fold in patients using concomitant CYP1A2 inhibitors).

AZMACORT INHALATION AEROSOL

(Triamcinolone Acetonide) 407

May interact with:

Prednisone (Potential for increased likelihood of HPA suppression).

No products indexed under this heading.

AZOPT OPHTHALMIC SUSPENSION

(Brinzolamide) 540

May interact with carbonic anhydrase inhibitors and salicylates. Compounds in these categories include:

Acetazolamide (There is a potential for an additive effect on the known systemic effects of carbonic anhydrase inhibition in patients receiving an oral carbonic anhydrase inhibitor and brinzolamide; co-administration is not recommended).

No products indexed under this heading.

Aspirin (Co-administration with high dose salicylate and oral carbonic anhydrase inhibitor has resulted in rare instances of drug interactions). Products include:

Aggrenox Capsules 819
Bayer Aspirin 750
Percodan Tablets 1130
St. Joseph 81 mg Aspirin Chewable and Enteric Coated Tablets 1903

Aspirin, Enteric Coated (Co-administration with high dose salicylate and oral carbonic anhydrase inhibitor has resulted in rare instances of drug interactions).

No products indexed under this heading.

Aspirin Buffered (Co-administration with high dose salicylate and oral carbonic anhydrase inhibitor has resulted in rare instances of drug interactions).

No products indexed under this heading.

Choline Magnesium Trisalicylate (Co-administration with high dose salicylate and oral carbonic anhydrase inhibitor has resulted in rare instances of drug interactions).

No products indexed under this heading.

Dichlorphenamide (There is a potential for an additive effect on the known systemic effects of carbonic anhydrase inhibition in patients receiving an oral carbonic anhydrase inhibitor and brinzolamide; co-administration is not recommended).

No products indexed under this heading.

Diflunisal (Co-administration with high dose salicylate and oral carbonic anhydrase inhibitor has resulted in rare instances of drug interactions).

No products indexed under this heading.

Dorzolamide Hydrochloride (There is a potential for an additive effect on the known systemic effects of carbonic anhydrase inhibition in patients receiving an oral carbonic anhydrase inhibitor and brinzolamide; co-administration is not recommended). Products include:

Cosopt Sterile Ophthalmic Solution 1969
Trusopt Sterile Ophthalmic Solution 2128

Magnesium Salicylate (Co-administration with high dose salicylate and oral carbonic anhydrase inhibitor has resulted in rare instances of drug interactions).

No products indexed under this heading.

Methazolamide (There is a potential for an additive effect on the known systemic effects of carbonic anhydrase inhibition in patients receiving an oral carbonic anhydrase inhibitor and brinzolamide; co-administration is not recommended).

No products indexed under this heading.

Salsalate (Co-administration with high dose salicylate and oral carbonic anhydrase inhibitor has resulted in rare instances of drug interactions).

No products indexed under this heading.

Torsemide (There is a potential for an additive effect on the known systemic effects of carbonic anhydrase inhibition in patients receiving an oral carbonic anhydrase inhibitor and brinzolamide; co-administration is not recommended). Products include:

Demadex Injection 2630
Demadex Tablets 2630

AZOR TABLETS

(Amlodipine Besylate, Olmesartan Medoxomil) 1005

None cited in PDR database.

BACTROBAN CREAM

(Mupirocin Calcium) 1366

None cited in PDR database.

BACTROBAN NASAL

(Mupirocin Calcium) 1367

None cited in PDR database.

BACTROBAN OINTMENT

(Mupirocin) 1368

None cited in PDR database.

BARACLUDE ORAL SOLUTION

(Entecavir) 900
See Baraclude Tablets

BARACLUDE TABLETS

(Entecavir) 900
May interact with nephrotoxic agents. Compounds in these categories include:

Abacavir Sulfate (Since entecavir is primarily eliminated by the kidneys co-administration of entecavir with drugs that reduce renal function or compete for active tubular secretion may increase serum concentrations of either entecavir or the co-administered drug). Products include:

Epzicom Tablets 1422
Trizivir Tablets 1622
Ziagen 1673

Acyclovir (Since entecavir is primarily eliminated by the kidneys co-administration of entecavir with drugs that reduce renal function or compete for active tubular secretion may increase serum concentrations of either entecavir or the co-administered drug). Products include:

Zovirax 1690
Zovirax Cream 817
Zovirax Ointment 819

Acyclovir Sodium (Since entecavir is primarily eliminated by the kidneys co-administration of entecavir with drugs that reduce renal function or compete for active tubular secretion may increase serum concentrations of either entecavir or the co-administered drug).
No products indexed under this heading.

Alatrofloxacin Mesylate (Since entecavir is primarily eliminated by the kidneys co-administration of entecavir with drugs that reduce renal function or compete for active tubular secretion may increase serum concentrations of either entecavir or the co-administered drug).
No products indexed under this heading.

Aldesleukin (Since entecavir is primarily eliminated by the kidneys co-administration of entecavir with drugs that reduce renal function or compete for active tubular secretion may increase serum concentrations of either entecavir or the co-administered drug). Products include:

Proleukin for Injection 2287

Amikacin Sulfate (Since entecavir is primarily eliminated by the kidneys co-administration of entecavir with drugs that reduce renal function or compete for active tubular secretion may increase serum concentrations of either entecavir or the co-administered drug).
No products indexed under this heading.

Amoxicillin (Since entecavir is primarily eliminated by the kidneys co-administration of entecavir with drugs that reduce renal function or compete for active tubular secretion may increase serum concentrations of either entecavir or the co-administered drug). Products include:

Amoxil Capsules 1305
Amoxil Chewable Tablets 1305
Amoxil Pediatric Drops for Oral Suspension 1305
Amoxil Powder for Oral Suspension 1305
Amoxil Tablets 1305
Augmentin 1323
Augmentin Tablets 1327
Augmentin XR Extended Release Tablets 1333
Augmentin ES-600 Powder for Oral Suspension 1329
Moxatag Tablets 2165

Amoxicillin Trihydrate (Since entecavir is primarily eliminated by the kidneys co-administration of entecavir with drugs that reduce renal function or compete for active tubular secretion may increase serum concentrations of either entecavir or the co-administered drug).
No products indexed under this heading.

Amphotericin B (Since entecavir is primarily eliminated by the kidneys co-administration of entecavir with drugs that reduce renal function or compete for active tubular secretion may increase serum concentrations of either entecavir or the co-administered drug).
No products indexed under this heading.

Amphotericin B, liposomal (Since entecavir is primarily eliminated by the kidneys co-administration of entecavir with drugs that reduce renal function or compete for active tubular secretion may increase serum concentrations of either entecavir or the co-administered drug). Products include:

AmBisome for Injection 606

Amphotericin B Cholesteryl Sulfate (Since entecavir is primarily eliminated by the kidneys co-administration of entecavir with drugs that reduce renal function or compete for active tubular secretion may increase serum concentrations of either entecavir or the co-administered drug).
No products indexed under this heading.

Amphotericin B Lipid Complex (Since entecavir is primarily eliminated by the kidneys co-administration of entecavir with drugs that reduce renal function or compete for active tubular secretion may increase serum concentrations of either entecavir or the co-administered drug). Products include:

Abelcet Injection 1134

Ampicillin (Since entecavir is primarily eliminated by the kidneys co-administration of entecavir with drugs that reduce renal function or compete for active tubular secretion may increase serum concentrations of either entecavir or the co-administered drug).
No products indexed under this heading.

Ampicillin Sodium (Since entecavir is primarily eliminated by the kidneys co-administration of entecavir with drugs that reduce renal function or compete for active tubular secretion may increase serum concentrations of either entecavir or the co-administered drug).
No products indexed under this heading.

Ampicillin Trihydrate (Since entecavir is primarily eliminated by the kidneys co-administration of entecavir with drugs that reduce renal function or compete for active tubular secretion may increase serum concentrations of either entecavir or the co-administered drug).
No products indexed under this heading.

Amprenavir (Since entecavir is primarily eliminated by the kidneys co-administration of entecavir with drugs that reduce renal function or compete for active tubular secretion may increase serum concentrations of either entecavir or the co-administered drug).
No products indexed under this heading.

Aspirin (Since entecavir is primarily eliminated by the kidneys co-administration of entecavir with drugs that reduce renal function or compete for active tubular secretion may increase serum concentrations of either entecavir or the co-administered drug). Products include:

Aggrenox Capsules 819
Bayer Aspirin 750
Percodan Tablets 1130
St. Joseph 81 mg Aspirin Chewable and Enteric Coated Tablets 1903

Atazanavir (Since entecavir is primarily eliminated by the kidneys co-administration of entecavir with drugs that reduce renal function or compete for active tubular secretion may increase serum concentrations of either entecavir or the co-administered drug).
No products indexed under this heading.

Atorvastatin Calcium (Since entecavir is primarily eliminated by the kidneys co-administration of entecavir with drugs that reduce renal function or compete for active tubular secretion may increase serum concentrations of either entecavir or the co-administered drug). Products include:

Lipitor Tablets 2501

Azithromycin Dihydrate (Since entecavir is primarily eliminated by the kidneys co-administration of entecavir with drugs that reduce renal function or compete for active tubular secretion may increase serum concentrations of either entecavir or the co-administered drug).
No products indexed under this heading.

Azlocillin Sodium (Since entecavir is primarily eliminated by the kidneys co-administration of entecavir with drugs that reduce renal function or compete for active tubular secretion may increase serum concentrations of either entecavir or the co-administered drug).
No products indexed under this heading.

Aztreonam (Since entecavir is primarily eliminated by the kidneys co-administration of entecavir with drugs that reduce renal function or compete for active tubular secretion may increase serum concentrations of either entecavir or the co-administered drug).
No products indexed under this heading.

Bacampicillin Hydrochloride (Since entecavir is primarily eliminated by the kidneys co-administration of entecavir with drugs that reduce renal function or compete for active tubular secretion may increase serum concentrations of either entecavir or the co-administered drug).
No products indexed under this heading.

Balsalazide Disodium (Since entecavir is primarily eliminated by the kidneys co-administration of entecavir with drugs that reduce renal function or compete for active tubular secretion may increase serum concentrations of either entecavir or the co-administered drug).
No products indexed under this heading.

Benazepril Hydrochloride (Since entecavir is primarily eliminated by the kidneys co-administration of entecavir with drugs that reduce renal function or compete for active tubular secretion may increase serum concentrations of either entecavir or the co-administered drug).
No products indexed under this heading.

Bendroflumethiazide (Since entecavir is primarily eliminated by the kidneys co-administration of entecavir with drugs that reduce renal function or compete for active tubular secretion may increase serum concentrations of either entecavir or the co-administered drug).
No products indexed under this heading.

Caffeine (Since entecavir is primarily eliminated by the kidneys co-administration of entecavir with drugs that reduce renal function or compete for active tubular secretion may increase serum concentrations of either entecavir or the co-administered drug). Products include:

BioLean Free Tablets .... ■ 635
BioLean II Tablets .... ■ 635
Winrgy Dietary Supplement .... ■ 642

Captopril (Since entecavir is primarily eliminated by the kidneys co-administration of entecavir with drugs that reduce renal function or compete for active tubular secretion may increase serum concentrations of either entecavir or the co-administered drug). Products include:

Captopril Tablets 2182

Carbenicillin Disodium (Since entecavir is primarily eliminated by the kidneys co-administration of entecavir with drugs that reduce renal function or compete for active tubular secretion may increase serum concentrations of either entecavir or the co-administered drug).
No products indexed under this heading.

Carbenicillin Indanyl Sodium (Since entecavir is primarily eliminated by the kidneys co-administration of entecavir with drugs that reduce renal function or compete for active tubular secretion may increase serum concentrations of either entecavir or the co-administered drug).
No products indexed under this heading.

Carboplatin (Since entecavir is primarily eliminated by the kidneys co-administration of entecavir with drugs that reduce renal function or compete for active tubular secretion may increase serum concentrations of either entecavir or the co-administered drug).
No products indexed under this heading.

Carmustine (BCNU) (Since entecavir is primarily eliminated by the kidneys co-administration of entecavir with drugs that reduce renal function or compete for active tubular secretion may increase serum concentrations of either entecavir or the co-administered drug).
No products indexed under this heading.

Cefaclor (Since entecavir is primarily eliminated by the kidneys co-administration of entecavir with drugs that reduce renal function or compete for active tubular secretion may increase serum concentrations of either entecavir or the co-administered drug).
No products indexed under this heading.

Cefadroxil (Since entecavir is primarily eliminated by the kidneys co-administration of entecavir with drugs that reduce renal function or compete for active tubular secretion may increase serum concentrations of either entecavir or the co-administered drug).
No products indexed under this heading.

Cefamandole Nafate (Since entecavir is primarily eliminated by the kidneys co-administration of entecavir with drugs that reduce renal function or compete for active tubular secretion may increase serum concentrations of either entecavir or the co-administered drug).
No products indexed under this heading.

Cefazolin Sodium (Since entecavir is primarily eliminated by the kidneys co-administration of entecavir with drugs that reduce renal function or compete for active tubular secretion may increase serum concentrations of either entecavir or the co-administered drug).
No products indexed under this heading.

Cefdinir (Since entecavir is primarily eliminated by the kidneys co-administration of entecavir with drugs that reduce renal function or compete for active tubular secretion may increase serum concentrations of either entecavir or the co-administered drug). Products include:
Omnicef Capsules **497**
Omnicef for Oral Suspension **497**

Cefepime Hydrochloride (Since entecavir is primarily eliminated by the kidneys co-administration of entecavir with drugs that reduce renal function or compete for active tubular secretion may increase serum concentrations of either entecavir or the co-administered drug).
No products indexed under this heading.

Cefixime (Since entecavir is primarily eliminated by the kidneys co-administration of entecavir with drugs that reduce renal function or compete for active tubular secretion may increase serum concentrations of either entecavir or the co-administered drug). Products include:
Suprax for Oral Suspension **1891**
Suprax Tablets **1891**

Cefmetazole Sodium (Since entecavir is primarily eliminated by the kidneys co-administration of entecavir with drugs that reduce renal function or compete for active tubular secretion may increase serum concentrations of either entecavir or the co-administered drug).
No products indexed under this heading.

Cefonicid Sodium (Since entecavir is primarily eliminated by the kidneys co-administration of entecavir with drugs that reduce renal function or compete for active tubular secretion may increase serum concentrations of either entecavir or the co-administered drug).
No products indexed under this heading.

Cefoperazone Sodium (Since entecavir is primarily eliminated by the kidneys co-administration of entecavir with drugs that reduce renal function or compete for active tubular secretion may increase serum concentrations of either entecavir or the co-administered drug).
No products indexed under this heading.

Ceforanide (Since entecavir is primarily eliminated by the kidneys co-administration of entecavir with drugs that reduce renal function or compete for active tubular secretion may increase serum concentrations of either entecavir or the co-administered drug).
No products indexed under this heading.

Cefotaxime Sodium (Since entecavir is primarily eliminated by the kidneys co-administration of entecavir with drugs that reduce renal function or compete for active tubular secretion may increase serum concentrations of either entecavir or the co-administered drug).
No products indexed under this heading.

Cefotetan (Since entecavir is primarily eliminated by the kidneys co-administration of entecavir with drugs that reduce renal function or compete for active tubular secretion may increase serum concentrations of either entecavir or the co-administered drug).
No products indexed under this heading.

Cefoxitin Sodium (Since entecavir is primarily eliminated by the kidneys co-administration of entecavir with drugs that reduce renal function or compete for active tubular secretion may increase serum concentrations of either entecavir or the co-administered drug).
No products indexed under this heading.

Cefpodoxime Proxetil (Since entecavir is primarily eliminated by the kidneys co-administration of entecavir with drugs that reduce renal function or compete for active tubular secretion may increase serum concentrations of either entecavir or the co-administered drug).
No products indexed under this heading.

Cefprozil (Since entecavir is primarily eliminated by the kidneys co-administration of entecavir with drugs that reduce renal function or compete for active tubular secretion may increase serum concentrations of either entecavir or the co-administered drug).
No products indexed under this heading.

Ceftazidime (Since entecavir is primarily eliminated by the kidneys co-administration of entecavir with drugs that reduce renal function or compete for active tubular secretion may increase serum concentrations of either entecavir or the co-administered drug). Products include:
Fortaz **1450**

Ceftizoxime Sodium (Since entecavir is primarily eliminated by the kidneys co-administration of entecavir with drugs that reduce renal function or compete for active tubular secretion may increase serum concentrations of either entecavir or the co-administered drug).
No products indexed under this heading.

Ceftriaxone Sodium (Since entecavir is primarily eliminated by the kidneys co-administration of entecavir with drugs that reduce renal function or compete for active tubular secretion may increase serum concentrations of either entecavir or the co-administered drug). Products include:
Rocephin Injectable Vials, ADD-Vantage, Galaxy, Bulk........... **2642**

Cefuroxime Axetil (Since entecavir is primarily eliminated by the kidneys co-administration of entecavir with drugs that reduce renal function or compete for active tubular secretion may increase serum concentrations of either entecavir or the co-administered drug). Products include:
Ceftin **1380**

Cefuroxime Sodium (Since entecavir is primarily eliminated by the kidneys co-administration of entecavir with drugs that reduce renal function or compete for active tubular secretion may increase serum concentrations of either entecavir or the co-administered drug).
No products indexed under this heading.

Celecoxib (Since entecavir is primarily eliminated by the kidneys co-administration of entecavir with drugs that reduce renal function or compete for active tubular secretion may increase serum concentrations of either entecavir or the co-administered drug). Products include:
Celebrex Capsules **2979**

Cephalexin (Since entecavir is primarily eliminated by the kidneys co-administration of entecavir with drugs that reduce renal function or compete for active tubular secretion may increase serum concentrations of either entecavir or the co-administered drug).
No products indexed under this heading.

Cephalothin Sodium (Since entecavir is primarily eliminated by the kidneys co-administration of entecavir with drugs that reduce renal function or compete for active tubular secretion may increase serum concentrations of either entecavir or the co-administered drug).
No products indexed under this heading.

Cephapirin Sodium (Since entecavir is primarily eliminated by the kidneys co-administration of entecavir with drugs that reduce renal function or compete for active tubular secretion may increase serum concentrations of either entecavir or the co-administered drug).
No products indexed under this heading.

Cephradine (Since entecavir is primarily eliminated by the kidneys co-administration of entecavir with drugs that reduce renal function or compete for active tubular secretion may increase serum concentrations of either entecavir or the co-administered drug).
No products indexed under this heading.

Cerivastatin Sodium (Since entecavir is primarily eliminated by the kidneys co-administration of entecavir with drugs that reduce renal function or compete for active tubular secretion may increase serum concentrations of either entecavir or the co-administered drug).
No products indexed under this heading.

Chlorothiazide (Since entecavir is primarily eliminated by the kidneys co-administration of entecavir with drugs that reduce renal function or compete for active tubular secretion may increase serum concentrations of either entecavir or the co-administered drug).
No products indexed under this heading.

Chlorothiazide Sodium (Since entecavir is primarily eliminated by the kidneys co-administration of entecavir with drugs that reduce renal function or compete for active tubular secretion may increase serum concentrations of either entecavir or the co-administered drug). Products include:
Intravenous Sodium Diuril **2490**

Chlorpropamide (Since entecavir is primarily eliminated by the kidneys co-administration of entecavir with drugs that reduce renal function or compete for active tubular secretion may increase serum concentrations of either entecavir or the co-administered drug).
No products indexed under this heading.

Cidofovir (Since entecavir is primarily eliminated by the kidneys co-administration of entecavir with drugs that reduce renal function or compete for active tubular secretion may increase serum concentrations of either entecavir or the co-administered drug).
No products indexed under this heading.

Cilastatin Sodium (Since entecavir is primarily eliminated by the kidneys co-administration of entecavir with drugs that reduce renal function or compete for active tubular secretion may increase serum concentrations

of either entecavir or the co-administered drug). Products include:

- Primaxin I.M. 2080
- Primaxin I.V. 2083

Cimetidine (Since entecavir is primarily eliminated by the kidneys co-administration of entecavir with drugs that reduce renal function or compete for active tubular secretion may increase serum concentrations of either entecavir or the co-administered drug).

No products indexed under this heading.

Cimetidine Hydrochloride (Since entecavir is primarily eliminated by the kidneys co-administration of entecavir with drugs that reduce renal function or compete for active tubular secretion may increase serum concentrations of either entecavir or the co-administered drug).

No products indexed under this heading.

Cisplatin (Since entecavir is primarily eliminated by the kidneys co-administration of entecavir with drugs that reduce renal function or compete for active tubular secretion may increase serum concentrations of either entecavir or the co-administered drug).

No products indexed under this heading.

Cladribine (Since entecavir is primarily eliminated by the kidneys co-administration of entecavir with drugs that reduce renal function or compete for active tubular secretion may increase serum concentrations of either entecavir or the co-administered drug). Products include:

- Leustatin Injection 2384

Clozapine (Since entecavir is primarily eliminated by the kidneys co-administration of entecavir with drugs that reduce renal function or compete for active tubular secretion may increase serum concentrations of either entecavir or the co-administered drug).

No products indexed under this heading.

Colistimethate Sodium (Since entecavir is primarily eliminated by the kidneys co-administration of entecavir with drugs that reduce renal function or compete for active tubular secretion may increase serum concentrations of either entecavir or the co-administered drug).

No products indexed under this heading.

Colistin Sulfate (Since entecavir is primarily eliminated by the kidneys co-administration of entecavir with drugs that reduce renal function or compete for active tubular secretion may increase serum concentrations of either entecavir or the co-administered drug).

No products indexed under this heading.

Cyclophosphamide (Since entecavir is primarily eliminated by the kidneys co-administration of entecavir with drugs that reduce renal function or compete for active tubular secretion may increase serum concentrations of either entecavir or the co-administered drug).

No products indexed under this heading.

Cyclosporine (Since entecavir is primarily eliminated by the kidneys co-administration of entecavir with drugs that reduce renal function or compete for active tubular secretion may increase serum concentrations of either entecavir or the co-administered drug). Products include:

- Gengraf Capsules 435
- Neoral Oral Solution 2280
- Neoral Soft Gelatin Capsules 2280
- Restasis Ophthalmic Emulsion 557
- Sandimmune 2296

Cytarabine (Since entecavir is primarily eliminated by the kidneys co-administration of entecavir with drugs that reduce renal function or compete for active tubular secretion may increase serum concentrations of either entecavir or the co-administered drug).

No products indexed under this heading.

Cytarabine Liposome (Since entecavir is primarily eliminated by the kidneys co-administration of entecavir with drugs that reduce renal function or compete for active tubular secretion may increase serum concentrations of either entecavir or the co-administered drug). Products include:

- DepoCyt Injection 1136

Delavirdine Mesylate (Since entecavir is primarily eliminated by the kidneys co-administration of entecavir with drugs that reduce renal function or compete for active tubular secretion may increase serum concentrations of either entecavir or the co-administered drug).

No products indexed under this heading.

Diatrizoate Meglumine (Since entecavir is primarily eliminated by the kidneys co-administration of entecavir with drugs that reduce renal function or compete for active tubular secretion may increase serum concentrations of either entecavir or the co-administered drug).

No products indexed under this heading.

Diatrizoate Sodium (Since entecavir is primarily eliminated by the kidneys co-administration of entecavir with drugs that reduce renal function or compete for active tubular secretion may increase serum concentrations of either entecavir or the co-administered drug).

No products indexed under this heading.

Diclofenac Potassium (Since entecavir is primarily eliminated by the kidneys co-administration of entecavir with drugs that reduce renal function or compete for active tubular secretion may increase serum concentrations of either entecavir or the co-administered drug).

No products indexed under this heading.

Diclofenac Sodium (Since entecavir is primarily eliminated by the kidneys co-administration of entecavir with drugs that reduce renal function or compete for active tubular secretion may increase serum concentrations of either entecavir or the co-administered drug). Products include:

- Diclofenac Sodium Ophthalmic Solution ⊙240
- Voltaren Ophthalmic Solution 2336
- Voltaren Tablets 2334
- Voltaren-XR Tablets 2337

Dicloxacillin Sodium (Since entecavir is primarily eliminated by the kidneys co-administration of entecavir with drugs that reduce renal function or compete for active tubular secretion may increase serum concentrations of either entecavir or the co-administered drug).

No products indexed under this heading.

Didanosine (Since entecavir is primarily eliminated by the kidneys co-administration of entecavir with drugs that reduce renal function or compete for active tubular secretion may increase serum concentrations of either entecavir or the co-administered drug).

No products indexed under this heading.

Efavirenz (Since entecavir is primarily eliminated by the kidneys co-administration of entecavir with drugs that reduce renal function or compete for active tubular secretion may increase serum concentrations of either entecavir or the co-administered drug). Products include:

- Atripla Tablets 938
- Sustiva Capsules 930
- Sustiva Tablets 930

Emtricitabine (Since entecavir is primarily eliminated by the kidneys co-administration of entecavir with drugs that reduce renal function or compete for active tubular secretion may increase serum concentrations of either entecavir or the co-administered drug). Products include:

- Atripla Tablets 938
- Emtriva Capsules 1246
- Emtriva Oral Solution 1246
- Truvada Tablets 1262

Enalapril Maleate (Since entecavir is primarily eliminated by the kidneys co-administration of entecavir with drugs that reduce renal function or compete for active tubular secretion may increase serum concentrations of either entecavir or the co-administered drug).

No products indexed under this heading.

Enalaprilat (Since entecavir is primarily eliminated by the kidneys co-administration of entecavir with drugs that reduce renal function or compete for active tubular secretion may increase serum concentrations of either entecavir or the co-administered drug).

No products indexed under this heading.

Enfuvirtide (Since entecavir is primarily eliminated by the kidneys co-administration of entecavir with drugs that reduce renal function or compete for active tubular secretion may increase serum concentrations of either entecavir or the co-administered drug).

No products indexed under this heading.

Ethiodized Oil (Since entecavir is primarily eliminated by the kidneys co-administration of entecavir with drugs that reduce renal function or compete for active tubular secretion may increase serum concentrations of either entecavir or the co-administered drug).

No products indexed under this heading.

Etodolac (Since entecavir is primarily eliminated by the kidneys co-administration of entecavir with drugs that reduce renal function or compete for active tubular secretion may increase serum concentrations of either entecavir or the co-administered drug).

No products indexed under this heading.

Fenoprofen Calcium (Since entecavir is primarily eliminated by the kidneys co-administration of entecavir with drugs that reduce renal function or compete for active tubular secretion may increase serum concentrations of either entecavir or the co-administered drug). Products include:

- Nalfon Capsules 2508

Filgrastim (Since entecavir is primarily eliminated by the kidneys co-administration of entecavir with drugs that reduce renal function or compete for active tubular secretion may increase serum concentrations of either entecavir or the co-administered drug). Products include:

- Neupogen for Injection 589

Fluorouracil (Since entecavir is primarily eliminated by the kidneys co-administration of entecavir with drugs that reduce renal function or compete for active tubular secretion may increase serum concentrations of either entecavir or the co-administered drug). Products include:

- Carac Cream 0.5% 2722

Flurbiprofen (Since entecavir is primarily eliminated by the kidneys co-administration of entecavir with drugs that reduce renal function or compete for active tubular secretion may increase serum concentrations of either entecavir or the co-administered drug).

No products indexed under this heading.

Fluvastatin Sodium (Since entecavir is primarily eliminated by the kidneys co-administration of entecavir with drugs that reduce renal function or compete for active tubular secretion may increase serum concentrations of either entecavir or the co-administered drug). Products include:

- Lescol Capsules 2268
- Lescol XL Tablets 2268

Foscarnet Sodium (Since entecavir is primarily eliminated by the kidneys co-administration of entecavir with drugs that reduce renal function or compete for active tubular secretion may increase serum concentrations of either entecavir or the co-administered drug).

No products indexed under this heading.

Fosinopril Sodium (Since entecavir is primarily eliminated by the kidneys co-administration of entecavir with drugs that reduce renal function or compete for active tubular secretion may increase serum concentrations of either entecavir or the co-administered drug).

No products indexed under this heading.

Furosemide (Since entecavir is primarily eliminated by the kidneys co-administration of entecavir with drugs that reduce renal function or compete for active tubular secretion may increase serum concentrations

of either entecavir or the co-administered drug). Products include:

Furosemide Tablets 2186

Gadopentetate Dimeglumine (Since entecavir is primarily eliminated by the kidneys co-administration of entecavir with drugs that reduce renal function or compete for active tubular secretion may increase serum concentrations of either entecavir or the co-administered drug).

No products indexed under this heading.

Gentamicin (Since entecavir is primarily eliminated by the kidneys co-administration of entecavir with drugs that reduce renal function or compete for active tubular secretion may increase serum concentrations of either entecavir or the co-administered drug).

No products indexed under this heading.

Gentamicin Sulfate (Since entecavir is primarily eliminated by the kidneys co-administration of entecavir with drugs that reduce renal function or compete for active tubular secretion may increase serum concentrations of either entecavir or the co-administered drug). Products include:

Pred-G Ophthalmic Ointment .... ⊙ 229
Pred-G Ophthalmic Suspension .... ⊙ 228

Glipizide (Since entecavir is primarily eliminated by the kidneys co-administration of entecavir with drugs that reduce renal function or compete for active tubular secretion may increase serum concentrations of either entecavir or the co-administered drug).

No products indexed under this heading.

Globulin, Immune (Human) (Since entecavir is primarily eliminated by the kidneys co-administration of entecavir with drugs that reduce renal function or compete for active tubular secretion may increase serum concentrations of either entecavir or the co-administered drug). Products include:

Flebogamma 5% 1715

Glyburide (Since entecavir is primarily eliminated by the kidneys co-administration of entecavir with drugs that reduce renal function or compete for active tubular secretion may increase serum concentrations of either entecavir or the co-administered drug).

No products indexed under this heading.

Gold Therapy (Since entecavir is primarily eliminated by the kidneys co-administration of entecavir with drugs that reduce renal function or compete for active tubular secretion may increase serum concentrations of either entecavir or the co-administered drug).

No products indexed under this heading.

HMG-CoA Reductase Inhibitors (Since entecavir is primarily eliminated by the kidneys co-administration of entecavir with drugs that reduce renal function or compete for active tubular secretion may increase serum concentrations of either entecavir or the co-administered drug).

No products indexed under this heading.

Hydrochlorothiazide (Since entecavir is primarily eliminated by the kidneys co-administration of entecavir with drugs that reduce renal function or compete for active tubular secretion may increase serum concentrations of either entecavir or the co-administered drug). Products include:

Atacand HCT 642
Avalide Tablets 892
Avalide Tablets 2713
Benicar HCT Tablets 1010
Diovan HCT Tablets 2216
Dyazide Capsules 1405
Micardis HCT Tablets 854
Prinzide Tablets 2092
Tekturna HCT Tablets 2324
Teveten HCT Tablets 517

Hydroflumethiazide (Since entecavir is primarily eliminated by the kidneys co-administration of entecavir with drugs that reduce renal function or compete for active tubular secretion may increase serum concentrations of either entecavir or the co-administered drug).

No products indexed under this heading.

Ibuprofen (Since entecavir is primarily eliminated by the kidneys co-administration of entecavir with drugs that reduce renal function or compete for active tubular secretion may increase serum concentrations of either entecavir or the co-administered drug). Products include:

Motrin IB Tablets and Caplets 1900
Children's Motrin Oral Suspension ... 1901
Children's Motrin Non-Staining Dye-Free Oral Suspension 1901
Children's Motrin Cold Oral Suspension 1899
Infants' Motrin Concentrated Drops 1901
Infants' Motrin Non-Staining Dye-Free Concentrated Drops 1901
Junior Strength Motrin Caplets and Chewable Tablets 1901
Vicoprofen Tablets 533

Idarubicin Hydrochloride (Since entecavir is primarily eliminated by the kidneys co-administration of entecavir with drugs that reduce renal function or compete for active tubular secretion may increase serum concentrations of either entecavir or the co-administered drug).

No products indexed under this heading.

Ifosfamide (Since entecavir is primarily eliminated by the kidneys co-administration of entecavir with drugs that reduce renal function or compete for active tubular secretion may increase serum concentrations of either entecavir or the co-administered drug).

No products indexed under this heading.

Imipenem (Since entecavir is primarily eliminated by the kidneys co-administration of entecavir with drugs that reduce renal function or compete for active tubular secretion may increase serum concentrations of either entecavir or the co-administered drug). Products include:

Primaxin I.M. 2080
Primaxin I.V. 2083

Immune Globulin Intravenous (Human) (Since entecavir is primarily eliminated by the kidneys co-administration of entecavir with drugs that reduce renal function or compete for active tubular secretion may increase serum concentrations of either entecavir or the co-administered drug). Products include:

Flebogamma 5% DIF 1718
Gammagard Liquid 730
Gammagard S/D 734
Gamunex 3094

Indinavir Sulfate (Since entecavir is primarily eliminated by the kidneys co-administration of entecavir with drugs that reduce renal function or compete for active tubular secretion may increase serum concentrations of either entecavir or the co-administered drug). Products include:

Crixivan Capsules 1979

Indomethacin (Since entecavir is primarily eliminated by the kidneys co-administration of entecavir with drugs that reduce renal function or compete for active tubular secretion may increase serum concentrations of either entecavir or the co-administered drug). Products include:

Indocin 2024

Indomethacin Sodium Trihydrate (Since entecavir is primarily eliminated by the kidneys co-administration of entecavir with drugs that reduce renal function or compete for active tubular secretion may increase serum concentrations of either entecavir or the co-administered drug). Products include:

Indocin I.V. 2489

Interferon Beta-1b (Since entecavir is primarily eliminated by the kidneys co-administration of entecavir with drugs that reduce renal function or compete for active tubular secretion may increase serum concentrations of either entecavir or the co-administered drug). Products include:

Betaseron for SC Injection 756

Interleuken-2 (Since entecavir is primarily eliminated by the kidneys co-administration of entecavir with drugs that reduce renal function or compete for active tubular secretion may increase serum concentrations of either entecavir or the co-administered drug).

No products indexed under this heading.

Iodamide Meglumine (Since entecavir is primarily eliminated by the kidneys co-administration of entecavir with drugs that reduce renal function or compete for active tubular secretion may increase serum concentrations of either entecavir or the co-administered drug).

No products indexed under this heading.

Iohexol (Since entecavir is primarily eliminated by the kidneys co-administration of entecavir with drugs that reduce renal function or compete for active tubular secretion may increase serum concentrations of either entecavir or the co-administered drug).

No products indexed under this heading.

Iopamidol (Since entecavir is primarily eliminated by the kidneys co-administration of entecavir with drugs that reduce renal function or compete for active tubular secretion may increase serum concentrations of either entecavir or the co-administered drug).

No products indexed under this heading.

Iopanoic Acid (Since entecavir is primarily eliminated by the kidneys co-administration of entecavir with drugs that reduce renal function or compete for active tubular secretion may increase serum concentrations of either entecavir or the co-administered drug).

No products indexed under this heading.

Iothalamate Meglumine (Since entecavir is primarily eliminated by the kidneys co-administration of entecavir with drugs that reduce renal function or compete for active tubular secretion may increase serum concentrations of either entecavir or the co-administered drug).

No products indexed under this heading.

Ioxaglate Meglumine (Since entecavir is primarily eliminated by the kidneys co-administration of entecavir with drugs that reduce renal function or compete for active tubular secretion may increase serum concentrations of either entecavir or the co-administered drug).

No products indexed under this heading.

Ioxaglate Sodium (Since entecavir is primarily eliminated by the kidneys co-administration of entecavir with drugs that reduce renal function or compete for active tubular secretion may increase serum concentrations of either entecavir or the co-administered drug).

No products indexed under this heading.

Kanamycin Sulfate (Since entecavir is primarily eliminated by the kidneys co-administration of entecavir with drugs that reduce renal function or compete for active tubular secretion may increase serum concentrations of either entecavir or the co-administered drug).

No products indexed under this heading.

Ketoprofen (Since entecavir is primarily eliminated by the kidneys co-administration of entecavir with drugs that reduce renal function or compete for active tubular secretion may increase serum concentrations of either entecavir or the co-administered drug).

No products indexed under this heading.

Ketorolac Tromethamine (Since entecavir is primarily eliminated by the kidneys co-administration of entecavir with drugs that reduce renal function or compete for active tubular secretion may increase serum concentrations of either entecavir or the co-administered drug).

No products indexed under this heading.

Lamium album (Since entecavir is primarily eliminated by the kidneys co-administration of entecavir with drugs that reduce renal function or compete for active tubular secretion may increase serum concentrations of either entecavir or the co-administered drug).

No products indexed under this heading.

Lisinopril (Since entecavir is primarily eliminated by the kidneys co-administration of entecavir with drugs that reduce renal function or compete for active tubular secretion may increase serum concentrations

of either entecavir or the co-administered drug). Products include:

Prinivil Tablets ... 2087
Prinzide Tablets ... 2092

Lithium (Since entecavir is primarily eliminated by the kidneys co-administration of entecavir with drugs that reduce renal function or compete for active tubular secretion may increase serum concentrations of either entecavir or the co-administered drug).

No products indexed under this heading.

Lithium Carbonate (Since entecavir is primarily eliminated by the kidneys co-administration of entecavir with drugs that reduce renal function or compete for active tubular secretion may increase serum concentrations of either entecavir or the co-administered drug).

No products indexed under this heading.

Lithium Citrate (Since entecavir is primarily eliminated by the kidneys co-administration of entecavir with drugs that reduce renal function or compete for active tubular secretion may increase serum concentrations of either entecavir or the co-administered drug).

No products indexed under this heading.

Lopinavir (Since entecavir is primarily eliminated by the kidneys co-administration of entecavir with drugs that reduce renal function or compete for active tubular secretion may increase serum concentrations of either entecavir or the co-administered drug). Products include:

Kaletra ... 452

Loracarbef (Since entecavir is primarily eliminated by the kidneys co-administration of entecavir with drugs that reduce renal function or compete for active tubular secretion may increase serum concentrations of either entecavir or the co-administered drug).

No products indexed under this heading.

Lovastatin (Since entecavir is primarily eliminated by the kidneys co-administration of entecavir with drugs that reduce renal function or compete for active tubular secretion may increase serum concentrations of either entecavir or the co-administered drug). Products include:

Advicor Tablets ... 402
Mevacor Tablets ... 2063

Meclofenamate Sodium (Since entecavir is primarily eliminated by the kidneys co-administration of entecavir with drugs that reduce renal function or compete for active tubular secretion may increase serum concentrations of either entecavir or the co-administered drug).

No products indexed under this heading.

Mefenamic Acid (Since entecavir is primarily eliminated by the kidneys co-administration of entecavir with drugs that reduce renal function or compete for active tubular secretion may increase serum concentrations of either entecavir or the co-administered drug).

No products indexed under this heading.

Meloxicam (Since entecavir is primarily eliminated by the kidneys co-administration of entecavir with drugs that reduce renal function or compete for active tubular secretion may increase serum concentrations of either entecavir or the co-administered drug). Products include:

Mobic Oral Suspension ... 863
Mobic Tablets ... 863

Melphalan Hydrochloride (Since entecavir is primarily eliminated by the kidneys co-administration of entecavir with drugs that reduce renal function or compete for active tubular secretion may increase serum concentrations of either entecavir or the co-administered drug).

No products indexed under this heading.

Mesalamine (Since entecavir is primarily eliminated by the kidneys co-administration of entecavir with drugs that reduce renal function or compete for active tubular secretion may increase serum concentrations of either entecavir or the co-administered drug). Products include:

Asacol Delayed-Release Tablets ... 2579
Canasa Rectal Suppositories ... 705
Lialda Tablets ... 3029
Pentasa Capsules ... 3030

Methimazole (Since entecavir is primarily eliminated by the kidneys co-administration of entecavir with drugs that reduce renal function or compete for active tubular secretion may increase serum concentrations of either entecavir or the co-administered drug).

No products indexed under this heading.

Methotrexate (Since entecavir is primarily eliminated by the kidneys co-administration of entecavir with drugs that reduce renal function or compete for active tubular secretion may increase serum concentrations of either entecavir or the co-administered drug).

No products indexed under this heading.

Methotrexate Sodium (Since entecavir is primarily eliminated by the kidneys co-administration of entecavir with drugs that reduce renal function or compete for active tubular secretion may increase serum concentrations of either entecavir or the co-administered drug).

No products indexed under this heading.

Methyclothiazide (Since entecavir is primarily eliminated by the kidneys co-administration of entecavir with drugs that reduce renal function or compete for active tubular secretion may increase serum concentrations of either entecavir or the co-administered drug).

No products indexed under this heading.

Mezlocillin Sodium (Since entecavir is primarily eliminated by the kidneys co-administration of entecavir with drugs that reduce renal function or compete for active tubular secretion may increase serum concentrations of either entecavir or the co-administered drug).

No products indexed under this heading.

Minocycline Hydrochloride (Since entecavir is primarily eliminated by the kidneys co-administration of entecavir with drugs that reduce renal function or compete for active tubular secretion may increase serum concentrations of either entecavir or the co-administered drug). Products include:

Solodyn Extended Release Tablets ... 1938

Mitomycin (Mitomycin-C) (Since entecavir is primarily eliminated by the kidneys co-administration of entecavir with drugs that reduce renal function or compete for active tubular secretion may increase serum concentrations of either entecavir or the co-administered drug).

No products indexed under this heading.

Moexipril Hydrochloride (Since entecavir is primarily eliminated by the kidneys co-administration of entecavir with drugs that reduce renal function or compete for active tubular secretion may increase serum concentrations of either entecavir or the co-administered drug).

No products indexed under this heading.

Muromonab-CD3 (Since entecavir is primarily eliminated by the kidneys co-administration of entecavir with drugs that reduce renal function or compete for active tubular secretion may increase serum concentrations of either entecavir or the co-administered drug). Products include:

Orthoclone OKT3 Sterile Solution ... 2387

Nabumetone (Since entecavir is primarily eliminated by the kidneys co-administration of entecavir with drugs that reduce renal function or compete for active tubular secretion may increase serum concentrations of either entecavir or the co-administered drug).

No products indexed under this heading.

Nafcillin Sodium (Since entecavir is primarily eliminated by the kidneys co-administration of entecavir with drugs that reduce renal function or compete for active tubular secretion may increase serum concentrations of either entecavir or the co-administered drug).

No products indexed under this heading.

Naproxen (Since entecavir is primarily eliminated by the kidneys co-administration of entecavir with drugs that reduce renal function or compete for active tubular secretion may increase serum concentrations of either entecavir or the co-administered drug). Products include:

EC-Naprosyn Delayed-Release Tablets ... 2632
Naprosyn Suspension ... 2632
Naprosyn Tablets ... 2632

Naproxen Sodium (Since entecavir is primarily eliminated by the kidneys co-administration of entecavir with drugs that reduce renal function or compete for active tubular secretion may increase serum concentrations of either entecavir or the co-administered drug). Products include:

Anaprox Tablets ... 2632
Anaprox DS Tablets ... 2632
Treximet Tablets ... 1616

Nelfinavir Mesylate (Since entecavir is primarily eliminated by the kidneys co-administration of entecavir with drugs that reduce renal function or compete for active tubular secretion may increase serum concentrations of either entecavir or the co-administered drug).

No products indexed under this heading.

Neomycin (Since entecavir is primarily eliminated by the kidneys co-administration of entecavir with drugs that reduce renal function or compete for active tubular secretion may increase serum concentrations of either entecavir or the co-administered drug).

No products indexed under this heading.

Neomycin, oral (Since entecavir is primarily eliminated by the kidneys co-administration of entecavir with drugs that reduce renal function or compete for active tubular secretion may increase serum concentrations of either entecavir or the co-administered drug).

No products indexed under this heading.

Neomycin Sulfate (Since entecavir is primarily eliminated by the kidneys co-administration of entecavir with drugs that reduce renal function or compete for active tubular secretion may increase serum concentrations of either entecavir or the co-administered drug). Products include:

Neosporin Ophthalmic Solution Sterile ... ⊙252

Nevirapine (Since entecavir is primarily eliminated by the kidneys co-administration of entecavir with drugs that reduce renal function or compete for active tubular secretion may increase serum concentrations of either entecavir or the co-administered drug). Products include:

Viramune Oral Suspension ... 873
Viramune Tablets ... 873

Norfloxacin (Since entecavir is primarily eliminated by the kidneys co-administration of entecavir with drugs that reduce renal function or compete for active tubular secretion may increase serum concentrations of either entecavir or the co-administered drug). Products include:

Noroxin Tablets ... 2069

Olsalazine Sodium (Since entecavir is primarily eliminated by the kidneys co-administration of entecavir with drugs that reduce renal function or compete for active tubular secretion may increase serum concentrations of either entecavir or the co-administered drug).

No products indexed under this heading.

Omeprazole (Since entecavir is primarily eliminated by the kidneys co-administration of entecavir with drugs that reduce renal function or compete for active tubular secretion may increase serum concentrations of either entecavir or the co-administered drug).

No products indexed under this heading.

Oxaprozin (Since entecavir is primarily eliminated by the kidneys co-administration of entecavir with drugs that reduce renal function or compete for active tubular secretion may increase serum concentrations of either entecavir or the co-administered drug).
No products indexed under this heading.

Pamidronate Disodium (Since entecavir is primarily eliminated by the kidneys co-administration of entecavir with drugs that reduce renal function or compete for active tubular secretion may increase serum concentrations of either entecavir or the co-administered drug).
No products indexed under this heading.

Paroxetine Hydrochloride (Since entecavir is primarily eliminated by the kidneys co-administration of entecavir with drugs that reduce renal function or compete for active tubular secretion may increase serum concentrations of either entecavir or the co-administered drug). Products include:
Paxil 1535
Paxil CR Controlled-Release Tablets 1544

Penicillamine (Since entecavir is primarily eliminated by the kidneys co-administration of entecavir with drugs that reduce renal function or compete for active tubular secretion may increase serum concentrations of either entecavir or the co-administered drug). Products include:
Cuprimine Capsules 1986

Penicillin G Benzathine (Since entecavir is primarily eliminated by the kidneys co-administration of entecavir with drugs that reduce renal function or compete for active tubular secretion may increase serum concentrations of either entecavir or the co-administered drug). Products include:
Bicillin C-R Injectable Suspension 1775
Bicillin L-A Injection 1777

Penicillin G Potassium (Since entecavir is primarily eliminated by the kidneys co-administration of entecavir with drugs that reduce renal function or compete for active tubular secretion may increase serum concentrations of either entecavir or the co-administered drug).
No products indexed under this heading.

Penicillin G Procaine (Since entecavir is primarily eliminated by the kidneys co-administration of entecavir with drugs that reduce renal function or compete for active tubular secretion may increase serum concentrations of either entecavir or the co-administered drug). Products include:
Bicillin C-R Injectable Suspension 1775
Bicillin L-A Injection 1777

Penicillin G Sodium (Since entecavir is primarily eliminated by the kidneys co-administration of entecavir with drugs that reduce renal function or compete for active tubular secretion may increase serum concentrations of either entecavir or the co-administered drug).
No products indexed under this heading.

Penicillin V Potassium (Since entecavir is primarily eliminated by the kidneys co-administration of entecavir with drugs that reduce renal function or compete for active tubular secretion may increase serum concentrations of either entecavir or the co-administered drug).
No products indexed under this heading.

Pentamidine Isethionate (Since entecavir is primarily eliminated by the kidneys co-administration of entecavir with drugs that reduce renal function or compete for active tubular secretion may increase serum concentrations of either entecavir or the co-administered drug).
No products indexed under this heading.

Perindopril Erbumine (Since entecavir is primarily eliminated by the kidneys co-administration of entecavir with drugs that reduce renal function or compete for active tubular secretion may increase serum concentrations of either entecavir or the co-administered drug). Products include:
Aceon Tablets (2 mg, 4 mg, 8 mg) 3038

Phenylbutazone (Since entecavir is primarily eliminated by the kidneys co-administration of entecavir with drugs that reduce renal function or compete for active tubular secretion may increase serum concentrations of either entecavir or the co-administered drug).
No products indexed under this heading.

Piroxicam (Since entecavir is primarily eliminated by the kidneys co-administration of entecavir with drugs that reduce renal function or compete for active tubular secretion may increase serum concentrations of either entecavir or the co-administered drug).
No products indexed under this heading.

Plicamycin (Since entecavir is primarily eliminated by the kidneys co-administration of entecavir with drugs that reduce renal function or compete for active tubular secretion may increase serum concentrations of either entecavir or the co-administered drug).
No products indexed under this heading.

Polymyxin (Since entecavir is primarily eliminated by the kidneys co-administration of entecavir with drugs that reduce renal function or compete for active tubular secretion may increase serum concentrations of either entecavir or the co-administered drug).
No products indexed under this heading.

Polymyxin B Sulfate (Since entecavir is primarily eliminated by the kidneys co-administration of entecavir with drugs that reduce renal function or compete for active tubular secretion may increase serum concentrations of either entecavir or the co-administered drug). Products include:
Neosporin Ophthalmic Solution Sterile .... ⊙252

Polythiazide (Since entecavir is primarily eliminated by the kidneys co-administration of entecavir with drugs that reduce renal function or compete for active tubular secretion may increase serum concentrations of either entecavir or the co-administered drug).
No products indexed under this heading.

Pravastatin Sodium (Since entecavir is primarily eliminated by the kidneys co-administration of entecavir with drugs that reduce renal function or compete for active tubular secretion may increase serum concentrations of either entecavir or the co-administered drug).
No products indexed under this heading.

Probenecid (Since entecavir is primarily eliminated by the kidneys co-administration of entecavir with drugs that reduce renal function or compete for active tubular secretion may increase serum concentrations of either entecavir or the co-administered drug).
No products indexed under this heading.

Quinapril Hydrochloride (Since entecavir is primarily eliminated by the kidneys co-administration of entecavir with drugs that reduce renal function or compete for active tubular secretion may increase serum concentrations of either entecavir or the co-administered drug).
No products indexed under this heading.

Rabeprazole Sodium (Since entecavir is primarily eliminated by the kidneys co-administration of entecavir with drugs that reduce renal function or compete for active tubular secretion may increase serum concentrations of either entecavir or the co-administered drug). Products include:
Aciphex Tablets 1053

Ramipril (Since entecavir is primarily eliminated by the kidneys co-administration of entecavir with drugs that reduce renal function or compete for active tubular secretion may increase serum concentrations of either entecavir or the co-administered drug).
No products indexed under this heading.

Rifampin (Since entecavir is primarily eliminated by the kidneys co-administration of entecavir with drugs that reduce renal function or compete for active tubular secretion may increase serum concentrations of either entecavir or the co-administered drug).
No products indexed under this heading.

Riluzole (Since entecavir is primarily eliminated by the kidneys co-administration of entecavir with drugs that reduce renal function or compete for active tubular secretion may increase serum concentrations of either entecavir or the co-administered drug). Products include:
Rilutek Tablets 2771

Ritonavir (Since entecavir is primarily eliminated by the kidneys co-administration of entecavir with drugs that reduce renal function or compete for active tubular secretion may increase serum concentrations of either entecavir or the co-administered drug). Products include:
Kaletra 452
Norvir 489

Rofecoxib (Since entecavir is primarily eliminated by the kidneys co-administration of entecavir with drugs that reduce renal function or compete for active tubular secretion may increase serum concentrations of either entecavir or the co-administered drug).
No products indexed under this heading.

Saquinavir (Since entecavir is primarily eliminated by the kidneys co-administration of entecavir with drugs that reduce renal function or compete for active tubular secretion may increase serum concentrations of either entecavir or the co-administered drug).
No products indexed under this heading.

Sibutramine Hydrochloride Monohydrate (Since entecavir is primarily eliminated by the kidneys co-administration of entecavir with drugs that reduce renal function or compete for active tubular secretion may increase serum concentrations of either entecavir or the co-administered drug). Products include:
Meridia Capsules 475

Simvastatin (Since entecavir is primarily eliminated by the kidneys co-administration of entecavir with drugs that reduce renal function or compete for active tubular secretion may increase serum concentrations of either entecavir or the co-administered drug). Products include:
Simcor Tablets 502
Vytorin 10/10 Tablets 2149
Vytorin 10/10 Tablets 2939
Vytorin 10/20 Tablets 2149
Vytorin 10/20 Tablets 2939
Vytorin 10/40 Tablets 2149
Vytorin 10/40 Tablets 2939
Vytorin 10/80 Tablets 2149
Vytorin 10/80 Tablets 2939
Zocor Tablets 2136

Spirapril Hydrochloride (Since entecavir is primarily eliminated by the kidneys co-administration of entecavir with drugs that reduce renal function or compete for active tubular secretion may increase serum concentrations of either entecavir or the co-administered drug).
No products indexed under this heading.

Stavudine (Since entecavir is primarily eliminated by the kidneys co-administration of entecavir with drugs that reduce renal function or compete for active tubular secretion may increase serum concentrations of either entecavir or the co-administered drug).
No products indexed under this heading.

Streptomycin Sulfate (Since entecavir is primarily eliminated by the kidneys co-administration of entecavir with drugs that reduce renal function or compete for active tubular secretion may increase serum concentrations of either entecavir or the co-administered drug).
No products indexed under this heading.

Streptozocin (Since entecavir is primarily eliminated by the kidneys co-administration of entecavir with drugs that reduce renal function or compete for active tubular secretion may increase serum concentrations of either entecavir or the co-administered drug).
No products indexed under this heading.

Sulfacytine (Since entecavir is primarily eliminated by the kidneys co-administration of entecavir with drugs that reduce renal function or compete for active tubular secretion may increase serum concentrations of either entecavir or the co-administered drug).
No products indexed under this heading.

Sulfamethizole (Since entecavir is primarily eliminated by the kidneys co-administration of entecavir with drugs that reduce renal function or compete for active tubular secretion may increase serum concentrations of either entecavir or the co-administered drug).
No products indexed under this heading.

Sulfamethoxazole (Since entecavir is primarily eliminated by the kidneys co-administration of entecavir with drugs that reduce renal function or compete for active tubular secretion may increase serum concentrations of either entecavir or the co-administered drug).
No products indexed under this heading.

Sulfasalazine (Since entecavir is primarily eliminated by the kidneys co-administration of entecavir with drugs that reduce renal function or compete for active tubular secretion may increase serum concentrations of either entecavir or the co-administered drug).
No products indexed under this heading.

Sulfinpyrazone (Since entecavir is primarily eliminated by the kidneys co-administration of entecavir with drugs that reduce renal function or compete for active tubular secretion may increase serum concentrations of either entecavir or the co-administered drug).
No products indexed under this heading.

Sulfisoxazole Acetyl (Since entecavir is primarily eliminated by the kidneys co-administration of entecavir with drugs that reduce renal function or compete for active tubular secretion may increase serum concentrations of either entecavir or the co-administered drug).
No products indexed under this heading.

Sulfisoxazole Diolamine (Since entecavir is primarily eliminated by the kidneys co-administration of entecavir with drugs that reduce renal function or compete for active tubular secretion may increase serum concentrations of either entecavir or the co-administered drug).
No products indexed under this heading.

Sulindac (Since entecavir is primarily eliminated by the kidneys co-administration of entecavir with drugs that reduce renal function or compete for active tubular secretion may increase serum concentrations of either entecavir or the co-administered drug). Products include:
Clinoril Tablets 1962

Tacrolimus (Since entecavir is primarily eliminated by the kidneys co-administration of entecavir with drugs that reduce renal function or compete for active tubular secretion may increase serum concentrations of either entecavir or the co-administered drug). Products include:
Prograf Capsules and Injection 622
Protopic Ointment 628

Tenofovir Disoproxil Fumarate (Since entecavir is primarily eliminated by the kidneys co-administration of entecavir with drugs that reduce renal function or compete for active tubular secretion may increase serum concentrations of either entecavir or the co-administered drug). Products include:
Atripla Tablets 938
Truvada Tablets 1262
Viread Tablets 1268

Thioguanine (Since entecavir is primarily eliminated by the kidneys co-administration of entecavir with drugs that reduce renal function or compete for active tubular secretion may increase serum concentrations of either entecavir or the co-administered drug). Products include:
Tabloid Tablets 1601

Ticarcillin Disodium (Since entecavir is primarily eliminated by the kidneys co-administration of entecavir with drugs that reduce renal function or compete for active tubular secretion may increase serum concentrations of either entecavir or the co-administered drug). Products include:
Timentin ADD-Vantage 1606
Timentin Injection Galaxy Container 1609
Timentin IV Infusion 1603
Timentin Pharmacy Bulk Package 1613

Tobramycin (Since entecavir is primarily eliminated by the kidneys co-administration of entecavir with drugs that reduce renal function or compete for active tubular secretion may increase serum concentrations of either entecavir or the co-administered drug). Products include:
Zylet Ophthalmic Suspension .... ⊙247

Tobramycin Sulfate (Since entecavir is primarily eliminated by the kidneys co-administration of entecavir with drugs that reduce renal function or compete for active tubular secretion may increase serum concentrations of either entecavir or the co-administered drug).
No products indexed under this heading.

Tolazamide (Since entecavir is primarily eliminated by the kidneys co-administration of entecavir with drugs that reduce renal function or compete for active tubular secretion may increase serum concentrations of either entecavir or the co-administered drug).
No products indexed under this heading.

Tolbutamide (Since entecavir is primarily eliminated by the kidneys co-administration of entecavir with drugs that reduce renal function or compete for active tubular secretion may increase serum concentrations of either entecavir or the co-administered drug).
No products indexed under this heading.

Tolmetin Sodium (Since entecavir is primarily eliminated by the kidneys co-administration of entecavir with drugs that reduce renal function or compete for active tubular secretion may increase serum concentrations of either entecavir or the co-administered drug).
No products indexed under this heading.

Trandolapril (Since entecavir is primarily eliminated by the kidneys co-administration of entecavir with drugs that reduce renal function or compete for active tubular secretion may increase serum concentrations of either entecavir or the co-administered drug). Products include:
Mavik Tablets 472
Tarka Tablets 511

Triamterene (Since entecavir is primarily eliminated by the kidneys co-administration of entecavir with drugs that reduce renal function or compete for active tubular secretion may increase serum concentrations of either entecavir or the co-administered drug). Products include:
Dyazide Capsules 1405
Dyrenium Capsules 3189

Trimethadione (Since entecavir is primarily eliminated by the kidneys co-administration of entecavir with drugs that reduce renal function or compete for active tubular secretion may increase serum concentrations of either entecavir or the co-administered drug).
No products indexed under this heading.

Trovafloxacin Mesylate (Since entecavir is primarily eliminated by the kidneys co-administration of entecavir with drugs that reduce renal function or compete for active tubular secretion may increase serum concentrations of either entecavir or the co-administered drug).
No products indexed under this heading.

Tyropanoate Sodium (Since entecavir is primarily eliminated by the kidneys co-administration of entecavir with drugs that reduce renal function or compete for active tubular secretion may increase serum concentrations of either entecavir or the co-administered drug).
No products indexed under this heading.

Valacyclovir Hydrochloride (Since entecavir is primarily eliminated by the kidneys co-administration of entecavir with drugs that reduce renal function or compete for active tubular secretion may increase serum concentrations of either entecavir or the co-administered drug). Products include:
Valtrex Caplets 1635

Valdecoxib (Since entecavir is primarily eliminated by the kidneys co-administration of entecavir with drugs that reduce renal function or compete for active tubular secretion may increase serum concentrations of either entecavir or the co-administered drug).
No products indexed under this heading.

Vancomycin Hydrochloride (Since entecavir is primarily eliminated by the kidneys co-administration of entecavir with drugs that reduce renal function or compete for active tubular secretion may increase serum concentrations of either entecavir or the co-administered drug).
No products indexed under this heading.

Voriconazole (Since entecavir is primarily eliminated by the kidneys co-administration of entecavir with drugs that reduce renal function or compete for active tubular secretion may increase serum concentrations of either entecavir or the co-administered drug).
No products indexed under this heading.

Zalcitabine (Since entecavir is primarily eliminated by the kidneys co-administration of entecavir with drugs that reduce renal function or compete for active tubular secretion may increase serum concentrations of either entecavir or the co-administered drug).
No products indexed under this heading.

Zidovudine (Since entecavir is primarily eliminated by the kidneys co-administration of entecavir with drugs that reduce renal function or compete for active tubular secretion may increase serum concentrations of either entecavir or the co-administered drug). Products include:
Combivir Tablets 1384
Retrovir 1574
Retrovir IV Infusion 1579
Trizivir Tablets 1622

Zoledronic acid (Since entecavir is primarily eliminated by the kidneys co-administration of entecavir with drugs that reduce renal function or compete for active tubular secretion may increase serum concentrations of either entecavir or the co-administered drug). Products include:
Reclast Injection 2291
Zometa for Intravenous Infusion 2341

BAUSCH & LOMB OCUVITE ADULT 50+ VITAMIN AND MINERAL SUPPLEMENT
(Copper, Lutein, Omega-3 Acids, Vitamin C, Vitamin E, Vitamins with Minerals, Zinc Oxide) .... ⊙237
None cited in PDR database.

BAUSCH & LOMB ALAWAY EYE DROPS
(Ketotifen Fumarate) .... ⊙237
None cited in PDR database.

BAUSCH & LOMB OCUVITE DF VITAMIN SUPPLEMENT
(Alpha Lipoic Acid, Genistein, Niacin, Vitamins, Multiple) .... ⊙238
None cited in PDR database.

BAUSCH & LOMB OCUVITE LUTEIN VITAMIN AND MINERAL SUPPLEMENT
(Lutein, Vitamins with Minerals) .... ⊙238
None cited in PDR database.

BAUSCH & LOMB OCUVITE PRESERVISION AREDS TABLETS
(Vitamins with Minerals) .... ⊙238
None cited in PDR database.

BAUSCH & LOMB PRESERVISION AREDS SOFTGELS
(Vitamins with Minerals) .... ⊙239
None cited in PDR database.

BAUSCH & LOMB PRESERVISION LUTEIN SOFTGELS
(Lutein, Vitamins with Minerals) .... ⊙239
None cited in PDR database.

BAYER ASPIRIN
(Aspirin) 750
May interact with ACE inhibitors, beta blockers, anticoagulants, diuretics, oral hypoglycemic agents, non-steroidal anti-inflammatory agents, phenytoin, valproate, and certain other agents. Compounds in these categories include:

Acarbose (Moderate doses of aspirin may increase the effectiveness of oral hypoglycemic drugs, leading to hypoglycemia). Products include:
Precose Tablets 792

Acebutolol Hydrochloride (The hypotensive effects of beta blockers may be diminished by the concomitant administration of aspirin due to inhibition of renal prostaglandins, leading to decreased renal blood flow, and salt and fluid retention).
No products indexed under this heading.

Acetazolamide (Concurrent use of aspirin and acetazolamide can lead to high serum concentrations of acetazolamide (and toxicity) due to competition at the renal tubule for secretion).
No products indexed under this heading.

Acetazolamide Sodium (Concurrent use of aspirin and acetazolamide can lead to high serum concentrations of acetazolamide (and toxicity) due to competition at the renal tubule for secretion).
No products indexed under this heading.

Amiloride Hydrochloride (The effectiveness of diuretics in patients with underlying renal or cardiovascular disease may be diminished by the concomitant administration of aspirin due to inhibition of renal prostaglandins, leading to decreased renal blood flow, and salt and fluidretention).
No products indexed under this heading.

Anisindione (Patients on anticoagulation therapy are at increased risk for bleeding because of drug-drug interactions and the effect on platelets. Aspirin can displace warfarin from protein binding sites, leading to prolongation of both the prothrombin time and bleeding time. Aspirin can increase the anticoagulant activity of heparin, increasing bleeding risk).
No products indexed under this heading.

Ardeparin Sodium (Patients on anticoagulation therapy are at increased risk for bleeding because of drug-drug interactions and the effect on platelets. Aspirin can displace warfarin from protein binding sites, leading to prolongation of both the prothrombin time and bleeding time. Aspirin can increase the anticoagulant activity of heparin, increasing bleeding risk).
No products indexed under this heading.

Atenolol (The hypotensive effects of beta blockers may be diminished by the concomitant administration of aspirin due to inhibition of renal prostaglandins, leading to decreased renal blood flow, and salt and fluid retention).
No products indexed under this heading.

Benazepril Hydrochloride (The hyponatremic and hypotensive effects of ACE inhibitors may be diminished by the concomitant administration of aspirin due to its indirect effect on the renin-angiotensin conversion pathway).
No products indexed under this heading.

Bendroflumethiazide (The effectiveness of diuretics in patients with underlying renal or cardiovascular disease may be diminished by the concomitant administration of aspirin due to inhibition of renal prostaglandins, leading to decreased renal blood flow, and salt and fluidretention).
No products indexed under this heading.

Betaxolol Hydrochloride (The hypotensive effects of beta blockers may be diminished by the concomitant administration of aspirin due to inhibition of renal prostaglandins, leading to decreased renal blood flow, and salt and fluid retention).
No products indexed under this heading.

Bisoprolol Fumarate (The hypotensive effects of beta blockers may be diminished by the concomitant administration of aspirin due to inhibition of renal prostaglandins, leading to decreased renal blood flow, and salt and fluid retention).
No products indexed under this heading.

Bumetanide (The effectiveness of diuretics in patients with underlying renal or cardiovascular disease may be diminished by the concomitant administration of aspirin due to inhibition of renal prostaglandins, leading to decreased renal blood flow, and salt and fluidretention).
No products indexed under this heading.

Captopril (The hyponatremic and hypotensive effects of ACE inhibitors may be diminished by the concomitant administration of aspirin due to its indirect effect on the renin-angiotensin conversion pathway). Products include:
Captopril Tablets 2182

Carteolol Hydrochloride (The hypotensive effects of beta blockers may be diminished by the concomitant administration of aspirin due to inhibition of renal prostaglandins, leading to decreased renal blood flow, and salt and fluid retention).
No products indexed under this heading.

Celecoxib (The concurrent use of aspirin with other NSAIDs should be avoided because this may increase bleeding or lead to decreased renal function). Products include:
Celebrex Capsules 2979

Chlorothiazide (The effectiveness of diuretics in patients with underlying renal or cardiovascular disease may be diminished by the concomitant administration of aspirin due to inhibition of renal prostaglandins, leading to decreased renal blood flow, and salt and fluidretention).
No products indexed under this heading.

Chlorothiazide Sodium (The effectiveness of diuretics in patients with underlying renal or cardiovascular disease may be diminished by the concomitant administration of aspirin due to inhibition of renal prostaglandins, leading to decreased renal blood flow, and salt and fluidretention). Products include:
Intravenous Sodium Diuril 2490

Chlorpropamide (Moderate doses of aspirin may increase the effectiveness of oral hypoglycemic drugs, leading to hypoglycemia).
No products indexed under this heading.

Chlorthalidone (The effectiveness of diuretics in patients with underlying renal or cardiovascular disease may be diminished by the concomitant administration of aspirin due to inhibition of renal prostaglandins, leading to decreased renal blood flow, and salt and fluidretention). Products include:
Clorpres Tablets 2185

Dalteparin Sodium (Patients on anticoagulation therapy are at increased risk for bleeding because of drug-drug interactions and the effect on platelets. Aspirin can displace warfarin from protein binding sites, leading to prolongation of both the prothrombin time and bleeding time. Aspirin can increase the anticoagulant activity of heparin, increasing bleeding risk). Products include:
Fragmin Injection 1070

Danaparoid Sodium (Patients on anticoagulation therapy are at increased risk for bleeding because of drug-drug interactions and the effect on platelets. Aspirin can displace warfarin from protein binding sites, leading to prolongation of both the prothrombin time and bleeding time. Aspirin can increase the anticoagulant activity of heparin, increasing bleeding risk).
No products indexed under this heading.

Diclofenac Epolamine (The concurrent use of aspirin with other NSAIDs should be avoided because this may increase bleeding or lead to decreased renal function). Products include:
Flector Patch 561

Diclofenac Potassium (The concurrent use of aspirin with other NSAIDs should be avoided because this may increase bleeding or lead to decreased renal function).
No products indexed under this heading.

Diclofenac Sodium (The concurrent use of aspirin with other NSAIDs should be avoided because this may increase bleeding or lead to decreased renal function). Products include:
Diclofenac Sodium Ophthalmic Solution.. ⊙240
Voltaren Ophthalmic Solution 2336
Voltaren Tablets 2334
Voltaren-XR Tablets......................... 2337

Dicumarol (Patients on anticoagulation therapy are at increased risk for bleeding because of drug-drug interactions and the effect on platelets. Aspirin can displace warfarin from protein binding sites, leading to prolongation of both the prothrombin time and bleeding time. Aspirin can increase the anticoagulant activity of heparin, increasing bleeding risk).
No products indexed under this heading.

Divalproex Sodium (Salicylate can displace protein-bound valproic acid, leading to an increase in serum valproic acid levels). Products include:
Depakote ER Tablets 423

Enalapril Maleate (The hyponatremic and hypotensive effects of ACE inhibitors may be diminished by the concomitant administration of aspirin due to its indirect effect on the renin-angiotensin conversion pathway).
No products indexed under this heading.

Enalaprilat (The hyponatremic and hypotensive effects of ACE inhibitors may be diminished by the concomitant administration of aspirin due to its indirect effect on the renin-angiotensin conversion pathway).
No products indexed under this heading.

Enoxaparin Sodium (Patients on anticoagulation therapy are at increased risk for bleeding because of drug-drug interactions and the effect on platelets. Aspirin can displace warfarin from protein binding sites, leading to prolongation of both the prothrombin time and bleeding time. Aspirin can increase the anticoagulant activity of heparin, increasing bleeding risk). Products include:
Lovenox Injection 2756

Esmolol Hydrochloride (The hypotensive effects of beta blockers may be diminished by the concomitant administration of aspirin due to inhibition of renal prostaglandins, leading to decreased renal blood flow, and salt and fluid retention).
No products indexed under this heading.

Ethacrynic Acid (The effectiveness of diuretics in patients with underlying renal or cardiovascular disease may be diminished by the concomitant administration of aspirin due to inhibition of renal prostaglandins, leading to decreased renal blood flow, and salt and fluidretention). Products include:
Edecrin Tablets 698

Etodolac (The concurrent use of aspirin with other NSAIDs should be avoided because this may increase bleeding or lead to decreased renal function).
No products indexed under this heading.

Fenoprofen Calcium (The concurrent use of aspirin with other NSAIDs should be avoided because this may increase bleeding or lead to decreased renal function). Products include:
Nalfon Capsules 2508

IMPORTANT NOTE: Always consult each drug listing in the patient's regimen for possible interactions.

Flurbiprofen (The concurrent use of aspirin with other NSAIDs should be avoided because this may increase bleeding or lead to decreased renal function).
No products indexed under this heading.

Fondaparinux Sodium (Patients on anticoagulation therapy are at increased risk for bleeding because of drug-drug interactions and the effect on platelets. Aspirin can displace warfarin from protein binding sites, leading to prolongation of both the prothrombin time and bleeding time. Aspirin can increase the anticoagulant activity of heparin, increasing bleeding risk). Products include:
Arixtra Injection 1313

Fosinopril Sodium (The hyponatremic and hypotensive effects of ACE inhibitors may be diminished by the concomitant administration of aspirin due to its indirect effect on the renin-angiotensin conversion pathway).
No products indexed under this heading.

Fosphenytoin Sodium (Salicylate can displace protein-bound phenytoin, leading to a decrease in the total concentration of phenytoin).
No products indexed under this heading.

Furosemide (The effectiveness of diuretics in patients with underlying renal or cardiovascular disease may be diminished by the concomitant administration of aspirin due to inhibition of renal prostaglandins, leading to decreased renal blood flow, and salt and fluidretention). Products include:
Furosemide Tablets 2186

Glimepiride (Moderate doses of aspirin may increase the effectiveness of oral hypoglycemic drugs, leading to hypoglycemia). Products include:
Avandaryl Tablets 1344
Duetact Tablets 3085

Glipizide (Moderate doses of aspirin may increase the effectiveness of oral hypoglycemic drugs, leading to hypoglycemia).
No products indexed under this heading.

Glyburide (Moderate doses of aspirin may increase the effectiveness of oral hypoglycemic drugs, leading to hypoglycemia).
No products indexed under this heading.

Heparin Calcium (Patients on anticoagulation therapy are at increased risk for bleeding because of drug-drug interactions and the effect on platelets. Aspirin can displace warfarin from protein binding sites, leading to prolongation of both the prothrombin time and bleeding time. Aspirin can increase the anticoagulant activity of heparin, increasing bleeding risk).
No products indexed under this heading.

Heparin Sodium (Patients on anticoagulation therapy are at increased risk for bleeding because of drug-drug interactions and the effect on platelets. Aspirin can displace warfarin from protein binding sites, leading to prolongation of both the prothrombin time and bleeding time. Aspirin can increase the anticoagulant activity of heparin, increasing bleeding risk).
No products indexed under this heading.

Hydrochlorothiazide (The effectiveness of diuretics in patients with underlying renal or cardiovascular disease may be diminished by the concomitant administration of aspirin due to inhibition of renal prostaglandins, leading to decreased renal blood flow, and salt and fluidretention). Products include:
Atacand HCT 642
Avalide Tablets 892
Avalide Tablets 2713
Benicar HCT Tablets 1010
Diovan HCT Tablets 2216
Dyazide Capsules 1405
Micardis HCT Tablets 854
Prinzide Tablets 2092
Tekturna HCT Tablets 2324
Teveten HCT Tablets 517

Hydroflumethiazide (The effectiveness of diuretics in patients with underlying renal or cardiovascular disease may be diminished by the concomitant administration of aspirin due to inhibition of renal prostaglandins, leading to decreased renal blood flow, and salt and fluidretention).
No products indexed under this heading.

Ibuprofen (The concurrent use of aspirin with other NSAIDs should be avoided because this may increase bleeding or lead to decreased renal function). Products include:
Motrin IB Tablets and Caplets 1900
Children's Motrin Oral Suspension 1901
Children's Motrin Non-Staining Dye-Free Oral Suspension 1901
Children's Motrin Cold Oral Suspension 1899
Infants' Motrin Concentrated Drops 1901
Infants' Motrin Non-Staining Dye-Free Concentrated Drops 1901
Junior Strength Motrin Caplets and Chewable Tablets 1901
Vicoprofen Tablets 533

Indapamide (The effectiveness of diuretics in patients with underlying renal or cardiovascular disease may be diminished by the concomitant administration of aspirin due to inhibition of renal prostaglandins, leading to decreased renal blood flow, and salt and fluidretention). Products include:
Indapamide Tablets 2188

Indomethacin (The concurrent use of aspirin with other NSAIDs should be avoided because this may increase bleeding or lead to decreased renal function). Products include:
Indocin 2024

Indomethacin Sodium Trihydrate (The concurrent use of aspirin with other NSAIDs should be avoided because this may increase bleeding or lead to decreased renal function). Products include:
Indocin I.V. 2489

Ketoprofen (The concurrent use of aspirin with other NSAIDs should be avoided because this may increase bleeding or lead to decreased renal function).
No products indexed under this heading.

Ketorolac Tromethamine (The concurrent use of aspirin with other NSAIDs should be avoided because this may increase bleeding or lead to decreased renal function).
No products indexed under this heading.

Labetalol Hydrochloride (The hypotensive effects of beta blockers may be diminished by the concomitant administration of aspirin due to inhibition of renal prostaglandins, leading to decreased renal blood flow, and salt and fluid retention).
No products indexed under this heading.

Levobunolol Hydrochloride (The hypotensive effects of beta blockers may be diminished by the concomitant administration of aspirin due to inhibition of renal prostaglandins, leading to decreased renal blood flow, and salt and fluid retention).
No products indexed under this heading.

Lisinopril (The hyponatremic and hypotensive effects of ACE inhibitors may be diminished by the concomitant administration of aspirin due to its indirect effect on the renin-angiotensin conversion pathway). Products include:
Prinivil Tablets 2087
Prinzide Tablets 2092

Low Molecular Weight Heparins (Patients on anticoagulation therapy are at increased risk for bleeding because of drug-drug interactions and the effect on platelets. Aspirin can displace warfarin from protein binding sites, leading to prolongation of both the prothrombin time and bleeding time. Aspirin can increase the anticoagulant activity of heparin, increasing bleeding risk).
No products indexed under this heading.

Meclofenamate Sodium (The concurrent use of aspirin with other NSAIDs should be avoided because this may increase bleeding or lead to decreased renal function).
No products indexed under this heading.

Mefenamic Acid (The concurrent use of aspirin with other NSAIDs should be avoided because this may increase bleeding or lead to decreased renal function).
No products indexed under this heading.

Meloxicam (The concurrent use of aspirin with other NSAIDs should be avoided because this may increase bleeding or lead to decreased renal function). Products include:
Mobic Oral Suspension 863
Mobic Tablets 863

Metformin Hydrochloride (Moderate doses of aspirin may increase the effectiveness of oral hypoglycemic drugs, leading to hypoglycemia). Products include:
ActoPlus Met Tablets 3071
Avandamet Tablets 1336
Janumet Tablets 2041
PrandiMet Tablets 2967

Methotrexate (Salicylate can inhibit renal clearance of methotrexate, leading to bone marrow toxicity, especially in the elderly or renal-impaired).
No products indexed under this heading.

Methotrexate Sodium (Salicylate can inhibit renal clearance of methotrexate, leading to bone marrow toxicity, especially in the elderly or renal-impaired).
No products indexed under this heading.

Methyclothiazide (The effectiveness of diuretics in patients with underlying renal or cardiovascular disease may be diminished by the concomitant administration of aspirin due to inhibition of renal prostaglandins, leading to decreased renal blood flow, and salt and fluidretention).
No products indexed under this heading.

Metipranolol Hydrochloride (The hypotensive effects of beta blockers may be diminished by the concomitant administration of aspirin due to inhibition of renal prostaglandins, leading to decreased renal blood flow, and salt and fluid retention).
No products indexed under this heading.

Metolazone (The effectiveness of diuretics in patients with underlying renal or cardiovascular disease may be diminished by the concomitant administration of aspirin due to inhibition of renal prostaglandins, leading to decreased renal blood flow, and salt and fluidretention).
No products indexed under this heading.

Metoprolol Succinate (The hypotensive effects of beta blockers may be diminished by the concomitant administration of aspirin due to inhibition of renal prostaglandins, leading to decreased renal blood flow, and salt and fluid retention). Products include:
Toprol-XL Tablets 666

Metoprolol Tartrate (The hypotensive effects of beta blockers may be diminished by the concomitant administration of aspirin due to inhibition of renal prostaglandins, leading to decreased renal blood flow, and salt and fluid retention).
No products indexed under this heading.

Miglitol (Moderate doses of aspirin may increase the effectiveness of oral hypoglycemic drugs, leading to hypoglycemia).
No products indexed under this heading.

Moexipril Hydrochloride (The hyponatremic and hypotensive effects of ACE inhibitors may be diminished by the concomitant administration of aspirin due to its indirect effect on the renin-angiotensin conversion pathway).
No products indexed under this heading.

Nabumetone (The concurrent use of aspirin with other NSAIDs should be avoided because this may increase bleeding or lead to decreased renal function).
No products indexed under this heading.

Nadolol (The hypotensive effects of beta blockers may be diminished by the concomitant administration of aspirin due to inhibition of renal prostaglandins, leading to decreased renal blood flow, and salt and fluid retention). Products include:
Nadolol Tablets 2191

Naproxen (The concurrent use of aspirin with other NSAIDs should be avoided because this may increase bleeding or lead to decreased renal function). Products include:
EC-Naprosyn Delayed-Release Tablets 2632
Naprosyn Suspension 2632
Naprosyn Tablets 2632

Naproxen Sodium (The concurrent use of aspirin with other NSAIDs should be avoided because this may increase bleeding or lead to decreased renal function). Products include:
Anaprox Tablets 2632
Anaprox DS Tablets 2632
Treximet Tablets 1616

Nateglinide (Moderate doses of aspirin may increase the effectiveness of oral hypoglycemic drugs, leading to hypoglycemia). Products include:
Starlix Tablets 2314

Nebivolol (The hypotensive effects of beta blockers may be diminished by the concomitant administration of aspirin due to inhibition of renal prostaglandins, leading to decreased renal blood flow, and salt and fluid retention). Products include:
Bystolic Tablets 1155

Oxaprozin (The concurrent use of aspirin with other NSAIDs should be avoided because this may increase bleeding or lead to decreased renal function).
No products indexed under this heading.

Penbutolol Sulfate (The hypotensive effects of beta blockers may be diminished by the concomitant administration of aspirin due to inhibition of renal prostaglandins, leading to decreased renal blood flow, and salt and fluid retention).
No products indexed under this heading.

Perindopril Erbumine (The hyponatremic and hypotensive effects of ACE inhibitors may be diminished by the concomitant administration of aspirin due to its indirect effect on the renin-angiotensin conversion pathway). Products include:
Aceon Tablets (2 mg, 4 mg, 8 mg) 3038

Phenylbutazone (The concurrent use of aspirin with other NSAIDs should be avoided because this may increase bleeding or lead to decreased renal function).
No products indexed under this heading.

Phenytoin (Salicylate can displace protein-bound phenytoin, leading to a decrease in the total concentration of phenytoin).
No products indexed under this heading.

Phenytoin Sodium (Salicylate can displace protein-bound phenytoin, leading to a decrease in the total concentration of phenytoin). Products include:
Phenytek Capsules 2192

Pindolol (The hypotensive effects of beta blockers may be diminished by the concomitant administration of aspirin due to inhibition of renal prostaglandins, leading to decreased renal blood flow, and salt and fluid retention).
No products indexed under this heading.

Pioglitazone Hydrochloride (Moderate doses of aspirin may increase the effectiveness of oral hypoglycemic drugs, leading to hypoglycemia). Products include:
ActoPlus Met Tablets 3071
Actos Tablets 3077
Duetact Tablets 3085

Piroxicam (The concurrent use of aspirin with other NSAIDs should be avoided because this may increase bleeding or lead to decreased renal function).
No products indexed under this heading.

Polythiazide (The effectiveness of diuretics in patients with underlying renal or cardiovascular disease may be diminished by the concomitant administration of aspirin due to inhibition of renal prostaglandins, leading to decreased renal blood flow, and salt and fluidretention).
No products indexed under this heading.

Probenecid (Salicylates antagonize the uricosuric action of uricosuric agents).
No products indexed under this heading.

Propranolol Hydrochloride (The hypotensive effects of beta blockers may be diminished by the concomitant administration of aspirin due to inhibition of renal prostaglandins, leading to decreased renal blood flow, and salt and fluid retention). Products include:
InnoPran XL Extended Release Capsules 1484

Quinapril Hydrochloride (The hyponatremic and hypotensive effects of ACE inhibitors may be diminished by the concomitant administration of aspirin due to its indirect effect on the renin-angiotensin conversion pathway).
No products indexed under this heading.

Ramipril (The hyponatremic and hypotensive effects of ACE inhibitors may be diminished by the concomitant administration of aspirin due to its indirect effect on the renin-angiotensin conversion pathway).
No products indexed under this heading.

Repaglinide (Moderate doses of aspirin may increase the effectiveness of oral hypoglycemic drugs, leading to hypoglycemia). Products include:
PrandiMet Tablets 2967
Prandin Tablets 2971

Rofecoxib (The concurrent use of aspirin with other NSAIDs should be avoided because this may increase bleeding or lead to decreased renal function).
No products indexed under this heading.

Rosiglitazone Maleate (Moderate doses of aspirin may increase the effectiveness of oral hypoglycemic drugs, leading to hypoglycemia). Products include:
Avandamet Tablets 1336
Avandaryl Tablets 1344
Avandia Tablets 1351

Sitagliptin Phosphate (Moderate doses of aspirin may increase the effectiveness of oral hypoglycemic drugs, leading to hypoglycemia). Products include:
Janumet Tablets 2041
Januvia Tablets 2048

Sotalol Hydrochloride (The hypotensive effects of beta blockers may be diminished by the concomitant administration of aspirin due to inhibition of renal prostaglandins, leading to decreased renal blood flow, and salt and fluid retention).
No products indexed under this heading.

Spirapril Hydrochloride (The hyponatremic and hypotensive effects of ACE inhibitors may be diminished by the concomitant administration of aspirin due to its indirect effect on the renin-angiotensin conversion pathway).
No products indexed under this heading.

Spironolactone (The effectiveness of diuretics in patients with underlying renal or cardiovascular disease may be diminished by the concomitant administration of aspirin due to inhibition of renal prostaglandins, leading to decreased renal blood flow, and salt and fluidretention).
No products indexed under this heading.

Sulfinpyrazone (Salicylates antagonize the uricosuric action of uricosuric agents).
No products indexed under this heading.

Sulindac (The concurrent use of aspirin with other NSAIDs should be avoided because this may increase bleeding or lead to decreased renal function). Products include:
Clinoril Tablets 1962

Timolol Hemihydrate (The hypotensive effects of beta blockers may be diminished by the concomitant administration of aspirin due to inhibition of renal prostaglandins, leading to decreased renal blood flow, and salt and fluid retention). Products include:
Betimol Ophthalmic Solution 3181

Timolol Maleate (The hypotensive effects of beta blockers may be diminished by the concomitant administration of aspirin due to inhibition of renal prostaglandins, leading to decreased renal blood flow, and salt and fluid retention). Products include:
Combigan Ophthalmic Solution 553
Cosopt Sterile Ophthalmic Solution 1969
Timoptic Sterile Ophthalmic Solution 2121
Timoptic in Ocudose 2124
Timoptic-XE Sterile Ophthalmic Gel Forming Solution 2125

Tinzaparin Sodium (Patients on anticoagulation therapy are at increased risk for bleeding because of drug-drug interactions and the effect on platelets. Aspirin can displace warfarin from protein binding sites, leading to prolongation of both the prothrombin time and bleeding time. Aspirin can increase the anticoagulant activity of heparin, increasing bleeding risk).
No products indexed under this heading.

Tolazamide (Moderate doses of aspirin may increase the effectiveness of oral hypoglycemic drugs, leading to hypoglycemia).
No products indexed under this heading.

Tolbutamide (Moderate doses of aspirin may increase the effectiveness of oral hypoglycemic drugs, leading to hypoglycemia).
No products indexed under this heading.

Tolmetin Sodium (The concurrent use of aspirin with other NSAIDs should be avoided because this may increase bleeding or lead to decreased renal function).
No products indexed under this heading.

Torsemide (The effectiveness of diuretics in patients with underlying renal or cardiovascular disease may be diminished by the concomitant administration of aspirin due to inhibition of renal prostaglandins, leading to decreased renal blood flow, and salt and fluidretention). Products include:
Demadex Injection 2630
Demadex Tablets 2630

Trandolapril (The hyponatremic and hypotensive effects of ACE inhibitors may be diminished by the concomitant administration of aspirin due to its indirect effect on the renin-angiotensin conversion pathway). Products include:
Mavik Tablets 472
Tarka Tablets 511

Triamterene (The effectiveness of diuretics in patients with underlying renal or cardiovascular disease may be diminished by the concomitant administration of aspirin due to inhibition of renal prostaglandins, leading to decreased renal blood flow, and salt and fluidretention). Products include:
Dyazide Capsules 1405
Dyrenium Capsules 3189

Troglitazone (Moderate doses of aspirin may increase the effectiveness of oral hypoglycemic drugs, leading to hypoglycemia).
No products indexed under this heading.

Valdecoxib (The concurrent use of aspirin with other NSAIDs should be avoided because this may increase bleeding or lead to decreased renal function).
No products indexed under this heading.

Valproate Sodium (Salicylate can displace protein-bound valproic acid, leading to an increase in serum valproic acid levels).
No products indexed under this heading.

Valproic Acid (Salicylate can displace protein-bound valproic acid, leading to an increase in serum valproic acid levels).
No products indexed under this heading.

Warfarin Sodium (Patients on anticoagulation therapy are at increased risk for bleeding because of drug-drug interactions and the effect on platelets. Aspirin can displace warfarin from protein binding sites, leading to prolongation of both the prothrombin time and bleeding time. Aspirin can increase the anticoagulant activity of heparin, increasing bleeding risk).
No products indexed under this heading.

BECONASE AQ NASAL SPRAY

(Beclomethasone Dipropionate Monohydrate) 1369
None cited in PDR database.

BEELITH TABLETS

(Magnesium Oxide, Vitamin B_6) 813
May interact with:

Prescription Drugs, unspecified (Concurrent use should be avoided).
No products indexed under this heading.

IMPORTANT NOTE: Always consult each drug listing in the patient's regimen for possible interactions.

BENADRYL ALLERGY & COLD KAPGELS
(Acetaminophen, Diphenhydramine Hydrochloride, Phenylephrine Hydrochloride)................................... 1895
May interact with hypnotics and sedatives, monoamine oxidase inhibitors, tranquilizers, and certain other agents. Compounds in these categories include:

Alprazolam (May increase drowsiness effect).
No products indexed under this heading.

Buspirone Hydrochloride (May increase drowsiness effect).
No products indexed under this heading.

Butabarbital (May increase drowsiness effect).
No products indexed under this heading.

Butabarbital Sodium (May increase drowsiness effect).
No products indexed under this heading.

Chloral Hydrate (May increase drowsiness effect).
No products indexed under this heading.

Chlordiazepoxide (May increase drowsiness effect).
No products indexed under this heading.

Chlordiazepoxide Hydrochloride (May increase drowsiness effect).
No products indexed under this heading.

Chlorpromazine (May increase drowsiness effect).
No products indexed under this heading.

Chlorpromazine Hydrochloride (May increase drowsiness effect).
No products indexed under this heading.

Chlorprothixene (May increase drowsiness effect).
No products indexed under this heading.

Chlorprothixene Hydrochloride (May increase drowsiness effect).
No products indexed under this heading.

Clorazepate Dipotassium (May increase drowsiness effect).
No products indexed under this heading.

Diazepam (May increase drowsiness effect). Products include:
Valium Tablets 2658

Droperidol (May increase drowsiness effect).
No products indexed under this heading.

Estazolam (May increase drowsiness effect).
No products indexed under this heading.

Ethchlorvynol (May increase drowsiness effect).
No products indexed under this heading.

Ethinamate (May increase drowsiness effect).
No products indexed under this heading.

Fluphenazine Decanoate (May increase drowsiness effect).
No products indexed under this heading.

Fluphenazine Enanthate (May increase drowsiness effect).
No products indexed under this heading.

Fluphenazine Hydrochloride (May increase drowsiness effect).
No products indexed under this heading.

Flurazepam Hydrochloride (May increase drowsiness effect).
No products indexed under this heading.

Glutethimide (May increase drowsiness effect).
No products indexed under this heading.

Haloperidol (May increase drowsiness effect).
No products indexed under this heading.

Haloperidol Decanoate (May increase drowsiness effect).
No products indexed under this heading.

Hydroxyzine Hydrochloride (May increase drowsiness effect).
No products indexed under this heading.

Isocarboxazid (Avoid use with monoamine oxidase inhibitors (MAOI) or for two weeks after stopping MAOI drug). Products include:
Marplan Tablets 3177

Lorazepam (May increase drowsiness effect).
No products indexed under this heading.

Loxapine Hydrochloride (May increase drowsiness effect).
No products indexed under this heading.

Loxapine Succinate (May increase drowsiness effect).
No products indexed under this heading.

Meprobamate (May increase drowsiness effect).
No products indexed under this heading.

Mesoridazine Besylate (May increase drowsiness effect).
No products indexed under this heading.

Midazolam Hydrochloride (May increase drowsiness effect).
No products indexed under this heading.

Moclobemide (Avoid use with monoamine oxidase inhibitors (MAOI) or for two weeks after stopping MAOI drug).
No products indexed under this heading.

Molindone Hydrochloride (May increase drowsiness effect). Products include:
Moban Tablets 1116

Oxazepam (May increase drowsiness effect).
No products indexed under this heading.

Pargyline Hydrochloride (Avoid use with monoamine oxidase inhibitors (MAOI) or for two weeks after stopping MAOI drug).
No products indexed under this heading.

Perphenazine (May increase drowsiness effect).
No products indexed under this heading.

Phenelzine Sulfate (Avoid use with monoamine oxidase inhibitors (MAOI) or for two weeks after stopping MAOI drug).
No products indexed under this heading.

Prazepam (May increase drowsiness effect).
No products indexed under this heading.

Procarbazine Hydrochloride (Avoid use with monoamine oxidase inhibitors (MAOI) or for two weeks after stopping MAOI drug).
No products indexed under this heading.

Prochlorperazine (May increase drowsiness effect).
No products indexed under this heading.

Promethazine Hydrochloride (May increase drowsiness effect).
No products indexed under this heading.

Propofol (May increase drowsiness effect).
No products indexed under this heading.

Quazepam (May increase drowsiness effect).
No products indexed under this heading.

Ramelteon (May increase drowsiness effect). Products include:
Rozerem Tablets 3091

Rasagiline Mesylate (Avoid use with monoamine oxidase inhibitors (MAOI) or for two weeks after stopping MAOI drug). Products include:
Azilect Tablets 3106

Secobarbital Sodium (May increase drowsiness effect).
No products indexed under this heading.

Selegiline (Avoid use with monoamine oxidase inhibitors (MAOI) or for two weeks after stopping MAOI drug). Products include:
Emsam Transdermal System 905

Selegiline Hydrochloride (Avoid use with monoamine oxidase inhibitors (MAOI) or for two weeks after stopping MAOI drug). Products include:
Eldepryl Capsules 3052

Sodium Butabarbital (May increase drowsiness effect).
No products indexed under this heading.

Temazepam (May increase drowsiness effect).
No products indexed under this heading.

Thioridazine Hydrochloride (May increase drowsiness effect). Products include:
Thioridazine Hydrochloride Tablets.. 2195

Thiothixene (May increase drowsiness effect). Products include:
Thiothixene Capsules 2197

Tranylcypromine Sulfate (Avoid use with monoamine oxidase inhibitors (MAOI) or for two weeks after stopping MAOI drug). Products include:
Parnate Tablets 1532

Triazolam (May increase drowsiness effect).
No products indexed under this heading.

Trifluoperazine Hydrochloride (May increase drowsiness effect).
No products indexed under this heading.

Zaleplon (May increase drowsiness effect).
No products indexed under this heading.

Zolpidem Tartrate (May increase drowsiness effect). Products include:
Ambien Tablets 2692
Ambien CR Tablets 2696

Food Interactions

Alcohol (Concurrent use may increase drowsiness).

BENADRYL ALLERGY & SINUS HEADACHE KAPGELS
(Acetaminophen, Diphenhydramine Hydrochloride, Phenylephrine Hydrochloride)................................... 1895
May interact with hypnotics and sedatives, monoamine oxidase inhibitors, tranquilizers, and certain other agents. Compounds in these categories include:

Alprazolam (May increase drowsiness effect).
No products indexed under this heading.

Buspirone Hydrochloride (May increase drowsiness effect).
No products indexed under this heading.

Butabarbital (May increase drowsiness effect).
No products indexed under this heading.

Butabarbital Sodium (May increase drowsiness effect).
No products indexed under this heading.

Chloral Hydrate (May increase drowsiness effect).
No products indexed under this heading.

Chlordiazepoxide (May increase drowsiness effect).
No products indexed under this heading.

Chlordiazepoxide Hydrochloride (May increase drowsiness effect).
No products indexed under this heading.

Chlorpromazine (May increase drowsiness effect).
No products indexed under this heading.

Chlorpromazine Hydrochloride (May increase drowsiness effect).
No products indexed under this heading.

Chlorprothixene (May increase drowsiness effect).
No products indexed under this heading.

Chlorprothixene Hydrochloride (May increase drowsiness effect).
No products indexed under this heading.

Clorazepate Dipotassium (May increase drowsiness effect).
No products indexed under this heading.

Diazepam (May increase drowsiness effect). Products include:
Valium Tablets 2658

Diphenhydramine (Concurrent use with other diphenhydramine containing products is not recommended).
No products indexed under this heading.

Droperidol (May increase drowsiness effect).
No products indexed under this heading.

Estazolam (May increase drowsiness effect).
No products indexed under this heading.

Ethchlorvynol (May increase drowsiness effect).
No products indexed under this heading.

Ethinamate (May increase drowsiness effect).
No products indexed under this heading.

Fluphenazine Decanoate (May increase drowsiness effect).
No products indexed under this heading.

Fluphenazine Enanthate (May increase drowsiness effect).
No products indexed under this heading.

Fluphenazine Hydrochloride (May increase drowsiness effect).
No products indexed under this heading.

Flurazepam Hydrochloride (May increase drowsiness effect).
No products indexed under this heading.

Glutethimide (May increase drowsiness effect).
No products indexed under this heading.

Haloperidol (May increase drowsiness effect).
No products indexed under this heading.

Haloperidol Decanoate (May increase drowsiness effect).
No products indexed under this heading.

Hydroxyzine Hydrochloride (May increase drowsiness effect).
No products indexed under this heading.

Isocarboxazid (Avoid use with monoamine oxidase inhibitor (MAOI) or for two weeks after stopping MAOI drug). Products include:
Marplan Tablets **3177**

Lorazepam (May increase drowsiness effect).
No products indexed under this heading.

Loxapine Hydrochloride (May increase drowsiness effect).
No products indexed under this heading.

Loxapine Succinate (May increase drowsiness effect).
No products indexed under this heading.

Meprobamate (May increase drowsiness effect).
No products indexed under this heading.

Mesoridazine Besylate (May increase drowsiness effect).
No products indexed under this heading.

Midazolam Hydrochloride (May increase drowsiness effect).
No products indexed under this heading.

Moclobemide (Avoid use with monoamine oxidase inhibitor (MAOI) or for two weeks after stopping MAOI drug).
No products indexed under this heading.

Molindone Hydrochloride (May increase drowsiness effect). Products include:
Moban Tablets **1116**

Oxazepam (May increase drowsiness effect).
No products indexed under this heading.

Pargyline Hydrochloride (Avoid use with monoamine oxidase inhibitor (MAOI) or for two weeks after stopping MAOI drug).
No products indexed under this heading.

Perphenazine (May increase drowsiness effect).
No products indexed under this heading.

Phenelzine Sulfate (Avoid use with monoamine oxidase inhibitor (MAOI) or for two weeks after stopping MAOI drug).
No products indexed under this heading.

Prazepam (May increase drowsiness effect).
No products indexed under this heading.

Procarbazine Hydrochloride (Avoid use with monoamine oxidase inhibitor (MAOI) or for two weeks after stopping MAOI drug).
No products indexed under this heading.

Prochlorperazine (May increase drowsiness effect).
No products indexed under this heading.

Promethazine Hydrochloride (May increase drowsiness effect).
No products indexed under this heading.

Propofol (May increase drowsiness effect).
No products indexed under this heading.

Quazepam (May increase drowsiness effect).
No products indexed under this heading.

Ramelteon (May increase drowsiness effect). Products include:
Rozerem Tablets **3091**

Rasagiline Mesylate (Avoid use with monoamine oxidase inhibitor (MAOI) or for two weeks after stopping MAOI drug). Products include:
Azilect Tablets **3106**

Secobarbital Sodium (May increase drowsiness effect).
No products indexed under this heading.

Selegiline (Avoid use with monoamine oxidase inhibitor (MAOI) or for two weeks after stopping MAOI drug). Products include:
Emsam Transdermal System **905**

Selegiline Hydrochloride (Avoid use with monoamine oxidase inhibitor (MAOI) or for two weeks after stopping MAOI drug). Products include:
Eldepryl Capsules **3052**

Sodium Butabarbital (May increase drowsiness effect).
No products indexed under this heading.

Temazepam (May increase drowsiness effect).
No products indexed under this heading.

Thioridazine Hydrochloride (May increase drowsiness effect). Products include:
Thioridazine Hydrochloride Tablets **2195**

Thiothixene (May increase drowsiness effect). Products include:
Thiothixene Capsules **2197**

Tranylcypromine Sulfate (Avoid use with monoamine oxidase inhibitor (MAOI) or for two weeks after stopping MAOI drug). Products include:
Parnate Tablets **1532**

Triazolam (May increase drowsiness effect).
No products indexed under this heading.

Trifluoperazine Hydrochloride (May increase drowsiness effect).
No products indexed under this heading.

Zaleplon (May increase drowsiness effect).
No products indexed under this heading.

Zolpidem Tartrate (May increase drowsiness effect). Products include:
Ambien Tablets **2692**
Ambien CR Tablets **2696**

Food Interactions

Alcohol (Increases drowsiness effect; avoid concomitant use).

BENADRYL SEVERE ALLERGY & SINUS HEADACHE CAPLETS

(Acetaminophen, Diphenhydramine Hydrochloride, Phenylephrine Hydrochloride) **1897**
May interact with hypnotics and sedatives, monoamine oxidase inhibitors, tranquilizers, and certain other agents. Compounds in these categories include:

Alprazolam (Concurrent use may increase drowsiness effect).
No products indexed under this heading.

Buspirone Hydrochloride (Concurrent use may increase drowsiness effect).
No products indexed under this heading.

Butabarbital (Concurrent use may increase drowsiness effect).
No products indexed under this heading.

Butabarbital Sodium (Concurrent use may increase drowsiness effect).
No products indexed under this heading.

Chloral Hydrate (Concurrent use may increase drowsiness effect).
No products indexed under this heading.

Chlordiazepoxide (Concurrent use may increase drowsiness effect).
No products indexed under this heading.

Chlordiazepoxide Hydrochloride (Concurrent use may increase drowsiness effect).
No products indexed under this heading.

Chlorpromazine (Concurrent use may increase drowsiness effect).
No products indexed under this heading.

Chlorpromazine Hydrochloride (Concurrent use may increase drowsiness effect).
No products indexed under this heading.

Chlorprothixene (Concurrent use may increase drowsiness effect).
No products indexed under this heading.

Chlorprothixene Hydrochloride (Concurrent use may increase drowsiness effect).
No products indexed under this heading.

Clorazepate Dipotassium (Concurrent use may increase drowsiness effect).
No products indexed under this heading.

Diazepam (Concurrent use may increase drowsiness effect). Products include:
Valium Tablets **2658**

Droperidol (Concurrent use may increase drowsiness effect).
No products indexed under this heading.

Estazolam (Concurrent use may increase drowsiness effect).
No products indexed under this heading.

Ethchlorvynol (Concurrent use may increase drowsiness effect).
No products indexed under this heading.

Ethinamate (Concurrent use may increase drowsiness effect).
No products indexed under this heading.

Fluphenazine Decanoate (Concurrent use may increase drowsiness effect).
No products indexed under this heading.

Fluphenazine Enanthate (Concurrent use may increase drowsiness effect).
No products indexed under this heading.

Fluphenazine Hydrochloride (Concurrent use may increase drowsiness effect).
No products indexed under this heading.

Flurazepam Hydrochloride (Concurrent use may increase drowsiness effect).
No products indexed under this heading.

Glutethimide (Concurrent use may increase drowsiness effect).
No products indexed under this heading.

Haloperidol (Concurrent use may increase drowsiness effect).
No products indexed under this heading.

Haloperidol Decanoate (Concurrent use may increase drowsiness effect).
No products indexed under this heading.

Hydroxyzine Hydrochloride (Concurrent use may increase drowsiness effect).
No products indexed under this heading.

Isocarboxazid (Concurrent and/or sequential use with MAO inhibitors is not recommended). Products include:
Marplan Tablets **3177**

Lorazepam (Concurrent use may increase drowsiness effect).
No products indexed under this heading.

Loxapine Hydrochloride (Concurrent use may increase drowsiness effect).
No products indexed under this heading.

Loxapine Succinate (Concurrent use may increase drowsiness effect).
No products indexed under this heading.

Meprobamate (Concurrent use may increase drowsiness effect).
No products indexed under this heading.

Mesoridazine Besylate (Concurrent use may increase drowsiness effect).
No products indexed under this heading.

Moclobemide (Concurrent and/or sequential use with MAO inhibitors is not recommended).
No products indexed under this heading.

Molindone Hydrochloride (Concurrent use may increase drowsiness effect). Products include:
Moban Tablets 1116

Oxazepam (Concurrent use may increase drowsiness effect).
No products indexed under this heading.

Pargyline Hydrochloride (Concurrent and/or sequential use with MAO inhibitors is not recommended).
No products indexed under this heading.

Perphenazine (Concurrent use may increase drowsiness effect).
No products indexed under this heading.

Phenelzine Sulfate (Concurrent and/or sequential use with MAO inhibitors is not recommended).
No products indexed under this heading.

Prazepam (Concurrent use may increase drowsiness effect).
No products indexed under this heading.

Procarbazine Hydrochloride (Concurrent and/or sequential use with MAO inhibitors is not recommended).
No products indexed under this heading.

Prochlorperazine (Concurrent use may increase drowsiness effect).
No products indexed under this heading.

Promethazine Hydrochloride (Concurrent use may increase drowsiness effect).
No products indexed under this heading.

Ramelteon (Concurrent use may increase drowsiness effect). Products include:
Rozerem Tablets 3091

Rasagiline Mesylate (Concurrent and/or sequential use with MAO inhibitors is not recommended). Products include:
Azilect Tablets 3106

Selegiline (Concurrent and/or sequential use with MAO inhibitors is not recommended). Products include:
Emsam Transdermal System 905

Selegiline Hydrochloride (Concurrent and/or sequential use with MAO inhibitors is not recommended). Products include:
Eldepryl Capsules 3052

Thioridazine Hydrochloride (Concurrent use may increase drowsiness effect). Products include:
Thioridazine Hydrochloride Tablets 2195

Thiothixene (Concurrent use may increase drowsiness effect). Products include:
Thiothixene Capsules 2197

Tranylcypromine Sulfate (Concurrent and/or sequential use with MAO inhibitors is not recommended). Products include:
Parnate Tablets 1532

Trifluoperazine Hydrochloride (Concurrent use may increase drowsiness effect).
No products indexed under this heading.

Food Interactions

Alcohol (Increases drowsiness effect; avoid concomitant use).

BENADRYL DYE-FREE ALLERGY LIQUI-GELS SOFTGELS

(Diphenhydramine Hydrochloride) 1897
May interact with hypnotics and sedatives, tranquilizers, and certain other agents. Compounds in these categories include:

Alprazolam (Concurrent use may increase drowsiness effect).
No products indexed under this heading.

Buspirone Hydrochloride (Concurrent use may increase drowsiness effect).
No products indexed under this heading.

Butabarbital (Concurrent use may increase drowsiness effect).
No products indexed under this heading.

Butabarbital Sodium (Concurrent use may increase drowsiness effect).
No products indexed under this heading.

Chloral Hydrate (Concurrent use may increase drowsiness effect).
No products indexed under this heading.

Chlordiazepoxide (Concurrent use may increase drowsiness effect).
No products indexed under this heading.

Chlordiazepoxide Hydrochloride (Concurrent use may increase drowsiness effect).
No products indexed under this heading.

Chlorpromazine (Concurrent use may increase drowsiness effect).
No products indexed under this heading.

Chlorpromazine Hydrochloride (Concurrent use may increase drowsiness effect).
No products indexed under this heading.

Chlorprothixene (Concurrent use may increase drowsiness effect).
No products indexed under this heading.

Chlorprothixene Hydrochloride (Concurrent use may increase drowsiness effect).
No products indexed under this heading.

Clorazepate Dipotassium (Concurrent use may increase drowsiness effect).
No products indexed under this heading.

Diazepam (Concurrent use may increase drowsiness effect). Products include:
Valium Tablets 2658

Droperidol (Concurrent use may increase drowsiness effect).
No products indexed under this heading.

Estazolam (Concurrent use may increase drowsiness effect).
No products indexed under this heading.

Ethchlorvynol (Concurrent use may increase drowsiness effect).
No products indexed under this heading.

Ethinamate (Concurrent use may increase drowsiness effect).
No products indexed under this heading.

Fluphenazine Decanoate (Concurrent use may increase drowsiness effect).
No products indexed under this heading.

Fluphenazine Enanthate (Concurrent use may increase drowsiness effect).
No products indexed under this heading.

Fluphenazine Hydrochloride (Concurrent use may increase drowsiness effect).
No products indexed under this heading.

Flurazepam Hydrochloride (Concurrent use may increase drowsiness effect).
No products indexed under this heading.

Glutethimide (Concurrent use may increase drowsiness effect).
No products indexed under this heading.

Haloperidol (Concurrent use may increase drowsiness effect).
No products indexed under this heading.

Haloperidol Decanoate (Concurrent use may increase drowsiness effect).
No products indexed under this heading.

Hydroxyzine Hydrochloride (Concurrent use may increase drowsiness effect).
No products indexed under this heading.

Lorazepam (Concurrent use may increase drowsiness effect).
No products indexed under this heading.

Loxapine Hydrochloride (Concurrent use may increase drowsiness effect).
No products indexed under this heading.

Loxapine Succinate (Concurrent use may increase drowsiness effect).
No products indexed under this heading.

Meprobamate (Concurrent use may increase drowsiness effect).
No products indexed under this heading.

Mesoridazine Besylate (Concurrent use may increase drowsiness effect).
No products indexed under this heading.

Midazolam Hydrochloride (Concurrent use may increase drowsiness effect).
No products indexed under this heading.

Molindone Hydrochloride (Concurrent use may increase drowsiness effect). Products include:
Moban Tablets 1116

Oxazepam (Concurrent use may increase drowsiness effect).
No products indexed under this heading.

Perphenazine (Concurrent use may increase drowsiness effect).
No products indexed under this heading.

Prazepam (Concurrent use may increase drowsiness effect).
No products indexed under this heading.

Prochlorperazine (Concurrent use may increase drowsiness effect).
No products indexed under this heading.

Promethazine Hydrochloride (Concurrent use may increase drowsiness effect).
No products indexed under this heading.

Propofol (Concurrent use may increase drowsiness effect).
No products indexed under this heading.

Quazepam (Concurrent use may increase drowsiness effect).
No products indexed under this heading.

Ramelteon (Concurrent use may increase drowsiness effect). Products include:
Rozerem Tablets 3091

Secobarbital Sodium (Concurrent use may increase drowsiness effect).
No products indexed under this heading.

Sodium Butabarbital (Concurrent use may increase drowsiness effect).
No products indexed under this heading.

Temazepam (Concurrent use may increase drowsiness effect).
No products indexed under this heading.

Thioridazine Hydrochloride (Concurrent use may increase drowsiness effect). Products include:
Thioridazine Hydrochloride Tablets 2195

Thiothixene (Concurrent use may increase drowsiness effect). Products include:
Thiothixene Capsules 2197

Triazolam (Concurrent use may increase drowsiness effect).
No products indexed under this heading.

Trifluoperazine Hydrochloride (Concurrent use may increase drowsiness effect).
No products indexed under this heading.

Zaleplon (Concurrent use may increase drowsiness effect).
No products indexed under this heading.

Zolpidem Tartrate (Concurrent use may increase drowsiness effect). Products include:
Ambien Tablets 2692
Ambien CR Tablets 2696

Food Interactions

Alcohol (Increases drowsiness effect; avoid concomitant use).

BENADRYL ALLERGY KAPGELS

(Diphenhydramine Hydrochloride) 1895
May interact with hypnotics and sedatives, tranquilizers, and certain other agents. Compounds in these categories include:

Alprazolam (Concurrent use may increase drowsiness effect).
No products indexed under this heading.

Buspirone Hydrochloride (Concurrent use may increase drowsiness effect).
No products indexed under this heading.

Butabarbital (Concurrent use may increase drowsiness effect).
No products indexed under this heading.

Butabarbital Sodium (Concurrent use may increase drowsiness effect).
No products indexed under this heading.

Chloral Hydrate (Concurrent use may increase drowsiness effect).
No products indexed under this heading.

Chlordiazepoxide (Concurrent use may increase drowsiness effect).
No products indexed under this heading.

Chlordiazepoxide Hydrochloride (Concurrent use may increase drowsiness effect).
No products indexed under this heading.

Chlorpromazine (Concurrent use may increase drowsiness effect).
No products indexed under this heading.

Chlorpromazine Hydrochloride (Concurrent use may increase drowsiness effect).
No products indexed under this heading.

Chlorprothixene (Concurrent use may increase drowsiness effect).
No products indexed under this heading.

Chlorprothixene Hydrochloride (Concurrent use may increase drowsiness effect).
No products indexed under this heading.

Clorazepate Dipotassium (Concurrent use may increase drowsiness effect).
No products indexed under this heading.

Diazepam (Concurrent use may increase drowsiness effect).
Products include:
Valium Tablets 2658

Droperidol (Concurrent use may increase drowsiness effect).
No products indexed under this heading.

Estazolam (Concurrent use may increase drowsiness effect).
No products indexed under this heading.

Ethchlorvynol (Concurrent use may increase drowsiness effect).
No products indexed under this heading.

Ethinamate (Concurrent use may increase drowsiness effect).
No products indexed under this heading.

Fluphenazine Decanoate (Concurrent use may increase drowsiness effect).
No products indexed under this heading.

Fluphenazine Enanthate (Concurrent use may increase drowsiness effect).
No products indexed under this heading.

Fluphenazine Hydrochloride (Concurrent use may increase drowsiness effect).
No products indexed under this heading.

Flurazepam Hydrochloride (Concurrent use may increase drowsiness effect).
No products indexed under this heading.

Glutethimide (Concurrent use may increase drowsiness effect).
No products indexed under this heading.

Haloperidol (Concurrent use may increase drowsiness effect).
No products indexed under this heading.

Haloperidol Decanoate (Concurrent use may increase drowsiness effect).
No products indexed under this heading.

Hydroxyzine Hydrochloride (Concurrent use may increase drowsiness effect).
No products indexed under this heading.

Lorazepam (Concurrent use may increase drowsiness effect).
No products indexed under this heading.

Midazolam Hydrochloride (Concurrent use may increase drowsiness effect).
No products indexed under this heading.

Propofol (Concurrent use may increase drowsiness effect).
No products indexed under this heading.

Quazepam (Concurrent use may increase drowsiness effect).
No products indexed under this heading.

Ramelteon (Concurrent use may increase drowsiness effect).
Products include:
Rozerem Tablets 3091

Secobarbital Sodium (Concurrent use may increase drowsiness effect).
No products indexed under this heading.

Sodium Butabarbital (Concurrent use may increase drowsiness effect).
No products indexed under this heading.

Temazepam (Concurrent use may increase drowsiness effect).
No products indexed under this heading.

Triazolam (Concurrent use may increase drowsiness effect).
No products indexed under this heading.

Zaleplon (Concurrent use may increase drowsiness effect).
No products indexed under this heading.

Zolpidem Tartrate (Concurrent use may increase drowsiness effect).
Products include:
Ambien Tablets 2692
Ambien CR Tablets 2696

Food Interactions

Alcohol (Increases drowsiness effect; avoid concomittant use).

BENADRYL ALLERGY QUICK DISSOLVE STRIPS
(Diphenhydramine Hydrochloride) 1896
May interact with hypnotics and sedatives, tranquilizers, and certain other agents. Compounds in these categories include:

Alprazolam (Concurrent use may increase drowsiness effect).
No products indexed under this heading.

Buspirone Hydrochloride (Concurrent use may increase drowsiness effect).
No products indexed under this heading.

Butabarbital (Concurrent use may increase drowsiness effect).
No products indexed under this heading.

Butabarbital Sodium (Concurrent use may increase drowsiness effect).
No products indexed under this heading.

Chloral Hydrate (Concurrent use may increase drowsiness effect).
No products indexed under this heading.

Chlordiazepoxide (Concurrent use may increase drowsiness effect).
No products indexed under this heading.

Chlordiazepoxide Hydrochloride (Concurrent use may increase drowsiness effect).
No products indexed under this heading.

Chlorpromazine (Concurrent use may increase drowsiness effect).
No products indexed under this heading.

Chlorpromazine Hydrochloride (Concurrent use may increase drowsiness effect).
No products indexed under this heading.

Chlorprothixene (Concurrent use may increase drowsiness effect).
No products indexed under this heading.

Chlorprothixene Hydrochloride (Concurrent use may increase drowsiness effect).
No products indexed under this heading.

Clorazepate Dipotassium (Concurrent use may increase drowsiness effect).
No products indexed under this heading.

Diazepam (Concurrent use may increase drowsiness effect).
Products include:
Valium Tablets 2658

Droperidol (Concurrent use may increase drowsiness effect).
No products indexed under this heading.

Estazolam (Concurrent use may increase drowsiness effect).
No products indexed under this heading.

Ethchlorvynol (Concurrent use may increase drowsiness effect).
No products indexed under this heading.

Ethinamate (Concurrent use may increase drowsiness effect).
No products indexed under this heading.

Fluphenazine Decanoate (Concurrent use may increase drowsiness effect).
No products indexed under this heading.

Fluphenazine Enanthate (Concurrent use may increase drowsiness effect).
No products indexed under this heading.

Fluphenazine Hydrochloride (Concurrent use may increase drowsiness effect).
No products indexed under this heading.

Flurazepam Hydrochloride (Concurrent use may increase drowsiness effect).
No products indexed under this heading.

Glutethimide (Concurrent use may increase drowsiness effect).
No products indexed under this heading.

Haloperidol (Concurrent use may increase drowsiness effect).
No products indexed under this heading.

Haloperidol Decanoate (Concurrent use may increase drowsiness effect).
No products indexed under this heading.

Hydroxyzine Hydrochloride (Concurrent use may increase drowsiness effect).
No products indexed under this heading.

Lorazepam (Concurrent use may increase drowsiness effect).
No products indexed under this heading.

Midazolam Hydrochloride (Concurrent use may increase drowsiness effect).
No products indexed under this heading.

Propofol (Concurrent use may increase drowsiness effect).
No products indexed under this heading.

Quazepam (Concurrent use may increase drowsiness effect).
No products indexed under this heading.

Ramelteon (Concurrent use may increase drowsiness effect).
Products include:
Rozerem Tablets 3091

Secobarbital Sodium (Concurrent use may increase drowsiness effect).
No products indexed under this heading.

Sodium Butabarbital (Concurrent use may increase drowsiness effect).
No products indexed under this heading.

Temazepam (Concurrent use may increase drowsiness effect).
No products indexed under this heading.

Triazolam (Concurrent use may increase drowsiness effect).
No products indexed under this heading.

Zaleplon (Concurrent use may increase drowsiness effect).
No products indexed under this heading.

Zolpidem Tartrate (Concurrent use may increase drowsiness effect).
Products include:

Ambien Tablets 2692
Ambien CR Tablets 2696

Food Interactions

Alcohol (Increases drowsiness effect; avoid concomitant use).

BENADRYL ALLERGY ULTRATAB TABLETS

(Diphenhydramine Hydrochloride) 1896
May interact with hypnotics and sedatives, tranquilizers, and certain other agents. Compounds in these categories include:

Alprazolam (Concurrent use may increase drowsiness effect).
No products indexed under this heading.

Buspirone Hydrochloride (Concurrent use may increase drowsiness effect).
No products indexed under this heading.

Butabarbital (Concurrent use may increase drowsiness effect).
No products indexed under this heading.

Butabarbital Sodium (Concurrent use may increase drowsiness effect).
No products indexed under this heading.

Chloral Hydrate (Concurrent use may increase drowsiness effect).
No products indexed under this heading.

Chlordiazepoxide (Concurrent use may increase drowsiness effect).
No products indexed under this heading.

Chlordiazepoxide Hydrochloride (Concurrent use may increase drowsiness effect).
No products indexed under this heading.

Chlorpromazine (Concurrent use may increase drowsiness effect).
No products indexed under this heading.

Chlorpromazine Hydrochloride (Concurrent use may increase drowsiness effect).
No products indexed under this heading.

Chlorprothixene (Concurrent use may increase drowsiness effect).
No products indexed under this heading.

Chlorprothixene Hydrochloride (Concurrent use may increase drowsiness effect).
No products indexed under this heading.

Clorazepate Dipotassium (Concurrent use may increase drowsiness effect).
No products indexed under this heading.

Diazepam (Concurrent use may increase drowsiness effect).
Products include:
Valium Tablets 2658

Droperidol (Concurrent use may increase drowsiness effect).
No products indexed under this heading.

Estazolam (Concurrent use may increase drowsiness effect).
No products indexed under this heading.

Ethchlorvynol (Concurrent use may increase drowsiness effect).
No products indexed under this heading.

Ethinamate (Concurrent use may increase drowsiness effect).
No products indexed under this heading.

Fluphenazine Decanoate (Concurrent use may increase drowsiness effect).
No products indexed under this heading.

Fluphenazine Enanthate (Concurrent use may increase drowsiness effect).
No products indexed under this heading.

Fluphenazine Hydrochloride (Concurrent use may increase drowsiness effect).
No products indexed under this heading.

Flurazepam Hydrochloride (Concurrent use may increase drowsiness effect).
No products indexed under this heading.

Glutethimide (Concurrent use may increase drowsiness effect).
No products indexed under this heading.

Haloperidol (Concurrent use may increase drowsiness effect).
No products indexed under this heading.

Haloperidol Decanoate (Concurrent use may increase drowsiness effect).
No products indexed under this heading.

Hydroxyzine Hydrochloride (Concurrent use may increase drowsiness effect).
No products indexed under this heading.

Lorazepam (Concurrent use may increase drowsiness effect).
No products indexed under this heading.

Loxapine Hydrochloride (Concurrent use may increase drowsiness effect).
No products indexed under this heading.

Loxapine Succinate (Concurrent use may increase drowsiness effect).
No products indexed under this heading.

Meprobamate (Concurrent use may increase drowsiness effect).
No products indexed under this heading.

Mesoridazine Besylate (Concurrent use may increase drowsiness effect).
No products indexed under this heading.

Midazolam Hydrochloride (Concurrent use may increase drowsiness effect).
No products indexed under this heading.

Molindone Hydrochloride (Concurrent use may increase drowsiness effect). Products include:
Moban Tablets 1116

Oxazepam (Concurrent use may increase drowsiness effect).
No products indexed under this heading.

Perphenazine (Concurrent use may increase drowsiness effect).
No products indexed under this heading.

Prazepam (Concurrent use may increase drowsiness effect).
No products indexed under this heading.

Prochlorperazine (Concurrent use may increase drowsiness effect).
No products indexed under this heading.

Promethazine Hydrochloride (Concurrent use may increase drowsiness effect).
No products indexed under this heading.

Propofol (Concurrent use may increase drowsiness effect).
No products indexed under this heading.

Quazepam (Concurrent use may increase drowsiness effect).
No products indexed under this heading.

Ramelteon (Concurrent use may increase drowsiness effect).
Products include:
Rozerem Tablets 3091

Secobarbital Sodium (Concurrent use may increase drowsiness effect).
No products indexed under this heading.

Sodium Butabarbital (Concurrent use may increase drowsiness effect).
No products indexed under this heading.

Temazepam (Concurrent use may increase drowsiness effect).
No products indexed under this heading.

Thioridazine Hydrochloride (Concurrent use may increase drowsiness effect). Products include:
Thioridazine Hydrochloride Tablets 2195

Thiothixene (Concurrent use may increase drowsiness effect).
Products include:
Thiothixene Capsules 2197

Triazolam (Concurrent use may increase drowsiness effect).
No products indexed under this heading.

Trifluoperazine Hydrochloride (Concurrent use may increase drowsiness effect).
No products indexed under this heading.

Zaleplon (Concurrent use may increase drowsiness effect).
No products indexed under this heading.

Zolpidem Tartrate (Concurrent use may increase drowsiness effect).
Products include:
Ambien Tablets 2692
Ambien CR Tablets 2696

Food Interactions

Alcohol (Increases drowsiness effect; avoid concomitant use).

CHILDREN'S BENADRYL DYE-FREE ALLERGY LIQUID

(Diphenhydramine Hydrochloride) 1897
May interact with hypnotics and sedatives and tranquilizers. Compounds in these categories include:

Alprazolam (Concurrent use may increase drowsiness effect).
No products indexed under this heading.

Buspirone Hydrochloride (Concurrent use may increase drowsiness effect).
No products indexed under this heading.

Butabarbital (Concurrent use may increase drowsiness effect).
No products indexed under this heading.

Butabarbital Sodium (Concurrent use may increase drowsiness effect).
No products indexed under this heading.

Chloral Hydrate (Concurrent use may increase drowsiness effect).
No products indexed under this heading.

Chlordiazepoxide (Concurrent use may increase drowsiness effect).
No products indexed under this heading.

Chlordiazepoxide Hydrochloride (Concurrent use may increase drowsiness effect).
No products indexed under this heading.

Chlorpromazine (Concurrent use may increase drowsiness effect).
No products indexed under this heading.

Chlorpromazine Hydrochloride (Concurrent use may increase drowsiness effect).
No products indexed under this heading.

Chlorprothixene (Concurrent use may increase drowsiness effect).
No products indexed under this heading.

Chlorprothixene Hydrochloride (Concurrent use may increase drowsiness effect).
No products indexed under this heading.

Clorazepate Dipotassium (Concurrent use may increase drowsiness effect).
No products indexed under this heading.

Diazepam (Concurrent use may increase drowsiness effect).
Products include:
Valium Tablets 2658

Droperidol (Concurrent use may increase drowsiness effect).
No products indexed under this heading.

Estazolam (Concurrent use may increase drowsiness effect).
No products indexed under this heading.

Ethchlorvynol (Concurrent use may increase drowsiness effect).
No products indexed under this heading.

Ethinamate (Concurrent use may increase drowsiness effect).
No products indexed under this heading.

Fluphenazine Decanoate (Concurrent use may increase drowsiness effect).
No products indexed under this heading.

Fluphenazine Enanthate (Concurrent use may increase drowsiness effect).
No products indexed under this heading.

Fluphenazine Hydrochloride (Concurrent use may increase drowsiness effect).
No products indexed under this heading.

Flurazepam Hydrochloride (Concurrent use may increase drowsiness effect).
No products indexed under this heading.

Glutethimide (Concurrent use may increase drowsiness effect).
No products indexed under this heading.

Haloperidol (Concurrent use may increase drowsiness effect).
No products indexed under this heading.

Haloperidol Decanoate (Concurrent use may increase drowsiness effect).
No products indexed under this heading.

Hydroxyzine Hydrochloride (Concurrent use may increase drowsiness effect).
No products indexed under this heading.

Lorazepam (Concurrent use may increase drowsiness effect).
No products indexed under this heading.

Loxapine Hydrochloride (Concurrent use may increase drowsiness effect).
No products indexed under this heading.

Loxapine Succinate (Concurrent use may increase drowsiness effect).
No products indexed under this heading.

Meprobamate (Concurrent use may increase drowsiness effect).
No products indexed under this heading.

Mesoridazine Besylate (Concurrent use may increase drowsiness effect).
No products indexed under this heading.

Midazolam Hydrochloride (Concurrent use may increase drowsiness effect).
No products indexed under this heading.

Molindone Hydrochloride (Concurrent use may increase drowsiness effect). Products include:
Moban Tablets **1116**

Oxazepam (Concurrent use may increase drowsiness effect).
No products indexed under this heading.

Perphenazine (Concurrent use may increase drowsiness effect).
No products indexed under this heading.

Prazepam (Concurrent use may increase drowsiness effect).
No products indexed under this heading.

Prochlorperazine (Concurrent use may increase drowsiness effect).
No products indexed under this heading.

Promethazine Hydrochloride (Concurrent use may increase drowsiness effect).
No products indexed under this heading.

Propofol (Concurrent use may increase drowsiness effect).
No products indexed under this heading.

Quazepam (Concurrent use may increase drowsiness effect).
No products indexed under this heading.

Ramelteon (Concurrent use may increase drowsiness effect).
Products include:
Rozerem Tablets **3091**

Secobarbital Sodium (Concurrent use may increase drowsiness effect).
No products indexed under this heading.

Sodium Butabarbital (Concurrent use may increase drowsiness effect).
No products indexed under this heading.

Temazepam (Concurrent use may increase drowsiness effect).
No products indexed under this heading.

Thioridazine Hydrochloride (Concurrent use may increase drowsiness effect). Products include:
Thioridazine Hydrochloride Tablets **2195**

Thiothixene (Concurrent use may increase drowsiness effect).
Products include:
Thiothixene Capsules **2197**

Triazolam (Concurrent use may increase drowsiness effect).
No products indexed under this heading.

Trifluoperazine Hydrochloride (Concurrent use may increase drowsiness effect).
No products indexed under this heading.

Zaleplon (Concurrent use may increase drowsiness effect).
No products indexed under this heading.

Zolpidem Tartrate (Concurrent use may increase drowsiness effect).
Products include:
Ambien Tablets **2692**
Ambien CR Tablets **2696**

CHILDREN'S BENADRYL ALLERGY FASTMELTS

(Diphenhydramine Hydrochloride) **1897**
May interact with hypnotics and sedatives, tranquilizers, and certain other agents. Compounds in these categories include:

Alprazolam (Concurrent use may increase drowsiness effect).
No products indexed under this heading.

Buspirone Hydrochloride (Concurrent use may increase drowsiness effect).
No products indexed under this heading.

Butabarbital (Concurrent use may increase drowsiness effect).
No products indexed under this heading.

Butabarbital Sodium (Concurrent use may increase drowsiness effect).
No products indexed under this heading.

Chloral Hydrate (Concurrent use may increase drowsiness effect).
No products indexed under this heading.

Chlordiazepoxide (Concurrent use may increase drowsiness effect).
No products indexed under this heading.

Chlordiazepoxide Hydrochloride (Concurrent use may increase drowsiness effect).
No products indexed under this heading.

Chlorpromazine (Concurrent use may increase drowsiness effect).
No products indexed under this heading.

Chlorpromazine Hydrochloride (Concurrent use may increase drowsiness effect).
No products indexed under this heading.

Chlorprothixene (Concurrent use may increase drowsiness effect).
No products indexed under this heading.

Chlorprothixene Hydrochloride (Concurrent use may increase drowsiness effect).
No products indexed under this heading.

Clorazepate Dipotassium (Concurrent use may increase drowsiness effect).
No products indexed under this heading.

Diazepam (Concurrent use may increase drowsiness effect).
Products include:
Valium Tablets **2658**

Droperidol (Concurrent use may increase drowsiness effect).
No products indexed under this heading.

Estazolam (Concurrent use may increase drowsiness effect).
No products indexed under this heading.

Ethchlorvynol (Concurrent use may increase drowsiness effect).
No products indexed under this heading.

Ethinamate (Concurrent use may increase drowsiness effect).
No products indexed under this heading.

Fluphenazine Decanoate (Concurrent use may increase drowsiness effect).
No products indexed under this heading.

Fluphenazine Enanthate (Concurrent use may increase drowsiness effect).
No products indexed under this heading.

Fluphenazine Hydrochloride (Concurrent use may increase drowsiness effect).
No products indexed under this heading.

Flurazepam Hydrochloride (Concurrent use may increase drowsiness effect).
No products indexed under this heading.

Glutethimide (Concurrent use may increase drowsiness effect).
No products indexed under this heading.

Haloperidol (Concurrent use may increase drowsiness effect).
No products indexed under this heading.

Haloperidol Decanoate (Concurrent use may increase drowsiness effect).
No products indexed under this heading.

Hydroxyzine Hydrochloride (Concurrent use may increase drowsiness effect).
No products indexed under this heading.

Lorazepam (Concurrent use may increase drowsiness effect).
No products indexed under this heading.

Midazolam Hydrochloride (Concurrent use may increase drowsiness effect).
No products indexed under this heading.

Propofol (Concurrent use may increase drowsiness effect).
No products indexed under this heading.

Quazepam (Concurrent use may increase drowsiness effect).
No products indexed under this heading.

Ramelteon (Concurrent use may increase drowsiness effect).
Products include:
Rozerem Tablets **3091**

Secobarbital Sodium (Concurrent use may increase drowsiness effect).
No products indexed under this heading.

Sodium Butabarbital (Concurrent use may increase drowsiness effect).
No products indexed under this heading.

Temazepam (Concurrent use may increase drowsiness effect).
No products indexed under this heading.

Triazolam (Concurrent use may increase drowsiness effect).
No products indexed under this heading.

Zaleplon (Concurrent use may increase drowsiness effect).
No products indexed under this heading.

Zolpidem Tartrate (Concurrent use may increase drowsiness effect).
Products include:
Ambien Tablets **2692**
Ambien CR Tablets **2696**

Food Interactions

Alcohol (Increases drowsiness effect; avoid concurrent use).

CHILDREN'S BENADRYL ALLERGY LIQUID

(Diphenhydramine Hydrochloride) **1898**
May interact with hypnotics and sedatives and tranquilizers. Compounds in these categories include:

Alprazolam (Concurrent use may increase drowsiness effect).
No products indexed under this heading.

Buspirone Hydrochloride (Concurrent use may increase drowsiness effect).
No products indexed under this heading.

Butabarbital (Concurrent use may increase drowsiness effect).
No products indexed under this heading.

Butabarbital Sodium (Concurrent use may increase drowsiness effect).
No products indexed under this heading.

Chloral Hydrate (Concurrent use may increase drowsiness effect).
No products indexed under this heading.

Chlordiazepoxide (Concurrent use may increase drowsiness effect).
No products indexed under this heading.

Chlordiazepoxide Hydrochloride (Concurrent use may increase drowsiness effect).
No products indexed under this heading.

Chlorpromazine (Concurrent use may increase drowsiness effect).
No products indexed under this heading.

Chlorpromazine Hydrochloride (Concurrent use may increase drowsiness effect).
No products indexed under this heading.

Chlorprothixene (Concurrent use may increase drowsiness effect).
No products indexed under this heading.

Chlorprothixene Hydrochloride (Concurrent use may increase drowsiness effect).
No products indexed under this heading.

Clorazepate Dipotassium (Concurrent use may increase drowsiness effect).
No products indexed under this heading.

Diazepam (Concurrent use may increase drowsiness effect). Products include:
Valium Tablets 2658

Droperidol (Concurrent use may increase drowsiness effect).
No products indexed under this heading.

Estazolam (Concurrent use may increase drowsiness effect).
No products indexed under this heading.

Ethchlorvynol (Concurrent use may increase drowsiness effect).
No products indexed under this heading.

Ethinamate (Concurrent use may increase drowsiness effect).
No products indexed under this heading.

Fluphenazine Decanoate (Concurrent use may increase drowsiness effect).
No products indexed under this heading.

Fluphenazine Enanthate (Concurrent use may increase drowsiness effect).
No products indexed under this heading.

Fluphenazine Hydrochloride (Concurrent use may increase drowsiness effect).
No products indexed under this heading.

Flurazepam Hydrochloride (Concurrent use may increase drowsiness effect).
No products indexed under this heading.

Glutethimide (Concurrent use may increase drowsiness effect).
No products indexed under this heading.

Haloperidol (Concurrent use may increase drowsiness effect).
No products indexed under this heading.

Haloperidol Decanoate (Concurrent use may increase drowsiness effect).
No products indexed under this heading.

Hydroxyzine Hydrochloride (Concurrent use may increase drowsiness effect).
No products indexed under this heading.

Lorazepam (Concurrent use may increase drowsiness effect).
No products indexed under this heading.

Loxapine Hydrochloride (Concurrent use may increase drowsiness effect).
No products indexed under this heading.

Loxapine Succinate (Concurrent use may increase drowsiness effect).
No products indexed under this heading.

Meprobamate (Concurrent use may increase drowsiness effect).
No products indexed under this heading.

Mesoridazine Besylate (Concurrent use may increase drowsiness effect).
No products indexed under this heading.

Midazolam Hydrochloride (Concurrent use may increase drowsiness effect).
No products indexed under this heading.

Molindone Hydrochloride (Concurrent use may increase drowsiness effect). Products include:
Moban Tablets 1116

Oxazepam (Concurrent use may increase drowsiness effect).
No products indexed under this heading.

Perphenazine (Concurrent use may increase drowsiness effect).
No products indexed under this heading.

Prazepam (Concurrent use may increase drowsiness effect).
No products indexed under this heading.

Prochlorperazine (Concurrent use may increase drowsiness effect).
No products indexed under this heading.

Promethazine Hydrochloride (Concurrent use may increase drowsiness effect).
No products indexed under this heading.

Propofol (Concurrent use may increase drowsiness effect).
No products indexed under this heading.

Quazepam (Concurrent use may increase drowsiness effect).
No products indexed under this heading.

Ramelteon (Concurrent use may increase drowsiness effect). Products include:
Rozerem Tablets 3091

Secobarbital Sodium (Concurrent use may increase drowsiness effect).
No products indexed under this heading.

Sodium Butabarbital (Concurrent use may increase drowsiness effect).
No products indexed under this heading.

Temazepam (Concurrent use may increase drowsiness effect).
No products indexed under this heading.

Thioridazine Hydrochloride (Concurrent use may increase drowsiness effect). Products include:
Thioridazine Hydrochloride Tablets 2195

Thiothixene (Concurrent use may increase drowsiness effect). Products include:
Thiothixene Capsules 2197

Triazolam (Concurrent use may increase drowsiness effect).
No products indexed under this heading.

Trifluoperazine Hydrochloride (Concurrent use may increase drowsiness effect).
No products indexed under this heading.

Zaleplon (Concurrent use may increase drowsiness effect).
No products indexed under this heading.

Zolpidem Tartrate (Concurrent use may increase drowsiness effect). Products include:
Ambien Tablets 2692
Ambien CR Tablets 2696

CHILDREN'S BENADRYL ALLERGY PERFECT MEASURE

(Diphenhydramine Hydrochloride) 1896
May interact with hypnotics and sedatives, tranquilizers, and certain other agents. Compounds in these categories include:

Alprazolam (Concurrent use may increase drowsiness).
No products indexed under this heading.

Buspirone Hydrochloride (Concurrent use may increase drowsiness).
No products indexed under this heading.

Butabarbital (Concurrent use may increase drowsiness).
No products indexed under this heading.

Butabarbital Sodium (Concurrent use may increase drowsiness).
No products indexed under this heading.

Chloral Hydrate (Concurrent use may increase drowsiness).
No products indexed under this heading.

Chlordiazepoxide (Concurrent use may increase drowsiness).
No products indexed under this heading.

Chlordiazepoxide Hydrochloride (Concurrent use may increase drowsiness).
No products indexed under this heading.

Chlorpromazine (Concurrent use may increase drowsiness).
No products indexed under this heading.

Chlorpromazine Hydrochloride (Concurrent use may increase drowsiness).
No products indexed under this heading.

Chlorprothixene (Concurrent use may increase drowsiness).
No products indexed under this heading.

Chlorprothixene Hydrochloride (Concurrent use may increase drowsiness).
No products indexed under this heading.

Clorazepate Dipotassium (Concurrent use may increase drowsiness).
No products indexed under this heading.

Diazepam (Concurrent use may increase drowsiness). Products include:
Valium Tablets 2658

Droperidol (Concurrent use may increase drowsiness).
No products indexed under this heading.

Estazolam (Concurrent use may increase drowsiness).
No products indexed under this heading.

Ethchlorvynol (Concurrent use may increase drowsiness).
No products indexed under this heading.

Ethinamate (Concurrent use may increase drowsiness).
No products indexed under this heading.

Fluphenazine Decanoate (Concurrent use may increase drowsiness).
No products indexed under this heading.

Fluphenazine Enanthate (Concurrent use may increase drowsiness).
No products indexed under this heading.

Fluphenazine Hydrochloride (Concurrent use may increase drowsiness).
No products indexed under this heading.

Flurazepam Hydrochloride (Concurrent use may increase drowsiness).
No products indexed under this heading.

Glutethimide (Concurrent use may increase drowsiness).
No products indexed under this heading.

Haloperidol (Concurrent use may increase drowsiness).
No products indexed under this heading.

Haloperidol Decanoate (Concurrent use may increase drowsiness).
No products indexed under this heading.

Hydroxyzine Hydrochloride (Concurrent use may increase drowsiness).
No products indexed under this heading.

Lorazepam (Concurrent use may increase drowsiness).
No products indexed under this heading.

Loxapine Hydrochloride (Concurrent use may increase drowsiness).
No products indexed under this heading.

Loxapine Succinate (Concurrent use may increase drowsiness).
No products indexed under this heading.

Meprobamate (Concurrent use may increase drowsiness).
No products indexed under this heading.

Mesoridazine Besylate (Concurrent use may increase drowsiness).
No products indexed under this heading.

Midazolam Hydrochloride (Concurrent use may increase drowsiness).
No products indexed under this heading.

Molindone Hydrochloride (Concurrent use may increase drowsiness). Products include:
Moban Tablets 1116

Oxazepam (Concurrent use may increase drowsiness).
No products indexed under this heading.

Perphenazine (Concurrent use may increase drowsiness).
No products indexed under this heading.

Prazepam (Concurrent use may increase drowsiness).
No products indexed under this heading.

Prochlorperazine (Concurrent use may increase drowsiness).
No products indexed under this heading.

Promethazine Hydrochloride (Concurrent use may increase drowsiness).
No products indexed under this heading.

Propofol (Concurrent use may increase drowsiness).
No products indexed under this heading.

Quazepam (Concurrent use may increase drowsiness).
No products indexed under this heading.

Ramelteon (Concurrent use may increase drowsiness). Products include:
Rozerem Tablets 3091

Secobarbital Sodium (Concurrent use may increase drowsiness).
No products indexed under this heading.

Sodium Butabarbital (Concurrent use may increase drowsiness).
No products indexed under this heading.

Temazepam (Concurrent use may increase drowsiness).
No products indexed under this heading.

Thioridazine Hydrochloride (Concurrent use may increase drowsiness). Products include:
Thioridazine Hydrochloride Tablets 2195

Thiothixene (Concurrent use may increase drowsiness). Products include:
Thiothixene Capsules 2197

Triazolam (Concurrent use may increase drowsiness).
No products indexed under this heading.

Trifluoperazine Hydrochloride (Concurrent use may increase drowsiness).
No products indexed under this heading.

Zaleplon (Concurrent use may increase drowsiness).
No products indexed under this heading.

Zolpidem Tartrate (Concurrent use may increase drowsiness). Products include:
Ambien Tablets 2692
Ambien CR Tablets 2696

Food Interactions

Alcohol (Concurrent use may increase drowsiness).

CHILDREN'S BENADRYL-D ALLERGY & SINUS LIQUID

(Diphenhydramine Hydrochloride, Phenylephrine Hydrochloride) 1896

May interact with hypnotics and sedatives, monoamine oxidase inhibitors, tranquilizers, and certain other agents. Compounds in these categories include:

Alprazolam (Concurrent use may increase drowsiness).
No products indexed under this heading.

Buspirone Hydrochloride (Concurrent use may increase drowsiness).
No products indexed under this heading.

Butabarbital (Concurrent use may increase drowsiness).
No products indexed under this heading.

Butabarbital Sodium (Concurrent use may increase drowsiness).
No products indexed under this heading.

Chloral Hydrate (Concurrent use may increase drowsiness).
No products indexed under this heading.

Chlordiazepoxide (Concurrent use may increase drowsiness).
No products indexed under this heading.

Chlordiazepoxide Hydrochloride (Concurrent use may increase drowsiness).
No products indexed under this heading.

Chlorpromazine (Concurrent use may increase drowsiness).
No products indexed under this heading.

Chlorpromazine Hydrochloride (Concurrent use may increase drowsiness).
No products indexed under this heading.

Chlorprothixene (Concurrent use may increase drowsiness).
No products indexed under this heading.

Chlorprothixene Hydrochloride (Concurrent use may increase drowsiness).
No products indexed under this heading.

Clorazepate Dipotassium (Concurrent use may increase drowsiness).
No products indexed under this heading.

Diazepam (Concurrent use may increase drowsiness). Products include:
Valium Tablets 2658

Droperidol (Concurrent use may increase drowsiness).
No products indexed under this heading.

Estazolam (Concurrent use may increase drowsiness).
No products indexed under this heading.

Ethchlorvynol (Concurrent use may increase drowsiness).
No products indexed under this heading.

Ethinamate (Concurrent use may increase drowsiness).
No products indexed under this heading.

Fluphenazine Decanoate (Concurrent use may increase drowsiness).
No products indexed under this heading.

Fluphenazine Enanthate (Concurrent use may increase drowsiness).
No products indexed under this heading.

Fluphenazine Hydrochloride (Concurrent use may increase drowsiness).
No products indexed under this heading.

Flurazepam Hydrochloride (Concurrent use may increase drowsiness).
No products indexed under this heading.

Glutethimide (Concurrent use may increase drowsiness).
No products indexed under this heading.

Haloperidol (Concurrent use may increase drowsiness).
No products indexed under this heading.

Haloperidol Decanoate (Concurrent use may increase drowsiness).
No products indexed under this heading.

Hydroxyzine Hydrochloride (Concurrent use may increase drowsiness).
No products indexed under this heading.

Isocarboxazid (Avoid use with monoamine oxidase inhibitor (MAOI) or for two weeks after stopping MAOI drug). Products include:
Marplan Tablets 3177

Lorazepam (Concurrent use may increase drowsiness).
No products indexed under this heading.

Loxapine Hydrochloride (Concurrent use may increase drowsiness).
No products indexed under this heading.

Loxapine Succinate (Concurrent use may increase drowsiness).
No products indexed under this heading.

Meprobamate (Concurrent use may increase drowsiness).
No products indexed under this heading.

Mesoridazine Besylate (Concurrent use may increase drowsiness).
No products indexed under this heading.

Midazolam Hydrochloride (Concurrent use may increase drowsiness).
No products indexed under this heading.

Moclobemide (Avoid use with monoamine oxidase inhibitor (MAOI) or for two weeks after stopping MAOI drug).
No products indexed under this heading.

Molindone Hydrochloride (Concurrent use may increase drowsiness). Products include:
Moban Tablets 1116

Oxazepam (Concurrent use may increase drowsiness).
No products indexed under this heading.

Pargyline Hydrochloride (Avoid use with monoamine oxidase inhibitor (MAOI) or for two weeks after stopping MAOI drug).
No products indexed under this heading.

Perphenazine (Concurrent use may increase drowsiness).
No products indexed under this heading.

Phenelzine Sulfate (Avoid use with monoamine oxidase inhibitor (MAOI) or for two weeks after stopping MAOI drug).
No products indexed under this heading.

Prazepam (Concurrent use may increase drowsiness).
No products indexed under this heading.

Procarbazine Hydrochloride (Avoid use with monoamine oxidase inhibitor (MAOI) or for two weeks after stopping MAOI drug).
No products indexed under this heading.

Prochlorperazine (Concurrent use may increase drowsiness).
No products indexed under this heading.

Promethazine Hydrochloride (Concurrent use may increase drowsiness).
No products indexed under this heading.

Propofol (Concurrent use may increase drowsiness).
No products indexed under this heading.

Quazepam (Concurrent use may increase drowsiness).
No products indexed under this heading.

Ramelteon (Concurrent use may increase drowsiness). Products include:
Rozerem Tablets 3091

Rasagiline Mesylate (Avoid use with monoamine oxidase inhibitor (MAOI) or for two weeks after stopping MAOI drug). Products include:
Azilect Tablets 3106

Secobarbital Sodium (Concurrent use may increase drowsiness).
No products indexed under this heading.

Selegiline (Avoid use with monoamine oxidase inhibitor (MAOI) or for two weeks after stopping MAOI drug). Products include:
Emsam Transdermal System 905

Selegiline Hydrochloride (Avoid use with monoamine oxidase inhibitor (MAOI) or for two weeks after stopping MAOI drug). Products include:
Eldepryl Capsules 3052

Sodium Butabarbital (Concurrent use may increase drowsiness).
No products indexed under this heading.

Temazepam (Concurrent use may increase drowsiness).
No products indexed under this heading.

Thioridazine Hydrochloride (Concurrent use may increase drowsiness). Products include:
Thioridazine Hydrochloride Tablets 2195

Thiothixene (Concurrent use may increase drowsiness). Products include:
Thiothixene Capsules 2197

Tranylcypromine Sulfate (Avoid use with monoamine oxidase inhibitor (MAOI) or for two weeks after stopping MAOI drug). Products include:
Parnate Tablets 1532

Triazolam (Concurrent use may increase drowsiness).
No products indexed under this heading.

Trifluoperazine Hydrochloride (Concurrent use may increase drowsiness).
No products indexed under this heading.

Zaleplon (Concurrent use may increase drowsiness).
No products indexed under this heading.

Zolpidem Tartrate (Concurrent use may increase drowsiness). Products include:

Ambien Tablets 2692
Ambien CR Tablets 2696

Food Interactions

Alcohol (Concurrent use may increase drowsiness).

BENADRYL-D ALLERGY & SINUS TABLET

(Diphenhydramine Hydrochloride, Phenylephrine Hydrochloride)............ 1896
May interact with hypnotics and sedatives, monoamine oxidase inhibitors, tranquilizers, and certain other agents. Compounds in these categories include:

Alprazolam (May increase drowsiness effect).
No products indexed under this heading.

Buspirone Hydrochloride (May increase drowsiness effect).
No products indexed under this heading.

Butabarbital (May increase drowsiness effect).
No products indexed under this heading.

Butabarbital Sodium (May increase drowsiness effect).
No products indexed under this heading.

Chloral Hydrate (May increase drowsiness effect).
No products indexed under this heading.

Chlordiazepoxide (May increase drowsiness effect).
No products indexed under this heading.

Chlordiazepoxide Hydrochloride (May increase drowsiness effect).
No products indexed under this heading.

Chlorpromazine (May increase drowsiness effect).
No products indexed under this heading.

Chlorpromazine Hydrochloride (May increase drowsiness effect).
No products indexed under this heading.

Chlorprothixene (May increase drowsiness effect).
No products indexed under this heading.

Chlorprothixene Hydrochloride (May increase drowsiness effect).
No products indexed under this heading.

Clorazepate Dipotassium (May increase drowsiness effect).
No products indexed under this heading.

Diazepam (May increase drowsiness effect). Products include:
Valium Tablets 2658

Droperidol (May increase drowsiness effect).
No products indexed under this heading.

Estazolam (May increase drowsiness effect).
No products indexed under this heading.

Ethchlorvynol (May increase drowsiness effect).
No products indexed under this heading.

Ethinamate (May increase drowsiness effect).
No products indexed under this heading.

Fluphenazine Decanoate (May increase drowsiness effect).
No products indexed under this heading.

Fluphenazine Enanthate (May increase drowsiness effect).
No products indexed under this heading.

Fluphenazine Hydrochloride (May increase drowsiness effect).
No products indexed under this heading.

Flurazepam Hydrochloride (May increase drowsiness effect).
No products indexed under this heading.

Glutethimide (May increase drowsiness effect).
No products indexed under this heading.

Haloperidol (May increase drowsiness effect).
No products indexed under this heading.

Haloperidol Decanoate (May increase drowsiness effect).
No products indexed under this heading.

Hydroxyzine Hydrochloride (May increase drowsiness effect).
No products indexed under this heading.

Isocarboxazid (Avoid use with monoamine oxidase inhibitor (MAOI) or for two weeks after stopping MAOI drug). Products include:
Marplan Tablets 3177

Lorazepam (May increase drowsiness effect).
No products indexed under this heading.

Loxapine Hydrochloride (May increase drowsiness effect).
No products indexed under this heading.

Loxapine Succinate (May increase drowsiness effect).
No products indexed under this heading.

Meprobamate (May increase drowsiness effect).
No products indexed under this heading.

Mesoridazine Besylate (May increase drowsiness effect).
No products indexed under this heading.

Midazolam Hydrochloride (May increase drowsiness effect).
No products indexed under this heading.

Moclobemide (Avoid use with monoamine oxidase inhibitor (MAOI) or for two weeks after stopping MAOI drug).
No products indexed under this heading.

Molindone Hydrochloride (May increase drowsiness effect). Products include:
Moban Tablets 1116

Oxazepam (May increase drowsiness effect).
No products indexed under this heading.

Pargyline Hydrochloride (Avoid use with monoamine oxidase inhibitor (MAOI) or for two weeks after stopping MAOI drug).
No products indexed under this heading.

Perphenazine (May increase drowsiness effect).
No products indexed under this heading.

Phenelzine Sulfate (Avoid use with monoamine oxidase inhibitor (MAOI) or for two weeks after stopping MAOI drug).
No products indexed under this heading.

Prazepam (May increase drowsiness effect).
No products indexed under this heading.

Procarbazine Hydrochloride (Avoid use with monoamine oxidase inhibitor (MAOI) or for two weeks after stopping MAOI drug).
No products indexed under this heading.

Prochlorperazine (May increase drowsiness effect).
No products indexed under this heading.

Promethazine Hydrochloride (May increase drowsiness effect).
No products indexed under this heading.

Propofol (May increase drowsiness effect).
No products indexed under this heading.

Quazepam (May increase drowsiness effect).
No products indexed under this heading.

Ramelteon (May increase drowsiness effect). Products include:
Rozerem Tablets 3091

Rasagiline Mesylate (Avoid use with monoamine oxidase inhibitor (MAOI) or for two weeks after stopping MAOI drug). Products include:
Azilect Tablets 3106

Secobarbital Sodium (May increase drowsiness effect).
No products indexed under this heading.

Selegiline (Avoid use with monoamine oxidase inhibitor (MAOI) or for two weeks after stopping MAOI drug). Products include:
Emsam Transdermal System 905

Selegiline Hydrochloride (Avoid use with monoamine oxidase inhibitor (MAOI) or for two weeks after stopping MAOI drug). Products include:
Eldepryl Capsules 3052

Sodium Butabarbital (May increase drowsiness effect).
No products indexed under this heading.

Temazepam (May increase drowsiness effect).
No products indexed under this heading.

Thioridazine Hydrochloride (May increase drowsiness effect). Products include:
Thioridazine Hydrochloride Tablets 2195

Thiothixene (May increase drowsiness effect). Products include:
Thiothixene Capsules 2197

Tranylcypromine Sulfate (Avoid use with monoamine oxidase inhibitor (MAOI) or for two weeks after stopping MAOI drug). Products include:
Parnate Tablets 1532

Triazolam (May increase drowsiness effect).
No products indexed under this heading.

Trifluoperazine Hydrochloride (May increase drowsiness effect).
No products indexed under this heading.

Zaleplon (May increase drowsiness effect).
No products indexed under this heading.

Zolpidem Tartrate (May increase drowsiness effect). Products include:
Ambien Tablets 2692
Ambien CR Tablets 2696

Food Interactions

Alcohol (Increases drowsiness effect; avoid concomitant use).

BENEFIX VIALS

(Antihemophilic Factor (Recombinant)) 3191
None cited in PDR database.

BENICAR TABLETS

(Olmesartan Medoxomil) 1009
None cited in PDR database.

BENICAR HCT TABLETS

(Hydrochlorothiazide, Olmesartan Medoxomil)............................ 1010
May interact with angiotensin-II receptor antagonists, antihypertensives, barbiturates, corticosteroids, curariform skeletal muscle relaxants, oral hypoglycemic agents, insulin, lithium preparations, narcotic analgesics, non-steroidal anti-inflammatory agents, vasopressors, and certain other agents. Compounds in these categories include:

Acarbose (Co-administration may require a dosage adjustment of the antidiabetic drug). Products include:
Precose Tablets 792

Acebutolol Hydrochloride (Co-administration could have additive effect or potentiation).
No products indexed under this heading.

ACTH (Co-administration could cause intensified electrolyte depletion, particularly hypokalemia).
No products indexed under this heading.

Alfentanil Hydrochloride (Concurrent administration could cause potentiation of orthostatic hypotension).
No products indexed under this heading.

Aliskiren (Co-administration could have additive effect or potentiation). Products include:
Tekturna Tablets 2321
Tekturna HCT Tablets 2324

Amlodipine Besylate (Co-administration could have additive effect or potentiation). Products include:
Azor Tablets 1005
Exforge Tablets 2238

Aprobarbital (Concurrent administration could cause potentiation of orthostatic hypotension).
No products indexed under this heading.

Atenolol (Co-administration could have additive effect or potentiation).
No products indexed under this heading.

Atracurium Besylate (Co-administration could cause possible increased responsiveness to the muscle relaxant).
No products indexed under this heading.

Benazepril Hydrochloride (Co-administration could have additive effect or potentiation).
No products indexed under this heading.

Bendroflumethiazide (Co-administration could have additive effect or potentiation).
No products indexed under this heading.

Betamethasone Acetate (Co-administration could cause intensified electrolyte depletion, particularly hypokalemia).
No products indexed under this heading.

Betamethasone Sodium Phosphate (Co-administration could cause intensified electrolyte depletion, particularly hypokalemia).
No products indexed under this heading.

Betaxolol Hydrochloride (Co-administration could have additive effect or potentiation).
No products indexed under this heading.

Bisoprolol Fumarate (Co-administration could have additive effect or potentiation).
No products indexed under this heading.

Budesonide (Co-administration could cause intensified electrolyte depletion, particularly hypokalemia). Products include:
- Pulmicort Flexhaler 654
- Symbicort 80/4.5 Inhalation Aerosol........ 659
- Symbicort 160/4.5 Inhalation Aerosol........ 659

Buprenorphine Hydrochloride (Concurrent administration could cause potentiation of orthostatic hypotension). Products include:
- Suboxone Tablets........ 2601
- Subutex Tablets 2601

Butabarbital (Concurrent administration could cause potentiation of orthostatic hypotension).
No products indexed under this heading.

Butalbital (Concurrent administration could cause potentiation of orthostatic hypotension).
No products indexed under this heading.

Candesartan Cilexetil (Co-administration could have additive effect or potentiation). Products include:
- Atacand Tablets 639
- Atacand HCT 642

Captopril (Co-administration could have additive effect or potentiation). Products include:
- Captopril Tablets 2182

Carteolol Hydrochloride (Co-administration could have additive effect or potentiation).
No products indexed under this heading.

Celecoxib (In some patients the administration of a non-steroidal anti-inflammatory agent can reduce the diuretic, natriuretic and antihypertensive effects of loop, potassium-sparing and thiazide diuretics). Products include:
- Celebrex Capsules 2979

Chlorothiazide (Co-administration could have additive effect or potentiation).
No products indexed under this heading.

Chlorothiazide Sodium (Co-administration could have additive effect or potentiation). Products include:
- Intravenous Sodium Diuril 2490

Chlorpropamide (Co-administration may require a dosage adjustment of the antidiabetic drug).
No products indexed under this heading.

Chlorthalidone (Co-administration could have additive effect or potentiation). Products include:
- Clorpres Tablets 2185

Cholestyramine (Absorption of hydrochlorothiazide is impaired in the presence of anionic exchange resins; single doses of cholestyramine bind the hydrochlorothiazide and reduce its absorption from the gastrointestinal tract by 85%).
No products indexed under this heading.

Ciclesonide (Co-administration could cause intensified electrolyte depletion, particularly hypokalemia). Products include:
- Alvesco Inhalation Aerosol 2985
- Omnaris Nasal Spray 2998

Cisatracurium Besylate (Co-administration could cause possible increased responsiveness to the muscle relaxant). Products include:
- Nimbex Injection 484

Clonidine (Co-administration could have additive effect or potentiation). Products include:
- Catapres-TTS 842

Clonidine Hydrochloride (Co-administration could have additive effect or potentiation). Products include:
- Catapres Tablets 841
- Clorpres Tablets 2185

Codeine Phosphate (Concurrent administration could cause potentiation of orthostatic hypotension). Products include:
- Tylenol with Codeine Tablets 2427

Colestipol (Absorption of hydrochlorothiazide is impaired in the presence of anionic exchange resins; single doses of colestipol bind the hydrochlorothiazide and reduce its absorption from the gastrointestinal tract by 43%).
No products indexed under this heading.

Colestipol Hydrochloride (Absorption of hydrochlorothiazide is impaired in the presence of anionic exchange resins; single doses of colestipol bind the hydrochlorothiazide and reduce its absorption from the gastrointestinal tract by 43%).
No products indexed under this heading.

Cortisone Acetate (Co-administration could cause intensified electrolyte depletion, particularly hypokalemia).
No products indexed under this heading.

Deserpidine (Co-administration could have additive effect or potentiation).
No products indexed under this heading.

Dexamethasone (Co-administration could cause intensified electrolyte depletion, particularly hypokalemia). Products include:
- Ciprodex Otic Suspension 541

Dexamethasone Acetate (Co-administration could cause intensified electrolyte depletion, particularly hypokalemia).
No products indexed under this heading.

Dexamethasone Sodium Phosphate (Co-administration could cause intensified electrolyte depletion, particularly hypokalemia).
No products indexed under this heading.

Dezocine (Concurrent administration could cause potentiation of orthostatic hypotension).
No products indexed under this heading.

Diazoxide (Co-administration could have additive effect or potentiation). Products include:
- Proglycem Capsules 1185
- Proglycem Suspension 1185

Diclofenac Epolamine (In some patients the administration of a non-steroidal anti-inflammatory agent can reduce the diuretic, natriuretic and antihypertensive effects of loop, potassium-sparing and thiazide diuretics). Products include:
- Flector Patch 561

Diclofenac Potassium (In some patients the administration of a non-steroidal anti-inflammatory agent can reduce the diuretic, natriuretic and antihypertensive effects of loop, potassium-sparing and thiazide diuretics).
No products indexed under this heading.

Diclofenac Sodium (In some patients the administration of a non-steroidal anti-inflammatory agent can reduce the diuretic, natriuretic and antihypertensive effects of loop, potassium-sparing and thiazide diuretics). Products include:
- Diclofenac Sodium Ophthalmic Solution........ ⊙ 240
- Voltaren Ophthalmic Solution 2336
- Voltaren Tablets 2334
- Voltaren-XR Tablets 2337

Diltiazem Hydrochloride (Co-administration could have additive effect or potentiation). Products include:
- Cardizem LA Extended Release Tablets........ 421

Dobutamine (Co-administration could cause possible decreased response to pressor amines but not sufficient to preclude their use).
No products indexed under this heading.

Dobutamine Hydrochloride (Co-administration could cause possible decreased response to pressor amines but not sufficient to preclude their use).
No products indexed under this heading.

Dopamine Hydrochloride (Co-administration could cause possible decreased response to pressor amines but not sufficient to preclude their use).
No products indexed under this heading.

Doxacurium Chloride (Co-administration could cause possible increased responsiveness to the muscle relaxant).
No products indexed under this heading.

Doxazosin Mesylate (Co-administration could have additive effect or potentiation).
No products indexed under this heading.

Enalapril Maleate (Co-administration could have additive effect or potentiation).
No products indexed under this heading.

Enalaprilat (Co-administration could have additive effect or potentiation).
No products indexed under this heading.

Ephedrine Sulfate (Co-administration could cause possible decreased response to pressor amines but not sufficient to preclude their use).
No products indexed under this heading.

Epinephrine Bitartrate (Co-administration could cause possible decreased response to pressor amines but not sufficient to preclude their use).
No products indexed under this heading.

Epinephrine Hydrochloride (Co-administration could cause possible decreased response to pressor amines but not sufficient to preclude their use).
No products indexed under this heading.

Eprosartan Mesylate (Co-administration could have additive effect or potentiation). Products include:
- Teveten Tablets 515
- Teveten HCT Tablets 517

Esmolol Hydrochloride (Co-administration could have additive effect or potentiation).
No products indexed under this heading.

Etodolac (In some patients the administration of a non-steroidal anti-inflammatory agent can reduce the diuretic, natriuretic and antihypertensive effects of loop, potassium-sparing and thiazide diuretics).
No products indexed under this heading.

Felodipine (Co-administration could have additive effect or potentiation).
No products indexed under this heading.

Fenoprofen Calcium (In some patients the administration of a non-steroidal anti-inflammatory agent can reduce the diuretic, natriuretic and antihypertensive effects of loop, potassium-sparing and thiazide diuretics). Products include:
- Nalfon Capsules 2508

Fentanyl (Concurrent administration could cause potentiation of orthostatic hypotension). Products include:
- Duragesic Transdermal System 2405
- Ionsys Transdermal System 2410

Fentanyl Citrate (Concurrent administration could cause potentiation of orthostatic hypotension). Products include:
- Actiq 959
- Fentora Tablets 968

Fludrocortisone Acetate (Co-administration could cause intensified electrolyte depletion, particularly hypokalemia).
No products indexed under this heading.

Flunisolide (Co-administration could cause intensified electrolyte depletion, particularly hypokalemia). Products include:
- Aerobid/Aerobid-M 1153

IMPORTANT NOTE: Always consult each drug listing in the patient's regimen for possible interactions.

Flurbiprofen (In some patients the administration of a non-steroidal anti-inflammatory agent can reduce the diuretic, natriuretic and antihypertensive effects of loop, potassium-sparing and thiazide diuretics).
No products indexed under this heading.

Fluticasone Propionate (Co-administration could cause intensified electrolyte depletion, particularly hypokalemia). Products include:
Advair Diskus 100/50 1276
Advair Diskus 250/50 1276
Advair Diskus 500/50 1276
Advair HFA 45/21 Inhalation Aerosol 1288
Advair HFA 115/21 Inhalation Aerosol 1288
Advair HFA 230/21 Inhalation Aerosol 1288
Flonase Nasal Spray 1431
Flovent Diskus 50 mcg 1435

Fluticasone Propionate HFA (Co-administration could cause intensified electrolyte depletion, particularly hypokalemia). Products include:
Flovent HFA 1440

Fosinopril Sodium (Co-administration could have additive effect or potentiation).
No products indexed under this heading.

Furosemide (Co-administration could have additive effect or potentiation). Products include:
Furosemide Tablets 2186

Glimepiride (Co-administration may require a dosage adjustment of the antidiabetic drug). Products include:
Avandaryl Tablets 1344
Duetact Tablets 3085

Glipizide (Co-administration may require a dosage adjustment of the antidiabetic drug).
No products indexed under this heading.

Glyburide (Co-administration may require a dosage adjustment of the antidiabetic drug).
No products indexed under this heading.

Guanabenz Acetate (Co-administration could have additive effect or potentiation).
No products indexed under this heading.

Guanethidine Monosulfate (Co-administration could have additive effect or potentiation).
No products indexed under this heading.

Hydralazine Hydrochloride (Co-administration could have additive effect or potentiation).
No products indexed under this heading.

Hydrocodone Bitartrate (Concurrent administration could cause potentiation of orthostatic hypotension). Products include:
Lortab 5/500 Tablets 3143
Lortab 7.5/500 Tablets 3144
Lortab 10/500 Tablets 3144
Vicodin Tablets 529
Vicodin ES Tablets 530
Vicodin HP Tablets 531
Vicoprofen Tablets 533
Zydone Tablets 1132

Hydrocodone Polistirex (Concurrent administration could cause potentiation of orthostatic hypotension). Products include:
Tussionex Pennkinetic Extended-Release Suspension 3154

Hydrocortisone (Co-administration could cause intensified electrolyte depletion, particularly hypokalemia).
No products indexed under this heading.

Hydrocortisone Acetate (Co-administration could cause intensified electrolyte depletion, particularly hypokalemia). Products include:
Analpram-HC 1140
Pramosone 1141

Hydrocortisone Sodium Phosphate (Co-administration could cause intensified electrolyte depletion, particularly hypokalemia).
No products indexed under this heading.

Hydrocortisone Sodium Succinate (Co-administration could cause intensified electrolyte depletion, particularly hypokalemia).
No products indexed under this heading.

Hydroflumethiazide (Co-administration could have additive effect or potentiation).
No products indexed under this heading.

Hydromorphone Hydrochloride (Concurrent administration could cause potentiation of orthostatic hypotension).
No products indexed under this heading.

Ibuprofen (In some patients the administration of a non-steroidal anti-inflammatory agent can reduce the diuretic, natriuretic and antihypertensive effects of loop, potassium-sparing and thiazide diuretics). Products include:
Motrin IB Tablets and Caplets 1900
Children's Motrin Oral Suspension 1901
Children's Motrin Non-Staining Dye-Free Oral Suspension 1901
Children's Motrin Cold Oral Suspension 1899
Infants' Motrin Concentrated Drops 1901
Infants' Motrin Non-Staining Dye-Free Concentrated Drops 1901
Junior Strength Motrin Caplets and Chewable Tablets 1901
Vicoprofen Tablets 533

Indapamide (Co-administration could have additive effect or potentiation). Products include:
Indapamide Tablets 2188

Indomethacin (In some patients the administration of a non-steroidal anti-inflammatory agent can reduce the diuretic, natriuretic and antihypertensive effects of loop, potassium-sparing and thiazide diuretics). Products include:
Indocin 2024

Indomethacin Sodium Trihydrate (In some patients the administration of a non-steroidal anti-inflammatory agent can reduce the diuretic, natriuretic and antihypertensive effects of loop, potassium-sparing and thiazide diuretics). Products include:
Indocin I.V. 2489

Insulin (Co-administration may require a dosage adjustment of the antidiabetic drug).
No products indexed under this heading.

Insulin, Human, Zinc Suspension (Co-administration may require a dosage adjustment of the antidiabetic drug).
No products indexed under this heading.

Insulin, Human (rDNA origin) (Co-administration may require a dosage adjustment of the antidiabetic drug). Products include:
Exubera Inhalation Powder 2515

Insulin, Human NPH (Co-administration may require a dosage adjustment of the antidiabetic drug). Products include:
Humulin N Vial 1846

Insulin, Human Regular (Co-administration may require a dosage adjustment of the antidiabetic drug). Products include:
Humulin R 1849
Humulin R (U-500) 1850

Insulin, Human Regular and Human NPH Mixture (Co-administration may require a dosage adjustment of the antidiabetic drug). Products include:
Humulin 50/50, 100 Units 1843
Humulin 70/30 Vial 1844

Insulin, NPH (Co-administration may require a dosage adjustment of the antidiabetic drug).
No products indexed under this heading.

Insulin, Regular (Co-administration may require a dosage adjustment of the antidiabetic drug).
No products indexed under this heading.

Insulin, Regular and NPH mixture (Co-administration may require a dosage adjustment of the antidiabetic drug).
No products indexed under this heading.

Insulin, Zinc Crystals (Co-administration may require a dosage adjustment of the antidiabetic drug).
No products indexed under this heading.

Insulin, Zinc Suspension (Co-administration may require a dosage adjustment of the antidiabetic drug).
No products indexed under this heading.

Insulin Aspart (Co-administration may require a dosage adjustment of the antidiabetic drug).
No products indexed under this heading.

Insulin Aspart, Human (Co-administration may require a dosage adjustment of the antidiabetic drug). Products include:
NovoLog Mix 70/30 2364

Insulin Aspart, Human Regular (Co-administration may require a dosage adjustment of the antidiabetic drug). Products include:
NovoLog Injection 2359

Insulin Aspart Protamine, Human (Co-administration may require a dosage adjustment of the antidiabetic drug). Products include:
NovoLog Mix 70/30 2364

Insulin Detemir (rDNA Origin) (Co-administration may require a dosage adjustment of the antidiabetic drug). Products include:
Levemir Injection 2352

Insulin glargine (Co-administration may require a dosage adjustment of the antidiabetic drug). Products include:
Lantus Injection 2749

Insulin Glulisine (Co-administration may require a dosage adjustment of the antidiabetic drug). Products include:
Apidra Injection 2706

Insulin Lispro, Human (Co-administration may require a dosage adjustment of the antidiabetic drug). Products include:
Humalog-Pen and KwikPen 1829
Humalog Mix 50/50-Pen and KwikPen 1833
Humalog Mix 75/25-Pen and KwikPen 1835

Insulin Lispro Protamine, Human (Co-administration may require a dosage adjustment of the antidiabetic drug). Products include:
Humalog Mix 50/50-Pen and KwikPen 1833
Humalog Mix 75/25-Pen and KwikPen 1835

Irbesartan (Co-administration could have additive effect or potentiation). Products include:
Avalide Tablets 892
Avalide Tablets 2713
Avapro Tablets 897
Avapro Tablets 2718

Isoproterenol Hydrochloride (Co-administration could cause possible decreased response to pressor amines but not sufficient to preclude their use).
No products indexed under this heading.

Isoproterenol Sulfate (Co-administration could cause possible decreased response to pressor amines but not sufficient to preclude their use).
No products indexed under this heading.

Isradipine (Co-administration could have additive effect or potentiation). Products include:
DynaCirc CR Controlled Release Tablets 1407

Ketoprofen (In some patients the administration of a non-steroidal anti-inflammatory agent can reduce the diuretic, natriuretic and antihypertensive effects of loop, potassium-sparing and thiazide diuretics).
No products indexed under this heading.

Ketorolac Tromethamine (In some patients the administration of a non-steroidal anti-inflammatory agent can reduce the diuretic, natriuretic and antihypertensive effects of loop, potassium-sparing and thiazide diuretics).
No products indexed under this heading.

Labetalol Hydrochloride (Co-administration could have additive effect or potentiation).
No products indexed under this heading.

Levorphanol Tartrate (Concurrent administration could cause potentiation of orthostatic hypotension).
No products indexed under this heading.

Lisinopril (Co-administration could have additive effect or potentiation). Products include:
Prinivil Tablets 2087
Prinzide Tablets 2092

Lithium (Lithium should not generally be given with diuretics; diuretic agents reduce the renal clearance of lithium and add a high risk of lithium toxicity).
No products indexed under this heading.

Lithium Carbonate (Lithium should not generally be given with diuretics; diuretic agents reduce the renal clearance of lithium and add a high risk of lithium toxicity).
No products indexed under this heading.

Lithium Citrate (Lithium should not generally be given with diuretics; diuretic agents reduce the renal clearance of lithium and add a high risk of lithium toxicity).
No products indexed under this heading.

Losartan Potassium (Co-administration could have additive effect or potentiation). Products include:
Cozaar Tablets ... 1973

Mecamylamine Hydrochloride (Co-administration could have additive effect or potentiation).
No products indexed under this heading.

Meclofenamate Sodium (In some patients the administration of a non-steroidal anti-inflammatory agent can reduce the diuretic, natriuretic and antihypertensive effects of loop, potassium-sparing and thiazide diuretics).
No products indexed under this heading.

Mefenamic Acid (In some patients the administration of a non-steroidal anti-inflammatory agent can reduce the diuretic, natriuretic and antihypertensive effects of loop, potassium-sparing and thiazide diuretics).
No products indexed under this heading.

Meloxicam (In some patients the administration of a non-steroidal anti-inflammatory agent can reduce the diuretic, natriuretic and antihypertensive effects of loop, potassium-sparing and thiazide diuretics). Products include:
Mobic Oral Suspension ... 863
Mobic Tablets ... 863

Meperidine Hydrochloride (Concurrent administration could cause potentiation of orthostatic hypotension).
No products indexed under this heading.

Mephentermine Sulfate (Co-administration could cause possible decreased response to pressor amines but not sufficient to preclude their use).
No products indexed under this heading.

Mephobarbital (Concurrent administration could cause potentiation of orthostatic hypotension).
No products indexed under this heading.

Metaraminol Bitartrate (Co-administration could cause possible decreased response to pressor amines but not sufficient to preclude their use).
No products indexed under this heading.

Metformin Hydrochloride (Co-administration may require a dosage adjustment of the antidiabetic drug). Products include:
ActoPlus Met Tablets ... 3071
Avandamet Tablets ... 1336
Janumet Tablets ... 2041
PrandiMet Tablets ... 2967

Methadone Hydrochloride (Concurrent administration could cause potentiation of orthostatic hypotension).
No products indexed under this heading.

Methoxamine Hydrochloride (Co-administration could cause possible decreased response to pressor amines but not sufficient to preclude their use).
No products indexed under this heading.

Methyclothiazide (Co-administration could have additive effect or potentiation).
No products indexed under this heading.

Methyldopa (Co-administration could have additive effect or potentiation).
No products indexed under this heading.

Methyldopate Hydrochloride (Co-administration could have additive effect or potentiation).
No products indexed under this heading.

Methylprednisolone Acetate (Co-administration could cause intensified electrolyte depletion, particularly hypokalemia).
No products indexed under this heading.

Methylprednisolone Sodium Succinate (Co-administration could cause intensified electrolyte depletion, particularly hypokalemia).
No products indexed under this heading.

Metocurine Iodide (Co-administration could cause possible increased responsiveness to the muscle relaxant).
No products indexed under this heading.

Metolazone (Co-administration could have additive effect or potentiation).
No products indexed under this heading.

Metoprolol Succinate (Co-administration could have additive effect or potentiation). Products include:
Toprol-XL Tablets ... 666

Metoprolol Tartrate (Co-administration could have additive effect or potentiation).
No products indexed under this heading.

Metyrosine (Co-administration could have additive effect or potentiation). Products include:
Demser Capsules ... 1989

Mibefradil Dihydrochloride (Co-administration could have additive effect or potentiation).
No products indexed under this heading.

Miglitol (Co-administration may require a dosage adjustment of the antidiabetic drug).
No products indexed under this heading.

Minoxidil (Co-administration could have additive effect or potentiation).
No products indexed under this heading.

Mivacurium Chloride (Co-administration could cause possible increased responsiveness to the muscle relaxant).
No products indexed under this heading.

Moexipril Hydrochloride (Co-administration could have additive effect or potentiation).
No products indexed under this heading.

Mometasone Furoate (Co-administration could cause intensified electrolyte depletion, particularly hypokalemia). Products include:
Asmanex Twisthaler ... 2797
Elocon Cream 0.1% ... 2840
Elocon Lotion 0.1% ... 2841
Elocon Ointment 0.1% ... 2842

Mometasone Furoate Monohydrate (Co-administration could cause intensified electrolyte depletion, particularly hypokalemia). Products include:
Nasonex Nasal Spray ... 2883

Morphine Sulfate (Concurrent administration could cause potentiation of orthostatic hypotension). Products include:
Avinza Capsules ... 1772
DepoDur Injection ... 1095
MS Contin Tablets ... 2585

Nabumetone (In some patients the administration of a non-steroidal anti-inflammatory agent can reduce the diuretic, natriuretic and antihypertensive effects of loop, potassium-sparing and thiazide diuretics).
No products indexed under this heading.

Nadolol (Co-administration could have additive effect or potentiation). Products include:
Nadolol Tablets ... 2191

Naproxen (In some patients the administration of a non-steroidal anti-inflammatory agent can reduce the diuretic, natriuretic and antihypertensive effects of loop, potassium-sparing and thiazide diuretics). Products include:
EC-Naprosyn Delayed-Release Tablets ... 2632
Naprosyn Suspension ... 2632
Naprosyn Tablets ... 2632

Naproxen Sodium (In some patients the administration of a non-steroidal anti-inflammatory agent can reduce the diuretic, natriuretic and antihypertensive effects of loop, potassium-sparing and thiazide diuretics). Products include:
Anaprox Tablets ... 2632
Anaprox DS Tablets ... 2632
Treximet Tablets ... 1616

Nateglinide (Co-administration may require a dosage adjustment of the antidiabetic drug). Products include:
Starlix Tablets ... 2314

Nebivolol (Co-administration could have additive effect or potentiation). Products include:
Bystolic Tablets ... 1155

Nicardipine Hydrochloride (Co-administration could have additive effect or potentiation). Products include:
Cardene I.V. ... 1093

Nifedipine (Co-administration could have additive effect or potentiation).
No products indexed under this heading.

Nisoldipine (Co-administration could have additive effect or potentiation). Products include:
Sular Extended Release Tablets ... 2975

Nitroglycerin (Co-administration could have additive effect or potentiation). Products include:
Nitro-Dur Transdermal Infusion System ... 2887
Nitrolingual Pumpspray ... 2965

Norepinephrine Bitartrate (Co-administration could cause possible decreased response to pressor amines but not sufficient to preclude their use).
No products indexed under this heading.

Oxaprozin (In some patients the administration of a non-steroidal anti-inflammatory agent can reduce the diuretic, natriuretic and antihypertensive effects of loop, potassium-sparing and thiazide diuretics).
No products indexed under this heading.

Oxycodone Hydrochloride (Concurrent administration could cause potentiation of orthostatic hypotension). Products include:
OxyContin Tablets ... 2589
OxyIR Capsules ... 2593
Percocet Tablets ... 1127
Percodan Tablets ... 1130

Pancuronium Bromide (Co-administration could cause possible increased responsiveness to the muscle relaxant).
No products indexed under this heading.

Penbutolol Sulfate (Co-administration could have additive effect or potentiation).
No products indexed under this heading.

Pentobarbital Sodium (Concurrent administration could cause potentiation of orthostatic hypotension). Products include:
Nembutal Sodium Solution, USP ... 2494

Perindopril Erbumine (Co-administration could have additive effect or potentiation). Products include:
Aceon Tablets (2 mg, 4 mg, 8 mg) ... 3038

Phenobarbital (Concurrent administration could cause potentiation of orthostatic hypotension). Products include:
Donnatal Extentabs ... 2507

Phenoxybenzamine Hydrochloride (Co-administration could have additive effect or potentiation). Products include:
Dibenzyline Capsules ... 3188

Phentolamine Mesylate (Co-administration could have additive effect or potentiation).
No products indexed under this heading.

Phenylbutazone (In some patients the administration of a non-steroidal anti-inflammatory agent can reduce the diuretic, natriuretic and antihypertensive effects of loop, potassium-sparing and thiazide diuretics).
No products indexed under this heading.

Phenylephrine Hydrochloride (Co-administration could cause possible decreased response to pressor amines but not sufficient to preclude their use). Products include:
Actifed Cold & Allergy Tablets ... 1895
Benadryl Allergy & Cold Kapgels ... 1895
Benadryl Allergy & Sinus Headache Kapgels ... 1895
Benadryl Severe Allergy & Sinus Headache Caplets ... 1897
Children's Benadryl-D Allergy & Sinus Liquid ... 1896
Benadryl-D Allergy & Sinus Tablet ... 1896
PediaCare Children's Allergy & Cold Liquid ... 1902
PediaCare Children's Decongestant Liquid ... 1902

PediaCare Children's Liquid Multi-Symptom Cold 1902
Sinutab Non-Drying Caplets 1905
Sinutab Sinus Caplets 1905
Children's Sudafed PE Cold & Cough Liquid 1907
Children's Sudafed PE Nasal Decongestant Liquid 1906
Sudafed PE Cold & Cough Caplets 1907
Sudafed PE Nasal Decongestant Tablets 1907
Sudafed PE Nighttime Cold Caplets 1907
Sudafed PE Non-Drying Sinus Caplets 1908
Sudafed PE Severe Cold Caplets 1908
Sudafed PE Sinus & Allergy Tablets 1908
Sudafed PE Sinus Headache Caplets 1908
Tylenol Allergy Multi-Symptom Caplets with Cool Burst and Rapid Release Gelcaps 1916
Tylenol Allergy Multi-Symptom Nighttime Caplets with Cool Burst 1916
Children's Tylenol Plus Cold Suspension Liquid 1912
Children's Tylenol Plus Cold & Allergy Suspension Liquid 1914
Children's Tylenol Plus Flu Suspension Liquid 1914
Children's Tylenol Plus Multi-Symptom Cold Suspension Liquid 1912
Tylenol Cold Head Congestion Daytime Caplets with Cool Burst 1910
Tylenol Cold Head Congestion Nighttime Caplets with Cool Burst 1910
Tylenol Cold Head Congestion Severe Daytime Caplets with Cool Burst 1910
Tylenol Cold Multi-Symptom Daytime Caplets with Cool Burst and Rapid Release Gels 1913
Tylenol Cold Multi-Symptom Daytime Liquid with Citrus Burst 1913
Tylenol Cold Multi-Symptom Nighttime Caplets with Cool Burst 1913
Tylenol Cold Multi-Symptom Nighttime Liquid with Cool Burst 1913
Tylenol Cold Multi-Symptom Severe Caplets with Cool Burst 1913
Tylenol Cold Multi-Symptom Severe Daytime Liquid with Citrus Burst 1913
Tylenol Sinus Congestion & Pain Daytime Caplets with Cool Burst and Gelcaps 1917
Tylenol Sinus Congestion & Pain Nighttime Caplets with Cool Burst 1917
Tylenol Sinus Congestion & Pain Severe Caplets with Cool Burst 1917
Vicks DayQuil Cold & Flu Multi-Symptom Relief ▣ 616
Vicks DayQuil LiquiCaps 2567
Vicks DayQuil Liquid 2567
Vicks DayQuil Multi-Symptom Cold/Flu Relief 2567

Pindolol (Co-administration could have additive effect or potentiation).
No products indexed under this heading.

Pioglitazone Hydrochloride (Co-administration may require a dosage adjustment of the antidiabetic drug). Products include:
ActoPlus Met Tablets 3071
Actos Tablets 3077
Duetact Tablets 3085

Pipecuronium Bromide (Co-administration could cause possible increased responsiveness to the muscle relaxant).
No products indexed under this heading.

Piroxicam (In some patients the administration of a non-steroidal anti-inflammatory agent can reduce the diuretic, natriuretic and antihypertensive effects of loop, potassium-sparing and thiazide diuretics).
No products indexed under this heading.

Polythiazide (Co-administration could have additive effect or potentiation).
No products indexed under this heading.

Prazosin Hydrochloride (Co-administration could have additive effect or potentiation).
No products indexed under this heading.

Prednisolone Acetate (Co-administration could cause intensified electrolyte depletion, particularly hypokalemia). Products include:
Pred Forte Ophthalmic Suspension ⊙ 227
Pred Mild Ophthalmic Suspension ⊙ 230
Pred-G Ophthalmic Ointment ⊙ 229
Pred-G Ophthalmic Suspension ⊙ 228

Prednisolone Sodium Phosphate (Co-administration could cause intensified electrolyte depletion, particularly hypokalemia).
No products indexed under this heading.

Prednisolone Tebutate (Co-administration could cause intensified electrolyte depletion, particularly hypokalemia).
No products indexed under this heading.

Prednisone (Co-administration could cause intensified electrolyte depletion, particularly hypokalemia).
No products indexed under this heading.

Propoxyphene Hydrochloride (Concurrent administration could cause potentiation of orthostatic hypotension).
No products indexed under this heading.

Propoxyphene Napsylate (Concurrent administration could cause potentiation of orthostatic hypotension).
No products indexed under this heading.

Propranolol Hydrochloride (Co-administration could have additive effect or potentiation). Products include:
InnoPran XL Extended Release Capsules 1484

Quinapril Hydrochloride (Co-administration could have additive effect or potentiation).
No products indexed under this heading.

Ramipril (Co-administration could have additive effect or potentiation).
No products indexed under this heading.

Rapacuronium Bromide (Co-administration could cause possible increased responsiveness to the muscle relaxant).
No products indexed under this heading.

Rauwolfia Serpentina (Co-administration could have additive effect or potentiation).
No products indexed under this heading.

Remifentanil Hydrochloride (Concurrent administration could cause potentiation of orthostatic hypotension).
No products indexed under this heading.

Repaglinide (Co-administration may require a dosage adjustment of the antidiabetic drug). Products include:
PrandiMet Tablets 2967
Prandin Tablets 2971

Rescinnamine (Co-administration could have additive effect or potentiation).
No products indexed under this heading.

Reserpine (Co-administration could have additive effect or potentiation).
No products indexed under this heading.

Rocuronium Bromide (Co-administration could cause possible increased responsiveness to the muscle relaxant). Products include:
Zemuron Injection 2947

Rofecoxib (In some patients the administration of a non-steroidal anti-inflammatory agent can reduce the diuretic, natriuretic and antihypertensive effects of loop, potassium-sparing and thiazide diuretics).
No products indexed under this heading.

Rosiglitazone Maleate (Co-administration may require a dosage adjustment of the antidiabetic drug). Products include:
Avandamet Tablets 1336
Avandaryl Tablets 1344
Avandia Tablets 1351

Secobarbital Sodium (Concurrent administration could cause potentiation of orthostatic hypotension).
No products indexed under this heading.

Sitagliptin Phosphate (Co-administration may require a dosage adjustment of the antidiabetic drug). Products include:
Janumet Tablets 2041
Januvia Tablets 2048

Sodium Nitroprusside (Co-administration could have additive effect or potentiation).
No products indexed under this heading.

Sotalol Hydrochloride (Co-administration could have additive effect or potentiation).
No products indexed under this heading.

Spirapril Hydrochloride (Co-administration could have additive effect or potentiation).
No products indexed under this heading.

Sufentanil Citrate (Concurrent administration could cause potentiation of orthostatic hypotension).
No products indexed under this heading.

Sulindac (In some patients the administration of a non-steroidal anti-inflammatory agent can reduce the diuretic, natriuretic and antihypertensive effects of loop, potassium-sparing and thiazide diuretics). Products include:
Clinoril Tablets 1962

Telmisartan (Co-administration could have additive effect or potentiation). Products include:
Micardis Tablets 852
Micardis HCT Tablets 854

Terazosin Hydrochloride (Co-administration could have additive effect or potentiation).
No products indexed under this heading.

Thiamylal Sodium (Concurrent administration could cause potentiation of orthostatic hypotension).
No products indexed under this heading.

Timolol Maleate (Co-administration could have additive effect or potentiation). Products include:
Combigan Ophthalmic Solution 553
Cosopt Sterile Ophthalmic Solution 1969
Timoptic Sterile Ophthalmic Solution 2121
Timoptic in Ocudose 2124
Timoptic-XE Sterile Ophthalmic Gel Forming Solution 2125

Tolazamide (Co-administration may require a dosage adjustment of the antidiabetic drug).
No products indexed under this heading.

Tolbutamide (Co-administration may require a dosage adjustment of the antidiabetic drug).
No products indexed under this heading.

Tolmetin Sodium (In some patients the administration of a non-steroidal anti-inflammatory agent can reduce the diuretic, natriuretic and antihypertensive effects of loop, potassium-sparing and thiazide diuretics).
No products indexed under this heading.

Torsemide (Co-administration could have additive effect or potentiation). Products include:
Demadex Injection 2630
Demadex Tablets 2630

Trandolapril (Co-administration could have additive effect or potentiation). Products include:
Mavik Tablets 472
Tarka Tablets 511

Triamcinolone (Co-administration could cause intensified electrolyte depletion, particularly hypokalemia).
No products indexed under this heading.

Triamcinolone Acetonide (Co-administration could cause intensified electrolyte depletion, particularly hypokalemia). Products include:
Azmacort Inhalation Aerosol 407
Nasacort AQ Nasal Spray 2765
Triesence Injectable Suspension ⊙ 209

Triamcinolone Diacetate (Co-administration could cause intensified electrolyte depletion, particularly hypokalemia).
No products indexed under this heading.

Triamcinolone Hexacetonide (Co-administration could cause intensified electrolyte depletion, particularly hypokalemia).
No products indexed under this heading.

Trimethaphan Camsylate (Co-administration could have additive effect or potentiation).
No products indexed under this heading.

Troglitazone (Co-administration may require a dosage adjustment of the antidiabetic drug).
No products indexed under this heading.

Tubocurarine Chloride (Co-administration could cause possible increased responsiveness to the muscle relaxant).
No products indexed under this heading.

Valdecoxib (In some patients the administration of a non-steroidal anti-inflammatory agent can reduce the diuretic, natriuretic and antihypertensive effects of loop, potassium-sparing and thiazide diuretics).
No products indexed under this heading.

Valsartan (Co-administration could have additive effect or potentiation). Products include:
Diovan Tablets ... 2212
Diovan HCT Tablets ... 2216
Exforge Tablets ... 2238

Vecuronium Bromide (Co-administration could cause possible increased responsiveness to the muscle relaxant).
No products indexed under this heading.

Verapamil Hydrochloride (Co-administration could have additive effect or potentiation). Products include:
Tarka Tablets ... 511

Food Interactions

Alcohol (Concurrent administration could cause potentiation of orthostatic hypotension).

BENTYL CAPSULES
(Dicyclomine Hydrochloride) ... 703
See Bentyl Tablets

BENTYL INJECTION
(Dicyclomine Hydrochloride) ... 703
See Bentyl Tablets

BENTYL SYRUP
(Dicyclomine Hydrochloride) ... 703
See Bentyl Tablets

BENTYL TABLETS
(Dicyclomine Hydrochloride) ... 703
May interact with agents used to treat achlorhydria and/or to test gastric secretion, antacids, antiglaucoma agents, antihistamines, benzodiazepines, corticosteroids, monoamine oxidase inhibitors, narcotic analgesics, antipsychotic agents, nitrates and nitrites, sympathomimetics, tricyclic antidepressants, type 1 antiarrhythmic drugs, and certain other agents. Compounds in these categories include:

Acetazolamide (Anticholinergics antagonize the effects of antiglaucoma agents).
No products indexed under this heading.

Acetylcholine Chloride (Anticholinergics antagonize the effects of antiglaucoma agents).
No products indexed under this heading.

Acrivastine (Antihistamines may increase certain actions or side effects of anticholinergic agents).
No products indexed under this heading.

Albuterol (Sympathomimetic agents may increase certain actions or side effects of anticholinergic agents).
No products indexed under this heading.

Albuterol Sulfate (Sympathomimetic agents may increase certain actions or side effects of anticholinergic agents). Products include:
Combivent Inhalation Aerosol ... 845
ProAir HFA Inhalation Aerosol ... 3113
Proventil HFA Inhalation Aerosol ... 2914
Ventolin HFA Inhalation Aerosol ... 1638

Alfentanil Hydrochloride (Narcotic analgesics may increase certain actions or side effects of anticholinergic agents).
No products indexed under this heading.

Alprazolam (Benzodiazepines may increase certain actions or side effects of anticholinergic agents).
No products indexed under this heading.

Aluminum Carbonate (Antacids may interfere with the absorption of anticholinergic agents; therefore, simultaneous use of these drugs should be avoided).
No products indexed under this heading.

Aluminum Hydroxide (Antacids may interfere with the absorption of anticholinergic agents; therefore, simultaneous use of these drugs should be avoided).
No products indexed under this heading.

Amantadine Hydrochloride (Amantadine may increase certain actions or side effects of anticholinergic agents).
No products indexed under this heading.

Amitriptyline Hydrochloride (Tricyclic antidepressants may increase certain actions or side effects of anticholinergic agents).
No products indexed under this heading.

Amoxapine (Tricyclic antidepressants may increase certain actions or side effects of anticholinergic agents).
No products indexed under this heading.

Amyl Nitrite (Nitrates and nitrites may increase certain actions or side effects of anticholinergic agents).
No products indexed under this heading.

Aripiprazole (Antipsychotic agents may increase certain actions or side effects of anticholinergic agents). Products include:
Abilify Injection ... 881
Abilify Injection ... 2466
Abilify Oral Solution ... 881
Abilify Oral Solution ... 2466
Abilify Discmelt Orally Disintegrating Tablets ... 881
Abilify Discmelt Orally Disintegrating Tablets ... 2466
Abilify Tablets ... 881
Abilify Tablets ... 2466

Astemizole (Antihistamines may increase certain actions or side effects of anticholinergic agents).
No products indexed under this heading.

Azatadine Maleate (Antihistamines may increase certain actions or side effects of anticholinergic agents).
No products indexed under this heading.

Betamethasone Acetate (Anticholinergic drugs in the presence of increased intraocular pressure may be hazardous when taken concurrently with agents such as corticosteroids).
No products indexed under this heading.

Betamethasone Sodium Phosphate (Anticholinergic drugs in the presence of increased intraocular pressure may be hazardous when taken concurrently with agents such as corticosteroids).
No products indexed under this heading.

Betaxolol Hydrochloride (Anticholinergics antagonize the effects of antiglaucoma agents).
No products indexed under this heading.

Bromodiphenhydramine Hydrochloride (Antihistamines may increase certain actions or side effects of anticholinergic agents).
No products indexed under this heading.

Brompheniramine Maleate (Antihistamines may increase certain actions or side effects of anticholinergic agents).
No products indexed under this heading.

Budesonide (Anticholinergic drugs in the presence of increased intraocular pressure may be hazardous when taken concurrently with agents such as corticosteroids). Products include:
Pulmicort Flexhaler ... 654
Symbicort 80/4.5 Inhalation Aerosol ... 659
Symbicort 160/4.5 Inhalation Aerosol ... 659

Buprenorphine Hydrochloride (Narcotic analgesics may increase certain actions or side effects of anticholinergic agents). Products include:
Suboxone Tablets ... 2601
Subutex Tablets ... 2601

Carbachol (Anticholinergics antagonize the effects of antiglaucoma agents).
No products indexed under this heading.

Cetirizine Hydrochloride (Antihistamines may increase certain actions or side effects of anticholinergic agents). Products include:
Zyrtec Allergy Tablets ... 1919
Zyrtec Chewable Tablets ... 1920
Children's Zyrtec Allergy Chewable Tablets ... 1922
Children's Zyrtec Allergy Syrup ... 1920
Children's Zyrtec Hives Relief Syrup ... 1920
Zyrtec Syrup ... 1920
Zyrtec Tablets ... 1920
Zyrtec-D 12 Hour Extended Release Tablets ... 1923
Zyrtec-D Allergy & Congestion Extended-Release Tablets ... 1923

Chlordiazepoxide (Benzodiazepines may increase certain actions or side effects of anticholinergic agents).
No products indexed under this heading.

Chlordiazepoxide Hydrochloride (Benzodiazepines may increase certain actions or side effects of anticholinergic agents).
No products indexed under this heading.

Chlorpheniramine Maleate (Antihistamines may increase certain actions or side effects of anticholinergic agents). Products include:
Actifed Cold & Allergy Tablets ... 1895
Sudafed PE Sinus & Allergy Tablets ... 1908
Tylenol Allergy Multi-Symptom Caplets with Cool Burst and Rapid Release Gelcaps ... 1916
Children's Tylenol Plus Cold Suspension Liquid ... 1912
Children's Tylenol Plus Cough & Runny Nose Suspension Liquid ... 1912
Children's Tylenol Plus Flu Suspension Liquid ... 1914
Children's Tylenol Plus Multi-Symptom Cold Suspension Liquid ... 1912
Tylenol Cold Head Congestion Nighttime Caplets with Cool Burst ... 1910
Tylenol Cold Multi-Symptom Nighttime Caplets with Cool Burst ... 1913
Tylenol Sinus Congestion & Pain Nighttime Caplets with Cool Burst ... 1917

Chlorpheniramine Polistirex (Antihistamines may increase certain actions or side effects of anticholinergic agents). Products include:
Tussionex Pennkinetic Extended-Release Suspension ... 3154

Chlorpheniramine Tannate (Antihistamines may increase certain actions or side effects of anticholinergic agents).
No products indexed under this heading.

Chlorpromazine (Antipsychotic agents may increase certain actions or side effects of anticholinergic agents).
No products indexed under this heading.

Chlorpromazine Hydrochloride (Antipsychotic agents may increase certain actions or side effects of anticholinergic agents).
No products indexed under this heading.

Chlorprothixene (Antipsychotic agents may increase certain actions or side effects of anticholinergic agents).
No products indexed under this heading.

Chlorprothixene Hydrochloride (Antipsychotic agents may increase certain actions or side effects of anticholinergic agents).
No products indexed under this heading.

Ciclesonide (Anticholinergic drugs in the presence of increased intraocular pressure may be hazardous when taken concurrently with agents such as corticosteroids). Products include:
Alvesco Inhalation Aerosol ... 2985
Omnaris Nasal Spray ... 2998

Cisapride (Anticholinergic drugs may antagonize the effects of drugs that alter gastrointestinal motility).
No products indexed under this heading.

Clemastine Fumarate (Antihistamines may increase certain actions or side effects of anticholinergic agents).
No products indexed under this heading.

Clomipramine Hydrochloride (Tricyclic antidepressants may increase certain actions or side effects of anticholinergic agents).
No products indexed under this heading.

Clorazepate Dipotassium (Benzodiazepines may increase certain actions or side effects of anticholinergic agents).
No products indexed under this heading.

IMPORTANT NOTE: Always consult each drug listing in the patient's regimen for possible interactions.

Clozapine (Antipsychotic agents may increase certain actions or side effects of anticholinergic agents).
No products indexed under this heading.

Codeine Phosphate (Narcotic analgesics may increase certain actions or side effects of anticholinergic agents). Products include:
Tylenol with Codeine Tablets 2427

Cortisone Acetate (Anticholinergic drugs in the presence of increased intraocular pressure may be hazardous when taken concurrently with agents such as corticosteroids).
No products indexed under this heading.

Cyproheptadine Hydrochloride (Antihistamines may increase certain actions or side effects of anticholinergic agents).
No products indexed under this heading.

Demecarium Bromide (Anticholinergics antagonize the effects of antiglaucoma agents).
No products indexed under this heading.

Desipramine Hydrochloride (Tricyclic antidepressants may increase certain actions or side effects of anticholinergic agents).
No products indexed under this heading.

Dexamethasone (Anticholinergic drugs in the presence of increased intraocular pressure may be hazardous when taken concurrently with agents such as corticosteroids). Products include:
Ciprodex Otic Suspension 541

Dexamethasone Acetate (Anticholinergic drugs in the presence of increased intraocular pressure may be hazardous when taken concurrently with agents such as corticosteroids).
No products indexed under this heading.

Dexamethasone Sodium Phosphate (Anticholinergic drugs in the presence of increased intraocular pressure may be hazardous when taken concurrently with agents such as corticosteroids).
No products indexed under this heading.

Dexchlorpheniramine Maleate (Antihistamines may increase certain actions or side effects of anticholinergic agents).
No products indexed under this heading.

Dexpanthenol (Anticholinergic drugs may antagonize the effects of drugs that alter gastrointestinal motility).
No products indexed under this heading.

Dezocine (Narcotic analgesics may increase certain actions or side effects of anticholinergic agents).
No products indexed under this heading.

Diazepam (Benzodiazepines may increase certain actions or side effects of anticholinergic agents). Products include:
Valium Tablets 2658

Dichlorphenamide (Anticholinergics antagonize the effects of antiglaucoma agents).
No products indexed under this heading.

Digoxin (Anticholinergic agents may affect gastrointestinal absorption of various drugs, such as slowly dissolving dosage forms of digoxin; increased serum digoxin concentrations may result). Products include:
Lanoxin Injection 1498
Lanoxin Injection Pediatric 1502
Lanoxin Tablets 1505

Diphenhydramine Citrate (Antihistamines may increase certain actions or side effects of anticholinergic agents).
No products indexed under this heading.

Diphenhydramine Hydrochloride (Antihistamines may increase certain actions or side effects of anticholinergic agents). Products include:
Benadryl Allergy & Cold Kapgels 1895
Benadryl Allergy & Sinus Headache Kapgels 1895
Benadryl Severe Allergy & Sinus Headache Caplets 1897
Benadryl Dye-Free Allergy Liqui-gels Softgels 1897
Benadryl Allergy Kapgels 1895
Benadryl Allergy Quick Dissolve Strips 1896
Benadryl Allergy Ultratab Tablets 1896
Children's Benadryl Dye-Free Allergy Liquid 1897
Children's Benadryl Allergy Fastmelts 1897
Children's Benadryl Allergy Liquid 1898
Children's Benadryl Allergy Perfect Measure 1896
Children's Benadryl-D Allergy & Sinus Liquid 1896
Benadryl-D Allergy & Sinus Tablet 1896
PediaCare Children's Allergy & Cold Liquid 1902
PediaCare Children's Allergy Liquid 1902
Simply Sleep Caplets 1905
Sudafed PE Nighttime Cold Caplets.. 1907
Sudafed PE Severe Cold Caplets 1908
Extra Strength Tylenol PM Caplets, Geltabs, Liquid, and Rapid Release Gels...................... 1915
Tylenol Allergy Multi-Symptom Nighttime Caplets with Cool Burst... 1916
Tylenol Severe Allergy Caplets 1916
Children's Tylenol Plus Cold & Allergy Suspension Liquid 1914
Tylenol Sore Throat Nighttime Liquid with Cool Burst.................. 1918

Diphenylpyraline Hydrochloride (Antihistamines may increase certain actions or side effects of anticholinergic agents).
No products indexed under this heading.

Dipivefrin Hydrochloride (Anticholinergics antagonize the effects of antiglaucoma agents).
No products indexed under this heading.

Disopyramide Phosphate (Class I antiarrhythmic agents may increase certain actions or side effects of anticholinergic agents).
No products indexed under this heading.

Dobutamine Hydrochloride (Sympathomimetic agents may increase certain actions or side effects of anticholinergic agents).
No products indexed under this heading.

Dopamine Hydrochloride (Sympathomimetic agents may increase certain actions or side effects of anticholinergic agents).
No products indexed under this heading.

Doxepin Hydrochloride (Tricyclic antidepressants may increase certain actions or side effects of anticholinergic agents).
No products indexed under this heading.

Echothiophate Iodide (Anticholinergics antagonize the effects of antiglaucoma agents).
No products indexed under this heading.

Ephedrine Hydrochloride (Sympathomimetic agents may increase certain actions or side effects of anticholinergic agents).
No products indexed under this heading.

Ephedrine Sulfate (Sympathomimetic agents may increase certain actions or side effects of anticholinergic agents).
No products indexed under this heading.

Ephedrine Tannate (Sympathomimetic agents may increase certain actions or side effects of anticholinergic agents).
No products indexed under this heading.

Epinephrine (Sympathomimetic agents may increase certain actions or side effects of anticholinergic agents). Products include:
EpiPen 1024

Epinephrine Bitartrate (Sympathomimetic agents may increase certain actions or side effects of anticholinergic agents).
No products indexed under this heading.

Epinephrine Hydrochloride (Sympathomimetic agents may increase certain actions or side effects of anticholinergic agents).
No products indexed under this heading.

Epinephryl Borate (Anticholinergics antagonize the effects of antiglaucoma agents).
No products indexed under this heading.

Erythrityl Tetranitrate (Nitrates and nitrites may increase certain actions or side effects of anticholinergic agents).
No products indexed under this heading.

Estazolam (Benzodiazepines may increase certain actions or side effects of anticholinergic agents).
No products indexed under this heading.

Fentanyl (Narcotic analgesics may increase certain actions or side effects of anticholinergic agents). Products include:
Duragesic Transdermal System 2405
Ionsys Transdermal System 2410

Fentanyl Citrate (Narcotic analgesics may increase certain actions or side effects of anticholinergic agents). Products include:
Actiq 959
Fentora Tablets 968

Fexofenadine Hydrochloride (Antihistamines may increase certain actions or side effects of anticholinergic agents). Products include:
Allegra Oral Solution 2684
Allegra Tablets 2684
Allegra-D 12 Hour Extended-Release Tablets............ 2687
Allegra-D 24 Hour Extended-Release Tablets............ 2690

Fludrocortisone Acetate (Anticholinergic drugs in the presence of increased intraocular pressure may be hazardous when taken concurrently with agents such as corticosteroids).
No products indexed under this heading.

Flunisolide (Anticholinergic drugs in the presence of increased intraocular pressure may be hazardous when taken concurrently with agents such as corticosteroids). Products include:
Aerobid/Aerobid-M 1153

Fluphenazine Decanoate (Antipsychotic agents may increase certain actions or side effects of anticholinergic agents).
No products indexed under this heading.

Fluphenazine Enanthate (Antipsychotic agents may increase certain actions or side effects of anticholinergic agents).
No products indexed under this heading.

Fluphenazine Hydrochloride (Antipsychotic agents may increase certain actions or side effects of anticholinergic agents).
No products indexed under this heading.

Flurazepam Hydrochloride (Benzodiazepines may increase certain actions or side effects of anticholinergic agents).
No products indexed under this heading.

Fluticasone Propionate (Anticholinergic drugs in the presence of increased intraocular pressure may be hazardous when taken concurrently with agents such as corticosteroids). Products include:
Advair Diskus 100/50 1276
Advair Diskus 250/50 1276
Advair Diskus 500/50 1276
Advair HFA 45/21 Inhalation Aerosol... 1288
Advair HFA 115/21 Inhalation Aerosol... 1288
Advair HFA 230/21 Inhalation Aerosol... 1288
Flonase Nasal Spray 1431
Flovent Diskus 50 mcg 1435

Fluticasone Propionate HFA (Anticholinergic drugs in the presence of increased intraocular pressure may be hazardous when taken concurrently with agents such as corticosteroids). Products include:
Flovent HFA 1440

Glutamic Acid Hydrochloride (The inhibiting effects of anticholinergic drugs on gastric hydrochloric acid secretion are antagonized by agents used to treat achlorhydria and those used to test gastric secretion).
No products indexed under this heading.

Halazepam (Benzodiazepines may increase certain actions or side effects of anticholinergic agents).
No products indexed under this heading.

Haloperidol (Antipsychotic agents may increase certain actions or side effects of anticholinergic agents).
No products indexed under this heading.

Haloperidol Decanoate (Antipsychotic agents may increase certain actions or side effects of anticholinergic agents).
No products indexed under this heading.

Hydrocodone Bitartrate (Narcotic analgesics may increase certain actions or side effects of anticholinergic agents). Products include:
Lortab 5/500 Tablets **3143**
Lortab 7.5/500 Tablets **3144**
Lortab 10/500 Tablets **3144**
Vicodin Tablets **529**
Vicodin ES Tablets **530**
Vicodin HP Tablets **531**
Vicoprofen Tablets **533**
Zydone Tablets **1132**

Hydrocodone Polistirex (Narcotic analgesics may increase certain actions or side effects of anticholinergic agents). Products include:
Tussionex Pennkinetic Extended-Release Suspension **3154**

Hydrocortisone (Anticholinergic drugs in the presence of increased intraocular pressure may be hazardous when taken concurrently with agents such as corticosteroids).
No products indexed under this heading.

Hydrocortisone Acetate (Anticholinergic drugs in the presence of increased intraocular pressure may be hazardous when taken concurrently with agents such as corticosteroids). Products include:
Analpram-HC **1140**
Pramosone **1141**

Hydrocortisone Sodium Phosphate (Anticholinergic drugs in the presence of increased intraocular pressure may be hazardous when taken concurrently with agents such as corticosteroids).
No products indexed under this heading.

Hydrocortisone Sodium Succinate (Anticholinergic drugs in the presence of increased intraocular pressure may be hazardous when taken concurrently with agents such as corticosteroids).
No products indexed under this heading.

Hydromorphone Hydrochloride (Narcotic analgesics may increase certain actions or side effects of anticholinergic agents).
No products indexed under this heading.

Imipramine Hydrochloride (Tricyclic antidepressants may increase certain actions or side effects of anticholinergic agents).
No products indexed under this heading.

Imipramine Pamoate (Tricyclic antidepressants may increase certain actions or side effects of anticholinergic agents).
No products indexed under this heading.

Isocarboxazid (MAO inhibitors may increase certain actions or side effects of anticholinergic agents). Products include:
Marplan Tablets **3177**

Isoflurophate (Anticholinergics antagonize the effects of antiglaucoma agents).
No products indexed under this heading.

Isoproterenol Hydrochloride (Sympathomimetic agents may increase certain actions or side effects of anticholinergic agents).
No products indexed under this heading.

Isoproterenol Sulfate (Sympathomimetic agents may increase certain actions or side effects of anticholinergic agents).
No products indexed under this heading.

Isosorbide Dinitrate (Nitrates and nitrites may increase certain actions or side effects of anticholinergic agents).
No products indexed under this heading.

Isosorbide Mononitrate (Nitrates and nitrites may increase certain actions or side effects of anticholinergic agents).
No products indexed under this heading.

Levalbuterol Hydrochloride (Sympathomimetic agents may increase certain actions or side effects of anticholinergic agents). Products include:
Xopenex Inhalation Solution **3001**
Xopenex Inhalation Solution Concentrate **3005**

Levobunolol Hydrochloride (Anticholinergics antagonize the effects of antiglaucoma agents).
No products indexed under this heading.

Levorphanol Tartrate (Narcotic analgesics may increase certain actions or side effects of anticholinergic agents).
No products indexed under this heading.

Lithium Carbonate (Antipsychotic agents may increase certain actions or side effects of anticholinergic agents).
No products indexed under this heading.

Lithium Citrate (Antipsychotic agents may increase certain actions or side effects of anticholinergic agents).
No products indexed under this heading.

Loratadine (Antihistamines may increase certain actions or side effects of anticholinergic agents).
No products indexed under this heading.

Lorazepam (Benzodiazepines may increase certain actions or side effects of anticholinergic agents).
No products indexed under this heading.

Loxapine Hydrochloride (Antipsychotic agents may increase certain actions or side effects of anticholinergic agents).
No products indexed under this heading.

Loxapine Succinate (Antipsychotic agents may increase certain actions or side effects of anticholinergic agents).
No products indexed under this heading.

Magaldrate (Antacids may interfere with the absorption of anticholinergic agents; therefore, simultaneous use of these drugs should be avoided).
No products indexed under this heading.

Magnesium Hydroxide (Antacids may interfere with the absorption of anticholinergic agents; therefore, simultaneous use of these drugs should be avoided). Products include:
Fleet Pedia-Lax Chewable Tablets **1145**
Pepcid Complete Chewable Tablets **1771**
Extra Strength Rolaids Freshmint Tablets **1903**
Rolaids Multi-Symptom Berry Tablets **1903**
Rolaids Original Peppermint Tablets **1903**

Magnesium Oxide (Antacids may interfere with the absorption of anticholinergic agents; therefore, simultaneous use of these drugs should be avoided). Products include:
Beelith Tablets **813**

Maprotiline Hydrochloride (Tricyclic antidepressants may increase certain actions or side effects of anticholinergic agents).
No products indexed under this heading.

Meperidine Hydrochloride (Narcotic analgesics may increase certain actions or side effects of anticholinergic agents).
No products indexed under this heading.

Mesoridazine Besylate (Antipsychotic agents may increase certain actions or side effects of anticholinergic agents).
No products indexed under this heading.

Metaproterenol Sulfate (Sympathomimetic agents may increase certain actions or side effects of anticholinergic agents).
No products indexed under this heading.

Metaraminol Bitartrate (Sympathomimetic agents may increase certain actions or side effects of anticholinergic agents).
No products indexed under this heading.

Methadone Hydrochloride (Narcotic analgesics may increase certain actions or side effects of anticholinergic agents).
No products indexed under this heading.

Methazolamide (Anticholinergics antagonize the effects of antiglaucoma agents).
No products indexed under this heading.

Methdilazine Hydrochloride (Antihistamines may increase certain actions or side effects of anticholinergic agents).
No products indexed under this heading.

Methotrimeprazine (Antipsychotic agents may increase certain actions or side effects of anticholinergic agents).
No products indexed under this heading.

Methoxamine Hydrochloride (Sympathomimetic agents may increase certain actions or side effects of anticholinergic agents).
No products indexed under this heading.

Methylprednisolone Acetate (Anticholinergic drugs in the presence of increased intraocular pressure may be hazardous when taken concurrently with agents such as corticosteroids).
No products indexed under this heading.

Methylprednisolone Sodium Succinate (Anticholinergic drugs in the presence of increased intraocular pressure may be hazardous when taken concurrently with agents such as corticosteroids).
No products indexed under this heading.

Metoclopramide Hydrochloride (Anticholinergic drugs may antagonize the effects of drugs that alter gastrointestinal motility).
No products indexed under this heading.

Midazolam Hydrochloride (Benzodiazepines may increase certain actions or side effects of anticholinergic agents).
No products indexed under this heading.

Moclobemide (MAO inhibitors may increase certain actions or side effects of anticholinergic agents).
No products indexed under this heading.

Molindone Hydrochloride (Antipsychotic agents may increase certain actions or side effects of anticholinergic agents). Products include:
Moban Tablets **1116**

Mometasone Furoate (Anticholinergic drugs in the presence of increased intraocular pressure may be hazardous when taken concurrently with agents such as corticosteroids). Products include:
Asmanex Twisthaler **2797**
Elocon Cream 0.1% **2840**
Elocon Lotion 0.1% **2841**
Elocon Ointment 0.1% **2842**

Mometasone Furoate Monohydrate (Anticholinergic drugs in the presence of increased intraocular pressure may be hazardous when taken concurrently with agents such as corticosteroids). Products include:
Nasonex Nasal Spray **2883**

Moricizine Hydrochloride (Class I antiarrhythmic agents may increase certain actions or side effects of anticholinergic agents).
No products indexed under this heading.

Morphine Sulfate (Narcotic analgesics may increase certain actions or side effects of anticholinergic agents). Products include:
Avinza Capsules **1772**
DepoDur Injection **1095**
MS Contin Tablets **2585**

Nitroglycerin (Nitrates and nitrites may increase certain actions or side effects of anticholinergic agents). Products include:
Nitro-Dur Transdermal Infusion System.. **2887**
Nitrolingual Pumpspray **2965**

Norepinephrine Bitartrate (Sympathomimetic agents may increase certain actions or side effects of anticholinergic agents).
No products indexed under this heading.

Nortriptyline Hydrochloride (Tricyclic antidepressants may increase certain actions or side effects of anticholinergic agents).
No products indexed under this heading.

Olanzapine (Antipsychotic agents may increase certain actions or side effects of anticholinergic agents). Products include:
Symbyax Capsules **1871**
Zyprexa Tablets **1883**
Zyprexa IntraMuscular **1883**
Zyprexa ZYDIS Orally Disintegrating Tablets.................. **1883**

Oxazepam (Benzodiazepines may increase certain actions or side effects of anticholinergic agents).
No products indexed under this heading.

Oxycodone Hydrochloride (Narcotic analgesics may increase certain actions or side effects of anticholinergic agents). Products include:
- OxyContin Tablets 2589
- OxyIR Capsules 2593
- Percocet Tablets 1127
- Percodan Tablets 1130

Paliperidone (Antipsychotic agents may increase certain actions or side effects of anticholinergic agents). Products include:
- Invega Extended-Release Tablets 1748

Pargyline Hydrochloride (MAO inhibitors may increase certain actions or side effects of anticholinergic agents).
No products indexed under this heading.

Pentaerythritol Tetranitrate (Nitrates and nitrites may increase certain actions or side effects of anticholinergic agents).
No products indexed under this heading.

Pentagastrin (The inhibiting effects of anticholinergic drugs on gastric hydrochloric acid secretion are antagonized by agents used to treat achlorhydria and those used to test gastric secretion).
No products indexed under this heading.

Perphenazine (Antipsychotic agents may increase certain actions or side effects of anticholinergic agents).
No products indexed under this heading.

Phenelzine Sulfate (MAO inhibitors may increase certain actions or side effects of anticholinergic agents).
No products indexed under this heading.

Phenylephrine Bitartrate (Sympathomimetic agents may increase certain actions or side effects of anticholinergic agents).
No products indexed under this heading.

Phenylephrine Hydrochloride (Sympathomimetic agents may increase certain actions or side effects of anticholinergic agents). Products include:
- Actifed Cold & Allergy Tablets 1895
- Benadryl Allergy & Cold Kapgels 1895
- Benadryl Allergy & Sinus Headache Kapgels 1895
- Benadryl Severe Allergy & Sinus Headache Caplets 1897
- Children's Benadryl-D Allergy & Sinus Liquid 1896
- Benadryl-D Allergy & Sinus Tablet 1896
- PediaCare Children's Allergy & Cold Liquid 1902
- PediaCare Children's Decongestant Liquid 1902
- PediaCare Children's Liquid Multi-Symptom Cold 1902
- Sinutab Non-Drying Caplets 1905
- Sinutab Sinus Caplets 1905
- Children's Sudafed PE Cold & Cough Liquid 1907
- Children's Sudafed PE Nasal Decongestant Liquid 1906
- Sudafed PE Cold & Cough Caplets 1907
- Sudafed PE Nasal Decongestant Tablets 1907
- Sudafed PE Nighttime Cold Caplets 1907
- Sudafed PE Non-Drying Sinus Caplets 1908
- Sudafed PE Severe Cold Caplets 1908
- Sudafed PE Sinus & Allergy Tablets 1908
- Sudafed PE Sinus Headache Caplets 1908
- Tylenol Allergy Multi-Symptom Caplets with Cool Burst and Rapid Release Gelcaps 1916
- Tylenol Allergy Multi-Symptom Nighttime Caplets with Cool Burst 1916
- Children's Tylenol Plus Cold Suspension Liquid 1912
- Children's Tylenol Plus Cold & Allergy Suspension Liquid 1914
- Children's Tylenol Plus Flu Suspension Liquid 1914
- Children's Tylenol Plus Multi-Symptom Cold Suspension Liquid 1912
- Tylenol Cold Head Congestion Daytime Caplets with Cool Burst 1910
- Tylenol Cold Head Congestion Nighttime Caplets with Cool Burst 1910
- Tylenol Cold Head Congestion Severe Daytime Caplets with Cool Burst 1910
- Tylenol Cold Multi-Symptom Daytime Caplets with Cool Burst and Rapid Release Gels 1913
- Tylenol Cold Multi-Symptom Daytime Liquid with Citrus Burst 1913
- Tylenol Cold Multi-Symptom Nighttime Caplets with Cool Burst 1913
- Tylenol Cold Multi-Symptom Nighttime Liquid with Cool Burst 1913
- Tylenol Cold Multi-Symptom Severe Caplets with Cool Burst 1913
- Tylenol Cold Multi-Symptom Severe Daytime Liquid with Citrus Burst 1913
- Tylenol Sinus Congestion & Pain Daytime Caplets with Cool Burst and Gelcaps 1917
- Tylenol Sinus Congestion & Pain Nighttime Caplets with Cool Burst 1917
- Tylenol Sinus Congestion & Pain Severe Caplets with Cool Burst 1917
- Vicks DayQuil Cold & Flu Multi-Symptom Relief .... ▣616
- Vicks DayQuil LiquiCaps 2567
- Vicks DayQuil Liquid 2567
- Vicks DayQuil Multi-Symptom Cold/Flu Relief 2567

Phenylephrine Tannate (Sympathomimetic agents may increase certain actions or side effects of anticholinergic agents).
No products indexed under this heading.

Phenylpropanolamine Hydrochloride (Sympathomimetic agents may increase certain actions or side effects of anticholinergic agents).
No products indexed under this heading.

Pilocarpine (Anticholinergics antagonize the effects of antiglaucoma agents).
No products indexed under this heading.

Pilocarpine Hydrochloride (Anticholinergics antagonize the effects of antiglaucoma agents). Products include:
- Salagen Tablets 1082

Pimozide (Antipsychotic agents may increase certain actions or side effects of anticholinergic agents).
No products indexed under this heading.

Pirbuterol Acetate (Sympathomimetic agents may increase certain actions or side effects of anticholinergic agents). Products include:
- Maxair Autohaler 1705

Prazepam (Benzodiazepines may increase certain actions or side effects of anticholinergic agents).
No products indexed under this heading.

Prednisolone Acetate (Anticholinergic drugs in the presence of increased intraocular pressure may be hazardous when taken concurrently with agents such as corticosteroids). Products include:
- Pred Forte Ophthalmic Suspension .... ⊙227
- Pred Mild Ophthalmic Suspension .... ⊙230
- Pred-G Ophthalmic Ointment .... ⊙229
- Pred-G Ophthalmic Suspension .... ⊙228

Prednisolone Sodium Phosphate (Anticholinergic drugs in the presence of increased intraocular pressure may be hazardous when taken concurrently with agents such as corticosteroids).
No products indexed under this heading.

Prednisolone Tebutate (Anticholinergic drugs in the presence of increased intraocular pressure may be hazardous when taken concurrently with agents such as corticosteroids).
No products indexed under this heading.

Prednisone (Anticholinergic drugs in the presence of increased intraocular pressure may be hazardous when taken concurrently with agents such as corticosteroids).
No products indexed under this heading.

Procainamide Hydrochloride (Class I antiarrhythmic agents may increase certain actions or side effects of anticholinergic agents).
No products indexed under this heading.

Procarbazine Hydrochloride (MAO inhibitors may increase certain actions or side effects of anticholinergic agents).
No products indexed under this heading.

Prochlorperazine (Antipsychotic agents may increase certain actions or side effects of anticholinergic agents).
No products indexed under this heading.

Promethazine Hydrochloride (Antihistamines may increase certain actions or side effects of anticholinergic agents).
No products indexed under this heading.

Propafenone Hydrochloride (Class I antiarrhythmic agents may increase certain actions or side effects of anticholinergic agents). Products include:
- Rythmol Tablets 1586
- Rythmol SR Capsules 1590

Propoxyphene Hydrochloride (Narcotic analgesics may increase certain actions or side effects of anticholinergic agents).
No products indexed under this heading.

Propoxyphene Napsylate (Narcotic analgesics may increase certain actions or side effects of anticholinergic agents).
No products indexed under this heading.

Protriptyline Hydrochloride (Tricyclic antidepressants may increase certain actions or side effects of anticholinergic agents).
No products indexed under this heading.

Pseudoephedrine Hydrochloride (Sympathomimetic agents may increase certain actions or side effects of anticholinergic agents). Products include:
- Allegra-D 12 Hour Extended-Release Tablets 2687
- Allegra-D 24 Hour Extended-Release Tablets 2690
- Children's Motrin Cold Oral Suspension 1899
- Sudafed 12 Hour Nasal Decongestant Non-Drowsy Caplets 1909
- Sudafed 24 Hour Non-Drowsy Nasal Decongestant Tablets 1906
- Children's Sudafed Nasal Decongestant Liquid 1906
- Sudafed Nasal Decongestant Tablets 1906
- Tylenol Cold Severe Congestion Daytime Caplets with Cool Burst 1912
- Tylenol Sinus Severe Congestion Caplets with Cool Burst 1917
- Vicks NyQuil LiquiCaps 2567
- Vicks NyQuil Liquid 2567
- Vicks NyQuil Multi-Symptom Cold/Flu Relief 2567
- Zyrtec-D 12 Hour Extended Release Tablets 1923
- Zyrtec-D Allergy & Congestion Extended-Release Tablets 1923

Pseudoephedrine Sulfate (Sympathomimetic agents may increase certain actions or side effects of anticholinergic agents). Products include:
- Clarinex-D 12-Hour Extended-Release Tablets 2831
- Clarinex-D 24-Hour Extended-Release Tablets 2834

Pyrilamine Maleate (Antihistamines may increase certain actions or side effects of anticholinergic agents).
No products indexed under this heading.

Pyrilamine Tannate (Antihistamines may increase certain actions or side effects of anticholinergic agents).
No products indexed under this heading.

Quazepam (Benzodiazepines may increase certain actions or side effects of anticholinergic agents).
No products indexed under this heading.

Quetiapine Fumarate (Antipsychotic agents may increase certain actions or side effects of anticholinergic agents).
No products indexed under this heading.

Quinidine Gluconate (Class I antiarrhythmic agents may increase certain actions or side effects of anticholinergic agents).
No products indexed under this heading.

Quinidine Polygalacturonate (Class I antiarrhythmic agents may increase certain actions or side effects of anticholinergic agents).
No products indexed under this heading.

Quinidine Sulfate (Class I antiarrhythmic agents may increase certain actions or side effects of anticholinergic agents).
No products indexed under this heading.

Rasagiline Mesylate (MAO inhibitors may increase certain actions or side effects of anticholinergic agents). Products include:
- Azilect Tablets 3106

Remifentanil Hydrochloride (Narcotic analgesics may increase certain actions or side effects of anticholinergic agents).
No products indexed under this heading.

Risperidone (Antipsychotic agents may increase certain actions or side effects of anticholinergic agents). Products include:
- Risperdal Consta Long-Acting Injection 1753

Salmeterol Xinafoate (Sympathomimetic agents may increase certain actions or side effects of anticholinergic agents). Products include:
- Advair Diskus 100/50 1276
- Advair Diskus 250/50 1276
- Advair Diskus 500/50 1276
- Advair HFA 45/21 Inhalation Aerosol 1288
- Advair HFA 115/21 Inhalation Aerosol 1288
- Advair HFA 230/21 Inhalation Aerosol 1288
- Serevent Diskus 1594

Selegiline (MAO inhibitors may increase certain actions or side effects of anticholinergic agents). Products include:
- Emsam Transdermal System 905

Selegiline Hydrochloride (MAO inhibitors may increase certain actions or side effects of anticholinergic agents). Products include:
- Eldepryl Capsules 3052

Sodium Bicarbonate (Antacids may interfere with the absorption of anticholinergic agents; therefore, simultaneous use of these drugs should be avoided). Products include:
- Ceo-Two Laxative Suppository 815

Sufentanil Citrate (Narcotic analgesics may increase certain actions or side effects of anticholinergic agents).
No products indexed under this heading.

Temazepam (Benzodiazepines may increase certain actions or side effects of anticholinergic agents).
No products indexed under this heading.

Terbutaline Sulfate (Sympathomimetic agents may increase certain actions or side effects of anticholinergic agents).
No products indexed under this heading.

Terfenadine (Antihistamines may increase certain actions or side effects of anticholinergic agents).
No products indexed under this heading.

Thioridazine Hydrochloride (Antipsychotic agents may increase certain actions or side effects of anticholinergic agents). Products include:
- Thioridazine Hydrochloride Tablets 2195

Thiothixene (Antipsychotic agents may increase certain actions or side effects of anticholinergic agents). Products include:
- Thiothixene Capsules 2197

Timolol Maleate (Anticholinergics antagonize the effects of antiglaucoma agents). Products include:
- Combigan Ophthalmic Solution 553
- Cosopt Sterile Ophthalmic Solution 1969
- Timoptic Sterile Ophthalmic Solution 2121
- Timoptic in Ocudose 2124
- Timoptic-XE Sterile Ophthalmic Gel Forming Solution 2125

Tranylcypromine Sulfate (MAO inhibitors may increase certain actions or side effects of anticholinergic agents). Products include:
- Parnate Tablets 1532

Triamcinolone (Anticholinergic drugs in the presence of increased intraocular pressure may be hazardous when taken concurrently with agents such as corticosteroids).
No products indexed under this heading.

Triamcinolone Acetonide (Anticholinergic drugs in the presence of increased intraocular pressure may be hazardous when taken concurrently with agents such as corticosteroids). Products include:
- Azmacort Inhalation Aerosol 407
- Nasacort AQ Nasal Spray 2765
- Triesence Injectable Suspension .... ⊙ 209

Triamcinolone Diacetate (Anticholinergic drugs in the presence of increased intraocular pressure may be hazardous when taken concurrently with agents such as corticosteroids).
No products indexed under this heading.

Triamcinolone Hexacetonide (Anticholinergic drugs in the presence of increased intraocular pressure may be hazardous when taken concurrently with agents such as corticosteroids).
No products indexed under this heading.

Triazolam (Benzodiazepines may increase certain actions or side effects of anticholinergic agents).
No products indexed under this heading.

Trifluoperazine Hydrochloride (Antipsychotic agents may increase certain actions or side effects of anticholinergic agents).
No products indexed under this heading.

Trimeprazine Tartrate (Antihistamines may increase certain actions or side effects of anticholinergic agents).
No products indexed under this heading.

Trimipramine Maleate (Tricyclic antidepressants may increase certain actions or side effects of anticholinergic agents).
No products indexed under this heading.

Tripelennamine Hydrochloride (Antihistamines may increase certain actions or side effects of anticholinergic agents).
No products indexed under this heading.

Triprolidine Hydrochloride (Antihistamines may increase certain actions or side effects of anticholinergic agents).
No products indexed under this heading.

Ziprasidone Hydrochloride (Antipsychotic agents may increase certain actions or side effects of anticholinergic agents). Products include:
- Geodon Capsules 2520

BENZACLIN TOPICAL GEL

(Benzoyl Peroxide, Clindamycin Phosphate) 2721
May interact with peeling/desquamating agents and certain other agents. Compounds in these categories include:

Acitretin (Concomitant topical acne therapy should be used with caution because a possible cumulative irritancy may occur, especially with the use of peeling, desquamating or abrasive agents). Products include:
- Soriatane Capsules 3062

Adapalene (Concomitant topical acne therapy should be used with caution because a possible cumulative irritancy may occur, especially with the use of peeling, desquamating or abrasive agents).
No products indexed under this heading.

Azelaic Acid (Concomitant topical acne therapy should be used with caution because a possible cumulative irritancy may occur, especially with the use of peeling, desquamating or abrasive agents). Products include:
- Finacea Gel 1742

Calcipotriene (Concomitant topical acne therapy should be used with caution because a possible cumulative irritancy may occur, especially with the use of peeling, desquamating or abrasive agents).
No products indexed under this heading.

Clindamycin, Topical (Concomitant topical acne therapy should be used with caution because a possible cumulative irritancy may occur, especially with the use of peeling, desquamating or abrasive agents).
No products indexed under this heading.

Clotrimazole, Topical (Concomitant topical acne therapy should be used with caution because a possible cumulative irritancy may occur, especially with the use of peeling, desquamating or abrasive agents).
No products indexed under this heading.

Coal Tar (Concomitant topical acne therapy should be used with caution because a possible cumulative irritancy may occur, especially with the use of peeling, desquamating or abrasive agents).
No products indexed under this heading.

Concomitant Topical Acne Therapy (Possible cumulative irritancy effect may occur, especially with the use of peeling, desquamating, or abrasive agents).
No products indexed under this heading.

Erythromycin, Topical (Concomitant topical acne therapy should be used with caution because a possible cumulative irritancy may occur, especially with the use of peeling, desquamating or abrasive agents).
No products indexed under this heading.

Fluorouracil, Topical (Concomitant topical acne therapy should be used with caution because a possible cumulative irritancy may occur, especially with the use of peeling, desquamating or abrasive agents).
No products indexed under this heading.

Hydroquinone (Concomitant topical acne therapy should be used with caution because a possible cumulative irritancy may occur, especially with the use of peeling, desquamating or abrasive agents).
No products indexed under this heading.

Isotretinoin (Concomitant topical acne therapy should be used with caution because a possible cumulative irritancy may occur, especially with the use of peeling, desquamating or abrasive agents). Products include:
- Accutane Capsules 2607

Mequinol (Concomitant topical acne therapy should be used with caution because a possible cumulative irritancy may occur, especially with the use of peeling, desquamating or abrasive agents).
No products indexed under this heading.

Podofilox (Concomitant topical acne therapy should be used with caution because a possible cumulative irritancy may occur, especially with the use of peeling, desquamating or abrasive agents).
No products indexed under this heading.

Salicylic Acid (Concomitant topical acne therapy should be used with caution because a possible cumulative irritancy may occur, especially with the use of peeling, desquamating or abrasive agents).
No products indexed under this heading.

Sulfur Preparations (Concomitant topical acne therapy should be used with caution because a possible cumulative irritancy may occur, especially with the use of peeling, desquamating or abrasive agents).
No products indexed under this heading.

Tazarotene (Concomitant topical acne therapy should be used with caution because a possible cumulative irritancy may occur, especially with the use of peeling, desquamating or abrasive agents).
No products indexed under this heading.

Tretinoin (Concomitant topical acne therapy should be used with caution because a possible cumulative irritancy may occur, especially with the use of peeling, desquamating or abrasive agents). Products include:
- Vesanoid Capsules 2660
- Ziana Gel 1942

Zalcitabine (Concomitant topical acne therapy should be used with caution because a possible cumulative irritancy may occur, especially with the use of peeling, desquamating or abrasive agents).
No products indexed under this heading.

BETADINE 5% OPHTHALMIC SOLUTION

(Povidone Iodine) .... ⊙202
None cited in PDR database.

BETASERON FOR SC INJECTION

(Interferon Beta-1b) 756
None cited in PDR database.

BETIMOL OPHTHALMIC SOLUTION

(Timolol Hemihydrate) 3181
May interact with beta blockers, calcium channel blockers, cardiac glycosides, and certain other agents. Compounds in these categories include:

Acebutolol Hydrochloride (Concurrent use with systemic beta blockers may result in additive effect either on the intraocular pressure or the known systemic effect of beta blockade).
No products indexed under this heading.

Amlodipine Besylate (Possible atrioventricular conduction disturbances, left ventricular failure, and hypotension). Products include:

Azor Tablets 1005
Exforge Tablets 2238

Atenolol (Concurrent use with systemic beta blockers may result in additive effect either on the intraocular pressure or the known systemic effect of beta blockade).
No products indexed under this heading.

Bepridil Hydrochloride (Possible atrioventricular conduction disturbances, left ventricular failure, and hypotension).
No products indexed under this heading.

Betaxolol Hydrochloride (Concurrent use with systemic beta blockers may result in additive effect either on the intraocular pressure or the known systemic effect of beta blockade).
No products indexed under this heading.

Bisoprolol Fumarate (Concurrent use with systemic beta blockers may result in additive effect either on the intraocular pressure or the known systemic effect of beta blockade).
No products indexed under this heading.

Carteolol Hydrochloride (Concurrent use with systemic beta blockers may result in additive effect either on the intraocular pressure or the known systemic effect of beta blockade).
No products indexed under this heading.

Deslanoside (Concomitant use of beta blockers with digitalis and calcium antagonists may have additive effects in prolonging atrioventricular conduction time).
No products indexed under this heading.

Digitalis Glycoside Preparations (Concomitant use of beta blockers with digitalis and calcium antagonists may have additive effects in prolonging atrioventricular conduction time).
No products indexed under this heading.

Digitoxin (Concomitant use of beta blockers with digitalis and calcium antagonists may have additive effects in prolonging atrioventricular conduction time).
No products indexed under this heading.

Digoxin (Concomitant use of beta blockers with digitalis and calcium antagonists may have additive effects in prolonging atrioventricular conduction time). Products include:
Lanoxin Injection 1498
Lanoxin Injection Pediatric 1502
Lanoxin Tablets 1505

Diltiazem Hydrochloride (Possible atrioventricular conduction disturbances, left ventricular failure, and hypotension). Products include:
Cardizem LA Extended Release Tablets 421

Epinephrine (Patients with a history of atopy or anaphylactic reactions to a variety of allergens may be unresponsive to the usual dose of injectable epinephrine used to treat allergic reactions). Products include:
EpiPen 1024

Epinephrine Bitartrate (Patients with a history of atopy or anaphylactic reactions to a variety of allergens may be unresponsive to the usual dose of injectable epinephrine used to treat allergic reactions).
No products indexed under this heading.

Esmolol Hydrochloride (Concurrent use with systemic beta blockers may result in additive effect either on the intraocular pressure or the known systemic effect of beta blockade).
No products indexed under this heading.

Felodipine (Possible atrioventricular conduction disturbances, left ventricular failure, and hypotension).
No products indexed under this heading.

Isradipine (Possible atrioventricular conduction disturbances, left ventricular failure, and hypotension). Products include:
DynaCirc CR Controlled Release Tablets 1407

Labetalol Hydrochloride (Concurrent use with systemic beta blockers may result in additive effect either on the intraocular pressure or the known systemic effect of beta blockade).
No products indexed under this heading.

Levobunolol Hydrochloride (Concurrent use with systemic beta blockers may result in additive effect either on the intraocular pressure or the known systemic effect of beta blockade).
No products indexed under this heading.

Metipranolol Hydrochloride (Concurrent use with systemic beta blockers may result in additive effect either on the intraocular pressure or the known systemic effect of beta blockade).
No products indexed under this heading.

Metoprolol Succinate (Concurrent use with systemic beta blockers may result in additive effect either on the intraocular pressure or the known systemic effect of beta blockade). Products include:
Toprol-XL Tablets 666

Metoprolol Tartrate (Concurrent use with systemic beta blockers may result in additive effect either on the intraocular pressure or the known systemic effect of beta blockade).
No products indexed under this heading.

Mibefradil Dihydrochloride (Possible atrioventricular conduction disturbances, left ventricular failure, and hypotension).
No products indexed under this heading.

Nadolol (Concurrent use with systemic beta blockers may result in additive effect either on the intraocular pressure or the known systemic effect of beta blockade). Products include:
Nadolol Tablets 2191

Nebivolol (Concurrent use with systemic beta blockers may result in additive effect either on the intraocular pressure or the known systemic effect of beta blockade). Products include:
Bystolic Tablets 1155

Nicardipine Hydrochloride (Possible atrioventricular conduction disturbances, left ventricular failure, and hypotension). Products include:
Cardene I.V. 1093

Nifedipine (Possible atrioventricular conduction disturbances, left ventricular failure, and hypotension).
No products indexed under this heading.

Nimodipine (Possible atrioventricular conduction disturbances, left ventricular failure, and hypotension). Products include:
Nimotop Capsules 790

Nisoldipine (Possible atrioventricular conduction disturbances, left ventricular failure, and hypotension). Products include:
Sular Extended Release Tablets 2975

Penbutolol Sulfate (Concurrent use with systemic beta blockers may result in additive effect either on the intraocular pressure or the known systemic effect of beta blockade).
No products indexed under this heading.

Pindolol (Concurrent use with systemic beta blockers may result in additive effect either on the intraocular pressure or the known systemic effect of beta blockade).
No products indexed under this heading.

Propranolol Hydrochloride (Concurrent use with systemic beta blockers may result in additive effect either on the intraocular pressure or the known systemic effect of beta blockade). Products include:
InnoPran XL Extended Release Capsules 1484

Sotalol Hydrochloride (Concurrent use with systemic beta blockers may result in additive effect either on the intraocular pressure or the known systemic effect of beta blockade).
No products indexed under this heading.

Timolol Maleate (Concurrent use with systemic beta blockers may result in additive effect either on the intraocular pressure or the known systemic effect of beta blockade). Products include:
Combigan Ophthalmic Solution 553
Cosopt Sterile Ophthalmic Solution 1969
Timoptic Sterile Ophthalmic Solution 2121
Timoptic in Ocudose 2124
Timoptic-XE Sterile Ophthalmic Gel Forming Solution 2125

Verapamil Hydrochloride (Possible atrioventricular conduction disturbances, left ventricular failure, and hypotension). Products include:
Tarka Tablets 511

BEVITAMEL TABLETS
(Folic Acid, Melatonin, Vitamin B_{12}) 3190
None cited in PDR database.

BEXXAR
(Iodine I 131 Tositumomab, Tositumomab)................................... 1371
May interact with anticoagulants, oral anticoagulants, and platelet inhibitors. Compounds in these categories include:

Anisindione (Due to the frequent occurrence of severe and prolonged thrombocytopenia, the potential benefits of medications that interfere with platelet function and/or anticoagulation should be weighed against the potential increased risk of bleeding and hemorrhage).
No products indexed under this heading.

Ardeparin Sodium (Due to the frequent occurrence of severe and prolonged thrombocytopenia, the potential benefits of medications that interfere with platelet function and/or anticoagulation should be weighed against the potential increased risk of bleeding and hemorrhage).
No products indexed under this heading.

Aspirin (Due to the frequent occurrence of severe and prolonged thrombocytopenia, the potential benefits of medications that interfere with platelet function and/or anticoagulation should be weighed against the potential increased risk of bleeding and hemorrhage). Products include:
Aggrenox Capsules 819
Bayer Aspirin 750
Percodan Tablets 1130
St. Joseph 81 mg Aspirin Chewable and Enteric Coated Tablets 1903

Aspirin, Enteric Coated (Due to the frequent occurrence of severe and prolonged thrombocytopenia, the potential benefits of medications that interfere with platelet function and/or anticoagulation should be weighed against the potential increased risk of bleeding and hemorrhage).
No products indexed under this heading.

Aspirin Buffered (Due to the frequent occurrence of severe and prolonged thrombocytopenia, the potential benefits of medications that interfere with platelet function and/or anticoagulation should be weighed against the potential increased risk of bleeding and hemorrhage).
No products indexed under this heading.

Azlocillin Sodium (Due to the frequent occurrence of severe and prolonged thrombocytopenia, the potential benefits of medications that interfere with platelet function and/or anticoagulation should be weighed against the potential increased risk of bleeding and hemorrhage).
No products indexed under this heading.

Carbenicillin Indanyl Sodium (Due to the frequent occurrence of severe and prolonged thrombocytopenia, the potential benefits of medications that interfere with platelet function and/or anticoagulation should be weighed against the potential increased risk of bleeding and hemorrhage).
No products indexed under this heading.

Choline Magnesium Trisalicylate (Due to the frequent occurrence of severe and prolonged thrombocytopenia, the potential benefits of medications that interfere with platelet function and/or anticoagulation should be weighed against the potential increased risk of bleeding and hemorrhage).
No products indexed under this heading.

Clopidogrel Bisulfate (Due to the frequent occurrence of severe and prolonged thrombocytopenia, the potential benefits of medications that interfere with platelet function and/or anticoagulation should be

weighed against the potential increased risk of bleeding and hemorrhage). Products include:

Plavix Tablets ... 926
Plavix Tablets ... 2767

Dalteparin Sodium (Due to the frequent occurrence of severe and prolonged thrombocytopenia, the potential benefits of medications that interfere with platelet function and/or anticoagulation should be weighed against the potential increased risk of bleeding and hemorrhage). Products include:

Fragmin Injection ... 1070

Danaparoid Sodium (Due to the frequent occurrence of severe and prolonged thrombocytopenia, the potential benefits of medications that interfere with platelet function and/or anticoagulation should be weighed against the potential increased risk of bleeding and hemorrhage).

No products indexed under this heading.

Diclofenac Potassium (Due to the frequent occurrence of severe and prolonged thrombocytopenia, the potential benefits of medications that interfere with platelet function and/or anticoagulation should be weighed against the potential increased risk of bleeding and hemorrhage).

No products indexed under this heading.

Diclofenac Sodium (Due to the frequent occurrence of severe and prolonged thrombocytopenia, the potential benefits of medications that interfere with platelet function and/or anticoagulation should be weighed against the potential increased risk of bleeding and hemorrhage). Products include:

Diclofenac Sodium Ophthalmic Solution ... ⊙ 240
Voltaren Ophthalmic Solution ... 2336
Voltaren Tablets ... 2334
Voltaren-XR Tablets ... 2337

Dicumarol (Due to the frequent occurrence of severe and prolonged thrombocytopenia, the potential benefits of medications that interfere with platelet function and/or anticoagulation should be weighed against the potential increased risk of bleeding and hemorrhage).

No products indexed under this heading.

Diflunisal (Due to the frequent occurrence of severe and prolonged thrombocytopenia, the potential benefits of medications that interfere with platelet function and/or anticoagulation should be weighed against the potential increased risk of bleeding and hemorrhage).

No products indexed under this heading.

Dipyridamole (Due to the frequent occurrence of severe and prolonged thrombocytopenia, the potential benefits of medications that interfere with platelet function and/or anticoagulation should be weighed against the potential increased risk of bleeding and hemorrhage). Products include:

Aggrenox Capsules ... 819
Persantine Tablets ... 869

Enoxaparin Sodium (Due to the frequent occurrence of severe and prolonged thrombocytopenia, the potential benefits of medications that interfere with platelet function and/or anticoagulation should be weighed against the potential increased risk of bleeding and hemorrhage). Products include:

Lovenox Injection ... 2756

Fenoprofen Calcium (Due to the frequent occurrence of severe and prolonged thrombocytopenia, the potential benefits of medications that interfere with platelet function and/or anticoagulation should be weighed against the potential increased risk of bleeding and hemorrhage). Products include:

Nalfon Capsules ... 2508

Flurbiprofen (Due to the frequent occurrence of severe and prolonged thrombocytopenia, the potential benefits of medications that interfere with platelet function and/or anticoagulation should be weighed against the potential increased risk of bleeding and hemorrhage).

No products indexed under this heading.

Fondaparinux Sodium (Due to the frequent occurrence of severe and prolonged thrombocytopenia, the potential benefits of medications that interfere with platelet function and/or anticoagulation should be weighed against the potential increased risk of bleeding and hemorrhage). Products include:

Arixtra Injection ... 1313

Heparin Calcium (Due to the frequent occurrence of severe and prolonged thrombocytopenia, the potential benefits of medications that interfere with platelet function and/or anticoagulation should be weighed against the potential increased risk of bleeding and hemorrhage).

No products indexed under this heading.

Heparin Sodium (Due to the frequent occurrence of severe and prolonged thrombocytopenia, the potential benefits of medications that interfere with platelet function and/or anticoagulation should be weighed against the potential increased risk of bleeding and hemorrhage).

No products indexed under this heading.

Ibuprofen (Due to the frequent occurrence of severe and prolonged thrombocytopenia, the potential benefits of medications that interfere with platelet function and/or anticoagulation should be weighed against the potential increased risk of bleeding and hemorrhage). Products include:

Motrin IB Tablets and Caplets ... 1900
Children's Motrin Oral Suspension ... 1901
Children's Motrin Non-Staining Dye-Free Oral Suspension ... 1901
Children's Motrin Cold Oral Suspension ... 1899
Infants' Motrin Concentrated Drops ... 1901
Infants' Motrin Non-Staining Dye-Free Concentrated Drops ... 1901
Junior Strength Motrin Caplets and Chewable Tablets ... 1901
Vicoprofen Tablets ... 533

Indomethacin (Due to the frequent occurrence of severe and prolonged thrombocytopenia, the potential benefits of medications that interfere with platelet function and/or anticoagulation should be weighed against the potential increased risk of bleeding and hemorrhage). Products include:

Indocin ... 2024

Indomethacin Sodium Trihydrate (Due to the frequent occurrence of severe and prolonged thrombocytopenia, the potential benefits of medications that interfere with platelet function and/or anticoagulation should be weighed against the potential increased risk of bleeding and hemorrhage). Products include:

Indocin I.V. ... 2489

Ketoprofen (Due to the frequent occurrence of severe and prolonged thrombocytopenia, the potential benefits of medications that interfere with platelet function and/or anticoagulation should be weighed against the potential increased risk of bleeding and hemorrhage).

No products indexed under this heading.

Low Molecular Weight Heparins (Due to the frequent occurrence of severe and prolonged thrombocytopenia, the potential benefits of medications that interfere with platelet function and/or anticoagulation should be weighed against the potential increased risk of bleeding and hemorrhage).

No products indexed under this heading.

Magnesium Salicylate (Due to the frequent occurrence of severe and prolonged thrombocytopenia, the potential benefits of medications that interfere with platelet function and/or anticoagulation should be weighed against the potential increased risk of bleeding and hemorrhage).

No products indexed under this heading.

Meclofenamate Sodium (Due to the frequent occurrence of severe and prolonged thrombocytopenia, the potential benefits of medications that interfere with platelet function and/or anticoagulation should be weighed against the potential increased risk of bleeding and hemorrhage).

No products indexed under this heading.

Mefenamic Acid (Due to the frequent occurrence of severe and prolonged thrombocytopenia, the potential benefits of medications that interfere with platelet function and/or anticoagulation should be weighed against the potential increased risk of bleeding and hemorrhage).

No products indexed under this heading.

Mezlocillin Sodium (Due to the frequent occurrence of severe and prolonged thrombocytopenia, the potential benefits of medications that interfere with platelet function and/or anticoagulation should be weighed against the potential increased risk of bleeding and hemorrhage).

No products indexed under this heading.

Nafcillin Sodium (Due to the frequent occurrence of severe and prolonged thrombocytopenia, the potential benefits of medications that interfere with platelet function and/or anticoagulation should be weighed against the potential increased risk of bleeding and hemorrhage).

No products indexed under this heading.

Naproxen (Due to the frequent occurrence of severe and prolonged thrombocytopenia, the potential benefits of medications that interfere with platelet function and/or anticoagulation should be weighed against the potential increased risk of bleeding and hemorrhage). Products include:

EC-Naprosyn Delayed-Release Tablets ... 2632
Naprosyn Suspension ... 2632
Naprosyn Tablets ... 2632

Naproxen Sodium (Due to the frequent occurrence of severe and prolonged thrombocytopenia, the potential benefits of medications that interfere with platelet function and/or anticoagulation should be weighed against the potential increased risk of bleeding and hemorrhage). Products include:

Anaprox Tablets ... 2632
Anaprox DS Tablets ... 2632
Treximet Tablets ... 1616

Penicillin G Benzathine (Due to the frequent occurrence of severe and prolonged thrombocytopenia, the potential benefits of medications that interfere with platelet function and/or anticoagulation should be weighed against the potential increased risk of bleeding and hemorrhage). Products include:

Bicillin C-R Injectable Suspension ... 1775
Bicillin L-A Injection ... 1777

Penicillin G Procaine (Due to the frequent occurrence of severe and prolonged thrombocytopenia, the potential benefits of medications that interfere with platelet function and/or anticoagulation should be weighed against the potential increased risk of bleeding and hemorrhage). Products include:

Bicillin C-R Injectable Suspension ... 1775
Bicillin L-A Injection ... 1777

Phenylbutazone (Due to the frequent occurrence of severe and prolonged thrombocytopenia, the potential benefits of medications that interfere with platelet function and/or anticoagulation should be weighed against the potential increased risk of bleeding and hemorrhage).

No products indexed under this heading.

Piroxicam (Due to the frequent occurrence of severe and prolonged thrombocytopenia, the potential benefits of medications that interfere with platelet function and/or anticoagulation should be weighed against the potential increased risk of bleeding and hemorrhage).

No products indexed under this heading.

Salsalate (Due to the frequent occurrence of severe and prolonged thrombocytopenia, the potential benefits of medications that interfere with platelet function and/or anticoagulation should be weighed against the potential increased risk of bleeding and hemorrhage).

No products indexed under this heading.

Sulindac (Due to the frequent occurrence of severe and prolonged thrombocytopenia, the potential benefits of medications that interfere with platelet function and/or anticoagulation should be weighed against the potential increased risk of bleeding and hemorrhage). Products include:

Clinoril Tablets ... 1962

Ticarcillin Disodium (Due to the frequent occurrence of severe and prolonged thrombocytopenia, the potential benefits of medications that interfere with platelet function and/ or anticoagulation should be weighed against the potential increased risk of bleeding and hemorrhage). Products include:

Timentin ADD-Vantage 1606
Timentin Injection Galaxy Container 1609
Timentin IV Infusion 1603
Timentin Pharmacy Bulk Package 1613

Ticlopidine Hydrochloride (Due to the frequent occurrence of severe and prolonged thrombocytopenia, the potential benefits of medications that interfere with platelet function and/or anticoagulation should be weighed against the potential increased risk of bleeding and hemorrhage).

No products indexed under this heading.

Tinzaparin Sodium (Due to the frequent occurrence of severe and prolonged thrombocytopenia, the potential benefits of medications that interfere with platelet function and/ or anticoagulation should be weighed against the potential increased risk of bleeding and hemorrhage).

No products indexed under this heading.

Tolmetin Sodium (Due to the frequent occurrence of severe and prolonged thrombocytopenia, the potential benefits of medications that interfere with platelet function and/ or anticoagulation should be weighed against the potential increased risk of bleeding and hemorrhage).

No products indexed under this heading.

Warfarin Sodium (Due to the frequent occurrence of severe and prolonged thrombocytopenia, the potential benefits of medications that interfere with platelet function and/ or anticoagulation should be weighed against the potential increased risk of bleeding and hemorrhage).

No products indexed under this heading.

BIAXIN FILMTAB TABLETS

(Clarithromycin) 411

May interact with oral anticoagulants, cytochrome p450 3a4 substrates (selected), HMG-CoA reductase inhibitors, oral hypoglycemic agents, insulin, phenytoin, quinidine, valproate, xanthines, and certain other agents. Compounds in these categories include:

Acarbose (Clarithromycin, in rare cases, causes hypoglycemia, some of which have occurred in patients taking oral hypoglycemic agents). Products include:

Precose Tablets 792

Alfentanil Hydrochloride (Concurrent use of erythromycin and/or clarithromycin in patients receiving drugs metabolized by the cytochrome P450 system may be associated with elevation in serum levels of alfentanil).

No products indexed under this heading.

Alprazolam (Co-administration of erythromycin or clarithromycin and a drug primarily metabolized by CYP3A may be associated with elevation in drug concentrations that could increase or prolong both the therapeutic and adverse effects of the concomitant drug).

No products indexed under this heading.

Aminophylline (Co-administration in patients who are receiving high doses of theophylline may be associated with an increase in serum theophylline levels and potential theophylline toxicity).

No products indexed under this heading.

Amiodarone Hydrochloride (Co-administration of erythromycin or clarithromycin and a drug primarily metabolized by CYP3A may be associated with elevation in drug concentrations that could increase or prolong both the therapeutic and adverse effects of the concomitant drug).

No products indexed under this heading.

Amitriptyline Hydrochloride (Co-administration of erythromycin or clarithromycin and a drug primarily metabolized by CYP3A may be associated with elevation in drug concentrations that could increase or prolong both the therapeutic and adverse effects of the concomitant drug).

No products indexed under this heading.

Amlodipine Besylate (Co-administration of erythromycin or clarithromycin and a drug primarily metabolized by CYP3A may be associated with elevation in drug concentrations that could increase or prolong both the therapeutic and adverse effects of the concomitant drug). Products include:

Azor Tablets 1005
Exforge Tablets 2238

Anisindione (Co-administration may result in the potentiation of oral anticoagulant effects).

No products indexed under this heading.

Aprepitant (Co-administration of erythromycin or clarithromycin and a drug primarily metabolized by CYP3A may be associated with elevation in drug concentrations that could increase or prolong both the therapeutic and adverse effects of the concomitant drug). Products include:

Emend Capsules 1992

Astemizole (Concurrent use of erythromycin in patients receiving astemizole has resulted in prolonged QT interval and torsade de pointes; because clarithromycin is metabolized by P450, co-administration is contraindicated).

No products indexed under this heading.

Atorvastatin Calcium (Co-administration of erythromycin or clarithromycin and a drug primarily metabolized by CYP3A may be associated with elevation in drug concentrations that could increase or prolong both the therapeutic and adverse effects of the concomitant drug). Products include:

Lipitor Tablets 2501

Belladonna Ergotamine (Co-administration of erythromycin or clarithromycin and a drug primarily metabolized by CYP3A may be associated with elevation in drug concentrations that could increase or prolong both the therapeutic and adverse effects of the concomitant drug).

No products indexed under this heading.

Bromocriptine Mesylate (Concurrent use of erythromycin and/or clarithromycin in patients receiving drugs metabolized by the cytochrome P450 system may be associated with elevation in serum levels of bromocriptine).

No products indexed under this heading.

Buspirone Hydrochloride (Co-administration of erythromycin or clarithromycin and a drug primarily metabolized by CYP3A may be associated with elevation in drug concentrations that could increase or prolong both the therapeutic and adverse effects of the concomitant drug).

No products indexed under this heading.

Busulfan (Co-administration of erythromycin or clarithromycin and a drug primarily metabolized by CYP3A may be associated with elevation in drug concentrations that could increase or prolong both the therapeutic and adverse effects of the concomitant drug). Products include:

Busulfex Injection 2477
Myleran Tablets 1530

Carbamazepine (Potential for increased serum concentration of carbamazepine). Products include:

Carbatrol Capsules 3019
Equetro Extended-Release Capsules 3174

Cerivastatin Sodium (Co-administration of erythromycin or clarithromycin and a drug primarily metabolized by CYP3A may be associated with elevation in drug concentrations that could increase or prolong both the therapeutic and adverse effects of the concomitant drug).

No products indexed under this heading.

Chlorpheniramine (Co-administration of erythromycin or clarithromycin and a drug primarily metabolized by CYP3A may be associated with elevation in drug concentrations that could increase or prolong both the therapeutic and adverse effects of the concomitant drug).

No products indexed under this heading.

Chlorpheniramine Maleate (Co-administration of erythromycin or clarithromycin and a drug primarily metabolized by CYP3A may be associated with elevation in drug concentrations that could increase or prolong both the therapeutic and adverse effects of the concomitant drug). Products include:

Actifed Cold & Allergy Tablets 1895
Sudafed PE Sinus & Allergy Tablets 1908
Tylenol Allergy Multi-Symptom Caplets with Cool Burst and Rapid Release Gelcaps 1916
Children's Tylenol Plus Cold Suspension Liquid 1912
Children's Tylenol Plus Cough & Runny Nose Suspension Liquid 1912
Children's Tylenol Plus Flu Suspension Liquid 1914
Children's Tylenol Plus Multi-Symptom Cold Suspension Liquid 1912
Tylenol Cold Head Congestion Nighttime Caplets with Cool Burst 1910
Tylenol Cold Multi-Symptom Nighttime Caplets with Cool Burst 1913
Tylenol Sinus Congestion & Pain Nighttime Caplets with Cool Burst 1917

Chlorpheniramine Polistirex (Co-administration of erythromycin or clarithromycin and a drug primarily metabolized by CYP3A may be associated with elevation in drug concentrations that could increase or prolong both the therapeutic and adverse effects of the concomitant drug). Products include:

Tussionex Pennkinetic Extended-Release Suspension 3154

Chlorpheniramine Tannate (Co-administration of erythromycin or clarithromycin and a drug primarily metabolized by CYP3A may be associated with elevation in drug concentrations that could increase or prolong both the therapeutic and adverse effects of the concomitant drug).

No products indexed under this heading.

Chlorpropamide (Clarithromycin, in rare cases, causes hypoglycemia, some of which have occurred in patients taking oral hypoglycemic agents).

No products indexed under this heading.

Cisapride (Concurrent use of erythromycin and/or clarithromycin in patients receiving cisapride has been reported to result in rare cases of cardiovascular adverse events including prolonged QT interval, ventricular tachycardia, ventricular fibrillation, and torsade de pointes, and death have been reported; co-administration is contraindicated).

No products indexed under this heading.

Colchicine (Concomitant administration may lead to increased exposure to colchicine. Patients should be monitored for clinical symptoms of colchicine toxicity).

No products indexed under this heading.

Cyclosporine (Concurrent use of erythromycin and/or clarithromycin in patients receiving drugs metabolized by the cytochrome P450 system may be associated with elevation in serum levels of cyclosporine). Products include:

Gengraf Capsules 435
Neoral Oral Solution 2280
Neoral Soft Gelatin Capsules 2280
Restasis Ophthalmic Emulsion 557
Sandimmune 2296

Desogestrel (Co-administration of erythromycin or clarithromycin and a drug primarily metabolized by CYP3A may be associated with elevation in drug concentrations that could increase or prolong both the therapeutic and adverse effects of the concomitant drug). Products include:

Mircette Tablets 1034

Diazepam (Co-administration of erythromycin or clarithromycin and a drug primarily metabolized by

CYP3A may be associated with elevation in drug concentrations that could increase or prolong both the therapeutic and adverse effects of the concomitant drug). Products include:

Valium Tablets **2658**

Dicumarol (Co-administration may result in the potentiation of oral anticoagulant effects).

No products indexed under this heading.

Digoxin (Concomitant use has resulted in elevated digoxin serum concentrations and some patients have shown signs of digoxin toxicity, including arrhythmias. Serum digoxin concentrations should be carefully monitored during co-administration). Products include:

Lanoxin Injection **1498**
Lanoxin Injection Pediatric **1502**
Lanoxin Tablets **1505**

Dihydroergotamine Mesylate (Post-marketing reports indicate that co-administration of clarithromycin with dihydroergotamine has been associated with acute ergot toxicity characterized by vasospasm and ischemia of the extremities and other tissues including the central nervous system. Concomitant administration of clarithromycin with dihydroergotamine is contraindicated).

No products indexed under this heading.

Diltiazem Hydrochloride (Co-administration of erythromycin or clarithromycin and a drug primarily metabolized by CYP3A may be associated with elevation in drug concentrations that could increase or prolong both the therapeutic and adverse effects of the concomitant drug). Products include:

Cardizem LA Extended Release Tablets **421**

Diltiazem Maleate (Co-administration of erythromycin or clarithromycin and a drug primarily metabolized by CYP3A may be associated with elevation in drug concentrations that could increase or prolong both the therapeutic and adverse effects of the concomitant drug).

No products indexed under this heading.

Disopyramide (There have been post-marketing reports of torsades de pointes occurring with the concurrent use of clarithromycin and quinidine or disopyramide. ECG should be monitored for QTc prolongation during co-administration of clarithromycin with these drugs. Serum concentrations of these medications should also be monitored).

No products indexed under this heading.

Disopyramide Phosphate (There have been post-marketing reports of torsades de pointes occurring with the concurrent use of clarithromycin and quinidine or disopyramide. ECG should be monitored for QTc prolongation during co-administration of clarithromycin with these drugs. Serum concentrations of these medications should also be monitored).

No products indexed under this heading.

Disulfiram (Co-administration of erythromycin or clarithromycin and a drug primarily metabolized by CYP3A may be associated with elevation in drug concentrations that could increase or prolong both the therapeutic and adverse effects of the concomitant drug).

No products indexed under this heading.

Divalproex Sodium (Concurrent use of erythromycin and/or clarithromycin in patients receiving drugs metabolized by the cytochrome P450 system may be associated with elevation in serum levels of valproate). Products include:

Depakote ER Tablets **423**

Doxorubicin Hydrochloride (Co-administration of erythromycin or clarithromycin and a drug primarily metabolized by CYP3A may be associated with elevation in drug concentrations that could increase or prolong both the therapeutic and adverse effects of the concomitant drug).

No products indexed under this heading.

Dronabinol (Co-administration of erythromycin or clarithromycin and a drug primarily metabolized by CYP3A may be associated with elevation in drug concentrations that could increase or prolong both the therapeutic and adverse effects of the concomitant drug). Products include:

Marinol Capsules **3163**

Dyphylline (Co-administration in patients who are receiving high doses of theophylline may be associated with an increase in serum theophylline levels and potential theophylline toxicity).

No products indexed under this heading.

Ergotamine Tartrate (Post-marketing reports indicate that co-administration of clarithromycin with ergotamine has been associated with acute ergot toxicity characterized by vasospasm and ischemia of the extremities and other tissues including the central nervous system. Concomitant administration of clarithromycin with ergotamine is contraindicated).

No products indexed under this heading.

Erythromycin (Co-administration of erythromycin or clarithromycin and a drug primarily metabolized by CYP3A may be associated with elevation in drug concentrations that could increase or prolong both the therapeutic and adverse effects of the concomitant drug).

No products indexed under this heading.

Erythromycin Estolate (Co-administration of erythromycin or clarithromycin and a drug primarily metabolized by CYP3A may be associated with elevation in drug concentrations that could increase or prolong both the therapeutic and adverse effects of the concomitant drug).

No products indexed under this heading.

Erythromycin Ethylsuccinate (Co-administration of erythromycin or clarithromycin and a drug primarily metabolized by CYP3A may be associated with elevation in drug concentrations that could increase or prolong both the therapeutic and adverse effects of the concomitant drug). Products include:

E.E.S. **433**
EryPed **431**

Erythromycin Gluceptate (Co-administration of erythromycin or clarithromycin and a drug primarily metabolized by CYP3A may be associated with elevation in drug concentrations that could increase or prolong both the therapeutic and adverse effects of the concomitant drug).

No products indexed under this heading.

Erythromycin Lactobionate (Co-administration of erythromycin or clarithromycin and a drug primarily metabolized by CYP3A may be associated with elevation in drug concentrations that could increase or prolong both the therapeutic and adverse effects of the concomitant drug).

No products indexed under this heading.

Erythromycin Stearate (Co-administration of erythromycin or clarithromycin and a drug primarily metabolized by CYP3A may be associated with elevation in drug concentrations that could increase or prolong both the therapeutic and adverse effects of the concomitant drug).

No products indexed under this heading.

Estradiol (Co-administration of erythromycin or clarithromycin and a drug primarily metabolized by CYP3A may be associated with elevation in drug concentrations that could increase or prolong both the therapeutic and adverse effects of the concomitant drug). Products include:

Activella Tablets **2347**
Angeliq Tablets **751**
Climara Transdermal System **763**
Climara Pro Transdermal System **768**
Divigel **3167**
Vagifem Tablets **2375**

Estradiol Benzoate (Co-administration of erythromycin or clarithromycin and a drug primarily metabolized by CYP3A may be associated with elevation in drug concentrations that could increase or prolong both the therapeutic and adverse effects of the concomitant drug).

No products indexed under this heading.

Estradiol Cypionate (Co-administration of erythromycin or clarithromycin and a drug primarily metabolized by CYP3A may be associated with elevation in drug concentrations that could increase or prolong both the therapeutic and adverse effects of the concomitant drug).

No products indexed under this heading.

Estradiol Valerate (Co-administration of erythromycin or clarithromycin and a drug primarily metabolized by CYP3A may be associated with elevation in drug concentrations that could increase or prolong both the therapeutic and adverse effects of the concomitant drug).

No products indexed under this heading.

Ethinyl Estradiol (Co-administration of erythromycin or clarithromycin and a drug primarily metabolized by CYP3A may be associated with elevation in drug concentrations that could increase or prolong both the therapeutic and adverse effects of the concomitant drug). Products include:

Lybrel Tablets **3204**
Mircette Tablets **1034**
NuvaRing **2897**
Ortho-Cyclen/Ortho Tri-Cyclen **2449**
Ortho Evra Transdermal System **2437**
Ortho Tri-Cyclen Lo Tablets **2458**
Seasonique Tablets **1046**
Yaz Tablets **805**

Ethosuximide (Co-administration of erythromycin or clarithromycin and a drug primarily metabolized by CYP3A may be associated with elevation in drug concentrations that could increase or prolong both the therapeutic and adverse effects of the concomitant drug).

No products indexed under this heading.

Ethynodiol Diacetate (Co-administration of erythromycin or clarithromycin and a drug primarily metabolized by CYP3A may be associated with elevation in drug concentrations that could increase or prolong both the therapeutic and adverse effects of the concomitant drug).

No products indexed under this heading.

Etoposide (Co-administration of erythromycin or clarithromycin and a drug primarily metabolized by CYP3A may be associated with elevation in drug concentrations that could increase or prolong both the therapeutic and adverse effects of the concomitant drug).

No products indexed under this heading.

Etoposide Phosphate (Co-administration of erythromycin or clarithromycin and a drug primarily metabolized by CYP3A may be associated with elevation in drug concentrations that could increase or prolong both the therapeutic and adverse effects of the concomitant drug).

No products indexed under this heading.

Felodipine (Co-administration of erythromycin or clarithromycin and a drug primarily metabolized by CYP3A may be associated with elevation in drug concentrations that could increase or prolong both the therapeutic and adverse effects of the concomitant drug).

No products indexed under this heading.

Fentanyl (Co-administration of erythromycin or clarithromycin and a drug primarily metabolized by CYP3A may be associated with elevation in drug concentrations that could increase or prolong both the therapeutic and adverse effects of the concomitant drug). Products include:

Duragesic Transdermal System **2405**
Ionsys Transdermal System **2410**

Fentanyl Citrate (Co-administration of erythromycin or clarithromycin and a drug primarily metabolized by CYP3A may be associated with elevation in drug concentrations that could increase or prolong both the therapeutic and adverse effects of the concomitant drug). Products include:

Actiq 959
Fentora Tablets 968

Fluconazole (Co-administration has resulted in increases in the mean steady-state clarithromycin Cmin and AUC).
No products indexed under this heading.

Fluvastatin Sodium (As with other macrolides, clarithromycin has been reported to increase concentrations of HMG-CoA reducatase inhibitors (eg, lovastatin, simvastatin). Rare reports of rhabdomyolysis have been reported in patients taking these drugs concomitantly). Products include:
Lescol Capsules 2268
Lescol XL Tablets 2268

Fosphenytoin Sodium (Concurrent use of erythromycin and/or clarithromycin in patients receiving drugs metabolized by the cytochrome P450 system may be associated with elevation in serum levels of phenytoin).
No products indexed under this heading.

Glimepiride (Clarithromycin, in rare cases, causes hypoglycemia, some of which have occurred in patients taking oral hypoglycemic agents). Products include:
Avandaryl Tablets 1344
Duetact Tablets 3085

Glipizide (Clarithromycin, in rare cases, causes hypoglycemia, some of which have occurred in patients taking oral hypoglycemic agents).
No products indexed under this heading.

Glyburide (Clarithromycin, in rare cases, causes hypoglycemia, some of which have occurred in patients taking oral hypoglycemic agents).
No products indexed under this heading.

Haloperidol (Co-administration of erythromycin or clarithromycin and a drug primarily metabolized by CYP3A may be associated with elevation in drug concentrations that could increase or prolong both the therapeutic and adverse effects of the concomitant drug).
No products indexed under this heading.

Haloperidol Decanoate (Co-administration of erythromycin or clarithromycin and a drug primarily metabolized by CYP3A may be associated with elevation in drug concentrations that could increase or prolong both the therapeutic and adverse effects of the concomitant drug).
No products indexed under this heading.

Haloperidol Lactate (Co-administration of erythromycin or clarithromycin and a drug primarily metabolized by CYP3A may be associated with elevation in drug concentrations that could increase or prolong both the therapeutic and adverse effects of the concomitant drug).
No products indexed under this heading.

Hexobarbital (Concurrent use of erythromycin and/or clarithromycin in patients receiving drugs metabolized by the cytochrome P450 system may be associated with elevation in serum levels of hexobarbital).
No products indexed under this heading.

Indinavir Sulfate (Co-administration of erythromycin or clarithromycin and a drug primarily metabolized by CYP3A may be associated with elevation in drug concentrations that could increase or prolong both the therapeutic and adverse effects of the concomitant drug). Products include:
Crixivan Capsules 1979

Insulin (Clarithromycin, in rare cases, causes hypoglycemia, some of which have occurred in patients taking insulin).
No products indexed under this heading.

Insulin, Human, Zinc Suspension (Clarithromycin, in rare cases, causes hypoglycemia, some of which have occurred in patients taking insulin).
No products indexed under this heading.

Insulin, Human (rDNA origin) (Clarithromycin, in rare cases, causes hypoglycemia, some of which have occurred in patients taking insulin). Products include:
Exubera Inhalation Powder 2515

Insulin, Human NPH (Clarithromycin, in rare cases, causes hypoglycemia, some of which have occurred in patients taking insulin). Products include:
Humulin N Vial 1846

Insulin, Human Regular (Clarithromycin, in rare cases, causes hypoglycemia, some of which have occurred in patients taking insulin). Products include:
Humulin R 1849
Humulin R (U-500) 1850

Insulin, Human Regular and Human NPH Mixture (Clarithromycin, in rare cases, causes hypoglycemia, some of which have occurred in patients taking insulin). Products include:
Humulin 50/50, 100 Units 1843
Humulin 70/30 Vial 1844

Insulin, NPH (Clarithromycin, in rare cases, causes hypoglycemia, some of which have occurred in patients taking insulin).
No products indexed under this heading.

Insulin, Regular (Clarithromycin, in rare cases, causes hypoglycemia, some of which have occurred in patients taking insulin).
No products indexed under this heading.

Insulin, Regular and NPH mixture (Clarithromycin, in rare cases, causes hypoglycemia, some of which have occurred in patients taking insulin).
No products indexed under this heading.

Insulin, Zinc Crystals (Clarithromycin, in rare cases, causes hypoglycemia, some of which have occurred in patients taking insulin).
No products indexed under this heading.

Insulin, Zinc Suspension (Clarithromycin, in rare cases, causes hypoglycemia, some of which have occurred in patients taking insulin).
No products indexed under this heading.

Insulin Aspart (Clarithromycin, in rare cases, causes hypoglycemia, some of which have occurred in patients taking insulin).
No products indexed under this heading.

Insulin Aspart, Human (Clarithromycin, in rare cases, causes hypoglycemia, some of which have occurred in patients taking insulin). Products include:
NovoLog Mix 70/30 2364

Insulin Aspart, Human Regular (Clarithromycin, in rare cases, causes hypoglycemia, some of which have occurred in patients taking insulin). Products include:
NovoLog Injection 2359

Insulin Aspart Protamine, Human (Clarithromycin, in rare cases, causes hypoglycemia, some of which have occurred in patients taking insulin). Products include:
NovoLog Mix 70/30 2364

Insulin Detemir (rDNA Origin) (Clarithromycin, in rare cases, causes hypoglycemia, some of which have occurred in patients taking insulin). Products include:
Levemir Injection 2352

Insulin glargine (Clarithromycin, in rare cases, causes hypoglycemia, some of which have occurred in patients taking insulin). Products include:
Lantus Injection 2749

Insulin Glulisine (Clarithromycin, in rare cases, causes hypoglycemia, some of which have occurred in patients taking insulin). Products include:
Apidra Injection 2706

Insulin Lispro, Human (Clarithromycin, in rare cases, causes hypoglycemia, some of which have occurred in patients taking insulin). Products include:
Humalog-Pen and KwikPen 1829
Humalog Mix 50/50-Pen and KwikPen 1833
Humalog Mix 75/25-Pen and KwikPen 1835

Insulin Lispro Protamine, Human (Clarithromycin, in rare cases, causes hypoglycemia, some of which have occurred in patients taking insulin). Products include:
Humalog Mix 50/50-Pen and KwikPen 1833
Humalog Mix 75/25-Pen and KwikPen 1835

Isradipine (Co-administration of erythromycin or clarithromycin and a drug primarily metabolized by CYP3A may be associated with elevation in drug concentrations that could increase or prolong both the therapeutic and adverse effects of the concomitant drug). Products include:
DynaCirc CR Controlled Release Tablets 1407

Itraconazole (Co-administration of erythromycin or clarithromycin and a drug primarily metabolized by CYP3A may be associated with elevation in drug concentrations that could increase or prolong both the therapeutic and adverse effects of the concomitant drug).
No products indexed under this heading.

Ixabepilone (Co-administration of erythromycin or clarithromycin and a drug primarily metabolized by CYP3A may be associated with elevation in drug concentrations that could increase or prolong both the therapeutic and adverse effects of the concomitant drug). Products include:
Ixempra Kit for Injection 915

Ketoconazole (Co-administration of erythromycin or clarithromycin and a drug primarily metabolized by CYP3A may be associated with elevation in drug concentrations that could increase or prolong both the therapeutic and adverse effects of the concomitant drug). Products include:
Extina Foam, 2% 3057
Nizoral A-D Shampoo 1901

Levonorgestrel (Co-administration of erythromycin or clarithromycin and a drug primarily metabolized by CYP3A may be associated with elevation in drug concentrations that could increase or prolong both the therapeutic and adverse effects of the concomitant drug). Products include:
Climara Pro Transdermal System 768
Lybrel Tablets 3204
Mirena Intrauterine System 779
Plan B Tablets 1044
Seasonique Tablets 1046

Lidocaine (Co-administration of erythromycin or clarithromycin and a drug primarily metabolized by CYP3A may be associated with elevation in drug concentrations that could increase or prolong both the therapeutic and adverse effects of the concomitant drug). Products include:
Lidoderm Patch 1114

Lidocaine Hydrochloride (Co-administration of erythromycin or clarithromycin and a drug primarily metabolized by CYP3A may be associated with elevation in drug concentrations that could increase or prolong both the therapeutic and adverse effects of the concomitant drug).
No products indexed under this heading.

Lovastatin (Co-administration of erythromycin or clarithromycin and a drug primarily metabolized by CYP3A may be associated with elevation in drug concentrations that could increase or prolong both the therapeutic and adverse effects of the concomitant drug). Products include:
Advicor Tablets 402
Mevacor Tablets 2063

Mestranol (Co-administration of erythromycin or clarithromycin and a drug primarily metabolized by CYP3A may be associated with elevation in drug concentrations that could increase or prolong both the therapeutic and adverse effects of the concomitant drug).
No products indexed under this heading.

Metformin Hydrochloride (Clarithromycin, in rare cases, causes hypoglycemia, some of which have occurred in patients taking oral hypoglycemic agents). Products include:
ActoPlus Met Tablets 3071
Avandamet Tablets 1336
Janumet Tablets 2041
PrandiMet Tablets 2967

Methadone Hydrochloride (Co-administration of erythromycin or clarithromycin and a drug primarily metabolized by CYP3A may be associated with elevation in drug concentrations that could increase or prolong both the therapeutic and adverse effects of the concomitant drug).
No products indexed under this heading.

Midazolam Hydrochloride (Erythromycin has been reported to decrease the clearance of midazolam and thus may increase its pharmacologic effects. There have been post-marketing reports of drug interactions and CNS effects (eg, somnolence, confusion) with the concomitant use of clarithromycin and triazolam).
No products indexed under this heading.

Miglitol (Clarithromycin, in rare cases, causes hypoglycemia, some of which have occurred in patients taking oral hypoglycemic agents).
No products indexed under this heading.

Nateglinide (Clarithromycin, in rare cases, causes hypoglycemia, some of which have occurred in patients taking oral hypoglycemic agents). Products include:
Starlix Tablets 2314

Nefazodone Hydrochloride (Co-administration of erythromycin or clarithromycin and a drug primarily metabolized by CYP3A may be associated with elevation in drug concentrations that could increase or prolong both the therapeutic and adverse effects of the concomitant drug).
No products indexed under this heading.

Nelfinavir Mesylate (Co-administration of erythromycin or clarithromycin and a drug primarily metabolized by CYP3A may be associated with elevation in drug concentrations that could increase or prolong both the therapeutic and adverse effects of the concomitant drug).
No products indexed under this heading.

Nicardipine Hydrochloride (Co-administration of erythromycin or clarithromycin and a drug primarily metabolized by CYP3A may be associated with elevation in drug concentrations that could increase or prolong both the therapeutic and adverse effects of the concomitant drug). Products include:
Cardene I.V. 1093

Nifedipine (Co-administration of erythromycin or clarithromycin and a drug primarily metabolized by CYP3A may be associated with elevation in drug concentrations that could increase or prolong both the therapeutic and adverse effects of the concomitant drug).
No products indexed under this heading.

Nimodipine (Co-administration of erythromycin or clarithromycin and a drug primarily metabolized by CYP3A may be associated with elevation in drug concentrations that could increase or prolong both the therapeutic and adverse effects of the concomitant drug). Products include:
Nimotop Capsules 790

Nisoldipine (Co-administration of erythromycin or clarithromycin and a drug primarily metabolized by CYP3A may be associated with elevation in drug concentrations that could increase or prolong both the therapeutic and adverse effects of the concomitant drug). Products include:
Sular Extended Release Tablets 2975

Nitrendipine (Co-administration of erythromycin or clarithromycin and a drug primarily metabolized by CYP3A may be associated with elevation in drug concentrations that could increase or prolong both the therapeutic and adverse effects of the concomitant drug).
No products indexed under this heading.

Norethindrone (Co-administration of erythromycin or clarithromycin and a drug primarily metabolized by CYP3A may be associated with elevation in drug concentrations that could increase or prolong both the therapeutic and adverse effects of the concomitant drug). Products include:
Ortho Micronor Tablets 2446

Norethindrone Acetate (Co-administration of erythromycin or clarithromycin and a drug primarily metabolized by CYP3A may be associated with elevation in drug concentrations that could increase or prolong both the therapeutic and adverse effects of the concomitant drug). Products include:
Activella Tablets 2347

Norgestrel (Co-administration of erythromycin or clarithromycin and a drug primarily metabolized by CYP3A may be associated with elevation in drug concentrations that could increase or prolong both the therapeutic and adverse effects of the concomitant drug).
No products indexed under this heading.

Omeprazole (Co-administration increases the steady-state plasma concentrations, Cmax, AUC 0-24, and T 1/2 of omeprazole).
No products indexed under this heading.

Ondansetron (Co-administration of erythromycin or clarithromycin and a drug primarily metabolized by CYP3A may be associated with elevation in drug concentrations that could increase or prolong both the therapeutic and adverse effects of the concomitant drug). Products include:
Zofran ODT Orally Disintegrating Tablets 1687

Ondansetron Hydrochloride (Co-administration of erythromycin or clarithromycin and a drug primarily metabolized by CYP3A may be associated with elevation in drug concentrations that could increase or prolong both the therapeutic and adverse effects of the concomitant drug). Products include:
Zofran Injection 1682
Zofran 1687

Paclitaxel (Co-administration of erythromycin or clarithromycin and a drug primarily metabolized by CYP3A may be associated with elevation in drug concentrations that could increase or prolong both the therapeutic and adverse effects of the concomitant drug).
No products indexed under this heading.

Phenytoin (Concurrent use of erythromycin and/or clarithromycin in patients receiving drugs metabolized by the cytochrome P450 system may be associated with elevation in serum levels of phenytoin).
No products indexed under this heading.

Phenytoin Sodium (Concurrent use of erythromycin and/or clarithromycin in patients receiving drugs metabolized by the cytochrome P450 system may be associated with elevation in serum levels of phenytoin). Products include:
Phenytek Capsules 2192

Pimozide (Concurrent use of erythromycin and/or clarithromycin in patients receiving pimozide has been reported to result in rare cases of cardiovascular adverse events including prolonged QT interval, ventricular tachycardia, ventricular fibrillation, and torsade de pointes, and death; co-administration is contraindicated).
No products indexed under this heading.

Pioglitazone Hydrochloride (Clarithromycin, in rare cases, causes hypoglycemia, some of which have occurred in patients taking oral hypoglycemic agents). Products include:
ActoPlus Met Tablets 3071
Actos Tablets 3077
Duetact Tablets 3085

Polyestradiol Phosphate (Co-administration of erythromycin or clarithromycin and a drug primarily metabolized by CYP3A may be associated with elevation in drug concentrations that could increase or prolong both the therapeutic and adverse effects of the concomitant drug).
No products indexed under this heading.

Pravastatin Sodium (As with other macrolides, clarithromycin has been reported to increase concentrations of HMG-CoA reducatase inhibitors (eg, lovastatin, simvastatin). Rare reports of rhabdomyolysis have been reported in patients taking these drugs concomitantly).
No products indexed under this heading.

Quinidine (There have been post-marketing reports of torsades de pointes occurring with the concurrent use of clarithromycin and quinidine or disopyramide. ECG should be monitored for QTc prolongation during co-administration of clarithromycin with these drugs. Serum concentrations of these medications should also be monitored).
No products indexed under this heading.

Quinidine Gluconate (Co-administration of erythromycin or clarithromycin and a drug primarily metabolized by CYP3A may be associated with elevation in drug concentrations that could increase or prolong both the therapeutic and adverse effects of the concomitant drug).
No products indexed under this heading.

Quinidine Hydrochloride (There have been post-marketing reports of torsades de pointes occurring with the concurrent use of clarithromycin and quinidine or disopyramide. ECG should be monitored for QTc prolongation during co-administration of clarithromycin with these drugs. Serum concentrations of these medications should also be monitored).
No products indexed under this heading.

Quinidine Polygalacturonate (Co-administration of erythromycin or clarithromycin and a drug primarily metabolized by CYP3A may be associated with elevation in drug concentrations that could increase or prolong both the therapeutic and adverse effects of the concomitant drug).
No products indexed under this heading.

Quinidine Sulfate (Co-administration of erythromycin or clarithromycin and a drug primarily metabolized by CYP3A may be associated with elevation in drug concentrations that could increase or prolong both the therapeutic and adverse effects of the concomitant drug).
No products indexed under this heading.

Ranitidine Bismuth Citrate (Co-administration has resulted in increased plasma ranitidine concentrations (57%), increased plasma bismuth trough concentrations (48%), and increased 14-hydroxy-clarithromycin plasma concentrations (31%); these effects are clinically insignificant).
No products indexed under this heading.

Repaglinide (Clarithromycin, in rare cases, causes hypoglycemia, some of which have occurred in patients taking oral hypoglycemic agents). Products include:
PrandiMet Tablets 2967
Prandin Tablets 2971

Rifabutin (Co-administration of erythromycin or clarithromycin and a drug primarily metabolized by CYP3A may be associated with elevation in drug concentrations that could increase or prolong both the therapeutic and adverse effects of the concomitant drug).
No products indexed under this heading.

Ritonavir (Co-administration has resulted in a 77% increase in clarithromycin AUC and a 100% decrease in the AUC of 14-OH clarithromycin; dosage adjustments may be needed if clarithromycin is administered to patients with renal impairment). Products include:
Kaletra 452
Norvir 489

Rosiglitazone Maleate (Clarithromycin, in rare cases, causes hypoglycemia, some of which have occurred in patients taking oral hypoglycemic agents). Products include:
Avandamet Tablets 1336
Avandaryl Tablets 1344
Avandia Tablets 1351

Rosuvastatin Calcium (As with other macrolides, clarithromycin has been reported to increase concentrations of HMG-CoA reducatase inhibitors (eg, lovastatin, simvastatin). Rare reports of rhabdomyolysis

have been reported in patients taking these drugs concomitantly). Products include:

Crestor Tablets 677

Saquinavir (Co-administration of erythromycin or clarithromycin and a drug primarily metabolized by CYP3A may be associated with elevation in drug concentrations that could increase or prolong both the therapeutic and adverse effects of the concomitant drug).

No products indexed under this heading.

Saquinavir Mesylate (Co-administration of erythromycin or clarithromycin and a drug primarily metabolized by CYP3A may be associated with elevation in drug concentrations that could increase or prolong both the therapeutic and adverse effects of the concomitant drug).

No products indexed under this heading.

Sertraline Hydrochloride (Co-administration of erythromycin or clarithromycin and a drug primarily metabolized by CYP3A may be associated with elevation in drug concentrations that could increase or prolong both the therapeutic and adverse effects of the concomitant drug).

No products indexed under this heading.

Sildenafil Citrate (Co-administration of erythromycin or clarithromycin and a drug primarily metabolized by CYP3A may be associated with elevation in drug concentrations that could increase or prolong both the therapeutic and adverse effects of the concomitant drug).

No products indexed under this heading.

Simvastatin (Co-administration of erythromycin or clarithromycin and a drug primarily metabolized by CYP3A may be associated with elevation in drug concentrations that could increase or prolong both the therapeutic and adverse effects of the concomitant drug). Products include:

Simcor Tablets 502
Vytorin 10/10 Tablets 2149
Vytorin 10/10 Tablets 2939
Vytorin 10/20 Tablets 2149
Vytorin 10/20 Tablets 2939
Vytorin 10/40 Tablets 2149
Vytorin 10/40 Tablets 2939
Vytorin 10/80 Tablets 2149
Vytorin 10/80 Tablets 2939
Zocor Tablets 2136

Sirolimus (Co-administration of erythromycin or clarithromycin and a drug primarily metabolized by CYP3A may be associated with elevation in drug concentrations that could increase or prolong both the therapeutic and adverse effects of the concomitant drug). Products include:

Rapamune 3260

Sitagliptin Phosphate (Clarithromycin, in rare cases, causes hypoglycemia, some of which have occurred in patients taking oral hypoglycemic agents). Products include:

Janumet Tablets 2041
Januvia Tablets 2048

Tacrolimus (Concurrent use of erythromycin and/or clarithromycin in patients receiving drugs metabolized by the cytochrome P450 system may be associated with elevation in serum levels of tacrolimus). Products include:

Prograf Capsules and Injection 622
Protopic Ointment 628

Tadalafil (Co-administration of erythromycin or clarithromycin and a drug primarily metabolized by CYP3A may be associated with elevation in drug concentrations that could increase or prolong both the therapeutic and adverse effects of the concomitant drug). Products include:

Cialis Tablets 1792

Tamoxifen Citrate (Co-administration of erythromycin or clarithromycin and a drug primarily metabolized by CYP3A may be associated with elevation in drug concentrations that could increase or prolong both the therapeutic and adverse effects of the concomitant drug).

No products indexed under this heading.

Terfenadine (Co-administration has resulted in increase in active metabolite of terfenadine by 3-fold; rare cases of cardiovascular adverse events including prolonged QT interval, ventricular tachycardia, ventricular fibrillation, and torsade de pointes, and death have been reported; co-administration is contraindicated).

No products indexed under this heading.

Theophylline (Co-administration in patients who are receiving high doses of theophylline may be associated with an increase in serum theophylline levels and potential theophylline toxicity).

No products indexed under this heading.

Theophylline Anhydrous (Co-administration in patients who are receiving high doses of theophylline may be associated with an increase in serum theophylline levels and potential theophylline toxicity). Products include:

Uniphyl Tablets 2595

Theophylline Calcium Salicylate (Co-administration in patients who are receiving high doses of theophylline may be associated with an increase in serum theophylline levels and potential theophylline toxicity).

No products indexed under this heading.

Theophylline Dihydroxypropyl (Glyceryl) (Co-administration in patients who are receiving high doses of theophylline may be associated with an increase in serum theophylline levels and potential theophylline toxicity).

No products indexed under this heading.

Theophylline Ethylenediamine (Co-administration in patients who are receiving high doses of theophylline may be associated with an increase in serum theophylline levels and potential theophylline toxicity).

No products indexed under this heading.

Theophylline Sodium Glycinate (Co-administration in patients who are receiving high doses of theophylline may be associated with an increase in serum theophylline levels and potential theophylline toxicity).

No products indexed under this heading.

Tiagabine Hydrochloride (Co-administration of erythromycin or clarithromycin and a drug primarily metabolized by CYP3A may be associated with elevation in drug concentrations that could increase or prolong both the therapeutic and adverse effects of the concomitant drug). Products include:

Gabitril Tablets 973

Tolazamide (Clarithromycin, in rare cases, causes hypoglycemia, some of which have occurred in patients taking oral hypoglycemic agents).

No products indexed under this heading.

Tolbutamide (Clarithromycin, in rare cases, causes hypoglycemia, some of which have occurred in patients taking oral hypoglycemic agents).

No products indexed under this heading.

Tolterodine Tartrate (Co-administration of erythromycin or clarithromycin and a drug primarily metabolized by CYP3A may be associated with elevation in drug concentrations that could increase or prolong both the therapeutic and adverse effects of the concomitant drug).

No products indexed under this heading.

Trazodone Hydrochloride (Co-administration of erythromycin or clarithromycin and a drug primarily metabolized by CYP3A may be associated with elevation in drug concentrations that could increase or prolong both the therapeutic and adverse effects of the concomitant drug).

No products indexed under this heading.

Triazolam (Erthromycin has been reported to decrease the clearance of triazolam and thus may increase it pharmacologic effects. There have been post-marketing reports of drug interactions and CNS effects (eg, somnolence, confusion) with the concomitant use of clarithromycin and triazolam).

No products indexed under this heading.

Troglitazone (Clarithromycin, in rare cases, causes hypoglycemia, some of which have occurred in patients taking oral hypoglycemic agents).

No products indexed under this heading.

Valproate Sodium (Concurrent use of erythromycin and/or clarithromycin in patients receiving drugs metabolized by the cytochrome P450 system may be associated with elevation in serum levels of valproate).

No products indexed under this heading.

Valproic Acid (Concurrent use of erythromycin and/or clarithromycin in patients receiving drugs metabolized by the cytochrome P450 system may be associated with elevation in serum levels of valproate).

No products indexed under this heading.

Vardenafil Hydrochloride (Co-administration of erythromycin or clarithromycin and a drug primarily metabolized by CYP3A may be associated with elevation in drug concentrations that could increase or prolong both the therapeutic and adverse effects of the concomitant drug). Products include:

Levitra Tablets 2876

Verapamil Hydrochloride (Co-administration of erythromycin or clarithromycin and a drug primarily metabolized by CYP3A may be associated with elevation in drug concentrations that could increase or prolong both the therapeutic and adverse effects of the concomitant drug). Products include:

Tarka Tablets 511

Vinblastine Sulfate (Co-administration of erythromycin or clarithromycin and a drug primarily metabolized by CYP3A may be associated with elevation in drug concentrations that could increase or prolong both the therapeutic and adverse effects of the concomitant drug).

No products indexed under this heading.

Vincristine Sulfate (Co-administration of erythromycin or clarithromycin and a drug primarily metabolized by CYP3A may be associated with elevation in drug concentrations that could increase or prolong both the therapeutic and adverse effects of the concomitant drug).

No products indexed under this heading.

Warfarin Sodium (Co-administration may result in the potentiation of oral anticoagulant effects).

No products indexed under this heading.

Zidovudine (Potential for decreased steady-state zidovudine concentration). Products include:

Combivir Tablets 1384
Retrovir 1574
Retrovir IV Infusion 1579
Trizivir Tablets 1622

Food Interactions

Food, unspecified (Food slightly delays both the onset of absorption and the formation of the active metabolite, but does not affect the extent of bioavailability; Biaxin may be administered without regard to food).

BIAXIN GRANULES

(Clarithromycin) 411
See Biaxin Filmtab Tablets

BIAXIN XL FILMTAB TABLETS

(Clarithromycin) 411
See Biaxin Filmtab Tablets

BICILLIN C-R INJECTABLE SUSPENSION

(Penicillin G Benzathine, Penicillin G Procaine)................................ 1775

May interact with bacteriostatic antibiotics, parenteral tetracyclines, tetracyclines, and certain other agents. Compounds in these categories include:

Chloramphenicol (A bacteriostatic antibiotic may antagonize the bactericidal effect of penicillin, and concurrent use of these drugs should be avoided).

No products indexed under this heading.

Chloramphenicol Palmitate (A bacteriostatic antibiotic may antagonize the bactericidal effect of penicillin, and concurrent use of these drugs should be avoided).
No products indexed under this heading.

Chloramphenicol Sodium Succinate (A bacteriostatic antibiotic may antagonize the bactericidal effect of penicillin, and concurrent use of these drugs should be avoided).
No products indexed under this heading.

Demeclocycline Hydrochloride (A bacteriostatic antibiotic may antagonize the bactericidal effect of penicillin, and concurrent use of these drugs should be avoided).
No products indexed under this heading.

Doxycycline Calcium (A bacteriostatic antibiotic may antagonize the bactericidal effect of penicillin, and concurrent use of these drugs should be avoided).
No products indexed under this heading.

Doxycycline Hyclate (A bacteriostatic antibiotic may antagonize the bactericidal effect of penicillin, and concurrent use of these drugs should be avoided).
No products indexed under this heading.

Doxycycline Monohydrate (A bacteriostatic antibiotic may antagonize the bactericidal effect of penicillin, and concurrent use of these drugs should be avoided).
No products indexed under this heading.

Erythromycin (A bacteriostatic antibiotic may antagonize the bactericidal effect of penicillin, and concurrent use of these drugs should be avoided).
No products indexed under this heading.

Erythromycin Estolate (A bacteriostatic antibiotic may antagonize the bactericidal effect of penicillin, and concurrent use of these drugs should be avoided).
No products indexed under this heading.

Erythromycin Ethylsuccinate (A bacteriostatic antibiotic may antagonize the bactericidal effect of penicillin, and concurrent use of these drugs should be avoided). Products include:
E.E.S. 433
EryPed 431

Erythromycin Gluceptate (A bacteriostatic antibiotic may antagonize the bactericidal effect of penicillin, and concurrent use of these drugs should be avoided).
No products indexed under this heading.

Erythromycin Stearate (A bacteriostatic antibiotic may antagonize the bactericidal effect of penicillin, and concurrent use of these drugs should be avoided).
No products indexed under this heading.

Methacycline Hydrochloride (A bacteriostatic antibiotic may antagonize the bactericidal effect of penicillin, and concurrent use of these drugs should be avoided).
No products indexed under this heading.

Minocycline Hydrochloride (A bacteriostatic antibiotic may antagonize the bactericidal effect of penicillin, and concurrent use of these drugs should be avoided). Products include:
Solodyn Extended Release Tablets 1938

Oxytetracycline (A bacteriostatic antibiotic may antagonize the bactericidal effect of penicillin, and concurrent use of these drugs should be avoided).
No products indexed under this heading.

Oxytetracycline Hydrochloride (A bacteriostatic antibiotic may antagonize the bactericidal effect of penicillin, and concurrent use of these drugs should be avoided).
No products indexed under this heading.

Probenecid (Concurrent administration of penicillin and probenecid increases and prolongs serum penicillin levels by decreasing the apparent volume of distribution and slowing the rate of excretion by competitively inhibiting renal tubular secretion of penicillin).
No products indexed under this heading.

Sulfamethizole (A bacteriostatic antibiotic may antagonize the bactericidal effect of penicillin, and concurrent use of these drugs should be avoided).
No products indexed under this heading.

Sulfamethoxazole (A bacteriostatic antibiotic may antagonize the bactericidal effect of penicillin, and concurrent use of these drugs should be avoided).
No products indexed under this heading.

Sulfisoxazole Acetyl (A bacteriostatic antibiotic may antagonize the bactericidal effect of penicillin, and concurrent use of these drugs should be avoided).
No products indexed under this heading.

Tetracycline Hydrochloride (A bacteriostatic antibiotic may antagonize the bactericidal effect of penicillin, and concurrent use of these drugs should be avoided). Products include:
Pylera Capsules 714

BICILLIN L-A INJECTION
(Penicillin G Benzathine, Penicillin G Procaine) 1777
May interact with bacteriostatic antibiotics, parenteral tetracyclines, tetracyclines, and certain other agents. Compounds in these categories include:

Chloramphenicol (A bacteriostatic antibiotic may antagonize the bactericidal effect of penicillin, and concurrent use of these drugs should be avoided).
No products indexed under this heading.

Chloramphenicol Palmitate (A bacteriostatic antibiotic may antagonize the bactericidal effect of penicillin, and concurrent use of these drugs should be avoided).
No products indexed under this heading.

Chloramphenicol Sodium Succinate (A bacteriostatic antibiotic may antagonize the bactericidal effect of penicillin, and concurrent use of these drugs should be avoided).
No products indexed under this heading.

Demeclocycline Hydrochloride (A bacteriostatic antibiotic may antagonize the bactericidal effect of penicillin, and concurrent use of these drugs should be avoided).
No products indexed under this heading.

Doxycycline Calcium (A bacteriostatic antibiotic may antagonize the bactericidal effect of penicillin, and concurrent use of these drugs should be avoided).
No products indexed under this heading.

Doxycycline Hyclate (A bacteriostatic antibiotic may antagonize the bactericidal effect of penicillin, and concurrent use of these drugs should be avoided).
No products indexed under this heading.

Doxycycline Monohydrate (A bacteriostatic antibiotic may antagonize the bactericidal effect of penicillin, and concurrent use of these drugs should be avoided).
No products indexed under this heading.

Erythromycin (A bacteriostatic antibiotic may antagonize the bactericidal effect of penicillin, and concurrent use of these drugs should be avoided).
No products indexed under this heading.

Erythromycin Estolate (A bacteriostatic antibiotic may antagonize the bactericidal effect of penicillin, and concurrent use of these drugs should be avoided).
No products indexed under this heading.

Erythromycin Ethylsuccinate (A bacteriostatic antibiotic may antagonize the bactericidal effect of penicillin, and concurrent use of these drugs should be avoided). Products include:
E.E.S. 433
EryPed 431

Erythromycin Gluceptate (A bacteriostatic antibiotic may antagonize the bactericidal effect of penicillin, and concurrent use of these drugs should be avoided).
No products indexed under this heading.

Erythromycin Stearate (A bacteriostatic antibiotic may antagonize the bactericidal effect of penicillin, and concurrent use of these drugs should be avoided).
No products indexed under this heading.

Methacycline Hydrochloride (A bacteriostatic antibiotic may antagonize the bactericidal effect of penicillin, and concurrent use of these drugs should be avoided).
No products indexed under this heading.

Minocycline Hydrochloride (A bacteriostatic antibiotic may antagonize the bactericidal effect of penicillin, and concurrent use of these drugs should be avoided). Products include:
Solodyn Extended Release Tablets 1938

Oxytetracycline (A bacteriostatic antibiotic may antagonize the bactericidal effect of penicillin, and concurrent use of these drugs should be avoided).
No products indexed under this heading.

Oxytetracycline Hydrochloride (A bacteriostatic antibiotic may antagonize the bactericidal effect of penicillin, and concurrent use of these drugs should be avoided).
No products indexed under this heading.

Probenecid (Concurrent administration of penicillin and probenecid increases and prolongs serum penicillin levels by decreasing the apparent volume of distribution and slowing the rate of excretion by competitively inhibiting renal tubular secretion of penicillin).
No products indexed under this heading.

Sulfamethizole (A bacteriostatic antibiotic may antagonize the bactericidal effect of penicillin, and concurrent use of these drugs should be avoided).
No products indexed under this heading.

Sulfamethoxazole (A bacteriostatic antibiotic may antagonize the bactericidal effect of penicillin, and concurrent use of these drugs should be avoided).
No products indexed under this heading.

Sulfisoxazole Acetyl (A bacteriostatic antibiotic may antagonize the bactericidal effect of penicillin, and concurrent use of these drugs should be avoided).
No products indexed under this heading.

Tetracycline Hydrochloride (A bacteriostatic antibiotic may antagonize the bactericidal effect of penicillin, and concurrent use of these drugs should be avoided). Products include:
Pylera Capsules 714

BIOLEAN FREE TABLETS
(Amino Acid Preparations, Caffeine, Ginkgo biloba, Ginseng, Green Tea Extract, Herbals with Vitamins & Minerals, Niacinamide, Potassium Citrate, Vitamin B_6) 635
May interact with monoamine oxidase inhibitors and certain other agents. Compounds in these categories include:

Caffeine-containing medications (Concurrent caffeine intake should be minimized).
No products indexed under this heading.

Isocarboxazid (Concurrent use with MAO inhibitors is not recommended). Products include:
Marplan Tablets 3177

Moclobemide (Concurrent use with MAO inhibitors is not recommended).
No products indexed under this heading.

Pargyline Hydrochloride (Concurrent use with MAO inhibitors is not recommended).
No products indexed under this heading.

Phenelzine Sulfate (Concurrent use with MAO inhibitors is not recommended).
No products indexed under this heading.

Procarbazine Hydrochloride (Concurrent use with MAO inhibitors is not recommended).
No products indexed under this heading.

Rasagiline Mesylate (Concurrent use with MAO inhibitors is not recommended). Products include:
Azilect Tablets 3106

Selegiline (Concurrent use with MAO inhibitors is not recommended). Products include:
Emsam Transdermal System 905

Selegiline Hydrochloride (Concurrent use with MAO inhibitors is not recommended). Products include:
Eldepryl Capsules 3052

Tranylcypromine Sulfate (Concurrent use with MAO inhibitors is not recommended). Products include:
Parnate Tablets 1532

BIOLEAN II TABLETS

(Amino Acid Preparations, Caffeine, Calcium Carbonate, Herbals, Multiple)................................ ▣635
May interact with monoamine oxidase inhibitors and certain other agents. Compounds in these categories include:

Isocarboxazid (If you are using a MAOI, consult a health professional before using this product). Products include:
Marplan Tablets 3177

Moclobemide (If you are using a MAOI, consult a health professional before using this product).
No products indexed under this heading.

Pargyline Hydrochloride (If you are using a MAOI, consult a health professional before using this product).
No products indexed under this heading.

Phenelzine Sulfate (If you are using a MAOI, consult a health professional before using this product).
No products indexed under this heading.

D-Phenylalanine (BioLean II contains 196 mg phenylalanine per AM serving. Not for use by children under the age of 18, pregnant or lactating women).
No products indexed under this heading.

L-Phenylalanine (BioLean II contains 196 mg phenylalanine per AM serving. Not for use by children under the age of 18, pregnant or lactating women).
No products indexed under this heading.

Procarbazine Hydrochloride (If you are using a MAOI, consult a health professional before using this product).
No products indexed under this heading.

Rasagiline Mesylate (If you are using a MAOI, consult a health professional before using this product). Products include:
Azilect Tablets 3106

Selegiline (If you are using a MAOI, consult a health professional before using this product). Products include:
Emsam Transdermal System 905

Selegiline Hydrochloride (If you are using a MAOI, consult a health professional before using this product). Products include:
Eldepryl Capsules 3052

Tranylcypromine Sulfate (If you are using a MAOI, consult a health professional before using this product). Products include:
Parnate Tablets 1532

BIOS LIFE DRINK MIX

(Fiber, Phytosterols, Vitamins with Minerals).. 3158
None cited in PDR database.

BLEPH-10 OPHTHALMIC SOLUTION 10%

(Sulfacetamide Sodium) .... ⊙215
May interact with silver preparations. Compounds in these categories include:

Silver Acetate (Incompatible).
No products indexed under this heading.

Silver Nitrate (Incompatible).
No products indexed under this heading.

Silver Sulfadiazine (Incompatible).
No products indexed under this heading.

BONIVA INJECTION

(Ibandronate Sodium) 2614
None cited in PDR database.

BONIVA TABLETS

(Ibandronate Sodium) 2618
May interact with antacids containing aluminum, calcium and magnesium, non-steroidal anti-inflammatory agents, and certain other agents. Compounds in these categories include:

Aluminum Carbonate (Products containing calcium and other multivalent cations (such as aluminum, magnesium, iron) are likely to interfere with absorption of ibandronate sodium. Ibandronate sodium should be taken at least 60 minutes before any oral medications containing multivalent cations (including antacids)).
No products indexed under this heading.

Aluminum Hydroxide (Products containing calcium and other multivalent cations (such as aluminum, magnesium, iron) are likely to interfere with absorption of ibandronate sodium. Ibandronate sodium should be taken at least 60 minutes before any oral medications containing multivalent cations (including antacids)).
No products indexed under this heading.

Aspirin (Since aspirin and bisphosphonates are associated with gastrointestinal irritation, caution should be exercised in the concomitant use of aspirin products with ibandronate sodium). Products include:
Aggrenox Capsules 819
Bayer Aspirin 750
Percodan Tablets 1130
St. Joseph 81 mg Aspirin Chewable and Enteric Coated Tablets 1903

Aspirin, Enteric Coated (Since aspirin and bisphosphonates are associated with gastrointestinal irritation, caution should be exercised in the concomitant use of aspirin products with ibandronate sodium).
No products indexed under this heading.

Aspirin Buffered (Since aspirin and bisphosphonates are associated with gastrointestinal irritation, caution should be exercised in the concomitant use of aspirin products with ibandronate sodium).
No products indexed under this heading.

Calcium (Products containing calcium and other multivalent cations (such as aluminum, magnesium, iron) are likely to interfere with absorption of ibandronate sodium. Ibandronate sodium should be taken at least 60 minutes before any oral medications containing multivalent cations (including supplements and vitamins)). Products include:
Phyto-Vite Tablets .... ▣639
Vibe Liquid Multi-Nutrient Supplement .... ▣626

Calcium (Oyster Shell) (Products containing calcium and other multivalent cations (such as aluminum, magnesium, iron) are likely to interfere with absorption of ibandronate sodium. Ibandronate sodium should be taken at least 60 minutes before any oral medications containing multivalent cations (including supplements and vitamins)).
No products indexed under this heading.

Calcium Carbonate (Products containing calcium and other multivalent cations (such as aluminum, magnesium, iron) are likely to interfere with absorption of ibandronate sodium. Ibandronate sodium should be taken at least 60 minutes before any oral medications containing multivalent cations (including supplements and vitamins)). Products include:
Accelerator Tablets .... ▣634
Actonel with Calcium Tablets 2574
BioLean II Tablets .... ▣635
Calcet Triple Calcium + Vitamin D Tablets.. ▣629
D-Cal Chewable Caplets .... ▣624
Elixir Capsules .... ▣636
Pepcid Complete Chewable Tablets 1771
Extra Strength Rolaids Plus Gas Relief Tropical Fruit Softchews...... 1903
Extra Strength Rolaids Softchews Vanilla Creme 1903
Extra Strength Rolaids Freshmint Tablets 1903
Rolaids Multi-Symptom Berry Tablets 1903
Rolaids Original Peppermint Tablets 1903

Calcium Citrate (Products containing calcium and other multivalent cations (such as aluminum, magnesium, iron) are likely to interfere with absorption of ibandronate sodium. Ibandronate sodium should be taken at least 60 minutes before any oral medications containing multivalent cations (including supplements and vitamins)). Products include:
Active Calcium Tablets 3173
CitraNatal DHA Tablets 2175
CitraNatal 90 DHA Tablets 2175

Celecoxib (Since NSAIDs and bisphosphonates are associated with gastrointestinal irritation, caution should be exercised in the concomitant use of NSAIDs with ibandronate sodium). Products include:
Celebrex Capsules 2979

Diclofenac Epolamine (Since NSAIDs and bisphosphonates are associated with gastrointestinal irritation, caution should be exercised in the concomitant use of NSAIDs with ibandronate sodium). Products include:
Flector Patch 561

Diclofenac Potassium (Since NSAIDs and bisphosphonates are associated with gastrointestinal irritation, caution should be exercised in the concomitant use of NSAIDs with ibandronate sodium).
No products indexed under this heading.

Diclofenac Sodium (Since NSAIDs and bisphosphonates are associated with gastrointestinal irritation, caution should be exercised in the concomitant use of NSAIDs with ibandronate sodium). Products include:
Diclofenac Sodium Ophthalmic Solution .... ⊙240
Voltaren Ophthalmic Solution 2336
Voltaren Tablets 2334
Voltaren-XR Tablets 2337

Etodolac (Since NSAIDs and bisphosphonates are associated with gastrointestinal irritation, caution should be exercised in the concomitant use of NSAIDs with ibandronate sodium).
No products indexed under this heading.

Fenoprofen Calcium (Since NSAIDs and bisphosphonates are associated with gastrointestinal irritation, caution should be exercised in the concomitant use of NSAIDs with ibandronate sodium). Products include:
Nalfon Capsules 2508

Flurbiprofen (Since NSAIDs and bisphosphonates are associated with gastrointestinal irritation, caution should be exercised in the concomitant use of NSAIDs with ibandronate sodium).
No products indexed under this heading.

Ibuprofen (Since NSAIDs and bisphosphonates are associated with gastrointestinal irritation, caution should be exercised in the concomitant use of NSAIDs with ibandronate sodium). Products include:
Motrin IB Tablets and Caplets 1900
Children's Motrin Oral Suspension ... 1901
Children's Motrin Non-Staining Dye-Free Oral Suspension............ 1901
Children's Motrin Cold Oral Suspension 1899
Infants' Motrin Concentrated Drops.. 1901
Infants' Motrin Non-Staining Dye-Free Concentrated Drops....... 1901
Junior Strength Motrin Caplets and Chewable Tablets.................. 1901
Vicoprofen Tablets 533

Indomethacin (Since NSAIDs and bisphosphonates are associated with gastrointestinal irritation, caution should be exercised in the concomitant use of NSAIDs with ibandronate sodium). Products include:
Indocin 2024

Indomethacin Sodium Trihydrate (Since NSAIDs and bisphosphonates are associated with gastrointestinal irritation, caution should be exercised in the concomitant use of NSAIDs with ibandronate sodium). Products include:
Indocin I.V. 2489

Iron (Products containing calcium and other multivalent cations (such as aluminum, magnesium, iron) are likely to interfere with absorption of ibandronate sodium. Ibandronate sodium should be taken at least 60 minutes before any oral medications containing multivalent cations (including supplements and vitamins)). Products include:
Phyto-Vite Tablets .... ▣639

Iron Supplements (Products containing calcium and other multivalent cations (such as aluminum, magnesium, iron) are likely to interfere with absorption of ibandronate sodium. Ibandronate sodium should be taken at least 60 minutes before any oral medications containing multivalent cations (including supplements and vitamins)).
No products indexed under this heading.

Ketoprofen (Since NSAIDs and bisphosphonates are associated with gastrointestinal irritation, caution should be exercised in the concomitant use of NSAIDs with ibandronate sodium).
No products indexed under this heading.

Ketorolac Tromethamine (Since NSAIDs and bisphosphonates are associated with gastrointestinal irritation, caution should be exercised in the concomitant use of NSAIDs with ibandronate sodium).
No products indexed under this heading.

Magaldrate (Products containing calcium and other multivalent cations (such as aluminum, magnesium, iron) are likely to interfere with absorption of ibandronate sodium. Ibandronate sodium should be taken at least 60 minutes before any oral medications containing multivalent cations (including antacids)).
No products indexed under this heading.

Magnesium Hydroxide (Products containing calcium and other multivalent cations (such as aluminum, magnesium, iron) are likely to interfere with absorption of ibandronate sodium. Ibandronate sodium should be taken at least 60 minutes before any oral medications containing multivalent cations (including antacids)).
Products include:
Fleet Pedia-Lax Chewable Tablets 1145
Pepcid Complete Chewable Tablets 1771
Extra Strength Rolaids Freshmint Tablets 1903
Rolaids Multi-Symptom Berry Tablets 1903
Rolaids Original Peppermint Tablets 1903

Magnesium Oxide (Products containing calcium and other multivalent cations (such as aluminum, magnesium, iron) are likely to interfere with absorption of ibandronate sodium. Ibandronate sodium should be taken at least 60 minutes before any oral medications containing multivalent cations (including antacids)).
Products include:
Beelith Tablets 813

Meclofenamate Sodium (Since NSAIDs and bisphosphonates are associated with gastrointestinal irritation, caution should be exercised in the concomitant use of NSAIDs with ibandronate sodium).
No products indexed under this heading.

Mefenamic Acid (Since NSAIDs and bisphosphonates are associated with gastrointestinal irritation, caution should be exercised in the concomitant use of NSAIDs with ibandronate sodium).
No products indexed under this heading.

Meloxicam (Since NSAIDs and bisphosphonates are associated with gastrointestinal irritation, caution should be exercised in the concomitant use of NSAIDs with ibandronate sodium). Products include:
Mobic Oral Suspension 863
Mobic Tablets 863

Multivitamins (Products containing calcium and other multivalent cations (such as aluminum, magnesium, iron) are likely to interfere with absorption of ibandronate sodium. Ibandronate sodium should be taken at least 60 minutes before any oral medications containing multivalent cations (including vitamins)).
No products indexed under this heading.

Multivitamins with Minerals (Products containing calcium and other multivalent cations (such as aluminum, magnesium, iron) are likely to interfere with absorption of ibandronate sodium. Ibandronate sodium should be taken at least 60 minutes before any oral medications containing multivalent cations (including vitamins)). Products include:
CitraNatal DHA Tablets 2175
CitraNatal 90 DHA Tablets 2175

Nabumetone (Since NSAIDs and bisphosphonates are associated with gastrointestinal irritation, caution should be exercised in the concomitant use of NSAIDs with ibandronate sodium).
No products indexed under this heading.

Naproxen (Since NSAIDs and bisphosphonates are associated with gastrointestinal irritation, caution should be exercised in the concomitant use of NSAIDs with ibandronate sodium). Products include:
EC-Naprosyn Delayed-Release Tablets 2632
Naprosyn Suspension 2632
Naprosyn Tablets 2632

Naproxen Sodium (Since NSAIDs and bisphosphonates are associated with gastrointestinal irritation, caution should be exercised in the concomitant use of NSAIDs with ibandronate sodium). Products include:
Anaprox Tablets 2632
Anaprox DS Tablets 2632
Treximet Tablets 1616

Oxaprozin (Since NSAIDs and bisphosphonates are associated with gastrointestinal irritation, caution should be exercised in the concomitant use of NSAIDs with ibandronate sodium).
No products indexed under this heading.

Phenylbutazone (Since NSAIDs and bisphosphonates are associated with gastrointestinal irritation, caution should be exercised in the concomitant use of NSAIDs with ibandronate sodium).
No products indexed under this heading.

Piroxicam (Since NSAIDs and bisphosphonates are associated with gastrointestinal irritation, caution should be exercised in the concomitant use of NSAIDs with ibandronate sodium).
No products indexed under this heading.

Rofecoxib (Since NSAIDs and bisphosphonates are associated with gastrointestinal irritation, caution should be exercised in the concomitant use of NSAIDs with ibandronate sodium).
No products indexed under this heading.

Sulindac (Since NSAIDs and bisphosphonates are associated with gastrointestinal irritation, caution should be exercised in the concomitant use of NSAIDs with ibandronate sodium). Products include:
Clinoril Tablets 1962

Tolmetin Sodium (Since NSAIDs and bisphosphonates are associated with gastrointestinal irritation, caution should be exercised in the concomitant use of NSAIDs with ibandronate sodium).
No products indexed under this heading.

Valdecoxib (Since NSAIDs and bisphosphonates are associated with gastrointestinal irritation, caution should be exercised in the concomitant use of NSAIDs with ibandronate sodium).
No products indexed under this heading.

Vitamins, Multiple (Products containing calcium and other multivalent cations (such as aluminum, magnesium, iron) are likely to interfere with absorption of ibandronate sodium. Ibandronate sodium should be taken at least 60 minutes before any oral medications containing multivalent cations (including vitamins)).
Products include:
Bausch & Lomb Ocuvite DF Vitamin Supplement .... ⊙238
Mega Antioxidant Tablets 3174
Vibe Liquid Multi-Nutrient Supplement .... ▣626

Vitamins with Iron (Products containing calcium and other multivalent cations (such as aluminum, magnesium, iron) are likely to interfere with absorption of ibandronate sodium. Ibandronate sodium should be taken at least 60 minutes before any oral medications containing multivalent cations (including vitamins)).
No products indexed under this heading.

BOOSTRIX

(Diphtheria & Tetanus Toxoids and Acellular Pertussis Vaccine Adsorbed) 1377

May interact with alkylating agents, antimetabolites, corticosteroids, cytotoxic drugs, immunosuppressive agents, and certain other agents. Compounds in these categories include:

Azathioprine (May reduce immune response to vaccines. When administered to patients who are receiving immunosuppressive therapy, who have an immunodeficiency disorder, or who have received a recent injection of immune globulin, an adequate immunologic response may not be obtained).
No products indexed under this heading.

Basiliximab (May reduce immune response to vaccines. When administered to patients who are receiving immunosuppressive therapy, who have an immunodeficiency disorder, or who have received a recent injection of immune globulin, an adequate immunologic response may not be obtained). Products include:
Simulect for Injection 2306

Betamethasone Acetate (May reduce immune response to vaccines when used concomitantly with corticosteroids (greater than physiologic doses). When administered to patients who are receiving immunosuppressive therapy, who have an immunodeficiency disorder, or who have received arecent injection of immune globulin, an adequate immunologic response may not be obtained).
No products indexed under this heading.

Betamethasone Sodium Phosphate (May reduce immune response to vaccines when used concomitantly with corticosteroids (greater than physiologic doses). When administered to patients who are receiving immunosuppressive therapy, who have an immunodeficiency disorder, or who have received arecent injection of immune globulin, an adequate immunologic response may not be obtained).
No products indexed under this heading.

Bleomycin Sulfate (May reduce immune response to vaccines. When administered to patients who are receiving immunosuppressive therapy, who have an immunodeficiency disorder, or who have received a recent injection of immune globulin, an adequate immunologic response may not be obtained).
No products indexed under this heading.

Budesonide (May reduce immune response to vaccines when used concomitantly with corticosteroids (greater than physiologic doses). When administered to patients who are receiving immunosuppressive therapy, who have an immunodeficiency disorder, or who have received arecent injection of immune globulin, an adequate immunologic response may not be obtained).
Products include:
Pulmicort Flexhaler 654
Symbicort 80/4.5 Inhalation Aerosol 659
Symbicort 160/4.5 Inhalation Aerosol 659

Busulfan (May reduce immune response to vaccines. When administered to patients who are receiving immunosuppressive therapy, who have an immunodeficiency disorder, or who have received a recent injection of immune globulin, an adequate immunologic response may not be obtained). Products include:
Busulfex Injection 2477
Myleran Tablets 1530

Capecitabine (May reduce immune response to vaccines. When administered to patients who are receiving immunosuppressive therapy, who have an immunodeficiency disorder, or who have received a recent injection of immune globulin, an adequate immunologic response may not be obtained). Products include:
Xeloda Tablets 2662

Carmustine (BCNU) (May reduce immune response to vaccines. When administered to patients who are receiving immunosuppressive therapy, who have an immunodeficiency disorder, or who have received a recent injection of immune globulin, an adequate immunologic response may not be obtained).
No products indexed under this heading.

Chlorambucil (May reduce immune response to vaccines. When administered to patients who are receiving immunosuppressive therapy, who have an immunodeficiency disorder, or who have received a recent injection of immune globulin, an adequate immunologic response may not be obtained). Products include:

Leukeran Tablets 1508

Ciclesonide (May reduce immune response to vaccines when used concomitantly with corticosteroids (greater than physiologic doses). When administered to patients who are receiving immunosuppressive therapy, who have an immunodeficiency disorder, or who have received arecent injection of immune globulin, an adequate immunologic response may not be obtained). Products include:

Alvesco Inhalation Aerosol 2985
Omnaris Nasal Spray 2998

Cladribine (May reduce immune response to vaccines. When administered to patients who are receiving immunosuppressive therapy, who have an immunodeficiency disorder, or who have received a recent injection of immune globulin, an adequate immunologic response may not be obtained). Products include:

Leustatin Injection 2384

Cortisone Acetate (May reduce immune response to vaccines when used concomitantly with corticosteroids (greater than physiologic doses). When administered to patients who are receiving immunosuppressive therapy, who have an immunodeficiency disorder, or who have received arecent injection of immune globulin, an adequate immunologic response may not be obtained).

No products indexed under this heading.

Cyclophosphamide (May reduce immune response to vaccines. When administered to patients who are receiving immunosuppressive therapy, who have an immunodeficiency disorder, or who have received a recent injection of immune globulin, an adequate immunologic response may not be obtained).

No products indexed under this heading.

Cyclosporine (May reduce immune response to vaccines. When administered to patients who are receiving immunosuppressive therapy, who have an immunodeficiency disorder, or who have received a recent injection of immune globulin, an adequate immunologic response may not be obtained). Products include:

Gengraf Capsules 435
Neoral Oral Solution 2280
Neoral Soft Gelatin Capsules 2280
Restasis Ophthalmic Emulsion 557
Sandimmune 2296

Cytarabine (May reduce immune response to vaccines. When administered to patients who are receiving immunosuppressive therapy, who have an immunodeficiency disorder, or who have received a recent injection of immune globulin, an adequate immunologic response may not be obtained).

No products indexed under this heading.

Dacarbazine (May reduce immune response to vaccines. When administered to patients who are receiving immunosuppressive therapy, who have an immunodeficiency disorder, or who have received a recent injection of immune globulin, an adequate immunologic response may not be obtained).

No products indexed under this heading.

Daunorubicin Hydrochloride (May reduce immune response to vaccines. When administered to patients who are receiving immunosuppressive therapy, who have an immunodeficiency disorder, or who have received a recent injection of immune globulin, an adequate immunologic response may not be obtained).

No products indexed under this heading.

Dexamethasone (May reduce immune response to vaccines when used concomitantly with corticosteroids (greater than physiologic doses). When administered to patients who are receiving immunosuppressive therapy, who have an immunodeficiency disorder, or who have received arecent injection of immune globulin, an adequate immunologic response may not be obtained). Products include:

Ciprodex Otic Suspension 541

Dexamethasone Acetate (May reduce immune response to vaccines when used concomitantly with corticosteroids (greater than physiologic doses). When administered to patients who are receiving immunosuppressive therapy, who have an immunodeficiency disorder, or who have received arecent injection of immune globulin, an adequate immunologic response may not be obtained).

No products indexed under this heading.

Dexamethasone Sodium Phosphate (May reduce immune response to vaccines when used concomitantly with corticosteroids (greater than physiologic doses). When administered to patients who are receiving immunosuppressive therapy, who have an immunodeficiency disorder, or who have received arecent injection of immune globulin, an adequate immunologic response may not be obtained).

No products indexed under this heading.

Doxorubicin Hydrochloride (May reduce immune response to vaccines. When administered to patients who are receiving immunosuppressive therapy, who have an immunodeficiency disorder, or who have received a recent injection of immune globulin, an adequate immunologic response may not be obtained).

No products indexed under this heading.

Epirubicin Hydrochloride (May reduce immune response to vaccines. When administered to patients who are receiving immunosuppressive therapy, who have an immunodeficiency disorder, or who have received a recent injection of immune globulin, an adequate immunologic response may not be obtained).

No products indexed under this heading.

Floxuridine (May reduce immune response to vaccines. When administered to patients who are receiving immunosuppressive therapy, who have an immunodeficiency disorder, or who have received a recent injection of immune globulin, an adequate immunologic response may not be obtained).

No products indexed under this heading.

Fludarabine Phosphate (May reduce immune response to vaccines. When administered to patients who are receiving immunosuppressive therapy, who have an immunodeficiency disorder, or who have received a recent injection of immune globulin, an adequate immunologic response may not be obtained).

No products indexed under this heading.

Fludrocortisone Acetate (May reduce immune response to vaccines when used concomitantly with corticosteroids (greater than physiologic doses). When administered to patients who are receiving immunosuppressive therapy, who have an immunodeficiency disorder, or who have received arecent injection of immune globulin, an adequate immunologic response may not be obtained).

No products indexed under this heading.

Flunisolide (May reduce immune response to vaccines when used concomitantly with corticosteroids (greater than physiologic doses). When administered to patients who are receiving immunosuppressive therapy, who have an immunodeficiency disorder, or who have received arecent injection of immune globulin, an adequate immunologic response may not be obtained). Products include:

Aerobid/Aerobid-M 1153

Fluorouracil (May reduce immune response to vaccines. When administered to patients who are receiving immunosuppressive therapy, who have an immunodeficiency disorder, or who have received a recent injection of immune globulin, an adequate immunologic response may not be obtained). Products include:

Carac Cream 0.5% 2722

Fluticasone Propionate (May reduce immune response to vaccines when used concomitantly with corticosteroids (greater than physiologic doses). When administered to patients who are receiving immunosuppressive therapy, who have an immunodeficiency disorder, or who have received arecent injection of immune globulin, an adequate immunologic response may not be obtained). Products include:

Advair Diskus 100/50 1276
Advair Diskus 250/50 1276
Advair Diskus 500/50 1276
Advair HFA 45/21 Inhalation Aerosol 1288
Advair HFA 115/21 Inhalation Aerosol 1288
Advair HFA 230/21 Inhalation Aerosol 1288
Flonase Nasal Spray 1431
Flovent Diskus 50 mcg 1435

Fluticasone Propionate HFA (May reduce immune response to vaccines when used concomitantly with corticosteroids (greater than physiologic doses). When administered to patients who are receiving immunosuppressive therapy, who have an immunodeficiency disorder, or who have received arecent injection of immune globulin, an adequate immunologic response may not be obtained). Products include:

Flovent HFA 1440

Gemcitabine Hydrochloride (May reduce immune response to vaccines. When administered to patients who are receiving immunosuppressive therapy, who have an immunodeficiency disorder, or who have received a recent injection of immune globulin, an adequate immunologic response may not be obtained). Products include:

Gemzar for Injection 1820

Hydrocortisone (May reduce immune response to vaccines when used concomitantly with corticosteroids (greater than physiologic doses). When administered to patients who are receiving immunosuppressive therapy, who have an immunodeficiency disorder, or who have received arecent injection of immune globulin, an adequate immunologic response may not be obtained).

No products indexed under this heading.

Hydrocortisone Acetate (May reduce immune response to vaccines when used concomitantly with corticosteroids (greater than physiologic doses). When administered to patients who are receiving immunosuppressive therapy, who have an immunodeficiency disorder, or who have received arecent injection of immune globulin, an adequate immunologic response may not be obtained). Products include:

Analpram-HC 1140
Pramosone 1141

Hydrocortisone Sodium Phosphate (May reduce immune response to vaccines when used concomitantly with corticosteroids (greater than physiologic doses). When administered to patients who are receiving immunosuppressive therapy, who have an immunodeficiency disorder, or who have received arecent injection of immune globulin, an adequate immunologic response may not be obtained).

No products indexed under this heading.

Hydrocortisone Sodium Succinate (May reduce immune response to vaccines when used concomitantly with corticosteroids (greater than physiologic doses). When administered to patients who are receiving immunosuppressive therapy, who have an immunodeficiency disorder, or who have received arecent injection of immune globulin, an adequate immunologic response may not be obtained).

No products indexed under this heading.

Hydroxyurea (May reduce immune response to vaccines. When administered to patients who are receiving immunosuppressive therapy, who have an immunodeficiency disorder, or who have received a recent injection of immune globulin, an adequate immunologic response may not be obtained).

No products indexed under this heading.

Immune Globulin Intravenous (Human) (May reduce immune response to vaccines. When administered to patients who are receiving immunosuppressive therapy, who have an immunodeficiency disorder, or who have received a recent injection of immune globulin, an adequate immunologic response may not be obtained). Products include:

Flebogamma 5% DIF 1718
Gammagard Liquid 730
Gammagard S/D 734
Gamunex 3094

Lomustine (CCNU) (May reduce immune response to vaccines. When administered to patients who are receiving immunosuppressive therapy, who have an immunodeficiency disorder, or who have received a recent injection of immune globulin, an adequate immunologic response may not be obtained).

No products indexed under this heading.

Mechlorethamine Hydrochloride (May reduce immune response to vaccines. When administered to patients who are receiving immunosuppressive therapy, who have an immunodeficiency disorder, or who have received a recent injection of immune globulin, an adequate immunologic response may not be obtained). Products include:

Mustargen for Injection 2492

Melphalan (May reduce immune response to vaccines. When administered to patients who are receiving immunosuppressive therapy, who have an immunodeficiency disorder, or who have received a recent injection of immune globulin, an adequate immunologic response may not be obtained).

No products indexed under this heading.

Mercaptopurine (May reduce immune response to vaccines. When administered to patients who are receiving immunosuppressive therapy, who have an immunodeficiency disorder, or who have received a recent injection of immune globulin, an adequate immunologic response may not be obtained).

No products indexed under this heading.

Methotrexate (May reduce immune response to vaccines. When administered to patients who are receiving immunosuppressive therapy, who have an immunodeficiency disorder, or who have received a recent injection of immune globulin, an adequate immunologic response may not be obtained).

No products indexed under this heading.

Methotrexate Sodium (May reduce immune response to vaccines. When administered to patients who are receiving immunosuppressive therapy, who have an immunodeficiency disorder, or who have received a recent injection of immune globulin, an adequate immunologic response may not be obtained).

No products indexed under this heading.

Methylprednisolone Acetate (May reduce immune response to vaccines when used concomitantly with corticosteroids (greater than physiologic doses). When administered to patients who are receiving immunosuppressive therapy, who have an immunodeficiency disorder, or who have received arecent injection of immune globulin, an adequate immunologic response may not be obtained).

No products indexed under this heading.

Methylprednisolone Sodium Succinate (May reduce immune response to vaccines when used concomitantly with corticosteroids (greater than physiologic doses). When administered to patients who are receiving immunosuppressive therapy, who have an immunodeficiency disorder, or who have received arecent injection of immune globulin, an adequate immunologic response may not be obtained).

No products indexed under this heading.

Mitotane (May reduce immune response to vaccines. When administered to patients who are receiving immunosuppressive therapy, who have an immunodeficiency disorder, or who have received a recent injection of immune globulin, an adequate immunologic response may not be obtained).

No products indexed under this heading.

Mitoxantrone Hydrochloride (May reduce immune response to vaccines. When administered to patients who are receiving immunosuppressive therapy, who have an immunodeficiency disorder, or who have received a recent injection of immune globulin, an adequate immunologic response may not be obtained). Products include:

Novantrone for Injection Concentrate 1100

Mometasone Furoate (May reduce immune response to vaccines when used concomitantly with corticosteroids (greater than physiologic doses). When administered to patients who are receiving immunosuppressive therapy, who have an immunodeficiency disorder, or who have received arecent injection of immune globulin, an adequate immunologic response may not be obtained). Products include:

Asmanex Twisthaler 2797
Elocon Cream 0.1% 2840
Elocon Lotion 0.1% 2841
Elocon Ointment 0.1% 2842

Mometasone Furoate Monohydrate (May reduce immune response to vaccines when used concomitantly with corticosteroids (greater than physiologic doses). When administered to patients who are receiving immunosuppressive therapy, who have an immunodeficiency disorder, or who have received arecent injection of immune globulin, an adequate immunologic response may not be obtained). Products include:

Nasonex Nasal Spray 2883

Muromonab-CD3 (May reduce immune response to vaccines. When administered to patients who are receiving immunosuppressive therapy, who have an immunodeficiency disorder, or who have received a recent injection of immune globulin, an adequate immunologic response may not be obtained). Products include:

Orthoclone OKT3 Sterile Solution 2387

Mycophenolate Mofetil (May reduce immune response to vaccines. When administered to patients who are receiving immunosuppressive therapy, who have an immunodeficiency disorder, or who have received a recent injection of immune globulin, an adequate immunologic response may not be obtained). Products include:

CellCept Capsules 2622
CellCept Oral Suspension 2622
CellCept Tablets 2622

Pentostatin (May reduce immune response to vaccines. When administered to patients who are receiving immunosuppressive therapy, who have an immunodeficiency disorder, or who have received a recent injection of immune globulin, an adequate immunologic response may not be obtained).

No products indexed under this heading.

Prednisolone Acetate (May reduce immune response to vaccines when used concomitantly with corticosteroids (greater than physiologic doses). When administered to patients who are receiving immunosuppressive therapy, who have an immunodeficiency disorder, or who have received arecent injection of immune globulin, an adequate immunologic response may not be obtained). Products include:

Pred Forte Ophthalmic Suspension .... ⊙ 227
Pred Mild Ophthalmic Suspension .... ⊙ 230
Pred-G Ophthalmic Ointment .... ⊙ 229
Pred-G Ophthalmic Suspension .... ⊙ 228

Prednisolone Sodium Phosphate (May reduce immune response to vaccines when used concomitantly with corticosteroids (greater than physiologic doses). When administered to patients who are receiving immunosuppressive therapy, who have an immunodeficiency disorder, or who have received arecent injection of immune globulin, an adequate immunologic response may not be obtained).

No products indexed under this heading.

Prednisolone Tebutate (May reduce immune response to vaccines when used concomitantly with corticosteroids (greater than physiologic doses). When administered to patients who are receiving immunosuppressive therapy, who have an immunodeficiency disorder, or who have received arecent injection of immune globulin, an adequate immunologic response may not be obtained).

No products indexed under this heading.

Prednisone (May reduce immune response to vaccines when used concomitantly with corticosteroids (greater than physiologic doses). When administered to patients who are receiving immunosuppressive therapy, who have an immunodeficiency disorder, or who have received arecent injection of immune globulin, an adequate immunologic response may not be obtained).

No products indexed under this heading.

Procarbazine Hydrochloride (May reduce immune response to vaccines. When administered to patients who are receiving immunosuppressive therapy, who have an immunodeficiency disorder, or who have received a recent injection of immune globulin, an adequate immunologic response may not be obtained).

No products indexed under this heading.

Sirolimus (May reduce immune response to vaccines. When administered to patients who are receiving immunosuppressive therapy, who have an immunodeficiency disorder, or who have received a recent injection of immune globulin, an adequate immunologic response may not be obtained). Products include:

Rapamune 3260

Tacrolimus (May reduce immune response to vaccines. When administered to patients who are receiving immunosuppressive therapy, who have an immunodeficiency disorder, or who have received a recent injection of immune globulin, an adequate immunologic response may not be obtained). Products include:

Prograf Capsules and Injection 622
Protopic Ointment 628

Tamoxifen Citrate (May reduce immune response to vaccines. When administered to patients who are receiving immunosuppressive therapy, who have an immunodeficiency disorder, or who have received a recent injection of immune globulin, an adequate immunologic response may not be obtained).

No products indexed under this heading.

Thioguanine (May reduce immune response to vaccines. When administered to patients who are receiving immunosuppressive therapy, who have an immunodeficiency disorder, or who have received a recent injection of immune globulin, an adequate immunologic response may not be obtained). Products include:

Tabloid Tablets 1601

Thiotepa (May reduce immune response to vaccines. When administered to patients who are receiving immunosuppressive therapy, who have an immunodeficiency disorder, or who have received a recent injection of immune globulin, an adequate immunologic response may not be obtained).

No products indexed under this heading.

Triamcinolone (May reduce immune response to vaccines when used concomitantly with corticosteroids (greater than physiologic doses). When administered to patients who are receiving immunosuppressive therapy, who have an immunodeficiency disorder, or who have received arecent injection of immune globulin, an adequate immunologic response may not be obtained).

No products indexed under this heading.

Triamcinolone Acetonide (May reduce immune response to vaccines when used concomitantly with corticosteroids (greater than physiologic doses). When administered to patients who are receiving immunosuppressive therapy, who have an immunodeficiency disorder, or who have received arecent injection of immune globulin, an adequate immunologic response may not be obtained). Products include:

Azmacort Inhalation Aerosol 407
Nasacort AQ Nasal Spray 2765
Triesence Injectable Suspension .... ⊙209

Triamcinolone Diacetate (May reduce immune response to vaccines when used concomitantly with corticosteroids (greater than physiologic doses). When administered to patients who are receiving immunosuppressive therapy, who have an immunodeficiency disorder, or who have received arecent injection of immune globulin, an adequate immunologic response may not be obtained).

No products indexed under this heading.

Triamcinolone Hexacetonide (May reduce immune response to vaccines when used concomitantly with corticosteroids (greater than physiologic doses). When administered to patients who are receiving immunosuppressive therapy, who have an immunodeficiency disorder, or who have received arecent injection of immune globulin, an adequate immunologic response may not be obtained).

No products indexed under this heading.

Vincristine Sulfate (May reduce immune response to vaccines. When administered to patients who are receiving immunosuppressive therapy, who have an immunodeficiency disorder, or who have received a recent injection of immune globulin, an adequate immunologic response may not be obtained).

No products indexed under this heading.

BOTOX PURIFIED NEUROTOXIN COMPLEX

(Botulinum Toxin Type A) 550

None cited in PDR database.

BREVOXYL-4 CREAMY WASH

(Benzoyl Peroxide) 3054

None cited in PDR database.

BREVOXYL-4 GEL

(Benzoyl Peroxide) 3054

None cited in PDR database.

BREVOXYL-8 CREAMY WASH

(Benzoyl Peroxide) 3054

None cited in PDR database.

BREVOXYL-8 GEL

(Benzoyl Peroxide) 3054

None cited in PDR database.

BROVANA INHALATION SOLUTION

(Arformoterol Tartrate) 2990

May interact with beta blockers, beta-adrenergic stimulating agents, corticosteroids, diuretics, loop diuretics, monoamine oxidase inhibitors, nonpotassium-sparing diuretics, xanthines, and certain other agents. Compounds in these categories include:

Acebutolol Hydrochloride (Beta-adrenergic receptor antagonists (beta-blockers) and aformoterol tartrate may interfere with the effect of each other when administered concurrently. Beta-blockers not only block the therapeutic effects of beta-agonists, but may produce severe bronchospasm in COPD patients. Therefore, patients with COPD should not normally be treated with beta-blockers. However, under certain circumstances, e.g., as prophylaxis after myocardial infarction, there may be no acceptable alternatives to the use of beta-blockers in patients with COPD. In this setting, cardioselective beta-blockers could be considered, although they should be administered with caution).

No products indexed under this heading.

Albuterol (If additional adrenergic drugs are to be administered by any route, they should be used with caution because the pharmacologically predictable sympathetic effects of aformoterol tartrate may be potentiated).

No products indexed under this heading.

Albuterol Sulfate (If additional adrenergic drugs are to be administered by any route, they should be used with caution because the pharmacologically predictable sympathetic effects of aformoterol tartrate may be potentiated). Products include:

Combivent Inhalation Aerosol 845
ProAir HFA Inhalation Aerosol 3113
Proventil HFA Inhalation Aerosol 2914
Ventolin HFA Inhalation Aerosol 1638

Amiloride Hydrochloride (The ECG changes and/or hypokalemia that may result from the administration of non-potassium sparing diuretics (such as loop or thiazide diuretics) can be acutely worsened by beta-agonists, especially when the recommended dose of the beta-agonist is exceeded. Although the clinical significance of these effects is not known, caution is advised in the co-administration of beta-agonists with non-potassium sparing diuretics. Concomitant treatment with diuretics may potentiate any hypokalemic effect of adrenergic agonists).

No products indexed under this heading.

Aminophylline (Concomitant treatment with methylxanthines (aminophylline, theophylline) may potentiate any hypokalemic effect of adrenergic agonists. In trials, heart rate and systolic blood pressure were approximately 2-3 bpm and 6-8 mm Hg higher, respectively, in subjects on concomitant theophylline compared with the overall population).

No products indexed under this heading.

Atenolol (Beta-adrenergic receptor antagonists (beta-blockers) and aformoterol tartrate may interfere with the effect of each other when administered concurrently. Beta-blockers not only block the therapeutic effects of beta-agonists, but may produce severe bronchospasm in COPD patients. Therefore, patients with COPD should not normally be treated with beta-blockers. However, under certain circumstances, e.g., as prophylaxis after myocardial infarction, there may be no acceptable alternatives to the use of beta-blockers in patients with COPD. In this setting, cardioselective beta-blockers could be considered, although they should be administered with caution).

No products indexed under this heading.

Bendroflumethiazide (The ECG changes and/or hypokalemia that may result from the administration of nonpotassium sparing diuretics (such as loop or thiazide diuretics) can be acutely worsened by beta-agonists, especially when the recommended dose of the beta-agonist is exceeded. Although the clinical significance of these effects is not known, caution is advised in the co-administration of beta-agonists with non-potassium sparing diuretics).

No products indexed under this heading.

Betamethasone Acetate (Concomitant treatment with steroids may potentiate any hypokalemic effect of adrenergic agonists).

No products indexed under this heading.

Betamethasone Sodium Phosphate (Concomitant treatment with steroids may potentiate any hypokalemic effect of adrenergic agonists).

No products indexed under this heading.

Betaxolol Hydrochloride (Beta-adrenergic receptor antagonists (beta-blockers) and aformoterol tartrate may interfere with the effect of each other when administered concurrently. Beta-blockers not only block the therapeutic effects of beta-agonists, but may produce severe bronchospasm in COPD patients. Therefore, patients with COPD should not normally be treated with beta-blockers. However, under certain circumstances, e.g., as prophylaxis after myocardial infarction, there may be no acceptable alternatives to the use of beta-blockers in patients with COPD. In this setting, cardioselective beta-blockers could be considered, although they should be administered with caution).

No products indexed under this heading.

Bisoprolol Fumarate (Beta-adrenergic receptor antagonists (beta-blockers) and aformoterol tartrate may interfere with the effect of each other when administered concurrently. Beta-blockers not only block the therapeutic effects of beta-agonists, but may produce severe bronchospasm in COPD patients. Therefore, patients with COPD should not normally be treated with beta-blockers. However, under certain circumstances, e.g., as prophylaxis after myocardial infarction, there may be no acceptable alternatives to the use of beta-blockers in patients with COPD. In this setting, cardioselective beta-blockers could be considered, although they should be administered with caution).

No products indexed under this heading.

Bitolterol Mesylate (If additional adrenergic drugs are to be administered by any route, they should be used with caution because the pharmacologically predictable sympathetic effects of aformoterol tartrate may be potentiated).

No products indexed under this heading.

Budesonide (Concomitant treatment with steroids may potentiate any hypokalemic effect of adrenergic agonists). Products include:

Pulmicort Flexhaler 654
Symbicort 80/4.5 Inhalation Aerosol.. 659
Symbicort 160/4.5 Inhalation Aerosol.. 659

Bumetanide (The ECG changes and/or hypokalemia that may result from the administration of nonpotassium sparing diuretics (such as loop or thiazide diuretics) can be acutely worsened by beta-agonists, especially when the recommended dose of the beta-agonist is exceeded. Although the clinical significance of these effects is not known, caution is advised in the co-administration of beta-agonists with non-potassium sparing diuretics).

No products indexed under this heading.

Carteolol Hydrochloride (Beta-adrenergic receptor antagonists (beta-blockers) and aformoterol tartrate may interfere with the effect of each other when administered concurrently. Beta-blockers not only block the therapeutic effects of beta-agonists, but may produce severe bronchospasm in COPD patients. Therefore, patients with COPD should not normally be treated with beta-blockers. However, under certain circumstances, e.g., as prophylaxis after myocardial infarction, there may be no acceptable alternatives to the use of beta-blockers in patients with COPD. In this setting, cardioselective beta-blockers could be considered, although they should be administered with caution).

No products indexed under this heading.

Chlorothiazide (The ECG changes and/or hypokalemia that may result from the administration of nonpotassium sparing diuretics (such as loop or thiazide diuretics) can be acutely worsened by beta-agonists, especially when the recommended dose of the beta-agonist is exceeded. Although the clinical significance of these effects is not known, caution is advised in the co-administration of beta-agonists with non-potassium sparing diuretics).

No products indexed under this heading.

Chlorothiazide Sodium (The ECG changes and/or hypokalemia that may result from the administration of nonpotassium sparing diuretics (such as loop or thiazide diuretics) can be acutely worsened by beta-agonists, especially when the recommended dose of the beta-agonist is exceeded. Although the clinical significance of these effects is not known, caution is advised in the co-administration of beta-agonists with non-potassium sparing diuretics). Products include:

Intravenous Sodium Diuril 2490

Chlorthalidone (The ECG changes and/or hypokalemia that may result from the administration of non-potassium sparing diuretics (such as loop or thiazide diuretics) can be acutely worsened by beta-agonists, especially when the recommended dose of the beta-agonist is exceeded. Although the clinical significance of these effects is not known, caution is advised in the co-administration of beta-agonists with non-potassium sparing diuretics. Concomitant treatment with diuretics may potentiate any hypokalemic effect of adrenergic agonists). Products include:

Clorpres Tablets 2185

Ciclesonide (Concomitant treatment with steroids may potentiate any hypokalemic effect of adrenergic agonists). Products include:

Alvesco Inhalation Aerosol 2985
Omnaris Nasal Spray 2998

Cortisone Acetate (Concomitant treatment with steroids may potentiate any hypokalemic effect of adrenergic agonists).

No products indexed under this heading.

Dexamethasone (Concomitant treatment with steroids may potentiate any hypokalemic effect of adrenergic agonists). Products include:

Ciprodex Otic Suspension 541

Dexamethasone Acetate (Concomitant treatment with steroids may potentiate any hypokalemic effect of adrenergic agonists).

No products indexed under this heading.

Dexamethasone Sodium Phosphate (Concomitant treatment with steroids may potentiate any hypokalemic effect of adrenergic agonists).

No products indexed under this heading.

Dobutamine (If additional adrenergic drugs are to be administered by any route, they should be used with caution because the pharmacologically predictable sympathetic effects of aformoterol tartrate may be potentiated).

No products indexed under this heading.

Dobutamine Hydrochloride (If additional adrenergic drugs are to be administered by any route, they should be used with caution because the pharmacologically predictable sympathetic effects of aformoterol tartrate may be potentiated).

No products indexed under this heading.

Dyphylline (Concomitant treatment with methylxanthines (aminophylline, theophylline) may potentiate any hypokalemic effect of adrenergic agonists. In trials, heart rate and systolic blood pressure were approximately 2-3 bpm and 6-8 mm Hg higher, respectively, in subjects on concomitant theophylline compared with the overall population).

No products indexed under this heading.

Ephedrine Hydrochloride (If additional adrenergic drugs are to be administered by any route, they should be used with caution because the pharmacologically predictable sympathetic effects of aformoterol tartrate may be potentiated).

No products indexed under this heading.

Ephedrine Sulfate (If additional adrenergic drugs are to be administered by any route, they should be used with caution because the pharmacologically predictable sympathetic effects of aformoterol tartrate may be potentiated).

No products indexed under this heading.

Ephedrine Tannate (If additional adrenergic drugs are to be administered by any route, they should be used with caution because the pharmacologically predictable sympathetic effects of aformoterol tartrate may be potentiated).

No products indexed under this heading.

Epinephrine (If additional adrenergic drugs are to be administered by any route, they should be used with caution because the pharmacologically predictable sympathetic effects of aformoterol tartrate may be potentiated). Products include:

EpiPen 1024

Epinephrine Hydrochloride (If additional adrenergic drugs are to be administered by any route, they should be used with caution because the pharmacologically predictable sympathetic effects of aformoterol tartrate may be potentiated).

No products indexed under this heading.

Esmolol Hydrochloride (Beta-adrenergic receptor antagonists (beta-blockers) and aformoterol tartrate may interfere with the effect of each other when administered concurrently. Beta-blockers not only block the therapeutic effects of beta-agonists, but may produce severe bronchospasm in COPD patients. Therefore, patients with COPD should not normally be treated with beta-blockers. However, under certain circumstances, e.g., as prophylaxis after myocardial infarction, there may be no acceptable alternatives to the use of beta-blockers in patients with COPD. In this setting, cardioselective beta-blockers could be considered, although they should be administered with caution).

No products indexed under this heading.

Ethacrynic Acid (The ECG changes and/or hypokalemia that may result from the administration of nonpotassium sparing diuretics (such as loop or thiazide diuretics) can be acutely worsened by beta-agonists, especially when the recommended dose of the beta-agonist is exceeded. Although the clinical significance of these effects is not known, caution is advised in the co-administration of beta-agonists with non-potassium sparing diuretics). Products include:

Edecrin Tablets 698

Fludrocortisone Acetate (Concomitant treatment with steroids may potentiate any hypokalemic effect of adrenergic agonists).

No products indexed under this heading.

Flunisolide (Concomitant treatment with steroids may potentiate any hypokalemic effect of adrenergic agonists). Products include:

Aerobid/Aerobid-M 1153

Fluticasone Propionate (Concomitant treatment with steroids may potentiate any hypokalemic effect of adrenergic agonists). Products include:

Advair Diskus 100/50 1276
Advair Diskus 250/50 1276
Advair Diskus 500/50 1276
Advair HFA 45/21 Inhalation Aerosol 1288
Advair HFA 115/21 Inhalation Aerosol 1288
Advair HFA 230/21 Inhalation Aerosol 1288
Flonase Nasal Spray 1431
Flovent Diskus 50 mcg 1435

Fluticasone Propionate HFA (Concomitant treatment with steroids may potentiate any hypokalemic effect of adrenergic agonists). Products include:

Flovent HFA 1440

Furosemide (The ECG changes and/or hypokalemia that may result from the administration of nonpotassium sparing diuretics (such as loop or thiazide diuretics) can be acutely worsened by beta-agonists, especially when the recommended dose of the beta-agonist is exceeded. Although the clinical significance of these effects is not known, caution is advised in the co-administration of beta-agonists with non-potassium sparing diuretics). Products include:

Furosemide Tablets 2186

Hydrochlorothiazide (The ECG changes and/or hypokalemia that may result from the administration of nonpotassium sparing diuretics (such as loop or thiazide diuretics) can be acutely worsened by beta-agonists, especially when the recommended dose of the beta-agonist is exceeded. Although the clinical significance of these effects is not known, caution is advised in the co-administration of beta-agonists with non-potassium sparing diuretics). Products include:

Atacand HCT 642
Avalide Tablets 892
Avalide Tablets 2713
Benicar HCT Tablets 1010
Diovan HCT Tablets 2216
Dyazide Capsules 1405
Micardis HCT Tablets 854
Prinzide Tablets 2092
Tekturna HCT Tablets 2324
Teveten HCT Tablets 517

Hydrocortisone (Concomitant treatment with steroids may potentiate any hypokalemic effect of adrenergic agonists).

No products indexed under this heading.

Hydrocortisone Acetate (Concomitant treatment with steroids may potentiate any hypokalemic effect of adrenergic agonists). Products include:

Analpram-HC 1140
Pramosone 1141

Hydrocortisone Sodium Phosphate (Concomitant treatment with steroids may potentiate any hypokalemic effect of adrenergic agonists).

No products indexed under this heading.

Hydrocortisone Sodium Succinate (Concomitant treatment with steroids may potentiate any hypokalemic effect of adrenergic agonists).

No products indexed under this heading.

Hydroflumethiazide (The ECG changes and/or hypokalemia that may result from the administration of nonpotassium sparing diuretics (such as loop or thiazide diuretics) can be acutely worsened by beta-agonists, especially when the recommended dose of the beta-agonist is exceeded. Although the clinical significance of these effects is not known, caution is advised in the co-administration of beta-agonists with non-potassium sparing diuretics).

No products indexed under this heading.

Indapamide (The ECG changes and/or hypokalemia that may result from the administration of non-potassium sparing diuretics (such as loop or thiazide diuretics) can be acutely worsened by beta-agonists, especially when the recommended dose of the beta-agonist is exceeded. Although the clinical significance of these effects is not known, caution is advised in the co-administration of beta-agonists with non-potassium sparing diuretics. Concomitant treatment with diuretics may potentiate any hypokalemic effect of adrenergic agonists). Products include:

Indapamide Tablets 2188

Isocarboxazid (Aformoterol tartrate, as with other beta2-agonists, should be administered with extreme caution to patients being treated with monoamine oxidase inhibitors, tricyclic antidepressants or drugs known to prolong the QTc interval because the action of adrenergic agonits on the cardiovascular system may be potentiated by these agents. Drugs that are known to prolong the QTc interval have an increased risk of ventricular arrhythmias). Products include:

Marplan Tablets 3177

Isoetharine (If additional adrenergic drugs are to be administered by any route, they should be used with caution because the pharmacologically predictable sympathetic effects of aformoterol tartrate may be potentiated).

No products indexed under this heading.

Isoproterenol Hydrochloride (If additional adrenergic drugs are to be administered by any route, they should be used with caution because the pharmacologically predictable sympathetic effects of aformoterol tartrate may be potentiated).

No products indexed under this heading.

Isoproterenol Sulfate (If additional adrenergic drugs are to be administered by any route, they should be used with caution because the pharmacologically predictable sympathetic effects of aformoterol tartrate may be potentiated).

No products indexed under this heading.

Labetalol Hydrochloride (Beta-adrenergic receptor antagonists (beta-blockers) and aformoterol tartrate may interfere with the effect of each other when administered concurrently. Beta-blockers not only block the therapeutic effects of beta-agonists, but may produce severe bronchospasm in COPD patients. Therefore, patients with COPD should not normally be treated with beta-blockers. However, under certain circumstances, e.g., as prophylaxis after myocardial infarction, there may be no acceptable alternatives to the use of beta-blockers in patients with COPD. In this setting, cardioselective beta-blockers could be considered, although they should be administered with caution).

No products indexed under this heading.

Levalbuterol Hydrochloride (If additional adrenergic drugs are to be administered by any route, they should be used with caution because the pharmacologically predictable sympathetic effects of aformoterol tartrate may be potentiated). Products include:

Xopenex Inhalation Solution 3001
Xopenex Inhalation Solution Concentrate 3005

Levobunolol Hydrochloride (Beta-adrenergic receptor antagonists (beta-blockers) and aformoterol tartrate may interfere with the effect of each other when administered concurrently. Beta-blockers not only block the therapeutic effects of beta-agonists, but may produce severe bronchospasm in COPD patients. Therefore, patients with COPD should not normally be treated with beta-blockers. However, under certain circumstances, e.g., as prophylaxis after myocardial infarction, there may be no acceptable alternatives to the use of beta-blockers in patients with COPD. In this setting, cardioselective beta-blockers could be considered, although they should be administered with caution).
No products indexed under this heading.

Metaproterenol Sulfate (If additional adrenergic drugs are to be administered by any route, they should be used with caution because the pharmacologically predictable sympathetic effects of aformoterol tartrate may be potentiated).
No products indexed under this heading.

Methyclothiazide (The ECG changes and/or hypokalemia that may result from the administration of non-potassium sparing diuretics (such as loop or thiazide diuretics) can be acutely worsened by beta-agonists, especially when the recommended dose of the beta-agonist is exceeded. Although the clinical significance of these effects is not known, caution is advised in the co-administration of beta-agonists with non-potassium sparing diuretics).
No products indexed under this heading.

Methylprednisolone Acetate (Concomitant treatment with steroids may potentiate any hypokalemic effect of adrenergic agonists).
No products indexed under this heading.

Methylprednisolone Sodium Succinate (Concomitant treatment with steroids may potentiate any hypokalemic effect of adrenergic agonists).
No products indexed under this heading.

Metipranolol Hydrochloride (Beta-adrenergic receptor antagonists (beta-blockers) and aformoterol tartrate may interfere with the effect of each other when administered concurrently. Beta-blockers not only block the therapeutic effects of beta-agonists, but may produce severe bronchospasm in COPD patients. Therefore, patients with COPD should not normally be treated with beta-blockers. However, under certain circumstances, e.g., as prophylaxis after myocardial infarction, there may be no acceptable alternatives to the use of beta-blockers in patients with COPD. In this setting, cardioselective beta-blockers could be considered, although they should be administered with caution).
No products indexed under this heading.

Metolazone (The ECG changes and/or hypokalemia that may result from the administration of non-potassium sparing diuretics (such as loop or thiazide diuretics) can be acutely worsened by beta-agonists, especially when the recommended dose of the beta-agonist is exceeded. Although the clinical significance of these effects is not known, caution is advised in the co-administration of beta-agonists with non-potassium sparing diuretics. Concomitant treatment with diuretics may potentiate any hypokalemic effect of adrenergic agonists).
No products indexed under this heading.

Metoprolol Succinate (Beta-adrenergic receptor antagonists (beta-blockers) and aformoterol tartrate may interfere with the effect of each other when administered concurrently. Beta-blockers not only block the therapeutic effects of beta-agonists, but may produce severe bronchospasm in COPD patients. Therefore, patients with COPD should not normally be treated with beta-blockers. However, under certain circumstances, e.g., as prophylaxis after myocardial infarction, there may be no acceptable alternatives to the use of beta-blockers in patients with COPD. In this setting, cardioselective beta-blockers could be considered, although they should be administered with caution). Products include:
Toprol-XL Tablets 666

Metoprolol Tartrate (Beta-adrenergic receptor antagonists (beta-blockers) and aformoterol tartrate may interfere with the effect of each other when administered concurrently. Beta-blockers not only block the therapeutic effects of beta-agonists, but may produce severe bronchospasm in COPD patients. Therefore, patients with COPD should not normally be treated with beta-blockers. However, under certain circumstances, e.g., as prophylaxis after myocardial infarction, there may be no acceptable alternatives to the use of beta-blockers in patients with COPD. In this setting, cardioselective beta-blockers could be considered, although they should be administered with caution).
No products indexed under this heading.

Moclobemide (Aformoterol tartrate, as with other beta2-agonists, should be administered with extreme caution to patients being treated with monoamine oxidase inhibitors, tricyclic antidepressants or drugs known to prolong the QTc interval because the action of adrenergic agonits on the cardiovascular system may be potentiated by these agents. Drugs that are known to prolong the QTc interval have an increased risk of ventricular arrhythmias).
No products indexed under this heading.

Mometasone Furoate (Concomitant treatment with steroids may potentiate any hypokalemic effect of adrenergic agonists). Products include:
Asmanex Twisthaler 2797
Elocon Cream 0.1% 2840
Elocon Lotion 0.1% 2841
Elocon Ointment 0.1% 2842

Mometasone Furoate Monohydrate (Concomitant treatment with steroids may potentiate any hypokalemic effect of adrenergic agonists). Products include:
Nasonex Nasal Spray 2883

Nadolol (Beta-adrenergic receptor antagonists (beta-blockers) and aformoterol tartrate may interfere with the effect of each other when administered concurrently. Beta-blockers not only block the therapeutic effects of beta-agonists, but may produce severe bronchospasm in COPD patients. Therefore, patients with COPD should not normally be treated with beta-blockers. However, under certain circumstances, e.g., as prophylaxis after myocardial infarction, there may be no acceptable alternatives to the use of beta-blockers in patients with COPD. In this setting, cardioselective beta-blockers could be considered, although they should be administered with caution). Products include:
Nadolol Tablets 2191

Nebivolol (Beta-adrenergic receptor antagonists (beta-blockers) and aformoterol tartrate may interfere with the effect of each other when administered concurrently. Beta-blockers not only block the therapeutic effects of beta-agonists, but may produce severe bronchospasm in COPD patients. Therefore, patients with COPD should not normally be treated with beta-blockers. However, under certain circumstances, e.g., as prophylaxis after myocardial infarction, there may be no acceptable alternatives to the use of beta-blockers in patients with COPD. In this setting, cardioselective beta-blockers could be considered, although they should be administered with caution). Products include:
Bystolic Tablets 1155

Pargyline Hydrochloride (Aformoterol tartrate, as with other beta2-agonists, should be administered with extreme caution to patients being treated with monoamine oxidase inhibitors, tricyclic antidepressants or drugs known to prolong the QTc interval because the action of adrenergic agonits on the cardiovascular system may be potentiated by these agents. Drugs that are known to prolong the QTc interval have an increased risk of ventricular arrhythmias).
No products indexed under this heading.

Paroxetine Hydrochloride (When paroxetine, a potent inhibitor of CYP2D6, was co-administered with arformoterol tartrate at steady-state, exposure to either drug was not altered. Dosage adjustments of arformoterol tartrate are not necessary when the drug is given concomitantly with potent CYP2D6 inhibitors). Products include:
Paxil 1535
Paxil CR Controlled-Release Tablets 1544

Paroxetine Mesylate (When paroxetine, a potent inhibitor of CYP2D6, was co-administered with arformoterol tartrate at steady-state, exposure to either drug was not altered. Dosage adjustments of arformoterol tartrate are not necessary when the drug is given concomitantly with potent CYP2D6 inhibitors).
No products indexed under this heading.

Penbutolol Sulfate (Beta-adrenergic receptor antagonists (beta-blockers) and aformoterol tartrate may interfere with the effect of each other when administered concurrently. Beta-blockers not only block the therapeutic effects of beta-agonists, but may produce severe bronchospasm in COPD patients. Therefore, patients with COPD should not normally be treated with beta-blockers. However, under certain circumstances, e.g., as prophylaxis after myocardial infarction, there may be no acceptable alternatives to the use of beta-blockers in patients with COPD. In this setting, cardioselective beta-blockers could be considered, although they should be administered with caution).
No products indexed under this heading.

Phenelzine Sulfate (Aformoterol tartrate, as with other beta2-agonists, should be administered with extreme caution to patients being treated with monoamine oxidase inhibitors, tricyclic antidepressants or drugs known to prolong the QTc interval because the action of adrenergic agonits on the cardiovascular system may be potentiated by these agents. Drugs that are known to prolong the QTc interval have an increased risk of ventricular arrhythmias).
No products indexed under this heading.

Pindolol (Beta-adrenergic receptor antagonists (beta-blockers) and aformoterol tartrate may interfere with the effect of each other when administered concurrently. Beta-blockers not only block the therapeutic effects of beta-agonists, but may produce severe bronchospasm in COPD patients. Therefore, patients with COPD should not normally be treated with beta-blockers. However, under certain circumstances, e.g., as prophylaxis after myocardial infarction, there may be no acceptable alternatives to the use of beta-blockers in patients with COPD. In this setting, cardioselective beta-blockers could be considered, although they should be administered with caution).
No products indexed under this heading.

Pirbuterol Acetate (If additional adrenergic drugs are to be administered by any route, they should be used with caution because the pharmacologically predictable sympathetic effects of aformoterol tartrate may be potentiated). Products include:
Maxair Autohaler 1705

Polythiazide (The ECG changes and/or hypokalemia that may result from the administration of nonpotassium sparing diuretics (such as loop or thiazide diuretics) can be acutely worsened by beta-agonists, especially when the recommended dose of the beta-agonist is exceeded. Although the clinical significance of these effects is not known, caution is advised in the co-administration of beta-agonists with non-potassium sparing diuretics).
No products indexed under this heading.

Prednisolone Acetate (Concomitant treatment with steroids may potentiate any hypokalemic effect of adrenergic agonists). Products include:
Pred Forte Ophthalmic Suspension .... ⊙ 227

Pred Mild Ophthalmic Suspension .... ⊙ **230**
Pred-G Ophthalmic Ointment .... ⊙ **229**
Pred-G Ophthalmic Suspension .... ⊙ **228**

Prednisolone Sodium Phosphate (Concomitant treatment with steroids may potentiate any hypokalemic effect of adrenergic agonists).
No products indexed under this heading.

Prednisolone Tebutate (Concomitant treatment with steroids may potentiate any hypokalemic effect of adrenergic agonists).
No products indexed under this heading.

Prednisone (Concomitant treatment with steroids may potentiate any hypokalemic effect of adrenergic agonists).
No products indexed under this heading.

Procarbazine Hydrochloride (Aformoterol tartrate, as with other beta2-agonists, should be administered with extreme caution to patients being treated with monoamine oxidase inhibitors, tricyclic antidepressants or drugs known to prolong the QTc interval because the action of adrenergic agonits on the cardiovascular system may be potentiated by these agents. Drugs that are known to prolong the QTc interval have an increased risk of ventricular arrhythmias).
No products indexed under this heading.

Propranolol Hydrochloride (Beta-adrenergic receptor antagonists (beta-blockers) and aformoterol tartrate may interfere with the effect of each other when administered concurrently. Beta-blockers not only block the therapeutic effects of beta-agonists, but may produce severe bronchospasm in COPD patients. Therefore, patients with COPD should not normally be treated with beta-blockers. However, under certain circumstances, e.g., as prophylaxis after myocardial infarction, there may be no acceptable alternatives to the use of beta-blockers in patients with COPD. In this setting, cardioselective beta-blockers could be considered, although they should be administered with caution). Products include:
InnoPran XL Extended Release Capsules **1484**

Rasagiline Mesylate (Aformoterol tartrate, as with other beta2-agonists, should be administered with extreme caution to patients being treated with monoamine oxidase inhibitors, tricyclic antidepressants or drugs known to prolong the QTc interval because the action of adrenergic agonits on the cardiovascular system may be potentiated by these agents. Drugs that are known to prolong the QTc interval have an increased risk of ventricular arrhythmias). Products include:
Azilect Tablets **3106**

Salmeterol Xinafoate (If additional adrenergic drugs are to be administered by any route, they should be used with caution because the pharmacologically predictable sympathetic effects of aformoterol tartrate may be potentiated). Products include:
Advair Diskus 100/50 .... **1276**
Advair Diskus 250/50 .... **1276**
Advair Diskus 500/50 .... **1276**
Advair HFA 45/21 Inhalation Aerosol **1288**
Advair HFA 115/21 Inhalation Aerosol **1288**
Advair HFA 230/21 Inhalation Aerosol **1288**
Serevent Diskus **1594**

Selegiline (Aformoterol tartrate, as with other beta2-agonists, should be administered with extreme caution to patients being treated with monoamine oxidase inhibitors, tricyclic antidepressants or drugs known to prolong the QTc interval because the action of adrenergic agonits on the cardiovascular system may be potentiated by these agents. Drugs that are known to prolong the QTc interval have an increased risk of ventricular arrhythmias). Products include:
Emsam Transdermal System **905**

Selegiline Hydrochloride (Aformoterol tartrate, as with other beta2-agonists, should be administered with extreme caution to patients being treated with monoamine oxidase inhibitors, tricyclic antidepressants or drugs known to prolong the QTc interval because the action of adrenergic agonits on the cardiovascular system may be potentiated by these agents. Drugs that are known to prolong the QTc interval have an increased risk of ventricular arrhythmias). Products include:
Eldepryl Capsules **3052**

Sotalol Hydrochloride (Beta-adrenergic receptor antagonists (beta-blockers) and aformoterol tartrate may interfere with the effect of each other when administered concurrently. Beta-blockers not only block the therapeutic effects of beta-agonists, but may produce severe bronchospasm in COPD patients. Therefore, patients with COPD should not normally be treated with beta-blockers. However, under certain circumstances, e.g., as prophylaxis after myocardial infarction, there may be no acceptable alternatives to the use of beta-blockers in patients with COPD. In this setting, cardioselective beta-blockers could be considered, although they should be administered with caution).
No products indexed under this heading.

Spironolactone (The ECG changes and/or hypokalemia that may result from the administration of non-potassium sparing diuretics (such as loop or thiazide diuretics) can be acutely worsened by beta-agonists, especially when the recommended dose of the beta-agonist is exceeded. Although the clinical significance of these effects is not known, caution is advised in the co-administration of beta-agonists with non-potassium sparing diuretics. Concomitant treatment with diuretics may potentiate any hypokalemic effect of adrenergic agonists).
No products indexed under this heading.

Terbutaline Sulfate (If additional adrenergic drugs are to be administered by any route, they should be used with caution because the pharmacologically predictable sympathetic effects of aformoterol tartrate may be potentiated).
No products indexed under this heading.

Theophylline (Concomitant treatment with methylxanthines (aminophylline, theophylline) may potentiate any hypokalemic effect of adrenergic agonists. In trials, heart rate and systolic blood pressure were approximately 2-3 bpm and 6-8 mm Hg higher, respectively, in subjects on concomitant theophylline compared with the overall population).
No products indexed under this heading.

Theophylline Anhydrous (Concomitant treatment with methylxanthines (aminophylline, theophylline) may potentiate any hypokalemic effect of adrenergic agonists. In trials, heart rate and systolic blood pressure were approximately 2-3 bpm and 6-8 mm Hg higher, respectively, in subjects on concomitant theophylline compared with the overall population). Products include:
Uniphyl Tablets **2595**

Theophylline Calcium Salicylate (Concomitant treatment with methylxanthines (aminophylline, theophylline) may potentiate any hypokalemic effect of adrenergic agonists. In trials, heart rate and systolic blood pressure were approximately 2-3 bpm and 6-8 mm Hg higher, respectively, in subjects on concomitant theophylline compared with the overall population).
No products indexed under this heading.

Theophylline Dihydroxypropyl (Glyceryl) (Concomitant treatment with methylxanthines (aminophylline, theophylline) may potentiate any hypokalemic effect of adrenergic agonists. In trials, heart rate and systolic blood pressure were approximately 2-3 bpm and 6-8 mm Hg higher, respectively, in subjects on concomitant theophylline compared with the overall population).
No products indexed under this heading.

Theophylline Ethylenediamine (Concomitant treatment with methylxanthines (aminophylline, theophylline) may potentiate any hypokalemic effect of adrenergic agonists. In trials, heart rate and systolic blood pressure were approximately 2-3 bpm and 6-8 mm Hg higher, respectively, in subjects on concomitant theophylline compared with the overall population).
No products indexed under this heading.

Theophylline Sodium Glycinate (Concomitant treatment with methylxanthines (aminophylline, theophylline) may potentiate any hypokalemic effect of adrenergic agonists. In trials, heart rate and systolic blood pressure were approximately 2-3 bpm and 6-8 mm Hg higher, respectively, in subjects on concomitant theophylline compared with the overall population).
No products indexed under this heading.

Timolol Hemihydrate (Beta-adrenergic receptor antagonists (beta-blockers) and aformoterol tartrate may interfere with the effect of each other when administered concurrently. Beta-blockers not only block the therapeutic effects of beta-agonists, but may produce severe bronchospasm in COPD patients. Therefore, patients with COPD should not normally be treated with beta-blockers. However, under certain circumstances, e.g., as prophylaxis after myocardial infarction, there may be no acceptable alternatives to the use of beta-blockers in patients with COPD. In this setting, cardioselective beta-blockers could be considered, although they should be administered with caution). Products include:
Betimol Ophthalmic Solution **3181**

Timolol Maleate (Beta-adrenergic receptor antagonists (beta-blockers) and aformoterol tartrate may interfere with the effect of each other when administered concurrently. Beta-blockers not only block the therapeutic effects of beta-agonists, but may produce severe bronchospasm in COPD patients. Therefore, patients with COPD should not normally be treated with beta-blockers. However, under certain circumstances, e.g., as prophylaxis after myocardial infarction, there may be no acceptable alternatives to the use of beta-blockers in patients with COPD. In this setting, cardioselective beta-blockers could be considered, although they should be administered with caution). Products include:
Combigan Ophthalmic Solution **553**
Cosopt Sterile Ophthalmic Solution **1969**
Timoptic Sterile Ophthalmic Solution **2121**
Timoptic in Ocudose **2124**
Timoptic-XE Sterile Ophthalmic Gel Forming Solution **2125**

Torsemide (The ECG changes and/or hypokalemia that may result from the administration of nonpotassium sparing diuretics (such as loop or thiazide diuretics) can be acutely worsened by beta-agonists, especially when the recommended dose of the beta-agonist is exceeded. Although the clinical significance of these effects is not known, caution is advised in the co-administration of beta-agonists with non-potassium sparing diuretics). Products include:
Demadex Injection **2630**
Demadex Tablets **2630**

Tranylcypromine Sulfate (Aformoterol tartrate, as with other beta2-agonists, should be administered with extreme caution to patients being treated with monoamine oxidase inhibitors, tricyclic antidepressants or drugs known to prolong the QTc interval because the action of adrenergic agonits on the cardiovascular system may be potentiated by these agents. Drugs that are known to prolong the QTc interval have an increased risk of ventricular arrhythmias). Products include:
Parnate Tablets **1532**

Triamcinolone (Concomitant treatment with steroids may potentiate any hypokalemic effect of adrenergic agonists).
No products indexed under this heading.

Triamcinolone Acetonide (Concomitant treatment with steroids may potentiate any hypokalemic effect of adrenergic agonists). Products include:
Azmacort Inhalation Aerosol **407**
Nasacort AQ Nasal Spray **2765**
Triesence Injectable Suspension .... ⊙ **209**

Triamcinolone Diacetate (Concomitant treatment with steroids may potentiate any hypokalemic effect of adrenergic agonists).
No products indexed under this heading.

Triamcinolone Hexacetonide (Concomitant treatment with steroids may potentiate any hypokalemic effect of adrenergic agonists).
No products indexed under this heading.

Triamterene (The ECG changes and/or hypokalemia that may result from the administration of non-potassium sparing diuretics (such as loop or thiazide diuretics) can be acutely worsened by beta-agonists, especially when the recommended dose of the beta-agonist is exceeded. Although the clinical significance of these effects is not known, caution is advised in the co-administration of beta-agonists with non-potassium sparing diuretics. Concomitant treatment with diuretics may potentiate any hypokalemic effect of adrenergic agonists).
Products include:
Dyazide Capsules **1405**
Dyrenium Capsules **3189**

BUSULFEX INJECTION

(Busulfan) **2477**
May interact with phenytoin and certain other agents. Compounds in these categories include:

Acetaminophen (Use of acetaminophen prior to (less than 72 hours) or concurrent with Busulfex may result in reduced busulfan clearance since acetaminophen decreases glutathione levels in the blood and tissues). Products include:
Benadryl Allergy & Cold Kapgels **1895**
Benadryl Allergy & Sinus Headache Kapgels **1895**
Benadryl Severe Allergy & Sinus Headache Caplets **1897**
Lortab 5/500 Tablets **3143**
Lortab 7.5/500 Tablets **3144**
Lortab 10/500 Tablets **3144**
Percocet Tablets **1127**
Sinutab Sinus Caplets **1905**
Sudafed PE Cold & Cough Caplets **1907**
Sudafed PE Nighttime Cold Caplets **1907**
Sudafed PE Severe Cold Caplets **1908**
Sudafed PE Sinus Headache Caplets **1908**
Regular Strength Tylenol Tablets **1915**
Tylenol 8 Hour Extended Release Caplets **1915**
Extra Strength Tylenol Caplets, Cool Caplets, and EZ Tabs **1915**
Extra Strength Tylenol Adult Rapid Blast Liquid **1915**
Extra Strength Tylenol PM Caplets, Geltabs, Liquid, and Rapid Release Gels **1915**
Extra Strength Tylenol Rapid Release Gels **1915**
Tylenol with Codeine Tablets **2427**
Tylenol Allergy Multi-Symptom Caplets with Cool Burst and Rapid Release Gelcaps **1916**
Tylenol Allergy Multi-Symptom Nighttime Caplets with Cool Burst **1916**
Tylenol Severe Allergy Caplets **1916**
Tylenol Arthritis Pain Extended Release Geltabs/Caplets **1915**
Tylenol Chest Congestion Caplets with Cool Burst **1910**
Tylenol Chest Congestion Liquid with Cool Burst **1910**
Children's Tylenol Plus Cold Suspension Liquid **1912**
Children's Tylenol Plus Cold & Allergy Suspension Liquid **1914**
Children's Tylenol Plus Cough & Runny Nose Suspension Liquid **1912**
Children's Tylenol Plus Cough & Sore Throat Suspension Liquid **1912**
Children's Tylenol Plus Flu Suspension Liquid **1914**
Children's Tylenol Suspension Liquid **1909**
Children's Tylenol Meltaways **1909**
Children's Tylenol Plus Multi-Symptom Cold Suspension Liquid **1912**
Tylenol Cold Severe Congestion Daytime Caplets with Cool Burst **1912**
Tylenol Cold Head Congestion Daytime Caplets with Cool Burst **1910**
Tylenol Cold Head Congestion Nighttime Caplets with Cool Burst **1910**
Tylenol Cold Head Congestion Severe Daytime Caplets with Cool Burst **1910**
Tylenol Cold Multi-Symptom Daytime Caplets with Cool Burst and Rapid Release Gels **1913**
Tylenol Cold Multi-Symptom Daytime Liquid with Citrus Burst **1913**
Tylenol Cold Multi-Symptom Nighttime Caplets with Cool Burst **1913**
Tylenol Cold Multi-Symptom Nighttime Liquid with Cool Burst **1913**
Tylenol Cold Multi-Symptom Severe Caplets with Cool Burst **1913**
Tylenol Cold Multi-Symptom Severe Daytime Liquid with Citrus Burst **1913**
Tylenol Cough & Sore Throat Daytime Liquid with Cool Burst **1918**
Tylenol Cough & Sore Throat Nighttime Liquid with Cool Burst **1918**
Concentrated Tylenol Infants' Drops **1909**
Jr. Tylenol Meltaways **1909**
Tylenol Sinus Congestion & Pain Daytime Caplets with Cool Burst and Gelcaps **1917**
Tylenol Sinus Congestion & Pain Nighttime Caplets with Cool Burst **1917**
Tylenol Sinus Congestion & Pain Severe Caplets with Cool Burst **1917**
Tylenol Sinus Severe Congestion Caplets with Cool Burst **1917**
Tylenol Sore Throat Daytime Liquid with Cool Burst **1918**
Tylenol Sore Throat Nighttime Liquid with Cool Burst **1918**
Women's Tylenol Menstrual Relief Caplets **1919**
Vicks DayQuil Cold & Flu Multi-Symptom Relief .... ▣**616**
Vicks DayQuil LiquiCaps **2567**
Vicks DayQuil Liquid **2567**
Vicks DayQuil Multi-Symptom Cold/Flu Relief **2567**
Vicks NyQuil Cold & Flu Multi-Symptom Relief .... ▣**617**
Vicks NyQuil LiquiCaps **2567**
Vicks NyQuil Liquid **2567**
Vicks NyQuil Multi-Symptom Cold/Flu Relief **2567**
Vicodin Tablets **529**
Vicodin ES Tablets **530**
Vicodin HP Tablets **531**
Zydone Tablets **1132**

Fosphenytoin Sodium (Phenytoin increases the clearance of busulfan by 15% or more, possibly due to the induction of glutathione-S-transferase).
No products indexed under this heading.

Itraconazole (Itraconazole decreases busulfan clearance by up to 25%).
No products indexed under this heading.

Phenytoin (Phenytoin increases the clearance of busulfan by 15% or more, possibly due to the induction of glutathione-S-transferase).
No products indexed under this heading.

Phenytoin Sodium (Phenytoin increases the clearance of busulfan by 15% or more, possibly due to the induction of glutathione-S-transferase). Products include:
Phenytek Capsules **2192**

BYETTA INJECTION

(Exenatide) **600**
May interact with bacteriostatic antibiotics, beta-lactams antibiotics, fluoroquinolone antibiotics, macrolide antibiotics, oral contraceptives, penicillins, tetracyclines, and certain other agents. Compounds in these categories include:

Acetaminophen (When 1000 mg acetaminophen exlixir was given with 10 mcg of exenatide (0 hours) and 1 hour, 2 hours, and 4 hours after exenatide, acetaminophen AUCs were decreased by 21%, 23%, 24%, and 14%, respectively; Cmax was decreased by 37%, 56%, 54%, and 41%, respectively; Tmax was increased from 0.6 hour in the control period to 0.9 hour, 4.2 hours, 3.3 hours, and 1.6 hours, respectively. Acetaminohpen AUC, Cmax and Tmax were not significantly changed when acetaminophen was given 1 hour before exenatide). Products include:
Benadryl Allergy & Cold Kapgels **1895**
Benadryl Allergy & Sinus Headache Kapgels **1895**
Benadryl Severe Allergy & Sinus Headache Caplets **1897**
Lortab 5/500 Tablets **3143**
Lortab 7.5/500 Tablets **3144**
Lortab 10/500 Tablets **3144**
Percocet Tablets **1127**
Sinutab Sinus Caplets **1905**
Sudafed PE Cold & Cough Caplets **1907**
Sudafed PE Nighttime Cold Caplets **1907**
Sudafed PE Severe Cold Caplets **1908**
Sudafed PE Sinus Headache Caplets **1908**
Regular Strength Tylenol Tablets **1915**
Tylenol 8 Hour Extended Release Caplets **1915**
Extra Strength Tylenol Caplets, Cool Caplets, and EZ Tabs **1915**
Extra Strength Tylenol Adult Rapid Blast Liquid **1915**
Extra Strength Tylenol PM Caplets, Geltabs, Liquid, and Rapid Release Gels **1915**
Extra Strength Tylenol Rapid Release Gels **1915**
Tylenol with Codeine Tablets **2427**
Tylenol Allergy Multi-Symptom Caplets with Cool Burst and Rapid Release Gelcaps **1916**
Tylenol Allergy Multi-Symptom Nighttime Caplets with Cool Burst **1916**
Tylenol Severe Allergy Caplets **1916**
Tylenol Arthritis Pain Extended Release Geltabs/Caplets **1915**
Tylenol Chest Congestion Caplets with Cool Burst **1910**
Tylenol Chest Congestion Liquid with Cool Burst **1910**
Children's Tylenol Plus Cold Suspension Liquid **1912**
Children's Tylenol Plus Cold & Allergy Suspension Liquid **1914**
Children's Tylenol Plus Cough & Runny Nose Suspension Liquid **1912**
Children's Tylenol Plus Cough & Sore Throat Suspension Liquid **1912**
Children's Tylenol Plus Flu Suspension Liquid **1914**
Children's Tylenol Suspension Liquid **1909**
Children's Tylenol Meltaways **1909**
Children's Tylenol Plus Multi-Symptom Cold Suspension Liquid **1912**
Tylenol Cold Severe Congestion Daytime Caplets with Cool Burst **1912**
Tylenol Cold Head Congestion Daytime Caplets with Cool Burst **1910**
Tylenol Cold Head Congestion Nighttime Caplets with Cool Burst **1910**
Tylenol Cold Head Congestion Severe Daytime Caplets with Cool Burst **1910**
Tylenol Cold Multi-Symptom Daytime Caplets with Cool Burst and Rapid Release Gels **1913**
Tylenol Cold Multi-Symptom Daytime Liquid with Citrus Burst **1913**
Tylenol Cold Multi-Symptom Nighttime Caplets with Cool Burst **1913**
Tylenol Cold Multi-Symptom Nighttime Liquid with Cool Burst **1913**
Tylenol Cold Multi-Symptom Severe Caplets with Cool Burst **1913**
Tylenol Cold Multi-Symptom Severe Daytime Liquid with Citrus Burst **1913**
Tylenol Cough & Sore Throat Daytime Liquid with Cool Burst **1918**
Tylenol Cough & Sore Throat Nighttime Liquid with Cool Burst **1918**
Concentrated Tylenol Infants' Drops **1909**
Jr. Tylenol Meltaways **1909**
Tylenol Sinus Congestion & Pain Daytime Caplets with Cool Burst and Gelcaps **1917**
Tylenol Sinus Congestion & Pain Nighttime Caplets with Cool Burst **1917**
Tylenol Sinus Congestion & Pain Severe Caplets with Cool Burst **1917**
Tylenol Sinus Severe Congestion Caplets with Cool Burst **1917**
Tylenol Sore Throat Daytime Liquid with Cool Burst **1918**
Tylenol Sore Throat Nighttime Liquid with Cool Burst **1918**
Women's Tylenol Menstrual Relief Caplets **1919**
Vicks DayQuil Cold & Flu Multi-Symptom Relief .... ▣**616**
Vicks DayQuil LiquiCaps **2567**
Vicks DayQuil Liquid **2567**
Vicks DayQuil Multi-Symptom Cold/Flu Relief **2567**
Vicks NyQuil Cold & Flu Multi-Symptom Relief .... ▣**617**
Vicks NyQuil LiquiCaps **2567**
Vicks NyQuil Liquid **2567**
Vicks NyQuil Multi-Symptom Cold/Flu Relief **2567**
Vicodin Tablets **529**
Vicodin ES Tablets **530**
Vicodin HP Tablets **531**
Zydone Tablets **1132**

Alatrofloxacin Mesylate (The effect of exenatide to slow gastric emptying may reduce the extent and rate of absorption of orally administered drugs. Exenatide should be used with caution in patients receiving oral medications that require rapid gastrointestinal absorption. For oral medications that are dependent on threshold concentrations for efficacy, such as antibiotics, patients should be advised to take those drugs at least 1 hr before exenatide injection. If such drugs are to be administered with food, patients should be advised to take them with a meal or snack when exenatide is not administered).
No products indexed under this heading.

5-Amino-Salicylic Acid (The effect of exenatide to slow gastric emptying may reduce the extent and rate of absorption of orally administered drugs. Exenatide should be used with caution in patients receiving oral medications that require rapid gastrointestinal absorption. For oral medications that are dependent

on threshold concentrations for efficacy, such as antibiotics, patients should be advised to take those drugs at least 1 hr before exenatide injection. If such drugs are to be administered with food, patients should be advised to take them with a meal or snack when exenatide is not administered).
No products indexed under this heading.

Amoxicillin (The effect of exenatide to slow gastric emptying may reduce the extent and rate of absorption of orally administered drugs. Exenatide should be used with caution in patients receiving oral medications that require rapid gastrointestinal absorption. For oral medications that are dependent on threshold concentrations for efficacy, such as antibiotics, patients should be advised to take those drugs at least 1 hr before exenatide injection. If such drugs are to be administered with food, patients should be advised to take them with a meal or snack when exenatide is not administered).
Products include:
Amoxil Capsules **1305**
Amoxil Chewable Tablets **1305**
Amoxil Pediatric Drops for Oral Suspension **1305**
Amoxil Powder for Oral Suspension **1305**
Amoxil Tablets **1305**
Augmentin **1323**
Augmentin Tablets **1327**
Augmentin XR Extended Release Tablets **1333**
Augmentin ES-600 Powder for Oral Suspension **1329**
Moxatag Tablets **2165**

Amoxicillin Trihydrate (The effect of exenatide to slow gastric emptying may reduce the extent and rate of absorption of orally administered drugs. Exenatide should be used with caution in patients receiving oral medications that require rapid gastrointestinal absorption. For oral medications that are dependent on threshold concentrations for efficacy, such as antibiotics, patients should be advised to take those drugs at least 1 hr before exenatide injection. If such drugs are to be administered with food, patients should be advised to take them with a meal or snack when exenatide is not administered).
No products indexed under this heading.

Ampicillin (The effect of exenatide to slow gastric emptying may reduce the extent and rate of absorption of orally administered drugs. Exenatide should be used with caution in patients receiving oral medications that require rapid gastrointestinal absorption. For oral medications that are dependent on threshold concentrations for efficacy, such as antibiotics, patients should be advised to take those drugs at least 1 hr before exenatide injection. If such drugs are to be administered with food, patients should be advised to take them with a meal or snack when exenatide is not administered).
No products indexed under this heading.

Ampicillin Sodium (The effect of exenatide to slow gastric emptying may reduce the extent and rate of absorption of orally administered drugs. Exenatide should be used with caution in patients receiving oral medications that require rapid gastrointestinal absorption. For oral medications that are dependent on threshold concentrations for efficacy, such as antibiotics, patients should be advised to take those drugs at least 1 hr before exenatide injection. If such drugs are to be administered with food, patients should be advised to take them with a meal or snack when exenatide is not administered).
No products indexed under this heading.

Ampicillin Trihydrate (The effect of exenatide to slow gastric emptying may reduce the extent and rate of absorption of orally administered drugs. Exenatide should be used with caution in patients receiving oral medications that require rapid gastrointestinal absorption. For oral medications that are dependent on threshold concentrations for efficacy, such as antibiotics, patients should be advised to take those drugs at least 1 hr before exenatide injection. If such drugs are to be administered with food, patients should be advised to take them with a meal or snack when exenatide is not administered).
No products indexed under this heading.

Azithromycin Dihydrate (The effect of exenatide to slow gastric emptying may reduce the extent and rate of absorption of orally administered drugs. Exenatide should be used with caution in patients receiving oral medications that require rapid gastrointestinal absorption. For oral medications that are dependent on threshold concentrations for efficacy, such as antibiotics, patients should be advised to take those drugs at least 1 hr before exenatide injection. If such drugs are to be administered with food, patients should be advised to take them with a meal or snack when exenatide is not administered).
No products indexed under this heading.

Azlocillin Sodium (The effect of exenatide to slow gastric emptying may reduce the extent and rate of absorption of orally administered drugs. Exenatide should be used with caution in patients receiving oral medications that require rapid gastrointestinal absorption. For oral medications that are dependent on threshold concentrations for efficacy, such as antibiotics, patients should be advised to take those drugs at least 1 hr before exenatide injection. If such drugs are to be administered with food, patients should be advised to take them with a meal or snack when exenatide is not administered).
No products indexed under this heading.

Aztreonam (The effect of exenatide to slow gastric emptying may reduce the extent and rate of absorption of orally administered drugs. Exenatide should be used with caution in patients receiving oral medications that require rapid gastrointestinal absorption. For oral medications that are dependent on threshold concentrations for efficacy, such as antibiotics, patients should be advised to take those drugs at least 1 hr before exenatide injection. If such drugs are to be administered with food, patients should be advised to take them with a meal or snack when exenatide is not administered).
No products indexed under this heading.

Bacampicillin Hydrochloride (The effect of exenatide to slow gastric emptying may reduce the extent and rate of absorption of orally administered drugs. Exenatide should be used with caution in patients receiving oral medications that require rapid gastrointestinal absorption. For oral medications that are dependent on threshold concentrations for efficacy, such as antibiotics, patients should be advised to take those drugs at least 1 hr before exenatide injection. If such drugs are to be administered with food, patients should be advised to take them with a meal or snack when exenatide is not administered).
No products indexed under this heading.

Carbenicillin Disodium (The effect of exenatide to slow gastric emptying may reduce the extent and rate of absorption of orally administered drugs. Exenatide should be used with caution in patients receiving oral medications that require rapid gastrointestinal absorption. For oral medications that are dependent on threshold concentrations for efficacy, such as antibiotics, patients should be advised to take those drugs at least 1 hr before exenatide injection. If such drugs are to be administered with food, patients should be advised to take them with a meal or snack when exenatide is not administered).
No products indexed under this heading.

Carbenicillin Indanyl Sodium (The effect of exenatide to slow gastric emptying may reduce the extent and rate of absorption of orally administered drugs. Exenatide should be used with caution in patients receiving oral medications that require rapid gastrointestinal absorption. For oral medications that are dependent on threshold concentrations for efficacy, such as antibiotics, patients should be advised to take those drugs at least 1 hr before exenatide injection. If such drugs are to be administered with food, patients should be advised to take them with a meal or snack when exenatide is not administered).
No products indexed under this heading.

Cefaclor (The effect of exenatide to slow gastric emptying may reduce the extent and rate of absorption of orally administered drugs. Exenatide should be used with caution in patients receiving oral medications that require rapid gastrointestinal absorption. For oral medications that are dependent on threshold concentrations for efficacy, such as antibiotics, patients should be advised to take those drugs at least 1 hr before exenatide injection. If such drugs are to be administered with food, patients should be advised to take them with a meal or snack when exenatide is not administered).
No products indexed under this heading.

Cefadroxil (The effect of exenatide to slow gastric emptying may reduce the extent and rate of absorption of orally administered drugs. Exenatide should be used with caution in patients receiving oral medications that require rapid gastrointestinal absorption. For oral medications that are dependent on threshold concentrations for efficacy, such as antibiotics, patients should be advised to take those drugs at least 1 hr before exenatide injection. If such drugs are to be administered with food, patients should be advised to take them with a meal or snack when exenatide is not administered).
No products indexed under this heading.

Cefamandole Nafate (The effect of exenatide to slow gastric emptying may reduce the extent and rate of absorption of orally administered drugs. Exenatide should be used with caution in patients receiving oral medications that require rapid gastrointestinal absorption. For oral medications that are dependent on threshold concentrations for efficacy, such as antibiotics, patients should be advised to take those drugs at least 1 hr before exenatide injection. If such drugs are to be administered with food, patients should be advised to take them with a meal or snack when exenatide is not administered).
No products indexed under this heading.

Cefazolin Sodium (The effect of exenatide to slow gastric emptying may reduce the extent and rate of absorption of orally administered drugs. Exenatide should be used with caution in patients receiving oral medications that require rapid gastrointestinal absorption. For oral medications that are dependent on threshold concentrations for efficacy, such as antibiotics, patients should be advised to take those drugs at least 1 hr before exenatide injection. If such drugs are to be administered with food, patients should be advised to take them with a meal or snack when exenatide is not administered).
No products indexed under this heading.

Cefixime (The effect of exenatide to slow gastric emptying may reduce the extent and rate of absorption of orally administered drugs. Exenatide should be used with caution in patients receiving oral medications that require rapid gastrointestinal absorption. For oral medications that are dependent on threshold concentrations for efficacy, such as antibiotics, patients should be advised to take those drugs at least 1 hr before exenatide injection. If such drugs are to be administered with food, patients should be advised to take them with a meal or snack when exenatide is not administered).
Products include:
Suprax for Oral Suspension **1891**
Suprax Tablets **1891**

Cefmetazole Sodium (The effect of exenatide to slow gastric emptying may reduce the extent and rate of absorption of orally administered drugs. Exenatide should be used with caution in patients receiving oral medications that require rapid gastrointestinal absorption. For oral medications that are dependent on threshold concentrations for efficacy, such as antibiotics, patients should be advised to take those drugs at least 1 hr before exenatide injection. If such drugs are to be administered with food, patients should be advised to take them with a meal or snack when exenatide is not administered).

No products indexed under this heading.

Cefonicid Sodium (The effect of exenatide to slow gastric emptying may reduce the extent and rate of absorption of orally administered drugs. Exenatide should be used with caution in patients receiving oral medications that require rapid gastrointestinal absorption. For oral medications that are dependent on threshold concentrations for efficacy, such as antibiotics, patients should be advised to take those drugs at least 1 hr before exenatide injection. If such drugs are to be administered with food, patients should be advised to take them with a meal or snack when exenatide is not administered).

No products indexed under this heading.

Cefoperazone Sodium (The effect of exenatide to slow gastric emptying may reduce the extent and rate of absorption of orally administered drugs. Exenatide should be used with caution in patients receiving oral medications that require rapid gastrointestinal absorption. For oral medications that are dependent on threshold concentrations for efficacy, such as antibiotics, patients should be advised to take those drugs at least 1 hr before exenatide injection. If such drugs are to be administered with food, patients should be advised to take them with a meal or snack when exenatide is not administered).

No products indexed under this heading.

Ceforanide (The effect of exenatide to slow gastric emptying may reduce the extent and rate of absorption of orally administered drugs. Exenatide should be used with caution in patients receiving oral medications that require rapid gastrointestinal absorption. For oral medications that are dependent on threshold concentrations for efficacy, such as antibiotics, patients should be advised to take those drugs at least 1 hr before exenatide injection. If such drugs are to be administered with food, patients should be advised to take them with a meal or snack when exenatide is not administered).

No products indexed under this heading.

Cefotaxime Sodium (The effect of exenatide to slow gastric emptying may reduce the extent and rate of absorption of orally administered drugs. Exenatide should be used with caution in patients receiving oral medications that require rapid gastrointestinal absorption. For oral medications that are dependent on threshold concentrations for efficacy, such as antibiotics, patients should be advised to take those drugs at least 1 hr before exenatide injection. If such drugs are to be administered with food, patients should be advised to take them with a meal or snack when exenatide is not administered).

No products indexed under this heading.

Cefotetan (The effect of exenatide to slow gastric emptying may reduce the extent and rate of absorption of orally administered drugs. Exenatide should be used with caution in patients receiving oral medications that require rapid gastrointestinal absorption. For oral medications that are dependent on threshold concentrations for efficacy, such as antibiotics, patients should be advised to take those drugs at least 1 hr before exenatide injection. If such drugs are to be administered with food, patients should be advised to take them with a meal or snack when exenatide is not administered).

No products indexed under this heading.

Cefoxitin Sodium (The effect of exenatide to slow gastric emptying may reduce the extent and rate of absorption of orally administered drugs. Exenatide should be used with caution in patients receiving oral medications that require rapid gastrointestinal absorption. For oral medications that are dependent on threshold concentrations for efficacy, such as antibiotics, patients should be advised to take those drugs at least 1 hr before exenatide injection. If such drugs are to be administered with food, patients should be advised to take them with a meal or snack when exenatide is not administered).

No products indexed under this heading.

Cefpodoxime Proxetil (The effect of exenatide to slow gastric emptying may reduce the extent and rate of absorption of orally administered drugs. Exenatide should be used with caution in patients receiving oral medications that require rapid gastrointestinal absorption. For oral medications that are dependent on threshold concentrations for efficacy, such as antibiotics, patients should be advised to take those drugs at least 1 hr before exenatide injection. If such drugs are to be administered with food, patients should be advised to take them with a meal or snack when exenatide is not administered).

No products indexed under this heading.

Cefprozil (The effect of exenatide to slow gastric emptying may reduce the extent and rate of absorption of orally administered drugs. Exenatide should be used with caution in patients receiving oral medications that require rapid gastrointestinal absorption. For oral medications that are dependent on threshold concentrations for efficacy, such as antibiotics, patients should be advised to take those drugs at least 1 hr before exenatide injection. If such drugs are to be administered with food, patients should be advised to take them with a meal or snack when exenatide is not administered).

No products indexed under this heading.

Ceftazidime (The effect of exenatide to slow gastric emptying may reduce the extent and rate of absorption of orally administered drugs. Exenatide should be used with caution in patients receiving oral medications that require rapid gastrointestinal absorption. For oral medications that are dependent on threshold concentrations for efficacy, such as antibiotics, patients should be advised to take those drugs at least 1 hr before exenatide injection. If such drugs are to be administered with food, patients should be advised to take them with a meal or snack when exenatide is not administered). Products include:

Fortaz 1450

Ceftizoxime Sodium (The effect of exenatide to slow gastric emptying may reduce the extent and rate of absorption of orally administered drugs. Exenatide should be used with caution in patients receiving oral medications that require rapid gastrointestinal absorption. For oral medications that are dependent on threshold concentrations for efficacy, such as antibiotics, patients should be advised to take those drugs at least 1 hr before exenatide injection. If such drugs are to be administered with food, patients should be advised to take them with a meal or snack when exenatide is not administered).

No products indexed under this heading.

Ceftriaxone Sodium (The effect of exenatide to slow gastric emptying may reduce the extent and rate of absorption of orally administered drugs. Exenatide should be used with caution in patients receiving oral medications that require rapid gastrointestinal absorption. For oral medications that are dependent on threshold concentrations for efficacy, such as antibiotics, patients should be advised to take those drugs at least 1 hr before exenatide injection. If such drugs are to be administered with food, patients should be advised to take them with a meal or snack when exenatide is not administered). Products include:

Rocephin Injectable Vials, ADD-Vantage, Galaxy, Bulk 2642

Cefuroxime Axetil (The effect of exenatide to slow gastric emptying may reduce the extent and rate of absorption of orally administered drugs. Exenatide should be used with caution in patients receiving oral medications that require rapid gastrointestinal absorption. For oral medications that are dependent on threshold concentrations for efficacy, such as antibiotics, patients should be advised to take those drugs at least 1 hr before exenatide injection. If such drugs are to be administered with food, patients should be advised to take them with a meal or snack when exenatide is not administered). Products include:

Ceftin 1380

Cefuroxime Sodium (The effect of exenatide to slow gastric emptying may reduce the extent and rate of absorption of orally administered drugs. Exenatide should be used with caution in patients receiving oral medications that require rapid gastrointestinal absorption. For oral medications that are dependent on threshold concentrations for efficacy, such as antibiotics, patients should be advised to take those drugs at least 1 hr before exenatide injection. If such drugs are to be administered with food, patients should be advised to take them with a meal or snack when exenatide is not administered).

No products indexed under this heading.

Cephalexin (The effect of exenatide to slow gastric emptying may reduce the extent and rate of absorption of orally administered drugs. Exenatide should be used with caution in patients receiving oral medications that require rapid gastrointestinal absorption. For oral medications that are dependent on threshold concentrations for efficacy, such as antibiotics, patients should be advised to take those drugs at least 1 hr before exenatide injection. If such drugs are to be administered with food, patients should be advised to take them with a meal or snack when exenatide is not administered).

No products indexed under this heading.

Cephalothin Sodium (The effect of exenatide to slow gastric emptying may reduce the extent and rate of absorption of orally administered drugs. Exenatide should be used with caution in patients receiving oral medications that require rapid gastrointestinal absorption. For oral medications that are dependent on threshold concentrations for efficacy, such as antibiotics, patients should be advised to take those drugs at least 1 hr before exenatide injection. If such drugs are to be administered with food, patients should be advised to take them with a meal or snack when exenatide is not administered).

No products indexed under this heading.

Cephapirin Sodium (The effect of exenatide to slow gastric emptying may reduce the extent and rate of absorption of orally administered drugs. Exenatide should be used with caution in patients receiving oral medications that require rapid gastrointestinal absorption. For oral medications that are dependent on threshold concentrations for efficacy, such as antibiotics, patients should be advised to take those drugs at least 1 hr before exenatide injection. If such drugs are to be administered with food, patients should be advised to take them with a meal or snack when exenatide is not administered).

No products indexed under this heading.

Cephradine (The effect of exenatide to slow gastric emptying may reduce the extent and rate of absorption of orally administered drugs. Exenatide should be used with caution in patients receiving oral medications that require rapid gastrointestinal absorption. For oral medications that are dependent on threshold concentrations for efficacy, such as antibiotics, patients should be advised to take those drugs at least 1 hr before exenatide injection. If such drugs are to be administered with food, patients should be advised to take them with a meal or snack when exenatide is not administered).

No products indexed under this heading.

Chloramphenicol (The effect of exenatide to slow gastric emptying may reduce the extent and rate of absorption of orally administered drugs. Exenatide should be used with caution in patients receiving oral medications that require rapid gastrointestinal absorption. For oral medications that are dependent on threshold concentrations for efficacy, such as antibiotics, patients should be advised to take those drugs at least 1 hr before exenatide injection. If such drugs are to be administered with food, patients should be advised to take them with a meal or snack when exenatide is not administered).

No products indexed under this heading.

Chloramphenicol Palmitate (The effect of exenatide to slow gastric emptying may reduce the extent and rate of absorption of orally administered drugs. Exenatide should be used with caution in patients receiving oral medications that require rapid gastrointestinal absorption. For oral medications that are dependent on threshold concentrations for efficacy, such as antibiotics, patients should be advised to take those drugs at least 1 hr before exenatide injection. If such drugs are to be administered with food, patients should be advised to take them with a meal or snack when exenatide is not administered).

No products indexed under this heading.

Chloramphenicol Sodium Succinate (The effect of exenatide to slow gastric emptying may reduce the extent and rate of absorption of orally administered drugs. Exenatide should be used with caution in patients receiving oral medications that require rapid gastrointestinal absorption. For oral medications that are dependent on threshold concentrations for efficacy, such as antibiotics, patients should be advised to take those drugs at least 1 hr before exenatide injection. If such drugs are to be administered with food, patients should be advised to take them with a meal or snack when exenatide is not administered).

No products indexed under this heading.

Cilastatin Sodium (The effect of exenatide to slow gastric emptying may reduce the extent and rate of absorption of orally administered drugs. Exenatide should be used with caution in patients receiving oral medications that require rapid gastrointestinal absorption. For oral medications that are dependent on threshold concentrations for efficacy, such as antibiotics, patients should be advised to take those drugs at least 1 hr before exenatide injection. If such drugs are to be administered with food, patients should be advised to take them with a meal or snack when exenatide is not administered). Products include:

Primaxin I.M. **2080**
Primaxin I.V. **2083**

Ciprofloxacin (The effect of exenatide to slow gastric emptying may reduce the extent and rate of absorption of orally administered drugs. Exenatide should be used with caution in patients receiving oral medications that require rapid gastrointestinal absorption. For oral medications that are dependent on threshold concentrations for efficacy, such as antibiotics, patients should be advised to take those drugs at least 1 hr before exenatide injection. If such drugs are to be administered with food, patients should be advised to take them with a meal or snack when exenatide is not administered). Products include:

Cipro I.V. **2817**
Cipro Oral Suspension **2810**
Cipro XR Tablets **2823**
Ciprodex Otic Suspension **541**

Ciprofloxacin Hydrochloride (The effect of exenatide to slow gastric emptying may reduce the extent and rate of absorption of orally administered drugs. Exenatide should be used with caution in patients receiving oral medications that require rapid gastrointestinal absorption. For oral medications that are dependent on threshold concentrations for efficacy, such as antibiotics, patients should be advised to take those drugs at least 1 hr before exenatide injection. If such drugs are to be administered with food, patients should be advised to take them with a meal or snack when exenatide is not administered). Products include:

Cipro Tablets **2810**

Clarithromycin (The effect of exenatide to slow gastric emptying may reduce the extent and rate of absorption of orally administered drugs. Exenatide should be used with caution in patients receiving oral medications that require rapid gastrointestinal absorption. For oral medications that are dependent on threshold concentrations for efficacy, such as antibiotics, patients should be advised to take those drugs at least 1 hr before exenatide injection. If such drugs are to be administered with food, patients should be advised to take them with a meal or snack when exenatide is not administered). Products include:

Biaxin/Biaxin XL **411**

Demeclocycline Hydrochloride (The effect of exenatide to slow gastric emptying may reduce the extent and rate of absorption of orally administered drugs. Exenatide should be used with caution in patients receiving oral medications that require rapid gastrointestinal absorption. For oral medications that are dependent on threshold concentrations for efficacy, such as antibiotics, patients should be advised to take those drugs at least 1 hr before exenatide injection. If such drugs are to be administered with food, patients should be advised to take them with a meal or snack when exenatide is not administered).

No products indexed under this heading.

Desogestrel (The effect of exenatide to slow gastric emptying may reduce the extent and rate of absorption of orally administered drugs. Exenatide should be used with caution in patients receiving oral medications that require rapid gastrointestinal absorption. For oral medications that are dependent on threshold concentrations for efficacy, such as contraceptives, patients should be advised to take those drugs at least 1 hr before exenatide injection. If such drugs are to be administered with food, patients should be advised to take them with a meal or snack when exenatide is not administered). Products include:

Mircette Tablets **1034**

Dicloxacillin Sodium (The effect of exenatide to slow gastric emptying may reduce the extent and rate of absorption of orally administered drugs. Exenatide should be used with caution in patients receiving oral medications that require rapid gastrointestinal absorption. For oral medications that are dependent on threshold concentrations for efficacy, such as antibiotics, patients should be advised to take those drugs at least 1 hr before exenatide injection. If such drugs are to be administered with food, patients should be advised to take them with a meal or snack when exenatide is not administered).

No products indexed under this heading.

Digoxin (Co-administration of repeated doses of exenatide (10 mcg BID) decreased the Cmax of oral digoxin (0.25 mg QD) by 17% and delayed the Tmax by approximately 2.5 hours; however, the overall steady-state pharmacokinetic exposure (AUC) was not changed). Products include:

Lanoxin Injection **1498**
Lanoxin Injection Pediatric **1502**
Lanoxin Tablets **1505**

Dirithromycin (The effect of exenatide to slow gastric emptying may reduce the extent and rate of absorption of orally administered drugs. Exenatide should be used with caution in patients receiving oral medications that require rapid gastrointestinal absorption. For oral medications that are dependent on threshold concentrations for efficacy, such as antibiotics, patients should be advised to take those drugs at least 1 hr before exenatide injection. If such drugs are to be administered with food, patients should be advised to take them with a meal or snack when exenatide is not administered).

No products indexed under this heading.

Doxycycline Calcium (The effect of exenatide to slow gastric emptying may reduce the extent and rate of absorption of orally administered drugs. Exenatide should be used with caution in patients receiving oral medications that require rapid gastrointestinal absorption. For oral medications that are dependent on threshold concentrations for efficacy, such as antibiotics, patients should be advised to take those drugs at least 1 hr before exenatide injection. If such drugs are to be administered with food, patients should be advised to take them with a meal or snack when exenatide is not administered).

No products indexed under this heading.

Doxycycline Hyclate (The effect of exenatide to slow gastric emptying may reduce the extent and rate of absorption of orally administered drugs. Exenatide should be used with caution in patients receiving oral medications that require rapid gastrointestinal absorption. For oral medications that are dependent on threshold concentrations for efficacy, such as antibiotics, patients should be advised to take those drugs at least 1 hr before exenatide injection. If such drugs are to be administered with food, patients should be advised to take them with a meal or snack when exenatide is not administered).

No products indexed under this heading.

Doxycycline Monohydrate (The effect of exenatide to slow gastric emptying may reduce the extent and rate of absorption of orally administered drugs. Exenatide should be used with caution in patients receiving oral medications that require rapid gastrointestinal absorption. For oral medications that are dependent on threshold concentrations for efficacy, such as antibiotics, patients should be advised to take those drugs at least 1 hr before exenatide injection. If such drugs are to be administered with food, patients should be advised to take them with a meal or snack when exenatide is not administered).

No products indexed under this heading.

Enoxacin (The effect of exenatide to slow gastric emptying may reduce the extent and rate of absorption of orally administered drugs. Exenatide should be used with caution in patients receiving oral medications that require rapid gastrointestinal absorption. For oral medications that are dependent on threshold concentrations for efficacy, such as antibiotics, patients should be advised to take those drugs at least 1 hr before exenatide injection. If such drugs are to be administered with food, patients should be advised to take them with a meal or snack when exenatide is not administered).

No products indexed under this heading.

Erythromycin (The effect of exenatide to slow gastric emptying may reduce the extent and rate of absorption of orally administered drugs. Exenatide should be used with caution in patients receiving oral medications that require rapid gastrointestinal absorption. For oral medications that are dependent on threshold concentrations for efficacy, such as antibiotics, patients should be advised to take those drugs at least 1 hr before exenatide injection. If such drugs are to be administered with food, patients should be advised to take them with a meal or snack when exenatide is not administered).

No products indexed under this heading.

Erythromycin Estolate (The effect of exenatide to slow gastric emptying may reduce the extent and rate of absorption of orally administered drugs. Exenatide should be used with caution in patients receiving oral medications that require rapid gastrointestinal absorption. For oral medications that are dependent on threshold concentrations for efficacy, such as antibiotics, patients should be advised to take those drugs at least 1 hr before exenatide injection. If such drugs are to be administered with food, patients should be advised to take them with a meal or snack when exenatide is not administered).

No products indexed under this heading.

Erythromycin Ethylsuccinate (The effect of exenatide to slow gastric emptying may reduce the extent and rate of absorption of orally administered drugs. Exenatide should be used with caution in patients receiving oral medications that require rapid gastrointestinal absorption. For oral medications that are dependent on threshold concentrations for efficacy, such as antibiotics, patients should be advised to take those drugs at least 1 hr before

exenatide injection. If such drugs are to be administered with food, patients should be advised to take them with a meal or snack when exenatide is not administered).
Products include:

E.E.S. 433
EryPed 431

Erythromycin Gluceptate (The effect of exenatide to slow gastric emptying may reduce the extent and rate of absorption of orally administered drugs. Exenatide should be used with caution in patients receiving oral medications that require rapid gastrointestinal absorption. For oral medications that are dependent on threshold concentrations for efficacy, such as antibiotics, patients should be advised to take those drugs at least 1 hr before exenatide injection. If such drugs are to be administered with food, patients should be advised to take them with a meal or snack when exenatide is not administered).

No products indexed under this heading.

Erythromycin Stearate (The effect of exenatide to slow gastric emptying may reduce the extent and rate of absorption of orally administered drugs. Exenatide should be used with caution in patients receiving oral medications that require rapid gastrointestinal absorption. For oral medications that are dependent on threshold concentrations for efficacy, such as antibiotics, patients should be advised to take those drugs at least 1 hr before exenatide injection. If such drugs are to be administered with food, patients should be advised to take them with a meal or snack when exenatide is not administered).

No products indexed under this heading.

Ethinyl Estradiol (The effect of exenatide to slow gastric emptying may reduce the extent and rate of absorption of orally administered drugs. Exenatide should be used with caution in patients receiving oral medications that require rapid gastrointestinal absorption. For oral medications that are dependent on threshold concentrations for efficacy, such as contraceptives, patients should be advised to take those drugs at least 1 hr before exenatide injection. If such drugs are to be administered with food, patients should be advised to take them with a meal or snack when exenatide is not administered). Products include:

Lybrel Tablets 3204
Mircette Tablets 1034
NuvaRing 2897
Ortho-Cyclen/Ortho Tri-Cyclen 2449
Ortho Evra Transdermal System 2437
Ortho Tri-Cyclen Lo Tablets 2458
Seasonique Tablets 1046
Yaz Tablets 805

Ethynodiol Diacetate (The effect of exenatide to slow gastric emptying may reduce the extent and rate of absorption of orally administered drugs. Exenatide should be used with caution in patients receiving oral medications that require rapid gastrointestinal absorption. For oral medications that are dependent on threshold concentrations for efficacy, such as contraceptives, patients should be advised to take those drugs at least 1 hr before exenatide injection. If such drugs are to be administered with food, patients should be advised to take them with a meal or snack when exenatide is not administered).

No products indexed under this heading.

Gatifloxacin (The effect of exenatide to slow gastric emptying may reduce the extent and rate of absorption of orally administered drugs. Exenatide should be used with caution in patients receiving oral medications that require rapid gastrointestinal absorption. For oral medications that are dependent on threshold concentrations for efficacy, such as antibiotics, patients should be advised to take those drugs at least 1 hr before exenatide injection. If such drugs are to be administered with food, patients should be advised to take them with a meal or snack when exenatide is not administered).

No products indexed under this heading.

Grepafloxacin Hydrochloride (The effect of exenatide to slow gastric emptying may reduce the extent and rate of absorption of orally administered drugs. Exenatide should be used with caution in patients receiving oral medications that require rapid gastrointestinal absorption. For oral medications that are dependent on threshold concentrations for efficacy, such as antibiotics, patients should be advised to take those drugs at least 1 hr before exenatide injection. If such drugs are to be administered with food, patients should be advised to take them with a meal or snack when exenatide is not administered).

No products indexed under this heading.

Imipenem (The effect of exenatide to slow gastric emptying may reduce the extent and rate of absorption of orally administered drugs. Exenatide should be used with caution in patients receiving oral medications that require rapid gastrointestinal absorption. For oral medications that are dependent on threshold concentrations for efficacy, such as antibiotics, patients should be advised to take those drugs at least 1 hr before exenatide injection. If such drugs are to be administered with food, patients should be advised to take them with a meal or snack when exenatide is not administered).
Products include:

Primaxin I.M. 2080
Primaxin I.V. 2083

Levofloxacin (The effect of exenatide to slow gastric emptying may reduce the extent and rate of absorption of orally administered drugs. Exenatide should be used with caution in patients receiving oral medications that require rapid gastrointestinal absorption. For oral medications that are dependent on threshold concentrations for efficacy, such as antibiotics, patients should be advised to take those drugs at least 1 hr before exenatide injection. If such drugs are to be administered with food, patients should be advised to take them with a meal or snack when exenatide is not administered). Products include:

Iquix Ophthalmic Solution 3183
Levaquin 2416
Levaquin in 5% Dextrose Injection 2416
Quixin Ophthalmic Solution 3184

Levonorgestrel (The effect of exenatide to slow gastric emptying may reduce the extent and rate of absorption of orally administered drugs. Exenatide should be used with caution in patients receiving oral medications that require rapid gastrointestinal absorption. For oral medications that are dependent on threshold concentrations for efficacy, such as contraceptives, patients should be advised to take those drugs at least 1 hr before exenatide injection. If such drugs are to be administered with food, patients should be advised to take them with a meal or snack when exenatide is not administered). Products include:

Climara Pro Transdermal System 768
Lybrel Tablets 3204
Mirena Intrauterine System 779
Plan B Tablets 1044
Seasonique Tablets 1046

Lisinopril (Lisinopril steady-state Tmax was delayed 2 hours).
Products include:

Prinivil Tablets 2087
Prinzide Tablets 2092

Lomefloxacin Hydrochloride (The effect of exenatide to slow gastric emptying may reduce the extent and rate of absorption of orally administered drugs. Exenatide should be used with caution in patients receiving oral medications that require rapid gastrointestinal absorption. For oral medications that are dependent on threshold concentrations for efficacy, such as antibiotics, patients should be advised to take those drugs at least 1 hr before exenatide injection. If such drugs are to be administered with food, patients should be advised to take them with a meal or snack when exenatide is not administered).

No products indexed under this heading.

Loracarbef (The effect of exenatide to slow gastric emptying may reduce the extent and rate of absorption of orally administered drugs. Exenatide should be used with caution in patients receiving oral medications that require rapid gastrointestinal absorption. For oral medications that are dependent on threshold concentrations for efficacy, such as antibiotics, patients should be advised to take those drugs at least 1 hr before exenatide injection. If such drugs are to be administered with food, patients should be advised to take them with a meal or snack when exenatide is not administered).

No products indexed under this heading.

Lovastatin (Lovastatin AUC and Cmax were decreased approximately 40% and 28%, respectively, and Tmax was delayed about 4 hours when exenatide was administered concomitantly with a single dose of lovastatin (40 mg) compared with lovastatin administered alone. In the30-week controlled clinical trials of exenatide, the use of exenatide in patients already receiving HMG CoA reductase inhibitors was not associated with consistent changes in lipid profiles compared to baseline).
Products include:

Advicor Tablets 402
Mevacor Tablets 2063

Mestranol (The effect of exenatide to slow gastric emptying may reduce the extent and rate of absorption of orally administered drugs. Exenatide should be used with caution in patients receiving oral medications that require rapid gastrointestinal absorption. For oral medications that are dependent on threshold concentrations for efficacy, such as contraceptives, patients should be advised to take those drugs at least 1 hr before exenatide injection. If such drugs are to be administered with food, patients should be advised to take them with a meal or snack when exenatide is not administered).

No products indexed under this heading.

Methacycline Hydrochloride (The effect of exenatide to slow gastric emptying may reduce the extent and rate of absorption of orally administered drugs. Exenatide should be used with caution in patients receiving oral medications that require rapid gastrointestinal absorption. For oral medications that are dependent on threshold concentrations for efficacy, such as antibiotics, patients should be advised to take those drugs at least 1 hr before exenatide injection. If such drugs are to be administered with food, patients should be advised to take them with a meal or snack when exenatide is not administered).

No products indexed under this heading.

Mezlocillin Sodium (The effect of exenatide to slow gastric emptying may reduce the extent and rate of absorption of orally administered drugs. Exenatide should be used with caution in patients receiving oral medications that require rapid gastrointestinal absorption. For oral medications that are dependent on threshold concentrations for efficacy, such as antibiotics, patients should be advised to take those drugs at least 1 hr before exenatide injection. If such drugs are to be administered with food, patients should be advised to take them with a meal or snack when exenatide is not administered).

No products indexed under this heading.

Minocycline Hydrochloride (The effect of exenatide to slow gastric emptying may reduce the extent and rate of absorption of orally administered drugs. Exenatide should be used with caution in patients receiving oral medications that require rapid gastrointestinal absorption. For oral medications that are dependent on threshold concentrations for efficacy, such as antibiotics, patients should be advised to take those drugs at least 1 hr before exenatide injection. If such drugs are to be administered with food, patients should be advised to take them with a meal or snack when exenatide is not administered). Products include:

Solodyn Extended Release Tablets 1938

Moxifloxacin Hydrochloride (The effect of exenatide to slow gastric emptying may reduce the extent and rate of absorption of orally administered drugs. Exenatide should be used with caution in patients receiving oral medications that require rapid gastrointestinal absorption. For oral medications that are dependent on threshold concentrations for efficacy, such as antibiotics, patients should be advised to take those drugs at least 1 hr before exenatide injection. If such drugs are to be administered with food, patients should be advised to take them with a meal or snack when exenatide is not administered). Products include:

Avelox 2803
Vigamox Ophthalmic Solution 548

Nafcillin Sodium (The effect of exenatide to slow gastric emptying may reduce the extent and rate of absorption of orally administered drugs. Exenatide should be used with caution in patients receiving oral medications that require rapid gastrointestinal absorption. For oral medications that are dependent on threshold concentrations for efficacy, such as antibiotics, patients should be advised to take those drugs at least 1 hr before exenatide injection. If such drugs are to be administered with food, patients should be advised to take them with a meal or snack when exenatide is not administered).

No products indexed under this heading.

Norethindrone (The effect of exenatide to slow gastric emptying may reduce the extent and rate of absorption of orally administered drugs. Exenatide should be used with caution in patients receiving oral medications that require rapid gastrointestinal absorption. For oral medications that are dependent on threshold concentrations for efficacy, such as contraceptives, patients should be advised to take those drugs at least 1 hr before exenatide injection. If such drugs are to be administered with food, patients should be advised to take them with a meal or snack when exenatide is not administered). Products include:

Ortho Micronor Tablets 2446

Norethynodrel (The effect of exenatide to slow gastric emptying may reduce the extent and rate of absorption of orally administered drugs. Exenatide should be used with caution in patients receiving oral medications that require rapid gastrointestinal absorption. For oral medications that are dependent on threshold concentrations for efficacy, such as contraceptives, patients should be advised to take those drugs at least 1 hr before exenatide injection. If such drugs are to be administered with food, patients should be advised to take them with a meal or snack when exenatide is not administered).

No products indexed under this heading.

Norfloxacin (The effect of exenatide to slow gastric emptying may reduce the extent and rate of absorption of orally administered drugs. Exenatide should be used with caution in patients receiving oral medications that require rapid gastrointestinal absorption. For oral medications that are dependent on threshold concentrations for efficacy, such as antibiotics, patients should be advised to take those drugs at least 1 hr before exenatide injection. If such drugs are to be administered with food, patients should be advised to take them with a meal or snack when exenatide is not administered). Products include:

Noroxin Tablets 2069

Norgestimate (The effect of exenatide to slow gastric emptying may reduce the extent and rate of absorption of orally administered drugs. Exenatide should be used with caution in patients receiving oral medications that require rapid gastrointestinal absorption. For oral medications that are dependent on threshold concentrations for efficacy, such as contraceptives, patients should be advised to take those drugs at least 1 hr before exenatide injection. If such drugs are to be administered with food, patients should be advised to take them with a meal or snack when exenatide is not administered). Products include:

Ortho-Cyclen/Ortho Tri-Cyclen 2449
Ortho Tri-Cyclen Lo Tablets 2458

Norgestrel (The effect of exenatide to slow gastric emptying may reduce the extent and rate of absorption of orally administered drugs. Exenatide should be used with caution in patients receiving oral medications that require rapid gastrointestinal absorption. For oral medications that are dependent on threshold concentrations for efficacy, such as contraceptives, patients should be advised to take those drugs at least 1 hr before exenatide injection. If such drugs are to be administered with food, patients should be advised to take them with a meal or snack when exenatide is not administered).

No products indexed under this heading.

Ofloxacin (The effect of exenatide to slow gastric emptying may reduce the extent and rate of absorption of orally administered drugs. Exenatide should be used with caution in patients receiving oral medications that require rapid gastrointestinal absorption. For oral medications that are dependent on threshold concentrations for efficacy, such as antibiotics, patients should be advised to take those drugs at least 1 hr before exenatide injection. If such drugs are to be administered with food, patients should be advised to take them with a meal or snack when exenatide is not administered). Products include:

Ofloxacin Ophthalmic Solution 0.3% .... ⊙ 243

Oral Medications, unspecified (The effect of exenatide to slow gastric emptying may reduce the extent and rate of absorption of orally administered drugs. Exenatide should be used with caution in patients receiving oral medications that require rapid gastrointestinal absorption).

No products indexed under this heading.

Oxytetracycline Hydrochloride (The effect of exenatide to slow gastric emptying may reduce the extent and rate of absorption of orally administered drugs. Exenatide should be used with caution in patients receiving oral medications that require rapid gastrointestinal absorption. For oral medications that are dependent on threshold concentrations for efficacy, such as antibiotics, patients should be advised to take those drugs at least 1 hr before exenatide injection. If such drugs are to be administered with food, patients should be advised to take them with a meal or snack when exenatide is not administered).

No products indexed under this heading.

Penicillin G Benzathine (The effect of exenatide to slow gastric emptying may reduce the extent and rate of absorption of orally administered drugs. Exenatide should be used with caution in patients receiving oral medications that require rapid gastrointestinal absorption. For oral medications that are dependent on threshold concentrations for efficacy, such as antibiotics, patients should be advised to take those drugs at least 1 hr before exenatide injection. If such drugs are to be administered with food, patients should be advised to take them with a meal or snack when exenatide is not administered). Products include:

Bicillin C-R Injectable Suspension 1775
Bicillin L-A Injection 1777

Penicillin G Potassium (The effect of exenatide to slow gastric emptying may reduce the extent and rate of absorption of orally administered drugs. Exenatide should be used with caution in patients receiving oral medications that require rapid gastrointestinal absorption. For oral medications that are dependent on threshold concentrations for efficacy, such as antibiotics, patients should be advised to take those drugs at least 1 hr before exenatide injection. If such drugs are to be administered with food, patients should be advised to take them with a meal or snack when exenatide is not administered).

No products indexed under this heading.

Penicillin G Procaine (The effect of exenatide to slow gastric emptying may reduce the extent and rate of absorption of orally administered drugs. Exenatide should be used with caution in patients receiving oral medications that require rapid gastrointestinal absorption. For oral medications that are dependent on threshold concentrations for efficacy, such as antibiotics, patients should be advised to take those drugs at least 1 hr before exenatide injection. If such drugs are to be administered with food, patients should be advised to take them with a meal or snack when exenatide is not administered). Products include:

Bicillin C-R Injectable Suspension 1775
Bicillin L-A Injection 1777

Penicillin G Sodium (The effect of exenatide to slow gastric emptying may reduce the extent and rate of absorption of orally administered drugs. Exenatide should be used with caution in patients receiving oral medications that require rapid gastrointestinal absorption. For oral medications that are dependent on threshold concentrations for efficacy, such as antibiotics, patients should be advised to take those drugs at least 1 hr before exenatide injection. If such drugs are to be administered with food, patients should be advised to take them with a meal or snack when exenatide is not administered).

No products indexed under this heading.

Penicillin V Potassium (The effect of exenatide to slow gastric emptying may reduce the extent and rate of absorption of orally administered drugs. Exenatide should be used with caution in patients receiving oral medications that require rapid gastrointestinal absorption. For oral medications that are dependent on threshold concentrations for efficacy, such as antibiotics, patients should be advised to take those drugs at least 1 hr before exenatide injection. If such drugs are to be administered with food, patients should be advised to take them with a meal or snack when exenatide is not administered).

No products indexed under this heading.

Sulfamethizole (The effect of exenatide to slow gastric emptying may reduce the extent and rate of absorption of orally administered drugs. Exenatide should be used with caution in patients receiving oral medications that require rapid gastrointestinal absorption. For oral medications that are dependent on threshold concentrations for efficacy, such as antibiotics, patients should be advised to take those drugs at least 1 hr before exenatide injection. If such drugs are to be administered with food, patients should be advised to take them with a meal or snack when exenatide is not administered).

No products indexed under this heading.

Sulfamethoxazole (The effect of exenatide to slow gastric emptying may reduce the extent and rate of absorption of orally administered drugs. Exenatide should be used with caution in patients receiving oral medications that require rapid gastrointestinal absorption. For oral medications that are dependent on threshold concentrations for efficacy, such as antibiotics, patients should be advised to take those drugs at least 1 hr before exenatide injection. If such drugs are to be administered with food, patients should be advised to take them with a meal or snack when exenatide is not administered).

No products indexed under this heading.

Sulfisoxazole Acetyl (The effect of exenatide to slow gastric emptying may reduce the extent and rate of absorption of orally administered drugs. Exenatide should be used with caution in patients receiving oral medications that require rapid gastrointestinal absorption. For oral medications that are dependent on threshold concentrations for efficacy, such as antibiotics, patients should be advised to take those drugs at least 1 hr before exenatide injection. If such drugs are to be administered with food, patients should be advised to take them with a meal or snack when exenatide is not administered).

No products indexed under this heading.

Tetracycline Hydrochloride (The effect of exenatide to slow gastric emptying may reduce the extent and rate of absorption of orally administered drugs. Exenatide should be used with caution in patients receiving oral medications that require rapid gastrointestinal absorption. For oral medications that are dependent on threshold concentrations for efficacy, such as antibiotics, patients should be advised to take those drugs at least 1 hr before exenatide injection. If such drugs are to be administered with food, patients should be advised to take them with a meal or snack when exenatide is not administered). Products include:

Pylera Capsules 714

Ticarcillin Disodium (The effect of exenatide to slow gastric emptying may reduce the extent and rate of absorption of orally administered drugs. Exenatide should be used with caution in patients receiving oral medications that require rapid gastrointestinal absorption. For oral medications that are dependent on threshold concentrations for efficacy, such as antibiotics, patients should be advised to take those drugs at least 1 hr before exenatide injection. If such drugs are to be administered with food, patients should be advised to take them with a meal or snack when exenatide is not administered). Products include:

Timentin ADD-Vantage 1606
Timentin Injection Galaxy Container 1609
Timentin IV Infusion 1603
Timentin Pharmacy Bulk Package 1613

Troleandomycin (The effect of exenatide to slow gastric emptying may reduce the extent and rate of absorption of orally administered drugs. Exenatide should be used with caution in patients receiving oral medications that require rapid gastrointestinal absorption. For oral medications that are dependent on threshold concentrations for efficacy, such as antibiotics, patients should be advised to take those drugs at least 1 hr before exenatide injection. If such drugs are to be administered with food, patients should be advised to take them with a meal or snack when exenatide is not administered).

No products indexed under this heading.

Trovafloxacin Mesylate (The effect of exenatide to slow gastric emptying may reduce the extent and rate of absorption of orally administered drugs. Exenatide should be used with caution in patients receiving oral medications that require rapid gastrointestinal absorption. For oral medications that are dependent on threshold concentrations for efficacy, such as antibiotics, patients should be advised to take those drugs at least 1 hr before exenatide injection. If such drugs are to be administered with food, patients should be advised to take them with a meal or snack when exenatide is not administered).

No products indexed under this heading.

Warfarin Sodium (In a controlled clinical pharmacology study in healthy volunteers, a delay in warfarin Tmax of about 2 hours was observed when warfarin was administered 30 min after exenatide. No clinically relevant effects on Cmax or AUC were observed. However, since market introduction there have been some spontaneously cases reported of increased INR with concomitant use of warfarin and exenatide, sometimes associated with bleeding).

No products indexed under this heading.

BYSTOLIC TABLETS

(Nebivolol) 1155

May interact with antiarrhythmics, catecholamine depleting drugs, calcium channel blockers, cytochrome p450 2d6 inducers (selected), cytochrome p450 2d6 inhibitors (selected), cardiac glycosides, oral hypoglycemic agents, insulin, and certain other agents. Compounds in these categories include:

Acarbose (Beta-blockers may mask some of the manifestations of hypoglycemia, particularly tachycardia. Nonselective beta-blockers may potentiate insulin-induced hypoglycemia and delay recovery of serum glucose levels. It is not known whether nebivolol has these effects. Patients subject to spontaneous hypoglycemia, or diabetic patients receiving insulin or oral hypoglycemic agents, should be advised about these possibilities and nebivolol should be used with caution). Products include:

Precose Tablets 792

Acebutolol Hydrochloride (Nebivolol should be used with care when myocardial depressants or inhibitors of AV-conduction, such as antiarrhythmic agents, such as disopyramide, are used concurrently).

No products indexed under this heading.

Adenosine (Nebivolol should be used with care when myocardial depressants or inhibitors of AV-conduction, such as antiarrhythmic agents, such as disopyramide, are used concurrently). Products include:

Adenocard IV Injection 603
Adenoscan 605

Amiodarone Hydrochloride (Nebivolol should be used with care when myocardial depressants or inhibitors of AV-conduction, such as antiarrhythmic agents, such as disopyramide, are used concurrently).

No products indexed under this heading.

Amitriptyline Hydrochloride (Drugs that inhibit CYP2D6 can be expected to increase plasma levels of nebivolol. When nebivolol is co-administered with an inhibitor of CYP2D6, patients should be closely monitored and the nebivolol dose adjusted according to blood pressure response. Use caution when nebivolol is co-administered with CYP2D6 inhibitors).

No products indexed under this heading.

Amlodipine Besylate (Because of significant negative inotropic and chronotropic effects in patients treated with beta-blockers and calcium channel blockers of the verapamil and diltiazem type, caution should be used in patients treated concomitantly with these agents and ECGand blood pressure should be monitored. Nebivolol should be used with care when myocardial depressants or inhibitors of AV-conduction, such as certain calcium antagonists (particularly of the phenylalkylamine [verapamil] and benzothiazepine [diltiazem] classes)). Products include:

Azor Tablets 1005
Exforge Tablets 2238

Amoxapine (Drugs that inhibit CYP2D6 can be expected to increase plasma levels of nebivolol. When nebivolol is co-administered with an inhibitor of CYP2D6, patients should be closely monitored and the nebivolol dose adjusted according to blood pressure response. Use caution when nebivolol is co-administered with CYP2D6 inhibitors).

No products indexed under this heading.

Bepridil Hydrochloride (Because of significant negative inotropic and chronotropic effects in patients treated with beta-blockers and calcium channel blockers of the verapamil and diltiazem type, caution should be used in patients treated concomitantly with these agents and ECGand blood pressure should be monitored. Nebivolol should be used with care when myocardial depressants or inhibitors of AV-conduction, such as certain calcium antagonists (particularly of the phenylalkylamine [verapamil] and benzothiazepine [diltiazem] classes)).

No products indexed under this heading.

Bretylium Tosylate (Nebivolol should be used with care when myocardial depressants or inhibitors of AV-conduction, such as antiarrhythmic agents, such as disopyramide, are used concurrently).

No products indexed under this heading.

Bupropion Hydrochloride (Drugs that inhibit CYP2D6 can be expected to increase plasma levels of nebivolol. When nebivolol is co-administered with an inhibitor of CYP2D6, patients should be closely monitored and the nebivolol dose adjusted according to blood pressure response. Use caution when nebivolol is co-administered with CYP2D6 inhibitors). Products include:

Wellbutrin Tablets 1648
Wellbutrin SR Sustained-Release Tablets 1653
Wellbutrin XL Extended-Release Tablets 1659
Zyban Sustained-Release Tablets 1692

Carbamazepine (When nebivolol is co-administered with an inducer of CYP2D6, patients should be closely monitored and the nebivolol dose adjusted according to blood pressure response). Products include:

Carbatrol Capsules 3019
Equetro Extended-Release Capsules 3174

Celecoxib (Drugs that inhibit CYP2D6 can be expected to increase plasma levels of nebivolol. When nebivolol is co-administered with an inhibitor of CYP2D6, patients should be closely monitored and the nebivolol dose adjusted according to blood pressure response. Use caution when nebivolol is co-administered with CYP2D6 inhibitors). Products include:

Celebrex Capsules 2979

Chloroquine Hydrochloride (Drugs that inhibit CYP2D6 can be expected to increase plasma levels of nebivolol. When nebivolol is co-administered with an inhibitor of CYP2D6, patients should be closely monitored and the nebivolol dose adjusted according to blood pressure response. Use caution when nebivolol is co-administered with CYP2D6 inhibitors).

No products indexed under this heading.

Chloroquine Phosphate (Drugs that inhibit CYP2D6 can be expected to increase plasma levels of nebivolol. When nebivolol is co-administered with an inhibitor of CYP2D6, patients should be closely monitored and the nebivolol dose adjusted according to blood pressure response. Use caution when nebivolol is co-administered with CYP2D6 inhibitors).

No products indexed under this heading.

Chlorpheniramine (Drugs that inhibit CYP2D6 can be expected to increase plasma levels of nebivolol. When nebivolol is co-administered with an inhibitor of CYP2D6, patients should be closely monitored and the nebivolol dose adjusted according to blood pressure response. Use caution when nebivolol is co-administered with CYP2D6 inhibitors).

No products indexed under this heading.

Chlorpheniramine Maleate (Drugs that inhibit CYP2D6 can be expected to increase plasma levels of nebivolol. When nebivolol is co-administered with an inhibitor of CYP2D6, patients should be closely monitored and the nebivolol dose adjusted according to blood pressure response. Use caution when nebivolol is co-administered with CYP2D6 inhibitors). Products include:

Actifed Cold & Allergy Tablets 1895
Sudafed PE Sinus & Allergy Tablets 1908
Tylenol Allergy Multi-Symptom Caplets with Cool Burst and Rapid Release Gelcaps 1916
Children's Tylenol Plus Cold Suspension Liquid 1912
Children's Tylenol Plus Cough & Runny Nose Suspension Liquid 1912
Children's Tylenol Plus Flu Suspension Liquid 1914
Children's Tylenol Plus Multi-Symptom Cold Suspension Liquid 1912
Tylenol Cold Head Congestion Nighttime Caplets with Cool Burst 1910
Tylenol Cold Multi-Symptom Nighttime Caplets with Cool Burst 1913
Tylenol Sinus Congestion & Pain Nighttime Caplets with Cool Burst 1917

Chlorpheniramine Polistirex (Drugs that inhibit CYP2D6 can be expected to increase plasma levels of nebivolol. When nebivolol is co-administered with an inhibitor of CYP2D6, patients should be closely monitored and the nebivolol dose adjusted according to blood pressure response. Use caution when nebivolol is co-administered with CYP2D6 inhibitors). Products include:

Tussionex Pennkinetic Extended-Release Suspension 3154

Chlorpheniramine Tannate (Drugs that inhibit CYP2D6 can be expected to increase plasma levels of nebivolol. When nebivolol is co-administered with an inhibitor of CYP2D6, patients should be closely monitored and the nebivolol dose adjusted according to blood pressure response. Use caution when nebivolol is co-administered with CYP2D6 inhibitors).

No products indexed under this heading.

Chlorpropamide (Beta-blockers may mask some of the manifestations of hypoglycemia, particularly tachycardia. Nonselective beta-blockers may potentiate insulin-induced hypoglycemia and delay recovery of serum glucose levels. It is not known whether nebivolol has these effects. Patients subject to spontaneous hypoglycemia, or diabetic patients receiving insulin or oral hypoglycemic agents, should be advised about these possibilities and nebivolol should be used with

caution).
No products indexed under this heading.

Cimetidine (Drugs that inhibit CYP2D6 can be expected to increase plasma levels of nebivolol. When nebivolol is co-administered with an inhibitor of CYP2D6, patients should be closely monitored and the nebivolol dose adjusted according to blood pressure response. Use caution when nebivolol is co-administered with CYP2D6 inhibitors).
No products indexed under this heading.

Cimetidine Hydrochloride (Drugs that inhibit CYP2D6 can be expected to increase plasma levels of nebivolol. When nebivolol is co-administered with an inhibitor of CYP2D6, patients should be closely monitored and the nebivolol dose adjusted according to blood pressure response. Use caution when nebivolol is co-administered with CYP2D6 inhibitors).
No products indexed under this heading.

Citalopram Hydrobromide (Drugs that inhibit CYP2D6 can be expected to increase plasma levels of nebivolol. When nebivolol is co-administered with an inhibitor of CYP2D6, patients should be closely monitored and the nebivolol dose adjusted according to blood pressure response. Use caution when nebivolol is co-administered with CYP2D6 inhibitors). Products include:
Celexa 1160

Clomipramine Hydrochloride (Drugs that inhibit CYP2D6 can be expected to increase plasma levels of nebivolol. When nebivolol is co-administered with an inhibitor of CYP2D6, patients should be closely monitored and the nebivolol dose adjusted according to blood pressure response. Use caution when nebivolol is co-administered with CYP2D6 inhibitors).
No products indexed under this heading.

Clonidine (In patients who are receiving nebivolol and clonidine, nebivolol should be discontinued for several days before the gradual tapering of clonidine). Products include:
Catapres-TTS 842

Cocaine Hydrochloride (Drugs that inhibit CYP2D6 can be expected to increase plasma levels of nebivolol. When nebivolol is co-administered with an inhibitor of CYP2D6, patients should be closely monitored and the nebivolol dose adjusted according to blood pressure response. Use caution when nebivolol is co-administered with CYP2D6 inhibitors).
No products indexed under this heading.

Deserpidine (Patients receiving catecholamine-depleting drugs, such as reserpine or guanethidine, should be closely monitored, because the added beta-blocking action of nebivolol may produce excessive reduction of sympathetic activity).
No products indexed under this heading.

Desipramine Hydrochloride (Drugs that inhibit CYP2D6 can be expected to increase plasma levels of nebivolol. When nebivolol is co-administered with an inhibitor of CYP2D6, patients should be closely monitored and the nebivolol dose adjusted according to blood pressure response. Use caution when nebivolol is co-administered with CYP2D6 inhibitors).
No products indexed under this heading.

Deslanoside (Both digitalis glycosides and beta-blockers slow atrioventricular conduction and decrease heart rate. Concomitant use can increase the risk of bradycardia).
No products indexed under this heading.

Digitalis Glycoside Preparations (Both digitalis glycosides and beta-blockers slow atrioventricular conduction and decrease heart rate. Concomitant use can increase the risk of bradycardia).
No products indexed under this heading.

Digitoxin (Both digitalis glycosides and beta-blockers slow atrioventricular conduction and decrease heart rate. Concomitant use can increase the risk of bradycardia).
No products indexed under this heading.

Digoxin (Both digitalis glycosides and beta-blockers slow atrioventricular conduction and decrease heart rate. Concomitant use can increase the risk of bradycardia). Products include:
Lanoxin Injection 1498
Lanoxin Injection Pediatric 1502
Lanoxin Tablets 1505

Diltiazem Hydrochloride (Because of significant negative inotropic and chronotropic effects in patients treated with beta-blockers and calcium channel blockers of the verapamil and diltiazem type, caution should be used in patients treated concomitantly with these agents and ECGand blood pressure should be monitored. Nebivolol should be used with care when myocardial depressants or inhibitors of AV-conduction, such as certain calcium antagonists (particularly of the phenylalkylamine [verapamil] and benzothiazepine [diltiazem] classes)). Products include:
Cardizem LA Extended Release Tablets 421

Diphenhydramine (Drugs that inhibit CYP2D6 can be expected to increase plasma levels of nebivolol. When nebivolol is co-administered with an inhibitor of CYP2D6, patients should be closely monitored and the nebivolol dose adjusted according to blood pressure response. Use caution when nebivolol is co-administered with CYP2D6 inhibitors).
No products indexed under this heading.

Diphenhydramine Hydrochloride (Drugs that inhibit CYP2D6 can be expected to increase plasma levels of nebivolol. When nebivolol is co-administered with an inhibitor of CYP2D6, patients should be closely monitored and the nebivolol dose adjusted according to blood pressure response. Use caution when nebivolol is co-administered with CYP2D6 inhibitors). Products include:
Benadryl Allergy & Cold Kapgels 1895
Benadryl Allergy & Sinus Headache Kapgels 1895
Benadryl Severe Allergy & Sinus Headache Caplets 1897
Benadryl Dye-Free Allergy Liqui-gels Softgels 1897
Benadryl Allergy Kapgels 1895
Benadryl Allergy Quick Dissolve Strips 1896
Benadryl Allergy Ultratab Tablets 1896
Children's Benadryl Dye-Free Allergy Liquid 1897
Children's Benadryl Allergy Fastmelts 1897
Children's Benadryl Allergy Liquid 1898
Children's Benadryl Allergy Perfect Measure 1896
Children's Benadryl-D Allergy & Sinus Liquid 1896
Benadryl-D Allergy & Sinus Tablet 1896
PediaCare Children's Allergy & Cold Liquid 1902
PediaCare Children's Allergy Liquid 1902
Simply Sleep Caplets 1905
Sudafed PE Nighttime Cold Caplets 1907
Sudafed PE Severe Cold Caplets 1908
Extra Strength Tylenol PM Caplets, Geltabs, Liquid, and Rapid Release Gels 1915
Tylenol Allergy Multi-Symptom Nighttime Caplets with Cool Burst 1916
Tylenol Severe Allergy Caplets 1916
Children's Tylenol Plus Cold & Allergy Suspension Liquid 1914
Tylenol Sore Throat Nighttime Liquid with Cool Burst 1918

Disopyramide Phosphate (Nebivolol should be used with care when myocardial depressants or inhibitors of AV-conduction, such as antiarrhythmic agents, such as disopyramide, are used concurrently).
No products indexed under this heading.

Dofetilide (Nebivolol should be used with care when myocardial depressants or inhibitors of AV-conduction, such as antiarrhythmic agents, such as disopyramide, are used concurrently).
No products indexed under this heading.

Doxepin Hydrochloride (Drugs that inhibit CYP2D6 can be expected to increase plasma levels of nebivolol. When nebivolol is co-administered with an inhibitor of CYP2D6, patients should be closely monitored and the nebivolol dose adjusted according to blood pressure response. Use caution when nebivolol is co-administered with CYP2D6 inhibitors).
No products indexed under this heading.

Escitalopram Oxalate (Drugs that inhibit CYP2D6 can be expected to increase plasma levels of nebivolol. When nebivolol is co-administered with an inhibitor of CYP2D6, patients should be closely monitored and the nebivolol dose adjusted according to blood pressure response. Use caution when nebivolol is co-administered with CYP2D6 inhibitors). Products include:
Lexapro Oral Suspension 1174
Lexapro Tablets 1174

Ethanol (When nebivolol is co-administered with an inducer of CYP2D6, patients should be closely monitored and the nebivolol dose adjusted according to blood pressure response).
No products indexed under this heading.

Felodipine (Because of significant negative inotropic and chronotropic effects in patients treated with beta-blockers and calcium channel blockers of the verapamil and diltiazem type, caution should be used in patients treated concomitantly with these agents and ECGand blood pressure should be monitored. Nebivolol should be used with care when myocardial depressants or inhibitors of AV-conduction, such as certain calcium antagonists (particularly of the phenylalkylamine [verapamil] and benzothiazepine [diltiazem] classes)).
No products indexed under this heading.

Flecainide Acetate (Nebivolol should be used with care when myocardial depressants or inhibitors of AV-conduction, such as antiarrhythmic agents, such as disopyramide, are used concurrently).
No products indexed under this heading.

Fluoxetine (Drugs that inhibit CYP2D6 can be expected to increase plasma levels of nebivolol. When nebivolol is co-administered with an inhibitor of CYP2D6, patients should be closely monitored and the nebivolol dose adjusted according to blood pressure response. Use caution when nebivolol is co-administered with CYP2D6 inhibitors).
No products indexed under this heading.

Fluoxetine Hydrochloride (Drugs that inhibit CYP2D6 can be expected to increase plasma levels of nebivolol. When nebivolol is co-administered with an inhibitor of CYP2D6, patients should be closely monitored and the nebivolol dose adjusted according to blood pressure response. Use caution when nebivolol is co-administered with CYP2D6 inhibitors). Products include:
Prozac Weekly Capsules 1852
Prozac Pulvules and Liquid 1852
Symbyax Capsules 1871

Fluphenazine Decanoate (Drugs that inhibit CYP2D6 can be expected to increase plasma levels of nebivolol. When nebivolol is co-administered with an inhibitor of CYP2D6, patients should be closely monitored and the nebivolol dose adjusted according to blood pressure response. Use caution when nebivolol is co-administered with CYP2D6 inhibitors).
No products indexed under this heading.

Fluphenazine Enanthate (Drugs that inhibit CYP2D6 can be expected to increase plasma levels of nebivolol. When nebivolol is co-administered with an inhibitor of CYP2D6, patients should be closely monitored and the nebivolol dose adjusted according to blood pressure response. Use caution when nebivolol is co-administered with CYP2D6 inhibitors).
No products indexed under this heading.

Fluphenazine Hydrochloride (Drugs that inhibit CYP2D6 can be expected to increase plasma levels of nebivolol. When nebivolol is co-administered with an inhibitor of CYP2D6, patients should be closely monitored and the nebivolol dose adjusted according to blood pressure response. Use caution when nebivolol is co-administered with CYP2D6 inhibitors).
No products indexed under this heading.

Fluvoxamine Maleate (Drugs that inhibit CYP2D6 can be expected to increase plasma levels of nebivolol. When nebivolol is co-administered with an inhibitor of CYP2D6, patients should be closely monitored and the nebivolol dose adjusted according to blood pressure response. Use caution when nebivolol is co-administered with CYP2D6 inhibitors). Products include:
Luvox CR Extended-Release Capsules **1759**

Glimepiride (Beta-blockers may mask some of the manifestations of hypoglycemia, particularly tachycardia. Nonselective beta-blockers may potentiate insulin-induced hypoglycemia and delay recovery of serum glucose levels. It is not known whether nebivolol has these effects. Patients subject to spontaneous hypoglycemia, or diabetic patients receiving insulin or oral hypoglycemic agents, should be advised about these possibilities and nebivolol should be used with caution). Products include:
Avandaryl Tablets **1344**
Duetact Tablets **3085**

Glipizide (Beta-blockers may mask some of the manifestations of hypoglycemia, particularly tachycardia. Nonselective beta-blockers may potentiate insulin-induced hypoglycemia and delay recovery of serum glucose levels. It is not known whether nebivolol has these effects. Patients subject to spontaneous hypoglycemia, or diabetic patients receiving insulin or oral hypoglycemic agents, should be advised about these possibilities and nebivolol should be used with caution).
No products indexed under this heading.

Glyburide (Beta-blockers may mask some of the manifestations of hypoglycemia, particularly tachycardia. Nonselective beta-blockers may potentiate insulin-induced hypoglycemia and delay recovery of serum glucose levels. It is not known whether nebivolol has these effects. Patients subject to spontaneous hypoglycemia, or diabetic patients receiving insulin or oral hypoglycemic agents, should be advised about these possibilities and nebivolol should be used with caution).
No products indexed under this heading.

Guanethidine Monosulfate (Patients receiving catecholamine-depleting drugs, such as reserpine or guanethidine, should be closely monitored, because the added beta-blocking action of nebivolol may produce excessive reduction of sympathetic activity).
No products indexed under this heading.

Halofantrine Hydrochloride (Drugs that inhibit CYP2D6 can be expected to increase plasma levels of nebivolol. When nebivolol is co-administered with an inhibitor of CYP2D6, patients should be closely monitored and the nebivolol dose adjusted according to blood pressure response. Use caution when nebivolol is co-administered with CYP2D6 inhibitors).
No products indexed under this heading.

Haloperidol (Drugs that inhibit CYP2D6 can be expected to increase plasma levels of nebivolol. When nebivolol is co-administered with an inhibitor of CYP2D6, patients should be closely monitored and the nebivolol dose adjusted according to blood pressure response. Use caution when nebivolol is co-administered with CYP2D6 inhibitors).
No products indexed under this heading.

Haloperidol Decanoate (Drugs that inhibit CYP2D6 can be expected to increase plasma levels of nebivolol. When nebivolol is co-administered with an inhibitor of CYP2D6, patients should be closely monitored and the nebivolol dose adjusted according to blood pressure response. Use caution when nebivolol is co-administered with CYP2D6 inhibitors).
No products indexed under this heading.

Hydroxychloroquine Sulfate (Drugs that inhibit CYP2D6 can be expected to increase plasma levels of nebivolol. When nebivolol is co-administered with an inhibitor of CYP2D6, patients should be closely monitored and the nebivolol dose adjusted according to blood pressure response. Use caution when nebivolol is co-administered with CYP2D6 inhibitors).
No products indexed under this heading.

Hypericum Perforatum (When nebivolol is co-administered with an inducer of CYP2D6, patients should be closely monitored and the nebivolol dose adjusted according to blood pressure response).
No products indexed under this heading.

Imatinib Mesylate (Drugs that inhibit CYP2D6 can be expected to increase plasma levels of nebivolol. When nebivolol is co-administered with an inhibitor of CYP2D6, patients should be closely monitored and the nebivolol dose adjusted according to blood pressure response. Use caution when nebivolol is co-administered with CYP2D6 inhibitors). Products include:
Gleevec Tablets **2255**

Imipramine Hydrochloride (Drugs that inhibit CYP2D6 can be expected to increase plasma levels of nebivolol. When nebivolol is co-administered with an inhibitor of CYP2D6, patients should be closely monitored and the nebivolol dose adjusted according to blood pressure response. Use caution when nebivolol is co-administered with CYP2D6 inhibitors).
No products indexed under this heading.

Imipramine Pamoate (Drugs that inhibit CYP2D6 can be expected to increase plasma levels of nebivolol. When nebivolol is co-administered with an inhibitor of CYP2D6, patients should be closely monitored and the nebivolol dose adjusted according to blood pressure response. Use caution when nebivolol is co-administered with CYP2D6 inhibitors).
No products indexed under this heading.

Insulin (Beta-blockers may mask some of the manifestations of hypoglycemia, partiuclarly tachycardia. Nonselective beta-blockers may potentiate insulin-induced hypoglycemia and delay recovery of serum glucose levels. It is not known whether nebivolol has these effects. Patients subject to spontaneous hypoglycemia, or diabetic patients receiving insulin or oral hypoglycemic agents, should be advised about these possibilities and nebivolol should be used with caution).
No products indexed under this heading.

Insulin, Human, Zinc Suspension (Beta-blockers may mask some of the manifestations of hypoglycemia, partiuclarly tachycardia. Nonselective beta-blockers may potentiate insulin-induced hypoglycemia and delay recovery of serum glucose levels. It is not known whether nebivolol has these effects. Patients subject to spontaneous hypoglycemia, or diabetic patients receiving insulin or oral hypoglycemic agents, should be advised about these possibilities and nebivolol should be used with caution).
No products indexed under this heading.

Insulin, Human (rDNA origin) (Beta-blockers may mask some of the manifestations of hypoglycemia, partiuclarly tachycardia. Nonselective beta-blockers may potentiate insulin-induced hypoglycemia and delay recovery of serum glucose levels. It is not known whether nebivolol has these effects. Patients subject to spontaneous hypoglycemia, or diabetic patients receiving insulin or oral hypoglycemic agents, should be advised about these possibilities and nebivolol should be used with caution). Products include:
Exubera Inhalation Powder **2515**

Insulin, Human NPH (Beta-blockers may mask some of the manifestations of hypoglycemia, particularly tachycardia. Nonselective beta-blockers may potentiate insulin-induced hypoglycemia and delay recovery of serum glucose levels. It is not known whether nebivolol has these effects. Patients subject to spontaneous hypoglycemia, or diabetic patients receiving insulin or oral hypoglycemic agents, should be advised about these possibilities and nebivolol should be used with caution). Products include:
Humulin N Vial **1846**

Insulin, Human Regular (Beta-blockers may mask some of the manifestations of hypoglycemia, particularly tachycardia. Nonselective beta-blockers may potentiate insulin-induced hypoglycemia and delay recovery of serum glucose levels. It is not known whether nebivolol has these effects. Patients subject to spontaneous hypoglycemia, or diabetic patients receiving insulin or oral hypoglycemic agents, should be advised about these possibilities and nebivolol should be used with caution). Products include:
Humulin R **1849**
Humulin R (U-500) **1850**

Insulin, Human Regular and Human NPH Mixture (Beta-blockers may mask some of the manifestations of hypoglycemia, partiuclarly tachycardia. Nonselective beta-blockers may potentiate insulin-induced hypoglycemia and delay recovery of serum glucose levels. It is not known whether nebivolol has these effects. Patients subject to spontaneous hypoglycemia, or diabetic patients receiving insulin or oral hypoglycemic agents, should be advised about these possibilities and nebivolol should be used with caution). Products include:
Humulin 50/50, 100 Units **1843**
Humulin 70/30 Vial **1844**

Insulin, NPH (Beta-blockers may mask some of the manifestations of hypoglycemia, partiuclarly tachycardia. Nonselective beta-blockers may potentiate insulin-induced hypoglycemia and delay recovery of serum glucose levels. It is not known whether nebivolol has these effects. Patients subject to spontaneous hypoglycemia, or diabetic patients receiving insulin or oral hypoglycemic agents, should be advised about these possibilities and nebivolol should be used with caution).
No products indexed under this heading.

Insulin, Regular (Beta-blockers may mask some of the manifestations of hypoglycemia, partiuclarly tachycardia. Nonselective beta-blockers may potentiate insulin-induced hypoglycemia and delay recovery of serum glucose levels. It is not known whether nebivolol has these effects. Patients subject to spontaneous hypoglycemia, or diabetic patients receiving insulin or oral hypoglycemic agents, should be advised about these possibilities and nebivolol should be used with caution).
No products indexed under this heading.

Insulin, Regular and NPH mixture (Beta-blockers may mask some of the manifestations of hypoglycemia, partiuclarly tachycardia. Nonselective beta-blockers may potentiate insulin-induced hypoglycemia and delay recovery of serum glucose levels. It is not known whether nebivolol has these effects. Patients subject to spontaneous hypoglycemia, or diabetic patients receiving insulin or oral hypoglycemic agents, should be advised about these possibilities and nebivolol should be used with caution).
No products indexed under this heading.

Insulin, Zinc Crystals (Beta-blockers may mask some of the manifestations of hypoglycemia, partiuclarly tachycardia. Nonselective beta-blockers may potentiate insulin-induced hypoglycemia and delay recovery of serum glucose levels. It is not known whether nebivolol has these effects. Patients subject to spontaneous hypoglycemia, or diabetic patients receiving insulin or oral hypoglycemic agents, should be advised about these possibilities

and nebivolol should be used with caution).
No products indexed under this heading.

Insulin, Zinc Suspension (Beta-blockers may mask some of the manifestations of hypoglycemia, partiuclarly tachycardia. Nonselective beta-blockers may potentiate insulin-induced hypoglycemia and delay recovery of serum glucose levels. It is not known whether nebivolol has these effects. Patients subject to spontaneous hypoglycemia, or diabetic patients receiving insulin or oral hypoglycemic agents, should be advised about these possibilities and nebivolol should be used with caution).
No products indexed under this heading.

Insulin Aspart (Beta-blockers may mask some of the manifestations of hypoglycemia, partiuclarly tachycardia. Nonselective beta-blockers may potentiate insulin-induced hypoglycemia and delay recovery of serum glucose levels. It is not known whether nebivolol has these effects. Patients subject to spontaneous hypoglycemia, or diabetic patients receiving insulin or oral hypoglycemic agents, should be advised about these possibilities and nebivolol should be used with caution).
No products indexed under this heading.

Insulin Aspart, Human (Beta-blockers may mask some of the manifestations of hypoglycemia, partiuclarly tachycardia. Nonselective beta-blockers may potentiate insulin-induced hypoglycemia and delay recovery of serum glucose levels. It is not known whether nebivolol has these effects. Patients subject to spontaneous hypoglycemia, or diabetic patients receiving insulin or oral hypoglycemic agents, should be advised about these possibilities and nebivolol should be used with caution). Products include:
NovoLog Mix 70/30 2364

Insulin Aspart, Human Regular (Beta-blockers may mask some of the manifestations of hypoglycemia, partiuclarly tachycardia. Nonselective beta-blockers may potentiate insulin-induced hypoglycemia and delay recovery of serum glucose levels. It is not known whether nebivolol has these effects. Patients subject to spontaneous hypoglycemia, or diabetic patients receiving insulin or oral hypoglycemic agents, should be advised about these possibilities and nebivolol should be used with caution). Products include:
NovoLog Injection 2359

Insulin Aspart Protamine, Human (Beta-blockers may mask some of the manifestations of hypoglycemia, particularly tachycardia. Nonselective beta-blockers may potentiate insulin-induced hypoglycemia and delay recovery of serum glucose levels. It is not known whether nebivolol has these effects. Patients subject to spontaneous hypoglycemia, or diabetic patients receiving insulin or oral hypoglycemic agents, should be advised about these possibilities and nebivolol should be used with caution). Products include:
NovoLog Mix 70/30 2364

Insulin Detemir (rDNA Origin) (Beta-blockers may mask some of the manifestations of hypoglycemia, partiuclarly tachycardia. Nonselective beta-blockers may potentiate insulin-induced hypoglycemia and delay recovery of serum glucose levels. It is not known whether nebivolol has these effects. Patients subject to spontaneous hypoglycemia, or diabetic patients receiving insulin or oral hypoglycemic agents, should be advised about these possibilities and nebivolol should be used with caution). Products include:
Levemir Injection 2352

Insulin glargine (Beta-blockers may mask some of the manifestations of hypoglycemia, partiuclarly tachycardia. Nonselective beta-blockers may potentiate insulin-induced hypoglycemia and delay recovery of serum glucose levels. It is not known whether nebivolol has these effects. Patients subject to spontaneous hypoglycemia, or diabetic patients receiving insulin or oral hypoglycemic agents, should be advised about these possibilities and nebivolol should be used with caution). Products include:
Lantus Injection 2749

Insulin Glulisine (Beta-blockers may mask some of the manifestations of hypoglycemia, partiuclarly tachycardia. Nonselective beta-blockers may potentiate insulin-induced hypoglycemia and delay recovery of serum glucose levels. It is not known whether nebivolol has these effects. Patients subject to spontaneous hypoglycemia, or diabetic patients receiving insulin or oral hypoglycemic agents, should be advised about these possibilities and nebivolol should be used with caution). Products include:
Apidra Injection 2706

Insulin Lispro, Human (Beta-blockers may mask some of the manifestations of hypoglycemia, partiuclarly tachycardia. Nonselective beta-blockers may potentiate insulin-induced hypoglycemia and delay recovery of serum glucose levels. It is not known whether nebivolol has these effects. Patients subject to spontaneous hypoglycemia, or diabetic patients receiving insulin or oral hypoglycemic agents, should be advised about these possibilities and nebivolol should be used with caution). Products include:
Humalog-Pen and KwikPen 1829
Humalog Mix 50/50-Pen and KwikPen 1833
Humalog Mix 75/25-Pen and KwikPen 1835

Insulin Lispro Protamine, Human (Beta-blockers may mask some of the manifestations of hypoglycemia, partiuclarly tachycardia. Nonselective beta-blockers may potentiate insulin-induced hypoglycemia and delay recovery of serum glucose levels. It is not known whether nebivolol has these effects. Patients subject to spontaneous hypoglycemia, or diabetic patients receiving insulin or oral hypoglycemic agents, should be advised about these possibilities and nebivolol should be used with caution). Products include:
Humalog Mix 50/50-Pen and KwikPen 1833
Humalog Mix 75/25-Pen and KwikPen 1835

Isradipine (Because of significant negative inotropic and chronotropic effects in patients treated with beta-blockers and calcium channel blockers of the verapamil and diltiazem type, caution should be used in patients treated concomitantly with these agents and ECGand blood pressure should be monitored. Nebivolol should be used with care when myocardial depressants or inhibitors of AV-conduction, such as certain calcium antagonists (particularly of the phenylalkylamine [verapamil] and benzothiazepine [diltiazem] classes)). Products include:
DynaCirc CR Controlled Release Tablets 1407

Lidocaine Hydrochloride (Nebivolol should be used with care when myocardial depressants or inhibitors of AV-conduction, such as antiarrhythmic agents, such as disopyramide, are used concurrently).
No products indexed under this heading.

Maprotiline Hydrochloride (Drugs that inhibit CYP2D6 can be expected to increase plasma levels of nebivolol. When nebivolol is co-administered with an inhibitor of CYP2D6, patients should be closely monitored and the nebivolol dose adjusted according to blood pressure response. Use caution when nebivolol is co-administered with CYP2D6 inhibitors).
No products indexed under this heading.

Metformin Hydrochloride (Beta-blockers may mask some of the manifestations of hypoglycemia, particularly tachycardia. Nonselective beta-blockers may potentiate insulin-induced hypoglycemia and delay recovery of serum glucose levels. It is not known whether nebivolol has these effects. Patients subject to spontaneous hypoglycemia, or diabetic patients receiving insulin or oral hypoglycemic agents, should be advised about these possibilities and nebivolol should be used with caution). Products include:
ActoPlus Met Tablets 3071
Avandamet Tablets 1336
Janumet Tablets 2041
PrandiMet Tablets 2967

Methadone Hydrochloride (Drugs that inhibit CYP2D6 can be expected to increase plasma levels of nebivolol. When nebivolol is co-administered with an inhibitor of CYP2D6, patients should be closely monitored and the nebivolol dose adjusted according to blood pressure response. Use caution when nebivolol is co-administered with CYP2D6 inhibitors).
No products indexed under this heading.

Mexiletine Hydrochloride (Nebivolol should be used with care when myocardial depressants or inhibitors of AV-conduction, such as antiarrhythmic agents, such as disopyramide, are used concurrently).
No products indexed under this heading.

Mibefradil Dihydrochloride (Because of significant negative inotropic and chronotropic effects in patients treated with beta-blockers and calcium channel blockers of the verapamil and diltiazem type, caution should be used in patients treated concomitantly with these agents and ECGand blood pressure should be monitored. Nebivolol should be used with care when myocardial depressants or inhibitors of AV-conduction, such as certain calcium antagonists (particularly of the phenylalkylamine [verapamil] and benzothiazepine [diltiazem] classes)).
No products indexed under this heading.

Miglitol (Beta-blockers may mask some of the manifestations of hypoglycemia, particularly tachycardia. Nonselective beta-blockers may potentiate insulin-induced hypoglycemia and delay recovery of serum glucose levels. It is not known whether nebivolol has these effects. Patients subject to spontaneous hypoglycemia, or diabetic patients receiving insulin or oral hypoglycemic agents, should be advised about these possibilities and nebivolol should be used with caution).
No products indexed under this heading.

Moclobemide (Drugs that inhibit CYP2D6 can be expected to increase plasma levels of nebivolol. When nebivolol is co-administered with an inhibitor of CYP2D6, patients should be closely monitored and the nebivolol dose adjusted according to blood pressure response. Use caution when nebivolol is co-administered with CYP2D6 inhibitors).
No products indexed under this heading.

Moricizine Hydrochloride (Nebivolol should be used with care when myocardial depressants or inhibitors of AV-conduction, such as antiarrhythmic agents, such as disopyramide, are used concurrently).
No products indexed under this heading.

Nateglinide (Beta-blockers may mask some of the manifestations of hypoglycemia, particularly tachycardia. Nonselective beta-blockers may potentiate insulin-induced hypoglycemia and delay recovery of serum glucose levels. It is not known whether nebivolol has these effects. Patients subject to spontaneous hypoglycemia, or diabetic patients receiving insulin or oral hypoglycemic agents, should be advised about these possibilities and nebivolol should be used with caution). Products include:
Starlix Tablets 2314

Nicardipine Hydrochloride (Because of significant negative inotropic and chronotropic effects in patients treated with beta-blockers and calcium channel blockers of the verapamil and diltiazem type, caution should be used in patients treated concomitantly with these agents and ECGand blood pressure should be monitored. Nebivolol should be used with care when myocardial depressants or inhibitors of AV-conduction, such as certain calcium antagonists (particularly of the phenylalkylamine [verapamil] and benzothiazepine [diltiazem] classes)). Products include:
Cardene I.V. 1093

Nifedipine (Because of significant negative inotropic and chronotropic effects in patients treated with beta-blockers and calcium channel blockers of the verapamil and diltiazem type, caution should be used in patients treated concomitantly with these agents and ECGand blood pressure should be monitored. Nebivolol should be used with care when myocardial depressants or

inhibitors of AV-conduction, such as certain calcium antagonists (particularly of the phenylalkylamine [verapamil] and benzothiazepine [diltiazem] classes)).

No products indexed under this heading.

Nimodipine (Because of significant negative inotropic and chronotropic effects in patients treated with beta-blockers and calcium channel blockers of the verapamil and diltiazem type, caution should be used in patients treated concomitantly with these agents and ECGand blood pressure should be monitored. Nebivolol should be used with care when myocardial depressants or inhibitors of AV-conduction, such as certain calcium antagonists (particularly of the phenylalkylamine [verapamil] and benzothiazepine [diltiazem] classes)). Products include:

Nimotop Capsules **790**

Nisoldipine (Because of significant negative inotropic and chronotropic effects in patients treated with beta-blockers and calcium channel blockers of the verapamil and diltiazem type, caution should be used in patients treated concomitantly with these agents and ECGand blood pressure should be monitored. Nebivolol should be used with care when myocardial depressants or inhibitors of AV-conduction, such as certain calcium antagonists (particularly of the phenylalkylamine [verapamil] and benzothiazepine [diltiazem] classes)). Products include:

Sular Extended Release Tablets **2975**

Nortriptyline Hydrochloride (Drugs that inhibit CYP2D6 can be expected to increase plasma levels of nebivolol. When nebivolol is co-administered with an inhibitor of CYP2D6, patients should be closely monitored and the nebivolol dose adjusted according to blood pressure response. Use caution when nebivolol is co-administered with CYP2D6 inhibitors).

No products indexed under this heading.

Paroxetine Hydrochloride (Drugs that inhibit CYP2D6 can be expected to increase plasma levels of nebivolol. When nebivolol is co-administered with an inhibitor of CYP2D6, patients should be closely monitored and the nebivolol dose adjusted according to blood pressure response. Use caution when nebivolol is co-administered with CYP2D6 inhibitors). Products include:

Paxil **1535**
Paxil CR Controlled-Release Tablets **1544**

Perphenazine (Drugs that inhibit CYP2D6 can be expected to increase plasma levels of nebivolol. When nebivolol is co-administered with an inhibitor of CYP2D6, patients should be closely monitored and the nebivolol dose adjusted according to blood pressure response. Use caution when nebivolol is co-administered with CYP2D6 inhibitors).

No products indexed under this heading.

Phenobarbital (When nebivolol is co-administered with an inducer of CYP2D6, patients should be closely monitored and the nebivolol dose adjusted according to blood pressure response). Products include:

Donnatal Extentabs **2507**

Phenobarbital Sodium (When nebivolol is co-administered with an inducer of CYP2D6, patients should be closely monitored and the nebivolol dose adjusted according to blood pressure response).

No products indexed under this heading.

Phenytoin (When nebivolol is co-administered with an inducer of CYP2D6, patients should be closely monitored and the nebivolol dose adjusted according to blood pressure response).

No products indexed under this heading.

Phenytoin Sodium (When nebivolol is co-administered with an inducer of CYP2D6, patients should be closely monitored and the nebivolol dose adjusted according to blood pressure response). Products include:

Phenytek Capsules **2192**

Pioglitazone Hydrochloride (Beta-blockers may mask some of the manifestations of hypoglycemia, particularly tachycardia. Nonselective beta-blockers may potentiate insulin-induced hypoglycemia and delay recovery of serum glucose levels. It is not known whether nebivolol has these effects. Patients subject to spontaneous hypoglycemia, or diabetic patients receiving insulin or oral hypoglycemic agents, should be advised about these possibilities and nebivolol should be used with caution). Products include:

ActoPlus Met Tablets **3071**
Actos Tablets **3077**
Duetact Tablets **3085**

Primidone (When nebivolol is co-administered with an inducer of CYP2D6, patients should be closely monitored and the nebivolol dose adjusted according to blood pressure response).

No products indexed under this heading.

Procainamide Hydrochloride (Nebivolol should be used with care when myocardial depressants or inhibitors of AV-conduction, such as antiarrhythmic agents, such as disopyramide, are used concurrently).

No products indexed under this heading.

Propafenone Hydrochloride (Nebivolol should be used with care when myocardial depressants or inhibitors of AV-conduction, such as antiarrhythmic agents, such as disopyramide, are used concurrently). Products include:

Rythmol Tablets **1586**
Rythmol SR Capsules **1590**

Propoxyphene Hydrochloride (Drugs that inhibit CYP2D6 can be expected to increase plasma levels of nebivolol. When nebivolol is co-administered with an inhibitor of CYP2D6, patients should be closely monitored and the nebivolol dose adjusted according to blood pressure response. Use caution when nebivolol is co-administered with CYP2D6 inhibitors).

No products indexed under this heading.

Propoxyphene Napsylate (Drugs that inhibit CYP2D6 can be expected to increase plasma levels of nebivolol. When nebivolol is co-administered with an inhibitor of CYP2D6, patients should be closely monitored and the nebivolol dose adjusted according to blood pressure response. Use caution when nebivolol is co-administered with CYP2D6 inhibitors).

No products indexed under this heading.

Propranolol Hydrochloride (Nebivolol should be used with care when myocardial depressants or inhibitors of AV-conduction, such as antiarrhythmic agents, such as disopyramide, are used concurrently). Products include:

InnoPran XL Extended Release Capsules **1484**

Protriptyline Hydrochloride (Drugs that inhibit CYP2D6 can be expected to increase plasma levels of nebivolol. When nebivolol is co-administered with an inhibitor of CYP2D6, patients should be closely monitored and the nebivolol dose adjusted according to blood pressure response. Use caution when nebivolol is co-administered with CYP2D6 inhibitors).

No products indexed under this heading.

Quinacrine Hydrochloride (Drugs that inhibit CYP2D6 can be expected to increase plasma levels of nebivolol. When nebivolol is co-administered with an inhibitor of CYP2D6, patients should be closely monitored and the nebivolol dose adjusted according to blood pressure response. Use caution when nebivolol is co-administered with CYP2D6 inhibitors).

No products indexed under this heading.

Quinidine Gluconate (Nebivolol should be used with care when myocardial depressants or inhibitors of AV-conduction, such as antiarrhythmic agents, such as disopyramide, are used concurrently).

No products indexed under this heading.

Quinidine Hydrochloride (Drugs that inhibit CYP2D6 can be expected to increase plasma levels of nebivolol. When nebivolol is co-administered with an inhibitor of CYP2D6, patients should be closely monitored and the nebivolol dose adjusted according to blood pressure response. Use caution when nebivolol is co-administered with CYP2D6 inhibitors).

No products indexed under this heading.

Quinidine Polygalacturonate (Nebivolol should be used with care when myocardial depressants or inhibitors of AV-conduction, such as antiarrhythmic agents, such as disopyramide, are used concurrently).

No products indexed under this heading.

Quinidine Sulfate (Nebivolol should be used with care when myocardial depressants or inhibitors of AV-conduction, such as antiarrhythmic agents, such as disopyramide, are used concurrently).

No products indexed under this heading.

Ranitidine Bismuth Citrate (Drugs that inhibit CYP2D6 can be expected to increase plasma levels of nebivolol. When nebivolol is co-administered with an inhibitor of CYP2D6, patients should be closely monitored and the nebivolol dose adjusted according to blood pressure response. Use caution when nebivolol is co-administered with CYP2D6 inhibitors).

No products indexed under this heading.

Ranitidine Hydrochloride (Drugs that inhibit CYP2D6 can be expected to increase plasma levels of nebivolol. When nebivolol is co-administered with an inhibitor of CYP2D6, patients should be closely monitored and the nebivolol dose adjusted according to blood pressure response. Use caution when nebivolol is co-administered with CYP2D6 inhibitors). Products include:

Zantac 75 Tablets .... ▣ **603**
Zantac **1670**
Zantac Injection **1666**
Zantac Injection Pharmacy Bulk Package **1668**
Maximum Strength Zantac 150 Tablets .... ▣ **603**
Maximum Strength Zantac 150 Cool Mint Tablets .... ▣ **603**

Rauwolfia Serpentina (Patients receiving catecholamine-depleting drugs, such as reserpine or guanethidine, should be closely monitored, because the added beta-blocking action of nebivolol may produce excessive reduction of sympathetic activity).

No products indexed under this heading.

Repaglinide (Beta-blockers may mask some of the manifestations of hypoglycemia, particularly tachycardia. Nonselective beta-blockers may potentiate insulin-induced hypoglycemia and delay recovery of serum glucose levels. It is not known whether nebivolol has these effects. Patients subject to spontaneous hypoglycemia, or diabetic patients receiving insulin or oral hypoglycemic agents, should be advised about these possibilities and nebivolol should be used with caution). Products include:

PrandiMet Tablets **2967**
Prandin Tablets **2971**

Rescinnamine (Patients receiving catecholamine-depleting drugs, such as reserpine or guanethidine, should be closely monitored, because the added beta-blocking action of nebivolol may produce excessive reduction of sympathetic activity).

No products indexed under this heading.

Reserpine (Patients receiving catecholamine-depleting drugs, such as reserpine or guanethidine, should be closely monitored, because the added beta-blocking action of nebivolol may produce excessive reduction of sympathetic activity).

No products indexed under this heading.

Rifampin (When nebivolol is co-administered with an inducer of CYP2D6, patients should be closely monitored and the nebivolol dose adjusted according to blood pressure response).

No products indexed under this heading.

Ritonavir (Drugs that inhibit CYP2D6 can be expected to increase plasma levels of nebivolol. When nebivolol is co-administered with an inhibitor of CYP2D6, patients should be closely monitored and the nebivolol dose adjusted according to blood pressure response. Use caution when nebivolol is co-administered with CYP2D6 inhibitors). Products include:
- Kaletra **452**
- Norvir **489**

Rosiglitazone Maleate (Beta-blockers may mask some of the manifestations of hypoglycemia, particularly tachycardia. Nonselective beta-blockers may potentiate insulin-induced hypoglycemia and delay recovery of serum glucose levels. It is not known whether nebivolol has these effects. Patients subject to spontaneous hypoglycemia, or diabetic patients receiving insulin or oral hypoglycemic agents, should be advised about these possibilities and nebivolol should be used with caution). Products include:
- Avandamet Tablets **1336**
- Avandaryl Tablets **1344**
- Avandia Tablets **1351**

Sertraline Hydrochloride (Drugs that inhibit CYP2D6 can be expected to increase plasma levels of nebivolol. When nebivolol is co-administered with an inhibitor of CYP2D6, patients should be closely monitored and the nebivolol dose adjusted according to blood pressure response. Use caution when nebivolol is co-administered with CYP2D6 inhibitors).
No products indexed under this heading.

Sildenafil Citrate (The co-administration of nebivolol and sildenafil decreased AUC and Cmax of sildenafil by 21 and 23%, respectively. The effect on the Cmax and AUC for d-nebivolol was also small (less than 20%). The effect on vital signs (e.g., pulse and blood pressure) was approximately the sum of the effects of sildenafil and nebivolol).
No products indexed under this heading.

Sitagliptin Phosphate (Beta-blockers may mask some of the manifestations of hypoglycemia, particularly tachycardia. Nonselective beta-blockers may potentiate insulin-induced hypoglycemia and delay recovery of serum glucose levels. It is not known whether nebivolol has these effects. Patients subject to spontaneous hypoglycemia, or diabetic patients receiving insulin or oral hypoglycemic agents, should be advised about these possibilities and nebivolol should be used with caution). Products include:
- Janumet Tablets **2041**
- Januvia Tablets **2048**

Sotalol Hydrochloride (Nebivolol should be used with care when myocardial depressants or inhibitors of AV-conduction, such as antiarrhythmic agents, such as disopyramide, are used concurrently).
No products indexed under this heading.

Terbinafine Hydrochloride (Drugs that inhibit CYP2D6 can be expected to increase plasma levels of nebivolol. When nebivolol is co-administered with an inhibitor of CYP2D6, patients should be closely monitored and the nebivolol dose adjusted according to blood pressure response. Use caution when nebivolol is co-administered with CYP2D6 inhibitors). Products include:
- Lamisil Oral Granules **2264**
- Lamisil Tablets **2266**

Thioridazine Hydrochloride (Drugs that inhibit CYP2D6 can be expected to increase plasma levels of nebivolol. When nebivolol is co-administered with an inhibitor of CYP2D6, patients should be closely monitored and the nebivolol dose adjusted according to blood pressure response. Use caution when nebivolol is co-administered with CYP2D6 inhibitors). Products include:
- Thioridazine Hydrochloride Tablets **2195**

Tocainide Hydrochloride (Nebivolol should be used with care when myocardial depressants or inhibitors of AV-conduction, such as antiarrhythmic agents, such as disopyramide, are used concurrently).
No products indexed under this heading.

Tolazamide (Beta-blockers may mask some of the manifestations of hypoglycemia, particularly tachycardia. Nonselective beta-blockers may potentiate insulin-induced hypoglycemia and delay recovery of serum glucose levels. It is not known whether nebivolol has these effects. Patients subject to spontaneous hypoglycemia, or diabetic patients receiving insulin or oral hypoglycemic agents, should be advised about these possibilities and nebivolol should be used with caution).
No products indexed under this heading.

Tolbutamide (Beta-blockers may mask some of the manifestations of hypoglycemia, particularly tachycardia. Nonselective beta-blockers may potentiate insulin-induced hypoglycemia and delay recovery of serum glucose levels. It is not known whether nebivolol has these effects. Patients subject to spontaneous hypoglycemia, or diabetic patients receiving insulin or oral hypoglycemic agents, should be advised about these possibilities and nebivolol should be used with caution).
No products indexed under this heading.

Trimipramine Maleate (Drugs that inhibit CYP2D6 can be expected to increase plasma levels of nebivolol. When nebivolol is co-administered with an inhibitor of CYP2D6, patients should be closely monitored and the nebivolol dose adjusted according to blood pressure response. Use caution when nebivolol is co-administered with CYP2D6 inhibitors).
No products indexed under this heading.

Troglitazone (Beta-blockers may mask some of the manifestations of hypoglycemia, particularly tachycardia. Nonselective beta-blockers may potentiate insulin-induced hypoglycemia and delay recovery of serum glucose levels. It is not known whether nebivolol has these effects. Patients subject to spontaneous hypoglycemia, or diabetic patients receiving insulin or oral hypoglycemic agents, should be advised about these possibilities and nebivolol should be used with caution).
No products indexed under this heading.

Vardenafil Hydrochloride (Drugs that inhibit CYP2D6 can be expected to increase plasma levels of nebivolol. When nebivolol is co-administered with an inhibitor of CYP2D6, patients should be closely monitored and the nebivolol dose adjusted according to blood pressure response. Use caution when nebivolol is co-administered with CYP2D6 inhibitors). Products include:
- Levitra Tablets **2876**

Verapamil Hydrochloride (Because of significant negative inotropic and chronotropic effects in patients treated with beta-blockers and calcium channel blockers of the verapamil and diltiazem type, caution should be used in patients treated concomitantly with these agents and ECGand blood pressure should be monitored. Nebivolol should be used with care when myocardial depressants or inhibitors of AV-conduction, such as certain calcium antagonists (particularly of the phenylalkylamine [verapamil] and benzothiazepine [diltiazem] classes)). Products include:
- Tarka Tablets **511**

CALCET TRIPLE CALCIUM + VITAMIN D TABLETS

(Calcium Carbonate, Calcium Gluconate, Calcium Lactate, Cholecalciferol) **629**
None cited in PDR database.

CALCIJEX INJECTION

(Calcitriol) **419**
May interact with:

Magnesium Carbonate (Co-administration with magnesium-containing antacids may lead to the development of hypermagnesemia; concurrent use should be avoided).
No products indexed under this heading.

Magnesium Hydroxide (Co-administration with magnesium-containing antacids may lead to the development of hypermagnesemia; concurrent use should be avoided). Products include:
- Fleet Pedia-Lax Chewable Tablets **1145**
- Pepcid Complete Chewable Tablets **1771**
- Extra Strength Rolaids Freshmint Tablets **1903**
- Rolaids Multi-Symptom Berry Tablets **1903**
- Rolaids Original Peppermint Tablets **1903**

Vitamin D (Since calcitriol is the most potent metabolite of vitamin D available, vitamin D and its derivatives should be withheld during treatment). Products include:
- Active Calcium Tablets **3173**
- D-Cal Chewable Caplets **624**
- Norwegian Cod Liver Oil **949**

CAMPATH AMPULES

(Alemtuzumab) **761**
May interact with:

Live Virus Vaccines (Patients who have recently received alemtuzumab, should not be immunized with live viral vaccines).
No products indexed under this heading.

CAMPRAL TABLETS

(Acamprosate Calcium) **1158**
May interact with antidepressant drugs and certain other agents. Compounds in these categories include:

Amitriptyline Hydrochloride (Patients taking acaprosate calcium concomitantly with antidepressants more commonly reported both weight gain and weight loss, compared with patients taking either medication alone).
No products indexed under this heading.

Amoxapine (Patients taking acaprosate calcium concomitantly with antidepressants more commonly reported both weight gain and weight loss, compared with patients taking either medication alone).
No products indexed under this heading.

Bupropion Hydrochloride (Patients taking acaprosate calcium concomitantly with antidepressants more commonly reported both weight gain and weight loss, compared with patients taking either medication alone). Products include:
- Wellbutrin Tablets **1648**
- Wellbutrin SR Sustained-Release Tablets **1653**
- Wellbutrin XL Extended-Release Tablets **1659**
- Zyban Sustained-Release Tablets **1692**

Citalopram Hydrobromide (Patients taking acaprosate calcium concomitantly with antidepressants more commonly reported both weight gain and weight loss, compared with patients taking either medication alone). Products include:
- Celexa **1160**

Desipramine Hydrochloride (Patients taking acaprosate calcium concomitantly with antidepressants more commonly reported both weight gain and weight loss, compared with patients taking either medication alone).
No products indexed under this heading.

Doxepin Hydrochloride (Patients taking acaprosate calcium concomitantly with antidepressants more commonly reported both weight gain and weight loss, compared with patients taking either medication alone).
No products indexed under this heading.

Escitalopram Oxalate (Patients taking acaprosate calcium concomitantly with antidepressants more commonly reported both weight gain and weight loss, compared with patients taking either medication alone). Products include:
- Lexapro Oral Suspension **1174**
- Lexapro Tablets **1174**

Fluoxetine Hydrochloride (Patients taking acaprosate calcium concomitantly with antidepressants more commonly reported both weight gain and weight loss, compared with patients taking either medication alone). Products include:
- Prozac Weekly Capsules **1852**
- Prozac Pulvules and Liquid **1852**
- Symbyax Capsules **1871**

Imipramine Hydrochloride (Patients taking acaprosate calcium concomitantly with antidepressants more commonly reported both weight gain and weight loss, compared with patients taking either medication alone).
No products indexed under this heading.

Imipramine Pamoate (Patients taking acaprosate calcium concomitantly with antidepressants more commonly reported both weight gain and weight loss, compared with patients taking either medication alone).
No products indexed under this heading.

Isocarboxazid (Patients taking acaprosate calcium concomitantly with antidepressants more commonly reported both weight gain and weight loss, compared with patients taking either medication alone). Products include:
Marplan Tablets 3177

Maprotiline Hydrochloride (Patients taking acaprosate calcium concomitantly with antidepressants more commonly reported both weight gain and weight loss, compared with patients taking either medication alone).
No products indexed under this heading.

Mirtazapine (Patients taking acaprosate calcium concomitantly with antidepressants more commonly reported both weight gain and weight loss, compared with patients taking either medication alone). Products include:
Remeron Tablets 2924
RemeronSolTab Tablets 2927

Naltrexone Hydrochloride (Co-administration of naltrexone with acamprosate calcium produced a 25% increase in AUC and a 33% increase in the Cmax of acamprosate. No adjustment of dosage is recommended in such patients).
No products indexed under this heading.

Nefazodone Hydrochloride (Patients taking acaprosate calcium concomitantly with antidepressants more commonly reported both weight gain and weight loss, compared with patients taking either medication alone).
No products indexed under this heading.

Nortriptyline Hydrochloride (Patients taking acaprosate calcium concomitantly with antidepressants more commonly reported both weight gain and weight loss, compared with patients taking either medication alone).
No products indexed under this heading.

Paroxetine Hydrochloride (Patients taking acaprosate calcium concomitantly with antidepressants more commonly reported both weight gain and weight loss, compared with patients taking either medication alone). Products include:
Paxil 1535
Paxil CR Controlled-Release Tablets 1544

Phenelzine Sulfate (Patients taking acaprosate calcium concomitantly with antidepressants more commonly reported both weight gain and weight loss, compared with patients taking either medication alone).
No products indexed under this heading.

Protriptyline Hydrochloride (Patients taking acaprosate calcium concomitantly with antidepressants more commonly reported both weight gain and weight loss, compared with patients taking either medication alone).
No products indexed under this heading.

Selegiline (Patients taking acaprosate calcium concomitantly with antidepressants more commonly reported both weight gain and weight loss, compared with patients taking either medication alone). Products include:
Emsam Transdermal System 905

Selegiline Hydrochloride (Patients taking acaprosate calcium concomitantly with antidepressants more commonly reported both weight gain and weight loss, compared with patients taking either medication alone). Products include:
Eldepryl Capsules 3052

Sertraline Hydrochloride (Patients taking acaprosate calcium concomitantly with antidepressants more commonly reported both weight gain and weight loss, compared with patients taking either medication alone).
No products indexed under this heading.

Tranylcypromine Sulfate (Patients taking acaprosate calcium concomitantly with antidepressants more commonly reported both weight gain and weight loss, compared with patients taking either medication alone). Products include:
Parnate Tablets 1532

Trazodone Hydrochloride (Patients taking acaprosate calcium concomitantly with antidepressants more commonly reported both weight gain and weight loss, compared with patients taking either medication alone).
No products indexed under this heading.

Trimipramine Maleate (Patients taking acaprosate calcium concomitantly with antidepressants more commonly reported both weight gain and weight loss, compared with patients taking either medication alone).
No products indexed under this heading.

Venlafaxine Hydrochloride (Patients taking acaprosate calcium concomitantly with antidepressants more commonly reported both weight gain and weight loss, compared with patients taking either medication alone). Products include:
Effexor XR Extended-Release Capsules.................................... 3195
Venlafaxine Hydrochloride Tablets ... 2199

CANASA RECTAL SUPPOSITORIES

(Mesalamine) 705
May interact with:

Sulfasalazine (Patients on concurrent oral products that contain or release mesalamine should be carefully monitored with urinalysis, BUN and creatinine testing).
No products indexed under this heading.

CANCIDAS FOR INJECTION

(Caspofungin acetate) 1953
May interact with dexamethasone, phenytoin, and certain other agents. Compounds in these categories include:

Carbamazepine (Results from regression analyses of adult patient pharmacokinetic data suggest that co-administration of other inducers of drug clearance, such as carbamazepine, with caspofungin may result in clinically meaningful reductions in caspofungin concentrations. It is not known which drug clearance mechanism involved in caspofungin disposition may be inducible. When caspofungin is co-administered to adults with inducers of drug clearance, such as carbamazepine, use of a daily dose of 70 mg of caspofungin should be considered. When caspofungin is co-administered to pediatric patients with inducers of drugs, such as carbamazepine, a caspofungin dose of 70 mg/m^2 daily (not to exceed an actual daily dose of 70 mg) should be considered). Products include:
Carbatrol Capsules 3019
Equetro Extended-Release Capsules 3174

Cyclosporine (In two adult clinical studies, cyclosporine (one 4 mg/kg dose or two 3 mg/kg doses) increased the AUC of caspofungin by approximately 35%. Caspofungin did not increase the plasma levels of cyclosporine. There were transient increases in liver ALT and AST when caspofungin and cyclosporine were co-administered. Caspofungin and cyclosporine should only be used concomitantly in those patients for whom the potential benefit outweighs the potential risk. Patients who develop adbormal liver function tests during concomitant therapy should be monitored and the risk/benefit of continuing therapy should be evaluated). Products include:
Gengraf Capsules 435
Neoral Oral Solution 2280
Neoral Soft Gelatin Capsules 2280
Restasis Ophthalmic Emulsion 557
Sandimmune 2296

Dexamethasone (Results from regression analyses of adult patient pharmacokinetic data suggest that co-administration of other inducers of drug clearance, such as dexamethasone, with caspofungin may result in clinically meaningful reductions in caspofungin concentrations. It is not known which drug clearance mechanism involved in caspofungin disposition may be inducible. When caspofungin is co-administered to adult patients with inducers of drug clearance, such as dexamethasone, use of a daily dose of 70 mg of caspofungin should be considered. When caspofungin is co-administered to pediatric patients with inducers of drug clearance, such as dexamethasone, a caspofungin dose of 70 mg/m^2 daily (do not exceed daily) should be considered). Products include:
Ciprodex Otic Suspension 541

Dexamethasone Acetate (Results from regression analyses of adult patient pharmacokinetic data suggest that co-administration of other inducers of drug clearance, such as dexamethasone, with caspofungin may result in clinically meaningful reductions in caspofungin concentrations. It is not known which drug clearance mechanism involved in caspofungin disposition may be inducible. When caspofungin is co-administered to adult patients with inducers of drug clearance, such as dexamethasone, use of a daily dose of 70 mg of caspofungin should be considered. When caspofungin is co-administered to pediatric patients with inducers of drug clearance, such as dexamethasone, a caspofungin dose of 70 mg/m^2 daily (do not exceed daily) should be considered).
No products indexed under this heading.

Dexamethasone Sodium Phosphate (Results from regression analyses of adult patient pharmacokinetic data suggest that co-administration of other inducers of drug clearance, such as dexamethasone, with caspofungin may result in clinically meaningful reductions in caspofungin concentrations. It is not known which drug clearance mechanism involved in caspofungin disposition may be inducible. When caspofungin is co-administered to adult patients with inducers of drug clearance, such as dexamethasone, use of a daily dose of 70 mg of caspofungin should be considered. When caspofungin is co-administered to pediatric patients with inducers of drug clearance, such as dexamethasone, a caspofungin dose of 70 mg/m^2 daily (do not exceed daily) should be considered).
No products indexed under this heading.

Efavirenz (Results from regression analyses of adult patient pharmacokinetic data suggest that co-administration of other inducers of drug clearance, such as efavirenz, with caspofungin may result in clinically meaningful reductions in caspofungin concentrations. It is not known which drug clearance mechanism involved in caspofungin disposition may be inducible. When caspofungin is co-administered to adults with inducers of drug clearance, such as efavirenz, use of a daily dose of 70 mg of caspofungin should be considered. When caspofungin is co-administered to pediatric patients with inducers of drugs, such as efavirenz, a caspofungin dose of 70 mg/m^2 daily (not to exceed an actual daily dose of 70 mg) should be considered). Products include:
Atripla Tablets 938
Sustiva Capsules 930
Sustiva Tablets 930

Fosphenytoin Sodium (Results from regression analyses of adult patient pharmacokinetic data suggest that co-administration of other inducers of drug clearance, such as phenytoin, with caspofungin may

result in clinically meaningful reductions in caspofungin concentrations. It is not known which drug clearance mechanism involved in caspofungin disposition may be inducible. When caspofungin is co-administered to adult patients with inducers of drug clearance, such as phenytoin, use of a daily dose of 70 mg of caspofungin should be considered. When caspofungin is co-administered to pediatric patients with inducers of drug clearance, such as phenytoin, a caspofungin dose of 70 mg/m^2 daily (not to exceed an actual daily dose of 70 mg) should be considered).
No products indexed under this heading.

Nevirapine (Results from regression analyses of adult patient pharmacokinetic data suggest that co-administration of other inducers of drug clearance, such as nevirapine, with caspofungin may result in clinically meaningful reductions in caspofungin concentrations. It is not known which drug clearance mechanism involved in caspofungin disposition may be inducible. When caspofungin is co-administered to adults with inducers of drug clearance, such as nevirapine, use of a daily dose of 70 mg of caspofungin should be considered. When caspofungin is co-administered to pediatric patients with inducers of drugs, such as neviraprine, a caspofungin dose of 70 mg/m^2 daily (not to exceed an actual daily dose of 70 mg) should be considered). Products include:
Viramune Oral Suspension 873
Viramune Tablets 873

Phenytoin (Results from regression analyses of adult patient pharmacokinetic data suggest that co-administration of other inducers of drug clearance, such as phenytoin, with caspofungin may result in clinically meaningful reductions in caspofungin concentrations. It is not known which drug clearance mechanism involved in caspofungin disposition may be inducible. When caspofungin is co-administered to adult patients with inducers of drug clearance, such as phenytoin, use of a daily dose of 70 mg of caspofungin should be considered. When caspofungin is co-administered to pediatric patients with inducers of drug clearance, such as phenytoin, a caspofungin dose of 70 mg/m^2 daily (not to exceed an actual daily dose of 70 mg) should be considered).
No products indexed under this heading.

Phenytoin Sodium (Results from regression analyses of adult patient pharmacokinetic data suggest that co-administration of other inducers of drug clearance, such as phenytoin, with caspofungin may result in clinically meaningful reductions in caspofungin concentrations. It is not known which drug clearance mechanism involved in caspofungin disposition may be inducible. When caspofungin is co-administered to adult patients with inducers of drug clearance, such as phenytoin, use of a daily dose of 70 mg of caspofungin should be considered. When caspofungin is co-administered to pediatric patients with inducers of drug clearance, such as phenytoin, a caspofungin dose of 70 mg/m^2 daily (not to exceed an actual daily dose of 70 mg) should be considered). Products include:
Phenytek Capsules 2192

Rifampin (A drug-drug interaction study with rifampin in adult healthy volunteers has shown a 30% decrease in caspofungin trough concentrations. Adult patients on rifampin should receive 70 mg of caspofungin daily. When caspofungin is co-administered to pediatric patients with inducers of drug clearance, such as rifampin, a caspofungin dose of 70 mg/m^2 daily (not to exceed an actual daily dose of 70 mg) should be considered).
No products indexed under this heading.

Tacrolimus (Caspofungin reduced the blood $AUC_{0\text{-}12}$ of tacrolimus by approximately 20%, peak blood concentration (Cmax) by 16%, and 12-hour blood concentration (C_{12hr}) by 26% in healthy adult subjects when tacrolimus (2 doses of 0.1 mg/kg 12 hours apart) was administered on the tenth day of caspofungin 70 mg daily, as comparted to results from a control period in which tacrolimus was administered alone. For patients receiving both therapies, standard monitoring of tacrolimus blood concentrations and appropriate tacrolimus dosage adjustments are recommended). Products include:
Prograf Capsules and Injection 622
Protopic Ointment 628

CAPASTAT SULFATE FOR INJECTION

(Capreomycin Sulfate) 1791
May interact with aminoglycosides, antituberculosis drugs, and certain other agents. Compounds in these categories include:

Amikacin Sulfate (Additive ototoxicity and/or nephrotoxicity).
No products indexed under this heading.

Aminosalicylic Acid (Potential for febrile reactions and abnormal liver function tests). Products include:
Paser Granules 1747

p-Aminosalicylic Acid (Potential for febrile reactions and abnormal liver function tests).
No products indexed under this heading.

Colistin Sulfate (Additive ototoxicity and/or nephrotoxicity).
No products indexed under this heading.

Cycloserine (Potential for febrile reactions and abnormal liver function tests). Products include:
Seromycin Capsules 1864

Ethambutol Hydrochloride (Potential for febrile reactions and abnormal liver function tests).
No products indexed under this heading.

Ether (May enhance the partial neuromuscular blockade caused by capreomycin).
No products indexed under this heading.

Gentamicin Sulfate (Additive ototoxicity and/or nephrotoxicity). Products include:
Pred-G Ophthalmic Ointment .... ⊙229
Pred-G Ophthalmic Suspension ...... ⊙228

Isoniazid (Potential for febrile reactions and abnormal liver function tests).
No products indexed under this heading.

Kanamycin Sulfate (Additive ototoxicity and/or nephrotoxicity).
No products indexed under this heading.

Neomycin, oral (Additive ototoxicity and/or nephrotoxicity).
No products indexed under this heading.

Neostigmine Bromide (May antagonize the partial neuromuscular blockade caused by capreomycin).
No products indexed under this heading.

Neostigmine Methylsulfate (May antagonize the partial neuromuscular blockade caused by capreomycin).
No products indexed under this heading.

Paromomycin Sulfate (Additive ototoxicity and/or nephrotoxicity).
No products indexed under this heading.

Polymyxin B Sulfate (Additive ototoxicity and/or nephrotoxicity). Products include:
Neosporin Ophthalmic Solution Sterile .... ⊙252

Pyrazinamide (Potential for febrile reactions and abnormal liver function tests).
No products indexed under this heading.

Rifampin (Potential for febrile reactions and abnormal liver function tests).
No products indexed under this heading.

Rifapentine (Potential for febrile reactions and abnormal liver function tests).
No products indexed under this heading.

Streptomycin Sulfate (Additive ototoxicity and/or nephrotoxicity).
No products indexed under this heading.

Tobramycin (Additive ototoxicity and/or nephrotoxicity). Products include:
Zylet Ophthalmic Suspension .... ⊙247

Tobramycin Sulfate (Additive ototoxicity and/or nephrotoxicity).
No products indexed under this heading.

Vancomycin Hydrochloride (Additive ototoxicity and/or nephrotoxicity).
No products indexed under this heading.

Viomycin (Additive ototoxicity and/or nephrotoxicity).
No products indexed under this heading.

CAPTOPRIL TABLETS

(Captopril) 2182
May interact with beta blockers, diuretics, ganglionic blocking agents, lithium preparations, nitrates and nitrites, non-steroidal anti-inflammatory agents, peripheral adrenergic blockers, potassium preparations, inhibitors of endogenous prostaglandin synthesis, potassium sparing diuretics, agents causing renin release, thiazides, vasodilators, and certain other agents. Compounds in these categories include:

Acebutolol Hydrochloride (Less than additive antihypertensive effect).
No products indexed under this heading.

Amiloride Hydrochloride (Hypotension; increased serum potassium).
No products indexed under this heading.

Amyl Nitrite (Discontinue before starting captopril; if resumed administer at lower dosage).
No products indexed under this heading.

Aspirin (Antihypertensive effects of captopril reduced). Products include:
Aggrenox Capsules 819
Bayer Aspirin 750
Percodan Tablets 1130
St. Joseph 81 mg Aspirin Chewable and Enteric Coated Tablets 1903

Atenolol (Less than additive antihypertensive effect).
No products indexed under this heading.

Bendroflumethiazide (Captopril's effect will be augmented).
No products indexed under this heading.

Betaxolol Hydrochloride (Less than additive antihypertensive effect).
No products indexed under this heading.

Bisoprolol Fumarate (Less than additive antihypertensive effect).
No products indexed under this heading.

Bumetanide (Captopril's effect will be augmented; hypotension).
No products indexed under this heading.

Carteolol Hydrochloride (Less than additive antihypertensive effect).
No products indexed under this heading.

Celecoxib (Antihypertensive effects of captopril reduced). Products include:
Celebrex Capsules 2979

Chlorothiazide (Captopril's effect will be augmented).
No products indexed under this heading.

Chlorothiazide Sodium (Captopril's effect will be augmented). Products include:
Intravenous Sodium Diuril 2490

Chlorthalidone (Captopril's effect will be augmented; hypotension; increased serum potassium). Products include:
Clorpres Tablets 2185

Deserpidine (Use with caution).
No products indexed under this heading.

Diazoxide (Drugs having vasodilator activity should, if possible, be discontinued before starting captopril). Products include:

Proglycem Capsules 1185
Proglycem Suspension 1185

Diclofenac Epolamine (Antihypertensive effects of captopril reduced). Products include:
Flector Patch 561

Diclofenac Potassium (Antihypertensive effects of captopril reduced).
No products indexed under this heading.

Diclofenac Sodium (Antihypertensive effects of captopril reduced). Products include:
Diclofenac Sodium Ophthalmic Solution .... ⊙240
Voltaren Ophthalmic Solution 2336
Voltaren Tablets 2334
Voltaren-XR Tablets 2337

Epoprostenol Sodium (Drugs having vasodilator activity should, if possible, be discontinued before starting captopril). Products include:
Flolan for Injection 1426

Erythrityl Tetranitrate (Discontinue before starting captopril; if resumed administer at lower dosage).
No products indexed under this heading.

Esmolol Hydrochloride (Less than additive antihypertensive effect).
No products indexed under this heading.

Ethacrynic Acid (Captopril's effect will be augmented; hypotension). Products include:
Edecrin Tablets 698

Ethaverine Hydrochloride (Drugs having vasodilator activity should, if possible, be discontinued before starting captopril).
No products indexed under this heading.

Etodolac (Antihypertensive effects of captopril reduced).
No products indexed under this heading.

Fenoprofen Calcium (Antihypertensive effects of captopril reduced). Products include:
Nalfon Capsules 2508

Flurbiprofen (Antihypertensive effects of captopril reduced).
No products indexed under this heading.

Furosemide (Captopril's effect will be augmented; hypotension). Products include:
Furosemide Tablets 2186

Guanethidine Monosulfate (Use with caution).
No products indexed under this heading.

Hydralazine Hydrochloride (Drugs having vasodilator activity should, if possible, be discontinued before starting captopril).
No products indexed under this heading.

Hydrochlorothiazide (Captopril's effect will be augmented). Products include:
Atacand HCT 642
Avalide Tablets 892
Avalide Tablets 2713
Benicar HCT Tablets 1010
Diovan HCT Tablets 2216
Dyazide Capsules 1405
Micardis HCT Tablets 854
Prinzide Tablets 2092
Tekturna HCT Tablets 2324
Teveten HCT Tablets 517

Hydroflumethiazide (Captopril's effect will be augmented).
No products indexed under this heading.

Ibuprofen (Antihypertensive effects of captopril reduced). Products include:
Motrin IB Tablets and Caplets 1900
Children's Motrin Oral Suspension ... 1901
Children's Motrin Non-Staining Dye-Free Oral Suspension 1901
Children's Motrin Cold Oral Suspension 1899
Infants' Motrin Concentrated Drops 1901
Infants' Motrin Non-Staining Dye-Free Concentrated Drops 1901
Junior Strength Motrin Caplets and Chewable Tablets 1901
Vicoprofen Tablets 533

Indapamide (Captopril's effect will be augmented; hypotension). Products include:
Indapamide Tablets 2188

Indomethacin (Antihypertensive effects of captopril reduced). Products include:
Indocin 2024

Indomethacin Sodium Trihydrate (Antihypertensive effects of captopril reduced). Products include:
Indocin I.V. 2489

Isosorbide Dinitrate (Discontinue before starting captopril; if resumed administer at lower dosage).
No products indexed under this heading.

Isosorbide Mononitrate (Discontinue before starting captopril; if resumed administer at lower dosage).
No products indexed under this heading.

Isoxsuprine Hydrochloride (Drugs having vasodilator activity should, if possible, be discontinued before starting captopril).
No products indexed under this heading.

Ketoprofen (Antihypertensive effects of captopril reduced).
No products indexed under this heading.

Ketorolac Tromethamine (Antihypertensive effects of captopril reduced).
No products indexed under this heading.

Labetalol Hydrochloride (Less than additive antihypertensive effect).
No products indexed under this heading.

Levobunolol Hydrochloride (Less than additive antihypertensive effect).
No products indexed under this heading.

Lithium (Increased serum lithium levels and symptoms of lithium toxicity).
No products indexed under this heading.

Lithium Carbonate (Increased serum lithium levels and symptoms of lithium toxicity).
No products indexed under this heading.

Lithium Citrate (Increased serum lithium levels and symptoms of lithium toxicity).
No products indexed under this heading.

Mecamylamine Hydrochloride (Use with caution).
No products indexed under this heading.

Meclofenamate Sodium (Antihypertensive effects of captopril reduced).
No products indexed under this heading.

Mefenamic Acid (Antihypertensive effects of captopril reduced).
No products indexed under this heading.

Meloxicam (Antihypertensive effects of captopril reduced). Products include:
Mobic Oral Suspension 863
Mobic Tablets 863

Methyclothiazide (Captopril's effect will be augmented).
No products indexed under this heading.

Metipranolol Hydrochloride (Less than additive antihypertensive effect).
No products indexed under this heading.

Metolazone (Captopril's effect will be augmented; hypotension).
No products indexed under this heading.

Metoprolol Succinate (Less than additive antihypertensive effect). Products include:
Toprol-XL Tablets 666

Metoprolol Tartrate (Less than additive antihypertensive effect).
No products indexed under this heading.

Minoxidil (Drugs having vasodilator activity should, if possible, be discontinued before starting captopril).
No products indexed under this heading.

Nabumetone (Antihypertensive effects of captopril reduced).
No products indexed under this heading.

Nadolol (Less than additive antihypertensive effect). Products include:
Nadolol Tablets 2191

Naproxen (Antihypertensive effects of captopril reduced). Products include:
EC-Naprosyn Delayed-Release Tablets 2632
Naprosyn Suspension 2632
Naprosyn Tablets 2632

Naproxen Sodium (Antihypertensive effects of captopril reduced). Products include:
Anaprox Tablets 2632
Anaprox DS Tablets 2632
Treximet Tablets 1616

Nebivolol (Less than additive antihypertensive effect). Products include:
Bystolic Tablets 1155

Nitroglycerin (Discontinue before starting captopril; if resumed administer at lower dosage). Products include:
Nitro-Dur Transdermal Infusion System 2887
Nitrolingual Pumpspray 2965

Nitroglycerin, long-acting formulations (Drugs having vasodilator activity should, if possible, be discontinued before starting captopril).
No products indexed under this heading.

Nitroglycerin Intravenous (Drugs having vasodilator activity should, if possible, be discontinued before starting captopril).
No products indexed under this heading.

Oxaprozin (Antihypertensive effects of captopril reduced).
No products indexed under this heading.

Papaverine (Drugs having vasodilator activity should, if possible, be discontinued before starting captopril).
No products indexed under this heading.

Papaverine Hydrochloride (Drugs having vasodilator activity should, if possible, be discontinued before starting captopril).
No products indexed under this heading.

Penbutolol Sulfate (Less than additive antihypertensive effect).
No products indexed under this heading.

Pentaerythritol Tetranitrate (Discontinue before starting captopril; if resumed administer at lower dosage).
No products indexed under this heading.

Phenylbutazone (Antihypertensive effects of captopril reduced).
No products indexed under this heading.

Pindolol (Less than additive antihypertensive effect).
No products indexed under this heading.

Piroxicam (Antihypertensive effects of captopril reduced).
No products indexed under this heading.

Polythiazide (Captopril's effect will be augmented).
No products indexed under this heading.

Potassium Acid Phosphate (Potential for significant increase in serum potassium). Products include:
K-Phos Original (Sodium Free) Tablets 814

Potassium Bicarbonate (Potential for significant increase in serum potassium).
No products indexed under this heading.

Potassium Chloride (Potential for significant increase in serum potassium). Products include:
MoviPrep Oral Solution 2679

Potassium Citrate (Potential for significant increase in serum potassium). Products include:
BioLean Free Tablets .... ◙635
Urocit-K Tablets 2176

Potassium Gluconate (Potential for significant increase in serum potassium).
No products indexed under this heading.

Potassium Phosphate (Potential for significant increase in serum potassium). Products include:
K-Phos Neutral Tablets 813

Prazosin Hydrochloride (Use with caution).
No products indexed under this heading.

Propranolol Hydrochloride (Less than additive antihypertensive effect). Products include:
InnoPran XL Extended Release Capsules 1484

Rauwolfia Serpentina (Use with caution).
No products indexed under this heading.

Rescinnamine (Use with caution).
No products indexed under this heading.

Reserpine (Use with caution).
No products indexed under this heading.

Rofecoxib (Antihypertensive effects of captopril reduced).
No products indexed under this heading.

Sotalol Hydrochloride (Less than additive antihypertensive effect).
No products indexed under this heading.

Spironolactone (Captopril's effect will be augmented; hypotension; increased serum potassium).
No products indexed under this heading.

Sulindac (Antihypertensive effects of captopril reduced). Products include:
Clinoril Tablets **1962**

Terazosin Hydrochloride (Use with caution).
No products indexed under this heading.

Timolol Hemihydrate (Less than additive antihypertensive effect). Products include:
Betimol Ophthalmic Solution **3181**

Timolol Maleate (Less than additive antihypertensive effect). Products include:
Combigan Ophthalmic Solution **553**
Cosopt Sterile Ophthalmic Solution **1969**
Timoptic Sterile Ophthalmic Solution **2121**
Timoptic in Ocudose **2124**
Timoptic-XE Sterile Ophthalmic Gel Forming Solution **2125**

Tolazoline Hydrochloride (Drugs having vasodilator activity should, if possible, be discontinued before starting captopril).
No products indexed under this heading.

Tolmetin Sodium (Antihypertensive effects of captopril reduced).
No products indexed under this heading.

Torsemide (Captopril's effect will be augmented; hypotension). Products include:
Demadex Injection **2630**
Demadex Tablets **2630**

Triamterene (Captopril's effect will be augmented; hypotension; increased serum potassium). Products include:
Dyazide Capsules **1405**
Dyrenium Capsules **3189**

Trimethaphan Camsylate (Use with caution).
No products indexed under this heading.

Valdecoxib (Antihypertensive effects of captopril reduced).
No products indexed under this heading.

Food Interactions

Alcohol (Drugs having vasodilator activity should, if possible, be discontinued before starting captopril).

Food, unspecified (Reduces absorption by about 30% to 40%; should be given one hour before meals).

CARAC CREAM 0.5%

(Fluorouracil) **2722**
None cited in PDR database.

CARAFATE SUSPENSION

(Sucralfate) **706**
May interact with fluoroquinolone antibiotics, quinidine, xanthines, and certain other agents. Compounds in these categories include:

Alatrofloxacin Mesylate (Potential for reduced extent of absorption (bioavailability) with concomitant oral administration; dosing the concomitant medication 2 hours before sucralfate eliminates the interaction).
No products indexed under this heading.

Aluminum Carbonate (Simultaneous administration within one-half hour before or after sucralfate should be avoided; may increase the total body burden of aluminum).
No products indexed under this heading.

Aluminum Hydroxide (Simultaneous administration within one-half hour before or after sucralfate should be avoided; may increase the total body burden of aluminum).
No products indexed under this heading.

Aminophylline (Simultaneous administration results in reduced oral absorption of theophylline).
No products indexed under this heading.

Cimetidine (Simultaneous administration results in reduced oral absorption of oral cimetidine; dosing the concomitant medication 2 hours before sucralfate eliminates the interaction).
No products indexed under this heading.

Cimetidine Hydrochloride (Simultaneous administration results in reduced oral absorption of oral cimetidine; dosing the concomitant medication 2 hours before sucralfate eliminates the interaction).
No products indexed under this heading.

Ciprofloxacin (Potential for reduced extent of absorption (bioavailability) with concomitant oral administration; dosing the concomitant medication 2 hours before sucralfate eliminates the interaction). Products include:
Cipro I.V. **2817**
Cipro Oral Suspension **2810**
Cipro XR Tablets **2823**
Ciprodex Otic Suspension **541**

Ciprofloxacin Hydrochloride (Potential for reduced extent of absorption (bioavailability) with concomitant oral administration; dosing the concomitant medication 2 hours before sucralfate eliminates the interaction). Products include:
Cipro Tablets **2810**

Digoxin (Simultaneous administration results in reduced oral absorption of oral digoxin; dosing the concomitant medication 2 hours before sucralfate eliminates the interaction). Products include:
Lanoxin Injection **1498**
Lanoxin Injection Pediatric **1502**
Lanoxin Tablets **1505**

Dyphylline (Simultaneous administration results in reduced oral absorption of theophylline).
No products indexed under this heading.

Enoxacin (Potential for reduced extent of absorption (bioavailability) with concomitant oral administration; dosing the concomitant medication 2 hours before sucralfate eliminates the interaction).
No products indexed under this heading.

Gatifloxacin (Potential for reduced extent of absorption (bioavailability) with concomitant oral administration; dosing the concomitant medication 2 hours before sucralfate eliminates the interaction).
No products indexed under this heading.

Grepafloxacin Hydrochloride (Potential for reduced extent of absorption (bioavailability) with concomitant oral administration; dosing the concomitant medication 2 hours before sucralfate eliminates the interaction).
No products indexed under this heading.

Ketoconazole (Simultaneous administration results in reduced oral absorption of oral ketoconazole). Products include:
Extina Foam, 2% **3057**
Nizoral A-D Shampoo **1901**

Levofloxacin (Potential for reduced extent of absorption (bioavailability) with concomitant oral administration; dosing the concomitant medication 2 hours before sucralfate eliminates the interaction). Products include:
Iquix Ophthalmic Solution **3183**
Levaquin **2416**
Levaquin in 5% Dextrose Injection **2416**
Quixin Ophthalmic Solution **3184**

Levothyroxine Sodium (Potential for reduced extent of absorption (bioavailability) with concomitant oral administration). Products include:
Levothroid Tablets **1170**
Levoxyl Tablets **1780**
Synthroid Tablets **507**

Lomefloxacin Hydrochloride (Potential for reduced extent of absorption (bioavailability) with concomitant oral administration; dosing the concomitant medication 2 hours before sucralfate eliminates the interaction).
No products indexed under this heading.

Magnesium Hydroxide (Simultaneous administration within one-half hour before or after sucralfate should be avoided; may increase the total body burden of aluminum). Products include:
Fleet Pedia-Lax Chewable Tablets **1145**
Pepcid Complete Chewable Tablets **1771**
Extra Strength Rolaids Freshmint Tablets **1903**
Rolaids Multi-Symptom Berry Tablets **1903**
Rolaids Original Peppermint Tablets **1903**

Magnesium Oxide (Simultaneous administration within one-half hour before or after sucralfate should be avoided; may increase the total body burden of aluminum). Products include:
Beelith Tablets **813**

Moxifloxacin Hydrochloride (Potential for reduced extent of absorption (bioavailability) with concomitant oral administration; dosing the concomitant medication 2 hours before sucralfate eliminates the interaction). Products include:
Avelox **2803**
Vigamox Ophthalmic Solution **548**

Norfloxacin (Potential for reduced extent of absorption (bioavailability) with concomitant oral administration; dosing the concomitant medication 2 hours before sucralfate eliminates the interaction). Products include:
Noroxin Tablets **2069**

Ofloxacin (Potential for reduced extent of absorption (bioavailability) with concomitant oral administration; dosing the concomitant medication 2 hours before sucralfate eliminates the interaction). Products include:
Ofloxacin Ophthalmic Solution 0.3% .... ⊙ **243**

Phenytoin (Simultaneous administration results in reduced oral absorption of oral phenytoin).
No products indexed under this heading.

Phenytoin Sodium (Simultaneous administration results in reduced oral absorption of oral phenytoin). Products include:
Phenytek Capsules **2192**

Quinidine (Potential for reduced extent of absorption (bioavailability) with concomitant oral administration).
No products indexed under this heading.

Quinidine Gluconate (Potential for reduced extent of absorption (bioavailability) with concomitant oral administration).
No products indexed under this heading.

Quinidine Hydrochloride (Potential for reduced extent of absorption (bioavailability) with concomitant oral administration).
No products indexed under this heading.

Quinidine Polygalacturonate (Potential for reduced extent of absorption (bioavailability) with concomitant oral administration).
No products indexed under this heading.

Quinidine Sulfate (Potential for reduced extent of absorption (bioavailability) with concomitant oral administration).
No products indexed under this heading.

Ranitidine Hydrochloride (Simultaneous administration results in reduced oral absorption of oral ranitidine; dosing the concomitant medication 2 hours before sucralfate eliminates the interaction). Products include:
Zantac 75 Tablets **603**
Zantac **1670**
Zantac Injection **1666**
Zantac Injection Pharmacy Bulk Package **1668**
Maximum Strength Zantac 150 Tablets **603**
Maximum Strength Zantac 150 Cool Mint Tablets **603**

Tetracycline Hydrochloride (Simultaneous administration results in reduced oral absorption of oral tetracycline). Products include:
Pylera Capsules **714**

Theophylline (Simultaneous administration results in reduced oral absorption of theophylline).
No products indexed under this heading.

Theophylline Anhydrous (Simultaneous administration results in reduced oral absorption of theophylline). Products include:
Uniphyl Tablets **2595**

IMPORTANT NOTE: Always consult each drug listing in the patient's regimen for possible interactions.

Theophylline Calcium Salicylate (Simultaneous administration results in reduced oral absorption of theophylline).
No products indexed under this heading.

Theophylline Dihydroxypropyl (Glyceryl) (Simultaneous administration results in reduced oral absorption of theophylline).
No products indexed under this heading.

Theophylline Ethylenediamine (Simultaneous administration results in reduced oral absorption of theophylline).
No products indexed under this heading.

Theophylline Sodium Glycinate (Simultaneous administration results in reduced oral absorption of theophylline).
No products indexed under this heading.

Trovafloxacin Mesylate (Potential for reduced extent of absorption (bioavailability) with concomitant oral administration; dosing the concomitant medication 2 hours before sucralfate eliminates the interaction).
No products indexed under this heading.

Warfarin Sodium (Subtherapeutic prothrombin times with concomitant warfarin and sucralfate have been reported in spontaneous and published reports; clinical studies have demonstrated no changes in the prothrombin time with the addition of sucralfate to chronic warfarin therapy).
No products indexed under this heading.

CARAFATE TABLETS

(Sucralfate) 707

May interact with fluoroquinolone antibiotics, quinidine, xanthines, and certain other agents. Compounds in these categories include:

Alatrofloxacin Mesylate (Potential for reduced extent of absorption (bioavailability) with concomitant oral administration; dosing the concomitant medication 2 hours before sucralfate eliminates the interaction).
No products indexed under this heading.

Aluminum Carbonate (Simultaneous administration within one-half hour before or after sucralfate should be avoided; may increase the total body burden of aluminum).
No products indexed under this heading.

Aluminum Hydroxide (Simultaneous administration within one-half hour before or after sucralfate should be avoided; may increase the total body burden of aluminum).
No products indexed under this heading.

Aminophylline (Simultaneous administration results in reduced oral absorption of theophylline).
No products indexed under this heading.

Cimetidine (Simultaneous administration results in reduced oral absorption of oral cimetidine; dosing the concomitant medication 2 hours before sucralfate eliminates the interaction).
No products indexed under this heading.

Cimetidine Hydrochloride (Simultaneous administration results in reduced oral absorption of oral cimetidine; dosing the concomitant medication 2 hours before sucralfate eliminates the interaction).
No products indexed under this heading.

Ciprofloxacin (Potential for reduced extent of absorption (bioavailability) with concomitant oral administration; dosing the concomitant medication 2 hours before sucralfate eliminates the interaction).
Products include:
Cipro I.V. 2817
Cipro Oral Suspension 2810
Cipro XR Tablets 2823
Ciprodex Otic Suspension 541

Ciprofloxacin Hydrochloride (Potential for reduced extent of absorption (bioavailability) with concomitant oral administration; dosing the concomitant medication 2 hours before sucralfate eliminates the interaction). Products include:
Cipro Tablets 2810

Digoxin (Simultaneous administration results in reduced oral absorption of oral digoxin; dosing the concomitant medication 2 hours before sucralfate eliminates the interaction).
Products include:
Lanoxin Injection 1498
Lanoxin Injection Pediatric 1502
Lanoxin Tablets 1505

Dyphylline (Simultaneous administration results in reduced oral absorption of theophylline).
No products indexed under this heading.

Enoxacin (Potential for reduced extent of absorption (bioavailability) with concomitant oral administration; dosing the concomitant medication 2 hours before sucralfate eliminates the interaction).
No products indexed under this heading.

Gatifloxacin (Potential for reduced extent of absorption (bioavailability) with concomitant oral administration; dosing the concomitant medication 2 hours before sucralfate eliminates the interaction).
No products indexed under this heading.

Grepafloxacin Hydrochloride (Potential for reduced extent of absorption (bioavailability) with concomitant oral administration; dosing the concomitant medication 2 hours before sucralfate eliminates the interaction).
No products indexed under this heading.

Ketoconazole (Simultaneous administration results in reduced oral absorption of oral ketoconazole). Products include:
Extina Foam, 2% 3057
Nizoral A-D Shampoo 1901

Levofloxacin (Potential for reduced extent of absorption (bioavailability) with concomitant oral administration; dosing the concomitant medication 2 hours before sucralfate eliminates the interaction). Products include:
Iquix Ophthalmic Solution 3183
Levaquin 2416
Levaquin in 5% Dextrose Injection 2416
Quixin Ophthalmic Solution 3184

Levothyroxine Sodium (Potential for reduced extent of absorption (bioavailability) with concomitant oral administration). Products include:
Levothroid Tablets 1170
Levoxyl Tablets 1780
Synthroid Tablets 507

Lomefloxacin Hydrochloride (Potential for reduced extent of absorption (bioavailability) with concomitant oral administration; dosing the concomitant medication 2 hours before sucralfate eliminates the interaction).
No products indexed under this heading.

Magnesium Hydroxide (Simultaneous administration within one-half hour before or after sucralfate should be avoided; may increase the total body burden of aluminum).
Products include:
Fleet Pedia-Lax Chewable Tablets 1145
Pepcid Complete Chewable Tablets 1771
Extra Strength Rolaids Freshmint Tablets 1903
Rolaids Multi-Symptom Berry Tablets 1903
Rolaids Original Peppermint Tablets 1903

Magnesium Oxide (Simultaneous administration within one-half hour before or after sucralfate should be avoided; may increase the total body burden of aluminum). Products include:
Beelith Tablets 813

Moxifloxacin Hydrochloride (Potential for reduced extent of absorption (bioavailability) with concomitant oral administration; dosing the concomitant medication 2 hours before sucralfate eliminates the interaction). Products include:
Avelox 2803
Vigamox Ophthalmic Solution 548

Norfloxacin (Potential for reduced extent of absorption (bioavailability) with concomitant oral administration; dosing the concomitant medication 2 hours before sucralfate eliminates the interaction). Products include:
Noroxin Tablets 2069

Ofloxacin (Potential for reduced extent of absorption (bioavailability) with concomitant oral administration; dosing the concomitant medication 2 hours before sucralfate eliminates the interaction). Products include:
Ofloxacin Ophthalmic Solution 0.3% .... ⊙243

Phenytoin (Simultaneous administration results in reduced oral absorption of oral phenytoin).
No products indexed under this heading.

Phenytoin Sodium (Simultaneous administration results in reduced oral absorption of oral phenytoin).
Products include:
Phenytek Capsules 2192

Quinidine (Potential for reduced extent of absorption (bioavailability) with concomitant oral administration).
No products indexed under this heading.

Quinidine Gluconate (Potential for reduced extent of absorption (bioavailability) with concomitant oral administration).
No products indexed under this heading.

Quinidine Hydrochloride (Potential for reduced extent of absorption (bioavailability) with concomitant oral administration).
No products indexed under this heading.

Quinidine Polygalacturonate (Potential for reduced extent of absorption (bioavailability) with concomitant oral administration).
No products indexed under this heading.

Quinidine Sulfate (Potential for reduced extent of absorption (bioavailability) with concomitant oral administration).
No products indexed under this heading.

Ranitidine Hydrochloride (Simultaneous administration results in reduced oral absorption of oral ranitidine; dosing the concomitant medication 2 hours before sucralfate eliminates the interaction). Products include:
Zantac 75 Tablets .... ▣603
Zantac 1670
Zantac Injection 1666
Zantac Injection Pharmacy Bulk Package 1668
Maximum Strength Zantac 150 Tablets .... ▣603
Maximum Strength Zantac 150 Cool Mint Tablets .... ▣603

Tetracycline Hydrochloride (Simultaneous administration results in reduced oral absorption of oral tetracycline). Products include:
Pylera Capsules 714

Theophylline (Simultaneous administration results in reduced oral absorption of theophylline).
No products indexed under this heading.

Theophylline Anhydrous (Simultaneous administration results in reduced oral absorption of theophylline). Products include:
Uniphyl Tablets 2595

Theophylline Calcium Salicylate (Simultaneous administration results in reduced oral absorption of theophylline).
No products indexed under this heading.

Theophylline Dihydroxypropyl (Glyceryl) (Simultaneous administration results in reduced oral absorption of theophylline).
No products indexed under this heading.

Theophylline Ethylenediamine (Simultaneous administration results in reduced oral absorption of theophylline).
No products indexed under this heading.

Theophylline Sodium Glycinate (Simultaneous administration results in reduced oral absorption of theophylline).
No products indexed under this heading.

Trovafloxacin Mesylate (Potential for reduced extent of absorption (bioavailability) with concomitant oral administration; dosing the concomitant medication 2 hours before sucralfate eliminates the interaction).
No products indexed under this heading.

Warfarin Sodium (Subtherapeutic prothrombin times with concomitant warfarin and sucralfate have been reported in spontaneous and published reports; clinical studies have demonstrated no changes in the prothrombin time with the addition of sucralfate to chronic warfarin therapy).
No products indexed under this heading.

CARBATROL CAPSULES

(Carbamazepine) 3019

May interact with antimalarials, cytochrome p450 1a2 substrates (selected), cytochrome p450 3a4 inducers (selected), cytochrome p450 3a4 inhibitors (selected), cytochrome p450 3a4 substrates (selected), doxycycline, anticonvulsants, erythromycin, lithium preparations, macrolide antibiotics, monoamine oxidase inhibitors, antipsychotic agents, oral contraceptives, phenytoin, valproate, xanthines, and certain other agents. Compounds in these categories include:

Acetaminophen (Carbamazepine induces hepatic CYP activity and causes or would be expected to decrease plasma levels of acetaminophen). Products include:

- Benadryl Allergy & Cold Kapgels 1895
- Benadryl Allergy & Sinus Headache Kapgels 1895
- Benadryl Severe Allergy & Sinus Headache Caplets 1897
- Lortab 5/500 Tablets 3143
- Lortab 7.5/500 Tablets 3144
- Lortab 10/500 Tablets 3144
- Percocet Tablets 1127
- Sinutab Sinus Caplets 1905
- Sudafed PE Cold & Cough Caplets 1907
- Sudafed PE Nighttime Cold Caplets 1907
- Sudafed PE Severe Cold Caplets 1908
- Sudafed PE Sinus Headache Caplets 1908
- Regular Strength Tylenol Tablets 1915
- Tylenol 8 Hour Extended Release Caplets 1915
- Extra Strength Tylenol Caplets, Cool Caplets, and EZ Tabs 1915
- Extra Strength Tylenol Adult Rapid Blast Liquid 1915
- Extra Strength Tylenol PM Caplets, Geltabs, Liquid, and Rapid Release Gels 1915
- Extra Strength Tylenol Rapid Release Gels 1915
- Tylenol with Codeine Tablets 2427
- Tylenol Allergy Multi-Symptom Caplets with Cool Burst and Rapid Release Gelcaps 1916
- Tylenol Allergy Multi-Symptom Nighttime Caplets with Cool Burst 1916
- Tylenol Severe Allergy Caplets 1916
- Tylenol Arthritis Pain Extended Release Geltabs/Caplets 1915
- Tylenol Chest Congestion Caplets with Cool Burst 1910
- Tylenol Chest Congestion Liquid with Cool Burst 1910
- Children's Tylenol Plus Cold Suspension Liquid 1912
- Children's Tylenol Plus Cold & Allergy Suspension Liquid 1914
- Children's Tylenol Plus Cough & Runny Nose Suspension Liquid 1912
- Children's Tylenol Plus Cough & Sore Throat Suspension Liquid 1912
- Children's Tylenol Plus Flu Suspension Liquid 1914
- Children's Tylenol Suspension Liquid 1909
- Children's Tylenol Meltaways 1909
- Children's Tylenol Plus Multi-Symptom Cold Suspension Liquid 1912
- Tylenol Cold Severe Congestion Daytime Caplets with Cool Burst 1912
- Tylenol Cold Head Congestion Daytime Caplets with Cool Burst 1910
- Tylenol Cold Head Congestion Nighttime Caplets with Cool Burst 1910
- Tylenol Cold Head Congestion Severe Daytime Caplets with Cool Burst 1910
- Tylenol Cold Multi-Symptom Daytime Caplets with Cool Burst and Rapid Release Gels 1913
- Tylenol Cold Multi-Symptom Daytime Liquid with Citrus Burst 1913
- Tylenol Cold Multi-Symptom Nighttime Caplets with Cool Burst 1913
- Tylenol Cold Multi-Symptom Nighttime Liquid with Cool Burst 1913
- Tylenol Cold Multi-Symptom Severe Caplets with Cool Burst 1913
- Tylenol Cold Multi-Symptom Severe Daytime Liquid with Citrus Burst 1913
- Tylenol Cough & Sore Throat Daytime Liquid with Cool Burst 1918
- Tylenol Cough & Sore Throat Nighttime Liquid with Cool Burst 1918
- Concentrated Tylenol Infants' Drops 1909
- Jr. Tylenol Meltaways 1909
- Tylenol Sinus Congestion & Pain Daytime Caplets with Cool Burst and Gelcaps 1917
- Tylenol Sinus Congestion & Pain Nighttime Caplets with Cool Burst 1917
- Tylenol Sinus Congestion & Pain Severe Caplets with Cool Burst 1917
- Tylenol Sinus Severe Congestion Caplets with Cool Burst 1917
- Tylenol Sore Throat Daytime Liquid with Cool Burst 1918
- Tylenol Sore Throat Nighttime Liquid with Cool Burst 1918
- Women's Tylenol Menstrual Relief Caplets 1919
- Vicks DayQuil Cold & Flu Multi-Symptom Relief 616
- Vicks DayQuil LiquiCaps 2567
- Vicks DayQuil Liquid 2567
- Vicks DayQuil Multi-Symptom Cold/Flu Relief 2567
- Vicks NyQuil Cold & Flu Multi-Symptom Relief 617
- Vicks NyQuil LiquiCaps 2567
- Vicks NyQuil Liquid 2567
- Vicks NyQuil Multi-Symptom Cold/Flu Relief 2567
- Vicodin Tablets 529
- Vicodin ES Tablets 530
- Vicodin HP Tablets 531
- Zydone Tablets 1132

Acetazolamide (Carbamazepine is metabolized mainly by cytochrome P450 (CYP) 3A4 to the active carbamazepine 10,11 -epoxide, which is further metabolized to the trans-diol by epoxide hydrolase. Therefore, the potential exists for interaction between carbamazepine and any agent that inhibits CYP3A4 and/ or epoxide hydrolase).

No products indexed under this heading.

Alatrofloxacin Mesylate (Carbamazepine is known to induce CYP1A2 and CYP3A4. Therefore, the potential exists for interaction between carbamazepine and any agent metabolized by one (or more) of these enzymes).

No products indexed under this heading.

Alfentanil Hydrochloride (Carbamazepine is known to induce CYP1A2 and CYP3A4. Therefore, the potential exists for interaction between carbamazepine and any agent metabolized by one (or more) of these enzymes).

No products indexed under this heading.

Allium sativum (Carbamazepine is metabolized by CYP3A4. Therefore, the potential exists for interaction between caramazepine and any agent that induces CYP3A4).

No products indexed under this heading.

Alprazolam (Carbamazepine induces hepatic CYP activity and causes or would be expected to decrease plasma levels of alprazolam).

No products indexed under this heading.

Aminophylline (Inducers of CYP3A4, such as theophylline, can increase the rate of carbamazepine metabolism and can thus decrease plasma carbamazepine levels; carbamazepine induces hepatic CYP activity and causes or would be expected to decrease plasma levels of theophylline).

No products indexed under this heading.

Amiodarone Hydrochloride (Carbamazepine is metabolized mainly by cytochrome P450 (CYP) 3A4 to the active carbamazepine 10,11 -epoxide, which is further metabolized to the trans-diol by epoxide hydrolase. Therefore, the potential exists for interaction between carbamazepine and any agent that inhibits its CYP3A4 and/or epoxide hydrolase).

No products indexed under this heading.

Amitriptyline Hydrochloride (Carbamazepine is known to induce CYP1A2 and CYP3A4. Therefore, the potential exists for interaction between carbamazepine and any agent metabolized by one (or more) of these enzymes).

No products indexed under this heading.

Amlodipine Besylate (Carbamazepine is known to induce CYP1A2 and CYP3A4. Therefore, the potential exists for interaction between carbamazepine and any agent metabolized by one (or more) of these enzymes). Products include:

- Azor Tablets 1005
- Exforge Tablets 2238

Amoxapine (Carbamazepine is known to induce CYP1A2 and CYP3A4. Therefore, the potential exists for interaction between carbamazepine and any agent metabolized by one (or more) of these enzymes).

No products indexed under this heading.

Amprenavir (Carbamazepine is metabolized mainly by cytochrome P450 (CYP) 3A4 to the active carbamazepine 10,11 -epoxide, which is further metabolized to the trans-diol by epoxide hydrolase. Therefore, the potential exists for interaction between carbamazepine and any agent that inhibits CYP3A4 and/ or epoxide hydrolase).

No products indexed under this heading.

Anagrelide Hydrochloride (Carbamazepine is known to induce CYP1A2 and CYP3A4. Therefore, the potential exists for interaction between carbamazepine and any agent metabolized by one (or more) of these enzymes). Products include:

- Agrylin Capsules 3017

Anastrozole (Carbamazepine is metabolized mainly by cytochrome P450 (CYP) 3A4 to the active carbamazepine 10,11 -epoxide, which is further metabolized to the trans-diol by epoxide hydrolase. Therefore, the potential exists for interaction between carbamazepine and any agent that inhibits CYP3A4 and/ or epoxide hydrolase). Products include:

- Arimidex Tablets 672

Aprepitant (Carbamazepine is metabolized mainly by cytochrome P450 (CYP) 3A4 to the active carbamazepine 10,11 -epoxide, which is further metabolized to the trans-diol by epoxide hydrolase. Therefore, the potential exists for interaction between carbamazepine and any agent that inhibits CYP3A4 and/ or epoxide hydrolase). Products include:

- Emend Capsules 1992

Aripiprazole (Co-administration with psychotropic agents has resulted in isolated cases of neuroleptic malignant syndrome). Products include:

- Abilify Injection 881
- Abilify Injection 2466
- Abilify Oral Solution 881
- Abilify Oral Solution 2466
- Abilify Discmelt Orally Disintegrating Tablets 881
- Abilify Discmelt Orally Disintegrating Tablets 2466
- Abilify Tablets 881
- Abilify Tablets 2466

Astemizole (Carbamazepine is known to induce CYP1A2 and CYP3A4. Therefore, the potential exists for interaction between carbamazepine and any agent metabolized by one (or more) of these enzymes).

No products indexed under this heading.

Atazanavir (Carbamazepine is metabolized mainly by cytochrome P450 (CYP) 3A4 to the active carbamazepine 10,11 -epoxide, which is further metabolized to the trans-diol by epoxide hydrolase. Therefore, the potential exists for interaction between carbamazepine and any agent that inhibits CYP3A4 and/ or epoxide hydrolase).

No products indexed under this heading.

Atazanavir Sulfate (Carbamazepine is metabolized mainly by cytochrome P450 (CYP) 3A4 to the active carbamazepine 10,11 -epoxide, which is further metabolized to the trans-diol by epoxide hydrolase. Therefore, the potential exists for interaction between carbamazepine and any agent that inhibits its CYP3A4 and/or epoxide hydrolase). Products include:

- Reyataz Capsules 3299

Atorvastatin Calcium (Carbamazepine is known to induce CYP1A2 and CYP3A4. Therefore, the potential exists for interaction between carbamazepine and any agent metabolized by one (or more) of these enzymes). Products include:

- Lipitor Tablets 2501

Azithromycin Dihydrate (Inhibitors of CYP3A4, such as macrolides, inhibit carbamazepine metabolism and thus increase plasma carbamazepine levels).

No products indexed under this heading.

Belladonna Ergotamine (Carbamazepine is known to induce CYP1A2 and CYP3A4. Therefore, the potential exists for interaction between carbamazepine and any agent metabolized by one (or more) of these enzymes).

No products indexed under this heading.

IMPORTANT NOTE: Always consult each drug listing in the patient's regimen for possible interactions.

Betamethasone Acetate (Carbamazepine is metabolized by CYP3A4. Therefore, the potential exists for interaction between caramazepine and any agent that induces CYP3A4).
No products indexed under this heading.

Betamethasone Sodium Phosphate (Carbamazepine is metabolized by CYP3A4. Therefore, the potential exists for interaction between caramazepine and any agent that induces CYP3A4).
No products indexed under this heading.

Buspirone Hydrochloride (Carbamazepine is known to induce CYP1A2 and CYP3A4. Therefore, the potential exists for interaction between carbamazepine and any agent metabolized by one (or more) of these enzymes).
No products indexed under this heading.

Busulfan (Carbamazepine is known to induce CYP1A2 and CYP3A4. Therefore, the potential exists for interaction between carbamazepine and any agent metabolized by one (or more) of these enzymes).
Products include:
Busulfex Injection 2477
Myleran Tablets 1530

Caffeine (Carbamazepine is known to induce CYP1A2 and CYP3A4. Therefore, the potential exists for interaction between carbamazepine and any agent metabolized by one (or more) of these enzymes).
Products include:
BioLean Free Tablets ..... ▣635
BioLean II Tablets ..... ▣635
Winrgy Dietary Supplement ..... ▣642

Caffeine Anhydrous (Carbamazepine is known to induce CYP1A2 and CYP3A4. Therefore, the potential exists for interaction between carbamazepine and any agent metabolized by one (or more) of these enzymes).
No products indexed under this heading.

Cerivastatin Sodium (Carbamazepine is known to induce CYP1A2 and CYP3A4. Therefore, the potential exists for interaction between carbamazepine and any agent metabolized by one (or more) of these enzymes).
No products indexed under this heading.

Chlordiazepoxide (Carbamazepine is known to induce CYP1A2 and CYP3A4. Therefore, the potential exists for interaction between carbamazepine and any agent metabolized by one (or more) of these enzymes).
No products indexed under this heading.

Chlordiazepoxide Hydrochloride (Carbamazepine is known to induce CYP1A2 and CYP3A4. Therefore, the potential exists for interaction between carbamazepine and any agent metabolized by one (or more) of these enzymes).
No products indexed under this heading.

Chloroquine Hydrochloride (Antimalarial drugs, such as chloroquine and mefloquine, may antagonize the activity of carbamazepine).
No products indexed under this heading.

Chloroquine Phosphate (Antimalarial drugs, such as chloroquine and mefloquine, may antagonize the activity of carbamazepine).
No products indexed under this heading.

Chlorpheniramine (Carbamazepine is known to induce CYP1A2 and CYP3A4. Therefore, the potential exists for interaction between carbamazepine and any agent metabolized by one (or more) of these enzymes).
No products indexed under this heading.

Chlorpheniramine Maleate (Carbamazepine is known to induce CYP1A2 and CYP3A4. Therefore, the potential exists for interaction between carbamazepine and any agent metabolized by one (or more) of these enzymes). Products include:
Actifed Cold & Allergy Tablets 1895
Sudafed PE Sinus & Allergy Tablets 1908
Tylenol Allergy Multi-Symptom Caplets with Cool Burst and Rapid Release Gelcaps 1916
Children's Tylenol Plus Cold Suspension Liquid 1912
Children's Tylenol Plus Cough & Runny Nose Suspension Liquid 1912
Children's Tylenol Plus Flu Suspension Liquid 1914
Children's Tylenol Plus Multi-Symptom Cold Suspension Liquid 1912
Tylenol Cold Head Congestion Nighttime Caplets with Cool Burst 1910
Tylenol Cold Multi-Symptom Nighttime Caplets with Cool Burst 1913
Tylenol Sinus Congestion & Pain Nighttime Caplets with Cool Burst 1917

Chlorpheniramine Polistirex (Carbamazepine is known to induce CYP1A2 and CYP3A4. Therefore, the potential exists for interaction between carbamazepine and any agent metabolized by one (or more) of these enzymes). Products include:
Tussionex Pennkinetic Extended-Release Suspension 3154

Chlorpheniramine Tannate (Carbamazepine is known to induce CYP1A2 and CYP3A4. Therefore, the potential exists for interaction between carbamazepine and any agent metabolized by one (or more) of these enzymes).
No products indexed under this heading.

Chlorpromazine (Co-administration with psychotropic agents has resulted in isolated cases of neuroleptic malignant syndrome).
No products indexed under this heading.

Chlorpromazine Hydrochloride (Co-administration with psychotropic agents has resulted in isolated cases of neuroleptic malignant syndrome).
No products indexed under this heading.

Chlorprothixene (Co-administration with psychotropic agents has resulted in isolated cases of neuroleptic malignant syndrome).
No products indexed under this heading.

Chlorprothixene Hydrochloride (Co-administration with psychotropic agents has resulted in isolated cases of neuroleptic malignant syndrome).
No products indexed under this heading.

Cimetidine (Inhibitors of CYP3A4, such as cimetidine, inhibit carbamazepine metabolism and thus increase plasma carbamazepine levels).
No products indexed under this heading.

Cimetidine Hydrochloride (Inhibitors of CYP3A4, such as cimetidine, inhibit carbamazepine metabolism and thus increase plasma carbamazepine levels).
No products indexed under this heading.

Ciprofloxacin (Carbamazepine is metabolized mainly by cytochrome P450 (CYP) 3A4 to the active carbamazepine 10,11 -epoxide, which is further metabolized to the trans-diol by epoxide hydrolase. Therefore, the potential exists for interaction between carbamazepine and any agent that inhibits CYP3A4 and/or epoxide hydrolase). Products include:
Cipro I.V. 2817
Cipro Oral Suspension 2810
Cipro XR Tablets 2823
Ciprodex Otic Suspension 541

Ciprofloxacin Hydrochloride (Carbamazepine is metabolized by CYP3A4. Therefore, the potential exists for interaction between caramazepine and any agent that induces CYP3A4). Products include:
Cipro Tablets 2810

Cisapride (Carbamazepine is known to induce CYP1A2 and CYP3A4. Therefore, the potential exists for interaction between carbamazepine and any agent metabolized by one (or more) of these enzymes).
No products indexed under this heading.

Cisplatin (Inducers of CYP3A4, such as cisplatin, can increase the rate of carbamazepine metabolism and can thus decrease plasma carbamazepine levels).
No products indexed under this heading.

Clarithromycin (Inhibitors of CYP3A4, such as clarithromycin, inhibit carbamazepine metabolism and thus increase plasma carbamazepine levels). Products include:
Biaxin/Biaxin XL 411

Clomipramine Hydrochloride (Carbamazepine can increase plasma levels of clomipramine).
No products indexed under this heading.

Clonazepam (Carbamazepine induces hepatic CYP activity and causes or would be expected to decrease plasma levels of clonazepine; alterations of thryoid function have been reported in combination therapy with other anticonvulsants). Products include:
Klonopin 2639

Clopidogrel Bisulfate (Carbamazepine is known to induce CYP1A2 and CYP3A4. Therefore, the potential exists for interaction between carbamazepine and any agent metabolized by one (or more) of these enzymes). Products include:
Plavix Tablets 926
Plavix Tablets 2767

Clotrimazole (Carbamazepine is metabolized mainly by cytochrome P450 (CYP) 3A4 to the active carbamazepine 10,11 -epoxide, which is further metabolized to the trans-diol by epoxide hydrolase. Therefore, the potential exists for interaction between carbamazepine and any agent that inhibits CYP3A4 and/or epoxide hydrolase). Products include:
Lotrisone 2881

Clozapine (Carbamazepine induces hepatic CYP activity and causes or would be expected to decrease plasma levels of clozapine).
No products indexed under this heading.

Cortisone Acetate (Carbamazepine is metabolized by CYP3A4. Therefore, the potential exists for interaction between caramazepine and any agent that induces CYP3A4).
No products indexed under this heading.

Cyclobenzaprine (Carbamazepine is known to induce CYP1A2 and CYP3A4. Therefore, the potential exists for interaction between carbamazepine and any agent metabolized by one (or more) of these enzymes).
No products indexed under this heading.

Cyclobenzaprine Hydrochloride (Carbamazepine is known to induce CYP1A2 and CYP3A4. Therefore, the potential exists for interaction between carbamazepine and any agent metabolized by one (or more) of these enzymes). Products include:
Amrix Capsules 966

Cyclosporine (Carbamazepine is metabolized mainly by cytochrome P450 (CYP) 3A4 to the active carbamazepine 10,11 -epoxide, which is further metabolized to the trans-diol by epoxide hydrolase. Therefore, the potential exists for interaction between carbamazepine and any agent that inhibits CYP3A4 and/or epoxide hydrolase). Products include:
Gengraf Capsules 435
Neoral Oral Solution 2280
Neoral Soft Gelatin Capsules 2280
Restasis Ophthalmic Emulsion 557
Sandimmune 2296

Dalfopristin (Carbamazepine is metabolized mainly by cytochrome P450 (CYP) 3A4 to the active carbamazepine 10,11 -epoxide, which is further metabolized to the trans-diol by epoxide hydrolase. Therefore, the potential exists for interaction between carbamazepine and any agent that inhibits CYP3A4 and/or epoxide hydrolase).
No products indexed under this heading.

Danazol (Inhibitors of CYP3A4, such as danazol, inhibit carbamazepine metabolism and thus increase plasma carbamazepine levels).
No products indexed under this heading.

Delavirdine Mesylate (Carbamazepine is metabolized mainly by cytochrome P450 (CYP) 3A4 to the active carbamazepine 10,11 -epoxide, which is further metabolized to the trans-diol by epoxide hydrolase. Therefore, the potential exists for interaction between carbamazepine and any agent that inhibits CYP3A4 and/or epoxide hydrolase).
No products indexed under this heading.

Desipramine Hydrochloride (Carbamazepine is known to induce CYP1A2 and CYP3A4. Therefore, the potential exists for interaction between carbamazepine and any agent metabolized by one (or more) of these enzymes).
No products indexed under this heading.

Desogestrel (Carbamazepine induces hepatic CYP activity and causes or would be expected to decrease plasma levels of oral contraceptives; breakthrough bleeding has been reported among patients receiving concomitant oral contraceptives and their reliability may be adversely affected). Products include:
Mircette Tablets ... 1034

Dexamethasone (Carbamazepine is metabolized by CYP3A4. Therefore, the potential exists for interaction between caramazepine and any agent that induces CYP3A4).
Products include:
Ciprodex Otic Suspension ... 541

Dexamethasone Acetate (Carbamazepine is metabolized by CYP3A4. Therefore, the potential exists for interaction between caramazepine and any agent that induces CYP3A4).
No products indexed under this heading.

Dexamethasone Sodium Phosphate (Carbamazepine is metabolized by CYP3A4. Therefore, the potential exists for interaction between caramazepine and any agent that induces CYP3A4).
No products indexed under this heading.

Diazepam (Carbamazepine is known to induce CYP1A2 and CYP3A4. Therefore, the potential exists for interaction between carbamazepine and any agent metabolized by one (or more) of these enzymes). Products include:
Valium Tablets ... 2658

Dicumarol (Carbamazepine induces hepatic CYP activity and causes or would be expected to decrease plasma levels of dicumarol).
No products indexed under this heading.

Dihydroergotamine Mesylate (Carbamazepine is known to induce CYP1A2 and CYP3A4. Therefore, the potential exists for interaction between carbamazepine and any agent metabolized by one (or more) of these enzymes).
No products indexed under this heading.

Diltiazem Hydrochloride (Inhibitors of CYP3A4, such as diltiazem, inhibit carbamazepine metabolism and thus increase plasma carbamazepine levels). Products include:
Cardizem LA Extended Release Tablets ... 421

Diltiazem Maleate (Carbamazepine is metabolized mainly by cytochrome P450 (CYP) 3A4 to the active carbamazepine 10,11 -epoxide, which is further metabolized to the trans-diol by epoxide hydrolase. Therefore, the potential exists for interaction between carbamazepine and any agent that inhibits CYP3A4 and/or epoxide hydrolase).
No products indexed under this heading.

Dirithromycin (Inhibitors of CYP3A4, such as macrolides, inhibit carbamazepine metabolism and thus increase plasma carbamazepine levels).
No products indexed under this heading.

Disopyramide (Carbamazepine is known to induce CYP1A2 and CYP3A4. Therefore, the potential exists for interaction between carbamazepine and any agent metabolized by one (or more) of these enzymes).
No products indexed under this heading.

Disopyramide Phosphate (Carbamazepine is known to induce CYP1A2 and CYP3A4. Therefore, the potential exists for interaction between carbamazepine and any agent metabolized by one (or more) of these enzymes).
No products indexed under this heading.

Disulfiram (Carbamazepine is known to induce CYP1A2 and CYP3A4. Therefore, the potential exists for interaction between carbamazepine and any agent metabolized by one (or more) of these enzymes).
No products indexed under this heading.

Divalproex Sodium (Inhibitors of CYP3A4, such as valproate, inhibit carbamazepine metabolism and thus increase plasma carbamazepine levels; carbamazepine induces hepatic CYP activity and causes or would be expected to decrease plasma levels of valproate; alterations of thyroid function have been reported in combination therapy with other anticonvulsants). Products include:
Depakote ER Tablets ... 423

Doxepin Hydrochloride (Carbamazepine is known to induce CYP1A2 and CYP3A4. Therefore, the potential exists for interaction between carbamazepine and any agent metabolized by one (or more) of these enzymes).
No products indexed under this heading.

Doxorubicin Hydrochloride (Inducers of CYP3A4, such as doxorubicin, can increase the rate of carbamazepine metabolism and can thus decrease plasma carbamazepine levels).
No products indexed under this heading.

Doxycycline Calcium (Carbamazepine induces hepatic CYP activity and causes or would be expected to decrease plasma levels of doxycycline).
No products indexed under this heading.

Doxycycline Hyclate (Carbamazepine induces hepatic CYP activity and causes or would be expected to decrease plasma levels of doxycycline).
No products indexed under this heading.

Doxycycline Monohydrate (Carbamazepine induces hepatic CYP activity and causes or would be expected to decrease plasma levels of doxycycline).
No products indexed under this heading.

Dronabinol (Carbamazepine is known to induce CYP1A2 and CYP3A4. Therefore, the potential exists for interaction between carbamazepine and any agent metabolized by one (or more) of these enzymes). Products include:
Marinol Capsules ... 3163

Dyphylline (Inducers of CYP3A4, such as theophylline, can increase the rate of carbamazepine metabolism and can thus decrease plasma carbamazepine levels; carbamazepine induces hepatic CYP activity and causes or would be expected to decrease plasma levels of theophylline).
No products indexed under this heading.

Efavirenz (Carbamazepine is metabolized mainly by cytochrome P450 (CYP) 3A4 to the active carbamazepine 10,11 -epoxide, which is further metabolized to the trans-diol by epoxide hydrolase. Therefore, the potential exists for interaction between carbamazepine and any agent that inhibits CYP3A4 and/ or epoxide hydrolase). Products include:
Atripla Tablets ... 938
Sustiva Capsules ... 930
Sustiva Tablets ... 930

Enoxacin (Carbamazepine is known to induce CYP1A2 and CYP3A4. Therefore, the potential exists for interaction between carbamazepine and any agent metabolized by one (or more) of these enzymes).
No products indexed under this heading.

Ergotamine Tartrate (Carbamazepine is known to induce CYP1A2 and CYP3A4. Therefore, the potential exists for interaction between carbamazepine and any agent metabolized by one (or more) of these enzymes).
No products indexed under this heading.

Erythromycin (Inhibitors of CYP3A4, such as erythromycin, inhibit carbamazepine metabolism and thus increase plasma carbamazepine levels).
No products indexed under this heading.

Erythromycin Estolate (Inhibitors of CYP3A4, such as erythromycin, inhibit carbamazepine metabolism and thus increase plasma carbamazepine levels).
No products indexed under this heading.

Erythromycin Ethylsuccinate (Inhibitors of CYP3A4, such as erythromycin, inhibit carbamazepine metabolism and thus increase plasma carbamazepine levels). Products include:
E.E.S. ... 433
EryPed ... 431

Erythromycin Gluceptate (Inhibitors of CYP3A4, such as erythromycin, inhibit carbamazepine metabolism and thus increase plasma carbamazepine levels).
No products indexed under this heading.

Erythromycin Lactobionate (Inhibitors of CYP3A4, such as erythromycin, inhibit carbamazepine metabolism and thus increase plasma carbamazepine levels).
No products indexed under this heading.

Erythromycin Stearate (Inhibitors of CYP3A4, such as erythromycin, inhibit carbamazepine metabolism and thus increase plasma carbamazepine levels).
No products indexed under this heading.

Esomeprazole Magnesium (Carbamazepine is metabolized mainly by cytochrome P450 (CYP) 3A4 to the active carbamazepine 10,11 -epoxide, which is further metabolized to the trans-diol by epoxide hydrolase. Therefore, the potential exists for interaction between carbamazepine and any agent that inhibits CYP3A4 and/or epoxide hydrolase). Products include:
Nexium Delayed-Release Capsules ... 645
Nexium Delayed-Release Oral Suspension ... 645

Estradiol (Carbamazepine is known to induce CYP1A2 and CYP3A4. Therefore, the potential exists for interaction between carbamazepine and any agent metabolized by one (or more) of these enzymes).
Products include:
Activella Tablets ... 2347
Angeliq Tablets ... 751
Climara Transdermal System ... 763
Climara Pro Transdermal System ... 768
Divigel ... 3167
Vagifem Tablets ... 2375

Estradiol Benzoate (Carbamazepine is known to induce CYP1A2 and CYP3A4. Therefore, the potential exists for interaction between carbamazepine and any agent metabolized by one (or more) of these enzymes).
No products indexed under this heading.

Estradiol Cypionate (Carbamazepine is known to induce CYP1A2 and CYP3A4. Therefore, the potential exists for interaction between carbamazepine and any agent metabolized by one (or more) of these enzymes).
No products indexed under this heading.

Estradiol Valerate (Carbamazepine is known to induce CYP1A2 and CYP3A4. Therefore, the potential exists for interaction between carbamazepine and any agent metabolized by one (or more) of these enzymes).
No products indexed under this heading.

Ethinyl Estradiol (Carbamazepine induces hepatic CYP activity and causes or would be expected to decrease plasma levels of oral contraceptives; breakthrough bleeding has been reported among patients receiving concomitant oral contraceptives and their reliability may be adversely affected). Products include:
Lybrel Tablets ... 3204

Mircette Tablets 1034
NuvaRing 2897
Ortho-Cyclen/Ortho Tri-Cyclen 2449
Ortho Evra Transdermal System 2437
Ortho Tri-Cyclen Lo Tablets 2458
Seasonique Tablets 1046
Yaz Tablets 805

Ethosuximide (Carbamazepine induces hepatic CYP activity and causes or would be expected to decrease plasma levels of ethosuximide; alterations of thyroid function have been reported in combination therapy with other anticonvulsants).
No products indexed under this heading.

Ethotoin (Alterations of thyroid function have been reported in combination therapy with other anticonvulsants).
No products indexed under this heading.

Ethynodiol Diacetate (Carbamazepine induces hepatic CYP activity and causes or would be expected to decrease plasma levels of oral contraceptives; breakthrough bleeding has been reported among patients receiving concomitant oral contraceptives and their reliability may be adversely affected).
No products indexed under this heading.

Etoposide (Carbamazepine is known to induce CYP1A2 and CYP3A4. Therefore, the potential exists for interaction between carbamazepine and any agent metabolized by one (or more) of these enzymes).
No products indexed under this heading.

Etoposide Phosphate (Carbamazepine is known to induce CYP1A2 and CYP3A4. Therefore, the potential exists for interaction between carbamazepine and any agent metabolized by one (or more) of these enzymes).
No products indexed under this heading.

Felbamate (Inducers of CYP3A4, such as felbamate, can increase the rate of carbamazepine metabolism and can thus decrease plasma carbamazepine levels; alterations of thryoid function have been reported in combination therapy with other anticonvulsants).
No products indexed under this heading.

Felodipine (Carbamazepine is known to induce CYP1A2 and CYP3A4. Therefore, the potential exists for interaction between carbamazepine and any agent metabolized by one (or more) of these enzymes).
No products indexed under this heading.

Fentanyl (Carbamazepine is known to induce CYP1A2 and CYP3A4. Therefore, the potential exists for interaction between carbamazepine and any agent metabolized by one (or more) of these enzymes). Products include:
Duragesic Transdermal System 2405
Ionsys Transdermal System 2410

Fentanyl Citrate (Carbamazepine is known to induce CYP1A2 and CYP3A4. Therefore, the potential exists for interaction between carbamazepine and any agent metabolized by one (or more) of these enzymes). Products include:
Actiq 959
Fentora Tablets 968

Fluconazole (Carbamazepine is metabolized mainly by cytochrome P450 (CYP) 3A4 to the active carbamazepine 10,11 -epoxide, which is further metabolized to the trans-diol by epoxide hydrolase. Therefore, the potential exists for interaction between carbamazepine and any agent that inhibits CYP3A4 and/or epoxide hydrolase).
No products indexed under this heading.

Fludrocortisone Acetate (Carbamazepine is metabolized by CYP3A4. Therefore, the potential exists for interaction between caramazepine and any agent that induces CYP3A4).
No products indexed under this heading.

Fluoxetine (Carbamazepine is metabolized mainly by cytochrome P450 (CYP) 3A4 to the active carbamazepine 10,11 -epoxide, which is further metabolized to the trans-diol by epoxide hydrolase. Therefore, the potential exists for interaction between carbamazepine and any agent that inhibits CYP3A4 and/or epoxide hydrolase).
No products indexed under this heading.

Fluoxetine Hydrochloride (Inhibitors of CYP3A4, such as fluoxetine, inhibit carbamazepine metabolism and thus increase plasma carbamazepine levels). Products include:
Prozac Weekly Capsules 1852
Prozac Pulvules and Liquid 1852
Symbyax Capsules 1871

Fluphenazine Decanoate (Coadministration with psychotropic agents has resulted in isolated cases of neuroleptic malignant syndrome).
No products indexed under this heading.

Fluphenazine Enanthate (Coadministration with psychotropic agents has resulted in isolated cases of neuroleptic malignant syndrome).
No products indexed under this heading.

Fluphenazine Hydrochloride (Coadministration with psychotropic agents has resulted in isolated cases of neuroleptic malignant syndrome).
No products indexed under this heading.

Flutamide (Carbamazepine is known to induce CYP1A2 and CYP3A4. Therefore, the potential exists for interaction between carbamazepine and any agent metabolized by one (or more) of these enzymes).
No products indexed under this heading.

Fluticasone Propionate (Carbamazepine is known to induce CYP1A2 and CYP3A4. Therefore, the potential exists for interaction between carbamazepine and any agent metabolized by one (or more) of these enzymes). Products include:
Advair Diskus 100/50 1276
Advair Diskus 250/50 1276
Advair Diskus 500/50 1276
Advair HFA 45/21 Inhalation Aerosol 1288
Advair HFA 115/21 Inhalation Aerosol 1288
Advair HFA 230/21 Inhalation Aerosol 1288
Flonase Nasal Spray 1431
Flovent Diskus 50 mcg 1435

Fluvoxamine Maleate (Carbamazepine is metabolized mainly by cytochrome P450 (CYP) 3A4 to the active carbamazepine 10,11 -epoxide, which is further metabolized to the trans-diol by epoxide hydrolase. Therefore, the potential exists for interaction between carbamazepine and any agent that inhibits CYP3A4 and/or epoxide hydrolase). Products include:
Luvox CR Extended-Release Capsules 1759

Fosamprenavir Calcium (Carbamazepine is metabolized mainly by cytochrome P450 (CYP) 3A4 to the active carbamazepine 10,11 -epoxide, which is further metabolized to the trans-diol by epoxide hydrolase. Therefore, the potential exists for interaction between carbamazepine and any agent that inhibits CYP3A4 and/or epoxide hydrolase). Products include:
Lexiva Oral Suspension 1510
Lexiva Tablets 1510

Fosphenytoin (Alterations of thyroid function have been reported in combination therapy with other anticonvulsants).
No products indexed under this heading.

Fosphenytoin Sodium (Inducers of CYP3A4, such as phenytoin, can increase the rate of carbamazepine metabolism and can thus decrease plasma carbamazepine levels; phenytoin levels have been reported to increase or decrease in the presence of carbamazepine; careful monitoring of phenytoin plasma levels following co-medication with carbamazepine is advised. Alterations of thyroid function have been reported in combination therapy with other anticonvulsants).
No products indexed under this heading.

Gabapentin (Alterations of thyroid function have been reported in combination therapy with other anticonvulsants).
No products indexed under this heading.

Garlic Extract (Carbamazepine is metabolized by CYP3A4. Therefore, the potential exists for interaction between caramazepine and any agent that induces CYP3A4).
No products indexed under this heading.

Garlic Oil (Carbamazepine is metabolized by CYP3A4. Therefore, the potential exists for interaction between caramazepine and any agent that induces CYP3A4).
No products indexed under this heading.

Grepafloxacin Hydrochloride (Carbamazepine is known to induce CYP1A2 and CYP3A4. Therefore, the potential exists for interaction between carbamazepine and any agent metabolized by one (or more) of these enzymes).
No products indexed under this heading.

Haloperidol (Carbamazepine induces hepatic CYP activity and causes or would be expected to decrease plasma levels of haloperidol).
No products indexed under this heading.

Haloperidol Decanoate (Carbamazepine induces hepatic CYP activity and causes or would be expected to decrease plasma levels of haloperidol).
No products indexed under this heading.

Haloperidol Lactate (Carbamazepine is known to induce CYP1A2 and CYP3A4. Therefore, the potential exists for interaction between carbamazepine and any agent metabolized by one (or more) of these enzymes).
No products indexed under this heading.

Hydrocortisone (Carbamazepine is metabolized by CYP3A4. Therefore, the potential exists for interaction between caramazepine and any agent that induces CYP3A4).
No products indexed under this heading.

Hydrocortisone Acetate (Carbamazepine is metabolized by CYP3A4. Therefore, the potential exists for interaction between caramazepine and any agent that induces CYP3A4). Products include:
Analpram-HC 1140
Pramosone 1141

Hydrocortisone Butyrate (Carbamazepine is metabolized by CYP3A4. Therefore, the potential exists for interaction between caramazepine and any agent that induces CYP3A4).
No products indexed under this heading.

Hydrocortisone Cypionate (Carbamazepine is metabolized by CYP3A4. Therefore, the potential exists for interaction between caramazepine and any agent that induces CYP3A4).
No products indexed under this heading.

Hydrocortisone Hemisuccinate (Carbamazepine is metabolized by CYP3A4. Therefore, the potential exists for interaction between caramazepine and any agent that induces CYP3A4).
No products indexed under this heading.

Hydrocortisone Probutate (Carbamazepine is metabolized by CYP3A4. Therefore, the potential exists for interaction between caramazepine and any agent that induces CYP3A4).
No products indexed under this heading.

Hydrocortisone Sodium Phosphate (Carbamazepine is metabolized by CYP3A4. Therefore, the potential exists for interaction between caramazepine and any agent that induces CYP3A4).
No products indexed under this heading.

Hydrocortisone Sodium Succinate (Carbamazepine is metabolized by CYP3A4. Therefore, the potential exists for interaction between caramazepine and any agent that induces CYP3A4).
No products indexed under this heading.

Hydrocortisone Valerate (Carbamazepine is metabolized by CYP3A4. Therefore, the potential exists for interaction between caramazepine and any agent that induces CYP3A4).
No products indexed under this heading.

Hypericum (Carbamazepine is metabolized by CYP3A4. Therefore, the potential exists for interaction between caramazepine and any agent that induces CYP3A4). Products include:
Satieté Tablets 640

Hypericum Perforatum (Carbamazepine is metabolized by CYP3A4. Therefore, the potential exists for interaction between caramazepine and any agent that induces CYP3A4).
No products indexed under this heading.

Imipramine Hydrochloride (Carbamazepine is known to induce CYP1A2 and CYP3A4. Therefore, the potential exists for interaction between carbamazepine and any agent metabolized by one (or more) of these enzymes).
No products indexed under this heading.

Imipramine Pamoate (Carbamazepine is known to induce CYP1A2 and CYP3A4. Therefore, the potential exists for interaction between carbamazepine and any agent metabolized by one (or more) of these enzymes).
No products indexed under this heading.

Indinavir Sulfate (Carbamazepine is metabolized mainly by cytochrome P450 (CYP) 3A4 to the active carbamazepine 10,11 -epoxide, which is further metabolized to the trans-diol by epoxide hydrolase. Therefore, the potential exists for interaction between carbamazepine and any agent that inhibits CYP3A4 and/or epoxide hydrolase). Products include:
Crixivan Capsules 1979

Isocarboxazid (Because of the relationship of carbamazepine to other tricyclic compounds, on theoretical grounds, co-administration with MAO inhibitors is contraindicated). Products include:
Marplan Tablets 3177

Isoniazid (Inhibitors of CYP3A4, such as isoniazid, inhibit carbamazepine metabolism and thus increase plasma carbamazepine levels).
No products indexed under this heading.

Isradipine (Carbamazepine is known to induce CYP1A2 and CYP3A4. Therefore, the potential exists for interaction between carbamazepine and any agent metabolized by one (or more) of these enzymes). Products include:
DynaCirc CR Controlled Release Tablets 1407

Itraconazole (Inhibitors of CYP3A4, such as itraconazole, inhibit carbamazepine metabolism and thus increase plasma carbamazepine levels).
No products indexed under this heading.

Ixabepilone (Carbamazepine is known to induce CYP1A2 and CYP3A4. Therefore, the potential exists for interaction between carbamazepine and any agent metabolized by one (or more) of these enzymes). Products include:
Ixempra Kit for Injection 915

Ketoconazole (Inhibitors of CYP3A4, such as ketoconazole, inhibit carbamazepine metabolism and thus increase plasma carbamazepine levels). Products include:
Extina Foam, 2% 3057
Nizoral A-D Shampoo 1901

Lamotrigine (Alterations of thyroid function have been reported in combination therapy with other anticonvulsants). Products include:
Lamictal 1488

Levetiracetam (Alterations of thyroid function have been reported in combination therapy with other anticonvulsants). Products include:
Keppra Injection 3137
Keppra Oral Solution 3131
Keppra Tablets 3131

Levobupivacaine Hydrochloride (Carbamazepine is known to induce CYP1A2 and CYP3A4. Therefore, the potential exists for interaction between carbamazepine and any agent metabolized by one (or more) of these enzymes).
No products indexed under this heading.

Levonorgestrel (Carbamazepine induces hepatic CYP activity and causes or would be expected to decrease plasma levels of oral contraceptives; breakthrough bleeding has been reported among patients receiving concomitant oral contraceptives and their reliability may be adversely affected). Products include:
Climara Pro Transdermal System 768
Lybrel Tablets 3204
Mirena Intrauterine System 779
Plan B Tablets 1044
Seasonique Tablets 1046

Lidocaine (Carbamazepine is known to induce CYP1A2 and CYP3A4. Therefore, the potential exists for interaction between carbamazepine and any agent metabolized by one (or more) of these enzymes). Products include:
Lidoderm Patch 1114

Lidocaine Hydrochloride (Carbamazepine is known to induce CYP1A2 and CYP3A4. Therefore, the potential exists for interaction between carbamazepine and any agent metabolized by one (or more) of these enzymes).
No products indexed under this heading.

Lithium (Co-administration may increase the risk of neurotoxic side effects).
No products indexed under this heading.

Lithium Carbonate (Co-administration with psychotropic agents has resulted in isolated cases of neuroleptic malignant syndrome).
No products indexed under this heading.

Lithium Citrate (Co-administration with psychotropic agents has resulted in isolated cases of neuroleptic malignant syndrome).
No products indexed under this heading.

Lomefloxacin Hydrochloride (Carbamazepine is known to induce CYP1A2 and CYP3A4. Therefore, the potential exists for interaction between carbamazepine and any agent metabolized by one (or more) of these enzymes).
No products indexed under this heading.

Lopinavir (Carbamazepine is metabolized mainly by cytochrome P450 (CYP) 3A4 to the active carbamazepine 10,11 -epoxide, which is further metabolized to the trans-diol by epoxide hydrolase. Therefore, the potential exists for interaction between carbamazepine and any agent that inhibits CYP3A4 and/or epoxide hydrolase). Products include:
Kaletra 452

Loratadine (Inhibitors of CYP3A4, such as loratadine, inhibit carbamazepine metabolism and thus increase plasma carbamazepine levels).
No products indexed under this heading.

Lovastatin (Carbamazepine is known to induce CYP1A2 and CYP3A4. Therefore, the potential exists for interaction between carbamazepine and any agent metabolized by one (or more) of these enzymes). Products include:
Advicor Tablets 402
Mevacor Tablets 2063

Loxapine Hydrochloride (Co-administration with psychotropic agents has resulted in isolated cases of neuroleptic malignant syndrome).
No products indexed under this heading.

Loxapine Succinate (Co-administration with psychotropic agents has resulted in isolated cases of neuroleptic malignant syndrome).
No products indexed under this heading.

Maprotiline Hydrochloride (Carbamazepine is known to induce CYP1A2 and CYP3A4. Therefore, the potential exists for interaction between carbamazepine and any agent metabolized by one (or more) of these enzymes).
No products indexed under this heading.

Mefloquine Hydrochloride (Antimalarial drugs, such as chloroquine and mefloquine, may antagonize the activity of carbamazepine).
No products indexed under this heading.

Mephenytoin (Alterations of thyroid function have been reported in combination therapy with other anticonvulsants).
No products indexed under this heading.

Mesoridazine Besylate (Co-administration with psychotropic agents has resulted in isolated cases of neuroleptic malignant syndrome).
No products indexed under this heading.

Mestranol (Carbamazepine induces hepatic CYP activity and causes or would be expected to decrease plasma levels of oral contraceptives; breakthrough bleeding has been reported among patients receiving concomitant oral contraceptives and their reliability may be adversely affected).
No products indexed under this heading.

Methadone Hydrochloride (Carbamazepine is known to induce CYP1A2 and CYP3A4. Therefore, the potential exists for interaction between carbamazepine and any agent metabolized by one (or more) of these enzymes).
No products indexed under this heading.

Methotrimeprazine (Co-administration with psychotropic agents has resulted in isolated cases of neuroleptic malignant syndrome).
No products indexed under this heading.

Methsuximide (Carbamezepine induces hepatic CYP activity and causes or would be expected to decrease plasma levels of methsuximide; alterations of thyroid function have been reported in combination therapy with other anticonvulsants).
No products indexed under this heading.

Methylprednisolone (Carbamazepine is metabolized by CYP3A4. Therefore, the potential exists for interaction between caramazepine and any agent that induces CYP3A4).
No products indexed under this heading.

Methylprednisolone Acetate (Carbamazepine is metabolized by CYP3A4. Therefore, the potential exists for interaction between caramazepine and any agent that induces CYP3A4).
No products indexed under this heading.

Methylprednisolone Sodium Succinate (Carbamazepine is metabolized by CYP3A4. Therefore, the potential exists for interaction between caramazepine and any agent that induces CYP3A4).
No products indexed under this heading.

Metronidazole (Carbamazepine is metabolized mainly by cytochrome P450 (CYP) 3A4 to the active carbamazepine 10,11 -epoxide, which is further metabolized to the trans-diol by epoxide hydrolase. Therefore, the potential exists for interaction between carbamazepine and any agent that inhibits CYP3A4 and/or epoxide hydrolase). Products include:
Pylera Capsules 714

Metronidazole Benzoate (Carbamazepine is metabolized mainly by cytochrome P450 (CYP) 3A4 to the active carbamazepine 10,11 -epoxide, which is further metabolized to the trans-diol by epoxide hydrolase. Therefore, the potential exists for interaction between carbamazepine and any agent that inhibits CYP3A4 and/or epoxide hydrolase).
No products indexed under this heading.

Metronidazole Hydrochloride (Carbamazepine is metabolized mainly by cytochrome P450 (CYP) 3A4 to the active carbamazepine 10,11 -epoxide, which is further metabolized to the trans-diol by epoxide hydrolase. Therefore, the potential exists for interaction between carbamazepine and any agent that inhibits CYP3A4 and/or epoxide hydrolase).
No products indexed under this heading.

Metronidazole Sodium (Carbamazepine is metabolized mainly by cytochrome P450 (CYP) 3A4 to the active carbamazepine 10,11 -epoxide, which is further metabolized to the trans-diol by epoxide hydrolase. Therefore, the potential exists for interaction between carbamazepine and any agent that inhibits its CYP3A4 and/or epoxide hydrolase).
No products indexed under this heading.

Mexiletine Hydrochloride (Carbamazepine is known to induce CYP1A2 and CYP3A4. Therefore, the potential exists for interaction between carbamazepine and any agent metabolized by one (or more) of these enzymes).
No products indexed under this heading.

Miconazole (Carbamazepine is metabolized mainly by cytochrome P450 (CYP) 3A4 to the active carbamazepine 10,11 -epoxide, which is further metabolized to the trans-diol by epoxide hydrolase. Therefore, the potential exists for interaction between carbamazepine and any agent that inhibits CYP3A4 and/or epoxide hydrolase).
No products indexed under this heading.

Miconazole Nitrate (Carbamazepine is metabolized mainly by cytochrome P450 (CYP) 3A4 to the active carbamazepine 10,11 -epoxide, which is further metabolized to the trans-diol by epoxide hydrolase. Therefore, the potential exists for interaction between carbamazepine and any agent that inhibits its CYP3A4 and/or epoxide hydrolase).
No products indexed under this heading.

Midazolam Hydrochloride (Carbamazepine is known to induce CYP1A2 and CYP3A4. Therefore, the potential exists for interaction between carbamazepine and any agent metabolized by one (or more) of these enzymes).
No products indexed under this heading.

Mirtazapine (Carbamazepine is known to induce CYP1A2 and CYP3A4. Therefore, the potential exists for interaction between carbamazepine and any agent metabolized by one (or more) of these enzymes). Products include:
Remeron Tablets **2924**
RemeronSolTab Tablets **2927**

Moclobemide (Because of the relationship of carbamazepine to other tricyclic compounds, on theoretical grounds, co-administration with MAO inhibitors is contraindicated).
No products indexed under this heading.

Modafinil (Carbamazepine is metabolized by CYP3A4. Therefore, the potential exists for interaction between caramazepine and any agent that induces CYP3A4). Products include:
Provigil Tablets **977**

Molindone Hydrochloride (Co-administration with psychotropic agents has resulted in isolated cases of neuroleptic malignant syndrome). Products include:
Moban Tablets **1116**

Moxifloxacin Hydrochloride (Carbamazepine is known to induce CYP1A2 and CYP3A4. Therefore, the potential exists for interaction between carbamazepine and any agent metabolized by one (or more) of these enzymes). Products include:
Avelox **2803**
Vigamox Ophthalmic Solution **548**

Nafcillin Sodium (Carbamazepine is known to induce CYP1A2 and CYP3A4. Therefore, the potential exists for interaction between carbamazepine and any agent metabolized by one (or more) of these enzymes).
No products indexed under this heading.

Naproxen (Carbamazepine is known to induce CYP1A2 and CYP3A4. Therefore, the potential exists for interaction between carbamazepine and any agent metabolized by one (or more) of these enzymes). Products include:
EC-Naprosyn Delayed-Release Tablets **2632**
Naprosyn Suspension **2632**
Naprosyn Tablets **2632**

Naproxen Sodium (Carbamazepine is known to induce CYP1A2 and CYP3A4. Therefore, the potential exists for interaction between carbamazepine and any agent metabolized by one (or more) of these enzymes). Products include:
Anaprox Tablets **2632**
Anaprox DS Tablets **2632**
Treximet Tablets **1616**

Nefazodone Hydrochloride (Carbamazepine is metabolized mainly by cytochrome P450 (CYP) 3A4 to the active carbamazepine 10,11 -epoxide, which is further metabolized to the trans-diol by epoxide hydrolase. Therefore, the potential exists for interaction between carbamazepine and any agent that inhibits its CYP3A4 and/or epoxide hydrolase).
No products indexed under this heading.

Nelfinavir Mesylate (Carbamazepine is metabolized mainly by cytochrome P450 (CYP) 3A4 to the active carbamazepine 10,11 -epoxide, which is further metabolized to the trans-diol by epoxide hydrolase. Therefore, the potential exists for interaction between carbamazepine and any agent that inhibits its CYP3A4 and/or epoxide hydrolase).
No products indexed under this heading.

Nevirapine (Carbamazepine is metabolized mainly by cytochrome P450 (CYP) 3A4 to the active carbamazepine 10,11 -epoxide, which is further metabolized to the trans-diol by epoxide hydrolase. Therefore, the potential exists for interaction between carbamazepine and any agent that inhibits CYP3A4 and/or epoxide hydrolase). Products include:
Viramune Oral Suspension **873**
Viramune Tablets **873**

Niacinamide (Inhibitors of CYP3A4, such as niacinamide, inhibit carbamazepine metabolism and thus increase plasma carbamazepine levels). Products include:
BioLean Free Tablets .... ■□**635**

Nicardipine Hydrochloride (Carbamazepine is known to induce CYP1A2 and CYP3A4. Therefore, the potential exists for interaction between carbamazepine and any agent metabolized by one (or more) of these enzymes). Products include:
Cardene I.V. **1093**

Nicotinamide (Inhibitors of CYP3A4, such as nicotinamide, inhibit carbamazepine metabolism and thus increase plasma carbamazepine levels).
No products indexed under this heading.

Nicotine Polacrilex (Carbamazepine is known to induce CYP1A2 and CYP3A4. Therefore, the potential exists for interaction between carbamazepine and any agent metabolized by one (or more) of these enzymes).
No products indexed under this heading.

Nicotine Salicylate (Carbamazepine is known to induce CYP1A2 and CYP3A4. Therefore, the potential exists for interaction between carbamazepine and any agent metabolized by one (or more) of these enzymes).
No products indexed under this heading.

Nicotine Sulfate (Carbamazepine is known to induce CYP1A2 and CYP3A4. Therefore, the potential exists for interaction between carbamazepine and any agent metabolized by one (or more) of these enzymes).
No products indexed under this heading.

Nifedipine (Carbamazepine is metabolized mainly by cytochrome P450 (CYP) 3A4 to the active carbamazepine 10,11 -epoxide, which is further metabolized to the trans-diol by epoxide hydrolase. Therefore, the potential exists for interaction between carbamazepine and any agent that inhibits CYP3A4 and/or epoxide hydrolase).
No products indexed under this heading.

Nimodipine (Carbamazepine is known to induce CYP1A2 and CYP3A4. Therefore, the potential exists for interaction between carbamazepine and any agent metabolized by one (or more) of these enzymes). Products include:
Nimotop Capsules **790**

Nisoldipine (Carbamazepine is known to induce CYP1A2 and CYP3A4. Therefore, the potential exists for interaction between carbamazepine and any agent metabolized by one (or more) of these enzymes). Products include:
Sular Extended Release Tablets **2975**

Nitrendipine (Carbamazepine is known to induce CYP1A2 and CYP3A4. Therefore, the potential exists for interaction between carbamazepine and any agent metabolized by one (or more) of these enzymes).
No products indexed under this heading.

Norethindrone (Carbamazepine induces hepatic CYP activity and causes or would be expected to decrease plasma levels of oral contraceptives; breakthrough bleeding has been reported among patients receiving concomitant oral contraceptives and their reliability may be adversely affected). Products include:
Ortho Micronor Tablets **2446**

Norethindrone Acetate (Carbamazepine is known to induce CYP1A2 and CYP3A4. Therefore, the potential exists for interaction between carbamazepine and any agent metabolized by one (or more) of these enzymes). Products include:
Activella Tablets **2347**

Norethynodrel (Carbamazepine induces hepatic CYP activity and causes or would be expected to decrease plasma levels of oral contraceptives; breakthrough bleeding has been reported among patients receiving concomitant oral contraceptives and their reliability may be adversely affected).
No products indexed under this heading.

Norfloxacin (Carbamazepine is metabolized mainly by cytochrome P450 (CYP) 3A4 to the active carbamazepine 10,11 -epoxide, which is further metabolized to the trans-diol by epoxide hydrolase. Therefore, the potential exists for interaction between carbamazepine and any agent that inhibits CYP3A4 and/or epoxide hydrolase). Products include:
Noroxin Tablets **2069**

Norgestimate (Carbamazepine induces hepatic CYP activity and causes or would be expected to decrease plasma levels of oral contraceptives; breakthrough bleeding has been reported among patients receiving concomitant oral contraceptives and their reliability may be adversely affected). Products include:
Ortho-Cyclen/Ortho Tri-Cyclen **2449**
Ortho Tri-Cyclen Lo Tablets **2458**

Norgestrel (Carbamazepine induces hepatic CYP activity and causes or would be expected to decrease plasma levels of oral contraceptives; breakthrough bleeding has been reported among patients receiving concomitant oral contraceptives and their reliability may be adversely affected).
No products indexed under this heading.

Nortriptyline Hydrochloride (Carbamazepine is known to induce CYP1A2 and CYP3A4. Therefore, the potential exists for interaction between carbamazepine and any agent metabolized by one (or more) of these enzymes).
No products indexed under this heading.

Ofloxacin (Carbamazepine is known to induce CYP1A2 and CYP3A4. Therefore, the potential exists for interaction between carbamazepine and any agent metabolized by one (or more) of these enzymes). Products include:
Ofloxacin Ophthalmic Solution 0.3% .... ⊙**243**

Olanzapine (Co-administration with psychotropic agents has resulted in isolated cases of neuroleptic malignant syndrome). Products include:
Symbyax Capsules **1871**
Zyprexa Tablets **1883**
Zyprexa IntraMuscular **1883**
Zyprexa ZYDIS Orally Disintegrating Tablets **1883**

Omeprazole (Carbamazepine is metabolized mainly by cytochrome P450 (CYP) 3A4 to the active carbamazepine 10,11 -epoxide, which is further metabolized to the trans-diol by epoxide hydrolase. Therefore, the potential exists for interaction between carbamazepine and any agent that inhibits CYP3A4 and/or epoxide hydrolase).
No products indexed under this heading.

Ondansetron (Carbamazepine is known to induce CYP1A2 and CYP3A4. Therefore, the potential exists for interaction between carbamazepine and any agent metabolized by one (or more) of these enzymes). Products include:
Zofran ODT Orally Disintegrating Tablets **1687**

Ondansetron Hydrochloride (Carbamazepine is known to induce CYP1A2 and CYP3A4. Therefore, the potential exists for interaction between carbamazepine and any agent metabolized by one (or more) of these enzymes). Products include:
Zofran Injection **1682**
Zofran **1687**

Oxcarbazepine (Alterations of thyroid function have been reported in combination therapy with other anticonvulsants).
No products indexed under this heading.

Paclitaxel (Carbamazepine is known to induce CYP1A2 and CYP3A4. Therefore, the potential exists for interaction between carbamazepine and any agent metabolized by one (or more) of these enzymes).
No products indexed under this heading.

Paliperidone (Co-administration with psychotropic agents has resulted in isolated cases of neuroleptic malignant syndrome). Products include:
Invega Extended-Release Tablets **1748**

Paramethadione (Alterations of thyroid function have been reported in combination therapy with other anticonvulsants).
No products indexed under this heading.

Pargyline Hydrochloride (Because of the relationship of carbamazepine to other tricyclic compounds, on theoretical grounds, co-administration with MAO inhibitors is contraindicated).
No products indexed under this heading.

Paroxetine Hydrochloride (Carbamazepine is metabolized mainly by cytochrome P450 (CYP) 3A4 to the active carbamazepine 10,11 -epoxide, which is further metabolized to the trans-diol by epoxide hydrolase. Therefore, the potential exists for interaction between carbamazepine and any agent that inhibits CYP3A4 and/or epoxide hydrolase). Products include:
Paxil **1535**
Paxil CR Controlled-Release Tablets **1544**

Perphenazine (Co-administration with psychotropic agents has resulted in isolated cases of neuroleptic malignant syndrome).
No products indexed under this heading.

Phenacemide (Alterations of thyroid function have been reported in combination therapy with other anticonvulsants).
No products indexed under this heading.

Phenelzine Sulfate (Because of the relationship of carbamazepine to other tricyclic compounds, on theoretical grounds, co-administration with MAO inhibitors is contraindicated).
No products indexed under this heading.

Phenobarbital (Inducers of CYP3A4, such as phenobarbital, can increase the rate of carbamazepine metabolism and can thus decrease plasma carbamazepine levels; alterations of thyroid function have been reported in combination therapy with other anticonvulsants). Products include:
Donnatal Extentabs **2507**

Phenobarbital Sodium (Carbamazepine is metabolized by CYP3A4. Therefore, the potential exists for interaction between caramazepine and any agent that induces CYP3A4).
No products indexed under this heading.

Phensuximide (Carbamezapine induces hepatic CYP activity and causes or would be expected to decrease plasma levels of phensuximide; alterations of thyroid function have been reported in combination therapy with other anticonvulsants).
No products indexed under this heading.

Phenytoin (Inducers of CYP3A4, such as phenytoin, can increase the rate of carbamazepine metabolism and can thus decrease plasma carbamazepine levels; phenytoin levels have been reported to increase or decrease in the presence of carbamazepine; careful monitoring of phenytoin plasma levels following co-medication with carbamazepine is advised. Alterations of thyroid function have been reported in combination therapy with other anticonvulsants).
No products indexed under this heading.

Phenytoin Sodium (Inducers of CYP3A4, such as phenytoin, can increase the rate of carbamazepine metabolism and can thus decrease plasma carbamazepine levels; phenytoin levels have been reported to increase or decrease in the presence of carbamazepine; careful monitoring of phenytoin plasma levels following co-medication with carbamazepine is advised. Alterations of thyroid function have been reported in combination therapy with other anticonvulsants). Products include:
Phenytek Capsules **2192**

Pimozide (Co-administration with psychotropic agents has resulted in isolated cases of neuroleptic malignant syndrome).
No products indexed under this heading.

Polyestradiol Phosphate (Carbamazepine is known to induce CYP1A2 and CYP3A4. Therefore, the potential exists for interaction between carbamazepine and any agent metabolized by one (or more) of these enzymes).
No products indexed under this heading.

Prednisolone Acetate (Carbamazepine is metabolized by CYP3A4. Therefore, the potential exists for interaction between caramazepine and any agent that induces CYP3A4). Products include:
Pred Forte Ophthalmic Suspension .... ⊙ **227**
Pred Mild Ophthalmic Suspension .... ⊙ **230**
Pred-G Ophthalmic Ointment .... ⊙ **229**
Pred-G Ophthalmic Suspension .... ⊙ **228**

Prednisolone Sodium Phosphate (Carbamazepine is metabolized by CYP3A4. Therefore, the potential exists for interaction between caramazepine and any agent that induces CYP3A4).
No products indexed under this heading.

Prednisolone Tebutate (Carbamazepine is metabolized by CYP3A4. Therefore, the potential exists for interaction between caramazepine and any agent that induces CYP3A4).
No products indexed under this heading.

Prednisone (Carbamazepine is metabolized by CYP3A4. Therefore, the potential exists for interaction between caramazepine and any agent that induces CYP3A4).
No products indexed under this heading.

Primidone (Inducers of CYP3A4, such as primidone, can increase the rate of carbamazepine metabolism and can thus decrease plasma carbamazepine levels; carbamazepine increases levels of primidone; alterations of thyroid function have been reported in combination therapy with other anticonvulsants).
No products indexed under this heading.

Procarbazine Hydrochloride (Because of the relationship of carbamazepine to other tricyclic compounds, on theoretical grounds, co-administration with MAO inhibitors is contraindicated).
No products indexed under this heading.

Prochlorperazine (Co-administration with psychotropic agents has resulted in isolated cases of neuroleptic malignant syndrome).
No products indexed under this heading.

Promethazine Hydrochloride (Co-administration with psychotropic agents has resulted in isolated cases of neuroleptic malignant syndrome).
No products indexed under this heading.

Propafenone Hydrochloride (Carbamazepine is known to induce CYP1A2 and CYP3A4. Therefore, the potential exists for interaction between carbamazepine and any agent metabolized by one (or more) of these enzymes). Products include:
Rythmol Tablets **1586**
Rythmol SR Capsules **1590**

Propoxyphene Hydrochloride (Inhibitors of CYP3A4, such as propoxyphene, inhibit carbamazepine metabolism and thus increase plasma carbamazepine levels).
No products indexed under this heading.

Propoxyphene Napsylate (Inhibitors of CYP3A4, such as propoxyphene, inhibit carbamazepine metabolism and thus increase plasma carbamazepine levels).
No products indexed under this heading.

Propranolol Hydrochloride (Carbamazepine is known to induce CYP1A2 and CYP3A4. Therefore, the potential exists for interaction between carbamazepine and any agent metabolized by one (or more) of these enzymes). Products include:
InnoPran XL Extended Release Capsules **1484**

Protriptyline Hydrochloride (Carbamazepine is known to induce CYP1A2 and CYP3A4. Therefore, the potential exists for interaction between carbamazepine and any agent metabolized by one (or more) of these enzymes).
No products indexed under this heading.

Pyrimethamine (Anti-malarial drugs, such as chloroquine and mefloquine, may antagonize the activity of carbamazepine). Products include:
Daraprim Tablets **1400**
Fansidar Tablets **2636**

Quetiapine Fumarate (Co-administration with psychotropic agents has resulted in isolated cases of neuroleptic malignant syndrome).
No products indexed under this heading.

Quinidine (Carbamazepine is metabolized mainly by cytochrome P450 (CYP) 3A4 to the active carbamazepine 10,11 -epoxide, which is further metabolized to the trans-diol by epoxide hydrolase. Therefore, the potential exists for interaction between carbamazepine and any agent that inhibits CYP3A4 and/or epoxide hydrolase).
No products indexed under this heading.

Quinidine Gluconate (Carbamazepine is known to induce CYP1A2 and CYP3A4. Therefore, the potential exists for interaction between carbamazepine and any agent metabolized by one (or more) of these enzymes).
No products indexed under this heading.

Quinidine Hydrochloride (Carbamazepine is metabolized mainly by cytochrome P450 (CYP) 3A4 to the active carbamazepine 10,11 -epoxide, which is further metabolized to the trans-diol by epoxide hydrolase. Therefore, the potential exists for interaction between carbamazepine and any agent that inhibits CYP3A4 and/or epoxide hydrolase).
No products indexed under this heading.

Quinidine Polygalacturonate (Carbamazepine is metabolized mainly by cytochrome P450 (CYP) 3A4 to the active carbamazepine 10,11 -epoxide, which is further metabolized to the trans-diol by epoxide hydrolase. Therefore, the potential exists for interaction between carbamazepine and any agent that inhibits CYP3A4 and/or epoxide hydrolase).
No products indexed under this heading.

Quinidine Sulfate (Carbamazepine is metabolized mainly by cytochrome P450 (CYP) 3A4 to the active carbamazepine 10,11 -epoxide, which is further metabolized to the trans-diol by epoxide hydrolase. Therefore, the potential exists for interaction between carbamazepine and any agent that inhibits CYP3A4 and/or epoxide hydrolase).
No products indexed under this heading.

Quinine (Carbamazepine is metabolized mainly by cytochrome P450 (CYP) 3A4 to the active carbamazepine 10,11 -epoxide, which is further metabolized to the trans-diol by epoxide hydrolase. Therefore, the potential exists for interaction between carbamazepine and any agent that inhibits CYP3A4 and/or epoxide hydrolase).
No products indexed under this heading.

Quinine Sulfate (Carbamazepine is metabolized mainly by cytochrome P450 (CYP) 3A4 to the active carbamazepine 10,11 -epoxide, which is further metabolized to the trans-diol by epoxide hydrolase. Therefore, the potential exists for interaction between carbamazepine and any agent that inhibits CYP3A4 and/or epoxide hydrolase).
No products indexed under this heading.

Quinupristin (Carbamazepine is metabolized mainly by cytochrome P450 (CYP) 3A4 to the active carbamazepine 10,11 -epoxide, which is further metabolized to the trans-diol by epoxide hydrolase. Therefore, the potential exists for interaction between carbamazepine and any agent that inhibits CYP3A4 and/or epoxide hydrolase).
No products indexed under this heading.

Ranitidine Bismuth Citrate (Carbamazepine is metabolized mainly by cytochrome P450 (CYP) 3A4 to the active carbamazepine 10,11 -epoxide, which is further metabolized to the trans-diol by epoxide hydrolase. Therefore, the potential exists for interaction between carbamazepine and any agent that inhibits CYP3A4 and/or epoxide hydrolase).
No products indexed under this heading.

Ranitidine Hydrochloride (Carbamazepine is metabolized mainly by cytochrome P450 (CYP) 3A4 to the active carbamazepine 10,11 -epoxide, which is further metabolized to the trans-diol by epoxide hydrolase. Therefore, the potential exists for interaction between carbamazepine and any agent that inhibits CYP3A4 and/or epoxide hydrolase). Products include:

- Zantac 75 Tablets .... ▪603
- Zantac 1670
- Zantac Injection 1666
- Zantac Injection Pharmacy Bulk Package 1668
- Maximum Strength Zantac 150 Tablets .... ▪603
- Maximum Strength Zantac 150 Cool Mint Tablets .... ▪603

Rasagiline Mesylate (Because of the relationship of carbamazepine to other tricyclic compounds, on theoretical grounds, co-administration with MAO inhibitors is contraindicated). Products include:

- Azilect Tablets 3106

Rifabutin (Carbamazepine is metabolized by CYP3A4. Therefore, the potential exists for interaction between caramazepine and any agent that induces CYP3A4).
No products indexed under this heading.

Rifampicin (Carbamazepine is metabolized by CYP3A4. Therefore, the potential exists for interaction between caramazepine and any agent that induces CYP3A4).
No products indexed under this heading.

Rifampin (Inducers of CYP3A4, such as rifampin, can increase the rate of carbamazepine metabolism and can thus decrease plasma carbamazepine levels).
No products indexed under this heading.

Rifapentine (Carbamazepine is metabolized by CYP3A4. Therefore, the potential exists for interaction between caramazepine and any agent that induces CYP3A4).
No products indexed under this heading.

Riluzole (Carbamazepine is known to induce CYP1A2 and CYP3A4. Therefore, the potential exists for interaction between carbamazepine and any agent metabolized by one (or more) of these enzymes). Products include:

- Rilutek Tablets 2771

Risperidone (Co-administration with psychotropic agents has resulted in isolated cases of neuroleptic malignant syndrome). Products include:

- Risperdal Consta Long-Acting Injection 1753

Ritonavir (Carbamazepine is metabolized mainly by cytochrome P450 (CYP) 3A4 to the active carbamazepine 10,11 -epoxide, which is further metabolized to the trans-diol by epoxide hydrolase. Therefore, the potential exists for interaction between carbamazepine and any agent that inhibits CYP3A4 and/or epoxide hydrolase). Products include:

- Kaletra 452
- Norvir 489

Ropinirole Hydrochloride (Carbamazepine is known to induce CYP1A2 and CYP3A4. Therefore, the potential exists for interaction between carbamazepine and any agent metabolized by one (or more) of these enzymes). Products include:

- Requip Tablets 1561
- Requip XL Tablets 1568

Ropivacaine Hydrochloride (Carbamazepine is known to induce CYP1A2 and CYP3A4. Therefore, the potential exists for interaction between carbamazepine and any agent metabolized by one (or more) of these enzymes).
No products indexed under this heading.

Saquinavir (Carbamazepine is metabolized mainly by cytochrome P450 (CYP) 3A4 to the active carbamazepine 10,11 -epoxide, which is further metabolized to the trans-diol by epoxide hydrolase. Therefore, the potential exists for interaction between carbamazepine and any agent that inhibits CYP3A4 and/or epoxide hydrolase).
No products indexed under this heading.

Saquinavir Mesylate (Carbamazepine is metabolized mainly by cytochrome P450 (CYP) 3A4 to the active carbamazepine 10,11 -epoxide, which is further metabolized to the trans-diol by epoxide hydrolase. Therefore, the potential exists for interaction between carbamazepine and any agent that inhibits CYP3A4 and/or epoxide hydrolase).
No products indexed under this heading.

Selegiline (Because of the relationship of carbamazepine to other tricyclic compounds, on theoretical grounds, co-administration with MAO inhibitors is contraindicated). Products include:

- Emsam Transdermal System 905

Selegiline Hydrochloride (Because of the relationship of carbamazepine to other tricyclic compounds, on theoretical grounds, co-administration with MAO inhibitors is contraindicated). Products include:

- Eldepryl Capsules 3052

Sertraline Hydrochloride (Carbamazepine is metabolized mainly by cytochrome P450 (CYP) 3A4 to the active carbamazepine 10,11 -epoxide, which is further metabolized to the trans-diol by epoxide hydrolase. Therefore, the potential exists for interaction between carbamazepine and any agent that inhibits CYP3A4 and/or epoxide hydrolase).
No products indexed under this heading.

Sildenafil Citrate (Carbamazepine is metabolized mainly by cytochrome P450 (CYP) 3A4 to the active carbamazepine 10,11 -epoxide, which is further metabolized to the trans-diol by epoxide hydrolase. Therefore, the potential exists for interaction between carbamazepine and any agent that inhibits CYP3A4 and/or epoxide hydrolase).
No products indexed under this heading.

Simvastatin (Carbamazepine is known to induce CYP1A2 and CYP3A4. Therefore, the potential exists for interaction between carbamazepine and any agent metabolized by one (or more) of these enzymes). Products include:

- Simcor Tablets 502
- Vytorin 10/10 Tablets 2149
- Vytorin 10/10 Tablets 2939
- Vytorin 10/20 Tablets 2149
- Vytorin 10/20 Tablets 2939
- Vytorin 10/40 Tablets 2149
- Vytorin 10/40 Tablets 2939
- Vytorin 10/80 Tablets 2149
- Vytorin 10/80 Tablets 2939
- Zocor Tablets 2136

Sirolimus (Carbamazepine is known to induce CYP1A2 and CYP3A4. Therefore, the potential exists for interaction between carbamazepine and any agent metabolized by one (or more) of these enzymes). Products include:

- Rapamune 3260

Sulfinpyrazone (Carbamazepine is metabolized by CYP3A4. Therefore, the potential exists for interaction between caramazepine and any agent that induces CYP3A4).
No products indexed under this heading.

Tacrine Hydrochloride (Carbamazepine is known to induce CYP1A2 and CYP3A4. Therefore, the potential exists for interaction between carbamazepine and any agent metabolized by one (or more) of these enzymes).
No products indexed under this heading.

Tacrolimus (Carbamazepine is known to induce CYP1A2 and CYP3A4. Therefore, the potential exists for interaction between carbamazepine and any agent metabolized by one (or more) of these enzymes). Products include:

- Prograf Capsules and Injection 622
- Protopic Ointment 628

Tadalafil (Carbamazepine is known to induce CYP1A2 and CYP3A4. Therefore, the potential exists for interaction between carbamazepine and any agent metabolized by one (or more) of these enzymes). Products include:

- Cialis Tablets 1792

Tamoxifen Citrate (Carbamazepine is known to induce CYP1A2 and CYP3A4. Therefore, the potential exists for interaction between carbamazepine and any agent metabolized by one (or more) of these enzymes).
No products indexed under this heading.

Telithromycin (Carbamazepine is metabolized mainly by cytochrome P450 (CYP) 3A4 to the active carbamazepine 10,11 -epoxide, which is further metabolized to the trans-diol by epoxide hydrolase. Therefore, the potential exists for interaction between carbamazepine and any agent that inhibits CYP3A4 and/or epoxide hydrolase). Products include:

- Ketek Tablets 2744

Terfenadine (Inhibitors of CYP3A4, such as terfenadine, inhibit carbamazepine metabolism and thus increase plasma carbamazepine levels).
No products indexed under this heading.

Theophylline (Inducers of CYP3A4, such as theophylline, can increase the rate of carbamazepine metabolism and can thus decrease plasma carbamazepine levels; carbamazepine induces hepatic CYP activity and causes or would be expected to decrease plasma levels of theophylline).
No products indexed under this heading.

Theophylline Anhydrous (Inducers of CYP3A4, such as theophylline, can increase the rate of carbamazepine metabolism and can thus decrease plasma carbamazepine levels; carbamazepine induces hepatic CYP activity and causes or would be expected to decrease plasma levels of theophylline). Products include:

- Uniphyl Tablets 2595

Theophylline Calcium Salicylate (Inducers of CYP3A4, such as theophylline, can increase the rate of carbamazepine metabolism and can thus decrease plasma carbamazepine levels; carbamazepine induces hepatic CYP activity and causes or would be expected to decrease plasma levels of theophylline).
No products indexed under this heading.

Theophylline Dihydroxypropyl (Glyceryl) (Inducers of CYP3A4, such as theophylline, can increase the rate of carbamazepine metabolism and can thus decrease plasma carbamazepine levels; carbamazepine induces hepatic CYP activity and causes or would be expected to decrease plasma levels of theophylline).
No products indexed under this heading.

Theophylline Ethylenediamine (Inducers of CYP3A4, such as theophylline, can increase the rate of carbamazepine metabolism and can thus decrease plasma carbamazepine levels; carbamazepine induces hepatic CYP activity and causes or would be expected to decrease plasma levels of theophylline).
No products indexed under this heading.

Theophylline Sodium Glycinate (Inducers of CYP3A4, such as theophylline, can increase the rate of carbamazepine metabolism and can thus decrease plasma carbamazepine levels; carbamazepine induces hepatic CYP activity and causes or would be expected to decrease plasma levels of theophylline).
No products indexed under this heading.

Thioridazine Hydrochloride (Co-administration with psychotropic agents has resulted in isolated cases of neuroleptic malignant syndrome). Products include:
Thioridazine Hydrochloride Tablets 2195

Thiothixene (Co-administration with psychotropic agents has resulted in isolated cases of neuroleptic malignant syndrome). Products include:
Thiothixene Capsules 2197

Tiagabine Hydrochloride (Alterations of thyroid function have been reported in combination therapy with other anticonvulsants). Products include:
Gabitril Tablets 973

Tolterodine Tartrate (Carbamazepine is known to induce CYP1A2 and CYP3A4. Therefore, the potential exists for interaction between carbamazepine and any agent metabolized by one (or more) of these enzymes).
No products indexed under this heading.

Topiramate (Alterations of thyroid function have been reported in combination therapy with other anticonvulsants).
No products indexed under this heading.

Tranylcypromine Sulfate (Because of the relationship of carbamazepine to other tricyclic compounds, on theoretical grounds, co-administration with MAO inhibitors is contraindicated). Products include:
Parnate Tablets 1532

Trazodone Hydrochloride (Carbamazepine is known to induce CYP1A2 and CYP3A4. Therefore, the potential exists for interaction between carbamazepine and any agent metabolized by one (or more) of these enzymes. Carbamazepine has been shown to reduce plasma levels of trazodone).
No products indexed under this heading.

Triamcinolone (Carbamazepine is metabolized by CYP3A4. Therefore, the potential exists for interaction between caramazepine and any agent that induces CYP3A4).
No products indexed under this heading.

Triamcinolone Acetonide (Carbamazepine is metabolized by CYP3A4. Therefore, the potential exists for interaction between caramazepine and any agent that induces CYP3A4). Products include:
Azmacort Inhalation Aerosol 407
Nasacort AQ Nasal Spray 2765
Triesence Injectable Suspension .... ⊙209

Triamcinolone Diacetate (Carbamazepine is metabolized by CYP3A4. Therefore, the potential exists for interaction between caramazepine and any agent that induces CYP3A4).
No products indexed under this heading.

Triamcinolone Hexacetonide (Carbamazepine is metabolized by CYP3A4. Therefore, the potential exists for interaction between caramazepine and any agent that induces CYP3A4).
No products indexed under this heading.

Triazolam (Carbamazepine is known to induce CYP1A2 and CYP3A4. Therefore, the potential exists for interaction between carbamazepine and any agent metabolized by one (or more) of these enzymes).
No products indexed under this heading.

Trifluoperazine Hydrochloride (Co-administration with psychotropic agents has resulted in isolated cases of neuroleptic malignant syndrome).
No products indexed under this heading.

Trimethadione (Alterations of thyroid function have been reported in combination therapy with other anticonvulsants).
No products indexed under this heading.

Trimethaphan Camsylate (Carbamazepine is known to induce CYP1A2 and CYP3A4. Therefore, the potential exists for interaction between carbamazepine and any agent metabolized by one (or more) of these enzymes).
No products indexed under this heading.

Trimipramine Maleate (Carbamazepine is known to induce CYP1A2 and CYP3A4. Therefore, the potential exists for interaction between carbamazepine and any agent metabolized by one (or more) of these enzymes).
No products indexed under this heading.

Troglitazone (Carbamazepine is metabolized mainly by cytochrome P450 (CYP) 3A4 to the active carbamazepine 10,11 -epoxide, which is further metabolized to the trans-diol by epoxide hydrolase. Therefore, the potential exists for interaction between carbamazepine and any agent that inhibits CYP3A4 and/or epoxide hydrolase).
No products indexed under this heading.

Troleandomycin (Inhibitors of CYP3A4, such as troleandomycin, inhibit carbamazepine metabolism and thus increase plasma carbamazepine levels).
No products indexed under this heading.

Trovafloxacin Mesylate (Carbamazepine is known to induce CYP1A2 and CYP3A4. Therefore, the potential exists for interaction between carbamazepine and any agent metabolized by one (or more) of these enzymes).
No products indexed under this heading.

Valproate Sodium (Inhibitors of CYP3A4, such as valproate, inhibit carbamazepine metabolism and thus increase plasma carbamazepine levels; carbamazepine induces hepatic CYP activity and causes or would be expected to decrease plasma levels of valproate; alterations of thyroid function have been reported in combination therapy with other anticonvulsants).
No products indexed under this heading.

Valproic Acid (Inhibitors of CYP3A4, such as valproate, inhibit carbamazepine metabolism and thus increase plasma carbamazepine levels; carbamazepine induces hepatic CYP activity and causes or would be expected to decrease plasma levels of valproate; alterations of thyroid function have been reported in combination therapy with other anticonvulsants).
No products indexed under this heading.

Vardenafil Hydrochloride (Carbamazepine is metabolized mainly by cytochrome P450 (CYP) 3A4 to the active carbamazepine 10,11 -epoxide, which is further metabolized to the trans-diol by epoxide hydrolase. Therefore, the potential exists for interaction between carbamazepine and any agent that inhibits CYP3A4 and/or epoxide hydrolase). Products include:
Levitra Tablets 2876

Verapamil Hydrochloride (Inhibitors of CYP3A4, such as verapamil, inhibit carbamazepine metabolism and thus increase plasma carbamazepine levels). Products include:
Tarka Tablets 511

Vinblastine Sulfate (Carbamazepine is known to induce CYP1A2 and CYP3A4. Therefore, the potential exists for interaction between carbamazepine and any agent metabolized by one (or more) of these enzymes).
No products indexed under this heading.

Vincristine Sulfate (Carbamazepine is known to induce CYP1A2 and CYP3A4. Therefore, the potential exists for interaction between carbamazepine and any agent metabolized by one (or more) of these enzymes).
No products indexed under this heading.

Voriconazole (Carbamazepine is metabolized mainly by cytochrome P450 (CYP) 3A4 to the active carbamazepine 10,11 -epoxide, which is further metabolized to the trans-diol by epoxide hydrolase. Therefore, the potential exists for interaction between carbamazepine and any agent that inhibits CYP3A4 and/or epoxide hydrolase).
No products indexed under this heading.

Warfarin Sodium (Carbemezapine induces hepatic CYP activity and causes or would be expected to decrease plasma levels of warfarin. Warfarin's anticoagulant effect can be reduced in the presence of carbamazepine).
No products indexed under this heading.

Zafirlukast (Carbamazepine is metabolized mainly by cytochrome P450 (CYP) 3A4 to the active carbamazepine 10,11 -epoxide, which is further metabolized to the trans-diol by epoxide hydrolase. Therefore, the potential exists for interaction between carbamazepine and any agent that inhibits CYP3A4 and/or epoxide hydrolase). Products include:
Accolate Tablets 669

Zileuton (Carbamazepine is metabolized mainly by cytochrome P450 (CYP) 3A4 to the active carbamazepine 10,11 -epoxide, which is further metabolized to the trans-diol by epoxide hydrolase. Therefore, the potential exists for interaction between carbamazepine and any agent that inhibits CYP3A4 and/or epoxide hydrolase).
No products indexed under this heading.

Ziprasidone Hydrochloride (Co-administration with psychotropic agents has resulted in isolated cases of neuroleptic malignant syndrome). Products include:
Geodon Capsules 2520

Zolmitriptan (Carbamazepine is known to induce CYP1A2 and CYP3A4. Therefore, the potential exists for interaction between carbamazepine and any agent metabolized by one (or more) of these enzymes). Products include:
Zomig Tablets 694
Zomig Nasal Spray 689
Zomig-ZMT Tablets 694

Zonisamide (Alterations of thyroid function have been reported in combination therapy with other anticonvulsants). Products include:
Zonegran Capsules 1089

Food Interactions

Food, unspecified (A high fat meal increased the rat of absorption of a single 400 mg dose but not the AUC; elimination half-life remains unchanged between fasting and fed states).

Grapefruit (Carbamazepine is metabolized mainly by cytochrome P450 (CYP) 3A4 to the active carbamazepine 10,11 -epoxide, which is further metabolized to the trans-diol by epoxide hydrolase. Therefore, the potential exists for interaction between carbamazepine and any agent that inhibits CYP3A4 and/or epoxide hydrolase).

Grapefruit Juice (Carbamazepine is metabolized mainly by cytochrome P450 (CYP) 3A4 to the active carbamazepine 10,11 -epoxide, which is further metabolized to the trans-diol by epoxide hydrolase. Therefore, the potential exists for interaction between carbamazepine and any agent that inhibits CYP3A4 and/or epoxide hydrolase).

CARDENE I.V.

(Nicardipine Hydrochloride) 1093

May interact with antihypertensives, beta blockers, and certain other agents. Compounds in these categories include:

Acebutolol Hydrochloride (In vitro and in some patients a negative inotropic effect has been observed with Cardene I.V., therefore, caution should be exercised when co-administered with beta blockers in patients with CHF or significant left ventricular dysfunction).
No products indexed under this heading.

Aliskiren (Careful monitoring of patients being treated with other medications, including other antihypertensive agents, is necessary to detect and promptly treat any undesired effects from concomitant administration). Products include:
Tekturna Tablets 2321
Tekturna HCT Tablets 2324

Amlodipine Besylate (Careful monitoring of patients being treated with other medications, including other antihypertensive agents, is necessary to detect and promptly treat any undesired effects from concomitant administration). Products include:
Azor Tablets 1005
Exforge Tablets 2238

Atenolol (In vitro and in some patients a negative inotropic effect has been observed with Cardene I.V., therefore, caution should be exercised when co-administered with beta blockers in patients with CHF or significant left ventricular dysfunction).
No products indexed under this heading.

Benazepril Hydrochloride (Careful monitoring of patients being treated with other medications, including other antihypertensive agents, is necessary to detect and promptly treat any undesired effects from concomitant administration).
No products indexed under this heading.

Bendroflumethiazide (Careful monitoring of patients being treated with other medications, including other antihypertensive agents, is necessary to detect and promptly treat any undesired effects from concomitant administration).
No products indexed under this heading.

Beta Blockers (Cardene I.V. may be safely used concomitantly with beta-blockers. However, exercise caution when using Cardene I.V. in combination with a beta-blocker in CHF patients).
No products indexed under this heading.

Betaxolol Hydrochloride (In vitro and in some patients a negative inotropic effect has been observed with Cardene I.V., therefore, caution should be exercised when co-administered with beta blockers in patients with CHF or significant left ventricular dysfunction).
No products indexed under this heading.

Bisoprolol Fumarate (In vitro and in some patients a negative inotropic effect has been observed with Cardene I.V., therefore, caution should be exercised when co-administered with beta blockers in patients with CHF or significant left ventricular dysfunction).
No products indexed under this heading.

Candesartan Cilexetil (Careful monitoring of patients being treated with other medications, including other antihypertensive agents, is necessary to detect and promptly treat any undesired effects from concomitant administration). Products include:
Atacand Tablets 639
Atacand HCT 642

Captopril (Careful monitoring of patients being treated with other medications, including other antihypertensive agents, is necessary to detect and promptly treat any undesired effects from concomitant administration). Products include:
Captopril Tablets 2182

Carteolol Hydrochloride (In vitro and in some patients a negative inotropic effect has been observed with Cardene I.V., therefore, caution should be exercised when co-administered with beta blockers in patients with CHF or significant left ventricular dysfunction).
No products indexed under this heading.

Chlorothiazide (Careful monitoring of patients being treated with other medications, including other antihypertensive agents, is necessary to detect and promptly treat any undesired effects from concomitant administration).
No products indexed under this heading.

Chlorothiazide Sodium (Careful monitoring of patients being treated with other medications, including other antihypertensive agents, is necessary to detect and promptly treat any undesired effects from concomitant administration). Products include:
Intravenous Sodium Diuril 2490

Chlorthalidone (Careful monitoring of patients being treated with other medications, including other antihypertensive agents, is necessary to detect and promptly treat any undesired effects from concomitant administration). Products include:
Clorpres Tablets 2185

Cimetidine (Co-administration of cimetidine with Cardene I.V. increases nicardipine plasma concentration. Carefully monitor).
No products indexed under this heading.

Cimetidine Hydrochloride (Co-administration of cimetidine with Cardene I.V. increases nicardipine plasma concentration).
No products indexed under this heading.

Clonidine (Careful monitoring of patients being treated with other medications, including other antihypertensive agents, is necessary to detect and promptly treat any undesired effects from concomitant administration). Products include:
Catapres-TTS 842

Clonidine Hydrochloride (Careful monitoring of patients being treated with other medications, including other antihypertensive agents, is necessary to detect and promptly treat any undesired effects from concomitant administration). Products include:
Catapres Tablets 841
Clorpres Tablets 2185

Cyclosporine (Co-administration of Cardene I.V. and cyclosporine results in elevated plasma cyclosporine levels. Closely monitor plasma concentrations of cyclosporine and reduce dose accordingly). Products include:
Gengraf Capsules 435
Neoral Oral Solution 2280
Neoral Soft Gelatin Capsules 2280
Restasis Ophthalmic Emulsion 557
Sandimmune 2296

Deserpidine (Careful monitoring of patients being treated with other medications, including other antihypertensive agents, is necessary to detect and promptly treat any undesired effects from concomitant administration).
No products indexed under this heading.

Diazoxide (Careful monitoring of patients being treated with other medications, including other antihypertensive agents, is necessary to detect and promptly treat any undesired effects from concomitant administration). Products include:
Proglycem Capsules 1185
Proglycem Suspension 1185

Digoxin (No alteration in digoxin plasma levels, however, as a precaution, digoxin levels should be evaluated when concomitant therapy is initiated). Products include:
Lanoxin Injection 1498
Lanoxin Injection Pediatric 1502
Lanoxin Tablets 1505

Diltiazem Hydrochloride (Careful monitoring of patients being treated with other medications, including other antihypertensive agents, is necessary to detect and promptly treat any undesired effects from concomitant administration). Products include:
Cardizem LA Extended Release Tablets 421

Doxazosin Mesylate (Careful monitoring of patients being treated with other medications, including other antihypertensive agents, is necessary to detect and promptly treat any undesired effects from concomitant administration).
No products indexed under this heading.

Enalapril Maleate (Careful monitoring of patients being treated with other medications, including other antihypertensive agents, is necessary to detect and promptly treat any undesired effects from concomitant administration).
No products indexed under this heading.

Enalaprilat (Careful monitoring of patients being treated with other medications, including other antihypertensive agents, is necessary to detect and promptly treat any undesired effects from concomitant administration).
No products indexed under this heading.

Eprosartan Mesylate (Careful monitoring of patients being treated with other medications, including other antihypertensive agents, is necessary to detect and promptly treat any undesired effects from concomitant administration). Products include:
Teveten Tablets 515
Teveten HCT Tablets 517

Esmolol Hydrochloride (In vitro and in some patients a negative inotropic effect has been observed with Cardene I.V., therefore, caution should be exercised when co-administered with beta blockers in patients with CHF or significant left ventricular dysfunction).
No products indexed under this heading.

Felodipine (Careful monitoring of patients being treated with other medications, including other antihypertensive agents, is necessary to detect and promptly treat any undesired effects from concomitant administration).
No products indexed under this heading.

Fentanyl (Potential for hypotension with fentanyl anesthesia when used with calcium channel blockers and beta blockers; such reaction has not been observed with Cardene I.V. during clinical trials). Products include:
Duragesic Transdermal System 2405
Ionsys Transdermal System 2410

Fentanyl Citrate (Potential for hypotension with fentanyl anesthesia when used with calcium channel blockers and beta blockers; such reaction has not been observed with Cardene I.V. during clinical trials). Products include:
Actiq 959
Fentora Tablets 968

Fosinopril Sodium (Careful monitoring of patients being treated with other medications, including other antihypertensive agents, is necessary to detect and promptly treat any undesired effects from concomitant administration).
No products indexed under this heading.

Furosemide (Careful monitoring of patients being treated with other medications, including other antihypertensive agents, is necessary to detect and promptly treat any undesired effects from concomitant administration). Products include:
Furosemide Tablets 2186

Guanabenz Acetate (Careful monitoring of patients being treated with other medications, including other antihypertensive agents, is necessary to detect and promptly treat any undesired effects from concomitant administration).
No products indexed under this heading.

Guanethidine Monosulfate (Careful monitoring of patients being treated with other medications, including other antihypertensive agents, is necessary to detect and promptly treat any undesired effects from concomitant administration).
No products indexed under this heading.

Hydralazine Hydrochloride (Careful monitoring of patients being treated with other medications, including other antihypertensive agents, is necessary to detect and promptly treat any undesired effects from concomitant administration).
No products indexed under this heading.

Hydrochlorothiazide (Careful monitoring of patients being treated with other medications, including other antihypertensive agents, is necessary to detect and promptly treat any undesired effects from concomitant administration). Products include:

Atacand HCT ... 642
Avalide Tablets ... 892
Avalide Tablets ... 2713
Benicar HCT Tablets ... 1010
Diovan HCT Tablets ... 2216
Dyazide Capsules ... 1405
Micardis HCT Tablets ... 854
Prinzide Tablets ... 2092
Tekturna HCT Tablets ... 2324
Teveten HCT Tablets ... 517

Hydroflumethiazide (Careful monitoring of patients being treated with other medications, including other antihypertensive agents, is necessary to detect and promptly treat any undesired effects from concomitant administration).

No products indexed under this heading.

Indapamide (Careful monitoring of patients being treated with other medications, including other antihypertensive agents, is necessary to detect and promptly treat any undesired effects from concomitant administration). Products include:

Indapamide Tablets ... 2188

Irbesartan (Careful monitoring of patients being treated with other medications, including other antihypertensive agents, is necessary to detect and promptly treat any undesired effects from concomitant administration). Products include:

Avalide Tablets ... 892
Avalide Tablets ... 2713
Avapro Tablets ... 897
Avapro Tablets ... 2718

Isradipine (Careful monitoring of patients being treated with other medications, including other antihypertensive agents, is necessary to detect and promptly treat any undesired effects from concomitant administration). Products include:

DynaCirc CR Controlled Release Tablets ... 1407

Labetalol Hydrochloride (In vitro and in some patients a negative inotropic effect has been observed with Cardene I.V., therefore, caution should be exercised when co-administered with beta blockers in patients with CHF or significant left ventricular dysfunction).

No products indexed under this heading.

Levobunolol Hydrochloride (In vitro and in some patients a negative inotropic effect has been observed with Cardene I.V., therefore, caution should be exercised when co-administered with beta blockers in patients with CHF or significant left ventricular dysfunction).

No products indexed under this heading.

Lisinopril (Careful monitoring of patients being treated with other medications, including other antihypertensive agents, is necessary to detect and promptly treat any undesired effects from concomitant administration). Products include:

Prinivil Tablets ... 2087
Prinzide Tablets ... 2092

Losartan Potassium (Careful monitoring of patients being treated with other medications, including other antihypertensive agents, is necessary to detect and promptly treat any undesired effects from concomitant administration). Products include:

Cozaar Tablets ... 1973

Mecamylamine Hydrochloride (Careful monitoring of patients being treated with other medications, including other antihypertensive agents, is necessary to detect and promptly treat any undesired effects from concomitant administration).

No products indexed under this heading.

Methyclothiazide (Careful monitoring of patients being treated with other medications, including other antihypertensive agents, is necessary to detect and promptly treat any undesired effects from concomitant administration).

No products indexed under this heading.

Methyldopa (Careful monitoring of patients being treated with other medications, including other antihypertensive agents, is necessary to detect and promptly treat any undesired effects from concomitant administration).

No products indexed under this heading.

Methyldopate Hydrochloride (Careful monitoring of patients being treated with other medications, including other antihypertensive agents, is necessary to detect and promptly treat any undesired effects from concomitant administration).

No products indexed under this heading.

Metipranolol Hydrochloride (In vitro and in some patients a negative inotropic effect has been observed with Cardene I.V., therefore, caution should be exercised when co-administered with beta blockers in patients with CHF or significant left ventricular dysfunction).

No products indexed under this heading.

Metolazone (Careful monitoring of patients being treated with other medications, including other antihypertensive agents, is necessary to detect and promptly treat any undesired effects from concomitant administration).

No products indexed under this heading.

Metoprolol Succinate (In vitro and in some patients a negative inotropic effect has been observed with Cardene I.V., therefore, caution should be exercised when co-administered with beta blockers in patients with CHF or significant left ventricular dysfunction). Products include:

Toprol-XL Tablets ... 666

Metoprolol Tartrate (In vitro and in some patients a negative inotropic effect has been observed with Cardene I.V., therefore, caution should be exercised when co-administered with beta blockers in patients with CHF or significant left ventricular dysfunction).

No products indexed under this heading.

Metyrosine (Careful monitoring of patients being treated with other medications, including other antihypertensive agents, is necessary to detect and promptly treat any undesired effects from concomitant administration). Products include:

Demser Capsules ... 1989

Mibefradil Dihydrochloride (Careful monitoring of patients being treated with other medications, including other antihypertensive agents, is necessary to detect and promptly treat any undesired effects from concomitant administration).

No products indexed under this heading.

Minoxidil (Careful monitoring of patients being treated with other medications, including other antihypertensive agents, is necessary to detect and promptly treat any undesired effects from concomitant administration).

No products indexed under this heading.

Moexipril Hydrochloride (Careful monitoring of patients being treated with other medications, including other antihypertensive agents, is necessary to detect and promptly treat any undesired effects from concomitant administration).

No products indexed under this heading.

Nadolol (In vitro and in some patients a negative inotropic effect has been observed with Cardene I.V., therefore, caution should be exercised when co-administered with beta blockers in patients with CHF or significant left ventricular dysfunction). Products include:

Nadolol Tablets ... 2191

Nebivolol (In vitro and in some patients a negative inotropic effect has been observed with Cardene I.V., therefore, caution should be exercised when co-administered with beta blockers in patients with CHF or significant left ventricular dysfunction). Products include:

Bystolic Tablets ... 1155

Nifedipine (Careful monitoring of patients being treated with other medications, including other antihypertensive agents, is necessary to detect and promptly treat any undesired effects from concomitant administration).

No products indexed under this heading.

Nisoldipine (Careful monitoring of patients being treated with other medications, including other antihypertensive agents, is necessary to detect and promptly treat any undesired effects from concomitant administration). Products include:

Sular Extended Release Tablets ... 2975

Nitroglycerin (Careful monitoring of patients being treated with other medications, including other antihypertensive agents, is necessary to detect and promptly treat any undesired effects from concomitant administration). Products include:

Nitro-Dur Transdermal Infusion System ... 2887
Nitrolingual Pumpspray ... 2965

Penbutolol Sulfate (In vitro and in some patients a negative inotropic effect has been observed with Cardene I.V., therefore, caution should be exercised when co-administered with beta blockers in patients with CHF or significant left ventricular dysfunction).

No products indexed under this heading.

Perindopril Erbumine (Careful monitoring of patients being treated with other medications, including other antihypertensive agents, is necessary to detect and promptly treat any undesired effects from concomitant administration). Products include:

Aceon Tablets (2 mg, 4 mg, 8 mg) ... 3038

Phenoxybenzamine Hydrochloride (Careful monitoring of patients being treated with other medications, including other antihypertensive agents, is necessary to detect and promptly treat any undesired effects from concomitant administration). Products include:

Dibenzyline Capsules ... 3188

Phentolamine Mesylate (Careful monitoring of patients being treated with other medications, including other antihypertensive agents, is necessary to detect and promptly treat any undesired effects from concomitant administration).

No products indexed under this heading.

Pindolol (In vitro and in some patients a negative inotropic effect has been observed with Cardene I.V., therefore, caution should be exercised when co-administered with beta blockers in patients with CHF or significant left ventricular dysfunction).

No products indexed under this heading.

Polythiazide (Careful monitoring of patients being treated with other medications, including other antihypertensive agents, is necessary to detect and promptly treat any undesired effects from concomitant administration).

No products indexed under this heading.

Prazosin Hydrochloride (Careful monitoring of patients being treated with other medications, including other antihypertensive agents, is necessary to detect and promptly treat any undesired effects from concomitant administration).

No products indexed under this heading.

Propranolol Hydrochloride (In vitro and in some patients a negative inotropic effect has been observed with Cardene I.V., therefore, caution should be exercised when co-administered with beta blockers in patients with CHF or significant left ventricular dysfunction). Products include:

InnoPran XL Extended Release Capsules ... 1484

Quinapril Hydrochloride (Careful monitoring of patients being treated with other medications, including other antihypertensive agents, is necessary to detect and promptly treat any undesired effects from concomitant administration).

No products indexed under this heading.

Ramipril (Careful monitoring of patients being treated with other medications, including other antihypertensive agents, is necessary to detect and promptly treat any undesired effects from concomitant administration).

No products indexed under this heading.

Rauwolfia Serpentina (Careful monitoring of patients being treated with other medications, including other antihypertensive agents, is necessary to detect and promptly treat any undesired effects from concomitant administration).
No products indexed under this heading.

Rescinnamine (Careful monitoring of patients being treated with other medications, including other antihypertensive agents, is necessary to detect and promptly treat any undesired effects from concomitant administration).
No products indexed under this heading.

Reserpine (Careful monitoring of patients being treated with other medications, including other antihypertensive agents, is necessary to detect and promptly treat any undesired effects from concomitant administration).
No products indexed under this heading.

Sodium Nitroprusside (Careful monitoring of patients being treated with other medications, including other antihypertensive agents, is necessary to detect and promptly treat any undesired effects from concomitant administration).
No products indexed under this heading.

Sotalol Hydrochloride (In vitro and in some patients a negative inotropic effect has been observed with Cardene I.V., therefore, caution should be exercised when co-administered with beta blockers in patients with CHF or significant left ventricular dysfunction).
No products indexed under this heading.

Spirapril Hydrochloride (Careful monitoring of patients being treated with other medications, including other antihypertensive agents, is necessary to detect and promptly treat any undesired effects from concomitant administration).
No products indexed under this heading.

Telmisartan (Careful monitoring of patients being treated with other medications, including other antihypertensive agents, is necessary to detect and promptly treat any undesired effects from concomitant administration). Products include:
Micardis Tablets ... 852
Micardis HCT Tablets ... 854

Terazosin Hydrochloride (Careful monitoring of patients being treated with other medications, including other antihypertensive agents, is necessary to detect and promptly treat any undesired effects from concomitant administration).
No products indexed under this heading.

Timolol Hemihydrate (In vitro and in some patients a negative inotropic effect has been observed with Cardene I.V., therefore, caution should be exercised when co-administered with beta blockers in patients with CHF or significant left ventricular dysfunction). Products include:
Betimol Ophthalmic Solution ... 3181

Timolol Maleate (In vitro and in some patients a negative inotropic effect has been observed with Cardene I.V., therefore, caution should be exercised when co-administered with beta blockers in patients with CHF or significant left ventricular dysfunction). Products include:
Combigan Ophthalmic Solution ... 553
Cosopt Sterile Ophthalmic Solution ... 1969
Timoptic Sterile Ophthalmic Solution ... 2121
Timoptic in Ocudose ... 2124
Timoptic-XE Sterile Ophthalmic Gel Forming Solution ... 2125

Torsemide (Careful monitoring of patients being treated with other medications, including other antihypertensive agents, is necessary to detect and promptly treat any undesired effects from concomitant administration). Products include:
Demadex Injection ... 2630
Demadex Tablets ... 2630

Trandolapril (Careful monitoring of patients being treated with other medications, including other antihypertensive agents, is necessary to detect and promptly treat any undesired effects from concomitant administration). Products include:
Mavik Tablets ... 472
Tarka Tablets ... 511

Trimethaphan Camsylate (Careful monitoring of patients being treated with other medications, including other antihypertensive agents, is necessary to detect and promptly treat any undesired effects from concomitant administration).
No products indexed under this heading.

Valsartan (Careful monitoring of patients being treated with other medications, including other antihypertensive agents, is necessary to detect and promptly treat any undesired effects from concomitant administration). Products include:
Diovan Tablets ... 2212
Diovan HCT Tablets ... 2216
Exforge Tablets ... 2238

Verapamil Hydrochloride (Careful monitoring of patients being treated with other medications, including other antihypertensive agents, is necessary to detect and promptly treat any undesired effects from concomitant administration). Products include:
Tarka Tablets ... 511

CARDIOESSENTIALS CAPSULES

(Coenzyme Q-10, Levocarnitine, Taurine) ... 3159
None cited in PDR database.

CARDIZEM LA EXTENDED RELEASE TABLETS

(Diltiazem Hydrochloride) ... 421
May interact with anesthetics, antihypertensives, benzodiazepines, beta blockers, cytochrome p450 3a4 inducers (selected), cytochrome p450 3a4 inhibitors (selected), cytochrome p450 3a4 substrates (selected), cardiac glycosides, quinidine, and certain other agents. Compounds in these categories include:

Acebutolol Hydrochloride (Pharmacologic studies indicate that there may be additive effects in prolonging A-V conduction when using beta-blockers or digitalis concomitantly with diltiazem).
No products indexed under this heading.

Acetazolamide (Diltiazem is both a substrate and an inhibitor of the CYP3A4 enzyme system. Other drugs that are specific substrates, inhibitors, or inducers of this enzyme system may have a significant impact on the efficacy and side effect profile of diltiazem).
No products indexed under this heading.

Alfentanil Hydrochloride (The depression of cardiac contractility, conductivity, and automaticity, as well as the vascular dilation associated with anesthetics, may be potentiated by calcium channel blockers).
No products indexed under this heading.

Aliskiren (Diltiazem has an additive effect when used with other antihypertensive agents. Therefore, the dosage of diltiazem or concomitant antihypertensives may need to be adjusted when adding one to the other). Products include:
Tekturna Tablets ... 2321
Tekturna HCT Tablets ... 2324

Allium sativum (Diltiazem is both a substrate and an inhibitor of the CYP3A4 enzyme system. Other drugs that are specific substrates, inhibitors, or inducers of this enzyme system may have a significant impact on the efficacy and side effect profile of diltiazem).
No products indexed under this heading.

Alprazolam (Studies showed that diltiazem increased the AUC of midazolam and triazolam by 3- to 4-fold and the Cmax by 2-fold, compared to placebo. The elimination half-life of midazolam and triazolam also increased during co-administration with diltiazem).
No products indexed under this heading.

Amiodarone Hydrochloride (Patients taking other drugs that are substrates of CYP450, especially patients with renal and/or hepatic impairment, may require dosage adjustment when starting or stopping concomitantly administered diltiazem in order to maintain optimum therapeutic blood levels).
No products indexed under this heading.

Amitriptyline Hydrochloride (Patients taking other drugs that are substrates of CYP450, especially patients with renal and/or hepatic impairment, may require dosage adjustment when starting or stopping concomitantly administered diltiazem in order to maintain optimum therapeutic blood levels).
No products indexed under this heading.

Amlodipine Besylate (Diltiazem has an additive effect when used with other antihypertensive agents. Therefore, the dosage of diltiazem or concomitant antihypertensives may need to be adjusted when adding one to the other). Products include:
Azor Tablets ... 1005
Exforge Tablets ... 2238

Amprenavir (Diltiazem is both a substrate and an inhibitor of the CYP3A4 enzyme system. Other drugs that are specific substrates, inhibitors, or inducers of this enzyme system may have a significant impact on the efficacy and side effect profile of diltiazem).
No products indexed under this heading.

Anastrozole (Diltiazem is both a substrate and an inhibitor of the CYP3A4 enzyme system. Other drugs that are specific substrates, inhibitors, or inducers of this enzyme system may have a significant impact on the efficacy and side effect profile of diltiazem). Products include:
Arimidex Tablets ... 672

Aprepitant (Patients taking other drugs that are substrates of CYP450, especially patients with renal and/or hepatic impairment, may require dosage adjustment when starting or stopping concomitantly administered diltiazem in order to maintain optimum therapeutic blood levels). Products include:
Emend Capsules ... 1992

Astemizole (Patients taking other drugs that are substrates of CYP450, especially patients with renal and/or hepatic impairment, may require dosage adjustment when starting or stopping concomitantly administered diltiazem in order to maintain optimum therapeutic blood levels).
No products indexed under this heading.

Atazanavir (Diltiazem is both a substrate and an inhibitor of the CYP3A4 enzyme system. Other drugs that are specific substrates, inhibitors, or inducers of this enzyme system may have a significant impact on the efficacy and side effect profile of diltiazem).
No products indexed under this heading.

Atazanavir Sulfate (Diltiazem is both a substrate and an inhibitor of the CYP3A4 enzyme system. Other drugs that are specific substrates, inhibitors, or inducers of this enzyme system may have a significant impact on the efficacy and side effect profile of diltiazem). Products include:
Reyataz Capsules ... 3299

Atenolol (Pharmacologic studies indicate that there may be additive effects in prolonging A-V conduction when using beta-blockers or digitalis concomitantly with diltiazem).
No products indexed under this heading.

Atorvastatin Calcium (Patients taking other drugs that are substrates of CYP450, especially patients with renal and/or hepatic impairment, may require dosage adjustment when starting or stopping concomitantly administered diltiazem in order to maintain optimum therapeutic blood levels). Products include:
Lipitor Tablets ... 2501

Belladonna Ergotamine (Patients taking other drugs that are substrates of CYP450, especially patients with renal and/or hepatic impairment, may require dosage adjustment when starting or stopping concomitantly administered diltiazem in order to maintain optimum therapeutic blood levels).
No products indexed under this heading.

Benazepril Hydrochloride (Diltiazem has an additive effect when used with other antihypertensive agents. Therefore, the dosage of diltiazem or concomitant antihypertensives may need to be adjusted when adding one to the other).
No products indexed under this heading.

Bendroflumethiazide (Diltiazem has an additive effect when used with other antihypertensive agents. Therefore, the dosage of diltiazem or concomitant antihypertensives may need to be adjusted when adding one to the other).
No products indexed under this heading.

Betamethasone Acetate (Diltiazem is both a substrate and an inhibitor of the CYP3A4 enzyme system. Other drugs that are specific substrates, inhibitors, or inducers of this enzyme system may have a significant impact on the efficacy and side effect profile of diltiazem).
No products indexed under this heading.

Betamethasone Sodium Phosphate (Diltiazem is both a substrate and an inhibitor of the CYP3A4 enzyme system. Other drugs that are specific substrates, inhibitors, or inducers of this enzyme system may have a significant impact on the efficacy and side effect profile of diltiazem).
No products indexed under this heading.

Betaxolol Hydrochloride (Pharmacologic studies indicate that there may be additive effects in prolonging A-V conduction when using beta-blockers or digitalis concomitantly with diltiazem).
No products indexed under this heading.

Bisoprolol Fumarate (Pharmacologic studies indicate that there may be additive effects in prolonging A-V conduction when using beta-blockers or digitalis concomitantly with diltiazem).
No products indexed under this heading.

Buspirone Hydrochloride (Studies showed that diltiazem increased the AUC of buspirone by 5.5 fold and the Cmax by 4.1 fold. Enhanced effects of buspirone may be possible).
No products indexed under this heading.

Busulfan (Patients taking other drugs that are substrates of CYP450, especially patients with renal and/or hepatic impairment, may require dosage adjustment when starting or stopping concomitantly administered diltiazem in order to maintain optimum therapeutic blood levels). Products include:
Busulfex Injection 2477
Myleran Tablets 1530

Candesartan Cilexetil (Diltiazem has an additive effect when used with other antihypertensive agents. Therefore, the dosage of diltiazem or concomitant antihypertensives may need to be adjusted when adding one to the other). Products include:
Atacand Tablets 639
Atacand HCT 642

Captopril (Diltiazem has an additive effect when used with other antihypertensive agents. Therefore, the dosage of diltiazem or concomitant antihypertensives may need to be adjusted when adding one to the other). Products include:
Captopril Tablets 2182

Carbamazepine (Concomitant administration of diltiazem with carbamazepine has been reported to result in elevated serum levels of carbamazepine (40% to 72% increase), resulting in toxicity in some cases). Products include:
Carbatrol Capsules 3019
Equetro Extended-Release Capsules 3174

Carteolol Hydrochloride (Pharmacologic studies indicate that there may be additive effects in prolonging A-V conduction when using beta-blockers or digitalis concomitantly with diltiazem).
No products indexed under this heading.

Cerivastatin Sodium (Patients taking other drugs that are substrates of CYP450, especially patients with renal and/or hepatic impairment, may require dosage adjustment when starting or stopping concomitantly administered diltiazem in order to maintain optimum therapeutic blood levels).
No products indexed under this heading.

Chlordiazepoxide (Studies showed that diltiazem increased the AUC of midazolam and triazolam by 3- to 4-fold and the Cmax by 2-fold, compared to placebo. The elimination half-life of midazolam and triazolam also increased during co-administration with diltiazem).
No products indexed under this heading.

Chlordiazepoxide Hydrochloride (Studies showed that diltiazem increased the AUC of midazolam and triazolam by 3- to 4-fold and the Cmax by 2-fold, compared to placebo. The elimination half-life of midazolam and triazolam also increased during co-administration with diltiazem).
No products indexed under this heading.

Chlorothiazide (Diltiazem has an additive effect when used with other antihypertensive agents. Therefore, the dosage of diltiazem or concomitant antihypertensives may need to be adjusted when adding one to the other).
No products indexed under this heading.

Chlorothiazide Sodium (Diltiazem has an additive effect when used with other antihypertensive agents. Therefore, the dosage of diltiazem or concomitant antihypertensives may need to be adjusted when adding one to the other). Products include:
Intravenous Sodium Diuril 2490

Chlorpheniramine (Patients taking other drugs that are substrates of CYP450, especially patients with renal and/or hepatic impairment, may require dosage adjustment when starting or stopping concomitantly administered diltiazem in order to maintain optimum therapeutic blood levels).
No products indexed under this heading.

Chlorpheniramine Maleate (Patients taking other drugs that are substrates of CYP450, especially patients with renal and/or hepatic impairment, may require dosage adjustment when starting or stopping concomitantly administered diltiazem in order to maintain optimum therapeutic blood levels). Products include:
Actifed Cold & Allergy Tablets 1895
Sudafed PE Sinus & Allergy Tablets 1908
Tylenol Allergy Multi-Symptom Caplets with Cool Burst and Rapid Release Gelcaps 1916
Children's Tylenol Plus Cold Suspension Liquid 1912
Children's Tylenol Plus Cough & Runny Nose Suspension Liquid 1912
Children's Tylenol Plus Flu Suspension Liquid 1914
Children's Tylenol Plus Multi-Symptom Cold Suspension Liquid 1912
Tylenol Cold Head Congestion Nighttime Caplets with Cool Burst 1910
Tylenol Cold Multi-Symptom Nighttime Caplets with Cool Burst 1913
Tylenol Sinus Congestion & Pain Nighttime Caplets with Cool Burst 1917

Chlorpheniramine Polistirex (Patients taking other drugs that are substrates of CYP450, especially patients with renal and/or hepatic impairment, may require dosage adjustment when starting or stopping concomitantly administered diltiazem in order to maintain optimum therapeutic blood levels). Products include:
Tussionex Pennkinetic Extended-Release Suspension 3154

Chlorpheniramine Tannate (Patients taking other drugs that are substrates of CYP450, especially patients with renal and/or hepatic impairment, may require dosage adjustment when starting or stopping concomitantly administered diltiazem in order to maintain optimum therapeutic blood levels).
No products indexed under this heading.

Chlorthalidone (Diltiazem has an additive effect when used with other antihypertensive agents. Therefore, the dosage of diltiazem or concomitant antihypertensives may need to be adjusted when adding one to the other). Products include:
Clorpres Tablets 2185

Cimetidine (A study in six healthy volunteers has shown a significant increase in peak diltiazem plasma levels (58%) and AUC (53%) after a 1-week course of cimetidine at 1200 mg per day and a single dose of diltiazem 60 mg).
No products indexed under this heading.

Cimetidine Hydrochloride (A study in six healthy volunteers has shown a significant increase in peak diltiazem plasma levels (58%) and AUC (53%) after a 1-week course of cimetidine at 1200 mg per day and a single dose of diltiazem 60 mg).
No products indexed under this heading.

Ciprofloxacin (Diltiazem is both a substrate and an inhibitor of the CYP3A4 enzyme system. Other drugs that are specific substrates, inhibitors, or inducers of this enzyme system may have a significant impact on the efficacy and side effect profile of diltiazem). Products include:
Cipro I.V. 2817
Cipro Oral Suspension 2810
Cipro XR Tablets 2823
Ciprodex Otic Suspension 541

Ciprofloxacin Hydrochloride (Diltiazem is both a substrate and an inhibitor of the CYP3A4 enzyme system. Other drugs that are specific substrates, inhibitors, or inducers of this enzyme system may have a significant impact on the efficacy and side effect profile of diltiazem). Products include:
Cipro Tablets 2810

Cisapride (Patients taking other drugs that are substrates of CYP450, especially patients with renal and/or hepatic impairment, may require dosage adjustment when starting or stopping concomitantly administered diltiazem in order to maintain optimum therapeutic blood levels).
No products indexed under this heading.

Cisplatin (Diltiazem is both a substrate and an inhibitor of the CYP3A4 enzyme system. Other drugs that are specific substrates, inhibitors, or inducers of this enzyme system may have a significant impact on the efficacy and side effect profile of diltiazem).
No products indexed under this heading.

Clarithromycin (Patients taking other drugs that are substrates of CYP450, especially patients with renal and/or hepatic impairment, may require dosage adjustment when starting or stopping concomitantly administered diltiazem in order to maintain optimum therapeutic blood levels). Products include:
Biaxin/Biaxin XL 411

Clonidine (Diltiazem has an additive effect when used with other antihypertensive agents. Therefore, the dosage of diltiazem or concomitant antihypertensives may need to be adjusted when adding one to the other). Products include:
Catapres-TTS 842

Clonidine Hydrochloride (Diltiazem has an additive effect when used with other antihypertensive agents. Therefore, the dosage of diltiazem or concomitant antihypertensives may need to be adjusted when adding one to the other). Products include:
Catapres Tablets 841
Clorpres Tablets 2185

Clorazepate Dipotassium (Studies showed that diltiazem increased the AUC of midazolam and triazolam by 3- to 4-fold and the Cmax by 2-fold, compared to placebo. The elimination half-life of midazolam and triazolam also increased during co-administration with diltiazem).
No products indexed under this heading.

Clotrimazole (Diltiazem is both a substrate and an inhibitor of the CYP3A4 enzyme system. Other drugs that are specific substrates, inhibitors, or inducers of this enzyme system may have a significant impact on the efficacy and side effect profile of diltiazem). Products include:
Lotrisone 2881

Cortisone Acetate (Diltiazem is both a substrate and an inhibitor of the CYP3A4 enzyme system. Other drugs that are specific substrates, inhibitors, or inducers of this enzyme system may have a significant impact on the efficacy and side effect profile of diltiazem).
No products indexed under this heading.

Cyclosporine (In renal and cardiac transplant recipients, a reduction of cyclosporine dose ranging from 15% to 48% was necessary to maintain cyclosporine trough concentrations similar to those seen prior to the addition of diltiazem. If these agents are to be administered concurrently, cyclosporine concentrations should be monitored, especially when diltiazem therapy is initiated, adjusted or discontinued). Products include:
Gengraf Capsules 435
Neoral Oral Solution 2280
Neoral Soft Gelatin Capsules 2280
Restasis Ophthalmic Emulsion 557
Sandimmune 2296

Dalfopristin (Diltiazem is both a substrate and an inhibitor of the CYP3A4 enzyme system. Other drugs that are specific substrates, inhibitors, or inducers of this enzyme system may have a significant impact on the efficacy and side effect profile of diltiazem).
No products indexed under this heading.

Danazol (Diltiazem is both a substrate and an inhibitor of the CYP3A4 enzyme system. Other drugs that are specific substrates, inhibitors, or inducers of this enzyme system may have a significant impact on the efficacy and side effect profile of diltiazem).
No products indexed under this heading.

Delavirdine Mesylate (Diltiazem is both a substrate and an inhibitor of the CYP3A4 enzyme system. Other drugs that are specific substrates, inhibitors, or inducers of this enzyme system may have a significant impact on the efficacy and side effect profile of diltiazem).
No products indexed under this heading.

Deserpidine (Diltiazem has an additive effect when used with other antihypertensive agents. Therefore, the dosage of diltiazem or concomitant antihypertensives may need to be adjusted when adding one to the other).
No products indexed under this heading.

Deslanoside (Pharmacologic studies indicate that there may be additive effects in prolonging A-V conduction when using beta-blockers or digitalis concomitantly with diltiazem).
No products indexed under this heading.

Desogestrel (Patients taking other drugs that are substrates of CYP450, especially patients with renal and/or hepatic impairment, may require dosage adjustment when starting or stopping concomitantly administered diltiazem in order to maintain optimum therapeutic blood levels). Products include:
Mircette Tablets 1034

Dexamethasone (Diltiazem is both a substrate and an inhibitor of the CYP3A4 enzyme system. Other drugs that are specific substrates, inhibitors, or inducers of this enzyme system may have a significant impact on the efficacy and side effect profile of diltiazem). Products include:
Ciprodex Otic Suspension 541

Dexamethasone Acetate (Diltiazem is both a substrate and an inhibitor of the CYP3A4 enzyme system. Other drugs that are specific substrates, inhibitors, or inducers of this enzyme system may have a significant impact on the efficacy and side effect profile of diltiazem).
No products indexed under this heading.

Dexamethasone Sodium Phosphate (Diltiazem is both a substrate and an inhibitor of the CYP3A4 enzyme system. Other drugs that are specific substrates, inhibitors, or inducers of this enzyme system may have a significant impact on the efficacy and side effect profile of diltiazem).
No products indexed under this heading.

Diazepam (Studies showed that diltiazem increased the AUC of midazolam and triazolam by 3- to 4-fold and the Cmax by 2-fold, compared to placebo. The elimination half-life of midazolam and triazolam also increased during co-administration with diltiazem). Products include:
Valium Tablets 2658

Diazoxide (Diltiazem has an additive effect when used with other antihypertensive agents. Therefore, the dosage of diltiazem or concomitant antihypertensives may need to be adjusted when adding one to the other). Products include:
Proglycem Capsules 1185
Proglycem Suspension 1185

Digitalis Glycoside Preparations (Pharmacologic studies indicate that there may be additive effects in prolonging A-V conduction when using beta-blockers or digitalis concomitantly with diltiazem).
No products indexed under this heading.

Digitoxin (Pharmacologic studies indicate that there may be additive effects in prolonging A-V conduction when using beta-blockers or digitalis concomitantly with diltiazem).
No products indexed under this heading.

Digoxin (Pharmacologic studies indicate that there may be additive effects in prolonging A-V conduction when using beta-blockers or digitalis concomitantly with diltiazem). Products include:
Lanoxin Injection 1498
Lanoxin Injection Pediatric 1502
Lanoxin Tablets 1505

Dihydroergotamine Mesylate (Patients taking other drugs that are substrates of CYP450, especially patients with renal and/or hepatic impairment, may require dosage adjustment when starting or stopping concomitantly administered diltiazem in order to maintain optimum therapeutic blood levels).
No products indexed under this heading.

Diltiazem Maleate (Patients taking other drugs that are substrates of CYP450, especially patients with renal and/or hepatic impairment, may require dosage adjustment when starting or stopping concomitantly administered diltiazem in order to maintain optimum therapeutic blood levels).
No products indexed under this heading.

Disopyramide (Patients taking other drugs that are substrates of CYP450, especially patients with renal and/or hepatic impairment, may require dosage adjustment when starting or stopping concomitantly administered diltiazem in order to maintain optimum therapeutic blood levels).
No products indexed under this heading.

Disopyramide Phosphate (Patients taking other drugs that are substrates of CYP450, especially patients with renal and/or hepatic impairment, may require dosage adjustment when starting or stopping concomitantly administered diltiazem in order to maintain optimum therapeutic blood levels).
No products indexed under this heading.

Disulfiram (Patients taking other drugs that are substrates of CYP450, especially patients with renal and/or hepatic impairment, may require dosage adjustment when starting or stopping concomitantly administered diltiazem in order to maintain optimum therapeutic blood levels).
No products indexed under this heading.

Doxazosin Mesylate (Diltiazem has an additive effect when used with other antihypertensive agents. Therefore, the dosage of diltiazem or concomitant antihypertensives may need to be adjusted when adding one to the other).
No products indexed under this heading.

Doxorubicin Hydrochloride (Patients taking other drugs that are substrates of CYP450, especially patients with renal and/or hepatic impairment, may require dosage adjustment when starting or stopping concomitantly administered diltiazem in order to maintain optimum therapeutic blood levels).
No products indexed under this heading.

Dronabinol (Patients taking other drugs that are substrates of CYP450, especially patients with renal and/or hepatic impairment, may require dosage adjustment when starting or stopping concomitantly administered diltiazem in order to maintain optimum therapeutic blood levels). Products include:
Marinol Capsules 3163

Efavirenz (Diltiazem is both a substrate and an inhibitor of the CYP3A4 enzyme system. Other drugs that are specific substrates, inhibitors, or inducers of this enzyme system may have a significant impact on the efficacy and side effect profile of diltiazem). Products include:
Atripla Tablets 938
Sustiva Capsules 930
Sustiva Tablets 930

Enalapril Maleate (Diltiazem has an additive effect when used with other antihypertensive agents. Therefore, the dosage of diltiazem or concomitant antihypertensives may need to be adjusted when adding one to the other).
No products indexed under this heading.

Enalaprilat (Diltiazem has an additive effect when used with other antihypertensive agents. Therefore, the dosage of diltiazem or concomitant antihypertensives may need to be adjusted when adding one to the other).
No products indexed under this heading.

Enflurane (The depression of cardiac contractility, conductivity, and automaticity, as well as the vascular dilation associated with anesthetics, may be potentiated by calcium channel blockers).
No products indexed under this heading.

Eprosartan Mesylate (Diltiazem has an additive effect when used with other antihypertensive agents. Therefore, the dosage of diltiazem or concomitant antihypertensives may need to be adjusted when adding one to the other). Products include:
Teveten Tablets 515
Teveten HCT Tablets 517

Ergotamine Tartrate (Patients taking other drugs that are substrates of CYP450, especially patients with renal and/or hepatic impairment, may require dosage adjustment when starting or stopping concomitantly administered diltiazem in order to maintain optimum therapeutic blood levels).
No products indexed under this heading.

Erythromycin (Patients taking other drugs that are substrates of CYP450, especially patients with renal and/or hepatic impairment, may require dosage adjustment when starting or stopping concomitantly administered diltiazem in order to maintain optimum therapeutic blood levels).
No products indexed under this heading.

Erythromycin Estolate (Patients taking other drugs that are substrates of CYP450, especially patients with renal and/or hepatic impairment, may require dosage adjustment when starting or stopping concomitantly administered diltiazem in order to maintain optimum therapeutic blood levels).
No products indexed under this heading.

Erythromycin Ethylsuccinate (Patients taking other drugs that are substrates of CYP450, especially patients with renal and/or hepatic impairment, may require dosage adjustment when starting or stopping concomitantly administered diltiazem in order to maintain optimum therapeutic blood levels). Products include:
E.E.S. 433
EryPed 431

Erythromycin Gluceptate (Patients taking other drugs that are substrates of CYP450, especially patients with renal and/or hepatic impairment, may require dosage adjustment when starting or stopping concomitantly administered diltiazem in order to maintain optimum therapeutic blood levels).
No products indexed under this heading.

Erythromycin Lactobionate (Patients taking other drugs that are substrates of CYP450, especially patients with renal and/or hepatic impairment, may require dosage adjustment when starting or stopping concomitantly administered diltiazem in order to maintain optimum therapeutic blood levels).
No products indexed under this heading.

Erythromycin Stearate (Patients taking other drugs that are substrates of CYP450, especially patients with renal and/or hepatic impairment, may require dosage adjustment when starting or stopping concomitantly administered diltiazem in order to maintain optimum therapeutic blood levels).
No products indexed under this heading.

Esmolol Hydrochloride (Pharmacologic studies indicate that there may be additive effects in prolonging A-V conduction when using beta-blockers or digitalis concomitantly with diltiazem).
No products indexed under this heading.

Esomeprazole Magnesium (Diltiazem is both a substrate and an inhibitor of the CYP3A4 enzyme system. Other drugs that are specific substrates, inhibitors, or inducers of this enzyme system may have a significant impact on the efficacy and side effect profile of diltiazem). Products include:
Nexium Delayed-Release Capsules 645
Nexium Delayed-Release Oral Suspension 645

Estazolam (Studies showed that diltiazem increased the AUC of midazolam and triazolam by 3- to 4-fold and the Cmax by 2-fold, compared to placebo. The elimination half-life of midazolam and triazolam also increased during co-administration with diltiazem).
No products indexed under this heading.

Estradiol (Patients taking other drugs that are substrates of CYP450, especially patients with renal and/or hepatic impairment, may require dosage adjustment when starting or stopping concomitantly administered diltiazem in order to maintain optimum therapeutic blood levels). Products include:
Activella Tablets 2347
Angeliq Tablets 751
Climara Transdermal System 763
Climara Pro Transdermal System 768
Divigel 3167
Vagifem Tablets 2375

Estradiol Benzoate (Patients taking other drugs that are substrates of CYP450, especially patients with renal and/or hepatic impairment, may require dosage adjustment when starting or stopping concomitantly administered diltiazem in order to maintain optimum therapeutic blood levels).
No products indexed under this heading.

Estradiol Cypionate (Patients taking other drugs that are substrates of CYP450, especially patients with renal and/or hepatic impairment, may require dosage adjustment when starting or stopping concomitantly administered diltiazem in order to maintain optimum therapeutic blood levels).
No products indexed under this heading.

Estradiol Valerate (Patients taking other drugs that are substrates of CYP450, especially patients with renal and/or hepatic impairment, may require dosage adjustment when starting or stopping concomitantly administered diltiazem in order to maintain optimum therapeutic blood levels).
No products indexed under this heading.

Ethinyl Estradiol (Patients taking other drugs that are substrates of CYP450, especially patients with renal and/or hepatic impairment, may require dosage adjustment when starting or stopping concomitantly administered diltiazem in order to maintain optimum therapeutic blood levels). Products include:
Lybrel Tablets 3204
Mircette Tablets 1034
NuvaRing 2897
Ortho-Cyclen/Ortho Tri-Cyclen 2449
Ortho Evra Transdermal System 2437
Ortho Tri-Cyclen Lo Tablets 2458
Seasonique Tablets 1046
Yaz Tablets 805

Ethosuximide (Patients taking other drugs that are substrates of CYP450, especially patients with renal and/or hepatic impairment, may require dosage adjustment when starting or stopping concomitantly administered diltiazem in order to maintain optimum therapeutic blood levels).
No products indexed under this heading.

Ethynodiol Diacetate (Patients taking other drugs that are substrates of CYP450, especially patients with renal and/or hepatic impairment, may require dosage adjustment when starting or stopping concomitantly administered diltiazem in order to maintain optimum therapeutic blood levels).
No products indexed under this heading.

Etoposide (Patients taking other drugs that are substrates of CYP450, especially patients with renal and/or hepatic impairment, may require dosage adjustment when starting or stopping concomitantly administered diltiazem in order to maintain optimum therapeutic blood levels).
No products indexed under this heading.

Etoposide Phosphate (Patients taking other drugs that are substrates of CYP450, especially patients with renal and/or hepatic impairment, may require dosage adjustment when starting or stopping concomitantly administered diltiazem in order to maintain optimum therapeutic blood levels).
No products indexed under this heading.

Felbamate (Diltiazem is both a substrate and an inhibitor of the CYP3A4 enzyme system. Other drugs that are specific substrates, inhibitors, or inducers of this enzyme system may have a significant impact on the efficacy and side effect profile of diltiazem).
No products indexed under this heading.

Felodipine (Diltiazem has an additive effect when used with other antihypertensive agents. Therefore, the dosage of diltiazem or concomitant antihypertensives may need to be adjusted when adding one to the other).
No products indexed under this heading.

Fentanyl (Patients taking other drugs that are substrates of CYP450, especially patients with renal and/or hepatic impairment, may require dosage adjustment when starting or stopping concomitantly administered diltiazem in order to maintain optimum therapeutic blood levels). Products include:
Duragesic Transdermal System 2405
Ionsys Transdermal System 2410

Fentanyl Citrate (The depression of cardiac contractility, conductivity, and automaticity, as well as the vascular dilation associated with anesthetics, may be potentiated by calcium channel blockers). Products include:
Actiq 959
Fentora Tablets 968

Fluconazole (Diltiazem is both a substrate and an inhibitor of the CYP3A4 enzyme system. Other drugs that are specific substrates, inhibitors, or inducers of this enzyme system may have a significant impact on the efficacy and side effect profile of diltiazem).
No products indexed under this heading.

Fludrocortisone Acetate (Diltiazem is both a substrate and an inhibitor of the CYP3A4 enzyme system. Other drugs that are specific substrates, inhibitors, or inducers of this enzyme system may have a significant impact on the efficacy and side effect profile of diltiazem).
No products indexed under this heading.

Fluoxetine (Diltiazem is both a substrate and an inhibitor of the CYP3A4 enzyme system. Other drugs that are specific substrates, inhibitors, or inducers of this enzyme system may have a significant impact on the efficacy and side effect profile of diltiazem).
No products indexed under this heading.

Fluoxetine Hydrochloride (Diltiazem is both a substrate and an inhibitor of the CYP3A4 enzyme system. Other drugs that are specific substrates, inhibitors, or inducers of this enzyme system may have a significant impact on the efficacy and side effect profile of diltiazem). Products include:
Prozac Weekly Capsules 1852
Prozac Pulvules and Liquid 1852
Symbyax Capsules 1871

Flurazepam Hydrochloride (Studies showed that diltiazem increased the AUC of midazolam and triazolam by 3- to 4-fold and the Cmax by 2-fold, compared to placebo. The elimination half-life of midazolam and triazolam also increased during co-administration with diltiazem).
No products indexed under this heading.

Fluvoxamine Maleate (Diltiazem is both a substrate and an inhibitor of the CYP3A4 enzyme system. Other drugs that are specific substrates, inhibitors, or inducers of this enzyme system may have a significant impact on the efficacy and side effect profile of diltiazem). Products include:
Luvox CR Extended-Release Capsules 1759

Fosamprenavir Calcium (Diltiazem is both a substrate and an inhibitor of the CYP3A4 enzyme system. Other drugs that are specific substrates, inhibitors, or inducers of this enzyme system may have a significant impact on the efficacy and side effect profile of diltiazem). Products include:
Lexiva Oral Suspension 1510
Lexiva Tablets 1510

Fosinopril Sodium (Diltiazem has an additive effect when used with other antihypertensive agents. Therefore, the dosage of diltiazem or concomitant antihypertensives may need to be adjusted when adding one to the other).
No products indexed under this heading.

Fosphenytoin Sodium (Diltiazem is both a substrate and an inhibitor of the CYP3A4 enzyme system. Other drugs that are specific substrates, inhibitors, or inducers of this enzyme system may have a significant impact on the efficacy and side effect profile of diltiazem).
No products indexed under this heading.

Furosemide (Diltiazem has an additive effect when used with other antihypertensive agents. Therefore, the dosage of diltiazem or concomitant antihypertensives may need to be adjusted when adding one to the other). Products include:
Furosemide Tablets 2186

Garlic Extract (Diltiazem is both a substrate and an inhibitor of the CYP3A4 enzyme system. Other drugs that are specific substrates, inhibitors, or inducers of this enzyme system may have a significant impact on the efficacy and side effect profile of diltiazem).
No products indexed under this heading.

Garlic Oil (Diltiazem is both a substrate and an inhibitor of the CYP3A4 enzyme system. Other drugs that are specific substrates, inhibitors, or inducers of this enzyme system may have a significant impact on the efficacy and side effect profile of diltiazem).
No products indexed under this heading.

Guanabenz Acetate (Diltiazem has an additive effect when used with other antihypertensive agents. Therefore, the dosage of diltiazem or concomitant antihypertensives may need to be adjusted when adding one to the other).
No products indexed under this heading.

Guanethidine Monosulfate (Diltiazem has an additive effect when used with other antihypertensive agents. Therefore, the dosage of diltiazem or concomitant antihypertensives may need to be adjusted when adding one to the other).
No products indexed under this heading.

Halazepam (Studies showed that diltiazem increased the AUC of midazolam and triazolam by 3- to 4-fold and the Cmax by 2-fold, compared to placebo. The elimination half-life of midazolam and triazolam also increased during co-administration with diltiazem).
No products indexed under this heading.

Haloperidol (Patients taking other drugs that are substrates of CYP450, especially patients with renal and/or hepatic impairment, may require dosage adjustment when starting or stopping concomitantly administered diltiazem in order to maintain optimum therapeutic blood levels).
No products indexed under this heading.

Haloperidol Decanoate (Patients taking other drugs that are substrates of CYP450, especially patients with renal and/or hepatic impairment, may require dosage adjustment when starting or stopping concomitantly administered diltiazem in order to maintain optimum therapeutic blood levels).
No products indexed under this heading.

Haloperidol Lactate (Patients taking other drugs that are substrates of CYP450, especially patients with renal and/or hepatic impairment, may require dosage adjustment when starting or stopping concomitantly administered diltiazem in order to maintain optimum therapeutic blood levels).
No products indexed under this heading.

Halothane (The depression of cardiac contractility, conductivity, and automaticity, as well as the vascular dilation associated with anesthetics, may be potentiated by calcium channel blockers).
No products indexed under this heading.

Hydralazine Hydrochloride (Diltiazem has an additive effect when used with other antihypertensive agents. Therefore, the dosage of diltiazem or concomitant antihypertensives may need to be adjusted when adding one to the other).
No products indexed under this heading.

Hydrochlorothiazide (Diltiazem has an additive effect when used with other antihypertensive agents. Therefore, the dosage of diltiazem or concomitant antihypertensives may need to be adjusted when adding one to the other). Products include:
Atacand HCT 642
Avalide Tablets 892
Avalide Tablets 2713
Benicar HCT Tablets 1010
Diovan HCT Tablets 2216
Dyazide Capsules 1405
Micardis HCT Tablets 854
Prinzide Tablets 2092
Tekturna HCT Tablets 2324
Teveten HCT Tablets 517

Hydrocortisone (Diltiazem is both a substrate and an inhibitor of the CYP3A4 enzyme system. Other drugs that are specific substrates, inhibitors, or inducers of this enzyme system may have a significant impact on the efficacy and side effect profile of diltiazem).
No products indexed under this heading.

Hydrocortisone Acetate (Diltiazem is both a substrate and an inhibitor of the CYP3A4 enzyme system. Other drugs that are specific substrates, inhibitors, or inducers of this enzyme system may have a significant impact on the efficacy and side effect profile of diltiazem). Products include:
Analpram-HC 1140
Pramosone 1141

Hydrocortisone Butyrate (Diltiazem is both a substrate and an inhibitor of the CYP3A4 enzyme system. Other drugs that are specific substrates, inhibitors, or inducers of this enzyme system may have a significant impact on the efficacy and side effect profile of diltiazem).
No products indexed under this heading.

Hydrocortisone Cypionate (Diltiazem is both a substrate and an inhibitor of the CYP3A4 enzyme system. Other drugs that are specific substrates, inhibitors, or inducers of this enzyme system may have a significant impact on the efficacy and side effect profile of diltiazem).
No products indexed under this heading.

Hydrocortisone Hemisuccinate (Diltiazem is both a substrate and an inhibitor of the CYP3A4 enzyme system. Other drugs that are specific substrates, inhibitors, or inducers of this enzyme system may have a significant impact on the efficacy and side effect profile of diltiazem).
No products indexed under this heading.

Hydrocortisone Probutate (Diltiazem is both a substrate and an inhibitor of the CYP3A4 enzyme system. Other drugs that are specific substrates, inhibitors, or inducers of this enzyme system may have a significant impact on the efficacy and side effect profile of diltiazem).
No products indexed under this heading.

Hydrocortisone Sodium Phosphate (Diltiazem is both a substrate and an inhibitor of the CYP3A4 enzyme system. Other drugs that are specific substrates, inhibitors, or inducers of this enzyme system may have a significant impact on the efficacy and side effect profile of diltiazem).
No products indexed under this heading.

Hydrocortisone Sodium Succinate (Diltiazem is both a substrate and an inhibitor of the CYP3A4 enzyme system. Other drugs that are specific substrates, inhibitors, or inducers of this enzyme system may have a significant impact on the efficacy and side effect profile of diltiazem).
No products indexed under this heading.

Hydrocortisone Valerate (Diltiazem is both a substrate and an inhibitor of the CYP3A4 enzyme system. Other drugs that are specific substrates, inhibitors, or inducers of this enzyme system may have a significant impact on the efficacy and side effect profile of diltiazem).
No products indexed under this heading.

Hydroflumethiazide (Diltiazem has an additive effect when used with other antihypertensive agents. Therefore, the dosage of diltiazem or concomitant antihypertensives may need to be adjusted when adding one to the other).
No products indexed under this heading.

Hypericum (Diltiazem is both a substrate and an inhibitor of the CYP3A4 enzyme system. Other drugs that are specific substrates, inhibitors, or inducers of this enzyme system may have a significant impact on the efficacy and side effect profile of diltiazem). Products include:
Satieté Tablets .... ▣ 640

Hypericum Perforatum (Diltiazem is both a substrate and an inhibitor of the CYP3A4 enzyme system. Other drugs that are specific substrates, inhibitors, or inducers of this enzyme system may have a significant impact on the efficacy and side effect profile of diltiazem).
No products indexed under this heading.

Indapamide (Diltiazem has an additive effect when used with other antihypertensive agents. Therefore, the dosage of diltiazem or concomitant antihypertensives may need to be adjusted when adding one to the other). Products include:
Indapamide Tablets 2188

Indinavir Sulfate (Patients taking other drugs that are substrates of CYP450, especially patients with renal and/or hepatic impairment, may require dosage adjustment when starting or stopping concomitantly administered diltiazem in order to maintain optimum therapeutic blood levels). Products include:
Crixivan Capsules 1979

Irbesartan (Diltiazem has an additive effect when used with other antihypertensive agents. Therefore, the dosage of diltiazem or concomitant antihypertensives may need to be adjusted when adding one to the other). Products include:
Avalide Tablets 892
Avalide Tablets 2713
Avapro Tablets 897
Avapro Tablets 2718

Isoflurane (The depression of cardiac contractility, conductivity, and automaticity, as well as the vascular dilation associated with anesthetics, may be potentiated by calcium channel blockers).
No products indexed under this heading.

Isoniazid (Diltiazem is both a substrate and an inhibitor of the CYP3A4 enzyme system. Other drugs that are specific substrates, inhibitors, or inducers of this enzyme system may have a significant impact on the efficacy and side effect profile of diltiazem).
No products indexed under this heading.

Isradipine (Diltiazem has an additive effect when used with other antihypertensive agents. Therefore, the dosage of diltiazem or concomitant antihypertensives may need to be adjusted when adding one to the other). Products include:
DynaCirc CR Controlled Release Tablets 1407

Itraconazole (Patients taking other drugs that are substrates of CYP450, especially patients with renal and/or hepatic impairment, may require dosage adjustment when starting or stopping concomitantly administered diltiazem in order to maintain optimum therapeutic blood levels).
No products indexed under this heading.

Ixabepilone (Patients taking other drugs that are substrates of CYP450, especially patients with renal and/or hepatic impairment, may require dosage adjustment when starting or stopping concomitantly administered diltiazem in order to maintain optimum therapeutic blood levels). Products include:
Ixempra Kit for Injection 915

Ketamine Hydrochloride (The depression of cardiac contractility, conductivity, and automaticity, as well as the vascular dilation associated with anesthetics, may be potentiated by calcium channel blockers).
No products indexed under this heading.

Ketoconazole (Patients taking other drugs that are substrates of CYP450, especially patients with renal and/or hepatic impairment, may require dosage adjustment when starting or stopping concomitantly administered diltiazem in order to maintain optimum therapeutic blood levels). Products include:
Extina Foam, 2% 3057
Nizoral A-D Shampoo 1901

Labetalol Hydrochloride (Pharmacologic studies indicate that there may be additive effects in prolonging A-V conduction when using beta-blockers or digitalis concomitantly with diltiazem).
No products indexed under this heading.

Levobunolol Hydrochloride (Pharmacologic studies indicate that there may be additive effects in prolonging A-V conduction when using beta-blockers or digitalis concomitantly with diltiazem).
No products indexed under this heading.

Levonorgestrel (Patients taking other drugs that are substrates of CYP450, especially patients with renal and/or hepatic impairment, may require dosage adjustment when starting or stopping concomitantly administered diltiazem in order to maintain optimum therapeutic blood levels). Products include:
Climara Pro Transdermal System 768
Lybrel Tablets 3204
Mirena Intrauterine System 779
Plan B Tablets 1044
Seasonique Tablets 1046

Lidocaine (Patients taking other drugs that are substrates of CYP450, especially patients with renal and/or hepatic impairment, may require dosage adjustment when starting or stopping concomitantly administered diltiazem in order to maintain optimum therapeutic blood levels). Products include:
Lidoderm Patch 1114

Lidocaine Hydrochloride (Patients taking other drugs that are substrates of CYP450, especially patients with renal and/or hepatic impairment, may require dosage adjustment when starting or stopping concomitantly administered diltiazem in order to maintain optimum therapeutic blood levels).
No products indexed under this heading.

Lisinopril (Diltiazem has an additive effect when used with other antihypertensive agents. Therefore, the dosage of diltiazem or concomitant antihypertensives may need to be adjusted when adding one to the other). Products include:
Prinivil Tablets 2087
Prinzide Tablets 2092

Lopinavir (Diltiazem is both a substrate and an inhibitor of the CYP3A4 enzyme system. Other drugs that are specific substrates, inhibitors, or inducers of this enzyme system may have a significant impact on the efficacy and side effect profile of diltiazem). Products include:
Kaletra 452

Loratadine (Diltiazem is both a substrate and an inhibitor of the CYP3A4 enzyme system. Other drugs that are specific substrates, inhibitors, or inducers of this enzyme system may have a significant impact on the efficacy and side effect profile of diltiazem).
No products indexed under this heading.

Lorazepam (Studies showed that diltiazem increased the AUC of midazolam and triazolam by 3- to 4-fold and the Cmax by 2-fold, compared to placebo. The elimination half-life of midazolam and triazolam also increased during co-administration with diltiazem).
No products indexed under this heading.

Losartan Potassium (Diltiazem has an additive effect when used with other antihypertensive agents. Therefore, the dosage of diltiazem or concomitant antihypertensives may need to be adjusted when adding one to the other). Products include:
Cozaar Tablets 1973

Lovastatin (In a ten-subject study, co-administration of diltiazem (120 mg bid diltiazem SR) with lovastatin resulted in a 3-4 times increase in mean lovastatin AUC and Cmax versus lovastatin alone). Products include:
Advicor Tablets 402
Mevacor Tablets 2063

Mecamylamine Hydrochloride (Diltiazem has an additive effect when used with other antihypertensive agents. Therefore, the dosage of diltiazem or concomitant antihypertensives may need to be adjusted when adding one to the other).
No products indexed under this heading.

Mephenytoin (Diltiazem is both a substrate and an inhibitor of the CYP3A4 enzyme system. Other drugs that are specific substrates, inhibitors, or inducers of this enzyme system may have a significant impact on the efficacy and side effect profile of diltiazem).
No products indexed under this heading.

Mestranol (Patients taking other drugs that are substrates of CYP450, especially patients with renal and/or hepatic impairment, may require dosage adjustment when starting or stopping concomitantly administered diltiazem in order to maintain optimum therapeutic blood levels).
No products indexed under this heading.

Methadone Hydrochloride (Patients taking other drugs that are substrates of CYP450, especially patients with renal and/or hepatic impairment, may require dosage adjustment when starting or stopping concomitantly administered diltiazem in order to maintain optimum therapeutic blood levels).
No products indexed under this heading.

Methohexital Sodium (The depression of cardiac contractility, conductivity, and automaticity, as well as the vascular dilation associated with anesthetics, may be potentiated by calcium channel blockers).
No products indexed under this heading.

Methsuximide (Diltiazem is both a substrate and an inhibitor of the CYP3A4 enzyme system. Other drugs that are specific substrates, inhibitors, or inducers of this enzyme system may have a significant impact on the efficacy and side effect profile of diltiazem).
No products indexed under this heading.

Methyclothiazide (Diltiazem has an additive effect when used with other antihypertensive agents. Therefore, the dosage of diltiazem or concomitant antihypertensives may need to be adjusted when adding one to the other).
No products indexed under this heading.

Methyldopa (Diltiazem has an additive effect when used with other antihypertensive agents. Therefore, the dosage of diltiazem or concomitant antihypertensives may need to be adjusted when adding one to the other).
No products indexed under this heading.

Methyldopate Hydrochloride (Diltiazem has an additive effect when used with other antihypertensive agents. Therefore, the dosage of diltiazem or concomitant antihypertensives may need to be adjusted when adding one to the other).
No products indexed under this heading.

Methylprednisolone (Diltiazem is both a substrate and an inhibitor of the CYP3A4 enzyme system. Other drugs that are specific substrates, inhibitors, or inducers of this enzyme system may have a significant impact on the efficacy and side effect profile of diltiazem).
No products indexed under this heading.

Methylprednisolone Acetate (Diltiazem is both a substrate and an inhibitor of the CYP3A4 enzyme system. Other drugs that are specific substrates, inhibitors, or inducers of this enzyme system may have a significant impact on the efficacy and side effect profile of diltiazem).
No products indexed under this heading.

Methylprednisolone Sodium Succinate (Diltiazem is both a substrate and an inhibitor of the CYP3A4 enzyme system. Other drugs that are specific substrates, inhibitors, or inducers of this enzyme system may have a significant impact on the efficacy and side effect profile of diltiazem).
No products indexed under this heading.

Metipranolol Hydrochloride (Pharmacologic studies indicate that there may be additive effects in prolonging A-V conduction when using beta-blockers or digitalis concomitantly with diltiazem).
No products indexed under this heading.

Metolazone (Diltiazem has an additive effect when used with other antihypertensive agents. Therefore, the dosage of diltiazem or concomitant antihypertensives may need to be adjusted when adding one to the other).
No products indexed under this heading.

Metoprolol Succinate (Pharmacologic studies indicate that there may be additive effects in prolonging A-V conduction when using beta-blockers or digitalis concomitantly with diltiazem). Products include:
Toprol-XL Tablets 666

Metoprolol Tartrate (Pharmacologic studies indicate that there may be additive effects in prolonging A-V conduction when using beta-blockers or digitalis concomitantly with diltiazem).
No products indexed under this heading.

Metronidazole (Diltiazem is both a substrate and an inhibitor of the CYP3A4 enzyme system. Other drugs that are specific substrates, inhibitors, or inducers of this enzyme system may have a significant impact on the efficacy and side effect profile of diltiazem). Products include:
Pylera Capsules 714

Metronidazole Benzoate (Diltiazem is both a substrate and an inhibitor of the CYP3A4 enzyme system. Other drugs that are specific substrates, inhibitors, or inducers of this enzyme system may have a significant impact on the efficacy and side effect profile of diltiazem).
No products indexed under this heading.

Metronidazole Hydrochloride (Diltiazem is both a substrate and an inhibitor of the CYP3A4 enzyme system. Other drugs that are specific substrates, inhibitors, or inducers of this enzyme system may have a significant impact on the efficacy and side effect profile of diltiazem).
No products indexed under this heading.

Metyrosine (Diltiazem has an additive effect when used with other antihypertensive agents. Therefore, the dosage of diltiazem or concomitant antihypertensives may need to be adjusted when adding one to the other). Products include:
Demser Capsules 1989

Mibefradil Dihydrochloride (Diltiazem has an additive effect when used with other antihypertensive agents. Therefore, the dosage of diltiazem or concomitant antihypertensives may need to be adjusted when adding one to the other).
No products indexed under this heading.

Miconazole (Diltiazem is both a substrate and an inhibitor of the CYP3A4 enzyme system. Other drugs that are specific substrates, inhibitors, or inducers of this enzyme system may have a significant impact on the efficacy and side effect profile of diltiazem).
No products indexed under this heading.

Miconazole Nitrate (Diltiazem is both a substrate and an inhibitor of the CYP3A4 enzyme system. Other drugs that are specific substrates, inhibitors, or inducers of this enzyme system may have a significant impact on the efficacy and side effect profile of diltiazem).
No products indexed under this heading.

Midazolam Hydrochloride (The depression of cardiac contractility, conductivity, and automaticity, as well as the vascular dilation associated with anesthetics, may be potentiated by calcium channel blockers).
No products indexed under this heading.

Minoxidil (Diltiazem has an additive effect when used with other antihypertensive agents. Therefore, the dosage of diltiazem or concomitant antihypertensives may need to be adjusted when adding one to the other).
No products indexed under this heading.

Modafinil (Diltiazem is both a substrate and an inhibitor of the CYP3A4 enzyme system. Other drugs that are specific substrates, inhibitors, or inducers of this enzyme system may have a significant impact on the efficacy and side effect profile of diltiazem). Products include:
Provigil Tablets 977

Moexipril Hydrochloride (Diltiazem has an additive effect when used with other antihypertensive agents. Therefore, the dosage of diltiazem or concomitant antihypertensives may need to be adjusted when adding one to the other).
No products indexed under this heading.

Nadolol (Pharmacologic studies indicate that there may be additive effects in prolonging A-V conduction when using beta-blockers or digitalis concomitantly with diltiazem).
Products include:
Nadolol Tablets 2191

Nebivolol (Pharmacologic studies indicate that there may be additive effects in prolonging A-V conduction when using beta-blockers or digitalis concomitantly with diltiazem).
Products include:
Bystolic Tablets 1155

Nefazodone Hydrochloride (Patients taking other drugs that are substrates of CYP450, especially patients with renal and/or hepatic impairment, may require dosage adjustment when starting or stopping concomitantly administered diltiazem in order to maintain optimum therapeutic blood levels).
No products indexed under this heading.

Nelfinavir Mesylate (Patients taking other drugs that are substrates of CYP450, especially patients with renal and/or hepatic impairment, may require dosage adjustment when starting or stopping concomitantly administered diltiazem in order to maintain optimum therapeutic blood levels).
No products indexed under this heading.

Nevirapine (Diltiazem is both a substrate and an inhibitor of the CYP3A4 enzyme system. Other drugs that are specific substrates, inhibitors, or inducers of this enzyme system may have a significant impact on the efficacy and side effect profile of diltiazem). Products include:
Viramune Oral Suspension 873
Viramune Tablets 873

Niacinamide (Diltiazem is both a substrate and an inhibitor of the CYP3A4 enzyme system. Other drugs that are specific substrates, inhibitors, or inducers of this enzyme system may have a significant impact on the efficacy and side effect profile of diltiazem). Products include:
BioLean Free Tablets .... ▣635

Nicardipine Hydrochloride (Diltiazem has an additive effect when used with other antihypertensive agents. Therefore, the dosage of diltiazem or concomitant antihypertensives may need to be adjusted when adding one to the other). Products include:
Cardene I.V. 1093

Nicotinamide (Diltiazem is both a substrate and an inhibitor of the CYP3A4 enzyme system. Other drugs that are specific substrates, inhibitors, or inducers of this enzyme system may have a significant impact on the efficacy and side effect profile of diltiazem).
No products indexed under this heading.

Nifedipine (Diltiazem has an additive effect when used with other antihypertensive agents. Therefore, the dosage of diltiazem or concomitant antihypertensives may need to be adjusted when adding one to the other).
No products indexed under this heading.

Nimodipine (Patients taking other drugs that are substrates of CYP450, especially patients with renal and/or hepatic impairment, may require dosage adjustment when starting or stopping concomitantly administered diltiazem in order to maintain optimum therapeutic blood levels). Products include:
Nimotop Capsules 790

Nisoldipine (Diltiazem has an additive effect when used with other antihypertensive agents. Therefore, the dosage of diltiazem or concomitant antihypertensives may need to be adjusted when adding one to the other). Products include:
Sular Extended Release Tablets 2975

Nitrendipine (Patients taking other drugs that are substrates of CYP450, especially patients with renal and/or hepatic impairment, may require dosage adjustment when starting or stopping concomitantly administered diltiazem in order to maintain optimum therapeutic blood levels).
No products indexed under this heading.

Nitroglycerin (Diltiazem has an additive effect when used with other antihypertensive agents. Therefore, the dosage of diltiazem or concomitant antihypertensives may need to be adjusted when adding one to the other). Products include:
Nitro-Dur Transdermal Infusion System.. 2887
Nitrolingual Pumpspray 2965

Norethindrone (Patients taking other drugs that are substrates of CYP450, especially patients with renal and/or hepatic impairment, may require dosage adjustment when starting or stopping concomitantly administered diltiazem in order to maintain optimum therapeutic blood levels). Products include:
Ortho Micronor Tablets 2446

Norethindrone Acetate (Patients taking other drugs that are substrates of CYP450, especially patients with renal and/or hepatic impairment, may require dosage adjustment when starting or stopping concomitantly administered diltiazem in order to maintain optimum therapeutic blood levels). Products include:
Activella Tablets 2347

Norfloxacin (Diltiazem is both a substrate and an inhibitor of the CYP3A4 enzyme system. Other drugs that are specific substrates, inhibitors, or inducers of this enzyme system may have a significant impact on the efficacy and side effect profile of diltiazem). Products include:
Noroxin Tablets 2069

Norgestrel (Patients taking other drugs that are substrates of CYP450, especially patients with renal and/or hepatic impairment, may require dosage adjustment when starting or stopping concomitantly administered diltiazem in order to maintain optimum therapeutic blood levels).
No products indexed under this heading.

Omeprazole (Diltiazem is both a substrate and an inhibitor of the CYP3A4 enzyme system. Other drugs that are specific substrates, inhibitors, or inducers of this enzyme system may have a significant impact on the efficacy and side effect profile of diltiazem).
No products indexed under this heading.

Ondansetron (Patients taking other drugs that are substrates of CYP450, especially patients with renal and/or hepatic impairment, may require dosage adjustment when starting or stopping concomitantly administered diltiazem in order to maintain optimum therapeutic blood levels). Products include:
Zofran ODT Orally Disintegrating Tablets.. 1687

Ondansetron Hydrochloride (Patients taking other drugs that are substrates of CYP450, especially patients with renal and/or hepatic impairment, may require dosage adjustment when starting or stopping concomitantly administered diltiazem in order to maintain optimum therapeutic blood levels). Products include:
Zofran Injection 1682
Zofran 1687

Oxazepam (Studies showed that diltiazem increased the AUC of midazolam and triazolam by 3- to 4-fold and the Cmax by 2-fold, compared to placebo. The elimination half-life of midazolam and triazolam also increased during co-administration with diltiazem).
No products indexed under this heading.

Oxcarbazepine (Diltiazem is both a substrate and an inhibitor of the CYP3A4 enzyme system. Other drugs that are specific substrates, inhibitors, or inducers of this enzyme system may have a significant impact on the efficacy and side effect profile of diltiazem).
No products indexed under this heading.

Paclitaxel (Patients taking other drugs that are substrates of CYP450, especially patients with renal and/or hepatic impairment, may require dosage adjustment when starting or stopping concomitantly administered diltiazem in order to maintain optimum therapeutic blood levels).
No products indexed under this heading.

Paroxetine Hydrochloride (Diltiazem is both a substrate and an inhibitor of the CYP3A4 enzyme system. Other drugs that are specific substrates, inhibitors, or inducers of this enzyme system may have a significant impact on the efficacy and side effect profile of diltiazem). Products include:
Paxil 1535
Paxil CR Controlled-Release Tablets.. 1544

Penbutolol Sulfate (Pharmacologic studies indicate that there may be additive effects in prolonging A-V conduction when using beta-blockers or digitalis concomitantly with diltiazem).
No products indexed under this heading.

Perindopril Erbumine (Diltiazem has an additive effect when used with other antihypertensive agents. Therefore, the dosage of diltiazem or concomitant antihypertensives may need to be adjusted when adding one to the other). Products include:
Aceon Tablets (2 mg, 4 mg, 8 mg).. 3038

Phenobarbital (Diltiazem is both a substrate and an inhibitor of the CYP3A4 enzyme system. Other drugs that are specific substrates, inhibitors, or inducers of this enzyme system may have a significant impact on the efficacy and side effect profile of diltiazem). Products include:
Donnatal Extentabs 2507

Phenobarbital Sodium (Diltiazem is both a substrate and an inhibitor of the CYP3A4 enzyme system. Other drugs that are specific substrates, inhibitors, or inducers of this enzyme system may have a significant impact on the efficacy and side effect profile of diltiazem).
No products indexed under this heading.

Phenoxybenzamine Hydrochloride (Diltiazem has an additive effect when used with other antihypertensive agents. Therefore, the dosage of diltiazem or concomitant antihypertensives may need to be adjusted when adding one to the other). Products include:
Dibenzyline Capsules 3188

Phentolamine Mesylate (Diltiazem has an additive effect when used with other antihypertensive agents. Therefore, the dosage of diltiazem or concomitant antihypertensives may need to be adjusted when adding one to the other).
No products indexed under this heading.

Phenytoin (Diltiazem is both a substrate and an inhibitor of the CYP3A4 enzyme system. Other drugs that are specific substrates, inhibitors, or inducers of this enzyme system may have a significant impact on the efficacy and side effect profile of diltiazem).
No products indexed under this heading.

Phenytoin Sodium (Diltiazem is both a substrate and an inhibitor of the CYP3A4 enzyme system. Other drugs that are specific substrates, inhibitors, or inducers of this enzyme system may have a significant impact on the efficacy and side effect profile of diltiazem). Products include:
Phenytek Capsules 2192

Pimozide (Patients taking other drugs that are substrates of CYP450, especially patients with renal and/or hepatic impairment, may require dosage adjustment when starting or stopping concomitantly administered diltiazem in order to maintain optimum therapeutic blood levels).
No products indexed under this heading.

Pindolol (Pharmacologic studies indicate that there may be additive effects in prolonging A-V conduction when using beta-blockers or digitalis concomitantly with diltiazem).
No products indexed under this heading.

Polyestradiol Phosphate (Patients taking other drugs that are substrates of CYP450, especially patients with renal and/or hepatic impairment, may require dosage adjustment when starting or stopping concomitantly administered diltiazem in order to maintain optimum therapeutic blood levels).
No products indexed under this heading.

Polythiazide (Diltiazem has an additive effect when used with other antihypertensive agents. Therefore, the dosage of diltiazem or concomitant antihypertensives may need to be adjusted when adding one to the other).
No products indexed under this heading.

Prazepam (Studies showed that diltiazem increased the AUC of midazolam and triazolam by 3- to 4-fold and the Cmax by 2-fold, compared to placebo. The elimination half-life of midazolam and triazolam also increased during co-administration with diltiazem).
No products indexed under this heading.

Prazosin Hydrochloride (Diltiazem has an additive effect when used with other antihypertensive agents. Therefore, the dosage of diltiazem or concomitant antihypertensives may need to be adjusted when adding one to the other).
No products indexed under this heading.

Prednisolone Acetate (Diltiazem is both a substrate and an inhibitor of the CYP3A4 enzyme system. Other drugs that are specific substrates, inhibitors, or inducers of this enzyme system may have a significant impact on the efficacy and side effect profile of diltiazem). Products include:
Pred Forte Ophthalmic Suspension .... ⊙ 227
Pred Mild Ophthalmic Suspension .... ⊙ 230
Pred-G Ophthalmic Ointment .... ⊙ 229
Pred-G Ophthalmic Suspension .... ⊙ 228

Prednisolone Sodium Phosphate (Diltiazem is both a substrate and an inhibitor of the CYP3A4 enzyme system. Other drugs that are specific substrates, inhibitors, or inducers of this enzyme system may have a significant impact on the efficacy and side effect profile of diltiazem).
No products indexed under this heading.

Prednisolone Tebutate (Diltiazem is both a substrate and an inhibitor of the CYP3A4 enzyme system. Other drugs that are specific substrates, inhibitors, or inducers of this enzyme system may have a significant impact on the efficacy and side effect profile of diltiazem).
No products indexed under this heading.

Prednisone (Diltiazem is both a substrate and an inhibitor of the CYP3A4 enzyme system. Other drugs that are specific substrates, inhibitors, or inducers of this enzyme system may have a significant impact on the efficacy and side effect profile of diltiazem).
No products indexed under this heading.

Primidone (Diltiazem is both a substrate and an inhibitor of the CYP3A4 enzyme system. Other drugs that are specific substrates, inhibitors, or inducers of this enzyme system may have a significant impact on the efficacy and side effect profile of diltiazem).
No products indexed under this heading.

Propofol (The depression of cardiac contractility, conductivity, and automaticity, as well as the vascular dilation associated with anesthetics, may be potentiated by calcium channel blockers).
No products indexed under this heading.

Propoxyphene Hydrochloride (Diltiazem is both a substrate and an inhibitor of the CYP3A4 enzyme system. Other drugs that are specific substrates, inhibitors, or inducers of this enzyme system may have a significant impact on the efficacy and side effect profile of diltiazem).
No products indexed under this heading.

Propoxyphene Napsylate (Diltiazem is both a substrate and an inhibitor of the CYP3A4 enzyme system. Other drugs that are specific substrates, inhibitors, or inducers of this enzyme system may have a significant impact on the efficacy and side effect profile of diltiazem).
No products indexed under this heading.

Propranolol Hydrochloride (Pharmacologic studies indicate that there may be additive effects in prolonging A-V conduction when using beta-blockers or digitalis concomitantly with diltiazem). Products include:
InnoPran XL Extended Release Capsules 1484

Quazepam (Studies showed that diltiazem increased the AUC of midazolam and triazolam by 3- to 4-fold and the Cmax by 2-fold, compared to placebo. The elimination half-life of midazolam and triazolam also increased during co-administration with diltiazem).
No products indexed under this heading.

Quinapril Hydrochloride (Diltiazem has an additive effect when used with other antihypertensive agents. Therefore, the dosage of diltiazem or concomitant antihypertensives may need to be adjusted when adding one to the other).
No products indexed under this heading.

Quinidine (Diltiazem significantly increases the AUC of quinidine by 51%, t1/2 by 36%, and decreases it Cloral by 33%. Monitoring for quinidine adverse effects may be warranted and the dose adjusted accordingly).
No products indexed under this heading.

Quinidine Gluconate (Diltiazem significantly increases the AUC of quinidine by 51%, t1/2 by 36%, and decreases it Cloral by 33%. Monitoring for quinidine adverse effects may be warranted and the dose adjusted accordingly).
No products indexed under this heading.

Quinidine Hydrochloride (Diltiazem significantly increases the AUC of quinidine by 51%, t1/2 by 36%, and decreases it Cloral by 33%. Monitoring for quinidine adverse effects may be warranted and the dose adjusted accordingly).
No products indexed under this heading.

Quinidine Polygalacturonate (Diltiazem significantly increases the AUC of quinidine by 51%, t1/2 by 36%, and decreases it Cloral by 33%. Monitoring for quinidine adverse effects may be warranted and the dose adjusted accordingly).
No products indexed under this heading.

Quinidine Sulfate (Diltiazem significantly increases the AUC of quinidine by 51%, t1/2 by 36%, and decreases it Cloral by 33%. Monitoring for quinidine adverse effects may be warranted and the dose adjusted accordingly).
No products indexed under this heading.

Quinine (Diltiazem is both a substrate and an inhibitor of the CYP3A4 enzyme system. Other drugs that are specific substrates, inhibitors, or inducers of this enzyme system may have a significant impact on the efficacy and side effect profile of diltiazem).
No products indexed under this heading.

Quinine Sulfate (Diltiazem is both a substrate and an inhibitor of the CYP3A4 enzyme system. Other drugs that are specific substrates, inhibitors, or inducers of this enzyme system may have a significant impact on the efficacy and side effect profile of diltiazem).
No products indexed under this heading.

Quinupristin (Diltiazem is both a substrate and an inhibitor of the CYP3A4 enzyme system. Other drugs that are specific substrates, inhibitors, or inducers of this enzyme system may have a significant impact on the efficacy and side effect profile of diltiazem).
No products indexed under this heading.

Ramipril (Diltiazem has an additive effect when used with other antihypertensive agents. Therefore, the dosage of diltiazem or concomitant antihypertensives may need to be adjusted when adding one to the other).
No products indexed under this heading.

Ranitidine Bismuth Citrate (Diltiazem is both a substrate and an inhibitor of the CYP3A4 enzyme system. Other drugs that are specific substrates, inhibitors, or inducers of this enzyme system may have a significant impact on the efficacy and side effect profile of diltiazem).
No products indexed under this heading.

Ranitidine Hydrochloride (Diltiazem is both a substrate and an inhibitor of the CYP3A4 enzyme system. Other drugs that are specific substrates, inhibitors, or inducers of this enzyme system may have a significant impact on the efficacy and side effect profile of diltiazem). Products include:
Zantac 75 Tablets 603
Zantac 1670
Zantac Injection 1666
Zantac Injection Pharmacy Bulk Package 1668
Maximum Strength Zantac 150 Tablets 603
Maximum Strength Zantac 150 Cool Mint Tablets 603

Rauwolfia Serpentina (Diltiazem has an additive effect when used with other antihypertensive agents. Therefore, the dosage of diltiazem or concomitant antihypertensives may need to be adjusted when adding one to the other).
No products indexed under this heading.

Remifentanil Hydrochloride (The depression of cardiac contractility, conductivity, and automaticity, as well as the vascular dilation associated with anesthetics, may be potentiated by calcium channel blockers).
No products indexed under this heading.

Rescinnamine (Diltiazem has an additive effect when used with other antihypertensive agents. Therefore, the dosage of diltiazem or concomitant antihypertensives may need to be adjusted when adding one to the other).
No products indexed under this heading.

Reserpine (Diltiazem has an additive effect when used with other antihypertensive agents. Therefore, the dosage of diltiazem or concomitant antihypertensives may need to be adjusted when adding one to the other).
No products indexed under this heading.

Rifabutin (Patients taking other drugs that are substrates of CYP450, especially patients with renal and/or hepatic impairment, may require dosage adjustment when starting or stopping concomitantly administered diltiazem in order to maintain optimum therapeutic blood levels).
No products indexed under this heading.

Rifampicin (Diltiazem is both a substrate and an inhibitor of the CYP3A4 enzyme system. Other drugs that are specific substrates, inhibitors, or inducers of this enzyme system may have a significant impact on the efficacy and side effect profile of diltiazem).
No products indexed under this heading.

Rifampin (Co-administration of rifampin with diltiazem lowered the diltiazem plasma concentrations to undetectable levels. Co-administration of diltiazem with rifampin or any known CYP3A4 inducer should be avoided when possible and alternative therapy considered).
No products indexed under this heading.

Rifapentine (Diltiazem is both a substrate and an inhibitor of the CYP3A4 enzyme system. Other drugs that are specific substrates, inhibitors, or inducers of this enzyme system may have a significant impact on the efficacy and side effect profile of diltiazem).
No products indexed under this heading.

Ritonavir (Patients taking other drugs that are substrates of CYP450, especially patients with renal and/or hepatic impairment, may require dosage adjustment when starting or stopping concomitantly administered diltiazem in order to maintain optimum therapeutic blood levels). Products include:
Kaletra 452
Norvir 489

Saquinavir (Patients taking other drugs that are substrates of CYP450, especially patients with renal and/or hepatic impairment, may require dosage adjustment when starting or stopping concomitantly administered diltiazem in order to maintain optimum therapeutic blood levels).
No products indexed under this heading.

Saquinavir Mesylate (Patients taking other drugs that are substrates of CYP450, especially patients with renal and/or hepatic impairment, may require dosage adjustment when starting or stopping concomitantly administered diltiazem in order to maintain optimum therapeutic blood levels).
No products indexed under this heading.

Sertraline Hydrochloride (Patients taking other drugs that are substrates of CYP450, especially patients with renal and/or hepatic impairment, may require dosage adjustment when starting or stopping concomitantly administered diltiazem in order to maintain optimum therapeutic blood levels).
No products indexed under this heading.

Sildenafil Citrate (Patients taking other drugs that are substrates of CYP450, especially patients with renal and/or hepatic impairment, may require dosage adjustment when starting or stopping concomitantly administered diltiazem in order to maintain optimum therapeutic blood levels).
No products indexed under this heading.

Simvastatin (Patients taking other drugs that are substrates of CYP450, especially patients with renal and/or hepatic impairment, may require dosage adjustment when starting or stopping concomitantly administered diltiazem in order to maintain optimum therapeutic blood levels). Products include:
Simcor Tablets ... 502
Vytorin 10/10 Tablets ... 2149
Vytorin 10/10 Tablets ... 2939
Vytorin 10/20 Tablets ... 2149
Vytorin 10/20 Tablets ... 2939
Vytorin 10/40 Tablets ... 2149
Vytorin 10/40 Tablets ... 2939
Vytorin 10/80 Tablets ... 2149
Vytorin 10/80 Tablets ... 2939
Zocor Tablets ... 2136

Sirolimus (Patients taking other drugs that are substrates of CYP450, especially patients with renal and/or hepatic impairment, may require dosage adjustment when starting or stopping concomitantly administered diltiazem in order to maintain optimum therapeutic blood levels). Products include:
Rapamune ... 3260

Sodium Nitroprusside (Diltiazem has an additive effect when used with other antihypertensive agents. Therefore, the dosage of diltiazem or concomitant antihypertensives may need to be adjusted when adding one to the other).
No products indexed under this heading.

Sotalol Hydrochloride (Pharmacologic studies indicate that there may be additive effects in prolonging A-V conduction when using beta-blockers or digitalis concomitantly with diltiazem).
No products indexed under this heading.

Spirapril Hydrochloride (Diltiazem has an additive effect when used with other antihypertensive agents. Therefore, the dosage of diltiazem or concomitant antihypertensives may need to be adjusted when adding one to the other).
No products indexed under this heading.

Sufentanil Citrate (The depression of cardiac contractility, conductivity, and automaticity, as well as the vascular dilation associated with anesthetics, may be potentiated by calcium channel blockers).
No products indexed under this heading.

Sulfinpyrazone (Diltiazem is both a substrate and an inhibitor of the CYP3A4 enzyme system. Other drugs that are specific substrates, inhibitors, or inducers of this enzyme system may have a significant impact on the efficacy and side effect profile of diltiazem).
No products indexed under this heading.

Tacrolimus (Patients taking other drugs that are substrates of CYP450, especially patients with renal and/or hepatic impairment, may require dosage adjustment when starting or stopping concomitantly administered diltiazem in order to maintain optimum therapeutic blood levels). Products include:
Prograf Capsules and Injection ... 622
Protopic Ointment ... 628

Tadalafil (Patients taking other drugs that are substrates of CYP450, especially patients with renal and/or hepatic impairment, may require dosage adjustment when starting or stopping concomitantly administered diltiazem in order to maintain optimum therapeutic blood levels). Products include:
Cialis Tablets ... 1792

Tamoxifen Citrate (Patients taking other drugs that are substrates of CYP450, especially patients with renal and/or hepatic impairment, may require dosage adjustment when starting or stopping concomitantly administered diltiazem in order to maintain optimum therapeutic blood levels).
No products indexed under this heading.

Telithromycin (Diltiazem is both a substrate and an inhibitor of the CYP3A4 enzyme system. Other drugs that are specific substrates, inhibitors, or inducers of this enzyme system may have a significant impact on the efficacy and side effect profile of diltiazem). Products include:
Ketek Tablets ... 2744

Telmisartan (Diltiazem has an additive effect when used with other antihypertensive agents. Therefore, the dosage of diltiazem or concomitant antihypertensives may need to be adjusted when adding one to the other). Products include:
Micardis Tablets ... 852
Micardis HCT Tablets ... 854

Temazepam (Studies showed that diltiazem increased the AUC of midazolam and triazolam by 3- to 4-fold and the Cmax by 2-fold, compared to placebo. The elimination half-life of midazolam and triazolam also increased during co-administration with diltiazem).
No products indexed under this heading.

Terazosin Hydrochloride (Diltiazem has an additive effect when used with other antihypertensive agents. Therefore, the dosage of diltiazem or concomitant antihypertensives may need to be adjusted when adding one to the other).
No products indexed under this heading.

Theophylline (Diltiazem is both a substrate and an inhibitor of the CYP3A4 enzyme system. Other drugs that are specific substrates, inhibitors, or inducers of this enzyme system may have a significant impact on the efficacy and side effect profile of diltiazem).
No products indexed under this heading.

Theophylline Anhydrous (Diltiazem is both a substrate and an inhibitor of the CYP3A4 enzyme system. Other drugs that are specific substrates, inhibitors, or inducers of this enzyme system may have a significant impact on the efficacy and side effect profile of diltiazem). Products include:
Uniphyl Tablets ... 2595

Theophylline Calcium Salicylate (Diltiazem is both a substrate and an inhibitor of the CYP3A4 enzyme system. Other drugs that are specific substrates, inhibitors, or inducers of this enzyme system may have a significant impact on the efficacy and side effect profile of diltiazem).
No products indexed under this heading.

Theophylline Dihydroxypropyl (Glyceryl) (Diltiazem is both a substrate and an inhibitor of the CYP3A4 enzyme system. Other drugs that are specific substrates, inhibitors, or inducers of this enzyme system may have a significant impact on the efficacy and side effect profile of diltiazem).
No products indexed under this heading.

Theophylline Ethylenediamine (Diltiazem is both a substrate and an inhibitor of the CYP3A4 enzyme system. Other drugs that are specific substrates, inhibitors, or inducers of this enzyme system may have a significant impact on the efficacy and side effect profile of diltiazem).
No products indexed under this heading.

Thiamylal Sodium (The depression of cardiac contractility, conductivity, and automaticity, as well as the vascular dilation associated with anesthetics, may be potentiated by calcium channel blockers).
No products indexed under this heading.

Tiagabine Hydrochloride (Patients taking other drugs that are substrates of CYP450, especially patients with renal and/or hepatic impairment, may require dosage adjustment when starting or stopping concomitantly administered diltiazem in order to maintain optimum therapeutic blood levels). Products include:
Gabitril Tablets ... 973

Timolol Hemihydrate (Pharmacologic studies indicate that there may be additive effects in prolonging A-V conduction when using beta-blockers or digitalis concomitantly with diltiazem). Products include:
Betimol Ophthalmic Solution ... 3181

Timolol Maleate (Pharmacologic studies indicate that there may be additive effects in prolonging A-V conduction when using beta-blockers or digitalis concomitantly with diltiazem). Products include:
Combigan Ophthalmic Solution ... 553
Cosopt Sterile Ophthalmic Solution ... 1969
Timoptic Sterile Ophthalmic Solution ... 2121
Timoptic in Ocudose ... 2124
Timoptic-XE Sterile Ophthalmic Gel Forming Solution ... 2125

Tolterodine Tartrate (Patients taking other drugs that are substrates of CYP450, especially patients with renal and/or hepatic impairment, may require dosage adjustment when starting or stopping concomitantly administered diltiazem in order to maintain optimum therapeutic blood levels).
No products indexed under this heading.

Torsemide (Diltiazem has an additive effect when used with other antihypertensive agents. Therefore, the dosage of diltiazem or concomitant antihypertensives may need to be adjusted when adding one to the other). Products include:
Demadex Injection ... 2630
Demadex Tablets ... 2630

Trandolapril (Diltiazem has an additive effect when used with other antihypertensive agents. Therefore, the dosage of diltiazem or concomitant antihypertensives may need to be adjusted when adding one to the other). Products include:
Mavik Tablets ... 472
Tarka Tablets ... 511

Trazodone Hydrochloride (Patients taking other drugs that are substrates of CYP450, especially patients with renal and/or hepatic impairment, may require dosage adjustment when starting or stopping concomitantly administered diltiazem in order to maintain optimum therapeutic blood levels).
No products indexed under this heading.

Triamcinolone (Diltiazem is both a substrate and an inhibitor of the CYP3A4 enzyme system. Other drugs that are specific substrates, inhibitors, or inducers of this enzyme system may have a significant impact on the efficacy and side effect profile of diltiazem).
No products indexed under this heading.

Triamcinolone Acetonide (Diltiazem is both a substrate and an inhibitor of the CYP3A4 enzyme system. Other drugs that are specific substrates, inhibitors, or inducers of this enzyme system may have a significant impact on the efficacy and side effect profile of diltiazem). Products include:
Azmacort Inhalation Aerosol ... 407
Nasacort AQ Nasal Spray ... 2765
Triesence Injectable Suspension ... ⊙209

Triamcinolone Diacetate (Diltiazem is both a substrate and an inhibitor of the CYP3A4 enzyme system. Other drugs that are specific substrates, inhibitors, or inducers of this enzyme system may have a significant impact on the efficacy and side effect profile of diltiazem).
No products indexed under this heading.

Triamcinolone Hexacetonide (Diltiazem is both a substrate and an inhibitor of the CYP3A4 enzyme system. Other drugs that are specific substrates, inhibitors, or inducers of this enzyme system may have a significant impact on the efficacy and side effect profile of diltiazem).
No products indexed under this heading.

Triazolam (Studies showed that diltiazem increased the AUC of midazolam and triazolam by 3- to 4-fold and the Cmax by 2-fold, compared to placebo. The elimination half-life of midazolam and triazolam also increased during co-administration with diltiazem).
No products indexed under this heading.

Trimethaphan Camsylate (Diltiazem has an additive effect when used with other antihypertensive agents. Therefore, the dosage of diltiazem or concomitant antihypertensives may need to be adjusted when adding one to the other).
No products indexed under this heading.

Troglitazone (Diltiazem is both a substrate and an inhibitor of the CYP3A4 enzyme system. Other drugs that are specific substrates, inhibitors, or inducers of this enzyme system may have a significant impact on the efficacy and side effect profile of diltiazem).
No products indexed under this heading.

Troleandomycin (Diltiazem is both a substrate and an inhibitor of the CYP3A4 enzyme system. Other drugs that are specific substrates, inhibitors, or inducers of this enzyme system may have a significant impact on the efficacy and side effect profile of diltiazem).
No products indexed under this heading.

Valproate Sodium (Diltiazem is both a substrate and an inhibitor of the CYP3A4 enzyme system. Other drugs that are specific substrates, inhibitors, or inducers of this enzyme system may have a significant impact on the efficacy and side effect profile of diltiazem).
No products indexed under this heading.

Valsartan (Diltiazem has an additive effect when used with other antihypertensive agents. Therefore, the dosage of diltiazem or concomitant antihypertensives may need to be adjusted when adding one to the other). Products include:
Diovan Tablets 2212
Diovan HCT Tablets 2216
Exforge Tablets 2238

Vardenafil Hydrochloride (Patients taking other drugs that are substrates of CYP450, especially patients with renal and/or hepatic impairment, may require dosage adjustment when starting or stopping concomitantly administered diltiazem in order to maintain optimum therapeutic blood levels). Products include:
Levitra Tablets 2876

Verapamil Hydrochloride (Diltiazem has an additive effect when used with other antihypertensive agents. Therefore, the dosage of diltiazem or concomitant antihypertensives may need to be adjusted when adding one to the other). Products include:
Tarka Tablets 511

Vinblastine Sulfate (Patients taking other drugs that are substrates of CYP450, especially patients with renal and/or hepatic impairment, may require dosage adjustment when starting or stopping concomitantly administered diltiazem in order to maintain optimum therapeutic blood levels).
No products indexed under this heading.

Vincristine Sulfate (Patients taking other drugs that are substrates of CYP450, especially patients with renal and/or hepatic impairment, may require dosage adjustment when starting or stopping concomitantly administered diltiazem in order to maintain optimum therapeutic blood levels).
No products indexed under this heading.

Voriconazole (Diltiazem is both a substrate and an inhibitor of the CYP3A4 enzyme system. Other drugs that are specific substrates, inhibitors, or inducers of this enzyme system may have a significant impact on the efficacy and side effect profile of diltiazem).
No products indexed under this heading.

Warfarin Sodium (Patients taking other drugs that are substrates of CYP450, especially patients with renal and/or hepatic impairment, may require dosage adjustment when starting or stopping concomitantly administered diltiazem in order to maintain optimum therapeutic blood levels).
No products indexed under this heading.

Zafirlukast (Diltiazem is both a substrate and an inhibitor of the CYP3A4 enzyme system. Other drugs that are specific substrates, inhibitors, or inducers of this enzyme system may have a significant impact on the efficacy and side effect profile of diltiazem). Products include:
Accolate Tablets 669

Zileuton (Diltiazem is both a substrate and an inhibitor of the CYP3A4 enzyme system. Other drugs that are specific substrates, inhibitors, or inducers of this enzyme system may have a significant impact on the efficacy and side effect profile of diltiazem).
No products indexed under this heading.

Food Interactions

Grapefruit (Diltiazem is both a substrate and an inhibitor of the CYP3A4 enzyme system. Other drugs that are specific substrates, inhibitors, or inducers of this enzyme system may have a significant impact on the efficacy and side effect profile of diltiazem).

Grapefruit Juice (Diltiazem is both a substrate and an inhibitor of the CYP3A4 enzyme system. Other drugs that are specific substrates, inhibitors, or inducers of this enzyme system may have a significant impact on the efficacy and side effect profile of diltiazem).

CATAPRES TABLETS

(Clonidine Hydrochloride) 841
May interact with barbiturates, beta blockers, calcium channel blockers, cardiac glycosides, hypnotics and sedatives, tricyclic antidepressants, and certain other agents. Compounds in these categories include:

Acebutolol Hydrochloride (Co-administration with agents known to affect sinus node function or AV nodal conduction, such as beta blockers, may result in additive effects such as bradycardia and AV block).
No products indexed under this heading.

Amitriptyline Hydrochloride (Co-administration may reduce the hypotensive effects; dosage adjustment may be necessary; concurrent use has resulted in corneal lesions in rats within 5 days).
No products indexed under this heading.

Amlodipine Besylate (Co-administration with agents known to affect sinus node function or AV nodal conduction, such as calcium channel blockers, may result in additive effects such as bradycardia and AV block). Products include:
Azor Tablets 1005
Exforge Tablets 2238

Amoxapine (Co-administration may reduce the hypotensive effects; dosage adjustment may be necessary).
No products indexed under this heading.

Aprobarbital (Clonidine may potentiate the CNS-depressive effects).
No products indexed under this heading.

Atenolol (Co-administration with agents known to affect sinus node function or AV nodal conduction, such as beta blockers, may result in additive effects such as bradycardia and AV block).
No products indexed under this heading.

Bepridil Hydrochloride (Co-administration with agents known to affect sinus node function or AV nodal conduction, such as calcium channel blockers, may result in additive effects such as bradycardia and AV block).
No products indexed under this heading.

Betaxolol Hydrochloride (Co-administration with agents known to affect sinus node function or AV nodal conduction, such as beta blockers, may result in additive effects such as bradycardia and AV block).
No products indexed under this heading.

Bisoprolol Fumarate (Co-administration with agents known to affect sinus node function or AV nodal conduction, such as beta blockers, may result in additive effects such as bradycardia and AV block).
No products indexed under this heading.

Butabarbital (Clonidine may potentiate the CNS-depressive effects).
No products indexed under this heading.

Butabarbital Sodium (Clonidine may potentiate the CNS-depressive effects).
No products indexed under this heading.

Butalbital (Clonidine may potentiate the CNS-depressive effects).
No products indexed under this heading.

Carteolol Hydrochloride (Co-administration with agents known to affect sinus node function or AV nodal conduction, such as beta blockers, may result in additive effects such as bradycardia and AV block).
No products indexed under this heading.

Chloral Hydrate (Clonidine may potentiate the CNS-depressive effects).
No products indexed under this heading.

Clomipramine Hydrochloride (Co-administration may reduce the hypotensive effects; dosage adjustment may be necessary).
No products indexed under this heading.

Desipramine Hydrochloride (Co-administration may reduce the hypotensive effects; dosage adjustment may be necessary).
No products indexed under this heading.

Deslanoside (Co-administration with agents known to affect sinus node function or AV nodal conduction, such as digitalis, may result in additive effects such as bradycardia and AV block).
No products indexed under this heading.

Digitalis Glycoside Preparations (Co-administration with agents known to affect sinus node function or AV nodal conduction, such as digitalis, may result in additive effects such as bradycardia and AV block).
No products indexed under this heading.

Digitoxin (Co-administration with agents known to affect sinus node function or AV nodal conduction, such as digitalis, may result in additive effects such as bradycardia and AV block).
No products indexed under this heading.

Digoxin (Co-administration with agents known to affect sinus node function or AV nodal conduction, such as digitalis, may result in additive effects such as bradycardia and AV block). Products include:
Lanoxin Injection 1498
Lanoxin Injection Pediatric 1502
Lanoxin Tablets 1505

Diltiazem Hydrochloride (Co-administration with agents known to affect sinus node function or AV nodal conduction, such as calcium channel blockers, may result in additive effects such as bradycardia and AV block). Products include:
Cardizem LA Extended Release Tablets 421

Doxepin Hydrochloride (Co-administration may reduce the hypotensive effects; dosage adjustment may be necessary).
No products indexed under this heading.

Esmolol Hydrochloride (Co-administration with agents known to affect sinus node function or AV nodal conduction, such as beta blockers, may result in additive effects such as bradycardia and AV block).
No products indexed under this heading.

Estazolam (Clonidine may potentiate the CNS-depressive effects).
No products indexed under this heading.

Ethchlorvynol (Clonidine may potentiate the CNS-depressive effects).
No products indexed under this heading.

Ethinamate (Clonidine may potentiate the CNS-depressive effects).
No products indexed under this heading.

Felodipine (Co-administration with agents known to affect sinus node function or AV nodal conduction, such as calcium channel blockers, may result in additive effects such as bradycardia and AV block).
No products indexed under this heading.

Flurazepam Hydrochloride (Clonidine may potentiate the CNS-depressive effects).
No products indexed under this heading.

Glutethimide (Clonidine may potentiate the CNS-depressive effects).
No products indexed under this heading.

Imipramine Hydrochloride (Co-administration may reduce the hypotensive effects; dosage adjustment may be necessary).
No products indexed under this heading.

Imipramine Pamoate (Co-administration may reduce the hypotensive effects; dosage adjustment may be necessary).
No products indexed under this heading.

Isradipine (Co-administration with agents known to affect sinus node function or AV nodal conduction, such as calcium channel blockers, may result in additive effects such as bradycardia and AV block).
Products include:
DynaCirc CR Controlled Release Tablets 1407

Labetalol Hydrochloride (Co-administration with agents known to affect sinus node function or AV nodal conduction, such as beta blockers, may result in additive effects such as bradycardia and AV block).
No products indexed under this heading.

Levobunolol Hydrochloride (Co-administration with agents known to affect sinus node function or AV nodal conduction, such as beta blockers, may result in additive effects such as bradycardia and AV block).
No products indexed under this heading.

Lorazepam (Clonidine may potentiate the CNS-depressive effects).
No products indexed under this heading.

Maprotiline Hydrochloride (Co-administration may reduce the hypotensive effects; dosage adjustment may be necessary).
No products indexed under this heading.

Mephobarbital (Clonidine may potentiate the CNS-depressive effects).
No products indexed under this heading.

Metipranolol Hydrochloride (Co-administration with agents known to affect sinus node function or AV nodal conduction, such as beta blockers, may result in additive effects such as bradycardia and AV block).
No products indexed under this heading.

Metoprolol Succinate (Co-administration with agents known to affect sinus node function or AV nodal conduction, such as beta blockers, may result in additive effects such as bradycardia and AV block). Products include:
Toprol-XL Tablets 666

Metoprolol Tartrate (Co-administration with agents known to affect sinus node function or AV nodal conduction, such as beta blockers, may result in additive effects such as bradycardia and AV block).
No products indexed under this heading.

Mibefradil Dihydrochloride (Co-administration with agents known to affect sinus node function or AV nodal conduction, such as calcium channel blockers, may result in additive effects such as bradycardia and AV block).
No products indexed under this heading.

Midazolam Hydrochloride (Clonidine may potentiate the CNS-depressive effects).
No products indexed under this heading.

Nadolol (Co-administration with agents known to affect sinus node function or AV nodal conduction, such as beta blockers, may result in additive effects such as bradycardia and AV block). Products include:
Nadolol Tablets 2191

Nebivolol (Co-administration with agents known to affect sinus node function or AV nodal conduction, such as beta blockers, may result in additive effects such as bradycardia and AV block). Products include:
Bystolic Tablets 1155

Nicardipine Hydrochloride (Co-administration with agents known to affect sinus node function or AV nodal conduction, such as calcium channel blockers, may result in additive effects such as bradycardia and AV block). Products include:
Cardene I.V. 1093

Nifedipine (Co-administration with agents known to affect sinus node function or AV nodal conduction, such as calcium channel blockers, may result in additive effects such as bradycardia and AV block).
No products indexed under this heading.

Nimodipine (Co-administration with agents known to affect sinus node function or AV nodal conduction, such as calcium channel blockers, may result in additive effects such as bradycardia and AV block). Products include:
Nimotop Capsules 790

Nisoldipine (Co-administration with agents known to affect sinus node function or AV nodal conduction, such as calcium channel blockers, may result in additive effects such as bradycardia and AV block). Products include:
Sular Extended Release Tablets 2975

Nortriptyline Hydrochloride (Co-administration may reduce the hypotensive effects; dosage adjustment may be necessary).
No products indexed under this heading.

Penbutolol Sulfate (Co-administration with agents known to affect sinus node function or AV nodal conduction, such as beta blockers, may result in additive effects such as bradycardia and AV block).
No products indexed under this heading.

Pentobarbital Sodium (Clonidine may potentiate the CNS-depressive effects). Products include:
Nembutal Sodium Solution, USP 2494

Phenobarbital (Clonidine may potentiate the CNS-depressive effects). Products include:
Donnatal Extentabs 2507

Pindolol (Co-administration with agents known to affect sinus node function or AV nodal conduction, such as beta blockers, may result in additive effects such as bradycardia and AV block).
No products indexed under this heading.

Propofol (Clonidine may potentiate the CNS-depressive effects).
No products indexed under this heading.

Propranolol Hydrochloride (Co-administration with agents known to affect sinus node function or AV nodal conduction, such as beta blockers, may result in additive effects such as bradycardia and AV block). Products include:
InnoPran XL Extended Release Capsules 1484

Protriptyline Hydrochloride (Co-administration may reduce the hypotensive effects; dosage adjustment may be necessary).
No products indexed under this heading.

Quazepam (Clonidine may potentiate the CNS-depressive effects).
No products indexed under this heading.

Ramelteon (Clonidine may potentiate the CNS-depressive effects).
Products include:
Rozerem Tablets 3091

Secobarbital Sodium (Clonidine may potentiate the CNS-depressive effects).
No products indexed under this heading.

Sodium Butabarbital (Clonidine may potentiate the CNS-depressive effects).
No products indexed under this heading.

Sotalol Hydrochloride (Co-administration with agents known to affect sinus node function or AV nodal conduction, such as beta blockers, may result in additive effects such as bradycardia and AV block).
No products indexed under this heading.

Temazepam (Clonidine may potentiate the CNS-depressive effects).
No products indexed under this heading.

Thiamylal Sodium (Clonidine may potentiate the CNS-depressive effects).
No products indexed under this heading.

Timolol Hemihydrate (Co-administration with agents known to affect sinus node function or AV nodal conduction, such as beta blockers, may result in additive effects such as bradycardia and AV block). Products include:
Betimol Ophthalmic Solution 3181

Timolol Maleate (Co-administration with agents known to affect sinus node function or AV nodal conduction, such as beta blockers, may result in additive effects such as bradycardia and AV block). Products include:
Combigan Ophthalmic Solution 553
Cosopt Sterile Ophthalmic Solution 1969
Timoptic Sterile Ophthalmic Solution 2121
Timoptic in Ocudose 2124
Timoptic-XE Sterile Ophthalmic Gel Forming Solution 2125

Triazolam (Clonidine may potentiate the CNS-depressive effects).
No products indexed under this heading.

Trimipramine Maleate (Co-administration may reduce the hypotensive effects; dosage adjustment may be necessary).
No products indexed under this heading.

Verapamil Hydrochloride (Co-administration with agents known to affect sinus node function or AV nodal conduction, such as calcium channel blockers, may result in additive effects such as bradycardia and AV block). Products include:
Tarka Tablets 511

Zaleplon (Clonidine may potentiate the CNS-depressive effects).
No products indexed under this heading.

Zolpidem Tartrate (Clonidine may potentiate the CNS-depressive effects). Products include:
Ambien Tablets 2692
Ambien CR Tablets 2696

Food Interactions

Alcohol (Clonidine may potentiate the CNS-depressive effects).

CATAPRES-TTS
(Clonidine) 842
May interact with barbiturates, beta blockers, calcium channel blockers, cardiac glycosides, hypnotics and sedatives, tricyclic antidepressants, and certain other agents. Compounds in these categories include:

Acebutolol Hydrochloride (Co-administration with agents known to affect sinus node function or AV nodal conduction, such as beta blockers, may result in additive effects such as bradycardia and AV block).
No products indexed under this heading.

Amitriptyline Hydrochloride (Co-administration may reduce the hypotensive effects; dosage adjustment may be necessary; concurrent use has resulted in corneal lesions in rats within 5 days).
No products indexed under this heading.

Amlodipine Besylate (Co-administration with agents known to affect sinus node function or AV nodal conduction, such as calcium channel blockers, may result in additive effects such as bradycardia and AV block). Products include:
Azor Tablets 1005
Exforge Tablets 2238

Amoxapine (Co-administration may reduce the hypotensive effects; dosage adjustment may be necessary).
No products indexed under this heading.

Aprobarbital (Clonidine may potentiate the CNS-depressive effects).
No products indexed under this heading.

Atenolol (Co-administration with agents known to affect sinus node function or AV nodal conduction, such as beta blockers, may result in additive effects such as bradycardia and AV block).
No products indexed under this heading.

Bepridil Hydrochloride (Co-administration with agents known to affect sinus node function or AV nodal conduction, such as calcium channel blockers, may result in additive effects such as bradycardia and AV block).
No products indexed under this heading.

Betaxolol Hydrochloride (Co-administration with agents known to affect sinus node function or AV nodal conduction, such as beta blockers, may result in additive effects such as bradycardia and AV block).
No products indexed under this heading.

Bisoprolol Fumarate (Co-administration with agents known to affect sinus node function or AV nodal conduction, such as beta blockers, may result in additive effects such as bradycardia and AV block).
No products indexed under this heading.

Butabarbital (Clonidine may potentiate the CNS-depressive effects).
No products indexed under this heading.

Butabarbital Sodium (Clonidine may potentiate the CNS-depressive effects).
No products indexed under this heading.

Butalbital (Clonidine may potentiate the CNS-depressive effects).
No products indexed under this heading.

Carteolol Hydrochloride (Co-administration with agents known to affect sinus node function or AV nodal conduction, such as beta blockers, may result in additive effects such as bradycardia and AV block).
No products indexed under this heading.

Chloral Hydrate (Clonidine may potentiate the CNS-depressive effects).
No products indexed under this heading.

Clomipramine Hydrochloride (Co-administration may reduce the hypotensive effects; dosage adjustment may be necessary).
No products indexed under this heading.

Desipramine Hydrochloride (Co-administration may reduce the hypotensive effects; dosage adjustment may be necessary).
No products indexed under this heading.

Deslanoside (Co-administration with agents known to affect sinus node function or AV nodal conduction, such as digitalis, may result in additive effects such as bradycardia and AV block).
No products indexed under this heading.

Digitalis Glycoside Preparations (Co-administration with agents known to affect sinus node function or AV nodal conduction, such as digitalis, may result in additive effects such as bradycardia and AV block).
No products indexed under this heading.

Digitoxin (Co-administration with agents known to affect sinus node function or AV nodal conduction, such as digitalis, may result in additive effects such as bradycardia and AV block).
No products indexed under this heading.

Digoxin (Co-administration with agents known to affect sinus node function or AV nodal conduction, such as digitalis, may result in additive effects such as bradycardia and AV block). Products include:
Lanoxin Injection 1498
Lanoxin Injection Pediatric 1502
Lanoxin Tablets 1505

Diltiazem Hydrochloride (Co-administration with agents known to affect sinus node function or AV nodal conduction, such as calcium channel blockers, may result in additive effects such as bradycardia and AV block). Products include:
Cardizem LA Extended Release Tablets 421

Doxepin Hydrochloride (Co-administration may reduce the hypotensive effects; dosage adjustment may be necessary).
No products indexed under this heading.

Esmolol Hydrochloride (Co-administration with agents known to affect sinus node function or AV nodal conduction, such as beta blockers, may result in additive effects such as bradycardia and AV block).
No products indexed under this heading.

Estazolam (Clonidine may potentiate the CNS-depressive effects).
No products indexed under this heading.

Ethchlorvynol (Clonidine may potentiate the CNS-depressive effects).
No products indexed under this heading.

Ethinamate (Clonidine may potentiate the CNS-depressive effects).
No products indexed under this heading.

Felodipine (Co-administration with agents known to affect sinus node function or AV nodal conduction, such as calcium channel blockers, may result in additive effects such as bradycardia and AV block).
No products indexed under this heading.

Flurazepam Hydrochloride (Clonidine may potentiate the CNS-depressive effects).
No products indexed under this heading.

Glutethimide (Clonidine may potentiate the CNS-depressive effects).
No products indexed under this heading.

Imipramine Hydrochloride (Co-administration may reduce the hypotensive effects; dosage adjustment may be necessary).
No products indexed under this heading.

Imipramine Pamoate (Co-administration may reduce the hypotensive effects; dosage adjustment may be necessary).
No products indexed under this heading.

Isradipine (Co-administration with agents known to affect sinus node function or AV nodal conduction, such as calcium channel blockers, may result in additive effects such as bradycardia and AV block). Products include:
DynaCirc CR Controlled Release Tablets 1407

Labetalol Hydrochloride (Co-administration with agents known to affect sinus node function or AV nodal conduction, such as beta blockers, may result in additive effects such as bradycardia and AV block).
No products indexed under this heading.

Levobunolol Hydrochloride (Co-administration with agents known to affect sinus node function or AV nodal conduction, such as beta blockers, may result in additive effects such as bradycardia and AV block).
No products indexed under this heading.

Lorazepam (Clonidine may potentiate the CNS-depressive effects).
No products indexed under this heading.

Maprotiline Hydrochloride (Co-administration may reduce the hypotensive effects; dosage adjustment may be necessary).
No products indexed under this heading.

Mephobarbital (Clonidine may potentiate the CNS-depressive effects).
No products indexed under this heading.

Metipranolol Hydrochloride (Co-administration with agents known to affect sinus node function or AV nodal conduction, such as beta blockers, may result in additive effects such as bradycardia and AV block).
No products indexed under this heading.

Metoprolol Succinate (Co-administration with agents known to affect sinus node function or AV nodal conduction, such as beta blockers, may result in additive effects such as bradycardia and AV block). Products include:
Toprol-XL Tablets 666

Metoprolol Tartrate (Co-administration with agents known to affect sinus node function or AV nodal conduction, such as beta blockers, may result in additive effects such as bradycardia and AV block).
No products indexed under this heading.

Mibefradil Dihydrochloride (Co-administration with agents known to affect sinus node function or AV nodal conduction, such as calcium channel blockers, may result in additive effects such as bradycardia and AV block).
No products indexed under this heading.

Midazolam Hydrochloride (Clonidine may potentiate the CNS-depressive effects).
No products indexed under this heading.

Nadolol (Co-administration with agents known to affect sinus node function or AV nodal conduction, such as beta blockers, may result in additive effects such as bradycardia and AV block). Products include:
Nadolol Tablets 2191

Nebivolol (Co-administration with agents known to affect sinus node function or AV nodal conduction, such as beta blockers, may result in additive effects such as bradycardia and AV block). Products include:
Bystolic Tablets 1155

Nicardipine Hydrochloride (Co-administration with agents known to affect sinus node function or AV nodal conduction, such as calcium channel blockers, may result in additive effects such as bradycardia and AV block). Products include:
Cardene I.V. 1093

Nifedipine (Co-administration with agents known to affect sinus node function or AV nodal conduction, such as calcium channel blockers, may result in additive effects such as bradycardia and AV block).
No products indexed under this heading.

Nimodipine (Co-administration with agents known to affect sinus node function or AV nodal conduction, such as calcium channel blockers, may result in additive effects such as bradycardia and AV block). Products include:
Nimotop Capsules 790

Nisoldipine (Co-administration with agents known to affect sinus node function or AV nodal conduction, such as calcium channel blockers, may result in additive effects such as bradycardia and AV block). Products include:
Sular Extended Release Tablets 2975

Nortriptyline Hydrochloride (Co-administration may reduce the hypotensive effects; dosage adjustment may be necessary).
No products indexed under this heading.

Penbutolol Sulfate (Co-administration with agents known to affect sinus node function or AV nodal conduction, such as beta blockers, may result in additive effects such as bradycardia and AV block).
No products indexed under this heading.

Pentobarbital Sodium (Clonidine may potentiate the CNS-depressive effects). Products include:
Nembutal Sodium Solution, USP 2494

Phenobarbital (Clonidine may potentiate the CNS-depressive effects). Products include:
Donnatal Extentabs 2507

Pindolol (Co-administration with agents known to affect sinus node function or AV nodal conduction, such as beta blockers, may result in additive effects such as bradycardia and AV block).
No products indexed under this heading.

Propofol (Clonidine may potentiate the CNS-depressive effects).
No products indexed under this heading.

Propranolol Hydrochloride (Co-administration with agents known to affect sinus node function or AV nodal conduction, such as beta blockers, may result in additive effects such as bradycardia and AV block). Products include:
InnoPran XL Extended Release Capsules 1484

Protriptyline Hydrochloride (Co-administration may reduce the hypotensive effects; dosage adjustment may be necessary).
No products indexed under this heading.

Quazepam (Clonidine may potentiate the CNS-depressive effects).
No products indexed under this heading.

Ramelteon (Clonidine may potentiate the CNS-depressive effects). Products include:
Rozerem Tablets 3091

Secobarbital Sodium (Clonidine may potentiate the CNS-depressive effects).
No products indexed under this heading.

Sodium Butabarbital (Clonidine may potentiate the CNS-depressive effects).
No products indexed under this heading.

Sotalol Hydrochloride (Co-administration with agents known to affect sinus node function or AV nodal conduction, such as beta blockers, may result in additive effects such as bradycardia and AV block).
No products indexed under this heading.

Temazepam (Clonidine may potentiate the CNS-depressive effects).
No products indexed under this heading.

Thiamylal Sodium (Clonidine may potentiate the CNS-depressive effects).
No products indexed under this heading.

Timolol Hemihydrate (Co-administration with agents known to affect sinus node function or AV nodal conduction, such as beta blockers, may result in additive effects such as bradycardia and AV block). Products include:
Betimol Ophthalmic Solution 3181

Timolol Maleate (Co-administration with agents known to affect sinus node function or AV nodal conduction, such as beta blockers, may result in additive effects such as bradycardia and AV block). Products include:
Combigan Ophthalmic Solution 553
Cosopt Sterile Ophthalmic Solution 1969
Timoptic Sterile Ophthalmic Solution 2121
Timoptic in Ocudose 2124
Timoptic-XE Sterile Ophthalmic Gel Forming Solution 2125

Triazolam (Clonidine may potentiate the CNS-depressive effects).
No products indexed under this heading.

Trimipramine Maleate (Co-administration may reduce the hypotensive effects; dosage adjustment may be necessary).
No products indexed under this heading.

Verapamil Hydrochloride (Co-administration with agents known to affect sinus node function or AV nodal conduction, such as calcium channel blockers, may result in additive effects such as bradycardia and AV block). Products include:
Tarka Tablets 511

Zaleplon (Clonidine may potentiate the CNS-depressive effects).
No products indexed under this heading.

Zolpidem Tartrate (Clonidine may potentiate the CNS-depressive effects). Products include:
Ambien Tablets 2692
Ambien CR Tablets 2696

Food Interactions

Alcohol (Clonidine may potentiate the CNS-depressive effects).

CATASOD-OCUXTRA MEGA-30 MG PLUS MCT DIETARY SUPPLEMENT

(Lutein, Medium-Chain Triglycerides, Vitamins with Minerals, Zeaxanthin) 995
None cited in PDR database.

CATHFLO ACTIVASE

(Alteplase) 1198
See Activase I.V.

CEFTIN FOR ORAL SUSPENSION

(Cefuroxime Axetil) 1380
See Ceftin Tablets

CEFTIN TABLETS

(Cefuroxime Axetil) 1380
May interact with oral anticoagulants, drugs that reduce gastric acidity, and certain other agents. Compounds in these categories include:

Aluminum Carbonate (Drugs that reduce gastric acidity may result in a lower bioavailability of Ceftin compared with that of fasting state and tend to cancel the effect of postprandial absorption).
No products indexed under this heading.

Aluminum Hydroxide (Drugs that reduce gastric acidity may result in a lower bioavailability of Ceftin compared with that of fasting state and tend to cancel the effect of postprandial absorption).
No products indexed under this heading.

Anisindione (Cephalosporins may be associated with a fall in prothrombin activity; those at risk include patients previously stabilized on anticoagulant therapy).
No products indexed under this heading.

Cimetidine (Drugs that reduce gastric acidity may result in a lower bioavailability of Ceftin compared with that of fasting state and tend to cancel the effect of postprandial absorption).
No products indexed under this heading.

Cimetidine Hydrochloride (Drugs that reduce gastric acidity may result in a lower bioavailability of Ceftin compared with that of fasting state and tend to cancel the effect of postprandial absorption).
No products indexed under this heading.

Dicumarol (Cephalosporins may be associated with a fall in prothrombin activity; those at risk include patients previously stabilized on anticoagulant therapy).
No products indexed under this heading.

Esomeprazole Magnesium (Drugs that reduce gastric acidity may result in a lower bioavailability of Ceftin compared with that of fasting state and tend to cancel the effect of postprandial absorption). Products include:
Nexium Delayed-Release Capsules 645
Nexium Delayed-Release Oral Suspension 645

Famotidine (Drugs that reduce gastric acidity may result in a lower bioavailability of Ceftin compared with that of fasting state and tend to cancel the effect of postprandial absorption). Products include:
Pepcid Tablets 2075
Original Strength Pepcid AC Gelcaps 1771
Original Strength Pepcid AC Tablets 1771
Maximum Strength Pepcid AC Tablets 1771
Pepcid Complete Chewable Tablets 1771

Lansoprazole (Drugs that reduce gastric acidity may result in a lower bioavailability of Ceftin compared with that of fasting state and tend to cancel the effect of postprandial absorption).
No products indexed under this heading.

Magnesium Hydroxide (Drugs that reduce gastric acidity may result in a lower bioavailability of Ceftin compared with that of fasting state and tend to cancel the effect of postprandial absorption). Products include:
Fleet Pedia-Lax Chewable Tablets 1145
Pepcid Complete Chewable Tablets 1771
Extra Strength Rolaids Freshmint Tablets 1903
Rolaids Multi-Symptom Berry Tablets 1903
Rolaids Original Peppermint Tablets 1903

Nizatidine (Drugs that reduce gastric acidity may result in a lower bioavailability of Ceftin compared with that of fasting state and tend to cancel the effect of postprandial absorption). Products include:
Axid Capsules 1364

Omeprazole (Drugs that reduce gastric acidity may result in a lower bioavailability of Ceftin compared with that of fasting state and tend to cancel the effect of postprandial absorption).
No products indexed under this heading.

Probenecid (Increases serum concentration of cefuroxime).
No products indexed under this heading.

Rabeprazole Sodium (Drugs that reduce gastric acidity may result in a lower bioavailability of Ceftin compared with that of fasting state and tend to cancel the effect of postprandial absorption). Products include:
Aciphex Tablets 1053

Ranitidine Hydrochloride (Drugs that reduce gastric acidity may result in a lower bioavailability of Ceftin compared with that of fasting state and tend to cancel the effect of postprandial absorption). Products include:
Zantac 75 Tablets .... ▣ 603
Zantac 1670
Zantac Injection 1666
Zantac Injection Pharmacy Bulk Package 1668
Maximum Strength Zantac 150 Tablets .... ▣ 603
Maximum Strength Zantac 150 Cool Mint Tablets .... ▣ 603

Warfarin Sodium (Cephalosporins may be associated with a fall in prothrombin activity; those at risk include patients previously stabilized on anticoagulant therapy).
No products indexed under this heading.

Food Interactions

Food, unspecified (Absorption is greater when taken after food).

CELEBREX CAPSULES

(Celecoxib) 2979
May interact with ACE inhibitors, antacids containing aluminum, calcium and magnesium, oral anticoagulants, lithium preparations, non-steroidal anti-inflammatory agents, thiazides, and certain other agents. Compounds in these categories include:

Aluminum Carbonate (Co-administration with an aluminum-and-magnesium-containing antacid resulted in a reduction in plasma celecoxib concentration with a decrease of 37% in Cmax and 10% in AUC).
No products indexed under this heading.

Aluminum Hydroxide (Co-administration with an aluminum-and-magnesium-containing antacid resulted in a reduction in plasma celecoxib concentration with a decrease of 37% in Cmax and 10% in AUC).
No products indexed under this heading.

Amiodarone Hydrochloride (Co-administration of celecoxib with drugs known to inhibit CYP4502C9, such as amiodarone, may result in increased plasma concentration; caution should be exercised if used concurrently).
No products indexed under this heading.

Anisindione (Serious bleeding events, some of which were fatal, have been reported, predominately in the elderly, in association with increases in prothrombin time in patients receiving celecoxib concurrently with warfarin. Anticoagulant activity should be monitored, particularly in the first few days, after initiating or changing celecoxib therapy in patients receiving warfarin or similar agents, since these patients are at an increased risk of bleeding complications).
No products indexed under this heading.

Aspirin (Co-administration may result in an increased rate of GI ulceration or other complications; low dose of aspirin can be used with celecoxib). Products include:
Aggrenox Capsules 819
Bayer Aspirin 750
Percodan Tablets 1130
St. Joseph 81 mg Aspirin Chewable and Enteric Coated Tablets 1903

Benazepril Hydrochloride (Co-administration of NSAIDs with ACE inhibitors may result in diminished antihypertensive effect of ACE inhibitors).
No products indexed under this heading.

Bendroflumethiazide (Co-administration of NSAIDs with thiazides may result in reduced natriuretic effect of thiazide diuretics).
No products indexed under this heading.

Captopril (Co-administration of NSAIDs with ACE inhibitors may result in diminished antihypertensive effect of ACE inhibitors). Products include:
Captopril Tablets 2182

Chlorothiazide (Co-administration of NSAIDs with thiazides may result in reduced natriuretic effect of thiazide diuretics).
No products indexed under this heading.

Chlorothiazide Sodium (Co-administration of NSAIDs with thiazides may result in reduced natriuretic effect of thiazide diuretics). Products include:
Intravenous Sodium Diuril 2490

Diclofenac Epolamine (Concomitant use of celecoxib with any dose of a non-aspirin NSAID should be avoided). Products include:
Flector Patch 561

Diclofenac Potassium (Concomitant use of celecoxib with any dose of a non-aspirin NSAID should be avoided).
No products indexed under this heading.

Diclofenac Sodium (Concomitant use of celecoxib with any dose of a non-aspirin NSAID should be avoided). Products include:
Diclofenac Sodium Ophthalmic Solution .... ⊙240
Voltaren Ophthalmic Solution 2336
Voltaren Tablets 2334
Voltaren-XR Tablets 2337

Dicumarol (Serious bleeding events, some of which were fatal, have been reported, predominately in the elderly, in association with increases in prothrombin time in patients receiving celecoxib concurrently with warfarin. Anticoagulant activity should be monitored, particularly in the first few days, after initiating or changing celecoxib therapy in patients receiving warfarin or similar agents, since these patients are at an increased risk of bleeding complications).
No products indexed under this heading.

Enalapril Maleate (Co-administration of NSAIDs with ACE inhibitors may result in diminished antihypertensive effect of ACE inhibitors).
No products indexed under this heading.

Enalaprilat (Co-administration of NSAIDs with ACE inhibitors may result in diminished antihypertensive effect of ACE inhibitors).
No products indexed under this heading.

Etodolac (Concomitant use of celecoxib with any dose of a non-aspirin NSAID should be avoided).
No products indexed under this heading.

Fenoprofen Calcium (Concomitant use of celecoxib with any dose of a non-aspirin NSAID should be avoided). Products include:
Nalfon Capsules 2508

Fluconazole (Co-administration has resulted in a two-fold increase in celecoxib plasma concentration due to inhibition of celecoxib metabolism via P4502C9).
No products indexed under this heading.

Flurbiprofen (Concomitant use of celecoxib with any dose of a non-aspirin NSAID should be avoided).
No products indexed under this heading.

Fosinopril Sodium (Co-administration of NSAIDs with ACE inhibitors may result in diminished antihypertensive effect of ACE inhibitors).
No products indexed under this heading.

Furosemide (Co-administration of NSAIDs with thiazides may result in reduced natriuretic effect of furosemide). Products include:
Furosemide Tablets 2186

Hydrochlorothiazide (Co-administration of NSAIDs with thiazides may result in reduced natriuretic effect of thiazide diuretics). Products include:
Atacand HCT 642
Avalide Tablets 892
Avalide Tablets 2713
Benicar HCT Tablets 1010
Diovan HCT Tablets 2216
Dyazide Capsules 1405
Micardis HCT Tablets 854
Prinzide Tablets 2092
Tekturna HCT Tablets 2324
Teveten HCT Tablets 517

Hydroflumethiazide (Co-administration of NSAIDs with thiazides may result in reduced natriuretic effect of thiazide diuretics).
No products indexed under this heading.

Ibuprofen (Concomitant use of celecoxib with any dose of a non-aspirin NSAID should be avoided). Products include:
Motrin IB Tablets and Caplets 1900
Children's Motrin Oral Suspension ... 1901
Children's Motrin Non-Staining Dye-Free Oral Suspension 1901
Children's Motrin Cold Oral Suspension 1899
Infants' Motrin Concentrated Drops 1901
Infants' Motrin Non-Staining Dye-Free Concentrated Drops 1901
Junior Strength Motrin Caplets and Chewable Tablets 1901
Vicoprofen Tablets 533

Indomethacin (Concomitant use of celecoxib with any dose of a non-aspirin NSAID should be avoided). Products include:
Indocin 2024

Indomethacin Sodium Trihydrate (Concomitant use of celecoxib with any dose of a non-aspirin NSAID should be avoided). Products include:
Indocin I.V. 2489

Itraconazole (Co-administration of celecoxib with drugs known to inhibit CYP4502C9, such as itraconazole, may result in increased plasma concentration; caution should be exercised if used concurrently).
No products indexed under this heading.

Ketoconazole (Co-administration of celecoxib with drugs known to inhibit CYP4502C9, such as ketoconazole, may result in increased plasma concentration; caution should be exercised if used concurrently). Products include:
Extina Foam, 2% 3057
Nizoral A-D Shampoo 1901

Ketoprofen (Concomitant use of celecoxib with any dose of a non-aspirin NSAID should be avoided).
No products indexed under this heading.

Ketorolac Tromethamine (Concomitant use of celecoxib with any dose of a non-aspirin NSAID should be avoided).
No products indexed under this heading.

Lisinopril (Co-administration of NSAIDs with ACE inhibitors may result in diminished antihypertensive effect of ACE inhibitors). Products include:
Prinivil Tablets 2087
Prinzide Tablets 2092

Lithium (Co-administration has resulted in increased steady-state lithium plasma levels).
No products indexed under this heading.

Lithium Carbonate (Co-administration has resulted in increased steady-state lithium plasma levels).
No products indexed under this heading.

Lithium Citrate (Co-administration has resulted in increased steady-state lithium plasma levels).
No products indexed under this heading.

Magaldrate (Co-administration with an aluminum-and-magnesium-containing antacid resulted in a reduction in plasma celecoxib concentration with a decrease of 37% in Cmax and 10% in AUC).
No products indexed under this heading.

Magnesium Hydroxide (Co-administration with an aluminum-and-magnesium-containing antacid resulted in a reduction in plasma celecoxib concentration with a decrease of 37% in Cmax and 10% in AUC). Products include:
Fleet Pedia-Lax Chewable Tablets 1145
Pepcid Complete Chewable Tablets 1771
Extra Strength Rolaids Freshmint Tablets 1903
Rolaids Multi-Symptom Berry Tablets 1903
Rolaids Original Peppermint Tablets 1903

Magnesium Oxide (Co-administration with an aluminum-and-magnesium-containing antacid resulted in a reduction in plasma celecoxib concentration with a decrease of 37% in Cmax and 10% in AUC). Products include:
Beelith Tablets 813

Meclofenamate Sodium (Concomitant use of celecoxib with any dose of a non-aspirin NSAID should be avoided).
No products indexed under this heading.

Mefenamic Acid (Concomitant use of celecoxib with any dose of a non-aspirin NSAID should be avoided).
No products indexed under this heading.

Meloxicam (Concomitant use of celecoxib with any dose of a non-aspirin NSAID should be avoided). Products include:
Mobic Oral Suspension 863
Mobic Tablets 863

Methyclothiazide (Co-administration of NSAIDs with thiazides may result in reduced natriuretic effect of thiazide diuretics).
No products indexed under this heading.

Moexipril Hydrochloride (Co-administration of NSAIDs with ACE inhibitors may result in diminished antihypertensive effect of ACE inhibitors).
No products indexed under this heading.

Nabumetone (Concomitant use of celecoxib with any dose of a non-aspirin NSAID should be avoided).
No products indexed under this heading.

Naproxen (Concomitant use of celecoxib with any dose of a non-aspirin NSAID should be avoided). Products include:
EC-Naprosyn Delayed-Release Tablets 2632
Naprosyn Suspension 2632
Naprosyn Tablets 2632

Naproxen Sodium (Concomitant use of celecoxib with any dose of a non-aspirin NSAID should be avoided). Products include:
Anaprox Tablets 2632
Anaprox DS Tablets 2632
Treximet Tablets 1616

Oxaprozin (Concomitant use of celecoxib with any dose of a non-aspirin NSAID should be avoided).
No products indexed under this heading.

Perindopril Erbumine (Co-administration of NSAIDs with ACE inhibitors may result in diminished antihypertensive effect of ACE inhibitors). Products include:
Aceon Tablets (2 mg, 4 mg, 8 mg) 3038

Phenylbutazone (Concomitant use of celecoxib with any dose of a non-aspirin NSAID should be avoided).
No products indexed under this heading.

Piroxicam (Concomitant use of celecoxib with any dose of a non-aspirin NSAID should be avoided).
No products indexed under this heading.

Polythiazide (Co-administration of NSAIDs with thiazides may result in reduced natriuretic effect of thiazide diuretics).
No products indexed under this heading.

Quinapril Hydrochloride (Co-administration of NSAIDs with ACE inhibitors may result in diminished antihypertensive effect of ACE inhibitors).
No products indexed under this heading.

Ramipril (Co-administration of NSAIDs with ACE inhibitors may result in diminished antihypertensive effect of ACE inhibitors).
No products indexed under this heading.

Rofecoxib (Concomitant use of celecoxib with any dose of a non-aspirin NSAID should be avoided).
No products indexed under this heading.

Spirapril Hydrochloride (Co-administration of NSAIDs with ACE inhibitors may result in diminished antihypertensive effect of ACE inhibitors).
No products indexed under this heading.

Sulindac (Concomitant use of celecoxib with any dose of a non-aspirin NSAID should be avoided). Products include:
Clinoril Tablets 1962

Tolmetin Sodium (Concomitant use of celecoxib with any dose of a non-aspirin NSAID should be avoided).
No products indexed under this heading.

Trandolapril (Co-administration of NSAIDs with ACE inhibitors may result in diminished antihypertensive effect of ACE inhibitors). Products include:
Mavik Tablets 472
Tarka Tablets 511

Valdecoxib (Concomitant use of celecoxib with any dose of a non-aspirin NSAID should be avoided).
No products indexed under this heading.

Warfarin Sodium (Serious bleeding events, some of which were fatal, have been reported, predominately in the elderly, in association with increases in prothrombin time in patients receiving celecoxib concurrently with warfarin. Anticoagulant activity should be monitored,particulary in the first few days, after initiating or changing celecoxib therapy in patients receiving warfarin or similar agents, since these patients are at an increased risk of bleeding complications).
No products indexed under this heading.

Food Interactions

Food, unspecified (Co-administration with a high-fat meal delayed peak plasma levels for about 1 to 2 hours with an increase in total absorption (AUC) of 10% to 20%; Celebrex can be administered without regard to the timing of meals).

CELEXA ORAL SOLUTION

(Citalopram Hydrobromide) 1160
See Celexa Tablets

CELEXA TABLETS

(Citalopram Hydrobromide) 1160
May interact with central nervous system depressants, central nervous system stimulants, anticoagulants, cytochrome p450 2c19 inhibitors (selected), cytochrome p450 3a4 inhibitors (selected), erythromycin, lithium preparations, macrolide antibiotics, monoamine oxidase inhibitors, non-steroidal anti-inflammatory agents, serotoninergic agents, tricyclic antidepressants, triptans, and certain other agents. Compounds in these categories include:

Acetazolamide (In vitro studies indicated that CYP3A4 and CYP2C19 are the primary enzymes involved in the metabolism of citalopram. However, co-administration of citalopram (40 mg) and ketoconazole (200 mg), a potent inhibitor of CYP3A4, did not significantly affect the pharmacokinetics of citalopram. Because citalopram is metabolized by multiple enzyme systems, inhibition of a single enzyme may not appreciably decrease citalopram clearance).
No products indexed under this heading.

Alfentanil Hydrochloride (Given the primary CNS effects of citalopram, caution should be used when it is taken in combination with other centrally acting drugs).
No products indexed under this heading.

Almotriptan Malate (There have been rare post-marketing reports of serotonin syndrome with the use of a SSRI and a triptan. If concomitant treatment of citalopram hydrobromide with a triptan is clinically warranted, careful observation of the patient is advised, particularly during treatment initiation and dose increases). Products include:
Axert Tablets 2431

Alprazolam (Given the primary CNS effects of citalopram, caution should be used when it is taken in combination with other centrally acting drugs).
No products indexed under this heading.

Amiodarone Hydrochloride (In vitro studies indicated that CYP3A4 and CYP2C19 are the primary enzymes involved in the metabolism of citalopram. However, co-administration of citalopram (40 mg) and ketoconazole (200 mg), a potent inhibitor of CYP3A4, did not significantly affect the pharmacokinetics of citalopram. Because citalopram is metabolized by multiple enzyme systems, inhibition of a single enzyme may not appreciably decrease citalopram clearance).
No products indexed under this heading.

Amitriptyline Hydrochloride (Co-administration of imipramine with citalopram has resulted in a 50% increase in active metabolite, desipramine concentration; the clinical significance of these findings is unknown; caution is indicated if tricyclic antidepressants are co-administered with citalopram, a relatively weak inhibitor of CYP2D6).
No products indexed under this heading.

Amoxapine (Co-administration of imipramine with citalopram has resulted in a 50% increase in active metabolite, desipramine concentration; the clinical significance of these findings is unknown; caution is indicated if tricyclic antidepressants are co-administered with citalopram, a relatively weak inhibitor of CYP2D6).
No products indexed under this heading.

Amphetamine Resins (Given the primary CNS effects of citalopram, caution should be used when it is taken in combination with other centrally acting drugs).
No products indexed under this heading.

Amprenavir (In vitro studies indicated that CYP3A4 and CYP2C19 are the primary enzymes involved in the metabolism of citalopram. However, co-administration of citalopram (40 mg) and ketoconazole (200 mg), a potent inhibitor of CYP3A4, did not significantly affect the pharmacokinetics of citalopram. Because citalopram is metabolized by multiple enzyme systems, inhibition of a single enzyme may not appreciably decrease citalopram clearance).
No products indexed under this heading.

Anastrozole (In vitro studies indicated that CYP3A4 and CYP2C19 are the primary enzymes involved in the metabolism of citalopram. However, co-administration of citalopram (40 mg) and ketoconazole (200 mg), a potent inhibitor of CYP3A4, did not significantly affect the pharmacokinetics of citalopram. Because citalopram is metabolized by multiple enzyme systems, inhibition of a single enzyme may not appreciably decrease citalopram clearance). Products include:
Arimidex Tablets 672

Anisindione (The combined use of psychotropic drugs that interfere with serotonin reuptake and drugs that affect coagulation has been associated with an increased risk of bleeding).
No products indexed under this heading.

Aprepitant (In vitro studies indicated that CYP3A4 and CYP2C19 are the primary enzymes involved in the metabolism of citalopram. However, co-administration of citalopram (40 mg) and ketoconazole (200 mg), a potent inhibitor of CYP3A4, did not significantly affect the pharmacokinetics of citalopram. Because citalopram is metabolized by multiple enzyme systems, inhibition of a single enzyme may not appreciably decrease citalopram clearance). Products include:
Emend Capsules 1992

Aprobarbital (Given the primary CNS effects of citalopram, caution should be used when it is taken in combination with other centrally acting drugs).
No products indexed under this heading.

Ardeparin Sodium (The combined use of psychotropic drugs that interfere with serotonin reuptake and drugs that affect coagulation has been associated with an increased risk of bleeding).
No products indexed under this heading.

Aspirin (The combined use of psycotropic drugs that interfere with serotonin reuptake and drugs that affect coagulation has been associated with an increased risk of bleeding; use caution when co-administering). Products include:
Aggrenox Capsules 819
Bayer Aspirin 750
Percodan Tablets 1130
St. Joseph 81 mg Aspirin Chewable and Enteric Coated Tablets 1903

Aspirin, Enteric Coated (The combined use of psycotropic drugs that interfere with serotonin reuptake and drugs that affect coagulation has been associated with an increased risk of bleeding; use caution when co-administering).
No products indexed under this heading.

Aspirin Buffered (The combined use of psycotropic drugs that interfere with serotonin reuptake and drugs that affect coagulation has been associated with an increased risk of bleeding; use caution when co-administering).
No products indexed under this heading.

Atazanavir (In vitro studies indicated that CYP3A4 and CYP2C19 are the primary enzymes involved in the metabolism of citalopram. However, co-administration of citalopram (40 mg) and ketoconazole (200 mg), a potent inhibitor of CYP3A4, did not significantly affect the pharmacokinetics of citalopram. Because citalopram is metabolized by multiple enzyme systems, inhibition of a single enzyme may not appreciably decrease citalopram clearance).
No products indexed under this heading.

Atazanavir Sulfate (In vitro studies indicated that CYP3A4 and CYP2C19 are the primary enzymes involved in the metabolism of citalopram. However, co-administration of citalopram (40 mg) and ketoconazole (200 mg), a potent inhibitor of CYP3A4, did not significantly affect the pharmacokinetics of citalopram. Because citalopram is metabolized by multiple enzyme systems, inhibition of a single enzyme may not appreciably decrease citalopram clearance). Products include:
Reyataz Capsules 3299

Azithromycin Dihydrate (Co-administration with potent inhibitors of CYP3A4, such as macrolide antibiotics, may decrease the clearance of citalopram).
No products indexed under this heading.

Buprenorphine Hydrochloride (Given the primary CNS effects of citalopram, caution should be used when it is taken in combination with other centrally acting drugs). Products include:
Suboxone Tablets 2601
Subutex Tablets 2601

Buspirone Hydrochloride (Given the primary CNS effects of citalopram, caution should be used when it is taken in combination with other centrally acting drugs).
No products indexed under this heading.

Butabarbital (Given the primary CNS effects of citalopram, caution should be used when it is taken in combination with other centrally acting drugs).
No products indexed under this heading.

Butalbital (Given the primary CNS effects of citalopram, caution should be used when it is taken in combination with other centrally acting drugs).
No products indexed under this heading.

Carbamazepine (Given the enzyme inducing properties of carbamazepine, the possibility that carbamazepine might increase the clearance of citalopram should be considered if the two drugs are co-administered; during pharmacokinetic studies, the citalopram levels were unaffected with concurrent use). Products include:
Carbatrol Capsules 3019
Equetro Extended-Release Capsules 3174

Celecoxib (The combined use of psycotropic drugs that interfere with serotonin reuptake and drugs that affect coagulation has been associated with an increased risk of bleeding; use caution when co-administering). Products include:
Celebrex Capsules 2979

Chlordiazepoxide (Given the primary CNS effects of citalopram, caution should be used when it is taken in combination with other centrally acting drugs).
No products indexed under this heading.

Chlordiazepoxide Hydrochloride (Given the primary CNS effects of citalopram, caution should be used when it is taken in combination with other centrally acting drugs).
No products indexed under this heading.

Chlorpromazine (Given the primary CNS effects of citalopram, caution should be used when it is taken in combination with other centrally acting drugs).
No products indexed under this heading.

Chlorpromazine Hydrochloride (Given the primary CNS effects of citalopram, caution should be used when it is taken in combination with other centrally acting drugs).
No products indexed under this heading.

Chlorprothixene (Given the primary CNS effects of citalopram, caution should be used when it is taken in combination with other centrally acting drugs).
No products indexed under this heading.

Chlorprothixene Hydrochloride (Given the primary CNS effects of citalopram, caution should be used when it is taken in combination with other centrally acting drugs).
No products indexed under this heading.

Chlorprothixene Lactate (Given the primary CNS effects of citalopram, caution should be used when it is taken in combination with other centrally acting drugs).
No products indexed under this heading.

Cimetidine (Co-administration has resulted in an increase in citalopram AUC and Cmax by 43% and 39% respectively; the clinical significance of these findings is unknown).
No products indexed under this heading.

Cimetidine Hydrochloride (Co-administration has resulted in an increase in citalopram AUC and Cmax by 43% and 39% respectively; the clinical significance of these findings is unknown).
No products indexed under this heading.

Ciprofloxacin (In vitro studies indicated that CYP3A4 and CYP2C19 are the primary enzymes involved in the metabolism of citalopram. However, co-administration of citalopram (40 mg) and ketoconazole (200 mg), a potent inhibitor of CYP3A4, did not significantly affect the pharmacokinetics of citalopram. Because citalopram is metabolized by multiple enzyme systems, inhibition of a single enzyme may not appreciably decrease citalopram clearance). Products include:
Cipro I.V. 2817
Cipro Oral Suspension 2810
Cipro XR Tablets 2823
Ciprodex Otic Suspension 541

Clarithromycin (Co-administration with potent inhibitors of CYP3A4, such as macrolide antibiotics, may decrease the clearance of citalopram). Products include:
Biaxin/Biaxin XL 411

Clomipramine Hydrochloride (Co-administration of imipramine with citalopram has resulted in a 50% increase in active metabolite, desipramine concentration; the clinical significance of these findings is unknown; caution is indicated if tricyclic antidepressants are co-administered with citalopram, a relatively weak inhibitor of CYP2D6).
No products indexed under this heading.

Clorazepate Dipotassium (Given the primary CNS effects of citalopram, caution should be used when it is taken in combination with other centrally acting drugs).
No products indexed under this heading.

Clotrimazole (In vitro studies indicated that CYP3A4 and CYP2C19 are the primary enzymes involved in the metabolism of citalopram. However, co-administration of citalopram (40 mg) and ketoconazole (200 mg), a potent inhibitor of CYP3A4, did not significantly affect the pharmacokinetics of citalopram. Because citalopram is metabolized by multiple enzyme systems, inhibition of a single enzyme may not appreciably decrease citalopram clearance). Products include:
Lotrisone 2881

Clozapine (Given the primary CNS effects of citalopram, caution should be used when it is taken in combination with other centrally acting drugs).
No products indexed under this heading.

Codeine Phosphate (Given the primary CNS effects of citalopram, caution should be used when it is taken in combination with other centrally acting drugs). Products include:
Tylenol with Codeine Tablets 2427

Cyclosporine (In vitro studies indicated that CYP3A4 and CYP2C19 are the primary enzymes involved in the metabolism of citalopram. However, co-administration of citalopram (40 mg) and ketoconazole (200 mg), a potent inhibitor of CYP3A4, did not significantly affect the pharmacokinetics of citalopram. Because citalopram is metabolized by multiple enzyme systems, inhibition of a single enzyme may not appreciably decrease citalopram clearance). Products include:
Gengraf Capsules 435
Neoral Oral Solution 2280
Neoral Soft Gelatin Capsules 2280
Restasis Ophthalmic Emulsion 557
Sandimmune 2296

Dalfopristin (In vitro studies indicated that CYP3A4 and CYP2C19 are the primary enzymes involved in the metabolism of citalopram. However, co-administration of citalopram (40 mg) and ketoconazole (200 mg), a potent inhibitor of CYP3A4, did not significantly affect the pharmacokinetics of citalopram. Because citalopram is metabolized by multiple enzyme systems, inhibition of a single enzyme may not appreciably decrease citalopram clearance).
No products indexed under this heading.

Dalteparin Sodium (The combined use of psychotropic drugs that interfere with serotonin reuptake and drugs that affect coagulation has been associated with an increased risk of bleeding). Products include:
Fragmin Injection 1070

Danaparoid Sodium (The combined use of psychotropic drugs that interfere with serotonin reuptake and drugs that affect coagulation has been associated with an increased risk of bleeding).
No products indexed under this heading.

Danazol (In vitro studies indicated that CYP3A4 and CYP2C19 are the primary enzymes involved in the metabolism of citalopram. However, co-administration of citalopram (40 mg) and ketoconazole (200 mg), a potent inhibitor of CYP3A4, did not significantly affect the pharmacokinetics of citalopram. Because citalopram is metabolized by multiple enzyme systems, inhibition of a single enzyme may not appreciably decrease citalopram clearance).
No products indexed under this heading.

Delavirdine Mesylate (In vitro studies indicated that CYP3A4 and CYP2C19 are the primary enzymes involved in the metabolism of citalopram. However, co-administration of citalopram (40 mg) and ketoconazole (200 mg), a potent inhibitor of CYP3A4, did not significantly affect the pharmacokinetics of citalopram. Because citalopram is metabolized by multiple enzyme systems, inhibition of a single enzyme may not appreciably decrease citalopram clearance).
No products indexed under this heading.

Desflurane (Given the primary CNS effects of citalopram, caution should be used when it is taken in combination with other centrally acting drugs).
No products indexed under this heading.

Desipramine Hydrochloride (Co-administration of imipramine with citalopram has resulted in a 50% increase in active metabolite, desipramine concentration; the clinical significance of these findings is unknown; caution is indicated if tricyclic antidepressants are co-administered with citalopram, a relatively weak inhibitor of CYP2D6).
No products indexed under this heading.

Desogestrel (In vitro studies indicated that CYP3A4 and CYP2C19 are the primary enzymes involved in the metabolism of citalopram. However, co-administration of citalopram (40 mg) and ketoconazole (200 mg), a potent inhibitor of CYP3A4, did not significantly affect the pharmacokinetics of citalopram. Because citalopram is metabolized by multiple enzyme systems, inhibition of a single enzyme may not appreciably decrease citalopram clearance). Products include:
Mircette Tablets 1034

Dextroamphetamine Sulfate (Given the primary CNS effects of citalopram, caution should be used when it is taken in combination with other centrally acting drugs). Products include:
Adderall XR Capsules 3012
Dexedrine 1401

Dezocine (Given the primary CNS effects of citalopram, caution should be used when it is taken in combination with other centrally acting drugs).
No products indexed under this heading.

Diazepam (Given the primary CNS effects of citalopram, caution should be used when it is taken in combination with other centrally acting drugs). Products include:
Valium Tablets 2658

Diclofenac Epolamine (The combined use of psycotropic drugs that interfere with serotonin reuptake and drugs that affect coagulation has been associated with an increased risk of bleeding; use caution when co-administering). Products include:
Flector Patch 561

Diclofenac Potassium (The combined use of psycotropic drugs that interfere with serotonin reuptake and drugs that affect coagulation has been associated with an increased risk of bleeding; use caution when co-administering).
No products indexed under this heading.

Diclofenac Sodium (The combined use of psycotropic drugs that interfere with serotonin reuptake and drugs that affect coagulation has been associated with an increased risk of bleeding; use caution when co-administering). Products include:
Diclofenac Sodium Ophthalmic Solution .... ⊙ 240
Voltaren Ophthalmic Solution 2336
Voltaren Tablets 2334
Voltaren-XR Tablets 2337

Dicumarol (The combined use of psychotropic drugs that interfere with serotonin reuptake and drugs that affect coagulation has been associated with an increased risk of bleeding).
No products indexed under this heading.

Digoxin (In subjects who had received 21 days of 40 mg/day citalopram hydrobromide, combined

administration of citalopram hydrobromide and digoxin (single dose of 1 mg) did not significantly affect the pharmacokinetics of either citalopram or digoxin). Products include:

Lanoxin Injection ... 1498
Lanoxin Injection Pediatric ... 1502
Lanoxin Tablets ... 1505

Diltiazem Hydrochloride (In vitro studies indicated that CYP3A4 and CYP2C19 are the primary enzymes involved in the metabolism of citalopram. However, co-administration of citalopram (40 mg) and ketoconazole (200 mg), a potent inhibitor of CYP3A4, did not significantly affect the pharmacokinetics of citalopram. Because citalopram is metabolized by multiple enzyme systems, inhibition of a single enzyme may not appreciably decrease citalopram clearance). Products include:

Cardizem LA Extended Release Tablets ... 421

Diltiazem Maleate (In vitro studies indicated that CYP3A4 and CYP2C19 are the primary enzymes involved in the metabolism of citalopram. However, co-administration of citalopram (40 mg) and ketoconazole (200 mg), a potent inhibitor of CYP3A4, did not significantly affect the pharmacokinetics of citalopram. Because citalopram is metabolized by multiple enzyme systems, inhibition of a single enzyme may not appreciably decrease citalopram clearance).

No products indexed under this heading.

Dirithromycin (Co-administration with potent inhibitors of CYP3A4, such as macrolide antibiotics, may decrease the clearance of citalopram).

No products indexed under this heading.

Doxepin Hydrochloride (Co-administration of imipramine with citalopram has resulted in a 50% increase in active metabolite, desipramine concentration; the clinical significance of these findings is unknown; caution is indicated if tricyclic antidepressants are co-administered with citalopram, a relatively weak inhibitor of CYP2D6).

No products indexed under this heading.

Droperidol (Given the primary CNS effects of citalopram, caution should be used when it is taken in combination with other centrally acting drugs).

No products indexed under this heading.

Efavirenz (In vitro studies indicated that CYP3A4 and CYP2C19 are the primary enzymes involved in the metabolism of citalopram. However, co-administration of citalopram (40 mg) and ketoconazole (200 mg), a potent inhibitor of CYP3A4, did not significantly affect the pharmacokinetics of citalopram. Because citalopram is metabolized by multiple enzyme systems, inhibition of a single enzyme may not appreciably decrease citalopram clearance). Products include:

Atripla Tablets ... 938
Sustiva Capsules ... 930
Sustiva Tablets ... 930

Eletriptan Hydrobromide (There have been rare post-marketing reports of serotonin syndrome with the use of a SSRI and a triptan. If concomitant treatment of citalopram hydrobromide with a triptan is clinically warranted, careful observation of the patient is advised, particularly during treatment initiation and dose increases).

No products indexed under this heading.

Enflurane (Given the primary CNS effects of citalopram, caution should be used when it is taken in combination with other centrally acting drugs).

No products indexed under this heading.

Enoxaparin Sodium (The combined use of psychotropic drugs that interfere with serotonin reuptake and drugs that affect coagulation has been associated with an increased risk of bleeding). Products include:

Lovenox Injection ... 2756

Erythromycin (Co-administration with potent inhibitors of CYP3A4, such as macrolide antibiotics, may decrease the clearance of citalopram).

No products indexed under this heading.

Erythromycin Estolate (Co-administration with potent inhibitors of CYP3A4, such as macrolide antibiotics, may decrease the clearance of citalopram).

No products indexed under this heading.

Erythromycin Ethylsuccinate (Co-administration with potent inhibitors of CYP3A4, such as macrolide antibiotics, may decrease the clearance of citalopram). Products include:

E.E.S. ... 433
EryPed ... 431

Erythromycin Gluceptate (Co-administration with potent inhibitors of CYP3A4, such as macrolide antibiotics, may decrease the clearance of citalopram).

No products indexed under this heading.

Erythromycin Lactobionate (Co-administration with potent inhibitors of CYP3A4, such as erythromycin, may decrease the clearance of citalopram).

No products indexed under this heading.

Erythromycin Stearate (Co-administration with potent inhibitors of CYP3A4, such as macrolide antibiotics, may decrease the clearance of citalopram).

No products indexed under this heading.

Escitalopram Oxalate (Development of a potentially life-threatening serotonin syndrome may occur with SSRIs, particularly with concomitant use of serotinergic drugs, including triptans. Caution is advised when citalopram hydrobromide is co-administered with other drugs that may affect the serotinergic neurotransmitter systems). Products include:

Lexapro Oral Suspension ... 1174
Lexapro Tablets ... 1174

Esomeprazole Magnesium (In vitro studies indicated that CYP3A4 and CYP2C19 are the primary enzymes involved in the metabolism of citalopram. However, co-administration of citalopram (40 mg) and ketoconazole (200 mg), a potent inhibitor of CYP3A4, did not significantly affect the pharmacokinetics of citalopram. Because citalopram is metabolized by multiple enzyme systems, inhibition of a single enzyme may not appreciably decrease citalopram clearance). Products include:

Nexium Delayed-Release Capsules ... 645
Nexium Delayed-Release Oral Suspension ... 645

Estazolam (Given the primary CNS effects of citalopram, caution should be used when it is taken in combination with other centrally acting drugs).

No products indexed under this heading.

Ethanol (Given the primary CNS effects of citalopram, caution should be used when it is taken in combination with other centrally acting drugs).

No products indexed under this heading.

Ethchlorvynol (Given the primary CNS effects of citalopram, caution should be used when it is taken in combination with other centrally acting drugs).

No products indexed under this heading.

Ethinamate (Given the primary CNS effects of citalopram, caution should be used when it is taken in combination with other centrally acting drugs).

No products indexed under this heading.

Ethinyl Estradiol (In vitro studies indicated that CYP3A4 and CYP2C19 are the primary enzymes involved in the metabolism of citalopram. However, co-administration of citalopram (40 mg) and ketoconazole (200 mg), a potent inhibitor of CYP3A4, did not significantly affect the pharmacokinetics of citalopram. Because citalopram is metabolized by multiple enzyme systems, inhibition of a single enzyme may not appreciably decrease citalopram clearance). Products include:

Lybrel Tablets ... 3204
Mircette Tablets ... 1034
NuvaRing ... 2897
Ortho-Cyclen/Ortho Tri-Cyclen ... 2449
Ortho Evra Transdermal System ... 2437
Ortho Tri-Cyclen Lo Tablets ... 2458
Seasonique Tablets ... 1046
Yaz Tablets ... 805

Ethyl Alcohol (Given the primary CNS effects of citalopram, caution should be used when it is taken in combination with other centrally acting drugs).

No products indexed under this heading.

Ethynodiol Diacetate (In vitro studies indicated that CYP3A4 and CYP2C19 are the primary enzymes involved in the metabolism of citalopram. However, co-administration of citalopram (40 mg) and ketoconazole (200 mg), a potent inhibitor of CYP3A4, did not significantly affect the pharmacokinetics of citalopram. Because citalopram is metabolized by multiple enzyme systems, inhibition of a single enzyme may not appreciably decrease citalopram clearance).

No products indexed under this heading.

Etodolac (The combined use of psycotropic drugs that interfere with serotonin reuptake and drugs that affect coagulation has been associated with an increased risk of bleeding; use caution when co-administering).

No products indexed under this heading.

Felbamate (In vitro studies indicated that CYP3A4 and CYP2C19 are the primary enzymes involved in the metabolism of citalopram. However, co-administration of citalopram (40 mg) and ketoconazole (200 mg), a potent inhibitor of CYP3A4, did not significantly affect the pharmacokinetics of citalopram. Because citalopram is metabolized by multiple enzyme systems, inhibition of a single enzyme may not appreciably decrease citalopram clearance).

No products indexed under this heading.

Fenoprofen Calcium (The combined use of psycotropic drugs that interfere with serotonin reuptake and drugs that affect coagulation has been associated with an increased risk of bleeding; use caution when co-administering). Products include:

Nalfon Capsules ... 2508

Fentanyl (Given the primary CNS effects of citalopram, caution should be used when it is taken in combination with other centrally acting drugs). Products include:

Duragesic Transdermal System ... 2405
Ionsys Transdermal System ... 2410

Fentanyl Citrate (Given the primary CNS effects of citalopram, caution should be used when it is taken in combination with other centrally acting drugs). Products include:

Actiq ... 959
Fentora Tablets ... 968

Fluconazole (Co-administration with potent inhibitors of CYP3A4, such as fluconazole, may decrease the clearance of citalopram).

No products indexed under this heading.

Fluoxetine (In vitro studies indicated that CYP3A4 and CYP2C19 are the primary enzymes involved in the metabolism of citalopram. However, co-administration of citalopram (40 mg) and ketoconazole (200 mg), a potent inhibitor of CYP3A4, did not significantly affect the pharmacokinetics of citalopram. Because citalopram is metabolized by multiple enzyme systems, inhibition of a single enzyme may not appreciably decrease citalopram clearance).

No products indexed under this heading.

Fluoxetine Hydrochloride (Development of a potentially life-threatening serotonin syndrome may occur with SSRIs, particularly with concomitant use of serotinergic drugs, including triptans. Caution is advised when citalopram hydrobromide is co-administered with other drugs that may affect the serotinergic neurotransmitter systems). Products include:

Prozac Weekly Capsules ... 1852
Prozac Pulvules and Liquid ... 1852
Symbyax Capsules ... 1871

Fluphenazine Decanoate (Given the primary CNS effects of citalopram, caution should be used when it is taken in combination with other centrally acting drugs).
No products indexed under this heading.

Fluphenazine Enanthate (Given the primary CNS effects of citalopram, caution should be used when it is taken in combination with other centrally acting drugs).
No products indexed under this heading.

Fluphenazine Hydrochloride (Given the primary CNS effects of citalopram, caution should be used when it is taken in combination with other centrally acting drugs).
No products indexed under this heading.

Flurazepam Hydrochloride (Given the primary CNS effects of citalopram, caution should be used when it is taken in combination with other centrally acting drugs).
No products indexed under this heading.

Flurbiprofen (The combined use of psycotropic drugs that interfere with serotonin reuptake and drugs that affect coagulation has been associated with an increased risk of bleeding; use caution when co-administering).
No products indexed under this heading.

Fluvastatin Sodium (In vitro studies indicated that CYP3A4 and CYP2C19 are the primary enzymes involved in the metabolism of citalopram. However, co-administration of citalopram (40 mg) and ketoconazole (200 mg), a potent inhibitor of CYP3A4, did not significantly affect the pharmacokinetics of citalopram. Because citalopram is metabolized by multiple enzyme systems, inhibition of a single enzyme may not appreciably decrease citalopram clearance). Products include:
Lescol Capsules ... 2268
Lescol XL Tablets ... 2268

Fluvoxamine (In vitro studies indicated that CYP3A4 and CYP2C19 are the primary enzymes involved in the metabolism of citalopram. However, co-administration of citalopram (40 mg) and ketoconazole (200 mg), a potent inhibitor of CYP3A4, did not significantly affect the pharmacokinetics of citalopram. Because citalopram is metabolized by multiple enzyme systems, inhibition of a single enzyme may not appreciably decrease citalopram clearance).
No products indexed under this heading.

Fluvoxamine Maleate (Development of a potentially life-threatening serotonin syndrome may occur with SSRIs, particularly with concomitant use of serotinergic drugs, including triptans. Caution is advised when citalopram hydrobromide is co-administered with other drugs that may affect the serotinergic neurotransmitter systems). Products include:
Luvox CR Extended-Release Capsules ... 1759

Fondaparinux Sodium (The combined use of psychotropic drugs that interfere with serotonin reuptake and drugs that affect coagulation has been associated with an increased risk of bleeding). Products include:
Arixtra Injection ... 1313

Fosamprenavir Calcium (In vitro studies indicated that CYP3A4 and CYP2C19 are the primary enzymes involved in the metabolism of citalopram. However, co-administration of citalopram (40 mg) and ketoconazole (200 mg), a potent inhibitor of CYP3A4, did not significantly affect the pharmacokinetics of citalopram. Because citalopram is metabolized by multiple enzyme systems, inhibition of a single enzyme may not appreciably decrease citalopram clearance). Products include:
Lexiva Oral Suspension ... 1510
Lexiva Tablets ... 1510

Frovatriptan Succinate (There have been rare post-marketing reports of serotonin syndrome with the use of a SSRI and a triptan. If concomitant treatment of citalopram hydrobromide with a triptan is clinically warranted, careful observation of the patient is advised, particularly during treatment initiation and dose increases). Products include:
Frova Tablets ... 1111

Glutethimide (Given the primary CNS effects of citalopram, caution should be used when it is taken in combination with other centrally acting drugs).
No products indexed under this heading.

Haloperidol (Given the primary CNS effects of citalopram, caution should be used when it is taken in combination with other centrally acting drugs).
No products indexed under this heading.

Haloperidol Decanoate (Given the primary CNS effects of citalopram, caution should be used when it is taken in combination with other centrally acting drugs).
No products indexed under this heading.

Heparin Calcium (The combined use of psychotropic drugs that interfere with serotonin reuptake and drugs that affect coagulation has been associated with an increased risk of bleeding).
No products indexed under this heading.

Heparin Sodium (The combined use of psychotropic drugs that interfere with serotonin reuptake and drugs that affect coagulation has been associated with an increased risk of bleeding).
No products indexed under this heading.

Hydrocodone Bitartrate (Given the primary CNS effects of citalopram, caution should be used when it is taken in combination with other centrally acting drugs). Products include:
Lortab 5/500 Tablets ... 3143
Lortab 7.5/500 Tablets ... 3144
Lortab 10/500 Tablets ... 3144
Vicodin Tablets ... 529
Vicodin ES Tablets ... 530
Vicodin HP Tablets ... 531
Vicoprofen Tablets ... 533
Zydone Tablets ... 1132

Hydrocodone Polistirex (Given the primary CNS effects of citalopram, caution should be used when it is taken in combination with other centrally acting drugs). Products include:
Tussionex Pennkinetic Extended-Release Suspension ... 3154

Hydromorphone Hydrochloride (Given the primary CNS effects of citalopram, caution should be used when it is taken in combination with other centrally acting drugs).
No products indexed under this heading.

Hydroxyzine Hydrochloride (Given the primary CNS effects of citalopram, caution should be used when it is taken in combination with other centrally acting drugs).
No products indexed under this heading.

Hypericum (There is a risk of serotonin syndrome with concomitant use of citalopram hydrobromide and tramadol. Caution is advised when citalopram hydrobromide is co-administered with other drugs that may affect the serotinergic neurotransmitter systems, such as St. John's Wort). Products include:
Satieté Tablets ... 640

Ibuprofen (The combined use of psycotropic drugs that interfere with serotonin reuptake and drugs that affect coagulation has been associated with an increased risk of bleeding; use caution when co-administering). Products include:
Motrin IB Tablets and Caplets ... 1900
Children's Motrin Oral Suspension ... 1901
Children's Motrin Non-Staining Dye-Free Oral Suspension ... 1901
Children's Motrin Cold Oral Suspension ... 1899
Infants' Motrin Concentrated Drops ... 1901
Infants' Motrin Non-Staining Dye-Free Concentrated Drops ... 1901
Junior Strength Motrin Caplets and Chewable Tablets ... 1901
Vicoprofen Tablets ... 533

Imipramine Hydrochloride (Co-administration of imipramine with citalopram has resulted in a 50% increase in active metabolite, desipramine concentration; the clinical significance of these findings is unknown; caution is indicated if tricyclic antidepressants are co-administered with citalopram, a relatively weak inhibitor of CYP2D6).
No products indexed under this heading.

Imipramine Pamoate (Co-administration of imipramine with citalopram has resulted in a 50% increase in active metabolite, desipramine concentration; the clinical significance of these findings is unknown; caution is indicated if tricyclic antidepressants are co-administered with citalopram, a relatively weak inhibitor of CYP2D6).
No products indexed under this heading.

Indinavir Sulfate (In vitro studies indicated that CYP3A4 and CYP2C19 are the primary enzymes involved in the metabolism of citalopram. However, co-administration of citalopram (40 mg) and ketoconazole (200 mg), a potent inhibitor of CYP3A4, did not significantly affect the pharmacokinetics of citalopram. Because citalopram is metabolized by multiple enzyme systems, inhibition of a single enzyme may not appreciably decrease citalopram clearance). Products include:
Crixivan Capsules ... 1979

Indomethacin (The combined use of psycotropic drugs that interfere with serotonin reuptake and drugs that affect coagulation has been associated with an increased risk of bleeding; use caution when co-administering). Products include:
Indocin ... 2024

Indomethacin Sodium Trihydrate (The combined use of psycotropic drugs that interfere with serotonin reuptake and drugs that affect coagulation has been associated with an increased risk of bleeding; use caution when co-administering). Products include:
Indocin I.V. ... 2489

Isocarboxazid (Co-administration of serotonin reuptake inhibitors and MAO inhibitors has resulted in serious, sometimes fatal, reactions including hyperthermia, rigidity, myoclonus, serotonin syndrome, and other potentially serious adverse reactions; concurrent and/or sequential use is contraindicated). Products include:
Marplan Tablets ... 3177

Isoflurane (Given the primary CNS effects of citalopram, caution should be used when it is taken in combination with other centrally acting drugs).
No products indexed under this heading.

Isoniazid (In vitro studies indicated that CYP3A4 and CYP2C19 are the primary enzymes involved in the metabolism of citalopram. However, co-administration of citalopram (40 mg) and ketoconazole (200 mg), a potent inhibitor of CYP3A4, did not significantly affect the pharmacokinetics of citalopram. Because citalopram is metabolized by multiple enzyme systems, inhibition of a single enzyme may not appreciably decrease citalopram clearance).
No products indexed under this heading.

Itraconazole (Co-administration with potent inhibitors of CYP3A4, such as itraconazole, may decrease the clearance of citalopram).
No products indexed under this heading.

Ketamine Hydrochloride (Given the primary CNS effects of citalopram, caution should be used when it is taken in combination with other centrally acting drugs).
No products indexed under this heading.

Ketoconazole (Co-administration resulted in decreased Cmax and AUC of ketoconazole by 21% and 10% respectively, and did not significantly affect the pharmacokinetics of citalopram). Products include:
Extina Foam, 2% ... 3057
Nizoral A-D Shampoo ... 1901

Ketoprofen (The combined use of psycotropic drugs that interfere with serotonin reuptake and drugs that affect coagulation has been associated with an increased risk of bleeding; use caution when co-administering).
No products indexed under this heading.

Ketorolac Tromethamine (The combined use of psycotropic drugs that interfere with serotonin reuptake and drugs that affect coagulation has been associated with an increased risk of bleeding; use caution when co-administering).
No products indexed under this heading.

Lansoprazole (In vitro studies indicated that CYP3A4 and CYP2C19

IMPORTANT NOTE: Always consult each drug listing in the patient's regimen for possible interactions.

are the primary enzymes involved in the metabolism of citalopram. However, co-administration of citalopram (40 mg) and ketoconazole (200 mg), a potent inhibitor of CYP3A4, did not significantly affect the pharmacokinetics of citalopram. Because citalopram is metabolized by multiple enzyme systems, inhibition of a single enzyme may not appreciably decrease citalopram clearance).
No products indexed under this heading.

Letrozole (In vitro studies indicated that CYP3A4 and CYP2C19 are the primary enzymes involved in the metabolism of citalopram. However, co-administration of citalopram (40 mg) and ketoconazole (200 mg), a potent inhibitor of CYP3A4, did not significantly affect the pharmacokinetics of citalopram. Because citalopram is metabolized by multiple enzyme systems, inhibition of a single enzyme may not appreciably decrease citalopram clearance). Products include:
Femara Tablets 2246

Levomethadyl Acetate Hydrochloride (Given the primary CNS effects of citalopram, caution should be used when it is taken in combination with other centrally acting drugs).
No products indexed under this heading.

Levonorgestrel (In vitro studies indicated that CYP3A4 and CYP2C19 are the primary enzymes involved in the metabolism of citalopram. However, co-administration of citalopram (40 mg) and ketoconazole (200 mg), a potent inhibitor of CYP3A4, did not significantly affect the pharmacokinetics of citalopram. Because citalopram is metabolized by multiple enzyme systems, inhibition of a single enzyme may not appreciably decrease citalopram clearance). Products include:
Climara Pro Transdermal System 768
Lybrel Tablets 3204
Mirena Intrauterine System 779
Plan B Tablets 1044
Seasonique Tablets 1046

Levorphanol Tartrate (Given the primary CNS effects of citalopram, caution should be used when it is taken in combination with other centrally acting drugs).
No products indexed under this heading.

Linezolid (There is a risk of serotonin syndrome with concomitant use of citalopram hydrobromide and tramadol. Caution is advised when citalopram hydrobromide is co-administered with other drugs that may affect the serotinergic neurotransmitter systems, such as linezolid). Products include:
Zyvox 2552

Lithium (There is a risk of serotonin syndrome with concomitant use of citalopram hydrobromide and tramadol. Caution is advised when citalopram hydrobromide is co-administered with other drugs that may affect the serotinergic neurotransmitter systems, such as lithium).
No products indexed under this heading.

Lithium Carbonate (There is a risk of serotonin syndrome with concomitant use of citalopram hydrobromide and tramadol. Caution is advised when citalopram hydrobromide is co-administered with other drugs that may affect the serotinergic neurotransmitter systems, such as lithium).
No products indexed under this heading.

Lithium Citrate (There is a risk of serotonin syndrome with concomitant use of citalopram hydrobromide and tramadol. Caution is advised when citalopram hydrobromide is co-administered with other drugs that may affect the serotinergic neurotransmitter systems, such as lithium).
No products indexed under this heading.

Lopinavir (In vitro studies indicated that CYP3A4 and CYP2C19 are the primary enzymes involved in the metabolism of citalopram. However, co-administration of citalopram (40 mg) and ketoconazole (200 mg), a potent inhibitor of CYP3A4, did not significantly affect the pharmacokinetics of citalopram. Because citalopram is metabolized by multiple enzyme systems, inhibition of a single enzyme may not appreciably decrease citalopram clearance). Products include:
Kaletra 452

Loratadine (In vitro studies indicated that CYP3A4 and CYP2C19 are the primary enzymes involved in the metabolism of citalopram. However, co-administration of citalopram (40 mg) and ketoconazole (200 mg), a potent inhibitor of CYP3A4, did not significantly affect the pharmacokinetics of citalopram. Because citalopram is metabolized by multiple enzyme systems, inhibition of a single enzyme may not appreciably decrease citalopram clearance).
No products indexed under this heading.

Lorazepam (Given the primary CNS effects of citalopram, caution should be used when it is taken in combination with other centrally acting drugs).
No products indexed under this heading.

Low Molecular Weight Heparins (The combined use of psychotropic drugs that interfere with serotonin reuptake and drugs that affect coagulation has been associated with an increased risk of bleeding).
No products indexed under this heading.

Loxapine Hydrochloride (Given the primary CNS effects of citalopram, caution should be used when it is taken in combination with other centrally acting drugs).
No products indexed under this heading.

Loxapine Succinate (Given the primary CNS effects of citalopram, caution should be used when it is taken in combination with other centrally acting drugs).
No products indexed under this heading.

Maprotiline Hydrochloride (Co-administration of imipramine with citalopram has resulted in a 50% increase in active metabolite, desipramine concentration; the clinical significance of these findings is unknown; caution is indicated if tricyclic antidepressants are co-administered with citalopram, a relatively weak inhibitor of CYP2D6).
No products indexed under this heading.

Meclofenamate Sodium (The combined use of psycotropic drugs that interfere with serotonin reuptake and drugs that affect coagulation has been associated with an increased risk of bleeding; use caution when co-administering).
No products indexed under this heading.

Mefenamic Acid (The combined use of psycotropic drugs that interfere with serotonin reuptake and drugs that affect coagulation has been associated with an increased risk of bleeding; use caution when co-administering).
No products indexed under this heading.

Meloxicam (The combined use of psycotropic drugs that interfere with serotonin reuptake and drugs that affect coagulation has been associated with an increased risk of bleeding; use caution when co-administering). Products include:
Mobic Oral Suspension 863
Mobic Tablets 863

Meperidine Hydrochloride (Given the primary CNS effects of citalopram, caution should be used when it is taken in combination with other centrally acting drugs).
No products indexed under this heading.

Mephobarbital (Given the primary CNS effects of citalopram, caution should be used when it is taken in combination with other centrally acting drugs).
No products indexed under this heading.

Meprobamate (Given the primary CNS effects of citalopram, caution should be used when it is taken in combination with other centrally acting drugs).
No products indexed under this heading.

Mesoridazine Besylate (Given the primary CNS effects of citalopram, caution should be used when it is taken in combination with other centrally acting drugs).
No products indexed under this heading.

Mestranol (In vitro studies indicated that CYP3A4 and CYP2C19 are the primary enzymes involved in the metabolism of citalopram. However, co-administration of citalopram (40 mg) and ketoconazole (200 mg), a potent inhibitor of CYP3A4, did not significantly affect the pharmacokinetics of citalopram. Because citalopram is metabolized by multiple enzyme systems, inhibition of a single enzyme may not appreciably decrease citalopram clearance).
No products indexed under this heading.

Methadone Hydrochloride (Given the primary CNS effects of citalopram, caution should be used when it is taken in combination with other centrally acting drugs).
No products indexed under this heading.

Methamphetamine Hydrochloride (Given the primary CNS effects of citalopram, caution should be used when it is taken in combination with other centrally acting drugs).
No products indexed under this heading.

Methohexital Sodium (Given the primary CNS effects of citalopram, caution should be used when it is taken in combination with other centrally acting drugs).
No products indexed under this heading.

Methotrimeprazine (Given the primary CNS effects of citalopram, caution should be used when it is taken in combination with other centrally acting drugs).
No products indexed under this heading.

Methoxyflurane (Given the primary CNS effects of citalopram, caution should be used when it is taken in combination with other centrally acting drugs).
No products indexed under this heading.

Methylphenidate (Given the primary CNS effects of citalopram, caution should be used when it is taken in combination with other centrally acting drugs). Products include:
Daytrana Transdermal Patch 3022

Methylphenidate Hydrochloride (Given the primary CNS effects of citalopram, caution should be used when it is taken in combination with other centrally acting drugs). Products include:
Concerta Extended-Release Tablets 1925
Metadate CD Capsules 3146

Metoprolol Succinate (Co-administration has resulted in a two-fold increase in the plasma levels of metoprolol; increased plasma levels of metoprolol have been associated with decreased cardioselectivity; no clinically significant effects on the blood pressure or heart rate have been reported with concurrent use). Products include:
Toprol-XL Tablets 666

Metoprolol Tartrate (Co-administration has resulted in a two-fold increase in the plasma levels of metoprolol; increased plasma levels of metoprolol have been associated with decreased cardioselectivity; no clinically significant effects on the blood pressure or heart rate have been reported with concurrent use).
No products indexed under this heading.

Metronidazole (In vitro studies indicated that CYP3A4 and CYP2C19 are the primary enzymes involved in the metabolism of citalopram. However, co-administration of citalopram (40 mg) and ketoconazole (200 mg), a potent inhibitor of CYP3A4, did not significantly affect the pharmacokinetics of citalopram. Because citalopram is metabolized by multiple enzyme systems, inhibition of a single enzyme may not appreciably decrease citalopram clearance). Products include:
Pylera Capsules 714

Metronidazole Benzoate (In vitro studies indicated that CYP3A4 and CYP2C19 are the primary enzymes involved in the metabolism of citalopram. However, co-administration of citalopram (40 mg) and ketoconazole (200 mg), a potent inhibitor of CYP3A4, did not significantly affect the pharmacokinetics of citalopram. Because citalopram is metabolized by multiple enzyme systems, inhibition of a single enzyme may not appreciably decrease citalopram clearance).

No products indexed under this heading.

Metronidazole Hydrochloride (In vitro studies indicated that CYP3A4 and CYP2C19 are the primary enzymes involved in the metabolism of citalopram. However, co-administration of citalopram (40 mg) and ketoconazole (200 mg), a potent inhibitor of CYP3A4, did not significantly affect the pharmacokinetics of citalopram. Because citalopram is metabolized by multiple enzyme systems, inhibition of a single enzyme may not appreciably decrease citalopram clearance).

No products indexed under this heading.

Metronidazole Sodium (In vitro studies indicated that CYP3A4 and CYP2C19 are the primary enzymes involved in the metabolism of citalopram. However, co-administration of citalopram (40 mg) and ketoconazole (200 mg), a potent inhibitor of CYP3A4, did not significantly affect the pharmacokinetics of citalopram. Because citalopram is metabolized by multiple enzyme systems, inhibition of a single enzyme may not appreciably decrease citalopram clearance).

No products indexed under this heading.

Miconazole (In vitro studies indicated that CYP3A4 and CYP2C19 are the primary enzymes involved in the metabolism of citalopram. However, co-administration of citalopram (40 mg) and ketoconazole (200 mg), a potent inhibitor of CYP3A4, did not significantly affect the pharmacokinetics of citalopram. Because citalopram is metabolized by multiple enzyme systems, inhibition of a single enzyme may not appreciably decrease citalopram clearance).

No products indexed under this heading.

Miconazole Nitrate (In vitro studies indicated that CYP3A4 and CYP2C19 are the primary enzymes involved in the metabolism of citalopram. However, co-administration of citalopram (40 mg) and ketoconazole (200 mg), a potent inhibitor of CYP3A4, did not significantly affect the pharmacokinetics of citalopram. Because citalopram is metabolized by multiple enzyme systems, inhibition of a single enzyme may not appreciably decrease citalopram clearance).

No products indexed under this heading.

Midazolam Hydrochloride (Given the primary CNS effects of citalopram, caution should be used when it is taken in combination with other centrally acting drugs).

No products indexed under this heading.

Moclobemide (Co-administration of serotonin reuptake inhibitors and MAO inhibitors has resulted in serious, sometimes fatal, reactions including hyperthermia, rigidity, myoclonus, serotonin syndrome, and other potentially serious adverse reactions; concurrent and/or sequential use is contraindicated).

No products indexed under this heading.

Modafinil (In vitro studies indicated that CYP3A4 and CYP2C19 are the primary enzymes involved in the metabolism of citalopram. However, co-administration of citalopram (40 mg) and ketoconazole (200 mg), a potent inhibitor of CYP3A4, did not significantly affect the pharmacokinetics of citalopram. Because citalopram is metabolized by multiple enzyme systems, inhibition of a single enzyme may not appreciably decrease citalopram clearance). Products include:

Provigil Tablets 977

Molindone Hydrochloride (Given the primary CNS effects of citalopram, caution should be used when it is taken in combination with other centrally acting drugs). Products include:

Moban Tablets 1116

Morphine Sulfate (Given the primary CNS effects of citalopram, caution should be used when it is taken in combination with other centrally acting drugs). Products include:

Avinza Capsules 1772
DepoDur Injection 1095
MS Contin Tablets 2585

Nabumetone (The combined use of psycotropic drugs that interfere with serotonin reuptake and drugs that affect coagulation has been associated with an increased risk of bleeding; use caution when co-administering).

No products indexed under this heading.

Naproxen (The combined use of psycotropic drugs that interfere with serotonin reuptake and drugs that affect coagulation has been associated with an increased risk of bleeding; use caution when co-administering). Products include:

EC-Naprosyn Delayed-Release Tablets 2632
Naprosyn Suspension 2632
Naprosyn Tablets 2632

Naproxen Sodium (The combined use of psycotropic drugs that interfere with serotonin reuptake and drugs that affect coagulation has been associated with an increased risk of bleeding; use caution when co-administering). Products include:

Anaprox Tablets 2632
Anaprox DS Tablets 2632
Treximet Tablets 1616

Naratriptan Hydrochloride (There have been rare post-marketing reports of serotonin syndrome with the use of a SSRI and a triptan. If concomitant treatment of citalopram hydrobromide with a triptan is clinically warranted, careful observation of the patient is advised, particularly during treatment initiation and dose increases). Products include:

Amerge Tablets 1301

Nefazodone Hydrochloride (In vitro studies indicated that CYP3A4 and CYP2C19 are the primary enzymes involved in the metabolism of citalopram. However, co-administration of citalopram (40 mg) and ketoconazole (200 mg), a potent inhibitor of CYP3A4, did not significantly affect the pharmacokinetics of citalopram. Because citalopram is metabolized by multiple enzyme systems, inhibition of a single enzyme may not appreciably decrease citalopram clearance).

No products indexed under this heading.

Nelfinavir Mesylate (In vitro studies indicated that CYP3A4 and CYP2C19 are the primary enzymes involved in the metabolism of citalopram. However, co-administration of citalopram (40 mg) and ketoconazole (200 mg), a potent inhibitor of CYP3A4, did not significantly affect the pharmacokinetics of citalopram. Because citalopram is metabolized by multiple enzyme systems, inhibition of a single enzyme may not appreciably decrease citalopram clearance).

No products indexed under this heading.

Nevirapine (In vitro studies indicated that CYP3A4 and CYP2C19 are the primary enzymes involved in the metabolism of citalopram. However, co-administration of citalopram (40 mg) and ketoconazole (200 mg), a potent inhibitor of CYP3A4, did not significantly affect the pharmacokinetics of citalopram. Because citalopram is metabolized by multiple enzyme systems, inhibition of a single enzyme may not appreciably decrease citalopram clearance). Products include:

Viramune Oral Suspension 873
Viramune Tablets 873

Niacinamide (In vitro studies indicated that CYP3A4 and CYP2C19 are the primary enzymes involved in the metabolism of citalopram. However, co-administration of citalopram (40 mg) and ketoconazole (200 mg), a potent inhibitor of CYP3A4, did not significantly affect the pharmacokinetics of citalopram. Because citalopram is metabolized by multiple enzyme systems, inhibition of a single enzyme may not appreciably decrease citalopram clearance). Products include:

BioLean Free Tablets 635

Nicotinamide (In vitro studies indicated that CYP3A4 and CYP2C19 are the primary enzymes involved in the metabolism of citalopram. However, co-administration of citalopram (40 mg) and ketoconazole (200 mg), a potent inhibitor of CYP3A4, did not significantly affect the pharmacokinetics of citalopram. Because citalopram is metabolized by multiple enzyme systems, inhibition of a single enzyme may not appreciably decrease citalopram clearance).

No products indexed under this heading.

Nifedipine (In vitro studies indicated that CYP3A4 and CYP2C19 are the primary enzymes involved in the metabolism of citalopram. However, co-administration of citalopram (40 mg) and ketoconazole (200 mg), a potent inhibitor of CYP3A4, did not significantly affect the pharmacokinetics of citalopram. Because citalopram is metabolized by multiple enzyme systems, inhibition of a single enzyme may not appreciably decrease citalopram clearance).

No products indexed under this heading.

Norethindrone (In vitro studies indicated that CYP3A4 and CYP2C19 are the primary enzymes involved in the metabolism of citalopram. However, co-administration of citalopram (40 mg) and ketoconazole (200 mg), a potent inhibitor of CYP3A4, did not significantly affect the pharmacokinetics of citalopram. Because citalopram is metabolized by multiple enzyme systems, inhibition of a single enzyme may not appreciably decrease citalopram clearance). Products include:

Ortho Micronor Tablets 2446

Norethynodrel (In vitro studies indicated that CYP3A4 and CYP2C19 are the primary enzymes involved in the metabolism of citalopram. However, co-administration of citalopram (40 mg) and ketoconazole (200 mg), a potent inhibitor of CYP3A4, did not significantly affect the pharmacokinetics of citalopram. Because citalopram is metabolized by multiple enzyme systems, inhibition of a single enzyme may not appreciably decrease citalopram clearance).

No products indexed under this heading.

Norfloxacin (In vitro studies indicated that CYP3A4 and CYP2C19 are the primary enzymes involved in the metabolism of citalopram. However, co-administration of citalopram (40 mg) and ketoconazole (200 mg), a potent inhibitor of CYP3A4, did not significantly affect the pharmacokinetics of citalopram. Because citalopram is metabolized by multiple enzyme systems, inhibition of a single enzyme may not appreciably decrease citalopram clearance). Products include:

Noroxin Tablets 2069

Norgestimate (In vitro studies indicated that CYP3A4 and CYP2C19 are the primary enzymes involved in the metabolism of citalopram. However, co-administration of citalopram (40 mg) and ketoconazole (200 mg), a potent inhibitor of CYP3A4, did not significantly affect the pharmacokinetics of citalopram. Because citalopram is metabolized by multiple enzyme systems, inhibition of a single enzyme may not appreciably decrease citalopram clearance). Products include:

Ortho-Cyclen/Ortho Tri-Cyclen 2449
Ortho Tri-Cyclen Lo Tablets 2458

Norgestrel (In vitro studies indicated that CYP3A4 and CYP2C19 are the primary enzymes involved in the metabolism of citalopram. However, co-administration of citalopram (40 mg) and ketoconazole (200 mg), a potent inhibitor of CYP3A4, did not significantly affect the pharmacokinetics of citalopram. Because citalopram is metabolized by multiple enzyme systems, inhibition of a single enzyme may not appreciably decrease citalopram clearance).

No products indexed under this heading.

Nortriptyline Hydrochloride (Co-administration of imipramine with citalopram has resulted in a 50% increase in active metabolite, desipramine concentration; the clinical significance of these findings is unknown; caution is indicated if tricyclic antidepressants are co-administered with citalopram, a relatively weak inhibitor of CYP2D6).

No products indexed under this heading.

Olanzapine (Given the primary CNS effects of citalopram, caution should be used when it is taken in combination with other centrally acting drugs). Products include:

Symbyax Capsules 1871
Zyprexa Tablets 1883
Zyprexa IntraMuscular 1883
Zyprexa ZYDIS Orally Disintegrating Tablets 1883

Omeprazole (Co-administration with potent inhibitors of CYP2C19, such as omeprazole, may decrease the clearance of citalopram).

No products indexed under this heading.

Oxaprozin (The combined use of psycotropic drugs that interfere with serotonin reuptake and drugs that affect coagulation has been associated with an increased risk of bleeding; use caution when co-administering).

No products indexed under this heading.

Oxazepam (Given the primary CNS effects of citalopram, caution should be used when it is taken in combination with other centrally acting drugs).

No products indexed under this heading.

Oxcarbazepine (In vitro studies indicated that CYP3A4 and CYP2C19 are the primary enzymes involved in the metabolism of citalopram. However, co-administration of citalopram (40 mg) and ketoconazole (200 mg), a potent inhibitor of CYP3A4, did not significantly affect the pharmacokinetics of citalopram. Because citalopram is metabolized by multiple enzyme systems, inhibition of a single enzyme may not appreciably decrease citalopram clearance).

No products indexed under this heading.

Oxycodone Hydrochloride (Given the primary CNS effects of citalopram, caution should be used when it is taken in combination with other centrally acting drugs). Products include:

OxyContin Tablets 2589
OxyIR Capsules 2593
Percocet Tablets 1127
Percodan Tablets 1130

Pargyline Hydrochloride (Co-administration of serotonin reuptake inhibitors and MAO inhibitors has resulted in serious, sometimes fatal, reactions including hyperthermia, rigidity, myoclonus, serotonin syndrome, and other potentially serious adverse reactions; concurrent and/or sequential use is contraindicated).

No products indexed under this heading.

Paroxetine Hydrochloride (Development of a potentially life-threatening serotonin syndrome may occur with SSRIs, particularly with concomitant use of serotinergic drugs, including triptans. Caution is advised when citalopram hydrobromide is co-administered with other drugs that may affect the serotinergic neurotransmitter systems). Products include:

Paxil 1535
Paxil CR Controlled-Release Tablets 1544

Pemoline (Given the primary CNS effects of citalopram, caution should be used when it is taken in combination with other centrally acting drugs).

No products indexed under this heading.

Pentobarbital Sodium (Given the primary CNS effects of citalopram, caution should be used when it is taken in combination with other centrally acting drugs). Products include:

Nembutal Sodium Solution, USP 2494

Perphenazine (Given the primary CNS effects of citalopram, caution should be used when it is taken in combination with other centrally acting drugs).

No products indexed under this heading.

Phenelzine Sulfate (Co-administration of serotonin reuptake inhibitors and MAO inhibitors has resulted in serious, sometimes fatal, reactions including hyperthermia, rigidity, myoclonus, serotonin syndrome, and other potentially serious adverse reactions; concurrent and/or sequential use is contraindicated).

No products indexed under this heading.

Phenobarbital (Given the primary CNS effects of citalopram, caution should be used when it is taken in combination with other centrally acting drugs). Products include:

Donnatal Extentabs 2507

Phenylbutazone (The combined use of psycotropic drugs that interfere with serotonin reuptake and drugs that affect coagulation has been associated with an increased risk of bleeding; use caution when co-administering).

No products indexed under this heading.

Pimozide (In a controlled study, a single dose of pimozide 2 mg co-administered with citalopram 40 mg given once daily for 11 days was associated with a mean increase in QTc values of approximately 10 msec. compared to pimozide given alone. Concomitant use in patients taking pimozide is contraindicated).

No products indexed under this heading.

Piroxicam (The combined use of psycotropic drugs that interfere with serotonin reuptake and drugs that affect coagulation has been associated with an increased risk of bleeding; use caution when co-administering).

No products indexed under this heading.

Prazepam (Given the primary CNS effects of citalopram, caution should be used when it is taken in combination with other centrally acting drugs).

No products indexed under this heading.

Procarbazine Hydrochloride (Co-administration of serotonin reuptake inhibitors and MAO inhibitors has resulted in serious, sometimes fatal, reactions including hyperthermia, rigidity, myoclonus, serotonin syndrome, and other potentially serious adverse reactions; concurrent and/or sequential use is contraindicated).

No products indexed under this heading.

Prochlorperazine (Given the primary CNS effects of citalopram, caution should be used when it is taken in combination with other centrally acting drugs).

No products indexed under this heading.

Promethazine Hydrochloride (Given the primary CNS effects of citalopram, caution should be used when it is taken in combination with other centrally acting drugs).

No products indexed under this heading.

Propofol (Given the primary CNS effects of citalopram, caution should be used when it is taken in combination with other centrally acting drugs).

No products indexed under this heading.

Propoxyphene Hydrochloride (Given the primary CNS effects of citalopram, caution should be used when it is taken in combination with other centrally acting drugs).

No products indexed under this heading.

Propoxyphene Napsylate (Given the primary CNS effects of citalopram, caution should be used when it is taken in combination with other centrally acting drugs).

No products indexed under this heading.

Protriptyline Hydrochloride (Co-administration of imipramine with citalopram has resulted in a 50% increase in active metabolite, desipramine concentration; the clinical significance of these findings is unknown; caution is indicated if tricyclic antidepressants are co-administered with citalopram, a relatively weak inhibitor of CYP2D6).

No products indexed under this heading.

Quazepam (Given the primary CNS effects of citalopram, caution should be used when it is taken in combination with other centrally acting drugs).

No products indexed under this heading.

Quetiapine Fumarate (Given the primary CNS effects of citalopram, caution should be used when it is taken in combination with other centrally acting drugs).

No products indexed under this heading.

Quinidine (In vitro studies indicated that CYP3A4 and CYP2C19 are the primary enzymes involved in the metabolism of citalopram. However, co-administration of citalopram (40 mg) and ketoconazole (200 mg), a potent inhibitor of CYP3A4, did not significantly affect the pharmacokinetics of citalopram. Because citalopram is metabolized by multiple enzyme systems, inhibition of a single enzyme may not appreciably decrease citalopram clearance).

No products indexed under this heading.

Quinidine Hydrochloride (In vitro studies indicated that CYP3A4 and CYP2C19 are the primary enzymes involved in the metabolism of citalopram. However, co-administration of citalopram (40 mg) and ketoconazole (200 mg), a potent inhibitor of CYP3A4, did not significantly affect the pharmacokinetics of citalopram. Because citalopram is metabolized by multiple enzyme systems, inhibition of a single enzyme may not appreciably decrease citalopram clearance).

No products indexed under this heading.

Quinidine Polygalacturonate (In vitro studies indicated that CYP3A4 and CYP2C19 are the primary enzymes involved in the metabolism of citalopram. However, co-administration of citalopram (40 mg) and ketoconazole (200 mg), a potent inhibitor of CYP3A4, did not significantly affect the pharmacokinetics of citalopram. Because citalopram is metabolized by multiple enzyme systems, inhibition of a single enzyme may not appreciably decrease citalopram clearance).

No products indexed under this heading.

Quinidine Sulfate (In vitro studies indicated that CYP3A4 and CYP2C19 are the primary enzymes involved in the metabolism of citalopram. However, co-administration of citalopram (40 mg) and ketoconazole (200 mg), a potent inhibitor of CYP3A4, did not significantly affect the pharmacokinetics of citalopram. Because citalopram is metabolized by multiple enzyme systems, inhibition of a single enzyme may not appreciably decrease citalopram clearance).

No products indexed under this heading.

Quinine (In vitro studies indicated that CYP3A4 and CYP2C19 are the primary enzymes involved in the metabolism of citalopram. However, co-administration of citalopram (40 mg) and ketoconazole (200 mg), a potent inhibitor of CYP3A4, did not significantly affect the pharmacokinetics of citalopram. Because citalopram is metabolized by multiple enzyme systems, inhibition of a single enzyme may not appreciably decrease citalopram clearance).

No products indexed under this heading.

Quinine Sulfate (In vitro studies indicated that CYP3A4 and CYP2C19 are the primary enzymes involved in the metabolism of citalopram. However, co-administration of citalopram (40 mg) and ketoconazole (200 mg), a potent inhibitor of CYP3A4, did not significantly affect the pharmacokinetics of citalopram. Because citalopram is metabolized by multiple enzyme systems, inhibition of a single enzyme may not appreciably decrease citalopram clearance).

No products indexed under this heading.

Quinupristin (In vitro studies indicated that CYP3A4 and CYP2C19 are the primary enzymes involved in the metabolism of citalopram. However, co-administration of citalopram (40 mg) and ketoconazole (200 mg), a potent inhibitor of CYP3A4, did not significantly affect the pharmacokinetics of citalopram. Because citalopram is metabolized by multiple enzyme systems, inhibition of a single enzyme may not appreciably decrease citalopram clearance).

No products indexed under this heading.

Ranitidine Bismuth Citrate (In vitro studies indicated that CYP3A4 and CYP2C19 are the primary enzymes involved in the metabolism of citalopram. However, co-

administration of citalopram (40 mg) and ketoconazole (200 mg), a potent inhibitor of CYP3A4, did not significantly affect the pharmacokinetics of citalopram. Because citalopram is metabolized by multiple enzyme systems, inhibition of a single enzyme may not appreciably decrease citalopram clearance).
No products indexed under this heading.

Ranitidine Hydrochloride (In vitro studies indicated that CYP3A4 and CYP2C19 are the primary enzymes involved in the metabolism of citalopram. However, co-administration of citalopram (40 mg) and ketoconazole (200 mg), a potent inhibitor of CYP3A4, did not significantly affect the pharmacokinetics of citalopram. Because citalopram is metabolized by multiple enzyme systems, inhibition of a single enzyme may not appreciably decrease citalopram clearance). Products include:
Zantac 75 Tablets 603
Zantac **1670**
Zantac Injection **1666**
Zantac Injection Pharmacy Bulk Package **1668**
Maximum Strength Zantac 150 Tablets 603
Maximum Strength Zantac 150 Cool Mint Tablets 603

Rasagiline Mesylate (Co-administration of serotonin reuptake inhibitors and MAO inhibitors has resulted in serious, sometimes fatal, reactions including hyperthermia, rigidity, myoclonus, serotonin syndrome, and other potentially serious adverse reactions; concurrent and/or sequential use is contraindicated). Products include:
Azilect Tablets **3106**

Remifentanil Hydrochloride (Given the primary CNS effects of citalopram, caution should be used when it is taken in combination with other centrally acting drugs).
No products indexed under this heading.

Risperidone (Given the primary CNS effects of citalopram, caution should be used when it is taken in combination with other centrally acting drugs). Products include:
Risperdal Consta Long-Acting Injection **1753**

Ritonavir (In vitro studies indicated that CYP3A4 and CYP2C19 are the primary enzymes involved in the metabolism of citalopram. However, co-administration of citalopram (40 mg) and ketoconazole (200 mg), a potent inhibitor of CYP3A4, did not significantly affect the pharmacokinetics of citalopram. Because citalopram is metabolized by multiple enzyme systems, inhibition of a single enzyme may not appreciably decrease citalopram clearance). Products include:
Kaletra **452**
Norvir **489**

Rizatriptan Benzoate (There have been rare post-marketing reports of serotonin syndrome with the use of a SSRI and a triptan. If concomitant treatment of citalopram hydrobromide with a triptan is clinically warranted, careful observation of the patient is advised, particularly during treatment initiation and dose increases). Products include:
Maxalt Tablets **2056**
Maxalt-MLT Orally Disintegrating Tablets **2056**

Rofecoxib (The combined use of psycotropic drugs that interfere with serotonin reuptake and drugs that affect coagulation has been associated with an increased risk of bleeding; use caution when co-administering).
No products indexed under this heading.

Saquinavir (In vitro studies indicated that CYP3A4 and CYP2C19 are the primary enzymes involved in the metabolism of citalopram. However, co-administration of citalopram (40 mg) and ketoconazole (200 mg), a potent inhibitor of CYP3A4, did not significantly affect the pharmacokinetics of citalopram. Because citalopram is metabolized by multiple enzyme systems, inhibition of a single enzyme may not appreciably decrease citalopram clearance).
No products indexed under this heading.

Saquinavir Mesylate (In vitro studies indicated that CYP3A4 and CYP2C19 are the primary enzymes involved in the metabolism of citalopram. However, co-administration of citalopram (40 mg) and ketoconazole (200 mg), a potent inhibitor of CYP3A4, did not significantly affect the pharmacokinetics of citalopram. Because citalopram is metabolized by multiple enzyme systems, inhibition of a single enzyme may not appreciably decrease citalopram clearance).
No products indexed under this heading.

Secobarbital Sodium (Given the primary CNS effects of citalopram, caution should be used when it is taken in combination with other centrally acting drugs).
No products indexed under this heading.

Selegiline (Co-administration of serotonin reuptake inhibitors and MAO inhibitors has resulted in serious, sometimes fatal, reactions including hyperthermia, rigidity, myoclonus, serotonin syndrome, and other potentially serious adverse reactions; concurrent and/or sequential use is contraindicated). Products include:
Emsam Transdermal System **905**

Selegiline Hydrochloride (Co-administration of serotonin reuptake inhibitors and MAO inhibitors has resulted in serious, sometimes fatal, reactions including hyperthermia, rigidity, myoclonus, serotonin syndrome, and other potentially serious adverse reactions; concurrent and/or sequential use is contraindicated). Products include:
Eldepryl Capsules **3052**

Sertraline Hydrochloride (Development of a potentially life-threatening serotonin syndrome may occur with SSRIs, particularly with concomitant use of serotinergic drugs, including triptans. Caution is advised when citalopram hydrobromide is co-administered with other drugs that may affect the serotinergic neurotransmitter systems).
No products indexed under this heading.

Sevoflurane (Given the primary CNS effects of citalopram, caution should be used when it is taken in combination with other centrally acting drugs). Products include:
Ultane Liquid for Inhalation **524**

Sildenafil Citrate (In vitro studies indicated that CYP3A4 and CYP2C19 are the primary enzymes involved in the metabolism of citalopram. However, co-administration of citalopram (40 mg) and ketoconazole (200 mg), a potent inhibitor of CYP3A4, did not significantly affect the pharmacokinetics of citalopram. Because citalopram is metabolized by multiple enzyme systems, inhibition of a single enzyme may not appreciably decrease citalopram clearance).
No products indexed under this heading.

Sodium Oxybate (Given the primary CNS effects of citalopram, caution should be used when it is taken in combination with other centrally acting drugs). Products include:
Xyrem Oral Solution **1766**

Sufentanil Citrate (Given the primary CNS effects of citalopram, caution should be used when it is taken in combination with other centrally acting drugs).
No products indexed under this heading.

Sulfaphenazole (In vitro studies indicated that CYP3A4 and CYP2C19 are the primary enzymes involved in the metabolism of citalopram. However, co-administration of citalopram (40 mg) and ketoconazole (200 mg), a potent inhibitor of CYP3A4, did not significantly affect the pharmacokinetics of citalopram. Because citalopram is metabolized by multiple enzyme systems, inhibition of a single enzyme may not appreciably decrease citalopram clearance).
No products indexed under this heading.

Sulindac (The combined use of psycotropic drugs that interfere with serotonin reuptake and drugs that affect coagulation has been associated with an increased risk of bleeding; use caution when co-administering). Products include:
Clinoril Tablets **1962**

Sumatriptan (Co-administration of SSRIs and sumatriptan has resulted in weakness, hyperreflexia, and incoordination). Products include:
Imitrex Nasal Spray **1470**

Sumatriptan Succinate (Co-administration of SSRIs and sumatriptan has resulted in weakness, hyperreflexia, and incoordination). Products include:
Imitrex Injection **1465**
Imitrex Tablets **1474**
Treximet Tablets **1616**

Telithromycin (In vitro studies indicated that CYP3A4 and CYP2C19 are the primary enzymes involved in the metabolism of citalopram. However, co-administration of citalopram (40 mg) and ketoconazole (200 mg), a potent inhibitor of CYP3A4, did not significantly affect the pharmacokinetics of citalopram. Because citalopram is metabolized by multiple enzyme systems, inhibition of a single enzyme may not appreciably decrease citalopram clearance). Products include:
Ketek Tablets **2744**

Telmisartan (In vitro studies indicated that CYP3A4 and CYP2C19 are the primary enzymes involved in the metabolism of citalopram. However, co-administration of citalopram (40 mg) and ketoconazole (200 mg), a potent inhibitor of CYP3A4, did not significantly affect the pharmacokinetics of citalopram. Because citalopram is metabolized by multiple enzyme systems, inhibition of a single enzyme may not appreciably decrease citalopram clearance). Products include:
Micardis Tablets **852**
Micardis HCT Tablets **854**

Temazepam (Given the primary CNS effects of citalopram, caution should be used when it is taken in combination with other centrally acting drugs).
No products indexed under this heading.

Theophylline (Combined administration of citalopram hydrobromide (40 mg/day for 21 days) and the CYP1A2 substrate theophylline (single dose of 300 mg) did not affect the pharmacokinetics of theophylline. The effect of theophylline on the pharmacokinetics of citalopram hydrobromide was not evaluated).
No products indexed under this heading.

Thiamylal Sodium (Given the primary CNS effects of citalopram, caution should be used when it is taken in combination with other centrally acting drugs).
No products indexed under this heading.

Thioridazine Hydrochloride (Given the primary CNS effects of citalopram, caution should be used when it is taken in combination with other centrally acting drugs). Products include:
Thioridazine Hydrochloride Tablets **2195**

Thiothixene (Given the primary CNS effects of citalopram, caution should be used when it is taken in combination with other centrally acting drugs). Products include:
Thiothixene Capsules **2197**

Ticlopidine Hydrochloride (In vitro studies indicated that CYP3A4 and CYP2C19 are the primary enzymes involved in the metabolism of citalopram. However, co-administration of citalopram (40 mg) and ketoconazole (200 mg), a potent inhibitor of CYP3A4, did not significantly affect the pharmacokinetics of citalopram. Because citalopram is metabolized by multiple enzyme systems, inhibition of a single enzyme may not appreciably decrease citalopram clearance).
No products indexed under this heading.

Tinzaparin Sodium (The combined use of psychotropic drugs that interfere with serotonin reuptake and drugs that affect coagulation has been associated with an increased risk of bleeding).
No products indexed under this heading.

Tolbutamide (In vitro studies indicated that CYP3A4 and CYP2C19 are the primary enzymes involved in the metabolism of citalopram. However, co-administration of citalopram (40 mg) and ketoconazole (200 mg), a potent inhibitor of CYP3A4, did not significantly affect the pharmacokinetics of citalopram. Because citalopram is metabolized by multiple enzyme systems, inhibition of a single enzyme may not appreciably decrease citalopram clearance).
No products indexed under this heading.

Tolbutamide Sodium (In vitro studies indicated that CYP3A4 and CYP2C19 are the primary enzymes involved in the metabolism of citalopram. However, co-administration of citalopram (40 mg) and ketoconazole (200 mg), a potent inhibitor of CYP3A4, did not significantly affect the pharmacokinetics of citalopram. Because citalopram is metabolized by multiple enzyme systems, inhibition of a single enzyme may not appreciably decrease citalopram clearance).

No products indexed under this heading.

Tolmetin Sodium (The combined use of psycotropic drugs that interfere with serotonin reuptake and drugs that affect coagulation has been associated with an increased risk of bleeding; use caution when co-administering).

No products indexed under this heading.

Topiramate (In vitro studies indicated that CYP3A4 and CYP2C19 are the primary enzymes involved in the metabolism of citalopram. However, co-administration of citalopram (40 mg) and ketoconazole (200 mg), a potent inhibitor of CYP3A4, did not significantly affect the pharmacokinetics of citalopram. Because citalopram is metabolized by multiple enzyme systems, inhibition of a single enzyme may not appreciably decrease citalopram clearance).

No products indexed under this heading.

Tramadol Hydrochloride (There is a risk of serotonin syndrome with concomitant use of citalopram hydrobromide and tramadol. Caution is advised when citalopram hydrobromide is co-administered with other drugs that may affect the serotinergic neurotransmitter systems, such as tramadol). Products include:

Ultram ER Extended-Release Tablets **2428**

Tranylcypromine Sulfate (Co-administration of serotonin reuptake inhibitors and MAO inhibitors has resulted in serious, sometimes fatal, reactions including hyperthermia, rigidity, myoclonus, serotonin syndrome, and other potentially serious adverse reactions; concurrent and/or sequential use is contraindicated). Products include:

Parnate Tablets **1532**

Triazolam (Combined administration of citalopram hydrobromide (Titrated to 40 mg/day for 28 days) and the CYP3A4 substrate triazolam (single dose of 0.25) did not significantly affect the pharmacokinetics of either citalopram hydrobromide or triazolam).

No products indexed under this heading.

Trifluoperazine Hydrochloride (Given the primary CNS effects of citalopram, caution should be used when it is taken in combination with other centrally acting drugs).

No products indexed under this heading.

Trimipramine Maleate (Co-administration of imipramine with citalopram has resulted in a 50% increase in active metabolite, desipramine concentration; the clinical significance of these findings is unknown; caution is indicated if tricyclic antidepressants are co-administered with citalopram, a relatively weak inhibitor of CYP2D6).

No products indexed under this heading.

Troglitazone (In vitro studies indicated that CYP3A4 and CYP2C19 are the primary enzymes involved in the metabolism of citalopram. However, co-administration of citalopram (40 mg) and ketoconazole (200 mg), a potent inhibitor of CYP3A4, did not significantly affect the pharmacokinetics of citalopram. Because citalopram is metabolized by multiple enzyme systems, inhibition of a single enzyme may not appreciably decrease citalopram clearance).

No products indexed under this heading.

Troleandomycin (Co-administration with potent inhibitors of CYP3A4, such as macrolide antibiotics, may decrease the clearance of citalopram).

No products indexed under this heading.

Valdecoxib (The combined use of psycotropic drugs that interfere with serotonin reuptake and drugs that affect coagulation has been associated with an increased risk of bleeding; use caution when co-administering).

No products indexed under this heading.

Valproate Sodium (In vitro studies indicated that CYP3A4 and CYP2C19 are the primary enzymes involved in the metabolism of citalopram. However, co-administration of citalopram (40 mg) and ketoconazole (200 mg), a potent inhibitor of CYP3A4, did not significantly affect the pharmacokinetics of citalopram. Because citalopram is metabolized by multiple enzyme systems, inhibition of a single enzyme may not appreciably decrease citalopram clearance).

No products indexed under this heading.

Vardenafil Hydrochloride (In vitro studies indicated that CYP3A4 and CYP2C19 are the primary enzymes involved in the metabolism of citalopram. However, co-administration of citalopram (40 mg) and ketoconazole (200 mg), a potent inhibitor of CYP3A4, did not significantly affect the pharmacokinetics of citalopram. Because citalopram is metabolized by multiple enzyme systems, inhibition of a single enzyme may not appreciably decrease citalopram clearance). Products include:

Levitra Tablets **2876**

Venlafaxine Hydrochloride (Development of a potentially life-threatening serotonin syndrome may occur with SSRIs, particularly with concomitant use of serotinergic drugs, including triptans. Caution is advised when citalopram hydrobromide is co-administered with other drugs that may affect the serotinergic neurotransmitter systems). Products include:

Effexor XR Extended-Release Capsules **3195**

Venlafaxine Hydrochloride Tablets ... **2199**

Verapamil Hydrochloride (In vitro studies indicated that CYP3A4 and CYP2C19 are the primary enzymes involved in the metabolism of citalopram. However, co-administration of citalopram (40 mg) and ketoconazole (200 mg), a potent inhibitor of CYP3A4, did not significantly affect the pharmacokinetics of citalopram. Because citalopram is metabolized by multiple enzyme systems, inhibition of a single enzyme may not appreciably decrease citalopram clearance). Products include:

Tarka Tablets **511**

Voriconazole (In vitro studies indicated that CYP3A4 and CYP2C19 are the primary enzymes involved in the metabolism of citalopram. However, co-administration of citalopram (40 mg) and ketoconazole (200 mg), a potent inhibitor of CYP3A4, did not significantly affect the pharmacokinetics of citalopram. Because citalopram is metabolized by multiple enzyme systems, inhibition of a single enzyme may not appreciably decrease citalopram clearance).

No products indexed under this heading.

Warfarin Sodium (Altered anticoagulant effects, including increased bleeding, have been reported when SSRIs and SNRIs are co-administered with warfarin. Patients receiving warfarin therapy should be carefully monitored when citalopram is initiated or discontinued).

No products indexed under this heading.

Zafirlukast (In vitro studies indicated that CYP3A4 and CYP2C19 are the primary enzymes involved in the metabolism of citalopram. However, co-administration of citalopram (40 mg) and ketoconazole (200 mg), a potent inhibitor of CYP3A4, did not significantly affect the pharmacokinetics of citalopram. Because citalopram is metabolized by multiple enzyme systems, inhibition of a single enzyme may not appreciably decrease citalopram clearance). Products include:

Accolate Tablets **669**

Zaleplon (Given the primary CNS effects of citalopram, caution should be used when it is taken in combination with other centrally acting drugs).

No products indexed under this heading.

Zileuton (In vitro studies indicated that CYP3A4 and CYP2C19 are the primary enzymes involved in the metabolism of citalopram. However, co-administration of citalopram (40 mg) and ketoconazole (200 mg), a potent inhibitor of CYP3A4, did not significantly affect the pharmacokinetics of citalopram. Because citalopram is metabolized by multiple enzyme systems, inhibition of a single enzyme may not appreciably decrease citalopram clearance).

No products indexed under this heading.

Ziprasidone Hydrochloride (Given the primary CNS effects of citalopram, caution should be used when it is taken in combination with other centrally acting drugs). Products include:

Geodon Capsules **2520**

Zolmitriptan (There have been rare post-marketing reports of serotonin syndrome with the use of a SSRI and a triptan. If concomitant treatment of citalopram hydrobromide with a triptan is clinically warranted, careful observation of the patient is advised, particularly during treatment initiation and dose increases). Products include:

Zomig Tablets **694**
Zomig Nasal Spray **689**
Zomig-ZMT Tablets **694**

Zolpidem Tartrate (Given the primary CNS effects of citalopram, caution should be used when it is taken in combination with other centrally acting drugs). Products include:

Ambien Tablets **2692**
Ambien CR Tablets **2696**

Food Interactions

Alcohol (Although citalopram did not potentiate cognitive and motor effects of alcohol, concurrent use is not recommended).

Grapefruit (In vitro studies indicated that CYP3A4 and CYP2C19 are the primary enzymes involved in the metabolism of citalopram. However, co-administration of citalopram (40 mg) and ketoconazole (200 mg), a potent inhibitor of CYP3A4, did not significantly affect the pharmacokinetics of citalopram. Because citalopram is metabolized by multiple enzyme systems, inhibition of a single enzyme may not appreciably decrease citalopram clearance).

Grapefruit Juice (In vitro studies indicated that CYP3A4 and CYP2C19 are the primary enzymes involved in the metabolism of citalopram. However, co-administration of citalopram (40 mg) and ketoconazole (200 mg), a potent inhibitor of CYP3A4, did not significantly affect the pharmacokinetics of citalopram. Because citalopram is metabolized by multiple enzyme systems, inhibition of a single enzyme may not appreciably decrease citalopram clearance).

CELLCEPT CAPSULES

(Mycophenolate Mofetil) **2622**

See CellCept Tablets

CELLCEPT INTRAVENOUS

(Mycophenolate Mofetil Hydrochloride) **2622**

May interact with antacids, oral contraceptives, vaccines, live, and certain other agents. Compounds in these categories include:

Acyclovir (Co-administration of mycophenolate mofetil (1 g) and acyclovir (800 mg) to 12 healthy volunteers resulted in no significant change in mycophenolic acid (MPA) AUC and Cmax. However the phenolic glucuronide of MPA (MPAG) and acyclovir plasma AUCs were increased 10.6% and 21.9% respectively. Because MPAG plasma concentrations are increased in the presence of renal impairment, as are acyclovir concentrations, the potential exists for mycophenolate and acyclovir or its prodrug (eg, valacyclovir) to compete for tubular secretion, further increasing the concentrations of both drugs). Products include:

Zovirax **1690**
Zovirax Cream **817**
Zovirax Ointment **819**

Acyclovir Sodium (Co-administration of mycophenolate mofetil (1 g) and acyclovir (800 mg) to 12 healthy volunteers resulted in no significant change in mycophenolic acid (MPA) AUC and Cmax. However the phenolic glucuronide of MPA (MPAG) and acyclovir plasma AUCs were increased 10.6% and 21.9% respectively. Because MPAG plasma concentrations are increased in the presence of renal impairment, as are acyclovir concentrations, the potential exists for mycophenolate and acyclovir or its prodrug (eg, valacyclovir) to compete for tubular secretion, further increasing the concentrations of both drugs).

No products indexed under this heading.

Aluminum Carbonate (Absorption of a single dose of mycophenolate mofetil (2 g) was decreased when administered to ten rheumatoid arthritis patients also taking Maalox TC (10 mL q.i.d.) The Cmax and AUC (0-24h) for MPA was 33% and 17% lower, respectively, than when mycophenolate mofetil was administered alone under fasting conditions. Mycophenolate mofetil may be administered to patients who are also taking antacids containing magnesium and aluminum hydroxides, however it is recommended that mycophenolate mofetil and the antacid not be administered simultaneously).

No products indexed under this heading.

Aluminum Hydroxide (Absorption of a single dose of mycophenolate mofetil (2 g) was decreased when administered to ten rheumatoid arthritis patients also taking Maalox TC (10 mL q.i.d.) The Cmax and AUC (0-24h) for MPA was 33% and 17% lower, respectively, than when mycophenolate mofetil was administered alone under fasting conditions. Mycophenolate mofetil may be administered to patients who are also taking antacids containing magnesium and aluminum hydroxides, however it is recommended that mycophenolate mofetil and the antacid not be administered simultaneously).

No products indexed under this heading.

Azathioprine (It is recommended that mycophenolate mofetil not be administered concomitantly with azathioprine because both have the potential to cause bone marrow suppression and such concomitant administration has not been studied clinically).

No products indexed under this heading.

Azathioprine Sodium (It is recommended that mycophenolate mofetil not be administered concomitantly with azathioprine because both have the potential to cause bone marrow suppression and such concomitant administration has not been studied clinically).

No products indexed under this heading.

BCG Vaccine (During treatment with mycophenolate mofetil, the use of live attenuated vaccines should be avoided and patients should be advised that vaccines may be less effective. Influenza vaccination may be of value. Prescribers should refer to national guidelines for influenza vaccination).

No products indexed under this heading.

Cholestyramine (Following single-dose administration of 1.5 g mycophenolate mofetil to 12 healthy volunteers pretreated with 4 g t.i.d. of cholestyramine for 4 days, MPA AUC decreased approximately 40%. This decrease is consistent with interruption of enterohepatic recirculation which may be due to binding of recirculating MPAG with cholestyramine in the intestine. Some degree of enterohepatic recirculation is also anticipated following intravenous administration of mycophenolate mofetil. Therefore, mycophenolate mofetil is not recommended to be given with cholestyramine or other agents that may interfere with enterohepatic recirculation).

No products indexed under this heading.

Cyclosporine (In renal transplant patients, mean MPA exposure (AUC 0-12h) was approximately 30% to 50% greater when mycophenolate mofetil is administered without cyclosporine compared with when mycophenolate mofetil is co-administered with cyclosporine. This interaction is due to cyclosporine inhibition of multidrug-resistance-associated protein 2 (MRP-2) transporter in the biliary tract, thereby preventing the excretion of MPAG into the bile that would lead to enterohepatic recirculation of MPA. This information should be taken into consideration when mycophenolate mofetil is used without cyclosporine). Products include:

Gengraf Capsules 435
Neoral Oral Solution 2280
Neoral Soft Gelatin Capsules 2280
Restasis Ophthalmic Emulsion 557
Sandimmune 2296

Desogestrel (A study of co-administration of mycophenolate mofetil and oral contraceptives containing ethinyl estradiol and levonorgestrel, desogestrel or gestodene was conducted in 18 women with psoriasis over 3 consecutive menstrual cycles. Mean AUC (0-24h) was similar for ethinyl estradiol and 3-keto desogestrel, however mean levonorgestrel AUC (0-24h) significantly decreased by about 15%. There was large inter-patient variability in the data. Mean serum levels of LH, FSH and progesterone were not significantlyaffected. Mycophenolate mofetil may not have any influence on the ovulation-suppressing action of the studied oral contraceptives. Concurrent use with oral contraceptives should be used with caution and additional birth control methods considered). Products include:

Mircette Tablets 1034

Ethinyl Estradiol (A study of co-administration of mycophenolate mofetil and oral contraceptives containing ethinyl estradiol and levonorgestrel, desogestrel or gestodene was conducted in 18 women with psoriasis over 3 consecutive menstrual cycles. Mean AUC (0-24h) was similar for ethinyl estradiol and 3-keto desogestrel, however mean levonorgestrel AUC (0-24h) significantly decreased by about 15%. There was large inter-patient variability in the data. Mean serum levels of LH, FSH and progesterone were not significantlyaffected. Mycophenolate mofetil may not have any influence on the ovulation-suppressing action of the studied oral contraceptives. Concurrent use with oral contraceptives should be used with caution and additional birth control methods considered). Products include:

Lybrel Tablets 3204
Mircette Tablets 1034
NuvaRing 2897
Ortho-Cyclen/Ortho Tri-Cyclen 2449
Ortho Evra Transdermal System 2437
Ortho Tri-Cyclen Lo Tablets 2458
Seasonique Tablets 1046
Yaz Tablets 805

Ethynodiol Diacetate (A study of co-administration of mycophenolate mofetil and oral contraceptives containing ethinyl estradiol and levonorgestrel, desogestrel or gestodene was conducted in 18 women with psoriasis over 3 consecutive menstrual cycles. Mean AUC (0-24h) was similar for ethinyl estradiol and 3-keto desogestrel, however mean levonorgestrel AUC (0-24h) significantly decreased by about 15%. There was large inter-patient variability in the data. Mean serum levels of LH, FSH and progesterone were not significantlyaffected. Mycophenolate mofetil may not have any influence on the ovulation-suppressing action of the studied oral contraceptives. Concurrent use with oral contraceptives should be used with caution and additional birth control methods considered).

No products indexed under this heading.

Ganciclovir (Because MPAG plasma concentrations are increased in the presence of renal impairment, as are ganciclovir concentrations, the two drugs will compete for tubular secretion and thus further increases in concentrations of both drugs may occur. In patients with renal impairment in which mycophenolate mofetil and ganciclovir or its prodrug (eg, valganciclovir) are co-administered, patients should be monitored carefully).

No products indexed under this heading.

Ganciclovir Sodium (Because MPAG plasma concentrations are increased in the presence of renal impairment, as are ganciclovir concentrations, the two drugs will compete for tubular secretion and thus further increases in concentrations of both drugs may occur. In patients with renal impairment in which mycophenolate mofetil and ganciclovir or its prodrug (eg, valganciclovir) are co-administered, patients should be monitored carefully).

No products indexed under this heading.

Influenza Vaccine, Live Attenuated (During treatment with mycophenolate mofetil, the use of live attenuated vaccines should be avoided and patients should be advised that vaccines may be less effective. Influenza vaccination may be of value. Prescribers should refer to national guidelines for influenza vaccination).

No products indexed under this heading.

Influenza Virus Vaccine Live, Intranasal (During treatment with mycophenolate mofetil, the use of live attenuated vaccines should be avoided and patients should be advised that vaccines may be less effective. Influenza vaccination may be of value. Prescribers should refer to national guidelines for influenza vaccination). Products include:

FluMist Vaccine 1945

Levonorgestrel (A study of co-administration of mycophenolate mofetil and oral contraceptives containing ethinyl estradiol and levonorgestrel, desogestrel or gestodene was conducted in 18 women with psoriasis over 3 consecutive menstrual cycles. Mean AUC (0-24h) was similar for ethinyl estradiol and 3-keto desogestrel, however mean levonorgestrel AUC (0-24h) significantly decreased by about 15%. There was large inter-patient variability in the data. Mean serum levels of LH, FSH and progesterone were not significantlyaffected. Mycophenolate mofetil may not have any influence on the ovulation-suppressing action of the studied oral contraceptives. Concurrent use with oral contraceptives should be used with caution and additional birth control methods considered). Products include:

Climara Pro Transdermal System 768
Lybrel Tablets 3204
Mirena Intrauterine System 779
Plan B Tablets 1044
Seasonique Tablets 1046

Magaldrate (Absorption of a single dose of mycophenolate mofetil (2 g) was decreased when administered to ten rheumatoid arthritis patients also taking Maalox TC (10 mL q.i.d.) The Cmax and AUC (0-24h) for MPA was 33% and 17% lower, respectively, than when mycophenolate mofetil was administered alone under fasting conditions. Mycophenolate mofetil may be administered to patients who are also taking antacids containing magnesium and aluminum hydroxides, however it is recommended that mycophenolate mofetil and the antacid not be administered simultaneously).

No products indexed under this heading.

Magnesium Hydroxide (Absorption of a single dose of mycophenolate mofetil (2 g) was decreased when administered to ten rheumatoid arthritis patients also taking Maalox TC (10 mL q.i.d.) The Cmax and AUC (0-24h) for MPA was 33% and 17% lower, respectively, than when mycophenolate mofetil was administered alone under fasting conditions. Mycophenolate mofetil may be administered to patients who are also taking antacids containing magnesium and aluminum hydroxides, however it is recommended that mycophenolate mofetil and the antacid not be administered simultaneously). Products include:

Fleet Pedia-Lax Chewable Tablets 1145
Pepcid Complete Chewable Tablets 1771
Extra Strength Rolaids Freshmint Tablets 1903
Rolaids Multi-Symptom Berry Tablets 1903
Rolaids Original Peppermint Tablets 1903

Magnesium Oxide (Absorption of a single dose of mycophenolate mofetil (2 g) was decreased when administered to ten rheumatoid arthritis patients also taking Maalox TC (10 mL q.i.d.) The Cmax and AUC (0-24h) for MPA was 33% and 17% lower, respectively, than when mycophenolate mofetil was administered alone under fasting conditions. Mycophenolate mofetil may be administered to patients who are also taking antacids containing magnesium and aluminum hydroxides, however it is recommended that mycophenolate mofetil and the antacid not be administered simultaneously). Products include:

Beelith Tablets 813

Measles, Mumps, Rubella and Varicella Virus Vaccine Live (During treatment with mycophenolate mofetil, the use of live attenuated vaccines should be avoided and patients should be advised that vaccines may be less effective. Influenza vaccination may be of value. Prescribers should refer to national guidelines for influenza vaccination). Products include:

ProQuad 2099

Measles, Mumps & Rubella Virus Vaccine, Live (During treatment with mycophenolate mofetil, the use of live attenuated vaccines should be avoided and patients should be advised that vaccines may be less effective. Influenza vaccination may be of value. Prescribers should refer to national guidelines for influenza vaccination). Products include:

M-M-R II 2054

Measles & Rubella Virus Vaccine Live (During treatment with mycophenolate mofetil, the use of live attenuated vaccines should be avoided and patients should be advised that vaccines may be less effective. Influenza vaccination may be of value. Prescribers should refer to national guidelines for influenza vaccination).

No products indexed under this heading.

Measles Virus Vaccine Live (During treatment with mycophenolate mofetil, the use of live attenuated vaccines should be avoided and patients should be advised that vaccines may be less effective. Influenza vaccination may be of value. Prescribers should refer to national guidelines for influenza vaccination). Products include:

Attenuvax 1951

Mestranol (A study of co-administration of mycophenolate mofetil and oral contraceptives containing ethinyl estradiol and levonorgestrel, desogestrel or gestodene was conducted in 18 women with psoriasis over 3 consecutive menstrual cycles. Mean AUC (0-24h) was similar for ethinyl estradiol and 3-keto desogestrel, however mean levonorgestrel AUC (0-24h) significantly decreased by about 15%. There was large inter-patient variability in the data. Mean serum levels of LH, FSH and progesterone were not significantlyaffected. Mycophenolate mofetil may not have any influence on the ovulation-suppressing action of the studied oral contraceptives. Concurrent use with oral contraceptives should be used with caution and additional birth control methods considered).

No products indexed under this heading.

Metronidazole (Following single-dose administration of mycophenolate mofetil (1 g) to 11 healthy volunteers on day 4 of a 5-day course of a combination of norfloxacin and metronidazole, the mean MPA AUC 0-48h was significantly reduced by 33% compared to the administration of mycophenolate mofetil alone (p<0.05). Therefore, mycophenolate mofetil is not recommended to be given with the combination of norfloxacin and metronidazole. There was no significant effect on mean MPA AUC 0-48h when mycophenolate mofetil was concomitantly administered with norfloxacin or metronidazole separately). Products include:

Pylera Capsules 714

Metronidazole Benzoate (Following single-dose administration of mycophenolate mofetil (1 g) to 11 healthy volunteers on day 4 of a 5-day course of a combination of norfloxacin and metronidazole, the mean MPA AUC 0-48h was significantly reduced by 33% compared to the administration of mycophenolate mofetil alone (p<0.05). Therefore, mycophenolate mofetil is not recommended to be given with the combination of norfloxacin and metronidazole. There was no significant effect on mean MPA AUC 0-48h when mycophenolate mofetil was concomitantly administered with norfloxacin or metronidazole separately).

No products indexed under this heading.

Metronidazole Hydrochloride (Following single-dose administration of mycophenolate mofetil (1 g) to 11 healthy volunteers on day 4 of a 5-day course of a combination of norfloxacin and metronidazole, the mean MPA AUC 0-48h was significantly reduced by 33% compared to the administration of mycophenolate mofetil alone (p<0.05). Therefore, mycophenolate mofetil is not recommended to be given with the combination of norfloxacin and metronidazole. There was no significant effect on mean MPA AUC 0-48h when mycophenolate mofetil was concomitantly administered with norfloxacin or metronidazole separately).

No products indexed under this heading.

Metronidazole Sodium (Following single-dose administration of mycophenolate mofetil (1 g) to 11 healthy volunteers on day 4 of a 5-day course of a combination of norfloxacin and metronidazole, the mean MPA AUC 0-48h was significantly reduced by 33% compared to the administration of mycophenolate mofetil alone (p<0.05). Therefore, mycophenolate mofetil is not recommended to be given with the combination of norfloxacin and metronidazole. There was no significant effect on mean MPA AUC 0-48h when mycophenolate mofetil was concomitantly administered with norfloxacin or metronidazole separately).

No products indexed under this heading.

Mumps Virus Vaccine, Live (During treatment with mycophenolate mofetil, the use of live attenuated vaccines should be avoided and patients should be advised that vaccines may be less effective. Influenza vaccination may be of value. Prescribers should refer to national guidelines for influenza vaccination). Products include:

Mumpsvax 2068

Norethindrone (A study of co-administration of mycophenolate mofetil and oral contraceptives containing ethinyl estradiol and levonorgestrel, desogestrel or gestodene was conducted in 18 women with psoriasis over 3 consecutive menstrual cycles. Mean AUC (0-24h) was similar for ethinyl estradiol and 3-keto desogestrel, however mean levonorgestrel AUC (0-24h) significantly decreased by about 15%. There was large inter-patient variability in the data. Mean serum levels of LH, FSH and progesterone were not significantlyaffected. Mycophenolate mofetil may not have any influence on the ovulation-suppressing action of the studied oral contraceptives. Concurrent use with oral contraceptives should be used with caution and additional birth control methods considered). Products include:

Ortho Micronor Tablets 2446

Norethynodrel (A study of co-administration of mycophenolate mofetil and oral contraceptives containing ethinyl estradiol and levonorgestrel, desogestrel or gestodene was conducted in 18 women with psoriasis over 3 consecutive menstrual cycles. Mean AUC (0-24h) was similar for ethinyl estradiol and 3-keto desogestrel, however mean levonorgestrel AUC (0-24h) significantly decreased by about 15%. There was large inter-patient variability in the data. Mean serum levels of LH, FSH and progesterone were not significantlyaffected. Mycophenolate mofetil may not have any influence on the ovulation-suppressing action of the studied oral contraceptives. Concurrent use with oral contraceptives should be used with caution and additional birth control methods considered).

No products indexed under this heading.

Norfloxacin (Following single-dose administration of mycophenolate mofetil (1 g) to 11 healthy volunteers on day 4 of a 5-day course of a combination of norfloxacin and metronidazole, the mean MPA AUC 0-48h was significantly reduced by 33% compared to the administration of mycophenolate mofetil alone (p<0.05). Therefore, mycophenolate mofetil is not recommended to be given with the combination of norfloxacin and metronidazole. There was no significant effect on mean MPA AUC 0-48h when mycophenolate mofetil was concomitantly administered with norfloxacin or metronidazole separately). Products include:

Noroxin Tablets 2069

Norgestimate (A study of co-administration of mycophenolate mofetil and oral contraceptives containing ethinyl estradiol and levonorgestrel, desogestrel or gestodene was conducted in 18 women with psoriasis over 3 consecutive menstrual cycles. Mean AUC (0-24h) was similar for ethinyl estradiol and 3-keto desogestrel, however mean levonorgestrel AUC (0-24h) significantly decreased by about 15%. There was large inter-patient variability in the data. Mean serum levels of LH, FSH and progesterone were not significantlyaffected. Mycophenolate mofetil may not have any influence on the ovulation-suppressing action of the studied oral contraceptives. Concurrent use with oral contraceptives should be used with caution and additional birth control methods considered). Products include:

Ortho-Cyclen/Ortho Tri-Cyclen 2449

Ortho Tri-Cyclen Lo Tablets 2458

Norgestrel (A study of co-administration of mycophenolate mofetil and oral contraceptives containing ethinyl estradiol and levonorgestrel, desogestrel or gestodene was conducted in 18 women with psoriasis over 3 consecutive menstrual cycles. Mean AUC (0-24h) was similar for ethinyl estradiol and 3-keto desogestrel, however mean levonorgestrel AUC (0-24h) significantly decreased by about 15%. There was large inter-patient variability in the data. Mean serum levels of LH, FSH and progesterone were not significantlyaffected. Mycophenolate mofetil may not have any influence on the ovulation-suppressing action of the studied oral contraceptives. Concurrent use with oral contraceptives should be used with caution and additional birth control methods considered).

No products indexed under this heading.

Poliovirus Vaccine, Live, Oral, Trivalent, Types 1,2,3 (Sabin) (During treatment with mycophenolate mofetil, the use of live attenuated vaccines should be avoided and patients should be advised that vaccines may be less effective. Influenza vaccination may be of value. Prescribers should refer to national guidelines for influenza vaccination).

No products indexed under this heading.

Polysorbate 80 (Mycophenolate mofetil hydrochloride for injection is contraindicated in patients who are allergic to polysorbate 80).

No products indexed under this heading.

Probenecid (The measured value for renal clearance of MPAG indicates removal occurs by renal tubular secretion as well as glomerular filtration. Other drugs known to undergo renal tubular secretion may compete with MPAG and thereby raise plasma concentrations of MPAG or the other drug undergoing tubular secretion).

No products indexed under this heading.

Rifampin (In a single heart-lung transplant patient, after correction for dose, a 67% decrease in MPA exposure (AUC 0-12h) has been observed with concomitant administration of mycophenolate mofetil and rifampin. Therefore, mycophenolate mofetil is not recommended to be given with rifampin concomitantly unless benefit outweighs the risk).

No products indexed under this heading.

Rotavirus Vaccine, Live, Oral, Tetravalent (During treatment with mycophenolate mofetil, the use of live attenuated vaccines should be avoided and patients should be advised that vaccines may be less effective. Influenza vaccination may be of value. Prescribers should refer to national guidelines for influenza vaccination).

No products indexed under this heading.

Rubella & Mumps Virus Vaccine Live (During treatment with mycophenolate mofetil, the use of live attenuated vaccines should be avoided and patients should be advised that vaccines may be less effective. Influenza vaccination may be of value. Prescribers should refer to national guidelines for influenza vaccination).
No products indexed under this heading.

Rubella Virus Vaccine Live (During treatment with mycophenolate mofetil, the use of live attenuated vaccines should be avoided and patients should be advised that vaccines may be less effective. Influenza vaccination may be of value. Prescribers should refer to national guidelines for influenza vaccination). Products include:
Meruvax II 2061

Sevelamer Hydrochloride (Concomitant administration of sevelamer and mycophenolate mofetil in adult and pediatric patients decreased the mean MPA Cmax and AUC 0-12h by 36% and 26% respectively. This data suggest that sevelamer and other calcium free phosphate binders should not be administered simultaneously with mycophenolate mofetil. Alternately, it is recommended that sevelamer and other calcium free phosphate binders preferentially could be given 2 hours after mycophenolate mofetil intake to minimize the impact of the absorption of MPA).
No products indexed under this heading.

Smallpox Vaccine (During treatment with mycophenolate mofetil, the use of live attenuated vaccines should be avoided and patients should be advised that vaccines may be less effective. Influenza vaccination may be of value. Prescribers should refer to national guidelines for influenza vaccination).
No products indexed under this heading.

Sodium Bicarbonate (Absorption of a single dose of mycophenolate mofetil (2 g) was decreased when administered to ten rheumatoid arthritis patients also taking Maalox TC (10 mL q.i.d.) The Cmax and AUC (0-24h) for MPA was 33% and 17% lower, respectively, than when mycophenolate mofetil was administered alone under fasting conditions. Mycophenolate mofetil may be administered to patients who are also taking antacids containing magnesium and aluminum hydroxides, however it is recommended that mycophenolate mofetil and the antacid not be administered simultaneously). Products include:
Ceo-Two Laxative Suppository 815

Sulfamethoxazole (Following single-dose administration of mycophenolate mofetil (1.5 g) to 12 healthy male volunteers on day 8 of a 10-day course of trimethoprim 160 mg/sulfamethoxazole 800 mg administered b.i.d., no effect on the bioavailability of MPA was observed. The mean (±SD) AUC and Cmax of MPA after concomitant administration were 75.2 (+/-19.8) µg•h/mL and 34.0 (+/-6.6) µg/mL, respectively compared to 79.2 (±27.9) µg•mL and 34.2 (+/-10.7 µg/mL, respectively, after administration of mycophenolate mofetil alone).
No products indexed under this heading.

Trimethoprim (Following single-dose administration of mycophenolate mofetil (1.5 g) to 12 healthy male volunteers on day 8 of a 10-day course of trimethoprim 160 mg/sulfamethoxazole 800 mg administered b.i.d., no effect on the bioavailability of MPA was observed. The mean (±SD) AUC and Cmax of MPA after concomitant administration were 75.2 (+/-19.8) µg•h/mL and 34.0 (+/-6.6) µg/mL, respectively compared to 79.2 (±27.9) µg•mL and 34.2 (+/-10.7 µg/mL, respectively, after administration of mycophenolate mofetil alone).
No products indexed under this heading.

Trimethoprim Hydrochloride (Following single-dose administration of mycophenolate mofetil (1.5 g) to 12 healthy male volunteers on day 8 of a 10-day course of trimethoprim 160 mg/sulfamethoxazole 800 mg administered b.i.d., no effect on the bioavailability of MPA was observed. The mean (±SD) AUC and Cmax of MPA after concomitant administration were 75.2 (+/-19.8) µg•h/mL and 34.0 (+/-6.6) µg/mL, respectively compared to 79.2 (±27.9) µg•mL and 34.2 (+/-10.7 µg/mL, respectively, after administration of mycophenolate mofetil alone).
No products indexed under this heading.

Trimethoprim Sulfate (Following single-dose administration of mycophenolate mofetil (1.5 g) to 12 healthy male volunteers on day 8 of a 10-day course of trimethoprim 160 mg/sulfamethoxazole 800 mg administered b.i.d., no effect on the bioavailability of MPA was observed. The mean (±SD) AUC and Cmax of MPA after concomitant administration were 75.2 (+/-19.8) µg•h/mL and 34.0 (+/-6.6) µg/mL, respectively compared to 79.2 (±27.9) µg•mL and 34.2 (+/-10.7 µg/mL, respectively, after administration of mycophenolate mofetil alone).
No products indexed under this heading.

Typhoid Vaccine (During treatment with mycophenolate mofetil, the use of live attenuated vaccines should be avoided and patients should be advised that vaccines may be less effective. Influenza vaccination may be of value. Prescribers should refer to national guidelines for influenza vaccination).
No products indexed under this heading.

Valacyclovir Hydrochloride (Co-administration of mycophenolate mofetil (1 g) and acyclovir (800 mg) to 12 healthy volunteers resulted in no significant change in mycophenolic acid (MPA) AUC and Cmax. However the phenolic glucuronide of MPA (MPAG) and acyclovir plasma AUCs were increased 10.6% and 21.9% respectively. Because MPAG plasma concentrations are increased in the presence of renal impairment, as are acyclovir concentrations, the potential exists for mycophenolate and acyclovir or its prodrug (eg, valacyclovir) to compete for tubular secretion, further increasing the concentrations of both drugs). Products include:
Valtrex Caplets 1635

Valganciclovir Hydrochloride (Because MPAG plasma concentrations are increased in the presence of renal impairment, as are ganciclovir concentrations, the two drugs will compete for tubular secretion and thus further increases in concentrations of both drugs may occur. In patients with renal impairment in which mycophenolate mofetil and ganciclovir or its prodrug (eg, valganciclovir) are co-administered, patients should be monitored carefully). Products include:
Valcyte Tablets 2654

Varicella Virus Vaccine Live (During treatment with mycophenolate mofetil, the use of live attenuated vaccines should be avoided and patients should be advised that vaccines may be less effective. Influenza vaccination may be of value. Prescribers should refer to national guidelines for influenza vaccination). Products include:
Varivax 2133

Yellow Fever Vaccine (During treatment with mycophenolate mofetil, the use of live attenuated vaccines should be avoided and patients should be advised that vaccines may be less effective. Influenza vaccination may be of value. Prescribers should refer to national guidelines for influenza vaccination).
No products indexed under this heading.

Zoster Vaccine Live (During treatment with mycophenolate mofetil, the use of live attenuated vaccines should be avoided and patients should be advised that vaccines may be less effective. Influenza vaccination may be of value. Prescribers should refer to national guidelines for influenza vaccination). Products include:
Zostavax Injection 2145

CELLCEPT ORAL SUSPENSION

(Mycophenolate Mofetil) 2622
May interact with antacids, oral contraceptives, vaccines, live, and certain other agents. Compounds in these categories include:

Acyclovir (Co-administration of mycophenolate mofetil (1 g) and acyclovir (800 mg) to 12 healthy volunteers resulted in no significant change in mycophenolic acid (MPA) AUC and Cmax. However the phenolic glucuronide of MPA (MPAG) and acyclovir plasma AUCs were increased 10.6% and 21.9% respectively. Because MPAG plasma concentrations are increased in the presence of renal impairment, as are acyclovir concentrations, the potential exists for mycophenolate and acyclovir or its prodrug (eg, valacyclovir) to compete for tubular secretion, further increasing the concentrations of both drugs). Products include:
Zovirax 1690
Zovirax Cream 817
Zovirax Ointment 819

Acyclovir Sodium (Co-administration of mycophenolate mofetil (1 g) and acyclovir (800 mg) to 12 healthy volunteers resulted in no significant change in mycophenolic acid (MPA) AUC and Cmax. However the phenolic glucuronide of MPA (MPAG) and acyclovir plasma AUCs were increased 10.6% and 21.9% respectively. Because MPAG plasma concentrations are increased in the presence of renal impairment, as are acyclovir concentrations, the potential exists for mycophenolate and acyclovir or its prodrug (eg, valacyclovir) to compete for tubular secretion, further increasing the concentrations of both drugs).
No products indexed under this heading.

Aluminum Carbonate (Absorption of a single dose of mycophenolate mofetil (2 g) was decreased when administered to ten rheumatoid arthritis patients also taking Maalox TC (10 mL q.i.d.) The Cmax and AUC (0-24h) for MPA was 33% and 17% lower, respectively, than when mycophenolate mofetil was administered alone under fasting conditions. Mycophenolate mofetil may be administered to patients who are also taking antacids containing magnesium and aluminum hydroxides, however it is recommended that mycophenolate mofetil and the antacid not be administered simultaneously).
No products indexed under this heading.

Aluminum Hydroxide (Absorption of a single dose of mycophenolate mofetil (2 g) was decreased when administered to ten rheumatoid arthritis patients also taking Maalox TC (10 mL q.i.d.) The Cmax and AUC (0-24h) for MPA was 33% and 17% lower, respectively, than when mycophenolate mofetil was administered alone under fasting conditions. Mycophenolate mofetil may be administered to patients who are also taking antacids containing magnesium and aluminum hydroxides, however it is recommended that mycophenolate mofetil and the antacid not be administered simultaneously).
No products indexed under this heading.

Azathioprine (It is recommended that mycophenolate mofetil not be administered concomitantly with azathioprine because both have the potential to cause bone marrow suppression and such concomitant administration has not been studied clinically).
No products indexed under this heading.

Azathioprine Sodium (It is recommended that mycophenolate mofetil not be administered concomitantly with azathioprine because both have the potential to cause bone marrow suppression and such concomitant administration has not been studied clinically).
No products indexed under this heading.

BCG Vaccine (During treatment with mycophenolate mofetil, the use of live attenuated vaccines should be avoided and patients should be advised that vaccines may be less effective. Influenza vaccination may be of value. Prescribers should refer to national guidelines for influenza vaccination).
No products indexed under this heading.

Cholestyramine (Following single-dose administration of 1.5 g mycophenolate mofetil to 12 healthy volunteers pretreated with 4 g t.i.d. of cholestyramine for 4 days, MPA AUC decreased approximately 40%. This decrease is consistent with interruption of enterohepatic recirculation which may be due to binding of recirculating MPAG with cholestyramine in the intestine. Some degree of enterohepatic recirculation is also anticipated following intravenous administration of mycophenolate mofetil. Therefore, mycophenolate mofetil is not recommended to be given with cholestyramine or other agents that may interfere with enterohepatic recirculation).

No products indexed under this heading.

Cyclosporine (In renal transplant patients, mean MPA exposure (AUC 0-12h) was approximately 30% to 50% greater when mycophenolate mofetil is administered without cyclosporine compared with when mycophenolate mofetil is co-administered with cyclosporine. This interaction is due to cyclosporine inhibition of multidrug-resistance-associated protein 2 (MRP-2) transporter in the biliary tract, thereby preventing the excretion of MPAG into the bile that would lead to enterohepatic recirculation of MPA. This information should be taken into consideration when mycophenolate mofetil is used without cyclosporine). Products include:

Gengraf Capsules 435
Neoral Oral Solution 2280
Neoral Soft Gelatin Capsules 2280
Restasis Ophthalmic Emulsion 557
Sandimmune 2296

Desogestrel (A study of co-administration of mycophenolate mofetil and oral contraceptives containing ethinyl estradiol and levonorgestrel, desogestrel or gestodene was conducted in 18 women with psoriasis over 3 consecutive menstrual cycles. Mean AUC (0-24h) was similar for ethinyl estradiol and 3-keto desogestrel, however mean levonorgestrel AUC (0-24h) significantly decreased by about 15%. There was large inter-patient variability in the data. Mean serum levels of LH, FSH and progesterone were not significantlyaffected. Mycophenolate mofetil may not have any influence on the ovulation-suppressing action of the studied oral contraceptives. Concurrent use with oral contraceptives should be used with caution and additional birth control methods considered). Products include:

Mircette Tablets 1034

Ethinyl Estradiol (A study of co-administration of mycophenolate mofetil and oral contraceptives containing ethinyl estradiol and levonorgestrel, desogestrel or gestodene was conducted in 18 women with psoriasis over 3 consecutive menstrual cycles. Mean AUC (0-24h) was similar for ethinyl estradiol and 3-keto desogestrel, however mean levonorgestrel AUC (0-24h) significantly decreased by about 15%. There was large inter-patient variability in the data. Mean serum levels of LH, FSH and progesterone were not significantlyaffected. Mycophenolate mofetil may not have any influence on the ovulation-suppressing action of the studied oral contraceptives. Concurrent use with oral contraceptives should be used with caution and additional birth control methods considered). Products include:

Lybrel Tablets 3204
Mircette Tablets 1034
NuvaRing 2897
Ortho-Cyclen/Ortho Tri-Cyclen 2449
Ortho Evra Transdermal System 2437
Ortho Tri-Cyclen Lo Tablets 2458
Seasonique Tablets 1046
Yaz Tablets 805

Ethynodiol Diacetate (A study of co-administration of mycophenolate mofetil and oral contraceptives containing ethinyl estradiol and levonorgestrel, desogestrel or gestodene was conducted in 18 women with psoriasis over 3 consecutive menstrual cycles. Mean AUC (0-24h) was similar for ethinyl estradiol and 3-keto desogestrel, however mean levonorgestrel AUC (0-24h) significantly decreased by about 15%. There was large inter-patient variability in the data. Mean serum levels of LH, FSH and progesterone were not significantlyaffected. Mycophenolate mofetil may not have any influence on the ovulation-suppressing action of the studied oral contraceptives. Concurrent use with oral contraceptives should be used with caution and additional birth control methods considered).

No products indexed under this heading.

Ganciclovir (Because MPAG plasma concentrations are increased in the presence of renal impairment, as are ganciclovir concentrations, the two drugs will compete for tubular secretion and thus further increases in concentrations of both drugs may occur. In patients with renal impairment in which mycophenolate mofetil and ganciclovir or its prodrug (eg, valganciclovir) are co-administered, patients should be monitored carefully).

No products indexed under this heading.

Ganciclovir Sodium (Because MPAG plasma concentrations are increased in the presence of renal impairment, as are ganciclovir concentrations, the two drugs will compete for tubular secretion and thus further increases in concentrations of both drugs may occur. In patients with renal impairment in which mycophenolate mofetil and ganciclovir or its prodrug (eg, valganciclovir) are co-administered, patients should be monitored carefully).

No products indexed under this heading.

Influenza Vaccine, Live Attenuated (During treatment with mycophenolate mofetil, the use of live attenuated vaccines should be avoided and patients should be advised that vaccines may be less effective. Influenza vaccination may be of value. Prescribers should refer to national guidelines for influenza vaccination).

No products indexed under this heading.

Influenza Virus Vaccine Live, Intranasal (During treatment with mycophenolate mofetil, the use of live attenuated vaccines should be avoided and patients should be advised that vaccines may be less effective. Influenza vaccination may be of value. Prescribers should refer to national guidelines for influenza vaccination). Products include:

FluMist Vaccine 1945

Levonorgestrel (A study of co-administration of mycophenolate mofetil and oral contraceptives containing ethinyl estradiol and levonorgestrel, desogestrel or gestodene was conducted in 18 women with psoriasis over 3 consecutive menstrual cycles. Mean AUC (0-24h) was similar for ethinyl estradiol and 3-keto desogestrel, however mean levonorgestrel AUC (0-24h) significantly decreased by about 15%. There was large inter-patient variability in the data. Mean serum levels of LH, FSH and progesterone were not significantlyaffected. Mycophenolate mofetil may not have any influence on the ovulation-suppressing action of the studied oral contraceptives. Concurrent use with oral contraceptives should be used with caution and additional birth control methods considered). Products include:

Climara Pro Transdermal System 768
Lybrel Tablets 3204
Mirena Intrauterine System 779
Plan B Tablets 1044
Seasonique Tablets 1046

Magaldrate (Absorption of a single dose of mycophenolate mofetil (2 g) was decreased when administered to ten rheumatoid arthritis patients also taking Maalox TC (10 mL q.i.d.) The Cmax and AUC (0-24h) for MPA was 33% and 17% lower, respectively, than when mycophenolate mofetil was administered alone under fasting conditions. Mycophenolate mofetil may be administered to patients who are also taking antacids containing magnesium and aluminum hydroxides, however it is recommended that mycophenolate mofetil and the antacid not be administered simultaneously).

No products indexed under this heading.

Magnesium Hydroxide (Absorption of a single dose of mycophenolate mofetil (2 g) was decreased when administered to ten rheumatoid arthritis patients also taking Maalox TC (10 mL q.i.d.) The Cmax and AUC (0-24h) for MPA was 33% and 17% lower, respectively, than when mycophenolate mofetil was administered alone under fasting conditions. Mycophenolate mofetil may be administered to patients who are also taking antacids containing magnesium and aluminum hydroxides, however it is recommended that mycophenolate mofetil and the antacid not be administered simultaneously). Products include:

Fleet Pedia-Lax Chewable Tablets 1145
Pepcid Complete Chewable Tablets 1771
Extra Strength Rolaids Freshmint Tablets 1903
Rolaids Multi-Symptom Berry Tablets 1903
Rolaids Original Peppermint Tablets 1903

Magnesium Oxide (Absorption of a single dose of mycophenolate mofetil (2 g) was decreased when administered to ten rheumatoid arthritis patients also taking Maalox TC (10 mL q.i.d.) The Cmax and AUC (0-24h) for MPA was 33% and 17% lower, respectively, than when mycophenolate mofetil was administered alone under fasting conditions. Mycophenolate mofetil may be administered to patients who are also taking antacids containing magnesium and aluminum hydroxides, however it is recommended that mycophenolate mofetil and the antacid not be administered simultaneously). Products include:

Beelith Tablets 813

Measles, Mumps, Rubella and Varicella Virus Vaccine Live (During treatment with mycophenolate mofetil, the use of live attenuated vaccines should be avoided and patients should be advised that vaccines may be less effective. Influenza vaccination may be of value. Prescribers should refer to national guidelines for influenza vaccination). Products include:

ProQuad 2099

Measles, Mumps & Rubella Virus Vaccine, Live (During treatment with mycophenolate mofetil, the use of live attenuated vaccines should be avoided and patients should be advised that vaccines may be less effective. Influenza vaccination may be of value. Prescribers should refer to national guidelines for influenza vaccination). Products include:

M-M-R II 2054

Measles & Rubella Virus Vaccine Live (During treatment with mycophenolate mofetil, the use of live attenuated vaccines should be avoided and patients should be advised that vaccines may be less effective. Influenza vaccination may be of value. Prescribers should refer to national guidelines for influenza vaccination).

No products indexed under this heading.

Measles Virus Vaccine Live (During treatment with mycophenolate mofetil, the use of live attenuated vaccines should be avoided and patients should be advised that vaccines may be less effective. Influenza vaccination may be of value. Prescribers should refer to national guidelines for influenza vaccination). Products include:

Attenuvax 1951

Mestranol (A study of co-administration of mycophenolate mofetil and oral contraceptives containing ethinyl estradiol and levonorgestrel, desogestrel or gestodene was conducted in 18 women with psoriasis over 3 consecutive menstrual cycles. Mean AUC (0-24h) was similar for ethinyl estradiol and 3-keto desogestrel, however mean levonorgestrel AUC (0-24h) significantly decreased by about 15%. There was large inter-patient variability in the data. Mean serum levels of LH, FSH and progesterone were not significantlyaffected. Mycophenolate mofetil may not have any influence on the ovulation-suppressing action of the studied oral contraceptives. Concurrent use with oral contraceptives should be used with caution and additional birth control methods considered).

No products indexed under this heading.

Metronidazole (Following single-dose administration of mycophenolate mofetil (1 g) to 11 healthy volunteers on day 4 of a 5-day course of a combination of norfloxacin and metronidazole, the mean MPA AUC 0-48h was significantly reduced by 33% compared to the administration of mycophenolate mofetil alone ($p<0.05$). Therefore, mycophenolate mofetil is not recommended to be given with the combination of norfloxacin and metronidazole. There was no significant effect on mean MPA AUC 0-48h when mycophenolate mofetil was concomitantly administered with norfloxacin or metronidazole separately). Products include:

Pylera Capsules 714

Metronidazole Benzoate (Following single-dose administration of mycophenolate mofetil (1 g) to 11 healthy volunteers on day 4 of a 5-day course of a combination of norfloxacin and metronidazole, the mean MPA AUC 0-48h was significantly reduced by 33% compared to the administration of mycophenolate mofetil alone (p<0.05). Therefore, mycophenolate mofetil is not recommended to be given with the combination of norfloxacin and metronidazole. There was no significant effect on mean MPA AUC 0-48h when mycophenolate mofetil was concomitantly administered with norfloxacin or metronidazole separately).

No products indexed under this heading.

Metronidazole Hydrochloride (Following single-dose administration of mycophenolate mofetil (1 g) to 11 healthy volunteers on day 4 of a 5-day course of a combination of norfloxacin and metronidazole, the mean MPA AUC 0-48h was significantly reduced by 33% compared to the administration of mycophenolate mofetil alone (p<0.05). Therefore, mycophenolate mofetil is not recommended to be given with the combination of norfloxacin and metronidazole. There was no significant effect on mean MPA AUC 0-48h when mycophenolate mofetil was concomitantly administered with norfloxacin or metronidazole separately).

No products indexed under this heading.

Metronidazole Sodium (Following single-dose administration of mycophenolate mofetil (1 g) to 11 healthy volunteers on day 4 of a 5-day course of a combination of norfloxacin and metronidazole, the mean MPA AUC 0-48h was significantly reduced by 33% compared to the administration of mycophenolate mofetil alone (p<0.05). Therefore, mycophenolate mofetil is not recommended to be given with the combination of norfloxacin and metronidazole. There was no significant effect on mean MPA AUC 0-48h when mycophenolate mofetil was concomitantly administered with norfloxacin or metronidazole separately).

No products indexed under this heading.

Mumps Virus Vaccine, Live (During treatment with mycophenolate mofetil, the use of live attenuated vaccines should be avoided and patients should be advised that vaccines may be less effective. Influenza vaccination may be of value. Prescribers should refer to national guidelines for influenza vaccination). Products include:

Mumpsvax 2068

Norethindrone (A study of co-administration of mycophenolate mofetil and oral contraceptives containing ethinyl estradiol and levonorgestrel, desogestrel or gestodene was conducted in 18 women with psoriasis over 3 consecutive menstrual cycles. Mean AUC (0-24h) was similar for ethinyl estradiol and 3-keto desogestrel, however mean levonorgestrel AUC (0-24h) significantly decreased by about 15%. There was large inter-patient variability in the data. Mean serum levels of LH, FSH and progesterone were not significantlyaffected. Mycophenolate mofetil may not have any influence on the ovulation-suppressing action of the studied oral contraceptives. Concurrent use with oral contraceptives should be used with caution and additional birth control methods considered). Products include:

Ortho Micronor Tablets 2446

Norethynodrel (A study of co-administration of mycophenolate mofetil and oral contraceptives containing ethinyl estradiol and levonorgestrel, desogestrel or gestodene was conducted in 18 women with psoriasis over 3 consecutive menstrual cycles. Mean AUC (0-24h) was similar for ethinyl estradiol and 3-keto desogestrel, however mean levonorgestrel AUC (0-24h) significantly decreased by about 15%. There was large inter-patient variability in the data. Mean serum levels of LH, FSH and progesterone were not significantlyaffected. Mycophenolate mofetil may not have any influence on the ovulation-suppressing action of the studied oral contraceptives. Concurrent use with oral contraceptives should be used with caution and additional birth control methods considered).

No products indexed under this heading.

Norfloxacin (Following single-dose administration of mycophenolate mofetil (1 g) to 11 healthy volunteers on day 4 of a 5-day course of a combination of norfloxacin and metronidazole, the mean MPA AUC 0-48h was significantly reduced by 33% compared to the administration of mycophenolate mofetil alone (p<0.05). Therefore, mycophenolate mofetil is not recommended to be given with the combination of norfloxacin and metronidazole. There was no significant effect on mean MPA AUC 0-48h when mycophenolate mofetil was concomitantly administered with norfloxacin or metronidazole separately). Products include:

Noroxin Tablets 2069

Norgestimate (A study of co-administration of mycophenolate mofetil and oral contraceptives containing ethinyl estradiol and levonorgestrel, desogestrel or gestodene was conducted in 18 women with psoriasis over 3 consecutive menstrual cycles. Mean AUC (0-24h) was similar for ethinyl estradiol and 3-keto desogestrel, however mean levonorgestrel AUC (0-24h) significantly decreased by about 15%. There was large inter-patient variability in the data. Mean serum levels of LH, FSH and progesterone were not significantlyaffected. Mycophenolate mofetil may not have any influence on the ovulation-suppressing action of the studied oral contraceptives. Concurrent use with oral contraceptives should be used with caution and additional birth control methods considered). Products include:

Ortho-Cyclen/Ortho Tri-Cyclen 2449
Ortho Tri-Cyclen Lo Tablets 2458

Norgestrel (A study of co-administration of mycophenolate mofetil and oral contraceptives containing ethinyl estradiol and levonorgestrel, desogestrel or gestodene was conducted in 18 women with psoriasis over 3 consecutive menstrual cycles. Mean AUC (0-24h) was similar for ethinyl estradiol and 3-keto desogestrel, however mean levonorgestrel AUC (0-24h) was significantly decreased by about 15%. There was large inter-patient variability in the data. Mean serum levels of LH, FSH and progesterone were not significantlyaffected. Mycophenolate mofetil may not have any influence on the ovulation-suppressing action of the studied oral contraceptives. Concurrent use with oral contraceptives should be used with caution and additional birth control methods considered).

No products indexed under this heading.

D-Phenylalanine (Mycophenolate mofetil oral suspension contains aspartame, a source of phenylalanine (0.56 mg phenylalanine/mL suspension). Therefore, care should be taken if mycophenolate mofetil oral suspension is administered to patients with phenylketonuria).

No products indexed under this heading.

L-Phenylalanine (Mycophenolate mofetil oral suspension contains aspartame, a source of phenylalanine (0.56 mg phenylalanine/mL suspension). Therefore, care should be taken if mycophenolate mofetil oral suspension is administered to patients with phenylketonuria).

No products indexed under this heading.

Poliovirus Vaccine, Live, Oral, Trivalent, Types 1,2,3 (Sabin) (During treatment with mycophenolate mofetil, the use of live attenuated vaccines should be avoided and patients should be advised that vaccines may be less effective. Influenza vaccination may be of value. Prescribers should refer to national guidelines for influenza vaccination).

No products indexed under this heading.

Probenecid (The measured value for renal clearance of MPAG indicates removal occurs by renal tubular secretion as well as glomerular filtration. Other drugs known to undergo renal tubular secretion may compete with MPAG and thereby raise plasma concentrations of MPAG or the other drug undergoing tubular secretion).

No products indexed under this heading.

Rifampin (In a single heart-lung transplant patient, after correction for dose, a 67% decrease in MPA exposure (AUC 0-12h) has been observed with concomitant administration of mycophenolate mofetil and rifampin. Therefore, mycophenolate mofetil is not recommended to be given with rifampin concomitantly unless benefit outweighs the risk).

No products indexed under this heading.

Rotavirus Vaccine, Live, Oral, Tetravalent (During treatment with mycophenolate mofetil, the use of live attenuated vaccines should be avoided and patients should be advised that vaccines may be less effective. Influenza vaccination may be of value. Prescribers should refer to national guidelines for influenza vaccination).

No products indexed under this heading.

Rubella & Mumps Virus Vaccine Live (During treatment with mycophenolate mofetil, the use of live attenuated vaccines should be avoided and patients should be advised that vaccines may be less effective. Influenza vaccination may be of value. Prescribers should refer to national guidelines for influenza vaccination).

No products indexed under this heading.

Rubella Virus Vaccine Live (During treatment with mycophenolate mofetil, the use of live attenuated vaccines should be avoided and patients should be advised that vaccines may be less effective. Influenza vaccination may be of value. Prescribers should refer to national guidelines for influenza vaccination). Products include:

Meruvax II 2061

Sevelamer Hydrochloride (Concomitant administration of sevelamer and mycophenolate mofetil in adult and pediatric patients decreased the mean MPA Cmax and AUC 0-12h by 36% and 26% respectively. This data suggest that sevelamer and other calcium free phosphate binders should not be administered simultaneously with mycophenolate mofetil. Alternately, it is recommended that sevelamer and other calcium free phosphate binders preferentially could be given 2 hours after mycophenolate mofetil intake to minimize the impact of the absorption of MPA).

No products indexed under this heading.

Smallpox Vaccine (During treatment with mycophenolate mofetil, the use of live attenuated vaccines should be avoided and patients should be advised that vaccines may be less effective. Influenza vaccination may be of value. Prescribers should refer to national guidelines for influenza vaccination).

No products indexed under this heading.

Sodium Bicarbonate (Absorption of a single dose of mycophenolate mofetil (2 g) was decreased when administered to ten rheumatoid arthritis patients also taking Maalox TC (10 mL q.i.d.) The Cmax and AUC (0-24h) for MPA was 33% and 17% lower, respectively, than when mycophenolate mofetil was administered alone under fasting conditions. Mycophenolate mofetil may be administered to patients who are also taking antacids containing magnesium and aluminum hydroxides, however it is recommended that mycophenolate mofetil and the antacid not be administered simultaneously). Products include:

Ceo-Two Laxative Suppository 815

Sulfamethoxazole (Following single-dose administration of mycophenolate mofetil (1.5 g) to 12 healthy male volunteers on day 8 of a 10-day course of trimethoprim 160 mg/sulfamethoxazole 800 mg administered b.i.d., no effect on the bioavailability of MPA was observed. The mean (±SD) AUC and Cmax of MPA after concomitant administration were 75.2 (+/-19.8) µg•h/mL and 34.0 (+/-6.6) µg/mL, respectively compared to 79.2 (±27.9) µg•mL and 34.2 (±10.7 µg/mL, respectively, after administration of

IMPORTANT NOTE: Always consult each drug listing in the patient's regimen for possible interactions.

mycophenolate mofetil alone).
No products indexed under this heading.

Trimethoprim (Following single-dose administration of mycophenolate mofetil (1.5 g) to 12 healthy male volunteers on day 8 of a 10-day course of trimethoprim 160 mg/sulfamethoxazole 800 mg administered b.i.d., no effect on the bioavailability of MPA was observed. The mean (+/-SD) AUC and Cmax of MPA after concomitant administration were 75.2 (+/-19.8) ug*h/mL and 34.0 (+/-6.6) ug/mL, respectively compared to 79.2 (+/-27.9) ug*mL and 34.2 (+/-10.7 ug/mL, respectively, after administration of mycophenolate mofetil alone).
No products indexed under this heading.

Trimethoprim Hydrochloride (Following single-dose administration of mycophenolate mofetil (1.5 g) to 12 healthy male volunteers on day 8 of a 10-day course of trimethoprim 160 mg/sulfamethoxazole 800 mg administered b.i.d., no effect on the bioavailability of MPA was observed. The mean (±SD) AUC and Cmax of MPA after concomitant administration were 75.2 (+/-19.8) µg•h/mL and 34.0 (+/-6.6) µg/mL, respectively compared to 79.2 (±27.9) µg•mL and 34.2 (±10.7 µg/mL, respectively, after administration of mycophenolate mofetil alone).
No products indexed under this heading.

Trimethoprim Sulfate (Following single-dose administration of mycophenolate mofetil (1.5 g) to 12 healthy male volunteers on day 8 of a 10-day course of trimethoprim 160 mg/sulfamethoxazole 800 mg administered b.i.d., no effect on the bioavailability of MPA was observed. The mean (±SD) AUC and Cmax of MPA after concomitant administration were 75.2 (+/-19.8) µg•h/mL and 34.0 (+/-6.6) µg/mL, respectively compared to 79.2 (±27.9) µg•mL and 34.2 (±10.7 µg/mL, respectively, after administration of mycophenolate mofetil alone).
No products indexed under this heading.

Typhoid Vaccine (During treatment with mycophenolate mofetil, the use of live attenuated vaccines should be avoided and patients should be advised that vaccines may be less effective. Influenza vaccination may be of value. Prescribers should refer to national guidelines for influenza vaccination).
No products indexed under this heading.

Valacyclovir Hydrochloride (Co-administration of mycophenolate mofetil (1 g) and acyclovir (800 mg) to 12 healthy volunteers resulted in no significant change in mycophenolic acid (MPA) AUC and Cmax. However the phenolic glucuronide of MPA (MPAG) and acyclovir plasma AUCs were increased 10.6% and 21.9% respectively. Because MPAG plasma concentrations are increased in the presence of renal impairment, as are acyclovir concentrations, the potential exists for mycophenolate and acyclovir or its prodrug (eg, valacyclovir) to compete for tubular secretion, further increasing the concentrations of both drugs). Products include:
Valtrex Caplets 1635

Valganciclovir Hydrochloride (Because MPAG plasma concentrations are increased in the presence of renal impairment, as are ganciclovir concentrations, the two drugs will compete for tubular secretion and thus further increases in concentrations of both drugs may occur. In patients with renal impairment in which mycophenolate mofetil and ganciclovir or its prodrug (eg, valganciclovir) are co-administered, patients should be monitored carefully). Products include:
Valcyte Tablets 2654

Varicella Virus Vaccine Live (During treatment with mycophenolate mofetil, the use of live attenuated vaccines should be avoided and patients should be advised that vaccines may be less effective. Influenza vaccination may be of value. Prescribers should refer to national guidelines for influenza vaccination). Products include:
Varivax 2133

Yellow Fever Vaccine (During treatment with mycophenolate mofetil, the use of live attenuated vaccines should be avoided and patients should be advised that vaccines may be less effective. Influenza vaccination may be of value. Prescribers should refer to national guidelines for influenza vaccination).
No products indexed under this heading.

Zoster Vaccine Live (During treatment with mycophenolate mofetil, the use of live attenuated vaccines should be avoided and patients should be advised that vaccines may be less effective. Influenza vaccination may be of value. Prescribers should refer to national guidelines for influenza vaccination). Products include:
Zostavax Injection 2145

CELLCEPT TABLETS

(Mycophenolate Mofetil) 2622
May interact with antacids, oral contraceptives, vaccines, live, and certain other agents. Compounds in these categories include:

Acyclovir (Co-administration of mycophenolate mofetil (1 g) and acyclovir (800 mg) to 12 healthy volunteers resulted in no significant change in mycophenolic acid (MPA) AUC and Cmax. However the phenolic glucuronide of MPA (MPAG) and acyclovir plasma AUCs were increased 10.6% and 21.9% respectively. Because MPAG plasma concentrations are increased in the presence of renal impairment, as are acyclovir concentrations, the potential exists for mycophenolate and acyclovir or its prodrug (eg, valacyclovir) to compete for tubular secretion, further increasing the concentrations of both drugs). Products include:
Zovirax 1690
Zovirax Cream 817
Zovirax Ointment 819

Acyclovir Sodium (Co-administration of mycophenolate mofetil (1 g) and acyclovir (800 mg) to 12 healthy volunteers resulted in no significant change in mycophenolic acid (MPA) AUC and Cmax. However the phenolic glucuronide of MPA (MPAG) and acyclovir plasma AUCs were increased 10.6% and 21.9% respectively. Because MPAG plasma concentrations are increased in the presence of renal impairment, as are acyclovir concentrations, the potential exists for mycophenolate and acyclovir or its prodrug (eg, valacyclovir) to compete for tubular secretion, further increasing the concentrations of both drugs).
No products indexed under this heading.

Aluminum Carbonate (Absorption of a single dose of mycophenolate mofetil (2 g) was decreased when administered to ten rheumatoid arthritis patients also taking Maalox TC (10 mL q.i.d.) The Cmax and AUC (0-24h) for MPA was 33% and 17% lower, respectively, than when mycophenolate mofetil was administered alone under fasting conditions. Mycophenolate mofetil may be administered to patients who are also taking antacids containing magnesium and aluminum hydroxides, however it is recommended that mycophenolate mofetil and the antacid not be administered simultaneously).
No products indexed under this heading.

Aluminum Hydroxide (Absorption of a single dose of mycophenolate mofetil (2 g) was decreased when administered to ten rheumatoid arthritis patients also taking Maalox TC (10 mL q.i.d.) The Cmax and AUC (0-24h) for MPA was 33% and 17% lower, respectively, than when mycophenolate mofetil was administered alone under fasting conditions. Mycophenolate mofetil may be administered to patients who are also taking antacids containing magnesium and aluminum hydroxides, however it is recommended that mycophenolate mofetil and the antacid not be administered simultaneously).
No products indexed under this heading.

Azathioprine (It is recommended that mycophenolate mofetil not be administered concomitantly with azathioprine because both have the potential to cause bone marrow suppression and such concomitant administration has not been studied clinically).
No products indexed under this heading.

Azathioprine Sodium (It is recommended that mycophenolate mofetil not be administered concomitantly with azathioprine because both have the potential to cause bone marrow suppression and such concomitant administration has not been studied clinically).
No products indexed under this heading.

BCG Vaccine (During treatment with mycophenolate mofetil, the use of live attenuated vaccines should be avoided and patients should be advised that vaccines may be less effective. Influenza vaccination may be of value. Prescribers should refer to national guidelines for influenza vaccination).
No products indexed under this heading.

Cholestyramine (Following single-dose administration of 1.5 g mycophenolate mofetil to 12 healthy volunteers pretreated with 4 g t.i.d. of cholestyramine for 4 days, MPA AUC decreased approximately 40%. This decrease is consistent with interruption of enterohepatic recirculation which may be due to binding of recirculating MPAG with cholestyramine in the intestine. Some degree of enterohepatic recirculation is also anticipated following intravenous administration of mycophenolate mofetil. Therefore, mycophenolate mofetil is not recommended to be given with cholestyramine or other agents that may interfere with enterohepatic recirculation).
No products indexed under this heading.

Cyclosporine (In renal transplant patients, mean MPA exposure (AUC 0-12h) was approximately 30% to 50% greater when mycophenolate mofetil is administered without cyclosporine compared with when mycophenolate mofetil is co-administered with cyclosporine. This interaction is due to cyclosporine inhibition of multidrug-resistance-associated protein 2 (MRP-2) transporter in the biliary tract, thereby preventing the excretion of MPAG into the bile that would lead to enterohepatic recirculation of MPA. This information should be taken into consideration when mycophenolate mofetil is used without cyclosporine). Products include:
Gengraf Capsules 435
Neoral Oral Solution 2280
Neoral Soft Gelatin Capsules 2280
Restasis Ophthalmic Emulsion 557
Sandimmune 2296

Desogestrel (A study of co-administration of mycophenolate mofetil and oral contraceptives containing ethinyl estradiol and levonorgestrel, desogestrel or gestodene was conducted in 18 women with psoriasis over 3 consecutive menstrual cycles. Mean AUC (0-24h) was similar for ethinyl estradiol and 3-keto desogestrel, however mean levonorgestrel AUC (0-24h) significantly decreased by about 15%. There was large inter-patient variability in the data. Mean serum levels of LH, FSH and progesterone were not significantlyaffected. Mycophenolate mofetil may not have any influence on the ovulation-suppressing action of the studied oral contraceptives. Concurrent use with oral contraceptives should be used with caution and additional birth control methods considered). Products include:
Mircette Tablets 1034

Ethinyl Estradiol (A study of co-administration of mycophenolate mofetil and oral contraceptives containing ethinyl estradiol and levonorgestrel, desogestrel or gestodene was conducted in 18 women with psoriasis over 3 consecutive menstrual cycles. Mean AUC (0-24h) was similar for ethinyl estradiol and 3-keto desogestrel, however mean levonorgestrel AUC (0-24h) significantly decreased by about 15%. There was large inter-patient variability in the data. Mean serum levels of LH, FSH and progesterone were not significantlyaffected. Mycophenolate mofetil may not have any influence on the ovulation-suppressing action of the studied oral contraceptives. Concurrent use with oral contraceptives should be used with caution and additional birth control methods considered). Products include:
Lybrel Tablets 3204
Mircette Tablets 1034
NuvaRing 2897

Ortho-Cyclen/Ortho Tri-Cyclen 2449
Ortho Evra Transdermal System 2437
Ortho Tri-Cyclen Lo Tablets 2458
Seasonique Tablets 1046
Yaz Tablets 805

Ethynodiol Diacetate (A study of co-administration of mycophenolate mofetil and oral contraceptives containing ethinyl estradiol and levonorgestrel, desogestrel or gestodene was conducted in 18 women with psoriasis over 3 consecutive menstrual cycles. Mean AUC (0-24h) was similar for ethinyl estradiol and 3-keto desogestrel, however mean levonorgestrel AUC (0-24h) significantly decreased by about 15%. There was large inter-patient variability in the data. Mean serum levels of LH, FSH and progesterone were not significantlyaffected. Mycophenolate mofetil may not have any influence on the ovulation-suppressing action of the studied oral contraceptives. Concurrent use with oral contraceptives should be used with caution and additional birth control methods considered).
No products indexed under this heading.

Ganciclovir (Because MPAG plasma concentrations are increased in the presence of renal impairment, as are ganciclovir concentrations, the two drugs will compete for tubular secretion and thus further increases in concentrations of both drugs may occur. In patients with renal impairment in which mycophenolate mofetil and ganciclovir or its prodrug (eg, valganciclovir) are co-administered, patients should be monitored carefully).
No products indexed under this heading.

Ganciclovir Sodium (Because MPAG plasma concentrations are increased in the presence of renal impairment, as are ganciclovir concentrations, the two drugs will compete for tubular secretion and thus further increases in concentrations of both drugs may occur. In patients with renal impairment in which mycophenolate mofetil and ganciclovir or its prodrug (eg, valganciclovir) are co-administered, patients should be monitored carefully).
No products indexed under this heading.

Influenza Vaccine, Live Attenuated (During treatment with mycophenolate mofetil, the use of live attenuated vaccines should be avoided and patients should be advised that vaccines may be less effective. Influenza vaccination may be of value. Prescribers should refer to national guidelines for influenza vaccination).
No products indexed under this heading.

Influenza Virus Vaccine Live, Intranasal (During treatment with mycophenolate mofetil, the use of live attenuated vaccines should be avoided and patients should be advised that vaccines may be less effective. Influenza vaccination may be of value. Prescribers should refer to national guidelines for influenza vaccination). Products include:
FluMist Vaccine 1945

Levonorgestrel (A study of co-administration of mycophenolate mofetil and oral contraceptives containing ethinyl estradiol and levonorgestrel, desogestrel or gestodene was conducted in 18 women with psoriasis over 3 consecutive menstrual cycles. Mean AUC (0-24h) was similar for ethinyl estradiol and 3-keto desogestrel, however mean levonorgestrel AUC (0-24h) significantly decreased by about 15%. There was large inter-patient variability in the data. Mean serum levels of LH, FSH and progesterone were not significantlyaffected. Mycophenolate mofetil may not have any influence on the ovulation-suppressing action of the studied oral contraceptives. Concurrent use with oral contraceptives should be used with caution and additional birth control methods considered). Products include:
Climara Pro Transdermal System 768
Lybrel Tablets 3204
Mirena Intrauterine System 779
Plan B Tablets 1044
Seasonique Tablets 1046

Magaldrate (Absorption of a single dose of mycophenolate mofetil (2 g) was decreased when administered to ten rheumatoid arthritis patients also taking Maalox TC (10 mL q.i.d.) The Cmax and AUC (0-24h) for MPA was 33% and 17% lower, respectively, than when mycophenolate mofetil was administered alone under fasting conditions. Mycophenolate mofetil may be administered to patients who are also taking antacids containing magnesium and aluminum hydroxides, however it is recommended that mycophenolate mofetil and the antacid not be administered simultaneously).
No products indexed under this heading.

Magnesium Hydroxide (Absorption of a single dose of mycophenolate mofetil (2 g) was decreased when administered to ten rheumatoid arthritis patients also taking Maalox TC (10 mL q.i.d.) The Cmax and AUC (0-24h) for MPA was 33% and 17% lower, respectively, than when mycophenolate mofetil was administered alone under fasting conditions. Mycophenolate mofetil may be administered to patients who are also taking antacids containing magnesium and aluminum hydroxides, however it is recommended that mycophenolate mofetil and the antacid not be administered simultaneously). Products include:
Fleet Pedia-Lax Chewable Tablets 1145
Pepcid Complete Chewable Tablets 1771
Extra Strength Rolaids Freshmint Tablets 1903
Rolaids Multi-Symptom Berry Tablets 1903
Rolaids Original Peppermint Tablets 1903

Magnesium Oxide (Absorption of a single dose of mycophenolate mofetil (2 g) was decreased when administered to ten rheumatoid arthritis patients also taking Maalox TC (10 mL q.i.d.) The Cmax and AUC (0-24h) for MPA was 33% and 17% lower, respectively, than when mycophenolate mofetil was administered alone under fasting conditions. Mycophenolate mofetil may be administered to patients who are also taking antacids containing magnesium and aluminum hydroxides, however it is recommended that mycophenolate mofetil and the antacid not be administered simultaneously). Products include:
Beelith Tablets 813

Measles, Mumps, Rubella and Varicella Virus Vaccine Live (During treatment with mycophenolate mofetil, the use of live attenuated vaccines should be avoided and patients should be advised that vaccines may be less effective. Influenza vaccination may be of value. Prescribers should refer to national guidelines for influenza vaccination). Products include:
ProQuad 2099

Measles, Mumps & Rubella Virus Vaccine, Live (During treatment with mycophenolate mofetil, the use of live attenuated vaccines should be avoided and patients should be advised that vaccines may be less effective. Influenza vaccination may be of value. Prescribers should refer to national guidelines for influenza vaccination). Products include:
M-M-R II 2054

Measles & Rubella Virus Vaccine Live (During treatment with mycophenolate mofetil, the use of live attenuated vaccines should be avoided and patients should be advised that vaccines may be less effective. Influenza vaccination may be of value. Prescribers should refer to national guidelines for influenza vaccination).
No products indexed under this heading.

Measles Virus Vaccine Live (During treatment with mycophenolate mofetil, the use of live attenuated vaccines should be avoided and patients should be advised that vaccines may be less effective. Influenza vaccination may be of value. Prescribers should refer to national guidelines for influenza vaccination). Products include:
Attenuvax 1951

Mestranol (A study of co-administration of mycophenolate mofetil and oral contraceptives containing ethinyl estradiol and levonorgestrel, desogestrel or gestodene was conducted in 18 women with psoriasis over 3 consecutive menstrual cycles. Mean AUC (0-24h) was similar for ethinyl estradiol and 3-keto desogestrel, however mean levonorgestrel AUC (0-24h) significantly decreased by about 15%. There was large inter-patient variability in the data. Mean serum levels of LH, FSH and progesterone were not significantlyaffected. Mycophenolate mofetil may not have any influence on the ovulation-suppressing action of the studied oral contraceptives. Concurrent use with oral contraceptives should be used with caution and additional birth control methods considered).
No products indexed under this heading.

Metronidazole (Following single-dose administration of mycophenolate mofetil (1 g) to 11 healthy volunteers on day 4 of a 5-day course of a combination of norfloxacin and metronidazole, the mean MPA AUC 0-48h was significantly reduced by 33% compared to the administration of mycophenolate mofetil alone ($p<0.05$). Therefore, mycophenolate mofetil is not recommended to be given with the combination of norfloxacin and metronidazole. There was no significant effect on mean MPA AUC 0-48h when mycophenolate mofetil was concomitantly administered with norfloxacin or metronidazole separately). Products include:
Pylera Capsules 714

Metronidazole Benzoate (Following single-dose administration of mycophenolate mofetil (1 g) to 11 healthy volunteers on day 4 of a 5-day course of a combination of norfloxacin and metronidazole, the mean MPA AUC 0-48h was significantly reduced by 33% compared to the administration of mycophenolate mofetil alone ($p<0.05$). Therefore, mycophenolate mofetil is not recommended to be given with the combination of norfloxacin and metronidazole. There was no significant effect on mean MPA AUC 0-48h when mycophenolate mofetil was concomitantly administered with norfloxacin or metronidazole separately).
No products indexed under this heading.

Metronidazole Hydrochloride (Following single-dose administration of mycophenolate mofetil (1 g) to 11 healthy volunteers on day 4 of a 5-day course of a combination of norfloxacin and metronidazole, the mean MPA AUC 0-48h was significantly reduced by 33% compared to the administration of mycophenolate mofetil alone ($p<0.05$). Therefore, mycophenolate mofetil is not recommended to be given with the combination of norfloxacin and metronidazole. There was no significant effect on mean MPA AUC 0-48h when mycophenolate mofetil was concomitantly administered with norfloxacin or metronidazole separately).
No products indexed under this heading.

Metronidazole Sodium (Following single-dose administration of mycophenolate mofetil (1 g) to 11 healthy volunteers on day 4 of a 5-day course of a combination of norfloxacin and metronidazole, the mean MPA AUC 0-48h was significantly reduced by 33% compared to the administration of mycophenolate mofetil alone ($p<0.05$). Therefore, mycophenolate mofetil is not recommended to be given with the combination of norfloxacin and metronidazole. There was no significant effect on mean MPA AUC 0-48h when mycophenolate mofetil was concomitantly administered with norfloxacin or metronidazole separately).
No products indexed under this heading.

Mumps Virus Vaccine, Live (During treatment with mycophenolate mofetil, the use of live attenuated vaccines should be avoided and patients should be advised that vaccines may be less effective. Influenza vaccination may be of value. Prescribers should refer to national guidelines for influenza vaccination). Products include:
Mumpsvax 2068

Norethindrone (A study of co-administration of mycophenolate mofetil and oral contraceptives containing ethinyl estradiol and levonorgestrel, desogestrel or gestodene was conducted in 18 women with psoriasis over 3 consecutive menstrual cycles. Mean AUC (0-24h) was similar for ethinyl estradiol and 3-keto desogestrel, however mean levonorgestrel AUC (0-24h) significantly decreased by about 15%. There was large inter-patient variabili-

ty in the data. Mean serum levels of LH, FSH and progesterone were not significantlyaffected. Mycophenolate mofetil may not have any influence on the ovulation-suppressing action of the studied oral contraceptives. Concurrent use with oral contraceptives should be used with caution and additional birth control methods considered). Products include:

Ortho Micronor Tablets 2446

Norethynodrel (A study of co-administration of mycophenolate mofetil and oral contraceptives containing ethinyl estradiol and levonorgestrel, desogestrel or gestodene was conducted in 18 women with psoriasis over 3 consecutive menstrual cycles. Mean AUC (0-24h) was similar for ethinyl estradiol and 3-keto desogestrel, however mean levonorgestrel AUC (0-24h) significantly decreased by about 15%. There was large inter-patient variability in the data. Mean serum levels of LH, FSH and progesterone were not significantlyaffected. Mycophenolate mofetil may not have any influence on the ovulation-suppressing action of the studied oral contraceptives. Concurrent use with oral contraceptives should be used with caution and additional birth control methods considered).

No products indexed under this heading.

Norfloxacin (Following single-dose administration of mycophenolate mofetil (1 g) to 11 healthy volunteers on day 4 of a 5-day course of a combination of norfloxacin and metronidazole, the mean MPA AUC 0-48h was significantly reduced by 33% compared to the administration of mycophenolate mofetil alone ($p<0.05$). Therefore, mycophenolate mofetil is not recommended to be given with the combination of norfloxacin and metronidazole. There was no significant effect on mean MPA AUC 0-48h when mycophenolate mofetil was concomitantly administered with norfloxacin or metronidazole separately). Products include:

Noroxin Tablets 2069

Norgestimate (A study of co-administration of mycophenolate mofetil and oral contraceptives containing ethinyl estradiol and levonorgestrel, desogestrel or gestodene was conducted in 18 women with psoriasis over 3 consecutive menstrual cycles. Mean AUC (0-24h) was similar for ethinyl estradiol and 3-keto desogestrel, however mean levonorgestrel AUC (0-24h) significantly decreased by about 15%. There was large inter-patient variability in the data. Mean serum levels of LH, FSH and progesterone were not significantlyaffected. Mycophenolate mofetil may not have any influence on the ovulation-suppressing action of the studied oral contraceptives. Concurrent use with oral contraceptives should be used with caution and additional birth control methods considered). Products include:

Ortho-Cyclen/Ortho Tri-Cyclen 2449
Ortho Tri-Cyclen Lo Tablets 2458

Norgestrel (A study of co-administration of mycophenolate mofetil and oral contraceptives containing ethinyl estradiol and levonorgestrel, desogestrel or gestodene was conducted in 18 women with psoriasis over 3 consecutive menstrual cycles. Mean AUC (0-24h) was similar for ethinyl estradiol and 3-keto desogestrel, however mean levonorgestrel AUC (0-24h) significantly decreased by about 15%. There was large inter-patient variability in the data. Mean serum levels of LH, FSH and progesterone were not significantlyaffected. Mycophenolate mofetil may not have any influence on the ovulation-suppressing action of the studied oral contraceptives. Concurrent use with oral contraceptives should be used with caution and additional birth control methods considered).

No products indexed under this heading.

Poliovirus Vaccine, Live, Oral, Trivalent, Types 1,2,3 (Sabin) (During treatment with mycophenolate mofetil, the use of live attenuated vaccines should be avoided and patients should be advised that vaccines may be less effective. Influenza vaccination may be of value. Prescribers should refer to national guidelines for influenza vaccination).

No products indexed under this heading.

Probenecid (The measured value for renal clearance of MPAG indicates removal occurs by renal tubular secretion as well as glomerular filtration. Other drugs known to undergo renal tubular secretion may compete with MPAG and thereby raise plasma concentrations of MPAG or the other drug undergoing tubular secretion).

No products indexed under this heading.

Rifampin (In a single heart-lung transplant patient, after correction for dose, a 67% decrease in MPA exposure (AUC 0-12h) has been observed with concomitant administration of mycophenolate mofetil and rifampin. Therefore, mycophenolate mofetil is not recommended to be given with rifampin concomitantly unless benefit outweighs the risk).

No products indexed under this heading.

Rotavirus Vaccine, Live, Oral, Tetravalent (During treatment with mycophenolate mofetil, the use of live attenuated vaccines should be avoided and patients should be advised that vaccines may be less effective. Influenza vaccination may be of value. Prescribers should refer to national guidelines for influenza vaccination).

No products indexed under this heading.

Rubella & Mumps Virus Vaccine Live (During treatment with mycophenolate mofetil, the use of live attenuated vaccines should be avoided and patients should be advised that vaccines may be less effective. Influenza vaccination may be of value. Prescribers should refer to national guidelines for influenza vaccination).

No products indexed under this heading.

Rubella Virus Vaccine Live (During treatment with mycophenolate mofetil, the use of live attenuated vaccines should be avoided and patients should be advised that vaccines may be less effective. Influenza vaccination may be of value. Prescribers should refer to national guidelines for influenza vaccination). Products include:

Meruvax II 2061

Sevelamer Hydrochloride (Concomitant administration of sevelamer and mycophenolate mofetil in adult and pediatric patients decreased the mean MPA Cmax and AUC 0-12h by 36% and 26% respectively. This data suggest that sevelamer and other calcium free phosphate binders should not be administered simultaneously with mycophenolate mofetil. Alternately, it is recommended that sevelamer and other calcium free phosphate binders preferentially could be given 2 hours after mycophenolate mofetil intake to minimize the impact of the absorption of MPA).

No products indexed under this heading.

Smallpox Vaccine (During treatment with mycophenolate mofetil, the use of live attenuated vaccines should be avoided and patients should be advised that vaccines may be less effective. Influenza vaccination may be of value. Prescribers should refer to national guidelines for influenza vaccination).

No products indexed under this heading.

Sodium Bicarbonate (Absorption of a single dose of mycophenolate mofetil (2 g) was decreased when administered to ten rheumatoid arthritis patients also taking Maalox TC (10 mL q.i.d.) The Cmax and AUC (0-24h) for MPA was 33% and 17% lower, respectively, than when mycophenolate mofetil was administered alone under fasting conditions. Mycophenolate mofetil may be administered to patients who are also taking antacids containing magnesium and aluminum hydroxides, however it is recommended that mycophenolate mofetil and the antacid not be administered simultaneously). Products include:

Ceo-Two Laxative Suppository 815

Sulfamethoxazole (Following single-dose administration of mycophenolate mofetil (1.5 g) to 12 healthy male volunteers on day 8 of a 10-day course of trimethoprim 160 mg/sulfamethoxazole 800 mg administered b.i.d., no effect on the bioavailability of MPA was observed. The mean (±SD) AUC and Cmax of MPA after concomitant administration were 75.2 (+/-19.8) µg•h/mL and 34.0 (+/-6.6) µg/mL, respectively compared to 79.2 (±27.9) µg•mL and 34.2 (±10.7 µg/mL, respectively, after administration of mycophenolate mofetil alone).

No products indexed under this heading.

Trimethoprim (Following single-dose administration of mycophenolate mofetil (1.5 g) to 12 healthy male volunteers on day 8 of a 10-day course of trimethoprim 160 mg/sulfamethoxazole 800 mg administered b.i.d., no effect on the bioavailability of MPA was observed. The mean (±SD) AUC and Cmax of MPA after concomitant administration were 75.2 (+/-19.8) µg•h/mL and 34.0 (+/-6.6) µg/mL, respectively compared to 79.2 (±27.9) µg•mL and 34.2 (±10.7 µg/mL, respectively, after administration of mycophenolate mofetil alone).

No products indexed under this heading.

Trimethoprim Hydrochloride (Following single-dose administration of mycophenolate mofetil (1.5 g) to 12 healthy male volunteers on day 8 of a 10-day course of trimethoprim 160 mg/sulfamethoxazole 800 mg administered b.i.d., no effect on the bioavailability of MPA was observed. The mean (±SD) AUC and Cmax of MPA after concomitant administration were 75.2 (±19.8) µg•h/mL and 34.0 (+/-6.6) µg/mL, respectively compared to 79.2 (±27.9) µg•mL and 34.2 (+/-10.7 µg/mL, respectively, after administration of mycophenolate mofetil alone).

No products indexed under this heading.

Trimethoprim Sulfate (Following single-dose administration of mycophenolate mofetil (1.5 g) to 12 healthy male volunteers on day 8 of a 10-day course of trimethoprim 160 mg/sulfamethoxazole 800 mg administered b.i.d., no effect on the bioavailability of MPA was observed. The mean (±SD) AUC and Cmax of MPA after concomitant administration were 75.2 (+/-19.8) µg•h/mL and 34.0 (+/-6.6) µg/mL, respectively compared to 79.2 (±27.9) µg•mL and 34.2 (±10.7 µg/mL, respectively, after administration of mycophenolate mofetil alone).

No products indexed under this heading.

Typhoid Vaccine (During treatment with mycophenolate mofetil, the use of live attenuated vaccines should be avoided and patients should be advised that vaccines may be less effective. Influenza vaccination may be of value. Prescribers should refer to national guidelines for influenza vaccination).

No products indexed under this heading.

Valacyclovir Hydrochloride (Co-administration of mycophenolate mofetil (1 g) and acyclovir (800 mg) to 12 healthy volunteers resulted in no significant change in mycophenolic acid (MPA) AUC and Cmax. However the phenolic glucuronide of MPA (MPAG) and acyclovir plasma AUCs were increased 10.6% and 21.9% respectively. Because MPAG plasma concentrations are increased in the presence of renal impairment, as are acyclovir concentrations, the potential exists for mycophenolate and acyclovir or its prodrug (eg, valacyclovir) to compete for tubular secretion, further increasing the concentrations of both drugs). Products include:

Valtrex Caplets 1635

Valganciclovir Hydrochloride (Because MPAG plasma concentrations are increased in the presence of renal impairment, as are ganciclovir concentrations, the two drugs will compete for tubular secretion and thus further increases in concentrations of both drugs may occur. In patients with renal impairment in which mycophenolate mofetil and ganciclovir or its prodrug (eg, valganciclovir) are co-administered, patients should be monitored carefully). Products include:

Valcyte Tablets 2654

Varicella Virus Vaccine Live (During treatment with mycophenolate mofetil, the use of live attenuated vaccines should be avoided and patients should be advised that vaccines may be less effective. Influenza vaccination may be of value. Prescribers should refer to national guidelines for influenza vaccination). Products include:

Varivax 2133

Yellow Fever Vaccine (During treatment with mycophenolate mofetil, the use of live attenuated vaccines should be avoided and patients should be advised that vaccines may be less effective. Influenza vaccination may be of value. Prescribers should refer to national guidelines for influenza vaccination).

No products indexed under this heading.

Zoster Vaccine Live (During treatment with mycophenolate mofetil, the use of live attenuated vaccines should be avoided and patients should be advised that vaccines may be less effective. Influenza vaccination may be of value. Prescribers should refer to national guidelines for influenza vaccination). Products include:

Zostavax Injection 2145

CEO-TWO LAXATIVE SUPPOSITORY

(Potassium Bitartrate, Sodium Bicarbonate).................................... 815

None cited in PDR database.

CEREZYME FOR INJECTION

(Imiglucerase) 1238

None cited in PDR database.

CERVIDIL VAGINAL INSERT

(Dinoprostone) 1165

May interact with oxytocic drugs. Compounds in these categories include:

Ergonovine Maleate (Dinoprostone may augment the activity of oxytocic agents and concomitant use is not recommended; a dosing interval of at least 30 minutes is recommended for sequential use).

No products indexed under this heading.

Methylergonovine Maleate (Dinoprostone may augment the activity of oxytocic agents and concomitant use is not recommended; a dosing interval of at least 30 minutes is recommended for sequential use).

No products indexed under this heading.

Oxytocin (Dinoprostone may augment the activity of oxytocic agents and concomitant use is not recommended; a dosing interval of at least 30 minutes is recommended for sequential use).

No products indexed under this heading.

CHANTIX TABLETS

(Varenicline Tartrate) 2511

May interact with:

Cimetidine (Co-administration of an OCT2 inhibitor, cimetidine (300 mg QID), with varenicline (2 mg single dose) to 12 smokers increased the systemic exposure of varenicline by 29% (90% CI: 21.5%, 36.9%) due to a reduction in varenicline renal clearance).

No products indexed under this heading.

Cimetidine Hydrochloride (Co-administration of an OCT2 inhibitor, cimetidine (300 mg QID), with varenicline (2 mg single dose) to 12 smokers increased the systemic exposure of varenicline by 29% (90% CI: 21.5%, 36.9%) due to a reduction in varenicline renal clearance).

No products indexed under this heading.

Nicotine (Co-administration of varenicline (1 mg BID) and transdermal nicotine (21 mg/day) for up to 12 days did not affect nicotine pharmacokinetics, the incidence of nausea, headache, vomiting, dizziness, dyspepsia and fatigue was greater for the combination than for NRT alone. In this study, eight of twenty-two (36%) subjects treated with the combination of varenicline and NRT prematurely discontinued treatment due to adverse events, compared to one of seventeen (6%) of subjects treated with NRT and placebo).

No products indexed under this heading.

Nicotine Polacrilex (Co-administration of varenicline (1 mg BID) and transdermal nicotine (21 mg/day) for up to 12 days did not affect nicotine pharmacokinetics, the incidence of nausea, headache, vomiting, dizziness, dyspepsia and fatigue was greater for the combination than for NRT alone. In this study, eight of twenty-two (36%) subjects treated with the combination of varenicline and NRT prematurely discontinued treatment due to adverse events, compared to one of seventeen (6%) of subjects treated with NRT and placebo).

No products indexed under this heading.

Nicotine Salicylate (Co-administration of varenicline (1 mg BID) and transdermal nicotine (21 mg/day) for up to 12 days did not affect nicotine pharmacokinetics, the incidence of nausea, headache, vomiting, dizziness, dyspepsia and fatigue was greater for the combination than for NRT alone. In this study, eight of twenty-two (36%) subjects treated with the combination of varenicline and NRT prematurely discontinued treatment due to adverse events, compared to one of seventeen (6%) of subjects treated with NRT and placebo).

No products indexed under this heading.

Nicotine Sulfate (Co-administration of varenicline (1 mg BID) and transdermal nicotine (21 mg/day) for up to 12 days did not affect nicotine pharmacokinetics, the incidence of nausea, headache, vomiting, dizziness, dyspepsia and fatigue was greater for the combination than for NRT alone. In this study, eight of twenty-two (36%) subjects treated with the combination of varenicline and NRT prematurely discontinued treatment due to adverse events, compared to one of seventeen (6%) of subjects treated with NRT and placebo).

No products indexed under this heading.

CHELATED MINERAL TABLETS

(Minerals, Multiple) 3173

None cited in PDR database.

CHEMET CAPSULES

(Succimer) 2484

May interact with:

Calcium Disodium Edetate (Concomitant administration is not recommended).

No products indexed under this heading.

CIALIS TABLETS

(Tadalafil) 1792

May interact with alpha adrenergic blockers, angiotensin-II receptor antagonists, antacids, antihypertensives, cytochrome p450 3a4 inducers (selected), cytochrome p450 3a4 inhibitors (selected), cytochrome p450 3a4 inhibitors, potent, erythromycin, nitrates and nitrites, phenytoin, protease inhibitors, and certain other agents. Compounds in these categories include:

Acebutolol Hydrochloride (PDE5 inhibitors, including tadalafil, are mild systemic vasodilators. Clinical pharmacology studies were conducted to assess the effect of tadalafil on the potentiation of the blood-pressure-lowering effects of selected antihypertensive medications (amlodipine, angiotensin II receptor blockers, bendrofluazide, enalapril, and metoprolol). Small reductions in blood pressure occurred following co-administration of tadalafil with these agents compared to placebo).

No products indexed under this heading.

Acetazolamide (Tadalafil is a substrate of and predominantly metabolized by CYP3A4. Studies have shown that drugs that inhibit CYP3A4 can increase tadalafil exposure. When tadalafil is used on an as-needed basis, patients taking concomitant potent inhibitors of CYP3A4, such as ketoconazole or ritonavir, the maximum recommended dose of tadalafil is 10 mg, not to exceed once every 72 hours. When tadalafil is used in a once-daily regimen, patients taking concomitant potent inhibitors of CYP3A4, such as ketoconazole or ritonavir, the dose should not exceed 2.5 mg).

No products indexed under this heading.

Aliskiren (PDE5 inhibitors, including tadalafil, are mild systemic vasodilators. Clinical pharmacology studies were conducted to assess the effect of tadalafil on the potentiation of the blood-pressure-lowering effects of selected antihypertensive medications (amlodipine, angiotesin II receptor blockers, bendrofluazide, enalapril, and metoprolol). Small reductions in blood pressure occurred following co-administration of tadalafil with these agents compared to placebo). Products include:

Tekturna Tablets 2321

Tekturna HCT Tablets 2324

Allium sativum (Studies have shown that drugs that induce CYP3A4 can decrease tadalafil exposure).

No products indexed under this heading.

Aluminum Carbonate (Simultaneous administration of an antacid (magnesium hydroxide/aluminum hydroxide) and tadalafil reduced the apparent rate of absorption of tadalafil without altering exposure (AUC) to tadalafil).

No products indexed under this heading.

Aluminum Hydroxide (Simultaneous administration of an antacid (magnesium hydroxide/aluminum hydroxide) and tadalafil reduced the apparent rate of absorption of tadalafil without altering exposure (AUC) to tadalafil).

No products indexed under this heading.

Amiodarone Hydrochloride (Tadalafil is a substrate of and predominantly metabolized by CYP3A4. Studies have shown that drugs that inhibit CYP3A4 can increase tadalafil exposure. When tadalafil is used on an as-needed basis, patients taking concomitant potent inhibitors of CYP3A4, such as ketoconazole or ritonavir, the maximum recommended dose of tadalafil is 10 mg, not to exceed once every 72 hours. When tadalafil is used in a once-daily regimen, patients taking concomitant potent inhibitors of CYP3A4, such as ketoconazole or ritonavir, the dose should not exceed 2.5 mg).

No products indexed under this heading.

Amlodipine Besylate (A study was conducted to assess the interaction of amlodipine (5mg daily) and tadalafil 10mg. There were no effects of tadalafil on amlodipine blood levels and no effect of amlodipine on tadalafil blood levels. The mean reduction in supine systolic/diastolic blood pressure due to tadalafil 10mg in subjects taking amlodipine was 3/2mm Hg, compare to placebo). Products include:

Azor Tablets 1005

Exforge Tablets 2238

Amprenavir (Tadalafil is metabolized predominantly by CYP3A4 in the liver. The dose of tadalafil should be limited to 10 mg no more than once every 72 hours in patients taking potent inhibitors of CYP3A4, such as ritonavir, ketoconazole, and itraconazole. In patients taking potent inhibitors of CYP3A4 and tadalafil for once-daily use, the dose of tadalafil should not exceed 2.5 mg).

No products indexed under this heading.

Amyl Nitrite (Administration of tadalafil to patients using any form of organic nitrate, either regularly and/or intermittently, is contraindicated).

No products indexed under this heading.

Anastrozole (Tadalafil is a substrate of and predominantly metabolized by CYP3A4. Studies have shown that drugs that inhibit CYP3A4 can increase tadalafil exposure. When tadalafil is used on an as-needed basis, patients taking concomitant potent inhibitors of CYP3A4, such as ketoconazole or ritonavir, the maximum recommended dose of tadalafil is 10 mg, not to exceed once every 72 hours. When tadalafil is used in a once-daily regimen, patients taking concomitant potent inhibitors of CYP3A4, such as ketoconazole or ritonavir, the dose should not exceed 2.5 mg). Products include:

Arimidex Tablets 672

Aprepitant (Tadalafil is a substrate of and predominantly metabolized by CYP3A4. Studies have shown that drugs that inhibit CYP3A4 can increase tadalafil exposure. When tadalafil is used on an as-needed basis, patients taking concomitant potent inhibitors of CYP3A4, such as

ketoconazole or ritonavir, the maximum recommended dose of tadalafil is 10 mg, not to exceed once every 72 hours. When tadalafil is used in a once-daily regimen, patients taking concomitant potent inhibitors of CYP3A4, such as ketoconazole or ritonavir, the dose should not exceed 2.5 mg). Products include:

Emend Capsules 1992

Atazanavir (Tadalafil is metabolized predominantly by CYP3A4 in the liver. The dose of tadalafil should be limited to 10 mg no more than once every 72 hours in patients taking potent inhibitors of CYP3A4, such as ritonavir, ketoconazole, and itraconazole. In patients taking potent inhibitors of CYP3A4 and tadalafil for once-daily use, the dose of tadalafil should not exceed 2.5 mg).

No products indexed under this heading.

Atazanavir Sulfate (Tadalafil is metabolized predominantly by CYP3A4 in the liver. The dose of tadalafil should be limited to 10 mg no more than once every 72 hours in patients taking potent inhibitors of CYP3A4, such as ritonavir, ketoconazole, and itraconazole. In patients taking potent inhibitors of CYP3A4 and tadalafil for once-daily use, the dose of tadalafil should not exceed 2.5 mg). Products include:

Reyataz Capsules 3299

Atenolol (PDE5 inhibitors, including tadalafil, are mild systemic vasodilators. Clinical pharmacology studies were conducted to assess the effect of tadalafil on the potentiation of the blood-pressure-lowering effects of selected antihypertensive medications (amlodipine, angiotesin II receptor blockers, bendrofluazide, enalapril, and metoprolol). Small reductions in blood pressure occurred following co-administration of tadalafil with these agents compared to placebo).

No products indexed under this heading.

Benazepril Hydrochloride (PDE5 inhibitors, including tadalafil, are mild systemic vasodilators. Clinical pharmacology studies were conducted to assess the effect of tadalafil on the potentiation of the blood-pressure-lowering effects of selected antihypertensive medications (amlodipine, angiotesin II receptor blockers, bendrofluazide, enalapril, and metoprolol). Small reductions in blood pressure occurred following co-administration of tadalafil with these agents compared to placebo).

No products indexed under this heading.

Bendrofluazide (A study was conducted to assess the interaction of bendrofluazide (2.5mg daily) and tadalafil 10mg. Following dosing, the mean reduction in supine systolic diastolic blood pressure due to tadalafil 10mg in subjects taking bendrofluazide was 6/4mm Hg, compared to placebo).

No products indexed under this heading.

Bendroflumethiazide (PDE5 inhibitors, including tadalafil, are mild systemic vasodilators. Clinical pharmacology studies were conducted to assess the effect of tadalafil on the potentiation of the blood-pressure-lowering effects of selected antihypertensive medications (amlodipine, angiotesin II receptor blockers, bendrofluazide, enalapril, and metoprolol). Small reductions in blood pressure occurred following co-administration of tadalafil with these agents compared to placebo).

No products indexed under this heading.

Betamethasone Acetate (Studies have shown that drugs that induce CYP3A4 can decrease tadalafil exposure).

No products indexed under this heading.

Betamethasone Sodium Phosphate (Studies have shown that drugs that induce CYP3A4 can decrease tadalafil exposure).

No products indexed under this heading.

Betaxolol Hydrochloride (PDE5 inhibitors, including tadalafil, are mild systemic vasodilators. Clinical pharmacology studies were conducted to assess the effect of tadalafil on the potentiation of the blood-pressure-lowering effects of selected antihypertensive medications (amlodipine, angiotesin II receptor blockers, bendrofluazide, enalapril, and metoprolol). Small reductions in blood pressure occurred following co-administration of tadalafil with these agents compared to placebo).

No products indexed under this heading.

Bisoprolol Fumarate (PDE5 inhibitors, including tadalafil, are mild systemic vasodilators. Clinical pharmacology studies were conducted to assess the effect of tadalafil on the potentiation of the blood-pressure-lowering effects of selected antihypertensive medications (amlodipine, angiotesin II receptor blockers, bendrofluazide, enalapril, and metoprolol). Small reductions in blood pressure occurred following co-administration of tadalafil with these agents compared to placebo).

No products indexed under this heading.

Candesartan Cilexetil (PDE5 inhibitors, including tadalafil, are mild systemic vasodilators. Clinical pharmacology studies were conducted to assess the effect of tadalafil on the potentiation of the blood-pressure-lowering effects of selected antihypertensive medications (amlodipine, angiotesin II receptor blockers, bendrofluazide, enalapril, and metoprolol). Small reductions in blood pressure occurred following co-administration of tadalafil with these agents compared to placebo). Products include:

Atacand Tablets 639
Atacand HCT 642

Captopril (PDE5 inhibitors, including tadalafil, are mild systemic vasodilators. Clinical pharmacology studies were conducted to assess the effect of tadalafil on the potentiation of the blood-pressure-lowering effects of selected antihypertensive medications (amlodipine, angiotesin II receptor blockers, bendrofluazide, enalapril, and metoprolol). Small reductions in blood pressure occurred following co-administration of tadalafil with these agents compared to placebo). Products include:

Captopril Tablets 2182

Carbamazepine (CYP3A4 inducers, such as carbamazepine, may decrease tadalafil exposure. No dose adjustment is warranted). Products include:

Carbatrol Capsules 3019
Equetro Extended-Release Capsules 3174

Carteolol Hydrochloride (PDE5 inhibitors, including tadalafil, are mild systemic vasodilators. Clinical pharmacology studies were conducted to assess the effect of tadalafil on the potentiation of the blood-pressure-lowering effects of selected antihypertensive medications (amlodipine, angiotesin II receptor blockers, bendrofluazide, enalapril, and metoprolol). Small reductions in blood pressure occurred following co-administration of tadalafil with these agents compared to placebo).

No products indexed under this heading.

Chlorothiazide (PDE5 inhibitors, including tadalafil, are mild systemic vasodilators. Clinical pharmacology studies were conducted to assess the effect of tadalafil on the potentiation of the blood-pressure-lowering effects of selected antihypertensive medications (amlodipine, angiotesin II receptor blockers, bendrofluazide, enalapril, and metoprolol). Small reductions in blood pressure occurred following co-administration of tadalafil with these agents compared to placebo).

No products indexed under this heading.

Chlorothiazide Sodium (PDE5 inhibitors, including tadalafil, are mild systemic vasodilators. Clinical pharmacology studies were conducted to assess the effect of tadalafil on the potentiation of the blood-pressure-lowering effects of selected antihypertensive medications (amlodipine, angiotesin II receptor blockers, bendrofluazide, enalapril, and metoprolol). Small reductions in blood pressure occurred following co-administration of tadalafil with these agents compared to placebo). Products include:

Intravenous Sodium Diuril 2490

Chlorthalidone (PDE5 inhibitors, including tadalafil, are mild systemic vasodilators. Clinical pharmacology studies were conducted to assess the effect of tadalafil on the potentiation of the blood-pressure-lowering effects of selected antihypertensive medications (amlodipine, angiotesin II receptor blockers, bendrofluazide, enalapril, and metoprolol). Small reductions in blood pressure occurred following co-administration of tadalafil with these agents compared to placebo). Products include:

Clorpres Tablets 2185

Cimetidine (Tadalafil is a substrate of and predominantly metabolized by CYP3A4. Studies have shown that drugs that inhibit CYP3A4 can increase tadalafil exposure. When tadalafil is used on an as-needed basis, patients taking concomitant potent inhibitors of CYP3A4, such as ketoconazole or ritonavir, the maximum recommended dose of tadalafil is 10 mg, not to exceed once every 72 hours. When tadalafil is used in a once-daily regimen, patients taking concomitant potent inhibitors of CYP3A4, such as ketoconazole or ritonavir, the dose should not exceed 2.5 mg).

No products indexed under this heading.

Cimetidine Hydrochloride (Tadalafil is a substrate of and predominantly metabolized by CYP3A4. Studies have shown that drugs that inhibit CYP3A4 can increase tadalafil exposure. When tadalafil is used on an as-needed basis, patients taking concomitant potent inhibitors of CYP3A4, such as ketoconazole or ritonavir, the maximum recommended dose of tadalafil is 10 mg, not to exceed once every 72 hours. When tadalafil is used in a once-daily regimen, patients taking concomitant potent inhibitors of CYP3A4, such as ketoconazole or ritonavir, the dose should not exceed 2.5 mg).

No products indexed under this heading.

Ciprofloxacin (Tadalafil is a substrate of and predominantly metabolized by CYP3A4. Studies have shown that drugs that inhibit CYP3A4 can increase tadalafil exposure. When tadalafil is used on an as-needed basis, patients taking concomitant potent inhibitors of CYP3A4, such as ketoconazole or ritonavir, the maximum recommended dose of tadalafil is 10 mg, not to exceed once every 72 hours. When tadalafil is used in a once-daily regimen, patients taking concomitant potent inhibitors of CYP3A4, such as ketoconazole or ritonavir, the dose should not exceed 2.5 mg). Products include:

Cipro I.V. 2817
Cipro Oral Suspension 2810
Cipro XR Tablets 2823
Ciprodex Otic Suspension 541

Ciprofloxacin Hydrochloride (Studies have shown that drugs that induce CYP3A4 can decrease tadalafil exposure). Products include:

Cipro Tablets 2810

Cisplatin (Studies have shown that drugs that induce CYP3A4 can decrease tadalafil exposure).

No products indexed under this heading.

Clarithromycin (Tadalafil is metabolized predominantly by CYP3A4 in the liver. The dose of tadalafil should be limited to 10 mg no more than once every 72 hours in patients taking potent inhibitors of CYP3A4, such as ritonavir, ketoconazole, and itraconazole. In patients taking potent inhibitors of CYP3A4 and tadalafil for once-daily use, the dose of tadalafil should not exceed 2.5 mg). Products include:

Biaxin/Biaxin XL 411

Clonidine (PDE5 inhibitors, including tadalafil, are mild systemic vasodilators. Clinical pharmacology studies were conducted to assess the effect of tadalafil on the potentiation of the blood-pressure-lowering effects of selected antihypertensive medications (amlodipine, angiotesin II receptor blockers, bendrofluazide, enalapril, and metoprolol). Small reductions in blood pressure occurred following co-administration of tadalafil with these agents compared to placebo). Products include:

Catapres-TTS 842

Clonidine Hydrochloride (PDE5 inhibitors, including tadalafil, are mild systemic vasodilators. Clinical pharmacology studies were conducted to assess the effect of tadalafil on the potentiation of the blood-pressure-lowering effects of selected antihypertensive medications (amlodipine, angiotesin II receptor blockers, bendrofluazide, enalapril, and metoprolol). Small reductions in blood pressure occurred following co-administration of tadalafil with these agents compared to placebo). Products include:

Catapres Tablets 841
Clorpres Tablets 2185

Clotrimazole (Tadalafil is a substrate of and predominantly metabolized by CYP3A4. Studies have shown that drugs that inhibit CYP3A4 can increase tadalafil exposure. When tadalafil is used on an as-needed basis, patients taking concomitant potent inhibitors of CYP3A4, such as ketoconazole or ritonavir, the maximum recommended dose of tadalafil is 10 mg, not to exceed once every 72 hours. When tadalafil is used in a once-daily regimen, patients taking concomitant potent inhibitors of CYP3A4, such as ketoconazole or ritonavir, the dose should not exceed 2.5 mg). Products include:

Lotrisone 2881

Cortisone Acetate (Studies have shown that drugs that induce CYP3A4 can decrease tadalafil exposure).

No products indexed under this heading.

Cyclosporine (Tadalafil is a substrate of and predominantly metabolized by CYP3A4. Studies have shown that drugs that inhibit CYP3A4 can increase tadalafil exposure. When tadalafil is used on an as-needed basis, patients taking concomitant potent inhibitors of CYP3A4, such as ketoconazole or ritonavir, the maximum recommended dose of tadalafil is 10 mg, not to exceed once every 72 hours. When tadalafil is used in a once-daily regimen, patients taking concomitant potent inhibitors of CYP3A4, such as ketoconazole or ritonavir, the dose should not exceed 2.5 mg). Products include:

Gengraf Capsules 435
Neoral Oral Solution 2280
Neoral Soft Gelatin Capsules 2280
Restasis Ophthalmic Emulsion 557
Sandimmune 2296

Dalfopristin (Tadalafil is a substrate of and predominantly metabolized by CYP3A4. Studies have shown that drugs that inhibit CYP3A4 can increase tadalafil exposure. When tadalafil is used on an as-needed basis, patients taking concomitant potent inhibitors of CYP3A4, such as ketoconazole or ritonavir, the maximum recommended dose of tadalafil is 10 mg, not to exceed once every 72 hours. When tadalafil is used in a once-daily regimen, patients taking concomitant potent inhibitors of CYP3A4, such as ketoconazole or ritonavir, the dose should not exceed 2.5 mg).

No products indexed under this heading.

Danazol (Tadalafil is a substrate of and predominantly metabolized by CYP3A4. Studies have shown that drugs that inhibit CYP3A4 can increase tadalafil exposure. When tadalafil is used on an as-needed basis, patients taking concomitant potent inhibitors of CYP3A4, such as ketoconazole or ritonavir, the maximum recommended dose of tadalafil is 10 mg, not to exceed once every 72 hours. When tadalafil is used in a once-daily regimen, patients taking concomitant potent inhibitors of CYP3A4, such as ketoconazole or ritonavir, the dose should not exceed 2.5 mg).

No products indexed under this heading.

Darunavir (Ritonavir (500 mg or 600 mg b.i.d. at steady state), an inhibitor of CYP3A4, CYP2C9, CYP2C19, and CYP2D6, increased tadalafil 20 mg single-dose exposure (AUC) by 32% with a 30% reduction in Cmax, relative to the values for tadalafil 20 mg alone. Ritonavir (200 mg b.i.d.), increased tadalafil 20 mg single-dose exposure (AUC) by 124% with no change in Cmax, relative to the values for tadalafil 20 mg alone. Although specific interactions have not been studied, other HIV protease inhibitors would likely increase tadalafil exposure).

No products indexed under this heading.

Delavirdine Mesylate (Tadalafil is metabolized predominantly by CYP3A4 in the liver. The dose of tadalafil should be limited to 10 mg no more than once every 72 hours in patients taking potent inhibitors of CYP3A4, such as ritonavir, ketoconazole, and itraconazole. In patients taking potent inhibitors of CYP3A4 and tadalafil for once-daily use, the dose of tadalafil should not exceed 2.5 mg).

No products indexed under this heading.

Delavirine (Tadalafil is metabolized predominantly by CYP3A4 in the liver. The dose of tadalafil should be limited to 10 mg no more than once every 72 hours in patients taking potent inhibitors of CYP3A4, such as ritonavir, ketoconazole, and itraconazole. In patients taking potent inhibitors of CYP3A4 and tadalafil for once-daily use, the dose of tadalafil should not exceed 2.5 mg).

No products indexed under this heading.

Deserpidine (PDE5 inhibitors, including tadalafil, are mild systemic vasodilators. Clinical pharmacology studies were conducted to assess the effect of tadalafil on the potentiation of the blood-pressure-lowering effects of selected antihypertensive medications (amlodipine, angiotesin II receptor blockers, bendrofluazide, enalapril, and metoprolol). Small reductions in blood pressure occurred following co-administration of tadalafil with these agents compared to placebo).

No products indexed under this heading.

Dexamethasone (Studies have shown that drugs that induce CYP3A4 can decrease tadalafil exposure). Products include:

Ciprodex Otic Suspension 541

Dexamethasone Acetate (Studies have shown that drugs that induce CYP3A4 can decrease tadalafil exposure).

No products indexed under this heading.

Dexamethasone Sodium Phosphate (Studies have shown that drugs that induce CYP3A4 can decrease tadalafil exposure).

No products indexed under this heading.

Diazoxide (PDE5 inhibitors, including tadalafil, are mild systemic vasodilators. Clinical pharmacology studies were conducted to assess the effect of tadalafil on the potentiation of the blood-pressure-lowering effects of selected antihypertensive medications (amlodipine, angiotesin II receptor blockers, bendrofluazide, enalapril, and metoprolol). Small reductions in blood pressure occurred following co-administration of tadalafil with these agents compared to placebo). Products include:

Proglycem Capsules 1185
Proglycem Suspension 1185

Diltiazem Hydrochloride (PDE5 inhibitors, including tadalafil, are mild systemic vasodilators. Clinical pharmacology studies were conducted to assess the effect of tadalafil on the potentiation of the blood-pressure-lowering effects of selected antihypertensive medications (amlodipine, angiotesin II receptor blockers, bendrofluazide, enalapril, and metoprolol). Small reductions in blood pressure occurred following co-administration of tadalafil with these agents compared to placebo). Products include:

Cardizem LA Extended Release Tablets 421

Diltiazem Maleate (Tadalafil is a substrate of and predominantly metabolized by CYP3A4. Studies have shown that drugs that inhibit CYP3A4 can increase tadalafil exposure. When tadalafil is used on an as-needed basis, patients taking concomitant potent inhibitors of CYP3A4, such as ketoconazole or ritonavir, the maximum recommended dose of tadalafil is 10 mg, not to exceed once every 72 hours. When tadalafil is used in a once-daily regimen, patients taking concomitant potent inhibitors of CYP3A4, such as ketoconazole or ritonavir, the dose should not exceed 2.5 mg).

No products indexed under this heading.

Doxazosin Mesylate (Caution is advised when PDE5 inhibitors are co-administered with alpha-blockers. PDE5 inhibitors, including tadalafil, and alpha-adrenergic blocking agents are both vasodilators with blood-pressure lowering effects. When vasodilators are used in combination, an additive effect on blood pressure may be anticipated. In some patients, concomitant use of these two drug classes can lower blood presure significantly, which may lead to symptomatic hypotension (e.g., fainting)).

No products indexed under this heading.

Doxorubicin Hydrochloride (Studies have shown that drugs that induce CYP3A4 can decrease tadalafil exposure).

No products indexed under this heading.

Efavirenz (Tadalafil is a substrate of and predominantly metabolized by CYP3A4. Studies have shown that drugs that inhibit CYP3A4 can increase tadalafil exposure. When tadalafil is used on an as-needed basis, patients taking concomitant potent inhibitors of CYP3A4, such as ketoconazole or ritonavir, the maximum recommended dose of tadalafil is 10 mg, not to exceed once every 72 hours. When tadalafil is used in a once-daily regimen, patients taking concomitant potent inhibitors of CYP3A4, such as ketoconazole or ritonavir, the dose should not exceed 2.5 mg). Products include:

Atripla Tablets 938
Sustiva Capsules 930
Sustiva Tablets 930

Enalapril Maleate (Following dosing with enalapril (10-20mg daily) and tadalafil 10mg, the mean reduction in supine systolic/diastolic blood pressure due to tadalafil 10mg in subjects taking analapril was 4/1mm Hg, compared to placebo).

No products indexed under this heading.

Enalaprilat (Following dosing with enalapril (10-20mg daily) and tadalafil 10mg, the mean reduction in supine systolic/diastolic blood pressure due to tadalafil 10mg in subjects taking analapril was 4/1mm Hg, compared to placebo).

No products indexed under this heading.

Eprosartan Mesylate (PDE5 inhibitors, including tadalafil, are mild systemic vasodilators. Clinical pharmacology studies were conducted to assess the effect of tadalafil on the potentiation of the blood-pressure-lowering effects of selected antihypertensive medications (amlodipine, angiotesin II receptor blockers, bendrofluazide, enalapril, and metoprolol). Small reductions in blood pressure occurred following co-administration of tadalafil with these agents compared to placebo). Products include:

Teveten Tablets 515
Teveten HCT Tablets 517

Erythrityl Tetranitrate (Administration of tadalafil to patients using any form of organic nitrate, either regularly and/or intermittently, is contraindicated).

No products indexed under this heading.

Erythromycin (CYP3A4 inhibitors such as erythromycin may likely increase tadalafil exposure).

No products indexed under this heading.

Erythromycin Estolate (CYP3A4 inhibitors such as erythromycin may likely increase tadalafil exposure).

No products indexed under this heading.

Erythromycin Ethylsuccinate (CYP3A4 inhibitors such as erythromycin may likely increase tadalafil exposure). Products include:

E.E.S. 433
EryPed 431

Erythromycin Gluceptate (CYP3A4 inhibitors such as erythromycin may likely increase tadalafil exposure).

No products indexed under this heading.

Erythromycin Lactobionate (CYP3A4 inhibitors such as erythromycin may likely increase tadalafil exposure).

No products indexed under this heading.

Erythromycin Stearate (CYP3A4 inhibitors such as erythromycin may likely increase tadalafil exposure).

No products indexed under this heading.

Esmolol Hydrochloride (PDE5 inhibitors, including tadalafil, are mild systemic vasodilators. Clinical pharmacology studies were conducted to assess the effect of tadalafil on the potentiation of the blood-pressure-

lowering effects of selected antihypertensive medications (amlodipine, angiotesin II receptor blockers, bendrofluazide, enalapril, and metoprolol). Small reductions in blood pressure occurred following co-administration of tadalafil with these agents compared to placebo).
No products indexed under this heading.

Esomeprazole Magnesium (Tadalafil is a substrate of and predominantly metabolized by CYP3A4. Studies have shown that drugs that inhibit CYP3A4 can increase tadalafil exposure. When tadalafil is used on an as-needed basis, patients taking concomitant potent inhibitors of CYP3A4, such as ketoconazole or ritonavir, the maximum recommended dose of tadalafil is 10 mg, not to exceed once every 72 hours. When tadalafil is used in a once-daily regimen, patients taking concomitant potent inhibitors of CYP3A4, such as ketoconazole or ritonavir, the dose should not exceed 2.5 mg). Products include:
Nexium Delayed-Release Capsules **645**
Nexium Delayed-Release Oral Suspension **645**

Ethosuximide (Studies have shown that drugs that induce CYP3A4 can decrease tadalafil exposure).
No products indexed under this heading.

Felbamate (Studies have shown that drugs that induce CYP3A4 can decrease tadalafil exposure).
No products indexed under this heading.

Felodipine (PDE5 inhibitors, including tadalafil, are mild systemic vasodilators. Clinical pharmacology studies were conducted to assess the effect of tadalafil on the potentiation of the blood-pressure-lowering effects of selected antihypertensive medications (amlodipine, angiotesin II receptor blockers, bendrofluazide, enalapril, and metoprolol). Small reductions in blood pressure occurred following co-administration of tadalafil with these agents compared to placebo).
No products indexed under this heading.

Fluconazole (Tadalafil is a substrate of and predominantly metabolized by CYP3A4. Studies have shown that drugs that inhibit CYP3A4 can increase tadalafil exposure. When tadalafil is used on an as-needed basis, patients taking concomitant potent inhibitors of CYP3A4, such as ketoconazole or ritonavir, the maximum recommended dose of tadalafil is 10 mg, not to exceed once every 72 hours. When tadalafil is used in a once-daily regimen, patients taking concomitant potent inhibitors of CYP3A4, such as ketoconazole or ritonavir, the dose should not exceed 2.5 mg).
No products indexed under this heading.

Fludrocortisone Acetate (Studies have shown that drugs that induce CYP3A4 can decrease tadalafil exposure).
No products indexed under this heading.

Fluoxetine (Tadalafil is a substrate of and predominantly metabolized by CYP3A4. Studies have shown that drugs that inhibit CYP3A4 can increase tadalafil exposure. When tadalafil is used on an as-needed basis, patients taking concomitant potent inhibitors of CYP3A4, such as ketoconazole or ritonavir, the maximum recommended dose of tadalafil is 10 mg, not to exceed once every 72 hours. When tadalafil is used in a once-daily regimen, patients taking concomitant potent inhibitors of CYP3A4, such as ketoconazole or ritonavir, the dose should not exceed 2.5 mg).
No products indexed under this heading.

Fluoxetine Hydrochloride (Tadalafil is a substrate of and predominantly metabolized by CYP3A4. Studies have shown that drugs that inhibit CYP3A4 can increase tadalafil exposure. When tadalafil is used on an as-needed basis, patients taking concomitant potent inhibitors of CYP3A4, such as ketoconazole or ritonavir, the maximum recommended dose of tadalafil is 10 mg, not to exceed once every 72 hours. When tadalafil is used in a once-daily regimen, patients taking concomitant potent inhibitors of CYP3A4, such as ketoconazole or ritonavir, the dose should not exceed 2.5 mg). Products include:
Prozac Weekly Capsules **1852**
Prozac Pulvules and Liquid **1852**
Symbyax Capsules **1871**

Fluvoxamine Maleate (Tadalafil is a substrate of and predominantly metabolized by CYP3A4. Studies have shown that drugs that inhibit CYP3A4 can increase tadalafil exposure. When tadalafil is used on an as-needed basis, patients taking concomitant potent inhibitors of CYP3A4, such as ketoconazole or ritonavir, the maximum recommended dose of tadalafil is 10 mg, not to exceed once every 72 hours. When tadalafil is used in a once-daily regimen, patients taking concomitant potent inhibitors of CYP3A4, such as ketoconazole or ritonavir, the dose should not exceed 2.5 mg). Products include:
Luvox CR Extended-Release Capsules **1759**

Fosamprenavir Calcium (Tadalafil is metabolized predominantly by CYP3A4 in the liver. The dose of tadalafil should be limited to 10 mg no more than once every 72 hours in patients taking potent inhibitors of CYP3A4, such as ritonavir, ketoconazole, and itraconazole. In patients taking potent inhibitors of CYP3A4 and tadalafil for once-daily use, the dose of tadalafil should not exceed 2.5 mg). Products include:
Lexiva Oral Suspension **1510**
Lexiva Tablets **1510**

Fosinopril Sodium (PDE5 inhibitors, including tadalafil, are mild systemic vasodilators. Clinical pharmacology studies were conducted to assess the effect of tadalafil on the potentiation of the blood-pressure-lowering effects of selected antihypertensive medications (amlodipine, angiotesin II receptor blockers, bendrofluazide, enalapril, and metoprolol). Small reductions in blood pressure occurred following co-administration of tadalafil with these agents compared to placebo).
No products indexed under this heading.

Fosphenytoin Sodium (CYP3A4 inducers, such as phenytoin, may decrease tadalafil exposure. No dose adjustment is warranted).
No products indexed under this heading.

Furosemide (PDE5 inhibitors, including tadalafil, are mild systemic vasodilators. Clinical pharmacology studies were conducted to assess the effect of tadalafil on the potentiation of the blood-pressure-lowering effects of selected antihypertensive medications (amlodipine, angiotesin II receptor blockers, bendrofluazide, enalapril, and metoprolol). Small reductions in blood pressure occurred following co-administration of tadalafil with these agents compared to placebo). Products include:
Furosemide Tablets **2186**

Garlic Extract (Studies have shown that drugs that induce CYP3A4 can decrease tadalafil exposure).
No products indexed under this heading.

Garlic Oil (Studies have shown that drugs that induce CYP3A4 can decrease tadalafil exposure).
No products indexed under this heading.

Guanabenz Acetate (PDE5 inhibitors, including tadalafil, are mild systemic vasodilators. Clinical pharmacology studies were conducted to assess the effect of tadalafil on the potentiation of the blood-pressure-lowering effects of selected antihypertensive medications (amlodipine, angiotesin II receptor blockers, bendrofluazide, enalapril, and metoprolol). Small reductions in blood pressure occurred following co-administration of tadalafil with these agents compared to placebo).
No products indexed under this heading.

Guanethidine Monosulfate (PDE5 inhibitors, including tadalafil, are mild systemic vasodilators. Clinical pharmacology studies were conducted to assess the effect of tadalafil on the potentiation of the blood-pressure-lowering effects of selected antihypertensive medications (amlodipine, angiotesin II receptor blockers, bendrofluazide, enalapril, and metoprolol). Small reductions in blood pressure occurred following co-administration of tadalafil with these agents compared to placebo).
No products indexed under this heading.

Hydralazine Hydrochloride (PDE5 inhibitors, including tadalafil, are mild systemic vasodilators. Clinical pharmacology studies were conducted to assess the effect of tadalafil on the potentiation of the blood-pressure-lowering effects of selected antihypertensive medications (amlodipine, angiotesin II receptor blockers, bendrofluazide, enalapril, and metoprolol). Small reductions in blood pressure occurred following co-administration of tadalafil with these agents compared to placebo).
No products indexed under this heading.

Hydrochlorothiazide (PDE5 inhibitors, including tadalafil, are mild systemic vasodilators. Clinical pharmacology studies were conducted to assess the effect of tadalafil on the potentiation of the blood-pressure-lowering effects of selected antihypertensive medications (amlodipine, angiotesin II receptor blockers, bendrofluazide, enalapril, and metoprolol). Small reductions in blood pressure occurred following co-administration of tadalafil with these agents compared to placebo). Products include:
Atacand HCT **642**
Avalide Tablets **892**
Avalide Tablets **2713**
Benicar HCT Tablets **1010**
Diovan HCT Tablets **2216**
Dyazide Capsules **1405**
Micardis HCT Tablets **854**
Prinzide Tablets **2092**
Tekturna HCT Tablets **2324**
Teveten HCT Tablets **517**

Hydrocortisone (Studies have shown that drugs that induce CYP3A4 can decrease tadalafil exposure).
No products indexed under this heading.

Hydrocortisone Acetate (Studies have shown that drugs that induce CYP3A4 can decrease tadalafil exposure). Products include:
Analpram-HC **1140**
Pramosone **1141**

Hydrocortisone Butyrate (Studies have shown that drugs that induce CYP3A4 can decrease tadalafil exposure).
No products indexed under this heading.

Hydrocortisone Cypionate (Studies have shown that drugs that induce CYP3A4 can decrease tadalafil exposure).
No products indexed under this heading.

Hydrocortisone Hemisuccinate (Studies have shown that drugs that induce CYP3A4 can decrease tadalafil exposure).
No products indexed under this heading.

Hydrocortisone Probutate (Studies have shown that drugs that induce CYP3A4 can decrease tadalafil exposure).
No products indexed under this heading.

Hydrocortisone Sodium Phosphate (Studies have shown that drugs that induce CYP3A4 can decrease tadalafil exposure).
No products indexed under this heading.

Hydrocortisone Sodium Succinate (Studies have shown that drugs that induce CYP3A4 can decrease tadalafil exposure).
No products indexed under this heading.

Hydrocortisone Valerate (Studies have shown that drugs that induce CYP3A4 can decrease tadalafil exposure).
No products indexed under this heading.

Hydroflumethiazide (PDE5 inhibitors, including tadalafil, are mild systemic vasodilators. Clinical pharmacology studies were conducted to assess the effect of tadalafil on the potentiation of the blood-pressure-lowering effects of selected antihypertensive medications (amlodipine, angiotesin II receptor blockers, bendrofluazide, enalapril, and metoprolol). Small reductions in blood pressure occurred following co-administration of tadalafil with these agents compared to placebo).
No products indexed under this heading.

Hypericum (Studies have shown that drugs that induce CYP3A4 can decrease tadalafil exposure). Products include:

Satieté Tablets 640

Hypericum Perforatum (Studies have shown that drugs that induce CYP3A4 can decrease tadalafil exposure).

No products indexed under this heading.

Indapamide (PDE5 inhibitors, including tadalafil, are mild systemic vasodilators. Clinical pharmacology studies were conducted to assess the effect of tadalafil on the potentiation of the blood-pressure-lowering effects of selected antihypertensive medications (amlodipine, angiotesin II receptor blockers, bendrofluazide, enalapril, and metoprolol). Small reductions in blood pressure occurred following co-administration of tadalafil with these agents compared to placebo). Products include:

Indapamide Tablets 2188

Indinavir Sulfate (Tadalafil is metabolized predominantly by CYP3A4 in the liver. The dose of tadalafil should be limited to 10 mg no more than once every 72 hours in patients taking potent inhibitors of CYP3A4, such as ritonavir, ketoconazole, and itraconazole. In patients taking potent inhibitors of CYP3A4 and tadalafil for once-daily use, the dose of tadalafil should not exceed 2.5 mg). Products include:

Crixivan Capsules 1979

Irbesartan (PDE5 inhibitors, including tadalafil, are mild systemic vasodilators. Clinical pharmacology studies were conducted to assess the effect of tadalafil on the potentiation of the blood-pressure-lowering effects of selected antihypertensive medications (amlodipine, angiotesin II receptor blockers, bendrofluazide, enalapril, and metoprolol). Small reductions in blood pressure occurred following co-administration of tadalafil with these agents compared to placebo). Products include:

Avalide Tablets 892
Avalide Tablets 2713
Avapro Tablets 897
Avapro Tablets 2718

Isoniazid (Tadalafil is a substrate of and predominantly metabolized by CYP3A4. Studies have shown that drugs that inhibit CYP3A4 can increase tadalafil exposure. When tadalafil is used on an as-needed basis, patients taking concomitant potent inhibitors of CYP3A4, such as ketoconazole or ritonavir, the maximum recommended dose of tadalafil is 10 mg, not to exceed once every 72 hours. When tadalafil is used in a once-daily regimen, patients taking concomitant potent inhibitors of CYP3A4, such as ketoconazole or ritonavir, the dose should not exceed 2.5 mg).

No products indexed under this heading.

Isosorbide Dinitrate (Administration of tadalafil to patients using any form of organic nitrate, either regularly and/or intermittently, is contraindicated).

No products indexed under this heading.

Isosorbide Mononitrate (Administration of tadalafil to patients using any form of organic nitrate, either regularly and/or intermittently, is contraindicated).

No products indexed under this heading.

Isradipine (PDE5 inhibitors, including tadalafil, are mild systemic vasodilators. Clinical pharmacology studies were conducted to assess the effect of tadalafil on the potentiation of the blood-pressure-lowering effects of selected antihypertensive medications (amlodipine, angiotesin II receptor blockers, bendrofluazide, enalapril, and metoprolol). Small reductions in blood pressure occurred following co-administration of tadalafil with these agents compared to placebo). Products include:

DynaCirc CR Controlled Release Tablets 1407

Itraconazole (CYP3A4 inhibitors such as itraconazole may likely increase tadalafil exposure).

No products indexed under this heading.

Ketoconazole (Ketoconazole increased tadalafil 20mg single dose exposure (AUC) by 312% and Cmax by 22%, relative to the values for tadalafil 20mg alone. Ketoconazole increased tadalafil 10mg single dose exposure (AUC) by 107% and Cmax by 15%, relative to the values for tadalafil 10mg alone. Based on these results, the dose of tadalafil should not exceed 10mg and tadalafil should not be taken more frequently than once in 72 hours). Products include:

Extina Foam, 2% 3057
Nizoral A-D Shampoo 1901

Labetalol Hydrochloride (PDE5 inhibitors, including tadalafil, are mild systemic vasodilators. Clinical pharmacology studies were conducted to assess the effect of tadalafil on the potentiation of the blood-pressure-lowering effects of selected antihypertensive medications (amlodipine, angiotesin II receptor blockers, bendrofluazide, enalapril, and metoprolol). Small reductions in blood pressure occurred following co-administration of tadalafil with these agents compared to placebo).

No products indexed under this heading.

Lisinopril (PDE5 inhibitors, including tadalafil, are mild systemic vasodilators. Clinical pharmacology studies were conducted to assess the effect of tadalafil on the potentiation of the blood-pressure-lowering effects of selected antihypertensive medications (amlodipine, angiotesin II receptor blockers, bendrofluazide, enalapril, and metoprolol). Small reductions in blood pressure occurred following co-administration of tadalafil with these agents compared to placebo). Products include:

Prinivil Tablets 2087
Prinzide Tablets 2092

Lopinavir (Tadalafil is metabolized predominantly by CYP3A4 in the liver. The dose of tadalafil should be limited to 10 mg no more than once every 72 hours in patients taking potent inhibitors of CYP3A4, such as ritonavir, ketoconazole, and itraconazole. In patients taking potent inhibitors of CYP3A4 and tadalafil for once-daily use, the dose of tadalafil should not exceed 2.5 mg). Products include:

Kaletra 452

Loratadine (Tadalafil is a substrate of and predominantly metabolized by CYP3A4. Studies have shown that drugs that inhibit CYP3A4 can increase tadalafil exposure. When tadalafil is used on an as-needed basis, patients taking concomitant potent inhibitors of CYP3A4, such as ketoconazole or ritonavir, the maximum recommended dose of tadalafil is 10 mg, not to exceed once every 72 hours. When tadalafil is used in a once-daily regimen, patients taking concomitant potent inhibitors of CYP3A4, such as ketoconazole or ritonavir, the dose should not exceed 2.5 mg).

No products indexed under this heading.

Losartan Potassium (PDE5 inhibitors, including tadalafil, are mild systemic vasodilators. Clinical pharmacology studies were conducted to assess the effect of tadalafil on the potentiation of the blood-pressure-lowering effects of selected antihypertensive medications (amlodipine, angiotesin II receptor blockers, bendrofluazide, enalapril, and metoprolol). Small reductions in blood pressure occurred following co-administration of tadalafil with these agents compared to placebo). Products include:

Cozaar Tablets 1973

Magaldrate (Simultaneous administration of an antacid (magnesium hydroxide/aluminum hydroxide) and tadalafil reduced the apparent rate of absorption of tadalafil without altering exposure (AUC) to tadalafil).

No products indexed under this heading.

Magnesium Hydroxide (Simultaneous administration of an antacid (magnesium hydroxide/aluminum hydroxide) and tadalafil reduced the apparent rate of absorption of tadalafil without altering exposure (AUC) to tadalafil). Products include:

Fleet Pedia-Lax Chewable Tablets 1145
Pepcid Complete Chewable Tablets 1771
Extra Strength Rolaids Freshmint Tablets 1903
Rolaids Multi-Symptom Berry Tablets 1903
Rolaids Original Peppermint Tablets 1903

Magnesium Oxide (Simultaneous administration of an antacid (magnesium hydroxide/aluminum hydroxide) and tadalafil reduced the apparent rate of absorption of tadalafil without altering exposure (AUC) to tadalafil). Products include:

Beelith Tablets 813

Mecamylamine Hydrochloride (PDE5 inhibitors, including tadalafil, are mild systemic vasodilators. Clinical pharmacology studies were conducted to assess the effect of tadalafil on the potentiation of the blood-pressure-lowering effects of selected antihypertensive medications (amlodipine, angiotesin II receptor blockers, bendrofluazide, enalapril, and metoprolol). Small reductions in blood pressure occurred following co-administration of tadalafil with these agents compared to placebo).

No products indexed under this heading.

Mephenytoin (Studies have shown that drugs that induce CYP3A4 can decrease tadalafil exposure).

No products indexed under this heading.

Methsuximide (Studies have shown that drugs that induce CYP3A4 can decrease tadalafil exposure).

No products indexed under this heading.

Methyclothiazide (PDE5 inhibitors, including tadalafil, are mild systemic vasodilators. Clinical pharmacology studies were conducted to assess the effect of tadalafil on the potentiation of the blood-pressure-lowering effects of selected antihypertensive medications (amlodipine, angiotesin II receptor blockers, bendrofluazide, enalapril, and metoprolol). Small reductions in blood pressure occurred following co-administration of tadalafil with these agents compared to placebo).

No products indexed under this heading.

Methyldopa (PDE5 inhibitors, including tadalafil, are mild systemic vasodilators. Clinical pharmacology studies were conducted to assess the effect of tadalafil on the potentiation of the blood-pressure-lowering effects of selected antihypertensive medications (amlodipine, angiotesin II receptor blockers, bendrofluazide, enalapril, and metoprolol). Small reductions in blood pressure occurred following co-administration of tadalafil with these agents compared to placebo).

No products indexed under this heading.

Methyldopate Hydrochloride (PDE5 inhibitors, including tadalafil, are mild systemic vasodilators. Clinical pharmacology studies were conducted to assess the effect of tadalafil on the potentiation of the blood-pressure-lowering effects of selected antihypertensive medications (amlodipine, angiotesin II receptor blockers, bendrofluazide, enalapril, and metoprolol). Small reductions in blood pressure occurred following co-administration of tadalafil with these agents compared to placebo).

No products indexed under this heading.

Methylprednisolone (Studies have shown that drugs that induce CYP3A4 can decrease tadalafil exposure).

No products indexed under this heading.

Methylprednisolone Acetate (Studies have shown that drugs that induce CYP3A4 can decrease tadalafil exposure).

No products indexed under this heading.

Methylprednisolone Sodium Succinate (Studies have shown that drugs that induce CYP3A4 can decrease tadalafil exposure).

No products indexed under this heading.

Metolazone (PDE5 inhibitors, including tadalafil, are mild systemic vasodilators. Clinical pharmacology studies were conducted to assess the effect of tadalafil on the potentiation of the blood-pressure-lowering effects of selected antihypertensive medications (amlodipine, angiotesin II receptor blockers, bendrofluazide, enalapril, and metoprolol). Small reductions in blood pressure occurred following co-administration of tadalafil with these agents compared to placebo).

No products indexed under this heading.

Metoprolol Succinate (Following dosing with sustained-release metoprolol (25-200mg daily) and tadalafil 10mg, the mean reduction in supine systolic/diastolic blood pressure due to tadalafil 10mg in subjects taking metoprolol was 5/3mm Hg, compared to placebo). Products include:

Toprol-XL Tablets 666

Metoprolol Tartrate (Following dosing with sustained-release metoprolol (25-200mg daily) and tadalafil 10mg, the mean reduction in supine systolic/diastolic blood pressure due to tadalafil 10mg in subjects taking metoprolol was 5/3mm Hg, compared to placebo).

No products indexed under this heading.

Metronidazole (Tadalafil is a substrate of and predominantly metabolized by CYP3A4. Studies have shown that drugs that inhibit CYP3A4 can increase tadalafil exposure. When tadalafil is used on an as-needed basis, patients taking concomitant potent inhibitors of CYP3A4, such as ketoconazole or ritonavir, the maximum recommended dose of tadalafil is 10 mg, not to exceed once every 72 hours. When tadalafil is used in a once-daily regimen, patients taking concomitant potent inhibitors of CYP3A4, such as ketoconazole or ritonavir, the dose should not exceed 2.5 mg). Products include:

Pylera Capsules 714

Metronidazole Benzoate (Tadalafil is a substrate of and predominantly metabolized by CYP3A4. Studies have shown that drugs that inhibit CYP3A4 can increase tadalafil exposure. When tadalafil is used on an as-needed basis, patients taking concomitant potent inhibitors of CYP3A4, such as ketoconazole or ritonavir, the maximum recommended dose of tadalafil is 10 mg, not to exceed once every 72 hours. When tadalafil is used in a once-daily regimen, patients taking concomitant potent inhibitors of CYP3A4, such as ketoconazole or ritonavir, the dose should not exceed 2.5 mg).

No products indexed under this heading.

Metronidazole Hydrochloride (Tadalafil is a substrate of and predominantly metabolized by CYP3A4. Studies have shown that drugs that inhibit CYP3A4 can increase tadalafil exposure. When tadalafil is used on an as-needed basis, patients taking concomitant potent inhibitors of CYP3A4, such as ketoconazole or ritonavir, the maximum recommended dose of tadalafil is 10 mg, not to exceed once every 72 hours. When tadalafil is used in a once-daily regimen, patients taking concomitant potent inhibitors of CYP3A4, such as ketoconazole or ritonavir, the dose should not exceed 2.5 mg).

No products indexed under this heading.

Metronidazole Sodium (Tadalafil is a substrate of and predominantly metabolized by CYP3A4. Studies have shown that drugs that inhibit CYP3A4 can increase tadalafil exposure. When tadalafil is used on an as-needed basis, patients taking concomitant potent inhibitors of CYP3A4, such as ketoconazole or ritonavir, the maximum recommended dose of tadalafil is 10 mg, not to exceed once every 72 hours. When tadalafil is used in a once-daily regimen, patients taking concomitant potent inhibitors of CYP3A4, such as ketoconazole or ritonavir, the dose should not exceed 2.5 mg).

No products indexed under this heading.

Metyrosine (PDE5 inhibitors, including tadalafil, are mild systemic vasodilators. Clinical pharmacology studies were conducted to assess the effect of tadalafil on the potentiation of the blood-pressure-lowering effects of selected antihypertensive medications (amlodipine, angiotesin II receptor blockers, bendrofluazide, enalapril, and metoprolol). Small reductions in blood pressure occurred following co-administration of tadalafil with these agents compared to placebo). Products include:

Demser Capsules 1989

Mibefradil Dihydrochloride (PDE5 inhibitors, including tadalafil, are mild systemic vasodilators. Clinical pharmacology studies were conducted to assess the effect of tadalafil on the potentiation of the blood-pressure-lowering effects of selected antihypertensive medications (amlodipine, angiotesin II receptor blockers, bendrofluazide, enalapril, and metoprolol). Small reductions in blood pressure occurred following co-administration of tadalafil with these agents compared to placebo).

No products indexed under this heading.

Miconazole (Tadalafil is a substrate of and predominantly metabolized by CYP3A4. Studies have shown that drugs that inhibit CYP3A4 can increase tadalafil exposure. When tadalafil is used on an as-needed basis, patients taking concomitant potent inhibitors of CYP3A4, such as ketoconazole or ritonavir, the maximum recommended dose of tadalafil is 10 mg, not to exceed once every 72 hours. When tadalafil is used in a once-daily regimen, patients taking concomitant potent inhibitors of CYP3A4, such as ketoconazole or ritonavir, the dose should not exceed 2.5 mg).

No products indexed under this heading.

Miconazole Nitrate (Tadalafil is a substrate of and predominantly metabolized by CYP3A4. Studies have shown that drugs that inhibit CYP3A4 can increase tadalafil exposure. When tadalafil is used on an as-needed basis, patients taking concomitant potent inhibitors of CYP3A4, such as ketoconazole or ritonavir, the maximum recommended dose of tadalafil is 10 mg, not to exceed once every 72 hours. When tadalafil is used in a once-daily regimen, patients taking concomitant potent inhibitors of CYP3A4, such as ketoconazole or ritonavir, the dose should not exceed 2.5 mg).

No products indexed under this heading.

Minoxidil (PDE5 inhibitors, including tadalafil, are mild systemic vasodilators. Clinical pharmacology studies were conducted to assess the effect of tadalafil on the potentiation of the blood-pressure-lowering effects of selected antihypertensive medications (amlodipine, angiotesin II receptor blockers, bendrofluazide, enalapril, and metoprolol). Small reductions in blood pressure occurred following co-administration of tadalafil with these agents compared to placebo).

No products indexed under this heading.

Modafinil (Studies have shown that drugs that induce CYP3A4 can decrease tadalafil exposure). Products include:

Provigil Tablets 977

Moexipril Hydrochloride (PDE5 inhibitors, including tadalafil, are mild systemic vasodilators. Clinical pharmacology studies were conducted to assess the effect of tadalafil on the potentiation of the blood-pressure-lowering effects of selected antihypertensive medications (amlodipine, angiotesin II receptor blockers, bendrofluazide, enalapril, and metoprolol). Small reductions in blood pressure occurred following co-administration of tadalafil with these agents compared to placebo).

No products indexed under this heading.

Nadolol (PDE5 inhibitors, including tadalafil, are mild systemic vasodilators. Clinical pharmacology studies were conducted to assess the effect of tadalafil on the potentiation of the blood-pressure-lowering effects of selected antihypertensive medications (amlodipine, angiotesin II receptor blockers, bendrofluazide, enalapril, and metoprolol). Small reductions in blood pressure occurred following co-administration of tadalafil with these agents compared to placebo). Products include:

Nadolol Tablets 2191

Nebivolol (PDE5 inhibitors, including tadalafil, are mild systemic vasodilators. Clinical pharmacology studies were conducted to assess the effect of tadalafil on the potentiation of the blood-pressure-lowering effects of selected antihypertensive medications (amlodipine, angiotesin II receptor blockers, bendrofluazide, enalapril, and metoprolol). Small reductions in blood pressure occurred following co-administration of tadalafil with these agents compared to placebo). Products include:

Bystolic Tablets 1155

Nefazodone Hydrochloride (Tadalafil is metabolized predominantly by CYP3A4 in the liver. The dose of tadalafil should be limited to 10 mg no more than once every 72 hours in patients taking potent inhibitors of CYP3A4, such as ritonavir, ketoconazole, and itraconazole. In patients taking potent inhibitors of CYP3A4 and tadalafil for once-daily use, the dose of tadalafil should not exceed 2.5 mg).

No products indexed under this heading.

Nelfinavir Mesylate (Tadalafil is metabolized predominantly by CYP3A4 in the liver. The dose of tadalafil should be limited to 10 mg no more than once every 72 hours in patients taking potent inhibitors of CYP3A4, such as ritonavir, ketoconazole, and itraconazole. In patients taking potent inhibitors of CYP3A4 and tadalafil for once-daily use, the dose of tadalafil should not exceed 2.5 mg).

No products indexed under this heading.

Nevirapine (Tadalafil is a substrate of and predominantly metabolized by CYP3A4. Studies have shown that drugs that inhibit CYP3A4 can increase tadalafil exposure. When tadalafil is used on an as-needed basis, patients taking concomitant potent inhibitors of CYP3A4, such as ketoconazole or ritonavir, the maximum recommended dose of tadalafil is 10 mg, not to exceed once every 72 hours. When tadalafil is used in a once-daily regimen, patients taking concomitant potent inhibitors of CYP3A4, such as ketoconazole or ritonavir, the dose should not exceed 2.5 mg). Products include:

Viramune Oral Suspension 873
Viramune Tablets 873

Niacinamide (Tadalafil is a substrate of and predominantly metabolized by CYP3A4. Studies have shown that drugs that inhibit CYP3A4 can increase tadalafil exposure. When tadalafil is used on an as-needed basis, patients taking concomitant potent inhibitors of CYP3A4, such as ketoconazole or ritonavir, the maximum recommended dose of tadalafil is 10 mg, not to exceed once every 72 hours. When tadalafil is used in a once-daily regimen, patients taking concomitant potent inhibitors of CYP3A4, such as ketoconazole or ritonavir, the dose should not exceed 2.5 mg). Products include:

BioLean Free Tablets .... ■635

Nicardipine Hydrochloride (PDE5 inhibitors, including tadalafil, are mild systemic vasodilators. Clinical pharmacology studies were conducted to assess the effect of tadalafil on the potentiation of the blood-pressure-lowering effects of selected antihypertensive medications (amlodipine, angiotesin II receptor blockers, bendrofluazide, enalapril, and metoprolol). Small reductions in blood pressure occurred following co-administration of tadalafil with these agents compared to placebo). Products include:

Cardene I.V. 1093

Nicotinamide (Tadalafil is a substrate of and predominantly metabolized by CYP3A4. Studies have shown that drugs that inhibit CYP3A4 can increase tadalafil exposure. When tadalafil is used on an as-needed basis, patients taking concomitant potent inhibitors of CYP3A4, such as ketoconazole or ritonavir, the maximum recommended dose of tadalafil is 10 mg, not to exceed once every 72 hours. When tadalafil is used in a once-daily regimen, patients taking concomitant potent inhibitors of CYP3A4, such as ketoconazole or ritonavir, the dose should not exceed 2.5 mg).

No products indexed under this heading.

Nifedipine (PDE5 inhibitors, including tadalafil, are mild systemic vasodilators. Clinical pharmacology studies were conducted to assess the effect of tadalafil on the potentiation of the blood-pressure-lowering effects of selected antihypertensive medications (amlodipine, angiotesin II receptor blockers, bendrofluazide, enalapril, and metoprolol). Small reductions in blood pressure occurred following co-administration

of tadalafil with these agents compared to placebo).
No products indexed under this heading.

Nisoldipine (PDE5 inhibitors, including tadalafil, are mild systemic vasodilators. Clinical pharmacology studies were conducted to assess the effect of tadalafil on the potentiation of the blood-pressure-lowering effects of selected antihypertensive medications (amlodipine, angiotesin II receptor blockers, bendrofluazide, enalapril, and metoprolol). Small reductions in blood pressure occurred following co-administration of tadalafil with these agents compared to placebo). Products include:
Sular Extended Release Tablets 2975

Nitroglycerin (Administration of tadalafil to patients using any form of organic nitrate, either regularly and/or intermittently, is contraindicated). Products include:
Nitro-Dur Transdermal Infusion System 2887
Nitrolingual Pumpspray 2965

Norfloxacin (Tadalafil is a substrate of and predominantly metabolized by CYP3A4. Studies have shown that drugs that inhibit CYP3A4 can increase tadalafil exposure. When tadalafil is used on an as-needed basis, patients taking concomitant potent inhibitors of CYP3A4, such as ketoconazole or ritonavir, the maximum recommended dose of tadalafil is 10 mg, not to exceed once every 72 hours. When tadalafil is used in a once-daily regimen, patients taking concomitant potent inhibitors of CYP3A4, such as ketoconazole or ritonavir, the dose should not exceed 2.5 mg). Products include:
Noroxin Tablets 2069

Omeprazole (Tadalafil is a substrate of and predominantly metabolized by CYP3A4. Studies have shown that drugs that inhibit CYP3A4 can increase tadalafil exposure. When tadalafil is used on an as-needed basis, patients taking concomitant potent inhibitors of CYP3A4, such as ketoconazole or ritonavir, the maximum recommended dose of tadalafil is 10 mg, not to exceed once every 72 hours. When tadalafil is used in a once-daily regimen, patients taking concomitant potent inhibitors of CYP3A4, such as ketoconazole or ritonavir, the dose should not exceed 2.5 mg).
No products indexed under this heading.

Oxcarbazepine (Studies have shown that drugs that induce CYP3A4 can decrease tadalafil exposure).
No products indexed under this heading.

Paroxetine Hydrochloride (Tadalafil is a substrate of and predominantly metabolized by CYP3A4. Studies have shown that drugs that inhibit CYP3A4 can increase tadalafil exposure. When tadalafil is used on an as-needed basis, patients taking concomitant potent inhibitors of CYP3A4, such as ketoconazole or ritonavir, the maximum recommended dose of tadalafil is 10 mg, not to exceed once every 72 hours. When tadalafil is used in a once-daily regimen, patients taking concomitant potent inhibitors of CYP3A4, such as ketoconazole or ritonavir, the dose should not exceed 2.5 mg). Products include:
Paxil 1535
Paxil CR Controlled-Release Tablets 1544

Penbutolol Sulfate (PDE5 inhibitors, including tadalafil, are mild systemic vasodilators. Clinical pharmacology studies were conducted to assess the effect of tadalafil on the potentiation of the blood-pressure-lowering effects of selected antihypertensive medications (amlodipine, angiotesin II receptor blockers, bendrofluazide, enalapril, and metoprolol). Small reductions in blood pressure occurred following co-administration of tadalafil with these agents compared to placebo).
No products indexed under this heading.

Pentaerythritol Tetranitrate (Administration of tadalafil to patients using any form of organic nitrate, either regularly and/or intermittently, is contraindicated).
No products indexed under this heading.

Perindopril Erbumine (PDE5 inhibitors, including tadalafil, are mild systemic vasodilators. Clinical pharmacology studies were conducted to assess the effect of tadalafil on the potentiation of the blood-pressure-lowering effects of selected antihypertensive medications (amlodipine, angiotesin II receptor blockers, bendrofluazide, enalapril, and metoprolol). Small reductions in blood pressure occurred following co-administration of tadalafil with these agents compared to placebo). Products include:
Aceon Tablets (2 mg, 4 mg, 8 mg) 3038

Phenobarbital (CYP3A4 inducers, such as phenobarbital, may decrease tadalafil exposure. No dose adjustment is warranted). Products include:
Donnatal Extentabs 2507

Phenobarbital Sodium (CYP3A4 inducers, such as phenobarbital, may decrease tadalafil exposure. No dose adjustment is warranted).
No products indexed under this heading.

Phenoxybenzamine Hydrochloride (PDE5 inhibitors, including tadalafil, are mild systemic vasodilators. Clinical pharmacology studies were conducted to assess the effect of tadalafil on the potentiation of the blood-pressure-lowering effects of selected antihypertensive medications (amlodipine, angiotesin II receptor blockers, bendrofluazide, enalapril, and metoprolol). Small reductions in blood pressure occurred following co-administration of tadalafil with these agents compared to placebo). Products include:
Dibenzyline Capsules 3188

Phentolamine Mesylate (PDE5 inhibitors, including tadalafil, are mild systemic vasodilators. Clinical pharmacology studies were conducted to assess the effect of tadalafil on the potentiation of the blood-pressure-lowering effects of selected antihypertensive medications (amlodipine, angiotesin II receptor blockers, bendrofluazide, enalapril, and metoprolol). Small reductions in blood pressure occurred following co-administration of tadalafil with these agents compared to placebo).
No products indexed under this heading.

Phenytoin (CYP3A4 inducers, such as phenytoin, may decrease tadalafil exposure. No dose adjustment is warranted).
No products indexed under this heading.

Phenytoin Sodium (CYP3A4 inducers, such as phenytoin, may decrease tadalafil exposure. No dose adjustment is warranted). Products include:
Phenytek Capsules 2192

Pindolol (PDE5 inhibitors, including tadalafil, are mild systemic vasodilators. Clinical pharmacology studies were conducted to assess the effect of tadalafil on the potentiation of the blood-pressure-lowering effects of selected antihypertensive medications (amlodipine, angiotesin II receptor blockers, bendrofluazide, enalapril, and metoprolol). Small reductions in blood pressure occurred following co-administration of tadalafil with these agents compared to placebo).
No products indexed under this heading.

Polythiazide (PDE5 inhibitors, including tadalafil, are mild systemic vasodilators. Clinical pharmacology studies were conducted to assess the effect of tadalafil on the potentiation of the blood-pressure-lowering effects of selected antihypertensive medications (amlodipine, angiotesin II receptor blockers, bendrofluazide, enalapril, and metoprolol). Small reductions in blood pressure occurred following co-administration of tadalafil with these agents compared to placebo).
No products indexed under this heading.

Prazosin Hydrochloride (Caution is advised when PDE5 inhibitors are co-administered with alpha-blockers. PDE5 inhibitors, including tadalafil, and alpha-adrenergic blocking agents are both vasodilators with blood-pressure lowering effects. When vasodilators are used in combination, an additive effect on blood pressure may be anticipated. In some patients, concomitant use of these two drug classes can lower blood presure significantly, which may lead to symptomatic hypotension (e.g., fainting)).
No products indexed under this heading.

Prednisolone Acetate (Studies have shown that drugs that induce CYP3A4 can decrease tadalafil exposure). Products include:
Pred Forte Ophthalmic Suspension .... ⊙ 227
Pred Mild Ophthalmic Suspension .... ⊙ 230
Pred-G Ophthalmic Ointment .... ⊙ 229
Pred-G Ophthalmic Suspension .... ⊙ 228

Prednisolone Sodium Phosphate (Studies have shown that drugs that induce CYP3A4 can decrease tadalafil exposure).
No products indexed under this heading.

Prednisolone Tebutate (Studies have shown that drugs that induce CYP3A4 can decrease tadalafil exposure).
No products indexed under this heading.

Prednisone (Studies have shown that drugs that induce CYP3A4 can decrease tadalafil exposure).
No products indexed under this heading.

Primidone (Studies have shown that drugs that induce CYP3A4 can decrease tadalafil exposure).
No products indexed under this heading.

Propoxyphene Hydrochloride (Tadalafil is a substrate of and predominantly metabolized by CYP3A4. Studies have shown that drugs that inhibit CYP3A4 can increase tadalafil exposure. When tadalafil is used on an as-needed basis, patients taking concomitant potent inhibitors of CYP3A4, such as ketoconazole or ritonavir, the maximum recommended dose of tadalafil is 10 mg, not to exceed once every 72 hours. When tadalafil is used in a once-daily regimen, patients taking concomitant potent inhibitors of CYP3A4, such as ketoconazole or ritonavir, the dose should not exceed 2.5 mg).
No products indexed under this heading.

Propoxyphene Napsylate (Tadalafil is a substrate of and predominantly metabolized by CYP3A4. Studies have shown that drugs that inhibit CYP3A4 can increase tadalafil exposure. When tadalafil is used on an as-needed basis, patients taking concomitant potent inhibitors of CYP3A4, such as ketoconazole or ritonavir, the maximum recommended dose of tadalafil is 10 mg, not to exceed once every 72 hours. When tadalafil is used in a once-daily regimen, patients taking concomitant potent inhibitors of CYP3A4, such as ketoconazole or ritonavir, the dose should not exceed 2.5 mg).
No products indexed under this heading.

Propranolol Hydrochloride (PDE5 inhibitors, including tadalafil, are mild systemic vasodilators. Clinical pharmacology studies were conducted to assess the effect of tadalafil on the potentiation of the blood-pressure-lowering effects of selected antihypertensive medications (amlodipine, angiotesin II receptor blockers, bendrofluazide, enalapril, and metoprolol). Small reductions in blood pressure occurred following co-administration of tadalafil with these agents compared to placebo). Products include:
InnoPran XL Extended Release Capsules 1484

Quinapril Hydrochloride (PDE5 inhibitors, including tadalafil, are mild systemic vasodilators. Clinical pharmacology studies were conducted to assess the effect of tadalafil on the potentiation of the blood-pressure-lowering effects of selected antihypertensive medications (amlodipine, angiotesin II receptor blockers, bendrofluazide, enalapril, and metoprolol). Small reductions in blood pressure occurred following co-administration of tadalafil with these agents compared to placebo).
No products indexed under this heading.

Quinidine (Tadalafil is a substrate of and predominantly metabolized by CYP3A4. Studies have shown that drugs that inhibit CYP3A4 can increase tadalafil exposure. When tadalafil is used on an as-needed basis, patients taking concomitant potent inhibitors of CYP3A4, such as ketoconazole or ritonavir, the maximum recommended dose of tadalafil is 10 mg, not to exceed once every 72 hours. When tadalafil is used in a once-daily regimen, patients taking concomitant potent inhibitors of CYP3A4, such as ketoconazole or ritonavir, the dose should not exceed 2.5 mg).

No products indexed under this heading.

Quinidine Hydrochloride (Tadalafil is a substrate of and predominantly metabolized by CYP3A4. Studies have shown that drugs that inhibit CYP3A4 can increase tadalafil exposure. When tadalafil is used on an as-needed basis, patients taking concomitant potent inhibitors of CYP3A4, such as ketoconazole or ritonavir, the maximum recommended dose of tadalafil is 10 mg, not to exceed once every 72 hours. When tadalafil is used in a once-daily regimen, patients taking concomitant potent inhibitors of CYP3A4, such as ketoconazole or ritonavir, the dose should not exceed 2.5 mg).

No products indexed under this heading.

Quinidine Polygalacturonate (Tadalafil is a substrate of and predominantly metabolized by CYP3A4. Studies have shown that drugs that inhibit CYP3A4 can increase tadalafil exposure. When tadalafil is used on an as-needed basis, patients taking concomitant potent inhibitors of CYP3A4, such as ketoconazole or ritonavir, the maximum recommended dose of tadalafil is 10 mg, not to exceed once every 72 hours. When tadalafil is used in a once-daily regimen, patients taking concomitant potent inhibitors of CYP3A4, such as ketoconazole or ritonavir, the dose should not exceed 2.5 mg).

No products indexed under this heading.

Quinidine Sulfate (Tadalafil is a substrate of and predominantly metabolized by CYP3A4. Studies have shown that drugs that inhibit CYP3A4 can increase tadalafil exposure. When tadalafil is used on an as-needed basis, patients taking concomitant potent inhibitors of CYP3A4, such as ketoconazole or ritonavir, the maximum recommended dose of tadalafil is 10 mg, not to exceed once every 72 hours. When tadalafil is used in a once-daily regimen, patients taking concomitant potent inhibitors of CYP3A4, such as ketoconazole or ritonavir, the dose should not exceed 2.5 mg).

No products indexed under this heading.

Quinine (Tadalafil is a substrate of and predominantly metabolized by CYP3A4. Studies have shown that drugs that inhibit CYP3A4 can increase tadalafil exposure. When tadalafil is used on an as-needed basis, patients taking concomitant potent inhibitors of CYP3A4, such as ketoconazole or ritonavir, the maximum recommended dose of tadalafil is 10 mg, not to exceed once every 72 hours. When tadalafil is used in a once-daily regimen, patients taking concomitant potent inhibitors of CYP3A4, such as ketoconazole or ritonavir, the dose should not exceed 2.5 mg).

No products indexed under this heading.

Quinine Sulfate (Tadalafil is a substrate of and predominantly metabolized by CYP3A4. Studies have shown that drugs that inhibit CYP3A4 can increase tadalafil exposure. When tadalafil is used on an as-needed basis, patients taking concomitant potent inhibitors of CYP3A4, such as ketoconazole or ritonavir, the maximum recommended dose of tadalafil is 10 mg, not to exceed once every 72 hours. When tadalafil is used in a once-daily regimen, patients taking concomitant potent inhibitors of CYP3A4, such as ketoconazole or ritonavir, the dose should not exceed 2.5 mg).

No products indexed under this heading.

Quinupristin (Tadalafil is a substrate of and predominantly metabolized by CYP3A4. Studies have shown that drugs that inhibit CYP3A4 can increase tadalafil exposure. When tadalafil is used on an as-needed basis, patients taking concomitant potent inhibitors of CYP3A4, such as ketoconazole or ritonavir, the maximum recommended dose of tadalafil is 10 mg, not to exceed once every 72 hours. When tadalafil is used in a once-daily regimen, patients taking concomitant potent inhibitors of CYP3A4, such as ketoconazole or ritonavir, the dose should not exceed 2.5 mg).

No products indexed under this heading.

Ramipril (PDE5 inhibitors, including tadalafil, are mild systemic vasodilators. Clinical pharmacology studies were conducted to assess the effect of tadalafil on the potentiation of the blood-pressure-lowering effects of selected antihypertensive medications (amlodipine, angiotesin II receptor blockers, bendrofluazide, enalapril, and metoprolol). Small reductions in blood pressure occurred following co-administration of tadalafil with these agents compared to placebo).

No products indexed under this heading.

Ranitidine Bismuth Citrate (Tadalafil is a substrate of and predominantly metabolized by CYP3A4. Studies have shown that drugs that inhibit CYP3A4 can increase tadalafil exposure. When tadalafil is used on an as-needed basis, patients taking concomitant potent inhibitors of CYP3A4, such as ketoconazole or ritonavir, the maximum recommended dose of tadalafil is 10 mg, not to exceed once every 72 hours. When tadalafil is used in a once-daily regimen, patients taking concomitant potent inhibitors of CYP3A4, such as ketoconazole or ritonavir, the dose should not exceed 2.5 mg).

No products indexed under this heading.

Ranitidine Hydrochloride (Tadalafil is a substrate of and predominantly metabolized by CYP3A4. Studies have shown that drugs that inhibit CYP3A4 can increase tadalafil exposure. When tadalafil is used on an as-needed basis, patients taking concomitant potent inhibitors of CYP3A4, such as ketoconazole or ritonavir, the maximum recommended dose of tadalafil is 10 mg, not to exceed once every 72 hours. When tadalafil is used in a once-daily regimen, patients taking concomitant potent inhibitors of CYP3A4, such as ketoconazole or ritonavir, the dose should not exceed 2.5 mg). Products include:

Zantac 75 Tablets .... ▣ 603
Zantac 1670
Zantac Injection 1666
Zantac Injection Pharmacy Bulk Package 1668
Maximum Strength Zantac 150 Tablets .... ▣ 603
Maximum Strength Zantac 150 Cool Mint Tablets .... ▣ 603

Rauwolfia Serpentina (PDE5 inhibitors, including tadalafil, are mild systemic vasodilators. Clinical pharmacology studies were conducted to assess the effect of tadalafil on the potentiation of the blood-pressure-lowering effects of selected antihypertensive medications (amlodipine, angiotesin II receptor blockers, bendrofluazide, enalapril, and metoprolol). Small reductions in blood pressure occurred following co-administration of tadalafil with these agents compared to placebo).

No products indexed under this heading.

Rescinnamine (PDE5 inhibitors, including tadalafil, are mild systemic vasodilators. Clinical pharmacology studies were conducted to assess the effect of tadalafil on the potentiation of the blood-pressure-lowering effects of selected antihypertensive medications (amlodipine, angiotesin II receptor blockers, bendrofluazide, enalapril, and metoprolol). Small reductions in blood pressure occurred following co-administration of tadalafil with these agents compared to placebo).

No products indexed under this heading.

Reserpine (PDE5 inhibitors, including tadalafil, are mild systemic vasodilators. Clinical pharmacology studies were conducted to assess the effect of tadalafil on the potentiation of the blood-pressure-lowering effects of selected antihypertensive medications (amlodipine, angiotesin II receptor blockers, bendrofluazide, enalapril, and metoprolol). Small reductions in blood pressure occurred following co-administration of tadalafil with these agents compared to placebo).

No products indexed under this heading.

Rifabutin (Studies have shown that drugs that induce CYP3A4 can decrease tadalafil exposure).

No products indexed under this heading.

Rifampicin (Studies have shown that drugs that induce CYP3A4 can decrease tadalafil exposure).

No products indexed under this heading.

Rifampin (Rifampin reduced tadalafil 10mg single dose exposure (AUC) by 88% and Cmax by 46% relative to the values for tadalafil 10mg alone. No dose adjustment is warranted).

No products indexed under this heading.

Rifapentine (Studies have shown that drugs that induce CYP3A4 can decrease tadalafil exposure).

No products indexed under this heading.

Ritonavir (Ritonavir increased tadalafil 20mg single dose exposure (AUC) by 124% with no change in Cmax, relative to the values for tadalafil 20mg alone. Based on these results, the dose of tadalafil should not exceed 10mg and tadalafil should not be taken more frequently than once in 72 hours). Products include:

Kaletra 452
Norvir 489

Saquinavir (Tadalafil is metabolized predominantly by CYP3A4 in the liver. The dose of tadalafil should be limited to 10 mg no more than once every 72 hours in patients taking potent inhibitors of CYP3A4, such as ritonavir, ketoconazole, and itraconazole. In patients taking potent inhibitors of CYP3A4 and tadalafil for once-daily use, the dose of tadalafil should not exceed 2.5 mg).

No products indexed under this heading.

Saquinavir Mesylate (Tadalafil is metabolized predominantly by CYP3A4 in the liver. The dose of tadalafil should be limited to 10 mg no more than once every 72 hours in patients taking potent inhibitors of CYP3A4, such as ritonavir, ketoconazole, and itraconazole. In patients taking potent inhibitors of CYP3A4 and tadalafil for once-daily use, the dose of tadalafil should not exceed 2.5 mg).

No products indexed under this heading.

Sertraline Hydrochloride (Tadalafil is a substrate of and predominantly metabolized by CYP3A4. Studies have shown that drugs that inhibit CYP3A4 can increase tadalafil exposure. When tadalafil is used on an as-needed basis, patients taking concomitant potent inhibitors of CYP3A4, such as ketoconazole or ritonavir, the maximum recommended dose of tadalafil is 10 mg, not to exceed once every 72 hours. When tadalafil is used in a once-daily regimen, patients taking concomitant potent inhibitors of CYP3A4, such as ketoconazole or ritonavir, the dose should not exceed 2.5 mg).

No products indexed under this heading.

Sildenafil Citrate (Tadalafil is a substrate of and predominantly metabolized by CYP3A4. Studies have shown that drugs that inhibit CYP3A4 can increase tadalafil exposure. When tadalafil is used on an as-needed basis, patients taking concomitant potent inhibitors of CYP3A4, such as ketoconazole or ritonavir, the maximum recommended dose of tadalafil is 10 mg, not to exceed once every 72 hours. When tadalafil is used in a once-daily regimen, patients taking concomitant potent inhibitors of CYP3A4, such as ketoconazole or ritonavir, the dose should not exceed 2.5 mg).

No products indexed under this heading.

Sodium Bicarbonate (Simultaneous administration of an antacid (magnesium hydroxide/aluminum hydroxide) and tadalafil reduced the apparent rate of absorption of tadalafil without altering exposure (AUC) to tadalafil). Products include:

Ceo-Two Laxative Suppository 815

Sodium Nitroprusside (PDE5 inhibitors, including tadalafil, are mild systemic vasodilators. Clinical pharmacology studies were conducted to assess the effect of tadalafil on the potentiation of the blood-pressure-lowering effects of selected antihypertensive medications (amlodipine, angiotesin II receptor blockers, bendrofluazide, enalapril, and metoprolol). Small reductions in blood pressure occurred following co-administration of tadalafil with these

agents compared to placebo).
No products indexed under this heading.

Sotalol Hydrochloride (PDE5 inhibitors, including tadalafil, are mild systemic vasodilators. Clinical pharmacology studies were conducted to assess the effect of tadalafil on the potentiation of the blood-pressure-lowering effects of selected antihypertensive medications (amlodipine, angiotesin II receptor blockers, bendrofluazide, enalapril, and metoprolol). Small reductions in blood pressure occurred following co-administration of tadalafil with these agents compared to placebo).
No products indexed under this heading.

Spirapril Hydrochloride (PDE5 inhibitors, including tadalafil, are mild systemic vasodilators. Clinical pharmacology studies were conducted to assess the effect of tadalafil on the potentiation of the blood-pressure-lowering effects of selected antihypertensive medications (amlodipine, angiotesin II receptor blockers, bendrofluazide, enalapril, and metoprolol). Small reductions in blood pressure occurred following co-administration of tadalafil with these agents compared to placebo).
No products indexed under this heading.

Sulfinpyrazone (Studies have shown that drugs that induce CYP3A4 can decrease tadalafil exposure).
No products indexed under this heading.

Tamsulosin Hydrochloride (Caution is advised when PDE5 inhibitors are co-administered with alpha-blockers. PDE5 inhibitors, including tadalafil, and alpha-adrenergic blocking agents are both vasodilators with blood-pressure lowering effects. When vasodilators are used in combination, an additive effect on blood pressure may be anticipated. In some patients, concomitant use of these two drug classes can lower blood presure significantly, which may lead to symptomatic hypotension (e.g., fainting)). Products include:
Flomax Capsules 848

Telithromycin (Tadalafil is metabolized predominantly by CYP3A4 in the liver. The dose of tadalafil should be limited to 10 mg no more than once every 72 hours in patients taking potent inhibitors of CYP3A4, such as ritonavir, ketoconazole, and itraconazole. In patients taking potent inhibitors of CYP3A4 and tadalafil for once-daily use, the dose of tadalafil should not exceed 2.5 mg). Products include:
Ketek Tablets 2744

Telmisartan (PDE5 inhibitors, including tadalafil, are mild systemic vasodilators. Clinical pharmacology studies were conducted to assess the effect of tadalafil on the potentiation of the blood-pressure-lowering effects of selected antihypertensive medications (amlodipine, angiotesin II receptor blockers, bendrofluazide, enalapril, and metoprolol). Small reductions in blood pressure occurred following co-administration of tadalafil with these agents compared to placebo). Products include:
Micardis Tablets 852
Micardis HCT Tablets 854

Terazosin Hydrochloride (Caution is advised when PDE5 inhibitors are co-administered with alpha-blockers. PDE5 inhibitors, including tadalafil, and alpha-adrenergic blocking agents are both vasodilators with blood-pressure lowering effects. When vasodilators are used in combination, an additive effect on blood pressure may be anticipated. In some patients, concomitant use of these two drug classes can lower blood presure significantly, which may lead to symptomatic hypotension (e.g., fainting)).
No products indexed under this heading.

Theophylline (Studies have shown that drugs that induce CYP3A4 can decrease tadalafil exposure).
No products indexed under this heading.

Theophylline Anhydrous (Studies have shown that drugs that induce CYP3A4 can decrease tadalafil exposure). Products include:
Uniphyl Tablets 2595

Theophylline Calcium Salicylate (Studies have shown that drugs that induce CYP3A4 can decrease tadalafil exposure).
No products indexed under this heading.

Theophylline Dihydroxypropyl (Glyceryl) (Studies have shown that drugs that induce CYP3A4 can decrease tadalafil exposure).
No products indexed under this heading.

Theophylline Ethylenediamine (Studies have shown that drugs that induce CYP3A4 can decrease tadalafil exposure).
No products indexed under this heading.

Timolol Maleate (PDE5 inhibitors, including tadalafil, are mild systemic vasodilators. Clinical pharmacology studies were conducted to assess the effect of tadalafil on the potentiation of the blood-pressure-lowering effects of selected antihypertensive medications (amlodipine, angiotesin II receptor blockers, bendrofluazide, enalapril, and metoprolol). Small reductions in blood pressure occurred following co-administration of tadalafil with these agents compared to placebo). Products include:
Combigan Ophthalmic Solution 553
Cosopt Sterile Ophthalmic Solution 1969
Timoptic Sterile Ophthalmic Solution 2121
Timoptic in Ocudose 2124
Timoptic-XE Sterile Ophthalmic Gel Forming Solution 2125

Tipranavir (Ritonavir (500 mg or 600 mg b.i.d. at steady state), an inhibitor of CYP3A4, CYP2C9, CYP2C19, and CYP2D6, increased tadalafil 20 mg single-dose exposure (AUC) by 32% with a 30% reduction in Cmax, relative to the values for tadalafil 20 mg alone. Ritonavir (200 mg b.i.d.), increased tadalafil 20 mg single-dose exposure (AUC) by 124% with no change in Cmax, relative to the values for tadalafil 20 mg alone. Although specific interactions have not been studied, other HIV protease inhibitors would likely increase tadalafil exposure). Products include:
Aptivus Capsules 823
Aptivus Oral Solution 823

Torsemide (PDE5 inhibitors, including tadalafil, are mild systemic vasodilators. Clinical pharmacology studies were conducted to assess the effect of tadalafil on the potentiation of the blood-pressure-lowering effects of selected antihypertensive medications (amlodipine, angiotesin II receptor blockers, bendrofluazide, enalapril, and metoprolol). Small reductions in blood pressure occurred following co-administration of tadalafil with these agents compared to placebo). Products include:
Demadex Injection 2630
Demadex Tablets 2630

Trandolapril (PDE5 inhibitors, including tadalafil, are mild systemic vasodilators. Clinical pharmacology studies were conducted to assess the effect of tadalafil on the potentiation of the blood-pressure-lowering effects of selected antihypertensive medications (amlodipine, angiotesin II receptor blockers, bendrofluazide, enalapril, and metoprolol). Small reductions in blood pressure occurred following co-administration of tadalafil with these agents compared to placebo). Products include:
Mavik Tablets 472
Tarka Tablets 511

Triamcinolone (Studies have shown that drugs that induce CYP3A4 can decrease tadalafil exposure).
No products indexed under this heading.

Triamcinolone Acetonide (Studies have shown that drugs that induce CYP3A4 can decrease tadalafil exposure). Products include:
Azmacort Inhalation Aerosol 407
Nasacort AQ Nasal Spray 2765
Triesence Injectable Suspension .... ⊙209

Triamcinolone Diacetate (Studies have shown that drugs that induce CYP3A4 can decrease tadalafil exposure).
No products indexed under this heading.

Triamcinolone Hexacetonide (Studies have shown that drugs that induce CYP3A4 can decrease tadalafil exposure).
No products indexed under this heading.

Trimethaphan Camsylate (PDE5 inhibitors, including tadalafil, are mild systemic vasodilators. Clinical pharmacology studies were conducted to assess the effect of tadalafil on the potentiation of the blood-pressure-lowering effects of selected antihypertensive medications (amlodipine, angiotesin II receptor blockers, bendrofluazide, enalapril, and metoprolol). Small reductions in blood pressure occurred following co-administration of tadalafil with these agents compared to placebo).
No products indexed under this heading.

Troglitazone (Tadalafil is a substrate of and predominantly metabolized by CYP3A4. Studies have shown that drugs that inhibit CYP3A4 can increase tadalafil exposure. When tadalafil is used on an as-needed basis, patients taking concomitant potent inhibitors of CYP3A4, such as ketoconazole or ritonavir, the maximum recommended dose of tadalafil is 10 mg, not to exceed once every 72 hours. When tadalafil is used in a once-daily regimen, patients taking concomitant potent inhibitors of CYP3A4, such as ketoconazole or ritonavir, the dose should not exceed 2.5 mg).
No products indexed under this heading.

Troleandomycin (Tadalafil is metabolized predominantly by CYP3A4 in the liver. The dose of tadalafil should be limited to 10 mg no more than once every 72 hours in patients taking potent inhibitors of CYP3A4, such as ritonavir, ketoconazole, and itraconazole. In patients taking potent inhibitors of CYP3A4 and tadalafil for once-daily use, the dose of tadalafil should not exceed 2.5 mg).
No products indexed under this heading.

Valproate Sodium (Tadalafil is a substrate of and predominantly metabolized by CYP3A4. Studies have shown that drugs that inhibit CYP3A4 can increase tadalafil exposure. When tadalafil is used on an as-needed basis, patients taking concomitant potent inhibitors of CYP3A4, such as ketoconazole or ritonavir, the maximum recommended dose of tadalafil is 10 mg, not to exceed once every 72 hours. When tadalafil is used in a once-daily regimen, patients taking concomitant potent inhibitors of CYP3A4, such as ketoconazole or ritonavir, the dose should not exceed 2.5 mg).
No products indexed under this heading.

Valsartan (PDE5 inhibitors, including tadalafil, are mild systemic vasodilators. Clinical pharmacology studies were conducted to assess the effect of tadalafil on the potentiation of the blood-pressure-lowering effects of selected antihypertensive medications (amlodipine, angiotesin II receptor blockers, bendrofluazide, enalapril, and metoprolol). Small reductions in blood pressure occurred following co-administration of tadalafil with these agents compared to placebo). Products include:
Diovan Tablets 2212
Diovan HCT Tablets 2216
Exforge Tablets 2238

Vardenafil Hydrochloride (Tadalafil is a substrate of and predominantly metabolized by CYP3A4. Studies have shown that drugs that inhibit CYP3A4 can increase tadalafil exposure. When tadalafil is used on an as-needed basis, patients taking concomitant potent inhibitors of CYP3A4, such as ketoconazole or ritonavir, the maximum recommended dose of tadalafil is 10 mg, not to exceed once every 72 hours. When tadalafil is used in a once-daily regimen, patients taking concomitant potent inhibitors of CYP3A4, such as ketoconazole or ritonavir, the dose should not exceed 2.5 mg). Products include:
Levitra Tablets 2876

Verapamil Hydrochloride (PDE5 inhibitors, including tadalafil, are mild systemic vasodilators. Clinical pharmacology studies were conducted to assess the effect of tadalafil on the potentiation of the blood-pressure-lowering effects of selected antihypertensive medications (amlodipine, angiotesin II receptor blockers, bendrofluazide, enalapril, and metoprolol). Small reductions in blood pressure occurred following co-administration of tadalafil with these agents compared to placebo). Products include:
Tarka Tablets 511

Voriconazole (Tadalafil is metabolized predominantly by CYP3A4 in the liver. The dose of tadalafil should be limited to 10 mg no more than once every 72 hours in patients taking potent inhibitors of CYP3A4, such as ritonavir, ketoconazole, and itraconazole. In patients taking potent inhibitors of CYP3A4 and tadalafil for once-daily use, the dose of tadalafil should not exceed 2.5 mg).

No products indexed under this heading.

Zafirlukast (Tadalafil is a substrate of and predominantly metabolized by CYP3A4. Studies have shown that drugs that inhibit CYP3A4 can increase tadalafil exposure. When tadalafil is used on an as-needed basis, patients taking concomitant potent inhibitors of CYP3A4, such as ketoconazole or ritonavir, the maximum recommended dose of tadalafil is 10 mg, not to exceed once every 72 hours. When tadalafil is used in a once-daily regimen, patients taking concomitant potent inhibitors of CYP3A4, such as ketoconazole or ritonavir, the dose should not exceed 2.5 mg). Products include:

Accolate Tablets 669

Zileuton (Tadalafil is a substrate of and predominantly metabolized by CYP3A4. Studies have shown that drugs that inhibit CYP3A4 can increase tadalafil exposure. When tadalafil is used on an as-needed basis, patients taking concomitant potent inhibitors of CYP3A4, such as ketoconazole or ritonavir, the maximum recommended dose of tadalafil is 10 mg, not to exceed once every 72 hours. When tadalafil is used in a once-daily regimen, patients taking concomitant potent inhibitors of CYP3A4, such as ketoconazole or ritonavir, the dose should not exceed 2.5 mg).

No products indexed under this heading.

Food Interactions

Alcohol (Both tadalafil and alcohol act as mild vasodilators. When mild vasodilators are taken in combination, blood-pressure lowering effects of each individual compound may be increased. Substantial consumption of alcohol in combination with tadalafil may increase the potential for orthostatic signs and symptoms, including increase in heart rate, decrease in standing blood pressure, dizziness, and headache).

Grapefruit (Tadalafil is a substrate of and predominantly metabolized by CYP3A4. Studies have shown that drugs that inhibit CYP3A4 can increase tadalafil exposure. When tadalafil is used on an as-needed basis, patients taking concomitant potent inhibitors of CYP3A4, such as ketoconazole or ritonavir, the maximum recommended dose of tadalafil is 10 mg, not to exceed once every 72 hours. When tadalafil is used in a once-daily regimen, patients taking concomitant potent inhibitors of CYP3A4, such as ketoconazole or ritonavir, the dose should not exceed 2.5 mg).

Grapefruit Juice (CYP3A4 inhibitors such as grapefruit juice may likely increase tadalafil exposure).

CIMZIA

(Certolizumab pegol) 3127

May interact with immunosuppressive agents, vaccines, live, and certain other agents. Compounds in these categories include:

Anakinra (Concurrent administration of anakinra (an interleukin-1 antagonist) and another TNF-blocker has shown an increased risk of serious infections, an increased risk of neutropenia and no added benefit compared to these medicinal products alone. Therefore, the combination of anakinra with other TNF-blockers, including certolizumab pegol, may also result in similar toxicities). Products include:

Kineret Injection 585

Azathioprine (Serious infections, sepsis and cases of opportunistic infections, including fatalities, have been reported in patients receiving TNF-blockers, including certolizumab pegol. Many of the serious infections reported have occurred in patients on concomitantimmunosuppressive therapy that, in addition to their Crohn's disease, could predispose them to infections. Infections have been reported in patients receiving certolizumab pegol alone or in conjunction with immunosuppressive agents. Exercise caution when considering the use of certolizumab pegol in patients with concomitant immunosuppressive therapy).

No products indexed under this heading.

Basiliximab (Serious infections, sepsis and cases of opportunistic infections, including fatalities, have been reported in patients receiving TNF-blockers, including certolizumab pegol. Many of the serious infections reported have occurred in patients on concomitantimmunosuppressive therapy that, in addition to their Crohn's disease, could predispose them to infections. Infections have been reported in patients receiving certolizumab pegol alone or in conjunction with immunosuppressive agents. Exercise caution when considering the use of certolizumab pegol in patients with concomitant immunosuppressive therapy). Products include:

Simulect for Injection 2306

BCG Vaccine (No data is available on the response to vaccinations or the secondary transmission of infection by live vaccines in patients receiving certolizumab pegol. Do not administer live vaccines or attenuated vaccines concurrently with certolizumab pegol).

No products indexed under this heading.

Cyclosporine (Serious infections, sepsis and cases of opportunistic infections, including fatalities, have been reported in patients receiving TNF-blockers, including certolizumab pegol. Many of the serious infections reported have occurred in patients on concomitantimmunosuppressive therapy that, in addition to their Crohn's disease, could predispose them to infections. Infections have been reported in patients receiving certolizumab pegol alone or in conjunction with immunosuppressive agents. Exercise caution when considering the use of certolizumab pegol in patients with concomitant immunosuppressive therapy). Products include:

Gengraf Capsules 435
Neoral Oral Solution 2280
Neoral Soft Gelatin Capsules 2280
Restasis Ophthalmic Emulsion 557
Sandimmune 2296

Influenza Vaccine, Live Attenuated (No data is available on the response to vaccinations or the secondary transmission of infection by live vaccines in patients receiving certolizumab pegol. Do not administer live vaccines or attenuated vaccines concurrently with certolizumab pegol).

No products indexed under this heading.

Influenza Virus Vaccine Live, Intranasal (No data is available on the response to vaccinations or the secondary transmission of infection by live vaccines in patients receiving certolizumab pegol. Do not administer live vaccines or attenuated vaccines concurrently with certolizumab pegol). Products include:

FluMist Vaccine 1945

Measles, Mumps, Rubella and Varicella Virus Vaccine Live (No data is available on the response to vaccinations or the secondary transmission of infection by live vaccines in patients receiving certolizumab pegol. Do not administer live vaccines or attenuated vaccines concurrently with certolizumab pegol). Products include:

ProQuad 2099

Measles, Mumps & Rubella Virus Vaccine, Live (No data is available on the response to vaccinations or the secondary transmission of infection by live vaccines in patients receiving certolizumab pegol. Do not administer live vaccines or attenuated vaccines concurrently with certolizumab pegol). Products include:

M-M-R II 2054

Measles & Rubella Virus Vaccine Live (No data is available on the response to vaccinations or the secondary transmission of infection by live vaccines in patients receiving certolizumab pegol. Do not administer live vaccines or attenuated vaccines concurrently with certolizumab pegol).

No products indexed under this heading.

Measles Virus Vaccine Live (No data is available on the response to vaccinations or the secondary transmission of infection by live vaccines in patients receiving certolizumab pegol. Do not administer live vaccines or attenuated vaccines concurrently with certolizumab pegol). Products include:

Attenuvax 1951

Mumps Virus Vaccine, Live (No data is available on the response to vaccinations or the secondary transmission of infection by live vaccines in patients receiving certolizumab pegol. Do not administer live vaccines or attenuated vaccines concurrently with certolizumab pegol). Products include:

Mumpsvax 2068

Muromonab-CD3 (Serious infections, sepsis and cases of opportunistic infections, including fatalities, have been reported in patients receiving TNF-blockers, including certolizumab pegol. Many of the serious infections reported have occurred in patients on concomitantimmunosuppressive therapy that, in addition to their Crohn's disease, could predispose them to infections. Infections have been reported in patients receiving certolizumab pegol alone or in conjunction with immunosuppressive agents. Exercise caution when considering the use of certolizumab pegol in patients with concomitant immunosuppressive therapy). Products include:

Orthoclone OKT3 Sterile Solution 2387

Mycophenolate Mofetil (Serious infections, sepsis and cases of opportunistic infections, including fatalities, have been reported in patients receiving TNF-blockers, including certolizumab pegol. Many of the serious infections reported have occurred in patients on concomitantimmunosuppressive therapy that, in addition to their Crohn's disease, could predispose them to infections. Infections have been reported in patients receiving certolizumab pegol alone or in conjunction with immunosuppressive agents. Exercise caution when considering the use of certolizumab pegol in patients with concomitant immunosuppressive therapy). Products include:

CellCept Capsules 2622
CellCept Oral Suspension 2622
CellCept Tablets 2622

Poliovirus Vaccine, Live, Oral, Trivalent, Types 1,2,3 (Sabin) (No data is available on the response to vaccinations or the secondary transmission of infection by live vaccines in patients receiving certolizumab pegol. Do not administer live vaccines or attenuated vaccines concurrently with certolizumab pegol).

No products indexed under this heading.

Rotavirus Vaccine, Live, Oral, Tetravalent (No data is available on the response to vaccinations or the secondary transmission of infection by live vaccines in patients receiving certolizumab pegol. Do not administer live vaccines or attenuated vaccines concurrently with certolizumab pegol).

No products indexed under this heading.

Rubella & Mumps Virus Vaccine Live (No data is available on the response to vaccinations or the secondary transmission of infection by live vaccines in patients receiving certolizumab pegol. Do not administer live vaccines or attenuated vaccines concurrently with certolizumab pegol).

No products indexed under this heading.

Rubella Virus Vaccine Live (No data is available on the response to vaccinations or the secondary transmission of infection by live vaccines in patients receiving certolizumab pegol. Do not administer live vaccines or attenuated vaccines concurrently with certolizumab pegol). Products include:

Meruvax II 2061

Sirolimus (Serious infections, sepsis and cases of opportunistic infections, including fatalities, have been reported in patients receiving TNF-blockers, including certolizumab pegol. Many of the serious infections reported have occurred in patients on concomitantimmunosuppressive therapy that, in addition to their Crohn's disease, could predispose them to infections. Infections have been reported in patients receiving certolizumab pegol alone or in conjunction with immunosuppressive agents. Exercise caution when considering the use of certolizumab pegol in patients with concomitant immunosuppressive therapy). Products include:

- Rapamune ... 3260

Smallpox Vaccine (No data is available on the response to vaccinations or the secondary transmission of infection by live vaccines in patients receiving certolizumab pegol. Do not administer live vaccines or attenuated vaccines concurrently with certolizumab pegol).

No products indexed under this heading.

Tacrolimus (Serious infections, sepsis and cases of opportunistic infections, including fatalities, have been reported in patients receiving TNF-blockers, including certolizumab pegol. Many of the serious infections reported have occurred in patients on concomitantimmunosuppressive therapy that, in addition to their Crohn's disease, could predispose them to infections. Infections have been reported in patients receiving certolizumab pegol alone or in conjunction with immunosuppressive agents. Exercise caution when considering the use of certolizumab pegol in patients with concomitant immunosuppressive therapy). Products include:

- Prograf Capsules and Injection ... 622
- Protopic Ointment ... 628

Typhoid Vaccine (No data is available on the response to vaccinations or the secondary transmission of infection by live vaccines in patients receiving certolizumab pegol. Do not administer live vaccines or attenuated vaccines concurrently with certolizumab pegol).

No products indexed under this heading.

Varicella Virus Vaccine Live (No data is available on the response to vaccinations or the secondary transmission of infection by live vaccines in patients receiving certolizumab pegol. Do not administer live vaccines or attenuated vaccines concurrently with certolizumab pegol). Products include:

- Varivax ... 2133

Yellow Fever Vaccine (No data is available on the response to vaccinations or the secondary transmission of infection by live vaccines in patients receiving certolizumab pegol. Do not administer live vaccines or attenuated vaccines concurrently with certolizumab pegol).

No products indexed under this heading.

Zoster Vaccine Live (No data is available on the response to vaccinations or the secondary transmission of infection by live vaccines in patients receiving certolizumab pegol. Do not administer live vaccines or attenuated vaccines concurrently with certolizumab pegol). Products include:

- Zostavax Injection ... 2145

CIPRO I.V.

(Ciprofloxacin) ... 2817

May interact with antacids containing aluminum, calcium and magnesium, class 1A antiarrhythmics, class III antiarrhythmics, calcium preparations, corticosteroids, oral anticoagulants, cytochrome p450 1a2 substrates (selected), iron containing oral preparations, non-steroidal anti-inflammatory agents, phenytoin, xanthines, and certain other agents. Compounds in these categories include:

Acetaminophen (Ciprofloxacin is a moderate inhibitor of CYP450 1A2 isoenzymes. Co-administration of ciprofloxacin and other drugs primarily metabolized by the CYP450 1A2 enzyme pathway may result in increased plasma concentrations of the co-administered drug and couldlead to clinically significant pharmacodynamic side effects). Products include:

- Benadryl Allergy & Cold Kapgels ... 1895
- Benadryl Allergy & Sinus Headache Kapgels ... 1895
- Benadryl Severe Allergy & Sinus Headache Caplets ... 1897
- Lortab 5/500 Tablets ... 3143
- Lortab 7.5/500 Tablets ... 3144
- Lortab 10/500 Tablets ... 3144
- Percocet Tablets ... 1127
- Sinutab Sinus Caplets ... 1905
- Sudafed PE Cold & Cough Caplets ... 1907
- Sudafed PE Nighttime Cold Caplets ... 1907
- Sudafed PE Severe Cold Caplets ... 1908
- Sudafed PE Sinus Headache Caplets ... 1908
- Regular Strength Tylenol Tablets ... 1915
- Tylenol 8 Hour Extended Release Caplets ... 1915
- Extra Strength Tylenol Caplets, Cool Caplets, and EZ Tabs ... 1915
- Extra Strength Tylenol Adult Rapid Blast Liquid ... 1915
- Extra Strength Tylenol PM Caplets, Geltabs, Liquid, and Rapid Release Gels ... 1915
- Extra Strength Tylenol Rapid Release Gels ... 1915
- Tylenol with Codeine Tablets ... 2427
- Tylenol Allergy Multi-Symptom Caplets with Cool Burst and Rapid Release Gelcaps ... 1916
- Tylenol Allergy Multi-Symptom Nighttime Caplets with Cool Burst ... 1916
- Tylenol Severe Allergy Caplets ... 1916
- Tylenol Arthritis Pain Extended Release Geltabs/Caplets ... 1915
- Tylenol Chest Congestion Caplets with Cool Burst ... 1910
- Tylenol Chest Congestion Liquid with Cool Burst ... 1910
- Children's Tylenol Plus Cold Suspension Liquid ... 1912
- Children's Tylenol Plus Cold & Allergy Suspension Liquid ... 1914
- Children's Tylenol Plus Cough & Runny Nose Suspension Liquid ... 1912
- Children's Tylenol Plus Cough & Sore Throat Suspension Liquid ... 1912
- Children's Tylenol Plus Flu Suspension Liquid ... 1914
- Children's Tylenol Suspension Liquid ... 1909
- Children's Tylenol Meltaways ... 1909
- Children's Tylenol Plus Multi-Symptom Cold Suspension Liquid ... 1912
- Tylenol Cold Severe Congestion Daytime Caplets with Cool Burst ... 1912
- Tylenol Cold Head Congestion Daytime Caplets with Cool Burst ... 1910
- Tylenol Cold Head Congestion Nighttime Caplets with Cool Burst ... 1910
- Tylenol Cold Head Congestion Severe Daytime Caplets with Cool Burst ... 1910
- Tylenol Cold Multi-Symptom Daytime Caplets with Cool Burst and Rapid Release Gels ... 1913
- Tylenol Cold Multi-Symptom Daytime Liquid with Citrus Burst ... 1913
- Tylenol Cold Multi-Symptom Nighttime Caplets with Cool Burst ... 1913
- Tylenol Cold Multi-Symptom Nighttime Liquid with Cool Burst ... 1913
- Tylenol Cold Multi-Symptom Severe Caplets with Cool Burst ... 1913
- Tylenol Cold Multi-Symptom Severe Daytime Liquid with Citrus Burst ... 1913
- Tylenol Cough & Sore Throat Daytime Liquid with Cool Burst ... 1918
- Tylenol Cough & Sore Throat Nighttime Liquid with Cool Burst ... 1918
- Concentrated Tylenol Infants' Drops ... 1909
- Jr. Tylenol Meltaways ... 1909
- Tylenol Sinus Congestion & Pain Daytime Caplets with Cool Burst and Gelcaps ... 1917
- Tylenol Sinus Congestion & Pain Nighttime Caplets with Cool Burst ... 1917
- Tylenol Sinus Congestion & Pain Severe Caplets with Cool Burst ... 1917
- Tylenol Sinus Severe Congestion Caplets with Cool Burst ... 1917
- Tylenol Sore Throat Daytime Liquid with Cool Burst ... 1918
- Tylenol Sore Throat Nighttime Liquid with Cool Burst ... 1918
- Women's Tylenol Menstrual Relief Caplets ... 1919
- Vicks DayQuil Cold & Flu Multi-Symptom Relief ... 616
- Vicks DayQuil LiquiCaps ... 2567
- Vicks DayQuil Liquid ... 2567
- Vicks DayQuil Multi-Symptom Cold/Flu Relief ... 2567
- Vicks NyQuil Cold & Flu Multi-Symptom Relief ... 617
- Vicks NyQuil LiquiCaps ... 2567
- Vicks NyQuil Liquid ... 2567
- Vicks NyQuil Multi-Symptom Cold/Flu Relief ... 2567
- Vicodin Tablets ... 529
- Vicodin ES Tablets ... 530
- Vicodin HP Tablets ... 531
- Zydone Tablets ... 1132

Alatrofloxacin Mesylate (Ciprofloxacin is a moderate inhibitor of CYP450 1A2 isoenzymes. Co-administration of ciprofloxacin and other drugs primarily metabolized by the CYP450 1A2 enzyme pathway may result in increased plasma concentrations of the co-administered drug and couldlead to clinically significant pharmacodynamic side effects).

No products indexed under this heading.

Aluminum Carbonate (Concurrent administration of these antacids may substantially interfere with the oral absorption of ciprofloxacin; antacids may be administered either two hours after or six hours before ciprofloxacin dosing without a significant decrease in bioavailability).

No products indexed under this heading.

Aluminum Hydroxide (Concurrent administration of these antacids may substantially interfere with the oral absorption of ciprofloxacin; antacids may be administered either two hours after or six hours before ciprofloxacin dosing without a significant decrease in bioavailability).

No products indexed under this heading.

Aminophylline (Potential for severe and fatal reactions including cardiac arrest, seizures, respiratory failure and status epilepticus; concurrent use should be avoided or serum levels of theophylline should be monitored carefully).

No products indexed under this heading.

Amiodarone Hydrochloride (In general, elderly patients may be more susceptible to drug-associated effects on the QT interval. Therefore, precaution should be taken when using ciprofloxacin with concomitant drugs that can result in prolongation of the QT interval (eg, class IA or class III antiarrhythmics)).

No products indexed under this heading.

Amitriptyline Hydrochloride (Ciprofloxacin is a moderate inhibitor of CYP450 1A2 isoenzymes. Co-administration of ciprofloxacin and other drugs primarily metabolized by the CYP450 1A2 enzyme pathway may result in increased plasma concentrations of the co-administered drug and couldlead to clinically significant pharmacodynamic side effects).

No products indexed under this heading.

Amoxapine (Ciprofloxacin is a moderate inhibitor of CYP450 1A2 isoenzymes. Co-administration of ciprofloxacin and other drugs primarily metabolized by the CYP450 1A2 enzyme pathway may result in increased plasma concentrations of the co-administered drug and couldlead to clinically significant pharmacodynamic side effects).

No products indexed under this heading.

Anagrelide Hydrochloride (Ciprofloxacin is a moderate inhibitor of CYP450 1A2 isoenzymes. Co-administration of ciprofloxacin and other drugs primarily metabolized by the CYP450 1A2 enzyme pathway may result in increased plasma concentrations of the co-administered drug and couldlead to clinically significant pharmacodynamic side effects). Products include:

- Agrylin Capsules ... 3017

Anisindione (Enhanced effects of anticoagulant).

No products indexed under this heading.

Betamethasone Acetate (Risk of ruptures of the shoulder, hand, Achilles tendon or other tendons may be increased in patients receiving concomitant corticosteroids, especially in the elderly).

No products indexed under this heading.

Betamethasone Sodium Phosphate (Risk of ruptures of the shoulder, hand, Achilles tendon or other tendons may be increased in patients receiving concomitant corticosteroids, especially in the elderly).

No products indexed under this heading.

Bretylium Tosylate (In general, elderly patients may be more susceptible to drug-associated effects on the QT interval. Therefore, precaution should be taken when using ciprofloxacin with concomitant drugs that can result in prolongation of the QT interval (eg, class IA or class III antiarrhythmics)).

No products indexed under this heading.

Budesonide (Risk of ruptures of the shoulder, hand, Achilles tendon or other tendons may be increased in patients receiving concomitant corticosteroids, especially in the elderly). Products include:

- Pulmicort Flexhaler ... 654
- Symbicort 80/4.5 Inhalation Aerosol ... 659
- Symbicort 160/4.5 Inhalation Aerosol ... 659

Caffeine (Reduced clearance of caffeine and a prolongation of its serum half-life). Products include:

- BioLean Free Tablets ... 635
- BioLean II Tablets ... 635
- Winrgy Dietary Supplement ... 642

Caffeine Anhydrous (Ciprofloxacin is a moderate inhibitor of CYP450 1A2 isoenzymes. Co-administration of ciprofloxacin and other drugs primarily metabolized by the CYP450 1A2 enzyme pathway may result in increased plasma concentrations of the co-administered drug and couldlead to clinically significant pharmacodynamic side effects).
No products indexed under this heading.

Caffeine Citrate (Reduced clearance of caffeine and a prolongation of its serum half-life).
No products indexed under this heading.

Calcium Carbonate (Co-administration with calcium-containing products may substantially interfere with the oral absorption of quinolones; these preparations may be taken six hours before or two hours after taking ciprofloxacin). Products include:
Accelerator Tablets ▣ 634
Actonel with Calcium Tablets 2574
BioLean II Tablets ▣ 635
Calcet Triple Calcium + Vitamin D Tablets ▣ 629
D-Cal Chewable Caplets ▣ 624
Elixir Capsules ▣ 636
Pepcid Complete Chewable Tablets 1771
Extra Strength Rolaids Plus Gas Relief Tropical Fruit Softchews 1903
Extra Strength Rolaids Softchews Vanilla Creme 1903
Extra Strength Rolaids Freshmint Tablets 1903
Rolaids Multi-Symptom Berry Tablets 1903
Rolaids Original Peppermint Tablets 1903

Calcium Chloride (Co-administration with calcium-containing products may substantially interfere with the oral absorption of quinolones; these preparations may be taken six hours before or two hours after taking ciprofloxacin).
No products indexed under this heading.

Calcium Citrate (Co-administration with calcium-containing products may substantially interfere with the oral absorption of quinolones; these preparations may be taken six hours before or two hours after taking ciprofloxacin). Products include:
Active Calcium Tablets 3173
CitraNatal DHA Tablets 2175
CitraNatal 90 DHA Tablets 2175

Calcium Glubionate (Co-administration with calcium-containing products may substantially interfere with the oral absorption of quinolones; these preparations may be taken six hours before or two hours after taking ciprofloxacin).
No products indexed under this heading.

Celecoxib (NSAIDs in combination with very high doses of quinolones have been shown to provoke convulsions in pre-clinical trials). Products include:
Celebrex Capsules 2979

Chlordiazepoxide (Ciprofloxacin is a moderate inhibitor of CYP450 1A2 isoenzymes. Co-administration of ciprofloxacin and other drugs primarily metabolized by the CYP450 1A2 enzyme pathway may result in increased plasma concentrations of the co-administered drug and couldlead to clinically significant pharmacodynamic side effects).
No products indexed under this heading.

Chlordiazepoxide Hydrochloride (Ciprofloxacin is a moderate inhibitor of CYP450 1A2 isoenzymes. Co-administration of ciprofloxacin and other drugs primarily metabolized by the CYP450 1A2 enzyme pathway may result in increased plasma concentrations of the co-administered drug and couldlead to clinically significant pharmacodynamic side effects).
No products indexed under this heading.

Ciclesonide (Risk of ruptures of the shoulder, hand, Achilles tendon or other tendons may be increased in patients receiving concomitant corticosteroids, especially in the elderly). Products include:
Alvesco Inhalation Aerosol 2985
Omnaris Nasal Spray 2998

Cimetidine Hydrochloride (Ciprofloxacin is a moderate inhibitor of CYP450 1A2 isoenzymes. Co-administration of ciprofloxacin and other drugs primarily metabolized by the CYP450 1A2 enzyme pathway may result in increased plasma concentrations of the co-administered drug and couldlead to clinically significant pharmacodynamic side effects).
No products indexed under this heading.

Ciprofloxacin Hydrochloride (Ciprofloxacin is a moderate inhibitor of CYP450 1A2 isoenzymes. Co-administration of ciprofloxacin and other drugs primarily metabolized by the CYP450 1A2 enzyme pathway may result in increased plasma concentrations of the co-administered drug and couldlead to clinically significant pharmacodynamic side effects). Products include:
Cipro Tablets 2810

Clomipramine Hydrochloride (Ciprofloxacin is a moderate inhibitor of CYP450 1A2 isoenzymes. Co-administration of ciprofloxacin and other drugs primarily metabolized by the CYP450 1A2 enzyme pathway may result in increased plasma concentrations of the co-administered drug and couldlead to clinically significant pharmacodynamic side effects).
No products indexed under this heading.

Clopidogrel Bisulfate (Ciprofloxacin is a moderate inhibitor of CYP450 1A2 isoenzymes. Co-administration of ciprofloxacin and other drugs primarily metabolized by the CYP450 1A2 enzyme pathway may result in increased plasma concentrations of the co-administered drug and couldlead to clinically significant pharmacodynamic side effects). Products include:
Plavix Tablets 926
Plavix Tablets 2767

Clozapine (Ciprofloxacin is a moderate inhibitor of CYP450 1A2 isoenzymes. Co-administration of ciprofloxacin and other drugs primarily metabolized by the CYP450 1A2 enzyme pathway may result in increased plasma concentrations of the co-administered drug and couldlead to clinically significant pharmacodynamic side effects).
No products indexed under this heading.

Cortisone Acetate (Risk of ruptures of the shoulder, hand, Achilles tendon or other tendons may be increased in patients receiving concomitant corticosteroids, especially in the elderly).
No products indexed under this heading.

Cyclobenzaprine (Ciprofloxacin is a moderate inhibitor of CYP450 1A2 isoenzymes. Co-administration of ciprofloxacin and other drugs primarily metabolized by the CYP450 1A2 enzyme pathway may result in increased plasma concentrations of the co-administered drug and couldlead to clinically significant pharmacodynamic side effects).
No products indexed under this heading.

Cyclobenzaprine Hydrochloride (Ciprofloxacin is a moderate inhibitor of CYP450 1A2 isoenzymes. Co-administration of ciprofloxacin and other drugs primarily metabolized by the CYP450 1A2 enzyme pathway may result in increased plasma concentrations of the co-administered drug and couldlead to clinically significant pharmacodynamic side effects). Products include:
Amrix Capsules 966

Cyclosporine (Transient elevations in serum creatinine). Products include:
Gengraf Capsules 435
Neoral Oral Solution 2280
Neoral Soft Gelatin Capsules 2280
Restasis Ophthalmic Emulsion 557
Sandimmune 2296

Desipramine Hydrochloride (Ciprofloxacin is a moderate inhibitor of CYP450 1A2 isoenzymes. Co-administration of ciprofloxacin and other drugs primarily metabolized by the CYP450 1A2 enzyme pathway may result in increased plasma concentrations of the co-administered drug and couldlead to clinically significant pharmacodynamic side effects).
No products indexed under this heading.

Dexamethasone (Risk of ruptures of the shoulder, hand, Achilles tendon or other tendons may be increased in patients receiving concomitant corticosteroids, especially in the elderly). Products include:
Ciprodex Otic Suspension 541

Dexamethasone Acetate (Risk of ruptures of the shoulder, hand, Achilles tendon or other tendons may be increased in patients receiving concomitant corticosteroids, especially in the elderly).
No products indexed under this heading.

Dexamethasone Sodium Phosphate (Risk of ruptures of the shoulder, hand, Achilles tendon or other tendons may be increased in patients receiving concomitant corticosteroids, especially in the elderly).
No products indexed under this heading.

Diazepam (Ciprofloxacin is a moderate inhibitor of CYP450 1A2 isoenzymes. Co-administration of ciprofloxacin and other drugs primarily metabolized by the CYP450 1A2 enzyme pathway may result in increased plasma concentrations of the co-administered drug and couldlead to clinically significant pharmacodynamic side effects). Products include:
Valium Tablets 2658

Diclofenac Epolamine (NSAIDs in combination with very high doses of quinolones have been shown to provoke convulsions in pre-clinical trials). Products include:
Flector Patch 561

Diclofenac Potassium (NSAIDs in combination with very high doses of quinolones have been shown to provoke convulsions in pre-clinical trials).
No products indexed under this heading.

Diclofenac Sodium (NSAIDs in combination with very high doses of quinolones have been shown to provoke convulsions in pre-clinical trials). Products include:
Diclofenac Sodium Ophthalmic Solution ⊙ 240
Voltaren Ophthalmic Solution 2336
Voltaren Tablets 2334
Voltaren-XR Tablets 2337

Dicumarol (Enhanced effects of anticoagulant).
No products indexed under this heading.

Didanosine (Didanosine (Videx) chewable tablets or pediatric powder for oral solution contains aluminum-magnesium-based antacid; co-administration may interfere with Cipro oral absorption; these preparations may be taken six hours before or two hours after taking ciprofloxacin).
No products indexed under this heading.

Diltiazem Hydrochloride (Ciprofloxacin is a moderate inhibitor of CYP450 1A2 isoenzymes. Co-administration of ciprofloxacin and other drugs primarily metabolized by the CYP450 1A2 enzyme pathway may result in increased plasma concentrations of the co-administered drug and couldlead to clinically significant pharmacodynamic side effects). Products include:
Cardizem LA Extended Release Tablets 421

Diltiazem Maleate (Ciprofloxacin is a moderate inhibitor of CYP450 1A2 isoenzymes. Co-administration of ciprofloxacin and other drugs primarily metabolized by the CYP450 1A2 enzyme pathway may result in increased plasma concentrations of the co-administered drug and couldlead to clinically significant pharmacodynamic side effects).
No products indexed under this heading.

Disopyramide (In general, elderly patients may be more susceptible to drug-associated effects on the QT interval. Therefore, precaution should be taken when using ciprofloxacin with concomitant drugs that can result in prolongation of the QT interval (eg, class IA or class III antiarrhythmics)).
No products indexed under this heading.

Doxepin Hydrochloride (Ciprofloxacin is a moderate inhibitor of CYP450 1A2 isoenzymes. Co-administration of ciprofloxacin and other drugs primarily metabolized by the CYP450 1A2 enzyme pathway may result in increased plasma concentrations of the co-administered drug and couldlead to clinically significant pharmacodynamic side effects).
No products indexed under this heading.

Dyphylline (Potential for severe and fatal reactions including cardiac arrest, seizures, respiratory failure and status epilepticus; concurrent use should be avoided or serum levels of theophylline should be monitored carefully).
No products indexed under this heading.

Enoxacin (Ciprofloxacin is a moderate inhibitor of CYP450 1A2 isoenzymes. Co-administration of ciprofloxacin and other drugs primarily metabolized by the CYP450 1A2 enzyme pathway may result in increased plasma concentrations of the co-administered drug and couldlead to clinically significant pharmacodynamic side effects).
No products indexed under this heading.

Erythromycin (Ciprofloxacin is a moderate inhibitor of CYP450 1A2 isoenzymes. Co-administration of ciprofloxacin and other drugs primarily metabolized by the CYP450 1A2 enzyme pathway may result in increased plasma concentrations of the co-administered drug and couldlead to clinically significant pharmacodynamic side effects).
No products indexed under this heading.

Erythromycin Estolate (Ciprofloxacin is a moderate inhibitor of CYP450 1A2 isoenzymes. Co-administration of ciprofloxacin and other drugs primarily metabolized by the CYP450 1A2 enzyme pathway may result in increased plasma concentrations of the co-administered drug and couldlead to clinically significant pharmacodynamic side effects).
No products indexed under this heading.

Erythromycin Ethylsuccinate (Ciprofloxacin is a moderate inhibitor of CYP450 1A2 isoenzymes. Co-administration of ciprofloxacin and other drugs primarily metabolized by the CYP450 1A2 enzyme pathway may result in increased plasma concentrations of the co-administered drug and couldlead to clinically significant pharmacodynamic side effects). Products include:
E.E.S. ... **433**
EryPed ... **431**

Erythromycin Gluceptate (Ciprofloxacin is a moderate inhibitor of CYP450 1A2 isoenzymes. Co-administration of ciprofloxacin and other drugs primarily metabolized by the CYP450 1A2 enzyme pathway may result in increased plasma concentrations of the co-administered drug and couldlead to clinically significant pharmacodynamic side effects).
No products indexed under this heading.

Erythromycin Lactobionate (Ciprofloxacin is a moderate inhibitor of CYP450 1A2 isoenzymes. Co-administration of ciprofloxacin and other drugs primarily metabolized by the CYP450 1A2 enzyme pathway may result in increased plasma concentrations of the co-administered drug and couldlead to clinically significant pharmacodynamic side effects).
No products indexed under this heading.

Erythromycin Stearate (Ciprofloxacin is a moderate inhibitor of CYP450 1A2 isoenzymes. Co-administration of ciprofloxacin and other drugs primarily metabolized by the CYP450 1A2 enzyme pathway may result in increased plasma concentrations of the co-administered drug and couldlead to clinically significant pharmacodynamic side effects).
No products indexed under this heading.

Estradiol (Ciprofloxacin is a moderate inhibitor of CYP450 1A2 isoenzymes. Co-administration of ciprofloxacin and other drugs primarily metabolized by the CYP450 1A2 enzyme pathway may result in increased plasma concentrations of the co-administered drug and couldlead to clinically significant pharmacodynamic side effects). Products include:
Activella Tablets ... **2347**
Angeliq Tablets ... **751**
Climara Transdermal System ... **763**
Climara Pro Transdermal System ... **768**
Divigel ... **3167**
Vagifem Tablets ... **2375**

Estradiol Benzoate (Ciprofloxacin is a moderate inhibitor of CYP450 1A2 isoenzymes. Co-administration of ciprofloxacin and other drugs primarily metabolized by the CYP450 1A2 enzyme pathway may result in increased plasma concentrations of the co-administered drug and couldlead to clinically significant pharmacodynamic side effects).
No products indexed under this heading.

Estradiol Cypionate (Ciprofloxacin is a moderate inhibitor of CYP450 1A2 isoenzymes. Co-administration of ciprofloxacin and other drugs primarily metabolized by the CYP450 1A2 enzyme pathway may result in increased plasma concentrations of the co-administered drug and couldlead to clinically significant pharmacodynamic side effects).
No products indexed under this heading.

Etodolac (NSAIDs in combination with very high doses of quinolones have been shown to provoke convulsions in pre-clinical trials).
No products indexed under this heading.

Fenoprofen Calcium (NSAIDs in combination with very high doses of quinolones have been shown to provoke convulsions in pre-clinical trials). Products include:
Nalfon Capsules ... **2508**

Ferrous Fumarate (Co-administration with iron-containing products may substantially interfere with the oral absorption of quinolones; these preparations may be taken six hours before or two hours after taking ciprofloxacin).
No products indexed under this heading.

Ferrous Gluconate (Co-administration with iron-containing products may substantially interfere with the oral absorption of quinolones; these preparations may be taken six hours before or two hours after taking ciprofloxacin). Products include:
CitraNatal DHA Tablets ... **2175**

Ferrous Sulfate (Co-administration with iron-containing products may substantially interfere with the oral absorption of quinolones; these preparations may be taken six hours before or two hours after taking ciprofloxacin).
No products indexed under this heading.

Fludrocortisone Acetate (Risk of ruptures of the shoulder, hand, Achilles tendon or other tendons may be increased in patients receiving concomitant corticosteroids, especially in the elderly).
No products indexed under this heading.

Flunisolide (Risk of ruptures of the shoulder, hand, Achilles tendon or other tendons may be increased in patients receiving concomitant corticosteroids, especially in the elderly). Products include:
Aerobid/Aerobid-M ... **1153**

Flurbiprofen (NSAIDs in combination with very high doses of quinolones have been shown to provoke convulsions in pre-clinical trials).
No products indexed under this heading.

Flutamide (Ciprofloxacin is a moderate inhibitor of CYP450 1A2 isoenzymes. Co-administration of ciprofloxacin and other drugs primarily metabolized by the CYP450 1A2 enzyme pathway may result in increased plasma concentrations of the co-administered drug and couldlead to clinically significant pharmacodynamic side effects).
No products indexed under this heading.

Fluticasone Propionate (Risk of ruptures of the shoulder, hand, Achilles tendon or other tendons may be increased in patients receiving concomitant corticosteroids, especially in the elderly). Products include:
Advair Diskus 100/50 ... **1276**
Advair Diskus 250/50 ... **1276**
Advair Diskus 500/50 ... **1276**
Advair HFA 45/21 Inhalation Aerosol ... **1288**
Advair HFA 115/21 Inhalation Aerosol ... **1288**
Advair HFA 230/21 Inhalation Aerosol ... **1288**
Flonase Nasal Spray ... **1431**
Flovent Diskus 50 mcg ... **1435**

Fluticasone Propionate HFA (Risk of ruptures of the shoulder, hand, Achilles tendon or other tendons may be increased in patients receiving concomitant corticosteroids, especially in the elderly). Products include:
Flovent HFA ... **1440**

Fluvoxamine Maleate (Ciprofloxacin is a moderate inhibitor of CYP450 1A2 isoenzymes. Co-administration of ciprofloxacin and other drugs primarily metabolized by the CYP450 1A2 enzyme pathway may result in increased plasma concentrations of the co-administered drug and couldlead to clinically significant pharmacodynamic side effects). Products include:
Luvox CR Extended-Release Capsules ... **1759**

Fosphenytoin Sodium (Potential for change in serum phenytoin levels).
No products indexed under this heading.

Glyburide (Co-administration, on rare occasions, has resulted in severe hypoglycemia).
No products indexed under this heading.

Grepafloxacin Hydrochloride (Ciprofloxacin is a moderate inhibitor of CYP450 1A2 isoenzymes. Co-administration of ciprofloxacin and other drugs primarily metabolized by the CYP450 1A2 enzyme pathway may result in increased plasma concentrations of the co-administered drug and couldlead to clinically significant pharmacodynamic side effects).
No products indexed under this heading.

Haloperidol (Ciprofloxacin is a moderate inhibitor of CYP450 1A2 isoenzymes. Co-administration of ciprofloxacin and other drugs primarily metabolized by the CYP450 1A2 enzyme pathway may result in increased plasma concentrations of the co-administered drug and couldlead to clinically significant pharmacodynamic side effects).
No products indexed under this heading.

Haloperidol Decanoate (Ciprofloxacin is a moderate inhibitor of CYP450 1A2 isoenzymes. Co-administration of ciprofloxacin and other drugs primarily metabolized by the CYP450 1A2 enzyme pathway may result in increased plasma concentrations of the co-administered drug and couldlead to clinically significant pharmacodynamic side effects).
No products indexed under this heading.

Haloperidol Lactate (Ciprofloxacin is a moderate inhibitor of CYP450 1A2 isoenzymes. Co-administration of ciprofloxacin and other drugs primarily metabolized by the CYP450 1A2 enzyme pathway may result in increased plasma concentrations of the co-administered drug and couldlead to clinically significant pharmacodynamic side effects).
No products indexed under this heading.

Hydrocortisone (Risk of ruptures of the shoulder, hand, Achilles tendon or other tendons may be increased in patients receiving concomitant corticosteroids, especially in the elderly).
No products indexed under this heading.

Hydrocortisone Acetate (Risk of ruptures of the shoulder, hand, Achilles tendon or other tendons may be increased in patients receiving concomitant corticosteroids, especially in the elderly). Products include:
Analpram-HC ... **1140**
Pramosone ... **1141**

Hydrocortisone Sodium Phosphate (Risk of ruptures of the shoulder, hand, Achilles tendon or other tendons may be increased in patients receiving concomitant corticosteroids, especially in the elderly).
No products indexed under this heading.

Hydrocortisone Sodium Succinate (Risk of ruptures of the shoulder, hand, Achilles tendon or other tendons may be increased in patients receiving concomitant corticosteroids, especially in the elderly).
No products indexed under this heading.

Ibuprofen (NSAIDs in combination with very high doses of quinolones have been shown to provoke convulsions in pre-clinical trials). Products include:
Motrin IB Tablets and Caplets 1900
Children's Motrin Oral Suspension ... 1901
Children's Motrin Non-Staining Dye-Free Oral Suspension............ 1901
Children's Motrin Cold Oral Suspension................................... 1899
Infants' Motrin Concentrated Drops... 1901
Infants' Motrin Non-Staining Dye-Free Concentrated Drops....... 1901
Junior Strength Motrin Caplets and Chewable Tablets.................. 1901
Vicoprofen Tablets 533

Imipramine Hydrochloride (Ciprofloxacin is a moderate inhibitor of CYP450 1A2 isoenzymes. Co-administration of ciprofloxacin and other drugs primarily metabolized by the CYP450 1A2 enzyme pathway may result in increased plasma concentrations of the co-administered drug and couldlead to clinically significant pharmacodynamic side effects).
No products indexed under this heading.

Imipramine Pamoate (Ciprofloxacin is a moderate inhibitor of CYP450 1A2 isoenzymes. Co-administration of ciprofloxacin and other drugs primarily metabolized by the CYP450 1A2 enzyme pathway may result in increased plasma concentrations of the co-administered drug and couldlead to clinically significant pharmacodynamic side effects).
No products indexed under this heading.

Indomethacin (NSAIDs in combination with very high doses of quinolones have been shown to provoke convulsions in pre-clinical trials). Products include:
Indocin 2024

Indomethacin Sodium Trihydrate (NSAIDs in combination with very high doses of quinolones have been shown to provoke convulsions in pre-clinical trials). Products include:
Indocin I.V. 2489

Iron (Co-administration with iron-containing products may substantially interfere with the oral absorption of quinolones; these preparations may be taken six hours before or two hours after taking ciprofloxacin). Products include:
Phyto-Vite Tablets .... ▣ 639

Ketoprofen (NSAIDs in combination with very high doses of quinolones have been shown to provoke convulsions in pre-clinical trials).
No products indexed under this heading.

Ketorolac Tromethamine (NSAIDs in combination with very high doses of quinolones have been shown to provoke convulsions in pre-clinical trials).
No products indexed under this heading.

Levobupivacaine Hydrochloride (Ciprofloxacin is a moderate inhibitor of CYP450 1A2 isoenzymes. Co-administration of ciprofloxacin and other drugs primarily metabolized by the CYP450 1A2 enzyme pathway may result in increased plasma concentrations of the co-administered drug and couldlead to clinically significant pharmacodynamic side effects).
No products indexed under this heading.

Lomefloxacin Hydrochloride (Ciprofloxacin is a moderate inhibitor of CYP450 1A2 isoenzymes. Co-administration of ciprofloxacin and other drugs primarily metabolized by the CYP450 1A2 enzyme pathway may result in increased plasma concentrations of the co-administered drug and couldlead to clinically significant pharmacodynamic side effects).
No products indexed under this heading.

Magaldrate (Concurrent administration of these antacids may substantially interfere with the oral absorption of ciprofloxacin; antacids may be administered either two hours after or six hours before ciprofloxacin dosing without a significant decrease in bioavailability).
No products indexed under this heading.

Magnesium Hydroxide (Concurrent administration of these antacids may substantially interfere with the oral absorption of ciprofloxacin; antacids may be administered either two hours after or six hours before ciprofloxacin dosing without a significant decrease in bioavailability). Products include:
Fleet Pedia-Lax Chewable Tablets 1145
Pepcid Complete Chewable Tablets.. 1771
Extra Strength Rolaids Freshmint Tablets.. 1903
Rolaids Multi-Symptom Berry Tablets.. 1903
Rolaids Original Peppermint Tablets.. 1903

Magnesium Oxide (Concurrent administration of these antacids may substantially interfere with the oral absorption of ciprofloxacin; antacids may be administered either two hours after or six hours before ciprofloxacin dosing without a significant decrease in bioavailability). Products include:
Beelith Tablets 813

Maprotiline Hydrochloride (Ciprofloxacin is a moderate inhibitor of CYP450 1A2 isoenzymes. Co-administration of ciprofloxacin and other drugs primarily metabolized by the CYP450 1A2 enzyme pathway may result in increased plasma concentrations of the co-administered drug and couldlead to clinically significant pharmacodynamic side effects).
No products indexed under this heading.

Meclofenamate Sodium (NSAIDs in combination with very high doses of quinolones have been shown to provoke convulsions in pre-clinical trials).
No products indexed under this heading.

Mefenamic Acid (NSAIDs in combination with very high doses of quinolones have been shown to provoke convulsions in pre-clinical trials).
No products indexed under this heading.

Meloxicam (NSAIDs in combination with very high doses of quinolones have been shown to provoke convulsions in pre-clinical trials). Products include:
Mobic Oral Suspension 863
Mobic Tablets 863

Methadone Hydrochloride (Ciprofloxacin is a moderate inhibitor of CYP450 1A2 isoenzymes. Co-administration of ciprofloxacin and other drugs primarily metabolized by the CYP450 1A2 enzyme pathway may result in increased plasma concentrations of the co-administered drug and couldlead to clinically significant pharmacodynamic side effects).
No products indexed under this heading.

Methotrexate (Renal tubular transport of methotrexate may be inhibited by concomitant administration of ciprofloxacin potentially leading to increased plasma levels of methotrexate).
No products indexed under this heading.

Methotrexate Sodium (Renal tubular transport of methotrexate may be inhibited by concomitant administration of ciprofloxacin potentially leading to increased plasma levels of methotrexate).
No products indexed under this heading.

Methylprednisolone Acetate (Risk of ruptures of the shoulder, hand, Achilles tendon or other tendons may be increased in patients receiving concomitant corticosteroids, especially in the elderly).
No products indexed under this heading.

Methylprednisolone Sodium Succinate (Risk of ruptures of the shoulder, hand, Achilles tendon or other tendons may be increased in patients receiving concomitant corticosteroids, especially in the elderly).
No products indexed under this heading.

Metoclopramide Hydrochloride (Metoclopramide significantly accelerates the absorption of oral ciprofloxacin resulting in a shorter time to reach maximum plasma concentrations).
No products indexed under this heading.

Mexiletine Hydrochloride (Ciprofloxacin is a moderate inhibitor of CYP450 1A2 isoenzymes. Co-administration of ciprofloxacin and other drugs primarily metabolized by the CYP450 1A2 enzyme pathway may result in increased plasma concentrations of the co-administered drug and couldlead to clinically significant pharmacodynamic side effects).
No products indexed under this heading.

Mirtazapine (Ciprofloxacin is a moderate inhibitor of CYP450 1A2 isoenzymes. Co-administration of ciprofloxacin and other drugs primarily metabolized by the CYP450 1A2 enzyme pathway may result in increased plasma concentrations of the co-administered drug and couldlead to clinically significant pharmacodynamic side effects). Products include:
Remeron Tablets 2924
RemeronSolTab Tablets 2927

Mometasone Furoate (Risk of ruptures of the shoulder, hand, Achilles tendon or other tendons may be increased in patients receiving concomitant corticosteroids, especially in the elderly). Products include:
Asmanex Twisthaler 2797
Elocon Cream 0.1% 2840
Elocon Lotion 0.1% 2841
Elocon Ointment 0.1% 2842

Mometasone Furoate Monohydrate (Risk of ruptures of the shoulder, hand, Achilles tendon or other tendons may be increased in patients receiving concomitant corticosteroids, especially in the elderly). Products include:
Nasonex Nasal Spray 2883

Moricizine Hydrochloride (In general, elderly patients may be more susceptible to drug-associated effects on the QT interval. Therefore, precaution should be taken when using ciprofloxacin with concomitant drugs that can result in prolongation of the QT interval (eg, class IA or class III antiarrhythmics)).
No products indexed under this heading.

Moxifloxacin Hydrochloride (Ciprofloxacin is a moderate inhibitor of CYP450 1A2 isoenzymes. Co-administration of ciprofloxacin and other drugs primarily metabolized by the CYP450 1A2 enzyme pathway may result in increased plasma concentrations of the co-administered drug and couldlead to clinically significant pharmacodynamic side effects). Products include:
Avelox 2803
Vigamox Ophthalmic Solution .... ⊙ 548

Nabumetone (NSAIDs in combination with very high doses of quinolones have been shown to provoke convulsions in pre-clinical trials).
No products indexed under this heading.

Nafcillin Sodium (Ciprofloxacin is a moderate inhibitor of CYP450 1A2 isoenzymes. Co-administration of ciprofloxacin and other drugs primarily metabolized by the CYP450 1A2 enzyme pathway may result in increased plasma concentrations of the co-administered drug and couldlead to clinically significant pharmacodynamic side effects).
No products indexed under this heading.

Naproxen (NSAIDs in combination with very high doses of quinolones have been shown to provoke convulsions in pre-clinical trials). Products include:
EC-Naprosyn Delayed-Release Tablets.. 2632
Naprosyn Suspension 2632
Naprosyn Tablets 2632

Naproxen Sodium (NSAIDs in combination with very high doses of quinolones have been shown to provoke convulsions in pre-clinical trials). Products include:
Anaprox Tablets 2632
Anaprox DS Tablets 2632
Treximet Tablets 1616

Nicotine Polacrilex (Ciprofloxacin is a moderate inhibitor of CYP450 1A2 isoenzymes. Co-administration of ciprofloxacin and other drugs primarily metabolized by the CYP450 1A2 enzyme pathway may result in increased plasma concentrations of the co-administered drug and couldlead to clinically significant pharmacodynamic side effects).
No products indexed under this heading.

Nicotine Salicylate (Ciprofloxacin is a moderate inhibitor of CYP450 1A2 isoenzymes. Co-administration of ciprofloxacin and other drugs primarily metabolized by the CYP450 1A2 enzyme pathway may result in increased plasma concentrations of the co-administered drug and couldlead to clinically significant pharmacodynamic side effects).
No products indexed under this heading.

Nicotine Sulfate (Ciprofloxacin is a moderate inhibitor of CYP450 1A2 isoenzymes. Co-administration of ciprofloxacin and other drugs primarily metabolized by the CYP450 1A2 enzyme pathway may result in increased plasma concentrations of the co-administered drug and couldlead to clinically significant pharmacodynamic side effects).
No products indexed under this heading.

Norethindrone Acetate (Ciprofloxacin is a moderate inhibitor of CYP450 1A2 isoenzymes. Co-administration of ciprofloxacin and other drugs primarily metabolized by the CYP450 1A2 enzyme pathway may result in increased plasma concentrations of the co-administered drug and couldlead to clinically significant pharmacodynamic side effects). Products include:
Activella Tablets **2347**

Norfloxacin (Ciprofloxacin is a moderate inhibitor of CYP450 1A2 isoenzymes. Co-administration of ciprofloxacin and other drugs primarily metabolized by the CYP450 1A2 enzyme pathway may result in increased plasma concentrations of the co-administered drug and couldlead to clinically significant pharmacodynamic side effects). Products include:
Noroxin Tablets **2069**

Nortriptyline Hydrochloride (Ciprofloxacin is a moderate inhibitor of CYP450 1A2 isoenzymes. Co-administration of ciprofloxacin and other drugs primarily metabolized by the CYP450 1A2 enzyme pathway may result in increased plasma concentrations of the co-administered drug and couldlead to clinically significant pharmacodynamic side effects).
No products indexed under this heading.

Ofloxacin (Ciprofloxacin is a moderate inhibitor of CYP450 1A2 isoenzymes. Co-administration of ciprofloxacin and other drugs primarily metabolized by the CYP450 1A2 enzyme pathway may result in increased plasma concentrations of the co-administered drug and couldlead to clinically significant pharmacodynamic side effects). Products include:
Ofloxacin Ophthalmic Solution 0.3% .... ⊙**243**

Olanzapine (Ciprofloxacin is a moderate inhibitor of CYP450 1A2 isoenzymes. Co-administration of ciprofloxacin and other drugs primarily metabolized by the CYP450 1A2 enzyme pathway may result in increased plasma concentrations of the co-administered drug and couldlead to clinically significant pharmacodynamic side effects). Products include:
Symbyax Capsules **1871**
Zyprexa Tablets **1883**
Zyprexa IntraMuscular **1883**
Zyprexa ZYDIS Orally Disintegrating Tablets **1883**

Ondansetron (Ciprofloxacin is a moderate inhibitor of CYP450 1A2 isoenzymes. Co-administration of ciprofloxacin and other drugs primarily metabolized by the CYP450 1A2 enzyme pathway may result in increased plasma concentrations of the co-administered drug and couldlead to clinically significant pharmacodynamic side effects). Products include:
Zofran ODT Orally Disintegrating Tablets **1687**

Ondansetron Hydrochloride (Ciprofloxacin is a moderate inhibitor of CYP450 1A2 isoenzymes. Co-administration of ciprofloxacin and other drugs primarily metabolized by the CYP450 1A2 enzyme pathway may result in increased plasma concentrations of the co-administered drug and couldlead to clinically significant pharmacodynamic side effects). Products include:
Zofran Injection **1682**
Zofran **1687**

Oxaprozin (NSAIDs in combination with very high doses of quinolones have been shown to provoke convulsions in pre-clinical trials).
No products indexed under this heading.

Phenobarbital Sodium (Ciprofloxacin is a moderate inhibitor of CYP450 1A2 isoenzymes. Co-administration of ciprofloxacin and other drugs primarily metabolized by the CYP450 1A2 enzyme pathway may result in increased plasma concentrations of the co-administered drug and couldlead to clinically significant pharmacodynamic side effects).
No products indexed under this heading.

Phenylbutazone (NSAIDs in combination with very high doses of quinolones have been shown to provoke convulsions in pre-clinical trials).
No products indexed under this heading.

Phenytoin (Potential for change in serum phenytoin levels).
No products indexed under this heading.

Phenytoin Sodium (Potential for change in serum phenytoin levels). Products include:
Phenytek Capsules **2192**

Piroxicam (NSAIDs in combination with very high doses of quinolones have been shown to provoke convulsions in pre-clinical trials).
No products indexed under this heading.

Polysaccharide Iron Complex (Co-administration with iron-containing products may substantially interfere with the oral absorption of quinolones; these preparations may be taken six hours before or two hours after taking ciprofloxacin). Products include:
Nu-Iron 150 Capsules **2165**

Prednisolone Acetate (Risk of ruptures of the shoulder, hand, Achilles tendon or other tendons may be increased in patients receiving concomitant corticosteroids, especially in the elderly). Products include:
Pred Forte Ophthalmic Suspension .... ⊙**227**
Pred Mild Ophthalmic Suspension .... ⊙**230**
Pred-G Ophthalmic Ointment .... ⊙**229**
Pred-G Ophthalmic Suspension .... ⊙**228**

Prednisolone Sodium Phosphate (Risk of ruptures of the shoulder, hand, Achilles tendon or other tendons may be increased in patients receiving concomitant corticosteroids, especially in the elderly).
No products indexed under this heading.

Prednisolone Tebutate (Risk of ruptures of the shoulder, hand, Achilles tendon or other tendons may be increased in patients receiving concomitant corticosteroids, especially in the elderly).
No products indexed under this heading.

Prednisone (Risk of ruptures of the shoulder, hand, Achilles tendon or other tendons may be increased in patients receiving concomitant corticosteroids, especially in the elderly).
No products indexed under this heading.

Probenecid (Interferes with renal tubular secretion of ciprofloxacin).
No products indexed under this heading.

Procainamide (In general, elderly patients may be more susceptible to drug-associated effects on the QT interval. Therefore, precaution should be taken when using ciprofloxacin with concomitant drugs that can result in prolongation of the QT interval (eg, class IA or class III antiarrhythmics)).
No products indexed under this heading.

Propafenone Hydrochloride (Ciprofloxacin is a moderate inhibitor of CYP450 1A2 isoenzymes. Co-administration of ciprofloxacin and other drugs primarily metabolized by the CYP450 1A2 enzyme pathway may result in increased plasma concentrations of the co-administered drug and couldlead to clinically significant pharmacodynamic side effects). Products include:
Rythmol Tablets **1586**
Rythmol SR Capsules **1590**

Propranolol Hydrochloride (Ciprofloxacin is a moderate inhibitor of CYP450 1A2 isoenzymes. Co-administration of ciprofloxacin and other drugs primarily metabolized by the CYP450 1A2 enzyme pathway may result in increased plasma concentrations of the co-administered drug and couldlead to clinically significant pharmacodynamic side effects). Products include:
InnoPran XL Extended Release Capsules **1484**

Protriptyline Hydrochloride (Ciprofloxacin is a moderate inhibitor of CYP450 1A2 isoenzymes. Co-administration of ciprofloxacin and other drugs primarily metabolized by the CYP450 1A2 enzyme pathway may result in increased plasma concentrations of the co-administered drug and couldlead to clinically significant pharmacodynamic side effects).
No products indexed under this heading.

Quinidine (In general, elderly patients may be more susceptible to drug-associated effects on the QT interval. Therefore, precaution should be taken when using ciprofloxacin with concomitant drugs that can result in prolongation of the QT interval (eg, class IA or class III antiarrhythmics)).
No products indexed under this heading.

Quinidine Gluconate (In general, elderly patients may be more susceptible to drug-associated effects on the QT interval. Therefore, precaution should be taken when using ciprofloxacin with concomitant drugs that can result in prolongation of the QT interval (eg, class IA or class III antiarrhythmics)).
No products indexed under this heading.

Quinidine Hydrochloride (In general, elderly patients may be more susceptible to drug-associated effects on the QT interval. Therefore, precaution should be taken when using ciprofloxacin with concomitant drugs that can result in prolongation of the QT interval (eg, class IA or class III antiarrhythmics)).
No products indexed under this heading.

Quinidine Polygalacturonate (In general, elderly patients may be more susceptible to drug-associated effects on the QT interval. Therefore, precaution should be taken when using ciprofloxacin with concomitant drugs that can result in prolongation of the QT interval (eg, class IA or class III antiarrhythmics)).
No products indexed under this heading.

Quinidine Sulfate (In general, elderly patients may be more susceptible to drug-associated effects on the QT interval. Therefore, precaution should be taken when using ciprofloxacin with concomitant drugs that can result in prolongation of the QT interval (eg, class IA or class III antiarrhythmics)).
No products indexed under this heading.

Riluzole (Ciprofloxacin is a moderate inhibitor of CYP450 1A2 isoenzymes. Co-administration of ciprofloxacin and other drugs primarily metabolized by the CYP450 1A2 enzyme pathway may result in increased plasma concentrations of the co-administered drug and couldlead to clinically significant pharmacodynamic side effects). Products include:
Rilutek Tablets **2771**

Ritonavir (Ciprofloxacin is a moderate inhibitor of CYP450 1A2 isoenzymes. Co-administration of ciprofloxacin and other drugs primarily metabolized by the CYP450 1A2 enzyme pathway may result in increased plasma concentrations of the co-administered drug and could-lead to clinically significant pharmacodynamic side effects). Products include:

Kaletra 452
Norvir 489

Rofecoxib (NSAIDs in combination with very high doses of quinolones have been shown to provoke convulsions in pre-clinical trials).

No products indexed under this heading.

Ropinirole Hydrochloride (Ciprofloxacin is a moderate inhibitor of CYP450 1A2 isoenzymes. Co-administration of ciprofloxacin and other drugs primarily metabolized by the CYP450 1A2 enzyme pathway may result in increased plasma concentrations of the co-administered drug and couldlead to clinically significant pharmacodynamic side effects). Products include:

Requip Tablets 1561
Requip XL Tablets 1568

Ropivacaine Hydrochloride (Ciprofloxacin is a moderate inhibitor of CYP450 1A2 isoenzymes. Co-administration of ciprofloxacin and other drugs primarily metabolized by the CYP450 1A2 enzyme pathway may result in increased plasma concentrations of the co-administered drug and couldlead to clinically significant pharmacodynamic side effects).

No products indexed under this heading.

Sotalol Hydrochloride (In general, elderly patients may be more susceptible to drug-associated effects on the QT interval. Therefore, precaution should be taken when using ciprofloxacin with concomitant drugs that can result in prolongation of the QT interval (eg, class IA or class III antiarrhythmics)).

No products indexed under this heading.

Sucralfate (Co-administration with sucralfate may substantially interfere with the oral absorption of quinolones; these preparations may be taken six hours before or two hours after taking ciprofloxacin). Products include:

Carafate Suspension 706
Carafate Tablets 707

Sulindac (NSAIDs in combination with very high doses of quinolones have been shown to provoke convulsions in pre-clinical trials). Products include:

Clinoril Tablets 1962

Tacrine Hydrochloride (Ciprofloxacin is a moderate inhibitor of CYP450 1A2 isoenzymes. Co-administration of ciprofloxacin and other drugs primarily metabolized by the CYP450 1A2 enzyme pathway may result in increased plasma concentrations of the co-administered drug and couldlead to clinically significant pharmacodynamic side effects).

No products indexed under this heading.

Tamoxifen Citrate (Ciprofloxacin is a moderate inhibitor of CYP450 1A2 isoenzymes. Co-administration of ciprofloxacin and other drugs primarily metabolized by the CYP450 1A2 enzyme pathway may result in increased plasma concentrations of the co-administered drug and could-lead to clinically significant pharmacodynamic side effects).

No products indexed under this heading.

Theophylline (Potential for severe and fatal reactions including cardiac arrest, seizures, respiratory failure and status epilepticus; concurrent use should be avoided or serum levels of theophylline should be monitored carefully).

No products indexed under this heading.

Theophylline Anhydrous (Potential for severe and fatal reactions including cardiac arrest, seizures, respiratory failure and status epilepticus; concurrent use should be avoided or serum levels of theophylline should be monitored carefully). Products include:

Uniphyl Tablets 2595

Theophylline Calcium Salicylate (Potential for severe and fatal reactions including cardiac arrest, seizures, respiratory failure and status epilepticus; concurrent use should be avoided or serum levels of theophylline should be monitored carefully).

No products indexed under this heading.

Theophylline Dihydroxypropyl (Glyceryl) (Potential for severe and fatal reactions including cardiac arrest, seizures, respiratory failure and status epilepticus; concurrent use should be avoided or serum levels of theophylline should be monitored carefully).

No products indexed under this heading.

Theophylline Ethylenediamine (Potential for severe and fatal reactions including cardiac arrest, seizures, respiratory failure and status epilepticus; concurrent use should be avoided or serum levels of theophylline should be monitored carefully).

No products indexed under this heading.

Theophylline Sodium Glycinate (Potential for severe and fatal reactions including cardiac arrest, seizures, respiratory failure and status epilepticus; concurrent use should be avoided or serum levels of theophylline should be monitored carefully).

No products indexed under this heading.

Tizanidine Hydrochloride (Concomitant administration is contraindicated).

No products indexed under this heading.

Tolmetin Sodium (NSAIDs in combination with very high doses of quinolones have been shown to provoke convulsions in pre-clinical trials).

No products indexed under this heading.

Triamcinolone (Risk of ruptures of the shoulder, hand, Achilles tendon or other tendons may be increased in patients receiving concomitant corticosteroids, especially in the elderly).

No products indexed under this heading.

Triamcinolone Acetonide (Risk of ruptures of the shoulder, hand, Achilles tendon or other tendons may be increased in patients receiving concomitant corticosteroids, especially in the elderly). Products include:

Azmacort Inhalation Aerosol 407
Nasacort AQ Nasal Spray 2765
Triesence Injectable Suspension .... ⊙209

Triamcinolone Diacetate (Risk of ruptures of the shoulder, hand, Achilles tendon or other tendons may be increased in patients receiving concomitant corticosteroids, especially in the elderly).

No products indexed under this heading.

Triamcinolone Hexacetonide (Risk of ruptures of the shoulder, hand, Achilles tendon or other tendons may be increased in patients receiving concomitant corticosteroids, especially in the elderly).

No products indexed under this heading.

Trimethaphan Camsylate (Ciprofloxacin is a moderate inhibitor of CYP450 1A2 isoenzymes. Co-administration of ciprofloxacin and other drugs primarily metabolized by the CYP450 1A2 enzyme pathway may result in increased plasma concentrations of the co-administered drug and couldlead to clinically significant pharmacodynamic side effects).

No products indexed under this heading.

Trimipramine Maleate (Ciprofloxacin is a moderate inhibitor of CYP450 1A2 isoenzymes. Co-administration of ciprofloxacin and other drugs primarily metabolized by the CYP450 1A2 enzyme pathway may result in increased plasma concentrations of the co-administered drug and couldlead to clinically significant pharmacodynamic side effects).

No products indexed under this heading.

Trovafloxacin Mesylate (Ciprofloxacin is a moderate inhibitor of CYP450 1A2 isoenzymes. Co-administration of ciprofloxacin and other drugs primarily metabolized by the CYP450 1A2 enzyme pathway may result in increased plasma concentrations of the co-administered drug and couldlead to clinically significant pharmacodynamic side effects).

No products indexed under this heading.

Valdecoxib (NSAIDs in combination with very high doses of quinolones have been shown to provoke convulsions in pre-clinical trials).

No products indexed under this heading.

Verapamil Hydrochloride (Ciprofloxacin is a moderate inhibitor of CYP450 1A2 isoenzymes. Co-administration of ciprofloxacin and other drugs primarily metabolized by the CYP450 1A2 enzyme pathway may result in increased plasma concentrations of the co-administered drug and couldlead to clinically significant pharmacodynamic side effects). Products include:

Tarka Tablets 511

Warfarin Sodium (Enhanced effects of anticoagulant).

No products indexed under this heading.

Zileuton (Ciprofloxacin is a moderate inhibitor of CYP450 1A2 isoenzymes. Co-administration of ciprofloxacin and other drugs primarily metabolized by the CYP450 1A2 enzyme pathway may result in increased plasma concentrations of the co-administered drug and could-lead to clinically significant pharmacodynamic side effects).

No products indexed under this heading.

Zinc Sulfate (Co-administration with zinc-containing products may substantially interfere with the oral absorption of quinolones; these preparations may be taken six hours before or two hours after taking ciprofloxacin). Products include:

Clear Eyes Itchy Eye Relief .... ⊙255
Zinc-220 Capsules 564

Zolmitriptan (Ciprofloxacin is a moderate inhibitor of CYP450 1A2 isoenzymes. Co-administration of ciprofloxacin and other drugs primarily metabolized by the CYP450 1A2 enzyme pathway may result in increased plasma concentrations of the co-administered drug and could-lead to clinically significant pharmacodynamic side effects). Products include:

Zomig Tablets 694
Zomig Nasal Spray 689
Zomig-ZMT Tablets 694

Food Interactions

Dairy products (Oral ciprofloxacin should not be taken concurrently with milk or yogurt alone, since absorption of ciprofloxacin may be significantly reduced; dietary calcium as part of a meal; however, does not significantly affect ciprofloxacin absorption).

Food, unspecified (Delays the oral absorption of the drug resulting in peak concentrations that are closer to two hours after dosing).

CIPRO ORAL SUSPENSION

(Ciprofloxacin) 2810

See Cipro Tablets

CIPRO TABLETS

(Ciprofloxacin Hydrochloride) 2810

May interact with antacids containing aluminum, calcium and magnesium, Class I antiarrhythmics, class III antiarrhythmics, calcium preparations, corticosteroids, oral anticoagulants, cytochrome p450 1a2 substrates (selected), iron containing oral preparations, non-steroidal anti-inflammatory agents, phenytoin, drugs that prolong the QT interval, theophyllines, xanthines, and certain other agents. Compounds in these categories include:

Acetaminophen (Ciprofloxacin is an inhibitor of the hepatic CYP1A2 enzyme pathway. Co-administration of ciprofloxacin and other drugs primarily metabolized by CYP1A2 results in increased plasma concentrations of the co-administered drug and could lead to clinically significant pharmacodynamic side effects of the co-administered drug). Products include:

Benadryl Allergy & Cold Kapgels 1895
Benadryl Allergy & Sinus Headache Kapgels 1895
Benadryl Severe Allergy & Sinus Headache Caplets 1897
Lortab 5/500 Tablets 3143
Lortab 7.5/500 Tablets 3144
Lortab 10/500 Tablets 3144
Percocet Tablets 1127
Sinutab Sinus Caplets 1905
Sudafed PE Cold & Cough Caplets 1907
Sudafed PE Nighttime Cold Caplets 1907
Sudafed PE Severe Cold Caplets 1908
Sudafed PE Sinus Headache Caplets 1908
Regular Strength Tylenol Tablets 1915
Tylenol 8 Hour Extended Release Caplets 1915
Extra Strength Tylenol Caplets, Cool Caplets, and EZ Tabs 1915
Extra Strength Tylenol Adult Rapid Blast Liquid 1915

Extra Strength Tylenol PM Caplets, Geltabs, Liquid, and Rapid Release Gels 1915
Extra Strength Tylenol Rapid Release Gels 1915
Tylenol with Codeine Tablets 2427
Tylenol Allergy Multi-Symptom Caplets with Cool Burst and Rapid Release Gelcaps 1916
Tylenol Allergy Multi-Symptom Nighttime Caplets with Cool Burst 1916
Tylenol Severe Allergy Caplets 1916
Tylenol Arthritis Pain Extended Release Geltabs/Caplets 1915
Tylenol Chest Congestion Caplets with Cool Burst 1910
Tylenol Chest Congestion Liquid with Cool Burst 1910
Children's Tylenol Plus Cold Suspension Liquid 1912
Children's Tylenol Plus Cold & Allergy Suspension Liquid 1914
Children's Tylenol Plus Cough & Runny Nose Suspension Liquid 1912
Children's Tylenol Plus Cough & Sore Throat Suspension Liquid 1912
Children's Tylenol Plus Flu Suspension Liquid 1914
Children's Tylenol Suspension Liquid 1909
Children's Tylenol Meltaways 1909
Children's Tylenol Plus Multi-Symptom Cold Suspension Liquid 1912
Tylenol Cold Severe Congestion Daytime Caplets with Cool Burst 1912
Tylenol Cold Head Congestion Daytime Caplets with Cool Burst 1910
Tylenol Cold Head Congestion Nighttime Caplets with Cool Burst 1910
Tylenol Cold Head Congestion Severe Daytime Caplets with Cool Burst 1910
Tylenol Cold Multi-Symptom Daytime Caplets with Cool Burst and Rapid Release Gels 1913
Tylenol Cold Multi-Symptom Daytime Liquid with Citrus Burst ... 1913
Tylenol Cold Multi-Symptom Nighttime Caplets with Cool Burst 1913
Tylenol Cold Multi-Symptom Nighttime Liquid with Cool Burst ... 1913
Tylenol Cold Multi-Symptom Severe Caplets with Cool Burst 1913
Tylenol Cold Multi-Symptom Severe Daytime Liquid with Citrus Burst 1913
Tylenol Cough & Sore Throat Daytime Liquid with Cool Burst 1918
Tylenol Cough & Sore Throat Nighttime Liquid with Cool Burst ... 1918
Concentrated Tylenol Infants' Drops 1909
Jr. Tylenol Meltaways 1909
Tylenol Sinus Congestion & Pain Daytime Caplets with Cool Burst and Gelcaps 1917
Tylenol Sinus Congestion & Pain Nighttime Caplets with Cool Burst 1917
Tylenol Sinus Congestion & Pain Severe Caplets with Cool Burst 1917
Tylenol Sinus Severe Congestion Caplets with Cool Burst 1917
Tylenol Sore Throat Daytime Liquid with Cool Burst 1918
Tylenol Sore Throat Nighttime Liquid with Cool Burst 1918
Women's Tylenol Menstrual Relief Caplets 1919
Vicks DayQuil Cold & Flu Multi-Symptom Relief 616
Vicks DayQuil LiquiCaps 2567
Vicks DayQuil Liquid 2567
Vicks DayQuil Multi-Symptom Cold/Flu Relief 2567
Vicks NyQuil Cold & Flu Multi-Symptom Relief 617
Vicks NyQuil LiquiCaps 2567
Vicks NyQuil Liquid 2567
Vicks NyQuil Multi-Symptom Cold/Flu Relief 2567
Vicodin Tablets 529
Vicodin ES Tablets 530
Vicodin HP Tablets 531
Zydone Tablets 1132

Alatrofloxacin Mesylate (Ciprofloxacin is an inhibitor of the hepatic CYP1A2 enzyme pathway. Co-administration of ciprofloxacin and other drugs primarily metabolized by CYP1A2 results in increased plasma concentrations of the co-administered drug and could lead to clinically significant pharmacodynamic side effects of the co-administered drug).
No products indexed under this heading.

Alprazolam (In general, elderly patients may be more susceptible to drug-associated effects on the QT interval. Therefore, precautions should be taken when using ciprofloxacin with concomitant drugs that can result in prolongation of the QT interval).
No products indexed under this heading.

Aluminum Carbonate (Concurrent administration of ciprofloxacin, with multivalent cation-containing products, such as magnesium/aluminum antacids, may substantially decrease its absorption, resulting in serum and urine levels considerably lower than desired. Ciprofloxacin may be taken two hours before or six hours after taking magnesium or aluminum containing antacids).
No products indexed under this heading.

Aluminum Hydroxide (Concurrent administration of ciprofloxacin, with multivalent cation-containing products, such as magnesium/aluminum antacids, may substantially decrease its absorption, resulting in serum and urine levels considerably lower than desired. Ciprofloxacin may be taken two hours before or six hours after taking magnesium or aluminum containing antacids).
No products indexed under this heading.

Aminophylline (Ciprofloxacin is an inhibitor of the hepatic CYP1A2 enzyme pathway. Co-administration of ciprofloxacin and other drugs primarily metabolized by CYP1A2 such as methylxanthines, results in increased plasma concentrations of co-administered drug and could lead to clinically significant pharmacodynamic side effects of the co-administered drug).
No products indexed under this heading.

Amiodarone Hydrochloride (In general, elderly patients may be more susceptible to drug-associated effects on the QT interval. Therefore, precautions should be taken when using ciprofloxacin with concomitant drugs that can result in prolongation of the QT interval).
No products indexed under this heading.

Amitriptyline Hydrochloride (In general, elderly patients may be more susceptible to drug-associated effects on the QT interval. Therefore, precautions should be taken when using ciprofloxacin with concomitant drugs that can result in prolongation of the QT interval).
No products indexed under this heading.

Amoxapine (In general, elderly patients may be more susceptible to drug-associated effects on the QT interval. Therefore, precautions should be taken when using ciprofloxacin with concomitant drugs that can result in prolongation of the QT interval).
No products indexed under this heading.

Anagrelide Hydrochloride (Ciprofloxacin is an inhibitor of the hepatic CYP1A2 enzyme pathway. Co-administration of ciprofloxacin and other drugs primarily metabolized by CYP1A2 results in increased plasma concentrations of the co-administered drug and could lead to clinically significant pharmacodynamic side effects of the co-administered drug). Products include:
Agrylin Capsules 3017

Anisindione (Ciprofloxacin has been reported to enhance the effects of the oral anticoagulant warfarin or its derivatives. When these products are administered concomitantly, prothrombin time or other suitable coagulant tests should be closely monitored).
No products indexed under this heading.

Astemizole (In general, elderly patients may be more susceptible to drug-associated effects on the QT interval. Therefore, precautions should be taken when using ciprofloxacin with concomitant drugs that can result in prolongation of the QT interval).
No products indexed under this heading.

Betamethasone Acetate (Ruptures of the shoulder, hand, Achilles tendon, or other tendons that required surgical repair or resulted in prolonged disability have been reported in patients receiving ciprofloxacin. Post-marketing surveillance reports indicate that this risk may be increased in patients receiving concomitant corticosteroids, especially the elderly).
No products indexed under this heading.

Betamethasone Sodium Phosphate (Ruptures of the shoulder, hand, Achilles tendon, or other tendons that required surgical repair or resulted in prolonged disability have been reported in patients receiving ciprofloxacin. Post-marketing surveillance reports indicate that this risk may be increased in patients receiving concomitant corticosteroids, especially the elderly).
No products indexed under this heading.

Bretylium Tosylate (In general, elderly patients may be more susceptible to drug-associated effects on the QT interval. Therefore, precautions should be taken when using ciprofloxacin with concomitant drugs that can result in prolongation of the QT interval).
No products indexed under this heading.

Budesonide (Ruptures of the shoulder, hand, Achilles tendon, or other tendons that required surgical repair or resulted in prolonged disability have been reported in patients receiving ciprofloxacin. Post-marketing surveillance reports indicate that this risk may be increased in patients receiving concomitant corticosteroids, especially the elderly). Products include:
Pulmicort Flexhaler 654
Symbicort 80/4.5 Inhalation Aerosol 659
Symbicort 160/4.5 Inhalation Aerosol 659

Buspirone Hydrochloride (In general, elderly patients may be more susceptible to drug-associated effects on the QT interval. Therefore, precautions should be taken when using ciprofloxacin with concomitant drugs that can result in prolongation of the QT interval).
No products indexed under this heading.

Caffeine (Ciprofloxacin has been shown to interfere with the metabolism of caffeine. This may lead to reduced clearance of caffeine and a prolongation of its serum half-life). Products include:
BioLean Free Tablets 635
BioLean II Tablets 635
Winrgy Dietary Supplement 642

Caffeine Anhydrous (Ciprofloxacin has been shown to interfere with the metabolism of caffeine. This may lead to reduced clearance of caffeine and a prolongation of its serum half-life).
No products indexed under this heading.

Caffeine Citrate (Ciprofloxacin has been shown to interfere with the metabolism of caffeine. This may lead to reduced clearance of caffeine and a prolongation of its serum half-life).
No products indexed under this heading.

Calcium Carbonate (Concurrent administration of ciprofloxacin with multivalent cation-containing products, such as products containing calcium, may substantially decrease its absorption, resulting in serum and urine levels considerably lower than desired. Ciprofloxacin should be administered at least 2 hours before or 6 hours after products containing calcium). Products include:
Accelerator Tablets 634
Actonel with Calcium Tablets 2574
BioLean II Tablets 635
Calcet Triple Calcium + Vitamin D Tablets 629
D-Cal Chewable Caplets 624
Elixir Capsules 636
Pepcid Complete Chewable Tablets 1771
Extra Strength Rolaids Plus Gas Relief Tropical Fruit Softchews 1903
Extra Strength Rolaids Softchews Vanilla Creme 1903
Extra Strength Rolaids Freshmint Tablets 1903
Rolaids Multi-Symptom Berry Tablets 1903
Rolaids Original Peppermint Tablets 1903

Calcium Chloride (Concurrent administration of ciprofloxacin with multivalent cation-containing products, such as products containing calcium, may substantially decrease its absorption, resulting in serum and urine levels considerably lower than desired. Ciprofloxacin should be administered at least 2 hours before or 6 hours after products containing calcium).
No products indexed under this heading.

Calcium Citrate (Concurrent administration of ciprofloxacin with multivalent cation-containing products, such as products containing calcium, may substantially decrease its absorption, resulting in serum and urine levels considerably lower than desired. Ciprofloxacin should be administered at least 2 hours before or 6 hours after products containing calcium). Products include:

Active Calcium Tablets 3173
CitraNatal DHA Tablets 2175
CitraNatal 90 DHA Tablets 2175

Calcium Glubionate (Concurrent administration of ciprofloxacin with multivalent cation-containing products, such as products containing calcium, may substantially decrease its absorption, resulting in serum and urine levels considerably lower than desired. Ciprofloxacin should be administered at least 2 hours before or 6 hours after products containing calcium).

No products indexed under this heading.

Celecoxib (Non-steroidal anti-inflammatory drugs in combination of very high doses of quinolones have been shown to provoke convulsions in pre-clinical studies). Products include:

Celebrex Capsules 2979

Chlordiazepoxide (In general, elderly patients may be more susceptible to drug-associated effects on the QT interval. Therefore, precautions should be taken when using ciprofloxacin with concomitant drugs that can result in prolongation of the QT interval).

No products indexed under this heading.

Chlordiazepoxide Hydrochloride (In general, elderly patients may be more susceptible to drug-associated effects on the QT interval. Therefore, precautions should be taken when using ciprofloxacin with concomitant drugs that can result in prolongation of the QT interval).

No products indexed under this heading.

Chlorpromazine (In general, elderly patients may be more susceptible to drug-associated effects on the QT interval. Therefore, precautions should be taken when using ciprofloxacin with concomitant drugs that can result in prolongation of the QT interval).

No products indexed under this heading.

Chlorpromazine Hydrochloride (In general, elderly patients may be more susceptible to drug-associated effects on the QT interval. Therefore, precautions should be taken when using ciprofloxacin with concomitant drugs that can result in prolongation of the QT interval).

No products indexed under this heading.

Chlorprothixene (In general, elderly patients may be more susceptible to drug-associated effects on the QT interval. Therefore, precautions should be taken when using ciprofloxacin with concomitant drugs that can result in prolongation of the QT interval).

No products indexed under this heading.

Chlorprothixene Hydrochloride (In general, elderly patients may be more susceptible to drug-associated effects on the QT interval. Therefore, precautions should be taken when using ciprofloxacin with concomitant drugs that can result in prolongation of the QT interval).

No products indexed under this heading.

Ciclesonide (Ruptures of the shoulder, hand, Achilles tendon, or other tendons that required surgical repair or resulted in prolonged disability have been reported in patients receiving ciprofloxacin. Post-marketing surveillance reports indicate that this risk may be increased in patients receiving concomitant corticosteroids, especially the elderly). Products include:

Alvesco Inhalation Aerosol 2985
Omnaris Nasal Spray 2998

Cimetidine Hydrochloride (Ciprofloxacin is an inhibitor of the hepatic CYP1A2 enzyme pathway. Co-administration of ciprofloxacin and other drugs primarily metabolized by CYP1A2 results in increased plasma concentrations of the co-administered drug and could lead to clinically significant pharmacodynamic side effects of the co-administered drug).

No products indexed under this heading.

Ciprofloxacin (Ciprofloxacin is an inhibitor of the hepatic CYP1A2 enzyme pathway. Co-administration of ciprofloxacin and other drugs primarily metabolized by CYP1A2 results in increased plasma concentrations of the co-administered drug and could lead to clinically significant pharmacodynamic side effects of the co-administered drug). Products include:

Cipro I.V. 2817
Cipro Oral Suspension 2810
Cipro XR Tablets 2823
Ciprodex Otic Suspension 541

Clomipramine Hydrochloride (In general, elderly patients may be more susceptible to drug-associated effects on the QT interval. Therefore, precautions should be taken when using ciprofloxacin with concomitant drugs that can result in prolongation of the QT interval).

No products indexed under this heading.

Clopidogrel Bisulfate (Ciprofloxacin is an inhibitor of the hepatic CYP1A2 enzyme pathway. Co-administration of ciprofloxacin and other drugs primarily metabolized by CYP1A2 results in increased plasma concentrations of the co-administered drug and could lead to clinically significant pharmacodynamic side effects of the co-administered drug). Products include:

Plavix Tablets 926
Plavix Tablets 2767

Clorazepate Dipotassium (In general, elderly patients may be more susceptible to drug-associated effects on the QT interval. Therefore, precautions should be taken when using ciprofloxacin with concomitant drugs that can result in prolongation of the QT interval).

No products indexed under this heading.

Clozapine (In general, elderly patients may be more susceptible to drug-associated effects on the QT interval. Therefore, precautions should be taken when using ciprofloxacin with concomitant drugs that can result in prolongation of the QT interval).

No products indexed under this heading.

Cortisone Acetate (Ruptures of the shoulder, hand, Achilles tendon, or other tendons that required surgical repair or resulted in prolonged disability have been reported in patients receiving ciprofloxacin. Post-marketing surveillance reports indicate that this risk may be increased in patients receiving concomitant corticosteroids, especially the elderly).

No products indexed under this heading.

Cyclobenzaprine (Ciprofloxacin is an inhibitor of the hepatic CYP1A2 enzyme pathway. Co-administration of ciprofloxacin and other drugs primarily metabolized by CYP1A2 results in increased plasma concentrations of the co-administered drug and could lead to clinically significant pharmacodynamic side effects of the co-administered drug).

No products indexed under this heading.

Cyclobenzaprine Hydrochloride (Ciprofloxacin is an inhibitor of the hepatic CYP1A2 enzyme pathway. Co-administration of ciprofloxacin and other drugs primarily metabolized by CYP1A2 results in increased plasma concentrations of the co-administered drug and could lead to clinically significant pharmacodynamic side effects of the co-administered drug). Products include:

Amrix Capsules 966

Cyclosporine (Ciprofloxacin has been associated with transient elevations in serum creatinine in patients receiving cyclosporine concomitantly). Products include:

Gengraf Capsules 435
Neoral Oral Solution 2280
Neoral Soft Gelatin Capsules 2280
Restasis Ophthalmic Emulsion 557
Sandimmune 2296

Desipramine Hydrochloride (In general, elderly patients may be more susceptible to drug-associated effects on the QT interval. Therefore, precautions should be taken when using ciprofloxacin with concomitant drugs that can result in prolongation of the QT interval).

No products indexed under this heading.

Dexamethasone (Ruptures of the shoulder, hand, Achilles tendon, or other tendons that required surgical repair or resulted in prolonged disability have been reported in patients receiving ciprofloxacin. Post-marketing surveillance reports indicate that this risk may be increased in patients receiving concomitant corticosteroids, especially the elderly). Products include:

Ciprodex Otic Suspension 541

Dexamethasone Acetate (Ruptures of the shoulder, hand, Achilles tendon, or other tendons that required surgical repair or resulted in prolonged disability have been reported in patients receiving ciprofloxacin. Post-marketing surveillance reports indicate that this risk may be increased in patients receiving concomitant corticosteroids, especially the elderly).

No products indexed under this heading.

Dexamethasone Sodium Phosphate (Ruptures of the shoulder, hand, Achilles tendon, or other tendons that required surgical repair or resulted in prolonged disability have been reported in patients receiving ciprofloxacin. Post-marketing surveillance reports indicate that this risk may be increased in patients receiving concomitant corticosteroids, especially the elderly).

No products indexed under this heading.

Diazepam (In general, elderly patients may be more susceptible to drug-associated effects on the QT interval. Therefore, precautions should be taken when using ciprofloxacin with concomitant drugs that can result in prolongation of the QT interval). Products include:

Valium Tablets 2658

Diclofenac Epolamine (Non-steroidal anti-inflammatory drugs in combination of very high doses of quinolones have been shown to provoke convulsions in pre-clinical studies). Products include:

Flector Patch 561

Diclofenac Potassium (Non-steroidal anti-inflammatory drugs in combination of very high doses of quinolones have been shown to provoke convulsions in pre-clinical studies).

No products indexed under this heading.

Diclofenac Sodium (Non-steroidal anti-inflammatory drugs in combination of very high doses of quinolones have been shown to provoke convulsions in pre-clinical studies). Products include:

Diclofenac Sodium Ophthalmic Solution.. ⊙240
Voltaren Ophthalmic Solution 2336
Voltaren Tablets 2334
Voltaren-XR Tablets 2337

Dicumarol (Ciprofloxacin has been reported to enhance the effects of the oral anticoagulant warfarin or its derivatives. When these products are administered concomitantly, prothrombin time or other suitable coagulant tests should be closely monitored).

No products indexed under this heading.

Didanosine (Concurrent administration of ciprofloxacin with multivalent cation-containing products, such as didanosine chewable/buffered tablets or pediatric powder, may substantially decrease its absorption, resulting in serum and urine levels considerably lower than desired. Ciprofloxacin should be administered at least 2 hours before or 6 hours after didanosine chewable/buffered tablets or pediatric powder for oral solution).

No products indexed under this heading.

Diltiazem Hydrochloride (Ciprofloxacin is an inhibitor of the hepatic CYP1A2 enzyme pathway. Co-administration of ciprofloxacin and other drugs primarily metabolized by CYP1A2 results in increased plasma concentrations of the co-administered drug and could lead to clinically significant pharmacodynamic side effects of the co-administered drug). Products include:

Cardizem LA Extended Release Tablets **421**

Diltiazem Maleate (Ciprofloxacin is an inhibitor of the hepatic CYP1A2 enzyme pathway. Co-administration of ciprofloxacin and other drugs primarily metabolized by CYP1A2 results in increased plasma concentrations of the co-administered drug and could lead to clinically significant pharmacodynamic side effects of the co-administered drug).

No products indexed under this heading.

Disopyramide (In general, eldery patients may be more susceptible to drug-associated effects on the QT interval. Therefore precautions should be taken when using ciprofloxacin with concomitant drugs that can result in prolongation of the QT interval (e.g., class IA antiarrhythmics)).

No products indexed under this heading.

Disopyramide Phosphate (In general, elderly patients may be more susceptible to drug-associated effects on the QT interval. Therefore, precautions should be taken when using ciprofloxacin with concomitant drugs that can result in prolongation of the QT interval).

No products indexed under this heading.

Dofetilide (In general, elderly patients may be more susceptible to drug-associated effects on the QT interval. Therefore, precautions should be taken when using ciprofloxacin with concomitant drugs that can result in prolongation of the QT interval).

No products indexed under this heading.

Doxepin Hydrochloride (In general, elderly patients may be more susceptible to drug-associated effects on the QT interval. Therefore, precautions should be taken when using ciprofloxacin with concomitant drugs that can result in prolongation of the QT interval).

No products indexed under this heading.

Droperidol (In general, elderly patients may be more susceptible to drug-associated effects on the QT interval. Therefore, precautions should be taken when using ciprofloxacin with concomitant drugs that can result in prolongation of the QT interval).

No products indexed under this heading.

Dyphylline (Ciprofloxacin is an inhibitor of the hepatic CYP1A2 enzyme pathway. Co-administration of ciprofloxacin and other drugs primarily metabolized by CYP1A2 such as methylxanthines, results in increased plasma concentrations of co-administered drug and could lead to clinically significant pharmacodynamic side effects of the co-administered drug).

No products indexed under this heading.

Enoxacin (Ciprofloxacin is an inhibitor of the hepatic CYP1A2 enzyme pathway. Co-administration of ciprofloxacin and other drugs primarily metabolized by CYP1A2 results in increased plasma concentrations of the co-administered drug and could lead to clinically significant pharmacodynamic side effects of the co-administered drug).

No products indexed under this heading.

Erythromycin (In general, elderly patients may be more susceptible to drug-associated effects on the QT interval. Therefore, precautions should be taken when using ciprofloxacin with concomitant drugs that can result in prolongation of the QT interval).

No products indexed under this heading.

Erythromycin Estolate (In general, elderly patients may be more susceptible to drug-associated effects on the QT interval. Therefore, precautions should be taken when using ciprofloxacin with concomitant drugs that can result in prolongation of the QT interval).

No products indexed under this heading.

Erythromycin Ethylsuccinate (In general, elderly patients may be more susceptible to drug-associated effects on the QT interval. Therefore, precautions should be taken when using ciprofloxacin with concomitant drugs that can result in prolongation of the QT interval). Products include:

E.E.S. **433**
EryPed **431**

Erythromycin Gluceptate (In general, elderly patients may be more susceptible to drug-associated effects on the QT interval. Therefore, precautions should be taken when using ciprofloxacin with concomitant drugs that can result in prolongation of the QT interval).

No products indexed under this heading.

Erythromycin Lactobionate (In general, elderly patients may be more susceptible to drug-associated effects on the QT interval. Therefore, precautions should be taken when using ciprofloxacin with concomitant drugs that can result in prolongation of the QT interval).

No products indexed under this heading.

Erythromycin Stearate (In general, elderly patients may be more susceptible to drug-associated effects on the QT interval. Therefore, precautions should be taken when using ciprofloxacin with concomitant drugs that can result in prolongation of the QT interval).

No products indexed under this heading.

Estradiol (Ciprofloxacin is an inhibitor of the hepatic CYP1A2 enzyme pathway. Co-administration of ciprofloxacin and other drugs primarily metabolized by CYP1A2 results in increased plasma concentrations of the co-administered drug and could lead to clinically significant pharmacodynamic side effects of the co-administered drug). Products include:

Activella Tablets **2347**
Angeliq Tablets **751**
Climara Transdermal System **763**
Climara Pro Transdermal System **768**
Divigel **3167**
Vagifem Tablets **2375**

Estradiol Benzoate (Ciprofloxacin is an inhibitor of the hepatic CYP1A2 enzyme pathway. Co-administration of ciprofloxacin and other drugs primarily metabolized by CYP1A2 results in increased plasma concentrations of the co-administered drug and could lead to clinically significant pharmacodynamic side effects of the co-administered drug).

No products indexed under this heading.

Estradiol Cypionate (Ciprofloxacin is an inhibitor of the hepatic CYP1A2 enzyme pathway. Co-administration of ciprofloxacin and other drugs primarily metabolized by CYP1A2 results in increased plasma concentrations of the co-administered drug and could lead to clinically significant pharmacodynamic side effects of the co-administered drug).

No products indexed under this heading.

Etodolac (Non-steroidal anti-inflammatory drugs in combination of very high doses of quinolones have been shown to provoke convulsions in pre-clinical studies).

No products indexed under this heading.

Fenoprofen Calcium (Non-steroidal anti-inflammatory drugs in combination of very high doses of quinolones have been shown to provoke convulsions in pre-clinical studies). Products include:

Nalfon Capsules **2508**

Ferrous Fumarate (Concurrent administration of ciprofloxacin with multivalent cation-containing products, such as products containing iron, may substantially decrease its absorption, resulting in serum and urine levels considerably lower than desired. Ciprofloxacin should be administered at least 2 hours before or 6 hours after products containing iron).

No products indexed under this heading.

Ferrous Gluconate (Concurrent administration of ciprofloxacin with multivalent cation-containing products, such as products containing iron, may substantially decrease its absorption, resulting in serum and urine levels considerably lower than desired. Ciprofloxacin should be administered at least 2 hours before or 6 hours after products containing iron). Products include:

CitraNatal DHA Tablets **2175**

Ferrous Sulfate (Concurrent administration of ciprofloxacin with multivalent cation-containing products, such as products containing iron, may substantially decrease its absorption, resulting in serum and urine levels considerably lower than desired. Ciprofloxacin should be administered at least 2 hours before or 6 hours after products containing iron).

No products indexed under this heading.

Flecainide Acetate (In general, elderly patients may be more susceptible to drug-associated effects on the QT interval. Therefore, precautions should be taken when using ciprofloxacin with concomitant drugs that can result in prolongation of the QT interval).

No products indexed under this heading.

Fludrocortisone Acetate (Ruptures of the shoulder, hand, Achilles tendon, or other tendons that required surgical repair or resulted in prolonged disability have been reported in patients receiving ciprofloxacin. Post-marketing surveillance reports indicate that this risk may be increased in patients receiving concomitant corticosteroids, especially the elderly).

No products indexed under this heading.

Flunisolide (Ruptures of the shoulder, hand, Achilles tendon, or other tendons that required surgical repair or resulted in prolonged disability have been reported in patients receiving ciprofloxacin. Post-marketing surveillance reports indicate that this risk may be increased in patients receiving concomitant corticosteroids, especially the elderly). Products include:

Aerobid/Aerobid-M **1153**

Fluphenazine Decanoate (In general, elderly patients may be more susceptible to drug-associated effects on the QT interval. Therefore, precautions should be taken when using ciprofloxacin with concomitant drugs that can result in prolongation of the QT interval).

No products indexed under this heading.

Fluphenazine Enanthate (In general, elderly patients may be more susceptible to drug-associated effects on the QT interval. Therefore, precautions should be taken when using ciprofloxacin with concomitant drugs that can result in prolongation of the QT interval).

No products indexed under this heading.

Fluphenazine Hydrochloride (In general, elderly patients may be more susceptible to drug-associated effects on the QT interval. Therefore, precautions should be taken when using ciprofloxacin with concomitant drugs that can result in prolongation of the QT interval).

No products indexed under this heading.

Flurbiprofen (Non-steroidal anti-inflammatory drugs in combination of very high doses of quinolones have been shown to provoke convulsions in pre-clinical studies).

No products indexed under this heading.

Flutamide (Ciprofloxacin is an inhibitor of the hepatic CYP1A2 enzyme pathway. Co-administration of ciprofloxacin and other drugs primarily metabolized by CYP1A2 results in increased plasma concentrations of the co-administered drug and could lead to clinically significant pharmacodynamic side effects of the co-administered drug).

No products indexed under this heading.

Fluticasone Propionate (Ruptures of the shoulder, hand, Achilles tendon, or other tendons that required surgical repair or resulted in prolonged disability have been reported in patients receiving ciprofloxacin. Post-marketing surveillance reports indicate that this risk may be increased in patients receiving concomitant corticosteroids, especially the elderly). Products include:

Advair Diskus 100/50 .... **1276**
Advair Diskus 250/50 .... **1276**

Advair Diskus 500/50 .... **1276**
Advair HFA 45/21 Inhalation Aerosol.. **1288**
Advair HFA 115/21 Inhalation Aerosol.. **1288**
Advair HFA 230/21 Inhalation Aerosol.. **1288**
Flonase Nasal Spray **1431**
Flovent Diskus 50 mcg **1435**

Fluticasone Propionate HFA (Ruptures of the shoulder, hand, Achilles tendon, or other tendons that required surgical repair or resulted in prolonged disability have been reported in patients receiving ciprofloxacin. Post-marketing surveillance reports indicate that this risk may be increased in patients receiving concomitant corticosteroids, especially the elderly). Products include:
Flovent HFA **1440**

Fluvoxamine Maleate (Ciprofloxacin is an inhibitor of the hepatic CYP1A2 enzyme pathway. Co-administration of ciprofloxacin and other drugs primarily metabolized by CYP1A2 results in increased plasma concentrations of the co-administered drug and could lead to clinically significant pharmacodynamic side effects of the co-administered drug). Products include:
Luvox CR Extended-Release Capsules..................................... **1759**

Fosphenytoin Sodium (Altered serum levels of phenytoin (increased and decreased) have been reported in patients receiving concomitant ciprofloxacin).
No products indexed under this heading.

Glyburide (The concomitant administration of ciprofloxacin with the sulfonylurea glyburide has, on rare occasions, resulted in severe hypoglycemia).
No products indexed under this heading.

Grepafloxacin Hydrochloride (Ciprofloxacin is an inhibitor of the hepatic CYP1A2 enzyme pathway. Co-administration of ciprofloxacin and other drugs primarily metabolized by CYP1A2 results in increased plasma concentrations of the co-administered drug and could lead to clinically significant pharmacodynamic side effects of the co-administered drug).
No products indexed under this heading.

Haloperidol (In general, elderly patients may be more susceptible to drug-associated effects on the QT interval. Therefore, precautions should be taken when using ciprofloxacin with concomitant drugs that can result in prolongation of the QT interval).
No products indexed under this heading.

Haloperidol Decanoate (In general, elderly patients may be more susceptible to drug-associated effects on the QT interval. Therefore, precautions should be taken when using ciprofloxacin with concomitant drugs that can result in prolongation of the QT interval).
No products indexed under this heading.

Haloperidol Lactate (Ciprofloxacin is an inhibitor of the hepatic CYP1A2 enzyme pathway. Co-administration of ciprofloxacin and other drugs primarily metabolized by CYP1A2 results in increased plasma concentrations of the co-administered drug and could lead to clinically significant pharmacodynamic side effects of the co-administered drug).
No products indexed under this heading.

Hydrocortisone (Ruptures of the shoulder, hand, Achilles tendon, or other tendons that required surgical repair or resulted in prolonged disability have been reported in patients receiving ciprofloxacin. Post-marketing surveillance reports indicate that this risk may be increased in patients receiving concomitant corticosteroids, especially the elderly).
No products indexed under this heading.

Hydrocortisone Acetate (Ruptures of the shoulder, hand, Achilles tendon, or other tendons that required surgical repair or resulted in prolonged disability have been reported in patients receiving ciprofloxacin. Post-marketing surveillance reports indicate that this risk may be increased in patients receiving concomitant corticosteroids, especially the elderly). Products include:
Analpram-HC **1140**
Pramosone **1141**

Hydrocortisone Sodium Phosphate (Ruptures of the shoulder, hand, Achilles tendon, or other tendons that required surgical repair or resulted in prolonged disability have been reported in patients receiving ciprofloxacin. Post-marketing surveillance reports indicate that this risk may be increased in patients receiving concomitant corticosteroids, especially the elderly).
No products indexed under this heading.

Hydrocortisone Sodium Succinate (Ruptures of the shoulder, hand, Achilles tendon, or other tendons that required surgical repair or resulted in prolonged disability have been reported in patients receiving ciprofloxacin. Post-marketing surveillance reports indicate that this risk may be increased in patients receiving concomitant corticosteroids, especially the elderly).
No products indexed under this heading.

Hydroxyzine Hydrochloride (In general, elderly patients may be more susceptible to drug-associated effects on the QT interval. Therefore, precautions should be taken when using ciprofloxacin with concomitant drugs that can result in prolongation of the QT interval).
No products indexed under this heading.

Ibuprofen (Non-steroidal anti-inflammatory drugs in combination of very high doses of quinolones have been shown to provoke convulsions in pre-clinical studies). Products include:
Motrin IB Tablets and Caplets **1900**
Children's Motrin Oral Suspension ... **1901**
Children's Motrin Non-Staining Dye-Free Oral Suspension............ **1901**
Children's Motrin Cold Oral Suspension **1899**
Infants' Motrin Concentrated Drops... **1901**
Infants' Motrin Non-Staining Dye-Free Concentrated Drops....... **1901**
Junior Strength Motrin Caplets and Chewable Tablets.................. **1901**
Vicoprofen Tablets **533**

Imipramine Hydrochloride (In general, elderly patients may be more susceptible to drug-associated effects on the QT interval. Therefore, precautions should be taken when using ciprofloxacin with concomitant drugs that can result in prolongation of the QT interval).
No products indexed under this heading.

Imipramine Pamoate (In general, elderly patients may be more susceptible to drug-associated effects on the QT interval. Therefore, precautions should be taken when using ciprofloxacin with concomitant drugs that can result in prolongation of the QT interval).
No products indexed under this heading.

Indomethacin (Non-steroidal anti-inflammatory drugs in combination of very high doses of quinolones have been shown to provoke convulsions in pre-clinical studies). Products include:
Indocin **2024**

Indomethacin Sodium Trihydrate (Non-steroidal anti-inflammatory drugs in combination of very high doses of quinolones have been shown to provoke convulsions in pre-clinical studies). Products include:
Indocin I.V. **2489**

Iron (Concurrent administration of ciprofloxacin with multivalent cation-containing products, such as products containing iron, may substantially decrease its absorption, resulting in serum and urine levels considerably lower than desired. Ciprofloxacin should be administered at least 2 hours before or 6 hours after products containing iron). Products include:
Phyto-Vite Tablets .... ▣ **639**

Isocarboxazid (In general, elderly patients may be more susceptible to drug-associated effects on the QT interval. Therefore, precautions should be taken when using ciprofloxacin with concomitant drugs that can result in prolongation of the QT interval). Products include:
Marplan Tablets **3177**

Ketoprofen (Non-steroidal anti-inflammatory drugs in combination of very high doses of quinolones have been shown to provoke convulsions in pre-clinical studies).
No products indexed under this heading.

Ketorolac Tromethamine (Non-steroidal anti-inflammatory drugs in combination of very high doses of quinolones have been shown to provoke convulsions in pre-clinical studies).
No products indexed under this heading.

Levobupivacaine Hydrochloride (Ciprofloxacin is an inhibitor of the hepatic CYP1A2 enzyme pathway. Co-administration of ciprofloxacin and other drugs primarily metabolized by CYP1A2 results in increased plasma concentrations of the co-administered drug and could lead to clinically significant pharmacodynamic side effects of the co-administered drug).
No products indexed under this heading.

Lidocaine (In general, elderly patients may be more susceptible to drug-associated effects on the QT interval. Therefore precautions should be taken when using ciprofloxacin with concomitant drugs that can result in prolongation of the QT interval (e.g., class IA antiarrhythmics)). Products include:
Lidoderm Patch **1114**

Lidocaine Hydrochloride (In general, elderly patients may be more susceptible to drug-associated effects on the QT interval. Therefore, precautions should be taken when using ciprofloxacin with concomitant drugs that can result in prolongation of the QT interval).
No products indexed under this heading.

Lithium Carbonate (In general, elderly patients may be more susceptible to drug-associated effects on the QT interval. Therefore, precautions should be taken when using ciprofloxacin with concomitant drugs that can result in prolongation of the QT interval).
No products indexed under this heading.

Lithium Citrate (In general, elderly patients may be more susceptible to drug-associated effects on the QT interval. Therefore, precautions should be taken when using ciprofloxacin with concomitant drugs that can result in prolongation of the QT interval).
No products indexed under this heading.

Lomefloxacin Hydrochloride (Ciprofloxacin is an inhibitor of the hepatic CYP1A2 enzyme pathway. Co-administration of ciprofloxacin and other drugs primarily metabolized by CYP1A2 results in increased plasma concentrations of the co-administered drug and could lead to clinically significant pharmacodynamic side effects of the co-administered drug).
No products indexed under this heading.

Lorazepam (In general, elderly patients may be more susceptible to drug-associated effects on the QT interval. Therefore, precautions should be taken when using ciprofloxacin with concomitant drugs that can result in prolongation of the QT interval).
No products indexed under this heading.

Loxapine Hydrochloride (In general, elderly patients may be more susceptible to drug-associated effects on the QT interval. Therefore, precautions should be taken when using ciprofloxacin with concomitant drugs that can result in prolongation of the QT interval).
No products indexed under this heading.

Loxapine Succinate (In general, elderly patients may be more susceptible to drug-associated effects on the QT interval. Therefore, precautions should be taken when using ciprofloxacin with concomitant drugs that can result in prolongation of the QT interval).
No products indexed under this heading.

Magaldrate (Concurrent administration of ciprofloxacin, with multivalent cation-containing products, such as magnesium/aluminum antacids, may substantially decrease its absorption, resulting in serum and urine levels considerably lower than desired. Ciprofloxacin may be taken two hours before or six hours after taking magnesium or aluminum containing antacids).
No products indexed under this heading.

Magnesium Hydroxide (Concurrent administration of ciprofloxacin, with multivalent cation-containing products, such as magnesium/aluminum antacids, may substantially decrease its absorption, resulting in serum and urine levels considerably lower than desired. Ciprofloxacin may be taken two hours before or six hours after taking magnesium or aluminum containing antacids). Products include:
Fleet Pedia-Lax Chewable Tablets **1145**
Pepcid Complete Chewable Tablets **1771**
Extra Strength Rolaids Freshmint Tablets **1903**
Rolaids Multi-Symptom Berry Tablets **1903**
Rolaids Original Peppermint Tablets **1903**

Magnesium Oxide (Concurrent administration of ciprofloxacin, with multivalent cation-containing products, such as magnesium/aluminum antacids, may substantially decrease its absorption, resulting in serum and urine levels considerably lower than desired. Ciprofloxacin may be taken two hours before or six hours after taking magnesium or aluminum containing antacids). Products include:
Beelith Tablets **813**

Maprotiline Hydrochloride (In general, elderly patients may be more susceptible to drug-associated effects on the QT interval. Therefore, precautions should be taken when using ciprofloxacin with concomitant drugs that can result in prolongation of the QT interval).
No products indexed under this heading.

Meclofenamate Sodium (Non-steroidal anti-inflammatory drugs in combination of very high doses of quinolones have been shown to provoke convulsions in pre-clinical studies).
No products indexed under this heading.

Mefenamic Acid (Non-steroidal anti-inflammatory drugs in combination of very high doses of quinolones have been shown to provoke convulsions in pre-clinical studies).
No products indexed under this heading.

Meloxicam (Non-steroidal anti-inflammatory drugs in combination of very high doses of quinolones have been shown to provoke convulsions in pre-clinical studies). Products include:
Mobic Oral Suspension **863**
Mobic Tablets **863**

Meprobamate (In general, elderly patients may be more susceptible to drug-associated effects on the QT interval. Therefore, precautions should be taken when using ciprofloxacin with concomitant drugs that can result in prolongation of the QT interval).
No products indexed under this heading.

Mesoridazine Besylate (In general, elderly patients may be more susceptible to drug-associated effects on the QT interval. Therefore, precautions should be taken when using ciprofloxacin with concomitant drugs that can result in prolongation of the QT interval).
No products indexed under this heading.

Methadone Hydrochloride (Ciprofloxacin is an inhibitor of the hepatic CYP1A2 enzyme pathway. Co-administration of ciprofloxacin and other drugs primarily metabolized by CYP1A2 results in increased plasma concentrations of the co-administered drug and could lead to clinically significant pharmacodynamic side effects of the co-administered drug).
No products indexed under this heading.

Methotrexate (Renal tubular transport of methotrexate may be inhibited by concomitant administration of ciprofloxacin potentially leading to increased plasma levels of methotrexate. This might increase the risk of methotrexate associated toxic reactions. Therefore, patients under methotrexate therapy should be carefully monitored when concomitant ciprofloxacin therapy is indicated).
No products indexed under this heading.

Methotrexate Sodium (Renal tubular transport of methotrexate may be inhibited by concomitant administration of ciprofloxacin potentially leading to increased plasma levels of methotrexate. This might increase the risk of methotrexate associated toxic reactions. Therefore, patients under methotrexate therapy should be carefully monitored when concomitant ciprofloxacin therapy is indicated).
No products indexed under this heading.

Methylprednisolone Acetate (Ruptures of the shoulder, hand, Achilles tendon, or other tendons that required surgical repair or resulted in prolonged disability have been reported in patients receiving ciprofloxacin. Post-marketing surveillance reports indicate that this risk may be increased in patients receiving concomitant corticosteroids, especially the elderly).
No products indexed under this heading.

Methylprednisolone Sodium Succinate (Ruptures of the shoulder, hand, Achilles tendon, or other tendons that required surgical repair or resulted in prolonged disability have been reported in patients receiving ciprofloxacin. Post-marketing surveillance reports indicate that this risk may be increased in patients receiving concomitant corticosteroids, especially the elderly).
No products indexed under this heading.

Metoclopramide Hydrochloride (Metoclopramide significantly accelerates the absorption of oral ciprofloxacin resulting in shorter time to reach maximum plasma concentrations. No significant effect was observed on the bioavailability of ciprofloxacin).
No products indexed under this heading.

Mexiletine Hydrochloride (In general, elderly patients may be more susceptible to drug-associated effects on the QT interval. Therefore, precautions should be taken when using ciprofloxacin with concomitant drugs that can result in prolongation of the QT interval).
No products indexed under this heading.

Midazolam Hydrochloride (In general, elderly patients may be more susceptible to drug-associated effects on the QT interval. Therefore, precautions should be taken when using ciprofloxacin with concomitant drugs that can result in prolongation of the QT interval).
No products indexed under this heading.

Mirtazapine (Ciprofloxacin is an inhibitor of the hepatic CYP1A2 enzyme pathway. Co-administration of ciprofloxacin and other drugs primarily metabolized by CYP1A2 results in increased plasma concentrations of the co-administered drug and could lead to clinically significant pharmacodynamic side effects of the co-administered drug). Products include:
Remeron Tablets **2924**
RemeronSolTab Tablets **2927**

Molindone Hydrochloride (In general, elderly patients may be more susceptible to drug-associated effects on the QT interval. Therefore, precautions should be taken when using ciprofloxacin with concomitant drugs that can result in prolongation of the QT interval). Products include:
Moban Tablets **1116**

Mometasone Furoate (Ruptures of the shoulder, hand, Achilles tendon, or other tendons that required surgical repair or resulted in prolonged disability have been reported in patients receiving ciprofloxacin. Post-marketing surveillance reports indicate that this risk may be increased in patients receiving concomitant corticosteroids, especially the elderly). Products include:
Asmanex Twisthaler **2797**
Elocon Cream 0.1% **2840**
Elocon Lotion 0.1% **2841**
Elocon Ointment 0.1% **2842**

Mometasone Furoate Monohydrate (Ruptures of the shoulder, hand, Achilles tendon, or other tendons that required surgical repair or resulted in prolonged disability have been reported in patients receiving ciprofloxacin. Post-marketing surveillance reports indicate that this risk may be increased in patients receiving concomitant corticosteroids, especially the elderly). Products include:
Nasonex Nasal Spray **2883**

Moricizine Hydrochloride (In general, eldery patients may be more susceptible to drug-associated effects on the QT interval. Therefore precautions should be taken when using ciprofloxacin with concomitant drugs that can result in prolongation of the QT interval (e.g., class IA antiarrhythmics)).
No products indexed under this heading.

Moxifloxacin Hydrochloride (Ciprofloxacin is an inhibitor of the hepatic CYP1A2 enzyme pathway. Co-administration of ciprofloxacin and other drugs primarily metabolized by CYP1A2 results in increased plasma concentrations of the co-administered drug and could lead to clinically significant pharmacodynamic side effects of the co-administered drug). Products include:
Avelox **2803**
Vigamox Ophthalmic Solution **548**

Nabumetone (Non-steroidal anti-inflammatory drugs in combination of very high doses of quinolones have been shown to provoke convulsions in pre-clinical studies).
No products indexed under this heading.

Nafcillin Sodium (Ciprofloxacin is an inhibitor of the hepatic CYP1A2 enzyme pathway. Co-administration of ciprofloxacin and other drugs primarily metabolized by CYP1A2 results in increased plasma concentrations of the co-administered drug and could lead to clinically significant pharmacodynamic side effects of the co-administered drug).
No products indexed under this heading.

Naproxen (Non-steroidal anti-inflammatory drugs in combination of very high doses of quinolones have been shown to provoke convulsions in pre-clinical studies). Products include:
EC-Naprosyn Delayed-Release Tablets **2632**
Naprosyn Suspension **2632**
Naprosyn Tablets **2632**

Naproxen Sodium (Non-steroidal anti-inflammatory drugs in combination of very high doses of quinolones have been shown to provoke convulsions in pre-clinical studies). Products include:
Anaprox Tablets **2632**
Anaprox DS Tablets **2632**
Treximet Tablets **1616**

Nicotine Polacrilex (Ciprofloxacin is an inhibitor of the hepatic CYP1A2 enzyme pathway. Co-administration of ciprofloxacin and other drugs primarily metabolized by CYP1A2 results in increased plasma concentrations of the co-administered drug and could lead to clinically significant pharmacodynamic side effects of the co-administered drug).
No products indexed under this heading.

Nicotine Salicylate (Ciprofloxacin is an inhibitor of the hepatic CYP1A2 enzyme pathway. Co-administration of ciprofloxacin and other drugs primarily metabolized by CYP1A2 results in increased plasma concentrations of the co-administered drug and could lead to clinically significant pharmacodynamic side effects of the co-administered drug).
No products indexed under this heading.

Nicotine Sulfate (Ciprofloxacin is an inhibitor of the hepatic CYP1A2 enzyme pathway. Co-administration of ciprofloxacin and other drugs primarily metabolized by CYP1A2 results in increased plasma concentrations of the co-administered drug and could lead to clinically significant pharmacodynamic side effects of the co-administered drug).
No products indexed under this heading.

Norethindrone Acetate (Ciprofloxacin is an inhibitor of the hepatic CYP1A2 enzyme pathway. Co-administration of ciprofloxacin and other drugs primarily metabolized by CYP1A2 results in increased plasma concentrations of the co-administered drug and could lead to clinically significant pharmacodynamic side effects of the co-administered drug). Products include:

Activella Tablets 2347

Norfloxacin (Ciprofloxacin is an inhibitor of the hepatic CYP1A2 enzyme pathway. Co-administration of ciprofloxacin and other drugs primarily metabolized by CYP1A2 results in increased plasma concentrations of the co-administered drug and could lead to clinically significant pharmacodynamic side effects of the co-administered drug). Products include:

Noroxin Tablets 2069

Nortriptyline Hydrochloride (In general, elderly patients may be more susceptible to drug-associated effects on the QT interval. Therefore, precautions should be taken when using ciprofloxacin with concomitant drugs that can result in prolongation of the QT interval).

No products indexed under this heading.

Ofloxacin (Ciprofloxacin is an inhibitor of the hepatic CYP1A2 enzyme pathway. Co-administration of ciprofloxacin and other drugs primarily metabolized by CYP1A2 results in increased plasma concentrations of the co-administered drug and could lead to clinically significant pharmacodynamic side effects of the co-administered drug). Products include:

Ofloxacin Ophthalmic Solution 0.3% .... ⊙ 243

Olanzapine (In general, elderly patients may be more susceptible to drug-associated effects on the QT interval. Therefore, precautions should be taken when using ciprofloxacin with concomitant drugs that can result in prolongation of the QT interval). Products include:

Symbyax Capsules 1871
Zyprexa Tablets 1883
Zyprexa IntraMuscular 1883
Zyprexa ZYDIS Orally Disintegrating Tablets 1883

Ondansetron (Ciprofloxacin is an inhibitor of the hepatic CYP1A2 enzyme pathway. Co-administration of ciprofloxacin and other drugs primarily metabolized by CYP1A2 results in increased plasma concentrations of the co-administered drug and could lead to clinically significant pharmacodynamic side effects of the co-administered drug). Products include:

Zofran ODT Orally Disintegrating Tablets 1687

Ondansetron Hydrochloride (Ciprofloxacin is an inhibitor of the hepatic CYP1A2 enzyme pathway. Co-administration of ciprofloxacin and other drugs primarily metabolized by CYP1A2 results in increased plasma concentrations of the co-administered drug and could lead to clinically significant pharmacodynamic side effects of the co-administered drug). Products include:

Zofran Injection 1682
Zofran 1687

Oxaprozin (Non-steroidal anti-inflammatory drugs in combination of very high doses of quinolones have been shown to provoke convulsions in pre-clinical studies).

No products indexed under this heading.

Oxazepam (In general, elderly patients may be more susceptible to drug-associated effects on the QT interval. Therefore, precautions should be taken when using ciprofloxacin with concomitant drugs that can result in prolongation of the QT interval).

No products indexed under this heading.

Perphenazine (In general, elderly patients may be more susceptible to drug-associated effects on the QT interval. Therefore, precautions should be taken when using ciprofloxacin with concomitant drugs that can result in prolongation of the QT interval).

No products indexed under this heading.

Phenelzine Sulfate (In general, elderly patients may be more susceptible to drug-associated effects on the QT interval. Therefore, precautions should be taken when using ciprofloxacin with concomitant drugs that can result in prolongation of the QT interval).

No products indexed under this heading.

Phenobarbital Sodium (Ciprofloxacin is an inhibitor of the hepatic CYP1A2 enzyme pathway. Co-administration of ciprofloxacin and other drugs primarily metabolized by CYP1A2 results in increased plasma concentrations of the co-administered drug and could lead to clinically significant pharmacodynamic side effects of the co-administered drug).

No products indexed under this heading.

Phenylbutazone (Non-steroidal anti-inflammatory drugs in combination of very high doses of quinolones have been shown to provoke convulsions in pre-clinical studies).

No products indexed under this heading.

Phenytoin (Altered serum levels of phenytoin (increased and decreased) have been reported in patients receiving concomitant ciprofloxacin).

No products indexed under this heading.

Phenytoin Sodium (Altered serum levels of phenytoin (increased and decreased) have been reported in patients receiving concomitant ciprofloxacin). Products include:

Phenytek Capsules 2192

Piroxicam (Non-steroidal anti-inflammatory drugs in combination of very high doses of quinolones have been shown to provoke convulsions in pre-clinical studies).

No products indexed under this heading.

Polysaccharide Iron Complex (Concurrent administration of ciprofloxacin with multivalent cation-containing products, such as products containing iron, may substantially decrease its absorption, resulting in serum and urine levels considerably lower than desired. Ciprofloxacin should be administered at least 2 hours before or 6 hours after products containing iron). Products include:

Nu-Iron 150 Capsules 2165

Prazepam (In general, elderly patients may be more susceptible to drug-associated effects on the QT interval. Therefore, precautions should be taken when using ciprofloxacin with concomitant drugs that can result in prolongation of the QT interval).

No products indexed under this heading.

Prednisolone Acetate (Ruptures of the shoulder, hand, Achilles tendon, or other tendons that required surgical repair or resulted in prolonged disability have been reported in patients receiving ciprofloxacin. Post-marketing surveillance reports indicate that this risk may be increased in patients receiving concomitant corticosteroids, especially the elderly). Products include:

Pred Forte Ophthalmic Suspension .... ⊙ 227
Pred Mild Ophthalmic Suspension .... ⊙ 230
Pred-G Ophthalmic Ointment .... ⊙ 229
Pred-G Ophthalmic Suspension .... ⊙ 228

Prednisolone Sodium Phosphate (Ruptures of the shoulder, hand, Achilles tendon, or other tendons that required surgical repair or resulted in prolonged disability have been reported in patients receiving ciprofloxacin. Post-marketing surveillance reports indicate that this risk may be increased in patients receiving concomitant corticosteroids, especially the elderly).

No products indexed under this heading.

Prednisolone Tebutate (Ruptures of the shoulder, hand, Achilles tendon, or other tendons that required surgical repair or resulted in prolonged disability have been reported in patients receiving ciprofloxacin. Post-marketing surveillance reports indicate that this risk may be increased in patients receiving concomitant corticosteroids, especially the elderly).

No products indexed under this heading.

Prednisone (Ruptures of the shoulder, hand, Achilles tendon, or other tendons that required surgical repair or resulted in prolonged disability have been reported in patients receiving ciprofloxacin. Post-marketing surveillance reports indicate that this risk may be increased in patients receiving concomitant corticosteroids, especially the elderly).

No products indexed under this heading.

Probenecid (Probenecid interferes with renal tubular secretion of ciprofloxacin and produces an increase in the level of ciprofloxacin in the serum. This should be considered if patients are receiving both drugs concomitantly).

No products indexed under this heading.

Procainamide (In general, eldery patients may be more susceptible to drug-associated effects on the QT interval. Therefore precautions should be taken when using ciprofloxacin with concomitant drugs that can result in prolongation of the QT interval (e.g., class IA antiarrhythmics)).

No products indexed under this heading.

Procainamide Hydrochloride (In general, elderly patients may be more susceptible to drug-associated effects on the QT interval. Therefore, precautions should be taken when using ciprofloxacin with concomitant drugs that can result in prolongation of the QT interval).

No products indexed under this heading.

Prochlorperazine (In general, elderly patients may be more susceptible to drug-associated effects on the QT interval. Therefore, precautions should be taken when using ciprofloxacin with concomitant drugs that can result in prolongation of the QT interval).

No products indexed under this heading.

Promethazine Hydrochloride (In general, elderly patients may be more susceptible to drug-associated effects on the QT interval. Therefore, precautions should be taken when using ciprofloxacin with concomitant drugs that can result in prolongation of the QT interval).

No products indexed under this heading.

Propafenone Hydrochloride (In general, elderly patients may be more susceptible to drug-associated effects on the QT interval. Therefore, precautions should be taken when using ciprofloxacin with concomitant drugs that can result in prolongation of the QT interval). Products include:

Rythmol Tablets 1586
Rythmol SR Capsules 1590

Propranolol Hydrochloride (Ciprofloxacin is an inhibitor of the hepatic CYP1A2 enzyme pathway. Co-administration of ciprofloxacin and other drugs primarily metabolized by CYP1A2 results in increased plasma concentrations of the co-administered drug and could lead to clinically significant pharmacodynamic side effects of the co-administered drug). Products include:

InnoPran XL Extended Release Capsules 1484

Protriptyline Hydrochloride (In general, elderly patients may be more susceptible to drug-associated effects on the QT interval. Therefore, precautions should be taken when using ciprofloxacin with concomitant drugs that can result in prolongation of the QT interval).

No products indexed under this heading.

Quetiapine Fumarate (In general, elderly patients may be more susceptible to drug-associated effects on the QT interval. Therefore, precautions should be taken when using ciprofloxacin with concomitant drugs that can result in prolongation of the QT interval).

No products indexed under this heading.

Quinidine (In general, eldery patients may be more susceptible to drug-associated effects on the QT interval. Therefore precautions should be taken when using ciprofloxacin with concomitant drugs that can result in prolongation of the QT interval (e.g., class IA antiarrhythmics)).

No products indexed under this heading.

Quinidine Gluconate (In general, elderly patients may be more susceptible to drug-associated effects on the QT interval. Therefore, precautions should be taken when using ciprofloxacin with concomitant drugs that can result in prolongation of the QT interval).
No products indexed under this heading.

Quinidine Polygalacturonate (In general, elderly patients may be more susceptible to drug-associated effects on the QT interval. Therefore, precautions should be taken when using ciprofloxacin with concomitant drugs that can result in prolongation of the QT interval).
No products indexed under this heading.

Quinidine Sulfate (In general, elderly patients may be more susceptible to drug-associated effects on the QT interval. Therefore, precautions should be taken when using ciprofloxacin with concomitant drugs that can result in prolongation of the QT interval).
No products indexed under this heading.

Riluzole (Ciprofloxacin is an inhibitor of the hepatic CYP1A2 enzyme pathway. Co-administration of ciprofloxacin and other drugs primarily metabolized by CYP1A2 results in increased plasma concentrations of the co-administered drug and could lead to clinically significant pharmacodynamic side effects of the co-administered drug). Products include:
Rilutek Tablets 2771

Risperidone (In general, elderly patients may be more susceptible to drug-associated effects on the QT interval. Therefore, precautions should be taken when using ciprofloxacin with concomitant drugs that can result in prolongation of the QT interval). Products include:
Risperdal Consta Long-Acting Injection 1753

Ritonavir (Ciprofloxacin is an inhibitor of the hepatic CYP1A2 enzyme pathway. Co-administration of ciprofloxacin and other drugs primarily metabolized by CYP1A2 results in increased plasma concentrations of the co-administered drug and could lead to clinically significant pharmacodynamic side effects of the co-administered drug). Products include:
Kaletra 452
Norvir 489

Rofecoxib (Non-steroidal anti-inflammatory drugs in combination of very high doses of quinolones have been shown to provoke convulsions in pre-clinical studies).
No products indexed under this heading.

Ropinirole Hydrochloride (Ciprofloxacin is an inhibitor of the hepatic CYP1A2 enzyme pathway. Co-administration of ciprofloxacin and other drugs primarily metabolized by CYP1A2 results in increased plasma concentrations of the co-administered drug and could lead to clinically significant pharmacodynamic side effects of the co-administered drug). Products include:
Requip Tablets 1561
Requip XL Tablets 1568

Ropivacaine Hydrochloride (Ciprofloxacin is an inhibitor of the hepatic CYP1A2 enzyme pathway. Co-administration of ciprofloxacin and other drugs primarily metabolized by CYP1A2 results in increased plasma concentrations of the co-administered drug and could lead to clinically significant pharmacodynamic side effects of the co-administered drug).
No products indexed under this heading.

Sotalol Hydrochloride (In general, elderly patients may be more susceptible to drug-associated effects on the QT interval. Therefore, precautions should be taken when using ciprofloxacin with concomitant drugs that can result in prolongation of the QT interval (e.g., class III antiarrhythmics)).
No products indexed under this heading.

Sucralfate (Concurrent administration of ciprofloxacin with multivalent cation-containing products, such as sucralfate, may substantially decrease its absorption, resulting in serum and urine levels considerably lower than desired. Ciprofloxacin should be administered at least 2 hours before or 6 hours after sucralfate). Products include:
Carafate Suspension 706
Carafate Tablets 707

Sulindac (Non-steroidal anti-inflammatory drugs in combination of very high doses of quinolones have been shown to provoke convulsions in pre-clinical studies). Products include:
Clinoril Tablets 1962

Tacrine Hydrochloride (Ciprofloxacin is an inhibitor of the hepatic CYP1A2 enzyme pathway. Co-administration of ciprofloxacin and other drugs primarily metabolized by CYP1A2 results in increased plasma concentrations of the co-administered drug and could lead to clinically significant pharmacodynamic side effects of the co-administered drug).
No products indexed under this heading.

Tamoxifen Citrate (Ciprofloxacin is an inhibitor of the hepatic CYP1A2 enzyme pathway. Co-administration of ciprofloxacin and other drugs primarily metabolized by CYP1A2 results in increased plasma concentrations of the co-administered drug and could lead to clinically significant pharmacodynamic side effects of the co-administered drug).
No products indexed under this heading.

Theophylline (Concurrent administration of ciprofloxacin with theophylline may lead to elevated serum concentrations of theophylline and prolongation of its elimination half-life. Serious and fatal reactions have been reported in patients receiving concurrent administration of ciprofloxacin and theophylline. These reactions have included cardiac arrest, seizures, status epilepticus, and respiratory failure. Although similar serious adverse effects have been reported in patients receiving theophylline alone, the possibility that these reactions may be potentiated by ciprofloxacin cannot be eliminated. If concomitant use cannot be avoided, serum levels of theophylline should be monitored and dosage adjustments made as appropriate).
No products indexed under this heading.

Theophylline Anhydrous (Concurrent administration of ciprofloxacin with theophylline may lead to elevated serum concentrations of theophylline and prolongation of its elimination half-life. Serious and fatal reactions have been reported in patients receiving concurrent administration of ciprofloxacin and theophylline. These reactions have included cardiac arrest, seizures, status epilepticus, and respiratory failure. Although similar serious adverse effects have been reported in patients receiving theophylline alone, the possibility that these reactions may be potentiated by ciprofloxacin cannot be eliminated. If concomitant use cannot be avoided, serum levels of theophylline should be monitored and dosage adjustments made as appropriate). Products include:
Uniphyl Tablets 2595

Theophylline Calcium Salicylate (Concurrent administration of ciprofloxacin with theophylline may lead to elevated serum concentrations of theophylline and prolongation of its elimination half-life. Serious and fatal reactions have been reported in patients receiving concurrent administration of ciprofloxacin and theophylline. These reactions have included cardiac arrest, seizures, status epilepticus, and respiratory failure. Although similar serious adverse effects have been reported in patients receiving theophylline alone, the possibility that these reactions may be potentiated by ciprofloxacin cannot be eliminated. If concomitant use cannot be avoided, serum levels of theophylline should be monitored and dosage adjustments made as appropriate).
No products indexed under this heading.

Theophylline Dihydroxypropyl (Glyceryl) (Concurrent administration of ciprofloxacin with theophylline may lead to elevated serum concentrations of theophylline and prolongation of its elimination half-life. Serious and fatal reactions have been reported in patients receiving concurrent administration of ciprofloxacin and theophylline. These reactions have included cardiac arrest, seizures, status epilepticus, and respiratory failure. Although similar serious adverse effects have been reported in patients receiving theophylline alone, the possibility that these reactions may be potentiated by ciprofloxacin cannot be eliminated. If concomitant use cannot be avoided, serum levels of theophylline should be monitored and dosage adjustments made as appropriate).
No products indexed under this heading.

Theophylline Ethylenediamine (Concurrent administration of ciprofloxacin with theophylline may lead to elevated serum concentrations of theophylline and prolongation of its elimination half-life. Serious and fatal reactions have been reported in patients receiving concurrent administration of ciprofloxacin and theophylline. These reactions have included cardiac arrest, seizures, status epilepticus, and respiratory failure. Although similar serious adverse effects have been reported in patients receiving theophylline alone, the possibility that these reactions may be potentiated by ciprofloxacin cannot be eliminated. If concomitant use cannot be avoided, serum levels of theophylline should be monitored and dosage adjustments made as appropriate).
No products indexed under this heading.

Theophylline Sodium Glycinate (Concurrent administration of ciprofloxacin with theophylline may lead to elevated serum concentrations of theophylline and prolongation of its elimination half-life. Serious and fatal reactions have been reported in patients receiving concurrent administration of ciprofloxacin and theophylline. These reactions have included cardiac arrest, seizures, status epilepticus, and respiratory failure. Although similar serious adverse effects have been reported in patients receiving theophylline alone, the possibility that these reactions may be potentiated by ciprofloxacin cannot be eliminated. If concomitant use cannot be avoided, serum levels of theophylline should be monitored and dosage adjustments made as appropriate).
No products indexed under this heading.

Thioridazine Hydrochloride (In general, elderly patients may be more susceptible to drug-associated effects on the QT interval. Therefore, precautions should be taken when using ciprofloxacin with concomitant drugs that can result in prolongation of the QT interval). Products include:
Thioridazine Hydrochloride Tablets 2195

Thiothixene (In general, elderly patients may be more susceptible to drug-associated effects on the QT interval. Therefore, precautions should be taken when using ciprofloxacin with concomitant drugs that can result in prolongation of the QT interval). Products include:
Thiothixene Capsules 2197

Tizanidine (In a pharmacokinetic study, systemic exposure of tizanidine (4 mg single dose) was significantly increased (Cmax 7-fold, AUC 10-fold) when the drug was given concomitantly with ciprofloxacin (500 mg b.i.d. for 3 days). The hypotensive and sedative effects to tizanidine were also potentiated. Concomitant administration of tizanidine and ciprofloxacin is contraindicated).
No products indexed under this heading.

Tizanidine Hydrochloride (In a pharmacokinetic study, systemic exposure of tizanidine (4 mg single dose) was significantly increased (Cmax 7-fold, AUC 10-fold) when the drug was given concomitantly with ciprofloxacin (500 mg b.i.d. for 3 days). The hypotensive and sedative effects to tizanidine were also potentiated. Concomitant administration of tizanidine and ciprofloxacin is contraindicated).
No products indexed under this heading.

Tocainide Hydrochloride (In general, elderly patients may be more susceptible to drug-associated effects on the QT interval. Therefore, precautions should be taken when using ciprofloxacin with concomitant drugs that can result in prolongation of the QT interval).
No products indexed under this heading.

Tolmetin Sodium (Non-steroidal anti-inflammatory drugs in combination of very high doses of quinolones have been shown to provoke convulsions in pre-clinical studies).
No products indexed under this heading.

Tranylcypromine Sulfate (In general, elderly patients may be more susceptible to drug-associated effects on the QT interval. Therefore, precautions should be taken when using ciprofloxacin with concomitant drugs that can result in prolongation of the QT interval). Products include:
Parnate Tablets 1532

Triamcinolone (Ruptures of the shoulder, hand, Achilles tendon, or other tendons that required surgical repair or resulted in prolonged disability have been reported in patients receiving ciprofloxacin. Post-marketing surveillance reports indicate that this risk may be increased in patients receiving concomitant corticosteroids, especially the elderly).
No products indexed under this heading.

Triamcinolone Acetonide (Ruptures of the shoulder, hand, Achilles tendon, or other tendons that required surgical repair or resulted in prolonged disability have been reported in patients receiving ciprofloxacin. Post-marketing surveillance reports indicate that this risk may be increased in patients receiving concomitant corticosteroids, especially the elderly). Products include:
Azmacort Inhalation Aerosol 407
Nasacort AQ Nasal Spray 2765
Triesence Injectable Suspension .... ⊙209

Triamcinolone Diacetate (Ruptures of the shoulder, hand, Achilles tendon, or other tendons that required surgical repair or resulted in prolonged disability have been reported in patients receiving ciprofloxacin. Post-marketing surveillance reports indicate that this risk may be increased in patients receiving concomitant corticosteroids, especially the elderly).
No products indexed under this heading.

Triamcinolone Hexacetonide (Ruptures of the shoulder, hand, Achilles tendon, or other tendons that required surgical repair or resulted in prolonged disability have been reported in patients receiving ciprofloxacin. Post-marketing surveillance reports indicate that this risk may be increased in patients receiving concomitant corticosteroids, especially the elderly).
No products indexed under this heading.

Trifluoperazine Hydrochloride (In general, elderly patients may be more susceptible to drug-associated effects on the QT interval. Therefore, precautions should be taken when using ciprofloxacin with concomitant drugs that can result in prolongation of the QT interval).
No products indexed under this heading.

Trimethaphan Camsylate (Ciprofloxacin is an inhibitor of the hepatic CYP1A2 enzyme pathway. Co-administration of ciprofloxacin and other drugs primarily metabolized by CYP1A2 results in increased plasma concentrations of the co-administered drug and could lead to clinically significant pharmacodynamic side effects of the co-administered drug).
No products indexed under this heading.

Trimipramine Maleate (In general, elderly patients may be more susceptible to drug-associated effects on the QT interval. Therefore, precautions should be taken when using ciprofloxacin with concomitant drugs that can result in prolongation of the QT interval).
No products indexed under this heading.

Trovafloxacin Mesylate (Ciprofloxacin is an inhibitor of the hepatic CYP1A2 enzyme pathway. Co-administration of ciprofloxacin and other drugs primarily metabolized by CYP1A2 results in increased plasma concentrations of the co-administered drug and could lead to clinically significant pharmacodynamic side effects of the co-administered drug).
No products indexed under this heading.

Valdecoxib (Non-steroidal anti-inflammatory drugs in combination of very high doses of quinolones have been shown to provoke convulsions in pre-clinical studies).
No products indexed under this heading.

Verapamil Hydrochloride (Ciprofloxacin is an inhibitor of the hepatic CYP1A2 enzyme pathway. Co-administration of ciprofloxacin and other drugs primarily metabolized by CYP1A2 results in increased plasma concentrations of the co-administered drug and could lead to clinically significant pharmacodynamic side effects of the co-administered drug). Products include:
Tarka Tablets 511

Warfarin Sodium (Ciprofloxacin has been reported to enhance the effects of the oral anticoagulant warfarin or its derivatives. When these products are administered concomitantly, prothrombin time or other suitable coagulant tests should be closely monitored).
No products indexed under this heading.

Zileuton (Ciprofloxacin is an inhibitor of the hepatic CYP1A2 enzyme pathway. Co-administration of ciprofloxacin and other drugs primarily metabolized by CYP1A2 results in increased plasma concentrations of the co-administered drug and could lead to clinically significant pharmacodynamic side effects of the co-administered drug).
No products indexed under this heading.

Zinc (Concurrent administration of ciprofloxacin with multivalent cation-containing products, such as products containing zinc, may substantially decrease its absorption, resulting in serum and urine levels considerably lower than desired. Ciprofloxacin should be administered at least 2 hours before or 6 hours after products containing iron). Products include:
Comax Dietary Supplement 995
Glaucofit Dietary Supplement 995
Glauma Dietary Supplement 995
Tonox Dietary Supplement 995
Vibe Liquid Multi-Nutrient Supplement .... ▣626
Visutein Capsules 3159

Ziprasidone Hydrochloride (In general, elderly patients may be more susceptible to drug-associated effects on the QT interval. Therefore, precautions should be taken when using ciprofloxacin with concomitant drugs that can result in prolongation of the QT interval). Products include:
Geodon Capsules 2520

Zolmitriptan (Ciprofloxacin is an inhibitor of the hepatic CYP1A2 enzyme pathway. Co-administration of ciprofloxacin and other drugs primarily metabolized by CYP1A2 results in increased plasma concentrations of the co-administered drug and could lead to clinically significant pharmacodynamic side effects of the co-administered drug). Products include:
Zomig Tablets 694
Zomig Nasal Spray 689
Zomig-ZMT Tablets 694

Food Interactions

Dairy products (Ciprofloxacin should not be taken with dairy products (like milk or yogurt) alone since absorption of ciprofloxacin may be significantly reduced; however, ciprofloxacin may be taken with a meal that contains these products).

Food, unspecified (When ciprofloxacin tablets are given concomitantly with food, there is a delay in the absorption of the drug, resulting in peak concentrations that occur closer to 2 hours after dosing rather than 1 hour, whereas there is no delay observed when ciprofloxacin suspension is given with food. The overall absorption of ciprofloxacin tablets or ciprofloxacin suspension, however, is not substantially affected. The pharmacokinetics of ciprofloxacin given as the suspension are also not affected by food).

Fruit juices, unspecified (Ciprofloxacin should not be taken with calcium-fortified juices alone since absorption of ciprofloxacin may be significantly reduced; however, ciprofloxacin may be taken with a meal that contains these products).

CIPRO XR TABLETS

(Ciprofloxacin) 2823

May interact with antacids containing aluminum, calcium and magnesium, nonabsorbable antacids, calcium preparations, cations, corticosteroids, oral anticoagulants, cytochrome p450 1a2 substrates (selected), iron containing oral preparations, non-steroidal anti-inflammatory agents, phenytoin, theophyllines, and certain other agents. Compounds in these categories include:

Acetaminophen (Ciprofloxacin is an inhibitor of the hepatic CYP1A2 enzyme pathway. Co-administration of ciprofloxacin and other drugs primarily metabolized by CYP1A2 results in increased plasma concentrations of the co-administered drug and could lead to clinically significant pharmacodynamic side effects of the co-administered drug). Products include:
Benadryl Allergy & Cold Kapgels 1895
Benadryl Allergy & Sinus Headache Kapgels 1895
Benadryl Severe Allergy & Sinus Headache Caplets 1897
Lortab 5/500 Tablets 3143
Lortab 7.5/500 Tablets 3144
Lortab 10/500 Tablets 3144
Percocet Tablets 1127
Sinutab Sinus Caplets 1905
Sudafed PE Cold & Cough Caplets 1907
Sudafed PE Nighttime Cold Caplets 1907
Sudafed PE Severe Cold Caplets 1908
Sudafed PE Sinus Headache Caplets 1908
Regular Strength Tylenol Tablets 1915
Tylenol 8 Hour Extended Release Caplets 1915
Extra Strength Tylenol Caplets, Cool Caplets, and EZ Tabs 1915
Extra Strength Tylenol Adult Rapid Blast Liquid 1915
Extra Strength Tylenol PM Caplets, Geltabs, Liquid, and Rapid Release Gels 1915
Extra Strength Tylenol Rapid Release Gels 1915
Tylenol with Codeine Tablets 2427
Tylenol Allergy Multi-Symptom Caplets with Cool Burst and Rapid Release Gelcaps 1916
Tylenol Allergy Multi-Symptom Nighttime Caplets with Cool Burst 1916
Tylenol Severe Allergy Caplets 1916
Tylenol Arthritis Pain Extended Release Geltabs/Caplets 1915
Tylenol Chest Congestion Caplets with Cool Burst 1910
Tylenol Chest Congestion Liquid with Cool Burst 1910
Children's Tylenol Plus Cold Suspension Liquid 1912
Children's Tylenol Plus Cold & Allergy Suspension Liquid 1914
Children's Tylenol Plus Cough & Runny Nose Suspension Liquid 1912
Children's Tylenol Plus Cough & Sore Throat Suspension Liquid 1912
Children's Tylenol Plus Flu Suspension Liquid 1914
Children's Tylenol Suspension Liquid 1909
Children's Tylenol Meltaways 1909
Children's Tylenol Plus Multi-Symptom Cold Suspension Liquid 1912
Tylenol Cold Severe Congestion Daytime Caplets with Cool Burst 1912
Tylenol Cold Head Congestion Daytime Caplets with Cool Burst 1910
Tylenol Cold Head Congestion Nighttime Caplets with Cool Burst 1910
Tylenol Cold Head Congestion Severe Daytime Caplets with Cool Burst 1910
Tylenol Cold Multi-Symptom Daytime Caplets with Cool Burst and Rapid Release Gels 1913
Tylenol Cold Multi-Symptom Daytime Liquid with Citrus Burst ... 1913
Tylenol Cold Multi-Symptom Nighttime Caplets with Cool Burst 1913
Tylenol Cold Multi-Symptom Nighttime Liquid with Cool Burst ... 1913
Tylenol Cold Multi-Symptom Severe Caplets with Cool Burst 1913
Tylenol Cold Multi-Symptom Severe Daytime Liquid with Citrus Burst 1913
Tylenol Cough & Sore Throat Daytime Liquid with Cool Burst 1918
Tylenol Cough & Sore Throat Nighttime Liquid with Cool Burst ... 1918
Concentrated Tylenol Infants' Drops 1909
Jr. Tylenol Meltaways 1909
Tylenol Sinus Congestion & Pain Daytime Caplets with Cool Burst and Gelcaps 1917

Tylenol Sinus Congestion & Pain Nighttime Caplets with Cool Burst........ 1917
Tylenol Sinus Congestion & Pain Severe Caplets with Cool Burst..... 1917
Tylenol Sinus Severe Congestion Caplets with Cool Burst........ 1917
Tylenol Sore Throat Daytime Liquid with Cool Burst........ 1918
Tylenol Sore Throat Nighttime Liquid with Cool Burst........ 1918
Women's Tylenol Menstrual Relief Caplets........ 1919
Vicks DayQuil Cold & Flu Multi-Symptom Relief........ 616
Vicks DayQuil LiquiCaps........ 2567
Vicks DayQuil Liquid........ 2567
Vicks DayQuil Multi-Symptom Cold/Flu Relief........ 2567
Vicks NyQuil Cold & Flu Multi-Symptom Relief........ 617
Vicks NyQuil LiquiCaps........ 2567
Vicks NyQuil Liquid........ 2567
Vicks NyQuil Multi-Symptom Cold/Flu Relief........ 2567
Vicodin Tablets........ 529
Vicodin ES Tablets........ 530
Vicodin HP Tablets........ 531
Zydone Tablets........ 1132

Alatrofloxacin Mesylate (Ciprofloxacin is an inhibitor of the hepatic CYP1A2 enzyme pathway. Co-administration of ciprofloxacin and other drugs primarily metabolized by CYP1A2 results in increased plasma concentrations of the co-administered drug and could lead to clinically significant pharmacodynamic side effects of the co-administered drug).
No products indexed under this heading.

Aluminum Carbonate (When ciprofloxacin extended release tablets, given as a single 1000 mg dose, were administered 2 hours before or 4 hours after a magnesium/aluminum-containing antacid (900 mg aluminum hydroxide and 600 mg magnesium hydroxide as a single oral dose) to 18 healthy volunteers, there was a 4% and 19% reduction, respectively, in the mean Cmax of ciprofloxacin. The reduction in the mean AUC was 24% and 26%, respectively. Ciprofloxacin extended release tablets should be administered at least 2 hours before or 6 hours after antacids containing magnesium or aluminum).
No products indexed under this heading.

Aluminum-containing Compounds, unspecified (Concurrent administration of ciprofloxacin with multivalent cation-containing products may substantially interfere with the absorption of ciprofloxacin, resulting in serum and urine levels considerably lower than desired. Ciprofloxacin extended release tablets should be administered at least 2 hours before or 6 hours after metal cations).
No products indexed under this heading.

Aluminum Hydroxide (When ciprofloxacin extended release tablets, given as a single 1000 mg dose, were administered 2 hours before or 4 hours after a magnesium/aluminum-containing antacid (900 mg aluminum hydroxide and 600 mg magnesium hydroxide as a single oral dose) to 18 healthy volunteers, there was a 4% and 19% reduction, respectively, in the mean Cmax of ciprofloxacin. The reduction in the mean AUC was 24% and 26%, respectively. Ciprofloxacin extended release tablets should be administered at least 2 hours before or 6 hours after antacids containing magnesium or aluminum).
No products indexed under this heading.

Amiodarone Hydrochloride (Ciprofloxacin is an inhibitor of the hepatic CYP1A2 enzyme pathway. Co-administration of ciprofloxacin and other drugs primarily metabolized by CYP1A2 results in increased plasma concentrations of the co-administered drug and could lead to clinically significant pharmacodynamic side effects of the co-administered drug).
No products indexed under this heading.

Amitriptyline Hydrochloride (Ciprofloxacin is an inhibitor of the hepatic CYP1A2 enzyme pathway. Co-administration of ciprofloxacin and other drugs primarily metabolized by CYP1A2 results in increased plasma concentrations of the co-administered drug and could lead to clinically significant pharmacodynamic side effects of the co-administered drug).
No products indexed under this heading.

Amoxapine (Ciprofloxacin is an inhibitor of the hepatic CYP1A2 enzyme pathway. Co-administration of ciprofloxacin and other drugs primarily metabolized by CYP1A2 results in increased plasma concentrations of the co-administered drug and could lead to clinically significant pharmacodynamic side effects of the co-administered drug).
No products indexed under this heading.

Anagrelide Hydrochloride (Ciprofloxacin is an inhibitor of the hepatic CYP1A2 enzyme pathway. Co-administration of ciprofloxacin and other drugs primarily metabolized by CYP1A2 results in increased plasma concentrations of the co-administered drug and could lead to clinically significant pharmacodynamic side effects of the co-administered drug). Products include:
Agrylin Capsules........ 3017

Anisindione (Ciprofloxacin has been reported to enhance the effects of the oral anticoagulant warfarin or its derivatives. When these products are administered concomitantly, prothrombin time or other suitable coagulation tests should be closely monitored).
No products indexed under this heading.

Betamethasone Acetate (The risk of serious tendon disorders with quinolones is higher in those over 65 years of age, especially those on corticosteroids).
No products indexed under this heading.

Betamethasone Sodium Phosphate (The risk of serious tendon disorders with quinolones is higher in those over 65 years of age, especially those on corticosteroids).
No products indexed under this heading.

Budesonide (The risk of serious tendon disorders with quinolones is higher in those over 65 years of age, especially those on corticosteroids). Products include:
Pulmicort Flexhaler........ 654
Symbicort 80/4.5 Inhalation Aerosol........ 659
Symbicort 160/4.5 Inhalation Aerosol........ 659

Caffeine (Ciprofloxacin has been shown to interfere with the metabolism of caffeine. This may lead to reduced clearance of caffeine and a prolongation of its serum half-life). Products include:
BioLean Free Tablets........ 635
BioLean II Tablets........ 635
Winrgy Dietary Supplement........ 642

Caffeine Anhydrous (Ciprofloxacin has been shown to interfere with the metabolism of caffeine. This may lead to reduced clearance of caffeine and a prolongation of its serum half-life).
No products indexed under this heading.

Caffeine Citrate (Ciprofloxacin has been shown to interfere with the metabolism of caffeine. This may lead to reduced clearance of caffeine and a prolongation of its serum half-life).
No products indexed under this heading.

Calcium (Concurrent administration of ciprofloxacin with multivalent cation-containing products may substantially interfere with the absorption of ciprofloxacin, resulting in serum and urine levels considerably lower than desired. Ciprofloxacin extended release tablets should be administered at least 2 hours before or 6 hours after metal cations). Products include:
Phyto-Vite Tablets........ 639
Vibe Liquid Multi-Nutrient Supplement........ 626

Calcium Carbonate (Concurrent administration of ciprofloxacin with multivalent cation-containing products, such as products containing calcium, may substantially interfere with the absorption of ciprofloxacin, resulting in serum and urine levels considerably lower than desired). Products include:
Accelerator Tablets........ 634
Actonel with Calcium Tablets........ 2574
BioLean II Tablets........ 635
Calcet Triple Calcium + Vitamin D Tablets........ 629
D-Cal Chewable Caplets........ 624
Elixir Capsules........ 636
Pepcid Complete Chewable Tablets........ 1771
Extra Strength Rolaids Plus Gas Relief Tropical Fruit Softchews........ 1903
Extra Strength Rolaids Softchews Vanilla Creme........ 1903
Extra Strength Rolaids Freshmint Tablets........ 1903
Rolaids Multi-Symptom Berry Tablets........ 1903
Rolaids Original Peppermint Tablets........ 1903

Calcium Chloride (Concurrent administration of ciprofloxacin with multivalent cation-containing products, such as products containing calcium, may substantially interfere with the absorption of ciprofloxacin, resulting in serum and urine levels considerably lower than desired).
No products indexed under this heading.

Calcium Citrate (Concurrent administration of ciprofloxacin with multivalent cation-containing products, such as products containing calcium, may substantially interfere with the absorption of ciprofloxacin, resulting in serum and urine levels considerably lower than desired). Products include:
Active Calcium Tablets........ 3173
CitraNatal DHA Tablets........ 2175
CitraNatal 90 DHA Tablets........ 2175

Calcium Glubionate (Concurrent administration of ciprofloxacin with multivalent cation-containing products, such as products containing calcium, may substantially interfere with the absorption of ciprofloxacin, resulting in serum and urine levels considerably lower than desired).
No products indexed under this heading.

Celecoxib (Non-steroidal anti-inflammatory drugs, in combination with very high doses of quinolones, have been shown to provoke convulsions in pre-clinical studies). Products include:
Celebrex Capsules........ 2979

Chlordiazepoxide (Ciprofloxacin is an inhibitor of the hepatic CYP1A2 enzyme pathway. Co-administration of ciprofloxacin and other drugs primarily metabolized by CYP1A2 results in increased plasma concentrations of the co-administered drug and could lead to clinically significant pharmacodynamic side effects of the co-administered drug).
No products indexed under this heading.

Chlordiazepoxide Hydrochloride (Ciprofloxacin is an inhibitor of the hepatic CYP1A2 enzyme pathway. Co-administration of ciprofloxacin and other drugs primarily metabolized by CYP1A2 results in increased plasma concentrations of the co-administered drug and could lead to clinically significant pharmacodynamic side effects of the co-administered drug).
No products indexed under this heading.

Ciclesonide (The risk of serious tendon disorders with quinolones is higher in those over 65 years of age, especially those on corticosteroids). Products include:
Alvesco Inhalation Aerosol........ 2985
Omnaris Nasal Spray........ 2998

Cimetidine Hydrochloride (Ciprofloxacin is an inhibitor of the hepatic CYP1A2 enzyme pathway. Co-administration of ciprofloxacin and other drugs primarily metabolized by CYP1A2 results in increased plasma concentrations of the co-administered drug and could lead to clinically significant pharmacodynamic side effects of the co-administered drug).
No products indexed under this heading.

Ciprofloxacin Hydrochloride (Ciprofloxacin is an inhibitor of the hepatic CYP1A2 enzyme pathway. Co-administration of ciprofloxacin and other drugs primarily metabolized by CYP1A2 results in increased plasma concentrations of the co-administered drug and could lead to clinically significant pharmacodynamic side effects of the co-administered drug). Products include:
Cipro Tablets........ 2810

Clomipramine Hydrochloride (Ciprofloxacin is an inhibitor of the hepatic CYP1A2 enzyme pathway. Co-administration of ciprofloxacin and other drugs primarily metabolized by CYP1A2 results in increased plasma concentrations of the co-administered drug and could lead to clinically significant pharmacodynamic side effects of the co-administered drug).
No products indexed under this heading.

Clopidogrel Bisulfate (Ciprofloxacin is an inhibitor of the hepatic CYP1A2 enzyme pathway. Co-administration of ciprofloxacin and other drugs primarily metabolized by CYP1A2 results in increased plasma concentrations of the co-administered drug and could lead to clinically significant pharmacodynamic side effects of the co-administered drug). Products include:

Plavix Tablets 926
Plavix Tablets 2767

Clozapine (Ciprofloxacin is an inhibitor of the hepatic CYP1A2 enzyme pathway. Co-administration of ciprofloxacin and other drugs primarily metabolized by CYP1A2 results in increased plasma concentrations of the co-administered drug and could lead to clinically significant pharmacodynamic side effects of the co-administered drug).

No products indexed under this heading.

Cortisone Acetate (The risk of serious tendon disorders with quinolones is higher in those over 65 years of age, especially those on corticosteroids).

No products indexed under this heading.

Cyclobenzaprine (Ciprofloxacin is an inhibitor of the hepatic CYP1A2 enzyme pathway. Co-administration of ciprofloxacin and other drugs primarily metabolized by CYP1A2 results in increased plasma concentrations of the co-administered drug and could lead to clinically significant pharmacodynamic side effects of the co-administered drug).

No products indexed under this heading.

Cyclobenzaprine Hydrochloride (Ciprofloxacin is an inhibitor of the hepatic CYP1A2 enzyme pathway. Co-administration of ciprofloxacin and other drugs primarily metabolized by CYP1A2 results in increased plasma concentrations of the co-administered drug and could lead to clinically significant pharmacodynamic side effects of the co-administered drug). Products include:

Amrix Capsules 966

Cyclosporine (Ciprofloxacin has been associated with transient elevations in serum creatinine in patients receiving cyclosporine concomitantly). Products include:

Gengraf Capsules 435
Neoral Oral Solution 2280
Neoral Soft Gelatin Capsules 2280
Restasis Ophthalmic Emulsion 557
Sandimmune 2296

Desipramine Hydrochloride (Ciprofloxacin is an inhibitor of the hepatic CYP1A2 enzyme pathway. Co-administration of ciprofloxacin and other drugs primarily metabolized by CYP1A2 results in increased plasma concentrations of the co-administered drug and could lead to clinically significant pharmacodynamic side effects of the co-administered drug).

No products indexed under this heading.

Dexamethasone (The risk of serious tendon disorders with quinolones is higher in those over 65 years of age, especially those on corticosteroids). Products include:

Ciprodex Otic Suspension 541

Dexamethasone Acetate (The risk of serious tendon disorders with quinolones is higher in those over 65 years of age, especially those on corticosteroids).

No products indexed under this heading.

Dexamethasone Sodium Phosphate (The risk of serious tendon disorders with quinolones is higher in those over 65 years of age, especially those on corticosteroids).

No products indexed under this heading.

Diazepam (Ciprofloxacin is an inhibitor of the hepatic CYP1A2 enzyme pathway. Co-administration of ciprofloxacin and other drugs primarily metabolized by CYP1A2 results in increased plasma concentrations of the co-administered drug and could lead to clinically significant pharmacodynamic side effects of the co-administered drug). Products include:

Valium Tablets 2658

Diclofenac Epolamine (Non-steroidal anti-inflammatory drugs, in combination with very high doses of quinolones, have been shown to provoke convulsions in pre-clinical studies). Products include:

Flector Patch 561

Diclofenac Potassium (Non-steroidal anti-inflammatory drugs, in combination with very high doses of quinolones, have been shown to provoke convulsions in pre-clinical studies).

No products indexed under this heading.

Diclofenac Sodium (Non-steroidal anti-inflammatory drugs, in combination with very high doses of quinolones, have been shown to provoke convulsions in pre-clinical studies). Products include:

Diclofenac Sodium Ophthalmic Solution .... ⊙240
Voltaren Ophthalmic Solution 2336
Voltaren Tablets 2334
Voltaren-XR Tablets 2337

Dicumarol (Ciprofloxacin has been reported to enhance the effects of the oral anticoagulant warfarin or its derivatives. When these products are administered concomitantly, prothrombin time or other suitable coagulation tests should be closely monitored).

No products indexed under this heading.

Didanosine (Concurrent administration of ciprofloxacin with multivalent cation-containing products, such as didanosine chewable/buffered tablets or pediatric powder, may substantially interfere with the absorption of ciprofloxacin, resulting in serum and urine levels considerably lower than desired. Ciprofloxacin extended release tablets should be administered at least 2 hours before or 6 hours after didanosine).

No products indexed under this heading.

Diltiazem Hydrochloride (Ciprofloxacin is an inhibitor of the hepatic CYP1A2 enzyme pathway. Co-administration of ciprofloxacin and other drugs primarily metabolized by CYP1A2 results in increased plasma concentrations of the co-administered drug and could lead to clinically significant pharmacodynamic side effects of the co-administered drug). Products include:

Cardizem LA Extended Release Tablets 421

Diltiazem Maleate (Ciprofloxacin is an inhibitor of the hepatic CYP1A2 enzyme pathway. Co-administration of ciprofloxacin and other drugs primarily metabolized by CYP1A2 results in increased plasma concentrations of the co-administered drug and could lead to clinically significant pharmacodynamic side effects of the co-administered drug).

No products indexed under this heading.

Doxepin Hydrochloride (Ciprofloxacin is an inhibitor of the hepatic CYP1A2 enzyme pathway. Co-administration of ciprofloxacin and other drugs primarily metabolized by CYP1A2 results in increased plasma concentrations of the co-administered drug and could lead to clinically significant pharmacodynamic side effects of the co-administered drug).

No products indexed under this heading.

Enoxacin (Ciprofloxacin is an inhibitor of the hepatic CYP1A2 enzyme pathway. Co-administration of ciprofloxacin and other drugs primarily metabolized by CYP1A2 results in increased plasma concentrations of the co-administered drug and could lead to clinically significant pharmacodynamic side effects of the co-administered drug).

No products indexed under this heading.

Erythromycin (Ciprofloxacin is an inhibitor of the hepatic CYP1A2 enzyme pathway. Co-administration of ciprofloxacin and other drugs primarily metabolized by CYP1A2 results in increased plasma concentrations of the co-administered drug and could lead to clinically significant pharmacodynamic side effects of the co-administered drug).

No products indexed under this heading.

Erythromycin Estolate (Ciprofloxacin is an inhibitor of the hepatic CYP1A2 enzyme pathway. Co-administration of ciprofloxacin and other drugs primarily metabolized by CYP1A2 results in increased plasma concentrations of the co-administered drug and could lead to clinically significant pharmacodynamic side effects of the co-administered drug).

No products indexed under this heading.

Erythromycin Ethylsuccinate (Ciprofloxacin is an inhibitor of the hepatic CYP1A2 enzyme pathway. Co-administration of ciprofloxacin and other drugs primarily metabolized by CYP1A2 results in increased plasma concentrations of the co-administered drug and could lead to clinically significant pharmacodynamic side effects of the co-administered drug). Products include:

E.E.S. 433
EryPed 431

Erythromycin Gluceptate (Ciprofloxacin is an inhibitor of the hepatic CYP1A2 enzyme pathway. Co-administration of ciprofloxacin and other drugs primarily metabolized by CYP1A2 results in increased plasma concentrations of the co-administered drug and could lead to clinically significant pharmacodynamic side effects of the co-administered drug).

No products indexed under this heading.

Erythromycin Lactobionate (Ciprofloxacin is an inhibitor of the hepatic CYP1A2 enzyme pathway. Co-administration of ciprofloxacin and other drugs primarily metabolized by CYP1A2 results in increased plasma concentrations of the co-administered drug and could lead to clinically significant pharmacodynamic side effects of the co-administered drug).

No products indexed under this heading.

Erythromycin Stearate (Ciprofloxacin is an inhibitor of the hepatic CYP1A2 enzyme pathway. Co-administration of ciprofloxacin and other drugs primarily metabolized by CYP1A2 results in increased plasma concentrations of the co-administered drug and could lead to clinically significant pharmacodynamic side effects of the co-administered drug).

No products indexed under this heading.

Estradiol (Ciprofloxacin is an inhibitor of the hepatic CYP1A2 enzyme pathway. Co-administration of ciprofloxacin and other drugs primarily metabolized by CYP1A2 results in increased plasma concentrations of the co-administered drug and could lead to clinically significant pharmacodynamic side effects of the co-administered drug). Products include:

Activella Tablets 2347
Angeliq Tablets 751
Climara Transdermal System 763
Climara Pro Transdermal System 768
Divigel 3167
Vagifem Tablets 2375

Estradiol Benzoate (Ciprofloxacin is an inhibitor of the hepatic CYP1A2 enzyme pathway. Co-administration of ciprofloxacin and other drugs primarily metabolized by CYP1A2 results in increased plasma concentrations of the co-administered drug and could lead to clinically significant pharmacodynamic side effects of the co-administered drug).

No products indexed under this heading.

Estradiol Cypionate (Ciprofloxacin is an inhibitor of the hepatic CYP1A2 enzyme pathway. Co-administration of ciprofloxacin and other drugs primarily metabolized by CYP1A2 results in increased plasma concentrations of the co-administered drug and could lead to clinically significant pharmacodynamic side effects of the co-administered drug).

No products indexed under this heading.

Etodolac (Non-steroidal anti-inflammatory drugs, in combination with very high doses of quinolones, have been shown to provoke convulsions in pre-clinical studies).

No products indexed under this heading.

Fenoprofen Calcium (Non-steroidal anti-inflammatory drugs, in combination with very high doses of quinolones, have been shown to provoke convulsions in pre-clinical studies). Products include:
Nalfon Capsules 2508

Ferrous Fumarate (Concurrent administration of ciprofloxacin with multivalent cation-containing products, such as products containing iron, may substantially interfere with the absorption of ciprofloxacin, resulting in serum and urine levels considerably lower than desired. Ciprofloxacin extended release tablets should be administered at least 2 hours before or 6 hours after metal cations such as iron).
No products indexed under this heading.

Ferrous Gluconate (Concurrent administration of ciprofloxacin with multivalent cation-containing products, such as products containing iron, may substantially interfere with the absorption of ciprofloxacin, resulting in serum and urine levels considerably lower than desired. Ciprofloxacin extended release tablets should be administered at least 2 hours before or 6 hours after metal cations such as iron). Products include:
CitraNatal DHA Tablets 2175

Ferrous Sulfate (Concurrent administration of ciprofloxacin with multivalent cation-containing products, such as products containing iron, may substantially interfere with the absorption of ciprofloxacin, resulting in serum and urine levels considerably lower than desired. Ciprofloxacin extended release tablets should be administered at least 2 hours before or 6 hours after metal cations such as iron).
No products indexed under this heading.

Fludrocortisone Acetate (The risk of serious tendon disorders with quinolones is higher in those over 65 years of age, especially those on corticosteroids).
No products indexed under this heading.

Flunisolide (The risk of serious tendon disorders with quinolones is higher in those over 65 years of age, especially those on corticosteroids). Products include:
Aerobid/Aerobid-M 1153

Flurbiprofen (Non-steroidal anti-inflammatory drugs, in combination with very high doses of quinolones, have been shown to provoke convulsions in pre-clinical studies).
No products indexed under this heading.

Flutamide (Ciprofloxacin is an inhibitor of the hepatic CYP1A2 enzyme pathway. Co-administration of ciprofloxacin and other drugs primarily metabolized by CYP1A2 results in increased plasma concentrations of the co-administered drug and could lead to clinically significant pharmacodynamic side effects of the co-administered drug).
No products indexed under this heading.

Fluticasone Propionate (The risk of serious tendon disorders with quinolones is higher in those over 65 years of age, especially those on corticosteroids). Products include:
Advair Diskus 100/50 1276
Advair Diskus 250/50 1276
Advair Diskus 500/50 1276
Advair HFA 45/21 Inhalation Aerosol 1288
Advair HFA 115/21 Inhalation Aerosol 1288
Advair HFA 230/21 Inhalation Aerosol 1288
Flonase Nasal Spray 1431
Flovent Diskus 50 mcg 1435

Fluticasone Propionate HFA (The risk of serious tendon disorders with quinolones is higher in those over 65 years of age, especially those on corticosteroids). Products include:
Flovent HFA 1440

Fluvoxamine Maleate (Ciprofloxacin is an inhibitor of the hepatic CYP1A2 enzyme pathway. Co-administration of ciprofloxacin and other drugs primarily metabolized by CYP1A2 results in increased plasma concentrations of the co-administered drug and could lead to clinically significant pharmacodynamic side effects of the co-administered drug). Products include:
Luvox CR Extended-Release Capsules 1759

Fosphenytoin Sodium (Altered serum levels of phenytoin (increased and decreased) have been reported in patients receiving concomitant ciprofloxacin).
No products indexed under this heading.

Glyburide (The concomitant administration of ciprofloxacin with the sulfonylurea glyburide has, on rare occasions, resulted in severe hypoglycemia).
No products indexed under this heading.

Grepafloxacin Hydrochloride (Ciprofloxacin is an inhibitor of the hepatic CYP1A2 enzyme pathway. Co-administration of ciprofloxacin and other drugs primarily metabolized by CYP1A2 results in increased plasma concentrations of the co-administered drug and could lead to clinically significant pharmacodynamic side effects of the co-administered drug).
No products indexed under this heading.

Haloperidol (Ciprofloxacin is an inhibitor of the hepatic CYP1A2 enzyme pathway. Co-administration of ciprofloxacin and other drugs primarily metabolized by CYP1A2 results in increased plasma concentrations of the co-administered drug and could lead to clinically significant pharmacodynamic side effects of the co-administered drug).
No products indexed under this heading.

Haloperidol Decanoate (Ciprofloxacin is an inhibitor of the hepatic CYP1A2 enzyme pathway. Co-administration of ciprofloxacin and other drugs primarily metabolized by CYP1A2 results in increased plasma concentrations of the co-administered drug and could lead to clinically significant pharmacodynamic side effects of the co-administered drug).
No products indexed under this heading.

Haloperidol Lactate (Ciprofloxacin is an inhibitor of the hepatic CYP1A2 enzyme pathway. Co-administration of ciprofloxacin and other drugs primarily metabolized by CYP1A2 results in increased plasma concentrations of the co-administered drug and could lead to clinically significant pharmacodynamic side effects of the co-administered drug).
No products indexed under this heading.

Hydrocortisone (The risk of serious tendon disorders with quinolones is higher in those over 65 years of age, especially those on corticosteroids).
No products indexed under this heading.

Hydrocortisone Acetate (The risk of serious tendon disorders with quinolones is higher in those over 65 years of age, especially those on corticosteroids). Products include:
Analpram-HC 1140
Pramosone 1141

Hydrocortisone Sodium Phosphate (The risk of serious tendon disorders with quinolones is higher in those over 65 years of age, especially those on corticosteroids).
No products indexed under this heading.

Hydrocortisone Sodium Succinate (The risk of serious tendon disorders with quinolones is higher in those over 65 years of age, especially those on corticosteroids).
No products indexed under this heading.

Ibuprofen (Non-steroidal anti-inflammatory drugs, in combination with very high doses of quinolones, have been shown to provoke convulsions in pre-clinical studies). Products include:
Motrin IB Tablets and Caplets 1900
Children's Motrin Oral Suspension 1901
Children's Motrin Non-Staining Dye-Free Oral Suspension 1901
Children's Motrin Cold Oral Suspension 1899
Infants' Motrin Concentrated Drops 1901
Infants' Motrin Non-Staining Dye-Free Concentrated Drops 1901
Junior Strength Motrin Caplets and Chewable Tablets 1901
Vicoprofen Tablets 533

Imipramine Hydrochloride (Ciprofloxacin is an inhibitor of the hepatic CYP1A2 enzyme pathway. Co-administration of ciprofloxacin and other drugs primarily metabolized by CYP1A2 results in increased plasma concentrations of the co-administered drug and could lead to clinically significant pharmacodynamic side effects of the co-administered drug).
No products indexed under this heading.

Imipramine Pamoate (Ciprofloxacin is an inhibitor of the hepatic CYP1A2 enzyme pathway. Co-administration of ciprofloxacin and other drugs primarily metabolized by CYP1A2 results in increased plasma concentrations of the co-administered drug and could lead to clinically significant pharmacodynamic side effects of the co-administered drug).
No products indexed under this heading.

Indomethacin (Non-steroidal anti-inflammatory drugs, in combination with very high doses of quinolones, have been shown to provoke convulsions in pre-clinical studies). Products include:
Indocin 2024

Indomethacin Sodium Trihydrate (Non-steroidal anti-inflammatory drugs, in combination with very high doses of quinolones, have been shown to provoke convulsions in pre-clinical studies). Products include:
Indocin I.V. 2489

Iron (Concurrent administration of ciprofloxacin with multivalent cation-containing products may substantially interfere with the absorption of ciprofloxacin, resulting in serum and urine levels considerably lower than desired. Ciprofloxacin extended release tablets should be administered at least 2 hours before or 6 hours after metal cations). Products include:
Phyto-Vite Tablets 639

Ketoprofen (Non-steroidal anti-inflammatory drugs, in combination with very high doses of quinolones, have been shown to provoke convulsions in pre-clinical studies).
No products indexed under this heading.

Ketorolac Tromethamine (Non-steroidal anti-inflammatory drugs, in combination with very high doses of quinolones, have been shown to provoke convulsions in pre-clinical studies).
No products indexed under this heading.

Levobupivacaine Hydrochloride (Ciprofloxacin is an inhibitor of the hepatic CYP1A2 enzyme pathway. Co-administration of ciprofloxacin and other drugs primarily metabolized by CYP1A2 results in increased plasma concentrations of the co-administered drug and could lead to clinically significant pharmacodynamic side effects of the co-administered drug).
No products indexed under this heading.

Lomefloxacin Hydrochloride (Ciprofloxacin is an inhibitor of the hepatic CYP1A2 enzyme pathway. Co-administration of ciprofloxacin and other drugs primarily metabolized by CYP1A2 results in increased plasma concentrations of the co-administered drug and could lead to clinically significant pharmacodynamic side effects of the co-administered drug).
No products indexed under this heading.

Magaldrate (When ciprofloxacin extended release tablets, given as a single 1000 mg dose, were administered 2 hours before or 4 hours after a magnesium/aluminum-containing antacid (900 mg aluminum hydroxide and 600 mg magnesium hydroxide as a single oral dose) to 18 healthy volunteers, there was a 4% and 19% reduction, respectively, in the mean Cmax of ciprofloxacin. The reduction in the mean AUC was 24% and 26%, respectively. Ciprofloxacin extended release tablets should be administered at least 2 hours before or 6 hours after antacids containing magnesium or aluminum).
No products indexed under this heading.

Magnesium (Concurrent administration of ciprofloxacin with multivalent cation-containing products may substantially interfere with the absorption of ciprofloxacin, resulting in serum and urine levels considerably lower than desired. Ciprofloxacin extended release tablets should be administered at least 2 hours before or 6 hours after metal cations). Products include:

Protector Capsules .... ▣639
Vibe Liquid Multi-Nutrient Supplement .... ▣626

Magnesium Carbonate (When ciprofloxacin extended release tablets, given as a single 1000 mg dose, were administered 2 hours before or 4 hours after a magnesium/aluminum-containing antacid (900 mg aluminum hydroxide and 600 mg magnesium hydroxide as a single oral dose) to 18 healthy volunteers, there was a 4% and 19% reduction, respectively, in the mean Cmax of ciprofloxacin. The reduction in the mean AUC was 24% and 26%, respectively. Ciprofloxacin extended release tablets should be administered at least 2 hours before or 6 hours after antacids containing magnesium or aluminum).
No products indexed under this heading.

Magnesium Hydroxide (When ciprofloxacin extended release tablets, given as a single 1000 mg dose, were administered 2 hours before or 4 hours after a magnesium/aluminum-containing antacid (900 mg aluminum hydroxide and 600 mg magnesium hydroxide as a single oral dose) to 18 healthy volunteers, there was a 4% and 19% reduction, respectively, in the mean Cmax of ciprofloxacin. The reduction in the mean AUC was 24% and 26%, respectively. Ciprofloxacin extended release tablets should be administered at least 2 hours before or 6 hours after antacids containing magnesium or aluminum). Products include:

Fleet Pedia-Lax Chewable Tablets 1145
Pepcid Complete Chewable Tablets 1771
Extra Strength Rolaids Freshmint Tablets 1903
Rolaids Multi-Symptom Berry Tablets 1903
Rolaids Original Peppermint Tablets 1903

Magnesium Oxide (When ciprofloxacin extended release tablets, given as a single 1000 mg dose, were administered 2 hours before or 4 hours after a magnesium/aluminum-containing antacid (900 mg aluminum hydroxide and 600 mg magnesium hydroxide as a single oral dose) to 18 healthy volunteers, there was a 4% and 19% reduction, respectively, in the mean Cmax of ciprofloxacin. The reduction in the mean AUC was 24% and 26%, respectively. Ciprofloxacin extended release tablets should be administered at least 2 hours before or 6 hours after antacids containing magnesium or aluminum). Products include:

Beelith Tablets 813

Maprotiline Hydrochloride (Ciprofloxacin is an inhibitor of the hepatic CYP1A2 enzyme pathway. Co-administration of ciprofloxacin and other drugs primarily metabolized by CYP1A2 results in increased plasma concentrations of the co-administered drug and could lead to clinically significant pharmacodynamic side effects of the co-administered drug).
No products indexed under this heading.

Meclofenamate Sodium (Non-steroidal anti-inflammatory drugs, in combination with very high doses of quinolones, have been shown to provoke convulsions in pre-clinical studies).
No products indexed under this heading.

Mefenamic Acid (Non-steroidal anti-inflammatory drugs, in combination with very high doses of quinolones, have been shown to provoke convulsions in pre-clinical studies).
No products indexed under this heading.

Meloxicam (Non-steroidal anti-inflammatory drugs, in combination with very high doses of quinolones, have been shown to provoke convulsions in pre-clinical studies). Products include:

Mobic Oral Suspension 863
Mobic Tablets 863

Methadone Hydrochloride (Ciprofloxacin is an inhibitor of the hepatic CYP1A2 enzyme pathway. Co-administration of ciprofloxacin and other drugs primarily metabolized by CYP1A2 results in increased plasma concentrations of the co-administered drug and could lead to clinically significant pharmacodynamic side effects of the co-administered drug).
No products indexed under this heading.

Methotrexate (Renal tubular transport of methotrexate may be inhibited by concomitant administration of ciprofloxacin, potentially leading to increased plasma levels of methotrexate. This might increase the risk of methotrexate-associated toxic reactions. Therefore, patients under methotrexate therapy should be carefully monitored when concomitant ciprofloxacin therapy is indicated).
No products indexed under this heading.

Methotrexate Sodium (Renal tubular transport of methotrexate may be inhibited by concomitant administration of ciprofloxacin, potentially leading to increased plasma levels of methotrexate. This might increase the risk of methotrexate-associated toxic reactions. Therefore, patients under methotrexate therapy should be carefully monitored when concomitant ciprofloxacin therapy is indicated).
No products indexed under this heading.

Methylprednisolone Acetate (The risk of serious tendon disorders with quinolones is higher in those over 65 years of age, especially those on corticosteroids).
No products indexed under this heading.

Methylprednisolone Sodium Succinate (The risk of serious tendon disorders with quinolones is higher in those over 65 years of age, especially those on corticosteroids).
No products indexed under this heading.

Metoclopramide Hydrochloride (Metoclopramide significantly accelerates the absorption of oral ciprofloxacin, resulting in a shorter time to reach maximum plasma concentrations. No significant effect was observed on the bioavailability of ciprofloxacin).
No products indexed under this heading.

Mexiletine Hydrochloride (Ciprofloxacin is an inhibitor of the hepatic CYP1A2 enzyme pathway. Co-administration of ciprofloxacin and other drugs primarily metabolized by CYP1A2 results in increased plasma concentrations of the co-administered drug and could lead to clinically significant pharmacodynamic side effects of the co-administered drug).
No products indexed under this heading.

Mirtazapine (Ciprofloxacin is an inhibitor of the hepatic CYP1A2 enzyme pathway. Co-administration of ciprofloxacin and other drugs primarily metabolized by CYP1A2 results in increased plasma concentrations of the co-administered drug and could lead to clinically significant pharmacodynamic side effects of the co-administered drug). Products include:

Remeron Tablets 2924
RemeronSolTab Tablets 2927

Mometasone Furoate (The risk of serious tendon disorders with quinolones is higher in those over 65 years of age, especially those on corticosteroids). Products include:

Asmanex Twisthaler 2797
Elocon Cream 0.1% 2840
Elocon Lotion 0.1% 2841
Elocon Ointment 0.1% 2842

Mometasone Furoate Monohydrate (The risk of serious tendon disorders with quinolones is higher in those over 65 years of age, especially those on corticosteroids). Products include:

Nasonex Nasal Spray 2883

Moxifloxacin Hydrochloride (Ciprofloxacin is an inhibitor of the hepatic CYP1A2 enzyme pathway. Co-administration of ciprofloxacin and other drugs primarily metabolized by CYP1A2 results in increased plasma concentrations of the co-administered drug and could lead to clinically significant pharmacodynamic side effects of the co-administered drug). Products include:

Avelox 2803
Vigamox Ophthalmic Solution .... ⊙548

Nabumetone (Non-steroidal anti-inflammatory drugs, in combination with very high doses of quinolones, have been shown to provoke convulsions in pre-clinical studies).
No products indexed under this heading.

Nafcillin Sodium (Ciprofloxacin is an inhibitor of the hepatic CYP1A2 enzyme pathway. Co-administration of ciprofloxacin and other drugs primarily metabolized by CYP1A2 results in increased plasma concentrations of the co-administered drug and could lead to clinically significant pharmacodynamic side effects of the co-administered drug).
No products indexed under this heading.

Naproxen (Non-steroidal anti-inflammatory drugs, in combination with very high doses of quinolones, have been shown to provoke convulsions in pre-clinical studies). Products include:

EC-Naprosyn Delayed-Release Tablets 2632
Naprosyn Suspension 2632
Naprosyn Tablets 2632

Naproxen Sodium (Non-steroidal anti-inflammatory drugs, in combination with very high doses of quinolones, have been shown to provoke convulsions in pre-clinical studies). Products include:

Anaprox Tablets 2632
Anaprox DS Tablets 2632
Treximet Tablets 1616

Nicotine Polacrilex (Ciprofloxacin is an inhibitor of the hepatic CYP1A2 enzyme pathway. Co-administration of ciprofloxacin and other drugs primarily metabolized by CYP1A2 results in increased plasma concentrations of the co-administered drug and could lead to clinically significant pharmacodynamic side effects of the co-administered drug).
No products indexed under this heading.

Nicotine Salicylate (Ciprofloxacin is an inhibitor of the hepatic CYP1A2 enzyme pathway. Co-administration of ciprofloxacin and other drugs primarily metabolized by CYP1A2 results in increased plasma concentrations of the co-administered drug and could lead to clinically significant pharmacodynamic side effects of the co-administered drug).
No products indexed under this heading.

Nicotine Sulfate (Ciprofloxacin is an inhibitor of the hepatic CYP1A2 enzyme pathway. Co-administration of ciprofloxacin and other drugs primarily metabolized by CYP1A2 results in increased plasma concentrations of the co-administered drug and could lead to clinically significant pharmacodynamic side effects of the co-administered drug).
No products indexed under this heading.

Norethindrone Acetate (Ciprofloxacin is an inhibitor of the hepatic CYP1A2 enzyme pathway. Co-administration of ciprofloxacin and other drugs primarily metabolized by CYP1A2 results in increased plasma concentrations of the co-administered drug and could lead to clinically significant pharmacodynamic side effects of the co-administered drug). Products include:

Activella Tablets 2347

Norfloxacin (Ciprofloxacin is an inhibitor of the hepatic CYP1A2 enzyme pathway. Co-administration of ciprofloxacin and other drugs primarily metabolized by CYP1A2 results in increased plasma concentrations of the co-administered drug and could lead to clinically significant pharmacodynamic side effects of the co-administered drug). Products include:

Noroxin Tablets 2069

Nortriptyline Hydrochloride (Ciprofloxacin is an inhibitor of the hepatic CYP1A2 enzyme pathway. Co-administration of ciprofloxacin and other drugs primarily metabolized by CYP1A2 results in increased plasma concentrations of the co-administered drug and could lead to clinically significant pharmacodynamic side effects of the co-administered drug).
No products indexed under this heading.

Ofloxacin (Ciprofloxacin is an inhibitor of the hepatic CYP1A2 enzyme pathway. Co-administration of ciprofloxacin and other drugs primarily metabolized by CYP1A2 results in increased plasma concentrations of the co-administered drug and could lead to clinically significant pharmacodynamic side effects of the co-administered drug). Products include:

Ofloxacin Ophthalmic Solution 0.3% .... ⊙243

Olanzapine (Ciprofloxacin is an inhibitor of the hepatic CYP1A2 enzyme pathway. Co-administration of ciprofloxacin and other drugs primarily metabolized by CYP1A2 results in increased plasma concentrations of the co-administered drug and could lead to clinically significant pharmacodynamic side effects of the co-administered drug). Products include:

Symbyax Capsules **1871**
Zyprexa Tablets **1883**
Zyprexa IntraMuscular **1883**
Zyprexa ZYDIS Orally Disintegrating Tablets **1883**

Omeprazole (When ciprofloxacin extended release tablets were administered as a single 1000 mg dose concomitantly with omeprazole (40 mg once daily for 3 days) to 18 healthy volunteers, the mean AUC and Cmax of ciprofloxacin were reduced by 20% and 23%, respectively. The clinical significance of this interaction has not been determined).

No products indexed under this heading.

Omeprazole Magnesium (When ciprofloxacin extended release tablets were administered as a single 1000 mg dose concomitantly with omeprazole (40 mg once daily for 3 days) to 18 healthy volunteers, the mean AUC and Cmax of ciprofloxacin were reduced by 20% and 23%, respectively. The clinical significance of this interaction has not been determined). Products include:

Prilosec OTC Tablets **2565**

Ondansetron (Ciprofloxacin is an inhibitor of the hepatic CYP1A2 enzyme pathway. Co-administration of ciprofloxacin and other drugs primarily metabolized by CYP1A2 results in increased plasma concentrations of the co-administered drug and could lead to clinically significant pharmacodynamic side effects of the co-administered drug). Products include:

Zofran ODT Orally Disintegrating Tablets **1687**

Ondansetron Hydrochloride (Ciprofloxacin is an inhibitor of the hepatic CYP1A2 enzyme pathway. Co-administration of ciprofloxacin and other drugs primarily metabolized by CYP1A2 results in increased plasma concentrations of the co-administered drug and could lead to clinically significant pharmacodynamic side effects of the co-administered drug). Products include:

Zofran Injection **1682**
Zofran **1687**

Oxaprozin (Non-steroidal anti-inflammatory drugs, in combination with very high doses of quinolones, have been shown to provoke convulsions in pre-clinical studies).

No products indexed under this heading.

Phenobarbital Sodium (Ciprofloxacin is an inhibitor of the hepatic CYP1A2 enzyme pathway. Co-administration of ciprofloxacin and other drugs primarily metabolized by CYP1A2 results in increased plasma concentrations of the co-administered drug and could lead to clinically significant pharmacodynamic side effects of the co-administered drug).

No products indexed under this heading.

Phenylbutazone (Non-steroidal anti-inflammatory drugs, in combination with very high doses of quinolones, have been shown to provoke convulsions in pre-clinical studies).

No products indexed under this heading.

Phenytoin (Altered serum levels of phenytoin (increased and decreased) have been reported in patients receiving concomitant ciprofloxacin).

No products indexed under this heading.

Phenytoin Sodium (Altered serum levels of phenytoin (increased and decreased) have been reported in patients receiving concomitant ciprofloxacin). Products include:

Phenytek Capsules **2192**

Piroxicam (Non-steroidal anti-inflammatory drugs, in combination with very high doses of quinolones, have been shown to provoke convulsions in pre-clinical studies).

No products indexed under this heading.

Polysaccharide Iron Complex (Concurrent administration of ciprofloxacin with multivalent cation-containing products, such as products containing iron, may substantially interfere with the absorption of ciprofloxacin, resulting in serum and urine levels considerably lower than desired. Ciprofloxacin extended release tablets should be administered at least 2 hours before or 6 hours after metal cations such as iron). Products include:

Nu-Iron 150 Capsules **2165**

Prednisolone Acetate (The risk of serious tendon disorders with quinolones is higher in those over 65 years of age, especially those on corticosteroids). Products include:

Pred Forte Ophthalmic Suspension .... ⊙227
Pred Mild Ophthalmic Suspension .... ⊙230
Pred-G Ophthalmic Ointment .... ⊙229
Pred-G Ophthalmic Suspension .... ⊙228

Prednisolone Sodium Phosphate (The risk of serious tendon disorders with quinolones is higher in those over 65 years of age, especially those on corticosteroids).

No products indexed under this heading.

Prednisolone Tebutate (The risk of serious tendon disorders with quinolones is higher in those over 65 years of age, especially those on corticosteroids).

No products indexed under this heading.

Prednisone (The risk of serious tendon disorders with quinolones is higher in those over 65 years of age, especially those on corticosteroids).

No products indexed under this heading.

Probenecid (Probenecid interferes with renal tubular secretion of ciprofloxacin and produces an increase in the level of ciprofloxacin in the serum. This should be considered if patients are receiving both drugs concomitantly).

No products indexed under this heading.

Propafenone Hydrochloride (Ciprofloxacin is an inhibitor of the hepatic CYP1A2 enzyme pathway. Co-administration of ciprofloxacin and other drugs primarily metabolized by CYP1A2 results in increased plasma concentrations of the co-administered drug and could lead to clinically significant pharmacodynamic side effects of the co-administered drug). Products include:

Rythmol Tablets **1586**
Rythmol SR Capsules **1590**

Propranolol Hydrochloride (Ciprofloxacin is an inhibitor of the hepatic CYP1A2 enzyme pathway. Co-administration of ciprofloxacin and other drugs primarily metabolized by CYP1A2 results in increased plasma concentrations of the co-administered drug and could lead to clinically significant pharmacodynamic side effects of the co-administered drug). Products include:

InnoPran XL Extended Release Capsules **1484**

Protriptyline Hydrochloride (Ciprofloxacin is an inhibitor of the hepatic CYP1A2 enzyme pathway. Co-administration of ciprofloxacin and other drugs primarily metabolized by CYP1A2 results in increased plasma concentrations of the co-administered drug and could lead to clinically significant pharmacodynamic side effects of the co-administered drug).

No products indexed under this heading.

Riluzole (Ciprofloxacin is an inhibitor of the hepatic CYP1A2 enzyme pathway. Co-administration of ciprofloxacin and other drugs primarily metabolized by CYP1A2 results in increased plasma concentrations of the co-administered drug and could lead to clinically significant pharmacodynamic side effects of the co-administered drug). Products include:

Rilutek Tablets **2771**

Ritonavir (Ciprofloxacin is an inhibitor of the hepatic CYP1A2 enzyme pathway. Co-administration of ciprofloxacin and other drugs primarily metabolized by CYP1A2 results in increased plasma concentrations of the co-administered drug and could lead to clinically significant pharmacodynamic side effects of the co-administered drug). Products include:

Kaletra **452**
Norvir **489**

Rofecoxib (Non-steroidal anti-inflammatory drugs, in combination with very high doses of quinolones, have been shown to provoke convulsions in pre-clinical studies).

No products indexed under this heading.

Ropinirole Hydrochloride (Ciprofloxacin is an inhibitor of the hepatic CYP1A2 enzyme pathway. Co-administration of ciprofloxacin and other drugs primarily metabolized by CYP1A2 results in increased plasma concentrations of the co-administered drug and could lead to clinically significant pharmacodynamic side effects of the co-administered drug). Products include:

Requip Tablets **1561**
Requip XL Tablets **1568**

Ropivacaine Hydrochloride (Ciprofloxacin is an inhibitor of the hepatic CYP1A2 enzyme pathway. Co-administration of ciprofloxacin and other drugs primarily metabolized by CYP1A2 results in increased plasma concentrations of the co-administered drug and could lead to clinically significant pharmacodynamic side effects of the co-administered drug).

No products indexed under this heading.

Sucralfate (Concurrent administration of ciprofloxacin with multivalent cation-containing products, such as sucralfate, may substantially interfere with the absorption of ciprofloxacin, resulting in serum and urine levels considerably lower than desired. Ciprofloxacin extended release tablets should be administered at least 2 hours before or 6 hours after sucralfate). Products include:

Carafate Suspension **706**
Carafate Tablets **707**

Sulindac (Non-steroidal anti-inflammatory drugs, in combination with very high doses of quinolones, have been shown to provoke convulsions in pre-clinical studies). Products include:

Clinoril Tablets **1962**

Tacrine Hydrochloride (Ciprofloxacin is an inhibitor of the hepatic CYP1A2 enzyme pathway. Co-administration of ciprofloxacin and other drugs primarily metabolized by CYP1A2 results in increased plasma concentrations of the co-administered drug and could lead to clinically significant pharmacodynamic side effects of the co-administered drug).

No products indexed under this heading.

Tamoxifen Citrate (Ciprofloxacin is an inhibitor of the hepatic CYP1A2 enzyme pathway. Co-administration of ciprofloxacin and other drugs primarily metabolized by CYP1A2 results in increased plasma concentrations of the co-administered drug and could lead to clinically significant pharmacodynamic side effects of the co-administered drug).

No products indexed under this heading.

Theophylline (Concurrent administration of ciprofloxacin with theophylline may lead to elevated serum concentrations of theophylline and prolongation of its elimination half-life. This may result in increased risk of theophylline-related adverse reactions. If concomitant use cannot be avoided, serum levels of theophylline should be monitored and dosage adjustments made as appropriate. Serious and fatal reactions have been reported in patients receiving concurrent administration of ciprofloxacin and theophylline).

No products indexed under this heading.

Theophylline Anhydrous (Concurrent administration of ciprofloxacin with theophylline may lead to elevated serum concentrations of theophylline and prolongation of its elimination half-life. This may result in increased risk of theophylline-related adverse reactions. If concomitant use cannot be avoided, serum levels of theophylline should be monitored and dosage adjustments made as appropriate. Serious and fatal reactions have been reported in patients receiving concurrent administration of ciprofloxacin and theophylline). Products include:

Uniphyl Tablets 2595

Theophylline Calcium Salicylate (Concurrent administration of ciprofloxacin with theophylline may lead to elevated serum concentrations of theophylline and prolongation of its elimination half-life. This may result in increased risk of theophylline-related adverse reactions. If concomitant use cannot be avoided, serum levels of theophylline should be monitored and dosage adjustments made as appropriate. Serious and fatal reactions have been reported in patients receiving concurrent administration of ciprofloxacin and theophylline).

No products indexed under this heading.

Theophylline Dihydroxypropyl (Glyceryl) (Concurrent administration of ciprofloxacin with theophylline may lead to elevated serum concentrations of theophylline and prolongation of its elimination half-life. This may result in increased risk of theophylline-related adverse reactions. If concomitant use cannot be avoided, serum levels of theophylline should be monitored and dosage adjustments made as appropriate. Serious and fatal reactions have been reported in patients receiving concurrent administration of ciprofloxacin and theophylline).

No products indexed under this heading.

Theophylline Ethylenediamine (Concurrent administration of ciprofloxacin with theophylline may lead to elevated serum concentrations of theophylline and prolongation of its elimination half-life. This may result in increased risk of theophylline-related adverse reactions. If concomitant use cannot be avoided, serum levels of theophylline should be monitored and dosage adjustments made as appropriate. Serious and fatal reactions have been reported in patients receiving concurrent administration of ciprofloxacin and theophylline).

No products indexed under this heading.

Theophylline Sodium Glycinate (Concurrent administration of ciprofloxacin with theophylline may lead to elevated serum concentrations of theophylline and prolongation of its elimination half-life. This may result in increased risk of theophylline-related adverse reactions. If concomitant use cannot be avoided, serum levels of theophylline should be monitored and dosage adjustments made as appropriate. Serious and fatal reactions have been reported in patients receiving concurrent administration of ciprofloxacin and theophylline).

No products indexed under this heading.

Tizanidine (In a pharmacokinetic study, systemic exposure of tizanidine (4 mg single dose) was significantly increased (Cmax 7-fold, AUC 10-fold) when the drug was given concomitantly with ciprofloxacin (500 mg b.i.d. for 3 days). The hypotensive and sedative effects of tizanidine were also potentiated. Concomitant administration of tizanidine and ciprofloxacin is contraindicated).

No products indexed under this heading.

Tizanidine Hydrochloride (In a pharmacokinetic study, systemic exposure of tizanidine (4 mg single dose) was significantly increased (Cmax 7-fold, AUC 10-fold) when the drug was given concomitantly with ciprofloxacin (500 mg b.i.d. for 3 days). The hypotensive and sedative effects of tizanidine were also potentiated. Concomitant administration of tizanidine and ciprofloxacin is contraindicated).

No products indexed under this heading.

Tolmetin Sodium (Non-steroidal anti-inflammatory drugs, in combination with very high doses of quinolones, have been shown to provoke convulsions in pre-clinical studies).

No products indexed under this heading.

Triamcinolone (The risk of serious tendon disorders with quinolones is higher in those over 65 years of age, especially those on corticosteroids).

No products indexed under this heading.

Triamcinolone Acetonide (The risk of serious tendon disorders with quinolones is higher in those over 65 years of age, especially those on corticosteroids). Products include:

Azmacort Inhalation Aerosol 407
Nasacort AQ Nasal Spray 2765
Triesence Injectable Suspension .... ⊙ 209

Triamcinolone Diacetate (The risk of serious tendon disorders with quinolones is higher in those over 65 years of age, especially those on corticosteroids).

No products indexed under this heading.

Triamcinolone Hexacetonide (The risk of serious tendon disorders with quinolones is higher in those over 65 years of age, especially those on corticosteroids).

No products indexed under this heading.

Trimethaphan Camsylate (Ciprofloxacin is an inhibitor of the hepatic CYP1A2 enzyme pathway. Co-administration of ciprofloxacin and other drugs primarily metabolized by CYP1A2 results in increased plasma concentrations of the co-administered drug and could lead to clinically significant pharmacodynamic side effects of the co-administered drug).

No products indexed under this heading.

Trimipramine Maleate (Ciprofloxacin is an inhibitor of the hepatic CYP1A2 enzyme pathway. Co-administration of ciprofloxacin and other drugs primarily metabolized by CYP1A2 results in increased plasma concentrations of the co-administered drug and could lead to clinically significant pharmacodynamic side effects of the co-administered drug).

No products indexed under this heading.

Trovafloxacin Mesylate (Ciprofloxacin is an inhibitor of the hepatic CYP1A2 enzyme pathway. Co-administration of ciprofloxacin and other drugs primarily metabolized by CYP1A2 results in increased plasma concentrations of the co-administered drug and could lead to clinically significant pharmacodynamic side effects of the co-administered drug).

No products indexed under this heading.

Valdecoxib (Non-steroidal anti-inflammatory drugs, in combination with very high doses of quinolones, have been shown to provoke convulsions in pre-clinical studies).

No products indexed under this heading.

Verapamil Hydrochloride (Ciprofloxacin is an inhibitor of the hepatic CYP1A2 enzyme pathway. Co-administration of ciprofloxacin and other drugs primarily metabolized by CYP1A2 results in increased plasma concentrations of the co-administered drug and could lead to clinically significant pharmacodynamic side effects of the co-administered drug). Products include:

Tarka Tablets 511

Warfarin Sodium (Ciprofloxacin has been reported to enhance the effects of the oral anticoagulant warfarin or its derivatives. When these products are administered concomitantly, prothrombin time or other suitable coagulation tests should be closely monitored).

No products indexed under this heading.

Zileuton (Ciprofloxacin is an inhibitor of the hepatic CYP1A2 enzyme pathway. Co-administration of ciprofloxacin and other drugs primarily metabolized by CYP1A2 results in increased plasma concentrations of the co-administered drug and could lead to clinically significant pharmacodynamic side effects of the co-administered drug).

No products indexed under this heading.

Zinc (Concurrent administration of ciprofloxacin with multivalent cation-containing products such as zinc may substantially interfere with the absorption of ciprofloxacin, resulting in serum and urine levels considerably lower than desired. Ciprofloxacin extended release tablets should be administered at least 2 hours before or 6 hours after metal cations such as zinc). Products include:

Comax Dietary Supplement 995
Glaucofit Dietary Supplement 995
Glauma Dietary Supplement 995
Tonox Dietary Supplement 995
Vibe Liquid Multi-Nutrient Supplement .... ▣ 626
Visutein Capsules 3159

Zinc Acetate (Concurrent administration of ciprofloxacin with multivalent cation-containing products such as zinc may substantially interfere with the absorption of ciprofloxacin, resulting in serum and urine levels considerably lower than desired. Ciprofloxacin extended release tablets should be administered at least 2 hours before or 6 hours after metal cations such as zinc).

No products indexed under this heading.

Zinc Chloride (Concurrent administration of ciprofloxacin with multivalent cation-containing products such as zinc may substantially interfere with the absorption of ciprofloxacin, resulting in serum and urine levels considerably lower than desired. Ciprofloxacin extended release tablets should be administered at least 2 hours before or 6 hours after metal cations such as zinc).

No products indexed under this heading.

Zinc Citrate (Concurrent administration of ciprofloxacin with multivalent cation-containing products such as zinc may substantially interfere with the absorption of ciprofloxacin, resulting in serum and urine levels considerably lower than desired. Ciprofloxacin extended release tablets should be administered at least 2 hours before or 6 hours after metal cations such as zinc).

No products indexed under this heading.

Zinc-Containing Multivitamins (Concurrent administration of ciprofloxacin with multivalent cation-containing products such as zinc may substantially interfere with the absorption of ciprofloxacin, resulting in serum and urine levels considerably lower than desired. Ciprofloxacin extended release tablets should be administered at least 2 hours before or 6 hours after multivitamin preparations with zinc).

No products indexed under this heading.

Zinc Gluconate (Concurrent administration of ciprofloxacin with multivalent cation-containing products such as zinc may substantially interfere with the absorption of ciprofloxacin, resulting in serum and urine levels considerably lower than desired. Ciprofloxacin extended release tablets should be administered at least 2 hours before or 6 hours after metal cations such as zinc).

No products indexed under this heading.

Zinc Oxide (Concurrent administration of ciprofloxacin with multivalent cation-containing products such as zinc may substantially interfere with the absorption of ciprofloxacin, resulting in serum and urine levels considerably lower than desired. Ciprofloxacin extended release tablets should be administered at least 2 hours before or 6 hours after metal cations such as zinc). Products include:

Bausch & Lomb Ocuvite Adult 50+ Vitamin and Mineral Supplement .... ⊙ 237
CitraNatal DHA Tablets 2175
CitraNatal 90 DHA Tablets 2175

Zinc Phenosulfonate (Concurrent administration of ciprofloxacin with multivalent cation-containing products such as zinc may substantially interfere with the absorption of ciprofloxacin, resulting in serum and urine levels considerably lower than desired. Ciprofloxacin extended release tablets should be administered at least 2 hours before or 6 hours after metal cations such as zinc).

No products indexed under this heading.

Zinc Pyrithione (Concurrent administration of ciprofloxacin with multivalent cation-containing products such as zinc may substantially interfere with the absorption of ciprofloxacin, resulting in serum and urine levels considerably lower than desired. Ciprofloxacin extended release tablets should be administered at least 2 hours before or 6 hours after metal cations such as zinc).
No products indexed under this heading.

Zinc Sulfate (Concurrent administration of ciprofloxacin with multivalent cation-containing products such as zinc may substantially interfere with the absorption of ciprofloxacin, resulting in serum and urine levels considerably lower than desired. Ciprofloxacin extended release tablets should be administered at least 2 hours before or 6 hours after metal cations such as zinc). Products include:
Clear Eyes Itchy Eye Relief .... ⊙ 255
Zinc-220 Capsules 564

Zinc Undecylenate (Concurrent administration of ciprofloxacin with multivalent cation-containing products such as zinc may substantially interfere with the absorption of ciprofloxacin, resulting in serum and urine levels considerably lower than desired. Ciprofloxacin extended release tablets should be administered at least 2 hours before or 6 hours after metal cations such as zinc).
No products indexed under this heading.

Zolmitriptan (Ciprofloxacin is an inhibitor of the hepatic CYP1A2 enzyme pathway. Co-administration of ciprofloxacin and other drugs primarily metabolized by CYP1A2 results in increased plasma concentrations of the co-administered drug and could lead to clinically significant pharmacodynamic side effects of the co-administered drug). Products include:
Zomig Tablets 694
Zomig Nasal Spray 689
Zomig-ZMT Tablets 694

Food Interactions

Dairy products (Although ciprofloxacin extended release tablets may be taken with meals that include milk, concomitant administration with dairy products should be avoided, since decreased absorption is possible).

Food, calcium-rich (Although ciprofloxacin extended release tablets may be taken with meals that include milk, concomitant administration with dairy products or with calcium-fortified juices alone should be avoided, since decreased absorption is possible).

CIPRODEX OTIC SUSPENSION

(Ciprofloxacin, Dexamethasone) 541
None cited in PDR database.

CITRANATAL DHA CAPSULES

(Docosahexaenoic Acid (DHA)) 2175
None cited in PDR database.

CITRANATAL DHA TABLETS

(Calcium Citrate, Copper, Docusate Sodium, Ferrous Gluconate, Folic Acid, Iron Carbonyl, Multivitamins with Minerals, Potassium Iodide, Zinc Oxide) 2175
None cited in PDR database.

CITRANATAL 90 DHA CAPSULES

(Docosahexaenoic Acid (DHA)) 2175
None cited in PDR database.

CITRANATAL 90 DHA TABLETS

(Calcium Citrate, Copper, Docusate Sodium, Folic Acid, Iron Carbonyl, Multivitamins with Minerals, Potassium Iodide, Zinc Oxide) 2175
None cited in PDR database.

CLARINEX SYRUP

(Desloratadine) 2828
See Clarinex Tablets

CLARINEX TABLETS

(Desloratadine) 2828
May interact with erythromycin and certain other agents. Compounds in these categories include:

Azithromycin Dihydrate (Co-administration resulted in increased Cmax and AUC of desloratadine by 15% and 5% respectively; Cmax and AUC of 3-hydroxydesloratadine increased by 15% and 4% respectively; there were no clinically relevant changes in the safety profile of desloratadine).
No products indexed under this heading.

Cimetidine (Co-administration resulted in increased Cmax and AUC of desloratadine by 12% and 19% respectively; Cmax and AUC of 3-hydroxydesloratadine decreased by 11% and 3% respectively; there were no clinically relevant changes in the safety profile of desloratadine).
No products indexed under this heading.

Cimetidine Hydrochloride (Co-administration resulted in increased Cmax and AUC of desloratadine by 12% and 19% respectively; Cmax and AUC of 3-hydroxydesloratadine decreased by 11% and 3% respectively; there were no clinically relevant changes in the safety profile of desloratadine).
No products indexed under this heading.

Erythromycin (Co-administration resulted in increased Cmax and AUC of desloratadine by 24% and 14% respectively; Cmax and AUC of 3-hydroxydesloratadine increased by 43% and 40% respectively; there were no clinically relevant changes in the safety profile of desloratadine).
No products indexed under this heading.

Erythromycin Estolate (Co-administration resulted in increased Cmax and AUC of desloratadine by 24% and 14% respectively; Cmax and AUC of 3-hydroxydesloratadine increased by 43% and 40% respectively; there were no clinically relevant changes in the safety profile of desloratadine).
No products indexed under this heading.

Erythromycin Ethylsuccinate (Co-administration resulted in increased Cmax and AUC of desloratadine by 24% and 14% respectively; Cmax and AUC of 3-hydroxydesloratadine increased by 43% and 40% respectively; there were no clinically relevant changes in the safety profile of desloratadine). Products include:
E.E.S. 433
EryPed 431

Erythromycin Gluceptate (Co-administration resulted in increased Cmax and AUC of desloratadine by 24% and 14% respectively; Cmax and AUC of 3-hydroxydesloratadine increased by 43% and 40% respectively; there were no clinically relevant changes in the safety profile of desloratadine).
No products indexed under this heading.

Erythromycin Lactobionate (Co-administration resulted in increased Cmax and AUC of desloratadine by 24% and 14% respectively; Cmax and AUC of 3-hydroxydesloratadine increased by 43% and 40% respectively; there were no clinically relevant changes in the safety profile of desloratadine).
No products indexed under this heading.

Erythromycin Stearate (Co-administration resulted in increased Cmax and AUC of desloratadine by 24% and 14% respectively; Cmax and AUC of 3-hydroxydesloratadine increased by 43% and 40% respectively; there were no clinically relevant changes in the safety profile of desloratadine).
No products indexed under this heading.

Fluoxetine Hydrochloride (Co-administration resulted in increased Cmax of desloratadine by 15%; Cmax and AUC of 3-hydroxydesloratadine increased by 17% and 13% respectively; there were no clinically relevant changes in the safety profile of desloratadine). Products include:
Prozac Weekly Capsules 1852
Prozac Pulvules and Liquid 1852
Symbyax Capsules 1871

Ketoconazole (Co-administration resulted in increased Cmax and AUC of desloratadine by 45% and 39% respectively; Cmax and AUC of 3-hydroxydesloratadine increased by 43% and 72% respectively; there were no clinically relevant changes in the safety profile of desloratadine). Products include:
Extina Foam, 2% 3057
Nizoral A-D Shampoo 1901

CLARINEX REDITABS TABLETS

(Desloratadine) 2828
See Clarinex Tablets

CLARINEX-D 12-HOUR EXTENDED-RELEASE TABLETS

(Desloratadine, Pseudoephedrine Sulfate) 2831
May interact with beta blockers, erythromycin, cardiac glycosides, monoamine oxidase inhibitors, veratrum alkaloids, and certain other agents. Compounds in these categories include:

Acebutolol Hydrochloride (The antihypertensive effects of beta-adrenergic blocking agents, methyldopa, mecamylamine, reserpine, and veratrum alkaloids may be reduced by sympathomimetics).
No products indexed under this heading.

Atenolol (The antihypertensive effects of beta-adrenergic blocking agents, methyldopa, mecamylamine, reserpine, and veratrum alkaloids may be reduced by sympathomimetics).
No products indexed under this heading.

Azithromycin (Although increased plasma concentrations (Cmax and AUC 0-24 hours) of desloratadine and/or 3-hydroxyloratadine were observed, there were no clinically relevant changes in the safety profile of desloratadine, as assessed by electrocardiographic parameters(including the corrected QT interval), clinical lab tests, vital signs, and adverse events). Products include:
AzaSite Ophthalmic Drops 1740

Azithromycin Dihydrate (Although increased plasma concentrations (Cmax and AUC 0-24 hours) of desloratadine and/or 3-hydroxyloratadine were observed, there were no clinically relevant changes in the safety profile of desloratadine, as assessed by electrocardiographic parameters (including the corrected QT interval), clinical lab tests, vital signs, and adverse events).
No products indexed under this heading.

Betaxolol Hydrochloride (The antihypertensive effects of beta-adrenergic blocking agents, methyldopa, mecamylamine, reserpine, and veratrum alkaloids may be reduced by sympathomimetics).
No products indexed under this heading.

Bisoprolol Fumarate (The antihypertensive effects of beta-adrenergic blocking agents, methyldopa, mecamylamine, reserpine, and veratrum alkaloids may be reduced by sympathomimetics).
No products indexed under this heading.

Carteolol Hydrochloride (The antihypertensive effects of beta-adrenergic blocking agents, methyldopa, mecamylamine, reserpine, and veratrum alkaloids may be reduced by sympathomimetics).
No products indexed under this heading.

Cimetidine (Although increased plasma concentrations (Cmax and AUC 0-24 hours) of desloratadine and/or 3-hydroxyloratadine were observed, there were no clinically relevant changes in the safety profile of desloratadine, as assessed by electrocardiographic parameters (including the corrected QT interval), clinical lab tests, vital signs, and adverse events).
No products indexed under this heading.

Cimetidine Hydrochloride (Although increased plasma concentrations (Cmax and AUC 0-24 hours) of desloratadine and/or 3-hydroxyloratadine were observed, there were no clinically relevant changes in the safety profile of desloratadine, as assessed by electrocardiographic parameters (including the corrected QT interval), clinical lab tests, vital signs, and adverse events).
No products indexed under this heading.

Cryptenamine Preparations (The antihypertensive effects of beta-adrenergic blocking agents, methyldopa, mecamylamine, reserpine, and veratrum alkaloids may be reduced by sympathomimetics).
No products indexed under this heading.

Deslanoside (Increased ectopic pacemaker activity can occur when pseudoephedrine is used concomitantly with digitalis).
No products indexed under this heading.

Digitalis Glycoside Preparations (Increased ectopic pacemaker activity can occur when pseudoephedrine is used concomitantly with digitalis).
No products indexed under this heading.

Digitoxin (Increased ectopic pacemaker activity can occur when pseudoephedrine is used concomitantly with digitalis).
No products indexed under this heading.

Digoxin (Increased ectopic pacemaker activity can occur when pseudoephedrine is used concomitantly with digitalis). Products include:
Lanoxin Injection **1498**
Lanoxin Injection Pediatric **1502**
Lanoxin Tablets **1505**

Erythromycin (Although increased plasma concentrations (Cmax and AUC 0-24 hours) of desloratadine and/or 3-hydroxydesloratadine were observed, there were no clinically relevant changes in the safety profile of desloratadine, as were assessed by electrocardiographic parameters (including the corrected QT interval), clinical lab tests, vital signs, and adverse events).
No products indexed under this heading.

Erythromycin Estolate (Although increased plasma concentrations (Cmax and AUC 0-24 hours) of desloratadine and/or 3-hydroxydesloratadine were observed, there were no clinically relevant changes in the safety profile of desloratadine, as were assessed by electrocardiographic parameters (including the corrected QT interval), clinical lab tests, vital signs, and adverse events).
No products indexed under this heading.

Erythromycin Ethylsuccinate (Although increased plasma concentrations (Cmax and AUC 0-24 hours) of desloratadine and/or 3-hydroxydesloratadine were observed, there were no clinically relevant changes in the safety profile of desloratadine, as were assessed by electrocardiographic parameters (including the corrected QT interval), clinical lab tests, vital signs, and adverse events). Products include:
E.E.S. **433**
EryPed **431**

Erythromycin Gluceptate (Although increased plasma concentrations (Cmax and AUC 0-24 hours) of desloratadine and/or 3-hydroxydesloratadine were observed, there were no clinically relevant changes in the safety profile of desloratadine, as were assessed by electrocardiographic parameters (including the corrected QT interval), clinical lab tests, vital signs, and adverse events).
No products indexed under this heading.

Erythromycin Lactobionate (Although increased plasma concentrations (Cmax and AUC 0-24 hours) of desloratadine and/or 3-hydroxydesloratadine were observed, there were no clinically relevant changes in the safety profile of desloratadine, as were assessed by electrocardiographic parameters (including the corrected QT interval), clinical lab tests, vital signs, and adverse events).
No products indexed under this heading.

Erythromycin Stearate (Although increased plasma concentrations (Cmax and AUC 0-24 hours) of desloratadine and/or 3-hydroxydesloratadine were observed, there were no clinically relevant changes in the safety profile of desloratadine, as were assessed by electrocardiographic parameters (including the corrected QT interval), clinical lab tests, vital signs, and adverse events).
No products indexed under this heading.

Esmolol Hydrochloride (The antihypertensive effects of beta-adrenergic blocking agents, methyldopa, mecamylamine, reserpine, and veratrum alkaloids may be reduced by sympathomimetics).
No products indexed under this heading.

Fluoxetine (Although increased plasma concentrations (Cmax and AUC 0-24 hours) of desloratadine and/or 3-hydroxyloratadine were observed, there were no clinically relevant changes in the safety profile of desloratadine, as assessed by electrocardiographic parameters (including the corrected QT interval), clinical lab tests, vital signs, and adverse events).
No products indexed under this heading.

Fluoxetine Hydrochloride (Although increased plasma concentrations (Cmax and AUC 0-24 hours) of desloratadine and/or 3-hydroxyloratadine were observed, there were no clinically relevant changes in the safety profile of desloratadine, as assessed by electrocardiographic parameters (including the corrected QT interval), clinical lab tests, vital signs, and adverse events). Products include:
Prozac Weekly Capsules **1852**
Prozac Pulvules and Liquid **1852**
Symbyax Capsules **1871**

Isocarboxazid (Due to the pseudoephedrine component, concomitant use with monoamine oxidase inhibitors (MAOIs) or within 14 days after stopping treatment with MAOIs is contraindicated). Products include:
Marplan Tablets **3177**

Ketoconazole (Although increased plasma concentrations (Cmax and AUC 0-24 hours) of desloratadine and/or 3-hydroxyloratadine were observed, there were no clinically relevant changes in the safety profile of desloratadine, as assessed by electrocardiographic parameters (including the corrected QT interval), clinical lab tests, vital signs, and adverse events). Products include:
Extina Foam, 2% **3057**
Nizoral A-D Shampoo **1901**

Labetalol Hydrochloride (The antihypertensive effects of beta-adrenergic blocking agents, methyldopa, mecamylamine, reserpine, and veratrum alkaloids may be reduced by sympathomimetics).
No products indexed under this heading.

Levobunolol Hydrochloride (The antihypertensive effects of beta-adrenergic blocking agents, methyldopa, mecamylamine, reserpine, and veratrum alkaloids may be reduced by sympathomimetics).
No products indexed under this heading.

Mecamylamine Hydrochloride (The antihypertensive effects of beta-adrenergic blocking agents, methyldopa, mecamylamine, reserpine, and veratrum alkaloids may be reduced by sympathomimetics).
No products indexed under this heading.

Methyldopa (The antihypertensive effects of beta-adrenergic blocking agents, methyldopa, mecamylamine, reserpine, and veratrum alkaloids may be reduced by sympathomimetics).
No products indexed under this heading.

Methyldopate Hydrochloride (The antihypertensive effects of beta-adrenergic blocking agents, methyldopa, mecamylamine, reserpine, and veratrum alkaloids may be reduced by sympathomimetics).
No products indexed under this heading.

Metipranolol Hydrochloride (The antihypertensive effects of beta-adrenergic blocking agents, methyldopa, mecamylamine, reserpine, and veratrum alkaloids may be reduced by sympathomimetics).
No products indexed under this heading.

Metoprolol Succinate (The antihypertensive effects of beta-adrenergic blocking agents, methyldopa, mecamylamine, reserpine, and veratrum alkaloids may be reduced by sympathomimetics). Products include:
Toprol-XL Tablets **666**

Metoprolol Tartrate (The antihypertensive effects of beta-adrenergic blocking agents, methyldopa, mecamylamine, reserpine, and veratrum alkaloids may be reduced by sympathomimetics).
No products indexed under this heading.

Moclobemide (Due to the pseudoephedrine component, concomitant use with monoamine oxidase inhibitors (MAOIs) or within 14 days after stopping treatment with MAOIs is contraindicated).
No products indexed under this heading.

Nadolol (The antihypertensive effects of beta-adrenergic blocking agents, methyldopa, mecamylamine, reserpine, and veratrum alkaloids may be reduced by sympathomimetics). Products include:
Nadolol Tablets **2191**

Nebivolol (The antihypertensive effects of beta-adrenergic blocking agents, methyldopa, mecamylamine, reserpine, and veratrum alkaloids may be reduced by sympathomimetics). Products include:
Bystolic Tablets **1155**

Pargyline Hydrochloride (Due to the pseudoephedrine component, concomitant use with monoamine oxidase inhibitors (MAOIs) or within 14 days after stopping treatment with MAOIs is contraindicated).
No products indexed under this heading.

Penbutolol Sulfate (The antihypertensive effects of beta-adrenergic blocking agents, methyldopa, mecamylamine, reserpine, and veratrum alkaloids may be reduced by sympathomimetics).
No products indexed under this heading.

Phenelzine Sulfate (Due to the pseudoephedrine component, concomitant use with monoamine oxidase inhibitors (MAOIs) or within 14 days after stopping treatment with MAOIs is contraindicated).
No products indexed under this heading.

Pindolol (The antihypertensive effects of beta-adrenergic blocking agents, methyldopa, mecamylamine, reserpine, and veratrum alkaloids may be reduced by sympathomimetics).
No products indexed under this heading.

Procarbazine Hydrochloride (Due to the pseudoephedrine component, concomitant use with monoamine oxidase inhibitors (MAOIs) or within 14 days after stopping treatment with MAOIs is contraindicated).
No products indexed under this heading.

Propranolol Hydrochloride (The antihypertensive effects of beta-adrenergic blocking agents, methyldopa, mecamylamine, reserpine, and veratrum alkaloids may be reduced by sympathomimetics). Products include:
InnoPran XL Extended Release Capsules **1484**

Rasagiline Mesylate (Due to the pseudoephedrine component, concomitant use with monoamine oxidase inhibitors (MAOIs) or within 14 days after stopping treatment with MAOIs is contraindicated). Products include:
Azilect Tablets **3106**

Selegiline (Due to the pseudoephedrine component, concomitant use with monoamine oxidase inhibitors (MAOIs) or within 14 days after stopping treatment with MAOIs is contraindicated). Products include:
Emsam Transdermal System **905**

Selegiline Hydrochloride (Due to the pseudoephedrine component, concomitant use with monoamine oxidase inhibitors (MAOIs) or within 14 days after stopping treatment with MAOIs is contraindicated). Products include:
Eldepryl Capsules **3052**

Sotalol Hydrochloride (The antihypertensive effects of beta-adrenergic blocking agents, methyldopa, mecamylamine, reserpine, and veratrum alkaloids may be reduced by sympathomimetics).
No products indexed under this heading.

Timolol Hemihydrate (The antihypertensive effects of beta-adrenergic blocking agents, methyldopa, mecamylamine, reserpine, and veratrum alkaloids may be reduced by sympathomimetics). Products include:

Betimol Ophthalmic Solution 3181

Timolol Maleate (The antihypertensive effects of beta-adrenergic blocking agents, methyldopa, mecamylamine, reserpine, and veratrum alkaloids may be reduced by sympathomimetics). Products include:

Combigan Ophthalmic Solution 553
Cosopt Sterile Ophthalmic Solution 1969
Timoptic Sterile Ophthalmic Solution 2121
Timoptic in Ocudose 2124
Timoptic-XE Sterile Ophthalmic Gel Forming Solution 2125

Tranylcypromine Sulfate (Due to the pseudoephedrine component, concomitant use with monoamine oxidase inhibitors (MAOIs) or within 14 days after stopping treatment with MAOIs is contraindicated). Products include:

Parnate Tablets 1532

CLARINEX-D 24-HOUR EXTENDED-RELEASE TABLETS

(Desloratadine, Pseudoephedrine Sulfate) 2834

May interact with beta blockers, cardiac glycosides, monoamine oxidase inhibitors, veratrum alkaloids, and certain other agents. Compounds in these categories include:

Acebutolol Hydrochloride (The antihypertensive effects of beta-adrenergic blocking agents may be reduced by sympathomimetics).
No products indexed under this heading.

Atenolol (The antihypertensive effects of beta-adrenergic blocking agents may be reduced by sympathomimetics).
No products indexed under this heading.

Betaxolol Hydrochloride (The antihypertensive effects of beta-adrenergic blocking agents may be reduced by sympathomimetics).
No products indexed under this heading.

Bisoprolol Fumarate (The antihypertensive effects of beta-adrenergic blocking agents may be reduced by sympathomimetics).
No products indexed under this heading.

Carteolol Hydrochloride (The antihypertensive effects of beta-adrenergic blocking agents may be reduced by sympathomimetics).
No products indexed under this heading.

Cryptenamine Preparations (The antihypertensive effects of veratrum alkaloids may be reduced by sympathomimetics).
No products indexed under this heading.

Deslanoside (Increased ectopic pacemaker activity can occur when pseudoephedrine is used concomitantly with digitalis).
No products indexed under this heading.

Digitalis Glycoside Preparations (Increased ectopic pacemaker activity can occur when pseudoephedrine is used concomitantly with digitalis).
No products indexed under this heading.

Digitoxin (Increased ectopic pacemaker activity can occur when pseudoephedrine is used concomitantly with digitalis).
No products indexed under this heading.

Digoxin (Increased ectopic pacemaker activity can occur when pseudoephedrine is used concomitantly with digitalis). Products include:

Lanoxin Injection 1498
Lanoxin Injection Pediatric 1502
Lanoxin Tablets 1505

Esmolol Hydrochloride (The antihypertensive effects of beta-adrenergic blocking agents may be reduced by sympathomimetics).
No products indexed under this heading.

Isocarboxazid (Due to the pseudoephedrine component, Clarinex-D 24 Hour extended-release tablets should not be used by patients taking monoamine oxidase inhibitors or within 14 days after stopping such treatment). Products include:

Marplan Tablets 3177

Labetalol Hydrochloride (The antihypertensive effects of beta-adrenergic blocking agents may be reduced by sympathomimetics).
No products indexed under this heading.

Levobunolol Hydrochloride (The antihypertensive effects of beta-adrenergic blocking agents may be reduced by sympathomimetics).
No products indexed under this heading.

Mecamylamine Hydrochloride (The antihypertensive effects of mecamylamine may be reduced by sympathomimetics).
No products indexed under this heading.

Methyldopa (The antihypertensive effects of methyldopa may be reduced by sympathomimetics).
No products indexed under this heading.

Methyldopate Hydrochloride (The antihypertensive effects of methyldopa may be reduced by sympathomimetics).
No products indexed under this heading.

Metipranolol Hydrochloride (The antihypertensive effects of beta-adrenergic blocking agents may be reduced by sympathomimetics).
No products indexed under this heading.

Metoprolol Succinate (The antihypertensive effects of beta-adrenergic blocking agents may be reduced by sympathomimetics). Products include:

Toprol-XL Tablets 666

Metoprolol Tartrate (The antihypertensive effects of beta-adrenergic blocking agents may be reduced by sympathomimetics).
No products indexed under this heading.

Moclobemide (Due to the pseudoephedrine component, Clarinex-D 24 Hour extended-release tablets should not be used by patients taking monoamine oxidase inhibitors or within 14 days after stopping such treatment).
No products indexed under this heading.

Nadolol (The antihypertensive effects of beta-adrenergic blocking agents may be reduced by sympathomimetics). Products include:

Nadolol Tablets 2191

Nebivolol (The antihypertensive effects of beta-adrenergic blocking agents may be reduced by sympathomimetics). Products include:

Bystolic Tablets 1155

Pargyline Hydrochloride (Due to the pseudoephedrine component, Clarinex-D 24 Hour extended-release tablets should not be used by patients taking monoamine oxidase inhibitors or within 14 days after stopping such treatment).
No products indexed under this heading.

Penbutolol Sulfate (The antihypertensive effects of beta-adrenergic blocking agents may be reduced by sympathomimetics).
No products indexed under this heading.

Phenelzine Sulfate (Due to the pseudoephedrine component, Clarinex-D 24 Hour extended-release tablets should not be used by patients taking monoamine oxidase inhibitors or within 14 days after stopping such treatment).
No products indexed under this heading.

Pindolol (The antihypertensive effects of beta-adrenergic blocking agents may be reduced by sympathomimetics).
No products indexed under this heading.

Procarbazine Hydrochloride (Due to the pseudoephedrine component, Clarinex-D 24 Hour extended-release tablets should not be used by patients taking monoamine oxidase inhibitors or within 14 days after stopping such treatment).
No products indexed under this heading.

Propranolol Hydrochloride (The antihypertensive effects of beta-adrenergic blocking agents may be reduced by sympathomimetics). Products include:

InnoPran XL Extended Release Capsules 1484

Rasagiline Mesylate (Due to the pseudoephedrine component, Clarinex-D 24 Hour extended-release tablets should not be used by patients taking monoamine oxidase inhibitors or within 14 days after stopping such treatment). Products include:

Azilect Tablets 3106

Reserpine (The antihypertensive effects of reserpine may be reduced by sympathomimetics).
No products indexed under this heading.

Selegiline (Due to the pseudoephedrine component, Clarinex-D 24 Hour extended-release tablets should not be used by patients taking monoamine oxidase inhibitors or within 14 days after stopping such treatment). Products include:

Emsam Transdermal System 905

Selegiline Hydrochloride (Due to the pseudoephedrine component, Clarinex-D 24 Hour extended-release tablets should not be used by patients taking monoamine oxidase inhibitors or within 14 days after stopping such treatment). Products include:

Eldepryl Capsules 3052

Sotalol Hydrochloride (The antihypertensive effects of beta-adrenergic blocking agents may be reduced by sympathomimetics).
No products indexed under this heading.

Timolol Hemihydrate (The antihypertensive effects of beta-adrenergic blocking agents may be reduced by sympathomimetics). Products include:

Betimol Ophthalmic Solution 3181

Timolol Maleate (The antihypertensive effects of beta-adrenergic blocking agents may be reduced by sympathomimetics). Products include:

Combigan Ophthalmic Solution 553
Cosopt Sterile Ophthalmic Solution 1969
Timoptic Sterile Ophthalmic Solution 2121
Timoptic in Ocudose 2124
Timoptic-XE Sterile Ophthalmic Gel Forming Solution 2125

Tranylcypromine Sulfate (Due to the pseudoephedrine component, Clarinex-D 24 Hour extended-release tablets should not be used by patients taking monoamine oxidase inhibitors or within 14 days after stopping such treatment). Products include:

Parnate Tablets 1532

CLARITY CAPSULES

(Amino Acid Preparations, Bee Pollen, Ginkgo biloba, Herbals with Vitamins & Minerals, Hydroxypropyl Methylcellulose, Lecithin) 636
None cited in PDR database.

CLEAR EYES FOR DRY EYES

(Carboxymethylcellulose Sodium, Glycerin) .... ⊙255
None cited in PDR database.

CLEAR EYES ITCHY EYE RELIEF

(Glycerin, Naphazoline Hydrochloride, Zinc Sulfate) .... ⊙255
None cited in PDR database.

CLEAR EYES TRIPLE ACTION RELIEF

(Polyvinyl Alcohol, Povidone, Tetrahydrozoline Hydrochloride) .... ⊙255
None cited in PDR database.

CLEVIPREX

(Clevidipine Butyrate) 1936
None cited in PDR database.

CLIMARA TRANSDERMAL SYSTEM

(Estradiol) 763

May interact with cytochrome p450 3a4 inducers (selected), cytochrome p450 3a4 inhibitors (selected), and certain other agents. Compounds in these categories include:

Acetazolamide (Inhibitors of CYP3A4 such as erythromycin, clarithromycin, ketoconazole, itraconazole, ritonavir and grapefruit juice may increase plasma concentrations of estrogens and may result in side effects).
No products indexed under this heading.

Allium sativum (Inducers of CYP3A4 may reduce plasma concentrations of estrogens, possibly resulting in a decrease in therapeutic effects and/or changes in the uterine bleeding profile).
No products indexed under this heading.

Nifedipine (Inhibitors of CYP3A4 such as erythromycin, clarithromycin, ketoconazole, itraconazole, ritonavir and grapefruit juice may increase plasma concentrations of estrogens and may result in side effects).
No products indexed under this heading.

Norfloxacin (Inhibitors of CYP3A4 such as erythromycin, clarithromycin, ketoconazole, itraconazole, ritonavir and grapefruit juice may increase plasma concentrations of estrogens and may result in side effects). Products include:
Noroxin Tablets 2069

Omeprazole (Inhibitors of CYP3A4 such as erythromycin, clarithromycin, ketoconazole, itraconazole, ritonavir and grapefruit juice may increase plasma concentrations of estrogens and may result in side effects).
No products indexed under this heading.

Oxcarbazepine (Inducers of CYP3A4 may reduce plasma concentrations of estrogens, possibly resulting in a decrease in therapeutic effects and/or changes in the uterine bleeding profile).
No products indexed under this heading.

Paroxetine Hydrochloride (Inhibitors of CYP3A4 such as erythromycin, clarithromycin, ketoconazole, itraconazole, ritonavir and grapefruit juice may increase plasma concentrations of estrogens and may result in side effects). Products include:
Paxil 1535
Paxil CR Controlled-Release Tablets 1544

Phenobarbital (Inducers of CYP3A4, such as phenobarbital, may be reduce plasma concentrations of estrogens, possibly resulting in a decrease in therapeutic effects and/or changes in uterine bleeding profile). Products include:
Donnatal Extentabs 2507

Phenobarbital Sodium (Inducers of CYP3A4 may reduce plasma concentrations of estrogens, possibly resulting in a decrease in therapeutic effects and/or changes in the uterine bleeding profile).
No products indexed under this heading.

Phenytoin (Inducers of CYP3A4 may reduce plasma concentrations of estrogens, possibly resulting in a decrease in therapeutic effects and/ or changes in the uterine bleeding profile).
No products indexed under this heading.

Phenytoin Sodium (Inducers of CYP3A4 may reduce plasma concentrations of estrogens, possibly resulting in a decrease in therapeutic effects and/or changes in the uterine bleeding profile). Products include:
Phenytek Capsules 2192

Prednisolone Acetate (Inducers of CYP3A4 may reduce plasma concentrations of estrogens, possibly resulting in a decrease in therapeutic effects and/or changes in the uterine bleeding profile). Products include:
Pred Forte Ophthalmic Suspension .... ⊙227
Pred Mild Ophthalmic Suspension .... ⊙230
Pred-G Ophthalmic Ointment .... ⊙229
Pred-G Ophthalmic Suspension .... ⊙228

Prednisolone Sodium Phosphate (Inducers of CYP3A4 may reduce plasma concentrations of estrogens, possibly resulting in a decrease in therapeutic effects and/or changes in the uterine bleeding profile).
No products indexed under this heading.

Prednisolone Tebutate (Inducers of CYP3A4 may reduce plasma concentrations of estrogens, possibly resulting in a decrease in therapeutic effects and/or changes in the uterine bleeding profile).
No products indexed under this heading.

Prednisone (Inducers of CYP3A4 may reduce plasma concentrations of estrogens, possibly resulting in a decrease in therapeutic effects and/ or changes in the uterine bleeding profile).
No products indexed under this heading.

Primidone (Inducers of CYP3A4 may reduce plasma concentrations of estrogens, possibly resulting in a decrease in therapeutic effects and/ or changes in the uterine bleeding profile).
No products indexed under this heading.

Propoxyphene Hydrochloride (Inhibitors of CYP3A4 such as erythromycin, clarithromycin, ketoconazole, itraconazole, ritonavir and grapefruit juice may increase plasma concentrations of estrogens and may result in side effects).
No products indexed under this heading.

Propoxyphene Napsylate (Inhibitors of CYP3A4 such as erythromycin, clarithromycin, ketoconazole, itraconazole, ritonavir and grapefruit juice may increase plasma concentrations of estrogens and may result in side effects).
No products indexed under this heading.

Quinidine (Inhibitors of CYP3A4 such as erythromycin, clarithromycin, ketoconazole, itraconazole, ritonavir and grapefruit juice may increase plasma concentrations of estrogens and may result in side effects).
No products indexed under this heading.

Quinidine Hydrochloride (Inhibitors of CYP3A4 such as erythromycin, clarithromycin, ketoconazole, itraconazole, ritonavir and grapefruit juice may increase plasma concentrations of estrogens and may result in side effects).
No products indexed under this heading.

Quinidine Polygalacturonate (Inhibitors of CYP3A4 such as erythromycin, clarithromycin, ketoconazole, itraconazole, ritonavir and grapefruit juice may increase plasma concentrations of estrogens and may result in side effects).
No products indexed under this heading.

Quinidine Sulfate (Inhibitors of CYP3A4 such as erythromycin, clarithromycin, ketoconazole, itraconazole, ritonavir and grapefruit juice may increase plasma concentrations of estrogens and may result in side effects).
No products indexed under this heading.

Quinine (Inhibitors of CYP3A4 such as erythromycin, clarithromycin, ketoconazole, itraconazole, ritonavir and grapefruit juice may increase plasma concentrations of estrogens and may result in side effects).
No products indexed under this heading.

Quinine Sulfate (Inhibitors of CYP3A4 such as erythromycin, clarithromycin, ketoconazole, itraconazole, ritonavir and grapefruit juice may increase plasma concentrations of estrogens and may result in side effects).
No products indexed under this heading.

Quinupristin (Inhibitors of CYP3A4 such as erythromycin, clarithromycin, ketoconazole, itraconazole, ritonavir and grapefruit juice may increase plasma concentrations of estrogens and may result in side effects).
No products indexed under this heading.

Ranitidine Bismuth Citrate (Inhibitors of CYP3A4 such as erythromycin, clarithromycin, ketoconazole, itraconazole, ritonavir and grapefruit juice may increase plasma concentrations of estrogens and may result in side effects).
No products indexed under this heading.

Ranitidine Hydrochloride (Inhibitors of CYP3A4 such as erythromycin, clarithromycin, ketoconazole, itraconazole, ritonavir and grapefruit juice may increase plasma concentrations of estrogens and may result in side effects). Products include:
Zantac 75 Tablets .... ▣603
Zantac 1670
Zantac Injection 1666
Zantac Injection Pharmacy Bulk Package 1668
Maximum Strength Zantac 150 Tablets .... ▣603
Maximum Strength Zantac 150 Cool Mint Tablets .... ▣603

Rifabutin (Inducers of CYP3A4 may reduce plasma concentrations of estrogens, possibly resulting in a decrease in therapeutic effects and/ or changes in the uterine bleeding profile).
No products indexed under this heading.

Rifampicin (Inducers of CYP3A4 may reduce plasma concentrations of estrogens, possibly resulting in a decrease in therapeutic effects and/ or changes in the uterine bleeding profile).
No products indexed under this heading.

Rifampin (Inducers of CYP3A4, such as rifampin, may reduce plasma concentrations of estrogens, possibly resulting in a decrease in therapuetic effects and/or changes in uterine bleeding profile).
No products indexed under this heading.

Rifapentine (Inducers of CYP3A4 may reduce plasma concentrations of estrogens, possibly resulting in a decrease in therapeutic effects and/ or changes in the uterine bleeding profile).
No products indexed under this heading.

Ritonavir (Inducers of CYP3A4, such as ritonavir, may increase plasma concentrations of estrogens and may result in side effects). Products include:
Kaletra 452
Norvir 489

Saquinavir (Inhibitors of CYP3A4 such as erythromycin, clarithromycin, ketoconazole, itraconazole, ritonavir and grapefruit juice may increase plasma concentrations of estrogens and may result in side effects).
No products indexed under this heading.

Saquinavir Mesylate (Inhibitors of CYP3A4 such as erythromycin, clarithromycin, ketoconazole, itraconazole, ritonavir and grapefruit juice may increase plasma concentrations of estrogens and may result in side effects).
No products indexed under this heading.

Sertraline Hydrochloride (Inhibitors of CYP3A4 such as erythromycin, clarithromycin, ketoconazole, itraconazole, ritonavir and grapefruit juice may increase plasma concentrations of estrogens and may result in side effects).
No products indexed under this heading.

Sildenafil Citrate (Inhibitors of CYP3A4 such as erythromycin, clarithromycin, ketoconazole, itraconazole, ritonavir and grapefruit juice may increase plasma concentrations of estrogens and may result in side effects).
No products indexed under this heading.

Sulfinpyrazone (Inducers of CYP3A4 may reduce plasma concentrations of estrogens, possibly resulting in a decrease in therapeutic effects and/or changes in the uterine bleeding profile).
No products indexed under this heading.

Telithromycin (Inhibitors of CYP3A4 such as erythromycin, clarithromycin, ketoconazole, itraconazole, ritonavir and grapefruit juice may increase plasma concentrations of estrogens and may result in side effects). Products include:
Ketek Tablets 2744

Theophylline (Inducers of CYP3A4 may reduce plasma concentrations of estrogens, possibly resulting in a decrease in therapeutic effects and/ or changes in the uterine bleeding profile).
No products indexed under this heading.

Theophylline Anhydrous (Inducers of CYP3A4 may reduce plasma concentrations of estrogens, possibly resulting in a decrease in therapeutic effects and/or changes in the uterine bleeding profile). Products include:
Uniphyl Tablets 2595

Theophylline Calcium Salicylate (Inducers of CYP3A4 may reduce plasma concentrations of estrogens, possibly resulting in a decrease in therapeutic effects and/or changes in the uterine bleeding profile).
No products indexed under this heading.

Theophylline Dihydroxypropyl (Glyceryl) (Inducers of CYP3A4 may reduce plasma concentrations of estrogens, possibly resulting in a decrease in therapeutic effects and/or changes in the uterine bleeding profile).
No products indexed under this heading.

Theophylline Ethylenediamine (Inducers of CYP3A4 may reduce plasma concentrations of estrogens, possibly resulting in a decrease in therapeutic effects and/or changes in the uterine bleeding profile).
No products indexed under this heading.

Triamcinolone (Inducers of CYP3A4 may reduce plasma concentrations of estrogens, possibly resulting in a decrease in therapeutic effects and/or changes in the uterine bleeding profile).
No products indexed under this heading.

Triamcinolone Acetonide (Inducers of CYP3A4 may reduce plasma concentrations of estrogens, possibly resulting in a decrease in therapeutic effects and/or changes in the uterine bleeding profile). Products include:
Azmacort Inhalation Aerosol 407
Nasacort AQ Nasal Spray 2765
Triesence Injectable Suspension .... ⊙209

Triamcinolone Diacetate (Inducers of CYP3A4 may reduce plasma concentrations of estrogens, possibly resulting in a decrease in therapeutic effects and/or changes in the uterine bleeding profile).
No products indexed under this heading.

Triamcinolone Hexacetonide (Inducers of CYP3A4 may reduce plasma concentrations of estrogens, possibly resulting in a decrease in therapeutic effects and/or changes in the uterine bleeding profile).
No products indexed under this heading.

Troglitazone (Inducers of CYP3A4 may reduce plasma concentrations of estrogens, possibly resulting in a decrease in therapeutic effects and/or changes in the uterine bleeding profile).
No products indexed under this heading.

Troleandomycin (Inhibitors of CYP3A4 such as erythromycin, clarithromycin, ketoconazole, itraconazole, ritonavir and grapefruit juice may increase plasma concentrations of estrogens and may result in side effects).
No products indexed under this heading.

Valproate Sodium (Inhibitors of CYP3A4 such as erythromycin, clarithromycin, ketoconazole, itraconazole, ritonavir and grapefruit juice may increase plasma concentrations of estrogens and may result in side effects).
No products indexed under this heading.

Vardenafil Hydrochloride (Inhibitors of CYP3A4 such as erythromycin, clarithromycin, ketoconazole, itraconazole, ritonavir and grapefruit juice may increase plasma concentrations of estrogens and may result in side effects). Products include:
Levitra Tablets 2876

Verapamil Hydrochloride (Inhibitors of CYP3A4 such as erythromycin, clarithromycin, ketoconazole, itraconazole, ritonavir and grapefruit juice may increase plasma concentrations of estrogens and may result in side effects). Products include:
Tarka Tablets 511

Voriconazole (Inhibitors of CYP3A4 such as erythromycin, clarithromycin, ketoconazole, itraconazole, ritonavir and grapefruit juice may increase plasma concentrations of estrogens and may result in side effects).
No products indexed under this heading.

Zafirlukast (Inhibitors of CYP3A4 such as erythromycin, clarithromycin, ketoconazole, itraconazole, ritonavir and grapefruit juice may increase plasma concentrations of estrogens and may result in side effects). Products include:
Accolate Tablets 669

Zileuton (Inhibitors of CYP3A4 such as erythromycin, clarithromycin, ketoconazole, itraconazole, ritonavir and grapefruit juice may increase plasma concentrations of estrogens and may result in side effects).
No products indexed under this heading.

Food Interactions

Grapefruit (Inhibitors of CYP3A4 such as erythromycin, clarithromycin, ketoconazole, itraconazole, ritonavir and grapefruit juice may increase plasma concentrations of estrogens and may result in side effects).

Grapefruit Juice (Inducers of CYP3A4, such as grapefruit juice, may increase plasma concentrations of estrogens and may result in side effects).

CLIMARA PRO TRANSDERMAL SYSTEM

(Estradiol, Levonorgestrel) 768
May interact with cytochrome p450 2c18 inhibitors (selected), cytochrome p450 2c19 inducers (selected), cytochrome p450 2c19 inhibitors (selected), cytochrome p450 2c8 inducers (selected), cytochrome p450 2c8 inhibitors (selected), cytochrome p450 2c9 inducers (selected), cytochrome p450 2c9 inhibitors (selected), cytochrome p450 3a4 inducers (selected), and cytochrome p450 3a4 inhibitors (selected). Compounds in these categories include:

Acetazolamide (Inhibitors of CYP3A4 such as erythromycin, clarithromycin, ketoconazole, itraconazole, ritonavir and grapefruit juice may increase plasma concentrations of estrogens and may result in side effects).
No products indexed under this heading.

Allium sativum (Inducers of CYP3A4 may reduce plasma concentrations of estrogens, possibly resulting in a decrease in therapeutic effects and/or changes in the uterine bleeding profile).
No products indexed under this heading.

Amiodarone Hydrochloride (Inhibitors of CYP3A4 such as erythromycin, clarithromycin, ketoconazole, itraconazole, ritonavir and grapefruit juice may increase plasma concentrations of estrogens and may result in side effects).
No products indexed under this heading.

Amprenavir (Inhibitors of CYP3A4 such as erythromycin, clarithromycin, ketoconazole, itraconazole, ritonavir and grapefruit juice may increase plasma concentrations of estrogens and may result in side effects).
No products indexed under this heading.

Anastrozole (Inhibitors of CYP3A4 such as erythromycin, clarithromycin, ketoconazole, itraconazole, ritonavir and grapefruit juice may increase plasma concentrations of estrogens and may result in side effects). Products include:
Arimidex Tablets 672

Aprepitant (Inducers of CYP3A4 may reduce plasma concentrations of estrogens, possibly resulting in a decrease in therapeutic effects and/or changes in the uterine bleeding profile). Products include:
Emend Capsules 1992

Atazanavir (Inhibitors of CYP3A4 such as erythromycin, clarithromycin, ketoconazole, itraconazole, ritonavir and grapefruit juice may increase plasma concentrations of estrogens and may result in side effects).
No products indexed under this heading.

Atazanavir Sulfate (Inhibitors of CYP3A4 such as erythromycin, clarithromycin, ketoconazole, itraconazole, ritonavir and grapefruit juice may increase plasma concentrations of estrogens and may result in side effects). Products include:
Reyataz Capsules 3299

Bendroflumethiazide (Based on in-vitro and in-vivo studies, it can be assumed that CYP3A, CYP2E and CYP2C are involved in the metabolism of levonorgestrel. Likewise, inducers or inhibitors of these enzymes may either, respectively, decrease the therapeutic effects or resultin side effects).
No products indexed under this heading.

Betamethasone Acetate (Inducers of CYP3A4 may reduce plasma concentrations of estrogens, possibly resulting in a decrease in therapeutic effects and/or changes in the uterine bleeding profile).
No products indexed under this heading.

Betamethasone Sodium Phosphate (Inducers of CYP3A4 may reduce plasma concentrations of estrogens, possibly resulting in a decrease in therapeutic effects and/or changes in the uterine bleeding profile).
No products indexed under this heading.

Carbamazepine (Inducers of CYP3A4 may reduce plasma concentrations of estrogens, possibly resulting in a decrease in therapeutic effects and/or changes in the uterine bleeding profile). Products include:
Carbatrol Capsules 3019
Equetro Extended-Release Capsules 3174

Chloramphenicol (Based on in-vitro and in-vivo studies, it can be assumed that CYP3A, CYP2E and CYP2C are involved in the metabolism of levonorgestrel. Likewise, inducers or inhibitors of these enzymes may either, respectively, decrease the therapeutic effects or resultin side effects).
No products indexed under this heading.

Chlorothiazide (Based on in-vitro and in-vivo studies, it can be assumed that CYP3A, CYP2E and CYP2C are involved in the metabolism of levonorgestrel. Likewise, inducers or inhibitors of these enzymes may either, respectively, decrease the therapeutic effects or resultin side effects).
No products indexed under this heading.

Chlorothiazide Sodium (Based on in-vitro and in-vivo studies, it can be assumed that CYP3A, CYP2E and CYP2C are involved in the metabolism of levonorgestrel. Likewise, inducers or inhibitors of these enzymes may either, respectively, decrease the therapeutic effects or resultin side effects). Products include:
Intravenous Sodium Diuril 2490

Chlorpropamide (Based on in-vitro and in-vivo studies, it can be assumed that CYP3A, CYP2E and CYP2C are involved in the metabolism of levonorgestrel. Likewise, inducers or inhibitors of these enzymes may either, respectively, decrease the therapeutic effects or resultin side effects).
No products indexed under this heading.

Cimetidine (Inhibitors of CYP3A4 such as erythromycin, clarithromycin, ketoconazole, itraconazole, ritonavir and grapefruit juice may increase plasma concentrations of estrogens and may result in side effects).
No products indexed under this heading.

Cimetidine Hydrochloride (Inhibitors of CYP3A4 such as erythromycin, clarithromycin, ketoconazole, itraconazole, ritonavir and grapefruit juice may increase plasma concentrations of estrogens and may result in side effects).
No products indexed under this heading.

Ciprofloxacin (Inhibitors of CYP3A4 such as erythromycin, clarithromycin, ketoconazole, itraconazole, ritonavir and grapefruit juice may increase plasma concentrations of estrogens and may result in side effects). Products include:
Cipro I.V. 2817
Cipro Oral Suspension 2810
Cipro XR Tablets 2823
Ciprodex Otic Suspension 541

Ciprofloxacin Hydrochloride (Inducers of CYP3A4 may reduce plasma concentrations of estrogens, possibly resulting in a decrease in therapeutic effects and/or changes in the uterine bleeding profile). Products include:
Cipro Tablets 2810

Cisplatin (Inducers of CYP3A4 may reduce plasma concentrations of estrogens, possibly resulting in a decrease in therapeutic effects and/or changes in the uterine bleeding profile).
No products indexed under this heading.

Citalopram Hydrobromide (Based on in-vitro and in-vivo studies, it can be assumed that CYP3A, CYP2E and CYP2C are involved in the metabolism of levonorgestrel. Likewise, inducers or inhibitors of these enzymes may either, respectively, decrease the therapeutic effects or resultin side effects). Products include:
Celexa 1160

Clarithromycin (Inhibitors of CYP3A4 such as erythromycin, clarithromycin, ketoconazole, itraconazole, ritonavir and grapefruit juice may increase plasma concentrations of estrogens and may result in side effects). Products include:
Biaxin/Biaxin XL 411

Clopidogrel Hydrogen Sulfate (Based on in-vitro and in-vivo studies, it can be assumed that CYP3A, CYP2E and CYP2C are involved in the metabolism of levonorgestrel. Likewise, inducers or inhibitors of these enzymes may either, respectively, decrease the therapeutic effects or resultin side effects).
No products indexed under this heading.

Clotrimazole (Inhibitors of CYP3A4 such as erythromycin, clarithromycin, ketoconazole, itraconazole, ritonavir and grapefruit juice may increase plasma concentrations of estrogens and may result in side effects). Products include:
Lotrisone 2881

Cortisone Acetate (Inducers of CYP3A4 may reduce plasma concentrations of estrogens, possibly resulting in a decrease in therapeutic effects and/or changes in the uterine bleeding profile).
No products indexed under this heading.

Cyclosporine (Inhibitors of CYP3A4 such as erythromycin, clarithromycin, ketoconazole, itraconazole, ritonavir and grapefruit juice may increase plasma concentrations of estrogens and may result in side effects). Products include:
Gengraf Capsules 435
Neoral Oral Solution 2280
Neoral Soft Gelatin Capsules 2280
Restasis Ophthalmic Emulsion 557
Sandimmune 2296

Dalfopristin (Inhibitors of CYP3A4 such as erythromycin, clarithromycin, ketoconazole, itraconazole, ritonavir and grapefruit juice may increase plasma concentrations of estrogens and may result in side effects).
No products indexed under this heading.

Danazol (Inhibitors of CYP3A4 such as erythromycin, clarithromycin, ketoconazole, itraconazole, ritonavir and grapefruit juice may increase plasma concentrations of estrogens and may result in side effects).
No products indexed under this heading.

Delavirdine Mesylate (Inhibitors of CYP3A4 such as erythromycin, clarithromycin, ketoconazole, itraconazole, ritonavir and grapefruit juice may increase plasma concentrations of estrogens and may result in side effects).
No products indexed under this heading.

Desogestrel (Based on in-vitro and in-vivo studies, it can be assumed that CYP3A, CYP2E and CYP2C are involved in the metabolism of levonorgestrel. Likewise, inducers or inhibitors of these enzymes may either, respectively, decrease the therapeutic effects or resultin side effects). Products include:
Mircette Tablets 1034

Dexamethasone (Inducers of CYP3A4 may reduce plasma concentrations of estrogens, possibly resulting in a decrease in therapeutic effects and/or changes in the uterine bleeding profile). Products include:
Ciprodex Otic Suspension 541

Dexamethasone Acetate (Inducers of CYP3A4 may reduce plasma concentrations of estrogens, possibly resulting in a decrease in therapeutic effects and/or changes in the uterine bleeding profile).
No products indexed under this heading.

Dexamethasone Sodium Phosphate (Inducers of CYP3A4 may reduce plasma concentrations of estrogens, possibly resulting in a decrease in therapeutic effects and/or changes in the uterine bleeding profile).
No products indexed under this heading.

Diclofenac Potassium (Based on in-vitro and in-vivo studies, it can be assumed that CYP3A, CYP2E and CYP2C are involved in the metabolism of levonorgestrel. Likewise, inducers or inhibitors of these enzymes may either, respectively, decrease the therapeutic effects or resultin side effects).
No products indexed under this heading.

Diclofenac Sodium (Based on in-vitro and in-vivo studies, it can be assumed that CYP3A, CYP2E and CYP2C are involved in the metabolism of levonorgestrel. Likewise, inducers or inhibitors of these enzymes may either, respectively, decrease the therapeutic effects or resultin side effects). Products include:
Diclofenac Sodium Ophthalmic Solution ..... ⊙ 240
Voltaren Ophthalmic Solution 2336
Voltaren Tablets 2334
Voltaren-XR Tablets 2337

Diltiazem Hydrochloride (Inhibitors of CYP3A4 such as erythromycin, clarithromycin, ketoconazole, itraconazole, ritonavir and grapefruit juice may increase plasma concentrations of estrogens and may result in side effects). Products include:
Cardizem LA Extended Release Tablets 421

Diltiazem Maleate (Inhibitors of CYP3A4 such as erythromycin, clarithromycin, ketoconazole, itraconazole, ritonavir and grapefruit juice may increase plasma concentrations of estrogens and may result in side effects).
No products indexed under this heading.

Disulfiram (Based on in-vitro and in-vivo studies, it can be assumed that CYP3A, CYP2E and CYP2C are involved in the metabolism of levonorgestrel. Likewise, inducers or inhibitors of these enzymes may either, respectively, decrease the therapeutic effects or resultin side effects).
No products indexed under this heading.

Doxorubicin Hydrochloride (Inducers of CYP3A4 may reduce plasma concentrations of estrogens, possibly resulting in a decrease in therapeutic effects and/or changes in the uterine bleeding profile).
No products indexed under this heading.

Efavirenz (Inducers of CYP3A4 may reduce plasma concentrations of estrogens, possibly resulting in a decrease in therapeutic effects and/or changes in the uterine bleeding profile). Products include:
Atripla Tablets 938
Sustiva Capsules 930
Sustiva Tablets 930

Erythromycin (Inhibitors of CYP3A4 such as erythromycin, clarithromycin, ketoconazole, itraconazole, ritonavir and grapefruit juice may increase plasma concentrations of estrogens and may result in side effects).
No products indexed under this heading.

Erythromycin Estolate (Inhibitors of CYP3A4 such as erythromycin, clarithromycin, ketoconazole, itraconazole, ritonavir and grapefruit juice may increase plasma concentrations of estrogens and may result in side effects).
No products indexed under this heading.

Erythromycin Ethylsuccinate (Inhibitors of CYP3A4 such as erythromycin, clarithromycin, ketoconazole, itraconazole, ritonavir and grapefruit juice may increase plasma concentrations of estrogens and may result in side effects). Products include:
E.E.S. 433
EryPed 431

Erythromycin Gluceptate (Inhibitors of CYP3A4 such as erythromycin, clarithromycin, ketoconazole, itraconazole, ritonavir and grapefruit juice may increase plasma concentrations of estrogens and may result in side effects).
No products indexed under this heading.

Erythromycin Lactobionate (Inhibitors of CYP3A4 such as erythromycin, clarithromycin, ketoconazole, itraconazole, ritonavir and grapefruit juice may increase plasma concentrations of estrogens and may result in side effects).
No products indexed under this heading.

Erythromycin Stearate (Inhibitors of CYP3A4 such as erythromycin, clarithromycin, ketoconazole, itraconazole, ritonavir and grapefruit juice may increase plasma concentrations of estrogens and may result in side effects).
No products indexed under this heading.

Esomeprazole Magnesium (Inhibitors of CYP3A4 such as erythromycin, clarithromycin, ketoconazole, itraconazole, ritonavir and grapefruit juice may increase plasma concentrations of estrogens and may result in side effects). Products include:
Nexium Delayed-Release Capsules 645
Nexium Delayed-Release Oral Suspension 645

Ethinyl Estradiol (Based on in-vitro and in-vivo studies, it can be assumed that CYP3A, CYP2E and CYP2C are involved in the metabolism of levonorgestrel. Likewise, inducers or inhibitors of these enzymes may either, respectively, decrease the therapeutic effects or resultin side effects). Products include:
Lybrel Tablets 3204
Mircette Tablets 1034
NuvaRing 2897
Ortho-Cyclen/Ortho Tri-Cyclen 2449
Ortho Evra Transdermal System 2437
Ortho Tri-Cyclen Lo Tablets 2458
Seasonique Tablets 1046
Yaz Tablets 805

Ethosuximide (Inducers of CYP3A4 may reduce plasma concentrations of estrogens, possibly resulting in a decrease in therapeutic effects and/or changes in the uterine bleeding profile).
No products indexed under this heading.

Ethynodiol Diacetate (Based on in-vitro and in-vivo studies, it can be assumed that CYP3A, CYP2E and CYP2C are involved in the metabolism of levonorgestrel. Likewise, inducers or inhibitors of these enzymes may either, respectively, decrease the therapeutic effects or resultin side effects).
No products indexed under this heading.

Felbamate (Inducers of CYP3A4 may reduce plasma concentrations of estrogens, possibly resulting in a decrease in therapeutic effects and/or changes in the uterine bleeding profile).
No products indexed under this heading.

Fenofibrate (Based on in-vitro and in-vivo studies, it can be assumed that CYP3A, CYP2E and CYP2C are involved in the metabolism of levonorgestrel. Likewise, inducers or inhibitors of these enzymes may either, respectively, decrease the therapeutic effects or resultin side effects). Products include:
Fenoglide Tablets 2960
Tricor Tablets 520

Fluconazole (Inhibitors of CYP3A4 such as erythromycin, clarithromycin, ketoconazole, itraconazole, ritonavir and grapefruit juice may increase plasma concentrations of estrogens and may result in side effects).
No products indexed under this heading.

Fludrocortisone Acetate (Inducers of CYP3A4 may reduce plasma concentrations of estrogens, possibly resulting in a decrease in therapeutic effects and/or changes in the uterine bleeding profile).
No products indexed under this heading.

Fluorouracil (Based on in-vitro and in-vivo studies, it can be assumed that CYP3A, CYP2E and CYP2C are involved in the metabolism of levonorgestrel. Likewise, inducers or inhibitors of these enzymes may

either, respectively, decrease the therapeutic effects or resultin side effects). Products include:
Carac Cream 0.5% **2722**

Fluoxetine (Inhibitors of CYP3A4 such as erythromycin, clarithromycin, ketoconazole, itraconazole, ritonavir and grapefruit juice may increase plasma concentrations of estrogens and may result in side effects).
No products indexed under this heading.

Fluoxetine Hydrochloride (Inhibitors of CYP3A4 such as erythromycin, clarithromycin, ketoconazole, itraconazole, ritonavir and grapefruit juice may increase plasma concentrations of estrogens and may result in side effects). Products include:
Prozac Weekly Capsules **1852**
Prozac Pulvules and Liquid **1852**
Symbyax Capsules **1871**

Flurbiprofen (Based on in-vitro and in-vivo studies, it can be assumed that CYP3A, CYP2E and CYP2C are involved in the metabolism of levonorgestrel. Likewise, inducers or inhibitors of these enzymes may either, respectively, decrease the therapeutic effects or resultin side effects).
No products indexed under this heading.

Flurbiprofen Sodium (Based on in-vitro and in-vivo studies, it can be assumed that CYP3A, CYP2E and CYP2C are involved in the metabolism of levonorgestrel. Likewise, inducers or inhibitors of these enzymes may either, respectively, decrease the therapeutic effects or resultin side effects).
No products indexed under this heading.

Fluvastatin Sodium (Based on in-vitro and in-vivo studies, it can be assumed that CYP3A, CYP2E and CYP2C are involved in the metabolism of levonorgestrel. Likewise, inducers or inhibitors of these enzymes may either, respectively, decrease the therapeutic effects or resultin side effects). Products include:
Lescol Capsules **2268**
Lescol XL Tablets **2268**

Fluvoxamine (Based on in-vitro and in-vivo studies, it can be assumed that CYP3A, CYP2E and CYP2C are involved in the metabolism of levonorgestrel. Likewise, inducers or inhibitors of these enzymes may either, respectively, decrease the therapeutic effects or resultin side effects).
No products indexed under this heading.

Fluvoxamine Maleate (Inhibitors of CYP3A4 such as erythromycin, clarithromycin, ketoconazole, itraconazole, ritonavir and grapefruit juice may increase plasma concentrations of estrogens and may result in side effects). Products include:
Luvox CR Extended-Release Capsules **1759**

Fosamprenavir Calcium (Inhibitors of CYP3A4 such as erythromycin, clarithromycin, ketoconazole, itraconazole, ritonavir and grapefruit juice may increase plasma concentrations of estrogens and may result in side effects). Products include:
Lexiva Oral Suspension **1510**
Lexiva Tablets **1510**

Fosphenytoin Sodium (Inducers of CYP3A4 may reduce plasma concentrations of estrogens, possibly resulting in a decrease in therapeutic effects and/or changes in the uterine bleeding profile).
No products indexed under this heading.

Garlic Extract (Inducers of CYP3A4 may reduce plasma concentrations of estrogens, possibly resulting in a decrease in therapeutic effects and/or changes in the uterine bleeding profile).
No products indexed under this heading.

Garlic Oil (Inducers of CYP3A4 may reduce plasma concentrations of estrogens, possibly resulting in a decrease in therapeutic effects and/or changes in the uterine bleeding profile).
No products indexed under this heading.

Gemfibrozil (Based on in-vitro and in-vivo studies, it can be assumed that CYP3A, CYP2E and CYP2C are involved in the metabolism of levonorgestrel. Likewise, inducers or inhibitors of these enzymes may either, respectively, decrease the therapeutic effects or resultin side effects).
No products indexed under this heading.

Glipizide (Based on in-vitro and in-vivo studies, it can be assumed that CYP3A, CYP2E and CYP2C are involved in the metabolism of levonorgestrel. Likewise, inducers or inhibitors of these enzymes may either, respectively, decrease the therapeutic effects or resultin side effects).
No products indexed under this heading.

Glyburide (Based on in-vitro and in-vivo studies, it can be assumed that CYP3A, CYP2E and CYP2C are involved in the metabolism of levonorgestrel. Likewise, inducers or inhibitors of these enzymes may either, respectively, decrease the therapeutic effects or resultin side effects).
No products indexed under this heading.

Hydrochlorothiazide (Based on in-vitro and in-vivo studies, it can be assumed that CYP3A, CYP2E and CYP2C are involved in the metabolism of levonorgestrel. Likewise, inducers or inhibitors of these enzymes may either, respectively, decrease the therapeutic effects or resultin side effects). Products include:
Atacand HCT **642**
Avalide Tablets **892**
Avalide Tablets **2713**
Benicar HCT Tablets **1010**
Diovan HCT Tablets **2216**
Dyazide Capsules **1405**
Micardis HCT Tablets **854**
Prinzide Tablets **2092**
Tekturna HCT Tablets **2324**
Teveten HCT Tablets **517**

Hydrocortisone (Inducers of CYP3A4 may reduce plasma concentrations of estrogens, possibly resulting in a decrease in therapeutic effects and/or changes in the uterine bleeding profile).
No products indexed under this heading.

Hydrocortisone Acetate (Inducers of CYP3A4 may reduce plasma concentrations of estrogens, possibly resulting in a decrease in therapeutic effects and/or changes in the uterine bleeding profile). Products include:
Analpram-HC **1140**
Pramosone **1141**

Hydrocortisone Butyrate (Inducers of CYP3A4 may reduce plasma concentrations of estrogens, possibly resulting in a decrease in therapeutic effects and/or changes in the uterine bleeding profile).
No products indexed under this heading.

Hydrocortisone Cypionate (Inducers of CYP3A4 may reduce plasma concentrations of estrogens, possibly resulting in a decrease in therapeutic effects and/or changes in the uterine bleeding profile).
No products indexed under this heading.

Hydrocortisone Hemisuccinate (Inducers of CYP3A4 may reduce plasma concentrations of estrogens, possibly resulting in a decrease in therapeutic effects and/or changes in the uterine bleeding profile).
No products indexed under this heading.

Hydrocortisone Probutate (Inducers of CYP3A4 may reduce plasma concentrations of estrogens, possibly resulting in a decrease in therapeutic effects and/or changes in the uterine bleeding profile).
No products indexed under this heading.

Hydrocortisone Sodium Phosphate (Inducers of CYP3A4 may reduce plasma concentrations of estrogens, possibly resulting in a decrease in therapeutic effects and/or changes in the uterine bleeding profile).
No products indexed under this heading.

Hydrocortisone Sodium Succinate (Inducers of CYP3A4 may reduce plasma concentrations of estrogens, possibly resulting in a decrease in therapeutic effects and/or changes in the uterine bleeding profile).
No products indexed under this heading.

Hydrocortisone Valerate (Inducers of CYP3A4 may reduce plasma concentrations of estrogens, possibly resulting in a decrease in therapeutic effects and/or changes in the uterine bleeding profile).
No products indexed under this heading.

Hydroflumethiazide (Based on in-vitro and in-vivo studies, it can be assumed that CYP3A, CYP2E and CYP2C are involved in the metabolism of levonorgestrel. Likewise, inducers or inhibitors of these enzymes may either, respectively, decrease the therapeutic effects or resultin side effects).
No products indexed under this heading.

Hypericum (Inducers of CYP3A4 may reduce plasma concentrations of estrogens, possibly resulting in a decrease in therapeutic effects and/or changes in the uterine bleeding profile). Products include:
Satieté Tablets **640**

Hypericum Perforatum (Inducers of CYP3A4 may reduce plasma concentrations of estrogens, possibly resulting in a decrease in therapeutic effects and/or changes in the uterine bleeding profile).
No products indexed under this heading.

Imatinib Mesylate (Based on in-vitro and in-vivo studies, it can be assumed that CYP3A, CYP2E and CYP2C are involved in the metabolism of levonorgestrel. Likewise, inducers or inhibitors of these enzymes may either, respectively, decrease the therapeutic effects or resultin side effects). Products include:
Gleevec Tablets **2255**

Indinavir Sulfate (Inhibitors of CYP3A4 such as erythromycin, clarithromycin, ketoconazole, itraconazole, ritonavir and grapefruit juice may increase plasma concentrations of estrogens and may result in side effects). Products include:
Crixivan Capsules **1979**

Indomethacin (Based on in-vitro and in-vivo studies, it can be assumed that CYP3A, CYP2E and CYP2C are involved in the metabolism of levonorgestrel. Likewise, inducers or inhibitors of these enzymes may either, respectively, decrease the therapeutic effects or resultin side effects). Products include:
Indocin **2024**

Indomethacin Sodium Trihydrate (Based on in-vitro and in-vivo studies, it can be assumed that CYP3A, CYP2E and CYP2C are involved in the metabolism of levonorgestrel. Likewise, inducers or inhibitors of these enzymes may either, respectively, decrease the therapeutic effects or resultin side effects). Products include:
Indocin I.V. **2489**

Isoniazid (Inhibitors of CYP3A4 such as erythromycin, clarithromycin, ketoconazole, itraconazole, ritonavir and grapefruit juice may increase plasma concentrations of estrogens and may result in side effects).
No products indexed under this heading.

Itraconazole (Inhibitors of CYP3A4 such as erythromycin, clarithromycin, ketoconazole, itraconazole, ritonavir and grapefruit juice may increase plasma concentrations of estrogens and may result in side effects).
No products indexed under this heading.

Ketoconazole (Inhibitors of CYP3A4 such as erythromycin, clarithromycin, ketoconazole, itraconazole, ritonavir and grapefruit juice may increase plasma concentrations of estrogens and may result in side effects). Products include:
Extina Foam, 2% **3057**
Nizoral A-D Shampoo **1901**

Ketoprofen (Based on in-vitro and in-vivo studies, it can be assumed that CYP3A, CYP2E and CYP2C are involved in the metabolism of levonorgestrel. Likewise, inducers or inhibitors of these enzymes may either, respectively, decrease the therapeutic effects or resultin side effects).
No products indexed under this heading.

Lansoprazole (Based on in-vitro and in-vivo studies, it can be assumed that CYP3A, CYP2E and CYP2C are involved in the metabolism of levonorgestrel. Likewise, inducers or inhibitors of these enzymes may either, respectively, decrease the therapeutic effects or resultin side effects).
No products indexed under this heading.

Leflunomide (Based on in-vitro and in-vivo studies, it can be assumed that CYP3A, CYP2E and CYP2C are involved in the metabolism of levonorgestrel. Likewise, inducers or inhibitors of these enzymes may either, respectively, decrease the therapeutic effects or resultin side effects).
No products indexed under this heading.

Letrozole (Based on in-vitro and in-vivo studies, it can be assumed that CYP3A, CYP2E and CYP2C are involved in the metabolism of levonorgestrel. Likewise, inducers or inhibitors of these enzymes may either, respectively, decrease the therapeutic effects or resultin side effects). Products include:
Femara Tablets **2246**

Lopinavir (Inhibitors of CYP3A4 such as erythromycin, clarithromycin, ketoconazole, itraconazole, ritonavir and grapefruit juice may increase plasma concentrations of estrogens and may result in side effects). Products include:
Kaletra **452**

Loratadine (Inhibitors of CYP3A4 such as erythromycin, clarithromycin, ketoconazole, itraconazole, ritonavir and grapefruit juice may increase plasma concentrations of estrogens and may result in side effects).
No products indexed under this heading.

Lovastatin (Based on in-vitro and in-vivo studies, it can be assumed that CYP3A, CYP2E and CYP2C are involved in the metabolism of levonorgestrel. Likewise, inducers or inhibitors of these enzymes may either, respectively, decrease the therapeutic effects or resultin side effects). Products include:
Advicor Tablets **402**
Mevacor Tablets **2063**

Mephenytoin (Inducers of CYP3A4 may reduce plasma concentrations of estrogens, possibly resulting in a decrease in therapeutic effects and/or changes in the uterine bleeding profile).
No products indexed under this heading.

Mestranol (Based on in-vitro and in-vivo studies, it can be assumed that CYP3A, CYP2E and CYP2C are involved in the metabolism of levonorgestrel. Likewise, inducers or inhibitors of these enzymes may either, respectively, decrease the therapeutic effects or resultin side effects).
No products indexed under this heading.

Methsuximide (Inducers of CYP3A4 may reduce plasma concentrations of estrogens, possibly resulting in a decrease in therapeutic effects and/or changes in the uterine bleeding profile).
No products indexed under this heading.

Methyclothiazide (Based on in-vitro and in-vivo studies, it can be assumed that CYP3A, CYP2E and CYP2C are involved in the metabolism of levonorgestrel. Likewise, inducers or inhibitors of these enzymes may either, respectively, decrease the therapeutic effects or resultin side effects).
No products indexed under this heading.

Methylprednisolone (Inducers of CYP3A4 may reduce plasma concentrations of estrogens, possibly resulting in a decrease in therapeutic effects and/or changes in the uterine bleeding profile).
No products indexed under this heading.

Methylprednisolone Acetate (Inducers of CYP3A4 may reduce plasma concentrations of estrogens, possibly resulting in a decrease in therapeutic effects and/or changes in the uterine bleeding profile).
No products indexed under this heading.

Methylprednisolone Sodium Succinate (Inducers of CYP3A4 may reduce plasma concentrations of estrogens, possibly resulting in a decrease in therapeutic effects and/or changes in the uterine bleeding profile).
No products indexed under this heading.

Metronidazole (Inhibitors of CYP3A4 such as erythromycin, clarithromycin, ketoconazole, itraconazole, ritonavir and grapefruit juice may increase plasma concentrations of estrogens and may result in side effects). Products include:
Pylera Capsules **714**

Metronidazole Benzoate (Inhibitors of CYP3A4 such as erythromycin, clarithromycin, ketoconazole, itraconazole, ritonavir and grapefruit juice may increase plasma concentrations of estrogens and may result in side effects).
No products indexed under this heading.

Metronidazole Hydrochloride (Inhibitors of CYP3A4 such as erythromycin, clarithromycin, ketoconazole, itraconazole, ritonavir and grapefruit juice may increase plasma concentrations of estrogens and may result in side effects).
No products indexed under this heading.

Miconazole (Inhibitors of CYP3A4 such as erythromycin, clarithromycin, ketoconazole, itraconazole, ritonavir and grapefruit juice may increase plasma concentrations of estrogens and may result in side effects).
No products indexed under this heading.

Miconazole Nitrate (Inhibitors of CYP3A4 such as erythromycin, clarithromycin, ketoconazole, itraconazole, ritonavir and grapefruit juice may increase plasma concentrations of estrogens and may result in side effects).
No products indexed under this heading.

Modafinil (Inducers of CYP3A4 may reduce plasma concentrations of estrogens, possibly resulting in a decrease in therapeutic effects and/or changes in the uterine bleeding profile). Products include:
Provigil Tablets **977**

Nefazodone Hydrochloride (Inhibitors of CYP3A4 such as erythromycin, clarithromycin, ketoconazole, itraconazole, ritonavir and grapefruit juice may increase plasma concentrations of estrogens and may result in side effects).
No products indexed under this heading.

Nelfinavir Mesylate (Inhibitors of CYP3A4 such as erythromycin, clarithromycin, ketoconazole, itraconazole, ritonavir and grapefruit juice may increase plasma concentrations of estrogens and may result in side effects).
No products indexed under this heading.

Nevirapine (Inducers of CYP3A4 may reduce plasma concentrations of estrogens, possibly resulting in a decrease in therapeutic effects and/or changes in the uterine bleeding profile). Products include:
Viramune Oral Suspension **873**
Viramune Tablets **873**

Niacinamide (Inhibitors of CYP3A4 such as erythromycin, clarithromycin, ketoconazole, itraconazole, ritonavir and grapefruit juice may increase plasma concentrations of estrogens and may result in side effects). Products include:
BioLean Free Tablets .... ▣**635**

Nicardipine Hydrochloride (Based on in-vitro and in-vivo studies, it can be assumed that CYP3A, CYP2E and CYP2C are involved in the metabolism of levonorgestrel. Likewise, inducers or inhibitors of these enzymes may either, respectively, decrease the therapeutic effects or resultin side effects). Products include:
Cardene I.V. **1093**

Nicotinamide (Inhibitors of CYP3A4 such as erythromycin, clarithromycin, ketoconazole, itraconazole, ritonavir and grapefruit juice may increase plasma concentrations of estrogens and may result in side effects).
No products indexed under this heading.

Nifedipine (Inhibitors of CYP3A4 such as erythromycin, clarithromycin, ketoconazole, itraconazole, ritonavir and grapefruit juice may increase plasma concentrations of estrogens and may result in side effects).
No products indexed under this heading.

Norethindrone (Based on in-vitro and in-vivo studies, it can be assumed that CYP3A, CYP2E and CYP2C are involved in the metabolism of levonorgestrel. Likewise, inducers or inhibitors of these enzymes may either, respectively, decrease the therapeutic effects or resultin side effects). Products include:
Ortho Micronor Tablets **2446**

Norethindrone Acetate (Based on in-vitro and in-vivo studies, it can be assumed that CYP3A, CYP2E and CYP2C are involved in the metabolism of levonorgestrel. Likewise, inducers or inhibitors of these enzymes may either, respectively, decrease the therapeutic effects or resultin side effects). Products include:
Activella Tablets **2347**

Norethynodrel (Based on in-vitro and in-vivo studies, it can be assumed that CYP3A, CYP2E and CYP2C are involved in the metabolism of levonorgestrel. Likewise, inducers or inhibitors of these enzymes may either, respectively, decrease the therapeutic effects or resultin side effects).
No products indexed under this heading.

Norfloxacin (Inhibitors of CYP3A4 such as erythromycin, clarithromycin, ketoconazole, itraconazole, ritonavir and grapefruit juice may increase plasma concentrations of estrogens and may result in side effects). Products include:
Noroxin Tablets **2069**

Norgestimate (Based on in-vitro and in-vivo studies, it can be assumed that CYP3A, CYP2E and CYP2C are involved in the metabolism of levonorgestrel. Likewise, inducers or inhibitors of these enzymes may either, respectively, decrease the therapeutic effects or resultin side effects). Products include:
Ortho-Cyclen/Ortho Tri-Cyclen **2449**
Ortho Tri-Cyclen Lo Tablets **2458**

Norgestrel (Based on in-vitro and in-vivo studies, it can be assumed that CYP3A, CYP2E and CYP2C are involved in the metabolism of levonorgestrel. Likewise, inducers or inhibitors of these enzymes may either, respectively, decrease the therapeutic effects or resultin side effects).
No products indexed under this heading.

Omeprazole (Inhibitors of CYP3A4 such as erythromycin, clarithromycin, ketoconazole, itraconazole, ritonavir and grapefruit juice may increase plasma concentrations of estrogens and may result in side effects).
No products indexed under this heading.

Oxcarbazepine (Inducers of CYP3A4 may reduce plasma concentrations of estrogens, possibly resulting in a decrease in therapeutic effects and/or changes in the uterine bleeding profile).
No products indexed under this heading.

Oxiconazole Nitrate (Based on in-vitro and in-vivo studies, it can be assumed that CYP3A, CYP2E and CYP2C are involved in the metabolism of levonorgestrel. Likewise, inducers or inhibitors of these enzymes may either, respectively, decrease the therapeutic effects or resultin side effects).
No products indexed under this heading.

Paroxetine Hydrochloride (Inhibitors of CYP3A4 such as erythromycin, clarithromycin, ketoconazole, itraconazole, ritonavir and grapefruit juice may increase plasma concentrations of estrogens and may result in side effects). Products include:
Paxil **1535**
Paxil CR Controlled-Release Tablets **1544**

Phenobarbital (Inducers of CYP3A4 may reduce plasma concentrations of estrogens, possibly resulting in a decrease in therapeutic effects and/or changes in the uterine bleeding profile). Products include:

Donnatal Extentabs **2507**

Phenobarbital Sodium (Inducers of CYP3A4 may reduce plasma concentrations of estrogens, possibly resulting in a decrease in therapeutic effects and/or changes in the uterine bleeding profile).
No products indexed under this heading.

Phenylbutazone (Based on in-vitro and in-vivo studies, it can be assumed that CYP3A, CYP2E and CYP2C are involved in the metabolism of levonorgestrel. Likewise, inducers or inhibitors of these enzymes may either, respectively, decrease the therapeutic effects or resultin side effects).
No products indexed under this heading.

Phenytoin (Inducers of CYP3A4 may reduce plasma concentrations of estrogens, possibly resulting in a decrease in therapeutic effects and/or changes in the uterine bleeding profile).
No products indexed under this heading.

Phenytoin Sodium (Inducers of CYP3A4 may reduce plasma concentrations of estrogens, possibly resulting in a decrease in therapeutic effects and/or changes in the uterine bleeding profile). Products include:
Phenytek Capsules **2192**

Polythiazide (Based on in-vitro and in-vivo studies, it can be assumed that CYP3A, CYP2E and CYP2C are involved in the metabolism of levonorgestrel. Likewise, inducers or inhibitors of these enzymes may either, respectively, decrease the therapeutic effects or resultin side effects).
No products indexed under this heading.

Prednisolone Acetate (Inducers of CYP3A4 may reduce plasma concentrations of estrogens, possibly resulting in a decrease in therapeutic effects and/or changes in the uterine bleeding profile). Products include:
Pred Forte Ophthalmic Suspension .... ⊙**227**
Pred Mild Ophthalmic Suspension .... ⊙**230**
Pred-G Ophthalmic Ointment .... ⊙**229**
Pred-G Ophthalmic Suspension ...... ⊙**228**

Prednisolone Sodium Phosphate (Inducers of CYP3A4 may reduce plasma concentrations of estrogens, possibly resulting in a decrease in therapeutic effects and/or changes in the uterine bleeding profile).
No products indexed under this heading.

Prednisolone Tebutate (Inducers of CYP3A4 may reduce plasma concentrations of estrogens, possibly resulting in a decrease in therapeutic effects and/or changes in the uterine bleeding profile).
No products indexed under this heading.

Prednisone (Inducers of CYP3A4 may reduce plasma concentrations of estrogens, possibly resulting in a decrease in therapeutic effects and/or changes in the uterine bleeding profile).
No products indexed under this heading.

Primidone (Inducers of CYP3A4 may reduce plasma concentrations of estrogens, possibly resulting in a decrease in therapeutic effects and/or changes in the uterine bleeding profile).
No products indexed under this heading.

Propoxyphene Hydrochloride (Inhibitors of CYP3A4 such as erythromycin, clarithromycin, ketoconazole, itraconazole, ritonavir and grapefruit juice may increase plasma concentrations of estrogens and may result in side effects).
No products indexed under this heading.

Propoxyphene Napsylate (Inhibitors of CYP3A4 such as erythromycin, clarithromycin, ketoconazole, itraconazole, ritonavir and grapefruit juice may increase plasma concentrations of estrogens and may result in side effects).
No products indexed under this heading.

Quercetin (Based on in-vitro and in-vivo studies, it can be assumed that CYP3A, CYP2E and CYP2C are involved in the metabolism of levonorgestrel. Likewise, inducers or inhibitors of these enzymes may either, respectively, decrease the therapeutic effects or resultin side effects).
No products indexed under this heading.

Quinidine (Inhibitors of CYP3A4 such as erythromycin, clarithromycin, ketoconazole, itraconazole, ritonavir and grapefruit juice may increase plasma concentrations of estrogens and may result in side effects).
No products indexed under this heading.

Quinidine Hydrochloride (Inhibitors of CYP3A4 such as erythromycin, clarithromycin, ketoconazole, itraconazole, ritonavir and grapefruit juice may increase plasma concentrations of estrogens and may result in side effects).
No products indexed under this heading.

Quinidine Polygalacturonate (Inhibitors of CYP3A4 such as erythromycin, clarithromycin, ketoconazole, itraconazole, ritonavir and grapefruit juice may increase plasma concentrations of estrogens and may result in side effects).
No products indexed under this heading.

Quinidine Sulfate (Inhibitors of CYP3A4 such as erythromycin, clarithromycin, ketoconazole, itraconazole, ritonavir and grapefruit juice may increase plasma concentrations of estrogens and may result in side effects).
No products indexed under this heading.

Quinine (Inhibitors of CYP3A4 such as erythromycin, clarithromycin, ketoconazole, itraconazole, ritonavir and grapefruit juice may increase plasma concentrations of estrogens and may result in side effects).
No products indexed under this heading.

Quinine Sulfate (Inhibitors of CYP3A4 such as erythromycin, clarithromycin, ketoconazole, itraconazole, ritonavir and grapefruit juice may increase plasma concentrations of estrogens and may result in side effects).
No products indexed under this heading.

Quinupristin (Inhibitors of CYP3A4 such as erythromycin, clarithromycin, ketoconazole, itraconazole, ritonavir and grapefruit juice may increase plasma concentrations of estrogens and may result in side effects).
No products indexed under this heading.

Ranitidine Bismuth Citrate (Inhibitors of CYP3A4 such as erythromycin, clarithromycin, ketoconazole, itraconazole, ritonavir and grapefruit juice may increase plasma concentrations of estrogens and may result in side effects).
No products indexed under this heading.

Ranitidine Hydrochloride (Inhibitors of CYP3A4 such as erythromycin, clarithromycin, ketoconazole, itraconazole, ritonavir and grapefruit juice may increase plasma concentrations of estrogens and may result in side effects). Products include:
Zantac 75 Tablets **603**
Zantac **1670**
Zantac Injection **1666**
Zantac Injection Pharmacy Bulk Package **1668**
Maximum Strength Zantac 150 Tablets **603**
Maximum Strength Zantac 150 Cool Mint Tablets **603**

Rifabutin (Inducers of CYP3A4 may reduce plasma concentrations of estrogens, possibly resulting in a decrease in therapeutic effects and/or changes in the uterine bleeding profile).
No products indexed under this heading.

Rifampicin (Inducers of CYP3A4 may reduce plasma concentrations of estrogens, possibly resulting in a decrease in therapeutic effects and/or changes in the uterine bleeding profile).
No products indexed under this heading.

Rifampin (Inducers of CYP3A4 may reduce plasma concentrations of estrogens, possibly resulting in a decrease in therapeutic effects and/or changes in the uterine bleeding profile).
No products indexed under this heading.

Rifapentine (Inducers of CYP3A4 may reduce plasma concentrations of estrogens, possibly resulting in a decrease in therapeutic effects and/or changes in the uterine bleeding profile).
No products indexed under this heading.

Ritonavir (Inhibitors of CYP3A4 such as erythromycin, clarithromycin, ketoconazole, itraconazole, ritonavir and grapefruit juice may increase plasma concentrations of estrogens and may result in side effects). Products include:
Kaletra **452**
Norvir **489**

Saquinavir (Inhibitors of CYP3A4 such as erythromycin, clarithromycin, ketoconazole, itraconazole, ritonavir and grapefruit juice may increase plasma concentrations of estrogens and may result in side effects).
No products indexed under this heading.

Saquinavir Mesylate (Inhibitors of CYP3A4 such as erythromycin, clarithromycin, ketoconazole, itraconazole, ritonavir and grapefruit juice may increase plasma concentrations of estrogens and may result in side effects).
No products indexed under this heading.

Secobarbital Sodium (Based on in-vitro and in-vivo studies, it can be assumed that CYP3A, CYP2E and CYP2C are involved in the metabolism of levonorgestrel. Likewise, inducers or inhibitors of these enzymes may either, respectively, decrease the therapeutic effects or resultin side effects).
No products indexed under this heading.

Sertraline Hydrochloride (Inhibitors of CYP3A4 such as erythromycin, clarithromycin, ketoconazole, itraconazole, ritonavir and grapefruit juice may increase plasma concentrations of estrogens and may result in side effects).
No products indexed under this heading.

Sildenafil Citrate (Inhibitors of CYP3A4 such as erythromycin, clarithromycin, ketoconazole, itraconazole, ritonavir and grapefruit juice may increase plasma concentrations of estrogens and may result in side effects).
No products indexed under this heading.

Sulfacytine (Based on in-vitro and in-vivo studies, it can be assumed that CYP3A, CYP2E and CYP2C are involved in the metabolism of levonorgestrel. Likewise, inducers or inhibitors of these enzymes may either, respectively, decrease the therapeutic effects or resultin side effects).
No products indexed under this heading.

Sulfamethizole (Based on in-vitro and in-vivo studies, it can be assumed that CYP3A, CYP2E and CYP2C are involved in the metabolism of levonorgestrel. Likewise, inducers or inhibitors of these enzymes may either, respectively, decrease the therapeutic effects or resultin side effects).
No products indexed under this heading.

Sulfamethoxazole (Based on in-vitro and in-vivo studies, it can be assumed that CYP3A, CYP2E and CYP2C are involved in the metabolism of levonorgestrel. Likewise, inducers or inhibitors of these enzymes may either, respectively, decrease the therapeutic effects or resultin side effects).
No products indexed under this heading.

Sulfaphenazole (Based on in-vitro and in-vivo studies, it can be assumed that CYP3A, CYP2E and CYP2C are involved in the metabolism of levonorgestrel. Likewise, inducers or inhibitors of these enzymes may either, respectively, decrease the therapeutic effects or resultin side effects).
No products indexed under this heading.

Sulfasalazine (Based on in-vitro and in-vivo studies, it can be assumed that CYP3A, CYP2E and CYP2C are involved in the metabolism of levonorgestrel. Likewise, inducers or inhibitors of these enzymes may either, respectively, decrease the therapeutic effects or resultin side effects).
No products indexed under this heading.

Sulfinpyrazone (Inducers of CYP3A4 may reduce plasma concentrations of estrogens, possibly resulting in a decrease in therapeutic effects and/or changes in the uterine bleeding profile).
No products indexed under this heading.

Sulfisoxazole Acetyl (Based on in-vitro and in-vivo studies, it can be assumed that CYP3A, CYP2E and CYP2C are involved in the metabolism of levonorgestrel. Likewise, inducers or inhibitors of these enzymes may either, respectively, decrease the therapeutic effects or resultin side effects).
No products indexed under this heading.

Sulfisoxazole Diolamine (Based on in-vitro and in-vivo studies, it can be assumed that CYP3A, CYP2E and CYP2C are involved in the metabolism of levonorgestrel. Likewise, inducers or inhibitors of these enzymes may either, respectively, decrease the therapeutic effects or resultin side effects).
No products indexed under this heading.

Telithromycin (Inhibitors of CYP3A4 such as erythromycin, clarithromycin, ketoconazole, itraconazole, ritonavir and grapefruit juice may increase plasma concentrations of estrogens and may result in side effects). Products include:
Ketek Tablets **2744**

Telmisartan (Based on in-vitro and in-vivo studies, it can be assumed that CYP3A, CYP2E and CYP2C are involved in the metabolism of levonorgestrel. Likewise, inducers or inhibitors of these enzymes may either, respectively, decrease the therapeutic effects or resultin side effects). Products include:
Micardis Tablets **852**
Micardis HCT Tablets **854**

Terconazole (Based on in-vitro and in-vivo studies, it can be assumed that CYP3A, CYP2E and CYP2C are involved in the metabolism of levonorgestrel. Likewise, inducers or inhibitors of these enzymes may either, respectively, decrease the therapeutic effects or resultin side effects).
No products indexed under this heading.

Theophylline (Inducers of CYP3A4 may reduce plasma concentrations of estrogens, possibly resulting in a decrease in therapeutic effects and/or changes in the uterine bleeding profile).
No products indexed under this heading.

Theophylline Anhydrous (Inducers of CYP3A4 may reduce plasma concentrations of estrogens, possibly resulting in a decrease in therapeutic effects and/or changes in the uterine bleeding profile). Products include:
Uniphyl Tablets **2595**

Theophylline Calcium Salicylate (Inducers of CYP3A4 may reduce plasma concentrations of estrogens, possibly resulting in a decrease in therapeutic effects and/or changes in the uterine bleeding profile).
No products indexed under this heading.

Theophylline Dihydroxypropyl (Glyceryl) (Inducers of CYP3A4 may reduce plasma concentrations of estrogens, possibly resulting in a decrease in therapeutic effects and/or changes in the uterine bleeding profile).
No products indexed under this heading.

Theophylline Ethylenediamine (Inducers of CYP3A4 may reduce plasma concentrations of estrogens, possibly resulting in a decrease in therapeutic effects and/or changes in the uterine bleeding profile).
No products indexed under this heading.

Ticlopidine Hydrochloride (Based on in-vitro and in-vivo studies, it can be assumed that CYP3A, CYP2E and CYP2C are involved in the metabolism of levonorgestrel. Likewise, inducers or inhibitors of these enzymes may either, respectively, decrease the therapeutic effects or resultin side effects).
No products indexed under this heading.

Tolazamide (Based on in-vitro and in-vivo studies, it can be assumed that CYP3A, CYP2E and CYP2C are involved in the metabolism of levonorgestrel. Likewise, inducers or inhibitors of these enzymes may either, respectively, decrease the therapeutic effects or resultin side effects).
No products indexed under this heading.

Tolbutamide (Based on in-vitro and in-vivo studies, it can be assumed that CYP3A, CYP2E and CYP2C are involved in the metabolism of levonorgestrel. Likewise, inducers or inhibitors of these enzymes may either, respectively, decrease the therapeutic effects or resultin side effects).
No products indexed under this heading.

Tolbutamide Sodium (Based on in-vitro and in-vivo studies, it can be assumed that CYP3A, CYP2E and CYP2C are involved in the metabolism of levonorgestrel. Likewise, inducers or inhibitors of these enzymes may either, respectively, decrease the therapeutic effects or resultin side effects).
No products indexed under this heading.

Topiramate (Based on in-vitro and in-vivo studies, it can be assumed that CYP3A, CYP2E and CYP2C are involved in the metabolism of levonorgestrel. Likewise, inducers or inhibitors of these enzymes may either, respectively, decrease the therapeutic effects or resultin side effects).
No products indexed under this heading.

Triamcinolone (Inducers of CYP3A4 may reduce plasma concentrations of estrogens, possibly resulting in a decrease in therapeutic effects and/or changes in the uterine bleeding profile).
No products indexed under this heading.

Triamcinolone Acetonide (Inducers of CYP3A4 may reduce plasma concentrations of estrogens, possibly resulting in a decrease in therapeutic effects and/or changes in the uterine bleeding profile). Products include:
Azmacort Inhalation Aerosol **407**
Nasacort AQ Nasal Spray **2765**
Triesence Injectable Suspension .... ⊙ **209**

Triamcinolone Diacetate (Inducers of CYP3A4 may reduce plasma concentrations of estrogens, possibly resulting in a decrease in therapeutic effects and/or changes in the uterine bleeding profile).
No products indexed under this heading.

Triamcinolone Hexacetonide (Inducers of CYP3A4 may reduce plasma concentrations of estrogens, possibly resulting in a decrease in therapeutic effects and/or changes in the uterine bleeding profile).
No products indexed under this heading.

Trimethoprim (Based on in-vitro and in-vivo studies, it can be assumed that CYP3A, CYP2E and CYP2C are involved in the metabolism of levonorgestrel. Likewise, inducers or inhibitors of these enzymes may either, respectively, decrease the therapeutic effects or resultin side effects).
No products indexed under this heading.

Trimethoprim Hydrochloride (Based on in-vitro and in-vivo studies, it can be assumed that CYP3A, CYP2E and CYP2C are involved in the metabolism of levonorgestrel. Likewise, inducers or inhibitors of these enzymes may either, respectively, decrease the therapeutic effects or resultin side effects).
No products indexed under this heading.

Troglitazone (Inducers of CYP3A4 may reduce plasma concentrations of estrogens, possibly resulting in a decrease in therapeutic effects and/or changes in the uterine bleeding profile).
No products indexed under this heading.

Troleandomycin (Inhibitors of CYP3A4 such as erythromycin, clarithromycin, ketoconazole, itraconazole, ritonavir and grapefruit juice may increase plasma concentrations of estrogens and may result in side effects).
No products indexed under this heading.

Valproate Sodium (Inhibitors of CYP3A4 such as erythromycin, clarithromycin, ketoconazole, itraconazole, ritonavir and grapefruit juice may increase plasma concentrations of estrogens and may result in side effects).
No products indexed under this heading.

Vardenafil Hydrochloride (Inhibitors of CYP3A4 such as erythromycin, clarithromycin, ketoconazole, itraconazole, ritonavir and grapefruit juice may increase plasma concentrations of estrogens and may result in side effects). Products include:
Levitra Tablets **2876**

Verapamil Hydrochloride (Inhibitors of CYP3A4 such as erythromycin, clarithromycin, ketoconazole, itraconazole, ritonavir and grapefruit juice may increase plasma concentrations of estrogens and may result in side effects). Products include:
Tarka Tablets **511**

Voriconazole (Inhibitors of CYP3A4 such as erythromycin, clarithromycin, ketoconazole, itraconazole, ritonavir and grapefruit juice may increase plasma concentrations of estrogens and may result in side effects).
No products indexed under this heading.

Zafirlukast (Inhibitors of CYP3A4 such as erythromycin, clarithromycin, ketoconazole, itraconazole, ritonavir and grapefruit juice may increase plasma concentrations of estrogens and may result in side effects). Products include:
Accolate Tablets **669**

Zileuton (Inhibitors of CYP3A4 such as erythromycin, clarithromycin, ketoconazole, itraconazole, ritonavir and grapefruit juice may increase plasma concentrations of estrogens and may result in side effects).
No products indexed under this heading.

Food Interactions

Grapefruit (Inhibitors of CYP3A4 such as erythromycin, clarithromycin, ketoconazole, itraconazole, ritonavir and grapefruit juice may increase plasma concentrations of estrogens and may result in side effects).

Grapefruit Juice (Inhibitors of CYP3A4 such as erythromycin, clarithromycin, ketoconazole, itraconazole, ritonavir and grapefruit juice may increase plasma concentrations of estrogens and may result in side effects).

CLINORIL TABLETS

(Sulindac) **1962**
May interact with ACE inhibitors, angiotensin-II receptor antagonists, oral anticoagulants, diuretics, oral hypoglycemic agents, lithium preparations, non-steroidal anti-inflammatory agents, and certain other agents. Compounds in these categories include:

Acarbose (Special attention should be paid to patients taking higher doses than those recommended and to patients with renal or metabolic impairment). Products include:
Precose Tablets **792**

Amiloride Hydrochloride (Sulindac can reduce the natriuretic effect of furosemide and thiazides in some patients. This response has been attributed to inhibition of renal prostaglandin synthesis. During concomitant therapy with NSAIDs, the patient should be observed closely for signs of renal failure, as well as to assure diuretic efficacy).
No products indexed under this heading.

Anisindione (Special attention should be paid to patients taking higher doses than those recommended and to patients with renal or metabolic impairment).
No products indexed under this heading.

Aspirin (Increased gastrointestinal reactions). Products include:
- Aggrenox Capsules ... **819**
- Bayer Aspirin ... **750**
- Percodan Tablets ... **1130**
- St. Joseph 81 mg Aspirin Chewable and Enteric Coated Tablets ... **1903**

Aspirin, Enteric Coated (Increased gastrointestinal reactions).
No products indexed under this heading.

Benazepril Hydrochloride (Reports suggest that NSAIDs may diminish the antihypertensive effect of ACE-inhibitors and angiotensin II antagonists. These interactions should be given consideration in patients taking NSAIDs concomitantly with ACE-inhibitors or angiotensin II antagonists. In some patients with compromised renal function, the co-administration of an NSAID and an ACE-inhibitor or an angiotensin II antagonist may result in further deterioration of renal function, including possible acute renal failure, which is usually reversible).
No products indexed under this heading.

Bendroflumethiazide (Sulindac can reduce the natriuretic effect of furosemide and thiazides in some patients. This response has been attributed to inhibition of renal prostaglandin synthesis. During concomitant therapy with NSAIDs, the patient should be observed closely for signs of renal failure, as well as to assure diuretic efficacy).
No products indexed under this heading.

Bumetanide (Sulindac can reduce the natriuretic effect of furosemide and thiazides in some patients. This response has been attributed to inhibition of renal prostaglandin synthesis. During concomitant therapy with NSAIDs, the patient should be observed closely for signs of renal failure, as well as to assure diuretic efficacy).
No products indexed under this heading.

Candesartan Cilexetil (Reports suggest that NSAIDs may diminish the antihypertensive effect of ACE-inhibitors and angiotensin II antagonists. These interactions should be given consideration in patients taking NSAIDs concomitantly with ACE-inhibitors or angiotensin II antagonists. In some patients with compromised renal function, the co-administration of an NSAID and an ACE-inhibitor or an angiotensin II antagonist may result in further deterioration of renal function, including possible acute renal failure, which is usually reversible). Products include:
- Atacand Tablets ... **639**
- Atacand HCT ... **642**

Captopril (Reports suggest that NSAIDs may diminish the antihypertensive effect of ACE-inhibitors and angiotensin II antagonists. These interactions should be given consideration in patients taking NSAIDs concomitantly with ACE-inhibitors or angiotensin II antagonists. In some patients with compromised renal function, the co-administration of an NSAID and an ACE-inhibitor or an angiotensin II antagonist may result in further deterioration of renal function, including possible acute renal failure, which is usually reversible). Products include:
- Captopril Tablets ... **2182**

Celecoxib (Concomitant use is not recommended due to the increased possibility of gastrointestinal toxicity, with little or no increase in efficacy). Products include:
- Celebrex Capsules ... **2979**

Chlorothiazide (Sulindac can reduce the natriuretic effect of furosemide and thiazides in some patients. This response has been attributed to inhibition of renal prostaglandin synthesis. During concomitant therapy with NSAIDs, the patient should be observed closely for signs of renal failure, as well as to assure diuretic efficacy).
No products indexed under this heading.

Chlorothiazide Sodium (Sulindac can reduce the natriuretic effect of furosemide and thiazides in some patients. This response has been attributed to inhibition of renal prostaglandin synthesis. During concomitant therapy with NSAIDs, the patient should be observed closely for signs of renal failure, as well as to assure diuretic efficacy). Products include:
- Intravenous Sodium Diuril ... **2490**

Chlorpropamide (Special attention should be paid to patients taking higher doses than those recommended and to patients with renal or metabolic impairment).
No products indexed under this heading.

Chlorthalidone (Sulindac can reduce the natriuretic effect of furosemide and thiazides in some patients. This response has been attributed to inhibition of renal prostaglandin synthesis. During concomitant therapy with NSAIDs, the patient should be observed closely for signs of renal failure, as well as to assure diuretic efficacy). Products include:
- Clorpres Tablets ... **2185**

Cyclosporine (Increased cyclosporine-induced toxicity). Products include:
- Gengraf Capsules ... **435**
- Neoral Oral Solution ... **2280**
- Neoral Soft Gelatin Capsules ... **2280**
- Restasis Ophthalmic Emulsion ... **557**
- Sandimmune ... **2296**

Diclofenac Epolamine (Concomitant use is not recommended due to the increased possibility of gastrointestinal toxicity, with little or no increase in efficacy). Products include:
- Flector Patch ... **561**

Diclofenac Potassium (Concomitant use is not recommended due to the increased possibility of gastrointestinal toxicity, with little or no increase in efficacy).
No products indexed under this heading.

Diclofenac Sodium (Concomitant use is not recommended due to the increased possibility of gastrointestinal toxicity, with little or no increase in efficacy). Products include:
- Diclofenac Sodium Ophthalmic Solution ... ⊙ **240**
- Voltaren Ophthalmic Solution ... **2336**
- Voltaren Tablets ... **2334**
- Voltaren-XR Tablets ... **2337**

Dicumarol (Special attention should be paid to patients taking higher doses than those recommended and to patients with renal or metabolic impairment).
No products indexed under this heading.

Diflunisal (Decreased plasma levels of sulindac).
No products indexed under this heading.

DMSO (Reduced efficacy of sulindac; peripheral neuropathy).
No products indexed under this heading.

Enalapril Maleate (Reports suggest that NSAIDs may diminish the antihypertensive effect of ACE-inhibitors and angiotensin II antagonists. These interactions should be given consideration in patients taking NSAIDs concomitantly with ACE-inhibitors or angiotensin II antagonists. In some patients with compromised renal function, the co-administration of an NSAID and an ACE-inhibitor or an angiotensin II antagonist may result in further deterioration of renal function, including possible acute renal failure, which is usually reversible).
No products indexed under this heading.

Enalaprilat (Reports suggest that NSAIDs may diminish the antihypertensive effect of ACE-inhibitors and angiotensin II antagonists. These interactions should be given consideration in patients taking NSAIDs concomitantly with ACE-inhibitors or angiotensin II antagonists. In some patients with compromised renal function, the co-administration of an NSAID and an ACE-inhibitor or an angiotensin II antagonist may result in further deterioration of renal function, including possible acute renal failure, which is usually reversible).
No products indexed under this heading.

Eprosartan Mesylate (Reports suggest that NSAIDs may diminish the antihypertensive effect of ACE-inhibitors and angiotensin II antagonists. These interactions should be given consideration in patients taking NSAIDs concomitantly with ACE-inhibitors or angiotensin II antagonists. In some patients with compromised renal function, the co-administration of an NSAID and an ACE-inhibitor or an angiotensin II antagonist may result in further deterioration of renal function, including possible acute renal failure, which is usually reversible). Products include:
- Teveten Tablets ... **515**
- Teveten HCT Tablets ... **517**

Ethacrynic Acid (Sulindac can reduce the natriuretic effect of furosemide and thiazides in some patients. This response has been attributed to inhibition of renal prostaglandin synthesis. During concomitant therapy with NSAIDs, the patient should be observed closely for signs of renal failure, as well as to assure diuretic efficacy). Products include:
- Edecrin Tablets ... **698**

Etodolac (Concomitant use is not recommended due to the increased possibility of gastrointestinal toxicity, with little or no increase in efficacy).
No products indexed under this heading.

Fenoprofen Calcium (Concomitant use is not recommended due to the increased possibility of gastrointestinal toxicity, with little or no increase in efficacy). Products include:
- Nalfon Capsules ... **2508**

Flurbiprofen (Concomitant use is not recommended due to the increased possibility of gastrointestinal toxicity, with little or no increase in efficacy).
No products indexed under this heading.

Fosinopril Sodium (Reports suggest that NSAIDs may diminish the antihypertensive effect of ACE-inhibitors and angiotensin II antagonists. These interactions should be given consideration in patients taking NSAIDs concomitantly with ACE-inhibitors or angiotensin II antagonists. In some patients with compromised renal function, the co-administration of an NSAID and an ACE-inhibitor or an angiotensin II antagonist may result in further deterioration of renal function, including possible acute renal failure, which is usually reversible).
No products indexed under this heading.

Furosemide (Clinoril may blunt the renal response to I.V. furosemide). Products include:
- Furosemide Tablets ... **2186**

Glimepiride (Special attention should be paid to patients taking higher doses than those recommended and to patients with renal or metabolic impairment). Products include:
- Avandaryl Tablets ... **1344**
- Duetact Tablets ... **3085**

Glipizide (Special attention should be paid to patients taking higher doses than those recommended and to patients with renal or metabolic impairment).
No products indexed under this heading.

Glyburide (Special attention should be paid to patients taking higher doses than those recommended and to patients with renal or metabolic impairment).
No products indexed under this heading.

Hydrochlorothiazide (Sulindac can reduce the natriuretic effect of furosemide and thiazides in some patients. This response has been attributed to inhibition of renal prostaglandin synthesis. During concomitant therapy with NSAIDs, the patient should be observed closely for signs of renal failure, as well as to assure diuretic efficacy). Products include:
- Atacand HCT ... **642**
- Avalide Tablets ... **892**
- Avalide Tablets ... **2713**
- Benicar HCT Tablets ... **1010**
- Diovan HCT Tablets ... **2216**
- Dyazide Capsules ... **1405**

Micardis HCT Tablets 854
Prinzide Tablets 2092
Tekturna HCT Tablets 2324
Teveten HCT Tablets 517

Hydroflumethiazide (Sulindac can reduce the natriuretic effect of furosemide and thiazides in some patients. This response has been attributed to inhibition of renal prostaglandin synthesis. During concomitant therapy with NSAIDs, the patient should be observed closely for signs of renal failure, as well as to assure diuretic efficacy).
No products indexed under this heading.

Ibuprofen (Concomitant use is not recommended due to the increased possibility of gastrointestinal toxicity, with little or no increase in efficacy). Products include:
Motrin IB Tablets and Caplets 1900
Children's Motrin Oral Suspension ... 1901
Children's Motrin Non-Staining Dye-Free Oral Suspension 1901
Children's Motrin Cold Oral Suspension 1899
Infants' Motrin Concentrated Drops 1901
Infants' Motrin Non-Staining Dye-Free Concentrated Drops 1901
Junior Strength Motrin Caplets and Chewable Tablets 1901
Vicoprofen Tablets 533

Indapamide (Sulindac can reduce the natriuretic effect of furosemide and thiazides in some patients. This response has been attributed to inhibition of renal prostaglandin synthesis. During concomitant therapy with NSAIDs, the patient should be observed closely for signs of renal failure, as well as to assure diuretic efficacy). Products include:
Indapamide Tablets 2188

Indomethacin (Concomitant use is not recommended due to the increased possibility of gastrointestinal toxicity, with little or no increase in efficacy). Products include:
Indocin 2024

Indomethacin Sodium Trihydrate (Concomitant use is not recommended due to the increased possibility of gastrointestinal toxicity, with little or no increase in efficacy). Products include:
Indocin I.V. 2489

Irbesartan (Reports suggest that NSAIDs may diminish the antihypertensive effect of ACE-inhibitors and angiotensin II antagonists. These interactions should be given consideration in patients taking NSAIDs concomitantly with ACE-inhibitors or angiotensin II antagonists. In some patients with compromised renal function, the co-administration of an NSAID and an ACE-inhibitor or an angiotensin II antagonist may result in further deterioration of renal function, including possible acute renal failure, which is usually reversible). Products include:
Avalide Tablets 892
Avalide Tablets 2713
Avapro Tablets 897
Avapro Tablets 2718

Ketoprofen (Concomitant use is not recommended due to the increased possibility of gastrointestinal toxicity, with little or no increase in efficacy).
No products indexed under this heading.

Ketorolac Tromethamine (Concomitant use is not recommended due to the increased possibility of gastrointestinal toxicity, with little or no increase in efficacy).
No products indexed under this heading.

Lisinopril (Reports suggest that NSAIDs may diminish the antihypertensive effect of ACE-inhibitors and angiotensin II antagonists. These interactions should be given consideration in patients taking NSAIDs concomitantly with ACE-inhibitors or angiotensin II antagonists. In some patients with compromised renal function, the co-administration of an NSAID and an ACE-inhibitor or an angiotensin II antagonist may result in further deterioration of renal function, including possible acute renal failure, which is usually reversible). Products include:
Prinivil Tablets 2087
Prinzide Tablets 2092

Lithium (NSAIDs have produced an elevation of plasma lithium levels and a reduction in renal lithium clearance. The mean minimum lithium concentration increased 15% and the renal clearance was decreased by approximately 20%. These effects have been attributed to inhibition of renal prostaglandin synthesis by the NSAID. Thus, when NSAIDs and lithium are administered concurrently, subject should be observed carefully for signs of lithium toxicity).
No products indexed under this heading.

Lithium Carbonate (NSAIDs have produced an elevation of plasma lithium levels and a reduction in renal lithium clearance. The mean minimum lithium concentration increased 15% and the renal clearance was decreased by approximately 20%. These effects have been attributed to inhibition of renal prostaglandin synthesis by the NSAID. Thus, when NSAIDs and lithium are administered concurrently, subject should be observed carefully for signs of lithium toxicity).
No products indexed under this heading.

Lithium Citrate (NSAIDs have produced an elevation of plasma lithium levels and a reduction in renal lithium clearance. The mean minimum lithium concentration increased 15% and the renal clearance was decreased by approximately 20%. These effects have been attributed to inhibition of renal prostaglandin synthesis by the NSAID. Thus, when NSAIDs and lithium are administered concurrently, subject should be observed carefully for signs of lithium toxicity).
No products indexed under this heading.

Losartan Potassium (Reports suggest that NSAIDs may diminish the antihypertensive effect of ACE-inhibitors and angiotensin II antagonists. These interactions should be given consideration in patients taking NSAIDs concomitantly with ACE-inhibitors or angiotensin II antagonists. In some patients with compromised renal function, the co-administration of an NSAID and an ACE-inhibitor or an angiotensin II antagonist may result in further deterioration of renal function, including possible acute renal failure, which is usually reversible). Products include:
Cozaar Tablets 1973

Meclofenamate Sodium (Concomitant use is not recommended due to the increased possibility of gastrointestinal toxicity, with little or no increase in efficacy).
No products indexed under this heading.

Mefenamic Acid (Concomitant use is not recommended due to the increased possibility of gastrointestinal toxicity, with little or no increase in efficacy).
No products indexed under this heading.

Meloxicam (Concomitant use is not recommended due to the increased possibility of gastrointestinal toxicity, with little or no increase in efficacy). Products include:
Mobic Oral Suspension 863
Mobic Tablets 863

Metformin Hydrochloride (Special attention should be paid to patients taking higher doses than those recommended and to patients with renal or metabolic impairment). Products include:
ActoPlus Met Tablets 3071
Avandamet Tablets 1336
Janumet Tablets 2041
PrandiMet Tablets 2967

Methotrexate Sodium (Decreased tubular secretion of methotrexate and potentiation of its toxicity).
No products indexed under this heading.

Methyclothiazide (Sulindac can reduce the natriuretic effect of furosemide and thiazides in some patients. This response has been attributed to inhibition of renal prostaglandin synthesis. During concomitant therapy with NSAIDs, the patient should be observed closely for signs of renal failure, as well as to assure diuretic efficacy).
No products indexed under this heading.

Metolazone (Sulindac can reduce the natriuretic effect of furosemide and thiazides in some patients. This response has been attributed to inhibition of renal prostaglandin synthesis. During concomitant therapy with NSAIDs, the patient should be observed closely for signs of renal failure, as well as to assure diuretic efficacy).
No products indexed under this heading.

Miglitol (Special attention should be paid to patients taking higher doses than those recommended and to patients with renal or metabolic impairment).
No products indexed under this heading.

Moexipril Hydrochloride (Reports suggest that NSAIDs may diminish the antihypertensive effect of ACE-inhibitors and angiotensin II antagonists. These interactions should be given consideration in patients taking NSAIDs concomitantly with ACE-inhibitors or angiotensin II antagonists. In some patients with compromised renal function, the co-administration of an NSAID and an ACE-inhibitor or an angiotensin II antagonist may result in further deterioration of renal function, including possible acute renal failure, which is usually reversible).
No products indexed under this heading.

Nabumetone (Concomitant use is not recommended due to the increased possibility of gastrointestinal toxicity, with little or no increase in efficacy).
No products indexed under this heading.

Naproxen (Concomitant use is not recommended due to the increased possibility of gastrointestinal toxicity, with little or no increase in efficacy). Products include:
EC-Naprosyn Delayed-Release Tablets 2632
Naprosyn Suspension 2632
Naprosyn Tablets 2632

Naproxen Sodium (Concomitant use is not recommended due to the increased possibility of gastrointestinal toxicity, with little or no increase in efficacy). Products include:
Anaprox Tablets 2632
Anaprox DS Tablets 2632
Treximet Tablets 1616

Nateglinide (Special attention should be paid to patients taking higher doses than those recommended and to patients with renal or metabolic impairment). Products include:
Starlix Tablets 2314

Oxaprozin (Concomitant use is not recommended due to the increased possibility of gastrointestinal toxicity, with little or no increase in efficacy).
No products indexed under this heading.

Perindopril Erbumine (Reports suggest that NSAIDs may diminish the antihypertensive effect of ACE-inhibitors and angiotensin II antagonists. These interactions should be given consideration in patients taking NSAIDs concomitantly with ACE-inhibitors or angiotensin II antagonists. In some patients with compromised renal function, the co-administration of an NSAID and an ACE-inhibitor or an angiotensin II antagonist may result in further deterioration of renal function, including possible acute renal failure, which is usually reversible). Products include:
Aceon Tablets (2 mg, 4 mg, 8 mg) 3038

Phenylbutazone (Concomitant use is not recommended due to the increased possibility of gastrointestinal toxicity, with little or no increase in efficacy).
No products indexed under this heading.

Pioglitazone Hydrochloride (Special attention should be paid to patients taking higher doses than those recommended and to patients with renal or metabolic impairment). Products include:
ActoPlus Met Tablets 3071
Actos Tablets 3077
Duetact Tablets 3085

Piroxicam (Concomitant use is not recommended due to the increased possibility of gastrointestinal toxicity, with little or no increase in efficacy).
No products indexed under this heading.

Polythiazide (Sulindac can reduce the natriuretic effect of furosemide and thiazides in some patients. This response has been attributed to inhibition of renal prostaglandin synthesis. During concomitant therapy with NSAIDs, the patient should be observed closely for signs of renal failure, as well as to assure diuretic efficacy).
No products indexed under this heading.

Probenecid (Increased plasma levels of sulindac; modest reduction in uricosuric action of probenecid).
No products indexed under this heading.

Quinapril Hydrochloride (Reports suggest that NSAIDs may diminish the antihypertensive effect of ACE-inhibitors and angiotensin II antagonists. These interactions should be given consideration in patients taking NSAIDs concomitantly with ACE-inhibitors or angiotensin II antagonists. In some patients with compromised renal function, the co-administration of an NSAID and an ACE-inhibitor or an angiotensin II antagonist may result in further deterioration of renal function, including possible acute renal failure, which is usually reversible).
No products indexed under this heading.

Ramipril (Reports suggest that NSAIDs may diminish the antihypertensive effect of ACE-inhibitors and angiotensin II antagonists. These interactions should be given consideration in patients taking NSAIDs concomitantly with ACE-inhibitors or angiotensin II antagonists. In some patients with compromised renal function, the co-administration of an NSAID and an ACE-inhibitor or an angiotensin II antagonist may result in further deterioration of renal function, including possible acute renal failure, which is usually reversible).
No products indexed under this heading.

Repaglinide (Special attention should be paid to patients taking higher doses than those recommended and to patients with renal or metabolic impairment). Products include:
PrandiMet Tablets 2967
Prandin Tablets 2971

Rofecoxib (Concomitant use is not recommended due to the increased possibility of gastrointestinal toxicity, with little or no increase in efficacy).
No products indexed under this heading.

Rosiglitazone Maleate (Special attention should be paid to patients taking higher doses than those recommended and to patients with renal or metabolic impairment). Products include:
Avandamet Tablets 1336
Avandaryl Tablets 1344
Avandia Tablets 1351

Sitagliptin Phosphate (Special attention should be paid to patients taking higher doses than those recommended and to patients with renal or metabolic impairment). Products include:
Janumet Tablets 2041
Januvia Tablets 2048

Spirapril Hydrochloride (Reports suggest that NSAIDs may diminish the antihypertensive effect of ACE-inhibitors and angiotensin II antagonists. These interactions should be given consideration in patients taking NSAIDs concomitantly with ACE-inhibitors or angiotensin II antagonists. In some patients with compromised renal function, the co-administration of an NSAID and an ACE-inhibitor or an angiotensin II antagonist may result in further deterioration of renal function, including possible acute renal failure, which is usually reversible).
No products indexed under this heading.

Spironolactone (Sulindac can reduce the natriuretic effect of furosemide and thiazides in some patients. This response has been attributed to inhibition of renal prostaglandin synthesis. During concomitant therapy with NSAIDs, the patient should be observed closely for signs of renal failure, as well as to assure diuretic efficacy).
No products indexed under this heading.

Telmisartan (Reports suggest that NSAIDs may diminish the antihypertensive effect of ACE-inhibitors and angiotensin II antagonists. These interactions should be given consideration in patients taking NSAIDs concomitantly with ACE-inhibitors or angiotensin II antagonists. In some patients with compromised renal function, the co-administration of an NSAID and an ACE-inhibitor or an angiotensin II antagonist may result in further deterioration of renal function, including possible acute renal failure, which is usually reversible). Products include:
Micardis Tablets 852
Micardis HCT Tablets 854

Tolazamide (Special attention should be paid to patients taking higher doses than those recommended and to patients with renal or metabolic impairment).
No products indexed under this heading.

Tolbutamide (Special attention should be paid to patients taking higher doses than those recommended and to patients with renal or metabolic impairment).
No products indexed under this heading.

Tolmetin Sodium (Concomitant use is not recommended due to the increased possibility of gastrointestinal toxicity, with little or no increase in efficacy).
No products indexed under this heading.

Torsemide (Sulindac can reduce the natriuretic effect of furosemide and thiazides in some patients. This response has been attributed to inhibition of renal prostaglandin synthesis. During concomitant therapy with NSAIDs, the patient should be observed closely for signs of renal failure, as well as to assure diuretic efficacy). Products include:
Demadex Injection 2630
Demadex Tablets 2630

Trandolapril (Reports suggest that NSAIDs may diminish the antihypertensive effect of ACE-inhibitors and angiotensin II antagonists. These interactions should be given consideration in patients taking NSAIDs concomitantly with ACE-inhibitors or angiotensin II antagonists. In some patients with compromised renal function, the co-administration of an NSAID and an ACE-inhibitor or an angiotensin II antagonist may result in further deterioration of renal function, including possible acute renal failure, which is usually reversible). Products include:
Mavik Tablets 472
Tarka Tablets 511

Triamterene (Sulindac can reduce the natriuretic effect of furosemide and thiazides in some patients. This response has been attributed to inhibition of renal prostaglandin synthesis. During concomitant therapy with NSAIDs, the patient should be observed closely for signs of renal failure, as well as to assure diuretic efficacy). Products include:
Dyazide Capsules 1405
Dyrenium Capsules 3189

Troglitazone (Special attention should be paid to patients taking higher doses than those recommended and to patients with renal or metabolic impairment).
No products indexed under this heading.

Valdecoxib (Concomitant use is not recommended due to the increased possibility of gastrointestinal toxicity, with little or no increase in efficacy).
No products indexed under this heading.

Valsartan (Reports suggest that NSAIDs may diminish the antihypertensive effect of ACE-inhibitors and angiotensin II antagonists. These interactions should be given consideration in patients taking NSAIDs concomitantly with ACE-inhibitors or angiotensin II antagonists. In some patients with compromised renal function, the co-administration of an NSAID and an ACE-inhibitor or an angiotensin II antagonist may result in further deterioration of renal function, including possible acute renal failure, which is usually reversible). Products include:
Diovan Tablets 2212
Diovan HCT Tablets 2216
Exforge Tablets 2238

Warfarin Sodium (Special attention should be paid to patients taking higher doses than those recommended and to patients with renal or metabolic impairment).
No products indexed under this heading.

Food Interactions

Food, unspecified (The peak plasma concentrations of biologically active sulfide metabolite is delayed slightly in the presence of food).

CLOLAR FOR INTRAVENOUS INFUSION

(Clofarabine) 1239
May interact with:

Cyclophosphamide (Patients who have previously received a hematopoetic stem cell transplant may be at higher risk for hepatotoxicity suggestive of veno-occlusive disease following treatment with clofarabine when used in combination with etoposide and cyclophosphamide).
No products indexed under this heading.

Etoposide (Patients who have previously received a hematopoetic stem cell transplant may be at higher risk for hepatotoxicity suggestive of veno-occlusive disease following treatment with clofarabine when used in combination with etoposide and cyclophosphamide).
No products indexed under this heading.

CLORPACTIN WCS-90

(Sodium Oxychlorosene) 1722
None cited in PDR database.

CLORPRES TABLETS

(Chlorthalidone, Clonidine Hydrochloride) 2185
May interact with antihypertensives, barbiturates, beta blockers, cardiac glycosides, oral hypoglycemic agents, hypnotics and sedatives, insulin, lithium preparations, narcotic analgesics, tricyclic antidepressants, and certain other agents. Compounds in these categories include:

Acarbose (Chlorthalidone causes hyperglycemia; higher dosage of oral hypoglycemic agents may be required). Products include:
Precose Tablets 792

Acebutolol Hydrochloride (Chlorthalidone may add to or potentiate the action of other antihypertensives; if therapy is to be discontinued in patients receiving clonidine and beta blockers concurrently, beta blockers should be discontinued several days before the gradual withdrawal of clonidine).
No products indexed under this heading.

Alfentanil Hydrochloride (Orthostatic hypotension may be aggravated by narcotics; orthostatic hypotension may be aggravated by barbiturates).
No products indexed under this heading.

Aliskiren (Chlorthalidone may add to or potentiate the action of other antihypertensives). Products include:
Tekturna Tablets 2321
Tekturna HCT Tablets 2324

Amitriptyline Hydrochloride (Co-administration of clonidine with tricyclic antidepressants may result in reduced effect of clonidine, necessitating an increase in dosage; concurrent use enhances the manifestation of corneal lesions in rats).
No products indexed under this heading.

Amlodipine Besylate (Chlorthalidone may add to or potentiate the action of other antihypertensives). Products include:
Azor Tablets 1005
Exforge Tablets 2238

Amoxapine (Co-administration of clonidine with tricyclic antidepressants may result in reduced effect of clonidine, necessitating an increase in dosage).
No products indexed under this heading.

Aprobarbital (Clonidine may enhance the CNS-depressive effects of barbiturates; orthostatic hypotension may be aggravated by barbiturates).
No products indexed under this heading.

Atenolol (Chlorthalidone may add to or potentiate the action of other antihypertensives; if therapy is to be discontinued in patients receiving clonidine and beta blockers concurrently, beta blockers should be discontinued several days before the gradual withdrawal of clonidine).
No products indexed under this heading.

Benazepril Hydrochloride (Chlorthalidone may add to or potentiate the action of other antihypertensives).
No products indexed under this heading.

Bendroflumethiazide (Chlorthalidone may add to or potentiate the action of other antihypertensives).
No products indexed under this heading.

Betaxolol Hydrochloride (Chlorthalidone may add to or potentiate the action of other antihypertensives; if therapy is to be discontinued in patients receiving clonidine and beta blockers concurrently, beta blockers should be discontinued several days before the gradual withdrawal of clonidine).
No products indexed under this heading.

Bisoprolol Fumarate (Chlorthalidone may add to or potentiate the action of other antihypertensives; if therapy is to be discontinued in patients receiving clonidine and beta blockers concurrently, beta blockers should be discontinued several days before the gradual withdrawal of clonidine).
No products indexed under this heading.

Buprenorphine Hydrochloride (Orthostatic hypotension may be aggravated by narcotics; orthostatic hypotension may be aggravated by barbiturates). Products include:
Suboxone Tablets ... 2601
Subutex Tablets ... 2601

Butabarbital (Clonidine may enhance the CNS-depressive effects of barbiturates; orthostatic hypotension may be aggravated by barbiturates).
No products indexed under this heading.

Butabarbital Sodium (Clonidine may enhance the CNS-depressive effects of other sedatives).
No products indexed under this heading.

Butalbital (Clonidine may enhance the CNS-depressive effects of barbiturates; orthostatic hypotension may be aggravated by barbiturates).
No products indexed under this heading.

Candesartan Cilexetil (Chlorthalidone may add to or potentiate the action of other antihypertensives). Products include:
Atacand Tablets ... 639
Atacand HCT ... 642

Captopril (Chlorthalidone may add to or potentiate the action of other antihypertensives). Products include:
Captopril Tablets ... 2182

Carteolol Hydrochloride (Chlorthalidone may add to or potentiate the action of other antihypertensives; if therapy is to be discontinued in patients receiving clonidine and beta blockers concurrently, beta blockers should be discontinued several days before the gradual withdrawal of clonidine).
No products indexed under this heading.

Chloral Hydrate (Clonidine may enhance the CNS-depressive effects of other sedatives).
No products indexed under this heading.

Chlorothiazide (Chlorthalidone may add to or potentiate the action of other antihypertensives).
No products indexed under this heading.

Chlorothiazide Sodium (Chlorthalidone may add to or potentiate the action of other antihypertensives). Products include:
Intravenous Sodium Diuril ... 2490

Chlorpropamide (Chlorthalidone causes hyperglycemia; higher dosage of oral hypoglycemic agents may be required).
No products indexed under this heading.

Clomipramine Hydrochloride (Co-administration of clonidine with tricyclic antidepressants may result in reduced effect of clonidine, necessitating an increase in dosage).
No products indexed under this heading.

Clonidine (Chlorthalidone may add to or potentiate the action of other antihypertensives). Products include:
Catapres-TTS ... 842

Codeine Phosphate (Orthostatic hypotension may be aggravated by narcotics; orthostatic hypotension may be aggravated by barbiturates). Products include:
Tylenol with Codeine Tablets ... 2427

Deserpidine (Chlorthalidone may add to or potentiate the action of other antihypertensives).
No products indexed under this heading.

Desipramine Hydrochloride (Co-administration of clonidine with tricyclic antidepressants may result in reduced effect of clonidine, necessitating an increase in dosage).
No products indexed under this heading.

Deslanoside (Digitalis therapy may exaggerate the metabolic effects of hypokalemia especially with reference to myocardial activity).
No products indexed under this heading.

Dezocine (Orthostatic hypotension may be aggravated by narcotics; orthostatic hypotension may be aggravated by barbiturates).
No products indexed under this heading.

Diazoxide (Chlorthalidone may add to or potentiate the action of other antihypertensives). Products include:
Proglycem Capsules ... 1185
Proglycem Suspension ... 1185

Digitalis Glycoside Preparations (Digitalis therapy may exaggerate the metabolic effects of hypokalemia especially with reference to myocardial activity).
No products indexed under this heading.

Digitoxin (Digitalis therapy may exaggerate the metabolic effects of hypokalemia especially with reference to myocardial activity).
No products indexed under this heading.

Digoxin (Digitalis therapy may exaggerate the metabolic effects of hypokalemia especially with reference to myocardial activity). Products include:
Lanoxin Injection ... 1498
Lanoxin Injection Pediatric ... 1502
Lanoxin Tablets ... 1505

Diltiazem Hydrochloride (Chlorthalidone may add to or potentiate the action of other antihypertensives). Products include:
Cardizem LA Extended Release Tablets ... 421

Doxazosin Mesylate (Chlorthalidone may add to or potentiate the action of other antihypertensives).
No products indexed under this heading.

Doxepin Hydrochloride (Co-administration of clonidine with tricyclic antidepressants may result in reduced effect of clonidine, necessitating an increase in dosage).
No products indexed under this heading.

Enalapril Maleate (Chlorthalidone may add to or potentiate the action of other antihypertensives).
No products indexed under this heading.

Enalaprilat (Chlorthalidone may add to or potentiate the action of other antihypertensives).
No products indexed under this heading.

Eprosartan Mesylate (Chlorthalidone may add to or potentiate the action of other antihypertensives). Products include:
Teveten Tablets ... 515
Teveten HCT Tablets ... 517

Esmolol Hydrochloride (Chlorthalidone may add to or potentiate the action of other antihypertensives; if therapy is to be discontinued in patients receiving clonidine and beta blockers concurrently, beta blockers should be discontinued several days before the gradual withdrawal of clonidine).
No products indexed under this heading.

Estazolam (Clonidine may enhance the CNS-depressive effects of other sedatives).
No products indexed under this heading.

Ethchlorvynol (Clonidine may enhance the CNS-depressive effects of other sedatives).
No products indexed under this heading.

Ethinamate (Clonidine may enhance the CNS-depressive effects of other sedatives).
No products indexed under this heading.

Felodipine (Chlorthalidone may add to or potentiate the action of other antihypertensives).
No products indexed under this heading.

Fentanyl (Orthostatic hypotension may be aggravated by narcotics; orthostatic hypotension may be aggravated by barbiturates). Products include:
Duragesic Transdermal System ... 2405
Ionsys Transdermal System ... 2410

Fentanyl Citrate (Orthostatic hypotension may be aggravated by narcotics; orthostatic hypotension may be aggravated by barbiturates). Products include:
Actiq ... 959
Fentora Tablets ... 968

Flurazepam Hydrochloride (Clonidine may enhance the CNS-depressive effects of other sedatives).
No products indexed under this heading.

Fosinopril Sodium (Chlorthalidone may add to or potentiate the action of other antihypertensives).
No products indexed under this heading.

Furosemide (Chlorthalidone may add to or potentiate the action of other antihypertensives). Products include:
Furosemide Tablets ... 2186

Glimepiride (Chlorthalidone causes hyperglycemia; higher dosage of oral hypoglycemic agents may be required). Products include:
Avandaryl Tablets ... 1344
Duetact Tablets ... 3085

Glipizide (Chlorthalidone causes hyperglycemia; higher dosage of oral hypoglycemic agents may be required).
No products indexed under this heading.

Glutethimide (Clonidine may enhance the CNS-depressive effects of other sedatives).
No products indexed under this heading.

Glyburide (Chlorthalidone causes hyperglycemia; higher dosage of oral hypoglycemic agents may be required).
No products indexed under this heading.

Guanabenz Acetate (Chlorthalidone may add to or potentiate the action of other antihypertensives).
No products indexed under this heading.

Guanethidine Monosulfate (Chlorthalidone may add to or potentiate the action of other antihypertensives).
No products indexed under this heading.

Hydralazine Hydrochloride (Chlorthalidone may add to or potentiate the action of other antihypertensives).
No products indexed under this heading.

Hydrochlorothiazide (Chlorthalidone may add to or potentiate the action of other antihypertensives). Products include:
Atacand HCT ... 642
Avalide Tablets ... 892
Avalide Tablets ... 2713
Benicar HCT Tablets ... 1010
Diovan HCT Tablets ... 2216
Dyazide Capsules ... 1405
Micardis HCT Tablets ... 854
Prinzide Tablets ... 2092
Tekturna HCT Tablets ... 2324
Teveten HCT Tablets ... 517

Hydrocodone Bitartrate (Orthostatic hypotension may be aggravated by narcotics; orthostatic hypotension may be aggravated by barbiturates). Products include:
Lortab 5/500 Tablets ... 3143
Lortab 7.5/500 Tablets ... 3144
Lortab 10/500 Tablets ... 3144
Vicodin Tablets ... 529
Vicodin ES Tablets ... 530
Vicodin HP Tablets ... 531
Vicoprofen Tablets ... 533
Zydone Tablets ... 1132

Hydrocodone Polistirex (Orthostatic hypotension may be aggravated by narcotics; orthostatic hypotension may be aggravated by barbiturates). Products include:
Tussionex Pennkinetic Extended-Release Suspension ... 3154

Hydroflumethiazide (Chlorthalidone may add to or potentiate the action of other antihypertensives).
No products indexed under this heading.

Hydromorphone Hydrochloride (Orthostatic hypotension may be aggravated by narcotics; orthostatic hypotension may be aggravated by barbiturates).
No products indexed under this heading.

Imipramine Hydrochloride (Co-administration of clonidine with tricyclic antidepressants may result in reduced effect of clonidine, necessitating an increase in dosage).
No products indexed under this heading.

Imipramine Pamoate (Co-administration of clonidine with tricyclic antidepressants may result in reduced effect of clonidine, necessitating an increase in dosage).
No products indexed under this heading.

Indapamide (Chlorthalidone may add to or potentiate the action of other antihypertensives). Products include:
Indapamide Tablets 2188

Insulin (Chlorthalidone causes hyperglycemia; insulin requirements may be increased, decreased, or unchanged).
No products indexed under this heading.

Insulin, Human, Zinc Suspension (Chlorthalidone causes hyperglycemia; insulin requirements may be increased, decreased, or unchanged).
No products indexed under this heading.

Insulin, Human (rDNA origin) (Chlorthalidone causes hyperglycemia; insulin requirements may be increased, decreased, or unchanged). Products include:
Exubera Inhalation Powder 2515

Insulin, Human NPH (Chlorthalidone causes hyperglycemia; insulin requirements may be increased, decreased, or unchanged). Products include:
Humulin N Vial 1846

Insulin, Human Regular (Chlorthalidone causes hyperglycemia; insulin requirements may be increased, decreased, or unchanged). Products include:
Humulin R 1849
Humulin R (U-500) 1850

Insulin, Human Regular and Human NPH Mixture (Chlorthalidone causes hyperglycemia; insulin requirements may be increased, decreased, or unchanged). Products include:
Humulin 50/50, 100 Units 1843
Humulin 70/30 Vial 1844

Insulin, NPH (Chlorthalidone causes hyperglycemia; insulin requirements may be increased, decreased, or unchanged).
No products indexed under this heading.

Insulin, Regular (Chlorthalidone causes hyperglycemia; insulin requirements may be increased, decreased, or unchanged).
No products indexed under this heading.

Insulin, Regular and NPH mixture (Chlorthalidone causes hyperglycemia; insulin requirements may be increased, decreased, or unchanged).
No products indexed under this heading.

Insulin, Zinc Crystals (Chlorthalidone causes hyperglycemia; insulin requirements may be increased, decreased, or unchanged).
No products indexed under this heading.

Insulin, Zinc Suspension (Chlorthalidone causes hyperglycemia; insulin requirements may be increased, decreased, or unchanged).
No products indexed under this heading.

Insulin Aspart (Chlorthalidone causes hyperglycemia; insulin requirements may be increased, decreased, or unchanged).
No products indexed under this heading.

Insulin Aspart, Human (Chlorthalidone causes hyperglycemia; insulin requirements may be increased, decreased, or unchanged). Products include:
NovoLog Mix 70/30 2364

Insulin Aspart, Human Regular (Chlorthalidone causes hyperglycemia; insulin requirements may be increased, decreased, or unchanged). Products include:
NovoLog Injection 2359

Insulin Aspart Protamine, Human (Chlorthalidone causes hyperglycemia; insulin requirements may be increased, decreased, or unchanged). Products include:
NovoLog Mix 70/30 2364

Insulin Detemir (rDNA Origin) (Chlorthalidone causes hyperglycemia; insulin requirements may be increased, decreased, or unchanged). Products include:
Levemir Injection 2352

Insulin glargine (Chlorthalidone causes hyperglycemia; insulin requirements may be increased, decreased, or unchanged). Products include:
Lantus Injection 2749

Insulin Glulisine (Chlorthalidone causes hyperglycemia; insulin requirements may be increased, decreased, or unchanged). Products include:
Apidra Injection 2706

Insulin Lispro, Human (Chlorthalidone causes hyperglycemia; insulin requirements may be increased, decreased, or unchanged). Products include:
Humalog-Pen and KwikPen 1829
Humalog Mix 50/50-Pen and KwikPen 1833
Humalog Mix 75/25-Pen and KwikPen 1835

Insulin Lispro Protamine, Human (Chlorthalidone causes hyperglycemia; insulin requirements may be increased, decreased, or unchanged). Products include:
Humalog Mix 50/50-Pen and KwikPen 1833
Humalog Mix 75/25-Pen and KwikPen 1835

Irbesartan (Chlorthalidone may add to or potentiate the action of other antihypertensives). Products include:
Avalide Tablets 892
Avalide Tablets 2713
Avapro Tablets 897
Avapro Tablets 2718

Isradipine (Chlorthalidone may add to or potentiate the action of other antihypertensives). Products include:
DynaCirc CR Controlled Release Tablets 1407

Labetalol Hydrochloride (Chlorthalidone may add to or potentiate the action of other antihypertensives; if therapy is to be discontinued in patients receiving clonidine and beta blockers concurrently, beta blockers should be discontinued several days before the gradual withdrawal of clonidine).
No products indexed under this heading.

Levobunolol Hydrochloride (Chlorthalidone may add to or potentiate the action of other antihypertensives; if therapy is to be discontinued in patients receiving clonidine and beta blockers concurrently, beta blockers should be discontinued several days before the gradual withdrawal of clonidine).
No products indexed under this heading.

Levorphanol Tartrate (Orthostatic hypotension may be aggravated by narcotics; orthostatic hypotension may be aggravated by barbiturates).
No products indexed under this heading.

Lisinopril (Chlorthalidone may add to or potentiate the action of other antihypertensives). Products include:
Prinivil Tablets 2087
Prinzide Tablets 2092

Lithium (Chlorthalidone reduces renal clearance of lithium, increasing the risk of lithium toxicity).
No products indexed under this heading.

Lithium Carbonate (Chlorthalidone reduces renal clearance of lithium, increasing the risk of lithium toxicity).
No products indexed under this heading.

Lithium Citrate (Chlorthalidone reduces renal clearance of lithium, increasing the risk of lithium toxicity).
No products indexed under this heading.

Lorazepam (Clonidine may enhance the CNS-depressive effects of other sedatives).
No products indexed under this heading.

Losartan Potassium (Chlorthalidone may add to or potentiate the action of other antihypertensives). Products include:
Cozaar Tablets 1973

Maprotiline Hydrochloride (Co-administration of clonidine with tricyclic antidepressants may result in reduced effect of clonidine, necessitating an increase in dosage).
No products indexed under this heading.

Mecamylamine Hydrochloride (Chlorthalidone may add to or potentiate the action of other antihypertensives).
No products indexed under this heading.

Meperidine Hydrochloride (Orthostatic hypotension may be aggravated by narcotics; orthostatic hypotension may be aggravated by barbiturates).
No products indexed under this heading.

Mephobarbital (Clonidine may enhance the CNS-depressive effects of barbiturates; orthostatic hypotension may be aggravated by barbiturates).
No products indexed under this heading.

Metformin Hydrochloride (Chlorthalidone causes hyperglycemia; higher dosage of oral hypoglycemic agents may be required). Products include:
ActoPlus Met Tablets 3071
Avandamet Tablets 1336
Janumet Tablets 2041
PrandiMet Tablets 2967

Methadone Hydrochloride (Orthostatic hypotension may be aggravated by narcotics; orthostatic hypotension may be aggravated by barbiturates).
No products indexed under this heading.

Methyclothiazide (Chlorthalidone may add to or potentiate the action of other antihypertensives).
No products indexed under this heading.

Methyldopa (Chlorthalidone may add to or potentiate the action of other antihypertensives).
No products indexed under this heading.

Methyldopate Hydrochloride (Chlorthalidone may add to or potentiate the action of other antihypertensives).
No products indexed under this heading.

Metipranolol Hydrochloride (Chlorthalidone may add to or potentiate the action of other antihypertensives; if therapy is to be discontinued in patients receiving clonidine and beta blockers concurrently, beta blockers should be discontinued several days before the gradual withdrawal of clonidine).
No products indexed under this heading.

Metolazone (Chlorthalidone may add to or potentiate the action of other antihypertensives).
No products indexed under this heading.

Metoprolol Succinate (Chlorthalidone may add to or potentiate the action of other antihypertensives; if therapy is to be discontinued in patients receiving clonidine and beta blockers concurrently, beta blockers should be discontinued several days before the gradual withdrawal of clonidine). Products include:
Toprol-XL Tablets 666

Metoprolol Tartrate (Chlorthalidone may add to or potentiate the action of other antihypertensives; if therapy is to be discontinued in patients receiving clonidine and beta blockers concurrently, beta blockers should be discontinued several days before the gradual withdrawal of clonidine).
No products indexed under this heading.

Metyrosine (Chlorthalidone may add to or potentiate the action of other antihypertensives). Products include:
Demser Capsules 1989

Mibefradil Dihydrochloride (Chlorthalidone may add to or potentiate the action of other antihypertensives).
No products indexed under this heading.

Midazolam Hydrochloride (Clonidine may enhance the CNS-depressive effects of other sedatives).
No products indexed under this heading.

Miglitol (Chlorthalidone causes hyperglycemia; higher dosage of oral hypoglycemic agents may be required).
No products indexed under this heading.

Minoxidil (Chlorthalidone may add to or potentiate the action of other antihypertensives).
No products indexed under this heading.

Moexipril Hydrochloride (Chlorthalidone may add to or potentiate the action of other antihypertensives).
No products indexed under this heading.

Morphine Sulfate (Orthostatic hypotension may be aggravated by narcotics; orthostatic hypotension may be aggravated by barbiturates). Products include:
Avinza Capsules 1772
DepoDur Injection 1095
MS Contin Tablets 2585

Nadolol (Chlorthalidone may add to or potentiate the action of other antihypertensives; if therapy is to be discontinued in patients receiving clonidine and beta blockers concurrently, beta blockers should be discontinued several days before the gradual withdrawal of clonidine). Products include:
Nadolol Tablets 2191

Nateglinide (Chlorthalidone causes hyperglycemia; higher dosage of oral hypoglycemic agents may be required). Products include:
Starlix Tablets 2314

Nebivolol (Chlorthalidone may add to or potentiate the action of other antihypertensives; if therapy is to be discontinued in patients receiving clonidine and beta blockers concurrently, beta blockers should be discontinued several days before the gradual withdrawal of clonidine). Products include:
Bystolic Tablets 1155

Nicardipine Hydrochloride (Chlorthalidone may add to or potentiate the action of other antihypertensives). Products include:
Cardene I.V. 1093

Nifedipine (Chlorthalidone may add to or potentiate the action of other antihypertensives).
No products indexed under this heading.

Nisoldipine (Chlorthalidone may add to or potentiate the action of other antihypertensives). Products include:
Sular Extended Release Tablets 2975

Nitroglycerin (Chlorthalidone may add to or potentiate the action of other antihypertensives). Products include:
Nitro-Dur Transdermal Infusion System 2887
Nitrolingual Pumpspray 2965

Norepinephrine Bitartrate (Chlorthalidone may decrease arterial responsiveness to norepinephrine).
No products indexed under this heading.

Nortriptyline Hydrochloride (Co-administration of clonidine with tricyclic antidepressants may result in reduced effect of clonidine, necessitating an increase in dosage).
No products indexed under this heading.

Oxycodone Hydrochloride (Orthostatic hypotension may be aggravated by narcotics; orthostatic hypotension may be aggravated by barbiturates). Products include:
OxyContin Tablets 2589
OxyIR Capsules 2593
Percocet Tablets 1127
Percodan Tablets 1130

Penbutolol Sulfate (Chlorthalidone may add to or potentiate the action of other antihypertensives; if therapy is to be discontinued in patients receiving clonidine and beta blockers concurrently, beta blockers should be discontinued several days before the gradual withdrawal of clonidine).
No products indexed under this heading.

Pentobarbital Sodium (Clonidine may enhance the CNS-depressive effects of barbiturates; orthostatic hypotension may be aggravated by barbiturates). Products include:
Nembutal Sodium Solution, USP 2494

Perindopril Erbumine (Chlorthalidone may add to or potentiate the action of other antihypertensives). Products include:
Aceon Tablets (2 mg, 4 mg, 8 mg) 3038

Phenobarbital (Clonidine may enhance the CNS-depressive effects of barbiturates; orthostatic hypotension may be aggravated by barbiturates). Products include:
Donnatal Extentabs 2507

Phenoxybenzamine Hydrochloride (Chlorthalidone may add to or potentiate the action of other antihypertensives). Products include:
Dibenzyline Capsules 3188

Phentolamine Mesylate (Chlorthalidone may add to or potentiate the action of other antihypertensives).
No products indexed under this heading.

Pindolol (Chlorthalidone may add to or potentiate the action of other antihypertensives; if therapy is to be discontinued in patients receiving clonidine and beta blockers concurrently, beta blockers should be discontinued several days before the gradual withdrawal of clonidine).
No products indexed under this heading.

Pioglitazone Hydrochloride (Chlorthalidone causes hyperglycemia; higher dosage of oral hypoglycemic agents may be required). Products include:
ActoPlus Met Tablets 3071
Actos Tablets 3077
Duetact Tablets 3085

Polythiazide (Chlorthalidone may add to or potentiate the action of other antihypertensives).
No products indexed under this heading.

Prazosin Hydrochloride (Chlorthalidone may add to or potentiate the action of other antihypertensives).
No products indexed under this heading.

Propofol (Clonidine may enhance the CNS-depressive effects of other sedatives).
No products indexed under this heading.

Propoxyphene Hydrochloride (Orthostatic hypotension may be aggravated by narcotics; orthostatic hypotension may be aggravated by barbiturates).
No products indexed under this heading.

Propoxyphene Napsylate (Orthostatic hypotension may be aggravated by narcotics; orthostatic hypotension may be aggravated by barbiturates).
No products indexed under this heading.

Propranolol Hydrochloride (Chlorthalidone may add to or potentiate the action of other antihypertensives; if therapy is to be discontinued in patients receiving clonidine and beta blockers concurrently, beta blockers should be discontinued several days before the gradual withdrawal of clonidine). Products include:
InnoPran XL Extended Release Capsules 1484

Protriptyline Hydrochloride (Co-administration of clonidine with tricyclic antidepressants may result in reduced effect of clonidine, necessitating an increase in dosage).
No products indexed under this heading.

Quazepam (Clonidine may enhance the CNS-depressive effects of other sedatives).
No products indexed under this heading.

Quinapril Hydrochloride (Chlorthalidone may add to or potentiate the action of other antihypertensives).
No products indexed under this heading.

Ramelteon (Clonidine may enhance the CNS-depressive effects of other sedatives). Products include:
Rozerem Tablets 3091

Ramipril (Chlorthalidone may add to or potentiate the action of other antihypertensives).
No products indexed under this heading.

Rauwolfia Serpentina (Chlorthalidone may add to or potentiate the action of other antihypertensives).
No products indexed under this heading.

Remifentanil Hydrochloride (Orthostatic hypotension may be aggravated by narcotics; orthostatic hypotension may be aggravated by barbiturates).
No products indexed under this heading.

Repaglinide (Chlorthalidone causes hyperglycemia; higher dosage of oral hypoglycemic agents may be required). Products include:
PrandiMet Tablets 2967
Prandin Tablets 2971

Rescinnamine (Chlorthalidone may add to or potentiate the action of other antihypertensives).
No products indexed under this heading.

Reserpine (Chlorthalidone may add to or potentiate the action of other antihypertensives).
No products indexed under this heading.

Rosiglitazone Maleate (Chlorthalidone causes hyperglycemia; higher dosage of oral hypoglycemic agents may be required). Products include:
Avandamet Tablets 1336
Avandaryl Tablets 1344
Avandia Tablets 1351

Secobarbital Sodium (Clonidine may enhance the CNS-depressive effects of barbiturates; orthostatic hypotension may be aggravated by barbiturates).
No products indexed under this heading.

Sitagliptin Phosphate (Chlorthalidone causes hyperglycemia; higher dosage of oral hypoglycemic agents may be required). Products include:
Janumet Tablets 2041
Januvia Tablets 2048

Sodium Butabarbital (Clonidine may enhance the CNS-depressive effects of other sedatives).
No products indexed under this heading.

Sodium Nitroprusside (Chlorthalidone may add to or potentiate the action of other antihypertensives).
No products indexed under this heading.

Sotalol Hydrochloride (Chlorthalidone may add to or potentiate the action of other antihypertensives; if therapy is to be discontinued in patients receiving clonidine and beta blockers concurrently, beta blockers should be discontinued several days before the gradual withdrawal of clonidine).
No products indexed under this heading.

Spirapril Hydrochloride (Chlorthalidone may add to or potentiate the action of other antihypertensives).
No products indexed under this heading.

Sufentanil Citrate (Orthostatic hypotension may be aggravated by narcotics; orthostatic hypotension may be aggravated by barbiturates).
No products indexed under this heading.

Telmisartan (Chlorthalidone may add to or potentiate the action of other antihypertensives). Products include:
Micardis Tablets 852
Micardis HCT Tablets 854

Temazepam (Clonidine may enhance the CNS-depressive effects of other sedatives).
No products indexed under this heading.

Terazosin Hydrochloride (Chlorthalidone may add to or potentiate the action of other antihypertensives).
No products indexed under this heading.

Thiamylal Sodium (Clonidine may enhance the CNS-depressive effects of barbiturates; orthostatic hypotension may be aggravated by barbiturates).
No products indexed under this heading.

Timolol Hemihydrate (Chlorthalidone may add to or potentiate the action of other antihypertensives; if therapy is to be discontinued in patients receiving clonidine and beta blockers concurrently, beta blockers should be discontinued several days before the gradual withdrawal of clonidine). Products include:
Betimol Ophthalmic Solution 3181

Timolol Maleate (Chlorthalidone may add to or potentiate the action of other antihypertensives; if therapy is to be discontinued in patients receiving clonidine and beta block-

ers concurrently, beta blockers should be discontinued several days before the gradual withdrawal of clonidine). Products include:
- Combigan Ophthalmic Solution 553
- Cosopt Sterile Ophthalmic Solution 1969
- Timoptic Sterile Ophthalmic Solution 2121
- Timoptic in Ocudose 2124
- Timoptic-XE Sterile Ophthalmic Gel Forming Solution 2125

Tolazamide (Chlorthalidone causes hyperglycemia; higher dosage of oral hypoglycemic agents may be required).
No products indexed under this heading.

Tolbutamide (Chlorthalidone causes hyperglycemia; higher dosage of oral hypoglycemic agents may be required).
No products indexed under this heading.

Torsemide (Chlorthalidone may add to or potentiate the action of other antihypertensives). Products include:
- Demadex Injection 2630
- Demadex Tablets 2630

Trandolapril (Chlorthalidone may add to or potentiate the action of other antihypertensives). Products include:
- Mavik Tablets 472
- Tarka Tablets 511

Triazolam (Clonidine may enhance the CNS-depressive effects of other sedatives).
No products indexed under this heading.

Trimethaphan Camsylate (Chlorthalidone may add to or potentiate the action of other antihypertensives).
No products indexed under this heading.

Trimipramine Maleate (Co-administration of clonidine with tricyclic antidepressants may result in reduced effect of clonidine, necessitating an increase in dosage).
No products indexed under this heading.

Troglitazone (Chlorthalidone causes hyperglycemia; higher dosage of oral hypoglycemic agents may be required).
No products indexed under this heading.

Tubocurarine Chloride (Chlorthalidone may increase responsiveness to tubocurarine).
No products indexed under this heading.

Valsartan (Chlorthalidone may add to or potentiate the action of other antihypertensives). Products include:
- Diovan Tablets 2212
- Diovan HCT Tablets 2216
- Exforge Tablets 2238

Verapamil Hydrochloride (Chlorthalidone may add to or potentiate the action of other antihypertensives). Products include:
- Tarka Tablets 511

Zaleplon (Clonidine may enhance the CNS-depressive effects of other sedatives).
No products indexed under this heading.

Zolpidem Tartrate (Clonidine may enhance the CNS-depressive effects of other sedatives). Products include:
- Ambien Tablets 2692
- Ambien CR Tablets 2696

Food Interactions

Alcohol (Clonidine may enhance the CNS-depressive effects of alcohol; orthostatic hypotension may be aggravated by alcohol).

CM PLEX CREAM

(Fatty Acids, Olive Oil) 3159
None cited in PDR database.

CM PLEX SOFTGELS

(Fatty Acids, Salmon Oil, Soy oil) 3159
None cited in PDR database.

COMAX DIETARY SUPPLEMENT

(Alpha Lipoic Acid, Lutein, Peptidase, Rutoside, Selenium, Vitamin B_{12}, Vitamin C, Vitamin E, Zeaxanthin, Zinc) 995
None cited in PDR database.

COMBIGAN OPHTHALMIC SOLUTION

(Brimonidine Tartrate, Timolol Maleate) 553
May interact with anesthetics, antihypertensives, barbiturates, beta blockers, catecholamine depleting drugs, calcium channel blockers, central nervous system depressants, cytochrome p450 2d6 inhibitors (selected), cardiac glycosides, oral hypoglycemic agents, hypnotics and sedatives, insulin, monoamine oxidase inhibitors, narcotic analgesics, tricyclic antidepressants, and certain other agents. Compounds in these categories include:

Acarbose (Beta-adrenergic blocking agents should be administered with caution in patients subject to spontaneous hypoglycemia or to diabetic patients (especially those with labile diabetes) who are receiving insulin or oral hypoglycemic agents. Beta-adrenergic receptor blocking agents may mask the signs and symptoms of acute hypoglycemia). Products include:
- Precose Tablets 792

Acebutolol Hydrochloride (Patients who are receiving a beta-adrenergic blocking agent orally and Combigan should be observed for potential additive effects of beta-blockade, both systemic and on intraocular pressure. The concomitant use of two topical beta-adrenergic blocking agents is not recommended).
No products indexed under this heading.

Alfentanil Hydrochloride (Although specific drug interaction studies have not been conducted with Combigan, the possibility of an additive or potentiating effect with CNS depressants (alcohol, barbiturates, opiates, sedatives or anesthetics) should be considered).
No products indexed under this heading.

Aliskiren (Because Combigan may reduce blood pressure, caution in using drugs such as antihypertensives with Combigan is advised). Products include:
- Tekturna Tablets 2321
- Tekturna HCT Tablets 2324

Alprazolam (Although specific drug interaction studies have not been conducted with Combigan, the possibility of an additive or potentiating effect with CNS depressants (alcohol, barbiturates, opiates, sedatives or anesthetics) should be considered).
No products indexed under this heading.

Amiodarone Hydrochloride (Potentiated systemic beta-blockade (e.g., decreased heart rate, depression) has been reported during combined treatment with CYP2D6 inhibitors (e.g., quinidine, SSRIs) and timolol).
No products indexed under this heading.

Amitriptyline Hydrochloride (Tricyclic antidepressants have been reported to blunt the hypotensive effect of systemic clonidine. It is not known whether the concurrent use of these agents with Combigan in humans can lead to resulting interference with the IOP lowering effect. Caution, however, is advised in patients taking tricyclic antidepressants which can affect the metabolism and uptake of circulating amines).
No products indexed under this heading.

Amlodipine Besylate (Caution should be used in the co-administration of beta-adrenergic blocking agents, such as Combigan, and oral or intravenous calcium antagonists because of possible atrioventricular conduction disturbances, left ventricular failure and hypotension. In patients with impaired cardiac function, co-administration should be avoided. The concomitant use of beta-adrenergic blocking agents with calcium antagonists may have additive effects in prolonging atrioventricular conduction time). Products include:
- Azor Tablets 1005
- Exforge Tablets 2238

Amoxapine (Tricyclic antidepressants have been reported to blunt the hypotensive effect of systemic clonidine. It is not known whether the concurrent use of these agents with Combigan in humans can lead to resulting interference with the IOP lowering effect. Caution, however, is advised in patients taking tricyclic antidepressants which can affect the metabolism and uptake of circulating amines).
No products indexed under this heading.

Aprobarbital (Although specific drug interaction studies have not been conducted with Combigan, the possibility of an additive or potentiating effect with CNS depressants (alcohol, barbiturates, opiates, sedatives or anesthetics) should be considered).
No products indexed under this heading.

Atenolol (Patients who are receiving a beta-adrenergic blocking agent orally and Combigan should be observed for potential additive effects of beta-blockade, both systemic and on intraocular pressure. The concomitant use of two topical beta-adrenergic blocking agents is not recommended).
No products indexed under this heading.

Benazepril Hydrochloride (Because Combigan may reduce blood pressure, caution in using drugs such as antihypertensives with Combigan is advised).
No products indexed under this heading.

Bendroflumethiazide (Because Combigan may reduce blood pressure, caution in using drugs such as antihypertensives with Combigan is advised).
No products indexed under this heading.

Bepridil Hydrochloride (Caution should be used in the co-administration of beta-adrenergic blocking agents, such as Combigan, and oral or intravenous calcium antagonists because of possible atrioventricular conduction disturbances, left ventricular failure and hypotension. In patients with impaired cardiac function, co-administration should be avoided. The concomitant use of beta-adrenergic blocking agents with calcium antagonists may have additive effects in proloning atrioventricular conduction time).
No products indexed under this heading.

Betaxolol Hydrochloride (Patients who are receiving a beta-adrenergic blocking agent orally and Combigan should be observed for potential additive effects of beta-blockade, both systemic and on intraocular pressure. The concomitant use of two topical beta-adrenergic blocking agents is not recommended).
No products indexed under this heading.

Bisoprolol Fumarate (Patients who are receiving a beta-adrenergic blocking agent orally and Combigan should be observed for potential additive effects of beta-blockade, both systemic and on intraocular pressure. The concomitant use of two topical beta-adrenergic blocking agents is not recommended).
No products indexed under this heading.

Buprenorphine Hydrochloride (Although specific drug interaction studies have not been conducted with Combigan, the possibility of an additive or potentiating effect with CNS depressants (alcohol, barbiturates, opiates, sedatives or anesthetics) should be considered). Products include:
- Suboxone Tablets 2601
- Subutex Tablets 2601

Bupropion Hydrochloride (Potentiated systemic beta-blockade (e.g., decreased heart rate, depression) has been reported during combined treatment with CYP2D6 inhibitors (e.g., quinidine, SSRIs) and timolol). Products include:
- Wellbutrin Tablets 1648
- Wellbutrin SR Sustained-Release Tablets 1653
- Wellbutrin XL Extended-Release Tablets 1659
- Zyban Sustained-Release Tablets 1692

Buspirone Hydrochloride (Although specific drug interaction studies have not been conducted with Combigan, the possibility of an additive or potentiating effect with CNS depressants (alcohol, barbiturates, opiates, sedatives or anesthetics) should be considered).
No products indexed under this heading.

Butabarbital (Although specific drug interaction studies have not been conducted with Combigan, the possibility of an additive or potentiating effect with CNS depressants (alcohol, barbiturates, opiates, sedatives or anesthetics) should be considered).
No products indexed under this heading.

Butabarbital Sodium (Although specific drug interaction studies have not been conducted with Combigan, the possibility of an additive or potentiating effect with CNS depressants (alcohol, barbiturates, opiates, sedatives or anesthetics) should be considered).
No products indexed under this heading.

Butalbital (Although specific drug interaction studies have not been conducted with Combigan, the possibility of an additive or potentiating effect with CNS depressants (alcohol, barbiturates, opiates, sedatives or anesthetics) should be considered).
No products indexed under this heading.

Candesartan Cilexetil (Because Combigan may reduce blood pressure, caution in using drugs such as antihypertensives with Combigan is advised). Products include:
Atacand Tablets ... 639
Atacand HCT ... 642

Captopril (Because Combigan may reduce blood pressure, caution in using drugs such as antihypertensives with Combigan is advised). Products include:
Captopril Tablets ... 2182

Carteolol Hydrochloride (Patients who are receiving a beta-adrenergic blocking agent orally and Combigan should be observed for potential additive effects of beta-blockade, both systemic and on intraocular pressure. The concomitant use of two topical beta-adrenergic blocking agents is not recommended).
No products indexed under this heading.

Celecoxib (Potentiated systemic beta-blockade (e.g., decreased heart rate, depression) has been reported during combined treatment with CYP2D6 inhibitors (e.g., quinidine, SSRIs) and timolol). Products include:
Celebrex Capsules ... 2979

Chloral Hydrate (Although specific drug interaction studies have not been conducted with Combigan, the possibility of an additive or potentiating effect with CNS depressants (alcohol, barbiturates, opiates, sedatives or anesthetics) should be considered).
No products indexed under this heading.

Chlordiazepoxide (Although specific drug interaction studies have not been conducted with Combigan, the possibility of an additive or potentiating effect with CNS depressants (alcohol, barbiturates, opiates, sedatives or anesthetics) should be considered).
No products indexed under this heading.

Chlordiazepoxide Hydrochloride (Although specific drug interaction studies have not been conducted with Combigan, the possibility of an additive or potentiating effect with CNS depressants (alcohol, barbiturates, opiates, sedatives or anesthetics) should be considered).
No products indexed under this heading.

Chloroquine Hydrochloride (Potentiated systemic beta-blockade (e.g., decreased heart rate, depression) has been reported during combined treatment with CYP2D6 inhibitors (e.g., quinidine, SSRIs) and timolol).
No products indexed under this heading.

Chloroquine Phosphate (Potentiated systemic beta-blockade (e.g., decreased heart rate, depression) has been reported during combined treatment with CYP2D6 inhibitors (e.g., quinidine, SSRIs) and timolol).
No products indexed under this heading.

Chlorothiazide (Because Combigan may reduce blood pressure, caution in using drugs such as antihypertensives with Combigan is advised).
No products indexed under this heading.

Chlorothiazide Sodium (Because Combigan may reduce blood pressure, caution in using drugs such as antihypertensives with Combigan is advised). Products include:
Intravenous Sodium Diuril ... 2490

Chlorpheniramine (Potentiated systemic beta-blockade (e.g., decreased heart rate, depression) has been reported during combined treatment with CYP2D6 inhibitors (e.g., quinidine, SSRIs) and timolol).
No products indexed under this heading.

Chlorpheniramine Maleate (Potentiated systemic beta-blockade (e.g., decreased heart rate, depression) has been reported during combined treatment with CYP2D6 inhibitors (e.g., quinidine, SSRIs) and timolol). Products include:
Actifed Cold & Allergy Tablets ... 1895
Sudafed PE Sinus & Allergy Tablets ... 1908
Tylenol Allergy Multi-Symptom Caplets with Cool Burst and Rapid Release Gelcaps ... 1916
Children's Tylenol Plus Cold Suspension Liquid ... 1912
Children's Tylenol Plus Cough & Runny Nose Suspension Liquid ... 1912
Children's Tylenol Plus Flu Suspension Liquid ... 1914
Children's Tylenol Plus Multi-Symptom Cold Suspension Liquid ... 1912
Tylenol Cold Head Congestion Nighttime Caplets with Cool Burst ... 1910
Tylenol Cold Multi-Symptom Nighttime Caplets with Cool Burst ... 1913
Tylenol Sinus Congestion & Pain Nighttime Caplets with Cool Burst ... 1917

Chlorpheniramine Polistirex (Potentiated systemic beta-blockade (e.g., decreased heart rate, depression) has been reported during combined treatment with CYP2D6 inhibitors (e.g., quinidine, SSRIs) and timolol). Products include:
Tussionex Pennkinetic Extended-Release Suspension ... 3154

Chlorpheniramine Tannate (Potentiated systemic beta-blockade (e.g., decreased heart rate, depression) has been reported during combined treatment with CYP2D6 inhibitors (e.g., quinidine, SSRIs) and timolol).
No products indexed under this heading.

Chlorpromazine (Although specific drug interaction studies have not been conducted with Combigan, the possibility of an additive or potentiating effect with CNS depressants (alcohol, barbiturates, opiates, sedatives or anesthetics) should be considered).
No products indexed under this heading.

Chlorpromazine Hydrochloride (Although specific drug interaction studies have not been conducted with Combigan, the possibility of an additive or potentiating effect with CNS depressants (alcohol, barbiturates, opiates, sedatives or anesthetics) should be considered).
No products indexed under this heading.

Chlorpropamide (Beta-adrenergic blocking agents should be administered with caution in patients subject to spontaneous hypoglycemia or to diabetic patients (especially those with labile diabetes) who are receiving insulin or oral hypoglycemic agents. Beta-adrenergic receptor blocking agents may mask the signs and symptoms of acute hypoglycemia).
No products indexed under this heading.

Chlorprothixene (Although specific drug interaction studies have not been conducted with Combigan, the possibility of an additive or potentiating effect with CNS depressants (alcohol, barbiturates, opiates, sedatives or anesthetics) should be considered).
No products indexed under this heading.

Chlorprothixene Hydrochloride (Although specific drug interaction studies have not been conducted with Combigan, the possibility of an additive or potentiating effect with CNS depressants (alcohol, barbiturates, opiates, sedatives or anesthetics) should be considered).
No products indexed under this heading.

Chlorprothixene Lactate (Although specific drug interaction studies have not been conducted with Combigan, the possibility of an additive or potentiating effect with CNS depressants (alcohol, barbiturates, opiates, sedatives or anesthetics) should be considered).
No products indexed under this heading.

Chlorthalidone (Because Combigan may reduce blood pressure, caution in using drugs such as antihypertensives with Combigan is advised). Products include:
Clorpres Tablets ... 2185

Cimetidine (Potentiated systemic beta-blockade (e.g., decreased heart rate, depression) has been reported during combined treatment with CYP2D6 inhibitors (e.g., quinidine, SSRIs) and timolol).
No products indexed under this heading.

Cimetidine Hydrochloride (Potentiated systemic beta-blockade (e.g., decreased heart rate, depression) has been reported during combined treatment with CYP2D6 inhibitors (e.g., quinidine, SSRIs) and timolol).
No products indexed under this heading.

Citalopram Hydrobromide (Potentiated systemic beta-blockade (e.g., decreased heart rate, depression) has been reported during combined treatment with CYP2D6 inhibitors (e.g., quinidine, SSRIs) and timolol). Products include:
Celexa ... 1160

Clomipramine Hydrochloride (Tricyclic antidepressants have been reported to blunt the hypotensive effect of systemic clonidine. It is not known whether the concurrent use of these agents with Combigan in humans can lead to resulting interference with the IOP lowering effect. Caution, however, is advised in patients taking tricyclic antidepressants which can affect the metabolism and uptake of circulating amines).
No products indexed under this heading.

Clonidine (Because Combigan may reduce blood pressure, caution in using drugs such as antihypertensives with Combigan is advised). Products include:
Catapres-TTS ... 842

Clonidine Hydrochloride (Because Combigan may reduce blood pressure, caution in using drugs such as antihypertensives with Combigan is advised). Products include:
Catapres Tablets ... 841
Clorpres Tablets ... 2185

Clorazepate Dipotassium (Although specific drug interaction studies have not been conducted with Combigan, the possibility of an additive or potentiating effect with CNS depressants (alcohol, barbiturates, opiates, sedatives or anesthetics) should be considered).
No products indexed under this heading.

Clozapine (Although specific drug interaction studies have not been conducted with Combigan, the possibility of an additive or potentiating effect with CNS depressants (alcohol, barbiturates, opiates, sedatives or anesthetics) should be considered).
No products indexed under this heading.

Cocaine Hydrochloride (Potentiated systemic beta-blockade (e.g., decreased heart rate, depression) has been reported during combined treatment with CYP2D6 inhibitors (e.g., quinidine, SSRIs) and timolol).
No products indexed under this heading.

Codeine Phosphate (Although specific drug interaction studies have not been conducted with Combigan, the possibility of an additive or potentiating effect with CNS depressants (alcohol, barbiturates, opiates, sedatives or anesthetics) should be considered). Products include:
Tylenol with Codeine Tablets ... 2427

Deserpidine (Because Combigan may reduce blood pressure, caution in using drugs such as antihypertensives with Combigan is advised).
No products indexed under this heading.

Desflurane (Although specific drug interaction studies have not been conducted with Combigan, the possibility of an additive or potentiating effect with CNS depressants (alcohol, barbiturates, opiates, sedatives or anesthetics) should be considered).
No products indexed under this heading.

Desipramine Hydrochloride (Tricyclic antidepressants have been reported to blunt the hypotensive effect of systemic clonidine. It is not known whether the concurrent use of these agents with Combigan in humans can lead to resulting interference with the IOP lowering effect. Caution, however, is advised in patients taking tricyclic antidepressants which can affect the metabolism and uptake of circulating amines).
No products indexed under this heading.

Deslanoside (Because Combigan may reduce blood pressure, caution in using drugs such as cardiac glycosides with Combigan is advised. The concomitant use of beta-adrenergic blocking agents with digitalis may have additive effects in prolonging atrioventricular conduction time).
No products indexed under this heading.

Dezocine (Although specific drug interaction studies have not been conducted with Combigan, the possibility of an additive or potentiating effect with CNS depressants (alcohol, barbiturates, opiates, sedatives or anesthetics) should be considered).
No products indexed under this heading.

Diazepam (Although specific drug interaction studies have not been conducted with Combigan, the possibility of an additive or potentiating effect with CNS depressants (alcohol, barbiturates, opiates, sedatives or anesthetics) should be considered). Products include:
Valium Tablets 2658

Diazoxide (Because Combigan may reduce blood pressure, caution in using drugs such as antihypertensives with Combigan is advised). Products include:
Proglycem Capsules 1185
Proglycem Suspension 1185

Digitalis Glycoside Preparations (Because Combigan may reduce blood pressure, caution in using drugs such as cardiac glycosides with Combigan is advised. The concomitant use of beta-adrenergic blocking agents with digitalis may have additive effects in prolonging atrioventricular conduction time).
No products indexed under this heading.

Digitoxin (Because Combigan may reduce blood pressure, caution in using drugs such as cardiac glycosides with Combigan is advised. The concomitant use of beta-adrenergic blocking agents with digitalis may have additive effects in prolonging atrioventricular conduction time).
No products indexed under this heading.

Digoxin (Because Combigan may reduce blood pressure, caution in using drugs such as cardiac glycosides with Combigan is advised. The concomitant use of beta-adrenergic blocking agents with digitalis may have additive effects in prolonging atrioventricular conduction time). Products include:
Lanoxin Injection 1498
Lanoxin Injection Pediatric 1502
Lanoxin Tablets 1505

Diltiazem Hydrochloride (Caution should be used in the co-administration of beta-adrenergic blocking agents, such as Combigan, and oral or intravenous calcium antagonists because of possible atrioventricular conduction disturbances, left ventricular failure and hypotension. In patients with impaired cardiac function, co-administration should be avoided. The concomitant use of beta-adrenergic blocking agents with calcium antagonists may have additive effects in proloning atrioventricular conduction time). Products include:
Cardizem LA Extended Release Tablets 421

Diphenhydramine (Potentiated systemic beta-blockade (e.g., decreased heart rate, depression) has been reported during combined treatment with CYP2D6 inhibitors (e.g., quinidine, SSRIs) and timolol).
No products indexed under this heading.

Diphenhydramine Hydrochloride (Potentiated systemic beta-blockade (e.g., decreased heart rate, depression) has been reported during combined treatment with CYP2D6 inhibitors (e.g., quinidine, SSRIs) and timolol). Products include:
Benadryl Allergy & Cold Kapgels 1895
Benadryl Allergy & Sinus Headache Kapgels 1895
Benadryl Severe Allergy & Sinus Headache Caplets 1897
Benadryl Dye-Free Allergy Liqui-gels Softgels 1897
Benadryl Allergy Kapgels 1895
Benadryl Allergy Quick Dissolve Strips 1896
Benadryl Allergy Ultratab Tablets 1896
Children's Benadryl Dye-Free Allergy Liquid 1897
Children's Benadryl Allergy Fastmelts 1897
Children's Benadryl Allergy Liquid 1898
Children's Benadryl Allergy Perfect Measure 1896
Children's Benadryl-D Allergy & Sinus Liquid 1896
Benadryl-D Allergy & Sinus Tablet 1896
PediaCare Children's Allergy & Cold Liquid 1902
PediaCare Children's Allergy Liquid 1902
Simply Sleep Caplets 1905
Sudafed PE Nighttime Cold Caplets 1907
Sudafed PE Severe Cold Caplets 1908
Extra Strength Tylenol PM Caplets, Geltabs, Liquid, and Rapid Release Gels 1915
Tylenol Allergy Multi-Symptom Nighttime Caplets with Cool Burst 1916
Tylenol Severe Allergy Caplets 1916
Children's Tylenol Plus Cold & Allergy Suspension Liquid 1914
Tylenol Sore Throat Nighttime Liquid with Cool Burst 1918

Doxazosin Mesylate (Because Combigan may reduce blood pressure, caution in using drugs such as antihypertensives with Combigan is advised).
No products indexed under this heading.

Doxepin Hydrochloride (Tricyclic antidepressants have been reported to blunt the hypotensive effect of systemic clonidine. It is not known whether the concurrent use of these agents with Combigan in humans can lead to resulting interference with the IOP lowering effect. Caution, however, is advised in patients taking tricyclic antidepressants which can affect the metabolism and uptake of circulating amines).
No products indexed under this heading.

Droperidol (Although specific drug interaction studies have not been conducted with Combigan, the possibility of an additive or potentiating effect with CNS depressants (alcohol, barbiturates, opiates, sedatives or anesthetics) should be considered).
No products indexed under this heading.

Enalapril Maleate (Because Combigan may reduce blood pressure, caution in using drugs such as antihypertensives with Combigan is advised).
No products indexed under this heading.

Enalaprilat (Because Combigan may reduce blood pressure, caution in using drugs such as antihypertensives with Combigan is advised).
No products indexed under this heading.

Enflurane (Although specific drug interaction studies have not been conducted with Combigan, the possibility of an additive or potentiating effect with CNS depressants (alcohol, barbiturates, opiates, sedatives or anesthetics) should be considered).
No products indexed under this heading.

Eprosartan Mesylate (Because Combigan may reduce blood pressure, caution in using drugs such as antihypertensives with Combigan is advised). Products include:
Teveten Tablets 515
Teveten HCT Tablets 517

Escitalopram Oxalate (Potentiated systemic beta-blockade (e.g., decreased heart rate, depression) has been reported during combined treatment with CYP2D6 inhibitors (e.g., quinidine, SSRIs) and timolol). Products include:
Lexapro Oral Suspension 1174
Lexapro Tablets 1174

Esmolol Hydrochloride (Patients who are receiving a beta-adrenergic blocking agent orally and Combigan should be observed for potential additive effects of beta-blockade, both systemic and on intraocular pressure. The concomitant use of two topical beta-adrenergic blocking agents is not recommended).
No products indexed under this heading.

Estazolam (Although specific drug interaction studies have not been conducted with Combigan, the possibility of an additive or potentiating effect with CNS depressants (alcohol, barbiturates, opiates, sedatives or anesthetics) should be considered).
No products indexed under this heading.

Ethanol (Although specific drug interaction studies have not been conducted with Combigan, the possibility of an additive or potentiating effect with CNS depressants (alcohol, barbiturates, opiates, sedatives or anesthetics) should be considered).
No products indexed under this heading.

Ethchlorvynol (Although specific drug interaction studies have not been conducted with Combigan, the possibility of an additive or potentiating effect with CNS depressants (alcohol, barbiturates, opiates, sedatives or anesthetics) should be considered).
No products indexed under this heading.

Ethinamate (Although specific drug interaction studies have not been conducted with Combigan, the possibility of an additive or potentiating effect with CNS depressants (alcohol, barbiturates, opiates, sedatives or anesthetics) should be considered).
No products indexed under this heading.

Ethyl Alcohol (Although specific drug interaction studies have not been conducted with Combigan, the possibility of an additive or potentiating effect with CNS depressants (alcohol, barbiturates, opiates, sedatives or anesthetics) should be considered).
No products indexed under this heading.

Felodipine (Caution should be used in the co-administration of beta-adrenergic blocking agents, such as Combigan, and oral or intravenous calcium antagonists because of possible atrioventricular conduction disturbances, left ventricular failure and hypotension. In patients with impaired cardiac function, co-administration should be avoided. The concomitant use of beta-adrenergic blocking agents with calcium antagonists may have additive effects in proloning atrioventricular conduction time).
No products indexed under this heading.

Fentanyl (Although specific drug interaction studies have not been conducted with Combigan, the possibility of an additive or potentiating effect with CNS depressants (alcohol, barbiturates, opiates, sedatives or anesthetics) should be considered). Products include:
Duragesic Transdermal System 2405
Ionsys Transdermal System 2410

Fentanyl Citrate (Although specific drug interaction studies have not been conducted with Combigan, the possibility of an additive or potentiating effect with CNS depressants (alcohol, barbiturates, opiates, sedatives or anesthetics) should be considered). Products include:
Actiq 959
Fentora Tablets 968

Fluoxetine (Potentiated systemic beta-blockade (e.g., decreased heart rate, depression) has been reported during combined treatment with CYP2D6 inhibitors (e.g., quinidine, SSRIs) and timolol).
No products indexed under this heading.

Fluoxetine Hydrochloride (Potentiated systemic beta-blockade (e.g., decreased heart rate, depression) has been reported during combined treatment with CYP2D6 inhibitors (e.g., quinidine, SSRIs) and timolol). Products include:

Prozac Weekly Capsules 1852
Prozac Pulvules and Liquid 1852
Symbyax Capsules 1871

Fluphenazine Decanoate (Although specific drug interaction studies have not been conducted with Combigan, the possibility of an additive or potentiating effect with CNS depressants (alcohol, barbiturates, opiates, sedatives or anesthetics) should be considered).

No products indexed under this heading.

Fluphenazine Enanthate (Although specific drug interaction studies have not been conducted with Combigan, the possibility of an additive or potentiating effect with CNS depressants (alcohol, barbiturates, opiates, sedatives or anesthetics) should be considered).

No products indexed under this heading.

Fluphenazine Hydrochloride (Although specific drug interaction studies have not been conducted with Combigan, the possibility of an additive or potentiating effect with CNS depressants (alcohol, barbiturates, opiates, sedatives or anesthetics) should be considered).

No products indexed under this heading.

Flurazepam Hydrochloride (Although specific drug interaction studies have not been conducted with Combigan, the possibility of an additive or potentiating effect with CNS depressants (alcohol, barbiturates, opiates, sedatives or anesthetics) should be considered).

No products indexed under this heading.

Fluvoxamine Maleate (Potentiated systemic beta-blockade (e.g., decreased heart rate, depression) has been reported during combined treatment with CYP2D6 inhibitors (e.g., quinidine, SSRIs) and timolol). Products include:

Luvox CR Extended-Release Capsules 1759

Fosinopril Sodium (Because Combigan may reduce blood pressure, caution in using drugs such as antihypertensives with Combigan is advised).

No products indexed under this heading.

Furosemide (Because Combigan may reduce blood pressure, caution in using drugs such as antihypertensives with Combigan is advised). Products include:

Furosemide Tablets 2186

Glimepiride (Beta-adrenergic blocking agents should be administered with caution in patients subject to spontaneous hypoglycemia or to diabetic patients (especially those with labile diabetes) who are receiving insulin or oral hypoglycemic agents. Beta-adrenergic receptor blocking agents may mask the signs and symptoms of acute hypoglycemia). Products include:

Avandaryl Tablets 1344
Duetact Tablets 3085

Glipizide (Beta-adrenergic blocking agents should be administered with caution in patients subject to spontaneous hypoglycemia or to diabetic patients (especially those with labile diabetes) who are receiving insulin or oral hypoglycemic agents. Beta-adrenergic receptor blocking agents may mask the signs and symptoms of acute hypoglycemia).

No products indexed under this heading.

Glutethimide (Although specific drug interaction studies have not been conducted with Combigan, the possibility of an additive or potentiating effect with CNS depressants (alcohol, barbiturates, opiates, sedatives or anesthetics) should be considered).

No products indexed under this heading.

Glyburide (Beta-adrenergic blocking agents should be administered with caution in patients subject to spontaneous hypoglycemia or to diabetic patients (especially those with labile diabetes) who are receiving insulin or oral hypoglycemic agents. Beta-adrenergic receptor blocking agents may mask the signs and symptoms of acute hypoglycemia).

No products indexed under this heading.

Guanabenz Acetate (Because Combigan may reduce blood pressure, caution in using drugs such as antihypertensives with Combigan is advised).

No products indexed under this heading.

Guanethidine Monosulfate (Because Combigan may reduce blood pressure, caution in using drugs such as antihypertensives with Combigan is advised).

No products indexed under this heading.

Halofantrine Hydrochloride (Potentiated systemic beta-blockade (e.g., decreased heart rate, depression) has been reported during combined treatment with CYP2D6 inhibitors (e.g., quinidine, SSRIs) and timolol).

No products indexed under this heading.

Haloperidol (Although specific drug interaction studies have not been conducted with Combigan, the possibility of an additive or potentiating effect with CNS depressants (alcohol, barbiturates, opiates, sedatives or anesthetics) should be considered).

No products indexed under this heading.

Haloperidol Decanoate (Although specific drug interaction studies have not been conducted with Combigan, the possibility of an additive or potentiating effect with CNS depressants (alcohol, barbiturates, opiates, sedatives or anesthetics) should be considered).

No products indexed under this heading.

Halothane (Although specific drug interaction studies have not been conducted with Combigan, the possibility of an additive or potentiating effect with CNS depressants (alcohol, barbiturates, opiates, sedatives or anesthetics) should be considered).

No products indexed under this heading.

Hydralazine Hydrochloride (Because Combigan may reduce blood pressure, caution in using drugs such as antihypertensives with Combigan is advised).

No products indexed under this heading.

Hydrochlorothiazide (Because Combigan may reduce blood pressure, caution in using drugs such as antihypertensives with Combigan is advised). Products include:

Atacand HCT 642
Avalide Tablets 892
Avalide Tablets 2713
Benicar HCT Tablets 1010
Diovan HCT Tablets 2216
Dyazide Capsules 1405
Micardis HCT Tablets 854
Prinzide Tablets 2092
Tekturna HCT Tablets 2324
Teveten HCT Tablets 517

Hydrocodone Bitartrate (Although specific drug interaction studies have not been conducted with Combigan, the possibility of an additive or potentiating effect with CNS depressants (alcohol, barbiturates, opiates, sedatives or anesthetics) should be considered). Products include:

Lortab 5/500 Tablets 3143
Lortab 7.5/500 Tablets 3144
Lortab 10/500 Tablets 3144
Vicodin Tablets 529
Vicodin ES Tablets 530
Vicodin HP Tablets 531
Vicoprofen Tablets 533
Zydone Tablets 1132

Hydrocodone Polistirex (Although specific drug interaction studies have not been conducted with Combigan, the possibility of an additive or potentiating effect with CNS depressants (alcohol, barbiturates, opiates, sedatives or anesthetics) should be considered). Products include:

Tussionex Pennkinetic Extended-Release Suspension 3154

Hydroflumethiazide (Because Combigan may reduce blood pressure, caution in using drugs such as antihypertensives with Combigan is advised).

No products indexed under this heading.

Hydromorphone Hydrochloride (Although specific drug interaction studies have not been conducted with Combigan, the possibility of an additive or potentiating effect with CNS depressants (alcohol, barbiturates, opiates, sedatives or anesthetics) should be considered).

No products indexed under this heading.

Hydroxychloroquine Sulfate (Potentiated systemic beta-blockade (e.g., decreased heart rate, depression) has been reported during combined treatment with CYP2D6 inhibitors (e.g., quinidine, SSRIs) and timolol).

No products indexed under this heading.

Hydroxyzine Hydrochloride (Although specific drug interaction studies have not been conducted with Combigan, the possibility of an additive or potentiating effect with CNS depressants (alcohol, barbiturates, opiates, sedatives or anesthetics) should be considered).

No products indexed under this heading.

Imatinib Mesylate (Potentiated systemic beta-blockade (e.g., decreased heart rate, depression) has been reported during combined treatment with CYP2D6 inhibitors (e.g., quinidine, SSRIs) and timolol). Products include:

Gleevec Tablets 2255

Imipramine Hydrochloride (Tricyclic antidepressants have been reported to blunt the hypotensive effect of systemic clonidine. It is not known whether the concurrent use of these agents with Combigan in humans can lead to resulting interference with the IOP lowering effect. Caution, however, is advised in patients taking tricyclic antidepressants which can affect the metabolism and uptake of circulating amines).

No products indexed under this heading.

Imipramine Pamoate (Tricyclic antidepressants have been reported to blunt the hypotensive effect of systemic clonidine. It is not known whether the concurrent use of these agents with Combigan in humans can lead to resulting interference with the IOP lowering effect. Caution, however, is advised in patients taking tricyclic antidepressants which can affect the metabolism and uptake of circulating amines).

No products indexed under this heading.

Indapamide (Because Combigan may reduce blood pressure, caution in using drugs such as antihypertensives with Combigan is advised). Products include:

Indapamide Tablets 2188

Insulin (Beta-adrenergic blocking agents should be administered with caution in patients subject to spontaneous hypoglycemia or to diabetic patients (especially those with labile diabetes) who are receiving insulin or oral hypoglycemic agents. Beta-adrenergic receptor blocking agents may mask the signs and symptoms of acute hypoglycemia).

No products indexed under this heading.

Insulin, Human, Zinc Suspension (Beta-adrenergic blocking agents should be administered with caution in patients subject to spontaneous hypoglycemia or to diabetic patients (especially those with labile diabetes) who are receiving insulin or oral hypoglycemic agents. Beta-adrenergic receptor blocking agents may mask the signs and symptoms of acute hypoglycemia).

No products indexed under this heading.

Insulin, Human (rDNA origin) (Beta-adrenergic blocking agents should be administered with caution in patients subject to spontaneous hypoglycemia or to diabetic patients (especially those with labile diabetes) who are receiving insulin or oral hypoglycemic agents. Beta-adrenergic receptor blocking agents may mask the signs and symptoms of acute hypoglycemia). Products include:

Exubera Inhalation Powder 2515

Insulin, Human NPH (Beta-adrenergic blocking agents should be administered with caution in patients subject to spontaneous hypoglycemia or to diabetic patients (especially those with labile diabetes) who are receiving insulin or oral hypoglycemic agents. Beta-adrenergic receptor blocking agents may mask the signs and symptoms of acute hypoglycemia). Products include:

Humulin N Vial 1846

Insulin, Human Regular (Beta-adrenergic blocking agents should be administered with caution in patients subject to spontaneous hypoglycemia or to diabetic patients (especially those with labile diabetes) who are receiving insulin or oral hypoglycemic agents. Beta-adrenergic receptor blocking agents may mask the signs and symptoms of acute hypoglycemia). Products include:

Humulin R 1849
Humulin R (U-500) 1850

Insulin, Human Regular and Human NPH Mixture (Beta-adrenergic blocking agents should be administered with caution in patients subject to spontaneous hypoglycemia or to diabetic patients (especially those with labile diabetes) who are receiving insulin or oral hypoglycemic agents. Beta-adrenergic receptor blocking agents may mask the signs and symptoms of acute hypoglycemia). Products include:

Humulin 50/50, 100 Units 1843
Humulin 70/30 Vial 1844

Insulin, NPH (Beta-adrenergic blocking agents should be administered with caution in patients subject to spontaneous hypoglycemia or to diabetic patients (especially those with labile diabetes) who are receiving insulin or oral hypoglycemic agents. Beta-adrenergic receptor blocking agents may mask the signs and symptoms of acute hypoglycemia).

No products indexed under this heading.

Insulin, Regular (Beta-adrenergic blocking agents should be administered with caution in patients subject to spontaneous hypoglycemia or to diabetic patients (especially those with labile diabetes) who are receiving insulin or oral hypoglycemic agents. Beta-adrenergic receptor blocking agents may mask the signs and symptoms of acute hypoglycemia).

No products indexed under this heading.

Insulin, Regular and NPH mixture (Beta-adrenergic blocking agents should be administered with caution in patients subject to spontaneous hypoglycemia or to diabetic patients (especially those with labile diabetes) who are receiving insulin or oral hypoglycemic agents. Beta-adrenergic receptor blocking agents may mask the signs and symptoms of acute hypoglycemia).

No products indexed under this heading.

Insulin, Zinc Crystals (Beta-adrenergic blocking agents should be administered with caution in patients subject to spontaneous hypoglycemia or to diabetic patients (especially those with labile diabetes) who are receiving insulin or oral hypoglycemic agents. Beta-adrenergic receptor blocking agents may mask the signs and symptoms of acute hypoglycemia).

No products indexed under this heading.

Insulin, Zinc Suspension (Beta-adrenergic blocking agents should be administered with caution in patients subject to spontaneous hypoglycemia or to diabetic patients (especially those with labile diabetes) who are receiving insulin or oral hypoglycemic agents. Beta-adrenergic receptor blocking agents may mask the signs and symptoms of acute hypoglycemia).

No products indexed under this heading.

Insulin Aspart (Beta-adrenergic blocking agents should be administered with caution in patients subject to spontaneous hypoglycemia or to diabetic patients (especially those with labile diabetes) who are receiving insulin or oral hypoglycemic agents. Beta-adrenergic receptor blocking agents may mask the signs and symptoms of acute hypoglycemia).

No products indexed under this heading.

Insulin Aspart, Human (Beta-adrenergic blocking agents should be administered with caution in patients subject to spontaneous hypoglycemia or to diabetic patients (especially those with labile diabetes) who are receiving insulin or oral hypoglycemic agents. Beta-adrenergic receptor blocking agents may mask the signs and symptoms of acute hypoglycemia). Products include:

NovoLog Mix 70/30 2364

Insulin Aspart, Human Regular (Beta-adrenergic blocking agents should be administered with caution in patients subject to spontaneous hypoglycemia or to diabetic patients (especially those with labile diabetes) who are receiving insulin or oral hypoglycemic agents. Beta-adrenergic receptor blocking agents may mask the signs and symptoms of acute hypoglycemia). Products include:

NovoLog Injection 2359

Insulin Aspart Protamine, Human (Beta-adrenergic blocking agents should be administered with caution in patients subject to spontaneous hypoglycemia or to diabetic patients (especially those with labile diabetes) who are receiving insulin or oral hypoglycemic agents. Beta-adrenergic receptor blocking agents may mask the signs and symptoms of acute hypoglycemia). Products include:

NovoLog Mix 70/30 2364

Insulin Detemir (rDNA Origin) (Beta-adrenergic blocking agents should be administered with caution in patients subject to spontaneous hypoglycemia or to diabetic patients (especially those with labile diabetes) who are receiving insulin or oral hypoglycemic agents. Beta-adrenergic receptor blocking agents may mask the signs and symptoms of acute hypoglycemia). Products include:

Levemir Injection 2352

Insulin glargine (Beta-adrenergic blocking agents should be administered with caution in patients subject to spontaneous hypoglycemia or to diabetic patients (especially those with labile diabetes) who are receiving insulin or oral hypoglycemic agents. Beta-adrenergic receptor blocking agents may mask the signs and symptoms of acute hypoglycemia). Products include:

Lantus Injection 2749

Insulin Glulisine (Beta-adrenergic blocking agents should be administered with caution in patients subject to spontaneous hypoglycemia or to diabetic patients (especially those with labile diabetes) who are receiving insulin or oral hypoglycemic agents. Beta-adrenergic receptor blocking agents may mask the signs and symptoms of acute hypoglycemia). Products include:

Apidra Injection 2706

Insulin Lispro, Human (Beta-adrenergic blocking agents should be administered with caution in patients subject to spontaneous hypoglycemia or to diabetic patients (especially those with labile diabetes) who are receiving insulin or oral hypoglycemic agents. Beta-adrenergic receptor blocking agents may mask the signs and symptoms of acute hypoglycemia). Products include:

Humalog-Pen and KwikPen 1829
Humalog Mix 50/50-Pen and KwikPen 1833
Humalog Mix 75/25-Pen and KwikPen 1835

Insulin Lispro Protamine, Human (Beta-adrenergic blocking agents should be administered with caution in patients subject to spontaneous hypoglycemia or to diabetic patients (especially those with labile diabetes) who are receiving insulin or oral hypoglycemic agents. Beta-adrenergic receptor blocking agents may mask the signs and symptoms of acute hypoglycemia). Products include:

Humalog Mix 50/50-Pen and KwikPen 1833
Humalog Mix 75/25-Pen and KwikPen 1835

Irbesartan (Because Combigan may reduce blood pressure, caution in using drugs such as antihypertensives with Combigan is advised). Products include:

Avalide Tablets 892
Avalide Tablets 2713
Avapro Tablets 897
Avapro Tablets 2718

Isocarboxazid (Monoamine oxidase (MAO) inhibitors may theoretically interfere with the metabolism of brimonidine and potentially result in an increased systemic side-effect such as hypotension. Caution is advised in patients taking MAO inhibitors which can affect the metabolism and uptake of circulating amines). Products include:

Marplan Tablets 3177

Isoflurane (Although specific drug interaction studies have not been conducted with Combigan, the possibility of an additive or potentiating effect with CNS depressants (alcohol, barbiturates, opiates, sedatives or anesthetics) should be considered).

No products indexed under this heading.

Isradipine (Caution should be used in the co-administration of beta-adrenergic blocking agents, such as Combigan, and oral or intravenous calcium antagonists because of possible atrioventricular conduction disturbances, left ventricular failure and hypotension. In patients with impaired cardiac function, co-administration should be avoided. The concomitant use of beta-adrenergic blocking agents with calcium antagonists may have additive effects in proloning atrioventricular conduction time). Products include:

DynaCirc CR Controlled Release Tablets 1407

Ketamine Hydrochloride (Although specific drug interaction studies have not been conducted with Combigan, the possibility of an additive or potentiating effect with CNS depressants (alcohol, barbiturates, opiates, sedatives or anesthetics) should be considered).

No products indexed under this heading.

Labetalol Hydrochloride (Patients who are receiving a beta-adrenergic blocking agent orally and Combigan should be observed for potential additive effects of beta-blockade, both systemic and on intraocular pressure. The concomitant use of two topical beta-adrenergic blocking agents is not recommended).

No products indexed under this heading.

Levobunolol Hydrochloride (Patients who are receiving a beta-adrenergic blocking agent orally and Combigan should be observed for potential additive effects of beta-blockade, both systemic and on intraocular pressure. The concomitant use of two topical beta-adrenergic blocking agents is not recommended).

No products indexed under this heading.

Levomethadyl Acetate Hydrochloride (Although specific drug interaction studies have not been conducted with Combigan, the possibility of an additive or potentiating effect with CNS depressants (alcohol, barbiturates, opiates, sedatives or anesthetics) should be considered).

No products indexed under this heading.

Levorphanol Tartrate (Although specific drug interaction studies have not been conducted with Combigan, the possibility of an additive or potentiating effect with CNS depressants (alcohol, barbiturates, opiates, sedatives or anesthetics) should be considered).

No products indexed under this heading.

Lisinopril (Because Combigan may reduce blood pressure, caution in using drugs such as antihypertensives with Combigan is advised). Products include:

Prinivil Tablets 2087
Prinzide Tablets 2092

Lorazepam (Although specific drug interaction studies have not been conducted with Combigan, the possibility of an additive or potentiating effect with CNS depressants (alcohol, barbiturates, opiates, sedatives or anesthetics) should be considered).

No products indexed under this heading.

Losartan Potassium (Because Combigan may reduce blood pressure, caution in using drugs such as antihypertensives with Combigan is advised). Products include:

Cozaar Tablets 1973

Loxapine Hydrochloride (Although specific drug interaction studies have not been conducted with Combigan, the possibility of an additive or potentiating effect with CNS depressants (alcohol, barbiturates, opiates, sedatives or anesthetics) should be considered).
No products indexed under this heading.

Loxapine Succinate (Although specific drug interaction studies have not been conducted with Combigan, the possibility of an additive or potentiating effect with CNS depressants (alcohol, barbiturates, opiates, sedatives or anesthetics) should be considered).
No products indexed under this heading.

Maprotiline Hydrochloride (Tricyclic antidepressants have been reported to blunt the hypotensive effect of systemic clonidine. It is not known whether the concurrent use of these agents with Combigan in humans can lead to resulting interference with the IOP lowering effect. Caution, however, is advised in patients taking tricyclic antidepressants which can affect the metabolism and uptake of circulating amines).
No products indexed under this heading.

Mecamylamine Hydrochloride (Because Combigan may reduce blood pressure, caution in using drugs such as antihypertensives with Combigan is advised).
No products indexed under this heading.

Meperidine Hydrochloride (Although specific drug interaction studies have not been conducted with Combigan, the possibility of an additive or potentiating effect with CNS depressants (alcohol, barbiturates, opiates, sedatives or anesthetics) should be considered).
No products indexed under this heading.

Mephobarbital (Although specific drug interaction studies have not been conducted with Combigan, the possibility of an additive or potentiating effect with CNS depressants (alcohol, barbiturates, opiates, sedatives or anesthetics) should be considered).
No products indexed under this heading.

Meprobamate (Although specific drug interaction studies have not been conducted with Combigan, the possibility of an additive or potentiating effect with CNS depressants (alcohol, barbiturates, opiates, sedatives or anesthetics) should be considered).
No products indexed under this heading.

Mesoridazine Besylate (Although specific drug interaction studies have not been conducted with Combigan, the possibility of an additive or potentiating effect with CNS depressants (alcohol, barbiturates, opiates, sedatives or anesthetics) should be considered).
No products indexed under this heading.

Metformin Hydrochloride (Beta-adrenergic blocking agents should be administered with caution in patients subject to spontaneous hypoglycemia or to diabetic patients (especially those with labile diabetes) who are receiving insulin or oral hypoglycemic agents. Beta-adrenergic receptor blocking agents may mask the signs and symptoms of acute hypoglycemia). Products include:
ActoPlus Met Tablets **3071**
Avandamet Tablets **1336**
Janumet Tablets **2041**
PrandiMet Tablets **2967**

Methadone Hydrochloride (Although specific drug interaction studies have not been conducted with Combigan, the possibility of an additive or potentiating effect with CNS depressants (alcohol, barbiturates, opiates, sedatives or anesthetics) should be considered).
No products indexed under this heading.

Methohexital Sodium (Although specific drug interaction studies have not been conducted with Combigan, the possibility of an additive or potentiating effect with CNS depressants (alcohol, barbiturates, opiates, sedatives or anesthetics) should be considered).
No products indexed under this heading.

Methotrimeprazine (Although specific drug interaction studies have not been conducted with Combigan, the possibility of an additive or potentiating effect with CNS depressants (alcohol, barbiturates, opiates, sedatives or anesthetics) should be considered).
No products indexed under this heading.

Methoxyflurane (Although specific drug interaction studies have not been conducted with Combigan, the possibility of an additive or potentiating effect with CNS depressants (alcohol, barbiturates, opiates, sedatives or anesthetics) should be considered).
No products indexed under this heading.

Methyclothiazide (Because Combigan may reduce blood pressure, caution in using drugs such as antihypertensives with Combigan is advised).
No products indexed under this heading.

Methyldopa (Because Combigan may reduce blood pressure, caution in using drugs such as antihypertensives with Combigan is advised).
No products indexed under this heading.

Methyldopate Hydrochloride (Because Combigan may reduce blood pressure, caution in using drugs such as antihypertensives with Combigan is advised).
No products indexed under this heading.

Metipranolol Hydrochloride (Patients who are receiving a beta-adrenergic blocking agent orally and Combigan should be observed for potential additive effects of beta-blockade, both systemic and on intraocular pressure. The concomitant use of two topical beta-adrenergic blocking agents is not recommended).
No products indexed under this heading.

Metolazone (Because Combigan may reduce blood pressure, caution in using drugs such as antihypertensives with Combigan is advised).
No products indexed under this heading.

Metoprolol Succinate (Patients who are receiving a beta-adrenergic blocking agent orally and Combigan should be observed for potential additive effects of beta-blockade, both systemic and on intraocular pressure. The concomitant use of two topical beta-adrenergic blocking agents is not recommended). Products include:
Toprol-XL Tablets **666**

Metoprolol Tartrate (Patients who are receiving a beta-adrenergic blocking agent orally and Combigan should be observed for potential additive effects of beta-blockade, both systemic and on intraocular pressure. The concomitant use of two topical beta-adrenergic blocking agents is not recommended).
No products indexed under this heading.

Metyrosine (Because Combigan may reduce blood pressure, caution in using drugs such as antihypertensives with Combigan is advised). Products include:
Demser Capsules **1989**

Mibefradil Dihydrochloride (Caution should be used in the co-administration of beta-adrenergic blocking agents, such as Combigan, and oral or intravenous calcium antagonists because of possible atrioventricular conduction disturbances, left ventricular failure and hypotension. In patients with impaired cardiac function, co-administration should be avoided. The concomitant use of beta-adrenergic blocking agents with calcium antagonists may have additive effects in proloning atrioventricular conduction time).
No products indexed under this heading.

Midazolam Hydrochloride (Although specific drug interaction studies have not been conducted with Combigan, the possibility of an additive or potentiating effect with CNS depressants (alcohol, barbiturates, opiates, sedatives or anesthetics) should be considered).
No products indexed under this heading.

Miglitol (Beta-adrenergic blocking agents should be administered with caution in patients subject to spontaneous hypoglycemia or to diabetic patients (especially those with labile diabetes) who are receiving insulin or oral hypoglycemic agents. Beta-adrenergic receptor blocking agents may mask the signs and symptoms of acute hypoglycemia).
No products indexed under this heading.

Minoxidil (Because Combigan may reduce blood pressure, caution in using drugs such as antihypertensives with Combigan is advised).
No products indexed under this heading.

Moclobemide (Monoamine oxidase (MAO) inhibitors may theoretically interfere with the metabolism of brimonidine and potentially result in an increased systemic side-effect such as hypotension. Caution is advised in patients taking MAO inhibitors which can affect the metabolism and uptake of circulating amines).
No products indexed under this heading.

Moexipril Hydrochloride (Because Combigan may reduce blood pressure, caution in using drugs such as antihypertensives with Combigan is advised).
No products indexed under this heading.

Molindone Hydrochloride (Although specific drug interaction studies have not been conducted with Combigan, the possibility of an additive or potentiating effect with CNS depressants (alcohol, barbiturates, opiates, sedatives or anesthetics) should be considered). Products include:
Moban Tablets **1116**

Morphine Sulfate (Although specific drug interaction studies have not been conducted with Combigan, the possibility of an additive or potentiating effect with CNS depressants (alcohol, barbiturates, opiates, sedatives or anesthetics) should be considered). Products include:
Avinza Capsules **1772**
DepoDur Injection **1095**
MS Contin Tablets **2585**

Nadolol (Patients who are receiving a beta-adrenergic blocking agent orally and Combigan should be observed for potential additive effects of beta-blockade, both systemic and on intraocular pressure. The concomitant use of two topical beta-adrenergic blocking agents is not recommended). Products include:
Nadolol Tablets **2191**

Nateglinide (Beta-adrenergic blocking agents should be administered with caution in patients subject to spontaneous hypoglycemia or to diabetic patients (especially those with labile diabetes) who are receiving insulin or oral hypoglycemic agents. Beta-adrenergic receptor blocking agents may mask the signs and symptoms of acute hypoglycemia). Products include:
Starlix Tablets **2314**

Nebivolol (Patients who are receiving a beta-adrenergic blocking agent orally and Combigan should be observed for potential additive effects of beta-blockade, both systemic and on intraocular pressure. The concomitant use of two topical beta-adrenergic blocking agents is not recommended). Products include:
Bystolic Tablets **1155**

Nicardipine Hydrochloride (Caution should be used in the co-administration of beta-adrenergic blocking agents, such as Combigan, and oral or intravenous calcium antagonists because of possible atrioventricular conduction disturbances, left ventricular failure and hypotension. In patients with impaired cardiac function, co-administration should be avoided. The concomitant use of beta-adrenergic blocking agents with calcium antagonists may have additive effects in proloning atrioventricular conduction time). Products include:

Cardene I.V. 1093

Nifedipine (Caution should be used in the co-administration of beta-adrenergic blocking agents, such as Combigan, and oral or intravenous calcium antagonists because of possible atrioventricular conduction disturbances, left ventricular failure and hypotension. In patients with impaired cardiac function, co-administration should be avoided. The concomitant use of beta-adrenergic blocking agents with calcium antagonists may have additive effects in proloning atrioventricular conduction time).

No products indexed under this heading.

Nimodipine (Caution should be used in the co-administration of beta-adrenergic blocking agents, such as Combigan, and oral or intravenous calcium antagonists because of possible atrioventricular conduction disturbances, left ventricular failure and hypotension. In patients with impaired cardiac function, co-administration should be avoided. The concomitant use of beta-adrenergic blocking agents with calcium antagonists may have additive effects in proloning atrioventricular conduction time). Products include:

Nimotop Capsules 790

Nisoldipine (Caution should be used in the co-administration of beta-adrenergic blocking agents, such as Combigan, and oral or intravenous calcium antagonists because of possible atrioventricular conduction disturbances, left ventricular failure and hypotension. In patients with impaired cardiac function, co-administration should be avoided. The concomitant use of beta-adrenergic blocking agents with calcium antagonists may have additive effects in proloning atrioventricular conduction time). Products include:

Sular Extended Release Tablets 2975

Nitroglycerin (Because Combigan may reduce blood pressure, caution in using drugs such as antihypertensives with Combigan is advised). Products include:

Nitro-Dur Transdermal Infusion System.. 2887
Nitrolingual Pumpspray 2965

Nortriptyline Hydrochloride (Tricyclic antidepressants have been reported to blunt the hypotensive effect of systemic clonidine. It is not known whether the concurrent use of these agents with Combigan in humans can lead to resulting interference with the IOP lowering effect. Caution, however, is advised in patients taking tricyclic antidepressants which can affect the metabolism and uptake of circulating amines).

No products indexed under this heading.

Olanzapine (Although specific drug interaction studies have not been conducted with Combigan, the possibility of an additive or potentiating effect with CNS depressants (alcohol, barbiturates, opiates, sedatives or anesthetics) should be considered). Products include:

Symbyax Capsules 1871
Zyprexa Tablets 1883
Zyprexa IntraMuscular 1883
Zyprexa ZYDIS Orally Disintegrating Tablets.................. 1883

Oxazepam (Although specific drug interaction studies have not been conducted with Combigan, the possibility of an additive or potentiating effect with CNS depressants (alcohol, barbiturates, opiates, sedatives or anesthetics) should be considered).

No products indexed under this heading.

Oxycodone Hydrochloride (Although specific drug interaction studies have not been conducted with Combigan, the possibility of an additive or potentiating effect with CNS depressants (alcohol, barbiturates, opiates, sedatives or anesthetics) should be considered). Products include:

OxyContin Tablets 2589
OxyIR Capsules 2593
Percocet Tablets 1127
Percodan Tablets 1130

Pargyline Hydrochloride (Monoamine oxidase (MAO) inhibitors may theoretically interfere with the metabolism of brimonidine and potentially result in an increased systemic side-effect such as hypotension. Caution is advised in patients taking MAO inhibitors which can affect the metabolism and uptake of circulating amines).

No products indexed under this heading.

Paroxetine Hydrochloride (Potentiated systemic beta-blockade (e.g., decreased heart rate, depression) has been reported during combined treatment with CYP2D6 inhibitors (e.g., quinidine, SSRIs) and timolol). Products include:

Paxil 1535
Paxil CR Controlled-Release Tablets... 1544

Penbutolol Sulfate (Patients who are receiving a beta-adrenergic blocking agent orally and Combigan should be observed for potential additive effects of beta-blockade, both systemic and on intraocular pressure. The concomitant use of two topical beta-adrenergic blocking agents is not recommended).

No products indexed under this heading.

Pentobarbital Sodium (Although specific drug interaction studies have not been conducted with Combigan, the possibility of an additive or potentiating effect with CNS depressants (alcohol, barbiturates, opiates, sedatives or anesthetics) should be considered). Products include:

Nembutal Sodium Solution, USP 2494

Perindopril Erbumine (Because Combigan may reduce blood pressure, caution in using drugs such as antihypertensives with Combigan is advised). Products include:

Aceon Tablets (2 mg, 4 mg, 8 mg)... 3038

Perphenazine (Although specific drug interaction studies have not been conducted with Combigan, the possibility of an additive or potentiating effect with CNS depressants (alcohol, barbiturates, opiates, sedatives or anesthetics) should be considered).

No products indexed under this heading.

Phenelzine Sulfate (Monoamine oxidase (MAO) inhibitors may theoretically interfere with the metabolism of brimonidine and potentially result in an increased systemic side-effect such as hypotension. Caution is advised in patients taking MAO inhibitors which can affect the metabolism and uptake of circulating amines).

No products indexed under this heading.

Phenobarbital (Although specific drug interaction studies have not been conducted with Combigan, the possibility of an additive or potentiating effect with CNS depressants (alcohol, barbiturates, opiates, sedatives or anesthetics) should be considered). Products include:

Donnatal Extentabs 2507

Phenoxybenzamine Hydrochloride (Because Combigan may reduce blood pressure, caution in using drugs such as antihypertensives with Combigan is advised). Products include:

Dibenzyline Capsules 3188

Phentolamine Mesylate (Because Combigan may reduce blood pressure, caution in using drugs such as antihypertensives with Combigan is advised).

No products indexed under this heading.

Pindolol (Patients who are receiving a beta-adrenergic blocking agent orally and Combigan should be observed for potential additive effects of beta-blockade, both systemic and on intraocular pressure. The concomitant use of two topical beta-adrenergic blocking agents is not recommended).

No products indexed under this heading.

Pioglitazone Hydrochloride (Beta-adrenergic blocking agents should be administered with caution in patients subject to spontaneous hypoglycemia or to diabetic patients (especially those with labile diabetes) who are receiving insulin or oral hypoglycemic agents. Beta-adrenergic receptor blocking agents may mask the signs and symptoms of acute hypoglycemia). Products include:

ActoPlus Met Tablets 3071
Actos Tablets 3077
Duetact Tablets 3085

Polythiazide (Because Combigan may reduce blood pressure, caution in using drugs such as antihypertensives with Combigan is advised).

No products indexed under this heading.

Prazepam (Although specific drug interaction studies have not been conducted with Combigan, the possibility of an additive or potentiating effect with CNS depressants (alcohol, barbiturates, opiates, sedatives or anesthetics) should be considered).

No products indexed under this heading.

Prazosin Hydrochloride (Because Combigan may reduce blood pressure, caution in using drugs such as antihypertensives with Combigan is advised).

No products indexed under this heading.

Procarbazine Hydrochloride (Monoamine oxidase (MAO) inhibitors may theoretically interfere with the metabolism of brimonidine and potentially result in an increased systemic side-effect such as hypotension. Caution is advised in patients taking MAO inhibitors which can affect the metabolism and uptake of circulating amines).

No products indexed under this heading.

Prochlorperazine (Although specific drug interaction studies have not been conducted with Combigan, the possibility of an additive or potentiating effect with CNS depressants (alcohol, barbiturates, opiates, sedatives or anesthetics) should be considered).

No products indexed under this heading.

Promethazine Hydrochloride (Although specific drug interaction studies have not been conducted with Combigan, the possibility of an additive or potentiating effect with CNS depressants (alcohol, barbiturates, opiates, sedatives or anesthetics) should be considered).

No products indexed under this heading.

Propafenone Hydrochloride (Potentiated systemic beta-blockade (e.g., decreased heart rate, depression) has been reported during combined treatment with CYP2D6 inhibitors (e.g., quinidine, SSRIs) and timolol). Products include:

Rythmol Tablets 1586
Rythmol SR Capsules 1590

Propofol (Although specific drug interaction studies have not been conducted with Combigan, the possibility of an additive or potentiating effect with CNS depressants (alcohol, barbiturates, opiates, sedatives or anesthetics) should be considered).

No products indexed under this heading.

Propoxyphene Hydrochloride (Although specific drug interaction studies have not been conducted with Combigan, the possibility of an additive or potentiating effect with CNS depressants (alcohol, barbiturates, opiates, sedatives or anesthetics) should be considered).

No products indexed under this heading.

Propoxyphene Napsylate (Although specific drug interaction studies have not been conducted with Combigan, the possibility of an additive or potentiating effect with CNS depressants (alcohol, barbiturates, opiates, sedatives or anesthetics) should be considered).

No products indexed under this heading.

Propranolol Hydrochloride (Patients who are receiving a beta-adrenergic blocking agent orally and Combigan should be observed for potential additive effects of beta-blockade, both systemic and on intraocular pressure. The concomitant use of two topical beta-adrenergic blocking agents is not recommended). Products include:

InnoPran XL Extended Release Capsules.................................... 1484

Protriptyline Hydrochloride (Tricyclic antidepressants have been reported to blunt the hypotensive effect of systemic clonidine. It is not

known whether the concurrent use of these agents with Combigan in humans can lead to resulting interference with the IOP lowering effect. Caution, however, is advised in patients taking tricyclic antidepressants which can affect the metabolism and uptake of circulating amines).
No products indexed under this heading.

Quazepam (Although specific drug interaction studies have not been conducted with Combigan, the possibility of an additive or potentiating effect with CNS depressants (alcohol, barbiturates, opiates, sedatives or anesthetics) should be considered).
No products indexed under this heading.

Quetiapine Fumarate (Although specific drug interaction studies have not been conducted with Combigan, the possibility of an additive or potentiating effect with CNS depressants (alcohol, barbiturates, opiates, sedatives or anesthetics) should be considered).
No products indexed under this heading.

Quinacrine Hydrochloride (Potentiated systemic beta-blockade (e.g., decreased heart rate, depression) has been reported during combined treatment with CYP2D6 inhibitors (e.g., quinidine, SSRIs) and timolol).
No products indexed under this heading.

Quinapril Hydrochloride (Because Combigan may reduce blood pressure, caution in using drugs such as antihypertensives with Combigan is advised).
No products indexed under this heading.

Quinidine Gluconate (Potentiated systemic beta-blockade (e.g., decreased heart rate, depression) has been reported during combined treatment with CYP2D6 inhibitors (e.g., quinidine, SSRIs) and timolol).
No products indexed under this heading.

Quinidine Hydrochloride (Potentiated systemic beta-blockade (e.g., decreased heart rate, depression) has been reported during combined treatment with CYP2D6 inhibitors (e.g., quinidine, SSRIs) and timolol).
No products indexed under this heading.

Quinidine Polygalacturonate (Potentiated systemic beta-blockade (e.g., decreased heart rate, depression) has been reported during combined treatment with CYP2D6 inhibitors (e.g., quinidine, SSRIs) and timolol).
No products indexed under this heading.

Quinidine Sulfate (Potentiated systemic beta-blockade (e.g., decreased heart rate, depression) has been reported during combined treatment with CYP2D6 inhibitors (e.g., quinidine, SSRIs) and timolol).
No products indexed under this heading.

Ramelteon (Although specific drug interaction studies have not been conducted with Combigan, the possibility of an additive or potentiating effect with CNS depressants (alcohol, barbiturates, opiates, sedatives or anesthetics) should be considered). Products include:
Rozerem Tablets **3091**

Ramipril (Because Combigan may reduce blood pressure, caution in using drugs such as antihypertensives with Combigan is advised).
No products indexed under this heading.

Ranitidine Bismuth Citrate (Potentiated systemic beta-blockade (e.g., decreased heart rate, depression) has been reported during combined treatment with CYP2D6 inhibitors (e.g., quinidine, SSRIs) and timolol).
No products indexed under this heading.

Ranitidine Hydrochloride (Potentiated systemic beta-blockade (e.g., decreased heart rate, depression) has been reported during combined treatment with CYP2D6 inhibitors (e.g., quinidine, SSRIs) and timolol). Products include:
Zantac 75 Tablets .... ▣ **603**
Zantac **1670**
Zantac Injection **1666**
Zantac Injection Pharmacy Bulk Package **1668**
Maximum Strength Zantac 150 Tablets .... ▣ **603**
Maximum Strength Zantac 150 Cool Mint Tablets .... ▣ **603**

Rasagiline Mesylate (Monoamine oxidase (MAO) inhibitors may theoretically interfere with the metabolism of brimonidine and potentially result in an increased systemic side-effect such as hypotension. Caution is advised in patients taking MAO inhibitors which can affect the metabolism and uptake of circulating amines). Products include:
Azilect Tablets **3106**

Rauwolfia Serpentina (Because Combigan may reduce blood pressure, caution in using drugs such as antihypertensives with Combigan is advised).
No products indexed under this heading.

Remifentanil Hydrochloride (Although specific drug interaction studies have not been conducted with Combigan, the possibility of an additive or potentiating effect with CNS depressants (alcohol, barbiturates, opiates, sedatives or anesthetics) should be considered).
No products indexed under this heading.

Repaglinide (Beta-adrenergic blocking agents should be administered with caution in patients subject to spontaneous hypoglycemia or to diabetic patients (especially those with labile diabetes) who are receiving insulin or oral hypoglycemic agents. Beta-adrenergic receptor blocking agents may mask the signs and symptoms of acute hypoglycemia). Products include:
PrandiMet Tablets **2967**
Prandin Tablets **2971**

Rescinnamine (Because Combigan may reduce blood pressure, caution in using drugs such as antihypertensives with Combigan is advised).
No products indexed under this heading.

Reserpine (Because Combigan may reduce blood pressure, caution in using drugs such as antihypertensives with Combigan is advised).
No products indexed under this heading.

Risperidone (Although specific drug interaction studies have not been conducted with Combigan, the possibility of an additive or potentiating effect with CNS depressants (alcohol, barbiturates, opiates, sedatives or anesthetics) should be considered). Products include:
Risperdal Consta Long-Acting Injection **1753**

Ritonavir (Potentiated systemic beta-blockade (e.g., decreased heart rate, depression) has been reported during combined treatment with CYP2D6 inhibitors (e.g., quinidine, SSRIs) and timolol). Products include:
Kaletra **452**
Norvir **489**

Rosiglitazone Maleate (Beta-adrenergic blocking agents should be administered with caution in patients subject to spontaneous hypoglycemia or to diabetic patients (especially those with labile diabetes) who are receiving insulin or oral hypoglycemic agents. Beta-adrenergic receptor blocking agents may mask the signs and symptoms of acute hypoglycemia). Products include:
Avandamet Tablets **1336**
Avandaryl Tablets **1344**
Avandia Tablets **1351**

Secobarbital Sodium (Although specific drug interaction studies have not been conducted with Combigan, the possibility of an additive or potentiating effect with CNS depressants (alcohol, barbiturates, opiates, sedatives or anesthetics) should be considered).
No products indexed under this heading.

Selegiline (Monoamine oxidase (MAO) inhibitors may theoretically interfere with the metabolism of brimonidine and potentially result in an increased systemic side-effect such as hypotension. Caution is advised in patients taking MAO inhibitors which can affect the metabolism and uptake of circulating amines). Products include:
Emsam Transdermal System **905**

Selegiline Hydrochloride (Monoamine oxidase (MAO) inhibitors may theoretically interfere with the metabolism of brimonidine and potentially result in an increased systemic side-effect such as hypotension. Caution is advised in patients taking MAO inhibitors which can affect the metabolism and uptake of circulating amines). Products include:
Eldepryl Capsules **3052**

Sertraline Hydrochloride (Potentiated systemic beta-blockade (e.g., decreased heart rate, depression) has been reported during combined treatment with CYP2D6 inhibitors (e.g., quinidine, SSRIs) and timolol).
No products indexed under this heading.

Sevoflurane (Although specific drug interaction studies have not been conducted with Combigan, the possibility of an additive or potentiating effect with CNS depressants (alcohol, barbiturates, opiates, sedatives or anesthetics) should be considered). Products include:
Ultane Liquid for Inhalation **524**

Sildenafil Citrate (Potentiated systemic beta-blockade (e.g., decreased heart rate, depression) has been reported during combined treatment with CYP2D6 inhibitors (e.g., quinidine, SSRIs) and timolol).
No products indexed under this heading.

Sitagliptin Phosphate (Beta-adrenergic blocking agents should be administered with caution in patients subject to spontaneous hypoglycemia or to diabetic patients (especially those with labile diabetes) who are receiving insulin or oral hypoglycemic agents. Beta-adrenergic receptor blocking agents may mask the signs and symptoms of acute hypoglycemia). Products include:
Janumet Tablets **2041**
Januvia Tablets **2048**

Sodium Butabarbital (Although specific drug interaction studies have not been conducted with Combigan, the possibility of an additive or potentiating effect with CNS depressants (alcohol, barbiturates, opiates, sedatives or anesthetics) should be considered).
No products indexed under this heading.

Sodium Nitroprusside (Because Combigan may reduce blood pressure, caution in using drugs such as antihypertensives with Combigan is advised).
No products indexed under this heading.

Sodium Oxybate (Although specific drug interaction studies have not been conducted with Combigan, the possibility of an additive or potentiating effect with CNS depressants (alcohol, barbiturates, opiates, sedatives or anesthetics) should be considered). Products include:
Xyrem Oral Solution **1766**

Sotalol Hydrochloride (Patients who are receiving a beta-adrenergic blocking agent orally and Combigan should be observed for potential additive effects of beta-blockade, both systemic and on intraocular pressure. The concomitant use of two topical beta-adrenergic blocking agents is not recommended).
No products indexed under this heading.

Spirapril Hydrochloride (Because Combigan may reduce blood pressure, caution in using drugs such as antihypertensives with Combigan is advised).
No products indexed under this heading.

Sufentanil Citrate (Although specific drug interaction studies have not been conducted with Combigan, the possibility of an additive or potentiating effect with CNS depressants (alcohol, barbiturates, opiates, sedatives or anesthetics) should be considered).
No products indexed under this heading.

Telmisartan (Because Combigan may reduce blood pressure, caution in using drugs such as antihypertensives with Combigan is advised). Products include:
Micardis Tablets **852**
Micardis HCT Tablets **854**

Temazepam (Although specific drug interaction studies have not been conducted with Combigan, the possibility of an additive or potentiating effect with CNS depressants (alcohol, barbiturates, opiates, sedatives or anesthetics) should be considered).
No products indexed under this heading.

Terazosin Hydrochloride (Because Combigan may reduce blood pressure, caution in using drugs such as antihypertensives with Combigan is advised).
No products indexed under this heading.

Terbinafine Hydrochloride (Potentiated systemic beta-blockade (e.g., decreased heart rate, depression) has been reported during combined treatment with CYP2D6 inhibitors (e.g., quinidine, SSRIs) and timolol). Products include:
Lamisil Oral Granules 2264
Lamisil Tablets 2266

Thiamylal Sodium (Although specific drug interaction studies have not been conducted with Combigan, the possibility of an additive or potentiating effect with CNS depressants (alcohol, barbiturates, opiates, sedatives or anesthetics) should be considered).
No products indexed under this heading.

Thioridazine Hydrochloride (Although specific drug interaction studies have not been conducted with Combigan, the possibility of an additive or potentiating effect with CNS depressants (alcohol, barbiturates, opiates, sedatives or anesthetics) should be considered). Products include:
Thioridazine Hydrochloride Tablets 2195

Thiothixene (Although specific drug interaction studies have not been conducted with Combigan, the possibility of an additive or potentiating effect with CNS depressants (alcohol, barbiturates, opiates, sedatives or anesthetics) should be considered). Products include:
Thiothixene Capsules 2197

Timolol Hemihydrate (Patients who are receiving a beta-adrenergic blocking agent orally and Combigan should be observed for potential additive effects of beta-blockade, both systemic and on intraocular pressure. The concomitant use of two topical beta-adrenergic blocking agents is not recommended). Products include:
Betimol Ophthalmic Solution 3181

Tolazamide (Beta-adrenergic blocking agents should be administered with caution in patients subject to spontaneous hypoglycemia or to diabetic patients (especially those with labile diabetes) who are receiving insulin or oral hypoglycemic agents. Beta-adrenergic receptor blocking agents may mask the signs and symptoms of acute hypoglycemia).
No products indexed under this heading.

Tolbutamide (Beta-adrenergic blocking agents should be administered with caution in patients subject to spontaneous hypoglycemia or to diabetic patients (especially those with labile diabetes) who are receiving insulin or oral hypoglycemic agents. Beta-adrenergic receptor blocking agents may mask the signs and symptoms of acute hypoglycemia).
No products indexed under this heading.

Torsemide (Because Combigan may reduce blood pressure, caution in using drugs such as antihypertensives with Combigan is advised). Products include:
Demadex Injection 2630
Demadex Tablets 2630

Trandolapril (Because Combigan may reduce blood pressure, caution in using drugs such as antihypertensives with Combigan is advised). Products include:
Mavik Tablets 472
Tarka Tablets 511

Tranylcypromine Sulfate (Monoamine oxidase (MAO) inhibitors may theoretically interfere with the metabolism of brimonidine and potentially result in an increased systemic side-effect such as hypotension. Caution is advised in patients taking MAO inhibitors which can affect the metabolism and uptake of circulating amines). Products include:
Parnate Tablets 1532

Triazolam (Although specific drug interaction studies have not been conducted with Combigan, the possibility of an additive or potentiating effect with CNS depressants (alcohol, barbiturates, opiates, sedatives or anesthetics) should be considered).
No products indexed under this heading.

Trifluoperazine Hydrochloride (Although specific drug interaction studies have not been conducted with Combigan, the possibility of an additive or potentiating effect with CNS depressants (alcohol, barbiturates, opiates, sedatives or anesthetics) should be considered).
No products indexed under this heading.

Trimethaphan Camsylate (Because Combigan may reduce blood pressure, caution in using drugs such as antihypertensives with Combigan is advised).
No products indexed under this heading.

Trimipramine Maleate (Tricyclic antidepressants have been reported to blunt the hypotensive effect of systemic clonidine. It is not known whether the concurrent use of these agents with Combigan in humans can lead to resulting interference with the IOP lowering effect. Caution, however, is advised in patients taking tricyclic antidepressants which can affect the metabolism and uptake of circulating amines).
No products indexed under this heading.

Troglitazone (Beta-adrenergic blocking agents should be administered with caution in patients subject to spontaneous hypoglycemia or to diabetic patients (especially those with labile diabetes) who are receiving insulin or oral hypoglycemic agents. Beta-adrenergic receptor blocking agents may mask the signs and symptoms of acute hypoglycemia).
No products indexed under this heading.

Valsartan (Because Combigan may reduce blood pressure, caution in using drugs such as antihypertensives with Combigan is advised). Products include:
Diovan Tablets 2212
Diovan HCT Tablets 2216
Exforge Tablets 2238

Vardenafil Hydrochloride (Potentiated systemic beta-blockade (e.g., decreased heart rate, depression) has been reported during combined treatment with CYP2D6 inhibitors (e.g., quinidine, SSRIs) and timolol). Products include:
Levitra Tablets 2876

Verapamil Hydrochloride (Caution should be used in the co-administration of beta-adrenergic blocking agents, such as Combigan, and oral or intravenous calcium antagonists because of possible atrioventricular conduction disturbances, left ventricular failure and hypotension. In patients with impaired cardiac function, co-administration should be avoided. The concomitant use of beta-adrenergic blocking agents with calcium antagonists may have additive effects in prolonging atrioventricular conduction time). Products include:
Tarka Tablets 511

Zaleplon (Although specific drug interaction studies have not been conducted with Combigan, the possibility of an additive or potentiating effect with CNS depressants (alcohol, barbiturates, opiates, sedatives or anesthetics) should be considered).
No products indexed under this heading.

Ziprasidone Hydrochloride (Although specific drug interaction studies have not been conducted with Combigan, the possibility of an additive or potentiating effect with CNS depressants (alcohol, barbiturates, opiates, sedatives or anesthetics) should be considered). Products include:
Geodon Capsules 2520

Zolpidem Tartrate (Although specific drug interaction studies have not been conducted with Combigan, the possibility of an additive or potentiating effect with CNS depressants (alcohol, barbiturates, opiates, sedatives or anesthetics) should be considered). Products include:
Ambien Tablets 2692
Ambien CR Tablets 2696

Food Interactions

Alcohol (Although specific drug interaction studies have not been conducted with Combigan, the possibility of an additive or potentiating effect with CNS depressants (alcohol, barbiturates, opiates, sedatives or anesthetics) should be considered).

COMBIVENT INHALATION AEROSOL

(Albuterol Sulfate, Ipratropium Bromide) 845

May interact with anticholinergics, beta blockers, monoamine oxidase inhibitors, nonpotassium-sparing diuretics, sympathomimetics, and tricyclic antidepressants. Compounds in these categories include:

Acebutolol Hydrochloride (Co-administration with beta blockers inhibits the effects of each other).
No products indexed under this heading.

Albuterol (Co-administration with other sympathomimetic agents increases the risk of adverse cardiovascular effects).
No products indexed under this heading.

Amitriptyline Hydrochloride (Co-administration with tricyclic antidepressant can potentiate the action of albuterol on the cardiovascular system).
No products indexed under this heading.

Amoxapine (Co-administration with tricyclic antidepressant can potentiate the action of albuterol on the cardiovascular system).
No products indexed under this heading.

Atenolol (Co-administration with beta blockers inhibits the effects of each other).
No products indexed under this heading.

Atropine Sulfate (Co-administration has some potential for additive anticholinergic effects; caution is advised). Products include:
Donnatal Extentabs 2507

Belladonna Alkaloids (Co-administration has some potential for additive anticholinergic effects; caution is advised). Products include:
Hyland's Teething Tablets 621

Bendroflumethiazide (Co-administration with non-potassium-sparing diuretics can result in acute worsening of ECG changes and/or hypokalemia, especially when recommended dose of the beta agonist is exceeded; clinical significance of this interaction is unknown).
No products indexed under this heading.

Benztropine Mesylate (Co-administration has some potential for additive anticholinergic effects; caution is advised).
No products indexed under this heading.

Betaxolol Hydrochloride (Co-administration with beta blockers inhibits the effects of each other).
No products indexed under this heading.

Biperiden Hydrochloride (Co-administration has some potential for additive anticholinergic effects; caution is advised).
No products indexed under this heading.

Bisoprolol Fumarate (Co-administration with beta blockers inhibits the effects of each other).
No products indexed under this heading.

Bumetanide (Co-administration with non-potassium-sparing diuretics can result in acute worsening of ECG changes and/or hypokalemia, especially when recommended dose of the beta agonist is exceeded; clinical significance of this interaction is unknown).
No products indexed under this heading.

Carteolol Hydrochloride (Co-administration with beta blockers inhibits the effects of each other).
No products indexed under this heading.

Chlorothiazide (Co-administration with non-potassium-sparing diuretics can result in acute worsening of ECG changes and/or hypokalemia, especially when recommended dose of the beta agonist is exceeded; clinical significance of this interaction is unknown).
No products indexed under this heading.

Chlorothiazide Sodium (Co-administration with non-potassium-sparing diuretics can result in acute worsening of ECG changes and/or hypokalemia, especially when recommended dose of the beta agonist is exceeded; clinical significance of this interaction is unknown). Products include:

Intravenous Sodium Diuril ... 2490

Clidinium Bromide (Co-administration has some potential for additive anticholinergic effects; caution is advised).

No products indexed under this heading.

Clomipramine Hydrochloride (Co-administration with tricyclic antidepressant can potentiate the action of albuterol on the cardiovascular system).

No products indexed under this heading.

Desipramine Hydrochloride (Co-administration with tricyclic antidepressant can potentiate the action of albuterol on the cardiovascular system).

No products indexed under this heading.

Dicyclomine Hydrochloride (Co-administration has some potential for additive anticholinergic effects; caution is advised). Products include:

Bentyl Capsules ... 703
Bentyl Injection ... 703
Bentyl Syrup ... 703
Bentyl Tablets ... 703

Dobutamine Hydrochloride (Co-administration with other sympathomimetic agents increases the risk of adverse cardiovascular effects).

No products indexed under this heading.

Dopamine Hydrochloride (Co-administration with other sympathomimetic agents increases the risk of adverse cardiovascular effects).

No products indexed under this heading.

Doxepin Hydrochloride (Co-administration with tricyclic antidepressant can potentiate the action of albuterol on the cardiovascular system).

No products indexed under this heading.

Ephedrine Hydrochloride (Co-administration with other sympathomimetic agents increases the risk of adverse cardiovascular effects).

No products indexed under this heading.

Ephedrine Sulfate (Co-administration with other sympathomimetic agents increases the risk of adverse cardiovascular effects).

No products indexed under this heading.

Ephedrine Tannate (Co-administration with other sympathomimetic agents increases the risk of adverse cardiovascular effects).

No products indexed under this heading.

Epinephrine (Co-administration with other sympathomimetic agents increases the risk of adverse cardiovascular effects). Products include:

EpiPen ... 1024

Epinephrine Bitartrate (Co-administration with other sympathomimetic agents increases the risk of adverse cardiovascular effects).

No products indexed under this heading.

Epinephrine Hydrochloride (Co-administration with other sympathomimetic agents increases the risk of adverse cardiovascular effects).

No products indexed under this heading.

Esmolol Hydrochloride (Co-administration with beta blockers inhibits the effects of each other).

No products indexed under this heading.

Ethacrynic Acid (Co-administration with non-potassium-sparing diuretics can result in acute worsening of ECG changes and/or hypokalemia, especially when recommended dose of the beta agonist is exceeded; clinical significance of this interaction is unknown). Products include:

Edecrin Tablets ... 698

Furosemide (Co-administration with non-potassium-sparing diuretics can result in acute worsening of ECG changes and/or hypokalemia, especially when recommended dose of the beta agonist is exceeded; clinical significance of this interaction is unknown). Products include:

Furosemide Tablets ... 2186

Glycopyrrolate (Co-administration has some potential for additive anticholinergic effects; caution is advised).

No products indexed under this heading.

Hydrochlorothiazide (Co-administration with non-potassium-sparing diuretics can result in acute worsening of ECG changes and/or hypokalemia, especially when recommended dose of the beta agonist is exceeded; clinical significance of this interaction is unknown). Products include:

Atacand HCT ... 642
Avalide Tablets ... 892
Avalide Tablets ... 2713
Benicar HCT Tablets ... 1010
Diovan HCT Tablets ... 2216
Dyazide Capsules ... 1405
Micardis HCT Tablets ... 854
Prinzide Tablets ... 2092
Tekturna HCT Tablets ... 2324
Teveten HCT Tablets ... 517

Hydroflumethiazide (Co-administration with non-potassium-sparing diuretics can result in acute worsening of ECG changes and/or hypokalemia, especially when recommended dose of the beta agonist is exceeded; clinical significance of this interaction is unknown).

No products indexed under this heading.

Hyoscyamine (Co-administration has some potential for additive anticholinergic effects; caution is advised).

No products indexed under this heading.

Hyoscyamine Sulfate (Co-administration has some potential for additive anticholinergic effects; caution is advised). Products include:

Donnatal Extentabs ... 2507

Imipramine Hydrochloride (Co-administration with tricyclic antidepressant can potentiate the action of albuterol on the cardiovascular system).

No products indexed under this heading.

Imipramine Pamoate (Co-administration with tricyclic antidepressant can potentiate the action of albuterol on the cardiovascular system).

No products indexed under this heading.

Isocarboxazid (Co-administration with MAO inhibitors can potentiate the action of albuterol on the cardiovascular system). Products include:

Marplan Tablets ... 3177

Isoproterenol Hydrochloride (Co-administration with other sympathomimetic agents increases the risk of adverse cardiovascular effects).

No products indexed under this heading.

Isoproterenol Sulfate (Co-administration with other sympathomimetic agents increases the risk of adverse cardiovascular effects).

No products indexed under this heading.

Labetalol Hydrochloride (Co-administration with beta blockers inhibits the effects of each other).

No products indexed under this heading.

Levalbuterol Hydrochloride (Co-administration with other sympathomimetic agents increases the risk of adverse cardiovascular effects). Products include:

Xopenex Inhalation Solution ... 3001
Xopenex Inhalation Solution Concentrate ... 3005

Levobunolol Hydrochloride (Co-administration with beta blockers inhibits the effects of each other).

No products indexed under this heading.

Maprotiline Hydrochloride (Co-administration with tricyclic antidepressant can potentiate the action of albuterol on the cardiovascular system).

No products indexed under this heading.

Mepenzolate Bromide (Co-administration has some potential for additive anticholinergic effects; caution is advised).

No products indexed under this heading.

Metaproterenol Sulfate (Co-administration with other sympathomimetic agents increases the risk of adverse cardiovascular effects).

No products indexed under this heading.

Metaraminol Bitartrate (Co-administration with other sympathomimetic agents increases the risk of adverse cardiovascular effects).

No products indexed under this heading.

Methoxamine Hydrochloride (Co-administration with other sympathomimetic agents increases the risk of adverse cardiovascular effects).

No products indexed under this heading.

Methyclothiazide (Co-administration with non-potassium-sparing diuretics can result in acute worsening of ECG changes and/or hypokalemia, especially when recommended dose of the beta agonist is exceeded; clinical significance of this interaction is unknown).

No products indexed under this heading.

Metipranolol Hydrochloride (Co-administration with beta blockers inhibits the effects of each other).

No products indexed under this heading.

Metoprolol Succinate (Co-administration with beta blockers inhibits the effects of each other). Products include:

Toprol-XL Tablets ... 666

Metoprolol Tartrate (Co-administration with beta blockers inhibits the effects of each other).

No products indexed under this heading.

Moclobemide (Co-administration with MAO inhibitors can potentiate the action of albuterol on the cardiovascular system).

No products indexed under this heading.

Nadolol (Co-administration with beta blockers inhibits the effects of each other). Products include:

Nadolol Tablets ... 2191

Nebivolol (Co-administration with beta blockers inhibits the effects of each other). Products include:

Bystolic Tablets ... 1155

Norepinephrine Bitartrate (Co-administration with other sympathomimetic agents increases the risk of adverse cardiovascular effects).

No products indexed under this heading.

Nortriptyline Hydrochloride (Co-administration with tricyclic antidepressant can potentiate the action of albuterol on the cardiovascular system).

No products indexed under this heading.

Oxybutynin Chloride (Co-administration has some potential for additive anticholinergic effects; caution is advised).

No products indexed under this heading.

Pargyline Hydrochloride (Co-administration with MAO inhibitors can potentiate the action of albuterol on the cardiovascular system).

No products indexed under this heading.

Penbutolol Sulfate (Co-administration with beta blockers inhibits the effects of each other).

No products indexed under this heading.

Phenelzine Sulfate (Co-administration with MAO inhibitors can potentiate the action of albuterol on the cardiovascular system).

No products indexed under this heading.

Phenylephrine Bitartrate (Co-administration with other sympathomimetic agents increases the risk of adverse cardiovascular effects).

No products indexed under this heading.

Phenylephrine Hydrochloride (Co-administration with other sympathomimetic agents increases the risk of adverse cardiovascular effects). Products include:

Actifed Cold & Allergy Tablets ... 1895
Benadryl Allergy & Cold Kapgels ... 1895
Benadryl Allergy & Sinus Headache Kapgels ... 1895
Benadryl Severe Allergy & Sinus Headache Caplets ... 1897
Children's Benadryl-D Allergy & Sinus Liquid ... 1896
Benadryl-D Allergy & Sinus Tablet ... 1896
PediaCare Children's Allergy & Cold Liquid ... 1902
PediaCare Children's Decongestant Liquid ... 1902
PediaCare Children's Liquid Multi-Symptom Cold ... 1902
Sinutab Non-Drying Caplets ... 1905
Sinutab Sinus Caplets ... 1905
Children's Sudafed PE Cold & Cough Liquid ... 1907
Children's Sudafed PE Nasal Decongestant Liquid ... 1906

Sudafed PE Cold & Cough Caplets 1907
Sudafed PE Nasal Decongestant Tablets 1907
Sudafed PE Nighttime Cold Caplets 1907
Sudafed PE Non-Drying Sinus Caplets 1908
Sudafed PE Severe Cold Caplets 1908
Sudafed PE Sinus & Allergy Tablets 1908
Sudafed PE Sinus Headache Caplets 1908
Tylenol Allergy Multi-Symptom Caplets with Cool Burst and Rapid Release Gelcaps 1916
Tylenol Allergy Multi-Symptom Nighttime Caplets with Cool Burst 1916
Children's Tylenol Plus Cold Suspension Liquid 1912
Children's Tylenol Plus Cold & Allergy Suspension Liquid 1914
Children's Tylenol Plus Flu Suspension Liquid 1914
Children's Tylenol Plus Multi-Symptom Cold Suspension Liquid 1912
Tylenol Cold Head Congestion Daytime Caplets with Cool Burst 1910
Tylenol Cold Head Congestion Nighttime Caplets with Cool Burst 1910
Tylenol Cold Head Congestion Severe Daytime Caplets with Cool Burst 1910
Tylenol Cold Multi-Symptom Daytime Caplets with Cool Burst and Rapid Release Gels 1913
Tylenol Cold Multi-Symptom Daytime Liquid with Citrus Burst 1913
Tylenol Cold Multi-Symptom Nighttime Caplets with Cool Burst 1913
Tylenol Cold Multi-Symptom Nighttime Liquid with Cool Burst 1913
Tylenol Cold Multi-Symptom Severe Caplets with Cool Burst 1913
Tylenol Cold Multi-Symptom Severe Daytime Liquid with Citrus Burst 1913
Tylenol Sinus Congestion & Pain Daytime Caplets with Cool Burst and Gelcaps 1917
Tylenol Sinus Congestion & Pain Nighttime Caplets with Cool Burst 1917
Tylenol Sinus Congestion & Pain Severe Caplets with Cool Burst 1917
Vicks DayQuil Cold & Flu Multi-Symptom Relief 616
Vicks DayQuil LiquiCaps 2567
Vicks DayQuil Liquid 2567
Vicks DayQuil Multi-Symptom Cold/Flu Relief 2567

Phenylephrine Tannate (Co-administration with other sympathomimetic agents increases the risk of adverse cardiovascular effects).
No products indexed under this heading.

Phenylpropanolamine Hydrochloride (Co-administration with other sympathomimetic agents increases the risk of adverse cardiovascular effects).
No products indexed under this heading.

Pindolol (Co-administration with beta blockers inhibits the effects of each other).
No products indexed under this heading.

Pirbuterol Acetate (Co-administration with other sympathomimetic agents increases the risk of adverse cardiovascular effects). Products include:
Maxair Autohaler 1705

Polythiazide (Co-administration with non-potassium-sparing diuretics can result in acute worsening of ECG changes and/or hypokalemia, especially when recommended dose of the beta agonist is exceeded; clinical significance of this interaction is unknown).
No products indexed under this heading.

Procarbazine Hydrochloride (Co-administration with MAO inhibitors can potentiate the action of albuterol on the cardiovascular system).
No products indexed under this heading.

Procyclidine Hydrochloride (Co-administration has some potential for additive anticholinergic effects; caution is advised).
No products indexed under this heading.

Propantheline Bromide (Co-administration has some potential for additive anticholinergic effects; caution is advised).
No products indexed under this heading.

Propranolol Hydrochloride (Co-administration with beta blockers inhibits the effects of each other). Products include:
InnoPran XL Extended Release Capsules 1484

Protriptyline Hydrochloride (Co-administration with tricyclic antidepressant can potentiate the action of albuterol on the cardiovascular system).
No products indexed under this heading.

Pseudoephedrine Hydrochloride (Co-administration with other sympathomimetic agents increases the risk of adverse cardiovascular effects). Products include:
Allegra-D 12 Hour Extended-Release Tablets 2687
Allegra-D 24 Hour Extended-Release Tablets 2690
Children's Motrin Cold Oral Suspension 1899
Sudafed 12 Hour Nasal Decongestant Non-Drowsy Caplets 1909
Sudafed 24 Hour Non-Drowsy Nasal Decongestant Tablets 1906
Children's Sudafed Nasal Decongestant Liquid 1906
Sudafed Nasal Decongestant Tablets 1906
Tylenol Cold Severe Congestion Daytime Caplets with Cool Burst 1912
Tylenol Sinus Severe Congestion Caplets with Cool Burst 1917
Vicks NyQuil LiquiCaps 2567
Vicks NyQuil Liquid 2567
Vicks NyQuil Multi-Symptom Cold/Flu Relief 2567
Zyrtec-D 12 Hour Extended Release Tablets 1923
Zyrtec-D Allergy & Congestion Extended-Release Tablets 1923

Pseudoephedrine Sulfate (Co-administration with other sympathomimetic agents increases the risk of adverse cardiovascular effects). Products include:
Clarinex-D 12-Hour Extended-Release Tablets 2831
Clarinex-D 24-Hour Extended-Release Tablets 2834

Rasagiline Mesylate (Co-administration with MAO inhibitors can potentiate the action of albuterol on the cardiovascular system). Products include:
Azilect Tablets 3106

Salmeterol Xinafoate (Co-administration with other sympathomimetic agents increases the risk of adverse cardiovascular effects). Products include:
Advair Diskus 100/50 1276
Advair Diskus 250/50 1276
Advair Diskus 500/50 1276
Advair HFA 45/21 Inhalation Aerosol 1288
Advair HFA 115/21 Inhalation Aerosol 1288
Advair HFA 230/21 Inhalation Aerosol 1288
Serevent Diskus 1594

Scopolamine (Co-administration has some potential for additive anticholinergic effects; caution is advised). Products include:
Transderm Scōp Transdermal Therapeutic System 2206

Scopolamine Hydrobromide (Co-administration has some potential for additive anticholinergic effects; caution is advised). Products include:
Donnatal Extentabs 2507

Selegiline (Co-administration with MAO inhibitors can potentiate the action of albuterol on the cardiovascular system). Products include:
Emsam Transdermal System 905

Selegiline Hydrochloride (Co-administration with MAO inhibitors can potentiate the action of albuterol on the cardiovascular system). Products include:
Eldepryl Capsules 3052

Sotalol Hydrochloride (Co-administration with beta blockers inhibits the effects of each other).
No products indexed under this heading.

Terbutaline Sulfate (Co-administration with other sympathomimetic agents increases the risk of adverse cardiovascular effects).
No products indexed under this heading.

Timolol Hemihydrate (Co-administration with beta blockers inhibits the effects of each other). Products include:
Betimol Ophthalmic Solution 3181

Timolol Maleate (Co-administration with beta blockers inhibits the effects of each other). Products include:
Combigan Ophthalmic Solution 553
Cosopt Sterile Ophthalmic Solution 1969
Timoptic Sterile Ophthalmic Solution 2121
Timoptic in Ocudose 2124
Timoptic-XE Sterile Ophthalmic Gel Forming Solution 2125

Tolterodine Tartrate (Co-administration has some potential for additive anticholinergic effects; caution is advised).
No products indexed under this heading.

Torsemide (Co-administration with non-potassium-sparing diuretics can result in acute worsening of ECG changes and/or hypokalemia, especially when recommended dose of the beta agonist is exceeded; clinical significance of this interaction is unknown). Products include:
Demadex Injection 2630
Demadex Tablets 2630

Tranylcypromine Sulfate (Co-administration with MAO inhibitors can potentiate the action of albuterol on the cardiovascular system). Products include:
Parnate Tablets 1532

Tridihexethyl Chloride (Co-administration has some potential for additive anticholinergic effects; caution is advised).
No products indexed under this heading.

Trihexyphenidyl Hydrochloride (Co-administration has some potential for additive anticholinergic effects; caution is advised).
No products indexed under this heading.

Trimipramine Maleate (Co-administration with tricyclic antidepressant can potentiate the action of albuterol on the cardiovascular system).
No products indexed under this heading.

COMBIVIR TABLETS

(Lamivudine, Zidovudine) 1384
May interact with cytotoxic drugs, Interferon alpha, and certain other agents. Compounds in these categories include:

Bleomycin Sulfate (May increase the hematologic toxicity of zidovudine).
No products indexed under this heading.

Bone Marrow Depressants, unspecified (May increase the hematologic toxicity of zidovudine).
No products indexed under this heading.

Cyclophosphamide (May increase the hematologic toxicity of zidovudine).
No products indexed under this heading.

Daunorubicin Hydrochloride (May increase the hematologic toxicity of zidovudine).
No products indexed under this heading.

Doxorubicin Hydrochloride (Co-administration should be avoided since an antagonistic relationship with zidovudine has been demonstrated in vitro; may increase the hematologic toxicity of zidovudine).
No products indexed under this heading.

Epirubicin Hydrochloride (May increase the hematologic toxicity of zidovudine).
No products indexed under this heading.

Fluorouracil (May increase the hematologic toxicity of zidovudine). Products include:
Carac Cream 0.5% 2722

Ganciclovir Sodium (May increase the hematologic toxicity of zidovudine).
No products indexed under this heading.

Hydroxyurea (May increase the hematologic toxicity of zidovudine).
No products indexed under this heading.

Interferon alfa-2a, Recombinant (Hepatic decompensation has occurred in HIV/HCV co-infected patients receiving combination antiretroviral therapy for HIV and interferon alpha with or without ribavirin. Patients receiving interferon alpha with or without ribavirin and Combivir should be closely monitored for treatment-associated toxicities, especially hepatic decompensation, neutropenia, and anemia. Discontinuation of Combivir should be considered as medically appropriate. Dis-

continuation of interferon alpha, ribavirin, or both shouldalso be considered if worsening clinical toxicities are observed, including hepatic decompensation (e.g., Childs Pugh greater than 6)).
No products indexed under this heading.

Interferon alfa-2b, Recombinant (Hepatic decompensation has occurred in HIV/HCV co-infected patients receiving combination antiretroviral therapy for HIV and interferon alpha with or without ribavirin. Patients receiving interferon alpha with or without ribavirin and Combivir should be closely monitored for treatment-associated toxicities, especially hepatic decompensation, neutropenia, and anemia. Discontinuation of Combivir should be considered as medically appropriate. Discontinuation of interferon alpha, ribavirin, or both shouldalso be considered if worsening clinical toxicities are observed, including hepatic decompensation (e.g., Childs Pugh greater than 6)). Products include:
Intron A for Injection 2859

Interferon alfa-N3 (Human Leukocyte Derived) (Hepatic decompensation has occurred in HIV/HCV co-infected patients receiving combination antiretroviral therapy for HIV and interferon alpha with or without ribavirin. Patients receiving interferon alpha with or without ribavirin and Combivir should be closely monitored for treatment-associated toxicities, especially hepatic decompensation, neutropenia, and anemia. Discontinuation of Combivir should be considered as medically appropriate. Discontinuation of interferon alpha, ribavirin, or both shouldalso be considered if worsening clinical toxicities are observed, including hepatic decompensation (e.g., Childs Pugh greater than 6)). Products include:
Alferon N Injection 1726

Methotrexate Sodium (May increase the hematologic toxicity of zidovudine).
No products indexed under this heading.

Mitotane (May increase the hematologic toxicity of zidovudine).
No products indexed under this heading.

Mitoxantrone Hydrochloride (May increase the hematologic toxicity of zidovudine). Products include:
Novantrone for Injection Concentrate 1100

Peginterferon Alfa-2b (Hepatic decompensation has occurred in HIV/HCV co-infected patients receiving combination antiretroviral therapy for HIV and interferon alpha with or without ribavirin. Patients receiving interferon alpha with or without ribavirin and Combivir should be closely monitored for treatment-associated toxicities, especially hepatic decompensation, neutropenia, and anemia. Discontinuation of Combivir should be considered as medically appropriate. Discontinuation of interferon alpha, ribavirin, or both shouldalso be considered if worsening clinical toxicities are observed, including hepatic decompensation (e.g., Childs Pugh greater than 6)). Products include:
PegIntron Powder for Injection 2903

Procarbazine Hydrochloride (May increase the hematologic toxicity of zidovudine).
No products indexed under this heading.

Ribavirin (Co-administration should be avoided since an antagonistic relationship with zidovudine has been demonstrated in vitro). Products include:
Rebetol 2917

Stavudine (Co-administration should be avoided since an antagonistic relationship with zidovudine has been demonstrated in vitro).
No products indexed under this heading.

Sulfamethoxazole (Co-administration with TMP/SMX has been shown to increase lamivudine exposure).
No products indexed under this heading.

Tamoxifen Citrate (May increase the hematologic toxicity of zidovudine).
No products indexed under this heading.

Trimethoprim (Co-administration with TMP/SMX has been shown to increase lamivudine exposure).
No products indexed under this heading.

Vincristine Sulfate (May increase the hematologic toxicity of zidovudine).
No products indexed under this heading.

Zalacitabine (Lamivudine and zalacitabine may inhibit the intracellular phosphorylation of one another; combination therapy is not recommended).
No products indexed under this heading.

COMTAN TABLETS

(Entacapone) 2208
May interact with central nervous system depressants, drugs metabolized by Catechol-O-methytransferase, erythromycin, nonselective MAO inhibitors, and certain other agents. Compounds in these categories include:

Alfentanil Hydrochloride (Possible additive sedative effects).
No products indexed under this heading.

Alprazolam (Possible additive sedative effects).
No products indexed under this heading.

Ampicillin Sodium (As most entacapone excretion is via bile, co-administration with drugs known to interfere with biliary excretion, glucuronidation, and intestinal beta-glucuronidation, such as ampicillin, requires caution).
No products indexed under this heading.

Apomorphine (Co-administration of drugs that are metabolized by catechol-O-methyltransferase (COMT) may result in increased heart rates, possibly arrhythmias, and excessive changes in blood pressure).
No products indexed under this heading.

Aprobarbital (Possible additive sedative effects).
No products indexed under this heading.

Bitolterol Mesylate (Co-administration of drugs that are metabolized by catechol-O-methyltransferase (COMT) may result in increased heart rates, possibly arrhythmias, and excessive changes in blood pressure).
No products indexed under this heading.

Buprenorphine Hydrochloride (Possible additive sedative effects). Products include:
Suboxone Tablets 2601
Subutex Tablets 2601

Buspirone Hydrochloride (Possible additive sedative effects).
No products indexed under this heading.

Butabarbital (Possible additive sedative effects).
No products indexed under this heading.

Butalbital (Possible additive sedative effects).
No products indexed under this heading.

Chloramphenicol Sodium Succinate (As most entacapone excretion is via bile, co-administration with drugs known to interfere with biliary excretion, glucuronidation, and intestinal beta-glucuronidation, such as chloramphenicol, requires caution).
No products indexed under this heading.

Chlordiazepoxide (Possible additive sedative effects).
No products indexed under this heading.

Chlordiazepoxide Hydrochloride (Possible additive sedative effects).
No products indexed under this heading.

Chlorpromazine (Possible additive sedative effects).
No products indexed under this heading.

Chlorpromazine Hydrochloride (Possible additive sedative effects).
No products indexed under this heading.

Chlorprothixene (Possible additive sedative effects).
No products indexed under this heading.

Chlorprothixene Hydrochloride (Possible additive sedative effects).
No products indexed under this heading.

Chlorprothixene Lactate (Possible additive sedative effects).
No products indexed under this heading.

Cholestyramine (As most entacapone excretion is via bile, co-administration with drugs known to interfere with biliary excretion, glucuronidation, and intestinal beta-glucuronidation, such as cholestyramine, requires caution).
No products indexed under this heading.

Clorazepate Dipotassium (Possible additive sedative effects).
No products indexed under this heading.

Clozapine (Possible additive sedative effects).
No products indexed under this heading.

Codeine Phosphate (Possible additive sedative effects). Products include:
Tylenol with Codeine Tablets 2427

Desflurane (Possible additive sedative effects).
No products indexed under this heading.

Dezocine (Possible additive sedative effects).
No products indexed under this heading.

Diazepam (Possible additive sedative effects). Products include:
Valium Tablets 2658

Dobutamine Hydrochloride (Co-administration of drugs that are metabolized by catechol-O-methyltransferase (COMT) may result in increased heart rates, possibly arrhythmias, and excessive changes in blood pressure).
No products indexed under this heading.

Dopamine Hydrochloride (Co-administration of drugs that are metabolized by catechol-O-methyltransferase (COMT) may result in increased heart rates, possibly arrhythmias, and excessive changes in blood pressure).
No products indexed under this heading.

Droperidol (Possible additive sedative effects).
No products indexed under this heading.

Enflurane (Possible additive sedative effects).
No products indexed under this heading.

Epinephrine (Co-administration of drugs that are metabolized by catechol-O-methyltransferase (COMT) may result in increased heart rates, possibly arrhythmias, and excessive changes in blood pressure; concurrent use of epinephrine infusion has resulted in a case report of ventricular tachycardia). Products include:
EpiPen 1024

Epinephrine Bitartrate (Co-administration of drugs that are metabolized by catechol-O-methyltransferase (COMT) may result in increased heart rates, possibly arrhythmias, and excessive changes in blood pressure; concurrent use of epinephrine infusion has resulted in a case report of ventricular tachycardia).
No products indexed under this heading.

Epinephrine Hydrochloride (Co-administration of drugs that are metabolized by catechol-O-methyltransferase (COMT) may result in increased heart rates, possibly arrhythmias, and excessive changes in blood pressure; concurrent use of epinephrine infusion has resulted in a case report of ventricular tachycardia).
No products indexed under this heading.

Erythromycin (As most entacapone excretion is via bile, co-administration with drugs known to interfere with biliary excretion, glucuronidation, and intestinal beta-glucuronidation, such as erythromycin, requires caution).
No products indexed under this heading.

Erythromycin Estolate (As most entacapone excretion is via bile, co-administration with drugs known to interfere with biliary excretion, glucuronidation, and intestinal beta-glucuronidation, such as erythromycin, requires caution).
No products indexed under this heading.

Erythromycin Ethylsuccinate (As most entacapone excretion is via bile, co-administration with drugs known to interfere with biliary excretion, glucuronidation, and intestinal beta-glucuronidation, such as erythromycin, requires caution). Products include:
E.E.S. 433
EryPed 431

Erythromycin Gluceptate (As most entacapone excretion is via bile, co-administration with drugs known to interfere with biliary excretion, glucuronidation, and intestinal beta-glucuronidation, such as erythromycin, requires caution).
No products indexed under this heading.

Erythromycin Lactobionate (As most entacapone excretion is via bile, co-administration with drugs known to interfere with biliary excretion, glucuronidation, and intestinal beta-glucuronidation, such as erythromycin, requires caution).
No products indexed under this heading.

Erythromycin Stearate (As most entacapone excretion is via bile, co-administration with drugs known to interfere with biliary excretion, glucuronidation, and intestinal beta-glucuronidation, such as erythromycin, requires caution).
No products indexed under this heading.

Estazolam (Possible additive sedative effects).
No products indexed under this heading.

Ethanol (Possible additive sedative effects).
No products indexed under this heading.

Ethchlorvynol (Possible additive sedative effects).
No products indexed under this heading.

Ethinamate (Possible additive sedative effects).
No products indexed under this heading.

Ethyl Alcohol (Possible additive sedative effects).
No products indexed under this heading.

Fentanyl (Possible additive sedative effects). Products include:
Duragesic Transdermal System 2405
Ionsys Transdermal System 2410

Fentanyl Citrate (Possible additive sedative effects). Products include:
Actiq 959
Fentora Tablets 968

Fluphenazine Decanoate (Possible additive sedative effects).
No products indexed under this heading.

Fluphenazine Enanthate (Possible additive sedative effects).
No products indexed under this heading.

Fluphenazine Hydrochloride (Possible additive sedative effects).
No products indexed under this heading.

Flurazepam Hydrochloride (Possible additive sedative effects).
No products indexed under this heading.

Glutethimide (Possible additive sedative effects).
No products indexed under this heading.

Haloperidol (Possible additive sedative effects).
No products indexed under this heading.

Haloperidol Decanoate (Possible additive sedative effects).
No products indexed under this heading.

Hydrocodone Bitartrate (Possible additive sedative effects). Products include:
Lortab 5/500 Tablets 3143
Lortab 7.5/500 Tablets 3144
Lortab 10/500 Tablets 3144
Vicodin Tablets 529
Vicodin ES Tablets 530
Vicodin HP Tablets 531
Vicoprofen Tablets 533
Zydone Tablets 1132

Hydrocodone Polistirex (Possible additive sedative effects). Products include:
Tussionex Pennkinetic Extended-Release Suspension 3154

Hydromorphone Hydrochloride (Possible additive sedative effects).
No products indexed under this heading.

Hydroxyzine Hydrochloride (Possible additive sedative effects).
No products indexed under this heading.

Isocarboxazid (Co-administration of non-selective MAO inhibitors with entacapone would result in inhibition of the majority of the pathways responsible for normal catecholamine metabolism; concurrent use should be avoided). Products include:
Marplan Tablets 3177

Isoetharine (Co-administration of drugs that are metabolized by catechol-O-methyltransferase (COMT) may result in increased heart rates, possibly arrhythmias, and excessive changes in blood pressure).
No products indexed under this heading.

Isoflurane (Possible additive sedative effects).
No products indexed under this heading.

Isoproterenol Hydrochloride (Co-administration of drugs that are metabolized by catechol-O-methyltransferase (COMT) may result in increased heart rates, possibly arrhythmias, and excessive changes in blood pressure).
No products indexed under this heading.

Isoproterenol Sulfate (Co-administration of drugs that are metabolized by catechol-O-methyltransferase (COMT) may result in increased heart rates, possibly arrhythmias, and excessive changes in blood pressure).
No products indexed under this heading.

Ketamine Hydrochloride (Possible additive sedative effects).
No products indexed under this heading.

Levodopa (Entacapone enhances levodopa bioavailability and, therefore, might be expected to increase the occurence of orthostatic hypotension). Products include:
Stalevo Tablets 2309

Levomethadyl Acetate Hydrochloride (Possible additive sedative effects).
No products indexed under this heading.

Levorphanol Tartrate (Possible additive sedative effects).
No products indexed under this heading.

Lorazepam (Possible additive sedative effects).
No products indexed under this heading.

Loxapine Hydrochloride (Possible additive sedative effects).
No products indexed under this heading.

Loxapine Succinate (Possible additive sedative effects).
No products indexed under this heading.

Meperidine Hydrochloride (Possible additive sedative effects).
No products indexed under this heading.

Mephobarbital (Possible additive sedative effects).
No products indexed under this heading.

Meprobamate (Possible additive sedative effects).
No products indexed under this heading.

Mesoridazine Besylate (Possible additive sedative effects).
No products indexed under this heading.

Methadone Hydrochloride (Possible additive sedative effects).
No products indexed under this heading.

Methohexital Sodium (Possible additive sedative effects).
No products indexed under this heading.

Methotrimeprazine (Possible additive sedative effects).
No products indexed under this heading.

Methoxyflurane (Possible additive sedative effects).
No products indexed under this heading.

Methyldopa (Co-administration of drugs that are metabolized by catechol-O-methyltransferase (COMT) may result in increased heart rates, possibly arrhythmias, and excessive changes in blood pressure).
No products indexed under this heading.

Midazolam Hydrochloride (Possible additive sedative effects).
No products indexed under this heading.

Molindone Hydrochloride (Possible additive sedative effects). Products include:
Moban Tablets 1116

Morphine Sulfate (Possible additive sedative effects). Products include:
Avinza Capsules 1772
DepoDur Injection 1095
MS Contin Tablets 2585

Norepinephrine Bitartrate (Co-administration of drugs that are metabolized by catechol-O-methyltransferase (COMT) may result in increased heart rates, possibly arrhythmias, and excessive changes in blood pressure).
No products indexed under this heading.

Olanzapine (Possible additive sedative effects). Products include:
Symbyax Capsules 1871
Zyprexa Tablets 1883
Zyprexa IntraMuscular 1883
Zyprexa ZYDIS Orally Disintegrating Tablets 1883

Oxazepam (Possible additive sedative effects).
No products indexed under this heading.

Oxycodone Hydrochloride (Possible additive sedative effects). Products include:
OxyContin Tablets 2589
OxyIR Capsules 2593
Percocet Tablets 1127
Percodan Tablets 1130

Pargyline Hydrochloride (Co-administration of non-selective MAO inhibitors with entacapone would result in inhibition of the majority of the pathways responsible for normal catecholamine metabolism; concurrent use should be avoided).
No products indexed under this heading.

Pentobarbital Sodium (Possible additive sedative effects). Products include:
Nembutal Sodium Solution, USP 2494

Perphenazine (Possible additive sedative effects).
No products indexed under this heading.

Phenelzine Sulfate (Co-administration of non-selective MAO inhibitors with entacapone would result in inhibition of the majority of the pathways responsible for normal catecholamine metabolism; concurrent use should be avoided).
No products indexed under this heading.

Phenobarbital (Possible additive sedative effects). Products include:
Donnatal Extentabs 2507

Prazepam (Possible additive sedative effects).
No products indexed under this heading.

Probenecid (As most entacapone excretion is via bile, co-administration with drugs known to interfere with biliary excretion, glucuronidation, and intestinal beta-glucuronidation, such as probenecid, requires caution).
No products indexed under this heading.

Procarbazine Hydrochloride (Co-administration of non-selective MAO inhibitors with entacapone would result in inhibition of the majority of the pathways responsible for normal catecholamine metabolism; concurrent use should be avoided).
No products indexed under this heading.

Prochlorperazine (Possible additive sedative effects).
No products indexed under this heading.

Promethazine Hydrochloride (Possible additive sedative effects).
No products indexed under this heading.

Propofol (Possible additive sedative effects).
No products indexed under this heading.

Propoxyphene Hydrochloride (Possible additive sedative effects).
No products indexed under this heading.

Propoxyphene Napsylate (Possible additive sedative effects).
No products indexed under this heading.

Quazepam (Possible additive sedative effects).
No products indexed under this heading.

Quetiapine Fumarate (Possible additive sedative effects).
No products indexed under this heading.

Remifentanil Hydrochloride (Possible additive sedative effects).
No products indexed under this heading.

Rifampin (As most entacapone excretion is via bile, co-administration with drugs known to interfere with biliary excretion, glucuronidation, and intestinal beta-glucuronidation, such as rifampin, requires caution).
No products indexed under this heading.

Risperidone (Possible additive sedative effects). Products include:
Risperdal Consta Long-Acting Injection 1753

Secobarbital Sodium (Possible additive sedative effects).
No products indexed under this heading.

Sevoflurane (Possible additive sedative effects). Products include:
Ultane Liquid for Inhalation 524

Sufentanil Citrate (Possible additive sedative effects).
No products indexed under this heading.

Temazepam (Possible additive sedative effects).
No products indexed under this heading.

Thiamylal Sodium (Possible additive sedative effects).
No products indexed under this heading.

Thioridazine Hydrochloride (Possible additive sedative effects). Products include:
Thioridazine Hydrochloride Tablets 2195

Thiothixene (Possible additive sedative effects). Products include:
Thiothixene Capsules 2197

Tranylcypromine Sulfate (Co-administration of non-selective MAO inhibitors with entacapone would result in inhibition of the majority of the pathways responsible for normal catecholamine metabolism; concurrent use should be avoided). Products include:
Parnate Tablets 1532

Triazolam (Possible additive sedative effects).
No products indexed under this heading.

Trifluoperazine Hydrochloride (Possible additive sedative effects).
No products indexed under this heading.

Zaleplon (Possible additive sedative effects).
No products indexed under this heading.

Ziprasidone Hydrochloride (Possible additive sedative effects). Products include:
Geodon Capsules 2520

Zolpidem Tartrate (Possible additive sedative effects). Products include:
Ambien Tablets 2692
Ambien CR Tablets 2696

Food Interactions

Alcohol (Possible additive sedative effects).

COMVAX

(Haemophilus B Conjugate Vaccine, Hepatitis B Vaccine, Recombinant) 1966
May interact with immunosuppressive agents. Compounds in these categories include:

Azathioprine (Deferral of immunization may be considered in individuals receiving immunosuppressive therapy).
No products indexed under this heading.

Basiliximab (Deferral of immunization may be considered in individuals receiving immunosuppressive therapy). Products include:
Simulect for Injection 2306

Cyclosporine (Deferral of immunization may be considered in individuals receiving immunosuppressive therapy). Products include:
Gengraf Capsules 435
Neoral Oral Solution 2280
Neoral Soft Gelatin Capsules 2280
Restasis Ophthalmic Emulsion 557
Sandimmune 2296

Muromonab-CD3 (Deferral of immunization may be considered in individuals receiving immunosuppressive therapy). Products include:
Orthoclone OKT3 Sterile Solution 2387

Mycophenolate Mofetil (Deferral of immunization may be considered in individuals receiving immunosuppressive therapy). Products include:
CellCept Capsules 2622
CellCept Oral Suspension 2622
CellCept Tablets 2622

Sirolimus (Deferral of immunization may be considered in individuals receiving immunosuppressive therapy). Products include:
Rapamune 3260

Tacrolimus (Deferral of immunization may be considered in individuals receiving immunosuppressive therapy). Products include:
Prograf Capsules and Injection 622
Protopic Ointment 628

CONCERTA EXTENDED-RELEASE TABLETS

(Methylphenidate Hydrochloride) 1925
May interact with oral anticoagulants, monoamine oxidase inhibitors, phenytoin, selective serotonin reuptake inhibitors, and tricyclic antidepressants. Compounds in these categories include:

Amitriptyline Hydrochloride (Studies have shown that methylphenidate may inhibit the metabolism of some antidepressants (eg, tricyclics). It may be necessary to downward dose adjust the dosage and monitor plasma drug concentrations when initiating or discontinuing concomitant methylphenidate).
No products indexed under this heading.

Amoxapine (Studies have shown that methylphenidate may inhibit the metabolism of some antidepressants (eg, tricyclics). It may be necessary to downward dose adjust the dosage and monitor plasma drug concentrations when initiating or discontinuing concomitant methylphenidate).
No products indexed under this heading.

Anisindione (Methylphenidate may inhibit the metabolism of coumarin anticoagulants; downward dosage adjustment of anticoagulants may be required. Dosage adjustment and plasma drug concentrations monitoring may be necessary when initiating or discontinuing concomitant methylphenidate).
No products indexed under this heading.

Citalopram Hydrobromide (Studies have shown that methylphenidate may inhibit the metabolism of antidepressants (eg, selective serotoinin reuptate inhibitors). It may be necessary to downward dose adjust the dosage and monitor plasma drug concentrations when initiating or discontinuing concomitant methylphenidate). Products include:
Celexa 1160

Clomipramine Hydrochloride (Studies have shown that methylphenidate may inhibit the metabolism of some antidepressants (eg, tricyclics). It may be necessary to downward dose adjust the dosage and monitor plasma drug concentrations when initiating or discontinuing concomitant methylphenidate).
No products indexed under this heading.

Clonidine (Serious adverse events have been reported in concomitant use with clonidine, although no causality for the combination has been established). Products include:
Catapres-TTS 842

Clonidine Hydrochloride (Serious adverse events have been reported in concomitant use with clonidine, although no causality for the combination has been established). Products include:
Catapres Tablets 841
Clorpres Tablets 2185

Desipramine Hydrochloride (Studies have shown that methylphenidate may inhibit the metabolism of some antidepressants (eg, tricyclics). It may be necessary to downward dose adjust the dosage and monitor plasma drug concentrations when initiating or discontinuing concomitant methylphenidate).
No products indexed under this heading.

Dicumarol (Methylphenidate may inhibit the metabolism of coumarin anticoagulants; downward dosage adjustment of anticoagulants may be required. Dosage adjustment and plasma drug concentrations monitoring may be necessary when initiating or discontinuing concomitant methylphenidate).
No products indexed under this heading.

Dobutamine (Methylphenidate causes a rise in blood pressure; co-administration with other pressor agents should be undertaken with caution).
No products indexed under this heading.

Dobutamine Hydrochloride (Methylphenidate causes a rise in blood pressure; co-administration with other pressor agents should be undertaken with caution).
No products indexed under this heading.

Dopamine Hydrochloride (Methylphenidate causes a rise in blood pressure; co-administration with other pressor agents should be undertaken with caution).
No products indexed under this heading.

Doxepin Hydrochloride (Studies have shown that methylphenidate may inhibit the metabolism of some antidepressants (eg, tricyclics). It may be necessary to downward dose adjust the dosage and monitor plasma drug concentrations when initiating or discontinuing concomitant methylphenidate).
No products indexed under this heading.

Ephedrine Sulfate (Methylphenidate causes a rise in blood pressure; co-administration with other pressor agents should be undertaken with caution).
No products indexed under this heading.

Epinephrine Bitartrate (Methylphenidate causes a rise in blood pressure; co-administration with other pressor agents should be undertaken with caution).
No products indexed under this heading.

Epinephrine Hydrochloride (Methylphenidate causes a rise in blood pressure; co-administration with other pressor agents should be undertaken with caution).
No products indexed under this heading.

Escitalopram Oxalate (Studies have shown that methylphenidate may inhibit the metabolism of antidepressants (eg, selective serotoinin reuptate inhibitors). It may be necessary to downward dose adjust the dosage and monitor plasma drug concentrations when initiating or discontinuing concomitant methylphenidate). Products include:
Lexapro Oral Suspension 1174
Lexapro Tablets 1174

Fluoxetine (Studies have shown that methylphenidate may inhibit the metabolism of antidepressants (eg, selective serotoinin reuptate inhibitors). It may be necessary to downward dose adjust the dosage and monitor plasma drug concentrations when initiating or discontinuing concomitant methylphenidate).
No products indexed under this heading.

Fluoxetine Hydrochloride (Studies have shown that methylphenidate may inhibit the metabolism of antidepressants (eg, selective serotoinin reuptate inhibitors). It may be necessary to downward dose adjust the dosage and monitor plasma drug concentrations when initiating or discontinuing concomitant methylphenidate). Products include:
Prozac Weekly Capsules 1852
Prozac Pulvules and Liquid 1852
Symbyax Capsules 1871

Fluvoxamine Maleate (Studies have shown that methylphenidate may inhibit the metabolism of antidepressants (eg, selective serotoinin reuptate inhibitors). It may be necessary to downward dose adjust the dosage and monitor plasma drug concentrations when initiating or discontinuing concomitant methylphenidate). Products include:

Luvox CR Extended-Release Capsules **1759**

Fosphenytoin Sodium (Studies have shown that methylphenidate may inhibit the metabolism of anticonvulsants (eg, phenytoin). It may be necessary to downward dose adjust the dosage and monitor plasma drug concentrations when initiating or discontinuing concomitant methylphenidate).

No products indexed under this heading.

Imipramine Hydrochloride (Studies have shown that methylphenidate may inhibit the metabolism of some antidepressants (eg, tricyclics). It may be necessary to downward dose adjust the dosage and monitor plasma drug concentrations when initiating or discontinuing concomitant methylphenidate).

No products indexed under this heading.

Imipramine Pamoate (Studies have shown that methylphenidate may inhibit the metabolism of some antidepressants (eg, tricyclics). It may be necessary to downward dose adjust the dosage and monitor plasma drug concentrations when initiating or discontinuing concomitant methylphenidate).

No products indexed under this heading.

Isocarboxazid (Co-administration with MOA inhibitors may result in hypertensive crises; concurrent and/or sequential use is contraindicated. Methylphenidate HCl is contraindicated during treatment with monoamine oxidase (MAO) inhibitors, and also with a minimum of 14 days following discontinuation of an MAO inhibitor. Co-administration is not recommended). Products include:

Marplan Tablets **3177**

Isoproterenol Hydrochloride (Methylphenidate causes a rise in blood pressure; co-administration with other pressor agents should be undertaken with caution).

No products indexed under this heading.

Isoproterenol Sulfate (Methylphenidate causes a rise in blood pressure; co-administration with other pressor agents should be undertaken with caution).

No products indexed under this heading.

Maprotiline Hydrochloride (Studies have shown that methylphenidate may inhibit the metabolism of some antidepressants (eg, tricyclics). It may be necessary to downward dose adjust the dosage and monitor plasma drug concentrations when initiating or discontinuing concomitant methylphenidate).

No products indexed under this heading.

Mephentermine Sulfate (Methylphenidate causes a rise in blood pressure; co-administration with other pressor agents should be undertaken with caution).

No products indexed under this heading.

Metaraminol Bitartrate (Methylphenidate causes a rise in blood pressure; co-administration with other pressor agents should be undertaken with caution).

No products indexed under this heading.

Methoxamine Hydrochloride (Methylphenidate causes a rise in blood pressure; co-administration with other pressor agents should be undertaken with caution).

No products indexed under this heading.

Moclobemide (Co-administration with MOA inhibitors may result in hypertensive crises; concurrent and/or sequential use is contraindicated. Methylphenidate HCl is contraindicated during treatment with monoamine oxidase (MAO) inhibitors, and also with a minimum of 14 days following discontinuation of an MAO inhibitor. Co-administration is not recommended).

No products indexed under this heading.

Norepinephrine Bitartrate (Methylphenidate causes a rise in blood pressure; co-administration with other pressor agents should be undertaken with caution).

No products indexed under this heading.

Nortriptyline Hydrochloride (Studies have shown that methylphenidate may inhibit the metabolism of some antidepressants (eg, tricyclics). It may be necessary to downward dose adjust the dosage and monitor plasma drug concentrations when initiating or discontinuing concomitant methylphenidate).

No products indexed under this heading.

Pargyline Hydrochloride (Co-administration with MOA inhibitors may result in hypertensive crises; concurrent and/or sequential use is contraindicated. Methylphenidate HCl is contraindicated during treatment with monoamine oxidase (MAO) inhibitors, and also with a minimum of 14 days following discontinuation of an MAO inhibitor. Co-administration is not recommended).

No products indexed under this heading.

Paroxetine Hydrochloride (Studies have shown that methylphenidate may inhibit the metabolism of antidepressants (eg, selective serotoinin reuptate inhibitors). It may be necessary to downward dose adjust the dosage and monitor plasma drug concentrations when initiating or discontinuing concomitant methylphenidate). Products include:

Paxil **1535**

Paxil CR Controlled-Release Tablets **1544**

Phenelzine Sulfate (Co-administration with MOA inhibitors may result in hypertensive crises; concurrent and/or sequential use is contraindicated. Methylphenidate HCl is contraindicated during treatment with monoamine oxidase (MAO) inhibitors, and also with a minimum of 14 days following discontinuation of an MAO inhibitor. Co-administration is not recommended).

No products indexed under this heading.

Phenobarbital (Studies have shown that methylphenidate may inhibit the metabolism of anticonvulsants (eg, phenobarbital). It may be necessary to downward dose adjust the dosage and monitor plasma drug concentrations when initiating or discontinuing concomitant methylphenidate). Products include:

Donnatal Extentabs **2507**

Phenylephrine Hydrochloride (Methylphenidate causes a rise in blood pressure; co-administration with other pressor agents should be undertaken with caution). Products include:

Actifed Cold & Allergy Tablets **1895**
Benadryl Allergy & Cold Kapgels **1895**
Benadryl Allergy & Sinus Headache Kapgels **1895**
Benadryl Severe Allergy & Sinus Headache Caplets **1897**
Children's Benadryl-D Allergy & Sinus Liquid **1896**
Benadryl-D Allergy & Sinus Tablet **1896**
PediaCare Children's Allergy & Cold Liquid **1902**
PediaCare Children's Decongestant Liquid **1902**
PediaCare Children's Liquid Multi-Symptom Cold **1902**
Sinutab Non-Drying Caplets **1905**
Sinutab Sinus Caplets **1905**
Children's Sudafed PE Cold & Cough Liquid **1907**
Children's Sudafed PE Nasal Decongestant Liquid **1906**
Sudafed PE Cold & Cough Caplets **1907**
Sudafed PE Nasal Decongestant Tablets **1907**
Sudafed PE Nighttime Cold Caplets **1907**
Sudafed PE Non-Drying Sinus Caplets **1908**
Sudafed PE Severe Cold Caplets **1908**
Sudafed PE Sinus & Allergy Tablets **1908**
Sudafed PE Sinus Headache Caplets **1908**
Tylenol Allergy Multi-Symptom Caplets with Cool Burst and Rapid Release Gelcaps **1916**
Tylenol Allergy Multi-Symptom Nighttime Caplets with Cool Burst **1916**
Children's Tylenol Plus Cold Suspension Liquid **1912**
Children's Tylenol Plus Cold & Allergy Suspension Liquid **1914**
Children's Tylenol Plus Flu Suspension Liquid **1914**
Children's Tylenol Plus Multi-Symptom Cold Suspension Liquid **1912**
Tylenol Cold Head Congestion Daytime Caplets with Cool Burst **1910**
Tylenol Cold Head Congestion Nighttime Caplets with Cool Burst **1910**
Tylenol Cold Head Congestion Severe Daytime Caplets with Cool Burst **1910**
Tylenol Cold Multi-Symptom Daytime Caplets with Cool Burst and Rapid Release Gels **1913**
Tylenol Cold Multi-Symptom Daytime Liquid with Citrus Burst **1913**
Tylenol Cold Multi-Symptom Nighttime Caplets with Cool Burst **1913**
Tylenol Cold Multi-Symptom Nighttime Liquid with Cool Burst **1913**
Tylenol Cold Multi-Symptom Severe Caplets with Cool Burst **1913**
Tylenol Cold Multi-Symptom Severe Daytime Liquid with Citrus Burst **1913**
Tylenol Sinus Congestion & Pain Daytime Caplets with Cool Burst and Gelcaps **1917**
Tylenol Sinus Congestion & Pain Nighttime Caplets with Cool Burst **1917**
Tylenol Sinus Congestion & Pain Severe Caplets with Cool Burst **1917**
Vicks DayQuil Cold & Flu Multi-Symptom Relief **616**
Vicks DayQuil LiquiCaps **2567**
Vicks DayQuil Liquid **2567**
Vicks DayQuil Multi-Symptom Cold/Flu Relief **2567**

Phenytoin (Studies have shown that methylphenidate may inhibit the metabolism of anticonvulsants (eg, phenytoin). It may be necessary to downward dose adjust the dosage and monitor plasma drug concentrations when initiating or discontinuing concomitant methylphenidate).

No products indexed under this heading.

Phenytoin Sodium (Studies have shown that methylphenidate may inhibit the metabolism of anticonvulsants (eg, phenytoin). It may be necessary to downward dose adjust the dosage and monitor plasma drug concentrations when initiating or discontinuing concomitant methylphenidate). Products include:

Phenytek Capsules **2192**

Primidone (Studies have shown that methylphenidate may inhibit the metabolism of anticonvulsants (eg, primidone). It may be necessary to downward dose adjust the dosage and monitor plasma drug concentrations when initiating or discontinuing concomitant methylphenidate).

No products indexed under this heading.

Procarbazine Hydrochloride (Co-administration with MOA inhibitors may result in hypertensive crises; concurrent and/or sequential use is contraindicated. Methylphenidate HCl is contraindicated during treatment with monoamine oxidase (MAO) inhibitors, and also with a minimum of 14 days following discontinuation of an MAO inhibitor. Co-administration is not recommended).

No products indexed under this heading.

Protriptyline Hydrochloride (Studies have shown that methylphenidate may inhibit the metabolism of some antidepressants (eg, tricyclics). It may be necessary to downward dose adjust the dosage and monitor plasma drug concentrations when initiating or discontinuing concomitant methylphenidate).

No products indexed under this heading.

Rasagiline Mesylate (Co-administration with MOA inhibitors may result in hypertensive crises; concurrent and/or sequential use is contraindicated. Methylphenidate HCl is contraindicated during treatment with monoamine oxidase (MAO) inhibitors, and also with a minimum of 14 days following discontinuation of an MAO inhibitor. Co-administration is not recommended). Products include:

Azilect Tablets **3106**

Selegiline (Co-administration with MOA inhibitors may result in hypertensive crises; concurrent and/or sequential use is contraindicated. Methylphenidate HCl is contraindicated during treatment with monoamine oxidase (MAO) inhibitors, and also with a minimum of 14 days following discontinuation of an MAO inhibitor. Co-administration is not recommended). Products include:

Emsam Transdermal System **905**

Selegiline Hydrochloride (Co-administration with MOA inhibitors may result in hypertensive crises; concurrent and/or sequential use is contraindicated. Methylphenidate

HCl is contraindicated during treatment with monoamine oxidase (MAO) inhibitors, and also with a minimum of 14 days following discontinuation of an MAO inhibitor. Co-administration is not recommended). Products include:

Eldepryl Capsules 3052

Sertraline Hydrochloride (Studies have shown that methylphenidate may inhibit the metabolism of antidepressants (eg, selective serotoinin reuptate inhibitors). It may be necessary to downward dose adjust the dosage and monitor plasma drug concentrations when initiating or discontinuing concomitant methylphenidate).

No products indexed under this heading.

Tranylcypromine Sulfate (Co-administration with MOA inhibitors may result in hypertensive crises; concurrent and/or sequential use is contraindicated. Methylphenidate HCl is contraindicated during treatment with monoamine oxidase (MAO) inhibitors, and also with a minimum of 14 days following discontinuation of an MAO inhibitor. Co-administration is not recommended). Products include:

Parnate Tablets 1532

Trimipramine Maleate (Studies have shown that methylphenidate may inhibit the metabolism of some antidepressants (eg, tricyclics). It may be necessary to downward dose adjust the dosage and monitor plasma drug concentrations when initiating or discontinuing concomitant methylphenidate).

No products indexed under this heading.

Warfarin Sodium (Methylphenidate may inhibit the metabolism of coumarin anticoagulants; downward dosage adjustment of anticoagulants may be required. Dosage adjustment and plasma drug concentrations monitoring may be necessary when initiating or discontinuing concomitant methylphenidate).

No products indexed under this heading.

COPAXONE FOR INJECTION

(Glatiramer Acetate) 3110

None cited in PDR database.

COQUINONE 30 CAPSULES

(Coenzyme Q-10, Lipoic Acid) 3173

None cited in PDR database.

CORDYMAX CS-4 CAPSULES

(Herbals, Multiple) 2560

May interact with oral anticoagulants and monoamine oxidase inhibitors. Compounds in these categories include:

Anisindione (Concurrent use with anticoagulants requires consultation with a physician).

No products indexed under this heading.

Dicumarol (Concurrent use with anticoagulants requires consultation with a physician).

No products indexed under this heading.

Isocarboxazid (Concurrent use with MAO inhibitors requires consultation with a physician). Products include:

Marplan Tablets 3177

Moclobemide (Concurrent use with MAO inhibitors requires consultation with a physician).

No products indexed under this heading.

Pargyline Hydrochloride (Concurrent use with MAO inhibitors requires consultation with a physician).

No products indexed under this heading.

Phenelzine Sulfate (Concurrent use with MAO inhibitors requires consultation with a physician).

No products indexed under this heading.

Procarbazine Hydrochloride (Concurrent use with MAO inhibitors requires consultation with a physician).

No products indexed under this heading.

Rasagiline Mesylate (Concurrent use with MAO inhibitors requires consultation with a physician). Products include:

Azilect Tablets 3106

Selegiline (Concurrent use with MAO inhibitors requires consultation with a physician). Products include:

Emsam Transdermal System 905

Selegiline Hydrochloride (Concurrent use with MAO inhibitors requires consultation with a physician). Products include:

Eldepryl Capsules 3052

Tranylcypromine Sulfate (Concurrent use with MAO inhibitors requires consultation with a physician). Products include:

Parnate Tablets 1532

Warfarin Sodium (Concurrent use with anticoagulants requires consultation with a physician).

No products indexed under this heading.

COREG TABLETS

(Carvedilol) 1387

May interact with catecholamine depleting drugs, cytochrome p450 2d6 inhibitors (selected), diuretics, epinephrine-containing products, oral hypoglycemic agents, insulin, monoamine oxidase inhibitors, quinidine, and certain other agents. Compounds in these categories include:

Acarbose (Beta-blockers may mask some of the manifestations of hypoglycemia, particularly tachycardia; nonselective beta-blockers may potentiate insulin-induced hypoglycemia and delay recovery of serum glucose levels; in congestive heart failure patients with diabetes, carvedilol therapy may lead to worsening of hyperglycemia, which responds to intensification of hypoglycemia). Products include:

Precose Tablets 792

Amiloride Hydrochloride (Concomitant administration with a diuretic can be expected to produce additive effects and exaggerate the orthostatic component of carvedilol action).

No products indexed under this heading.

Amiodarone Hydrochloride (Interactions of carvedilol with strong inhibitors of CYP2D6, such as quinidine, have not been studied, but these drugs would be expected to increase blood levels of the R(+) enantiomer of carvedilol. Analysis of side effects showed that poor 2D6 metabolizers had a higher rate of dizziness during up-titration, presumably resulting from vasodilating effects of the higher concentrations of the alpha-blocking R(+) enantiomer).

No products indexed under this heading.

Amitriptyline Hydrochloride (Interactions of carvedilol with strong inhibitors of CYP2D6, such as quinidine, have not been studied, but these drugs would be expected to increase blood levels of the R(+) enantiomer of carvedilol. Analysis of side effects showed that poor 2D6 metabolizers had a higher rate of dizziness during up-titration, presumably resulting from vasodilating effects of the higher concentrations of the alpha-blocking R(+) enantiomer).

No products indexed under this heading.

Amoxapine (Interactions of carvedilol with strong inhibitors of CYP2D6, such as quinidine, have not been studied, but these drugs would be expected to increase blood levels of the R(+) enantiomer of carvedilol. Analysis of side effects showed that poor 2D6 metabolizers had a higher rate of dizziness during up-titration, presumably resulting from vasodilating effects of the higher concentrations of the alpha-blocking R(+) enantiomer).

No products indexed under this heading.

Bendroflumethiazide (Concomitant administration with a diuretic can be expected to produce additive effects and exaggerate the orthostatic component of carvedilol action).

No products indexed under this heading.

Bumetanide (Concomitant administration with a diuretic can be expected to produce additive effects and exaggerate the orthostatic component of carvedilol action).

No products indexed under this heading.

Bupropion Hydrochloride (Interactions of carvedilol with strong inhibitors of CYP2D6, such as quinidine, have not been studied, but these drugs would be expected to increase blood levels of the R(+) enantiomer of carvedilol. Analysis of side effects showed that poor 2D6 metabolizers had a higher rate of dizziness during up-titration, presumably resulting from vasodilating effects of the higher concentrations of the alpha-blocking R(+) enantiomer). Products include:

Wellbutrin Tablets 1648

Wellbutrin SR Sustained-Release Tablets 1653

Wellbutrin XL Extended-Release Tablets 1659

Zyban Sustained-Release Tablets 1692

Celecoxib (Interactions of carvedilol with strong inhibitors of CYP2D6, such as quinidine, have not been studied, but these drugs would be expected to increase blood levels of the R(+) enantiomer of carvedilol. Analysis of side effects showed that poor 2D6 metabolizers had a higher rate of dizziness during up-titration, presumably resulting from vasodilating effects of the higher concentrations of the alpha-blocking R(+) enantiomer). Products include:

Celebrex Capsules 2979

Chloroquine Hydrochloride (Interactions of carvedilol with strong inhibitors of CYP2D6, such as quinidine, have not been studied, but these drugs would be expected to increase blood levels of the R(+) enantiomer of carvedilol. Analysis of side effects showed that poor 2D6 metabolizers had a higher rate of dizziness during up-titration, presumably resulting from vasodilating effects of the higher concentrations of the alpha-blocking R(+) enantiomer).

No products indexed under this heading.

Chloroquine Phosphate (Interactions of carvedilol with strong inhibitors of CYP2D6, such as quinidine, have not been studied, but these drugs would be expected to increase blood levels of the R(+) enantiomer of carvedilol. Analysis of side effects showed that poor 2D6 metabolizers had a higher rate of dizziness during up-titration, presumably resulting from vasodilating effects of the higher concentrations of the alpha-blocking R(+) enantiomer).

No products indexed under this heading.

Chlorothiazide (Concomitant administration with a diuretic can be expected to produce additive effects and exaggerate the orthostatic component of carvedilol action).

No products indexed under this heading.

Chlorothiazide Sodium (Concomitant administration with a diuretic can be expected to produce additive effects and exaggerate the orthostatic component of carvedilol action). Products include:

Intravenous Sodium Diuril 2490

Chlorpheniramine (Interactions of carvedilol with strong inhibitors of CYP2D6, such as quinidine, have not been studied, but these drugs would be expected to increase blood levels of the R(+) enantiomer of carvedilol. Analysis of side effects showed that poor 2D6 metabolizers had a higher rate of dizziness during up-titration, presumably resulting from vasodilating effects of the higher concentrations of the alpha-blocking R(+) enantiomer).

No products indexed under this heading.

Chlorpheniramine Maleate (Interactions of carvedilol with strong inhibitors of CYP2D6, such as quinidine, have not been studied, but these drugs would be expected to increase blood levels of the R(+) enantiomer of carvedilol. Analysis of side effects showed that poor 2D6 metabolizers had a higher rate of dizziness during up-titration, presumably resulting from vasodilating effects of the higher concentrations of the alpha-blocking R(+) enantiomer). Products include:

Actifed Cold & Allergy Tablets 1895

Sudafed PE Sinus & Allergy Tablets 1908

Tylenol Allergy Multi-Symptom Caplets with Cool Burst and Rapid Release Gelcaps 1916

Children's Tylenol Plus Cold Suspension Liquid 1912

Children's Tylenol Plus Cough & Runny Nose Suspension Liquid 1912

Children's Tylenol Plus Flu Suspension Liquid 1914

Children's Tylenol Plus Multi-Symptom Cold Suspension Liquid 1912
Tylenol Cold Head Congestion Nighttime Caplets with Cool Burst 1910
Tylenol Cold Multi-Symptom Nighttime Caplets with Cool Burst 1913
Tylenol Sinus Congestion & Pain Nighttime Caplets with Cool Burst 1917

Chlorpheniramine Polistirex (Interactions of carvedilol with strong inhibitors of CYP2D6, such as quinidine, have not been studied, but these drugs would be expected to increase blood levels of the R(+) enantiomer of carvedilol. Analysis of side effects showed that poor 2D6 metabolizers had a higher rate of dizziness during up-titration, presumably resulting from vasodilating effects of the higher concentrations of the alpha-blocking R(+) enantiomer). Products include:
Tussionex Pennkinetic Extended-Release Suspension 3154

Chlorpheniramine Tannate (Interactions of carvedilol with strong inhibitors of CYP2D6, such as quinidine, have not been studied, but these drugs would be expected to increase blood levels of the R(+) enantiomer of carvedilol. Analysis of side effects showed that poor 2D6 metabolizers had a higher rate of dizziness during up-titration, presumably resulting from vasodilating effects of the higher concentrations of the alpha-blocking R(+) enantiomer).
No products indexed under this heading.

Chlorpropamide (Beta-blockers may mask some of the manifestations of hypoglycemia, particularly tachycardia; nonselective beta-blockers may potentiate insulin-induced hypoglycemia and delay recovery of serum glucose levels; in congestive heart failure patients with diabetes, carvedilol therapy may lead to worsening of hyperglycemia, which responds to intensification of hypoglycemia).
No products indexed under this heading.

Chlorthalidone (Concomitant administration with a diuretic can be expected to produce additive effects and exaggerate the orthostatic component of carvedilol action). Products include:
Clorpres Tablets 2185

Cimetidine (Carvedilol undergoes substantial oxidative metabolism; co-administration has resulted in increased steady-state AUC of carvedilol by about 30% with no change in Cmax).
No products indexed under this heading.

Cimetidine Hydrochloride (Carvedilol undergoes substantial oxidative metabolism; co-administration has resulted in increased steady-state AUC of carvedilol by about 30% with no change in Cmax).
No products indexed under this heading.

Citalopram Hydrobromide (Interactions of carvedilol with strong inhibitors of CYP2D6, such as quinidine, have not been studied, but these drugs would be expected to increase blood levels of the R(+) enantiomer of carvedilol. Analysis of side effects showed that poor 2D6 metabolizers had a higher rate of dizziness during up-titration, presumably resulting from vasodilating effects of the higher concentrations of the alpha-blocking R(+) enantiomer). Products include:
Celexa 1160

Clomipramine Hydrochloride (Interactions of carvedilol with strong inhibitors of CYP2D6, such as quinidine, have not been studied, but these drugs would be expected to increase blood levels of the R(+) enantiomer of carvedilol. Analysis of side effects showed that poor 2D6 metabolizers had a higher rate of dizziness during up-titration, presumably resulting from vasodilating effects of the higher concentrations of the alpha-blocking R(+) enantiomer).
No products indexed under this heading.

Clonidine (Concomitant administration of clonidine with agents with beta-blocking properties may potentiate blood-pressure- and heart-rate-lowering effects. When concomitant treatment with agents with beta-blocking properties and clonidine is to be terminated, the beta-blocking agent should be discontinued first. Clonidine therapy can then be discontinued several days later by gradually decreasing the dosage). Products include:
Catapres-TTS 842

Clonidine Hydrochloride (Concomitant administration of clonidine with agents with beta-blocking properties may potentiate blood-pressure- and heart-rate-lowering effects. When concomitant treatment with agents with beta-blocking properties and clonidine is to be terminated, thebeta-blocking agent should be discontinued first. Clonidine therapy can then be discontinued several days later by gradually decreasing the dosage). Products include:
Catapres Tablets 841
Clorpres Tablets 2185

Cocaine Hydrochloride (Interactions of carvedilol with strong inhibitors of CYP2D6, such as quinidine, have not been studied, but these drugs would be expected to increase blood levels of the R(+) enantiomer of carvedilol. Analysis of side effects showed that poor 2D6 metabolizers had a higher rate of dizziness during up-titration, presumably resulting from vasodilating effects of the higher concentrations of the alpha-blocking R(+) enantiomer).
No products indexed under this heading.

Cyclosporine (Co-administration in renal transplant patients has resulted in a modest increase in mean trough cyclosporine concentrations; dose of cyclosporine may need to be reduced in some patients). Products include:
Gengraf Capsules 435
Neoral Oral Solution 2280
Neoral Soft Gelatin Capsules 2280
Restasis Ophthalmic Emulsion 557
Sandimmune 2296

Deserpidine (Patients receiving agents with beta-blocking properties and a drug that may deplete catecholamines should be observed closely for signs of hypotension and/or severe bradycardia).
No products indexed under this heading.

Desipramine Hydrochloride (Interactions of carvedilol with strong inhibitors of CYP2D6, such as quinidine, have not been studied, but these drugs would be expected to increase blood levels of the R(+) enantiomer of carvedilol. Analysis of side effects showed that poor 2D6 metabolizers had a higher rate of dizziness during up-titration, presumably resulting from vasodilating effects of the higher concentrations of the alpha-blocking R(+) enantiomer).
No products indexed under this heading.

Digoxin (Co-administration increases digoxin concentraton by 15%. Both digoxin and carvedilol slow AV conduction. Therefore, increased monitoring of digoxin is recommended when initiating, adjusting or discontinuing carvedilol). Products include:
Lanoxin Injection 1498
Lanoxin Injection Pediatric 1502
Lanoxin Tablets 1505

Diltiazem Hydrochloride (Co-administration has resulted in isolated cases of conduction disturbances, rarely with hemodynamic. Monitoring of ECG and blood pressure is recommended). Products include:
Cardizem LA Extended Release Tablets 421

Diphenhydramine (Interactions of carvedilol with strong inhibitors of CYP2D6, such as quinidine, have not been studied, but these drugs would be expected to increase blood levels of the R(+) enantiomer of carvedilol. Analysis of side effects showed that poor 2D6 metabolizers had a higher rate of dizziness during up-titration, presumably resulting from vasodilating effects of the higher concentrations of the alpha-blocking R(+) enantiomer).
No products indexed under this heading.

Diphenhydramine Hydrochloride (Interactions of carvedilol with strong inhibitors of CYP2D6, such as quinidine, have not been studied, but these drugs would be expected to increase blood levels of the R(+) enantiomer of carvedilol. Analysis of side effects showed that poor 2D6 metabolizers had a higher rate of dizziness during up-titration, presumably resulting from vasodilating effects of the higher concentrations of the alpha-blocking R(+) enantiomer). Products include:
Benadryl Allergy & Cold Kapgels 1895
Benadryl Allergy & Sinus Headache Kapgels 1895
Benadryl Severe Allergy & Sinus Headache Caplets 1897
Benadryl Dye-Free Allergy Liqui-gels Softgels 1897
Benadryl Allergy Kapgels 1895
Benadryl Allergy Quick Dissolve Strips 1896
Benadryl Allergy Ultratab Tablets 1896
Children's Benadryl Dye-Free Allergy Liquid 1897
Children's Benadryl Allergy Fastmelts 1897
Children's Benadryl Allergy Liquid 1898
Children's Benadryl Allergy Perfect Measure 1896
Children's Benadryl-D Allergy & Sinus Liquid 1896
Benadryl-D Allergy & Sinus Tablet 1896
PediaCare Children's Allergy & Cold Liquid 1902
PediaCare Children's Allergy Liquid 1902
Simply Sleep Caplets 1905
Sudafed PE Nighttime Cold Caplets 1907
Sudafed PE Severe Cold Caplets 1908
Extra Strength Tylenol PM Caplets, Geltabs, Liquid, and Rapid Release Gels 1915
Tylenol Allergy Multi-Symptom Nighttime Caplets with Cool Burst 1916
Tylenol Severe Allergy Caplets 1916
Children's Tylenol Plus Cold & Allergy Suspension Liquid 1914
Tylenol Sore Throat Nighttime Liquid with Cool Burst 1918

Doxepin Hydrochloride (Interactions of carvedilol with strong inhibitors of CYP2D6, such as quinidine, have not been studied, but these drugs would be expected to increase blood levels of the R(+) enantiomer of carvedilol. Analysis of side effects showed that poor 2D6 metabolizers had a higher rate of dizziness during up-titration, presumably resulting from vasodilating effects of the higher concentrations of the alpha-blocking R(+) enantiomer).
No products indexed under this heading.

Epinephrine (Patients on beta-blocker therapy and with a history of severe anaphylactic reactions to a variety of allergens may be unresponsive to the usual doses of epinephrine used to treat allergic reactions). Products include:
EpiPen 1024

Epinephrine Bitartrate (Patients on beta-blocker therapy and with a history of severe anaphylactic reactions to a variety of allergens may be unresponsive to the usual doses of epinephrine used to treat allergic reactions).
No products indexed under this heading.

Epinephrine Hydrochloride (Potential for unresponsiveness to the usual dose of epinephrine used to treat allergic reactions).
No products indexed under this heading.

Escitalopram Oxalate (Interactions of carvedilol with strong inhibitors of CYP2D6, such as quinidine, have not been studied, but these drugs would be expected to increase blood levels of the R(+) enantiomer of carvedilol. Analysis of side effects showed that poor 2D6 metabolizers had a higher rate of dizziness during up-titration, presumably resulting from vasodilating effects of the higher concentrations of the alpha-blocking R(+) enantiomer). Products include:
Lexapro Oral Suspension 1174
Lexapro Tablets 1174

Ethacrynic Acid (Concomitant administration with a diuretic can be expected to produce additive effects and exaggerate the orthostatic component of carvedilol action). Products include:
Edecrin Tablets 698

Fluoxetine (Interactions of carvedilol with strong inhibitors of CYP2D6, such as quinidine, have not been studied, but these drugs would be expected to increase blood levels of the R(+) enantiomer of carvedilol. Analysis of side effects showed that poor 2D6 metabolizers had a higher rate of dizziness during up-titration, presumably resulting from vasodilating effects of the higher concentrations of the alpha-blocking R(+)

enantiomer).
No products indexed under this heading.

Fluoxetine Hydrochloride (Interactions of carvedilol with strong inhibitors of CYP2D6, such as fluoxetine, have not been studied, but these drugs would be expected to increase blood levels of the R(+) enantiomer of carvedilol. Analysis of side effects showed that poor 2D6 metabolizers had a higher rate of dizziness during up-titration, presumably resulting from vasodilating effects of the higher concentrations of the alpha-blocking R(+) enantiomer). Products include:
Prozac Weekly Capsules 1852
Prozac Pulvules and Liquid 1852
Symbyax Capsules 1871

Fluphenazine Decanoate (Interactions of carvedilol with strong inhibitors of CYP2D6, such as quinidine, have not been studied, but these drugs would be expected to increase blood levels of the R(+) enantiomer of carvedilol. Analysis of side effects showed that poor 2D6 metabolizers had a higher rate of dizziness during up-titration, presumably resulting from vasodilating effects of the higher concentrations of the alpha-blocking R(+) enantiomer).
No products indexed under this heading.

Fluphenazine Enanthate (Interactions of carvedilol with strong inhibitors of CYP2D6, such as quinidine, have not been studied, but these drugs would be expected to increase blood levels of the R(+) enantiomer of carvedilol. Analysis of side effects showed that poor 2D6 metabolizers had a higher rate of dizziness during up-titration, presumably resulting from vasodilating effects of the higher concentrations of the alpha-blocking R(+) enantiomer).
No products indexed under this heading.

Fluphenazine Hydrochloride (Interactions of carvedilol with strong inhibitors of CYP2D6, such as quinidine, have not been studied, but these drugs would be expected to increase blood levels of the R(+) enantiomer of carvedilol. Analysis of side effects showed that poor 2D6 metabolizers had a higher rate of dizziness during up-titration, presumably resulting from vasodilating effects of the higher concentrations of the alpha-blocking R(+) enantiomer).
No products indexed under this heading.

Fluvoxamine Maleate (Interactions of carvedilol with strong inhibitors of CYP2D6, such as quinidine, have not been studied, but these drugs would be expected to increase blood levels of the R(+) enantiomer of carvedilol. Analysis of side effects showed that poor 2D6 metabolizers had a higher rate of dizziness during up-titration, presumably resulting from vasodilating effects of the higher concentrations of the alpha-blocking R(+) enantiomer). Products include:
Luvox CR Extended-Release Capsules 1759

Furosemide (Concomitant administration with a diuretic can be expected to produce additive effects and exaggerate the orthostatic component of carvedilol action). Products include:
Furosemide Tablets 2186

Glimepiride (Beta-blockers may mask some of the manifestations of hypoglycemia, particularly tachycardia; nonselective beta-blockers may potentiate insulin-induced hypoglycemia and delay recovery of serum glucose levels; in congestive heart failure patients with diabetes, carvedilol therapy may lead to worsening of hyperglycemia, which responds to intensification of hypoglycemia). Products include:
Avandaryl Tablets 1344
Duetact Tablets 3085

Glipizide (Beta-blockers may mask some of the manifestations of hypoglycemia, particularly tachycardia; nonselective beta-blockers may potentiate insulin-induced hypoglycemia and delay recovery of serum glucose levels; in congestive heart failure patients with diabetes, carvedilol therapy may lead to worsening of hyperglycemia, which responds to intensification of hypoglycemia).
No products indexed under this heading.

Glyburide (Beta-blockers may mask some of the manifestations of hypoglycemia, particularly tachycardia; nonselective beta-blockers may potentiate insulin-induced hypoglycemia and delay recovery of serum glucose levels; in congestive heart failure patients with diabetes, carvedilol therapy may lead to worsening of hyperglycemia, which responds to intensification of hypoglycemia).
No products indexed under this heading.

Guanethidine Monosulfate (Patients receiving agents with beta-blocking properties and a drug that may deplete catecholamines should be observed closely for signs of hypotension and/or severe bradycardia).
No products indexed under this heading.

Halofantrine Hydrochloride (Interactions of carvedilol with strong inhibitors of CYP2D6, such as quinidine, have not been studied, but these drugs would be expected to increase blood levels of the R(+) enantiomer of carvedilol. Analysis of side effects showed that poor 2D6 metabolizers had a higher rate of dizziness during up-titration, presumably resulting from vasodilating effects of the higher concentrations of the alpha-blocking R(+) enantiomer).
No products indexed under this heading.

Haloperidol (Interactions of carvedilol with strong inhibitors of CYP2D6, such as quinidine, have not been studied, but these drugs would be expected to increase blood levels of the R(+) enantiomer of carvedilol. Analysis of side effects showed that poor 2D6 metabolizers had a higher rate of dizziness during up-titration, presumably resulting from vasodilating effects of the higher concentrations of the alpha-blocking R(+) enantiomer).
No products indexed under this heading.

Haloperidol Decanoate (Interactions of carvedilol with strong inhibitors of CYP2D6, such as quinidine, have not been studied, but these drugs would be expected to increase blood levels of the R(+) enantiomer of carvedilol. Analysis of side effects showed that poor 2D6 metabolizers had a higher rate of dizziness during up-titration, presumably resulting from vasodilating effects of the higher concentrations of the alpha-blocking R(+) enantiomer).
No products indexed under this heading.

Hydrochlorothiazide (Concomitant administration with a diuretic can be expected to produce additive effects and exaggerate the orthostatic component of carvedilol action). Products include:
Atacand HCT 642
Avalide Tablets 892
Avalide Tablets 2713
Benicar HCT Tablets 1010
Diovan HCT Tablets 2216
Dyazide Capsules 1405
Micardis HCT Tablets 854
Prinzide Tablets 2092
Tekturna HCT Tablets 2324
Teveten HCT Tablets 517

Hydroflumethiazide (Concomitant administration with a diuretic can be expected to produce additive effects and exaggerate the orthostatic component of carvedilol action).
No products indexed under this heading.

Hydroxychloroquine Sulfate (Interactions of carvedilol with strong inhibitors of CYP2D6, such as quinidine, have not been studied, but these drugs would be expected to increase blood levels of the R(+) enantiomer of carvedilol. Analysis of side effects showed that poor 2D6 metabolizers had a higher rate of dizziness during up-titration, presumably resulting from vasodilating effects of the higher concentrations of the alpha-blocking R(+) enantiomer).
No products indexed under this heading.

Imatinib Mesylate (Interactions of carvedilol with strong inhibitors of CYP2D6, such as quinidine, have not been studied, but these drugs would be expected to increase blood levels of the R(+) enantiomer of carvedilol. Analysis of side effects showed that poor 2D6 metabolizers had a higher rate of dizziness during up-titration, presumably resulting from vasodilating effects of the higher concentrations of the alpha-blocking R(+) enantiomer). Products include:
Gleevec Tablets 2255

Imipramine Hydrochloride (Interactions of carvedilol with strong inhibitors of CYP2D6, such as quinidine, have not been studied, but these drugs would be expected to increase blood levels of the R(+) enantiomer of carvedilol. Analysis of side effects showed that poor 2D6 metabolizers had a higher rate of dizziness during up-titration, presumably resulting from vasodilating effects of the higher concentrations of the alpha-blocking R(+) enantiomer).
No products indexed under this heading.

Imipramine Pamoate (Interactions of carvedilol with strong inhibitors of CYP2D6, such as quinidine, have not been studied, but these drugs would be expected to increase blood levels of the R(+) enantiomer of carvedilol. Analysis of side effects showed that poor 2D6 metabolizers had a higher rate of dizziness during up-titration, presumably resulting from vasodilating effects of the higher concentrations of the alpha-blocking R(+) enantiomer).
No products indexed under this heading.

Indapamide (Concomitant administration with a diuretic can be expected to produce additive effects and exaggerate the orthostatic component of carvedilol action). Products include:
Indapamide Tablets 2188

Insulin (Beta-blockers may mask some of the manifestations of hypoglycemia, particularly tachycardia; nonselective beta-blockers may potentiate insulin-induced hypoglycemia and delay recovery of serum glucose levels; in congestive heart failure patients with diabetes, carvedilol therapy may lead to worsening of hyperglycemia, which responds to intensification of hypoglycemia).
No products indexed under this heading.

Insulin, Human, Zinc Suspension (Beta-blockers may mask some of the manifestations of hypoglycemia, particularly tachycardia; nonselective beta-blockers may potentiate insulin-induced hypoglycemia and delay recovery of serum glucose levels; in congestive heart failure patients with diabetes, carvedilol therapy may lead to worsening of hyperglycemia, which responds to intensification of hypoglycemia).
No products indexed under this heading.

Insulin, Human (rDNA origin) (Beta-blockers may mask some of the manifestations of hypoglycemia, particularly tachycardia; nonselective beta-blockers may potentiate insulin-induced hypoglycemia and delay recovery of serum glucose levels; in congestive heart failure patients with diabetes, carvedilol therapy may lead to worsening of hyperglycemia, which responds to intensification of hypoglycemia). Products include:
Exubera Inhalation Powder 2515

Insulin, Human NPH (Beta-blockers may mask some of the manifestations of hypoglycemia, particularly tachycardia; nonselective beta-blockers may potentiate insulin-induced hypoglycemia and delay recovery of serum glucose levels; in congestive heart failure patients with diabetes, carvedilol therapy may lead to worsening of hyperglycemia, which responds to intensification of hypoglycemia). Products include:
Humulin N Vial 1846

Insulin, Human Regular (Beta-blockers may mask some of the manifestations of hypoglycemia, particularly tachycardia; nonselective beta-blockers may potentiate insulin-induced hypoglycemia and delay recovery of serum glucose levels; in congestive heart failure patients with diabetes, carvedilol therapy may lead to worsening of hyperglycemia, which responds to intensification of hypoglycemia). Products include:
Humulin R 1849

Humulin R (U-500) 1850

Insulin, Human Regular and Human NPH Mixture (Beta-blockers may mask some of the manifestations of hypoglycemia, particularly tachycardia; nonselective beta-blockers may potentiate insulin-induced hypoglycemia and delay recovery of serum glucose levels; in congestive heart failure patients with diabetes, carvedilol therapy may lead to worsening of hyperglycemia, which responds to intensification of hypoglycemia). Products include:

Humulin 50/50, 100 Units 1843
Humulin 70/30 Vial 1844

Insulin, NPH (Beta-blockers may mask some of the manifestations of hypoglycemia, particularly tachycardia; nonselective beta-blockers may potentiate insulin-induced hypoglycemia and delay recovery of serum glucose levels; in congestive heart failure patients with diabetes, carvedilol therapy may lead to worsening of hyperglycemia, which responds to intensification of hypoglycemia).

No products indexed under this heading.

Insulin, Regular (Beta-blockers may mask some of the manifestations of hypoglycemia, particularly tachycardia; nonselective beta-blockers may potentiate insulin-induced hypoglycemia and delay recovery of serum glucose levels; in congestive heart failure patients with diabetes, carvedilol therapy may lead to worsening of hyperglycemia, which responds to intensification of hypoglycemia).

No products indexed under this heading.

Insulin, Regular and NPH mixture (Beta-blockers may mask some of the manifestations of hypoglycemia, particularly tachycardia; nonselective beta-blockers may potentiate insulin-induced hypoglycemia and delay recovery of serum glucose levels; in congestive heart failure patients with diabetes, carvedilol therapy may lead to worsening of hyperglycemia, which responds to intensification of hypoglycemia).

No products indexed under this heading.

Insulin, Zinc Crystals (Beta-blockers may mask some of the manifestations of hypoglycemia, particularly tachycardia; nonselective beta-blockers may potentiate insulin-induced hypoglycemia and delay recovery of serum glucose levels; in congestive heart failure patients with diabetes, carvedilol therapy may lead to worsening of hyperglycemia, which responds to intensification of hypoglycemia).

No products indexed under this heading.

Insulin, Zinc Suspension (Beta-blockers may mask some of the manifestations of hypoglycemia, particularly tachycardia; nonselective beta-blockers may potentiate insulin-induced hypoglycemia and delay recovery of serum glucose levels; in congestive heart failure patients with diabetes, carvedilol therapy may lead to worsening of hyperglycemia, which responds to intensification of hypoglycemia).

No products indexed under this heading.

Insulin Aspart (Beta-blockers may mask some of the manifestations of hypoglycemia, particularly tachycardia; nonselective beta-blockers may potentiate insulin-induced hypoglycemia and delay recovery of serum glucose levels; in congestive heart failure patients with diabetes, carvedilol therapy may lead to worsening of hyperglycemia, which responds to intensification of hypoglycemia).

No products indexed under this heading.

Insulin Aspart, Human (Beta-blockers may mask some of the manifestations of hypoglycemia, particularly tachycardia; nonselective beta-blockers may potentiate insulin-induced hypoglycemia and delay recovery of serum glucose levels; in congestive heart failure patients with diabetes, carvedilol therapy may lead to worsening of hyperglycemia, which responds to intensification of hypoglycemia). Products include:

NovoLog Mix 70/30 2364

Insulin Aspart, Human Regular (Beta-blockers may mask some of the manifestations of hypoglycemia, particularly tachycardia; nonselective beta-blockers may potentiate insulin-induced hypoglycemia and delay recovery of serum glucose levels; in congestive heart failure patients with diabetes, carvedilol therapy may lead to worsening of hyperglycemia, which responds to intensification of hypoglycemia). Products include:

NovoLog Injection 2359

Insulin Aspart Protamine, Human (Beta-blockers may mask some of the manifestations of hypoglycemia, particularly tachycardia; nonselective beta-blockers may potentiate insulin-induced hypoglycemia and delay recovery of serum glucose levels; in congestive heart failure patients with diabetes, carvedilol therapy may lead to worsening of hyperglycemia, which responds to intensification of hypoglycemia). Products include:

NovoLog Mix 70/30 2364

Insulin Detemir (rDNA Origin) (Beta-blockers may mask some of the manifestations of hypoglycemia, particularly tachycardia; nonselective beta-blockers may potentiate insulin-induced hypoglycemia and delay recovery of serum glucose levels; in congestive heart failure patients with diabetes, carvedilol therapy may lead to worsening of hyperglycemia, which responds to intensification of hypoglycemia). Products include:

Levemir Injection 2352

Insulin glargine (Beta-blockers may mask some of the manifestations of hypoglycemia, particularly tachycardia; nonselective beta-blockers may potentiate insulin-induced hypoglycemia and delay recovery of serum glucose levels; in congestive heart failure patients with diabetes, carvedilol therapy may lead to worsening of hyperglycemia, which responds to intensification of hypoglycemia). Products include:

Lantus Injection 2749

Insulin Glulisine (Beta-blockers may mask some of the manifestations of hypoglycemia, particularly tachycardia; nonselective beta-blockers may potentiate insulin-induced hypoglycemia and delay recovery of serum glucose levels; in congestive heart failure patients with diabetes, carvedilol therapy may lead to worsening of hyperglycemia, which responds to intensification of hypoglycemia). Products include:

Apidra Injection 2706

Insulin Lispro, Human (Beta-blockers may mask some of the manifestations of hypoglycemia, particularly tachycardia; nonselective beta-blockers may potentiate insulin-induced hypoglycemia and delay recovery of serum glucose levels; in congestive heart failure patients with diabetes, carvedilol therapy may lead to worsening of hyperglycemia, which responds to intensification of hypoglycemia). Products include:

Humalog-Pen and KwikPen 1829
Humalog Mix 50/50-Pen and KwikPen 1833
Humalog Mix 75/25-Pen and KwikPen 1835

Insulin Lispro Protamine, Human (Beta-blockers may mask some of the manifestations of hypoglycemia, particularly tachycardia; nonselective beta-blockers may potentiate insulin-induced hypoglycemia and delay recovery of serum glucose levels; in congestive heart failure patients with diabetes, carvedilol therapy may lead to worsening of hyperglycemia, which responds to intensification of hypoglycemia). Products include:

Humalog Mix 50/50-Pen and KwikPen 1833
Humalog Mix 75/25-Pen and KwikPen 1835

Isocarboxazid (Patients receiving agents with beta-blocking properties and a drug that may deplete catecholamines (e.g., MAO Inhibitors) should be observed closely for signs of hypotension and/or severe bradycardia). Products include:

Marplan Tablets 3177

Maprotiline Hydrochloride (Interactions of carvedilol with strong inhibitors of CYP2D6, such as quinidine, have not been studied, but these drugs would be expected to increase blood levels of the R(+) enantiomer of carvedilol. Analysis of side effects showed that poor 2D6 metabolizers had a higher rate of dizziness during up-titration, presumably resulting from vasodilating effects of the higher concentrations of the alpha-blocking R(+) enantiomer).

No products indexed under this heading.

Metformin Hydrochloride (Beta-blockers may mask some of the manifestations of hypoglycemia, particularly tachycardia; nonselective beta-blockers may potentiate insulin-induced hypoglycemia and delay recovery of serum glucose levels; in congestive heart failure patients with diabetes, carvedilol therapy may lead to worsening of hyperglycemia, which responds to intensification of hypoglycemia). Products include:

ActoPlus Met Tablets 3071
Avandamet Tablets 1336
Janumet Tablets 2041
PrandiMet Tablets 2967

Methadone Hydrochloride (Interactions of carvedilol with strong inhibitors of CYP2D6, such as quinidine, have not been studied, but these drugs would be expected to increase blood levels of the R(+) enantiomer of carvedilol. Analysis of side effects showed that poor 2D6 metabolizers had a higher rate of dizziness during up-titration, presumably resulting from vasodilating effects of the higher concentrations of the alpha-blocking R(+) enantiomer).

No products indexed under this heading.

Methyclothiazide (Concomitant administration with a diuretic can be expected to produce additive effects and exaggerate the orthostatic component of carvedilol action).

No products indexed under this heading.

Metolazone (Concomitant administration with a diuretic can be expected to produce additive effects and exaggerate the orthostatic component of carvedilol action).

No products indexed under this heading.

Mibefradil Dihydrochloride (Interactions of carvedilol with strong inhibitors of CYP2D6, such as quinidine, have not been studied, but these drugs would be expected to increase blood levels of the R(+) enantiomer of carvedilol. Analysis of side effects showed that poor 2D6 metabolizers had a higher rate of dizziness during up-titration, presumably resulting from vasodilating effects of the higher concentrations of the alpha-blocking R(+) enantiomer).

No products indexed under this heading.

Miglitol (Beta-blockers may mask some of the manifestations of hypoglycemia, particularly tachycardia; nonselective beta-blockers may potentiate insulin-induced hypoglycemia and delay recovery of serum glucose levels; in congestive heart failure patients with diabetes, carvedilol therapy may lead to worsening of hyperglycemia, which responds to intensification of hypoglycemia).

No products indexed under this heading.

Moclobemide (Patients receiving agents with beta-blocking properties and a drug that may deplete catecholamines (e.g., MAO Inhibitors) should be observed closely for signs of hypotension and/or severe bradycardia).

No products indexed under this heading.

Nateglinide (Beta-blockers may mask some of the manifestations of hypoglycemia, particularly tachycardia; nonselective beta-blockers may potentiate insulin-induced hypoglycemia and delay recovery of serum glucose levels; in congestive heart failure patients with diabetes, carvedilol therapy may lead to worsening of hyperglycemia, which responds to intensification of hypoglycemia). Products include:

Starlix Tablets 2314

Nortriptyline Hydrochloride (Interactions of carvedilol with strong inhibitors of CYP2D6, such as quinidine, have not been studied, but these drugs would be expected to increase blood levels of the R(+) enantiomer of carvedilol. Analysis of side effects showed that poor 2D6 metabolizers had a higher rate of

dizziness during up-titration, presumably resulting from vasodilating effects of the higher concentrations of the alpha-blocking R(+) enantiomer).
No products indexed under this heading.

Pargyline Hydrochloride (Patients receiving agents with beta-blocking properties and a drug that may deplete catecholamines (e.g., MAO Inhibitors) should be observed closely for signs of hypotension and/or severe bradycardia).
No products indexed under this heading.

Paroxetine Hydrochloride (Interactions of carvedilol with strong inhibitors of CYP2D6, such as paroxetine, have not been studied, but these drugs would be expected to increase blood levels of the R(+) enantiomer of carvedilol. Analysis of side effects showed that poor 2D6 metabolizers had a higher rate of dizziness during up-titration, presumably resulting from vasodilating effects of the higher concentrations of the alpha-blocking R(+) enantiomer). Products include:
Paxil 1535
Paxil CR Controlled-Release Tablets 1544

Perphenazine (Interactions of carvedilol with strong inhibitors of CYP2D6, such as quinidine, have not been studied, but these drugs would be expected to increase blood levels of the R(+) enantiomer of carvedilol. Analysis of side effects showed that poor 2D6 metabolizers had a higher rate of dizziness during up-titration, presumably resulting from vasodilating effects of the higher concentrations of the alpha-blocking R(+) enantiomer).
No products indexed under this heading.

Phenelzine Sulfate (Patients receiving agents with beta-blocking properties and a drug that may deplete catecholamines (e.g., MAO Inhibitors) should be observed closely for signs of hypotension and/or severe bradycardia).
No products indexed under this heading.

Pioglitazone Hydrochloride (Beta-blockers may mask some of the manifestations of hypoglycemia, particularly tachycardia; nonselective beta-blockers may potentiate insulin-induced hypoglycemia and delay recovery of serum glucose levels; in congestive heart failure patients with diabetes, carvedilol therapy may lead to worsening of hyperglycemia, which responds to intensification of hypoglycemia). Products include:
ActoPlus Met Tablets 3071
Actos Tablets 3077
Duetact Tablets 3085

Polythiazide (Concomitant administration with a diuretic can be expected to produce additive effects and exaggerate the orthostatic component of carvedilol action).
No products indexed under this heading.

Procarbazine Hydrochloride (Patients receiving agents with beta-blocking properties and a drug that may deplete catecholamines (e.g., MAO Inhibitors) should be observed closely for signs of hypotension and/or severe bradycardia).
No products indexed under this heading.

Propafenone Hydrochloride (Interactions of carvedilol with strong inhibitors of CYP2D6, such as propafenone, have not been studied, but these drugs would be expected to increase blood levels of the R(+) enantiomer of carvedilol. Analysis of side effects showed that poor 2D6 metabolizers had a higher rate of dizziness during up-titration, presumably resulting from vasodilating effects of the higher concentrations of the alpha-blocking R(+) enantiomer). Products include:
Rythmol Tablets 1586
Rythmol SR Capsules 1590

Propoxyphene Hydrochloride (Interactions of carvedilol with strong inhibitors of CYP2D6, such as quinidine, have not been studied, but these drugs would be expected to increase blood levels of the R(+) enantiomer of carvedilol. Analysis of side effects showed that poor 2D6 metabolizers had a higher rate of dizziness during up-titration, presumably resulting from vasodilating effects of the higher concentrations of the alpha-blocking R(+) enantiomer).
No products indexed under this heading.

Propoxyphene Napsylate (Interactions of carvedilol with strong inhibitors of CYP2D6, such as quinidine, have not been studied, but these drugs would be expected to increase blood levels of the R(+) enantiomer of carvedilol. Analysis of side effects showed that poor 2D6 metabolizers had a higher rate of dizziness during up-titration, presumably resulting from vasodilating effects of the higher concentrations of the alpha-blocking R(+) enantiomer).
No products indexed under this heading.

Protriptyline Hydrochloride (Interactions of carvedilol with strong inhibitors of CYP2D6, such as quinidine, have not been studied, but these drugs would be expected to increase blood levels of the R(+) enantiomer of carvedilol. Analysis of side effects showed that poor 2D6 metabolizers had a higher rate of dizziness during up-titration, presumably resulting from vasodilating effects of the higher concentrations of the alpha-blocking R(+) enantiomer).
No products indexed under this heading.

Quinacrine Hydrochloride (Interactions of carvedilol with strong inhibitors of CYP2D6, such as quinidine, have not been studied, but these drugs would be expected to increase blood levels of the R(+) enantiomer of carvedilol. Analysis of side effects showed that poor 2D6 metabolizers had a higher rate of dizziness during up-titration, presumably resulting from vasodilating effects of the higher concentrations of the alpha-blocking R(+) enantiomer).
No products indexed under this heading.

Quinidine (Co-administration of carvedilol with strong inhibitors of CYP2D6, such as quinidine, have not been studied, but quinidine would be expected to increase blood levels).
No products indexed under this heading.

Quinidine Gluconate (Co-administration of carvedilol with strong inhibitors of CYP2D6, such as quinidine, have not been studied, but quinidine would be expected to increase blood levels).
No products indexed under this heading.

Quinidine Hydrochloride (Co-administration of carvedilol with strong inhibitors of CYP2D6, such as quinidine, have not been studied, but quinidine would be expected to increase blood levels).
No products indexed under this heading.

Quinidine Polygalacturonate (Co-administration of carvedilol with strong inhibitors of CYP2D6, such as quinidine, have not been studied, but quinidine would be expected to increase blood levels).
No products indexed under this heading.

Quinidine Sulfate (Co-administration of carvedilol with strong inhibitors of CYP2D6, such as quinidine, have not been studied, but quinidine would be expected to increase blood levels).
No products indexed under this heading.

Ranitidine Bismuth Citrate (Interactions of carvedilol with strong inhibitors of CYP2D6, such as quinidine, have not been studied, but these drugs would be expected to increase blood levels of the R(+) enantiomer of carvedilol. Analysis of side effects showed that poor 2D6 metabolizers had a higher rate of dizziness during up-titration, presumably resulting from vasodilating effects of the higher concentrations of the alpha-blocking R(+) enantiomer).
No products indexed under this heading.

Ranitidine Hydrochloride (Interactions of carvedilol with strong inhibitors of CYP2D6, such as quinidine, have not been studied, but these drugs would be expected to increase blood levels of the R(+) enantiomer of carvedilol. Analysis of side effects showed that poor 2D6 metabolizers had a higher rate of dizziness during up-titration, presumably resulting from vasodilating effects of the higher concentrations of the alpha-blocking R(+) enantiomer). Products include:
Zantac 75 Tablets .... ▣603
Zantac 1670
Zantac Injection 1666
Zantac Injection Pharmacy Bulk Package 1668
Maximum Strength Zantac 150 Tablets .... ▣603
Maximum Strength Zantac 150 Cool Mint Tablets .... ▣603

Rasagiline Mesylate (Patients receiving agents with beta-blocking properties and a drug that may deplete catecholamines (e.g., MAO Inhibitors) should be observed closely for signs of hypotension and/or severe bradycardia). Products include:
Azilect Tablets 3106

Rauwolfia Serpentina (Patients receiving agents with beta-blocking properties and a drug that may deplete catecholamines should be observed closely for signs of hypotension and/or severe bradycardia).
No products indexed under this heading.

Repaglinide (Beta-blockers may mask some of the manifestations of hypoglycemia, particularly tachycardia; nonselective beta-blockers may potentiate insulin-induced hypoglycemia and delay recovery of serum glucose levels; in congestive heart failure patients with diabetes, carvedilol therapy may lead to worsening of hyperglycemia, which responds to intensification of hypoglycemia). Products include:
PrandiMet Tablets 2967
Prandin Tablets 2971

Rescinnamine (Patients receiving agents with beta-blocking properties and a drug that may deplete catecholamines should be observed closely for signs of hypotension and/or severe bradycardia).
No products indexed under this heading.

Reserpine (Co-administration of agents with beta-blocking properties and a drug that can deplete catecholamines, such as reserpine, may result in hypotension and/or severe bradycardia).
No products indexed under this heading.

Rifampin (Carvedilol undergoes substantial oxidative metabolism, co-administration has resulted in decreased AUC and Cmax of carvedilol by about 70%).
No products indexed under this heading.

Ritonavir (Interactions of carvedilol with strong inhibitors of CYP2D6, such as quinidine, have not been studied, but these drugs would be expected to increase blood levels of the R(+) enantiomer of carvedilol. Analysis of side effects showed that poor 2D6 metabolizers had a higher rate of dizziness during up-titration, presumably resulting from vasodilating effects of the higher concentrations of the alpha-blocking R(+) enantiomer). Products include:
Kaletra 452
Norvir 489

Rosiglitazone Maleate (Beta-blockers may mask some of the manifestations of hypoglycemia, particularly tachycardia; nonselective beta-blockers may potentiate insulin-induced hypoglycemia and delay recovery of serum glucose levels; in congestive heart failure patients with diabetes, carvedilol therapy may lead to worsening of hyperglycemia, which responds to intensification of hypoglycemia). Products include:
Avandamet Tablets 1336
Avandaryl Tablets 1344
Avandia Tablets 1351

Selegiline (Patients receiving agents with beta-blocking properties and a drug that may deplete catecholamines (e.g., MAO Inhibitors) should be observed closely for signs of hypotension and/or severe bradycardia). Products include:
Emsam Transdermal System 905

Selegiline Hydrochloride (Patients receiving agents with beta-blocking properties and a drug that may deplete catecholamines (e.g., MAO Inhibitors) should be observed closely for signs of hypotension and/or severe bradycardia). Products include:
Eldepryl Capsules 3052

Sertraline Hydrochloride (Interactions of carvedilol with strong inhibi-

tors of CYP2D6, such as quinidine, have not been studied, but these drugs would be expected to increase blood levels of the R(+) enantiomer of carvedilol. Analysis of side effects showed that poor 2D6 metabolizers had a higher rate of dizziness during up-titration, presumably resulting from vasodilating effects of the higher concentrations of the alpha-blocking R(+) enantiomer).

No products indexed under this heading.

Sildenafil Citrate (Interactions of carvedilol with strong inhibitors of CYP2D6, such as quinidine, have not been studied, but these drugs would be expected to increase blood levels of the R(+) enantiomer of carvedilol. Analysis of side effects showed that poor 2D6 metabolizers had a higher rate of dizziness during up-titration, presumably resulting from vasodilating effects of the higher concentrations of the alpha-blocking R(+) enantiomer).

No products indexed under this heading.

Sitagliptin Phosphate (Beta-blockers may mask some of the manifestations of hypoglycemia, particularly tachycardia; nonselective beta-blockers may potentiate insulin-induced hypoglycemia and delay recovery of serum glucose levels; in congestive heart failure patients with diabetes, carvedilol therapy may lead to worsening of hyperglycemia, which responds to intensification of hypoglycemia). Products include:

Janumet Tablets 2041
Januvia Tablets 2048

Spironolactone (Concomitant administration with a diuretic can be expected to produce additive effects and exaggerate the orthostatic component of carvedilol action).

No products indexed under this heading.

Terbinafine Hydrochloride (Interactions of carvedilol with strong inhibitors of CYP2D6, such as quinidine, have not been studied, but these drugs would be expected to increase blood levels of the R(+) enantiomer of carvedilol. Analysis of side effects showed that poor 2D6 metabolizers had a higher rate of dizziness during up-titration, presumably resulting from vasodilating effects of the higher concentrations of the alpha-blocking R(+) enantiomer). Products include:

Lamisil Oral Granules 2264
Lamisil Tablets 2266

Thioridazine Hydrochloride (Interactions of carvedilol with strong inhibitors of CYP2D6, such as quinidine, have not been studied, but these drugs would be expected to increase blood levels of the R(+) enantiomer of carvedilol. Analysis of side effects showed that poor 2D6 metabolizers had a higher rate of dizziness during up-titration, presumably resulting from vasodilating effects of the higher concentrations of the alpha-blocking R(+) enantiomer). Products include:

Thioridazine Hydrochloride Tablets 2195

Tolazamide (Beta-blockers may mask some of the manifestations of hypoglycemia, particularly tachycardia; nonselective beta-blockers may potentiate insulin-induced hypoglycemia and delay recovery of serum glucose levels; in congestive heart failure patients with diabetes, carvedilol therapy may lead to worsening of hyperglycemia, which responds to intensification of hypoglycemia).

No products indexed under this heading.

Tolbutamide (Beta-blockers may mask some of the manifestations of hypoglycemia, particularly tachycardia; nonselective beta-blockers may potentiate insulin-induced hypoglycemia and delay recovery of serum glucose levels; in congestive heart failure patients with diabetes, carvedilol therapy may lead to worsening of hyperglycemia, which responds to intensification of hypoglycemia).

No products indexed under this heading.

Torsemide (Concomitant administration with a diuretic can be expected to produce additive effects and exaggerate the orthostatic component of carvedilol action). Products include:

Demadex Injection 2630
Demadex Tablets 2630

Tranylcypromine Sulfate (Patients receiving agents with beta-blocking properties and a drug that may deplete catecholamines (e.g., MAO Inhibitors) should be observed closely for signs of hypotension and/or severe bradycardia). Products include:

Parnate Tablets 1532

Triamterene (Concomitant administration with a diuretic can be expected to produce additive effects and exaggerate the orthostatic component of carvedilol action). Products include:

Dyazide Capsules 1405
Dyrenium Capsules 3189

Trimipramine Maleate (Interactions of carvedilol with strong inhibitors of CYP2D6, such as quinidine, have not been studied, but these drugs would be expected to increase blood levels of the R(+) enantiomer of carvedilol. Analysis of side effects showed that poor 2D6 metabolizers had a higher rate of dizziness during up-titration, presumably resulting from vasodilating effects of the higher concentrations of the alpha-blocking R(+) enantiomer).

No products indexed under this heading.

Troglitazone (Beta-blockers may mask some of the manifestations of hypoglycemia, particularly tachycardia; nonselective beta-blockers may potentiate insulin-induced hypoglycemia and delay recovery of serum glucose levels; in congestive heart failure patients with diabetes, carvedilol therapy may lead to worsening of hyperglycemia, which responds to intensification of hypoglycemia).

No products indexed under this heading.

Vardenafil Hydrochloride (Interactions of carvedilol with strong inhibitors of CYP2D6, such as quinidine, have not been studied, but these drugs would be expected to increase blood levels of the R(+) enantiomer of carvedilol. Analysis of side effects showed that poor 2D6 metabolizers had a higher rate of dizziness during up-titration, presumably resulting from vasodilating effects of the higher concentrations of the alpha-blocking R(+) enantiomer). Products include:

Levitra Tablets 2876

Verapamil Hydrochloride (Co-administration has resulted in isolated cases of conduction disturbances, rarely with hemodynamic. Monitoring of ECG and blood pressure is recommended). Products include:

Tarka Tablets 511

Food Interactions

Food, unspecified (When carvedilol is administered with food, the rate of absorption is slowed, as evidenced by a delay in the time to reach peak plasma levels, with no significant difference in extent of bioavailability; patients should be instructed to take Coreg with food in order to minimize the risk of hypotension).

COREG CR EXTENDED-RELEASE CAPSULES

(Carvedilol Phosphate) 1393

May interact with beta blockers, catecholamine depleting drugs, cytochrome p450 2d6 inhibitors (selected), epinephrine-containing products, oral hypoglycemic agents, insulin, monoamine oxidase inhibitors, quinidine, and certain other agents. Compounds in these categories include:

Acarbose (Agents with beta-blocking properties may enhance the blood sugar-reducing effect of insulin and oral hypoglycemics. Therefore, in patients taking insulin or hypoglycemics, regular monitoring of blood glucose is recommended). Products include:

Precose Tablets 792

Acebutolol Hydrochloride (Beta blockers slow atrioventricular conduction and decrease heart rate. Concomitant use can increase the risk of bradycardia).

No products indexed under this heading.

Amiodarone Hydrochloride (Interactions of carvedilol with strong inhibitors of CYP2D6, such as quinidine, have not been studied, but these drugs would be expected to increase blood levels of the R(+) enantiomer of carvedilol. Analysis of side effects showed that poor 2D6 metabolizers had a higher rate of dizziness during up-titration, presumably resulting from vasodilating effects of the higher concentrations of the alpha-blocking R(+) enantiomer).

No products indexed under this heading.

Amitriptyline Hydrochloride (Interactions of carvedilol with strong inhibitors of CYP2D6, such as quinidine, have not been studied, but these drugs would be expected to increase blood levels of the R(+) enantiomer of carvedilol. Analysis of side effects showed that poor 2D6 metabolizers had a higher rate of dizziness during up-titration, presumably resulting from vasodilating effects of the higher concentrations of the alpha-blocking R(+) enantiomer).

No products indexed under this heading.

Amoxapine (Interactions of carvedilol with strong inhibitors of CYP2D6, such as quinidine, have not been studied, but these drugs would be expected to increase blood levels of the R(+) enantiomer of carvedilol. Analysis of side effects showed that poor 2D6 metabolizers had a higher rate of dizziness during up-titration, presumably resulting from vasodilating effects of the higher concentrations of the alpha-blocking R(+) enantiomer).

No products indexed under this heading.

Atenolol (Beta blockers slow atrioventricular conduction and decrease heart rate. Concomitant use can increase the risk of bradycardia).

No products indexed under this heading.

Betaxolol Hydrochloride (Beta blockers slow atrioventricular conduction and decrease heart rate. Concomitant use can increase the risk of bradycardia).

No products indexed under this heading.

Bisoprolol Fumarate (Beta blockers slow atrioventricular conduction and decrease heart rate. Concomitant use can increase the risk of bradycardia).

No products indexed under this heading.

Bupropion Hydrochloride (Interactions of carvedilol with strong inhibitors of CYP2D6, such as quinidine, have not been studied, but these drugs would be expected to increase blood levels of the R(+) enantiomer of carvedilol. Analysis of side effects showed that poor 2D6 metabolizers had a higher rate of dizziness during up-titration, presumably resulting from vasodilating effects of the higher concentrations of the alpha-blocking R(+) enantiomer). Products include:

Wellbutrin Tablets 1648
Wellbutrin SR Sustained-Release Tablets 1653
Wellbutrin XL Extended-Release Tablets 1659
Zyban Sustained-Release Tablets 1692

Carteolol Hydrochloride (Beta blockers slow atrioventricular conduction and decrease heart rate. Concomitant use can increase the risk of bradycardia).

No products indexed under this heading.

Celecoxib (Interactions of carvedilol with strong inhibitors of CYP2D6, such as quinidine, have not been studied, but these drugs would be expected to increase blood levels of the R(+) enantiomer of carvedilol. Analysis of side effects showed that poor 2D6 metabolizers had a higher rate of dizziness during up-titration, presumably resulting from vasodilating effects of the higher concentrations of the alpha-blocking R(+) enantiomer). Products include:

Celebrex Capsules 2979

Chloroquine Hydrochloride (Interactions of carvedilol with strong inhibitors of CYP2D6, such as quinidine, have not been studied, but these drugs would be expected to increase blood levels of the R(+) enantiomer of carvedilol. Analysis of side effects showed that poor 2D6

metabolizers had a higher rate of dizziness during up-titration, presumably resulting from vasodilating effects of the higher concentrations of the alpha-blocking R(+) enantiomer).
No products indexed under this heading.

Chloroquine Phosphate (Interactions of carvedilol with strong inhibitors of CYP2D6, such as quinidine, have not been studied, but these drugs would be expected to increase blood levels of the R(+) enantiomer of carvedilol. Analysis of side effects showed that poor 2D6 metabolizers had a higher rate of dizziness during up-titration, presumably resulting from vasodilating effects of the higher concentrations of the alpha-blocking R(+) enantiomer).
No products indexed under this heading.

Chlorpheniramine (Interactions of carvedilol with strong inhibitors of CYP2D6, such as quinidine, have not been studied, but these drugs would be expected to increase blood levels of the R(+) enantiomer of carvedilol. Analysis of side effects showed that poor 2D6 metabolizers had a higher rate of dizziness during up-titration, presumably resulting from vasodilating effects of the higher concentrations of the alpha-blocking R(+) enantiomer).
No products indexed under this heading.

Chlorpheniramine Maleate (Interactions of carvedilol with strong inhibitors of CYP2D6, such as quinidine, have not been studied, but these drugs would be expected to increase blood levels of the R(+) enantiomer of carvedilol. Analysis of side effects showed that poor 2D6 metabolizers had a higher rate of dizziness during up-titration, presumably resulting from vasodilating effects of the higher concentrations of the alpha-blocking R(+) enantiomer). Products include:
Actifed Cold & Allergy Tablets 1895
Sudafed PE Sinus & Allergy Tablets 1908
Tylenol Allergy Multi-Symptom Caplets with Cool Burst and Rapid Release Gelcaps 1916
Children's Tylenol Plus Cold Suspension Liquid 1912
Children's Tylenol Plus Cough & Runny Nose Suspension Liquid 1912
Children's Tylenol Plus Flu Suspension Liquid 1914
Children's Tylenol Plus Multi-Symptom Cold Suspension Liquid 1912
Tylenol Cold Head Congestion Nighttime Caplets with Cool Burst 1910
Tylenol Cold Multi-Symptom Nighttime Caplets with Cool Burst 1913
Tylenol Sinus Congestion & Pain Nighttime Caplets with Cool Burst 1917

Chlorpheniramine Polistirex (Interactions of carvedilol with strong inhibitors of CYP2D6, such as quinidine, have not been studied, but these drugs would be expected to increase blood levels of the R(+) enantiomer of carvedilol. Analysis of side effects showed that poor 2D6 metabolizers had a higher rate of dizziness during up-titration, presumably resulting from vasodilating effects of the higher concentrations of the alpha-blocking R(+) enantiomer). Products include:
Tussionex Pennkinetic Extended-Release Suspension 3154

Chlorpheniramine Tannate (Interactions of carvedilol with strong inhibitors of CYP2D6, such as quinidine, have not been studied, but these drugs would be expected to increase blood levels of the R(+) enantiomer of carvedilol. Analysis of side effects showed that poor 2D6 metabolizers had a higher rate of dizziness during up-titration, presumably resulting from vasodilating effects of the higher concentrations of the alpha-blocking R(+) enantiomer).
No products indexed under this heading.

Chlorpropamide (Agents with beta-blocking properties may enhance the blood sugar-reducing effect of insulin and oral hypoglycemics. Therefore, in patients taking insulin or hypoglycemics, regular monitoring of blood glucose is recommended).
No products indexed under this heading.

Cimetidine (Carvedilol undergoes substantial oxidative metabolism; co-administration has resulted in increased steady-state AUC of carvedilol by about 30% with no change in Cmax).
No products indexed under this heading.

Cimetidine Hydrochloride (Carvedilol undergoes substantial oxidative metabolism; co-administration has resulted in increased steady-state AUC of carvedilol by about 30% with no change in Cmax).
No products indexed under this heading.

Citalopram Hydrobromide (Interactions of carvedilol with strong inhibitors of CYP2D6, such as quinidine, have not been studied, but these drugs would be expected to increase blood levels of the R(+) enantiomer of carvedilol. Analysis of side effects showed that poor 2D6 metabolizers had a higher rate of dizziness during up-titration, presumably resulting from vasodilating effects of the higher concentrations of the alpha-blocking R(+) enantiomer). Products include:
Celexa 1160

Clomipramine Hydrochloride (Interactions of carvedilol with strong inhibitors of CYP2D6, such as quinidine, have not been studied, but these drugs would be expected to increase blood levels of the R(+) enantiomer of carvedilol. Analysis of side effects showed that poor 2D6 metabolizers had a higher rate of dizziness during up-titration, presumably resulting from vasodilating effects of the higher concentrations of the alpha-blocking R(+) enantiomer).
No products indexed under this heading.

Clonidine (Concomitant administration of clonidine with agents with beta-blocking properties may potentiate blood pressure and heart rate-lowering effects. When concomitant treatment with agents with beta-blocking properties and clonidine is to be terminated, the beta-blocking agent should be discontinued first. Clonidine therapy can then be discontinued several days later by gradually decreasing the dosage). Products include:
Catapres-TTS 842

Clonidine Hydrochloride (Concomitant administration of clonidine with agents with beta-blocking properties may potentiate blood pressure and heart rate-lowering effects. When concomitant treatment with agents with β-blocking properties and clonidine is to be terminated, the β-blocking agent should be discontinued first. Clonidine therapy can then be discontinued several days later by gradually decreasing the dosage). Products include:
Catapres Tablets 841
Clorpres Tablets 2185

Cocaine Hydrochloride (Interactions of carvedilol with strong inhibitors of CYP2D6, such as quinidine, have not been studied, but these drugs would be expected to increase blood levels of the R(+) enantiomer of carvedilol. Analysis of side effects showed that poor 2D6 metabolizers had a higher rate of dizziness during up-titration, presumably resulting from vasodilating effects of the higher concentrations of the alpha-blocking R(+) enantiomer).
No products indexed under this heading.

Cyclosporine (Co-administration in renal transplant patients has resulted in a modest increase in mean trough cyclosporine concentrations; dose of cyclosporine may need to be reduced in some patients. Due to wide interindividual variablility in the dose adjustment required, it is recommended that cyclosporine concentrations be monitored closely after initiation of carvedilol therapy and that the dose of cyclosporine be adjusted as appropriate). Products include:
Gengraf Capsules 435
Neoral Oral Solution 2280
Neoral Soft Gelatin Capsules 2280
Restasis Ophthalmic Emulsion 557
Sandimmune 2296

Deserpidine (Patients receiving agents with beta-blocking properties and a drug that may deplete catecholamines should be observed closely for signs of hypotension and/or severe bradycardia).
No products indexed under this heading.

Desipramine Hydrochloride (Interactions of carvedilol with strong inhibitors of CYP2D6, such as quinidine, have not been studied, but these drugs would be expected to increase blood levels of the R(+) enantiomer of carvedilol. Analysis of side effects showed that poor 2D6 metabolizers had a higher rate of dizziness during up-titration, presumably resulting from vasodilating effects of the higher concentrations of the alpha-blocking R(+) enantiomer).
No products indexed under this heading.

Digoxin (Digitalis glycosides slow atrioventricular conduction and decrease heart rate. Concomitant use can increase the risk of bradycardia. Co-administration increases digoxin concentraton by 15%. Therefore, increased monitoring of digoxin is recommended when initiating, adjusting or discontinuing carvedilol). Products include:
Lanoxin Injection 1498
Lanoxin Injection Pediatric 1502
Lanoxin Tablets 1505

Diltiazem Hydrochloride (Isolated cases of conduction disturbances (rarely with hemodynamic compromise) have been observed when carvedilol is co-administered with diltiazem. As with other agents with beta-blocking properties, if carvedilol is to be administered orally with calcium channel blockers of the verapamil or diltiazem type, it is recommended that ECG and blood pressure be monitored). Products include:
Cardizem LA Extended Release Tablets 421

Diltiazem Maleate (Isolated cases of conduction disturbances (rarely with hemodynamic compromise) have been observed when carvedilol is co-administered with diltiazem. As with other agents with beta-blocking properties, if carvedilol is to be administered orally with calcium channel blockers of the verapamil or diltiazem type, it is recommended that ECG and blood pressure be monitored).
No products indexed under this heading.

Diphenhydramine (Interactions of carvedilol with strong inhibitors of CYP2D6, such as quinidine, have not been studied, but these drugs would be expected to increase blood levels of the R(+) enantiomer of carvedilol. Analysis of side effects showed that poor 2D6 metabolizers had a higher rate of dizziness during up-titration, presumably resulting from vasodilating effects of the higher concentrations of the alpha-blocking R(+) enantiomer).
No products indexed under this heading.

Diphenhydramine Hydrochloride (Interactions of carvedilol with strong inhibitors of CYP2D6, such as quinidine, have not been studied, but these drugs would be expected to increase blood levels of the R(+) enantiomer of carvedilol. Analysis of side effects showed that poor 2D6 metabolizers had a higher rate of dizziness during up-titration, presumably resulting from vasodilating effects of the higher concentrations of the alpha-blocking R(+) enantiomer). Products include:
Benadryl Allergy & Cold Kapgels 1895
Benadryl Allergy & Sinus Headache Kapgels 1895
Benadryl Severe Allergy & Sinus Headache Caplets 1897
Benadryl Dye-Free Allergy Liqui-gels Softgels 1897
Benadryl Allergy Kapgels 1895
Benadryl Allergy Quick Dissolve Strips 1896
Benadryl Allergy Ultratab Tablets 1896
Children's Benadryl Dye-Free Allergy Liquid 1897
Children's Benadryl Allergy Fastmelts 1897
Children's Benadryl Allergy Liquid 1898
Children's Benadryl Allergy Perfect Measure 1896
Children's Benadryl-D Allergy & Sinus Liquid 1896
Benadryl-D Allergy & Sinus Tablet 1896
PediaCare Children's Allergy & Cold Liquid 1902
PediaCare Children's Allergy Liquid 1902
Simply Sleep Caplets 1905
Sudafed PE Nighttime Cold Caplets 1907
Sudafed PE Severe Cold Caplets 1908

Extra Strength Tylenol PM Caplets, Geltabs, Liquid, and Rapid Release Gels 1915
Tylenol Allergy Multi-Symptom Nighttime Caplets with Cool Burst 1916
Tylenol Severe Allergy Caplets 1916
Children's Tylenol Plus Cold & Allergy Suspension Liquid 1914
Tylenol Sore Throat Nighttime Liquid with Cool Burst 1918

Doxepin Hydrochloride (Interactions of carvedilol with strong inhibitors of CYP2D6, such as quinidine, have not been studied, but these drugs would be expected to increase blood levels of the R(+) enantiomer of carvedilol. Analysis of side effects showed that poor 2D6 metabolizers had a higher rate of dizziness during up-titration, presumably resulting from vasodilating effects of the higher concentrations of the alpha-blocking R(+) enantiomer).
No products indexed under this heading.

Epinephrine (Patients on beta-blocker therapy and with a history of severe anaphylactic reactions to a variety of allergens may be unresponsive to the usual doses of epinephrine used to treat allergic reactions). Products include:
EpiPen 1024

Epinephrine Bitartrate (Patients on beta-blocker therapy and with a history of severe anaphylactic reactions to a variety of allergens may be unresponsive to the usual doses of epinephrine used to treat allergic reactions).
No products indexed under this heading.

Epinephrine Hydrochloride (Potential for unresponsiveness to the usual dose of epinephrine used to treat allergic reactions).
No products indexed under this heading.

Escitalopram Oxalate (Interactions of carvedilol with strong inhibitors of CYP2D6, such as quinidine, have not been studied, but these drugs would be expected to increase blood levels of the R(+) enantiomer of carvedilol. Analysis of side effects showed that poor 2D6 metabolizers had a higher rate of dizziness during up-titration, presumably resulting from vasodilating effects of the higher concentrations of the alpha-blocking R(+) enantiomer). Products include:
Lexapro Oral Suspension 1174
Lexapro Tablets 1174

Esmolol Hydrochloride (Beta blockers slow atrioventricular conduction and decrease heart rate. Concomitant use can increase the risk of bradycardia).
No products indexed under this heading.

Ethanol (Concomitant administration of Coreg CR with alcohol may affect the modified release properties of Coreg CR, potentially resulting in a faster rate of release and higher than expected peak and lower than expected trough plasma concentrations of carvedilol phosphate. To avoid the potential for this interaction, the administration of Coreg CR with alcohol (including prescription and OTC medications that contain ethanol) should be separated by at least two hours).
No products indexed under this heading.

Ethyl Alcohol (Concomitant administration of Coreg CR with alcohol may affect the modified release properties of Coreg CR, potentially resulting in a faster rate of release and higher than expected peak and lower than expected trough plasma concentrations of carvedilol phosphate. To avoid the potential for this interaction, the administration of Coreg CR with alcohol (including prescription and OTC medications that contain ethanol) should be separated by at least two hours).
No products indexed under this heading.

Fluoxetine (Interactions of carvedilol with strong inhibitors of CYP2D6, such as quinidine, have not been studied, but these drugs would be expected to increase blood levels of the R(+) enantiomer of carvedilol. Analysis of side effects showed that poor 2D6 metabolizers had a higher rate of dizziness during up-titration, presumably resulting from vasodilating effects of the higher concentrations of the alpha-blocking R(+) enantiomer).
No products indexed under this heading.

Fluoxetine Hydrochloride (Interactions of carvedilol with strong inhibitors of CYP2D6, such as fluoxetine, have not been studied, but these drugs would be expected to increase blood levels of the R(+) enantiomer of carvedilol. Analysis of side effects showed that poor 2D6 metabolizers had a higher rate of dizziness during up-titration, presumably resulting from vasodilating effects of the higher concentrations of the alpha-blocking R(+) enantiomer). Products include:
Prozac Weekly Capsules 1852
Prozac Pulvules and Liquid 1852
Symbyax Capsules 1871

Fluphenazine Decanoate (Interactions of carvedilol with strong inhibitors of CYP2D6, such as quinidine, have not been studied, but these drugs would be expected to increase blood levels of the R(+) enantiomer of carvedilol. Analysis of side effects showed that poor 2D6 metabolizers had a higher rate of dizziness during up-titration, presumably resulting from vasodilating effects of the higher concentrations of the alpha-blocking R(+) enantiomer).
No products indexed under this heading.

Fluphenazine Enanthate (Interactions of carvedilol with strong inhibitors of CYP2D6, such as quinidine, have not been studied, but these drugs would be expected to increase blood levels of the R(+) enantiomer of carvedilol. Analysis of side effects showed that poor 2D6 metabolizers had a higher rate of dizziness during up-titration, presumably resulting from vasodilating effects of the higher concentrations of the alpha-blocking R(+) enantiomer).
No products indexed under this heading.

Fluphenazine Hydrochloride (Interactions of carvedilol with strong inhibitors of CYP2D6, such as quinidine, have not been studied, but these drugs would be expected to increase blood levels of the R(+) enantiomer of carvedilol. Analysis of side effects showed that poor 2D6 metabolizers had a higher rate of dizziness during up-titration, presumably resulting from vasodilating effects of the higher concentrations of the alpha-blocking R(+) enantiomer).
No products indexed under this heading.

Fluvoxamine Maleate (Interactions of carvedilol with strong inhibitors of CYP2D6, such as quinidine, have not been studied, but these drugs would be expected to increase blood levels of the R(+) enantiomer of carvedilol. Analysis of side effects showed that poor 2D6 metabolizers had a higher rate of dizziness during up-titration, presumably resulting from vasodilating effects of the higher concentrations of the alpha-blocking R(+) enantiomer). Products include:
Luvox CR Extended-Release Capsules 1759

Glimepiride (Agents with beta-blocking properties may enhance the blood sugar-reducing effect of insulin and oral hypoglycemics. Therefore, in patients taking insulin or hypoglycemics, regular monitoring of blood glucose is recommended). Products include:
Avandaryl Tablets 1344
Duetact Tablets 3085

Glipizide (Agents with beta-blocking properties may enhance the blood sugar-reducing effect of insulin and oral hypoglycemics. Therefore, in patients taking insulin or hypoglycemics, regular monitoring of blood glucose is recommended).
No products indexed under this heading.

Glyburide (Agents with beta-blocking properties may enhance the blood sugar-reducing effect of insulin and oral hypoglycemics. Therefore, in patients taking insulin or hypoglycemics, regular monitoring of blood glucose is recommended).
No products indexed under this heading.

Guanethidine Monosulfate (Patients receiving agents with beta-blocking properties and a drug that may deplete catecholamines should be observed closely for signs of hypotension and/or severe bradycardia).
No products indexed under this heading.

Halofantrine Hydrochloride (Interactions of carvedilol with strong inhibitors of CYP2D6, such as quinidine, have not been studied, but these drugs would be expected to increase blood levels of the R(+) enantiomer of carvedilol. Analysis of side effects showed that poor 2D6 metabolizers had a higher rate of dizziness during up-titration, presumably resulting from vasodilating effects of the higher concentrations of the alpha-blocking R(+) enantiomer).
No products indexed under this heading.

Haloperidol (Interactions of carvedilol with strong inhibitors of CYP2D6, such as quinidine, have not been studied, but these drugs would be expected to increase blood levels of the R(+) enantiomer of carvedilol. Analysis of side effects showed that poor 2D6 metabolizers had a higher rate of dizziness during up-titration, presumably resulting from vasodilating effects of the higher concentrations of the alpha-blocking R(+) enantiomer).
No products indexed under this heading.

Haloperidol Decanoate (Interactions of carvedilol with strong inhibitors of CYP2D6, such as quinidine, have not been studied, but these drugs would be expected to increase blood levels of the R(+) enantiomer of carvedilol. Analysis of side effects showed that poor 2D6 metabolizers had a higher rate of dizziness during up-titration, presumably resulting from vasodilating effects of the higher concentrations of the alpha-blocking R(+) enantiomer).
No products indexed under this heading.

Hydroxychloroquine Sulfate (Interactions of carvedilol with strong inhibitors of CYP2D6, such as quinidine, have not been studied, but these drugs would be expected to increase blood levels of the R(+) enantiomer of carvedilol. Analysis of side effects showed that poor 2D6 metabolizers had a higher rate of dizziness during up-titration, presumably resulting from vasodilating effects of the higher concentrations of the alpha-blocking R(+) enantiomer).
No products indexed under this heading.

Imatinib Mesylate (Interactions of carvedilol with strong inhibitors of CYP2D6, such as quinidine, have not been studied, but these drugs would be expected to increase blood levels of the R(+) enantiomer of carvedilol. Analysis of side effects showed that poor 2D6 metabolizers had a higher rate of dizziness during up-titration, presumably resulting from vasodilating effects of the higher concentrations of the alpha-blocking R(+) enantiomer). Products include:
Gleevec Tablets 2255

Imipramine Hydrochloride (Interactions of carvedilol with strong inhibitors of CYP2D6, such as quinidine, have not been studied, but these drugs would be expected to increase blood levels of the R(+) enantiomer of carvedilol. Analysis of side effects showed that poor 2D6 metabolizers had a higher rate of dizziness during up-titration, presumably resulting from vasodilating effects of the higher concentrations of the alpha-blocking R(+) enantiomer).
No products indexed under this heading.

Imipramine Pamoate (Interactions of carvedilol with strong inhibitors of CYP2D6, such as quinidine, have not been studied, but these drugs would be expected to increase blood levels of the R(+) enantiomer of carvedilol. Analysis of side effects showed that poor 2D6 metabolizers had a higher rate of dizziness during up-titration, presumably resulting from vasodilating effects of the higher concentrations of the alpha-blocking R(+) enantiomer).
No products indexed under this heading.

Insulin (Agents with beta-blocking properties may enhance the blood sugar-reducing effect of insulin and oral hypoglycemics. Therefore, in patients taking insulin or hypoglycemics, regular monitoring of blood glucose is recommended).
 No products indexed under this heading.

Insulin, Human, Zinc Suspension (Agents with beta-blocking properties may enhance the blood sugar-reducing effect of insulin and oral hypoglycemics. Therefore, in patients taking insulin or hypoglycemics, regular monitoring of blood glucose is recommended).
 No products indexed under this heading.

Insulin, Human (rDNA origin) (Agents with beta-blocking properties may enhance the blood sugar-reducing effect of insulin and oral hypoglycemics. Therefore, in patients taking insulin or hypoglycemics, regular monitoring of blood glucose is recommended). Products include:
 Exubera Inhalation Powder 2515

Insulin, Human NPH (Agents with beta-blocking properties may enhance the blood sugar-reducing effect of insulin and oral hypoglycemics. Therefore, in patients taking insulin or hypoglycemics, regular monitoring of blood glucose is recommended). Products include:
 Humulin N Vial 1846

Insulin, Human Regular (Agents with beta-blocking properties may enhance the blood sugar-reducing effect of insulin and oral hypoglycemics. Therefore, in patients taking insulin or hypoglycemics, regular monitoring of blood glucose is recommended). Products include:
 Humulin R 1849
 Humulin R (U-500) 1850

Insulin, Human Regular and Human NPH Mixture (Agents with beta-blocking properties may enhance the blood sugar-reducing effect of insulin and oral hypoglycemics. Therefore, in patients taking insulin or hypoglycemics, regular monitoring of blood glucose is recommended). Products include:
 Humulin 50/50, 100 Units 1843
 Humulin 70/30 Vial 1844

Insulin, NPH (Agents with beta-blocking properties may enhance the blood sugar-reducing effect of insulin and oral hypoglycemics. Therefore, in patients taking insulin or hypoglycemics, regular monitoring of blood glucose is recommended).
 No products indexed under this heading.

Insulin, Regular (Agents with beta-blocking properties may enhance the blood sugar-reducing effect of insulin and oral hypoglycemics. Therefore, in patients taking insulin or hypoglycemics, regular monitoring of blood glucose is recommended).
 No products indexed under this heading.

Insulin, Regular and NPH mixture (Agents with beta-blocking properties may enhance the blood sugar-reducing effect of insulin and oral hypoglycemics. Therefore, in patients taking insulin or hypoglycemics, regular monitoring of blood glucose is recommended).
 No products indexed under this heading.

Insulin, Zinc Crystals (Agents with beta-blocking properties may enhance the blood sugar-reducing effect of insulin and oral hypoglycemics. Therefore, in patients taking insulin or hypoglycemics, regular monitoring of blood glucose is recommended).
 No products indexed under this heading.

Insulin, Zinc Suspension (Agents with beta-blocking properties may enhance the blood sugar-reducing effect of insulin and oral hypoglycemics. Therefore, in patients taking insulin or hypoglycemics, regular monitoring of blood glucose is recommended).
 No products indexed under this heading.

Insulin Aspart (Agents with beta-blocking properties may enhance the blood sugar-reducing effect of insulin and oral hypoglycemics. Therefore, in patients taking insulin or hypoglycemics, regular monitoring of blood glucose is recommended).
 No products indexed under this heading.

Insulin Aspart, Human (Agents with beta-blocking properties may enhance the blood sugar-reducing effect of insulin and oral hypoglycemics. Therefore, in patients taking insulin or hypoglycemics, regular monitoring of blood glucose is recommended). Products include:
 NovoLog Mix 70/30 2364

Insulin Aspart, Human Regular (Agents with beta-blocking properties may enhance the blood sugar-reducing effect of insulin and oral hypoglycemics. Therefore, in patients taking insulin or hypoglycemics, regular monitoring of blood glucose is recommended). Products include:
 NovoLog Injection 2359

Insulin Aspart Protamine, Human (Agents with beta-blocking properties may enhance the blood sugar-reducing effect of insulin and oral hypoglycemics. Therefore, in patients taking insulin or hypoglycemics, regular monitoring of blood glucose is recommended). Products include:
 NovoLog Mix 70/30 2364

Insulin Detemir (rDNA Origin) (Agents with beta-blocking properties may enhance the blood sugar-reducing effect of insulin and oral hypoglycemics. Therefore, in patients taking insulin or hypoglycemics, regular monitoring of blood glucose is recommended). Products include:
 Levemir Injection 2352

Insulin glargine (Agents with beta-blocking properties may enhance the blood sugar-reducing effect of insulin and oral hypoglycemics. Therefore, in patients taking insulin or hypoglycemics, regular monitoring of blood glucose is recommended). Products include:
 Lantus Injection 2749

Insulin Glulisine (Agents with beta-blocking properties may enhance the blood sugar-reducing effect of insulin and oral hypoglycemics. Therefore, in patients taking insulin or hypoglycemics, regular monitoring of blood glucose is recommended). Products include:
 Apidra Injection 2706

Insulin Lispro, Human (Agents with beta-blocking properties may enhance the blood sugar-reducing effect of insulin and oral hypoglycemics. Therefore, in patients taking insulin or hypoglycemics, regular monitoring of blood glucose is recommended). Products include:
 Humalog-Pen and KwikPen 1829
 Humalog Mix 50/50-Pen and KwikPen 1833
 Humalog Mix 75/25-Pen and KwikPen 1835

Insulin Lispro Protamine, Human (Agents with beta-blocking properties may enhance the blood sugar-reducing effect of insulin and oral hypoglycemics. Therefore, in patients taking insulin or hypoglycemics, regular monitoring of blood glucose is recommended). Products include:
 Humalog Mix 50/50-Pen and KwikPen 1833
 Humalog Mix 75/25-Pen and KwikPen 1835

Isocarboxazid (Patients receiving agents with beta-blocking properties and a drug that may deplete catecholamines should be observed closely for signs of hypotension and/or severe bradycardia). Products include:
 Marplan Tablets 3177

Labetalol Hydrochloride (Beta blockers slow atrioventricular conduction and decrease heart rate. Concomitant use can increase the risk of bradycardia).
 No products indexed under this heading.

Levobunolol Hydrochloride (Beta blockers slow atrioventricular conduction and decrease heart rate. Concomitant use can increase the risk of bradycardia).
 No products indexed under this heading.

Maprotiline Hydrochloride (Interactions of carvedilol with strong inhibitors of CYP2D6, such as quinidine, have not been studied, but these drugs would be expected to increase blood levels of the R(+) enantiomer of carvedilol. Analysis of side effects showed that poor 2D6 metabolizers had a higher rate of dizziness during up-titration, presumably resulting from vasodilating effects of the higher concentrations of the alpha-blocking R(+) enantiomer).
 No products indexed under this heading.

Metformin Hydrochloride (Agents with beta-blocking properties may enhance the blood sugar-reducing effect of insulin and oral hypoglycemics. Therefore, in patients taking insulin or hypoglycemics, regular monitoring of blood glucose is recommended). Products include:
 ActoPlus Met Tablets 3071
 Avandamet Tablets 1336
 Janumet Tablets 2041
 PrandiMet Tablets 2967

Methadone Hydrochloride (Interactions of carvedilol with strong inhibitors of CYP2D6, such as quinidine, have not been studied, but these drugs would be expected to increase blood levels of the R(+) enantiomer of carvedilol. Analysis of side effects showed that poor 2D6 metabolizers had a higher rate of dizziness during up-titration, presumably resulting from vasodilating effects of the higher concentrations of the alpha-blocking R(+) enantiomer).
 No products indexed under this heading.

Metipranolol Hydrochloride (Beta blockers slow atrioventricular conduction and decrease heart rate. Concomitant use can increase the risk of bradycardia).
 No products indexed under this heading.

Metoprolol Succinate (Beta blockers slow atrioventricular conduction and decrease heart rate. Concomitant use can increase the risk of bradycardia). Products include:
 Toprol-XL Tablets 666

Metoprolol Tartrate (Beta blockers slow atrioventricular conduction and decrease heart rate. Concomitant use can increase the risk of bradycardia).
 No products indexed under this heading.

Mibefradil Dihydrochloride (Interactions of carvedilol with strong inhibitors of CYP2D6, such as quinidine, have not been studied, but these drugs would be expected to increase blood levels of the R(+) enantiomer of carvedilol. Analysis of side effects showed that poor 2D6 metabolizers had a higher rate of dizziness during up-titration, presumably resulting from vasodilating effects of the higher concentrations of the alpha-blocking R(+) enantiomer).
 No products indexed under this heading.

Miglitol (Agents with beta-blocking properties may enhance the blood sugar-reducing effect of insulin and oral hypoglycemics. Therefore, in patients taking insulin or hypoglycemics, regular monitoring of blood glucose is recommended).
 No products indexed under this heading.

Moclobemide (Patients receiving agents with beta-blocking properties and a drug that may deplete catecholamines should be observed closely for signs of hypotension and/or severe bradycardia).
 No products indexed under this heading.

Nadolol (Beta blockers slow atrioventricular conduction and decrease heart rate. Concomitant use can increase the risk of bradycardia). Products include:
 Nadolol Tablets 2191

Nateglinide (Agents with beta-blocking properties may enhance the blood sugar-reducing effect of insulin and oral hypoglycemics. Therefore, in patients taking insulin or hypoglycemics, regular monitoring of blood glucose is recommended). Products include:
 Starlix Tablets 2314

Nebivolol (Beta blockers slow atrioventricular conduction and decrease heart rate. Concomitant use can increase the risk of bradycardia). Products include:
 Bystolic Tablets 1155

Nortriptyline Hydrochloride (Interactions of carvedilol with strong inhibitors of CYP2D6, such as quinidine, have not been studied, but these drugs would be expected to increase blood levels of the R(+) enantiomer of carvedilol. Analysis of side effects showed that poor 2D6 metabolizers had a higher rate of dizziness during up-titration, presumably resulting from vasodilating effects of the higher concentrations of the alpha-blocking R(+) enantiomer).

No products indexed under this heading.

Pargyline Hydrochloride (Patients receiving agents with beta-blocking properties and a drug that may deplete catecholamines should be observed closely for signs of hypotension and/or severe bradycardia).

No products indexed under this heading.

Paroxetine Hydrochloride (Interactions of carvedilol with strong inhibitors of CYP2D6, such as paroxetine, have not been studied, but these drugs would be expected to increase blood levels of the R(+) enantiomer of carvedilol. Analysis of side effects showed that poor 2D6 metabolizers had a higher rate of dizziness during up-titration, presumably resulting from vasodilating effects of the higher concentrations of the alpha-blocking R(+) enantiomer). Products include:

Paxil 1535
Paxil CR Controlled-Release Tablets 1544

Penbutolol Sulfate (Beta blockers slow atrioventricular conduction and decrease heart rate. Concomitant use can increase the risk of bradycardia).

No products indexed under this heading.

Perphenazine (Interactions of carvedilol with strong inhibitors of CYP2D6, such as quinidine, have not been studied, but these drugs would be expected to increase blood levels of the R(+) enantiomer of carvedilol. Analysis of side effects showed that poor 2D6 metabolizers had a higher rate of dizziness during up-titration, presumably resulting from vasodilating effects of the higher concentrations of the alpha-blocking R(+) enantiomer).

No products indexed under this heading.

Phenelzine Sulfate (Patients receiving agents with beta-blocking properties and a drug that may deplete catecholamines should be observed closely for signs of hypotension and/or severe bradycardia).

No products indexed under this heading.

Pindolol (Beta blockers slow atrioventricular conduction and decrease heart rate. Concomitant use can increase the risk of bradycardia).

No products indexed under this heading.

Pioglitazone Hydrochloride (Agents with beta-blocking properties may enhance the blood sugar-reducing effect of insulin and oral hypoglycemics. Therefore, in patients taking insulin or hypoglycemics, regular monitoring of blood glucose is recommended). Products include:

ActoPlus Met Tablets 3071
Actos Tablets 3077
Duetact Tablets 3085

Procarbazine Hydrochloride (Patients receiving agents with beta-blocking properties and a drug that may deplete catecholamines should be observed closely for signs of hypotension and/or severe bradycardia).

No products indexed under this heading.

Propafenone Hydrochloride (Interactions of carvedilol with strong inhibitors of CYP2D6, such as propafenone, have not been studied, but these drugs would be expected to increase blood levels of the R(+) enantiomer of carvedilol. Analysis of side effects showed that poor 2D6 metabolizers had a higher rate of dizziness during up-titration, presumably resulting from vasodilating effects of the higher concentrations of the alpha-blocking R(+) enantiomer). Products include:

Rythmol Tablets 1586
Rythmol SR Capsules 1590

Propoxyphene Hydrochloride (Interactions of carvedilol with strong inhibitors of CYP2D6, such as quinidine, have not been studied, but these drugs would be expected to increase blood levels of the R(+) enantiomer of carvedilol. Analysis of side effects showed that poor 2D6 metabolizers had a higher rate of dizziness during up-titration, presumably resulting from vasodilating effects of the higher concentrations of the alpha-blocking R(+) enantiomer).

No products indexed under this heading.

Propoxyphene Napsylate (Interactions of carvedilol with strong inhibitors of CYP2D6, such as quinidine, have not been studied, but these drugs would be expected to increase blood levels of the R(+) enantiomer of carvedilol. Analysis of side effects showed that poor 2D6 metabolizers had a higher rate of dizziness during up-titration, presumably resulting from vasodilating effects of the higher concentrations of the alpha-blocking R(+) enantiomer).

No products indexed under this heading.

Propranolol Hydrochloride (Beta blockers slow atrioventricular conduction and decrease heart rate. Concomitant use can increase the risk of bradycardia). Products include:

InnoPran XL Extended Release Capsules 1484

Protriptyline Hydrochloride (Interactions of carvedilol with strong inhibitors of CYP2D6, such as quinidine, have not been studied, but these drugs would be expected to increase blood levels of the R(+) enantiomer of carvedilol. Analysis of side effects showed that poor 2D6 metabolizers had a higher rate of dizziness during up-titration, presumably resulting from vasodilating effects of the higher concentrations of the alpha-blocking R(+) enantiomer).

No products indexed under this heading.

Quinacrine Hydrochloride (Interactions of carvedilol with strong inhibitors of CYP2D6, such as quinidine, have not been studied, but these drugs would be expected to increase blood levels of the R(+) enantiomer of carvedilol. Analysis of side effects showed that poor 2D6 metabolizers had a higher rate of dizziness during up-titration, presumably resulting from vasodilating effects of the higher concentrations of the alpha-blocking R(+) enantiomer).

No products indexed under this heading.

Quinidine (Co-administration of carvedilol with strong inhibitors of CYP2D6, such as quinidine, have not been studied, but quinidine would be expected to increase blood levels).

No products indexed under this heading.

Quinidine Gluconate (Co-administration of carvedilol with strong inhibitors of CYP2D6, such as quinidine, have not been studied, but quinidine would be expected to increase blood levels).

No products indexed under this heading.

Quinidine Hydrochloride (Co-administration of carvedilol with strong inhibitors of CYP2D6, such as quinidine, have not been studied, but quinidine would be expected to increase blood levels).

No products indexed under this heading.

Quinidine Polygalacturonate (Co-administration of carvedilol with strong inhibitors of CYP2D6, such as quinidine, have not been studied, but quinidine would be expected to increase blood levels).

No products indexed under this heading.

Quinidine Sulfate (Co-administration of carvedilol with strong inhibitors of CYP2D6, such as quinidine, have not been studied, but quinidine would be expected to increase blood levels).

No products indexed under this heading.

Ranitidine Bismuth Citrate (Interactions of carvedilol with strong inhibitors of CYP2D6, such as quinidine, have not been studied, but these drugs would be expected to increase blood levels of the R(+) enantiomer of carvedilol. Analysis of side effects showed that poor 2D6 metabolizers had a higher rate of dizziness during up-titration, presumably resulting from vasodilating effects of the higher concentrations of the alpha-blocking R(+) enantiomer).

No products indexed under this heading.

Ranitidine Hydrochloride (Interactions of carvedilol with strong inhibitors of CYP2D6, such as quinidine, have not been studied, but these drugs would be expected to increase blood levels of the R(+) enantiomer of carvedilol. Analysis of side effects showed that poor 2D6 metabolizers had a higher rate of dizziness during up-titration, presumably resulting from vasodilating effects of the higher concentrations of the alpha-blocking R(+) enantiomer). Products include:

Zantac 75 Tablets 603
Zantac 1670
Zantac Injection 1666
Zantac Injection Pharmacy Bulk Package 1668
Maximum Strength Zantac 150 Tablets 603
Maximum Strength Zantac 150 Cool Mint Tablets 603

Rasagiline Mesylate (Patients receiving agents with beta-blocking properties and a drug that may deplete catecholamines should be observed closely for signs of hypotension and/or severe bradycardia). Products include:

Azilect Tablets 3106

Rauwolfia Serpentina (Patients receiving agents with beta-blocking properties and a drug that may deplete catecholamines should be observed closely for signs of hypotension and/or severe bradycardia).

No products indexed under this heading.

Repaglinide (Agents with beta-blocking properties may enhance the blood sugar-reducing effect of insulin and oral hypoglycemics. Therefore, in patients taking insulin or hypoglycemics, regular monitoring of blood glucose is recommended). Products include:

PrandiMet Tablets 2967
Prandin Tablets 2971

Rescinnamine (Patients receiving agents with beta-blocking properties and a drug that may deplete catecholamines should be observed closely for signs of hypotension and/or severe bradycardia).

No products indexed under this heading.

Reserpine (Co-administration of agents with beta-blocking properties and a drug that can deplete catecholamines, such as reserpine, may result in hypotension and/or severe bradycardia).

No products indexed under this heading.

Rifampin (Carvedilol undergoes substantial oxidative metabolism, co-administration has resulted in decreased AUC and Cmax of carvedilol by about 70%).

No products indexed under this heading.

Ritonavir (Interactions of carvedilol with strong inhibitors of CYP2D6, such as quinidine, have not been studied, but these drugs would be expected to increase blood levels of the R(+) enantiomer of carvedilol. Analysis of side effects showed that poor 2D6 metabolizers had a higher rate of dizziness during up-titration, presumably resulting from vasodilating effects of the higher concentrations of the alpha-blocking R(+) enantiomer). Products include:

Kaletra 452
Norvir 489

Rosiglitazone Maleate (Agents with beta-blocking properties may enhance the blood sugar-reducing effect of insulin and oral hypoglycemics. Therefore, in patients taking insulin or hypoglycemics, regular monitoring of blood glucose is recommended). Products include:

Avandamet Tablets 1336
Avandaryl Tablets 1344
Avandia Tablets 1351

Selegiline (Patients receiving agents with beta-blocking properties and a drug that may deplete catecholamines should be observed closely for signs of hypotension and/or severe bradycardia). Products include:

Emsam Transdermal System 905

Selegiline Hydrochloride (Patients receiving agents with beta-blocking properties and a drug that may deplete catecholamines should be observed closely for signs of hypotension and/or severe bradycardia). Products include:

Eldepryl Capsules 3052

Sertraline Hydrochloride (Interactions of carvedilol with strong inhibitors of CYP2D6, such as quinidine, have not been studied, but these drugs would be expected to increase blood levels of the R(+) enantiomer of carvedilol. Analysis of side effects showed that poor 2D6 metabolizers had a higher rate of dizziness during up-titration, presumably resulting from vasodilating effects of the higher concentrations of the alpha-blocking R(+) enantiomer).

No products indexed under this heading.

Sildenafil Citrate (Interactions of carvedilol with strong inhibitors of CYP2D6, such as quinidine, have not been studied, but these drugs would be expected to increase blood levels of the R(+) enantiomer of carvedilol. Analysis of side effects showed that poor 2D6 metabolizers had a higher rate of dizziness during up-titration, presumably resulting from vasodilating effects of the higher concentrations of the alpha-blocking R(+) enantiomer).

No products indexed under this heading.

Sitagliptin Phosphate (Agents with beta-blocking properties may enhance the blood sugar-reducing effect of insulin and oral hypoglycemics. Therefore, in patients taking insulin or hypoglycemics, regular monitoring of blood glucose is recommended). Products include:

Janumet Tablets 2041
Januvia Tablets 2048

Sotalol Hydrochloride (Beta blockers slow atrioventricular conduction and decrease heart rate. Concomitant use can increase the risk of bradycardia).

No products indexed under this heading.

Terbinafine Hydrochloride (Interactions of carvedilol with strong inhibitors of CYP2D6, such as quinidine, have not been studied, but these drugs would be expected to increase blood levels of the R(+) enantiomer of carvedilol. Analysis of side effects showed that poor 2D6 metabolizers had a higher rate of dizziness during up-titration, presumably resulting from vasodilating effects of the higher concentrations of the alpha-blocking R(+) enantiomer). Products include:

Lamisil Oral Granules 2264
Lamisil Tablets 2266

Thioridazine Hydrochloride (Interactions of carvedilol with strong inhibitors of CYP2D6, such as quinidine, have not been studied, but these drugs would be expected to increase blood levels of the R(+) enantiomer of carvedilol. Analysis of side effects showed that poor 2D6 metabolizers had a higher rate of dizziness during up-titration, presumably resulting from vasodilating effects of the higher concentrations of the alpha-blocking R(+) enantiomer). Products include:

Thioridazine Hydrochloride Tablets 2195

Timolol Hemihydrate (Beta blockers slow atrioventricular conduction and decrease heart rate. Concomitant use can increase the risk of bradycardia). Products include:

Betimol Ophthalmic Solution 3181

Timolol Maleate (Beta blockers slow atrioventricular conduction and decrease heart rate. Concomitant use can increase the risk of bradycardia). Products include:

Combigan Ophthalmic Solution 553
Cosopt Sterile Ophthalmic Solution 1969
Timoptic Sterile Ophthalmic Solution 2121
Timoptic in Ocudose 2124
Timoptic-XE Sterile Ophthalmic Gel Forming Solution 2125

Tolazamide (Agents with beta-blocking properties may enhance the blood sugar-reducing effect of insulin and oral hypoglycemics. Therefore, in patients taking insulin or hypoglycemics, regular monitoring of blood glucose is recommended).

No products indexed under this heading.

Tolbutamide (Agents with beta-blocking properties may enhance the blood sugar-reducing effect of insulin and oral hypoglycemics. Therefore, in patients taking insulin or hypoglycemics, regular monitoring of blood glucose is recommended).

No products indexed under this heading.

Tranylcypromine Sulfate (Patients receiving agents with beta-blocking properties and a drug that may deplete catecholamines should be observed closely for signs of hypotension and/or severe bradycardia). Products include:

Parnate Tablets 1532

Trimipramine Maleate (Interactions of carvedilol with strong inhibitors of CYP2D6, such as quinidine, have not been studied, but these drugs would be expected to increase blood levels of the R(+) enantiomer of carvedilol. Analysis of side effects showed that poor 2D6 metabolizers had a higher rate of dizziness during up-titration, presumably resulting from vasodilating effects of the higher concentrations of the alpha-blocking R(+) enantiomer).

No products indexed under this heading.

Troglitazone (Agents with beta-blocking properties may enhance the blood sugar-reducing effect of insulin and oral hypoglycemics. Therefore, in patients taking insulin or hypoglycemics, regular monitoring of blood glucose is recommended).

No products indexed under this heading.

Vardenafil Hydrochloride (Interactions of carvedilol with strong inhibitors of CYP2D6, such as quinidine, have not been studied, but these drugs would be expected to increase blood levels of the R(+) enantiomer of carvedilol. Analysis of side effects showed that poor 2D6 metabolizers had a higher rate of dizziness during up-titration, presumably resulting from vasodilating effects of the higher concentrations of the alpha-blocking R(+) enantiomer). Products include:

Levitra Tablets 2876

Verapamil Hydrochloride (Isolated cases of conduction disturbances (rarely with hemodynamic compromise) have been observed when carvedilol is co-administered with diltiazem. As with other agents with beta-blocking properties, if carvedilol is to be administered orally with calcium channel blockers of the verapamil or diltiazem type, it is recommended that ECG and blood pressure be monitored). Products include:

Tarka Tablets 511

Food Interactions

Alcohol (Concomitant administration of Coreg CR with alcohol may affect the modified release properties of Coreg CR, potentially resulting in a faster rate of release and higher than expected peak and lower than expected trough plasma concentrations of carvedilol phosphate. To avoid the potential for this interaction, the administration of Coreg CR with alcohol (including prescription and OTC medications that contain ethanol) should be separated by at least two hours).

Food, unspecified (Administration of Coreg CR with a high-fat meal resulted in increases in AUC (~20%) and Cmax compared to Coreg CR administered with a standard meal. Decreases in AUC (27%) and Cmax (43%) were observed when Coreg CR was administered in the fasting state compared to administration after a standard meal. Coreg CR should be taken with food).

COSMEGEN FOR INJECTION

(Dactinomycin) 2485

May interact with vaccines, live. Compounds in these categories include:

BCG Vaccine (Live virus vaccines should not be administered during drug therapy with dactinomycin).

No products indexed under this heading.

Influenza Vaccine, Live Attenuated (Live virus vaccines should not be administered during drug therapy with dactinomycin).

No products indexed under this heading.

Influenza Virus Vaccine Live, Intranasal (Live virus vaccines should not be administered during drug therapy with dactinomycin). Products include:

FluMist Vaccine 1945

Measles, Mumps, Rubella and Varicella Virus Vaccine Live (Live virus vaccines should not be administered during drug therapy with dactinomycin). Products include:

ProQuad 2099

Measles, Mumps & Rubella Virus Vaccine, Live (Live virus vaccines should not be administered during drug therapy with dactinomycin). Products include:

M-M-R II 2054

Measles & Rubella Virus Vaccine Live (Live virus vaccines should not be administered during drug therapy with dactinomycin).

No products indexed under this heading.

Measles Virus Vaccine Live (Live virus vaccines should not be administered during drug therapy with dactinomycin). Products include:

Attenuvax 1951

Mumps Virus Vaccine, Live (Live virus vaccines should not be administered during drug therapy with dactinomycin). Products include:

Mumpsvax 2068

Poliovirus Vaccine, Live, Oral, Trivalent, Types 1,2,3 (Sabin) (Live virus vaccines should not be administered during drug therapy with dactinomycin).

No products indexed under this heading.

Rotavirus Vaccine, Live, Oral, Tetravalent (Live virus vaccines should not be administered during drug therapy with dactinomycin).

No products indexed under this heading.

Rubella & Mumps Virus Vaccine Live (Live virus vaccines should not be administered during drug therapy with dactinomycin).

No products indexed under this heading.

Rubella Virus Vaccine Live (Live virus vaccines should not be administered during drug therapy with dactinomycin). Products include:

Meruvax II 2061

Smallpox Vaccine (Live virus vaccines should not be administered during drug therapy with dactinomycin).

No products indexed under this heading.

Typhoid Vaccine (Live virus vaccines should not be administered during drug therapy with dactinomycin).

No products indexed under this heading.

Varicella Virus Vaccine Live (Live virus vaccines should not be administered during drug therapy with dactinomycin). Products include:

Varivax 2133

Yellow Fever Vaccine (Live virus vaccines should not be administered during drug therapy with dactinomycin).

No products indexed under this heading.

Zoster Vaccine Live (Live virus vaccines should not be administered during drug therapy with dactinomycin). Products include:

Zostavax Injection 2145

COSOPT STERILE OPHTHALMIC SOLUTION

(Dorzolamide Hydrochloride, Timolol Maleate) 1969

May interact with beta blockers, carbonic anhydrase inhibitors, calcium channel blockers, cardiac glycosides, quinidine, salicylates, and certain other agents. Compounds in these categories include:

Acebutolol Hydrochloride (Co-administration of oral beta-adrenergic blockers and Cosopt may result in potential additive effects of beta-blockade, both systemic and on intraocular pressure).

No products indexed under this heading.

Acetazolamide (Co-administration with oral carbonic anhydrase inhibitor may result in additive carbonic anhydrase inhibition).

No products indexed under this heading.

Amlodipine Besylate (Co-administration of beta-adrenergic blockers and calcium channel blockers may result in possible atrioventricular conduction disturbances, left ventricular failure, and hypotension). Products include:

Azor Tablets 1005
Exforge Tablets 2238

Aspirin (Potential for acid-base and electrolyte disturbances with high-dose salicylate therapy). Products include:

Aggrenox Capsules 819
Bayer Aspirin 750
Percodan Tablets 1130

St. Joseph 81 mg Aspirin Chewable and Enteric Coated Tablets 1903

Aspirin, Enteric Coated (Potential for acid-base and electrolyte disturbances with high-dose salicylate therapy).
No products indexed under this heading.

Aspirin Buffered (Potential for acid-base and electrolyte disturbances with high-dose salicylate therapy).
No products indexed under this heading.

Atenolol (Co-administration of oral beta-adrenergic blockers and Cosopt may result in potential additive effects of beta-blockade, both systemic and on intraocular pressure).
No products indexed under this heading.

Bepridil Hydrochloride (Co-administration of beta-adrenergic blockers and calcium channel blockers may result in possible atrioventricular conduction disturbances, left ventricular failure, and hypotension).
No products indexed under this heading.

Betaxolol Hydrochloride (Co-administration of oral beta-adrenergic blockers and Cosopt may result in potential additive effects of beta-blockade, both systemic and on intraocular pressure; the concomitant use of two topical beta-adrenergic agents is not recommended).
No products indexed under this heading.

Carteolol Hydrochloride (Co-administration of oral beta-adrenergic blockers and Cosopt may result in potential additive effects of beta-blockade, both systemic and on intraocular pressure; the concomitant use of two topical beta-adrenergic agents is not recommended).
No products indexed under this heading.

Choline Magnesium Trisalicylate (Potential for acid-base and electrolyte disturbances with high-dose salicylate therapy).
No products indexed under this heading.

Clonidine (Oral beta-adrenergic blocking agents may exacerbate the rebound hypertension which can follow withdrawal of clonidine; there have been no reports of exacerbation of rebound hypertension with ophthalmic timolol). Products include:
Catapres-TTS 842

Clonidine Hydrochloride (Oral beta-adrenergic blocking agents may exacerbate the rebound hypertension which can follow withdrawal of clonidine; there have been no reports of exacerbation of rebound hypertension with ophthalmic timolol). Products include:
Catapres Tablets 841
Clorpres Tablets 2185

Deslanoside (The concomitant use of beta-adrenergic blocking agents with digitalis and calcium antagonists may have additive effects in prolonging atrioventricular conduction time).
No products indexed under this heading.

Dichlorphenamide (Co-administration with oral carbonic anhydrase inhibitor may result in additive carbonic anhydrase inhibition).
No products indexed under this heading.

Diflunisal (Potential for acid-base and electrolyte disturbances with high-dose salicylate therapy).
No products indexed under this heading.

Digitalis Glycoside Preparations (The concomitant use of beta-adrenergic blocking agents with digitalis and calcium antagonists may have additive effects in prolonging atrioventricular conduction time).
No products indexed under this heading.

Digitoxin (The concomitant use of beta-adrenergic blocking agents with digitalis and calcium antagonists may have additive effects in prolonging atrioventricular conduction time).
No products indexed under this heading.

Digoxin (The concomitant use of beta-adrenergic blocking agents with digitalis and calcium antagonists may have additive effects in prolonging atrioventricular conduction time). Products include:
Lanoxin Injection 1498
Lanoxin Injection Pediatric 1502
Lanoxin Tablets 1505

Diltiazem Hydrochloride (Co-administration of beta-adrenergic blockers and calcium channel blockers may result in possible atrioventricular conduction disturbances, left ventricular failure, and hypotension). Products include:
Cardizem LA Extended Release Tablets 421

Epinephrine (Patients with a history of atopy or anaphylactic reactions to a variety of allergens may be unresponsive to the usual dose of injectable epinephrine used to treat allergic reactions). Products include:
EpiPen 1024

Epinephrine Hydrochloride (Patients with a history of atopy or anaphylactic reactions to a variety of allergens may be unresponsive to the usual dose of injectable epinephrine used to treat allergic reactions).
No products indexed under this heading.

Felodipine (Co-administration of beta-adrenergic blockers and calcium channel blockers may result in possible atrioventricular conduction disturbances, left ventricular failure, and hypotension).
No products indexed under this heading.

Isradipine (Co-administration of beta-adrenergic blockers and calcium channel blockers may result in possible atrioventricular conduction disturbances, left ventricular failure, and hypotension). Products include:
DynaCirc CR Controlled Release Tablets 1407

Levobunolol Hydrochloride (Co-administration of oral beta-adrenergic blockers and Cosopt may result in potential additive effects of beta-blockade, both systemic and on intraocular pressure; the concomitant use of two topical beta-adrenergic agents is not recommended).
No products indexed under this heading.

Magnesium Salicylate (Potential for acid-base and electrolyte disturbances with high-dose salicylate therapy).
No products indexed under this heading.

Methazolamide (Co-administration with oral carbonic anhydrase inhibitor may result in additive carbonic anhydrase inhibition).
No products indexed under this heading.

Metipranolol Hydrochloride (Co-administration of oral beta-adrenergic blockers and Cosopt may result in potential additive effects of beta-blockade, both systemic and on intraocular pressure; the concomitant use of two topical beta-adrenergic agents is not recommended).
No products indexed under this heading.

Mibefradil Dihydrochloride (Co-administration of beta-adrenergic blockers and calcium channel blockers may result in possible atrioventricular conduction disturbances, left ventricular failure, and hypotension).
No products indexed under this heading.

Nebivolol (Co-administration of oral beta-adrenergic blockers and Cosopt may result in potential additive effects of beta-blockade, both systemic and on intraocular pressure). Products include:
Bystolic Tablets 1155

Nicardipine Hydrochloride (Co-administration of beta-adrenergic blockers and calcium channel blockers may result in possible atrioventricular conduction disturbances, left ventricular failure, and hypotension). Products include:
Cardene I.V. 1093

Nifedipine (Co-administration of beta-adrenergic blockers and calcium channel blockers may result in possible atrioventricular conduction disturbances, left ventricular failure, and hypotension).
No products indexed under this heading.

Nimodipine (Co-administration of beta-adrenergic blockers and calcium channel blockers may result in possible atrioventricular conduction disturbances, left ventricular failure, and hypotension). Products include:
Nimotop Capsules 790

Nisoldipine (Co-administration of beta-adrenergic blockers and calcium channel blockers may result in possible atrioventricular conduction disturbances, left ventricular failure, and hypotension). Products include:
Sular Extended Release Tablets 2975

Quinidine (Potentiated systemic beta-blockade has been reported during combined treatment with quinidine and timolol).
No products indexed under this heading.

Quinidine Gluconate (Potentiated systemic beta-blockade has been reported during combined treatment with quinidine and timolol).
No products indexed under this heading.

Quinidine Hydrochloride (Potentiated systemic beta-blockade has been reported during combined treatment with quinidine and timolol).
No products indexed under this heading.

Quinidine Polygalacturonate (Potentiated systemic beta-blockade has been reported during combined treatment with quinidine and timolol).
No products indexed under this heading.

Quinidine Sulfate (Potentiated systemic beta-blockade has been reported during combined treatment with quinidine and timolol).
No products indexed under this heading.

Reserpine (Co-administration of catecholamine-depleting drugs and beta-adrenergic blocker may result in possible additive effects and the production of hypotension and/or marked bradycardia).
No products indexed under this heading.

Salsalate (Potential for acid-base and electrolyte disturbances with high-dose salicylate therapy).
No products indexed under this heading.

Timolol Hemihydrate (Co-administration of oral beta-adrenergic blockers and Cosopt may result in potential additive effects of beta-blockade, both systemic and on intraocular pressure; the concomitant use of two topical beta-adrenergic agents is not recommended). Products include:
Betimol Ophthalmic Solution 3181

Verapamil Hydrochloride (Co-administration of beta-adrenergic blockers and calcium channel blockers may result in possible atrioventricular conduction disturbances, left ventricular failure, and hypotension). Products include:
Tarka Tablets 511

COZAAR TABLETS

(Losartan Potassium) 1973
May interact with lithium preparations, non-steroidal anti-inflammatory agents, potassium preparations, potassium sparing diuretics, and certain other agents. Compounds in these categories include:

Amiloride Hydrochloride (Concomitant use with potassium-sparing diuretics may lead to hyperkalemia).
No products indexed under this heading.

Celecoxib (In some patients with compromised renal function who are being treated with non-steroidal anti-inflammatory drugs (NSAIDs), including those that selectively inhibit cyclooxygenase-2 inhibitors (COX-2 inhibitors), the co-administration of angiotensin II receptor antagonists including losartan may result in a further deterioration of renal function. These effects are usually reversible. Reports suggest that NSAIDs, including selective COX-2 inhibitors, may diminish the antihypertensive effect of angiotensin II receptor antagonists, including losartan. This interaction should be given consideration in patients taking NSAIDs, including selective COX-2 inhibitors, concomitantly with angiotensin II receptor antagonists). Products include:
Celebrex Capsules 2979

Cimetidine (Co-administration leads to an increase of about 18% in AUC of losartan with no effect on pharmacokinetics of its active metabolites).
No products indexed under this heading.

Cimetidine Hydrochloride (Co-administration leads to an increase of about 18% in AUC of losartan with no effect on pharmacokinetics of its active metabolites).
No products indexed under this heading.

Diclofenac Epolamine (In some patients with compromised renal function who are being treated with non-steroidal anti-inflammatory drugs (NSAIDs), including those that selectively inhibit cyclooxygenase-2 inhibitors (COX-2 inhibitors), the co-administration of angiotensin II receptor antagonists including losartan may result in a further deterioration of renal function. These effects are usually reversible. Reports suggest that NSAIDs, including selective COX-2 inhibitors, may diminish the antihypertensive effect of angiotensin II receptor antagonists, including losartan. This interaction should be given consideration in patients taking NSAIDs, including selective COX-2 inhibitors, concomitantly with angiotensin II receptor antagonists). Products include:
Flector Patch 561

Diclofenac Potassium (In some patients with compromised renal function who are being treated with non-steroidal anti-inflammatory drugs (NSAIDs), including those that selectively inhibit cyclooxygenase-2 inhibitors (COX-2 inhibitors), the co-administration of angiotensin II receptor antagonists including losartan may result in a further deterioration of renal function. These effects are usually reversible. Reports suggest that NSAIDs, including selective COX-2 inhibitors, may diminish the antihypertensive effect of angiotensin II receptor antagonists, including losartan. This interaction should be given consideration in patients taking NSAIDs, including selective COX-2 inhibitors, concomitantly with angiotensin II receptor antagonists).
No products indexed under this heading.

Diclofenac Sodium (In some patients with compromised renal function who are being treated with non-steroidal anti-inflammatory drugs (NSAIDs), including those that selectively inhibit cyclooxygenase-2 inhibitors (COX-2 inhibitors), the co-administration of angiotensin II receptor antagonists including losartan may result in a further deterioration of renal function. These effects are usually reversible. Reports suggest that NSAIDs, including selective COX-2 inhibitors, may diminish the antihypertensive effect of angiotensin II receptor antagonists, including losartan. This interaction should be given consideration in patients taking NSAIDs, including selective COX-2 inhibitors, concomitantly with angiotensin II receptor antagonists). Products include:
Diclofenac Sodium Ophthalmic Solution .... ⊙240
Voltaren Ophthalmic Solution 2336
Voltaren Tablets 2334
Voltaren-XR Tablets 2337

Etodolac (In some patients with compromised renal function who are being treated with non-steroidal anti-inflammatory drugs (NSAIDs), including those that selectively inhibit cyclooxygenase-2 inhibitors (COX-2 inhibitors), the co-administration of angiotensin II receptor antagonists including losartan may result in a further deterioration of renal function. These effects are usually reversible. Reports suggest that NSAIDs, including selective COX-2 inhibitors, may diminish the antihypertensive effect of angiotensin II receptor antagonists, including losartan. This interaction should be given consideration in patients taking NSAIDs, including selective COX-2 inhibitors, concomitantly with angiotensin II receptor antagonists).
No products indexed under this heading.

Fenoprofen Calcium (In some patients with compromised renal function who are being treated with non-steroidal anti-inflammatory drugs (NSAIDs), including those that selectively inhibit cyclooxygenase-2 inhibitors (COX-2 inhibitors), the co-administration of angiotensin II receptor antagonists including losartan may result in a further deterioration of renal function. These effects are usually reversible. Reports suggest that NSAIDs, including selective COX-2 inhibitors, may diminish the antihypertensive effect of angiotensin II receptor antagonists, including losartan. This interaction should be given consideration in patients taking NSAIDs, including selective COX-2 inhibitors, concomitantly with angiotensin II receptor antagonists). Products include:
Nalfon Capsules 2508

Fluconazole (Fluconazole, an inhibitor of cytochrome P450 2C, decreased the AUC of the active metabolite by approximately 40%, but increased the AUC of losartan by approximately 70% following multiple doses).
No products indexed under this heading.

Flurbiprofen (In some patients with compromised renal function who are being treated with non-steroidal anti-inflammatory drugs (NSAIDs), including those that selectively inhibit cyclooxygenase-2 inhibitors (COX-2 inhibitors), the co-administration of angiotensin II receptor antagonists including losartan may result in a further deterioration of renal function. These effects are usually reversible. Reports suggest that NSAIDs, including selective COX-2 inhibitors, may diminish the antihypertensive effect of angiotensin II receptor antagonists, including losartan. This interaction should be given consideration in patients taking NSAIDs, including selective COX-2 inhibitors, concomitantly with angiotensin II receptor antagonists).
No products indexed under this heading.

Gestodene (*in vitro* studies show significant inhibition of the formation of the active metabolite by inhibitors of P450 3A4 such as gestodene; pharmacodynamic consequences of concomitant use is undefined).
No products indexed under this heading.

Ibuprofen (In some patients with compromised renal function who are being treated with non-steroidal anti-inflammatory drugs (NSAIDs), including those that selectively inhibit cyclooxygenase-2 inhibitors (COX-2 inhibitors), the co-administration of angiotensin II receptor antagonists including losartan may result in a further deterioration of renal function. These effects are usually reversible. Reports suggest that NSAIDs, including selective COX-2 inhibitors, may diminish the antihypertensive effect of angiotensin II receptor antagonists, including losartan. This interaction should be given consideration in patients taking NSAIDs, including selective COX-2 inhibitors, concomitantly with angiotensin II receptor antagonists). Products include:
Motrin IB Tablets and Caplets 1900
Children's Motrin Oral Suspension ... 1901
Children's Motrin Non-Staining Dye-Free Oral Suspension............. 1901
Children's Motrin Cold Oral Suspension 1899
Infants' Motrin Concentrated Drops 1901
Infants' Motrin Non-Staining Dye-Free Concentrated Drops....... 1901
Junior Strength Motrin Caplets and Chewable Tablets.................. 1901
Vicoprofen Tablets 533

Indomethacin (Antihypertensive effect of losartan may be blunted by indomethacin). Products include:
Indocin 2024

Indomethacin Sodium Trihydrate (Antihypertensive effect of losartan may be blunted by indomethacin). Products include:
Indocin I.V. 2489

Ketoconazole (*in vitro* studies show significant inhibition of the formation of the active metabolite by inhibitors of P450 3A4 such as ketoconazole or complete inhibition by the combination of ketoconazole and sulfaphenazole; pharmacodynamic consequences of concomitant use is undefined). Products include:
Extina Foam, 2% 3057
Nizoral A-D Shampoo 1901

Ketoprofen (In some patients with compromised renal function who are being treated with non-steroidal anti-inflammatory drugs (NSAIDs), including those that selectively inhibit cyclooxygenase-2 inhibitors (COX-2 inhibitors), the co-administration of angiotensin II receptor antagonists including losartan may result in a further deterioration of renal function. These effects are usually reversible. Reports suggest that NSAIDs, including selective COX-2 inhibitors, may diminish the antihypertensive effect of angiotensin II receptor antagonists, including losartan. This interaction should be given consideration in patients taking NSAIDs, including selective COX-2 inhibitors, concomitantly with angiotensin II receptor antagonists).
No products indexed under this heading.

Ketorolac Tromethamine (In some patients with compromised renal function who are being treated with non-steroidal anti-inflammatory drugs (NSAIDs), including those that selectively inhibit cyclooxygenase-2 inhibitors (COX-2 inhibitors), the co-administration of angiotensin II receptor antagonists including losartan may result in a further deterioration of renal function. These effects are usually reversible. Reports suggest that NSAIDs, including selective COX-2 inhibitors, may diminish the antihypertensive effect of angiotensin II receptor antagonists, including losartan. This interaction should be given consideration in patients taking NSAIDs, including selective COX-2 inhibitors, concomitantly with angiotensin II receptor antagonists).
No products indexed under this heading.

Lithium (As with other drugs which affect the excretion of sodium, lithium excretion may be reduced. Therefore, serum lithium levels should be monitored carefully if lithium salts are to be co-administered with angiotensin II receptor antagonists).
No products indexed under this heading.

Lithium Carbonate (As with other drugs which affect the excretion of sodium, lithium excretion may be reduced. Therefore, serum lithium levels should be monitored carefully if lithium salts are to be co-administered with angiotensin II receptor antagonists).
No products indexed under this heading.

Lithium Citrate (As with other drugs which affect the excretion of sodium, lithium excretion may be reduced. Therefore, serum lithium levels should be monitored carefully if lithium salts are to be co-administered with angiotensin II receptor antagonists).
No products indexed under this heading.

Meclofenamate Sodium (In some patients with compromised renal function who are being treated with non-steroidal anti-inflammatory drugs (NSAIDs), including those that selectively inhibit cyclooxygenase-2 inhibitors (COX-2 inhibitors), the co-administration of angiotensin II receptor antagonists including losartan may result in a further deterioration of renal function. These effects are usually reversible. Reports suggest that NSAIDs, including selective COX-2 inhibitors, may diminish the antihypertensive effect of angiotensin II receptor antagonists, including losartan. This interaction should be given consideration in patients taking NSAIDs, including selective COX-2 inhibitors, concomitantly with angiotensin II receptor antagonists).
No products indexed under this heading.

Mefenamic Acid (In some patients with compromised renal function who are being treated with non-steroidal anti-inflammatory drugs (NSAIDs), including those that selectively inhibit cyclooxygenase-2 inhibitors (COX-2 inhibitors), the co-administration of angiotensin II receptor antagonists including losartan may result in a further deterioration of renal function. These effects are usually reversible. Reports suggest that NSAIDs, including selective COX-2 inhibitors, may diminish the antihypertensive effect of angiotensin II receptor antagonists, including losartan. This interaction should be given consideration in patients taking NSAIDs, including selective COX-2 inhibitors, concomitantly with angiotensin II receptor antagonists).
No products indexed under this heading.

Meloxicam (In some patients with compromised renal function who are being treated with non-steroidal anti-inflammatory drugs (NSAIDs), including those that selectively inhibit cyclooxygenase-2 inhibitors (COX-2 inhibitors), the co-administration of angiotensin II receptor antagonists including losartan may result in a further deterioration of renal function. These effects are usually reversible. Reports suggest that NSAIDs, including selective COX-2 inhibitors, may diminish the antihypertensive effect of angiotensin II receptor antagonists, including losartan. This interaction should be given consideration in patients taking NSAIDs, including selective COX-2 inhibitors, concomitantly with angiotensin II receptor antagonists). Products include:

Mobic Oral Suspension **863**
Mobic Tablets **863**

Nabumetone (In some patients with compromised renal function who are being treated with non-steroidal anti-inflammatory drugs (NSAIDs), including those that selectively inhibit cyclooxygenase-2 inhibitors (COX-2 inhibitors), the co-administration of angiotensin II receptor antagonists including losartan may result in a further deterioration of renal function. These effects are usually reversible. Reports suggest that NSAIDs, including selective COX-2 inhibitors, may diminish the antihypertensive effect of angiotensin II receptor antagonists, including losartan. This interaction should be given consideration in patients taking NSAIDs, including selective COX-2 inhibitors, concomitantly with angiotensin II receptor antagonists).

No products indexed under this heading.

Naproxen (In some patients with compromised renal function who are being treated with non-steroidal anti-inflammatory drugs (NSAIDs), including those that selectively inhibit cyclooxygenase-2 inhibitors (COX-2 inhibitors), the co-administration of angiotensin II receptor antagonists including losartan may result in a further deterioration of renal function. These effects are usually reversible. Reports suggest that NSAIDs, including selective COX-2 inhibitors, may diminish the antihypertensive effect of angiotensin II receptor antagonists, including losartan. This interaction should be given consideration in patients taking NSAIDs, including selective COX-2 inhibitors, concomitantly with angiotensin II receptor antagonists). Products include:

EC-Naprosyn Delayed-Release Tablets **2632**
Naprosyn Suspension **2632**
Naprosyn Tablets **2632**

Naproxen Sodium (In some patients with compromised renal function who are being treated with non-steroidal anti-inflammatory drugs (NSAIDs), including those that selectively inhibit cyclooxygenase-2 inhibitors (COX-2 inhibitors), the co-administration of angiotensin II receptor antagonists including losartan may result in a further deterioration of renal function. These effects are usually reversible. Reports suggest that NSAIDs, including selective COX-2 inhibitors, may diminish the antihypertensive effect of angiotensin II receptor antagonists, including losartan. This interaction should be given consideration in patients taking NSAIDs, including selective COX-2 inhibitors, concomitantly with angiotensin II receptor antagonists). Products include:

Anaprox Tablets **2632**
Anaprox DS Tablets **2632**

Treximet Tablets **1616**

Oxaprozin (In some patients with compromised renal function who are being treated with non-steroidal anti-inflammatory drugs (NSAIDs), including those that selectively inhibit cyclooxygenase-2 inhibitors (COX-2 inhibitors), the co-administration of angiotensin II receptor antagonists including losartan may result in a further deterioration of renal function. These effects are usually reversible. Reports suggest that NSAIDs, including selective COX-2 inhibitors, may diminish the antihypertensive effect of angiotensin II receptor antagonists, including losartan. This interaction should be given consideration in patients taking NSAIDs, including selective COX-2 inhibitors, concomitantly with angiotensin II receptor antagonists).

No products indexed under this heading.

Phenobarbital (Co-administration leads to a reduction of about 20% in AUC of losartan and that of its active metabolites). Products include:

Donnatal Extentabs **2507**

Phenylbutazone (In some patients with compromised renal function who are being treated with non-steroidal anti-inflammatory drugs (NSAIDs), including those that selectively inhibit cyclooxygenase-2 inhibitors (COX-2 inhibitors), the co-administration of angiotensin II receptor antagonists including losartan may result in a further deterioration of renal function. These effects are usually reversible. Reports suggest that NSAIDs, including selective COX-2 inhibitors, may diminish the antihypertensive effect of angiotensin II receptor antagonists, including losartan. This interaction should be given consideration in patients taking NSAIDs, including selective COX-2 inhibitors, concomitantly with angiotensin II receptor antagonists).

No products indexed under this heading.

Piroxicam (In some patients with compromised renal function who are being treated with non-steroidal anti-inflammatory drugs (NSAIDs), including those that selectively inhibit cyclooxygenase-2 inhibitors (COX-2 inhibitors), the co-administration of angiotensin II receptor antagonists including losartan may result in a further deterioration of renal function. These effects are usually reversible. Reports suggest that NSAIDs, including selective COX-2 inhibitors, may diminish the antihypertensive effect of angiotensin II receptor antagonists, including losartan. This interaction should be given consideration in patients taking NSAIDs, including selective COX-2 inhibitors, concomitantly with angiotensin II receptor antagonists).

No products indexed under this heading.

Potassium Acid Phosphate (Concomitant use with potassium supplements or salt substitute containing potassium may lead to hyperkalemia; patients should be advised to avoid these potassium-containing preparations). Products include:

K-Phos Original (Sodium Free) Tablets **814**

Potassium Bicarbonate (Concomitant use with potassium supplements or salt substitute containing potassium may lead to hyperkalemia; patients should be advised to avoid these potassium-containing preparations).

No products indexed under this heading.

Potassium Chloride (Concomitant use with potassium supplements or salt substitute containing potassium may lead to hyperkalemia; patients should be advised to avoid these potassium-containing preparations). Products include:

MoviPrep Oral Solution **2679**

Potassium Citrate (Concomitant use with potassium supplements or salt substitute containing potassium may lead to hyperkalemia; patients should be advised to avoid these potassium-containing preparations). Products include:

BioLean Free Tablets **635**
Urocit-K Tablets **2176**

Potassium Gluconate (Concomitant use with potassium supplements or salt substitute containing potassium may lead to hyperkalemia; patients should be advised to avoid these potassium-containing preparations).

No products indexed under this heading.

Potassium Phosphate (Concomitant use with potassium supplements or salt substitute containing potassium may lead to hyperkalemia; patients should be advised to avoid these potassium-containing preparations). Products include:

K-Phos Neutral Tablets **813**

Rifampin (Approximately 40% reduction in the AUC of losartan has been reported with rifampin).

No products indexed under this heading.

Rofecoxib (In some patients with compromised renal function who are being treated with non-steroidal anti-inflammatory drugs (NSAIDs), including those that selectively inhibit cyclooxygenase-2 inhibitors (COX-2 inhibitors), the co-administration of angiotensin II receptor antagonists including losartan may result in a further deterioration of renal function. These effects are usually reversible. Reports suggest that NSAIDs, including selective COX-2 inhibitors, may diminish the antihypertensive effect of angiotensin II receptor antagonists, including losartan. This interaction should be given consideration in patients taking NSAIDs, including selective COX-2 inhibitors, concomitantly with angiotensin II receptor antagonists).

No products indexed under this heading.

Salt Substitutes (Concomitant use with salt substitutes may lead to hyperkalemia).

No products indexed under this heading.

Spironolactone (Concomitant use with potassium-sparing diuretics may lead to hyperkalemia).

No products indexed under this heading.

Sulfaphenazole (*in vitro* studies show significant inhibition of the formation of the active metabolite by inhibitors of P450 3A4 such as sulfaphenazole; pharmacodynamic consequences of concomitant use is undefined).

No products indexed under this heading.

Sulindac (In some patients with compromised renal function who are being treated with non-steroidal anti-inflammatory drugs (NSAIDs), including those that selectively inhibit cyclooxygenase-2 inhibitors (COX-2 inhibitors), the co-administration of angiotensin II receptor antagonists including losartan may result in a further deterioration of renal function. These effects are usually reversible. Reports suggest that NSAIDs, including selective COX-2 inhibitors, may diminish the antihypertensive effect of angiotensin II receptor antagonists, including losartan. This interaction should be given consideration in patients taking NSAIDs, including selective COX-2 inhibitors, concomitantly with angiotensin II receptor antagonists). Products include:

Clinoril Tablets **1962**

Tolmetin Sodium (In some patients with compromised renal function who are being treated with non-steroidal anti-inflammatory drugs (NSAIDs), including those that selectively inhibit cyclooxygenase-2 inhibitors (COX-2 inhibitors), the co-administration of angiotensin II receptor antagonists including losartan may result in a further deterioration of renal function. These effects are usually reversible. Reports suggest that NSAIDs, including selective COX-2 inhibitors, may diminish the antihypertensive effect of angiotensin II receptor antagonists, including losartan. This interaction should be given consideration in patients taking NSAIDs, including selective COX-2 inhibitors, concomitantly with angiotensin II receptor antagonists).

No products indexed under this heading.

Triamterene (Concomitant use with potassium-sparing diuretics may lead to hyperkalemia). Products include:

Dyazide Capsules **1405**
Dyrenium Capsules **3189**

Troleandomycin (*in vitro* studies show significant inhibition of the formation of the active metabolite by inhibitors of P450 3A4 such as troleandomycin; pharmacodynamic consequences of concomitant use is undefined).

No products indexed under this heading.

Valdecoxib (In some patients with compromised renal function who are being treated with non-steroidal anti-inflammatory drugs (NSAIDs), including those that selectively inhibit cyclooxygenase-2 inhibitors (COX-2 inhibitors), the co-administration of angiotensin II receptor antagonists including losartan may result in a further deterioration of renal function. These effects are usually reversible. Reports suggest that NSAIDs, including selective COX-2 inhibitors, may diminish the antihypertensive effect of angiotensin II receptor antagonists, including losartan. This interaction should be given consideration in patients taking

NSAIDs, including selective COX-2 inhibitors, concomitantly with angiotensin II receptor antagonists).

No products indexed under this heading.

Food Interactions

Meal, unspecified (A meal slows absorption and decreases Cmax, but has minor effects on losartan AUC or on the AUC of the metabolite).

CREON 5 CAPSULES

(Pancrelipase) **3041**

Food Interactions

Food having a pH greater than 5.5 (Can dissolve the protective coating resulting in early release of enzymes, irritation of oral mucosa, and/or loss of enzyme activity).

CREON 10 CAPSULES

(Pancrelipase) **3042**

See Creon 5 Capsules

CREON 20 CAPSULES

(Pancrelipase) **3042**

See Creon 5 Capsules

CRESTOR TABLETS

(Rosuvastatin Calcium) **677**

May interact with antacids, oral anticoagulants, erythromycin, fibrates, oral contraceptives, and certain other agents. Compounds in these categories include:

Aluminum Carbonate (When taking rosuvastatin calcium with an aluminum and magnesium hydroxide combination antacid, the antacid should be taken at least 2 hours after rosuvastatin calcium administration).

No products indexed under this heading.

Aluminum Hydroxide (When taking rosuvastatin calcium with an aluminum and magnesium hydroxide combination antacid, the antacid should be taken at least 2 hours after rosuvastatin calcium administration).

No products indexed under this heading.

Anisindione (Rosuvastatin calcium significantly increased INR in patients receiving coumarin anticoagulants. Therefore caution should be exercised when coumarin anticoagulants are given in conjunction with rosuvastatin calcium. In patients taking coumarin anticoagulants and rosuvastatin calcium concomitantly, INR should be determined before starting rosuvastatin calcium and frequently enough during early therapy to ensure that no significant alteration of INR occurs).

No products indexed under this heading.

Cimetidine (Although clinical studies have shown that rosuvastatin calcium alone does not reduce basal plasma cortisol concentration or impair adrenal reserve, caution should be exercised if rosuvastatin calcium is administered concomitantly with drugs that may decrease the levels or activity of endogenous steroid hormones such as ketoconazole, spironolactone, and cimetidine).

No products indexed under this heading.

Cimetidine Hydrochloride (Although clinical studies have shown that rosuvastatin calcium alone does not reduce basal plasma cortisol concentration or impair adrenal reserve, caution should be exercised if rosuvastatin calcium is administered concomitantly with drugs that may decrease the levels or activity of endogenous steroid hormones such as ketoconazole, spironolactone, and cimetidine).

No products indexed under this heading.

Clofibrate (When rosuvastatin calcium was co-administered with fenofibrate, no clinically significant increase in the AUC of rosuvastatin or fenofibrate was observed. The benefit of further alterations in lipid levels by the combined use of rosuvastatin calcium withfibrates should be carefully weighed against the potential risks of this combination).

No products indexed under this heading.

Cyclosporine (Cyclosporine significantly increased rosuvastatin exposure. Therefore, in patients taking cyclosporine, therapy should be limited to rosuvastatin calcium 5 mg once daily). Products include:

Gengraf Capsules **435**
Neoral Oral Solution **2280**
Neoral Soft Gelatin Capsules **2280**
Restasis Ophthalmic Emulsion **557**
Sandimmune **2296**

Desogestrel (Co-administration may lead to increased ethinyl estradiol and norgestrel levels). Products include:

Mircette Tablets **1034**

Dicumarol (Rosuvastatin calcium significantly increased INR in patients receiving coumarin anticoagulants. Therefore caution should be exercised when coumarin anticoagulants are given in conjunction with rosuvastatin calcium. In patients taking coumarin anticoagulants and rosuvastatin calcium concomitantly, INR should be determined before starting rosuvastatin calcium and frequently enough during early therapy to ensure that no significant alteration of INR occurs).

No products indexed under this heading.

Erythromycin (Co-administration may lead to decreased rosuvastatin calcium levels).

No products indexed under this heading.

Erythromycin Estolate (Co-administration may lead to decreased rosuvastatin calcium levels).

No products indexed under this heading.

Erythromycin Ethylsuccinate (Co-administration may lead to decreased rosuvastatin calcium levels). Products include:

E.E.S. **433**
EryPed **431**

Erythromycin Gluceptate (Co-administration may lead to decreased rosuvastatin calcium levels).

No products indexed under this heading.

Erythromycin Lactobionate (Co-administration may lead to decreased rosuvastatin calcium levels).

No products indexed under this heading.

Erythromycin Stearate (Co-administration may lead to decreased rosuvastatin calcium levels).

No products indexed under this heading.

Ethinyl Estradiol (Co-administration may lead to increased ethinyl estradiol and norgestrel levels). Products include:

Lybrel Tablets **3204**
Mircette Tablets **1034**
NuvaRing **2897**
Ortho-Cyclen/Ortho Tri-Cyclen **2449**
Ortho Evra Transdermal System **2437**
Ortho Tri-Cyclen Lo Tablets **2458**
Seasonique Tablets **1046**
Yaz Tablets **805**

Ethynodiol Diacetate (Co-administration may lead to increased ethinyl estradiol and norgestrel levels).

No products indexed under this heading.

Fenofibrate (When rosuvastatin calcium was co-administered with fenofibrate, no clinically significant increase in the AUC of rosuvastatin or fenofibrate was observed. The benefit of further alterations in lipid levels by the combined use of rosuvastatin calcium withfibrates should be carefully weighed against the potential risks of this combination). Products include:

Fenoglide Tablets **2960**
Tricor Tablets **520**

Gemfibrozil (Gemfibrozil significantly increased rosuvastatin exposure. Therefore, combination therapy with rosuvastatin calcium and gemfibrozil should be avoided. If used, do not exceed rosuvastatin calcium 10 mg once daily).

No products indexed under this heading.

Itraconazole (Co-administration may lead to increased rosuvastatin calcium levels).

No products indexed under this heading.

Ketoconazole (Although clinical studies have shown that rosuvastatin calcium alone does not reduce basal plasma cortisol concentration or impair adrenal reserve, caution should be exercised if rosuvastatin calcium is administered concomitantly with drugs that may decrease the levels or activity of endogenous steroid hormones such as ketoconazole, spironolactone, and cimetidine). Products include:

Extina Foam, 2% **3057**
Nizoral A-D Shampoo **1901**

Levonorgestrel (Co-administration may lead to increased ethinyl estradiol and norgestrel levels). Products include:

Climara Pro Transdermal System **768**
Lybrel Tablets **3204**
Mirena Intrauterine System **779**
Plan B Tablets **1044**
Seasonique Tablets **1046**

Lopinavir (The combination of lopinavir and ritonavir significantly increased rosuvastatin exposure. Therefore, in patients taking a combination of lopinavir and ritonavir, the dose of rosuvastatin calcium should be limited to 10 mg once daily. The effect of other protease inhibitors on rosuvastatin pharmacokinetics has not been examined). Products include:

Kaletra **452**

Magaldrate (When taking rosuvastatin calcium with an aluminum and magnesium hydroxide combination antacid, the antacid should be taken at least 2 hours after rosuvastatin calcium administration).

No products indexed under this heading.

Magnesium Hydroxide (When taking rosuvastatin calcium with an aluminum and magnesium hydroxide combination antacid, the antacid should be taken at least 2 hours after rosuvastatin calcium administration). Products include:

Fleet Pedia-Lax Chewable Tablets **1145**
Pepcid Complete Chewable Tablets **1771**
Extra Strength Rolaids Freshmint Tablets **1903**
Rolaids Multi-Symptom Berry Tablets **1903**
Rolaids Original Peppermint Tablets **1903**

Magnesium Oxide (When taking rosuvastatin calcium with an aluminum and magnesium hydroxide combination antacid, the antacid should be taken at least 2 hours after rosuvastatin calcium administration). Products include:

Beelith Tablets **813**

Mestranol (Co-administration may lead to increased ethinyl estradiol and norgestrel levels).

No products indexed under this heading.

Niacin (The risk of skeletal muscle effects may be enhanced when rosuvastatin calcium is used in combination with niacin; a reduction in rosuvastatin calcium dosage should be considered in this setting). Products include:

Advicor Tablets **402**
Bausch & Lomb Ocuvite DF Vitamin Supplement .... ⊙**238**
Dismutax Dietary Supplement **995**
Niaspan Extended-Release Tablets **480**
NT-Kinase Dietary Supplement **995**
Simcor Tablets **502**

Niacinamide (The risk of skeletal muscle effects may be enhanced when rosuvastatin calcium is used in combination with niacin; a reduction in rosuvastatin calcium dosage should be considered in this setting). Products include:

BioLean Free Tablets .... ▣**635**

Norethindrone (Co-administration may lead to increased ethinyl estradiol and norgestrel levels). Products include:

Ortho Micronor Tablets **2446**

Norethynodrel (Co-administration may lead to increased ethinyl estradiol and norgestrel levels).

No products indexed under this heading.

Norgestimate (Co-administration may lead to increased ethinyl estradiol and norgestrel levels). Products include:

Ortho-Cyclen/Ortho Tri-Cyclen **2449**
Ortho Tri-Cyclen Lo Tablets **2458**

Norgestrel (Co-administration may lead to increased ethinyl estradiol and norgestrel levels).

No products indexed under this heading.

Ritonavir (The combination of lopinavir and ritonavir significantly increased rosuvastatin exposure. Therefore, in patients taking a combination of lopinavir and ritonavir, the dose of rosuvastatin calcium should be limited to 10 mg once daily. The effect of other protease inhibitors on rosuvastatin pharmacokinetics has not been examined). Products include:

Kaletra 452
Norvir 489

Sodium Bicarbonate (When taking rosuvastatin calcium with an aluminum and magnesium hydroxide combination antacid, the antacid should be taken at least 2 hours after rosuvastatin calcium administration). Products include:

Ceo-Two Laxative Suppository 815

Spironolactone (Although clinical studies have shown that rosuvastatin calcium alone does not reduce basal plasma cortisol concentration or impair adrenal reserve, caution should be exercised if rosuvastatin calcium is administered concomitantly with drugs that may decrease the levels or activity of endogenous steroid hormones such as ketoconazole, spironolactone, and cimetidine).

No products indexed under this heading.

Warfarin Sodium (Rosuvastatin calcium significantly increased INR in patients receiving coumarin anticoagulants. Therefore caution should be exercised when coumarin anticoagulants are given in conjunction with rosuvastatin calcium. In patients taking coumarin anticoagulants and rosuvastatin calcium concomitantly, INR should be determined before starting rosuvastatin calcium and frequently enough during early therapy to ensure that no significant alteration of INR occurs).

No products indexed under this heading.

CRINONE 4% GEL

(Progesterone) 992

None cited in PDR database.

CRINONE 8% GEL

(Progesterone) 992

None cited in PDR database.

CRIXIVAN CAPSULES

(Indinavir Sulfate) 1979

May interact with calcium channel blockers, cytochrome p450 3a4 inducers (selected), cytochrome p450 3a4 inhibitors (selected), cytochrome p450 3a4 substrates (selected), dexamethasone, ergot-containing drugs, phenytoin, and certain other agents. Compounds in these categories include:

Acetazolamide (Co-administration of indinavir and other drugs that inhibit CYP3A4 may decrease the clearance of indinavir and may result in increased plasma concentrations of indinavir).

No products indexed under this heading.

Alfentanil Hydrochloride (Co-administration of indinavir and drugs primarily metabolized by CYP3A4 may result in increased plasma concentrations of the other drug, which could increase or prolong its therapeutic and adverse effects).

No products indexed under this heading.

Allium sativum (Drugs that induce CYP3A4 activity would be expected to increase the clearance of indinavir, resulting in lowered plasma concentrations of indinavir).

No products indexed under this heading.

Alprazolam (Concomitant use with alprazolam is contraindicated due to potential for serious and/or life-threatening reactions such as prolonged or increased sedation or respiratory depression).

No products indexed under this heading.

Amiodarone Hydrochloride (Inhibition of CYP3A4 by indinavir could result in elevated plasma concentrations of amiodarone potentially causing serious or life-threatening reactions; co-administration is contraindicated).

No products indexed under this heading.

Amitriptyline Hydrochloride (Co-administration of indinavir and drugs primarily metabolized by CYP3A4 may result in increased plasma concentrations of the other drug, which could increase or prolong its therapeutic and adverse effects).

No products indexed under this heading.

Amlodipine Besylate (Co-administration of calcium channel blockers with indinavir may result in increased plasma concentrations of the dihydropyridine calcium channel blockers which could increase or prolong their therapeutic and adverse effects. Caution is warranted and clinical monitoring is recommended). Products include:

Azor Tablets 1005
Exforge Tablets 2238

Amprenavir (Co-administration of indinavir and other drugs that inhibit CYP3A4 may decrease the clearance of indinavir and may result in increased plasma concentrations of indinavir).

No products indexed under this heading.

Anastrozole (Co-administration of indinavir and other drugs that inhibit CYP3A4 may decrease the clearance of indinavir and may result in increased plasma concentrations of indinavir). Products include:

Arimidex Tablets 672

Aprepitant (Co-administration of indinavir and drugs primarily metabolized by CYP3A4 may result in increased plasma concentrations of the other drug, which could increase or prolong its therapeutic and adverse effects). Products include:

Emend Capsules 1992

Astemizole (Inhibition of CYP3A4 by indinavir could result in elevated plasma concentrations of astemizole potentially causing serious or life-threatening reactions; co-administration is contraindicated).

No products indexed under this heading.

Atazanavir (Both indinavir sulfate and atazanavir are associated with indirect (unconjugated) hyperbilirubinemia. Combinations of these drugs have not been studied and co-administration of indinavir sulfate and atazanavir is not recommended).

No products indexed under this heading.

Atazanavir Sulfate (Both indinavir sulfate and atazanavir are associated with indirect (unconjugated) hyperbilirubinemia. Combinations of these drugs have not been studied and co-administration of indinavir sulfate and atazanavir is not recommended). Products include:

Reyataz Capsules 3299

Atorvastatin Calcium (Co-administration of indinavir and atorvastatin may lead to increased atorvastatin concentrations. The risk of myopathy, including rhabdomyolysis, may be increased when protease inhibitors, including indinavir, are used in combination with HMG-CoA inhibitors that are metabolized by the CYP3A4 pathway. Use lowest possible dose of atorvastatin with careful monitoring, or consider HMG-CoA reductase inhibitors that are not primarily metabolized by CYP3A, such as pravastatin or fluvastatin in combination with indinavir). Products include:

Lipitor Tablets 2501

Belladonna Ergotamine (Co-administration of indinavir and drugs primarily metabolized by CYP3A4 may result in increased plasma concentrations of the other drug, which could increase or prolong its therapeutic and adverse effects).

No products indexed under this heading.

Bepridil Hydrochloride (Co-administration may lead to increased bepridil concentrations. Caution is warranted and therapeutic concentration monitoring is recommended for antiarrhythmics when co-administered with indinavir).

No products indexed under this heading.

Betamethasone Acetate (Drugs that induce CYP3A4 activity would be expected to increase the clearance of indinavir, resulting in lowered plasma concentrations of indinavir).

No products indexed under this heading.

Betamethasone Sodium Phosphate (Drugs that induce CYP3A4 activity would be expected to increase the clearance of indinavir, resulting in lowered plasma concentrations of indinavir).

No products indexed under this heading.

Buspirone Hydrochloride (Co-administration of indinavir and drugs primarily metabolized by CYP3A4 may result in increased plasma concentrations of the other drug, which could increase or prolong its therapeutic and adverse effects).

No products indexed under this heading.

Busulfan (Co-administration of indinavir and drugs primarily metabolized by CYP3A4 may result in increased plasma concentrations of the other drug, which could increase or prolong its therapeutic and adverse effects). Products include:

Busulfex Injection 2477
Myleran Tablets 1530

Carbamazepine (Could diminish plasma concentrations of indinavir because carbamazepine is an inducer of P450 3A4; caution is advised if co-administered). Products include:

Carbatrol Capsules 3019
Equetro Extended-Release Capsules 3174

Cerivastatin Sodium (The risk of myopathy including rhabdomyolysis may be increased when protease inhibitors, including indinavir, are used in combination with HMG-CoA inhibitors that are metabolized by the CYP3A4 pathway).

No products indexed under this heading.

Chlorpheniramine (Co-administration of indinavir and drugs primarily metabolized by CYP3A4 may result in increased plasma concentrations of the other drug, which could increase or prolong its therapeutic and adverse effects).

No products indexed under this heading.

Chlorpheniramine Maleate (Co-administration of indinavir and drugs primarily metabolized by CYP3A4 may result in increased plasma concentrations of the other drug, which could increase or prolong its therapeutic and adverse effects). Products include:

Actifed Cold & Allergy Tablets 1895
Sudafed PE Sinus & Allergy Tablets 1908
Tylenol Allergy Multi-Symptom Caplets with Cool Burst and Rapid Release Gelcaps 1916
Children's Tylenol Plus Cold Suspension Liquid 1912
Children's Tylenol Plus Cough & Runny Nose Suspension Liquid 1912
Children's Tylenol Plus Flu Suspension Liquid 1914
Children's Tylenol Plus Multi-Symptom Cold Suspension Liquid 1912
Tylenol Cold Head Congestion Nighttime Caplets with Cool Burst 1910
Tylenol Cold Multi-Symptom Nighttime Caplets with Cool Burst 1913
Tylenol Sinus Congestion & Pain Nighttime Caplets with Cool Burst 1917

Chlorpheniramine Polistirex (Co-administration of indinavir and drugs primarily metabolized by CYP3A4 may result in increased plasma concentrations of the other drug, which could increase or prolong its therapeutic and adverse effects). Products include:

Tussionex Pennkinetic Extended-Release Suspension 3154

Chlorpheniramine Tannate (Co-administration of indinavir and drugs primarily metabolized by CYP3A4 may result in increased plasma concentrations of the other drug, which could increase or prolong its therapeutic and adverse effects).

No products indexed under this heading.

Cimetidine (Co-administration of indinavir and other drugs that inhibit CYP3A4 may decrease the clearance of indinavir and may result in increased plasma concentrations of indinavir).

No products indexed under this heading.

Cimetidine Hydrochloride (Co-administration of indinavir and other drugs that inhibit CYP3A4 may decrease the clearance of indinavir and may result in increased plasma concentrations of indinavir).

No products indexed under this heading.

Ciprofloxacin (Co-administration of indinavir and other drugs that inhibit CYP3A4 may decrease the clearance of indinavir and may result in increased plasma concentrations of indinavir). Products include:

Cipro I.V. 2817
Cipro Oral Suspension 2810
Cipro XR Tablets 2823
Ciprodex Otic Suspension 541

Ciprofloxacin Hydrochloride (Drugs that induce CYP3A4 activity would be expected to increase the clearance of indinavir, resulting in lowered plasma concentrations of indinavir). Products include:

Cipro Tablets **2810**

Cisapride (Inhibition of CYP3A4 by indinavir could result in elevated plasma concentrations of cisapride, potentially causing serious or life-threatening reactions; co-administration is contraindicated).

No products indexed under this heading.

Cisplatin (Drugs that induce CYP3A4 activity would be expected to increase the clearance of indinavir, resulting in lowered plasma concentrations of indinavir).

No products indexed under this heading.

Clarithromycin (Co-administration of indinavir and clarithromycin may lead to increased clarithromycin and indinvair concentrations. The appropriate doses for this combination, with respect to safety and efficacy, have not been established). Products include:

Biaxin/Biaxin XL **411**

Clotrimazole (Co-administration of indinavir and other drugs that inhibit CYP3A4 may decrease the clearance of indinavir and may result in increased plasma concentrations of indinavir). Products include:

Lotrisone **2881**

Cortisone Acetate (Drugs that induce CYP3A4 activity would be expected to increase the clearance of indinavir, resulting in lowered plasma concentrations of indinavir).

No products indexed under this heading.

Cyclosporine (Co-administration of indinavir and cyclosporine may lead to increased cyclosporine concentrations). Products include:

Gengraf Capsules **435**
Neoral Oral Solution **2280**
Neoral Soft Gelatin Capsules **2280**
Restasis Ophthalmic Emulsion **557**
Sandimmune **2296**

Dalfopristin (Co-administration of indinavir and other drugs that inhibit CYP3A4 may decrease the clearance of indinavir and may result in increased plasma concentrations of indinavir).

No products indexed under this heading.

Danazol (Co-administration of indinavir and other drugs that inhibit CYP3A4 may decrease the clearance of indinavir and may result in increased plasma concentrations of indinavir).

No products indexed under this heading.

Delavirdine Mesylate (Co-administration results in inhibition of indinavir metabolism producing an increase in indinavir concentrations; a reduction of indinavir dosage should be considered when used concurrently).

No products indexed under this heading.

Desogestrel (Co-administration of indinavir and drugs primarily metabolized by CYP3A4 may result in increased plasma concentrations of the other drug, which could increase or prolong its therapeutic and adverse effects). Products include:

Mircette Tablets **1034**

Dexamethasone (Could diminish plasma concentrations of indinavir because dexamethasone is an inducer of P450 3A4; caution is advised if co-administered). Products include:

Ciprodex Otic Suspension **541**

Dexamethasone Acetate (Could diminish plasma concentrations of indinavir because dexamethasone is an inducer of P450 3A4; caution is advised if co-administered).

No products indexed under this heading.

Dexamethasone Sodium Phosphate (Could diminish plasma concentrations of indinavir because dexamethasone is an inducer of P450 3A4; caution is advised if co-administered).

No products indexed under this heading.

Diazepam (Co-administration of indinavir and drugs primarily metabolized by CYP3A4 may result in increased plasma concentrations of the other drug, which could increase or prolong its therapeutic and adverse effects). Products include:

Valium Tablets **2658**

Didanosine (Gastric acid rapidly degrades didanosine and a normal (acidic) gastric pH may be necessary for the optimum absorption of indinavir; if administered concomitantly, they should be administered at least one hour apart on an empty stomach).

No products indexed under this heading.

Dihydroergotamine Mesylate (Inhibition of CYP3A4 by indinavir could result in elevated plasma concentrations of ergot derivatives, potentially causing serious or life-threatening reactions; co-administration is contraindicated).

No products indexed under this heading.

Diltiazem Hydrochloride (Co-administration of calcium channel blockers with indinavir may result in increased plasma concentrations of the dihydropyridine calcium channel blockers which could increase or prolong their therapeutic and adverse effects. Caution is warranted and clinical monitoring is recommended). Products include:

Cardizem LA Extended Release Tablets **421**

Diltiazem Maleate (Co-administration of indinavir and drugs primarily metabolized by CYP3A4 may result in increased plasma concentrations of the other drug, which could increase or prolong its therapeutic and adverse effects).

No products indexed under this heading.

Disopyramide (Co-administration of indinavir and drugs primarily metabolized by CYP3A4 may result in increased plasma concentrations of the other drug, which could increase or prolong its therapeutic and adverse effects).

No products indexed under this heading.

Disopyramide Phosphate (Co-administration of indinavir and drugs primarily metabolized by CYP3A4 may result in increased plasma concentrations of the other drug, which could increase or prolong its therapeutic and adverse effects).

No products indexed under this heading.

Disulfiram (Co-administration of indinavir and drugs primarily metabolized by CYP3A4 may result in increased plasma concentrations of the other drug, which could increase or prolong its therapeutic and adverse effects).

No products indexed under this heading.

Doxorubicin Hydrochloride (Co-administration of indinavir and drugs primarily metabolized by CYP3A4 may result in increased plasma concentrations of the other drug, which could increase or prolong its therapeutic and adverse effects).

No products indexed under this heading.

Dronabinol (Co-administration of indinavir and drugs primarily metabolized by CYP3A4 may result in increased plasma concentrations of the other drug, which could increase or prolong its therapeutic and adverse effects). Products include:

Marinol Capsules **3163**

Efavirenz (Co-administration results in a decrease in the plasma concentrations of indinavir; a dosage increase of indinavir is recommended when used concurrently). Products include:

Atripla Tablets **938**
Sustiva Capsules **930**
Sustiva Tablets **930**

Ergonovine Maleate (Inhibition of CYP3A4 by indinavir could result in elevated plasma concentrations of ergot derivatives, potentially causing serious or life-threatening reactions; co-administration is contraindicated).

No products indexed under this heading.

Ergotamine Tartrate (Inhibition of CYP3A4 by indinavir could result in elevated plasma concentrations of ergot derivatives, potentially causing serious or life-threatening reactions; co-administration is contraindicated).

No products indexed under this heading.

Erythromycin (Co-administration of indinavir and drugs primarily metabolized by CYP3A4 may result in increased plasma concentrations of the other drug, which could increase or prolong its therapeutic and adverse effects).

No products indexed under this heading.

Erythromycin Estolate (Co-administration of indinavir and drugs primarily metabolized by CYP3A4 may result in increased plasma concentrations of the other drug, which could increase or prolong its therapeutic and adverse effects).

No products indexed under this heading.

Erythromycin Ethylsuccinate (Co-administration of indinavir and drugs primarily metabolized by CYP3A4 may result in increased plasma concentrations of the other drug, which could increase or prolong its therapeutic and adverse effects). Products include:

E.E.S. **433**
EryPed **431**

Erythromycin Gluceptate (Co-administration of indinavir and drugs primarily metabolized by CYP3A4 may result in increased plasma concentrations of the other drug, which could increase or prolong its therapeutic and adverse effects).

No products indexed under this heading.

Erythromycin Lactobionate (Co-administration of indinavir and drugs primarily metabolized by CYP3A4 may result in increased plasma concentrations of the other drug, which could increase or prolong its therapeutic and adverse effects).

No products indexed under this heading.

Erythromycin Stearate (Co-administration of indinavir and drugs primarily metabolized by CYP3A4 may result in increased plasma concentrations of the other drug, which could increase or prolong its therapeutic and adverse effects).

No products indexed under this heading.

Esomeprazole Magnesium (Co-administration of indinavir and other drugs that inhibit CYP3A4 may decrease the clearance of indinavir and may result in increased plasma concentrations of indinavir). Products include:

Nexium Delayed-Release Capsules **645**
Nexium Delayed-Release Oral Suspension **645**

Estradiol (Co-administration of indinavir and drugs primarily metabolized by CYP3A4 may result in increased plasma concentrations of the other drug, which could increase or prolong its therapeutic and adverse effects). Products include:

Activella Tablets **2347**
Angeliq Tablets **751**
Climara Transdermal System **763**
Climara Pro Transdermal System **768**
Divigel **3167**
Vagifem Tablets **2375**

Estradiol Benzoate (Co-administration of indinavir and drugs primarily metabolized by CYP3A4 may result in increased plasma concentrations of the other drug, which could increase or prolong its therapeutic and adverse effects).

No products indexed under this heading.

Estradiol Cypionate (Co-administration of indinavir and drugs primarily metabolized by CYP3A4 may result in increased plasma concentrations of the other drug, which could increase or prolong its therapeutic and adverse effects).

No products indexed under this heading.

Estradiol Valerate (Co-administration of indinavir and drugs primarily metabolized by CYP3A4 may result in increased plasma concentrations of the other drug, which could increase or prolong its therapeutic and adverse effects).

No products indexed under this heading.

Ethinyl Estradiol (Co-administration with Ortho-Novum 1/35 has resulted in an increase in ethinyl estradiol AUC). Products include:

Lybrel Tablets **3204**
Mircette Tablets **1034**
NuvaRing **2897**
Ortho-Cyclen/Ortho Tri-Cyclen **2449**
Ortho Evra Transdermal System **2437**

Ortho Tri-Cyclen Lo Tablets 2458
Seasonique Tablets 1046
Yaz Tablets 805

Ethosuximide (Co-administration of indinavir and drugs primarily metabolized by CYP3A4 may result in increased plasma concentrations of the other drug, which could increase or prolong its therapeutic and adverse effects).
No products indexed under this heading.

Ethynodiol Diacetate (Co-administration of indinavir and drugs primarily metabolized by CYP3A4 may result in increased plasma concentrations of the other drug, which could increase or prolong its therapeutic and adverse effects).
No products indexed under this heading.

Etoposide (Co-administration of indinavir and drugs primarily metabolized by CYP3A4 may result in increased plasma concentrations of the other drug, which could increase or prolong its therapeutic and adverse effects).
No products indexed under this heading.

Etoposide Phosphate (Co-administration of indinavir and drugs primarily metabolized by CYP3A4 may result in increased plasma concentrations of the other drug, which could increase or prolong its therapeutic and adverse effects).
No products indexed under this heading.

Felbamate (Drugs that induce CYP3A4 activity would be expected to increase the clearance of indinavir, resulting in lowered plasma concentrations of indinavir).
No products indexed under this heading.

Felodipine (Co-administration of calcium channel blockers with indinavir may result in increased plasma concentrations of the dihydropyridine calcium channel blockers which could increase or prolong their therapeutic and adverse effects. Caution is warranted and clinical monitoring is recommended).
No products indexed under this heading.

Fentanyl (Co-administration of indinavir and drugs primarily metabolized by CYP3A4 may result in increased plasma concentrations of the other drug, which could increase or prolong its therapeutic and adverse effects). Products include:
Duragesic Transdermal System 2405
Ionsys Transdermal System 2410

Fentanyl Citrate (Co-administration of indinavir and drugs primarily metabolized by CYP3A4 may result in increased plasma concentrations of the other drug, which could increase or prolong its therapeutic and adverse effects). Products include:
Actiq 959
Fentora Tablets 968

Fluconazole (Co-administration has resulted in a 19% ± 33% decrease in indinavir AUC).
No products indexed under this heading.

Fludrocortisone Acetate (Drugs that induce CYP3A4 activity would be expected to increase the clearance of indinavir, resulting in lowered plasma concentrations of indinavir).
No products indexed under this heading.

Fluoxetine (Co-administration of indinavir and other drugs that inhibit CYP3A4 may decrease the clearance of indinavir and may result in increased plasma concentrations of indinavir).
No products indexed under this heading.

Fluoxetine Hydrochloride (Co-administration of indinavir and other drugs that inhibit CYP3A4 may decrease the clearance of indinavir and may result in increased plasma concentrations of indinavir).
Products include:
Prozac Weekly Capsules 1852
Prozac Pulvules and Liquid 1852
Symbyax Capsules 1871

Fluticasone Propionate (Concomitant use of fluticasone propionate and indinavir sulfate may increase plasma concentrations of fluticasone propionate; co-administer with caution. Consider alternatives to fluticasone propionate, particularly for long-term use). Products include:
Advair Diskus 100/50 1276
Advair Diskus 250/50 1276
Advair Diskus 500/50 1276
Advair HFA 45/21 Inhalation Aerosol.. 1288
Advair HFA 115/21 Inhalation Aerosol.. 1288
Advair HFA 230/21 Inhalation Aerosol.. 1288
Flonase Nasal Spray 1431
Flovent Diskus 50 mcg 1435

Fluticasone Propionate HFA (Concomitant use of fluticasone propionate and indinavir sulfate may increase plasma concentrations of fluticasone propionate; co-administer with caution. Consider alternatives to fluticasone propionate, particularly for long-term use). Products include:
Flovent HFA 1440

Fluvoxamine Maleate (Co-administration of indinavir and other drugs that inhibit CYP3A4 may decrease the clearance of indinavir and may result in increased plasma concentrations of indinavir).
Products include:
Luvox CR Extended-Release Capsules....................................... 1759

Fosamprenavir Calcium (Co-administration of indinavir and other drugs that inhibit CYP3A4 may decrease the clearance of indinavir and may result in increased plasma concentrations of indinavir).
Products include:
Lexiva Oral Suspension 1510
Lexiva Tablets 1510

Fosphenytoin Sodium (Could diminish plasma concentrations of indinavir because phenytoin is an inducer of P450 3A4; caution is advised if co-administered).
No products indexed under this heading.

Garlic Extract (Drugs that induce CYP3A4 activity would be expected to increase the clearance of indinavir, resulting in lowered plasma concentrations of indinavir).
No products indexed under this heading.

Garlic Oil (Drugs that induce CYP3A4 activity would be expected to increase the clearance of indinavir, resulting in lowered plasma concentrations of indinavir).
No products indexed under this heading.

Haloperidol (Co-administration of indinavir and drugs primarily metabolized by CYP3A4 may result in increased plasma concentrations of the other drug, which could increase or prolong its therapeutic and adverse effects).
No products indexed under this heading.

Haloperidol Decanoate (Co-administration of indinavir and drugs primarily metabolized by CYP3A4 may result in increased plasma concentrations of the other drug, which could increase or prolong its therapeutic and adverse effects).
No products indexed under this heading.

Haloperidol Lactate (Co-administration of indinavir and drugs primarily metabolized by CYP3A4 may result in increased plasma concentrations of the other drug, which could increase or prolong its therapeutic and adverse effects).
No products indexed under this heading.

Hydrocortisone (Drugs that induce CYP3A4 activity would be expected to increase the clearance of indinavir, resulting in lowered plasma concentrations of indinavir).
No products indexed under this heading.

Hydrocortisone Acetate (Drugs that induce CYP3A4 activity would be expected to increase the clearance of indinavir, resulting in lowered plasma concentrations of indinavir).
Products include:
Analpram-HC 1140
Pramosone 1141

Hydrocortisone Butyrate (Drugs that induce CYP3A4 activity would be expected to increase the clearance of indinavir, resulting in lowered plasma concentrations of indinavir).
No products indexed under this heading.

Hydrocortisone Cypionate (Drugs that induce CYP3A4 activity would be expected to increase the clearance of indinavir, resulting in lowered plasma concentrations of indinavir).
No products indexed under this heading.

Hydrocortisone Hemisuccinate (Drugs that induce CYP3A4 activity would be expected to increase the clearance of indinavir, resulting in lowered plasma concentrations of indinavir).
No products indexed under this heading.

Hydrocortisone Probutate (Drugs that induce CYP3A4 activity would be expected to increase the clearance of indinavir, resulting in lowered plasma concentrations of indinavir).
No products indexed under this heading.

Hydrocortisone Sodium Phosphate (Drugs that induce CYP3A4 activity would be expected to increase the clearance of indinavir, resulting in lowered plasma concentrations of indinavir).
No products indexed under this heading.

Hydrocortisone Sodium Succinate (Drugs that induce CYP3A4 activity would be expected to increase the clearance of indinavir, resulting in lowered plasma concentrations of indinavir).
No products indexed under this heading.

Hydrocortisone Valerate (Drugs that induce CYP3A4 activity would be expected to increase the clearance of indinavir, resulting in lowered plasma concentrations of indinavir).
No products indexed under this heading.

Hypericum (Co-administration of indinavir and St. John's Wort (hypericum perforatum) or products containing St. John's Wort has been shown to substantially decrease indinavir concentrations and may lead to loss of virologic response and possible resistance to indinavir or to the class of protease inhibitors; co-administration is not recommended).
Products include:
Satiété Tablets 640

Hypericum Perforatum (Drugs that induce CYP3A4 activity would be expected to increase the clearance of indinavir, resulting in lowered plasma concentrations of indinavir).
No products indexed under this heading.

Isoniazid (Co-administration has resulted in a 13% ± 15% increase in isoniazid AUC).
No products indexed under this heading.

Isradipine (Co-administration of calcium channel blockers with indinavir may result in increased plasma concentrations of the dihydropyridine calcium channel blockers which could increase or prolong their therapeutic and adverse effects. Caution is warranted and clinical monitoring is recommended). Products include:
DynaCirc CR Controlled Release Tablets....................................... 1407

Itraconazole (Co-administration of indinavir and itraconzole may lead to increased indinvair concentrations. Dose reduction of indinavir to 600 mg every 8 hours is recommended when administering itraconzole concomitantly).
No products indexed under this heading.

Ixabepilone (Co-administration of indinavir and drugs primarily metabolized by CYP3A4 may result in increased plasma concentrations of the other drug, which could increase or prolong its therapeutic and adverse effects). Products include:
Ixempra Kit for Injection 915

Ketoconazole (Co-administration of indinavir and ketoconazole may lead to increased indinvair concentrations. Dose reduction of indinavir to 600 mg every 8 hours is recommended when administering ketoconazole concomitantly). Products include:
Extina Foam, 2% 3057
Nizoral A-D Shampoo 1901

Levonorgestrel (Co-administration of indinavir and drugs primarily metabolized by CYP3A4 may result in increased plasma concentrations of the other drug, which could increase or prolong its therapeutic and adverse effects). Products include:
Climara Pro Transdermal System 768
Lybrel Tablets 3204

IMPORTANT NOTE: Always consult each drug listing in the patient's regimen for possible interactions.

Mirena Intrauterine System 779
Plan B Tablets 1044
Seasonique Tablets 1046

Lidocaine (Co-administration may lead to increased lidocaine concentrations. Caution is warranted and therapeutic concentration monitoring is recommended for antiarrhythmics when co-administered with indinavir). Products include:
Lidoderm Patch 1114

Lidocaine Hydrochloride (Co-administration may lead to increased lidocaine concentrations. Caution is warranted and therapeutic concentration monitoring is recommended for antiarrhythmics when co-administered with indinavir).
No products indexed under this heading.

Lopinavir (Co-administration of indinavir and other drugs that inhibit CYP3A4 may decrease the clearance of indinavir and may result in increased plasma concentrations of indinavir). Products include:
Kaletra 452

Loratadine (Co-administration of indinavir and other drugs that inhibit CYP3A4 may decrease the clearance of indinavir and may result in increased plasma concentrations of indinavir).
No products indexed under this heading.

Lovastatin (The risk of myopathy including rhabdomyolysis may be increased when protease inhibitors, including indinavir, are used in combination with HMG-CoA inhibitors that are metabolized by the CYP3A4 pathway; concomitant use is not recommended). Products include:
Advicor Tablets 402
Mevacor Tablets 2063

Mephenytoin (Drugs that induce CYP3A4 activity would be expected to increase the clearance of indinavir, resulting in lowered plasma concentrations of indinavir).
No products indexed under this heading.

Mestranol (Co-administration of indinavir and drugs primarily metabolized by CYP3A4 may result in increased plasma concentrations of the other drug, which could increase or prolong its therapeutic and adverse effects).
No products indexed under this heading.

Methadone Hydrochloride (Co-administration of indinavir and drugs primarily metabolized by CYP3A4 may result in increased plasma concentrations of the other drug, which could increase or prolong its therapeutic and adverse effects).
No products indexed under this heading.

Methsuximide (Drugs that induce CYP3A4 activity would be expected to increase the clearance of indinavir, resulting in lowered plasma concentrations of indinavir).
No products indexed under this heading.

Methylergonovine Maleate (Inhibition of CYP3A4 by indinavir could result in elevated plasma concentrations of ergot derivatives, potentially causing serious or life-threatening reactions; co-administration is contraindicated).
No products indexed under this heading.

Methylprednisolone (Drugs that induce CYP3A4 activity would be expected to increase the clearance of indinavir, resulting in lowered plasma concentrations of indinavir).
No products indexed under this heading.

Methylprednisolone Acetate (Drugs that induce CYP3A4 activity would be expected to increase the clearance of indinavir, resulting in lowered plasma concentrations of indinavir).
No products indexed under this heading.

Methylprednisolone Sodium Succinate (Drugs that induce CYP3A4 activity would be expected to increase the clearance of indinavir, resulting in lowered plasma concentrations of indinavir).
No products indexed under this heading.

Methysergide Maleate (Inhibition of CYP3A4 by indinavir could result in elevated plasma concentrations of ergot derivatives, potentially causing serious or life-threatening reactions; co-administration is contraindicated).
No products indexed under this heading.

Metronidazole (Co-administration of indinavir and other drugs that inhibit CYP3A4 may decrease the clearance of indinavir and may result in increased plasma concentrations of indinavir). Products include:
Pylera Capsules 714

Metronidazole Benzoate (Co-administration of indinavir and other drugs that inhibit CYP3A4 may decrease the clearance of indinavir and may result in increased plasma concentrations of indinavir).
No products indexed under this heading.

Metronidazole Hydrochloride (Co-administration of indinavir and other drugs that inhibit CYP3A4 may decrease the clearance of indinavir and may result in increased plasma concentrations of indinavir).
No products indexed under this heading.

Mibefradil Dihydrochloride (Co-administration of calcium channel blockers with indinavir may result in increased plasma concentrations of the dihydropyridine calcium channel blockers which could increase or prolong their therapeutic and adverse effects. Caution is warranted and clinical monitoring is recommended).
No products indexed under this heading.

Miconazole (Co-administration of indinavir and other drugs that inhibit CYP3A4 may decrease the clearance of indinavir and may result in increased plasma concentrations of indinavir).
No products indexed under this heading.

Miconazole Nitrate (Co-administration of indinavir and other drugs that inhibit CYP3A4 may decrease the clearance of indinavir and may result in increased plasma concentrations of indinavir).
No products indexed under this heading.

Midazolam Hydrochloride (Inhibition of CYP3A4 by indinavir could result in elevated plasma concentrations of midazolam potentially causing serious or life-threatening reactions; co-administration is contraindicated).
No products indexed under this heading.

Modafinil (Drugs that induce CYP3A4 activity would be expected to increase the clearance of indinavir, resulting in lowered plasma concentrations of indinavir). Products include:
Provigil Tablets 977

Nefazodone Hydrochloride (Co-administration of indinavir and drugs primarily metabolized by CYP3A4 may result in increased plasma concentrations of the other drug, which could increase or prolong its therapeutic and adverse effects).
No products indexed under this heading.

Nelfinavir Mesylate (Co-administration of indinavir and nelfinavir may lead to increased indinavir concentrations. The appropriate doses for this combination, with respect to safety and efficacy, have not been established).
No products indexed under this heading.

Nevirapine (Co-administration of indinavir and nevirapine may lead to decreased indinavir concentrations. The appropriate doses for this combination, with respect to saftey and efficacy, have not been established). Products include:
Viramune Oral Suspension 873
Viramune Tablets 873

Niacinamide (Co-administration of indinavir and other drugs that inhibit CYP3A4 may decrease the clearance of indinavir and may result in increased plasma concentrations of indinavir). Products include:
BioLean Free Tablets .... ■□635

Nicardipine Hydrochloride (Co-administration of calcium channel blockers with indinavir may result in increased plasma concentrations of the dihydropyridine calcium channel blockers which could increase or prolong their therapeutic and adverse effects. Caution is warranted and clinical monitoring is recommended). Products include:
Cardene I.V. 1093

Nicotinamide (Co-administration of indinavir and other drugs that inhibit CYP3A4 may decrease the clearance of indinavir and may result in increased plasma concentrations of indinavir).
No products indexed under this heading.

Nifedipine (Co-administration of calcium channel blockers with indinavir may result in increased plasma concentrations of the dihydropyridine calcium channel blockers which could increase or prolong their therapeutic and adverse effects. Caution is warranted and clinical monitoring is recommended).
No products indexed under this heading.

Nimodipine (Co-administration of calcium channel blockers with indinavir may result in increased plasma concentrations of the dihydropyridine calcium channel blockers which could increase or prolong their therapeutic and adverse effects. Caution is warranted and clinical monitoring is recommended). Products include:
Nimotop Capsules 790

Nisoldipine (Co-administration of calcium channel blockers with indinavir may result in increased plasma concentrations of the dihydropyridine calcium channel blockers which could increase or prolong their therapeutic and adverse effects. Caution is warranted and clinical monitoring is recommended). Products include:
Sular Extended Release Tablets 2975

Nitrendipine (Co-administration of indinavir and drugs primarily metabolized by CYP3A4 may result in increased plasma concentrations of the other drug, which could increase or prolong its therapeutic and adverse effects).
No products indexed under this heading.

Norethindrone (Co-administration with Ortho-Novum 1/35 has resulted in an increase in norethindrone AUC). Products include:
Ortho Micronor Tablets 2446

Norethindrone Acetate (Co-administration of indinavir and drugs primarily metabolized by CYP3A4 may result in increased plasma concentrations of the other drug, which could increase or prolong its therapeutic and adverse effects). Products include:
Activella Tablets 2347

Norfloxacin (Co-administration of indinavir and other drugs that inhibit CYP3A4 may decrease the clearance of indinavir and may result in increased plasma concentrations of indinavir). Products include:
Noroxin Tablets 2069

Norgestrel (Co-administration of indinavir and drugs primarily metabolized by CYP3A4 may result in increased plasma concentrations of the other drug, which could increase or prolong its therapeutic and adverse effects).
No products indexed under this heading.

Omeprazole (Co-administration of indinavir and other drugs that inhibit CYP3A4 may decrease the clearance of indinavir and may result in increased plasma concentrations of indinavir).
No products indexed under this heading.

Ondansetron (Co-administration of indinavir and drugs primarily metabolized by CYP3A4 may result in increased plasma concentrations of the other drug, which could increase or prolong its therapeutic and adverse effects). Products include:
Zofran ODT Orally Disintegrating Tablets 1687

Ondansetron Hydrochloride (Co-administration of indinavir and drugs primarily metabolized by CYP3A4 may result in increased plasma concentrations of the other drug, which could increase or prolong its therapeutic and adverse effects). Products include:
Zofran Injection 1682
Zofran 1687

Oxcarbazepine (Drugs that induce CYP3A4 activity would be expected to increase the clearance of indinavir, resulting in lowered plasma concentrations of indinavir).
No products indexed under this heading.

Paclitaxel (Co-administration of indinavir and drugs primarily metabolized by CYP3A4 may result in increased plasma concentrations of the other drug, which could increase or prolong its therapeutic and adverse effects).
No products indexed under this heading.

Paroxetine Hydrochloride (Co-administration of indinavir and other drugs that inhibit CYP3A4 may decrease the clearance of indinavir and may result in increased plasma concentrations of indinavir).
Products include:
Paxil 1535
Paxil CR Controlled-Release Tablets 1544

Phenobarbital (Could diminish plasma concentrations of indinavir because phenobarbital is an inducer of P450 3A4; caution is advised if co-administered). Products include:
Donnatal Extentabs 2507

Phenobarbital Sodium (Drugs that induce CYP3A4 activity would be expected to increase the clearance of indinavir, resulting in lowered plasma concentrations of indinavir).
No products indexed under this heading.

Phenytoin (Could diminish plasma concentrations of indinavir because phenytoin is an inducer of P450 3A4; caution is advised if co-administered).
No products indexed under this heading.

Phenytoin Sodium (Could diminish plasma concentrations of indinavir because phenytoin is an inducer of P450 3A4; caution is advised if co-administered). Products include:
Phenytek Capsules 2192

Pimozide (Inhibition of CYP3A4 by indinavir could result in elevated plasma concentrations of pimozide potentially causing serious or life-threatening reactions; co-administration is contraindicated).
No products indexed under this heading.

Polyestradiol Phosphate (Co-administration of indinavir and drugs primarily metabolized by CYP3A4 may result in increased plasma concentrations of the other drug, which could increase or prolong its therapeutic and adverse effects).
No products indexed under this heading.

Prednisolone Acetate (Drugs that induce CYP3A4 activity would be expected to increase the clearance of indinavir, resulting in lowered plasma concentrations of indinavir).
Products include:
Pred Forte Ophthalmic Suspension .... ⊙227
Pred Mild Ophthalmic Suspension .... ⊙230
Pred-G Ophthalmic Ointment .... ⊙229
Pred-G Ophthalmic Suspension .... ⊙228

Prednisolone Sodium Phosphate (Drugs that induce CYP3A4 activity would be expected to increase the clearance of indinavir, resulting in lowered plasma concentrations of indinavir).
No products indexed under this heading.

Prednisolone Tebutate (Drugs that induce CYP3A4 activity would be expected to increase the clearance of indinavir, resulting in lowered plasma concentrations of indinavir).
No products indexed under this heading.

Prednisone (Drugs that induce CYP3A4 activity would be expected to increase the clearance of indinavir, resulting in lowered plasma concentrations of indinavir).
No products indexed under this heading.

Primidone (Drugs that induce CYP3A4 activity would be expected to increase the clearance of indinavir, resulting in lowered plasma concentrations of indinavir).
No products indexed under this heading.

Propoxyphene Hydrochloride (Co-administration of indinavir and other drugs that inhibit CYP3A4 may decrease the clearance of indinavir and may result in increased plasma concentrations of indinavir).
No products indexed under this heading.

Propoxyphene Napsylate (Co-administration of indinavir and other drugs that inhibit CYP3A4 may decrease the clearance of indinavir and may result in increased plasma concentrations of indinavir).
No products indexed under this heading.

Quinidine (Co-administration of indinavir and quinidine may lead to increased quinidine concentrations. Caution is warranted and therapeutic concentration monitoring is recommended for antiarrhythmics when co-administered with indinavir).
No products indexed under this heading.

Quinidine Gluconate (Co-administration of indinavir and quinidine may lead to increased quinidine concentrations. Caution is warranted and therapeutic concentration monitoring is recommended for antiarrhythmics when co-administered with indinavir).
No products indexed under this heading.

Quinidine Hydrochloride (Co-administration of indinavir and quinidine may lead to increased quinidine concentrations. Caution is warranted and therapeutic concentration monitoring is recommended for antiarrhythmics when co-administered with indinavir).
No products indexed under this heading.

Quinidine Polygalacturonate (Co-administration of indinavir and quinidine lead to increased quinidine, concentrations. Caution is warranted and therapeutic concentration monitoring is recommended for antiarrhythmics when co-administered with indinavir).
No products indexed under this heading.

Quinidine Sulfate (Co-administration of indinavir and quinidine lead to increased quinidine, concentrations. Caution is warranted and therapeutic concentration monitoring is recommended for antiarrhythmics when co-administered with indinavir).
No products indexed under this heading.

Quinine (Co-administration of indinavir and other drugs that inhibit CYP3A4 may decrease the clearance of indinavir and may result in increased plasma concentrations of indinavir).
No products indexed under this heading.

Quinine Sulfate (Co-administration of indinavir and other drugs that inhibit CYP3A4 may decrease the clearance of indinavir and may result in increased plasma concentrations of indinavir).
No products indexed under this heading.

Quinupristin (Co-administration of indinavir and other drugs that inhibit CYP3A4 may decrease the clearance of indinavir and may result in increased plasma concentrations of indinavir).
No products indexed under this heading.

Ranitidine Bismuth Citrate (Co-administration of indinavir and other drugs that inhibit CYP3A4 may decrease the clearance of indinavir and may result in increased plasma concentrations of indinavir).
No products indexed under this heading.

Ranitidine Hydrochloride (Co-administration of indinavir and other drugs that inhibit CYP3A4 may decrease the clearance of indinavir and may result in increased plasma concentrations of indinavir).
Products include:
Zantac 75 Tablets 603
Zantac 1670
Zantac Injection 1666
Zantac Injection Pharmacy Bulk Package 1668
Maximum Strength Zantac 150 Tablets 603
Maximum Strength Zantac 150 Cool Mint Tablets 603

Rifabutin (Co-administration of indinavir and rifabutin may lead to decreased indinavir and increased rifabutin concentrations. Dose reduction of rifabutin to half the standard dose and a dose increase of indinavir to 1000 mg (three 333-mg capsules) every 8 hours are recommended when rifabutin and indinavir are co-administered).
No products indexed under this heading.

Rifampicin (Drugs that induce CYP3A4 activity would be expected to increase the clearance of indinavir, resulting in lowered plasma concentrations of indinavir).
No products indexed under this heading.

Rifampin (Markedly diminishes plasma concentrations of indinavir because rifampin is a potent inducer of P450 3A4; co-administration is not recommended).
No products indexed under this heading.

Rifapentine (Drugs that induce CYP3A4 activity would be expected to increase the clearance of indinavir, resulting in lowered plasma concentrations of indinavir).
No products indexed under this heading.

Ritonavir (Co-administration of indinavir and ritonavir may lead to increased indinavir and ritonavir concentrations. The appropriate doses for this combination, with respect to saftey and efficacy, have not been established. Preliminary clinical data suggest that the incidence of nephrolithiasis is higher in patients receiving indinavir in combination with ritonavir than those receiving indinavir 800 mg q8h). Products include:
Kaletra 452
Norvir 489

Rosuvastatin Calcium (Co-administration of indinavir and rosuvastatin may lead to increased rosuvastatin concentrations. The risk of myopathy, including rhabdomyolysis, may be increased when protease inhibitors, including indinavir, are used in combination with HMG-CoA inhibitors that are metabolized by the CYP3A4 pathway. Use lowest possible dose of rosuvastatin with careful monitoring, or consider HMG-CoA reductase inhibitors that are not primarily metabolized by CYP3A, such as pravastatin or fluvastatinin combination with indinavir). Products include:
Crestor Tablets 677

Saquinavir (Co-administration of indinavir and saquinavir may lead to increased saquinavir concentrations).
No products indexed under this heading.

Saquinavir Mesylate (Co-administration of indinavir and saquinavir may lead to increased saquinavir concentrations).
No products indexed under this heading.

Sertraline Hydrochloride (Co-administration of indinavir and drugs primarily metabolized by CYP3A4 may result in increased plasma concentrations of the other drug, which could increase or prolong its therapeutic and adverse effects).
No products indexed under this heading.

Sildenafil Citrate (Co-administration has resulted in increased sildenafil AUC by 340%; this may result in an increase in sildenafil-associated adverse events, including hypotension, priapism, and visual changes; based on this result the dose of sildenafil should not exceed 25 mg in a 48-hour period).
No products indexed under this heading.

Simvastatin (The risk of myopathy including rhabdomyolysis may be increased when protease inhibitors, including indinavir, are used in combination with HMG-CoA inhibitors that are metabolized by the CYP3A4 pathway; concomitant use is not recommended). Products include:
Simcor Tablets 502
Vytorin 10/10 Tablets 2149
Vytorin 10/10 Tablets 2939
Vytorin 10/20 Tablets 2149
Vytorin 10/20 Tablets 2939
Vytorin 10/40 Tablets 2149
Vytorin 10/40 Tablets 2939
Vytorin 10/80 Tablets 2149
Vytorin 10/80 Tablets 2939
Zocor Tablets 2136

Sirolimus (Co-administration of indinavir and sirolimus may lead to increased sirolimus concentrations).
Products include:
Rapamune 3260

Stavudine (Co-administration has resulted in a 25% ± 26% increase in stavudine AUC and no change in indinavir AUC; co-administration does not require dose modification).
No products indexed under this heading.

Sulfinpyrazone (Drugs that induce CYP3A4 activity would be expected to increase the clearance of indinavir, resulting in lowered plasma concentrations of indinavir).

No products indexed under this heading.

Tacrolimus (Co-administration of indinavir and tacrolimus may lead to increased tacrolimus concentrations). Products include:

Prograf Capsules and Injection 622
Protopic Ointment 628

Tadalafil (Co-administration of indinavir and tadalafil is expected to substantially increase plasma concentrations of tadalafil and may result in an increase in adverse events. Tadalafil dose should not exceed a maximum of 10 mg in a 72-hour period in patients receiving concomitant indinavir therapy). Products include:

Cialis Tablets 1792

Tamoxifen Citrate (Co-administration of indinavir and drugs primarily metabolized by CYP3A4 may result in increased plasma concentrations of the other drug, which could increase or prolong its therapeutic and adverse effects).

No products indexed under this heading.

Telithromycin (Co-administration of indinavir and other drugs that inhibit CYP3A4 may decrease the clearance of indinavir and may result in increased plasma concentrations of indinavir). Products include:

Ketek Tablets 2744

Terfenadine (Inhibition of CYP3A4 by indinavir could result in elevated plasma concentrations of terfenadine potentially causing serious or life-threatening reactions; co-administration is contraindicated).

No products indexed under this heading.

Theophylline (Drugs that induce CYP3A4 activity would be expected to increase the clearance of indinavir, resulting in lowered plasma concentrations of indinavir).

No products indexed under this heading.

Theophylline Anhydrous (Drugs that induce CYP3A4 activity would be expected to increase the clearance of indinavir, resulting in lowered plasma concentrations of indinavir). Products include:

Uniphyl Tablets 2595

Theophylline Calcium Salicylate (Drugs that induce CYP3A4 activity would be expected to increase the clearance of indinavir, resulting in lowered plasma concentrations of indinavir).

No products indexed under this heading.

Theophylline Dihydroxypropyl (Glyceryl) (Drugs that induce CYP3A4 activity would be expected to increase the clearance of indinavir, resulting in lowered plasma concentrations of indinavir).

No products indexed under this heading.

Theophylline Ethylenediamine (Drugs that induce CYP3A4 activity would be expected to increase the clearance of indinavir, resulting in lowered plasma concentrations of indinavir).

No products indexed under this heading.

Tiagabine Hydrochloride (Co-administration of indinavir and drugs primarily metabolized by CYP3A4 may result in increased plasma concentrations of the other drug, which could increase or prolong its therapeutic and adverse effects). Products include:

Gabitril Tablets 973

Tolterodine Tartrate (Co-administration of indinavir and drugs primarily metabolized by CYP3A4 may result in increased plasma concentrations of the other drug, which could increase or prolong its therapeutic and adverse effects).

No products indexed under this heading.

Trazodone Hydrochloride (Concomitant use of trazodone hydrochloride and indinavir sulfate may increase plasma concentrations of trazodone. If trazodone is used with a CYP3A4 inhibitor such as indinavir sulfate, the combinatin should be used with caution and a lower dose of trazodone should be considered).

No products indexed under this heading.

Triamcinolone (Drugs that induce CYP3A4 activity would be expected to increase the clearance of indinavir, resulting in lowered plasma concentrations of indinavir).

No products indexed under this heading.

Triamcinolone Acetonide (Drugs that induce CYP3A4 activity would be expected to increase the clearance of indinavir, resulting in lowered plasma concentrations of indinavir). Products include:

Azmacort Inhalation Aerosol 407
Nasacort AQ Nasal Spray 2765
Triesence Injectable Suspension .... ⊙209

Triamcinolone Diacetate (Drugs that induce CYP3A4 activity would be expected to increase the clearance of indinavir, resulting in lowered plasma concentrations of indinavir).

No products indexed under this heading.

Triamcinolone Hexacetonide (Drugs that induce CYP3A4 activity would be expected to increase the clearance of indinavir, resulting in lowered plasma concentrations of indinavir).

No products indexed under this heading.

Triazolam (Inhibition of CYP3A4 by indinavir could result in elevated plasma concentrations of triazolam potentially causing serious or life-threatening reactions; co-administration is contraindicated).

No products indexed under this heading.

Trimethoprim (Co-administration with trimethoprim/sulfamethoxazole tablets has resulted in a 19% ± 31% increase in trimethoprim AUC).

No products indexed under this heading.

Troglitazone (Drugs that induce CYP3A4 activity would be expected to increase the clearance of indinavir, resulting in lowered plasma concentrations of indinavir).

No products indexed under this heading.

Troleandomycin (Co-administration of indinavir and other drugs that inhibit CYP3A4 may decrease the clearance of indinavir and may result in increased plasma concentrations of indinavir).

No products indexed under this heading.

Valproate Sodium (Co-administration of indinavir and other drugs that inhibit CYP3A4 may decrease the clearance of indinavir and may result in increased plasma concentrations of indinavir).

No products indexed under this heading.

Vardenafil Hydrochloride (Co-administration of indinavir and vardenafil is expected to substantially increase plasma concentrations of vardenafil and may result in an increase in adverse events. Vardenafil dose should not exceed a maximum of 2.5 mg in a 24-hour period in patient receiving concomitant indinavir therapy). Products include:

Levitra Tablets 2876

Venlafaxine Hydrochloride (In a study, venlafaxine administered under steady-state conditions at 150 mg/day resulted in a 28% decrease in the AUC of a single 800 mg oral dose of indinavir and a 36% decrease in indinavir Cmax. Indinavir did not affect the pharmacokinetics of venlafaxine). Products include:

Effexor XR Extended-Release Capsules 3195
Venlafaxine Hydrochloride Tablets ... 2199

Verapamil Hydrochloride (Co-administration of calcium channel blockers with indinavir may result in increased plasma concentrations of the dihydropyridine calcium channel blockers which could increase or prolong their therapeutic and adverse effects. Caution is warranted and clinical monitoring is recommended). Products include:

Tarka Tablets 511

Vinblastine Sulfate (Co-administration of indinavir and drugs primarily metabolized by CYP3A4 may result in increased plasma concentrations of the other drug, which could increase or prolong its therapeutic and adverse effects).

No products indexed under this heading.

Vincristine Sulfate (Co-administration of indinavir and drugs primarily metabolized by CYP3A4 may result in increased plasma concentrations of the other drug, which could increase or prolong its therapeutic and adverse effects).

No products indexed under this heading.

Voriconazole (Co-administration of indinavir and other drugs that inhibit CYP3A4 may decrease the clearance of indinavir and may result in increased plasma concentrations of indinavir).

No products indexed under this heading.

Warfarin Sodium (Co-administration of indinavir and drugs primarily metabolized by CYP3A4 may result in increased plasma concentrations of the other drug, which could increase or prolong its therapeutic and adverse effects).

No products indexed under this heading.

Zafirlukast (Co-administration of indinavir and other drugs that inhibit CYP3A4 may decrease the clearance of indinavir and may result in increased plasma concentrations of indinavir). Products include:

Accolate Tablets 669

Zidovudine (Co-administration has resulted in a 13% ±- 48% increase in indinavir AUC and a 17% ± 23% increase in zidovudine AUC; co-administration does not require dose modification). Products include:

Combivir Tablets 1384
Retrovir 1574
Retrovir IV Infusion 1579
Trizivir Tablets 1622

Zileuton (Co-administration of indinavir and other drugs that inhibit CYP3A4 may decrease the clearance of indinavir and may result in increased plasma concentrations of indinavir).

No products indexed under this heading.

Food Interactions

Food, unspecified (Co-administration with a meal high in calories, fat, and protein has resulted in a 77% ± 8% reduction in AUC and an 84% ± 7% reduction in Cmax; administer without food 1 hour before or 2 hours after a meal).

Grapefruit (Co-administration of indinavir and other drugs that inhibit CYP3A4 may decrease the clearance of indinavir and may result in increased plasma concentrations of indinavir).

Grapefruit Juice (Potential for decrease in indinavir AUC).

CUBICIN FOR INJECTION

(Daptomycin) 995

May interact with aminoglycosides, beta-lactams antibiotics, HMG-CoA reductase inhibitors, and certain other agents. Compounds in these categories include:

Amikacin Sulfate (In vitro synergistic interactions of daptomycin with aminoglycosides, beta-lactam antibiotics, and rifampin have been shown against some isolates of staphylococci and enterococci).

No products indexed under this heading.

Atorvastatin Calcium (Experience with co-administration of HMG-CoA reductase inhibitors and Cubicin is limited, therefore, considerations should be given to temporarily suspending use of HMG-CoA reductase inhibitors in patients recieving Cubicin). Products include:

Lipitor Tablets 2501

Aztreonam (In vitro synergistic interactions of daptomycin with aminoglycosides, beta-lactam antibiotics, and rifampin have been shown against some isolates of staphylococci and enterococci).

No products indexed under this heading.

Cefaclor (In vitro synergistic interactions of daptomycin with aminoglycosides, beta-lactam antibiotics, and rifampin have been shown against some isolates of staphylococci and enterococci).

No products indexed under this heading.

Cefadroxil (In vitro synergistic interactions of daptomycin with aminoglycosides, beta-lactam antibiotics, and rifampin have been shown against some isolates of staphylococci and enterococci).

No products indexed under this heading.

Cefamandole Nafate (In vitro synergistic interactions of daptomycin with aminoglycosides, beta-lactam antibiotics, and rifampin have been shown against some isolates of staphylococci and enterococci).
No products indexed under this heading.

Cefazolin Sodium (In vitro synergistic interactions of daptomycin with aminoglycosides, beta-lactam antibiotics, and rifampin have been shown against some isolates of staphylococci and enterococci).
No products indexed under this heading.

Cefixime (In vitro synergistic interactions of daptomycin with aminoglycosides, beta-lactam antibiotics, and rifampin have been shown against some isolates of staphylococci and enterococci). Products include:
Suprax for Oral Suspension **1891**
Suprax Tablets **1891**

Cefmetazole Sodium (In vitro synergistic interactions of daptomycin with aminoglycosides, beta-lactam antibiotics, and rifampin have been shown against some isolates of staphylococci and enterococci).
No products indexed under this heading.

Cefonicid Sodium (In vitro synergistic interactions of daptomycin with aminoglycosides, beta-lactam antibiotics, and rifampin have been shown against some isolates of staphylococci and enterococci).
No products indexed under this heading.

Cefoperazone Sodium (In vitro synergistic interactions of daptomycin with aminoglycosides, beta-lactam antibiotics, and rifampin have been shown against some isolates of staphylococci and enterococci).
No products indexed under this heading.

Ceforanide (In vitro synergistic interactions of daptomycin with aminoglycosides, beta-lactam antibiotics, and rifampin have been shown against some isolates of staphylococci and enterococci).
No products indexed under this heading.

Cefotaxime Sodium (In vitro synergistic interactions of daptomycin with aminoglycosides, beta-lactam antibiotics, and rifampin have been shown against some isolates of staphylococci and enterococci).
No products indexed under this heading.

Cefotetan (In vitro synergistic interactions of daptomycin with aminoglycosides, beta-lactam antibiotics, and rifampin have been shown against some isolates of staphylococci and enterococci).
No products indexed under this heading.

Cefoxitin Sodium (In vitro synergistic interactions of daptomycin with aminoglycosides, beta-lactam antibiotics, and rifampin have been shown against some isolates of staphylococci and enterococci).
No products indexed under this heading.

Cefpodoxime Proxetil (In vitro synergistic interactions of daptomycin with aminoglycosides, beta-lactam antibiotics, and rifampin have been shown against some isolates of staphylococci and enterococci).
No products indexed under this heading.

Cefprozil (In vitro synergistic interactions of daptomycin with aminoglycosides, beta-lactam antibiotics, and rifampin have been shown against some isolates of staphylococci and enterococci).
No products indexed under this heading.

Ceftazidime (In vitro synergistic interactions of daptomycin with aminoglycosides, beta-lactam antibiotics, and rifampin have been shown against some isolates of staphylococci and enterococci). Products include:
Fortaz **1450**

Ceftizoxime Sodium (In vitro synergistic interactions of daptomycin with aminoglycosides, beta-lactam antibiotics, and rifampin have been shown against some isolates of staphylococci and enterococci).
No products indexed under this heading.

Ceftriaxone Sodium (In vitro synergistic interactions of daptomycin with aminoglycosides, beta-lactam antibiotics, and rifampin have been shown against some isolates of staphylococci and enterococci). Products include:
Rocephin Injectable Vials, ADD-Vantage, Galaxy, Bulk........... **2642**

Cefuroxime Axetil (In vitro synergistic interactions of daptomycin with aminoglycosides, beta-lactam antibiotics, and rifampin have been shown against some isolates of staphylococci and enterococci). Products include:
Ceftin **1380**

Cefuroxime Sodium (In vitro synergistic interactions of daptomycin with aminoglycosides, beta-lactam antibiotics, and rifampin have been shown against some isolates of staphylococci and enterococci).
No products indexed under this heading.

Cephalexin (In vitro synergistic interactions of daptomycin with aminoglycosides, beta-lactam antibiotics, and rifampin have been shown against some isolates of staphylococci and enterococci).
No products indexed under this heading.

Cephalothin Sodium (In vitro synergistic interactions of daptomycin with aminoglycosides, beta-lactam antibiotics, and rifampin have been shown against some isolates of staphylococci and enterococci).
No products indexed under this heading.

Cephapirin Sodium (In vitro synergistic interactions of daptomycin with aminoglycosides, beta-lactam antibiotics, and rifampin have been shown against some isolates of staphylococci and enterococci).
No products indexed under this heading.

Cephradine (In vitro synergistic interactions of daptomycin with aminoglycosides, beta-lactam antibiotics, and rifampin have been shown against some isolates of staphylococci and enterococci).
No products indexed under this heading.

Cerivastatin Sodium (Experience with co-administration of HMG-CoA reductase inhibitors and Cubicin is limited, therefore, considerations should be given to temporarily suspending use of HMG-CoA reductase inhibitors in patients recieving Cubicin).
No products indexed under this heading.

Cilastatin Sodium (In vitro synergistic interactions of daptomycin with aminoglycosides, beta-lactam antibiotics, and rifampin have been shown against some isolates of staphylococci and enterococci). Products include:
Primaxin I.M. **2080**
Primaxin I.V. **2083**

Fluvastatin Sodium (Experience with co-administration of HMG-CoA reductase inhibitors and Cubicin is limited, therefore, considerations should be given to temporarily suspending use of HMG-CoA reductase inhibitors in patients recieving Cubicin). Products include:
Lescol Capsules **2268**
Lescol XL Tablets **2268**

Gentamicin Sulfate (In vitro synergistic interactions of daptomycin with aminoglycosides, beta-lactam antibiotics, and rifampin have been shown against some isolates of staphylococci and enterococci). Products include:
Pred-G Ophthalmic Ointment .... ⊙**229**
Pred-G Ophthalmic Suspension ...... ⊙**228**

Imipenem (In vitro synergistic interactions of daptomycin with aminoglycosides, beta-lactam antibiotics, and rifampin have been shown against some isolates of staphylococci and enterococci). Products include:
Primaxin I.M. **2080**
Primaxin I.V. **2083**

Kanamycin Sulfate (In vitro synergistic interactions of daptomycin with aminoglycosides, beta-lactam antibiotics, and rifampin have been shown against some isolates of staphylococci and enterococci).
No products indexed under this heading.

Loracarbef (In vitro synergistic interactions of daptomycin with aminoglycosides, beta-lactam antibiotics, and rifampin have been shown against some isolates of staphylococci and enterococci).
No products indexed under this heading.

Lovastatin (Experience with co-administration of HMG-CoA reductase inhibitors and Cubicin is limited, therefore, considerations should be given to temporarily suspending use of HMG-CoA reductase inhibitors in patients recieving Cubicin). Products include:
Advicor Tablets **402**
Mevacor Tablets **2063**

Pravastatin Sodium (Experience with co-administration of HMG-CoA reductase inhibitors and Cubicin is limited, therefore, considerations should be given to temporarily suspending use of HMG-CoA reductase inhibitors in patients recieving Cubicin).
No products indexed under this heading.

Rifampin (In vitro synergistic interactions of daptomycin with aminoglycosides, beta-lactam antibiotics, and rifampin have been shown against some isolates of staphylococci and enterococci).
No products indexed under this heading.

Rosuvastatin Calcium (Experience with co-administration of HMG-CoA reductase inhibitors and Cubicin is limited, therefore, considerations should be given to temporarily suspending use of HMG-CoA reductase inhibitors in patients recieving Cubicin). Products include:
Crestor Tablets **677**

Simvastatin (Experience with co-administration of HMG-CoA reductase inhibitors and Cubicin is limited, therefore, considerations should be given to temporarily suspending use of HMG-CoA reductase inhibitors in patients recieving Cubicin). Products include:
Simcor Tablets **502**
Vytorin 10/10 Tablets **2149**
Vytorin 10/10 Tablets **2939**
Vytorin 10/20 Tablets **2149**
Vytorin 10/20 Tablets **2939**
Vytorin 10/40 Tablets **2149**
Vytorin 10/40 Tablets **2939**
Vytorin 10/80 Tablets **2149**
Vytorin 10/80 Tablets **2939**
Zocor Tablets **2136**

Streptomycin Sulfate (In vitro synergistic interactions of daptomycin with aminoglycosides, beta-lactam antibiotics, and rifampin have been shown against some isolates of staphylococci and enterococci).
No products indexed under this heading.

Tobramycin (In vitro synergistic interactions of daptomycin with aminoglycosides, beta-lactam antibiotics, and rifampin have been shown against some isolates of staphylococci and enterococci). Products include:
Zylet Ophthalmic Suspension .... ⊙**247**

Tobramycin Sulfate (Mean Cmax and AUC 0-∞ of daptomycin increased when administered with tobramycin, and the mean Cmax and AUC 0-∞ of tobramycin decreased when administered with daptomycin. Therefore, caution is warranted when daptomycin is co-administered with tobramycin).
No products indexed under this heading.

CUPRIMINE CAPSULES

(Penicillamine) **1986**
None cited in PDR database.

CYANOKIT 5G ANTIDOTE

(Hydroxocobalamin) **1021**
None cited in PDR database.

IMPORTANT NOTE: Always consult each drug listing in the patient's regimen for possible interactions.

CYMBALTA DELAYED-RELEASE CAPSULES
(Duloxetine Hydrochloride) 1801
May interact with aspirin-acetylsalicylic acid, central nervous system depressants, central nervous system stimulants, anticoagulants, cytochrome p450 1a2 inhibitors (selected), cytochrome p450 2d6 inhibitors (selected), cytochrome p450 2d6 substrates (selected), drugs that reduce gastric acidity, monoamine oxidase inhibitors, nonsteroidal anti-inflammatory agents, phenothiazines, quinolones, serotoninergic agents, tricyclic antidepressants, triptans, and certain other agents. Compounds in these categories include:

Alatrofloxacin Mesylate (Some quinolones, inhibitors of CYP1A2, would be expected to increase the AUC and Cmax of duloxetine; co-administration should be avoided).
No products indexed under this heading.

Alfentanil Hydrochloride (Given the primary CNS effects of duloxetine, it should be used with caution when it is taken in combination with or substituted for other centrally acting drugs, including those with a similar mechanism of action).
No products indexed under this heading.

Almotriptan Malate (Development of a potentially life-threatening serotonin syndrome may occur with concomitant use of duloxetine HCl and triptans. If concomitant treatment is clinically warranted, careful observation of the patient is advised, particularly during treatment initiation and dose increases). Products include:
Axert Tablets 2431

Alprazolam (Given the primary CNS effects of duloxetine, it should be used with caution when it is taken in combination with or substituted for other centrally acting drugs, including those with a similar mechanism of action).
No products indexed under this heading.

Aluminum Carbonate (Duloxetine has an enteric coating that resists dissolution until reaching a segment of the gastrointestinal tract where the pH exceeds 5.5. Drugs that raise the gastrointestinal pH may lead to an earlier release of duloxetine).
No products indexed under this heading.

Aluminum Hydroxide (Duloxetine has an enteric coating that resists dissolution until reaching a segment of the gastrointestinal tract where the pH exceeds 5.5. Drugs that raise the gastrointestinal pH may lead to an earlier release of duloxetine).
No products indexed under this heading.

Amiodarone Hydrochloride (Because CYP2D6 is involved in duloxetine metabolism, concomitant use of duloxetine with potent inhibitors of CYP2D6 would be expected to, and does, result in higher concentrations of duloxetine).
No products indexed under this heading.

Amitriptyline Hydrochloride (Duloxetine is a moderate inhibitor of CYP2D6. Co-administration of duloxetine with other drugs that are extensively metabolized by this isoenzyme, and which have a narrow therapeutic window, should be approached with caution. Plasma tricyclic antidepressant (TCA) concentrations may need to be monitored, and the dose of the TCA may need to be reduced, if a TCA is co-administered with duloxetine).
No products indexed under this heading.

Amoxapine (Duloxetine is a moderate inhibitor of CYP2D6. Co-administration of duloxetine with other drugs that are extensively metabolized by this isoenzyme, and which have a narrow therapeutic window, should be approached with caution. Plasma tricyclic antidepressant (TCA) concentrations may need to be monitored, and the dose of the TCA may need to be reduced, if a TCA is co-administered with duloxetine).
No products indexed under this heading.

Amphetamine Aspartate (Duloxetine is a moderate inhibitor of CYP2D6. Co-administration of duloxetine with other drugs that are extensively metabolized by this isoenzyme, and which have a narrow therapeutic window, should be approached with caution). Products include:
Adderall XR Capsules 3012

Amphetamine Aspartate Monohydrate (Duloxetine is a moderate inhibitor of CYP2D6. Co-administration of duloxetine with other drugs that are extensively metabolized by this isoenzyme, and which have a narrow therapeutic window, should be approached with caution).
No products indexed under this heading.

Amphetamine Resins (Given the primary CNS effects of duloxetine, it should be used with caution when it is taken in combination with or substituted for other centrally acting drugs, including those with a similar mechanism of action).
No products indexed under this heading.

Amphetamine Sulfate (Duloxetine is a moderate inhibitor of CYP2D6. Co-administration of duloxetine with other drugs that are extensively metabolized by this isoenzyme, and which have a narrow therapeutic window, should be approached with caution). Products include:
Adderall XR Capsules 3012

Anastrozole (Concomitant use of duloxetine with fluvoxamine, an inhibitor of CYP1A2, results in a 6-fold increase in AUC, about 2.5-fold increase in Cmax, and an approximately 3-fold increase in t1/2 of duloxetine. Since duloxetine is metabolized in part by CYP1A2, concomitant use of duloxetine with other inhibitors of CYP1A2, would be expected to have the same effects; these combinations should be avoided). Products include:
Arimidex Tablets 672

Anisindione (SSRIs and SNRIs, including duloxetine, may increase the risk of bleeding events. Concomitant use of aspirin, non-steroidal anti-inflammatory drugs, warfarin, and other anti-coagulants may add to this risk).
No products indexed under this heading.

Aprobarbital (Given the primary CNS effects of duloxetine, it should be used with caution when it is taken in combination with or substituted for other centrally acting drugs, including those with a similar mechanism of action).
No products indexed under this heading.

Ardeparin Sodium (SSRIs and SNRIs, including duloxetine, may increase the risk of bleeding events. Concomitant use of aspirin, non-steroidal anti-inflammatory drugs, warfarin, and other anti-coagulants may add to this risk).
No products indexed under this heading.

Aspirin (Studies that have demonstrated an association between the use of psychotropic drugs that interfere with serotonin reuptake and the occurrence of upper gastrointestinal bleeding have shown that concurrent use of aspirin may potentiate the risk of bleeding). Products include:
Aggrenox Capsules 819
Bayer Aspirin 750
Percodan Tablets 1130
St. Joseph 81 mg Aspirin Chewable and Enteric Coated Tablets 1903

Aspirin, Enteric Coated (SSRIs and SNRIs, including duloxetine, may increase the risk of bleeding events. Concomitant use of aspirin, non-steroidal anti-inflammatory drugs, warfarin, and other anti-coagulants may add to this risk).
No products indexed under this heading.

Aspirin Buffered (Studies that have demonstrated an association between the use of psychotropic drugs that interfere with serotonin reuptake and the occurrence of upper gastrointestinal bleeding have shown that concurrent use of aspirin may potentiate the risk of bleeding).
No products indexed under this heading.

Atomoxetine Hydrochloride (Duloxetine is a moderate inhibitor of CYP2D6. Co-administration of duloxetine with other drugs that are extensively metabolized by this isoenzyme, and which have a narrow therapeutic window, should be approached with caution). Products include:
Strattera Capsules 1864

Bisoprolol Fumarate (Duloxetine is a moderate inhibitor of CYP2D6. Co-administration of duloxetine with other drugs that are extensively metabolized by this isoenzyme, and which have a narrow therapeutic window, should be approached with caution).
No products indexed under this heading.

Buprenorphine Hydrochloride (Given the primary CNS effects of duloxetine, it should be used with caution when it is taken in combination with or substituted for other centrally acting drugs, including those with a similar mechanism of action). Products include:
Suboxone Tablets 2601
Subutex Tablets 2601

Bupropion Hydrochloride (Because CYP2D6 is involved in duloxetine metabolism, concomitant use of duloxetine with potent inhibitors of CYP2D6 would be expected to, and does, result in higher concentrations of duloxetine). Products include:
Wellbutrin Tablets 1648
Wellbutrin SR Sustained-Release Tablets 1653
Wellbutrin XL Extended-Release Tablets 1659
Zyban Sustained-Release Tablets 1692

Buspirone Hydrochloride (Given the primary CNS effects of duloxetine, it should be used with caution when it is taken in combination with or substituted for other centrally acting drugs, including those with a similar mechanism of action).
No products indexed under this heading.

Butabarbital (Given the primary CNS effects of duloxetine, it should be used with caution when it is taken in combination with or substituted for other centrally acting drugs, including those with a similar mechanism of action).
No products indexed under this heading.

Butalbital (Given the primary CNS effects of duloxetine, it should be used with caution when it is taken in combination with or substituted for other centrally acting drugs, including those with a similar mechanism of action).
No products indexed under this heading.

Captopril (Duloxetine is a moderate inhibitor of CYP2D6. Co-administration of duloxetine with other drugs that are extensively metabolized by this isoenzyme, and which have a narrow therapeutic window, should be approached with caution). Products include:
Captopril Tablets 2182

Carvedilol (Duloxetine is a moderate inhibitor of CYP2D6. Co-administration of duloxetine with other drugs that are extensively metabolized by this isoenzyme, and which have a narrow therapeutic window, should be approached with caution). Products include:
Coreg Tablets 1387

Celecoxib (SSRIs and SNRIs, including duloxetine, may increase the risk of bleeding events. Concomitant use of aspirin, non-steroidal anti-inflammatory drugs, warfarin, and other anti-coagulants may add to this risk). Products include:
Celebrex Capsules 2979

Cevimeline Hydrochloride (Duloxetine is a moderate inhibitor of CYP2D6. Co-administration of duloxetine with other drugs that are extensively metabolized by this isoenzyme, and which have a narrow therapeutic window, should be approached with caution). Products include:
Evoxac Capsules 1013

Chlordiazepoxide (Given the primary CNS effects of duloxetine, it should be used with caution when it is taken in combination with or substituted for other centrally acting drugs, including those with a similar mechanism of action).
No products indexed under this heading.

Chlordiazepoxide Hydrochloride (Given the primary CNS effects of duloxetine, it should be used with caution when it is taken in combination with or substituted for other centrally acting drugs, including those with a similar mechanism of action).
No products indexed under this heading.

Chloroquine Hydrochloride (Because CYP2D6 is involved in duloxetine metabolism, concomitant use of duloxetine with potent inhibitors of CYP2D6 would be expected to, and does, result in higher concentrations of duloxetine).
No products indexed under this heading.

Chloroquine Phosphate (Because CYP2D6 is involved in duloxetine metabolism, concomitant use of duloxetine with potent inhibitors of CYP2D6 would be expected to, and does, result in higher concentrations of duloxetine).
No products indexed under this heading.

Chlorpheniramine (Because CYP2D6 is involved in duloxetine metabolism, concomitant use of duloxetine with potent inhibitors of CYP2D6 would be expected to, and does, result in higher concentrations of duloxetine).
No products indexed under this heading.

Chlorpheniramine Maleate (Because CYP2D6 is involved in duloxetine metabolism, concomitant use of duloxetine with potent inhibitors of CYP2D6 would be expected to, and does, result in higher concentrations of duloxetine). Products include:
Actifed Cold & Allergy Tablets 1895
Sudafed PE Sinus & Allergy Tablets 1908
Tylenol Allergy Multi-Symptom Caplets with Cool Burst and Rapid Release Gelcaps 1916
Children's Tylenol Plus Cold Suspension Liquid 1912
Children's Tylenol Plus Cough & Runny Nose Suspension Liquid 1912
Children's Tylenol Plus Flu Suspension Liquid 1914
Children's Tylenol Plus Multi-Symptom Cold Suspension Liquid 1912
Tylenol Cold Head Congestion Nighttime Caplets with Cool Burst 1910
Tylenol Cold Multi-Symptom Nighttime Caplets with Cool Burst 1913
Tylenol Sinus Congestion & Pain Nighttime Caplets with Cool Burst 1917

Chlorpheniramine Polistirex (Because CYP2D6 is involved in duloxetine metabolism, concomitant use of duloxetine with potent inhibitors of CYP2D6 would be expected to, and does, result in higher concentrations of duloxetine). Products include:
Tussionex Pennkinetic Extended-Release Suspension 3154

Chlorpheniramine Tannate (Because CYP2D6 is involved in duloxetine metabolism, concomitant use of duloxetine with potent inhibitors of CYP2D6 would be expected to, and does, result in higher concentrations of duloxetine).
No products indexed under this heading.

Chlorpromazine (Duloxetine is a moderate inhibitor of CYP2D6. Co-administration of duloxetine with other drugs that are extensively metabolized by this isoenzyme, and which have a narrow therapeutic window, should be approached with caution).
No products indexed under this heading.

Chlorpromazine Hydrochloride (Duloxetine is a moderate inhibitor of CYP2D6. Co-administration of duloxetine with other drugs that are extensively metabolized by this isoenzyme, and which have a narrow therapeutic window, should be approached with caution).
No products indexed under this heading.

Chlorpropamide (Duloxetine is a moderate inhibitor of CYP2D6. Co-administration of duloxetine with other drugs that are extensively metabolized by this isoenzyme, and which have a narrow therapeutic window, should be approached with caution).
No products indexed under this heading.

Chlorprothixene (Given the primary CNS effects of duloxetine, it should be used with caution when it is taken in combination with or substituted for other centrally acting drugs, including those with a similar mechanism of action).
No products indexed under this heading.

Chlorprothixene Hydrochloride (Given the primary CNS effects of duloxetine, it should be used with caution when it is taken in combination with or substituted for other centrally acting drugs, including those with a similar mechanism of action).
No products indexed under this heading.

Chlorprothixene Lactate (Given the primary CNS effects of duloxetine, it should be used with caution when it is taken in combination with or substituted for other centrally acting drugs, including those with a similar mechanism of action).
No products indexed under this heading.

Cimetidine (Duloxetine has an enteric coating that resists dissolution until reaching a segment of the gastrointestinal tract where the pH exceeds 5.5. Drugs that raise the gastrointestinal pH may lead to an earlier release of duloxetine).
No products indexed under this heading.

Cimetidine Hydrochloride (Duloxetine has an enteric coating that resists dissolution until reaching a segment of the gastrointestinal tract where the pH exceeds 5.5. Drugs that raise the gastrointestinal pH may lead to an earlier release of duloxetine).
No products indexed under this heading.

Ciprofloxacin (Some quinolones, inhibitors of CYP1A2, would be expected to increase the AUC and Cmax of duloxetine; co-administration should be avoided). Products include:
Cipro I.V. 2817
Cipro Oral Suspension 2810
Cipro XR Tablets 2823
Ciprodex Otic Suspension 541

Ciprofloxacin Hydrochloride (Some quinolones, inhibitors of CYP1A2, would be expected to increase the AUC and Cmax of duloxetine; co-administration should be avoided). Products include:
Cipro Tablets 2810

Citalopram Hydrobromide (Development of a potentially life-threatening serotonin syndrome may occur with concomitant use of duloxetine HCl and serotonergic drugs. Concomitant use of duloxetine hydrochloride with serotonin precursors is not recommended). Products include:
Celexa 1160

Clarithromycin (Concomitant use of duloxetine with fluvoxamine, an inhibitor of CYP1A2, results in a 6-fold increase in AUC, about 2.5-fold increase in Cmax, and an approximately 3-fold increase in t1/2 of duloxetine. Since duloxetine is metabolized in part by CYP1A2, concomitant use of duloxetine with other inhibitors of CYP1A2, would be expected to have the same effects; these combinations should be avoided). Products include:
Biaxin/Biaxin XL 411

Clomipramine Hydrochloride (Duloxetine is a moderate inhibitor of CYP2D6. Co-administration of duloxetine with other drugs that are extensively metabolized by this isoenzyme, and which have a narrow therapeutic window, should be approached with caution. Plasma tricyclic antidepressant (TCA) concentrations may need to be monitored, and the dose of the TCA may need to be reduced, if a TCA is co-administered with duloxetine).
No products indexed under this heading.

Clorazepate Dipotassium (Given the primary CNS effects of duloxetine, it should be used with caution when it is taken in combination with or substituted for other centrally acting drugs, including those with a similar mechanism of action).
No products indexed under this heading.

Clozapine (Duloxetine is a moderate inhibitor of CYP2D6. Co-administration of duloxetine with other drugs that are extensively metabolized by this isoenzyme, and which have a narrow therapeutic window, should be approached with caution).
No products indexed under this heading.

Cocaine Hydrochloride (Because CYP2D6 is involved in duloxetine metabolism, concomitant use of duloxetine with potent inhibitors of CYP2D6 would be expected to, and does, result in higher concentrations of duloxetine).
No products indexed under this heading.

Codeine Phosphate (Duloxetine is a moderate inhibitor of CYP2D6. Co-administration of duloxetine with other drugs that are extensively metabolized by this isoenzyme, and which have a narrow therapeutic window, should be approached with caution). Products include:
Tylenol with Codeine Tablets 2427

Codeine Sulfate (Duloxetine is a moderate inhibitor of CYP2D6. Co-administration of duloxetine with other drugs that are extensively metabolized by this isoenzyme, and which have a narrow therapeutic window, should be approached with caution).
No products indexed under this heading.

Cyclobenzaprine Hydrochloride (Duloxetine is a moderate inhibitor of CYP2D6. Co-administration of duloxetine with other drugs that are extensively metabolized by this isoenzyme, and which have a narrow therapeutic window, should be approached with caution). Products include:
Amrix Capsules 966

Dalteparin Sodium (SSRIs and SNRIs, including duloxetine, may increase the risk of bleeding events. Concomitant use of aspirin, nonsteroidal anti-inflammatory drugs, warfarin, and other anti-coagulants may add to this risk). Products include:
Fragmin Injection 1070

Danaparoid Sodium (SSRIs and SNRIs, including duloxetine, may increase the risk of bleeding events. Concomitant use of aspirin, nonsteroidal anti-inflammatory drugs, warfarin, and other anti-coagulants may add to this risk).
No products indexed under this heading.

Desflurane (Given the primary CNS effects of duloxetine, it should be used with caution when it is taken in combination with or substituted for other centrally acting drugs, including those with a similar mechanism of action).
No products indexed under this heading.

Desipramine Hydrochloride (Duloxetine is a moderate inhibitor of CYP2D6. Co-administration of duloxetine with other drugs that are extensively metabolized by this isoenzyme, and which have a narrow therapeutic window, should be approached with caution. Plasma tricyclic antidepressant (TCA) concentrations may need to be monitored, and the dose of the TCA may need to be reduced, if a TCA is co-administered with duloxetine).
No products indexed under this heading.

Desogestrel (Concomitant use of duloxetine with fluvoxamine, an inhibitor of CYP1A2, results in a 6-fold increase in AUC, about 2.5-fold increase in Cmax, and an approximately 3-fold increase in t1/2 of duloxetine. Since duloxetine is metabolized in part by CYP1A2, concomitant use of duloxetine with other inhibitors of CYP1A2, would be expected to have the same effects; these combinations should be avoided). Products include:
Mircette Tablets 1034

Dexfenfluramine Hydrochloride (Duloxetine is a moderate inhibitor of CYP2D6. Co-administration of duloxetine with other drugs that are extensively metabolized by this isoenzyme, and which have a narrow therapeutic window, should be approached with caution).
No products indexed under this heading.

Dextroamphetamine Sulfate (Given the primary CNS effects of dulox-

etine, it should be used with caution when it is taken in combination with or substituted for other centrally acting drugs, including those with a similar mechanism of action). Products include:

- Adderall XR Capsules 3012
- Dexedrine 1401

Dextromethorphan Hydrobromide (Duloxetine is a moderate inhibitor of CYP2D6. Co-administration of duloxetine with other drugs that are extensively metabolized by this isoenzyme, and which have a narrow therapeutic window, should be approached with caution). Products include:

- PediaCare Children's Liquid Multi-Symptom Cold.................... 1902
- PediaCare Children's Long-Acting Cough.................... 1902
- Children's Sudafed PE Cold & Cough Liquid.................... 1907
- Sudafed PE Cold & Cough Caplets.................... 1907
- Children's Tylenol Plus Cough & Runny Nose Suspension Liquid..... 1912
- Children's Tylenol Plus Cough & Sore Throat Suspension Liquid..... 1912
- Children's Tylenol Plus Flu Suspension Liquid.................... 1914
- Children's Tylenol Plus Multi-Symptom Cold Suspension Liquid.................... 1912
- Tylenol Cold Severe Congestion Daytime Caplets with Cool Burst.................... 1912
- Tylenol Cold Head Congestion Daytime Caplets with Cool Burst.................... 1910
- Tylenol Cold Head Congestion Nighttime Caplets with Cool Burst.................... 1910
- Tylenol Cold Head Congestion Severe Daytime Caplets with Cool Burst.................... 1910
- Tylenol Cold Multi-Symptom Daytime Caplets with Cool Burst and Rapid Release Gels....... 1913
- Tylenol Cold Multi-Symptom Daytime Liquid with Citrus Burst... 1913
- Tylenol Cold Multi-Symptom Nighttime Caplets with Cool Burst.................... 1913
- Tylenol Cold Multi-Symptom Nighttime Liquid with Cool Burst... 1913
- Tylenol Cold Multi-Symptom Severe Caplets with Cool Burst..... 1913
- Tylenol Cold Multi-Symptom Severe Daytime Liquid with Citrus Burst.................... 1913
- Tylenol Cough & Sore Throat Daytime Liquid with Cool Burst...... 1918
- Tylenol Cough & Sore Throat Nighttime Liquid with Cool Burst... 1918
- Vicks DayQuil Cold & Flu Multi-Symptom Relief.................... ⊡616
- Vicks DayQuil LiquiCaps.................... 2567
- Vicks DayQuil Liquid.................... 2567
- Vicks DayQuil Multi-Symptom Cold/Flu Relief.................... 2567
- Vicks NyQuil Cold & Flu Multi-Symptom Relief.................... ⊡617
- Vicks NyQuil LiquiCaps.................... 2567
- Vicks NyQuil Liquid.................... 2567
- Vicks NyQuil Multi-Symptom Cold/Flu Relief.................... 2567

Dextromethorphan Polistirex (Duloxetine is a moderate inhibitor of CYP2D6. Co-administration of duloxetine with other drugs that are extensively metabolized by this isoenzyme, and which have a narrow therapeutic window, should be approached with caution).

No products indexed under this heading.

Dezocine (Given the primary CNS effects of duloxetine, it should be used with caution when it is taken in combination with or substituted for other centrally acting drugs, including those with a similar mechanism of action).

No products indexed under this heading.

Diazepam (Given the primary CNS effects of duloxetine, it should be used with caution when it is taken in combination with or substituted for other centrally acting drugs, including those with a similar mechanism of action). Products include:

- Valium Tablets.................... 2658

Diclofenac Epolamine (SSRIs and SNRIs, including duloxetine, may increase the risk of bleeding events. Concomitant use of aspirin, nonsteroidal anti-inflammatory drugs, warfarin, and other anti-coagulants may add to this risk). Products include:

- Flector Patch.................... 561

Diclofenac Potassium (SSRIs and SNRIs, including duloxetine, may increase the risk of bleeding events. Concomitant use of aspirin, nonsteroidal anti-inflammatory drugs, warfarin, and other anti-coagulants may add to this risk).

No products indexed under this heading.

Diclofenac Sodium (SSRIs and SNRIs, including duloxetine, may increase the risk of bleeding events. Concomitant use of aspirin, nonsteroidal anti-inflammatory drugs, warfarin, and other anti-coagulants may add to this risk). Products include:

- Diclofenac Sodium Ophthalmic Solution.................... ⊙240
- Voltaren Ophthalmic Solution.................... 2336
- Voltaren Tablets.................... 2334
- Voltaren-XR Tablets.................... 2337

Dicumarol (SSRIs and SNRIs, including duloxetine, may increase the risk of bleeding events. Concomitant use of aspirin, non-steroidal anti-inflammatory drugs, warfarin, and other anti-coagulants may add to this risk).

No products indexed under this heading.

Diphenhydramine (Because CYP2D6 is involved in duloxetine metabolism, concomitant use of duloxetine with potent inhibitors of CYP2D6 would be expected to, and does, result in higher concentrations of duloxetine).

No products indexed under this heading.

Diphenhydramine Hydrochloride (Because CYP2D6 is involved in duloxetine metabolism, concomitant use of duloxetine with potent inhibitors of CYP2D6 would be expected to, and does, result in higher concentrations of duloxetine). Products include:

- Benadryl Allergy & Cold Kapgels...... 1895
- Benadryl Allergy & Sinus Headache Kapgels.................... 1895
- Benadryl Severe Allergy & Sinus Headache Caplets.................... 1897
- Benadryl Dye-Free Allergy Liqui-gels Softgels.................... 1897
- Benadryl Allergy Kapgels.................... 1895
- Benadryl Allergy Quick Dissolve Strips.................... 1896
- Benadryl Allergy Ultratab Tablets..... 1896
- Children's Benadryl Dye-Free Allergy Liquid.................... 1897
- Children's Benadryl Allergy Fastmelts.................... 1897
- Children's Benadryl Allergy Liquid.... 1898
- Children's Benadryl Allergy Perfect Measure.................... 1896
- Children's Benadryl-D Allergy & Sinus Liquid.................... 1896
- Benadryl-D Allergy & Sinus Tablet.... 1896
- PediaCare Children's Allergy & Cold Liquid.................... 1902
- PediaCare Children's Allergy Liquid.................... 1902
- Simply Sleep Caplets.................... 1905
- Sudafed PE Nighttime Cold Caplets.................... 1907
- Sudafed PE Severe Cold Caplets..... 1908
- Extra Strength Tylenol PM Caplets, Geltabs, Liquid, and Rapid Release Gels.................... 1915
- Tylenol Allergy Multi-Symptom Nighttime Caplets with Cool Burst.................... 1916
- Tylenol Severe Allergy Caplets......... 1916
- Children's Tylenol Plus Cold & Allergy Suspension Liquid............ 1914
- Tylenol Sore Throat Nighttime Liquid with Cool Burst.................... 1918

Dolasetron Mesylate (Duloxetine is a moderate inhibitor of CYP2D6. Co-administration of duloxetine with other drugs that are extensively metabolized by this isoenzyme, and which have a narrow therapeutic window, should be approached with caution). Products include:

- Anzemet Injection.................... 2701
- Anzemet Tablets.................... 2704

Donepezil Hydrochloride (Duloxetine is a moderate inhibitor of CYP2D6. Co-administration of duloxetine with other drugs that are extensively metabolized by this isoenzyme, and which have a narrow therapeutic window, should be approached with caution). Products include:

- Aricept Tablets.................... 1062
- Aricept ODT Tablets.................... 1062

Doxepin Hydrochloride (Duloxetine is a moderate inhibitor of CYP2D6. Co-administration of duloxetine with other drugs that are extensively metabolized by this isoenzyme, and which have a narrow therapeutic window, should be approached with caution. Plasma tricyclic antidepressant (TCA) concentrations may need to be monitored, and the dose of the TCA may need to be reduced, if a TCA is co-administered with duloxetine).

No products indexed under this heading.

Droperidol (Given the primary CNS effects of duloxetine, it should be used with caution when it is taken in combination with or substituted for other centrally acting drugs, including those with a similar mechanism of action).

No products indexed under this heading.

Eletriptan Hydrobromide (Development of a potentially life-threatening serotonin syndrome may occur with concomitant use of duloxetine HCl and triptans. If concomitant treatment is clinically warranted, careful observation of the patient is advised, particularly during treatment initiation and dose increases).

No products indexed under this heading.

Encainide Hydrochloride (Duloxetine is a moderate inhibitor of CYP2D6. Co-administration of duloxetine with other drugs that are extensively metabolized by this isoenzyme, and which have a narrow therapeutic window, should be approached with caution).

No products indexed under this heading.

Enflurane (Given the primary CNS effects of duloxetine, it should be used with caution when it is taken in combination with or substituted for other centrally acting drugs, including those with a similar mechanism of action).

No products indexed under this heading.

Enoxacin (Some quinolones, inhibitors of CYP1A2, would be expected to increase the AUC and Cmax of duloxetine; co-administration should be avoided).

No products indexed under this heading.

Enoxaparin Sodium (SSRIs and SNRIs, including duloxetine, may increase the risk of bleeding events. Concomitant use of aspirin, nonsteroidal anti-inflammatory drugs, warfarin, and other anti-coagulants may add to this risk). Products include:

- Lovenox Injection.................... 2756

Escitalopram Oxalate (Development of a potentially life-threatening serotonin syndrome may occur with concomitant use of duloxetine HCl and serotonergic drugs. Concomitant use of duloxetine hydrochloride with serotonin precursors is not recommended). Products include:

- Lexapro Oral Suspension.................... 1174
- Lexapro Tablets.................... 1174

Esomeprazole Magnesium (Duloxetine has an enteric coating that resists dissolution until reaching a segment of the gastrointestinal tract where the pH exceeds 5.5. Drugs that raise the gastrointestinal pH may lead to an earlier release of duloxetine). Products include:

- Nexium Delayed-Release Capsules.................... 645
- Nexium Delayed-Release Oral Suspension.................... 645

Estazolam (Given the primary CNS effects of duloxetine, it should be used with caution when it is taken in combination with or substituted for other centrally acting drugs, including those with a similar mechanism of action).

No products indexed under this heading.

Ethanol (Given the primary CNS effects of duloxetine, it should be used with caution when it is taken in combination with or substituted for other centrally acting drugs, including those with a similar mechanism of action).

No products indexed under this heading.

Ethchlorvynol (Given the primary CNS effects of duloxetine, it should be used with caution when it is taken in combination with or substituted for other centrally acting drugs, including those with a similar mechanism of action).

No products indexed under this heading.

Ethinamate (Given the primary CNS effects of duloxetine, it should be used with caution when it is taken in combination with or substituted for other centrally acting drugs, including those with a similar mechanism of action).

No products indexed under this heading.

Ethinyl Estradiol (Concomitant use of duloxetine with fluvoxamine, an inhibitor of CYP1A2, results in a 6-fold increase in AUC, about 2.5-fold increase in Cmax, and an approximately 3-fold increase in t1/2 of duloxetine. Since duloxetine is metabolized in part by CYP1A2, concomitant use of duloxetine with other inhibitors of CYP1A2, would be expected to have the same effects; these combinations should be avoided). Products include:

Lybrel Tablets 3204
Mircette Tablets 1034
NuvaRing 2897
Ortho-Cyclen/Ortho Tri-Cyclen 2449
Ortho Evra Transdermal System 2437
Ortho Tri-Cyclen Lo Tablets 2458
Seasonique Tablets 1046
Yaz Tablets 805

Ethyl Alcohol (Use of duloxetine concomitantly with heavy alcohol intake may be associated with severe liver injury; for this reason, duloxetine should ordinarily not be prescribed for patients with substantial alcohol use).
No products indexed under this heading.

Etodolac (SSRIs and SNRIs, including duloxetine, may increase the risk of bleeding events. Concomitant use of aspirin, non-steroidal anti-inflammatory drugs, warfarin, and other anti-coagulants may add to this risk).
No products indexed under this heading.

Famotidine (Duloxetine has an enteric coating that resists dissolution until reaching a segment of the gastrointestinal tract where the pH exceeds 5.5. Drugs that raise the gastrointestinal pH may lead to an earlier release of duloxetine). Products include:

Pepcid Tablets 2075
Original Strength Pepcid AC Gelcaps 1771
Original Strength Pepcid AC Tablets 1771
Maximum Strength Pepcid AC Tablets 1771
Pepcid Complete Chewable Tablets 1771

Fenoprofen Calcium (SSRIs and SNRIs, including duloxetine, may increase the risk of bleeding events. Concomitant use of aspirin, non-steroidal anti-inflammatory drugs, warfarin, and other anti-coagulants may add to this risk). Products include:

Nalfon Capsules 2508

Fentanyl (Duloxetine is a moderate inhibitor of CYP2D6. Co-administration of duloxetine with other drugs that are extensively metabolized by this isoenzyme, and which have a narrow therapeutic window, should be approached with caution). Products include:

Duragesic Transdermal System 2405
Ionsys Transdermal System 2410

Fentanyl Citrate (Duloxetine is a moderate inhibitor of CYP2D6. Co-administration of duloxetine with other drugs that are extensively metabolized by this isoenzyme, and which have a narrow therapeutic window, should be approached with caution). Products include:

Actiq 959
Fentora Tablets 968

Flecainide Acetate (Duloxetine is a moderate inhibitor of CYP2D6. Co-administration of duloxetine with other drugs that are extensively metabolized by this isoenzyme, and which have a narrow therapeutic window, should be approached with caution).
No products indexed under this heading.

Fluoxetine (Duloxetine is a moderate inhibitor of CYP2D6. Co-administration of duloxetine with other drugs that are extensively metabolized by this isoenzyme, and which have a narrow therapeutic window, should be approached with caution).
No products indexed under this heading.

Fluoxetine Hydrochloride (Development of a potentially life-threatening serotonin syndrome may occur with concomitant use of duloxetine HCl and serotonergic drugs. Concomitant use of duloxetine hydrochloride with serotonin precursors is not recommended). Products include:

Prozac Weekly Capsules 1852
Prozac Pulvules and Liquid 1852
Symbyax Capsules 1871

Fluphenazine Decanoate (Duloxetine is a moderate inhibitor of CYP2D6. Co-administration of duloxetine with other drugs that are extensively metabolized by this isoenzyme, and which have a narrow therapeutic window, should be approached with caution).
No products indexed under this heading.

Fluphenazine Enanthate (Duloxetine is a moderate inhibitor of CYP2D6. Co-administration of duloxetine with other drugs that are extensively metabolized by this isoenzyme, and which have a narrow therapeutic window, should be approached with caution).
No products indexed under this heading.

Fluphenazine Hydrochloride (Duloxetine is a moderate inhibitor of CYP2D6. Co-administration of duloxetine with other drugs that are extensively metabolized by this isoenzyme, and which have a narrow therapeutic window, should be approached with caution).
No products indexed under this heading.

Flurazepam Hydrochloride (Given the primary CNS effects of duloxetine, it should be used with caution when it is taken in combination with or substituted for other centrally acting drugs, including those with a similar mechanism of action).
No products indexed under this heading.

Flurbiprofen (SSRIs and SNRIs, including duloxetine, may increase the risk of bleeding events. Concomitant use of aspirin, non-steroidal anti-inflammatory drugs, warfarin, and other anti-coagulants may add to this risk).
No products indexed under this heading.

Fluvoxamine (Concomitant use of duloxetine with fluvoxamine, a potent inhibitor of CYP1A2, results in approximately a 6-fold increase in AUC and about a 2.5-fold increase in Cmax of duloxetine; co-administration should be avoided).
No products indexed under this heading.

Fluvoxamine Maleate (Concomitant use of duloxetine with fluvoxamine, a potent inhibitor of CYP1A2, results in approximately a 6-fold increase in AUC and about a 2.5-fold increase in Cmax of duloxetine; co-administration should be avoided). Products include:

Luvox CR Extended-Release Capsules 1759

Fondaparinux Sodium (SSRIs and SNRIs, including duloxetine, may increase the risk of bleeding events. Concomitant use of aspirin, non-steroidal anti-inflammatory drugs, warfarin, and other anti-coagulants may add to this risk). Products include:

Arixtra Injection 1313

Formoterol Fumarate (Duloxetine is a moderate inhibitor of CYP2D6. Co-administration of duloxetine with other drugs that are extensively metabolized by this isoenzyme, and which have a narrow therapeutic window, should be approached with caution). Products include:

Foradil Aerolizer 2849
Perforomist Inhalation Solution 1025

Frovatriptan Succinate (Development of a potentially life-threatening serotonin syndrome may occur with concomitant use of duloxetine HCl and triptans. If concomitant treatment is clinically warranted, careful observation of the patient is advised, particularly during treatment initiation and dose increases). Products include:

Frova Tablets 1111

Galantamine Hydrobromide (Duloxetine is a moderate inhibitor of CYP2D6. Co-administration of duloxetine with other drugs that are extensively metabolized by this isoenzyme, and which have a narrow therapeutic window, should be approached with caution).
No products indexed under this heading.

Gatifloxacin (Concomitant use of duloxetine with fluvoxamine, an inhibitor of CYP1A2, results in a 6-fold increase in AUC, about 2.5-fold increase in Cmax, and an approximately 3-fold increase in t1/2 of duloxetine. Since duloxetine is metabolized in part by CYP1A2, concomitant use of duloxetine with other inhibitors of CYP1A2, would be expected to have the same effects; these combinations should be avoided).
No products indexed under this heading.

Gemifloxacin Mesylate (Concomitant use of duloxetine with fluvoxamine, an inhibitor of CYP1A2, results in a 6-fold increase in AUC, about 2.5-fold increase in Cmax, and an approximately 3-fold increase in t1/2 of duloxetine. Since duloxetine is metabolized in part by CYP1A2, concomitant use of duloxetine with other inhibitors of CYP1A2, would be expected to have the same effects; these combinations should be avoided).
No products indexed under this heading.

Glutethimide (Given the primary CNS effects of duloxetine, it should be used with caution when it is taken in combination with or substituted for other centrally acting drugs, including those with a similar mechanism of action).
No products indexed under this heading.

Grepafloxacin Hydrochloride (Some quinolones, inhibitors of CYP1A2, would be expected to increase the AUC and Cmax of duloxetine; co-administration should be avoided).
No products indexed under this heading.

Halofantrine Hydrochloride (Because CYP2D6 is involved in duloxetine metabolism, concomitant use of duloxetine with potent inhibitors of CYP2D6 would be expected to, and does, result in higher concentrations of duloxetine).
No products indexed under this heading.

Haloperidol (Duloxetine is a moderate inhibitor of CYP2D6. Co-administration of duloxetine with other drugs that are extensively metabolized by this isoenzyme, and which have a narrow therapeutic window, should be approached with caution).
No products indexed under this heading.

Haloperidol Decanoate (Duloxetine is a moderate inhibitor of CYP2D6. Co-administration of duloxetine with other drugs that are extensively metabolized by this isoenzyme, and which have a narrow therapeutic window, should be approached with caution).
No products indexed under this heading.

Heparin Calcium (SSRIs and SNRIs, including duloxetine, may increase the risk of bleeding events. Concomitant use of aspirin, non-steroidal anti-inflammatory drugs, warfarin, and other anti-coagulants may add to this risk).
No products indexed under this heading.

Heparin Sodium (SSRIs and SNRIs, including duloxetine, may increase the risk of bleeding events. Concomitant use of aspirin, non-steroidal anti-inflammatory drugs, warfarin, and other anti-coagulants may add to this risk).
No products indexed under this heading.

Hydrocodone Bitartrate (Duloxetine is a moderate inhibitor of CYP2D6. Co-administration of duloxetine with other drugs that are extensively metabolized by this isoenzyme, and which have a narrow therapeutic window, should be approached with caution). Products include:

Lortab 5/500 Tablets 3143
Lortab 7.5/500 Tablets 3144
Lortab 10/500 Tablets 3144
Vicodin Tablets 529
Vicodin ES Tablets 530
Vicodin HP Tablets 531
Vicoprofen Tablets 533
Zydone Tablets 1132

Hydrocodone Polistirex (Given the primary CNS effects of duloxetine, it should be used with caution when it is taken in combination with or substituted for other centrally acting drugs, including those with a similar mechanism of action). Products include:

Tussionex Pennkinetic Extended-Release Suspension 3154

Hydromorphone Hydrochloride (Given the primary CNS effects of duloxetine, it should be used with caution when it is taken in combination with or substituted for other centrally acting drugs, including those with a similar mechanism of action).
No products indexed under this heading.

Hydroxychloroquine Sulfate (Because CYP2D6 is involved in duloxetine metabolism, concomitant use of duloxetine with potent inhibitors of CYP2D6 would be expected to, and does, result in higher concentrations of duloxetine).
No products indexed under this heading.

Hydroxyzine Hydrochloride (Given the primary CNS effects of duloxetine, it should be used with caution when it is taken in combination with or substituted for other centrally acting drugs, including those with a similar mechanism of action).
No products indexed under this heading.

Hypericum (Caution is advised with co-administration of duloxetine with drugs that may affect the serotonergic neurotransmitter systems such as St. John's Wort because of potential development of serotonin syndrome). Products include:
Satieté Tablets 640

Hypericum Perforatum (Caution is advised with co-administration of duloxetine with drugs that may affect the serotonergic neurotransmitter systems such as St. John's Wort because of potential development of serotonin syndrome).
No products indexed under this heading.

Ibuprofen (SSRIs and SNRIs, including duloxetine, may increase the risk of bleeding events. Concomitant use of aspirin, non-steroidal anti-inflammatory drugs, warfarin, and other anti-coagulants may add to this risk). Products include:
Motrin IB Tablets and Caplets 1900
Children's Motrin Oral Suspension 1901
Children's Motrin Non-Staining Dye-Free Oral Suspension............ 1901
Children's Motrin Cold Oral Suspension 1899
Infants' Motrin Concentrated Drops.. 1901
Infants' Motrin Non-Staining Dye-Free Concentrated Drops....... 1901
Junior Strength Motrin Caplets and Chewable Tablets.................. 1901
Vicoprofen Tablets 533

Imatinib Mesylate (Because CYP2D6 is involved in duloxetine metabolism, concomitant use of duloxetine with potent inhibitors of CYP2D6 would be expected to, and does, result in higher concentrations of duloxetine). Products include:
Gleevec Tablets 2255

Imipramine Hydrochloride (Duloxetine is a moderate inhibitor of CYP2D6. Co-administration of duloxetine with other drugs that are extensively metabolized by this isoenzyme, and which have a narrow therapeutic window, should be approached with caution. Plasma tricyclic antidepressant (TCA) concentrations may need to be monitored, and the dose of the TCA may need to be reduced, if a TCA is co-administered with duloxetine).
No products indexed under this heading.

Imipramine Pamoate (Duloxetine is a moderate inhibitor of CYP2D6. Co-administration of duloxetine with other drugs that are extensively metabolized by this isoenzyme, and which have a narrow therapeutic window, should be approached with caution. Plasma tricyclic antidepressant (TCA) concentrations may need to be monitored, and the dose of the TCA may need to be reduced, if a TCA is co-administered with duloxetine).
No products indexed under this heading.

Indomethacin (SSRIs and SNRIs, including duloxetine, may increase the risk of bleeding events. Concomitant use of aspirin, non-steroidal anti-inflammatory drugs, warfarin, and other anti-coagulants may add to this risk). Products include:
Indocin 2024

Indomethacin Sodium Trihydrate (SSRIs and SNRIs, including duloxetine, may increase the risk of bleeding events. Concomitant use of aspirin, non-steroidal anti-inflammatory drugs, warfarin, and other anti-coagulants may add to this risk). Products include:
Indocin I.V. 2489

Indoramin Hydrochloride (Duloxetine is a moderate inhibitor of CYP2D6. Co-administration of duloxetine with other drugs that are extensively metabolized by this isoenzyme, and which have a narrow therapeutic window, should be approached with caution).
No products indexed under this heading.

Isocarboxazid (There have been reports of serious, sometimes fatal, reactions in patients receiving a serotonin reuptake inhibitor in combination with a monoamine oxidase inhibitor (MAOI). These reactions have also been reported in patients who have recently discontinued serotonin reuptake inhibitors and are started on an MAOI. Therefore, duloxetine use is contraindicated in combination with an MAOI, or within at least 14 days of discontinuing treatment with an MAOI. Based on the half-life of duloxetine, at least 5 days should be allowed after stopping duloxetine before starting an MAOI. Development of a potentially life-threatening serotonin syndrome may occur with concomitant use of duloxetine HCl and drugs which impair the metabolism of serotonin (e.g., MAOIs)). Products include:
Marplan Tablets 3177

Isoflurane (Given the primary CNS effects of duloxetine, it should be used with caution when it is taken in combination with or substituted for other centrally acting drugs, including those with a similar mechanism of action).
No products indexed under this heading.

Isoniazid (Concomitant use of duloxetine with fluvoxamine, an inhibitor of CYP1A2, results in a 6-fold increase in AUC, about 2.5-fold increase in Cmax, and an approximately 3-fold increase in t1/2 of duloxetine. Since duloxetine is metabolized in part by CYP1A2, concomitant use of duloxetine with other inhibitors of CYP1A2, would be expected to have the same effects; these combinations should be avoided).
No products indexed under this heading.

Isopropyl Alcohol (Use of duloxetine concomitantly with heavy alcohol intake may be associated with severe liver injury; for this reason, duloxetine should ordinarily not be prescribed for patients with substantial alcohol use).
No products indexed under this heading.

Ketamine Hydrochloride (Given the primary CNS effects of duloxetine, it should be used with caution when it is taken in combination with or substituted for other centrally acting drugs, including those with a similar mechanism of action).
No products indexed under this heading.

Ketoconazole (Concomitant use of duloxetine with fluvoxamine, an inhibitor of CYP1A2, results in a 6-fold increase in AUC, about 2.5-fold increase in Cmax, and an approximately 3-fold increase in t1/2 of duloxetine. Since duloxetine is metabolized in part by CYP1A2, concomitant use of duloxetine with other inhibitors of CYP1A2, would be expected to have the same effects; these combinations should be avoided). Products include:
Extina Foam, 2% 3057
Nizoral A-D Shampoo 1901

Ketoprofen (SSRIs and SNRIs, including duloxetine, may increase the risk of bleeding events. Concomitant use of aspirin, non-steroidal anti-inflammatory drugs, warfarin, and other anti-coagulants may add to this risk).
No products indexed under this heading.

Ketorolac Tromethamine (SSRIs and SNRIs, including duloxetine, may increase the risk of bleeding events. Concomitant use of aspirin, non-steroidal anti-inflammatory drugs, warfarin, and other anti-coagulants may add to this risk).
No products indexed under this heading.

Labetalol Hydrochloride (Duloxetine is a moderate inhibitor of CYP2D6. Co-administration of duloxetine with other drugs that are extensively metabolized by this isoenzyme, and which have a narrow therapeutic window, should be approached with caution).
No products indexed under this heading.

Lansoprazole (Duloxetine has an enteric coating that resists dissolution until reaching a segment of the gastrointestinal tract where the pH exceeds 5.5. Drugs that raise the gastrointestinal pH may lead to an earlier release of duloxetine).
No products indexed under this heading.

Levofloxacin (Concomitant use of duloxetine with fluvoxamine, an inhibitor of CYP1A2, results in a 6-fold increase in AUC, about 2.5-fold increase in Cmax, and an approximately 3-fold increase in t1/2 of duloxetine. Since duloxetine is metabolized in part by CYP1A2, concomitant use of duloxetine with other inhibitors of CYP1A2, would be expected to have the same effects; these combinations should be avoided). Products include:
Iquix Ophthalmic Solution 3183
Levaquin 2416
Levaquin in 5% Dextrose Injection 2416
Quixin Ophthalmic Solution 3184

Levomethadyl Acetate Hydrochloride (Given the primary CNS effects of duloxetine, it should be used with caution when it is taken in combination with or substituted for other centrally acting drugs, including those with a similar mechanism of action).
No products indexed under this heading.

Levonorgestrel (Concomitant use of duloxetine with fluvoxamine, an inhibitor of CYP1A2, results in a 6-fold increase in AUC, about 2.5-fold increase in Cmax, and an approximately 3-fold increase in t1/2 of duloxetine. Since duloxetine is metabolized in part by CYP1A2, concomitant use of duloxetine with other inhibitors of CYP1A2, would be expected to have the same effects; these combinations should be avoided). Products include:
Climara Pro Transdermal System 768
Lybrel Tablets 3204
Mirena Intrauterine System 779
Plan B Tablets 1044
Seasonique Tablets 1046

Levorphanol Tartrate (Given the primary CNS effects of duloxetine, it should be used with caution when it is taken in combination with or substituted for other centrally acting drugs, including those with a similar mechanism of action).
No products indexed under this heading.

Lidocaine (Duloxetine is a moderate inhibitor of CYP2D6. Co-administration of duloxetine with other drugs that are extensively metabolized by this isoenzyme, and which have a narrow therapeutic window, should be approached with caution). Products include:
Lidoderm Patch 1114

Lidocaine Hydrochloride (Duloxetine is a moderate inhibitor of CYP2D6. Co-administration of duloxetine with other drugs that are extensively metabolized by this isoenzyme, and which have a narrow therapeutic window, should be approached with caution).
No products indexed under this heading.

Lithium (Caution is advised with co-administration of duloxetine with drugs that may affect the serotonergic neurotransmitter systems such as lithium because of potential development of serotonin syndrome).
No products indexed under this heading.

Lithium Carbonate (Caution is advised with co-administration of duloxetine with drugs that may affect the serotonergic neurotransmitter systems such as lithium because of potential development of serotonin syndrome).
No products indexed under this heading.

Lithium Citrate (Caution is advised with co-administration of duloxetine with drugs that may affect the serotonergic neurotransmitter systems such as lithium because of potential development of serotonin syndrome).
No products indexed under this heading.

Lomefloxacin Hydrochloride (Some quinolones, inhibitors of CYP1A2, would be expected to increase the AUC and Cmax of duloxetine; co-administration should be avoided).
No products indexed under this heading.

Lorazepam (Given the primary CNS effects of duloxetine, it should be used with caution when it is taken in combination with or substituted for other centrally acting drugs, including those with a similar mechanism of action).
No products indexed under this heading.

Low Molecular Weight Heparins (SSRIs and SNRIs, including duloxetine, may increase the risk of bleeding events. Concomitant use of aspirin, non-steroidal anti-inflammatory drugs, warfarin, and other anti-coagulants may add to this risk).
No products indexed under this heading.

Loxapine Hydrochloride (Given the primary CNS effects of duloxetine, it should be used with caution when it is taken in combination with or substituted for other centrally acting drugs, including those with a similar mechanism of action).
No products indexed under this heading.

Loxapine Succinate (Given the primary CNS effects of duloxetine, it should be used with caution when it is taken in combination with or substituted for other centrally acting drugs, including those with a similar mechanism of action).
No products indexed under this heading.

Magnesium Hydroxide (Duloxetine has an enteric coating that resists dissolution until reaching a segment of the gastrointestinal tract where the pH exceeds 5.5. Drugs that raise the gastrointestinal pH may lead to an earlier release of duloxetine). Products include:
Fleet Pedia-Lax Chewable Tablets 1145
Pepcid Complete Chewable Tablets 1771
Extra Strength Rolaids Freshmint Tablets 1903
Rolaids Multi-Symptom Berry Tablets 1903
Rolaids Original Peppermint Tablets 1903

Maprotiline Hydrochloride (Duloxetine is a moderate inhibitor of CYP2D6. Co-administration of duloxetine with other drugs that are extensively metabolized by this isoenzyme, and which have a narrow therapeutic window, should be approached with caution. Plasma tricyclic antidepressant (TCA) concentrations may need to be monitored, and the dose of the TCA may need to be reduced, if a TCA is co-administered with duloxetine).
No products indexed under this heading.

Meclofenamate Sodium (SSRIs and SNRIs, including duloxetine, may increase the risk of bleeding events. Concomitant use of aspirin, non-steroidal anti-inflammatory drugs, warfarin, and other anti-coagulants may add to this risk).
No products indexed under this heading.

Mefenamic Acid (SSRIs and SNRIs, including duloxetine, may increase the risk of bleeding events. Concomitant use of aspirin, non-steroidal anti-inflammatory drugs, warfarin, and other anti-coagulants may add to this risk).
No products indexed under this heading.

Meloxicam (SSRIs and SNRIs, including duloxetine, may increase the risk of bleeding events. Concomitant use of aspirin, non-steroidal anti-inflammatory drugs, warfarin, and other anti-coagulants may add to this risk). Products include:
Mobic Oral Suspension 863
Mobic Tablets 863

Meperidine Hydrochloride (Duloxetine is a moderate inhibitor of CYP2D6. Co-administration of duloxetine with other drugs that are extensively metabolized by this isoenzyme, and which have a narrow therapeutic window, should be approached with caution).
No products indexed under this heading.

Mephobarbital (Given the primary CNS effects of duloxetine, it should be used with caution when it is taken in combination with or substituted for other centrally acting drugs, including those with a similar mechanism of action).
No products indexed under this heading.

Meprobamate (Given the primary CNS effects of duloxetine, it should be used with caution when it is taken in combination with or substituted for other centrally acting drugs, including those with a similar mechanism of action).
No products indexed under this heading.

Mesoridazine Besylate (Duloxetine is a moderate inhibitor of CYP2D6. Co-administration of duloxetine with other drugs that are extensively metabolized by this isoenzyme, and which have a narrow therapeutic window, should be approached with caution).
No products indexed under this heading.

Mestranol (Concomitant use of duloxetine with fluvoxamine, an inhibitor of CYP1A2, results in a 6-fold increase in AUC, about 2.5-fold increase in Cmax, and an approximately 3-fold increase in t1/2 of duloxetine. Since duloxetine is metabolized in part by CYP1A2, concomitant use of duloxetine with other inhibitors of CYP1A2, would be expected to have the same effects; these combinations should be avoided).
No products indexed under this heading.

Methadone Hydrochloride (Duloxetine is a moderate inhibitor of CYP2D6. Co-administration of duloxetine with other drugs that are extensively metabolized by this isoenzyme, and which have a narrow therapeutic window, should be approached with caution).
No products indexed under this heading.

Methamphetamine Hydrochloride (Duloxetine is a moderate inhibitor of CYP2D6. Co-administration of duloxetine with other drugs that are extensively metabolized by this isoenzyme, and which have a narrow therapeutic window, should be approached with caution).
No products indexed under this heading.

Methohexital Sodium (Given the primary CNS effects of duloxetine, it should be used with caution when it is taken in combination with or substituted for other centrally acting drugs, including those with a similar mechanism of action).
No products indexed under this heading.

Methotrimeprazine (Duloxetine is a moderate inhibitor of CYP2D6. Co-administration of duloxetine with other drugs that are extensively metabolized by this isoenzyme, and which have a narrow therapeutic window, should be approached with caution).
No products indexed under this heading.

Methoxsalen (Concomitant use of duloxetine with fluvoxamine, an inhibitor of CYP1A2, results in a 6-fold increase in AUC, about 2.5-fold increase in Cmax, and an approximately 3-fold increase in t1/2 of duloxetine. Since duloxetine is metabolized in part by CYP1A2, concomitant use of duloxetine with other inhibitors of CYP1A2, would be expected to have the same effects; these combinations should be avoided).
No products indexed under this heading.

Methoxyflurane (Given the primary CNS effects of duloxetine, it should be used with caution when it is taken in combination with or substituted for other centrally acting drugs, including those with a similar mechanism of action).
No products indexed under this heading.

Methylphenidate (Given the primary CNS effects of duloxetine, it should be used with caution when it is taken in combination with or substituted for other centrally acting drugs, including those with a similar mechanism of action). Products include:
Daytrana Transdermal Patch 3022

Methylphenidate Hydrochloride (Given the primary CNS effects of duloxetine, it should be used with caution when it is taken in combination with or substituted for other centrally acting drugs, including those with a similar mechanism of action). Products include:
Concerta Extended-Release Tablets 1925
Metadate CD Capsules 3146

Metoprolol Succinate (Duloxetine is a moderate inhibitor of CYP2D6. Co-administration of duloxetine with other drugs that are extensively metabolized by this isoenzyme, and which have a narrow therapeutic window, should be approached with caution). Products include:
Toprol-XL Tablets 666

Metoprolol Tartrate (Duloxetine is a moderate inhibitor of CYP2D6. Co-administration of duloxetine with other drugs that are extensively metabolized by this isoenzyme, and which have a narrow therapeutic window, should be approached with caution).
No products indexed under this heading.

Mexiletine Hydrochloride (Duloxetine is a moderate inhibitor of CYP2D6. Co-administration of duloxetine with other drugs that are extensively metabolized by this isoenzyme, and which have a narrow therapeutic window, should be approached with caution).
No products indexed under this heading.

Mibefradil Dihydrochloride (Because CYP2D6 is involved in duloxetine metabolism, concomitant use of duloxetine with potent inhibitors of CYP2D6 would be expected to, and does, result in higher concentrations of duloxetine).
No products indexed under this heading.

Midazolam Hydrochloride (Given the primary CNS effects of duloxetine, it should be used with caution when it is taken in combination with or substituted for other centrally acting drugs, including those with a similar mechanism of action).
No products indexed under this heading.

Mirtazapine (Duloxetine is a moderate inhibitor of CYP2D6. Co-administration of duloxetine with other drugs that are extensively metabolized by this isoenzyme, and which have a narrow therapeutic window, should be approached with caution). Products include:
Remeron Tablets 2924
RemeronSolTab Tablets 2927

Moclobemide (There have been reports of serious, sometimes fatal, reactions in patients receiving a serotonin reuptake inhibitor in combination with a monoamine oxidase inhibitor (MAOI). These reactions have also been reported in patients who have recently discontinued serotonin reuptake inhibitors and are started on an MAOI. Therefore, duloxetine use is contraindicated in combination with an MAOI, or within at least 14 days of discontinuing treatment with an MAOI. Based on the half-life of duloxetine, at least 5 days should be allowed after stopping duloxetine before starting an MAOI. Development of a potentially life-threatening serotonin syndrome may occur with concomitant use of duloxetine HCl and drugs which impair the metabolism of serotonin (e.g., MAOIs)).
No products indexed under this heading.

Molindone Hydrochloride (Given the primary CNS effects of duloxetine, it should be used with caution when it is taken in combination with or substituted for other centrally acting drugs, including those with a similar mechanism of action). Products include:
Moban Tablets 1116

Morphine Sulfate (Duloxetine is a moderate inhibitor of CYP2D6. Co-administration of duloxetine with other drugs that are extensively metabolized by this isoenzyme, and which have a narrow therapeutic window, should be approached with caution). Products include:

Avinza Capsules 1772
DepoDur Injection 1095
MS Contin Tablets 2585

Moxifloxacin Hydrochloride (Some quinolones, inhibitors of CYP1A2, would be expected to increase the AUC and Cmax of duloxetine; co-administration should be avoided). Products include:

Avelox 2803
Vigamox Ophthalmic Solution 548

Nabumetone (SSRIs and SNRIs, including duloxetine, may increase the risk of bleeding events. Concomitant use of aspirin, non-steroidal anti-inflammatory drugs, warfarin, and other anti-coagulants may add to this risk).

No products indexed under this heading.

Nalidixic Acid (Concomitant use of duloxetine with fluvoxamine, an inhibitor of CYP1A2, results in a 6-fold increase in AUC, about 2.5-fold increase in Cmax, and an approximately 3-fold increase in t1/2 of duloxetine. Since duloxetine is metabolized in part by CYP1A2, concomitant use of duloxetine with other inhibitors of CYP1A2, would be expected to have the same effects; these combinations should be avoided).

No products indexed under this heading.

Naproxen (SSRIs and SNRIs, including duloxetine, may increase the risk of bleeding events. Concomitant use of aspirin, non-steroidal anti-inflammatory drugs, warfarin, and other anti-coagulants may add to this risk). Products include:

EC-Naprosyn Delayed-Release Tablets 2632
Naprosyn Suspension 2632
Naprosyn Tablets 2632

Naproxen Sodium (SSRIs and SNRIs, including duloxetine, may increase the risk of bleeding events. Concomitant use of aspirin, non-steroidal anti-inflammatory drugs, warfarin, and other anti-coagulants may add to this risk). Products include:

Anaprox Tablets 2632
Anaprox DS Tablets 2632
Treximet Tablets 1616

Naratriptan Hydrochloride (Development of a potentially life-threatening serotonin syndrome may occur with concomitant use of duloxetine HCl and triptans. If concomitant treatment is clinically warranted, careful observation of the patient is advised, particularly during treatment initiation and dose increases). Products include:

Amerge Tablets 1301

Nelfinavir Mesylate (Duloxetine is a moderate inhibitor of CYP2D6. Co-administration of duloxetine with other drugs that are extensively metabolized by this isoenzyme, and which have a narrow therapeutic window, should be approached with caution).

No products indexed under this heading.

Nizatidine (Duloxetine has an enteric coating that resists dissolution until reaching a segment of the gastrointestinal tract where the pH exceeds 5.5. Drugs that raise the gastrointestinal pH may lead to an earlier release of duloxetine). Products include:

Axid Capsules 1364

Norethindrone (Concomitant use of duloxetine with fluvoxamine, an inhibitor of CYP1A2, results in a 6-fold increase in AUC, about 2.5-fold increase in Cmax, and an approximately 3-fold increase in t1/2 of duloxetine. Since duloxetine is metabolized in part by CYP1A2, concomitant use of duloxetine with other inhibitors of CYP1A2, would be expected to have the same effects; these combinations should be avoided). Products include:

Ortho Micronor Tablets 2446

Norfloxacin (Some quinolones, inhibitors of CYP1A2, would be expected to increase the AUC and Cmax of duloxetine; co-administration should be avoided). Products include:

Noroxin Tablets 2069

Norgestrel (Concomitant use of duloxetine with fluvoxamine, an inhibitor of CYP1A2, results in a 6-fold increase in AUC, about 2.5-fold increase in Cmax, and an approximately 3-fold increase in t1/2 of duloxetine. Since duloxetine is metabolized in part by CYP1A2, concomitant use of duloxetine with other inhibitors of CYP1A2, would be expected to have the same effects; these combinations should be avoided).

No products indexed under this heading.

Nortriptyline Hydrochloride (Duloxetine is a moderate inhibitor of CYP2D6. Co-administration of duloxetine with other drugs that are extensively metabolized by this isoenzyme, and which have a narrow therapeutic window, should be approached with caution. Plasma tricyclic antidepressant (TCA) concentrations may need to be monitored, and the dose of the TCA may need to be reduced, if a TCA is co-administered with duloxetine).

No products indexed under this heading.

Ofloxacin (Some quinolones, inhibitors of CYP1A2, would be expected to increase the AUC and Cmax of duloxetine; co-administration should be avoided). Products include:

Ofloxacin Ophthalmic Solution 0.3% .... ⊙243

Olanzapine (Duloxetine is a moderate inhibitor of CYP2D6. Co-administration of duloxetine with other drugs that are extensively metabolized by this isoenzyme, and which have a narrow therapeutic window, should be approached with caution). Products include:

Symbyax Capsules 1871
Zyprexa Tablets 1883
Zyprexa IntraMuscular 1883
Zyprexa ZYDIS Orally Disintegrating Tablets 1883

Omeprazole (Duloxetine is a moderate inhibitor of CYP2D6. Co-administration of duloxetine with other drugs that are extensively metabolized by this isoenzyme, and which have a narrow therapeutic window, should be approached with caution).

No products indexed under this heading.

Ondansetron (Duloxetine is a moderate inhibitor of CYP2D6. Co-administration of duloxetine with other drugs that are extensively metabolized by this isoenzyme, and which have a narrow therapeutic window, should be approached with caution). Products include:

Zofran ODT Orally Disintegrating Tablets 1687

Ondansetron Hydrochloride (Duloxetine is a moderate inhibitor of CYP2D6. Co-administration of duloxetine with other drugs that are extensively metabolized by this isoenzyme, and which have a narrow therapeutic window, should be approached with caution). Products include:

Zofran Injection 1682
Zofran 1687

Oxaprozin (SSRIs and SNRIs, including duloxetine, may increase the risk of bleeding events. Concomitant use of aspirin, non-steroidal anti-inflammatory drugs, warfarin, and other anti-coagulants may add to this risk).

No products indexed under this heading.

Oxazepam (Given the primary CNS effects of duloxetine, it should be used with caution when it is taken in combination with or substituted for other centrally acting drugs, including those with a similar mechanism of action).

No products indexed under this heading.

Oxycodone Hydrochloride (Duloxetine is a moderate inhibitor of CYP2D6. Co-administration of duloxetine with other drugs that are extensively metabolized by this isoenzyme, and which have a narrow therapeutic window, should be approached with caution). Products include:

OxyContin Tablets 2589
OxyIR Capsules 2593
Percocet Tablets 1127
Percodan Tablets 1130

Paclitaxel (Duloxetine is a moderate inhibitor of CYP2D6. Co-administration of duloxetine with other drugs that are extensively metabolized by this isoenzyme, and which have a narrow therapeutic window, should be approached with caution).

No products indexed under this heading.

Pargyline Hydrochloride (There have been reports of serious, sometimes fatal, reactions in patients receiving a serotonin reuptake inhibitor in combination with a monoamine oxidase inhibitor (MAOI). These reactions have also been reported in patients who have recently discontinued serotonin reuptake inhibitors and are started on an MAOI. Therefore, duloxetine use is contraindicated in combination with an MAOI, or within at least 14 days of discontinuing treatment with an MAOI. Based on the half-life of duloxetine, at least 5 days should be allowed after stopping duloxetine before starting an MAOI. Development of a potentially life-threatening serotonin syndrome may occur with concomitant use of duloxetine HCl and drugs which impair the metabolism of serotonin (e.g., MAOIs)).

No products indexed under this heading.

Paroxetine Hydrochloride (Paroxetine (20mg qd) increased the concentration of duloxetine (40mg qd) by about 60% and greater degrees of inhibition are expected with higher doses of paroxetine). Products include:

Paxil 1535
Paxil CR Controlled-Release Tablets 1544

Pemoline (Given the primary CNS effects of duloxetine, it should be used with caution when it is taken in combination with or substituted for other centrally acting drugs, including those with a similar mechanism of action).

No products indexed under this heading.

Pentobarbital Sodium (Given the primary CNS effects of duloxetine, it should be used with caution when it is taken in combination with or substituted for other centrally acting drugs, including those with a similar mechanism of action). Products include:

Nembutal Sodium Solution, USP 2494

Perphenazine (Duloxetine is a moderate inhibitor of CYP2D6. Co-administration of duloxetine with other drugs that are extensively metabolized by this isoenzyme, and which have a narrow therapeutic window, should be approached with caution).

No products indexed under this heading.

Phenelzine Sulfate (There have been reports of serious, sometimes fatal, reactions in patients receiving a serotonin reuptake inhibitor in combination with a monoamine oxidase inhibitor (MAOI). These reactions have also been reported in patients who have recently discontinued serotonin reuptake inhibitors and are started on an MAOI. Therefore, duloxetine use is contraindicated in combination with an MAOI, or within at least 14 days of discontinuing treatment with an MAOI. Based on the half-life of duloxetine, at least 5 days should be allowed after stopping duloxetine before starting an MAOI. Development of a potentially life-threatening serotonin syndrome may occur with concomitant use of duloxetine HCl and drugs which impair the metabolism of serotonin (e.g., MAOIs)).

No products indexed under this heading.

Phenobarbital (Given the primary CNS effects of duloxetine, it should be used with caution when it is taken in combination with or substituted for other centrally acting drugs, including those with a similar mechanism of action). Products include:

Donnatal Extentabs 2507

Phenylbutazone (SSRIs and SNRIs, including duloxetine, may increase the risk of bleeding events. Concomitant use of aspirin, non-steroidal anti-inflammatory drugs, warfarin, and other anti-coagulants may add to this risk).

No products indexed under this heading.

Pindolol (Duloxetine is a moderate inhibitor of CYP2D6. Co-administration of duloxetine with other drugs that are extensively metabolized by this isoenzyme, and which have a narrow therapeutic window, should be approached with caution).

No products indexed under this heading.

Piroxicam (SSRIs and SNRIs, including duloxetine, may increase the risk of bleeding events. Concomitant use of aspirin, non-steroidal anti-inflammatory drugs, warfarin, and other anti-coagulants may add to this risk).
No products indexed under this heading.

Prazepam (Given the primary CNS effects of duloxetine, it should be used with caution when it is taken in combination with or substituted for other centrally acting drugs, including those with a similar mechanism of action).
No products indexed under this heading.

Procarbazine Hydrochloride (There have been reports of serious, sometimes fatal, reactions in patients receiving a serotonin reuptake inhibitor in combination with a monoamine oxidase inhibitor (MAOI). These reactions have also been reported in patients who have recently discontinued serotonin reuptake inhibitors and are started on an MAOI. Therefore, duloxetine use is contraindicated in combination with an MAOI, or within at least 14 days of discontinuing treatment with an MAOI. Based on the half-life of duloxetine, at least 5 days should be allowed after stopping duloxetine before starting an MAOI. Development of a potentially life-threatening serotonin syndrome may occur with concomitant use of duloxetine HCl and drugs which impair the metabolism of serotonin (e.g., MAOIs)).
No products indexed under this heading.

Prochlorperazine (Duloxetine is a moderate inhibitor of CYP2D6. Co-administration of duloxetine with other drugs that are extensively metabolized by this isoenzyme, and which have a narrow therapeutic window, should be approached with caution).
No products indexed under this heading.

Promethazine Hydrochloride (Duloxetine is a moderate inhibitor of CYP2D6. Co-administration of duloxetine with other drugs that are extensively metabolized by this isoenzyme, and which have a narrow therapeutic window, should be approached with caution).
No products indexed under this heading.

Propafenone Hydrochloride (Duloxetine is a moderate inhibitor of CYP2D6. Co-administration of duloxetine with other drugs that are extensively metabolized by this isoenzyme, and which have a narrow therapeutic window, should be approached with caution). Products include:
Rythmol Tablets 1586
Rythmol SR Capsules 1590

Propofol (Given the primary CNS effects of duloxetine, it should be used with caution when it is taken in combination with or substituted for other centrally acting drugs, including those with a similar mechanism of action).
No products indexed under this heading.

Propoxyphene Hydrochloride (Duloxetine is a moderate inhibitor of CYP2D6. Co-administration of duloxetine with other drugs that are extensively metabolized by this isoenzyme, and which have a narrow therapeutic window, should be approached with caution).
No products indexed under this heading.

Propoxyphene Napsylate (Duloxetine is a moderate inhibitor of CYP2D6. Co-administration of duloxetine with other drugs that are extensively metabolized by this isoenzyme, and which have a narrow therapeutic window, should be approached with caution).
No products indexed under this heading.

Propranolol Hydrochloride (Duloxetine is a moderate inhibitor of CYP2D6. Co-administration of duloxetine with other drugs that are extensively metabolized by this isoenzyme, and which have a narrow therapeutic window, should be approached with caution). Products include:
InnoPran XL Extended Release Capsules 1484

Protriptyline Hydrochloride (Duloxetine is a moderate inhibitor of CYP2D6. Co-administration of duloxetine with other drugs that are extensively metabolized by this isoenzyme, and which have a narrow therapeutic window, should be approached with caution. Plasma tricyclic antidepressant (TCA) concentrations may need to be monitored, and the dose of the TCA may need to be reduced, if a TCA is co-administered with duloxetine).
No products indexed under this heading.

Quazepam (Given the primary CNS effects of duloxetine, it should be used with caution when it is taken in combination with or substituted for other centrally acting drugs, including those with a similar mechanism of action).
No products indexed under this heading.

Quetiapine Fumarate (Duloxetine is a moderate inhibitor of CYP2D6. Co-administration of duloxetine with other drugs that are extensively metabolized by this isoenzyme, and which have a narrow therapeutic window, should be approached with caution).
No products indexed under this heading.

Quinacrine Hydrochloride (Because CYP2D6 is involved in duloxetine metabolism, concomitant use of duloxetine with potent inhibitors of CYP2D6 would be expected to, and does, result in higher concentrations of duloxetine).
No products indexed under this heading.

Quinidine Gluconate (Duloxetine is a moderate inhibitor of CYP2D6. Co-administration of duloxetine with other drugs that are extensively metabolized by this isoenzyme, and which have a narrow therapeutic window, should be approached with caution).
No products indexed under this heading.

Quinidine Hydrochloride (Duloxetine is a moderate inhibitor of CYP2D6. Co-administration of duloxetine with other drugs that are extensively metabolized by this isoenzyme, and which have a narrow therapeutic window, should be approached with caution).
No products indexed under this heading.

Quinidine Polygalacturonate (Duloxetine is a moderate inhibitor of CYP2D6. Co-administration of duloxetine with other drugs that are extensively metabolized by this isoenzyme, and which have a narrow therapeutic window, should be approached with caution).
No products indexed under this heading.

Quinidine Sulfate (Duloxetine is a moderate inhibitor of CYP2D6. Co-administration of duloxetine with other drugs that are extensively metabolized by this isoenzyme, and which have a narrow therapeutic window, should be approached with caution).
No products indexed under this heading.

Rabeprazole Sodium (Duloxetine has an enteric coating that resists dissolution until reaching a segment of the gastrointestinal tract where the pH exceeds 5.5. Drugs that raise the gastrointestinal pH may lead to an earlier release of duloxetine). Products include:
Aciphex Tablets 1053

Ranitidine Bismuth Citrate (Because CYP2D6 is involved in duloxetine metabolism, concomitant use of duloxetine with potent inhibitors of CYP2D6 would be expected to, and does, result in higher concentrations of duloxetine).
No products indexed under this heading.

Ranitidine Hydrochloride (Duloxetine has an enteric coating that resists dissolution until reaching a segment of the gastrointestinal tract where the pH exceeds 5.5. Drugs that raise the gastrointestinal pH may lead to an earlier release of duloxetine). Products include:
Zantac 75 Tablets 603
Zantac 1670
Zantac Injection 1666
Zantac Injection Pharmacy Bulk Package 1668
Maximum Strength Zantac 150 Tablets 603
Maximum Strength Zantac 150 Cool Mint Tablets 603

Rasagiline Mesylate (There have been reports of serious, sometimes fatal, reactions in patients receiving a serotonin reuptake inhibitor in combination with a monoamine oxidase inhibitor (MAOI). These reactions have also been reported in patients who have recently discontinued serotonin reuptake inhibitors and are started on an MAOI. Therefore, duloxetine use is contraindicated in combination with an MAOI, or within at least 14 days of discontinuing treatment with an MAOI. Based on the half-life of duloxetine, at least 5 days should be allowed after stopping duloxetine before starting an MAOI. Development of a potentially life-threatening serotonin syndrome may occur with concomitant use of duloxetine HCl and drugs which impair the metabolism of serotonin (e.g., MAOIs)). Products include:
Azilect Tablets 3106

Remifentanil Hydrochloride (Given the primary CNS effects of duloxetine, it should be used with caution when it is taken in combination with or substituted for other centrally acting drugs, including those with a similar mechanism of action).
No products indexed under this heading.

Risperidone (Duloxetine is a moderate inhibitor of CYP2D6. Co-administration of duloxetine with other drugs that are extensively metabolized by this isoenzyme, and which have a narrow therapeutic window, should be approached with caution). Products include:
Risperdal Consta Long-Acting Injection 1753

Ritonavir (Duloxetine is a moderate inhibitor of CYP2D6. Co-administration of duloxetine with other drugs that are extensively metabolized by this isoenzyme, and which have a narrow therapeutic window, should be approached with caution). Products include:
Kaletra 452
Norvir 489

Rizatriptan Benzoate (Development of a potentially life-threatening serotonin syndrome may occur with concomitant use of duloxetine HCl and triptans. If concomitant treatment is clinically warranted, careful observation of the patient is advised, particularly during treatment initiation and dose increases). Products include:
Maxalt Tablets 2056
Maxalt-MLT Orally Disintegrating Tablets 2056

Rofecoxib (SSRIs and SNRIs, including duloxetine, may increase the risk of bleeding events. Concomitant use of aspirin, non-steroidal anti-inflammatory drugs, warfarin, and other anti-coagulants may add to this risk).
No products indexed under this heading.

Secobarbital Sodium (Given the primary CNS effects of duloxetine, it should be used with caution when it is taken in combination with or substituted for other centrally acting drugs, including those with a similar mechanism of action).
No products indexed under this heading.

Selegiline (There have been reports of serious, sometimes fatal, reactions in patients receiving a serotonin reuptake inhibitor in combination with a monoamine oxidase inhibitor (MAOI). These reactions have also been reported in patients who have recently discontinued serotonin reuptake inhibitors and are started on an MAOI. Therefore, duloxetine use is contraindicated in combination with an MAOI, or within at least 14 days of discontinuing treatment with an MAOI. Based on the half-life of duloxetine, at least 5 days should be allowed after stopping duloxetine before starting an MAOI. Development of a potentially life-threatening serotonin syndrome may occur with concomitant use of duloxetine HCl and drugs which impair the metabolism of serotonin (e.g., MAOIs)). Products include:
Emsam Transdermal System 905

Selegiline Hydrochloride (There have been reports of serious, sometimes fatal, reactions in patients receiving a serotonin reuptake inhibitor in combination with a monoamine oxidase inhibitor (MAOI). These reactions have also been reported in patients who have recently discontinued serotonin reuptake inhibitors and are started on an MAOI. Therefore, duloxetine use is contraindicated in combination with an MAOI, or within at least 14 days of discontinuing treatment with an MAOI. Based on the half-life of duloxetine, at least 5 days should be allowed after stopping duloxetine before starting an MAOI. Development of a potentially life-threatening serotonin syndrome may occur with concomitant use of duloxetine HCl and drugs which impair the metabolism of serotonin (e.g., MAOIs)). Products include:

Eldepryl Capsules 3052

Sertraline Hydrochloride (Development of a potentially life-threatening serotonin syndrome may occur with concomitant use of duloxetine HCl and serotonergic drugs. Concomitant use of duloxetine hydrochloride with serotonin precursors is not recommended).

No products indexed under this heading.

Sevoflurane (Given the primary CNS effects of duloxetine, it should be used with caution when it is taken in combination with or substituted for other centrally acting drugs, including those with a similar mechanism of action). Products include:

Ultane Liquid for Inhalation 524

Sildenafil Citrate (Because CYP2D6 is involved in duloxetine metabolism, concomitant use of duloxetine with potent inhibitors of CYP2D6 would be expected to, and does, result in higher concentrations of duloxetine).

No products indexed under this heading.

Sodium Oxybate (Given the primary CNS effects of duloxetine, it should be used with caution when it is taken in combination with or substituted for other centrally acting drugs, including those with a similar mechanism of action). Products include:

Xyrem Oral Solution 1766

Sparfloxacin (Concomitant use of duloxetine with fluvoxamine, an inhibitor of CYP1A2, results in a 6-fold increase in AUC, about 2.5-fold increase in Cmax, and an approximately 3-fold increase in t1/2 of duloxetine. Since duloxetine is metabolized in part by CYP1A2, concomitant use of duloxetine with other inhibitors of CYP1A2, would be expected to have the same effects; these combinations should be avoided).

No products indexed under this heading.

Sufentanil Citrate (Given the primary CNS effects of duloxetine, it should be used with caution when it is taken in combination with or substituted for other centrally acting drugs, including those with a similar mechanism of action).

No products indexed under this heading.

Sulindac (SSRIs and SNRIs, including duloxetine, may increase the risk of bleeding events. Concomitant use of aspirin, non-steroidal anti-inflammatory drugs, warfarin, and other anti-coagulants may add to this risk). Products include:

Clinoril Tablets 1962

Sumatriptan (Development of a potentially life-threatening serotonin syndrome may occur with concomitant use of duloxetine HCl and triptans. If concomitant treatment is clinically warranted, careful observation of the patient is advised, particularly during treatment initiation and dose increases). Products include:

Imitrex Nasal Spray 1470

Sumatriptan Succinate (Development of a potentially life-threatening serotonin syndrome may occur with concomitant use of duloxetine HCl and triptans. If concomitant treatment is clinically warranted, careful observation of the patient is advised, particularly during treatment initiation and dose increases). Products include:

Imitrex Injection 1465
Imitrex Tablets 1474
Treximet Tablets 1616

Tacrine Hydrochloride (Concomitant use of duloxetine with fluvoxamine, an inhibitor of CYP1A2, results in a 6-fold increase in AUC, about 2.5-fold increase in Cmax, and an approximately 3-fold increase in t1/2 of duloxetine. Since duloxetine is metabolized in part by CYP1A2, concomitant use of duloxetine with other inhibitors of CYP1A2, would be expected to have the same effects; these combinations should be avoided).

No products indexed under this heading.

Tamoxifen Citrate (Duloxetine is a moderate inhibitor of CYP2D6. Co-administration of duloxetine with other drugs that are extensively metabolized by this isoenzyme, and which have a narrow therapeutic window, should be approached with caution).

No products indexed under this heading.

Temazepam (Given the primary CNS effects of duloxetine, it should be used with caution when it is taken in combination with or substituted for other centrally acting drugs, including those with a similar mechanism of action).

No products indexed under this heading.

Teniposide (Duloxetine is a moderate inhibitor of CYP2D6. Co-administration of duloxetine with other drugs that are extensively metabolized by this isoenzyme, and which have a narrow therapeutic window, should be approached with caution).

No products indexed under this heading.

Terbinafine Hydrochloride (Because CYP2D6 is involved in duloxetine metabolism, concomitant use of duloxetine with potent inhibitors of CYP2D6 would be expected to, and does, result in higher concentrations of duloxetine). Products include:

Lamisil Oral Granules 2264
Lamisil Tablets 2266

Testosterone (Duloxetine is a moderate inhibitor of CYP2D6. Co-administration of duloxetine with other drugs that are extensively metabolized by this isoenzyme, and which have a narrow therapeutic window, should be approached with caution). Products include:

AndroGel 3159
Testim 1% Gel 701

Testosterone Cypionate (Duloxetine is a moderate inhibitor of CYP2D6. Co-administration of duloxetine with other drugs that are extensively metabolized by this isoenzyme, and which have a narrow therapeutic window, should be approached with caution).

No products indexed under this heading.

Testosterone Enanthate (Duloxetine is a moderate inhibitor of CYP2D6. Co-administration of duloxetine with other drugs that are extensively metabolized by this isoenzyme, and which have a narrow therapeutic window, should be approached with caution). Products include:

Delatestryl Injection 1730

Testosterone Propionate (Duloxetine is a moderate inhibitor of CYP2D6. Co-administration of duloxetine with other drugs that are extensively metabolized by this isoenzyme, and which have a narrow therapeutic window, should be approached with caution).

No products indexed under this heading.

Thiamylal Sodium (Given the primary CNS effects of duloxetine, it should be used with caution when it is taken in combination with or substituted for other centrally acting drugs, including those with a similar mechanism of action).

No products indexed under this heading.

Thioridazine (Duloxetine is a moderate inhibitor of CYP2D6. Co-administration of duloxetine with other drugs that are extensively metabolized by this isoenzyme, and which have a narrow therapeutic window, should be approached with caution. Because of the risk of serious ventricular arrhythmias and sudden death potentially associated with elevated plasma levels of thioridazine, duloxetine and thioridazine should not be co-administered).

No products indexed under this heading.

Thioridazine Hydrochloride (Duloxetine is a moderate inhibitor of CYP2D6. Co-administration of duloxetine with other drugs that are extensively metabolized by this isoenzyme, and which have a narrow therapeutic window, should be approached with caution. Because of the risk of serious ventricular arrhythmias and sudden death potentially associated with elevated plasma levels of thioridazine, duloxetine and thioridazine should not be co-administered). Products include:

Thioridazine Hydrochloride Tablets 2195

Thiothixene (Given the primary CNS effects of duloxetine, it should be used with caution when it is taken in combination with or substituted for other centrally acting drugs, including those with a similar mechanism of action). Products include:

Thiothixene Capsules 2197

Ticlopidine Hydrochloride (Concomitant use of duloxetine with fluvoxamine, an inhibitor of CYP1A2, results in a 6-fold increase in AUC, about 2.5-fold increase in Cmax, and an approximately 3-fold increase in t1/2 of duloxetine. Since duloxetine is metabolized in part by CYP1A2, concomitant use of duloxetine with other inhibitors of CYP1A2, would be expected to have the same effects; these combinations should be avoided).

No products indexed under this heading.

Timolol Maleate (Duloxetine is a moderate inhibitor of CYP2D6. Co-administration of duloxetine with other drugs that are extensively metabolized by this isoenzyme, and which have a narrow therapeutic window, should be approached with caution). Products include:

Combigan Ophthalmic Solution 553
Cosopt Sterile Ophthalmic Solution 1969
Timoptic Sterile Ophthalmic Solution 2121
Timoptic in Ocudose 2124
Timoptic-XE Sterile Ophthalmic Gel Forming Solution 2125

Tinzaparin Sodium (SSRIs and SNRIs, including duloxetine, may increase the risk of bleeding events. Concomitant use of aspirin, non-steroidal anti-inflammatory drugs, warfarin, and other anti-coagulants may add to this risk).

No products indexed under this heading.

Tolmetin Sodium (SSRIs and SNRIs, including duloxetine, may increase the risk of bleeding events. Concomitant use of aspirin, non-steroidal anti-inflammatory drugs, warfarin, and other anti-coagulants may add to this risk).

No products indexed under this heading.

Tolterodine Tartrate (Duloxetine is a moderate inhibitor of CYP2D6. Co-administration of duloxetine with other drugs that are extensively metabolized by this isoenzyme, and which have a narrow therapeutic window, should be approached with caution).

No products indexed under this heading.

Tramadol Hydrochloride (Caution is advised with co-administration of duloxetine with drugs that may affect the serotonergic neurotransmitter systems such as tramadol because of potential development of serotonin syndrome). Products include:

Ultram ER Extended-Release Tablets 2428

Tranylcypromine Sulfate (There have been reports of serious, sometimes fatal, reactions in patients receiving a serotonin reuptake inhibitor in combination with a monoamine oxidase inhibitor (MAOI). These reactions have also been reported in patients who have recently discontinued serotonin reuptake inhibitors and are started on an MAOI. Therefore, duloxetine use is contraindicated in combination with an MAOI, or within at least 14 days of discontinuing treatment with an MAOI. Based on the half-life of duloxetine, at least 5 days should be allowed after stopping duloxetine before starting an MAOI. Development of a potentially life-threatening serotonin syndrome may occur with concomitant use of duloxetine HCl and drugs which impair the metabolism of serotonin (e.g., MAOIs)). Products include:

Parnate Tablets 1532

Trazodone Hydrochloride (Duloxetine is a moderate inhibitor of CYP2D6. Co-administration of duloxetine with other drugs that are extensively metabolized by this isoenzyme, and which have a narrow therapeutic window, should be approached with caution).
No products indexed under this heading.

Triazolam (Duloxetine is a moderate inhibitor of CYP2D6. Co-administration of duloxetine with other drugs that are extensively metabolized by this isoenzyme, and which have a narrow therapeutic window, should be approached with caution).
No products indexed under this heading.

Trifluoperazine Hydrochloride (Duloxetine is a moderate inhibitor of CYP2D6. Co-administration of duloxetine with other drugs that are extensively metabolized by this isoenzyme, and which have a narrow therapeutic window, should be approached with caution).
No products indexed under this heading.

Trimipramine Maleate (Duloxetine is a moderate inhibitor of CYP2D6. Co-administration of duloxetine with other drugs that are extensively metabolized by this isoenzyme, and which have a narrow therapeutic window, should be approached with caution. Plasma tricyclic antidepressant (TCA) concentrations may need to be monitored, and the dose of the TCA may need to be reduced, if a TCA is co-administered with duloxetine).
No products indexed under this heading.

Troleandomycin (Concomitant use of duloxetine with fluvoxamine, an inhibitor of CYP1A2, results in a 6-fold increase in AUC, about 2.5-fold increase in Cmax, and an approximately 3-fold increase in t1/2 of duloxetine. Since duloxetine is metabolized in part by CYP1A2, concomitant use of duloxetine with other inhibitors of CYP1A2, would be expected to have the same effects; these combinations should be avoided).
No products indexed under this heading.

Trovafloxacin Mesylate (Some quinolones, inhibitors of CYP1A2, would be expected to increase the AUC and Cmax of duloxetine; co-administration should be avoided).
No products indexed under this heading.

Tryptophan (Concomitant use of duloxetine with serotonin precursors (e.g., tryptophan) is not recommended).
No products indexed under this heading.

Valdecoxib (SSRIs and SNRIs, including duloxetine, may increase the risk of bleeding events. Concomitant use of aspirin, non-steroidal anti-inflammatory drugs, warfarin, and other anti-coagulants may add to this risk).
No products indexed under this heading.

Vardenafil Hydrochloride (Because CYP2D6 is involved in duloxetine metabolism, concomitant use of duloxetine with potent inhibitors of CYP2D6 would be expected to, and does, result in higher concentrations of duloxetine). Products include:

Levitra Tablets **2876**

Venlafaxine Hydrochloride (Development of a potentially life-threatening serotonin syndrome may occur with concomitant use of duloxetine HCl and serotonergic drugs. Concomitant use of duloxetine hydrochloride with serotonin precursors is not recommended). Products include:

Effexor XR Extended-Release Capsules **3195**
Venlafaxine Hydrochloride Tablets ... **2199**

Vinblastine Sulfate (Duloxetine is a moderate inhibitor of CYP2D6. Co-administration of duloxetine with other drugs that are extensively metabolized by this isoenzyme, and which have a narrow therapeutic window, should be approached with caution).
No products indexed under this heading.

Warfarin Sodium (Altered anticoagulant effects, including increased bleeding have been reported when SSRIs or SNRIs are co-administered with warfarin. Patients receiving warfarin therapy should be carefully monitored when duloxetine is initiated or discontinued).
No products indexed under this heading.

Zaleplon (Given the primary CNS effects of duloxetine, it should be used with caution when it is taken in combination with or substituted for other centrally acting drugs, including those with a similar mechanism of action).
No products indexed under this heading.

Zileuton (Concomitant use of duloxetine with fluvoxamine, an inhibitor of CYP1A2, results in a 6-fold increase in AUC, about 2.5-fold increase in Cmax, and an approximately 3-fold increase in t1/2 of duloxetine. Since duloxetine is metabolized in part by CYP1A2, concomitant use of duloxetine with other inhibitors of CYP1A2, would be expected to have the same effects; these combinations should be avoided).
No products indexed under this heading.

Ziprasidone Hydrochloride (Given the primary CNS effects of duloxetine, it should be used with caution when it is taken in combination with or substituted for other centrally acting drugs, including those with a similar mechanism of action). Products include:

Geodon Capsules **2520**

Zolmitriptan (Development of a potentially life-threatening serotonin syndrome may occur with concomitant use of duloxetine HCl and triptans. If concomitant treatment is clinically warranted, careful observation of the patient is advised, particularly during treatment initiation and dose increases). Products include:

Zomig Tablets **694**
Zomig Nasal Spray **689**
Zomig-ZMT Tablets **694**

Zolpidem Tartrate (Given the primary CNS effects of duloxetine, it should be used with caution when it is taken in combination with or substituted for other centrally acting drugs, including those with a similar mechanism of action). Products include:

Ambien Tablets **2692**
Ambien CR Tablets **2696**

Zonisamide (Duloxetine is a moderate inhibitor of CYP2D6. Co-administration of duloxetine with other drugs that are extensively metabolized by this isoenzyme, and which have a narrow therapeutic window, should be approached with caution). Products include:

Zonegran Capsules **1089**

Food Interactions

Alcohol (Use of duloxetine concomitantly with heavy alcohol intake may be associated with severe liver injury; for this reason, duloxetine should ordinarily not be prescribed for patients with substantial alcohol use).

Grapefruit Juice (Concomitant use of duloxetine with fluvoxamine, an inhibitor of CYP1A2, results in a 6-fold increase in AUC, about 2.5-fold increase in Cmax, and an approximately 3-fold increase in t1/2 of duloxetine. Since duloxetine is metabolized in part by CYP1A2, concomitant use of duloxetine with other inhibitors of CYP1A2, would be expected to have the same effects; these combinations should be avoided).

CYTOMEL TABLETS

(Liothyronine Sodium) **1778**

May interact with oral anticoagulants, estrogens, cardiac glycosides, oral hypoglycemic agents, insulin, tricyclic antidepressants, and certain other agents. Compounds in these categories include:

Acarbose (Initiating thyroid replacement therapy may cause increases in oral hypoglycemic requirements). Products include:

Precose Tablets **792**

Amitriptyline Hydrochloride (Use of thyroid hormones may increase receptor sensitivity and enhance antidepressant activity; transient cardiac arrhythmias; thyroid hormone activity may also be enhanced).
No products indexed under this heading.

Amoxapine (Use of thyroid hormones may increase receptor sensitivity and enhance antidepressant activity; transient cardiac arrhythmias; thyroid hormone activity may also be enhanced).
No products indexed under this heading.

Anisindione (Thyroid hormones appear to increase catabolism of vitamin K-dependent clotting factor; if oral anticoagulants are also given compensatory increases in clotting factor synthesis are impaired).
No products indexed under this heading.

Chlorotrianisene (Estrogens tend to increase serum thyroxine-binding globulin in a patient with a nonfunctioning thyroid gland who is receiving thyroid replacement therapy; patients without functioning thyroid gland who are on thyroid replacement therapy may need to increase their thyroid dose if estrogens or estrogen-containing oral contraceptives are given).
No products indexed under this heading.

Chlorpropamide (Initiating thyroid replacement therapy may cause increases in oral hypoglycemic requirements).
No products indexed under this heading.

Cholestyramine (Binds both T4 and T3 in the intestine thus impairing absorption of thyroid hormones; 4 to 5 hours should elapse between administration of thyroid hormone and cholestyramine).
No products indexed under this heading.

Clomipramine Hydrochloride (Use of thyroid hormones may increase receptor sensitivity and enhance antidepressant activity; transient cardiac arrhythmias; thyroid hormone activity may also be enhanced).
No products indexed under this heading.

Desipramine Hydrochloride (Use of thyroid hormones may increase receptor sensitivity and enhance antidepressant activity; transient cardiac arrhythmias; thyroid hormone activity may also be enhanced).
No products indexed under this heading.

Deslanoside (Thyroid preparations may potentiate the toxic effects of digitalis; thyroid hormone increase metabolic rate which requires an increase in digitalis dosage).
No products indexed under this heading.

Dicumarol (Thyroid hormones appear to increase catabolism of vitamin K-dependent clotting factor; if oral anticoagulants are also given compensatory increases in clotting factor synthesis are impaired).
No products indexed under this heading.

Dienestrol (Estrogens tend to increase serum thyroxine-binding globulin in a patient with a nonfunctioning thyroid gland who is receiving thyroid replacement therapy; patients without functioning thyroid gland who are on thyroid replacement therapy may need to increase their thyroid dose if estrogens or estrogen-containing oral contraceptives are given).
No products indexed under this heading.

Diethylstilbestrol (Estrogens tend to increase serum thyroxine-binding globulin in a patient with a nonfunctioning thyroid gland who is receiving thyroid replacement therapy; patients without functioning thyroid gland who are on thyroid replacement therapy may need to increase their thyroid dose if estrogens or estrogen-containing oral contraceptives are given).
No products indexed under this heading.

Digitalis Glycoside Preparations (Thyroid preparations may potentiate the toxic effects of digitalis; thyroid hormone increase metabolic rate which requires an increase in digitalis dosage).
No products indexed under this heading.

Digitoxin (Thyroid preparations may potentiate the toxic effects of digitalis; thyroid hormone increase metabolic rate which requires an increase in digitalis dosage).
No products indexed under this heading.

Digoxin (Thyroid preparations may potentiate the toxic effects of digitalis; thyroid hormone increase meta-

bolic rate which requires an increase in digitalis dosage). Products include:
Lanoxin Injection 1498
Lanoxin Injection Pediatric 1502
Lanoxin Tablets 1505

Doxepin Hydrochloride (Use of thyroid hormones may increase receptor sensitivity and enhance antidepressant activity; transient cardiac arrhythmias; thyroid hormone activity may also be enhanced).
No products indexed under this heading.

Epinephrine (Thyroxine increases the adrenergic effect of catecholamines, such as epinephrine). Products include:
EpiPen 1024

Epinephrine Bitartrate (Thyroxine increases the adrenergic effect of catecholamines, such as epinephrine).
No products indexed under this heading.

Epinephrine Hydrochloride (Thyroxine increases the adrenergic effect of catecholamines, such as epinephrine).
No products indexed under this heading.

Estradiol (Estrogens tend to increase serum thyroxine-binding globulin in a patient with a nonfunctioning thyroid gland who is receiving thyroid replacement therapy; patients without functioning thyroid gland who are on thyroid replacement therapy may need to increase their thyroid dose if estrogens or estrogen-containing oral contraceptives are given). Products include:
Activella Tablets 2347
Angeliq Tablets 751
Climara Transdermal System 763
Climara Pro Transdermal System 768
Divigel 3167
Vagifem Tablets 2375

Estrogens, Conjugated (Estrogens tend to increase serum thyroxine-binding globulin in a patient with a nonfunctioning thyroid gland who is receiving thyroid replacement therapy; patients without functioning thyroid gland who are on thyroid replacement therapy may need to increase their thyroid dose if estrogens or estrogen-containing oral contraceptives are given). Products include:
Premarin Intravenous 3217
Premarin Tablets 3221
Premarin Vaginal Cream 3228
Premphase Tablets 3232
Prempro Tablets 3232

Estrogens, Esterified (Estrogens tend to increase serum thyroxine-binding globulin in a patient with a nonfunctioning thyroid gland who is receiving thyroid replacement therapy; patients without functioning thyroid gland who are on thyroid replacement therapy may need to increase their thyroid dose if estrogens or estrogen-containing oral contraceptives are given). Products include:
Estratest Tablets 3043
Estratest H.S. Tablets 3043

Estropipate (Estrogens tend to increase serum thyroxine-binding globulin in a patient with a nonfunctioning thyroid gland who is receiving thyroid replacement therapy; patients without functioning thyroid gland who are on thyroid replacement therapy may need to increase their thyroid dose if estrogens or estrogen-containing oral contraceptives are given).
No products indexed under this heading.

Ethinyl Estradiol (Estrogens tend to increase serum thyroxine-binding globulin in a patient with a nonfunctioning thyroid gland who is receiving thyroid replacement therapy; patients without functioning thyroid gland who are on thyroid replacement therapy may need to increase their thyroid dose if estrogens or estrogen-containing oral contraceptives are given). Products include:
Lybrel Tablets 3204
Mircette Tablets 1034
NuvaRing 2897
Ortho-Cyclen/Ortho Tri-Cyclen 2449
Ortho Evra Transdermal System 2437
Ortho Tri-Cyclen Lo Tablets 2458
Seasonique Tablets 1046
Yaz Tablets 805

Glimepiride (Initiating thyroid replacement therapy may cause increases in oral hypoglycemic requirements). Products include:
Avandaryl Tablets 1344
Duetact Tablets 3085

Glipizide (Initiating thyroid replacement therapy may cause increases in oral hypoglycemic requirements).
No products indexed under this heading.

Glyburide (Initiating thyroid replacement therapy may cause increases in oral hypoglycemic requirements).
No products indexed under this heading.

Imipramine Hydrochloride (Use of thyroid hormones may increase receptor sensitivity and enhance antidepressant activity; transient cardiac arrhythmias; thyroid hormone activity may also be enhanced).
No products indexed under this heading.

Imipramine Pamoate (Use of thyroid hormones may increase receptor sensitivity and enhance antidepressant activity; transient cardiac arrhythmias; thyroid hormone activity may also be enhanced).
No products indexed under this heading.

Insulin (Initiating thyroid replacement therapy may cause increases in insulin requirements).
No products indexed under this heading.

Insulin, Human, Zinc Suspension (Initiating thyroid replacement therapy may cause increases in insulin requirements).
No products indexed under this heading.

Insulin, Human (rDNA origin) (Initiating thyroid replacement therapy may cause increases in insulin requirements). Products include:
Exubera Inhalation Powder 2515

Insulin, Human NPH (Initiating thyroid replacement therapy may cause increases in insulin requirements). Products include:
Humulin N Vial 1846

Insulin, Human Regular (Initiating thyroid replacement therapy may cause increases in insulin requirements). Products include:
Humulin R 1849
Humulin R (U-500) 1850

Insulin, Human Regular and Human NPH Mixture (Initiating thyroid replacement therapy may cause increases in insulin requirements). Products include:
Humulin 50/50, 100 Units 1843
Humulin 70/30 Vial 1844

Insulin, NPH (Initiating thyroid replacement therapy may cause increases in insulin requirements).
No products indexed under this heading.

Insulin, Regular (Initiating thyroid replacement therapy may cause increases in insulin requirements).
No products indexed under this heading.

Insulin, Regular and NPH mixture (Initiating thyroid replacement therapy may cause increases in insulin requirements).
No products indexed under this heading.

Insulin, Zinc Crystals (Initiating thyroid replacement therapy may cause increases in insulin requirements).
No products indexed under this heading.

Insulin, Zinc Suspension (Initiating thyroid replacement therapy may cause increases in insulin requirements).
No products indexed under this heading.

Insulin Aspart (Initiating thyroid replacement therapy may cause increases in insulin requirements).
No products indexed under this heading.

Insulin Aspart, Human (Initiating thyroid replacement therapy may cause increases in insulin requirements). Products include:
NovoLog Mix 70/30 2364

Insulin Aspart, Human Regular (Initiating thyroid replacement therapy may cause increases in insulin requirements). Products include:
NovoLog Injection 2359

Insulin Aspart Protamine, Human (Initiating thyroid replacement therapy may cause increases in insulin requirements). Products include:
NovoLog Mix 70/30 2364

Insulin Detemir (rDNA Origin) (Initiating thyroid replacement therapy may cause increases in insulin requirements). Products include:
Levemir Injection 2352

Insulin glargine (Initiating thyroid replacement therapy may cause increases in insulin requirements). Products include:
Lantus Injection 2749

Insulin Glulisine (Initiating thyroid replacement therapy may cause increases in insulin requirements). Products include:
Apidra Injection 2706

Insulin Lispro, Human (Initiating thyroid replacement therapy may cause increases in insulin requirements). Products include:
Humalog-Pen and KwikPen 1829
Humalog Mix 50/50-Pen and KwikPen 1833
Humalog Mix 75/25-Pen and KwikPen 1835

Insulin Lispro Protamine, Human (Initiating thyroid replacement therapy may cause increases in insulin requirements). Products include:
Humalog Mix 50/50-Pen and KwikPen 1833
Humalog Mix 75/25-Pen and KwikPen 1835

Ketamine Hydrochloride (Co-administration may cause hypertension and tachycardia).
No products indexed under this heading.

Maprotiline Hydrochloride (Use of thyroid hormones may increase receptor sensitivity and enhance antidepressant activity; transient cardiac arrhythmias; thyroid hormone activity may also be enhanced).
No products indexed under this heading.

Metformin Hydrochloride (Initiating thyroid replacement therapy may cause increases in oral hypoglycemic requirements). Products include:
ActoPlus Met Tablets 3071
Avandamet Tablets 1336
Janumet Tablets 2041
PrandiMet Tablets 2967

Miglitol (Initiating thyroid replacement therapy may cause increases in oral hypoglycemic requirements).
No products indexed under this heading.

Nateglinide (Initiating thyroid replacement therapy may cause increases in oral hypoglycemic requirements). Products include:
Starlix Tablets 2314

Norepinephrine Hydrochloride (Thyroxine increases the adrenergic effect of catecholamines, such as norepinephrine).
No products indexed under this heading.

Nortriptyline Hydrochloride (Use of thyroid hormones may increase receptor sensitivity and enhance antidepressant activity; transient cardiac arrhythmias; thyroid hormone activity may also be enhanced).
No products indexed under this heading.

Pioglitazone Hydrochloride (Initiating thyroid replacement therapy may cause increases in oral hypoglycemic requirements). Products include:
ActoPlus Met Tablets 3071
Actos Tablets 3077
Duetact Tablets 3085

Polyestradiol Phosphate (Estrogens tend to increase serum thyroxine-binding globulin in a patient with a nonfunctioning thyroid gland who is receiving thyroid replacement therapy; patients without functioning thyroid gland who are on thyroid replacement therapy may need to increase their thyroid dose if estrogens or estrogen-containing oral contraceptives are given).
No products indexed under this heading.

Protriptyline Hydrochloride (Use of thyroid hormones may increase receptor sensitivity and enhance antidepressant activity; transient cardiac arrhythmias; thyroid hormone activity may also be enhanced).
No products indexed under this heading.

Quinestrol (Estrogens tend to increase serum thyroxine-binding globulin in a patient with a nonfunctioning thyroid gland who is receiving thyroid replacement therapy; patients without functioning thyroid gland who are on thyroid replacement therapy may need to increase their thyroid dose if estrogens or estrogen-containing oral contraceptives are given).
No products indexed under this heading.

Repaglinide (Initiating thyroid replacement therapy may cause increases in oral hypoglycemic requirements). Products include:
PrandiMet Tablets 2967
Prandin Tablets 2971

Rosiglitazone Maleate (Initiating thyroid replacement therapy may cause increases in oral hypoglycemic requirements). Products include:
Avandamet Tablets 1336
Avandaryl Tablets 1344
Avandia Tablets 1351

Sitagliptin Phosphate (Initiating thyroid replacement therapy may cause increases in oral hypoglycemic requirements). Products include:
Janumet Tablets 2041
Januvia Tablets 2048

Tolazamide (Initiating thyroid replacement therapy may cause increases in oral hypoglycemic requirements).
No products indexed under this heading.

Tolbutamide (Initiating thyroid replacement therapy may cause increases in oral hypoglycemic requirements).
No products indexed under this heading.

Trimipramine Maleate (Use of thyroid hormones may increase receptor sensitivity and enhance antidepressant activity; transient cardiac arrhythmias; thyroid hormone activity may also be enhanced).
No products indexed under this heading.

Troglitazone (Initiating thyroid replacement therapy may cause increases in oral hypoglycemic requirements).
No products indexed under this heading.

Warfarin Sodium (Thyroid hormones appear to increase catabolism of vitamin K-dependent clotting factor; if oral anticoagulants are also given compensatory increases in clotting factor synthesis are impaired).
No products indexed under this heading.

DACOGEN INJECTION

(Decitabine) 1066
None cited in PDR database.

DAILY COMPLETE LIQUID

(Amino Acid Preparations, Antioxidants, Herbals with Vitamins & Minerals) 624
None cited in PDR database.

DANTRIUM CAPSULES

(Dantrolene Sodium) 2580
May interact with calcium channel blockers, central nervous system depressants, estrogens, hypnotics and sedatives, tranquilizers, and certain other agents. Compounds in these categories include:

Alfentanil Hydrochloride (Co-administration may result in increased drowsiness; caution should be exercised).
No products indexed under this heading.

Alprazolam (Co-administration may result in increased drowsiness; caution should be exercised).
No products indexed under this heading.

Amlodipine Besylate (Due to interaction between verapamil and dantrolene, combination of dantrolene and calcium channel blockers is not recommended during the management of malignant hyperthermia). Products include:
Azor Tablets 1005
Exforge Tablets 2238

Aprobarbital (Co-administration may result in increased drowsiness; caution should be exercised).
No products indexed under this heading.

Bepridil Hydrochloride (Due to interaction between verapamil and dantrolene, combination of dantrolene and calcium channel blockers is not recommended during the management of malignant hyperthermia).
No products indexed under this heading.

Buprenorphine Hydrochloride (Co-administration may result in increased drowsiness; caution should be exercised). Products include:
Suboxone Tablets 2601
Subutex Tablets 2601

Buspirone Hydrochloride (Co-administration may result in increased drowsiness; caution should be exercised).
No products indexed under this heading.

Butabarbital (Co-administration may result in increased drowsiness; caution should be exercised).
No products indexed under this heading.

Butabarbital Sodium (Co-administration may result in increased drowsiness; caution should be exercised).
No products indexed under this heading.

Butalbital (Co-administration may result in increased drowsiness; caution should be exercised).
No products indexed under this heading.

Chloral Hydrate (Co-administration may result in increased drowsiness; caution should be exercised).
No products indexed under this heading.

Chlordiazepoxide (Co-administration may result in increased drowsiness; caution should be exercised).
No products indexed under this heading.

Chlordiazepoxide Hydrochloride (Co-administration may result in increased drowsiness; caution should be exercised).
No products indexed under this heading.

Chlorotrianisene (Hepatotoxicity has occurred more often in women over 35 years of age receiving concomitant estrogen therapy).
No products indexed under this heading.

Chlorpromazine (Co-administration may result in increased drowsiness; caution should be exercised).
No products indexed under this heading.

Chlorpromazine Hydrochloride (Co-administration may result in increased drowsiness; caution should be exercised).
No products indexed under this heading.

Chlorprothixene (Co-administration may result in increased drowsiness; caution should be exercised).
No products indexed under this heading.

Chlorprothixene Hydrochloride (Co-administration may result in increased drowsiness; caution should be exercised).
No products indexed under this heading.

Chlorprothixene Lactate (Co-administration may result in increased drowsiness; caution should be exercised).
No products indexed under this heading.

Clorazepate Dipotassium (Co-administration may result in increased drowsiness; caution should be exercised).
No products indexed under this heading.

Clozapine (Co-administration may result in increased drowsiness; caution should be exercised).
No products indexed under this heading.

Codeine Phosphate (Co-administration may result in increased drowsiness; caution should be exercised). Products include:
Tylenol with Codeine Tablets 2427

Desflurane (Co-administration may result in increased drowsiness; caution should be exercised).
No products indexed under this heading.

Dezocine (Co-administration may result in increased drowsiness; caution should be exercised).
No products indexed under this heading.

Diazepam (Co-administration may result in increased drowsiness; caution should be exercised). Products include:
Valium Tablets 2658

Dienestrol (Hepatotoxicity has occurred more often in women over 35 years of age receiving concomitant estrogen therapy).
No products indexed under this heading.

Diethylstilbestrol (Hepatotoxicity has occurred more often in women over 35 years of age receiving concomitant estrogen therapy).
No products indexed under this heading.

Diltiazem Hydrochloride (Due to interaction between verapamil and dantrolene, combination of dantrolene and calcium channel blockers is not recommended during the management of malignant hyperthermia). Products include:
Cardizem LA Extended Release Tablets 421

Droperidol (Co-administration may result in increased drowsiness; caution should be exercised).
No products indexed under this heading.

Enflurane (Co-administration may result in increased drowsiness; caution should be exercised).
No products indexed under this heading.

Estazolam (Co-administration may result in increased drowsiness; caution should be exercised).
No products indexed under this heading.

Estradiol (Hepatotoxicity has occurred more often in women over 35 years of age receiving concomitant estrogen therapy). Products include:
Activella Tablets 2347
Angeliq Tablets 751
Climara Transdermal System 763
Climara Pro Transdermal System 768
Divigel 3167
Vagifem Tablets 2375

Estrogens, Conjugated (Hepatotoxicity has occurred more often in women over 35 years of age receiving concomitant estrogen therapy). Products include:
Premarin Intravenous 3217
Premarin Tablets 3221
Premarin Vaginal Cream 3228
Premphase Tablets 3232
Prempro Tablets 3232

Estrogens, Esterified (Hepatotoxicity has occurred more often in women over 35 years of age receiving concomitant estrogen therapy). Products include:
Estratest Tablets 3043
Estratest H.S. Tablets 3043

Estropipate (Hepatotoxicity has occurred more often in women over 35 years of age receiving concomitant estrogen therapy).
No products indexed under this heading.

Ethanol (Co-administration may result in increased drowsiness; caution should be exercised).
No products indexed under this heading.

Ethchlorvynol (Co-administration may result in increased drowsiness; caution should be exercised).
No products indexed under this heading.

Ethinamate (Co-administration may result in increased drowsiness; caution should be exercised).
No products indexed under this heading.

Ethinyl Estradiol (Hepatotoxicity has occurred more often in women over 35 years of age receiving concomitant estrogen therapy). Products include:
Lybrel Tablets 3204
Mircette Tablets 1034
NuvaRing 2897
Ortho-Cyclen/Ortho Tri-Cyclen 2449
Ortho Evra Transdermal System 2437
Ortho Tri-Cyclen Lo Tablets 2458
Seasonique Tablets 1046
Yaz Tablets 805

Ethyl Alcohol (Co-administration may result in increased drowsiness; caution should be exercised).
No products indexed under this heading.

Felodipine (Due to interaction between verapamil and dantrolene, combination of dantrolene and calcium channel blockers is not recommended during the management of malignant hyperthermia).
No products indexed under this heading.

Fentanyl (Co-administration may result in increased drowsiness; caution should be exercised). Products include:
Duragesic Transdermal System 2405
Ionsys Transdermal System 2410

Fentanyl Citrate (Co-administration may result in increased drowsiness; caution should be exercised). Products include:
Actiq 959
Fentora Tablets 968

Fluphenazine Decanoate (Co-administration may result in increased drowsiness; caution should be exercised).
No products indexed under this heading.

Fluphenazine Enanthate (Co-administration may result in increased drowsiness; caution should be exercised).
No products indexed under this heading.

Fluphenazine Hydrochloride (Co-administration may result in increased drowsiness; caution should be exercised).
No products indexed under this heading.

Flurazepam Hydrochloride (Co-administration may result in increased drowsiness; caution should be exercised).
No products indexed under this heading.

Glutethimide (Co-administration may result in increased drowsiness; caution should be exercised).
No products indexed under this heading.

Haloperidol (Co-administration may result in increased drowsiness; caution should be exercised).
No products indexed under this heading.

Haloperidol Decanoate (Co-administration may result in increased drowsiness; caution should be exercised).
No products indexed under this heading.

Hydrocodone Bitartrate (Co-administration may result in increased drowsiness; caution should be exercised). Products include:
Lortab 5/500 Tablets 3143
Lortab 7.5/500 Tablets 3144
Lortab 10/500 Tablets 3144
Vicodin Tablets 529
Vicodin ES Tablets 530
Vicodin HP Tablets 531
Vicoprofen Tablets 533
Zydone Tablets 1132

Hydrocodone Polistirex (Co-administration may result in increased drowsiness; caution should be exercised). Products include:
Tussionex Pennkinetic Extended-Release Suspension 3154

Hydromorphone Hydrochloride (Co-administration may result in increased drowsiness; caution should be exercised).
No products indexed under this heading.

Hydroxyzine Hydrochloride (Co-administration may result in increased drowsiness; caution should be exercised).
No products indexed under this heading.

Isoflurane (Co-administration may result in increased drowsiness; caution should be exercised).
No products indexed under this heading.

Isradipine (Due to interaction between verapamil and dantrolene, combination of dantrolene and calcium channel blockers is not recommended during the management of malignant hyperthermia). Products include:
DynaCirc CR Controlled Release Tablets 1407

Ketamine Hydrochloride (Co-administration may result in increased drowsiness; caution should be exercised).
No products indexed under this heading.

Levomethadyl Acetate Hydrochloride (Co-administration may result in increased drowsiness; caution should be exercised).
No products indexed under this heading.

Levorphanol Tartrate (Co-administration may result in increased drowsiness; caution should be exercised).
No products indexed under this heading.

Lorazepam (Co-administration may result in increased drowsiness; caution should be exercised).
No products indexed under this heading.

Loxapine Hydrochloride (Co-administration may result in increased drowsiness; caution should be exercised).
No products indexed under this heading.

Loxapine Succinate (Co-administration may result in increased drowsiness; caution should be exercised).
No products indexed under this heading.

Meperidine Hydrochloride (Co-administration may result in increased drowsiness; caution should be exercised).
No products indexed under this heading.

Mephobarbital (Co-administration may result in increased drowsiness; caution should be exercised).
No products indexed under this heading.

Meprobamate (Co-administration may result in increased drowsiness; caution should be exercised).
No products indexed under this heading.

Mesoridazine Besylate (Co-administration may result in increased drowsiness; caution should be exercised).
No products indexed under this heading.

Methadone Hydrochloride (Co-administration may result in increased drowsiness; caution should be exercised).
No products indexed under this heading.

Methohexital Sodium (Co-administration may result in increased drowsiness; caution should be exercised).
No products indexed under this heading.

Methotrimeprazine (Co-administration may result in increased drowsiness; caution should be exercised).
No products indexed under this heading.

Methoxyflurane (Co-administration may result in increased drowsiness; caution should be exercised).
No products indexed under this heading.

Mibefradil Dihydrochloride (Due to interaction between verapamil and dantrolene, combination of dantrolene and calcium channel blockers is not recommended during the management of malignant hyperthermia).
No products indexed under this heading.

Midazolam Hydrochloride (Co-administration may result in increased drowsiness; caution should be exercised).
No products indexed under this heading.

Molindone Hydrochloride (Co-administration may result in increased drowsiness; caution should be exercised). Products include:
Moban Tablets 1116

Morphine Sulfate (Co-administration may result in increased drowsiness; caution should be exercised). Products include:
Avinza Capsules 1772
DepoDur Injection 1095
MS Contin Tablets 2585

Nicardipine Hydrochloride (Due to interaction between verapamil and dantrolene, combination of dantrolene and calcium channel blockers is not recommended during the management of malignant hyperthermia). Products include:
Cardene I.V. 1093

Nifedipine (Due to interaction between verapamil and dantrolene, combination of dantrolene and calcium channel blockers is not recommended during the management of malignant hyperthermia).
No products indexed under this heading.

Nimodipine (Due to interaction between verapamil and dantrolene, combination of dantrolene and calcium channel blockers is not recommended during the management of malignant hyperthermia). Products include:
Nimotop Capsules 790

Nisoldipine (Due to interaction between verapamil and dantrolene, combination of dantrolene and calcium channel blockers is not recommended during the management of malignant hyperthermia). Products include:
Sular Extended Release Tablets 2975

Olanzapine (Co-administration may result in increased drowsiness; caution should be exercised). Products include:
Symbyax Capsules 1871
Zyprexa Tablets 1883
Zyprexa IntraMuscular 1883
Zyprexa ZYDIS Orally Disintegrating Tablets 1883

Oxazepam (Co-administration may result in increased drowsiness; caution should be exercised).
No products indexed under this heading.

Oxycodone Hydrochloride (Co-administration may result in increased drowsiness; caution should be exercised). Products include:
OxyContin Tablets 2589
OxyIR Capsules 2593
Percocet Tablets 1127
Percodan Tablets 1130

Pentobarbital Sodium (Co-administration may result in increased drowsiness; caution should be exercised). Products include:
Nembutal Sodium Solution, USP 2494

Perphenazine (Co-administration may result in increased drowsiness; caution should be exercised).
No products indexed under this heading.

Phenobarbital (Co-administration may result in increased drowsiness; caution should be exercised). Products include:
Donnatal Extentabs 2507

Polyestradiol Phosphate (Hepatotoxicity has occurred more often in women over 35 years of age receiving concomitant estrogen therapy).
No products indexed under this heading.

Prazepam (Co-administration may result in increased drowsiness; caution should be exercised).
No products indexed under this heading.

Prochlorperazine (Co-administration may result in increased drowsiness; caution should be exercised).
No products indexed under this heading.

Promethazine Hydrochloride (Co-administration may result in increased drowsiness; caution should be exercised).
No products indexed under this heading.

Propofol (Co-administration may result in increased drowsiness; caution should be exercised).
No products indexed under this heading.

Propoxyphene Hydrochloride (Co-administration may result in increased drowsiness; caution should be exercised).
No products indexed under this heading.

Propoxyphene Napsylate (Co-administration may result in increased drowsiness; caution should be exercised).
No products indexed under this heading.

Quazepam (Co-administration may result in increased drowsiness; caution should be exercised).
No products indexed under this heading.

Quetiapine Fumarate (Co-administration may result in increased drowsiness; caution should be exercised).
No products indexed under this heading.

Quinestrol (Hepatotoxicity has occurred more often in women over 35 years of age receiving concomitant estrogen therapy).
No products indexed under this heading.

Ramelteon (Co-administration may result in increased drowsiness; caution should be exercised). Products include:

Rozerem Tablets 3091

Remifentanil Hydrochloride (Co-administration may result in increased drowsiness; caution should be exercised).

No products indexed under this heading.

Risperidone (Co-administration may result in increased drowsiness; caution should be exercised). Products include:

Risperdal Consta Long-Acting Injection 1753

Secobarbital Sodium (Co-administration may result in increased drowsiness; caution should be exercised).

No products indexed under this heading.

Sevoflurane (Co-administration may result in increased drowsiness; caution should be exercised). Products include:

Ultane Liquid for Inhalation 524

Sodium Butabarbital (Co-administration may result in increased drowsiness; caution should be exercised).

No products indexed under this heading.

Sufentanil Citrate (Co-administration may result in increased drowsiness; caution should be exercised).

No products indexed under this heading.

Temazepam (Co-administration may result in increased drowsiness; caution should be exercised).

No products indexed under this heading.

Thiamylal Sodium (Co-administration may result in increased drowsiness; caution should be exercised).

No products indexed under this heading.

Thioridazine Hydrochloride (Co-administration may result in increased drowsiness; caution should be exercised). Products include:

Thioridazine Hydrochloride Tablets 2195

Thiothixene (Co-administration may result in increased drowsiness; caution should be exercised). Products include:

Thiothixene Capsules 2197

Triazolam (Co-administration may result in increased drowsiness; caution should be exercised).

No products indexed under this heading.

Trifluoperazine Hydrochloride (Co-administration may result in increased drowsiness; caution should be exercised).

No products indexed under this heading.

Vecuronium Bromide (Co-administration may result in potentiation of vecuronium-induced neuromuscular block).

No products indexed under this heading.

Verapamil Hydrochloride (Simultaneous use has resulted in rare cases of cardiovascular collapse). Products include:

Tarka Tablets 511

Zaleplon (Co-administration may result in increased drowsiness; caution should be exercised).

No products indexed under this heading.

Ziprasidone Hydrochloride (Co-administration may result in increased drowsiness; caution should be exercised). Products include:

Geodon Capsules 2520

Zolpidem Tartrate (Co-administration may result in increased drowsiness; caution should be exercised). Products include:

Ambien Tablets 2692
Ambien CR Tablets 2696

Food Interactions

Alcohol (Co-administration may result in increased drowsiness; caution should be exercised).

DANTRIUM INTRAVENOUS

(Dantrolene Sodium) 2582

May interact with:

Clofibrate (Reduces binding of dantrolene to plasma proteins).

No products indexed under this heading.

Tolbutamide (Increases binding of dantrolene to plasma proteins).

No products indexed under this heading.

Vecuronium Bromide (Administration of dantrolene may potentiate vecuronium-induced neuromuscular block).

No products indexed under this heading.

Verapamil Hydrochloride (The combination of therapeutic doses of intravenous dantrolene sodium and verapamil in halothane/alpha-chloralose anesthetized swine has resulted in ventricular fibrillation and cardiovascular collapse in association with hyperkalemia; it is recommended that this combination should not be used during the management of malignant hyperthermia crisis until the human data is available). Products include:

Tarka Tablets 511

Warfarin Sodium (Reduces binding of dantrolene to plasma proteins).

No products indexed under this heading.

DAPSONE TABLETS USP

(Dapsone) 1746

May interact with:

Pyrimethamine (Agranulocytosis; increased likelihood of hematological reactions). Products include:

Daraprim Tablets 1400
Fansidar Tablets 2636

Rifampin (Rifampin lowers dapsone 7- to 10-fold by accelerating plasma clearance).

No products indexed under this heading.

Trimethoprim (Mutual interaction between Dapsone and trimethoprim in which each raises the level of the other about 1.5 times).

No products indexed under this heading.

DARAPRIM TABLETS

(Pyrimethamine) 1400

May interact with cytotoxic drugs, dihydrofolate reductase inhibitors, agents associated with myelosuppression, phenytoin, sulfonamides, and certain other agents. Compounds in these categories include:

Altretamine (The concomitant use of other antifolic drugs or agents associated with myelosuppression including cytostatic agents while the patient is receiving pyrimethamine, may increase the risk of bone marrow suppression). Products include:

Hexalen Capsules 1078

Bendroflumethiazide (Co-administration of other antifolic drugs, such as sulfonamides, may increase the risk of bone marrow suppression; potential for hypersensitivity reactions such as Stevens-Johnson syndrome, toxic epidermal necrolysis, erythema multiforme, and anaphylaxis).

No products indexed under this heading.

Bleomycin Sulfate (The concomitant use of other antifolic drugs or agents associated with myelosuppression including cytostatic agents while the patient is receiving pyrimethamine, may increase the risk of bone marrow suppression).

No products indexed under this heading.

Busulfan (The concomitant use of other antifolic drugs or agents associated with myelosuppression including cytostatic agents while the patient is receiving pyrimethamine, may increase the risk of bone marrow suppression). Products include:

Busulfex Injection 2477
Myleran Tablets 1530

Chlorambucil (The concomitant use of other antifolic drugs or agents associated with myelosuppression including cytostatic agents while the patient is receiving pyrimethamine, may increase the risk of bone marrow suppression). Products include:

Leukeran Tablets 1508

Chlorothiazide (Co-administration of other antifolic drugs, such as sulfonamides, may increase the risk of bone marrow suppression; potential for hypersensitivity reactions such as Stevens-Johnson syndrome, toxic epidermal necrolysis, erythema multiforme, and anaphylaxis).

No products indexed under this heading.

Chlorothiazide Sodium (Co-administration of other antifolic drugs, such as sulfonamides, may increase the risk of bone marrow suppression; potential for hypersensitivity reactions such as Stevens-Johnson syndrome, toxic epidermal necrolysis, erythema multiforme, and anaphylaxis). Products include:

Intravenous Sodium Diuril 2490

Chlorpropamide (Co-administration of other antifolic drugs, such as sulfonamides, may increase the risk of bone marrow suppression; potential for hypersensitivity reactions such as Stevens-Johnson syndrome, toxic epidermal necrolysis, erythema multiforme, and anaphylaxis).

No products indexed under this heading.

Cladribine (The concomitant use of other antifolic drugs or agents associated with myelosuppression including cytostatic agents while the patient is receiving pyrimethamine, may increase the risk of bone marrow suppression). Products include:

Leustatin Injection 2384

Cyclophosphamide (The concomitant use of other antifolic drugs or agents associated with myelosuppression including cytostatic agents while the patient is receiving pyrimethamine, may increase the risk of bone marrow suppression).

No products indexed under this heading.

Daunorubicin Citrate Liposome (The concomitant use of other antifolic drugs or agents associated with myelosuppression including cytostatic agents while the patient is receiving pyrimethamine, may increase the risk of bone marrow suppression).

No products indexed under this heading.

Daunorubicin Hydrochloride (The concomitant use of other antifolic drugs or agents associated with myelosuppression including cytostatic agents while the patient is receiving pyrimethamine, may increase the risk of bone marrow suppression).

No products indexed under this heading.

Dexrazoxane (The concomitant use of other antifolic drugs or agents associated with myelosuppression including cytostatic agents while the patient is receiving pyrimethamine, may increase the risk of bone marrow suppression).

No products indexed under this heading.

Doxorubicin Hydrochloride (The concomitant use of other antifolic drugs or agents associated with myelosuppression including cytostatic agents while the patient is receiving pyrimethamine, may increase the risk of bone marrow suppression).

No products indexed under this heading.

Doxorubicin Hydrochloride Liposome (The concomitant use of other antifolic drugs or agents associated with myelosuppression including cytostatic agents while the patient is receiving pyrimethamine, may increase the risk of bone marrow suppression). Products include:

Doxil Injection 2378

Epirubicin Hydrochloride (The concomitant use of other antifolic drugs or agents associated with myelosuppression including cytostatic agents while the patient is receiving pyrimethamine, may increase the risk of bone marrow suppression).

No products indexed under this heading.

Fludarabine Phosphate (The concomitant use of other antifolic drugs or agents associated with myelosuppression including cytostatic agents while the patient is receiving pyrimethamine, may increase the risk of bone marrow suppression).

No products indexed under this heading.

Fluorouracil (The concomitant use of other antifolic drugs or agents associated with myelosuppression including cytostatic agents while the patient is receiving pyrimethamine, may increase the risk of bone marrow suppression). Products include:

Carac Cream 0.5% 2722

Fosphenytoin Sodium (Co-administration with agents that affect folate levels, such as phenytoin, should be undertaken with caution).
No products indexed under this heading.

Gemcitabine Hydrochloride (The concomitant use of other antifolic drugs or agents associated with myelosuppression including cytostatic agents while the patient is receiving pyrimethamine, may increase the risk of bone marrow suppression). Products include:
Gemzar for Injection 1820

Gemtuzumab Ozogamicin (The concomitant use of other antifolic drugs or agents associated with myelosuppression including cytostatic agents while the patient is receiving pyrimethamine, may increase the risk of bone marrow suppression). Products include:
Mylotarg for Injection 3212

Glipizide (Co-administration of other antifolic drugs, such as sulfonamides, may increase the risk of bone marrow suppression; potential for hypersensitivity reactions such as Stevens-Johnson syndrome, toxic epidermal necrolysis, erythema multiforme, and anaphylaxis).
No products indexed under this heading.

Glyburide (Co-administration of other antifolic drugs, such as sulfonamides, may increase the risk of bone marrow suppression; potential for hypersensitivity reactions such as Stevens-Johnson syndrome, toxic epidermal necrolysis, erythema multiforme, and anaphylaxis).
No products indexed under this heading.

Hydrochlorothiazide (Co-administration of other antifolic drugs, such as sulfonamides, may increase the risk of bone marrow suppression; potential for hypersensitivity reactions such as Stevens-Johnson syndrome, toxic epidermal necrolysis, erythema multiforme, and anaphylaxis). Products include:
Atacand HCT 642
Avalide Tablets 892
Avalide Tablets 2713
Benicar HCT Tablets 1010
Diovan HCT Tablets 2216
Dyazide Capsules 1405
Micardis HCT Tablets 854
Prinzide Tablets 2092
Tekturna HCT Tablets 2324
Teveten HCT Tablets 517

Hydroflumethiazide (Co-administration of other antifolic drugs, such as sulfonamides, may increase the risk of bone marrow suppression; potential for hypersensitivity reactions such as Stevens-Johnson syndrome, toxic epidermal necrolysis, erythema multiforme, and anaphylaxis).
No products indexed under this heading.

Hydroxyurea (The concomitant use of other antifolic drugs or agents associated with myelosuppression including cytostatic agents while the patient is receiving pyrimethamine, may increase the risk of bone marrow suppression).
No products indexed under this heading.

Idarubicin Hydrochloride (The concomitant use of other antifolic drugs or agents associated with myelosuppression including cytostatic agents while the patient is receiving pyrimethamine, may increase the risk of bone marrow suppression).
No products indexed under this heading.

Interferon alfa-2a, Recombinant (The concomitant use of other antifolic drugs or agents associated with myelosuppression including cytostatic agents while the patient is receiving pyrimethamine, may increase the risk of bone marrow suppression).
No products indexed under this heading.

Irinotecan Hydrochloride (The concomitant use of other antifolic drugs or agents associated with myelosuppression including cytostatic agents while the patient is receiving pyrimethamine, may increase the risk of bone marrow suppression).
No products indexed under this heading.

Lamotrigine (The concomitant use of other antifolic drugs, while the patient is receiving pyrimethamine, may increase the risk of bone marrow suppression). Products include:
Lamictal 1488

Lorazepam (Concomitant therapy may result in mild hepatotoxicity).
No products indexed under this heading.

Melphalan Hydrochloride (The concomitant use of other antifolic drugs or agents associated with myelosuppression including cytostatic agents while the patient is receiving pyrimethamine, may increase the risk of bone marrow suppression).
No products indexed under this heading.

Mercaptopurine (The concomitant use of other antifolic drugs or agents associated with myelosuppression including cytostatic agents while the patient is receiving pyrimethamine, may increase the risk of bone marrow suppression).
No products indexed under this heading.

Methotrexate Sodium (The concomitant use of other antifolic drugs or agents associated with myelosuppression including cytostatic agents while the patient is receiving pyrimethamine, may increase the risk of bone marrow suppression).
No products indexed under this heading.

Methyclothiazide (Co-administration of other antifolic drugs, such as sulfonamides, may increase the risk of bone marrow suppression; potential for hypersensitivity reactions such as Stevens-Johnson syndrome, toxic epidermal necrolysis, erythema multiforme, and anaphylaxis).
No products indexed under this heading.

Mitotane (The concomitant use of other antifolic drugs or agents associated with myelosuppression including cytostatic agents while the patient is receiving pyrimethamine, may increase the risk of bone marrow suppression).
No products indexed under this heading.

Mitoxantrone Hydrochloride (The concomitant use of other antifolic drugs or agents associated with myelosuppression including cytostatic agents while the patient is receiving pyrimethamine, may increase the risk of bone marrow suppression). Products include:
Novantrone for Injection Concentrate 1100

Phenytoin (Co-administration with agents that affect folate levels, such as phenytoin, should be undertaken with caution).
No products indexed under this heading.

Phenytoin Sodium (Co-administration with agents that affect folate levels, such as phenytoin, should be undertaken with caution). Products include:
Phenytek Capsules 2192

Polythiazide (Co-administration of other antifolic drugs, such as sulfonamides, may increase the risk of bone marrow suppression; potential for hypersensitivity reactions such as Stevens-Johnson syndrome, toxic epidermal necrolysis, erythema multiforme, and anaphylaxis).
No products indexed under this heading.

Procarbazine Hydrochloride (The concomitant use of other antifolic drugs or agents associated with myelosuppression including cytostatic agents while the patient is receiving pyrimethamine, may increase the risk of bone marrow suppression).
No products indexed under this heading.

Proguanil (May increase risk of bone marrow suppression).
No products indexed under this heading.

Sulfacytine (Co-administration of other antifolic drugs, such as sulfonamides, may increase the risk of bone marrow suppression; potential for hypersensitivity reactions such as Stevens-Johnson syndrome, toxic epidermal necrolysis, erythema multiforme, and anaphylaxis).
No products indexed under this heading.

Sulfamethizole (Co-administration of other antifolic drugs, such as sulfonamides, may increase the risk of bone marrow suppression; potential for hypersensitivity reactions such as Stevens-Johnson syndrome, toxic epidermal necrolysis, erythema multiforme, and anaphylaxis).
No products indexed under this heading.

Sulfamethoxazole (Co-administration of other antifolic drugs, such as sulfonamides, may increase the risk of bone marrow suppression; potential for hypersensitivity reactions such as Stevens-Johnson syndrome, toxic epidermal necrolysis, erythema multiforme, and anaphylaxis).
No products indexed under this heading.

Sulfasalazine (Co-administration of other antifolic drugs, such as sulfonamides, may increase the risk of bone marrow suppression; potential for hypersensitivity reactions such as Stevens-Johnson syndrome, toxic epidermal necrolysis, erythema multiforme, and anaphylaxis).
No products indexed under this heading.

Sulfinpyrazone (Co-administration of other antifolic drugs, such as sulfonamides, may increase the risk of bone marrow suppression; potential for hypersensitivity reactions such as Stevens-Johnson syndrome, toxic epidermal necrolysis, erythema multiforme, and anaphylaxis).
No products indexed under this heading.

Sulfisoxazole Acetyl (Co-administration of other antifolic drugs, such as sulfonamides, may increase the risk of bone marrow suppression; potential for hypersensitivity reactions such as Stevens-Johnson syndrome, toxic epidermal necrolysis, erythema multiforme, and anaphylaxis).
No products indexed under this heading.

Sulfisoxazole Diolamine (Co-administration of other antifolic drugs, such as sulfonamides, may increase the risk of bone marrow suppression; potential for hypersensitivity reactions such as Stevens-Johnson syndrome, toxic epidermal necrolysis, erythema multiforme, and anaphylaxis).
No products indexed under this heading.

Tamoxifen Citrate (The concomitant use of other antifolic drugs or agents associated with myelosuppression including cytostatic agents while the patient is receiving pyrimethamine, may increase the risk of bone marrow suppression).
No products indexed under this heading.

Temozolomide (The concomitant use of other antifolic drugs or agents associated with myelosuppression including cytostatic agents while the patient is receiving pyrimethamine, may increase the risk of bone marrow suppression). Products include:
Temodar Capsules 2931

Thioguanine (The concomitant use of other antifolic drugs or agents associated with myelosuppression including cytostatic agents while the patient is receiving pyrimethamine, may increase the risk of bone marrow suppression). Products include:
Tabloid Tablets 1601

Tolazamide (Co-administration of other antifolic drugs, such as sulfonamides, may increase the risk of bone marrow suppression; potential for hypersensitivity reactions such as Stevens-Johnson syndrome, toxic epidermal necrolysis, erythema multiforme, and anaphylaxis).
No products indexed under this heading.

Tolbutamide (Co-administration of other antifolic drugs, such as sulfonamides, may increase the risk of bone marrow suppression; potential for hypersensitivity reactions such as Stevens-Johnson syndrome, toxic epidermal necrolysis, erythema multiforme, and anaphylaxis).
No products indexed under this heading.

Trimethoprim (Co-administration of other antifolic drugs, such as sulfonamides or trimethoprim-sulfamethoxazole combinations, may increase the risk of bone marrow suppression; potential for hypersensitivity reactions such as Stevens-Johnson syndrome, toxic epidermal necrolysis, erythema multiforme, and anaphylaxis).
No products indexed under this heading.

Trimetrexate Glucuronate (The concomitant use of other antifolic drugs, while the patient is receiving pyrimethamine, may increase the risk of bone marrow suppression).
No products indexed under this heading.

Vincristine Sulfate (The concomitant use of other antifolic drugs or agents associated with myelosuppression including cytostatic agents while the patient is receiving pyrimethamine, may increase the risk of bone marrow suppression).
No products indexed under this heading.

Vinorelbine Tartrate (The concomitant use of other antifolic drugs or agents associated with myelosuppression including cytostatic agents while the patient is receiving pyrimethamine, may increase the risk of bone marrow suppression).
No products indexed under this heading.

Zidovudine (May increase risk of bone marrow suppression). Products include:
Combivir Tablets 1384
Retrovir 1574
Retrovir IV Infusion 1579
Trizivir Tablets 1622

DAYTRANA TRANSDERMAL PATCH
(Methylphenidate) 3022
May interact with antihypertensives, oral anticoagulants, anticonvulsants, monoamine oxidase inhibitors, selective serotonin reuptake inhibitors, tricyclic antidepressants, vasopressors, and certain other agents. Compounds in these categories include:

Acebutolol Hydrochloride (Methylphenidate may decrease the effectiveness of drugs used to treat hypertension).
No products indexed under this heading.

Aliskiren (Methylphenidate may decrease the effectiveness of drugs used to treat hypertension).
Products include:
Tekturna Tablets 2321
Tekturna HCT Tablets 2324

Amitriptyline Hydrochloride (Human pharmacologic studies have shown that methylphenidate may inhibit the metabolism of some tricyclic drugs (eg, imipramine, clomipramine, desipramine). Downward dose adjustments of these drugs may be required when given concomitantly with methylphenidate. It may be necessary to adjust the dosage and monitor plasma drug concentrations when initiating or discontinuing methylphenidate).
No products indexed under this heading.

Amlodipine Besylate (Methylphenidate may decrease the effectiveness of drugs used to treat hypertension).
Products include:
Azor Tablets 1005
Exforge Tablets 2238

Amoxapine (Human pharmacologic studies have shown that methylphenidate may inhibit the metabolism of some tricyclic drugs (eg, imipramine, clomipramine, desipramine). Downward dose adjustments of these drugs may be required when given concomitantly with methylphenidate. It may be necessary to adjust the dosage and monitor plasma drug concentrations when initiating or discontinuing methylphenidate).
No products indexed under this heading.

Anisindione (Human pharmacologic studies have shown that methylphenidate may inhibit the metabolism of coumarin anticoagulants. Downward dose adjustments of these drugs may be required when given concomitantly with methylphenidate. It may be necessary to adjust the dosage and monitor plasma drug concentrations or coagulation times when initiating or discontinuing methylphenidate).
No products indexed under this heading.

Atenolol (Methylphenidate may decrease the effectiveness of drugs used to treat hypertension).
No products indexed under this heading.

Benazepril Hydrochloride (Methylphenidate may decrease the effectiveness of drugs used to treat hypertension).
No products indexed under this heading.

Bendroflumethiazide (Methylphenidate may decrease the effectiveness of drugs used to treat hypertension).
No products indexed under this heading.

Betaxolol Hydrochloride (Methylphenidate may decrease the effectiveness of drugs used to treat hypertension).
No products indexed under this heading.

Bisoprolol Fumarate (Methylphenidate may decrease the effectiveness of drugs used to treat hypertension).
No products indexed under this heading.

Candesartan Cilexetil (Methylphenidate may decrease the effectiveness of drugs used to treat hypertension). Products include:
Atacand Tablets 639
Atacand HCT 642

Captopril (Methylphenidate may decrease the effectiveness of drugs used to treat hypertension).
Products include:
Captopril Tablets 2182

Carbamazepine (Human pharmacologic studies have shown that methylphenidate may inhibit the metabolism of anticonvulsants (eg, phenobarbital, phenytoin, primidone). Downward dose adjustments of these drugs may be required when given concomitantly with methylphenidate. It may be necessary to adjust the dosage and monitor plasma drug concentrations when initiating or discontinuing methylphenidate). Products include:
Carbatrol Capsules 3019
Equetro Extended-Release Capsules 3174

Carteolol Hydrochloride (Methylphenidate may decrease the effectiveness of drugs used to treat hypertension).
No products indexed under this heading.

Chlorothiazide (Methylphenidate may decrease the effectiveness of drugs used to treat hypertension).
No products indexed under this heading.

Chlorothiazide Sodium (Methylphenidate may decrease the effectiveness of drugs used to treat hypertension). Products include:
Intravenous Sodium Diuril 2490

Chlorthalidone (Methylphenidate may decrease the effectiveness of drugs used to treat hypertension).
Products include:
Clorpres Tablets 2185

Citalopram Hydrobromide (Human pharmacologic studies have shown that methylphenidate may inhibit the metabolism of selective serotonin reuptake inhibitors. Downward dose adjustments of these drugs may be required when given concomitantly with methylphenidate. It may be necessary to adjust the dosage and monitor plasma drug concentrations when initiating or discontinuing methylphenidate).
Products include:
Celexa 1160

Clomipramine Hydrochloride (Human pharmacologic studies have shown that methylphenidate may inhibit the metabolism of some tricyclic drugs (eg, imipramine, clomipramine, desipramine). Downward dose adjustments of these drugs may be required when given concomitantly with methylphenidate. It may be necessary to adjust the dosage and monitor plasma drug concentrations when initiating or discontinuing methylphenidate).
No products indexed under this heading.

Clonidine (Serious adverse events have been reported in concomitant use of methylphenidate with clonidine, although no causality for the combination has been established).
Products include:
Catapres-TTS 842

Clonidine Hydrochloride (Serious adverse events have been reported in concomitant use of methylphenidate with clonidine, although no causality for the combination has been established). Products include:
Catapres Tablets 841
Clorpres Tablets 2185

Deserpidine (Methylphenidate may decrease the effectiveness of drugs used to treat hypertension).
No products indexed under this heading.

Desipramine Hydrochloride (Human pharmacologic studies have shown that methylphenidate may inhibit the metabolism of some tricyclic drugs (eg, imipramine, clomipramine, desipramine). Downward dose adjustments of these drugs may be required when given concomitantly with methylphenidate. It may be necessary to adjust the dosage and monitor plasma drug concentrations when initiating or discontinuing methylphenidate).
No products indexed under this heading.

Diazoxide (Methylphenidate may decrease the effectiveness of drugs used to treat hypertension).
Products include:
Proglycem Capsules 1185
Proglycem Suspension 1185

Dicumarol (Human pharmacologic studies have shown that methylphenidate may inhibit the metabolism of coumarin anticoagulants. Downward dose adjustments of these drugs may be required when given concomitantly with methylphenidate. It may be necessary to adjust the dosage and monitor plasma drug concentrations or coagulation times when initiating or discontinuing methylphenidate).
No products indexed under this heading.

Diltiazem Hydrochloride (Methylphenidate may decrease the effectiveness of drugs used to treat hypertension). Products include:
Cardizem LA Extended Release Tablets 421

Divalproex Sodium (Human pharmacologic studies have shown that methylphenidate may inhibit the metabolism of anticonvulsants (eg, phenobarbital, phenytoin, primidone). Downward dose adjustments of these drugs may be required when given concomitantly with methylphenidate. It may be necessary to adjust the dosage and monitor plasma drug concentrations when initiating or discontinuing methylphenidate). Products include:
Depakote ER Tablets 423

Dobutamine (Because of a possible effect on blood pressure, methylphenidate transdermal system should be used cautiously with pressor agents).
No products indexed under this heading.

Dobutamine Hydrochloride (Because of a possible effect on blood pressure, methylphenidate transdermal system should be used cautiously with pressor agents).
No products indexed under this heading.

Dopamine Hydrochloride (Because of a possible effect on blood pressure, methylphenidate transdermal system should be used cautiously with pressor agents).
No products indexed under this heading.

Doxazosin Mesylate (Methylphenidate may decrease the effectiveness of drugs used to treat hypertension).
No products indexed under this heading.

Doxepin Hydrochloride (Human pharmacologic studies have shown that methylphenidate may inhibit the metabolism of some tricyclic drugs (eg, imipramine, clomipramine, desipramine). Downward dose adjustments of these drugs may be required when given concomitantly with methylphenidate. It may be necessary to adjust the dosage and monitor plasma drug concentrations when initiating or discontinuing methylphenidate).
No products indexed under this heading.

Enalapril Maleate (Methylphenidate may decrease the effectiveness of drugs used to treat hypertension).
No products indexed under this heading.

Enalaprilat (Methylphenidate may decrease the effectiveness of drugs used to treat hypertension).
No products indexed under this heading.

Ephedrine Sulfate (Because of a possible effect on blood pressure, methylphenidate transdermal system should be used cautiously with pressor agents).
No products indexed under this heading.

Epinephrine Bitartrate (Because of a possible effect on blood pressure, methylphenidate transdermal system should be used cautiously with pressor agents).
No products indexed under this heading.

Epinephrine Hydrochloride (Because of a possible effect on blood pressure, methylphenidate transdermal system should be used cautiously with pressor agents).
No products indexed under this heading.

Eprosartan Mesylate (Methylphenidate may decrease the effectiveness of drugs used to treat hypertension). Products include:
Teveten Tablets 515
Teveten HCT Tablets 517

Escitalopram Oxalate (Human pharmacologic studies have shown that methylphenidate may inhibit the metabolism of selective serotonin reuptake inhibitors. Downward dose adjustments of these drugs may be required when given concomitantly with methylphenidate. It may be necessary to adjust the dosage and monitor plasma drug concentrations when initiating or discontinuing methylphenidate). Products include:
Lexapro Oral Suspension 1174
Lexapro Tablets 1174

Esmolol Hydrochloride (Methylphenidate may decrease the effectiveness of drugs used to treat hypertension).
No products indexed under this heading.

Ethosuximide (Human pharmacologic studies have shown that methylphenidate may inhibit the metabolism of anticonvulsants (eg, phenobarbital, phenytoin, primidone). Downward dose adjustments of these drugs may be required when given concomitantly with methylphenidate. It may be necessary to adjust the dosage and monitor plasma drug concentrations when initiating or discontinuing methylphenidate).
No products indexed under this heading.

Ethotoin (Human pharmacologic studies have shown that methylphenidate may inhibit the metabolism of anticonvulsants (eg, phenobarbital, phenytoin, primidone). Downward dose adjustments of these drugs may be required when given concomitantly with methylphenidate. It may be necessary to adjust the dosage and monitor plasma drug concentrations when initiating or discontinuing methylphenidate).
No products indexed under this heading.

Felbamate (Human pharmacologic studies have shown that methylphenidate may inhibit the metabolism of anticonvulsants (eg, phenobarbital, phenytoin, primidone). Downward dose adjustments of these drugs may be required when given concomitantly with methylphenidate. It may be necessary to adjust the dosage and monitor plasma drug concentrations when initiating or discontinuing methylphenidate).
No products indexed under this heading.

Felodipine (Methylphenidate may decrease the effectiveness of drugs used to treat hypertension).
No products indexed under this heading.

Fluoxetine (Human pharmacologic studies have shown that methylphenidate may inhibit the metabolism of selective serotonin reuptake inhibitors. Downward dose adjustments of these drugs may be required when given concomitantly with methylphenidate. It may be necessary to adjust the dosage and monitor plasma drug concentrations when initiating or discontinuing methylphenidate).
No products indexed under this heading.

Fluoxetine Hydrochloride (Human pharmacologic studies have shown that methylphenidate may inhibit the metabolism of selective serotonin reuptake inhibitors. Downward dose adjustments of these drugs may be required when given concomitantly with methylphenidate. It may be necessary to adjust the dosage and monitor plasma drug concentrations when initiating or discontinuing methylphenidate). Products include:
Prozac Weekly Capsules 1852
Prozac Pulvules and Liquid 1852
Symbyax Capsules 1871

Fluvoxamine Maleate (Human pharmacologic studies have shown that methylphenidate may inhibit the metabolism of selective serotonin reuptake inhibitors. Downward dose adjustments of these drugs may be required when given concomitantly with methylphenidate. It may be necessary to adjust the dosage and monitor plasma drug concentrations when initiating or discontinuing methylphenidate). Products include:
Luvox CR Extended-Release Capsules 1759

Fosinopril Sodium (Methylphenidate may decrease the effectiveness of drugs used to treat hypertension).
No products indexed under this heading.

Fosphenytoin (Human pharmacologic studies have shown that methylphenidate may inhibit the metabolism of anticonvulsants (eg, phenobarbital, phenytoin, primidone). Downward dose adjustments of these drugs may be required when given concomitantly with methylphenidate. It may be necessary to adjust the dosage and monitor plasma drug concentrations when initiating or discontinuing methylphenidate).
No products indexed under this heading.

Fosphenytoin Sodium (Human pharmacologic studies have shown that methylphenidate may inhibit the metabolism of anticonvulsants (eg, phenobarbital, phenytoin, primidone). Downward dose adjustments of these drugs may be required when given concomitantly with methylphenidate. It may be necessary to adjust the dosage and monitor plasma drug concentrations when initiating or discontinuing methylphenidate).
No products indexed under this heading.

Furosemide (Methylphenidate may decrease the effectiveness of drugs used to treat hypertension). Products include:
Furosemide Tablets 2186

Gabapentin (Human pharmacologic studies have shown that methylphenidate may inhibit the metabolism of anticonvulsants (eg, phenobarbital, phenytoin, primidone). Downward dose adjustments of these drugs may be required when given concomitantly with methylphenidate. It may be necessary to adjust the dosage and monitor plasma drug concentrations when initiating or discontinuing methylphenidate).
No products indexed under this heading.

Guanabenz Acetate (Methylphenidate may decrease the effectiveness of drugs used to treat hypertension).
No products indexed under this heading.

Guanethidine Monosulfate (Methylphenidate may decrease the effectiveness of drugs used to treat hypertension).
No products indexed under this heading.

Hydralazine Hydrochloride (Methylphenidate may decrease the effectiveness of drugs used to treat hypertension).
No products indexed under this heading.

Hydrochlorothiazide (Methylphenidate may decrease the effectiveness of drugs used to treat hypertension). Products include:
Atacand HCT 642
Avalide Tablets 892
Avalide Tablets 2713
Benicar HCT Tablets 1010
Diovan HCT Tablets 2216
Dyazide Capsules 1405
Micardis HCT Tablets 854
Prinzide Tablets 2092
Tekturna HCT Tablets 2324
Teveten HCT Tablets 517

Hydroflumethiazide (Methylphenidate may decrease the effectiveness of drugs used to treat hypertension).
No products indexed under this heading.

Imipramine Hydrochloride (Human pharmacologic studies have shown that methylphenidate may inhibit the metabolism of some tricyclic drugs (eg, imipramine, clomipramine, desipramine). Downward dose adjustments of these drugs may be required when given concomitantly with methylphenidate. It may be necessary to adjust the dosage and monitor plasma drug concentrations when initiating or discontinuing methylphenidate).
No products indexed under this heading.

Imipramine Pamoate (Human pharmacologic studies have shown that methylphenidate may inhibit the metabolism of some tricyclic drugs (eg, imipramine, clomipramine, desipramine). Downward dose adjustments of these drugs may be required when given concomitantly with methylphenidate. It may be necessary to adjust the dosage and monitor plasma drug concentrations when initiating or discontinuing methylphenidate).
No products indexed under this heading.

Indapamide (Methylphenidate may decrease the effectiveness of drugs used to treat hypertension). Products include:
Indapamide Tablets 2188

Irbesartan (Methylphenidate may decrease the effectiveness of drugs used to treat hypertension). Products include:
Avalide Tablets 892
Avalide Tablets 2713
Avapro Tablets 897
Avapro Tablets 2718

Isocarboxazid (Methylphenidate transdermal system is contraindicated during treatment with monoamine oxidase inhibitors and also within a minimum of 14 days following discontinuation of treatment with a MAO inhibitor (hypertensive crises may occur)). Products include:
Marplan Tablets 3177

Isoproterenol Hydrochloride (Because of a possible effect on blood pressure, methylphenidate transdermal system should be used cautiously with pressor agents).
No products indexed under this heading.

Isoproterenol Sulfate (Because of a possible effect on blood pressure, methylphenidate transdermal system should be used cautiously with pressor agents).
No products indexed under this heading.

Isradipine (Methylphenidate may decrease the effectiveness of drugs used to treat hypertension). Products include:
DynaCirc CR Controlled Release Tablets 1407

Labetalol Hydrochloride (Methylphenidate may decrease the effectiveness of drugs used to treat hypertension).
No products indexed under this heading.

Lamotrigine (Human pharmacologic studies have shown that methylphenidate may inhibit the metabolism of anticonvulsants (eg, phenobarbital, phenytoin, primidone). Downward dose adjustments of these drugs may be required when given concomitantly with methylphenidate. It may be necessary to adjust the dosage and monitor plasma drug concentrations when initiating or discontinuing methylphenidate). Products include:
Lamictal 1488

Levetiracetam (Human pharmacologic studies have shown that methylphenidate may inhibit the metabolism of anticonvulsants (eg, phenobarbital, phenytoin, primidone). Downward dose adjustments of these drugs may be required when given concomitantly with methylphenidate. It may be necessary to adjust the dosage and monitor plasma drug concentrations when initiating or discontinuing methylphenidate). Products include:
Keppra Injection 3137
Keppra Oral Solution 3131
Keppra Tablets 3131

Lisinopril (Methylphenidate may decrease the effectiveness of drugs used to treat hypertension). Products include:
Prinivil Tablets 2087
Prinzide Tablets 2092

Losartan Potassium (Methylphenidate may decrease the effectiveness of drugs used to treat hypertension). Products include:
Cozaar Tablets 1973

Maprotiline Hydrochloride (Human pharmacologic studies have shown that methylphenidate may inhibit the metabolism of some tricyclic drugs (eg, imipramine, clomipramine, desipramine). Downward dose adjustments of these drugs may be required when given concomitantly with methylphenidate. It may be necessary to adjust the dosage and monitor plasma drug concentrations when initiating or discontinuing methylphenidate).
No products indexed under this heading.

Mecamylamine Hydrochloride (Methylphenidate may decrease the effectiveness of drugs used to treat hypertension).
No products indexed under this heading.

Mephentermine Sulfate (Because of a possible effect on blood pressure, methylphenidate transdermal system should be used cautiously with pressor agents).
No products indexed under this heading.

Mephenytoin (Human pharmacologic studies have shown that methylphenidate may inhibit the metabolism of anticonvulsants (eg, phenobarbital, phenytoin, primidone). Downward dose adjustments of these drugs may be required when given concomitantly with methylphenidate. It may be necessary to adjust the dosage and monitor plasma drug concentrations when initiating or discontinuing methylphenidate).
No products indexed under this heading.

Metaraminol Bitartrate (Because of a possible effect on blood pressure, methylphenidate transdermal system should be used cautiously with pressor agents).
No products indexed under this heading.

Methoxamine Hydrochloride (Because of a possible effect on blood pressure, methylphenidate transdermal system should be used cautiously with pressor agents).
No products indexed under this heading.

Methsuximide (Human pharmacologic studies have shown that methylphenidate may inhibit the metabolism of anticonvulsants (eg, phenobarbital, phenytoin, primidone). Downward dose adjustments of these drugs may be required when given concomitantly with methylphenidate. It may be necessary to adjust the dosage and monitor plasma drug concentrations when initiating or discontinuing methylphenidate).
No products indexed under this heading.

Methyclothiazide (Methylphenidate may decrease the effectiveness of drugs used to treat hypertension).
No products indexed under this heading.

Methyldopa (Methylphenidate may decrease the effectiveness of drugs used to treat hypertension).
No products indexed under this heading.

Methyldopate Hydrochloride (Methylphenidate may decrease the effectiveness of drugs used to treat hypertension).
No products indexed under this heading.

Metolazone (Methylphenidate may decrease the effectiveness of drugs used to treat hypertension).
No products indexed under this heading.

Metoprolol Succinate (Methylphenidate may decrease the effectiveness of drugs used to treat hypertension). Products include:
Toprol-XL Tablets 666

Metoprolol Tartrate (Methylphenidate may decrease the effectiveness of drugs used to treat hypertension).
No products indexed under this heading.

Metyrosine (Methylphenidate may decrease the effectiveness of drugs used to treat hypertension).
Products include:
Demser Capsules 1989

Mibefradil Dihydrochloride (Methylphenidate may decrease the effectiveness of drugs used to treat hypertension).
No products indexed under this heading.

Minoxidil (Methylphenidate may decrease the effectiveness of drugs used to treat hypertension).
No products indexed under this heading.

Moclobemide (Methylphenidate transdermal system is contraindicated during treatment with monoamine oxidase inhibitors and also within a minimum of 14 days following discontinuation of treatment with a MAO inhibitor (hypertensive crises may occur)).
No products indexed under this heading.

Moexipril Hydrochloride (Methylphenidate may decrease the effectiveness of drugs used to treat hypertension).
No products indexed under this heading.

Nadolol (Methylphenidate may decrease the effectiveness of drugs used to treat hypertension).
Products include:
Nadolol Tablets 2191

Nebivolol (Methylphenidate may decrease the effectiveness of drugs used to treat hypertension).
Products include:
Bystolic Tablets 1155

Nicardipine Hydrochloride (Methylphenidate may decrease the effectiveness of drugs used to treat hypertension). Products include:
Cardene I.V. 1093

Nifedipine (Methylphenidate may decrease the effectiveness of drugs used to treat hypertension).
No products indexed under this heading.

Nisoldipine (Methylphenidate may decrease the effectiveness of drugs used to treat hypertension).
Products include:
Sular Extended Release Tablets 2975

Nitroglycerin (Methylphenidate may decrease the effectiveness of drugs used to treat hypertension).
Products include:
Nitro-Dur Transdermal Infusion System 2887
Nitrolingual Pumpspray 2965

Norepinephrine Bitartrate (Because of a possible effect on blood pressure, methylphenidate transdermal system should be used cautiously with pressor agents).
No products indexed under this heading.

Nortriptyline Hydrochloride (Human pharmacologic studies have shown that methylphenidate may inhibit the metabolism of some tricyclic drugs (eg, imipramine, clomipramine, desipramine). Downward dose adjustments of these drugs may be required when given concomitantly with methylphenidate. It may be necessary to adjust the dosage and monitor plasma drug concentrations when initiating or discontinuing methylphenidate).
No products indexed under this heading.

Oxcarbazepine (Human pharmacologic studies have shown that methylphenidate may inhibit the metabolism of anticonvulsants (eg, phenobarbital, phenytoin, primidone). Downward dose adjustments of these drugs may be required when given concomitantly with methylphenidate. It may be necessary to adjust the dosage and monitor plasma drug concentrations when initiating or discontinuing methylphenidate).
No products indexed under this heading.

Paramethadione (Human pharmacologic studies have shown that methylphenidate may inhibit the metabolism of anticonvulsants (eg, phenobarbital, phenytoin, primidone). Downward dose adjustments of these drugs may be required when given concomitantly with methylphenidate. It may be necessary to adjust the dosage and monitor plasma drug concentrations when initiating or discontinuing methylphenidate).
No products indexed under this heading.

Pargyline Hydrochloride (Methylphenidate transdermal system is contraindicated during treatment with monoamine oxidase inhibitors and also within a minimum of 14 days following discontinuation of treatment with a MAO inhibitor (hypertensive crises may occur)).
No products indexed under this heading.

Paroxetine Hydrochloride (Human pharmacologic studies have shown that methylphenidate may inhibit the metabolism of selective serotonin reuptake inhibitors. Downward dose adjustments of these drugs may be required when given concomitantly with methylphenidate. It may be necessary to adjust the dosage and monitor plasma drug concentrations when initiating or discontinuing methylphenidate).
Products include:
Paxil 1535
Paxil CR Controlled-Release Tablets 1544

Penbutolol Sulfate (Methylphenidate may decrease the effectiveness of drugs used to treat hypertension).
No products indexed under this heading.

Perindopril Erbumine (Methylphenidate may decrease the effectiveness of drugs used to treat hypertension). Products include:
Aceon Tablets (2 mg, 4 mg, 8 mg) 3038

Phenacemide (Human pharmacologic studies have shown that methylphenidate may inhibit the metabolism of anticonvulsants (eg, phenobarbital, phenytoin, primidone). Downward dose adjustments of these drugs may be required when given concomitantly with methylphenidate. It may be necessary to adjust the dosage and monitor plasma drug concentrations when initiating or discontinuing methylphenidate).
No products indexed under this heading.

Phenelzine Sulfate (Methylphenidate transdermal system is contraindicated during treatment with monoamine oxidase inhibitors and also within a minimum of 14 days following discontinuation of treatment with a MAO inhibitor (hypertensive crises may occur)).
No products indexed under this heading.

Phenobarbital (Human pharmacologic studies have shown that methylphenidate may inhibit the metabolism of anticonvulsants (eg, phenobarbital, phenytoin, primidone). Downward dose adjustments of these drugs may be required when given concomitantly with methylphenidate. It may be necessary to adjust the dosage and monitor plasma drug concentrations when initiating or discontinuing methylphenidate). Products include:
Donnatal Extentabs 2507

Phenoxybenzamine Hydrochloride (Methylphenidate may decrease the effectiveness of drugs used to treat hypertension). Products include:
Dibenzyline Capsules 3188

Phensuximide (Human pharmacologic studies have shown that methylphenidate may inhibit the metabolism of anticonvulsants (eg, phenobarbital, phenytoin, primidone). Downward dose adjustments of these drugs may be required when given concomitantly with methylphenidate. It may be necessary to adjust the dosage and monitor plasma drug concentrations when initiating or discontinuing methylphenidate).
No products indexed under this heading.

Phentolamine Mesylate (Methylphenidate may decrease the effectiveness of drugs used to treat hypertension).
No products indexed under this heading.

Phenylephrine Hydrochloride (Because of a possible effect on blood pressure, methylphenidate transdermal system should be used cautiously with pressor agents).
Products include:
Actifed Cold & Allergy Tablets 1895
Benadryl Allergy & Cold Kapgels 1895
Benadryl Allergy & Sinus Headache Kapgels 1895
Benadryl Severe Allergy & Sinus Headache Caplets 1897
Children's Benadryl-D Allergy & Sinus Liquid 1896
Benadryl-D Allergy & Sinus Tablet 1896
PediaCare Children's Allergy & Cold Liquid 1902
PediaCare Children's Decongestant Liquid 1902

IMPORTANT NOTE: Always consult each drug listing in the patient's regimen for possible interactions.

PediaCare Children's Liquid Multi-Symptom Cold 1902
Sinutab Non-Drying Caplets 1905
Sinutab Sinus Caplets 1905
Children's Sudafed PE Cold & Cough Liquid 1907
Children's Sudafed PE Nasal Decongestant Liquid 1906
Sudafed PE Cold & Cough Caplets 1907
Sudafed PE Nasal Decongestant Tablets 1907
Sudafed PE Nighttime Cold Caplets 1907
Sudafed PE Non-Drying Sinus Caplets 1908
Sudafed PE Severe Cold Caplets 1908
Sudafed PE Sinus & Allergy Tablets 1908
Sudafed PE Sinus Headache Caplets 1908
Tylenol Allergy Multi-Symptom Caplets with Cool Burst and Rapid Release Gelcaps 1916
Tylenol Allergy Multi-Symptom Nighttime Caplets with Cool Burst 1916
Children's Tylenol Plus Cold Suspension Liquid 1912
Children's Tylenol Plus Cold & Allergy Suspension Liquid 1914
Children's Tylenol Plus Flu Suspension Liquid 1914
Children's Tylenol Plus Multi-Symptom Cold Suspension Liquid 1912
Tylenol Cold Head Congestion Daytime Caplets with Cool Burst 1910
Tylenol Cold Head Congestion Nighttime Caplets with Cool Burst 1910
Tylenol Cold Head Congestion Severe Daytime Caplets with Cool Burst 1910
Tylenol Cold Multi-Symptom Daytime Caplets with Cool Burst and Rapid Release Gels 1913
Tylenol Cold Multi-Symptom Daytime Liquid with Citrus Burst 1913
Tylenol Cold Multi-Symptom Nighttime Caplets with Cool Burst 1913
Tylenol Cold Multi-Symptom Nighttime Liquid with Cool Burst 1913
Tylenol Cold Multi-Symptom Severe Caplets with Cool Burst 1913
Tylenol Cold Multi-Symptom Severe Daytime Liquid with Citrus Burst 1913
Tylenol Sinus Congestion & Pain Daytime Caplets with Cool Burst and Gelcaps 1917
Tylenol Sinus Congestion & Pain Nighttime Caplets with Cool Burst 1917
Tylenol Sinus Congestion & Pain Severe Caplets with Cool Burst 1917
Vicks DayQuil Cold & Flu Multi-Symptom Relief 616
Vicks DayQuil LiquiCaps 2567
Vicks DayQuil Liquid 2567
Vicks DayQuil Multi-Symptom Cold/Flu Relief 2567

Phenytoin (Human pharmacologic studies have shown that methylphenidate may inhibit the metabolism of anticonvulsants (eg, phenobarbital, phenytoin, primidone). Downward dose adjustments of these drugs may be required when given concomitantly with methylphenidate. It may be necessary to adjust the dosage and monitor plasma drug concentrations when initiating or discontinuing methylphenidate).
No products indexed under this heading.

Phenytoin Sodium (Human pharmacologic studies have shown that methylphenidate may inhibit the metabolism of anticonvulsants (eg, phenobarbital, phenytoin, primidone). Downward dose adjustments of these drugs may be required when given concomitantly with methylphenidate. It may be necessary to adjust the dosage and monitor plasma drug concentrations when initiating or discontinuing methylphenidate). Products include:
Phenytek Capsules 2192

Pindolol (Methylphenidate may decrease the effectiveness of drugs used to treat hypertension).
No products indexed under this heading.

Polythiazide (Methylphenidate may decrease the effectiveness of drugs used to treat hypertension).
No products indexed under this heading.

Prazosin Hydrochloride (Methylphenidate may decrease the effectiveness of drugs used to treat hypertension).
No products indexed under this heading.

Primidone (Human pharmacologic studies have shown that methylphenidate may inhibit the metabolism of anticonvulsants (eg, phenobarbital, phenytoin, primidone). Downward dose adjustments of these drugs may be required when given concomitantly with methylphenidate. It may be necessary to adjust the dosage and monitor plasma drug concentrations when initiating or discontinuing methylphenidate).
No products indexed under this heading.

Procarbazine Hydrochloride (Methylphenidate transdermal system is contraindicated during treatment with monoamine oxidase inhibitors and also within a minimum of 14 days following discontinuation of treatment with a MAO inhibitor (hypertensive crises may occur)).
No products indexed under this heading.

Propranolol Hydrochloride (Methylphenidate may decrease the effectiveness of drugs used to treat hypertension). Products include:
InnoPran XL Extended Release Capsules 1484

Protriptyline Hydrochloride (Human pharmacologic studies have shown that methylphenidate may inhibit the metabolism of some tricyclic drugs (eg, imipramine, clomipramine, desipramine). Downward dose adjustments of these drugs may be required when given concomitantly with methylphenidate. It may be necessary to adjust the dosage and monitor plasma drug concentrations when initiating or discontinuing methylphenidate).
No products indexed under this heading.

Quinapril Hydrochloride (Methylphenidate may decrease the effectiveness of drugs used to treat hypertension).
No products indexed under this heading.

Ramipril (Methylphenidate may decrease the effectiveness of drugs used to treat hypertension).
No products indexed under this heading.

Rasagiline Mesylate (Methylphenidate transdermal system is contraindicated during treatment with monoamine oxidase inhibitors and also within a minimum of 14 days following discontinuation of treatment with a MAO inhibitor (hypertensive crises may occur)). Products include:
Azilect Tablets 3106

Rauwolfia Serpentina (Methylphenidate may decrease the effectiveness of drugs used to treat hypertension).
No products indexed under this heading.

Rescinnamine (Methylphenidate may decrease the effectiveness of drugs used to treat hypertension).
No products indexed under this heading.

Reserpine (Methylphenidate may decrease the effectiveness of drugs used to treat hypertension).
No products indexed under this heading.

Selegiline (Methylphenidate transdermal system is contraindicated during treatment with monoamine oxidase inhibitors and also within a minimum of 14 days following discontinuation of treatment with a MAO inhibitor (hypertensive crises may occur)). Products include:
Emsam Transdermal System 905

Selegiline Hydrochloride (Methylphenidate transdermal system is contraindicated during treatment with monoamine oxidase inhibitors and also within a minimum of 14 days following discontinuation of treatment with a MAO inhibitor (hypertensive crises may occur)). Products include:
Eldepryl Capsules 3052

Sertraline Hydrochloride (Human pharmacologic studies have shown that methylphenidate may inhibit the metabolism of selective serotonin reuptake inhibitors. Downward dose adjustments of these drugs may be required when given concomitantly with methylphenidate. It may be necessary to adjust the dosage and monitor plasma drug concentrations when initiating or discontinuing methylphenidate).
No products indexed under this heading.

Sodium Nitroprusside (Methylphenidate may decrease the effectiveness of drugs used to treat hypertension).
No products indexed under this heading.

Sotalol Hydrochloride (Methylphenidate may decrease the effectiveness of drugs used to treat hypertension).
No products indexed under this heading.

Spirapril Hydrochloride (Methylphenidate may decrease the effectiveness of drugs used to treat hypertension).
No products indexed under this heading.

Telmisartan (Methylphenidate may decrease the effectiveness of drugs used to treat hypertension). Products include:
Micardis Tablets 852
Micardis HCT Tablets 854

Terazosin Hydrochloride (Methylphenidate may decrease the effectiveness of drugs used to treat hypertension).
No products indexed under this heading.

Tiagabine Hydrochloride (Human pharmacologic studies have shown that methylphenidate may inhibit the metabolism of anticonvulsants (eg, phenobarbital, phenytoin, primidone). Downward dose adjustments of these drugs may be required when given concomitantly with methylphenidate. It may be necessary to adjust the dosage and monitor plasma drug concentrations when initiating or discontinuing methylphenidate). Products include:
Gabitril Tablets 973

Timolol Maleate (Methylphenidate may decrease the effectiveness of drugs used to treat hypertension). Products include:
Combigan Ophthalmic Solution 553
Cosopt Sterile Ophthalmic Solution 1969
Timoptic Sterile Ophthalmic Solution 2121
Timoptic in Ocudose 2124
Timoptic-XE Sterile Ophthalmic Gel Forming Solution 2125

Topiramate (Human pharmacologic studies have shown that methylphenidate may inhibit the metabolism of anticonvulsants (eg, phenobarbital, phenytoin, primidone). Downward dose adjustments of these drugs may be required when given concomitantly with methylphenidate. It may be necessary to adjust the dosage and monitor plasma drug concentrations when initiating or discontinuing methylphenidate).
No products indexed under this heading.

Torsemide (Methylphenidate may decrease the effectiveness of drugs used to treat hypertension). Products include:
Demadex Injection 2630
Demadex Tablets 2630

Trandolapril (Methylphenidate may decrease the effectiveness of drugs used to treat hypertension). Products include:
Mavik Tablets 472
Tarka Tablets 511

Tranylcypromine Sulfate (Methylphenidate transdermal system is contraindicated during treatment with monoamine oxidase inhibitors and also within a minimum of 14 days following discontinuation of treatment with a MAO inhibitor (hypertensive crises may occur)). Products include:
Parnate Tablets 1532

Trimethadione (Human pharmacologic studies have shown that methylphenidate may inhibit the metabolism of anticonvulsants (eg, phenobarbital, phenytoin, primidone). Downward dose adjustments of these drugs may be required when given concomitantly with methylphenidate. It may be necessary to adjust the dosage and monitor plasma drug concentrations when initiating or discontinuing methylphenidate).
No products indexed under this heading.

Trimethaphan Camsylate (Methylphenidate may decrease the effectiveness of drugs used to treat hypertension).
No products indexed under this heading.

Trimipramine Maleate (Human pharmacologic studies have shown that methylphenidate may inhibit the metabolism of some tricyclic drugs (eg, imipramine, clomipramine, desipramine). Downward dose adjustments of these drugs may be required when given concomitantly with methylphenidate. It may be necessary to adjust the dosage and monitor plasma drug concentrations when initiating or discontinuing

methylphenidate).
No products indexed under this heading.

Valproate Sodium (Human pharmacologic studies have shown that methylphenidate may inhibit the metabolism of anticonvulsants (eg, phenobarbital, phenytoin, primidone). Downward dose adjustments of these drugs may be required when given concomitantly with methylphenidate. It may be necessary to adjust the dosage and monitor plasma drug concentrations when initiating or discontinuing methylphenidate).
No products indexed under this heading.

Valproic Acid (Human pharmacologic studies have shown that methylphenidate may inhibit the metabolism of anticonvulsants (eg, phenobarbital, phenytoin, primidone). Downward dose adjustments of these drugs may be required when given concomitantly with methylphenidate. It may be necessary to adjust the dosage and monitor plasma drug concentrations when initiating or discontinuing methylphenidate).
No products indexed under this heading.

Valsartan (Methylphenidate may decrease the effectiveness of drugs used to treat hypertension). Products include:
Diovan Tablets 2212
Diovan HCT Tablets 2216
Exforge Tablets 2238

Verapamil Hydrochloride (Methylphenidate may decrease the effectiveness of drugs used to treat hypertension). Products include:
Tarka Tablets 511

Warfarin Sodium (Human pharmacologic studies have shown that methylphenidate may inhibit the metabolism of coumarin anticoagulants. Downward dose adjustments of these drugs may be required when given concomitantly with methylphenidate. It may be necessary to adjust the dosage and monitor plasma drug concentrations or coagulation times when initiating or discontinuing methylphenidate).
No products indexed under this heading.

Zonisamide (Human pharmacologic studies have shown that methylphenidate may inhibit the metabolism of anticonvulsants (eg, phenobarbital, phenytoin, primidone). Downward dose adjustments of these drugs may be required when given concomitantly with methylphenidate. It may be necessary to adjust the dosage and monitor plasma drug concentrations when initiating or discontinuing methylphenidate). Products include:
Zonegran Capsules 1089

D-CAL CHEWABLE CAPLETS

(Calcium Carbonate, Vitamin D) .... ▣624
None cited in PDR database.

DDS-ACIDOPHILUS CAPSULES, TABLETS, AND POWDER

(Lactobacillus Acidophilus) .... ▣634
None cited in PDR database.

DELATESTRYL INJECTION

(Testosterone Enanthate) 1730
May interact with corticosteroids, oral anticoagulants, oral hypoglycemic agents, insulin, and certain other agents. Compounds in these categories include:

Acarbose (In diabetic patients, the metabolic effects of androgens may decrease blood glucose and, therefore, antidiabetic drug requirements). Products include:
Precose Tablets 792

ACTH (Co-administration of testosterone with ACTH may enhance edema formation).
No products indexed under this heading.

Anisindione (Co-administration of C-17 substituted derivatives of testosterone, such as methandrostenolone, have been reported to decrease the anticoagulant requirements; concomitant therapy has resulted in bleeding).
No products indexed under this heading.

Betamethasone Acetate (Co-administration of testosterone with corticosteroids may enhance edema formation).
No products indexed under this heading.

Betamethasone Sodium Phosphate (Co-administration of testosterone with corticosteroids may enhance edema formation).
No products indexed under this heading.

Budesonide (Co-administration of testosterone with corticosteroids may enhance edema formation). Products include:
Pulmicort Flexhaler 654
Symbicort 80/4.5 Inhalation Aerosol 659
Symbicort 160/4.5 Inhalation Aerosol 659

Chlorpropamide (In diabetic patients, the metabolic effects of androgens may decrease blood glucose and, therefore, antidiabetic drug requirements).
No products indexed under this heading.

Ciclesonide (Co-administration of testosterone with corticosteroids may enhance edema formation). Products include:
Alvesco Inhalation Aerosol 2985
Omnaris Nasal Spray 2998

Cortisone Acetate (Co-administration of testosterone with corticosteroids may enhance edema formation).
No products indexed under this heading.

Dexamethasone (Co-administration of testosterone with corticosteroids may enhance edema formation). Products include:
Ciprodex Otic Suspension 541

Dexamethasone Acetate (Co-administration of testosterone with corticosteroids may enhance edema formation).
No products indexed under this heading.

Dexamethasone Sodium Phosphate (Co-administration of testosterone with corticosteroids may enhance edema formation).
No products indexed under this heading.

Dicumarol (Co-administration of C-17 substituted derivatives of testosterone, such as methandrostenolone, have been reported to decrease the anticoagulant requirements; concomitant therapy has resulted in bleeding).
No products indexed under this heading.

Fludrocortisone Acetate (Co-administration of testosterone with corticosteroids may enhance edema formation).
No products indexed under this heading.

Flunisolide (Co-administration of testosterone with corticosteroids may enhance edema formation). Products include:
Aerobid/Aerobid-M 1153

Fluticasone Propionate (Co-administration of testosterone with corticosteroids may enhance edema formation). Products include:
Advair Diskus 100/50 1276
Advair Diskus 250/50 1276
Advair Diskus 500/50 1276
Advair HFA 45/21 Inhalation Aerosol 1288
Advair HFA 115/21 Inhalation Aerosol 1288
Advair HFA 230/21 Inhalation Aerosol 1288
Flonase Nasal Spray 1431
Flovent Diskus 50 mcg 1435

Fluticasone Propionate HFA (Co-administration of testosterone with corticosteroids may enhance edema formation). Products include:
Flovent HFA 1440

Glimepiride (In diabetic patients, the metabolic effects of androgens may decrease blood glucose and, therefore, antidiabetic drug requirements). Products include:
Avandaryl Tablets 1344
Duetact Tablets 3085

Glipizide (In diabetic patients, the metabolic effects of androgens may decrease blood glucose and, therefore, antidiabetic drug requirements).
No products indexed under this heading.

Glyburide (In diabetic patients, the metabolic effects of androgens may decrease blood glucose and, therefore, antidiabetic drug requirements).
No products indexed under this heading.

Hydrocortisone (Co-administration of testosterone with corticosteroids may enhance edema formation).
No products indexed under this heading.

Hydrocortisone Acetate (Co-administration of testosterone with corticosteroids may enhance edema formation). Products include:
Analpram-HC 1140
Pramosone 1141

Hydrocortisone Sodium Phosphate (Co-administration of testosterone with corticosteroids may enhance edema formation).
No products indexed under this heading.

Hydrocortisone Sodium Succinate (Co-administration of testosterone with corticosteroids may enhance edema formation).
No products indexed under this heading.

Insulin (In diabetic patients, the metabolic effects of androgens may decrease blood glucose and, therefore, insulin requirements).
No products indexed under this heading.

Insulin, Human, Zinc Suspension (In diabetic patients, the metabolic effects of androgens may decrease blood glucose and, therefore, insulin requirements).
No products indexed under this heading.

Insulin, Human (rDNA origin) (In diabetic patients, the metabolic effects of androgens may decrease blood glucose and, therefore, insulin requirements). Products include:
Exubera Inhalation Powder 2515

Insulin, Human NPH (In diabetic patients, the metabolic effects of androgens may decrease blood glucose and, therefore, insulin requirements). Products include:
Humulin N Vial 1846

Insulin, Human Regular (In diabetic patients, the metabolic effects of androgens may decrease blood glucose and, therefore, insulin requirements). Products include:
Humulin R 1849
Humulin R (U-500) 1850

Insulin, Human Regular and Human NPH Mixture (In diabetic patients, the metabolic effects of androgens may decrease blood glucose and, therefore, insulin requirements). Products include:
Humulin 50/50, 100 Units 1843
Humulin 70/30 Vial 1844

Insulin, NPH (In diabetic patients, the metabolic effects of androgens may decrease blood glucose and, therefore, insulin requirements).
No products indexed under this heading.

Insulin, Regular (In diabetic patients, the metabolic effects of androgens may decrease blood glucose and, therefore, insulin requirements).
No products indexed under this heading.

Insulin, Regular and NPH mixture (In diabetic patients, the metabolic effects of androgens may decrease blood glucose and, therefore, insulin requirements).
No products indexed under this heading.

Insulin, Zinc Crystals (In diabetic patients, the metabolic effects of androgens may decrease blood glucose and, therefore, insulin requirements).
No products indexed under this heading.

Insulin, Zinc Suspension (In diabetic patients, the metabolic effects of androgens may decrease blood glucose and, therefore, insulin requirements).
No products indexed under this heading.

Insulin Aspart (In diabetic patients, the metabolic effects of androgens may decrease blood glucose and, therefore, insulin requirements).
No products indexed under this heading.

Insulin Aspart, Human (In diabetic patients, the metabolic effects of androgens may decrease blood glucose and, therefore, insulin requirements). Products include:
NovoLog Mix 70/30 2364

IMPORTANT NOTE: Always consult each drug listing in the patient's regimen for possible interactions.

Insulin Aspart, Human Regular (In diabetic patients, the metabolic effects of androgens may decrease blood glucose and, therefore, insulin requirements). Products include:
NovoLog Injection 2359

Insulin Aspart Protamine, Human (In diabetic patients, the metabolic effects of androgens may decrease blood glucose and, therefore, insulin requirements). Products include:
NovoLog Mix 70/30 2364

Insulin Detemir (rDNA Origin) (In diabetic patients, the metabolic effects of androgens may decrease blood glucose and, therefore, insulin requirements). Products include:
Levemir Injection 2352

Insulin glargine (In diabetic patients, the metabolic effects of androgens may decrease blood glucose and, therefore, insulin requirements). Products include:
Lantus Injection 2749

Insulin Glulisine (In diabetic patients, the metabolic effects of androgens may decrease blood glucose and, therefore, insulin requirements). Products include:
Apidra Injection 2706

Insulin Lispro, Human (In diabetic patients, the metabolic effects of androgens may decrease blood glucose and, therefore, insulin requirements). Products include:
Humalog-Pen and KwikPen 1829
Humalog Mix 50/50-Pen and KwikPen 1833
Humalog Mix 75/25-Pen and KwikPen 1835

Insulin Lispro Protamine, Human (In diabetic patients, the metabolic effects of androgens may decrease blood glucose and, therefore, insulin requirements). Products include:
Humalog Mix 50/50-Pen and KwikPen 1833
Humalog Mix 75/25-Pen and KwikPen 1835

Metformin Hydrochloride (In diabetic patients, the metabolic effects of androgens may decrease blood glucose and, therefore, antidiabetic drug requirements). Products include:
ActoPlus Met Tablets 3071
Avandamet Tablets 1336
Janumet Tablets 2041
PrandiMet Tablets 2967

Methylprednisolone Acetate (Co-administration of testosterone with corticosteroids may enhance edema formation).
No products indexed under this heading.

Methylprednisolone Sodium Succinate (Co-administration of testosterone with corticosteroids may enhance edema formation).
No products indexed under this heading.

Miglitol (In diabetic patients, the metabolic effects of androgens may decrease blood glucose and, therefore, antidiabetic drug requirements).
No products indexed under this heading.

Mometasone Furoate (Co-administration of testosterone with corticosteroids may enhance edema formation). Products include:
Asmanex Twisthaler 2797
Elocon Cream 0.1% 2840
Elocon Lotion 0.1% 2841
Elocon Ointment 0.1% 2842

Mometasone Furoate Monohydrate (Co-administration of testosterone with corticosteroids may enhance edema formation). Products include:
Nasonex Nasal Spray 2883

Nateglinide (In diabetic patients, the metabolic effects of androgens may decrease blood glucose and, therefore, antidiabetic drug requirements). Products include:
Starlix Tablets 2314

Oxyphenbutazone (Co-administration of androgens and oxyphenbutazone may result in elevated serum levels of oxyphenbutazone).
No products indexed under this heading.

Pioglitazone Hydrochloride (In diabetic patients, the metabolic effects of androgens may decrease blood glucose and, therefore, antidiabetic drug requirements). Products include:
ActoPlus Met Tablets 3071
Actos Tablets 3077
Duetact Tablets 3085

Prednisolone Acetate (Co-administration of testosterone with corticosteroids may enhance edema formation). Products include:
Pred Forte Ophthalmic Suspension .... ⊙227
Pred Mild Ophthalmic Suspension .... ⊙230
Pred-G Ophthalmic Ointment .... ⊙229
Pred-G Ophthalmic Suspension .... ⊙228

Prednisolone Sodium Phosphate (Co-administration of testosterone with corticosteroids may enhance edema formation).
No products indexed under this heading.

Prednisolone Tebutate (Co-administration of testosterone with corticosteroids may enhance edema formation).
No products indexed under this heading.

Prednisone (Co-administration of testosterone with corticosteroids may enhance edema formation).
No products indexed under this heading.

Repaglinide (In diabetic patients, the metabolic effects of androgens may decrease blood glucose and, therefore, antidiabetic drug requirements). Products include:
PrandiMet Tablets 2967
Prandin Tablets 2971

Rosiglitazone Maleate (In diabetic patients, the metabolic effects of androgens may decrease blood glucose and, therefore, antidiabetic drug requirements). Products include:
Avandamet Tablets 1336
Avandaryl Tablets 1344
Avandia Tablets 1351

Sitagliptin Phosphate (In diabetic patients, the metabolic effects of androgens may decrease blood glucose and, therefore, antidiabetic drug requirements). Products include:
Janumet Tablets 2041
Januvia Tablets 2048

Tolazamide (In diabetic patients, the metabolic effects of androgens may decrease blood glucose and, therefore, antidiabetic drug requirements).
No products indexed under this heading.

Tolbutamide (In diabetic patients, the metabolic effects of androgens may decrease blood glucose and, therefore, antidiabetic drug requirements).
No products indexed under this heading.

Triamcinolone (Co-administration of testosterone with corticosteroids may enhance edema formation).
No products indexed under this heading.

Triamcinolone Acetonide (Co-administration of testosterone with corticosteroids may enhance edema formation). Products include:
Azmacort Inhalation Aerosol 407
Nasacort AQ Nasal Spray 2765
Triesence Injectable Suspension .... ⊙209

Triamcinolone Diacetate (Co-administration of testosterone with corticosteroids may enhance edema formation).
No products indexed under this heading.

Triamcinolone Hexacetonide (Co-administration of testosterone with corticosteroids may enhance edema formation).
No products indexed under this heading.

Troglitazone (In diabetic patients, the metabolic effects of androgens may decrease blood glucose and, therefore, antidiabetic drug requirements).
No products indexed under this heading.

Warfarin Sodium (Co-administration of C-17 substituted derivatives of testosterone, such as methandrostenolone, have been reported to decrease the anticoagulant requirements; concomitant therapy has resulted in bleeding).
No products indexed under this heading.

DEMADEX INJECTION

(Torsemide) 2630
See Demadex Tablets

DEMADEX TABLETS

(Torsemide) 2630
May interact with aminoglycosides, lithium preparations, non-steroidal anti-inflammatory agents, salicylates, and certain other agents. Compounds in these categories include:

Amikacin Sulfate (Co-administration of other diuretics has been reported to increase the ototoxic potential of aminoglycoside antibiotics, especially in the presence of impaired renal function; concurrent use of aminoglycoside and torsemide has not been studied, however, such combined therapy should be undertaken with great caution).
No products indexed under this heading.

Aspirin (Co-administration in patients receiving high dose of salicylates may be associated with salicylate toxicity due to competition for secretion by renal tubule). Products include:
Aggrenox Capsules 819
Bayer Aspirin 750
Percodan Tablets 1130
St. Joseph 81 mg Aspirin Chewable and Enteric Coated Tablets 1903

Aspirin, Enteric Coated (Co-administration in patients receiving high dose of salicylates may be associated with salicylate toxicity due to competition for secretion by renal tubule).
No products indexed under this heading.

Aspirin Buffered (Co-administration in patients receiving high dose of salicylates may be associated with salicylate toxicity due to competition for secretion by renal tubule).
No products indexed under this heading.

Celecoxib (Co-administration of another loop diuretic and nonsteroidal anti-inflammatory agents has been associated with renal dysfunction; concurrent use of torsemide and these agents has not been studied, however, such combined therapy should be undertaken with great caution). Products include:
Celebrex Capsules 2979

Cholestyramine (Possibility of decreased oral absorption of torsemide; simultaneous administration is not recommended).
No products indexed under this heading.

Choline Magnesium Trisalicylate (Co-administration in patients receiving high dose of salicylates may be associated with salicylate toxicity due to competition for secretion by renal tubule).
No products indexed under this heading.

Diclofenac Epolamine (Co-administration of another loop diuretic and nonsteroidal anti-inflammatory agents has been associated with renal dysfunction; concurrent use of torsemide and these agents has not been studied, however, such combined therapy should be undertaken with great caution). Products include:
Flector Patch 561

Diclofenac Potassium (Co-administration of another loop diuretic and nonsteroidal anti-inflammatory agents has been associated with renal dysfunction; concurrent use of torsemide and these agents has not been studied, however, such combined therapy should be undertaken with great caution).
No products indexed under this heading.

Diclofenac Sodium (Co-administration of another loop diuretic and nonsteroidal anti-inflammatory agents has been associated with renal dysfunction; concurrent use of torsemide and these agents has not been studied, however, such combined therapy should be undertaken with great caution). Products include:
Diclofenac Sodium Ophthalmic Solution .... ⊙240
Voltaren Ophthalmic Solution 2336
Voltaren Tablets 2334
Voltaren-XR Tablets 2337

Diflunisal (Co-administration in patients receiving high dose of salicylates may be associated with salicylate toxicity due to competition for secretion by renal tubule).
No products indexed under this heading.

Digoxin (Co-administration of digoxin is reported to increase the AUC for torsemide by 50%, but dose adjustment of torsemide is not necessary). Products include:

Lanoxin Injection ... 1498
Lanoxin Injection Pediatric ... 1502
Lanoxin Tablets ... 1505

Etodolac (Co-administration of another loop diuretic and nonsteroidal anti-inflammatory agents has been associated with renal dysfunction; concurrent use of torsemide and these agents has not been studied, however, such combined therapy should be undertaken with great caution).

No products indexed under this heading.

Fenoprofen Calcium (Co-administration of another loop diuretic and nonsteroidal anti-inflammatory agents has been associated with renal dysfunction; concurrent use of torsemide and these agents has not been studied, however, such combined therapy should be undertaken with great caution). Products include:

Nalfon Capsules ... 2508

Flurbiprofen (Co-administration of another loop diuretic and nonsteroidal anti-inflammatory agents has been associated with renal dysfunction; concurrent use of torsemide and these agents has not been studied, however, such combined therapy should be undertaken with great caution).

No products indexed under this heading.

Gentamicin Sulfate (Co-administration of other diuretics has been reported to increase the ototoxic potential of aminoglycoside antibiotics, especially in the presence of impaired renal function; concurrent use of aminoglycoside and torsemide has not been studied, however, such combined therapy should be undertaken with great caution). Products include:

Pred-G Ophthalmic Ointment ... ⊙229
Pred-G Ophthalmic Suspension ... ⊙228

Ibuprofen (Co-administration of another loop diuretic and nonsteroidal anti-inflammatory agents has been associated with renal dysfunction; concurrent use of torsemide and these agents has not been studied, however, such combined therapy should be undertaken with great caution). Products include:

Motrin IB Tablets and Caplets ... 1900
Children's Motrin Oral Suspension ... 1901
Children's Motrin Non-Staining Dye-Free Oral Suspension ... 1901
Children's Motrin Cold Oral Suspension ... 1899
Infants' Motrin Concentrated Drops ... 1901
Infants' Motrin Non-Staining Dye-Free Concentrated Drops ... 1901
Junior Strength Motrin Caplets and Chewable Tablets ... 1901
Vicoprofen Tablets ... 533

Indomethacin (The natriuretic effect of torsemide is partially inhibited by the concomitant administration of indomethacin). Products include:

Indocin ... 2024

Indomethacin Sodium Trihydrate (The natriuretic effect of torsemide is partially inhibited by the concomitant administration of indomethacin). Products include:

Indocin I.V. ... 2489

Kanamycin Sulfate (Co-administration of other diuretics has been reported to increase the ototoxic potential of aminoglycoside antibiotics, especially in the presence of impaired renal function; concurrent use of aminoglycoside and torsemide has not been studied, however, such combined therapy should be undertaken with great caution).

No products indexed under this heading.

Ketoprofen (Co-administration of another loop diuretic and nonsteroidal anti-inflammatory agents has been associated with renal dysfunction; concurrent use of torsemide and these agents has not been studied, however, such combined therapy should be undertaken with great caution).

No products indexed under this heading.

Ketorolac Tromethamine (Co-administration of another loop diuretic and nonsteroidal anti-inflammatory agents has been associated with renal dysfunction; concurrent use of torsemide and these agents has not been studied, however, such combined therapy should be undertaken with great caution).

No products indexed under this heading.

Lithium (Co-administration of other diuretics are known to reduce the renal clearance of lithium, inducing a high risk of lithium toxicity; concurrent use of lithium and torsemide has not been studied, however, such combined therapy should be undertaken with great caution).

No products indexed under this heading.

Lithium Carbonate (Co-administration of other diuretics are known to reduce the renal clearance of lithium, inducing a high risk of lithium toxicity; concurrent use of lithium and torsemide has not been studied, however, such combined therapy should be undertaken with great caution).

No products indexed under this heading.

Lithium Citrate (Co-administration of other diuretics are known to reduce the renal clearance of lithium, inducing a high risk of lithium toxicity; concurrent use of lithium and torsemide has not been studied, however, such combined therapy should be undertaken with great caution).

No products indexed under this heading.

Magnesium Salicylate (Co-administration in patients receiving high dose of salicylates may be associated with salicylate toxicity due to competition for secretion by renal tubule).

No products indexed under this heading.

Meclofenamate Sodium (Co-administration of another loop diuretic and nonsteroidal anti-inflammatory agents has been associated with renal dysfunction; concurrent use of torsemide and these agents has not been studied, however, such combined therapy should be undertaken with great caution).

No products indexed under this heading.

Mefenamic Acid (Co-administration of another loop diuretic and nonsteroidal anti-inflammatory agents has been associated with renal dysfunction; concurrent use of torsemide and these agents has not been studied, however, such combined therapy should be undertaken with great caution).

No products indexed under this heading.

Meloxicam (Co-administration of another loop diuretic and nonsteroidal anti-inflammatory agents has been associated with renal dysfunction; concurrent use of torsemide and these agents has not been studied, however, such combined therapy should be undertaken with great caution). Products include:

Mobic Oral Suspension ... 863
Mobic Tablets ... 863

Nabumetone (Co-administration of another loop diuretic and nonsteroidal anti-inflammatory agents has been associated with renal dysfunction; concurrent use of torsemide and these agents has not been studied, however, such combined therapy should be undertaken with great caution).

No products indexed under this heading.

Naproxen (Co-administration of another loop diuretic and nonsteroidal anti-inflammatory agents has been associated with renal dysfunction; concurrent use of torsemide and these agents has not been studied, however, such combined therapy should be undertaken with great caution). Products include:

EC-Naprosyn Delayed-Release Tablets ... 2632
Naprosyn Suspension ... 2632
Naprosyn Tablets ... 2632

Naproxen Sodium (Co-administration of another loop diuretic and nonsteroidal anti-inflammatory agents has been associated with renal dysfunction; concurrent use of torsemide and these agents has not been studied, however, such combined therapy should be undertaken with great caution). Products include:

Anaprox Tablets ... 2632
Anaprox DS Tablets ... 2632
Treximet Tablets ... 1616

Oxaprozin (Co-administration of another loop diuretic and nonsteroidal anti-inflammatory agents has been associated with renal dysfunction; concurrent use of torsemide and these agents has not been studied, however, such combined therapy should be undertaken with great caution).

No products indexed under this heading.

Phenylbutazone (Co-administration of another loop diuretic and nonsteroidal anti-inflammatory agents has been associated with renal dysfunction; concurrent use of torsemide and these agents has not been studied, however, such combined therapy should be undertaken with great caution).

No products indexed under this heading.

Piroxicam (Co-administration of another loop diuretic and nonsteroidal anti-inflammatory agents has been associated with renal dysfunction; concurrent use of torsemide and these agents has not been studied, however, such combined therapy should be undertaken with great caution).

No products indexed under this heading.

Probenecid (Reduces secretion of torsemide into the proximal tubule and thereby decreases diuretic effect).

No products indexed under this heading.

Rofecoxib (Co-administration of another loop diuretic and nonsteroidal anti-inflammatory agents has been associated with renal dysfunction; concurrent use of torsemide and these agents has not been studied, however, such combined therapy should be undertaken with great caution).

No products indexed under this heading.

Salsalate (Co-administration in patients receiving high dose of salicylates may be associated with salicylate toxicity due to competition for secretion by renal tubule).

No products indexed under this heading.

Spironolactone (Co-administration may be associated with significant reduction in the renal clearance of spironolactone, with corresponding increase in the AUC).

No products indexed under this heading.

Streptomycin Sulfate (Co-administration of other diuretics has been reported to increase the ototoxic potential of aminoglycoside antibiotics, especially in the presence of impaired renal function; concurrent use of aminoglycoside and torsemide has not been studied, however, such combined therapy should be undertaken with great caution).

No products indexed under this heading.

Sulindac (Co-administration of another loop diuretic and nonsteroidal anti-inflammatory agents has been associated with renal dysfunction; concurrent use of torsemide and these agents has not been studied, however, such combined therapy should be undertaken with great caution). Products include:

Clinoril Tablets ... 1962

Tobramycin (Co-administration of other diuretics has been reported to increase the ototoxic potential of aminoglycoside antibiotics, especially in the presence of impaired renal function; concurrent use of aminoglycoside and torsemide has not been studied, however, such combined therapy should be undertaken with great caution). Products include:

Zylet Ophthalmic Suspension ... ⊙247

Tobramycin Sulfate (Co-administration of other diuretics has been reported to increase the ototoxic potential of aminoglycoside antibiotics, especially in the presence of impaired renal function; concurrent use of aminoglycoside and torsemide has not been studied, however, such combined therapy should be undertaken with great caution).

No products indexed under this heading.

Tolmetin Sodium (Co-administration of another loop diuretic and nonsteroidal anti-inflammatory agents has been associated with renal dysfunction; concurrent use of torsemide and these agents has not been studied, however, such combined therapy should be undertaken with great caution).
No products indexed under this heading.

Valdecoxib (Co-administration of another loop diuretic and nonsteroidal anti-inflammatory agents has been associated with renal dysfunction; concurrent use of torsemide and these agents has not been studied, however, such combined therapy should be undertaken with great caution).
No products indexed under this heading.

Food Interactions

Food, unspecified (Simultaneous food intake delays the time to Cmax by about 30 minutes, but overall bioavailability (AUC) and diuretic activity are unchanged).

DEMSER CAPSULES

(Metyrosine) 1989

May interact with central nervous system depressants, hypnotics and sedatives, phenothiazines, tranquilizers, and certain other agents. Compounds in these categories include:

Alfentanil Hydrochloride (Concurrent use of metyrosine with alcohol or other CNS depressants can increase their sedative effects).
No products indexed under this heading.

Alprazolam (Concurrent use of metyrosine with alcohol or other CNS depressants can increase their sedative effects).
No products indexed under this heading.

Aprobarbital (Concurrent use of metyrosine with alcohol or other CNS depressants can increase their sedative effects).
No products indexed under this heading.

Buprenorphine Hydrochloride (Concurrent use of metyrosine with alcohol or other CNS depressants can increase their sedative effects).
Products include:
Suboxone Tablets 2601
Subutex Tablets 2601

Buspirone Hydrochloride (Concurrent use of metyrosine with alcohol or other CNS depressants can increase their sedative effects).
No products indexed under this heading.

Butabarbital (Concurrent use of metyrosine with alcohol or other CNS depressants can increase their sedative effects).
No products indexed under this heading.

Butabarbital Sodium (Metyrosine may add to the sedative effects of alcohol and other CNS depressants, (e.g., hypnotics and sedatives)).
No products indexed under this heading.

Butalbital (Concurrent use of metyrosine with alcohol or other CNS depressants can increase their sedative effects).
No products indexed under this heading.

Chloral Hydrate (Metyrosine may add to the sedative effects of alcohol and other CNS depressants, (e.g., hypnotics and sedatives)).
No products indexed under this heading.

Chlordiazepoxide (Concurrent use of metyrosine with alcohol or other CNS depressants can increase their sedative effects).
No products indexed under this heading.

Chlordiazepoxide Hydrochloride (Concurrent use of metyrosine with alcohol or other CNS depressants can increase their sedative effects).
No products indexed under this heading.

Chlorpromazine (Caution should be observed in administering metyrosine to patients receiving phenothiazines or haloperidol because the extrapyramidal effects of these drugs can be expected to be potentiated by inhibition of catecholamine synthesis).
No products indexed under this heading.

Chlorpromazine Hydrochloride (Caution should be observed in administering metyrosine to patients receiving phenothiazines or haloperidol because the extrapyramidal effects of these drugs can be expected to be potentiated by inhibition of catecholamine synthesis).
No products indexed under this heading.

Chlorprothixene (Concurrent use of metyrosine with alcohol or other CNS depressants can increase their sedative effects).
No products indexed under this heading.

Chlorprothixene Hydrochloride (Concurrent use of metyrosine with alcohol or other CNS depressants can increase their sedative effects).
No products indexed under this heading.

Chlorprothixene Lactate (Additive sedative effects).
No products indexed under this heading.

Clorazepate Dipotassium (Concurrent use of metyrosine with alcohol or other CNS depressants can increase their sedative effects).
No products indexed under this heading.

Clozapine (Concurrent use of metyrosine with alcohol or other CNS depressants can increase their sedative effects).
No products indexed under this heading.

Codeine Phosphate (Concurrent use of metyrosine with alcohol or other CNS depressants can increase their sedative effects). Products include:
Tylenol with Codeine Tablets 2427

Desflurane (Concurrent use of metyrosine with alcohol or other CNS depressants can increase their sedative effects).
No products indexed under this heading.

Dezocine (Concurrent use of metyrosine with alcohol or other CNS depressants can increase their sedative effects).
No products indexed under this heading.

Diazepam (Concurrent use of metyrosine with alcohol or other CNS depressants can increase their sedative effects). Products include:
Valium Tablets 2658

Droperidol (Concurrent use of metyrosine with alcohol or other CNS depressants can increase their sedative effects).
No products indexed under this heading.

Enflurane (Concurrent use of metyrosine with alcohol or other CNS depressants can increase their sedative effects).
No products indexed under this heading.

Estazolam (Concurrent use of metyrosine with alcohol or other CNS depressants can increase their sedative effects).
No products indexed under this heading.

Ethanol (Concurrent use of metyrosine with alcohol or other CNS depressants can increase their sedative effects).
No products indexed under this heading.

Ethchlorvynol (Concurrent use of metyrosine with alcohol or other CNS depressants can increase their sedative effects).
No products indexed under this heading.

Ethinamate (Concurrent use of metyrosine with alcohol or other CNS depressants can increase their sedative effects).
No products indexed under this heading.

Ethyl Alcohol (Concurrent use of metyrosine with alcohol or other CNS depressants can increase their sedative effects).
No products indexed under this heading.

Fentanyl (Concurrent use of metyrosine with alcohol or other CNS depressants can increase their sedative effects). Products include:
Duragesic Transdermal System 2405
Ionsys Transdermal System 2410

Fentanyl Citrate (Concurrent use of metyrosine with alcohol or other CNS depressants can increase their sedative effects). Products include:
Actiq 959
Fentora Tablets 968

Fluphenazine Decanoate (Caution should be observed in administering metyrosine to patients receiving phenothiazines or haloperidol because the extrapyramidal effects of these drugs can be expected to be potentiated by inhibition of catecholamine synthesis).
No products indexed under this heading.

Fluphenazine Enanthate (Caution should be observed in administering metyrosine to patients receiving phenothiazines or haloperidol because the extrapyramidal effects of these drugs can be expected to be potentiated by inhibition of catecholamine synthesis).
No products indexed under this heading.

Fluphenazine Hydrochloride (Caution should be observed in administering metyrosine to patients receiving phenothiazines or haloperidol because the extrapyramidal effects of these drugs can be expected to be potentiated by inhibition of catecholamine synthesis).
No products indexed under this heading.

Flurazepam Hydrochloride (Concurrent use of metyrosine with alcohol or other CNS depressants can increase their sedative effects).
No products indexed under this heading.

Glutethimide (Concurrent use of metyrosine with alcohol or other CNS depressants can increase their sedative effects).
No products indexed under this heading.

Haloperidol (Caution should be observed in administering metyrosine to patients receiving phenothiazines or haloperidol because the extrapyramidal effects of these drugs can be expected to be potentiated by inhibition of catecholamine synthesis).
No products indexed under this heading.

Haloperidol Decanoate (Caution should be observed in administering metyrosine to patients receiving phenothiazines or haloperidol because the extrapyramidal effects of these drugs can be expected to be potentiated by inhibition of catecholamine synthesis).
No products indexed under this heading.

Haloperidol Lactate (Caution should be observed in administering metyrosine to patients receiving phenothiazines or haloperidol because the extrapyramidal effects of these drugs can be expected to be potentiated by inhibition of catecholamine synthesis).
No products indexed under this heading.

Hydrocodone Bitartrate (Concurrent use of metyrosine with alcohol or other CNS depressants can increase their sedative effects).
Products include:
Lortab 5/500 Tablets 3143
Lortab 7.5/500 Tablets 3144
Lortab 10/500 Tablets 3144
Vicodin Tablets 529
Vicodin ES Tablets 530
Vicodin HP Tablets 531
Vicoprofen Tablets 533
Zydone Tablets 1132

Hydrocodone Polistirex (Concurrent use of metyrosine with alcohol or other CNS depressants can increase their sedative effects).
Products include:
Tussionex Pennkinetic
Extended-Release Suspension...... 3154

Hydromorphone Hydrochloride (Concurrent use of metyrosine with alcohol or other CNS depressants can increase their sedative effects).
No products indexed under this heading.

Hydroxyzine Hydrochloride (Concurrent use of metyrosine with alcohol or other CNS depressants can increase their sedative effects).
No products indexed under this heading.

Isoflurane (Concurrent use of metyrosine with alcohol or other CNS depressants can increase their sedative effects).
No products indexed under this heading.

Ketamine Hydrochloride (Concurrent use of metyrosine with alcohol or other CNS depressants can increase their sedative effects).
No products indexed under this heading.

Levomethadyl Acetate Hydrochloride (Concurrent use of metyrosine with alcohol or other CNS depressants can increase their sedative effects).
No products indexed under this heading.

Levorphanol Tartrate (Concurrent use of metyrosine with alcohol or other CNS depressants can increase their sedative effects).
No products indexed under this heading.

Lorazepam (Concurrent use of metyrosine with alcohol or other CNS depressants can increase their sedative effects).
No products indexed under this heading.

Loxapine Hydrochloride (Concurrent use of metyrosine with alcohol or other CNS depressants can increase their sedative effects).
No products indexed under this heading.

Loxapine Succinate (Concurrent use of metyrosine with alcohol or other CNS depressants can increase their sedative effects).
No products indexed under this heading.

Meperidine Hydrochloride (Concurrent use of metyrosine with alcohol or other CNS depressants can increase their sedative effects).
No products indexed under this heading.

Mephobarbital (Concurrent use of metyrosine with alcohol or other CNS depressants can increase their sedative effects).
No products indexed under this heading.

Meprobamate (Concurrent use of metyrosine with alcohol or other CNS depressants can increase their sedative effects).
No products indexed under this heading.

Mesoridazine Besylate (Caution should be observed in administering metyrosine to patients receiving phenothiazines or haloperidol because the extrapyramidal effects of these drugs can be expected to be potentiated by inhibition of catecholamine synthesis).
No products indexed under this heading.

Methadone Hydrochloride (Concurrent use of metyrosine with alcohol or other CNS depressants can increase their sedative effects).
No products indexed under this heading.

Methohexital Sodium (Concurrent use of metyrosine with alcohol or other CNS depressants can increase their sedative effects).
No products indexed under this heading.

Methotrimeprazine (Caution should be observed in administering metyrosine to patients receiving phenothiazines or haloperidol because the extrapyramidal effects of these drugs can be expected to be potentiated by inhibition of catecholamine synthesis).
No products indexed under this heading.

Methoxyflurane (Concurrent use of metyrosine with alcohol or other CNS depressants can increase their sedative effects).
No products indexed under this heading.

Midazolam Hydrochloride (Concurrent use of metyrosine with alcohol or other CNS depressants can increase their sedative effects).
No products indexed under this heading.

Molindone Hydrochloride (Concurrent use of metyrosine with alcohol or other CNS depressants can increase their sedative effects). Products include:
Moban Tablets ... 1116

Morphine Sulfate (Concurrent use of metyrosine with alcohol or other CNS depressants can increase their sedative effects). Products include:
Avinza Capsules ... 1772
DepoDur Injection ... 1095
MS Contin Tablets ... 2585

Olanzapine (Concurrent use of metyrosine with alcohol or other CNS depressants can increase their sedative effects). Products include:
Symbyax Capsules ... 1871
Zyprexa Tablets ... 1883
Zyprexa IntraMuscular ... 1883
Zyprexa ZYDIS Orally Disintegrating Tablets ... 1883

Oxazepam (Concurrent use of metyrosine with alcohol or other CNS depressants can increase their sedative effects).
No products indexed under this heading.

Oxycodone Hydrochloride (Concurrent use of metyrosine with alcohol or other CNS depressants can increase their sedative effects). Products include:
OxyContin Tablets ... 2589
OxyIR Capsules ... 2593
Percocet Tablets ... 1127
Percodan Tablets ... 1130

Pentobarbital Sodium (Concurrent use of metyrosine with alcohol or other CNS depressants can increase their sedative effects). Products include:
Nembutal Sodium Solution, USP ... 2494

Perphenazine (Possible potentiation of extrapyramidal effects of perphenazine; additive sedative effects).
No products indexed under this heading.

Phenobarbital (Concurrent use of metyrosine with alcohol or other CNS depressants can increase their sedative effects). Products include:
Donnatal Extentabs ... 2507

Prazepam (Concurrent use of metyrosine with alcohol or other CNS depressants can increase their sedative effects).
No products indexed under this heading.

Prochlorperazine (Caution should be observed in administering metyrosine to patients receiving phenothiazines or haloperidol because the extrapyramidal effects of these drugs can be expected to be potentiated by inhibition of catecholamine synthesis).
No products indexed under this heading.

Promethazine Hydrochloride (Caution should be observed in administering metyrosine to patients receiving phenothiazines or haloperidol because the extrapyramidal effects of these drugs can be expected to be potentiated by inhibition of catecholamine synthesis).
No products indexed under this heading.

Propofol (Concurrent use of metyrosine with alcohol or other CNS depressants can increase their sedative effects).
No products indexed under this heading.

Propoxyphene Hydrochloride (Concurrent use of metyrosine with alcohol or other CNS depressants can increase their sedative effects).
No products indexed under this heading.

Propoxyphene Napsylate (Concurrent use of metyrosine with alcohol or other CNS depressants can increase their sedative effects).
No products indexed under this heading.

Quazepam (Concurrent use of metyrosine with alcohol or other CNS depressants can increase their sedative effects).
No products indexed under this heading.

Quetiapine Fumarate (Concurrent use of metyrosine with alcohol or other CNS depressants can increase their sedative effects).
No products indexed under this heading.

Ramelteon (Metyrosine may add to the sedative effects of alcohol and other CNS depressants, (e.g., hypnotics and sedatives)). Products include:
Rozerem Tablets ... 3091

Remifentanil Hydrochloride (Concurrent use of metyrosine with alcohol or other CNS depressants can increase their sedative effects).
No products indexed under this heading.

Risperidone (Concurrent use of metyrosine with alcohol or other CNS depressants can increase their sedative effects). Products include:
Risperdal Consta Long-Acting Injection ... 1753

Secobarbital Sodium (Concurrent use of metyrosine with alcohol or other CNS depressants can increase their sedative effects).
No products indexed under this heading.

Sevoflurane (Concurrent use of metyrosine with alcohol or other CNS depressants can increase their sedative effects). Products include:
Ultane Liquid for Inhalation ... 524

Sodium Butabarbital (Metyrosine may add to the sedative effects of alcohol and other CNS depressants, (e.g., hypnotics and sedatives)).
No products indexed under this heading.

Sodium Oxybate (Concurrent use of metyrosine with alcohol or other CNS depressants can increase their sedative effects). Products include:
Xyrem Oral Solution ... 1766

Sufentanil Citrate (Concurrent use of metyrosine with alcohol or other CNS depressants can increase their sedative effects).
No products indexed under this heading.

Temazepam (Concurrent use of metyrosine with alcohol or other CNS depressants can increase their sedative effects).
No products indexed under this heading.

Thiamylal Sodium (Concurrent use of metyrosine with alcohol or other CNS depressants can increase their sedative effects).
No products indexed under this heading.

Thioridazine Hydrochloride (Caution should be observed in administering metyrosine to patients receiving phenothiazines or haloperidol because the extrapyramidal effects of these drugs can be expected to be potentiated by inhibition of catecholamine synthesis). Products include:
Thioridazine Hydrochloride Tablets ... 2195

Thiothixene (Concurrent use of metyrosine with alcohol or other CNS depressants can increase their sedative effects). Products include:
Thiothixene Capsules ... 2197

Triazolam (Concurrent use of metyrosine with alcohol or other CNS depressants can increase their sedative effects).
No products indexed under this heading.

Trifluoperazine Hydrochloride (Caution should be observed in administering metyrosine to patients receiving phenothiazines or haloperidol because the extrapyramidal effects of these drugs can be expected to be potentiated by inhibition of catecholamine synthesis).
No products indexed under this heading.

Zaleplon (Concurrent use of metyrosine with alcohol or other CNS depressants can increase their sedative effects).
No products indexed under this heading.

Ziprasidone Hydrochloride (Concurrent use of metyrosine with alcohol or other CNS depressants can increase their sedative effects). Products include:
Geodon Capsules ... 2520

Zolpidem Tartrate (Concurrent use of metyrosine with alcohol or other CNS depressants can increase their sedative effects). Products include:
Ambien Tablets ... 2692
Ambien CR Tablets ... 2696

Food Interactions

Alcohol (Concurrent use of metyrosine with alcohol or other CNS depressants can increase their sedative effects).

DENAVIR CREAM

(Penciclovir) ... 2205
None cited in PDR database.

IMPORTANT NOTE: Always consult each drug listing in the patient's regimen for possible interactions.

DEPAKOTE ER TABLETS
(Divalproex Sodium) 423
May interact with central nervous system depressants, phenytoin, and certain other agents. Compounds in these categories include:

Alfentanil Hydrochloride (Valproate produces CNS depression, especially when combined with another CNS depressant).
No products indexed under this heading.

Alprazolam (Valproate produces CNS depression, especially when combined with another CNS depressant).
No products indexed under this heading.

Amitriptyline Hydrochloride (Co-administration has resulted in a decrease in plasma clearance of amitriptyline; rare postmarketing reports of increased amitriptyline levels).
No products indexed under this heading.

Aprobarbital (Valproate produces CNS depression, especially when combined with another CNS depressant).
No products indexed under this heading.

Aspirin (Co-administration has resulted in a decrease in protein binding and an inhibition of metabolism of valproate; valproate free fraction was increased 4-fold in the presence of aspirin compared to valproate alone). Products include:
Aggrenox Capsules 819
Bayer Aspirin 750
Percodan Tablets 1130
St. Joseph 81 mg Aspirin Chewable and Enteric Coated Tablets 1903

Buprenorphine Hydrochloride (Valproate produces CNS depression, especially when combined with another CNS depressant). Products include:
Suboxone Tablets 2601
Subutex Tablets 2601

Buspirone Hydrochloride (Valproate produces CNS depression, especially when combined with another CNS depressant).
No products indexed under this heading.

Butabarbital (Valproate produces CNS depression, especially when combined with another CNS depressant).
No products indexed under this heading.

Butalbital (Valproate produces CNS depression, especially when combined with another CNS depressant).
No products indexed under this heading.

Carbamazepine (Co-administration has resulted in decreased serum levels of carbamazepine and increased serum levels of carbamazepine 10,11-epoxide; drugs that affect the levels of expression of hepatic enzymes, particularly those that elevate levels of glucuronosyltransferases, such as carbamazepine, may increase the clearance of valproate). Products include:
Carbatrol Capsules 3019
Equetro Extended-Release Capsules 3174

Chlordiazepoxide (Valproate produces CNS depression, especially when combined with another CNS depressant).
No products indexed under this heading.

Chlordiazepoxide Hydrochloride (Valproate produces CNS depression, especially when combined with another CNS depressant).
No products indexed under this heading.

Chlorpromazine (Co-administration has resulted in an increase in trough plasma levels of valproate).
No products indexed under this heading.

Chlorpromazine Hydrochloride (Co-administration has resulted in an increase in trough plasma levels of valproate).
No products indexed under this heading.

Chlorprothixene (Valproate produces CNS depression, especially when combined with another CNS depressant).
No products indexed under this heading.

Chlorprothixene Hydrochloride (Valproate produces CNS depression, especially when combined with another CNS depressant).
No products indexed under this heading.

Chlorprothixene Lactate (Valproate produces CNS depression, especially when combined with another CNS depressant).
No products indexed under this heading.

Clonazepam (Co-administration may induce absence status in patients with a history of absence type seizures). Products include:
Klonopin 2639

Clorazepate Dipotassium (Valproate produces CNS depression, especially when combined with another CNS depressant).
No products indexed under this heading.

Clozapine (Valproate produces CNS depression, especially when combined with another CNS depressant).
No products indexed under this heading.

Codeine Phosphate (Valproate produces CNS depression, especially when combined with another CNS depressant). Products include:
Tylenol with Codeine Tablets 2427

Desflurane (Valproate produces CNS depression, especially when combined with another CNS depressant).
No products indexed under this heading.

Dezocine (Valproate produces CNS depression, especially when combined with another CNS depressant).
No products indexed under this heading.

Diazepam (Co-administration increases the free fraction of diazepam by 90% in healthy volunteers; plasma clearance and volume of distribution for diazepam were reduced by 25% and 20%, respectively, in the presence of valproate). Products include:
Valium Tablets 2658

Droperidol (Valproate produces CNS depression, especially when combined with another CNS depressant).
No products indexed under this heading.

Enflurane (Valproate produces CNS depression, especially when combined with another CNS depressant).
No products indexed under this heading.

Ertapenem (A clinically significant reduction in serum valproic acid concentration has been reported in patients receiving carbapenem antibiotics such as ertapenem, and may result in loss of seizure control. Alternative antibacterial or anticonvulsant therapy should be considered if serum valproic acid concentrations drop significantly or seizure control deteriorates). Products include:
Invanz for Injection 2029

Estazolam (Valproate produces CNS depression, especially when combined with another CNS depressant).
No products indexed under this heading.

Ethanol (Valproate produces CNS depression, especially when combined with another CNS depressant).
No products indexed under this heading.

Ethchlorvynol (Valproate produces CNS depression, especially when combined with another CNS depressant).
No products indexed under this heading.

Ethinamate (Valproate produces CNS depression, especially when combined with another CNS depressant).
No products indexed under this heading.

Ethosuximide (Valproate inhibits the metabolism of ethosuximide; co-administration was accompanied by a 25% increase in elimination half-life of ethosuximide and a 15% decrease in its total clearance as compared to ethosuximide alone).
No products indexed under this heading.

Ethyl Alcohol (Valproate produces CNS depression, especially when combined with another CNS depressant).
No products indexed under this heading.

Felbamate (Co-administration has resulted in an increase in mean valproate peak concentration).
No products indexed under this heading.

Fentanyl (Valproate produces CNS depression, especially when combined with another CNS depressant). Products include:
Duragesic Transdermal System 2405
Ionsys Transdermal System 2410

Fentanyl Citrate (Valproate produces CNS depression, especially when combined with another CNS depressant). Products include:
Actiq 959
Fentora Tablets 968

Fluphenazine Decanoate (Valproate produces CNS depression, especially when combined with another CNS depressant).
No products indexed under this heading.

Fluphenazine Enanthate (Valproate produces CNS depression, especially when combined with another CNS depressant).
No products indexed under this heading.

Fluphenazine Hydrochloride (Valproate produces CNS depression, especially when combined with another CNS depressant).
No products indexed under this heading.

Flurazepam Hydrochloride (Valproate produces CNS depression, especially when combined with another CNS depressant).
No products indexed under this heading.

Fosphenytoin Sodium (Co-administration with drugs that affect the levels of expression of hepatic enzymes, particularly those that elevate levels of glucuronosyltransferases, such as phenytoin, may increase the clearance of valproate; valproate displaces phenytoin from its plasma binding sites and inhibits its hepatic metabolism; concurrent use has resulted in breakthrough seizures).
No products indexed under this heading.

Glutethimide (Valproate produces CNS depression, especially when combined with another CNS depressant).
No products indexed under this heading.

Haloperidol (Valproate produces CNS depression, especially when combined with another CNS depressant).
No products indexed under this heading.

Haloperidol Decanoate (Valproate produces CNS depression, especially when combined with another CNS depressant).
No products indexed under this heading.

Hydrocodone Bitartrate (Valproate produces CNS depression, especially when combined with another CNS depressant). Products include:
Lortab 5/500 Tablets 3143
Lortab 7.5/500 Tablets 3144
Lortab 10/500 Tablets 3144
Vicodin Tablets 529
Vicodin ES Tablets 530
Vicodin HP Tablets 531
Vicoprofen Tablets 533
Zydone Tablets 1132

Hydrocodone Polistirex (Valproate produces CNS depression, especially when combined with another CNS depressant). Products include:
Tussionex Pennkinetic Extended-Release Suspension 3154

Hydromorphone Hydrochloride (Valproate produces CNS depression, especially when combined with another CNS depressant).
No products indexed under this heading.

Hydroxyzine Hydrochloride (Valproate produces CNS depression, especially when combined with another CNS depressant).
No products indexed under this heading.

Imipenem (A clinically significant reduction in serum valproic acid concentration has been reported in patients receiving carbapenem antibiotics such as imipenem, and may result in loss of seizure control. Alternative antibacterial or anticonvulsant therapy should be considered if serum valproic acid concentrations drop significantly or seizure control deteriorates). Products include:

Primaxin I.M. **2080**
Primaxin I.V. **2083**

Isoflurane (Valproate produces CNS depression, especially when combined with another CNS depressant).
No products indexed under this heading.

Ketamine Hydrochloride (Valproate produces CNS depression, especially when combined with another CNS depressant).
No products indexed under this heading.

Lamotrigine (Co-administration has resulted in increased elimination half-life of lamotrigine from 26 to 72 hours and serious skin reactions, such as Stevens-Johnson syndrome and toxic epidermal necrolysis). Products include:

Lamictal **1488**

Levomethadyl Acetate Hydrochloride (Valproate produces CNS depression, especially when combined with another CNS depressant).
No products indexed under this heading.

Levorphanol Tartrate (Valproate produces CNS depression, especially when combined with another CNS depressant).
No products indexed under this heading.

Lorazepam (Co-administration was accompanied by a 17% decrease in the plasma clearance of lorazepam).
No products indexed under this heading.

Loxapine Hydrochloride (Valproate produces CNS depression, especially when combined with another CNS depressant).
No products indexed under this heading.

Loxapine Succinate (Valproate produces CNS depression, especially when combined with another CNS depressant).
No products indexed under this heading.

Meperidine Hydrochloride (Valproate produces CNS depression, especially when combined with another CNS depressant).
No products indexed under this heading.

Mephobarbital (Valproate produces CNS depression, especially when combined with another CNS depressant).
No products indexed under this heading.

Meprobamate (Valproate produces CNS depression, especially when combined with another CNS depressant).
No products indexed under this heading.

Meropenem (A clinically significant reduction in serum valproic acid concentration has been reported in patients receiving carbapenem antibiotics such as meropenem, and may result in loss of seizure control. Alternative antibacterial or anticonvulsant therapy should be considered if serum valproic acid concentrations drop significantly or seizure control deteriorates). Products include:

Merrem I.V. **684**

Mesoridazine Besylate (Valproate produces CNS depression, especially when combined with another CNS depressant).
No products indexed under this heading.

Methadone Hydrochloride (Valproate produces CNS depression, especially when combined with another CNS depressant).
No products indexed under this heading.

Methohexital Sodium (Valproate produces CNS depression, especially when combined with another CNS depressant).
No products indexed under this heading.

Methotrimeprazine (Valproate produces CNS depression, especially when combined with another CNS depressant).
No products indexed under this heading.

Methoxyflurane (Valproate produces CNS depression, especially when combined with another CNS depressant).
No products indexed under this heading.

Midazolam Hydrochloride (Valproate produces CNS depression, especially when combined with another CNS depressant).
No products indexed under this heading.

Molindone Hydrochloride (Valproate produces CNS depression, especially when combined with another CNS depressant). Products include:

Moban Tablets **1116**

Morphine Sulfate (Valproate produces CNS depression, especially when combined with another CNS depressant). Products include:

Avinza Capsules **1772**
DepoDur Injection **1095**
MS Contin Tablets **2585**

Nortriptyline Hydrochloride (Co-administration has resulted in a decrease in the net clearance of nortriptyline).
No products indexed under this heading.

Olanzapine (Valproate produces CNS depression, especially when combined with another CNS depressant). Products include:

Symbyax Capsules **1871**
Zyprexa Tablets **1883**
Zyprexa IntraMuscular **1883**
Zyprexa ZYDIS Orally Disintegrating Tablets **1883**

Oxazepam (Valproate produces CNS depression, especially when combined with another CNS depressant).
No products indexed under this heading.

Oxycodone Hydrochloride (Valproate produces CNS depression, especially when combined with another CNS depressant). Products include:

OxyContin Tablets **2589**
OxyIR Capsules **2593**
Percocet Tablets **1127**
Percodan Tablets **1130**

Pentobarbital Sodium (Valproate produces CNS depression, especially when combined with another CNS depressant). Products include:

Nembutal Sodium Solution, USP **2494**

Perphenazine (Valproate produces CNS depression, especially when combined with another CNS depressant).
No products indexed under this heading.

Phenobarbital (Co-administration with drugs that affect the levels of expression of hepatic enzymes, particularly those that elevate levels of glucuronosyltransferases, such as phenobarbital, may increase the clearance of valproate; valproate inhibits the metabolism of phenobarbital; co-administration has resulted in an increase in half-life and a decrease in plasma clearance of phenobarbital; all patients should be monitored for neurological toxicity because of severe CNS depression). Products include:

Donnatal Extentabs **2507**

Phenytoin (Co-administration with drugs that affect the levels of expression of hepatic enzymes, particularly those that elevate levels of glucuronosyltransferases, such as phenytoin, may increase the clearance of valproate; valproate displaces phenytoin from its plasma binding sites and inhibits its hepatic metabolism; concurrent use has resulted in breakthrough seizures).
No products indexed under this heading.

Phenytoin Sodium (Co-administration with drugs that affect the levels of expression of hepatic enzymes, particularly those that elevate levels of glucuronosyltransferases, such as phenytoin, may increase the clearance of valproate; valproate displaces phenytoin from its plasma binding sites and inhibits its hepatic metabolism; concurrent use has resulted in breakthrough seizures). Products include:

Phenytek Capsules **2192**

Prazepam (Valproate produces CNS depression, especially when combined with another CNS depressant).
No products indexed under this heading.

Primidone (Co-administration may result in severe CNS depression because primidone is metabolized to a barbiturate; potential for same interaction as phenobarbital and valproate).
No products indexed under this heading.

Prochlorperazine (Valproate produces CNS depression, especially when combined with another CNS depressant).
No products indexed under this heading.

Promethazine Hydrochloride (Valproate produces CNS depression, especially when combined with another CNS depressant).
No products indexed under this heading.

Propofol (Valproate produces CNS depression, especially when combined with another CNS depressant).
No products indexed under this heading.

Propoxyphene Hydrochloride (Valproate produces CNS depression, especially when combined with another CNS depressant).
No products indexed under this heading.

Propoxyphene Napsylate (Valproate produces CNS depression, especially when combined with another CNS depressant).
No products indexed under this heading.

Quazepam (Valproate produces CNS depression, especially when combined with another CNS depressant).
No products indexed under this heading.

Quetiapine Fumarate (Valproate produces CNS depression, especially when combined with another CNS depressant).
No products indexed under this heading.

Remifentanil Hydrochloride (Valproate produces CNS depression, especially when combined with another CNS depressant).
No products indexed under this heading.

Rifampin (Co-administration has resulted in an increase in the oral clearance of valproate. Valproate dosage adjustment may be necessary when it is co-administered with rifampin).
No products indexed under this heading.

Risperidone (Valproate produces CNS depression, especially when combined with another CNS depressant). Products include:

Risperdal Consta Long-Acting Injection **1753**

Secobarbital Sodium (Valproate produces CNS depression, especially when combined with another CNS depressant).
No products indexed under this heading.

Sevoflurane (Valproate produces CNS depression, especially when combined with another CNS depressant). Products include:

Ultane Liquid for Inhalation **524**

Sodium Oxybate (Valproate produces CNS depression, especially when combined with another CNS depressant). Products include:

Xyrem Oral Solution **1766**

Sufentanil Citrate (Valproate produces CNS depression, especially when combined with another CNS depressant).
No products indexed under this heading.

Temazepam (Valproate produces CNS depression, especially when combined with another CNS depressant).
No products indexed under this heading.

Thiamylal Sodium (Valproate produces CNS depression, especially when combined with another CNS depressant).
No products indexed under this heading.

Thioridazine Hydrochloride (Valproate produces CNS depression, especially when combined with another CNS depressant). Products include:

Thioridazine Hydrochloride Tablets **2195**

Thiothixene (Valproate produces CNS depression, especially when combined with another CNS depressant). Products include:
Thiothixene Capsules 2197

Tolbutamide (Co-administration in in vitro experiments has resulted in increased unbound fraction of tolbutamide).
No products indexed under this heading.

Topiramate (Concomitant administration of topiramate and valproic acid has been associated with hyperammonemia with or without encephalopathy in patients who have tolerated either drug alone).
No products indexed under this heading.

Triazolam (Valproate produces CNS depression, especially when combined with another CNS depressant).
No products indexed under this heading.

Trifluoperazine Hydrochloride (Valproate produces CNS depression, especially when combined with another CNS depressant).
No products indexed under this heading.

Warfarin Sodium (Co-administration in in vitro experiments has resulted in increased unbound fraction of warfarin).
No products indexed under this heading.

Zaleplon (Valproate produces CNS depression, especially when combined with another CNS depressant).
No products indexed under this heading.

Zidovudine (Co-administration has resulted in decreased clearance of zidovudine; the half-life of zidovudine was unaffected). Products include:
Combivir Tablets 1384
Retrovir 1574
Retrovir IV Infusion 1579
Trizivir Tablets 1622

Ziprasidone Hydrochloride (Valproate produces CNS depression, especially when combined with another CNS depressant). Products include:
Geodon Capsules 2520

Zolpidem Tartrate (Valproate produces CNS depression, especially when combined with another CNS depressant). Products include:
Ambien Tablets 2692
Ambien CR Tablets 2696

Food Interactions

Alcohol (Valproate produces CNS depression, especially when combined with another CNS depressant, such as alcohol).

DEPOCYT INJECTION
(Cytarabine Liposome) 1136
May interact with cytotoxic drugs. Compounds in these categories include:

Bleomycin Sulfate (Co-administration of intrathecal cytarabine and other cytotoxic agents administered intrathecally may enhance neurotoxicity).
No products indexed under this heading.

Cyclophosphamide (Co-administration of intrathecal cytarabine and other cytotoxic agents administered intrathecally may enhance neurotoxicity).
No products indexed under this heading.

Daunorubicin Hydrochloride (Co-administration of intrathecal cytarabine and other cytotoxic agents administered intrathecally may enhance neurotoxicity).
No products indexed under this heading.

Doxorubicin Hydrochloride (Co-administration of intrathecal cytarabine and other cytotoxic agents administered intrathecally may enhance neurotoxicity).
No products indexed under this heading.

Epirubicin Hydrochloride (Co-administration of intrathecal cytarabine and other cytotoxic agents administered intrathecally may enhance neurotoxicity).
No products indexed under this heading.

Fluorouracil (Co-administration of intrathecal cytarabine and other cytotoxic agents administered intrathecally may enhance neurotoxicity). Products include:
Carac Cream 0.5% 2722

Hydroxyurea (Co-administration of intrathecal cytarabine and other cytotoxic agents administered intrathecally may enhance neurotoxicity).
No products indexed under this heading.

Methotrexate Sodium (Co-administration of intrathecal cytarabine and other cytotoxic agents administered intrathecally may enhance neurotoxicity).
No products indexed under this heading.

Mitotane (Co-administration of intrathecal cytarabine and other cytotoxic agents administered intrathecally may enhance neurotoxicity).
No products indexed under this heading.

Mitoxantrone Hydrochloride (Co-administration of intrathecal cytarabine and other cytotoxic agents administered intrathecally may enhance neurotoxicity). Products include:
Novantrone for Injection Concentrate 1100

Procarbazine Hydrochloride (Co-administration of intrathecal cytarabine and other cytotoxic agents administered intrathecally may enhance neurotoxicity).
No products indexed under this heading.

Tamoxifen Citrate (Co-administration of intrathecal cytarabine and other cytotoxic agents administered intrathecally may enhance neurotoxicity).
No products indexed under this heading.

Vincristine Sulfate (Co-administration of intrathecal cytarabine and other cytotoxic agents administered intrathecally may enhance neurotoxicity).
No products indexed under this heading.

DEPODUR INJECTION
(Morphine Sulfate) 1095
May interact with anesthetics, central nervous system depressants, hypnotics and sedatives, local anesthetics, monoamine oxidase inhibitors, muscle relaxants, phenothiazines, and certain other agents. Compounds in these categories include:

Alfentanil Hydrochloride (The concurrent use of other central nervous system (CNS) depressants increase the risk of respiratory depression, hypotension, profound sedation, or coma. Use with caution and with vigilant monitoring in patients taking these agents).
No products indexed under this heading.

Alprazolam (The concurrent use of other central nervous system (CNS) depressants increase the risk of respiratory depression, hypotension, profound sedation, or coma. Use with caution and with vigilant monitoring in patients taking these agents).
No products indexed under this heading.

Aprobarbital (The concurrent use of other central nervous system (CNS) depressants increase the risk of respiratory depression, hypotension, profound sedation, or coma. Use with caution and with vigilant monitoring in patients taking these agents).
No products indexed under this heading.

Atracurium Besylate (Respiratory depression associated with morphine may delay recovery of spontaneous pulmonary ventilation when neuromuscular blocking agents are co-administered).
No products indexed under this heading.

Baclofen (Respiratory depression associated with morphine may delay recovery of spontaneous pulmonary ventilation when neuromuscular blocking agents are co-administered).
No products indexed under this heading.

Bupivacaine Hydrochloride (Administration of morphine sulfate ER injection three minutes after a test dose increases peak serum concentrations of morphine. Increasing the interval between the test dose and administration of morphine sulfate liposomal injection administration to at least 15 minutes minimizes this pharmacokinetic interaction. Safety and efficacy of morphine sulfate ER injection when used in conjunction with therapeutic epidural doses of lidocaine with epinephrine (for conduction anesthesia) have not been studied in clinical trials. Epidural local anesthetics should not be used before or after morphine sulfate ER injection except in the form of a test dose. Co-administration of morphine sulfate ER liposomal injection with any local anesthetic is not recommended).
No products indexed under this heading.

Buprenorphine Hydrochloride (The concurrent use of other central nervous system (CNS) depressants increase the risk of respiratory depression, hypotension, profound sedation, or coma. Use with caution and with vigilant monitoring in patients taking these agents). Products include:
Suboxone Tablets 2601
Subutex Tablets 2601

Buspirone Hydrochloride (The concurrent use of other central nervous system (CNS) depressants increase the risk of respiratory depression, hypotension, profound sedation, or coma. Use with caution and with vigilant monitoring in patients taking these agents).
No products indexed under this heading.

Butabarbital (The concurrent use of other central nervous system (CNS) depressants increase the risk of respiratory depression, hypotension, profound sedation, or coma. Use with caution and with vigilant monitoring in patients taking these agents).
No products indexed under this heading.

Butabarbital Sodium (The concurrent use of other central nervous system (CNS) depressants increase the risk of respiratory depression, hypotension, profound sedation, or coma. Use with caution and with vigilant monitoring in patients taking these agents).
No products indexed under this heading.

Butalbital (The concurrent use of other central nervous system (CNS) depressants increase the risk of respiratory depression, hypotension, profound sedation, or coma. Use with caution and with vigilant monitoring in patients taking these agents).
No products indexed under this heading.

Carisoprodol (Respiratory depression associated with morphine may delay recovery of spontaneous pulmonary ventilation when neuromuscular blocking agents are co-administered). Products include:
Soma Tablets 1931

Chloral Hydrate (The concurrent use of other central nervous system (CNS) depressants increase the risk of respiratory depression, hypotension, profound sedation, or coma. Use with caution and with vigilant monitoring in patients taking these agents).
No products indexed under this heading.

Chlordiazepoxide (The concurrent use of other central nervous system (CNS) depressants increase the risk of respiratory depression, hypotension, profound sedation, or coma. Use with caution and with vigilant monitoring in patients taking these agents).
No products indexed under this heading.

Chlordiazepoxide Hydrochloride (The concurrent use of other central nervous system (CNS) depressants increase the risk of respiratory depression, hypotension, profound sedation, or coma. Use with caution and with vigilant monitoring in patients taking these agents).
No products indexed under this heading.

Chloroprocaine Hydrochloride (Administration of morphine sulfate ER injection three minutes after a test dose increases peak serum concentrations of morphine. Increasing

the interval between the test dose and administration of morphine sulfate liposomal injection administration to at least 15 minutes minimizes this pharmacokinetic interaction. Safety and efficacy of morphine sulfate ER injection when used in conjunction with therapeutic epidural doses of lidocaine with epinephrine (for conduction anesthesia) have not been studied in clinical trials. Epidural local anesthetics should not be used before or after morphine sulfate ER injection except in the form of a test dose. Co-administration of morphine sulfate ER liposomal injection with any local anesthetic is not recommended).
No products indexed under this heading.

Chlorpromazine (The concurrent use of other central nervous system (CNS) depressants increase the risk of respiratory depression, hypotension, profound sedation, or coma. Use with caution and with vigilant monitoring in patients taking these agents).
No products indexed under this heading.

Chlorpromazine Hydrochloride (The concurrent use of other central nervous system (CNS) depressants increase the risk of respiratory depression, hypotension, profound sedation, or coma. Use with caution and with vigilant monitoring in patients taking these agents).
No products indexed under this heading.

Chlorprothixene (The concurrent use of other central nervous system (CNS) depressants increase the risk of respiratory depression, hypotension, profound sedation, or coma. Use with caution and with vigilant monitoring in patients taking these agents).
No products indexed under this heading.

Chlorprothixene Hydrochloride (The concurrent use of other central nervous system (CNS) depressants increase the risk of respiratory depression, hypotension, profound sedation, or coma. Use with caution and with vigilant monitoring in patients taking these agents).
No products indexed under this heading.

Chlorprothixene Lactate (The concurrent use of other central nervous system (CNS) depressants increase the risk of respiratory depression, hypotension, profound sedation, or coma. Use with caution and with vigilant monitoring in patients taking these agents).
No products indexed under this heading.

Chlorzoxazone (Respiratory depression associated with morphine may delay recovery of spontaneous pulmonary ventilation when neuromuscular blocking agents are co-administered).
No products indexed under this heading.

Cisatracurium Besylate (Respiratory depression associated with morphine may delay recovery of spontaneous pulmonary ventilation when neuromuscular blocking agents are co-administered). Products include:
Nimbex Injection 484

Clorazepate Dipotassium (The concurrent use of other central nervous system (CNS) depressants increase the risk of respiratory depression, hypotension, profound sedation, or coma. Use with caution and with vigilant monitoring in patients taking these agents).
No products indexed under this heading.

Clozapine (The concurrent use of other central nervous system (CNS) depressants increase the risk of respiratory depression, hypotension, profound sedation, or coma. Use with caution and with vigilant monitoring in patients taking these agents).
No products indexed under this heading.

Codeine Phosphate (The concurrent use of other central nervous system (CNS) depressants increase the risk of respiratory depression, hypotension, profound sedation, or coma. Use with caution and with vigilant monitoring in patients taking these agents). Products include:
Tylenol with Codeine Tablets 2427

Cyclobenzaprine Hydrochloride (Respiratory depression associated with morphine may delay recovery of spontaneous pulmonary ventilation when neuromuscular blocking agents are co-administered).
Products include:
Amrix Capsules 966

Dantrolene Sodium (Respiratory depression associated with morphine may delay recovery of spontaneous pulmonary ventilation when neuromuscular blocking agents are co-administered). Products include:
Dantrium Capsules 2580
Dantrium Intravenous 2582

Desflurane (The concurrent use of other central nervous system (CNS) depressants increase the risk of respiratory depression, hypotension, profound sedation, or coma. Use with caution and with vigilant monitoring in patients taking these agents).
No products indexed under this heading.

Dezocine (The concurrent use of other central nervous system (CNS) depressants increase the risk of respiratory depression, hypotension, profound sedation, or coma. Use with caution and with vigilant monitoring in patients taking these agents).
No products indexed under this heading.

Diazepam (The concurrent use of other central nervous system (CNS) depressants increase the risk of respiratory depression, hypotension, profound sedation, or coma. Use with caution and with vigilant monitoring in patients taking these agents). Products include:
Valium Tablets 2658

Doxacurium Chloride (Respiratory depression associated with morphine may delay recovery of spontaneous pulmonary ventilation when neuromuscular blocking agents are co-administered).
No products indexed under this heading.

Droperidol (The concurrent use of other central nervous system (CNS) depressants including droperidol, increases the risk of respiratory depression, hypotension, profound sedation, or coma. Use with caution and with vigilant monitoring in patients taking droperidol).
No products indexed under this heading.

Enflurane (The concurrent use of other central nervous system (CNS) depressants increase the risk of respiratory depression, hypotension, profound sedation, or coma. Use with caution and with vigilant monitoring in patients taking these agents).
No products indexed under this heading.

Estazolam (The concurrent use of other central nervous system (CNS) depressants increase the risk of respiratory depression, hypotension, profound sedation, or coma. Use with caution and with vigilant monitoring in patients taking these agents).
No products indexed under this heading.

Ethanol (The concurrent use of other central nervous system (CNS) depressants increase the risk of respiratory depression, hypotension, profound sedation, or coma. Use with caution and with vigilant monitoring in patients taking these agents).
No products indexed under this heading.

Ethchlorvynol (The concurrent use of other central nervous system (CNS) depressants increase the risk of respiratory depression, hypotension, profound sedation, or coma. Use with caution and with vigilant monitoring in patients taking these agents).
No products indexed under this heading.

Ethinamate (The concurrent use of other central nervous system (CNS) depressants increase the risk of respiratory depression, hypotension, profound sedation, or coma. Use with caution and with vigilant monitoring in patients taking these agents).
No products indexed under this heading.

Ethyl Alcohol (The concurrent use of other central nervous system (CNS) depressants increase the risk of respiratory depression, hypotension, profound sedation, or coma. Use with caution and with vigilant monitoring in patients taking these agents).
No products indexed under this heading.

Etidocaine Hydrochloride (Administration of morphine sulfate ER injection three minutes after a test dose increases peak serum concentrations of morphine. Increasing the interval between the test dose and administration of morphine sulfate liposomal injection administration to at least 15 minutes minimizes this pharmacokinetic interaction. Safety and efficacy of morphine sulfate ER injection when used in conjunction with therapeutic epidural doses of lidocaine with epinephrine (for conduction anesthesia) have not been studied in clinical trials. Epidural local anesthetics should not be used before or after morphine sulfate ER injection except in the form of a test dose. Co-administration of morphine sulfate ER liposomal injection with any local anesthetic is not recommended).
No products indexed under this heading.

Fentanyl (The concurrent use of other central nervous system (CNS) depressants increase the risk of respiratory depression, hypotension, profound sedation, or coma. Use with caution and with vigilant monitoring in patients taking these agents). Products include:
Duragesic Transdermal System 2405
Ionsys Transdermal System 2410

Fentanyl Citrate (The concurrent use of other central nervous system (CNS) depressants increase the risk of respiratory depression, hypotension, profound sedation, or coma. Use with caution and with vigilant monitoring in patients taking these agents). Products include:
Actiq 959
Fentora Tablets 968

Fluphenazine Decanoate (The concurrent use of other central nervous system (CNS) depressants increase the risk of respiratory depression, hypotension, profound sedation, or coma. Use with caution and with vigilant monitoring in patients taking these agents).
No products indexed under this heading.

Fluphenazine Enanthate (The concurrent use of other central nervous system (CNS) depressants increase the risk of respiratory depression, hypotension, profound sedation, or coma. Use with caution and with vigilant monitoring in patients taking these agents).
No products indexed under this heading.

Fluphenazine Hydrochloride (The concurrent use of other central nervous system (CNS) depressants increase the risk of respiratory depression, hypotension, profound sedation, or coma. Use with caution and with vigilant monitoring in patients taking these agents).
No products indexed under this heading.

Flurazepam Hydrochloride (The concurrent use of other central nervous system (CNS) depressants increase the risk of respiratory depression, hypotension, profound sedation, or coma. Use with caution and with vigilant monitoring in patients taking these agents).
No products indexed under this heading.

Glutethimide (The concurrent use of other central nervous system (CNS) depressants increase the risk of respiratory depression, hypotension, profound sedation, or coma. Use with caution and with vigilant monitoring in patients taking these agents).
No products indexed under this heading.

Haloperidol (The concurrent use of other central nervous system (CNS) depressants increase the risk of respiratory depression, hypotension, profound sedation, or coma. Use with caution and with vigilant monitoring in patients taking these agents).
No products indexed under this heading.

Haloperidol Decanoate (The concurrent use of other central nervous system (CNS) depressants increase the risk of respiratory depression, hypotension, profound sedation, or coma. Use with caution and with vigilant monitoring in patients taking these agents).

No products indexed under this heading.

Halothane (The concurrent use of other central nervous system (CNS) depressants increase the risk of respiratory depression, hypotension, profound sedation, or coma. Use with caution and with vigilant monitoring in patients taking these agents).

No products indexed under this heading.

Hydrocodone Bitartrate (The concurrent use of other central nervous system (CNS) depressants increase the risk of respiratory depression, hypotension, profound sedation, or coma. Use with caution and with vigilant monitoring in patients taking these agents). Products include:

Lortab 5/500 Tablets **3143**
Lortab 7.5/500 Tablets **3144**
Lortab 10/500 Tablets **3144**
Vicodin Tablets **529**
Vicodin ES Tablets **530**
Vicodin HP Tablets **531**
Vicoprofen Tablets **533**
Zydone Tablets **1132**

Hydrocodone Polistirex (The concurrent use of other central nervous system (CNS) depressants increase the risk of respiratory depression, hypotension, profound sedation, or coma. Use with caution and with vigilant monitoring in patients taking these agents). Products include:

Tussionex Pennkinetic
Extended-Release Suspension **3154**

Hydromorphone Hydrochloride (The concurrent use of other central nervous system (CNS) depressants increase the risk of respiratory depression, hypotension, profound sedation, or coma. Use with caution and with vigilant monitoring in patients taking these agents).

No products indexed under this heading.

Hydroxyzine Hydrochloride (The concurrent use of other central nervous system (CNS) depressants increase the risk of respiratory depression, hypotension, profound sedation, or coma. Use with caution and with vigilant monitoring in patients taking these agents).

No products indexed under this heading.

Isocarboxazid (MAOIs markedly potentiate the action of morphine. Morphine sulfate extended release liposomal injection should not be used in patients taking MAOIs or within 14 days of stopping such treatment). Products include:

Marplan Tablets **3177**

Isoflurane (The concurrent use of other central nervous system (CNS) depressants increase the risk of respiratory depression, hypotension, profound sedation, or coma. Use with caution and with vigilant monitoring in patients taking these agents).

No products indexed under this heading.

Ketamine Hydrochloride (The concurrent use of other central nervous system (CNS) depressants increase the risk of respiratory depression, hypotension, profound sedation, or coma. Use with caution and with vigilant monitoring in patients taking these agents).

No products indexed under this heading.

Levobupivacaine Hydrochloride (Administration of morphine sulfate ER injection three minutes after a test dose increases peak serum concentrations of morphine. Increasing the interval between the test dose and administration of morphine sulfate liposomal injection administration to at least 15 minutes minimizes this pharmacokinetic interaction. Safety and efficacy of morphine sulfate ER injection when used in conjunction with therapeutic epidural doses of lidocaine with epinephrine (for conduction anesthesia) have not been studied in clinical trials. Epidural local anesthetics should not be used before or after morphine sulfate ER injection except in the form of a test dose. Co-administration of morphine sulfate ER liposomal injection with any local anesthetic is not recommended).

No products indexed under this heading.

Levomethadyl Acetate Hydrochloride (The concurrent use of other central nervous system (CNS) depressants increase the risk of respiratory depression, hypotension, profound sedation, or coma. Use with caution and with vigilant monitoring in patients taking these agents).

No products indexed under this heading.

Levorphanol Tartrate (The concurrent use of other central nervous system (CNS) depressants increase the risk of respiratory depression, hypotension, profound sedation, or coma. Use with caution and with vigilant monitoring in patients taking these agents).

No products indexed under this heading.

Lidocaine Hydrochloride (Administration of morphine sulfate ER injection three minutes after a test dose increases peak serum concentrations of morphine. Increasing the interval between the test dose and administration of morphine sulfate liposomal injection administration to at least 15 minutes minimizes this pharmacokinetic interaction. Safety and efficacy of morphine sulfate ER injection when used in conjunction with therapeutic epidural doses of lidocaine with epinephrine (for conduction anesthesia) have not been studied in clinical trials. Epidural local anesthetics should not be used before or after morphine sulfate ER injection except in the form of a test dose. Co-administration of morphine sulfate ER liposomal injection with any local anesthetic is not recommended).

No products indexed under this heading.

Lorazepam (The concurrent use of other central nervous system (CNS) depressants increase the risk of respiratory depression, hypotension, profound sedation, or coma. Use with caution and with vigilant monitoring in patients taking these agents).

No products indexed under this heading.

Loxapine Hydrochloride (The concurrent use of other central nervous system (CNS) depressants increase the risk of respiratory depression, hypotension, profound sedation, or coma. Use with caution and with vigilant monitoring in patients taking these agents).

No products indexed under this heading.

Loxapine Succinate (The concurrent use of other central nervous system (CNS) depressants increase the risk of respiratory depression, hypotension, profound sedation, or coma. Use with caution and with vigilant monitoring in patients taking these agents).

No products indexed under this heading.

Meperidine Hydrochloride (The concurrent use of other central nervous system (CNS) depressants increase the risk of respiratory depression, hypotension, profound sedation, or coma. Use with caution and with vigilant monitoring in patients taking these agents).

No products indexed under this heading.

Mephobarbital (The concurrent use of other central nervous system (CNS) depressants increase the risk of respiratory depression, hypotension, profound sedation, or coma. Use with caution and with vigilant monitoring in patients taking these agents).

No products indexed under this heading.

Mepivacaine Hydrochloride (Administration of morphine sulfate ER injection three minutes after a test dose increases peak serum concentrations of morphine. Increasing the interval between the test dose and administration of morphine sulfate liposomal injection administration to at least 15 minutes minimizes this pharmacokinetic interaction. Safety and efficacy of morphine sulfate ER injection when used in conjunction with therapeutic epidural doses of lidocaine with epinephrine (for conduction anesthesia) have not been studied in clinical trials. Epidural local anesthetics should not be used before or after morphine sulfate ER injection except in the form of a test dose. Co-administration of morphine sulfate ER liposomal injection with any local anesthetic is not recommended).

No products indexed under this heading.

Meprobamate (The concurrent use of other central nervous system (CNS) depressants increase the risk of respiratory depression, hypotension, profound sedation, or coma. Use with caution and with vigilant monitoring in patients taking these agents).

No products indexed under this heading.

Mesoridazine Besylate (The concurrent use of other central nervous system (CNS) depressants increase the risk of respiratory depression, hypotension, profound sedation, or coma. Use with caution and with vigilant monitoring in patients taking these agents).

No products indexed under this heading.

Metaxalone (Respiratory depression associated with morphine may delay recovery of spontaneous pulmonary ventilation when neuromuscular blocking agents are co-administered). Products include:

Skelaxin Tablets **1784**

Methadone Hydrochloride (The concurrent use of other central nervous system (CNS) depressants increase the risk of respiratory depression, hypotension, profound sedation, or coma. Use with caution and with vigilant monitoring in patients taking these agents).

No products indexed under this heading.

Methocarbamol (Respiratory depression associated with morphine may delay recovery of spontaneous pulmonary ventilation when neuromuscular blocking agents are co-administered).

No products indexed under this heading.

Methohexital Sodium (The concurrent use of other central nervous system (CNS) depressants increase the risk of respiratory depression, hypotension, profound sedation, or coma. Use with caution and with vigilant monitoring in patients taking these agents).

No products indexed under this heading.

Methotrimeprazine (The concurrent use of other central nervous system (CNS) depressants increase the risk of respiratory depression, hypotension, profound sedation, or coma. Use with caution and with vigilant monitoring in patients taking these agents).

No products indexed under this heading.

Methoxyflurane (The concurrent use of other central nervous system (CNS) depressants increase the risk of respiratory depression, hypotension, profound sedation, or coma. Use with caution and with vigilant monitoring in patients taking these agents).

No products indexed under this heading.

Metocurine Iodide (Respiratory depression associated with morphine may delay recovery of spontaneous pulmonary ventilation when neuromuscular blocking agents are co-administered).

No products indexed under this heading.

Midazolam Hydrochloride (The concurrent use of other central nervous system (CNS) depressants increase the risk of respiratory depression, hypotension, profound sedation, or coma. Use with caution and with vigilant monitoring in patients taking these agents).

No products indexed under this heading.

Mivacurium Chloride (Respiratory depression associated with morphine may delay recovery of spontaneous pulmonary ventilation when neuromuscular blocking agents are co-administered).
No products indexed under this heading.

Moclobemide (MAOIs markedly potentiate the action of morphine. Morphine sulfate extended release liposomal injection should not be used in patients taking MAOIs or within 14 days of stopping such treatment).
No products indexed under this heading.

Molindone Hydrochloride (The concurrent use of other central nervous system (CNS) depressants increase the risk of respiratory depression, hypotension, profound sedation, or coma. Use with caution and with vigilant monitoring in patients taking these agents). Products include:
Moban Tablets ... 1116

Olanzapine (The concurrent use of other central nervous system (CNS) depressants increase the risk of respiratory depression, hypotension, profound sedation, or coma. Use with caution and with vigilant monitoring in patients taking these agents). Products include:
Symbyax Capsules ... 1871
Zyprexa Tablets ... 1883
Zyprexa IntraMuscular ... 1883
Zyprexa ZYDIS Orally Disintegrating Tablets ... 1883

Orphenadrine Citrate (Respiratory depression associated with morphine may delay recovery of spontaneous pulmonary ventilation when neuromuscular blocking agents are co-administered).
No products indexed under this heading.

Oxazepam (The concurrent use of other central nervous system (CNS) depressants increase the risk of respiratory depression, hypotension, profound sedation, or coma. Use with caution and with vigilant monitoring in patients taking these agents).
No products indexed under this heading.

Oxycodone Hydrochloride (The concurrent use of other central nervous system (CNS) depressants increase the risk of respiratory depression, hypotension, profound sedation, or coma. Use with caution and with vigilant monitoring in patients taking these agents). Products include:
OxyContin Tablets ... 2589
OxyIR Capsules ... 2593
Percocet Tablets ... 1127
Percodan Tablets ... 1130

Pancuronium Bromide (Respiratory depression associated with morphine may delay recovery of spontaneous pulmonary ventilation when neuromuscular blocking agents are co-administered).
No products indexed under this heading.

Pargyline Hydrochloride (MAOIs markedly potentiate the action of morphine. Morphine sulfate extended release liposomal injection should not be used in patients taking MAOIs or within 14 days of stopping such treatment).
No products indexed under this heading.

Pentobarbital Sodium (The concurrent use of other central nervous system (CNS) depressants increase the risk of respiratory depression, hypotension, profound sedation, or coma. Use with caution and with vigilant monitoring in patients taking these agents). Products include:
Nembutal Sodium Solution, USP ... 2494

Perphenazine (The concurrent use of other central nervous system (CNS) depressants increase the risk of respiratory depression, hypotension, profound sedation, or coma. Use with caution and with vigilant monitoring in patients taking these agents).
No products indexed under this heading.

Phenelzine Sulfate (MAOIs markedly potentiate the action of morphine. Morphine sulfate extended release liposomal injection should not be used in patients taking MAOIs or within 14 days of stopping such treatment).
No products indexed under this heading.

Phenobarbital (The concurrent use of other central nervous system (CNS) depressants increase the risk of respiratory depression, hypotension, profound sedation, or coma. Use with caution and with vigilant monitoring in patients taking these agents). Products include:
Donnatal Extentabs ... 2507

Prazepam (The concurrent use of other central nervous system (CNS) depressants increase the risk of respiratory depression, hypotension, profound sedation, or coma. Use with caution and with vigilant monitoring in patients taking these agents).
No products indexed under this heading.

Procaine Hydrochloride (Administration of morphine sulfate ER injection three minutes after a test dose increases peak serum concentrations of morphine. Increasing the interval between the test dose and administration of morphine sulfate liposomal injection administration to at least 15 minutes minimizes this pharmacokinetic interaction. Safety and efficacy of morphine sulfate ER injection when used in conjunction with therapeutic epidural doses of lidocaine with epinephrine (for conduction anesthesia) have not been studied in clinical trials. Epidural local anesthetics should not be used before or after morphine sulfate ER injection except in the form of a test dose. Co-administration of morphine sulfate ER liposomal injection with any local anesthetic is not recommended).
No products indexed under this heading.

Procarbazine Hydrochloride (MAOIs markedly potentiate the action of morphine. Morphine sulfate extended release liposomal injection should not be used in patients taking MAOIs or within 14 days of stopping such treatment).
No products indexed under this heading.

Prochlorperazine (The concurrent use of other central nervous system (CNS) depressants increase the risk of respiratory depression, hypotension, profound sedation, or coma. Use with caution and with vigilant monitoring in patients taking these agents).
No products indexed under this heading.

Promethazine Hydrochloride (The concurrent use of other central nervous system (CNS) depressants increase the risk of respiratory depression, hypotension, profound sedation, or coma. Use with caution and with vigilant monitoring in patients taking these agents).
No products indexed under this heading.

Propofol (The concurrent use of other central nervous system (CNS) depressants increase the risk of respiratory depression, hypotension, profound sedation, or coma. Use with caution and with vigilant monitoring in patients taking these agents).
No products indexed under this heading.

Propoxyphene Hydrochloride (The concurrent use of other central nervous system (CNS) depressants increase the risk of respiratory depression, hypotension, profound sedation, or coma. Use with caution and with vigilant monitoring in patients taking these agents).
No products indexed under this heading.

Propoxyphene Napsylate (The concurrent use of other central nervous system (CNS) depressants increase the risk of respiratory depression, hypotension, profound sedation, or coma. Use with caution and with vigilant monitoring in patients taking these agents).
No products indexed under this heading.

Quazepam (The concurrent use of other central nervous system (CNS) depressants increase the risk of respiratory depression, hypotension, profound sedation, or coma. Use with caution and with vigilant monitoring in patients taking these agents).
No products indexed under this heading.

Quetiapine Fumarate (The concurrent use of other central nervous system (CNS) depressants increase the risk of respiratory depression, hypotension, profound sedation, or coma. Use with caution and with vigilant monitoring in patients taking these agents).
No products indexed under this heading.

Ramelteon (The concurrent use of other central nervous system (CNS) depressants increase the risk of respiratory depression, hypotension, profound sedation, or coma. Use with caution and with vigilant monitoring in patients taking these agents). Products include:
Rozerem Tablets ... 3091

Rapacuronium Bromide (Respiratory depression associated with morphine may delay recovery of spontaneous pulmonary ventilation when neuromuscular blocking agents are co-administered).
No products indexed under this heading.

Rasagiline Mesylate (MAOIs markedly potentiate the action of morphine. Morphine sulfate extended release liposomal injection should not be used in patients taking MAOIs or within 14 days of stopping such treatment). Products include:
Azilect Tablets ... 3106

Remifentanil Hydrochloride (The concurrent use of other central nervous system (CNS) depressants increase the risk of respiratory depression, hypotension, profound sedation, or coma. Use with caution and with vigilant monitoring in patients taking these agents).
No products indexed under this heading.

Risperidone (The concurrent use of other central nervous system (CNS) depressants increase the risk of respiratory depression, hypotension, profound sedation, or coma. Use with caution and with vigilant monitoring in patients taking these agents). Products include:
Risperdal Consta Long-Acting Injection ... 1753

Rocuronium Bromide (Respiratory depression associated with morphine may delay recovery of spontaneous pulmonary ventilation when neuromuscular blocking agents are co-administered). Products include:
Zemuron Injection ... 2947

Secobarbital Sodium (The concurrent use of other central nervous system (CNS) depressants increase the risk of respiratory depression, hypotension, profound sedation, or coma. Use with caution and with vigilant monitoring in patients taking these agents).
No products indexed under this heading.

Selegiline (MAOIs markedly potentiate the action of morphine. Morphine sulfate extended release liposomal injection should not be used in patients taking MAOIs or within 14 days of stopping such treatment). Products include:
Emsam Transdermal System ... 905

Selegiline Hydrochloride (MAOIs markedly potentiate the action of morphine. Morphine sulfate extended release liposomal injection should not be used in patients taking MAOIs or within 14 days of stopping such treatment). Products include:
Eldepryl Capsules ... 3052

Sevoflurane (The concurrent use of other central nervous system (CNS) depressants increase the risk of respiratory depression, hypotension, profound sedation, or coma. Use with caution and with vigilant monitoring in patients taking these agents). Products include:
Ultane Liquid for Inhalation ... 524

Sodium Butabarbital (The concurrent use of other central nervous system (CNS) depressants increase the risk of respiratory depression, hypotension, profound sedation, or coma. Use with caution and with vigilant monitoring in patients taking these agents).
No products indexed under this heading.

Sodium Oxybate (The concurrent use of other central nervous system (CNS) depressants increase the risk of respiratory depression, hypotension, profound sedation, or coma.

Use with caution and with vigilant monitoring in patients taking these agents). Products include:
Xyrem Oral Solution 1766

Succinylcholine Chloride (Respiratory depression associated with morphine may delay recovery of spontaneous pulmonary ventilation when neuromuscular blocking agents are co-administered).
No products indexed under this heading.

Sufentanil Citrate (The concurrent use of other central nervous system (CNS) depressants increase the risk of respiratory depression, hypotension, profound sedation, or coma. Use with caution and with vigilant monitoring in patients taking these agents).
No products indexed under this heading.

Temazepam (The concurrent use of other central nervous system (CNS) depressants increase the risk of respiratory depression, hypotension, profound sedation, or coma. Use with caution and with vigilant monitoring in patients taking these agents).
No products indexed under this heading.

Tetracaine Hydrochloride (Administration of morphine sulfate ER injection three minutes after a test dose increases peak serum concentrations of morphine. Increasing the interval between the test dose and administration of morphine sulfate liposomal injection administration to at least 15 minutes minimizes this pharmacokinetic interaction. Safety and efficacy of morphine sulfate ER injection when used in conjunction with therapeutic epidural doses of lidocaine with epinephrine (for conduction anesthesia) have not been studied in clinical trials. Epidural local anesthetics should not be used before or after morphine sulfate ER injection except in the form of a test dose. Co-administration of morphine sulfate ER liposomal injection with any local anesthetic is not recommended).
No products indexed under this heading.

Thiamylal Sodium (The concurrent use of other central nervous system (CNS) depressants increase the risk of respiratory depression, hypotension, profound sedation, or coma. Use with caution and with vigilant monitoring in patients taking these agents).
No products indexed under this heading.

Thioridazine Hydrochloride (The concurrent use of other central nervous system (CNS) depressants increase the risk of respiratory depression, hypotension, profound sedation, or coma. Use with caution and with vigilant monitoring in patients taking these agents). Products include:
Thioridazine Hydrochloride Tablets 2195

Thiothixene (The concurrent use of other central nervous system (CNS) depressants increase the risk of respiratory depression, hypotension, profound sedation, or coma. Use with caution and with vigilant monitoring in patients taking these agents). Products include:
Thiothixene Capsules 2197

Tranylcypromine Sulfate (MAOIs markedly potentiate the action of morphine. Morphine sulfate extended release liposomal injection should not be used in patients taking MAOIs or within 14 days of stopping such treatment). Products include:
Parnate Tablets 1532

Triazolam (The concurrent use of other central nervous system (CNS) depressants increase the risk of respiratory depression, hypotension, profound sedation, or coma. Use with caution and with vigilant monitoring in patients taking these agents).
No products indexed under this heading.

Trifluoperazine Hydrochloride (The concurrent use of other central nervous system (CNS) depressants increase the risk of respiratory depression, hypotension, profound sedation, or coma. Use with caution and with vigilant monitoring in patients taking these agents).
No products indexed under this heading.

Vecuronium Bromide (Respiratory depression associated with morphine may delay recovery of spontaneous pulmonary ventilation when neuromuscular blocking agents are co-administered).
No products indexed under this heading.

Zaleplon (The concurrent use of other central nervous system (CNS) depressants increase the risk of respiratory depression, hypotension, profound sedation, or coma. Use with caution and with vigilant monitoring in patients taking these agents).
No products indexed under this heading.

Ziprasidone Hydrochloride (The concurrent use of other central nervous system (CNS) depressants increase the risk of respiratory depression, hypotension, profound sedation, or coma. Use with caution and with vigilant monitoring in patients taking these agents). Products include:
Geodon Capsules 2520

Zolpidem Tartrate (The concurrent use of other central nervous system (CNS) depressants increase the risk of respiratory depression, hypotension, profound sedation, or coma. Use with caution and with vigilant monitoring in patients taking these agents). Products include:
Ambien Tablets 2692
Ambien CR Tablets 2696

Food Interactions

Alcohol (The concurrent use of other central nervous system (CNS) depressants increase the risk of respiratory depression, hypotension, profound sedation, or coma. Use with caution and with vigilant monitoring in patients taking these agents).

DEXEDRINE SPANSULE SUSTAINED-RELEASE CAPSULES

(Dextroamphetamine Sulfate) 1401
May interact with antihistamines, antihypertensives, beta blockers, monoamine oxidase inhibitors, phenytoin, thiazides, tricyclic antidepressants, urinary alkalinizing agents, veratrum alkaloids, and certain other agents. Compounds in these categories include:

Acebutolol Hydrochloride (Amphetamine may antagonize the hypotensive effects of antihypertensives; adrenergic blockers are inhibited by amphetamines).
No products indexed under this heading.

Acetazolamide (Increases the concentration of the non-ionized species of the amphetamine molecule, thereby decreasing urinary excretion; increases amphetamines blood levels and thereby potentiates the actions of amphetamines).
No products indexed under this heading.

Acetazolamide Sodium (Increases the concentration of the non-ionized species of the amphetamine molecule, thereby decreasing urinary excretion; increases amphetamines blood levels and thereby potentiates the actions of amphetamines).
No products indexed under this heading.

Acrivastine (Amphetamines may counteract the sedative effect of antihistamine).
No products indexed under this heading.

Aliskiren (Amphetamine may antagonize the hypotensive effects of antihypertensives). Products include:
Tekturna Tablets 2321
Tekturna HCT Tablets 2324

Amitriptyline Hydrochloride (Enhanced activity of tricyclic or sympathomimetics; possible increases in the brain concentration of d-amphetamine in the brain; cardiovascular effect may be potentiated).
No products indexed under this heading.

Amlodipine Besylate (Amphetamine may antagonize the hypotensive effects of antihypertensives). Products include:
Azor Tablets 1005
Exforge Tablets 2238

Ammonium Chloride (Increases the concentration of the ionized species of the amphetamine molecule, thereby increasing urinary excretion; lowers amphetamines blood levels and efficacy).
No products indexed under this heading.

Amoxapine (Enhanced activity of tricyclic or sympathomimetics; possible increases in the brain concentration of d-amphetamine in the brain; cardiovascular effect may be potentiated).
No products indexed under this heading.

Astemizole (Amphetamines may counteract the sedative effect of antihistamine).
No products indexed under this heading.

Atenolol (Amphetamine may antagonize the hypotensive effects of antihypertensives; adrenergic blockers are inhibited by amphetamines).
No products indexed under this heading.

Azatadine Maleate (Amphetamines may counteract the sedative effect of antihistamine).
No products indexed under this heading.

Benazepril Hydrochloride (Amphetamine may antagonize the hypotensive effects of antihypertensives).
No products indexed under this heading.

Bendroflumethiazide (Increases the concentration of the non-ionized species of the amphetamine molecule, thereby decreasing urinary excretion; increases amphetamines blood levels and thereby potentiates the actions of amphetamines).
No products indexed under this heading.

Betaxolol Hydrochloride (Amphetamine may antagonize the hypotensive effects of antihypertensives; adrenergic blockers are inhibited by amphetamines).
No products indexed under this heading.

Bisoprolol Fumarate (Amphetamine may antagonize the hypotensive effects of antihypertensives; adrenergic blockers are inhibited by amphetamines).
No products indexed under this heading.

Bromodiphenhydramine Hydrochloride (Amphetamines may counteract the sedative effect of antihistamine).
No products indexed under this heading.

Brompheniramine Maleate (Amphetamines may counteract the sedative effect of antihistamine).
No products indexed under this heading.

Candesartan Cilexetil (Amphetamine may antagonize the hypotensive effects of antihypertensives). Products include:
Atacand Tablets 639
Atacand HCT 642

Captopril (Amphetamine may antagonize the hypotensive effects of antihypertensives). Products include:
Captopril Tablets 2182

Carteolol Hydrochloride (Amphetamine may antagonize the hypotensive effects of antihypertensives; adrenergic blockers are inhibited by amphetamines).
No products indexed under this heading.

Cetirizine Hydrochloride (Amphetamines may counteract the sedative effect of antihistamine). Products include:
Zyrtec Allergy Tablets 1919
Zyrtec Chewable Tablets 1920
Children's Zyrtec Allergy Chewable Tablets 1922
Children's Zyrtec Allergy Syrup 1920
Children's Zyrtec Hives Relief Syrup 1920
Zyrtec Syrup 1920
Zyrtec Tablets 1920
Zyrtec-D 12 Hour Extended Release Tablets 1923
Zyrtec-D Allergy & Congestion Extended-Release Tablets 1923

Chlorothiazide (Increases the concentration of the non-ionized species of the amphetamine molecule, thereby decreasing urinary excretion; increases amphetamines blood levels and thereby potentiates the actions of amphetamines).
No products indexed under this heading.

Chlorothiazide Sodium (Increases the concentration of the non-ionized species of the amphetamine molecule, thereby decreasing urinary excretion; increases amphetamines blood levels and thereby potentiates the actions of amphetamines).
Products include:
- Intravenous Sodium Diuril 2490

Chlorpheniramine Maleate (Amphetamines may counteract the sedative effect of antihistamine).
Products include:
- Actifed Cold & Allergy Tablets 1895
- Sudafed PE Sinus & Allergy Tablets 1908
- Tylenol Allergy Multi-Symptom Caplets with Cool Burst and Rapid Release Gelcaps 1916
- Children's Tylenol Plus Cold Suspension Liquid 1912
- Children's Tylenol Plus Cough & Runny Nose Suspension Liquid 1912
- Children's Tylenol Plus Flu Suspension Liquid 1914
- Children's Tylenol Plus Multi-Symptom Cold Suspension Liquid 1912
- Tylenol Cold Head Congestion Nighttime Caplets with Cool Burst 1910
- Tylenol Cold Multi-Symptom Nighttime Caplets with Cool Burst 1913
- Tylenol Sinus Congestion & Pain Nighttime Caplets with Cool Burst 1917

Chlorpheniramine Polistirex (Amphetamines may counteract the sedative effect of antihistamine).
Products include:
- Tussionex Pennkinetic Extended-Release Suspension 3154

Chlorpheniramine Tannate (Amphetamines may counteract the sedative effect of antihistamine).
No products indexed under this heading.

Chlorpromazine (Blocks dopamine and norepinephrine reuptake resulting in inhibition of central stimulating effects).
No products indexed under this heading.

Chlorpromazine Hydrochloride (Blocks dopamine and norepinephrine reuptake resulting in inhibition of central stimulating effects).
No products indexed under this heading.

Chlorthalidone (Amphetamine may antagonize the hypotensive effects of antihypertensives). Products include:
- Clorpres Tablets 2185

Clemastine Fumarate (Amphetamines may counteract the sedative effect of antihistamine).
No products indexed under this heading.

Clomipramine Hydrochloride (Enhanced activity of tricyclic or sympathomimetics; possible increases in the brain concentration of d-amphetamine in the brain; cardiovascular effect may be potentiated).
No products indexed under this heading.

Clonidine (Amphetamine may antagonize the hypotensive effects of antihypertensives). Products include:
- Catapres-TTS 842

Clonidine Hydrochloride (Amphetamine may antagonize the hypotensive effects of antihypertensives).
Products include:
- Catapres Tablets 841
- Clorpres Tablets 2185

Cryptenamine Preparations (Amphetamines inhibit the hypotensive effect of veratrum alkaloids).
No products indexed under this heading.

Cyproheptadine Hydrochloride (Amphetamines may counteract the sedative effect of antihistamine).
No products indexed under this heading.

Deserpidine (Amphetamine may antagonize the hypotensive effects of antihypertensives).
No products indexed under this heading.

Desipramine Hydrochloride (Enhanced activity of tricyclic or sympathomimetics; possible increases in the brain concentration of d-amphetamine in the brain; cardiovascular effect may be potentiated).
No products indexed under this heading.

Dexchlorpheniramine Maleate (Amphetamines may counteract the sedative effect of antihistamine).
No products indexed under this heading.

Diazoxide (Amphetamine may antagonize the hypotensive effects of antihypertensives). Products include:
- Proglycem Capsules 1185
- Proglycem Suspension 1185

Diltiazem Hydrochloride (Amphetamine may antagonize the hypotensive effects of antihypertensives).
Products include:
- Cardizem LA Extended Release Tablets 421

Diphenhydramine Citrate (Amphetamines may counteract the sedative effect of antihistamine).
No products indexed under this heading.

Diphenhydramine Hydrochloride (Amphetamines may counteract the sedative effect of antihistamine).
Products include:
- Benadryl Allergy & Cold Kapgels 1895
- Benadryl Allergy & Sinus Headache Kapgels 1895
- Benadryl Severe Allergy & Sinus Headache Caplets 1897
- Benadryl Dye-Free Allergy Liqui-gels Softgels 1897
- Benadryl Allergy Kapgels 1895
- Benadryl Allergy Quick Dissolve Strips 1896
- Benadryl Allergy Ultratab Tablets 1896
- Children's Benadryl Dye-Free Allergy Liquid 1897
- Children's Benadryl Allergy Fastmelts 1897
- Children's Benadryl Allergy Liquid 1898
- Children's Benadryl Allergy Perfect Measure 1896
- Children's Benadryl-D Allergy & Sinus Liquid 1896
- Benadryl-D Allergy & Sinus Tablet 1896
- PediaCare Children's Allergy & Cold Liquid 1902
- PediaCare Children's Allergy Liquid 1902
- Simply Sleep Caplets 1905
- Sudafed PE Nighttime Cold Caplets 1907
- Sudafed PE Severe Cold Caplets 1908
- Extra Strength Tylenol PM Caplets, Geltabs, Liquid, and Rapid Release Gels 1915
- Tylenol Allergy Multi-Symptom Nighttime Caplets with Cool Burst 1916
- Tylenol Severe Allergy Caplets 1916
- Children's Tylenol Plus Cold & Allergy Suspension Liquid 1914
- Tylenol Sore Throat Nighttime Liquid with Cool Burst 1918

Diphenylpyraline Hydrochloride (Amphetamines may counteract the sedative effect of antihistamine).
No products indexed under this heading.

Doxazosin Mesylate (Amphetamine may antagonize the hypotensive effects of antihypertensives).
No products indexed under this heading.

Doxepin Hydrochloride (Enhanced activity of tricyclic or sympathomimetics; possible increases in the brain concentration of d-amphetamine in the brain; cardiovascular effect may be potentiated).
No products indexed under this heading.

Enalapril Maleate (Amphetamine may antagonize the hypotensive effects of antihypertensives).
No products indexed under this heading.

Enalaprilat (Amphetamine may antagonize the hypotensive effects of antihypertensives).
No products indexed under this heading.

Eprosartan Mesylate (Amphetamine may antagonize the hypotensive effects of antihypertensives).
Products include:
- Teveten Tablets 515
- Teveten HCT Tablets 517

Esmolol Hydrochloride (Amphetamine may antagonize the hypotensive effects of antihypertensives; adrenergic blockers are inhibited by amphetamines).
No products indexed under this heading.

Ethosuximide (Amphetamine may delay intestinal absorption of ethosuximide).
No products indexed under this heading.

Felodipine (Amphetamine may antagonize the hypotensive effects of antihypertensives).
No products indexed under this heading.

Fexofenadine Hydrochloride (Amphetamines may counteract the sedative effect of antihistamine).
Products include:
- Allegra Oral Solution 2684
- Allegra Tablets 2684
- Allegra-D 12 Hour Extended-Release Tablets 2687
- Allegra-D 24 Hour Extended-Release Tablets 2690

Fosinopril Sodium (Amphetamine may antagonize the hypotensive effects of antihypertensives).
No products indexed under this heading.

Fosphenytoin Sodium (Amphetamine delays intestinal absorption of phenytoin; co-administration may produce synergestic anticonvulsant action).
No products indexed under this heading.

Furosemide (Amphetamine may antagonize the hypotensive effects of antihypertensives). Products include:
- Furosemide Tablets 2186

Glutamic Acid Hydrochloride (Lowers absorption of amphetamines).
No products indexed under this heading.

Guanabenz Acetate (Amphetamine may antagonize the hypotensive effects of antihypertensives).
No products indexed under this heading.

Guanethidine Monosulfate (Lowers absorption of amphetamines).
No products indexed under this heading.

Haloperidol (Blocks dopamine and norepinephrine reuptake resulting in inhibition of central stimulating effects).
No products indexed under this heading.

Haloperidol Decanoate (Blocks dopamine and norepinephrine reuptake resulting in inhibition of central stimulating effects).
No products indexed under this heading.

Hydralazine Hydrochloride (Amphetamine may antagonize the hypotensive effects of antihypertensives).
No products indexed under this heading.

Hydrochlorothiazide (Increases the concentration of the non-ionized species of the amphetamine molecule, thereby decreasing urinary excretion; increases amphetamines blood levels and thereby potentiates the actions of amphetamines).
Products include:
- Atacand HCT 642
- Avalide Tablets 892
- Avalide Tablets 2713
- Benicar HCT Tablets 1010
- Diovan HCT Tablets 2216
- Dyazide Capsules 1405
- Micardis HCT Tablets 854
- Prinzide Tablets 2092
- Tekturna HCT Tablets 2324
- Teveten HCT Tablets 517

Hydroflumethiazide (Increases the concentration of the non-ionized species of the amphetamine molecule, thereby decreasing urinary excretion; increases amphetamines blood levels and thereby potentiates the actions of amphetamines).
No products indexed under this heading.

Imipramine Hydrochloride (Enhanced activity of tricyclic or sympathomimetics; possible increases in the brain concentration of d-amphetamine in the brain; cardiovascular effect may be potentiated).
No products indexed under this heading.

Imipramine Pamoate (Enhanced activity of tricyclic or sympathomimetics; possible increases in the brain concentration of d-amphetamine in the brain; cardiovascular effect may be potentiated).
No products indexed under this heading.

Indapamide (Amphetamine may antagonize the hypotensive effects of antihypertensives). Products include:
- Indapamide Tablets 2188

IMPORTANT NOTE: Always consult each drug listing in the patient's regimen for possible interactions.

Irbesartan (Amphetamine may antagonize the hypotensive effects of antihypertensives). Products include:
- Avalide Tablets 892
- Avalide Tablets 2713
- Avapro Tablets 897
- Avapro Tablets 2718

Isocarboxazid (Concurrent and/or sequential use with MAO inhibitors is contraindicated; hypertensive crisis may occur). Products include:
- Marplan Tablets 3177

Isradipine (Amphetamine may antagonize the hypotensive effects of antihypertensives). Products include:
- DynaCirc CR Controlled Release Tablets 1407

Labetalol Hydrochloride (Amphetamine may antagonize the hypotensive effects of antihypertensives; adrenergic blockers are inhibited by amphetamines).
No products indexed under this heading.

Levobunolol Hydrochloride (Amphetamine may antagonize the hypotensive effects of antihypertensives; adrenergic blockers are inhibited by amphetamines).
No products indexed under this heading.

Lisinopril (Amphetamine may antagonize the hypotensive effects of antihypertensives). Products include:
- Prinivil Tablets 2087
- Prinzide Tablets 2092

Lithium Carbonate (Inhibits stimulatory effects of amphetamines).
No products indexed under this heading.

Loratadine (Amphetamines may counteract the sedative effect of antihistamine).
No products indexed under this heading.

Losartan Potassium (Amphetamine may antagonize the hypotensive effects of antihypertensives). Products include:
- Cozaar Tablets 1973

Maprotiline Hydrochloride (Enhanced activity of tricyclic or sympathomimetics; possible increases in the brain concentration of d-amphetamine in the brain; cardiovascular effect may be potentiated).
No products indexed under this heading.

Mecamylamine Hydrochloride (Amphetamine may antagonize the hypotensive effects of antihypertensives).
No products indexed under this heading.

Meperidine Hydrochloride (Amphetamine potentiates the analgesic effect of meperidine).
No products indexed under this heading.

Methdilazine Hydrochloride (Amphetamines may counteract the sedative effect of antihistamine).
No products indexed under this heading.

Methenamine (Acidifying agents used in methenamine therapy increases the urinary excretion and reduces the efficacy of amphetamine).
No products indexed under this heading.

Methenamine Hippurate (Acidifying agents used in methenamine therapy increases the urinary excretion and reduces the efficacy of amphetamine).
No products indexed under this heading.

Methenamine Mandelate (Acidifying agents used in methenamine therapy increases the urinary excretion and reduces the efficacy of amphetamine). Products include:
- Uroqid-Acid No. 2 Tablets 814

Methyclothiazide (Increases the concentration of the non-ionized species of the amphetamine molecule, thereby decreasing urinary excretion; increases amphetamines blood levels and thereby potentiates the actions of amphetamines).
No products indexed under this heading.

Methyldopa (Amphetamine may antagonize the hypotensive effects of antihypertensives).
No products indexed under this heading.

Methyldopate Hydrochloride (Amphetamine may antagonize the hypotensive effects of antihypertensives).
No products indexed under this heading.

Metipranolol Hydrochloride (Amphetamine may antagonize the hypotensive effects of antihypertensives; adrenergic blockers are inhibited by amphetamines).
No products indexed under this heading.

Metolazone (Amphetamine may antagonize the hypotensive effects of antihypertensives).
No products indexed under this heading.

Metoprolol Succinate (Amphetamine may antagonize the hypotensive effects of antihypertensives; adrenergic blockers are inhibited by amphetamines). Products include:
- Toprol-XL Tablets 666

Metoprolol Tartrate (Amphetamine may antagonize the hypotensive effects of antihypertensives; adrenergic blockers are inhibited by amphetamines).
No products indexed under this heading.

Metyrosine (Amphetamine may antagonize the hypotensive effects of antihypertensives). Products include:
- Demser Capsules 1989

Mibefradil Dihydrochloride (Amphetamine may antagonize the hypotensive effects of antihypertensives).
No products indexed under this heading.

Minoxidil (Amphetamine may antagonize the hypotensive effects of antihypertensives).
No products indexed under this heading.

Moclobemide (Concurrent and/or sequential use with MAO inhibitors is contraindicated; hypertensive crisis may occur).
No products indexed under this heading.

Moexipril Hydrochloride (Amphetamine may antagonize the hypotensive effects of antihypertensives).
No products indexed under this heading.

Nadolol (Amphetamine may antagonize the hypotensive effects of antihypertensives; adrenergic blockers are inhibited by amphetamines). Products include:
- Nadolol Tablets 2191

Nebivolol (Amphetamine may antagonize the hypotensive effects of antihypertensives; adrenergic blockers are inhibited by amphetamines). Products include:
- Bystolic Tablets 1155

Nicardipine Hydrochloride (Amphetamine may antagonize the hypotensive effects of antihypertensives). Products include:
- Cardene I.V. 1093

Nifedipine (Amphetamine may antagonize the hypotensive effects of antihypertensives).
No products indexed under this heading.

Nisoldipine (Amphetamine may antagonize the hypotensive effects of antihypertensives). Products include:
- Sular Extended Release Tablets 2975

Nitroglycerin (Amphetamine may antagonize the hypotensive effects of antihypertensives). Products include:
- Nitro-Dur Transdermal Infusion System 2887
- Nitrolingual Pumpspray 2965

Norepinephrine Hydrochloride (Enhances adenergic effect of norepinephrine).
No products indexed under this heading.

Nortriptyline Hydrochloride (Enhanced activity of tricyclic or sympathomimetics; possible increases in the brain concentration of d-amphetamine in the brain; cardiovascular effect may be potentiated).
No products indexed under this heading.

Pargyline Hydrochloride (Concurrent and/or sequential use with MAO inhibitors is contraindicated; hypertensive crisis may occur).
No products indexed under this heading.

Penbutolol Sulfate (Amphetamine may antagonize the hypotensive effects of antihypertensives; adrenergic blockers are inhibited by amphetamines).
No products indexed under this heading.

Perindopril Erbumine (Amphetamine may antagonize the hypotensive effects of antihypertensives). Products include:
- Aceon Tablets (2 mg, 4 mg, 8 mg) 3038

Phenelzine Sulfate (Concurrent and/or sequential use with MAO inhibitors is contraindicated; hypertensive crisis may occur).
No products indexed under this heading.

Phenobarbital (Amphetamine delays intestinal absorption of phenobarbital; co-administration may produce synergistic anticonvulsant action). Products include:
- Donnatal Extentabs 2507

Phenoxybenzamine Hydrochloride (Amphetamine may antagonize the hypotensive effects of antihypertensives). Products include:
- Dibenzyline Capsules 3188

Phentolamine Mesylate (Amphetamine may antagonize the hypotensive effects of antihypertensives).
No products indexed under this heading.

Phenytoin (Amphetamine delays intestinal absorption of phenytoin; co-administration may produce synergistic anticonvulsant action).
No products indexed under this heading.

Phenytoin Sodium (Amphetamine delays intestinal absorption of phenytoin; co-administration may produce synergistic anticonvulsant action). Products include:
- Phenytek Capsules 2192

Pindolol (Amphetamine may antagonize the hypotensive effects of antihypertensives; adrenergic blockers are inhibited by amphetamines).
No products indexed under this heading.

Polythiazide (Increases the concentration of the non-ionized species of the amphetamine molecule, thereby decreasing urinary excretion; increases amphetamines blood levels and thereby potentiates the actions of amphetamines).
No products indexed under this heading.

Potassium Citrate (Increases the concentration of the non-ionized species of the amphetamine molecule, thereby decreasing urinary excretion; increases amphetamines blood levels and thereby potentiates the actions of amphetamines). Products include:
- BioLean Free Tablets ..... ▣ 635
- Urocit-K Tablets 2176

Prazosin Hydrochloride (Amphetamine may antagonize the hypotensive effects of antihypertensives).
No products indexed under this heading.

Procarbazine Hydrochloride (Concurrent and/or sequential use with MAO inhibitors is contraindicated; hypertensive crisis may occur).
No products indexed under this heading.

Promethazine Hydrochloride (Amphetamines may counteract the sedative effect of antihistamine).
No products indexed under this heading.

Propoxyphene Hydrochloride (In cases of propoxyphene overdosage, amphetamine CNS stimulation is potentiated and fatal convulsions can occur).
No products indexed under this heading.

Propoxyphene Napsylate (In cases of propoxyphene overdosage, amphetamine CNS stimulation is potentiated and fatal convulsions can occur).
No products indexed under this heading.

Propranolol Hydrochloride (Amphetamine may antagonize the hypotensive effects of antihypertensives; adrenergic blockers are inhibited by amphetamines). Products include:
- InnoPran XL Extended Release Capsules 1484

Protriptyline Hydrochloride (Enhanced activity of tricyclic or sympathomimetics; possible increases in the brain concentration of d-amphetamine in the brain; cardiovascular effect may be potentiated).
No products indexed under this heading.

Pyrilamine Maleate (Amphetamines may counteract the sedative effect of antihistamine).
No products indexed under this heading.

Pyrilamine Tannate (Amphetamines may counteract the sedative effect of antihistamine).
No products indexed under this heading.

Quinapril Hydrochloride (Amphetamine may antagonize the hypotensive effects of antihypertensives).
No products indexed under this heading.

Ramipril (Amphetamine may antagonize the hypotensive effects of antihypertensives).
No products indexed under this heading.

Rasagiline Mesylate (Concurrent and/or sequential use with MAO inhibitors is contraindicated; hypertensive crisis may occur). Products include:
Azilect Tablets 3106

Rauwolfia Serpentina (Amphetamine may antagonize the hypotensive effects of antihypertensives).
No products indexed under this heading.

Rescinnamine (Amphetamine may antagonize the hypotensive effects of antihypertensives).
No products indexed under this heading.

Reserpine (Lowers absorption of amphetamines).
No products indexed under this heading.

Selegiline (Concurrent and/or sequential use with MAO inhibitors is contraindicated; hypertensive crisis may occur). Products include:
Emsam Transdermal System 905

Selegiline Hydrochloride (Concurrent and/or sequential use with MAO inhibitors is contraindicated; hypertensive crisis may occur). Products include:
Eldepryl Capsules 3052

Sodium Acid Phosphate (Increases the concentration of the ionized species of the amphetamine molecule, thereby increasing urinary excretion; lowers amphetamines blood levels and efficacy). Products include:
Uroqid-Acid No. 2 Tablets 814

Sodium Bicarbonate (Increases absorption of amphetamines). Products include:
Ceo-Two Laxative Suppository 815

Sodium Citrate (Increases the concentration of the non-ionized species of the amphetamine molecule, thereby decreasing urinary excretion; increases amphetamines blood levels and thereby potentiates the actions of amphetamines).
No products indexed under this heading.

Sodium Nitroprusside (Amphetamine may antagonize the hypotensive effects of antihypertensives).
No products indexed under this heading.

Sotalol Hydrochloride (Amphetamine may antagonize the hypotensive effects of antihypertensives; adrenergic blockers are inhibited by amphetamines).
No products indexed under this heading.

Spirapril Hydrochloride (Amphetamine may antagonize the hypotensive effects of antihypertensives).
No products indexed under this heading.

Telmisartan (Amphetamine may antagonize the hypotensive effects of antihypertensives). Products include:
Micardis Tablets 852
Micardis HCT Tablets 854

Terazosin Hydrochloride (Amphetamine may antagonize the hypotensive effects of antihypertensives).
No products indexed under this heading.

Terfenadine (Amphetamines may counteract the sedative effect of antihistamine).
No products indexed under this heading.

Timolol Hemihydrate (Amphetamine may antagonize the hypotensive effects of antihypertensives; adrenergic blockers are inhibited by amphetamines). Products include:
Betimol Ophthalmic Solution 3181

Timolol Maleate (Amphetamine may antagonize the hypotensive effects of antihypertensives; adrenergic blockers are inhibited by amphetamines). Products include:
Combigan Ophthalmic Solution 553
Cosopt Sterile Ophthalmic Solution 1969
Timoptic Sterile Ophthalmic Solution 2121
Timoptic in Ocudose 2124
Timoptic-XE Sterile Ophthalmic Gel Forming Solution 2125

Torsemide (Amphetamine may antagonize the hypotensive effects of antihypertensives). Products include:
Demadex Injection 2630
Demadex Tablets 2630

Trandolapril (Amphetamine may antagonize the hypotensive effects of antihypertensives). Products include:
Mavik Tablets 472
Tarka Tablets 511

Tranylcypromine Sulfate (Concurrent and/or sequential use with MAO inhibitors is contraindicated; hypertensive crisis may occur). Products include:
Parnate Tablets 1532

Trimeprazine Tartrate (Amphetamines may counteract the sedative effect of antihistamine).
No products indexed under this heading.

Trimethaphan Camsylate (Amphetamine may antagonize the hypotensive effects of antihypertensives).
No products indexed under this heading.

Trimipramine Maleate (Enhanced activity of tricyclic or sympathomimetics; possible increases in the brain concentration of d-amphetamine in the brain; cardiovascular effect may be potentiated).
No products indexed under this heading.

Tripelennamine Hydrochloride (Amphetamines may counteract the sedative effect of antihistamine).
No products indexed under this heading.

Triprolidine Hydrochloride (Amphetamines may counteract the sedative effect of antihistamine).
No products indexed under this heading.

Valsartan (Amphetamine may antagonize the hypotensive effects of antihypertensives). Products include:
Diovan Tablets 2212
Diovan HCT Tablets 2216
Exforge Tablets 2238

Verapamil Hydrochloride (Amphetamine may antagonize the hypotensive effects of antihypertensives). Products include:
Tarka Tablets 511

Vitamin C (Lowers absorption of amphetamines). Products include:
Bausch & Lomb Ocuvite Adult 50+ Vitamin and Mineral Supplement .... ⊙237
Comax Dietary Supplement 995
Ferralet 90 Tablets 2175
Glaucofit Dietary Supplement 995
Glauma Dietary Supplement 995
MoviPrep Oral Solution 2679
Procosa II Tablets 3174
Proflavanol 90 Tablets 3174
Tonox Dietary Supplement 995
Vibe Liquid Multi-Nutrient Supplement 626

Food Interactions

Fruit juices, unspecified (Lowers absorption of amphetamines).

DEXEDRINE TABLETS

(Dextroamphetamine Sulfate) 1401
See Dexedrine Spansule Sustained-Release Capsules

DHEA PLUS TABLETS

(Dihydroepiandrosterone (DHEA), Ginkgo biloba) 636
None cited in PDR database.

DIBENZYLINE CAPSULES

(Phenoxybenzamine Hydrochloride) ... 3188
May interact with:

Alpha and Beta Adrenergic Stimulators (Exaggerated hypotensive response; tachycardia).
No products indexed under this heading.

Epinephrine (Exaggerated hypotensive response; tachycardia). Products include:
EpiPen 1024

Epinephrine Bitartrate (Exaggerated hypotensive response; tachycardia).
No products indexed under this heading.

Norepinephrine Bitartrate (Hyperthermia production of levarterenol blocked by dibenzyline).
No products indexed under this heading.

Reserpine (Hypothermia production of reserpine blocked by dibenzyline).
No products indexed under this heading.

DICLOFENAC SODIUM OPHTHALMIC SOLUTION

(Diclofenac Sodium) .... ⊙240
May interact with aspirin-acetylsalicylic acid, anticoagulants, corticosteroids, and phenothiazines. Compounds in these categories include:

Anisindione (It is recommended that diclofenac sodium ophthalmic solution, like other NSAIDs, be used with caution in patients with known bleeding tendencies or who are receiving other medications which may prolong bleeding time).
No products indexed under this heading.

Ardeparin Sodium (It is recommended that diclofenac sodium ophthalmic solution, like other NSAIDs, be used with caution in patients with known bleeding tendencies or who are receiving other medications which may prolong bleeding time).
No products indexed under this heading.

Aspirin (There is the possibility of cross sensitivity to acetylsalicylic acid; caution should be used when treating individuals who have previously exhibited sensitivity to acetylsalicylic acid). Products include:
Aggrenox Capsules 819
Bayer Aspirin 750
Percodan Tablets 1130
St. Joseph 81 mg Aspirin Chewable and Enteric Coated Tablets 1903

Aspirin, Enteric Coated (There is the possibility of cross sensitivity to acetylsalicylic acid; caution should be used when treating individuals who have previously exhibited sensitivity to acetylsalicylic acid).
No products indexed under this heading.

Aspirin Buffered (There is the possibility of cross sensitivity to acetylsalicylic acid; caution should be used when treating individuals who have previously exhibited sensitivity to acetylsalicylic acid).
No products indexed under this heading.

Betamethasone Acetate (All topical NSAIDs may slow or delay healing. Topical corticosteroids are also known to slow or delay healing. Concomitant use of topical NSAIDs and topical steroids may increase the potential for healing problems).
No products indexed under this heading.

Betamethasone Sodium Phosphate (All topical NSAIDs may slow or delay healing. Topical corticosteroids are also known to slow or delay healing. Concomitant use of topical NSAIDs and topical steroids may increase the potential for healing problems).
No products indexed under this heading.

Budesonide (All topical NSAIDs may slow or delay healing. Topical corticosteroids are also known to slow or delay healing. Concomitant use of topical NSAIDs and topical steroids may increase the potential for healing problems). Products include:
Pulmicort Flexhaler 654
Symbicort 80/4.5 Inhalation Aerosol 659
Symbicort 160/4.5 Inhalation Aerosol 659

IMPORTANT NOTE: Always consult each drug listing in the patient's regimen for possible interactions.

Chlorpromazine (There is the possibility of cross sensitivity to phenylacetic acid derivatives; caution should be used when treating individuals who have previously exhibited sensitivity to phenylacetic acid derivatives).
No products indexed under this heading.

Chlorpromazine Hydrochloride (There is the possibility of cross sensitivity to phenylacetic acid derivatives; caution should be used when treating individuals who have previously exhibited sensitivity to phenylacetic acid derivatives).
No products indexed under this heading.

Ciclesonide (All topical NSAIDs may slow or delay healing. Topical corticosteroids are also known to slow or delay healing. Concomitant use of topical NSAIDs and topical steroids may increase the potential for healing problems). Products include:
Alvesco Inhalation Aerosol **2985**
Omnaris Nasal Spray **2998**

Cortisone Acetate (All topical NSAIDs may slow or delay healing. Topical corticosteroids are also known to slow or delay healing. Concomitant use of topical NSAIDs and topical steroids may increase the potential for healing problems).
No products indexed under this heading.

Dalteparin Sodium (It is recommended that diclofenac sodium ophthalmic solution, like other NSAIDs, be used with caution in patients with known bleeding tendencies or who are receiving other medications which may prolong bleeding time). Products include:
Fragmin Injection **1070**

Danaparoid Sodium (It is recommended that diclofenac sodium ophthalmic solution, like other NSAIDs, be used with caution in patients with known bleeding tendencies or who are receiving other medications which may prolong bleeding time).
No products indexed under this heading.

Dexamethasone (All topical NSAIDs may slow or delay healing. Topical corticosteroids are also known to slow or delay healing. Concomitant use of topical NSAIDs and topical steroids may increase the potential for healing problems). Products include:
Ciprodex Otic Suspension **541**

Dexamethasone Acetate (All topical NSAIDs may slow or delay healing. Topical corticosteroids are also known to slow or delay healing. Concomitant use of topical NSAIDs and topical steroids may increase the potential for healing problems).
No products indexed under this heading.

Dexamethasone Sodium Phosphate (All topical NSAIDs may slow or delay healing. Topical corticosteroids are also known to slow or delay healing. Concomitant use of topical NSAIDs and topical steroids may increase the potential for healing problems).
No products indexed under this heading.

Dicumarol (It is recommended that diclofenac sodium ophthalmic solution, like other NSAIDs, be used with caution in patients with known bleeding tendencies or who are receiving other medications which may prolong bleeding time).
No products indexed under this heading.

Enoxaparin Sodium (It is recommended that diclofenac sodium ophthalmic solution, like other NSAIDs, be used with caution in patients with known bleeding tendencies or who are receiving other medications which may prolong bleeding time). Products include:
Lovenox Injection **2756**

Fludrocortisone Acetate (All topical NSAIDs may slow or delay healing. Topical corticosteroids are also known to slow or delay healing. Concomitant use of topical NSAIDs and topical steroids may increase the potential for healing problems).
No products indexed under this heading.

Flunisolide (All topical NSAIDs may slow or delay healing. Topical corticosteroids are also known to slow or delay healing. Concomitant use of topical NSAIDs and topical steroids may increase the potential for healing problems). Products include:
Aerobid/Aerobid-M **1153**

Fluphenazine Decanoate (There is the possibility of cross sensitivity to phenylacetic acid derivatives; caution should be used when treating individuals who have previously exhibited sensitivity to phenylacetic acid derivatives).
No products indexed under this heading.

Fluphenazine Enanthate (There is the possibility of cross sensitivity to phenylacetic acid derivatives; caution should be used when treating individuals who have previously exhibited sensitivity to phenylacetic acid derivatives).
No products indexed under this heading.

Fluphenazine Hydrochloride (There is the possibility of cross sensitivity to phenylacetic acid derivatives; caution should be used when treating individuals who have previously exhibited sensitivity to phenylacetic acid derivatives).
No products indexed under this heading.

Fluticasone Propionate (All topical NSAIDs may slow or delay healing. Topical corticosteroids are also known to slow or delay healing. Concomitant use of topical NSAIDs and topical steroids may increase the potential for healing problems). Products include:
Advair Diskus 100/50 .... **1276**
Advair Diskus 250/50 .... **1276**
Advair Diskus 500/50 .... **1276**
Advair HFA 45/21 Inhalation Aerosol... **1288**
Advair HFA 115/21 Inhalation Aerosol... **1288**
Advair HFA 230/21 Inhalation Aerosol... **1288**
Flonase Nasal Spray **1431**
Flovent Diskus 50 mcg **1435**

Fluticasone Propionate HFA (All topical NSAIDs may slow or delay healing. Topical corticosteroids are also known to slow or delay healing. Concomitant use of topical NSAIDs and topical steroids may increase the potential for healing problems). Products include:
Flovent HFA **1440**

Fondaparinux Sodium (It is recommended that diclofenac sodium ophthalmic solution, like other NSAIDs, be used with caution in patients with known bleeding tendencies or who are receiving other medications which may prolong bleeding time). Products include:
Arixtra Injection **1313**

Heparin Calcium (It is recommended that diclofenac sodium ophthalmic solution, like other NSAIDs, be used with caution in patients with known bleeding tendencies or who are receiving other medications which may prolong bleeding time).
No products indexed under this heading.

Heparin Sodium (It is recommended that diclofenac sodium ophthalmic solution, like other NSAIDs, be used with caution in patients with known bleeding tendencies or who are receiving other medications which may prolong bleeding time).
No products indexed under this heading.

Hydrocortisone (All topical NSAIDs may slow or delay healing. Topical corticosteroids are also known to slow or delay healing. Concomitant use of topical NSAIDs and topical steroids may increase the potential for healing problems).
No products indexed under this heading.

Hydrocortisone Acetate (All topical NSAIDs may slow or delay healing. Topical corticosteroids are also known to slow or delay healing. Concomitant use of topical NSAIDs and topical steroids may increase the potential for healing problems). Products include:
Analpram-HC **1140**
Pramosone **1141**

Hydrocortisone Sodium Phosphate (All topical NSAIDs may slow or delay healing. Topical corticosteroids are also known to slow or delay healing. Concomitant use of topical NSAIDs and topical steroids may increase the potential for healing problems).
No products indexed under this heading.

Hydrocortisone Sodium Succinate (All topical NSAIDs may slow or delay healing. Topical corticosteroids are also known to slow or delay healing. Concomitant use of topical NSAIDs and topical steroids may increase the potential for healing problems).
No products indexed under this heading.

Low Molecular Weight Heparins (It is recommended that diclofenac sodium ophthalmic solution, like other NSAIDs, be used with caution in patients with known bleeding tendencies or who are receiving other medications which may prolong bleeding time).
No products indexed under this heading.

Mesoridazine Besylate (There is the possibility of cross sensitivity to phenylacetic acid derivatives; caution should be used when treating individuals who have previously exhibited sensitivity to phenylacetic acid derivatives).
No products indexed under this heading.

Methotrimeprazine (There is the possibility of cross sensitivity to phenylacetic acid derivatives; caution should be used when treating individuals who have previously exhibited sensitivity to phenylacetic acid derivatives).
No products indexed under this heading.

Methylprednisolone Acetate (All topical NSAIDs may slow or delay healing. Topical corticosteroids are also known to slow or delay healing. Concomitant use of topical NSAIDs and topical steroids may increase the potential for healing problems).
No products indexed under this heading.

Methylprednisolone Sodium Succinate (All topical NSAIDs may slow or delay healing. Topical corticosteroids are also known to slow or delay healing. Concomitant use of topical NSAIDs and topical steroids may increase the potential for healing problems).
No products indexed under this heading.

Mometasone Furoate (All topical NSAIDs may slow or delay healing. Topical corticosteroids are also known to slow or delay healing. Concomitant use of topical NSAIDs and topical steroids may increase the potential for healing problems). Products include:
Asmanex Twisthaler **2797**
Elocon Cream 0.1% **2840**
Elocon Lotion 0.1% **2841**
Elocon Ointment 0.1% **2842**

Mometasone Furoate Monohydrate (All topical NSAIDs may slow or delay healing. Topical corticosteroids are also known to slow or delay healing. Concomitant use of topical NSAIDs and topical steroids may increase the potential for healing problems). Products include:
Nasonex Nasal Spray **2883**

Perphenazine (There is the possibility of cross sensitivity to phenylacetic acid derivatives; caution should be used when treating individuals who have previously exhibited sensitivity to phenylacetic acid derivatives).
No products indexed under this heading.

Prednisolone Acetate (All topical NSAIDs may slow or delay healing. Topical corticosteroids are also known to slow or delay healing. Concomitant use of topical NSAIDs and topical steroids may increase the potential for healing problems). Products include:
Pred Forte Ophthalmic Suspension.............................. ⊙**227**
Pred Mild Ophthalmic Suspension.............................. ⊙**230**
Pred-G Ophthalmic Ointment .... ⊙**229**
Pred-G Ophthalmic Suspension ...... ⊙**228**

Prednisolone Sodium Phosphate (All topical NSAIDs may slow or delay healing. Topical corticosteroids are also known to slow or delay healing. Concomitant use of topical NSAIDs and topical steroids may increase the potential for healing problems).
No products indexed under this heading.

Prednisolone Tebutate (All topical NSAIDs may slow or delay healing. Topical corticosteroids are also known to slow or delay healing. Concomitant use of topical NSAIDs and topical steroids may increase the potential for healing problems).
No products indexed under this heading.

Prednisone (All topical NSAIDs may slow or delay healing. Topical corticosteroids are also known to slow or delay healing. Concomitant use of topical NSAIDs and topical steroids may increase the potential for healing problems).
No products indexed under this heading.

Prochlorperazine (There is the possibility of cross sensitivity to phenylacetic acid derivatives; caution should be used when treating individuals who have previously exhibited sensitivity to phenylacetic acid derivatives).
No products indexed under this heading.

Promethazine Hydrochloride (There is the possibility of cross sensitivity to phenylacetic acid derivatives; caution should be used when treating individuals who have previously exhibited sensitivity to phenylacetic acid derivatives).
No products indexed under this heading.

Thioridazine Hydrochloride (There is the possibility of cross sensitivity to phenylacetic acid derivatives; caution should be used when treating individuals who have previously exhibited sensitivity to phenylacetic acid derivatives). Products include:
Thioridazine Hydrochloride Tablets 2195

Tinzaparin Sodium (It is recommended that diclofenac sodium ophthalmic solution, like other NSAIDs, be used with caution in patients with known bleeding tendencies or who are receiving other medications which may prolong bleeding time).
No products indexed under this heading.

Triamcinolone (All topical NSAIDs may slow or delay healing. Topical corticosteroids are also known to slow or delay healing. Concomitant use of topical NSAIDs and topical steroids may increase the potential for healing problems).
No products indexed under this heading.

Triamcinolone Acetonide (All topical NSAIDs may slow or delay healing. Topical corticosteroids are also known to slow or delay healing. Concomitant use of topical NSAIDs and topical steroids may increase the potential for healing problems). Products include:
Azmacort Inhalation Aerosol 407
Nasacort AQ Nasal Spray 2765
Triesence Injectable Suspension .... ⊙ 209

Triamcinolone Diacetate (All topical NSAIDs may slow or delay healing. Topical corticosteroids are also known to slow or delay healing. Concomitant use of topical NSAIDs and topical steroids may increase the potential for healing problems).
No products indexed under this heading.

Triamcinolone Hexacetonide (All topical NSAIDs may slow or delay healing. Topical corticosteroids are also known to slow or delay healing. Concomitant use of topical NSAIDs and topical steroids may increase the potential for healing problems).
No products indexed under this heading.

Trifluoperazine Hydrochloride (There is the possibility of cross sensitivity to phenylacetic acid derivatives; caution should be used when treating individuals who have previously exhibited sensitivity to phenylacetic acid derivatives).
No products indexed under this heading.

Warfarin Sodium (It is recommended that diclofenac sodium ophthalmic solution, like other NSAIDs, be used with caution in patients with known bleeding tendencies or who are receiving other medications which may prolong bleeding time).
No products indexed under this heading.

DIDRONEL TABLETS

(Etidronate Disodium) 2583
May interact with:

Warfarin Sodium (Co-administration has resulted in isolated reports of increase in prothrombin time without clinically significant sequelae).
No products indexed under this heading.

DIGIBIND FOR INJECTION

(Digoxin Immune Fab (Ovine)) 1403
None cited in PDR database.

DIOVAN TABLETS

(Valsartan) 2212
May interact with potassium preparations, potassium sparing diuretics, and certain other agents. Compounds in these categories include:

Amiloride Hydrochloride (Concurrent use may lead to hyperkalemia; potential for increase in serum creatinine in heart failure patients if used concurrently).
No products indexed under this heading.

Atenolol (Combination therapy is more antihypertensive than either component, but does not lower the heart rate more than atenolol alone).
No products indexed under this heading.

Potassium Acid Phosphate (Concurrent use may lead to hyperkalemia; potential for increase in serum creatinine in heart failure patients if used concurrently). Products include:
K-Phos Original (Sodium Free) Tablets 814

Potassium Bicarbonate (Concurrent use may lead to hyperkalemia; potential for increase in serum creatinine in heart failure patients if used concurrently).
No products indexed under this heading.

Potassium Chloride (Concurrent use may lead to hyperkalemia; potential for increase in serum creatinine in heart failure patients if used concurrently). Products include:
MoviPrep Oral Solution 2679

Potassium Citrate (Concurrent use may lead to hyperkalemia; potential for increase in serum creatinine in heart failure patients if used concurrently). Products include:
BioLean Free Tablets 635
Urocit-K Tablets 2176

Potassium Gluconate (Concurrent use may lead to hyperkalemia; potential for increase in serum creatinine in heart failure patients if used concurrently).
No products indexed under this heading.

Potassium Phosphate (Concurrent use may lead to hyperkalemia; potential for increase in serum creatinine in heart failure patients if used concurrently). Products include:
K-Phos Neutral Tablets 813

Salt Substitutes (Concurrent use may lead to hyperkalemia; potential for increase in serum creatinine in heart failure patients if used concurrently).
No products indexed under this heading.

Spironolactone (Concurrent use may lead to hyperkalemia; potential for increase in serum creatinine in heart failure patients if used concurrently).
No products indexed under this heading.

Triamterene (Concurrent use may lead to hyperkalemia; potential for increase in serum creatinine in heart failure patients if used concurrently). Products include:
Dyazide Capsules 1405
Dyrenium Capsules 3189

Food Interactions

Food, unspecified (Decreases the exposure (as measured by AUC) to valsartan about 40% and peak plasma concentration by about 50%).

DIOVAN HCT TABLETS

(Hydrochlorothiazide, Valsartan) 2216
May interact with antihypertensives, barbiturates, corticosteroids, cardiac glycosides, oral hypoglycemic agents, insulin, lithium preparations, narcotic analgesics, nondepolarizing neuromuscular blocking agents, nonsteroidal anti-inflammatory agents, potassium preparations, and certain other agents. Compounds in these categories include:

Acarbose (Dosage adjustment of the antidiabetic drug may be required). Products include:
Precose Tablets 792

Acebutolol Hydrochloride (Co-administration with other antihypertensives may result in additive effect or potentiation).
No products indexed under this heading.

ACTH (Co-administration of thiazide diuretics and ACTH may intensify electrolyte depletion, particularly hypokalemia).
No products indexed under this heading.

Alfentanil Hydrochloride (Co-administration of thiazide diuretics and narcotics may result in potentiation of orthostatic hypotension).
No products indexed under this heading.

Aliskiren (Co-administration with other antihypertensives may result in additive effect or potentiation). Products include:
Tekturna Tablets 2321
Tekturna HCT Tablets 2324

Amlodipine Besylate (Co-administration with other antihypertensives may result in additive effect or potentiation). Products include:
Azor Tablets 1005
Exforge Tablets 2238

Aprobarbital (Co-administration of thiazide diuretics and barbiturates may result in potentiation of orthostatic hypotension).
No products indexed under this heading.

Atenolol (Co-administration with other antihypertensives may result in additive effect or potentiation).
No products indexed under this heading.

Atracurium Besylate (Co-administration of thiazide diuretics and nondepolarizing skeletal muscle relaxants increases responsiveness to the muscle relaxants).
No products indexed under this heading.

Benazepril Hydrochloride (Co-administration with other antihypertensives may result in additive effect or potentiation).
No products indexed under this heading.

Bendroflumethiazide (Co-administration with other antihypertensives may result in additive effect or potentiation).
No products indexed under this heading.

Betamethasone Acetate (Co-administration of thiazide diuretics and corticosteroids may intensify electrolyte depletion, particularly hypokalemia).
No products indexed under this heading.

Betamethasone Sodium Phosphate (Co-administration of thiazide diuretics and corticosteroids may intensify electrolyte depletion, particularly hypokalemia).
No products indexed under this heading.

Betaxolol Hydrochloride (Co-administration with other antihypertensives may result in additive effect or potentiation).
No products indexed under this heading.

Bisoprolol Fumarate (Co-administration with other antihypertensives may result in additive effect or potentiation).
No products indexed under this heading.

Budesonide (Co-administration of thiazide diuretics and corticosteroids may intensify electrolyte depletion, particularly hypokalemia). Products include:
Pulmicort Flexhaler 654
Symbicort 80/4.5 Inhalation Aerosol 659
Symbicort 160/4.5 Inhalation Aerosol 659

Buprenorphine Hydrochloride (Co-administration of thiazide diuretics and narcotics may result in potentiation of orthostatic hypotension). Products include:
Suboxone Tablets 2601
Subutex Tablets 2601

Butabarbital (Co-administration of thiazide diuretics and barbiturates may result in potentiation of orthostatic hypotension).
No products indexed under this heading.

Butalbital (Co-administration of thiazide diuretics and barbiturates may result in potentiation of orthostatic hypotension).
No products indexed under this heading.

Candesartan Cilexetil (Co-administration with other antihypertensives may result in additive effect or potentiation). Products include:
Atacand Tablets 639
Atacand HCT 642

Captopril (Co-administration with other antihypertensives may result in additive effect or potentiation). Products include:
Captopril Tablets 2182

Carteolol Hydrochloride (Co-administration with other antihypertensives may result in additive effect or potentiation).
No products indexed under this heading.

Celecoxib (Co-administration of thiazide diuretics and non-steroidal anti-inflammatory agents can reduce the diuretic, natiuretic, and antihypertensive effects). Products include:
Celebrex Capsules 2979

Chlorothiazide (Co-administration with other antihypertensives may result in additive effect or potentiation).
No products indexed under this heading.

Chlorothiazide Sodium (Co-administration with other antihypertensives may result in additive effect or potentiation). Products include:
Intravenous Sodium Diuril 2490

Chlorpropamide (Dosage adjustment of the antidiabetic drug may be required).
No products indexed under this heading.

Chlorthalidone (Co-administration with other antihypertensives may result in additive effect or potentiation). Products include:
Clorpres Tablets 2185

Cholestyramine (Absorption of hydrochlorothiazide is impaired in the presence of anionic exchange resins, such as cholestyramine resulting in binding of the hydrochlorothiazide resulting in reduced absorption from GI tract by up to 85%).
No products indexed under this heading.

Ciclesonide (Co-administration of thiazide diuretics and corticosteroids may intensify electrolyte depletion, particularly hypokalemia). Products include:
Alvesco Inhalation Aerosol 2985
Omnaris Nasal Spray 2998

Cisatracurium Besylate (Co-administration of thiazide diuretics and nondepolarizing skeletal muscle relaxants increases responsiveness to the muscle relaxants). Products include:
Nimbex Injection 484

Clonidine (Co-administration with other antihypertensives may result in additive effect or potentiation). Products include:
Catapres-TTS 842

Clonidine Hydrochloride (Co-administration with other antihypertensives may result in additive effect or potentiation). Products include:
Catapres Tablets 841
Clorpres Tablets 2185

Codeine Phosphate (Co-administration of thiazide diuretics and narcotics may result in potentiation of orthostatic hypotension). Products include:
Tylenol with Codeine Tablets 2427

Colestipol Hydrochloride (Absorption of hydrochlorothiazide is impaired in the presence of anionic exchange resins, such as colestipol resulting in binding of the hydrochlorothiazide resulting in reduced absorption from GI tract by up to 43%).
No products indexed under this heading.

Cortisone Acetate (Co-administration of thiazide diuretics and corticosteroids may intensify electrolyte depletion, particularly hypokalemia).
No products indexed under this heading.

Deserpidine (Co-administration with other antihypertensives may result in additive effect or potentiation).
No products indexed under this heading.

Deslanoside (Hypokalemia induced by thiazides may cause cardiac arrhythmia and may sensitize or exaggerate the response of the heart to the toxic effects of digitalis, such as increased ventricular irritability).
No products indexed under this heading.

Dexamethasone (Co-administration of thiazide diuretics and corticosteroids may intensify electrolyte depletion, particularly hypokalemia). Products include:
Ciprodex Otic Suspension 541

Dexamethasone Acetate (Co-administration of thiazide diuretics and corticosteroids may intensify electrolyte depletion, particularly hypokalemia).
No products indexed under this heading.

Dexamethasone Sodium Phosphate (Co-administration of thiazide diuretics and corticosteroids may intensify electrolyte depletion, particularly hypokalemia).
No products indexed under this heading.

Dezocine (Co-administration of thiazide diuretics and narcotics may result in potentiation of orthostatic hypotension).
No products indexed under this heading.

Diazoxide (Co-administration with other antihypertensives may result in additive effect or potentiation). Products include:
Proglycem Capsules 1185
Proglycem Suspension 1185

Diclofenac Epolamine (Co-administration of thiazide diuretics and non-steroidal anti-inflammatory agents can reduce the diuretic, natiuretic, and antihypertensive effects). Products include:
Flector Patch 561

Diclofenac Potassium (Co-administration of thiazide diuretics and non-steroidal anti-inflammatory agents can reduce the diuretic, natiuretic, and antihypertensive effects).
No products indexed under this heading.

Diclofenac Sodium (Co-administration of thiazide diuretics and non-steroidal anti-inflammatory agents can reduce the diuretic, natiuretic, and antihypertensive effects). Products include:
Diclofenac Sodium Ophthalmic Solution .... ⊙ 240
Voltaren Ophthalmic Solution 2336
Voltaren Tablets 2334
Voltaren-XR Tablets 2337

Digitalis Glycoside Preparations (Hypokalemia induced by thiazides may cause cardiac arrhythmia and may sensitize or exaggerate the response of the heart to the toxic effects of digitalis, such as increased ventricular irritability).
No products indexed under this heading.

Digitoxin (Hypokalemia induced by thiazides may cause cardiac arrhythmia and may sensitize or exaggerate the response of the heart to the toxic effects of digitalis, such as increased ventricular irritability).
No products indexed under this heading.

Digoxin (Hypokalemia induced by thiazides may cause cardiac arrhythmia and may sensitize or exaggerate the response of the heart to the toxic effects of digitalis, such as increased ventricular irritability). Products include:
Lanoxin Injection 1498
Lanoxin Injection Pediatric 1502
Lanoxin Tablets 1505

Diltiazem Hydrochloride (Co-administration with other antihypertensives may result in additive effect or potentiation). Products include:
Cardizem LA Extended Release Tablets 421

Doxazosin Mesylate (Co-administration with other antihypertensives may result in additive effect or potentiation).
No products indexed under this heading.

Enalapril Maleate (Co-administration with other antihypertensives may result in additive effect or potentiation).
No products indexed under this heading.

Enalaprilat (Co-administration with other antihypertensives may result in additive effect or potentiation).
No products indexed under this heading.

Eprosartan Mesylate (Co-administration with other antihypertensives may result in additive effect or potentiation). Products include:
Teveten Tablets 515
Teveten HCT Tablets 517

Esmolol Hydrochloride (Co-administration with other antihypertensives may result in additive effect or potentiation).
No products indexed under this heading.

Etodolac (Co-administration of thiazide diuretics and non-steroidal anti-inflammatory agents can reduce the diuretic, natiuretic, and antihypertensive effects).
No products indexed under this heading.

Felodipine (Co-administration with other antihypertensives may result in additive effect or potentiation).
No products indexed under this heading.

Fenoprofen Calcium (Co-administration of thiazide diuretics and non-steroidal anti-inflammatory agents can reduce the diuretic, natiuretic, and antihypertensive effects). Products include:
Nalfon Capsules 2508

Fentanyl (Co-administration of thiazide diuretics and narcotics may result in potentiation of orthostatic hypotension). Products include:
Duragesic Transdermal System 2405
Ionsys Transdermal System 2410

Fentanyl Citrate (Co-administration of thiazide diuretics and narcotics may result in potentiation of orthostatic hypotension). Products include:
Actiq 959
Fentora Tablets 968

Fludrocortisone Acetate (Co-administration of thiazide diuretics and corticosteroids may intensify electrolyte depletion, particularly hypokalemia).
No products indexed under this heading.

Flunisolide (Co-administration of thiazide diuretics and corticosteroids may intensify electrolyte depletion, particularly hypokalemia). Products include:
Aerobid/Aerobid-M 1153

Flurbiprofen (Co-administration of thiazide diuretics and non-steroidal anti-inflammatory agents can reduce the diuretic, natiuretic, and antihypertensive effects).
No products indexed under this heading.

Fluticasone Propionate (Co-administration of thiazide diuretics and corticosteroids may intensify electrolyte depletion, particularly hypokalemia). Products include:
Advair Diskus 100/50 1276
Advair Diskus 250/50 1276
Advair Diskus 500/50 1276
Advair HFA 45/21 Inhalation Aerosol 1288
Advair HFA 115/21 Inhalation Aerosol 1288
Advair HFA 230/21 Inhalation Aerosol 1288
Flonase Nasal Spray 1431
Flovent Diskus 50 mcg 1435

Fluticasone Propionate HFA (Co-administration of thiazide diuretics and corticosteroids may intensify electrolyte depletion, particularly hypokalemia). Products include:
Flovent HFA 1440

Fosinopril Sodium (Co-administration with other antihypertensives may result in additive effect or potentiation).
No products indexed under this heading.

Furosemide (Co-administration with other antihypertensives may result in additive effect or potentiation). Products include:
Furosemide Tablets 2186

Glimepiride (Dosage adjustment of the antidiabetic drug may be required). Products include:
Avandaryl Tablets 1344
Duetact Tablets 3085

Glipizide (Dosage adjustment of the antidiabetic drug may be required).
No products indexed under this heading.

Glyburide (Dosage adjustment of the antidiabetic drug may be required).
No products indexed under this heading.

Guanabenz Acetate (Co-administration with other antihypertensives may result in additive effect or potentiation).
No products indexed under this heading.

Guanethidine Monosulfate (Co-administration with other antihypertensives may result in additive effect or potentiation).
No products indexed under this heading.

Hydralazine Hydrochloride (Co-administration with other antihypertensives may result in additive effect or potentiation).
No products indexed under this heading.

Hydrocodone Bitartrate (Co-administration of thiazide diuretics and narcotics may result in potentiation of orthostatic hypotension). Products include:
Lortab 5/500 Tablets 3143
Lortab 7.5/500 Tablets 3144
Lortab 10/500 Tablets 3144
Vicodin Tablets 529
Vicodin ES Tablets 530
Vicodin HP Tablets 531
Vicoprofen Tablets 533
Zydone Tablets 1132

Hydrocodone Polistirex (Co-administration of thiazide diuretics and narcotics may result in potentiation of orthostatic hypotension). Products include:
Tussionex Pennkinetic Extended-Release Suspension 3154

Hydrocortisone (Co-administration of thiazide diuretics and corticosteroids may intensify electrolyte depletion, particularly hypokalemia).
No products indexed under this heading.

Hydrocortisone Acetate (Co-administration of thiazide diuretics and corticosteroids may intensify electrolyte depletion, particularly hypokalemia). Products include:
Analpram-HC 1140
Pramosone 1141

Hydrocortisone Sodium Phosphate (Co-administration of thiazide diuretics and corticosteroids may intensify electrolyte depletion, particularly hypokalemia).
No products indexed under this heading.

Hydrocortisone Sodium Succinate (Co-administration of thiazide diuretics and corticosteroids may intensify electrolyte depletion, particularly hypokalemia).
No products indexed under this heading.

Hydroflumethiazide (Co-administration with other antihypertensives may result in additive effect or potentiation).
No products indexed under this heading.

Hydromorphone Hydrochloride (Co-administration of thiazide diuretics and narcotics may result in potentiation of orthostatic hypotension).
No products indexed under this heading.

Ibuprofen (Co-administration of thiazide diuretics and non-steroidal anti-inflammatory agents can reduce the diuretic, natiuretic, and antihypertensive effects). Products include:
Motrin IB Tablets and Caplets 1900
Children's Motrin Oral Suspension 1901
Children's Motrin Non-Staining Dye-Free Oral Suspension 1901
Children's Motrin Cold Oral Suspension 1899
Infants' Motrin Concentrated Drops 1901
Infants' Motrin Non-Staining Dye-Free Concentrated Drops 1901
Junior Strength Motrin Caplets and Chewable Tablets 1901
Vicoprofen Tablets 533

Indapamide (Co-administration with other antihypertensives may result in additive effect or potentiation). Products include:
Indapamide Tablets 2188

Indomethacin (Co-administration of thiazide diuretics and non-steroidal anti-inflammatory agents can reduce the diuretic, natiuretic, and antihypertensive effects). Products include:
Indocin 2024

Indomethacin Sodium Trihydrate (Co-administration of thiazide diuretics and non-steroidal anti-inflammatory agents can reduce the diuretic, natiuretic, and antihypertensive effects). Products include:
Indocin I.V. 2489

Insulin (Dosage adjustment of the antidiabetic drug may be required).
No products indexed under this heading.

Insulin, Human, Zinc Suspension (Dosage adjustment of the antidiabetic drug may be required).
No products indexed under this heading.

Insulin, Human (rDNA origin) (Dosage adjustment of the antidiabetic drug may be required). Products include:
Exubera Inhalation Powder 2515

Insulin, Human NPH (Dosage adjustment of the antidiabetic drug may be required). Products include:
Humulin N Vial 1846

Insulin, Human Regular (Dosage adjustment of the antidiabetic drug may be required). Products include:
Humulin R 1849
Humulin R (U-500) 1850

Insulin, Human Regular and Human NPH Mixture (Dosage adjustment of the antidiabetic drug may be required). Products include:
Humulin 50/50, 100 Units 1843
Humulin 70/30 Vial 1844

Insulin, NPH (Dosage adjustment of the antidiabetic drug may be required).
No products indexed under this heading.

Insulin, Regular (Dosage adjustment of the antidiabetic drug may be required).
No products indexed under this heading.

Insulin, Regular and NPH mixture (Dosage adjustment of the antidiabetic drug may be required).
No products indexed under this heading.

Insulin, Zinc Crystals (Dosage adjustment of the antidiabetic drug may be required).
No products indexed under this heading.

Insulin, Zinc Suspension (Dosage adjustment of the antidiabetic drug may be required).
No products indexed under this heading.

Insulin Aspart (Dosage adjustment of the antidiabetic drug may be required).
No products indexed under this heading.

Insulin Aspart, Human (Dosage adjustment of the antidiabetic drug may be required). Products include:
NovoLog Mix 70/30 2364

Insulin Aspart, Human Regular (Dosage adjustment of the antidiabetic drug may be required). Products include:
NovoLog Injection 2359

Insulin Aspart Protamine, Human (Dosage adjustment of the antidiabetic drug may be required). Products include:
NovoLog Mix 70/30 2364

Insulin Detemir (rDNA Origin) (Dosage adjustment of the antidiabetic drug may be required). Products include:
Levemir Injection 2352

Insulin glargine (Dosage adjustment of the antidiabetic drug may be required). Products include:
Lantus Injection 2749

Insulin Glulisine (Dosage adjustment of the antidiabetic drug may be required). Products include:
Apidra Injection 2706

Insulin Lispro, Human (Dosage adjustment of the antidiabetic drug may be required). Products include:
Humalog-Pen and KwikPen 1829
Humalog Mix 50/50-Pen and KwikPen 1833
Humalog Mix 75/25-Pen and KwikPen 1835

Insulin Lispro Protamine, Human (Dosage adjustment of the antidiabetic drug may be required). Products include:
Humalog Mix 50/50-Pen and KwikPen 1833
Humalog Mix 75/25-Pen and KwikPen 1835

Irbesartan (Co-administration with other antihypertensives may result in additive effect or potentiation). Products include:
Avalide Tablets 892
Avalide Tablets 2713
Avapro Tablets 897
Avapro Tablets 2718

Isradipine (Co-administration with other antihypertensives may result in additive effect or potentiation). Products include:
DynaCirc CR Controlled Release Tablets 1407

Ketoprofen (Co-administration of thiazide diuretics and non-steroidal anti-inflammatory agents can reduce the diuretic, natiuretic, and antihypertensive effects).
No products indexed under this heading.

Ketorolac Tromethamine (Co-administration of thiazide diuretics and non-steroidal anti-inflammatory agents can reduce the diuretic, natiuretic, and antihypertensive effects).
No products indexed under this heading.

Labetalol Hydrochloride (Co-administration with other antihypertensives may result in additive effect or potentiation).
No products indexed under this heading.

Levorphanol Tartrate (Co-administration of thiazide diuretics and narcotics may result in potentiation of orthostatic hypotension).
No products indexed under this heading.

Lisinopril (Co-administration with other antihypertensives may result in additive effect or potentiation). Products include:
Prinivil Tablets 2087
Prinzide Tablets 2092

Lithium (Diuretics reduce the renal clearance of lithium and add a high risk of lithium toxicity; concurrent use should be avoided).
No products indexed under this heading.

Lithium Carbonate (Diuretics reduce the renal clearance of lithium and add a high risk of lithium toxicity; concurrent use should be avoided).
No products indexed under this heading.

Lithium Citrate (Diuretics reduce the renal clearance of lithium and add a high risk of lithium toxicity; concurrent use should be avoided).
No products indexed under this heading.

Losartan Potassium (Co-administration with other antihypertensives may result in additive effect or potentiation). Products include:
Cozaar Tablets 1973

Mecamylamine Hydrochloride (Co-administration with other antihypertensives may result in additive effect or potentiation).
No products indexed under this heading.

Meclofenamate Sodium (Co-administration of thiazide diuretics and non-steroidal anti-inflammatory agents can reduce the diuretic, natiuretic, and antihypertensive effects).
No products indexed under this heading.

Mefenamic Acid (Co-administration of thiazide diuretics and non-steroidal anti-inflammatory agents can reduce the diuretic, natiuretic, and antihypertensive effects).
No products indexed under this heading.

Meloxicam (Co-administration of thiazide diuretics and non-steroidal anti-inflammatory agents can reduce the diuretic, natiuretic, and antihypertensive effects). Products include:
Mobic Oral Suspension 863
Mobic Tablets 863

Meperidine Hydrochloride (Co-administration of thiazide diuretics and narcotics may result in potentiation of orthostatic hypotension).
No products indexed under this heading.

Mephobarbital (Co-administration of thiazide diuretics and barbiturates may result in potentiation of orthostatic hypotension).
No products indexed under this heading.

Metformin Hydrochloride (Dosage adjustment of the antidiabetic drug may be required). Products include:
ActoPlus Met Tablets 3071
Avandamet Tablets 1336
Janumet Tablets 2041
PrandiMet Tablets 2967

Methadone Hydrochloride (Co-administration of thiazide diuretics and narcotics may result in potentiation of orthostatic hypotension).
No products indexed under this heading.

Methyclothiazide (Co-administration with other antihypertensives may result in additive effect or potentiation).
No products indexed under this heading.

Methyldopa (Co-administration with other antihypertensives may result in additive effect or potentiation).
No products indexed under this heading.

Methyldopate Hydrochloride (Co-administration with other antihypertensives may result in additive effect or potentiation).
No products indexed under this heading.

Methylprednisolone Acetate (Co-administration of thiazide diuretics and corticosteroids may intensify electrolyte depletion, particularly hypokalemia).
No products indexed under this heading.

Methylprednisolone Sodium Succinate (Co-administration of thiazide diuretics and corticosteroids may intensify electrolyte depletion, particularly hypokalemia).
No products indexed under this heading.

Metocurine Iodide (Co-administration of thiazide diuretics and nondepolarizing skeletal muscle relaxants increases responsiveness to the muscle relaxants).
No products indexed under this heading.

Metolazone (Co-administration with other antihypertensives may result in additive effect or potentiation).
No products indexed under this heading.

Metoprolol Succinate (Co-administration with other antihypertensives may result in additive effect or potentiation). Products include:
Toprol-XL Tablets 666

Metoprolol Tartrate (Co-administration with other antihypertensives may result in additive effect or potentiation).
No products indexed under this heading.

Metyrosine (Co-administration with other antihypertensives may result in additive effect or potentiation). Products include:
Demser Capsules 1989

Mibefradil Dihydrochloride (Co-administration with other antihypertensives may result in additive effect or potentiation).
No products indexed under this heading.

Miglitol (Dosage adjustment of the antidiabetic drug may be required).
No products indexed under this heading.

Minoxidil (Co-administration with other antihypertensives may result in additive effect or potentiation).
No products indexed under this heading.

Mivacurium Chloride (Co-administration of thiazide diuretics and nondepolarizing skeletal muscle relaxants increases responsiveness to the muscle relaxants).
No products indexed under this heading.

Moexipril Hydrochloride (Co-administration with other antihypertensives may result in additive effect or potentiation).
No products indexed under this heading.

Mometasone Furoate (Co-administration of thiazide diuretics and corticosteroids may intensify electrolyte depletion, particularly hypokalemia). Products include:
Asmanex Twisthaler 2797
Elocon Cream 0.1% 2840
Elocon Lotion 0.1% 2841
Elocon Ointment 0.1% 2842

Mometasone Furoate Monohydrate (Co-administration of thiazide diuretics and corticosteroids may intensify electrolyte depletion, particularly hypokalemia). Products include:
Nasonex Nasal Spray 2883

Morphine Sulfate (Co-administration of thiazide diuretics and narcotics may result in potentiation of orthostatic hypotension). Products include:
Avinza Capsules 1772
DepoDur Injection 1095
MS Contin Tablets 2585

Nabumetone (Co-administration of thiazide diuretics and non-steroidal anti-inflammatory agents can reduce the diuretic, natiuretic, and antihypertensive effects).
No products indexed under this heading.

Nadolol (Co-administration with other antihypertensives may result in additive effect or potentiation). Products include:
Nadolol Tablets 2191

Naproxen (Co-administration of thiazide diuretics and non-steroidal anti-inflammatory agents can reduce the diuretic, natiuretic, and antihypertensive effects). Products include:
EC-Naprosyn Delayed-Release Tablets 2632
Naprosyn Suspension 2632
Naprosyn Tablets 2632

Naproxen Sodium (Co-administration of thiazide diuretics and non-steroidal anti-inflammatory agents can reduce the diuretic, natiuretic, and antihypertensive effects). Products include:
Anaprox Tablets 2632
Anaprox DS Tablets 2632
Treximet Tablets 1616

Nateglinide (Dosage adjustment of the antidiabetic drug may be required). Products include:
Starlix Tablets 2314

Nebivolol (Co-administration with other antihypertensives may result in additive effect or potentiation). Products include:
Bystolic Tablets 1155

Nicardipine Hydrochloride (Co-administration with other antihypertensives may result in additive effect or potentiation). Products include:
Cardene I.V. 1093

Nifedipine (Co-administration with other antihypertensives may result in additive effect or potentiation).
No products indexed under this heading.

Nisoldipine (Co-administration with other antihypertensives may result in additive effect or potentiation). Products include:
Sular Extended Release Tablets 2975

Nitroglycerin (Co-administration with other antihypertensives may result in additive effect or potentiation). Products include:
Nitro-Dur Transdermal Infusion System 2887
Nitrolingual Pumpspray 2965

Norepinephrine Bitartrate (Co-administration with pressor amines (e.g. norepinephrine) may result in decreased response to pressor amines but not sufficient to preclude their use).
No products indexed under this heading.

Oxaprozin (Co-administration of thiazide diuretics and non-steroidal anti-inflammatory agents can reduce the diuretic, natiuretic, and antihypertensive effects).
No products indexed under this heading.

Oxycodone Hydrochloride (Co-administration of thiazide diuretics and narcotics may result in potentiation of orthostatic hypotension). Products include:
OxyContin Tablets 2589
OxyIR Capsules 2593
Percocet Tablets 1127
Percodan Tablets 1130

Pancuronium Bromide (Co-administration of thiazide diuretics and nondepolarizing skeletal muscle relaxants increases responsiveness to the muscle relaxants).
No products indexed under this heading.

Penbutolol Sulfate (Co-administration with other antihypertensives may result in additive effect or potentiation).
No products indexed under this heading.

Pentobarbital Sodium (Co-administration of thiazide diuretics and barbiturates may result in potentiation of orthostatic hypotension). Products include:
Nembutal Sodium Solution, USP 2494

Perindopril Erbumine (Co-administration with other antihypertensives may result in additive effect or potentiation). Products include:
Aceon Tablets (2 mg, 4 mg, 8 mg) 3038

Phenobarbital (Co-administration of thiazide diuretics and barbiturates may result in potentiation of orthostatic hypotension). Products include:
Donnatal Extentabs 2507

Phenoxybenzamine Hydrochloride (Co-administration with other antihypertensives may result in additive effect or potentiation). Products include:
Dibenzyline Capsules 3188

Phentolamine Mesylate (Co-administration with other antihypertensives may result in additive effect or potentiation).
No products indexed under this heading.

Phenylbutazone (Co-administration of thiazide diuretics and non-steroidal anti-inflammatory agents can reduce the diuretic, natiuretic, and antihypertensive effects).
No products indexed under this heading.

Pindolol (Co-administration with other antihypertensives may result in additive effect or potentiation).
No products indexed under this heading.

Pioglitazone Hydrochloride (Dosage adjustment of the antidiabetic drug may be required). Products include:
ActoPlus Met Tablets 3071
Actos Tablets 3077
Duetact Tablets 3085

Piroxicam (Co-administration of thiazide diuretics and non-steroidal anti-inflammatory agents can reduce the diuretic, natiuretic, and antihypertensive effects).
No products indexed under this heading.

Polythiazide (Co-administration with other antihypertensives may result in additive effect or potentiation).
No products indexed under this heading.

Potassium Acid Phosphate (Concurrent use with potassium salt substitutes or potassium supplements should be avoided unless directed by a prescriber). Products include:
K-Phos Original (Sodium Free) Tablets 814

Potassium Bicarbonate (Concurrent use with potassium salt substitutes or potassium supplements should be avoided unless directed by a prescriber).
No products indexed under this heading.

Potassium Chloride (Concurrent use with potassium salt substitutes or potassium supplements should be avoided unless directed by a prescriber). Products include:
MoviPrep Oral Solution 2679

Potassium Citrate (Concurrent use with potassium salt substitutes or potassium supplements should be avoided unless directed by a prescriber). Products include:
BioLean Free Tablets .... ▣635
Urocit-K Tablets 2176

Potassium Gluconate (Concurrent use with potassium salt substitutes or potassium supplements should be avoided unless directed by a prescriber).
No products indexed under this heading.

Potassium Phosphate (Concurrent use with potassium salt substitutes or potassium supplements should be avoided unless directed by a prescriber). Products include:
K-Phos Neutral Tablets 813

Prazosin Hydrochloride (Co-administration with other antihypertensives may result in additive effect or potentiation).
No products indexed under this heading.

Prednisolone Acetate (Co-administration of thiazide diuretics and corticosteroids may intensify electrolyte depletion, particularly hypokalemia). Products include:
Pred Forte Ophthalmic Suspension .... ⊙227
Pred Mild Ophthalmic Suspension .... ⊙230
Pred-G Ophthalmic Ointment .... ⊙229
Pred-G Ophthalmic Suspension .... ⊙228

Prednisolone Sodium Phosphate (Co-administration of thiazide diuretics and corticosteroids may intensify electrolyte depletion, particularly hypokalemia).
No products indexed under this heading.

Prednisolone Tebutate (Co-administration of thiazide diuretics and corticosteroids may intensify electrolyte depletion, particularly hypokalemia).
No products indexed under this heading.

Prednisone (Co-administration of thiazide diuretics and corticosteroids may intensify electrolyte depletion, particularly hypokalemia).
No products indexed under this heading.

Propoxyphene Hydrochloride (Co-administration of thiazide diuretics and narcotics may result in potentiation of orthostatic hypotension).
No products indexed under this heading.

Propoxyphene Napsylate (Co-administration of thiazide diuretics and narcotics may result in potentiation of orthostatic hypotension).
No products indexed under this heading.

Propranolol Hydrochloride (Co-administration with other antihypertensives may result in additive effect or potentiation). Products include:
InnoPran XL Extended Release Capsules 1484

Quinapril Hydrochloride (Co-administration with other antihypertensives may result in additive effect or potentiation).
No products indexed under this heading.

Ramipril (Co-administration with other antihypertensives may result in additive effect or potentiation).
No products indexed under this heading.

Rapacuronium Bromide (Co-administration of thiazide diuretics and nondepolarizing skeletal muscle relaxants increases responsiveness to the muscle relaxants).
No products indexed under this heading.

Rauwolfia Serpentina (Co-administration with other antihypertensives may result in additive effect or potentiation).
No products indexed under this heading.

Remifentanil Hydrochloride (Co-administration of thiazide diuretics and narcotics may result in potentiation of orthostatic hypotension).
No products indexed under this heading.

Repaglinide (Dosage adjustment of the antidiabetic drug may be required). Products include:
PrandiMet Tablets 2967
Prandin Tablets 2971

Rescinnamine (Co-administration with other antihypertensives may result in additive effect or potentiation).
No products indexed under this heading.

Reserpine (Co-administration with other antihypertensives may result in additive effect or potentiation).
No products indexed under this heading.

Rocuronium Bromide (Co-administration of thiazide diuretics and nondepolarizing skeletal muscle relaxants increases responsiveness to the muscle relaxants). Products include:
Zemuron Injection 2947

Rofecoxib (Co-administration of thiazide diuretics and non-steroidal anti-inflammatory agents can reduce the diuretic, natiuretic, and antihypertensive effects).
No products indexed under this heading.

Rosiglitazone Maleate (Dosage adjustment of the antidiabetic drug may be required). Products include:
Avandamet Tablets 1336
Avandaryl Tablets 1344
Avandia Tablets 1351

Secobarbital Sodium (Co-administration of thiazide diuretics and barbiturates may result in potentiation of orthostatic hypotension).
No products indexed under this heading.

Sitagliptin Phosphate (Dosage adjustment of the antidiabetic drug may be required). Products include:
Janumet Tablets 2041
Januvia Tablets 2048

Sodium Nitroprusside (Co-administration with other antihypertensives may result in additive effect or potentiation).
No products indexed under this heading.

Sotalol Hydrochloride (Co-administration with other antihypertensives may result in additive effect or potentiation).
No products indexed under this heading.

Spirapril Hydrochloride (Co-administration with other antihypertensives may result in additive effect or potentiation).
No products indexed under this heading.

Sufentanil Citrate (Co-administration of thiazide diuretics and narcotics may result in potentiation of orthostatic hypotension).
No products indexed under this heading.

Sulindac (Co-administration of thiazide diuretics and non-steroidal anti-inflammatory agents can reduce the diuretic, natiuretic, and antihypertensive effects). Products include:
Clinoril Tablets 1962

Telmisartan (Co-administration with other antihypertensives may result in additive effect or potentiation). Products include:
Micardis Tablets 852
Micardis HCT Tablets 854

Terazosin Hydrochloride (Co-administration with other antihypertensives may result in additive effect or potentiation).
No products indexed under this heading.

Thiamylal Sodium (Co-administration of thiazide diuretics and barbiturates may result in potentiation of orthostatic hypotension).
No products indexed under this heading.

Timolol Maleate (Co-administration with other antihypertensives may result in additive effect or potentiation). Products include:
Combigan Ophthalmic Solution 553
Cosopt Sterile Ophthalmic Solution 1969
Timoptic Sterile Ophthalmic Solution 2121
Timoptic in Ocudose 2124
Timoptic-XE Sterile Ophthalmic Gel Forming Solution 2125

Tolazamide (Dosage adjustment of the antidiabetic drug may be required).
No products indexed under this heading.

Tolbutamide (Dosage adjustment of the antidiabetic drug may be required).
No products indexed under this heading.

Tolmetin Sodium (Co-administration of thiazide diuretics and non-steroidal anti-inflammatory agents can reduce the diuretic, natiuretic, and antihypertensive effects).
No products indexed under this heading.

Torsemide (Co-administration with other antihypertensives may result in additive effect or potentiation). Products include:
Demadex Injection 2630
Demadex Tablets 2630

Trandolapril (Co-administration with other antihypertensives may result in additive effect or potentiation). Products include:
Mavik Tablets 472
Tarka Tablets 511

Triamcinolone (Co-administration of thiazide diuretics and corticosteroids may intensify electrolyte depletion, particularly hypokalemia).
No products indexed under this heading.

Triamcinolone Acetonide (Co-administration of thiazide diuretics and corticosteroids may intensify electrolyte depletion, particularly hypokalemia). Products include:
Azmacort Inhalation Aerosol 407
Nasacort AQ Nasal Spray 2765
Triesence Injectable Suspension .... ⊙209

Triamcinolone Diacetate (Co-administration of thiazide diuretics and corticosteroids may intensify electrolyte depletion, particularly hypokalemia).
No products indexed under this heading.

Triamcinolone Hexacetonide (Co-administration of thiazide diuretics and corticosteroids may intensify electrolyte depletion, particularly hypokalemia).
No products indexed under this heading.

Trimethaphan Camsylate (Co-administration with other antihypertensives may result in additive effect or potentiation).
No products indexed under this heading.

Troglitazone (Dosage adjustment of the antidiabetic drug may be required).
No products indexed under this heading.

Tubocurarine Chloride (Co-administration of thiazide diuretics and nondepolarizing skeletal muscle relaxants increases responsiveness to the muscle relaxants).
No products indexed under this heading.

Valdecoxib (Co-administration of thiazide diuretics and non-steroidal anti-inflammatory agents can reduce the diuretic, natiuretic, and antihypertensive effects).
No products indexed under this heading.

Vecuronium Bromide (Co-administration of thiazide diuretics and nondepolarizing skeletal muscle relaxants increases responsiveness to the muscle relaxants).
No products indexed under this heading.

Verapamil Hydrochloride (Co-administration with other antihypertensives may result in additive effect or potentiation). Products include:
Tarka Tablets 511

Food Interactions

Alcohol (Co-administration of thiazide diuretics and alcohol may result in potentiation of orthostatic hypotension).

DIPROLENE LOTION 0.05%

(Betamethasone Dipropionate) 2838
None cited in PDR database.

DIPROLENE OINTMENT 0.05%

(Betamethasone Dipropionate) 2839
None cited in PDR database.

DIPROLENE AF CREAM 0.05%

(Betamethasone Dipropionate) 2837
None cited in PDR database.

DISMUTAX DIETARY SUPPLEMENT

(Coenzyme Q-10, L-Arginine, Minerals, Niacin, Superoxide Dismutase) 995
None cited in PDR database.

DIVIGEL

(Estradiol) 3167
May interact with cytochrome p450 3a4 inducers (selected), cytochrome p450 3a4 inhibitors (selected), and certain other agents. Compounds in these categories include:

Acetazolamide (Inhibitors of CYP3A4, such as erythromycin, clarithromycin, ketoconazole, itraconazole, ritonavir, and grapefruit juice, may increase plasma concentrations of estrogens and result in side effects).
No products indexed under this heading.

Allium sativum (Inducers of CYP3A4, such as St. John's Wort preparations (Hypericum perforatum), phenobarbital and rifampin, may reduce plasma concentrations of estrogens, possibly resulting in a decrease in therapeutic effects and/or changes in the uterine bleeding profile).
No products indexed under this heading.

Amiodarone Hydrochloride (Inhibitors of CYP3A4, such as erythromycin, clarithromycin, ketoconazole, itraconazole, ritonavir, and grapefruit juice, may increase plasma concentrations of estrogens and result in side effects).
No products indexed under this heading.

Amprenavir (Inhibitors of CYP3A4, such as erythromycin, clarithromycin, ketoconazole, itraconazole, ritonavir, and grapefruit juice, may increase plasma concentrations of estrogens and result in side effects).
No products indexed under this heading.

Anastrozole (Inhibitors of CYP3A4, such as erythromycin, clarithromy-

cin, ketoconazole, itraconazole, ritonavir, and grapefruit juice, may increase plasma concentrations of estrogens and result in side effects). Products include:

Arimidex Tablets 672

Aprepitant (Inhibitors of CYP3A4, such as erythromycin, clarithromycin, ketoconazole, itraconazole, ritonavir, and grapefruit juice, may increase plasma concentrations of estrogens and result in side effects). Products include:

Emend Capsules 1992

Atazanavir (Inhibitors of CYP3A4, such as erythromycin, clarithromycin, ketoconazole, itraconazole, ritonavir, and grapefruit juice, may increase plasma concentrations of estrogens and result in side effects).

No products indexed under this heading.

Atazanavir Sulfate (Inhibitors of CYP3A4, such as erythromycin, clarithromycin, ketoconazole, itraconazole, ritonavir, and grapefruit juice, may increase plasma concentrations of estrogens and result in side effects). Products include:

Reyataz Capsules 3299

Betamethasone Acetate (Inducers of CYP3A4, such as St. John's Wort preparations (Hypericum perforatum), phenobarbital and rifampin, may reduce plasma concentrations of estrogens, possibly resulting in a decrease in therapeutic effects and/or changes in the uterine bleeding profile).

No products indexed under this heading.

Betamethasone Sodium Phosphate (Inducers of CYP3A4, such as St. John's Wort preparations (Hypericum perforatum), phenobarbital and rifampin, may reduce plasma concentrations of estrogens, possibly resulting in a decrease in therapeutic effects and/or changes in the uterine bleeding profile).

No products indexed under this heading.

Carbamazepine (Inducers of CYP3A4, such as carbamazepine may reduce plasma concentrations of estrogens, possibly resulting in a decrease in therapeutic effects and/or changes in the uterine bleeding profile). Products include:

Carbatrol Capsules 3019

Equetro Extended-Release Capsules 3174

Cimetidine (Inhibitors of CYP3A4, such as erythromycin, clarithromycin, ketoconazole, itraconazole, ritonavir, and grapefruit juice, may increase plasma concentrations of estrogens and result in side effects).

No products indexed under this heading.

Cimetidine Hydrochloride (Inhibitors of CYP3A4, such as erythromycin, clarithromycin, ketoconazole, itraconazole, ritonavir, and grapefruit juice, may increase plasma concentrations of estrogens and result in side effects).

No products indexed under this heading.

Ciprofloxacin (Inhibitors of CYP3A4, such as erythromycin, clarithromycin, ketoconazole, itraconazole, ritonavir, and grapefruit juice, may increase plasma concentrations of estrogens and result in side effects). Products include:

Cipro I.V. 2817

Cipro Oral Suspension 2810

Cipro XR Tablets 2823

Ciprodex Otic Suspension 541

Ciprofloxacin Hydrochloride (Inducers of CYP3A4, such as St. John's Wort preparations (Hypericum perforatum), phenobarbital and rifampin, may reduce plasma concentrations of estrogens, possibly resulting in a decrease in therapeutic effects and/or changes in the uterine bleeding profile). Products include:

Cipro Tablets 2810

Cisplatin (Inducers of CYP3A4, such as St. John's Wort preparations (Hypericum perforatum), phenobarbital and rifampin, may reduce plasma concentrations of estrogens, possibly resulting in a decrease in therapeutic effects and/or changes in the uterine bleeding profile).

No products indexed under this heading.

Clarithromycin (Inhibitors of CYP3A4, such as erythromycin, clarithromycin, ketoconazole, itraconazole, ritonavir, and grapefruit juice, may increase plasma concentrations of estrogens and result in side effects). Products include:

Biaxin/Biaxin XL 411

Clotrimazole (Inhibitors of CYP3A4, such as erythromycin, clarithromycin, ketoconazole, itraconazole, ritonavir, and grapefruit juice, may increase plasma concentrations of estrogens and result in side effects). Products include:

Lotrisone 2881

Cortisone Acetate (Inducers of CYP3A4, such as St. John's Wort preparations (Hypericum perforatum), phenobarbital and rifampin, may reduce plasma concentrations of estrogens, possibly resulting in a decrease in therapeutic effects and/or changes in the uterine bleeding profile).

No products indexed under this heading.

Cyclosporine (Inhibitors of CYP3A4, such as erythromycin, clarithromycin, ketoconazole, itraconazole, ritonavir, and grapefruit juice, may increase plasma concentrations of estrogens and result in side effects). Products include:

Gengraf Capsules 435

Neoral Oral Solution 2280

Neoral Soft Gelatin Capsules 2280

Restasis Ophthalmic Emulsion 557

Sandimmune 2296

Dalfopristin (Inhibitors of CYP3A4, such as erythromycin, clarithromycin, ketoconazole, itraconazole, ritonavir, and grapefruit juice, may increase plasma concentrations of estrogens and result in side effects).

No products indexed under this heading.

Danazol (Inhibitors of CYP3A4, such as erythromycin, clarithromycin, ketoconazole, itraconazole, ritonavir, and grapefruit juice, may increase plasma concentrations of estrogens and result in side effects).

No products indexed under this heading.

Delavirdine Mesylate (Inhibitors of CYP3A4, such as erythromycin, clarithromycin, ketoconazole, itraconazole, ritonavir, and grapefruit juice, may increase plasma concentrations of estrogens and result in side effects).

No products indexed under this heading.

Dexamethasone (Inducers of CYP3A4, such as St. John's Wort preparations (Hypericum perforatum), phenobarbital and rifampin, may reduce plasma concentrations of estrogens, possibly resulting in a decrease in therapeutic effects and/or changes in the uterine bleeding profile). Products include:

Ciprodex Otic Suspension 541

Dexamethasone Acetate (Inducers of CYP3A4, such as St. John's Wort preparations (Hypericum perforatum), phenobarbital and rifampin, may reduce plasma concentrations of estrogens, possibly resulting in a decrease in therapeutic effects and/or changes in the uterine bleeding profile).

No products indexed under this heading.

Dexamethasone Sodium Phosphate (Inducers of CYP3A4, such as St. John's Wort preparations (Hypericum perforatum), phenobarbital and rifampin, may reduce plasma concentrations of estrogens, possibly resulting in a decrease in therapeutic effects and/or changes in the uterine bleeding profile).

No products indexed under this heading.

Diltiazem Hydrochloride (Inhibitors of CYP3A4, such as erythromycin, clarithromycin, ketoconazole, itraconazole, ritonavir, and grapefruit juice, may increase plasma concentrations of estrogens and result in side effects). Products include:

Cardizem LA Extended Release Tablets 421

Diltiazem Maleate (Inhibitors of CYP3A4, such as erythromycin, clarithromycin, ketoconazole, itraconazole, ritonavir, and grapefruit juice, may increase plasma concentrations of estrogens and result in side effects).

No products indexed under this heading.

Doxorubicin Hydrochloride (Inducers of CYP3A4, such as St. John's Wort preparations (Hypericum perforatum), phenobarbital and rifampin, may reduce plasma concentrations of estrogens, possibly resulting in a decrease in therapeutic effects and/or changes in the uterine bleeding profile).

No products indexed under this heading.

Efavirenz (Inhibitors of CYP3A4, such as erythromycin, clarithromycin, ketoconazole, itraconazole, ritonavir, and grapefruit juice, may increase plasma concentrations of estrogens and result in side effects). Products include:

Atripla Tablets 938

Sustiva Capsules 930

Sustiva Tablets 930

Erythromycin (Inhibitors of CYP3A4, such as erythromycin, clarithromycin, ketoconazole, itraconazole, ritonavir, and grapefruit juice, may increase plasma concentrations of estrogens and result in side effects).

No products indexed under this heading.

Erythromycin Estolate (Inhibitors of CYP3A4, such as erythromycin, clarithromycin, ketoconazole, itraconazole, ritonavir, and grapefruit juice, may increase plasma concentrations of estrogens and result in side effects).

No products indexed under this heading.

Erythromycin Ethylsuccinate (Inhibitors of CYP3A4, such as erythromycin, clarithromycin, ketoconazole, itraconazole, ritonavir, and grapefruit juice, may increase plasma concentrations of estrogens and result in side effects). Products include:

E.E.S. 433

EryPed 431

Erythromycin Gluceptate (Inhibitors of CYP3A4, such as erythromycin, clarithromycin, ketoconazole, itraconazole, ritonavir, and grapefruit juice, may increase plasma concentrations of estrogens and result in side effects).

No products indexed under this heading.

Erythromycin Lactobionate (Inhibitors of CYP3A4, such as erythromycin, clarithromycin, ketoconazole, itraconazole, ritonavir, and grapefruit juice, may increase plasma concentrations of estrogens and result in side effects).

No products indexed under this heading.

Erythromycin Stearate (Inhibitors of CYP3A4, such as erythromycin, clarithromycin, ketoconazole, itraconazole, ritonavir, and grapefruit juice, may increase plasma concentrations of estrogens and result in side effects).

No products indexed under this heading.

Esomeprazole Magnesium (Inhibitors of CYP3A4, such as erythromycin, clarithromycin, ketoconazole, itraconazole, ritonavir, and grapefruit juice, may increase plasma concentrations of estrogens and result in side effects). Products include:

Nexium Delayed-Release Capsules 645

Nexium Delayed-Release Oral Suspension 645

Ethosuximide (Inducers of CYP3A4, such as St. John's Wort preparations (Hypericum perforatum), phenobarbital and rifampin, may reduce plasma concentrations of estrogens, possibly resulting in a decrease in therapeutic effects and/or changes in the uterine bleeding profile).

No products indexed under this heading.

Felbamate (Inducers of CYP3A4, such as St. John's Wort preparations (Hypericum perforatum), phenobarbital and rifampin, may reduce plasma concentrations of estrogens, possibly resulting in a decrease in therapeutic effects and/or changes in the uterine bleeding profile).

No products indexed under this heading.

Fluconazole (Inhibitors of CYP3A4, such as erythromycin, clarithromycin, ketoconazole, itraconazole, ritonavir, and grapefruit juice, may increase plasma concentrations of estrogens and result in side effects).

No products indexed under this heading.

Fludrocortisone Acetate (Inducers of CYP3A4, such as St. John's Wort preparations (Hypericum perforatum), phenobarbital and rifampin, may reduce plasma concentrations of estrogens, possibly resulting in a decrease in therapeutic effects and/or changes in the uterine bleeding profile).

No products indexed under this heading.

Fluoxetine (Inhibitors of CYP3A4, such as erythromycin, clarithromycin, ketoconazole, itraconazole, ritonavir, and grapefruit juice, may increase plasma concentrations of estrogens and result in side effects).
No products indexed under this heading.

Fluoxetine Hydrochloride (Inhibitors of CYP3A4, such as erythromycin, clarithromycin, ketoconazole, itraconazole, ritonavir, and grapefruit juice, may increase plasma concentrations of estrogens and result in side effects). Products include:
Prozac Weekly Capsules 1852
Prozac Pulvules and Liquid 1852
Symbyax Capsules 1871

Fluvoxamine Maleate (Inhibitors of CYP3A4, such as erythromycin, clarithromycin, ketoconazole, itraconazole, ritonavir, and grapefruit juice, may increase plasma concentrations of estrogens and result in side effects). Products include:
Luvox CR Extended-Release Capsules 1759

Fosamprenavir Calcium (Inhibitors of CYP3A4, such as erythromycin, clarithromycin, ketoconazole, itraconazole, ritonavir, and grapefruit juice, may increase plasma concentrations of estrogens and result in side effects). Products include:
Lexiva Oral Suspension 1510
Lexiva Tablets 1510

Fosphenytoin Sodium (Inducers of CYP3A4, such as St. John's Wort preparations (Hypericum perforatum), phenobarbital and rifampin, may reduce plasma concentrations of estrogens, possibly resulting in a decrease in therapeutic effects and/ or changes in the uterine bleeding profile).
No products indexed under this heading.

Garlic Extract (Inducers of CYP3A4, such as St. John's Wort preparations (Hypericum perforatum), phenobarbital and rifampin, may reduce plasma concentrations of estrogens, possibly resulting in a decrease in therapeutic effects and/ or changes in the uterine bleeding profile).
No products indexed under this heading.

Garlic Oil (Inducers of CYP3A4, such as St. John's Wort preparations (Hypericum perforatum), phenobarbital and rifampin, may reduce plasma concentrations of estrogens, possibly resulting in a decrease in therapeutic effects and/or changes in the uterine bleeding profile).
No products indexed under this heading.

Hydrocortisone (Inducers of CYP3A4, such as St. John's Wort preparations (Hypericum perforatum), phenobarbital and rifampin, may reduce plasma concentrations of estrogens, possibly resulting in a decrease in therapeutic effects and/ or changes in the uterine bleeding profile).
No products indexed under this heading.

Hydrocortisone Acetate (Inducers of CYP3A4, such as St. John's Wort preparations (Hypericum perforatum), phenobarbital and rifampin, may reduce plasma concentrations of estrogens, possibly resulting in a decrease in therapeutic effects and/ or changes in the uterine bleeding profile). Products include:
Analpram-HC 1140
Pramosone 1141

Hydrocortisone Butyrate (Inducers of CYP3A4, such as St. John's Wort preparations (Hypericum perforatum), phenobarbital and rifampin, may reduce plasma concentrations of estrogens, possibly resulting in a decrease in therapeutic effects and/ or changes in the uterine bleeding profile).
No products indexed under this heading.

Hydrocortisone Cypionate (Inducers of CYP3A4, such as St. John's Wort preparations (Hypericum perforatum), phenobarbital and rifampin, may reduce plasma concentrations of estrogens, possibly resulting in a decrease in therapeutic effects and/ or changes in the uterine bleeding profile).
No products indexed under this heading.

Hydrocortisone Hemisuccinate (Inducers of CYP3A4, such as St. John's Wort preparations (Hypericum perforatum), phenobarbital and rifampin, may reduce plasma concentrations of estrogens, possibly resulting in a decrease in therapeutic effects and/or changes in the uterine bleeding profile).
No products indexed under this heading.

Hydrocortisone Probutate (Inducers of CYP3A4, such as St. John's Wort preparations (Hypericum perforatum), phenobarbital and rifampin, may reduce plasma concentrations of estrogens, possibly resulting in a decrease in therapeutic effects and/ or changes in the uterine bleeding profile).
No products indexed under this heading.

Hydrocortisone Sodium Phosphate (Inducers of CYP3A4, such as St. John's Wort preparations (Hypericum perforatum), phenobarbital and rifampin, may reduce plasma concentrations of estrogens, possibly resulting in a decrease in therapeutic effects and/or changes in the uterine bleeding profile).
No products indexed under this heading.

Hydrocortisone Sodium Succinate (Inducers of CYP3A4, such as St. John's Wort preparations (Hypericum perforatum), phenobarbital and rifampin, may reduce plasma concentrations of estrogens, possibly resulting in a decrease in therapeutic effects and/or changes in the uterine bleeding profile).
No products indexed under this heading.

Hydrocortisone Valerate (Inducers of CYP3A4, such as St. John's Wort preparations (Hypericum perforatum), phenobarbital and rifampin, may reduce plasma concentrations of estrogens, possibly resulting in a decrease in therapeutic effects and/ or changes in the uterine bleeding profile).
No products indexed under this heading.

Hypericum (Inducers of CYP3A4, such as St. John's Wort preparations (Hypericum perforatum), phenobarbital and rifampin, may reduce plasma concentrations of estrogens, possibly resulting in a decrease in therapeutic effects and/or changes in the uterine bleeding profile). Products include:
Satieté Tablets 640

Hypericum Perforatum (Inducers of CYP3A4, such as St. John's Wort preparations (Hypericum perforatum), phenobarbital and rifampin, may reduce plasma concentrations of estrogens, possibly resulting in a decrease in therapeutic effects and/ or changes in the uterine bleeding profile).
No products indexed under this heading.

Indinavir Sulfate (Inhibitors of CYP3A4, such as erythromycin, clarithromycin, ketoconazole, itraconazole, ritonavir, and grapefruit juice, may increase plasma concentrations of estrogens and result in side effects). Products include:
Crixivan Capsules 1979

Isoniazid (Inhibitors of CYP3A4, such as erythromycin, clarithromycin, ketoconazole, itraconazole, ritonavir, and grapefruit juice, may increase plasma concentrations of estrogens and result in side effects).
No products indexed under this heading.

Itraconazole (Inhibitors of CYP3A4, such as erythromycin, clarithromycin, ketoconazole, itraconazole, ritonavir, and grapefruit juice, may increase plasma concentrations of estrogens and result in side effects).
No products indexed under this heading.

Ketoconazole (Inhibitors of CYP3A4, such as erythromycin, clarithromycin, ketoconazole, itraconazole, ritonavir, and grapefruit juice, may increase plasma concentrations of estrogens and result in side effects). Products include:
Extina Foam, 2% 3057
Nizoral A-D Shampoo 1901

Lopinavir (Inhibitors of CYP3A4, such as erythromycin, clarithromycin, ketoconazole, itraconazole, ritonavir, and grapefruit juice, may increase plasma concentrations of estrogens and result in side effects). Products include:
Kaletra 452

Loratadine (Inhibitors of CYP3A4, such as erythromycin, clarithromycin, ketoconazole, itraconazole, ritonavir, and grapefruit juice, may increase plasma concentrations of estrogens and result in side effects).
No products indexed under this heading.

Mephenytoin (Inducers of CYP3A4, such as St. John's Wort preparations (Hypericum perforatum), phenobarbital and rifampin, may reduce plasma concentrations of estrogens, possibly resulting in a decrease in therapeutic effects and/or changes in the uterine bleeding profile).
No products indexed under this heading.

Methsuximide (Inducers of CYP3A4, such as St. John's Wort preparations (Hypericum perforatum), phenobarbital and rifampin, may reduce plasma concentrations of estrogens, possibly resulting in a decrease in therapeutic effects and/ or changes in the uterine bleeding profile).
No products indexed under this heading.

Methylprednisolone (Inducers of CYP3A4, such as St. John's Wort preparations (Hypericum perforatum), phenobarbital and rifampin, may reduce plasma concentrations of estrogens, possibly resulting in a decrease in therapeutic effects and/ or changes in the uterine bleeding profile).
No products indexed under this heading.

Methylprednisolone Acetate (Inducers of CYP3A4, such as St. John's Wort preparations (Hypericum perforatum), phenobarbital and rifampin, may reduce plasma concentrations of estrogens, possibly resulting in a decrease in therapeutic effects and/or changes in the uterine bleeding profile).
No products indexed under this heading.

Methylprednisolone Sodium Succinate (Inducers of CYP3A4, such as St. John's Wort preparations (Hypericum perforatum), phenobarbital and rifampin, may reduce plasma concentrations of estrogens, possibly resulting in a decrease in therapeutic effects and/or changes in the uterine bleeding profile).
No products indexed under this heading.

Metronidazole (Inhibitors of CYP3A4, such as erythromycin, clarithromycin, ketoconazole, itraconazole, ritonavir, and grapefruit juice, may increase plasma concentrations of estrogens and result in side effects). Products include:
Pylera Capsules 714

Metronidazole Benzoate (Inhibitors of CYP3A4, such as erythromycin, clarithromycin, ketoconazole, itraconazole, ritonavir, and grapefruit juice, may increase plasma concentrations of estrogens and result in side effects).
No products indexed under this heading.

Metronidazole Hydrochloride (Inhibitors of CYP3A4, such as erythromycin, clarithromycin, ketoconazole, itraconazole, ritonavir, and grapefruit juice, may increase plasma concentrations of estrogens and result in side effects).
No products indexed under this heading.

Miconazole (Inhibitors of CYP3A4, such as erythromycin, clarithromycin, ketoconazole, itraconazole, ritonavir, and grapefruit juice, may increase plasma concentrations of estrogens and result in side effects).
No products indexed under this heading.

Miconazole Nitrate (Inhibitors of CYP3A4, such as erythromycin, clarithromycin, ketoconazole, itraconazole, ritonavir, and grapefruit juice, may increase plasma concentrations of estrogens and result in side effects).
No products indexed under this heading.

Modafinil (Inducers of CYP3A4, such as St. John's Wort preparations (Hypericum perforatum), phenobarbital and rifampin, may reduce plasma concentrations of estrogens, possibly resulting in a decrease in therapeutic effects and/or changes in the uterine bleeding profile). Products include:
Provigil Tablets 977

Nefazodone Hydrochloride (Inhibitors of CYP3A4, such as erythromycin, clarithromycin, ketoconazole, itraconazole, ritonavir, and grapefruit juice, may increase plasma concentrations of estrogens and result in side effects).
No products indexed under this heading.

Nelfinavir Mesylate (Inhibitors of CYP3A4, such as erythromycin, clarithromycin, ketoconazole, itraconazole, ritonavir, and grapefruit juice, may increase plasma concentrations of estrogens and result in side effects).
No products indexed under this heading.

Nevirapine (Inhibitors of CYP3A4, such as erythromycin, clarithromycin, ketoconazole, itraconazole, ritonavir, and grapefruit juice, may increase plasma concentrations of estrogens and result in side effects). Products include:
Viramune Oral Suspension 873
Viramune Tablets 873

Niacinamide (Inhibitors of CYP3A4, such as erythromycin, clarithromycin, ketoconazole, itraconazole, ritonavir, and grapefruit juice, may increase plasma concentrations of estrogens and result in side effects). Products include:
BioLean Free Tablets .... ■635

Nicotinamide (Inhibitors of CYP3A4, such as erythromycin, clarithromycin, ketoconazole, itraconazole, ritonavir, and grapefruit juice, may increase plasma concentrations of estrogens and result in side effects).
No products indexed under this heading.

Nifedipine (Inhibitors of CYP3A4, such as erythromycin, clarithromycin, ketoconazole, itraconazole, ritonavir, and grapefruit juice, may increase plasma concentrations of estrogens and result in side effects).
No products indexed under this heading.

Norfloxacin (Inhibitors of CYP3A4, such as erythromycin, clarithromycin, ketoconazole, itraconazole, ritonavir, and grapefruit juice, may increase plasma concentrations of estrogens and result in side effects). Products include:
Noroxin Tablets 2069

Omeprazole (Inhibitors of CYP3A4, such as erythromycin, clarithromycin, ketoconazole, itraconazole, ritonavir, and grapefruit juice, may increase plasma concentrations of estrogens and result in side effects).
No products indexed under this heading.

Oxcarbazepine (Inducers of CYP3A4, such as St. John's Wort preparations (Hypericum perforatum), phenobarbital and rifampin, may reduce plasma concentrations of estrogens, possibly resulting in a decrease in therapeutic effects and/or changes in the uterine bleeding profile).
No products indexed under this heading.

Paroxetine Hydrochloride (Inhibitors of CYP3A4, such as erythromycin, clarithromycin, ketoconazole, itraconazole, ritonavir, and grapefruit juice, may increase plasma concentrations of estrogens and result in side effects). Products include:
Paxil 1535
Paxil CR Controlled-Release Tablets 1544

Phenobarbital (Inducers of CYP3A4, such as St. John's Wort preparations (Hypericum perforatum), phenobarbital and rifampin, may reduce plasma concentrations of estrogens, possibly resulting in a decrease in therapeutic effects and/or changes in the uterine bleeding profile). Products include:
Donnatal Extentabs 2507

Phenobarbital Sodium (Inducers of CYP3A4, such as St. John's Wort preparations (Hypericum perforatum), phenobarbital and rifampin, may reduce plasma concentrations of estrogens, possibly resulting in a decrease in therapeutic effects and/or changes in the uterine bleeding profile).
No products indexed under this heading.

Phenytoin (Inducers of CYP3A4, such as St. John's Wort preparations (Hypericum perforatum), phenobarbital and rifampin, may reduce plasma concentrations of estrogens, possibly resulting in a decrease in therapeutic effects and/or changes in the uterine bleeding profile).
No products indexed under this heading.

Phenytoin Sodium (Inducers of CYP3A4, such as St. John's Wort preparations (Hypericum perforatum), phenobarbital and rifampin, may reduce plasma concentrations of estrogens, possibly resulting in a decrease in therapeutic effects and/or changes in the uterine bleeding profile). Products include:
Phenytek Capsules 2192

Prednisolone Acetate (Inducers of CYP3A4, such as St. John's Wort preparations (Hypericum perforatum), phenobarbital and rifampin, may reduce plasma concentrations of estrogens, possibly resulting in a decrease in therapeutic effects and/or changes in the uterine bleeding profile). Products include:
Pred Forte Ophthalmic Suspension .... ⊙227
Pred Mild Ophthalmic Suspension .... ⊙230
Pred-G Ophthalmic Ointment .... ⊙229
Pred-G Ophthalmic Suspension ...... ⊙228

Prednisolone Sodium Phosphate (Inducers of CYP3A4, such as St. John's Wort preparations (Hypericum perforatum), phenobarbital and rifampin, may reduce plasma concentrations of estrogens, possibly resulting in a decrease in therapeutic effects and/or changes in the uterine bleeding profile).
No products indexed under this heading.

Prednisolone Tebutate (Inducers of CYP3A4, such as St. John's Wort preparations (Hypericum perforatum), phenobarbital and rifampin, may reduce plasma concentrations of estrogens, possibly resulting in a decrease in therapeutic effects and/or changes in the uterine bleeding profile).
No products indexed under this heading.

Prednisone (Inducers of CYP3A4, such as St. John's Wort preparations (Hypericum perforatum), phenobarbital and rifampin, may reduce plasma concentrations of estrogens, possibly resulting in a decrease in therapeutic effects and/or changes in the uterine bleeding profile).
No products indexed under this heading.

Primidone (Inducers of CYP3A4, such as St. John's Wort preparations (Hypericum perforatum), phenobarbital and rifampin, may reduce plasma concentrations of estrogens, possibly resulting in a decrease in therapeutic effects and/or changes in the uterine bleeding profile).
No products indexed under this heading.

Propoxyphene Hydrochloride (Inhibitors of CYP3A4, such as erythromycin, clarithromycin, ketoconazole, itraconazole, ritonavir, and grapefruit juice, may increase plasma concentrations of estrogens and result in side effects).
No products indexed under this heading.

Propoxyphene Napsylate (Inhibitors of CYP3A4, such as erythromycin, clarithromycin, ketoconazole, itraconazole, ritonavir, and grapefruit juice, may increase plasma concentrations of estrogens and result in side effects).
No products indexed under this heading.

Quinidine (Inhibitors of CYP3A4, such as erythromycin, clarithromycin, ketoconazole, itraconazole, ritonavir, and grapefruit juice, may increase plasma concentrations of estrogens and result in side effects).
No products indexed under this heading.

Quinidine Hydrochloride (Inhibitors of CYP3A4, such as erythromycin, clarithromycin, ketoconazole, itraconazole, ritonavir, and grapefruit juice, may increase plasma concentrations of estrogens and result in side effects).
No products indexed under this heading.

Quinidine Polygalacturonate (Inhibitors of CYP3A4, such as erythromycin, clarithromycin, ketoconazole, itraconazole, ritonavir, and grapefruit juice, may increase plasma concentrations of estrogens and result in side effects).
No products indexed under this heading.

Quinidine Sulfate (Inhibitors of CYP3A4, such as erythromycin, clarithromycin, ketoconazole, itraconazole, ritonavir, and grapefruit juice, may increase plasma concentrations of estrogens and result in side effects).
No products indexed under this heading.

Quinine (Inhibitors of CYP3A4, such as erythromycin, clarithromycin, ketoconazole, itraconazole, ritonavir, and grapefruit juice, may increase plasma concentrations of estrogens and result in side effects).
No products indexed under this heading.

Quinine Sulfate (Inhibitors of CYP3A4, such as erythromycin, clarithromycin, ketoconazole, itraconazole, ritonavir, and grapefruit juice, may increase plasma concentrations of estrogens and result in side effects).
No products indexed under this heading.

Quinupristin (Inhibitors of CYP3A4, such as erythromycin, clarithromycin, ketoconazole, itraconazole, ritonavir, and grapefruit juice, may increase plasma concentrations of estrogens and result in side effects).
No products indexed under this heading.

Ranitidine Bismuth Citrate (Inhibitors of CYP3A4, such as erythromycin, clarithromycin, ketoconazole, itraconazole, ritonavir, and grapefruit juice, may increase plasma concentrations of estrogens and result in side effects).
No products indexed under this heading.

Ranitidine Hydrochloride (Inhibitors of CYP3A4, such as erythromycin, clarithromycin, ketoconazole, itraconazole, ritonavir, and grapefruit juice, may increase plasma concentrations of estrogens and result in side effects). Products include:
Zantac 75 Tablets .... ■603
Zantac 1670
Zantac Injection 1666
Zantac Injection Pharmacy Bulk Package 1668
Maximum Strength Zantac 150 Tablets .... ■603
Maximum Strength Zantac 150 Cool Mint Tablets .... ■603

Rifabutin (Inducers of CYP3A4, such as St. John's Wort preparations (Hypericum perforatum), phenobarbital and rifampin, may reduce plasma concentrations of estrogens, possibly resulting in a decrease in therapeutic effects and/or changes in the uterine bleeding profile).
No products indexed under this heading.

Rifampicin (Inducers of CYP3A4, such as St. John's Wort preparations (Hypericum perforatum), phenobarbital and rifampin, may reduce plasma concentrations of estrogens, possibly resulting in a decrease in therapeutic effects and/or changes in the uterine bleeding profile).
No products indexed under this heading.

Rifampin (Inducers of CYP3A4, such as St. John's Wort preparations (Hypericum perforatum), phenobarbital and rifampin, may reduce plasma concentrations of estrogens, possibly resulting in a decrease in therapeutic effects and/or changes in the uterine bleeding profile).
No products indexed under this heading.

Rifapentine (Inducers of CYP3A4, such as St. John's Wort preparations (Hypericum perforatum), phenobarbital and rifampin, may reduce plasma concentrations of estrogens, possibly resulting in a decrease in therapeutic effects and/or changes in the uterine bleeding profile).
No products indexed under this heading.

Ritonavir (Inhibitors of CYP3A4, such as erythromycin, clarithromycin, ketoconazole, itraconazole, ritonavir, and grapefruit juice, may

increase plasma concentrations of estrogens and result in side effects). Products include:

Kaletra 452
Norvir 489

Saquinavir (Inhibitors of CYP3A4, such as erythromycin, clarithromycin, ketoconazole, itraconazole, ritonavir, and grapefruit juice, may increase plasma concentrations of estrogens and result in side effects).

No products indexed under this heading.

Saquinavir Mesylate (Inhibitors of CYP3A4, such as erythromycin, clarithromycin, ketoconazole, itraconazole, ritonavir, and grapefruit juice, may increase plasma concentrations of estrogens and result in side effects).

No products indexed under this heading.

Sertraline Hydrochloride (Inhibitors of CYP3A4, such as erythromycin, clarithromycin, ketoconazole, itraconazole, ritonavir, and grapefruit juice, may increase plasma concentrations of estrogens and result in side effects).

No products indexed under this heading.

Sildenafil Citrate (Inhibitors of CYP3A4, such as erythromycin, clarithromycin, ketoconazole, itraconazole, ritonavir, and grapefruit juice, may increase plasma concentrations of estrogens and result in side effects).

No products indexed under this heading.

Sulfinpyrazone (Inducers of CYP3A4, such as St. John's Wort preparations (Hypericum perforatum), phenobarbital and rifampin, may reduce plasma concentrations of estrogens, possibly resulting in a decrease in therapeutic effects and/or changes in the uterine bleeding profile).

No products indexed under this heading.

Telithromycin (Inhibitors of CYP3A4, such as erythromycin, clarithromycin, ketoconazole, itraconazole, ritonavir, and grapefruit juice, may increase plasma concentrations of estrogens and result in side effects). Products include:

Ketek Tablets 2744

Theophylline (Inducers of CYP3A4, such as St. John's Wort preparations (Hypericum perforatum), phenobarbital and rifampin, may reduce plasma concentrations of estrogens, possibly resulting in a decrease in therapeutic effects and/or changes in the uterine bleeding profile).

No products indexed under this heading.

Theophylline Anhydrous (Inducers of CYP3A4, such as St. John's Wort preparations (Hypericum perforatum), phenobarbital and rifampin, may reduce plasma concentrations of estrogens, possibly resulting in a decrease in therapeutic effects and/or changes in the uterine bleeding profile). Products include:

Uniphyl Tablets 2595

Theophylline Calcium Salicylate (Inducers of CYP3A4, such as St. John's Wort preparations (Hypericum perforatum), phenobarbital and rifampin, may reduce plasma concentrations of estrogens, possibly resulting in a decrease in therapeutic effects and/or changes in the uterine bleeding profile).

No products indexed under this heading.

Theophylline Dihydroxypropyl (Glyceryl) (Inducers of CYP3A4, such as St. John's Wort preparations (Hypericum perforatum), phenobarbital and rifampin, may reduce plasma concentrations of estrogens, possibly resulting in a decrease in therapeutic effects and/or changes in the uterine bleeding profile).

No products indexed under this heading.

Theophylline Ethylenediamine (Inducers of CYP3A4, such as St. John's Wort preparations (Hypericum perforatum), phenobarbital and rifampin, may reduce plasma concentrations of estrogens, possibly resulting in a decrease in therapeutic effects and/or changes in the uterine bleeding profile).

No products indexed under this heading.

Triamcinolone (Inducers of CYP3A4, such as St. John's Wort preparations (Hypericum perforatum), phenobarbital and rifampin, may reduce plasma concentrations of estrogens, possibly resulting in a decrease in therapeutic effects and/or changes in the uterine bleeding profile).

No products indexed under this heading.

Triamcinolone Acetonide (Inducers of CYP3A4, such as St. John's Wort preparations (Hypericum perforatum), phenobarbital and rifampin, may reduce plasma concentrations of estrogens, possibly resulting in a decrease in therapeutic effects and/or changes in the uterine bleeding profile). Products include:

Azmacort Inhalation Aerosol 407
Nasacort AQ Nasal Spray 2765
Triesence Injectable Suspension .... ⊙ 209

Triamcinolone Diacetate (Inducers of CYP3A4, such as St. John's Wort preparations (Hypericum perforatum), phenobarbital and rifampin, may reduce plasma concentrations of estrogens, possibly resulting in a decrease in therapeutic effects and/or changes in the uterine bleeding profile).

No products indexed under this heading.

Triamcinolone Hexacetonide (Inducers of CYP3A4, such as St. John's Wort preparations (Hypericum perforatum), phenobarbital and rifampin, may reduce plasma concentrations of estrogens, possibly resulting in a decrease in therapeutic effects and/or changes in the uterine bleeding profile).

No products indexed under this heading.

Troglitazone (Inhibitors of CYP3A4, such as erythromycin, clarithromycin, ketoconazole, itraconazole, ritonavir, and grapefruit juice, may increase plasma concentrations of estrogens and result in side effects).

No products indexed under this heading.

Troleandomycin (Inhibitors of CYP3A4, such as erythromycin, clarithromycin, ketoconazole, itraconazole, ritonavir, and grapefruit juice, may increase plasma concentrations of estrogens and result in side effects).

No products indexed under this heading.

Valproate Sodium (Inhibitors of CYP3A4, such as erythromycin, clarithromycin, ketoconazole, itraconazole, ritonavir, and grapefruit juice, may increase plasma concentrations of estrogens and result in side effects).

No products indexed under this heading.

Vardenafil Hydrochloride (Inhibitors of CYP3A4, such as erythromycin, clarithromycin, ketoconazole, itraconazole, ritonavir, and grapefruit juice, may increase plasma concentrations of estrogens and result in side effects). Products include:

Levitra Tablets 2876

Verapamil Hydrochloride (Inhibitors of CYP3A4, such as erythromycin, clarithromycin, ketoconazole, itraconazole, ritonavir, and grapefruit juice, may increase plasma concentrations of estrogens and result in side effects). Products include:

Tarka Tablets 511

Voriconazole (Inhibitors of CYP3A4, such as erythromycin, clarithromycin, ketoconazole, itraconazole, ritonavir, and grapefruit juice, may increase plasma concentrations of estrogens and result in side effects).

No products indexed under this heading.

Zafirlukast (Inhibitors of CYP3A4, such as erythromycin, clarithromycin, ketoconazole, itraconazole, ritonavir, and grapefruit juice, may increase plasma concentrations of estrogens and result in side effects). Products include:

Accolate Tablets 669

Zileuton (Inhibitors of CYP3A4, such as erythromycin, clarithromycin, ketoconazole, itraconazole, ritonavir, and grapefruit juice, may increase plasma concentrations of estrogens and result in side effects).

No products indexed under this heading.

Food Interactions

Grapefruit (Inhibitors of CYP3A4, such as erythromycin, clarithromycin, ketoconazole, itraconazole, ritonavir, and grapefruit juice, may increase plasma concentrations of estrogens and result in side effects).

Grapefruit Juice (Inhibitors of CYP3A4, such as erythromycin, clarithromycin, ketoconazole, itraconazole, ritonavir, and grapefruit juice, may increase plasma concentrations of estrogens and result in side effects).

DONNATAL EXTENTABS
(Atropine Sulfate, Hyoscyamine Sulfate, Phenobarbital, Scopolamine Hydrobromide).............. 2507
May interact with anticoagulants. Compounds in these categories include:

Anisindione (Phenobarbital may decrease the effect of anticoagulants and necessitate larger doses of the anticoagulant for optimal effect. When phenobarbital is discontinued, the dose of the anticoagulant may have to be decreased).

No products indexed under this heading.

Ardeparin Sodium (Phenobarbital may decrease the effect of anticoagulants and necessitate larger doses of the anticoagulant for optimal effect. When phenobarbital is discontinued, the dose of the anticoagulant may have to be decreased).

No products indexed under this heading.

Dalteparin Sodium (Phenobarbital may decrease the effect of anticoagulants and necessitate larger doses of the anticoagulant for optimal effect. When phenobarbital is discontinued, the dose of the anticoagulant may have to be decreased). Products include:

Fragmin Injection 1070

Danaparoid Sodium (Phenobarbital may decrease the effect of anticoagulants and necessitate larger doses of the anticoagulant for optimal effect. When phenobarbital is discontinued, the dose of the anticoagulant may have to be decreased).

No products indexed under this heading.

Dicumarol (Phenobarbital may decrease the effect of anticoagulants and necessitate larger doses of the anticoagulant for optimal effect. When phenobarbital is discontinued, the dose of the anticoagulant may have to be decreased).

No products indexed under this heading.

Enoxaparin Sodium (Phenobarbital may decrease the effect of anticoagulants and necessitate larger doses of the anticoagulant for optimal effect. When phenobarbital is discontinued, the dose of the anticoagulant may have to be decreased). Products include:

Lovenox Injection 2756

Fondaparinux Sodium (Phenobarbital may decrease the effect of anticoagulants and necessitate larger doses of the anticoagulant for optimal effect. When phenobarbital is discontinued, the dose of the anticoagulant may have to be decreased). Products include:

Arixtra Injection 1313

Heparin Calcium (Phenobarbital may decrease the effect of anticoagulants and necessitate larger doses of the anticoagulant for optimal effect. When phenobarbital is discontinued, the dose of the anticoagulant may have to be decreased).

No products indexed under this heading.

Heparin Sodium (Phenobarbital may decrease the effect of anticoagulants and necessitate larger doses of the anticoagulant for optimal effect. When phenobarbital is discontinued, the dose of the anticoagulant may have to be decreased).

No products indexed under this heading.

Low Molecular Weight Heparins (Phenobarbital may decrease the effect of anticoagulants and necessitate larger doses of the anticoagulant for optimal effect. When phenobarbital is discontinued, the dose of the anticoagulant may have to be decreased).

No products indexed under this heading.

Tinzaparin Sodium (Phenobarbital may decrease the effect of anticoagulants and necessitate larger doses of the anticoagulant for optimal effect. When phenobarbital is discontinued, the dose of the anticoagulant may have to be decreased).

No products indexed under this heading.

Warfarin Sodium (Phenobarbital may decrease the effect of anticoagulants and necessitate larger doses of the anticoagulant for optimal effect. When phenobarbital is discontinued, the dose of the anticoagulant may have to be decreased).
No products indexed under this heading.

DORIBAX INJECTION
(Doripenem) 2400
May interact with valproate and certain other agents. Compounds in these categories include:

Divalproex Sodium (Carbapenems may reduce serum valproic acid concentrations to subtherapeutic levels, resulting in loss of seizure control. Serum valproic acid concentrations should be monitored frequently after initiating carbapenem therapy. Alternative antibacterial or anticonvulsant therapy should be considered if serum valproic acid concentrations cannot be maintained in the therapeutic range or seizures occur). Products include:
Depakote ER Tablets 423

Probenecid (Probenecid interferes with the active tubular secretion of doripenem, resulting in increased plasma concentrations of doripenem. Co-administration of probenecid with doripenem is not recommended).
No products indexed under this heading.

Valproate Sodium (Carbapenems may reduce serum valproic acid concentrations to subtherapeutic levels, resulting in loss of seizure control. Serum valproic acid concentrations should be monitored frequently after initiating carbapenem therapy. Alternative antibacterial or anticonvulsant therapy should be considered if serum valproic acid concentrations cannot be maintained in the therapeutic range or seizures occur).
No products indexed under this heading.

Valproic Acid (Carbapenems may reduce serum valproic acid concentrations to subtherapeutic levels, resulting in loss of seizure control. Serum valproic acid concentrations should be monitored frequently after initiating carbapenem therapy. Alternative antibacterial or anticonvulsant therapy should be considered if serum valproic acid concentrations cannot be maintained in the therapeutic range or seizures occur).
No products indexed under this heading.

DOXIL INJECTION
(Doxorubicin Hydrochloride Liposome).. 2378
May interact with antineoplastics and certain other agents. Compounds in these categories include:

Altretamine (Co-administration with the conventional formulation of doxorubicin results in potentiation of the toxicity of other anti-cancer therapies; this interaction may occur with Doxil). Products include:
Hexalen Capsules 1078

Anastrozole (Co-administration with the conventional formulation of doxorubicin results in potentiation of the toxicity of other anti-cancer therapies; this interaction may occur with Doxil). Products include:
Arimidex Tablets 672

Asparaginase (Co-administration with the conventional formulation of doxorubicin results in potentiation of the toxicity of other anti-cancer therapies; this interaction may occur with Doxil). Products include:
Elspar for Injection 1990
Elspar for Injection 2488

Bicalutamide (Co-administration with the conventional formulation of doxorubicin results in potentiation of the toxicity of other anti-cancer therapies; this interaction may occur with Doxil). Products include:
No products indexed under this heading.

Bleomycin Sulfate (Co-administration with the conventional formulation of doxorubicin results in potentiation of the toxicity of other anti-cancer therapies; this interaction may occur with Doxil).
No products indexed under this heading.

Busulfan (Co-administration with the conventional formulation of doxorubicin results in potentiation of the toxicity of other anti-cancer therapies; this interaction may occur with Doxil). Products include:
Busulfex Injection 2477
Myleran Tablets 1530

Carboplatin (Co-administration with the conventional formulation of doxorubicin results in potentiation of the toxicity of other anti-cancer therapies; this interaction may occur with Doxil).
No products indexed under this heading.

Carmustine (BCNU) (Co-administration with the conventional formulation of doxorubicin results in potentiation of the toxicity of other anti-cancer therapies; this interaction may occur with Doxil).
No products indexed under this heading.

Chlorambucil (Co-administration with the conventional formulation of doxorubicin results in potentiation of the toxicity of other anti-cancer therapies; this interaction may occur with Doxil). Products include:
Leukeran Tablets 1508

Cisplatin (Co-administration with the conventional formulation of doxorubicin results in potentiation of the toxicity of other anti-cancer therapies; this interaction may occur with Doxil).
No products indexed under this heading.

Cyclophosphamide (Co-administration of conventional formulation of doxorubicin with cyclophosphamide has resulted in exacerbation of cyclophosphamide-induced hemorrhagic cystitis; cardiac toxicity may occur at lower cumulative doses in patients who are receiving cyclophosphamide).
No products indexed under this heading.

Cyclosporine (Co-administration of conventional formulation of doxorubicin may result in increases in AUC for both doxorubicin and doxorubicinol possibly due to a decrease in clearance of parent drug and a decrease in metabolism of doxorubicin; potential for more profound and prolonged hematologic toxicity is associated with combined use; coma and seizures have also been reported). Products include:
Gengraf Capsules 435
Neoral Oral Solution 2280
Neoral Soft Gelatin Capsules 2280
Restasis Ophthalmic Emulsion 557
Sandimmune 2296

Dacarbazine (Co-administration with the conventional formulation of doxorubicin results in potentiation of the toxicity of other anti-cancer therapies; this interaction may occur with Doxil).
No products indexed under this heading.

Daunorubicin Citrate (Co-administration with the conventional formulation of doxorubicin results in potentiation of the toxicity of other anti-cancer therapies; this interaction may occur with Doxil).
No products indexed under this heading.

Daunorubicin Hydrochloride (Co-administration with the conventional formulation of doxorubicin results in potentiation of the toxicity of other anti-cancer therapies; this interaction may occur with Doxil).
No products indexed under this heading.

Denileukin Diftitox (Co-administration with the conventional formulation of doxorubicin results in potentiation of the toxicity of other anti-cancer therapies; this interaction may occur with Doxil). Products include:
Ontak Vials 1079

Docetaxel (Co-administration with the conventional formulation of doxorubicin results in potentiation of the toxicity of other anti-cancer therapies; this interaction may occur with Doxil). Products include:
Taxotere Injection Concentrate 2773

Doxorubicin Hydrochloride (Co-administration with the conventional formulation of doxorubicin results in potentiation of the toxicity of other anti-cancer therapies; this interaction may occur with Doxil).
No products indexed under this heading.

Epirubicin Hydrochloride (Co-administration with the conventional formulation of doxorubicin results in potentiation of the toxicity of other anti-cancer therapies; this interaction may occur with Doxil).
No products indexed under this heading.

Estramustine Phosphate Sodium (Co-administration with the conventional formulation of doxorubicin results in potentiation of the toxicity of other anti-cancer therapies; this interaction may occur with Doxil).
No products indexed under this heading.

Etoposide (Co-administration with the conventional formulation of doxorubicin results in potentiation of the toxicity of other anti-cancer therapies; this interaction may occur with Doxil).
No products indexed under this heading.

Exemestane (Co-administration with the conventional formulation of doxorubicin results in potentiation of the toxicity of other anti-cancer therapies; this interaction may occur with Doxil).
No products indexed under this heading.

Floxuridine (Co-administration with the conventional formulation of doxorubicin results in potentiation of the toxicity of other anti-cancer therapies; this interaction may occur with Doxil).
No products indexed under this heading.

Fluorouracil (Co-administration with the conventional formulation of doxorubicin results in potentiation of the toxicity of other anti-cancer therapies; this interaction may occur with Doxil). Products include:
Carac Cream 0.5% 2722

Flutamide (Co-administration with the conventional formulation of doxorubicin results in potentiation of the toxicity of other anti-cancer therapies; this interaction may occur with Doxil).
No products indexed under this heading.

Gemcitabine Hydrochloride (Co-administration with the conventional formulation of doxorubicin results in potentiation of the toxicity of other anti-cancer therapies; this interaction may occur with Doxil). Products include:
Gemzar for Injection 1820

Hydroxyurea (Co-administration with the conventional formulation of doxorubicin results in potentiation of the toxicity of other anti-cancer therapies; this interaction may occur with Doxil).
No products indexed under this heading.

Idarubicin Hydrochloride (Co-administration with the conventional formulation of doxorubicin results in potentiation of the toxicity of other anti-cancer therapies; this interaction may occur with Doxil).
No products indexed under this heading.

Ifosfamide (Co-administration with the conventional formulation of doxorubicin results in potentiation of the toxicity of other anti-cancer therapies; this interaction may occur with Doxil).
No products indexed under this heading.

Interferon alfa-2a, Recombinant (Co-administration with the conventional formulation of doxorubicin results in potentiation of the toxicity of other anti-cancer therapies; this interaction may occur with Doxil).
No products indexed under this heading.

Interferon alfa-2b, Recombinant (Co-administration with the conventional formulation of doxorubicin results in potentiation of the toxicity of other anti-cancer therapies; this interaction may occur with Doxil). Products include:
Intron A for Injection 2859

Irinotecan Hydrochloride (Co-administration with the conventional formulation of doxorubicin results in potentiation of the toxicity of other anti-cancer therapies; this interaction may occur with Doxil).
No products indexed under this heading.

Levamisole Hydrochloride (Co-administration with the conventional formulation of doxorubicin results in potentiation of the toxicity of other anti-cancer therapies; this interaction may occur with Doxil).
No products indexed under this heading.

Lomustine (CCNU) (Co-administration with the conventional formulation of doxorubicin results in potentiation of the toxicity of other anti-cancer therapies; this interaction may occur with Doxil).

No products indexed under this heading.

Mechlorethamine Hydrochloride (Co-administration with the conventional formulation of doxorubicin results in potentiation of the toxicity of other anti-cancer therapies; this interaction may occur with Doxil). Products include:

Mustargen for Injection 2492

Medroxyprogesterone Acetate (Co-administration of intravenous progesterone to patients with advanced malignancies at high doses with conventional formulation of fixed doxorubicin dose via bolus enhances doxorubicin-induced neutropenia and thrombocytopenia; this interaction may occur with Doxil). Products include:

Premphase Tablets 3232
Prempro Tablets 3232

Megestrol Acetate (Co-administration with the conventional formulation of doxorubicin results in potentiation of the toxicity of other anti-cancer therapies; this interaction may occur with Doxil). Products include:

Megace ES Oral Suspension 2499

Melphalan (Co-administration with the conventional formulation of doxorubicin results in potentiation of the toxicity of other anti-cancer therapies; this interaction may occur with Doxil).

No products indexed under this heading.

Mercaptopurine (Co-administration of conventional formulation of doxorubicin with 6-mercaptopurine has resulted in enhancement of hepatotoxicity of 6-mercaptopurine).

No products indexed under this heading.

Methotrexate Sodium (Co-administration with the conventional formulation of doxorubicin results in potentiation of the toxicity of other anti-cancer therapies; this interaction may occur with Doxil).

No products indexed under this heading.

Mitomycin (Mitomycin-C) (Co-administration with the conventional formulation of doxorubicin results in potentiation of the toxicity of other anti-cancer therapies; this interaction may occur with Doxil).

No products indexed under this heading.

Mitotane (Co-administration with the conventional formulation of doxorubicin results in potentiation of the toxicity of other anti-cancer therapies; this interaction may occur with Doxil).

No products indexed under this heading.

Mitoxantrone Hydrochloride (Co-administration with the conventional formulation of doxorubicin results in potentiation of the toxicity of other anti-cancer therapies; this interaction may occur with Doxil). Products include:

Novantrone for Injection Concentrate 1100

Oxaliplatin (Co-administration with the conventional formulation of doxorubicin results in potentiation of the toxicity of other anti-cancer therapies; this interaction may occur with Doxil). Products include:

Eloxatin for Injection 2731

Paclitaxel (Administration of paclitaxel infused over 24 hours followed by conventional formulation of doxorubicin administered over 48 hours resulted in a significant decrease in doxorubicin clearance with more profound neutropenic and stomatitis episodes than the reverse sequence of administration; this interaction may occur with Doxil).

No products indexed under this heading.

Phenobarbital (Co-administration with the conventional formulation of doxorubicin results in increased elimination of doxorubicin; this interaction may occur with Doxil). Products include:

Donnatal Extentabs 2507

Phenytoin (Co-administration with the conventional formulation of doxorubicin results in decreased phenytoin levels; this interaction may occur with Doxil).

No products indexed under this heading.

Phenytoin Sodium (Co-administration with the conventional formulation of doxorubicin results in decreased phenytoin levels; this interaction may occur with Doxil). Products include:

Phenytek Capsules 2192

Procarbazine Hydrochloride (Co-administration with the conventional formulation of doxorubicin results in potentiation of the toxicity of other anti-cancer therapies; this interaction may occur with Doxil).

No products indexed under this heading.

Progesterone (Co-administration of intravenous progesterone to patients with advanced malignancies at high doses with conventional formulation of fixed doxorubicin dose via bolus enhances doxorubicin-induced neutropenia and thrombocytopenia; this interaction may occur with Doxil). Products include:

Crinone 4% Gel 992
Crinone 8% Gel 992
Prometrium Capsules (100 mg, 200 mg) 3047

Streptozocin (Co-administration with the conventional formulation of doxorubicin results in inhibition of hepatic metabolism; this interaction may occur with Doxil).

No products indexed under this heading.

Tamoxifen Citrate (Co-administration with the conventional formulation of doxorubicin results in potentiation of the toxicity of other anti-cancer therapies; this interaction may occur with Doxil).

No products indexed under this heading.

Teniposide (Co-administration with the conventional formulation of doxorubicin results in potentiation of the toxicity of other anti-cancer therapies; this interaction may occur with Doxil).

No products indexed under this heading.

Thioguanine (Co-administration with the conventional formulation of doxorubicin results in potentiation of the toxicity of other anti-cancer therapies; this interaction may occur with Doxil). Products include:

Tabloid Tablets 1601

Thiotepa (Co-administration with the conventional formulation of doxorubicin results in potentiation of the toxicity of other anti-cancer therapies; this interaction may occur with Doxil).

No products indexed under this heading.

Topotecan Hydrochloride (Co-administration with the conventional formulation of doxorubicin results in potentiation of the toxicity of other anti-cancer therapies; this interaction may occur with Doxil). Products include:

Hycamtin for Injection 1459
Hycamtin Capsules 1456

Toremifene Citrate (Co-administration with the conventional formulation of doxorubicin results in potentiation of the toxicity of other anti-cancer therapies; this interaction may occur with Doxil).

No products indexed under this heading.

Valrubicin (Co-administration with the conventional formulation of doxorubicin results in potentiation of the toxicity of other anti-cancer therapies; this interaction may occur with Doxil). Products include:

Valstar Sterile Solution for Intravesical Instillation 1735

Verapamil Hydrochloride (Co-administration of conventional formulation of doxorubicin in animal studies has resulted in higher initial peak concentrations of doxorubicin in the heart with a higher incidence and severity of degenerative changes in cardiac tissue resulting in a shorter survival; this interaction may occur with Doxil). Products include:

Tarka Tablets 511

Vincristine Sulfate (Co-administration with the conventional formulation of doxorubicin results in potentiation of the toxicity of other anti-cancer therapies; this interaction may occur with Doxil).

No products indexed under this heading.

Vinorelbine Tartrate (Co-administration with the conventional formulation of doxorubicin results in potentiation of the toxicity of other anti-cancer therapies; this interaction may occur with Doxil).

No products indexed under this heading.

DRAMAMINE CHEWABLE TABLETS

(Dimenhydrinate) 1898
See Dramamine Original Tablets

DRAMAMINE LESS DROWSY TABLETS

(Meclizine Hydrochloride) 1898
See Dramamine Original Tablets

DRAMAMINE ORIGINAL TABLETS

(Dimenhydrinate) 1898

May interact with hypnotics and sedatives, tranquilizers, and certain other agents. Compounds in these categories include:

Alprazolam (May increase drowsiness effect).

No products indexed under this heading.

Buspirone Hydrochloride (May increase drowsiness effect).

No products indexed under this heading.

Butabarbital (May increase drowsiness effect).

No products indexed under this heading.

Butabarbital Sodium (May increase drowsiness effect).

No products indexed under this heading.

Chloral Hydrate (May increase drowsiness effect).

No products indexed under this heading.

Chlordiazepoxide (May increase drowsiness effect).

No products indexed under this heading.

Chlordiazepoxide Hydrochloride (May increase drowsiness effect).

No products indexed under this heading.

Chlorpromazine (May increase drowsiness effect).

No products indexed under this heading.

Chlorpromazine Hydrochloride (May increase drowsiness effect).

No products indexed under this heading.

Chlorprothixene (May increase drowsiness effect).

No products indexed under this heading.

Chlorprothixene Hydrochloride (May increase drowsiness effect).

No products indexed under this heading.

Clorazepate Dipotassium (May increase drowsiness effect).

No products indexed under this heading.

Diazepam (May increase drowsiness effect). Products include:

Valium Tablets 2658

Droperidol (May increase drowsiness effect).

No products indexed under this heading.

Estazolam (May increase drowsiness effect).

No products indexed under this heading.

Ethchlorvynol (May increase drowsiness effect).

No products indexed under this heading.

Ethinamate (May increase drowsiness effect).

No products indexed under this heading.

Fluphenazine Decanoate (May increase drowsiness effect).

No products indexed under this heading.

Fluphenazine Enanthate (May increase drowsiness effect).

No products indexed under this heading.

Fluphenazine Hydrochloride (May increase drowsiness effect).

No products indexed under this heading.

Flurazepam Hydrochloride (May increase drowsiness effect).

No products indexed under this heading.

Glutethimide (May increase drowsiness effect).

No products indexed under this heading.

Haloperidol (May increase drowsiness effect).

No products indexed under this heading.

IMPORTANT NOTE: Always consult each drug listing in the patient's regimen for possible interactions.

Haloperidol Decanoate (May increase drowsiness effect).
No products indexed under this heading.

Hydroxyzine Hydrochloride (May increase drowsiness effect).
No products indexed under this heading.

Lorazepam (May increase drowsiness effect).
No products indexed under this heading.

Loxapine Hydrochloride (May increase drowsiness effect).
No products indexed under this heading.

Loxapine Succinate (May increase drowsiness effect).
No products indexed under this heading.

Meprobamate (May increase drowsiness effect).
No products indexed under this heading.

Mesoridazine Besylate (May increase drowsiness effect).
No products indexed under this heading.

Midazolam Hydrochloride (May increase drowsiness effect).
No products indexed under this heading.

Molindone Hydrochloride (May increase drowsiness effect). Products include:
Moban Tablets 1116

Oxazepam (May increase drowsiness effect).
No products indexed under this heading.

Perphenazine (May increase drowsiness effect).
No products indexed under this heading.

Prazepam (May increase drowsiness effect).
No products indexed under this heading.

Prochlorperazine (May increase drowsiness effect).
No products indexed under this heading.

Promethazine Hydrochloride (May increase drowsiness effect).
No products indexed under this heading.

Propofol (May increase drowsiness effect).
No products indexed under this heading.

Quazepam (May increase drowsiness effect).
No products indexed under this heading.

Ramelteon (May increase drowsiness effect). Products include:
Rozerem Tablets 3091

Secobarbital Sodium (May increase drowsiness effect).
No products indexed under this heading.

Sodium Butabarbital (May increase drowsiness effect).
No products indexed under this heading.

Temazepam (May increase drowsiness effect).
No products indexed under this heading.

Thioridazine Hydrochloride (May increase drowsiness effect). Products include:
Thioridazine Hydrochloride Tablets 2195

Thiothixene (May increase drowsiness effect). Products include:
Thiothixene Capsules 2197

Triazolam (May increase drowsiness effect).
No products indexed under this heading.

Trifluoperazine Hydrochloride (May increase drowsiness effect).
No products indexed under this heading.

Zaleplon (May increase drowsiness effect).
No products indexed under this heading.

Zolpidem Tartrate (May increase drowsiness effect). Products include:
Ambien Tablets 2692
Ambien CR Tablets 2696

Food Interactions

Alcohol (May increase drowsiness effect).

DUAC TOPICAL GEL

(Benzoyl Peroxide, Clindamycin) 3054
May interact with erythromycin and certain other agents. Compounds in these categories include:

Concomitant Topical Acne Therapy (Concomitant topical acne therapy should be used with caution because a possible cumulative irritancy effect may occur, especially with the use of peeling, desquamating, or abrasive agents).
No products indexed under this heading.

Erythromycin (Clindamycin- and erythromycin-containing products should not be used in combination. In vitro studies have shown antagonism between these two antimicrobials. The clinical significance of this in vitro antagonism is not known).
No products indexed under this heading.

Erythromycin Estolate (Clindamycin- and erythromycin-containing products should not be used in combination. In vitro studies have shown antagonism between these two antimicrobials. The clinical significance of this in vitro antagonism is not known).
No products indexed under this heading.

Erythromycin Ethylsuccinate (Clindamycin- and erythromycin-containing products should not be used in combination. In vitro studies have shown antagonism between these two antimicrobials. The clinical significance of this in vitro antagonism is not known). Products include:
E.E.S. 433
EryPed 431

Erythromycin Gluceptate (Clindamycin- and erythromycin-containing products should not be used in combination. In vitro studies have shown antagonism between these two antimicrobials. The clinical significance of this in vitro antagonism is not known).
No products indexed under this heading.

Erythromycin Lactobionate (Clindamycin- and erythromycin-containing products should not be used in combination. In vitro studies have shown antagonism between these two antimicrobials. The clinical significance of this in vitro antagonism is not known).
No products indexed under this heading.

Erythromycin Stearate (Clindamycin- and erythromycin-containing products should not be used in combination. In vitro studies have shown antagonism between these two antimicrobials. The clinical significance of this in vitro antagonism is not known).
No products indexed under this heading.

DUETACT TABLETS

(Glimepiride, Pioglitazone Hydrochloride).................................. 3085
May interact with beta blockers, corticosteroids, oral anticoagulants, cytochrome p450 2c9 inducers (selected), cytochrome p450 2c9 inhibitors (selected), cytochrome p450 3a4 substrates (selected), diuretics, estrogens, monoamine oxidase inhibitors, non-steroidal anti-inflammatory agents, oral contraceptives, phenothiazines, phenytoin, salicylates, sulfonamides, sympathomimetics, thiazides, thyroid preparations, and certain other agents. Compounds in these categories include:

Acebutolol Hydrochloride (The hypoglycemic action of sulfonylureas may be potentiated by certain drugs, including beta adrenergic blocking agents. Due to the potential drug interaction between these drugs and glimepiride, the patient should be observed closely for hypoglycemia when these drugs are co-administered. Conversely, when these drugs are withdrawn, the patient should be observed closely for loss of glycemic control. If beta-blockers are used, caution should be exercised and patients should be warned about the potential for hypoglycemia).
No products indexed under this heading.

Albuterol (Certain drugs tend to produce hyperglycemia and may lead to loss of control. These drugs include the sympathomimetics. Due to the potential drug interaction between these drugs and glimepiride, the patient should be observed closely for loss of glycemic control when these drugs are co-administered. Conversely, when these drugs are withdrawn, the patient should be observed closely for hypoglycemia).
No products indexed under this heading.

Albuterol Sulfate (Certain drugs tend to produce hyperglycemia and may lead to loss of control. These drugs include the sympathomimetics. Due to the potential drug interaction between these drugs and glimepiride, the patient should be observed closely for loss of glycemic control when these drugs are co-administered. Conversely, when these drugs are withdrawn, the patient should be observed closely for hypoglycemia). Products include:
Combivent Inhalation Aerosol 845
ProAir HFA Inhalation Aerosol 3113
Proventil HFA Inhalation Aerosol 2914
Ventolin HFA Inhalation Aerosol 1638

Alfentanil Hydrochloride (In vivo drug-drug interaction studies have suggested that pioglitazone may be a weak inducer of CYP 450 isoform 3A4 substrate).
No products indexed under this heading.

Alprazolam (In vivo drug-drug interaction studies have suggested that pioglitazone may be a weak inducer of CYP 450 isoform 3A4 substrate).
No products indexed under this heading.

Amiloride Hydrochloride (Certain drugs tend to produce hyperglycemia and may lead to loss of control. These drugs include the thiazides and other diuretics. Due to the potential drug interaction between these drugs and glimepiride, the patient should be observed closely for loss of glycemic control when these drugs are co-administered. Conversely, when these drugs are withdrawn, the patient should be observed closely for hypoglycemia).
No products indexed under this heading.

Amiodarone Hydrochloride (There is a potential interaction of glimepiride with inhibitors (e.g., fluconazole) of cytochrome P450 2C9).
No products indexed under this heading.

Amitriptyline Hydrochloride (In vivo drug-drug interaction studies have suggested that pioglitazone may be a weak inducer of CYP 450 isoform 3A4 substrate).
No products indexed under this heading.

Amlodipine Besylate (In vivo drug-drug interaction studies have suggested that pioglitazone may be a weak inducer of CYP 450 isoform 3A4 substrate). Products include:
Azor Tablets 1005
Exforge Tablets 2238

Anastrozole (There is a potential interaction of glimepiride with inhibitors (e.g., fluconazole) of cytochrome P450 2C9). Products include:
Arimidex Tablets 672

Anisindione (The hypoglycemic action of sulfonylureas may be potentiated by certain drugs, including coumarins. Due to the potential drug interaction between these drugs and glimepiride, the patient should be observed closely for hypoglycemia when these drugs are co-administered. Conversely, when these drugs are withdrawn, the patient should be observed closely for loss of glycemic control).
No products indexed under this heading.

Aprepitant (There is a potential interaction of glimepiride with inducers (e.g., rifampicin) of cytochrome P450 2C9). Products include:
Emend Capsules 1992

Aspirin (The hypoglycemic action of sulfonylureas may be potentiated by certain drugs, included salicylates. Due to the potential drug interaction between these drugs and glimepiride, the patient should be observed closely for hypoglycemia when these drugs are co-administered. Conversely, when these drugs are withdrawn, the patient should be observed closely for loss of glycemic control). Products include:

- Aggrenox Capsules **819**
- Bayer Aspirin **750**
- Percodan Tablets **1130**
- St. Joseph 81 mg Aspirin Chewable and Enteric Coated Tablets **1903**

Aspirin, Enteric Coated (The hypoglycemic action of sulfonylureas may be potentiated by certain drugs, included salicylates. Due to the potential drug interaction between these drugs and glimepiride, the patient should be observed closely for hypoglycemia when these drugs are co-administered. Conversely, when these drugs are withdrawn, the patient should be observed closely for loss of glycemic control).
No products indexed under this heading.

Aspirin Buffered (The hypoglycemic action of sulfonylureas may be potentiated by certain drugs, included salicylates. Due to the potential drug interaction between these drugs and glimepiride, the patient should be observed closely for hypoglycemia when these drugs are co-administered. Conversely, when these drugs are withdrawn, the patient should be observed closely for loss of glycemic control).
No products indexed under this heading.

Astemizole (In vivo drug-drug interaction studies have suggested that pioglitazone may be a weak inducer of CYP 450 isoform 3A4 substrate).
No products indexed under this heading.

Atenolol (The hypoglycemic action of sulfonylureas may be potentiated by certain drugs, including beta adrenergic blocking agents. Due to the potential drug interaction between these drugs and glimepiride, the patient should be observed closely for hypoglycemia when these drugs are co-administered. Conversely, when these drugs are withdrawn, the patient should be observed closely for loss of glycemic control. If beta-blockers are used, caution should be exercised and patients should be warned about the potential for hypoglycemia).
No products indexed under this heading.

Atorvastatin Calcium (Co-administration of pioglitazone for 7 days with atorvastatin calcium 80 mg once daily resulted in a ratio of least square mean (90% CI) values for unchanged pioglitazone of 0.69 (0.57-0.85) for Cmax, 0.76 (0.65-0.88) for AUC, and 0.96 (0.87-1.05) for Cmin. For unchanged atorvastatin, the ratio of least square mean (90% CI) values were 0.77 (0.66-0.90) for Cmax, 0.86 (0.78-0.94) for AUC and 0.92 (0.82-1.02) for Cmin). Products include:

- Lipitor Tablets **2501**

Belladonna Ergotamine (In vivo drug-drug interaction studies have suggested that pioglitazone may be a weak inducer of CYP 450 isoform 3A4 substrate).
No products indexed under this heading.

Bendroflumethiazide (The hypoglycemic action of sulfonylureas may be potentiated by certain drugs, including sulfonamides. Due to the potential drug interaction between these drugs and glimepiride, the patient should be observed closely for hypoglycemia when these drugs are co-administered. Conversely when these drugs are withdrawn, the patient should be observed closely for loss of glycemic control).
No products indexed under this heading.

Betamethasone Acetate (Certain drugs tend to produce hyperglycemia and may lead to loss of control. These drugs include the corticosteroids. Due to the potential drug interaction between these drugs and glimepiride, the patient should be observed closely for loss of glycemic control when these drugs are co-administered. Conversely, when these drugs are withdrawn, the patient should be observed closely for hypoglycemia).
No products indexed under this heading.

Betamethasone Sodium Phosphate (Certain drugs tend to produce hyperglycemia and may lead to loss of control. These drugs include the corticosteroids. Due to the potential drug interaction between these drugs and glimepiride, the patient should be observed closely for loss of glycemic control when these drugs are co-administered. Conversely, when these drugs are withdrawn, the patient should be observed closely for hypoglycemia).
No products indexed under this heading.

Betaxolol Hydrochloride (The hypoglycemic action of sulfonylureas may be potentiated by certain drugs, including beta adrenergic blocking agents. Due to the potential drug interaction between these drugs and glimepiride, the patient should be observed closely for hypoglycemia when these drugs are co-administered. Conversely, when these drugs are withdrawn, the patient should be observed closely for loss of glycemic control. If beta-blockers are used, caution should be exercised and patients should be warned about the potential for hypoglycemia).
No products indexed under this heading.

Bisoprolol Fumarate (The hypoglycemic action of sulfonylureas may be potentiated by certain drugs, including beta adrenergic blocking agents. Due to the potential drug interaction between these drugs and glimepiride, the patient should be observed closely for hypoglycemia when these drugs are co-administered. Conversely, when these drugs are withdrawn, the patient should be observed closely for loss of glycemic control. If beta-blockers are used, caution should be exercised and patients should be warned about the potential for hypoglycemia).
No products indexed under this heading.

Budesonide (Certain drugs tend to produce hyperglycemia and may lead to loss of control. These drugs include the corticosteroids. Due to the potential drug interaction between these drugs and glimepiride, the patient should be observed closely for loss of glycemic control when these drugs are co-administered. Conversely, when these drugs are withdrawn, the patient should be observed closely for hypoglycemia). Products include:

- Pulmicort Flexhaler **654**
- Symbicort 80/4.5 Inhalation Aerosol **659**
- Symbicort 160/4.5 Inhalation Aerosol **659**

Bumetanide (Certain drugs tend to produce hyperglycemia and may lead to loss of control. These drugs include the thiazides and other diuretics. Due to the potential drug interaction between these drugs and glimepiride, the patient should be observed closely for loss of glycemic control when these drugs are co-administered. Conversely, when these drugs are withdrawn, the patient should be observed closely for hypoglycemia).
No products indexed under this heading.

Buspirone Hydrochloride (In vivo drug-drug interaction studies have suggested that pioglitazone may be a weak inducer of CYP 450 isoform 3A4 substrate).
No products indexed under this heading.

Busulfan (In vivo drug-drug interaction studies have suggested that pioglitazone may be a weak inducer of CYP 450 isoform 3A4 substrate). Products include:

- Busulfex Injection **2477**
- Myleran Tablets **1530**

Carbamazepine (There is a potential interaction of glimepiride with inducers (e.g., rifampicin) of cytochrome P450 2C9). Products include:

- Carbatrol Capsules **3019**
- Equetro Extended-Release Capsules **3174**

Carteolol Hydrochloride (The hypoglycemic action of sulfonylureas may be potentiated by certain drugs, including beta adrenergic blocking agents. Due to the potential drug interaction between these drugs and glimepiride, the patient should be observed closely for hypoglycemia when these drugs are co-administered. Conversely, when these drugs are withdrawn, the patient should be observed closely for loss of glycemic control. If beta-blockers are used, caution should be exercised and patients should be warned about the potential for hypoglycemia).
No products indexed under this heading.

Celecoxib (The hypoglycemic action of sulfonylureas may be potentiated by certain drugs, including nonsteroidial anti-inflammatory drugs. Due to the potential drug interaction between these drugs and glimepiride, the patient should be observed closely for hypoglycemia when these drugs are co-administered. Conversely, when these drugs are withdrawn, the patient should be observed closely for loss of glycemic control). Products include:

- Celebrex Capsules **2979**

Cerivastatin Sodium (In vivo drug-drug interaction studies have suggested that pioglitazone may be a weak inducer of CYP 450 isoform 3A4 substrate).
No products indexed under this heading.

Chloramphenicol (The hypoglycemic action of sulfonylureas may be potentiated by certain drugs, including chloramphenicol. Due to the potential drug interaction between these drugs and glimepiride, the patient should be observed closely for hypoglycemia when these drugs are co-administered. Conversely, when these drugs are withdrawn, the patient should be observed closely for loss of glycemic control).
No products indexed under this heading.

Chlorothiazide (The hypoglycemic action of sulfonylureas may be potentiated by certain drugs, including sulfonamides. Due to the potential drug interaction between these drugs and glimepiride, the patient should be observed closely for hypoglycemia when these drugs are co-administered. Conversely when these drugs are withdrawn, the patient should be observed closely for loss of glycemic control).
No products indexed under this heading.

Chlorothiazide Sodium (The hypoglycemic action of sulfonylureas may be potentiated by certain drugs, including sulfonamides. Due to the potential drug interaction between these drugs and glimepiride, the patient should be observed closely for hypoglycemia when these drugs are co-administered. Conversely when these drugs are withdrawn, the patient should be observed closely for loss of glycemic control). Products include:

- Intravenous Sodium Diuril **2490**

Chlorotrianisene (Certain drugs tend to produce hyperglycemia and may lead to loss of control. These drugs include the estrogens. Due to the potential drug interaction between these drugs and glimepiride, the patient should be observed closely for loss of glycemic control when these drugs are co-administered. Conversely, when these drugs are withdrawn, the patient should be observed closely for hypoglycemia).
No products indexed under this heading.

Chlorpheniramine (In vivo drug-drug interaction studies have suggested that pioglitazone may be a weak inducer of CYP 450 isoform 3A4 substrate).
No products indexed under this heading.

Chlorpheniramine Maleate (In vivo drug-drug interaction studies have suggested that pioglitazone may be a weak inducer of CYP 450 isoform 3A4 substrate). Products include:

- Actifed Cold & Allergy Tablets **1895**
- Sudafed PE Sinus & Allergy Tablets **1908**
- Tylenol Allergy Multi-Symptom Caplets with Cool Burst and Rapid Release Gelcaps **1916**
- Children's Tylenol Plus Cold Suspension Liquid **1912**
- Children's Tylenol Plus Cough & Runny Nose Suspension Liquid **1912**
- Children's Tylenol Plus Flu Suspension Liquid **1914**
- Children's Tylenol Plus Multi-Symptom Cold Suspension Liquid **1912**
- Tylenol Cold Head Congestion Nighttime Caplets with Cool Burst **1910**

Tylenol Cold Multi-Symptom Nighttime Caplets with Cool Burst 1913
Tylenol Sinus Congestion & Pain Nighttime Caplets with Cool Burst 1917

Chlorpheniramine Polistirex (In vivo drug-drug interaction studies have suggested that pioglitazone may be a weak inducer of CYP 450 isoform 3A4 substrate). Products include:
Tussionex Pennkinetic Extended-Release Suspension 3154

Chlorpheniramine Tannate (In vivo drug-drug interaction studies have suggested that pioglitazone may be a weak inducer of CYP 450 isoform 3A4 substrate).
No products indexed under this heading.

Chlorpromazine (Certain drugs tend to produce hyperglycemia and may lead to loss of control. These drugs include the phenothiazines. Due to the potential drug interaction between these drugs and glimepiride, the patient should be observed closely for loss of glycemic control when these drugs are co-administered. Conversely, when these drugs are withdrawn, the patient should be observed closely for hypoglycemia).
No products indexed under this heading.

Chlorpromazine Hydrochloride (Certain drugs tend to produce hyperglycemia and may lead to loss of control. These drugs include the phenothiazines. Due to the potential drug interaction between these drugs and glimepiride, the patient should be observed closely for loss of glycemic control when these drugs are co-administered. Conversely, when these drugs are withdrawn, the patient should be observed closely for hypoglycemia).
No products indexed under this heading.

Chlorpropamide (The hypoglycemic action of sulfonylureas may be potentiated by certain drugs, including sulfonamides. Due to the potential drug interaction between these drugs and glimepiride, the patient should be observed closely for hypoglycemia when these drugs are co-administered. Conversely when these drugs are withdrawn, the patient should be observed closely for loss of glycemic control).
No products indexed under this heading.

Chlorthalidone (Certain drugs tend to produce hyperglycemia and may lead to loss of control. These drugs include the thiazides and other diuretics. Due to the potential drug interaction between these drugs and glimepiride, the patient should be observed closely for loss of glycemic control when these drugs are co-administered. Conversely, when these drugs are withdrawn, the patient should be observed closely for hypoglycemia). Products include:
Clorpres Tablets 2185

Choline Magnesium Trisalicylate (The hypoglycemic action of sulfonylureas may be potentiated by certain drugs, included salicylates. Due to the potential drug interaction between these drugs and glimepiride, the patient should be observed closely for hypoglycemia when these drugs are co-administered. Conversely, when these drugs are withdrawn, the patient should be observed closely for loss of glycemic control).
No products indexed under this heading.

Ciclesonide (Certain drugs tend to produce hyperglycemia and may lead to loss of control. These drugs include the corticosteroids. Due to the potential drug interaction between these drugs and glimepiride, the patient should be observed closely for loss of glycemic control when these drugs are co-administered. Conversely, when these drugs are withdrawn, the patient should be observed closely for hypoglycemia). Products include:
Alvesco Inhalation Aerosol 2985
Omnaris Nasal Spray 2998

Cimetidine (There is a potential interaction of glimepiride with inhibitors (e.g., fluconazole) of cytochrome P450 2C9).
No products indexed under this heading.

Cimetidine Hydrochloride (There is a potential interaction of glimepiride with inhibitors (e.g., fluconazole) of cytochrome P450 2C9).
No products indexed under this heading.

Cisapride (In vivo drug-drug interaction studies have suggested that pioglitazone may be a weak inducer of CYP 450 isoform 3A4 substrate).
No products indexed under this heading.

Clarithromycin (In vivo drug-drug interaction studies have suggested that pioglitazone may be a weak inducer of CYP 450 isoform 3A4 substrate). Products include:
Biaxin/Biaxin XL 411

Clopidogrel Hydrogen Sulfate (There is a potential interaction of glimepiride with inhibitors (e.g., fluconazole) of cytochrome P450 2C9).
No products indexed under this heading.

Clotrimazole (There is a potential interaction of glimepiride with inhibitors (e.g., fluconazole) of cytochrome P450 2C9). Products include:
Lotrisone 2881

Cortisone Acetate (Certain drugs tend to produce hyperglycemia and may lead to loss of control. These drugs include the corticosteroids. Due to the potential drug interaction between these drugs and glimepiride, the patient should be observed closely for loss of glycemic control when these drugs are co-administered. Conversely, when these drugs are withdrawn, the patient should be observed closely for hypoglycemia).
No products indexed under this heading.

Cyclosporine (In vivo drug-drug interaction studies have suggested that pioglitazone may be a weak inducer of CYP 450 isoform 3A4 substrate). Products include:
Gengraf Capsules 435
Neoral Oral Solution 2280
Neoral Soft Gelatin Capsules 2280
Restasis Ophthalmic Emulsion 557
Sandimmune 2296

Desogestrel (Certain drugs tend to produce hyperglycemia and may lead to loss of control. These drugs include oral contraceptives. Due to the potential drug interaction between these drugs and glimepiride, the patient should be observed closely for loss of glycemic control when these drugs are co-administered. Conversely, when these drugs are withdrawn, the patient should be observed closely for hypoglycemia). Products include:
Mircette Tablets 1034

Dexamethasone (Certain drugs tend to produce hyperglycemia and may lead to loss of control. These drugs include the corticosteroids. Due to the potential drug interaction between these drugs and glimepiride, the patient should be observed closely for loss of glycemic control when these drugs are co-administered. Conversely, when these drugs are withdrawn, the patient should be observed closely for hypoglycemia). Products include:
Ciprodex Otic Suspension 541

Dexamethasone Acetate (Certain drugs tend to produce hyperglycemia and may lead to loss of control. These drugs include the corticosteroids. Due to the potential drug interaction between these drugs and glimepiride, the patient should be observed closely for loss of glycemic control when these drugs are co-administered. Conversely, when these drugs are withdrawn, the patient should be observed closely for hypoglycemia).
No products indexed under this heading.

Dexamethasone Sodium Phosphate (Certain drugs tend to produce hyperglycemia and may lead to loss of control. These drugs include the corticosteroids. Due to the potential drug interaction between these drugs and glimepiride, the patient should be observed closely for loss of glycemic control when these drugs are co-administered. Conversely, when these drugs are withdrawn, the patient should be observed closely for hypoglycemia).
No products indexed under this heading.

Diazepam (In vivo drug-drug interaction studies have suggested that pioglitazone may be a weak inducer of CYP 450 isoform 3A4 substrate). Products include:
Valium Tablets 2658

Diclofenac Epolamine (The hypoglycemic action of sulfonylureas may be potentiated by certain drugs, including nonsteroidial anti-inflammatory drugs. Due to the potential drug interaction between these drugs and glimepiride, the patient should be observed closely for hypoglycemia when these drugs are co-administered. Conversely, when these drugs are withdrawn, the patient should be observed closely for loss of glycemic control). Products include:
Flector Patch 561

Diclofenac Potassium (The hypoglycemic action of sulfonylureas may be potentiated by certain drugs, including nonsteroidial anti-inflammatory drugs. Due to the potential drug interaction between these drugs and glimepiride, the patient should be observed closely for hypoglycemia when these drugs are co-administered. Conversely, when these drugs are withdrawn, the patient should be observed closely for loss of glycemic control).
No products indexed under this heading.

Diclofenac Sodium (The hypoglycemic action of sulfonylureas may be potentiated by certain drugs, including nonsteroidial anti-inflammatory drugs. Due to the potential drug interaction between these drugs and glimepiride, the patient should be observed closely for hypoglycemia when these drugs are co-administered. Conversely, when these drugs are withdrawn, the patient should be observed closely for loss of glycemic control). Products include:
Diclofenac Sodium Ophthalmic Solution .... ⊙240
Voltaren Ophthalmic Solution 2336
Voltaren Tablets 2334
Voltaren-XR Tablets 2337

Dicumarol (The hypoglycemic action of sulfonylureas may be potentiated by certain drugs, including coumarins. Due to the potential drug interaction between these drugs and glimepiride, the patient should be observed closely for hypoglycemia when these drugs are co-administered. Conversely, when these drugs are withdrawn, the patient should be observed closely for loss of glycemic control).
No products indexed under this heading.

Dienestrol (Certain drugs tend to produce hyperglycemia and may lead to loss of control. These drugs include the estrogens. Due to the potential drug interaction between these drugs and glimepiride, the patient should be observed closely for loss of glycemic control when these drugs are co-administered. Conversely, when these drugs are withdrawn, the patient should be observed closely for hypoglycemia).
No products indexed under this heading.

Diethylstilbestrol (Certain drugs tend to produce hyperglycemia and may lead to loss of control. These drugs include the estrogens. Due to the potential drug interaction between these drugs and glimepiride, the patient should be observed closely for loss of glycemic control when these drugs are co-administered. Conversely, when these drugs are withdrawn, the patient should be observed closely for hypoglycemia).
No products indexed under this heading.

Diflunisal (The hypoglycemic action of sulfonylureas may be potentiated by certain drugs, included salicylates. Due to the potential drug interaction between these drugs and glimepiride, the patient should be observed closely for hypoglycemia when these drugs are co-administered. Conversely, when these drugs are withdrawn, the patient should be observed closely for loss of glycemic control).
No products indexed under this heading.

Dihydroergotamine Mesylate (In vivo drug-drug interaction studies have suggested that pioglitazone may be a weak inducer of CYP 450 isoform 3A4 substrate).
No products indexed under this heading.

Diltiazem Hydrochloride (In vivo drug-drug interaction studies have suggested that pioglitazone may be a weak inducer of CYP 450 isoform 3A4 substrate). Products include:

Cardizem LA Extended Release Tablets 421

Diltiazem Maleate (In vivo drug-drug interaction studies have suggested that pioglitazone may be a weak inducer of CYP 450 isoform 3A4 substrate).

No products indexed under this heading.

Disopyramide (In vivo drug-drug interaction studies have suggested that pioglitazone may be a weak inducer of CYP 450 isoform 3A4 substrate).

No products indexed under this heading.

Disopyramide Phosphate (In vivo drug-drug interaction studies have suggested that pioglitazone may be a weak inducer of CYP 450 isoform 3A4 substrate).

No products indexed under this heading.

Disulfiram (There is a potential interaction of glimepiride with inhibitors (e.g., fluconazole) of cytochrome P450 2C9).

No products indexed under this heading.

Dobutamine Hydrochloride (Certain drugs tend to produce hyperglycemia and may lead to loss of control. These drugs include the sympathomimetics. Due to the potential drug interaction between these drugs and glimepiride, the patient should be observed closely for loss of glycemic control when these drugs are co-administered. Conversely, when these drugs are withdrawn, the patient should be observed closely for hypoglycemia).

No products indexed under this heading.

Dopamine Hydrochloride (Certain drugs tend to produce hyperglycemia and may lead to loss of control. These drugs include the sympathomimetics. Due to the potential drug interaction between these drugs and glimepiride, the patient should be observed closely for loss of glycemic control when these drugs are co-administered. Conversely, when these drugs are withdrawn, the patient should be observed closely for hypoglycemia).

No products indexed under this heading.

Doxorubicin Hydrochloride (In vivo drug-drug interaction studies have suggested that pioglitazone may be a weak inducer of CYP 450 isoform 3A4 substrate).

No products indexed under this heading.

Dronabinol (In vivo drug-drug interaction studies have suggested that pioglitazone may be a weak inducer of CYP 450 isoform 3A4 substrate). Products include:

Marinol Capsules 3163

Efavirenz (There is a potential interaction of glimepiride with inhibitors (e.g., fluconazole) of cytochrome P450 2C9). Products include:

Atripla Tablets 938
Sustiva Capsules 930
Sustiva Tablets 930

Ephedrine Hydrochloride (Certain drugs tend to produce hyperglycemia and may lead to loss of control. These drugs include the sympathomimetics. Due to the potential drug interaction between these drugs and glimepiride, the patient should be observed closely for loss of glycemic control when these drugs are co-administered. Conversely, when these drugs are withdrawn, the patient should be observed closely for hypoglycemia).

No products indexed under this heading.

Ephedrine Sulfate (Certain drugs tend to produce hyperglycemia and may lead to loss of control. These drugs include the sympathomimetics. Due to the potential drug interaction between these drugs and glimepiride, the patient should be observed closely for loss of glycemic control when these drugs are co-administered. Conversely, when these drugs are withdrawn, the patient should be observed closely for hypoglycemia).

No products indexed under this heading.

Ephedrine Tannate (Certain drugs tend to produce hyperglycemia and may lead to loss of control. These drugs include the sympathomimetics. Due to the potential drug interaction between these drugs and glimepiride, the patient should be observed closely for loss of glycemic control when these drugs are co-administered. Conversely, when these drugs are withdrawn, the patient should be observed closely for hypoglycemia).

No products indexed under this heading.

Epinephrine (Certain drugs tend to produce hyperglycemia and may lead to loss of control. These drugs include the sympathomimetics. Due to the potential drug interaction between these drugs and glimepiride, the patient should be observed closely for loss of glycemic control when these drugs are co-administered. Conversely, when these drugs are withdrawn, the patient should be observed closely for hypoglycemia). Products include:

EpiPen 1024

Epinephrine Bitartrate (Certain drugs tend to produce hyperglycemia and may lead to loss of control. These drugs include the sympathomimetics. Due to the potential drug interaction between these drugs and glimepiride, the patient should be observed closely for loss of glycemic control when these drugs are co-administered. Conversely, when these drugs are withdrawn, the patient should be observed closely for hypoglycemia).

No products indexed under this heading.

Epinephrine Hydrochloride (Certain drugs tend to produce hyperglycemia and may lead to loss of control. These drugs include the sympathomimetics. Due to the potential drug interaction between these drugs and glimepiride, the patient should be observed closely for loss of glycemic control when these drugs are co-administered. Conversely, when these drugs are withdrawn, the patient should be observed closely for hypoglycemia).

No products indexed under this heading.

Ergotamine Tartrate (In vivo drug-drug interaction studies have suggested that pioglitazone may be a weak inducer of CYP 450 isoform 3A4 substrate).

No products indexed under this heading.

Erythromycin (In vivo drug-drug interaction studies have suggested that pioglitazone may be a weak inducer of CYP 450 isoform 3A4 substrate).

No products indexed under this heading.

Erythromycin Estolate (In vivo drug-drug interaction studies have suggested that pioglitazone may be a weak inducer of CYP 450 isoform 3A4 substrate).

No products indexed under this heading.

Erythromycin Ethylsuccinate (In vivo drug-drug interaction studies have suggested that pioglitazone may be a weak inducer of CYP 450 isoform 3A4 substrate). Products include:

E.E.S. 433
EryPed 431

Erythromycin Gluceptate (In vivo drug-drug interaction studies have suggested that pioglitazone may be a weak inducer of CYP 450 isoform 3A4 substrate).

No products indexed under this heading.

Erythromycin Lactobionate (In vivo drug-drug interaction studies have suggested that pioglitazone may be a weak inducer of CYP 450 isoform 3A4 substrate).

No products indexed under this heading.

Erythromycin Stearate (In vivo drug-drug interaction studies have suggested that pioglitazone may be a weak inducer of CYP 450 isoform 3A4 substrate).

No products indexed under this heading.

Esmolol Hydrochloride (The hypoglycemic action of sulfonylureas may be potentiated by certain drugs, including beta adrenergic blocking agents. Due to the potential drug interaction between these drugs and glimepiride, the patient should be observed closely for hypoglycemia when these drugs are co-administered. Conversely, when these drugs are withdrawn, the patient should be observed closely for loss of glycemic control. If beta-blockers are used, caution should be exercised and patients should be warned about the potential for hypoglycemia).

No products indexed under this heading.

Estradiol (Certain drugs tend to produce hyperglycemia and may lead to loss of control. These drugs include the estrogens. Due to the potential drug interaction between these drugs and glimepiride, the patient should be observed closely for loss of glycemic control when these drugs are co-administered. Conversely, when these drugs are withdrawn, the patient should be observed closely for hypoglycemia). Products include:

Activella Tablets 2347
Angeliq Tablets 751
Climara Transdermal System 763
Climara Pro Transdermal System 768
Divigel 3167
Vagifem Tablets 2375

Estradiol Benzoate (In vivo drug-drug interaction studies have suggested that pioglitazone may be a weak inducer of CYP 450 isoform 3A4 substrate).

No products indexed under this heading.

Estradiol Cypionate (In vivo drug-drug interaction studies have suggested that pioglitazone may be a weak inducer of CYP 450 isoform 3A4 substrate).

No products indexed under this heading.

Estradiol Valerate (In vivo drug-drug interaction studies have suggested that pioglitazone may be a weak inducer of CYP 450 isoform 3A4 substrate).

No products indexed under this heading.

Estrogens, Conjugated (Certain drugs tend to produce hyperglycemia and may lead to loss of control. These drugs include the estrogens. Due to the potential drug interaction between these drugs and glimepiride, the patient should be observed closely for loss of glycemic control when these drugs are co-administered. Conversely, when these drugs are withdrawn, the patient should be observed closely for hypoglycemia). Products include:

Premarin Intravenous 3217
Premarin Tablets 3221
Premarin Vaginal Cream 3228
Premphase Tablets 3232
Prempro Tablets 3232

Estrogens, Esterified (Certain drugs tend to produce hyperglycemia and may lead to loss of control. These drugs include the estrogens. Due to the potential drug interaction between these drugs and glimepiride, the patient should be observed closely for loss of glycemic control when these drugs are co-administered. Conversely, when these drugs are withdrawn, the patient should be observed closely for hypoglycemia). Products include:

Estratest Tablets 3043
Estratest H.S. Tablets 3043

Estropipate (Certain drugs tend to produce hyperglycemia and may lead to loss of control. These drugs include the estrogens. Due to the potential drug interaction between these drugs and glimepiride, the patient should be observed closely for loss of glycemic control when these drugs are co-administered. Conversely, when these drugs are withdrawn, the patient should be observed closely for hypoglycemia).

No products indexed under this heading.

Ethacrynic Acid (Certain drugs tend to produce hyperglycemia and may lead to loss of control. These drugs include the thiazides and other diuretics. Due to the potential drug interaction between these drugs and glimepiride, the patient should be observed closely for loss of glycemic control when these drugs are co-administered. Conversely, when these drugs are withdrawn, the patient should be observed closely for hypoglycemia). Products include:

Edecrin Tablets 698

Ethinyl Estradiol (Certain drugs tend to produce hyperglycemia and may lead to loss of control. These drugs include the estrogens. Due to

the potential drug interaction between these drugs and glimepiride, the patient should be observed closely for loss of glycemic control when these drugs are co-administered. Conversely, when these drugs are withdrawn, the patient should be observed closely for hypoglycemia). Products include:

Lybrel Tablets 3204
Mircette Tablets 1034
NuvaRing 2897
Ortho-Cyclen/Ortho Tri-Cyclen 2449
Ortho Evra Transdermal System 2437
Ortho Tri-Cyclen Lo Tablets 2458
Seasonique Tablets 1046
Yaz Tablets 805

Ethosuximide (In vivo drug-drug interaction studies have suggested that pioglitazone may be a weak inducer of CYP 450 isoform 3A4 substrate).

No products indexed under this heading.

Ethynodiol Diacetate (Certain drugs tend to produce hyperglycemia and may lead to loss of control. These drugs include oral contraceptives. Due to the potential drug interaction between these drugs and glimepiride, the patient should be observed closely for loss of glycemic control when these drugs are co-administered. Conversely, when these drugs are withdrawn, the patient should be observed closely for hypoglycemia).

No products indexed under this heading.

Etodolac (The hypoglycemic action of sulfonylureas may be potentiated by certain drugs, including nonsteroidial anti-inflammatory drugs. Due to the potential drug interaction between these drugs and glimepiride, the patient should be observed closely for hypoglycemia when these drugs are co-administered. Conversely, when these drugs are withdrawn, the patient should be observed closely for loss of glycemic control).

No products indexed under this heading.

Etoposide (In vivo drug-drug interaction studies have suggested that pioglitazone may be a weak inducer of CYP 450 isoform 3A4 substrate).

No products indexed under this heading.

Etoposide Phosphate (In vivo drug-drug interaction studies have suggested that pioglitazone may be a weak inducer of CYP 450 isoform 3A4 substrate).

No products indexed under this heading.

Felodipine (In vivo drug-drug interaction studies have suggested that pioglitazone may be a weak inducer of CYP 450 isoform 3A4 substrate).

No products indexed under this heading.

Fenofibrate (There is a potential interaction of glimepiride with inhibitors (e.g., fluconazole) of cytochrome P450 2C9). Products include:

Fenoglide Tablets 2960
Tricor Tablets 520

Fenoprofen Calcium (The hypoglycemic action of sulfonylureas may be potentiated by certain drugs, including nonsteroidial anti-inflammatory drugs. Due to the potential drug interaction between these drugs and glimepiride, the patient should be observed closely for hypoglycemia when these drugs are co-administered. Conversely, when these drugs are withdrawn, the patient should be observed closely for loss of glycemic control). Products include:

Nalfon Capsules 2508

Fentanyl (In vivo drug-drug interaction studies have suggested that pioglitazone may be a weak inducer of CYP 450 isoform 3A4 substrate). Products include:

Duragesic Transdermal System 2405
Ionsys Transdermal System 2410

Fentanyl Citrate (In vivo drug-drug interaction studies have suggested that pioglitazone may be a weak inducer of CYP 450 isoform 3A4 substrate). Products include:

Actiq 959
Fentora Tablets 968

Fluconazole (There is a potential interaction of glimepiride with inhibitors (e.g., fluconazole) of cytochrome P450 2C9).

No products indexed under this heading.

Fludrocortisone Acetate (Certain drugs tend to produce hyperglycemia and may lead to loss of control. These drugs include the corticosteroids. Due to the potential drug interaction between these drugs and glimepiride, the patient should be observed closely for loss of glycemic control when these drugs are co-administered. Conversely, when these drugs are withdrawn, the patient should be observed closely for hypoglycemia).

No products indexed under this heading.

Flunisolide (Certain drugs tend to produce hyperglycemia and may lead to loss of control. These drugs include the corticosteroids. Due to the potential drug interaction between these drugs and glimepiride, the patient should be observed closely for loss of glycemic control when these drugs are co-administered. Conversely, when these drugs are withdrawn, the patient should be observed closely for hypoglycemia). Products include:

Aerobid/Aerobid-M 1153

Fluorouracil (There is a potential interaction of glimepiride with inhibitors (e.g., fluconazole) of cytochrome P450 2C9). Products include:

Carac Cream 0.5% 2722

Fluoxetine Hydrochloride (There is a potential interaction of glimepiride with inhibitors (e.g., fluconazole) of cytochrome P450 2C9). Products include:

Prozac Weekly Capsules 1852
Prozac Pulvules and Liquid 1852
Symbyax Capsules 1871

Fluphenazine Decanoate (Certain drugs tend to produce hyperglycemia and may lead to loss of control. These drugs include the phenothiazines. Due to the potential drug interaction between these drugs and glimepiride, the patient should be observed closely for loss of glycemic control when these drugs are co-administered. Conversely, when these drugs are withdrawn, the patient should be observed closely for hypoglycemia).

No products indexed under this heading.

Fluphenazine Enanthate (Certain drugs tend to produce hyperglycemia and may lead to loss of control. These drugs include the phenothiazines. Due to the potential drug interaction between these drugs and glimepiride, the patient should be observed closely for loss of glycemic control when these drugs are co-administered. Conversely, when these drugs are withdrawn, the patient should be observed closely for hypoglycemia).

No products indexed under this heading.

Fluphenazine Hydrochloride (Certain drugs tend to produce hyperglycemia and may lead to loss of control. These drugs include the phenothiazines. Due to the potential drug interaction between these drugs and glimepiride, the patient should be observed closely for loss of glycemic control when these drugs are co-administered. Conversely, when these drugs are withdrawn, the patient should be observed closely for hypoglycemia).

No products indexed under this heading.

Flurbiprofen (The hypoglycemic action of sulfonylureas may be potentiated by certain drugs, including nonsteroidial anti-inflammatory drugs. Due to the potential drug interaction between these drugs and glimepiride, the patient should be observed closely for hypoglycemia when these drugs are co-administered. Conversely, when these drugs are withdrawn, the patient should be observed closely for loss of glycemic control).

No products indexed under this heading.

Flurbiprofen Sodium (There is a potential interaction of glimepiride with inhibitors (e.g., fluconazole) of cytochrome P450 2C9).

No products indexed under this heading.

Fluticasone Propionate (Certain drugs tend to produce hyperglycemia and may lead to loss of control. These drugs include the corticosteroids. Due to the potential drug interaction between these drugs and glimepiride, the patient should be observed closely for loss of glycemic control when these drugs are co-administered. Conversely, when these drugs are withdrawn, the patient should be observed closely for hypoglycemia). Products include:

Advair Diskus 100/50 1276
Advair Diskus 250/50 1276
Advair Diskus 500/50 1276
Advair HFA 45/21 Inhalation Aerosol 1288
Advair HFA 115/21 Inhalation Aerosol 1288
Advair HFA 230/21 Inhalation Aerosol 1288
Flonase Nasal Spray 1431
Flovent Diskus 50 mcg 1435

Fluticasone Propionate HFA (Certain drugs tend to produce hyperglycemia and may lead to loss of control. These drugs include the corticosteroids. Due to the potential drug interaction between these drugs and glimepiride, the patient should be observed closely for loss of glycemic control when these drugs are co-administered. Conversely, when these drugs are withdrawn, the patient should be observed closely for hypoglycemia). Products include:

Flovent HFA 1440

Fluvastatin Sodium (There is a potential interaction of glimepiride with inhibitors (e.g., fluconazole) of cytochrome P450 2C9). Products include:

Lescol Capsules 2268
Lescol XL Tablets 2268

Fluvoxamine Maleate (There is a potential interaction of glimepiride with inhibitors (e.g., fluconazole) of cytochrome P450 2C9). Products include:

Luvox CR Extended-Release Capsules 1759

Fosphenytoin Sodium (Certain drugs tend to produce hyperglycemia and may lead to loss of control. These drugs include phenytoin. Due to the potential drug interaction between these drugs and glimepiride, the patient should be observed closely for loss of glycemic control when these drugs are co-administered. Conversely, when these drugs are withdrawn, the patient should be observed closely for hypoglycemia).

No products indexed under this heading.

Furosemide (Certain drugs tend to produce hyperglycemia and may lead to loss of control. These drugs include the thiazides and other diuretics. Due to the potential drug interaction between these drugs and glimepiride, the patient should be observed closely for loss of glycemic control when these drugs are co-administered. Conversely, when these drugs are withdrawn, the patient should be observed closely for hypoglycemia). Products include:

Furosemide Tablets 2186

Gemfibrozil (Concomitant administration of gemfibrozil (oral 600 mg twice daily), an inhibitor of CYP2C8, with pioglitazone (oral 30 mg) in 10 healthy volunteers pre-treated for 2 days prior with gemfibrozil (oral 600 mg twice daily) resulted in pioglitazone exposure(AUC0-24) being 226% of the pioglitazone exposure in the absence of gemfibrozil).

No products indexed under this heading.

Glipizide (The hypoglycemic action of sulfonylureas may be potentiated by certain drugs, including sulfonamides. Due to the potential drug interaction between these drugs and glimepiride, the patient should be observed closely for hypoglycemia when these drugs are co-administered. Conversely when these drugs are withdrawn, the patient should be observed closely for loss of glycemic control).

No products indexed under this heading.

Glyburide (The hypoglycemic action of sulfonylureas may be potentiated by certain drugs, including sulfonamides. Due to the potential drug interaction between these drugs and glimepiride, the patient should be observed closely for hypoglycemia when these drugs are co-administered. Conversely when these drugs are withdrawn, the patient should be observed closely for loss of glycemic control).

No products indexed under this heading.

Haloperidol (In vivo drug-drug interaction studies have suggested that pioglitazone may be a weak inducer of CYP 450 isoform 3A4 substrate).
No products indexed under this heading.

Haloperidol Decanoate (In vivo drug-drug interaction studies have suggested that pioglitazone may be a weak inducer of CYP 450 isoform 3A4 substrate).
No products indexed under this heading.

Haloperidol Lactate (In vivo drug-drug interaction studies have suggested that pioglitazone may be a weak inducer of CYP 450 isoform 3A4 substrate).
No products indexed under this heading.

Hydrochlorothiazide (The hypoglycemic action of sulfonylureas may be potentiated by certain drugs, including sulfonamides. Due to the potential drug interaction between these drugs and glimepiride, the patient should be observed closely for hypoglycemia when these drugs are co-administered. Conversely when these drugs are withdrawn, the patient should be observed closely for loss of glycemic control).
Products include:
Atacand HCT 642
Avalide Tablets 892
Avalide Tablets 2713
Benicar HCT Tablets 1010
Diovan HCT Tablets 2216
Dyazide Capsules 1405
Micardis HCT Tablets 854
Prinzide Tablets 2092
Tekturna HCT Tablets 2324
Teveten HCT Tablets 517

Hydrocortisone (Certain drugs tend to produce hyperglycemia and may lead to loss of control. These drugs include the corticosteroids. Due to the potential drug interaction between these drugs and glimepiride, the patient should be observed closely for loss of glycemic control when these drugs are co-administered. Conversely, when these drugs are withdrawn, the patient should be observed closely for hypoglycemia).
No products indexed under this heading.

Hydrocortisone Acetate (Certain drugs tend to produce hyperglycemia and may lead to loss of control. These drugs include the corticosteroids. Due to the potential drug interaction between these drugs and glimepiride, the patient should be observed closely for loss of glycemic control when these drugs are co-administered. Conversely, when these drugs are withdrawn, the patient should be observed closely for hypoglycemia). Products include:
Analpram-HC 1140
Pramosone 1141

Hydrocortisone Sodium Phosphate (Certain drugs tend to produce hyperglycemia and may lead to loss of control. These drugs include the corticosteroids. Due to the potential drug interaction between these drugs and glimepiride, the patient should be observed closely for loss of glycemic control when these drugs are co-administered. Conversely, when these drugs are withdrawn, the patient should be observed closely for hypoglycemia).
No products indexed under this heading.

Hydrocortisone Sodium Succinate (Certain drugs tend to produce hyperglycemia and may lead to loss of control. These drugs include the corticosteroids. Due to the potential drug interaction between these drugs and glimepiride, the patient should be observed closely for loss of glycemic control when these drugs are co-administered. Conversely, when these drugs are withdrawn, the patient should be observed closely for hypoglycemia).
No products indexed under this heading.

Hydroflumethiazide (The hypoglycemic action of sulfonylureas may be potentiated by certain drugs, including sulfonamides. Due to the potential drug interaction between these drugs and glimepiride, the patient should be observed closely for hypoglycemia when these drugs are co-administered. Conversely when these drugs are withdrawn, the patient should be observed closely for loss of glycemic control).
No products indexed under this heading.

Ibuprofen (The hypoglycemic action of sulfonylureas may be potentiated by certain drugs, including nonsteroidial anti-inflammatory drugs. Due to the potential drug interaction between these drugs and glimepiride, the patient should be observed closely for hypoglycemia when these drugs are co-administered. Conversely, when these drugs are withdrawn, the patient should be observed closely for loss of glycemic control).
Products include:
Motrin IB Tablets and Caplets 1900
Children's Motrin Oral Suspension ... 1901
Children's Motrin Non-Staining Dye-Free Oral Suspension 1901
Children's Motrin Cold Oral Suspension 1899
Infants' Motrin Concentrated Drops 1901
Infants' Motrin Non-Staining Dye-Free Concentrated Drops 1901
Junior Strength Motrin Caplets and Chewable Tablets 1901
Vicoprofen Tablets 533

Imatinib Mesylate (There is a potential interaction of glimepiride with inhibitors (e.g., fluconazole) of cytochrome P450 2C9). Products include:
Gleevec Tablets 2255

Indapamide (Certain drugs tend to produce hyperglycemia and may lead to loss of control. These drugs include the thiazides and other diuretics. Due to the potential drug interaction between these drugs and glimepiride, the patient should be observed closely for loss of glycemic control when these drugs are co-administered. Conversely, when these drugs are withdrawn, the patient should be observed closely for hypoglycemia). Products include:
Indapamide Tablets 2188

Indinavir Sulfate (In vivo drug-drug interaction studies have suggested that pioglitazone may be a weak inducer of CYP 450 isoform 3A4 substrate). Products include:
Crixivan Capsules 1979

Indomethacin (The hypoglycemic action of sulfonylureas may be potentiated by certain drugs, including nonsteroidial anti-inflammatory drugs. Due to the potential drug interaction between these drugs and glimepiride, the patient should be observed closely for hypoglycemia when these drugs are co-administered. Conversely, when these drugs are withdrawn, the patient should be observed closely for loss of glycemic control).
Products include:
Indocin 2024

Indomethacin Sodium Trihydrate (The hypoglycemic action of sulfonylureas may be potentiated by certain drugs, including nonsteroidial anti-inflammatory drugs. Due to the potential drug interaction between these drugs and glimepiride, the patient should be observed closely for hypoglycemia when these drugs are co-administered. Conversely, when these drugs are withdrawn, the patient should be observed closely for loss of glycemic control).
Products include:
Indocin I.V. 2489

Isocarboxazid (The hypoglycemic action of sulfonylureas may be potentiated by certain drugs, including monoamine oxidase inhibitors. Due to the potential drug interaction between these drugs and glimepiride, the patient should be observed closely for hypoglycemia when these drugs are co-administered. Conversely, when these drugs are withdrawn, the patient should be observed closely for loss of glycemic control).
Products include:
Marplan Tablets 3177

Isoniazid (Certain drugs tend to produce hyperglycemia and may lead to loss of control. These drugs include isoniazid. Due to the potential drug interaction between this drug and glimepiride, the patient should be observed closely for loss of glycemic control when these drugs are co-administered. Conversely, when this drug is withdrawn, the patient should be observed closely for hypoglycemia).
No products indexed under this heading.

Isoproterenol Hydrochloride (Certain drugs tend to produce hyperglycemia and may lead to loss of control. These drugs include the sympathomimetics. Due to the potential drug interaction between these drugs and glimepiride, the patient should be observed closely for loss of glycemic control when these drugs are co-administered. Conversely, when these drugs are withdrawn, the patient should be observed closely for hypoglycemia).
No products indexed under this heading.

Isoproterenol Sulfate (Certain drugs tend to produce hyperglycemia and may lead to loss of control. These drugs include the sympathomimetics. Due to the potential drug interaction between these drugs and glimepiride, the patient should be observed closely for loss of glycemic control when these drugs are co-administered. Conversely, when these drugs are withdrawn, the patient should be observed closely for hypoglycemia).
No products indexed under this heading.

Isradipine (In vivo drug-drug interaction studies have suggested that pioglitazone may be a weak inducer of CYP 450 isoform 3A4 substrate).
Products include:
DynaCirc CR Controlled Release Tablets 1407

Itraconazole (There is a potential interaction of glimepiride with inhibitors (e.g., fluconazole) of cytochrome P450 2C9).
No products indexed under this heading.

Ixabepilone (In vivo drug-drug interaction studies have suggested that pioglitazone may be a weak inducer of CYP 450 isoform 3A4 substrate).
Products include:
Ixempra Kit for Injection 915

Ketoconazole (Co-administration of pioglitazone for 7 days with ketoconazole 200 mg administered twice daily resulted in a ratio of least square mean (90% CI) values for unchanged pioglitazone of 1.14 (1.06-1.23) for Cmax, 1.34 (1.26-1.41) for AUC and 1.87 (1.71-2.04)for Cmin). Products include:
Extina Foam, 2% 3057
Nizoral A-D Shampoo 1901

Ketoprofen (The hypoglycemic action of sulfonylureas may be potentiated by certain drugs, including nonsteroidial anti-inflammatory drugs. Due to the potential drug interaction between these drugs and glimepiride, the patient should be observed closely for hypoglycemia when these drugs are co-administered. Conversely, when these drugs are withdrawn, the patient should be observed closely for loss of glycemic control).
No products indexed under this heading.

Ketorolac Tromethamine (The hypoglycemic action of sulfonylureas may be potentiated by certain drugs, including nonsteroidial anti-inflammatory drugs. Due to the potential drug interaction between these drugs and glimepiride, the patient should be observed closely for hypoglycemia when these drugs are co-administered. Conversely, when these drugs are withdrawn, the patient should be observed closely for loss of glycemic control).
No products indexed under this heading.

Labetalol Hydrochloride (The hypoglycemic action of sulfonylureas may be potentiated by certain drugs, including beta adrenergic blocking agents. Due to the potential drug interaction between these drugs and glimepiride, the patient should be observed closely for hypoglycemia when these drugs are co-administered. Conversely, when these drugs are withdrawn, the patient should be observed closely for loss of glycemic control. If beta-blockers are used, caution should be exercised and patients should be warned about the potential for hypoglycemia).
No products indexed under this heading.

Leflunomide (There is a potential interaction of glimepiride with inhibitors (e.g., fluconazole) of cytochrome P450 2C9).
No products indexed under this heading.

Levalbuterol Hydrochloride (Certain drugs tend to produce hyperglycemia and may lead to loss of control. These drugs include the sympathomimetics. Due to the potential drug interaction between these drugs and glimepiride, the patient should be observed closely for loss of glycemic control when these drugs are co-administered. Conversely, when these drugs are withdrawn, the patient should be observed closely for hypoglycemia). Products include:

Xopenex Inhalation Solution **3001**
Xopenex Inhalation Solution Concentrate **3005**

Levobunolol Hydrochloride (The hypoglycemic action of sulfonylureas may be potentiated by certain drugs, including beta adrenergic blocking agents. Due to the potential drug interaction between these drugs and glimepiride, the patient should be observed closely for hypoglycemia when these drugs are co-administered. Conversely, when these drugs are withdrawn, the patient should be observed closely for loss of glycemic control. If beta-blockers are used, caution should be exercised and patients should be warned about the potential for hypoglycemia).

No products indexed under this heading.

Levonorgestrel (Certain drugs tend to produce hyperglycemia and may lead to loss of control. These drugs include oral contraceptives. Due to the potential drug interaction between these drugs and glimepiride, the patient should be observed closely for loss of glycemic control when these drugs are co-administered. Conversely, when these drugs are withdrawn, the patient should be observed closely for hypoglycemia). Products include:

Climara Pro Transdermal System **768**
Lybrel Tablets **3204**
Mirena Intrauterine System **779**
Plan B Tablets **1044**
Seasonique Tablets **1046**

Levothyroxine Sodium (Certain drugs tend to produce hyperglycemia and may lead to loss of control. These drugs include thyroid products. Due to the potential drug interaction between these drugs and glimepiride, the patient should be observed closely for loss of glycemic control when these drugs are co-administered. Conversely, when these drugs are withdrawn, the patient should be observed closely for hypoglycemia). Products include:

Levothroid Tablets **1170**
Levoxyl Tablets **1780**
Synthroid Tablets **507**

Lidocaine (In vivo drug-drug interaction studies have suggested that pioglitazone may be a weak inducer of CYP 450 isoform 3A4 substrate). Products include:

Lidoderm Patch **1114**

Lidocaine Hydrochloride (In vivo drug-drug interaction studies have suggested that pioglitazone may be a weak inducer of CYP 450 isoform 3A4 substrate).

No products indexed under this heading.

Liothyronine Sodium (Certain drugs tend to produce hyperglycemia and may lead to loss of control. These drugs include thyroid products. Due to the potential drug interaction between these drugs and glimepiride, the patient should be observed closely for loss of glycemic control when these drugs are co-administered. Conversely, when these drugs are withdrawn, the patient should be observed closely for hypoglycemia). Products include:

Cytomel Tablets **1778**

Liotrix (Certain drugs tend to produce hyperglycemia and may lead to loss of control. These drugs include thyroid products. Due to the potential drug interaction between these drugs and glimepiride, the patient should be observed closely for loss of glycemic control when these drugs are co-administered. Conversely, when these drugs are withdrawn, the patient should be observed closely for hypoglycemia).

No products indexed under this heading.

Lovastatin (There is a potential interaction of glimepiride with inhibitors (e.g., fluconazole) of cytochrome P450 2C9). Products include:

Advicor Tablets **402**
Mevacor Tablets **2063**

Magnesium Salicylate (The hypoglycemic action of sulfonylureas may be potentiated by certain drugs, included salicylates. Due to the potential drug interaction between these drugs and glimepiride, the patient should be observed closely for hypoglycemia when these drugs are co-administered. Conversely, when these drugs are withdrawn, the patient should be observed closely for loss of glycemic control).

No products indexed under this heading.

Meclofenamate Sodium (The hypoglycemic action of sulfonylureas may be potentiated by certain drugs, including nonsteroidial anti-inflammatory drugs. Due to the potential drug interaction between these drugs and glimepiride, the patient should be observed closely for hypoglycemia when these drugs are co-administered. Conversely, when these drugs are withdrawn, the patient should be observed closely for loss of glycemic control).

No products indexed under this heading.

Mefenamic Acid (The hypoglycemic action of sulfonylureas may be potentiated by certain drugs, including nonsteroidial anti-inflammatory drugs. Due to the potential drug interaction between these drugs and glimepiride, the patient should be observed closely for hypoglycemia when these drugs are co-administered. Conversely, when these drugs are withdrawn, the patient should be observed closely for loss of glycemic control).

No products indexed under this heading.

Meloxicam (The hypoglycemic action of sulfonylureas may be potentiated by certain drugs, including nonsteroidial anti-inflammatory drugs. Due to the potential drug interaction between these drugs and glimepiride, the patient should be observed closely for hypoglycemia when these drugs are co-administered. Conversely, when these drugs are withdrawn, the patient should be observed closely for loss of glycemic control). Products include:

Mobic Oral Suspension **863**
Mobic Tablets **863**

Mesoridazine Besylate (Certain drugs tend to produce hyperglycemia and may lead to loss of control. These drugs include the phenothiazines. Due to the potential drug interaction between these drugs and glimepiride, the patient should be observed closely for loss of glycemic control when these drugs are co-administered. Conversely, when these drugs are withdrawn, the patient should be observed closely for hypoglycemia).

No products indexed under this heading.

Mestranol (Certain drugs tend to produce hyperglycemia and may lead to loss of control. These drugs include oral contraceptives. Due to the potential drug interaction between these drugs and glimepiride, the patient should be observed closely for loss of glycemic control when these drugs are co-administered. Conversely, when these drugs are withdrawn, the patient should be observed closely for hypoglycemia).

No products indexed under this heading.

Metaproterenol Sulfate (Certain drugs tend to produce hyperglycemia and may lead to loss of control. These drugs include the sympathomimetics. Due to the potential drug interaction between these drugs and glimepiride, the patient should be observed closely for loss of glycemic control when these drugs are co-administered. Conversely, when these drugs are withdrawn, the patient should be observed closely for hypoglycemia).

No products indexed under this heading.

Metaraminol Bitartrate (Certain drugs tend to produce hyperglycemia and may lead to loss of control. These drugs include the sympathomimetics. Due to the potential drug interaction between these drugs and glimepiride, the patient should be observed closely for loss of glycemic control when these drugs are co-administered. Conversely, when these drugs are withdrawn, the patient should be observed closely for hypoglycemia).

No products indexed under this heading.

Methadone Hydrochloride (In vivo drug-drug interaction studies have suggested that pioglitazone may be a weak inducer of CYP 450 isoform 3A4 substrate).

No products indexed under this heading.

Methotrimeprazine (Certain drugs tend to produce hyperglycemia and may lead to loss of control. These drugs include the phenothiazines. Due to the potential drug interaction between these drugs and glimepiride, the patient should be observed closely for loss of glycemic control when these drugs are co-administered. Conversely, when these drugs are withdrawn, the patient should be observed closely for hypoglycemia).

No products indexed under this heading.

Methoxamine Hydrochloride (Certain drugs tend to produce hyperglycemia and may lead to loss of control. These drugs include the sympathomimetics. Due to the potential drug interaction between these drugs and glimepiride, the patient should be observed closely for loss of glycemic control when these drugs are co-administered. Conversely, when these drugs are withdrawn, the patient should be observed closely for hypoglycemia).

No products indexed under this heading.

Methyclothiazide (The hypoglycemic action of sulfonylureas may be potentiated by certain drugs, including sulfonamides. Due to the potential drug interaction between these drugs and glimepiride, the patient should be observed closely for hypoglycemia when these drugs are co-administered. Conversely when these drugs are withdrawn, the patient should be observed closely for loss of glycemic control).

No products indexed under this heading.

Methylprednisolone Acetate (Certain drugs tend to produce hyperglycemia and may lead to loss of control. These drugs include the corticosteroids. Due to the potential drug interaction between these drugs and glimepiride, the patient should be observed closely for loss of glycemic control when these drugs are co-administered. Conversely, when these drugs are withdrawn, the patient should be observed closely for hypoglycemia).

No products indexed under this heading.

Methylprednisolone Sodium Succinate (Certain drugs tend to produce hyperglycemia and may lead to loss of control. These drugs include the corticosteroids. Due to the potential drug interaction between these drugs and glimepiride, the patient should be observed closely for loss of glycemic control when these drugs are co-administered. Conversely, when these drugs are withdrawn, the patient should be observed closely for hypoglycemia).

No products indexed under this heading.

Metipranolol Hydrochloride (The hypoglycemic action of sulfonylureas may be potentiated by certain drugs, including beta adrenergic blocking agents. Due to the potential drug interaction between these drugs and glimepiride, the patient should be observed closely for hypoglycemia when these drugs are co-administered. Conversely, when these drugs are withdrawn, the patient should be observed closely for loss of glycemic control. If beta-blockers are used, caution should be exercised and patients should be warned about the potential for hypoglycemia).

No products indexed under this heading.

Metolazone (Certain drugs tend to produce hyperglycemia and may lead to loss of control. These drugs include the thiazides and other diuretics. Due to the potential drug interaction between these drugs and glimepiride, the patient should be observed closely for loss of glycemic control when these drugs are co-administered. Conversely, when these drugs are withdrawn, the patient should be observed closely for hypoglycemia).

No products indexed under this heading.

Metoprolol Succinate (The hypoglycemic action of sulfonylureas may be potentiated by certain drugs, including beta adrenergic blocking agents. Due to the potential drug interaction between these drugs and glimepiride, the patient should be observed closely for hypoglycemia when these drugs are co-administered. Conversely, when these drugs are withdrawn, the patient should be observed closely for loss of glycemic control. If beta-blockers are used, caution should be exercised and patients should be warned about the potential for hypoglycemia). Products include:

Toprol-XL Tablets 666

Metoprolol Tartrate (The hypoglycemic action of sulfonylureas may be potentiated by certain drugs, including beta adrenergic blocking agents. Due to the potential drug interaction between these drugs and glimepiride, the patient should be observed closely for hypoglycemia when these drugs are co-administered. Conversely, when these drugs are withdrawn, the patient should be observed closely for loss of glycemic control. If beta-blockers are used, caution should be exercised and patients should be warned about the potential for hypoglycemia).

No products indexed under this heading.

Metronidazole (There is a potential interaction of glimepiride with inhibitors (e.g., fluconazole) of cytochrome P450 2C9). Products include:

Pylera Capsules 714

Metronidazole Benzoate (There is a potential interaction of glimepiride with inhibitors (e.g., fluconazole) of cytochrome P450 2C9).

No products indexed under this heading.

Metronidazole Hydrochloride (There is a potential interaction of glimepiride with inhibitors (e.g., fluconazole) of cytochrome P450 2C9).

No products indexed under this heading.

Miconazole (A potential interaction between oral miconazole and oral hypoglycemic agents leading to severe hpyoglycemia has been reported. Whether this interaction also occurs with the intravenous, topical, or vaginal preparations of miconazole is not known).

No products indexed under this heading.

Miconazole Nitrate (A potential interaction between oral miconazole and oral hypoglycemic agents leading to severe hypoglycemia has been reported. Whether this interaction also occurs with intravenous, topical, or vaginal preparations of miconazole is not known).

No products indexed under this heading.

Midazolam Hydrochloride (Administration of pioglitazone for 15 days followed by a single 7.5 mg dose of midazolam syrup resulted in a 26% reduction in midazolam Cmax and AUC).

No products indexed under this heading.

Moclobemide (The hypoglycemic action of sulfonylureas may be potentiated by certain drugs, including monoamine oxidase inhibitors. Due to the potential drug interaction between these drugs and glimepiride, the patient should be observed closely for hypoglycemia when these drugs are co-administered. Conversely, when these drugs are withdrawn, the patient should be observed closely for loss of glycemic control).

No products indexed under this heading.

Modafinil (There is a potential interaction of glimepiride with inhibitors (e.g., fluconazole) of cytochrome P450 2C9). Products include:

Provigil Tablets 977

Mometasone Furoate (Certain drugs tend to produce hyperglycemia and may lead to loss of control. These drugs include the corticosteroids. Due to the potential drug interaction between these drugs and glimepiride, the patient should be observed closely for loss of glycemic control when these drugs are co-administered. Conversely, when these drugs are withdrawn, the patient should be observed closely for hypoglycemia). Products include:

Asmanex Twisthaler 2797
Elocon Cream 0.1% 2840
Elocon Lotion 0.1% 2841
Elocon Ointment 0.1% 2842

Mometasone Furoate Monohydrate (Certain drugs tend to produce hyperglycemia and may lead to loss of control. These drugs include the corticosteroids. Due to the potential drug interaction between these drugs and glimepiride, the patient should be observed closely for loss of glycemic control when these drugs are co-administered. Conversely, when these drugs are withdrawn, the patient should be observed closely for hypoglycemia). Products include:

Nasonex Nasal Spray 2883

Nabumetone (The hypoglycemic action of sulfonylureas may be potentiated by certain drugs, including nonsteroidial anti-inflammatory drugs. Due to the potential drug interaction between these drugs and glimepiride, the patient should be observed closely for hypoglycemia when these drugs are co-administered. Conversely, when these drugs are withdrawn, the patient should be observed closely for loss of glycemic control).

No products indexed under this heading.

Nadolol (The hypoglycemic action of sulfonylureas may be potentiated by certain drugs, including beta adrenergic blocking agents. Due to the potential drug interaction between these drugs and glimepiride, the patient should be observed closely for hypoglycemia when these drugs are co-administered. Conversely, when these drugs are withdrawn, the patient should be observed closely for loss of glycemic control. If beta-blockers are used, caution should be exercised and patients should be warned about the potential for hypoglycemia). Products include:

Nadolol Tablets 2191

Naproxen (The hypoglycemic action of sulfonylureas may be potentiated by certain drugs, including nonsteroidial anti-inflammatory drugs. Due to the potential drug interaction between these drugs and glimepiride, the patient should be observed closely for hypoglycemia when these drugs are co-administered. Conversely, when these drugs are withdrawn, the patient should be observed closely for loss of glycemic control). Products include:

EC-Naprosyn Delayed-Release Tablets 2632
Naprosyn Suspension 2632
Naprosyn Tablets 2632

Naproxen Sodium (The hypoglycemic action of sulfonylureas may be potentiated by certain drugs, including nonsteroidial anti-inflammatory drugs. Due to the potential drug interaction between these drugs and glimepiride, the patient should be observed closely for hypoglycemia when these drugs are co-administered. Conversely, when these drugs are withdrawn, the patient should be observed closely for loss of glycemic control). Products include:

Anaprox Tablets 2632
Anaprox DS Tablets 2632
Treximet Tablets 1616

Nebivolol (The hypoglycemic action of sulfonylureas may be potentiated by certain drugs, including beta adrenergic blocking agents. Due to the potential drug interaction between these drugs and glimepiride, the patient should be observed closely for hypoglycemia when these drugs are co-administered. Conversely, when these drugs are withdrawn, the patient should be observed closely for loss of glycemic control. If beta-blockers are used, caution should be exercised and patients should be warned about the potential for hypoglycemia). Products include:

Bystolic Tablets 1155

Nefazodone Hydrochloride (In vivo drug-drug interaction studies have suggested that pioglitazone may be a weak inducer of CYP 450 isoform 3A4 substrate).

No products indexed under this heading.

Nelfinavir Mesylate (In vivo drug-drug interaction studies have suggested that pioglitazone may be a weak inducer of CYP 450 isoform 3A4 substrate).

No products indexed under this heading.

Nicardipine Hydrochloride (In vivo drug-drug interaction studies have suggested that pioglitazone may be a weak inducer of CYP 450 isoform 3A4 substrate). Products include:

Cardene I.V. 1093

Nicotinic Acid (Certain drugs tend to produce hyperglycemia and may lead to loss of control. These drugs include nicotinic acid. Due to the potential drug interaction between this drug and glimepiride, the patient should be observed closely for loss of glycemic control when these drugs are co-administered. Conversely, when these drugs are withdrawn, the patient should be observed closely for hypoglycemia).

No products indexed under this heading.

Nifedipine (Co-administration of pioglitazone for 7 days with 30 mg nifedipine ER administered orally once daily for 4 days to male and female volunteers resulted in a ratio of least square mean (90% CI) values for unchanged nifedipine of 0.83 (0.73-0.95) for Cmax and clinical significance of this finding is unknown).

No products indexed under this heading.

Nimodipine (In vivo drug-drug interaction studies have suggested that pioglitazone may be a weak inducer of CYP 450 isoform 3A4 substrate). Products include:

Nimotop Capsules 790

Nisoldipine (In vivo drug-drug interaction studies have suggested that pioglitazone may be a weak inducer of CYP 450 isoform 3A4 substrate). Products include:

Sular Extended Release Tablets 2975

Nitrendipine (In vivo drug-drug interaction studies have suggested that pioglitazone may be a weak inducer of CYP 450 isoform 3A4 substrate).

No products indexed under this heading.

Norepinephrine Bitartrate (Certain drugs tend to produce hyperglycemia and may lead to loss of control. These drugs include the sympathomimetics. Due to the potential drug interaction between these drugs and glimepiride, the patient should be observed closely for loss of glycemic control when these drugs are co-administered. Conversely, when these drugs are withdrawn, the patient should be observed closely for hypoglycemia).

No products indexed under this heading.

Norethindrone (Certain drugs tend to produce hyperglycemia and may lead to loss of control. These drugs include oral contraceptives. Due to the potential drug interaction between these drugs and glimepiride, the patient should be observed closely for loss of glycemic control when these drugs are co-administered. Conversely, when these drugs are withdrawn, the patient should be observed closely for hypoglycemia). Products include:

Ortho Micronor Tablets 2446

Norethindrone Acetate (In vivo drug-drug interaction studies have suggested that pioglitazone may be a weak inducer of CYP 450 isoform 3A4 substrate). Products include:

Activella Tablets 2347

Norethynodrel (Certain drugs tend to produce hyperglycemia and may lead to loss of control. These drugs include oral contraceptives. Due to the potential drug interaction between these drugs and glimepiride, the patient should be observed closely for loss of glycemic control when these drugs are co-administered. Conversely, when these drugs are withdrawn, the patient should be observed closely for hypoglycemia).

No products indexed under this heading.

Norgestimate (Certain drugs tend to produce hyperglycemia and may lead to loss of control. These drugs include oral contraceptives. Due to the potential drug interaction between these drugs and glimepiride, the patient should be observed closely for loss of glycemic control when these drugs are co-administered. Conversely, when these drugs are withdrawn, the patient should be observed closely for hypoglycemia). Products include:

Ortho-Cyclen/Ortho Tri-Cyclen 2449
Ortho Tri-Cyclen Lo Tablets 2458

Norgestrel (Certain drugs tend to produce hyperglycemia and may lead to loss of control. These drugs include oral contraceptives. Due to the potential drug interaction between these drugs and glimepiride, the patient should be observed closely for loss of glycemic control when these drugs are co-administered. Conversely, when these drugs are withdrawn, the patient should be observed closely for hypoglycemia).

No products indexed under this heading.

Omeprazole (There is a potential interaction of glimepiride with inhibitors (e.g., fluconazole) of cytochrome P450 2C9).

No products indexed under this heading.

Ondansetron (In vivo drug-drug interaction studies have suggested that pioglitazone may be a weak inducer of CYP 450 isoform 3A4 substrate). Products include:

Zofran ODT Orally Disintegrating Tablets 1687

Ondansetron Hydrochloride (In vivo drug-drug interaction studies have suggested that pioglitazone may be a weak inducer of CYP 450 isoform 3A4 substrate). Products include:

Zofran Injection 1682
Zofran 1687

Oxaprozin (The hypoglycemic action of sulfonylureas may be potentiated by certain drugs, including nonsteroidial anti-inflammatory drugs. Due to the potential drug interaction between these drugs and glimepiride, the patient should be observed closely for hypoglycemia when these drugs are co-administered. Conversely, when these drugs are withdrawn, the patient should be observed closely for loss of glycemic control).

No products indexed under this heading.

Oxiconazole Nitrate (There is a potential interaction of glimepiride with inhibitors (e.g., fluconazole) of cytochrome P450 2C9).

No products indexed under this heading.

Paclitaxel (In vivo drug-drug interaction studies have suggested that pioglitazone may be a weak inducer of CYP 450 isoform 3A4 substrate).

No products indexed under this heading.

Pargyline Hydrochloride (The hypoglycemic action of sulfonylureas may be potentiated by certain drugs, including monoamine oxidase inhibitors. Due to the potential drug interaction between these drugs and glimepiride, the patient should be observed closely for hypoglycemia when these drugs are co-administered. Conversely, when these drugs are withdrawn, the patient should be observed closely for loss of glycemic control).

No products indexed under this heading.

Paroxetine Hydrochloride (There is a potential interaction of glimepiride with inhibitors (e.g., fluconazole) of cytochrome P450 2C9). Products include:

Paxil 1535
Paxil CR Controlled-Release Tablets 1544

Penbutolol Sulfate (The hypoglycemic action of sulfonylureas may be potentiated by certain drugs, including beta adrenergic blocking agents. Due to the potential drug interaction between these drugs and glimepiride, the patient should be observed closely for hypoglycemia when these drugs are co-administered. Conversely, when these drugs are withdrawn, the patient should be observed closely for loss of glycemic control. If beta-blockers are used, caution should be exercised and patients should be warned about the potential for hypoglycemia).

No products indexed under this heading.

Perphenazine (Certain drugs tend to produce hyperglycemia and may lead to loss of control. These drugs include the phenothiazines. Due to the potential drug interaction between these drugs and glimepiride, the patient should be observed closely for loss of glycemic control when these drugs are co-administered. Conversely, when these drugs are withdrawn, the patient should be observed closely for hypoglycemia).

No products indexed under this heading.

Phenelzine Sulfate (The hypoglycemic action of sulfonylureas may be potentiated by certain drugs, including monoamine oxidase inhibitors. Due to the potential drug interaction between these drugs and glimepiride, the patient should be observed closely for hypoglycemia when these drugs are co-administered. Conversely, when these drugs are withdrawn, the patient should be observed closely for loss of glycemic control).

No products indexed under this heading.

Phenobarbital (There is a potential interaction of glimepiride with inducers (e.g., rifampicin) of cytochrome P450 2C9). Products include:

Donnatal Extentabs 2507

Phenobarbital Sodium (There is a potential interaction of glimepiride with inducers (e.g., rifampicin) of cytochrome P450 2C9).

No products indexed under this heading.

Phenylbutazone (The hypoglycemic action of sulfonylureas may be potentiated by certain drugs, including nonsteroidial anti-inflammatory drugs. Due to the potential drug interaction between these drugs and glimepiride, the patient should be observed closely for hypoglycemia when these drugs are co-administered. Conversely, when these drugs are withdrawn, the patient should be observed closely for loss of glycemic control).

No products indexed under this heading.

Phenylephrine Bitartrate (Certain drugs tend to produce hyperglycemia and may lead to loss of control. These drugs include the sympathomimetics. Due to the potential drug interaction between these drugs and glimepiride, the patient should be observed closely for loss of glycemic control when these drugs are co-administered. Conversely, when these drugs are withdrawn, the patient should be observed closely for hypoglycemia).

No products indexed under this heading.

Phenylephrine Hydrochloride (Certain drugs tend to produce hyperglycemia and may lead to loss of control. These drugs include the sympathomimetics. Due to the potential drug interaction between these drugs and glimepiride, the patient should be observed closely for loss of glycemic control when these drugs are co-administered. Conversely, when these drugs are withdrawn, the patient should be observed closely for hypoglycemia). Products include:

Actifed Cold & Allergy Tablets 1895
Benadryl Allergy & Cold Kapgels 1895
Benadryl Allergy & Sinus Headache Kapgels 1895
Benadryl Severe Allergy & Sinus Headache Caplets 1897
Children's Benadryl-D Allergy & Sinus Liquid 1896
Benadryl-D Allergy & Sinus Tablet 1896
PediaCare Children's Allergy & Cold Liquid 1902
PediaCare Children's Decongestant Liquid..................... 1902
PediaCare Children's Liquid Multi-Symptom Cold..................... 1902
Sinutab Non-Drying Caplets 1905
Sinutab Sinus Caplets 1905
Children's Sudafed PE Cold & Cough Liquid 1907
Children's Sudafed PE Nasal Decongestant Liquid.................... 1906
Sudafed PE Cold & Cough Caplets.. 1907
Sudafed PE Nasal Decongestant Tablets 1907
Sudafed PE Nighttime Cold Caplets.. 1907
Sudafed PE Non-Drying Sinus Caplets.. 1908
Sudafed PE Severe Cold Caplets 1908
Sudafed PE Sinus & Allergy Tablets 1908
Sudafed PE Sinus Headache Caplets.. 1908
Tylenol Allergy Multi-Symptom Caplets with Cool Burst and Rapid Release Gelcaps................ 1916
Tylenol Allergy Multi-Symptom Nighttime Caplets with Cool Burst.. 1916
Children's Tylenol Plus Cold Suspension Liquid 1912
Children's Tylenol Plus Cold & Allergy Suspension Liquid............ 1914
Children's Tylenol Plus Flu Suspension Liquid 1914
Children's Tylenol Plus Multi-Symptom Cold Suspension Liquid 1912
Tylenol Cold Head Congestion Daytime Caplets with Cool Burst.. 1910
Tylenol Cold Head Congestion Nighttime Caplets with Cool Burst.. 1910
Tylenol Cold Head Congestion Severe Daytime Caplets with Cool Burst..................................... 1910
Tylenol Cold Multi-Symptom Daytime Caplets with Cool Burst and Rapid Release Gels....... 1913
Tylenol Cold Multi-Symptom Daytime Liquid with Citrus Burst ... 1913
Tylenol Cold Multi-Symptom Nighttime Caplets with Cool Burst.. 1913
Tylenol Cold Multi-Symptom Nighttime Liquid with Cool Burst ... 1913
Tylenol Cold Multi-Symptom Severe Caplets with Cool Burst..... 1913
Tylenol Cold Multi-Symptom Severe Daytime Liquid with Citrus Burst 1913
Tylenol Sinus Congestion & Pain Daytime Caplets with Cool Burst and Gelcaps.................... 1917
Tylenol Sinus Congestion & Pain Nighttime Caplets with Cool Burst.. 1917
Tylenol Sinus Congestion & Pain Severe Caplets with Cool Burst..... 1917
Vicks DayQuil Cold & Flu Multi-Symptom Relief .... ▣616
Vicks DayQuil LiquiCaps 2567
Vicks DayQuil Liquid 2567
Vicks DayQuil Multi-Symptom Cold/Flu Relief............................. 2567

Phenylephrine Tannate (Certain drugs tend to produce hyperglycemia and may lead to loss of control. These drugs include the sympathomimetics. Due to the potential drug interaction between these drugs and glimepiride, the patient should be observed closely for loss of glycemic control when these drugs are co-administered. Conversely, when these drugs are withdrawn, the patient should be observed closely for hypoglycemia).

No products indexed under this heading.

Phenylpropanolamine Hydrochloride (Certain drugs tend to produce hyperglycemia and may lead to loss of control. These drugs include the sympathomimetics. Due to the potential drug interaction between these drugs and glimepiride, the patient should be observed closely for loss of glycemic control when these drugs are co-administered. Conversely, when these drugs are withdrawn, the patient should be observed closely for hypoglycemia).

No products indexed under this heading.

Phenytoin (Certain drugs tend to produce hyperglycemia and may lead to loss of control. These drugs include phenytoin. Due to the potential drug interaction between these drugs and glimepiride, the patient should be observed closely for loss of glycemic control when these drugs are co-administered. Conversely, when these drugs are withdrawn, the patient should be observed closely for hypoglycemia).

No products indexed under this heading.

Phenytoin Sodium (Certain drugs tend to produce hyperglycemia and may lead to loss of control. These drugs include phenytoin. Due to the potential drug interaction between these drugs and glimepiride, the patient should be observed closely for loss of glycemic control when these drugs are co-administered. Conversely, when these drugs are withdrawn, the patient should be observed closely for hypoglycemia). Products include:

Phenytek Capsules 2192

Pimozide (In vivo drug-drug interaction studies have suggested that pioglitazone may be a weak inducer of CYP 450 isoform 3A4 substrate).

No products indexed under this heading.

Pindolol (The hypoglycemic action of sulfonylureas may be potentiated by certain drugs, including beta adrenergic blocking agents. Due to the potential drug interaction between these drugs and glimepiride, the patient should be observed closely for hypoglycemia

when these drugs are co-administered. Conversely, when these drugs are withdrawn, the patient should be observed closely for loss of glycemic control. If beta-blockers are used, caution should be exercised and patients should be warned about the potential for hypoglycemia).
No products indexed under this heading.

Pirbuterol Acetate (Certain drugs tend to produce hyperglycemia and may lead to loss of control. These drugs include the sympathomimetics. Due to the potential drug interaction between these drugs and glimepiride, the patient should be observed closely for loss of glycemic control when these drugs are co-administered. Conversely, when these drugs are withdrawn, the patient should be observed closely for hypoglycemia). Products include:
Maxair Autohaler 1705

Piroxicam (The hypoglycemic action of sulfonylureas may be potentiated by certain drugs, including nonsteroidial anti-inflammatory drugs. Due to the potential drug interaction between these drugs and glimepiride, the patient should be observed closely for hypoglycemia when these drugs are co-administered. Conversely, when these drugs are withdrawn, the patient should be observed closely for loss of glycemic control).
No products indexed under this heading.

Polyestradiol Phosphate (Certain drugs tend to produce hyperglycemia and may lead to loss of control. These drugs include the estrogens. Due to the potential drug interaction between these drugs and glimepiride, the patient should be observed closely for loss of glycemic control when these drugs are co-administered. Conversely, when these drugs are withdrawn, the patient should be observed closely for hypoglycemia).
No products indexed under this heading.

Polythiazide (The hypoglycemic action of sulfonylureas may be potentiated by certain drugs, including sulfonamides. Due to the potential drug interaction between these drugs and glimepiride, the patient should be observed closely for hypoglycemia when these drugs are co-administered. Conversely when these drugs are withdrawn, the patient should be observed closely for loss of glycemic control).
No products indexed under this heading.

Prednisolone Acetate (Certain drugs tend to produce hyperglycemia and may lead to loss of control. These drugs include the corticosteroids. Due to the potential drug interaction between these drugs and glimepiride, the patient should be observed closely for loss of glycemic control when these drugs are co-administered. Conversely, when these drugs are withdrawn, the patient should be observed closely for hypoglycemia). Products include:
Pred Forte Ophthalmic Suspension .... ⊙ 227
Pred Mild Ophthalmic Suspension .... ⊙ 230
Pred-G Ophthalmic Ointment .... ⊙ 229
Pred-G Ophthalmic Suspension ...... ⊙ 228

Prednisolone Sodium Phosphate (Certain drugs tend to produce hyperglycemia and may lead to loss of control. These drugs include the corticosteroids. Due to the potential drug interaction between these drugs and glimepiride, the patient should be observed closely for loss of glycemic control when these drugs are co-administered. Conversely, when these drugs are withdrawn, the patient should be observed closely for hypoglycemia).
No products indexed under this heading.

Prednisolone Tebutate (Certain drugs tend to produce hyperglycemia and may lead to loss of control. These drugs include the corticosteroids. Due to the potential drug interaction between these drugs and glimepiride, the patient should be observed closely for loss of glycemic control when these drugs are co-administered. Conversely, when these drugs are withdrawn, the patient should be observed closely for hypoglycemia).
No products indexed under this heading.

Prednisone (Certain drugs tend to produce hyperglycemia and may lead to loss of control. These drugs include the corticosteroids. Due to the potential drug interaction between these drugs and glimepiride, the patient should be observed closely for loss of glycemic control when these drugs are co-administered. Conversely, when these drugs are withdrawn, the patient should be observed closely for hypoglycemia).
No products indexed under this heading.

Primidone (There is a potential interaction of glimepiride with inducers (e.g., rifampicin) of cytochrome P450 2C9).
No products indexed under this heading.

Probenecid (The hypoglycemic action of sulfonylureas may be potentiated by certain drugs, including probenecid. Due to the potential drug interaction between these drugs and glimepiride, the patient should be observed closely for hypoglycemia when these drugs are co-administered. Conversely, when these drugs are withdrawn, the patient should be observed closely for loss of glycemic control).
No products indexed under this heading.

Procarbazine Hydrochloride (The hypoglycemic action of sulfonylureas may be potentiated by certain drugs, including monoamine oxidase inhibitors. Due to the potential drug interaction between these drugs and glimepiride, the patient should be observed closely for hypoglycemia when these drugs are co-administered. Conversely, when these drugs are withdrawn, the patient should be observed closely for loss of glycemic control).
No products indexed under this heading.

Prochlorperazine (Certain drugs tend to produce hyperglycemia and may lead to loss of control. These drugs include the phenothiazines. Due to the potential drug interaction between these drugs and glimepiride, the patient should be observed closely for loss of glycemic control when these drugs are co-administered. Conversely, when these drugs are withdrawn, the patient should be observed closely for hypoglycemia).
No products indexed under this heading.

Promethazine Hydrochloride (Certain drugs tend to produce hyperglycemia and may lead to loss of control. These drugs include the phenothiazines. Due to the potential drug interaction between these drugs and glimepiride, the patient should be observed closely for loss of glycemic control when these drugs are co-administered. Conversely, when these drugs are withdrawn, the patient should be observed closely for hypoglycemia).
No products indexed under this heading.

Propranolol Hydrochloride (Concomitant administration of propranolol (40 mg three times daily) and glimepiride significantly increased Cmax, AUC, and T 1/2 of glimepiride by 23%, 22%, and 15% respectively, and it decreased CL/f by 18%. Pooled data from clinical trials in patientswith type 2 diabetes showed no evidence of clinically significant adverse interactions with uncontrolled concurrent administration of beta-blockers. However, if beta-clockers are used, caution should be exercised and patients should be warned about the potential for hypoglycemia). Products include:
InnoPran XL Extended Release Capsules.................................... 1484

Pseudoephedrine Hydrochloride (Certain drugs tend to produce hyperglycemia and may lead to loss of control. These drugs include the sympathomimetics. Due to the potential drug interaction between these drugs and glimepiride, the patient should be observed closely for loss of glycemic control when these drugs are co-administered. Conversely, when these drugs are withdrawn, the patient should be observed closely for hypoglycemia). Products include:
Allegra-D 12 Hour Extended-Release Tablets............ 2687
Allegra-D 24 Hour Extended-Release Tablets............ 2690
Children's Motrin Cold Oral Suspension.................................. 1899
Sudafed 12 Hour Nasal Decongestant Non-Drowsy Caplets.. 1909
Sudafed 24 Hour Non-Drowsy Nasal Decongestant Tablets......... 1906
Children's Sudafed Nasal Decongestant Liquid.................... 1906
Sudafed Nasal Decongestant Tablets.. 1906
Tylenol Cold Severe Congestion Daytime Caplets with Cool Burst.. 1912
Tylenol Sinus Severe Congestion Caplets with Cool Burst............... 1917
Vicks NyQuil LiquiCaps 2567
Vicks NyQuil Liquid 2567
Vicks NyQuil Multi-Symptom Cold/Flu Relief................................... 2567
Zyrtec-D 12 Hour Extended Release Tablets........................... 1923
Zyrtec-D Allergy & Congestion Extended-Release Tablets............ 1923

Pseudoephedrine Sulfate (Certain drugs tend to produce hyperglycemia and may lead to loss of control. These drugs include the sympathomimetics. Due to the potential drug interaction between these drugs and glimepiride, the patient should be observed closely for loss of glycemic control when these drugs are co-administered. Conversely, when these drugs are withdrawn, the patient should be observed closely for hypoglycemia). Products include:
Clarinex-D 12-Hour Extended-Release Tablets............. 2831
Clarinex-D 24-Hour Extended-Release Tablets............. 2834

Quinestrol (Certain drugs tend to produce hyperglycemia and may lead to loss of control. These drugs include the estrogens. Due to the potential drug interaction between these drugs and glimepiride, the patient should be observed closely for loss of glycemic control when these drugs are co-administered. Conversely, when these drugs are withdrawn, the patient should be observed closely for hypoglycemia).
No products indexed under this heading.

Quinidine Gluconate (In vivo drug-drug interaction studies have suggested that pioglitazone may be a weak inducer of CYP 450 isoform 3A4 substrate).
No products indexed under this heading.

Quinidine Polygalacturonate (In vivo drug-drug interaction studies have suggested that pioglitazone may be a weak inducer of CYP 450 isoform 3A4 substrate).
No products indexed under this heading.

Quinidine Sulfate (In vivo drug-drug interaction studies have suggested that pioglitazone may be a weak inducer of CYP 450 isoform 3A4 substrate).
No products indexed under this heading.

Rasagiline Mesylate (The hypoglycemic action of sulfonylureas may be potentiated by certain drugs, including monoamine oxidase inhibitors. Due to the potential drug interaction between these drugs and glimepiride, the patient should be observed closely for hypoglycemia when these drugs are co-administered. Conversely, when these drugs are withdrawn, the patient should be observed closely for loss of glycemic control). Products include:
Azilect Tablets 3106

Rifabutin (In vivo drug-drug interaction studies have suggested that pioglitazone may be a weak inducer of CYP 450 isoform 3A4 substrate).
No products indexed under this heading.

Rifampin (Concomitant administration of rifampin (oral 600 mg once daily), an dinducer of CYP2C8 with pioglitazone (oral 30 mg) in 10 healthy volunteers pre-treated for 5 days prior with rifampin (oral 600 mg once daily) resulted in a decrease in the AUC of pioglitazone by 54%).
No products indexed under this heading.

Rifapentine (There is a potential interaction of glimepiride with inducers (e.g., rifampicin) of cytochrome P450 2C9).
No products indexed under this heading.

Ritonavir (There is a potential interaction of glimepiride with inhibitors (e.g., fluconazole) of cytochrome P450 2C9). Products include:

IMPORTANT NOTE: Always consult each drug listing in the patient's regimen for possible interactions.

Kaletra 452
Norvir 489

Rofecoxib (The hypoglycemic action of sulfonylureas may be potentiated by certain drugs, including nonsteroidial anti-inflammatory drugs. Due to the potential drug interaction between these drugs and glimepiride, the patient should be observed closely for hypoglycemia when these drugs are co-administered. Conversely, when these drugs are withdrawn, the patient should be observed closely for loss of glycemic control).

No products indexed under this heading.

Salmeterol Xinafoate (Certain drugs tend to produce hyperglycemia and may lead to loss of control. These drugs include the sympathomimetics. Due to the potential drug interaction between these drugs and glimepiride, the patient should be observed closely for loss of glycemic control when these drugs are co-administered. Conversely, when these drugs are withdrawn, the patient should be observed closely for hypoglycemia). Products include:

Advair Diskus 100/50 1276
Advair Diskus 250/50 1276
Advair Diskus 500/50 1276
Advair HFA 45/21 Inhalation Aerosol.. 1288
Advair HFA 115/21 Inhalation Aerosol.. 1288
Advair HFA 230/21 Inhalation Aerosol.. 1288
Serevent Diskus 1594

Salsalate (The hypoglycemic action of sulfonylureas may be potentiated by certain drugs, included salicylates. Due to the potential drug interaction between these drugs and glimepiride, the patient should be observed closely for hypoglycemia when these drugs are co-administered. Conversely, when these drugs are withdrawn, the patient should be observed closely for loss of glycemic control).

No products indexed under this heading.

Saquinavir (In vivo drug-drug interaction studies have suggested that pioglitazone may be a weak inducer of CYP 450 isoform 3A4 substrate).

No products indexed under this heading.

Saquinavir Mesylate (In vivo drug-drug interaction studies have suggested that pioglitazone may be a weak inducer of CYP 450 isoform 3A4 substrate).

No products indexed under this heading.

Secobarbital Sodium (There is a potential interaction of glimepiride with inducers (e.g., rifampicin) of cytochrome P450 2C9).

No products indexed under this heading.

Selegiline (The hypoglycemic action of sulfonylureas may be potentiated by certain drugs, including monoamine oxidase inhibitors. Due to the potential drug interaction between these drugs and glimepiride, the patient should be observed closely for hypoglycemia when these drugs are co-administered. Conversely, when these drugs are withdrawn, the patient should be observed closely for loss of glycemic control). Products include:

Emsam Transdermal System 905

Selegiline Hydrochloride (The hypoglycemic action of sulfonylureas may be potentiated by certain drugs, including monoamine oxidase inhibitors. Due to the potential drug interaction between these drugs and glimepiride, the patient should be observed closely for hypoglycemia when these drugs are co-administered. Conversely, when these drugs are withdrawn, the patient should be observed closely for loss of glycemic control). Products include:

Eldepryl Capsules 3052

Sertraline Hydrochloride (There is a potential interaction of glimepiride with inhibitors (e.g., fluconazole) of cytochrome P450 2C9).

No products indexed under this heading.

Sildenafil Citrate (There is a potential interaction of glimepiride with inhibitors (e.g., fluconazole) of cytochrome P450 2C9).

No products indexed under this heading.

Simvastatin (In vivo drug-drug interaction studies have suggested that pioglitazone may be a weak inducer of CYP 450 isoform 3A4 substrate). Products include:

Simcor Tablets 502
Vytorin 10/10 Tablets 2149
Vytorin 10/10 Tablets 2939
Vytorin 10/20 Tablets 2149
Vytorin 10/20 Tablets 2939
Vytorin 10/40 Tablets 2149
Vytorin 10/40 Tablets 2939
Vytorin 10/80 Tablets 2149
Vytorin 10/80 Tablets 2939
Zocor Tablets 2136

Sirolimus (In vivo drug-drug interaction studies have suggested that pioglitazone may be a weak inducer of CYP 450 isoform 3A4 substrate). Products include:

Rapamune 3260

Sotalol Hydrochloride (The hypoglycemic action of sulfonylureas may be potentiated by certain drugs, including beta adrenergic blocking agents. Due to the potential drug interaction between these drugs and glimepiride, the patient should be observed closely for hypoglycemia when these drugs are co-administered. Conversely, when these drugs are withdrawn, the patient should be observed closely for loss of glycemic control. If beta-blockers are used, caution should be exercised and patients should be warned about the potential for hypoglycemia).

No products indexed under this heading.

Spironolactone (Certain drugs tend to produce hyperglycemia and may lead to loss of control. These drugs include the thiazides and other diuretics. Due to the potential drug interaction between these drugs and glimepiride, the patient should be observed closely for loss of glycemic control when these drugs are co-administered. Conversely, when these drugs are withdrawn, the patient should be observed closely for hypoglycemia).

No products indexed under this heading.

Sulfacytine (The hypoglycemic action of sulfonylureas may be potentiated by certain drugs, including sulfonamides. Due to the potential drug interaction between these drugs and glimepiride, the patient should be observed closely for hypoglycemia when these drugs are co-administered. Conversely when these drugs are withdrawn, the patient should be observed closely for loss of glycemic control).

No products indexed under this heading.

Sulfamethizole (The hypoglycemic action of sulfonylureas may be potentiated by certain drugs, including sulfonamides. Due to the potential drug interaction between these drugs and glimepiride, the patient should be observed closely for hypoglycemia when these drugs are co-administered. Conversely when these drugs are withdrawn, the patient should be observed closely for loss of glycemic control).

No products indexed under this heading.

Sulfamethoxazole (The hypoglycemic action of sulfonylureas may be potentiated by certain drugs, including sulfonamides. Due to the potential drug interaction between these drugs and glimepiride, the patient should be observed closely for hypoglycemia when these drugs are co-administered. Conversely when these drugs are withdrawn, the patient should be observed closely for loss of glycemic control).

No products indexed under this heading.

Sulfasalazine (The hypoglycemic action of sulfonylureas may be potentiated by certain drugs, including sulfonamides. Due to the potential drug interaction between these drugs and glimepiride, the patient should be observed closely for hypoglycemia when these drugs are co-administered. Conversely when these drugs are withdrawn, the patient should be observed closely for loss of glycemic control).

No products indexed under this heading.

Sulfinpyrazone (The hypoglycemic action of sulfonylureas may be potentiated by certain drugs, including sulfonamides. Due to the potential drug interaction between these drugs and glimepiride, the patient should be observed closely for hypoglycemia when these drugs are co-administered. Conversely when these drugs are withdrawn, the patient should be observed closely for loss of glycemic control).

No products indexed under this heading.

Sulfisoxazole Acetyl (The hypoglycemic action of sulfonylureas may be potentiated by certain drugs, including sulfonamides. Due to the potential drug interaction between these drugs and glimepiride, the patient should be observed closely for hypoglycemia when these drugs are co-administered. Conversely when these drugs are withdrawn, the patient should be observed closely for loss of glycemic control).

No products indexed under this heading.

Sulfisoxazole Diolamine (The hypoglycemic action of sulfonylureas may be potentiated by certain drugs, including sulfonamides. Due to the potential drug interaction between these drugs and glimepiride, the patient should be observed closely for hypoglycemia when these drugs are co-administered. Conversely when these drugs are withdrawn, the patient should be observed closely for loss of glycemic control).

No products indexed under this heading.

Sulindac (The hypoglycemic action of sulfonylureas may be potentiated by certain drugs, including non-steroidial anti-inflammatory drugs. Due to the potential drug interaction between these drugs and glimepiride, the patient should be observed closely for hypoglycemia when these drugs are co-administered. Conversely, when these drugs are withdrawn, the patient should be observed closely for loss of glycemic control). Products include:

Clinoril Tablets 1962

Tacrolimus (In vivo drug-drug interaction studies have suggested that pioglitazone may be a weak inducer of CYP 450 isoform 3A4 substrate). Products include:

Prograf Capsules and Injection 622
Protopic Ointment 628

Tadalafil (In vivo drug-drug interaction studies have suggested that pioglitazone may be a weak inducer of CYP 450 isoform 3A4 substrate). Products include:

Cialis Tablets 1792

Tamoxifen Citrate (In vivo drug-drug interaction studies have suggested that pioglitazone may be a weak inducer of CYP 450 isoform 3A4 substrate).

No products indexed under this heading.

Terbutaline Sulfate (Certain drugs tend to produce hyperglycemia and may lead to loss of control. These drugs include the sympathomimetics. Due to the potential drug interaction between these drugs and glimepiride, the patient should be observed closely for loss of glycemic control when these drugs are co-administered. Conversely, when these drugs are withdrawn, the patient should be observed closely for hypoglycemia).

No products indexed under this heading.

Terconazole (There is a potential interaction of glimepiride with inhibitors (e.g., fluconazole) of cytochrome P450 2C9).

No products indexed under this heading.

Thioridazine Hydrochloride (Certain drugs tend to produce hyperglycemia and may lead to loss of control. These drugs include the phenothiazines. Due to the potential drug interaction between these drugs and glimepiride, the patient should be observed closely for loss of glycemic control when these drugs are co-administered. Conversely, when these drugs are withdrawn, the patient should be observed closely for hypoglycemia). Products include:

Thioridazine Hydrochloride Tablets 2195

Thyroglobulin (Certain drugs tend to produce hyperglycemia and may lead to loss of control. These drugs include thyroid products. Due to the potential drug interaction between these drugs and glimepiride, the patient should be observed closely for loss of glycemic control when these drugs are co-administered. Conversely, when these drugs are withdrawn, the patient should be

observed closely for hypoglycemia).
No products indexed under this heading.

Thyroid (Certain drugs tend to produce hyperglycemia and may lead to loss of control. These drugs include thyroid products. Due to the potential drug interaction between these drugs and glimepiride, the patient should be observed closely for loss of glycemic control when these drugs are co-administered. Conversely, when these drugs are withdrawn, the patient should be observed closely for hypoglycemia). Products include:
Naturethroid Tablets 2605

Thyroxine (Certain drugs tend to produce hyperglycemia and may lead to loss of control. These drugs include thyroid products. Due to the potential drug interaction between these drugs and glimepiride, the patient should be observed closely for loss of glycemic control when these drugs are co-administered. Conversely, when these drugs are withdrawn, the patient should be observed closely for hypoglycemia).
No products indexed under this heading.

Thyroxine Sodium (Certain drugs tend to produce hyperglycemia and may lead to loss of control. These drugs include thyroid products. Due to the potential drug interaction between these drugs and glimepiride, the patient should be observed closely for loss of glycemic control when these drugs are co-administered. Conversely, when these drugs are withdrawn, the patient should be observed closely for hypoglycemia).
No products indexed under this heading.

Tiagabine Hydrochloride (In vivo drug-drug interaction studies have suggested that pioglitazone may be a weak inducer of CYP 450 isoform 3A4 substrate). Products include:
Gabitril Tablets 973

Ticlopidine Hydrochloride (There is a potential interaction of glimepiride with inhibitors (e.g., fluconazole) of cytochrome P450 2C9).
No products indexed under this heading.

Timolol Hemihydrate (The hypoglycemic action of sulfonylureas may be potentiated by certain drugs, including beta adrenergic blocking agents. Due to the potential drug interaction between these drugs and glimepiride, the patient should be observed closely for hypoglycemia when these drugs are co-administered. Conversely, when these drugs are withdrawn, the patient should be observed closely for loss of glycemic control. If beta-blockers are used, caution should be exercised and patients should be warned about the potential for hypoglycemia). Products include:
Betimol Ophthalmic Solution 3181

Timolol Maleate (The hypoglycemic action of sulfonylureas may be potentiated by certain drugs, including beta adrenergic blocking agents. Due to the potential drug interaction between these drugs and glimepiride, the patient should be observed closely for hypoglycemia when these drugs are co-administered. Conversely, when these drugs are withdrawn, the patient should be observed closely for loss of glycemic control. If beta-blockers are used, caution should be exercised and patients should be warned about the potential for hypoglycemia). Products include:
Combigan Ophthalmic Solution 553
Cosopt Sterile Ophthalmic Solution 1969
Timoptic Sterile Ophthalmic Solution 2121
Timoptic in Ocudose 2124
Timoptic-XE Sterile Ophthalmic Gel Forming Solution 2125

Tolazamide (The hypoglycemic action of sulfonylureas may be potentiated by certain drugs, including sulfonamides. Due to the potential drug interaction between these drugs and glimepiride, the patient should be observed closely for hypoglycemia when these drugs are co-administered. Conversely when these drugs are withdrawn, the patient should be observed closely for loss of glycemic control).
No products indexed under this heading.

Tolbutamide (The hypoglycemic action of sulfonylureas may be potentiated by certain drugs, including sulfonamides. Due to the potential drug interaction between these drugs and glimepiride, the patient should be observed closely for hypoglycemia when these drugs are co-administered. Conversely when these drugs are withdrawn, the patient should be observed closely for loss of glycemic control).
No products indexed under this heading.

Tolbutamide Sodium (There is a potential interaction of glimepiride with inhibitors (e.g., fluconazole) of cytochrome P450 2C9).
No products indexed under this heading.

Tolmetin Sodium (The hypoglycemic action of sulfonylureas may be potentiated by certain drugs, including nonsteroidial anti-inflammatory drugs. Due to the potential drug interaction between these drugs and glimepiride, the patient should be observed closely for hypoglycemia when these drugs are co-administered. Conversely, when these drugs are withdrawn, the patient should be observed closely for loss of glycemic control).
No products indexed under this heading.

Tolterodine Tartrate (In vivo drug-drug interaction studies have suggested that pioglitazone may be a weak inducer of CYP 450 isoform 3A4 substrate).
No products indexed under this heading.

Torsemide (Certain drugs tend to produce hyperglycemia and may lead to loss of control. These drugs include the thiazides and other diuretics. Due to the potential drug interaction between these drugs and glimepiride, the patient should be observed closely for loss of glycemic control when these drugs are co-administered. Conversely, when these drugs are withdrawn, the patient should be observed closely for hypoglycemia). Products include:
Demadex Injection 2630
Demadex Tablets 2630

Tranylcypromine Sulfate (The hypoglycemic action of sulfonylureas may be potentiated by certain drugs, including monoamine oxidase inhibitors. Due to the potential drug interaction between these drugs and glimepiride, the patient should be observed closely for hypoglycemia when these drugs are co-administered. Conversely, when these drugs are withdrawn, the patient should be observed closely for loss of glycemic control). Products include:
Parnate Tablets 1532

Trazodone Hydrochloride (In vivo drug-drug interaction studies have suggested that pioglitazone may be a weak inducer of CYP 450 isoform 3A4 substrate).
No products indexed under this heading.

Triamcinolone (Certain drugs tend to produce hyperglycemia and may lead to loss of control. These drugs include the corticosteroids. Due to the potential drug interaction between these drugs and glimepiride, the patient should be observed closely for loss of glycemic control when these drugs are co-administered. Conversely, when these drugs are withdrawn, the patient should be observed closely for hypoglycemia).
No products indexed under this heading.

Triamcinolone Acetonide (Certain drugs tend to produce hyperglycemia and may lead to loss of control. These drugs include the corticosteroids. Due to the potential drug interaction between these drugs and glimepiride, the patient should be observed closely for loss of glycemic control when these drugs are co-administered. Conversely, when these drugs are withdrawn, the patient should be observed closely for hypoglycemia). Products include:
Azmacort Inhalation Aerosol 407
Nasacort AQ Nasal Spray 2765
Triesence Injectable Suspension .... ⊙209

Triamcinolone Diacetate (Certain drugs tend to produce hyperglycemia and may lead to loss of control. These drugs include the corticosteroids. Due to the potential drug interaction between these drugs and glimepiride, the patient should be observed closely for loss of glycemic control when these drugs are co-administered. Conversely, when these drugs are withdrawn, the patient should be observed closely for hypoglycemia).
No products indexed under this heading.

Triamcinolone Hexacetonide (Certain drugs tend to produce hyperglycemia and may lead to loss of control. These drugs include the corticosteroids. Due to the potential drug interaction between these drugs and glimepiride, the patient should be observed closely for loss of glycemic control when these drugs are co-administered. Conversely, when these drugs are withdrawn, the patient should be observed closely for hypoglycemia).
No products indexed under this heading.

Triamterene (Certain drugs tend to produce hyperglycemia and may lead to loss of control. These drugs include the thiazides and other diuretics. Due to the potential drug interaction between these drugs and glimepiride, the patient should be observed closely for loss of glycemic control when these drugs are co-administered. Conversely, when these drugs are withdrawn, the patient should be observed closely for hypoglycemia). Products include:
Dyazide Capsules 1405
Dyrenium Capsules 3189

Triazolam (In vivo drug-drug interaction studies have suggested that pioglitazone may be a weak inducer of CYP 450 isoform 3A4 substrate).
No products indexed under this heading.

Trifluoperazine Hydrochloride (Certain drugs tend to produce hyperglycemia and may lead to loss of control. These drugs include the phenothiazines. Due to the potential drug interaction between these drugs and glimepiride, the patient should be observed closely for loss of glycemic control when these drugs are co-administered. Conversely, when these drugs are withdrawn, the patient should be observed closely for hypoglycemia).
No products indexed under this heading.

Troglitazone (There is a potential interaction of glimepiride with inhibitors (e.g., fluconazole) of cytochrome P450 2C9).
No products indexed under this heading.

Valdecoxib (The hypoglycemic action of sulfonylureas may be potentiated by certain drugs, including nonsteroidial anti-inflammatory drugs. Due to the potential drug interaction between these drugs and glimepiride, the patient should be observed closely for hypoglycemia when these drugs are co-administered. Conversely, when these drugs are withdrawn, the patient should be observed closely for loss of glycemic control).
No products indexed under this heading.

Vardenafil Hydrochloride (There is a potential interaction of glimepiride with inhibitors (e.g., fluconazole) of cytochrome P450 2C9). Products include:
Levitra Tablets 2876

Verapamil Hydrochloride (In vivo drug-drug interaction studies have suggested that pioglitazone may be a weak inducer of CYP 450 isoform 3A4 substrate). Products include:
Tarka Tablets 511

Vinblastine Sulfate (In vivo drug-drug interaction studies have suggested that pioglitazone may be a weak inducer of CYP 450 isoform 3A4 substrate).
No products indexed under this heading.

Vincristine Sulfate (In vivo drug-drug interaction studies have suggested that pioglitazone may be a weak inducer of CYP 450 isoform 3A4 substrate).
No products indexed under this heading.

Voriconazole (There is a potential interaction of glimepiride with inhibitors (e.g., fluconazole) of cytochrome P450 2C9).
No products indexed under this heading.

Warfarin Sodium (The hypoglycemic action of sulfonylureas may be potentiated by certain drugs, including coumarins. Due to the potential drug interaction between these drugs and glimepiride, the patient

should be observed closely for hypoglycemia when these drugs are co-administered. Conversely, when these drugs are withdrawn, the patient should be observed closely for loss of glycemic control).
No products indexed under this heading.

Zafirlukast (There is a potential interaction of glimepiride with inhibitors (e.g., fluconazole) of cytochrome P450 2C9). Products include:
Accolate Tablets 669

DULCOLAX STOOL SOFTENER
(Docusate Sodium) .... ▣602
None cited in PDR database.

DULCOLAX SUPPOSITORIES
(Bisacodyl) .... ▣602
None cited in PDR database.

DULCOLAX TABLETS
(Bisacodyl) .... ▣602
May interact with antacids and certain other agents. Compounds in these categories include:

Aluminum Carbonate (Dulcolax should not be taken within one hour of taking an antacid).
No products indexed under this heading.

Aluminum Hydroxide (Dulcolax should not be taken within one hour of taking an antacid).
No products indexed under this heading.

Magaldrate (Dulcolax should not be taken within one hour of taking an antacid).
No products indexed under this heading.

Magnesium Hydroxide (Dulcolax should not be taken within one hour of taking an antacid). Products include:
Fleet Pedia-Lax Chewable Tablets 1145
Pepcid Complete Chewable Tablets 1771
Extra Strength Rolaids Freshmint Tablets 1903
Rolaids Multi-Symptom Berry Tablets 1903
Rolaids Original Peppermint Tablets 1903

Magnesium Oxide (Dulcolax should not be taken within one hour of taking an antacid). Products include:
Beelith Tablets 813

Sodium Bicarbonate (Dulcolax should not be taken within one hour of taking an antacid). Products include:
Ceo-Two Laxative Suppository 815

Food Interactions

Dairy products (Dulcolax should not be taken within one hour of taking milk).

DURAGESIC TRANSDERMAL SYSTEM
(Fentanyl) 2405
May interact with monoamine oxidase inhibitors, narcotic analgesics, phenothiazines, skeletal muscle relaxants, tranquilizers, and certain other agents. Compounds in these categories include:

Acetazolamide (The concomitant use of fentanyl with all CYP3A4 inhibitors (such as ritonavir, ketoconazole, itraconazole, troleandomycin, clarithromycin, nelfinavir, nefazodone, amiodarone, amprenavir, aprepitant, diltiazem, erythromycin, fluconazole, fosamprenavir, grapefruit juice, and verapamil) may result in an increase in fentanyl plasma concentrations, which could increase or prolong adverse drug effects and may cause potentially fatal respiratory depression. Patients receiving fentanyl and any CYP3A4 inhibitor should be monitored for an extended period of time and dosage adjustments should be made if warranted).
No products indexed under this heading.

Alfentanil Hydrochloride (The comcomitant use of fentanyl with other CNS depressants may cause respiratory depression, hypotension, and profound sedation or potentially result in coma. When such combined therapy is contemplated, the dose of one or both agents should be significantly reduced).
No products indexed under this heading.

Allium sativum (Fentanyl is metabolized mainly via the human cytochrome P450 3A4 isoenzyme system (CYP3A4). Co-administration with agents that induce CYP 3A4 activity may reduce the efficacy of fentanyl).
No products indexed under this heading.

Alprazolam (The comcomitant use of fentanyl with other CNS depressants may cause respiratory depression, hypotension, and profound sedation or potentially result in coma. When such combined therapy is contemplated, the dose of one or both agents should be significantly reduced).
No products indexed under this heading.

Amiodarone Hydrochloride (The concomitant use of fentanyl with all CYP3A4 inhibitors (such as ritonavir, ketoconazole, itraconazole, troleandomycin, clarithromycin, nelfinavir, nefazodone, amiodarone, amprenavir, aprepitant, diltiazem, erythromycin, fluconazole, fosamprenavir, grapefruit juice, and verapamil) may result in an increase in fentanyl plasma concentrations, which could increase or prolong adverse drug effects and may cause potentially fatal respiratory depression. Patients receiving fentanyl and any CYP3A4 inhibitor should be monitored for an extended period of time and dosage adjustments should be made if warranted).
No products indexed under this heading.

Amprenavir (The concomitant use of fentanyl with potent cytochrome P450 3A4 inhibitors may result in an increase in fentanyl plasma concentrations, which could increase or prolong adverse drug effects and may cause potentially fatal respiratory depression. Patients receiving fentanyl and potent CYP3A4 inhibitors should be carefully monitored for an extended period of time and dosage adjustments should be made if warranted).
No products indexed under this heading.

Anastrozole (The concomitant use of fentanyl with all CYP3A4 inhibitors (such as ritonavir, ketoconazole, itraconazole, troleandomycin, clarithromycin, nelfinavir, nefazodone, amiodarone, amprenavir, aprepitant, diltiazem, erythromycin, fluconazole, fosamprenavir, grapefruit juice, and verapamil) may result in an increase in fentanyl plasma concentrations, which could increase or prolong adverse drug effects and may cause potentially fatal respiratory depression. Patients receiving fentanyl and any CYP3A4 inhibitor should be monitored for an extended period of time and dosage adjustments should be made if warranted). Products include:
Arimidex Tablets 672

Aprepitant (The concomitant use of fentanyl with all CYP3A4 inhibitors (such as ritonavir, ketoconazole, itraconazole, troleandomycin, clarithromycin, nelfinavir, nefazodone, amiodarone, amprenavir, aprepitant, diltiazem, erythromycin, fluconazole, fosamprenavir, grapefruit juice, and verapamil) may result in an increase in fentanyl plasma concentrations, which could increase or prolong adverse drug effects and may cause potentially fatal respiratory depression. Patients receiving fentanyl and any CYP3A4 inhibitor should be monitored for an extended period of time and dosage adjustments should be made if warranted). Products include:
Emend Capsules 1992

Aprobarbital (The comcomitant use of fentanyl with other CNS depressants may cause respiratory depression, hypotension, and profound sedation or potentially result in coma. When such combined therapy is contemplated, the dose of one or both agents should be significantly reduced).
No products indexed under this heading.

Atazanavir (The concomitant use of fentanyl with potent cytochrome P450 3A4 inhibitors may result in an increase in fentanyl plasma concentrations, which could increase or prolong adverse drug effects and may cause potentially fatal respiratory depression. Patients receiving fentanyl and potent CYP3A4 inhibitors should be carefully monitored for an extended period of time and dosage adjustments should be made if warranted).
No products indexed under this heading.

Atazanavir Sulfate (The concomitant use of fentanyl with potent cytochrome P450 3A4 inhibitors may result in an increase in fentanyl plasma concentrations, which could increase or prolong adverse drug effects and may cause potentially fatal respiratory depression. Patients receiving fentanyl and potent CYP3A4 inhibitors should be carefully monitored for an extended period of time and dosage adjustments should be made if warranted). Products include:
Reyataz Capsules 3299

Baclofen (The concomitant use of fentanyl with other CNS depressants, including skeletal muscle relaxants, may cause respiratory depression, hypotension, and profound sedation or potentially result in coma. When such combined therapy is contemplated, the dose of one or both agents should be significantly reduced).
No products indexed under this heading.

Betamethasone Acetate (Fentanyl is metabolized mainly via the human cytochrome P450 3A4 isoenzyme system (CYP3A4). Co-administration with agents that induce CYP 3A4 activity may reduce the efficacy of fentanyl).
No products indexed under this heading.

Betamethasone Sodium Phosphate (Fentanyl is metabolized mainly via the human cytochrome P450 3A4 isoenzyme system (CYP3A4). Co-administration with agents that induce CYP 3A4 activity may reduce the efficacy of fentanyl).
No products indexed under this heading.

Buprenorphine Hydrochloride (The comcomitant use of fentanyl with other CNS depressants may cause respiratory depression, hypotension, and profound sedation or potentially result in coma. When such combined therapy is contemplated, the dose of one or both agents should be significantly reduced). Products include:
Suboxone Tablets 2601
Subutex Tablets 2601

Buspirone Hydrochloride (The comcomitant use of fentanyl with other CNS depressants may cause respiratory depression, hypotension, and profound sedation or potentially result in coma. When such combined therapy is contemplated, the dose of one or both agents should be significantly reduced).
No products indexed under this heading.

Butabarbital (The comcomitant use of fentanyl with other CNS depressants may cause respiratory depression, hypotension, and profound sedation or potentially result in coma. When such combined therapy is contemplated, the dose of one or both agents should be significantly reduced).
No products indexed under this heading.

Butabarbital Sodium (The concomitant use of fentanyl with other CNS depressants, including sedatives and hypnotics, may cause respiratory depression, hypotension, and profound sedation or potentially result in coma. When such combined therapy is contemplated, the dose of oneor both agents should be significantly reduced).
No products indexed under this heading.

Butalbital (The comcomitant use of fentanyl with other CNS depressants may cause respiratory depression, hypotension, and profound sedation or potentially result in coma. When such combined therapy is contemplated, the dose of one or both agents should be significantly reduced).
No products indexed under this heading.

Carbamazepine (Fentanyl is metabolized mainly via the human cytochrome P450 3A4 isoenzyme system (CYP3A4). Co-administration with agents that induce CYP 3A4 activity may reduce the efficacy of fentanyl). Products include:
Carbatrol Capsules 3019
Equetro Extended-Release Capsules 3174

Carisoprodol (The concomitant use of fentanyl with other CNS depressants, including skeletal muscle relaxants, may cause respiratory depression, hypotension, and profound sedation or potentially result in coma. When such combined therapy is contemplated, the dose of one or both agents should be significantly reduced). Products include:

Soma Tablets 1931

Chloral Hydrate (The concomitant use of fentanyl with other CNS depressants, including sedatives and hypnotics, may cause respiratory depression, hypotension, and profound sedation or potentially result in coma. When such combined therapy is contemplated, the dose of oneor both agents should be significantly reduced).

No products indexed under this heading.

Chlordiazepoxide (The concomitant use of fentanyl with other CNS depressants may cause respiratory depression, hypotension, and profound sedation or potentially result in coma. When such combined therapy is contemplated, the dose of one or both agents should be significantly reduced).

No products indexed under this heading.

Chlordiazepoxide Hydrochloride (The concomitant use of fentanyl with other CNS depressants may cause respiratory depression, hypotension, and profound sedation or potentially result in coma. When such combined therapy is contemplated, the dose of one or both agents should be significantly reduced).

No products indexed under this heading.

Chlorpromazine (The concomitant use of fentanyl with other CNS depressants may cause respiratory depression, hypotension, and profound sedation or potentially result in coma. When such combined therapy is contemplated, the dose of one or both agents should be significantly reduced).

No products indexed under this heading.

Chlorpromazine Hydrochloride (The concomitant use of fentanyl with other CNS depressants may cause respiratory depression, hypotension, and profound sedation or potentially result in coma. When such combined therapy is contemplated, the dose of one or both agents should be significantly reduced).

No products indexed under this heading.

Chlorprothixene (The concomitant use of fentanyl with other CNS depressants may cause respiratory depression, hypotension, and profound sedation or potentially result in coma. When such combined therapy is contemplated, the dose of one or both agents should be significantly reduced).

No products indexed under this heading.

Chlorprothixene Hydrochloride (The comcomitant use of fentanyl with other CNS depressants may cause respiratory depression, hypotension, and profound sedation or potentially result in coma. When such combined therapy is contemplated, the dose of one or both agents should be significantly reduced).

No products indexed under this heading.

Chlorprothixene Lactate (The comcomitant use of fentanyl with other CNS depressants may cause respiratory depression, hypotension, and profound sedation or potentially result in coma. When such combined therapy is contemplated, the dose of one or both agents should be significantly reduced).

No products indexed under this heading.

Chlorzoxazone (The concomitant use of fentanyl with other CNS depressants, including skeletal muscle relaxants, may cause respiratory depression, hypotension, and profound sedation or potentially result in coma. When such combined therapy is contemplated, the dose of one or both agents should be significantly reduced).

No products indexed under this heading.

Cimetidine (The concomitant use of fentanyl with all CYP3A4 inhibitors (such as ritonavir, ketoconazole, itraconazole, troleandomycin, clarithromycin, nelfinavir, nefazodone, amiodarone, amprenavir, aprepitant, diltiazem, erythromycin, fluconazole, fosamprenavir, grapefruit juice, and verapamil) may result in an increase in fentanyl plasma concentrations, which could increase or prolong adverse drug effects and may cause potentially fatal respiratory depression. Patients receiving fentanyl and any CYP3A4 inhibitor should be monitored for an extended period of time and dosage adjustments should be made if warranted).

No products indexed under this heading.

Cimetidine Hydrochloride (The concomitant use of fentanyl with all CYP3A4 inhibitors (such as ritonavir, ketoconazole, itraconazole, troleandomycin, clarithromycin, nelfinavir, nefazodone, amiodarone, amprenavir, aprepitant, diltiazem, erythromycin, fluconazole, fosamprenavir, grapefruit juice, and verapamil) may result in an increase in fentanyl plasma concentrations, which could increase or prolong adverse drug effects and may cause potentially fatal respiratory depression. Patients receiving fentanyl and any CYP3A4 inhibitor should be monitored for an extended period of time and dosage adjustments should be made if warranted).

No products indexed under this heading.

Ciprofloxacin (The concomitant use of fentanyl with all CYP3A4 inhibitors (such as ritonavir, ketoconazole, itraconazole, troleandomycin, clarithromycin, nelfinavir, nefazodone, amiodarone, amprenavir, aprepitant, diltiazem, erythromycin, fluconazole, fosamprenavir, grapefruit juice, and verapamil) may result in an increase in fentanyl plasma concentrations, which could increase or prolong adverse drug effects and may cause potentially fatal respiratory depression. Patients receiving fentanyl and any CYP3A4 inhibitor should be monitored for an extended period of time and dosage adjustments should be made if warranted). Products include:

Cipro I.V. 2817
Cipro Oral Suspension 2810
Cipro XR Tablets 2823
Ciprodex Otic Suspension 541

Ciprofloxacin Hydrochloride (Fentanyl is metabolized mainly via the human cytochrome P450 3A4 isoenzyme system (CYP3A4). Co-administration with agents that induce CYP 3A4 activity may reduce the efficacy of fentanyl). Products include:

Cipro Tablets 2810

Cisplatin (Fentanyl is metabolized mainly via the human cytochrome P450 3A4 isoenzyme system (CYP3A4). Co-administration with agents that induce CYP 3A4 activity may reduce the efficacy of fentanyl).

No products indexed under this heading.

Clarithromycin (The concomitant use of fentanyl with potent cytochrome P450 3A4 inhibitors may result in an increase in fentanyl plasma concentrations, which could increase or prolong adverse drug effects and may cause potentially fatal respiratory depression. Patients receiving fentanyl and potent CYP3A4 inhibitors should be carefully monitored for an extended period of time and dosage adjustments should be made if warranted). Products include:

Biaxin/Biaxin XL 411

Clorazepate Dipotassium (The comcomitant use of fentanyl with other CNS depressants may cause respiratory depression, hypotension, and profound sedation or potentially result in coma. When such combined therapy is contemplated, the dose of one or both agents should be significantly reduced).

No products indexed under this heading.

Clotrimazole (The concomitant use of fentanyl with all CYP3A4 inhibitors (such as ritonavir, ketoconazole, itraconazole, troleandomycin, clarithromycin, nelfinavir, nefazodone, amiodarone, amprenavir, aprepitant, diltiazem, erythromycin, fluconazole, fosamprenavir, grapefruit juice, and verapamil) may result in an increase in fentanyl plasma concentrations, which could increase or prolong adverse drug effects and may cause potentially fatal respiratory depression. Patients receiving fentanyl and any CYP3A4 inhibitor should be monitored for an extended period of time and dosage adjustments should be made if warranted). Products include:

Lotrisone 2881

Clozapine (The comcomitant use of fentanyl with other CNS depressants may cause respiratory depression, hypotension, and profound sedation or potentially result in coma. When such combined therapy is contemplated, the dose of one or both agents should be significantly reduced).

No products indexed under this heading.

Codeine Phosphate (The comcomitant use of fentanyl with other CNS depressants may cause respiratory depression, hypotension, and profound sedation or potentially result in coma. When such combined therapy is contemplated, the dose of one or both agents should be significantly reduced). Products include:

Tylenol with Codeine Tablets 2427

Cortisone Acetate (Fentanyl is metabolized mainly via the human cytochrome P450 3A4 isoenzyme system (CYP3A4). Co-administration with agents that induce CYP 3A4 activity may reduce the efficacy of fentanyl).

No products indexed under this heading.

Cyclobenzaprine Hydrochloride (The concomitant use of fentanyl with other CNS depressants, including skeletal muscle relaxants, may cause respiratory depression, hypotension, and profound sedation or potentially result in coma. When such combined therapy is contemplated, the dose of one or both agents should be significantly reduced). Products include:

Amrix Capsules 966

Cyclosporine (The concomitant use of fentanyl with all CYP3A4 inhibitors (such as ritonavir, ketoconazole, itraconazole, troleandomycin, clarithromycin, nelfinavir, nefazodone, amiodarone, amprenavir, aprepitant, diltiazem, erythromycin, fluconazole, fosamprenavir, grapefruit juice, and verapamil) may result in an increase in fentanyl plasma concentrations, which could increase or prolong adverse drug effects and may cause potentially fatal respiratory depression. Patients receiving fentanyl and any CYP3A4 inhibitor should be monitored for an extended period of time and dosage adjustments should be made if warranted). Products include:

Gengraf Capsules 435
Neoral Oral Solution 2280
Neoral Soft Gelatin Capsules 2280
Restasis Ophthalmic Emulsion 557
Sandimmune 2296

Dalfopristin (The concomitant use of fentanyl with all CYP3A4 inhibitors (such as ritonavir, ketoconazole, itraconazole, troleandomycin, clarithromycin, nelfinavir, nefazodone, amiodarone, amprenavir, aprepitant, diltiazem, erythromycin, fluconazole, fosamprenavir, grapefruit juice, and verapamil) may result in an increase in fentanyl plasma concentrations, which could increase or prolong adverse drug effects and may cause potentially fatal respiratory depression. Patients receiving fentanyl and any CYP3A4 inhibitor should be monitored for an extended period of time and dosage adjustments should be made if warranted).

No products indexed under this heading.

Danazol (The concomitant use of fentanyl with all CYP3A4 inhibitors (such as ritonavir, ketoconazole, itraconazole, troleandomycin, clarithromycin, nelfinavir, nefazodone, amiodarone, amprenavir, aprepitant, diltiazem, erythromycin, fluconazole, fosamprenavir, grapefruit juice, and verapamil) may result in an increase in fentanyl plasma concentrations, which could increase or prolong adverse drug effects and may cause potentially fatal respiratory depression. Patients receiving fentanyl and any CYP3A4 inhibitor should be monitored for an extended period of time and dosage adjustments should be made if warranted).

No products indexed under this heading.

Dantrolene Sodium (The concomitant use of fentanyl with other CNS depressants, including skeletal muscle relaxants, may cause respiratory depression, hypotension, and profound sedation or potentially result in coma. When such combined therapy is contemplated, the dose of one or both agents should be significantly reduced). Products include:

Dantrium Capsules **2580**
Dantrium Intravenous **2582**

Delavirdine Mesylate (The concomitant use of fentanyl with potent cytochrome P450 3A4 inhibitors may result in an increase in fentanyl plasma concentrations, which could increase or prolong adverse drug effects and may cause potentially fatal respiratory depression. Patients receiving fentanyl and potent CYP3A4 inhibitors should be carefully monitored for an extended period of time and dosage adjustments should be made if warranted).

No products indexed under this heading.

Delavirine (The concomitant use of fentanyl with potent cytochrome P450 3A4 inhibitors may result in an increase in fentanyl plasma concentrations, which could increase or prolong adverse drug effects and may cause potentially fatal respiratory depression. Patients receiving fentanyl and potent CYP3A4 inhibitors should be carefully monitored for an extended period of time and dosage adjustments should be made if warranted).

No products indexed under this heading.

Desflurane (The comcomitant use of fentanyl with other CNS depressants may cause respiratory depression, hypotension, and profound sedation or potentially result in coma. When such combined therapy is contemplated, the dose of one or both agents should be significantly reduced).

No products indexed under this heading.

Dexamethasone (Fentanyl is metabolized mainly via the human cytochrome P450 3A4 isoenzyme system (CYP3A4). Co-administration with agents that induce CYP 3A4 activity may reduce the efficacy of fentanyl). Products include:

Ciprodex Otic Suspension **541**

Dexamethasone Acetate (Fentanyl is metabolized mainly via the human cytochrome P450 3A4 isoenzyme system (CYP3A4). Co-administration with agents that induce CYP 3A4 activity may reduce the efficacy of fentanyl).

No products indexed under this heading.

Dexamethasone Sodium Phosphate (Fentanyl is metabolized mainly via the human cytochrome P450 3A4 isoenzyme system (CYP3A4). Co-administration with agents that induce CYP 3A4 activity may reduce the efficacy of fentanyl).

No products indexed under this heading.

Dezocine (The comcomitant use of fentanyl with other CNS depressants may cause respiratory depression, hypotension, and profound sedation or potentially result in coma. When such combined therapy is contemplated, the dose of one or both agents should be significantly reduced).

No products indexed under this heading.

Diazepam (The comcomitant use of fentanyl with other CNS depressants may cause respiratory depression, hypotension, and profound sedation or potentially result in coma. When such combined therapy is contemplated, the dose of one or both agents should be significantly reduced). Products include:

Valium Tablets **2658**

Diltiazem Hydrochloride (The concomitant use of fentanyl with all CYP3A4 inhibitors (such as ritonavir, ketoconazole, itraconazole, troleandomycin, clarithromycin, nelfinavir, nefazodone, amiodarone, amprenavir, aprepitant, diltiazem, erythromycin, fluconazole, fosamprenavir, grapefruit juice, and verapamil) may result in an increase in fentanyl plasma concentrations, which could increase or prolong adverse drug effects and may cause potentially fatal respiratory depression. Patients receiving fentanyl and any CYP3A4 inhibitor should be monitored for an extended period of time and dosage adjustments should be made if warranted). Products include:

Cardizem LA Extended Release Tablets **421**

Diltiazem Maleate (The concomitant use of fentanyl with all CYP3A4 inhibitors (such as ritonavir, ketoconazole, itraconazole, troleandomycin, clarithromycin, nelfinavir, nefazodone, amiodarone, amprenavir, aprepitant, diltiazem, erythromycin, fluconazole, fosamprenavir, grapefruit juice, and verapamil) may result in an increase in fentanyl plasma concentrations, which could increase or prolong adverse drug effects and may cause potentially fatal respiratory depression. Patients receiving fentanyl and any CYP3A4 inhibitor should be monitored for an extended period of time and dosage adjustments should be made if warranted).

No products indexed under this heading.

Doxorubicin Hydrochloride (Fentanyl is metabolized mainly via the human cytochrome P450 3A4 isoenzyme system (CYP3A4). Co-administration with agents that induce CYP 3A4 activity may reduce the efficacy of fentanyl).

No products indexed under this heading.

Droperidol (The comcomitant use of fentanyl with other CNS depressants may cause respiratory depression, hypotension, and profound sedation or potentially result in coma. When such combined therapy is contemplated, the dose of one or both agents should be significantly reduced).

No products indexed under this heading.

Efavirenz (The concomitant use of fentanyl with all CYP3A4 inhibitors (such as ritonavir, ketoconazole, itraconazole, troleandomycin, clarithromycin, nelfinavir, nefazodone, amiodarone, amprenavir, aprepitant, diltiazem, erythromycin, fluconazole, fosamprenavir, grapefruit juice, and verapamil) may result in an increase in fentanyl plasma concentrations, which could increase or prolong adverse drug effects and may cause potentially fatal respiratory depression. Patients receiving fentanyl and any CYP3A4 inhibitor should be monitored for an extended period of time and dosage adjustments should be made if warranted). Products include:

Atripla Tablets **938**
Sustiva Capsules **930**
Sustiva Tablets **930**

Enflurane (The comcomitant use of fentanyl with other CNS depressants may cause respiratory depression, hypotension, and profound sedation or potentially result in coma. When such combined therapy is contemplated, the dose of one or both agents should be significantly reduced).

No products indexed under this heading.

Erythromycin (The concomitant use of fentanyl with all CYP3A4 inhibitors (such as ritonavir, ketoconazole, itraconazole, troleandomycin, clarithromycin, nelfinavir, nefazodone, amiodarone, amprenavir, aprepitant, diltiazem, erythromycin, fluconazole, fosamprenavir, grapefruit juice, and verapamil) may result in an increase in fentanyl plasma concentrations, which could increase or prolong adverse drug effects and may cause potentially fatal respiratory depression. Patients receiving fentanyl and any CYP3A4 inhibitor should be monitored for an extended period of time and dosage adjustments should be made if warranted).

No products indexed under this heading.

Erythromycin Estolate (The concomitant use of fentanyl with all CYP3A4 inhibitors (such as ritonavir, ketoconazole, itraconazole, troleandomycin, clarithromycin, nelfinavir, nefazodone, amiodarone, amprenavir, aprepitant, diltiazem, erythromycin, fluconazole, fosamprenavir, grapefruit juice, and verapamil) may result in an increase in fentanyl plasma concentrations, which could increase or prolong adverse drug effects and may cause potentially fatal respiratory depression. Patients receiving fentanyl and any CYP3A4 inhibitor should be monitored for an extended period of time and dosage adjustments should be made if warranted).

No products indexed under this heading.

Erythromycin Ethylsuccinate (The concomitant use of fentanyl with all CYP3A4 inhibitors (such as ritonavir, ketoconazole, itraconazole, troleandomycin, clarithromycin, nelfinavir, nefazodone, amiodarone, amprenavir, aprepitant, diltiazem, erythromycin, fluconazole, fosamprenavir, grapefruit juice, and verapamil) may result in an increase in fentanyl plasma concentrations, which could increase or prolong adverse drug effects and may cause potentially fatal respiratory depression. Patients receiving fentanyl and any CYP3A4 inhibitor should be monitored for an extended period of time and dosage adjustments should be made if warranted). Products include:

E.E.S. **433**
EryPed **431**

Erythromycin Gluceptate (The concomitant use of fentanyl with all CYP3A4 inhibitors (such as ritonavir, ketoconazole, itraconazole, troleandomycin, clarithromycin, nelfinavir, nefazodone, amiodarone, amprenavir, aprepitant, diltiazem, erythromycin, fluconazole, fosamprenavir, grapefruit juice, and verapamil) may result in an increase in fentanyl plasma concentrations, which could increase or prolong adverse drug effects and may cause potentially fatal respiratory depression. Patients receiving fentanyl and any CYP3A4 inhibitor should be monitored for an extended period of time and dosage adjustments should be made if warranted).

No products indexed under this heading.

Erythromycin Lactobionate (The concomitant use of fentanyl with all CYP3A4 inhibitors (such as ritonavir, ketoconazole, itraconazole, troleandomycin, clarithromycin, nelfinavir, nefazodone, amiodarone, amprenavir, aprepitant, diltiazem, erythromycin, fluconazole, fosamprenavir, grapefruit juice, and verapamil) may result in an increase in fentanyl plasma concentrations, which could increase or prolong adverse drug effects and may cause potentially fatal respiratory depression. Patients receiving fentanyl and any CYP3A4 inhibitor should be monitored for an extended period of time and dosage adjustments should be made if warranted).

No products indexed under this heading.

Erythromycin Stearate (The concomitant use of fentanyl with all CYP3A4 inhibitors (such as ritonavir, ketoconazole, itraconazole, troleandomycin, clarithromycin, nelfinavir, nefazodone, amiodarone, amprenavir, aprepitant, diltiazem, erythromycin, fluconazole, fosamprenavir, grapefruit juice, and verapamil) may result in an increase in fentanyl plasma concentrations, which could increase or prolong adverse drug effects and may cause potentially fatal respiratory depression. Patients receiving fentanyl and any CYP3A4 inhibitor should be monitored for an extended period of time and dosage adjustments should be made if warranted).

No products indexed under this heading.

Esomeprazole Magnesium (The concomitant use of fentanyl with all CYP3A4 inhibitors (such as ritonavir, ketoconazole, itraconazole, troleandomycin, clarithromycin, nelfinavir, nefazodone, amiodarone, amprenavir, aprepitant, diltiazem, erythromycin, fluconazole, fosamprenavir, grapefruit juice, and verapamil) may result in an increase in fentanyl plasma concentrations, which could increase or prolong adverse drug effects and may cause potentially fatal respiratory depression. Patients receiving fentanyl and any CYP3A4 inhibitor should be monitored for an extended period of time and dosage adjustments should be made if warranted). Products include:

Nexium Delayed-Release Capsules 645
Nexium Delayed-Release Oral Suspension 645

Estazolam (The comcomitant use of fentanyl with other CNS depressants may cause respiratory depression, hypotension, and profound sedation or potentially result in coma. When such combined therapy is contemplated, the dose of one or both agents should be significantly reduced).
No products indexed under this heading.

Ethanol (The comcomitant use of fentanyl with other CNS depressants may cause respiratory depression, hypotension, and profound sedation or potentially result in coma. When such combined therapy is contemplated, the dose of one or both agents should be significantly reduced).
No products indexed under this heading.

Ethchlorvynol (The comcomitant use of fentanyl with other CNS depressants may cause respiratory depression, hypotension, and profound sedation or potentially result in coma. When such combined therapy is contemplated, the dose of one or both agents should be significantly reduced).
No products indexed under this heading.

Ethinamate (The comcomitant use of fentanyl with other CNS depressants may cause respiratory depression, hypotension, and profound sedation or potentially result in coma. When such combined therapy is contemplated, the dose of one or both agents should be significantly reduced).
No products indexed under this heading.

Ethosuximide (Fentanyl is metabolized mainly via the human cytochrome P450 3A4 isoenzyme system (CYP3A4). Co-administration with agents that induce CYP 3A4 activity may reduce the efficacy of fentanyl).
No products indexed under this heading.

Ethyl Alcohol (The comcomitant use of fentanyl with other CNS depressants may cause respiratory depression, hypotension, and profound sedation or potentially result in coma. When such combined therapy is contemplated, the dose of one or both agents should be significantly reduced).
No products indexed under this heading.

Felbamate (Fentanyl is metabolized mainly via the human cytochrome P450 3A4 isoenzyme system (CYP3A4). Co-administration with agents that induce CYP 3A4 activity may reduce the efficacy of fentanyl).
No products indexed under this heading.

Fentanyl Citrate (The comcomitant use of fentanyl with other CNS depressants may cause respiratory depression, hypotension, and profound sedation or potentially result in coma. When such combined therapy is contemplated, the dose of one or both agents should be significantly reduced). Products include:

Actiq 959
Fentora Tablets 968

Fluconazole (The concomitant use of fentanyl with all CYP3A4 inhibitors (such as ritonavir, ketoconazole, itraconazole, troleandomycin, clarithromycin, nelfinavir, nefazodone, amiodarone, amprenavir, aprepitant, diltiazem, erythromycin, fluconazole, fosamprenavir, grapefruit juice, and verapamil) may result in an increase in fentanyl plasma concentrations, which could increase or prolong adverse drug effects and may cause potentially fatal respiratory depression. Patients receiving fentanyl and any CYP3A4 inhibitor should be monitored for an extended period of time and dosage adjustments should be made if warranted).
No products indexed under this heading.

Fludrocortisone Acetate (Fentanyl is metabolized mainly via the human cytochrome P450 3A4 isoenzyme system (CYP3A4). Co-administration with agents that induce CYP 3A4 activity may reduce the efficacy of fentanyl).
No products indexed under this heading.

Fluoxetine (The concomitant use of fentanyl with all CYP3A4 inhibitors (such as ritonavir, ketoconazole, itraconazole, troleandomycin, clarithromycin, nelfinavir, nefazodone, amiodarone, amprenavir, aprepitant, diltiazem, erythromycin, fluconazole, fosamprenavir, grapefruit juice, and verapamil) may result in an increase in fentanyl plasma concentrations, which could increase or prolong adverse drug effects and may cause potentially fatal respiratory depression. Patients receiving fentanyl and any CYP3A4 inhibitor should be monitored for an extended period of time and dosage adjustments should be made if warranted).
No products indexed under this heading.

Fluoxetine Hydrochloride (The concomitant use of fentanyl with all CYP3A4 inhibitors (such as ritonavir, ketoconazole, itraconazole, troleandomycin, clarithromycin, nelfinavir, nefazodone, amiodarone, amprenavir, aprepitant, diltiazem, erythromycin, fluconazole, fosamprenavir, grapefruit juice, and verapamil) may result in an increase in fentanyl plasma concentrations, which could increase or prolong adverse drug effects and may cause potentially fatal respiratory depression. Patients receiving fentanyl and any CYP3A4 inhibitor should be monitored for an extended period of time and dosage adjustments should be made if warranted). Products include:

Prozac Weekly Capsules 1852
Prozac Pulvules and Liquid 1852
Symbyax Capsules 1871

Fluphenazine Decanoate (The comcomitant use of fentanyl with other CNS depressants may cause respiratory depression, hypotension, and profound sedation or potentially result in coma. When such combined therapy is contemplated, the dose of one or both agents should be significantly reduced).
No products indexed under this heading.

Fluphenazine Enanthate (The comcomitant use of fentanyl with other CNS depressants may cause respiratory depression, hypotension, and profound sedation or potentially result in coma. When such combined therapy is contemplated, the dose of one or both agents should be significantly reduced).
No products indexed under this heading.

Fluphenazine Hydrochloride (The comcomitant use of fentanyl with other CNS depressants may cause respiratory depression, hypotension, and profound sedation or potentially result in coma. When such combined therapy is contemplated, the dose of one or both agents should be significantly reduced).
No products indexed under this heading.

Flurazepam Hydrochloride (The comcomitant use of fentanyl with other CNS depressants may cause respiratory depression, hypotension, and profound sedation or potentially result in coma. When such combined therapy is contemplated, the dose of one or both agents should be significantly reduced).
No products indexed under this heading.

Fluvoxamine Maleate (The concomitant use of fentanyl with all CYP3A4 inhibitors (such as ritonavir, ketoconazole, itraconazole, troleandomycin, clarithromycin, nelfinavir, nefazodone, amiodarone, amprenavir, aprepitant, diltiazem, erythromycin, fluconazole, fosamprenavir, grapefruit juice, and verapamil) may result in an increase in fentanyl plasma concentrations, which could increase or prolong adverse drug effects and may cause potentially fatal respiratory depression. Patients receiving fentanyl and any CYP3A4 inhibitor should be monitored for an extended period of time and dosage adjustments should be made if warranted). Products include:

Luvox CR Extended-Release Capsules 1759

Fosamprenavir Calcium (The concomitant use of fentanyl with potent cytochrome P450 3A4 inhibitors may result in an increase in fentanyl plasma concentrations, which could increase or prolong adverse drug effects and may cause potentially fatal respiratory depression. Patients receiving fentanyl and potent CYP3A4 inhibitors should be carefully monitored for an extended period of time and dosage adjustments should be made if warranted). Products include:

Lexiva Oral Suspension 1510
Lexiva Tablets 1510

Fosphenytoin Sodium (Fentanyl is metabolized mainly via the human cytochrome P450 3A4 isoenzyme system (CYP3A4). Co-administration with agents that induce CYP 3A4 activity may reduce the efficacy of fentanyl).
No products indexed under this heading.

Garlic Extract (Fentanyl is metabolized mainly via the human cytochrome P450 3A4 isoenzyme system (CYP3A4). Co-administration with agents that induce CYP 3A4 activity may reduce the efficacy of fentanyl).
No products indexed under this heading.

Garlic Oil (Fentanyl is metabolized mainly via the human cytochrome P450 3A4 isoenzyme system (CYP3A4). Co-administration with agents that induce CYP 3A4 activity may reduce the efficacy of fentanyl).
No products indexed under this heading.

Glutethimide (The comcomitant use of fentanyl with other CNS depressants may cause respiratory depression, hypotension, and profound sedation or potentially result in coma. When such combined therapy is contemplated, the dose of one or both agents should be significantly reduced).
No products indexed under this heading.

Haloperidol (The comcomitant use of fentanyl with other CNS depressants may cause respiratory depression, hypotension, and profound sedation or potentially result in coma. When such combined therapy is contemplated, the dose of one or both agents should be significantly reduced).
No products indexed under this heading.

Haloperidol Decanoate (The comcomitant use of fentanyl with other CNS depressants may cause respiratory depression, hypotension, and profound sedation or potentially result in coma. When such combined therapy is contemplated, the dose of one or both agents should be significantly reduced).
No products indexed under this heading.

Hydrocodone Bitartrate (The comcomitant use of fentanyl with other CNS depressants may cause respiratory depression, hypotension, and profound sedation or potentially result in coma. When such combined therapy is contemplated, the dose of one or both agents should be significantly reduced). Products include:

Lortab 5/500 Tablets 3143
Lortab 7.5/500 Tablets 3144
Lortab 10/500 Tablets 3144
Vicodin Tablets 529
Vicodin ES Tablets 530
Vicodin HP Tablets 531
Vicoprofen Tablets 533
Zydone Tablets 1132

Hydrocodone Polistirex (The comcomitant use of fentanyl with other CNS depressants may cause respiratory depression, hypotension, and profound sedation or potentially result in coma. When such combined therapy is contemplated, the dose of one or both agents should be significantly reduced). Products include:

Tussionex Pennkinetic Extended-Release Suspension 3154

Hydrocortisone (Fentanyl is metabolized mainly via the human cytochrome P450 3A4 isoenzyme system (CYP3A4). Co-administration with agents that induce CYP 3A4 activity may reduce the efficacy of fentanyl).
No products indexed under this heading.

Hydrocortisone Acetate (Fentanyl is metabolized mainly via the human cytochrome P450 3A4 isoenzyme system (CYP3A4). Co-administration with agents that induce CYP 3A4 activity may reduce the efficacy of fentanyl). Products include:

Analpram-HC 1140
Pramosone 1141

Hydrocortisone Butyrate (Fentanyl is metabolized mainly via the human cytochrome P450 3A4 isoenzyme system (CYP3A4). Co-administration with agents that induce CYP 3A4 activity may reduce the efficacy of fentanyl).
No products indexed under this heading.

Hydrocortisone Cypionate (Fentanyl is metabolized mainly via the human cytochrome P450 3A4 isoenzyme system (CYP3A4). Co-administration with agents that induce CYP 3A4 activity may reduce the efficacy of fentanyl).
No products indexed under this heading.

Hydrocortisone Hemisuccinate (Fentanyl is metabolized mainly via the human cytochrome P450 3A4 isoenzyme system (CYP3A4). Co-administration with agents that induce CYP 3A4 activity may reduce the efficacy of fentanyl).
No products indexed under this heading.

Hydrocortisone Probutate (Fentanyl is metabolized mainly via the human cytochrome P450 3A4 isoenzyme system (CYP3A4). Co-administration with agents that induce CYP 3A4 activity may reduce the efficacy of fentanyl).
No products indexed under this heading.

Hydrocortisone Sodium Phosphate (Fentanyl is metabolized mainly via the human cytochrome P450 3A4 isoenzyme system (CYP3A4). Co-administration with agents that induce CYP 3A4 activity may reduce the efficacy of fentanyl).
No products indexed under this heading.

Hydrocortisone Sodium Succinate (Fentanyl is metabolized mainly via the human cytochrome P450 3A4 isoenzyme system (CYP3A4). Co-administration with agents that induce CYP 3A4 activity may reduce the efficacy of fentanyl).
No products indexed under this heading.

Hydrocortisone Valerate (Fentanyl is metabolized mainly via the human cytochrome P450 3A4 isoenzyme system (CYP3A4). Co-administration with agents that induce CYP 3A4 activity may reduce the efficacy of fentanyl).
No products indexed under this heading.

Hydromorphone Hydrochloride (The comcomitant use of fentanyl with other CNS depressants may cause respiratory depression, hypotension, and profound sedation or potentially result in coma. When such combined therapy is contemplated, the dose of one or both agents should be significantly reduced).
No products indexed under this heading.

Hydroxyzine Hydrochloride (The comcomitant use of fentanyl with other CNS depressants may cause respiratory depression, hypotension, and profound sedation or potentially result in coma. When such combined therapy is contemplated, the dose of one or both agents should be significantly reduced).
No products indexed under this heading.

Hypericum (Fentanyl is metabolized mainly via the human cytochrome P450 3A4 isoenzyme system (CYP3A4). Co-administration with agents that induce CYP 3A4 activity may reduce the efficacy of fentanyl). Products include:
Satieté Tablets .... ▣ 640

Hypericum Perforatum (Fentanyl is metabolized mainly via the human cytochrome P450 3A4 isoenzyme system (CYP3A4). Co-administration with agents that induce CYP 3A4 activity may reduce the efficacy of fentanyl).
No products indexed under this heading.

Indinavir Sulfate (The concomitant use of fentanyl with potent cytochrome P450 3A4 inhibitors may result in an increase in fentanyl plasma concentrations, which could increase or prolong adverse drug effects and may cause potentially fatal respiratory depression. Patients receiving fentanyl and potent CYP3A4 inhibitors should be carefully monitored for an extended period of time and dosage adjustments should be made if warranted). Products include:
Crixivan Capsules 1979

Isocarboxazid (Fentanyl is not recommended for use in patients who have received monoamine oxidase (MAO) inhibitors within 14 days because severe and unpredictable potentiation by MAO inhibitors has been reported with opioid analgesics). Products include:
Marplan Tablets 3177

Isoflurane (The comcomitant use of fentanyl with other CNS depressants may cause respiratory depression, hypotension, and profound sedation or potentially result in coma. When such combined therapy is contemplated, the dose of one or both agents should be significantly reduced).
No products indexed under this heading.

Isoniazid (The concomitant use of fentanyl with all CYP3A4 inhibitors (such as ritonavir, ketoconazole, itraconazole, troleandomycin, clarithromycin, nelfinavir, nefazodone, amiodarone, amprenavir, aprepitant, diltiazem, erythromycin, fluconazole, fosamprenavir, grapefruit juice, and verapamil) may result in an increase in fentanyl plasma concentrations, which could increase or prolong adverse drug effects and may cause potentially fatal respiratory depression. Patients receiving fentanyl and any CYP3A4 inhibitor should be monitored for an extended period of time and dosage adjustments should be made if warranted).
No products indexed under this heading.

Itraconazole (The concomitant use of fentanyl with potent cytochrome P450 3A4 inhibitors may result in an increase in fentanyl plasma concentrations, which could increase or prolong adverse drug effects and may cause potentially fatal respiratory depression. Patients receiving fentanyl and potent CYP3A4 inhibitors should be carefully monitored for an extended period of time and dosage adjustments should be made if warranted).
No products indexed under this heading.

Ketamine Hydrochloride (The comcomitant use of fentanyl with other CNS depressants may cause respiratory depression, hypotension, and profound sedation or potentially result in coma. When such combined therapy is contemplated, the dose of one or both agents should be significantly reduced).
No products indexed under this heading.

Ketoconazole (The concomitant use of fentanyl with potent cytochrome P450 3A4 inhibitors may result in an increase in fentanyl plasma concentrations, which could increase or prolong adverse drug effects and may cause potentially fatal respiratory depression. Patients receiving fentanyl and potent CYP3A4 inhibitors should be carefully monitored for an extended period of time and dosage adjustments should be made if warranted). Products include:
Extina Foam, 2% 3057
Nizoral A-D Shampoo 1901

Levomethadyl Acetate Hydrochloride (The comcomitant use of fentanyl with other CNS depressants may cause respiratory depression, hypotension, and profound sedation or potentially result in coma. When such combined therapy is contemplated, the dose of one or both agents should be significantly reduced).
No products indexed under this heading.

Levorphanol Tartrate (The comcomitant use of fentanyl with other CNS depressants may cause respiratory depression, hypotension, and profound sedation or potentially result in coma. When such combined therapy is contemplated, the dose of one or both agents should be significantly reduced).
No products indexed under this heading.

Lopinavir (The concomitant use of fentanyl with potent cytochrome P450 3A4 inhibitors may result in an increase in fentanyl plasma concentrations, which could increase or prolong adverse drug effects and may cause potentially fatal respiratory depression. Patients receiving fentanyl and potent CYP3A4 inhibitors should be carefully monitored for an extended period of time and dosage adjustments should be made if warranted). Products include:
Kaletra 452

Loratadine (The concomitant use of fentanyl with all CYP3A4 inhibitors (such as ritonavir, ketoconazole, itraconazole, troleandomycin, clarithromycin, nelfinavir, nefazodone, amiodarone, amprenavir, aprepitant, diltiazem, erythromycin, fluconazole, fosamprenavir, grapefruit juice, and verapamil) may result in an increase in fentanyl plasma concentrations, which could increase or prolong adverse drug effects and may cause potentially fatal respiratory depression. Patients receiving fentanyl and any CYP3A4 inhibitor should be monitored for an extended period of time and dosage adjustments should be made if warranted).
No products indexed under this heading.

Lorazepam (The comcomitant use of fentanyl with other CNS depressants may cause respiratory depression, hypotension, and profound sedation or potentially result in coma. When such combined therapy is contemplated, the dose of one or both agents should be significantly reduced).
No products indexed under this heading.

Loxapine Hydrochloride (The comcomitant use of fentanyl with other CNS depressants may cause respiratory depression, hypotension, and profound sedation or potentially result in coma. When such combined therapy is contemplated, the dose of one or both agents should be significantly reduced).
No products indexed under this heading.

Loxapine Succinate (The comcomitant use of fentanyl with other CNS depressants may cause respiratory depression, hypotension, and profound sedation or potentially result in coma. When such combined therapy is contemplated, the dose of one or both agents should be significantly reduced).
No products indexed under this heading.

Meperidine Hydrochloride (The comcomitant use of fentanyl with other CNS depressants may cause respiratory depression, hypotension, and profound sedation or potentially result in coma. When such combined therapy is contemplated, the dose of one or both agents should be significantly reduced).
No products indexed under this heading.

Mephenytoin (Fentanyl is metabolized mainly via the human cytochrome P450 3A4 isoenzyme system (CYP3A4). Co-administration with agents that induce CYP 3A4 activity may reduce the efficacy of fentanyl).
No products indexed under this heading.

Mephobarbital (The comcomitant use of fentanyl with other CNS depressants may cause respiratory depression, hypotension, and profound sedation or potentially result in coma. When such combined therapy is contemplated, the dose of one or both agents should be significantly reduced).
No products indexed under this heading.

Meprobamate (The comcomitant use of fentanyl with other CNS depressants may cause respiratory depression, hypotension, and profound sedation or potentially result in coma. When such combined therapy is contemplated, the dose of one or both agents should be significantly reduced).
No products indexed under this heading.

Mesoridazine Besylate (The comcomitant use of fentanyl with other CNS depressants may cause respiratory depression, hypotension, and profound sedation or potentially result in coma. When such combined therapy is contemplated, the dose of one or both agents should be significantly reduced).
No products indexed under this heading.

Metaxalone (The comcomitant use of fentanyl with other CNS depres-

BioLean Free Tablets .... ■635

Nicotinamide (The concomitant use of fentanyl with all CYP3A4 inhibitors (such as ritonavir, ketoconazole, itraconazole, troleandomycin, clarithromycin, nelfinavir, nefazodone, amiodarone, amprenavir, aprepitant, diltiazem, erythromycin, fluconazole, fosamprenavir, grapefruit juice, and verapamil) may result in an increase in fentanyl plasma concentrations, which could increase or prolong adverse drug effects and may cause potentially fatal respiratory depression. Patients receiving fentanyl and any CYP3A4 inhibitor should be monitored for an extended period of time and dosage adjustments should be made if warranted).
No products indexed under this heading.

Nifedipine (The concomitant use of fentanyl with all CYP3A4 inhibitors (such as ritonavir, ketoconazole, itraconazole, troleandomycin, clarithromycin, nelfinavir, nefazodone, amiodarone, amprenavir, aprepitant, diltiazem, erythromycin, fluconazole, fosamprenavir, grapefruit juice, and verapamil) may result in an increase in fentanyl plasma concentrations, which could increase or prolong adverse drug effects and may cause potentially fatal respiratory depression. Patients receiving fentanyl and any CYP3A4 inhibitor should be monitored for an extended period of time and dosage adjustments should be made if warranted).
No products indexed under this heading.

Norfloxacin (The concomitant use of fentanyl with all CYP3A4 inhibitors (such as ritonavir, ketoconazole, itraconazole, troleandomycin, clarithromycin, nelfinavir, nefazodone, amiodarone, amprenavir, aprepitant, diltiazem, erythromycin, fluconazole, fosamprenavir, grapefruit juice, and verapamil) may result in an increase in fentanyl plasma concentrations, which could increase or prolong adverse drug effects and may cause potentially fatal respiratory depression. Patients receiving fentanyl and any CYP3A4 inhibitor should be monitored for an extended period of time and dosage adjustments should be made if warranted). Products include:
Noroxin Tablets 2069

Olanzapine (The comcomitant use of fentanyl with other CNS depressants may cause respiratory depression, hypotension, and profound sedation or potentially result in coma. When such combined therapy is contemplated, the dose of one or both agents should be significantly reduced). Products include:
Symbyax Capsules 1871
Zyprexa Tablets 1883
Zyprexa IntraMuscular 1883
Zyprexa ZYDIS Orally Disintegrating Tablets 1883

Omeprazole (The concomitant use of fentanyl with all CYP3A4 inhibitors (such as ritonavir, ketoconazole, itraconazole, troleandomycin, clarithromycin, nelfinavir, nefazodone, amiodarone, amprenavir, aprepitant, diltiazem, erythromycin, fluconazole, fosamprenavir, grapefruit juice, and verapamil) may result in an increase in fentanyl plasma concentrations, which could increase or prolong adverse drug effects and may cause potentially fatal respiratory depression. Patients receiving fentanyl and any CYP3A4 inhibitor should be monitored for an extended period of time and dosage adjustments should be made if warranted).
No products indexed under this heading.

Orphenadrine Citrate (The concomitant use of fentanyl with other CNS depressants, including skeletal muscle relaxants, may cause respiratory depression, hypotension, and profound sedation or potentially result in coma. When such combined therapy is contemplated, the dose of one or both agents should be significantly reduced).
No products indexed under this heading.

Oxazepam (The comcomitant use of fentanyl with other CNS depressants may cause respiratory depression, hypotension, and profound sedation or potentially result in coma. When such combined therapy is contemplated, the dose of one or both agents should be significantly reduced).
No products indexed under this heading.

Oxcarbazepine (Fentanyl is metabolized mainly via the human cytochrome P450 3A4 isoenzyme system (CYP3A4). Co-administration with agents that induce CYP 3A4 activity may reduce the efficacy of fentanyl).
No products indexed under this heading.

Oxycodone Hydrochloride (The comcomitant use of fentanyl with other CNS depressants may cause respiratory depression, hypotension, and profound sedation or potentially result in coma. When such combined therapy is contemplated, the dose of one or both agents should be significantly reduced). Products include:
OxyContin Tablets 2589
OxyIR Capsules 2593
Percocet Tablets 1127
Percodan Tablets 1130

Pargyline Hydrochloride (Fentanyl is not recommended for use in patients who have received monoamine oxidase (MAO) inhibitors within 14 days because severe and unpredictable potentiation by MAO inhibitors has been reported with opioid analgesics).
No products indexed under this heading.

Paroxetine Hydrochloride (The concomitant use of fentanyl with all CYP3A4 inhibitors (such as ritonavir, ketoconazole, itraconazole, troleandomycin, clarithromycin, nelfinavir, nefazodone, amiodarone, amprenavir, aprepitant, diltiazem, erythromycin, fluconazole, fosamprenavir, grapefruit juice, and verapamil) may result in an increase in fentanyl plasma concentrations, which could increase or prolong adverse drug effects and may cause potentially fatal respiratory depression. Patients receiving fentanyl and any CYP3A4 inhibitor should be monitored for an extended period of time and dosage adjustments should be made if warranted). Products include:
Paxil 1535
Paxil CR Controlled-Release Tablets 1544

Pentobarbital Sodium (The comcomitant use of fentanyl with other CNS depressants may cause respiratory depression, hypotension, and profound sedation or potentially result in coma. When such combined therapy is contemplated, the dose of one or both agents should be significantly reduced). Products include:
Nembutal Sodium Solution, USP 2494

Perphenazine (The comcomitant use of fentanyl with other CNS depressants may cause respiratory depression, hypotension, and profound sedation or potentially result in coma. When such combined therapy is contemplated, the dose of one or both agents should be significantly reduced).
No products indexed under this heading.

Phenelzine Sulfate (Fentanyl is not recommended for use in patients who have received monoamine oxidase (MAO) inhibitors within 14 days because severe and unpredictable potentiation by MAO inhibitors has been reported with opioid analgesics).
No products indexed under this heading.

Phenobarbital (The comcomitant use of fentanyl with other CNS depressants may cause respiratory depression, hypotension, and profound sedation or potentially result in coma. When such combined therapy is contemplated, the dose of one or both agents should be significantly reduced). Products include:
Donnatal Extentabs 2507

Phenobarbital Sodium (Fentanyl is metabolized mainly via the human cytochrome P450 3A4 isoenzyme system (CYP3A4). Co-administration with agents that induce CYP 3A4 activity may reduce the efficacy of fentanyl).
No products indexed under this heading.

Phenytoin (Fentanyl is metabolized mainly via the human cytochrome P450 3A4 isoenzyme system (CYP3A4). Co-administration with agents that induce CYP 3A4 activity may reduce the efficacy of fentanyl).
No products indexed under this heading.

Phenytoin Sodium (Fentanyl is metabolized mainly via the human cytochrome P450 3A4 isoenzyme system (CYP3A4). Co-administration with agents that induce CYP 3A4 activity may reduce the efficacy of fentanyl). Products include:
Phenytek Capsules 2192

Prazepam (The comcomitant use of fentanyl with other CNS depressants may cause respiratory depression, hypotension, and profound sedation or potentially result in coma. When such combined therapy is contemplated, the dose of one or both agents should be significantly reduced).
No products indexed under this heading.

Prednisolone Acetate (Fentanyl is metabolized mainly via the human cytochrome P450 3A4 isoenzyme system (CYP3A4). Co-administration with agents that induce CYP 3A4 activity may reduce the efficacy of fentanyl). Products include:
Pred Forte Ophthalmic Suspension .... ⊙227
Pred Mild Ophthalmic Suspension .... ⊙230
Pred-G Ophthalmic Ointment .... ⊙229
Pred-G Ophthalmic Suspension ...... ⊙228

Prednisolone Sodium Phosphate (Fentanyl is metabolized mainly via the human cytochrome P450 3A4 isoenzyme system (CYP3A4). Co-administration with agents that induce CYP 3A4 activity may reduce the efficacy of fentanyl).
No products indexed under this heading.

Prednisolone Tebutate (Fentanyl is metabolized mainly via the human cytochrome P450 3A4 isoenzyme system (CYP3A4). Co-administration with agents that induce CYP 3A4 activity may reduce the efficacy of fentanyl).
No products indexed under this heading.

Prednisone (Fentanyl is metabolized mainly via the human cytochrome P450 3A4 isoenzyme system (CYP3A4). Co-administration with agents that induce CYP 3A4 activity may reduce the efficacy of fentanyl).
No products indexed under this heading.

Primidone (Fentanyl is metabolized mainly via the human cytochrome P450 3A4 isoenzyme system (CYP3A4). Co-administration with agents that induce CYP 3A4 activity may reduce the efficacy of fentanyl).
No products indexed under this heading.

Procarbazine Hydrochloride (Fentanyl is not recommended for use in patients who have received monoamine oxidase (MAO) inhibitors within 14 days because severe and unpredictable potentiation by MAO inhibitors has been reported with opioid analgesics).
No products indexed under this heading.

Prochlorperazine (The comcomitant use of fentanyl with other CNS depressants may cause respiratory depression, hypotension, and profound sedation or potentially result in coma. When such combined therapy is contemplated, the dose of one or both agents should be significantly reduced).
No products indexed under this heading.

Promethazine Hydrochloride (The comcomitant use of fentanyl with other CNS depressants may cause respiratory depression, hypotension, and profound sedation or potentially result in coma. When such combined therapy is contemplated, the dose of one or both agents should be significantly reduced).
No products indexed under this heading.

Propofol (The comcomitant use of fentanyl with other CNS depressants may cause respiratory depression, hypotension, and profound sedation or potentially result in coma. When such combined therapy is contemplated, the dose of one or both agents should be significantly reduced).
No products indexed under this heading.

cytochrome P450 3A4 inhibitors may result in an increase in fentanyl plasma concentrations, which could increase or prolong adverse drug effects and may cause potentially fatal respiratory depression. Patients receiving fentanyl and potent CYP3A4 inhibitors should be carefully monitored for an extended period of time and dosage adjustments should be made if warranted).
No products indexed under this heading.

Secobarbital Sodium (The concomitant use of fentanyl with other CNS depressants may cause respiratory depression, hypotension, and profound sedation or potentially result in coma. When such combined therapy is contemplated, the dose of one or both agents should be significantly reduced).
No products indexed under this heading.

Selegiline (Fentanyl is not recommended for use in patients who have received monoamine oxidase (MAO) inhibitors within 14 days because severe and unpredictable potentiation by MAO inhibitors has been reported with opioid analgesics). Products include:
Emsam Transdermal System 905

Selegiline Hydrochloride (Fentanyl is not recommended for use in patients who have received monoamine oxidase (MAO) inhibitors within 14 days because severe and unpredictable potentiation by MAO inhibitors has been reported with opioid analgesics). Products include:
Eldepryl Capsules 3052

Sertraline Hydrochloride (The concomitant use of fentanyl with all CYP3A4 inhibitors (such as ritonavir, ketoconazole, itraconazole, troleandomycin, clarithromycin, nelfinavir, nefazodone, amiodarone, amprenavir, aprepitant, diltiazem, erythromycin, fluconazole, fosamprenavir, grapefruit juice, and verapamil) may result in an increase in fentanyl plasma concentrations, which could increase or prolong adverse drug effects and may cause potentially fatal respiratory depression. Patients receiving fentanyl and any CYP3A4 inhibitor should be monitored for an extended period of time and dosage adjustments should be made if warranted).
No products indexed under this heading.

Sevoflurane (The comcomitant use of fentanyl with other CNS depressants may cause respiratory depression, hypotension, and profound sedation or potentially result in coma. When such combined therapy is contemplated, the dose of one or both agents should be significantly reduced). Products include:
Ultane Liquid for Inhalation 524

Sildenafil Citrate (The concomitant use of fentanyl with all CYP3A4 inhibitors (such as ritonavir, ketoconazole, itraconazole, troleandomycin, clarithromycin, nelfinavir, nefazodone, amiodarone, amprenavir, aprepitant, diltiazem, erythromycin, fluconazole, fosamprenavir, grapefruit juice, and verapamil) may result in an increase in fentanyl plasma concentrations, which could increase or prolong adverse drug effects and may cause potentially fatal respiratory depression. Patients receiving fentanyl and any CYP3A4 inhibitor should be monitored for an extended period of time and dosage adjustments should be made if warranted).
No products indexed under this heading.

Sodium Butabarbital (The concomitant use of fentanyl with other CNS depressants, including sedatives and hypnotics, may cause respiratory depression, hypotension, and profound sedation or potentially result in coma. When such combined therapy is contemplated, the dose of oneor both agents should be significantly reduced).
No products indexed under this heading.

Sodium Oxybate (The comcomitant use of fentanyl with other CNS depressants may cause respiratory depression, hypotension, and profound sedation or potentially result in coma. When such combined therapy is contemplated, the dose of one or both agents should be significantly reduced). Products include:
Xyrem Oral Solution 1766

Sufentanil Citrate (The comcomitant use of fentanyl with other CNS depressants may cause respiratory depression, hypotension, and profound sedation or potentially result in coma. When such combined therapy is contemplated, the dose of one or both agents should be significantly reduced).
No products indexed under this heading.

Sulfinpyrazone (Fentanyl is metabolized mainly via the human cytochrome P450 3A4 isoenzyme system (CYP3A4). Co-administration with agents that induce CYP 3A4 activity may reduce the efficacy of fentanyl).
No products indexed under this heading.

Telithromycin (The concomitant use of fentanyl with potent cytochrome P450 3A4 inhibitors may result in an increase in fentanyl plasma concentrations, which could increase or prolong adverse drug effects and may cause potentially fatal respiratory depression. Patients receiving fentanyl and potent CYP3A4 inhibitors should be carefully monitored for an extended period of time and dosage adjustments should be made if warranted). Products include:
Ketek Tablets 2744

Temazepam (The comcomitant use of fentanyl with other CNS depressants may cause respiratory depression, hypotension, and profound sedation or potentially result in coma. When such combined therapy is contemplated, the dose of one or both agents should be significantly reduced).
No products indexed under this heading.

Theophylline (Fentanyl is metabolized mainly via the human cytochrome P450 3A4 isoenzyme system (CYP3A4). Co-administration with agents that induce CYP 3A4 activity may reduce the efficacy of fentanyl).
No products indexed under this heading.

Theophylline Anhydrous (Fentanyl is metabolized mainly via the human cytochrome P450 3A4 isoenzyme system (CYP3A4). Co-administration with agents that induce CYP 3A4 activity may reduce the efficacy of fentanyl). Products include:
Uniphyl Tablets 2595

Theophylline Calcium Salicylate (Fentanyl is metabolized mainly via the human cytochrome P450 3A4 isoenzyme system (CYP3A4). Co-administration with agents that induce CYP 3A4 activity may reduce the efficacy of fentanyl).
No products indexed under this heading.

Theophylline Dihydroxypropyl (Glyceryl) (Fentanyl is metabolized mainly via the human cytochrome P450 3A4 isoenzyme system (CYP3A4). Co-administration with agents that induce CYP 3A4 activity may reduce the efficacy of fentanyl).
No products indexed under this heading.

Theophylline Ethylenediamine (Fentanyl is metabolized mainly via the human cytochrome P450 3A4 isoenzyme system (CYP3A4). Co-administration with agents that induce CYP 3A4 activity may reduce the efficacy of fentanyl).
No products indexed under this heading.

Thiamylal Sodium (The comcomitant use of fentanyl with other CNS depressants may cause respiratory depression, hypotension, and profound sedation or potentially result in coma. When such combined therapy is contemplated, the dose of one or both agents should be significantly reduced).
No products indexed under this heading.

Thioridazine Hydrochloride (The comcomitant use of fentanyl with other CNS depressants may cause respiratory depression, hypotension, and profound sedation or potentially result in coma. When such combined therapy is contemplated, the dose of one or both agents should be significantly reduced). Products include:
Thioridazine Hydrochloride Tablets 2195

Thiothixene (The comcomitant use of fentanyl with other CNS depressants may cause respiratory depression, hypotension, and profound sedation or potentially result in coma. When such combined therapy is contemplated, the dose of one or both agents should be significantly reduced). Products include:
Thiothixene Capsules 2197

Tranylcypromine Sulfate (Fentanyl is not recommended for use in patients who have received monoamine oxidase (MAO) inhibitors within 14 days because severe and unpredictable potentiation by MAO inhibitors has been reported with opioid analgesics). Products include:
Parnate Tablets 1532

Triamcinolone (Fentanyl is metabolized mainly via the human cytochrome P450 3A4 isoenzyme system (CYP3A4). Co-administration with agents that induce CYP 3A4 activity may reduce the efficacy of fentanyl).
No products indexed under this heading.

Triamcinolone Acetonide (Fentanyl is metabolized mainly via the human cytochrome P450 3A4 isoenzyme system (CYP3A4). Co-administration with agents that induce CYP 3A4 activity may reduce the efficacy of fentanyl). Products include:
Azmacort Inhalation Aerosol 407
Nasacort AQ Nasal Spray 2765
Triesence Injectable Suspension .... ⊙209

Triamcinolone Diacetate (Fentanyl is metabolized mainly via the human cytochrome P450 3A4 isoenzyme system (CYP3A4). Co-administration with agents that induce CYP 3A4 activity may reduce the efficacy of fentanyl).
No products indexed under this heading.

Triamcinolone Hexacetonide (Fentanyl is metabolized mainly via the human cytochrome P450 3A4 isoenzyme system (CYP3A4). Co-administration with agents that induce CYP 3A4 activity may reduce the efficacy of fentanyl).
No products indexed under this heading.

Triazolam (The comcomitant use of fentanyl with other CNS depressants may cause respiratory depression, hypotension, and profound sedation or potentially result in coma. When such combined therapy is contemplated, the dose of one or both agents should be significantly reduced).
No products indexed under this heading.

Trifluoperazine Hydrochloride (The comcomitant use of fentanyl with other CNS depressants may cause respiratory depression, hypotension, and profound sedation or potentially result in coma. When such combined therapy is contemplated, the dose of one or both agents should be significantly reduced).
No products indexed under this heading.

Troglitazone (The concomitant use of fentanyl with all CYP3A4 inhibitors (such as ritonavir, ketoconazole, itraconazole, troleandomycin, clarithromycin, nelfinavir, nefazodone, amiodarone, amprenavir, aprepitant, diltiazem, erythromycin, fluconazole, fosamprenavir, grapefruit juice, and verapamil) may result in an increase in fentanyl plasma concentrations, which could increase or prolong adverse drug effects and may cause potentially fatal respiratory depression. Patients receiving fentanyl and any CYP3A4 inhibitor should be monitored for an extended period of time and dosage adjustments should be made if warranted).
No products indexed under this heading.

Troleandomycin (The concomitant use of fentanyl with potent cytochrome P450 3A4 inhibitors may result in an increase in fentanyl plasma concentrations, which could increase or prolong adverse drug effects and may cause potentially fatal respiratory depression. Patients receiving fentanyl and potent CYP3A4 inhibitors should be carefully monitored for an extended period of time and dosage adjustments should be made if warranted).
No products indexed under this heading.

Valproate Sodium (The concomitant use of fentanyl with all CYP3A4 inhibitors (such as ritonavir, ketoconazole, itraconazole, troleandomy-

cin, clarithromycin, nelfinavir, nefazodone, amiodarone, amprenavir, aprepitant, diltiazem, erythromycin, fluconazole, fosamprenavir, grapefruit juice, and verapamil) may result in an increase in fentanyl plasma concentrations, which could increase or prolong adverse drug effects and may cause potentially fatal respiratory depression. Patients receiving fentanyl and any CYP3A4 inhibitor should be monitored for an extended period of time and dosage adjustments should be made if warranted).

No products indexed under this heading.

Vardenafil Hydrochloride (The concomitant use of fentanyl with all CYP3A4 inhibitors (such as ritonavir, ketoconazole, itraconazole, troleandomycin, clarithromycin, nelfinavir, nefazodone, amiodarone, amprenavir, aprepitant, diltiazem, erythromycin, fluconazole, fosamprenavir, grapefruit juice, and verapamil) may result in an increase in fentanyl plasma concentrations, which could increase or prolong adverse drug effects and may cause potentially fatal respiratory depression. Patients receiving fentanyl and any CYP3A4 inhibitor should be monitored for an extended period of time and dosage adjustments should be made if warranted). Products include:

Levitra Tablets 2876

Verapamil Hydrochloride (The concomitant use of fentanyl with all CYP3A4 inhibitors (such as ritonavir, ketoconazole, itraconazole, troleandomycin, clarithromycin, nelfinavir, nefazodone, amiodarone, amprenavir, aprepitant, diltiazem, erythromycin, fluconazole, fosamprenavir, grapefruit juice, and verapamil) may result in an increase in fentanyl plasma concentrations, which could increase or prolong adverse drug effects and may cause potentially fatal respiratory depression. Patients receiving fentanyl and any CYP3A4 inhibitor should be monitored for an extended period of time and dosage adjustments should be made if warranted). Products include:

Tarka Tablets 511

Voriconazole (The concomitant use of fentanyl with potent cytochrome P450 3A4 inhibitors may result in an increase in fentanyl plasma concentrations, which could increase or prolong adverse drug effects and may cause potentially fatal respiratory depression. Patients receiving fentanyl and potent CYP3A4 inhibitors should be carefully monitored for an extended period of time and dosage adjustments should be made if warranted).

No products indexed under this heading.

Zafirlukast (The concomitant use of fentanyl with all CYP3A4 inhibitors (such as ritonavir, ketoconazole, itraconazole, troleandomycin, clarithromycin, nelfinavir, nefazodone, amiodarone, amprenavir, aprepitant, diltiazem, erythromycin, fluconazole, fosamprenavir, grapefruit juice, and verapamil) may result in an increase in fentanyl plasma concentrations, which could increase or prolong adverse drug effects and may cause potentially fatal respiratory depression. Patients receiving fentanyl and any CYP3A4 inhibitor should be monitored for an extended period of time and dosage adjustments should be made if warranted). Products include:

Accolate Tablets 669

Zaleplon (The comcomitant use of fentanyl with other CNS depressants may cause respiratory depression, hypotension, and profound sedation or potentially result in coma. When such combined therapy is contemplated, the dose of one or both agents should be significantly reduced).

No products indexed under this heading.

Zileuton (The concomitant use of fentanyl with all CYP3A4 inhibitors (such as ritonavir, ketoconazole, itraconazole, troleandomycin, clarithromycin, nelfinavir, nefazodone, amiodarone, amprenavir, aprepitant, diltiazem, erythromycin, fluconazole, fosamprenavir, grapefruit juice, and verapamil) may result in an increase in fentanyl plasma concentrations, which could increase or prolong adverse drug effects and may cause potentially fatal respiratory depression. Patients receiving fentanyl and any CYP3A4 inhibitor should be monitored for an extended period of time and dosage adjustments should be made if warranted).

No products indexed under this heading.

Ziprasidone Hydrochloride (The comcomitant use of fentanyl with other CNS depressants may cause respiratory depression, hypotension, and profound sedation or potentially result in coma. When such combined therapy is contemplated, the dose of one or both agents should be significantly reduced). Products include:

Geodon Capsules 2520

Zolpidem Tartrate (The comcomitant use of fentanyl with other CNS depressants may cause respiratory depression, hypotension, and profound sedation or potentially result in coma. When such combined therapy is contemplated, the dose of one or both agents should be significantly reduced). Products include:

Ambien Tablets 2692
Ambien CR Tablets 2696

Food Interactions

Alcohol (The concomitant use of fentanyl with other CNS depressants, including alcohol, may cause respiratory depression, hypotension, and profound sedation or potentially result in coma. When such combined therapy is contemplated, the dose of one or both agents should be significantly reduced).

Grapefruit (The concomitant use of fentanyl with all CYP3A4 inhibitors (such as ritonavir, ketoconazole, itraconazole, troleandomycin, clarithromycin, nelfinavir, nefazodone, amiodarone, amprenavir, aprepitant, diltiazem, erythromycin, fluconazole, fosamprenavir, grapefruit juice, and verapamil) may result in an increase in fentanyl plasma concentrations, which could increase or prolong adverse drug effects and may cause potentially fatal respiratory depression. Patients receiving fentanyl and any CYP3A4 inhibitor should be monitored for an extended period of time and dosage adjustments should be made if warranted).

Grapefruit Juice (The concomitant use of fentanyl with all CYP3A4 inhibitors (such as ritonavir, ketoconazole, itraconazole, troleandomycin, clarithromycin, nelfinavir, nefazodone, amiodarone, amprenavir, aprepitant, diltiazem, erythromycin, fluconazole, fosamprenavir, grapefruit juice, and verapamil) may result in an increase in fentanyl plasma concentrations, which could increase or prolong adverse drug effects and may cause potentially fatal respiratory depression. Patients receiving fentanyl and any CYP3A4 inhibitor should be monitored for an extended period of time and dosage adjustments should be made if warranted).

DUREZOL OPHTHALMIC EMULSION

(Difluprednate) .... ⊙275

May interact with corticosteroids. Compounds in these categories include:

Betamethasone Acetate (Corticosteroid use may result in glaucoma with damage to the optic nerve, defects in visual acuity and fields of vision, and in posterior subcapsular cataract formation. Steroids should be used with caution in the presence of glaucoma and thus increase the hazard of secondary ocular infections. Employment of a corticosteroid medication in the treatment of patients with a history of herpes simplex requires great caution. The use of steroids after cataract surgery may delay healing and increase the incidence of bleb formation).

No products indexed under this heading.

Betamethasone Sodium Phosphate (Corticosteroid use may result in glaucoma with damage to the optic nerve, defects in visual acuity and fields of vision, and in posterior subcapsular cataract formation. Steroids should be used with caution in the presence of glaucoma and thus increase the hazard of secondary ocular infections. Employment of a corticosteroid medication in the treatment of patients with a history of herpes simplex requires great caution. The use of steroids after cataract surgery may delay healing and increase the incidence of bleb formation).

No products indexed under this heading.

Budesonide (Corticosteroid use may result in glaucoma with damage to the optic nerve, defects in visual acuity and fields of vision, and in posterior subcapsular cataract formation. Steroids should be used with caution in the presence of glaucoma and thus increase the hazard of secondary ocular infections. Employment of a corticosteroid medication in the treatment of patients with a history of herpes simplex requires great caution. The use of steroids after cataract surgery may delay healing and increase the incidence of bleb formation). Products include:

Pulmicort Flexhaler 654
Symbicort 80/4.5 Inhalation Aerosol 659
Symbicort 160/4.5 Inhalation Aerosol 659

Ciclesonide (Corticosteroid use may result in glaucoma with damage to the optic nerve, defects in visual acuity and fields of vision, and in posterior subcapsular cataract formation. Steroids should be used with caution in the presence of glaucoma and thus increase the hazard of secondary ocular infections. Employment of a corticosteroid medication in the treatment of patients with a history of herpes simplex requires great caution. The use of steroids after cataract surgery may delay healing and increase the incidence of bleb formation). Products include:

Alvesco Inhalation Aerosol 2985
Omnaris Nasal Spray 2998

Cortisone Acetate (Corticosteroid use may result in glaucoma with damage to the optic nerve, defects in visual acuity and fields of vision, and in posterior subcapsular cataract formation. Steroids should be used with caution in the presence of glaucoma and thus increase the hazard of secondary ocular infections. Employment of a corticosteroid medication in the treatment of patients with a history of herpes simplex requires great caution. The use of steroids after cataract surgery may delay healing and increase the incidence of bleb formation).

No products indexed under this heading.

Dexamethasone (Corticosteroid use may result in glaucoma with damage to the optic nerve, defects in visual acuity and fields of vision, and in posterior subcapsular cataract formation. Steroids should be used with caution in the presence of glaucoma and thus increase the hazard of secondary ocular infections. Employment of a corticosteroid medication in the treatment of patients with a history of herpes simplex requires great caution. The use of steroids after cataract surgery may delay healing and increase the incidence of bleb formation). Products include:

Ciprodex Otic Suspension 541

Dexamethasone Acetate (Corticosteroid use may result in glaucoma with damage to the optic nerve, defects in visual acuity and fields of vision, and in posterior subcapsular cataract formation. Steroids should be used with caution in the presence of glaucoma and thus increase the hazard of secondary ocular infections. Employment of a corticosteroid medication in the treatment of patients with a history of herpes simplex requires great caution. The use of steroids after cataract surgery may delay healing and increase the incidence of bleb formation).

No products indexed under this heading.

Dexamethasone Sodium Phosphate (Corticosteroid use may result in glaucoma with damage to the optic nerve, defects in visual acuity and fields of vision, and in posterior subcapsular cataract formation. Steroids should be used with caution in the presence of glaucoma and thus increase the hazard of secondary ocular infections. Employment of a corticosteroid medication in the treatment of patients with a history of herpes simplex requires great caution. The use of steroids after cataract surgery may delay healing and increase the incidence of bleb formation).

No products indexed under this heading.

Fludrocortisone Acetate (Corticosteroid use may result in glaucoma with damage to the optic nerve, defects in visual acuity and fields of vision, and in posterior subcapsular cataract formation. Steroids should be used with caution in the presence of glaucoma and thus increase the hazard of secondary ocular infections. Employment of a corticosteroid medication in the treatment of patients with a history of herpes simplex requires great caution. The use of steroids after cataract surgery may delay healing and increase the incidence of bleb formation).

No products indexed under this heading.

Flunisolide (Corticosteroid use may result in glaucoma with damage to the optic nerve, defects in visual acuity and fields of vision, and in posterior subcapsular cataract formation. Steroids should be used with caution in the presence of glaucoma and thus increase the hazard of secondary ocular infections. Employment of a corticosteroid medication in the treatment of patients with a history of herpes simplex requires great caution. The use of steroids after cataract surgery may delay healing and increase the incidence of bleb formation). Products include:

Aerobid/Aerobid-M **1153**

Fluticasone Propionate (Corticosteroid use may result in glaucoma with damage to the optic nerve, defects in visual acuity and fields of vision, and in posterior subcapsular cataract formation. Steroids should be used with caution in the presence of glaucoma and thus increase the hazard of secondary ocular infections. Employment of a corticosteroid medication in the treatment of patients with a history of herpes simplex requires great caution. The use of steroids after cataract surgery may delay healing and increase the incidence of bleb formation).
Products include:

Advair Diskus 100/50 .... **1276**
Advair Diskus 250/50 .... **1276**
Advair Diskus 500/50 .... **1276**
Advair HFA 45/21 Inhalation Aerosol **1288**
Advair HFA 115/21 Inhalation Aerosol **1288**
Advair HFA 230/21 Inhalation Aerosol **1288**
Flonase Nasal Spray **1431**
Flovent Diskus 50 mcg **1435**

Fluticasone Propionate HFA (Corticosteroid use may result in glaucoma with damage to the optic nerve, defects in visual acuity and fields of vision, and in posterior subcapsular cataract formation. Steroids should be used with caution in the presence of glaucoma and thus increase the hazard of secondary ocular infections. Employment of a corticosteroid medication in the treatment of patients with a history of herpes simplex requires great caution. The use of steroids after cataract surgery may delay healing and increase the incidence of bleb formation).
Products include:

Flovent HFA **1440**

Hydrocortisone (Corticosteroid use may result in glaucoma with damage to the optic nerve, defects in visual acuity and fields of vision, and in posterior subcapsular cataract formation. Steroids should be used with caution in the presence of glaucoma and thus increase the hazard of secondary ocular infections. Employment of a corticosteroid medication in the treatment of patients with a history of herpes simplex requires great caution. The use of steroids after cataract surgery may delay healing and increase the incidence of bleb formation).

No products indexed under this heading.

Hydrocortisone Acetate (Corticosteroid use may result in glaucoma with damage to the optic nerve, defects in visual acuity and fields of vision, and in posterior subcapsular cataract formation. Steroids should be used with caution in the presence of glaucoma and thus increase the hazard of secondary ocular infections. Employment of a corticosteroid medication in the treatment of patients with a history of herpes simplex requires great caution. The use of steroids after cataract surgery may delay healing and increase the incidence of bleb formation).
Products include:

Analpram-HC **1140**
Pramosone **1141**

Hydrocortisone Sodium Phosphate (Corticosteroid use may result in glaucoma with damage to the optic nerve, defects in visual acuity and fields of vision, and in posterior subcapsular cataract formation. Steroids should be used with caution in the presence of glaucoma and thus increase the hazard of secondary ocular infections. Employment of a corticosteroid medication in the treatment of patients with a history of herpes simplex requires great caution. The use of steroids after cataract surgery may delay healing and increase the incidence of bleb formation).

No products indexed under this heading.

Hydrocortisone Sodium Succinate (Corticosteroid use may result in glaucoma with damage to the optic nerve, defects in visual acuity and fields of vision, and in posterior subcapsular cataract formation. Steroids should be used with caution in the presence of glaucoma and thus increase the hazard of secondary ocular infections. Employment of a corticosteroid medication in the treatment of patients with a history of herpes simplex requires great caution. The use of steroids after cataract surgery may delay healing and increase the incidence of bleb formation).

No products indexed under this heading.

Methylprednisolone Acetate (Corticosteroid use may result in glaucoma with damage to the optic nerve, defects in visual acuity and fields of vision, and in posterior subcapsular cataract formation. Steroids should be used with caution in the presence of glaucoma and thus increase the hazard of secondary ocular infections. Employment of a corticosteroid medication in the treatment of patients with a history of herpes simplex requires great caution. The use of steroids after cataract surgery may delay healing and increase the incidence of bleb formation).

No products indexed under this heading.

Methylprednisolone Sodium Succinate (Corticosteroid use may result in glaucoma with damage to the optic nerve, defects in visual acuity and fields of vision, and in posterior subcapsular cataract formation. Steroids should be used with caution in the presence of glaucoma and thus increase the hazard of secondary ocular infections. Employment of a corticosteroid medication in the treatment of patients with a history of herpes simplex requires great caution. The use of steroids after cataract surgery may delay healing and increase the incidence of bleb formation).

No products indexed under this heading.

Mometasone Furoate (Corticosteroid use may result in glaucoma with damage to the optic nerve, defects in visual acuity and fields of vision, and in posterior subcapsular cataract formation. Steroids should be used with caution in the presence of glaucoma and thus increase the hazard of secondary ocular infections. Employment of a corticosteroid medication in the treatment of patients with a history of herpes simplex requires great caution. The use of steroids after cataract surgery may delay healing and increase the incidence of bleb formation).
Products include:

Asmanex Twisthaler **2797**
Elocon Cream 0.1% **2840**
Elocon Lotion 0.1% **2841**
Elocon Ointment 0.1% **2842**

Mometasone Furoate Monohydrate (Corticosteroid use may result in glaucoma with damage to the optic nerve, defects in visual acuity and fields of vision, and in posterior subcapsular cataract formation. Steroids should be used with caution in the presence of glaucoma and thus increase the hazard of secondary ocular infections. Employment of a corticosteroid medication in the treatment of patients with a history of herpes simplex requires great caution. The use of steroids after cataract surgery may delay healing and increase the incidence of bleb formation). Products include:

Nasonex Nasal Spray **2883**

Prednisolone Acetate (Corticosteroid use may result in glaucoma with damage to the optic nerve, defects in visual acuity and fields of vision, and in posterior subcapsular cataract formation. Steroids should be used with caution in the presence of glaucoma and thus increase the hazard of secondary ocular infections. Employment of a corticosteroid medication in the treatment of patients with a history of herpes simplex requires great caution. The use of steroids after cataract surgery may delay healing and increase the incidence of bleb formation).
Products include:

Pred Forte Ophthalmic Suspension .... ⊙ **227**
Pred Mild Ophthalmic Suspension .... ⊙ **230**
Pred-G Ophthalmic Ointment .... ⊙ **229**
Pred-G Ophthalmic Suspension .... ⊙ **228**

Prednisolone Sodium Phosphate (Corticosteroid use may result in glaucoma with damage to the optic nerve, defects in visual acuity and fields of vision, and in posterior subcapsular cataract formation. Steroids should be used with caution in the presence of glaucoma and thus increase the hazard of secondary ocular infections. Employment of a corticosteroid medication in the treatment of patients with a history of herpes simplex requires great caution. The use of steroids after cataract surgery may delay healing and increase the incidence of bleb formation).

No products indexed under this heading.

Prednisolone Tebutate (Corticosteroid use may result in glaucoma with damage to the optic nerve, defects in visual acuity and fields of vision, and in posterior subcapsular cataract formation. Steroids should be used with caution in the presence of glaucoma and thus increase the hazard of secondary ocular infections. Employment of a corticosteroid medication in the treatment of patients with a history of herpes simplex requires great caution. The use of steroids after cataract surgery may delay healing and increase the incidence of bleb formation).

No products indexed under this heading.

Prednisone (Corticosteroid use may result in glaucoma with damage to the optic nerve, defects in visual acuity and fields of vision, and in posterior subcapsular cataract formation. Steroids should be used with caution in the presence of glaucoma and thus increase the hazard of secondary ocular infections. Employment of a corticosteroid medication in the treatment of patients with a history of herpes simplex requires great caution. The use of steroids after cataract surgery may delay healing and increase the incidence of bleb formation).

No products indexed under this heading.

Triamcinolone (Corticosteroid use may result in glaucoma with damage to the optic nerve, defects in visual acuity and fields of vision, and in posterior subcapsular cataract formation. Steroids should be used with caution in the presence of glaucoma and thus increase the hazard of secondary ocular infections. Employment of a corticosteroid medication in the treatment of patients with a history of herpes simplex requires great caution. The use of steroids after cataract surgery may delay healing and increase the incidence of bleb formation).

No products indexed under this heading.

Triamcinolone Acetonide (Corticosteroid use may result in glaucoma with damage to the optic nerve, defects in visual acuity and fields of vision, and in posterior subcapsular cataract formation. Steroids should be used with caution in the presence of glaucoma and thus increase the hazard of secondary ocular infections. Employment of a corticosteroid medication in the treatment of patients with a history of herpes simplex requires great caution. The use of steroids after cataract surgery may delay healing and increase the incidence of bleb formation).
Products include:

Azmacort Inhalation Aerosol **407**
Nasacort AQ Nasal Spray **2765**
Triesence Injectable Suspension .... ⊙ **209**

Triamcinolone Diacetate (Corticosteroid use may result in glaucoma with damage to the optic nerve, defects in visual acuity and fields of vision, and in posterior subcapsular cataract formation. Steroids should be used with caution in the presence of glaucoma and thus increase the

hazard of secondary ocular infections. Employment of a corticosteroid medication in the treatment of patients with a history of herpes simplex requires great caution. The use of steroids after cataract surgery may delay healing and increase the incidence of bleb formation).
No products indexed under this heading.

Triamcinolone Hexacetonide (Corticosteroid use may result in glaucoma with damage to the optic nerve, defects in visual acuity and fields of vision, and in posterior subcapsular cataract formation. Steroids should be used with caution in the presence of glaucoma and thus increase the hazard of secondary ocular infections. Employment of a corticosteroid medication in the treatment of patients with a history of herpes simplex requires great caution. The use of steroids after cataract surgery may delay healing and increase the incidence of bleb formation).
No products indexed under this heading.

DYAZIDE CAPSULES

(Hydrochlorothiazide, Triamterene) **1405**
May interact with ACE inhibitors, antihypertensives, corticosteroids, oral anticoagulants, antigout agents, oral hypoglycemic agents, insulin, lithium preparations, nondepolarizing neuromuscular blocking agents, nonsteroidal anti-inflammatory agents, potassium preparations, potassium sparing diuretics, and certain other agents. Compounds in these categories include:

Acarbose (Increased risk of severe hyponatremia). Products include:
Precose Tablets **792**

Acebutolol Hydrochloride (May add to potentiate the action of other hypertensives).
No products indexed under this heading.

ACTH (May intensify electrolyte imbalance, particularly hypokalemia).
No products indexed under this heading.

Aliskiren (May add to potentiate the action of other hypertensives). Products include:
Tekturna Tablets **2321**
Tekturna HCT Tablets **2324**

Allopurinol (Dyazide may raise the level of blood uric acid; may require dosage adjustment of antigout agent).
No products indexed under this heading.

Amiloride Hydrochloride (Concurrent use is contraindicated).
No products indexed under this heading.

Amlodipine Besylate (May add to potentiate the action of other hypertensives). Products include:
Azor Tablets **1005**
Exforge Tablets **2238**

Amphotericin B (May intensify electrolyte imbalance, particularly hypokalemia).
No products indexed under this heading.

Anisindione (Effects of oral anticoagulants may be decreased).
No products indexed under this heading.

Atenolol (May add to potentiate the action of other hypertensives).
No products indexed under this heading.

Atracurium Besylate (Increased paralyzing effect).
No products indexed under this heading.

Benazepril Hydrochloride (May add to potentiate the action of other hypertensives; increased risk of hyperkalemia).
No products indexed under this heading.

Bendroflumethiazide (May add to potentiate the action of other hypertensives).
No products indexed under this heading.

Betamethasone Acetate (May intensify electrolyte imbalance, particularly hypokalemia).
No products indexed under this heading.

Betamethasone Sodium Phosphate (May intensify electrolyte imbalance, particularly hypokalemia).
No products indexed under this heading.

Betaxolol Hydrochloride (May add to potentiate the action of other hypertensives).
No products indexed under this heading.

Bisoprolol Fumarate (May add to potentiate the action of other hypertensives).
No products indexed under this heading.

Blood, whole (Concurrent use of whole blood from blood bank with triamterene may result in hyperkalemia, especially in patients with renal insufficiency).
No products indexed under this heading.

Budesonide (May intensify electrolyte imbalance, particularly hypokalemia). Products include:
Pulmicort Flexhaler **654**
Symbicort 80/4.5 Inhalation Aerosol.. **659**
Symbicort 160/4.5 Inhalation Aerosol.. **659**

Candesartan Cilexetil (May add to potentiate the action of other hypertensives). Products include:
Atacand Tablets **639**
Atacand HCT **642**

Captopril (May add to potentiate the action of other hypertensives; increased risk of hyperkalemia). Products include:
Captopril Tablets **2182**

Carteolol Hydrochloride (May add to potentiate the action of other hypertensives).
No products indexed under this heading.

Celecoxib (Potential for acute renal failure). Products include:
Celebrex Capsules **2979**

Chlorothiazide (May add to potentiate the action of other hypertensives).
No products indexed under this heading.

Chlorothiazide Sodium (May add to potentiate the action of other hypertensives). Products include:
Intravenous Sodium Diuril **2490**

Chlorpropamide (Increased risk of severe hyponatremia).
No products indexed under this heading.

Chlorthalidone (May add to potentiate the action of other hypertensives). Products include:
Clorpres Tablets **2185**

Ciclesonide (May intensify electrolyte imbalance, particularly hypokalemia). Products include:
Alvesco Inhalation Aerosol **2985**
Omnaris Nasal Spray **2998**

Cisatracurium Besylate (Increased paralyzing effect). Products include:
Nimbex Injection **484**

Clonidine (May add to potentiate the action of other hypertensives). Products include:
Catapres-TTS **842**

Clonidine Hydrochloride (May add to potentiate the action of other hypertensives). Products include:
Catapres Tablets **841**
Clorpres Tablets **2185**

Cortisone Acetate (May intensify electrolyte imbalance, particularly hypokalemia).
No products indexed under this heading.

Deserpidine (May add to potentiate the action of other hypertensives).
No products indexed under this heading.

Dexamethasone (May intensify electrolyte imbalance, particularly hypokalemia). Products include:
Ciprodex Otic Suspension **541**

Dexamethasone Acetate (May intensify electrolyte imbalance, particularly hypokalemia).
No products indexed under this heading.

Dexamethasone Sodium Phosphate (May intensify electrolyte imbalance, particularly hypokalemia).
No products indexed under this heading.

Diazoxide (May add to potentiate the action of other hypertensives). Products include:
Proglycem Capsules **1185**
Proglycem Suspension **1185**

Diclofenac Epolamine (Potential for acute renal failure). Products include:
Flector Patch **561**

Diclofenac Potassium (Potential for acute renal failure).
No products indexed under this heading.

Diclofenac Sodium (Potential for acute renal failure). Products include:
Diclofenac Sodium Ophthalmic Solution.. ⊙**240**
Voltaren Ophthalmic Solution **2336**
Voltaren Tablets **2334**
Voltaren-XR Tablets **2337**

Dicumarol (Effects of oral anticoagulants may be decreased).
No products indexed under this heading.

Diltiazem Hydrochloride (May add to potentiate the action of other hypertensives). Products include:
Cardizem LA Extended Release Tablets **421**

Doxazosin Mesylate (May add to potentiate the action of other hypertensives).
No products indexed under this heading.

Enalapril Maleate (May add to potentiate the action of other hypertensives; increased risk of hyperkalemia).
No products indexed under this heading.

Enalaprilat (May add to potentiate the action of other hypertensives; increased risk of hyperkalemia).
No products indexed under this heading.

Eprosartan Mesylate (May add to potentiate the action of other hypertensives). Products include:
Teveten Tablets **515**
Teveten HCT Tablets **517**

Esmolol Hydrochloride (May add to potentiate the action of other hypertensives).
No products indexed under this heading.

Etodolac (Potential for acute renal failure).
No products indexed under this heading.

Felodipine (May add to potentiate the action of other hypertensives).
No products indexed under this heading.

Fenoprofen Calcium (Potential for acute renal failure). Products include:
Nalfon Capsules **2508**

Fludrocortisone Acetate (May intensify electrolyte imbalance, particularly hypokalemia).
No products indexed under this heading.

Flunisolide (May intensify electrolyte imbalance, particularly hypokalemia). Products include:
Aerobid/Aerobid-M **1153**

Flurbiprofen (Potential for acute renal failure).
No products indexed under this heading.

Fluticasone Propionate (May intensify electrolyte imbalance, particularly hypokalemia). Products include:
Advair Diskus 100/50 .... **1276**
Advair Diskus 250/50 .... **1276**
Advair Diskus 500/50 .... **1276**
Advair HFA 45/21 Inhalation Aerosol.. **1288**
Advair HFA 115/21 Inhalation Aerosol.. **1288**
Advair HFA 230/21 Inhalation Aerosol.. **1288**
Flonase Nasal Spray **1431**
Flovent Diskus 50 mcg **1435**

Fluticasone Propionate HFA (May intensify electrolyte imbalance, particularly hypokalemia). Products include:
Flovent HFA **1440**

Fosinopril Sodium (May add to potentiate the action of other hypertensives; increased risk of hyperkalemia).
No products indexed under this heading.

Furosemide (May add to potentiate the action of other hypertensives). Products include:
Furosemide Tablets **2186**

Glimepiride (Thiazides may cause hyperglycemia and glycosuria; dosage alteration of oral antidiabetic agents may be required). Products include:
Avandaryl Tablets **1344**
Duetact Tablets **3085**

Glipizide (Thiazides may cause hyperglycemia and glycosuria; dosage alteration of oral antidiabetic agents may be required).
No products indexed under this heading.

Glyburide (Thiazides may cause hyperglycemia and glycosuria; dosage alteration of oral antidiabetic agents may be required).
No products indexed under this heading.

IMPORTANT NOTE: Always consult each drug listing in the patient's regimen for possible interactions.

Guanabenz Acetate (May add to potentiate the action of other hypertensives).
No products indexed under this heading.

Guanethidine Monosulfate (May add to potentiate the action of other hypertensives).
No products indexed under this heading.

Hydralazine Hydrochloride (May add to potentiate the action of other hypertensives).
No products indexed under this heading.

Hydrocortisone (May intensify electrolyte imbalance, particularly hypokalemia).
No products indexed under this heading.

Hydrocortisone Acetate (May intensify electrolyte imbalance, particularly hypokalemia). Products include:
Analpram-HC 1140
Pramosone 1141

Hydrocortisone Sodium Phosphate (May intensify electrolyte imbalance, particularly hypokalemia).
No products indexed under this heading.

Hydrocortisone Sodium Succinate (May intensify electrolyte imbalance, particularly hypokalemia).
No products indexed under this heading.

Hydroflumethiazide (May add to potentiate the action of other hypertensives).
No products indexed under this heading.

Ibuprofen (Potential for acute renal failure). Products include:
Motrin IB Tablets and Caplets 1900
Children's Motrin Oral Suspension ... 1901
Children's Motrin Non-Staining Dye-Free Oral Suspension 1901
Children's Motrin Cold Oral Suspension 1899
Infants' Motrin Concentrated Drops 1901
Infants' Motrin Non-Staining Dye-Free Concentrated Drops 1901
Junior Strength Motrin Caplets and Chewable Tablets 1901
Vicoprofen Tablets 533

Indapamide (May add to potentiate the action of other hypertensives). Products include:
Indapamide Tablets 2188

Indomethacin (Potential for acute renal failure). Products include:
Indocin 2024

Indomethacin Sodium Trihydrate (Potential for acute renal failure). Products include:
Indocin I.V. 2489

Insulin (Thiazides may cause hyperglycemia, glycosuria and alter insulin requirements in diabetes; diabetes mellitus may become manifest during thiazide administration).
No products indexed under this heading.

Insulin, Human, Zinc Suspension (Thiazides may cause hyperglycemia, glycosuria and alter insulin requirements in diabetes; diabetes mellitus may become manifest during thiazide administration).
No products indexed under this heading.

Insulin, Human (rDNA origin) (Thiazides may cause hyperglycemia, glycosuria and alter insulin requirements in diabetes; diabetes mellitus may become manifest during thiazide administration). Products include:
Exubera Inhalation Powder 2515

Insulin, Human NPH (Thiazides may cause hyperglycemia, glycosuria and alter insulin requirements in diabetes; diabetes mellitus may become manifest during thiazide administration). Products include:
Humulin N Vial 1846

Insulin, Human Regular (Thiazides may cause hyperglycemia, glycosuria and alter insulin requirements in diabetes; diabetes mellitus may become manifest during thiazide administration). Products include:
Humulin R 1849
Humulin R (U-500) 1850

Insulin, Human Regular and Human NPH Mixture (Thiazides may cause hyperglycemia, glycosuria and alter insulin requirements in diabetes; diabetes mellitus may become manifest during thiazide administration). Products include:
Humulin 50/50, 100 Units 1843
Humulin 70/30 Vial 1844

Insulin, NPH (Thiazides may cause hyperglycemia, glycosuria and alter insulin requirements in diabetes; diabetes mellitus may become manifest during thiazide administration).
No products indexed under this heading.

Insulin, Regular (Thiazides may cause hyperglycemia, glycosuria and alter insulin requirements in diabetes; diabetes mellitus may become manifest during thiazide administration).
No products indexed under this heading.

Insulin, Regular and NPH mixture (Thiazides may cause hyperglycemia, glycosuria and alter insulin requirements in diabetes; diabetes mellitus may become manifest during thiazide administration).
No products indexed under this heading.

Insulin, Zinc Crystals (Thiazides may cause hyperglycemia, glycosuria and alter insulin requirements in diabetes; diabetes mellitus may become manifest during thiazide administration).
No products indexed under this heading.

Insulin, Zinc Suspension (Thiazides may cause hyperglycemia, glycosuria and alter insulin requirements in diabetes; diabetes mellitus may become manifest during thiazide administration).
No products indexed under this heading.

Insulin Aspart (Thiazides may cause hyperglycemia, glycosuria and alter insulin requirements in diabetes; diabetes mellitus may become manifest during thiazide administration).
No products indexed under this heading.

Insulin Aspart, Human (Thiazides may cause hyperglycemia, glycosuria and alter insulin requirements in diabetes; diabetes mellitus may become manifest during thiazide administration). Products include:
NovoLog Mix 70/30 2364

Insulin Aspart, Human Regular (Thiazides may cause hyperglycemia, glycosuria and alter insulin requirements in diabetes; diabetes mellitus may become manifest during thiazide administration). Products include:
NovoLog Injection 2359

Insulin Aspart Protamine, Human (Thiazides may cause hyperglycemia, glycosuria and alter insulin requirements in diabetes; diabetes mellitus may become manifest during thiazide administration). Products include:
NovoLog Mix 70/30 2364

Insulin Detemir (rDNA Origin) (Thiazides may cause hyperglycemia, glycosuria and alter insulin requirements in diabetes; diabetes mellitus may become manifest during thiazide administration). Products include:
Levemir Injection 2352

Insulin glargine (Thiazides may cause hyperglycemia, glycosuria and alter insulin requirements in diabetes; diabetes mellitus may become manifest during thiazide administration). Products include:
Lantus Injection 2749

Insulin Glulisine (Thiazides may cause hyperglycemia, glycosuria and alter insulin requirements in diabetes; diabetes mellitus may become manifest during thiazide administration). Products include:
Apidra Injection 2706

Insulin Lispro, Human (Thiazides may cause hyperglycemia, glycosuria and alter insulin requirements in diabetes; diabetes mellitus may become manifest during thiazide administration). Products include:
Humalog-Pen and KwikPen 1829
Humalog Mix 50/50-Pen and KwikPen 1833
Humalog Mix 75/25-Pen and KwikPen 1835

Insulin Lispro Protamine, Human (Thiazides may cause hyperglycemia, glycosuria and alter insulin requirements in diabetes; diabetes mellitus may become manifest during thiazide administration). Products include:
Humalog Mix 50/50-Pen and KwikPen 1833
Humalog Mix 75/25-Pen and KwikPen 1835

Irbesartan (May add to potentiate the action of other hypertensives). Products include:
Avalide Tablets 892
Avalide Tablets 2713
Avapro Tablets 897
Avapro Tablets 2718

Isradipine (May add to potentiate the action of other hypertensives). Products include:
DynaCirc CR Controlled Release Tablets 1407

Ketoprofen (Potential for acute renal failure).
No products indexed under this heading.

Ketorolac Tromethamine (Potential for acute renal failure).
No products indexed under this heading.

Labetalol Hydrochloride (May add to potentiate the action of other hypertensives).
No products indexed under this heading.

Laxatives, unspecified (Interferes with the potassium-retaining effects of triamterene; chronic or overuse of laxatives may reduce serum potassium).
No products indexed under this heading.

Lisinopril (May add to potentiate the action of other hypertensives; increased risk of hyperkalemia). Products include:
Prinivil Tablets 2087
Prinzide Tablets 2092

Lithium (Reduced renal clearance and increased risk of lithium toxicity).
No products indexed under this heading.

Lithium Carbonate (Reduced renal clearance and increased risk of lithium toxicity).
No products indexed under this heading.

Lithium Citrate (Reduced renal clearance and increased risk of lithium toxicity).
No products indexed under this heading.

Losartan Potassium (May add to potentiate the action of other hypertensives). Products include:
Cozaar Tablets 1973

Mecamylamine Hydrochloride (May add to potentiate the action of other hypertensives).
No products indexed under this heading.

Meclofenamate Sodium (Potential for acute renal failure).
No products indexed under this heading.

Mefenamic Acid (Potential for acute renal failure).
No products indexed under this heading.

Meloxicam (Potential for acute renal failure). Products include:
Mobic Oral Suspension 863
Mobic Tablets 863

Metformin Hydrochloride (Increased risk of severe hyponatremia). Products include:
ActoPlus Met Tablets 3071
Avandamet Tablets 1336
Janumet Tablets 2041
PrandiMet Tablets 2967

Methenamine (Decreased effectiveness of methenamine due to alkalinization of urine).
No products indexed under this heading.

Methenamine Hippurate (Decreased effectiveness of methenamine due to alkalinization of urine).
No products indexed under this heading.

Methenamine Mandelate (Decreased effectiveness of methenamine due to alkalinization of urine). Products include:
Uroqid-Acid No. 2 Tablets 814

Methyclothiazide (May add to potentiate the action of other hypertensives).
No products indexed under this heading.

Methyldopa (May add to potentiate the action of other hypertensives).
No products indexed under this heading.

Methyldopate Hydrochloride (May add to potentiate the action of other hypertensives).
No products indexed under this heading.

Methylprednisolone Acetate (May intensify electrolyte imbalance, particularly hypokalemia).
No products indexed under this heading.

Methylprednisolone Sodium Succinate (May intensify electrolyte imbalance, particularly hypokalemia).
No products indexed under this heading.

Metocurine Iodide (Increased paralyzing effect).
No products indexed under this heading.

Metolazone (May add to potentiate the action of other hypertensives).
No products indexed under this heading.

Metoprolol Succinate (May add to potentiate the action of other hypertensives). Products include:
Toprol-XL Tablets 666

Metoprolol Tartrate (May add to potentiate the action of other hypertensives).
No products indexed under this heading.

Metyrosine (May add to potentiate the action of other hypertensives). Products include:
Demser Capsules 1989

Mibefradil Dihydrochloride (May add to potentiate the action of other hypertensives).
No products indexed under this heading.

Miglitol (Thiazides may cause hyperglycemia and glycosuria; dosage alteration of oral antidiabetic agents may be required).
No products indexed under this heading.

Minoxidil (May add to potentiate the action of other hypertensives).
No products indexed under this heading.

Mivacurium Chloride (Increased paralyzing effect).
No products indexed under this heading.

Moexipril Hydrochloride (May add to potentiate the action of other hypertensives; increased risk of hyperkalemia).
No products indexed under this heading.

Mometasone Furoate (May intensify electrolyte imbalance, particularly hypokalemia). Products include:
Asmanex Twisthaler 2797
Elocon Cream 0.1% 2840
Elocon Lotion 0.1% 2841
Elocon Ointment 0.1% 2842

Mometasone Furoate Monohydrate (May intensify electrolyte imbalance, particularly hypokalemia). Products include:
Nasonex Nasal Spray 2883

Nabumetone (Potential for acute renal failure).
No products indexed under this heading.

Nadolol (May add to potentiate the action of other hypertensives). Products include:
Nadolol Tablets 2191

Naproxen (Potential for acute renal failure). Products include:
EC-Naprosyn Delayed-Release Tablets 2632
Naprosyn Suspension 2632
Naprosyn Tablets 2632

Naproxen Sodium (Potential for acute renal failure). Products include:
Anaprox Tablets 2632
Anaprox DS Tablets 2632
Treximet Tablets 1616

Nateglinide (Thiazides may cause hyperglycemia and glycosuria; dosage alteration of oral antidiabetic agents may be required). Products include:
Starlix Tablets 2314

Nebivolol (May add to potentiate the action of other hypertensives). Products include:
Bystolic Tablets 1155

Nicardipine Hydrochloride (May add to potentiate the action of other hypertensives). Products include:
Cardene I.V. 1093

Nifedipine (May add to potentiate the action of other hypertensives).
No products indexed under this heading.

Nisoldipine (May add to potentiate the action of other hypertensives). Products include:
Sular Extended Release Tablets 2975

Nitroglycerin (May add to potentiate the action of other hypertensives). Products include:
Nitro-Dur Transdermal Infusion System 2887
Nitrolingual Pumpspray 2965

Norepinephrine Bitartrate (Decreased arterial responsiveness to norepinephrine).
No products indexed under this heading.

Oxaprozin (Potential for acute renal failure).
No products indexed under this heading.

Pancuronium Bromide (Increased paralyzing effect).
No products indexed under this heading.

Penbutolol Sulfate (May add to potentiate the action of other hypertensives).
No products indexed under this heading.

Penicillin G Potassium (Concurrent use of parenteral penicillin G potassium with triamterene may result in hyperkalemia, especially in patients with renal insufficiency).
No products indexed under this heading.

Perindopril Erbumine (May add to potentiate the action of other hypertensives; increased risk of hyperkalemia). Products include:
Aceon Tablets (2 mg, 4 mg, 8 mg) 3038

Phenoxybenzamine Hydrochloride (May add to potentiate the action of other hypertensives). Products include:
Dibenzyline Capsules 3188

Phentolamine Mesylate (May add to potentiate the action of other hypertensives).
No products indexed under this heading.

Phenylbutazone (Potential for acute renal failure).
No products indexed under this heading.

Pindolol (May add to potentiate the action of other hypertensives).
No products indexed under this heading.

Pioglitazone Hydrochloride (Thiazides may cause hyperglycemia and glycosuria; dosage alteration of oral antidiabetic agents may be required). Products include:
ActoPlus Met Tablets 3071
Actos Tablets 3077
Duetact Tablets 3085

Piroxicam (Potential for acute renal failure).
No products indexed under this heading.

Polythiazide (May add to potentiate the action of other hypertensives).
No products indexed under this heading.

Potassium Acid Phosphate (Potential for hyperkalemia; concomitant use should be avoided). Products include:
K-Phos Original (Sodium Free) Tablets 814

Potassium Bicarbonate (Potential for hyperkalemia; concomitant use should be avoided).
No products indexed under this heading.

Potassium Chloride (Potential for hyperkalemia; concomitant use should be avoided). Products include:
MoviPrep Oral Solution 2679

Potassium Citrate (Potential for hyperkalemia; concomitant use should be avoided). Products include:
BioLean Free Tablets 635
Urocit-K Tablets 2176

Potassium Gluconate (Potential for hyperkalemia; concomitant use should be avoided).
No products indexed under this heading.

Potassium Phosphate (Potential for hyperkalemia; concomitant use should be avoided). Products include:
K-Phos Neutral Tablets 813

Prazosin Hydrochloride (May add to potentiate the action of other hypertensives).
No products indexed under this heading.

Prednisolone Acetate (May intensify electrolyte imbalance, particularly hypokalemia). Products include:
Pred Forte Ophthalmic Suspension .... ⊙ 227
Pred Mild Ophthalmic Suspension .... ⊙ 230
Pred-G Ophthalmic Ointment .... ⊙ 229
Pred-G Ophthalmic Suspension .... ⊙ 228

Prednisolone Sodium Phosphate (May intensify electrolyte imbalance, particularly hypokalemia).
No products indexed under this heading.

Prednisolone Tebutate (May intensify electrolyte imbalance, particularly hypokalemia).
No products indexed under this heading.

Prednisone (May intensify electrolyte imbalance, particularly hypokalemia).
No products indexed under this heading.

Probenecid (Dyazide may raise the level of blood uric acid; may require dosage adjustment of antigout agent).
No products indexed under this heading.

Propranolol Hydrochloride (May add to potentiate the action of other hypertensives). Products include:
InnoPran XL Extended Release Capsules 1484

Quinapril Hydrochloride (May add to potentiate the action of other hypertensives; increased risk of hyperkalemia).
No products indexed under this heading.

Ramipril (May add to potentiate the action of other hypertensives; increased risk of hyperkalemia).
No products indexed under this heading.

Rapacuronium Bromide (Increased paralyzing effect).
No products indexed under this heading.

Rauwolfia Serpentina (May add to potentiate the action of other hypertensives).
No products indexed under this heading.

Repaglinide (Thiazides may cause hyperglycemia and glycosuria; dosage alteration of oral antidiabetic agents may be required). Products include:
PrandiMet Tablets 2967
Prandin Tablets 2971

Rescinnamine (May add to potentiate the action of other hypertensives).
No products indexed under this heading.

Reserpine (May add to potentiate the action of other hypertensives).
No products indexed under this heading.

Rocuronium Bromide (Increased paralyzing effect). Products include:
Zemuron Injection 2947

Rofecoxib (Potential for acute renal failure).
No products indexed under this heading.

Rosiglitazone Maleate (Thiazides may cause hyperglycemia and glycosuria; dosage alteration of oral antidiabetic agents may be required). Products include:
Avandamet Tablets 1336
Avandaryl Tablets 1344
Avandia Tablets 1351

Salt Substitutes (Concurrent use of salt substitues with triamterene may result in hyperkalemia, especially in patients with renal insufficiency).
No products indexed under this heading.

Sitagliptin Phosphate (Thiazides may cause hyperglycemia and glycosuria; dosage alteration of oral antidiabetic agents may be required). Products include:
Janumet Tablets 2041
Januvia Tablets 2048

Sodium Nitroprusside (May add to potentiate the action of other hypertensives).
No products indexed under this heading.

Sodium Polystyrene Sulfonate (May result in fluid retention).
No products indexed under this heading.

Sotalol Hydrochloride (May add to potentiate the action of other hypertensives).
No products indexed under this heading.

Spirapril Hydrochloride (May add to potentiate the action of other hypertensives; increased risk of hyperkalemia).
No products indexed under this heading.

Spironolactone (Concurrent use is contraindicated).
No products indexed under this heading.

Sulfinpyrazone (Dyazide may raise the level of blood uric acid; may require dosage adjustment of anti-gout agent).
No products indexed under this heading.

Sulindac (Potential for acute renal failure). Products include:
Clinoril Tablets 1962

Telmisartan (May add to potentiate the action of other hypertensives). Products include:
Micardis Tablets 852
Micardis HCT Tablets 854

Terazosin Hydrochloride (May add to potentiate the action of other hypertensives).
No products indexed under this heading.

Timolol Maleate (May add to potentiate the action of other hypertensives). Products include:
Combigan Ophthalmic Solution 553
Cosopt Sterile Ophthalmic Solution 1969
Timoptic Sterile Ophthalmic Solution 2121
Timoptic in Ocudose 2124
Timoptic-XE Sterile Ophthalmic Gel Forming Solution 2125

Tolazamide (Thiazides may cause hyperglycemia and glycosuria; dosage alteration of oral antidiabetic agents may be required).
No products indexed under this heading.

Tolbutamide (Thiazides may cause hyperglycemia and glycosuria; dosage alteration of oral antidiabetic agents may be required).
No products indexed under this heading.

Tolmetin Sodium (Potential for acute renal failure).
No products indexed under this heading.

Torsemide (May add to potentiate the action of other hypertensives). Products include:
Demadex Injection 2630
Demadex Tablets 2630

Trandolapril (May add to potentiate the action of other hypertensives; increased risk of hyperkalemia). Products include:
Mavik Tablets 472
Tarka Tablets 511

Triamcinolone (May intensify electrolyte imbalance, particularly hypokalemia).
No products indexed under this heading.

Triamcinolone Acetonide (May intensify electrolyte imbalance, particularly hypokalemia). Products include:
Azmacort Inhalation Aerosol 407
Nasacort AQ Nasal Spray 2765
Triesence Injectable Suspension ..... ⊙209

Triamcinolone Diacetate (May intensify electrolyte imbalance, particularly hypokalemia).
No products indexed under this heading.

Triamcinolone Hexacetonide (May intensify electrolyte imbalance, particularly hypokalemia).
No products indexed under this heading.

Trimethaphan Camsylate (May add to potentiate the action of other hypertensives).
No products indexed under this heading.

Troglitazone (Thiazides may cause hyperglycemia and glycosuria; dosage alteration of oral antidiabetic agents may be required).
No products indexed under this heading.

Tubocurarine Chloride (Increased paralyzing effect).
No products indexed under this heading.

Valdecoxib (Potential for acute renal failure).
No products indexed under this heading.

Valsartan (May add to potentiate the action of other hypertensives). Products include:
Diovan Tablets 2212
Diovan HCT Tablets 2216
Exforge Tablets 2238

Vecuronium Bromide (Increased paralyzing effect).
No products indexed under this heading.

Verapamil Hydrochloride (May add to potentiate the action of other hypertensives). Products include:
Tarka Tablets 511

Warfarin Sodium (Effects of oral anticoagulants may be decreased).
No products indexed under this heading.

Food Interactions

Milk, low fat (Concurrent use of low-salt milk with triamterene may result in hyperkalemia, especially in patients with renal insufficiency).

DYNACIRC CR CONTROLLED RELEASE TABLETS

(Isradipine) 1407
May interact with:

Cimetidine (Co-administration has resulted in increase in isradipine mean peak plasma concentrations and significant increase in the AUC).
No products indexed under this heading.

Cimetidine Hydrochloride (Co-administration has resulted in increase in isradipine mean peak plasma concentrations and significant increase in the AUC).
No products indexed under this heading.

Fentanyl (Severe hypotension has been reported during fentanyl anesthesia with concomitant use of beta-blocker and a calcium channel blocker). Products include:
Duragesic Transdermal System 2405
Ionsys Transdermal System 2410

Fentanyl Citrate (Severe hypotension has been reported during fentanyl anesthesia with concomitant use of beta-blocker and a calcium channel blocker). Products include:
Actiq 959
Fentora Tablets 968

Hydrochlorothiazide (Additive antihypertensive effect). Products include:
Atacand HCT 642
Avalide Tablets 892
Avalide Tablets 2713
Benicar HCT Tablets 1010
Diovan HCT Tablets 2216
Dyazide Capsules 1405
Micardis HCT Tablets 854
Prinzide Tablets 2092
Tekturna HCT Tablets 2324
Teveten HCT Tablets 517

Propranolol Hydrochloride (Co-administration has resulted in a small effect on the rate but no effect on the extent of isradipine bioavailability; significant increases in AUC and Cmax and decreases in tmax of propranolol were noted). Products include:
InnoPran XL Extended Release Capsules 1484

Rifampin (Co-administration has resulted in increased metabolism and higher clearance of isradipine; a reduction in isradipine levels to below the detectable limits has been noted).
No products indexed under this heading.

DYRENIUM CAPSULES

(Triamterene) 3189
May interact with ACE inhibitors, anesthetics, antihypertensives, diuretics, oral hypoglycemic agents, lithium preparations, nondepolarizing neuromuscular blocking agents, potassium preparations, preanesthetic medications, potassium sparing diuretics, and certain other agents. Compounds in these categories include:

Acarbose (Triamterene may raise blood glucose levels; for adult onset diabetes, dosage adjustments of hypoglycemic agents may be necessary during and after therapy). Products include:
Precose Tablets 792

Acebutolol Hydrochloride (The effects of antihypertensive agents may be potentiated when given concurrently).
No products indexed under this heading.

Alfentanil Hydrochloride (The effects of anesthetics may be potentiated when given concurrently).
No products indexed under this heading.

Aliskiren (The effects of antihypertensive agents may be potentiated when given concurrently). Products include:
Tekturna Tablets 2321
Tekturna HCT Tablets 2324

Amiloride Hydrochloride (Co-administration with other potassium-sparing agents has resulted in fatalities; these agents should not be given concomitantly).
No products indexed under this heading.

Amlodipine Besylate (The effects of antihypertensive agents may be potentiated when given concurrently). Products include:
Azor Tablets 1005
Exforge Tablets 2238

Atenolol (The effects of antihypertensive agents may be potentiated when given concurrently).
No products indexed under this heading.

Atracurium Besylate (The effects of nondepolarizing skeletal muscle relaxants may be potentiated when given concurrently).
No products indexed under this heading.

Benazepril Hydrochloride (Co-administration with potassium-sparing agents and angiotensin-coverting enzyme inhibitors increases the risk of hyperkalemia).
No products indexed under this heading.

Bendroflumethiazide (The effects of other diuretics may be potentiated when given concurrently).
No products indexed under this heading.

Betaxolol Hydrochloride (The effects of antihypertensive agents may be potentiated when given concurrently).
No products indexed under this heading.

Bisoprolol Fumarate (The effects of antihypertensive agents may be potentiated when given concurrently).
No products indexed under this heading.

Blood, whole (Co-administration with blood from blood banks may promote serum potassium accumulation and possibly result in hyperkalemia).
No products indexed under this heading.

Bumetanide (The effects of other diuretics may be potentiated when given concurrently).
No products indexed under this heading.

Candesartan Cilexetil (The effects of antihypertensive agents may be potentiated when given concurrently). Products include:
Atacand Tablets 639
Atacand HCT 642

Captopril (Co-administration with potassium-sparing agents and angiotensin-coverting enzyme inhibitors increases the risk of hyperkalemia). Products include:
Captopril Tablets 2182

Carteolol Hydrochloride (The effects of antihypertensive agents may be potentiated when given concurrently).
No products indexed under this heading.

Chlorothiazide (The effects of other diuretics may be potentiated when given concurrently).
No products indexed under this heading.

Chlorothiazide Sodium (The effects of other diuretics may be potentiated when given concurrently). Products include:
Intravenous Sodium Diuril 2490

Chlorpropamide (Triamterene may raise blood glucose levels; for adult onset diabetes, dosage adjustments of hypoglycemic agents may be necessary during and after therapy; increased risk of severe hyponatremia with concurrent use).
No products indexed under this heading.

Chlorthalidone (The effects of other diuretics may be potentiated when given concurrently). Products include:
Clorpres Tablets 2185

Cisatracurium Besylate (The effects of nondepolarizing skeletal muscle relaxants may be potentiated when given concurrently). Products include:
Nimbex Injection 484

Clonidine (The effects of antihypertensive agents may be potentiated when given concurrently). Products include:
Catapres-TTS 842

Clonidine Hydrochloride (The effects of antihypertensive agents may be potentiated when given concurrently). Products include:

Catapres Tablets ... 841
Clorpres Tablets ... 2185

Deserpidine (The effects of antihypertensive agents may be potentiated when given concurrently).
No products indexed under this heading.

Diazepam (The effects of pre-anesthetic agents may be potentiated when given concurrently). Products include:
Valium Tablets ... 2658

Diazoxide (The effects of antihypertensive agents may be potentiated when given concurrently). Products include:
Proglycem Capsules ... 1185
Proglycem Suspension ... 1185

Diltiazem Hydrochloride (The effects of antihypertensive agents may be potentiated when given concurrently). Products include:
Cardizem LA Extended Release Tablets ... 421

Doxazosin Mesylate (The effects of antihypertensive agents may be potentiated when given concurrently).
No products indexed under this heading.

Droperidol (The effects of pre-anesthetic agents may be potentiated when given concurrently).
No products indexed under this heading.

Enalapril Maleate (Co-administration with potassium-sparing agents and angiotensin-coverting enzyme inhibitors increases the risk of hyperkalemia).
No products indexed under this heading.

Enalaprilat (Co-administration with potassium-sparing agents and angiotensin-coverting enzyme inhibitors increases the risk of hyperkalemia).
No products indexed under this heading.

Enflurane (The effects of anesthetics may be potentiated when given concurrently).
No products indexed under this heading.

Eprosartan Mesylate (The effects of antihypertensive agents may be potentiated when given concurrently). Products include:
Teveten Tablets ... 515
Teveten HCT Tablets ... 517

Esmolol Hydrochloride (The effects of antihypertensive agents may be potentiated when given concurrently).
No products indexed under this heading.

Ethacrynic Acid (The effects of other diuretics may be potentiated when given concurrently). Products include:
Edecrin Tablets ... 698

Felodipine (The effects of antihypertensive agents may be potentiated when given concurrently).
No products indexed under this heading.

Fentanyl Citrate (The effects of anesthetics may be potentiated when given concurrently). Products include:
Actiq ... 959
Fentora Tablets ... 968

Fosinopril Sodium (Co-administration with potassium-sparing agents and angiotensin-coverting enzyme inhibitors increases the risk of hyperkalemia).
No products indexed under this heading.

Furosemide (The effects of other diuretics may be potentiated when given concurrently). Products include:
Furosemide Tablets ... 2186

Glimepiride (Triamterene may raise blood glucose levels; for adult onset diabetes, dosage adjustments of hypoglycemic agents may be necessary during and after therapy). Products include:
Avandaryl Tablets ... 1344
Duetact Tablets ... 3085

Glipizide (Triamterene may raise blood glucose levels; for adult onset diabetes, dosage adjustments of hypoglycemic agents may be necessary during and after therapy).
No products indexed under this heading.

Glyburide (Triamterene may raise blood glucose levels; for adult onset diabetes, dosage adjustments of hypoglycemic agents may be necessary during and after therapy).
No products indexed under this heading.

Guanabenz Acetate (The effects of antihypertensive agents may be potentiated when given concurrently).
No products indexed under this heading.

Guanethidine Monosulfate (The effects of antihypertensive agents may be potentiated when given concurrently).
No products indexed under this heading.

Halothane (The effects of anesthetics may be potentiated when given concurrently).
No products indexed under this heading.

Hydralazine Hydrochloride (The effects of antihypertensive agents may be potentiated when given concurrently).
No products indexed under this heading.

Hydrochlorothiazide (The effects of other diuretics may be potentiated when given concurrently). Products include:
Atacand HCT ... 642
Avalide Tablets ... 892
Avalide Tablets ... 2713
Benicar HCT Tablets ... 1010
Diovan HCT Tablets ... 2216
Dyazide Capsules ... 1405
Micardis HCT Tablets ... 854
Prinzide Tablets ... 2092
Tekturna HCT Tablets ... 2324
Teveten HCT Tablets ... 517

Hydroflumethiazide (The effects of other diuretics may be potentiated when given concurrently).
No products indexed under this heading.

Hydroxyzine Hydrochloride (The effects of pre-anesthetic agents may be potentiated when given concurrently).
No products indexed under this heading.

Indapamide (The effects of other diuretics may be potentiated when given concurrently). Products include:
Indapamide Tablets ... 2188

Indomethacin (Co-administration has resulted in acute renal failure). Products include:
Indocin ... 2024

Irbesartan (The effects of antihypertensive agents may be potentiated when given concurrently). Products include:
Avalide Tablets ... 892
Avalide Tablets ... 2713
Avapro Tablets ... 897
Avapro Tablets ... 2718

Isoflurane (The effects of anesthetics may be potentiated when given concurrently).
No products indexed under this heading.

Isradipine (The effects of antihypertensive agents may be potentiated when given concurrently). Products include:
DynaCirc CR Controlled Release Tablets ... 1407

Ketamine Hydrochloride (The effects of anesthetics may be potentiated when given concurrently).
No products indexed under this heading.

Labetalol Hydrochloride (The effects of antihypertensive agents may be potentiated when given concurrently).
No products indexed under this heading.

Lisinopril (Co-administration with potassium-sparing agents and angiotensin-coverting enzyme inhibitors increases the risk of hyperkalemia). Products include:
Prinivil Tablets ... 2087
Prinzide Tablets ... 2092

Lithium (Co-administration of lithium and diuretics results in diuretic-induced sodium loss that may reduce renal clearance of lithium and increase serum lithium levels with risk of lithium toxicity).
No products indexed under this heading.

Lithium Carbonate (Co-administration of lithium and diuretics results in diuretic-induced sodium loss that may reduce renal clearance of lithium and increase serum lithium levels with risk of lithium toxicity).
No products indexed under this heading.

Lithium Citrate (Co-administration of lithium and diuretics results in diuretic-induced sodium loss that may reduce renal clearance of lithium and increase serum lithium levels with risk of lithium toxicity).
No products indexed under this heading.

Lorazepam (The effects of pre-anesthetic agents may be potentiated when given concurrently).
No products indexed under this heading.

Losartan Potassium (The effects of antihypertensive agents may be potentiated when given concurrently). Products include:
Cozaar Tablets ... 1973

Mecamylamine Hydrochloride (The effects of antihypertensive agents may be potentiated when given concurrently).
No products indexed under this heading.

Meperidine Hydrochloride (The effects of pre-anesthetic agents may be potentiated when given concurrently).
No products indexed under this heading.

Metformin Hydrochloride (Triamterene may raise blood glucose levels; for adult onset diabetes, dosage adjustments of hypoglycemic agents may be necessary during and after therapy). Products include:
ActoPlus Met Tablets ... 3071
Avandamet Tablets ... 1336
Janumet Tablets ... 2041
PrandiMet Tablets ... 2967

Methohexital Sodium (The effects of anesthetics may be potentiated when given concurrently).
No products indexed under this heading.

Methyclothiazide (The effects of other diuretics may be potentiated when given concurrently).
No products indexed under this heading.

Methyldopa (The effects of antihypertensive agents may be potentiated when given concurrently).
No products indexed under this heading.

Methyldopate Hydrochloride (The effects of antihypertensive agents may be potentiated when given concurrently).
No products indexed under this heading.

Metocurine Iodide (The effects of nondepolarizing skeletal muscle relaxants may be potentiated when given concurrently).
No products indexed under this heading.

Metolazone (The effects of other diuretics may be potentiated when given concurrently).
No products indexed under this heading.

Metoprolol Succinate (The effects of antihypertensive agents may be potentiated when given concurrently). Products include:
Toprol-XL Tablets ... 666

Metoprolol Tartrate (The effects of antihypertensive agents may be potentiated when given concurrently).
No products indexed under this heading.

Metyrosine (The effects of antihypertensive agents may be potentiated when given concurrently). Products include:
Demser Capsules ... 1989

Mibefradil Dihydrochloride (The effects of antihypertensive agents may be potentiated when given concurrently).
No products indexed under this heading.

Midazolam Hydrochloride (The effects of anesthetics may be potentiated when given concurrently).
No products indexed under this heading.

Miglitol (Triamterene may raise blood glucose levels; for adult onset diabetes, dosage adjustments of hypoglycemic agents may be necessary during and after therapy).
No products indexed under this heading.

Minoxidil (The effects of antihypertensive agents may be potentiated when given concurrently).
No products indexed under this heading.

IMPORTANT NOTE: Always consult each drug listing in the patient's regimen for possible interactions.

Mivacurium Chloride (The effects of nondepolarizing skeletal muscle relaxants may be potentiated when given concurrently).
No products indexed under this heading.

Moexipril Hydrochloride (Co-administration with potassium-sparing agents and angiotensin-coverting enzyme inhibitors increases the risk of hyperkalemia).
No products indexed under this heading.

Morphine Sulfate (The effects of pre-anesthetic agents may be potentiated when given concurrently). Products include:
Avinza Capsules 1772
DepoDur Injection 1095
MS Contin Tablets 2585

Nadolol (The effects of antihypertensive agents may be potentiated when given concurrently). Products include:
Nadolol Tablets 2191

Nateglinide (Triamterene may raise blood glucose levels; for adult onset diabetes, dosage adjustments of hypoglycemic agents may be necessary during and after therapy). Products include:
Starlix Tablets 2314

Nebivolol (The effects of antihypertensive agents may be potentiated when given concurrently). Products include:
Bystolic Tablets 1155

Nicardipine Hydrochloride (The effects of antihypertensive agents may be potentiated when given concurrently). Products include:
Cardene I.V. 1093

Nifedipine (The effects of antihypertensive agents may be potentiated when given concurrently).
No products indexed under this heading.

Nisoldipine (The effects of antihypertensive agents may be potentiated when given concurrently). Products include:
Sular Extended Release Tablets 2975

Nitroglycerin (The effects of antihypertensive agents may be potentiated when given concurrently). Products include:
Nitro-Dur Transdermal Infusion System 2887
Nitrolingual Pumpspray 2965

Pancuronium Bromide (The effects of nondepolarizing skeletal muscle relaxants may be potentiated when given concurrently).
No products indexed under this heading.

Penbutolol Sulfate (The effects of antihypertensive agents may be potentiated when given concurrently).
No products indexed under this heading.

Penicillin G Potassium (Co-administration may promote serum potassium accumulation and possibly result in hyperkalemia).
No products indexed under this heading.

Pentobarbital Sodium (The effects of pre-anesthetic agents may be potentiated when given concurrently). Products include:
Nembutal Sodium Solution, USP 2494

Perindopril Erbumine (Co-administration with potassium-sparing agents and angiotensin-coverting enzyme inhibitors increases the risk of hyperkalemia). Products include:
Aceon Tablets (2 mg, 4 mg, 8 mg) 3038

Phenoxybenzamine Hydrochloride (The effects of antihypertensive agents may be potentiated when given concurrently). Products include:
Dibenzyline Capsules 3188

Phentolamine Mesylate (The effects of antihypertensive agents may be potentiated when given concurrently).
No products indexed under this heading.

Pindolol (The effects of antihypertensive agents may be potentiated when given concurrently).
No products indexed under this heading.

Pioglitazone Hydrochloride (Triamterene may raise blood glucose levels; for adult onset diabetes, dosage adjustments of hypoglycemic agents may be necessary during and after therapy). Products include:
ActoPlus Met Tablets 3071
Actos Tablets 3077
Duetact Tablets 3085

Polythiazide (The effects of other diuretics may be potentiated when given concurrently).
No products indexed under this heading.

Potassium Acid Phosphate (Co-administration with dietary potassium supplements increases the risk of hyperkalemia; concurrent use is contraindicated). Products include:
K-Phos Original (Sodium Free) Tablets 814

Potassium Bicarbonate (Co-administration with dietary potassium supplements increases the risk of hyperkalemia; concurrent use is contraindicated).
No products indexed under this heading.

Potassium Chloride (Co-administration with dietary potassium supplements increases the risk of hyperkalemia; concurrent use is contraindicated). Products include:
MoviPrep Oral Solution 2679

Potassium Citrate (Co-administration with dietary potassium supplements increases the risk of hyperkalemia; concurrent use is contraindicated). Products include:
BioLean Free Tablets .... ■ 635
Urocit-K Tablets 2176

Potassium Gluconate (Co-administration with dietary potassium supplements increases the risk of hyperkalemia; concurrent use is contraindicated).
No products indexed under this heading.

Potassium Phosphate (Co-administration with dietary potassium supplements increases the risk of hyperkalemia; concurrent use is contraindicated). Products include:
K-Phos Neutral Tablets 813

Prazosin Hydrochloride (The effects of antihypertensive agents may be potentiated when given concurrently).
No products indexed under this heading.

Promethazine Hydrochloride (The effects of pre-anesthetic agents may be potentiated when given concurrently).
No products indexed under this heading.

Propofol (The effects of anesthetics may be potentiated when given concurrently).
No products indexed under this heading.

Propranolol Hydrochloride (The effects of antihypertensive agents may be potentiated when given concurrently). Products include:
InnoPran XL Extended Release Capsules 1484

Quinapril Hydrochloride (Co-administration with potassium-sparing agents and angiotensin-coverting enzyme inhibitors increases the risk of hyperkalemia).
No products indexed under this heading.

Ramipril (Co-administration with potassium-sparing agents and angiotensin-coverting enzyme inhibitors increases the risk of hyperkalemia).
No products indexed under this heading.

Rapacuronium Bromide (The effects of nondepolarizing skeletal muscle relaxants may be potentiated when given concurrently).
No products indexed under this heading.

Rauwolfia Serpentina (The effects of antihypertensive agents may be potentiated when given concurrently).
No products indexed under this heading.

Remifentanil Hydrochloride (The effects of anesthetics may be potentiated when given concurrently).
No products indexed under this heading.

Repaglinide (Triamterene may raise blood glucose levels; for adult onset diabetes, dosage adjustments of hypoglycemic agents may be necessary during and after therapy). Products include:
PrandiMet Tablets 2967
Prandin Tablets 2971

Rescinnamine (The effects of antihypertensive agents may be potentiated when given concurrently).
No products indexed under this heading.

Reserpine (The effects of antihypertensive agents may be potentiated when given concurrently).
No products indexed under this heading.

Rocuronium Bromide (The effects of nondepolarizing skeletal muscle relaxants may be potentiated when given concurrently). Products include:
Zemuron Injection 2947

Rosiglitazone Maleate (Triamterene may raise blood glucose levels; for adult onset diabetes, dosage adjustments of hypoglycemic agents may be necessary during and after therapy). Products include:
Avandamet Tablets 1336
Avandaryl Tablets 1344
Avandia Tablets 1351

Secobarbital Sodium (The effects of pre-anesthetic agents may be potentiated when given concurrently).
No products indexed under this heading.

Sitagliptin Phosphate (Triamterene may raise blood glucose levels; for adult onset diabetes, dosage adjustments of hypoglycemic agents may be necessary during and after therapy). Products include:
Janumet Tablets 2041
Januvia Tablets 2048

Sodium Nitroprusside (The effects of antihypertensive agents may be potentiated when given concurrently).
No products indexed under this heading.

Sotalol Hydrochloride (The effects of antihypertensive agents may be potentiated when given concurrently).
No products indexed under this heading.

Spirapril Hydrochloride (Co-administration with potassium-sparing agents and angiotensin-coverting enzyme inhibitors increases the risk of hyperkalemia).
No products indexed under this heading.

Spironolactone (Co-administration with other potassium-sparing agents has resulted in fatalities; these agents should not be given concomitantly).
No products indexed under this heading.

Sufentanil Citrate (The effects of anesthetics may be potentiated when given concurrently).
No products indexed under this heading.

Telmisartan (The effects of antihypertensive agents may be potentiated when given concurrently). Products include:
Micardis Tablets 852
Micardis HCT Tablets 854

Terazosin Hydrochloride (The effects of antihypertensive agents may be potentiated when given concurrently).
No products indexed under this heading.

Thiamylal Sodium (The effects of anesthetics may be potentiated when given concurrently).
No products indexed under this heading.

Timolol Maleate (The effects of antihypertensive agents may be potentiated when given concurrently). Products include:
Combigan Ophthalmic Solution 553
Cosopt Sterile Ophthalmic Solution 1969
Timoptic Sterile Ophthalmic Solution 2121
Timoptic in Ocudose 2124
Timoptic-XE Sterile Ophthalmic Gel Forming Solution 2125

Tolazamide (Triamterene may raise blood glucose levels; for adult onset diabetes, dosage adjustments of hypoglycemic agents may be necessary during and after therapy).
No products indexed under this heading.

Tolbutamide (Triamterene may raise blood glucose levels; for adult onset diabetes, dosage adjustments of hypoglycemic agents may be necessary during and after therapy).
No products indexed under this heading.

Torsemide (The effects of other diuretics may be potentiated when given concurrently). Products include:
Demadex Injection 2630
Demadex Tablets 2630

Trandolapril (Co-administration with potassium-sparing agents and angiotensin-coverting enzyme inhibitors increases the risk of hyperkalemia). Products include:
Mavik Tablets 472
Tarka Tablets 511

Trimethaphan Camsylate (The effects of antihypertensive agents may be potentiated when given concurrently).
No products indexed under this heading.

Troglitazone (Triamterene may raise blood glucose levels; for adult onset diabetes, dosage adjustments of hypoglycemic agents may be necessary during and after therapy).
No products indexed under this heading.

Valsartan (The effects of antihypertensive agents may be potentiated when given concurrently). Products include:
Diovan Tablets 2212
Diovan HCT Tablets 2216
Exforge Tablets 2238

Vecuronium Bromide (The effects of nondepolarizing skeletal muscle relaxants may be potentiated when given concurrently).
No products indexed under this heading.

Verapamil Hydrochloride (The effects of antihypertensive agents may be potentiated when given concurrently). Products include:
Tarka Tablets 511

Food Interactions

Milk, low salt (Co-administration may promote serum potassium accumulation and possibly result in hyperkalemia).

EC-NAPROSYN DELAYED-RELEASE TABLETS

(Naproxen) 2632
May interact with ACE inhibitors, antacids containing aluminum, calcium and magnesium, beta blockers, oral anticoagulants, histamine H_2-receptor antagonists, hydantoin anticonvulsants, lithium preparations, selective serotonin reuptake inhibitors, sulfonylureas, thiazides, and certain other agents. Compounds in these categories include:

Acebutolol Hydrochloride (Reduced antihypertensive effect of beta blockers).
No products indexed under this heading.

Aluminum Carbonate (Due to the gastric pH elevating effects of intensive antacids therapy, concomitant administration of EC-Naprosyn is not recommended).
No products indexed under this heading.

Aluminum Hydroxide (Due to the gastric pH elevating effects of intensive antacids therapy, concomitant administration of EC-Naprosyn is not recommended).
No products indexed under this heading.

Anisindione (Short-term studies have failed to show any significant effect of concurrent use on prothrombin time; caution is advised since interactions have been seen with other NSAIDs).
No products indexed under this heading.

Aspirin (Naproxen is displaced from its binding sites during the concomitant administration of aspirin resulting in lower plasma concentrations and peak plasma levels; concurrent use is not recommended). Products include:
Aggrenox Capsules 819
Bayer Aspirin 750
Percodan Tablets 1130
St. Joseph 81 mg Aspirin Chewable and Enteric Coated Tablets 1903

Atenolol (Reduced antihypertensive effect of beta blockers).
No products indexed under this heading.

Benazepril Hydrochloride (Reports suggest that NSAIDs may diminish the antihypertensive effect of ACE-inhibitors. The use of NSAIDs in patients who are receiving ACE-inhibitors may potentiate renal dise states).
No products indexed under this heading.

Bendroflumethiazide (Clinical studies, as well as postmarketing observations, have shown that Naproxen can reduce the natriuretic effect of furosemide and thiazides in some patients. Response has been attributed to inhibition of renal prostaglandin synthesis. Patients should be observed closely for signs of renal failure, as well as to assure diuretic efficacy).
No products indexed under this heading.

Betaxolol Hydrochloride (Reduced antihypertensive effect of beta blockers).
No products indexed under this heading.

Bisoprolol Fumarate (Reduced antihypertensive effect of beta blockers).
No products indexed under this heading.

Captopril (Reports suggest that NSAIDs may diminish the antihypertensive effect of ACE-inhibitors. The use of NSAIDs in patients who are receiving ACE-inhibitors may potentiate renal dise states). Products include:
Captopril Tablets 2182

Carteolol Hydrochloride (Reduced antihypertensive effect of beta blockers).
No products indexed under this heading.

Chlorothiazide (Clinical studies, as well as postmarketing observations, have shown that Naproxen can reduce the natriuretic effect of furosemide and thiazides in some patients. Response has been attributed to inhibition of renal prostaglandin synthesis. Patients should be observed closely for signs of renal failure, as well as to assure diuretic efficacy).
No products indexed under this heading.

Chlorothiazide Sodium (Clinical studies, as well as postmarketing observations, have shown that Naproxen can reduce the natriuretic effect of furosemide and thiazides in some patients. Response has been attributed to inhibition of renal prostaglandin synthesis. Patients should be observed closely for signs of renal failure, as well as to assure diuretic efficacy). Products include:
Intravenous Sodium Diuril 2490

Chlorpropamide (Potential for sulfonylurea toxicity).
No products indexed under this heading.

Cholestyramine (Concomitant administration of cholestyramine can delay the absorption of naproxen).
No products indexed under this heading.

Cimetidine (Due to the gastric pH elevating effects of H_2-blockers concomitant administration of EC-Naprosyn is not recommended).
No products indexed under this heading.

Cimetidine Hydrochloride (Due to the gastric pH elevating effects of H_2-blockers concomitant administration of EC-Naprosyn is not recommended).
No products indexed under this heading.

Citalopram Hydrobromide (There is an increased risk of GI bleeding when selective serotonin reuptake inhibitors (SSRIs) are combined with NSAIDs. Caution should be used when NSAIDs are administered concomitantly with SSRIs). Products include:
Celexa 1160

Dicumarol (Short-term studies have failed to show any significant effect of concurrent use on prothrombin time; caution is advised since interactions have been seen with other NSAIDs).
No products indexed under this heading.

Enalapril Maleate (Reports suggest that NSAIDs may diminish the antihypertensive effect of ACE-inhibitors. The use of NSAIDs in patients who are receiving ACE-inhibitors may potentiate renal dise states).
No products indexed under this heading.

Enalaprilat (Reports suggest that NSAIDs may diminish the antihypertensive effect of ACE-inhibitors. The use of NSAIDs in patients who are receiving ACE-inhibitors may potentiate renal dise states).
No products indexed under this heading.

Escitalopram Oxalate (There is an increased risk of GI bleeding when selective serotonin reuptake inhibitors (SSRIs) are combined with NSAIDs. Caution should be used when NSAIDs are administered concomitantly with SSRIs). Products include:
Lexapro Oral Suspension 1174
Lexapro Tablets 1174

Esmolol Hydrochloride (Reduced antihypertensive effect of beta blockers).
No products indexed under this heading.

Ethotoin (Potential for hydantoin toxicity).
No products indexed under this heading.

Famotidine (Due to the gastric pH elevating effects of H_2-blockers concomitant administration of EC-Naprosyn is not recommended). Products include:
Pepcid Tablets 2075
Original Strength Pepcid AC Gelcaps 1771
Original Strength Pepcid AC Tablets 1771
Maximum Strength Pepcid AC Tablets 1771
Pepcid Complete Chewable Tablets 1771

Fluoxetine (There is an increased risk of GI bleeding when selective serotonin reuptake inhibitors (SSRIs) are combined with NSAIDs. Caution should be used when NSAIDs are administered concomitantly with SSRIs).
No products indexed under this heading.

Fluoxetine Hydrochloride (There is an increased risk of GI bleeding when selective serotonin reuptake inhibitors (SSRIs) are combined with NSAIDs. Caution should be used when NSAIDs are administered concomitantly with SSRIs). Products include:
Prozac Weekly Capsules 1852
Prozac Pulvules and Liquid 1852
Symbyax Capsules 1871

Fluvoxamine Maleate (There is an increased risk of GI bleeding when selective serotonin reuptake inhibitors (SSRIs) are combined with NSAIDs. Caution should be used when NSAIDs are administered concomitantly with SSRIs). Products include:
Luvox CR Extended-Release Capsules 1759

Fosinopril Sodium (Reports suggest that NSAIDs may diminish the antihypertensive effect of ACE-inhibitors. The use of NSAIDs in patients who are receiving ACE-inhibitors may potentiate renal dise states).
No products indexed under this heading.

Fosphenytoin Sodium (Potential for hydantoin toxicity).
No products indexed under this heading.

Furosemide (Clinical studies, as well as postmarketing observations, have shown that Naproxen can reduce the natriuretic effect of furosemide and thiazides in some patients. Response has been attributed to inhibition of renal prostaglandin synthesis. Patients should be observed closely for signs of renal failure, as well as to assure diuretic efficacy). Products include:
Furosemide Tablets 2186

Glimepiride (Potential for sulfonylurea toxicity). Products include:
Avandaryl Tablets 1344
Duetact Tablets 3085

Glipizide (Potential for sulfonylurea toxicity).
No products indexed under this heading.

Glyburide (Potential for sulfonylurea toxicity).
No products indexed under this heading.

Hydrochlorothiazide (Clinical studies, as well as postmarketing observations, have shown that Naproxen can reduce the natriuretic effect of furosemide and thiazides in some patients. Response has been attributed to inhibition of renal prostaglandin synthesis. Patients should be observed closely for signs of renal failure, as well as to assure diuretic efficacy). Products include:
Atacand HCT ... 642
Avalide Tablets ... 892
Avalide Tablets ... 2713
Benicar HCT Tablets ... 1010
Diovan HCT Tablets ... 2216
Dyazide Capsules ... 1405
Micardis HCT Tablets ... 854
Prinzide Tablets ... 2092
Tekturna HCT Tablets ... 2324
Teveten HCT Tablets ... 517

Hydroflumethiazide (Clinical studies, as well as postmarketing observations, have shown that Naproxen can reduce the natriuretic effect of furosemide and thiazides in some patients. Response has been attributed to inhibition of renal prostaglandin synthesis. Patients should be observed closely for signs of renal failure, as well as to assure diuretic efficacy).
No products indexed under this heading.

Labetalol Hydrochloride (Reduced antihypertensive effect of beta blockers).
No products indexed under this heading.

Levobunolol Hydrochloride (Reduced antihypertensive effect of beta blockers).
No products indexed under this heading.

Lisinopril (Reports suggest that NSAIDs may diminish the antihypertensive effect of ACE-inhibitors. The use of NSAIDs in patients who are receiving ACE-inhibitors may potentiate renal dise states). Products include:
Prinivil Tablets ... 2087
Prinzide Tablets ... 2092

Lithium (Inhibition of lithium renal clearance leading to increase in plasma lithium concentrations).
No products indexed under this heading.

Lithium Carbonate (Inhibition of lithium renal clearance leading to increase in plasma lithium concentrations).
No products indexed under this heading.

Lithium Citrate (Inhibition of lithium renal clearance leading to increase in plasma lithium concentrations).
No products indexed under this heading.

Magaldrate (Due to the gastric pH elevating effects of intensive antacids therapy, concomitant administration of EC-Naprosyn is not recommended).
No products indexed under this heading.

Magnesium Hydroxide (Due to the gastric pH elevating effects of intensive antacids therapy, concomitant administration of EC-Naprosyn is not recommended). Products include:
Fleet Pedia-Lax Chewable Tablets ... 1145
Pepcid Complete Chewable Tablets ... 1771
Extra Strength Rolaids Freshmint Tablets ... 1903
Rolaids Multi-Symptom Berry Tablets ... 1903
Rolaids Original Peppermint Tablets ... 1903

Magnesium Oxide (Due to the gastric pH elevating effects of intensive antacids therapy, concomitant administration of EC-Naprosyn is not recommended). Products include:
Beelith Tablets ... 813

Mephenytoin (Potential for hydantoin toxicity).
No products indexed under this heading.

Methotrexate Sodium (Potential for reduced tubular secretion of methotrexate and possible increased methotrexate toxicity as shown in animal model; caution is recommended).
No products indexed under this heading.

Methyclothiazide (Clinical studies, as well as postmarketing observations, have shown that Naproxen can reduce the natriuretic effect of furosemide and thiazides in some patients. Response has been attributed to inhibition of renal prostaglandin synthesis. Patients should be observed closely for signs of renal failure, as well as to assure diuretic efficacy).
No products indexed under this heading.

Metipranolol Hydrochloride (Reduced antihypertensive effect of beta blockers).
No products indexed under this heading.

Metoprolol Succinate (Reduced antihypertensive effect of beta blockers). Products include:
Toprol-XL Tablets ... 666

Metoprolol Tartrate (Reduced antihypertensive effect of beta blockers).
No products indexed under this heading.

Moexipril Hydrochloride (Reports suggest that NSAIDs may diminish the antihypertensive effect of ACE-inhibitors. The use of NSAIDs in patients who are receiving ACE-inhibitors may potentiate renal dise states).
No products indexed under this heading.

Nadolol (Reduced antihypertensive effect of beta blockers). Products include:
Nadolol Tablets ... 2191

Naproxen Sodium (Concurrent use of naproxen or naproxen sodium in any dosage form is not recommended since they all circulate in the plasma as the naproxen anion). Products include:
Anaprox Tablets ... 2632
Anaprox DS Tablets ... 2632
Treximet Tablets ... 1616

Nebivolol (Reduced antihypertensive effect of beta blockers). Products include:
Bystolic Tablets ... 1155

Nizatidine (Due to the gastric pH elevating effects of H_2-blockers concomitant administration of EC-Naprosyn is not recommended). Products include:
Axid Capsules ... 1364

Paroxetine Hydrochloride (There is an increased risk of GI bleeding when selective serotonin reuptake inhibitors (SSRIs) are combined with NSAIDs. Caution should be used when NSAIDs are administered concomitantly with SSRIs). Products include:
Paxil ... 1535
Paxil CR Controlled-Release Tablets ... 1544

Penbutolol Sulfate (Reduced antihypertensive effect of beta blockers).
No products indexed under this heading.

Perindopril Erbumine (Reports suggest that NSAIDs may diminish the antihypertensive effect of ACE-inhibitors. The use of NSAIDs in patients who are receiving ACE-inhibitors may potentiate renal dise states). Products include:
Aceon Tablets (2 mg, 4 mg, 8 mg) ... 3038

Phenytoin (Potential for hydantoin toxicity).
No products indexed under this heading.

Phenytoin Sodium (Potential for hydantoin toxicity). Products include:
Phenytek Capsules ... 2192

Pindolol (Reduced antihypertensive effect of beta blockers).
No products indexed under this heading.

Polythiazide (Clinical studies, as well as postmarketing observations, have shown that Naproxen can reduce the natriuretic effect of furosemide and thiazides in some patients. Response has been attributed to inhibition of renal prostaglandin synthesis. Patients should be observed closely for signs of renal failure, as well as to assure diuretic efficacy).
No products indexed under this heading.

Probenecid (Probenecid given concurrently increases naproxen anion plasma levels and extends its plasma half-life significantly).
No products indexed under this heading.

Propranolol Hydrochloride (Reduced antihypertensive effect of beta blockers). Products include:
InnoPran XL Extended Release Capsules ... 1484

Quinapril Hydrochloride (Reports suggest that NSAIDs may diminish the antihypertensive effect of ACE-inhibitors. The use of NSAIDs in patients who are receiving ACE-inhibitors may potentiate renal dise states).
No products indexed under this heading.

Ramipril (Reports suggest that NSAIDs may diminish the antihypertensive effect of ACE-inhibitors. The use of NSAIDs in patients who are receiving ACE-inhibitors may potentiate renal dise states).
No products indexed under this heading.

Ranitidine Bismuth Citrate (Due to the gastric pH elevating effects of H_2-blockers concomitant administration of EC-Naprosyn is not recommended).
No products indexed under this heading.

Ranitidine Hydrochloride (Due to the gastric pH elevating effects of H_2-blockers concomitant administration of EC-Naprosyn is not recommended). Products include:
Zantac 75 Tablets ... ▣603
Zantac ... 1670
Zantac Injection ... 1666
Zantac Injection Pharmacy Bulk Package ... 1668
Maximum Strength Zantac 150 Tablets ... ▣603
Maximum Strength Zantac 150 Cool Mint Tablets ... ▣603

Sertraline Hydrochloride (There is an increased risk of GI bleeding when selective serotonin reuptake inhibitors (SSRIs) are combined with NSAIDs. Caution should be used when NSAIDs are administered concomitantly with SSRIs).
No products indexed under this heading.

Sotalol Hydrochloride (Reduced antihypertensive effect of beta blockers).
No products indexed under this heading.

Spirapril Hydrochloride (Reports suggest that NSAIDs may diminish the antihypertensive effect of ACE-inhibitors. The use of NSAIDs in patients who are receiving ACE-inhibitors may potentiate renal dise states).
No products indexed under this heading.

Sucralfate (Due to the gastric pH elevating effects of sucralfate, concomitant administration of EC-Naprosyn is not recommended). Products include:
Carafate Suspension ... 706
Carafate Tablets ... 707

Sulfamethoxazole (Potential for sulfonamide toxicity).
No products indexed under this heading.

Sulfisoxazole Acetyl (Potential for sulfonamide toxicity).
No products indexed under this heading.

Timolol Hemihydrate (Reduced antihypertensive effect of beta blockers). Products include:
Betimol Ophthalmic Solution ... 3181

Timolol Maleate (Reduced antihypertensive effect of beta blockers). Products include:
Combigan Ophthalmic Solution ... 553
Cosopt Sterile Ophthalmic Solution ... 1969
Timoptic Sterile Ophthalmic Solution ... 2121
Timoptic in Ocudose ... 2124
Timoptic-XE Sterile Ophthalmic Gel Forming Solution ... 2125

Tolazamide (Potential for sulfonylurea toxicity).
No products indexed under this heading.

Tolbutamide (Potential for sulfonylurea toxicity).
No products indexed under this heading.

Trandolapril (Co-administration of NSAIDs and ACE inhibitors may potentiate renal disease states). Products include:
Mavik Tablets ... 472

Tarka Tablets 511

Warfarin Sodium (Short-term studies have failed to show any significant effect of concurrent use on prothrombin time; caution is advised since interactions have been seen with other NSAIDs).
No products indexed under this heading.

Food Interactions

Food, unspecified (The presence of food prolonged the time the EC-Naprosyn remained in the stomach, time to first detectable serum naproxen levels, and time to maximal naproxen levels (Tmax), but did not affect peak naproxen levels (Cmax)).

EDECRIN TABLETS

(Ethacrynic Acid) 698
See Edecrin Sodium Intravenous

EDECRIN SODIUM INTRAVENOUS

(Ethacrynate Sodium) 698
May interact with aminoglycosides, cephalosporins, cardiac glycosides, non-steroidal anti-inflammatory agents, and certain other agents. Compounds in these categories include:

Amikacin Sulfate (Increased ototoxic potential of aminoglycosides).
No products indexed under this heading.

Cefaclor (Increased ototoxic potential of cephalosporins).
No products indexed under this heading.

Cefadroxil (Increased ototoxic potential of cephalosporins).
No products indexed under this heading.

Cefamandole Nafate (Increased ototoxic potential of cephalosporins).
No products indexed under this heading.

Cefazolin Sodium (Increased ototoxic potential of cephalosporins).
No products indexed under this heading.

Cefdinir (Increased ototoxic potential of cephalosporins). Products include:
Omnicef Capsules 497
Omnicef for Oral Suspension 497

Cefepime Hydrochloride (Increased ototoxic potential of cephalosporins).
No products indexed under this heading.

Cefixime (Increased ototoxic potential of cephalosporins). Products include:
Suprax for Oral Suspension 1891
Suprax Tablets 1891

Cefmetazole Sodium (Increased ototoxic potential of cephalosporins).
No products indexed under this heading.

Cefonicid Sodium (Increased ototoxic potential of cephalosporins).
No products indexed under this heading.

Cefoperazone Sodium (Increased ototoxic potential of cephalosporins).
No products indexed under this heading.

Ceforanide (Increased ototoxic potential of cephalosporins).
No products indexed under this heading.

Cefotaxime Sodium (Increased ototoxic potential of cephalosporins).
No products indexed under this heading.

Cefotetan (Increased ototoxic potential of cephalosporins).
No products indexed under this heading.

Cefoxitin Sodium (Increased ototoxic potential of cephalosporins).
No products indexed under this heading.

Cefpodoxime Proxetil (Increased ototoxic potential of cephalosporins).
No products indexed under this heading.

Cefprozil (Increased ototoxic potential of cephalosporins).
No products indexed under this heading.

Ceftazidime (Increased ototoxic potential of cephalosporins). Products include:
Fortaz 1450

Ceftizoxime Sodium (Increased ototoxic potential of cephalosporins).
No products indexed under this heading.

Ceftriaxone Sodium (Increased ototoxic potential of cephalosporins). Products include:
Rocephin Injectable Vials, ADD-Vantage, Galaxy, Bulk........... 2642

Cefuroxime Axetil (Increased ototoxic potential of cephalosporins). Products include:
Ceftin 1380

Cefuroxime Sodium (Increased ototoxic potential of cephalosporins).
No products indexed under this heading.

Celecoxib (Reduces diuretic, natriuretic, and antihypertensive effects). Products include:
Celebrex Capsules 2979

Cephalexin (Increased ototoxic potential of cephalosporins).
No products indexed under this heading.

Cephalothin Sodium (Increased ototoxic potential of cephalosporins).
No products indexed under this heading.

Cephapirin Sodium (Increased ototoxic potential of cephalosporins).
No products indexed under this heading.

Cephradine (Increased ototoxic potential of cephalosporins).
No products indexed under this heading.

Deslanoside (Excessive potassium loss may precipitate digitalis toxicity).
No products indexed under this heading.

Diclofenac Epolamine (Reduces diuretic, natriuretic, and antihypertensive effects). Products include:
Flector Patch 561

Diclofenac Potassium (Reduces diuretic, natriuretic, and antihypertensive effects).
No products indexed under this heading.

Diclofenac Sodium (Reduces diuretic, natriuretic, and antihypertensive effects). Products include:
Diclofenac Sodium Ophthalmic Solution...................................... ⊙240
Voltaren Ophthalmic Solution 2336
Voltaren Tablets 2334
Voltaren-XR Tablets 2337

Digitalis Glycoside Preparations (Excessive potassium loss may precipitate digitalis toxicity).
No products indexed under this heading.

Digitoxin (Excessive potassium loss may precipitate digitalis toxicity).
No products indexed under this heading.

Digoxin (Excessive potassium loss may precipitate digitalis toxicity). Products include:
Lanoxin Injection 1498
Lanoxin Injection Pediatric 1502
Lanoxin Tablets 1505

Etodolac (Reduces diuretic, natriuretic, and antihypertensive effects).
No products indexed under this heading.

Fenoprofen Calcium (Reduces diuretic, natriuretic, and antihypertensive effects). Products include:
Nalfon Capsules 2508

Flurbiprofen (Reduces diuretic, natriuretic, and antihypertensive effects).
No products indexed under this heading.

Gentamicin Sulfate (Increased ototoxic potential of aminoglycosides). Products include:
Pred-G Ophthalmic Ointment .... ⊙229
Pred-G Ophthalmic Suspension ...... ⊙228

Ibuprofen (Reduces diuretic, natriuretic, and antihypertensive effects). Products include:
Motrin IB Tablets and Caplets 1900
Children's Motrin Oral Suspension ... 1901
Children's Motrin Non-Staining Dye-Free Oral Suspension............ 1901
Children's Motrin Cold Oral Suspension...................................... 1899
Infants' Motrin Concentrated Drops.. 1901
Infants' Motrin Non-Staining Dye-Free Concentrated Drops....... 1901
Junior Strength Motrin Caplets and Chewable Tablets.................... 1901
Vicoprofen Tablets 533

Indomethacin (Reduces diuretic, natriuretic, and antihypertensive effects). Products include:
Indocin 2024

Indomethacin Sodium Trihydrate (Reduces diuretic, natriuretic, and antihypertensive effects). Products include:
Indocin I.V. 2489

Isoproterenol Hydrochloride (Careful adjustment of dosages required).
No products indexed under this heading.

Kanamycin Sulfate (Increased ototoxic potential of aminoglycosides).
No products indexed under this heading.

Ketoprofen (Reduces diuretic, natriuretic, and antihypertensive effects).
No products indexed under this heading.

Ketorolac Tromethamine (Reduces diuretic, natriuretic, and antihypertensive effects).
No products indexed under this heading.

Lithium Carbonate (High risk of lithium toxicity).
No products indexed under this heading.

Lithium Citrate (High risk of lithium toxicity).
No products indexed under this heading.

Loracarbef (Increased ototoxic potential of cephalosporins).
No products indexed under this heading.

Meclofenamate Sodium (Reduces diuretic, natriuretic, and antihypertensive effects).
No products indexed under this heading.

Mefenamic Acid (Reduces diuretic, natriuretic, and antihypertensive effects).
No products indexed under this heading.

Meloxicam (Reduces diuretic, natriuretic, and antihypertensive effects). Products include:
Mobic Oral Suspension 863
Mobic Tablets 863

Nabumetone (Reduces diuretic, natriuretic, and antihypertensive effects).
No products indexed under this heading.

Naproxen (Reduces diuretic, natriuretic, and antihypertensive effects). Products include:
EC-Naprosyn Delayed-Release Tablets.. 2632
Naprosyn Suspension 2632
Naprosyn Tablets 2632

Naproxen Sodium (Reduces diuretic, natriuretic, and antihypertensive effects). Products include:
Anaprox Tablets 2632
Anaprox DS Tablets 2632
Treximet Tablets 1616

Oxaprozin (Reduces diuretic, natriuretic, and antihypertensive effects).
No products indexed under this heading.

Phenylbutazone (Reduces diuretic, natriuretic, and antihypertensive effects).
No products indexed under this heading.

Piroxicam (Reduces diuretic, natriuretic, and antihypertensive effects).
No products indexed under this heading.

Rofecoxib (Reduces diuretic, natriuretic, and antihypertensive effects).
No products indexed under this heading.

Streptomycin Sulfate (Increased ototoxic potential of aminoglycosides).
No products indexed under this heading.

Sulindac (Reduces diuretic, natriuretic, and antihypertensive effects). Products include:
Clinoril Tablets 1962

Tobramycin (Increased ototoxic potential of aminoglycosides). Products include:
Zylet Ophthalmic Suspension .... ⊙247

Tobramycin Sulfate (Increased ototoxic potential of aminoglycosides).
No products indexed under this heading.

Tolmetin Sodium (Reduces diuretic, natriuretic, and antihypertensive effects).
No products indexed under this heading.

Valdecoxib (Reduces diuretic, natriuretic, and antihypertensive effects).
No products indexed under this heading.

Warfarin Sodium (Warfarin displaced from plasma protein; reduction in warfarin dosage may be required).
No products indexed under this heading.

EDEX INJECTION
(Alprostadil) 2957
May interact with:

Dalteparin Sodium (The pharmacodynamic interaction between heparin (5,000 IU) and alprostadil intravenous infusion (90 mcg over 3 hours) was investigated. The results indicate significant changes in partial thromboplastin time (140% increase) and thrombint ime (120% increase). Therefore, caution should be exercised with concomitant administration of heparin and alprostadil).
Products include:
Fragmin Injection 1070

Enoxaparin Sodium (The pharmacodynamic interaction between heparin (5,000 IU) and alprostadil intravenous infusion (90 mcg over 3 hours) was investigated. The results indicate significant changes in partial thromboplastin time (140% increase) and thrombint ime (120% increase). Therefore, caution should be exercised with concomitant administration of heparin and alprostadil).
Products include:
Lovenox Injection 2756

Heparin (The pharmacodynamic interaction between heparin (5,000 IU) and alprostadil intravenous infusion (90 mcg over 3 hours) was investigated. The results indicate significant changes in partial thromboplastin time (140% increase) and thrombint ime (120% increase). Therefore, caution should be exercised with concomitant administration of heparin and alprostadil).
No products indexed under this heading.

Heparin Calcium (The pharmacodynamic interaction between heparin (5,000 IU) and alprostadil intravenous infusion (90 mcg over 3 hours) was investigated. The results indicate significant changes in partial thromboplastin time (140% increase) and thrombint ime (120% increase). Therefore, caution should be exercised with concomitant administration of heparin and alprostadil).
No products indexed under this heading.

Heparin Sodium (The pharmacodynamic interaction between heparin (5,000 IU) and alprostadil intravenous infusion (90 mcg over 3 hours) was investigated. The results indicate significant changes in partial thromboplastin time (140% increase) and thrombin time (120% increase). Therefore, caution should be exercised with concomitant administration of heparin and alprostadil).
No products indexed under this heading.

Low Molecular Weight Heparins (The pharmacodynamic interaction between heparin (5,000 IU) and alprostadil intravenous infusion (90 mcg over 3 hours) was investigated. The results indicate significant changes in partial thromboplastin time (140% increase) and thrombint ime (120% increase). Therefore, caution should be exercised with concomitant administration of heparin and alprostadil).
No products indexed under this heading.

E.E.S. 200 LIQUID
(Erythromycin Ethylsuccinate) 433
See E.E.S. 400 Filmtab Tablets

E.E.S. 400 LIQUID
(Erythromycin Ethylsuccinate) 433
See E.E.S. 400 Filmtab Tablets

E.E.S. 400 FILMTAB TABLETS
(Erythromycin Ethylsuccinate) 433
May interact with oral anticoagulants, HMG-CoA reductase inhibitors, phenytoin, triazolobenzodiazepines, valproate, xanthines, and certain other agents. Compounds in these categories include:

Alfentanil Hydrochloride (Concurrent use of erythromycin in patients receiving drugs metabolized by the cytochrome P450 system may be associated with elevation in serum levels of alfentanil).
No products indexed under this heading.

Alprazolam (Erythromycin has been reported to decrease the clearance of triazolam and midazolam; may increase the pharmacologic effect of these benzodiazepines).
No products indexed under this heading.

Aminophylline (Co-administration in patients who are receiving high doses of theophylline may be associated with an increase in serum theophylline levels and potential theophylline toxicity).
No products indexed under this heading.

Anisindione (Co-administration has resulted in increased anticoagulant effects).
No products indexed under this heading.

Astemizole (Concurrent use of erythromycin in patients receiving astemizole has been reported to significantly alter the metabolism of astemizole; rare cases of cardiovascular adverse events, including prolonged QT interval, cardiac arrest, torsade de pointes, and other ventricular arrhythmias have been reported; co-administration is contraindicated).
No products indexed under this heading.

Atorvastatin Calcium (Erythromycin has been reported to increase concentrations of HMG-CoA reductase inhibitors (e.g. lovastatin and simvastatin); rare reports of rhabdomyolysis have been reported in patients taking these drugs concomitantly). Products include:
Lipitor Tablets 2501

Bromocriptine Mesylate (Concurrent use of erythromycin in patients receiving drugs metabolized by the cytochrome P450 system may be associated with elevation in serum levels of bromocriptine).
No products indexed under this heading.

Carbamazepine (Concurrent use of erythromycin in patients receiving drugs metabolized by the cytochrome P450 system may be associated with elevation in serum levels of carbamazepine). Products include:
Carbatrol Capsules 3019
Equetro Extended-Release Capsules 3174

Cerivastatin Sodium (Erythromycin has been reported to increase concentrations of HMG-CoA reductase inhibitors (e.g. lovastatin and simvastatin); rare reports of rhabdomyolysis have been reported in patients taking these drugs concomitantly).
No products indexed under this heading.

Cisapride (Concurrent use of erythromycin in patients receiving cisapride has been reported to inhibit the metabolism of cisapride; cases of cardiovascular adverse events, including prolonged QT interval, torsade de pointes, ventricular tachycardia, and ventricular fibrillation have been reported; co-administration is contraindicated).
No products indexed under this heading.

Cyclosporine (Concurrent use of erythromycin in patients receiving drugs metabolized by the cytochrome P450 system may be associated with elevation in serum levels of cyclosporine). Products include:
Gengraf Capsules 435
Neoral Oral Solution 2280
Neoral Soft Gelatin Capsules 2280
Restasis Ophthalmic Emulsion 557
Sandimmune 2296

Dicumarol (Co-administration has resulted in increased anticoagulant effects).
No products indexed under this heading.

Digoxin (Co-administration has been reported to result in elevated digoxin serum levels). Products include:
Lanoxin Injection 1498
Lanoxin Injection Pediatric 1502
Lanoxin Tablets 1505

Dihydroergotamine Mesylate (Co-administration has been associated in some patients with acute ergot toxicity characterized by severe peripheral vasospasm and dysesthesia).
No products indexed under this heading.

Disopyramide Phosphate (Concurrent use of erythromycin in patients receiving drugs metabolized by the cytochrome P450 system may be associated with elevation in serum levels of disopyramide).
No products indexed under this heading.

Divalproex Sodium (There have been reports of interactions of erythromycin with drugs not thought to be metabolized by CYP3A, including valproate). Products include:
Depakote ER Tablets 423

Dyphylline (Co-administration in patients who are receiving high doses of theophylline may be associated with an increase in serum theophylline levels and potential theophylline toxicity).
No products indexed under this heading.

Ergotamine Tartrate (Co-administration has been associated in some patients with acute ergot toxicity characterized by severe peripheral vasospasm and dysesthesia).
No products indexed under this heading.

Fluvastatin Sodium (Erythromycin has been reported to increase concentrations of HMG-CoA reductase inhibitors (e.g. lovastatin and simvastatin); rare reports of rhabdomyolysis have been reported in patients taking these drugs concomitantly).
Products include:
Lescol Capsules 2268
Lescol XL Tablets 2268

Fosphenytoin Sodium (There have been reports of interactions of erythromycin with drugs not thought to be metabolized by CYP3A, including phenytoin).
No products indexed under this heading.

Hexobarbital (There have been reports of interactions of erythromycin with drugs not thought to be metabolized by CYP3A, including hexobarbital).
No products indexed under this heading.

Lovastatin (Erythromycin has been reported to increase concentrations of HMG-CoA reductase inhibitors (e.g. lovastatin and simvastatin); rare reports of rhabdomyolysis have been reported in patients taking these drugs concomitantly).
Products include:
Advicor Tablets 402
Mevacor Tablets 2063

Midazolam Hydrochloride (Erythromycin has been reported to decrease the clearance of triazolam and midazolam; may increase the pharmacologic effect of these benzodiazepines).
No products indexed under this heading.

Phenytoin (There have been reports of interactions of erythromycin with drugs not thought to be metabolized by CYP3A, including phenytoin).
No products indexed under this heading.

Phenytoin Sodium (There have been reports of interactions of erythromycin with drugs not thought to be metabolized by CYP3A, including phenytoin). Products include:
Phenytek Capsules 2192

Pimozide (Concurrent use of erythromycin in patients receiving drugs metabolized by the cytochrome P450 system may be associated with elevation in serum levels of pimozide; co-administration is contraindicated).
No products indexed under this heading.

Pravastatin Sodium (Erythromycin has been reported to increase concentrations of HMG-CoA reductase inhibitors (e.g. lovastatin and simvastatin); rare reports of rhabdomyolysis have been reported in patients taking these drugs concomitantly).
No products indexed under this heading.

Rosuvastatin Calcium (Erythromycin has been reported to increase concentrations of HMG-CoA reductase inhibitors (e.g. lovastatin and simvastatin); rare reports of rhabdomyolysis have been reported in patients taking these drugs concomitantly). Products include:
Crestor Tablets 677

Sildenafil Citrate (Erythromycin has been reported to increase the systemic exposure (AUC) of sildenafil).
No products indexed under this heading.

Simvastatin (Erythromycin has been reported to increase concentrations of HMG-CoA reductase inhibitors (e.g. lovastatin and simvastatin); rare reports of rhabdomyolysis have been reported in patients taking these drugs concomitantly). Products include:

- Simcor Tablets ... 502
- Vytorin 10/10 Tablets ... 2149
- Vytorin 10/10 Tablets ... 2939
- Vytorin 10/20 Tablets ... 2149
- Vytorin 10/20 Tablets ... 2939
- Vytorin 10/40 Tablets ... 2149
- Vytorin 10/40 Tablets ... 2939
- Vytorin 10/80 Tablets ... 2149
- Vytorin 10/80 Tablets ... 2939
- Zocor Tablets ... 2136

Tacrolimus (Concurrent use of erythromycin in patients receiving drugs metabolized by the cytochrome P450 system may be associated with elevation in serum levels of tacrolimus). Products include:

- Prograf Capsules and Injection ... 622
- Protopic Ointment ... 628

Terfenadine (Concurrent use of erythromycin in patients receiving terfenadine has been reported to significantly alter the metabolism of terfenadine; rare cases of cardiovascular adverse events, including prolonged QT interval, cardiac arrest, torsade de pointes, other ventricular arrhythmias, and death have been reported; co-administration is contraindicated).
No products indexed under this heading.

Theophylline (Co-administration in patients who are receiving high doses of theophylline may be associated with an increase in serum theophylline levels and potential theophylline toxicity).
No products indexed under this heading.

Theophylline Anhydrous (Co-administration in patients who are receiving high doses of theophylline may be associated with an increase in serum theophylline levels and potential theophylline toxicity). Products include:

- Uniphyl Tablets ... 2595

Theophylline Calcium Salicylate (Co-administration in patients who are receiving high doses of theophylline may be associated with an increase in serum theophylline levels and potential theophylline toxicity).
No products indexed under this heading.

Theophylline Dihydroxypropyl (Glyceryl) (Co-administration in patients who are receiving high doses of theophylline may be associated with an increase in serum theophylline levels and potential theophylline toxicity).
No products indexed under this heading.

Theophylline Ethylenediamine (Co-administration in patients who are receiving high doses of theophylline may be associated with an increase in serum theophylline levels and potential theophylline toxicity).
No products indexed under this heading.

Theophylline Sodium Glycinate (Co-administration in patients who are receiving high doses of theophylline may be associated with an increase in serum theophylline levels and potential theophylline toxicity).
No products indexed under this heading.

Triazolam (Erythromycin has been reported to decrease the clearance of triazolam and, thus, may increase the pharmacologic effect of the benzodiazepine).
No products indexed under this heading.

Valproate Sodium (There have been reports of interactions of erythromycin with drugs not thought to be metabolized by CYP3A, including valproate).
No products indexed under this heading.

Valproic Acid (There have been reports of interactions of erythromycin with drugs not thought to be metabolized by CYP3A, including valproate).
No products indexed under this heading.

Warfarin Sodium (Co-administration has resulted in increased anticoagulant effects).
No products indexed under this heading.

E.E.S. GRANULES

(Erythromycin Ethylsuccinate) ... 433
See E.E.S. 400 Filmtab Tablets

EFACOR DIETARY SUPPLEMENT

(Dietary Supplement, Docosahexaenoic Acid (DHA), Eicosapentaenoic Acid (EPA), Essential Fatty Acids, Fish Oils, Omega-3 Acids) ... 626
None cited in PDR database.

EFFEXOR XR EXTENDED-RELEASE CAPSULES

(Venlafaxine Hydrochloride) ... 3195
May interact with 5HT1-receptor agonists, aspirin-acetylsalicylic acid, central nervous system depressants, central nervous system stimulants, cytochrome p450 3a4 inhibitors (selected), diuretics, monoamine oxidase inhibitors, nonsteroidal anti-inflammatory agents, quinidine, selective serotonin reuptake inhibitors, and certain other agents. Compounds in these categories include:

5-hydroxytryptophan (Caution is advised when velafaxine is co-administered with other drugs that may affect serotonergic neurotransmitter systems).
No products indexed under this heading.

Acetazolamide (Concomitant use of CYP3A4 inhibitors and venlafaxine may increase levels of venlafaxine and O-desmethylvenlafaxine (ODV). Therefore, caution is advised if venlafaxine is used concomitantly with CYP3A4 inhibitors).
No products indexed under this heading.

Alfentanil Hydrochloride (Caution is advised if the concomitant administration of venlafaxine and CNS-active drugs is required).
No products indexed under this heading.

Almotriptan Malate (Based on the mechanism of action of venlafaxine and the potential for serotonin syndrome, caution is advised when velafaxine is co-administered with other drugs that may affect the serotonergic neurotransmitter systems, such as triptans). Products include:

- Axert Tablets ... 2431

Alprazolam (Caution is advised if the concomitant administration of venlafaxine and CNS-active drugs is required).
No products indexed under this heading.

Amiloride Hydrochloride (Hyponatremia may occur as a result of treatment with SSRIs and SNRIs, including venlafaxine hydrochloride. In many cases, this hyponatremia appears to be the result of the syndrome of inappropriate antidiuretic hormone secretion (SIADH). Patients taking diuretics or who are otherwise volume depleted may be at greater risk. Discontinuation of venlafaxine hydrochloride should be considered in patients with symptomatic hyponatremia and appropriate medical intervention should be instituted).
No products indexed under this heading.

Amiodarone Hydrochloride (Concomitant use of CYP3A4 inhibitors and venlafaxine may increase levels of venlafaxine and O-desmethylvenlafaxine (ODV). Therefore, caution is advised if venlafaxine is used concomitantly with CYP3A4 inhibitors).
No products indexed under this heading.

Amphetamine Resins (Caution is advised if the concomitant administration of venlafaxine and CNS-active drugs is required).
No products indexed under this heading.

Amprenavir (Concomitant use of CYP3A4 inhibitors and venlafaxine may increase levels of venlafaxine and O-desmethylvenlafaxine (ODV). Therefore, caution is advised if venlafaxine is used concomitantly with CYP3A4 inhibitors).
No products indexed under this heading.

Anastrozole (Concomitant use of CYP3A4 inhibitors and venlafaxine may increase levels of venlafaxine and O-desmethylvenlafaxine (ODV). Therefore, caution is advised if venlafaxine is used concomitantly with CYP3A4 inhibitors). Products include:

- Arimidex Tablets ... 672

Aprepitant (Concomitant use of CYP3A4 inhibitors and venlafaxine may increase levels of venlafaxine and O-desmethylvenlafaxine (ODV). Therefore, caution is advised if venlafaxine is used concomitantly with CYP3A4 inhibitors). Products include:

- Emend Capsules ... 1992

Aprobarbital (Caution is advised if the concomitant administration of venlafaxine and CNS-active drugs is required).
No products indexed under this heading.

Aspirin (Use of venlafaxine may increase the risk of bleeding events. Concomitant use of aspirin may potentiate the risk of bleeding. Case reports and studies have shown an association between use of drugs that interfere with serotonin reuptake and the occurrence of gastrointestinal bleeding. Bleeding events related to SSRIs and SNRIs used have ranged from ecchymoses, hematomas, epistaxis, and petechiae to life-threatening hemorrhages. Caution about the risk of bleeding associated with the concomitant use of venlafaxine and aspirin should be taken). Products include:

- Aggrenox Capsules ... 819
- Bayer Aspirin ... 750
- Percodan Tablets ... 1130
- St. Joseph 81 mg Aspirin Chewable and Enteric Coated Tablets ... 1903

Aspirin, Enteric Coated (Use of venlafaxine may increase the risk of bleeding events. Concomitant use of aspirin may potentiate the risk of bleeding. Case reports and studies have shown an association between use of drugs that interfere with serotonin reuptake and the occurrence of gastrointestinal bleeding. Bleeding events related to SSRIs and SNRIs used have ranged from ecchymoses, hematomas, epistaxis, and petechiae to life-threatening hemorrhages. Caution about the risk of bleeding associated with the concomitant use of venlafaxine and aspirin should be taken).
No products indexed under this heading.

Aspirin Buffered (Use of venlafaxine may increase the risk of bleeding events. Concomitant use of aspirin may potentiate the risk of bleeding. Case reports and studies have shown an association between use of drugs that interfere with serotonin reuptake and the occurrence of gastrointestinal bleeding. Bleeding events related to SSRIs and SNRIs used have ranged from ecchymoses, hematomas, epistaxis, and petechiae to life-threatening hemorrhages. Caution about the risk of bleeding associated with the concomitant use of venlafaxine and aspirin should be taken).
No products indexed under this heading.

Atazanavir (Concomitant use of CYP3A4 inhibitors and venlafaxine may increase levels of venlafaxine and O-desmethylvenlafaxine (ODV). Therefore, caution is advised if venlafaxine is used concomitantly with CYP3A4 inhibitors).
No products indexed under this heading.

Atazanavir Sulfate (Concomitant use of CYP3A4 inhibitors and venlafaxine may increase levels of venlafaxine and O-desmethylvenlafaxine (ODV). Therefore, caution is advised if venlafaxine is used concomitantly with CYP3A4 inhibitors). Products include:

- Reyataz Capsules ... 3299

Bendroflumethiazide (Hyponatremia may occur as a result of treatment with SSRIs and SNRIs, including venlafaxine hydrochloride. In many cases, this hyponatremia appears to be the result of the syndrome of inappropriate antidiuretic hormone secretion (SIADH). Patients taking diuretics or who are otherwise volume depleted may be at greater risk. Discontinuation of venlafaxine hydrochloride should be considered in patients with symptomatic hyponatremia and appropriate medical intervention should be instituted).
No products indexed under this heading.

Bumetanide (Hyponatremia may occur as a result of treatment with SSRIs and SNRIs, including venlafaxine hydrochloride. In many cases, this hyponatremia appears to be the result of the syndrome of inappropri-

ate antidiuretic hormone secretion (SIADH). Patients taking diuretics or who are otherwise volume depleted may be at greater risk. Discontinuation of venlafaxine hydrochloride should be considered in patients with symptomatic hyponatremia and appropriate medical intervention should be instituted).
No products indexed under this heading.

Buprenorphine Hydrochloride (Caution is advised if the concomitant administration of venlafaxine and CNS-active drugs is required). Products include:
Suboxone Tablets 2601
Subutex Tablets 2601

Buspirone Hydrochloride (Caution is advised if the concomitant administration of venlafaxine and CNS-active drugs is required).
No products indexed under this heading.

Butabarbital (Caution is advised if the concomitant administration of venlafaxine and CNS-active drugs is required).
No products indexed under this heading.

Butalbital (Caution is advised if the concomitant administration of venlafaxine and CNS-active drugs is required).
No products indexed under this heading.

Celecoxib (Use of venlafaxine may increase the risk of bleeding events. Concomitant use of nonsteroidal anti-inflammatory drugs (NSAIDs) may potentiate this risk of bleeding. Case reports and studies have shown an association between use of drugs that interfere with serotonin reuptake and the occurrence of gastrointestinal bleeding. Bleeding events related to SSRIs and SNRIs used have ranged from ecchymoses, hematomas, epistaxis and petechiae to life-threatening hemorrhages. Caution about the risk of bleeding associated with the concomitant use of venlafaxine and NSAIDs should be taken). Products include:
Celebrex Capsules 2979

Chlordiazepoxide (Caution is advised if the concomitant administration of venlafaxine and CNS-active drugs is required).
No products indexed under this heading.

Chlordiazepoxide Hydrochloride (Caution is advised if the concomitant administration of venlafaxine and CNS-active drugs is required).
No products indexed under this heading.

Chlorothiazide (Hyponatremia may occur as a result of treatment with SSRIs and SNRIs, including venlafaxine hydrochloride. In many cases, this hyponatremia appears to be the result of the syndrome of inappropriate antidiuretic hormone secretion (SIADH). Patients taking diuretics or who are otherwise volume depleted may be at greater risk. Discontinuation of venlafaxine hydrochloride should be considered in patients with symptomatic hyponatremia and appropriate medical intervention should be instituted).
No products indexed under this heading.

Chlorothiazide Sodium (Hyponatremia may occur as a result of treatment with SSRIs and SNRIs, including venlafaxine hydrochloride. In many cases, this hyponatremia appears to be the result of the syndrome of inappropriate antidiuretic hormone secretion (SIADH). Patients taking diuretics or who are otherwise volume depleted may be at greater risk. Discontinuation of venlafaxine hydrochloride should be considered in patients with symptomatic hyponatremia and appropriate medical intervention should be instituted). Products include:
Intravenous Sodium Diuril 2490

Chlorpromazine (Caution is advised if the concomitant administration of venlafaxine and CNS-active drugs is required).
No products indexed under this heading.

Chlorpromazine Hydrochloride (Caution is advised if the concomitant administration of venlafaxine and CNS-active drugs is required).
No products indexed under this heading.

Chlorprothixene (Caution is advised if the concomitant administration of venlafaxine and CNS-active drugs is required).
No products indexed under this heading.

Chlorprothixene Hydrochloride (Caution is advised if the concomitant administration of venlafaxine and CNS-active drugs is required).
No products indexed under this heading.

Chlorprothixene Lactate (Caution is advised if the concomitant administration of venlafaxine and CNS-active drugs is required).
No products indexed under this heading.

Chlorthalidone (Hyponatremia may occur as a result of treatment with SSRIs and SNRIs, including venlafaxine hydrochloride. In many cases, this hyponatremia appears to be the result of the syndrome of inappropriate antidiuretic hormone secretion (SIADH). Patients taking diuretics or who are otherwise volume depleted may be at greater risk. Discontinuation of venlafaxine hydrochloride should be considered in patients with symptomatic hyponatremia and appropriate medical intervention should be instituted). Products include:
Clorpres Tablets 2185

Cimetidine (Co-administration in a steady-state study for both drugs has resulted in inhibition of first-pass metabolism of venlafaxine; the oral clearance of venlafaxine was reduced by 43% and AUC and Cmax were increased by about 60%).
No products indexed under this heading.

Cimetidine Hydrochloride (Co-administration in a steady-state study for both drugs has resulted in inhibition of first-pass metabolism of venlafaxine; the oral clearance of venlafaxine was reduced by 43% and AUC and Cmax were increased by about 60%).
No products indexed under this heading.

Ciprofloxacin (Concomitant use of CYP3A4 inhibitors and venlafaxine may increase levels of venlafaxine and O-desmethylvenlafaxine (ODV). Therefore, caution is advised if venlafaxine is used concomitantly with CYP3A4 inhibitors). Products include:
Cipro I.V. 2817
Cipro Oral Suspension 2810
Cipro XR Tablets 2823
Ciprodex Otic Suspension 541

Citalopram Hydrobromide (Based on the mechanism of action of venlafaxine and the potential for serotonin syndrome, caution is advised when velafaxine is co-administered with other drugs that may affect the serotonergic neurotransmitter systems, such as serotonin reuptake inhibitors). Products include:
Celexa 1160

Clarithromycin (Concomitant use of CYP3A4 inhibitors and venlafaxine may increase levels of venlafaxine and O-desmethylvenlafaxine (ODV). Therefore, caution is advised if venlafaxine is used concomitantly with CYP3A4 inhibitors). Products include:
Biaxin/Biaxin XL 411

Clorazepate Dipotassium (Caution is advised if the concomitant administration of venlafaxine and CNS-active drugs is required).
No products indexed under this heading.

Clotrimazole (Concomitant use of CYP3A4 inhibitors and venlafaxine may increase levels of venlafaxine and O-desmethylvenlafaxine (ODV). Therefore, caution is advised if venlafaxine is used concomitantly with CYP3A4 inhibitors). Products include:
Lotrisone 2881

Clozapine (There have been reports of elevated clozapine levels that were temporarily associated with adverse events including seizures, following the addition of venlafaxine).
No products indexed under this heading.

Codeine Phosphate (Caution is advised if the concomitant administration of venlafaxine and CNS-active drugs is required). Products include:
Tylenol with Codeine Tablets 2427

Cyclosporine (Concomitant use of CYP3A4 inhibitors and venlafaxine may increase levels of venlafaxine and O-desmethylvenlafaxine (ODV). Therefore, caution is advised if venlafaxine is used concomitantly with CYP3A4 inhibitors). Products include:
Gengraf Capsules 435
Neoral Oral Solution 2280
Neoral Soft Gelatin Capsules 2280
Restasis Ophthalmic Emulsion 557
Sandimmune 2296

Dalfopristin (Concomitant use of CYP3A4 inhibitors and venlafaxine may increase levels of venlafaxine and O-desmethylvenlafaxine (ODV). Therefore, caution is advised if venlafaxine is used concomitantly with CYP3A4 inhibitors).
No products indexed under this heading.

Danazol (Concomitant use of CYP3A4 inhibitors and venlafaxine may increase levels of venlafaxine and O-desmethylvenlafaxine (ODV). Therefore, caution is advised if venlafaxine is used concomitantly with CYP3A4 inhibitors).
No products indexed under this heading.

Delavirdine Mesylate (Concomitant use of CYP3A4 inhibitors and venlafaxine may increase levels of venlafaxine and O-desmethylvenlafaxine (ODV). Therefore, caution is advised if venlafaxine is used concomitantly with CYP3A4 inhibitors).
No products indexed under this heading.

Desflurane (Caution is advised if the concomitant administration of venlafaxine and CNS-active drugs is required).
No products indexed under this heading.

Desipramine Hydrochloride (Based on the mechanism of action of venlafaxine and the potential for serotonin syndrome, caution is advised when venlafaxine is co-administered with other drugs that may affect serotonergic neurotransmitter systems, such as serotonin-norepinephrine reuptake inhibitors).
No products indexed under this heading.

Dextroamphetamine Sulfate (Caution is advised if the concomitant administration of venlafaxine and CNS-active drugs is required). Products include:
Adderall XR Capsules 3012
Dexedrine 1401

Dezocine (Caution is advised if the concomitant administration of venlafaxine and CNS-active drugs is required).
No products indexed under this heading.

Diazepam (Caution is advised if the concomitant administration of venlafaxine and CNS-active drugs is required). Products include:
Valium Tablets 2658

Diclofenac Epolamine (Use of venlafaxine may increase the risk of bleeding events. Concomitant use of nonsteroidal anti-inflammatory drugs (NSAIDs) may potentiate this risk of bleeding. Case reports and studies have shown an association between use of drugs that interfere with serotonin reuptake and the occurrence of gastrointestinal bleeding. Bleeding events related to SSRIs and SNRIs used have ranged from ecchymoses, hematomas, epistaxis and petechiae to life-threatening hemorrhages. Caution about the risk of bleeding associated with the concomitant use of venlafaxine and NSAIDs should be taken). Products include:
Flector Patch 561

Diclofenac Potassium (Use of venlafaxine may increase the risk of bleeding events. Concomitant use of nonsteroidal anti-inflammatory drugs (NSAIDs) may potentiate this risk of bleeding. Case reports and studies have shown an association between use of drugs that interfere with serotonin reuptake and the occurrence of gastrointestinal bleeding. Bleeding events related to SSRIs and SNRIs used have ranged from ecchymoses, hematomas, epistaxis and petechiae to life-threatening hemorrhages. Caution about the risk of bleeding associated with the concomitant use of venlafaxine and NSAIDs should be taken).
No products indexed under this heading.

Diclofenac Sodium (Use of venlafaxine may increase the risk of

bleeding events. Concomitant use of nonsteroidal anti-inflammatory drugs (NSAIDs) may potentiate this risk of bleeding. Case reports and studies have shown an association between use of drugs that interfere with serotonin reuptake and the occurrence of gastrointestinal bleeding. Bleeding events related to SSRIs and SNRIs used have ranged from ecchymoses, hematomas, epistaxis and petechiae to life-threatening hemorrhages. Caution about the risk of bleeding associated with the concomitant use of venlafaxine and NSAIDs should be taken). Products include:

Diclofenac Sodium Ophthalmic Solution .... ⊙ 240
Voltaren Ophthalmic Solution 2336
Voltaren Tablets 2334
Voltaren-XR Tablets 2337

Diltiazem Hydrochloride (Concomitant use of CYP3A4 inhibitors and venlafaxine may increase levels of venlafaxine and O-desmethylvenlafaxine (ODV). Therefore, caution is advised if venlafaxine is used concomitantly with CYP3A4 inhibitors). Products include:

Cardizem LA Extended Release Tablets 421

Diltiazem Maleate (Concomitant use of CYP3A4 inhibitors and venlafaxine may increase levels of venlafaxine and O-desmethylvenlafaxine (ODV). Therefore, caution is advised if venlafaxine is used concomitantly with CYP3A4 inhibitors).

No products indexed under this heading.

Droperidol (Caution is advised if the concomitant administration of venlafaxine and CNS-active drugs is required).

No products indexed under this heading.

Duloxetine Hydrochloride (Based on the mechanism of action of venlafaxine and the potential for serotonin syndrome, caution is advised when venlafaxine is co-administered with other drugs that may affect serotonergic neurotransmitter systems, such as serotonin-norepinephrine reuptake inhibitors). Products include:

Cymbalta Delayed-Release Capsules 1801

Efavirenz (Concomitant use of CYP3A4 inhibitors and venlafaxine may increase levels of venlafaxine and O-desmethylvenlafaxine (ODV). Therefore, caution is advised if venlafaxine is used concomitantly with CYP3A4 inhibitors). Products include:

Atripla Tablets 938
Sustiva Capsules 930
Sustiva Tablets 930

Eletriptan Hydrobromide (Based on the mechanism of action of venlafaxine and the potential for serotonin syndrome, caution is advised when velafaxine is co-administered with other drugs that may affect the serotonergic neurotransmitter systems, such as triptans).

No products indexed under this heading.

Enflurane (Caution is advised if the concomitant administration of venlafaxine and CNS-active drugs is required).

No products indexed under this heading.

Erythromycin (Concomitant use of CYP3A4 inhibitors and venlafaxine may increase levels of venlafaxine and O-desmethylvenlafaxine (ODV). Therefore, caution is advised if venlafaxine is used concomitantly with CYP3A4 inhibitors).

No products indexed under this heading.

Erythromycin Estolate (Concomitant use of CYP3A4 inhibitors and venlafaxine may increase levels of venlafaxine and O-desmethylvenlafaxine (ODV). Therefore, caution is advised if venlafaxine is used concomitantly with CYP3A4 inhibitors).

No products indexed under this heading.

Erythromycin Ethylsuccinate (Concomitant use of CYP3A4 inhibitors and venlafaxine may increase levels of venlafaxine and O-desmethylvenlafaxine (ODV). Therefore, caution is advised if venlafaxine is used concomitantly with CYP3A4 inhibitors). Products include:

E.E.S. 433
EryPed 431

Erythromycin Gluceptate (Concomitant use of CYP3A4 inhibitors and venlafaxine may increase levels of venlafaxine and O-desmethylvenlafaxine (ODV). Therefore, caution is advised if venlafaxine is used concomitantly with CYP3A4 inhibitors).

No products indexed under this heading.

Erythromycin Lactobionate (Concomitant use of CYP3A4 inhibitors and venlafaxine may increase levels of venlafaxine and O-desmethylvenlafaxine (ODV). Therefore, caution is advised if venlafaxine is used concomitantly with CYP3A4 inhibitors).

No products indexed under this heading.

Erythromycin Stearate (Concomitant use of CYP3A4 inhibitors and venlafaxine may increase levels of venlafaxine and O-desmethylvenlafaxine (ODV). Therefore, caution is advised if venlafaxine is used concomitantly with CYP3A4 inhibitors).

No products indexed under this heading.

Escitalopram Oxalate (Based on the mechanism of action of venlafaxine and the potential for serotonin syndrome, caution is advised when velafaxine is co-administered with other drugs that may affect the serotonergic neurotransmitter systems, such as serotonin reuptake inhibitors). Products include:

Lexapro Oral Suspension 1174
Lexapro Tablets 1174

Esomeprazole Magnesium (Concomitant use of CYP3A4 inhibitors and venlafaxine may increase levels of venlafaxine and O-desmethylvenlafaxine (ODV). Therefore, caution is advised if venlafaxine is used concomitantly with CYP3A4 inhibitors). Products include:

Nexium Delayed-Release Capsules 645
Nexium Delayed-Release Oral Suspension 645

Estazolam (Caution is advised if the concomitant administration of venlafaxine and CNS-active drugs is required).

No products indexed under this heading.

Ethacrynic Acid (Hyponatremia may occur as a result of treatment with SSRIs and SNRIs, including venlafaxine hydrochloride. In many cases, this hyponatremia appears to be the result of the syndrome of inappropriate antidiuretic hormone secretion (SIADH). Patients taking diuretics or who are otherwise volume depleted may be at greater risk. Discontinuation of venlafaxine hydrochloride should be considered in patients with symptomatic hyponatremia and appropriate medical intervention should be instituted). Products include:

Edecrin Tablets 698

Ethanol (Caution is advised if the concomitant administration of venlafaxine and CNS-active drugs is required).

No products indexed under this heading.

Ethchlorvynol (Caution is advised if the concomitant administration of venlafaxine and CNS-active drugs is required).

No products indexed under this heading.

Ethinamate (Caution is advised if the concomitant administration of venlafaxine and CNS-active drugs is required).

No products indexed under this heading.

Ethyl Alcohol (Caution is advised if the concomitant administration of venlafaxine and CNS-active drugs is required).

No products indexed under this heading.

Etodolac (Use of venlafaxine may increase the risk of bleeding events. Concomitant use of nonsteroidal anti-inflammatory drugs (NSAIDs) may potentiate this risk of bleeding. Case reports and studies have shown an association between use of drugs that interfere with serotonin reuptake and the occurrence of gastrointestinal bleeding. Bleeding events related to SSRIs and SNRIs used have ranged from ecchymoses, hematomas, epistaxis and petechiae to life-threatening hemorrhages. Caution about the risk of bleeding associated with the concomitant use of venlafaxine and NSAIDs should be taken).

No products indexed under this heading.

Fenoprofen Calcium (Use of venlafaxine may increase the risk of bleeding events. Concomitant use of nonsteroidal anti-inflammatory drugs (NSAIDs) may potentiate this risk of bleeding. Case reports and studies have shown an association between use of drugs that interfere with serotonin reuptake and the occurrence of gastrointestinal bleeding. Bleeding events related to SSRIs and SNRIs used have ranged from ecchymoses, hematomas, epistaxis and petechiae to life-threatening hemorrhages. Caution about the risk of bleeding associated with the concomitant use of venlafaxine and NSAIDs should be taken). Products include:

Nalfon Capsules 2508

Fentanyl (Caution is advised if the concomitant administration of venlafaxine and CNS-active drugs is required). Products include:

Duragesic Transdermal System 2405
Ionsys Transdermal System 2410

Fentanyl Citrate (Caution is advised if the concomitant administration of venlafaxine and CNS-active drugs is required). Products include:

Actiq 959
Fentora Tablets 968

Fluconazole (Concomitant use of CYP3A4 inhibitors and venlafaxine may increase levels of venlafaxine and O-desmethylvenlafaxine (ODV). Therefore, caution is advised if venlafaxine is used concomitantly with CYP3A4 inhibitors).

No products indexed under this heading.

Fluoxetine (Based on the mechanism of action of venlafaxine and the potential for serotonin syndrome, caution is advised when velafaxine is co-administered with other drugs that may affect the serotonergic neurotransmitter systems, such as serotonin reuptake inhibitors).

No products indexed under this heading.

Fluoxetine Hydrochloride (Based on the mechanism of action of venlafaxine and the potential for serotonin syndrome, caution is advised when velafaxine is co-administered with other drugs that may affect the serotonergic neurotransmitter systems, such as serotonin reuptake inhibitors). Products include:

Prozac Weekly Capsules 1852
Prozac Pulvules and Liquid 1852
Symbyax Capsules 1871

Fluphenazine Decanoate (Caution is advised if the concomitant administration of venlafaxine and CNS-active drugs is required).

No products indexed under this heading.

Fluphenazine Enanthate (Caution is advised if the concomitant administration of venlafaxine and CNS-active drugs is required).

No products indexed under this heading.

Fluphenazine Hydrochloride (Caution is advised if the concomitant administration of venlafaxine and CNS-active drugs is required).

No products indexed under this heading.

Flurazepam Hydrochloride (Caution is advised if the concomitant administration of venlafaxine and CNS-active drugs is required).

No products indexed under this heading.

Flurbiprofen (Use of venlafaxine may increase the risk of bleeding events. Concomitant use of nonsteroidal anti-inflammatory drugs (NSAIDs) may potentiate this risk of bleeding. Case reports and studies have shown an association between use of drugs that interfere with serotonin reuptake and the occurrence of gastrointestinal bleeding. Bleeding events related to SSRIs and SNRIs used have ranged from ecchymoses, hematomas, epistaxis and petechiae to life-threatening hemorrhages. Caution about the risk of bleeding associated with the concomitant use of venlafaxine and NSAIDs should be taken).

No products indexed under this heading.

Fluvoxamine Maleate (Based on the mechanism of action of venlafaxine and the potential for serotonin syndrome, caution is advised when velafaxine is co-administered with other drugs that may affect the serotonergic neurotransmitter systems, such as serotonin reuptake inhibitors). Products include:
- Luvox CR Extended-Release Capsules ... 1759

Fosamprenavir Calcium (Concomitant use of CYP3A4 inhibitors and venlafaxine may increase levels of venlafaxine and O-desmethylvenlafaxine (ODV). Therefore, caution is advised if venlafaxine is used concomitantly with CYP3A4 inhibitors). Products include:
- Lexiva Oral Suspension ... 1510
- Lexiva Tablets ... 1510

Frovatriptan Succinate (Based on the mechanism of action of venlafaxine and the potential for serotonin syndrome, caution is advised when velafaxine is co-administered with other drugs that may affect the serotonergic neurotransmitter systems, such as triptans). Products include:
- Frova Tablets ... 1111

Furosemide (Hyponatremia may occur as a result of treatment with SSRIs and SNRIs, including venlafaxine hydrochloride. In many cases, this hyponatremia appears to be the result of the syndrome of inappropriate antidiuretic hormone secretion (SIADH). Patients taking diuretics or who are otherwise volume depleted may be at greater risk. Discontinuation of venlafaxine hydrochloride should be considered in patients with symptomatic hyponatremia and appropriate medical intervention should be instituted). Products include:
- Furosemide Tablets ... 2186

Glutethimide (Caution is advised if the concomitant administration of venlafaxine and CNS-active drugs is required).
No products indexed under this heading.

Haloperidol (Venlafaxine administered under steady-state conditions in healthy subjects decreased total oral-dose clearance of a single dose of haloperidol by 42%, which resulted in a 70% increase in haloperidol AUC and an 88% increase in Cmax).
No products indexed under this heading.

Haloperidol Decanoate (Venlafaxine administered under steady-state conditions in healthy subjects decreased total oral-dose clearance of a single dose of haloperidol by 42%, which resulted in a 70% increase in haloperidol AUC and an 88% increase in Cmax).
No products indexed under this heading.

Hydrochlorothiazide (Hyponatremia may occur as a result of treatment with SSRIs and SNRIs, including venlafaxine hydrochloride. In many cases, this hyponatremia appears to be the result of the syndrome of inappropriate antidiuretic hormone secretion (SIADH). Patients taking diuretics or who are otherwise volume depleted may be at greater risk. Discontinuation of venlafaxine hydrochloride should be considered in patients with symptomatic hyponatremia and appropriate medical intervention should be instituted). Products include:
- Atacand HCT ... 642
- Avalide Tablets ... 892
- Avalide Tablets ... 2713
- Benicar HCT Tablets ... 1010
- Diovan HCT Tablets ... 2216
- Dyazide Capsules ... 1405
- Micardis HCT Tablets ... 854
- Prinzide Tablets ... 2092
- Tekturna HCT Tablets ... 2324
- Teveten HCT Tablets ... 517

Hydrocodone Bitartrate (Caution is advised if the concomitant administration of venlafaxine and CNS-active drugs is required). Products include:
- Lortab 5/500 Tablets ... 3143
- Lortab 7.5/500 Tablets ... 3144
- Lortab 10/500 Tablets ... 3144
- Vicodin Tablets ... 529
- Vicodin ES Tablets ... 530
- Vicodin HP Tablets ... 531
- Vicoprofen Tablets ... 533
- Zydone Tablets ... 1132

Hydrocodone Polistirex (Caution is advised if the concomitant administration of venlafaxine and CNS-active drugs is required). Products include:
- Tussionex Pennkinetic Extended-Release Suspension ... 3154

Hydroflumethiazide (Hyponatremia may occur as a result of treatment with SSRIs and SNRIs, including venlafaxine hydrochloride. In many cases, this hyponatremia appears to be the result of the syndrome of inappropriate antidiuretic hormone secretion (SIADH). Patients taking diuretics or who are otherwise volume depleted may be at greater risk. Discontinuation of venlafaxine hydrochloride should be considered in patients with symptomatic hyponatremia and appropriate medical intervention should be instituted).
No products indexed under this heading.

Hydromorphone Hydrochloride (Caution is advised if the concomitant administration of venlafaxine and CNS-active drugs is required).
No products indexed under this heading.

Hydroxyzine Hydrochloride (Caution is advised if the concomitant administration of venlafaxine and CNS-active drugs is required).
No products indexed under this heading.

Hypericum (Caution is advised when velafaxine is co-administered with other drugs that may affect serotonergic neurotransmitter systems). Products include:
- Satieté Tablets ... ▣ 640

Hypericum Perforatum (Caution is advised when velafaxine is co-administered with other drugs that may affect serotonergic neurotransmitter systems).
No products indexed under this heading.

Ibuprofen (Use of venlafaxine may increase the risk of bleeding events. Concomitant use of nonsteroidal anti-inflammatory drugs (NSAIDs) may potentiate this risk of bleeding. Case reports and studies have shown an association between use of drugs that interfere with serotonin reuptake and the occurrence of gastrointestinal bleeding. Bleeding events related to SSRIs and SNRIs used have ranged from ecchymoses, hematomas, epistaxis and petechiae to life-threatening hemorrhages. Caution about the risk of bleeding associated with the concomitant use of venlafaxine and NSAIDs should be taken). Products include:
- Motrin IB Tablets and Caplets ... 1900
- Children's Motrin Oral Suspension ... 1901
- Children's Motrin Non-Staining Dye-Free Oral Suspension ... 1901
- Children's Motrin Cold Oral Suspension ... 1899
- Infants' Motrin Concentrated Drops ... 1901
- Infants' Motrin Non-Staining Dye-Free Concentrated Drops ... 1901
- Junior Strength Motrin Caplets and Chewable Tablets ... 1901
- Vicoprofen Tablets ... 533

Indapamide (Hyponatremia may occur as a result of treatment with SSRIs and SNRIs, including venlafaxine hydrochloride. In many cases, this hyponatremia appears to be the result of the syndrome of inappropriate antidiuretic hormone secretion (SIADH). Patients taking diuretics or who are otherwise volume depleted may be at greater risk. Discontinuation of venlafaxine hydrochloride should be considered in patients with symptomatic hyponatremia and appropriate medical intervention should be instituted). Products include:
- Indapamide Tablets ... 2188

Indinavir Sulfate (Co-administration has resulted in a 28% decrease in the AUC and 36% decrease in the indinavir Cmax; the clinical significance of these findings is unknown). Products include:
- Crixivan Capsules ... 1979

Indomethacin (Use of venlafaxine may increase the risk of bleeding events. Concomitant use of nonsteroidal anti-inflammatory drugs (NSAIDs) may potentiate this risk of bleeding. Case reports and studies have shown an association between use of drugs that interfere with serotonin reuptake and the occurrence of gastrointestinal bleeding. Bleeding events related to SSRIs and SNRIs used have ranged from ecchymoses, hematomas, epistaxis and petechiae to life-threatening hemorrhages. Caution about the risk of bleeding associated with the concomitant use of venlafaxine and NSAIDs should be taken). Products include:
- Indocin ... 2024

Indomethacin Sodium Trihydrate (Use of venlafaxine may increase the risk of bleeding events. Concomitant use of nonsteroidal anti-inflammatory drugs (NSAIDs) may potentiate this risk of bleeding. Case reports and studies have shown an association between use of drugs that interfere with serotonin reuptake and the occurrence of gastrointestinal bleeding. Bleeding events related to SSRIs and SNRIs used have ranged from ecchymoses, hematomas, epistaxis and petechiae to life-threatening hemorrhages. Caution about the risk of bleeding associated with the concomitant use of venlafaxine and NSAIDs should be taken). Products include:
- Indocin I.V. ... 2489

Isocarboxazid (Adverse reactions, some of which were serious, have been reported in patients who have recently been discontinued from an MAO inhibitor and started on venlafaxine, or who have recently had venlafaxine therapy discontinued prior to initiation of an MAO inhibitor; concurrent and/or sequential use is contraindicated). Products include:
- Marplan Tablets ... 3177

Isoflurane (Caution is advised if the concomitant administration of venlafaxine and CNS-active drugs is required).
No products indexed under this heading.

Isoniazid (Concomitant use of CYP3A4 inhibitors and venlafaxine may increase levels of venlafaxine and O-desmethylvenlafaxine (ODV). Therefore, caution is advised if venlafaxine is used concomitantly with CYP3A4 inhibitors).
No products indexed under this heading.

Itraconazole (Concomitant use of CYP3A4 inhibitors and venlafaxine may increase levels of venlafaxine and O-desmethylvenlafaxine (ODV). Therefore, caution is advised if venlafaxine is used concomitantly with CYP3A4 inhibitors).
No products indexed under this heading.

Ketamine Hydrochloride (Caution is advised if the concomitant administration of venlafaxine and CNS-active drugs is required).
No products indexed under this heading.

Ketoconazole (Co-administration may lead to increased levels of venlafaxine and/or ketaconazole). Products include:
- Extina Foam, 2% ... 3057
- Nizoral A-D Shampoo ... 1901

Ketoprofen (Use of venlafaxine may increase the risk of bleeding events. Concomitant use of nonsteroidal anti-inflammatory drugs (NSAIDs) may potentiate this risk of bleeding. Case reports and studies have shown an association between use of drugs that interfere with serotonin reuptake and the occurrence of gastrointestinal bleeding. Bleeding events related to SSRIs and SNRIs used have ranged from ecchymoses, hematomas, epistaxis and petechiae to life-threatening hemorrhages. Caution about the risk of bleeding associated with the concomitant use of venlafaxine and NSAIDs should be taken).
No products indexed under this heading.

Ketorolac Tromethamine (Use of venlafaxine may increase the risk of bleeding events. Concomitant use of nonsteroidal anti-inflammatory drugs (NSAIDs) may potentiate this risk of bleeding. Case reports and studies have shown an association between use of drugs that interfere with serotonin reuptake and the occurrence of gastrointestinal bleeding. Bleeding events related to SSRIs and SNRIs used have ranged from ecchymoses, hematomas, epistaxis and petechiae to life-threatening hemorrhages. Caution about the risk of bleeding associated with the concomitant use of venlafaxine and NSAIDs should be taken).
No products indexed under this heading.

Levomethadyl Acetate Hydrochloride (Caution is advised if the concomitant administration of venlafaxine and CNS-active drugs is required).
No products indexed under this heading.

Levorphanol Tartrate (Caution is advised if the concomitant administration of venlafaxine and CNS-active drugs is required).
No products indexed under this heading.

Lithium Carbonate (Based on the mechanism of action of venlafaxine and the potential for serotonin syndrome, caution is advised when velafaxine is co-administered with other drugs that may affect the serotonergic neurotransmitter systems, such as lithium).
No products indexed under this heading.

Lithium Citrate (Based on the mechanism of action of venlafaxine and the potential for serotonin syndrome, caution is advised when velafaxine is co-administered with other drugs that may affect the serotonergic neurotransmitter systems, such as lithium).
No products indexed under this heading.

Lopinavir (Concomitant use of CYP3A4 inhibitors and venlafaxine may increase levels of venlafaxine and O-desmethylvenlafaxine (ODV). Therefore, caution is advised if venlafaxine is used concomitantly with CYP3A4 inhibitors). Products include:
Kaletra 452

Loratadine (Concomitant use of CYP3A4 inhibitors and venlafaxine may increase levels of venlafaxine and O-desmethylvenlafaxine (ODV). Therefore, caution is advised if venlafaxine is used concomitantly with CYP3A4 inhibitors).
No products indexed under this heading.

Lorazepam (Caution is advised if the concomitant administration of venlafaxine and CNS-active drugs is required).
No products indexed under this heading.

Loxapine Hydrochloride (Caution is advised if the concomitant administration of venlafaxine and CNS-active drugs is required).
No products indexed under this heading.

Loxapine Succinate (Caution is advised if the concomitant administration of venlafaxine and CNS-active drugs is required).
No products indexed under this heading.

Meclofenamate Sodium (Use of venlafaxine may increase the risk of bleeding events. Concomitant use of nonsteroidal anti-inflammatory drugs (NSAIDs) may potentiate this risk of bleeding. Case reports and studies have shown an association between use of drugs that interfere with serotonin reuptake and the occurrence of gastrointestinal bleeding. Bleeding events related to SSRIs and SNRIs used have ranged from ecchymoses, hematomas, epistaxis and petechiae to life-threatening hemorrhages. Caution about the risk of bleeding associated with the concomitant use of venlafaxine and NSAIDs should be taken).
No products indexed under this heading.

Mefenamic Acid (Use of venlafaxine may increase the risk of bleeding events. Concomitant use of nonsteroidal anti-inflammatory drugs (NSAIDs) may potentiate this risk of bleeding. Case reports and studies have shown an association between use of drugs that interfere with serotonin reuptake and the occurrence of gastrointestinal bleeding. Bleeding events related to SSRIs and SNRIs used have ranged from ecchymoses, hematomas, epistaxis and petechiae to life-threatening hemorrhages. Caution about the risk of bleeding associated with the concomitant use of venlafaxine and NSAIDs should be taken).
No products indexed under this heading.

Meloxicam (Use of venlafaxine may increase the risk of bleeding events. Concomitant use of nonsteroidal anti-inflammatory drugs (NSAIDs) may potentiate this risk of bleeding. Case reports and studies have shown an association between use of drugs that interfere with serotonin reuptake and the occurrence of gastrointestinal bleeding. Bleeding events related to SSRIs and SNRIs used have ranged from ecchymoses, hematomas, epistaxis and petechiae to life-threatening hemorrhages. Caution about the risk of bleeding associated with the concomitant use of venlafaxine and NSAIDs should be taken). Products include:
Mobic Oral Suspension 863
Mobic Tablets 863

Meperidine Hydrochloride (Caution is advised if the concomitant administration of venlafaxine and CNS-active drugs is required).
No products indexed under this heading.

Mephobarbital (Caution is advised if the concomitant administration of venlafaxine and CNS-active drugs is required).
No products indexed under this heading.

Meprobamate (Caution is advised if the concomitant administration of venlafaxine and CNS-active drugs is required).
No products indexed under this heading.

Mesoridazine Besylate (Caution is advised if the concomitant administration of venlafaxine and CNS-active drugs is required).
No products indexed under this heading.

Methadone Hydrochloride (Caution is advised if the concomitant administration of venlafaxine and CNS-active drugs is required).
No products indexed under this heading.

Methamphetamine Hydrochloride (Caution is advised if the concomitant administration of venlafaxine and CNS-active drugs is required).
No products indexed under this heading.

Methohexital Sodium (Caution is advised if the concomitant administration of venlafaxine and CNS-active drugs is required).
No products indexed under this heading.

Methotrimeprazine (Caution is advised if the concomitant administration of venlafaxine and CNS-active drugs is required).
No products indexed under this heading.

Methoxyflurane (Caution is advised if the concomitant administration of venlafaxine and CNS-active drugs is required).
No products indexed under this heading.

Methyclothiazide (Hyponatremia may occur as a result of treatment with SSRIs and SNRIs, including venlafaxine hydrochloride. In many cases, this hyponatremia appears to be the result of the syndrome of inappropriate antidiuretic hormone secretion (SIADH). Patients taking diuretics or who are otherwise volume depleted may be at greater risk. Discontinuation of venlafaxine hydrochloride should be considered in patients with symptomatic hyponatremia and appropriate medical intervention should be instituted).
No products indexed under this heading.

Methylphenidate (Caution is advised if the concomitant administration of venlafaxine and CNS-active drugs is required). Products include:
Daytrana Transdermal Patch 3022

Methylphenidate Hydrochloride (Caution is advised if the concomitant administration of venlafaxine and CNS-active drugs is required). Products include:
Concerta Extended-Release Tablets 1925
Metadate CD Capsules 3146

Metolazone (Hyponatremia may occur as a result of treatment with SSRIs and SNRIs, including venlafaxine hydrochloride. In many cases, this hyponatremia appears to be the result of the syndrome of inappropriate antidiuretic hormone secretion (SIADH). Patients taking diuretics or who are otherwise volume depleted may be at greater risk. Discontinuation of venlafaxine hydrochloride should be considered in patients with symptomatic hyponatremia and appropriate medical intervention should be instituted).
No products indexed under this heading.

Metoprolol Succinate (Venlafaxine appeared to reduce the blood pressure lowering effect of metoprolol. Caution should be exercised with co-administration of venlafaxine and metoprolol. Venlafaxine treatment has been associated with dose-related increases in blood pressure in some patients. It is recommended that patients receiving venlafaxine extended-release have regular monitoring of blood pressure). Products include:
Toprol-XL Tablets 666

Metoprolol Tartrate (Venlafaxine appeared to reduce the blood pressure lowering effect of metoprolol. Caution should be exercised with co-administration of venlafaxine and metoprolol. Venlafaxine treatment has been associated with dose-related increases in blood pressure in some patients. It is recommended that patients receiving venlafaxine extended-release have regular monitoring of blood pressure).
No products indexed under this heading.

Metronidazole (Concomitant use of CYP3A4 inhibitors and venlafaxine may increase levels of venlafaxine and O-desmethylvenlafaxine (ODV). Therefore, caution is advised if venlafaxine is used concomitantly with CYP3A4 inhibitors). Products include:
Pylera Capsules 714

Metronidazole Benzoate (Concomitant use of CYP3A4 inhibitors and venlafaxine may increase levels of venlafaxine and O-desmethylvenlafaxine (ODV). Therefore, caution is advised if venlafaxine is used concomitantly with CYP3A4 inhibitors).
No products indexed under this heading.

Metronidazole Hydrochloride (Concomitant use of CYP3A4 inhibitors and venlafaxine may increase levels of venlafaxine and O-desmethylvenlafaxine (ODV). Therefore, caution is advised if venlafaxine is used concomitantly with CYP3A4 inhibitors).
No products indexed under this heading.

Metronidazole Sodium (Concomitant use of CYP3A4 inhibitors and venlafaxine may increase levels of venlafaxine and O-desmethylvenlafaxine (ODV). Therefore, caution is advised if venlafaxine is used concomitantly with CYP3A4 inhibitors).
No products indexed under this heading.

Miconazole (Concomitant use of CYP3A4 inhibitors and venlafaxine may increase levels of venlafaxine and O-desmethylvenlafaxine (ODV). Therefore, caution is advised if venlafaxine is used concomitantly with CYP3A4 inhibitors).
No products indexed under this heading.

Miconazole Nitrate (Concomitant use of CYP3A4 inhibitors and venlafaxine may increase levels of venlafaxine and O-desmethylvenlafaxine (ODV). Therefore, caution is advised if venlafaxine is used concomitantly with CYP3A4 inhibitors).
No products indexed under this heading.

Midazolam Hydrochloride (Caution is advised if the concomitant administration of venlafaxine and CNS-active drugs is required).
No products indexed under this heading.

Moclobemide (Adverse reactions, some of which were serious, have been reported in patients who have recently been discontinued from an MAO inhibitor and started on venlafaxine, or who have recently had venlafaxine therapy discontinued prior to initiation of an MAO inhibitor; concurrent and/or sequential use is contraindicated).
No products indexed under this heading.

Molindone Hydrochloride (Caution is advised if the concomitant administration of venlafaxine and CNS-active drugs is required). Products include:
Moban Tablets 1116

Morphine Sulfate (Caution is advised if the concomitant administration of venlafaxine and CNS-active drugs is required). Products include:
Avinza Capsules 1772
DepoDur Injection 1095

MS Contin Tablets 2585

Nabumetone (Use of venlafaxine may increase the risk of bleeding events. Concomitant use of nonsteroidal anti-inflammatory drugs (NSAIDs) may potentiate this risk of bleeding. Case reports and studies have shown an association between use of drugs that interfere with serotonin reuptake and the occurrence of gastrointestinal bleeding. Bleeding events related to SSRIs and SNRIs used have ranged from ecchymoses, hematomas, epistaxis and petechiae to life-threatening hemorrhages. Caution about the risk of bleeding associated with the concomitant use of venlafaxine and NSAIDs should be taken).
No products indexed under this heading.

Naproxen (Use of venlafaxine may increase the risk of bleeding events. Concomitant use of nonsteroidal anti-inflammatory drugs (NSAIDs) may potentiate this risk of bleeding. Case reports and studies have shown an association between use of drugs that interfere with serotonin reuptake and the occurrence of gastrointestinal bleeding. Bleeding events related to SSRIs and SNRIs used have ranged from ecchymoses, hematomas, epistaxis and petechiae to life-threatening hemorrhages. Caution about the risk of bleeding associated with the concomitant use of venlafaxine and NSAIDs should be taken). Products include:
EC-Naprosyn Delayed-Release Tablets 2632
Naprosyn Suspension 2632
Naprosyn Tablets 2632

Naproxen Sodium (Use of venlafaxine may increase the risk of bleeding events. Concomitant use of nonsteroidal anti-inflammatory drugs (NSAIDs) may potentiate this risk of bleeding. Case reports and studies have shown an association between use of drugs that interfere with serotonin reuptake and the occurrence of gastrointestinal bleeding. Bleeding events related to SSRIs and SNRIs used have ranged from ecchymoses, hematomas, epistaxis and petechiae to life-threatening hemorrhages. Caution about the risk of bleeding associated with the concomitant use of venlafaxine and NSAIDs should be taken). Products include:
Anaprox Tablets 2632
Anaprox DS Tablets 2632
Treximet Tablets 1616

Naratriptan Hydrochloride (Based on the mechanism of action of venlafaxine and the potential for serotonin syndrome, caution is advised when velafaxine is co-administered with other drugs that may affect the serotonergic neurotransmitter systems, such as triptans). Products include:
Amerge Tablets 1301

Nefazodone Hydrochloride (Based on the mechanism of action of venlafaxine and the potential for serotonin syndrome, caution is advised when venlafaxine is co-administered with other drugs that may affect serotonergic neurotransmitter systems, such as serotonin-norepinephrine reuptake inhibitors).
No products indexed under this heading.

Nelfinavir Mesylate (Concomitant use of CYP3A4 inhibitors and venlafaxine may increase levels of venlafaxine and O-desmethylvenlafaxine (ODV). Therefore, caution is advised if venlafaxine is used concomitantly with CYP3A4 inhibitors).
No products indexed under this heading.

Nevirapine (Concomitant use of CYP3A4 inhibitors and venlafaxine may increase levels of venlafaxine and O-desmethylvenlafaxine (ODV). Therefore, caution is advised if venlafaxine is used concomitantly with CYP3A4 inhibitors). Products include:
Viramune Oral Suspension 873
Viramune Tablets 873

Niacinamide (Concomitant use of CYP3A4 inhibitors and venlafaxine may increase levels of venlafaxine and O-desmethylvenlafaxine (ODV). Therefore, caution is advised if venlafaxine is used concomitantly with CYP3A4 inhibitors). Products include:
BioLean Free Tablets .... ▣ 635

Nicotinamide (Concomitant use of CYP3A4 inhibitors and venlafaxine may increase levels of venlafaxine and O-desmethylvenlafaxine (ODV). Therefore, caution is advised if venlafaxine is used concomitantly with CYP3A4 inhibitors).
No products indexed under this heading.

Nifedipine (Concomitant use of CYP3A4 inhibitors and venlafaxine may increase levels of venlafaxine and O-desmethylvenlafaxine (ODV). Therefore, caution is advised if venlafaxine is used concomitantly with CYP3A4 inhibitors).
No products indexed under this heading.

Norfloxacin (Concomitant use of CYP3A4 inhibitors and venlafaxine may increase levels of venlafaxine and O-desmethylvenlafaxine (ODV). Therefore, caution is advised if venlafaxine is used concomitantly with CYP3A4 inhibitors). Products include:
Noroxin Tablets 2069

Olanzapine (Caution is advised if the concomitant administration of venlafaxine and CNS-active drugs is required). Products include:
Symbyax Capsules 1871
Zyprexa Tablets 1883
Zyprexa IntraMuscular 1883
Zyprexa ZYDIS Orally Disintegrating Tablets 1883

Omeprazole (Concomitant use of CYP3A4 inhibitors and venlafaxine may increase levels of venlafaxine and O-desmethylvenlafaxine (ODV). Therefore, caution is advised if venlafaxine is used concomitantly with CYP3A4 inhibitors).
No products indexed under this heading.

Oxaprozin (Use of venlafaxine may increase the risk of bleeding events. Concomitant use of nonsteroidal anti-inflammatory drugs (NSAIDs) may potentiate this risk of bleeding. Case reports and studies have shown an association between use of drugs that interfere with serotonin reuptake and the occurrence of gastrointestinal bleeding. Bleeding events related to SSRIs and SNRIs used have ranged from ecchymoses, hematomas, epistaxis and petechiae to life-threatening hemorrhages. Caution about the risk of bleeding associated with the concomitant use of venlafaxine and NSAIDs should be taken).
No products indexed under this heading.

Oxazepam (Caution is advised if the concomitant administration of venlafaxine and CNS-active drugs is required).
No products indexed under this heading.

Oxycodone Hydrochloride (Caution is advised if the concomitant administration of venlafaxine and CNS-active drugs is required). Products include:
OxyContin Tablets 2589
OxyIR Capsules 2593
Percocet Tablets 1127
Percodan Tablets 1130

Pargyline Hydrochloride (Adverse reactions, some of which were serious, have been reported in patients who have recently been discontinued from an MAO inhibitor and started on venlafaxine, or who have recently had venlafaxine therapy discontinued prior to initiation of an MAO inhibitor; concurrent and/or sequential use is contraindicated).
No products indexed under this heading.

Paroxetine Hydrochloride (Based on the mechanism of action of venlafaxine and the potential for serotonin syndrome, caution is advised when velafaxine is co-administered with other drugs that may affect the serotonergic neurotransmitter systems, such as serotonin reuptake inhibitors). Products include:
Paxil 1535
Paxil CR Controlled-Release Tablets 1544

Pemoline (Caution is advised if the concomitant administration of venlafaxine and CNS-active drugs is required).
No products indexed under this heading.

Pentobarbital Sodium (Caution is advised if the concomitant administration of venlafaxine and CNS-active drugs is required). Products include:
Nembutal Sodium Solution, USP 2494

Perphenazine (Caution is advised if the concomitant administration of venlafaxine and CNS-active drugs is required).
No products indexed under this heading.

Phenelzine Sulfate (Adverse reactions, some of which were serious, have been reported in patients who have recently been discontinued from an MAO inhibitor and started on venlafaxine, or who have recently had venlafaxine therapy discontinued prior to initiation of an MAO inhibitor; concurrent and/or sequential use is contraindicated).
No products indexed under this heading.

Phenobarbital (Caution is advised if the concomitant administration of venlafaxine and CNS-active drugs is required). Products include:
Donnatal Extentabs 2507

Phenylbutazone (Use of venlafaxine may increase the risk of bleeding events. Concomitant use of nonsteroidal anti-inflammatory drugs (NSAIDs) may potentiate this risk of bleeding. Case reports and studies have shown an association between use of drugs that interfere with serotonin reuptake and the occurrence of gastrointestinal bleeding. Bleeding events related to SSRIs and SNRIs used have ranged from ecchymoses, hematomas, epistaxis and petechiae to life-threatening hemorrhages. Caution about the risk of bleeding associated with the concomitant use of venlafaxine and NSAIDs should be taken).
No products indexed under this heading.

Piroxicam (Use of venlafaxine may increase the risk of bleeding events. Concomitant use of nonsteroidal anti-inflammatory drugs (NSAIDs) may potentiate this risk of bleeding. Case reports and studies have shown an association between use of drugs that interfere with serotonin reuptake and the occurrence of gastrointestinal bleeding. Bleeding events related to SSRIs and SNRIs used have ranged from ecchymoses, hematomas, epistaxis and petechiae to life-threatening hemorrhages. Caution about the risk of bleeding associated with the concomitant use of venlafaxine and NSAIDs should be taken).
No products indexed under this heading.

Polythiazide (Hyponatremia may occur as a result of treatment with SSRIs and SNRIs, including venlafaxine hydrochloride. In many cases, this hyponatremia appears to be the result of the syndrome of inappropriate antidiuretic hormone secretion (SIADH). Patients taking diuretics or who are otherwise volume depleted may be at greater risk. Discontinuation of venlafaxine hydrochloride should be considered in patients with symptomatic hyponatremia and appropriate medical intervention should be instituted).
No products indexed under this heading.

Prazepam (Caution is advised if the concomitant administration of venlafaxine and CNS-active drugs is required).
No products indexed under this heading.

Procarbazine Hydrochloride (Adverse reactions, some of which were serious, have been reported in patients who have recently been discontinued from an MAO inhibitor and started on venlafaxine, or who have recently had venlafaxine therapy discontinued prior to initiation of an MAO inhibitor; concurrent and/or sequential use is contraindicated).
No products indexed under this heading.

Prochlorperazine (Caution is advised if the concomitant administration of venlafaxine and CNS-active drugs is required).
No products indexed under this heading.

Promethazine Hydrochloride (Caution is advised if the concomitant administration of venlafaxine and CNS-active drugs is required).
No products indexed under this heading.

Propofol (Caution is advised if the concomitant administration of venlafaxine and CNS-active drugs is required).
No products indexed under this heading.

Propoxyphene Hydrochloride (Caution is advised if the concomitant administration of venlafaxine and CNS-active drugs is required).
No products indexed under this heading.

Propoxyphene Napsylate (Caution is advised if the concomitant administration of venlafaxine and CNS-active drugs is required).
No products indexed under this heading.

Quazepam (Caution is advised if the concomitant administration of venlafaxine and CNS-active drugs is required).
No products indexed under this heading.

Quetiapine Fumarate (Caution is advised if the concomitant administration of venlafaxine and CNS-active drugs is required).
No products indexed under this heading.

Quinidine (Venlafaxine is metabolized to its active metabolite, ODV, by CYP2D6; therefore, the potential exists for a drug interaction between the inhibitors of CYP2D6, such as quinidine and venlafaxine, resulting in increased plasma concentrations of venlafaxine and decreased concentrations of the active metabolite).
No products indexed under this heading.

Quinidine Gluconate (Venlafaxine is metabolized to its active metabolite, ODV, by CYP2D6; therefore, the potential exists for a drug interaction between the inhibitors of CYP2D6, such as quinidine and venlafaxine, resulting in increased plasma concentrations of venlafaxine and decreased concentrations of the active metabolite).
No products indexed under this heading.

Quinidine Hydrochloride (Venlafaxine is metabolized to its active metabolite, ODV, by CYP2D6; therefore, the potential exists for a drug interaction between the inhibitors of CYP2D6, such as quinidine and venlafaxine, resulting in increased plasma concentrations of venlafaxine and decreased concentrations of the active metabolite).
No products indexed under this heading.

Quinidine Polygalacturonate (Venlafaxine is metabolized to its active metabolite, ODV, by CYP2D6; therefore, the potential exists for a drug interaction between the inhibitors of CYP2D6, such as quinidine and venlafaxine, resulting in increased plasma concentrations of venlafaxine and decreased concentrations of the active metabolite).
No products indexed under this heading.

Quinidine Sulfate (Venlafaxine is metabolized to its active metabolite, ODV, by CYP2D6; therefore, the potential exists for a drug interaction between the inhibitors of CYP2D6, such as quinidine and venlafaxine, resulting in increased plasma concentrations of venlafaxine and decreased concentrations of the active metabolite).
No products indexed under this heading.

Quinine (Concomitant use of CYP3A4 inhibitors and venlafaxine may increase levels of venlafaxine and O-desmethylvenlafaxine (ODV). Therefore, caution is advised if venlafaxine is used concomitantly with CYP3A4 inhibitors).
No products indexed under this heading.

Quinine Sulfate (Concomitant use of CYP3A4 inhibitors and venlafaxine may increase levels of venlafaxine and O-desmethylvenlafaxine (ODV). Therefore, caution is advised if venlafaxine is used concomitantly with CYP3A4 inhibitors).
No products indexed under this heading.

Quinupristin (Concomitant use of CYP3A4 inhibitors and venlafaxine may increase levels of venlafaxine and O-desmethylvenlafaxine (ODV). Therefore, caution is advised if venlafaxine is used concomitantly with CYP3A4 inhibitors).
No products indexed under this heading.

Ranitidine Bismuth Citrate (Concomitant use of CYP3A4 inhibitors and venlafaxine may increase levels of venlafaxine and O-desmethylvenlafaxine (ODV). Therefore, caution is advised if venlafaxine is used concomitantly with CYP3A4 inhibitors).
No products indexed under this heading.

Ranitidine Hydrochloride (Concomitant use of CYP3A4 inhibitors and venlafaxine may increase levels of venlafaxine and O-desmethylvenlafaxine (ODV). Therefore, caution is advised if venlafaxine is used concomitantly with CYP3A4 inhibitors). Products include:
Zantac 75 Tablets 603
Zantac 1670
Zantac Injection 1666
Zantac Injection Pharmacy Bulk Package 1668
Maximum Strength Zantac 150 Tablets 603
Maximum Strength Zantac 150 Cool Mint Tablets 603

Rasagiline Mesylate (Adverse reactions, some of which were serious, have been reported in patients who have recently been discontinued from an MAO inhibitor and started on venlafaxine, or who have recently had venlafaxine therapy discontinued prior to initiation of an MAO inhibitor; concurrent and/or sequential use is contraindicated). Products include:
Azilect Tablets 3106

Remifentanil Hydrochloride (Caution is advised if the concomitant administration of venlafaxine and CNS-active drugs is required).
No products indexed under this heading.

Risperidone (Venlafaxine slightly inhibits the CYP2D6-mediated metabolism of risperidone resulting in an approximate 32% increase in risperidone AUC). Products include:
Risperdal Consta Long-Acting Injection 1753

Ritonavir (Concomitant use of CYP3A4 inhibitors and venlafaxine may increase levels of venlafaxine and O-desmethylvenlafaxine (ODV). Therefore, caution is advised if venlafaxine is used concomitantly with CYP3A4 inhibitors). Products include:
Kaletra 452
Norvir 489

Rizatriptan Benzoate (Based on the mechanism of action of venlafaxine and the potential for serotonin syndrome, caution is advised when velafaxine is co-administered with other drugs that may affect the serotonergic neurotransmitter systems, such as triptans). Products include:
Maxalt Tablets 2056
Maxalt-MLT Orally Disintegrating Tablets 2056

Rofecoxib (Use of venlafaxine may increase the risk of bleeding events. Concomitant use of nonsteroidal anti-inflammatory drugs (NSAIDs) may potentiate this risk of bleeding. Case reports and studies have shown an association between use of drugs that interfere with serotonin reuptake and the occurrence of gastrointestinal bleeding. Bleeding events related to SSRIs and SNRIs used have ranged from ecchymoses, hematomas, epistaxis and petechiae to life-threatening hemorrhages. Caution about the risk of bleeding associated with the concomitant use of venlafaxine and NSAIDs should be taken).
No products indexed under this heading.

Saquinavir (Concomitant use of CYP3A4 inhibitors and venlafaxine may increase levels of venlafaxine and O-desmethylvenlafaxine (ODV). Therefore, caution is advised if venlafaxine is used concomitantly with CYP3A4 inhibitors).
No products indexed under this heading.

Saquinavir Mesylate (Concomitant use of CYP3A4 inhibitors and venlafaxine may increase levels of venlafaxine and O-desmethylvenlafaxine (ODV). Therefore, caution is advised if venlafaxine is used concomitantly with CYP3A4 inhibitors).
No products indexed under this heading.

Secobarbital Sodium (Caution is advised if the concomitant administration of venlafaxine and CNS-active drugs is required).
No products indexed under this heading.

Selegiline (Adverse reactions, some of which were serious, have been reported in patients who have recently been discontinued from an MAO inhibitor and started on venlafaxine, or who have recently had venlafaxine therapy discontinued prior to initiation of an MAO inhibitor; concurrent and/or sequential use is contraindicated). Products include:
Emsam Transdermal System 905

Selegiline Hydrochloride (Adverse reactions, some of which were serious, have been reported in patients who have recently been discontinued from an MAO inhibitor and started on venlafaxine, or who have recently had venlafaxine therapy discontinued prior to initiation of an MAO inhibitor; concurrent and/or sequential use is contraindicated). Products include:
Eldepryl Capsules 3052

Sertraline Hydrochloride (Based on the mechanism of action of venlafaxine and the potential for serotonin syndrome, caution is advised when velafaxine is co-administered with other drugs that may affect the serotonergic neurotransmitter systems, such as serotonin reuptake inhibitors).
No products indexed under this heading.

Sevoflurane (Caution is advised if the concomitant administration of venlafaxine and CNS-active drugs is required). Products include:
Ultane Liquid for Inhalation 524

Sildenafil Citrate (Concomitant use of CYP3A4 inhibitors and venlafaxine may increase levels of venlafaxine and O-desmethylvenlafaxine (ODV). Therefore, caution is advised if venlafaxine is used concomitantly with CYP3A4 inhibitors).
No products indexed under this heading.

Sodium Oxybate (Caution is advised if the concomitant administration of venlafaxine and CNS-active drugs is required). Products include:
Xyrem Oral Solution 1766

Spironolactone (Hyponatremia may occur as a result of treatment with SSRIs and SNRIs, including venlafaxine hydrochloride. In many cases, this hyponatremia appears to be the result of the syndrome of inappropriate antidiuretic hormone secretion (SIADH). Patients taking diuretics or who are otherwise volume depleted may be at greater risk. Discontinuation of venlafaxine hydrochloride should be considered in patients with symptomatic hyponatremia and appropriate medical intervention should be instituted).
No products indexed under this heading.

Sufentanil Citrate (Caution is advised if the concomitant administration of venlafaxine and CNS-active drugs is required).
No products indexed under this heading.

Sulindac (Use of venlafaxine may increase the risk of bleeding events. Concomitant use of nonsteroidal anti-inflammatory drugs (NSAIDs) may potentiate this risk of bleeding. Case reports and studies have shown an association between use of drugs that interfere with serotonin reuptake and the occurrence of gastrointestinal bleeding. Bleeding events related to SSRIs and SNRIs used have ranged from ecchymoses, hematomas, epistaxis and petechiae to life-threatening hemorrhages. Caution about the risk of bleeding associated with the concomitant use of venlafaxine and NSAIDs should be taken). Products include:
Clinoril Tablets 1962

Sumatriptan (Based on the mechanism of action of venlafaxine and the potential for serotonin syndrome, caution is advised when velafaxine is co-administered with other drugs that may affect the serotonergic neurotransmitter systems, such as triptans). Products include:
Imitrex Nasal Spray 1470

Sumatriptan Succinate (Based on the mechanism of action of venlafaxine and the potential for serotonin syndrome, caution is advised when velafaxine is co-administered with

other drugs that may affect the serotonergic neurotransmitter systems, such as triptans). Products include:
Imitrex Injection 1465
Imitrex Tablets 1474
Treximet Tablets 1616

Telithromycin (Concomitant use of CYP3A4 inhibitors and venlafaxine may increase levels of venlafaxine and O-desmethylvenlafaxine (ODV). Therefore, caution is advised if venlafaxine is used concomitantly with CYP3A4 inhibitors). Products include:
Ketek Tablets 2744

Temazepam (Caution is advised if the concomitant administration of venlafaxine and CNS-active drugs is required).
No products indexed under this heading.

Thiamylal Sodium (Caution is advised if the concomitant administration of venlafaxine and CNS-active drugs is required).
No products indexed under this heading.

Thioridazine Hydrochloride (Caution is advised if the concomitant administration of venlafaxine and CNS-active drugs is required). Products include:
Thioridazine Hydrochloride Tablets 2195

Thiothixene (Caution is advised if the concomitant administration of venlafaxine and CNS-active drugs is required). Products include:
Thiothixene Capsules 2197

Tolmetin Sodium (Use of venlafaxine may increase the risk of bleeding events. Concomitant use of nonsteroidal anti-inflammatory drugs (NSAIDs) may potentiate this risk of bleeding. Case reports and studies have shown an association between use of drugs that interfere with serotonin reuptake and the occurrence of gastrointestinal bleeding. Bleeding events related to SSRIs and SNRIs used have ranged from ecchymoses, hematomas, epistaxis and petechiae to life-threatening hemorrhages. Caution about the risk of bleeding associated with the concomitant use of venlafaxine and NSAIDs should be taken).
No products indexed under this heading.

Torsemide (Hyponatremia may occur as a result of treatment with SSRIs and SNRIs, including venlafaxine hydrochloride. In many cases, this hyponatremia appears to be the result of the syndrome of inappropriate antidiuretic hormone secretion (SIADH). Patients taking diuretics or who are otherwise volume depleted may be at greater risk. Discontinuation of venlafaxine hydrochloride should be considered in patients with symptomatic hyponatremia and appropriate medical intervention should be instituted). Products include:
Demadex Injection 2630
Demadex Tablets 2630

Tramadol Hydrochloride (Caution is advised when velafaxine is co-administered with other drugs that may affect serotonergic neurotransmitter systems). Products include:
Ultram ER Extended-Release Tablets 2428

Tranylcypromine Sulfate (Adverse reactions, some of which were serious, have been reported in patients who have recently been discontinued from an MAO inhibitor and started on venlafaxine, or who have recently had venlafaxine therapy discontinued prior to initiation of an MAO inhibitor; concurrent and/or sequential use is contraindicated). Products include:
Parnate Tablets 1532

Triamterene (Hyponatremia may occur as a result of treatment with SSRIs and SNRIs, including venlafaxine hydrochloride. In many cases, this hyponatremia appears to be the result of the syndrome of inappropriate antidiuretic hormone secretion (SIADH). Patients taking diuretics or who are otherwise volume depleted may be at greater risk. Discontinuation of venlafaxine hydrochloride should be considered in patients with symptomatic hyponatremia and appropriate medical intervention should be instituted). Products include:
Dyazide Capsules 1405
Dyrenium Capsules 3189

Triazolam (Caution is advised if the concomitant administration of venlafaxine and CNS-active drugs is required).
No products indexed under this heading.

Trifluoperazine Hydrochloride (Caution is advised if the concomitant administration of venlafaxine and CNS-active drugs is required).
No products indexed under this heading.

Troglitazone (Concomitant use of CYP3A4 inhibitors and venlafaxine may increase levels of venlafaxine and O-desmethylvenlafaxine (ODV). Therefore, caution is advised if venlafaxine is used concomitantly with CYP3A4 inhibitors).
No products indexed under this heading.

Troleandomycin (Concomitant use of CYP3A4 inhibitors and venlafaxine may increase levels of venlafaxine and O-desmethylvenlafaxine (ODV). Therefore, caution is advised if venlafaxine is used concomitantly with CYP3A4 inhibitors).
No products indexed under this heading.

Tryptophan (Caution is advised when velafaxine is co-administered with other drugs that may affect serotonergic neurotransmitter systems).
No products indexed under this heading.

L-Tryptophan (Caution is advised when velafaxine is co-administered with other drugs that may affect serotonergic neurotransmitter systems).
No products indexed under this heading.

Valdecoxib (Use of venlafaxine may increase the risk of bleeding events. Concomitant use of nonsteroidal anti-inflammatory drugs (NSAIDs) may potentiate this risk of bleeding. Case reports and studies have shown an association between use of drugs that interfere with serotonin reuptake and the occurrence of gastrointestinal bleeding. Bleeding events related to SSRIs and SNRIs used have ranged from ecchymoses, hematomas, epistaxis and petechiae to life-threatening hemorrhages. Caution about the risk of bleeding associated with the concomitant use of venlafaxine and NSAIDs should be taken).
No products indexed under this heading.

Valproate Sodium (Concomitant use of CYP3A4 inhibitors and venlafaxine may increase levels of venlafaxine and O-desmethylvenlafaxine (ODV). Therefore, caution is advised if venlafaxine is used concomitantly with CYP3A4 inhibitors).
No products indexed under this heading.

Vardenafil Hydrochloride (Concomitant use of CYP3A4 inhibitors and venlafaxine may increase levels of venlafaxine and O-desmethylvenlafaxine (ODV). Therefore, caution is advised if venlafaxine is used concomitantly with CYP3A4 inhibitors). Products include:
Levitra Tablets 2876

Verapamil Hydrochloride (Concomitant use of CYP3A4 inhibitors and venlafaxine may increase levels of venlafaxine and O-desmethylvenlafaxine (ODV). Therefore, caution is advised if venlafaxine is used concomitantly with CYP3A4 inhibitors). Products include:
Tarka Tablets 511

Voriconazole (Concomitant use of CYP3A4 inhibitors and venlafaxine may increase levels of venlafaxine and O-desmethylvenlafaxine (ODV). Therefore, caution is advised if venlafaxine is used concomitantly with CYP3A4 inhibitors).
No products indexed under this heading.

Warfarin Sodium (Use of venlafaxine may increase the risk of bleeding events. Concomitant use of warfarin may potentiate this risk of bleeding. Case reports and studies have shown an association between use of drugs that interfere with serotonin reuptake and the occurrence of gastrointestinal bleeding. Bleeding events related to SSRIs and SNRIs used have ranged from ecchymoses, hematomas, epistaxis, and petechiae to life-threatening hemorrhages. Caution about the risk of bleeding associated with the concomitant use of venlafaxine and other drugs that affect coagulation should be taken).
No products indexed under this heading.

Zafirlukast (Concomitant use of CYP3A4 inhibitors and venlafaxine may increase levels of venlafaxine and O-desmethylvenlafaxine (ODV). Therefore, caution is advised if venlafaxine is used concomitantly with CYP3A4 inhibitors). Products include:
Accolate Tablets 669

Zaleplon (Caution is advised if the concomitant administration of venlafaxine and CNS-active drugs is required).
No products indexed under this heading.

Zileuton (Concomitant use of CYP3A4 inhibitors and venlafaxine may increase levels of venlafaxine and O-desmethylvenlafaxine (ODV). Therefore, caution is advised if venlafaxine is used concomitantly with CYP3A4 inhibitors).
No products indexed under this heading.

Ziprasidone Hydrochloride (Caution is advised if the concomitant administration of venlafaxine and CNS-active drugs is required). Products include:
Geodon Capsules 2520

Zolmitriptan (Based on the mechanism of action of venlafaxine and the potential for serotonin syndrome, caution is advised when velafaxine is co-administered with other drugs that may affect the serotonergic neurotransmitter systems, such as triptans). Products include:
Zomig Tablets 694
Zomig Nasal Spray 689
Zomig-ZMT Tablets 694

Zolpidem Tartrate (Caution is advised if the concomitant administration of venlafaxine and CNS-active drugs is required). Products include:
Ambien Tablets 2692
Ambien CR Tablets 2696

Food Interactions

Alcohol (Co-administration of venlafaxine as a stable regimen did not exaggerate the psychomotor and psychometric effects of alcohol; however, patients should be advised to avoid alcohol while taking venlafaxine).

Grapefruit (Concomitant use of CYP3A4 inhibitors and venlafaxine may increase levels of venlafaxine and O-desmethylvenlafaxine (ODV). Therefore, caution is advised if venlafaxine is used concomitantly with CYP3A4 inhibitors).

Grapefruit Juice (Concomitant use of CYP3A4 inhibitors and venlafaxine may increase levels of venlafaxine and O-desmethylvenlafaxine (ODV). Therefore, caution is advised if venlafaxine is used concomitantly with CYP3A4 inhibitors).

ELASTICITY CAPSULES

(Amino Acid Preparations, Herbals with Vitamins & Minerals) .... ▣636
None cited in PDR database.

ELDEPRYL CAPSULES

(Selegiline Hydrochloride) 3052
May interact with narcotic analgesics, selective serotonin reuptake inhibitors, tricyclic antidepressants, and certain other agents. Compounds in these categories include:

Alfentanil Hydrochloride (Contraindication warning for meperidine is extended to other opioids).
No products indexed under this heading.

Amitriptyline Hydrochloride (Co-administraton has resulted in severe CNS toxicity associated with hyperpyrexia and fatality; concurrent use in some patients may result in hypertension, syncope, asystole, diaphoresis seizures, changes in behavioral and mental status, and muscular rigidity; concurrent and/or sequential use is not recommended).
No products indexed under this heading.

Amoxapine (Co-administration may result in hypertension, syncope, asystole, diaphoresis seizures, changes in behavioral and mental status, and muscular rigidity; concurrent and/or sequential use is not recommended).
No products indexed under this heading.

Buprenorphine Hydrochloride (Contraindication warning for meperidine is extended to other opioids). Products include:

Suboxone Tablets 2601
Subutex Tablets 2601

Citalopram Hydrobromide (Potential for serious, sometimes fatal, reactions including hyperthermia, rigidity, myoclonus, autonomic instability, extreme agitation progressing to delirium and coma; concurrent and/or sequential use is not recommended). Products include:
Celexa 1160

Clomipramine Hydrochloride (Co-administration may result in hypertension, syncope, asystole, diaphoresis seizures, changes in behavioral and mental status, and muscular rigidity; concurrent and/or sequential use is not recommended).
No products indexed under this heading.

Codeine Phosphate (Contraindication warning for meperidine is extended to other opioids). Products include:
Tylenol with Codeine Tablets 2427

Desipramine Hydrochloride (Co-administration may result in hypertension, syncope, asystole, diaphoresis seizures, changes in behavioral and mental status, and muscular rigidity; concurrent and/or sequential use is not recommended).
No products indexed under this heading.

Dezocine (Contraindication warning for meperidine is extended to other opioids).
No products indexed under this heading.

Doxepin Hydrochloride (Co-administration may result in hypertension, syncope, asystole, diaphoresis seizures, changes in behavioral and mental status, and muscular rigidity; concurrent and/or sequential use is not recommended).
No products indexed under this heading.

Ephedrine Hydrochloride (Co-administration has resulted in one case of hypertensive crisis).
No products indexed under this heading.

Ephedrine Sulfate (Co-administration has resulted in one case of hypertensive crisis).
No products indexed under this heading.

Ephedrine Tannate (Co-administration has resulted in one case of hypertensive crisis).
No products indexed under this heading.

Fentanyl (Contraindication warning for meperidine is extended to other opioids). Products include:
Duragesic Transdermal System 2405
Ionsys Transdermal System 2410

Fentanyl Citrate (Contraindication warning for meperidine is extended to other opioids). Products include:
Actiq 959
Fentora Tablets 968

Fluoxetine (Potential for serious, sometimes fatal, reactions including hyperthermia, rigidity, myoclonus, autonomic instability, extreme agitation progressing to delirium and coma; concurrent and/or sequential use is not recommended).
No products indexed under this heading.

Fluoxetine Hydrochloride (Co-administration has resulted in serious, sometimes fatal, reactions including hyperthermia, rigidity, myoclonus, autonomic instability, extreme agitation progressing to delirium and coma; concurrent and/or sequential use is not recommended; because of long half-life of fluoxetine, at least 5 weeks or longer should elapse between discontinuation of fluoxetine and initiation of Eldepryl). Products include:
Prozac Weekly Capsules 1852
Prozac Pulvules and Liquid 1852
Symbyax Capsules 1871

Fluvoxamine Maleate (Potential for serious, sometimes fatal, reactions including hyperthermia, rigidity, myoclonus, autonomic instability, extreme agitation progressing to delirium and coma; concurrent and/or sequential use is not recommended). Products include:
Luvox CR Extended-Release Capsules 1759

Hydrocodone Bitartrate (Contraindication warning for meperidine is extended to other opioids). Products include:
Lortab 5/500 Tablets 3143
Lortab 7.5/500 Tablets 3144
Lortab 10/500 Tablets 3144
Vicodin Tablets 529
Vicodin ES Tablets 530
Vicodin HP Tablets 531
Vicoprofen Tablets 533
Zydone Tablets 1132

Hydrocodone Polistirex (Contraindication warning for meperidine is extended to other opioids). Products include:
Tussionex Pennkinetic Extended-Release Suspension 3154

Hydromorphone Hydrochloride (Contraindication warning for meperidine is extended to other opioids).
No products indexed under this heading.

Imipramine Hydrochloride (Co-administration may result in hypertension, syncope, asystole, diaphoresis seizures, changes in behavioral and mental status, and muscular rigidity; concurrent and/or sequential use is not recommended).
No products indexed under this heading.

Imipramine Pamoate (Co-administration may result in hypertension, syncope, asystole, diaphoresis seizures, changes in behavioral and mental status, and muscular rigidity; concurrent and/or sequential use is not recommended).
No products indexed under this heading.

Levodopa (Co-administration in some patients may exacerbate levodopa-associated side effects). Products include:
Stalevo Tablets 2309

Levorphanol Tartrate (Contraindication warning for meperidine is extended to other opioids).
No products indexed under this heading.

Maprotiline Hydrochloride (Co-administration may result in hypertension, syncope, asystole, diaphoresis seizures, changes in behavioral and mental status, and muscular rigidity; concurrent and/or sequential use is not recommended).
No products indexed under this heading.

Meperidine Hydrochloride (Co-administration has resulted in stupor, muscular rigidity, severe agitation, hallucination, and hyperpyrexia; concurrent use is contraindicated).
No products indexed under this heading.

Methadone Hydrochloride (Contraindication warning for meperidine is extended to other opioids).
No products indexed under this heading.

Morphine Sulfate (Contraindication warning for meperidine is extended to other opioids). Products include:
Avinza Capsules 1772
DepoDur Injection 1095
MS Contin Tablets 2585

Nortriptyline Hydrochloride (Co-administration may result in hypertension, syncope, asystole, diaphoresis seizures, changes in behavioral and mental status, and muscular rigidity; concurrent and/or sequential use is not recommended).
No products indexed under this heading.

Oxycodone Hydrochloride (Contraindication warning for meperidine is extended to other opioids). Products include:
OxyContin Tablets 2589
OxyIR Capsules 2593
Percocet Tablets 1127
Percodan Tablets 1130

Paroxetine Hydrochloride (Potential for serious, sometimes fatal, reactions including hyperthermia, rigidity, myoclonus, autonomic instability, extreme agitation progressing to delirium and coma; concurrent and/or sequential use is not recommended). Products include:
Paxil 1535
Paxil CR Controlled-Release Tablets 1544

Propoxyphene Hydrochloride (Contraindication warning for meperidine is extended to other opioids).
No products indexed under this heading.

Propoxyphene Napsylate (Contraindication warning for meperidine is extended to other opioids).
No products indexed under this heading.

Protriptyline Hydrochloride (Co-administration has resulted in tremors, agitation, and restlessness followed by unresponsiveness and fatality; concurrent use in some patients may result in hypertension, syncope, asystole, diaphoresis seizures, changes in behavioral and mental status, and muscular rigidity; concurrent and/or sequential use is not recommended).
No products indexed under this heading.

Sertraline Hydrochloride (Potential for serious, sometimes fatal, reactions including hyperthermia, rigidity, myoclonus, autonomic instability, extreme agitation progressing to delirium and coma; concurrent and/or sequential use is not recommended).
No products indexed under this heading.

Sufentanil Citrate (Contraindication warning for meperidine is extended to other opioids).
No products indexed under this heading.

Trimipramine Maleate (Co-administration may result in hypertension, syncope, asystole, diaphoresis seizures, changes in behavioral and mental status, and muscular rigidity; concurrent and/or sequential use is not recommended).
No products indexed under this heading.

Venlafaxine Hydrochloride (Potential for serious, sometimes fatal, reactions including hyperthermia, rigidity, myoclonus, autonomic instability, extreme agitation progressing to delirium and coma; concurrent and/or sequential use is not recommended). Products include:
Effexor XR Extended-Release Capsules 3195
Venlafaxine Hydrochloride Tablets 2199

Food Interactions

Food, unspecified (The bioavailability of selegiline is increased 3 to 4 fold when it is taken with food).

ELDERTONIC

(Vitamins with Minerals) 2163
None cited in PDR database.

ELESTAT OPHTHALMIC SOLUTION

(Epinastine Hydrochloride) 1741
None cited in PDR database.

ELIDEL CREAM 1%

(Pimecrolimus) 2221
May interact with cytochrome p450 3a inhibitors (selected). Compounds in these categories include:

Amiodarone Hydrochloride (The concomitant administration of known CYP3A family of inhibitors in patients with widespread and/or erythrodermic disease should be done with caution).
No products indexed under this heading.

Amprenavir (The concomitant administration of known CYP3A family of inhibitors in patients with widespread and/or erythrodermic disease should be done with caution).
No products indexed under this heading.

Aprepitant (The concomitant administration of known CYP3A family of inhibitors in patients with widespread and/or erythrodermic disease should be done with caution). Products include:
Emend Capsules 1992

Cimetidine (The concomitant administration of known CYP3A family of inhibitors in patients with widespread and/or erythrodermic disease should be done with caution).
No products indexed under this heading.

Cimetidine Hydrochloride (The concomitant administration of known CYP3A family of inhibitors in patients with widespread and/or erythrodermic disease should be done with caution).
No products indexed under this heading.

Ciprofloxacin (The concomitant administration of known CYP3A family of inhibitors in patients with widespread and/or erythrodermic disease should be done with caution). Products include:
Cipro I.V. 2817
Cipro Oral Suspension 2810
Cipro XR Tablets 2823
Ciprodex Otic Suspension 541

Ciprofloxacin Hydrochloride (The concomitant administration of known CYP3A family of inhibitors in patients with widespread and/or erythrodermic disease should be done with caution). Products include:
Cipro Tablets 2810

Clarithromycin (The concomitant administration of known CYP3A family of inhibitors in patients with widespread and/or erythrodermic disease should be done with caution). Products include:

Biaxin/Biaxin XL 411

Cyclosporine (The concomitant administration of known CYP3A family of inhibitors in patients with widespread and/or erythrodermic disease should be done with caution). Products include:

Gengraf Capsules 435
Neoral Oral Solution 2280
Neoral Soft Gelatin Capsules 2280
Restasis Ophthalmic Emulsion 557
Sandimmune 2296

Delavirdine Mesylate (The concomitant administration of known CYP3A family of inhibitors in patients with widespread and/or erythrodermic disease should be done with caution).

No products indexed under this heading.

Diltiazem Hydrochloride (The concomitant administration of known CYP3A family of inhibitors in patients with widespread and/or erythrodermic disease should be done with caution). Products include:

Cardizem LA Extended Release Tablets 421

Diltiazem Maleate (The concomitant administration of known CYP3A family of inhibitors in patients with widespread and/or erythrodermic disease should be done with caution).

No products indexed under this heading.

Efavirenz (The concomitant administration of known CYP3A family of inhibitors in patients with widespread and/or erythrodermic disease should be done with caution). Products include:

Atripla Tablets 938
Sustiva Capsules 930
Sustiva Tablets 930

Erythromycin (The concomitant administration of known CYP3A family of inhibitors in patients with widespread and/or erythrodermic disease should be done with caution).

No products indexed under this heading.

Fluconazole (The concomitant administration of known CYP3A family of inhibitors in patients with widespread and/or erythrodermic disease should be done with caution).

No products indexed under this heading.

Fluoxetine (The concomitant administration of known CYP3A family of inhibitors in patients with widespread and/or erythrodermic disease should be done with caution).

No products indexed under this heading.

Fluoxetine Hydrochloride (The concomitant administration of known CYP3A family of inhibitors in patients with widespread and/or erythrodermic disease should be done with caution). Products include:

Prozac Weekly Capsules 1852
Prozac Pulvules and Liquid 1852
Symbyax Capsules 1871

Fluvoxamine Maleate (The concomitant administration of known CYP3A family of inhibitors in patients with widespread and/or erythrodermic disease should be done with caution). Products include:

Luvox CR Extended-Release Capsules 1759

Indinavir Sulfate (The concomitant administration of known CYP3A family of inhibitors in patients with widespread and/or erythrodermic disease should be done with caution). Products include:

Crixivan Capsules 1979

Isoniazid (The concomitant administration of known CYP3A family of inhibitors in patients with widespread and/or erythrodermic disease should be done with caution).

No products indexed under this heading.

Itraconazole (The concomitant administration of known CYP3A family of inhibitors in patients with widespread and/or erythrodermic disease should be done with caution).

No products indexed under this heading.

Ketoconazole (The concomitant administration of known CYP3A family of inhibitors in patients with widespread and/or erythrodermic disease should be done with caution). Products include:

Extina Foam, 2% 3057
Nizoral A-D Shampoo 1901

Lopinavir (The concomitant administration of known CYP3A family of inhibitors in patients with widespread and/or erythrodermic disease should be done with caution). Products include:

Kaletra 452

Metronidazole (The concomitant administration of known CYP3A family of inhibitors in patients with widespread and/or erythrodermic disease should be done with caution). Products include:

Pylera Capsules 714

Metronidazole Benzoate (The concomitant administration of known CYP3A family of inhibitors in patients with widespread and/or erythrodermic disease should be done with caution).

No products indexed under this heading.

Metronidazole Hydrochloride (The concomitant administration of known CYP3A family of inhibitors in patients with widespread and/or erythrodermic disease should be done with caution).

No products indexed under this heading.

Miconazole (The concomitant administration of known CYP3A family of inhibitors in patients with widespread and/or erythrodermic disease should be done with caution).

No products indexed under this heading.

Nefazodone Hydrochloride (The concomitant administration of known CYP3A family of inhibitors in patients with widespread and/or erythrodermic disease should be done with caution).

No products indexed under this heading.

Nelfinavir Mesylate (The concomitant administration of known CYP3A family of inhibitors in patients with widespread and/or erythrodermic disease should be done with caution).

No products indexed under this heading.

Nifedipine (The concomitant administration of known CYP3A family of inhibitors in patients with widespread and/or erythrodermic disease should be done with caution).

No products indexed under this heading.

Norfloxacin (The concomitant administration of known CYP3A family of inhibitors in patients with widespread and/or erythrodermic disease should be done with caution). Products include:

Noroxin Tablets 2069

Paroxetine Hydrochloride (The concomitant administration of known CYP3A family of inhibitors in patients with widespread and/or erythrodermic disease should be done with caution). Products include:

Paxil 1535
Paxil CR Controlled-Release Tablets 1544

Quinine (The concomitant administration of known CYP3A family of inhibitors in patients with widespread and/or erythrodermic disease should be done with caution).

No products indexed under this heading.

Quinine Sulfate (The concomitant administration of known CYP3A family of inhibitors in patients with widespread and/or erythrodermic disease should be done with caution).

No products indexed under this heading.

Ritonavir (The concomitant administration of known CYP3A family of inhibitors in patients with widespread and/or erythrodermic disease should be done with caution). Products include:

Kaletra 452
Norvir 489

Saquinavir (The concomitant administration of known CYP3A family of inhibitors in patients with widespread and/or erythrodermic disease should be done with caution).

No products indexed under this heading.

Saquinavir Mesylate (The concomitant administration of known CYP3A family of inhibitors in patients with widespread and/or erythrodermic disease should be done with caution).

No products indexed under this heading.

Sertraline Hydrochloride (The concomitant administration of known CYP3A family of inhibitors in patients with widespread and/or erythrodermic disease should be done with caution).

No products indexed under this heading.

Troleandomycin (The concomitant administration of known CYP3A family of inhibitors in patients with widespread and/or erythrodermic disease should be done with caution).

No products indexed under this heading.

Venlafaxine Hydrochloride (The concomitant administration of known CYP3A family of inhibitors in patients with widespread and/or erythrodermic disease should be done with caution). Products include:

Effexor XR Extended-Release Capsules 3195
Venlafaxine Hydrochloride Tablets ... 2199

Verapamil Hydrochloride (The concomitant administration of known CYP3A family of inhibitors in patients with widespread and/or erythrodermic disease should be done with caution). Products include:

Tarka Tablets 511

Voriconazole (The concomitant administration of known CYP3A family of inhibitors in patients with widespread and/or erythrodermic disease should be done with caution).

No products indexed under this heading.

Zafirlukast (The concomitant administration of known CYP3A family of inhibitors in patients with widespread and/or erythrodermic disease should be done with caution). Products include:

Accolate Tablets 669

Zileuton (The concomitant administration of known CYP3A family of inhibitors in patients with widespread and/or erythrodermic disease should be done with caution).

No products indexed under this heading.

Food Interactions

Grapefruit (The concomitant administration of known CYP3A family of inhibitors in patients with widespread and/or erythrodermic disease should be done with caution).

ELIGARD 7.5 MG

(Leuprolide Acetate) 2724
None cited in PDR database.

ELIGARD 22.5 MG

(Leuprolide Acetate) 2724
None cited in PDR database.

ELIGARD 30 MG

(Leuprolide Acetate) 2724
None cited in PDR database.

ELIGARD 45 MG

(Leuprolide Acetate) 2724
None cited in PDR database.

ELITEK

(Rasburicase) 2729
None cited in PDR database.

ELIXIR CAPSULES

(Amino Acid Preparations, Bee Pollen, Calcium Carbonate, Folic Acid, Ginkgo biloba, Herbals with Vitamins & Minerals, Iron Amino Acid Chelate) .... ▣636
None cited in PDR database.

ELMIRON CAPSULES

(Pentosan Polysulfate Sodium) 2435

May interact with aspirin-acetylsalicylic acid, anticoagulants, oral anticoagulants, non-steroidal anti-inflammatory agents, and certain other agents. Compounds in these categories include:

Anisindione (Pentosan polysulfate sodium is a weak anticoagulant. At a daily dose of 300 mg, rectal hemorrhage was reported as an adverse event in 6.3% of patients. Bleeding complications of ecchymosis, epistaxis, and gum hemorrhage have been reported. Patients at increased risk of bleeding due to other therapies such as anticoagulants, should be evaluated for hemorrhage).

No products indexed under this heading.

Ardeparin Sodium (Pentosan polysulfate sodium is a weak anticoagulant. At a daily dose of 300 mg, rectal hemorrhage was reported as an adverse event in 6.3% of patients. Bleeding complications of ecchymosis, epistaxis, and gum hemorrhage have been reported. Patients at increased risk of bleeding due to other therapies such as anticoagulants, should be evaluated for hemorrhage).

No products indexed under this heading.

Aspirin (Pentosan polysulfate sodium is a weak anticoagulant. At a daily dose of 300 mg, rectal hemorrhage was reported as an adverse event in 6.3% of patients. Bleeding complications of ecchymosis, epistaxis, and gum hemorrhage have been reported. Patients at increased risk of bleeding due to other therapies such as high dose aspirin, should be evaluated for hemorrhage). Products include:

Aggrenox Capsules 819
Bayer Aspirin 750
Percodan Tablets 1130
St. Joseph 81 mg Aspirin Chewable and Enteric Coated Tablets 1903

Aspirin, Enteric Coated (Pentosan polysulfate sodium is a weak anticoagulant. At a daily dose of 300 mg, rectal hemorrhage was reported as an adverse event in 6.3% of patients. Bleeding complications of ecchymosis, epistaxis, and gum hemorrhage have been reported. Patients at increased risk of bleeding due to other therapies such as high dose aspirin, should be evaluated for hemorrhage).

No products indexed under this heading.

Aspirin Buffered (Pentosan polysulfate sodium is a weak anticoagulant. At a daily dose of 300 mg, rectal hemorrhage was reported as an adverse event in 6.3% of patients. Bleeding complications of ecchymosis, epistaxis, and gum hemorrhage have been reported. Patients at increased risk of bleeding due to other therapies such as high dose aspirin, should be evaluated for hemorrhage).

No products indexed under this heading.

Celecoxib (Pentosan polysulfate sodium is a weak anticoagulant. At a daily dose of 300 mg, rectal hemorrhage was reported as an adverse event in 6.3% of patients. Bleeding complications of ecchymosis, epistaxis, and gum hemorrhage have been reported. Patients at increased risk of bleeding due to other therapies such non-steroidal anti-inflammatory drugs, should be evaluated for hemorrhage). Products include:

Celebrex Capsules 2979

Dalteparin Sodium (Pentosan polysulfate sodium is a weak anticoagulant. At a daily dose of 300 mg, rectal hemorrhage was reported as an adverse event in 6.3% of patients. Bleeding complications of ecchymosis, epistaxis, and gum hemorrhage have been reported. Patients at increased risk of bleeding due to other therapies such as anticoagulants, should be evaluated for hemorrhage). Products include:

Fragmin Injection 1070

Danaparoid Sodium (Pentosan polysulfate sodium is a weak anticoagulant. At a daily dose of 300 mg, rectal hemorrhage was reported as an adverse event in 6.3% of patients. Bleeding complications of ecchymosis, epistaxis, and gum hemorrhage have been reported. Patients at increased risk of bleeding due to other therapies such as anticoagulants, should be evaluated for hemorrhage).

No products indexed under this heading.

Diclofenac Epolamine (Pentosan polysulfate sodium is a weak anticoagulant. At a daily dose of 300 mg, rectal hemorrhage was reported as an adverse event in 6.3% of patients. Bleeding complications of ecchymosis, epistaxis, and gum hemorrhage have been reported. Patients at increased risk of bleeding due to other therapies such non-steroidal anti-inflammatory drugs, should be evaluated for hemorrhage). Products include:

Flector Patch 561

Diclofenac Potassium (Pentosan polysulfate sodium is a weak anticoagulant. At a daily dose of 300 mg, rectal hemorrhage was reported as an adverse event in 6.3% of patients. Bleeding complications of ecchymosis, epistaxis, and gum hemorrhage have been reported. Patients at increased risk of bleeding due to other therapies such non-steroidal anti-inflammatory drugs, should be evaluated for hemorrhage).

No products indexed under this heading.

Diclofenac Sodium (Pentosan polysulfate sodium is a weak anticoagulant. At a daily dose of 300 mg, rectal hemorrhage was reported as an adverse event in 6.3% of patients. Bleeding complications of ecchymosis, epistaxis, and gum hemorrhage have been reported. Patients at increased risk of bleeding due to other therapies such non-steroidal anti-inflammatory drugs, should be evaluated for hemorrhage). Products include:

Diclofenac Sodium Ophthalmic Solution .... ⊙ 240
Voltaren Ophthalmic Solution 2336
Voltaren Tablets 2334
Voltaren-XR Tablets 2337

Dicumarol (Pentosan polysulfate sodium is a weak anticoagulant. At a daily dose of 300 mg, rectal hemorrhage was reported as an adverse event in 6.3% of patients. Bleeding complications of ecchymosis, epistaxis, and gum hemorrhage have been reported. Patients at increased risk of bleeding due to other therapies such as anticoagulants, should be evaluated for hemorrhage).

No products indexed under this heading.

Enoxaparin Sodium (Pentosan polysulfate sodium is a weak anticoagulant. At a daily dose of 300 mg, rectal hemorrhage was reported as an adverse event in 6.3% of patients. Bleeding complications of ecchymosis, epistaxis, and gum hemorrhage have been reported. Patients at increased risk of bleeding due to other therapies such as anticoagulants, should be evaluated for hemorrhage). Products include:

Lovenox Injection 2756

Etodolac (Pentosan polysulfate sodium is a weak anticoagulant. At a daily dose of 300 mg, rectal hemorrhage was reported as an adverse event in 6.3% of patients. Bleeding complications of ecchymosis, epistaxis, and gum hemorrhage have been reported. Patients at increased risk of bleeding due to other therapies such non-steroidal anti-inflammatory drugs, should be evaluated for hemorrhage).

No products indexed under this heading.

Fenoprofen Calcium (Pentosan polysulfate sodium is a weak anticoagulant. At a daily dose of 300 mg, rectal hemorrhage was reported as an adverse event in 6.3% of patients. Bleeding complications of ecchymosis, epistaxis, and gum hemorrhage have been reported. Patients at increased risk of bleeding due to other therapies such non-steroidal anti-inflammatory drugs, should be evaluated for hemorrhage). Products include:

Nalfon Capsules 2508

Flurbiprofen (Pentosan polysulfate sodium is a weak anticoagulant. At a daily dose of 300 mg, rectal hemorrhage was reported as an adverse event in 6.3% of patients. Bleeding complications of ecchymosis, epistaxis, and gum hemorrhage have been reported. Patients at increased risk of bleeding due to other therapies such non-steroidal anti-inflammatory drugs, should be evaluated for hemorrhage).

No products indexed under this heading.

Fondaparinux Sodium (Pentosan polysulfate sodium is a weak anticoagulant. At a daily dose of 300 mg, rectal hemorrhage was reported as an adverse event in 6.3% of patients. Bleeding complications of ecchymosis, epistaxis, and gum hemorrhage have been reported. Patients at increased risk of bleeding due to other therapies such as anticoagulants, should be evaluated for hemorrhage). Products include:

Arixtra Injection 1313

Heparin Calcium (Pentosan polysulfate sodium is a weak anticoagulant. At a daily dose of 300 mg, rectal hemorrhage was reported as an adverse event in 6.3% of patients. Bleeding complications of ecchymosis, epistaxis, and gum hemorrhage have been reported. Patients at increased risk of bleeding due to other therapies such as anticoagulants, should be evaluated for hemorrhage).

No products indexed under this heading.

Heparin Sodium (Pentosan polysulfate sodium is a weak anticoagulant. At a daily dose of 300 mg, rectal hemorrhage was reported as an adverse event in 6.3% of patients. Bleeding complications of ecchymosis, epistaxis, and gum hemorrhage have been reported. Patients at increased risk of bleeding due to other therapies such as anticoagulants, should be evaluated for hemorrhage).

No products indexed under this heading.

Ibuprofen (Pentosan polysulfate sodium is a weak anticoagulant. At a daily dose of 300 mg, rectal hemorrhage was reported as an adverse event in 6.3% of patients. Bleeding complications of ecchymosis, epistaxis, and gum hemorrhage have been reported. Patients at increased risk of bleeding due to other therapies such non-steroidal anti-inflammatory drugs, should be evaluated for hemorrhage). Products include:

Motrin IB Tablets and Caplets 1900
Children's Motrin Oral Suspension ... 1901
Children's Motrin Non-Staining Dye-Free Oral Suspension 1901
Children's Motrin Cold Oral Suspension 1899
Infants' Motrin Concentrated Drops 1901
Infants' Motrin Non-Staining Dye-Free Concentrated Drops 1901
Junior Strength Motrin Caplets and Chewable Tablets 1901
Vicoprofen Tablets 533

Indomethacin (Pentosan polysulfate sodium is a weak anticoagulant. At a daily dose of 300 mg, rectal hemorrhage was reported as an adverse event in 6.3% of patients. Bleeding complications of ecchymosis, epistaxis, and gum hemorrhage have been reported. Patients at increased risk of bleeding due to other therapies such non-steroidal anti-inflammatory drugs, should be evaluated for hemorrhage). Products include:

Indocin 2024

Indomethacin Sodium Trihydrate (Pentosan polysulfate sodium is a weak anticoagulant. At a daily dose of 300 mg, rectal hemorrhage was reported as an adverse event in 6.3% of patients. Bleeding complications of ecchymosis, epistaxis, and gum hemorrhage have been reported. Patients at increased risk of bleeding due to other therapies such non-steroidal anti-inflammatory drugs, should be evaluated for hemorrhage). Products include:

Indocin I.V. 2489

Ketoprofen (Pentosan polysulfate sodium is a weak anticoagulant. At a daily dose of 300 mg, rectal hemorrhage was reported as an adverse event in 6.3% of patients. Bleeding complications of ecchymosis, epistaxis, and gum hemorrhage have been reported. Patients at increased risk of bleeding due to other therapies such non-steroidal anti-inflammatory drugs, should be evaluated for hemorrhage).

No products indexed under this heading.

Ketorolac Tromethamine (Pentosan polysulfate sodium is a weak anticoagulant. At a daily dose of 300 mg, rectal hemorrhage was reported as an adverse event in 6.3% of patients. Bleeding complications of ecchymosis, epistaxis, and gum hemorrhage have been reported. Patients at increased risk of bleeding due to other therapies such non-steroidal anti-inflammatory drugs, should be evaluated for hemorrhage).

No products indexed under this heading.

Low Molecular Weight Heparins (Pentosan polysulfate sodium is a weak anticoagulant. At a daily dose of 300 mg, rectal hemorrhage was reported as an adverse event in 6.3% of patients. Bleeding complications of ecchymosis, epistaxis, and gum hemorrhage have been reported. Patients at increased risk of bleeding due to other therapies such as anticoagulants, should be evaluat-

ed for hemorrhage).
No products indexed under this heading.

Meclofenamate Sodium (Pentosan polysulfate sodium is a weak anticoagulant. At a daily dose of 300 mg, rectal hemorrhage was reported as an adverse event in 6.3% of patients. Bleeding complications of ecchymosis, epistaxis, and gum hemorrhage have been reported. Patients at increased risk of bleeding due to other therapies such non-steroidal anti-inflammatory drugs, should be evaluated for hemorrhage).
No products indexed under this heading.

Mefenamic Acid (Pentosan polysulfate sodium is a weak anticoagulant. At a daily dose of 300 mg, rectal hemorrhage was reported as an adverse event in 6.3% of patients. Bleeding complications of ecchymosis, epistaxis, and gum hemorrhage have been reported. Patients at increased risk of bleeding due to other therapies such non-steroidal anti-inflammatory drugs, should be evaluated for hemorrhage).
No products indexed under this heading.

Meloxicam (Pentosan polysulfate sodium is a weak anticoagulant. At a daily dose of 300 mg, rectal hemorrhage was reported as an adverse event in 6.3% of patients. Bleeding complications of ecchymosis, epistaxis, and gum hemorrhage have been reported. Patients at increased risk of bleeding due to other therapies such non-steroidal anti-inflammatory drugs, should be evaluated for hemorrhage). Products include:
Mobic Oral Suspension 863
Mobic Tablets 863

Nabumetone (Pentosan polysulfate sodium is a weak anticoagulant. At a daily dose of 300 mg, rectal hemorrhage was reported as an adverse event in 6.3% of patients. Bleeding complications of ecchymosis, epistaxis, and gum hemorrhage have been reported. Patients at increased risk of bleeding due to other therapies such non-steroidal anti-inflammatory drugs, should be evaluated for hemorrhage).
No products indexed under this heading.

Naproxen (Pentosan polysulfate sodium is a weak anticoagulant. At a daily dose of 300 mg, rectal hemorrhage was reported as an adverse event in 6.3% of patients. Bleeding complications of ecchymosis, epistaxis, and gum hemorrhage have been reported. Patients at increased risk of bleeding due to other therapies such non-steroidal anti-inflammatory drugs, should be evaluated for hemorrhage). Products include:
EC-Naprosyn Delayed-Release Tablets 2632
Naprosyn Suspension 2632
Naprosyn Tablets 2632

Naproxen Sodium (Pentosan polysulfate sodium is a weak anticoagulant. At a daily dose of 300 mg, rectal hemorrhage was reported as an adverse event in 6.3% of patients. Bleeding complications of ecchymosis, epistaxis, and gum hemorrhage have been reported. Patients at increased risk of bleeding due to other therapies such non-steroidal anti-inflammatory drugs, should be evaluated for hemorrhage). Products include:
Anaprox Tablets 2632
Anaprox DS Tablets 2632
Treximet Tablets 1616

Oxaprozin (Pentosan polysulfate sodium is a weak anticoagulant. At a daily dose of 300 mg, rectal hemorrhage was reported as an adverse event in 6.3% of patients. Bleeding complications of ecchymosis, epistaxis, and gum hemorrhage have been reported. Patients at increased risk of bleeding due to other therapies such non-steroidal anti-inflammatory drugs, should be evaluated for hemorrhage).
No products indexed under this heading.

Phenylbutazone (Pentosan polysulfate sodium is a weak anticoagulant. At a daily dose of 300 mg, rectal hemorrhage was reported as an adverse event in 6.3% of patients. Bleeding complications of ecchymosis, epistaxis, and gum hemorrhage have been reported. Patients at increased risk of bleeding due to other therapies such non-steroidal anti-inflammatory drugs, should be evaluated for hemorrhage).
No products indexed under this heading.

Piroxicam (Pentosan polysulfate sodium is a weak anticoagulant. At a daily dose of 300 mg, rectal hemorrhage was reported as an adverse event in 6.3% of patients. Bleeding complications of ecchymosis, epistaxis, and gum hemorrhage have been reported. Patients at increased risk of bleeding due to other therapies such non-steroidal anti-inflammatory drugs, should be evaluated for hemorrhage).
No products indexed under this heading.

Rofecoxib (Pentosan polysulfate sodium is a weak anticoagulant. At a daily dose of 300 mg, rectal hemorrhage was reported as an adverse event in 6.3% of patients. Bleeding complications of ecchymosis, epistaxis, and gum hemorrhage have been reported. Patients at increased risk of bleeding due to other therapies such non-steroidal anti-inflammatory drugs, should be evaluated for hemorrhage).
No products indexed under this heading.

Streptokinase (Pentosan polysulfate sodium is a weak anticoagulant. At a daily dose of 300 mg, rectal hemorrhage was reported as an adverse event in 6.3% of patients. Bleeding complications of ecchymosis, epistaxis, and gum hemorrhage have been reported. Patients at increased risk of bleeding due to other therapies such as streptokinase, should be evaluated for hemorrhage).
No products indexed under this heading.

Sulindac (Pentosan polysulfate sodium is a weak anticoagulant. At a daily dose of 300 mg, rectal hemorrhage was reported as an adverse event in 6.3% of patients. Bleeding complications of ecchymosis, epistaxis, and gum hemorrhage have been reported. Patients at increased risk of bleeding due to other therapies such non-steroidal anti-inflammatory drugs, should be evaluated for hemorrhage). Products include:
Clinoril Tablets 1962

Tinzaparin Sodium (Pentosan polysulfate sodium is a weak anticoagulant. At a daily dose of 300 mg, rectal hemorrhage was reported as an adverse event in 6.3% of patients. Bleeding complications of ecchymosis, epistaxis, and gum hemorrhage have been reported. Patients at increased risk of bleeding due to other therapies such as anticoagulants, should be evaluated for hemorrhage).
No products indexed under this heading.

Tolmetin Sodium (Pentosan polysulfate sodium is a weak anticoagulant. At a daily dose of 300 mg, rectal hemorrhage was reported as an adverse event in 6.3% of patients. Bleeding complications of ecchymosis, epistaxis, and gum hemorrhage have been reported. Patients at increased risk of bleeding due to other therapies such non-steroidal anti-inflammatory drugs, should be evaluated for hemorrhage).
No products indexed under this heading.

Valdecoxib (Pentosan polysulfate sodium is a weak anticoagulant. At a daily dose of 300 mg, rectal hemorrhage was reported as an adverse event in 6.3% of patients. Bleeding complications of ecchymosis, epistaxis, and gum hemorrhage have been reported. Patients at increased risk of bleeding due to other therapies such non-steroidal anti-inflammatory drugs, should be evaluated for hemorrhage).
No products indexed under this heading.

Warfarin Sodium (Pentosan polysulfate sodium is a weak anticoagulant. At 300 mg QD, rectal hemorrhage was reported as an adverse event in 6.3% of patients. Bleeding complications of ecchymosis, epistaxis, and gum hemorrhage have been reported. Patients at increased risk of bleeding due to other therapies such as coumarin angicoagulants, should be evaluated for hemorrhage. However, in a study in which healthy subjects received pentosan polysulfate sodium 100 mg capsule or placebo every 8 hours for 7 days, and were titrated with warfarin to an INR of 1.4 to 1.8, the pharmacokinetic parameters of R-warfarin and S-warfarin were similar in the absence and presence of pentosan polysulfate sodium. INR for warfarin + placebo and warfarin + pentosan polysulfate were comparable).
No products indexed under this heading.

ELOCON CREAM 0.1%

(Mometasone Furoate) 2840
None cited in PDR database.

ELOCON LOTION 0.1%

(Mometasone Furoate) 2841
None cited in PDR database.

ELOCON OINTMENT 0.1%

(Mometasone Furoate) 2842
None cited in PDR database.

ELOXATIN FOR INJECTION

(Oxaliplatin) 2731
May interact with anticoagulants, nephrotoxic agents, and certain other agents. Compounds in these categories include:

Abacavir Sulfate (Because platinum-containing species are eliminated primarily through the kidney, clearance of these products may be decreased by co-administration of potentially nephrotoxic compounds, although this has not been specifically studied). Products include:
Epzicom Tablets 1422
Trizivir Tablets 1622
Ziagen 1673

Acyclovir (Because platinum-containing species are eliminated primarily through the kidney, clearance of these products may be decreased by co-administration of potentially nephrotoxic compounds, although this has not been specifically studied). Products include:
Zovirax 1690
Zovirax Cream 817
Zovirax Ointment 819

Acyclovir Sodium (Because platinum-containing species are eliminated primarily through the kidney, clearance of these products may be decreased by co-administration of potentially nephrotoxic compounds, although this has not been specifically studied).
No products indexed under this heading.

Alatrofloxacin Mesylate (Because platinum-containing species are eliminated primarily through the kidney, clearance of these products may be decreased by co-administration of potentially nephrotoxic compounds, although this has not been specifically studied).
No products indexed under this heading.

Aldesleukin (Because platinum-containing species are eliminated primarily through the kidney, clearance of these products may be decreased by co-administration of potentially nephrotoxic compounds, although this has not been specifically studied). Products include:
Proleukin for Injection 2287

Amikacin Sulfate (Because platinum-containing species are eliminated primarily through the kidney, clearance of these products may be decreased by co-administration of potentially nephrotoxic compounds, although this has not been specifically studied).
No products indexed under this heading.

Amoxicillin (Because platinum-containing species are eliminated primarily through the kidney, clearance of these products may be decreased by co-administration of potentially nephrotoxic compounds, although this has not been specifically studied). Products include:
Amoxil Capsules 1305
Amoxil Chewable Tablets 1305
Amoxil Pediatric Drops for Oral Suspension 1305
Amoxil Powder for Oral Suspension 1305
Amoxil Tablets 1305
Augmentin 1323
Augmentin Tablets 1327
Augmentin XR Extended Release Tablets 1333

Augmentin ES-600 Powder for Oral Suspension 1329
Moxatag Tablets 2165

Amoxicillin Trihydrate (Because platinum-containing species are eliminated primarily through the kidney, clearance of these products may be decreased by co-administration of potentially nephrotoxic compounds, although this has not been specifically studied).
No products indexed under this heading.

Amphotericin B (Because platinum-containing species are eliminated primarily through the kidney, clearance of these products may be decreased by co-administration of potentially nephrotoxic compounds, although this has not been specifically studied).
No products indexed under this heading.

Amphotericin B, liposomal (Because platinum-containing species are eliminated primarily through the kidney, clearance of these products may be decreased by co-administration of potentially nephrotoxic compounds, although this has not been specifically studied).
Products include:
AmBisome for Injection 606

Amphotericin B Cholesteryl Sulfate (Because platinum-containing species are eliminated primarily through the kidney, clearance of these products may be decreased by co-administration of potentially nephrotoxic compounds, although this has not been specifically studied).
No products indexed under this heading.

Amphotericin B Lipid Complex (Because platinum-containing species are eliminated primarily through the kidney, clearance of these products may be decreased by co-administration of potentially nephrotoxic compounds, although this has not been specifically studied).
Products include:
Abelcet Injection 1134

Ampicillin (Because platinum-containing species are eliminated primarily through the kidney, clearance of these products may be decreased by co-administration of potentially nephrotoxic compounds, although this has not been specifically studied).
No products indexed under this heading.

Ampicillin Sodium (Because platinum-containing species are eliminated primarily through the kidney, clearance of these products may be decreased by co-administration of potentially nephrotoxic compounds, although this has not been specifically studied).
No products indexed under this heading.

Ampicillin Trihydrate (Because platinum-containing species are eliminated primarily through the kidney, clearance of these products may be decreased by co-administration of potentially nephrotoxic compounds, although this has not been specifically studied).
No products indexed under this heading.

Amprenavir (Because platinum-containing species are eliminated primarily through the kidney, clearance of these products may be decreased by co-administration of potentially nephrotoxic compounds, although this has not been specifically studied).
No products indexed under this heading.

Anisindione (There have been reports while on study and from post-marketing surveillance of prolonged prothrombin time and INR occasionally associated with hemorrhage in patients who received oxaliplatin plus 5-FU/LV while on anticoagulants. Patients receiving oxaliplatin plus 5-FU/LV and requiring oral anticoagulants may require closer monitoring).
No products indexed under this heading.

Ardeparin Sodium (There have been reports while on study and from post-marketing surveillance of prolonged prothrombin time and INR occasionally associated with hemorrhage in patients who received oxaliplatin plus 5-FU/LV while on anticoagulants. Patients receiving oxaliplatin plus 5-FU/LV and requiring oral anticoagulants may require closer monitoring).
No products indexed under this heading.

Aspirin (Because platinum-containing species are eliminated primarily through the kidney, clearance of these products may be decreased by co-administration of potentially nephrotoxic compounds, although this has not been specifically studied). Products include:
Aggrenox Capsules 819
Bayer Aspirin 750
Percodan Tablets 1130
St. Joseph 81 mg Aspirin Chewable and Enteric Coated Tablets 1903

Atazanavir (Because platinum-containing species are eliminated primarily through the kidney, clearance of these products may be decreased by co-administration of potentially nephrotoxic compounds, although this has not been specifically studied).
No products indexed under this heading.

Atorvastatin Calcium (Because platinum-containing species are eliminated primarily through the kidney, clearance of these products may be decreased by co-administration of potentially nephrotoxic compounds, although this has not been specifically studied). Products include:
Lipitor Tablets 2501

Azithromycin Dihydrate (Because platinum-containing species are eliminated primarily through the kidney, clearance of these products may be decreased by co-administration of potentially nephrotoxic compounds, although this has not been specifically studied).
No products indexed under this heading.

Azlocillin Sodium (Because platinum-containing species are eliminated primarily through the kidney, clearance of these products may be decreased by co-administration of potentially nephrotoxic compounds, although this has not been specifically studied).
No products indexed under this heading.

Aztreonam (Because platinum-containing species are eliminated primarily through the kidney, clearance of these products may be decreased by co-administration of potentially nephrotoxic compounds, although this has not been specifically studied).
No products indexed under this heading.

Bacampicillin Hydrochloride (Because platinum-containing species are eliminated primarily through the kidney, clearance of these products may be decreased by co-administration of potentially nephrotoxic compounds, although this has not been specifically studied).
No products indexed under this heading.

Balsalazide Disodium (Because platinum-containing species are eliminated primarily through the kidney, clearance of these products may be decreased by co-administration of potentially nephrotoxic compounds, although this has not been specifically studied).
No products indexed under this heading.

Benazepril Hydrochloride (Because platinum-containing species are eliminated primarily through the kidney, clearance of these products may be decreased by co-administration of potentially nephrotoxic compounds, although this has not been specifically studied).
No products indexed under this heading.

Bendroflumethiazide (Because platinum-containing species are eliminated primarily through the kidney, clearance of these products may be decreased by co-administration of potentially nephrotoxic compounds, although this has not been specifically studied).
No products indexed under this heading.

Caffeine (Because platinum-containing species are eliminated primarily through the kidney, clearance of these products may be decreased by co-administration of potentially nephrotoxic compounds, although this has not been specifically studied). Products include:
BioLean Free Tablets 635
BioLean II Tablets 635
Winrgy Dietary Supplement 642

Captopril (Because platinum-containing species are eliminated primarily through the kidney, clearance of these products may be decreased by co-administration of potentially nephrotoxic compounds, although this has not been specifically studied). Products include:
Captopril Tablets 2182

Carbenicillin Disodium (Because platinum-containing species are eliminated primarily through the kidney, clearance of these products may be decreased by co-administration of potentially nephrotoxic compounds, although this has not been specifically studied).
No products indexed under this heading.

Carbenicillin Indanyl Sodium (Because platinum-containing species are eliminated primarily through the kidney, clearance of these products may be decreased by co-administration of potentially nephrotoxic compounds, although this has not been specifically studied).
No products indexed under this heading.

Carboplatin (Because platinum-containing species are eliminated primarily through the kidney, clearance of these products may be decreased by co-administration of potentially nephrotoxic compounds, although this has not been specifically studied).
No products indexed under this heading.

Carmustine (BCNU) (Because platinum-containing species are eliminated primarily through the kidney, clearance of these products may be decreased by co-administration of potentially nephrotoxic compounds, although this has not been specifically studied).
No products indexed under this heading.

Cefaclor (Because platinum-containing species are eliminated primarily through the kidney, clearance of these products may be decreased by co-administration of potentially nephrotoxic compounds, although this has not been specifically studied).
No products indexed under this heading.

Cefadroxil (Because platinum-containing species are eliminated primarily through the kidney, clearance of these products may be decreased by co-administration of potentially nephrotoxic compounds, although this has not been specifically studied).
No products indexed under this heading.

Cefamandole Nafate (Because platinum-containing species are eliminated primarily through the kidney, clearance of these products may be decreased by co-administration of potentially nephrotoxic compounds, although this has not been specifically studied).
No products indexed under this heading.

Cefazolin Sodium (Because platinum-containing species are eliminated primarily through the kidney, clearance of these products may be decreased by co-administration of potentially nephrotoxic compounds, although this has not been specifically studied).
No products indexed under this heading.

Cefdinir (Because platinum-containing species are eliminated primarily through the kidney, clearance of these products may be decreased by co-administration of potentially nephrotoxic compounds, although this has not been specifically studied). Products include:
Omnicef Capsules 497
Omnicef for Oral Suspension 497

Cefepime Hydrochloride (Because platinum-containing species are eliminated primarily through the kidney, clearance of these products may be decreased by co-administration of potentially nephrotoxic compounds, although this has not been specifically studied).

No products indexed under this heading.

Cefixime (Because platinum-containing species are eliminated primarily through the kidney, clearance of these products may be decreased by co-administration of potentially nephrotoxic compounds, although this has not been specifically studied). Products include:

Suprax for Oral Suspension **1891**

Suprax Tablets **1891**

Cefmetazole Sodium (Because platinum-containing species are eliminated primarily through the kidney, clearance of these products may be decreased by co-administration of potentially nephrotoxic compounds, although this has not been specifically studied).

No products indexed under this heading.

Cefonicid Sodium (Because platinum-containing species are eliminated primarily through the kidney, clearance of these products may be decreased by co-administration of potentially nephrotoxic compounds, although this has not been specifically studied).

No products indexed under this heading.

Cefoperazone Sodium (Because platinum-containing species are eliminated primarily through the kidney, clearance of these products may be decreased by co-administration of potentially nephrotoxic compounds, although this has not been specifically studied).

No products indexed under this heading.

Ceforanide (Because platinum-containing species are eliminated primarily through the kidney, clearance of these products may be decreased by co-administration of potentially nephrotoxic compounds, although this has not been specifically studied).

No products indexed under this heading.

Cefotaxime Sodium (Because platinum-containing species are eliminated primarily through the kidney, clearance of these products may be decreased by co-administration of potentially nephrotoxic compounds, although this has not been specifically studied).

No products indexed under this heading.

Cefotetan (Because platinum-containing species are eliminated primarily through the kidney, clearance of these products may be decreased by co-administration of potentially nephrotoxic compounds, although this has not been specifically studied).

No products indexed under this heading.

Cefoxitin Sodium (Because platinum-containing species are eliminated primarily through the kidney, clearance of these products may be decreased by co-administration of potentially nephrotoxic compounds, although this has not been specifically studied).

No products indexed under this heading.

Cefpodoxime Proxetil (Because platinum-containing species are eliminated primarily through the kidney, clearance of these products may be decreased by co-administration of potentially nephrotoxic compounds, although this has not been specifically studied).

No products indexed under this heading.

Cefprozil (Because platinum-containing species are eliminated primarily through the kidney, clearance of these products may be decreased by co-administration of potentially nephrotoxic compounds, although this has not been specifically studied).

No products indexed under this heading.

Ceftazidime (Because platinum-containing species are eliminated primarily through the kidney, clearance of these products may be decreased by co-administration of potentially nephrotoxic compounds, although this has not been specifically studied). Products include:

Fortaz **1450**

Ceftizoxime Sodium (Because platinum-containing species are eliminated primarily through the kidney, clearance of these products may be decreased by co-administration of potentially nephrotoxic compounds, although this has not been specifically studied).

No products indexed under this heading.

Ceftriaxone Sodium (Because platinum-containing species are eliminated primarily through the kidney, clearance of these products may be decreased by co-administration of potentially nephrotoxic compounds, although this has not been specifically studied). Products include:

Rocephin Injectable Vials, ADD-Vantage, Galaxy, Bulk........... **2642**

Cefuroxime Axetil (Because platinum-containing species are eliminated primarily through the kidney, clearance of these products may be decreased by co-administration of potentially nephrotoxic compounds, although this has not been specifically studied). Products include:

Ceftin **1380**

Cefuroxime Sodium (Because platinum-containing species are eliminated primarily through the kidney, clearance of these products may be decreased by co-administration of potentially nephrotoxic compounds, although this has not been specifically studied).

No products indexed under this heading.

Celecoxib (Because platinum-containing species are eliminated primarily through the kidney, clearance of these products may be decreased by co-administration of potentially nephrotoxic compounds, although this has not been specifically studied). Products include:

Celebrex Capsules **2979**

Cephalexin (Because platinum-containing species are eliminated primarily through the kidney, clearance of these products may be decreased by co-administration of potentially nephrotoxic compounds, although this has not been specifically studied).

No products indexed under this heading.

Cephalothin Sodium (Because platinum-containing species are eliminated primarily through the kidney, clearance of these products may be decreased by co-administration of potentially nephrotoxic compounds, although this has not been specifically studied).

No products indexed under this heading.

Cephapirin Sodium (Because platinum-containing species are eliminated primarily through the kidney, clearance of these products may be decreased by co-administration of potentially nephrotoxic compounds, although this has not been specifically studied).

No products indexed under this heading.

Cephradine (Because platinum-containing species are eliminated primarily through the kidney, clearance of these products may be decreased by co-administration of potentially nephrotoxic compounds, although this has not been specifically studied).

No products indexed under this heading.

Cerivastatin Sodium (Because platinum-containing species are eliminated primarily through the kidney, clearance of these products may be decreased by co-administration of potentially nephrotoxic compounds, although this has not been specifically studied).

No products indexed under this heading.

Chlorothiazide (Because platinum-containing species are eliminated primarily through the kidney, clearance of these products may be decreased by co-administration of potentially nephrotoxic compounds, although this has not been specifically studied).

No products indexed under this heading.

Chlorothiazide Sodium (Because platinum-containing species are eliminated primarily through the kidney, clearance of these products may be decreased by co-administration of potentially nephrotoxic compounds, although this has not been specifically studied). Products include:

Intravenous Sodium Diuril **2490**

Chlorpropamide (Because platinum-containing species are eliminated primarily through the kidney, clearance of these products may be decreased by co-administration of potentially nephrotoxic compounds, although this has not been specifically studied).

No products indexed under this heading.

Cidofovir (Because platinum-containing species are eliminated primarily through the kidney, clearance of these products may be decreased by co-administration of potentially nephrotoxic compounds, although this has not been specifically studied).

No products indexed under this heading.

Cilastatin Sodium (Because platinum-containing species are eliminated primarily through the kidney, clearance of these products may be decreased by co-administration of potentially nephrotoxic compounds, although this has not been specifically studied). Products include:

Primaxin I.M. **2080**

Primaxin I.V. **2083**

Cimetidine (Because platinum-containing species are eliminated primarily through the kidney, clearance of these products may be decreased by co-administration of potentially nephrotoxic compounds, although this has not been specifically studied).

No products indexed under this heading.

Cimetidine Hydrochloride (Because platinum-containing species are eliminated primarily through the kidney, clearance of these products may be decreased by co-administration of potentially nephrotoxic compounds, although this has not been specifically studied).

No products indexed under this heading.

Cisplatin (Because platinum-containing species are eliminated primarily through the kidney, clearance of these products may be decreased by co-administration of potentially nephrotoxic compounds, although this has not been specifically studied).

No products indexed under this heading.

Cladribine (Because platinum-containing species are eliminated primarily through the kidney, clearance of these products may be decreased by co-administration of potentially nephrotoxic compounds, although this has not been specifically studied). Products include:

Leustatin Injection **2384**

Clozapine (Because platinum-containing species are eliminated primarily through the kidney, clearance of these products may be decreased by co-administration of potentially nephrotoxic compounds, although this has not been specifically studied).

No products indexed under this heading.

Colistimethate Sodium (Because platinum-containing species are eliminated primarily through the kidney, clearance of these products may be decreased by co-administration of potentially nephrotoxic compounds, although this has not been specifically studied).

No products indexed under this heading.

Colistin Sulfate (Because platinum-containing species are eliminated primarily through the kidney, clearance of these products may be decreased by co-administration of potentially nephrotoxic compounds, although this has not been specifically studied).

No products indexed under this heading.

Cyclophosphamide (Because platinum-containing species are eliminated primarily through the kidney, clearance of these products may be decreased by co-administration of potentially nephrotoxic compounds, although this has not been specifically studied).

No products indexed under this heading.

Cyclosporine (Because platinum-containing species are eliminated primarily through the kidney, clearance of these products may be decreased by co-administration of potentially nephrotoxic compounds, although this has not been specifically studied). Products include:

Gengraf Capsules 435
Neoral Oral Solution 2280
Neoral Soft Gelatin Capsules 2280
Restasis Ophthalmic Emulsion 557
Sandimmune 2296

Cytarabine (Because platinum-containing species are eliminated primarily through the kidney, clearance of these products may be decreased by co-administration of potentially nephrotoxic compounds, although this has not been specifically studied).

No products indexed under this heading.

Cytarabine Liposome (Because platinum-containing species are eliminated primarily through the kidney, clearance of these products may be decreased by co-administration of potentially nephrotoxic compounds, although this has not been specifically studied). Products include:

DepoCyt Injection 1136

Dalteparin Sodium (There have been reports while on study and from post-marketing surveillance of prolonged prothrombin time and INR occasionally associated with hemorrhage in patients who received oxaliplatin plus 5-FU/LV while on anticoagulants. Patients receiving oxaliplatin plus 5-FU/LV and requiring oral anticoagulants may require closer monitoring). Products include:

Fragmin Injection 1070

Danaparoid Sodium (There have been reports while on study and from post-marketing surveillance of prolonged prothrombin time and INR occasionally associated with hemorrhage in patients who received oxaliplatin plus 5-FU/LV while on anticoagulants. Patients receiving oxaliplatin plus 5-FU/LV and requiring oral anticoagulants may require closer monitoring).

No products indexed under this heading.

Delavirdine Mesylate (Because platinum-containing species are eliminated primarily through the kidney, clearance of these products may be decreased by co-administration of potentially nephrotoxic compounds, although this has not been specifically studied).

No products indexed under this heading.

Diatrizoate Meglumine (Because platinum-containing species are eliminated primarily through the kidney, clearance of these products may be decreased by co-administration of potentially nephrotoxic compounds, although this has not been specifically studied).

No products indexed under this heading.

Diatrizoate Sodium (Because platinum-containing species are eliminated primarily through the kidney, clearance of these products may be decreased by co-administration of potentially nephrotoxic compounds, although this has not been specifically studied).

No products indexed under this heading.

Diclofenac Potassium (Because platinum-containing species are eliminated primarily through the kidney, clearance of these products may be decreased by co-administration of potentially nephrotoxic compounds, although this has not been specifically studied).

No products indexed under this heading.

Diclofenac Sodium (Because platinum-containing species are eliminated primarily through the kidney, clearance of these products may be decreased by co-administration of potentially nephrotoxic compounds, although this has not been specifically studied). Products include:

Diclofenac Sodium Ophthalmic Solution.. ⊙240
Voltaren Ophthalmic Solution 2336
Voltaren Tablets 2334
Voltaren-XR Tablets 2337

Dicloxacillin Sodium (Because platinum-containing species are eliminated primarily through the kidney, clearance of these products may be decreased by co-administration of potentially nephrotoxic compounds, although this has not been specifically studied).

No products indexed under this heading.

Dicumarol (There have been reports while on study and from post-marketing surveillance of prolonged prothrombin time and INR occasionally associated with hemorrhage in patients who received oxaliplatin plus 5-FU/LV while on anticoagulants. Patients receiving oxaliplatin plus 5-FU/LV and requiring oral anticoagulants may require closer monitoring).

No products indexed under this heading.

Didanosine (Because platinum-containing species are eliminated primarily through the kidney, clearance of these products may be decreased by co-administration of potentially nephrotoxic compounds, although this has not been specifically studied).

No products indexed under this heading.

Efavirenz (Because platinum-containing species are eliminated primarily through the kidney, clearance of these products may be decreased by co-administration of potentially nephrotoxic compounds, although this has not been specifically studied). Products include:

Atripla Tablets 938
Sustiva Capsules 930
Sustiva Tablets 930

Emtricitabine (Because platinum-containing species are eliminated primarily through the kidney, clearance of these products may be decreased by co-administration of potentially nephrotoxic compounds, although this has not been specifically studied). Products include:

Atripla Tablets 938
Emtriva Capsules 1246
Emtriva Oral Solution 1246
Truvada Tablets 1262

Enalapril Maleate (Because platinum-containing species are eliminated primarily through the kidney, clearance of these products may be decreased by co-administration of potentially nephrotoxic compounds, although this has not been specifically studied).

No products indexed under this heading.

Enalaprilat (Because platinum-containing species are eliminated primarily through the kidney, clearance of these products may be decreased by co-administration of potentially nephrotoxic compounds, although this has not been specifically studied).

No products indexed under this heading.

Enfuvirtide (Because platinum-containing species are eliminated primarily through the kidney, clearance of these products may be decreased by co-administration of potentially nephrotoxic compounds, although this has not been specifically studied).

No products indexed under this heading.

Enoxaparin Sodium (There have been reports while on study and from post-marketing surveillance of prolonged prothrombin time and INR occasionally associated with hemorrhage in patients who received oxaliplatin plus 5-FU/LV while on anticoagulants. Patients receiving oxaliplatin plus 5-FU/LV and requiring oral anticoagulants may require closer monitoring). Products include:

Lovenox Injection 2756

Ethiodized Oil (Because platinum-containing species are eliminated primarily through the kidney, clearance of these products may be decreased by co-administration of potentially nephrotoxic compounds, although this has not been specifically studied).

No products indexed under this heading.

Etodolac (Because platinum-containing species are eliminated primarily through the kidney, clearance of these products may be decreased by co-administration of potentially nephrotoxic compounds, although this has not been specifically studied).

No products indexed under this heading.

Fenoprofen Calcium (Because platinum-containing species are eliminated primarily through the kidney, clearance of these products may be decreased by co-administration of potentially nephrotoxic compounds, although this has not been specifically studied). Products include:

Nalfon Capsules 2508

Filgrastim (Because platinum-containing species are eliminated primarily through the kidney, clearance of these products may be decreased by co-administration of potentially nephrotoxic compounds, although this has not been specifically studied). Products include:

Neupogen for Injection 589

Fluorouracil (Because platinum-containing species are eliminated primarily through the kidney, clearance of these products may be decreased by co-administration of potentially nephrotoxic compounds, although this has not been specifically studied). Products include:

Carac Cream 0.5% 2722

Flurbiprofen (Because platinum-containing species are eliminated primarily through the kidney, clearance of these products may be decreased by co-administration of potentially nephrotoxic compounds, although this has not been specifically studied).

No products indexed under this heading.

Fluvastatin Sodium (Because platinum-containing species are eliminated primarily through the kidney, clearance of these products may be decreased by co-administration of potentially nephrotoxic compounds, although this has not been specifically studied). Products include:

Lescol Capsules 2268
Lescol XL Tablets 2268

Fondaparinux Sodium (There have been reports while on study and from post-marketing surveillance of prolonged prothrombin time and INR occasionally associated with hemorrhage in patients who received oxaliplatin plus 5-FU/LV while on anticoagulants. Patients receiving oxaliplatin plus 5-FU/LV and requiring oral anticoagulants may require closer monitoring). Products include:

Arixtra Injection 1313

Foscarnet Sodium (Because platinum-containing species are eliminated primarily through the kidney, clearance of these products may be decreased by co-administration of potentially nephrotoxic compounds, although this has not been specifically studied).

No products indexed under this heading.

Fosinopril Sodium (Because platinum-containing species are eliminated primarily through the kidney, clearance of these products may be decreased by co-administration of potentially nephrotoxic compounds, although this has not been specifically studied).

No products indexed under this heading.

Furosemide (Because platinum-containing species are eliminated primarily through the kidney, clearance of these products may be decreased by co-administration of potentially nephrotoxic compounds, although this has not been specifically studied). Products include:

Furosemide Tablets 2186

Gadopentetate Dimeglumine (Because platinum-containing species are eliminated primarily through the kidney, clearance of these products may be decreased by co-administration of potentially nephrotoxic compounds, although this has not been specifically studied).

No products indexed under this heading.

Gentamicin (Because platinum-containing species are eliminated primarily through the kidney, clearance of these products may be decreased by co-administration of potentially nephrotoxic compounds, although this has not been specifically studied).

No products indexed under this heading.

Gentamicin Sulfate (Because platinum-containing species are eliminated primarily through the kidney, clearance of these products may be decreased by co-administration of potentially nephrotoxic compounds, although this has not been specifically studied). Products include:

Pred-G Ophthalmic Ointment .... ⊙229
Pred-G Ophthalmic Suspension ...... ⊙228

Glipizide (Because platinum-containing species are eliminated primarily through the kidney, clearance of these products may be decreased by co-administration of potentially nephrotoxic compounds, although this has not been specifically studied).

No products indexed under this heading.

Globulin, Immune (Human) (Because platinum-containing species are eliminated primarily through the kidney, clearance of these products may be decreased by co-administration of potentially nephrotoxic compounds, although this has not been specifically studied). Products include:

Flebogamma 5% 1715

Glyburide (Because platinum-containing species are eliminated primarily through the kidney, clearance of these products may be decreased by co-administration of potentially nephrotoxic compounds, although this has not been specifically studied).

No products indexed under this heading.

Gold Therapy (Because platinum-containing species are eliminated primarily through the kidney, clearance of these products may be decreased by co-administration of potentially nephrotoxic compounds, although this has not been specifically studied).

No products indexed under this heading.

Heparin Calcium (There have been reports while on study and from post-marketing surveillance of prolonged prothrombin time and INR occasionally associated with hemorrhage in patients who received oxaliplatin plus 5-FU/LV while on anticoagulants. Patients receiving oxaliplatin plus 5-FU/LV and requiring oral anticoagulants may require closer monitoring).

No products indexed under this heading.

Heparin Sodium (There have been reports while on study and from post-marketing surveillance of prolonged prothrombin time and INR occasionally associated with hemorrhage in patients who received oxaliplatin plus 5-FU/LV while on anticoagulants. Patients receiving oxaliplatin plus 5-FU/LV and requiring oral anticoagulants may require closer monitoring).

No products indexed under this heading.

HMG-CoA Reductase Inhibitors (Because platinum-containing species are eliminated primarily through the kidney, clearance of these products may be decreased by co-administration of potentially nephrotoxic compounds, although this has not been specifically studied).

No products indexed under this heading.

Hydrochlorothiazide (Because platinum-containing species are eliminated primarily through the kidney, clearance of these products may be decreased by co-administration of potentially nephrotoxic compounds, although this has not been specifically studied). Products include:

Atacand HCT 642
Avalide Tablets 892
Avalide Tablets 2713
Benicar HCT Tablets 1010
Diovan HCT Tablets 2216
Dyazide Capsules 1405
Micardis HCT Tablets 854
Prinzide Tablets 2092
Tekturna HCT Tablets 2324
Teveten HCT Tablets 517

Hydroflumethiazide (Because platinum-containing species are eliminated primarily through the kidney, clearance of these products may be decreased by co-administration of potentially nephrotoxic compounds, although this has not been specifically studied).

No products indexed under this heading.

Ibuprofen (Because platinum-containing species are eliminated primarily through the kidney, clearance of these products may be decreased by co-administration of potentially nephrotoxic compounds, although this has not been specifically studied). Products include:

Motrin IB Tablets and Caplets 1900
Children's Motrin Oral Suspension ... 1901
Children's Motrin Non-Staining Dye-Free Oral Suspension 1901
Children's Motrin Cold Oral Suspension 1899
Infants' Motrin Concentrated Drops 1901
Infants' Motrin Non-Staining Dye-Free Concentrated Drops 1901
Junior Strength Motrin Caplets and Chewable Tablets 1901
Vicoprofen Tablets 533

Idarubicin Hydrochloride (Because platinum-containing species are eliminated primarily through the kidney, clearance of these products may be decreased by co-administration of potentially nephrotoxic compounds, although this has not been specifically studied).

No products indexed under this heading.

Ifosfamide (Because platinum-containing species are eliminated primarily through the kidney, clearance of these products may be decreased by co-administration of potentially nephrotoxic compounds, although this has not been specifically studied).

No products indexed under this heading.

Imipenem (Because platinum-containing species are eliminated primarily through the kidney, clearance of these products may be decreased by co-administration of potentially nephrotoxic compounds, although this has not been specifically studied). Products include:

Primaxin I.M. 2080
Primaxin I.V. 2083

Immune Globulin Intravenous (Human) (Because platinum-containing species are eliminated primarily through the kidney, clearance of these products may be decreased by co-administration of potentially nephrotoxic compounds, although this has not been specifically studied). Products include:

Flebogamma 5% DIF 1718
Gammagard Liquid 730
Gammagard S/D 734
Gamunex 3094

Indinavir Sulfate (Because platinum-containing species are eliminated primarily through the kidney, clearance of these products may be decreased by co-administration of potentially nephrotoxic compounds, although this has not been specifically studied). Products include:

Crixivan Capsules 1979

Indomethacin (Because platinum-containing species are eliminated primarily through the kidney, clearance of these products may be decreased by co-administration of potentially nephrotoxic compounds, although this has not been specifically studied). Products include:

Indocin 2024

Indomethacin Sodium Trihydrate (Because platinum-containing species are eliminated primarily through the kidney, clearance of these products may be decreased by co-administration of potentially nephrotoxic compounds, although this has not been specifically studied). Products include:

Indocin I.V. 2489

Interferon Beta-1b (Because platinum-containing species are eliminated primarily through the kidney, clearance of these products may be decreased by co-administration of potentially nephrotoxic compounds, although this has not been specifically studied). Products include:

Betaseron for SC Injection 756

Interleukin-2 (Because platinum-containing species are eliminated primarily through the kidney, clearance of these products may be decreased by co-administration of potentially nephrotoxic compounds, although this has not been specifically studied).

No products indexed under this heading.

Iodamide Meglumine (Because platinum-containing species are eliminated primarily through the kidney, clearance of these products may be decreased by co-administration of potentially nephrotoxic compounds, although this has not been specifically studied).

No products indexed under this heading.

Iohexol (Because platinum-containing species are eliminated primarily through the kidney, clearance of these products may be decreased by co-administration of potentially nephrotoxic compounds, although this has not been specifically studied).

No products indexed under this heading.

Iopamidol (Because platinum-containing species are eliminated primarily through the kidney, clearance of these products may be decreased by co-administration of potentially nephrotoxic compounds, although this has not been specifically studied).

No products indexed under this heading.

Iopanoic Acid (Because platinum-containing species are eliminated primarily through the kidney, clearance of these products may be decreased by co-administration of potentially nephrotoxic compounds, although this has not been specifically studied).

No products indexed under this heading.

Iothalamate Meglumine (Because platinum-containing species are eliminated primarily through the kidney, clearance of these products may be decreased by co-administration of potentially nephrotoxic compounds, although this has not been specifically studied).

No products indexed under this heading.

Ioxaglate Meglumine (Because platinum-containing species are eliminated primarily through the kidney, clearance of these products may be decreased by co-administration of potentially nephrotoxic compounds, although this has not been specifically studied).

No products indexed under this heading.

Ioxaglate Sodium (Because platinum-containing species are eliminated primarily through the kidney, clearance of these products may be decreased by co-administration of potentially nephrotoxic compounds, although this has not been specifically studied).

No products indexed under this heading.

Kanamycin Sulfate (Because platinum-containing species are eliminated primarily through the kidney, clearance of these products may be decreased by co-administration of potentially nephrotoxic compounds, although this has not been specifically studied).

No products indexed under this heading.

Ketoprofen (Because platinum-containing species are eliminated primarily through the kidney, clearance of these products may be decreased by co-administration of potentially nephrotoxic compounds, although this has not been specifically studied).

No products indexed under this heading.

Ketorolac Tromethamine (Because platinum-containing species are eliminated primarily through the kidney, clearance of these products may be decreased by co-administration of potentially nephrotoxic compounds, although this has not been specifically studied).

No products indexed under this heading.

Lamium album (Because platinum-containing species are eliminated primarily through the kidney, clearance of these products may be decreased by co-administration of potentially nephrotoxic compounds, although this has not been specifically studied).

No products indexed under this heading.

Lisinopril (Because platinum-containing species are eliminated primarily through the kidney, clearance of these products may be decreased by co-administration of potentially nephrotoxic compounds, although this has not been specifically studied). Products include:

Prinivil Tablets 2087
Prinzide Tablets 2092

Lithium (Because platinum-containing species are eliminated primarily through the kidney, clearance of these products may be decreased by co-administration of potentially nephrotoxic compounds, although this has not been specifically studied).
No products indexed under this heading.

Lithium Carbonate (Because platinum-containing species are eliminated primarily through the kidney, clearance of these products may be decreased by co-administration of potentially nephrotoxic compounds, although this has not been specifically studied).
No products indexed under this heading.

Lithium Citrate (Because platinum-containing species are eliminated primarily through the kidney, clearance of these products may be decreased by co-administration of potentially nephrotoxic compounds, although this has not been specifically studied).
No products indexed under this heading.

Lopinavir (Because platinum-containing species are eliminated primarily through the kidney, clearance of these products may be decreased by co-administration of potentially nephrotoxic compounds, although this has not been specifically studied). Products include:
Kaletra 452

Loracarbef (Because platinum-containing species are eliminated primarily through the kidney, clearance of these products may be decreased by co-administration of potentially nephrotoxic compounds, although this has not been specifically studied).
No products indexed under this heading.

Lovastatin (Because platinum-containing species are eliminated primarily through the kidney, clearance of these products may be decreased by co-administration of potentially nephrotoxic compounds, although this has not been specifically studied). Products include:
Advicor Tablets 402
Mevacor Tablets 2063

Low Molecular Weight Heparins (There have been reports while on study and from post-marketing surveillance of prolonged prothrombin time and INR occasionally associated with hemorrhage in patients who received oxaliplatin plus 5-FU/LV while on anticoagulants. Patients receiving oxaliplatin plus 5-FU/LV and requiring oral anticoagulants may require closer monitoring).
No products indexed under this heading.

Meclofenamate Sodium (Because platinum-containing species are eliminated primarily through the kidney, clearance of these products may be decreased by co-administration of potentially nephrotoxic compounds, although this has not been specifically studied).
No products indexed under this heading.

Mefenamic Acid (Because platinum-containing species are eliminated primarily through the kidney, clearance of these products may be decreased by co-administration of potentially nephrotoxic compounds, although this has not been specifically studied).
No products indexed under this heading.

Meloxicam (Because platinum-containing species are eliminated primarily through the kidney, clearance of these products may be decreased by co-administration of potentially nephrotoxic compounds, although this has not been specifically studied). Products include:
Mobic Oral Suspension 863
Mobic Tablets 863

Melphalan Hydrochloride (Because platinum-containing species are eliminated primarily through the kidney, clearance of these products may be decreased by co-administration of potentially nephrotoxic compounds, although this has not been specifically studied).
No products indexed under this heading.

Mesalamine (Because platinum-containing species are eliminated primarily through the kidney, clearance of these products may be decreased by co-administration of potentially nephrotoxic compounds, although this has not been specifically studied). Products include:
Asacol Delayed-Release Tablets 2579
Canasa Rectal Suppositories 705
Lialda Tablets 3029
Pentasa Capsules 3030

Methimazole (Because platinum-containing species are eliminated primarily through the kidney, clearance of these products may be decreased by co-administration of potentially nephrotoxic compounds, although this has not been specifically studied).
No products indexed under this heading.

Methotrexate (Because platinum-containing species are eliminated primarily through the kidney, clearance of these products may be decreased by co-administration of potentially nephrotoxic compounds, although this has not been specifically studied).
No products indexed under this heading.

Methotrexate Sodium (Because platinum-containing species are eliminated primarily through the kidney, clearance of these products may be decreased by co-administration of potentially nephrotoxic compounds, although this has not been specifically studied).
No products indexed under this heading.

Methyclothiazide (Because platinum-containing species are eliminated primarily through the kidney, clearance of these products may be decreased by co-administration of potentially nephrotoxic compounds, although this has not been specifically studied).
No products indexed under this heading.

Mezlocillin Sodium (Because platinum-containing species are eliminated primarily through the kidney, clearance of these products may be decreased by co-administration of potentially nephrotoxic compounds, although this has not been specifically studied).
No products indexed under this heading.

Minocycline Hydrochloride (Because platinum-containing species are eliminated primarily through the kidney, clearance of these products may be decreased by co-administration of potentially nephrotoxic compounds, although this has not been specifically studied). Products include:
Solodyn Extended Release Tablets 1938

Mitomycin (Mitomycin-C) (Because platinum-containing species are eliminated primarily through the kidney, clearance of these products may be decreased by co-administration of potentially nephrotoxic compounds, although this has not been specifically studied).
No products indexed under this heading.

Moexipril Hydrochloride (Because platinum-containing species are eliminated primarily through the kidney, clearance of these products may be decreased by co-administration of potentially nephrotoxic compounds, although this has not been specifically studied).
No products indexed under this heading.

Muromonab-CD3 (Because platinum-containing species are eliminated primarily through the kidney, clearance of these products may be decreased by co-administration of potentially nephrotoxic compounds, although this has not been specifically studied). Products include:
Orthoclone OKT3 Sterile Solution 2387

Nabumetone (Because platinum-containing species are eliminated primarily through the kidney, clearance of these products may be decreased by co-administration of potentially nephrotoxic compounds, although this has not been specifically studied).
No products indexed under this heading.

Nafcillin Sodium (Because platinum-containing species are eliminated primarily through the kidney, clearance of these products may be decreased by co-administration of potentially nephrotoxic compounds, although this has not been specifically studied).
No products indexed under this heading.

Naproxen (Because platinum-containing species are eliminated primarily through the kidney, clearance of these products may be decreased by co-administration of potentially nephrotoxic compounds, although this has not been specifically studied). Products include:
EC-Naprosyn Delayed-Release Tablets 2632
Naprosyn Suspension 2632
Naprosyn Tablets 2632

Naproxen Sodium (Because platinum-containing species are eliminated primarily through the kidney, clearance of these products may be decreased by co-administration of potentially nephrotoxic compounds, although this has not been specifically studied). Products include:
Anaprox Tablets 2632
Anaprox DS Tablets 2632
Treximet Tablets 1616

Nelfinavir Mesylate (Because platinum-containing species are eliminated primarily through the kidney, clearance of these products may be decreased by co-administration of potentially nephrotoxic compounds, although this has not been specifically studied).
No products indexed under this heading.

Neomycin (Because platinum-containing species are eliminated primarily through the kidney, clearance of these products may be decreased by co-administration of potentially nephrotoxic compounds, although this has not been specifically studied).
No products indexed under this heading.

Neomycin, oral (Because platinum-containing species are eliminated primarily through the kidney, clearance of these products may be decreased by co-administration of potentially nephrotoxic compounds, although this has not been specifically studied).
No products indexed under this heading.

Neomycin Sulfate (Because platinum-containing species are eliminated primarily through the kidney, clearance of these products may be decreased by co-administration of potentially nephrotoxic compounds, although this has not been specifically studied). Products include:
Neosporin Ophthalmic Solution Sterile .... ⊙252

Nephrotoxic Drugs (Because platinum-containing species are eliminated primarily through the kidney, clearance of these products may be decreased by co-administration of potentially nephrotoxic compounds, although this has not been specifically studied).
No products indexed under this heading.

Nevirapine (Because platinum-containing species are eliminated primarily through the kidney, clearance of these products may be decreased by co-administration of potentially nephrotoxic compounds, although this has not been specifically studied). Products include:
Viramune Oral Suspension 873
Viramune Tablets 873

Norfloxacin (Because platinum-containing species are eliminated primarily through the kidney, clearance of these products may be decreased by co-administration of potentially nephrotoxic compounds, although this has not been specifically studied). Products include:
Noroxin Tablets 2069

Olsalazine Sodium (Because platinum-containing species are eliminated primarily through the kidney, clearance of these products may be decreased by co-administration of potentially nephrotoxic compounds, although this has not been specifically studied).
No products indexed under this heading.

IMPORTANT NOTE: Always consult each drug listing in the patient's regimen for possible interactions.

Omeprazole (Because platinum-containing species are eliminated primarily through the kidney, clearance of these products may be decreased by co-administration of potentially nephrotoxic compounds, although this has not been specifically studied).
No products indexed under this heading.

Oxaprozin (Because platinum-containing species are eliminated primarily through the kidney, clearance of these products may be decreased by co-administration of potentially nephrotoxic compounds, although this has not been specifically studied).
No products indexed under this heading.

Pamidronate Disodium (Because platinum-containing species are eliminated primarily through the kidney, clearance of these products may be decreased by co-administration of potentially nephrotoxic compounds, although this has not been specifically studied).
No products indexed under this heading.

Paroxetine Hydrochloride (Because platinum-containing species are eliminated primarily through the kidney, clearance of these products may be decreased by co-administration of potentially nephrotoxic compounds, although this has not been specifically studied). Products include:
Paxil 1535
Paxil CR Controlled-Release Tablets 1544

Penicillamine (Because platinum-containing species are eliminated primarily through the kidney, clearance of these products may be decreased by co-administration of potentially nephrotoxic compounds, although this has not been specifically studied). Products include:
Cuprimine Capsules 1986

Penicillin G Benzathine (Because platinum-containing species are eliminated primarily through the kidney, clearance of these products may be decreased by co-administration of potentially nephrotoxic compounds, although this has not been specifically studied). Products include:
Bicillin C-R Injectable Suspension 1775
Bicillin L-A Injection 1777

Penicillin G Potassium (Because platinum-containing species are eliminated primarily through the kidney, clearance of these products may be decreased by co-administration of potentially nephrotoxic compounds, although this has not been specifically studied).
No products indexed under this heading.

Penicillin G Procaine (Because platinum-containing species are eliminated primarily through the kidney, clearance of these products may be decreased by co-administration of potentially nephrotoxic compounds, although this has not been specifically studied). Products include:
Bicillin C-R Injectable Suspension 1775
Bicillin L-A Injection 1777

Penicillin G Sodium (Because platinum-containing species are eliminated primarily through the kidney, clearance of these products may be decreased by co-administration of potentially nephrotoxic compounds, although this has not been specifically studied).
No products indexed under this heading.

Penicillin V Potassium (Because platinum-containing species are eliminated primarily through the kidney, clearance of these products may be decreased by co-administration of potentially nephrotoxic compounds, although this has not been specifically studied).
No products indexed under this heading.

Pentamidine Isethionate (Because platinum-containing species are eliminated primarily through the kidney, clearance of these products may be decreased by co-administration of potentially nephrotoxic compounds, although this has not been specifically studied).
No products indexed under this heading.

Perindopril Erbumine (Because platinum-containing species are eliminated primarily through the kidney, clearance of these products may be decreased by co-administration of potentially nephrotoxic compounds, although this has not been specifically studied). Products include:
Aceon Tablets (2 mg, 4 mg, 8 mg) 3038

Phenylbutazone (Because platinum-containing species are eliminated primarily through the kidney, clearance of these products may be decreased by co-administration of potentially nephrotoxic compounds, although this has not been specifically studied).
No products indexed under this heading.

Piroxicam (Because platinum-containing species are eliminated primarily through the kidney, clearance of these products may be decreased by co-administration of potentially nephrotoxic compounds, although this has not been specifically studied).
No products indexed under this heading.

Plicamycin (Because platinum-containing species are eliminated primarily through the kidney, clearance of these products may be decreased by co-administration of potentially nephrotoxic compounds, although this has not been specifically studied).
No products indexed under this heading.

Polymyxin (Because platinum-containing species are eliminated primarily through the kidney, clearance of these products may be decreased by co-administration of potentially nephrotoxic compounds, although this has not been specifically studied).
No products indexed under this heading.

Polymyxin B Sulfate (Because platinum-containing species are eliminated primarily through the kidney, clearance of these products may be decreased by co-administration of potentially nephrotoxic compounds, although this has not been specifically studied). Products include:
Neosporin Ophthalmic Solution Sterile .... ⊙ 252

Polythiazide (Because platinum-containing species are eliminated primarily through the kidney, clearance of these products may be decreased by co-administration of potentially nephrotoxic compounds, although this has not been specifically studied).
No products indexed under this heading.

Pravastatin Sodium (Because platinum-containing species are eliminated primarily through the kidney, clearance of these products may be decreased by co-administration of potentially nephrotoxic compounds, although this has not been specifically studied).
No products indexed under this heading.

Probenecid (Because platinum-containing species are eliminated primarily through the kidney, clearance of these products may be decreased by co-administration of potentially nephrotoxic compounds, although this has not been specifically studied).
No products indexed under this heading.

Quinapril Hydrochloride (Because platinum-containing species are eliminated primarily through the kidney, clearance of these products may be decreased by co-administration of potentially nephrotoxic compounds, although this has not been specifically studied).
No products indexed under this heading.

Rabeprazole Sodium (Because platinum-containing species are eliminated primarily through the kidney, clearance of these products may be decreased by co-administration of potentially nephrotoxic compounds, although this has not been specifically studied). Products include:
Aciphex Tablets 1053

Ramipril (Because platinum-containing species are eliminated primarily through the kidney, clearance of these products may be decreased by co-administration of potentially nephrotoxic compounds, although this has not been specifically studied).
No products indexed under this heading.

Rifampin (Because platinum-containing species are eliminated primarily through the kidney, clearance of these products may be decreased by co-administration of potentially nephrotoxic compounds, although this has not been specifically studied).
No products indexed under this heading.

Riluzole (Because platinum-containing species are eliminated primarily through the kidney, clearance of these products may be decreased by co-administration of potentially nephrotoxic compounds, although this has not been specifically studied). Products include:
Rilutek Tablets 2771

Ritonavir (Because platinum-containing species are eliminated primarily through the kidney, clearance of these products may be decreased by co-administration of potentially nephrotoxic compounds, although this has not been specifically studied). Products include:
Kaletra 452
Norvir 489

Rofecoxib (Because platinum-containing species are eliminated primarily through the kidney, clearance of these products may be decreased by co-administration of potentially nephrotoxic compounds, although this has not been specifically studied).
No products indexed under this heading.

Saquinavir (Because platinum-containing species are eliminated primarily through the kidney, clearance of these products may be decreased by co-administration of potentially nephrotoxic compounds, although this has not been specifically studied).
No products indexed under this heading.

Sibutramine Hydrochloride Monohydrate (Because platinum-containing species are eliminated primarily through the kidney, clearance of these products may be decreased by co-administration of potentially nephrotoxic compounds, although this has not been specifically studied). Products include:
Meridia Capsules 475

Simvastatin (Because platinum-containing species are eliminated primarily through the kidney, clearance of these products may be decreased by co-administration of potentially nephrotoxic compounds, although this has not been specifically studied). Products include:
Simcor Tablets 502
Vytorin 10/10 Tablets 2149
Vytorin 10/10 Tablets 2939
Vytorin 10/20 Tablets 2149
Vytorin 10/20 Tablets 2939
Vytorin 10/40 Tablets 2149
Vytorin 10/40 Tablets 2939
Vytorin 10/80 Tablets 2149
Vytorin 10/80 Tablets 2939
Zocor Tablets 2136

Spirapril Hydrochloride (Because platinum-containing species are eliminated primarily through the kidney, clearance of these products may be decreased by co-administration of potentially nephrotoxic compounds, although this has not been specifically studied).
No products indexed under this heading.

Stavudine (Because platinum-containing species are eliminated primarily through the kidney, clearance of these products may be decreased by co-administration of potentially nephrotoxic compounds, although this has not been specifically studied).
No products indexed under this heading.

Streptomycin Sulfate (Because platinum-containing species are eliminated primarily through the kidney, clearance of these products may be decreased by co-administration of potentially nephrotoxic compounds, although this has not been specifically studied).
No products indexed under this heading.

Streptozocin (Because platinum-containing species are eliminated primarily through the kidney, clearance of these products may be decreased by co-administration of potentially nephrotoxic compounds, although this has not been specifically studied).
No products indexed under this heading.

Sulfacytine (Because platinum-containing species are eliminated primarily through the kidney, clearance of these products may be decreased by co-administration of potentially nephrotoxic compounds, although this has not been specifically studied).
No products indexed under this heading.

Sulfamethizole (Because platinum-containing species are eliminated primarily through the kidney, clearance of these products may be decreased by co-administration of potentially nephrotoxic compounds, although this has not been specifically studied).
No products indexed under this heading.

Sulfamethoxazole (Because platinum-containing species are eliminated primarily through the kidney, clearance of these products may be decreased by co-administration of potentially nephrotoxic compounds, although this has not been specifically studied).
No products indexed under this heading.

Sulfasalazine (Because platinum-containing species are eliminated primarily through the kidney, clearance of these products may be decreased by co-administration of potentially nephrotoxic compounds, although this has not been specifically studied).
No products indexed under this heading.

Sulfinpyrazone (Because platinum-containing species are eliminated primarily through the kidney, clearance of these products may be decreased by co-administration of potentially nephrotoxic compounds, although this has not been specifically studied).
No products indexed under this heading.

Sulfisoxazole Acetyl (Because platinum-containing species are eliminated primarily through the kidney, clearance of these products may be decreased by co-administration of potentially nephrotoxic compounds, although this has not been specifically studied).
No products indexed under this heading.

Sulfisoxazole Diolamine (Because platinum-containing species are eliminated primarily through the kidney, clearance of these products may be decreased by co-administration of potentially nephrotoxic compounds, although this has not been specifically studied).
No products indexed under this heading.

Sulindac (Because platinum-containing species are eliminated primarily through the kidney, clearance of these products may be decreased by co-administration of potentially nephrotoxic compounds, although this has not been specifically studied). Products include:
Clinoril Tablets 1962

Tacrolimus (Because platinum-containing species are eliminated primarily through the kidney, clearance of these products may be decreased by co-administration of potentially nephrotoxic compounds, although this has not been specifically studied). Products include:
Prograf Capsules and Injection 622
Protopic Ointment 628

Tenofovir Disoproxil Fumarate (Because platinum-containing species are eliminated primarily through the kidney, clearance of these products may be decreased by co-administration of potentially nephrotoxic compounds, although this has not been specifically studied). Products include:
Atripla Tablets 938
Truvada Tablets 1262
Viread Tablets 1268

Thioguanine (Because platinum-containing species are eliminated primarily through the kidney, clearance of these products may be decreased by co-administration of potentially nephrotoxic compounds, although this has not been specifically studied). Products include:
Tabloid Tablets 1601

Ticarcillin Disodium (Because platinum-containing species are eliminated primarily through the kidney, clearance of these products may be decreased by co-administration of potentially nephrotoxic compounds, although this has not been specifically studied). Products include:
Timentin ADD-Vantage 1606
Timentin Injection Galaxy Container 1609
Timentin IV Infusion 1603
Timentin Pharmacy Bulk Package 1613

Tinzaparin Sodium (There have been reports while on study and from post-marketing surveillance of prolonged prothrombin time and INR occasionally associated with hemorrhage in patients who received oxaliplatin plus 5-FU/LV while on anticoagulants. Patients receiving oxaliplatin plus 5-FU/LV and requiring oral anticoagulants may require closer monitoring).
No products indexed under this heading.

Tobramycin (Because platinum-containing species are eliminated primarily through the kidney, clearance of these products may be decreased by co-administration of potentially nephrotoxic compounds, although this has not been specifically studied). Products include:
Zylet Ophthalmic Suspension .... ⊙247

Tobramycin Sulfate (Because platinum-containing species are eliminated primarily through the kidney, clearance of these products may be decreased by co-administration of potentially nephrotoxic compounds, although this has not been specifically studied).
No products indexed under this heading.

Tolazamide (Because platinum-containing species are eliminated primarily through the kidney, clearance of these products may be decreased by co-administration of potentially nephrotoxic compounds, although this has not been specifically studied).
No products indexed under this heading.

Tolbutamide (Because platinum-containing species are eliminated primarily through the kidney, clearance of these products may be decreased by co-administration of potentially nephrotoxic compounds, although this has not been specifically studied).
No products indexed under this heading.

Tolmetin Sodium (Because platinum-containing species are eliminated primarily through the kidney, clearance of these products may be decreased by co-administration of potentially nephrotoxic compounds, although this has not been specifically studied).
No products indexed under this heading.

Trandolapril (Because platinum-containing species are eliminated primarily through the kidney, clearance of these products may be decreased by co-administration of potentially nephrotoxic compounds, although this has not been specifically studied). Products include:
Mavik Tablets 472
Tarka Tablets 511

Triamterene (Because platinum-containing species are eliminated primarily through the kidney, clearance of these products may be decreased by co-administration of potentially nephrotoxic compounds, although this has not been specifically studied). Products include:
Dyazide Capsules 1405
Dyrenium Capsules 3189

Trimethadione (Because platinum-containing species are eliminated primarily through the kidney, clearance of these products may be decreased by co-administration of potentially nephrotoxic compounds, although this has not been specifically studied).
No products indexed under this heading.

Trovafloxacin Mesylate (Because platinum-containing species are eliminated primarily through the kidney, clearance of these products may be decreased by co-administration of potentially nephrotoxic compounds, although this has not been specifically studied).
No products indexed under this heading.

Tyropanoate Sodium (Because platinum-containing species are eliminated primarily through the kidney, clearance of these products may be decreased by co-administration of potentially nephrotoxic compounds, although this has not been specifically studied).
No products indexed under this heading.

Valacyclovir Hydrochloride (Because platinum-containing species are eliminated primarily through the kidney, clearance of these products may be decreased by co-administration of potentially nephrotoxic compounds, although this has not been specifically studied). Products include:
Valtrex Caplets 1635

Valdecoxib (Because platinum-containing species are eliminated primarily through the kidney, clearance of these products may be decreased by co-administration of potentially nephrotoxic compounds, although this has not been specifically studied).
No products indexed under this heading.

Vancomycin Hydrochloride (Because platinum-containing species are eliminated primarily through the kidney, clearance of these products may be decreased by co-administration of potentially nephrotoxic compounds, although this has not been specifically studied).
No products indexed under this heading.

Voriconazole (Because platinum-containing species are eliminated primarily through the kidney, clearance of these products may be decreased by co-administration of potentially nephrotoxic compounds, although this has not been specifically studied).
No products indexed under this heading.

Warfarin Sodium (There have been reports while on study and from post-marketing surveillance of prolonged prothrombin time and INR occasionally associated with hemorrhage in patients who received oxaliplatin plus 5-FU/LV while on anticoagulants. Patients receiving oxaliplatin plus 5-FU/LV and requiring oral anticoagulants may require closer monitoring).
No products indexed under this heading.

Zalcitabine (Because platinum-containing species are eliminated primarily through the kidney, clearance of these products may be decreased by co-administration of potentially nephrotoxic compounds, although this has not been specifically studied).
No products indexed under this heading.

Zidovudine (Because platinum-containing species are eliminated primarily through the kidney, clearance of these products may be decreased by co-administration of potentially nephrotoxic compounds, although this has not been specifically studied). Products include:
Combivir Tablets 1384
Retrovir 1574
Retrovir IV Infusion 1579
Trizivir Tablets 1622

Zoledronic acid (Because platinum-containing species are eliminated primarily through the kidney, clearance of these products may be decreased by co-administration of potentially nephrotoxic compounds, although this has not been specifically studied). Products include:
Reclast Injection 2291
Zometa for Intravenous Infusion 2341

ELSPAR FOR INJECTION

(Asparaginase) 1990
May interact with:

Methotrexate Sodium (Tissue culture and animal studies indicate that asparaginase can diminish or abolish the effect of methotrexate on malignant cells).
No products indexed under this heading.

IMPORTANT NOTE: Always consult each drug listing in the patient's regimen for possible interactions.

Prednisone (The administration of asparaginase intravenously and concurrently with or immediately before a course of prednisone may be associated with increased toxicity).
No products indexed under this heading.

Vincristine Sulfate (The administration of asparaginase intravenouosly and concurrently with or immediately before a course of prednisone may be associated with increased toxicity).
No products indexed under this heading.

ELSPAR FOR INJECTION

(Asparaginase) 2488
None cited in PDR database.

EMEND CAPSULES

(Aprepitant) 1992
May interact with benzodiazepine that are metabolized by CYP3A4, cytochrome p450 2c9 substrates (selected), cytochrome p450 3a4 inducers (selected), cytochrome p450 3a4 inhibitors (selected), cytochrome p450 3a4 inhibitors, potent, cytochrome p450 3a4 substrates (selected), dexamethasone, methylprednisolone, oral contraceptives, phenytoin, and certain other agents. Compounds in these categories include:

Acarbose (Co-administration of fosaprepitant or oral aprepitant with drugs that are known to be metabolized by CYP2C9 may result in lower plasma concentrations of these drugs). Products include:
Precose Tablets 792

Acetazolamide (Aprepitant is a substrate for CYP3A4; therefore, co-administration of fosaprepitant or aprepitant with drugs that inhibit CYP3A4 activity may result in increased plasma concentrations of aprepitant. Consequently, concomitant administration of fosaprepitant or aprepitant with strong CYP3A4 inhibitors (e.g., ketoconazole, itraconazole, nefazodone, troleandomycin, clarithromycin, ritonavir, nelfinavir) should be approached with caution. Because moderate CYP3A4 inhibitors (e.g., diltiazem) result in a 2-fold increase in plasma concentrations of aprepitant, concomitant administration should also be approached with caution).
No products indexed under this heading.

Alfentanil Hydrochloride (As a moderate inhibitor of CYP3A4, aprepitant can increase plasma concentrations of orally co-administered medicinal products that are metabolized through CYP3A4).
No products indexed under this heading.

Allium sativum (Aprepitant is substrate for CYP3A4; therefore, co-administration of fosaprepitant or aprepitant with drugs that strongly induce CYP3A4 activity (e.g., rifampin, carbamazepine, phenytoin) may result in reduced plasma concentrations and decreased efficacy).
No products indexed under this heading.

Alprazolam (Fosaprepitant and oral aprepitant may increase the AUC of midazolam. The potential effects of increased plasma concentrations of midazolam or other benzodiazepines metabolized via CYP3A4 (alprazolam, triazolam) should be considered when co-administeringthese agents with a 3-day regimen of fosaprepitant followed by aprepitant).
No products indexed under this heading.

Amiodarone Hydrochloride (Aprepitant is a substrate for CYP3A4; therefore, co-administration of fosaprepitant or aprepitant with drugs that inhibit CYP3A4 activity may result in increased plasma concentrations of aprepitant. Consequently, concomitant administration of fosaprepitant or aprepitant with strong CYP3A4 inhibitors (e.g., ketoconazole, itraconazole, nefazodone, troleandomycin, clarithromycin, ritonavir, nelfinavir) should be approached with caution. Because moderate CYP3A4 inhibitors (e.g., diltiazem) result in a 2-fold increase in plasma concentrations of aprepitant, concomitant administration should also be approached with caution).
No products indexed under this heading.

Amitriptyline Hydrochloride (Co-administration of fosaprepitant or oral aprepitant with drugs that are known to be metabolized by CYP2C9 may result in lower plasma concentrations of these drugs).
No products indexed under this heading.

Amlodipine Besylate (As a moderate inhibitor of CYP3A4, aprepitant can increase plasma concentrations of orally co-administered medicinal products that are metabolized through CYP3A4). Products include:
Azor Tablets 1005
Exforge Tablets 2238

Amprenavir (Aprepitant is a substrate for CYP3A4; therefore, co-administration of fosaprepitant or aprepitant with drugs that inhibit CYP3A4 activity may result in increased plasma concentrations of aprepitant. Consequently, concomitant administration of fosaprepitant or apreitant with strong CYP3A4 inhibitors (e.g., ketoconazole, itraconzole, nefazodone, troleandomycin, clarithromycin, ritonavir, nelfinavir) should be approached with caution).
No products indexed under this heading.

Anastrozole (Aprepitant is a substrate for CYP3A4; therefore, co-administration of fosaprepitant or aprepitant with drugs that inhibit CYP3A4 activity may result in increased plasma concentrations of aprepitant. Consequently, concomitant administration of fosaprepitant or aprepitant with strong CYP3A4 inhibitors (e.g., ketoconazole, itraconazole, nefazodone, troleandomycin, clarithromycin, ritonavir, nelfinavir) should be approached with caution. Because moderate CYP3A4 inhibitors (e.g., diltiazem) result in a 2-fold increase in plasma concentrations of aprepitant, concomitant administration should also be approached with caution). Products include:
Arimidex Tablets 672

Astemizole (EMEND is a moderate CYP3A4 inhibitor; concurrent use with EMEND could result in elevated plasma concentrations of astemizole, potentially causing serious or life-threatening reactions, and is contraindicated).
No products indexed under this heading.

Atazanavir (Aprepitant is a substrate for CYP3A4; therefore, co-administration of fosaprepitant or aprepitant with drugs that inhibit CYP3A4 activity may result in increased plasma concentrations of aprepitant. Consequently, concomitant administration of fosaprepitant or apreitant with strong CYP3A4 inhibitors (e.g., ketoconazole, itraconzole, nefazodone, troleandomycin, clarithromycin, ritonavir, nelfinavir) should be approached with caution).
No products indexed under this heading.

Atazanavir Sulfate (Aprepitant is a substrate for CYP3A4; therefore, co-administration of fosaprepitant or aprepitant with drugs that inhibit CYP3A4 activity may result in increased plasma concentrations of aprepitant. Consequently, concomitant administration of fosaprepitant or apreitant with strong CYP3A4 inhibitors (e.g., ketoconazole, itraconzole, nefazodone, troleandomycin, clarithromycin, ritonavir, nelfinavir) should be approached with caution). Products include:
Reyataz Capsules 3299

Atorvastatin Calcium (As a moderate inhibitor of CYP3A4, aprepitant can increase plasma concentrations of orally co-administered medicinal products that are metabolized through CYP3A4). Products include:
Lipitor Tablets 2501

Belladonna Ergotamine (As a moderate inhibitor of CYP3A4, aprepitant can increase plasma concentrations of orally co-administered medicinal products that are metabolized through CYP3A4).
No products indexed under this heading.

Betamethasone Acetate (Aprepitant is substrate for CYP3A4; therefore, co-administration of fosaprepitant or aprepitant with drugs that strongly induce CYP3A4 activity (e.g., rifampin, carbamazepine, phenytoin) may result in reduced plasma concentrations and decreased efficacy).
No products indexed under this heading.

Betamethasone Sodium Phosphate (Aprepitant is substrate for CYP3A4; therefore, co-administration of fosaprepitant or aprepitant with drugs that strongly induce CYP3A4 activity (e.g., rifampin, carbamazepine, phenytoin) may result in reduced plasma concentrations and decreased efficacy).
No products indexed under this heading.

Buspirone Hydrochloride (As a moderate inhibitor of CYP3A4, aprepitant can increase plasma concentrations of orally co-administered medicinal products that are metabolized through CYP3A4).
No products indexed under this heading.

Busulfan (As a moderate inhibitor of CYP3A4, aprepitant can increase plasma concentrations of orally co-administered medicinal products that are metabolized through CYP3A4). Products include:
Busulfex Injection 2477
Myleran Tablets 1530

Candesartan Cilexetil (Co-administration of fosaprepitant or oral aprepitant with drugs that are known to be metabolized by CYP2C9 may result in lower plasma concentrations of these drugs). Products include:
Atacand Tablets 639
Atacand HCT 642

Carbamazepine (Aprepitant is substrate for CYP3A4; therefore, co-administration of fosaprepitant or aprepitant with drugs that strongly induce CYP3A4 activity (e.g., rifampin, carbamazepine, phenytoin) may result in reduced plasma concentrations and decreased efficacy). Products include:
Carbatrol Capsules 3019
Equetro Extended-Release Capsules 3174

Carvedilol (Co-administration of fosaprepitant or oral aprepitant with drugs that are known to be metabolized by CYP2C9 may result in lower plasma concentrations of these drugs). Products include:
Coreg Tablets 1387

Celecoxib (Co-administration of fosaprepitant or oral aprepitant with drugs that are known to be metabolized by CYP2C9 may result in lower plasma concentrations of these drugs). Products include:
Celebrex Capsules 2979

Cerivastatin Sodium (As a moderate inhibitor of CYP3A4, aprepitant can increase plasma concentrations of orally co-administered medicinal products that are metabolized through CYP3A4).
No products indexed under this heading.

Chlorpheniramine (As a moderate inhibitor of CYP3A4, aprepitant can increase plasma concentrations of orally co-administered medicinal products that are metabolized through CYP3A4).
No products indexed under this heading.

Chlorpheniramine Maleate (As a moderate inhibitor of CYP3A4, aprepitant can increase plasma concentrations of orally co-administered medicinal products that are metabolized through CYP3A4). Products include:
Actifed Cold & Allergy Tablets 1895
Sudafed PE Sinus & Allergy Tablets 1908
Tylenol Allergy Multi-Symptom Caplets with Cool Burst and Rapid Release Gelcaps 1916
Children's Tylenol Plus Cold Suspension Liquid 1912
Children's Tylenol Plus Cough & Runny Nose Suspension Liquid 1912
Children's Tylenol Plus Flu Suspension Liquid 1914
Children's Tylenol Plus Multi-Symptom Cold Suspension Liquid 1912
Tylenol Cold Head Congestion Nighttime Caplets with Cool Burst 1910
Tylenol Cold Multi-Symptom Nighttime Caplets with Cool Burst 1913
Tylenol Sinus Congestion & Pain Nighttime Caplets with Cool Burst 1917

Chlorpheniramine Polistirex (As a moderate inhibitor of CYP3A4, aprepitant can increase plasma concentrations of orally co-administered medicinal products that are metabolized through CYP3A4). Products include:

Tussionex Pennkinetic Extended-Release Suspension 3154

Chlorpheniramine Tannate (As a moderate inhibitor of CYP3A4, aprepitant can increase plasma concentrations of orally co-administered medicinal products that are metabolized through CYP3A4).

No products indexed under this heading.

Chlorpropamide (Co-administration of fosaprepitant or oral aprepitant with drugs that are known to be metabolized by CYP2C9 may result in lower plasma concentrations of these drugs).

No products indexed under this heading.

Cimetidine (Aprepitant is a substrate for CYP3A4; therefore, co-administration of fosaprepitant or aprepitant with drugs that inhibit CYP3A4 activity may result in increased plasma concentrations of aprepitant. Consequently, concomitant administration of fosaprepitant or aprepitant with strong CYP3A4 inhibitors (e.g., ketoconazole, itraconazole, nefazodone, troleandomycin, clarithromycin, ritonavir, nelfinavir) should be approached with caution. Because moderate CYP3A4 inhibitors (e.g., diltiazem) result in a 2-fold increase in plasma concentrations of aprepitant, concomitant administration should also be approached with caution).

No products indexed under this heading.

Cimetidine Hydrochloride (Aprepitant is a substrate for CYP3A4; therefore, co-administration of fosaprepitant or aprepitant with drugs that inhibit CYP3A4 activity may result in increased plasma concentrations of aprepitant. Consequently, concomitant administration of fosaprepitant or aprepitant with strong CYP3A4 inhibitors (e.g., ketoconazole, itraconazole, nefazodone, troleandomycin, clarithromycin, ritonavir, nelfinavir) should be approached with caution. Because moderate CYP3A4 inhibitors (e.g., diltiazem) result in a 2-fold increase in plasma concentrations of aprepitant, concomitant administration should also be approached with caution).

No products indexed under this heading.

Ciprofloxacin (Aprepitant is a substrate for CYP3A4; therefore, co-administration of fosaprepitant or aprepitant with drugs that inhibit CYP3A4 activity may result in increased plasma concentrations of aprepitant. Consequently, concomitant administration of fosaprepitant or aprepitant with strong CYP3A4 inhibitors (e.g., ketoconazole, itraconazole, nefazodone, troleandomycin, clarithromycin, ritonavir, nelfinavir) should be approached with caution. Because moderate CYP3A4 inhibitors (e.g., diltiazem) result in a 2-fold increase in plasma concentrations of aprepitant, concomitant administration should also be approached with caution). Products include:

Cipro I.V. 2817
Cipro Oral Suspension 2810
Cipro XR Tablets 2823
Ciprodex Otic Suspension 541

Ciprofloxacin Hydrochloride (Aprepitant is substrate for CYP3A4; therefore, co-administration of fosaprepitant or aprepitant with drugs that strongly induce CYP3A4 activity (e.g., rifampin, carbamazepine, phenytoin) may result in reduced plasma concentrations and decreased efficacy). Products include:

Cipro Tablets 2810

Cisapride (EMEND is a moderate CYP3A4 inhibitor; concurrent use with EMEND could result in elevated plasma concentrations of cisapride, potentially causing serious or life-threatening reactions, and is contraindicated).

No products indexed under this heading.

Cisplatin (Aprepitant is substrate for CYP3A4; therefore, co-administration of fosaprepitant or aprepitant with drugs that strongly induce CYP3A4 activity (e.g., rifampin, carbamazepine, phenytoin) may result in reduced plasma concentrations and decreased efficacy).

No products indexed under this heading.

Clarithromycin (Aprepitant is a substrate for CYP3A4; therefore, co-administration of fosaprepitant or aprepitant with drugs that inhibit CYP3A4 activity may result in increased plasma concentrations of aprepitant. Consequently, concomitant administration of fosaprepitant or apreitant with strong CYP3A4 inhibitors (e.g., ketoconazole, itraconzole, nefazodone, troleandomycin, clarithromycin, ritonavir, nelfinavir) should be approached with caution). Products include:

Biaxin/Biaxin XL 411

Clomipramine Hydrochloride (Co-administration of fosaprepitant or oral aprepitant with drugs that are known to be metabolized by CYP2C9 may result in lower plasma concentrations of these drugs).

No products indexed under this heading.

Clotrimazole (Aprepitant is a substrate for CYP3A4; therefore, co-administration of fosaprepitant or aprepitant with drugs that inhibit CYP3A4 activity may result in increased plasma concentrations of aprepitant. Consequently, concomitant administration of fosaprepitant or aprepitant with strong CYP3A4 inhibitors (e.g., ketoconazole, itraconazole, nefazodone, troleandomycin, clarithromycin, ritonavir, nelfinavir) should be approached with caution. Because moderate CYP3A4 inhibitors (e.g., diltiazem) result in a 2-fold increase in plasma concentrations of aprepitant, concomitant administration should also be approached with caution). Products include:

Lotrisone 2881

Cortisone Acetate (Aprepitant is substrate for CYP3A4; therefore, co-administration of fosaprepitant or aprepitant with drugs that strongly induce CYP3A4 activity (e.g., rifampin, carbamazepine, phenytoin) may result in reduced plasma concentrations and decreased efficacy).

No products indexed under this heading.

Cyclosporine (Aprepitant is a substrate for CYP3A4; therefore, co-administration of fosaprepitant or aprepitant with drugs that inhibit CYP3A4 activity may result in increased plasma concentrations of aprepitant. Consequently, concomitant administration of fosaprepitant or aprepitant with strong CYP3A4 inhibitors (e.g., ketoconazole, itraconazole, nefazodone, troleandomycin, clarithromycin, ritonavir, nelfinavir) should be approached with caution. Because moderate CYP3A4 inhibitors (e.g., diltiazem) result in a 2-fold increase in plasma concentrations of aprepitant, concomitant administration should also be approached with caution). Products include:

Gengraf Capsules 435
Neoral Oral Solution 2280
Neoral Soft Gelatin Capsules 2280
Restasis Ophthalmic Emulsion 557
Sandimmune 2296

Dalfopristin (Aprepitant is a substrate for CYP3A4; therefore, co-administration of fosaprepitant or aprepitant with drugs that inhibit CYP3A4 activity may result in increased plasma concentrations of aprepitant. Consequently, concomitant administration of fosaprepitant or aprepitant with strong CYP3A4 inhibitors (e.g., ketoconazole, itraconazole, nefazodone, troleandomycin, clarithromycin, ritonavir, nelfinavir) should be approached with caution. Because moderate CYP3A4 inhibitors (e.g., diltiazem) result in a 2-fold increase in plasma concentrations of aprepitant, concomitant administration should also be approached with caution).

No products indexed under this heading.

Danazol (Aprepitant is a substrate for CYP3A4; therefore, co-administration of fosaprepitant or aprepitant with drugs that inhibit CYP3A4 activity may result in increased plasma concentrations of aprepitant. Consequently, concomitant administration of fosaprepitant or aprepitant with strong CYP3A4 inhibitors (e.g., ketoconazole, itraconazole, nefazodone, troleandomycin, clarithromycin, ritonavir, nelfinavir) should be approached with caution. Because moderate CYP3A4 inhibitors (e.g., diltiazem) result in a 2-fold increase in plasma concentrations of aprepitant, concomitant administration should also be approached with caution).

No products indexed under this heading.

Delavirdine Mesylate (Aprepitant is a substrate for CYP3A4; therefore, co-administration of fosaprepitant or aprepitant with drugs that inhibit CYP3A4 activity may result in increased plasma concentrations of aprepitant. Consequently, concomitant administration of fosaprepitant or apreitant with strong CYP3A4 inhibitors (e.g., ketoconazole, itraconzole, nefazodone, troleandomycin, clarithromycin, ritonavir, nelfinavir) should be approached with caution).

No products indexed under this heading.

Delavirine (Aprepitant is a substrate for CYP3A4; therefore, co-administration of fosaprepitant or aprepitant with drugs that inhibit CYP3A4 activity may result in increased plasma concentrations of aprepitant. Consequently, concomitant administration of fosaprepitant or apreitant with strong CYP3A4 inhibitors (e.g., ketoconazole, itraconzole, nefazodone, troleandomycin, clarithromycin, ritonavir, nelfinavir) should be approached with caution).

No products indexed under this heading.

Desogestrel (The co-administration of fosaprepitant or aprepitant may reduce the efficacy of hormonal contraceptives during and for 28 days after administration of the last dose of either. Alternative or back-up methods of contraception should be used during treatment with fosaprepitant or aprepitant and for one month following the last dose of aprepitant). Products include:

Mircette Tablets 1034

Dexamethasone (Oral aprepitant may increase the AUC of dexamethasone, a CYP3A4 substrate. The oral dexamethasone should be reduced by approximately 50% when co-administered with regimen of fosaprepitant followed by aprepitant, to achieve exposures of dexamethasone similar to those obtained when dexamethasone is given without aprepitant). Products include:

Ciprodex Otic Suspension 541

Dexamethasone Acetate (Oral aprepitant may increase the AUC of dexamethasone, a CYP3A4 substrate. The oral dexamethasone should be reduced by approximately 50% when co-administered with regimen of fosaprepitant followed by aprepitant, to achieve exposures of dexamethasone similar to those obtained when dexamethasone is given without aprepitant).

No products indexed under this heading.

Dexamethasone Sodium Phosphate (Oral aprepitant may increase the AUC of dexamethasone, a CYP3A4 substrate. The oral dexamethasone should be reduced by approximately 50% when co-administered with regimen of fosaprepitant followed by aprepitant, to achieve exposures of dexamethasone similar to those obtained when dexamethasone is given without aprepitant).

No products indexed under this heading.

Dextromethorphan (Co-administration of fosaprepitant or oral aprepitant with drugs that are known to be metabolized by CYP2C9 may result in lower plasma concentrations of these drugs).

No products indexed under this heading.

Diazepam (Fosaprepitant and oral aprepitant may increase the AUC of midazolam. The potential effects of increased plasma concentrations of midazolam or other benzodiazepines metabolized via CYP3A4 (alprazolam, triazolam) should be considered when co-administeringthese agents with a 3-day regimen of fosaprepitant followed by aprepitant). Products include:

Valium Tablets 2658

Diclofenac Potassium (Co-administration of fosaprepitant or oral aprepitant with drugs that are known to be metabolized by CYP2C9 may result in lower plasma concentrations of these drugs).

No products indexed under this heading.

Diclofenac Sodium (Co-administration of fosaprepitant or oral aprepitant with drugs that are known to be metabolized by CYP2C9 may result in lower plasma concentrations of these drugs). Products include:
Diclofenac Sodium Ophthalmic Solution .... ⊙240
Voltaren Ophthalmic Solution 2336
Voltaren Tablets 2334
Voltaren-XR Tablets 2337

Dihydroergotamine Mesylate (As a moderate inhibitor of CYP3A4, aprepitant can increase plasma concentrations of orally co-administered medicinal products that are metabolized through CYP3A4).
No products indexed under this heading.

Diltiazem Hydrochloride (Aprepitant is a substrate for CYP3A4; therefore, co-administration of fosaprepitant or aprepitant with drugs that inhibit CYP3A4 activity may result in increased plasma concentrations of aprepitant. Consequently, concomitant administration of fosaprepitant or aprepitant with strong CYP3A4 inhibitors (e.g., ketoconazole, itraconazole, nefazodone, troleandomycin, clarithromycin, ritonavir, nelfinavir) should be approached with caution. Because moderate CYP3A4 inhibitors (e.g., diltiazem) result in a 2-fold increase in plasma concentrations of aprepitant, concomitant administration should also be approached with caution). Products include:
Cardizem LA Extended Release Tablets 421

Diltiazem Maleate (Aprepitant is a substrate for CYP3A4; therefore, co-administration of fosaprepitant or aprepitant with drugs that inhibit CYP3A4 activity may result in increased plasma concentrations of aprepitant. Consequently, concomitant administration of fosaprepitant or aprepitant with strong CYP3A4 inhibitors (e.g., ketoconazole, itraconazole, nefazodone, troleandomycin, clarithromycin, ritonavir, nelfinavir) should be approached with caution. Because moderate CYP3A4 inhibitors (e.g., diltiazem) result in a 2-fold increase in plasma concentrations of aprepitant, concomitant administration should also be approached with caution).
No products indexed under this heading.

Disopyramide (As a moderate inhibitor of CYP3A4, aprepitant can increase plasma concentrations of orally co-administered medicinal products that are metabolized through CYP3A4).
No products indexed under this heading.

Disopyramide Phosphate (As a moderate inhibitor of CYP3A4, aprepitant can increase plasma concentrations of orally co-administered medicinal products that are metabolized through CYP3A4).
No products indexed under this heading.

Disulfiram (As a moderate inhibitor of CYP3A4, aprepitant can increase plasma concentrations of orally co-administered medicinal products that are metabolized through CYP3A4).
No products indexed under this heading.

Docetaxel (Particular caution and careful monitoring are advised in patients receiving chemotherapy agents metabolized primarily by CYP3A4, like docetaxel). Products include:
Taxotere Injection Concentrate 2773

Doxorubicin Hydrochloride (Aprepitant is substrate for CYP3A4; therefore, co-administration of fosaprepitant or aprepitant with drugs that strongly induce CYP3A4 activity (e.g., rifampin, carbamazepine, phenytoin) may result in reduced plasma concentrations and decreased efficacy).
No products indexed under this heading.

Dronabinol (Co-administration of fosaprepitant or oral aprepitant with drugs that are known to be metabolized by CYP2C9 may result in lower plasma concentrations of these drugs). Products include:
Marinol Capsules 3163

Efavirenz (Aprepitant is a substrate for CYP3A4; therefore, co-administration of fosaprepitant or aprepitant with drugs that inhibit CYP3A4 activity may result in increased plasma concentrations of aprepitant. Consequently, concomitant administration of fosaprepitant or aprepitant with strong CYP3A4 inhibitors (e.g., ketoconazole, itraconazole, nefazodone, troleandomycin, clarithromycin, ritonavir, nelfinavir) should be approached with caution. Because moderate CYP3A4 inhibitors (e.g., diltiazem) result in a 2-fold increase in plasma concentrations of aprepitant, concomitant administration should also be approached with caution). Products include:
Atripla Tablets 938
Sustiva Capsules 930
Sustiva Tablets 930

Eprosartan Mesylate (Co-administration of fosaprepitant or oral aprepitant with drugs that are known to be metabolized by CYP2C9 may result in lower plasma concentrations of these drugs). Products include:
Teveten Tablets 515
Teveten HCT Tablets 517

Ergotamine Tartrate (As a moderate inhibitor of CYP3A4, aprepitant can increase plasma concentrations of orally co-administered medicinal products that are metabolized through CYP3A4).
No products indexed under this heading.

Erythromycin (Aprepitant is a substrate for CYP3A4; therefore, co-administration of fosaprepitant or aprepitant with drugs that inhibit CYP3A4 activity may result in increased plasma concentrations of aprepitant. Consequently, concomitant administration of fosaprepitant or aprepitant with strong CYP3A4 inhibitors (e.g., ketoconazole, itraconazole, nefazodone, troleandomycin, clarithromycin, ritonavir, nelfinavir) should be approached with caution. Because moderate CYP3A4 inhibitors (e.g., diltiazem) result in a 2-fold increase in plasma concentrations of aprepitant, concomitant administration should also be approached with caution).
No products indexed under this heading.

Erythromycin Estolate (Aprepitant is a substrate for CYP3A4; therefore, co-administration of fosaprepitant or aprepitant with drugs that inhibit CYP3A4 activity may result in increased plasma concentrations of aprepitant. Consequently, concomitant administration of fosaprepitant or aprepitant with strong CYP3A4 inhibitors (e.g., ketoconazole, itraconazole, nefazodone, troleandomycin, clarithromycin, ritonavir, nelfinavir) should be approached with caution. Because moderate CYP3A4 inhibitors (e.g., diltiazem) result in a 2-fold increase in plasma concentrations of aprepitant, concomitant administration should also be approached with caution).
No products indexed under this heading.

Erythromycin Ethylsuccinate (Aprepitant is a substrate for CYP3A4; therefore, co-administration of fosaprepitant or aprepitant with drugs that inhibit CYP3A4 activity may result in increased plasma concentrations of aprepitant. Consequently, concomitant administration of fosaprepitant or aprepitant with strong CYP3A4 inhibitors (e.g., ketoconazole, itraconazole, nefazodone, troleandomycin, clarithromycin, ritonavir, nelfinavir) should be approached with caution. Because moderate CYP3A4 inhibitors (e.g., diltiazem) result in a 2-fold increase in plasma concentrations of aprepitant, concomitant administration should also be approached with caution). Products include:
E.E.S. 433
EryPed 431

Erythromycin Gluceptate (Aprepitant is a substrate for CYP3A4; therefore, co-administration of fosaprepitant or aprepitant with drugs that inhibit CYP3A4 activity may result in increased plasma concentrations of aprepitant. Consequently, concomitant administration of fosaprepitant or aprepitant with strong CYP3A4 inhibitors (e.g., ketoconazole, itraconazole, nefazodone, troleandomycin, clarithromycin, ritonavir, nelfinavir) should be approached with caution. Because moderate CYP3A4 inhibitors (e.g., diltiazem) result in a 2-fold increase in plasma concentrations of aprepitant, concomitant administration should also be approached with caution).
No products indexed under this heading.

Erythromycin Lactobionate (Aprepitant is a substrate for CYP3A4; therefore, co-administration of fosaprepitant or aprepitant with drugs that inhibit CYP3A4 activity may result in increased plasma concentrations of aprepitant. Consequently, concomitant administration of fosaprepitant or aprepitant with strong CYP3A4 inhibitors (e.g., ketoconazole, itraconazole, nefazodone, troleandomycin, clarithromycin, ritonavir, nelfinavir) should be approached with caution. Because moderate CYP3A4 inhibitors (e.g., diltiazem) result in a 2-fold increase in plasma concentrations of aprepitant, concomitant administration should also be approached with caution).
No products indexed under this heading.

Erythromycin Stearate (Aprepitant is a substrate for CYP3A4; therefore, co-administration of fosaprepitant or aprepitant with drugs that inhibit CYP3A4 activity may result in increased plasma concentrations of aprepitant. Consequently, concomitant administration of fosaprepitant or aprepitant with strong CYP3A4 inhibitors (e.g., ketoconazole, itraconazole, nefazodone, troleandomycin, clarithromycin, ritonavir, nelfinavir) should be approached with caution. Because moderate CYP3A4 inhibitors (e.g., diltiazem) result in a 2-fold increase in plasma concentrations of aprepitant, concomitant administration should also be approached with caution).
No products indexed under this heading.

Esomeprazole Magnesium (Aprepitant is a substrate for CYP3A4; therefore, co-administration of fosaprepitant or aprepitant with drugs that inhibit CYP3A4 activity may result in increased plasma concentrations of aprepitant. Consequently, concomitant administration of fosaprepitant or aprepitant with strong CYP3A4 inhibitors (e.g., ketoconazole, itraconazole, nefazodone, troleandomycin, clarithromycin, ritonavir, nelfinavir) should be approached with caution. Because moderate CYP3A4 inhibitors (e.g., diltiazem) result in a 2-fold increase in plasma concentrations of aprepitant, concomitant administration should also be approached with caution). Products include:
Nexium Delayed-Release Capsules 645
Nexium Delayed-Release Oral Suspension 645

Estradiol (As a moderate inhibitor of CYP3A4, aprepitant can increase plasma concentrations of orally co-administered medicinal products that are metabolized through CYP3A4). Products include:
Activella Tablets 2347
Angeliq Tablets 751
Climara Transdermal System 763
Climara Pro Transdermal System 768
Divigel 3167
Vagifem Tablets 2375

Estradiol Benzoate (As a moderate inhibitor of CYP3A4, aprepitant can increase plasma concentrations of orally co-administered medicinal products that are metabolized through CYP3A4).
No products indexed under this heading.

Estradiol Cypionate (As a moderate inhibitor of CYP3A4, aprepitant can increase plasma concentrations of orally co-administered medicinal products that are metabolized through CYP3A4).
No products indexed under this heading.

Estradiol Valerate (As a moderate inhibitor of CYP3A4, aprepitant can increase plasma concentrations of orally co-administered medicinal products that are metabolized through CYP3A4).
No products indexed under this heading.

Ethinyl Estradiol (The co-administration of fosaprepitant or aprepitant may reduce the efficacy of hormonal contraceptives during and for 28 days after administration of the last dose of either. Alternative or back-up methods of contraception should be used during treatment with fosaprepitant or aprepitant and

for one month following the last dose of aprepitant). Products include:

Lybrel Tablets 3204
Mircette Tablets 1034
NuvaRing 2897
Ortho-Cyclen/Ortho Tri-Cyclen 2449
Ortho Evra Transdermal System 2437
Ortho Tri-Cyclen Lo Tablets 2458
Seasonique Tablets 1046
Yaz Tablets 805

Ethosuximide (Aprepitant is substrate for CYP3A4; therefore, co-administration of fosaprepitant or aprepitant with drugs that strongly induce CYP3A4 activity (e.g., rifampin, carbamazepine, phenytoin) may result in reduced plasma concentrations and decreased efficacy).
No products indexed under this heading.

Ethynodiol Diacetate (The co-administration of fosaprepitant or aprepitant may reduce the efficacy of hormonal contraceptives during and for 28 days after administration of the last dose of either. Alternative or back-up methods of contraception should be used during treatment with fosaprepitant or aprepitant and for one month following the last dose of aprepitant).
No products indexed under this heading.

Etodolac (Co-administration of fosaprepitant or oral aprepitant with drugs that are known to be metabolized by CYP2C9 may result in lower plasma concentrations of these drugs).
No products indexed under this heading.

Etoposide (Particular caution and careful monitoring are advised in patients receiving chemotherapy agents metabolized primarily by CYP3A4, like etoposide).
No products indexed under this heading.

Etoposide Phosphate (As a moderate inhibitor of CYP3A4, aprepitant can increase plasma concentrations of orally co-administered medicinal products that are metabolized through CYP3A4).
No products indexed under this heading.

Felbamate (Aprepitant is substrate for CYP3A4; therefore, co-administration of fosaprepitant or aprepitant with drugs that strongly induce CYP3A4 activity (e.g., rifampin, carbamazepine, phenytoin) may result in reduced plasma concentrations and decreased efficacy).
No products indexed under this heading.

Felodipine (As a moderate inhibitor of CYP3A4, aprepitant can increase plasma concentrations of orally co-administered medicinal products that are metabolized through CYP3A4).
No products indexed under this heading.

Fenoprofen Calcium (Co-administration of fosaprepitant or oral aprepitant with drugs that are known to be metabolized by CYP2C9 may result in lower plasma concentrations of these drugs). Products include:

Nalfon Capsules 2508

Fentanyl (As a moderate inhibitor of CYP3A4, aprepitant can increase plasma concentrations of orally co-administered medicinal products that are metabolized through CYP3A4). Products include:

Duragesic Transdermal System 2405
Ionsys Transdermal System 2410

Fentanyl Citrate (As a moderate inhibitor of CYP3A4, aprepitant can increase plasma concentrations of orally co-administered medicinal products that are metabolized through CYP3A4). Products include:

Actiq 959
Fentora Tablets 968

Fluconazole (Aprepitant is a substrate for CYP3A4; therefore, co-administration of fosaprepitant or aprepitant with drugs that inhibit CYP3A4 activity may result in increased plasma concentrations of aprepitant. Consequently, concomitant administration of fosaprepitant or aprepitant with strong CYP3A4 inhibitors (e.g., ketoconazole, itraconazole, nefazodone, troleandomycin, clarithromycin, ritonavir, nelfinavir) should be approached with caution. Because moderate CYP3A4 inhibitors (e.g., diltiazem) result in a 2-fold increase in plasma concentrations of aprepitant, concomitant administration should also be approached with caution).
No products indexed under this heading.

Fludrocortisone Acetate (Aprepitant is substrate for CYP3A4; therefore, co-administration of fosaprepitant or aprepitant with drugs that strongly induce CYP3A4 activity (e.g., rifampin, carbamazepine, phenytoin) may result in reduced plasma concentrations and decreased efficacy).
No products indexed under this heading.

Fluoxetine (Aprepitant is a substrate for CYP3A4; therefore, co-administration of fosaprepitant or aprepitant with drugs that inhibit CYP3A4 activity may result in increased plasma concentrations of aprepitant. Consequently, concomitant administration of fosaprepitant or aprepitant with strong CYP3A4 inhibitors (e.g., ketoconazole, itraconazole, nefazodone, troleandomycin, clarithromycin, ritonavir, nelfinavir) should be approached with caution. Because moderate CYP3A4 inhibitors (e.g., diltiazem) result in a 2-fold increase in plasma concentrations of aprepitant, concomitant administration should also be approached with caution).
No products indexed under this heading.

Fluoxetine Hydrochloride (Aprepitant is a substrate for CYP3A4; therefore, co-administration of fosaprepitant or aprepitant with drugs that inhibit CYP3A4 activity may result in increased plasma concentrations of aprepitant. Consequently, concomitant administration of fosaprepitant or aprepitant with strong CYP3A4 inhibitors (e.g., ketoconazole, itraconazole, nefazodone, troleandomycin, clarithromycin, ritonavir, nelfinavir) should be approached with caution. Because moderate CYP3A4 inhibitors (e.g., diltiazem) result in a 2-fold increase in plasma concentrations of aprepitant, concomitant administration should also be approached with caution). Products include:

Prozac Weekly Capsules 1852
Prozac Pulvules and Liquid 1852
Symbyax Capsules 1871

Flurbiprofen (Co-administration of fosaprepitant or oral aprepitant with drugs that are known to be metabolized by CYP2C9 may result in lower plasma concentrations of these drugs).
No products indexed under this heading.

Flurbiprofen Sodium (Co-administration of fosaprepitant or oral aprepitant with drugs that are known to be metabolized by CYP2C9 may result in lower plasma concentrations of these drugs).
No products indexed under this heading.

Fluvastatin Sodium (Co-administration of fosaprepitant or oral aprepitant with drugs that are known to be metabolized by CYP2C9 may result in lower plasma concentrations of these drugs). Products include:

Lescol Capsules 2268
Lescol XL Tablets 2268

Fluvoxamine Maleate (Aprepitant is a substrate for CYP3A4; therefore, co-administration of fosaprepitant or aprepitant with drugs that inhibit CYP3A4 activity may result in increased plasma concentrations of aprepitant. Consequently, concomitant administration of fosaprepitant or aprepitant with strong CYP3A4 inhibitors (e.g., ketoconazole, itraconazole, nefazodone, troleandomycin, clarithromycin, ritonavir, nelfinavir) should be approached with caution. Because moderate CYP3A4 inhibitors (e.g., diltiazem) result in a 2-fold increase in plasma concentrations of aprepitant, concomitant administration should also be approached with caution). Products include:

Luvox CR Extended-Release Capsules 1759

Fosamprenavir Calcium (Aprepitant is a substrate for CYP3A4; therefore, co-administration of fosaprepitant or aprepitant with drugs that inhibit CYP3A4 activity may result in increased plasma concentrations of aprepitant. Consequently, concomitant administration of fosaprepitant or apreitant with strong CYP3A4 inhibitors (e.g., ketoconazole, itraconzole, nefazodone, troleandomycin, clarithromycin, ritonavir, nelfinavir) should be approached with caution). Products include:

Lexiva Oral Suspension 1510
Lexiva Tablets 1510

Fosphenytoin Sodium (Aprepitant has been shown to induce the metabolism of S(-) warfarin and tolbutamide, which are metabolized through CYP2C9. Co-administration of aprepitant with these drugs or other drugs that are known to be metabolized by CYP2C9, such as phenytoin, may result in lower plasma concentrations of these drugs).
No products indexed under this heading.

Garlic Extract (Aprepitant is substrate for CYP3A4; therefore, co-administration of fosaprepitant or aprepitant with drugs that strongly induce CYP3A4 activity (e.g., rifampin, carbamazepine, phenytoin) may result in reduced plasma concentrations and decreased efficacy).
No products indexed under this heading.

Garlic Oil (Aprepitant is substrate for CYP3A4; therefore, co-administration of fosaprepitant or aprepitant with drugs that strongly induce CYP3A4 activity (e.g., rifampin, carbamazepine, phenytoin) may result in reduced plasma concentrations and decreased efficacy).
No products indexed under this heading.

Glimepiride (Co-administration of fosaprepitant or oral aprepitant with drugs that are known to be metabolized by CYP2C9 may result in lower plasma concentrations of these drugs). Products include:

Avandaryl Tablets 1344
Duetact Tablets 3085

Glipizide (Co-administration of fosaprepitant or oral aprepitant with drugs that are known to be metabolized by CYP2C9 may result in lower plasma concentrations of these drugs).
No products indexed under this heading.

Haloperidol (As a moderate inhibitor of CYP3A4, aprepitant can increase plasma concentrations of orally co-administered medicinal products that are metabolized through CYP3A4).
No products indexed under this heading.

Haloperidol Decanoate (As a moderate inhibitor of CYP3A4, aprepitant can increase plasma concentrations of orally co-administered medicinal products that are metabolized through CYP3A4).
No products indexed under this heading.

Haloperidol Lactate (As a moderate inhibitor of CYP3A4, aprepitant can increase plasma concentrations of orally co-administered medicinal products that are metabolized through CYP3A4).
No products indexed under this heading.

Hydrocortisone (Aprepitant is substrate for CYP3A4; therefore, co-administration of fosaprepitant or aprepitant with drugs that strongly induce CYP3A4 activity (e.g., rifampin, carbamazepine, phenytoin) may result in reduced plasma concentrations and decreased efficacy).
No products indexed under this heading.

Hydrocortisone Acetate (Aprepitant is substrate for CYP3A4; therefore, co-administration of fosaprepitant or aprepitant with drugs that strongly induce CYP3A4 activity (e.g., rifampin, carbamazepine, phenytoin) may result in reduced plasma concentrations and decreased efficacy). Products include:

Analpram-HC 1140
Pramosone 1141

Hydrocortisone Butyrate (Aprepitant is substrate for CYP3A4; therefore, co-administration of fosaprepitant or aprepitant with drugs that strongly induce CYP3A4 activity (e.g., rifampin, carbamazepine, phenytoin) may result in reduced plasma concentrations and decreased efficacy).
No products indexed under this heading.

Hydrocortisone Cypionate (Aprepitant is substrate for CYP3A4; therefore, co-administration of fosaprepitant or aprepitant with drugs that strongly induce CYP3A4 activity (e.g., rifampin, carbamazepine, phenytoin) may result in reduced plasma concentrations and decreased efficacy).
No products indexed under this heading.

Hydrocortisone Hemisuccinate (Aprepitant is substrate for CYP3A4; therefore, co-administration of fosaprepitant or aprepitant with drugs that strongly induce CYP3A4 activity (e.g., rifampin, carbamazepine, phenytoin) may result in reduced plasma concentrations and decreased efficacy).
No products indexed under this heading.

Hydrocortisone Probutate (Aprepitant is substrate for CYP3A4; therefore, co-administration of fosaprepitant or aprepitant with drugs that strongly induce CYP3A4 activity (e.g., rifampin, carbamazepine, phenytoin) may result in reduced plasma concentrations and decreased efficacy).
No products indexed under this heading.

Hydrocortisone Sodium Phosphate (Aprepitant is substrate for CYP3A4; therefore, co-administration of fosaprepitant or aprepitant with drugs that strongly induce CYP3A4 activity (e.g., rifampin, carbamazepine, phenytoin) may result in reduced plasma concentrations and decreased efficacy).
No products indexed under this heading.

Hydrocortisone Sodium Succinate (Aprepitant is substrate for CYP3A4; therefore, co-administration of fosaprepitant or aprepitant with drugs that strongly induce CYP3A4 activity (e.g., rifampin, carbamazepine, phenytoin) may result in reduced plasma concentrations and decreased efficacy).
No products indexed under this heading.

Hydrocortisone Valerate (Aprepitant is substrate for CYP3A4; therefore, co-administration of fosaprepitant or aprepitant with drugs that strongly induce CYP3A4 activity (e.g., rifampin, carbamazepine, phenytoin) may result in reduced plasma concentrations and decreased efficacy).
No products indexed under this heading.

Hypericum (Aprepitant is substrate for CYP3A4; therefore, co-administration of fosaprepitant or aprepitant with drugs that strongly induce CYP3A4 activity (e.g., rifampin, carbamazepine, phenytoin) may result in reduced plasma concentrations and decreased efficacy). Products include:
Satieté Tablets .... ■ 640

Hypericum Perforatum (Aprepitant is substrate for CYP3A4; therefore, co-administration of fosaprepitant or aprepitant with drugs that strongly induce CYP3A4 activity (e.g., rifampin, carbamazepine, phenytoin) may result in reduced plasma concentrations and decreased efficacy).
No products indexed under this heading.

Ibuprofen (Co-administration of fosaprepitant or oral aprepitant with drugs that are known to be metabolized by CYP2C9 may result in lower plasma concentrations of these drugs). Products include:
Motrin IB Tablets and Caplets 1900
Children's Motrin Oral Suspension ... 1901
Children's Motrin Non-Staining Dye-Free Oral Suspension............ 1901
Children's Motrin Cold Oral Suspension 1899
Infants' Motrin Concentrated Drops.. 1901
Infants' Motrin Non-Staining Dye-Free Concentrated Drops....... 1901
Junior Strength Motrin Caplets and Chewable Tablets................. 1901
Vicoprofen Tablets 533

Ifosfamide (Particular caution and careful monitoring are advised in patients receiving chemotherapy agents metabolized primarily by CYP3A4, like ifosfamide).
No products indexed under this heading.

Imatinib Mesylate (Particular caution and careful monitoring are advised in patients receiving chemotherapy agents metabolized primarily by CYP3A4, like imatinib). Products include:
Gleevec Tablets 2255

Imipramine Hydrochloride (Co-administration of fosaprepitant or oral aprepitant with drugs that are known to be metabolized by CYP2C9 may result in lower plasma concentrations of these drugs).
No products indexed under this heading.

Indinavir Sulfate (Aprepitant is a substrate for CYP3A4; therefore, co-administration of fosaprepitant or aprepitant with drugs that inhibit CYP3A4 activity may result in increased plasma concentrations of aprepitant. Consequently, concomitant administration of fosaprepitant or apreitant with strong CYP3A4 inhibitors (e.g., ketoconazole, itraconzole, nefazodone, troleandomycin, clarithromycin, ritonavir, nelfinavir) should be approached with caution). Products include:
Crixivan Capsules 1979

Indomethacin (Co-administration of fosaprepitant or oral aprepitant with drugs that are known to be metabolized by CYP2C9 may result in lower plasma concentrations of these drugs). Products include:
Indocin 2024

Indomethacin Sodium Trihydrate (Co-administration of fosaprepitant or oral aprepitant with drugs that are known to be metabolized by CYP2C9 may result in lower plasma concentrations of these drugs). Products include:
Indocin I.V. 2489

Irbesartan (Co-administration of fosaprepitant or oral aprepitant with drugs that are known to be metabolized by CYP2C9 may result in lower plasma concentrations of these drugs). Products include:
Avalide Tablets 892
Avalide Tablets 2713
Avapro Tablets 897
Avapro Tablets 2718

Irinotecan Hydrochloride (Particular caution and careful monitoring are advised in patients receiving chemotherapy agents metabolized primarily by CYP3A4, like irinotecan).
No products indexed under this heading.

Isoniazid (Aprepitant is a substrate for CYP3A4; therefore, co-administration of fosaprepitant or aprepitant with drugs that inhibit CYP3A4 activity may result in increased plasma concentrations of aprepitant. Consequently, concomitant administration of fosaprepitant or aprepitant with strong CYP3A4 inhibitors (e.g., ketoconazole, itraconazole, nefazodone, troleandomycin, clarithromycin, ritonavir, nelfinavir) should be approached with caution. Because moderate CYP3A4 inhibitors (e.g., diltiazem) result in a 2-fold increase in plasma concentrations of aprepitant, concomitant administration should also be approached with caution).
No products indexed under this heading.

Isradipine (As a moderate inhibitor of CYP3A4, aprepitant can increase plasma concentrations of orally co-administered medicinal products that are metabolized through CYP3A4). Products include:
DynaCirc CR Controlled Release Tablets 1407

Itraconazole (Aprepitant is a substrate for CYP3A4; therefore, co-administration of fosaprepitant or aprepitant with drugs that inhibit CYP3A4 activity may result in increased plasma concentrations of aprepitant. Consequently, concomitant administration of fosaprepitant or apreitant with strong CYP3A4 inhibitors (e.g., ketoconazole, itraconzole, nefazodone, troleandomycin, clarithromycin, ritonavir, nelfinavir) should be approached with caution).
No products indexed under this heading.

Ixabepilone (As a moderate inhibitor of CYP3A4, aprepitant can increase plasma concentrations of orally co-administered medicinal products that are metabolized through CYP3A4). Products include:
Ixempra Kit for Injection 915

Ketoconazole (Aprepitant is a substrate for CYP3A4; therefore, co-administration of fosaprepitant or aprepitant with drugs that inhibit CYP3A4 activity may result in increased plasma concentrations of aprepitant. Consequently, concomitant administration of fosaprepitant or apreitant with strong CYP3A4 inhibitors (e.g., ketoconazole, itraconzole, nefazodone, troleandomycin, clarithromycin, ritonavir, nelfinavir) should be approached with caution). Products include:
Extina Foam, 2% 3057
Nizoral A-D Shampoo 1901

Ketoprofen (Co-administration of fosaprepitant or oral aprepitant with drugs that are known to be metabolized by CYP2C9 may result in lower plasma concentrations of these drugs).
No products indexed under this heading.

Ketorolac Tromethamine (Co-administration of fosaprepitant or oral aprepitant with drugs that are known to be metabolized by CYP2C9 may result in lower plasma concentrations of these drugs).
No products indexed under this heading.

Lansoprazole (Co-administration of fosaprepitant or oral aprepitant with drugs that are known to be metabolized by CYP2C9 may result in lower plasma concentrations of these drugs).
No products indexed under this heading.

Levonorgestrel (The co-administration of fosaprepitant or aprepitant may reduce the efficacy of hormonal contraceptives during and for 28 days after administration of the last dose of either. Alternative or back-up methods of contraception should be used during treatment with fosaprepitant or aprepitant and for one month following the last dose of aprepitant). Products include:
Climara Pro Transdermal System 768
Lybrel Tablets 3204
Mirena Intrauterine System 779
Plan B Tablets 1044
Seasonique Tablets 1046

Lidocaine (As a moderate inhibitor of CYP3A4, aprepitant can increase plasma concentrations of orally co-administered medicinal products that are metabolized through CYP3A4). Products include:
Lidoderm Patch 1114

Lidocaine Hydrochloride (As a moderate inhibitor of CYP3A4, aprepitant can increase plasma concentrations of orally co-administered medicinal products that are metabolized through CYP3A4).
No products indexed under this heading.

Lopinavir (Aprepitant is a substrate for CYP3A4; therefore, co-administration of fosaprepitant or aprepitant with drugs that inhibit CYP3A4 activity may result in increased plasma concentrations of aprepitant. Consequently, concomitant administration of fosaprepitant or apreitant with strong CYP3A4 inhibitors (e.g., ketoconazole, itraconzole, nefazodone, troleandomycin, clarithromycin, ritonavir, nelfinavir) should be approached with caution). Products include:
Kaletra 452

Loratadine (Aprepitant is a substrate for CYP3A4; therefore, co-administration of fosaprepitant or aprepitant with drugs that inhibit CYP3A4 activity may result in increased plasma concentrations of aprepitant. Consequently, concomitant administration of fosaprepitant or aprepitant with strong CYP3A4 inhibitors (e.g., ketoconazole, itraconazole, nefazodone, troleandomycin, clarithromycin, ritonavir, nelfinavir) should be approached with caution. Because moderate CYP3A4 inhibitors (e.g., diltiazem) result in a 2-fold increase in plasma concentrations of aprepitant, concomitant administration should also be approached with caution).
No products indexed under this heading.

Losartan Potassium (Co-administration of fosaprepitant or oral aprepitant with drugs that are known to be metabolized by CYP2C9 may result in lower plasma concentrations of these drugs).
Products include:
Cozaar Tablets 1973

Lovastatin (As a moderate inhibitor of CYP3A4, aprepitant can increase plasma concentrations of orally co-administered medicinal products that are metabolized through CYP3A4).
Products include:
Advicor Tablets 402
Mevacor Tablets 2063

Meclofenamate Sodium (Co-administration of fosaprepitant or oral aprepitant with drugs that are known to be metabolized by CYP2C9 may result in lower plasma concentrations of these drugs).
No products indexed under this heading.

Mefenamic Acid (Co-administration of fosaprepitant or oral aprepitant with drugs that are known to be metabolized by CYP2C9 may result in lower plasma concentrations of these drugs).
No products indexed under this heading.

Meloxicam (Co-administration of fosaprepitant or oral aprepitant with drugs that are known to be metabolized by CYP2C9 may result in lower plasma concentrations of these drugs). Products include:
Mobic Oral Suspension 863
Mobic Tablets 863

Mephenytoin (Aprepitant is substrate for CYP3A4; therefore, co-administration of fosaprepitant or aprepitant with drugs that strongly induce CYP3A4 activity (e.g., rifampin, carbamazepine, phenytoin) may result in reduced plasma concentrations and decreased efficacy).
No products indexed under this heading.

Mestranol (The co-administration of fosaprepitant or aprepitant may reduce the efficacy of hormonal contraceptives during and for 28 days after administration of the last dose of either. Alternative or back-up methods of contraception should be used during treatment with fosaprepitant or aprepitant and for one month following the last dose of aprepitant).
No products indexed under this heading.

Metformin Hydrochloride (Co-administration of fosaprepitant or oral aprepitant with drugs that are known to be metabolized by CYP2C9 may result in lower plasma concentrations of these drugs).
Products include:
ActoPlus Met Tablets 3071
Avandamet Tablets 1336
Janumet Tablets 2041
PrandiMet Tablets 2967

Methadone Hydrochloride (As a moderate inhibitor of CYP3A4, aprepitant can increase plasma concentrations of orally co-administered medicinal products that are metabolized through CYP3A4).
No products indexed under this heading.

Methsuximide (Aprepitant is substrate for CYP3A4; therefore, co-administration of fosaprepitant or aprepitant with drugs that strongly induce CYP3A4 activity (e.g., rifampin, carbamazepine, phenytoin) may result in reduced plasma concentrations and decreased efficacy).
No products indexed under this heading.

Methylprednisolone (Oral aprepitant may increase the AUC of methylprednisolone, a CYP3A4 substrate. The IV methylprednisolone doses should be reduced by approximately 25% and the oral methylprednisolone dose should be reduced by approximately 50% when co-administered with a regimen of fosaprepitant followed by aprepitant to achieve exposures of methylprednisolone similar to those obtained when it is given without aprepitant).
No products indexed under this heading.

Methylprednisolone Acetate (Oral aprepitant may increase the AUC of methylprednisolone, a CYP3A4 substrate. The IV methylprednisolone doses should be reduced by approximately 25% and the oral methylprednisolone dose should be reduced by approximately 50% when co-administered with a regimen of fosaprepitant followed by aprepitant to achieve exposures of methylprednisolone similar to those obtained when it is given without aprepitant).
No products indexed under this heading.

Methylprednisolone Sodium Succinate (Oral aprepitant may increase the AUC of methylprednisolone, a CYP3A4 substrate. The IV methylprednisolone doses should be reduced by approximately 25% and the oral methylprednisolone dose should be reduced by approximately 50% when co-administered with a regimen of fosaprepitant followed by aprepitant to achieve exposures of methylprednisolone similar to those obtained when it is given without aprepitant).
No products indexed under this heading.

Metronidazole (Aprepitant is a substrate for CYP3A4; therefore, co-administration of fosaprepitant or aprepitant with drugs that inhibit CYP3A4 activity may result in increased plasma concentrations of aprepitant. Consequently, concomitant administration of fosaprepitant or aprepitant with strong CYP3A4 inhibitors (e.g., ketoconazole, itraconazole, nefazodone, troleandomycin, clarithromycin, ritonavir, nelfinavir) should be approached with caution. Because moderate CYP3A4 inhibitors (e.g., diltiazem) result in a 2-fold increase in plasma concentrations of aprepitant, concomitant administration should also be approached with caution). Products include:
Pylera Capsules 714

Metronidazole Benzoate (Aprepitant is a substrate for CYP3A4; therefore, co-administration of fosaprepitant or aprepitant with drugs that inhibit CYP3A4 activity may result in increased plasma concentrations of aprepitant. Consequently, concomitant administration of fosaprepitant or aprepitant with strong CYP3A4 inhibitors (e.g., ketoconazole, itraconazole, nefazodone, troleandomycin, clarithromycin, ritonavir, nelfinavir) should be approached with caution. Because moderate CYP3A4 inhibitors (e.g., diltiazem) result in a 2-fold increase in plasma concentrations of aprepitant, concomitant administration should also be approached with caution).
No products indexed under this heading.

Metronidazole Hydrochloride (Aprepitant is a substrate for CYP3A4; therefore, co-administration of fosaprepitant or aprepitant with drugs that inhibit CYP3A4 activity may result in increased plasma concentrations of aprepitant. Consequently, concomitant administration of fosaprepitant or aprepitant with strong CYP3A4 inhibitors (e.g., ketoconazole, itraconazole, nefazodone, troleandomycin, clarithromycin, ritonavir, nelfinavir) should be approached with caution. Because moderate CYP3A4 inhibitors (e.g., diltiazem) result in a 2-fold increase in plasma concentrations of aprepitant, concomitant administration should also be approached with caution).
No products indexed under this heading.

Metronidazole Sodium (Aprepitant is a substrate for CYP3A4; therefore, co-administration of fosaprepitant or aprepitant with drugs that inhibit CYP3A4 activity may result in increased plasma concentrations of aprepitant. Consequently, concomitant administration of fosaprepitant or aprepitant with strong CYP3A4 inhibitors (e.g., ketoconazole, itraconazole, nefazodone, troleandomycin, clarithromycin, ritonavir, nelfinavir) should be approached with caution. Because moderate CYP3A4 inhibitors (e.g., diltiazem) result in a 2-fold increase in plasma concentrations of aprepitant, concomitant administration should also be approached with caution).
No products indexed under this heading.

Miconazole (Aprepitant is a substrate for CYP3A4; therefore, co-administration of fosaprepitant or aprepitant with drugs that inhibit CYP3A4 activity may result in increased plasma concentrations of aprepitant. Consequently, concomitant administration of fosaprepitant or aprepitant with strong CYP3A4 inhibitors (e.g., ketoconazole, itraconazole, nefazodone, troleandomycin, clarithromycin, ritonavir, nelfinavir) should be approached with caution. Because moderate CYP3A4 inhibitors (e.g., diltiazem) result in a 2-fold increase in plasma concentrations of aprepitant, concomitant administration should also be approached with caution).
No products indexed under this heading.

Miconazole Nitrate (Aprepitant is a substrate for CYP3A4; therefore, co-administration of fosaprepitant or aprepitant with drugs that inhibit CYP3A4 activity may result in increased plasma concentrations of aprepitant. Consequently, concomitant administration of fosaprepitant or aprepitant with strong CYP3A4 inhibitors (e.g., ketoconazole, itraconazole, nefazodone, troleandomycin, clarithromycin, ritonavir, nelfinavir) should be approached with caution. Because moderate CYP3A4 inhibitors (e.g., diltiazem) result in a 2-fold increase in plasma concentrations of aprepitant, concomitant administration should also be approached with caution).
No products indexed under this heading.

Midazolam Hydrochloride (Fosaprepitant and oral aprepitant may increase the AUC of midazolam. The potential effects of increased plasma concentrations of midazolam or other benzodiazepines metabolized via CYP3A4 (alprazolam, triazolam) should be considered when co-administeringthese agents with a 3-day regimen of fosaprepitant followed by aprepitant).
No products indexed under this heading.

Miglitol (Co-administration of fosaprepitant or oral aprepitant with drugs that are known to be metabolized by CYP2C9 may result in lower plasma concentrations of these drugs).
No products indexed under this heading.

Mirtazapine (Co-administration of fosaprepitant or oral aprepitant with drugs that are known to be metabolized by CYP2C9 may result in lower plasma concentrations of these drugs). Products include:
Remeron Tablets 2924
RemeronSolTab Tablets 2927

Modafinil (Aprepitant is substrate for CYP3A4; therefore, co-administration of fosaprepitant or aprepitant with drugs that strongly induce CYP3A4 activity (e.g., rifampin, carbamazepine, phenytoin) may result in reduced plasma concentrations and decreased efficacy).
Products include:
Provigil Tablets 977

Montelukast Sodium (Co-administration of fosaprepitant or oral aprepitant with drugs that are known to be metabolized by CYP2C9 may result in lower plasma concentrations of these drugs).
Products include:
Singulair 2114

Nabumetone (Co-administration of fosaprepitant or oral aprepitant with drugs that are known to be metabolized by CYP2C9 may result in lower plasma concentrations of these drugs).
No products indexed under this heading.

Naproxen (Co-administration of fosaprepitant or oral aprepitant with drugs that are known to be metabolized by CYP2C9 may result in lower plasma concentrations of these drugs). Products include:
EC-Naprosyn Delayed-Release Tablets 2632
Naprosyn Suspension 2632
Naprosyn Tablets 2632

Naproxen Sodium (Co-administration of fosaprepitant or oral aprepitant with drugs that are known to be metabolized by CYP2C9 may result in lower plasma concentrations of these drugs).
Products include:
Anaprox Tablets 2632
Anaprox DS Tablets 2632
Treximet Tablets 1616

Nateglinide (Co-administration of fosaprepitant or oral aprepitant with drugs that are known to be metabolized by CYP2C9 may result in lower plasma concentrations of these drugs). Products include:
Starlix Tablets 2314

Nefazodone Hydrochloride (Aprepitant is a substrate for CYP3A4; therefore, co-administration of fosaprepitant or aprepitant with drugs that inhibit CYP3A4 activity may result in increased plasma concentrations of aprepitant. Consequently, concomitant administration of fosaprepitant or apreitant with strong CYP3A4 inhibitors (e.g., ketoconazole, itraconzole, nefazodone, troleandomycin, clarithromycin, ritonavir, nelfinavir) should be approached with caution).

No products indexed under this heading.

Nelfinavir Mesylate (Aprepitant is a substrate for CYP3A4; therefore, co-administration of fosaprepitant or aprepitant with drugs that inhibit CYP3A4 activity may result in increased plasma concentrations of aprepitant. Consequently, concomitant administration of fosaprepitant or apreitant with strong CYP3A4 inhibitors (e.g., ketoconazole, itraconzole, nefazodone, troleandomycin, clarithromycin, ritonavir, nelfinavir) should be approached with caution).

No products indexed under this heading.

Nevirapine (Aprepitant is a substrate for CYP3A4; therefore, co-administration of fosaprepitant or aprepitant with drugs that inhibit CYP3A4 activity may result in increased plasma concentrations of aprepitant. Consequently, concomitant administration of fosaprepitant or aprepitant with strong CYP3A4 inhibitors (e.g., ketoconazole, itraconazole, nefazodone, troleandomycin, clarithromycin, ritonavir, nelfinavir) should be approached with caution. Because moderate CYP3A4 inhibitors (e.g., diltiazem) result in a 2-fold increase in plasma concentrations of aprepitant, concomitant administration should also be approached with caution). Products include:

Viramune Oral Suspension 873
Viramune Tablets 873

Niacinamide (Aprepitant is a substrate for CYP3A4; therefore, co-administration of fosaprepitant or aprepitant with drugs that inhibit CYP3A4 activity may result in increased plasma concentrations of aprepitant. Consequently, concomitant administration of fosaprepitant or aprepitant with strong CYP3A4 inhibitors (e.g., ketoconazole, itraconazole, nefazodone, troleandomycin, clarithromycin, ritonavir, nelfinavir) should be approached with caution. Because moderate CYP3A4 inhibitors (e.g., diltiazem) result in a 2-fold increase in plasma concentrations of aprepitant, concomitant administration should also be approached with caution). Products include:

BioLean Free Tablets .... ▣635

Nicardipine Hydrochloride (As a moderate inhibitor of CYP3A4, aprepitant can increase plasma concentrations of orally co-administered medicinal products that are metabolized through CYP3A4). Products include:

Cardene I.V. 1093

Nicotinamide (Aprepitant is a substrate for CYP3A4; therefore, co-administration of fosaprepitant or aprepitant with drugs that inhibit CYP3A4 activity may result in increased plasma concentrations of aprepitant. Consequently, concomitant administration of fosaprepitant or aprepitant with strong CYP3A4 inhibitors (e.g., ketoconazole, itraconazole, nefazodone, troleandomycin, clarithromycin, ritonavir, nelfinavir) should be approached with caution. Because moderate CYP3A4 inhibitors (e.g., diltiazem) result in a 2-fold increase in plasma concentrations of aprepitant, concomitant administration should also be approached with caution).

No products indexed under this heading.

Nifedipine (Aprepitant is a substrate for CYP3A4; therefore, co-administration of fosaprepitant or aprepitant with drugs that inhibit CYP3A4 activity may result in increased plasma concentrations of aprepitant. Consequently, concomitant administration of fosaprepitant or aprepitant with strong CYP3A4 inhibitors (e.g., ketoconazole, itraconazole, nefazodone, troleandomycin, clarithromycin, ritonavir, nelfinavir) should be approached with caution. Because moderate CYP3A4 inhibitors (e.g., diltiazem) result in a 2-fold increase in plasma concentrations of aprepitant, concomitant administration should also be approached with caution).

No products indexed under this heading.

Nimodipine (As a moderate inhibitor of CYP3A4, aprepitant can increase plasma concentrations of orally co-administered medicinal products that are metabolized through CYP3A4). Products include:

Nimotop Capsules 790

Nisoldipine (As a moderate inhibitor of CYP3A4, aprepitant can increase plasma concentrations of orally co-administered medicinal products that are metabolized through CYP3A4). Products include:

Sular Extended Release Tablets 2975

Nitrendipine (As a moderate inhibitor of CYP3A4, aprepitant can increase plasma concentrations of orally co-administered medicinal products that are metabolized through CYP3A4).

No products indexed under this heading.

Norethindrone (The co-administration of fosaprepitant or aprepitant may reduce the efficacy of hormonal contraceptives during and for 28 days after administration of the last dose of either. Alternative or back-up methods of contraception should be used during treatment with fosaprepitant or aprepitant and for one month following the last dose of aprepitant). Products include:

Ortho Micronor Tablets 2446

Norethindrone Acetate (As a moderate inhibitor of CYP3A4, aprepitant can increase plasma concentrations of orally co-administered medicinal products that are metabolized through CYP3A4). Products include:

Activella Tablets 2347

Norethynodrel (The co-administration of fosaprepitant or aprepitant may reduce the efficacy of hormonal contraceptives during and for 28 days after administration of the last dose of either. Alternative or back-up methods of contraception should be used during treatment with fosaprepitant or aprepitant and for one month following the last dose of aprepitant).

No products indexed under this heading.

Norfloxacin (Aprepitant is a substrate for CYP3A4; therefore, co-administration of fosaprepitant or aprepitant with drugs that inhibit CYP3A4 activity may result in increased plasma concentrations of aprepitant. Consequently, concomitant administration of fosaprepitant or aprepitant with strong CYP3A4 inhibitors (e.g., ketoconazole, itraconazole, nefazodone, troleandomycin, clarithromycin, ritonavir, nelfinavir) should be approached with caution. Because moderate CYP3A4 inhibitors (e.g., diltiazem) result in a 2-fold increase in plasma concentrations of aprepitant, concomitant administration should also be approached with caution). Products include:

Noroxin Tablets 2069

Norgestimate (The co-administration of fosaprepitant or aprepitant may reduce the efficacy of hormonal contraceptives during and for 28 days after administration of the last dose of either. Alternative or back-up methods of contraception should be used during treatment with fosaprepitant or aprepitant and for one month following the last dose of aprepitant). Products include:

Ortho-Cyclen/Ortho Tri-Cyclen 2449
Ortho Tri-Cyclen Lo Tablets 2458

Norgestrel (The co-administration of fosaprepitant or aprepitant may reduce the efficacy of hormonal contraceptives during and for 28 days after administration of the last dose of either. Alternative or back-up methods of contraception should be used during treatment with fosaprepitant or aprepitant and for one month following the last dose of aprepitant).

No products indexed under this heading.

Omeprazole (Aprepitant is a substrate for CYP3A4; therefore, co-administration of fosaprepitant or aprepitant with drugs that inhibit CYP3A4 activity may result in increased plasma concentrations of aprepitant. Consequently, concomitant administration of fosaprepitant or aprepitant with strong CYP3A4 inhibitors (e.g., ketoconazole, itraconazole, nefazodone, troleandomycin, clarithromycin, ritonavir, nelfinavir) should be approached with caution. Because moderate CYP3A4 inhibitors (e.g., diltiazem) result in a 2-fold increase in plasma concentrations of aprepitant, concomitant administration should also be approached with caution).

No products indexed under this heading.

Ondansetron (As a moderate inhibitor of CYP3A4, aprepitant can increase plasma concentrations of orally co-administered medicinal products that are metabolized through CYP3A4). Products include:

Zofran ODT Orally Disintegrating Tablets 1687

Ondansetron Hydrochloride (As a moderate inhibitor of CYP3A4, aprepitant can increase plasma concentrations of orally co-administered medicinal products that are metabolized through CYP3A4). Products include:

Zofran Injection 1682
Zofran 1687

Oxaprozin (Co-administration of fosaprepitant or oral aprepitant with drugs that are known to be metabolized by CYP2C9 may result in lower plasma concentrations of these drugs).

No products indexed under this heading.

Oxcarbazepine (Aprepitant is substrate for CYP3A4; therefore, co-administration of fosaprepitant or aprepitant with drugs that strongly induce CYP3A4 activity (e.g., rifampin, carbamazepine, phenytoin) may result in reduced plasma concentrations and decreased efficacy).

No products indexed under this heading.

Paclitaxel (Particular caution and careful monitoring are advised in patients receiving chemotherapy agents metabolized primarily by CYP3A4, like paclitaxel).

No products indexed under this heading.

Paroxetine Hydrochloride (Co-administration resulted in a decrease in AUC by approximately 25% and Cmax by approximately 20% of both aprepitant and paroxetine). Products include:

Paxil 1535
Paxil CR Controlled-Release Tablets 1544

Phenobarbital (Aprepitant is substrate for CYP3A4; therefore, co-administration of fosaprepitant or aprepitant with drugs that strongly induce CYP3A4 activity (e.g., rifampin, carbamazepine, phenytoin) may result in reduced plasma concentrations and decreased efficacy). Products include:

Donnatal Extentabs 2507

Phenobarbital Sodium (Aprepitant is substrate for CYP3A4; therefore, co-administration of fosaprepitant or aprepitant with drugs that strongly induce CYP3A4 activity (e.g., rifampin, carbamazepine, phenytoin) may result in reduced plasma concentrations and decreased efficacy).

No products indexed under this heading.

Phenylbutazone (Co-administration of fosaprepitant or oral aprepitant with drugs that are known to be metabolized by CYP2C9 may result in lower plasma concentrations of these drugs).

No products indexed under this heading.

Phenytoin (Aprepitant has been shown to induce the metabolism of S(-) warfarin and tolbutamide, which are metabolized through CYP2C9. Co-administration of aprepitant with these drugs or other drugs that are known to be metabolized by CYP2C9, such as phenytoin, may result in lower plasma concentrations of these drugs).

No products indexed under this heading.

Phenytoin Sodium (Aprepitant has been shown to induce the metabolism of S(-) warfarin and tolbutamide, which are metabolized through CYP2C9. Co-administration of aprepitant with these drugs or other drugs that are known to be metabolized by CYP2C9, such as phenytoin, may result in lower plasma concentrations of these drugs). Products include:

Phenytek Capsules **2192**

Pimozide (EMEND is a moderate CYP3A4 inhibitor; concurrent use with EMEND could result in elevated plasma concentrations of pimozide, potentially causing serious or life-threatening reactions, and is contraindicated).

No products indexed under this heading.

Pioglitazone Hydrochloride (Co-administration of fosaprepitant or oral aprepitant with drugs that are known to be metabolized by CYP2C9 may result in lower plasma concentrations of these drugs). Products include:

ActoPlus Met Tablets **3071**
Actos Tablets **3077**
Duetact Tablets **3085**

Piroxicam (Co-administration of fosaprepitant or oral aprepitant with drugs that are known to be metabolized by CYP2C9 may result in lower plasma concentrations of these drugs).

No products indexed under this heading.

Polyestradiol Phosphate (As a moderate inhibitor of CYP3A4, aprepitant can increase plasma concentrations of orally co-administered medicinal products that are metabolized through CYP3A4).

No products indexed under this heading.

Prednisolone Acetate (Aprepitant is substrate for CYP3A4; therefore, co-administration of fosaprepitant or aprepitant with drugs that strongly induce CYP3A4 activity (e.g., rifampin, carbamazepine, phenytoin) may result in reduced plasma concentrations and decreased efficacy). Products include:

Pred Forte Ophthalmic Suspension .... ⊙ **227**
Pred Mild Ophthalmic Suspension .... ⊙ **230**
Pred-G Ophthalmic Ointment .... ⊙ **229**
Pred-G Ophthalmic Suspension ...... ⊙ **228**

Prednisolone Sodium Phosphate (Aprepitant is substrate for CYP3A4; therefore, co-administration of fosaprepitant or aprepitant with drugs that strongly induce CYP3A4 activity (e.g., rifampin, carbamazepine, phenytoin) may result in reduced plasma concentrations and decreased efficacy).

No products indexed under this heading.

Prednisolone Tebutate (Aprepitant is substrate for CYP3A4; therefore, co-administration of fosaprepitant or aprepitant with drugs that strongly induce CYP3A4 activity (e.g., rifampin, carbamazepine, phenytoin) may result in reduced plasma concentrations and decreased efficacy).

No products indexed under this heading.

Prednisone (Aprepitant is substrate for CYP3A4; therefore, co-administration of fosaprepitant or aprepitant with drugs that strongly induce CYP3A4 activity (e.g., rifampin, carbamazepine, phenytoin) may result in reduced plasma concentrations and decreased efficacy).

No products indexed under this heading.

Primidone (Aprepitant is substrate for CYP3A4; therefore, co-administration of fosaprepitant or aprepitant with drugs that strongly induce CYP3A4 activity (e.g., rifampin, carbamazepine, phenytoin) may result in reduced plasma concentrations and decreased efficacy).

No products indexed under this heading.

Propoxyphene Hydrochloride (Aprepitant is a substrate for CYP3A4; therefore, co-administration of fosaprepitant or aprepitant with drugs that inhibit CYP3A4 activity may result in increased plasma concentrations of aprepitant. Consequently, concomitant administration of fosaprepitant or aprepitant with strong CYP3A4 inhibitors (e.g., ketoconazole, itraconazole, nefazodone, troleandomycin, clarithromycin, ritonavir, nelfinavir) should be approached with caution. Because moderate CYP3A4 inhibitors (e.g., diltiazem) result in a 2-fold increase in plasma concentrations of aprepitant, concomitant administration should also be approached with caution).

No products indexed under this heading.

Propoxyphene Napsylate (Aprepitant is a substrate for CYP3A4; therefore, co-administration of fosaprepitant or aprepitant with drugs that inhibit CYP3A4 activity may result in increased plasma concentrations of aprepitant. Consequently, concomitant administration of fosaprepitant or aprepitant with strong CYP3A4 inhibitors (e.g., ketoconazole, itraconazole, nefazodone, troleandomycin, clarithromycin, ritonavir, nelfinavir) should be approached with caution. Because moderate CYP3A4 inhibitors (e.g., diltiazem) result in a 2-fold increase in plasma concentrations of aprepitant, concomitant administration should also be approached with caution).

No products indexed under this heading.

Quinidine (Aprepitant is a substrate for CYP3A4; therefore, co-administration of fosaprepitant or aprepitant with drugs that inhibit CYP3A4 activity may result in increased plasma concentrations of aprepitant. Consequently, concomitant administration of fosaprepitant or aprepitant with strong CYP3A4 inhibitors (e.g., ketoconazole, itraconazole, nefazodone, troleandomycin, clarithromycin, ritonavir, nelfinavir) should be approached with caution. Because moderate CYP3A4 inhibitors (e.g., diltiazem) result in a 2-fold increase in plasma concentrations of aprepitant, concomitant administration should also be approached with caution).

No products indexed under this heading.

Quinidine Gluconate (As a moderate inhibitor of CYP3A4, aprepitant can increase plasma concentrations of orally co-administered medicinal products that are metabolized through CYP3A4).

No products indexed under this heading.

Quinidine Hydrochloride (Aprepitant is a substrate for CYP3A4; therefore, co-administration of fosaprepitant or aprepitant with drugs that inhibit CYP3A4 activity may result in increased plasma concentrations of aprepitant. Consequently, concomitant administration of fosaprepitant or aprepitant with strong CYP3A4 inhibitors (e.g., ketoconazole, itraconazole, nefazodone, troleandomycin, clarithromycin, ritonavir, nelfinavir) should be approached with caution. Because moderate CYP3A4 inhibitors (e.g., diltiazem) result in a 2-fold increase in plasma concentrations of aprepitant, concomitant administration should also be approached with caution).

No products indexed under this heading.

Quinidine Polygalacturonate (Aprepitant is a substrate for CYP3A4; therefore, co-administration of fosaprepitant or aprepitant with drugs that inhibit CYP3A4 activity may result in increased plasma concentrations of aprepitant. Consequently, concomitant administration of fosaprepitant or aprepitant with strong CYP3A4 inhibitors (e.g., ketoconazole, itraconazole, nefazodone, troleandomycin, clarithromycin, ritonavir, nelfinavir) should be approached with caution. Because moderate CYP3A4 inhibitors (e.g., diltiazem) result in a 2-fold increase in plasma concentrations of aprepitant, concomitant administration should also be approached with caution).

No products indexed under this heading.

Quinidine Sulfate (Aprepitant is a substrate for CYP3A4; therefore, co-administration of fosaprepitant or aprepitant with drugs that inhibit CYP3A4 activity may result in increased plasma concentrations of aprepitant. Consequently, concomitant administration of fosaprepitant or aprepitant with strong CYP3A4 inhibitors (e.g., ketoconazole, itraconazole, nefazodone, troleandomycin, clarithromycin, ritonavir, nelfinavir) should be approached with caution. Because moderate CYP3A4 inhibitors (e.g., diltiazem) result in a 2-fold increase in plasma concentrations of aprepitant, concomitant administration should also be approached with caution).

No products indexed under this heading.

Quinine (Aprepitant is a substrate for CYP3A4; therefore, co-administration of fosaprepitant or aprepitant with drugs that inhibit CYP3A4 activity may result in increased plasma concentrations of aprepitant. Consequently, concomitant administration of fosaprepitant or aprepitant with strong CYP3A4 inhibitors (e.g., ketoconazole, itraconazole, nefazodone, troleandomycin, clarithromycin, ritonavir, nelfinavir) should be approached with caution. Because moderate CYP3A4 inhibitors (e.g., diltiazem) result in a 2-fold increase in plasma concentrations of aprepitant, concomitant administration should also be approached with caution).

No products indexed under this heading.

Quinine Sulfate (Aprepitant is a substrate for CYP3A4; therefore, co-administration of fosaprepitant or aprepitant with drugs that inhibit CYP3A4 activity may result in increased plasma concentrations of aprepitant. Consequently, concomitant administration of fosaprepitant or aprepitant with strong CYP3A4 inhibitors (e.g., ketoconazole, itraconazole, nefazodone, troleandomycin, clarithromycin, ritonavir, nelfinavir) should be approached with caution. Because moderate CYP3A4 inhibitors (e.g., diltiazem) result in a 2-fold increase in plasma concentrations of aprepitant, concomitant administration should also be approached with caution).

No products indexed under this heading.

Quinupristin (Aprepitant is a substrate for CYP3A4; therefore, co-administration of fosaprepitant or aprepitant with drugs that inhibit CYP3A4 activity may result in increased plasma concentrations of aprepitant. Consequently, concomitant administration of fosaprepitant or aprepitant with strong CYP3A4 inhibitors (e.g., ketoconazole, itraconazole, nefazodone, troleandomycin, clarithromycin, ritonavir, nelfinavir) should be approached with caution. Because moderate CYP3A4 inhibitors (e.g., diltiazem) result in a 2-fold increase in plasma concentrations of aprepitant, concomitant administration should also be approached with caution).

No products indexed under this heading.

Ranitidine Bismuth Citrate (Aprepitant is a substrate for CYP3A4; therefore, co-administration of fosaprepitant or aprepitant with drugs that inhibit CYP3A4 activity may result in increased plasma concentrations of aprepitant. Consequently, concomitant administration of fosaprepitant or aprepitant with strong CYP3A4 inhibitors (e.g., ketoconazole, itraconazole, nefazodone, troleandomycin, clarithromycin, ritonavir, nelfinavir) should be approached with caution. Because moderate CYP3A4 inhibitors (e.g., diltiazem) result in a 2-fold increase in plasma concentrations of aprepitant, concomitant administration should also be approached with caution).

No products indexed under this heading.

Ranitidine Hydrochloride (Aprepitant is a substrate for CYP3A4; therefore, co-administration of fosaprepitant or aprepitant with drugs that inhibit CYP3A4 activity may result in increased plasma concentrations of aprepitant. Consequently, concomitant administration of fosaprepitant or aprepitant with strong CYP3A4 inhibitors (e.g., ketoconazole, itraconazole, nefazodone, troleandomycin, clarithromycin, ritonavir, nelfinavir) should be approached with caution. Because moderate CYP3A4 inhibitors (e.g., diltiazem) result in a 2-fold increase in plasma concentrations of aprepitant, concomitant administration should also be approached with caution). Products include:

Zantac 75 Tablets ▣ 603
Zantac 1670
Zantac Injection 1666
Zantac Injection Pharmacy Bulk Package 1668
Maximum Strength Zantac 150 Tablets ▣ 603
Maximum Strength Zantac 150 Cool Mint Tablets ▣ 603

Repaglinide (Co-administration of fosaprepitant or oral aprepitant with drugs that are known to be metabolized by CYP2C9 may result in lower plasma concentrations of these drugs). Products include:

PrandiMet Tablets 2967
Prandin Tablets 2971

Rifabutin (Aprepitant is substrate for CYP3A4; therefore, co-administration of fosaprepitant or aprepitant with drugs that strongly induce CYP3A4 activity (e.g., rifampin, carbamazepine, phenytoin) may result in reduced plasma concentrations and decreased efficacy).

No products indexed under this heading.

Rifampicin (Aprepitant is substrate for CYP3A4; therefore, co-administration of fosaprepitant or aprepitant with drugs that strongly induce CYP3A4 activity (e.g., rifampin, carbamazepine, phenytoin) may result in reduced plasma concentrations and decreased efficacy).

No products indexed under this heading.

Rifampin (Aprepitant is substrate for CYP3A4; therefore, co-administration of fosaprepitant or aprepitant with drugs that strongly induce CYP3A4 activity (e.g., rifampin, carbamazepine, phenytoin) may result in reduced plasma concentrations and decreased efficacy).

No products indexed under this heading.

Rifapentine (Aprepitant is substrate for CYP3A4; therefore, co-administration of fosaprepitant or aprepitant with drugs that strongly induce CYP3A4 activity (e.g., rifampin, carbamazepine, phenytoin) may result in reduced plasma concentrations and decreased efficacy).

No products indexed under this heading.

Ritonavir (Aprepitant is a substrate for CYP3A4; therefore, co-administration of fosaprepitant or aprepitant with drugs that inhibit CYP3A4 activity may result in increased plasma concentrations of aprepitant. Consequently, concomitant administration of fosaprepitant or apreitant with strong CYP3A4 inhibitors (e.g., ketoconazole, itraconzole, nefazodone, troleandomycin, clarithromycin, ritonavir, nelfinavir) should be approached with caution). Products include:

Kaletra 452
Norvir 489

Rofecoxib (Co-administration of fosaprepitant or oral aprepitant with drugs that are known to be metabolized by CYP2C9 may result in lower plasma concentrations of these drugs).

No products indexed under this heading.

Rosiglitazone Maleate (Co-administration of fosaprepitant or oral aprepitant with drugs that are known to be metabolized by CYP2C9 may result in lower plasma concentrations of these drugs). Products include:

Avandamet Tablets 1336
Avandaryl Tablets 1344
Avandia Tablets 1351

Saquinavir (Aprepitant is a substrate for CYP3A4; therefore, co-administration of fosaprepitant or aprepitant with drugs that inhibit CYP3A4 activity may result in increased plasma concentrations of aprepitant. Consequently, concomitant administration of fosaprepitant or apreitant with strong CYP3A4 inhibitors (e.g., ketoconazole, itraconzole, nefazodone, troleandomycin, clarithromycin, ritonavir, nelfinavir) should be approached with caution).

No products indexed under this heading.

Saquinavir Mesylate (Aprepitant is a substrate for CYP3A4; therefore, co-administration of fosaprepitant or aprepitant with drugs that inhibit CYP3A4 activity may result in increased plasma concentrations of aprepitant. Consequently, concomitant administration of fosaprepitant or apreitant with strong CYP3A4 inhibitors (e.g., ketoconazole, itraconzole, nefazodone, troleandomycin, clarithromycin, ritonavir, nelfinavir) should be approached with caution).

No products indexed under this heading.

Sertraline Hydrochloride (Aprepitant is a substrate for CYP3A4; therefore, co-administration of fosaprepitant or aprepitant with drugs that inhibit CYP3A4 activity may result in increased plasma concentrations of aprepitant. Consequently, concomitant administration of fosaprepitant or aprepitant with strong CYP3A4 inhibitors (e.g., ketoconazole, itraconazole, nefazodone, troleandomycin, clarithromycin, ritonavir, nelfinavir) should be approached with caution. Because moderate CYP3A4 inhibitors (e.g., diltiazem) result in a 2-fold increase in plasma concentrations of aprepitant, concomitant administration should also be approached with caution).

No products indexed under this heading.

Sildenafil Citrate (Aprepitant is a substrate for CYP3A4; therefore, co-administration of fosaprepitant or aprepitant with drugs that inhibit CYP3A4 activity may result in increased plasma concentrations of aprepitant. Consequently, concomitant administration of fosaprepitant or apreitant with strong CYP3A4 inhibitors (e.g., ketoconazole, itraconazole, nefazodone, troleandomycin, clarithromycin, ritonavir, nelfinavir) should be approached with caution. Because moderate CYP3A4 inhibitors (e.g., diltiazem) result in a 2-fold increase in plasma concentrations of aprepitant, concomitant administration should also be approached with caution).

No products indexed under this heading.

Simvastatin (As a moderate inhibitor of CYP3A4, aprepitant can increase plasma concentrations of orally co-administered medicinal products that are metabolized through CYP3A4). Products include:

Simcor Tablets 502
Vytorin 10/10 Tablets 2149
Vytorin 10/10 Tablets 2939
Vytorin 10/20 Tablets 2149
Vytorin 10/20 Tablets 2939
Vytorin 10/40 Tablets 2149
Vytorin 10/40 Tablets 2939
Vytorin 10/80 Tablets 2149
Vytorin 10/80 Tablets 2939
Zocor Tablets 2136

Sirolimus (As a moderate inhibitor of CYP3A4, aprepitant can increase plasma concentrations of orally co-administered medicinal products that are metabolized through CYP3A4). Products include:

Rapamune 3260

Sulfamethoxazole (Co-administration of fosaprepitant or oral aprepitant with drugs that are known to be metabolized by CYP2C9 may result in lower plasma concentrations of these drugs).

No products indexed under this heading.

Sulfinpyrazone (Aprepitant is substrate for CYP3A4; therefore, co-administration of fosaprepitant or aprepitant with drugs that strongly induce CYP3A4 activity (e.g., rifampin, carbamazepine, phenytoin) may result in reduced plasma concentrations and decreased efficacy).

No products indexed under this heading.

Sulindac (Co-administration of fosaprepitant or oral aprepitant with drugs that are known to be metabolized by CYP2C9 may result in lower plasma concentrations of these drugs). Products include:

Clinoril Tablets 1962

Suprofen (Co-administration of fosaprepitant or oral aprepitant with drugs that are known to be metabolized by CYP2C9 may result in lower plasma concentrations of these drugs).

No products indexed under this heading.

Tacrolimus (As a moderate inhibitor of CYP3A4, aprepitant can increase plasma concentrations of orally co-administered medicinal products that are metabolized through CYP3A4). Products include:

Prograf Capsules and Injection 622
Protopic Ointment 628

Tadalafil (As a moderate inhibitor of CYP3A4, aprepitant can increase plasma concentrations of orally co-administered medicinal products that are metabolized through CYP3A4). Products include:

Cialis Tablets 1792

Tamoxifen Citrate (Co-administration of fosaprepitant or oral aprepitant with drugs that are known to be metabolized by CYP2C9 may result in lower plasma concentrations of these drugs).

No products indexed under this heading.

Telithromycin (Aprepitant is a substrate for CYP3A4; therefore, co-administration of fosaprepitant or aprepitant with drugs that inhibit CYP3A4 activity may result in increased plasma concentrations of aprepitant. Consequently, concomitant administration of fosaprepitant or apreitant with strong CYP3A4 inhibitors (e.g., ketoconazole, itraconzole, nefazodone, troleandomycin, clarithromycin, ritonavir, nelfinavir) should be approached with caution). Products include:

Ketek Tablets 2744

Telmisartan (Co-administration of fosaprepitant or oral aprepitant with drugs that are known to be metabolized by CYP2C9 may result in lower plasma concentrations of these drugs). Products include:

Micardis Tablets 852
Micardis HCT Tablets 854

Terfenadine (EMEND is a moderate CYP3A4 inhibitor; concurrent use with EMEND could result in elevated plasma concentrations of terfenadine, potentially causing serious or life-threatening reactions, and is contraindicated).

No products indexed under this heading.

Theophylline (Aprepitant is substrate for CYP3A4; therefore, co-administration of fosaprepitant or aprepitant with drugs that strongly induce CYP3A4 activity (e.g., rifampin, carbamazepine, phenytoin) may result in reduced plasma concentrations and decreased efficacy).

No products indexed under this heading.

Theophylline Anhydrous (Aprepitant is substrate for CYP3A4; therefore, co-administration of fosaprepitant or aprepitant with drugs that strongly induce CYP3A4 activity (e.g., rifampin, carbamazepine, phenytoin) may result in reduced plasma concentrations and decreased efficacy). Products include:

Uniphyl Tablets 2595

Theophylline Calcium Salicylate (Aprepitant is substrate for CYP3A4; therefore, co-administration of fosaprepitant or aprepitant with drugs that strongly induce CYP3A4 activity (e.g., rifampin, carbamazepine, phenytoin) may result in reduced plasma concentrations and decreased efficacy).

No products indexed under this heading.

Theophylline Dihydroxypropyl (Glyceryl) (Aprepitant is substrate for CYP3A4; therefore, co-administration of fosaprepitant or aprepitant with drugs that strongly induce CYP3A4 activity (e.g., rifampin, carbamazepine, phenytoin) may result in reduced plasma concentrations and decreased efficacy).

No products indexed under this heading.

Theophylline Ethylenediamine (Aprepitant is substrate for CYP3A4; therefore, co-administration of fosaprepitant or aprepitant with drugs that strongly induce CYP3A4 activity (e.g., rifampin, carbamazepine, phenytoin) may result in reduced plasma concentrations and decreased efficacy).

No products indexed under this heading.

Tiagabine Hydrochloride (As a moderate inhibitor of CYP3A4, aprepitant can increase plasma concentrations of orally co-administered medicinal products that are metabolized through CYP3A4). Products include:

Gabitril Tablets 973

Tolazamide (Co-administration of fosaprepitant or oral aprepitant with drugs that are known to be metabolized by CYP2C9 may result in lower plasma concentrations of these drugs).

No products indexed under this heading.

Tolbutamide (Aprepitant is an inducer of CYP2C9; co-administration has been shown to induce the metabolism of tolbutamide which is metabolized through CYP2C9).

No products indexed under this heading.

Tolbutamide Sodium (Co-administration of fosaprepitant or oral aprepitant with drugs that are known to be metabolized by CYP2C9 may result in lower plasma concentrations of these drugs).

No products indexed under this heading.

Tolmetin Sodium (Co-administration of fosaprepitant or oral aprepitant with drugs that are known to be metabolized by CYP2C9 may result in lower plasma concentrations of these drugs).

No products indexed under this heading.

Tolterodine Tartrate (As a moderate inhibitor of CYP3A4, aprepitant can increase plasma concentrations of orally co-administered medicinal products that are metabolized through CYP3A4).

No products indexed under this heading.

Torsemide (Co-administration of fosaprepitant or oral aprepitant with drugs that are known to be metabolized by CYP2C9 may result in lower plasma concentrations of these drugs). Products include:

Demadex Injection 2630
Demadex Tablets 2630

Trazodone Hydrochloride (As a moderate inhibitor of CYP3A4, aprepitant can increase plasma concentrations of orally co-administered medicinal products that are metabolized through CYP3A4).

No products indexed under this heading.

Triamcinolone (Aprepitant is substrate for CYP3A4; therefore, co-administration of fosaprepitant or aprepitant with drugs that strongly induce CYP3A4 activity (e.g., rifampin, carbamazepine, phenytoin) may result in reduced plasma concentrations and decreased efficacy).

No products indexed under this heading.

Triamcinolone Acetonide (Aprepitant is substrate for CYP3A4; therefore, co-administration of fosaprepitant or aprepitant with drugs that strongly induce CYP3A4 activity (e.g., rifampin, carbamazepine, phenytoin) may result in reduced plasma concentrations and decreased efficacy). Products include:

Azmacort Inhalation Aerosol 407
Nasacort AQ Nasal Spray 2765
Triesence Injectable Suspension .... ⊙ 209

Triamcinolone Diacetate (Aprepitant is substrate for CYP3A4; therefore, co-administration of fosaprepitant or aprepitant with drugs that strongly induce CYP3A4 activity (e.g., rifampin, carbamazepine, phenytoin) may result in reduced plasma concentrations and decreased efficacy).

No products indexed under this heading.

Triamcinolone Hexacetonide (Aprepitant is substrate for CYP3A4; therefore, co-administration of fosaprepitant or aprepitant with drugs that strongly induce CYP3A4 activity (e.g., rifampin, carbamazepine, phenytoin) may result in reduced plasma concentrations and decreased efficacy).

No products indexed under this heading.

Triazolam (Fosaprepitant and oral aprepitant may increase the AUC of midazolam. The potential effects of increased plasma concentrations of midazolam or other benzodiazepines metabolized via CYP3A4 (alprazolam, triazolam) should be considered when co-administeringthese agents with a 3-day regimen of fosaprepitant followed by aprepitant).

No products indexed under this heading.

Troglitazone (Aprepitant is a substrate for CYP3A4; therefore, co-administration of fosaprepitant or aprepitant with drugs that inhibit CYP3A4 activity may result in increased plasma concentrations of aprepitant. Consequently, concomitant administration of fosaprepitant or aprepitant with strong CYP3A4 inhibitors (e.g., ketoconazole, itraconazole, nefazodone, troleandomycin, clarithromycin, ritonavir, nelfinavir) should be approached with caution. Because moderate CYP3A4 inhibitors (e.g., diltiazem) result in a 2-fold increase in plasma concentrations of aprepitant, concomitant administration should also be approached with caution).

No products indexed under this heading.

Troleandomycin (Aprepitant is a substrate for CYP3A4; therefore, co-administration of fosaprepitant or aprepitant with drugs that inhibit CYP3A4 activity may result in increased plasma concentrations of aprepitant. Consequently, concomitant administration of fosaprepitant or apreitant with strong CYP3A4 inhibitors (e.g., ketoconazole, itraconzole, nefazodone, troleandomycin, clarithromycin, ritonavir, nelfinavir) should be approached with caution).

No products indexed under this heading.

Valdecoxib (Co-administration of fosaprepitant or oral aprepitant with drugs that are known to be metabolized by CYP2C9 may result in lower plasma concentrations of these drugs).

No products indexed under this heading.

Valproate Sodium (Aprepitant is a substrate for CYP3A4; therefore, co-administration of fosaprepitant or aprepitant with drugs that inhibit CYP3A4 activity may result in increased plasma concentrations of aprepitant. Consequently, concomitant administration of fosaprepitant or aprepitant with strong CYP3A4 inhibitors (e.g., ketoconazole, itraconazole, nefazodone, troleandomycin, clarithromycin, ritonavir, nelfinavir) should be approached with caution. Because moderate CYP3A4 inhibitors (e.g., diltiazem) result in a 2-fold increase in plasma concentrations of aprepitant, concomitant administration should also be approached with caution).

No products indexed under this heading.

Valsartan (Co-administration of fosaprepitant or oral aprepitant with drugs that are known to be metabolized by CYP2C9 may result in lower plasma concentrations of these drugs). Products include:

Diovan Tablets 2212
Diovan HCT Tablets 2216
Exforge Tablets 2238

Vardenafil Hydrochloride (Aprepitant is a substrate for CYP3A4; therefore, co-administration of fosaprepitant or aprepitant with drugs that inhibit CYP3A4 activity may result in increased plasma concentrations of aprepitant. Consequently, concomitant administration of fosaprepitant or aprepitant with strong CYP3A4 inhibitors (e.g., ketoconazole, itraconazole, nefazodone, troleandomycin, clarithromycin, ritonavir, nelfinavir) should be approached with caution. Because moderate CYP3A4 inhibitors (e.g., diltiazem) result in a 2-fold increase in plasma concentrations of aprepitant, concomitant administration should also be approached with caution). Products include:

Levitra Tablets 2876

Verapamil Hydrochloride (Aprepitant is a substrate for CYP3A4; therefore, co-administration of fosaprepitant or aprepitant with drugs that inhibit CYP3A4 activity may result in increased plasma concentrations of aprepitant. Consequently, concomitant administration of fosaprepitant or aprepitant with strong CYP3A4 inhibitors (e.g., ketoconazole, itraconazole, nefazodone, troleandomycin, clarithromycin, ritonavir, nelfinavir) should be approached with caution. Because moderate CYP3A4 inhibitors (e.g., diltiazem) result in a 2-fold increase in plasma concentrations of aprepitant, concomitant administration should also be approached with caution). Products include:

Tarka Tablets 511

Vinblastine Sulfate (Particular caution and careful monitoring are advised in patients receiving chemotherapy agents metabolized primarily by CYP3A4, like vinblastine).

No products indexed under this heading.

Vincristine Sulfate (Particular caution and careful monitoring are advised in patients receiving chemotherapy agents metabolized primarily by CYP3A4, like vincristine).

No products indexed under this heading.

Voriconazole (Aprepitant is a substrate for CYP3A4; therefore, co-administration of fosaprepitant or aprepitant with drugs that inhibit CYP3A4 activity may result in increased plasma concentrations of aprepitant. Consequently, concomitant administration of fosaprepitant or apreitant with strong CYP3A4 inhibitors (e.g., ketoconazole, itraconzole, nefazodone, troleandomycin, clarithromycin, ritonavir, nelfinavir) should be approached with caution).

No products indexed under this heading.

Warfarin Sodium (Aprepitant is an inducer of CYP2C9; co-administration has been shown to induce the metabolism of S(-) warfarin which is metabolized through CYP2C9; may result in a clinically significant decrease in INR of prothrombin time. In patients on chronic warfarin therapy, prothrombin time (INR) should be closely monitored in the 2-week period, particularly at 7-10 days, following initiation of the 3-day regimen of fosaprepitant followed by aprepitant with each chemotherapy cycle).

No products indexed under this heading.

Zafirlukast (Aprepitant is a substrate for CYP3A4; therefore, co-administration of fosaprepitant or aprepitant with drugs that inhibit CYP3A4 activity may result in increased plasma concentrations of aprepitant. Consequently, concomitant administration of fosaprepitant or aprepitant with strong CYP3A4 inhibitors (e.g., ketoconazole, itraconazole, nefazodone, troleandomycin, clarithromycin, ritonavir, nelfinavir) should be approached with caution. Because moderate CYP3A4 inhibitors (e.g., diltiazem) result in a 2-fold increase in plasma concentrations of aprepitant, concomitant administration should also be approached with caution). Products include:

Accolate Tablets 669

Zileuton (Aprepitant is a substrate for CYP3A4; therefore, co-administration of fosaprepitant or aprepitant with drugs that inhibit CYP3A4 activity may result in increased plasma concentrations of aprepitant. Consequently, concomitant administration of fosaprepitant or aprepitant with strong CYP3A4 inhibitors (e.g., ketoconazole, itraconazole, nefazodone, troleandomycin, clarithromycin, ritonavir, nelfinavir) should be approached with caution. Because moderate CYP3A4 inhibitors (e.g., diltiazem) result in a 2-fold increase in plasma concentrations of aprepitant, concomitant administration should also be approached with caution).

No products indexed under this heading.

Food Interactions

Grapefruit (Aprepitant is a substrate for CYP3A4; therefore, co-administration of fosaprepitant or aprepitant with drugs that inhibit CYP3A4 activity may result in increased plasma concentrations of aprepitant. Consequently, concomitant administration of fosaprepitant or aprepitant with strong CYP3A4 inhibitors (e.g., ketoconazole, itraconazole, nefazodone, troleandomycin, clarithromycin, ritonavir, nelfinavir) should be approached with caution. Because moderate CYP3A4 inhibitors (e.g., diltiazem) result in a 2-fold increase in plasma concentrations of aprepitant, concomitant administration should also be approached with caution).

Grapefruit Juice (Aprepitant is a substrate for CYP3A4; therefore, co-administration of fosaprepitant or aprepitant with drugs that inhibit CYP3A4 activity may result in increased plasma concentrations of aprepitant. Consequently, concomitant administration of fosaprepitant or aprepitant with strong CYP3A4 inhibitors (e.g., ketoconazole, itraconazole, nefazodone, troleandomycin, clarithromycin, ritonavir, nelfinavir) should be approached with caution. Because moderate CYP3A4 inhibitors (e.g., diltiazem) result in a 2-fold increase in plasma concentrations of

aprepitant, concomitant administration should also be approached with caution).

EMEND FOR INJECTION

(Fosaprepitant Dimeglumine) 1999
See Emend Capsules

EMSAM TRANSDERMAL SYSTEM

(Selegiline) 905

May interact with amphetamines, general anesthetics, local anesthetics, monoamine oxidase inhibitors, narcotic analgesics, Serotonin and Norepinephrine Reuptake Inhibitors, selective serotonin reuptake inhibitors, sympathomimetics, tricyclic antidepressants, vasopressors, and certain other agents. Compounds in these categories include:

Albuterol (Avoid concomitant use of sympathomimetic agents with selegiline transdermal system).
No products indexed under this heading.

Albuterol Sulfate (Avoid concomitant use of sympathomimetic agents with selegiline transdermal system). Products include:
Combivent Inhalation Aerosol 845
ProAir HFA Inhalation Aerosol 3113
Proventil HFA Inhalation Aerosol 2914
Ventolin HFA Inhalation Aerosol 1638

Alfentanil Hydrochloride (Selegiline transdermal system is contraindicated with analgesic agents such as tramadol, methadone, and propoxyphene).
No products indexed under this heading.

Amitriptyline Hydrochloride (Selegiline transdermal system is contraindicated with tricyclic antidepressants).
No products indexed under this heading.

Amoxapine (Selegiline transdermal system is contraindicated with tricyclic antidepressants).
No products indexed under this heading.

Amphetamine Resins (Selegiline transdermal system is contraindicated for use with sympathomimetic amines, including amphetamines).
No products indexed under this heading.

Amphetamine Sulfate (Selegiline transdermal system is contraindicated for use with sympathomimetic amines, including amphetamines). Products include:
Adderall XR Capsules 3012

Bupivacaine Hydrochloride (Patients taking selegiline transdermal system should not be given local anesthesia containing sympathomimetic vasoconstrictors).
No products indexed under this heading.

Buprenorphine Hydrochloride (Selegiline transdermal system is contraindicated with analgesic agents such as tramadol, methadone, and propoxyphene). Products include:
Suboxone Tablets 2601
Subutex Tablets 2601

Bupropion (Selegiline transdermal system is contraindicated with bupropion hydrochloride. Concomitant use of selegiline transdermal system and buspirone hydrochloride is not advised since several cases of elevated blood pressure have been reported in patients taking MAO inhibitors who were then given buspirone hydrochloride).
No products indexed under this heading.

Bupropion Hydrochloride (Selegiline transdermal system is contraindicated with bupropion hydrochloride. Concomitant use of selegiline transdermal system and buspirone hydrochloride is not advised since several cases of elevated blood pressure have been reported in patients taking MAO inhibitors who were then given buspirone hydrochloride). Products include:
Wellbutrin Tablets 1648
Wellbutrin SR Sustained-Release Tablets 1653
Wellbutrin XL Extended-Release Tablets 1659
Zyban Sustained-Release Tablets 1692

Carbamazepine (Carbamazepine is contraindicated in patients taking selegiline). Products include:
Carbatrol Capsules 3019
Equetro Extended-Release Capsules 3174

Chloroprocaine Hydrochloride (Patients taking selegiline transdermal system should not be given local anesthesia containing sympathomimetic vasoconstrictors).
No products indexed under this heading.

Citalopram Hydrobromide (Selegiline transdermal system is contraindicated with selective serotonin reuptake inhibitors). Products include:
Celexa 1160

Clomipramine Hydrochloride (Selegiline transdermal system is contraindicated with tricyclic antidepressants).
No products indexed under this heading.

Cocaine Hydrochloride (Patients taking selegiline transdermal system should not be given cocaine).
No products indexed under this heading.

Codeine Phosphate (Selegiline transdermal system is contraindicated with analgesic agents such as tramadol, methadone, and propoxyphene). Products include:
Tylenol with Codeine Tablets 2427

Cyclobenzaprine (Selegiline transdermal system is contraindicated with cyclobenzaprine).
No products indexed under this heading.

Cyclobenzaprine Hydrochloride (Selegiline transdermal system is contraindicated with cyclobenzaprine). Products include:
Amrix Capsules 966

Desipramine Hydrochloride (Selegiline transdermal system is contraindicated with tricyclic antidepressants).
No products indexed under this heading.

Desvenlafaxine Succinate (Selegiline transdermal system is contraindicated with dual serotonin and norepinephrine reuptake inhibitors). Products include:
Pristiq Extended-Release Tablets 3247

Dextroamphetamine Sulfate (Selegiline transdermal system is contraindicated for use with sympathomimetic amines, including amphetamines). Products include:
Adderall XR Capsules 3012
Dexedrine 1401

Dextromethorphan (Selegiline transdermal system is contraindicated with the antitussive agent dextromethorphan).
No products indexed under this heading.

Dextromethorphan Hydrobromide (Selegiline transdermal system is contraindicated with the antitussive agent dextromethorphan). Products include:
PediaCare Children's Liquid Multi-Symptom Cold...................... 1902
PediaCare Children's Long-Acting Cough 1902
Children's Sudafed PE Cold & Cough Liquid 1907
Sudafed PE Cold & Cough Caplets.......................... 1907
Children's Tylenol Plus Cough & Runny Nose Suspension Liquid 1912
Children's Tylenol Plus Cough & Sore Throat Suspension Liquid 1912
Children's Tylenol Plus Flu Suspension Liquid 1914
Children's Tylenol Plus Multi-Symptom Cold Suspension Liquid 1912
Tylenol Cold Severe Congestion Daytime Caplets with Cool Burst.......................... 1912
Tylenol Cold Head Congestion Daytime Caplets with Cool Burst.......................... 1910
Tylenol Cold Head Congestion Nighttime Caplets with Cool Burst.......................... 1910
Tylenol Cold Head Congestion Severe Daytime Caplets with Cool Burst.......................... 1910
Tylenol Cold Multi-Symptom Daytime Caplets with Cool Burst and Rapid Release Gels....... 1913
Tylenol Cold Multi-Symptom Daytime Liquid with Citrus Burst... 1913
Tylenol Cold Multi-Symptom Nighttime Caplets with Cool Burst.......................... 1913
Tylenol Cold Multi-Symptom Nighttime Liquid with Cool Burst... 1913
Tylenol Cold Multi-Symptom Severe Caplets with Cool Burst..... 1913
Tylenol Cold Multi-Symptom Severe Daytime Liquid with Citrus Burst.......................... 1913
Tylenol Cough & Sore Throat Daytime Liquid with Cool Burst...... 1918
Tylenol Cough & Sore Throat Nighttime Liquid with Cool Burst... 1918
Vicks DayQuil Cold & Flu Multi-Symptom Relief .... ▣ 616
Vicks DayQuil LiquiCaps 2567
Vicks DayQuil Liquid 2567
Vicks DayQuil Multi-Symptom Cold/Flu Relief.......................... 2567
Vicks NyQuil Cold & Flu Multi-Symptom Relief................ ▣ 617
Vicks NyQuil LiquiCaps 2567
Vicks NyQuil Liquid 2567
Vicks NyQuil Multi-Symptom Cold/Flu Relief.......................... 2567

Dextromethorphan Polistirex (Selegiline transdermal system is contraindicated with the antitussive agent dextromethorphan).
No products indexed under this heading.

Dextromethorphan tannate (Selegiline transdermal system is contraindicated with the antitussive agent dextromethorphan).
No products indexed under this heading.

Dezocine (Selegiline transdermal system is contraindicated with analgesic agents such as tramadol, methadone, and propoxyphene).
No products indexed under this heading.

Dobutamine Hydrochloride (Avoid concomitant use of sympathomimetic agents with selegiline transdermal system).
No products indexed under this heading.

Dopamine Hydrochloride (Avoid concomitant use of sympathomimetic agents with selegiline transdermal system).
No products indexed under this heading.

Doxepin Hydrochloride (Selegiline transdermal system is contraindicated with tricyclic antidepressants).
No products indexed under this heading.

Duloxetine Hydrochloride (Selegiline transdermal system is contraindicated with dual serotonin and norepinephrine reuptake inhibitors). Products include:
Cymbalta Delayed-Release Capsules.......................... 1801

Enflurane (Patients taking selegiline transdermal system should not undergo elective surgery requiring general anesthesia).
No products indexed under this heading.

Ephedrine Hydrochloride (Selegiline transdermal system is contraindicated for use with ephedrine).
No products indexed under this heading.

Ephedrine Sulfate (Selegiline transdermal system is contraindicated for use with ephedrine).
No products indexed under this heading.

Ephedrine Tannate (Selegiline transdermal system is contraindicated for use with ephedrine).
No products indexed under this heading.

Epinephrine (Avoid concomitant use of sympathomimetic agents with selegiline transdermal system). Products include:
EpiPen 1024

Epinephrine Bitartrate (Avoid concomitant use of sympathomimetic agents with selegiline transdermal system).
No products indexed under this heading.

Epinephrine Hydrochloride (Avoid concomitant use of sympathomimetic agents with selegiline transdermal system).
No products indexed under this heading.

Escitalopram Oxalate (Selegiline transdermal system is contraindicated with selective serotonin reuptake inhibitors). Products include:
Lexapro Oral Suspension 1174
Lexapro Tablets 1174

Ethanol (The use of alcohol is not recommended while using selegiline transdermal system).
No products indexed under this heading.

Ethyl Alcohol (The use of alcohol is not recommended while using selegiline transdermal system).
No products indexed under this heading.

Etidocaine Hydrochloride (Patients taking selegiline transdermal system should not be given local anesthesia containing sympathomimetic vasoconstrictors).
No products indexed under this heading.

Fentanyl (Selegiline transdermal system is contraindicated with analgesic agents such as tramadol, methadone, and propoxyphene). Products include:
Duragesic Transdermal System 2405
Ionsys Transdermal System 2410

Fentanyl Citrate (Selegiline transdermal system is contraindicated with analgesic agents such as tramadol, methadone, and propoxyphene). Products include:
Actiq 959
Fentora Tablets 968

Fluoxetine (Selegiline transdermal system is contraindicated with selective serotonin reuptake inhibitors).
No products indexed under this heading.

Fluoxetine Hydrochloride (Selegiline transdermal system is contraindicated with selective serotonin reuptake inhibitors). Products include:
Prozac Weekly Capsules 1852
Prozac Pulvules and Liquid 1852
Symbyax Capsules 1871

Fluvoxamine Maleate (Selegiline transdermal system is contraindicated with selective serotonin reuptake inhibitors). Products include:
Luvox CR Extended-Release Capsules 1759

Hydrocodone Bitartrate (Selegiline transdermal system is contraindicated with analgesic agents such as tramadol, methadone, and propoxyphene). Products include:
Lortab 5/500 Tablets 3143
Lortab 7.5/500 Tablets 3144
Lortab 10/500 Tablets 3144
Vicodin Tablets 529
Vicodin ES Tablets 530
Vicodin HP Tablets 531
Vicoprofen Tablets 533
Zydone Tablets 1132

Hydrocodone Polistirex (Selegiline transdermal system is contraindicated with analgesic agents such as tramadol, methadone, and propoxyphene). Products include:
Tussionex Pennkinetic Extended-Release Suspension 3154

Hydromorphone Hydrochloride (Selegiline transdermal system is contraindicated with analgesic agents such as tramadol, methadone, and propoxyphene).
No products indexed under this heading.

Hypericum (Selegiline transdermal system is contraindicated with St. John's wort). Products include:
Satieté Tablets 640

Hypericum Perforatum (Selegiline transdermal system is contraindicated with St. John's wort).
No products indexed under this heading.

Imipramine Hydrochloride (Selegiline transdermal system is contraindicated with tricyclic antidepressants).
No products indexed under this heading.

Imipramine Pamoate (Selegiline transdermal system is contraindicated with tricyclic antidepressants).
No products indexed under this heading.

Isocarboxazid (Selegiline transdermal system should not be used with oral selegiline or other MAO inhibitors). Products include:
Marplan Tablets 3177

Isoflurane (Patients taking selegiline transdermal system should not undergo elective surgery requiring general anesthesia).
No products indexed under this heading.

Isoproterenol Hydrochloride (Avoid concomitant use of sympathomimetic agents with selegiline transdermal system).
No products indexed under this heading.

Isoproterenol Sulfate (Avoid concomitant use of sympathomimetic agents with selegiline transdermal system).
No products indexed under this heading.

Ketamine Hydrochloride (Patients taking selegiline transdermal system should not undergo elective surgery requiring general anesthesia).
No products indexed under this heading.

Levalbuterol Hydrochloride (Avoid concomitant use of sympathomimetic agents with selegiline transdermal system). Products include:
Xopenex Inhalation Solution 3001
Xopenex Inhalation Solution Concentrate 3005

Levobupivacaine Hydrochloride (Patients taking selegiline transdermal system should not be given local anesthesia containing sympathomimetic vasoconstrictors).
No products indexed under this heading.

Levorphanol Tartrate (Selegiline transdermal system is contraindicated with analgesic agents such as tramadol, methadone, and propoxyphene).
No products indexed under this heading.

Lidocaine Hydrochloride (Patients taking selegiline transdermal system should not be given local anesthesia containing sympathomimetic vasoconstrictors).
No products indexed under this heading.

Maprotiline Hydrochloride (Selegiline transdermal system is contraindicated with tricyclic antidepressants).
No products indexed under this heading.

Meperidine Hydrochloride (Selegiline transdermal system is contraindicated with bupropion hydrochloride).
No products indexed under this heading.

Mepivacaine Hydrochloride (Patients taking selegiline transdermal system should not be given local anesthesia containing sympathomimetic vasoconstrictors).
No products indexed under this heading.

Metaproterenol Sulfate (Avoid concomitant use of sympathomimetic agents with selegiline transdermal system).
No products indexed under this heading.

Metaraminol Bitartrate (Avoid concomitant use of sympathomimetic agents with selegiline transdermal system).
No products indexed under this heading.

Methadone Hydrochloride (Selegiline transdermal system is contraindicated with analgesic agents such as tramadol, methadone, and propoxyphene).
No products indexed under this heading.

Methamphetamine Hydrochloride (Selegiline transdermal system is contraindicated for use with sympathomimetic amines, including amphetamines).
No products indexed under this heading.

Methohexital Sodium (Patients taking selegiline transdermal system should not undergo elective surgery requiring general anesthesia).
No products indexed under this heading.

Methoxamine Hydrochloride (Avoid concomitant use of sympathomimetic agents with selegiline transdermal system).
No products indexed under this heading.

Methoxyflurane (Patients taking selegiline transdermal system should not undergo elective surgery requiring general anesthesia).
No products indexed under this heading.

Mirtazapine (Selegiline transdermal system is contraindicated with mirtazapine). Products include:
Remeron Tablets 2924
RemeronSolTab Tablets 2927

Moclobemide (Selegiline transdermal system should not be used with oral selegiline or other MAO inhibitors).
No products indexed under this heading.

Morphine Sulfate (Selegiline transdermal system is contraindicated with analgesic agents such as tramadol, methadone, and propoxyphene). Products include:
Avinza Capsules 1772
DepoDur Injection 1095
MS Contin Tablets 2585

Norepinephrine Bitartrate (Avoid concomitant use of sympathomimetic agents with selegiline transdermal system).
No products indexed under this heading.

Nortriptyline Hydrochloride (Selegiline transdermal system is contraindicated with tricyclic antidepressants).
No products indexed under this heading.

Oxcarbazepine (Oxcarbazepine is contraindicated in patients taking selegiline).
No products indexed under this heading.

Oxycodone Hydrochloride (Selegiline transdermal system is contraindicated with analgesic agents such as tramadol, methadone, and propoxyphene). Products include:
OxyContin Tablets 2589
OxyIR Capsules 2593
Percocet Tablets 1127
Percodan Tablets 1130

Pargyline Hydrochloride (Selegiline transdermal system should not be used with oral selegiline or other MAO inhibitors).
No products indexed under this heading.

Paroxetine Hydrochloride (Selegiline transdermal system is contraindicated with selective serotonin reuptake inhibitors). Products include:
Paxil 1535
Paxil CR Controlled-Release Tablets 1544

Phenelzine Sulfate (Selegiline transdermal system should not be used with oral selegiline or other MAO inhibitors).
No products indexed under this heading.

Phenylephrine (Selegiline transdermal system is contraindicated for use with phenylephrine).
No products indexed under this heading.

Phenylephrine Bitartrate (Selegiline transdermal system is contraindicated for use with phenylephrine).
No products indexed under this heading.

Phenylephrine Hydrobromide (Selegiline transdermal system is contraindicated for use with phenylephrine).
No products indexed under this heading.

Phenylephrine Hydrochloride (Selegiline transdermal system is contraindicated for use with phenylephrine). Products include:
Actifed Cold & Allergy Tablets 1895
Benadryl Allergy & Cold Kapgels 1895
Benadryl Allergy & Sinus Headache Kapgels 1895
Benadryl Severe Allergy & Sinus Headache Caplets 1897
Children's Benadryl-D Allergy & Sinus Liquid 1896
Benadryl-D Allergy & Sinus Tablet 1896
PediaCare Children's Allergy & Cold Liquid 1902
PediaCare Children's Decongestant Liquid 1902
PediaCare Children's Liquid Multi-Symptom Cold 1902
Sinutab Non-Drying Caplets 1905
Sinutab Sinus Caplets 1905
Children's Sudafed PE Cold & Cough Liquid 1907
Children's Sudafed PE Nasal Decongestant Liquid 1906
Sudafed PE Cold & Cough Caplets 1907
Sudafed PE Nasal Decongestant Tablets 1907
Sudafed PE Nighttime Cold Caplets 1907
Sudafed PE Non-Drying Sinus Caplets 1908
Sudafed PE Severe Cold Caplets 1908
Sudafed PE Sinus & Allergy Tablets 1908
Sudafed PE Sinus Headache Caplets 1908
Tylenol Allergy Multi-Symptom Caplets with Cool Burst and Rapid Release Gelcaps 1916
Tylenol Allergy Multi-Symptom Nighttime Caplets with Cool Burst 1916
Children's Tylenol Plus Cold Suspension Liquid 1912
Children's Tylenol Plus Cold & Allergy Suspension Liquid 1914
Children's Tylenol Plus Flu Suspension Liquid 1914
Children's Tylenol Plus Multi-Symptom Cold Suspension Liquid 1912

Tylenol Cold Head Congestion Daytime Caplets with Cool Burst 1910
Tylenol Cold Head Congestion Nighttime Caplets with Cool Burst 1910
Tylenol Cold Head Congestion Severe Daytime Caplets with Cool Burst 1910
Tylenol Cold Multi-Symptom Daytime Caplets with Cool Burst and Rapid Release Gels 1913
Tylenol Cold Multi-Symptom Daytime Liquid with Citrus Burst ... 1913
Tylenol Cold Multi-Symptom Nighttime Caplets with Cool Burst 1913
Tylenol Cold Multi-Symptom Nighttime Liquid with Cool Burst ... 1913
Tylenol Cold Multi-Symptom Severe Caplets with Cool Burst 1913
Tylenol Cold Multi-Symptom Severe Daytime Liquid with Citrus Burst 1913
Tylenol Sinus Congestion & Pain Daytime Caplets with Cool Burst and Gelcaps 1917
Tylenol Sinus Congestion & Pain Nighttime Caplets with Cool Burst 1917
Tylenol Sinus Congestion & Pain Severe Caplets with Cool Burst 1917
Vicks DayQuil Cold & Flu Multi-Symptom Relief .... ▣616
Vicks DayQuil LiquiCaps 2567
Vicks DayQuil Liquid 2567
Vicks DayQuil Multi-Symptom Cold/Flu Relief 2567

Phenylephrine Tannate (Selegiline transdermal system is contraindicated for use with phenylephrine).
No products indexed under this heading.

Phenylpropanolamine (Selegiline transdermal system is contraindicated for use with phenylpropanolamine).
No products indexed under this heading.

Phenylpropanolamine Bitartrate (Selegiline transdermal system is contraindicated for use with phenylpropanolamine).
No products indexed under this heading.

Phenylpropanolamine Containing Anorectics (Selegiline transdermal system is contraindicated for use with phenylpropanolamine).
No products indexed under this heading.

Phenylpropanolamine Hydrochloride (Selegiline transdermal system is contraindicated for use with phenylpropanolamine).
No products indexed under this heading.

Phenylpropanolamine Polistirex (Selegiline transdermal system is contraindicated for use with phenylpropanolamine).
No products indexed under this heading.

Pirbuterol Acetate (Avoid concomitant use of sympathomimetic agents with selegiline transdermal system). Products include:
Maxair Autohaler 1705

Procaine Hydrochloride (Patients taking selegiline transdermal system should not be given local anesthesia containing sympathomimetic vasoconstrictors).
No products indexed under this heading.

Procarbazine Hydrochloride (Selegiline transdermal system should not be used with oral selegiline or other MAO inhibitors).
No products indexed under this heading.

Propofol (Patients taking selegiline transdermal system should not undergo elective surgery requiring general anesthesia).
No products indexed under this heading.

Propoxyphene Hydrochloride (Selegiline transdermal system is contraindicated with analgesic agents such as tramadol, methadone, and propoxyphene).
No products indexed under this heading.

Propoxyphene Napsylate (Selegiline transdermal system is contraindicated with analgesic agents such as tramadol, methadone, and propoxyphene).
No products indexed under this heading.

Protriptyline Hydrochloride (Selegiline transdermal system is contraindicated with tricyclic antidepressants).
No products indexed under this heading.

Pseudoephedrine (Selegiline transdermal system is contraindicated for use with pseudoephedrine).
No products indexed under this heading.

Pseudoephedrine Hydrochloride (Selegiline transdermal system is contraindicated for use with pseudoephedrine). Products include:
Allegra-D 12 Hour Extended-Release Tablets 2687
Allegra-D 24 Hour Extended-Release Tablets 2690
Children's Motrin Cold Oral Suspension 1899
Sudafed 12 Hour Nasal Decongestant Non-Drowsy Caplets 1909
Sudafed 24 Hour Non-Drowsy Nasal Decongestant Tablets 1906
Children's Sudafed Nasal Decongestant Liquid 1906
Sudafed Nasal Decongestant Tablets 1906
Tylenol Cold Severe Congestion Daytime Caplets with Cool Burst 1912
Tylenol Sinus Severe Congestion Caplets with Cool Burst 1917
Vicks NyQuil LiquiCaps 2567
Vicks NyQuil Liquid 2567
Vicks NyQuil Multi-Symptom Cold/Flu Relief 2567
Zyrtec-D 12 Hour Extended Release Tablets 1923
Zyrtec-D Allergy & Congestion Extended-Release Tablets 1923

Pseudoephedrine Preparations (Selegiline transdermal system is contraindicated for use with pseudoephedrine).
No products indexed under this heading.

Pseudoephedrine Sulfate (Selegiline transdermal system is contraindicated for use with pseudoephedrine). Products include:
Clarinex-D 12-Hour Extended-Release Tablets 2831
Clarinex-D 24-Hour Extended-Release Tablets 2834

Pseudoephedrine Tannate (Selegiline transdermal system is contraindicated for use with pseudoephedrine).
No products indexed under this heading.

Rasagiline Mesylate (Selegiline transdermal system should not be used with oral selegiline or other MAO inhibitors). Products include:
Azilect Tablets 3106

Remifentanil Hydrochloride (Selegiline transdermal system is contraindicated with analgesic agents such as tramadol, methadone, and propoxyphene).
No products indexed under this heading.

Salmeterol Xinafoate (Avoid concomitant use of sympathomimetic agents with selegiline transdermal system). Products include:
Advair Diskus 100/50 1276
Advair Diskus 250/50 1276
Advair Diskus 500/50 1276
Advair HFA 45/21 Inhalation Aerosol 1288
Advair HFA 115/21 Inhalation Aerosol 1288
Advair HFA 230/21 Inhalation Aerosol 1288
Serevent Diskus 1594

Selegiline Hydrochloride (Selegiline transdermal system should not be used with oral selegiline or other MAO inhibitors). Products include:
Eldepryl Capsules 3052

Sertraline Hydrochloride (Selegiline transdermal system is contraindicated with selective serotonin reuptake inhibitors).
No products indexed under this heading.

Sevoflurane (Patients taking selegiline transdermal system should not undergo elective surgery requiring general anesthesia). Products include:
Ultane Liquid for Inhalation 524

Sufentanil Citrate (Selegiline transdermal system is contraindicated with analgesic agents such as tramadol, methadone, and propoxyphene).
No products indexed under this heading.

Terbutaline Sulfate (Avoid concomitant use of sympathomimetic agents with selegiline transdermal system).
No products indexed under this heading.

Tetracaine Hydrochloride (Patients taking selegiline transdermal system should not be given local anesthesia containing sympathomimetic vasoconstrictors).
No products indexed under this heading.

Tramadol Hydrochloride (Selegiline transdermal system is contraindicated with analgesic agents such as tramadol, methadone, and propoxyphene). Products include:
Ultram ER Extended-Release Tablets 2428

Tranylcypromine Sulfate (Selegiline transdermal system should not be used with oral selegiline or other MAO inhibitors). Products include:
Parnate Tablets 1532

Trimipramine Maleate (Selegiline transdermal system is contraindicated with tricyclic antidepressants).
No products indexed under this heading.

Tyramine (As a class, MAO inhibitors have been associated with hypertensive crises caused by the ingestion of foods with a high concentration of tyramine).
No products indexed under this heading.

Venlafaxine Hydrochloride (Selegiline transdermal system is contraindicated with dual serotonin and norepinephrine reuptake inhibitors). Products include:
Effexor XR Extended-Release Capsules 3195
Venlafaxine Hydrochloride Tablets ... 2199

Food Interactions

Alcohol (The use of alcohol is not recommended while using selegiline transdermal system).

Beverages with high tyramine (As a class, MAO inhibitors have been associated with hypertensive crises caused by the ingestion of foods with a high concentration of tyramine).

Food high in tyramine (As a class, MAO inhibitors have been associated with hypertensive crises caused by the ingestion of foods with a high concentration of tyramine).

Food with high concentration of tyramine (As a class, MAO inhibitors have been associated with hypertensive crises caused by the ingestion of foods with a high concentration of tyramine).

EMTRIVA CAPSULES

(Emtricitabine) 1246
May interact with:

Lamivudine (Emtricitabine should not be co-administered with lamivudine-containing products). Products include:
Combivir Tablets 1384
Epivir 1412
Epivir-HBV 1417
Epzicom Tablets 1422
Trizivir Tablets 1622

EMTRIVA ORAL SOLUTION

(Emtricitabine) 1246
May interact with:

See (Emtriva Capsules).
No products indexed under this heading.

ENABLEX EXTENDED-RELEASE TABLETS

(Darifenacin) 2225
May interact with anticholinergics, cytochrome p450 2d6 substrates (selected), cytochrome p450 3a4 inducers (selected), cytochrome p450 3a4 inhibitors, potent, tricyclic antidepressants, and certain other agents. Compounds in these categories include:

Allium sativum (Darifenacin metabolism is primarily mediated by the cytochrome P450 enzymes CYP2D6 and CYP3A4. Therefore, inducers of CYP3A4 may alter darifenacin pharmacokinetics).
No products indexed under this heading.

Amitriptyline Hydrochloride (Caution should be taken when darifenacin is used concomitantly with medications that are predominantly metabolized by CYP2D6 and which have a narrow therapeutic window, such as tricyclic antidepressants).
No products indexed under this heading.

Amoxapine (Caution should be taken when darifenacin is used concomitantly with medications that are predominantly metabolized by CYP2D6 and which have a narrow therapeutic window, such as tricyclic antidepressants).
No products indexed under this heading.

Amphetamine Aspartate (Caution should be taken when darifenacin is

used concomitantly with medications that are predominantly metabolized by CYP2D6 and that have a narrow therapeutic window). Products include:

Adderall XR Capsules 3012

Amphetamine Aspartate Monohydrate (Caution should be taken when darifenacin is used concomitantly with medications that are predominantly metabolized by CYP2D6 and that have a narrow therapeutic window).

No products indexed under this heading.

Amphetamine Sulfate (Caution should be taken when darifenacin is used concomitantly with medications that are predominantly metabolized by CYP2D6 and that have a narrow therapeutic window). Products include:

Adderall XR Capsules 3012

Amprenavir (The daily dose of darifenacin should not exceed 7.5 mg when co-administered with potent CYP3A4 inhibitors).

No products indexed under this heading.

Aprepitant (Darifenacin metabolism is primarily mediated by the cytochrome P450 enzymes CYP2D6 and CYP3A4. Therefore, inducers of CYP3A4 may alter darifenacin pharmacokinetics). Products include:

Emend Capsules 1992

Atazanavir (The daily dose of darifenacin should not exceed 7.5 mg when co-administered with potent CYP3A4 inhibitors).

No products indexed under this heading.

Atazanavir Sulfate (The daily dose of darifenacin should not exceed 7.5 mg when co-administered with potent CYP3A4 inhibitors). Products include:

Reyataz Capsules 3299

Atomoxetine Hydrochloride (Caution should be taken when darifenacin is used concomitantly with medications that are predominantly metabolized by CYP2D6 and that have a narrow therapeutic window). Products include:

Strattera Capsules 1864

Atropine Sulfate (The concomitant use of darifenacin with other anticholinergic agents may increase the frequency and/or severity of dry mouth, constipation, blurred vision and other anticholinergic pharmacological effects. Anticholinergic agents may potentially alter the absorption of some concomitantly administered drugs due to effects on gastrointestinal motility). Products include:

Donnatal Extentabs 2507

Belladonna Alkaloids (The concomitant use of darifenacin with other anticholinergic agents may increase the frequency and/or severity of dry mouth, constipation, blurred vision and other anticholinergic pharmacological effects. Anticholinergic agents may potentially alter the absorption of some concomitantly administered drugs due to effects on gastrointestinal motility). Products include:

Hyland's Teething Tablets .... ▣621

Benztropine Mesylate (The concomitant use of darifenacin with other anticholinergic agents may increase the frequency and/or severity of dry mouth, constipation, blurred vision and other anticholinergic pharmacological effects. Anticholinergic agents may potentially alter the absorption of some concomitantly administered drugs due to effects on gastrointestinal motility).

No products indexed under this heading.

Betamethasone Acetate (Darifenacin metabolism is primarily mediated by the cytochrome P450 enzymes CYP2D6 and CYP3A4. Therefore, inducers of CYP3A4 may alter darifenacin pharmacokinetics).

No products indexed under this heading.

Betamethasone Sodium Phosphate (Darifenacin metabolism is primarily mediated by the cytochrome P450 enzymes CYP2D6 and CYP3A4. Therefore, inducers of CYP3A4 may alter darifenacin pharmacokinetics).

No products indexed under this heading.

Biperiden Hydrochloride (The concomitant use of darifenacin with other anticholinergic agents may increase the frequency and/or severity of dry mouth, constipation, blurred vision and other anticholinergic pharmacological effects. Anticholinergic agents may potentially alter the absorption of some concomitantly administered drugs due to effects on gastrointestinal motility).

No products indexed under this heading.

Bisoprolol Fumarate (Caution should be taken when darifenacin is used concomitantly with medications that are predominantly metabolized by CYP2D6 and that have a narrow therapeutic window).

No products indexed under this heading.

Captopril (Caution should be taken when darifenacin is used concomitantly with medications that are predominantly metabolized by CYP2D6 and that have a narrow therapeutic window). Products include:

Captopril Tablets 2182

Carbamazepine (Darifenacin metabolism is primarily mediated by the cytochrome P450 enzymes CYP2D6 and CYP3A4. Therefore, inducers of CYP3A4 may alter darifenacin pharmacokinetics). Products include:

Carbatrol Capsules 3019

Equetro Extended-Release Capsules.................................... 3174

Carvedilol (Caution should be taken when darifenacin is used concomitantly with medications that are predominantly metabolized by CYP2D6 and that have a narrow therapeutic window). Products include:

Coreg Tablets 1387

Cevimeline Hydrochloride (Caution should be taken when darifenacin is used concomitantly with medications that are predominantly metabolized by CYP2D6 and that have a narrow therapeutic window). Products include:

Evoxac Capsules 1013

Chlorpromazine (Caution should be taken when darifenacin is used concomitantly with medications that are predominantly metabolized by CYP2D6 and that have a narrow therapeutic window).

No products indexed under this heading.

Chlorpromazine Hydrochloride (Caution should be taken when darifenacin is used concomitantly with medications that are predominantly metabolized by CYP2D6 and that have a narrow therapeutic window).

No products indexed under this heading.

Chlorpropamide (Caution should be taken when darifenacin is used concomitantly with medications that are predominantly metabolized by CYP2D6 and that have a narrow therapeutic window).

No products indexed under this heading.

Cimetidine (The mean Cmax and AUC of darifenacin following 30 mg once daily at steady state were 42% and 34% higher, respectively, in the presence of cimetidine, a mixed CYP P450 enzyme inhibitor).

No products indexed under this heading.

Cimetidine Hydrochloride (The mean Cmax and AUC of darifenacin following 30 mg once daily at steady state were 42% and 34% higher, respectively, in the presence of cimetidine, a mixed CYP P450 enzyme inhibitor).

No products indexed under this heading.

Ciprofloxacin Hydrochloride (Darifenacin metabolism is primarily mediated by the cytochrome P450 enzymes CYP2D6 and CYP3A4. Therefore, inducers of CYP3A4 may alter darifenacin pharmacokinetics). Products include:

Cipro Tablets 2810

Cisplatin (Darifenacin metabolism is primarily mediated by the cytochrome P450 enzymes CYP2D6 and CYP3A4. Therefore, inducers of CYP3A4 may alter darifenacin pharmacokinetics).

No products indexed under this heading.

Clarithromycin (The daily dose of darifenacin should not exceed 7.5 mg when co-administered with potent CYP3A4 inhibitors). Products include:

Biaxin/Biaxin XL 411

Clidinium Bromide (The concomitant use of darifenacin with other anticholinergic agents may increase the frequency and/or severity of dry mouth, constipation, blurred vision and other anticholinergic pharmacological effects. Anticholinergic agents may potentially alter the absorption of some concomitantly administered drugs due to effects on gastrointestinal motility).

No products indexed under this heading.

Clomipramine Hydrochloride (Caution should be taken when darifenacin is used concomitantly with medications that are predominantly metabolized by CYP2D6 and which have a narrow therapeutic window, such as tricyclic antidepressants).

No products indexed under this heading.

Clozapine (Caution should be taken when darifenacin is used concomitantly with medications that are predominantly metabolized by CYP2D6 and that have a narrow therapeutic window).

No products indexed under this heading.

Codeine Phosphate (Caution should be taken when darifenacin is used concomitantly with medications that are predominantly metabolized by CYP2D6 and that have a narrow therapeutic window). Products include:

Tylenol with Codeine Tablets 2427

Codeine Sulfate (Caution should be taken when darifenacin is used concomitantly with medications that are predominantly metabolized by CYP2D6 and that have a narrow therapeutic window).

No products indexed under this heading.

Cortisone Acetate (Darifenacin metabolism is primarily mediated by the cytochrome P450 enzymes CYP2D6 and CYP3A4. Therefore, inducers of CYP3A4 may alter darifenacin pharmacokinetics).

No products indexed under this heading.

Cyclobenzaprine Hydrochloride (Caution should be taken when darifenacin is used concomitantly with medications that are predominantly metabolized by CYP2D6 and that have a narrow therapeutic window). Products include:

Amrix Capsules 966

Delavirdine Mesylate (The daily dose of darifenacin should not exceed 7.5 mg when co-administered with potent CYP3A4 inhibitors).

No products indexed under this heading.

Delavirine (The daily dose of darifenacin should not exceed 7.5 mg when co-administered with potent CYP3A4 inhibitors).

No products indexed under this heading.

Desipramine Hydrochloride (Caution should be taken when darifenacin is used concomitantly with medications that are predominantly metabolized by CYP2D6 and which have a narrow therapeutic window, such as tricyclic antidepressants).

No products indexed under this heading.

Dexamethasone (Darifenacin metabolism is primarily mediated by the cytochrome P450 enzymes CYP2D6 and CYP3A4. Therefore, inducers of CYP3A4 may alter darifenacin pharmacokinetics). Products include:

Ciprodex Otic Suspension 541

Dexamethasone Acetate (Darifenacin metabolism is primarily mediated by the cytochrome P450 enzymes CYP2D6 and CYP3A4. Therefore, inducers of CYP3A4 may alter darifenacin pharmacokinetics).

No products indexed under this heading.

Dexamethasone Sodium Phosphate (Darifenacin metabolism is primarily mediated by the cytochrome P450 enzymes CYP2D6 and CYP3A4. Therefore, inducers of CYP3A4 may alter darifenacin pharmacokinetics).

No products indexed under this heading.

Dexfenfluramine Hydrochloride (Caution should be taken when darifenacin is used concomitantly with medications that are predominantly metabolized by CYP2D6 and that have a narrow therapeutic window).
No products indexed under this heading.

Dextromethorphan Hydrobromide (Caution should be taken when darifenacin is used concomitantly with medications that are predominantly metabolized by CYP2D6 and that have a narrow therapeutic window). Products include:
PediaCare Children's Liquid Multi-Symptom Cold 1902
PediaCare Children's Long-Acting Cough 1902
Children's Sudafed PE Cold & Cough Liquid 1907
Sudafed PE Cold & Cough Caplets 1907
Children's Tylenol Plus Cough & Runny Nose Suspension Liquid 1912
Children's Tylenol Plus Cough & Sore Throat Suspension Liquid 1912
Children's Tylenol Plus Flu Suspension Liquid 1914
Children's Tylenol Plus Multi-Symptom Cold Suspension Liquid 1912
Tylenol Cold Severe Congestion Daytime Caplets with Cool Burst 1912
Tylenol Cold Head Congestion Daytime Caplets with Cool Burst 1910
Tylenol Cold Head Congestion Nighttime Caplets with Cool Burst 1910
Tylenol Cold Head Congestion Severe Daytime Caplets with Cool Burst 1910
Tylenol Cold Multi-Symptom Daytime Caplets with Cool Burst and Rapid Release Gels 1913
Tylenol Cold Multi-Symptom Daytime Liquid with Citrus Burst 1913
Tylenol Cold Multi-Symptom Nighttime Caplets with Cool Burst 1913
Tylenol Cold Multi-Symptom Nighttime Liquid with Cool Burst 1913
Tylenol Cold Multi-Symptom Severe Caplets with Cool Burst 1913
Tylenol Cold Multi-Symptom Severe Daytime Liquid with Citrus Burst 1913
Tylenol Cough & Sore Throat Daytime Liquid with Cool Burst 1918
Tylenol Cough & Sore Throat Nighttime Liquid with Cool Burst 1918
Vicks DayQuil Cold & Flu Multi-Symptom Relief .... ▣616
Vicks DayQuil LiquiCaps 2567
Vicks DayQuil Liquid 2567
Vicks DayQuil Multi-Symptom Cold/Flu Relief 2567
Vicks NyQuil Cold & Flu Multi-Symptom Relief .... ▣617
Vicks NyQuil LiquiCaps 2567
Vicks NyQuil Liquid 2567
Vicks NyQuil Multi-Symptom Cold/Flu Relief 2567

Dextromethorphan Polistirex (Caution should be taken when darifenacin is used concomitantly with medications that are predominantly metabolized by CYP2D6 and that have a narrow therapeutic window).
No products indexed under this heading.

Dicyclomine Hydrochloride (The concomitant use of darifenacin with other anticholinergic agents may increase the frequency and/or severity of dry mouth, constipation, blurred vision and other anticholinergic pharmacological effects. Anticholinergic agents may potentially alter the absorption of some concomitantly administered drugs due to effects on gastrointestinal motility). Products include:
Bentyl Capsules 703
Bentyl Injection 703
Bentyl Syrup 703
Bentyl Tablets 703

Digoxin (Darifenacin (30 mg daily) co-administered with digoxin (0.25 mg) at steady state resulted in a 16% increase in digoxin exposure. Routine therapeutic drug monitoring for digoxin should be continued). Products include:
Lanoxin Injection 1498
Lanoxin Injection Pediatric 1502
Lanoxin Tablets 1505

Dolasetron Mesylate (Caution should be taken when darifenacin is used concomitantly with medications that are predominantly metabolized by CYP2D6 and that have a narrow therapeutic window). Products include:
Anzemet Injection 2701
Anzemet Tablets 2704

Donepezil Hydrochloride (Caution should be taken when darifenacin is used concomitantly with medications that are predominantly metabolized by CYP2D6 and that have a narrow therapeutic window). Products include:
Aricept Tablets 1062
Aricept ODT Tablets 1062

Doxepin Hydrochloride (Caution should be taken when darifenacin is used concomitantly with medications that are predominantly metabolized by CYP2D6 and which have a narrow therapeutic window, such as tricyclic antidepressants).
No products indexed under this heading.

Doxorubicin Hydrochloride (Darifenacin metabolism is primarily mediated by the cytochrome P450 enzymes CYP2D6 and CYP3A4. Therefore, inducers of CYP3A4 may alter darifenacin pharmacokinetics).
No products indexed under this heading.

Efavirenz (Darifenacin metabolism is primarily mediated by the cytochrome P450 enzymes CYP2D6 and CYP3A4. Therefore, inducers of CYP3A4 may alter darifenacin pharmacokinetics). Products include:
Atripla Tablets 938
Sustiva Capsules 930
Sustiva Tablets 930

Encainide Hydrochloride (Caution should be taken when darifenacin is used concomitantly with medications that are predominantly metabolized by CYP2D6 and that have a narrow therapeutic window).
No products indexed under this heading.

Ethosuximide (Darifenacin metabolism is primarily mediated by the cytochrome P450 enzymes CYP2D6 and CYP3A4. Therefore, inducers of CYP3A4 may alter darifenacin pharmacokinetics).
No products indexed under this heading.

Felbamate (Darifenacin metabolism is primarily mediated by the cytochrome P450 enzymes CYP2D6 and CYP3A4. Therefore, inducers of CYP3A4 may alter darifenacin pharmacokinetics).
No products indexed under this heading.

Fentanyl (Caution should be taken when darifenacin is used concomitantly with medications that are predominantly metabolized by CYP2D6 and that have a narrow therapeutic window). Products include:
Duragesic Transdermal System 2405
Ionsys Transdermal System 2410

Fentanyl Citrate (Caution should be taken when darifenacin is used concomitantly with medications that are predominantly metabolized by CYP2D6 and that have a narrow therapeutic window). Products include:
Actiq 959
Fentora Tablets 968

Flecainide Acetate (Caution should be taken when darifenacin is used concomitantly with medications that are predominantly metabolized by CYP2D6 and which have a narrow therapeutic window, such as flecainide).
No products indexed under this heading.

Fludrocortisone Acetate (Darifenacin metabolism is primarily mediated by the cytochrome P450 enzymes CYP2D6 and CYP3A4. Therefore, inducers of CYP3A4 may alter darifenacin pharmacokinetics).
No products indexed under this heading.

Fluoxetine (Caution should be taken when darifenacin is used concomitantly with medications that are predominantly metabolized by CYP2D6 and that have a narrow therapeutic window).
No products indexed under this heading.

Fluoxetine Hydrochloride (Caution should be taken when darifenacin is used concomitantly with medications that are predominantly metabolized by CYP2D6 and that have a narrow therapeutic window). Products include:
Prozac Weekly Capsules 1852
Prozac Pulvules and Liquid 1852
Symbyax Capsules 1871

Fluphenazine Decanoate (Caution should be taken when darifenacin is used concomitantly with medications that are predominantly metabolized by CYP2D6 and that have a narrow therapeutic window).
No products indexed under this heading.

Fluphenazine Enanthate (Caution should be taken when darifenacin is used concomitantly with medications that are predominantly metabolized by CYP2D6 and that have a narrow therapeutic window).
No products indexed under this heading.

Fluphenazine Hydrochloride (Caution should be taken when darifenacin is used concomitantly with medications that are predominantly metabolized by CYP2D6 and that have a narrow therapeutic window).
No products indexed under this heading.

Fluvoxamine Maleate (Caution should be taken when darifenacin is used concomitantly with medications that are predominantly metabolized by CYP2D6 and that have a narrow therapeutic window). Products include:
Luvox CR Extended-Release Capsules 1759

Formoterol Fumarate (Caution should be taken when darifenacin is used concomitantly with medications that are predominantly metabolized by CYP2D6 and that have a narrow therapeutic window). Products include:
Foradil Aerolizer 2849
Perforomist Inhalation Solution 1025

Fosamprenavir Calcium (The daily dose of darifenacin should not exceed 7.5 mg when co-administered with potent CYP3A4 inhibitors). Products include:
Lexiva Oral Suspension 1510
Lexiva Tablets 1510

Fosphenytoin Sodium (Darifenacin metabolism is primarily mediated by the cytochrome P450 enzymes CYP2D6 and CYP3A4. Therefore, inducers of CYP3A4 may alter darifenacin pharmacokinetics).
No products indexed under this heading.

Galantamine Hydrobromide (Caution should be taken when darifenacin is used concomitantly with medications that are predominantly metabolized by CYP2D6 and that have a narrow therapeutic window).
No products indexed under this heading.

Garlic Extract (Darifenacin metabolism is primarily mediated by the cytochrome P450 enzymes CYP2D6 and CYP3A4. Therefore, inducers of CYP3A4 may alter darifenacin pharmacokinetics).
No products indexed under this heading.

Garlic Oil (Darifenacin metabolism is primarily mediated by the cytochrome P450 enzymes CYP2D6 and CYP3A4. Therefore, inducers of CYP3A4 may alter darifenacin pharmacokinetics).
No products indexed under this heading.

Glycopyrrolate (The concomitant use of darifenacin with other anticholinergic agents may increase the frequency and/or severity of dry mouth, constipation, blurred vision and other anticholinergic pharmacological effects. Anticholinergic agents may potentially alter the absorption of some concomitantly administered drugs due to effects on gastrointestinal motility).
No products indexed under this heading.

Haloperidol (Caution should be taken when darifenacin is used concomitantly with medications that are predominantly metabolized by CYP2D6 and that have a narrow therapeutic window).
No products indexed under this heading.

Haloperidol Decanoate (Caution should be taken when darifenacin is used concomitantly with medications that are predominantly metabolized by CYP2D6 and that have a narrow therapeutic window).
No products indexed under this heading.

Hydrocodone Bitartrate (Caution should be taken when darifenacin is used concomitantly with medications that are predominantly metabolized by CYP2D6 and that have a narrow therapeutic window). Products include:
Lortab 5/500 Tablets 3143
Lortab 7.5/500 Tablets 3144
Lortab 10/500 Tablets 3144
Vicodin Tablets 529
Vicodin ES Tablets 530
Vicodin HP Tablets 531
Vicoprofen Tablets 533

Zydone Tablets 1132

Hydrocortisone (Darifenacin metabolism is primarily mediated by the cytochrome P450 enzymes CYP2D6 and CYP3A4. Therefore, inducers of CYP3A4 may alter darifenacin pharmacokinetics).
No products indexed under this heading.

Hydrocortisone Acetate (Darifenacin metabolism is primarily mediated by the cytochrome P450 enzymes CYP2D6 and CYP3A4. Therefore, inducers of CYP3A4 may alter darifenacin pharmacokinetics). Products include:
Analpram-HC 1140
Pramosone 1141

Hydrocortisone Butyrate (Darifenacin metabolism is primarily mediated by the cytochrome P450 enzymes CYP2D6 and CYP3A4. Therefore, inducers of CYP3A4 may alter darifenacin pharmacokinetics).
No products indexed under this heading.

Hydrocortisone Cypionate (Darifenacin metabolism is primarily mediated by the cytochrome P450 enzymes CYP2D6 and CYP3A4. Therefore, inducers of CYP3A4 may alter darifenacin pharmacokinetics).
No products indexed under this heading.

Hydrocortisone Hemisuccinate (Darifenacin metabolism is primarily mediated by the cytochrome P450 enzymes CYP2D6 and CYP3A4. Therefore, inducers of CYP3A4 may alter darifenacin pharmacokinetics).
No products indexed under this heading.

Hydrocortisone Probutate (Darifenacin metabolism is primarily mediated by the cytochrome P450 enzymes CYP2D6 and CYP3A4. Therefore, inducers of CYP3A4 may alter darifenacin pharmacokinetics).
No products indexed under this heading.

Hydrocortisone Sodium Phosphate (Darifenacin metabolism is primarily mediated by the cytochrome P450 enzymes CYP2D6 and CYP3A4. Therefore, inducers of CYP3A4 may alter darifenacin pharmacokinetics).
No products indexed under this heading.

Hydrocortisone Sodium Succinate (Darifenacin metabolism is primarily mediated by the cytochrome P450 enzymes CYP2D6 and CYP3A4. Therefore, inducers of CYP3A4 may alter darifenacin pharmacokinetics).
No products indexed under this heading.

Hydrocortisone Valerate (Darifenacin metabolism is primarily mediated by the cytochrome P450 enzymes CYP2D6 and CYP3A4. Therefore, inducers of CYP3A4 may alter darifenacin pharmacokinetics).
No products indexed under this heading.

Hyoscyamine (The concomitant use of darifenacin with other anticholinergic agents may increase the frequency and/or severity of dry mouth, constipation, blurred vision and other anticholinergic pharmacological effects. Anticholinergic agents may potentially alter the absorption of some concomitantly administered drugs due to effects on gastrointestinal motility).
No products indexed under this heading.

Hyoscyamine Sulfate (The concomitant use of darifenacin with other anticholinergic agents may increase the frequency and/or severity of dry mouth, constipation, blurred vision and other anticholinergic pharmacological effects. Anticholinergic agents may potentially alter the absorption of some concomitantly administered drugs due to effects on gastrointestinal motility). Products include:
Donnatal Extentabs 2507

Hypericum (Darifenacin metabolism is primarily mediated by the cytochrome P450 enzymes CYP2D6 and CYP3A4. Therefore, inducers of CYP3A4 may alter darifenacin pharmacokinetics). Products include:
Satieté Tablets 640

Hypericum Perforatum (Darifenacin metabolism is primarily mediated by the cytochrome P450 enzymes CYP2D6 and CYP3A4. Therefore, inducers of CYP3A4 may alter darifenacin pharmacokinetics).
No products indexed under this heading.

Imipramine Hydrochloride (Caution should be taken when darifenacin is used concomitantly with medications that are predominantly metabolized by CYP2D6 and which have a narrow therapeutic window, such as tricyclic antidepressants. The mean Cmax and AUC of imipramine, a CYP2D6 substrate, were increased 57% and 70%, respectively, in the presence of steady-state darifenacin 30 mg once daily. This was accompanied by a 3.6-fold increase in the mean Cmax and AUC of desipramine, the active metabolite of imipramine).
No products indexed under this heading.

Imipramine Pamoate (Caution should be taken when darifenacin is used concomitantly with medications that are predominantly metabolized by CYP2D6 and which have a narrow therapeutic window, such as tricyclic antidepressants. The mean Cmax and AUC of imipramine, a CYP2D6 substrate, were increased 57% and 70%, respectively, in the presence of steady-state darifenacin 30 mg once daily. This was accompanied by a 3.6-fold increase in the mean Cmax and AUC of desipramine, the active metabolite of imipramine).
No products indexed under this heading.

Indinavir Sulfate (The daily dose of darifenacin should not exceed 7.5 mg when co-administered with potent CYP3A4 inhibitors). Products include:
Crixivan Capsules 1979

Indoramin Hydrochloride (Caution should be taken when darifenacin is used concomitantly with medications that are predominantly metabolized by CYP2D6 and that have a narrow therapeutic window).
No products indexed under this heading.

Ipratropium Bromide (The concomitant use of darifenacin with other anticholinergic agents may increase the frequency and/or severity of dry mouth, constipation, blurred vision and other anticholinergic pharmacological effects. Anticholinergic agents may potentially alter the absorption of some concomitantly administered drugs due to effects on gastrointestinal motility). Products include:
Atrovent HFA Inhalation Aerosol 839
Atrovent Nasal Spray 0.03% 834
Atrovent Nasal Spray 0.06% 836
Combivent Inhalation Aerosol 845

Itraconazole (The daily dose of darifenacin should not exceed 7.5 mg when co-administered with potent CYP3A4 inhibitors).
No products indexed under this heading.

Ketoconazole (The daily dose of darifenacin should not exceed 7.5 mg when co-administered with potent CYP3A4 inhibitors. In a drug interaction study, when a 7.5 mg q.d. dose of darifenacin was given to steady state and co-administered with the potent CYP3A4 inhibitor ketoconazole 400 mg, mean darifenacin Cmax increased to 11.2 ng/mL for extensive metabolizers (EM) (n=10) and 55.4 ng/mL for one poor metabolizer (PM) subject (n=1). Mean AUC increased to 143 and 939 ng.h/mL for EMs and for one PM subject, respectively. When a 15 mg daily dose of darifenacin was given with ketoconazole, mean darifenacin Cmax increased to 67.6 ng/mL and 58.9 ng.mL for EMs (n=3)). Products include:
Extina Foam, 2% 3057
Nizoral A-D Shampoo 1901

Labetalol Hydrochloride (Caution should be taken when darifenacin is used concomitantly with medications that are predominantly metabolized by CYP2D6 and that have a narrow therapeutic window).
No products indexed under this heading.

Lidocaine (Caution should be taken when darifenacin is used concomitantly with medications that are predominantly metabolized by CYP2D6 and that have a narrow therapeutic window). Products include:
Lidoderm Patch 1114

Lidocaine Hydrochloride (Caution should be taken when darifenacin is used concomitantly with medications that are predominantly metabolized by CYP2D6 and that have a narrow therapeutic window).
No products indexed under this heading.

Lopinavir (The daily dose of darifenacin should not exceed 7.5 mg when co-administered with potent CYP3A4 inhibitors). Products include:
Kaletra 452

Maprotiline Hydrochloride (Caution should be taken when darifenacin is used concomitantly with medications that are predominantly metabolized by CYP2D6 and which have a narrow therapeutic window, such as tricyclic antidepressants).
No products indexed under this heading.

Mepenzolate Bromide (The concomitant use of darifenacin with other anticholinergic agents may increase the frequency and/or severity of dry mouth, constipation, blurred vision and other anticholinergic pharmacological effects. Anticholinergic agents may potentially alter the absorption of some concomitantly administered drugs due to effects on gastrointestinal motility).
No products indexed under this heading.

Meperidine Hydrochloride (Caution should be taken when darifenacin is used concomitantly with medications that are predominantly metabolized by CYP2D6 and that have a narrow therapeutic window).
No products indexed under this heading.

Mephenytoin (Darifenacin metabolism is primarily mediated by the cytochrome P450 enzymes CYP2D6 and CYP3A4. Therefore, inducers of CYP3A4 may alter darifenacin pharmacokinetics).
No products indexed under this heading.

Methadone Hydrochloride (Caution should be taken when darifenacin is used concomitantly with medications that are predominantly metabolized by CYP2D6 and that have a narrow therapeutic window).
No products indexed under this heading.

Methamphetamine Hydrochloride (Caution should be taken when darifenacin is used concomitantly with medications that are predominantly metabolized by CYP2D6 and that have a narrow therapeutic window).
No products indexed under this heading.

Methsuximide (Darifenacin metabolism is primarily mediated by the cytochrome P450 enzymes CYP2D6 and CYP3A4. Therefore, inducers of CYP3A4 may alter darifenacin pharmacokinetics).
No products indexed under this heading.

Methylprednisolone (Darifenacin metabolism is primarily mediated by the cytochrome P450 enzymes CYP2D6 and CYP3A4. Therefore, inducers of CYP3A4 may alter darifenacin pharmacokinetics).
No products indexed under this heading.

Methylprednisolone Acetate (Darifenacin metabolism is primarily mediated by the cytochrome P450 enzymes CYP2D6 and CYP3A4. Therefore, inducers of CYP3A4 may alter darifenacin pharmacokinetics).
No products indexed under this heading.

Methylprednisolone Sodium Succinate (Darifenacin metabolism is primarily mediated by the cytochrome P450 enzymes CYP2D6 and CYP3A4. Therefore, inducers of CYP3A4 may alter darifenacin pharmacokinetics).
No products indexed under this heading.

Metoprolol Succinate (Caution should be taken when darifenacin is used concomitantly with medications that are predominantly metabolized by CYP2D6 and that have a narrow therapeutic window). Products include:
Toprol-XL Tablets 666

Metoprolol Tartrate (Caution should be taken when darifenacin is used concomitantly with medications that are predominantly metabolized by CYP2D6 and that have a narrow therapeutic window).
No products indexed under this heading.

Mexiletine Hydrochloride (Caution should be taken when darifenacin is used concomitantly with medications that are predominantly metabolized by CYP2D6 and that have a narrow therapeutic window).
No products indexed under this heading.

Midazolam Hydrochloride (Darifenacin (30 mg daily) co-administered with a single oral dose of midazolam 7.5 mg resulted in a 17% increase in midazolam exposure).
No products indexed under this heading.

Mirtazapine (Caution should be taken when darifenacin is used concomitantly with medications that are predominantly metabolized by CYP2D6 and that have a narrow therapeutic window). Products include:
Remeron Tablets 2924
RemeronSolTab Tablets 2927

Modafinil (Darifenacin metabolism is primarily mediated by the cytochrome P450 enzymes CYP2D6 and CYP3A4. Therefore, inducers of CYP3A4 may alter darifenacin pharmacokinetics). Products include:
Provigil Tablets 977

Morphine Sulfate (Caution should be taken when darifenacin is used concomitantly with medications that are predominantly metabolized by CYP2D6 and that have a narrow therapeutic window). Products include:
Avinza Capsules 1772
DepoDur Injection 1095
MS Contin Tablets 2585

Nefazodone Hydrochloride (The daily dose of darifenacin should not exceed 7.5 mg when co-administered with potent CYP3A4 inhibitors).
No products indexed under this heading.

Nelfinavir Mesylate (The daily dose of darifenacin should not exceed 7.5 mg when co-administered with potent CYP3A4 inhibitors).
No products indexed under this heading.

Nevirapine (Darifenacin metabolism is primarily mediated by the cytochrome P450 enzymes CYP2D6 and CYP3A4. Therefore, inducers of CYP3A4 may alter darifenacin pharmacokinetics). Products include:
Viramune Oral Suspension 873
Viramune Tablets 873

Nortriptyline Hydrochloride (Caution should be taken when darifenacin is used concomitantly with medications that are predominantly metabolized by CYP2D6 and which have a narrow therapeutic window, such as tricyclic antidepressants).
No products indexed under this heading.

Olanzapine (Caution should be taken when darifenacin is used concomitantly with medications that are predominantly metabolized by CYP2D6 and that have a narrow therapeutic window). Products include:
Symbyax Capsules 1871
Zyprexa Tablets 1883
Zyprexa IntraMuscular 1883
Zyprexa ZYDIS Orally Disintegrating Tablets 1883

Omeprazole (Caution should be taken when darifenacin is used concomitantly with medications that are predominantly metabolized by CYP2D6 and that have a narrow therapeutic window).
No products indexed under this heading.

Ondansetron (Caution should be taken when darifenacin is used concomitantly with medications that are predominantly metabolized by CYP2D6 and that have a narrow therapeutic window). Products include:
Zofran ODT Orally Disintegrating Tablets 1687

Ondansetron Hydrochloride (Caution should be taken when darifenacin is used concomitantly with medications that are predominantly metabolized by CYP2D6 and that have a narrow therapeutic window). Products include:
Zofran Injection 1682
Zofran 1687

Oxcarbazepine (Darifenacin metabolism is primarily mediated by the cytochrome P450 enzymes CYP2D6 and CYP3A4. Therefore, inducers of CYP3A4 may alter darifenacin pharmacokinetics).
No products indexed under this heading.

Oxybutynin Chloride (The concomitant use of darifenacin with other anticholinergic agents may increase the frequency and/or severity of dry mouth, constipation, blurred vision and other anticholinergic pharmacological effects. Anticholinergic agents may potentially alter the absorption of some concomitantly administered drugs due to effects on gastrointestinal motility).
No products indexed under this heading.

Oxycodone Hydrochloride (Caution should be taken when darifenacin is used concomitantly with medications that are predominantly metabolized by CYP2D6 and that have a narrow therapeutic window). Products include:
OxyContin Tablets 2589
OxyIR Capsules 2593
Percocet Tablets 1127
Percodan Tablets 1130

Paclitaxel (Caution should be taken when darifenacin is used concomitantly with medications that are predominantly metabolized by CYP2D6 and that have a narrow therapeutic window).
No products indexed under this heading.

Paroxetine Hydrochloride (Caution should be taken when darifenacin is used concomitantly with medications that are predominantly metabolized by CYP2D6 and that have a narrow therapeutic window). Products include:
Paxil 1535
Paxil CR Controlled-Release Tablets 1544

Phenobarbital (Darifenacin metabolism is primarily mediated by the cytochrome P450 enzymes CYP2D6 and CYP3A4. Therefore, inducers of CYP3A4 may alter darifenacin pharmacokinetics). Products include:
Donnatal Extentabs 2507

Phenobarbital Sodium (Darifenacin metabolism is primarily mediated by the cytochrome P450 enzymes CYP2D6 and CYP3A4. Therefore, inducers of CYP3A4 may alter darifenacin pharmacokinetics).
No products indexed under this heading.

Phenytoin (Darifenacin metabolism is primarily mediated by the cytochrome P450 enzymes CYP2D6 and CYP3A4. Therefore, inducers of CYP3A4 may alter darifenacin pharmacokinetics).
No products indexed under this heading.

Phenytoin Sodium (Darifenacin metabolism is primarily mediated by the cytochrome P450 enzymes CYP2D6 and CYP3A4. Therefore, inducers of CYP3A4 may alter darifenacin pharmacokinetics). Products include:
Phenytek Capsules 2192

Pindolol (Caution should be taken when darifenacin is used concomitantly with medications that are predominantly metabolized by CYP2D6 and that have a narrow therapeutic window).
No products indexed under this heading.

Prednisolone Acetate (Darifenacin metabolism is primarily mediated by the cytochrome P450 enzymes CYP2D6 and CYP3A4. Therefore, inducers of CYP3A4 may alter darifenacin pharmacokinetics). Products include:
Pred Forte Ophthalmic Suspension .... ⊙227
Pred Mild Ophthalmic Suspension .... ⊙230
Pred-G Ophthalmic Ointment .... ⊙229
Pred-G Ophthalmic Suspension .... ⊙228

Prednisolone Sodium Phosphate (Darifenacin metabolism is primarily mediated by the cytochrome P450 enzymes CYP2D6 and CYP3A4. Therefore, inducers of CYP3A4 may alter darifenacin pharmacokinetics).
No products indexed under this heading.

Prednisolone Tebutate (Darifenacin metabolism is primarily mediated by the cytochrome P450 enzymes CYP2D6 and CYP3A4. Therefore, inducers of CYP3A4 may alter darifenacin pharmacokinetics).
No products indexed under this heading.

Prednisone (Darifenacin metabolism is primarily mediated by the cytochrome P450 enzymes CYP2D6 and CYP3A4. Therefore, inducers of CYP3A4 may alter darifenacin pharmacokinetics).
No products indexed under this heading.

Primidone (Darifenacin metabolism is primarily mediated by the cytochrome P450 enzymes CYP2D6 and CYP3A4. Therefore, inducers of CYP3A4 may alter darifenacin pharmacokinetics).
No products indexed under this heading.

Procyclidine Hydrochloride (The concomitant use of darifenacin with other anticholinergic agents may increase the frequency and/or severity of dry mouth, constipation, blurred vision and other anticholinergic pharmacological effects. Anticholinergic agents may potentially alter the absorption of some concomitantly administered drugs due to effects on gastrointestinal motility).
No products indexed under this heading.

Propafenone Hydrochloride (Caution should be taken when darifenacin is used concomitantly with medications that are predominantly metabolized by CYP2D6 and that have a narrow therapeutic window). Products include:
Rythmol Tablets 1586
Rythmol SR Capsules 1590

Propantheline Bromide (The concomitant use of darifenacin with other anticholinergic agents may increase the frequency and/or severity of dry mouth, constipation, blurred vision and other anticholinergic pharmacological effects. Anticholinergic agents may potentially alter the absorption of some concomitantly administered drugs due to effects on gastrointestinal motility).
No products indexed under this heading.

Propoxyphene Hydrochloride (Caution should be taken when darifenacin is used concomitantly with medications that are predominantly metabolized by CYP2D6 and that have a narrow therapeutic window).
No products indexed under this heading.

Propoxyphene Napsylate (Caution should be taken when darifenacin is used concomitantly with medications that are predominantly metabolized by CYP2D6 and that have a narrow therapeutic window).
No products indexed under this heading.

Propranolol Hydrochloride (Caution should be taken when darifenacin is used concomitantly with medications that are predominantly metabolized by CYP2D6 and that have a narrow therapeutic window). Products include:
InnoPran XL Extended Release Capsules 1484

Protriptyline Hydrochloride (Caution should be taken when darifenacin is used concomitantly with medications that are predominantly metabolized by CYP2D6 and which have a narrow therapeutic window, such as tricyclic antidepressants).
No products indexed under this heading.

Quetiapine Fumarate (Caution should be taken when darifenacin is used concomitantly with medications that are predominantly metabolized by CYP2D6 and that have a narrow therapeutic window).
No products indexed under this heading.

Quinidine Gluconate (Caution should be taken when darifenacin is used concomitantly with medications that are predominantly metabolized by CYP2D6 and that have a narrow therapeutic window).
No products indexed under this heading.

Quinidine Hydrochloride (Caution should be taken when darifenacin is used concomitantly with medications that are predominantly metabolized by CYP2D6 and that have a narrow therapeutic window).
No products indexed under this heading.

Quinidine Polygalacturonate (Caution should be taken when darifenacin is used concomitantly with medications that are predominantly metabolized by CYP2D6 and that have a narrow therapeutic window).
No products indexed under this heading.

Quinidine Sulfate (Caution should be taken when darifenacin is used concomitantly with medications that are predominantly metabolized by CYP2D6 and that have a narrow therapeutic window).
No products indexed under this heading.

Rifabutin (Darifenacin metabolism is primarily mediated by the cytochrome P450 enzymes CYP2D6 and CYP3A4. Therefore, inducers of CYP3A4 may alter darifenacin pharmacokinetics).
No products indexed under this heading.

Rifampicin (Darifenacin metabolism is primarily mediated by the cytochrome P450 enzymes CYP2D6 and CYP3A4. Therefore, inducers of CYP3A4 may alter darifenacin pharmacokinetics).
No products indexed under this heading.

Rifampin (Darifenacin metabolism is primarily mediated by the cytochrome P450 enzymes CYP2D6 and CYP3A4. Therefore, inducers of CYP3A4 may alter darifenacin pharmacokinetics).
No products indexed under this heading.

Rifapentine (Darifenacin metabolism is primarily mediated by the cytochrome P450 enzymes CYP2D6 and CYP3A4. Therefore, inducers of CYP3A4 may alter darifenacin pharmacokinetics).
No products indexed under this heading.

Risperidone (Caution should be taken when darifenacin is used concomitantly with medications that are predominantly metabolized by CYP2D6 and that have a narrow therapeutic window). Products include:
Risperdal Consta Long-Acting Injection 1753

Ritonavir (The daily dose of darifenacin should not exceed 7.5 mg when co-administered with potent CYP3A4 inhibitors). Products include:
Kaletra 452
Norvir 489

Saquinavir (The daily dose of darifenacin should not exceed 7.5 mg when co-administered with potent CYP3A4 inhibitors).
No products indexed under this heading.

Saquinavir Mesylate (The daily dose of darifenacin should not exceed 7.5 mg when co-administered with potent CYP3A4 inhibitors).
No products indexed under this heading.

Scopolamine (The concomitant use of darifenacin with other anticholinergic agents may increase the frequency and/or severity of dry mouth, constipation, blurred vision and other anticholinergic pharmacological effects. Anticholinergic agents may potentially alter the absorption of some concomitantly administered drugs due to effects on gastrointestinal motility). Products include:
Transderm Scōp Transdermal Therapeutic System 2206

Scopolamine Hydrobromide (The concomitant use of darifenacin with other anticholinergic agents may increase the frequency and/or severity of dry mouth, constipation, blurred vision and other anticholinergic pharmacological effects. Anticholinergic agents may potentially alter the absorption of some concomitantly administered drugs due to effects on gastrointestinal motility). Products include:
Donnatal Extentabs 2507

Sulfinpyrazone (Darifenacin metabolism is primarily mediated by the cytochrome P450 enzymes CYP2D6 and CYP3A4. Therefore, inducers of CYP3A4 may alter darifenacin pharmacokinetics).
No products indexed under this heading.

Tamoxifen Citrate (Caution should be taken when darifenacin is used concomitantly with medications that are predominantly metabolized by CYP2D6 and that have a narrow therapeutic window).
No products indexed under this heading.

Telithromycin (The daily dose of darifenacin should not exceed 7.5 mg when co-administered with potent CYP3A4 inhibitors). Products include:
Ketek Tablets 2744

Teniposide (Caution should be taken when darifenacin is used concomitantly with medications that are predominantly metabolized by CYP2D6 and that have a narrow therapeutic window).
No products indexed under this heading.

Testosterone (Caution should be taken when darifenacin is used concomitantly with medications that are predominantly metabolized by CYP2D6 and that have a narrow therapeutic window). Products include:
AndroGel 3159
Testim 1% Gel 701

Testosterone Cypionate (Caution should be taken when darifenacin is used concomitantly with medications that are predominantly metabolized by CYP2D6 and that have a narrow therapeutic window).
No products indexed under this heading.

Testosterone Enanthate (Caution should be taken when darifenacin is used concomitantly with medications that are predominantly metabolized by CYP2D6 and that have a narrow therapeutic window). Products include:
Delatestryl Injection 1730

Testosterone Propionate (Caution should be taken when darifenacin is used concomitantly with medications that are predominantly metabolized by CYP2D6 and that have a narrow therapeutic window).
No products indexed under this heading.

Theophylline (Darifenacin metabolism is primarily mediated by the cytochrome P450 enzymes CYP2D6 and CYP3A4. Therefore, inducers of CYP3A4 may alter darifenacin pharmacokinetics).
No products indexed under this heading.

Theophylline Anhydrous (Darifenacin metabolism is primarily mediated by the cytochrome P450 enzymes CYP2D6 and CYP3A4. Therefore, inducers of CYP3A4 may alter darifenacin pharmacokinetics). Products include:
Uniphyl Tablets 2595

Theophylline Calcium Salicylate (Darifenacin metabolism is primarily mediated by the cytochrome P450 enzymes CYP2D6 and CYP3A4. Therefore, inducers of CYP3A4 may alter darifenacin pharmacokinetics).
No products indexed under this heading.

Theophylline Dihydroxypropyl (Glyceryl) (Darifenacin metabolism is primarily mediated by the cytochrome P450 enzymes CYP2D6 and CYP3A4. Therefore, inducers of CYP3A4 may alter darifenacin pharmacokinetics).
No products indexed under this heading.

Theophylline Ethylenediamine (Darifenacin metabolism is primarily mediated by the cytochrome P450 enzymes CYP2D6 and CYP3A4. Therefore, inducers of CYP3A4 may alter darifenacin pharmacokinetics).
No products indexed under this heading.

Thioridazine (Caution should be taken when darifenacin is used concomitantly with medications that are predominantly metabolized by CYP2D6 and which have a narrow therapeutic window, such as thioridazine).
No products indexed under this heading.

Thioridazine Hydrochloride (Caution should be taken when darifenacin is used concomitantly with medications that are predominantly metabolized by CYP2D6 and which have a narrow therapeutic window, such as thioridazine). Products include:
Thioridazine Hydrochloride Tablets 2195

Timolol Maleate (Caution should be taken when darifenacin is used concomitantly with medications that are predominantly metabolized by CYP2D6 and that have a narrow therapeutic window). Products include:
Combigan Ophthalmic Solution 553
Cosopt Sterile Ophthalmic Solution 1969
Timoptic Sterile Ophthalmic Solution 2121
Timoptic in Ocudose 2124
Timoptic-XE Sterile Ophthalmic Gel Forming Solution 2125

Tolterodine Tartrate (The concomitant use of darifenacin with other anticholinergic agents may increase the frequency and/or severity of dry mouth, constipation, blurred vision and other anticholinergic pharmacological effects. Anticholinergic agents may potentially alter the absorption of some concomitantly administered drugs due to effects on gastrointestinal motility).
No products indexed under this heading.

Tramadol Hydrochloride (Caution should be taken when darifenacin is used concomitantly with medications that are predominantly metabolized by CYP2D6 and that have a narrow therapeutic window). Products include:
Ultram ER Extended-Release Tablets 2428

Trazodone Hydrochloride (Caution should be taken when darifenacin is used concomitantly with medications that are predominantly metabolized by CYP2D6 and that have a narrow therapeutic window).
No products indexed under this heading.

Triamcinolone (Darifenacin metabolism is primarily mediated by the cytochrome P450 enzymes CYP2D6 and CYP3A4. Therefore, inducers of CYP3A4 may alter darifenacin pharmacokinetics).
No products indexed under this heading.

Triamcinolone Acetonide (Darifenacin metabolism is primarily mediated by the cytochrome P450 enzymes CYP2D6 and CYP3A4. Therefore, inducers of CYP3A4 may alter darifenacin pharmacokinetics). Products include:
Azmacort Inhalation Aerosol 407
Nasacort AQ Nasal Spray 2765
Triesence Injectable Suspension .... ⊙209

Triamcinolone Diacetate (Darifenacin metabolism is primarily mediated by the cytochrome P450 enzymes CYP2D6 and CYP3A4. Therefore, inducers of CYP3A4 may alter darifenacin pharmacokinetics).
No products indexed under this heading.

Triamcinolone Hexacetonide (Darifenacin metabolism is primarily mediated by the cytochrome P450 enzymes CYP2D6 and CYP3A4. Therefore, inducers of CYP3A4 may alter darifenacin pharmacokinetics).
No products indexed under this heading.

Triazolam (Caution should be taken when darifenacin is used concomitantly with medications that are predominantly metabolized by CYP2D6 and that have a narrow therapeutic window).
No products indexed under this heading.

Tridihexethyl Chloride (The concomitant use of darifenacin with other anticholinergic agents may increase the frequency and/or severity of dry mouth, constipation, blurred vision and other anticholinergic pharmacological effects. Anticholinergic agents may potentially alter the absorption of some concomitantly administered drugs due to effects on gastrointestinal motility).
No products indexed under this heading.

Trihexyphenidyl Hydrochloride (The concomitant use of darifenacin with other anticholinergic agents may increase the frequency and/or severity of dry mouth, constipation, blurred vision and other anticholinergic pharmacological effects. Anticholinergic agents may potentially alter the absorption of some concomitantly administered drugs due to effects on gastrointestinal motility).
No products indexed under this heading.

Trimipramine Maleate (Caution should be taken when darifenacin is used concomitantly with medications that are predominantly metabolized by CYP2D6 and which have a narrow therapeutic window, such as tricyclic antidepressants).
No products indexed under this heading.

Troglitazone (Darifenacin metabolism is primarily mediated by the cytochrome P450 enzymes CYP2D6 and CYP3A4. Therefore, inducers of CYP3A4 may alter darifenacin pharmacokinetics).
No products indexed under this heading.

Troleandomycin (The daily dose of darifenacin should not exceed 7.5 mg when co-administered with potent CYP3A4 inhibitors).
No products indexed under this heading.

Venlafaxine Hydrochloride (Caution should be taken when darifenacin is used concomitantly with medications that are predominantly metabolized by CYP2D6 and that have a narrow therapeutic window). Products include:
Effexor XR Extended-Release Capsules 3195
Venlafaxine Hydrochloride Tablets ... 2199

Vinblastine Sulfate (Caution should be taken when darifenacin is used concomitantly with medications that are predominantly metabolized by CYP2D6 and that have a narrow therapeutic window).
No products indexed under this heading.

Voriconazole (The daily dose of darifenacin should not exceed 7.5 mg when co-administered with potent CYP3A4 inhibitors).
No products indexed under this heading.

Zonisamide (Caution should be taken when darifenacin is used concomitantly with medications that are predominantly metabolized by CYP2D6 and that have a narrow therapeutic window). Products include:
Zonegran Capsules 1089

ENBREL FOR INJECTION

(Etanercept) 569
May interact with vaccines, live and certain other agents. Compounds in these categories include:

Anakinra (Co-administration results in a 7% rate of serious infections and 2% of the patients develop neutropenia). Products include:
Kineret Injection 585

BCG Vaccine (Patients receiving etanercept may receive concurrent vaccinations, except for live vaccines).
No products indexed under this heading.

Cyclophosphamide (Concurrent cyclophosphamide therapy is not recommended).
No products indexed under this heading.

Influenza Vaccine, Live Attenuated (Patients receiving etanercept may receive concurrent vaccinations, except for live vaccines).
No products indexed under this heading.

Influenza Virus Vaccine Live, Intranasal (Patients receiving etanercept may receive concurrent vaccinations, except for live vaccines). Products include:
FluMist Vaccine 1945

Measles, Mumps, Rubella and Varicella Virus Vaccine Live (Patients receiving etanercept may receive concurrent vaccinations, except for live vaccines). Products include:
ProQuad 2099

Measles, Mumps & Rubella Virus Vaccine, Live (Patients receiving etanercept may receive concurrent vaccinations, except for live vaccines). Products include:
M-M-R II 2054

Measles & Rubella Virus Vaccine Live (Patients receiving etanercept may receive concurrent vaccinations, except for live vaccines).
No products indexed under this heading.

Measles Virus Vaccine Live (Patients receiving etanercept may receive concurrent vaccinations, except for live vaccines). Products include:
Attenuvax 1951

Mumps Virus Vaccine, Live (Patients receiving etanercept may receive concurrent vaccinations, except for live vaccines). Products include:
Mumpsvax 2068

Poliovirus Vaccine, Live, Oral, Trivalent, Types 1,2,3 (Sabin) (Patients receiving etanercept may receive concurrent vaccinations, except for live vaccines).
No products indexed under this heading.

Rotavirus Vaccine, Live, Oral, Tetravalent (Patients receiving etanercept may receive concurrent vaccinations, except for live vaccines).
No products indexed under this heading.

Rubella & Mumps Virus Vaccine Live (Patients receiving etanercept may receive concurrent vaccinations, except for live vaccines).
No products indexed under this heading.

Rubella Virus Vaccine Live (Patients receiving etanercept may receive concurrent vaccinations, except for live vaccines). Products include:
Meruvax II 2061

Smallpox Vaccine (Patients receiving etanercept may receive concurrent vaccinations, except for live vaccines).
No products indexed under this heading.

Sulfasalazine (Co-administration results in a mild decrease in mean neutrophil count).
No products indexed under this heading.

Typhoid Vaccine (Patients receiving etanercept may receive concurrent vaccinations, except for live vaccines).
No products indexed under this heading.

Varicella Virus Vaccine Live (Patients receiving etanercept may receive concurrent vaccinations, except for live vaccines). Products include:
Varivax 2133

Yellow Fever Vaccine (Patients receiving etanercept may receive concurrent vaccinations, except for live vaccines).
No products indexed under this heading.

Zoster Vaccine Live (Patients receiving etanercept may receive concurrent vaccinations, except for live vaccines). Products include:
Zostavax Injection 2145

ENGERIX-B VACCINE

(Hepatitis B Vaccine, Recombinant) ... 1409
None cited in PDR database.

ENJUVIA TABLETS

(Estrogens, Conjugated, Synthetic B) 1029
May interact with cytochrome p450 3a4 inducers (selected), cytochrome p450 3a4 inhibitors (selected), and thyroid preparations. Compounds in these categories include:

Acetazolamide (Inhibitors of CYP3A4 such as erythromycin, clarithromycin, ketoconazole, itraconazole, ritonavir and grapefruit juice may increase plasma concentrations of estrogens and may result in side effects).
No products indexed under this heading.

Allium sativum (Inducers of CYP3A4 such as St. John's Wort preparations (hypericum perforatum), phenobarbital, carbamazepine and rifampin may reduce plasma concentrations of estrogens, possibly resulting in a decrease in therapeutic effects and/or changes in the uterine bleeding profile).
No products indexed under this heading.

Amiodarone Hydrochloride (Inhibitors of CYP3A4 such as erythromycin, clarithromycin, ketoconazole, itraconazole, ritonavir and grapefruit juice may increase plasma concentrations of estrogens and may result in side effects).
No products indexed under this heading.

Amprenavir (Inhibitors of CYP3A4 such as erythromycin, clarithromycin, ketoconazole, itraconazole, ritonavir and grapefruit juice may increase plasma concentrations of estrogens and may result in side effects).
No products indexed under this heading.

Anastrozole (Inhibitors of CYP3A4 such as erythromycin, clarithromycin, ketoconazole, itraconazole, ritonavir and grapefruit juice may increase plasma concentrations of estrogens and may result in side effects). Products include:
Arimidex Tablets 672

Aprepitant (Inducers of CYP3A4 such as St. John's Wort preparations (hypericum perforatum), phenobarbital, carbamazepine and rifampin may reduce plasma concentrations of estrogens, possibly resulting in a decrease in therapeutic effects and/or changes in the uterine bleeding profile). Products include:
Emend Capsules 1992

Atazanavir (Inhibitors of CYP3A4 such as erythromycin, clarithromycin, ketoconazole, itraçonazole, ritonavir and grapefruit juice may increase plasma concentrations of estrogens and may result in side effects).
No products indexed under this heading.

Atazanavir Sulfate (Inhibitors of CYP3A4 such as erythromycin, clarithromycin, ketoconazole, itraconazole, ritonavir and grapefruit juice may increase plasma concentrations of estrogens and may result in side effects). Products include:
Reyataz Capsules 3299

Betamethasone Acetate (Inducers of CYP3A4 such as St. John's Wort preparations (hypericum perforatum), phenobarbital, carbamazepine and rifampin may reduce plasma concentrations of estrogens, possibly resulting in a decrease in therapeutic effects and/or changes in the uterine bleeding profile).
No products indexed under this heading.

Betamethasone Sodium Phosphate (Inducers of CYP3A4 such as St. John's Wort preparations (hypericum perforatum), phenobarbital, carbamazepine and rifampin may reduce plasma concentrations of estrogens, possibly resulting in a decrease in therapeutic effects and/or changes in the uterine bleeding profile).
No products indexed under this heading.

Carbamazepine (Inducers of CYP3A4 such as St. John's Wort preparations (hypericum perforatum), phenobarbital, carbamazepine and rifampin may reduce plasma concentrations of estrogens, possibly resulting in a decrease in therapeutic effects and/or changes in the uterine bleeding profile). Products include:
Carbatrol Capsules 3019
Equetro Extended-Release Capsules 3174

Cimetidine (Inhibitors of CYP3A4 such as erythromycin, clarithromycin, ketoconazole, itraconazole, ritonavir and grapefruit juice may increase plasma concentrations of estrogens and may result in side effects).
No products indexed under this heading.

Cimetidine Hydrochloride (Inhibitors of CYP3A4 such as erythromycin, clarithromycin, ketoconazole, itraconazole, ritonavir and grapefruit juice may increase plasma concentrations of estrogens and may result in side effects).
No products indexed under this heading.

Ciprofloxacin (Inhibitors of CYP3A4 such as erythromycin, clarithromycin, ketoconazole, itraconazole, ritonavir and grapefruit juice may increase plasma concentrations of estrogens and may result in side effects). Products include:
Cipro I.V. 2817
Cipro Oral Suspension 2810
Cipro XR Tablets 2823

Ciprodex Otic Suspension 541

Ciprofloxacin Hydrochloride (Inducers of CYP3A4 such as St. John's Wort preparations (hypericum perforatum), phenobarbital, carbamazepine and rifampin may reduce plasma concentrations of estrogens, possibly resulting in a decrease in therapeutic effects and/or changes in the uterine bleeding profile). Products include:
Cipro Tablets 2810

Cisplatin (Inducers of CYP3A4 such as St. John's Wort preparations (hypericum perforatum), phenobarbital, carbamazepine and rifampin may reduce plasma concentrations of estrogens, possibly resulting in a decrease in therapeutic effects and/ or changes in the uterine bleeding profile).
No products indexed under this heading.

Clarithromycin (Inhibitors of CYP3A4 such as erythromycin, clarithromycin, ketoconazole, itraconazole, ritonavir and grapefruit juice may increase plasma concentrations of estrogens and may result in side effects). Products include:
Biaxin/Biaxin XL 411

Clotrimazole (Inhibitors of CYP3A4 such as erythromycin, clarithromycin, ketoconazole, itraconazole, ritonavir and grapefruit juice may increase plasma concentrations of estrogens and may result in side effects). Products include:
Lotrisone 2881

Cortisone Acetate (Inducers of CYP3A4 such as St. John's Wort preparations (hypericum perforatum), phenobarbital, carbamazepine and rifampin may reduce plasma concentrations of estrogens, possibly resulting in a decrease in therapeutic effects and/or changes in the uterine bleeding profile).
No products indexed under this heading.

Cyclosporine (Inhibitors of CYP3A4 such as erythromycin, clarithromycin, ketoconazole, itraconazole, ritonavir and grapefruit juice may increase plasma concentrations of estrogens and may result in side effects). Products include:
Gengraf Capsules 435
Neoral Oral Solution 2280
Neoral Soft Gelatin Capsules 2280
Restasis Ophthalmic Emulsion 557
Sandimmune 2296

Dalfopristin (Inhibitors of CYP3A4 such as erythromycin, clarithromycin, ketoconazole, itraconazole, ritonavir and grapefruit juice may increase plasma concentrations of estrogens and may result in side effects).
No products indexed under this heading.

Danazol (Inhibitors of CYP3A4 such as erythromycin, clarithromycin, ketoconazole, itraconazole, ritonavir and grapefruit juice may increase plasma concentrations of estrogens and may result in side effects).
No products indexed under this heading.

Delavirdine Mesylate (Inhibitors of CYP3A4 such as erythromycin, clarithromycin, ketoconazole, itraconazole, ritonavir and grapefruit juice may increase plasma concentrations of estrogens and may result in side effects).
No products indexed under this heading.

Dexamethasone (Inducers of CYP3A4 such as St. John's Wort preparations (hypericum perforatum), phenobarbital, carbamazepine and rifampin may reduce plasma concentrations of estrogens, possibly resulting in a decrease in therapeutic effects and/or changes in the uterine bleeding profile). Products include:
Ciprodex Otic Suspension 541

Dexamethasone Acetate (Inducers of CYP3A4 such as St. John's Wort preparations (hypericum perforatum), phenobarbital, carbamazepine and rifampin may reduce plasma concentrations of estrogens, possibly resulting in a decrease in therapeutic effects and/or changes in the uterine bleeding profile).
No products indexed under this heading.

Dexamethasone Sodium Phosphate (Inducers of CYP3A4 such as St. John's Wort preparations (hypericum perforatum), phenobarbital, carbamazepine and rifampin may reduce plasma concentrations of estrogens, possibly resulting in a decrease in therapeutic effects and/ or changes in the uterine bleeding profile).
No products indexed under this heading.

Diltiazem Hydrochloride (Inhibitors of CYP3A4 such as erythromycin, clarithromycin, ketoconazole, itraconazole, ritonavir and grapefruit juice may increase plasma concentrations of estrogens and may result in side effects). Products include:
Cardizem LA Extended Release Tablets 421

Diltiazem Maleate (Inhibitors of CYP3A4 such as erythromycin, clarithromycin, ketoconazole, itraconazole, ritonavir and grapefruit juice may increase plasma concentrations of estrogens and may result in side effects).
No products indexed under this heading.

Doxorubicin Hydrochloride (Inducers of CYP3A4 such as St. John's Wort preparations (hypericum perforatum), phenobarbital, carbamazepine and rifampin may reduce plasma concentrations of estrogens, possibly resulting in a decrease in therapeutic effects and/or changes in the uterine bleeding profile).
No products indexed under this heading.

Efavirenz (Inducers of CYP3A4 such as St. John's Wort preparations (hypericum perforatum), phenobarbital, carbamazepine and rifampin may reduce plasma concentrations of estrogens, possibly resulting in a decrease in therapeutic effects and/ or changes in the uterine bleeding profile). Products include:
Atripla Tablets 938
Sustiva Capsules 930
Sustiva Tablets 930

Erythromycin (Inhibitors of CYP3A4 such as erythromycin, clarithromycin, ketoconazole, itraconazole, ritonavir and grapefruit juice may increase plasma concentrations of estrogens and may result in side effects).
No products indexed under this heading.

Erythromycin Estolate (Inhibitors of CYP3A4 such as erythromycin, clarithromycin, ketoconazole, itraconazole, ritonavir and grapefruit juice may increase plasma concentrations of estrogens and may result in side effects).
No products indexed under this heading.

Erythromycin Ethylsuccinate (Inhibitors of CYP3A4 such as erythromycin, clarithromycin, ketoconazole, itraconazole, ritonavir and grapefruit juice may increase plasma concentrations of estrogens and may result in side effects). Products include:
E.E.S. 433
EryPed 431

Erythromycin Gluceptate (Inhibitors of CYP3A4 such as erythromycin, clarithromycin, ketoconazole, itraconazole, ritonavir and grapefruit juice may increase plasma concentrations of estrogens and may result in side effects).
No products indexed under this heading.

Erythromycin Lactobionate (Inhibitors of CYP3A4 such as erythromycin, clarithromycin, ketoconazole, itraconazole, ritonavir and grapefruit juice may increase plasma concentrations of estrogens and may result in side effects).
No products indexed under this heading.

Erythromycin Stearate (Inhibitors of CYP3A4 such as erythromycin, clarithromycin, ketoconazole, itraconazole, ritonavir and grapefruit juice may increase plasma concentrations of estrogens and may result in side effects).
No products indexed under this heading.

Esomeprazole Magnesium (Inhibitors of CYP3A4 such as erythromycin, clarithromycin, ketoconazole, itraconazole, ritonavir and grapefruit juice may increase plasma concentrations of estrogens and may result in side effects). Products include:
Nexium Delayed-Release Capsules 645
Nexium Delayed-Release Oral Suspension...................................... 645

Ethosuximide (Inducers of CYP3A4 such as St. John's Wort preparations (hypericum perforatum), phenobarbital, carbamazepine and rifampin may reduce plasma concentrations of estrogens, possibly resulting in a decrease in therapeutic effects and/ or changes in the uterine bleeding profile).
No products indexed under this heading.

Felbamate (Inducers of CYP3A4 such as St. John's Wort preparations (hypericum perforatum), phenobarbital, carbamazepine and rifampin may reduce plasma concentrations of estrogens, possibly resulting in a decrease in therapeutic effects and/ or changes in the uterine bleeding profile).
No products indexed under this heading.

Fluconazole (Inhibitors of CYP3A4 such as erythromycin, clarithromycin, ketoconazole, itraconazole, ritonavir and grapefruit juice may increase plasma concentrations of estrogens and may result in side effects).
No products indexed under this heading.

Fludrocortisone Acetate (Inducers of CYP3A4 such as St. John's Wort preparations (hypericum perforatum), phenobarbital, carbamazepine and rifampin may reduce plasma concentrations of estrogens, possibly resulting in a decrease in therapeutic effects and/or changes in the uterine bleeding profile).
No products indexed under this heading.

Fluoxetine (Inhibitors of CYP3A4 such as erythromycin, clarithromycin, ketoconazole, itraconazole, ritonavir and grapefruit juice may increase plasma concentrations of estrogens and may result in side effects).
No products indexed under this heading.

Fluoxetine Hydrochloride (Inhibitors of CYP3A4 such as erythromycin, clarithromycin, ketoconazole, itraconazole, ritonavir and grapefruit juice may increase plasma concentrations of estrogens and may result in side effects). Products include:
Prozac Weekly Capsules 1852
Prozac Pulvules and Liquid 1852
Symbyax Capsules 1871

Fluvoxamine Maleate (Inhibitors of CYP3A4 such as erythromycin, clarithromycin, ketoconazole, itraconazole, ritonavir and grapefruit juice may increase plasma concentrations of estrogens and may result in side effects). Products include:
Luvox CR Extended-Release Capsules 1759

Fosamprenavir Calcium (Inhibitors of CYP3A4 such as erythromycin, clarithromycin, ketoconazole, itraconazole, ritonavir and grapefruit juice may increase plasma concentrations of estrogens and may result in side effects). Products include:
Lexiva Oral Suspension 1510
Lexiva Tablets 1510

Fosphenytoin Sodium (Inducers of CYP3A4 such as St. John's Wort preparations (hypericum perforatum), phenobarbital, carbamazepine and rifampin may reduce plasma concentrations of estrogens, possibly resulting in a decrease in therapeutic effects and/or changes in the uterine bleeding profile).
No products indexed under this heading.

Garlic Extract (Inducers of CYP3A4 such as St. John's Wort preparations (hypericum perforatum), phenobarbital, carbamazepine and rifampin may reduce plasma concentrations of estrogens, possibly resulting in a decrease in therapeutic effects and/or changes in the uterine bleeding profile).
No products indexed under this heading.

Garlic Oil (Inducers of CYP3A4 such as St. John's Wort preparations (hypericum perforatum), phenobarbital, carbamazepine and rifampin may reduce plasma concentrations of estrogens, possibly resulting in a decrease in therapeutic effects and/ or changes in the uterine bleeding profile).
No products indexed under this heading.

Hydrocortisone (Inducers of CYP3A4 such as St. John's Wort preparations (hypericum perforatum), phenobarbital, carbamazepine and rifampin may reduce plasma concentrations of estrogens, possibly resulting in a decrease in therapeutic effects and/or changes in the uterine bleeding profile).
No products indexed under this heading.

Hydrocortisone Acetate (Inducers of CYP3A4 such as St. John's Wort preparations (hypericum perforatum), phenobarbital, carbamazepine and rifampin may reduce plasma concentrations of estrogens, possibly resulting in a decrease in therapeutic effects and/or changes in the uterine bleeding profile). Products include:
Analpram-HC 1140
Pramosone 1141

Hydrocortisone Butyrate (Inducers of CYP3A4 such as St. John's Wort preparations (hypericum perforatum), phenobarbital, carbamazepine and rifampin may reduce plasma concentrations of estrogens, possibly resulting in a decrease in therapeutic effects and/or changes in the uterine bleeding profile).
No products indexed under this heading.

Hydrocortisone Cypionate (Inducers of CYP3A4 such as St. John's Wort preparations (hypericum perforatum), phenobarbital, carbamazepine and rifampin may reduce plasma concentrations of estrogens, possibly resulting in a decrease in therapeutic effects and/or changes in the uterine bleeding profile).
No products indexed under this heading.

Hydrocortisone Hemisuccinate (Inducers of CYP3A4 such as St. John's Wort preparations (hypericum perforatum), phenobarbital, carbamazepine and rifampin may reduce plasma concentrations of estrogens, possibly resulting in a decrease in therapeutic effects and/or changes in the uterine bleeding profile).
No products indexed under this heading.

Hydrocortisone Probutate (Inducers of CYP3A4 such as St. John's Wort preparations (hypericum perforatum), phenobarbital, carbamazepine and rifampin may reduce plasma concentrations of estrogens, possibly resulting in a decrease in therapeutic effects and/or changes in the uterine bleeding profile).
No products indexed under this heading.

Hydrocortisone Sodium Phosphate (Inducers of CYP3A4 such as St. John's Wort preparations (hypericum perforatum), phenobarbital, carbamazepine and rifampin may reduce plasma concentrations of estrogens, possibly resulting in a decrease in therapeutic effects and/or changes in the uterine bleeding profile).
No products indexed under this heading.

Hydrocortisone Sodium Succinate (Inducers of CYP3A4 such as St. John's Wort preparations (hypericum perforatum), phenobarbital, carbamazepine and rifampin may reduce plasma concentrations of estrogens, possibly resulting in a decrease in therapeutic effects and/or changes in the uterine bleeding profile).
No products indexed under this heading.

Hydrocortisone Valerate (Inducers of CYP3A4 such as St. John's Wort preparations (hypericum perforatum), phenobarbital, carbamazepine and rifampin may reduce plasma concentrations of estrogens, possibly resulting in a decrease in therapeutic effects and/or changes in the uterine bleeding profile).
No products indexed under this heading.

Hypericum (Inducers of CYP3A4 such as St. John's Wort preparations (hypericum perforatum), phenobarbital, carbamazepine and rifampin may reduce plasma concentrations of estrogens, possibly resulting in a decrease in therapeutic effects and/or changes in the uterine bleeding profile). Products include:
Satieté Tablets .... ▣640

Hypericum Perforatum (Inducers of CYP3A4 such as St. John's Wort preparations (hypericum perforatum), phenobarbital, carbamazepine and rifampin may reduce plasma concentrations of estrogens, possibly resulting in a decrease in therapeutic effects and/or changes in the uterine bleeding profile).
No products indexed under this heading.

Indinavir Sulfate (Inhibitors of CYP3A4 such as erythromycin, clarithromycin, ketoconazole, itraconazole, ritonavir and grapefruit juice may increase plasma concentrations of estrogens and may result in side effects). Products include:
Crixivan Capsules 1979

Isoniazid (Inhibitors of CYP3A4 such as erythromycin, clarithromycin, ketoconazole, itraconazole, ritonavir and grapefruit juice may increase plasma concentrations of estrogens and may result in side effects).
No products indexed under this heading.

Itraconazole (Inhibitors of CYP3A4 such as erythromycin, clarithromycin, ketoconazole, itraconazole, ritonavir and grapefruit juice may increase plasma concentrations of estrogens and may result in side effects).
No products indexed under this heading.

Ketoconazole (Inhibitors of CYP3A4 such as erythromycin, clarithromycin, ketoconazole, itraconazole, ritonavir and grapefruit juice may increase plasma concentrations of estrogens and may result in side effects). Products include:
Extina Foam, 2% 3057
Nizoral A-D Shampoo 1901

Levothyroxine Sodium (Patients on thyroid replacement therapy may require higher doses of thyroid hormone). Products include:
Levothroid Tablets 1170
Levoxyl Tablets 1780
Synthroid Tablets 507

Liothyronine Sodium (Patients on thyroid replacement therapy may require higher doses of thyroid hormone). Products include:
Cytomel Tablets 1778

Liotrix (Patients on thyroid replacement therapy may require higher doses of thyroid hormone).
No products indexed under this heading.

Lopinavir (Inhibitors of CYP3A4 such as erythromycin, clarithromycin, ketoconazole, itraconazole, ritonavir and grapefruit juice may increase plasma concentrations of estrogens and may result in side effects). Products include:
Kaletra 452

Loratadine (Inhibitors of CYP3A4 such as erythromycin, clarithromycin, ketoconazole, itraconazole, ritonavir and grapefruit juice may increase plasma concentrations of estrogens and may result in side effects).
No products indexed under this heading.

Mephenytoin (Inducers of CYP3A4 such as St. John's Wort preparations (hypericum perforatum), phenobarbital, carbamazepine and rifampin may reduce plasma concentrations of estrogens, possibly resulting in a decrease in therapeutic effects and/or changes in the uterine bleeding profile).
No products indexed under this heading.

Methsuximide (Inducers of CYP3A4 such as St. John's Wort preparations (hypericum perforatum), phenobarbital, carbamazepine and rifampin may reduce plasma concentrations of estrogens, possibly resulting in a decrease in therapeutic effects and/or changes in the uterine bleeding profile).
No products indexed under this heading.

Methylprednisolone (Inducers of CYP3A4 such as St. John's Wort preparations (hypericum perforatum), phenobarbital, carbamazepine and rifampin may reduce plasma concentrations of estrogens, possibly resulting in a decrease in therapeutic effects and/or changes in the uterine bleeding profile).
No products indexed under this heading.

Methylprednisolone Acetate (Inducers of CYP3A4 such as St. John's Wort preparations (hypericum perforatum), phenobarbital, carbamazepine and rifampin may reduce plasma concentrations of estrogens, possibly resulting in a decrease in therapeutic effects and/or changes in the uterine bleeding profile).
No products indexed under this heading.

Methylprednisolone Sodium Succinate (Inducers of CYP3A4 such as St. John's Wort preparations (hypericum perforatum), phenobarbital, carbamazepine and rifampin may reduce plasma concentrations of estrogens, possibly resulting in a decrease in therapeutic effects and/or changes in the uterine bleeding profile).
No products indexed under this heading.

Metronidazole (Inhibitors of CYP3A4 such as erythromycin, clarithromycin, ketoconazole, itraconazole, ritonavir and grapefruit juice may increase plasma concentrations of estrogens and may result in side effects). Products include:
Pylera Capsules 714

Metronidazole Benzoate (Inhibitors of CYP3A4 such as erythromycin, clarithromycin, ketoconazole, itraconazole, ritonavir and grapefruit juice may increase plasma concentrations of estrogens and may result in side effects).
No products indexed under this heading.

Metronidazole Hydrochloride (Inhibitors of CYP3A4 such as erythromycin, clarithromycin, ketoconazole, itraconazole, ritonavir and grapefruit juice may increase plasma concentrations of estrogens and may result in side effects).
No products indexed under this heading.

Miconazole (Inhibitors of CYP3A4 such as erythromycin, clarithromycin, ketoconazole, itraconazole, ritonavir and grapefruit juice may increase plasma concentrations of estrogens and may result in side effects).
No products indexed under this heading.

Miconazole Nitrate (Inhibitors of CYP3A4 such as erythromycin, clarithromycin, ketoconazole, itraconazole, ritonavir and grapefruit juice may increase plasma concentrations of estrogens and may result in side effects).
No products indexed under this heading.

Modafinil (Inducers of CYP3A4 such as St. John's Wort preparations (hypericum perforatum), phenobarbital, carbamazepine and rifampin may reduce plasma concentrations of estrogens, possibly resulting in a decrease in therapeutic effects and/or changes in the uterine bleeding profile). Products include:
Provigil Tablets 977

Nefazodone Hydrochloride (Inhibitors of CYP3A4 such as erythromycin, clarithromycin, ketoconazole, itraconazole, ritonavir and grapefruit juice may increase plasma concentrations of estrogens and may result in side effects).
No products indexed under this heading.

Nelfinavir Mesylate (Inhibitors of CYP3A4 such as erythromycin, clarithromycin, ketoconazole, itraconazole, ritonavir and grapefruit juice may increase plasma concentrations of estrogens and may result in side effects).
No products indexed under this heading.

Nevirapine (Inducers of CYP3A4 such as St. John's Wort preparations (hypericum perforatum), phenobarbital, carbamazepine and rifampin may reduce plasma concentrations of estrogens, possibly resulting in a decrease in therapeutic effects and/or changes in the uterine bleeding profile). Products include:
Viramune Oral Suspension 873
Viramune Tablets 873

Niacinamide (Inhibitors of CYP3A4 such as erythromycin, clarithromycin, ketoconazole, itraconazole, ritonavir and grapefruit juice may increase plasma concentrations of estrogens and may result in side effects). Products include:

Saquinavir Mesylate (Inhibitors of CYP3A4 such as erythromycin, clarithromycin, ketoconazole, itraconazole, ritonavir and grapefruit juice may increase plasma concentrations of estrogens and may result in side effects).
No products indexed under this heading.

Sertraline Hydrochloride (Inhibitors of CYP3A4 such as erythromycin, clarithromycin, ketoconazole, itraconazole, ritonavir and grapefruit juice may increase plasma concentrations of estrogens and may result in side effects).
No products indexed under this heading.

Sildenafil Citrate (Inhibitors of CYP3A4 such as erythromycin, clarithromycin, ketoconazole, itraconazole, ritonavir and grapefruit juice may increase plasma concentrations of estrogens and may result in side effects).
No products indexed under this heading.

Sulfinpyrazone (Inducers of CYP3A4 such as St. John's Wort preparations (hypericum perforatum), phenobarbital, carbamazepine and rifampin may reduce plasma concentrations of estrogens, possibly resulting in a decrease in therapeutic effects and/or changes in the uterine bleeding profile).
No products indexed under this heading.

Telithromycin (Inhibitors of CYP3A4 such as erythromycin, clarithromycin, ketoconazole, itraconazole, ritonavir and grapefruit juice may increase plasma concentrations of estrogens and may result in side effects). Products include:
Ketek Tablets 2744

Theophylline (Inducers of CYP3A4 such as St. John's Wort preparations (hypericum perforatum), phenobarbital, carbamazepine and rifampin may reduce plasma concentrations of estrogens, possibly resulting in a decrease in therapeutic effects and/or changes in the uterine bleeding profile).
No products indexed under this heading.

Theophylline Anhydrous (Inducers of CYP3A4 such as St. John's Wort preparations (hypericum perforatum), phenobarbital, carbamazepine and rifampin may reduce plasma concentrations of estrogens, possibly resulting in a decrease in therapeutic effects and/or changes in the uterine bleeding profile). Products include:
Uniphyl Tablets 2595

Theophylline Calcium Salicylate (Inducers of CYP3A4 such as St. John's Wort preparations (hypericum perforatum), phenobarbital, carbamazepine and rifampin may reduce plasma concentrations of estrogens, possibly resulting in a decrease in therapeutic effects and/or changes in the uterine bleeding profile).
No products indexed under this heading.

Theophylline Dihydroxypropyl (Glyceryl) (Inducers of CYP3A4 such as St. John's Wort preparations (hypericum perforatum), phenobarbital, carbamazepine and rifampin may reduce plasma concentrations of estrogens, possibly resulting in a decrease in therapeutic effects and/or changes in the uterine bleeding profile).
No products indexed under this heading.

Theophylline Ethylenediamine (Inducers of CYP3A4 such as St. John's Wort preparations (hypericum perforatum), phenobarbital, carbamazepine and rifampin may reduce plasma concentrations of estrogens, possibly resulting in a decrease in therapeutic effects and/or changes in the uterine bleeding profile).
No products indexed under this heading.

Thyroglobulin (Patients on thyroid replacement therapy may require higher doses of thryoid hormone).
No products indexed under this heading.

Thyroid (Patients on thyroid replacement therapy may require higher doses of thryoid hormone). Products include:
Naturethroid Tablets 2605

Thyroxine (Patients on thyroid replacement therapy may require higher doses of thryoid hormone).
No products indexed under this heading.

Thyroxine Sodium (Patients on thyroid replacement therapy may require higher doses of thryoid hormone).
No products indexed under this heading.

Triamcinolone (Inducers of CYP3A4 such as St. John's Wort preparations (hypericum perforatum), phenobarbital, carbamazepine and rifampin may reduce plasma concentrations of estrogens, possibly resulting in a decrease in therapeutic effects and/or changes in the uterine bleeding profile).
No products indexed under this heading.

Triamcinolone Acetonide (Inducers of CYP3A4 such as St. John's Wort preparations (hypericum perforatum), phenobarbital, carbamazepine and rifampin may reduce plasma concentrations of estrogens, possibly resulting in a decrease in therapeutic effects and/or changes in the uterine bleeding profile). Products include:
Azmacort Inhalation Aerosol 407
Nasacort AQ Nasal Spray 2765
Triesence Injectable Suspension .... ⊙209

Triamcinolone Diacetate (Inducers of CYP3A4 such as St. John's Wort preparations (hypericum perforatum), phenobarbital, carbamazepine and rifampin may reduce plasma concentrations of estrogens, possibly resulting in a decrease in therapeutic effects and/or changes in the uterine bleeding profile).
No products indexed under this heading.

Triamcinolone Hexacetonide (Inducers of CYP3A4 such as St. John's Wort preparations (hypericum perforatum), phenobarbital, carbamazepine and rifampin may reduce plasma concentrations of estrogens, possibly resulting in a decrease in therapeutic effects and/or changes in the uterine bleeding profile).
No products indexed under this heading.

Troglitazone (Inducers of CYP3A4 such as St. John's Wort preparations (hypericum perforatum), phenobarbital, carbamazepine and rifampin may reduce plasma concentrations of estrogens, possibly resulting in a decrease in therapeutic effects and/or changes in the uterine bleeding profile).
No products indexed under this heading.

Troleandomycin (Inhibitors of CYP3A4 such as erythromycin, clarithromycin, ketoconazole, itraconazole, ritonavir and grapefruit juice may increase plasma concentrations of estrogens and may result in side effects).
No products indexed under this heading.

Valproate Sodium (Inhibitors of CYP3A4 such as erythromycin, clarithromycin, ketoconazole, itraconazole, ritonavir and grapefruit juice may increase plasma concentrations of estrogens and may result in side effects).
No products indexed under this heading.

Vardenafil Hydrochloride (Inhibitors of CYP3A4 such as erythromycin, clarithromycin, ketoconazole, itraconazole, ritonavir and grapefruit juice may increase plasma concentrations of estrogens and may result in side effects). Products include:
Levitra Tablets 2876

Verapamil Hydrochloride (Inhibitors of CYP3A4 such as erythromycin, clarithromycin, ketoconazole, itraconazole, ritonavir and grapefruit juice may increase plasma concentrations of estrogens and may result in side effects). Products include:
Tarka Tablets 511

Voriconazole (Inhibitors of CYP3A4 such as erythromycin, clarithromycin, ketoconazole, itraconazole, ritonavir and grapefruit juice may increase plasma concentrations of estrogens and may result in side effects).
No products indexed under this heading.

Zafirlukast (Inhibitors of CYP3A4 such as erythromycin, clarithromycin, ketoconazole, itraconazole, ritonavir and grapefruit juice may increase plasma concentrations of estrogens and may result in side effects). Products include:
Accolate Tablets 669

Zileuton (Inhibitors of CYP3A4 such as erythromycin, clarithromycin, ketoconazole, itraconazole, ritonavir and grapefruit juice may increase plasma concentrations of estrogens and may result in side effects).
No products indexed under this heading.

Food Interactions

Grapefruit (Inhibitors of CYP3A4 such as erythromycin, clarithromycin, ketoconazole, itraconazole, ritonavir and grapefruit juice may increase plasma concentrations of estrogens and may result in side effects).

Grapefruit Juice (Inhibitors of CYP3A4 such as erythromycin, clarithromycin, ketoconazole, itraconazole, ritonavir and grapefruit juice may increase plasma concentrations of estrogens and may result in side effects).

ENTEREG CAPSULES

(Alvimopan) 3293
None cited in PDR database.

EPIPEN AUTO-INJECTOR

(Epinephrine) 1024
May interact with cardiac glycosides, monoamine oxidase inhibitors, quinidine, tricyclic antidepressants, and certain other agents. Compounds in these categories include:

Amitriptyline Hydrochloride (Co-administration with tricylcic antidepressants may potentiate the effects of epinephrine).
No products indexed under this heading.

Amoxapine (Co-administration with tricylcic antidepressants may potentiate the effects of epinephrine).
No products indexed under this heading.

Clomipramine Hydrochloride (Co-administration with tricylcic antidepressants may potentiate the effects of epinephrine).
No products indexed under this heading.

Desipramine Hydrochloride (Co-administration with tricylcic antidepressants may potentiate the effects of epinephrine).
No products indexed under this heading.

Deslanoside (Co-administration with drugs that may sensitize the heart to arrhythmias, such as digitalis, is not recommended).
No products indexed under this heading.

Digitalis Glycoside Preparations (Co-administration with drugs that may sensitize the heart to arrhythmias, such as digitalis, is not recommended).
No products indexed under this heading.

Digitoxin (Co-administration with drugs that may sensitize the heart to arrhythmias, such as digitalis, is not recommended).
No products indexed under this heading.

Digoxin (Co-administration with drugs that may sensitize the heart to arrhythmias, such as digitalis, is not recommended). Products include:
Lanoxin Injection 1498
Lanoxin Injection Pediatric 1502
Lanoxin Tablets 1505

Doxepin Hydrochloride (Co-administration with tricylcic antidepressants may potentiate the effects of epinephrine).
No products indexed under this heading.

Imipramine Hydrochloride (Co-administration with tricylcic antidepressants may potentiate the effects of epinephrine).
No products indexed under this heading.

Imipramine Pamoate (Co-administration with tricylcic antidepressants may potentiate the effects of epinephrine).
No products indexed under this heading.

Isocarboxazid (Co-administration with MAO inhibitors may potentiate the effects of epinephrine). Products include:
Marplan Tablets 3177

Maprotiline Hydrochloride (Co-administration with tricylcic antidepressants may potentiate the effects of epinephrine).
No products indexed under this heading.

Mercurial Diuretics (Co-administration with drugs that may sensitize the heart to arrhythmias, such as mercurial diuretics, is not recommended).
No products indexed under this heading.

Moclobemide (Co-administration with MAO inhibitors may potentiate the effects of epinephrine).
No products indexed under this heading.

Nortriptyline Hydrochloride (Co-administration with tricylcic antidepressants may potentiate the effects of epinephrine).
No products indexed under this heading.

Pargyline Hydrochloride (Co-administration with MAO inhibitors may potentiate the effects of epinephrine).
No products indexed under this heading.

Phenelzine Sulfate (Co-administration with MAO inhibitors may potentiate the effects of epinephrine).
No products indexed under this heading.

Procarbazine Hydrochloride (Co-administration with MAO inhibitors may potentiate the effects of epinephrine).
No products indexed under this heading.

Protriptyline Hydrochloride (Co-administration with tricylcic antidepressants may potentiate the effects of epinephrine).
No products indexed under this heading.

Quinidine (Co-administration with drugs that may sensitize the heart to arrhythmias, such as quinidine, is not recommended).
No products indexed under this heading.

Quinidine Gluconate (Co-administration with drugs that may sensitize the heart to arrhythmias, such as quinidine, is not recommended).
No products indexed under this heading.

Quinidine Hydrochloride (Co-administration with drugs that may sensitize the heart to arrhythmias, such as quinidine, is not recommended).
No products indexed under this heading.

Quinidine Polygalacturonate (Co-administration with drugs that may sensitize the heart to arrhythmias, such as quinidine, is not recommended).
No products indexed under this heading.

Quinidine Sulfate (Co-administration with drugs that may sensitize the heart to arrhythmias, such as quinidine, is not recommended).
No products indexed under this heading.

Rasagiline Mesylate (Co-administration with MAO inhibitors may potentiate the effects of epinephrine). Products include:
Azilect Tablets 3106

Selegiline (Co-administration with MAO inhibitors may potentiate the effects of epinephrine). Products include:
Emsam Transdermal System 905

Selegiline Hydrochloride (Co-administration with MAO inhibitors may potentiate the effects of epinephrine). Products include:
Eldepryl Capsules 3052

Tranylcypromine Sulfate (Co-administration with MAO inhibitors may potentiate the effects of epinephrine). Products include:
Parnate Tablets 1532

Trimipramine Maleate (Co-administration with tricylcic antidepressants may potentiate the effects of epinephrine).
No products indexed under this heading.

EPIPEN JR. AUTO-INJECTOR

(Epinephrine) 1024
See EpiPen Auto-Injector

EPIVIR ORAL SOLUTION

(Lamivudine) 1412
See Epivir Tablets

EPIVIR TABLETS

(Lamivudine) 1412
May interact with cationic drugs that are eliminated by renal tubular, Interferon alpha, and certain other agents. Compounds in these categories include:

Amiloride Hydrochloride (Lamivudine is predominantly eliminated in the urine by active organic secretion; therefore, the possibility of interactions with other drugs whose main route of elimination is active renal secretion via the organic cationic transport system should be considered).
No products indexed under this heading.

Digoxin (Lamivudine is predominantly eliminated in the urine by active organic secretion; therefore, the possibility of interactions with other drugs whose main route of elimination is active renal secretion via the organic cationic transport system should be considered). Products include:
Lanoxin Injection 1498
Lanoxin Injection Pediatric 1502
Lanoxin Tablets 1505

Emtricitabine (Lamivudine should not be administered concomitanty with emtricitabine-containing products). Products include:
Atripla Tablets 938
Emtriva Capsules 1246
Emtriva Oral Solution 1246
Truvada Tablets 1262

Interferon alfa-2a, Recombinant (Hepatic decompensation has occurred in HIV/HCV co-infected patients receiving combination antiretroviral therapy for HIV and interferon alpha with or withour ribavirin. Patients receiving interferon alpha with or without ribavirin and lamivudine should be closely monitored for treatment-associated toxicities, especially hepatic decompensation. Discontinuation of lamivudine should be considered as medically appropriate. Discontinuation of interferon alpha, ribavirin, or both should also be considered if worsening clinical toxicities are observed, including hepatic decompensation (e.g., Childs Pugh greater than 6)).
No products indexed under this heading.

Interferon alfa-2b, Recombinant (Hepatic decompensation has occurred in HIV/HCV co-infected patients receiving combination antiretroviral therapy for HIV and interferon alpha with or withour ribavirin. Patients receiving interferon alpha with or without ribavirin and lamivudine should be closely monitored for treatment-associated toxicities, especially hepatic decompensation. Discontinuation of lamivudine should be considered as medically appropriate. Discontinuation of interferon alpha, ribavirin, or both should also be considered if worsening clinical toxicities are observed, including hepatic decompensation (e.g., Childs Pugh greater than 6)). Products include:
Intron A for Injection 2859

Interferon alfa-N3 (Human Leukocyte Derived) (Hepatic decompensation has occurred in HIV/HCV co-infected patients receiving combination antiretroviral therapy for HIV and interferon alpha with or withour ribavirin. Patients receiving interferon alpha with or without ribavirin and lamivudine should be closely monitored for treatment-associated toxicities, especially hepatic decompensation. Discontinuation of lamivudine should be considered as medically appropriate. Discontinuation of interferon alpha, ribavirin, or both should also be considered if worsening clinical toxicities are observed, including hepatic decompensation (e.g., Childs Pugh greater than 6)). Products include:
Alferon N Injection 1726

Morphine Sulfate (Lamivudine is predominantly eliminated in the urine by active organic secretion; therefore, the possibility of interactions with other drugs whose main route of elimination is active renal secretion via the organic cationic transport system should be considered). Products include:
Avinza Capsules 1772
DepoDur Injection 1095
MS Contin Tablets 2585

Peginterferon Alfa-2b (Hepatic decompensation has occurred in HIV/HCV co-infected patients receiving combination antiretroviral therapy for HIV and interferon alpha with or withour ribavirin. Patients receiving interferon alpha with or without ribavirin and lamivudine should be closely monitored for treatment-associated toxicities, especially hepatic decompensation. Discontinuation of lamivudine should be considered as medically appropriate. Discontinuation of interferon alpha, ribavirin, or both should also be considered if worsening clinical toxicities are observed, including hepatic decompensation (e.g., Childs Pugh greater than 6)). Products include:
PegIntron Powder for Injection 2903

Procainamide Hydrochloride (Lamivudine is predominantly eliminated in the urine by active organic secretion; therefore, the possibility of interactions with other drugs whose main route of elimination is active renal secretion via the organic cationic transport system should be considered).
No products indexed under this heading.

Quinidine Gluconate (Lamivudine is predominantly eliminated in the urine by active organic secretion; therefore, the possibility of interactions with other drugs whose main route of elimination is active renal secretion via the organic cationic transport system should be considered).
No products indexed under this heading.

Quinidine Polygalacturonate (Lamivudine is predominantly eliminated in the urine by active organic secretion; therefore, the possibility of interactions with other drugs whose main route of elimination is active renal secretion via the organic cationic transport system should be considered).
No products indexed under this heading.

Quinidine Sulfate (Lamivudine is predominantly eliminated in the urine by active organic secretion; therefore, the possibility of interactions with other drugs whose main route of elimination is active renal secretion via the organic cationic transport system should be considered).
No products indexed under this heading.

Quinine Sulfate (Lamivudine is predominantly eliminated in the urine by active organic secretion; therefore, the possibility of interactions with other drugs whose main route of elimination is active renal secretion via the organic cationic transport system should be considered).
No products indexed under this heading.

Ranitidine Hydrochloride (Lamivudine is predominantly eliminated in the urine by active organic secretion; therefore, the possibility of interactions with other drugs whose main route of elimination is active renal secretion via the organic cationic transport system should be considered). Products include:
Zantac 75 Tablets .... ▣ 603
Zantac 1670
Zantac Injection 1666
Zantac Injection Pharmacy Bulk Package 1668
Maximum Strength Zantac 150 Tablets .... ▣ 603
Maximum Strength Zantac 150 Cool Mint Tablets .... ▣ 603

Sulfamethoxazole (Co-administration of lamivudine with 160 mg of trimethoprim and 800 mg of sulfamethoxazole once daily has been shown to increase lamivudine exposure (AUC); the effect of higher doses of TMP/SMX on lamivudine pharmacokinetics has not been investigated; no change in dose of either drug is recommended).
No products indexed under this heading.

Triamterene (Lamivudine is predominantly eliminated in the urine by active organic secretion; therefore,

IMPORTANT NOTE: Always consult each drug listing in the patient's regimen for possible interactions.

the possibility of interactions with other drugs whose main route of elimination is active renal secretion via the organic cationic transport system should be considered). Products include:

Dyazide Capsules 1405
Dyrenium Capsules 3189

Trimethoprim (Co-administration of lamivudine with 160 mg of trimethoprim and 800 mg of sulfamethoxazole once daily has been shown to increase lamivudine exposure (AUC); the effect of higher doses of TMP/SMX on lamivudine pharmacokinetics has not been investigated; no change in dose of either drug is recommended).
No products indexed under this heading.

Trimethoprim Sulfate (Lamivudine is predominantly eliminated in the urine by active organic secretion; therefore, the possibility of interactions with other drugs whose main route of elimination is active renal secretion via the organic cationic transport system should be considered).
No products indexed under this heading.

Vancomycin Hydrochloride (Lamivudine is predominantly eliminated in the urine by active organic secretion; therefore, the possibility of interactions with other drugs whose main route of elimination is active renal secretion via the organic cationic transport system should be considered).
No products indexed under this heading.

Zalcitabine (Lamivudine and zalcitabine may inhibit the intracellular phosphorylation of one another; concurrent use is not recommended).
No products indexed under this heading.

Food Interactions

Food, unspecified (Absorption of lamivudine was slower in the fed state compared with fasted state; there was no significant difference in systemic exposure in the fed state and fasted states; Epivir may be given with or without food).

EPIVIR-HBV ORAL SOLUTION

(Lamivudine) 1417
See Epivir-HBV Tablets

EPIVIR-HBV TABLETS

(Lamivudine) 1417
May interact with cationic drugs that are eliminated by renal tubular and certain other agents. Compounds in these categories include:

Amiloride Hydrochloride (Lamivudine is predominantly eliminated in the urine by active organic secretion; therefore, the possibility of interactions with other drugs whose main route of elimination is active renal secretion via the organic cationic transport system should be considered).
No products indexed under this heading.

Digoxin (Lamivudine is predominantly eliminated in the urine by active organic secretion; therefore, the possibility of interactions with other drugs whose main route of elimination is active renal secretion via the organic cationic transport system should be considered). Products include:

Lanoxin Injection 1498
Lanoxin Injection Pediatric 1502
Lanoxin Tablets 1505

Morphine Sulfate (Lamivudine is predominantly eliminated in the urine by active organic secretion; therefore, the possibility of interactions with other drugs whose main route of elimination is active renal secretion via the organic cationic transport system should be considered). Products include:

Avinza Capsules 1772
DepoDur Injection 1095
MS Contin Tablets 2585

Procainamide Hydrochloride (Lamivudine is predominantly eliminated in the urine by active organic secretion; therefore, the possibility of interactions with other drugs whose main route of elimination is active renal secretion via the organic cationic transport system should be considered).
No products indexed under this heading.

Quinidine Gluconate (Lamivudine is predominantly eliminated in the urine by active organic secretion; therefore, the possibility of interactions with other drugs whose main route of elimination is active renal secretion via the organic cationic transport system should be considered).
No products indexed under this heading.

Quinidine Polygalacturonate (Lamivudine is predominantly eliminated in the urine by active organic secretion; therefore, the possibility of interactions with other drugs whose main route of elimination is active renal secretion via the organic cationic transport system should be considered).
No products indexed under this heading.

Quinidine Sulfate (Lamivudine is predominantly eliminated in the urine by active organic secretion; therefore, the possibility of interactions with other drugs whose main route of elimination is active renal secretion via the organic cationic transport system should be considered).
No products indexed under this heading.

Quinine Sulfate (Lamivudine is predominantly eliminated in the urine by active organic secretion; therefore, the possibility of interactions with other drugs whose main route of elimination is active renal secretion via the organic cationic transport system should be considered).
No products indexed under this heading.

Ranitidine Hydrochloride (Lamivudine is predominantly eliminated in the urine by active organic secretion; therefore, the possibility of interactions with other drugs whose main route of elimination is active renal secretion via the organic cationic transport system should be considered). Products include:

Zantac 75 Tablets .... ▣603
Zantac 1670
Zantac Injection 1666
Zantac Injection Pharmacy Bulk Package 1668
Maximum Strength Zantac 150 Tablets .... ▣603
Maximum Strength Zantac 150 Cool Mint Tablets .... ▣603

Sulfamethoxazole (Co-administration of lamivudine with 160 mg of trimethoprim and 800 mg of sulfamethoxazole once daily has been shown to increase lamivudine exposure (AUC); the effect of higher doses of TMP/SMX on lamivudine pharmacokinetics has not been investigated; no change in dose of either drug is recommended).
No products indexed under this heading.

Triamterene (Lamivudine is predominantly eliminated in the urine by active organic secretion; therefore, the possibility of interactions with other drugs whose main route of elimination is active renal secretion via the organic cationic transport system should be considered). Products include:

Dyazide Capsules 1405
Dyrenium Capsules 3189

Trimethoprim (Co-administration of lamivudine with 160 mg of trimethoprim and 800 mg of sulfamethoxazole once daily has been shown to increase lamivudine exposure (AUC); the effect of higher doses of TMP/SMX on lamivudine pharmacokinetics has not been investigated; no change in dose of either drug is recommended).
No products indexed under this heading.

Trimethoprim Sulfate (Lamivudine is predominantly eliminated in the urine by active organic secretion; therefore, the possibility of interactions with other drugs whose main route of elimination is active renal secretion via the organic cationic transport system should be considered).
No products indexed under this heading.

Vancomycin Hydrochloride (Lamivudine is predominantly eliminated in the urine by active organic secretion; therefore, the possibility of interactions with other drugs whose main route of elimination is active renal secretion via the organic cationic transport system should be considered).
No products indexed under this heading.

Zalcitabine (Lamivudine and zalcitabine may inhibit the intracellular phosphorylation of one another; co-administration is not recommended).
No products indexed under this heading.

EPOGEN FOR INJECTION

(Epoetin Alfa) 576
None cited in PDR database.

EPZICOM TABLETS

(Abacavir Sulfate, Lamivudine) 1422
May interact with Interferon alpha and certain other agents. Compounds in these categories include:

Ethanol (Ethanol decreased the elimination of abacavir causing an increase in overall exposure).
No products indexed under this heading.

Interferon alfa-2a, Recombinant (Hepatic decompensation has occurred in HIV/HCV co-infected patients receiving combination antiretroviral therapy for HIV and interferon alpha with or without ribavirin. Patients receiving interferon alpha with or without ribavirin and Epzicom should be closely monitored for treatment-associated toxicities, especially hepatic decompensation. Discontinuation of Epzicom should be considered as medically appropriate. Discontinuation of interferon alpha, ribavirin, or both should also be considered if worsening clinical toxicities are observed, including hepatic decompensation (e.g., Childs Pugh greater than 6)).
No products indexed under this heading.

Interferon alfa-2b, Recombinant (Hepatic decompensation has occurred in HIV/HCV co-infected patients receiving combination antiretroviral therapy for HIV and interferon alpha with or without ribavirin. Patients receiving interferon alpha with or without ribavirin and Epzicom should be closely monitored for treatment-associated toxicities, especially hepatic decompensation. Discontinuation of Epzicom should be considered as medically appropriate. Discontinuation of interferon alpha, ribavirin, or both should also be considered if worsening clinical toxicities are observed, including hepatic decompensation (e.g., Childs Pugh greater than 6)). Products include:

Intron A for Injection 2859

Interferon alfa-N3 (Human Leukocyte Derived) (Hepatic decompensation has occurred in HIV/HCV co-infected patients receiving combination antiretroviral therapy for HIV and interferon alpha with or without ribavirin. Patients receiving interferon alpha with or without ribavirin and Epzicom should be closely monitored for treatment-associated toxicities, especially hepatic decompensation. Discontinuation of Epzicom should be considered as medically appropriate. Discontinuation of interferon alpha, ribavirin, or both should also be considered if worsening clinical toxicities are observed, including hepatic decompensation (e.g., Childs Pugh greater than 6)). Products include:

Alferon N Injection 1726

Methadone Hydrochloride (Co-administration in patients on methadone-maintenance therapy had increased methadone clearance by 22%. This alteration will not result in a methadone dose modification in the majority of patients; however, an increased methadone dose may be required in a small number of patients).
No products indexed under this heading.

Nelfinavir Mesylate (Co-administration of lamivudine with nelfinavir has been shown to increase the AUC of lamivudine by 10%).
No products indexed under this heading.

Peginterferon Alfa-2b (Hepatic decompensation has occurred in HIV/HCV co-infected patients receiving combination antiretroviral therapy for HIV and interferon alpha with or without ribavirin. Patients receiving interferon alpha with or without ribavirin and Epzicom should be closely monitored for treatment-associated toxicities, especially hepatic decompensation. Discontinuation of Epzicom should be considered as medically appropriate. Discontinuation of interferon alpha, ribavirin, or both should also be considered if worsening clinical toxicities are observed, including hepatic decompensation (e.g., Childs Pugh greater than 6)). Products include:

PegIntron Powder for Injection 2903

Sulfamethoxazole (Co-administration of lamivudine with 160mg of trimethoprim and 800mg of sulfamethoxazole once daily has been shown to increase lamivudine exposure (AUC). The effect of higher doses of TMP/SMX on lamivudine pharmacokinetics has not been investigated; no change in dose of either drug is recommended).

No products indexed under this heading.

Trimethoprim (Co-administration of lamivudine with 160mg of trimethoprim and 800mg of sulfamethoxazole once daily has been shown to increase lamivudine exposure (AUC). The effect of higher doses of TMP/SMX on lamivudine pharmacokinetics has not been investigated; no change in dose of either drug is recommended).

No products indexed under this heading.

Zalcitabine (Lamivudine and zalcitabine may inhibit the intracellular phosphorylation of one another; concurrent use is not recommended).

No products indexed under this heading.

EQUETRO EXTENDED-RELEASE CAPSULES

(Carbamazepine) 3174

May interact with antimalarials, central nervous system depressants, cytochrome p450 1a2 substrates (selected), cytochrome p450 3a4 inducers (selected), cytochrome p450 3a4 inhibitors (selected), cytochrome p450 3a4 substrates (selected), monoamine oxidase inhibitors, oral contraceptives, phenytoin, tricyclic antidepressants, and certain other agents. Compounds in these categories include:

Acetaminophen (Carbamazepine is known to induce CYP1A2 and CYP3A4. Therefore, the potential exists for interaction between carbamazepine and any agent metabolized by one (or more) of these enzymes. Agents that are metabolized by CYP1A2 and CYP3A4 may have decreased plasma levels when administered concomitantly with carbamazepine. Thus, if a patient has been titrated to a stable dosage on one of the agents in these categories, and then begins a course of treatment with carbamazepine, it is reasonable to expect that a dose increase for the concomitant agent may be necessary). Products include:

Benadryl Allergy & Cold Kapgels 1895
Benadryl Allergy & Sinus Headache Kapgels 1895
Benadryl Severe Allergy & Sinus Headache Caplets 1897
Lortab 5/500 Tablets 3143
Lortab 7.5/500 Tablets 3144
Lortab 10/500 Tablets 3144
Percocet Tablets 1127
Sinutab Sinus Caplets 1905
Sudafed PE Cold & Cough Caplets 1907
Sudafed PE Nighttime Cold Caplets 1907
Sudafed PE Severe Cold Caplets 1908
Sudafed PE Sinus Headache Caplets 1908
Regular Strength Tylenol Tablets 1915
Tylenol 8 Hour Extended Release Caplets 1915
Extra Strength Tylenol Caplets, Cool Caplets, and EZ Tabs 1915
Extra Strength Tylenol Adult Rapid Blast Liquid 1915
Extra Strength Tylenol PM Caplets, Geltabs, Liquid, and Rapid Release Gels 1915
Extra Strength Tylenol Rapid Release Gels 1915
Tylenol with Codeine Tablets 2427
Tylenol Allergy Multi-Symptom Caplets with Cool Burst and Rapid Release Gelcaps 1916
Tylenol Allergy Multi-Symptom Nighttime Caplets with Cool Burst 1916
Tylenol Severe Allergy Caplets 1916
Tylenol Arthritis Pain Extended Release Geltabs/Caplets 1915
Tylenol Chest Congestion Caplets with Cool Burst 1910
Tylenol Chest Congestion Liquid with Cool Burst 1910
Children's Tylenol Plus Cold Suspension Liquid 1912
Children's Tylenol Plus Cold & Allergy Suspension Liquid 1914
Children's Tylenol Plus Cough & Runny Nose Suspension Liquid 1912
Children's Tylenol Plus Cough & Sore Throat Suspension Liquid 1912
Children's Tylenol Plus Flu Suspension Liquid 1914
Children's Tylenol Suspension Liquid 1909
Children's Tylenol Meltaways 1909
Children's Tylenol Plus Multi-Symptom Cold Suspension Liquid 1912
Tylenol Cold Severe Congestion Daytime Caplets with Cool Burst 1912
Tylenol Cold Head Congestion Daytime Caplets with Cool Burst 1910
Tylenol Cold Head Congestion Nighttime Caplets with Cool Burst 1910
Tylenol Cold Head Congestion Severe Daytime Caplets with Cool Burst 1910
Tylenol Cold Multi-Symptom Daytime Caplets with Cool Burst and Rapid Release Gels 1913
Tylenol Cold Multi-Symptom Daytime Liquid with Citrus Burst ... 1913
Tylenol Cold Multi-Symptom Nighttime Caplets with Cool Burst 1913
Tylenol Cold Multi-Symptom Nighttime Liquid with Cool Burst ... 1913
Tylenol Cold Multi-Symptom Severe Caplets with Cool Burst 1913
Tylenol Cold Multi-Symptom Severe Daytime Liquid with Citrus Burst 1913
Tylenol Cough & Sore Throat Daytime Liquid with Cool Burst 1918
Tylenol Cough & Sore Throat Nighttime Liquid with Cool Burst ... 1918
Concentrated Tylenol Infants' Drops 1909
Jr. Tylenol Meltaways 1909
Tylenol Sinus Congestion & Pain Daytime Caplets with Cool Burst and Gelcaps 1917
Tylenol Sinus Congestion & Pain Nighttime Caplets with Cool Burst 1917
Tylenol Sinus Congestion & Pain Severe Caplets with Cool Burst 1917
Tylenol Sinus Severe Congestion Caplets with Cool Burst 1917
Tylenol Sore Throat Daytime Liquid with Cool Burst 1918
Tylenol Sore Throat Nighttime Liquid with Cool Burst 1918
Women's Tylenol Menstrual Relief Caplets 1919
Vicks DayQuil Cold & Flu Multi-Symptom Relief 616
Vicks DayQuil LiquiCaps 2567
Vicks DayQuil Liquid 2567
Vicks DayQuil Multi-Symptom Cold/Flu Relief 2567
Vicks NyQuil Cold & Flu Multi-Symptom Relief 617
Vicks NyQuil LiquiCaps 2567
Vicks NyQuil Liquid 2567
Vicks NyQuil Multi-Symptom Cold/Flu Relief 2567
Vicodin Tablets 529
Vicodin ES Tablets 530
Vicodin HP Tablets 531
Zydone Tablets 1132

Acetazolamide (Carbamazepine is metabolized mainly by CYP3A4 the active carbamazepine 10,11-epoxide, which is futher metabolized to the trans-diol by epoxide hydrolase. Therefore, the potential exists for interaction between carbamazepine and any agent that inhibits CYP3A4 and/or epoxide hydrolase. Agents that are CYP3A4 inhibitors may increase the plasma levels of carbamazepine. Thus, if a patient has been titrated to a stable dosage of carbamazepine, and then begins a course of treatment with a CYP3A4 or epoxide hydrolase inhibitor, it is reasonable to expect that a dose reduction for carbamazepine may be necessary).

No products indexed under this heading.

Alatrofloxacin Mesylate (Carbamazepine is known to induce CYP1A2 and CYP3A4. Therefore, the potential exists for interaction between carbamazepine and any agent metabolized by one (or more) of these enzymes. Agents that are metabolized by CYP1A2 and CYP3A4 may have decreased plasma levels when administered concomitantly with carbamazepine. Thus, if a patient has been titrated to a stable dosage on one of the agents in these categories, and then begins a course of treatment with carbamazepine, it is reasonable to expect that a dose increase for the concomitant agent may be necessary).

No products indexed under this heading.

Alfentanil Hydrochloride (Because of its primary CNS effect, caution should be used when carbamazepine is taken with other centrally-acting drugs).

No products indexed under this heading.

Allium sativum (Carbamazepine is metabolized by CYP3A4. Therefore, the potential exists for interaction between carbamazepine and any agent that induces CYP3A4. Agents that are CYP3A4 inducers may decrease plasma levels of carbamazepine. Thus, if a patient has been titrated to a stable dosage on carbamazepine, and then begins a course of treatment with a CYP3A4 inducers, it is reasonable to expect that a dose increase for carbamazepine may be necessary).

No products indexed under this heading.

Alprazolam (Because of its primary CNS effect, caution should be used when carbamazepine is taken with other centrally-acting drugs).

No products indexed under this heading.

Amiodarone Hydrochloride (Carbamazepine is metabolized mainly by CYP3A4 the active carbamazepine 10,11-epoxide, which is futher metabolized to the trans-diol by epoxide hydrolase. Therefore, the potential exists for interaction between carbamazepine and any agent that inhibits CYP3A4 and/or epoxide hydrolase. Agents that are CYP3A4 inhibitors may increase the plasma levels of carbamazepine. Thus, if a patient has been titrated to a stable dosage of carbamazepine, and then begins a course of treatment with a CYP3A4 or epoxide hydrolase inhibitor, it is reasonable to expect that a dose reduction for carbamazepine may be necessary).

No products indexed under this heading.

Amitriptyline Hydrochloride (Use is not recommended if known sensitivity to any of the tricyclic compounds).

No products indexed under this heading.

Amlodipine Besylate (Carbamazepine is known to induce CYP1A2 and CYP3A4. Therefore, the potential exists for interaction between carbamazepine and any agent metabolized by one (or more) of these enzymes. Agents that are metabolized by CYP1A2 and CYP3A4 may have decreased plasma levels when administered concomitantly with carbamazepine. Thus, if a patient has been titrated to a stable dosage on one of the agents in these categories, and then begins a course of treatment with carbamazepine, it is reasonable to expect that a dose increase for the concomitant agent may be necessary). Products include:

Azor Tablets 1005
Exforge Tablets 2238

Amoxapine (Use is not recommended if known sensitivity to any of the tricyclic compounds).

No products indexed under this heading.

Amprenavir (Carbamazepine is metabolized mainly by CYP3A4 the active carbamazepine 10,11-epoxide, which is futher metabolized to the trans-diol by epoxide hydrolase. Therefore, the potential exists for interaction between carbamazepine and any agent that inhibits CYP3A4 and/or epoxide hydrolase. Agents that are CYP3A4 inhibitors may increase the plasma levels of carbamazepine. Thus, if a patient has been titrated to a stable dosage of carbamazepine, and then begins a course of treatment with a CYP3A4 or epoxide hydrolase inhibitor, it is reasonable to expect that a dose reduction for carbamazepine may be necessary).

No products indexed under this heading.

Anagrelide Hydrochloride (Carbamazepine is known to induce CYP1A2 and CYP3A4. Therefore, the potential exists for interaction between carbamazepine and any agent metabolized by one (or more) of these enzymes. Agents that are metabolized by CYP1A2 and CYP3A4 may have decreased plasma levels when administered concomitantly with carbamazepine. Thus, if a patient has been titrated to a stable dosage on one of the agents in these categories, and then begins a course of treatment with carbamazepine, it is reasonable to expect that a dose increase for the concomitant agent may be necessary). Products include:

Agrylin Capsules 3017

Anastrozole (Carbamazepine is metabolized mainly by CYP3A4 the active carbamazepine 10,11-epoxide, which is futher metabolized to the trans-diol by epoxide hydrolase. Therefore, the potential exists for interaction between carbamazepine and any agent that inhibits CYP3A4 and/or epoxide hydrolase. Agents that are CYP3A4 inhibitors may increase the plasma levels of carbamazepine. Thus, if a patient has been titrated to a stable dosage of carbamazepine, and then begins a course of treatment with a CYP3A4 or epoxide hydrolase inhibitor, it is reasonable to expect that a dose reduction for carbamazepine may be necessary). Products include:

Arimidex Tablets 672

Aprepitant (Carbamazepine is metabolized mainly by CYP3A4 the active carbamazepine 10,11-epoxide, which is futher metabolized to the trans-diol by epoxide hydrolase. Therefore, the potential exists for interaction between carbamazepine and any agent that inhibits CYP3A4 and/or epoxide hydrolase. Agents that are CYP3A4 inhibitors may increase the plasma levels of carbamazepine. Thus, if a patient has been titrated to a stable dosage of carbamazepine, and then begins a course of treatment with a CYP3A4 or epoxide hydrolase inhibitor, it is reasonable to expect that a dose reduction for carbamazepine may be necessary). Products include:

Emend Capsules 1992

Aprobarbital (Because of its primary CNS effect, caution should be used when carbamazepine is taken with other centrally-acting drugs).

No products indexed under this heading.

Astemizole (Carbamazepine is known to induce CYP1A2 and CYP3A4. Therefore, the potential exists for interaction between carbamazepine and any agent metabolized by one (or more) of these enzymes. Agents that are metabolized by CYP1A2 and CYP3A4 may have decreased plasma levels when administered concomitantly with carbamazepine. Thus, if a patient has been titrated to a stable dosage on one of the agents in these categories, and then begins a course of treatment with carbamazepine, it is reasonable to expect that a dose increase for the concomitant agent may be necessary).

No products indexed under this heading.

Atazanavir (Carbamazepine is metabolized mainly by CYP3A4 the active carbamazepine 10,11-epoxide, which is futher metabolized to the trans-diol by epoxide hydrolase. Therefore, the potential exists for interaction between carbamazepine and any agent that inhibits CYP3A4 and/or epoxide hydrolase. Agents that are CYP3A4 inhibitors may increase the plasma levels of carbamazepine. Thus, if a patient has been titrated to a stable dosage of carbamazepine, and then begins a course of treatment with a CYP3A4 or epoxide hydrolase inhibitor, it is reasonable to expect that a dose reduction for carbamazepine may be necessary).

No products indexed under this heading.

Atazanavir Sulfate (Carbamazepine is metabolized mainly by CYP3A4 the active carbamazepine 10,11-epoxide, which is futher metabolized to the trans-diol by epoxide hydrolase. Therefore, the potential exists for interaction between carbamazepine and any agent that inhibits CYP3A4 and/or epoxide hydrolase. Agents that are CYP3A4 inhibitors may increase the plasma levels of carbamazepine. Thus, if a patient has been titrated to a stable dosage of carbamazepine, and then begins a course of treatment with a CYP3A4 or epoxide hydrolase inhibitor, it is reasonable to expect that a dose reduction for carbamazepine may be necessary). Products include:

Reyataz Capsules 3299

Atorvastatin Calcium (Carbamazepine is known to induce CYP1A2 and CYP3A4. Therefore, the potential exists for interaction between carbamazepine and any agent metabolized by one (or more) of these enzymes. Agents that are metabolized by CYP1A2 and CYP3A4 may have decreased plasma levels when administered concomitantly with carbamazepine. Thus, if a patient has been titrated to a stable dosage on one of the agents in these categories, and then begins a course of treatment with carbamazepine, it is reasonable to expect that a dose increase for the concomitant agent may be necessary). Products include:

Lipitor Tablets 2501

Belladonna Ergotamine (Carbamazepine is known to induce CYP1A2 and CYP3A4. Therefore, the potential exists for interaction between carbamazepine and any agent metabolized by one (or more) of these enzymes. Agents that are metabolized by CYP1A2 and CYP3A4 may have decreased plasma levels when administered concomitantly with carbamazepine. Thus, if a patient has been titrated to a stable dosage on one of the agents in these categories, and then begins a course of treatment with carbamazepine, it is reasonable to expect that a dose increase for the concomitant agent may be necessary).

No products indexed under this heading.

Betamethasone Acetate (Carbamazepine is metabolized by CYP3A4. Therefore, the potential exists for interaction between carbamazepine and any agent that induces CYP3A4. Agents that are CYP3A4 inducers may decrease plasma levels of carbamazepine. Thus, if a patient has been titrated to a stable dosage on carbamazepine, and then begins a course of treatment with a CYP3A4 inducers, it is reasonable to expect that a dose increase for carbamazepine may be necessary).

No products indexed under this heading.

Betamethasone Sodium Phosphate (Carbamazepine is metabolized by CYP3A4. Therefore, the potential exists for interaction between carbamazepine and any agent that induces CYP3A4. Agents that are CYP3A4 inducers may decrease plasma levels of carbamazepine. Thus, if a patient has been titrated to a stable dosage on carbamazepine, and then begins a course of treatment with a CYP3A4 inducers, it is reasonable to expect that a dose increase for carbamazepine may be necessary).

No products indexed under this heading.

Buprenorphine Hydrochloride (Because of its primary CNS effect, caution should be used when carbamazepine is taken with other centrally-acting drugs). Products include:

Suboxone Tablets 2601
Subutex Tablets 2601

Buspirone Hydrochloride (Because of its primary CNS effect, caution should be used when carbamazepine is taken with other centrally-acting drugs).

No products indexed under this heading.

Busulfan (Carbamazepine is known to induce CYP1A2 and CYP3A4. Therefore, the potential exists for interaction between carbamazepine and any agent metabolized by one (or more) of these enzymes. Agents that are metabolized by CYP1A2 and CYP3A4 may have decreased plasma levels when administered concomitantly with carbamazepine. Thus, if a patient has been titrated to a stable dosage on one of the agents in these categories, and then begins a course of treatment with carbamazepine, it is reasonable to expect that a dose increase for the concomitant agent may be necessary). Products include:

Busulfex Injection 2477
Myleran Tablets 1530

Butabarbital (Because of its primary CNS effect, caution should be used when carbamazepine is taken with other centrally-acting drugs).

No products indexed under this heading.

Butalbital (Because of its primary CNS effect, caution should be used when carbamazepine is taken with other centrally-acting drugs).

No products indexed under this heading.

Caffeine (Carbamazepine is known to induce CYP1A2 and CYP3A4. Therefore, the potential exists for interaction between carbamazepine and any agent metabolized by one (or more) of these enzymes. Agents that are metabolized by CYP1A2 and CYP3A4 may have decreased plasma levels when administered concomitantly with carbamazepine. Thus, if a patient has been titrated to a stable dosage on one of the agents in these categories, and then begins a course of treatment with carbamazepine, it is reasonable to expect that a dose increase for the concomitant agent may be necessary). Products include:

BioLean Free Tablets .... ■ 635
BioLean II Tablets .... ■ 635
Winrgy Dietary Supplement .... ■ 642

Caffeine Anhydrous (Carbamazepine is known to induce CYP1A2 and CYP3A4. Therefore, the potential exists for interaction between carbamazepine and any agent metabolized by one (or more) of these enzymes. Agents that are metabolized by CYP1A2 and CYP3A4 may have decreased plasma levels when administered concomitantly with carbamazepine. Thus, if a patient has been titrated to a stable dosage on one of the agents in these categories, and then begins a course of treatment with carbamazepine, it is reasonable to expect that a dose increase for the concomitant agent may be necessary).

No products indexed under this heading.

Cerivastatin Sodium (Carbamazepine is known to induce CYP1A2 and CYP3A4. Therefore, the potential exists for interaction between carbamazepine and any agent metabolized by one (or more) of these enzymes. Agents that are metabolized by CYP1A2 and CYP3A4 may have decreased plasma levels when administered concomitantly with carbamazepine. Thus, if a patient has been titrated to a stable dosage on one of the agents in these categories, and then begins a course of treatment with carbamazepine, it is reasonable to expect that a dose increase for the concomitant agent may be necessary).

No products indexed under this heading.

Chlordiazepoxide (Because of its primary CNS effect, caution should be used when carbamazepine is taken with other centrally-acting drugs).

No products indexed under this heading.

Chlordiazepoxide Hydrochloride (Because of its primary CNS effect, caution should be used when carbamazepine is taken with other centrally-acting drugs).

No products indexed under this heading.

Chloroquine Hydrochloride (Antimalarial drugs, such as chloroquine and mefloquine, may antagonize the activity of carbamazepine).

No products indexed under this heading.

Chloroquine Phosphate (Antimalarial drugs, such as chloroquine and mefloquine, may antagonize the activity of carbamazepine).

No products indexed under this heading.

Chlorpheniramine (Carbamazepine is known to induce CYP1A2 and CYP3A4. Therefore, the potential exists for interaction between carbamazepine and any agent metabolized by one (or more) of these enzymes. Agents that are metabolized by CYP1A2 and CYP3A4 may have decreased plasma levels when administered concomitantly with carbamazepine. Thus, if a patient has been titrated to a stable dosage on one of the agents in these categories, and then begins a course of treatment with carbamazepine, it is reasonable to expect that a dose increase for the concomitant agent may be necessary).

No products indexed under this heading.

Chlorpheniramine Maleate (Carbamazepine is known to induce CYP1A2 and CYP3A4. Therefore, the potential exists for interaction between carbamazepine and any agent metabolized by one (or more) of these enzymes. Agents that are metabolized by CYP1A2 and CYP3A4 may have decreased plasma levels when administered concomitantly with carbamazepine. Thus, if a patient has been titrated to a stable dosage on one of the agents in these categories, and then begins a course of treatment with carbamazepine, it is reasonable to expect that a dose increase for the concomitant agent may be necessary). Products include:

Actifed Cold & Allergy Tablets 1895
Sudafed PE Sinus & Allergy Tablets 1908
Tylenol Allergy Multi-Symptom Caplets with Cool Burst and Rapid Release Gelcaps 1916
Children's Tylenol Plus Cold Suspension Liquid 1912
Children's Tylenol Plus Cough & Runny Nose Suspension Liquid 1912
Children's Tylenol Plus Flu Suspension Liquid 1914
Children's Tylenol Plus Multi-Symptom Cold Suspension Liquid 1912
Tylenol Cold Head Congestion Nighttime Caplets with Cool Burst 1910
Tylenol Cold Multi-Symptom Nighttime Caplets with Cool Burst 1913
Tylenol Sinus Congestion & Pain Nighttime Caplets with Cool Burst 1917

Chlorpheniramine Polistirex (Carbamazepine is known to induce CYP1A2 and CYP3A4. Therefore, the potential exists for interaction between carbamazepine and any agent metabolized by one (or more) of these enzymes. Agents that are metabolized by CYP1A2 and CYP3A4 may have decreased plasma levels when administered concomitantly with carbamazepine. Thus, if a patient has been titrated to a stable dosage on one of the agents in these categories, and then begins a course of treatment with carbamazepine, it is reasonable to expect that a dose increase for the concomitant agent may be necessary). Products include:

Tussionex Pennkinetic Extended-Release Suspension 3154

Chlorpheniramine Tannate (Carbamazepine is known to induce CYP1A2 and CYP3A4. Therefore, the potential exists for interaction between carbamazepine and any agent metabolized by one (or more) of these enzymes. Agents that are metabolized by CYP1A2 and CYP3A4 may have decreased plasma levels when administered concomitantly with carbamazepine. Thus, if a patient has been titrated to a stable dosage on one of the agents in these categories, and then begins a course of treatment with carbamazepine, it is reasonable to expect that a dose increase for the concomitant agent may be necessary).

No products indexed under this heading.

Chlorpromazine (Because of its primary CNS effect, caution should be used when carbamazepine is taken with other centrally-acting drugs).

No products indexed under this heading.

Chlorpromazine Hydrochloride (Because of its primary CNS effect, caution should be used when carbamazepine is taken with other centrally-acting drugs).

No products indexed under this heading.

Chlorprothixene (Because of its primary CNS effect, caution should be used when carbamazepine is taken with other centrally-acting drugs).

No products indexed under this heading.

Chlorprothixene Hydrochloride (Because of its primary CNS effect, caution should be used when carbamazepine is taken with other centrally-acting drugs).

No products indexed under this heading.

Chlorprothixene Lactate (Because of its primary CNS effect, caution should be used when carbamazepine is taken with other centrally-acting drugs).

No products indexed under this heading.

Cimetidine (Carbamazepine is metabolized mainly by CYP3A4 the active carbamazepine 10,11-epoxide, which is futher metabolized to the trans-diol by epoxide hydrolase. Therefore, the potential exists for interaction between carbamazepine and any agent that inhibits CYP3A4 and/or epoxide hydrolase. Agents that are CYP3A4 inhibitors may increase the plasma levels of carbamazepine. Thus, if a patient has been titrated to a stable dosage of carbamazepine, and then begins a course of treatment with a CYP3A4 or epoxide hydrolase inhibitor, it is reasonable to expect that a dose reduction for carbamazepine may be necessary).

No products indexed under this heading.

Cimetidine Hydrochloride (Carbamazepine is metabolized mainly by CYP3A4 the active carbamazepine 10,11-epoxide, which is futher metabolized to the trans-diol by epoxide hydrolase. Therefore, the potential exists for interaction between carbamazepine and any agent that inhibits CYP3A4 and/or epoxide hydrolase. Agents that are CYP3A4 inhibitors may increase the plasma levels of carbamazepine. Thus, if a patient has been titrated to a stable dosage of carbamazepine, and then begins a course of treatment with a CYP3A4 or epoxide hydrolase inhibitor, it is reasonable to expect that a dose reduction for carbamazepine may be necessary).

No products indexed under this heading.

Ciprofloxacin (Carbamazepine is metabolized mainly by CYP3A4 the active carbamazepine 10,11-epoxide, which is futher metabolized to the trans-diol by epoxide hydrolase. Therefore, the potential exists for interaction between carbamazepine and any agent that inhibits CYP3A4 and/or epoxide hydrolase. Agents that are CYP3A4 inhibitors may increase the plasma levels of carbamazepine. Thus, if a patient has been titrated to a stable dosage of carbamazepine, and then begins a course of treatment with a CYP3A4 or epoxide hydrolase inhibitor, it is reasonable to expect that a dose reduction for carbamazepine may be necessary). Products include:

Cipro I.V. 2817
Cipro Oral Suspension 2810
Cipro XR Tablets 2823
Ciprodex Otic Suspension 541

Ciprofloxacin Hydrochloride (Carbamazepine is metabolized by CYP3A4. Therefore, the potential exists for interaction between carbamazepine and any agent that induces CYP3A4. Agents that are CYP3A4 inducers may decrease plasma levels of carbamazepine. Thus, if a patient has been titrated to a stable dosage on carbamazepine, and then begins a course of treatment with a CYP3A4 inducers, it is reasonable to expect that a dose increase for carbamazepine may be necessary). Products include:

Cipro Tablets 2810

Cisapride (Carbamazepine is known to induce CYP1A2 and CYP3A4. Therefore, the potential exists for interaction between carbamazepine and any agent metabolized by one (or more) of these enzymes. Agents that are metabolized by CYP1A2 and CYP3A4 may have decreased plasma levels when administered concomitantly with carbamazepine. Thus, if a patient has been titrated to a stable dosage on one of the agents in these categories, and then begins a course of treatment with carbamazepine, it is reasonable to expect that a dose increase for the concomitant agent may be necessary).

No products indexed under this heading.

Cisplatin (Carbamazepine is metabolized by CYP3A4. Therefore, the potential exists for interaction between carbamazepine and any agent that induces CYP3A4. Agents that are CYP3A4 inducers may decrease plasma levels of carbamazepine. Thus, if a patient has been titrated to a stable dosage on carbamazepine, and then begins a course of treatment with a CYP3A4 inducers, it is reasonable to expect that a dose increase for carbamazepine may be necessary).

No products indexed under this heading.

Clarithromycin (Carbamazepine is metabolized mainly by CYP3A4 the active carbamazepine 10,11-epoxide, which is futher metabolized to the trans-diol by epoxide hydrolase. Therefore, the potential exists for interaction between carbamazepine and any agent that inhibits CYP3A4 and/or epoxide hydrolase. Agents that are CYP3A4 inhibitors may increase the plasma levels of carbamazepine. Thus, if a patient has been titrated to a stable dosage of carbamazepine, and then begins a course of treatment with a CYP3A4 or epoxide hydrolase inhibitor, it is reasonable to expect that a dose reduction for carbamazepine may be necessary). Products include:

Biaxin/Biaxin XL 411

Clomipramine Hydrochloride (Carbamazepine increases the plasma levels of clomipramine HCl).

No products indexed under this heading.

Clopidogrel Bisulfate (Carbamazepine is known to induce CYP1A2 and CYP3A4. Therefore, the potential exists for interaction between carbamazepine and any agent metabolized by one (or more) of these enzymes. Agents that are metabolized by CYP1A2 and CYP3A4 may have decreased plasma levels when administered concomitantly with carbamazepine. Thus, if a patient has been titrated to a stable dosage on one of the agents in these categories, and then begins a course of treatment with carbamazepine, it is reasonable to expect that a dose increase for the concomitant agent may be necessary). Products include:

Plavix Tablets 926
Plavix Tablets 2767

Clorazepate Dipotassium (Because of its primary CNS effect, caution should be used when carbamazepine is taken with other centrally-acting drugs).

No products indexed under this heading.

Clotrimazole (Carbamazepine is metabolized mainly by CYP3A4 the active carbamazepine 10,11-epoxide, which is futher metabolized to the trans-diol by epoxide hydrolase. Therefore, the potential exists for interaction between carbamazepine and any agent that inhibits CYP3A4 and/or epoxide hydrolase. Agents that are CYP3A4 inhibitors may increase the plasma levels of carbamazepine. Thus, if a patient has been titrated to a stable dosage of carbamazepine, and then begins a course of treatment with a CYP3A4 or epoxide hydrolase inhibitor, it is reasonable to expect that a dose reduction for carbamazepine may be necessary). Products include:

Lotrisone 2881

Clozapine (Because of its primary CNS effect, caution should be used when carbamazepine is taken with other centrally-acting drugs).

No products indexed under this heading.

Codeine Phosphate (Because of its primary CNS effect, caution should be used when carbamazepine is taken with other centrally-acting drugs). Products include:

Tylenol with Codeine Tablets 2427

Cortisone Acetate (Carbamazepine is metabolized by CYP3A4. Therefore, the potential exists for interaction between carbamazepine and any agent that induces CYP3A4. Agents that are CYP3A4 inducers may decrease plasma levels of carbamazepine. Thus, if a patient has been titrated to a stable dosage on carbamazepine, and then begins a course of treatment with a CYP3A4 inducers, it is reasonable to expect that a dose increase for carbamazepine may be necessary).

No products indexed under this heading.

Cyclobenzaprine (Carbamazepine is known to induce CYP1A2 and CYP3A4. Therefore, the potential exists for interaction between carbamazepine and any agent metabolized by one (or more) of these enzymes. Agents that are metabolized by CYP1A2 and CYP3A4 may have decreased plasma levels when administered concomitantly with carbamazepine. Thus, if a patient has been titrated to a stable dosage on one of the agents in these categories, and then begins a course of treatment with carbamazepine, it is reasonable to expect that a dose increase for the concomitant agent may be necessary).

No products indexed under this heading.

Cyclobenzaprine Hydrochloride (Carbamazepine is known to induce CYP1A2 and CYP3A4. Therefore, the potential exists for interaction between carbamazepine and any agent metabolized by one (or more) of these enzymes. Agents that are metabolized by CYP1A2 and CYP3A4 may have decreased plasma levels when administered concomitantly with carbamazepine. Thus, if a patient has been titrated to a stable dosage on one of the agents in these categories, and then begins a course of treatment with carbamazepine, it is reasonable to expect that a dose increase for the concomitant agent may be necessary). Products include:

Amrix Capsules 966

Cyclosporine (Carbamazepine is metabolized mainly by CYP3A4 the active carbamazepine 10,11-epoxide, which is futher metabolized to the trans-diol by epoxide hydrolase. Therefore, the potential exists for interaction between carbamazepine and any agent that inhibits CYP3A4 and/or epoxide hydrolase. Agents that are CYP3A4 inhibitors may increase the plasma levels of carbamazepine. Thus, if a patient has been titrated to a stable dosage of carbamazepine, and then begins a course of treatment with a CYP3A4 or epoxide hydrolase inhibitor, it is reasonable to expect that a dose reduction for carbamazepine may be necessary). Products include:

Gengraf Capsules 435
Neoral Oral Solution 2280
Neoral Soft Gelatin Capsules 2280
Restasis Ophthalmic Emulsion 557
Sandimmune 2296

Dalfopristin (Carbamazepine is metabolized mainly by CYP3A4 the active carbamazepine 10,11-epoxide, which is futher metabolized to the trans-diol by epoxide hydrolase. Therefore, the potential exists for interaction between carbamazepine and any agent that inhibits CYP3A4 and/or epoxide hydrolase. Agents that are CYP3A4 inhibitors may increase the plasma levels of carbamazepine. Thus, if a patient has been titrated to a stable dosage of carbamazepine, and then begins a course of treatment with a CYP3A4 or epoxide hydrolase inhibitor, it is reasonable to expect that a dose reduction for carbamazepine may be necessary).

No products indexed under this heading.

Danazol (Carbamazepine is metabolized mainly by CYP3A4 the active carbamazepine 10,11-epoxide, which is futher metabolized to the trans-diol by epoxide hydrolase. Therefore, the potential exists for interaction between carbamazepine and any agent that inhibits CYP3A4 and/or epoxide hydrolase. Agents that are CYP3A4 inhibitors may increase the plasma levels of carbamazepine. Thus, if a patient has been titrated to a stable dosage of carbamazepine, and then begins a course of treatment with a CYP3A4 or epoxide hydrolase inhibitor, it is reasonable to expect that a dose reduction for carbamazepine may be necessary).

No products indexed under this heading.

Delavirdine Mesylate (Carbamazepine is metabolized mainly by CYP3A4 the active carbamazepine 10,11-epoxide, which is futher metabolized to the trans-diol by epoxide hydrolase. Therefore, the potential exists for interaction between carbamazepine and any agent that inhibits CYP3A4 and/or epoxide hydrolase. Agents that are CYP3A4 inhibitors may increase the plasma levels of carbamazepine. Thus, if a patient has been titrated to a stable dosage of carbamazepine, and then begins a course of treatment with a CYP3A4 or epoxide hydrolase inhibitor, it is reasonable to expect that a dose reduction for carbamazepine may be necessary).

No products indexed under this heading.

Desflurane (Because of its primary CNS effect, caution should be used when carbamazepine is taken with other centrally-acting drugs).

No products indexed under this heading.

Desipramine Hydrochloride (Use is not recommended if known sensitivity to any of the tricyclic compounds).

No products indexed under this heading.

Desogestrel (Carbamazepine is known to induce CYP1A2 and CYP3A4. Therefore, the potential exists for interaction between carbamazepine and any agent metabolized by one (or more) of these enzymes. Agents that are metabolized by CYP1A2 or CYP3A4 may have decreased plasma levels when administered concomitantly with carbamazepine. Breakthrough bleeding has been reported among patients receiving concomitant oral contraceptives and their reliability may be adversely affected). Products include:

Mircette Tablets 1034

Dexamethasone (Carbamazepine is metabolized by CYP3A4. Therefore, the potential exists for interaction between carbamazepine and any agent that induces CYP3A4. Agents that are CYP3A4 inducers may decrease plasma levels of carbamazepine. Thus, if a patient has been titrated to a stable dosage on carbamazepine, and then begins a course of treatment with a CYP3A4 inducers, it is reasonable to expect that a dose increase for carbamazepine may be necessary). Products include:

Ciprodex Otic Suspension 541

Dexamethasone Acetate (Carbamazepine is metabolized by CYP3A4. Therefore, the potential exists for interaction between carbamazepine and any agent that induces CYP3A4. Agents that are CYP3A4 inducers may decrease plasma levels of carbamazepine. Thus, if a patient has been titrated to a stable dosage on carbamazepine, and then begins a course of treatment with a CYP3A4 inducers, it is reasonable to expect that a dose increase for carbamazepine may be necessary).

No products indexed under this heading.

Dexamethasone Sodium Phosphate (Carbamazepine is metabolized by CYP3A4. Therefore, the potential exists for interaction between carbamazepine and any agent that induces CYP3A4. Agents that are CYP3A4 inducers may decrease plasma levels of carbamazepine. Thus, if a patient has been titrated to a stable dosage on carbamazepine, and then begins a course of treatment with a CYP3A4 inducers, it is reasonable to expect that a dose increase for carbamazepine may be necessary).

No products indexed under this heading.

Dezocine (Because of its primary CNS effect, caution should be used when carbamazepine is taken with other centrally-acting drugs).

No products indexed under this heading.

Diazepam (Because of its primary CNS effect, caution should be used when carbamazepine is taken with other centrally-acting drugs). Products include:

Valium Tablets 2658

Dihydroergotamine Mesylate (Carbamazepine is known to induce CYP1A2 and CYP3A4. Therefore, the potential exists for interaction between carbamazepine and any agent metabolized by one (or more) of these enzymes. Agents that are metabolized by CYP1A2 and CYP3A4 may have decreased plasma levels when administered concomitantly with carbamazepine. Thus, if a patient has been titrated to a stable dosage on one of the agents in these categories, and then begins a course of treatment with carbamazepine, it is reasonable to expect that a dose increase for the concomitant agent may be necessary).

No products indexed under this heading.

Diltiazem Hydrochloride (Carbamazepine is metabolized mainly by CYP3A4 the active carbamazepine 10,11-epoxide, which is futher metabolized to the trans-diol by epoxide hydrolase. Therefore, the potential exists for interaction between carbamazepine and any agent that inhibits CYP3A4 and/or epoxide hydrolase. Agents that are CYP3A4 inhibitors may increase the plasma levels of carbamazepine. Thus, if a patient has been titrated to a stable dosage of carbamazepine, and then begins a course of treatment with a CYP3A4 or epoxide hydrolase inhibitor, it is reasonable to expect that a dose reduction for carbamazepine may be necessary). Products include:

Cardizem LA Extended Release Tablets 421

Diltiazem Maleate (Carbamazepine is metabolized mainly by CYP3A4 the active carbamazepine 10,11-epoxide, which is futher metabolized to the trans-diol by epoxide hydrolase. Therefore, the potential exists for interaction between carbamazepine and any agent that inhibits CYP3A4 and/or epoxide hydrolase. Agents that are CYP3A4 inhibitors may increase the plasma levels of carbamazepine. Thus, if a patient has been titrated to a stable dosage of carbamazepine, and then begins a course of treatment with a CYP3A4 or epoxide hydrolase inhibitor, it is reasonable to expect that a dose reduction for carbamazepine may be necessary).

No products indexed under this heading.

Disopyramide (Carbamazepine is known to induce CYP1A2 and CYP3A4. Therefore, the potential exists for interaction between carbamazepine and any agent metabolized by one (or more) of these enzymes. Agents that are metabolized by CYP1A2 and CYP3A4 may have decreased plasma levels when administered concomitantly with carbamazepine. Thus, if a patient has been titrated to a stable dosage on one of the agents in these categories, and then begins a course of treatment with carbamazepine, it is reasonable to expect that a dose increase for the concomitant agent may be necessary).

No products indexed under this heading.

Disopyramide Phosphate (Carbamazepine is known to induce CYP1A2 and CYP3A4. Therefore, the potential exists for interaction between carbamazepine and any agent metabolized by one (or more) of these enzymes. Agents that are metabolized by CYP1A2 and CYP3A4 may have decreased plasma levels when administered concomitantly with carbamazepine. Thus, if a patient has been titrated to a stable dosage on one of the agents in these categories, and then begins a course of treatment with carbamazepine, it is reasonable to expect that a dose increase for the concomitant agent may be necessary).

No products indexed under this heading.

Disulfiram (Carbamazepine is known to induce CYP1A2 and CYP3A4. Therefore, the potential exists for interaction between carbamazepine and any agent metabolized by one (or more) of these enzymes. Agents that are metabolized by CYP1A2 and CYP3A4 may have decreased plasma levels when administered concomitantly with carbamazepine. Thus, if a patient has been titrated to a stable dosage on one of the agents in these categories, and then begins a course of treatment with carbamazepine, it is reasonable to expect that a dose increase for the concomitant agent may be necessary).

No products indexed under this heading.

Doxepin Hydrochloride (Use is not recommended if known sensitivity to any of the tricyclic compounds).

No products indexed under this heading.

Doxorubicin Hydrochloride (Carbamazepine is metabolized by CYP3A4. Therefore, the potential exists for interaction between carbamazepine and any agent that induces CYP3A4. Agents that are CYP3A4 inducers may decrease plasma levels of carbamazepine. Thus, if a patient has been titrated to a stable dosage on carbamazepine, and then begins a course of treatment with a CYP3A4 inducers, it is reasonable to expect that a dose increase for carbamazepine may be necessary).

No products indexed under this heading.

Dronabinol (Carbamazepine is known to induce CYP1A2 and CYP3A4. Therefore, the potential exists for interaction between car-

bamazepine and any agent metabolized by one (or more) of these enzymes. Agents that are metabolized by CYP1A2 and CYP3A4 may have decreased plasma levels when administered concomitantly with carbamazepine. Thus, if a patient has been titrated to a stable dosage on one of the agents in these categories, and then begins a course of treatment with carbamazepine, it is reasonable to expect that a dose increase for the concomitant agent may be necessary). Products include:

Marinol Capsules 3163

Droperidol (Because of its primary CNS effect, caution should be used when carbamazepine is taken with other centrally-acting drugs).

No products indexed under this heading.

Efavirenz (Carbamazepine is metabolized mainly by CYP3A4 the active carbamazepine 10,11-epoxide, which is futher metabolized to the trans-diol by epoxide hydrolase. Therefore, the potential exists for interaction between carbamazepine and any agent that inhibits CYP3A4 and/or epoxide hydrolase. Agents that are CYP3A4 inhibitors may increase the plasma levels of carbamazepine. Thus, if a patient has been titrated to a stable dosage of carbamazepine, and then begins a course of treatment with a CYP3A4 or epoxide hydrolase inhibitor, it is reasonable to expect that a dose reduction for carbamazepine may be necessary). Products include:

Atripla Tablets 938
Sustiva Capsules 930
Sustiva Tablets 930

Enflurane (Because of its primary CNS effect, caution should be used when carbamazepine is taken with other centrally-acting drugs).

No products indexed under this heading.

Enoxacin (Carbamazepine is known to induce CYP1A2 and CYP3A4. Therefore, the potential exists for interaction between carbamazepine and any agent metabolized by one (or more) of these enzymes. Agents that are metabolized by CYP1A2 and CYP3A4 may have decreased plasma levels when administered concomitantly with carbamazepine. Thus, if a patient has been titrated to a stable dosage on one of the agents in these categories, and then begins a course of treatment with carbamazepine, it is reasonable to expect that a dose increase for the concomitant agent may be necessary).

No products indexed under this heading.

Ergotamine Tartrate (Carbamazepine is known to induce CYP1A2 and CYP3A4. Therefore, the potential exists for interaction between carbamazepine and any agent metabolized by one (or more) of these enzymes. Agents that are metabolized by CYP1A2 and CYP3A4 may have decreased plasma levels when administered concomitantly with carbamazepine. Thus, if a patient has been titrated to a stable dosage on one of the agents in these categories, and then begins a course of treatment with carbamazepine, it is reasonable to expect that a dose increase for the concomitant agent may be necessary).

No products indexed under this heading.

Erythromycin (Carbamazepine is metabolized mainly by CYP3A4 the active carbamazepine 10,11-epoxide, which is futher metabolized to the trans-diol by epoxide hydrolase. Therefore, the potential exists for interaction between carbamazepine and any agent that inhibits CYP3A4 and/or epoxide hydrolase. Agents that are CYP3A4 inhibitors may increase the plasma levels of carbamazepine. Thus, if a patient has been titrated to a stable dosage of carbamazepine, and then begins a course of treatment with a CYP3A4 or epoxide hydrolase inhibitor, it is reasonable to expect that a dose reduction for carbamazepine may be necessary).

No products indexed under this heading.

Erythromycin Estolate (Carbamazepine is metabolized mainly by CYP3A4 the active carbamazepine 10,11-epoxide, which is futher metabolized to the trans-diol by epoxide hydrolase. Therefore, the potential exists for interaction between carbamazepine and any agent that inhibits CYP3A4 and/or epoxide hydrolase. Agents that are CYP3A4 inhibitors may increase the plasma levels of carbamazepine. Thus, if a patient has been titrated to a stable dosage of carbamazepine, and then begins a course of treatment with a CYP3A4 or epoxide hydrolase inhibitor, it is reasonable to expect that a dose reduction for carbamazepine may be necessary).

No products indexed under this heading.

Erythromycin Ethylsuccinate (Carbamazepine is metabolized mainly by CYP3A4 the active carbamazepine 10,11-epoxide, which is futher metabolized to the trans-diol by epoxide hydrolase. Therefore, the potential exists for interaction between carbamazepine and any agent that inhibits CYP3A4 and/or epoxide hydrolase. Agents that are CYP3A4 inhibitors may increase the plasma levels of carbamazepine. Thus, if a patient has been titrated to a stable dosage of carbamazepine, and then begins a course of treatment with a CYP3A4 or epoxide hydrolase inhibitor, it is reasonable to expect that a dose reduction for carbamazepine may be necessary). Products include:

E.E.S. 433
EryPed 431

Erythromycin Gluceptate (Carbamazepine is metabolized mainly by CYP3A4 the active carbamazepine 10,11-epoxide, which is futher metabolized to the trans-diol by epoxide hydrolase. Therefore, the potential exists for interaction between carbamazepine and any agent that inhibits CYP3A4 and/or epoxide hydrolase. Agents that are CYP3A4 inhibitors may increase the plasma levels of carbamazepine. Thus, if a patient has been titrated to a stable dosage of carbamazepine, and then begins a course of treatment with a CYP3A4 or epoxide hydrolase inhibitor, it is reasonable to expect that a dose reduction for carbamazepine may be necessary).

No products indexed under this heading.

Erythromycin Lactobionate (Carbamazepine is metabolized mainly by CYP3A4 the active carbamazepine 10,11-epoxide, which is futher metabolized to the trans-diol by epoxide hydrolase. Therefore, the potential exists for interaction between carbamazepine and any agent that inhibits CYP3A4 and/or epoxide hydrolase. Agents that are CYP3A4 inhibitors may increase the plasma levels of carbamazepine. Thus, if a patient has been titrated to a stable dosage of carbamazepine, and then begins a course of treatment with a CYP3A4 or epoxide hydrolase inhibitor, it is reasonable to expect that a dose reduction for carbamazepine may be necessary).

No products indexed under this heading.

Erythromycin Stearate (Carbamazepine is metabolized mainly by CYP3A4 the active carbamazepine 10,11-epoxide, which is futher metabolized to the trans-diol by epoxide hydrolase. Therefore, the potential exists for interaction between carbamazepine and any agent that inhibits CYP3A4 and/or epoxide hydrolase. Agents that are CYP3A4 inhibitors may increase the plasma levels of carbamazepine. Thus, if a patient has been titrated to a stable dosage of carbamazepine, and then begins a course of treatment with a CYP3A4 or epoxide hydrolase inhibitor, it is reasonable to expect that a dose reduction for carbamazepine may be necessary).

No products indexed under this heading.

Esomeprazole Magnesium (Carbamazepine is metabolized mainly by CYP3A4 the active carbamazepine 10,11-epoxide, which is futher metabolized to the trans-diol by epoxide hydrolase. Therefore, the potential exists for interaction between carbamazepine and any agent that inhibits CYP3A4 and/or epoxide hydrolase. Agents that are CYP3A4 inhibitors may increase the plasma levels of carbamazepine. Thus, if a patient has been titrated to a stable dosage of carbamazepine, and then begins a course of treatment with a CYP3A4 or epoxide hydrolase inhibitor, it is reasonable to expect that a dose reduction for carbamazepine may be necessary). Products include:

Nexium Delayed-Release Capsules 645
Nexium Delayed-Release Oral Suspension 645

Estazolam (Because of its primary CNS effect, caution should be used when carbamazepine is taken with other centrally-acting drugs).

No products indexed under this heading.

Estradiol (Carbamazepine is known to induce CYP1A2 and CYP3A4. Therefore, the potential exists for interaction between carbamazepine and any agent metabolized by one (or more) of these enzymes. Agents that are metabolized by CYP1A2 and CYP3A4 may have decreased plasma levels when administered concomitantly with carbamazepine. Thus, if a patient has been titrated to a stable dosage on one of the agents in these categories, and then begins a course of treatment with carbamazepine, it is reasonable to expect that a dose increase for the concomitant agent may be necessary). Products include:

Activella Tablets 2347
Angeliq Tablets 751
Climara Transdermal System 763
Climara Pro Transdermal System 768
Divigel 3167
Vagifem Tablets 2375

Estradiol Benzoate (Carbamazepine is known to induce CYP1A2 and CYP3A4. Therefore, the potential exists for interaction between carbamazepine and any agent metabolized by one (or more) of these enzymes. Agents that are metabolized by CYP1A2 and CYP3A4 may have decreased plasma levels when administered concomitantly with carbamazepine. Thus, if a patient has been titrated to a stable dosage on one of the agents in these categories, and then begins a course of treatment with carbamazepine, it is reasonable to expect that a dose increase for the concomitant agent may be necessary).

No products indexed under this heading.

Estradiol Cypionate (Carbamazepine is known to induce CYP1A2 and CYP3A4. Therefore, the potential exists for interaction between carbamazepine and any agent metabolized by one (or more) of these enzymes. Agents that are metabolized by CYP1A2 and CYP3A4 may have decreased plasma levels when administered concomitantly with carbamazepine. Thus, if a patient has been titrated to a stable dosage on one of the agents in these categories, and then begins a course of treatment with carbamazepine, it is reasonable to expect that a dose increase for the concomitant agent may be necessary).

No products indexed under this heading.

Estradiol Valerate (Carbamazepine is known to induce CYP1A2 and CYP3A4. Therefore, the potential exists for interaction between carbamazepine and any agent metabolized by one (or more) of these enzymes. Agents that are metabolized by CYP1A2 and CYP3A4 may have decreased plasma levels when administered concomitantly with carbamazepine. Thus, if a patient has been titrated to a stable dosage on one of the agents in these categories, and then begins a course of treatment with carbamazepine, it is reasonable to expect that a dose increase for the concomitant agent may be necessary).

No products indexed under this heading.

Ethanol (Because of its primary CNS effect, caution should be used when carbamazepine is taken with alcohol).

No products indexed under this heading.

Ethchlorvynol (Because of its primary CNS effect, caution should be used when carbamazepine is taken with other centrally-acting drugs).

No products indexed under this heading.

Ethinamate (Because of its primary CNS effect, caution should be used when carbamazepine is taken with other centrally-acting drugs).

No products indexed under this heading.

Ethinyl Estradiol (Carbamazepine is known to induce CYP1A2 and CYP3A4. Therefore, the potential exists for interaction between carbamazepine and any agent metabolized by one (or more) of these enzymes. Agents that are metabolized by CYP1A2 or CYP3A4 may have decreased plasma levels when administered concomitantly with carbamazepine. Breakthrough bleeding has been reported among patients receiving concomitant oral contraceptives and their reliability may be adversely affected). Products include:

Lybrel Tablets **3204**
Mircette Tablets **1034**
NuvaRing **2897**
Ortho-Cyclen/Ortho Tri-Cyclen **2449**
Ortho Evra Transdermal System **2437**
Ortho Tri-Cyclen Lo Tablets **2458**
Seasonique Tablets **1046**
Yaz Tablets **805**

Ethosuximide (Carbamazepine is metabolized by CYP3A4. Therefore, the potential exists for interaction between carbamazepine and any agent that induces CYP3A4. Agents that are CYP3A4 inducers may decrease plasma levels of carbamazepine. Thus, if a patient has been titrated to a stable dosage on carbamazepine, and then begins a course of treatment with a CYP3A4 inducers, it is reasonable to expect that a dose increase for carbamazepine may be necessary).
No products indexed under this heading.

Ethyl Alcohol (Because of its primary CNS effect, caution should be used when carbamazepine is taken with other centrally-acting drugs).
No products indexed under this heading.

Ethynodiol Diacetate (Carbamazepine is known to induce CYP1A2 and CYP3A4. Therefore, the potential exists for interaction between carbamazepine and any agent metabolized by one (or more) of these enzymes. Agents that are metabolized by CYP1A2 or CYP3A4 may have decreased plasma levels when administered concomitantly with carbamazepine. Breakthrough bleeding has been reported among patients receiving concomitant oral contraceptives and their reliability may be adversely affected).
No products indexed under this heading.

Etoposide (Carbamazepine is known to induce CYP1A2 and CYP3A4. Therefore, the potential exists for interaction between carbamazepine and any agent metabolized by one (or more) of these enzymes. Agents that are metabolized by CYP1A2 and CYP3A4 may have decreased plasma levels when administered concomitantly with carbamazepine. Thus, if a patient has been titrated to a stable dosage on one of the agents in these categories, and then begins a course of treatment with carbamazepine, it is reasonable to expect that a dose increase for the concomitant agent may be necessary).
No products indexed under this heading.

Etoposide Phosphate (Carbamazepine is known to induce CYP1A2 and CYP3A4. Therefore, the potential exists for interaction between carbamazepine and any agent metabolized by one (or more) of these enzymes. Agents that are metabolized by CYP1A2 and CYP3A4 may have decreased plasma levels when administered concomitantly with carbamazepine. Thus, if a patient has been titrated to a stable dosage on one of the agents in these categories, and then begins a course of treatment with carbamazepine, it is reasonable to expect that a dose increase for the concomitant agent may be necessary).
No products indexed under this heading.

Felbamate (Carbamazepine is metabolized by CYP3A4. Therefore, the potential exists for interaction between carbamazepine and any agent that induces CYP3A4. Agents that are CYP3A4 inducers may decrease plasma levels of carbamazepine. Thus, if a patient has been titrated to a stable dosage on carbamazepine, and then begins a course of treatment with a CYP3A4 inducers, it is reasonable to expect that a dose increase for carbamazepine may be necessary).
No products indexed under this heading.

Felodipine (Carbamazepine is known to induce CYP1A2 and CYP3A4. Therefore, the potential exists for interaction between carbamazepine and any agent metabolized by one (or more) of these enzymes. Agents that are metabolized by CYP1A2 and CYP3A4 may have decreased plasma levels when administered concomitantly with carbamazepine. Thus, if a patient has been titrated to a stable dosage on one of the agents in these categories, and then begins a course of treatment with carbamazepine, it is reasonable to expect that a dose increase for the concomitant agent may be necessary).
No products indexed under this heading.

Fentanyl (Because of its primary CNS effect, caution should be used when carbamazepine is taken with other centrally-acting drugs). Products include:

Duragesic Transdermal System **2405**
Ionsys Transdermal System **2410**

Fentanyl Citrate (Because of its primary CNS effect, caution should be used when carbamazepine is taken with other centrally-acting drugs). Products include:

Actiq **959**
Fentora Tablets **968**

Fluconazole (Carbamazepine is metabolized mainly by CYP3A4 the active carbamazepine 10,11-epoxide, which is futher metabolized to the trans-diol by epoxide hydrolase. Therefore, the potential exists for interaction between carbamazepine and any agent that inhibits CYP3A4 and/or epoxide hydrolase. Agents that are CYP3A4 inhibitors may increase the plasma levels of carbamazepine. Thus, if a patient has been titrated to a stable dosage of carbamazepine, and then begins a course of treatment with a CYP3A4 or epoxide hydrolase inhibitor, it is reasonable to expect that a dose reduction for carbamazepine may be necessary).
No products indexed under this heading.

Fludrocortisone Acetate (Carbamazepine is metabolized by CYP3A4. Therefore, the potential exists for interaction between carbamazepine and any agent that induces CYP3A4. Agents that are CYP3A4 inducers may decrease plasma levels of carbamazepine. Thus, if a patient has been titrated to a stable dosage on carbamazepine, and then begins a course of treatment with a CYP3A4 inducers, it is reasonable to expect that a dose increase for carbamazepine may be necessary).
No products indexed under this heading.

Fluoxetine (Carbamazepine is metabolized mainly by CYP3A4 the active carbamazepine 10,11-epoxide, which is futher metabolized to the trans-diol by epoxide hydrolase. Therefore, the potential exists for interaction between carbamazepine and any agent that inhibits CYP3A4 and/or epoxide hydrolase. Agents that are CYP3A4 inhibitors may increase the plasma levels of carbamazepine. Thus, if a patient has been titrated to a stable dosage of carbamazepine, and then begins a course of treatment with a CYP3A4 or epoxide hydrolase inhibitor, it is reasonable to expect that a dose reduction for carbamazepine may be necessary).
No products indexed under this heading.

Fluoxetine Hydrochloride (Carbamazepine is metabolized mainly by CYP3A4 the active carbamazepine 10,11-epoxide, which is futher metabolized to the trans-diol by epoxide hydrolase. Therefore, the potential exists for interaction between carbamazepine and any agent that inhibits CYP3A4 and/or epoxide hydrolase. Agents that are CYP3A4 inhibitors may increase the plasma levels of carbamazepine. Thus, if a patient has been titrated to a stable dosage of carbamazepine, and then begins a course of treatment with a CYP3A4 or epoxide hydrolase inhibitor, it is reasonable to expect that a dose reduction for carbamazepine may be necessary). Products include:

Prozac Weekly Capsules **1852**
Prozac Pulvules and Liquid **1852**
Symbyax Capsules **1871**

Fluphenazine Decanoate (Because of its primary CNS effect, caution should be used when carbamazepine is taken with other centrally-acting drugs).
No products indexed under this heading.

Fluphenazine Enanthate (Because of its primary CNS effect, caution should be used when carbamazepine is taken with other centrally-acting drugs).
No products indexed under this heading.

Fluphenazine Hydrochloride (Because of its primary CNS effect, caution should be used when carbamazepine is taken with other centrally-acting drugs).
No products indexed under this heading.

Flurazepam Hydrochloride (Because of its primary CNS effect, caution should be used when carbamazepine is taken with other centrally-acting drugs).
No products indexed under this heading.

Flutamide (Carbamazepine is known to induce CYP1A2 and CYP3A4. Therefore, the potential exists for interaction between carbamazepine and any agent metabolized by one (or more) of these enzymes. Agents that are metabolized by CYP1A2 and CYP3A4 may have decreased plasma levels when administered concomitantly with carbamazepine. Thus, if a patient has been titrated to a stable dosage on one of the agents in these categories, and then begins a course of treatment with carbamazepine, it is reasonable to expect that a dose increase for the concomitant agent may be necessary).
No products indexed under this heading.

Fluticasone Propionate (Carbamazepine is known to induce CYP1A2 and CYP3A4. Therefore, the potential exists for interaction between carbamazepine and any agent metabolized by one (or more) of these enzymes. Agents that are metabolized by CYP1A2 and CYP3A4 may have decreased plasma levels when administered concomitantly with carbamazepine. Thus, if a patient has been titrated to a stable dosage on one of the agents in these categories, and then begins a course of treatment with carbamazepine, it is reasonable to expect that a dose increase for the concomitant agent may be necessary). Products include:

Advair Diskus 100/50 .... **1276**
Advair Diskus 250/50 .... **1276**
Advair Diskus 500/50 .... **1276**
Advair HFA 45/21 Inhalation Aerosol **1288**
Advair HFA 115/21 Inhalation Aerosol **1288**
Advair HFA 230/21 Inhalation Aerosol **1288**
Flonase Nasal Spray **1431**
Flovent Diskus 50 mcg **1435**

Fluvoxamine Maleate (Carbamazepine is metabolized mainly by CYP3A4 the active carbamazepine 10,11-epoxide, which is futher metabolized to the trans-diol by epoxide hydrolase. Therefore, the potential exists for interaction between carbamazepine and any agent that inhibits CYP3A4 and/or epoxide hydrolase. Agents that are CYP3A4 inhibitors may increase the plasma levels of carbamazepine. Thus, if a patient has been titrated to a stable dosage of carbamazepine, and then begins a course of treatment with a CYP3A4 or epoxide hydrolase inhibitor, it is reasonable to expect that a dose reduction for carbamazepine may be necessary). Products include:

Luvox CR Extended-Release Capsules **1759**

Fosamprenavir Calcium (Carbamazepine is metabolized mainly by CYP3A4 the active carbamazepine 10,11-epoxide, which is futher metabolized to the trans-diol by epoxide hydrolase. Therefore, the potential exists for interaction between carbamazepine and any agent that inhibits CYP3A4 and/or epoxide hydrolase. Agents that are CYP3A4 inhibitors may increase the plasma levels of carbamazepine. Thus, if a patient has been titrated to a stable dosage of carbamazepine, and then begins a course of treatment with a CYP3A4 or epoxide hydrolase inhibitor, it is reasonable

to expect that a dose reduction for carbamazepine may be necessary). Products include:

Lexiva Oral Suspension **1510**
Lexiva Tablets **1510**

Fosphenytoin Sodium (Phenytoin levels may increase or decrease in the presence of carbamazepine. Careful monitoring of phenytoin plasma levels following co-administration with carbamazepine is advised).
No products indexed under this heading.

Garlic Extract (Carbamazepine is metabolized by CYP3A4. Therefore, the potential exists for interaction between carbamazepine and any agent that induces CYP3A4. Agents that are CYP3A4 inducers may decrease plasma levels of carbamazepine. Thus, if a patient has been titrated to a stable dosage on carbamazepine, and then begins a course of treatment with a CYP3A4 inducers, it is reasonable to expect that a dose increase for carbamazepine may be necessary).
No products indexed under this heading.

Garlic Oil (Carbamazepine is metabolized by CYP3A4. Therefore, the potential exists for interaction between carbamazepine and any agent that induces CYP3A4. Agents that are CYP3A4 inducers may decrease plasma levels of carbamazepine. Thus, if a patient has been titrated to a stable dosage on carbamazepine, and then begins a course of treatment with a CYP3A4 inducers, it is reasonable to expect that a dose increase for carbamazepine may be necessary).
No products indexed under this heading.

Glutethimide (Because of its primary CNS effect, caution should be used when carbamazepine is taken with other centrally-acting drugs).
No products indexed under this heading.

Grepafloxacin Hydrochloride (Carbamazepine is known to induce CYP1A2 and CYP3A4. Therefore, the potential exists for interaction between carbamazepine and any agent metabolized by one (or more) of these enzymes. Agents that are metabolized by CYP1A2 and CYP3A4 may have decreased plasma levels when administered concomitantly with carbamazepine. Thus, if a patient has been titrated to a stable dosage on one of the agents in these categories, and then begins a course of treatment with carbamazepine, it is reasonable to expect that a dose increase for the concomitant agent may be necessary).
No products indexed under this heading.

Haloperidol (Because of its primary CNS effect, caution should be used when carbamazepine is taken with other centrally-acting drugs).
No products indexed under this heading.

Haloperidol Decanoate (Because of its primary CNS effect, caution should be used when carbamazepine is taken with other centrally-acting drugs).
No products indexed under this heading.

Haloperidol Lactate (Carbamazepine is known to induce CYP1A2 and CYP3A4. Therefore, the potential exists for interaction between carbamazepine and any agent metabolized by one (or more) of these enzymes. Agents that are metabolized by CYP1A2 and CYP3A4 may have decreased plasma levels when administered concomitantly with carbamazepine. Thus, if a patient has been titrated to a stable dosage on one of the agents in these categories, and then begins a course of treatment with carbamazepine, it is reasonable to expect that a dose increase for the concomitant agent may be necessary).
No products indexed under this heading.

Hydrocodone Bitartrate (Because of its primary CNS effect, caution should be used when carbamazepine is taken with other centrally-acting drugs). Products include:

Lortab 5/500 Tablets **3143**
Lortab 7.5/500 Tablets **3144**
Lortab 10/500 Tablets **3144**
Vicodin Tablets **529**
Vicodin ES Tablets **530**
Vicodin HP Tablets **531**
Vicoprofen Tablets **533**
Zydone Tablets **1132**

Hydrocodone Polistirex (Because of its primary CNS effect, caution should be used when carbamazepine is taken with other centrally-acting drugs). Products include:

Tussionex Pennkinetic
Extended-Release Suspension **3154**

Hydrocortisone (Carbamazepine is metabolized by CYP3A4. Therefore, the potential exists for interaction between carbamazepine and any agent that induces CYP3A4. Agents that are CYP3A4 inducers may decrease plasma levels of carbamazepine. Thus, if a patient has been titrated to a stable dosage on carbamazepine, and then begins a course of treatment with a CYP3A4 inducers, it is reasonable to expect that a dose increase for carbamazepine may be necessary).
No products indexed under this heading.

Hydrocortisone Acetate (Carbamazepine is metabolized by CYP3A4. Therefore, the potential exists for interaction between carbamazepine and any agent that induces CYP3A4. Agents that are CYP3A4 inducers may decrease plasma levels of carbamazepine. Thus, if a patient has been titrated to a stable dosage on carbamazepine, and then begins a course of treatment with a CYP3A4 inducers, it is reasonable to expect that a dose increase for carbamazepine may be necessary). Products include:

Analpram-HC **1140**
Pramosone **1141**

Hydrocortisone Butyrate (Carbamazepine is metabolized by CYP3A4. Therefore, the potential exists for interaction between carbamazepine and any agent that induces CYP3A4. Agents that are CYP3A4 inducers may decrease plasma levels of carbamazepine. Thus, if a patient has been titrated to a stable dosage on carbamazepine, and then begins a course of treatment with a CYP3A4 inducers, it is reasonable to expect that a dose increase for carbamazepine may be necessary).
No products indexed under this heading.

Hydrocortisone Cypionate (Carbamazepine is metabolized by CYP3A4. Therefore, the potential exists for interaction between carbamazepine and any agent that induces CYP3A4. Agents that are CYP3A4 inducers may decrease plasma levels of carbamazepine. Thus, if a patient has been titrated to a stable dosage on carbamazepine, and then begins a course of treatment with a CYP3A4 inducers, it is reasonable to expect that a dose increase for carbamazepine may be necessary).
No products indexed under this heading.

Hydrocortisone Hemisuccinate (Carbamazepine is metabolized by CYP3A4. Therefore, the potential exists for interaction between carbamazepine and any agent that induces CYP3A4. Agents that are CYP3A4 inducers may decrease plasma levels of carbamazepine. Thus, if a patient has been titrated to a stable dosage on carbamazepine, and then begins a course of treatment with a CYP3A4 inducers, it is reasonable to expect that a dose increase for carbamazepine may be necessary).
No products indexed under this heading.

Hydrocortisone Probutate (Carbamazepine is metabolized by CYP3A4. Therefore, the potential exists for interaction between carbamazepine and any agent that induces CYP3A4. Agents that are CYP3A4 inducers may decrease plasma levels of carbamazepine. Thus, if a patient has been titrated to a stable dosage on carbamazepine, and then begins a course of treatment with a CYP3A4 inducers, it is reasonable to expect that a dose increase for carbamazepine may be necessary).
No products indexed under this heading.

Hydrocortisone Sodium Phosphate (Carbamazepine is metabolized by CYP3A4. Therefore, the potential exists for interaction between carbamazepine and any agent that induces CYP3A4. Agents that are CYP3A4 inducers may decrease plasma levels of carbamazepine. Thus, if a patient has been titrated to a stable dosage on carbamazepine, and then begins a course of treatment with a CYP3A4 inducers, it is reasonable to expect that a dose increase for carbamazepine may be necessary).
No products indexed under this heading.

Hydrocortisone Sodium Succinate (Carbamazepine is metabolized by CYP3A4. Therefore, the potential exists for interaction between carbamazepine and any agent that induces CYP3A4. Agents that are CYP3A4 inducers may decrease plasma levels of carbamazepine. Thus, if a patient has been titrated to a stable dosage on carbamazepine, and then begins a course of treatment with a CYP3A4 inducers, it is reasonable to expect that a dose increase for carbamazepine may be necessary).
No products indexed under this heading.

Hydrocortisone Valerate (Carbamazepine is metabolized by CYP3A4. Therefore, the potential exists for interaction between carbamazepine and any agent that induces CYP3A4. Agents that are CYP3A4 inducers may decrease plasma levels of carbamazepine. Thus, if a patient has been titrated to a stable dosage on carbamazepine, and then begins a course of treatment with a CYP3A4 inducers, it is reasonable to expect that a dose increase for carbamazepine may be necessary).
No products indexed under this heading.

Hydromorphone Hydrochloride (Because of its primary CNS effect, caution should be used when carbamazepine is taken with other centrally-acting drugs).
No products indexed under this heading.

Hydroxyzine Hydrochloride (Because of its primary CNS effect, caution should be used when carbamazepine is taken with other centrally-acting drugs).
No products indexed under this heading.

Hypericum (Carbamazepine is metabolized by CYP3A4. Therefore, the potential exists for interaction between carbamazepine and any agent that induces CYP3A4. Agents that are CYP3A4 inducers may decrease plasma levels of carbamazepine. Thus, if a patient has been titrated to a stable dosage on carbamazepine, and then begins a course of treatment with a CYP3A4 inducers, it is reasonable to expect that a dose increase for carbamazepine may be necessary). Products include:

Satieté Tablets **640**

Hypericum Perforatum (Carbamazepine is metabolized by CYP3A4. Therefore, the potential exists for interaction between carbamazepine and any agent that induces CYP3A4. Agents that are CYP3A4 inducers may decrease plasma levels of carbamazepine. Thus, if a patient has been titrated to a stable dosage on carbamazepine, and then begins a course of treatment with a CYP3A4 inducers, it is reasonable to expect that a dose increase for carbamazepine may be necessary).
No products indexed under this heading.

Imipramine Hydrochloride (Use is not recommended if known sensitivity to any of the tricyclic compounds).
No products indexed under this heading.

Imipramine Pamoate (Use is not recommended if known sensitivity to any of the tricyclic compounds).
No products indexed under this heading.

Indinavir Sulfate (Carbamazepine is metabolized mainly by CYP3A4 the active carbamazepine 10,11-epoxide, which is futher metabolized to the trans-diol by epoxide hydrolase. Therefore, the potential exists for interaction between carbamazepine and any agent that inhibits CYP3A4 and/or epoxide hydrolase. Agents that are CYP3A4 inhibitors may increase the plasma levels of carbamazepine. Thus, if a patient has been titrated to a stable dosage of carbamazepine, and then begins a course of treatment with a CYP3A4 or epoxide hydrolase inhibitor, it is reasonable

IMPORTANT NOTE: Always consult each drug listing in the patient's regimen for possible interactions.

to expect that a dose reduction for carbamazepine may be necessary). Products include:

Crixivan Capsules ... 1979

Isocarboxazid (Co-administration with, or for 14 days after discontinuing MAO inhibitors is not recommended). Products include:

Marplan Tablets ... 3177

Isoflurane (Because of its primary CNS effect, caution should be used when carbamazepine is taken with other centrally-acting drugs).

No products indexed under this heading.

Isoniazid (Carbamazepine is metabolized mainly by CYP3A4 the active carbamazepine 10,11-epoxide, which is futher metabolized to the trans-diol by epoxide hydrolase. Therefore, the potential exists for interaction between carbamazepine and any agent that inhibits CYP3A4 and/or epoxide hydrolase. Agents that are CYP3A4 inhibitors may increase the plasma levels of carbamazepine. Thus, if a patient has been titrated to a stable dosage of carbamazepine, and then begins a course of treatment with a CYP3A4 or epoxide hydrolase inhibitor, it is reasonable to expect that a dose reduction for carbamazepine may be necessary).

No products indexed under this heading.

Isradipine (Carbamazepine is known to induce CYP1A2 and CYP3A4. Therefore, the potential exists for interaction between carbamazepine and any agent metabolized by one (or more) of these enzymes. Agents that are metabolized by CYP1A2 and CYP3A4 may have decreased plasma levels when administered concomitantly with carbamazepine. Thus, if a patient has been titrated to a stable dosage on one of the agents in these categories, and then begins a course of treatment with carbamazepine, it is reasonable to expect that a dose increase for the concomitant agent may be necessary). Products include:

DynaCirc CR Controlled Release Tablets ... 1407

Itraconazole (Carbamazepine is metabolized mainly by CYP3A4 the active carbamazepine 10,11-epoxide, which is futher metabolized to the trans-diol by epoxide hydrolase. Therefore, the potential exists for interaction between carbamazepine and any agent that inhibits CYP3A4 and/or epoxide hydrolase. Agents that are CYP3A4 inhibitors may increase the plasma levels of carbamazepine. Thus, if a patient has been titrated to a stable dosage of carbamazepine, and then begins a course of treatment with a CYP3A4 or epoxide hydrolase inhibitor, it is reasonable to expect that a dose reduction for carbamazepine may be necessary).

No products indexed under this heading.

Ixabepilone (Carbamazepine is known to induce CYP1A2 and CYP3A4. Therefore, the potential exists for interaction between carbamazepine and any agent metabolized by one (or more) of these enzymes. Agents that are metabolized by CYP1A2 and CYP3A4 may have decreased plasma levels when administered concomitantly with carbamazepine. Thus, if a patient has been titrated to a stable dosage on one of the agents in these categories, and then begins a course of treatment with carbamazepine, it is reasonable to expect that a dose increase for the concomitant agent may be necessary). Products include:

Ixempra Kit for Injection ... 915

Ketamine Hydrochloride (Because of its primary CNS effect, caution should be used when carbamazepine is taken with other centrally-acting drugs).

No products indexed under this heading.

Ketoconazole (Carbamazepine is metabolized mainly by CYP3A4 the active carbamazepine 10,11-epoxide, which is futher metabolized to the trans-diol by epoxide hydrolase. Therefore, the potential exists for interaction between carbamazepine and any agent that inhibits CYP3A4 and/or epoxide hydrolase. Agents that are CYP3A4 inhibitors may increase the plasma levels of carbamazepine. Thus, if a patient has been titrated to a stable dosage of carbamazepine, and then begins a course of treatment with a CYP3A4 or epoxide hydrolase inhibitor, it is reasonable to expect that a dose reduction for carbamazepine may be necessary). Products include:

Extina Foam, 2% ... 3057
Nizoral A-D Shampoo ... 1901

Levobupivacaine Hydrochloride (Carbamazepine is known to induce CYP1A2 and CYP3A4. Therefore, the potential exists for interaction between carbamazepine and any agent metabolized by one (or more) of these enzymes. Agents that are metabolized by CYP1A2 and CYP3A4 may have decreased plasma levels when administered concomitantly with carbamazepine. Thus, if a patient has been titrated to a stable dosage on one of the agents in these categories, and then begins a course of treatment with carbamazepine, it is reasonable to expect that a dose increase for the concomitant agent may be necessary).

No products indexed under this heading.

Levomethadyl Acetate Hydrochloride (Because of its primary CNS effect, caution should be used when carbamazepine is taken with other centrally-acting drugs).

No products indexed under this heading.

Levonorgestrel (Carbamazepine is known to induce CYP1A2 and CYP3A4. Therefore, the potential exists for interaction between carbamazepine and any agent metabolized by one (or more) of these enzymes. Agents that are metabolized by CYP1A2 or CYP3A4 may have decreased plasma levels when administered concomitantly with carbamazepine. Breakthrough bleeding has been reported among patients receiving concomitant oral contraceptives and their reliability may be adversely affected). Products include:

Climara Pro Transdermal System ... 768
Lybrel Tablets ... 3204
Mirena Intrauterine System ... 779
Plan B Tablets ... 1044
Seasonique Tablets ... 1046

Levorphanol Tartrate (Because of its primary CNS effect, caution should be used when carbamazepine is taken with other centrally-acting drugs).

No products indexed under this heading.

Lidocaine (Carbamazepine is known to induce CYP1A2 and CYP3A4. Therefore, the potential exists for interaction between carbamazepine and any agent metabolized by one (or more) of these enzymes. Agents that are metabolized by CYP1A2 and CYP3A4 may have decreased plasma levels when administered concomitantly with carbamazepine. Thus, if a patient has been titrated to a stable dosage on one of the agents in these categories, and then begins a course of treatment with carbamazepine, it is reasonable to expect that a dose increase for the concomitant agent may be necessary). Products include:

Lidoderm Patch ... 1114

Lidocaine Hydrochloride (Carbamazepine is known to induce CYP1A2 and CYP3A4. Therefore, the potential exists for interaction between carbamazepine and any agent metabolized by one (or more) of these enzymes. Agents that are metabolized by CYP1A2 and CYP3A4 may have decreased plasma levels when administered concomitantly with carbamazepine. Thus, if a patient has been titrated to a stable dosage on one of the agents in these categories, and then begins a course of treatment with carbamazepine, it is reasonable to expect that a dose increase for the concomitant agent may be necessary).

No products indexed under this heading.

Lithium (Concomitant administration of carbamazepine and lithium may increase the risk of neurotoxic side effects).

No products indexed under this heading.

Lithium Carbonate (Concomitant administration of carbamazepine and lithium may increase the risk of neurotoxic side effects).

No products indexed under this heading.

Lithium Citrate (Concomitant administration of carbamazepine and lithium may increase the risk of neurotoxic side effects).

No products indexed under this heading.

Lomefloxacin Hydrochloride (Carbamazepine is known to induce CYP1A2 and CYP3A4. Therefore, the potential exists for interaction between carbamazepine and any agent metabolized by one (or more) of these enzymes. Agents that are metabolized by CYP1A2 and CYP3A4 may have decreased plasma levels when administered concomitantly with carbamazepine. Thus, if a patient has been titrated to a stable dosage on one of the agents in these categories, and then begins a course of treatment with carbamazepine, it is reasonable to expect that a dose increase for the concomitant agent may be necessary).

No products indexed under this heading.

Lopinavir (Carbamazepine is metabolized mainly by CYP3A4 the active carbamazepine 10,11-epoxide, which is futher metabolized to the trans-diol by epoxide hydrolase. Therefore, the potential exists for interaction between carbamazepine and any agent that inhibits CYP3A4 and/or epoxide hydrolase. Agents that are CYP3A4 inhibitors may increase the plasma levels of carbamazepine. Thus, if a patient has been titrated to a stable dosage of carbamazepine, and then begins a course of treatment with a CYP3A4 or epoxide hydrolase inhibitor, it is reasonable to expect that a dose reduction for carbamazepine may be necessary). Products include:

Kaletra ... 452

Loratadine (Carbamazepine is metabolized mainly by CYP3A4 the active carbamazepine 10,11-epoxide, which is futher metabolized to the trans-diol by epoxide hydrolase. Therefore, the potential exists for interaction between carbamazepine and any agent that inhibits CYP3A4 and/or epoxide hydrolase. Agents that are CYP3A4 inhibitors may increase the plasma levels of carbamazepine. Thus, if a patient has been titrated to a stable dosage of carbamazepine, and then begins a course of treatment with a CYP3A4 or epoxide hydrolase inhibitor, it is reasonable to expect that a dose reduction for carbamazepine may be necessary).

No products indexed under this heading.

Lorazepam (Because of its primary CNS effect, caution should be used when carbamazepine is taken with other centrally-acting drugs).

No products indexed under this heading.

Lovastatin (Carbamazepine is known to induce CYP1A2 and CYP3A4. Therefore, the potential exists for interaction between carbamazepine and any agent metabolized by one (or more) of these enzymes. Agents that are metabolized by CYP1A2 and CYP3A4 may have decreased plasma levels when administered concomitantly with carbamazepine. Thus, if a patient has been titrated to a stable dosage on one of the agents in these categories, and then begins a course of treatment with carbamazepine, it is reasonable to expect that a dose increase for the concomitant agent may be necessary). Products include:

Advicor Tablets ... 402
Mevacor Tablets ... 2063

Loxapine Hydrochloride (Because of its primary CNS effect, caution should be used when carbamazepine is taken with other centrally-acting drugs).

No products indexed under this heading.

Loxapine Succinate (Because of its primary CNS effect, caution should be used when carbamazepine is taken with other centrally-acting drugs).

No products indexed under this heading.

Maprotiline Hydrochloride (Use is not recommended if known sensitivity to any of the tricyclic compounds).
No products indexed under this heading.

Mefloquine Hydrochloride (Antimalarial drugs, such as chloroquine and mefloquine, may antagonize the activity of carbamazepine).
No products indexed under this heading.

Meperidine Hydrochloride (Because of its primary CNS effect, caution should be used when carbamazepine is taken with other centrally-acting drugs).
No products indexed under this heading.

Mephenytoin (Carbamazepine is metabolized by CYP3A4. Therefore, the potential exists for interaction between carbamazepine and any agent that induces CYP3A4. Agents that are CYP3A4 inducers may decrease plasma levels of carbamazepine. Thus, if a patient has been titrated to a stable dosage on carbamazepine, and then begins a course of treatment with a CYP3A4 inducers, it is reasonable to expect that a dose increase for carbamazepine may be necessary).
No products indexed under this heading.

Mephobarbital (Because of its primary CNS effect, caution should be used when carbamazepine is taken with other centrally-acting drugs).
No products indexed under this heading.

Meprobamate (Because of its primary CNS effect, caution should be used when carbamazepine is taken with other centrally-acting drugs).
No products indexed under this heading.

Mesoridazine Besylate (Because of its primary CNS effect, caution should be used when carbamazepine is taken with other centrally-acting drugs).
No products indexed under this heading.

Mestranol (Carbamazepine is known to induce CYP1A2 and CYP3A4. Therefore, the potential exists for interaction between carbamazepine and any agent metabolized by one (or more) of these enzymes. Agents that are metabolized by CYP1A2 or CYP3A4 may have decreased plasma levels when administered concomitantly with carbamazepine. Breakthrough bleeding has been reported among patients receiving concomitant oral contraceptives and their reliability may be adversely affected).
No products indexed under this heading.

Methadone Hydrochloride (Because of its primary CNS effect, caution should be used when carbamazepine is taken with other centrally-acting drugs).
No products indexed under this heading.

Methohexital Sodium (Because of its primary CNS effect, caution should be used when carbamazepine is taken with other centrally-acting drugs).
No products indexed under this heading.

Methotrimeprazine (Because of its primary CNS effect, caution should be used when carbamazepine is taken with other centrally-acting drugs).
No products indexed under this heading.

Methoxyflurane (Because of its primary CNS effect, caution should be used when carbamazepine is taken with other centrally-acting drugs).
No products indexed under this heading.

Methsuximide (Carbamazepine is metabolized by CYP3A4. Therefore, the potential exists for interaction between carbamazepine and any agent that induces CYP3A4. Agents that are CYP3A4 inducers may decrease plasma levels of carbamazepine. Thus, if a patient has been titrated to a stable dosage on carbamazepine, and then begins a course of treatment with a CYP3A4 inducers, it is reasonable to expect that a dose increase for carbamazepine may be necessary).
No products indexed under this heading.

Methylprednisolone (Carbamazepine is metabolized by CYP3A4. Therefore, the potential exists for interaction between carbamazepine and any agent that induces CYP3A4. Agents that are CYP3A4 inducers may decrease plasma levels of carbamazepine. Thus, if a patient has been titrated to a stable dosage on carbamazepine, and then begins a course of treatment with a CYP3A4 inducers, it is reasonable to expect that a dose increase for carbamazepine may be necessary).
No products indexed under this heading.

Methylprednisolone Acetate (Carbamazepine is metabolized by CYP3A4. Therefore, the potential exists for interaction between carbamazepine and any agent that induces CYP3A4. Agents that are CYP3A4 inducers may decrease plasma levels of carbamazepine. Thus, if a patient has been titrated to a stable dosage on carbamazepine, and then begins a course of treatment with a CYP3A4 inducers, it is reasonable to expect that a dose increase for carbamazepine may be necessary).
No products indexed under this heading.

Methylprednisolone Sodium Succinate (Carbamazepine is metabolized by CYP3A4. Therefore, the potential exists for interaction between carbamazepine and any agent that induces CYP3A4. Agents that are CYP3A4 inducers may decrease plasma levels of carbamazepine. Thus, if a patient has been titrated to a stable dosage on carbamazepine, and then begins a course of treatment with a CYP3A4 inducers, it is reasonable to expect that a dose increase for carbamazepine may be necessary).
No products indexed under this heading.

Metronidazole (Carbamazepine is metabolized mainly by CYP3A4 the active carbamazepine 10,11-epoxide, which is futher metabolized to the trans-diol by epoxide hydrolase. Therefore, the potential exists for interaction between carbamazepine and any agent that inhibits CYP3A4 and/or epoxide hydrolase. Agents that are CYP3A4 inhibitors may increase the plasma levels of carbamazepine. Thus, if a patient has been titrated to a stable dosage of carbamazepine, and then begins a course of treatment with a CYP3A4 or epoxide hydrolase inhibitor, it is reasonable to expect that a dose reduction for carbamazepine may be necessary). Products include:
Pylera Capsules 714

Metronidazole Benzoate (Carbamazepine is metabolized mainly by CYP3A4 the active carbamazepine 10,11-epoxide, which is futher metabolized to the trans-diol by epoxide hydrolase. Therefore, the potential exists for interaction between carbamazepine and any agent that inhibits CYP3A4 and/or epoxide hydrolase. Agents that are CYP3A4 inhibitors may increase the plasma levels of carbamazepine. Thus, if a patient has been titrated to a stable dosage of carbamazepine, and then begins a course of treatment with a CYP3A4 or epoxide hydrolase inhibitor, it is reasonable to expect that a dose reduction for carbamazepine may be necessary).
No products indexed under this heading.

Metronidazole Hydrochloride (Carbamazepine is metabolized mainly by CYP3A4 the active carbamazepine 10,11-epoxide, which is futher metabolized to the trans-diol by epoxide hydrolase. Therefore, the potential exists for interaction between carbamazepine and any agent that inhibits CYP3A4 and/or epoxide hydrolase. Agents that are CYP3A4 inhibitors may increase the plasma levels of carbamazepine. Thus, if a patient has been titrated to a stable dosage of carbamazepine, and then begins a course of treatment with a CYP3A4 or epoxide hydrolase inhibitor, it is reasonable to expect that a dose reduction for carbamazepine may be necessary).
No products indexed under this heading.

Mexiletine Hydrochloride (Carbamazepine is known to induce CYP1A2 and CYP3A4. Therefore, the potential exists for interaction between carbamazepine and any agent metabolized by one (or more) of these enzymes. Agents that are metabolized by CYP1A2 and CYP3A4 may have decreased plasma levels when administered concomitantly with carbamazepine. Thus, if a patient has been titrated to a stable dosage on one of the agents in these categories, and then begins a course of treatment with carbamazepine, it is reasonable to expect that a dose increase for the concomitant agent may be necessary).
No products indexed under this heading.

Miconazole (Carbamazepine is metabolized mainly by CYP3A4 the active carbamazepine 10,11-epoxide, which is futher metabolized to the trans-diol by epoxide hydrolase. Therefore, the potential exists for interaction between carbamazepine and any agent that inhibits CYP3A4 and/or epoxide hydrolase. Agents that are CYP3A4 inhibitors may increase the plasma levels of carbamazepine. Thus, if a patient has been titrated to a stable dosage of carbamazepine, and then begins a course of treatment with a CYP3A4 or epoxide hydrolase inhibitor, it is reasonable to expect that a dose reduction for carbamazepine may be necessary).
No products indexed under this heading.

Miconazole Nitrate (Carbamazepine is metabolized mainly by CYP3A4 the active carbamazepine 10,11-epoxide, which is futher metabolized to the trans-diol by epoxide hydrolase. Therefore, the potential exists for interaction between carbamazepine and any agent that inhibits CYP3A4 and/or epoxide hydrolase. Agents that are CYP3A4 inhibitors may increase the plasma levels of carbamazepine. Thus, if a patient has been titrated to a stable dosage of carbamazepine, and then begins a course of treatment with a CYP3A4 or epoxide hydrolase inhibitor, it is reasonable to expect that a dose reduction for carbamazepine may be necessary).
No products indexed under this heading.

Midazolam Hydrochloride (Because of its primary CNS effect, caution should be used when carbamazepine is taken with other centrally-acting drugs).
No products indexed under this heading.

Mirtazapine (Carbamazepine is known to induce CYP1A2 and CYP3A4. Therefore, the potential exists for interaction between carbamazepine and any agent metabolized by one (or more) of these enzymes. Agents that are metabolized by CYP1A2 and CYP3A4 may have decreased plasma levels when administered concomitantly with carbamazepine. Thus, if a patient has been titrated to a stable dosage on one of the agents in these categories, and then begins a course of treatment with carbamazepine, it is reasonable to expect that a dose increase for the concomitant agent may be necessary). Products include:
Remeron Tablets 2924
RemeronSolTab Tablets 2927

Moclobemide (Co-administration with, or for 14 days after discontinuing MAO inhibitors is not recommended).
No products indexed under this heading.

Modafinil (Carbamazepine is metabolized by CYP3A4. Therefore, the potential exists for interaction between carbamazepine and any agent that induces CYP3A4. Agents that are CYP3A4 inducers may decrease plasma levels of carbamazepine. Thus, if a patient has been titrated to a stable dosage on carbamazepine, and then begins a course of treatment with a CYP3A4 inducers, it is reasonable to expect that a dose increase for carbamazepine may be necessary). Products include:
Provigil Tablets 977

Molindone Hydrochloride (Because of its primary CNS effect, caution should be used when carbamazepine is taken with other centrally-acting drugs). Products include:
Moban Tablets 1116

Morphine Sulfate (Because of its primary CNS effect, caution should be used when carbamazepine is taken with other centrally-acting drugs). Products include:

Avinza Capsules 1772
DepoDur Injection 1095
MS Contin Tablets 2585

Moxifloxacin Hydrochloride (Carbamazepine is known to induce CYP1A2 and CYP3A4. Therefore, the potential exists for interaction between carbamazepine and any agent metabolized by one (or more) of these enzymes. Agents that are metabolized by CYP1A2 and CYP3A4 may have decreased plasma levels when administered concomitantly with carbamazepine. Thus, if a patient has been titrated to a stable dosage on one of the agents in these categories, and then begins a course of treatment with carbamazepine, it is reasonable to expect that a dose increase for the concomitant agent may be necessary). Products include:

Avelox 2803
Vigamox Ophthalmic Solution 548

Nafcillin Sodium (Carbamazepine is known to induce CYP1A2 and CYP3A4. Therefore, the potential exists for interaction between carbamazepine and any agent metabolized by one (or more) of these enzymes. Agents that are metabolized by CYP1A2 and CYP3A4 may have decreased plasma levels when administered concomitantly with carbamazepine. Thus, if a patient has been titrated to a stable dosage on one of the agents in these categories, and then begins a course of treatment with carbamazepine, it is reasonable to expect that a dose increase for the concomitant agent may be necessary).

No products indexed under this heading.

Naproxen (Carbamazepine is known to induce CYP1A2 and CYP3A4. Therefore, the potential exists for interaction between carbamazepine and any agent metabolized by one (or more) of these enzymes. Agents that are metabolized by CYP1A2 and CYP3A4 may have decreased plasma levels when administered concomitantly with carbamazepine. Thus, if a patient has been titrated to a stable dosage on one of the agents in these categories, and then begins a course of treatment with carbamazepine, it is reasonable to expect that a dose increase for the concomitant agent may be necessary). Products include:

EC-Naprosyn Delayed-Release Tablets 2632
Naprosyn Suspension 2632
Naprosyn Tablets 2632

Naproxen Sodium (Carbamazepine is known to induce CYP1A2 and CYP3A4. Therefore, the potential exists for interaction between carbamazepine and any agent metabolized by one (or more) of these enzymes. Agents that are metabolized by CYP1A2 and CYP3A4 may have decreased plasma levels when administered concomitantly with carbamazepine. Thus, if a patient has been titrated to a stable dosage on one of the agents in these categories, and then begins a course of treatment with carbamazepine, it is reasonable to expect that a dose increase for the concomitant agent may be necessary). Products include:

Anaprox Tablets 2632
Anaprox DS Tablets 2632
Treximet Tablets 1616

Nefazodone Hydrochloride (Carbamazepine is metabolized mainly by CYP3A4 the active carbamazepine 10,11-epoxide, which is futher metabolized to the trans-diol by epoxide hydrolase. Therefore, the potential exists for interaction between carbamazepine and any agent that inhibits CYP3A4 and/or epoxide hydrolase. Agents that are CYP3A4 inhibitors may increase the plasma levels of carbamazepine. Thus, if a patient has been titrated to a stable dosage of carbamazepine, and then begins a course of treatment with a CYP3A4 or epoxide hydrolase inhibitor, it is reasonable to expect that a dose reduction for carbamazepine may be necessary).

No products indexed under this heading.

Nelfinavir Mesylate (Carbamazepine is metabolized mainly by CYP3A4 the active carbamazepine 10,11-epoxide, which is futher metabolized to the trans-diol by epoxide hydrolase. Therefore, the potential exists for interaction between carbamazepine and any agent that inhibits CYP3A4 and/or epoxide hydrolase. Agents that are CYP3A4 inhibitors may increase the plasma levels of carbamazepine. Thus, if a patient has been titrated to a stable dosage of carbamazepine, and then begins a course of treatment with a CYP3A4 or epoxide hydrolase inhibitor, it is reasonable to expect that a dose reduction for carbamazepine may be necessary).

No products indexed under this heading.

Nevirapine (Carbamazepine is metabolized mainly by CYP3A4 the active carbamazepine 10,11-epoxide, which is futher metabolized to the trans-diol by epoxide hydrolase. Therefore, the potential exists for interaction between carbamazepine and any agent that inhibits CYP3A4 and/or epoxide hydrolase. Agents that are CYP3A4 inhibitors may increase the plasma levels of carbamazepine. Thus, if a patient has been titrated to a stable dosage of carbamazepine, and then begins a course of treatment with a CYP3A4 or epoxide hydrolase inhibitor, it is reasonable to expect that a dose reduction for carbamazepine may be necessary). Products include:

Viramune Oral Suspension 873
Viramune Tablets 873

Niacinamide (Carbamazepine is metabolized mainly by CYP3A4 the active carbamazepine 10,11-epoxide, which is futher metabolized to the trans-diol by epoxide hydrolase. Therefore, the potential exists for interaction between carbamazepine and any agent that inhibits CYP3A4 and/or epoxide hydrolase. Agents that are CYP3A4 inhibitors may increase the plasma levels of carbamazepine. Thus, if a patient has been titrated to a stable dosage of carbamazepine, and then begins a course of treatment with a CYP3A4 or epoxide hydrolase inhibitor, it is reasonable to expect that a dose reduction for carbamazepine may be necessary). Products include:

BioLean Free Tablets .... ▣ 635

Nicardipine Hydrochloride (Carbamazepine is known to induce CYP1A2 and CYP3A4. Therefore, the potential exists for interaction between carbamazepine and any agent metabolized by one (or more) of these enzymes. Agents that are metabolized by CYP1A2 and CYP3A4 may have decreased plasma levels when administered concomitantly with carbamazepine. Thus, if a patient has been titrated to a stable dosage on one of the agents in these categories, and then begins a course of treatment with carbamazepine, it is reasonable to expect that a dose increase for the concomitant agent may be necessary). Products include:

Cardene I.V. 1093

Nicotinamide (Carbamazepine is metabolized mainly by CYP3A4 the active carbamazepine 10,11-epoxide, which is futher metabolized to the trans-diol by epoxide hydrolase. Therefore, the potential exists for interaction between carbamazepine and any agent that inhibits CYP3A4 and/or epoxide hydrolase. Agents that are CYP3A4 inhibitors may increase the plasma levels of carbamazepine. Thus, if a patient has been titrated to a stable dosage of carbamazepine, and then begins a course of treatment with a CYP3A4 or epoxide hydrolase inhibitor, it is reasonable to expect that a dose reduction for carbamazepine may be necessary).

No products indexed under this heading.

Nicotine Polacrilex (Carbamazepine is known to induce CYP1A2 and CYP3A4. Therefore, the potential exists for interaction between carbamazepine and any agent metabolized by one (or more) of these enzymes. Agents that are metabolized by CYP1A2 and CYP3A4 may have decreased plasma levels when administered concomitantly with carbamazepine. Thus, if a patient has been titrated to a stable dosage on one of the agents in these categories, and then begins a course of treatment with carbamazepine, it is reasonable to expect that a dose increase for the concomitant agent may be necessary).

No products indexed under this heading.

Nicotine Salicylate (Carbamazepine is known to induce CYP1A2 and CYP3A4. Therefore, the potential exists for interaction between carbamazepine and any agent metabolized by one (or more) of these enzymes. Agents that are metabolized by CYP1A2 and CYP3A4 may have decreased plasma levels when administered concomitantly with carbamazepine. Thus, if a patient has been titrated to a stable dosage on one of the agents in these categories, and then begins a course of treatment with carbamazepine, it is reasonable to expect that a dose increase for the concomitant agent may be necessary).

No products indexed under this heading.

Nicotine Sulfate (Carbamazepine is known to induce CYP1A2 and CYP3A4. Therefore, the potential exists for interaction between carbamazepine and any agent metabolized by one (or more) of these enzymes. Agents that are metabolized by CYP1A2 and CYP3A4 may have decreased plasma levels when administered concomitantly with carbamazepine. Thus, if a patient has been titrated to a stable dosage on one of the agents in these categories, and then begins a course of treatment with carbamazepine, it is reasonable to expect that a dose increase for the concomitant agent may be necessary).

No products indexed under this heading.

Nifedipine (Carbamazepine is metabolized mainly by CYP3A4 the active carbamazepine 10,11-epoxide, which is futher metabolized to the trans-diol by epoxide hydrolase. Therefore, the potential exists for interaction between carbamazepine and any agent that inhibits CYP3A4 and/or epoxide hydrolase. Agents that are CYP3A4 inhibitors may increase the plasma levels of carbamazepine. Thus, if a patient has been titrated to a stable dosage of carbamazepine, and then begins a course of treatment with a CYP3A4 or epoxide hydrolase inhibitor, it is reasonable to expect that a dose reduction for carbamazepine may be necessary).

No products indexed under this heading.

Nimodipine (Carbamazepine is known to induce CYP1A2 and CYP3A4. Therefore, the potential exists for interaction between carbamazepine and any agent metabolized by one (or more) of these enzymes. Agents that are metabolized by CYP1A2 and CYP3A4 may have decreased plasma levels when administered concomitantly with carbamazepine. Thus, if a patient has been titrated to a stable dosage on one of the agents in these categories, and then begins a course of treatment with carbamazepine, it is reasonable to expect that a dose increase for the concomitant agent may be necessary). Products include:

Nimotop Capsules 790

Nisoldipine (Carbamazepine is known to induce CYP1A2 and CYP3A4. Therefore, the potential exists for interaction between carbamazepine and any agent metabolized by one (or more) of these enzymes. Agents that are metabolized by CYP1A2 and CYP3A4 may have decreased plasma levels when administered concomitantly with carbamazepine. Thus, if a patient has been titrated to a stable dosage on one of the agents in these categories, and then begins a course of treatment with carbamazepine, it is reasonable to expect that a dose increase for the concomitant agent may be necessary). Products include:

Sular Extended Release Tablets 2975

Nitrendipine (Carbamazepine is known to induce CYP1A2 and CYP3A4. Therefore, the potential exists for interaction between carbamazepine and any agent metabolized by one (or more) of these enzymes. Agents that are metabolized by CYP1A2 and CYP3A4 may have decreased plasma levels when administered concomitantly with carbamazepine. Thus, if a patient has been titrated to a stable dosage on one of the agents in these categories, and then begins a course of treatment with carbamazepine, it is reasonable to expect that a dose increase for the concomitant agent may be necessary).

No products indexed under this heading.

Norethindrone (Carbamazepine is known to induce CYP1A2 and CYP3A4. Therefore, the potential exists for interaction between carbamazepine and any agent metabolized by one (or more) of these enzymes. Agents that are metabolized by CYP1A2 or CYP3A4 may have decreased plasma levels when administered concomitantly with carbamazepine. Breakthrough bleeding has been reported among patients receiving concomitant oral contraceptives and their reliability may be adversely affected). Products include:

Ortho Micronor Tablets **2446**

Norethindrone Acetate (Carbamazepine is known to induce CYP1A2 and CYP3A4. Therefore, the potential exists for interaction between carbamazepine and any agent metabolized by one (or more) of these enzymes. Agents that are metabolized by CYP1A2 and CYP3A4 may have decreased plasma levels when administered concomitantly with carbamazepine. Thus, if a patient has been titrated to a stable dosage on one of the agents in these categories, and then begins a course of treatment with carbamazepine, it is reasonable to expect that a dose increase for the concomitant agent may be necessary). Products include:

Activella Tablets **2347**

Norethynodrel (Carbamazepine is known to induce CYP1A2 and CYP3A4. Therefore, the potential exists for interaction between carbamazepine and any agent metabolized by one (or more) of these enzymes. Agents that are metabolized by CYP1A2 or CYP3A4 may have decreased plasma levels when administered concomitantly with carbamazepine. Breakthrough bleeding has been reported among patients receiving concomitant oral contraceptives and their reliability may be adversely affected).

No products indexed under this heading.

Norfloxacin (Carbamazepine is metabolized mainly by CYP3A4 the active carbamazepine 10,11-epoxide, which is futher metabolized to the trans-diol by epoxide hydrolase. Therefore, the potential exists for interaction between carbamazepine and any agent that inhibits CYP3A4 and/or epoxide hydrolase. Agents that are CYP3A4 inhibitors may increase the plasma levels of carbamazepine. Thus, if a patient has been titrated to a stable dosage of carbamazepine, and then begins a course of treatment with a CYP3A4 or epoxide hydrolase inhibitor, it is reasonable to expect that a dose reduction for carbamazepine may be necessary). Products include:

Noroxin Tablets **2069**

Norgestimate (Carbamazepine is known to induce CYP1A2 and CYP3A4. Therefore, the potential exists for interaction between carbamazepine and any agent metabolized by one (or more) of these enzymes. Agents that are metabolized by CYP1A2 or CYP3A4 may have decreased plasma levels when administered concomitantly with carbamazepine. Breakthrough bleeding has been reported among patients receiving concomitant oral contraceptives and their reliability may be adversely affected). Products include:

Ortho-Cyclen/Ortho Tri-Cyclen **2449**
Ortho Tri-Cyclen Lo Tablets **2458**

Norgestrel (Carbamazepine is known to induce CYP1A2 and CYP3A4. Therefore, the potential exists for interaction between carbamazepine and any agent metabolized by one (or more) of these enzymes. Agents that are metabolized by CYP1A2 or CYP3A4 may have decreased plasma levels when administered concomitantly with carbamazepine. Breakthrough bleeding has been reported among patients receiving concomitant oral contraceptives and their reliability may be adversely affected).

No products indexed under this heading.

Nortriptyline Hydrochloride (Use is not recommended if known sensitivity to any of the tricyclic compounds).

No products indexed under this heading.

Ofloxacin (Carbamazepine is known to induce CYP1A2 and CYP3A4. Therefore, the potential exists for interaction between carbamazepine and any agent metabolized by one (or more) of these enzymes. Agents that are metabolized by CYP1A2 and CYP3A4 may have decreased plasma levels when administered concomitantly with carbamazepine. Thus, if a patient has been titrated to a stable dosage on one of the agents in these categories, and then begins a course of treatment with carbamazepine, it is reasonable to expect that a dose increase for the concomitant agent may be necessary). Products include:

Ofloxacin Ophthalmic Solution
0.3% .... ⊙**243**

Olanzapine (Because of its primary CNS effect, caution should be used when carbamazepine is taken with other centrally-acting drugs). Products include:

Symbyax Capsules **1871**
Zyprexa Tablets **1883**
Zyprexa IntraMuscular **1883**
Zyprexa ZYDIS Orally
Disintegrating Tablets.................. **1883**

Omeprazole (Carbamazepine is metabolized mainly by CYP3A4 the active carbamazepine 10,11-epoxide, which is futher metabolized to the trans-diol by epoxide hydrolase. Therefore, the potential exists for interaction between carbamazepine and any agent that inhibits CYP3A4 and/or epoxide hydrolase. Agents that are CYP3A4 inhibitors may increase the plasma levels of carbamazepine. Thus, if a patient has been titrated to a stable dosage of carbamazepine, and then begins a course of treatment with a CYP3A4 or epoxide hydrolase inhibitor, it is reasonable to expect that a dose reduction for carbamazepine may be necessary).

No products indexed under this heading.

Ondansetron (Carbamazepine is known to induce CYP1A2 and CYP3A4. Therefore, the potential exists for interaction between carbamazepine and any agent metabolized by one (or more) of these enzymes. Agents that are metabolized by CYP1A2 and CYP3A4 may have decreased plasma levels when administered concomitantly with carbamazepine. Thus, if a patient has been titrated to a stable dosage on one of the agents in these categories, and then begins a course of treatment with carbamazepine, it is reasonable to expect that a dose increase for the concomitant agent may be necessary). Products include:

Zofran ODT Orally Disintegrating
Tablets **1687**

Ondansetron Hydrochloride (Carbamazepine is known to induce CYP1A2 and CYP3A4. Therefore, the potential exists for interaction between carbamazepine and any agent metabolized by one (or more) of these enzymes. Agents that are metabolized by CYP1A2 and CYP3A4 may have decreased plasma levels when administered concomitantly with carbamazepine. Thus, if a patient has been titrated to a stable dosage on one of the agents in these categories, and then begins a course of treatment with carbamazepine, it is reasonable to expect that a dose increase for the concomitant agent may be necessary). Products include:

Zofran Injection **1682**
Zofran **1687**

Oxazepam (Because of its primary CNS effect, caution should be used when carbamazepine is taken with other centrally-acting drugs).

No products indexed under this heading.

Oxcarbazepine (Carbamazepine is metabolized by CYP3A4. Therefore, the potential exists for interaction between carbamazepine and any agent that induces CYP3A4. Agents that are CYP3A4 inducers may decrease plasma levels of carbamazepine. Thus, if a patient has been titrated to a stable dosage on carbamazepine, and then begins a course of treatment with a CYP3A4 inducers, it is reasonable to expect that a dose increase for carbamazepine may be necessary).

No products indexed under this heading.

Oxycodone Hydrochloride (Because of its primary CNS effect, caution should be used when carbamazepine is taken with other centrally-acting drugs). Products include:

OxyContin Tablets **2589**
OxyIR Capsules **2593**
Percocet Tablets **1127**
Percodan Tablets **1130**

Paclitaxel (Carbamazepine is known to induce CYP1A2 and CYP3A4. Therefore, the potential exists for interaction between carbamazepine and any agent metabolized by one (or more) of these enzymes. Agents that are metabolized by CYP1A2 and CYP3A4 may have decreased plasma levels when administered concomitantly with carbamazepine. Thus, if a patient has been titrated to a stable dosage on one of the agents in these categories, and then begins a course of treatment with carbamazepine, it is reasonable to expect that a dose increase for the concomitant agent may be necessary).

No products indexed under this heading.

Pargyline Hydrochloride (Co-administration with, or for 14 days after discontinuing MAO inhibitors is not recommended).

No products indexed under this heading.

Paroxetine Hydrochloride (Carbamazepine is metabolized mainly by CYP3A4 the active carbamazepine 10,11-epoxide, which is futher metabolized to the trans-diol by epoxide hydrolase. Therefore, the potential exists for interaction between carbamazepine and any agent that inhibits CYP3A4 and/or epoxide hydrolase. Agents that are CYP3A4 inhibitors may increase the plasma levels of carbamazepine. Thus, if a patient has been titrated to a stable dosage of carbamazepine, and then begins a course of treatment with a CYP3A4 or epoxide hydrolase inhibitor, it is reasonable to expect that a dose reduction for carbamazepine may be necessary). Products include:

Paxil **1535**
Paxil CR Controlled-Release
Tablets **1544**

Pentobarbital Sodium (Because of its primary CNS effect, caution should be used when carbamazepine is taken with other centrally-acting drugs). Products include:

Nembutal Sodium Solution, USP **2494**

Perphenazine (Because of its primary CNS effect, caution should be used when carbamazepine is taken with other centrally-acting drugs).

No products indexed under this heading.

Phenelzine Sulfate (Co-administration with, or for 14 days after discontinuing MAO inhibitors is not recommended).

No products indexed under this heading.

Phenobarbital (Because of its primary CNS effect, caution should be used when carbamazepine is taken with other centrally-acting drugs). Products include:

Donnatal Extentabs **2507**

Phenobarbital Sodium (Carbamazepine is metabolized by CYP3A4. Therefore, the potential exists for interaction between carbamazepine and any agent that induces CYP3A4. Agents that are CYP3A4 inducers may decrease plasma levels of carbamazepine. Thus, if a patient has been titrated to a stable dosage on carbamazepine, and then begins a course of treatment with a CYP3A4 inducers, it is reasonable to expect that a dose increase for carbamazepine may be necessary).

No products indexed under this heading.

Phenytoin (Carbamazepine is metabolized by CYP3A4. Therefore, the potential exists for interaction between carbamazepine and any agent that induces CYP3A4. Agents that are CYP3A4 inducers may decrease plasma levels of carbamazepine. Thus, if a patient has been titrated to a stable dosage on carbamazepine, and then begins a course of treatment with a CYP3A4 inducers, it is reasonable to expect that a dose increase for carbamazepine may be necessary. Carbamazepine may increase the plasma levels of phenytoin; careful monitoring of phenytoin plasma levels following co-medication with carbamazepine is advised).

No products indexed under this heading.

Phenytoin Sodium (Carbamazepine is metabolized by CYP3A4. Therefore, the potential exists for interaction between carbamazepine and any agent that induces CYP3A4. Agents that are CYP3A4 inducers may decrease plasma levels of carbamazepine. Thus, if a patient has been titrated to a stable dosage on carbamazepine, and then begins a course of treatment with a CYP3A4 inducers, it is reasonable to expect that a dose increase for carbamazepine may be necessary. Carbamazepine may increase the plasma levels of phenytoin; careful monitoring of phenytoin plasma levels following co-medication with carbamazepine is advised). Products include:

Phenytek Capsules 2192

Pimozide (Carbamazepine is known to induce CYP1A2 and CYP3A4. Therefore, the potential exists for interaction between carbamazepine and any agent metabolized by one (or more) of these enzymes. Agents that are metabolized by CYP1A2 and CYP3A4 may have decreased plasma levels when administered concomitantly with carbamazepine. Thus, if a patient has been titrated to a stable dosage on one of the agents in these categories, and then begins a course of treatment with carbamazepine, it is reasonable to expect that a dose increase for the concomitant agent may be necessary).

No products indexed under this heading.

Polyestradiol Phosphate (Carbamazepine is known to induce CYP1A2 and CYP3A4. Therefore, the potential exists for interaction between carbamazepine and any agent metabolized by one (or more) of these enzymes. Agents that are metabolized by CYP1A2 and CYP3A4 may have decreased plasma levels when administered concomitantly with carbamazepine. Thus, if a patient has been titrated to a stable dosage on one of the agents in these categories, and then begins a course of treatment with carbamazepine, it is reasonable to expect that a dose increase for the concomitant agent may be necessary).

No products indexed under this heading.

Prazepam (Because of its primary CNS effect, caution should be used when carbamazepine is taken with other centrally-acting drugs).

No products indexed under this heading.

Prednisolone Acetate (Carbamazepine is metabolized by CYP3A4. Therefore, the potential exists for interaction between carbamazepine and any agent that induces CYP3A4. Agents that are CYP3A4 inducers may decrease plasma levels of carbamazepine. Thus, if a patient has been titrated to a stable dosage on carbamazepine, and then begins a course of treatment with a CYP3A4 inducers, it is reasonable to expect that a dose increase for carbamazepine may be necessary). Products include:

Pred Forte Ophthalmic Suspension .... ⊙227
Pred Mild Ophthalmic Suspension .... ⊙230
Pred-G Ophthalmic Ointment .... ⊙229
Pred-G Ophthalmic Suspension ...... ⊙228

Prednisolone Sodium Phosphate (Carbamazepine is metabolized by CYP3A4. Therefore, the potential exists for interaction between carbamazepine and any agent that induces CYP3A4. Agents that are CYP3A4 inducers may decrease plasma levels of carbamazepine. Thus, if a patient has been titrated to a stable dosage on carbamazepine, and then begins a course of treatment with a CYP3A4 inducers, it is reasonable to expect that a dose increase for carbamazepine may be necessary).

No products indexed under this heading.

Prednisolone Tebutate (Carbamazepine is metabolized by CYP3A4. Therefore, the potential exists for interaction between carbamazepine and any agent that induces CYP3A4. Agents that are CYP3A4 inducers may decrease plasma levels of carbamazepine. Thus, if a patient has been titrated to a stable dosage on carbamazepine, and then begins a course of treatment with a CYP3A4 inducers, it is reasonable to expect that a dose increase for carbamazepine may be necessary).

No products indexed under this heading.

Prednisone (Carbamazepine is metabolized by CYP3A4. Therefore, the potential exists for interaction between carbamazepine and any agent that induces CYP3A4. Agents that are CYP3A4 inducers may decrease plasma levels of carbamazepine. Thus, if a patient has been titrated to a stable dosage on carbamazepine, and then begins a course of treatment with a CYP3A4 inducers, it is reasonable to expect that a dose increase for carbamazepine may be necessary).

No products indexed under this heading.

Primidone (Carbamazepine increases the plasma levels of primidone).

No products indexed under this heading.

Procarbazine Hydrochloride (Co-administration with, or for 14 days after discontinuing MAO inhibitors is not recommended).

No products indexed under this heading.

Prochlorperazine (Because of its primary CNS effect, caution should be used when carbamazepine is taken with other centrally-acting drugs).

No products indexed under this heading.

Promethazine Hydrochloride (Because of its primary CNS effect, caution should be used when carbamazepine is taken with other centrally-acting drugs).

No products indexed under this heading.

Propafenone Hydrochloride (Carbamazepine is known to induce CYP1A2 and CYP3A4. Therefore, the potential exists for interaction between carbamazepine and any agent metabolized by one (or more) of these enzymes. Agents that are metabolized by CYP1A2 and CYP3A4 may have decreased plasma levels when administered concomitantly with carbamazepine. Thus, if a patient has been titrated to a stable dosage on one of the agents in these categories, and then begins a course of treatment with carbamazepine, it is reasonable to expect that a dose increase for the concomitant agent may be necessary). Products include:

Rythmol Tablets 1586
Rythmol SR Capsules 1590

Propofol (Because of its primary CNS effect, caution should be used when carbamazepine is taken with other centrally-acting drugs).

No products indexed under this heading.

Propoxyphene Hydrochloride (Because of its primary CNS effect, caution should be used when carbamazepine is taken with other centrally-acting drugs).

No products indexed under this heading.

Propoxyphene Napsylate (Because of its primary CNS effect, caution should be used when carbamazepine is taken with other centrally-acting drugs).

No products indexed under this heading.

Propranolol Hydrochloride (Carbamazepine is known to induce CYP1A2 and CYP3A4. Therefore, the potential exists for interaction between carbamazepine and any agent metabolized by one (or more) of these enzymes. Agents that are metabolized by CYP1A2 and CYP3A4 may have decreased plasma levels when administered concomitantly with carbamazepine. Thus, if a patient has been titrated to a stable dosage on one of the agents in these categories, and then begins a course of treatment with carbamazepine, it is reasonable to expect that a dose increase for the concomitant agent may be necessary). Products include:

InnoPran XL Extended Release Capsules 1484

Protriptyline Hydrochloride (Use is not recommended if known sensitivity to any of the tricyclic compounds).

No products indexed under this heading.

Pyrimethamine (Anti-malarial drugs, such as chloroquine and mefloquine, may antagonize the activity of carbamazepine). Products include:

Daraprim Tablets 1400
Fansidar Tablets 2636

Quazepam (Because of its primary CNS effect, caution should be used when carbamazepine is taken with other centrally-acting drugs).

No products indexed under this heading.

Quetiapine Fumarate (Because of its primary CNS effect, caution should be used when carbamazepine is taken with other centrally-acting drugs).

No products indexed under this heading.

Quinidine (Carbamazepine is metabolized mainly by CYP3A4 the active carbamazepine 10,11-epoxide, which is futher metabolized to the trans-diol by epoxide hydrolase. Therefore, the potential exists for interaction between carbamazepine and any agent that inhibits CYP3A4 and/or epoxide hydrolase. Agents that are CYP3A4 inhibitors may increase the plasma levels of carbamazepine. Thus, if a patient has been titrated to a stable dosage of carbamazepine, and then begins a course of treatment with a CYP3A4 or epoxide hydrolase inhibitor, it is reasonable to expect that a dose reduction for carbamazepine may be necessary).

No products indexed under this heading.

Quinidine Gluconate (Carbamazepine is known to induce CYP1A2 and CYP3A4. Therefore, the potential exists for interaction between carbamazepine and any agent metabolized by one (or more) of these enzymes. Agents that are metabolized by CYP1A2 and CYP3A4 may have decreased plasma levels when administered concomitantly with carbamazepine. Thus, if a patient has been titrated to a stable dosage on one of the agents in these categories, and then begins a course of treatment with carbamazepine, it is reasonable to expect that a dose increase for the concomitant agent may be necessary).

No products indexed under this heading.

Quinidine Hydrochloride (Carbamazepine is metabolized mainly by CYP3A4 the active carbamazepine 10,11-epoxide, which is futher metabolized to the trans-diol by epoxide hydrolase. Therefore, the potential exists for interaction between carbamazepine and any agent that inhibits CYP3A4 and/or epoxide hydrolase. Agents that are CYP3A4 inhibitors may increase the plasma levels of carbamazepine. Thus, if a patient has been titrated to a stable dosage of carbamazepine, and then begins a course of treatment with a CYP3A4 or epoxide hydrolase inhibitor, it is reasonable to expect that a dose reduction for carbamazepine may be necessary).

No products indexed under this heading.

Quinidine Polygalacturonate (Carbamazepine is metabolized mainly by CYP3A4 the active carbamazepine 10,11-epoxide, which is futher metabolized to the trans-diol by epoxide hydrolase. Therefore, the potential exists for interaction between carbamazepine and any agent that inhibits CYP3A4 and/or epoxide hydrolase. Agents that are CYP3A4 inhibitors may increase the plasma levels of carbamazepine. Thus, if a patient has been titrated to a stable dosage of carbamazepine, and then begins a course of treatment with a CYP3A4 or epoxide hydrolase inhibitor, it is reasonable to expect that a dose reduction for carbamazepine may be necessary).

No products indexed under this heading.

Quinidine Sulfate (Carbamazepine is metabolized mainly by CYP3A4 the active carbamazepine 10,11-epoxide, which is futher metabolized to the trans-diol by epoxide hydrolase. Therefore, the potential exists for interaction between carbamazepine and any agent that inhibits CYP3A4 and/or epoxide hydrolase. Agents that are CYP3A4 inhibitors may increase the plasma levels of carbamazepine. Thus, if a patient has been titrated to a stable dosage of carbamazepine, and then begins a course of treatment with a CYP3A4 or epoxide hydrolase inhibitor, it is reasonable to expect that a dose reduction for carbamazepine may be necessary).

No products indexed under this heading.

Quinine (Carbamazepine is metabolized mainly by CYP3A4 the active carbamazepine 10,11-epoxide, which is futher metabolized to the trans-diol by epoxide hydrolase. Therefore, the potential exists for interaction between carbamazepine and any agent that inhibits CYP3A4 and/or epoxide hydrolase. Agents that are CYP3A4 inhibitors may increase the plasma levels of carbamazepine. Thus, if a patient has been titrated to a stable dosage of carbamazepine, and then begins a course of treatment with a CYP3A4 or epoxide hydrolase inhibitor, it is reasonable to expect that a dose reduction for carbamazepine may be necessary).

No products indexed under this heading.

Quinine Sulfate (Carbamazepine is metabolized mainly by CYP3A4 the active carbamazepine 10,11-epoxide, which is futher metabolized to the trans-diol by epoxide hydrolase. Therefore, the potential exists for interaction between carbamazepine and any agent that inhibits CYP3A4 and/or epoxide hydrolase. Agents that are CYP3A4 inhibitors may increase the plasma levels of carbamazepine. Thus, if a patient has been titrated to a stable dosage of carbamazepine, and then begins a course of treatment with a CYP3A4 or epoxide hydrolase inhibitor, it is reasonable to expect that a dose reduction for carbamazepine may be necessary).

No products indexed under this heading.

Quinupristin (Carbamazepine is metabolized mainly by CYP3A4 the active carbamazepine 10,11-epoxide, which is futher metabolized to the trans-diol by epoxide hydrolase. Therefore, the potential exists for interaction between carbamazepine and any agent that inhibits CYP3A4 and/or epoxide hydrolase. Agents that are CYP3A4 inhibitors may increase the plasma levels of carbamazepine. Thus, if a patient has been titrated to a stable dosage of carbamazepine, and then begins a course of treatment with a CYP3A4 or epoxide hydrolase inhibitor, it is reasonable to expect that a dose reduction for carbamazepine may be necessary).

No products indexed under this heading.

Ranitidine Bismuth Citrate (Carbamazepine is metabolized mainly by CYP3A4 the active carbamazepine 10,11-epoxide, which is futher metabolized to the trans-diol by epoxide hydrolase. Therefore, the potential exists for interaction between carbamazepine and any agent that inhibits CYP3A4 and/or epoxide hydrolase. Agents that are CYP3A4 inhibitors may increase the plasma levels of carbamazepine. Thus, if a patient has been titrated to a stable dosage of carbamazepine, and then begins a course of treatment with a CYP3A4 or epoxide hydrolase inhibitor, it is reasonable to expect that a dose reduction for carbamazepine may be necessary).

No products indexed under this heading.

Ranitidine Hydrochloride (Carbamazepine is metabolized mainly by CYP3A4 the active carbamazepine 10,11-epoxide, which is futher metabolized to the trans-diol by epoxide hydrolase. Therefore, the potential exists for interaction between carbamazepine and any agent that inhibits CYP3A4 and/or epoxide hydrolase. Agents that are CYP3A4 inhibitors may increase the plasma levels of carbamazepine. Thus, if a patient has been titrated to a stable dosage of carbamazepine, and then begins a course of treatment with a CYP3A4 or epoxide hydrolase inhibitor, it is reasonable to expect that a dose reduction for carbamazepine may be necessary). Products include:

Zantac 75 Tablets 603
Zantac **1670**
Zantac Injection **1666**
Zantac Injection Pharmacy Bulk Package **1668**
Maximum Strength Zantac 150 Tablets 603
Maximum Strength Zantac 150 Cool Mint Tablets 603

Rasagiline Mesylate (Co-administration with, or for 14 days after discontinuing MAO inhibitors is not recommended). Products include:

Azilect Tablets **3106**

Remifentanil Hydrochloride (Because of its primary CNS effect, caution should be used when carbamazepine is taken with other centrally-acting drugs).

No products indexed under this heading.

Rifabutin (Carbamazepine is metabolized by CYP3A4. Therefore, the potential exists for interaction between carbamazepine and any agent that induces CYP3A4. Agents that are CYP3A4 inducers may decrease plasma levels of carbamazepine. Thus, if a patient has been titrated to a stable dosage on carbamazepine, and then begins a course of treatment with a CYP3A4 inducers, it is reasonable to expect that a dose increase for carbamazepine may be necessary).

No products indexed under this heading.

Rifampicin (Carbamazepine is metabolized by CYP3A4. Therefore, the potential exists for interaction between carbamazepine and any agent that induces CYP3A4. Agents that are CYP3A4 inducers may decrease plasma levels of carbamazepine. Thus, if a patient has been titrated to a stable dosage on carbamazepine, and then begins a course of treatment with a CYP3A4 inducers, it is reasonable to expect that a dose increase for carbamazepine may be necessary).

No products indexed under this heading.

Rifampin (Carbamazepine is metabolized by CYP3A4. Therefore, the potential exists for interaction between carbamazepine and any agent that induces CYP3A4. Agents that are CYP3A4 inducers may decrease plasma levels of carbamazepine. Thus, if a patient has been titrated to a stable dosage on carbamazepine, and then begins a course of treatment with a CYP3A4 inducers, it is reasonable to expect that a dose increase for carbamazepine may be necessary).

No products indexed under this heading.

Rifapentine (Carbamazepine is metabolized by CYP3A4. Therefore, the potential exists for interaction between carbamazepine and any agent that induces CYP3A4. Agents that are CYP3A4 inducers may decrease plasma levels of carbamazepine. Thus, if a patient has been titrated to a stable dosage on carbamazepine, and then begins a course of treatment with a CYP3A4 inducers, it is reasonable to expect that a dose increase for carbamazepine may be necessary).

No products indexed under this heading.

Riluzole (Carbamazepine is known to induce CYP1A2 and CYP3A4. Therefore, the potential exists for interaction between carbamazepine and any agent metabolized by one (or more) of these enzymes. Agents that are metabolized by CYP1A2 and CYP3A4 may have decreased plasma levels when administered concomitantly with carbamazepine. Thus, if a patient has been titrated to a stable dosage on one of the agents in these categories, and then begins a course of treatment with carbamazepine, it is reasonable to expect that a dose increase for the concomitant agent may be necessary). Products include:

Rilutek Tablets **2771**

Risperidone (Because of its primary CNS effect, caution should be used when carbamazepine is taken with other centrally-acting drugs). Products include:

Risperdal Consta Long-Acting Injection **1753**

Ritonavir (Carbamazepine is metabolized mainly by CYP3A4 the active carbamazepine 10,11-epoxide, which is futher metabolized to the trans-diol by epoxide hydrolase. Therefore, the potential exists for interaction between carbamazepine and any agent that inhibits CYP3A4 and/or epoxide hydrolase. Agents that are CYP3A4 inhibitors may increase the plasma levels of carbamazepine. Thus, if a patient has been titrated to a stable dosage of carbamazepine, and then begins a course of treatment with a CYP3A4 or epoxide hydrolase inhibitor, it is reasonable to expect that a dose reduction for carbamazepine may be necessary). Products include:

Kaletra **452**
Norvir **489**

Ropinirole Hydrochloride (Carbamazepine is known to induce CYP1A2 and CYP3A4. Therefore, the potential exists for interaction between carbamazepine and any agent metabolized by one (or more) of these enzymes. Agents that are metabolized by CYP1A2 and CYP3A4 may have decreased plasma levels when administered concomitantly with carbamazepine. Thus, if a patient has been titrated to a stable dosage on one of the agents in these categories, and then begins a course of treatment with carbamazepine, it is reasonable to expect that a dose increase for the concomitant agent may be necessary). Products include:

Requip Tablets **1561**
Requip XL Tablets **1568**

Ropivacaine Hydrochloride (Carbamazepine is known to induce CYP1A2 and CYP3A4. Therefore, the potential exists for interaction between carbamazepine and any agent metabolized by one (or more) of these enzymes. Agents that are metabolized by CYP1A2 and CYP3A4 may have decreased plasma levels when administered concomitantly with carbamazepine. Thus, if a patient has been titrated to a stable dosage on one of the agents in these categories, and then begins a course of treatment with carbamazepine, it is reasonable to expect that a dose increase for the concomitant agent may be necessary).

No products indexed under this heading.

Saquinavir (Carbamazepine is metabolized mainly by CYP3A4 the active carbamazepine 10,11-epoxide, which is futher metabolized to the trans-diol by epoxide hydrolase. Therefore, the potential exists for interaction between carbamazepine and any agent that inhibits CYP3A4 and/or epoxide hydrolase. Agents that are CYP3A4 inhibitors may increase the plasma levels of carbamazepine. Thus, if a patient has been titrated to a stable dosage of carbamazepine, and then begins a course of treatment with a CYP3A4 or epoxide hydrolase inhibitor, it is reasonable to expect that a dose reduction for carbamazepine may be necessary).

No products indexed under this heading.

Saquinavir Mesylate (Carbamazepine is metabolized mainly by CYP3A4 the active carbamazepine 10,11-epoxide, which is futher metabolized to the trans-diol by epoxide hydrolase. Therefore, the potential exists for interaction between carbamazepine and any agent that inhibits CYP3A4 and/or epoxide hydrolase. Agents that are CYP3A4 inhibitors may increase the plasma levels of carbamazepine. Thus, if a patient has been titrated to a stable dosage of carbamazepine, and then begins a course of treatment with a CYP3A4 or epoxide hydrolase inhibitor, it is reasonable to expect that a dose reduction for carbamazepine may be necessary).

No products indexed under this heading.

Secobarbital Sodium (Because of its primary CNS effect, caution should be used when carbamazepine is taken with other centrally-acting drugs).

No products indexed under this heading.

Selegiline (Co-administration with, or for 14 days after discontinuing MAO inhibitors is not recommended). Products include:

Emsam Transdermal System **905**

Selegiline Hydrochloride (Co-administration with, or for 14 days after discontinuing MAO inhibitors is not recommended). Products include:

Eldepryl Capsules 3052

Sertraline Hydrochloride (Carbamazepine is metabolized mainly by CYP3A4 the active carbamazepine 10,11-epoxide, which is futher metabolized to the trans-diol by epoxide hydrolase. Therefore, the potential exists for interaction between carbamazepine and any agent that inhibits CYP3A4 and/or epoxide hydrolase. Agents that are CYP3A4 inhibitors may increase the plasma levels of carbamazepine. Thus, if a patient has been titrated to a stable dosage of carbamazepine, and then begins a course of treatment with a CYP3A4 or epoxide hydrolase inhibitor, it is reasonable to expect that a dose reduction for carbamazepine may be necessary).

No products indexed under this heading.

Sevoflurane (Because of its primary CNS effect, caution should be used when carbamazepine is taken with other centrally-acting drugs). Products include:

Ultane Liquid for Inhalation 524

Sildenafil Citrate (Carbamazepine is metabolized mainly by CYP3A4 the active carbamazepine 10,11-epoxide, which is futher metabolized to the trans-diol by epoxide hydrolase. Therefore, the potential exists for interaction between carbamazepine and any agent that inhibits CYP3A4 and/or epoxide hydrolase. Agents that are CYP3A4 inhibitors may increase the plasma levels of carbamazepine. Thus, if a patient has been titrated to a stable dosage of carbamazepine, and then begins a course of treatment with a CYP3A4 or epoxide hydrolase inhibitor, it is reasonable to expect that a dose reduction for carbamazepine may be necessary).

No products indexed under this heading.

Simvastatin (Carbamazepine is known to induce CYP1A2 and CYP3A4. Therefore, the potential exists for interaction between carbamazepine and any agent metabolized by one (or more) of these enzymes. Agents that are metabolized by CYP1A2 and CYP3A4 may have decreased plasma levels when administered concomitantly with carbamazepine. Thus, if a patient has been titrated to a stable dosage on one of the agents in these categories, and then begins a course of treatment with carbamazepine, it is reasonable to expect that a dose increase for the concomitant agent may be necessary). Products include:

Simcor Tablets 502
Vytorin 10/10 Tablets 2149
Vytorin 10/10 Tablets 2939
Vytorin 10/20 Tablets 2149
Vytorin 10/20 Tablets 2939
Vytorin 10/40 Tablets 2149
Vytorin 10/40 Tablets 2939
Vytorin 10/80 Tablets 2149
Vytorin 10/80 Tablets 2939
Zocor Tablets 2136

Sirolimus (Carbamazepine is known to induce CYP1A2 and CYP3A4. Therefore, the potential exists for interaction between carbamazepine and any agent metabolized by one (or more) of these enzymes. Agents that are metabolized by CYP1A2 and CYP3A4 may have decreased plasma levels when administered concomitantly with carbamazepine. Thus, if a patient has been titrated to a stable dosage on one of the agents in these categories, and then begins a course of treatment with carbamazepine, it is reasonable to expect that a dose increase for the concomitant agent may be necessary). Products include:

Rapamune 3260

Sodium Oxybate (Because of its primary CNS effect, caution should be used when carbamazepine is taken with other centrally-acting drugs). Products include:

Xyrem Oral Solution 1766

Sufentanil Citrate (Because of its primary CNS effect, caution should be used when carbamazepine is taken with other centrally-acting drugs).

No products indexed under this heading.

Sulfinpyrazone (Carbamazepine is metabolized by CYP3A4. Therefore, the potential exists for interaction between carbamazepine and any agent that induces CYP3A4. Agents that are CYP3A4 inducers may decrease plasma levels of carbamazepine. Thus, if a patient has been titrated to a stable dosage on carbamazepine, and then begins a course of treatment with a CYP3A4 inducers, it is reasonable to expect that a dose increase for carbamazepine may be necessary).

No products indexed under this heading.

Tacrine Hydrochloride (Carbamazepine is known to induce CYP1A2 and CYP3A4. Therefore, the potential exists for interaction between carbamazepine and any agent metabolized by one (or more) of these enzymes. Agents that are metabolized by CYP1A2 and CYP3A4 may have decreased plasma levels when administered concomitantly with carbamazepine. Thus, if a patient has been titrated to a stable dosage on one of the agents in these categories, and then begins a course of treatment with carbamazepine, it is reasonable to expect that a dose increase for the concomitant agent may be necessary).

No products indexed under this heading.

Tacrolimus (Carbamazepine is known to induce CYP1A2 and CYP3A4. Therefore, the potential exists for interaction between carbamazepine and any agent metabolized by one (or more) of these enzymes. Agents that are metabolized by CYP1A2 and CYP3A4 may have decreased plasma levels when administered concomitantly with carbamazepine. Thus, if a patient has been titrated to a stable dosage on one of the agents in these categories, and then begins a course of treatment with carbamazepine, it is reasonable to expect that a dose increase for the concomitant agent may be necessary). Products include:

Prograf Capsules and Injection 622
Protopic Ointment 628

Tadalafil (Carbamazepine is known to induce CYP1A2 and CYP3A4. Therefore, the potential exists for interaction between carbamazepine and any agent metabolized by one (or more) of these enzymes. Agents that are metabolized by CYP1A2 and CYP3A4 may have decreased plasma levels when administered concomitantly with carbamazepine. Thus, if a patient has been titrated to a stable dosage on one of the agents in these categories, and then begins a course of treatment with carbamazepine, it is reasonable to expect that a dose increase for the concomitant agent may be necessary). Products include:

Cialis Tablets 1792

Tamoxifen Citrate (Carbamazepine is known to induce CYP1A2 and CYP3A4. Therefore, the potential exists for interaction between carbamazepine and any agent metabolized by one (or more) of these enzymes. Agents that are metabolized by CYP1A2 and CYP3A4 may have decreased plasma levels when administered concomitantly with carbamazepine. Thus, if a patient has been titrated to a stable dosage on one of the agents in these categories, and then begins a course of treatment with carbamazepine, it is reasonable to expect that a dose increase for the concomitant agent may be necessary).

No products indexed under this heading.

Telithromycin (Carbamazepine is metabolized mainly by CYP3A4 the active carbamazepine 10,11-epoxide, which is futher metabolized to the trans-diol by epoxide hydrolase. Therefore, the potential exists for interaction between carbamazepine and any agent that inhibits CYP3A4 and/or epoxide hydrolase. Agents that are CYP3A4 inhibitors may increase the plasma levels of carbamazepine. Thus, if a patient has been titrated to a stable dosage of carbamazepine, and then begins a course of treatment with a CYP3A4 or epoxide hydrolase inhibitor, it is reasonable to expect that a dose reduction for carbamazepine may be necessary). Products include:

Ketek Tablets 2744

Temazepam (Because of its primary CNS effect, caution should be used when carbamazepine is taken with other centrally-acting drugs).

No products indexed under this heading.

Theophylline (Carbamazepine is metabolized by CYP3A4. Therefore, the potential exists for interaction between carbamazepine and any agent that induces CYP3A4. Agents that are CYP3A4 inducers may decrease plasma levels of carbamazepine. Thus, if a patient has been titrated to a stable dosage on carbamazepine, and then begins a course of treatment with a CYP3A4 inducers, it is reasonable to expect that a dose increase for carbamazepine may be necessary).

No products indexed under this heading.

Theophylline Anhydrous (Carbamazepine is metabolized by CYP3A4. Therefore, the potential exists for interaction between carbamazepine and any agent that induces CYP3A4. Agents that are CYP3A4 inducers may decrease plasma levels of carbamazepine. Thus, if a patient has been titrated to a stable dosage on carbamazepine, and then begins a course of treatment with a CYP3A4 inducers, it is reasonable to expect that a dose increase for carbamazepine may be necessary). Products include:

Uniphyl Tablets 2595

Theophylline Calcium Salicylate (Carbamazepine is metabolized by CYP3A4. Therefore, the potential exists for interaction between carbamazepine and any agent that induces CYP3A4. Agents that are CYP3A4 inducers may decrease plasma levels of carbamazepine. Thus, if a patient has been titrated to a stable dosage on carbamazepine, and then begins a course of treatment with a CYP3A4 inducers, it is reasonable to expect that a dose increase for carbamazepine may be necessary).

No products indexed under this heading.

Theophylline Dihydroxypropyl (Glyceryl) (Carbamazepine is metabolized by CYP3A4. Therefore, the potential exists for interaction between carbamazepine and any agent that induces CYP3A4. Agents that are CYP3A4 inducers may decrease plasma levels of carbamazepine. Thus, if a patient has been titrated to a stable dosage on carbamazepine, and then begins a course of treatment with a CYP3A4 inducers, it is reasonable to expect that a dose increase for carbamazepine may be necessary).

No products indexed under this heading.

Theophylline Ethylenediamine (Carbamazepine is metabolized by CYP3A4. Therefore, the potential exists for interaction between carbamazepine and any agent that induces CYP3A4. Agents that are CYP3A4 inducers may decrease plasma levels of carbamazepine. Thus, if a patient has been titrated to a stable dosage on carbamazepine, and then begins a course of treatment with a CYP3A4 inducers, it is reasonable to expect that a dose increase for carbamazepine may be necessary).

No products indexed under this heading.

Thiamylal Sodium (Because of its primary CNS effect, caution should be used when carbamazepine is taken with other centrally-acting drugs).

No products indexed under this heading.

Thioridazine Hydrochloride (Because of its primary CNS effect, caution should be used when carbamazepine is taken with other centrally-acting drugs). Products include:

Thioridazine Hydrochloride Tablets 2195

Thiothixene (Because of its primary CNS effect, caution should be used when carbamazepine is taken with other centrally-acting drugs). Products include:

Thiothixene Capsules 2197

Tiagabine Hydrochloride (Carbamazepine is known to induce CYP1A2 and CYP3A4. Therefore, the potential exists for interaction between carbamazepine and any agent metabolized by one (or more) of these enzymes. Agents that are metabolized by CYP1A2 and CYP3A4 may have decreased plasma levels when administered concomitantly with carbamazepine.

Thus, if a patient has been titrated to a stable dosage on one of the agents in these categories, and then begins a course of treatment with carbamazepine, it is reasonable to expect that a dose increase for the concomitant agent may be necessary). Products include:

Gabitril Tablets 973

Tolterodine Tartrate (Carbamazepine is known to induce CYP1A2 and CYP3A4. Therefore, the potential exists for interaction between carbamazepine and any agent metabolized by one (or more) of these enzymes. Agents that are metabolized by CYP1A2 and CYP3A4 may have decreased plasma levels when administered concomitantly with carbamazepine. Thus, if a patient has been titrated to a stable dosage on one of the agents in these categories, and then begins a course of treatment with carbamazepine, it is reasonable to expect that a dose increase for the concomitant agent may be necessary).

No products indexed under this heading.

Tranylcypromine Sulfate (Coadministration with, or for 14 days after discontinuing MAO inhibitors is not recommended). Products include:

Parnate Tablets 1532

Trazodone Hydrochloride (Carbamazepine is known to induce CYP1A2 and CYP3A4. Therefore, the potential exists for interaction between carbamazepine and any agent metabolized by one (or more) of these enzymes. Agents that are metabolized by CYP1A2 and CYP3A4 may have decreased plasma levels when administered concomitantly with carbamazepine. Thus, if a patient has been titrated to a stable dosage on one of the agents in these categories, and then begins a course of treatment with carbamazepine, it is reasonable to expect that a dose increase for the concomitant agent may be necessary).

No products indexed under this heading.

Triamcinolone (Carbamazepine is metabolized by CYP3A4. Therefore, the potential exists for interaction between carbamazepine and any agent that induces CYP3A4. Agents that are CYP3A4 inducers may decrease plasma levels of carbamazepine. Thus, if a patient has been titrated to a stable dosage on carbamazepine, and then begins a course of treatment with a CYP3A4 inducers, it is reasonable to expect that a dose increase for carbamazepine may be necessary).

No products indexed under this heading.

Triamcinolone Acetonide (Carbamazepine is metabolized by CYP3A4. Therefore, the potential exists for interaction between carbamazepine and any agent that induces CYP3A4. Agents that are CYP3A4 inducers may decrease plasma levels of carbamazepine. Thus, if a patient has been titrated to a stable dosage on carbamazepine, and then begins a course of treatment with a CYP3A4 inducers, it is reasonable to expect that a dose increase for carbamazepine may be necessary). Products include:

Azmacort Inhalation Aerosol 407
Nasacort AQ Nasal Spray 2765
Triesence Injectable Suspension .... ⊙ 209

Triamcinolone Diacetate (Carbamazepine is metabolized by CYP3A4. Therefore, the potential exists for interaction between carbamazepine and any agent that induces CYP3A4. Agents that are CYP3A4 inducers may decrease plasma levels of carbamazepine. Thus, if a patient has been titrated to a stable dosage on carbamazepine, and then begins a course of treatment with a CYP3A4 inducers, it is reasonable to expect that a dose increase for carbamazepine may be necessary).

No products indexed under this heading.

Triamcinolone Hexacetonide (Carbamazepine is metabolized by CYP3A4. Therefore, the potential exists for interaction between carbamazepine and any agent that induces CYP3A4. Agents that are CYP3A4 inducers may decrease plasma levels of carbamazepine. Thus, if a patient has been titrated to a stable dosage on carbamazepine, and then begins a course of treatment with a CYP3A4 inducers, it is reasonable to expect that a dose increase for carbamazepine may be necessary).

No products indexed under this heading.

Triazolam (Because of its primary CNS effect, caution should be used when carbamazepine is taken with other centrally-acting drugs).

No products indexed under this heading.

Trifluoperazine Hydrochloride (Because of its primary CNS effect, caution should be used when carbamazepine is taken with other centrally-acting drugs).

No products indexed under this heading.

Trimethaphan Camsylate (Carbamazepine is known to induce CYP1A2 and CYP3A4. Therefore, the potential exists for interaction between carbamazepine and any agent metabolized by one (or more) of these enzymes. Agents that are metabolized by CYP1A2 and CYP3A4 may have decreased plasma levels when administered concomitantly with carbamazepine. Thus, if a patient has been titrated to a stable dosage on one of the agents in these categories, and then begins a course of treatment with carbamazepine, it is reasonable to expect that a dose increase for the concomitant agent may be necessary).

No products indexed under this heading.

Trimipramine Maleate (Use is not recommended if known sensitivity to any of the tricyclic compounds).

No products indexed under this heading.

Troglitazone (Carbamazepine is metabolized mainly by CYP3A4 the active carbamazepine 10,11-epoxide, which is futher metabolized to the trans-diol by epoxide hydrolase. Therefore, the potential exists for interaction between carbamazepine and any agent that inhibits CYP3A4 and/or epoxide hydrolase. Agents that are CYP3A4 inhibitors may increase the plasma levels of carbamazepine. Thus, if a patient has been titrated to a stable dosage of carbamazepine, and then begins a course of treatment with a CYP3A4 or epoxide hydrolase inhibitor, it is reasonable to expect that a dose reduction for carbamazepine may be necessary).

No products indexed under this heading.

Troleandomycin (Carbamazepine is metabolized mainly by CYP3A4 the active carbamazepine 10,11-epoxide, which is futher metabolized to the trans-diol by epoxide hydrolase. Therefore, the potential exists for interaction between carbamazepine and any agent that inhibits CYP3A4 and/or epoxide hydrolase. Agents that are CYP3A4 inhibitors may increase the plasma levels of carbamazepine. Thus, if a patient has been titrated to a stable dosage of carbamazepine, and then begins a course of treatment with a CYP3A4 or epoxide hydrolase inhibitor, it is reasonable to expect that a dose reduction for carbamazepine may be necessary).

No products indexed under this heading.

Trovafloxacin Mesylate (Carbamazepine is known to induce CYP1A2 and CYP3A4. Therefore, the potential exists for interaction between carbamazepine and any agent metabolized by one (or more) of these enzymes. Agents that are metabolized by CYP1A2 and CYP3A4 may have decreased plasma levels when administered concomitantly with carbamazepine. Thus, if a patient has been titrated to a stable dosage on one of the agents in these categories, and then begins a course of treatment with carbamazepine, it is reasonable to expect that a dose increase for the concomitant agent may be necessary).

No products indexed under this heading.

Valproate Sodium (Carbamazepine is metabolized mainly by CYP3A4 the active carbamazepine 10,11-epoxide, which is futher metabolized to the trans-diol by epoxide hydrolase. Therefore, the potential exists for interaction between carbamazepine and any agent that inhibits CYP3A4 and/or epoxide hydrolase. Agents that are CYP3A4 inhibitors may increase the plasma levels of carbamazepine. Thus, if a patient has been titrated to a stable dosage of carbamazepine, and then begins a course of treatment with a CYP3A4 or epoxide hydrolase inhibitor, it is reasonable to expect that a dose reduction for carbamazepine may be necessary).

No products indexed under this heading.

Vardenafil Hydrochloride (Carbamazepine is metabolized mainly by CYP3A4 the active carbamazepine 10,11-epoxide, which is futher metabolized to the trans-diol by epoxide hydrolase. Therefore, the potential exists for interaction between carbamazepine and any agent that inhibits CYP3A4 and/or epoxide hydrolase. Agents that are CYP3A4 inhibitors may increase the plasma levels of carbamazepine. Thus, if a patient has been titrated to a stable dosage of carbamazepine, and then begins a course of treatment with a CYP3A4 or epoxide hydrolase inhibitor, it is reasonable to expect that a dose reduction for carbamazepine may be necessary). Products include:

Levitra Tablets 2876

Verapamil Hydrochloride (Carbamazepine is metabolized mainly by CYP3A4 the active carbamazepine 10,11-epoxide, which is futher metabolized to the trans-diol by epoxide hydrolase. Therefore, the potential exists for interaction between carbamazepine and any agent that inhibits CYP3A4 and/or epoxide hydrolase. Agents that are CYP3A4 inhibitors may increase the plasma levels of carbamazepine. Thus, if a patient has been titrated to a stable dosage of carbamazepine, and then begins a course of treatment with a CYP3A4 or epoxide hydrolase inhibitor, it is reasonable to expect that a dose reduction for carbamazepine may be necessary). Products include:

Tarka Tablets 511

Vinblastine Sulfate (Carbamazepine is known to induce CYP1A2 and CYP3A4. Therefore, the potential exists for interaction between carbamazepine and any agent metabolized by one (or more) of these enzymes. Agents that are metabolized by CYP1A2 and CYP3A4 may have decreased plasma levels when administered concomitantly with carbamazepine. Thus, if a patient has been titrated to a stable dosage on one of the agents in these categories, and then begins a course of treatment with carbamazepine, it is reasonable to expect that a dose increase for the concomitant agent may be necessary).

No products indexed under this heading.

Vincristine Sulfate (Carbamazepine is known to induce CYP1A2 and CYP3A4. Therefore, the potential exists for interaction between carbamazepine and any agent metabolized by one (or more) of these enzymes. Agents that are metabolized by CYP1A2 and CYP3A4 may have decreased plasma levels when administered concomitantly with carbamazepine. Thus, if a patient has been titrated to a stable dosage on one of the agents in these categories, and then begins a course of treatment with carbamazepine, it is reasonable to expect that a dose increase for the concomitant agent may be necessary).

No products indexed under this heading.

Voriconazole (Carbamazepine is metabolized mainly by CYP3A4 the active carbamazepine 10,11-epoxide, which is futher metabolized to the trans-diol by epoxide hydrolase. Therefore, the potential exists for interaction between carbamazepine and any agent that inhibits CYP3A4 and/or epoxide hydrolase. Agents that are CYP3A4 inhibitors may increase the plasma levels of carbamazepine. Thus, if a patient has been titrated to a stable dosage of carbamazepine, and then begins a course of treatment with a CYP3A4 or epoxide hydrolase inhibitor, it is reasonable to expect that a dose reduction for carbamazepine may be necessary).

No products indexed under this heading.

Warfarin Sodium (Carbamazepine is known to induce CYP1A2 and CYP3A4. Therefore, the potential exists for interaction between carbamazepine and any agent metabolized by one (or more) of these enzymes. Agents that are metabolized by CYP1A2 or CYP3A4 may have decreased plasma levels when administered concomitantly with carbamazepine. Thus, if a patient has been titrated to a stable dosage on one of the agents in these categories, and then begins a course of treatment with carbamazepine, it is reasonable to expect that a dose increase for the concomitant agent may be necessary. Therefore, warfarin's anticoagulant effect may be reduced in the presence of carbamazepine and dosage adjustment may be necessary).
No products indexed under this heading.

Zafirlukast (Carbamazepine is metabolized mainly by CYP3A4 the active carbamazepine 10,11-epoxide, which is futher metabolized to the trans-diol by epoxide hydrolase. Therefore, the potential exists for interaction between carbamazepine and any agent that inhibits CYP3A4 and/or epoxide hydrolase. Agents that are CYP3A4 inhibitors may increase the plasma levels of carbamazepine. Thus, if a patient has been titrated to a stable dosage of carbamazepine, and then begins a course of treatment with a CYP3A4 or epoxide hydrolase inhibitor, it is reasonable to expect that a dose reduction for carbamazepine may be necessary). Products include:
Accolate Tablets **669**

Zaleplon (Because of its primary CNS effect, caution should be used when carbamazepine is taken with other centrally-acting drugs).
No products indexed under this heading.

Zileuton (Carbamazepine is metabolized mainly by CYP3A4 the active carbamazepine 10,11-epoxide, which is futher metabolized to the trans-diol by epoxide hydrolase. Therefore, the potential exists for interaction between carbamazepine and any agent that inhibits CYP3A4 and/or epoxide hydrolase. Agents that are CYP3A4 inhibitors may increase the plasma levels of carbamazepine. Thus, if a patient has been titrated to a stable dosage of carbamazepine, and then begins a course of treatment with a CYP3A4 or epoxide hydrolase inhibitor, it is reasonable to expect that a dose reduction for carbamazepine may be necessary).
No products indexed under this heading.

Ziprasidone Hydrochloride (Because of its primary CNS effect, caution should be used when carbamazepine is taken with other centrally-acting drugs). Products include:
Geodon Capsules **2520**

Zolmitriptan (Carbamazepine is known to induce CYP1A2 and CYP3A4. Therefore, the potential exists for interaction between carbamazepine and any agent metabolized by one (or more) of these enzymes. Agents that are metabolized by CYP1A2 and CYP3A4 may have decreased plasma levels when administered concomitantly with carbamazepine. Thus, if a patient has been titrated to a stable dosage on one of the agents in these categories, and then begins a course of treatment with carbamazepine, it is reasonable to expect that a dose increase for the concomitant agent may be necessary). Products include:
Zomig Tablets **694**
Zomig Nasal Spray **689**
Zomig-ZMT Tablets **694**

Zolpidem Tartrate (Because of its primary CNS effect, caution should be used when carbamazepine is taken with other centrally-acting drugs). Products include:
Ambien Tablets **2692**
Ambien CR Tablets **2696**

Food Interactions

Alcohol (Because of its primary CNS effect, caution should be used when carbamazepine is taken with alcohol).

Grapefruit (Carbamazepine is metabolized mainly by CYP3A4 the active carbamazepine 10,11-epoxide, which is futher metabolized to the trans-diol by epoxide hydrolase. Therefore, the potential exists for interaction between carbamazepine and any agent that inhibits CYP3A4 and/or epoxide hydrolase. Agents that are CYP3A4 inhibitors may increase the plasma levels of carbamazepine. Thus, if a patient has been titrated to a stable dosage of carbamazepine, and then begins a course of treatment with a CYP3A4 or epoxide hydrolase inhibitor, it is reasonable to expect that a dose reduction for carbamazepine may be necessary).

Grapefruit Juice (Carbamazepine is metabolized mainly by CYP3A4 the active carbamazepine 10,11-epoxide, which is futher metabolized to the trans-diol by epoxide hydrolase. Therefore, the potential exists for interaction between carbamazepine and any agent that inhibits CYP3A4 and/or epoxide hydrolase. Agents that are CYP3A4 inhibitors may increase the plasma levels of carbamazepine. Thus, if a patient has been titrated to a stable dosage of carbamazepine, and then begins a course of treatment with a CYP3A4 or epoxide hydrolase inhibitor, it is reasonable to expect that a dose reduction for carbamazepine may be necessary).

ERBITUX

(Cetuximab) **912**
None cited in PDR database.

ERYPED 200 & ERYPED 400 ORAL SUSPENSION

(Erythromycin Ethylsuccinate) **431**
See EryPed Drops

ERYPED DROPS

(Erythromycin Ethylsuccinate) **431**
May interact with oral anticoagulants, cytochrome p450 3a substrates (selected), HMG-CoA reductase inhibitors, phenytoin, triazolobenzodiazepines, valproate, xanthines, and certain other agents. Compounds in these categories include:

Alfentanil Hydrochloride (Concurrent use of erythromycin in patients receiving drugs metabolized by the cytochrome P450 system may be associated with elevation in serum levels of alfentanil).
No products indexed under this heading.

Alprazolam (Erythromycin has been reported to decrease the clearance of triazolam and midazolam; may increase the pharmacologic effect of these benzodiazepines).
No products indexed under this heading.

Aminophylline (Co-administration in patients who are receiving high doses of theophylline may be associated with an increase in serum theophylline levels and potential theophylline toxicity).
No products indexed under this heading.

Anisindione (Co-administration has resulted in increased anticoagulant effects).
No products indexed under this heading.

Astemizole (Concurrent use of erythromycin in patients receiving drugs metabolized by the cytochrome P450 system may be associated with elevation in serum levels of astemizole; co-administration is contraindicated).
No products indexed under this heading.

Atorvastatin Calcium (Erythromycin has been reported to increase concentrations of HMG-CoA reductase inhibitors (e.g. lovastatin and simvastatin); rare reports of rhabdomyolysis have been reported in patients taking these drugs concomitantly). Products include:
Lipitor Tablets **2501**

Bromocriptine Mesylate (Concurrent use of erythromycin in patients receiving drugs metabolized by the cytochrome P450 system may be associated with elevation in serum levels of bromocriptine).
No products indexed under this heading.

Carbamazepine (Concurrent use of erythromycin in patients receiving drugs metabolized by the cytochrome P450 system may be associated with elevation in serum levels of carbamazepine). Products include:
Carbatrol Capsules **3019**
Equetro Extended-Release Capsules **3174**

Cerivastatin Sodium (Erythromycin has been reported to increase concentrations of HMG-CoA reductase inhibitors (e.g. lovastatin and simvastatin); rare reports of rhabdomyolysis have been reported in patients taking these drugs concomitantly).
No products indexed under this heading.

Cilostazol (Concurrent use of erythromycin in patients receiving drugs metabolized by the cytochrome P450 system may be associated with elevation in serum levels of cilostazol). Products include:
Pletal Tablets **2481**

Cisapride (Post-marketing reports have shown concurrent use of erythromycin and cisapride may result in QT prolongation, cardiac arrhythmias, ventricular tachycardia, ventricular fibrillation, and torsade de pointes; most likely due to the inhibition of hepatic metabolism of cisapride by erythromycin; co-administration is contraindicated).
No products indexed under this heading.

Cyclosporine (Concurrent use of erythromycin in patients receiving drugs metabolized by the cytochrome P450 system may be associated with elevation in serum levels of cyclosporine). Products include:
Gengraf Capsules **435**
Neoral Oral Solution **2280**
Neoral Soft Gelatin Capsules **2280**
Restasis Ophthalmic Emulsion **557**
Sandimmune **2296**

Dicumarol (Co-administration has resulted in increased anticoagulant effects).
No products indexed under this heading.

Digoxin (Co-administration has been reported to result in elevated digoxin serum levels). Products include:
Lanoxin Injection **1498**
Lanoxin Injection Pediatric **1502**
Lanoxin Tablets **1505**

Dihydroergotamine Mesylate (Co-administration has been associated in some patients with acute ergot toxicity characterized by severe peripheral vasospasm and dysesthesia).
No products indexed under this heading.

Disopyramide Phosphate (Concurrent use of erythromycin in patients receiving drugs metabolized by the cytochrome P450 system may be associated with elevation in serum levels of disopyramide).
No products indexed under this heading.

Divalproex Sodium (There have been reports of interactions of erythromycin with drugs not thought to be metabolized by CYP3A, including valproate). Products include:
Depakote ER Tablets **423**

Dyphylline (Co-administration in patients who are receiving high doses of theophylline may be associated with an increase in serum theophylline levels and potential theophylline toxicity).
No products indexed under this heading.

Ergotamine Tartrate (Co-administration has been associated in some patients with acute ergot toxicity characterized by severe peripheral vasospasm and dysesthesia).
No products indexed under this heading.

Fluvastatin Sodium (Erythromycin has been reported to increase concentrations of HMG-CoA reductase inhibitors (e.g. lovastatin and simvastatin); rare reports of rhabdomyolysis have been reported in patients taking these drugs concomitantly). Products include:
Lescol Capsules **2268**
Lescol XL Tablets **2268**

Fosphenytoin Sodium (There have been reports of interactions of erythromycin with drugs not thought to be metabolized by CYP3A, including phenytoin).
No products indexed under this heading.

Hexobarbital (There have been reports of interactions of erythromycin with drugs not thought to be metabolized by CYP3A, including hexobarbital).
No products indexed under this heading.

Lovastatin (Erythromycin has been reported to increase concentrations of HMG-CoA reductase inhibitors (e.g. lovastatin and simvastatin); rare reports of rhabdomyolysis have been reported in patients taking these drugs concomitantly). Products include:

Advicor Tablets 402
Mevacor Tablets 2063

Midazolam Hydrochloride (Erythromycin has been reported to decrease the clearance of triazolam and midazolam; may increase the pharmacologic effect of these benzodiazepines).

No products indexed under this heading.

Phenytoin (There have been reports of interactions of erythromycin with drugs not thought to be metabolized by CYP3A, including phenytoin).

No products indexed under this heading.

Phenytoin Sodium (There have been reports of interactions of erythromycin with drugs not thought to be metabolized by CYP3A, including phenytoin). Products include:

Phenytek Capsules 2192

Pimozide (Concurrent use of erythromycin in patients receiving drugs metabolized by the cytochrome P450 system may be associated with elevation in serum levels of pimozide; co-administration is contraindicated).

No products indexed under this heading.

Pravastatin Sodium (Erythromycin has been reported to increase concentrations of HMG-CoA reductase inhibitors (e.g. lovastatin and simvastatin); rare reports of rhabdomyolysis have been reported in patients taking these drugs concomitantly).

No products indexed under this heading.

Rosuvastatin Calcium (Erythromycin has been reported to increase concentrations of HMG-CoA reductase inhibitors (e.g. lovastatin and simvastatin); rare reports of rhabdomyolysis have been reported in patients taking these drugs concomitantly). Products include:

Crestor Tablets 677

Sildenafil Citrate (Erythromycin has been reported to increase the systemic exposure (AUC) of sildenafil).

No products indexed under this heading.

Simvastatin (Erythromycin has been reported to increase concentrations of HMG-CoA reductase inhibitors (e.g. lovastatin and simvastatin); rare reports of rhabdomyolysis have been reported in patients taking these drugs concomitantly). Products include:

Simcor Tablets 502
Vytorin 10/10 Tablets 2149
Vytorin 10/10 Tablets 2939
Vytorin 10/20 Tablets 2149
Vytorin 10/20 Tablets 2939
Vytorin 10/40 Tablets 2149
Vytorin 10/40 Tablets 2939
Vytorin 10/80 Tablets 2149
Vytorin 10/80 Tablets 2939
Zocor Tablets 2136

Tacrolimus (Concurrent use of erythromycin in patients receiving drugs metabolized by the cytochrome P450 system may be associated with elevation in serum levels of tacrolimus). Products include:

Prograf Capsules and Injection 622
Protopic Ointment 628

Terfenadine (Erythromycin has been reported to significantly alter the metabolism of the nonsedating antihistamine terfenadine when taken concomitantly; rare cases of electrocardiographic QT/QTc interval prolongation, cardiac arrest, torsade de pointes, and other ventricular arrhythmias have been observed; co-administration is contraindicated).

No products indexed under this heading.

Theophylline (Co-administration in patients who are receiving high doses of theophylline may be associated with an increase in serum theophylline levels and potential theophylline toxicity).

No products indexed under this heading.

Theophylline Anhydrous (Co-administration in patients who are receiving high doses of theophylline may be associated with an increase in serum theophylline levels and potential theophylline toxicity). Products include:

Uniphyl Tablets 2595

Theophylline Calcium Salicylate (Co-administration in patients who are receiving high doses of theophylline may be associated with an increase in serum theophylline levels and potential theophylline toxicity).

No products indexed under this heading.

Theophylline Dihydroxypropyl (Glyceryl) (Co-administration in patients who are receiving high doses of theophylline may be associated with an increase in serum theophylline levels and potential theophylline toxicity).

No products indexed under this heading.

Theophylline Ethylenediamine (Co-administration in patients who are receiving high doses of theophylline may be associated with an increase in serum theophylline levels and potential theophylline toxicity).

No products indexed under this heading.

Theophylline Sodium Glycinate (Co-administration in patients who are receiving high doses of theophylline may be associated with an increase in serum theophylline levels and potential theophylline toxicity).

No products indexed under this heading.

Tiagabine Hydrochloride (Co-administration of erythromycin and a drug primarily metabolized by CYP3A may be associated with elevations in drug concentrations that could increase or prolong both the therapeutic and adverse effects of the concomitant drug). Products include:

Gabitril Tablets 973

Triazolam (Erythromycin has been reported to decrease the clearance of triazolam and midazolam; may increase the pharmacologic effect of these benzodiazepines).

No products indexed under this heading.

Valproate Sodium (There have been reports of interactions of erythromycin with drugs not thought to be metabolized by CYP3A, including valproate).

No products indexed under this heading.

Valproic Acid (There have been reports of interactions of erythromycin with drugs not thought to be metabolized by CYP3A, including valproate).

No products indexed under this heading.

Warfarin Sodium (Co-administration has resulted in increased anticoagulant effects).

No products indexed under this heading.

ESSENTIAL CAPSULES

(Amino Acid Preparations, Bee Pollen, Herbals with Vitamins & Minerals, Hydroxypropyl Methylcellulose, Soy-containing dietary supplements) 637
None cited in PDR database.

ESTRATEST TABLETS

(Estrogens, Esterified, Methyltestosterone) 3043
See Estratest H.S. Tablets

ESTRATEST H.S. TABLETS

(Estrogens, Esterified, Methyltestosterone) 3043
May interact with oral anticoagulants, cytochrome p450 3a4 inducers (selected), cytochrome p450 3a4 inhibitors (selected), insulin, and certain other agents. Compounds in these categories include:

Acetazolamide (Co-administration with inhibitors of CYP3A4 may increase plasma concentrations of estrogens and may result in side effects).

No products indexed under this heading.

Allium sativum (Co-administration with inducers of CYP3A4 may reduce plasma concentrations of estrogens, possibly resulting in a decrease in therapeutic effects and/or changes in uterine bleeding profile).

No products indexed under this heading.

Amiodarone Hydrochloride (Co-administration with inhibitors of CYP3A4 may increase plasma concentrations of estrogens and may result in side effects).

No products indexed under this heading.

Amprenavir (Co-administration with inhibitors of CYP3A4 may increase plasma concentrations of estrogens and may result in side effects).

No products indexed under this heading.

Anastrozole (Co-administration with inhibitors of CYP3A4 may increase plasma concentrations of estrogens and may result in side effects). Products include:

Arimidex Tablets 672

Anisindione (Decreased anticoagulant requirements).

No products indexed under this heading.

Aprepitant (Co-administration with inducers of CYP3A4 may reduce plasma concentrations of estrogens, possibly resulting in a decrease in therapeutic effects and/or changes in uterine bleeding profile). Products include:

Emend Capsules 1992

Atazanavir (Co-administration with inhibitors of CYP3A4 may increase plasma concentrations of estrogens and may result in side effects).

No products indexed under this heading.

Atazanavir Sulfate (Co-administration with inhibitors of CYP3A4 may increase plasma concentrations of estrogens and may result in side effects). Products include:

Reyataz Capsules 3299

Betamethasone Acetate (Co-administration with inducers of CYP3A4 may reduce plasma concentrations of estrogens, possibly resulting in a decrease in therapeutic effects and/or changes in uterine bleeding profile).

No products indexed under this heading.

Betamethasone Sodium Phosphate (Co-administration with inducers of CYP3A4 may reduce plasma concentrations of estrogens, possibly resulting in a decrease in therapeutic effects and/or changes in uterine bleeding profile).

No products indexed under this heading.

Carbamazepine (Co-administration with inducers of CYP3A4 may reduce plasma concentrations of estrogens, possibly resulting in a decrease in therapeutic effects and/or changes in uterine bleeding profile). Products include:

Carbatrol Capsules 3019
Equetro Extended-Release Capsules 3174

Cimetidine (Co-administration with inhibitors of CYP3A4 may increase plasma concentrations of estrogens and may result in side effects).

No products indexed under this heading.

Cimetidine Hydrochloride (Co-administration with inhibitors of CYP3A4 may increase plasma concentrations of estrogens and may result in side effects).

No products indexed under this heading.

Ciprofloxacin (Co-administration with inhibitors of CYP3A4 may increase plasma concentrations of estrogens and may result in side effects). Products include:

Cipro I.V. 2817
Cipro Oral Suspension 2810
Cipro XR Tablets 2823
Ciprodex Otic Suspension 541

Ciprofloxacin Hydrochloride (Co-administration with inducers of CYP3A4 may reduce plasma concentrations of estrogens, possibly resulting in a decrease in therapeutic effects and/or changes in uterine bleeding profile). Products include:

Cipro Tablets 2810

Cisplatin (Co-administration with inducers of CYP3A4 may reduce plasma concentrations of estrogens, possibly resulting in a decrease in therapeutic effects and/or changes in uterine bleeding profile).

No products indexed under this heading.

Clarithromycin (Co-administration with inhibitors of CYP3A4 may increase plasma concentrations of estrogens and may result in side effects). Products include:

Biaxin/Biaxin XL 411

Clotrimazole (Co-administration with inhibitors of CYP3A4 may

therapeutic effects and/or changes in uterine bleeding profile). Products include:

Satieté Tablets 640

Hypericum Perforatum (Co-administration with inducers of CYP3A4 may reduce plasma concentrations of estrogens, possibly resulting in a decrease in therapeutic effects and/or changes in uterine bleeding profile).

No products indexed under this heading.

Indinavir Sulfate (Co-administration with inhibitors of CYP3A4 may increase plasma concentrations of estrogens and may result in side effects). Products include:

Crixivan Capsules 1979

Insulin (Decreased blood glucose and insulin requirements).

No products indexed under this heading.

Insulin, Human, Zinc Suspension (Decreased blood glucose and insulin requirements).

No products indexed under this heading.

Insulin, Human (rDNA origin) (Decreased blood glucose and insulin requirements). Products include:

Exubera Inhalation Powder 2515

Insulin, Human NPH (Decreased blood glucose and insulin requirements). Products include:

Humulin N Vial 1846

Insulin, Human Regular (Decreased blood glucose and insulin requirements). Products include:

Humulin R 1849
Humulin R (U-500) 1850

Insulin, Human Regular and Human NPH Mixture (Decreased blood glucose and insulin requirements). Products include:

Humulin 50/50, 100 Units 1843
Humulin 70/30 Vial 1844

Insulin, NPH (Decreased blood glucose and insulin requirements).

No products indexed under this heading.

Insulin, Regular (Decreased blood glucose and insulin requirements).

No products indexed under this heading.

Insulin, Regular and NPH mixture (Decreased blood glucose and insulin requirements).

No products indexed under this heading.

Insulin, Zinc Crystals (Decreased blood glucose and insulin requirements).

No products indexed under this heading.

Insulin, Zinc Suspension (Decreased blood glucose and insulin requirements).

No products indexed under this heading.

Insulin Aspart (Decreased blood glucose and insulin requirements).

No products indexed under this heading.

Insulin Aspart, Human (Decreased blood glucose and insulin requirements). Products include:

NovoLog Mix 70/30 2364

Insulin Aspart, Human Regular (Decreased blood glucose and insulin requirements). Products include:

NovoLog Injection 2359

Insulin Aspart Protamine, Human (Decreased blood glucose and insulin requirements). Products include:

NovoLog Mix 70/30 2364

Insulin Detemir (rDNA Origin) (Decreased blood glucose and insulin requirements). Products include:

Levemir Injection 2352

Insulin glargine (Decreased blood glucose and insulin requirements). Products include:

Lantus Injection 2749

Insulin Glulisine (Decreased blood glucose and insulin requirements). Products include:

Apidra Injection 2706

Insulin Lispro, Human (Decreased blood glucose and insulin requirements). Products include:

Humalog-Pen and KwikPen 1829
Humalog Mix 50/50-Pen and KwikPen 1833
Humalog Mix 75/25-Pen and KwikPen 1835

Insulin Lispro Protamine, Human (Decreased blood glucose and insulin requirements). Products include:

Humalog Mix 50/50-Pen and KwikPen 1833
Humalog Mix 75/25-Pen and KwikPen 1835

Isoniazid (Co-administration with inhibitors of CYP3A4 may increase plasma concentrations of estrogens and may result in side effects).

No products indexed under this heading.

Itraconazole (Co-administration with inhibitors of CYP3A4 may increase plasma concentrations of estrogens and may result in side effects).

No products indexed under this heading.

Ketoconazole (Co-administration with inhibitors of CYP3A4 may increase plasma concentrations of estrogens and may result in side effects). Products include:

Extina Foam, 2% 3057
Nizoral A-D Shampoo 1901

Lopinavir (Co-administration with inhibitors of CYP3A4 may increase plasma concentrations of estrogens and may result in side effects). Products include:

Kaletra 452

Loratadine (Co-administration with inhibitors of CYP3A4 may increase plasma concentrations of estrogens and may result in side effects).

No products indexed under this heading.

Mephenytoin (Co-administration with inducers of CYP3A4 may reduce plasma concentrations of estrogens, possibly resulting in a decrease in therapeutic effects and/or changes in uterine bleeding profile).

No products indexed under this heading.

Methsuximide (Co-administration with inducers of CYP3A4 may reduce plasma concentrations of estrogens, possibly resulting in a decrease in therapeutic effects and/or changes in uterine bleeding profile).

No products indexed under this heading.

Methylprednisolone (Co-administration with inducers of CYP3A4 may reduce plasma concentrations of estrogens, possibly resulting in a decrease in therapeutic effects and/or changes in uterine bleeding profile).

No products indexed under this heading.

Methylprednisolone Acetate (Co-administration with inducers of CYP3A4 may reduce plasma concentrations of estrogens, possibly resulting in a decrease in therapeutic effects and/or changes in uterine bleeding profile).

No products indexed under this heading.

Methylprednisolone Sodium Succinate (Co-administration with inducers of CYP3A4 may reduce plasma concentrations of estrogens, possibly resulting in a decrease in therapeutic effects and/or changes in uterine bleeding profile).

No products indexed under this heading.

Metronidazole (Co-administration with inhibitors of CYP3A4 may increase plasma concentrations of estrogens and may result in side effects). Products include:

Pylera Capsules 714

Metronidazole Benzoate (Co-administration with inhibitors of CYP3A4 may increase plasma concentrations of estrogens and may result in side effects).

No products indexed under this heading.

Metronidazole Hydrochloride (Co-administration with inhibitors of CYP3A4 may increase plasma concentrations of estrogens and may result in side effects).

No products indexed under this heading.

Miconazole (Co-administration with inhibitors of CYP3A4 may increase plasma concentrations of estrogens and may result in side effects).

No products indexed under this heading.

Miconazole Nitrate (Co-administration with inhibitors of CYP3A4 may increase plasma concentrations of estrogens and may result in side effects).

No products indexed under this heading.

Modafinil (Co-administration with inducers of CYP3A4 may reduce plasma concentrations of estrogens, possibly resulting in a decrease in therapeutic effects and/or changes in uterine bleeding profile). Products include:

Provigil Tablets 977

Nefazodone Hydrochloride (Co-administration with inhibitors of CYP3A4 may increase plasma concentrations of estrogens and may result in side effects).

No products indexed under this heading.

Nelfinavir Mesylate (Co-administration with inhibitors of CYP3A4 may increase plasma concentrations of estrogens and may result in side effects).

No products indexed under this heading.

Nevirapine (Co-administration with inducers of CYP3A4 may reduce plasma concentrations of estrogens, possibly resulting in a decrease in therapeutic effects and/or changes in uterine bleeding profile). Products include:

Viramune Oral Suspension 873
Viramune Tablets 873

Niacinamide (Co-administration with inhibitors of CYP3A4 may increase plasma concentrations of estrogens and may result in side effects). Products include:

BioLean Free Tablets 635

Nicotinamide (Co-administration with inhibitors of CYP3A4 may increase plasma concentrations of estrogens and may result in side effects).

No products indexed under this heading.

Nifedipine (Co-administration with inhibitors of CYP3A4 may increase plasma concentrations of estrogens and may result in side effects).

No products indexed under this heading.

Norfloxacin (Co-administration with inhibitors of CYP3A4 may increase plasma concentrations of estrogens and may result in side effects). Products include:

Noroxin Tablets 2069

Omeprazole (Co-administration with inhibitors of CYP3A4 may increase plasma concentrations of estrogens and may result in side effects).

No products indexed under this heading.

Oxcarbazepine (Co-administration with inducers of CYP3A4 may reduce plasma concentrations of estrogens, possibly resulting in a decrease in therapeutic effects and/or changes in uterine bleeding profile).

No products indexed under this heading.

Oxyphenbutazone (Concurrent use may result in elevated serum levels of oxyphenbutazone).

No products indexed under this heading.

Paroxetine Hydrochloride (Co-administration with inhibitors of CYP3A4 may increase plasma concentrations of estrogens and may result in side effects). Products include:

Paxil 1535
Paxil CR Controlled-Release Tablets 1544

Phenobarbital (Co-administration with inducers of CYP3A4 may reduce plasma concentrations of estrogens, possibly resulting in a decrease in therapeutic effects and/or changes in uterine bleeding profile). Products include:

Donnatal Extentabs 2507

Phenobarbital Sodium (Co-administration with inducers of CYP3A4 may reduce plasma concentrations of estrogens, possibly resulting in a decrease in therapeutic effects and/or changes in uterine bleeding profile).

No products indexed under this heading.

Phenytoin (Co-administration with inducers of CYP3A4 may reduce plasma concentrations of estrogens, possibly resulting in a decrease in therapeutic effects and/or changes in uterine bleeding profile).

No products indexed under this heading.

Phenytoin Sodium (Co-administration with inducers of

CYP3A4 may reduce plasma concentrations of estrogens, possibly resulting in a decrease in therapeutic effects and/or changes in uterine bleeding profile). Products include:

Phenytek Capsules 2192

Prednisolone Acetate (Co-administration with inducers of CYP3A4 may reduce plasma concentrations of estrogens, possibly resulting in a decrease in therapeutic effects and/or changes in uterine bleeding profile). Products include:

Pred Forte Ophthalmic Suspension .... ⊙ 227
Pred Mild Ophthalmic Suspension .... ⊙ 230
Pred-G Ophthalmic Ointment .... ⊙ 229
Pred-G Ophthalmic Suspension ...... ⊙ 228

Prednisolone Sodium Phosphate (Co-administration with inducers of CYP3A4 may reduce plasma concentrations of estrogens, possibly resulting in a decrease in therapeutic effects and/or changes in uterine bleeding profile).

No products indexed under this heading.

Prednisolone Tebutate (Co-administration with inducers of CYP3A4 may reduce plasma concentrations of estrogens, possibly resulting in a decrease in therapeutic effects and/or changes in uterine bleeding profile).

No products indexed under this heading.

Prednisone (Co-administration with inducers of CYP3A4 may reduce plasma concentrations of estrogens, possibly resulting in a decrease in therapeutic effects and/or changes in uterine bleeding profile).

No products indexed under this heading.

Primidone (Co-administration with inducers of CYP3A4 may reduce plasma concentrations of estrogens, possibly resulting in a decrease in therapeutic effects and/or changes in uterine bleeding profile).

No products indexed under this heading.

Propoxyphene Hydrochloride (Co-administration with inhibitors of CYP3A4 may increase plasma concentrations of estrogens and may result in side effects).

No products indexed under this heading.

Propoxyphene Napsylate (Co-administration with inhibitors of CYP3A4 may increase plasma concentrations of estrogens and may result in side effects).

No products indexed under this heading.

Quinidine (Co-administration with inhibitors of CYP3A4 may increase plasma concentrations of estrogens and may result in side effects).

No products indexed under this heading.

Quinidine Hydrochloride (Co-administration with inhibitors of CYP3A4 may increase plasma concentrations of estrogens and may result in side effects).

No products indexed under this heading.

Quinidine Polygalacturonate (Co-administration with inhibitors of CYP3A4 may increase plasma concentrations of estrogens and may result in side effects).

No products indexed under this heading.

Quinidine Sulfate (Co-administration with inhibitors of CYP3A4 may increase plasma concentrations of estrogens and may result in side effects).

No products indexed under this heading.

Quinine (Co-administration with inhibitors of CYP3A4 may increase plasma concentrations of estrogens and may result in side effects).

No products indexed under this heading.

Quinine Sulfate (Co-administration with inhibitors of CYP3A4 may increase plasma concentrations of estrogens and may result in side effects).

No products indexed under this heading.

Quinupristin (Co-administration with inhibitors of CYP3A4 may increase plasma concentrations of estrogens and may result in side effects).

No products indexed under this heading.

Ranitidine Bismuth Citrate (Co-administration with inhibitors of CYP3A4 may increase plasma concentrations of estrogens and may result in side effects).

No products indexed under this heading.

Ranitidine Hydrochloride (Co-administration with inhibitors of CYP3A4 may increase plasma concentrations of estrogens and may result in side effects). Products include:

Zantac 75 Tablets .... ▣ 603
Zantac 1670
Zantac Injection 1666
Zantac Injection Pharmacy Bulk Package 1668
Maximum Strength Zantac 150 Tablets .... ▣ 603
Maximum Strength Zantac 150 Cool Mint Tablets .... ▣ 603

Rifabutin (Co-administration with inducers of CYP3A4 may reduce plasma concentrations of estrogens, possibly resulting in a decrease in therapeutic effects and/or changes in uterine bleeding profile).

No products indexed under this heading.

Rifampicin (Co-administration with inducers of CYP3A4 may reduce plasma concentrations of estrogens, possibly resulting in a decrease in therapeutic effects and/or changes in uterine bleeding profile).

No products indexed under this heading.

Rifampin (Co-administration with inducers of CYP3A4 may reduce plasma concentrations of estrogens, possibly resulting in a decrease in therapeutic effects and/or changes in uterine bleeding profile).

No products indexed under this heading.

Rifapentine (Co-administration with inducers of CYP3A4 may reduce plasma concentrations of estrogens, possibly resulting in a decrease in therapeutic effects and/or changes in uterine bleeding profile).

No products indexed under this heading.

Ritonavir (Co-administration with inhibitors of CYP3A4 may increase plasma concentrations of estrogens and may result in side effects). Products include:

Kaletra 452
Norvir 489

Saquinavir (Co-administration with inhibitors of CYP3A4 may increase plasma concentrations of estrogens and may result in side effects).

No products indexed under this heading.

Saquinavir Mesylate (Co-administration with inhibitors of CYP3A4 may increase plasma concentrations of estrogens and may result in side effects).

No products indexed under this heading.

Sertraline Hydrochloride (Co-administration with inhibitors of CYP3A4 may increase plasma concentrations of estrogens and may result in side effects).

No products indexed under this heading.

Sildenafil Citrate (Co-administration with inhibitors of CYP3A4 may increase plasma concentrations of estrogens and may result in side effects).

No products indexed under this heading.

Sulfinpyrazone (Co-administration with inducers of CYP3A4 may reduce plasma concentrations of estrogens, possibly resulting in a decrease in therapeutic effects and/or changes in uterine bleeding profile).

No products indexed under this heading.

Telithromycin (Co-administration with inhibitors of CYP3A4 may increase plasma concentrations of estrogens and may result in side effects). Products include:

Ketek Tablets 2744

Theophylline (Co-administration with inducers of CYP3A4 may reduce plasma concentrations of estrogens, possibly resulting in a decrease in therapeutic effects and/or changes in uterine bleeding profile).

No products indexed under this heading.

Theophylline Anhydrous (Co-administration with inducers of CYP3A4 may reduce plasma concentrations of estrogens, possibly resulting in a decrease in therapeutic effects and/or changes in uterine bleeding profile). Products include:

Uniphyl Tablets 2595

Theophylline Calcium Salicylate (Co-administration with inducers of CYP3A4 may reduce plasma concentrations of estrogens, possibly resulting in a decrease in therapeutic effects and/or changes in uterine bleeding profile).

No products indexed under this heading.

Theophylline Dihydroxypropyl (Glyceryl) (Co-administration with inducers of CYP3A4 may reduce plasma concentrations of estrogens, possibly resulting in a decrease in therapeutic effects and/or changes in uterine bleeding profile).

No products indexed under this heading.

Theophylline Ethylenediamine (Co-administration with inducers of CYP3A4 may reduce plasma concentrations of estrogens, possibly resulting in a decrease in therapeutic effects and/or changes in uterine bleeding profile).

No products indexed under this heading.

Triamcinolone (Co-administration with inducers of CYP3A4 may reduce plasma concentrations of estrogens, possibly resulting in a decrease in therapeutic effects and/or changes in uterine bleeding profile).

No products indexed under this heading.

Triamcinolone Acetonide (Co-administration with inducers of CYP3A4 may reduce plasma concentrations of estrogens, possibly resulting in a decrease in therapeutic effects and/or changes in uterine bleeding profile). Products include:

Azmacort Inhalation Aerosol 407
Nasacort AQ Nasal Spray 2765
Triesence Injectable Suspension .... ⊙ 209

Triamcinolone Diacetate (Co-administration with inducers of CYP3A4 may reduce plasma concentrations of estrogens, possibly resulting in a decrease in therapeutic effects and/or changes in uterine bleeding profile).

No products indexed under this heading.

Triamcinolone Hexacetonide (Co-administration with inducers of CYP3A4 may reduce plasma concentrations of estrogens, possibly resulting in a decrease in therapeutic effects and/or changes in uterine bleeding profile).

No products indexed under this heading.

Troglitazone (Co-administration with inducers of CYP3A4 may reduce plasma concentrations of estrogens, possibly resulting in a decrease in therapeutic effects and/or changes in uterine bleeding profile).

No products indexed under this heading.

Troleandomycin (Co-administration with inhibitors of CYP3A4 may increase plasma concentrations of estrogens and may result in side effects).

No products indexed under this heading.

Valproate Sodium (Co-administration with inhibitors of CYP3A4 may increase plasma concentrations of estrogens and may result in side effects).

No products indexed under this heading.

Vardenafil Hydrochloride (Co-administration with inhibitors of CYP3A4 may increase plasma concentrations of estrogens and may result in side effects). Products include:

Levitra Tablets 2876

Verapamil Hydrochloride (Co-administration with inhibitors of CYP3A4 may increase plasma concentrations of estrogens and may result in side effects). Products include:

Tarka Tablets 511

Voriconazole (Co-administration with inhibitors of CYP3A4 may increase plasma concentrations of estrogens and may result in side effects).

No products indexed under this heading.

Warfarin Sodium (Decreased anticoagulant requirements).

No products indexed under this heading.

Zafirlukast (Co-administration with inhibitors of CYP3A4 may increase

plasma concentrations of estrogens and may result in side effects). Products include:
Accolate Tablets 669

Zileuton (Co-administration with inhibitors of CYP3A4 may increase plasma concentrations of estrogens and may result in side effects).
No products indexed under this heading.

Food Interactions

Grapefruit (Co-administration with inhibitors of CYP3A4 may increase plasma concentrations of estrogens and may result in side effects).

Grapefruit Juice (Co-administration with inhibitors of CYP3A4 may increase plasma concentrations of estrogens and may result in side effects).

EVISTA TABLETS

(Raloxifene Hydrochloride) 1810
May interact with estrogens and certain other agents. Compounds in these categories include:

Chlorotrianisene (The safety and concomitant use of raloxifene hydrochloride with systemic estrogens has not been established and its use is not recommended).
No products indexed under this heading.

Cholestyramine (Co-administration causes a 60% reduction in the absorption and enterohepatic cycling of raloxifene; concurrent use should be avoided).
No products indexed under this heading.

Diazepam (Raloxifene might affect the protein binding of other highly protein-bound drugs such as diazepam; caution should be exercised). Products include:
Valium Tablets 2658

Diazoxide (Raloxifene might affect the protein binding of other highly protein-bound drugs such as diazoxide; caution should be exercised). Products include:
Proglycem Capsules 1185
Proglycem Suspension 1185

Dienestrol (The safety and concomitant use of raloxifene hydrochloride with systemic estrogens has not been established and its use is not recommended).
No products indexed under this heading.

Diethylstilbestrol (The safety and concomitant use of raloxifene hydrochloride with systemic estrogens has not been established and its use is not recommended).
No products indexed under this heading.

Estradiol (The safety and concomitant use of raloxifene hydrochloride with systemic estrogens has not been established and its use is not recommended). Products include:
Activella Tablets 2347
Angeliq Tablets 751
Climara Transdermal System 763
Climara Pro Transdermal System 768
Divigel 3167
Vagifem Tablets 2375

Estrogens, Conjugated (The safety and concomitant use of raloxifene hydrochloride with systemic estrogens has not been established and its use is not recommended). Products include:
Premarin Intravenous 3217
Premarin Tablets 3221
Premarin Vaginal Cream 3228
Premphase Tablets 3232
Prempro Tablets 3232

Estrogens, Esterified (The safety and concomitant use of raloxifene hydrochloride with systemic estrogens has not been established and its use is not recommended). Products include:
Estratest Tablets 3043
Estratest H.S. Tablets 3043

Estropipate (The safety and concomitant use of raloxifene hydrochloride with systemic estrogens has not been established and its use is not recommended).
No products indexed under this heading.

Ethinyl Estradiol (The safety and concomitant use of raloxifene hydrochloride with systemic estrogens has not been established and its use is not recommended). Products include:
Lybrel Tablets 3204
Mircette Tablets 1034
NuvaRing 2897
Ortho-Cyclen/Ortho Tri-Cyclen 2449
Ortho Evra Transdermal System 2437
Ortho Tri-Cyclen Lo Tablets 2458
Seasonique Tablets 1046
Yaz Tablets 805

Lidocaine Hydrochloride (Raloxifene might affect the protein binding of other highly protein-bound drugs such as lidocaine; caution should be exercised).
No products indexed under this heading.

Polyestradiol Phosphate (The safety and concomitant use of raloxifene hydrochloride with systemic estrogens has not been established and its use is not recommended).
No products indexed under this heading.

Quinestrol (The safety and concomitant use of raloxifene hydrochloride with systemic estrogens has not been established and its use is not recommended).
No products indexed under this heading.

Warfarin Sodium (Co-administration has resulted in a 10% decrease in prothrombin time in single-dose studies; if used concurrently, prothrombin time should be monitored).
No products indexed under this heading.

Food Interactions

Food, unspecified (Administration of raloxifene with a standardized, high fat meal increases the absorption of raloxifene, but does not lead to clinically meaningful changes in systemic exposure; Evista can be administered without regard to meals).

EVOCLIN FOAM, 1%

(Clindamycin Phosphate) 3056
May interact with neuromuscular blocking agents and certain other agents. Compounds in these categories include:

Atracurium Besylate (Clindamycin has been shown to have neuromuscular blocking properties that may enhance the action of other neuromuscular blocking agents; therefore, it should be used with caution in patients receiving such agents).
No products indexed under this heading.

Cisatracurium Besylate (Clindamycin has been shown to have neuromuscular blocking properties that may enhance the action of other neuromuscular blocking agents; therefore, it should be used with caution in patients receiving such agents). Products include:
Nimbex Injection 484

Doxacurium Chloride (Clindamycin has been shown to have neuromuscular blocking properties that may enhance the action of other neuromuscular blocking agents; therefore, it should be used with caution in patients receiving such agents).
No products indexed under this heading.

Metocurine Iodide (Clindamycin has been shown to have neuromuscular blocking properties that may enhance the action of other neuromuscular blocking agents; therefore, it should be used with caution in patients receiving such agents).
No products indexed under this heading.

Mivacurium Chloride (Clindamycin has been shown to have neuromuscular blocking properties that may enhance the action of other neuromuscular blocking agents; therefore, it should be used with caution in patients receiving such agents).
No products indexed under this heading.

Pancuronium Bromide (Clindamycin has been shown to have neuromuscular blocking properties that may enhance the action of other neuromuscular blocking agents; therefore, it should be used with caution in patients receiving such agents).
No products indexed under this heading.

Rapacuronium Bromide (Clindamycin has been shown to have neuromuscular blocking properties that may enhance the action of other neuromuscular blocking agents; therefore, it should be used with caution in patients receiving such agents).
No products indexed under this heading.

Rocuronium Bromide (Clindamycin has been shown to have neuromuscular blocking properties that may enhance the action of other neuromuscular blocking agents; therefore, it should be used with caution in patients receiving such agents). Products include:
Zemuron Injection 2947

Succinylcholine Chloride (Clindamycin has been shown to have neuromuscular blocking properties that may enhance the action of other neuromuscular blocking agents; therefore, it should be used with caution in patients receiving such agents).
No products indexed under this heading.

Vecuronium Bromide (Clindamycin has been shown to have neuromuscular blocking properties that may enhance the action of other neuromuscular blocking agents; therefore, it should be used with caution in patients receiving such agents).
No products indexed under this heading.

EVOXAC CAPSULES

(Cevimeline Hydrochloride) 1013
May interact with antimuscarinic drugs, beta blockers, cytochrome p450 2d6 inhibitors (selected), cytochrome p450 3a4 inhibitors (selected), parasympathomimetics, and certain other agents. Compounds in these categories include:

Acebutolol Hydrochloride (Possibility of conduction disturbances; co-administration with beta adrenergic antagonists requires caution).
No products indexed under this heading.

Acetazolamide (Drugs which inhibit CYP3A3/4 also inhibit the metabolism of cevimeline).
No products indexed under this heading.

Amiodarone Hydrochloride (Co-administration with drugs which inhibit CYP2D6, such as amiodarone, may inhibit the metabolism of cevimeline resulting in a higher risk of adverse events).
No products indexed under this heading.

Amitriptyline Hydrochloride (Drugs which inhibit CYP2D6 also inhibit the metabolism of cevimeline. Cevimeline should be used with caution in individuals known or suspected to be deficient in CYP2D6 activity, as they may be at a higher risk of adverse events).
No products indexed under this heading.

Amoxapine (Drugs which inhibit CYP2D6 also inhibit the metabolism of cevimeline. Cevimeline should be used with caution in individuals known or suspected to be deficient in CYP2D6 activity, as they may be at a higher risk of adverse events).
No products indexed under this heading.

Amprenavir (Drugs which inhibit CYP3A3/4 also inhibit the metabolism of cevimeline).
No products indexed under this heading.

Anastrozole (Drugs which inhibit CYP3A3/4 also inhibit the metabolism of cevimeline). Products include:
Arimidex Tablets 672

Aprepitant (Drugs which inhibit CYP3A3/4 also inhibit the metabolism of cevimeline). Products include:
Emend Capsules 1992

Atazanavir (Drugs which inhibit CYP3A3/4 also inhibit the metabolism of cevimeline).
No products indexed under this heading.

Atazanavir Sulfate (Drugs which inhibit CYP3A3/4 also inhibit the metabolism of cevimeline). Products include:
Reyataz Capsules 3299

Atenolol (Possibility of conduction disturbances; co-administration with beta adrenergic antagonists requires caution).
No products indexed under this heading.

Atropine Sulfate (Cevimeline might interfere with the desirable antimuscarinic effects of drugs used concomitantly). Products include:
Donnatal Extentabs 2507

Belladonna Alkaloids (Cevimeline might interfere with the desirable antimuscarinic effects of drugs used concomitantly). Products include:

Hyland's Teething Tablets .... ▣621

Betaxolol Hydrochloride (Possibility of conduction disturbances; co-administration with beta adrenergic antagonists requires caution).
No products indexed under this heading.

Bisoprolol Fumarate (Possibility of conduction disturbances; co-administration with beta adrenergic antagonists requires caution).
No products indexed under this heading.

Bupropion Hydrochloride (Drugs which inhibit CYP2D6 also inhibit the metabolism of cevimeline. Cevimeline should be used with caution in individuals known or suspected to be deficient in CYP2D6 activity, as they may be at a higher risk of adverse events). Products include:
Wellbutrin Tablets **1648**
Wellbutrin SR Sustained-Release Tablets **1653**
Wellbutrin XL Extended-Release Tablets **1659**
Zyban Sustained-Release Tablets **1692**

Carteolol Hydrochloride (Possibility of conduction disturbances; co-administration with beta adrenergic antagonists requires caution).
No products indexed under this heading.

Celecoxib (Drugs which inhibit CYP2D6 also inhibit the metabolism of cevimeline. Cevimeline should be used with caution in individuals known or suspected to be deficient in CYP2D6 activity, as they may be at a higher risk of adverse events). Products include:
Celebrex Capsules **2979**

Chloroquine Hydrochloride (Drugs which inhibit CYP2D6 also inhibit the metabolism of cevimeline. Cevimeline should be used with caution in individuals known or suspected to be deficient in CYP2D6 activity, as they may be at a higher risk of adverse events).
No products indexed under this heading.

Chloroquine Phosphate (Drugs which inhibit CYP2D6 also inhibit the metabolism of cevimeline. Cevimeline should be used with caution in individuals known or suspected to be deficient in CYP2D6 activity, as they may be at a higher risk of adverse events).
No products indexed under this heading.

Chlorpheniramine (Drugs which inhibit CYP2D6 also inhibit the metabolism of cevimeline. Cevimeline should be used with caution in individuals known or suspected to be deficient in CYP2D6 activity, as they may be at a higher risk of adverse events).
No products indexed under this heading.

Chlorpheniramine Maleate (Drugs which inhibit CYP2D6 also inhibit the metabolism of cevimeline. Cevimeline should be used with caution in individuals known or suspected to be deficient in CYP2D6 activity, as they may be at a higher risk of adverse events). Products include:
Actifed Cold & Allergy Tablets **1895**
Sudafed PE Sinus & Allergy Tablets **1908**
Tylenol Allergy Multi-Symptom Caplets with Cool Burst and Rapid Release Gelcaps **1916**
Children's Tylenol Plus Cold Suspension Liquid **1912**
Children's Tylenol Plus Cough & Runny Nose Suspension Liquid **1912**
Children's Tylenol Plus Flu Suspension Liquid **1914**
Children's Tylenol Plus Multi-Symptom Cold Suspension Liquid **1912**
Tylenol Cold Head Congestion Nighttime Caplets with Cool Burst **1910**
Tylenol Cold Multi-Symptom Nighttime Caplets with Cool Burst **1913**
Tylenol Sinus Congestion & Pain Nighttime Caplets with Cool Burst **1917**

Chlorpheniramine Polistirex (Drugs which inhibit CYP2D6 also inhibit the metabolism of cevimeline. Cevimeline should be used with caution in individuals known or suspected to be deficient in CYP2D6 activity, as they may be at a higher risk of adverse events). Products include:
Tussionex Pennkinetic Extended-Release Suspension...... **3154**

Chlorpheniramine Tannate (Drugs which inhibit CYP2D6 also inhibit the metabolism of cevimeline. Cevimeline should be used with caution in individuals known or suspected to be deficient in CYP2D6 activity, as they may be at a higher risk of adverse events).
No products indexed under this heading.

Cimetidine (Co-administration with drugs which inhibit CYP2D6, such as cimetidine, may inhibit the metabolism of cevimeline resulting in a higher risk of adverse events).
No products indexed under this heading.

Cimetidine Hydrochloride (Co-administration with drugs which inhibit CYP2D6, such as cimetidine, may inhibit the metabolism of cevimeline resulting in a higher risk of adverse events).
No products indexed under this heading.

Ciprofloxacin (Drugs which inhibit CYP3A3/4 also inhibit the metabolism of cevimeline). Products include:
Cipro I.V. **2817**
Cipro Oral Suspension **2810**
Cipro XR Tablets **2823**
Ciprodex Otic Suspension **541**

Citalopram Hydrobromide (Drugs which inhibit CYP2D6 also inhibit the metabolism of cevimeline. Cevimeline should be used with caution in individuals known or suspected to be deficient in CYP2D6 activity, as they may be at a higher risk of adverse events). Products include:
Celexa **1160**

Clarithromycin (Co-administration with drugs which inhibit CYP3A3/4, such as clarithromycin, may inhibit the metabolism of cevimeline resulting in a higher risk of adverse events). Products include:
Biaxin/Biaxin XL **411**

Clidinium Bromide (Cevimeline might interfere with the desirable antimuscarinic effects of drugs used concomitantly).
No products indexed under this heading.

Clomipramine Hydrochloride (Drugs which inhibit CYP2D6 also inhibit the metabolism of cevimeline. Cevimeline should be used with caution in individuals known or suspected to be deficient in CYP2D6 activity, as they may be at a higher risk of adverse events).
No products indexed under this heading.

Clotrimazole (Drugs which inhibit CYP3A3/4 also inhibit the metabolism of cevimeline). Products include:
Lotrisone **2881**

Cocaine Hydrochloride (Drugs which inhibit CYP2D6 also inhibit the metabolism of cevimeline. Cevimeline should be used with caution in individuals known or suspected to be deficient in CYP2D6 activity, as they may be at a higher risk of adverse events).
No products indexed under this heading.

Cyclosporine (Drugs which inhibit CYP3A3/4 also inhibit the metabolism of cevimeline). Products include:
Gengraf Capsules **435**
Neoral Oral Solution **2280**
Neoral Soft Gelatin Capsules **2280**
Restasis Ophthalmic Emulsion **557**
Sandimmune **2296**

Dalfopristin (Drugs which inhibit CYP3A3/4 also inhibit the metabolism of cevimeline).
No products indexed under this heading.

Danazol (Drugs which inhibit CYP3A3/4 also inhibit the metabolism of cevimeline).
No products indexed under this heading.

Delavirdine Mesylate (Drugs which inhibit CYP3A3/4 also inhibit the metabolism of cevimeline).
No products indexed under this heading.

Desipramine Hydrochloride (Drugs which inhibit CYP2D6 also inhibit the metabolism of cevimeline. Cevimeline should be used with caution in individuals known or suspected to be deficient in CYP2D6 activity, as they may be at a higher risk of adverse events).
No products indexed under this heading.

Dicyclomine Hydrochloride (Cevimeline might interfere with the desirable antimuscarinic effects of drugs used concomitantly). Products include:
Bentyl Capsules **703**
Bentyl Injection **703**
Bentyl Syrup **703**
Bentyl Tablets **703**

Diltiazem Hydrochloride (Co-administration with drugs which inhibit CYP3A3/4, such as diltiazem, may inhibit the metabolism of cevimeline resulting in a higher risk of adverse events). Products include:
Cardizem LA Extended Release Tablets **421**

Diltiazem Maleate (Drugs which inhibit CYP3A3/4 also inhibit the metabolism of cevimeline).
No products indexed under this heading.

Diphenhydramine (Drugs which inhibit CYP2D6 also inhibit the metabolism of cevimeline. Cevimeline should be used with caution in individuals known or suspected to be deficient in CYP2D6 activity, as they may be at a higher risk of adverse events).
No products indexed under this heading.

Diphenhydramine Hydrochloride (Drugs which inhibit CYP2D6 also inhibit the metabolism of cevimeline. Cevimeline should be used with caution in individuals known or suspected to be deficient in CYP2D6 activity, as they may be at a higher risk of adverse events). Products include:
Benadryl Allergy & Cold Kapgels **1895**
Benadryl Allergy & Sinus Headache Kapgels **1895**
Benadryl Severe Allergy & Sinus Headache Caplets **1897**
Benadryl Dye-Free Allergy Liqui-gels Softgels **1897**
Benadryl Allergy Kapgels **1895**
Benadryl Allergy Quick Dissolve Strips **1896**
Benadryl Allergy Ultratab Tablets **1896**
Children's Benadryl Dye-Free Allergy Liquid **1897**
Children's Benadryl Allergy Fastmelts **1897**
Children's Benadryl Allergy Liquid **1898**
Children's Benadryl Allergy Perfect Measure **1896**
Children's Benadryl-D Allergy & Sinus Liquid **1896**
Benadryl-D Allergy & Sinus Tablet **1896**
PediaCare Children's Allergy & Cold Liquid **1902**
PediaCare Children's Allergy Liquid **1902**
Simply Sleep Caplets **1905**
Sudafed PE Nighttime Cold Caplets **1907**
Sudafed PE Severe Cold Caplets **1908**
Extra Strength Tylenol PM Caplets, Geltabs, Liquid, and Rapid Release Gels **1915**
Tylenol Allergy Multi-Symptom Nighttime Caplets with Cool Burst **1916**
Tylenol Severe Allergy Caplets **1916**
Children's Tylenol Plus Cold & Allergy Suspension Liquid **1914**
Tylenol Sore Throat Nighttime Liquid with Cool Burst **1918**

Doxepin Hydrochloride (Drugs which inhibit CYP2D6 also inhibit the metabolism of cevimeline. Cevimeline should be used with caution in individuals known or suspected to be deficient in CYP2D6 activity, as they may be at a higher risk of adverse events).
No products indexed under this heading.

Edrophonium Chloride (Co-administration with parasympathomimetic drugs can be expected to have additive effects).
No products indexed under this heading.

Efavirenz (Drugs which inhibit CYP3A3/4 also inhibit the metabolism of cevimeline). Products include:
Atripla Tablets **938**
Sustiva Capsules **930**
Sustiva Tablets **930**

Erythromycin (Drugs which inhibit CYP3A3/4 also inhibit the metabolism of cevimeline).
No products indexed under this heading.

Erythromycin Estolate (Drugs which inhibit CYP3A3/4 also inhibit the metabolism of cevimeline).
No products indexed under this heading.

Erythromycin Ethylsuccinate (Drugs which inhibit CYP3A3/4 also inhibit the metabolism of cevimeline). Products include:
E.E.S. 433
EryPed 431

Erythromycin Gluceptate (Drugs which inhibit CYP3A3/4 also inhibit the metabolism of cevimeline).
No products indexed under this heading.

Erythromycin Lactobionate (Drugs which inhibit CYP3A3/4 also inhibit the metabolism of cevimeline).
No products indexed under this heading.

Erythromycin Stearate (Drugs which inhibit CYP3A3/4 also inhibit the metabolism of cevimeline).
No products indexed under this heading.

Escitalopram Oxalate (Drugs which inhibit CYP2D6 also inhibit the metabolism of cevimeline. Cevimeline should be used with caution in individuals known or suspected to be deficient in CYP2D6 activity, as they may be at a higher risk of adverse events). Products include:
Lexapro Oral Suspension 1174
Lexapro Tablets 1174

Esmolol Hydrochloride (Possibility of conduction disturbances; co-administration with beta adrenergic antagonists requires caution).
No products indexed under this heading.

Esomeprazole Magnesium (Drugs which inhibit CYP3A3/4 also inhibit the metabolism of cevimeline). Products include:
Nexium Delayed-Release Capsules 645
Nexium Delayed-Release Oral Suspension 645

Fluconazole (Drugs which inhibit CYP3A3/4 also inhibit the metabolism of cevimeline).
No products indexed under this heading.

Fluoxetine (Drugs which inhibit CYP2D6 also inhibit the metabolism of cevimeline. Cevimeline should be used with caution in individuals known or suspected to be deficient in CYP2D6 activity, as they may be at a higher risk of adverse events).
No products indexed under this heading.

Fluoxetine Hydrochloride (Co-administration with drugs which inhibit CYP2D6, such as fluoxetine, may inhibit the metabolism of cevimeline resulting in a higher risk of adverse events). Products include:
Prozac Weekly Capsules 1852
Prozac Pulvules and Liquid 1852
Symbyax Capsules 1871

Fluphenazine Decanoate (Drugs which inhibit CYP2D6 also inhibit the metabolism of cevimeline. Cevimeline should be used with caution in individuals known or suspected to be deficient in CYP2D6 activity, as they may be at a higher risk of adverse events).
No products indexed under this heading.

Fluphenazine Enanthate (Drugs which inhibit CYP2D6 also inhibit the metabolism of cevimeline. Cevimeline should be used with caution in individuals known or suspected to be deficient in CYP2D6 activity, as they may be at a higher risk of adverse events).
No products indexed under this heading.

Fluphenazine Hydrochloride (Drugs which inhibit CYP2D6 also inhibit the metabolism of cevimeline. Cevimeline should be used with caution in individuals known or suspected to be deficient in CYP2D6 activity, as they may be at a higher risk of adverse events).
No products indexed under this heading.

Fluvoxamine Maleate (Drugs which inhibit CYP2D6 also inhibit the metabolism of cevimeline. Cevimeline should be used with caution in individuals known or suspected to be deficient in CYP2D6 activity, as they may be at a higher risk of adverse events). Products include:
Luvox CR Extended-Release Capsules 1759

Fosamprenavir Calcium (Drugs which inhibit CYP3A3/4 also inhibit the metabolism of cevimeline). Products include:
Lexiva Oral Suspension 1510
Lexiva Tablets 1510

Glycopyrrolate (Cevimeline might interfere with the desirable antimuscarinic effects of drugs used concomitantly).
No products indexed under this heading.

Halofantrine Hydrochloride (Drugs which inhibit CYP2D6 also inhibit the metabolism of cevimeline. Cevimeline should be used with caution in individuals known or suspected to be deficient in CYP2D6 activity, as they may be at a higher risk of adverse events).
No products indexed under this heading.

Haloperidol (Drugs which inhibit CYP2D6 also inhibit the metabolism of cevimeline. Cevimeline should be used with caution in individuals known or suspected to be deficient in CYP2D6 activity, as they may be at a higher risk of adverse events).
No products indexed under this heading.

Haloperidol Decanoate (Drugs which inhibit CYP2D6 also inhibit the metabolism of cevimeline. Cevimeline should be used with caution in individuals known or suspected to be deficient in CYP2D6 activity, as they may be at a higher risk of adverse events).
No products indexed under this heading.

Hydroxychloroquine Sulfate (Drugs which inhibit CYP2D6 also inhibit the metabolism of cevimeline. Cevimeline should be used with caution in individuals known or suspected to be deficient in CYP2D6 activity, as they may be at a higher risk of adverse events).
No products indexed under this heading.

Hyoscyamine (Cevimeline might interfere with the desirable antimuscarinic effects of drugs used concomitantly).
No products indexed under this heading.

Hyoscyamine Sulfate (Cevimeline might interfere with the desirable antimuscarinic effects of drugs used concomitantly). Products include:
Donnatal Extentabs 2507

Imatinib Mesylate (Drugs which inhibit CYP2D6 also inhibit the metabolism of cevimeline. Cevimeline should be used with caution in individuals known or suspected to be deficient in CYP2D6 activity, as they may be at a higher risk of adverse events). Products include:
Gleevec Tablets 2255

Imipramine Hydrochloride (Drugs which inhibit CYP2D6 also inhibit the metabolism of cevimeline. Cevimeline should be used with caution in individuals known or suspected to be deficient in CYP2D6 activity, as they may be at a higher risk of adverse events).
No products indexed under this heading.

Imipramine Pamoate (Drugs which inhibit CYP2D6 also inhibit the metabolism of cevimeline. Cevimeline should be used with caution in individuals known or suspected to be deficient in CYP2D6 activity, as they may be at a higher risk of adverse events).
No products indexed under this heading.

Indinavir Sulfate (Co-administration with drugs which inhibit CYP3A3/4, such as indinavir, may inhibit the metabolism of cevimeline resulting in a higher risk of adverse events). Products include:
Crixivan Capsules 1979

Ipratropium Bromide (Cevimeline might interfere with the desirable antimuscarinic effects of drugs used concomitantly). Products include:
Atrovent HFA Inhalation Aerosol 839
Atrovent Nasal Spray 0.03% 834
Atrovent Nasal Spray 0.06% 836
Combivent Inhalation Aerosol 845

Isoniazid (Drugs which inhibit CYP3A3/4 also inhibit the metabolism of cevimeline).
No products indexed under this heading.

Itraconazole (Co-administration with drugs which inhibit CYP3A3/4, such as itraconazole, may inhibit the metabolism of cevimeline resulting in a higher risk of adverse events).
No products indexed under this heading.

Ketoconazole (Co-administration with drugs which inhibit CYP3A3/4, such as ketoconazole, may inhibit the metabolism of cevimeline resulting in a higher risk of adverse events). Products include:
Extina Foam, 2% 3057
Nizoral A-D Shampoo 1901

Labetalol Hydrochloride (Possibility of conduction disturbances; co-administration with beta adrenergic antagonists requires caution).
No products indexed under this heading.

Levobunolol Hydrochloride (Possibility of conduction disturbances; co-administration with beta adrenergic antagonists requires caution).
No products indexed under this heading.

Lopinavir (Drugs which inhibit CYP3A3/4 also inhibit the metabolism of cevimeline). Products include:
Kaletra 452

Loratadine (Drugs which inhibit CYP3A3/4 also inhibit the metabolism of cevimeline).
No products indexed under this heading.

Maprotiline Hydrochloride (Drugs which inhibit CYP2D6 also inhibit the metabolism of cevimeline. Cevimeline should be used with caution in individuals known or suspected to be deficient in CYP2D6 activity, as they may be at a higher risk of adverse events).
No products indexed under this heading.

Mepenzolate Bromide (Cevimeline might interfere with the desirable antimuscarinic effects of drugs used concomitantly).
No products indexed under this heading.

Methadone Hydrochloride (Drugs which inhibit CYP2D6 also inhibit the metabolism of cevimeline. Cevimeline should be used with caution in individuals known or suspected to be deficient in CYP2D6 activity, as they may be at a higher risk of adverse events).
No products indexed under this heading.

Metipranolol Hydrochloride (Possibility of conduction disturbances; co-administration with beta adrenergic antagonists requires caution).
No products indexed under this heading.

Metoprolol Succinate (Possibility of conduction disturbances; co-administration with beta adrenergic antagonists requires caution). Products include:
Toprol-XL Tablets 666

Metoprolol Tartrate (Possibility of conduction disturbances; co-administration with beta adrenergic antagonists requires caution).
No products indexed under this heading.

Metronidazole (Drugs which inhibit CYP3A3/4 also inhibit the metabolism of cevimeline). Products include:
Pylera Capsules 714

Metronidazole Benzoate (Drugs which inhibit CYP3A3/4 also inhibit the metabolism of cevimeline).
No products indexed under this heading.

Metronidazole Hydrochloride (Drugs which inhibit CYP3A3/4 also inhibit the metabolism of cevimeline).
No products indexed under this heading.

Mibefradil Dihydrochloride (Drugs which inhibit CYP2D6 also inhibit the metabolism of cevimeline. Cevimeline should be used with caution in individuals known or suspected to be deficient in CYP2D6 activity, as they may be at a higher risk of adverse events).
No products indexed under this heading.

Miconazole (Drugs which inhibit CYP3A3/4 also inhibit the metabolism of cevimeline).
No products indexed under this heading.

Miconazole Nitrate (Drugs which inhibit CYP3A3/4 also inhibit the metabolism of cevimeline).
No products indexed under this heading.

Moclobemide (Drugs which inhibit CYP2D6 also inhibit the metabolism of cevimeline. Cevimeline should be used with caution in individuals known or suspected to be deficient in CYP2D6 activity, as they may be at a higher risk of adverse events).
No products indexed under this heading.

Nadolol (Possibility of conduction disturbances; co-administration with beta adrenergic antagonists requires caution). Products include:
Nadolol Tablets **2191**

Nebivolol (Possibility of conduction disturbances; co-administration with beta adrenergic antagonists requires caution). Products include:
Bystolic Tablets **1155**

Nefazodone Hydrochloride (Co-administration with drugs which inhibit CYP3A3/4, such as nefazodone, may inhibit the metabolism of cevimeline resulting in a higher risk of adverse events).
No products indexed under this heading.

Nelfinavir Mesylate (Co-administration with drugs which inhibit CYP3A3/4, such as nelfinavir, may inhibit the metabolism of cevimeline resulting in a higher risk of adverse events).
No products indexed under this heading.

Neostigmine Bromide (Co-administration with parasympathomimetic drugs can be expected to have additive effects).
No products indexed under this heading.

Neostigmine Methylsulfate (Co-administration with parasympathomimetic drugs can be expected to have additive effects).
No products indexed under this heading.

Nevirapine (Drugs which inhibit CYP3A3/4 also inhibit the metabolism of cevimeline). Products include:
Viramune Oral Suspension **873**
Viramune Tablets **873**

Niacinamide (Drugs which inhibit CYP3A3/4 also inhibit the metabolism of cevimeline). Products include:
BioLean Free Tablets .... ▣**635**

Nicotinamide (Drugs which inhibit CYP3A3/4 also inhibit the metabolism of cevimeline).
No products indexed under this heading.

Nifedipine (Drugs which inhibit CYP3A3/4 also inhibit the metabolism of cevimeline).
No products indexed under this heading.

Norfloxacin (Drugs which inhibit CYP3A3/4 also inhibit the metabolism of cevimeline). Products include:
Noroxin Tablets **2069**

Nortriptyline Hydrochloride (Drugs which inhibit CYP2D6 also inhibit the metabolism of cevimeline. Cevimeline should be used with caution in individuals known or suspected to be deficient in CYP2D6 activity, as they may be at a higher risk of adverse events).
No products indexed under this heading.

Omeprazole (Drugs which inhibit CYP3A3/4 also inhibit the metabolism of cevimeline).
No products indexed under this heading.

Oxyphenonium Bromide (Cevimeline might interfere with the desirable antimuscarinic effects of drugs used concomitantly).
No products indexed under this heading.

Paroxetine Hydrochloride (Co-administration with drugs which inhibit CYP2D6, such as paroxetine, may inhibit the metabolism of cevimeline resulting in a higher risk of adverse events). Products include:
Paxil **1535**
Paxil CR Controlled-Release Tablets **1544**

Penbutolol Sulfate (Possibility of conduction disturbances; co-administration with beta adrenergic antagonists requires caution).
No products indexed under this heading.

Perphenazine (Drugs which inhibit CYP2D6 also inhibit the metabolism of cevimeline. Cevimeline should be used with caution in individuals known or suspected to be deficient in CYP2D6 activity, as they may be at a higher risk of adverse events).
No products indexed under this heading.

Pindolol (Possibility of conduction disturbances; co-administration with beta adrenergic antagonists requires caution).
No products indexed under this heading.

Propafenone Hydrochloride (Drugs which inhibit CYP2D6 also inhibit the metabolism of cevimeline. Cevimeline should be used with caution in individuals known or suspected to be deficient in CYP2D6 activity, as they may be at a higher risk of adverse events). Products include:
Rythmol Tablets **1586**
Rythmol SR Capsules **1590**

Propantheline Bromide (Cevimeline might interfere with the desirable antimuscarinic effects of drugs used concomitantly).
No products indexed under this heading.

Propoxyphene Hydrochloride (Drugs which inhibit CYP2D6 also inhibit the metabolism of cevimeline. Cevimeline should be used with caution in individuals known or suspected to be deficient in CYP2D6 activity, as they may be at a higher risk of adverse events).
No products indexed under this heading.

Propoxyphene Napsylate (Drugs which inhibit CYP2D6 also inhibit the metabolism of cevimeline. Cevimeline should be used with caution in individuals known or suspected to be deficient in CYP2D6 activity, as they may be at a higher risk of adverse events).
No products indexed under this heading.

Propranolol Hydrochloride (Possibility of conduction disturbances; co-administration with beta adrenergic antagonists requires caution). Products include:
InnoPran XL Extended Release Capsules **1484**

Protriptyline Hydrochloride (Drugs which inhibit CYP2D6 also inhibit the metabolism of cevimeline. Cevimeline should be used with caution in individuals known or suspected to be deficient in CYP2D6 activity, as they may be at a higher risk of adverse events).
No products indexed under this heading.

Pyridostigmine Bromide (Co-administration with parasympathomimetic drugs can be expected to have additive effects).
No products indexed under this heading.

Quinacrine Hydrochloride (Drugs which inhibit CYP2D6 also inhibit the metabolism of cevimeline. Cevimeline should be used with caution in individuals known or suspected to be deficient in CYP2D6 activity, as they may be at a higher risk of adverse events).
No products indexed under this heading.

Quinidine (Drugs which inhibit CYP3A3/4 also inhibit the metabolism of cevimeline).
No products indexed under this heading.

Quinidine Gluconate (Drugs which inhibit CYP2D6 also inhibit the metabolism of cevimeline. Cevimeline should be used with caution in individuals known or suspected to be deficient in CYP2D6 activity, as they may be at a higher risk of adverse events).
No products indexed under this heading.

Quinidine Hydrochloride (Drugs which inhibit CYP2D6 also inhibit the metabolism of cevimeline. Cevimeline should be used with caution in individuals known or suspected to be deficient in CYP2D6 activity, as they may be at a higher risk of adverse events).
No products indexed under this heading.

Quinidine Polygalacturonate (Drugs which inhibit CYP2D6 also inhibit the metabolism of cevimeline. Cevimeline should be used with caution in individuals known or suspected to be deficient in CYP2D6 activity, as they may be at a higher risk of adverse events).
No products indexed under this heading.

Quinidine Sulfate (Drugs which inhibit CYP2D6 also inhibit the metabolism of cevimeline. Cevimeline should be used with caution in individuals known or suspected to be deficient in CYP2D6 activity, as they may be at a higher risk of adverse events).
No products indexed under this heading.

Quinine (Drugs which inhibit CYP3A3/4 also inhibit the metabolism of cevimeline).
No products indexed under this heading.

Quinine Sulfate (Drugs which inhibit CYP3A3/4 also inhibit the metabolism of cevimeline).
No products indexed under this heading.

Quinupristin (Drugs which inhibit CYP3A3/4 also inhibit the metabolism of cevimeline).
No products indexed under this heading.

Ranitidine Bismuth Citrate (Drugs which inhibit CYP2D6 also inhibit the metabolism of cevimeline. Cevimeline should be used with caution in individuals known or suspected to be deficient in CYP2D6 activity, as they may be at a higher risk of adverse events).
No products indexed under this heading.

Ranitidine Hydrochloride (Drugs which inhibit CYP2D6 also inhibit the metabolism of cevimeline. Cevimeline should be used with caution in individuals known or suspected to be deficient in CYP2D6 activity, as they may be at a higher risk of adverse events). Products include:
Zantac 75 Tablets .... ▣**603**
Zantac **1670**
Zantac Injection **1666**
Zantac Injection Pharmacy Bulk Package **1668**
Maximum Strength Zantac 150 Tablets .... ▣**603**
Maximum Strength Zantac 150 Cool Mint Tablets .... ▣**603**

Ritonavir (Co-administration with drugs which inhibit CYP2D6 and/or CYP3A3/4, such as ritonavir, may inhibit the metabolism of cevimeline resulting in a higher risk of adverse events). Products include:
Kaletra **452**
Norvir **489**

Saquinavir (Drugs which inhibit CYP3A3/4 also inhibit the metabolism of cevimeline).
No products indexed under this heading.

Saquinavir Mesylate (Drugs which inhibit CYP3A3/4 also inhibit the metabolism of cevimeline).
No products indexed under this heading.

Scopolamine (Cevimeline might interfere with the desirable antimuscarinic effects of drugs used concomitantly). Products include:
Transderm Scōp Transdermal Therapeutic System **2206**

Scopolamine Hydrobromide (Cevimeline might interfere with the desirable antimuscarinic effects of drugs used concomitantly). Products include:
Donnatal Extentabs **2507**

Sertraline Hydrochloride (Co-administration with drugs which inhibit CYP2D6, such as sertraline, may inhibit the metabolism of cevimeline resulting in a higher risk of adverse events).
No products indexed under this heading.

Sildenafil Citrate (Drugs which inhibit CYP2D6 also inhibit the metabolism of cevimeline. Cevimeline should be used with caution in individuals known or suspected to be deficient in CYP2D6 activity, as they may be at a higher risk of adverse events).
No products indexed under this heading.

Sotalol Hydrochloride (Possibility of conduction disturbances; co-administration with beta adrenergic antagonists requires caution).
No products indexed under this heading.

Telithromycin (Drugs which inhibit CYP3A3/4 also inhibit the metabolism of cevimeline). Products include:
Ketek Tablets **2744**

Terbinafine Hydrochloride (Drugs which inhibit CYP2D6 also inhibit the

metabolism of cevimeline. Cevimeline should be used with caution in individuals known or suspected to be deficient in CYP2D6 activity, as they may be at a higher risk of adverse events). Products include:
Lamisil Oral Granules 2264
Lamisil Tablets 2266

Thioridazine Hydrochloride (Drugs which inhibit CYP2D6 also inhibit the metabolism of cevimeline. Cevimeline should be used with caution in individuals known or suspected to be deficient in CYP2D6 activity, as they may be at a higher risk of adverse events). Products include:
Thioridazine Hydrochloride Tablets 2195

Timolol Hemihydrate (Possibility of conduction disturbances; co-administration with beta adrenergic antagonists requires caution). Products include:
Betimol Ophthalmic Solution 3181

Timolol Maleate (Possibility of conduction disturbances; co-administration with beta adrenergic antagonists requires caution). Products include:
Combigan Ophthalmic Solution 553
Cosopt Sterile Ophthalmic Solution 1969
Timoptic Sterile Ophthalmic Solution 2121
Timoptic in Ocudose 2124
Timoptic-XE Sterile Ophthalmic Gel Forming Solution 2125

Tolterodine Tartrate (Cevimeline might interfere with the desirable antimuscarinic effects of drugs used concomitantly).
No products indexed under this heading.

Tridihexethyl Chloride (Cevimeline might interfere with the desirable antimuscarinic effects of drugs used concomitantly).
No products indexed under this heading.

Trimipramine Maleate (Drugs which inhibit CYP2D6 also inhibit the metabolism of cevimeline. Cevimeline should be used with caution in individuals known or suspected to be deficient in CYP2D6 activity, as they may be at a higher risk of adverse events).
No products indexed under this heading.

Troglitazone (Drugs which inhibit CYP3A3/4 also inhibit the metabolism of cevimeline).
No products indexed under this heading.

Troleandomycin (Drugs which inhibit CYP3A3/4 also inhibit the metabolism of cevimeline).
No products indexed under this heading.

Valproate Sodium (Drugs which inhibit CYP3A3/4 also inhibit the metabolism of cevimeline).
No products indexed under this heading.

Vardenafil Hydrochloride (Drugs which inhibit CYP2D6 also inhibit the metabolism of cevimeline. Cevimeline should be used with caution in individuals known or suspected to be deficient in CYP2D6 activity, as they may be at a higher risk of adverse events). Products include:
Levitra Tablets 2876

Verapamil Hydrochloride (Co-administration with drugs which inhibit CYP3A3/4, such as verapamil, may inhibit the metabolism of cevimeline resulting in a higher risk of adverse events). Products include:
Tarka Tablets 511

Voriconazole (Drugs which inhibit CYP3A3/4 also inhibit the metabolism of cevimeline).
No products indexed under this heading.

Zafirlukast (Drugs which inhibit CYP3A3/4 also inhibit the metabolism of cevimeline). Products include:
Accolate Tablets 669

Zileuton (Drugs which inhibit CYP3A3/4 also inhibit the metabolism of cevimeline).
No products indexed under this heading.

Food Interactions

Food, unspecified (Co-administration with food decreases the rate of absorption, with a fasting Tmax of 1.53 hours and a Tmax of 2.86 hours after a meal; the peak concentration is reduced by 17.3%).

Grapefruit (Drugs which inhibit CYP3A3/4 also inhibit the metabolism of cevimeline).

Grapefruit Juice (Co-administration with drugs which inhibit CYP3A3/4, such as grapefruit juice, may inhibit the metabolism of cevimeline resulting in a higher risk of adverse events).

EXELON CAPSULES

(Rivastigmine Tartrate) 2229
May interact with anticholinergics and certain other agents. Compounds in these categories include:

Atropine Sulfate (Rivastigmine, a cholinesterase inhibitor, has the potential to interfere with the activity of anticholinergic medications). Products include:
Donnatal Extentabs 2507

Belladonna Alkaloids (Rivastigmine, a cholinesterase inhibitor, has the potential to interfere with the activity of anticholinergic medications). Products include:
Hyland's Teething Tablets .... ◘ 621

Benztropine Mesylate (Rivastigmine, a cholinesterase inhibitor, has the potential to interfere with the activity of anticholinergic medications).
No products indexed under this heading.

Bethanechol Chloride (Co-administration with cholinergic agonist, such as bethanechol, can be expected to result in a synergistic effect).
No products indexed under this heading.

Biperiden Hydrochloride (Rivastigmine, a cholinesterase inhibitor, has the potential to interfere with the activity of anticholinergic medications).
No products indexed under this heading.

Clidinium Bromide (Rivastigmine, a cholinesterase inhibitor, has the potential to interfere with the activity of anticholinergic medications).
No products indexed under this heading.

Dicyclomine Hydrochloride (Rivastigmine, a cholinesterase inhibitor, has the potential to interfere with the activity of anticholinergic medications). Products include:
Bentyl Capsules 703
Bentyl Injection 703
Bentyl Syrup 703
Bentyl Tablets 703

Glycopyrrolate (Rivastigmine, a cholinesterase inhibitor, has the potential to interfere with the activity of anticholinergic medications).
No products indexed under this heading.

Hyoscyamine (Rivastigmine, a cholinesterase inhibitor, has the potential to interfere with the activity of anticholinergic medications).
No products indexed under this heading.

Hyoscyamine Sulfate (Rivastigmine, a cholinesterase inhibitor, has the potential to interfere with the activity of anticholinergic medications). Products include:
Donnatal Extentabs 2507

Ipratropium Bromide (Rivastigmine, a cholinesterase inhibitor, has the potential to interfere with the activity of anticholinergic medications). Products include:
Atrovent HFA Inhalation Aerosol 839
Atrovent Nasal Spray 0.03% 834
Atrovent Nasal Spray 0.06% 836
Combivent Inhalation Aerosol 845

Mepenzolate Bromide (Rivastigmine, a cholinesterase inhibitor, has the potential to interfere with the activity of anticholinergic medications).
No products indexed under this heading.

Oxybutynin Chloride (Rivastigmine, a cholinesterase inhibitor, has the potential to interfere with the activity of anticholinergic medications).
No products indexed under this heading.

Procyclidine Hydrochloride (Rivastigmine, a cholinesterase inhibitor, has the potential to interfere with the activity of anticholinergic medications).
No products indexed under this heading.

Propantheline Bromide (Rivastigmine, a cholinesterase inhibitor, has the potential to interfere with the activity of anticholinergic medications).
No products indexed under this heading.

Scopolamine (Rivastigmine, a cholinesterase inhibitor, has the potential to interfere with the activity of anticholinergic medications). Products include:
Transderm Scōp Transdermal Therapeutic System 2206

Scopolamine Hydrobromide (Rivastigmine, a cholinesterase inhibitor, has the potential to interfere with the activity of anticholinergic medications). Products include:
Donnatal Extentabs 2507

Succinylcholine Chloride (Co-administration with succinylcholine can be expected to result in a synergistic effect).
No products indexed under this heading.

Tolterodine Tartrate (Rivastigmine, a cholinesterase inhibitor, has the potential to interfere with the activity of anticholinergic medications).
No products indexed under this heading.

Tridihexethyl Chloride (Rivastigmine, a cholinesterase inhibitor, has the potential to interfere with the activity of anticholinergic medications).
No products indexed under this heading.

Trihexyphenidyl Hydrochloride (Rivastigmine, a cholinesterase inhibitor, has the potential to interfere with the activity of anticholinergic medications).
No products indexed under this heading.

Food Interactions

Food, unspecified (Co-administration with food delays absorption (Tmax) by 90 minutes, lowers Cmax by approximately 30% and increases AUC by approximately 30%).

EXELON ORAL SOLUTION

(Rivastigmine Tartrate) 2229
See Exelon Capsules

EXELON PATCH

(Rivastigmine Tartrate) 2233
None cited in PDR database.

EXFORGE TABLETS

(Amlodipine Besylate, Valsartan) 2238
May interact with potassium preparations, potassium sparing diuretics, and certain other agents. Compounds in these categories include:

Amiloride Hydrochloride (As with other drugs that block angiotensin II or its effects, concomitant use of potassium sparing diuretics (eg, amiloride), may lead to increases in serum potassium and in heart failure patients to increases in serum creatinine).
No products indexed under this heading.

Potassium Acid Phosphate (As with other drugs that block angiotensin II or its effects, concomitant use of potassium potassium supplements, or salt substitutes containing potassium may lead to increases in serum potassium and in heart failure patients to increases in serum creatinine). Products include:
K-Phos Original (Sodium Free) Tablets 814

Potassium Bicarbonate (As with other drugs that block angiotensin II or its effects, concomitant use of potassium potassium supplements, or salt substitutes containing potassium may lead to increases in serum potassium and in heart failure patients to increases in serum creatinine).
No products indexed under this heading.

Potassium Chloride (As with other drugs that block angiotensin II or its effects, concomitant use of potassium potassium supplements, or salt substitutes containing potassium may lead to increases in serum potassium and in heart failure patients to increases in serum creatinine). Products include:
MoviPrep Oral Solution 2679

Potassium Citrate (As with other drugs that block angiotensin II or its effects, concomitant use of potassium potassium supplements, or salt substitutes containing potassium may lead to increases in serum potassium and in heart failure patients to increases in serum creatinine). Products include:

BioLean Free Tablets .... ▭635
Urocit-K Tablets 2176

Potassium Gluconate (As with other drugs that block angiotensin II or its effects, concomitant use of potassium potassium supplements, or salt substitutes containing potassium may lead to increases in serum potassium and in heart failure patients to increases in serum creatinine).
No products indexed under this heading.

Potassium Iodide (As with other drugs that block angiotensin II or its effects, concomitant use of potassium sparing diuretics (eg, spironolactone, triamterene, amiloride), potassium supplements, or salt substitutes containing potassium may lead to increases in serum potassium. In heart failure patients may lead to increases in serum creatinine). Products include:
CitraNatal DHA Tablets 2175
CitraNatal 90 DHA Tablets 2175

Potassium Phosphate (As with other drugs that block angiotensin II or its effects, concomitant use of potassium potassium supplements, or salt substitutes containing potassium may lead to increases in serum potassium and in heart failure patients to increases in serum creatinine). Products include:
K-Phos Neutral Tablets 813

Sildenafil Citrate (A single 100 mg dose of sildenafil in subjects with essential hypertension had no effect on the pharmacokinetic parameters of amlodipine. When amlodipine and sildenafil were used in combination, each agent independently exerted its own blood pressure lowering effect).
No products indexed under this heading.

Spironolactone (As with other drugs that block angiotensin II or its effects, concomitant use of potassium sparing diuretics (eg, spironolactone), may lead to increases in serum potassium and in heart failure patients to increases in serum creatinine).
No products indexed under this heading.

Triamterene (As with other drugs that block angiotensin II or its effects, concomitant use of potassium sparing diuretics (eg, triamterene), may lead to increases in serum potassium and in heart failure patients to increases in serum creatinine). Products include:
Dyazide Capsules 1405
Dyrenium Capsules 3189

EXJADE TABLETS

(Deferasirox) 2244
May interact with antacids containing aluminum, calcium and magnesium and certain other agents. Compounds in these categories include:

Aluminum Carbonate (Although deferasirox has a lower affinity for aluminum than for iron, deferasirox should not be taken with aluminum-containing antacid preparations).
No products indexed under this heading.

Aluminum Hydroxide (Although deferasirox has a lower affinity for aluminum than for iron, deferasirox should not be taken with aluminum-containing antacid preparations).
No products indexed under this heading.

Deferoxamine Mesylate (Deferasirox should not be combined with other iron chelator therapies, as safety of such combination has not been established).
No products indexed under this heading.

Magaldrate (Although deferasirox has a lower affinity for aluminum than for iron, deferasirox should not be taken with aluminum-containing antacid preparations).
No products indexed under this heading.

Magnesium Hydroxide (Although deferasirox has a lower affinity for aluminum than for iron, deferasirox should not be taken with aluminum-containing antacid preparations). Products include:
Fleet Pedia-Lax Chewable Tablets 1145
Pepcid Complete Chewable Tablets 1771
Extra Strength Rolaids Freshmint Tablets 1903
Rolaids Multi-Symptom Berry Tablets 1903
Rolaids Original Peppermint Tablets 1903

Magnesium Oxide (Although deferasirox has a lower affinity for aluminum than for iron, deferasirox should not be taken with aluminum-containing antacid preparations). Products include:
Beelith Tablets 813

EXPERIENCE CAPSULES

(Herbals, Multiple, Psyllium Preparations).................................... ▭624
None cited in PDR database.

EXTINA FOAM, 2%

(Ketoconazole) 3057
None cited in PDR database.

EXUBERA INHALATION POWDER

(Insulin, Human (rDNA origin)) 2515
May interact with ACE inhibitors, beta blockers, corticosteroids, diuretics, estrogens, fibrates, oral hypoglycemic agents, lithium preparations, monoamine oxidase inhibitors, oral contraceptives, phenothiazines, progestins, protease inhibitors, salicylates, sympathomimetic bronchodilators, sympathomimetics, sympathomimetic aerosol bronchodilators, thyroid preparations, and certain other agents. Compounds in these categories include:

Acarbose (Oral antidiabetic products may increase the blood glucose-lowering effect of insulin and susceptibility to hypoglycemia. Co-administration may require insulin dose adjustment and particularly close monitoring). Products include:
Precose Tablets 792

Acebutolol Hydrochloride (Beta-blockers may either increase or reduce the blood glucose-lowering effect of insulin. In addition, under the influence of sympatholytic medicinal products such as beta-blockers, the signs and symptoms of hypoglycemia may be reduced or absent. Co-administration may require insulin dose adjustment and particularly close monitoring).
No products indexed under this heading.

Albuterol (Sympathomimetics may reduce the blood glucose-lowering effect of insulin, which may result in hyperglycemia. Co-administration may require insulin dose adjustment and particularly close monitoring).
No products indexed under this heading.

Albuterol Sulfate (Sympathomimetics may reduce the blood glucose-lowering effect of insulin, which may result in hyperglycemia. Co-administration may require insulin dose adjustment and particularly close monitoring). Products include:
Combivent Inhalation Aerosol 845
ProAir HFA Inhalation Aerosol 3113
Proventil HFA Inhalation Aerosol 2914
Ventolin HFA Inhalation Aerosol 1638

Amiloride Hydrochloride (Diuretics may reduce the blood glucose-lowering effect of insulin, which may result in hyperglycemia. Co-administration may require insulin dose adjustment and particularly close monitoring).
No products indexed under this heading.

Amprenavir (Protease inhibitors may reduce the blood glucose-lowering effect of insulin, which may result in hyperglycemia. Co-administration may require insulin dose adjustment and particularly close monitoring).
No products indexed under this heading.

Aspirin (Salicylates may increase the blood glucose-lowering effect of insulin and susceptibility to hypoglycemia. Co-administration may require insulin dose adjustment and particularly close monitoring). Products include:
Aggrenox Capsules 819
Bayer Aspirin 750
Percodan Tablets 1130
St. Joseph 81 mg Aspirin Chewable and Enteric Coated Tablets 1903

Aspirin, Enteric Coated (Salicylates may increase the blood glucose-lowering effect of insulin and susceptibility to hypoglycemia. Co-administration may require insulin dose adjustment and particularly close monitoring).
No products indexed under this heading.

Aspirin Buffered (Salicylates may increase the blood glucose-lowering effect of insulin and susceptibility to hypoglycemia. Co-administration may require insulin dose adjustment and particularly close monitoring).
No products indexed under this heading.

Atenolol (Beta-blockers may either increase or reduce the blood glucose-lowering effect of insulin. In addition, under the influence of sympatholytic medicinal products such as beta-blockers, the signs and symptoms of hypoglycemia may be reduced or absent. Co-administration may require insulin dose adjustment and particularly close monitoring).
No products indexed under this heading.

Benazepril Hydrochloride (ACE inhibitors may increase the blood glucose-lowering effect of insulin and susceptibility to hypoglycemia. Co-administration may require insulin dose adjustment and particularly close monitoring).
No products indexed under this heading.

Bendroflumethiazide (Diuretics may reduce the blood glucose-lowering effect of insulin, which may result in hyperglycemia. Co-administration may require insulin dose adjustment and particularly close monitoring).
No products indexed under this heading.

Betamethasone Acetate (Corticosteroids may reduce the blood glucose-lowering effect of insulin, which may result in hyperglycemia. Co-administration may require insulin dose adjustment and particularly close monitoring).
No products indexed under this heading.

Betamethasone Sodium Phosphate (Corticosteroids may reduce the blood glucose-lowering effect of insulin, which may result in hyperglycemia. Co-administration may require insulin dose adjustment and particularly close monitoring).
No products indexed under this heading.

Betaxolol Hydrochloride (Beta-blockers may either increase or reduce the blood glucose-lowering effect of insulin. In addition, under the influence of sympatholytic medicinal products such as beta-blockers, the signs and symptoms of hypoglycemia may be reduced or absent. Co-administration may require insulin dose adjustment and particularly close monitoring).
No products indexed under this heading.

Bisoprolol Fumarate (Beta-blockers may either increase or reduce the blood glucose-lowering effect of insulin. In addition, under the influence of sympatholytic medicinal products such as beta-blockers, the signs and symptoms of hypoglycemia may be reduced or absent. Co-administration may require insulin dose adjustment and particularly close monitoring).
No products indexed under this heading.

Bitolterol Mesylate (Bronchodilators and other inhaled products may alter the absorption of inhaled human insulin. Consistent timing of dosing of bronchodilators relative to Exubera administration, close monitoring of blood glucose concentrations, and dose titration as appropriate are recommended. Co-administration may require insulin dose adjustment and particularly close monitoring).
No products indexed under this heading.

Budesonide (Corticosteroids may reduce the blood glucose-lowering effect of insulin, which may result in hyperglycemia. Co-administration may require insulin dose adjustment and particularly close monitoring). Products include:
Pulmicort Flexhaler 654
Symbicort 80/4.5 Inhalation Aerosol.. 659

Symbicort 160/4.5 Inhalation Aerosol ... 659

Bumetanide (Diuretics may reduce the blood glucose-lowering effect of insulin, which may result in hyperglycemia. Co-administration may require insulin dose adjustment and particularly close monitoring).
No products indexed under this heading.

Captopril (ACE inhibitors may increase the blood glucose-lowering effect of insulin and susceptibility to hypoglycemia. Co-administration may require insulin dose adjustment and particularly close monitoring). Products include:
Captopril Tablets ... 2182

Carteolol Hydrochloride (Beta-blockers may either increase or reduce the blood glucose-lowering effect of insulin. In addition, under the influence of sympatholytic medicinal products such as beta-blockers, the signs and symptoms of hypoglycemia may be reduced or absent. Co-administration may require insulin dose adjustment and particularly close monitoring).
No products indexed under this heading.

Chlorothiazide (Diuretics may reduce the blood glucose-lowering effect of insulin, which may result in hyperglycemia. Co-administration may require insulin dose adjustment and particularly close monitoring).
No products indexed under this heading.

Chlorothiazide Sodium (Diuretics may reduce the blood glucose-lowering effect of insulin, which may result in hyperglycemia. Co-administration may require insulin dose adjustment and particularly close monitoring). Products include:
Intravenous Sodium Diuril ... 2490

Chlorotrianisene (Estrogents may reduce the blood glucose-lowering effect of insulin, which may result in hyperglycemia. Co-administration may require insulin dose adjustment and particularly close monitoring).
No products indexed under this heading.

Chlorpromazine (Phenothiazine derivatives may reduce the blood glucose-lowering effect of insulin, which may result in hyperglycemia. Co-administration may require insulin dose adjustment and particularly close monitoring).
No products indexed under this heading.

Chlorpromazine Hydrochloride (Phenothiazine derivatives may reduce the blood glucose-lowering effect of insulin, which may result in hyperglycemia. Co-administration may require insulin dose adjustment and particularly close monitoring).
No products indexed under this heading.

Chlorpropamide (Oral antidiabetic products may increase the blood glucose-lowering effect of insulin and susceptibility to hypoglycemia. Co-administration may require insulin dose adjustment and particularly close monitoring).
No products indexed under this heading.

Chlorthalidone (Diuretics may reduce the blood glucose-lowering effect of insulin, which may result in hyperglycemia. Co-administration may require insulin dose adjustment and particularly close monitoring). Products include:
Clorpres Tablets ... 2185

Choline Magnesium Trisalicylate (Salicylates may increase the blood glucose-lowering effect of insulin and susceptibility to hypoglycemia. Co-administration may require insulin dose adjustment and particularly close monitoring).
No products indexed under this heading.

Ciclesonide (Corticosteroids may reduce the blood glucose-lowering effect of insulin, which may result in hyperglycemia. Co-administration may require insulin dose adjustment and particularly close monitoring). Products include:
Alvesco Inhalation Aerosol ... 2985
Omnaris Nasal Spray ... 2998

Clofibrate (Fibrates may increase the blood glucose-lowering effect of insulin and susceptibility to hypoglycemia. Co-administration may require insulin dose adjustment and particularly close monitoring).
No products indexed under this heading.

Clonidine (Clonidine may either increase or reduce the blood glucose-lowering effect of insulin. In addition, under the influence of sympatholytic medicinal products such as clonidine, the signs and symptoms of hypoglycemia may be reduced or absent. In addition, under the influence of clonidine, the signs and symptoms of hypoglycemia may be reduced or absent. Co-administration may require insulin dose adjustment and particularly close monitoring). Products include:
Catapres-TTS ... 842

Clonidine Hydrochloride (Clonidine may either increase or reduce the blood glucose-lowering effect of insulin. In addition, under the influence of sympatholytic medicinal products such as clonidine, the signs and symptoms of hypoglycemia may be reduced or absent. In addition, under the influence of clonidine, the signs and symptoms of hypoglycemia may be reduced or absent. Co-administration may require insulin dose adjustment and particularly close monitoring). Products include:
Catapres Tablets ... 841
Clorpres Tablets ... 2185

Clozapine (Atypical antipsychotics, such as clozapine, may reduce the blood glucose-lowering effect of insulin, which may result in hyperglycemia. Co-administration may require insulin dose adjustment and particularly close monitoring).
No products indexed under this heading.

Cortisone Acetate (Corticosteroids may reduce the blood glucose-lowering effect of insulin, which may result in hyperglycemia. Co-administration may require insulin dose adjustment and particularly close monitoring).
No products indexed under this heading.

Danazol (Danazol may reduce the blood glucose-lowering effect of insulin, which may result in hyperglycemia. Co-administration may require insulin dose adjustment and particularly close monitoring).
No products indexed under this heading.

Darunavir (Protease inhibitors may reduce the blood glucose-lowering effect of insulin, which may result in hyperglycemia. Co-administration may require insulin dose adjustment and particularly close monitoring).
No products indexed under this heading.

Desogestrel (Oral contraceptives may reduce the blood glucose-lowering effect of insulin, which may result in hyperglycemia. Co-administration may require insulin dose adjustment and particularly close monitoring). Products include:
Mircette Tablets ... 1034

Dexamethasone (Corticosteroids may reduce the blood glucose-lowering effect of insulin, which may result in hyperglycemia. Co-administration may require insulin dose adjustment and particularly close monitoring). Products include:
Ciprodex Otic Suspension ... 541

Dexamethasone Acetate (Corticosteroids may reduce the blood glucose-lowering effect of insulin, which may result in hyperglycemia. Co-administration may require insulin dose adjustment and particularly close monitoring).
No products indexed under this heading.

Dexamethasone Sodium Phosphate (Corticosteroids may reduce the blood glucose-lowering effect of insulin, which may result in hyperglycemia. Co-administration may require insulin dose adjustment and particularly close monitoring).
No products indexed under this heading.

Diazoxide (Diazoxide may reduce the blood glucose-lowering effect of insulin, which may result in hyperglycemia. Co-administration may require insulin dose adjustment and particularly close monitoring). Products include:
Proglycem Capsules ... 1185
Proglycem Suspension ... 1185

Dienestrol (Estrogents may reduce the blood glucose-lowering effect of insulin, which may result in hyperglycemia. Co-administration may require insulin dose adjustment and particularly close monitoring).
No products indexed under this heading.

Diethylstilbestrol (Estrogents may reduce the blood glucose-lowering effect of insulin, which may result in hyperglycemia. Co-administration may require insulin dose adjustment and particularly close monitoring).
No products indexed under this heading.

Diflunisal (Salicylates may increase the blood glucose-lowering effect of insulin and susceptibility to hypoglycemia. Co-administration may require insulin dose adjustment and particularly close monitoring).
No products indexed under this heading.

Disopyramide (Disopyramide may increase the blood glucose-lowering effect of insulin and susceptibility to hypoglycemia. Co-administration may require insulin dose adjustment and particularly close monitoring).
No products indexed under this heading.

Disopyramide Phosphate (Disopyramide may increase the blood glucose-lowering effect of insulin and susceptibility to hypoglycemia. Co-administration may require insulin dose adjustment and particularly close monitoring).
No products indexed under this heading.

Dobutamine Hydrochloride (Sympathomimetics may reduce the blood glucose-lowering effect of insulin, which may result in hyperglycemia. Co-administration may require insulin dose adjustment and particularly close monitoring).
No products indexed under this heading.

Dopamine Hydrochloride (Sympathomimetics may reduce the blood glucose-lowering effect of insulin, which may result in hyperglycemia. Co-administration may require insulin dose adjustment and particularly close monitoring).
No products indexed under this heading.

Enalapril Maleate (ACE inhibitors may increase the blood glucose-lowering effect of insulin and susceptibility to hypoglycemia. Co-administration may require insulin dose adjustment and particularly close monitoring).
No products indexed under this heading.

Enalaprilat (ACE inhibitors may increase the blood glucose-lowering effect of insulin and susceptibility to hypoglycemia. Co-administration may require insulin dose adjustment and particularly close monitoring).
No products indexed under this heading.

Ephedrine Hydrochloride (Sympathomimetics may reduce the blood glucose-lowering effect of insulin, which may result in hyperglycemia. Co-administration may require insulin dose adjustment and particularly close monitoring).
No products indexed under this heading.

Ephedrine Sulfate (Sympathomimetics may reduce the blood glucose-lowering effect of insulin, which may result in hyperglycemia. Co-administration may require insulin dose adjustment and particularly close monitoring).
No products indexed under this heading.

Ephedrine Tannate (Sympathomimetics may reduce the blood glucose-lowering effect of insulin, which may result in hyperglycemia. Co-administration may require insulin dose adjustment and particularly close monitoring).
No products indexed under this heading.

Epinephrine (Sympathomimetics may reduce the blood glucose-lowering effect of insulin, which may result in hyperglycemia. Co-administration may require insulin dose adjustment and particularly close monitoring). Products include:
EpiPen ... 1024

Epinephrine Bitartrate (Sympathomimetics may reduce the blood glucose-lowering effect of insulin, which may result in hyperglycemia. Co-administration may require insulin dose adjustment and particularly close monitoring).
No products indexed under this heading.

Epinephrine Hydrochloride (Sympathomimetics may reduce the blood glucose-lowering effect of insulin, which may result in hyperglycemia. Co-administration may require insulin dose adjustment and particularly close monitoring).
No products indexed under this heading.

Esmolol Hydrochloride (Beta-blockers may either increase or reduce the blood glucose-lowering effect of insulin. In addition, under the influence of sympatholytic medicinal products such as beta-blockers, the signs and symptoms of hypoglycemia may be reduced or absent. Co-administration may require insulin dose adjustment and particularly close monitoring).
No products indexed under this heading.

Estradiol (Estrogens may reduce the blood glucose-lowering effect of insulin, which may result in hyperglycemia. Co-administration may require insulin dose adjustment and particularly close monitoring).
Products include:
Activella Tablets 2347
Angeliq Tablets 751
Climara Transdermal System 763
Climara Pro Transdermal System 768
Divigel 3167
Vagifem Tablets 2375

Estrogens, Conjugated (Estrogens may reduce the blood glucose-lowering effect of insulin, which may result in hyperglycemia. Co-administration may require insulin dose adjustment and particularly close monitoring). Products include:
Premarin Intravenous 3217
Premarin Tablets 3221
Premarin Vaginal Cream 3228
Premphase Tablets 3232
Prempro Tablets 3232

Estrogens, Esterified (Estrogens may reduce the blood glucose-lowering effect of insulin, which may result in hyperglycemia. Co-administration may require insulin dose adjustment and particularly close monitoring). Products include:
Estratest Tablets 3043
Estratest H.S. Tablets 3043

Estropipate (Estrogens may reduce the blood glucose-lowering effect of insulin, which may result in hyperglycemia. Co-administration may require insulin dose adjustment and particularly close monitoring).
No products indexed under this heading.

Ethacrynic Acid (Diuretics may reduce the blood glucose-lowering effect of insulin, which may result in hyperglycemia. Co-administration may require insulin dose adjustment and particularly close monitoring).
Products include:
Edecrin Tablets 698

Ethanol (Alcohol may either increase or reduce the blood glucose-lowering effect of insulin. Co-administration may require insulin dose adjustment and particularly close monitoring).
No products indexed under this heading.

Ethinyl Estradiol (Oral contraceptives may reduce the blood glucose-lowering effect of insulin, which may result in hyperglycemia. Co-administration may require insulin dose adjustment and particularly close monitoring). Products include:
Lybrel Tablets 3204
Mircette Tablets 1034
NuvaRing 2897
Ortho-Cyclen/Ortho Tri-Cyclen 2449
Ortho Evra Transdermal System 2437
Ortho Tri-Cyclen Lo Tablets 2458
Seasonique Tablets 1046
Yaz Tablets 805

Ethynodiol Diacetate (Oral contraceptives may reduce the blood glucose-lowering effect of insulin, which may result in hyperglycemia. Co-administration may require insulin dose adjustment and particularly close monitoring).
No products indexed under this heading.

Fenofibrate (Fibrates may increase the blood glucose-lowering effect of insulin and susceptibility to hypoglycemia. Co-administration may require insulin dose adjustment and particularly close monitoring).
Products include:
Fenoglide Tablets 2960
Tricor Tablets 520

Fludrocortisone Acetate (Corticosteroids may reduce the blood glucose-lowering effect of insulin, which may result in hyperglycemia. Co-administration may require insulin dose adjustment and particularly close monitoring).
No products indexed under this heading.

Flunisolide (Corticosteroids may reduce the blood glucose-lowering effect of insulin, which may result in hyperglycemia. Co-administration may require insulin dose adjustment and particularly close monitoring).
Products include:
Aerobid/Aerobid-M 1153

Fluoxetine (Fluoxetine may increase the blood glucose-lowering effect of insulin and susceptibility to hypoglycemia. Co-administration may require insulin dose adjustment and particularly close monitoring).
No products indexed under this heading.

Fluoxetine Hydrochloride (Fluoxetine may increase the blood glucose-lowering effect of insulin and susceptibility to hypoglycemia. Co-administration may require insulin dose adjustment and particularly close monitoring). Products include:
Prozac Weekly Capsules 1852
Prozac Pulvules and Liquid 1852
Symbyax Capsules 1871

Fluphenazine Decanoate (Phenothiazine derivatives may reduce the blood glucose-lowering effect of insulin, which may result in hyperglycemia. Co-administration may require insulin dose adjustment and particularly close monitoring).
No products indexed under this heading.

Fluphenazine Enanthate (Phenothiazine derivatives may reduce the blood glucose-lowering effect of insulin, which may result in hyperglycemia. Co-administration may require insulin dose adjustment and particularly close monitoring).
No products indexed under this heading.

Fluphenazine Hydrochloride (Phenothiazine derivatives may reduce the blood glucose-lowering effect of insulin, which may result in hyperglycemia. Co-administration may require insulin dose adjustment and particularly close monitoring).
No products indexed under this heading.

Fluticasone Propionate (Corticosteroids may reduce the blood glucose-lowering effect of insulin, which may result in hyperglycemia. Co-administration may require insulin dose adjustment and particularly close monitoring). Products include:
Advair Diskus 100/50 1276
Advair Diskus 250/50 1276
Advair Diskus 500/50 1276
Advair HFA 45/21 Inhalation Aerosol 1288
Advair HFA 115/21 Inhalation Aerosol 1288
Advair HFA 230/21 Inhalation Aerosol 1288
Flonase Nasal Spray 1431
Flovent Diskus 50 mcg 1435

Fluticasone Propionate HFA (Corticosteroids may reduce the blood glucose-lowering effect of insulin, which may result in hyperglycemia. Co-administration may require insulin dose adjustment and particularly close monitoring). Products include:
Flovent HFA 1440

Fosamprenavir Calcium (Protease inhibitors may reduce the blood glucose-lowering effect of insulin, which may result in hyperglycemia. Co-administration may require insulin dose adjustment and particularly close monitoring). Products include:
Lexiva Oral Suspension 1510
Lexiva Tablets 1510

Fosinopril Sodium (ACE inhibitors may increase the blood glucose-lowering effect of insulin and susceptibility to hypoglycemia. Co-administration may require insulin dose adjustment and particularly close monitoring).
No products indexed under this heading.

Furosemide (Diuretics may reduce the blood glucose-lowering effect of insulin, which may result in hyperglycemia. Co-administration may require insulin dose adjustment and particularly close monitoring).
Products include:
Furosemide Tablets 2186

Gemfibrozil (Fibrates may increase the blood glucose-lowering effect of insulin and susceptibility to hypoglycemia. Co-administration may require insulin dose adjustment and particularly close monitoring).
No products indexed under this heading.

Glimepiride (Oral antidiabetic products may increase the blood glucose-lowering effect of insulin and susceptibility to hypoglycemia. Co-administration may require insulin dose adjustment and particularly close monitoring). Products include:
Avandaryl Tablets 1344
Duetact Tablets 3085

Glipizide (Oral antidiabetic products may increase the blood glucose-lowering effect of insulin and susceptibility to hypoglycemia. Co-administration may require insulin dose adjustment and particularly close monitoring).
No products indexed under this heading.

Glucagon (Glucagon may reduce the blood glucose-lowering effect of insulin, which may result in hyperglycemia. Co-administration may require insulin dose adjustment and particularly close monitoring).
Products include:
Glucagon for Injection Vials and Emergency Kit 1827

Glyburide (Oral antidiabetic products may increase the blood glucose-lowering effect of insulin and susceptibility to hypoglycemia. Co-administration may require insulin dose adjustment and particularly close monitoring).
No products indexed under this heading.

Guanethidine (Under the influence of sympatholytic medicinal products, such as guanethidine, the signs and symptoms of hypoglycemia may be reduced or absent. Co-administration may require insulin dose adjustment and particularly close monitoring).
No products indexed under this heading.

Guanethidine Monosulfate (Under the influence of sympatholytic medicinal products, such as guanethidine, the signs and symptoms of hypoglycemia may be reduced or absent. Co-administration may require insulin dose adjustment and particularly close monitoring).
No products indexed under this heading.

Guanethidine Sulfate (Under the influence of sympatholytic medicinal products, such as guanethidine, the signs and symptoms of hypoglycemia may be reduced or absent. Co-administration may require insulin dose adjustment and particularly close monitoring).
No products indexed under this heading.

Hydrochlorothiazide (Diuretics may reduce the blood glucose-lowering effect of insulin, which may result in hyperglycemia. Co-administration may require insulin dose adjustment and particularly close monitoring). Products include:
Atacand HCT 642
Avalide Tablets 892
Avalide Tablets 2713
Benicar HCT Tablets 1010
Diovan HCT Tablets 2216
Dyazide Capsules 1405
Micardis HCT Tablets 854
Prinzide Tablets 2092
Tekturna HCT Tablets 2324
Teveten HCT Tablets 517

Hydrocortisone (Corticosteroids may reduce the blood glucose-lowering effect of insulin, which may result in hyperglycemia. Co-administration may require insulin dose adjustment and particularly close monitoring).
No products indexed under this heading.

Hydrocortisone Acetate (Corticosteroids may reduce the blood glucose-lowering effect of insulin, which may result in hyperglycemia. Co-administration may require insulin dose adjustment and particularly close monitoring). Products include:

Analpram-HC **1140**
Pramosone **1141**

Hydrocortisone Sodium Phosphate (Corticosteroids may reduce the blood glucose-lowering effect of insulin, which may result in hyperglycemia. Co-administration may require insulin dose adjustment and particularly close monitoring).

No products indexed under this heading.

Hydrocortisone Sodium Succinate (Corticosteroids may reduce the blood glucose-lowering effect of insulin, which may result in hyperglycemia. Co-administration may require insulin dose adjustment and particularly close monitoring).

No products indexed under this heading.

Hydroflumethiazide (Diuretics may reduce the blood glucose-lowering effect of insulin, which may result in hyperglycemia. Co-administration may require insulin dose adjustment and particularly close monitoring).

No products indexed under this heading.

Indapamide (Diuretics may reduce the blood glucose-lowering effect of insulin, which may result in hyperglycemia. Co-administration may require insulin dose adjustment and particularly close monitoring). Products include:

Indapamide Tablets **2188**

Indinavir Sulfate (Protease inhibitors may reduce the blood glucose-lowering effect of insulin, which may result in hyperglycemia. Co-administration may require insulin dose adjustment and particularly close monitoring). Products include:

Crixivan Capsules **1979**

Isocarboxazid (MAO inhibitors may increase the blood glucose-lowering effect of insulin and susceptibility to hypoglycemia. Co-administration may require insulin dose adjustment and particularly close monitoring). Products include:

Marplan Tablets **3177**

Isoetharine (Bronchodilators and other inhaled products may alter the absorption of inhaled human insulin. Consistent timing of dosing of bronchodilators relative to Exubera administration, close monitoring of blood glucose concentrations, and dose titration as appropriate are recommended. Co-administration may require insulin dose adjustment and particularly close monitoring).

No products indexed under this heading.

Isoniazid (Isoniazid may reduce the blood glucose-lowering effect of insulin, which may result in hyperglycemia. Co-administration may require insulin dose adjustment and particularly close monitoring).

No products indexed under this heading.

Isoproterenol Hydrochloride (Sympathomimetics may reduce the blood glucose-lowering effect of insulin, which may result in hyperglycemia. Co-administration may require insulin dose adjustment and particularly close monitoring).

No products indexed under this heading.

Isoproterenol Sulfate (Sympathomimetics may reduce the blood glucose-lowering effect of insulin, which may result in hyperglycemia. Co-administration may require insulin dose adjustment and particularly close monitoring).

No products indexed under this heading.

Labetalol Hydrochloride (Beta-blockers may either increase or reduce the blood glucose-lowering effect of insulin. In addition, under the influence of sympatholytic medicinal products such as beta-blockers, the signs and symptoms of hypoglycemia may be reduced or absent. Co-administration may require insulin dose adjustment and particularly close monitoring).

No products indexed under this heading.

Levalbuterol Hydrochloride (Sympathomimetics may reduce the blood glucose-lowering effect of insulin, which may result in hyperglycemia. Co-administration may require insulin dose adjustment and particularly close monitoring). Products include:

Xopenex Inhalation Solution **3001**
Xopenex Inhalation Solution Concentrate **3005**

Levobunolol Hydrochloride (Beta-blockers may either increase or reduce the blood glucose-lowering effect of insulin. In addition, under the influence of sympatholytic medicinal products such as beta-blockers, the signs and symptoms of hypoglycemia may be reduced or absent. Co-administration may require insulin dose adjustment and particularly close monitoring).

No products indexed under this heading.

Levonorgestrel (Oral contraceptives may reduce the blood glucose-lowering effect of insulin, which may result in hyperglycemia. Co-administration may require insulin dose adjustment and particularly close monitoring). Products include:

Climara Pro Transdermal System **768**
Lybrel Tablets **3204**
Mirena Intrauterine System **779**
Plan B Tablets **1044**
Seasonique Tablets **1046**

Levothyroxine Sodium (Thyroid hormones may reduce the blood glucose-lowering effect of insulin, which may result in hyperglycemia. Co-administration may require insulin dose adjustment and particularly close monitoring). Products include:

Levothroid Tablets **1170**
Levoxyl Tablets **1780**
Synthroid Tablets **507**

Liothyronine Sodium (Thyroid hormones may reduce the blood glucose-lowering effect of insulin, which may result in hyperglycemia. Co-administration may require insulin dose adjustment and particularly close monitoring). Products include:

Cytomel Tablets **1778**

Liotrix (Thyroid hormones may reduce the blood glucose-lowering effect of insulin, which may result in hyperglycemia. Co-administration may require insulin dose adjustment and particularly close monitoring).

No products indexed under this heading.

Lisinopril (ACE inhibitors may increase the blood glucose-lowering effect of insulin and susceptibility to hypoglycemia. Co-administration may require insulin dose adjustment and particularly close monitoring). Products include:

Prinivil Tablets **2087**
Prinzide Tablets **2092**

Lithium (Lithium salts may either increase or reduce the blood glucose-lowering effect of insulin. Co-administration may require insulin dose adjustment and particularly close monitoring).

No products indexed under this heading.

Lithium Carbonate (Lithium salts may either increase or reduce the blood glucose-lowering effect of insulin. Co-administration may require insulin dose adjustment and particularly close monitoring).

No products indexed under this heading.

Lithium Citrate (Lithium salts may either increase or reduce the blood glucose-lowering effect of insulin. Co-administration may require insulin dose adjustment and particularly close monitoring).

No products indexed under this heading.

Lopinavir (Protease inhibitors may reduce the blood glucose-lowering effect of insulin, which may result in hyperglycemia. Co-administration may require insulin dose adjustment and particularly close monitoring). Products include:

Kaletra **452**

Magnesium Salicylate (Salicylates may increase the blood glucose-lowering effect of insulin and susceptibility to hypoglycemia. Co-administration may require insulin dose adjustment and particularly close monitoring).

No products indexed under this heading.

Medroxyprogesterone Acetate (Progestogens may reduce the blood glucose-lowering effect of insulin, which may result in hyperglycemia. Co-administration may require insulin dose adjustment and particularly close monitoring). Products include:

Premphase Tablets **3232**
Prempro Tablets **3232**

Megestrol Acetate (Progestogens may reduce the blood glucose-lowering effect of insulin, which may result in hyperglycemia. Co-administration may require insulin dose adjustment and particularly close monitoring). Products include:

Megace ES Oral Suspension **2499**

Mesoridazine Besylate (Phenothiazine derivatives may reduce the blood glucose-lowering effect of insulin, which may result in hyperglycemia. Co-administration may require insulin dose adjustment and particularly close monitoring).

No products indexed under this heading.

Mestranol (Oral contraceptives may reduce the blood glucose-lowering effect of insulin, which may result in hyperglycemia. Co-administration may require insulin dose adjustment and particularly close monitoring).

No products indexed under this heading.

Metaproterenol Sulfate (Sympathomimetics may reduce the blood glucose-lowering effect of insulin, which may result in hyperglycemia. Co-administration may require insulin dose adjustment and particularly close monitoring).

No products indexed under this heading.

Metaraminol Bitartrate (Sympathomimetics may reduce the blood glucose-lowering effect of insulin, which may result in hyperglycemia. Co-administration may require insulin dose adjustment and particularly close monitoring).

No products indexed under this heading.

Metformin Hydrochloride (Oral antidiabetic products may increase the blood glucose-lowering effect of insulin and susceptibility to hypoglycemia. Co-administration may require insulin dose adjustment and particularly close monitoring). Products include:

ActoPlus Met Tablets **3071**
Avandamet Tablets **1336**
Janumet Tablets **2041**
PrandiMet Tablets **2967**

Methotrimeprazine (Phenothiazine derivatives may reduce the blood glucose-lowering effect of insulin, which may result in hyperglycemia. Co-administration may require insulin dose adjustment and particularly close monitoring).

No products indexed under this heading.

Methoxamine Hydrochloride (Sympathomimetics may reduce the blood glucose-lowering effect of insulin, which may result in hyperglycemia. Co-administration may require insulin dose adjustment and particularly close monitoring).

No products indexed under this heading.

Methyclothiazide (Diuretics may reduce the blood glucose-lowering effect of insulin, which may result in hyperglycemia. Co-administration may require insulin dose adjustment and particularly close monitoring).

No products indexed under this heading.

Methylprednisolone Acetate (Corticosteroids may reduce the blood glucose-lowering effect of insulin, which may result in hyperglycemia. Co-administration may require insulin dose adjustment and particularly close monitoring).

No products indexed under this heading.

Methylprednisolone Sodium Succinate (Corticosteroids may reduce the blood glucose-lowering effect of insulin, which may result in hyperglycemia. Co-administration may require insulin dose adjustment and particularly close monitoring).

No products indexed under this heading.

Metipranolol Hydrochloride (Beta-blockers may either increase or reduce the blood glucose-lowering effect of insulin. In addition, under the influence of sympatholytic medicinal products such as beta-blockers, the signs and symptoms of hypoglycemia may be reduced or absent. Co-administration may require insulin dose adjustment and particularly close monitoring).

No products indexed under this heading.

Metolazone (Diuretics may reduce the blood glucose-lowering effect of insulin, which may result in hyperglycemia. Co-administration may require insulin dose adjustment and particularly close monitoring).
No products indexed under this heading.

Metoprolol Succinate (Beta-blockers may either increase or reduce the blood glucose-lowering effect of insulin. In addition, under the influence of sympatholytic medicinal products such as beta-blockers, the signs and symptoms of hypoglycemia may be reduced or absent. Co-administration may require insulin dose adjustment and particularly close monitoring). Products include:
Toprol-XL Tablets 666

Metoprolol Tartrate (Beta-blockers may either increase or reduce the blood glucose-lowering effect of insulin. In addition, under the influence of sympatholytic medicinal products such as beta-blockers, the signs and symptoms of hypoglycemia may be reduced or absent. Co-administration may require insulin dose adjustment and particularly close monitoring).
No products indexed under this heading.

Miglitol (Oral antidiabetic products may increase the blood glucose-lowering effect of insulin and susceptibility to hypoglycemia. Co-administration may require insulin dose adjustment and particularly close monitoring).
No products indexed under this heading.

Moclobemide (MAO inhibitors may increase the blood glucose-lowering effect of insulin and susceptibility to hypoglycemia. Co-administration may require insulin dose adjustment and particularly close monitoring).
No products indexed under this heading.

Moexipril Hydrochloride (ACE inhibitors may increase the blood glucose-lowering effect of insulin and susceptibility to hypoglycemia. Co-administration may require insulin dose adjustment and particularly close monitoring).
No products indexed under this heading.

Mometasone Furoate (Corticosteroids may reduce the blood glucose-lowering effect of insulin, which may result in hyperglycemia. Co-administration may require insulin dose adjustment and particularly close monitoring). Products include:
Asmanex Twisthaler 2797
Elocon Cream 0.1% 2840
Elocon Lotion 0.1% 2841
Elocon Ointment 0.1% 2842

Mometasone Furoate Monohydrate (Corticosteroids may reduce the blood glucose-lowering effect of insulin, which may result in hyperglycemia. Co-administration may require insulin dose adjustment and particularly close monitoring).
Products include:
Nasonex Nasal Spray 2883

Nadolol (Beta-blockers may either increase or reduce the blood glucose-lowering effect of insulin. In addition, under the influence of sympatholytic medicinal products such as beta-blockers, the signs and symptoms of hypoglycemia may be reduced or absent. Co-administration may require insulin dose adjustment and particularly close monitoring). Products include:
Nadolol Tablets 2191

Nateglinide (Oral antidiabetic products may increase the blood glucose-lowering effect of insulin and susceptibility to hypoglycemia. Co-administration may require insulin dose adjustment and particularly close monitoring). Products include:
Starlix Tablets 2314

Nebivolol (Beta-blockers may either increase or reduce the blood glucose-lowering effect of insulin. In addition, under the influence of sympatholytic medicinal products such as beta-blockers, the signs and symptoms of hypoglycemia may be reduced or absent. Co-administration may require insulin dose adjustment and particularly close monitoring). Products include:
Bystolic Tablets 1155

Nelfinavir Mesylate (Protease inhibitors may reduce the blood glucose-lowering effect of insulin, which may result in hyperglycemia. Co-administration may require insulin dose adjustment and particularly close monitoring).
No products indexed under this heading.

Norepinephrine Bitartrate (Sympathomimetics may reduce the blood glucose-lowering effect of insulin, which may result in hyperglycemia. Co-administration may require insulin dose adjustment and particularly close monitoring).
No products indexed under this heading.

Norethindrone (Oral contraceptives may reduce the blood glucose-lowering effect of insulin, which may result in hyperglycemia. Co-administration may require insulin dose adjustment and particularly close monitoring). Products include:
Ortho Micronor Tablets 2446

Norethynodrel (Oral contraceptives may reduce the blood glucose-lowering effect of insulin, which may result in hyperglycemia. Co-administration may require insulin dose adjustment and particularly close monitoring).
No products indexed under this heading.

Norgestimate (Oral contraceptives may reduce the blood glucose-lowering effect of insulin, which may result in hyperglycemia. Co-administration may require insulin dose adjustment and particularly close monitoring). Products include:
Ortho-Cyclen/Ortho Tri-Cyclen 2449
Ortho Tri-Cyclen Lo Tablets 2458

Norgestrel (Oral contraceptives may reduce the blood glucose-lowering effect of insulin, which may result in hyperglycemia. Co-administration may require insulin dose adjustment and particularly close monitoring).
No products indexed under this heading.

Olanzapine (Atypical antipsychotics, such as olanzapine, may reduce the blood glucose-lowering effect of insulin, which may result in hyperglycemia. Co-administration may require insulin dose adjustment and particularly close monitoring).
Products include:
Symbyax Capsules 1871
Zyprexa Tablets 1883
Zyprexa IntraMuscular 1883
Zyprexa ZYDIS Orally Disintegrating Tablets 1883

Pargyline Hydrochloride (MAO inhibitors may increase the blood glucose-lowering effect of insulin and susceptibility to hypoglycemia. Co-administration may require insulin dose adjustment and particularly close monitoring).
No products indexed under this heading.

Penbutolol Sulfate (Beta-blockers may either increase or reduce the blood glucose-lowering effect of insulin. In addition, under the influence of sympatholytic medicinal products such as beta-blockers, the signs and symptoms of hypoglycemia may be reduced or absent. Co-administration may require insulin dose adjustment and particularly close monitoring).
No products indexed under this heading.

Pentamidine Isethionate (Pentamidine may cause hypoglycemia, which may sometimes be followed by hyperglycemia. Co-administration may require insulin dose adjustment and particularly close monitoring).
No products indexed under this heading.

Pentoxifylline (Pentoxifylline may increase the blood glucose-lowering effect of insulin and susceptibility to hypoglycemia. Co-administration may require insulin dose adjustment and particularly close monitoring).
No products indexed under this heading.

Perindopril Erbumine (ACE inhibitors may increase the blood glucose-lowering effect of insulin and susceptibility to hypoglycemia. Co-administration may require insulin dose adjustment and particularly close monitoring). Products include:
Aceon Tablets (2 mg, 4 mg, 8 mg) 3038

Perphenazine (Phenothiazine derivatives may reduce the blood glucose-lowering effect of insulin, which may result in hyperglycemia. Co-administration may require insulin dose adjustment and particularly close monitoring).
No products indexed under this heading.

Phenelzine Sulfate (MAO inhibitors may increase the blood glucose-lowering effect of insulin and susceptibility to hypoglycemia. Co-administration may require insulin dose adjustment and particularly close monitoring).
No products indexed under this heading.

Phenylephrine Bitartrate (Sympathomimetics may reduce the blood glucose-lowering effect of insulin, which may result in hyperglycemia. Co-administration may require insulin dose adjustment and particularly close monitoring).
No products indexed under this heading.

Phenylephrine Hydrochloride (Sympathomimetics may reduce the blood glucose-lowering effect of insulin, which may result in hyperglycemia. Co-administration may require insulin dose adjustment and particularly close monitoring).
Products include:
Actifed Cold & Allergy Tablets 1895
Benadryl Allergy & Cold Kapgels 1895
Benadryl Allergy & Sinus Headache Kapgels 1895
Benadryl Severe Allergy & Sinus Headache Caplets 1897
Children's Benadryl-D Allergy & Sinus Liquid 1896
Benadryl-D Allergy & Sinus Tablet 1896
PediaCare Children's Allergy & Cold Liquid 1902
PediaCare Children's Decongestant Liquid 1902
PediaCare Children's Liquid Multi-Symptom Cold 1902
Sinutab Non-Drying Caplets 1905
Sinutab Sinus Caplets 1905
Children's Sudafed PE Cold & Cough Liquid 1907
Children's Sudafed PE Nasal Decongestant Liquid 1906
Sudafed PE Cold & Cough Caplets 1907
Sudafed PE Nasal Decongestant Tablets 1907
Sudafed PE Nighttime Cold Caplets 1907
Sudafed PE Non-Drying Sinus Caplets 1908
Sudafed PE Severe Cold Caplets 1908
Sudafed PE Sinus & Allergy Tablets 1908
Sudafed PE Sinus Headache Caplets 1908
Tylenol Allergy Multi-Symptom Caplets with Cool Burst and Rapid Release Gelcaps 1916
Tylenol Allergy Multi-Symptom Nighttime Caplets with Cool Burst 1916
Children's Tylenol Plus Cold Suspension Liquid 1912
Children's Tylenol Plus Cold & Allergy Suspension Liquid 1914
Children's Tylenol Plus Flu Suspension Liquid 1914
Children's Tylenol Plus Multi-Symptom Cold Suspension Liquid 1912
Tylenol Cold Head Congestion Daytime Caplets with Cool Burst 1910
Tylenol Cold Head Congestion Nighttime Caplets with Cool Burst 1910
Tylenol Cold Head Congestion Severe Daytime Caplets with Cool Burst 1910
Tylenol Cold Multi-Symptom Daytime Caplets with Cool Burst and Rapid Release Gels 1913
Tylenol Cold Multi-Symptom Daytime Liquid with Citrus Burst 1913
Tylenol Cold Multi-Symptom Nighttime Caplets with Cool Burst 1913
Tylenol Cold Multi-Symptom Nighttime Liquid with Cool Burst 1913
Tylenol Cold Multi-Symptom Severe Caplets with Cool Burst 1913
Tylenol Cold Multi-Symptom Severe Daytime Liquid with Citrus Burst 1913
Tylenol Sinus Congestion & Pain Daytime Caplets with Cool Burst and Gelcaps 1917
Tylenol Sinus Congestion & Pain Nighttime Caplets with Cool Burst 1917
Tylenol Sinus Congestion & Pain Severe Caplets with Cool Burst 1917
Vicks DayQuil Cold & Flu Multi-Symptom Relief 616
Vicks DayQuil LiquiCaps 2567
Vicks DayQuil Liquid 2567
Vicks DayQuil Multi-Symptom Cold/Flu Relief 2567

Phenylephrine Tannate (Sympathomimetics may reduce the blood glucose-lowering effect of insulin, which may result in hyperglycemia. Co-administration may require insulin dose adjustment and particularly close monitoring).
No products indexed under this heading.

Phenylpropanolamine Hydrochloride (Sympathomimetics may reduce the blood glucose-lowering effect of insulin, which may result in hyperglycemia. Co-administration may require insulin dose adjustment and particularly close monitoring).
No products indexed under this heading.

Pindolol (Beta-blockers may either increase or reduce the blood glucose-lowering effect of insulin. In addition, under the influence of sympatholytic medicinal products such as beta-blockers, the signs and symptoms of hypoglycemia may be reduced or absent. Co-administration may require insulin dose adjustment and particularly close monitoring).
No products indexed under this heading.

Pioglitazone Hydrochloride (Oral antidiabetic products may increase the blood glucose-lowering effect of insulin and susceptibility to hypoglycemia. Co-administration may require insulin dose adjustment and particularly close monitoring).
Products include:
ActoPlus Met Tablets 3071
Actos Tablets 3077
Duetact Tablets 3085

Pirbuterol Acetate (Sympathomimetics may reduce the blood glucose-lowering effect of insulin, which may result in hyperglycemia. Co-administration may require insulin dose adjustment and particularly close monitoring). Products include:
Maxair Autohaler 1705

Polyestradiol Phosphate (Estrogens may reduce the blood glucose-lowering effect of insulin, which may result in hyperglycemia. Co-administration may require insulin dose adjustment and particularly close monitoring).
No products indexed under this heading.

Polythiazide (Diuretics may reduce the blood glucose-lowering effect of insulin, which may result in hyperglycemia. Co-administration may require insulin dose adjustment and particularly close monitoring).
No products indexed under this heading.

Prednisolone Acetate (Corticosteroids may reduce the blood glucose-lowering effect of insulin, which may result in hyperglycemia. Co-administration may require insulin dose adjustment and particularly close monitoring). Products include:
Pred Forte Ophthalmic Suspension .... ⊙227
Pred Mild Ophthalmic Suspension .... ⊙230
Pred-G Ophthalmic Ointment .... ⊙229
Pred-G Ophthalmic Suspension .... ⊙228

Prednisolone Sodium Phosphate (Corticosteroids may reduce the blood glucose-lowering effect of insulin, which may result in hyperglycemia. Co-administration may require insulin dose adjustment and particularly close monitoring).
No products indexed under this heading.

Prednisolone Tebutate (Corticosteroids may reduce the blood glucose-lowering effect of insulin, which may result in hyperglycemia. Co-administration may require insulin dose adjustment and particularly close monitoring).
No products indexed under this heading.

Prednisone (Corticosteroids may reduce the blood glucose-lowering effect of insulin, which may result in hyperglycemia. Co-administration may require insulin dose adjustment and particularly close monitoring).
No products indexed under this heading.

Procarbazine Hydrochloride (MAO inhibitors may increase the blood glucose-lowering effect of insulin and susceptibility to hypoglycemia. Co-administration may require insulin dose adjustment and particularly close monitoring).
No products indexed under this heading.

Prochlorperazine (Phenothiazine derivatives may reduce the blood glucose-lowering effect of insulin, which may result in hyperglycemia. Co-administration may require insulin dose adjustment and particularly close monitoring).
No products indexed under this heading.

Promethazine Hydrochloride (Phenothiazine derivatives may reduce the blood glucose-lowering effect of insulin, which may result in hyperglycemia. Co-administration may require insulin dose adjustment and particularly close monitoring).
No products indexed under this heading.

Propoxyphene Hydrochloride (Propoxyphene may increase the blood glucose-lowering effect of insulin and susceptibility to hypoglycemia.Co-administration may require insulin dose adjustment and particularly close monitoring).
No products indexed under this heading.

Propoxyphene Napsylate (Propoxyphene may increase the blood glucose-lowering effect of insulin and susceptibility to hypoglycemia. Co-administration may require insulin dose adjustment and particularly close monitoring).
No products indexed under this heading.

Propranolol Hydrochloride (Beta-blockers may either increase or reduce the blood glucose-lowering effect of insulin. In addition, under the influence of sympatholytic medicinal products such as beta-blockers, the signs and symptoms of hypoglycemia may be reduced or absent. Co-administration may require insulin dose adjustment and particularly close monitoring). Products include:
InnoPran XL Extended Release Capsules 1484

Pseudoephedrine Hydrochloride (Sympathomimetics may reduce the blood glucose-lowering effect of insulin, which may result in hyperglycemia. Co-administration may require insulin dose adjustment and particularly close monitoring).
Products include:
Allegra-D 12 Hour Extended-Release Tablets 2687
Allegra-D 24 Hour Extended-Release Tablets 2690
Children's Motrin Cold Oral Suspension 1899
Sudafed 12 Hour Nasal Decongestant Non-Drowsy Caplets 1909
Sudafed 24 Hour Non-Drowsy Nasal Decongestant Tablets 1906
Children's Sudafed Nasal Decongestant Liquid 1906
Sudafed Nasal Decongestant Tablets 1906
Tylenol Cold Severe Congestion Daytime Caplets with Cool Burst 1912
Tylenol Sinus Severe Congestion Caplets with Cool Burst 1917
Vicks NyQuil LiquiCaps 2567
Vicks NyQuil Liquid 2567
Vicks NyQuil Multi-Symptom Cold/Flu Relief 2567
Zyrtec-D 12 Hour Extended Release Tablets 1923
Zyrtec-D Allergy & Congestion Extended-Release Tablets 1923

Pseudoephedrine Sulfate (Sympathomimetics may reduce the blood glucose-lowering effect of insulin, which may result in hyperglycemia. Co-administration may require insulin dose adjustment and particularly close monitoring).
Products include:
Clarinex-D 12-Hour Extended-Release Tablets 2831
Clarinex-D 24-Hour Extended-Release Tablets 2834

Quinapril Hydrochloride (ACE inhibitors may increase the blood glucose-lowering effect of insulin and susceptibility to hypoglycemia. Co-administration may require insulin dose adjustment and particularly close monitoring).
No products indexed under this heading.

Quinestrol (Estrogens may reduce the blood glucose-lowering effect of insulin, which may result in hyperglycemia. Co-administration may require insulin dose adjustment and particularly close monitoring).
No products indexed under this heading.

Ramipril (ACE inhibitors may increase the blood glucose-lowering effect of insulin and susceptibility to hypoglycemia. Co-administration may require insulin dose adjustment and particularly close monitoring).
No products indexed under this heading.

Rasagiline Mesylate (MAO inhibitors may increase the blood glucose-lowering effect of insulin and susceptibility to hypoglycemia.
Co-administration may require insulin dose adjustment and particularly close monitoring). Products include:
Azilect Tablets 3106

Repaglinide (Oral antidiabetic products may increase the blood glucose-lowering effect of insulin and susceptibility to hypoglycemia. Co-administration may require insulin dose adjustment and particularly close monitoring). Products include:
PrandiMet Tablets 2967
Prandin Tablets 2971

Reserpine (Under the influence of sympatholytic medicinal products, such as reserpine, the signs and symptoms of hypoglycemia may be reduced or absent. Co-administration may require insulin dose adjustment and particularly close monitoring).
No products indexed under this heading.

Ritonavir (Protease inhibitors may reduce the blood glucose-lowering effect of insulin, which may result in hyperglycemia. Co-administration may require insulin dose adjustment and particularly close monitoring).
Products include:
Kaletra 452
Norvir 489

Rosiglitazone Maleate (Oral antidiabetic products may increase the blood glucose-lowering effect of insulin and susceptibility to hypoglycemia. Co-administration may require insulin dose adjustment and particularly close monitoring).
Products include:
Avandamet Tablets 1336
Avandaryl Tablets 1344
Avandia Tablets 1351

Salmeterol Xinafoate (Sympathomimetics may reduce the blood glucose-lowering effect of insulin, which may result in hyperglycemia. Co-administration may require insulin dose adjustment and particularly close monitoring). Products include:
Advair Diskus 100/50 1276
Advair Diskus 250/50 1276
Advair Diskus 500/50 1276
Advair HFA 45/21 Inhalation Aerosol 1288
Advair HFA 115/21 Inhalation Aerosol 1288
Advair HFA 230/21 Inhalation Aerosol 1288
Serevent Diskus 1594

Salsalate (Salicylates may increase the blood glucose-lowering effect of insulin and susceptibility to hypoglycemia. Co-administration may require insulin dose adjustment and particularly close monitoring).
No products indexed under this heading.

Saquinavir (Protease inhibitors may reduce the blood glucose-lowering effect of insulin, which may result in hyperglycemia. Co-administration may require insulin dose adjustment and particularly close monitoring).
No products indexed under this heading.

Saquinavir Mesylate (Protease inhibitors may reduce the blood glucose-lowering effect of insulin, which may result in hyperglycemia. Co-administration may require insulin dose adjustment and particularly close monitoring).
No products indexed under this heading.

Selegiline (MAO inhibitors may increase the blood glucose-lowering effect of insulin and susceptibility to hypoglycemia. Co-administration may require insulin dose adjustment and particularly close monitoring).
Products include:
Emsam Transdermal System 905

Selegiline Hydrochloride (MAO inhibitors may increase the blood glucose-lowering effect of insulin and susceptibility to hypoglycemia. Co-administration may require insulin dose adjustment and particularly close monitoring). Products include:
Eldepryl Capsules 3052

Silver Sulfadiazine (Sulfonamide antibiotics may increase the blood glucose-lowering effect of insulin and susceptibility to hypoglycemia. Co-administration may require insulin dose adjustment and particularly close monitoring).
No products indexed under this heading.

Sitagliptin Phosphate (Oral antidiabetic products may increase the blood glucose-lowering effect of

insulin and susceptibility to hypoglycemia. Co-administration may require insulin dose adjustment and particularly close monitoring). Products include:
Janumet Tablets 2041
Januvia Tablets 2048

Somatropin (Somatropin may reduce the blood glucose-lowering effect of insulin, which may result in hyperglycemia. Co-administration may require insulin dose adjustment and particularly close monitoring). Products include:
Genotropin Lyophilized Powder 2547
Humatrope Vials and Cartridges 1838
Nutropin for Injection 1208
Nutropin AQ Injection 1212
Nutropin AQ NuSpin Injection 1212
Nutropin AQ Pen 1212
Nutropin AQ Pen Cartridge 1212

Somatropin (rDNA Origin) (Somatropin may reduce the blood glucose-lowering effect of insulin, which may result in hyperglycemia. Co-administration may require insulin dose adjustment and particularly close monitoring). Products include:
Norditropin Cartridges 2354
Tev-Tropin for Injection 1187

Sotalol Hydrochloride (Beta-blockers may either increase or reduce the blood glucose-lowering effect of insulin. In addition, under the influence of sympatholytic medicinal products such as beta-blockers, the signs and symptoms of hypoglycemia may be reduced or absent. Co-administration may require insulin dose adjustment and particularly close monitoring).
No products indexed under this heading.

Spirapril Hydrochloride (ACE inhibitors may increase the blood glucose-lowering effect of insulin and susceptibility to hypoglycemia. Co-administration may require insulin dose adjustment and particularly close monitoring).
No products indexed under this heading.

Spironolactone (Diuretics may reduce the blood glucose-lowering effect of insulin, which may result in hyperglycemia. Co-administration may require insulin dose adjustment and particularly close monitoring).
No products indexed under this heading.

Sulfadiazine (Sulfonamide antibiotics may increase the blood glucose-lowering effect of insulin and susceptibility to hypoglycemia. Co-administration may require insulin dose adjustment and particularly close monitoring).
No products indexed under this heading.

Sulfamethizole (Sulfonamide antibiotics may increase the blood glucose-lowering effect of insulin and susceptibility to hypoglycemia. Co-administration may require insulin dose adjustment and particularly close monitoring).
No products indexed under this heading.

Sulfamethoprim (Sulfonamide antibiotics may increase the blood glucose-lowering effect of insulin and susceptibility to hypoglycemia. Co-administration may require insulin dose adjustment and particularly close monitoring).
No products indexed under this heading.

Sulfamethoxazole (Sulfonamide antibiotics may increase the blood glucose-lowering effect of insulin and susceptibility to hypoglycemia. Co-administration may require insulin dose adjustment and particularly close monitoring).
No products indexed under this heading.

Sulfisoxazole Acetyl (Sulfonamide antibiotics may increase the blood glucose-lowering effect of insulin and susceptibility to hypoglycemia. Co-administration may require insulin dose adjustment and particularly close monitoring).
No products indexed under this heading.

Sulfisoxazole Diolamine (Sulfonamide antibiotics may increase the blood glucose-lowering effect of insulin and susceptibility to hypoglycemia. Co-administration may require insulin dose adjustment and particularly close monitoring).
No products indexed under this heading.

Terbutaline Sulfate (Sympathomimetics may reduce the blood glucose-lowering effect of insulin, which may result in hyperglycemia. Co-administration may require insulin dose adjustment and particularly close monitoring).
No products indexed under this heading.

Thioridazine Hydrochloride (Phenothiazine derivatives may reduce the blood glucose-lowering effect of insulin, which may result in hyperglycemia. Co-administration may require insulin dose adjustment and particularly close monitoring). Products include:
Thioridazine Hydrochloride Tablets 2195

Thyroglobulin (Thyroid hormones may reduce the blood glucose-lowering effect of insulin, which may result in hyperglycemia. Co-administration may require insulin dose adjustment and particularly close monitoring).
No products indexed under this heading.

Thyroid (Thyroid hormones may reduce the blood glucose-lowering effect of insulin, which may result in hyperglycemia. Co-administration may require insulin dose adjustment and particularly close monitoring). Products include:
Naturethroid Tablets 2605

Thyroxine (Thyroid hormones may reduce the blood glucose-lowering effect of insulin, which may result in hyperglycemia. Co-administration may require insulin dose adjustment and particularly close monitoring).
No products indexed under this heading.

Thyroxine Sodium (Thyroid hormones may reduce the blood glucose-lowering effect of insulin, which may result in hyperglycemia. Co-administration may require insulin dose adjustment and particularly close monitoring).
No products indexed under this heading.

Timolol Hemihydrate (Beta-blockers may either increase or reduce the blood glucose-lowering effect of insulin. In addition, under the influence of sympatholytic medicinal products such as beta-blockers, the signs and symptoms of hypoglycemia may be reduced or absent. Co-administration may require insulin dose adjustment and particularly close monitoring). Products include:
Betimol Ophthalmic Solution 3181

Timolol Maleate (Beta-blockers may either increase or reduce the blood glucose-lowering effect of insulin. In addition, under the influence of sympatholytic medicinal products such as beta-blockers, the signs and symptoms of hypoglycemia may be reduced or absent. Co-administration may require insulin dose adjustment and particularly close monitoring). Products include:
Combigan Ophthalmic Solution 553
Cosopt Sterile Ophthalmic Solution 1969
Timoptic Sterile Ophthalmic Solution 2121
Timoptic in Ocudose 2124
Timoptic-XE Sterile Ophthalmic Gel Forming Solution 2125

Tipranavir (Protease inhibitors may reduce the blood glucose-lowering effect of insulin, which may result in hyperglycemia. Co-administration may require insulin dose adjustment and particularly close monitoring). Products include:
Aptivus Capsules 823
Aptivus Oral Solution 823

Tolazamide (Oral antidiabetic products may increase the blood glucose-lowering effect of insulin and susceptibility to hypoglycemia. Co-administration may require insulin dose adjustment and particularly close monitoring).
No products indexed under this heading.

Tolbutamide (Oral antidiabetic products may increase the blood glucose-lowering effect of insulin and susceptibility to hypoglycemia. Co-administration may require insulin dose adjustment and particularly close monitoring).
No products indexed under this heading.

Torsemide (Diuretics may reduce the blood glucose-lowering effect of insulin, which may result in hyperglycemia. Co-administration may require insulin dose adjustment and particularly close monitoring). Products include:
Demadex Injection 2630
Demadex Tablets 2630

Trandolapril (ACE inhibitors may increase the blood glucose-lowering effect of insulin and susceptibility to hypoglycemia. Co-administration may require insulin dose adjustment and particularly close monitoring). Products include:
Mavik Tablets 472
Tarka Tablets 511

Tranylcypromine Sulfate (MAO inhibitors may increase the blood glucose-lowering effect of insulin and susceptibility to hypoglycemia. Co-administration may require insulin dose adjustment and particularly close monitoring). Products include:
Parnate Tablets 1532

Triamcinolone (Corticosteroids may reduce the blood glucose-lowering effect of insulin, which may result in hyperglycemia. Co-administration may require insulin dose adjustment and particularly close monitoring).
No products indexed under this heading.

Triamcinolone Acetonide (Corticosteroids may reduce the blood glucose-lowering effect of insulin, which may result in hyperglycemia. Co-administration may require insulin dose adjustment and particularly close monitoring). Products include:
Azmacort Inhalation Aerosol 407
Nasacort AQ Nasal Spray 2765
Triesence Injectable Suspension .... ⊙ 209

Triamcinolone Diacetate (Corticosteroids may reduce the blood glucose-lowering effect of insulin, which may result in hyperglycemia. Co-administration may require insulin dose adjustment and particularly close monitoring).
No products indexed under this heading.

Triamcinolone Hexacetonide (Corticosteroids may reduce the blood glucose-lowering effect of insulin, which may result in hyperglycemia. Co-administration may require insulin dose adjustment and particularly close monitoring).
No products indexed under this heading.

Triamterene (Diuretics may reduce the blood glucose-lowering effect of insulin, which may result in hyperglycemia. Co-administration may require insulin dose adjustment and particularly close monitoring). Products include:
Dyazide Capsules 1405
Dyrenium Capsules 3189

Trifluoperazine Hydrochloride (Phenothiazine derivatives may reduce the blood glucose-lowering effect of insulin, which may result in hyperglycemia. Co-administration may require insulin dose adjustment and particularly close monitoring).
No products indexed under this heading.

Troglitazone (Oral antidiabetic products may increase the blood glucose-lowering effect of insulin and susceptibility to hypoglycemia. Co-administration may require insulin dose adjustment and particularly close monitoring).
No products indexed under this heading.

Food Interactions

Alcohol (Alcohol may either increase or reduce the blood glucose-lowering effect of insulin. Co-administration may require insulin dose adjustment and particularly close monitoring).

FABRAZYME FOR INTRAVENOUS INFUSION

(Agalsidase beta) 1241
None cited in PDR database.

FANSIDAR TABLETS

(Pyrimethamine, Sulfadoxine) 2636
May interact with sulfonamides and certain other agents. Compounds in these categories include:

Bendroflumethiazide (Antifolic drugs such as sulfonamides or trimethoprim-sulfamethoxazole should not be used while the patient is receiving Fansidar for antimalarial prophylaxis).
No products indexed under this heading.

Chloroquine (Reports may indicate an increase in incidence and severity of adverse reactions when chloroquine is used with Fansidar as compared to the use of Fansidar alone).
No products indexed under this heading.

Chloroquine Hydrochloride (Reports may indicate an increase in incidence and severity of adverse reactions when chloroquine is used with Fansidar as compared to the use of Fansidar alone).
No products indexed under this heading.

Chloroquine Phosphate (Reports may indicate an increase in incidence and severity of adverse reactions when chloroquine is used with Fansidar as compared to the use of Fansidar alone).
No products indexed under this heading.

Chlorothiazide (Antifolic drugs such as sulfonamides or trimethoprim-sulfamethoxazole should not be used while the patient is receiving Fansidar for antimalarial prophylaxis).
No products indexed under this heading.

Chlorothiazide Sodium (Antifolic drugs such as sulfonamides or trimethoprim-sulfamethoxazole should not be used while the patient is receiving Fansidar for antimalarial prophylaxis). Products include:
- Intravenous Sodium Diuril ... 2490

Chlorpropamide (Antifolic drugs such as sulfonamides or trimethoprim-sulfamethoxazole should not be used while the patient is receiving Fansidar for antimalarial prophylaxis).
No products indexed under this heading.

Glipizide (Antifolic drugs such as sulfonamides or trimethoprim-sulfamethoxazole should not be used while the patient is receiving Fansidar for antimalarial prophylaxis).
No products indexed under this heading.

Glyburide (Antifolic drugs such as sulfonamides or trimethoprim-sulfamethoxazole should not be used while the patient is receiving Fansidar for antimalarial prophylaxis).
No products indexed under this heading.

Hydrochlorothiazide (Antifolic drugs such as sulfonamides or trimethoprim-sulfamethoxazole should not be used while the patient is receiving Fansidar for antimalarial prophylaxis). Products include:
- Atacand HCT ... 642
- Avalide Tablets ... 892
- Avalide Tablets ... 2713
- Benicar HCT Tablets ... 1010
- Diovan HCT Tablets ... 2216
- Dyazide Capsules ... 1405
- Micardis HCT Tablets ... 854
- Prinzide Tablets ... 2092
- Tekturna HCT Tablets ... 2324
- Teveten HCT Tablets ... 517

Hydroflumethiazide (Antifolic drugs such as sulfonamides or trimethoprim-sulfamethoxazole should not be used while the patient is receiving Fansidar for antimalarial prophylaxis).
No products indexed under this heading.

Methyclothiazide (Antifolic drugs such as sulfonamides or trimethoprim-sulfamethoxazole should not be used while the patient is receiving Fansidar for antimalarial prophylaxis).
No products indexed under this heading.

Polythiazide (Antifolic drugs such as sulfonamides or trimethoprim-sulfamethoxazole should not be used while the patient is receiving Fansidar for antimalarial prophylaxis).
No products indexed under this heading.

Sulfacytine (Antifolic drugs such as sulfonamides or trimethoprim-sulfamethoxazole should not be used while the patient is receiving Fansidar for antimalarial prophylaxis).
No products indexed under this heading.

Sulfamethizole (Antifolic drugs such as sulfonamides or trimethoprim-sulfamethoxazole should not be used while the patient is receiving Fansidar for antimalarial prophylaxis).
No products indexed under this heading.

Sulfamethoxazole (Antifolic drugs such as sulfonamides or trimethoprim-sulfamethoxazole should not be used while the patient is receiving Fansidar for antimalarial prophylaxis).
No products indexed under this heading.

Sulfasalazine (Antifolic drugs such as sulfonamides or trimethoprim-sulfamethoxazole should not be used while the patient is receiving Fansidar for antimalarial prophylaxis).
No products indexed under this heading.

Sulfinpyrazone (Antifolic drugs such as sulfonamides or trimethoprim-sulfamethoxazole should not be used while the patient is receiving Fansidar for antimalarial prophylaxis).
No products indexed under this heading.

Sulfisoxazole Acetyl (Antifolic drugs such as sulfonamides or trimethoprim-sulfamethoxazole should not be used while the patient is receiving Fansidar for antimalarial prophylaxis).
No products indexed under this heading.

Sulfisoxazole Diolamine (Antifolic drugs such as sulfonamides or trimethoprim-sulfamethoxazole should not be used while the patient is receiving Fansidar for antimalarial prophylaxis).
No products indexed under this heading.

Tolazamide (Antifolic drugs such as sulfonamides or trimethoprim-sulfamethoxazole should not be used while the patient is receiving Fansidar for antimalarial prophylaxis).
No products indexed under this heading.

Tolbutamide (Antifolic drugs such as sulfonamides or trimethoprim-sulfamethoxazole should not be used while the patient is receiving Fansidar for antimalarial prophylaxis).
No products indexed under this heading.

Trimethoprim (Antifolic drugs such as sulfonamides or trimethoprim-sulfamethoxazole should not be used while the patient is receiving Fansidar for antimalarial prophylaxis).
No products indexed under this heading.

Trimethoprim Hydrochloride (Antifolic drugs such as sulfonamides or trimethoprim-sulfamethoxazole should not be used while the patient is receiving Fansidar for antimalarial prophylaxis).
No products indexed under this heading.

Trimethoprim Sulfate (Antifolic drugs such as sulfonamides or trimethoprim-sulfamethoxazole should not be used while the patient is receiving Fansidar for antimalarial prophylaxis).
No products indexed under this heading.

FASLODEX INJECTION

(Fulvestrant) ... 682
None cited in PDR database.

FEIBA VH

(Anti-Inhibitor Coagulant Complex) ... 728
None cited in PDR database.

FEMARA TABLETS

(Letrozole) ... 2246
May interact with:

Tamoxifen Citrate (Co-administration of Femara and tamoxifen 20 mg daily resulted in a reduction of letrozole plasma levels of 38% on average. Clinical experience in the second-line breast cancer pivotal trials indicates that the therapeutic effect of Femara therapy is notimpaired if Femara is administered immediately after tamoxifen).
No products indexed under this heading.

FEMININE CAPSULES

(Amino Acid Preparations, Hydroxypropyl Methylcellulose, Minerals, Multiple, Soy-containing dietary supplements) ... 637
None cited in PDR database.

FENOGLIDE TABLETS

(Fenofibrate) ... 2960
May interact with bile acid sequestering agents, oral anticoagulants, HMG-CoA reductase inhibitors, immunosuppressive agents, nephrotoxic agents, and certain other agents. Compounds in these categories include:

Abacavir Sulfate (The benefits and risks of using fenofibrate with immunosuppressants and other potentially nephrotoxic agents should be carefully considered, and the lowest effective dose employed). Products include:
- Epzicom Tablets ... 1422
- Trizivir Tablets ... 1622
- Ziagen ... 1673

Acyclovir (The benefits and risks of using fenofibrate with immunosuppressants and other potentially nephrotoxic agents should be carefully considered, and the lowest effective dose employed). Products include:
- Zovirax ... 1690
- Zovirax Cream ... 817
- Zovirax Ointment ... 819

Acyclovir Sodium (The benefits and risks of using fenofibrate with immunosuppressants and other potentially nephrotoxic agents should be carefully considered, and the lowest effective dose employed).
No products indexed under this heading.

Alatrofloxacin Mesylate (The benefits and risks of using fenofibrate with immunosuppressants and other potentially nephrotoxic agents should be carefully considered, and the lowest effective dose employed).
No products indexed under this heading.

Aldesleukin (The benefits and risks of using fenofibrate with immunosuppressants and other potentially nephrotoxic agents should be carefully considered, and the lowest effective dose employed). Products include:
- Proleukin for Injection ... 2287

Amikacin Sulfate (The benefits and risks of using fenofibrate with immunosuppressants and other potentially nephrotoxic agents should be carefully considered, and the lowest effective dose employed).
No products indexed under this heading.

Amoxicillin (The benefits and risks of using fenofibrate with immunosuppressants and other potentially nephrotoxic agents should be carefully considered, and the lowest effective dose employed). Products include:
- Amoxil Capsules ... 1305
- Amoxil Chewable Tablets ... 1305
- Amoxil Pediatric Drops for Oral Suspension ... 1305
- Amoxil Powder for Oral Suspension ... 1305
- Amoxil Tablets ... 1305
- Augmentin ... 1323
- Augmentin Tablets ... 1327
- Augmentin XR Extended Release Tablets ... 1333
- Augmentin ES-600 Powder for Oral Suspension ... 1329
- Moxatag Tablets ... 2165

Amoxicillin Trihydrate (The benefits and risks of using fenofibrate with immunosuppressants and other potentially nephrotoxic agents should be carefully considered, and the lowest effective dose employed).
No products indexed under this heading.

Amphotericin B (The benefits and risks of using fenofibrate with immunosuppressants and other potentially nephrotoxic agents should be carefully considered, and the lowest effective dose employed).
No products indexed under this heading.

Amphotericin B, liposomal (The benefits and risks of using fenofibrate with immunosuppressants and other potentially nephrotoxic agents should be carefully considered, and the lowest effective dose employed). Products include:
- AmBisome for Injection ... 606

Amphotericin B Cholesteryl Sulfate (The benefits and risks of using fenofibrate with immunosuppressants and other potentially nephrotoxic agents should be carefully considered, and the lowest effective dose employed).
No products indexed under this heading.

Amphotericin B Lipid Complex (The benefits and risks of using fenofibrate with immunosuppressants and other potentially nephro-

toxic agents should be carefully considered, and the lowest effective dose employed). Products include:

Abelcet Injection 1134

Ampicillin (The benefits and risks of using fenofibrate with immunosuppressants and other potentially nephrotoxic agents should be carefully considered, and the lowest effective dose employed).

No products indexed under this heading.

Ampicillin Sodium (The benefits and risks of using fenofibrate with immunosuppressants and other potentially nephrotoxic agents should be carefully considered, and the lowest effective dose employed).

No products indexed under this heading.

Ampicillin Trihydrate (The benefits and risks of using fenofibrate with immunosuppressants and other potentially nephrotoxic agents should be carefully considered, and the lowest effective dose employed).

No products indexed under this heading.

Amprenavir (The benefits and risks of using fenofibrate with immunosuppressants and other potentially nephrotoxic agents should be carefully considered, and the lowest effective dose employed).

No products indexed under this heading.

Anisindione (Caution should be exercised when anticoagulants are given in conjunction with fenofibrate because of the potentiation of coumarin-type anticoagulants in prolonging the prothrombin time/INR. The dosage of the anticoagulant should be reduced to maintain the prothrombin/INR at the desired level to prevent bleeding complications. Frequent prothrombin time/INR determinations are advisable until it has been definitely determined that the prothrombin time/INR has stabilized).

No products indexed under this heading.

Aspirin (The benefits and risks of using fenofibrate with immunosuppressants and other potentially nephrotoxic agents should be carefully considered, and the lowest effective dose employed). Products include:

Aggrenox Capsules 819
Bayer Aspirin 750
Percodan Tablets 1130
St. Joseph 81 mg Aspirin Chewable and Enteric Coated Tablets 1903

Atazanavir (The benefits and risks of using fenofibrate with immunosuppressants and other potentially nephrotoxic agents should be carefully considered, and the lowest effective dose employed).

No products indexed under this heading.

Atorvastatin Calcium (The combined use of fenofibric acid derivatives, particularly gemfibrozil, and HMG-CoA reductase inhibitors results in an increased risk of rhabdomyolysis and myoglobinuria leading in a high proportion of cases to acute renal failure. The combined use of fenofibrate and HMG-CoA reductase inhibitors should be avoided unless the benefit of further alterations in lipid levels is likely to outweigh the increased risk of this drug combination). Products include:

Lipitor Tablets 2501

Azathioprine (The benefits and risks of using fenofibrate with immunosuppressants and other potentially nephrotoxic agents should be carefully considered, and the lowest effective dose employed).

No products indexed under this heading.

Azithromycin Dihydrate (The benefits and risks of using fenofibrate with immunosuppressants and other potentially nephrotoxic agents should be carefully considered, and the lowest effective dose employed).

No products indexed under this heading.

Azlocillin Sodium (The benefits and risks of using fenofibrate with immunosuppressants and other potentially nephrotoxic agents should be carefully considered, and the lowest effective dose employed).

No products indexed under this heading.

Aztreonam (The benefits and risks of using fenofibrate with immunosuppressants and other potentially nephrotoxic agents should be carefully considered, and the lowest effective dose employed).

No products indexed under this heading.

Bacampicillin Hydrochloride (The benefits and risks of using fenofibrate with immunosuppressants and other potentially nephrotoxic agents should be carefully considered, and the lowest effective dose employed).

No products indexed under this heading.

Balsalazide Disodium (The benefits and risks of using fenofibrate with immunosuppressants and other potentially nephrotoxic agents should be carefully considered, and the lowest effective dose employed).

No products indexed under this heading.

Basiliximab (The benefits and risks of using fenofibrate with immunosuppressants and other potentially nephrotoxic agents should be carefully considered, and the lowest effective dose employed). Products include:

Simulect for Injection 2306

Benazepril Hydrochloride (The benefits and risks of using fenofibrate with immunosuppressants and other potentially nephrotoxic agents should be carefully considered, and the lowest effective dose employed).

No products indexed under this heading.

Bendroflumethiazide (The benefits and risks of using fenofibrate with immunosuppressants and other potentially nephrotoxic agents should be carefully considered, and the lowest effective dose employed).

No products indexed under this heading.

Caffeine (The benefits and risks of using fenofibrate with immunosuppressants and other potentially nephrotoxic agents should be carefully considered, and the lowest effective dose employed). Products include:

BioLean Free Tablets .... ▣635
BioLean II Tablets .... ▣635
Winrgy Dietary Supplement .... ▣642

Captopril (The benefits and risks of using fenofibrate with immunosuppressants and other potentially nephrotoxic agents should be carefully considered, and the lowest effective dose employed). Products include:

Captopril Tablets 2182

Carbenicillin Disodium (The benefits and risks of using fenofibrate with immunosuppressants and other potentially nephrotoxic agents should be carefully considered, and the lowest effective dose employed).

No products indexed under this heading.

Carbenicillin Indanyl Sodium (The benefits and risks of using fenofibrate with immunosuppressants and other potentially nephrotoxic agents should be carefully considered, and the lowest effective dose employed).

No products indexed under this heading.

Carboplatin (The benefits and risks of using fenofibrate with immunosuppressants and other potentially nephrotoxic agents should be carefully considered, and the lowest effective dose employed).

No products indexed under this heading.

Carmustine (BCNU) (The benefits and risks of using fenofibrate with immunosuppressants and other potentially nephrotoxic agents should be carefully considered, and the lowest effective dose employed).

No products indexed under this heading.

Cefaclor (The benefits and risks of using fenofibrate with immunosuppressants and other potentially nephrotoxic agents should be carefully considered, and the lowest effective dose employed).

No products indexed under this heading.

Cefadroxil (The benefits and risks of using fenofibrate with immunosuppressants and other potentially nephrotoxic agents should be carefully considered, and the lowest effective dose employed).

No products indexed under this heading.

Cefamandole Nafate (The benefits and risks of using fenofibrate with immunosuppressants and other potentially nephrotoxic agents should be carefully considered, and the lowest effective dose employed).

No products indexed under this heading.

Cefazolin Sodium (The benefits and risks of using fenofibrate with immunosuppressants and other potentially nephrotoxic agents should be carefully considered, and the lowest effective dose employed).

No products indexed under this heading.

Cefdinir (The benefits and risks of using fenofibrate with immunosuppressants and other potentially nephrotoxic agents should be carefully considered, and the lowest effective dose employed). Products include:

Omnicef Capsules 497
Omnicef for Oral Suspension 497

Cefepime Hydrochloride (The benefits and risks of using fenofibrate with immunosuppressants and other potentially nephrotoxic agents should be carefully considered, and the lowest effective dose employed).

No products indexed under this heading.

Cefixime (The benefits and risks of using fenofibrate with immunosuppressants and other potentially nephrotoxic agents should be carefully considered, and the lowest effective dose employed). Products include:

Suprax for Oral Suspension 1891
Suprax Tablets 1891

Cefmetazole Sodium (The benefits and risks of using fenofibrate with immunosuppressants and other potentially nephrotoxic agents should be carefully considered, and the lowest effective dose employed).

No products indexed under this heading.

Cefonicid Sodium (The benefits and risks of using fenofibrate with immunosuppressants and other potentially nephrotoxic agents should be carefully considered, and the lowest effective dose employed).

No products indexed under this heading.

Cefoperazone Sodium (The benefits and risks of using fenofibrate with immunosuppressants and other potentially nephrotoxic agents should be carefully considered, and the lowest effective dose employed).

No products indexed under this heading.

Ceforanide (The benefits and risks of using fenofibrate with immunosuppressants and other potentially nephrotoxic agents should be carefully considered, and the lowest effective dose employed).

No products indexed under this heading.

Cefotaxime Sodium (The benefits and risks of using fenofibrate with immunosuppressants and other potentially nephrotoxic agents should be carefully considered, and the lowest effective dose employed).

No products indexed under this heading.

Cefotetan (The benefits and risks of using fenofibrate with immunosuppressants and other potentially nephrotoxic agents should be carefully considered, and the lowest effective dose employed).

No products indexed under this heading.

Cefoxitin Sodium (The benefits and risks of using fenofibrate with immunosuppressants and other potentially nephrotoxic agents should be carefully considered, and the lowest effective dose employed).

No products indexed under this heading.

Cefpodoxime Proxetil (The benefits and risks of using fenofibrate with immunosuppressants and other potentially nephrotoxic agents should be carefully considered, and the lowest effective dose employed).

No products indexed under this heading.

Cefprozil (The benefits and risks of using fenofibrate with immunosuppressants and other potentially nephrotoxic agents should be carefully considered, and the lowest effective dose employed).

No products indexed under this heading.

Ceftazidime (The benefits and risks of using fenofibrate with immunosuppressants and other potentially nephrotoxic agents should be carefully considered, and the lowest effective dose employed). Products include:

Fortaz 1450

Ceftizoxime Sodium (The benefits and risks of using fenofibrate with immunosuppressants and other potentially nephrotoxic agents should be carefully considered, and the lowest effective dose employed).
No products indexed under this heading.

Ceftriaxone Sodium (The benefits and risks of using fenofibrate with immunosuppressants and other potentially nephrotoxic agents should be carefully considered, and the lowest effective dose employed). Products include:
Rocephin Injectable Vials, ADD-Vantage, Galaxy, Bulk 2642

Cefuroxime Axetil (The benefits and risks of using fenofibrate with immunosuppressants and other potentially nephrotoxic agents should be carefully considered, and the lowest effective dose employed). Products include:
Ceftin 1380

Cefuroxime Sodium (The benefits and risks of using fenofibrate with immunosuppressants and other potentially nephrotoxic agents should be carefully considered, and the lowest effective dose employed).
No products indexed under this heading.

Celecoxib (The benefits and risks of using fenofibrate with immunosuppressants and other potentially nephrotoxic agents should be carefully considered, and the lowest effective dose employed). Products include:
Celebrex Capsules 2979

Cephalexin (The benefits and risks of using fenofibrate with immunosuppressants and other potentially nephrotoxic agents should be carefully considered, and the lowest effective dose employed).
No products indexed under this heading.

Cephalothin Sodium (The benefits and risks of using fenofibrate with immunosuppressants and other potentially nephrotoxic agents should be carefully considered, and the lowest effective dose employed).
No products indexed under this heading.

Cephapirin Sodium (The benefits and risks of using fenofibrate with immunosuppressants and other potentially nephrotoxic agents should be carefully considered, and the lowest effective dose employed).
No products indexed under this heading.

Cephradine (The benefits and risks of using fenofibrate with immunosuppressants and other potentially nephrotoxic agents should be carefully considered, and the lowest effective dose employed).
No products indexed under this heading.

Cerivastatin Sodium (The combined use of fenofibric acid derivatives, particularly gemfibrozil, and HMG-CoA reductase inhibitors results in an increased risk of rhabdomyolysis and myoglobinuria leading in a high proportion of cases to acute renal failure. The combined use of fenofibrate and HMG-CoA reductase inhibitors should be avoided unless the benefit of further alterations in lipid levels is likely to outweigh the increased risk of this drug combination).
No products indexed under this heading.

Chlorothiazide (The benefits and risks of using fenofibrate with immunosuppressants and other potentially nephrotoxic agents should be carefully considered, and the lowest effective dose employed).
No products indexed under this heading.

Chlorothiazide Sodium (The benefits and risks of using fenofibrate with immunosuppressants and other potentially nephrotoxic agents should be carefully considered, and the lowest effective dose employed). Products include:
Intravenous Sodium Diuril 2490

Chlorpropamide (The benefits and risks of using fenofibrate with immunosuppressants and other potentially nephrotoxic agents should be carefully considered, and the lowest effective dose employed).
No products indexed under this heading.

Cholestyramine (Since bile acid sequestrants may bind other drugs give concurrently, patients should take fenofibrate at least 1 hour before or 4 to 6 hours after a bile acid binding resin to avoid impeding its absorption).
No products indexed under this heading.

Cidofovir (The benefits and risks of using fenofibrate with immunosuppressants and other potentially nephrotoxic agents should be carefully considered, and the lowest effective dose employed).
No products indexed under this heading.

Cilastatin Sodium (The benefits and risks of using fenofibrate with immunosuppressants and other potentially nephrotoxic agents should be carefully considered, and the lowest effective dose employed). Products include:
Primaxin I.M. 2080
Primaxin I.V. 2083

Cimetidine (The benefits and risks of using fenofibrate with immunosuppressants and other potentially nephrotoxic agents should be carefully considered, and the lowest effective dose employed).
No products indexed under this heading.

Cimetidine Hydrochloride (The benefits and risks of using fenofibrate with immunosuppressants and other potentially nephrotoxic agents should be carefully considered, and the lowest effective dose employed).
No products indexed under this heading.

Cisplatin (The benefits and risks of using fenofibrate with immunosuppressants and other potentially nephrotoxic agents should be carefully considered, and the lowest effective dose employed).
No products indexed under this heading.

Cladribine (The benefits and risks of using fenofibrate with immunosuppressants and other potentially nephrotoxic agents should be carefully considered, and the lowest effective dose employed). Products include:
Leustatin Injection 2384

Clozapine (The benefits and risks of using fenofibrate with immunosuppressants and other potentially nephrotoxic agents should be carefully considered, and the lowest effective dose employed).
No products indexed under this heading.

Colesevelam Hydrochloride (Since bile acid sequestrants may bind other drugs give concurrently, patients should take fenofibrate at least 1 hour before or 4 to 6 hours after a bile acid binding resin to avoid impeding its absorption). Products include:
WelChol Tablets 1015

Colestipol Hydrochloride (Since bile acid sequestrants may bind other drugs give concurrently, patients should take fenofibrate at least 1 hour before or 4 to 6 hours after a bile acid binding resin to avoid impeding its absorption).
No products indexed under this heading.

Colistimethate Sodium (The benefits and risks of using fenofibrate with immunosuppressants and other potentially nephrotoxic agents should be carefully considered, and the lowest effective dose employed).
No products indexed under this heading.

Colistin Sulfate (The benefits and risks of using fenofibrate with immunosuppressants and other potentially nephrotoxic agents should be carefully considered, and the lowest effective dose employed).
No products indexed under this heading.

Cyclophosphamide (The benefits and risks of using fenofibrate with immunosuppressants and other potentially nephrotoxic agents should be carefully considered, and the lowest effective dose employed).
No products indexed under this heading.

Cyclosporine (Because cyclosporine can product nephrotoxicity with decreases in creatinine clearance and rises in serum creatinine, and because renal excretion is the primary elimination route of fibrate drugs including fenofibrate, there is a risk that an interaction will lead to deterioration of renal function. The benefits and risks of using fenofibrate with immunosuppressants and other potentially nephrotoxic agents should be carefully considered, and the lowest effective dose employed). Products include:
Gengraf Capsules 435
Neoral Oral Solution 2280
Neoral Soft Gelatin Capsules 2280
Restasis Ophthalmic Emulsion 557
Sandimmune 2296

Cytarabine (The benefits and risks of using fenofibrate with immunosuppressants and other potentially nephrotoxic agents should be carefully considered, and the lowest effective dose employed).
No products indexed under this heading.

Cytarabine Liposome (The benefits and risks of using fenofibrate with immunosuppressants and other potentially nephrotoxic agents should be carefully considered, and the lowest effective dose employed). Products include:
DepoCyt Injection 1136

Delavirdine Mesylate (The benefits and risks of using fenofibrate with immunosuppressants and other potentially nephrotoxic agents should be carefully considered, and the lowest effective dose employed).
No products indexed under this heading.

Diatrizoate Meglumine (The benefits and risks of using fenofibrate with immunosuppressants and other potentially nephrotoxic agents should be carefully considered, and the lowest effective dose employed).
No products indexed under this heading.

Diatrizoate Sodium (The benefits and risks of using fenofibrate with immunosuppressants and other potentially nephrotoxic agents should be carefully considered, and the lowest effective dose employed).
No products indexed under this heading.

Diclofenac Potassium (The benefits and risks of using fenofibrate with immunosuppressants and other potentially nephrotoxic agents should be carefully considered, and the lowest effective dose employed).
No products indexed under this heading.

Diclofenac Sodium (The benefits and risks of using fenofibrate with immunosuppressants and other potentially nephrotoxic agents should be carefully considered, and the lowest effective dose employed). Products include:
Diclofenac Sodium Ophthalmic Solution .... ⊙ 240
Voltaren Ophthalmic Solution 2336
Voltaren Tablets 2334
Voltaren-XR Tablets 2337

Dicloxacillin Sodium (The benefits and risks of using fenofibrate with immunosuppressants and other potentially nephrotoxic agents should be carefully considered, and the lowest effective dose employed).
No products indexed under this heading.

Dicumarol (Caution should be exercised when anticoagulants are given in conjunction with fenofibrate because of the potentiation of coumarin-type anticoagulants in prolonging the prothrombin time/INR. The dosage of the anticoagulant should be reduced to maintain the prothrombin/INR at the desired level to prevent bleeding complications. Frequent prothrombin time/INR determinations are advisable until it has been definitely determined that the prothrombin time/INR has stabilized).
No products indexed under this heading.

Didanosine (The benefits and risks of using fenofibrate with immunosuppressants and other potentially nephrotoxic agents should be carefully considered, and the lowest effective dose employed).
No products indexed under this heading.

Efavirenz (The benefits and risks of using fenofibrate with immunosuppressants and other potentially nephrotoxic agents should be carefully considered, and the lowest effective dose employed). Products include:
Atripla Tablets 938
Sustiva Capsules 930
Sustiva Tablets 930

Emtricitabine (The benefits and risks of using fenofibrate with immunosuppressants and other potentially nephrotoxic agents should be carefully considered, and the lowest effective dose employed). Products include:

- Atripla Tablets ... 938
- Emtriva Capsules ... 1246
- Emtriva Oral Solution ... 1246
- Truvada Tablets ... 1262

Enalapril Maleate (The benefits and risks of using fenofibrate with immunosuppressants and other potentially nephrotoxic agents should be carefully considered, and the lowest effective dose employed).
No products indexed under this heading.

Enalaprilat (The benefits and risks of using fenofibrate with immunosuppressants and other potentially nephrotoxic agents should be carefully considered, and the lowest effective dose employed).
No products indexed under this heading.

Enfuvirtide (The benefits and risks of using fenofibrate with immunosuppressants and other potentially nephrotoxic agents should be carefully considered, and the lowest effective dose employed).
No products indexed under this heading.

Ethiodized Oil (The benefits and risks of using fenofibrate with immunosuppressants and other potentially nephrotoxic agents should be carefully considered, and the lowest effective dose employed).
No products indexed under this heading.

Etodolac (The benefits and risks of using fenofibrate with immunosuppressants and other potentially nephrotoxic agents should be carefully considered, and the lowest effective dose employed).
No products indexed under this heading.

Fenoprofen Calcium (The benefits and risks of using fenofibrate with immunosuppressants and other potentially nephrotoxic agents should be carefully considered, and the lowest effective dose employed). Products include:

- Nalfon Capsules ... 2508

Filgrastim (The benefits and risks of using fenofibrate with immunosuppressants and other potentially nephrotoxic agents should be carefully considered, and the lowest effective dose employed). Products include:

- Neupogen for Injection ... 589

Fluorouracil (The benefits and risks of using fenofibrate with immunosuppressants and other potentially nephrotoxic agents should be carefully considered, and the lowest effective dose employed). Products include:

- Carac Cream 0.5% ... 2722

Flurbiprofen (The benefits and risks of using fenofibrate with immunosuppressants and other potentially nephrotoxic agents should be carefully considered, and the lowest effective dose employed).
No products indexed under this heading.

Fluvastatin Sodium (The combined use of fenofibric acid derivatives, particularly gemfibrozil, and HMG-CoA reductase inhibitors results in an increased risk of rhabdomyolysis and myoglobinuria leading in a high proportion of cases to acute renal failure. The combined use of fenofibrate and HMG-CoA reductase inhibitors should be avoided unless the benefit of further alterations in lipid levels is likely to outweigh the increased risk of this drug combination). Products include:

- Lescol Capsules ... 2268
- Lescol XL Tablets ... 2268

Foscarnet Sodium (The benefits and risks of using fenofibrate with immunosuppressants and other potentially nephrotoxic agents should be carefully considered, and the lowest effective dose employed).
No products indexed under this heading.

Fosinopril Sodium (The benefits and risks of using fenofibrate with immunosuppressants and other potentially nephrotoxic agents should be carefully considered, and the lowest effective dose employed).
No products indexed under this heading.

Furosemide (The benefits and risks of using fenofibrate with immunosuppressants and other potentially nephrotoxic agents should be carefully considered, and the lowest effective dose employed). Products include:

- Furosemide Tablets ... 2186

Gadopentetate Dimeglumine (The benefits and risks of using fenofibrate with immunosuppressants and other potentially nephrotoxic agents should be carefully considered, and the lowest effective dose employed).
No products indexed under this heading.

Gentamicin (The benefits and risks of using fenofibrate with immunosuppressants and other potentially nephrotoxic agents should be carefully considered, and the lowest effective dose employed).
No products indexed under this heading.

Gentamicin Sulfate (The benefits and risks of using fenofibrate with immunosuppressants and other potentially nephrotoxic agents should be carefully considered, and the lowest effective dose employed). Products include:

- Pred-G Ophthalmic Ointment ... ⊙229
- Pred-G Ophthalmic Suspension ... ⊙228

Glipizide (The benefits and risks of using fenofibrate with immunosuppressants and other potentially nephrotoxic agents should be carefully considered, and the lowest effective dose employed).
No products indexed under this heading.

Globulin, Immune (Human) (The benefits and risks of using fenofibrate with immunosuppressants and other potentially nephrotoxic agents should be carefully considered, and the lowest effective dose employed). Products include:

- Flebogamma 5% ... 1715

Glyburide (The benefits and risks of using fenofibrate with immunosuppressants and other potentially nephrotoxic agents should be carefully considered, and the lowest effective dose employed).
No products indexed under this heading.

Gold Therapy (The benefits and risks of using fenofibrate with immunosuppressants and other potentially nephrotoxic agents should be carefully considered, and the lowest effective dose employed).
No products indexed under this heading.

HMG-CoA Reductase Inhibitors (The benefits and risks of using fenofibrate with immunosuppressants and other potentially nephrotoxic agents should be carefully considered, and the lowest effective dose employed).
No products indexed under this heading.

Hydrochlorothiazide (The benefits and risks of using fenofibrate with immunosuppressants and other potentially nephrotoxic agents should be carefully considered, and the lowest effective dose employed). Products include:

- Atacand HCT ... 642
- Avalide Tablets ... 892
- Avalide Tablets ... 2713
- Benicar HCT Tablets ... 1010
- Diovan HCT Tablets ... 2216
- Dyazide Capsules ... 1405
- Micardis HCT Tablets ... 854
- Prinzide Tablets ... 2092
- Tekturna HCT Tablets ... 2324
- Teveten HCT Tablets ... 517

Hydroflumethiazide (The benefits and risks of using fenofibrate with immunosuppressants and other potentially nephrotoxic agents should be carefully considered, and the lowest effective dose employed).
No products indexed under this heading.

Ibuprofen (The benefits and risks of using fenofibrate with immunosuppressants and other potentially nephrotoxic agents should be carefully considered, and the lowest effective dose employed). Products include:

- Motrin IB Tablets and Caplets ... 1900
- Children's Motrin Oral Suspension ... 1901
- Children's Motrin Non-Staining Dye-Free Oral Suspension ... 1901
- Children's Motrin Cold Oral Suspension ... 1899
- Infants' Motrin Concentrated Drops ... 1901
- Infants' Motrin Non-Staining Dye-Free Concentrated Drops ... 1901
- Junior Strength Motrin Caplets and Chewable Tablets ... 1901
- Vicoprofen Tablets ... 533

Idarubicin Hydrochloride (The benefits and risks of using fenofibrate with immunosuppressants and other potentially nephrotoxic agents should be carefully considered, and the lowest effective dose employed).
No products indexed under this heading.

Ifosfamide (The benefits and risks of using fenofibrate with immunosuppressants and other potentially nephrotoxic agents should be carefully considered, and the lowest effective dose employed).
No products indexed under this heading.

Imipenem (The benefits and risks of using fenofibrate with immunosuppressants and other potentially nephrotoxic agents should be carefully considered, and the lowest effective dose employed). Products include:

- Primaxin I.M. ... 2080
- Primaxin I.V. ... 2083

Immune Globulin Intravenous (Human) (The benefits and risks of using fenofibrate with immunosuppressants and other potentially nephrotoxic agents should be carefully considered, and the lowest effective dose employed). Products include:

- Flebogamma 5% DIF ... 1718
- Gammagard Liquid ... 730
- Gammagard S/D ... 734
- Gamunex ... 3094

Indinavir Sulfate (The benefits and risks of using fenofibrate with immunosuppressants and other potentially nephrotoxic agents should be carefully considered, and the lowest effective dose employed). Products include:

- Crixivan Capsules ... 1979

Indomethacin (The benefits and risks of using fenofibrate with immunosuppressants and other potentially nephrotoxic agents should be carefully considered, and the lowest effective dose employed). Products include:

- Indocin ... 2024

Indomethacin Sodium Trihydrate (The benefits and risks of using fenofibrate with immunosuppressants and other potentially nephrotoxic agents should be carefully considered, and the lowest effective dose employed). Products include:

- Indocin I.V. ... 2489

Interferon Beta-1b (The benefits and risks of using fenofibrate with immunosuppressants and other potentially nephrotoxic agents should be carefully considered, and the lowest effective dose employed). Products include:

- Betaseron for SC Injection ... 756

Interleuken-2 (The benefits and risks of using fenofibrate with immunosuppressants and other potentially nephrotoxic agents should be carefully considered, and the lowest effective dose employed).
No products indexed under this heading.

Iodamide Meglumine (The benefits and risks of using fenofibrate with immunosuppressants and other potentially nephrotoxic agents should be carefully considered, and the lowest effective dose employed).
No products indexed under this heading.

Iohexol (The benefits and risks of using fenofibrate with immunosuppressants and other potentially nephrotoxic agents should be carefully considered, and the lowest effective dose employed).
No products indexed under this heading.

Iopamidol (The benefits and risks of using fenofibrate with immunosuppressants and other potentially nephrotoxic agents should be carefully considered, and the lowest effective dose employed).
No products indexed under this heading.

Iopanoic Acid (The benefits and risks of using fenofibrate with immunosuppressants and other potentially nephrotoxic agents should be carefully considered, and the lowest effective dose employed).
No products indexed under this heading.

Iothalamate Meglumine (The benefits and risks of using fenofibrate with immunosuppressants and other potentially nephrotoxic agents should be carefully considered, and the lowest effective dose employed).
No products indexed under this heading.

Ioxaglate Meglumine (The benefits and risks of using fenofibrate with immunosuppressants and other potentially nephrotoxic agents should be carefully considered, and the lowest effective dose employed).
No products indexed under this heading.

Ioxaglate Sodium (The benefits and risks of using fenofibrate with immunosuppressants and other potentially nephrotoxic agents should be carefully considered, and the lowest effective dose employed).
No products indexed under this heading.

Kanamycin Sulfate (The benefits and risks of using fenofibrate with immunosuppressants and other potentially nephrotoxic agents should be carefully considered, and the lowest effective dose employed).
No products indexed under this heading.

Ketoprofen (The benefits and risks of using fenofibrate with immunosuppressants and other potentially nephrotoxic agents should be carefully considered, and the lowest effective dose employed).
No products indexed under this heading.

Ketorolac Tromethamine (The benefits and risks of using fenofibrate with immunosuppressants and other potentially nephrotoxic agents should be carefully considered, and the lowest effective dose employed).
No products indexed under this heading.

Lamium album (The benefits and risks of using fenofibrate with immunosuppressants and other potentially nephrotoxic agents should be carefully considered, and the lowest effective dose employed).
No products indexed under this heading.

Lisinopril (The benefits and risks of using fenofibrate with immunosuppressants and other potentially nephrotoxic agents should be carefully considered, and the lowest effective dose employed). Products include:
Prinivil Tablets **2087**
Prinzide Tablets **2092**

Lithium (The benefits and risks of using fenofibrate with immunosuppressants and other potentially nephrotoxic agents should be carefully considered, and the lowest effective dose employed).
No products indexed under this heading.

Lithium Carbonate (The benefits and risks of using fenofibrate with immunosuppressants and other potentially nephrotoxic agents should be carefully considered, and the lowest effective dose employed).
No products indexed under this heading.

Lithium Citrate (The benefits and risks of using fenofibrate with immunosuppressants and other potentially nephrotoxic agents should be carefully considered, and the lowest effective dose employed).
No products indexed under this heading.

Lopinavir (The benefits and risks of using fenofibrate with immunosuppressants and other potentially nephrotoxic agents should be carefully considered, and the lowest effective dose employed). Products include:
Kaletra **452**

Loracarbef (The benefits and risks of using fenofibrate with immunosuppressants and other potentially nephrotoxic agents should be carefully considered, and the lowest effective dose employed).
No products indexed under this heading.

Lovastatin (The combined use of fenofibric acid derivatives, particularly gemfibrozil, and HMG-CoA reductase inhibitors results in an increased risk of rhabdomyolysis and myoglobinuria leading in a high proportion of cases to acute renal failure. The combined use of fenofibrate and HMG-CoA reductase inhibitors should be avoided unless the benefit of further alterations in lipid levels is likely to outweigh the increased risk of this drug combination). Products include:
Advicor Tablets **402**
Mevacor Tablets **2063**

Meclofenamate Sodium (The benefits and risks of using fenofibrate with immunosuppressants and other potentially nephrotoxic agents should be carefully considered, and the lowest effective dose employed).
No products indexed under this heading.

Mefenamic Acid (The benefits and risks of using fenofibrate with immunosuppressants and other potentially nephrotoxic agents should be carefully considered, and the lowest effective dose employed).
No products indexed under this heading.

Meloxicam (The benefits and risks of using fenofibrate with immunosuppressants and other potentially nephrotoxic agents should be carefully considered, and the lowest effective dose employed). Products include:
Mobic Oral Suspension **863**
Mobic Tablets **863**

Melphalan Hydrochloride (The benefits and risks of using fenofibrate with immunosuppressants and other potentially nephrotoxic agents should be carefully considered, and the lowest effective dose employed).
No products indexed under this heading.

Mesalamine (The benefits and risks of using fenofibrate with immunosuppressants and other potentially nephrotoxic agents should be carefully considered, and the lowest effective dose employed). Products include:
Asacol Delayed-Release Tablets **2579**
Canasa Rectal Suppositories **705**
Lialda Tablets **3029**
Pentasa Capsules **3030**

Methimazole (The benefits and risks of using fenofibrate with immunosuppressants and other potentially nephrotoxic agents should be carefully considered, and the lowest effective dose employed).
No products indexed under this heading.

Methotrexate (The benefits and risks of using fenofibrate with immunosuppressants and other potentially nephrotoxic agents should be carefully considered, and the lowest effective dose employed).
No products indexed under this heading.

Methotrexate Sodium (The benefits and risks of using fenofibrate with immunosuppressants and other potentially nephrotoxic agents should be carefully considered, and the lowest effective dose employed).
No products indexed under this heading.

Methyclothiazide (The benefits and risks of using fenofibrate with immunosuppressants and other potentially nephrotoxic agents should be carefully considered, and the lowest effective dose employed).
No products indexed under this heading.

Mezlocillin Sodium (The benefits and risks of using fenofibrate with immunosuppressants and other potentially nephrotoxic agents should be carefully considered, and the lowest effective dose employed).
No products indexed under this heading.

Minocycline Hydrochloride (The benefits and risks of using fenofibrate with immunosuppressants and other potentially nephrotoxic agents should be carefully considered, and the lowest effective dose employed). Products include:
Solodyn Extended Release Tablets **1938**

Mitomycin (Mitomycin-C) (The benefits and risks of using fenofibrate with immunosuppressants and other potentially nephrotoxic agents should be carefully considered, and the lowest effective dose employed).
No products indexed under this heading.

Moexipril Hydrochloride (The benefits and risks of using fenofibrate with immunosuppressants and other potentially nephrotoxic agents should be carefully considered, and the lowest effective dose employed).
No products indexed under this heading.

Muromonab-CD3 (The benefits and risks of using fenofibrate with immunosuppressants and other potentially nephrotoxic agents should be carefully considered, and the lowest effective dose employed). Products include:
Orthoclone OKT3 Sterile Solution **2387**

Mycophenolate Mofetil (The benefits and risks of using fenofibrate with immunosuppressants and other potentially nephrotoxic agents should be carefully considered, and the lowest effective dose employed). Products include:
CellCept Capsules **2622**
CellCept Oral Suspension **2622**
CellCept Tablets **2622**

Nabumetone (The benefits and risks of using fenofibrate with immunosuppressants and other potentially nephrotoxic agents should be carefully considered, and the lowest effective dose employed).
No products indexed under this heading.

Nafcillin Sodium (The benefits and risks of using fenofibrate with immunosuppressants and other potentially nephrotoxic agents should be carefully considered, and the lowest effective dose employed).
No products indexed under this heading.

Naproxen (The benefits and risks of using fenofibrate with immunosuppressants and other potentially nephrotoxic agents should be carefully considered, and the lowest effective dose employed). Products include:
EC-Naprosyn Delayed-Release Tablets **2632**
Naprosyn Suspension **2632**
Naprosyn Tablets **2632**

Naproxen Sodium (The benefits and risks of using fenofibrate with immunosuppressants and other potentially nephrotoxic agents should be carefully considered, and the lowest effective dose employed). Products include:
Anaprox Tablets **2632**
Anaprox DS Tablets **2632**
Treximet Tablets **1616**

Nelfinavir Mesylate (The benefits and risks of using fenofibrate with immunosuppressants and other potentially nephrotoxic agents should be carefully considered, and the lowest effective dose employed).
No products indexed under this heading.

Neomycin (The benefits and risks of using fenofibrate with immunosuppressants and other potentially nephrotoxic agents should be carefully considered, and the lowest effective dose employed).
No products indexed under this heading.

Neomycin, oral (The benefits and risks of using fenofibrate with immunosuppressants and other potentially nephrotoxic agents should be carefully considered, and the lowest effective dose employed).
No products indexed under this heading.

Neomycin Sulfate (The benefits and risks of using fenofibrate with immunosuppressants and other potentially nephrotoxic agents should be carefully considered, and the lowest effective dose employed). Products include:
Neosporin Ophthalmic Solution Sterile .... ⊙**252**

Nevirapine (The benefits and risks of using fenofibrate with immunosuppressants and other potentially nephrotoxic agents should be carefully considered, and the lowest effective dose employed). Products include:
Viramune Oral Suspension **873**
Viramune Tablets **873**

Norfloxacin (The benefits and risks of using fenofibrate with immunosuppressants and other potentially nephrotoxic agents should be carefully considered, and the lowest effective dose employed). Products include:
Noroxin Tablets **2069**

Olsalazine Sodium (The benefits and risks of using fenofibrate with immunosuppressants and other potentially nephrotoxic agents should be carefully considered, and the lowest effective dose employed).
No products indexed under this heading.

Omeprazole (The benefits and risks of using fenofibrate with immunosuppressants and other potentially nephrotoxic agents should be carefully considered, and the lowest effective dose employed).
No products indexed under this heading.

Oxaprozin (The benefits and risks of using fenofibrate with immunosuppressants and other potentially nephrotoxic agents should be carefully considered, and the lowest effective dose employed).

No products indexed under this heading.

Pamidronate Disodium (The benefits and risks of using fenofibrate with immunosuppressants and other potentially nephrotoxic agents should be carefully considered, and the lowest effective dose employed).

No products indexed under this heading.

Paroxetine Hydrochloride (The benefits and risks of using fenofibrate with immunosuppressants and other potentially nephrotoxic agents should be carefully considered, and the lowest effective dose employed). Products include:

Paxil 1535
Paxil CR Controlled-Release Tablets 1544

Penicillamine (The benefits and risks of using fenofibrate with immunosuppressants and other potentially nephrotoxic agents should be carefully considered, and the lowest effective dose employed). Products include:

Cuprimine Capsules 1986

Penicillin G Benzathine (The benefits and risks of using fenofibrate with immunosuppressants and other potentially nephrotoxic agents should be carefully considered, and the lowest effective dose employed). Products include:

Bicillin C-R Injectable Suspension 1775
Bicillin L-A Injection 1777

Penicillin G Potassium (The benefits and risks of using fenofibrate with immunosuppressants and other potentially nephrotoxic agents should be carefully considered, and the lowest effective dose employed).

No products indexed under this heading.

Penicillin G Procaine (The benefits and risks of using fenofibrate with immunosuppressants and other potentially nephrotoxic agents should be carefully considered, and the lowest effective dose employed). Products include:

Bicillin C-R Injectable Suspension 1775
Bicillin L-A Injection 1777

Penicillin G Sodium (The benefits and risks of using fenofibrate with immunosuppressants and other potentially nephrotoxic agents should be carefully considered, and the lowest effective dose employed).

No products indexed under this heading.

Penicillin V Potassium (The benefits and risks of using fenofibrate with immunosuppressants and other potentially nephrotoxic agents should be carefully considered, and the lowest effective dose employed).

No products indexed under this heading.

Pentamidine Isethionate (The benefits and risks of using fenofibrate with immunosuppressants and other potentially nephrotoxic agents should be carefully considered, and the lowest effective dose employed).

No products indexed under this heading.

Perindopril Erbumine (The benefits and risks of using fenofibrate with immunosuppressants and other potentially nephrotoxic agents should be carefully considered, and the lowest effective dose employed). Products include:

Aceon Tablets (2 mg, 4 mg, 8 mg) 3038

Phenylbutazone (The benefits and risks of using fenofibrate with immunosuppressants and other potentially nephrotoxic agents should be carefully considered, and the lowest effective dose employed).

No products indexed under this heading.

Piroxicam (The benefits and risks of using fenofibrate with immunosuppressants and other potentially nephrotoxic agents should be carefully considered, and the lowest effective dose employed).

No products indexed under this heading.

Plicamycin (The benefits and risks of using fenofibrate with immunosuppressants and other potentially nephrotoxic agents should be carefully considered, and the lowest effective dose employed).

No products indexed under this heading.

Polymyxin (The benefits and risks of using fenofibrate with immunosuppressants and other potentially nephrotoxic agents should be carefully considered, and the lowest effective dose employed).

No products indexed under this heading.

Polymyxin B Sulfate (The benefits and risks of using fenofibrate with immunosuppressants and other potentially nephrotoxic agents should be carefully considered, and the lowest effective dose employed). Products include:

Neosporin Ophthalmic Solution Sterile .... ⊙ 252

Polythiazide (The benefits and risks of using fenofibrate with immunosuppressants and other potentially nephrotoxic agents should be carefully considered, and the lowest effective dose employed).

No products indexed under this heading.

Pravastatin Sodium (The combined use of fenofibric acid derivatives, particularly gemfibrozil, and HMG-CoA reductase inhibitors results in an increased risk of rhabdomyolysis and myoglobinuria leading in a high proportion of cases to acute renal failure. The combined use of fenofibrate and HMG-CoA reductase inhibitors should be avoided unless the benefit of further alterations in lipid levels is likely to outweigh the increased risk of this drug combination).

No products indexed under this heading.

Probenecid (The benefits and risks of using fenofibrate with immunosuppressants and other potentially nephrotoxic agents should be carefully considered, and the lowest effective dose employed).

No products indexed under this heading.

Quinapril Hydrochloride (The benefits and risks of using fenofibrate with immunosuppressants and other potentially nephrotoxic agents should be carefully considered, and the lowest effective dose employed).

No products indexed under this heading.

Rabeprazole Sodium (The benefits and risks of using fenofibrate with immunosuppressants and other potentially nephrotoxic agents should be carefully considered, and the lowest effective dose employed). Products include:

Aciphex Tablets 1053

Ramipril (The benefits and risks of using fenofibrate with immunosuppressants and other potentially nephrotoxic agents should be carefully considered, and the lowest effective dose employed).

No products indexed under this heading.

Rifampin (The benefits and risks of using fenofibrate with immunosuppressants and other potentially nephrotoxic agents should be carefully considered, and the lowest effective dose employed).

No products indexed under this heading.

Riluzole (The benefits and risks of using fenofibrate with immunosuppressants and other potentially nephrotoxic agents should be carefully considered, and the lowest effective dose employed). Products include:

Rilutek Tablets 2771

Ritonavir (The benefits and risks of using fenofibrate with immunosuppressants and other potentially nephrotoxic agents should be carefully considered, and the lowest effective dose employed). Products include:

Kaletra 452
Norvir 489

Rofecoxib (The benefits and risks of using fenofibrate with immunosuppressants and other potentially nephrotoxic agents should be carefully considered, and the lowest effective dose employed).

No products indexed under this heading.

Rosuvastatin Calcium (The combined use of fenofibric acid derivatives, particularly gemfibrozil, and HMG-CoA reductase inhibitors results in an increased risk of rhabdomyolysis and myoglobinuria leading in a high proportion of cases to acute renal failure. The combined use of fenofibrate and HMG-CoA reductase inhibitors should be avoided unless the benefit of further alterations in lipid levels is likely to outweigh the increased risk of this drug combination). Products include:

Crestor Tablets 677

Saquinavir (The benefits and risks of using fenofibrate with immunosuppressants and other potentially nephrotoxic agents should be carefully considered, and the lowest effective dose employed).

No products indexed under this heading.

Sibutramine Hydrochloride Monohydrate (The benefits and risks of using fenofibrate with immunosuppressants and other potentially nephrotoxic agents should be carefully considered, and the lowest effective dose employed). Products include:

Meridia Capsules 475

Simvastatin (The combined use of fenofibric acid derivatives, particularly gemfibrozil, and HMG-CoA reductase inhibitors results in an increased risk of rhabdomyolysis and myoglobinuria leading in a high proportion of cases to acute renal failure. The combined use of fenofibrate and HMG-CoA reductase inhibitors should be avoided unless the benefit of further alterations in lipid levels is likely to outweigh the increased risk of this drug combination). Products include:

Simcor Tablets 502
Vytorin 10/10 Tablets 2149
Vytorin 10/10 Tablets 2939
Vytorin 10/20 Tablets 2149
Vytorin 10/20 Tablets 2939
Vytorin 10/40 Tablets 2149
Vytorin 10/40 Tablets 2939
Vytorin 10/80 Tablets 2149
Vytorin 10/80 Tablets 2939
Zocor Tablets 2136

Sirolimus (The benefits and risks of using fenofibrate with immunosuppressants and other potentially nephrotoxic agents should be carefully considered, and the lowest effective dose employed). Products include:

Rapamune 3260

Spirapril Hydrochloride (The benefits and risks of using fenofibrate with immunosuppressants and other potentially nephrotoxic agents should be carefully considered, and the lowest effective dose employed).

No products indexed under this heading.

Stavudine (The benefits and risks of using fenofibrate with immunosuppressants and other potentially nephrotoxic agents should be carefully considered, and the lowest effective dose employed).

No products indexed under this heading.

Streptomycin Sulfate (The benefits and risks of using fenofibrate with immunosuppressants and other potentially nephrotoxic agents should be carefully considered, and the lowest effective dose employed).

No products indexed under this heading.

Streptozocin (The benefits and risks of using fenofibrate with immunosuppressants and other potentially nephrotoxic agents should be carefully considered, and the lowest effective dose employed).

No products indexed under this heading.

Sulfacytine (The benefits and risks of using fenofibrate with immunosuppressants and other potentially nephrotoxic agents should be carefully considered, and the lowest effective dose employed).

No products indexed under this heading.

Sulfamethizole (The benefits and risks of using fenofibrate with immunosuppressants and other potentially nephrotoxic agents should be carefully considered, and the lowest effective dose employed).

No products indexed under this heading.

Sulfamethoxazole (The benefits and risks of using fenofibrate with immunosuppressants and other potentially nephrotoxic agents should be carefully considered, and the lowest effective dose employed).

No products indexed under this heading.

Sulfasalazine (The benefits and risks of using fenofibrate with immunosuppressants and other potentially nephrotoxic agents should be carefully considered, and the lowest effective dose employed).

No products indexed under this heading.

Sulfinpyrazone (The benefits and risks of using fenofibrate with immunosuppressants and other potentially nephrotoxic agents should be carefully considered, and the lowest effective dose employed).
No products indexed under this heading.

Sulfisoxazole Acetyl (The benefits and risks of using fenofibrate with immunosuppressants and other potentially nephrotoxic agents should be carefully considered, and the lowest effective dose employed).
No products indexed under this heading.

Sulfisoxazole Diolamine (The benefits and risks of using fenofibrate with immunosuppressants and other potentially nephrotoxic agents should be carefully considered, and the lowest effective dose employed).
No products indexed under this heading.

Sulindac (The benefits and risks of using fenofibrate with immunosuppressants and other potentially nephrotoxic agents should be carefully considered, and the lowest effective dose employed). Products include:
Clinoril Tablets **1962**

Tacrolimus (The benefits and risks of using fenofibrate with immunosuppressants and other potentially nephrotoxic agents should be carefully considered, and the lowest effective dose employed). Products include:
Prograf Capsules and Injection **622**
Protopic Ointment **628**

Tenofovir Disoproxil Fumarate (The benefits and risks of using fenofibrate with immunosuppressants and other potentially nephrotoxic agents should be carefully considered, and the lowest effective dose employed). Products include:
Atripla Tablets **938**
Truvada Tablets **1262**
Viread Tablets **1268**

Thioguanine (The benefits and risks of using fenofibrate with immunosuppressants and other potentially nephrotoxic agents should be carefully considered, and the lowest effective dose employed). Products include:
Tabloid Tablets **1601**

Ticarcillin Disodium (The benefits and risks of using fenofibrate with immunosuppressants and other potentially nephrotoxic agents should be carefully considered, and the lowest effective dose employed). Products include:
Timentin ADD-Vantage **1606**
Timentin Injection Galaxy Container **1609**
Timentin IV Infusion **1603**
Timentin Pharmacy Bulk Package **1613**

Tobramycin (The benefits and risks of using fenofibrate with immunosuppressants and other potentially nephrotoxic agents should be carefully considered, and the lowest effective dose employed). Products include:
Zylet Ophthalmic Suspension .... ⊙**247**

Tobramycin Sulfate (The benefits and risks of using fenofibrate with immunosuppressants and other potentially nephrotoxic agents should be carefully considered, and the lowest effective dose employed).
No products indexed under this heading.

Tolazamide (The benefits and risks of using fenofibrate with immunosuppressants and other potentially nephrotoxic agents should be carefully considered, and the lowest effective dose employed).
No products indexed under this heading.

Tolbutamide (The benefits and risks of using fenofibrate with immunosuppressants and other potentially nephrotoxic agents should be carefully considered, and the lowest effective dose employed).
No products indexed under this heading.

Tolmetin Sodium (The benefits and risks of using fenofibrate with immunosuppressants and other potentially nephrotoxic agents should be carefully considered, and the lowest effective dose employed).
No products indexed under this heading.

Trandolapril (The benefits and risks of using fenofibrate with immunosuppressants and other potentially nephrotoxic agents should be carefully considered, and the lowest effective dose employed). Products include:
Mavik Tablets **472**
Tarka Tablets **511**

Triamterene (The benefits and risks of using fenofibrate with immunosuppressants and other potentially nephrotoxic agents should be carefully considered, and the lowest effective dose employed). Products include:
Dyazide Capsules **1405**
Dyrenium Capsules **3189**

Trimethadione (The benefits and risks of using fenofibrate with immunosuppressants and other potentially nephrotoxic agents should be carefully considered, and the lowest effective dose employed).
No products indexed under this heading.

Trovafloxacin Mesylate (The benefits and risks of using fenofibrate with immunosuppressants and other potentially nephrotoxic agents should be carefully considered, and the lowest effective dose employed).
No products indexed under this heading.

Tyropanoate Sodium (The benefits and risks of using fenofibrate with immunosuppressants and other potentially nephrotoxic agents should be carefully considered, and the lowest effective dose employed).
No products indexed under this heading.

Valacyclovir Hydrochloride (The benefits and risks of using fenofibrate with immunosuppressants and other potentially nephrotoxic agents should be carefully considered, and the lowest effective dose employed). Products include:
Valtrex Caplets **1635**

Valdecoxib (The benefits and risks of using fenofibrate with immunosuppressants and other potentially nephrotoxic agents should be carefully considered, and the lowest effective dose employed).
No products indexed under this heading.

Vancomycin Hydrochloride (The benefits and risks of using fenofibrate with immunosuppressants and other potentially nephrotoxic agents should be carefully considered, and the lowest effective dose employed).
No products indexed under this heading.

Voriconazole (The benefits and risks of using fenofibrate with immunosuppressants and other potentially nephrotoxic agents should be carefully considered, and the lowest effective dose employed).
No products indexed under this heading.

Warfarin Sodium (Caution should be exercised when anticoagulants are given in conjunction with fenofibrate because of the potentiation of coumarin-type anticoagulants in prolonging the prothrombin time/INR. The dosage of the anticoagulant should be reduced to maintain the prothrombin/INR at the desired level to prevent bleeding complications. Frequent prothrombin time/INR determinations are advisable until it has been definitely determined that the prothrombin time/INR has stabilized).
No products indexed under this heading.

Zalcitabine (The benefits and risks of using fenofibrate with immunosuppressants and other potentially nephrotoxic agents should be carefully considered, and the lowest effective dose employed).
No products indexed under this heading.

Zidovudine (The benefits and risks of using fenofibrate with immunosuppressants and other potentially nephrotoxic agents should be carefully considered, and the lowest effective dose employed). Products include:
Combivir Tablets **1384**
Retrovir **1574**
Retrovir IV Infusion **1579**
Trizivir Tablets **1622**

Zoledronic acid (The benefits and risks of using fenofibrate with immunosuppressants and other potentially nephrotoxic agents should be carefully considered, and the lowest effective dose employed). Products include:
Reclast Injection **2291**
Zometa for Intravenous Infusion **2341**

FENTORA TABLETS

(Fentanyl Citrate) **968**

May interact with antihistamines, central nervous system depressants, cytochrome p450 3a4 inducers (selected), cytochrome p450 3a4 inhibitors (selected), cytochrome p450 3a4 inhibitors, potent, general anesthetics, hypnotics and sedatives, monoamine oxidase inhibitors, narcotic analgesics, phenothiazines, skeletal muscle relaxants, tranquilizers, and certain other agents. Compounds in these categories include:

Acetazolamide (The concomitant use of moderate CYP3A4 inhibitors such as amprenavir, aprepitant, diltiazem, erythromycin, fluconazole, fosamprenavir, grapefruit juice, and verapamil with fentanyl citrate may result in an increase in fentanyl plasma concentrations, which could increase or prolong adverse drug effects and may cause potentially fatal respiratory depression. Patients receiving fentanyl citrate and moderate CYP3A4 inhibitors should be carefully monitored for an extended period of time and dosage increase should be done conservatively).
No products indexed under this heading.

Acrivastine (The concomitant use of other CNS depressants, including sedating antihistamines, may produce increased depressant effects. Hypoventilation, hypotension, and profound sedation may occur).
No products indexed under this heading.

Alfentanil Hydrochloride (The concomitant use of other CNS depressants, including other opioids, sedatives or hypnotics, general anesthetics, phenothiazines, tranquilizers, skeletal muscle relaxants, sedating antihistamines, potent inhibitors of cytochrome P450 3A4 isoform (e.g.,erythromycin, ketoconazole, and certain protease inhibitors), and alcoholic beverages may produce increased depressant effects. Hypoventilation, hypotension, and profound sedation may occur).
No products indexed under this heading.

Allium sativum (Co-administration with agents that induce CYP3A4 activity may reduce the efficacy of fentanyl citrate).
No products indexed under this heading.

Alprazolam (The concomitant use of other CNS depressants, including other opioids, sedatives or hypnotics, general anesthetics, phenothiazines, tranquilizers, skeletal muscle relaxants, sedating antihistamines, potent inhibitors of cytochrome P450 3A4 isoform (e.g.,erythromycin, ketoconazole, and certain protease inhibitors), and alcoholic beverages may produce increased depressant effects. Hypoventilation, hypotension, and profound sedation may occur).
No products indexed under this heading.

Amiodarone Hydrochloride (The concomitant use of moderate CYP3A4 inhibitors such as amprenavir, aprepitant, diltiazem, erythromycin, fluconazole, fosamprenavir, grapefruit juice, and verapamil with fentanyl citrate may result in an increase in fentanyl plasma concentrations, which could increase or prolong adverse drug effects and may cause potentially fatal respiratory depression. Patients receiving fentanyl citrate and moderate CYP3A4 inhibitors should be carefully monitored for an extended period of time and dosage increase should be done conservatively).
No products indexed under this heading.

Amprenavir (The concomitant use of fentanyl citrate with ritonavir or other strong CYP3A4 inhibitors such as ketoconazole, itraconazole, troleandomycin, clarithromycin, nelfinavir, and nefazadone may result in a potentially dangerous increase in fentanyl plasma concentrations. Patients receiving fentanyl citrate and potent CYP3A4 inhibitors should be carefully monitored for an extended period of time and dosage increase should be done conservatively).
No products indexed under this heading.

Anastrozole (The concomitant use of moderate CYP3A4 inhibitors such as amprenavir, aprepitant, diltiazem, erythromycin, fluconazole, fosamprenavir, grapefruit juice, and verapamil with fentanyl citrate may result in an increase in fentanyl plasma concentrations, which could increase or prolong adverse drug effects and may cause potentially fatal respiratory depression. Patients receiving fentanyl citrate and moderate CYP3A4 inhibitors should be carefully monitored for an extended period of time and dosage increase should be done conservatively). Products include:
Arimidex Tablets 672

Aprepitant (The concomitant use of moderate CYP3A4 inhibitors such as amprenavir, aprepitant, diltiazem, erythromycin, fluconazole, fosamprenavir, grapefruit juice, and verapamil with fentanyl citrate may result in an increase in fentanyl plasma concentrations, which could increase or prolong adverse drug effects and may cause potentially fatal respiratory depression. Patients receiving fentanyl citrate and moderate CYP3A4 inhibitors should be carefully monitored for an extended period of time and dosage increase should be done conservatively). Products include:
Emend Capsules 1992

Aprobarbital (The concomitant use of other CNS depressants, including other opioids, sedatives or hypnotics, general anesthetics, phenothiazines, tranquilizers, skeletal muscle relaxants, sedating antihistamines, potent inhibitors of cytochrome P450 3A4 isoform (e.g.,erythromycin, ketoconazole, and certain protease inhibitors), and alcoholic beverages may produce increased depressant effects. Hypoventilation, hypotension, and profound sedation may occur).
No products indexed under this heading.

Astemizole (The concomitant use of other CNS depressants, including sedating antihistamines, may produce increased depressant effects. Hypoventilation, hypotension, and profound sedation may occur).
No products indexed under this heading.

Atazanavir (The concomitant use of fentanyl citrate with ritonavir or other strong CYP3A4 inhibitors such as ketoconazole, itraconazole, troleandomycin, clarithromycin, nelfinavir, and nefazadone may result in a potentially dangerous increase in fentanyl plasma concentrations. Patients receiving fentanyl citrate and potent CYP3A4 inhibitors should be carefully monitored for an extended period of time and dosage increase should be done conservatively).
No products indexed under this heading.

Atazanavir Sulfate (The concomitant use of fentanyl citrate with ritonavir or other strong CYP3A4 inhibitors such as ketoconazole, itraconazole, troleandomycin, clarithromycin, nelfinavir, and nefazadone may result in a potentially dangerous increase in fentanyl plasma concentrations. Patients receiving fentanyl citrate and potent CYP3A4 inhibitors should be carefully monitored for an extended period of time and dosage increase should be done conservatively). Products include:
Reyataz Capsules 3299

Azatadine Maleate (The concomitant use of other CNS depressants, including sedating antihistamines, may produce increased depressant effects. Hypoventilation, hypotension, and profound sedation may occur).
No products indexed under this heading.

Baclofen (The concomitant use of other CNS depressants, including skeletal muscle relaxants, may produce increased depressant effects. Hypoventilation, hypotension, and profound sedation may occur).
No products indexed under this heading.

Betamethasone Acetate (Co-administration with agents that induce CYP3A4 activity may reduce the efficacy of fentanyl citrate).
No products indexed under this heading.

Betamethasone Sodium Phosphate (Co-administration with agents that induce CYP3A4 activity may reduce the efficacy of fentanyl citrate).
No products indexed under this heading.

Bromodiphenhydramine Hydrochloride (The concomitant use of other CNS depressants, including sedating antihistamines, may produce increased depressant effects. Hypoventilation, hypotension, and profound sedation may occur).
No products indexed under this heading.

Brompheniramine Maleate (The concomitant use of other CNS depressants, including sedating antihistamines, may produce increased depressant effects. Hypoventilation, hypotension, and profound sedation may occur).
No products indexed under this heading.

Buprenorphine Hydrochloride (The concomitant use of other CNS depressants, including other opioids, sedatives or hypnotics, general anesthetics, phenothiazines, tranquilizers, skeletal muscle relaxants, sedating antihistamines, potent inhibitors of cytochrome P450 3A4 isoform (e.g.,erythromycin, ketoconazole, and certain protease inhibitors), and alcoholic beverages may produce increased depressant effects. Hypoventilation, hypotension, and profound sedation may occur). Products include:
Suboxone Tablets 2601
Subutex Tablets 2601

Buspirone Hydrochloride (The concomitant use of other CNS depressants, including other opioids, sedatives or hypnotics, general anesthetics, phenothiazines, tranquilizers, skeletal muscle relaxants, sedating antihistamines, potent inhibitors of cytochrome P450 3A4 isoform (e.g.,erythromycin, ketoconazole, and certain protease inhibitors), and alcoholic beverages may produce increased depressant effects. Hypoventilation, hypotension, and profound sedation may occur).
No products indexed under this heading.

Butabarbital (The concomitant use of other CNS depressants, including other opioids, sedatives or hypnotics, general anesthetics, phenothiazines, tranquilizers, skeletal muscle relaxants, sedating antihistamines, potent inhibitors of cytochrome P450 3A4 isoform (e.g.,erythromycin, ketoconazole, and certain protease inhibitors), and alcoholic beverages may produce increased depressant effects. Hypoventilation, hypotension, and profound sedation may occur).
No products indexed under this heading.

Butabarbital Sodium (The concomitant use of other CNS depressants, including sedatives or hypnotics, may produce increased depressant effects. Hypoventilation, hypotension, and profound sedation may occur).
No products indexed under this heading.

Butalbital (The concomitant use of other CNS depressants, including other opioids, sedatives or hypnotics, general anesthetics, phenothiazines, tranquilizers, skeletal muscle relaxants, sedating antihistamines, potent inhibitors of cytochrome P450 3A4 isoform (e.g.,erythromycin, ketoconazole, and certain protease inhibitors), and alcoholic beverages may produce increased depressant effects. Hypoventilation, hypotension, and profound sedation may occur).
No products indexed under this heading.

Carbamazepine (Co-administration with agents that induce CYP3A4 activity may reduce the efficacy of fentanyl citrate). Products include:
Carbatrol Capsules 3019
Equetro Extended-Release Capsules 3174

Carisoprodol (The concomitant use of other CNS depressants, including skeletal muscle relaxants, may produce increased depressant effects. Hypoventilation, hypotension, and profound sedation may occur). Products include:
Soma Tablets 1931

Cetirizine Hydrochloride (The concomitant use of other CNS depressants, including sedating antihistamines, may produce increased depressant effects. Hypoventilation, hypotension, and profound sedation may occur). Products include:
Zyrtec Allergy Tablets 1919
Zyrtec Chewable Tablets 1920
Children's Zyrtec Allergy Chewable Tablets 1922
Children's Zyrtec Allergy Syrup 1920
Children's Zyrtec Hives Relief Syrup 1920
Zyrtec Syrup 1920
Zyrtec Tablets 1920
Zyrtec-D 12 Hour Extended Release Tablets 1923
Zyrtec-D Allergy & Congestion Extended-Release Tablets 1923

Chloral Hydrate (The concomitant use of other CNS depressants, including sedatives or hypnotics, may produce increased depressant effects. Hypoventilation, hypotension, and profound sedation may occur).
No products indexed under this heading.

Chlordiazepoxide (The concomitant use of other CNS depressants, including other opioids, sedatives or hypnotics, general anesthetics, phenothiazines, tranquilizers, skeletal muscle relaxants, sedating antihistamines, potent inhibitors of cytochrome P450 3A4 isoform (e.g.,erythromycin, ketoconazole, and certain protease inhibitors), and alcoholic beverages may produce increased depressant effects. Hypoventilation, hypotension, and profound sedation may occur).
No products indexed under this heading.

Chlordiazepoxide Hydrochloride (The concomitant use of other CNS depressants, including other opioids, sedatives or hypnotics, general anesthetics, phenothiazines, tranquilizers, skeletal muscle relaxants, sedating antihistamines, potent inhibitors of cytochrome P450 3A4 isoform (e.g.,erythromycin, ketoconazole, and certain protease inhibitors), and alcoholic beverages may produce increased depressant effects. Hypoventilation, hypotension, and profound sedation may occur).
No products indexed under this heading.

Chlorpheniramine Maleate (The concomitant use of other CNS depressants, including sedating antihistamines, may produce increased depressant effects. Hypoventilation, hypotension, and profound sedation may occur). Products include:
Actifed Cold & Allergy Tablets 1895
Sudafed PE Sinus & Allergy Tablets 1908
Tylenol Allergy Multi-Symptom Caplets with Cool Burst and Rapid Release Gelcaps 1916
Children's Tylenol Plus Cold Suspension Liquid 1912
Children's Tylenol Plus Cough & Runny Nose Suspension Liquid 1912
Children's Tylenol Plus Flu Suspension Liquid 1914
Children's Tylenol Plus Multi-Symptom Cold Suspension Liquid 1912
Tylenol Cold Head Congestion Nighttime Caplets with Cool Burst 1910
Tylenol Cold Multi-Symptom Nighttime Caplets with Cool Burst 1913
Tylenol Sinus Congestion & Pain Nighttime Caplets with Cool Burst 1917

Chlorpheniramine Polistirex (The concomitant use of other CNS depressants, including sedating antihistamines, may produce increased depressant effects. Hypoventilation, hypotension, and profound sedation may occur). Products include:
Tussionex Pennkinetic Extended-Release Suspension 3154

Chlorpheniramine Tannate (The concomitant use of other CNS depressants, including sedating antihistamines, may produce increased depressant effects. Hypoventilation, hypotension, and profound sedation may occur).
No products indexed under this heading.

Chlorpromazine (The concomitant use of other CNS depressants, including other opioids, sedatives or hypnotics, general anesthetics, phenothiazines, tranquilizers, skeletal muscle relaxants, sedating antihistamines, potent inhibitors of cytochrome P450 3A4 isoform (e.g.,erythromycin, ketoconazole, and certain protease inhibitors), and alcoholic beverages may produce increased depressant effects. Hypoventilation, hypotension, and profound sedation may occur).

No products indexed under this heading.

Chlorpromazine Hydrochloride (The concomitant use of other CNS depressants, including other opioids, sedatives or hypnotics, general anesthetics, phenothiazines, tranquilizers, skeletal muscle relaxants, sedating antihistamines, potent inhibitors of cytochrome P450 3A4 isoform (e.g.,erythromycin, ketoconazole, and certain protease inhibitors), and alcoholic beverages may produce increased depressant effects. Hypoventilation, hypotension, and profound sedation may occur).

No products indexed under this heading.

Chlorprothixene (The concomitant use of other CNS depressants, including other opioids, sedatives or hypnotics, general anesthetics, phenothiazines, tranquilizers, skeletal muscle relaxants, sedating antihistamines, potent inhibitors of cytochrome P450 3A4 isoform (e.g.,erythromycin, ketoconazole, and certain protease inhibitors), and alcoholic beverages may produce increased depressant effects. Hypoventilation, hypotension, and profound sedation may occur).

No products indexed under this heading.

Chlorprothixene Hydrochloride (The concomitant use of other CNS depressants, including other opioids, sedatives or hypnotics, general anesthetics, phenothiazines, tranquilizers, skeletal muscle relaxants, sedating antihistamines, potent inhibitors of cytochrome P450 3A4 isoform (e.g.,erythromycin, ketoconazole, and certain protease inhibitors), and alcoholic beverages may produce increased depressant effects. Hypoventilation, hypotension, and profound sedation may occur).

No products indexed under this heading.

Chlorprothixene Lactate (The concomitant use of other CNS depressants, including other opioids, sedatives or hypnotics, general anesthetics, phenothiazines, tranquilizers, skeletal muscle relaxants, sedating antihistamines, potent inhibitors of cytochrome P450 3A4 isoform (e.g.,erythromycin, ketoconazole, and certain protease inhibitors), and alcoholic beverages may produce increased depressant effects. Hypoventilation, hypotension, and profound sedation may occur).

No products indexed under this heading.

Chlorzoxazone (The concomitant use of other CNS depressants, including skeletal muscle relaxants, may produce increased depressant effects. Hypoventilation, hypotension, and profound sedation may occur).

No products indexed under this heading.

Cimetidine (The concomitant use of moderate CYP3A4 inhibitors such as amprenavir, aprepitant, diltiazem, erythromycin, fluconazole, fosamprenavir, grapefruit juice, and verapamil with fentanyl citrate may result in an increase in fentanyl plasma concentrations, which could increase or prolong adverse drug effects and may cause potentially fatal respiratory depression. Patients receiving fentanyl citrate and moderate CYP3A4 inhibitors should be carefully monitored for an extended period of time and dosage increase should be done conservatively).

No products indexed under this heading.

Cimetidine Hydrochloride (The concomitant use of moderate CYP3A4 inhibitors such as amprenavir, aprepitant, diltiazem, erythromycin, fluconazole, fosamprenavir, grapefruit juice, and verapamil with fentanyl citrate may result in an increase in fentanyl plasma concentrations, which could increase or prolong adverse drug effects and may cause potentially fatal respiratory depression. Patients receiving fentanyl citrate and moderate CYP3A4 inhibitors should be carefully monitored for an extended period of time and dosage increase should be done conservatively).

No products indexed under this heading.

Ciprofloxacin (The concomitant use of moderate CYP3A4 inhibitors such as amprenavir, aprepitant, diltiazem, erythromycin, fluconazole, fosamprenavir, grapefruit juice, and verapamil with fentanyl citrate may result in an increase in fentanyl plasma concentrations, which could increase or prolong adverse drug effects and may cause potentially fatal respiratory depression. Patients receiving fentanyl citrate and moderate CYP3A4 inhibitors should be carefully monitored for an extended period of time and dosage increase should be done conservatively). Products include:

Cipro I.V. **2817**
Cipro Oral Suspension **2810**
Cipro XR Tablets **2823**
Ciprodex Otic Suspension **541**

Ciprofloxacin Hydrochloride (Co-administration with agents that induce CYP3A4 activity may reduce the efficacy of fentanyl citrate). Products include:

Cipro Tablets **2810**

Cisplatin (Co-administration with agents that induce CYP3A4 activity may reduce the efficacy of fentanyl citrate).

No products indexed under this heading.

Clarithromycin (The concomitant use of fentanyl citrate with ritonavir or other strong CYP3A4 inhibitors such as ketoconazole, itraconazole, troleandomycin, clarithromycin, nelfinavir, and nefazadone may result in a potentially dangerous increase in fentanyl plasma concentrations. Patients receiving fentanyl citrate and potent CYP3A4 inhibitors should be carefully monitored for an extended period of time and dosage increase should be done conservatively). Products include:

Biaxin/Biaxin XL **411**

Clemastine Fumarate (The concomitant use of other CNS depressants, including sedating antihistamines, may produce increased depressant effects. Hypoventilation, hypotension, and profound sedation may occur).

No products indexed under this heading.

Clorazepate Dipotassium (The concomitant use of other CNS depressants, including other opioids, sedatives or hypnotics, general anesthetics, phenothiazines, tranquilizers, skeletal muscle relaxants, sedating antihistamines, potent inhibitors of cytochrome P450 3A4 isoform (e.g.,erythromycin, ketoconazole, and certain protease inhibitors), and alcoholic beverages may produce increased depressant effects. Hypoventilation, hypotension, and profound sedation may occur).

No products indexed under this heading.

Clotrimazole (The concomitant use of moderate CYP3A4 inhibitors such as amprenavir, aprepitant, diltiazem, erythromycin, fluconazole, fosamprenavir, grapefruit juice, and verapamil with fentanyl citrate may result in an increase in fentanyl plasma concentrations, which could increase or prolong adverse drug effects and may cause potentially fatal respiratory depression. Patients receiving fentanyl citrate and moderate CYP3A4 inhibitors should be carefully monitored for an extended period of time and dosage increase should be done conservatively). Products include:

Lotrisone **2881**

Clozapine (The concomitant use of other CNS depressants, including other opioids, sedatives or hypnotics, general anesthetics, phenothiazines, tranquilizers, skeletal muscle relaxants, sedating antihistamines, potent inhibitors of cytochrome P450 3A4 isoform (e.g.,erythromycin, ketoconazole, and certain protease inhibitors), and alcoholic beverages may produce increased depressant effects. Hypoventilation, hypotension, and profound sedation may occur).

No products indexed under this heading.

Codeine Phosphate (The concomitant use of other CNS depressants, including other opioids, sedatives or hypnotics, general anesthetics, phenothiazines, tranquilizers, skeletal muscle relaxants, sedating antihistamines, potent inhibitors of cytochrome P450 3A4 isoform (e.g.,erythromycin, ketoconazole, and certain protease inhibitors), and alcoholic beverages may produce increased depressant effects. Hypoventilation, hypotension, and profound sedation may occur). Products include:

Tylenol with Codeine Tablets **2427**

Cortisone Acetate (Co-administration with agents that induce CYP3A4 activity may reduce the efficacy of fentanyl citrate).

No products indexed under this heading.

Cyclobenzaprine Hydrochloride (The concomitant use of other CNS depressants, including skeletal muscle relaxants, may produce increased depressant effects. Hypoventilation, hypotension, and profound sedation may occur). Products include:

Amrix Capsules **966**

Cyclosporine (The concomitant use of moderate CYP3A4 inhibitors such as amprenavir, aprepitant, diltiazem, erythromycin, fluconazole, fosamprenavir, grapefruit juice, and verapamil with fentanyl citrate may result in an increase in fentanyl plasma concentrations, which could increase or prolong adverse drug effects and may cause potentially fatal respiratory depression. Patients receiving fentanyl citrate and moderate CYP3A4 inhibitors should be carefully monitored for an extended period of time and dosage increase should be done conservatively). Products include:

Gengraf Capsules **435**
Neoral Oral Solution **2280**
Neoral Soft Gelatin Capsules **2280**
Restasis Ophthalmic Emulsion **557**
Sandimmune **2296**

Cyproheptadine Hydrochloride (The concomitant use of other CNS depressants, including sedating antihistamines, may produce increased depressant effects. Hypoventilation, hypotension, and profound sedation may occur).

No products indexed under this heading.

Dalfopristin (The concomitant use of moderate CYP3A4 inhibitors such as amprenavir, aprepitant, diltiazem, erythromycin, fluconazole, fosamprenavir, grapefruit juice, and verapamil with fentanyl citrate may result in an increase in fentanyl plasma concentrations, which could increase or prolong adverse drug effects and may cause potentially fatal respiratory depression. Patients receiving fentanyl citrate and moderate CYP3A4 inhibitors should be carefully monitored for an extended period of time and dosage increase should be done conservatively).

No products indexed under this heading.

Danazol (The concomitant use of moderate CYP3A4 inhibitors such as amprenavir, aprepitant, diltiazem, erythromycin, fluconazole, fosamprenavir, grapefruit juice, and verapamil with fentanyl citrate may result in an increase in fentanyl plasma concentrations, which could increase or prolong adverse drug effects and may cause potentially fatal respiratory depression. Patients receiving fentanyl citrate and moderate CYP3A4 inhibitors should be carefully monitored for an extended period of time and dosage increase should be done conservatively).

No products indexed under this heading.

Dantrolene Sodium (The concomitant use of other CNS depressants, including skeletal muscle relaxants, may produce increased depressant effects. Hypoventilation, hypotension, and profound sedation may occur). Products include:

Dantrium Capsules **2580**
Dantrium Intravenous **2582**

Delavirdine Mesylate (The concomitant use of moderate CYP3A4 inhibitors such as amprenavir, aprepitant, diltiazem, erythromycin, fluconazole, fosamprenavir, grapefruit juice, and verapamil with fentanyl citrate may result in an increase in fentanyl plasma concentrations, which could increase or prolong adverse drug effects and may cause potentially fatal respiratory depression. Patients receiving fentanyl citrate and moderate CYP3A4 inhibitors should be carefully monitored for an extended period of time and dosage increase should be done

conservatively).
No products indexed under this heading.

Delavirdine Mesylate (The concomitant use of fentanyl citrate with ritonavir or other strong CYP3A4 inhibitors such as ketoconazole, itraconazole, troleandomycin, clarithromycin, nelfinavir, and nefazadone may result in a potentially dangerous increase in fentanyl plasma concentrations. Patients receiving fentanyl citrate and potent CYP3A4 inhibitors should be carefully monitored for an extended period of time and dosage increase should be done conservatively).
No products indexed under this heading.

Delavirine (The concomitant use of fentanyl citrate with ritonavir or other strong CYP3A4 inhibitors such as ketoconazole, itraconazole, troleandomycin, clarithromycin, nelfinavir, and nefazadone may result in a potentially dangerous increase in fentanyl plasma concentrations. Patients receiving fentanyl citrate and potent CYP3A4 inhibitors should be carefully monitored for an extended period of time and dosage increase should be done conservatively).
No products indexed under this heading.

Desflurane (The concomitant use of other CNS depressants, including other opioids, sedatives or hypnotics, general anesthetics, phenothiazines, tranquilizers, skeletal muscle relaxants, sedating antihistamines, potent inhibitors of cytochrome P450 3A4 isoform (e.g.,erythromycin, ketoconazole, and certain protease inhibitors), and alcoholic beverages may produce increased depressant effects. Hypoventilation, hypotension, and profound sedation may occur).
No products indexed under this heading.

Dexamethasone (Co-administration with agents that induce CYP3A4 activity may reduce the efficacy of fentanyl citrate). Products include:
Ciprodex Otic Suspension 541

Dexamethasone Acetate (Co-administration with agents that induce CYP3A4 activity may reduce the efficacy of fentanyl citrate).
No products indexed under this heading.

Dexamethasone Sodium Phosphate (Co-administration with agents that induce CYP3A4 activity may reduce the efficacy of fentanyl citrate).
No products indexed under this heading.

Dexchlorpheniramine Maleate (The concomitant use of other CNS depressants, including sedating antihistamines, may produce increased depressant effects. Hypoventilation, hypotension, and profound sedation may occur).
No products indexed under this heading.

Dezocine (The concomitant use of other CNS depressants, including other opioids, sedatives or hypnotics, general anesthetics, phenothiazines, tranquilizers, skeletal muscle relaxants, sedating antihistamines, potent inhibitors of cytochrome P450 3A4 isoform (e.g.,erythromycin, ketoconazole, and certain protease inhibitors), and alcoholic beverages may produce increased depressant effects. Hypoventilation, hypotension, and profound sedation may occur).
No products indexed under this heading.

Diazepam (The concomitant use of other CNS depressants, including other opioids, sedatives or hypnotics, general anesthetics, phenothiazines, tranquilizers, skeletal muscle relaxants, sedating antihistamines, potent inhibitors of cytochrome P450 3A4 isoform (e.g.,erythromycin, ketoconazole, and certain protease inhibitors), and alcoholic beverages may produce increased depressant effects. Hypoventilation, hypotension, and profound sedation may occur). Products include:
Valium Tablets 2658

Diltiazem Hydrochloride (The concomitant use of moderate CYP3A4 inhibitors such as amprenavir, aprepitant, diltiazem, erythromycin, fluconazole, fosamprenavir, grapefruit juice, and verapamil with fentanyl citrate may result in an increase in fentanyl plasma concentrations, which could increase or prolong adverse drug effects and may cause potentially fatal respiratory depression. Patients receiving fentanyl citrate and moderate CYP3A4 inhibitors should be carefully monitored for an extended period of time and dosage increase should be done conservatively). Products include:
Cardizem LA Extended Release Tablets 421

Diltiazem Maleate (The concomitant use of moderate CYP3A4 inhibitors such as amprenavir, aprepitant, diltiazem, erythromycin, fluconazole, fosamprenavir, grapefruit juice, and verapamil with fentanyl citrate may result in an increase in fentanyl plasma concentrations, which could increase or prolong adverse drug effects and may cause potentially fatal respiratory depression. Patients receiving fentanyl citrate and moderate CYP3A4 inhibitors should be carefully monitored for an extended period of time and dosage increase should be done conservatively).
No products indexed under this heading.

Diphenhydramine Citrate (The concomitant use of other CNS depressants, including sedating antihistamines, may produce increased depressant effects. Hypoventilation, hypotension, and profound sedation may occur).
No products indexed under this heading.

Diphenhydramine Hydrochloride (The concomitant use of other CNS depressants, including sedating antihistamines, may produce increased depressant effects. Hypoventilation, hypotension, and profound sedation may occur). Products include:
Benadryl Allergy & Cold Kapgels 1895
Benadryl Allergy & Sinus Headache Kapgels 1895
Benadryl Severe Allergy & Sinus Headache Caplets 1897
Benadryl Dye-Free Allergy Liqui-gels Softgels 1897
Benadryl Allergy Kapgels 1895
Benadryl Allergy Quick Dissolve Strips 1896
Benadryl Allergy Ultratab Tablets 1896
Children's Benadryl Dye-Free Allergy Liquid 1897
Children's Benadryl Allergy Fastmelts 1897
Children's Benadryl Allergy Liquid 1898
Children's Benadryl Allergy Perfect Measure 1896
Children's Benadryl-D Allergy & Sinus Liquid 1896
Benadryl-D Allergy & Sinus Tablet 1896
PediaCare Children's Allergy & Cold Liquid 1902
PediaCare Children's Allergy Liquid 1902
Simply Sleep Caplets 1905
Sudafed PE Nighttime Cold Caplets 1907
Sudafed PE Severe Cold Caplets 1908
Extra Strength Tylenol PM Caplets, Geltabs, Liquid, and Rapid Release Gels 1915
Tylenol Allergy Multi-Symptom Nighttime Caplets with Cool Burst 1916
Tylenol Severe Allergy Caplets 1916
Children's Tylenol Plus Cold & Allergy Suspension Liquid 1914
Tylenol Sore Throat Nighttime Liquid with Cool Burst 1918

Diphenylpyraline Hydrochloride (The concomitant use of other CNS depressants, including sedating antihistamines, may produce increased depressant effects. Hypoventilation, hypotension, and profound sedation may occur).
No products indexed under this heading.

Doxorubicin Hydrochloride (Co-administration with agents that induce CYP3A4 activity may reduce the efficacy of fentanyl citrate).
No products indexed under this heading.

Droperidol (The concomitant use of other CNS depressants, including other opioids, sedatives or hypnotics, general anesthetics, phenothiazines, tranquilizers, skeletal muscle relaxants, sedating antihistamines, potent inhibitors of cytochrome P450 3A4 isoform (e.g.,erythromycin, ketoconazole, and certain protease inhibitors), and alcoholic beverages may produce increased depressant effects. Hypoventilation, hypotension, and profound sedation may occur).
No products indexed under this heading.

Efavirenz (The concomitant use of moderate CYP3A4 inhibitors such as amprenavir, aprepitant, diltiazem, erythromycin, fluconazole, fosamprenavir, grapefruit juice, and verapamil with fentanyl citrate may result in an increase in fentanyl plasma concentrations, which could increase or prolong adverse drug effects and may cause potentially fatal respiratory depression. Patients receiving fentanyl citrate and moderate CYP3A4 inhibitors should be carefully monitored for an extended period of time and dosage increase should be done conservatively). Products include:
Atripla Tablets 938
Sustiva Capsules 930
Sustiva Tablets 930

Enflurane (The concomitant use of other CNS depressants, including other opioids, sedatives or hypnotics, general anesthetics, phenothiazines, tranquilizers, skeletal muscle relaxants, sedating antihistamines, potent inhibitors of cytochrome P450 3A4 isoform (e.g.,erythromycin, ketoconazole, and certain protease inhibitors), and alcoholic beverages may produce increased depressant effects. Hypoventilation, hypotension, and profound sedation may occur).
No products indexed under this heading.

Erythromycin (The concomitant use of moderate CYP3A4 inhibitors such as amprenavir, aprepitant, diltiazem, erythromycin, fluconazole, fosamprenavir, grapefruit juice, and verapamil with fentanyl citrate may result in an increase in fentanyl plasma concentrations, which could increase or prolong adverse drug effects and may cause potentially fatal respiratory depression. Patients receiving fentanyl citrate and moderate CYP3A4 inhibitors should be carefully monitored for an extended period of time and dosage increase should be done conservatively).
No products indexed under this heading.

Erythromycin Estolate (The concomitant use of moderate CYP3A4 inhibitors such as amprenavir, aprepitant, diltiazem, erythromycin, fluconazole, fosamprenavir, grapefruit juice, and verapamil with fentanyl citrate may result in an increase in fentanyl plasma concentrations, which could increase or prolong adverse drug effects and may cause potentially fatal respiratory depression. Patients receiving fentanyl citrate and moderate CYP3A4 inhibitors should be carefully monitored for an extended period of time and dosage increase should be done conservatively).
No products indexed under this heading.

Erythromycin Ethylsuccinate (The concomitant use of moderate CYP3A4 inhibitors such as amprenavir, aprepitant, diltiazem, erythromycin, fluconazole, fosamprenavir, grapefruit juice, and verapamil with fentanyl citrate may result in an increase in fentanyl plasma concentrations, which could increase or prolong adverse drug effects and may cause potentially fatal respiratory depression. Patients receiving fentanyl citrate and moderate CYP3A4 inhibitors should be carefully monitored for an extended period of time and dosage increase should be done conservatively). Products include:
E.E.S. 433
EryPed 431

Erythromycin Gluceptate (The concomitant use of moderate CYP3A4 inhibitors such as amprenavir, aprepitant, diltiazem, erythromycin, fluconazole, fosamprenavir, grapefruit juice, and verapamil with fentanyl citrate may result in an increase in fentanyl plasma concentrations, which could increase or prolong adverse drug effects and may cause potentially fatal respiratory depression. Patients receiving fentanyl citrate and moderate CYP3A4 inhibitors should be carefully monitored for an extended period of time and dosage increase should be done conservatively).
No products indexed under this heading.

Erythromycin Lactobionate (The concomitant use of moderate CYP3A4 inhibitors such as amprenavir, aprepitant, diltiazem, erythromycin, fluconazole, fosamprenavir, grapefruit juice, and verapamil with fentanyl citrate may result in an increase in fentanyl plasma concentrations, which could increase or prolong adverse drug effects and may cause potentially fatal respiratory depression. Patients receiving fentanyl citrate and moderate CYP3A4 inhibitors should be carefully monitored for an extended period of time and dosage increase should be done conservatively).

No products indexed under this heading.

Erythromycin Stearate (The concomitant use of moderate CYP3A4 inhibitors such as amprenavir, aprepitant, diltiazem, erythromycin, fluconazole, fosamprenavir, grapefruit juice, and verapamil with fentanyl citrate may result in an increase in fentanyl plasma concentrations, which could increase or prolong adverse drug effects and may cause potentially fatal respiratory depression. Patients receiving fentanyl citrate and moderate CYP3A4 inhibitors should be carefully monitored for an extended period of time and dosage increase should be done conservatively).

No products indexed under this heading.

Esomeprazole Magnesium (The concomitant use of moderate CYP3A4 inhibitors such as amprenavir, aprepitant, diltiazem, erythromycin, fluconazole, fosamprenavir, grapefruit juice, and verapamil with fentanyl citrate may result in an increase in fentanyl plasma concentrations, which could increase or prolong adverse drug effects and may cause potentially fatal respiratory depression. Patients receiving fentanyl citrate and moderate CYP3A4 inhibitors should be carefully monitored for an extended period of time and dosage increase should be done conservatively). Products include:

Nexium Delayed-Release Capsules **645**
Nexium Delayed-Release Oral Suspension **645**

Estazolam (The concomitant use of other CNS depressants, including other opioids, sedatives or hypnotics, general anesthetics, phenothiazines, tranquilizers, skeletal muscle relaxants, sedating antihistamines, potent inhibitors of cytochrome P450 3A4 isoform (e.g.,erythromycin, ketoconazole, and certain protease inhibitors), and alcoholic beverages may produce increased depressant effects. Hypoventilation, hypotension, and profound sedation may occur).

No products indexed under this heading.

Ethanol (The concomitant use of other CNS depressants, including alcoholic beverages, may produce increased depressant effects. Hypoventilation, hypotension, and profound sedation may occur).

No products indexed under this heading.

Ethchlorvynol (The concomitant use of other CNS depressants, including other opioids, sedatives or hypnotics, general anesthetics, phenothiazines, tranquilizers, skeletal muscle relaxants, sedating antihistamines, potent inhibitors of cytochrome P450 3A4 isoform (e.g.,erythromycin, ketoconazole, and certain protease inhibitors), and alcoholic beverages may produce increased depressant effects. Hypoventilation, hypotension, and profound sedation may occur).

No products indexed under this heading.

Ethinamate (The concomitant use of other CNS depressants, including other opioids, sedatives or hypnotics, general anesthetics, phenothiazines, tranquilizers, skeletal muscle relaxants, sedating antihistamines, potent inhibitors of cytochrome P450 3A4 isoform (e.g.,erythromycin, ketoconazole, and certain protease inhibitors), and alcoholic beverages may produce increased depressant effects. Hypoventilation, hypotension, and profound sedation may occur).

No products indexed under this heading.

Ethosuximide (Co-administration with agents that induce CYP3A4 activity may reduce the efficacy of fentanyl citrate).

No products indexed under this heading.

Ethyl Alcohol (The concomitant use of other CNS depressants, including alcoholic beverages, may produce increased depressant effects. Hypoventilation, hypotension, and profound sedation may occur).

No products indexed under this heading.

Felbamate (Co-administration with agents that induce CYP3A4 activity may reduce the efficacy of fentanyl citrate).

No products indexed under this heading.

Fentanyl (The concomitant use of other CNS depressants, including other opioids, sedatives or hypnotics, general anesthetics, phenothiazines, tranquilizers, skeletal muscle relaxants, sedating antihistamines, potent inhibitors of cytochrome P450 3A4 isoform (e.g.,erythromycin, ketoconazole, and certain protease inhibitors), and alcoholic beverages may produce increased depressant effects. Hypoventilation, hypotension, and profound sedation may occur). Products include:

Duragesic Transdermal System **2405**
Ionsys Transdermal System **2410**

Fentanyl Citrate (The concomitant use of other CNS depressants, including other opioids, sedatives or hypnotics, general anesthetics, phenothiazines, tranquilizers, skeletal muscle relaxants, sedating antihistamines, potent inhibitors of cytochrome P450 3A4 isoform (e.g.,erythromycin, ketoconazole, and certain protease inhibitors), and alcoholic beverages may produce increased depressant effects. Hypoventilation, hypotension, and profound sedation may occur). Products include:

Actiq **959**
Fentora Tablets **968**

Fexofenadine Hydrochloride (The concomitant use of other CNS depressants, including sedating antihistamines, may produce increased depressant effects. Hypoventilation, hypotension, and profound sedation may occur). Products include:

Allegra Oral Solution **2684**
Allegra Tablets **2684**
Allegra-D 12 Hour Extended-Release Tablets **2687**
Allegra-D 24 Hour Extended-Release Tablets **2690**

Fluconazole (The concomitant use of moderate CYP3A4 inhibitors such as amprenavir, aprepitant, diltiazem, erythromycin, fluconazole, fosamprenavir, grapefruit juice, and verapamil with fentanyl citrate may result in an increase in fentanyl plasma concentrations, which could increase or prolong adverse drug effects and may cause potentially fatal respiratory depression. Patients receiving fentanyl citrate and moderate CYP3A4 inhibitors should be carefully monitored for an extended period of time and dosage increase should be done conservatively).

No products indexed under this heading.

Fludrocortisone Acetate (Co-administration with agents that induce CYP3A4 activity may reduce the efficacy of fentanyl citrate).

No products indexed under this heading.

Fluoxetine (The concomitant use of moderate CYP3A4 inhibitors such as amprenavir, aprepitant, diltiazem, erythromycin, fluconazole, fosamprenavir, grapefruit juice, and verapamil with fentanyl citrate may result in an increase in fentanyl plasma concentrations, which could increase or prolong adverse drug effects and may cause potentially fatal respiratory depression. Patients receiving fentanyl citrate and moderate CYP3A4 inhibitors should be carefully monitored for an extended period of time and dosage increase should be done conservatively).

No products indexed under this heading.

Fluoxetine Hydrochloride (The concomitant use of moderate CYP3A4 inhibitors such as amprenavir, aprepitant, diltiazem, erythromycin, fluconazole, fosamprenavir, grapefruit juice, and verapamil with fentanyl citrate may result in an increase in fentanyl plasma concentrations, which could increase or prolong adverse drug effects and may cause potentially fatal respiratory depression. Patients receiving fentanyl citrate and moderate CYP3A4 inhibitors should be carefully monitored for an extended period of time and dosage increase should be done conservatively). Products include:

Prozac Weekly Capsules **1852**
Prozac Pulvules and Liquid **1852**
Symbyax Capsules **1871**

Fluphenazine Decanoate (The concomitant use of other CNS depressants, including other opioids, sedatives or hypnotics, general anesthetics, phenothiazines, tranquilizers, skeletal muscle relaxants, sedating antihistamines, potent inhibitors of cytochrome P450 3A4 isoform (e.g.,erythromycin, ketoconazole, and certain protease inhibitors), and alcoholic beverages may produce increased depressant effects. Hypoventilation, hypotension, and profound sedation may occur).

No products indexed under this heading.

Fluphenazine Enanthate (The concomitant use of other CNS depressants, including other opioids, sedatives or hypnotics, general anesthetics, phenothiazines, tranquilizers, skeletal muscle relaxants, sedating antihistamines, potent inhibitors of cytochrome P450 3A4 isoform (e.g.,erythromycin, ketoconazole, and certain protease inhibitors), and alcoholic beverages may produce increased depressant effects. Hypoventilation, hypotension, and profound sedation may occur).

No products indexed under this heading.

Fluphenazine Hydrochloride (The concomitant use of other CNS depressants, including other opioids, sedatives or hypnotics, general anesthetics, phenothiazines, tranquilizers, skeletal muscle relaxants, sedating antihistamines, potent inhibitors of cytochrome P450 3A4 isoform (e.g.,erythromycin, ketoconazole, and certain protease inhibitors), and alcoholic beverages may produce increased depressant effects. Hypoventilation, hypotension, and profound sedation may occur).

No products indexed under this heading.

Flurazepam Hydrochloride (The concomitant use of other CNS depressants, including other opioids, sedatives or hypnotics, general anesthetics, phenothiazines, tranquilizers, skeletal muscle relaxants, sedating antihistamines, potent inhibitors of cytochrome P450 3A4 isoform (e.g.,erythromycin, ketoconazole, and certain protease inhibitors), and alcoholic beverages may produce increased depressant effects. Hypoventilation, hypotension, and profound sedation may occur).

No products indexed under this heading.

Fluvoxamine Maleate (The concomitant use of moderate CYP3A4 inhibitors such as amprenavir, aprepitant, diltiazem, erythromycin, fluconazole, fosamprenavir, grapefruit juice, and verapamil with fentanyl citrate may result in an increase in fentanyl plasma concentrations, which could increase or prolong adverse drug effects and may cause potentially fatal respiratory depression. Patients receiving fentanyl citrate and moderate CYP3A4 inhibitors should be carefully monitored for an extended period of time and dosage increase should be done conservatively). Products include:

Luvox CR Extended-Release Capsules **1759**

Fosamprenavir Calcium (The concomitant use of fentanyl citrate with ritonavir or other strong CYP3A4 inhibitors such as ketoconazole, itraconazole, troleandomycin, clarithromycin, nelfinavir, and nefazadone may result in a potentially dangerous increase in fentanyl plasma concentrations. Patients receiving fentanyl citrate and potent CYP3A4 inhibitors should be carefully monitored for an extended period of time and dosage increase should be done conservatively). Products include:

Lexiva Oral Suspension **1510**
Lexiva Tablets **1510**

Fosphenytoin Sodium (Co-administration with agents that induce CYP3A4 activity may reduce the efficacy of fentanyl citrate).

No products indexed under this heading.

Garlic Extract (Co-administration with agents that induce CYP3A4 activity may reduce the efficacy of fentanyl citrate).
No products indexed under this heading.

Garlic Oil (Co-administration with agents that induce CYP3A4 activity may reduce the efficacy of fentanyl citrate).
No products indexed under this heading.

Glutethimide (The concomitant use of other CNS depressants, including other opioids, sedatives or hypnotics, general anesthetics, phenothiazines, tranquilizers, skeletal muscle relaxants, sedating antihistamines, potent inhibitors of cytochrome P450 3A4 isoform (e.g.,erythromycin, ketoconazole, and certain protease inhibitors), and alcoholic beverages may produce increased depressant effects. Hypoventilation, hypotension, and profound sedation may occur).
No products indexed under this heading.

Haloperidol (The concomitant use of other CNS depressants, including other opioids, sedatives or hypnotics, general anesthetics, phenothiazines, tranquilizers, skeletal muscle relaxants, sedating antihistamines, potent inhibitors of cytochrome P450 3A4 isoform (e.g.,erythromycin, ketoconazole, and certain protease inhibitors), and alcoholic beverages may produce increased depressant effects. Hypoventilation, hypotension, and profound sedation may occur).
No products indexed under this heading.

Haloperidol Decanoate (The concomitant use of other CNS depressants, including other opioids, sedatives or hypnotics, general anesthetics, phenothiazines, tranquilizers, skeletal muscle relaxants, sedating antihistamines, potent inhibitors of cytochrome P450 3A4 isoform (e.g.,erythromycin, ketoconazole, and certain protease inhibitors), and alcoholic beverages may produce increased depressant effects. Hypoventilation, hypotension, and profound sedation may occur).
No products indexed under this heading.

Hydrocodone Bitartrate (The concomitant use of other CNS depressants, including other opioids, sedatives or hypnotics, general anesthetics, phenothiazines, tranquilizers, skeletal muscle relaxants, sedating antihistamines, potent inhibitors of cytochrome P450 3A4 isoform (e.g.,erythromycin, ketoconazole, and certain protease inhibitors), and alcoholic beverages may produce increased depressant effects. Hypoventilation, hypotension, and profound sedation may occur). Products include:
Lortab 5/500 Tablets **3143**
Lortab 7.5/500 Tablets **3144**
Lortab 10/500 Tablets **3144**
Vicodin Tablets **529**
Vicodin ES Tablets **530**
Vicodin HP Tablets **531**
Vicoprofen Tablets **533**
Zydone Tablets **1132**

Hydrocodone Polistirex (The concomitant use of other CNS depressants, including other opioids, sedatives or hypnotics, general anesthetics, phenothiazines, tranquilizers, skeletal muscle relaxants, sedating antihistamines, potent inhibitors of cytochrome P450 3A4 isoform (e.g.,erythromycin, ketoconazole, and certain protease inhibitors), and alcoholic beverages may produce increased depressant effects. Hypoventilation, hypotension, and profound sedation may occur). Products include:
Tussionex Pennkinetic Extended-Release Suspension...... **3154**

Hydrocortisone (Co-administration with agents that induce CYP3A4 activity may reduce the efficacy of fentanyl citrate).
No products indexed under this heading.

Hydrocortisone Acetate (Co-administration with agents that induce CYP3A4 activity may reduce the efficacy of fentanyl citrate). Products include:
Analpram-HC **1140**
Pramosone **1141**

Hydrocortisone Butyrate (Co-administration with agents that induce CYP3A4 activity may reduce the efficacy of fentanyl citrate).
No products indexed under this heading.

Hydrocortisone Cypionate (Co-administration with agents that induce CYP3A4 activity may reduce the efficacy of fentanyl citrate).
No products indexed under this heading.

Hydrocortisone Hemisuccinate (Co-administration with agents that induce CYP3A4 activity may reduce the efficacy of fentanyl citrate).
No products indexed under this heading.

Hydrocortisone Probutate (Co-administration with agents that induce CYP3A4 activity may reduce the efficacy of fentanyl citrate).
No products indexed under this heading.

Hydrocortisone Sodium Phosphate (Co-administration with agents that induce CYP3A4 activity may reduce the efficacy of fentanyl citrate).
No products indexed under this heading.

Hydrocortisone Sodium Succinate (Co-administration with agents that induce CYP3A4 activity may reduce the efficacy of fentanyl citrate).
No products indexed under this heading.

Hydrocortisone Valerate (Co-administration with agents that induce CYP3A4 activity may reduce the efficacy of fentanyl citrate).
No products indexed under this heading.

Hydromorphone Hydrochloride (The concomitant use of other CNS depressants, including other opioids, sedatives or hypnotics, general anesthetics, phenothiazines, tranquilizers, skeletal muscle relaxants, sedating antihistamines, potent inhibitors of cytochrome P450 3A4 isoform (e.g.,erythromycin, ketoconazole, and certain protease inhibitors), and alcoholic beverages may produce increased depressant effects. Hypoventilation, hypotension, and profound sedation may occur).
No products indexed under this heading.

Hydroxyzine Hydrochloride (The concomitant use of other CNS depressants, including other opioids, sedatives or hypnotics, general anesthetics, phenothiazines, tranquilizers, skeletal muscle relaxants, sedating antihistamines, potent inhibitors of cytochrome P450 3A4 isoform (e.g.,erythromycin, ketoconazole, and certain protease inhibitors), and alcoholic beverages may produce increased depressant effects. Hypoventilation, hypotension, and profound sedation may occur).
No products indexed under this heading.

Hypericum (Co-administration with agents that induce CYP3A4 activity may reduce the efficacy of fentanyl citrate). Products include:
Satieté Tablets .... ▣ **640**

Hypericum Perforatum (Co-administration with agents that induce CYP3A4 activity may reduce the efficacy of fentanyl citrate).
No products indexed under this heading.

Indinavir Sulfate (The concomitant use of fentanyl citrate with ritonavir or other strong CYP3A4 inhibitors such as ketoconazole, itraconazole, troleandomycin, clarithromycin, nelfinavir, and nefazadone may result in a potentially dangerous increase in fentanyl plasma concentrations. Patients receiving fentanyl citrate and potent CYP3A4 inhibitors should be carefully monitored for an extended period of time and dosage increase should be done conservatively). Products include:
Crixivan Capsules **1979**

Isocarboxazid (Fentanyl citrate is not recommended for use in patients who are receiving or have received MAO inhibitors within 14 days, because severe and unpredictable potentiation by MAO inhibitors has been reported with opioid analgesics). Products include:
Marplan Tablets **3177**

Isoflurane (The concomitant use of other CNS depressants, including other opioids, sedatives or hypnotics, general anesthetics, phenothiazines, tranquilizers, skeletal muscle relaxants, sedating antihistamines, potent inhibitors of cytochrome P450 3A4 isoform (e.g.,erythromycin, ketoconazole, and certain protease inhibitors), and alcoholic beverages may produce increased depressant effects. Hypoventilation, hypotension, and profound sedation may occur).
No products indexed under this heading.

Isoniazid (The concomitant use of moderate CYP3A4 inhibitors such as amprenavir, aprepitant, diltiazem, erythromycin, fluconazole, fosamprenavir, grapefruit juice, and verapamil with fentanyl citrate may result in an increase in fentanyl plasma concentrations, which could increase or prolong adverse drug effects and may cause potentially fatal respiratory depression. Patients receiving fentanyl citrate and moderate CYP3A4 inhibitors should be carefully monitored for an extended period of time and dosage increase should be done conservatively).
No products indexed under this heading.

Itraconazole (The concomitant use of fentanyl citrate with ritonavir or other strong CYP3A4 inhibitors such as ketoconazole, itraconazole, troleandomycin, clarithromycin, nelfinavir, and nefazadone may result in a potentially dangerous increase in fentanyl plasma concentrations. Patients receiving fentanyl citrate and potent CYP3A4 inhibitors should be carefully monitored for an extended period of time and dosage increase should be done conservatively).
No products indexed under this heading.

Ketamine Hydrochloride (The concomitant use of other CNS depressants, including other opioids, sedatives or hypnotics, general anesthetics, phenothiazines, tranquilizers, skeletal muscle relaxants, sedating antihistamines, potent inhibitors of cytochrome P450 3A4 isoform (e.g.,erythromycin, ketoconazole, and certain protease inhibitors), and alcoholic beverages may produce increased depressant effects. Hypoventilation, hypotension, and profound sedation may occur).
No products indexed under this heading.

Ketoconazole (The concomitant use of fentanyl citrate with ritonavir or other strong CYP3A4 inhibitors such as ketoconazole, itraconazole, troleandomycin, clarithromycin, nelfinavir, and nefazadone may result in a potentially dangerous increase in fentanyl plasma concentrations. Patients receiving fentanyl citrate and potent CYP3A4 inhibitors should be carefully monitored for an extended period of time and dosage increase should be done conservatively). Products include:
Extina Foam, 2% **3057**
Nizoral A-D Shampoo **1901**

Levomethadyl Acetate Hydrochloride (The concomitant use of other CNS depressants, including other opioids, sedatives or hypnotics, general anesthetics, phenothiazines, tranquilizers, skeletal muscle relaxants, sedating antihistamines, potent inhibitors of cytochrome P450 3A4 isoform (e.g.,erythromycin, ketoconazole, and certain protease inhibitors), and alcoholic beverages may produce increased depressant effects. Hypoventilation, hypotension, and profound sedation may occur).
No products indexed under this heading.

Levorphanol Tartrate (The concomitant use of other CNS depressants, including other opioids, sedatives or hypnotics, general anesthetics, phenothiazines, tranquilizers, skeletal muscle relaxants, sedating antihistamines, potent inhibitors of cytochrome P450 3A4 isoform (e.g.,erythromycin, ketoconazole, and certain protease inhibitors), and alcoholic beverages may produce increased depressant effects. Hypoventilation, hypotension, and profound sedation may occur).
No products indexed under this heading.

Lopinavir (The concomitant use of fentanyl citrate with ritonavir or other strong CYP3A4 inhibitors such as ketoconazole, itraconazole, troleandomycin, clarithromycin, nelfinavir, and nefazadone may result in a potentially dangerous increase in fentanyl plasma concentrations. Patients receiving fentanyl citrate and potent CYP3A4 inhibitors should be carefully monitored for an extended period of time and dosage increase should be done conservatively). Products include:

Kaletra 452

Loratadine (The concomitant use of moderate CYP3A4 inhibitors such as amprenavir, aprepitant, diltiazem, erythromycin, fluconazole, fosamprenavir, grapefruit juice, and verapamil with fentanyl citrate may result in an increase in fentanyl plasma concentrations, which could increase or prolong adverse drug effects and may cause potentially fatal respiratory depression. Patients receiving fentanyl citrate and moderate CYP3A4 inhibitors should be carefully monitored for an extended period of time and dosage increase should be done conservatively).

No products indexed under this heading.

Lorazepam (The concomitant use of other CNS depressants, including other opioids, sedatives or hypnotics, general anesthetics, phenothiazines, tranquilizers, skeletal muscle relaxants, sedating antihistamines, potent inhibitors of cytochrome P450 3A4 isoform (e.g.,erythromycin, ketoconazole, and certain protease inhibitors), and alcoholic beverages may produce increased depressant effects. Hypoventilation, hypotension, and profound sedation may occur).

No products indexed under this heading.

Loxapine Hydrochloride (The concomitant use of other CNS depressants, including other opioids, sedatives or hypnotics, general anesthetics, phenothiazines, tranquilizers, skeletal muscle relaxants, sedating antihistamines, potent inhibitors of cytochrome P450 3A4 isoform (e.g.,erythromycin, ketoconazole, and certain protease inhibitors), and alcoholic beverages may produce increased depressant effects. Hypoventilation, hypotension, and profound sedation may occur).

No products indexed under this heading.

Loxapine Succinate (The concomitant use of other CNS depressants, including other opioids, sedatives or hypnotics, general anesthetics, phenothiazines, tranquilizers, skeletal muscle relaxants, sedating antihistamines, potent inhibitors of cytochrome P450 3A4 isoform (e.g.,erythromycin, ketoconazole, and certain protease inhibitors), and alcoholic beverages may produce increased depressant effects. Hypoventilation, hypotension, and profound sedation may occur).

No products indexed under this heading.

Meperidine Hydrochloride (The concomitant use of other CNS depressants, including other opioids, sedatives or hypnotics, general anesthetics, phenothiazines, tranquilizers, skeletal muscle relaxants, sedating antihistamines, potent inhibitors of cytochrome P450 3A4 isoform (e.g.,erythromycin, ketoconazole, and certain protease inhibitors), and alcoholic beverages may produce increased depressant effects. Hypoventilation, hypotension, and profound sedation may occur).

No products indexed under this heading.

Mephenytoin (Co-administration with agents that induce CYP3A4 activity may reduce the efficacy of fentanyl citrate).

No products indexed under this heading.

Mephobarbital (The concomitant use of other CNS depressants, including other opioids, sedatives or hypnotics, general anesthetics, phenothiazines, tranquilizers, skeletal muscle relaxants, sedating antihistamines, potent inhibitors of cytochrome P450 3A4 isoform (e.g.,erythromycin, ketoconazole, and certain protease inhibitors), and alcoholic beverages may produce increased depressant effects. Hypoventilation, hypotension, and profound sedation may occur).

No products indexed under this heading.

Meprobamate (The concomitant use of other CNS depressants, including other opioids, sedatives or hypnotics, general anesthetics, phenothiazines, tranquilizers, skeletal muscle relaxants, sedating antihistamines, potent inhibitors of cytochrome P450 3A4 isoform (e.g.,erythromycin, ketoconazole, and certain protease inhibitors), and alcoholic beverages may produce increased depressant effects. Hypoventilation, hypotension, and profound sedation may occur).

No products indexed under this heading.

Mesoridazine Besylate (The concomitant use of other CNS depressants, including other opioids, sedatives or hypnotics, general anesthetics, phenothiazines, tranquilizers, skeletal muscle relaxants, sedating antihistamines, potent inhibitors of cytochrome P450 3A4 isoform (e.g.,erythromycin, ketoconazole, and certain protease inhibitors), and alcoholic beverages may produce increased depressant effects. Hypoventilation, hypotension, and profound sedation may occur).

No products indexed under this heading.

Metaxalone (The concomitant use of other CNS depressants, including skeletal muscle relaxants, may produce increased depressant effects. Hypoventilation, hypotension, and profound sedation may occur). Products include:

Skelaxin Tablets 1784

Methadone Hydrochloride (The concomitant use of other CNS depressants, including other opioids, sedatives or hypnotics, general anesthetics, phenothiazines, tranquilizers, skeletal muscle relaxants, sedating antihistamines, potent inhibitors of cytochrome P450 3A4 isoform (e.g.,erythromycin, ketoconazole, and certain protease inhibitors), and alcoholic beverages may produce increased depressant effects. Hypoventilation, hypotension, and profound sedation may occur).

No products indexed under this heading.

Methdilazine Hydrochloride (The concomitant use of other CNS depressants, including sedating antihistamines, may produce increased depressant effects. Hypoventilation, hypotension, and profound sedation may occur).

No products indexed under this heading.

Methocarbamol (The concomitant use of other CNS depressants, including skeletal muscle relaxants, may produce increased depressant effects. Hypoventilation, hypotension, and profound sedation may occur).

No products indexed under this heading.

Methohexital Sodium (The concomitant use of other CNS depressants, including other opioids, sedatives or hypnotics, general anesthetics, phenothiazines, tranquilizers, skeletal muscle relaxants, sedating antihistamines, potent inhibitors of cytochrome P450 3A4 isoform (e.g.,erythromycin, ketoconazole, and certain protease inhibitors), and alcoholic beverages may produce increased depressant effects. Hypoventilation, hypotension, and profound sedation may occur).

No products indexed under this heading.

Methotrimeprazine (The concomitant use of other CNS depressants, including other opioids, sedatives or hypnotics, general anesthetics, phenothiazines, tranquilizers, skeletal muscle relaxants, sedating antihistamines, potent inhibitors of cytochrome P450 3A4 isoform (e.g.,erythromycin, ketoconazole, and certain protease inhibitors), and alcoholic beverages may produce increased depressant effects. Hypoventilation, hypotension, and profound sedation may occur).

No products indexed under this heading.

Methoxyflurane (The concomitant use of other CNS depressants, including other opioids, sedatives or hypnotics, general anesthetics, phenothiazines, tranquilizers, skeletal muscle relaxants, sedating antihistamines, potent inhibitors of cytochrome P450 3A4 isoform (e.g.,erythromycin, ketoconazole, and certain protease inhibitors), and alcoholic beverages may produce increased depressant effects. Hypoventilation, hypotension, and profound sedation may occur).

No products indexed under this heading.

Methsuximide (Co-administration with agents that induce CYP3A4 activity may reduce the efficacy of fentanyl citrate).

No products indexed under this heading.

Methylprednisolone (Co-administration with agents that induce CYP3A4 activity may reduce the efficacy of fentanyl citrate).

No products indexed under this heading.

Methylprednisolone Acetate (Co-administration with agents that induce CYP3A4 activity may reduce the efficacy of fentanyl citrate).

No products indexed under this heading.

Methylprednisolone Sodium Succinate (Co-administration with agents that induce CYP3A4 activity may reduce the efficacy of fentanyl citrate).

No products indexed under this heading.

Metronidazole (The concomitant use of moderate CYP3A4 inhibitors such as amprenavir, aprepitant, diltiazem, erythromycin, fluconazole, fosamprenavir, grapefruit juice, and verapamil with fentanyl citrate may result in an increase in fentanyl plasma concentrations, which could increase or prolong adverse drug effects and may cause potentially fatal respiratory depression. Patients receiving fentanyl citrate and moderate CYP3A4 inhibitors should be carefully monitored for an extended period of time and dosage increase should be done conservatively). Products include:

Pylera Capsules 714

Metronidazole Benzoate (The concomitant use of moderate CYP3A4 inhibitors such as amprenavir, aprepitant, diltiazem, erythromycin, fluconazole, fosamprenavir, grapefruit juice, and verapamil with fentanyl citrate may result in an increase in fentanyl plasma concentrations, which could increase or prolong adverse drug effects and may cause potentially fatal respiratory depression. Patients receiving fentanyl citrate and moderate CYP3A4 inhibitors should be carefully monitored for an extended period of time and dosage increase should be done conservatively).

No products indexed under this heading.

Metronidazole Hydrochloride (The concomitant use of moderate CYP3A4 inhibitors such as amprenavir, aprepitant, diltiazem, erythromycin, fluconazole, fosamprenavir, grapefruit juice, and verapamil with fentanyl citrate may result in an increase in fentanyl plasma concentrations, which could increase or prolong adverse drug effects and may cause potentially fatal respiratory depression. Patients receiving fentanyl citrate and moderate CYP3A4 inhibitors should be carefully monitored for an extended period of time and dosage increase should be done conservatively).

No products indexed under this heading.

Miconazole (The concomitant use of moderate CYP3A4 inhibitors such as amprenavir, aprepitant, diltiazem, erythromycin, fluconazole, fosamprenavir, grapefruit juice, and verapamil with fentanyl citrate may result in an increase in fentanyl plasma concentrations, which could increase or prolong adverse drug effects and may cause potentially fatal respiratory depression. Patients receiving fentanyl citrate and moderate CYP3A4 inhibitors should be carefully monitored for an extended period of time and dosage increase should be done conservatively).

No products indexed under this heading.

Miconazole Nitrate (The concomitant use of moderate CYP3A4 inhibitors such as amprenavir, aprepitant, diltiazem, erythromycin, fluconazole, fosamprenavir, grapefruit juice, and verapamil with fentanyl citrate may result in an increase in fentanyl plas-

ma concentrations, which could increase or prolong adverse drug effects and may cause potentially fatal respiratory depression. Patients receiving fentanyl citrate and moderate CYP3A4 inhibitors should be carefully monitored for an extended period of time and dosage increase should be done conservatively).
No products indexed under this heading.

Midazolam Hydrochloride (The concomitant use of other CNS depressants, including other opioids, sedatives or hypnotics, general anesthetics, phenothiazines, tranquilizers, skeletal muscle relaxants, sedating antihistamines, potent inhibitors of cytochrome P450 3A4 isoform (e.g.,erythromycin, ketoconazole, and certain protease inhibitors), and alcoholic beverages may produce increased depressant effects. Hypoventilation, hypotension, and profound sedation may occur).
No products indexed under this heading.

Moclobemide (Fentanyl citrate is not recommended for use in patients who are receiving or have received MAO inhibitors within 14 days, because severe and unpredictable potentiation by MAO inhibitors has been reported with opioid analgesics).
No products indexed under this heading.

Modafinil (Co-administration with agents that induce CYP3A4 activity may reduce the efficacy of fentanyl citrate). Products include:
Provigil Tablets **977**

Molindone Hydrochloride (The concomitant use of other CNS depressants, including other opioids, sedatives or hypnotics, general anesthetics, phenothiazines, tranquilizers, skeletal muscle relaxants, sedating antihistamines, potent inhibitors of cytochrome P450 3A4 isoform (e.g.,erythromycin, ketoconazole, and certain protease inhibitors), and alcoholic beverages may produce increased depressant effects. Hypoventilation, hypotension, and profound sedation may occur). Products include:
Moban Tablets **1116**

Morphine Sulfate (The concomitant use of other CNS depressants, including other opioids, sedatives or hypnotics, general anesthetics, phenothiazines, tranquilizers, skeletal muscle relaxants, sedating antihistamines, potent inhibitors of cytochrome P450 3A4 isoform (e.g.,erythromycin, ketoconazole, and certain protease inhibitors), and alcoholic beverages may produce increased depressant effects. Hypoventilation, hypotension, and profound sedation may occur). Products include:
Avinza Capsules **1772**
DepoDur Injection **1095**
MS Contin Tablets **2585**

Nefazodone Hydrochloride (The concomitant use of fentanyl citrate with ritonavir or other strong CYP3A4 inhibitors such as ketoconazole, itraconazole, troleandomycin, clarithromycin, nelfinavir, and nefazadone may result in a potentially dangerous increase in fentanyl plasma concentrations. Patients receiving fentanyl citrate and potent CYP3A4 inhibitors should be carefully monitored for an extended period of time and dosage increase should be done conservatively).
No products indexed under this heading.

Nelfinavir Mesylate (The concomitant use of fentanyl citrate with ritonavir or other strong CYP3A4 inhibitors such as ketoconazole, itraconazole, troleandomycin, clarithromycin, nelfinavir, and nefazadone may result in a potentially dangerous increase in fentanyl plasma concentrations. Patients receiving fentanyl citrate and potent CYP3A4 inhibitors should be carefully monitored for an extended period of time and dosage increase should be done conservatively).
No products indexed under this heading.

Nevirapine (The concomitant use of moderate CYP3A4 inhibitors such as amprenavir, aprepitant, diltiazem, erythromycin, fluconazole, fosamprenavir, grapefruit juice, and verapamil with fentanyl citrate may result in an increase in fentanyl plasma concentrations, which could increase or prolong adverse drug effects and may cause potentially fatal respiratory depression. Patients receiving fentanyl citrate and moderate CYP3A4 inhibitors should be carefully monitored for an extended period of time and dosage increase should be done conservatively).
Products include:
Viramune Oral Suspension **873**
Viramune Tablets **873**

Niacinamide (The concomitant use of moderate CYP3A4 inhibitors such as amprenavir, aprepitant, diltiazem, erythromycin, fluconazole, fosamprenavir, grapefruit juice, and verapamil with fentanyl citrate may result in an increase in fentanyl plasma concentrations, which could increase or prolong adverse drug effects and may cause potentially fatal respiratory depression. Patients receiving fentanyl citrate and moderate CYP3A4 inhibitors should be carefully monitored for an extended period of time and dosage increase should be done conservatively).
Products include:
BioLean Free Tablets .... ▣ **635**

Nicotinamide (The concomitant use of moderate CYP3A4 inhibitors such as amprenavir, aprepitant, diltiazem, erythromycin, fluconazole, fosamprenavir, grapefruit juice, and verapamil with fentanyl citrate may result in an increase in fentanyl plasma concentrations, which could increase or prolong adverse drug effects and may cause potentially fatal respiratory depression. Patients receiving fentanyl citrate and moderate CYP3A4 inhibitors should be carefully monitored for an extended period of time and dosage increase should be done conservatively).
No products indexed under this heading.

Nifedipine (The concomitant use of moderate CYP3A4 inhibitors such as amprenavir, aprepitant, diltiazem, erythromycin, fluconazole, fosamprenavir, grapefruit juice, and verapamil with fentanyl citrate may result in an increase in fentanyl plasma concentrations, which could increase or prolong adverse drug effects and may cause potentially fatal respiratory depression. Patients receiving fentanyl citrate and moderate CYP3A4 inhibitors should be carefully monitored for an extended period of time and dosage increase should be done conservatively).
No products indexed under this heading.

Norfloxacin (The concomitant use of moderate CYP3A4 inhibitors such as amprenavir, aprepitant, diltiazem, erythromycin, fluconazole, fosamprenavir, grapefruit juice, and verapamil with fentanyl citrate may result in an increase in fentanyl plasma concentrations, which could increase or prolong adverse drug effects and may cause potentially fatal respiratory depression. Patients receiving fentanyl citrate and moderate CYP3A4 inhibitors should be carefully monitored for an extended period of time and dosage increase should be done conservatively).
Products include:
Noroxin Tablets **2069**

Olanzapine (The concomitant use of other CNS depressants, including other opioids, sedatives or hypnotics, general anesthetics, phenothiazines, tranquilizers, skeletal muscle relaxants, sedating antihistamines, potent inhibitors of cytochrome P450 3A4 isoform (e.g.,erythromycin, ketoconazole, and certain protease inhibitors), and alcoholic beverages may produce increased depressant effects. Hypoventilation, hypotension, and profound sedation may occur). Products include:
Symbyax Capsules **1871**
Zyprexa Tablets **1883**
Zyprexa IntraMuscular **1883**
Zyprexa ZYDIS Orally Disintegrating Tablets **1883**

Omeprazole (The concomitant use of moderate CYP3A4 inhibitors such as amprenavir, aprepitant, diltiazem, erythromycin, fluconazole, fosamprenavir, grapefruit juice, and verapamil with fentanyl citrate may result in an increase in fentanyl plasma concentrations, which could increase or prolong adverse drug effects and may cause potentially fatal respiratory depression. Patients receiving fentanyl citrate and moderate CYP3A4 inhibitors should be carefully monitored for an extended period of time and dosage increase should be done conservatively).
No products indexed under this heading.

Orphenadrine Citrate (The concomitant use of other CNS depressants, including skeletal muscle relaxants, may produce increased depressant effects. Hypoventilation, hypotension, and profound sedation may occur).
No products indexed under this heading.

Oxazepam (The concomitant use of other CNS depressants, including other opioids, sedatives or hypnotics, general anesthetics, phenothiazines, tranquilizers, skeletal muscle relaxants, sedating antihistamines, potent inhibitors of cytochrome P450 3A4 isoform (e.g.,erythromycin, ketoconazole, and certain protease inhibitors), and alcoholic beverages may produce increased depressant effects. Hypoventilation, hypotension, and profound sedation may occur).
No products indexed under this heading.

Oxcarbazepine (Co-administration with agents that induce CYP3A4 activity may reduce the efficacy of fentanyl citrate).
No products indexed under this heading.

Oxycodone Hydrochloride (The concomitant use of other CNS depressants, including other opioids, sedatives or hypnotics, general anesthetics, phenothiazines, tranquilizers, skeletal muscle relaxants, sedating antihistamines, potent inhibitors of cytochrome P450 3A4 isoform (e.g.,erythromycin, ketoconazole, and certain protease inhibitors), and alcoholic beverages may produce increased depressant effects. Hypoventilation, hypotension, and profound sedation may occur). Products include:
OxyContin Tablets **2589**
OxyIR Capsules **2593**
Percocet Tablets **1127**
Percodan Tablets **1130**

Pargyline Hydrochloride (Fentanyl citrate is not recommended for use in patients who are receiving or have received MAO inhibitors within 14 days, because severe and unpredictable potentiation by MAO inhibitors has been reported with opioid analgesics).
No products indexed under this heading.

Paroxetine Hydrochloride (The concomitant use of moderate CYP3A4 inhibitors such as amprenavir, aprepitant, diltiazem, erythromycin, fluconazole, fosamprenavir, grapefruit juice, and verapamil with fentanyl citrate may result in an increase in fentanyl plasma concentrations, which could increase or prolong adverse drug effects and may cause potentially fatal respiratory depression. Patients receiving fentanyl citrate and moderate CYP3A4 inhibitors should be carefully monitored for an extended period of time and dosage increase should be done conservatively).
Products include:
Paxil **1535**
Paxil CR Controlled-Release Tablets **1544**

Pentobarbital Sodium (The concomitant use of other CNS depressants, including other opioids, sedatives or hypnotics, general anesthetics, phenothiazines, tranquilizers, skeletal muscle relaxants, sedating antihistamines, potent inhibitors of cytochrome P450 3A4 isoform (e.g.,erythromycin, ketoconazole, and certain protease inhibitors), and alcoholic beverages may produce increased depressant effects. Hypoventilation, hypotension, and profound sedation may occur). Products include:
Nembutal Sodium Solution, USP **2494**

Perphenazine (The concomitant use of other CNS depressants, including other opioids, sedatives or hypnotics, general anesthetics, phenothiazines, tranquilizers, skeletal muscle relaxants, sedating antihistamines, potent inhibitors of cytochrome P450 3A4 isoform (e.g.,erythromycin, ketoconazole, and certain protease inhibitors), and alcoholic beverages may produce increased depressant effects. Hypoventilation, hypotension, and profound sedation may occur).
No products indexed under this heading.

in an increase in fentanyl plasma concentrations, which could increase or prolong adverse drug effects and may cause potentially fatal respiratory depression. Patients receiving fentanyl citrate and moderate CYP3A4 inhibitors should be carefully monitored for an extended period of time and dosage increase should be done conservatively).

No products indexed under this heading.

Ramelteon (The concomitant use of other CNS depressants, including sedatives or hypnotics, may produce increased depressant effects. Hypoventilation, hypotension, and profound sedation may occur). Products include:

Rozerem Tablets **3091**

Ranitidine Bismuth Citrate (The concomitant use of moderate CYP3A4 inhibitors such as amprenavir, aprepitant, diltiazem, erythromycin, fluconazole, fosamprenavir, grapefruit juice, and verapamil with fentanyl citrate may result in an increase in fentanyl plasma concentrations, which could increase or prolong adverse drug effects and may cause potentially fatal respiratory depression. Patients receiving fentanyl citrate and moderate CYP3A4 inhibitors should be carefully monitored for an extended period of time and dosage increase should be done conservatively).

No products indexed under this heading.

Ranitidine Hydrochloride (The concomitant use of moderate CYP3A4 inhibitors such as amprenavir, aprepitant, diltiazem, erythromycin, fluconazole, fosamprenavir, grapefruit juice, and verapamil with fentanyl citrate may result in an increase in fentanyl plasma concentrations, which could increase or prolong adverse drug effects and may cause potentially fatal respiratory depression. Patients receiving fentanyl citrate and moderate CYP3A4 inhibitors should be carefully monitored for an extended period of time and dosage increase should be done conservatively). Products include:

Zantac 75 Tablets .... ■ **603**
Zantac **1670**
Zantac Injection **1666**
Zantac Injection Pharmacy Bulk Package **1668**
Maximum Strength Zantac 150 Tablets .... ■ **603**
Maximum Strength Zantac 150 Cool Mint Tablets .... ■ **603**

Rasagiline Mesylate (Fentanyl citrate is not recommended for use in patients who are receiving or have received MAO inhibitors within 14 days, because severe and unpredictable potentiation by MAO inhibitors has been reported with opioid analgesics). Products include:

Azilect Tablets **3106**

Remifentanil Hydrochloride (The concomitant use of other CNS depressants, including other opioids, sedatives or hypnotics, general anesthetics, phenothiazines, tranquilizers, skeletal muscle relaxants, sedating antihistamines, potent inhibitors of cytochrome P450 3A4 isoform (e.g.,erythromycin, ketoconazole, and certain protease inhibitors), and alcoholic beverages may produce increased depressant effects. Hypoventilation, hypotension, and profound sedation may occur).

No products indexed under this heading.

Rifabutin (Co-administration with agents that induce CYP3A4 activity may reduce the efficacy of fentanyl citrate).

No products indexed under this heading.

Rifampicin (Co-administration with agents that induce CYP3A4 activity may reduce the efficacy of fentanyl citrate).

No products indexed under this heading.

Rifampin (Co-administration with agents that induce CYP3A4 activity may reduce the efficacy of fentanyl citrate).

No products indexed under this heading.

Rifapentine (Co-administration with agents that induce CYP3A4 activity may reduce the efficacy of fentanyl citrate).

No products indexed under this heading.

Risperidone (The concomitant use of other CNS depressants, including other opioids, sedatives or hypnotics, general anesthetics, phenothiazines, tranquilizers, skeletal muscle relaxants, sedating antihistamines, potent inhibitors of cytochrome P450 3A4 isoform (e.g.,erythromycin, ketoconazole, and certain protease inhibitors), and alcoholic beverages may produce increased depressant effects. Hypoventilation, hypotension, and profound sedation may occur). Products include:

Risperdal Consta Long-Acting Injection **1753**

Ritonavir (The concomitant use of fentanyl citrate with ritonavir or other strong CYP3A4 inhibitors such as ketoconazole, itraconazole, troleandomycin, clarithromycin, nelfinavir, and nefazadone may result in a potentially dangerous increase in fentanyl plasma concentrations. Patients receiving fentanyl citrate and potent CYP3A4 inhibitors should be carefully monitored for an extended period of time and dosage increase should be done conservatively). Products include:

Kaletra **452**
Norvir **489**

Saquinavir (The concomitant use of fentanyl citrate with ritonavir or other strong CYP3A4 inhibitors such as ketoconazole, itraconazole, troleandomycin, clarithromycin, nelfinavir, and nefazadone may result in a potentially dangerous increase in fentanyl plasma concentrations. Patients receiving fentanyl citrate and potent CYP3A4 inhibitors should be carefully monitored for an extended period of time and dosage increase should be done conservatively).

No products indexed under this heading.

Saquinavir Mesylate (The concomitant use of fentanyl citrate with ritonavir or other strong CYP3A4 inhibitors such as ketoconazole, itraconazole, troleandomycin, clarithromycin, nelfinavir, and nefazadone may result in a potentially dangerous increase in fentanyl plasma concentrations. Patients receiving fentanyl citrate and potent CYP3A4 inhibitors should be carefully monitored for an extended period of time and dosage increase should be done conservatively).

No products indexed under this heading.

Secobarbital Sodium (The concomitant use of other CNS depressants, including other opioids, sedatives or hypnotics, general anesthetics, phenothiazines, tranquilizers, skeletal muscle relaxants, sedating antihistamines, potent inhibitors of cytochrome P450 3A4 isoform (e.g.,erythromycin, ketoconazole, and certain protease inhibitors), and alcoholic beverages may produce increased depressant effects. Hypoventilation, hypotension, and profound sedation may occur).

No products indexed under this heading.

Selegiline (Fentanyl citrate is not recommended for use in patients who are receiving or have received MAO inhibitors within 14 days, because severe and unpredictable potentiation by MAO inhibitors has been reported with opioid analgesics). Products include:

Emsam Transdermal System **905**

Selegiline Hydrochloride (Fentanyl citrate is not recommended for use in patients who are receiving or have received MAO inhibitors within 14 days, because severe and unpredictable potentiation by MAO inhibitors has been reported with opioid analgesics). Products include:

Eldepryl Capsules **3052**

Sertraline Hydrochloride (The concomitant use of moderate CYP3A4 inhibitors such as amprenavir, aprepitant, diltiazem, erythromycin, fluconazole, fosamprenavir, grapefruit juice, and verapamil with fentanyl citrate may result in an increase in fentanyl plasma concentrations, which could increase or prolong adverse drug effects and may cause potentially fatal respiratory depression. Patients receiving fentanyl citrate and moderate CYP3A4 inhibitors should be carefully monitored for an extended period of time and dosage increase should be done conservatively).

No products indexed under this heading.

Sevoflurane (The concomitant use of other CNS depressants, including other opioids, sedatives or hypnotics, general anesthetics, phenothiazines, tranquilizers, skeletal muscle relaxants, sedating antihistamines, potent inhibitors of cytochrome P450 3A4 isoform (e.g.,erythromycin, ketoconazole, and certain protease inhibitors), and alcoholic beverages may produce increased depressant effects. Hypoventilation, hypotension, and profound sedation may occur). Products include:

Ultane Liquid for Inhalation **524**

Sildenafil Citrate (The concomitant use of moderate CYP3A4 inhibitors such as amprenavir, aprepitant, diltiazem, erythromycin, fluconazole, fosamprenavir, grapefruit juice, and verapamil with fentanyl citrate may result in an increase in fentanyl plasma concentrations, which could increase or prolong adverse drug effects and may cause potentially fatal respiratory depression. Patients receiving fentanyl citrate and moderate CYP3A4 inhibitors should be carefully monitored for an extended period of time and dosage increase should be done conservatively).

No products indexed under this heading.

Sodium Butabarbital (The concomitant use of other CNS depressants, including sedatives or hypnotics, may produce increased depressant effects. Hypoventilation, hypotension, and profound sedation may occur).

No products indexed under this heading.

Sodium Oxybate (The concomitant use of other CNS depressants, including other opioids, sedatives or hypnotics, general anesthetics, phenothiazines, tranquilizers, skeletal muscle relaxants, sedating antihistamines, potent inhibitors of cytochrome P450 3A4 isoform (e.g.,erythromycin, ketoconazole, and certain protease inhibitors), and alcoholic beverages may produce increased depressant effects. Hypoventilation, hypotension, and profound sedation may occur). Products include:

Xyrem Oral Solution **1766**

Sufentanil Citrate (The concomitant use of other CNS depressants, including other opioids, sedatives or hypnotics, general anesthetics, phenothiazines, tranquilizers, skeletal muscle relaxants, sedating antihistamines, potent inhibitors of cytochrome P450 3A4 isoform (e.g.,erythromycin, ketoconazole, and certain protease inhibitors), and alcoholic beverages may produce increased depressant effects. Hypoventilation, hypotension, and profound sedation may occur).

No products indexed under this heading.

Sulfinpyrazone (Co-administration with agents that induce CYP3A4 activity may reduce the efficacy of fentanyl citrate).

No products indexed under this heading.

Telithromycin (The concomitant use of fentanyl citrate with ritonavir or other strong CYP3A4 inhibitors such as ketoconazole, itraconazole, troleandomycin, clarithromycin, nelfinavir, and nefazadone may result in a potentially dangerous increase in fentanyl plasma concentrations. Patients receiving fentanyl citrate and potent CYP3A4 inhibitors should be carefully monitored for an extended period of time and dosage increase should be done conservatively). Products include:

Ketek Tablets **2744**

Temazepam (The concomitant use of other CNS depressants, including other opioids, sedatives or hypnotics, general anesthetics, phenothiazines, tranquilizers, skeletal muscle relaxants, sedating antihistamines, potent inhibitors of cytochrome P450 3A4 isoform (e.g.,erythromycin, ketoconazole, and certain protease inhibitors), and alcoholic beverages may produce increased depressant effects. Hypoventilation, hypotension, and profound sedation may occur).

No products indexed under this heading.

Terfenadine (The concomitant use of other CNS depressants, including sedating antihistamines, may produce increased depressant effects. Hypoventilation, hypotension, and profound sedation may occur).
No products indexed under this heading.

Theophylline (Co-administration with agents that induce CYP3A4 activity may reduce the efficacy of fentanyl citrate).
No products indexed under this heading.

Theophylline Anhydrous (Co-administration with agents that induce CYP3A4 activity may reduce the efficacy of fentanyl citrate). Products include:
Uniphyl Tablets 2595

Theophylline Calcium Salicylate (Co-administration with agents that induce CYP3A4 activity may reduce the efficacy of fentanyl citrate).
No products indexed under this heading.

Theophylline Dihydroxypropyl (Glyceryl) (Co-administration with agents that induce CYP3A4 activity may reduce the efficacy of fentanyl citrate).
No products indexed under this heading.

Theophylline Ethylenediamine (Co-administration with agents that induce CYP3A4 activity may reduce the efficacy of fentanyl citrate).
No products indexed under this heading.

Thiamylal Sodium (The concomitant use of other CNS depressants, including other opioids, sedatives or hypnotics, general anesthetics, phenothiazines, tranquilizers, skeletal muscle relaxants, sedating antihistamines, potent inhibitors of cytochrome P450 3A4 isoform (e.g.,erythromycin, ketoconazole, and certain protease inhibitors), and alcoholic beverages may produce increased depressant effects. Hypoventilation, hypotension, and profound sedation may occur).
No products indexed under this heading.

Thioridazine Hydrochloride (The concomitant use of other CNS depressants, including other opioids, sedatives or hypnotics, general anesthetics, phenothiazines, tranquilizers, skeletal muscle relaxants, sedating antihistamines, potent inhibitors of cytochrome P450 3A4 isoform (e.g.,erythromycin, ketoconazole, and certain protease inhibitors), and alcoholic beverages may produce increased depressant effects. Hypoventilation, hypotension, and profound sedation may occur). Products include:
Thioridazine Hydrochloride Tablets 2195

Thiothixene (The concomitant use of other CNS depressants, including other opioids, sedatives or hypnotics, general anesthetics, phenothiazines, tranquilizers, skeletal muscle relaxants, sedating antihistamines, potent inhibitors of cytochrome P450 3A4 isoform (e.g.,erythromycin, ketoconazole, and certain protease inhibitors), and alcoholic beverages may produce increased depressant effects. Hypoventilation, hypotension, and profound sedation may occur). Products include:
Thiothixene Capsules 2197

Tranylcypromine Sulfate (Fentanyl citrate is not recommended for use in patients who are receiving or have received MAO inhibitors within 14 days, because severe and unpredictable potentiation by MAO inhibitors has been reported with opioid analgesics). Products include:
Parnate Tablets 1532

Triamcinolone (Co-administration with agents that induce CYP3A4 activity may reduce the efficacy of fentanyl citrate).
No products indexed under this heading.

Triamcinolone Acetonide (Co-administration with agents that induce CYP3A4 activity may reduce the efficacy of fentanyl citrate). Products include:
Azmacort Inhalation Aerosol 407
Nasacort AQ Nasal Spray 2765
Triesence Injectable Suspension .... ⊙ 209

Triamcinolone Diacetate (Co-administration with agents that induce CYP3A4 activity may reduce the efficacy of fentanyl citrate).
No products indexed under this heading.

Triamcinolone Hexacetonide (Co-administration with agents that induce CYP3A4 activity may reduce the efficacy of fentanyl citrate).
No products indexed under this heading.

Triazolam (The concomitant use of other CNS depressants, including other opioids, sedatives or hypnotics, general anesthetics, phenothiazines, tranquilizers, skeletal muscle relaxants, sedating antihistamines, potent inhibitors of cytochrome P450 3A4 isoform (e.g.,erythromycin, ketoconazole, and certain protease inhibitors), and alcoholic beverages may produce increased depressant effects. Hypoventilation, hypotension, and profound sedation may occur).
No products indexed under this heading.

Trifluoperazine Hydrochloride (The concomitant use of other CNS depressants, including other opioids, sedatives or hypnotics, general anesthetics, phenothiazines, tranquilizers, skeletal muscle relaxants, sedating antihistamines, potent inhibitors of cytochrome P450 3A4 isoform (e.g.,erythromycin, ketoconazole, and certain protease inhibitors), and alcoholic beverages may produce increased depressant effects. Hypoventilation, hypotension, and profound sedation may occur).
No products indexed under this heading.

Trimeprazine Tartrate (The concomitant use of other CNS depressants, including sedating antihistamines, may produce increased depressant effects. Hypoventilation, hypotension, and profound sedation may occur).
No products indexed under this heading.

Tripelennamine Hydrochloride (The concomitant use of other CNS depressants, including sedating antihistamines, may produce increased depressant effects. Hypoventilation, hypotension, and profound sedation may occur).
No products indexed under this heading.

Triprolidine Hydrochloride (The concomitant use of other CNS depressants, including sedating antihistamines, may produce increased depressant effects. Hypoventilation, hypotension, and profound sedation may occur).
No products indexed under this heading.

Troglitazone (The concomitant use of moderate CYP3A4 inhibitors such as amprenavir, aprepitant, diltiazem, erythromycin, fluconazole, fosamprenavir, grapefruit juice, and verapamil with fentanyl citrate may result in an increase in fentanyl plasma concentrations, which could increase or prolong adverse drug effects and may cause potentially fatal respiratory depression. Patients receiving fentanyl citrate and moderate CYP3A4 inhibitors should be carefully monitored for an extended period of time and dosage increase should be done conservatively).
No products indexed under this heading.

Troleandomycin (The concomitant use of fentanyl citrate with ritonavir or other strong CYP3A4 inhibitors such as ketoconazole, itraconazole, troleandomycin, clarithromycin, nelfinavir, and nefazadone may result in a potentially dangerous increase in fentanyl plasma concentrations. Patients receiving fentanyl citrate and potent CYP3A4 inhibitors should be carefully monitored for an extended period of time and dosage increase should be done conservatively).
No products indexed under this heading.

Valproate Sodium (The concomitant use of moderate CYP3A4 inhibitors such as amprenavir, aprepitant, diltiazem, erythromycin, fluconazole, fosamprenavir, grapefruit juice, and verapamil with fentanyl citrate may result in an increase in fentanyl plasma concentrations, which could increase or prolong adverse drug effects and may cause potentially fatal respiratory depression. Patients receiving fentanyl citrate and moderate CYP3A4 inhibitors should be carefully monitored for an extended period of time and dosage increase should be done conservatively).
No products indexed under this heading.

Vardenafil Hydrochloride (The concomitant use of moderate CYP3A4 inhibitors such as amprenavir, aprepitant, diltiazem, erythromycin, fluconazole, fosamprenavir, grapefruit juice, and verapamil with fentanyl citrate may result in an increase in fentanyl plasma concentrations, which could increase or prolong adverse drug effects and may cause potentially fatal respiratory depression. Patients receiving fentanyl citrate and moderate CYP3A4 inhibitors should be carefully monitored for an extended period of time and dosage increase should be done conservatively). Products include:
Levitra Tablets 2876

Verapamil Hydrochloride (The concomitant use of moderate CYP3A4 inhibitors such as amprenavir, aprepitant, diltiazem, erythromycin, fluconazole, fosamprenavir, grapefruit juice, and verapamil with fentanyl citrate may result in an increase in fentanyl plasma concentrations, which could increase or prolong adverse drug effects and may cause potentially fatal respiratory depression. Patients receiving fentanyl citrate and moderate CYP3A4 inhibitors should be carefully monitored for an extended period of time and dosage increase should be done conservatively). Products include:
Tarka Tablets 511

Voriconazole (The concomitant use of fentanyl citrate with ritonavir or other strong CYP3A4 inhibitors such as ketoconazole, itraconazole, troleandomycin, clarithromycin, nelfinavir, and nefazadone may result in a potentially dangerous increase in fentanyl plasma concentrations. Patients receiving fentanyl citrate and potent CYP3A4 inhibitors should be carefully monitored for an extended period of time and dosage increase should be done conservatively).
No products indexed under this heading.

Zafirlukast (The concomitant use of moderate CYP3A4 inhibitors such as amprenavir, aprepitant, diltiazem, erythromycin, fluconazole, fosamprenavir, grapefruit juice, and verapamil with fentanyl citrate may result in an increase in fentanyl plasma concentrations, which could increase or prolong adverse drug effects and may cause potentially fatal respiratory depression. Patients receiving fentanyl citrate and moderate CYP3A4 inhibitors should be carefully monitored for an extended period of time and dosage increase should be done conservatively). Products include:
Accolate Tablets 669

Zaleplon (The concomitant use of other CNS depressants, including other opioids, sedatives or hypnotics, general anesthetics, phenothiazines, tranquilizers, skeletal muscle relaxants, sedating antihistamines, potent inhibitors of cytochrome P450 3A4 isoform (e.g.,erythromycin, ketoconazole, and certain protease inhibitors), and alcoholic beverages may produce increased depressant effects. Hypoventilation, hypotension, and profound sedation may occur).
No products indexed under this heading.

Zileuton (The concomitant use of moderate CYP3A4 inhibitors such as amprenavir, aprepitant, diltiazem, erythromycin, fluconazole, fosamprenavir, grapefruit juice, and verapamil with fentanyl citrate may result in an increase in fentanyl plasma concentrations, which could increase or prolong adverse drug effects and may cause potentially fatal respiratory depression. Patients receiving fentanyl citrate and moderate CYP3A4 inhibitors should be carefully monitored for an extended period of time and dosage increase should be done conservatively).
No products indexed under this heading.

Ziprasidone Hydrochloride (The concomitant use of other CNS depressants, including other opioids, sedatives or hypnotics, general anesthetics, phenothiazines, tranquilizers, skeletal muscle relaxants, sedating antihistamines, potent inhibitors of cytochrome P450 3A4 isoform (e.g.,erythromycin, ketoconazole, and certain protease inhibitors), and alcoholic beverages may produce increased depressant effects. Hypoventilation, hypotension, and profound sedation may occur). Products include:

Geodon Capsules **2520**

Zolpidem Tartrate (The concomitant use of other CNS depressants, including other opioids, sedatives or hypnotics, general anesthetics, phenothiazines, tranquilizers, skeletal muscle relaxants, sedating antihistamines, potent inhibitors of cytochrome P450 3A4 isotorm (e.g.,erythromycin, ketoconazole, and certain protease inhibitors), and alcoholic beverages may produce increased depressant effects. Hypoventilation, hypotension, and profound sedation may occur). Products include:

Ambien Tablets **2692**
Ambien CR Tablets **2696**

Food Interactions

Alcohol (The concomitant use of other CNS depressants, including alcoholic beverages, may produce increased depressant effects. Hypoventilation, hypotension, and profound sedation may occur).

Grapefruit (The concomitant use of moderate CYP3A4 inhibitors such as amprenavir, aprepitant, diltiazem, erythromycin, fluconazole, fosamprenavir, grapefruit juice, and verapamil with fentanyl citrate may result in an increase in fentanyl plasma concentrations, which could increase or prolong adverse drug effects and may cause potentially fatal respiratory depression. Patients receiving fentanyl citrate and moderate CYP3A4 inhibitors should be carefully monitored for an extended period of time and dosage increase should be done conservatively).

Grapefruit Juice (The concomitant use of moderate CYP3A4 inhibitors such as amprenavir, aprepitant, diltiazem, erythromycin, fluconazole, fosamprenavir, grapefruit juice, and verapamil with fentanyl citrate may result in an increase in fentanyl plasma concentrations, which could increase or prolong adverse drug effects and may cause potentially fatal respiratory depression. Patients receiving fentanyl citrate and moderate CYP3A4 inhibitors should be carefully monitored for an extended period of time and dosage increase should be done conservatively).

FERRALET 90 TABLETS

(Docusate Sodium, Folic Acid, Iron Carbonyl, Vitamin B_{12}, Vitamin C)........ **2175**
None cited in PDR database.

FIBRINASE DIETARY SUPPLEMENT

(Dehydroepiandrosterone, Herbal Medicines, unspecified, Vitex agnus-castus).................................. **995**
None cited in PDR database.

FINACEA GEL

(Azelaic Acid) **1742**
None cited in PDR database.

FLEBOGAMMA 5%

(Globulin, Immune (Human)) **1715**
May interact with vaccines, live. Compounds in these categories include:

BCG Vaccine (Antibodies in immune globulin intravenous (Human) may interfere with the responses to live viral vaccines, such as measles, mumps, and rubella. Physicians should be informed of recent therapy with immune globulin intravenous (Human) so that administration of live viral vaccines, if indicated, can be appropriately delayed 3 or more months from the time of IGIV administration).

No products indexed under this heading.

Influenza Vaccine, Live Attenuated (Antibodies in immune globulin intravenous (Human) may interfere with the responses to live viral vaccines, such as measles, mumps, and rubella. Physicians should be informed of recent therapy with immune globulin intravenous (Human) so that administration of live viral vaccines, if indicated, can be appropriately delayed 3 or more months from the time of IGIV administration).

No products indexed under this heading.

Influenza Virus Vaccine Live, Intranasal (Antibodies in immune globulin intravenous (Human) may interfere with the responses to live viral vaccines, such as measles, mumps, and rubella. Physicians should be informed of recent therapy with immune globulin intravenous (Human) so that administration of live viral vaccines, if indicated, can be appropriately delayed 3 or more months from the time of IGIV administration). Products include:

FluMist Vaccine **1945**

Measles, Mumps, Rubella and Varicella Virus Vaccine Live (Antibodies in immune globulin intravenous (Human) may interfere with the responses to live viral vaccines, such as measles, mumps, and rubella. Physicians should be informed of recent therapy with immune globulin intravenous (Human) so that administration of live viral vaccines, if indicated, can be appropriately delayed 3 or more months from the time of IGIV administration). Products include:

ProQuad **2099**

Measles, Mumps & Rubella Virus Vaccine, Live (Antibodies in immune globulin intravenous (Human) may interfere with the responses to live viral vaccines, such as measles, mumps, and rubella. Physicians should be informed of recent therapy with immune globulin intravenous (Human) so that administration of live viral vaccines, if indicated, can be appropriately delayed 3 or more months from the time of IGIV administration). Products include:

M-M-R II **2054**

Measles & Rubella Virus Vaccine Live (Antibodies in immune globulin intravenous (Human) may interfere with the responses to live viral vaccines, such as measles, mumps, and rubella. Physicians should be informed of recent therapy with immune globulin intravenous (Human) so that administration of live viral vaccines, if indicated, can be appropriately delayed 3 or more months from the time of IGIV administration).

No products indexed under this heading.

Measles Virus Vaccine Live (Antibodies in immune globulin intravenous (Human) may interfere with the responses to live viral vaccines, such as measles, mumps, and rubella. Physicians should be informed of recent therapy with immune globulin intravenous (Human) so that administration of live viral vaccines, if indicated, can be appropriately delayed 3 or more months from the time of IGIV administration). Products include:

Attenuvax **1951**

Mumps Virus Vaccine, Live (Antibodies in immune globulin intravenous (Human) may interfere with the responses to live viral vaccines, such as measles, mumps, and rubella. Physicians should be informed of recent therapy with immune globulin intravenous (Human) so that administration of live viral vaccines, if indicated, can be appropriately delayed 3 or more months from the time of IGIV administration). Products include:

Mumpsvax **2068**

Poliovirus Vaccine, Live, Oral, Trivalent, Types 1,2,3 (Sabin) (Antibodies in immune globulin intravenous (Human) may interfere with the responses to live viral vaccines, such as measles, mumps, and rubella. Physicians should be informed of recent therapy with immune globulin intravenous (Human) so that administration of live viral vaccines, if indicated, can be appropriately delayed 3 or more months from the time of IGIV administration).

No products indexed under this heading.

Rotavirus Vaccine, Live, Oral, Tetravalent (Antibodies in immune globulin intravenous (Human) may interfere with the responses to live viral vaccines, such as measles, mumps, and rubella. Physicians should be informed of recent therapy with immune globulin intravenous (Human) so that administration of live viral vaccines, if indicated, can be appropriately delayed 3 or more months from the time of IGIV administration).

No products indexed under this heading.

Rubella & Mumps Virus Vaccine Live (Antibodies in immune globulin intravenous (Human) may interfere with the responses to live viral vaccines, such as measles, mumps, and rubella. Physicians should be informed of recent therapy with immune globulin intravenous (Human) so that administration of live viral vaccines, if indicated, can be appropriately delayed 3 or more months from the time of IGIV administration).

No products indexed under this heading.

Rubella Virus Vaccine Live (Antibodies in immune globulin intravenous (Human) may interfere with the responses to live viral vaccines, such as measles, mumps, and rubella. Physicians should be informed of recent therapy with immune globulin intravenous (Human) so that administration of live viral vaccines, if indicated, can be appropriately delayed 3 or more months from the time of IGIV administration). Products include:

Meruvax II **2061**

Smallpox Vaccine (Antibodies in immune globulin intravenous (Human) may interfere with the responses to live viral vaccines, such as measles, mumps, and rubella. Physicians should be informed of recent therapy with immune globulin intravenous (Human) so that administration of live viral vaccines, if indicated, can be appropriately delayed 3 or more months from the time of IGIV administration).

No products indexed under this heading.

Typhoid Vaccine (Antibodies in immune globulin intravenous (Human) may interfere with the responses to live viral vaccines, such as measles, mumps, and rubella. Physicians should be informed of recent therapy with immune globulin intravenous (Human) so that administration of live viral vaccines, if indicated, can be appropriately delayed 3 or more months from the time of IGIV administration).

No products indexed under this heading.

Varicella Virus Vaccine Live (Antibodies in immune globulin intravenous (Human) may interfere with the responses to live viral vaccines, such as measles, mumps, and rubella. Physicians should be informed of recent therapy with immune globulin intravenous (Human) so that administration of live viral vaccines, if indicated, can be appropriately delayed 3 or more months from the time of IGIV administration). Products include:

Varivax **2133**

Yellow Fever Vaccine (Antibodies in immune globulin intravenous (Human) may interfere with the responses to live viral vaccines, such as measles, mumps, and rubella. Physicians should be informed of recent therapy with immune globulin intravenous (Human) so that administration of live viral vaccines, if indicated, can be appropriately delayed 3 or more months from the time of IGIV administration).

No products indexed under this heading.

Zoster Vaccine Live (Antibodies in immune globulin intravenous (Human) may interfere with the responses to live viral vaccines, such as measles, mumps, and rubella. Physicians should be informed of recent therapy with immune globulin intravenous (Human) so that administration of live viral vaccines, if indicated, can be appropriately delayed 3 or more months from the time of IGIV administration). Products include:

Zostavax Injection **2145**

FLEBOGAMMA 5% DIF

(Immune Globulin Intravenous (Human))... **1718**
May interact with vaccines, live. Compounds in these categories include:

BCG Vaccine (Antibodies in immune globulin intravenous (Human) may interfere with the responses to live viral vaccines, such as measles, mumps, and rubella. Physicians should be informed of recent therapy with immune globulin intravenous (Human) so that administration of live viral vaccines, if indicated, can be appropriately delayed 3 or more months from the time of IGIV administration).

No products indexed under this heading.

Influenza Vaccine, Live Attenuated (Antibodies in immune globulin intravenous (Human) may interfere with the responses to live viral vaccines, such as measles, mumps, and rubella. Physicians should be informed of recent therapy with immune globulin intravenous (Human) so that administration of live viral vaccines, if indicated, can be appropriately delayed 3 or more months from the time of IGIV administration).

No products indexed under this heading.

Influenza Virus Vaccine Live, Intranasal (Antibodies in immune globulin intravenous (Human) may interfere with the responses to live viral vaccines, such as measles, mumps, and rubella. Physicians should be informed of recent therapy with immune globulin intravenous (Human) so that administration of live viral vaccines, if indicated, can be appropriately delayed 3 or more months from the time of IGIV administration). Products include:

FluMist Vaccine 1945

Measles, Mumps, Rubella and Varicella Virus Vaccine Live (Antibodies in immune globulin intravenous (Human) may interfere with the responses to live viral vaccines, such as measles, mumps, and rubella. Physicians should be informed of recent therapy with immune globulin intravenous (Human) so that administration of live viral vaccines, if indicated, can be appropriately delayed 3 or more months from the time of IGIV administration). Products include:

ProQuad 2099

Measles, Mumps & Rubella Virus Vaccine, Live (Antibodies in immune globulin intravenous (Human) may interfere with the responses to live viral vaccines, such as measles, mumps, and rubella. Physicians should be informed of recent therapy with immune globulin intravenous (Human) so that administration of live viral vaccines, if indicated, can be appropriately delayed 3 or more months from the time of IGIV administration). Products include:

M-M-R II 2054

Measles & Rubella Virus Vaccine Live (Antibodies in immune globulin intravenous (Human) may interfere with the responses to live viral vaccines, such as measles, mumps, and rubella. Physicians should be informed of recent therapy with immune globulin intravenous (Human) so that administration of live viral vaccines, if indicated, can be appropriately delayed 3 or more months from the time of IGIV administration).

No products indexed under this heading.

Measles Virus Vaccine Live (Antibodies in immune globulin intravenous (Human) may interfere with the responses to live viral vaccines, such as measles, mumps, and rubella. Physicians should be informed of recent therapy with immune globulin intravenous (Human) so that administration of live viral vaccines, if indicated, can be appropriately delayed 3 or more months from the time of IGIV administration). Products include:

Attenuvax 1951

Mumps Virus Vaccine, Live (Antibodies in immune globulin intravenous (Human) may interfere with the responses to live viral vaccines, such as measles, mumps, and rubella. Physicians should be informed of recent therapy with immune globulin intravenous (Human) so that administration of live viral vaccines, if indicated, can be appropriately delayed 3 or more months from the time of IGIV administration). Products include:

Mumpsvax 2068

Poliovirus Vaccine, Live, Oral, Trivalent, Types 1,2,3 (Sabin) (Antibodies in immune globulin intravenous (Human) may interfere with the responses to live viral vaccines, such as measles, mumps, and rubella. Physicians should be informed of recent therapy with immune globulin intravenous (Human) so that administration of live viral vaccines, if indicated, can be appropriately delayed 3 or more months from the time of IGIV administration).

No products indexed under this heading.

Rotavirus Vaccine, Live, Oral, Tetravalent (Antibodies in immune globulin intravenous (Human) may interfere with the responses to live viral vaccines, such as measles, mumps, and rubella. Physicians should be informed of recent therapy with immune globulin intravenous (Human) so that administration of live viral vaccines, if indicated, can be appropriately delayed 3 or more months from the time of IGIV administration).

No products indexed under this heading.

Rubella & Mumps Virus Vaccine Live (Antibodies in immune globulin intravenous (Human) may interfere with the responses to live viral vaccines, such as measles, mumps, and rubella. Physicians should be informed of recent therapy with immune globulin intravenous (Human) so that administration of live viral vaccines, if indicated, can be appropriately delayed 3 or more months from the time of IGIV administration).

No products indexed under this heading.

Rubella Virus Vaccine Live (Antibodies in immune globulin intravenous (Human) may interfere with the responses to live viral vaccines, such as measles, mumps, and rubella. Physicians should be informed of recent therapy with immune globulin intravenous (Human) so that administration of live viral vaccines, if indicated, can be appropriately delayed 3 or more months from the time of IGIV administration). Products include:

Meruvax II 2061

Smallpox Vaccine (Antibodies in immune globulin intravenous (Human) may interfere with the responses to live viral vaccines, such as measles, mumps, and rubella. Physicians should be informed of recent therapy with immune globulin intravenous (Human) so that administration of live viral vaccines, if indicated, can be appropriately delayed 3 or more months from the time of IGIV administration).

No products indexed under this heading.

Typhoid Vaccine (Antibodies in immune globulin intravenous (Human) may interfere with the responses to live viral vaccines, such as measles, mumps, and rubella. Physicians should be informed of recent therapy with immune globulin intravenous (Human) so that administration of live viral vaccines, if indicated, can be appropriately delayed 3 or more months from the time of IGIV administration).

No products indexed under this heading.

Varicella Virus Vaccine Live (Antibodies in immune globulin intravenous (Human) may interfere with the responses to live viral vaccines, such as measles, mumps, and rubella. Physicians should be informed of recent therapy with immune globulin intravenous (Human) so that administration of live viral vaccines, if indicated, can be appropriately delayed 3 or more months from the time of IGIV administration). Products include:

Varivax 2133

Yellow Fever Vaccine (Antibodies in immune globulin intravenous (Human) may interfere with the responses to live viral vaccines, such as measles, mumps, and rubella. Physicians should be informed of recent therapy with immune globulin intravenous (Human) so that administration of live viral vaccines, if indicated, can be appropriately delayed 3 or more months from the time of IGIV administration).

No products indexed under this heading.

Zoster Vaccine Live (Antibodies in immune globulin intravenous (Human) may interfere with the responses to live viral vaccines, such as measles, mumps, and rubella. Physicians should be informed of recent therapy with immune globulin intravenous (Human) so that administration of live viral vaccines, if indicated, can be appropriately delayed 3 or more months from the time of IGIV administration). Products include:

Zostavax Injection 2145

FLECTOR PATCH

(Diclofenac Epolamine) 561

May interact with ACE inhibitors, aspirin-acetylsalicylic acid, lithium preparations, thiazides, and certain other agents. Compounds in these categories include:

Aspirin (When diclofenac epolamine is administered with aspirin, the binding of diclofenac to protein is reduced, although the clearance of free diclofenac is not altered. The clinical significance of this interaction is not known; however, as with other NSAIDs, concomitant administration of diclofenac and aspirin is not generally recommended because of the potential of increased adverse effects). Products include:

Aggrenox Capsules 819
Bayer Aspirin 750
Percodan Tablets 1130
St. Joseph 81 mg Aspirin Chewable and Enteric Coated Tablets 1903

Aspirin, Enteric Coated (When diclofenac epolamine is administered with aspirin, the binding of diclofenac to protein is reduced, although the clearance of free diclofenac is not altered. The clinical significance of this interaction is not known; however, as with other NSAIDs, concomitant administration of diclofenac and aspirin is not generally recommended because of the potential of increased adverse effects).

No products indexed under this heading.

Aspirin Buffered (When diclofenac epolamine is administered with aspirin, the binding of diclofenac to protein is reduced, although the clearance of free diclofenac is not altered. The clinical significance of this interaction is not known; however, as with other NSAIDs, concomitant administration of diclofenac and aspirin is not generally recommended because of the potential of increased adverse effects).

No products indexed under this heading.

Benazepril Hydrochloride (Reports suggest that NSAIDs may diminish the antihypertensive effect of ACE-inhibitors. This interaction should be given consideration in patients taking NSAIDs concomitantly with ACE-inhibitors).

No products indexed under this heading.

Bendroflumethiazide (Clinical studies, as well as post-marketing observations, have shown that diclofenac epolamine may reduce the natriuretic effect of furosemide and thiazides in some patients. This response has been attributed to inhibition of renal prostaglandin synthesis. During concomitant therapy with NSAIDs, the patient should be ovserved clsoely for signs of renal failure, as well as to assure diuretic efficacy).

No products indexed under this heading.

Captopril (Reports suggest that NSAIDs may diminish the antihypertensive effect of ACE-inhibitors. This interaction should be given consideration in patients taking NSAIDs concomitantly with ACE-inhibitors). Products include:

Captopril Tablets 2182

Chlorothiazide (Clinical studies, as well as post-marketing observations, have shown that diclofenac epolamine may reduce the natriuretic effect of furosemide and thiazides in some patients. This response has been attributed to inhibition of renal prostaglandin synthesis. During concomitant therapy with NSAIDs, the patient should be ovserved clsoely for signs of renal failure, as well as to assure diuretic efficacy).

No products indexed under this heading.

Chlorothiazide Sodium (Clinical studies, as well as post-marketing observations, have shown that diclofenac epolamine may reduce the natriuretic effect of furosemide and thiazides in some patients. This response has been attributed to inhibition of renal prostaglandin synthesis. During concomitant therapy with NSAIDs, the patient should be ovserved clsoely for signs of renal failure, as well as to assure diuretic efficacy). Products include:

Intravenous Sodium Diuril 2490

Enalapril Maleate (Reports suggest that NSAIDs may diminish the antihypertensive effect of ACE-inhibitors. This interaction should be given consideration in patients taking NSAIDs concomitantly with ACE-inhibitors).

No products indexed under this heading.

Enalaprilat (Reports suggest that NSAIDs may diminish the antihypertensive effect of ACE-inhibitors. This interaction should be given consideration in patients taking NSAIDs concomitantly with ACE-inhibitors).

No products indexed under this heading.

Fosinopril Sodium (Reports suggest that NSAIDs may diminish the antihypertensive effect of ACE-inhibitors. This interaction should be given consideration in patients taking NSAIDs concomitantly with ACE-inhibitors).

No products indexed under this heading.

Furosemide (Clinical studies, as well as post-marketing observations, have shown that diclofenac epolamine may reduce the natriuretic effect of furosemide and thiazides in some patients. This response has been attributed to inhibition of renal prostaglandin synthesis. During concomitant therapy with NSAIDs, the patient should be observed closely for signs of renal failure, as well as to assure diuretic efficacy). Products include:

Furosemide Tablets 2186

Hydrochlorothiazide (Clinical studies, as well as post-marketing observations, have shown that diclofenac epolamine may reduce the natriuretic effect of furosemide and thiazides in some patients. This response has been attributed to inhibition of renal prostaglandin synthesis. During concomitant therapy with NSAIDs, the patient should be ovserved clsoely for signs of renal failure, as well as to assure diuretic efficacy). Products include:

Atacand HCT 642
Avalide Tablets 892
Avalide Tablets 2713
Benicar HCT Tablets 1010
Diovan HCT Tablets 2216
Dyazide Capsules 1405
Micardis HCT Tablets 854
Prinzide Tablets 2092
Tekturna HCT Tablets 2324
Teveten HCT Tablets 517

Hydroflumethiazide (Clinical studies, as well as post-marketing observations, have shown that diclofenac epolamine may reduce the natriuretic effect of furosemide and thiazides in some patients. This response has been attributed to inhibition of renal prostaglandin synthesis. During concomitant therapy with NSAIDs, the patient should be ovserved clsoely for signs of renal failure, as well as to assure diuretic efficacy).

No products indexed under this heading.

Lisinopril (Reports suggest that NSAIDs may diminish the antihypertensive effect of ACE-inhibitors. This interaction should be given consideration in patients taking NSAIDs concomitantly with ACE-inhibitors). Products include:

Prinivil Tablets 2087
Prinzide Tablets 2092

Lithium (NSAIDs have produced an elevation of plasma lithium levels and a reduction in renal lithium clearance. The mean minimum lithium concentration increased 15% and the renal clearance was decreased by approximately 20%. These effects have been attributed to inhibition of renal prostaglandin synthesis by the NSAID. Thus, when NSAIDs and lithium are administered concurrently, subjects should be observed carefully for signs of lithium toxicity).

No products indexed under this heading.

Lithium Carbonate (NSAIDs have produced an elevation of plasma lithium levels and a reduction in renal lithium clearance. The mean minimum lithium concentration increased 15% and the renal clearance was decreased by approximately 20%. These effects have been attributed to inhibition of renal prostaglandin synthesis by the NSAID. Thus, when NSAIDs and lithium are administered concurrently, subjects should be observed carefully for signs of lithium toxicity).

No products indexed under this heading.

Lithium Citrate (NSAIDs have produced an elevation of plasma lithium levels and a reduction in renal lithium clearance. The mean minimum lithium concentration increased 15% and the renal clearance was decreased by approximately 20%. These effects have been attributed to inhibition of renal prostaglandin synthesis by the NSAID. Thus, when NSAIDs and lithium are administered concurrently, subjects should be observed carefully for signs of lithium toxicity).

No products indexed under this heading.

Methotrexate (NSAIDs have been reported to competitively inhibit methotrexate accumulation in rabbit kidney slices. This may indicate that they could enhance the toxicity of methotrexate. Caution should be used when NSAIDs are administered concomitantly with methotrexate).

No products indexed under this heading.

Methotrexate Sodium (NSAIDs have been reported to competitively inhibit methotrexate accumulation in rabbit kidney slices. This may indicate that they could enhance the toxicity of methotrexate. Caution should be used when NSAIDs are administered concomitantly with methotrexate).

No products indexed under this heading.

Methyclothiazide (Clinical studies, as well as post-marketing observations, have shown that diclofenac epolamine may reduce the natriuretic effect of furosemide and thiazides in some patients. This response has been attributed to inhibition of renal prostaglandin synthesis. During concomitant therapy with NSAIDs, the patient should be ovserved clsoely for signs of renal failure, as well as to assure diuretic efficacy).

No products indexed under this heading.

Moexipril Hydrochloride (Reports suggest that NSAIDs may diminish the antihypertensive effect of ACE-inhibitors. This interaction should be given consideration in patients taking NSAIDs concomitantly with ACE-inhibitors).

No products indexed under this heading.

Perindopril Erbumine (Reports suggest that NSAIDs may diminish the antihypertensive effect of ACE-inhibitors. This interaction should be given consideration in patients taking NSAIDs concomitantly with ACE-inhibitors). Products include:

Aceon Tablets (2 mg, 4 mg, 8 mg) 3038

Polythiazide (Clinical studies, as well as post-marketing observations, have shown that diclofenac epolamine may reduce the natriuretic effect of furosemide and thiazides in some patients. This response has been attributed to inhibition of renal prostaglandin synthesis. During concomitant therapy with NSAIDs, the patient should be ovserved clsoely for signs of renal failure, as well as to assure diuretic efficacy).

No products indexed under this heading.

Quinapril Hydrochloride (Reports suggest that NSAIDs may diminish the antihypertensive effect of ACE-inhibitors. This interaction should be given consideration in patients taking NSAIDs concomitantly with ACE-inhibitors).

No products indexed under this heading.

Ramipril (Reports suggest that NSAIDs may diminish the antihypertensive effect of ACE-inhibitors. This interaction should be given consideration in patients taking NSAIDs concomitantly with ACE-inhibitors).

No products indexed under this heading.

Spirapril Hydrochloride (Reports suggest that NSAIDs may diminish the antihypertensive effect of ACE-inhibitors. This interaction should be given consideration in patients taking NSAIDs concomitantly with ACE-inhibitors).

No products indexed under this heading.

Trandolapril (Reports suggest that NSAIDs may diminish the antihypertensive effect of ACE-inhibitors. This interaction should be given consideration in patients taking NSAIDs concomitantly with ACE-inhibitors). Products include:

Mavik Tablets 472
Tarka Tablets 511

Warfarin Sodium (The effects of warfarin and NSAIDS of GI bleeding are synergistic, such that users of both drugs together have a risk of serious GI bleeding higher than users of either drug alone).

No products indexed under this heading.

FLEET BABYLAX SUPPOSITORIES

(Glycerin) 1142

None cited in PDR database.

FLEET BISACODYL LAXATIVES

(Bisacodyl) 1143

None cited in PDR database.

FLEET ENEMA

(Sodium Phosphate) 1143

May interact with ACE inhibitors, angiotensin-II receptor antagonists, diuretics, lithium preparations, nonsteroidal anti-inflammatory agents, and oral phosphate supplements. Compounds in these categories include:

Amiloride Hydrochloride (Electrolyte disturbances are a risk associated with this product; concurrent use in patients taking agents known to disturb electrolytes balance requires caution).

No products indexed under this heading.

Benazepril Hydrochloride (Electrolyte disturbances are a risk associated with this product; concurrent use in patients taking agents known to disturb electrolytes balance requires caution).

No products indexed under this heading.

Bendroflumethiazide (Electrolyte disturbances are a risk associated with this product; concurrent use in patients taking agents known to disturb electrolytes balance requires caution).

No products indexed under this heading.

Bumetanide (Electrolyte disturbances are a risk associated with this product; concurrent use in patients taking agents known to disturb electrolytes balance requires caution).

No products indexed under this heading.

Candesartan Cilexetil (Electrolyte disturbances are a risk associated with this product; concurrent use in patients taking agents known to disturb electrolytes balance requires caution). Products include:

Atacand Tablets 639
Atacand HCT 642

Captopril (Electrolyte disturbances are a risk associated with this product; concurrent use in patients taking agents known to disturb electrolytes balance requires caution). Products include:

Captopril Tablets 2182

Celecoxib (Electrolyte disturbances are a risk associated with this product; concurrent use in patients taking agents known to disturb electrolytes balance requires caution). Products include:

Celebrex Capsules 2979

Chlorothiazide (Electrolyte disturbances are a risk associated with this product; concurrent use in patients taking agents known to disturb electrolytes balance requires caution).

No products indexed under this heading.

Chlorothiazide Sodium (Electrolyte disturbances are a risk associated with this product; concurrent use in patients taking agents known to disturb electrolytes balance requires caution). Products include:

Intravenous Sodium Diuril 2490

Chlorthalidone (Electrolyte disturbances are a risk associated with this product; concurrent use in patients taking agents known to disturb electrolytes balance requires caution). Products include:

Clorpres Tablets 2185

Diclofenac Epolamine (Electrolyte disturbances are a risk associated with this product; concurrent use in

patients taking agents known to disturb electrolytes balance requires caution). Products include:
- Flector Patch 561

Diclofenac Potassium (Electrolyte disturbances are a risk associated with this product; concurrent use in patients taking agents known to disturb electrolytes balance requires caution).
- No products indexed under this heading.

Diclofenac Sodium (Electrolyte disturbances are a risk associated with this product; concurrent use in patients taking agents known to disturb electrolytes balance requires caution). Products include:
- Diclofenac Sodium Ophthalmic Solution .... ⊙ 240
- Voltaren Ophthalmic Solution 2336
- Voltaren Tablets 2334
- Voltaren-XR Tablets 2337

Enalapril Maleate (Electrolyte disturbances are a risk associated with this product; concurrent use in patients taking agents known to disturb electrolytes balance requires caution).
- No products indexed under this heading.

Enalaprilat (Electrolyte disturbances are a risk associated with this product; concurrent use in patients taking agents known to disturb electrolytes balance requires caution).
- No products indexed under this heading.

Eprosartan Mesylate (Electrolyte disturbances are a risk associated with this product; concurrent use in patients taking agents known to disturb electrolytes balance requires caution). Products include:
- Teveten Tablets 515
- Teveten HCT Tablets 517

Ethacrynic Acid (Electrolyte disturbances are a risk associated with this product; concurrent use in patients taking agents known to disturb electrolytes balance requires caution). Products include:
- Edecrin Tablets 698

Etodolac (Electrolyte disturbances are a risk associated with this product; concurrent use in patients taking agents known to disturb electrolytes balance requires caution).
- No products indexed under this heading.

Fenoprofen Calcium (Electrolyte disturbances are a risk associated with this product; concurrent use in patients taking agents known to disturb electrolytes balance requires caution). Products include:
- Nalfon Capsules 2508

Flurbiprofen (Electrolyte disturbances are a risk associated with this product; concurrent use in patients taking agents known to disturb electrolytes balance requires caution).
- No products indexed under this heading.

Fosinopril Sodium (Electrolyte disturbances are a risk associated with this product; concurrent use in patients taking agents known to disturb electrolytes balance requires caution).
- No products indexed under this heading.

Furosemide (Electrolyte disturbances are a risk associated with this product; concurrent use in patients taking agents known to disturb electrolytes balance requires caution). Products include:
- Furosemide Tablets 2186

Hydrochlorothiazide (Electrolyte disturbances are a risk associated with this product; concurrent use in patients taking agents known to disturb electrolytes balance requires caution). Products include:
- Atacand HCT 642
- Avalide Tablets 892
- Avalide Tablets 2713
- Benicar HCT Tablets 1010
- Diovan HCT Tablets 2216
- Dyazide Capsules 1405
- Micardis HCT Tablets 854
- Prinzide Tablets 2092
- Tekturna HCT Tablets 2324
- Teveten HCT Tablets 517

Hydroflumethiazide (Electrolyte disturbances are a risk associated with this product; concurrent use in patients taking agents known to disturb electrolytes balance requires caution).
- No products indexed under this heading.

Ibuprofen (Electrolyte disturbances are a risk associated with this product; concurrent use in patients taking agents known to disturb electrolytes balance requires caution). Products include:
- Motrin IB Tablets and Caplets 1900
- Children's Motrin Oral Suspension 1901
- Children's Motrin Non-Staining Dye-Free Oral Suspension 1901
- Children's Motrin Cold Oral Suspension 1899
- Infants' Motrin Concentrated Drops 1901
- Infants' Motrin Non-Staining Dye-Free Concentrated Drops 1901
- Junior Strength Motrin Caplets and Chewable Tablets 1901
- Vicoprofen Tablets 533

Indapamide (Electrolyte disturbances are a risk associated with this product; concurrent use in patients taking agents known to disturb electrolytes balance requires caution). Products include:
- Indapamide Tablets 2188

Indomethacin (Electrolyte disturbances are a risk associated with this product; concurrent use in patients taking agents known to disturb electrolytes balance requires caution). Products include:
- Indocin 2024

Indomethacin Sodium Trihydrate (Electrolyte disturbances are a risk associated with this product; concurrent use in patients taking agents known to disturb electrolytes balance requires caution). Products include:
- Indocin I.V. 2489

Irbesartan (Electrolyte disturbances are a risk associated with this product; concurrent use in patients taking agents known to disturb electrolytes balance requires caution). Products include:
- Avalide Tablets 892
- Avalide Tablets 2713
- Avapro Tablets 897
- Avapro Tablets 2718

Ketoprofen (Electrolyte disturbances are a risk associated with this product; concurrent use in patients taking agents known to disturb electrolytes balance requires caution).
- No products indexed under this heading.

Ketorolac Tromethamine (Electrolyte disturbances are a risk associated with this product; concurrent use in patients taking agents known to disturb electrolytes balance requires caution).
- No products indexed under this heading.

Lisinopril (Electrolyte disturbances are a risk associated with this product; concurrent use in patients taking agents known to disturb electrolytes balance requires caution). Products include:
- Prinivil Tablets 2087
- Prinzide Tablets 2092

Lithium (Electrolyte disturbances are a risk associated with this product; concurrent use in patients taking agents known to disturb electrolytes balance requires caution).
- No products indexed under this heading.

Lithium Carbonate (Electrolyte disturbances are a risk associated with this product; concurrent use in patients taking agents known to disturb electrolytes balance requires caution).
- No products indexed under this heading.

Lithium Citrate (Electrolyte disturbances are a risk associated with this product; concurrent use in patients taking agents known to disturb electrolytes balance requires caution).
- No products indexed under this heading.

Losartan Potassium (Electrolyte disturbances are a risk associated with this product; concurrent use in patients taking agents known to disturb electrolytes balance requires caution). Products include:
- Cozaar Tablets 1973

Meclofenamate Sodium (Electrolyte disturbances are a risk associated with this product; concurrent use in patients taking agents known to disturb electrolytes balance requires caution).
- No products indexed under this heading.

Mefenamic Acid (Electrolyte disturbances are a risk associated with this product; concurrent use in patients taking agents known to disturb electrolytes balance requires caution).
- No products indexed under this heading.

Meloxicam (Electrolyte disturbances are a risk associated with this product; concurrent use in patients taking agents known to disturb electrolytes balance requires caution). Products include:
- Mobic Oral Suspension 863
- Mobic Tablets 863

Methyclothiazide (Electrolyte disturbances are a risk associated with this product; concurrent use in patients taking agents known to disturb electrolytes balance requires caution).
- No products indexed under this heading.

Metolazone (Electrolyte disturbances are a risk associated with this product; concurrent use in patients taking agents known to disturb electrolytes balance requires caution).
- No products indexed under this heading.

Moexipril Hydrochloride (Electrolyte disturbances are a risk associated with this product; concurrent use in patients taking agents known to disturb electrolytes balance requires caution).
- No products indexed under this heading.

Nabumetone (Electrolyte disturbances are a risk associated with this product; concurrent use in patients taking agents known to disturb electrolytes balance requires caution).
- No products indexed under this heading.

Naproxen (Electrolyte disturbances are a risk associated with this product; concurrent use in patients taking agents known to disturb electrolytes balance requires caution). Products include:
- EC-Naprosyn Delayed-Release Tablets 2632
- Naprosyn Suspension 2632
- Naprosyn Tablets 2632

Naproxen Sodium (Electrolyte disturbances are a risk associated with this product; concurrent use in patients taking agents known to disturb electrolytes balance requires caution). Products include:
- Anaprox Tablets 2632
- Anaprox DS Tablets 2632
- Treximet Tablets 1616

Oxaprozin (Electrolyte disturbances are a risk associated with this product; concurrent use in patients taking agents known to disturb electrolytes balance requires caution).
- No products indexed under this heading.

Perindopril Erbumine (Electrolyte disturbances are a risk associated with this product; concurrent use in patients taking agents known to disturb electrolytes balance requires caution). Products include:
- Aceon Tablets (2 mg, 4 mg, 8 mg) 3038

Phenylbutazone (Electrolyte disturbances are a risk associated with this product; concurrent use in patients taking agents known to disturb electrolytes balance requires caution).
- No products indexed under this heading.

Piroxicam (Electrolyte disturbances are a risk associated with this product; concurrent use in patients taking agents known to disturb electrolytes balance requires caution).
- No products indexed under this heading.

Polythiazide (Electrolyte disturbances are a risk associated with this product; concurrent use in patients taking agents known to disturb electrolytes balance requires caution).
- No products indexed under this heading.

Potassium Phosphate (No oral phosphate supplements or other sodium preparations including sodium phosphates-based enemas or tablets should be given concomitantly). Products include:
- K-Phos Neutral Tablets 813

Quinapril Hydrochloride (Electrolyte disturbances are a risk associated with this product; concurrent use in patients taking agents known to disturb electrolytes balance requires caution).
- No products indexed under this heading.

Ramipril (Electrolyte disturbances are a risk associated with this product; concurrent use in patients taking agents known to disturb electrolytes balance requires caution).
No products indexed under this heading.

Rofecoxib (Electrolyte disturbances are a risk associated with this product; concurrent use in patients taking agents known to disturb electrolytes balance requires caution).
No products indexed under this heading.

Spirapril Hydrochloride (Electrolyte disturbances are a risk associated with this product; concurrent use in patients taking agents known to disturb electrolytes balance requires caution).
No products indexed under this heading.

Spironolactone (Electrolyte disturbances are a risk associated with this product; concurrent use in patients taking agents known to disturb electrolytes balance requires caution).
No products indexed under this heading.

Sulindac (Electrolyte disturbances are a risk associated with this product; concurrent use in patients taking agents known to disturb electrolytes balance requires caution). Products include:
Clinoril Tablets 1962

Telmisartan (Electrolyte disturbances are a risk associated with this product; concurrent use in patients taking agents known to disturb electrolytes balance requires caution). Products include:
Micardis Tablets 852
Micardis HCT Tablets 854

Tolmetin Sodium (Electrolyte disturbances are a risk associated with this product; concurrent use in patients taking agents known to disturb electrolytes balance requires caution).
No products indexed under this heading.

Torsemide (Electrolyte disturbances are a risk associated with this product; concurrent use in patients taking agents known to disturb electrolytes balance requires caution). Products include:
Demadex Injection 2630
Demadex Tablets 2630

Trandolapril (Electrolyte disturbances are a risk associated with this product; concurrent use in patients taking agents known to disturb electrolytes balance requires caution). Products include:
Mavik Tablets 472
Tarka Tablets 511

Triamterene (Electrolyte disturbances are a risk associated with this product; concurrent use in patients taking agents known to disturb electrolytes balance requires caution). Products include:
Dyazide Capsules 1405
Dyrenium Capsules 3189

Valdecoxib (Electrolyte disturbances are a risk associated with this product; concurrent use in patients taking agents known to disturb electrolytes balance requires caution).
No products indexed under this heading.

Valsartan (Electrolyte disturbances are a risk associated with this product; concurrent use in patients taking agents known to disturb electrolytes balance requires caution). Products include:
Diovan Tablets 2212
Diovan HCT Tablets 2216
Exforge Tablets 2238

FLEET ENEMA EXTRA
(Sodium Phosphate) 1143
See Fleet Enema

FLEET ENEMA FOR CHILDREN
(Sodium Phosphate) 1143
See Fleet Enema

FLEET GLYCERIN LAXATIVES
(Glycerin) 1142
None cited in PDR database.

FLEET GLYCERIN SUPPOSITORIES
(Glycerin) 1142
None cited in PDR database.

FLEET MINERAL OIL ENEMA
(Mineral Oil) 1144
None cited in PDR database.

FLEET PEDIA-LAX CHEWABLE TABLETS
(Magnesium Hydroxide) 1145
None cited in PDR database.

FLEET PEDIA-LAX ENEMA
(Dibasic Sodium Phosphate, Monobasic Sodium Phosphate).......... ▣606
None cited in PDR database.

FLEET PEDIA-LAX ENEMA
(Sodium Phosphate) 1143
May interact with ACE inhibitors, angiotensin-II receptor antagonists, diuretics, lithium preparations, nonsteroidal anti-inflammatory agents, and oral phosphate supplements. Compounds in these categories include:

Amiloride Hydrochloride (Electrolyte disturbances are a risk associated with this product. Concurrent use of medications that may affect electrolyte levels, such as diuretics, may be associated with acute renal failure and requires caution).
No products indexed under this heading.

Benazepril Hydrochloride (Electrolyte disturbances are a risk associated with this product. Concurrent use of medications that may affect electrolyte levels, such as angiotensen converting enzyme inhibitors (ACE-Is), may be associated with acute renal failure and requires caution).
No products indexed under this heading.

Bendroflumethiazide (Electrolyte disturbances are a risk associated with this product. Concurrent use of medications that may affect electrolyte levels, such as diuretics, may be associated with acute renal failure and requires caution).
No products indexed under this heading.

Bumetanide (Electrolyte disturbances are a risk associated with this product. Concurrent use of medications that may affect electrolyte levels, such as diuretics, may be associated with acute renal failure and requires caution).
No products indexed under this heading.

Candesartan Cilexetil (Electrolyte disturbances are a risk associated with this product. Concurrent use of medications that may affect electrolyte levels, such as angiotensen receptor blockers (ARBs), may be associated with acute renal failure and requires caution). Products include:
Atacand Tablets 639
Atacand HCT 642

Captopril (Electrolyte disturbances are a risk associated with this product. Concurrent use of medications that may affect electrolyte levels, such as angiotensen converting enzyme inhibitors (ACE-Is), may be associated with acute renal failure and requires caution). Products include:
Captopril Tablets 2182

Celecoxib (Electrolyte disturbances are a risk associated with this product. Concurrent use of medications that may affect electrolyte levels, such as NSAIDs, may be associated with acute renal failure). Products include:
Celebrex Capsules 2979

Chlorothiazide (Electrolyte disturbances are a risk associated with this product. Concurrent use of medications that may affect electrolyte levels, such as diuretics, may be associated with acute renal failure and requires caution).
No products indexed under this heading.

Chlorothiazide Sodium (Electrolyte disturbances are a risk associated with this product. Concurrent use of medications that may affect electrolyte levels, such as diuretics, may be associated with acute renal failure and requires caution). Products include:
Intravenous Sodium Diuril 2490

Chlorthalidone (Electrolyte disturbances are a risk associated with this product. Concurrent use of medications that may affect electrolyte levels, such as diuretics, may be associated with acute renal failure and requires caution). Products include:
Clorpres Tablets 2185

Diclofenac Epolamine (Electrolyte disturbances are a risk associated with this product. Concurrent use of medications that may affect electrolyte levels, such as NSAIDs, may be associated with acute renal failure). Products include:
Flector Patch 561

Diclofenac Potassium (Electrolyte disturbances are a risk associated with this product. Concurrent use of medications that may affect electrolyte levels, such as NSAIDs, may be associated with acute renal failure).
No products indexed under this heading.

Diclofenac Sodium (Electrolyte disturbances are a risk associated with this product. Concurrent use of medications that may affect electrolyte levels, such as NSAIDs, may be associated with acute renal failure). Products include:
Diclofenac Sodium Ophthalmic Solution .... ⊙240
Voltaren Ophthalmic Solution 2336
Voltaren Tablets 2334
Voltaren-XR Tablets 2337

Enalapril Maleate (Electrolyte disturbances are a risk associated with this product. Concurrent use of medications that may affect electrolyte levels, such as angiotensen converting enzyme inhibitors (ACE-Is), may be associated with acute renal failure and requires caution).
No products indexed under this heading.

Enalaprilat (Electrolyte disturbances are a risk associated with this product. Concurrent use of medications that may affect electrolyte levels, such as angiotensen converting enzyme inhibitors (ACE-Is), may be associated with acute renal failure and requires caution).
No products indexed under this heading.

Eprosartan Mesylate (Electrolyte disturbances are a risk associated with this product. Concurrent use of medications that may affect electrolyte levels, such as angiotensen receptor blockers (ARBs), may be associated with acute renal failure and requires caution). Products include:
Teveten Tablets 515
Teveten HCT Tablets 517

Ethacrynic Acid (Electrolyte disturbances are a risk associated with this product. Concurrent use of medications that may affect electrolyte levels, such as diuretics, may be associated with acute renal failure and requires caution). Products include:
Edecrin Tablets 698

Etodolac (Electrolyte disturbances are a risk associated with this product. Concurrent use of medications that may affect electrolyte levels, such as NSAIDs, may be associated with acute renal failure).
No products indexed under this heading.

Fenoprofen Calcium (Electrolyte disturbances are a risk associated with this product. Concurrent use of medications that may affect electrolyte levels, such as NSAIDs, may be associated with acute renal failure). Products include:
Nalfon Capsules 2508

Flurbiprofen (Electrolyte disturbances are a risk associated with this product. Concurrent use of medications that may affect electrolyte levels, such as NSAIDs, may be associated with acute renal failure).
No products indexed under this heading.

Fosinopril Sodium (Electrolyte disturbances are a risk associated with this product. Concurrent use of medications that may affect electrolyte levels, such as angiotensen converting enzyme inhibitors (ACE-Is), may be associated with acute renal failure and requires caution).
No products indexed under this heading.

Furosemide (Electrolyte disturbances are a risk associated with this product. Concurrent use of medications that may affect electrolyte levels, such as diuretics, may be associated with acute renal failure and requires caution). Products include:
Furosemide Tablets 2186

Hydrochlorothiazide (Electrolyte disturbances are a risk associated with this product. Concurrent use of medications that may affect electrolyte levels, such as diuretics, may be associated with acute renal failure and requires caution). Products include:

Atacand HCT 642
Avalide Tablets 892
Avalide Tablets 2713
Benicar HCT Tablets 1010
Diovan HCT Tablets 2216
Dyazide Capsules 1405
Micardis HCT Tablets 854
Prinzide Tablets 2092
Tekturna HCT Tablets 2324
Teveten HCT Tablets 517

Hydroflumethiazide (Electrolyte disturbances are a risk associated with this product. Concurrent use of medications that may affect electrolyte levels, such as diuretics, may be associated with acute renal failure and requires caution).

No products indexed under this heading.

Ibuprofen (Electrolyte disturbances are a risk associated with this product. Concurrent use of medications that may affect electrolyte levels, such as NSAIDs, may be associated with acute renal failure). Products include:

Motrin IB Tablets and Caplets 1900
Children's Motrin Oral Suspension ... 1901
Children's Motrin Non-Staining Dye-Free Oral Suspension............ 1901
Children's Motrin Cold Oral Suspension 1899
Infants' Motrin Concentrated Drops 1901
Infants' Motrin Non-Staining Dye-Free Concentrated Drops....... 1901
Junior Strength Motrin Caplets and Chewable Tablets................ 1901
Vicoprofen Tablets 533

Indapamide (Electrolyte disturbances are a risk associated with this product. Concurrent use of medications that may affect electrolyte levels, such as diuretics, may be associated with acute renal failure and requires caution). Products include:

Indapamide Tablets 2188

Indomethacin (Electrolyte disturbances are a risk associated with this product. Concurrent use of medications that may affect electrolyte levels, such as NSAIDs, may be associated with acute renal failure). Products include:

Indocin 2024

Indomethacin Sodium Trihydrate (Electrolyte disturbances are a risk associated with this product. Concurrent use of medications that may affect electrolyte levels, such as NSAIDs, may be associated with acute renal failure). Products include:

Indocin I.V. 2489

Irbesartan (Electrolyte disturbances are a risk associated with this product. Concurrent use of medications that may affect electrolyte levels, such as angiotensin receptor blockers (ARBs), may be associated with acute renal failure and requires caution). Products include:

Avalide Tablets 892
Avalide Tablets 2713
Avapro Tablets 897
Avapro Tablets 2718

Ketoprofen (Electrolyte disturbances are a risk associated with this product. Concurrent use of medications that may affect electrolyte levels, such as NSAIDs, may be associated with acute renal failure).

No products indexed under this heading.

Ketorolac Tromethamine (Electrolyte disturbances are a risk associated with this product. Concurrent use of medications that may affect electrolyte levels, such as NSAIDs, may be associated with acute renal failure).

No products indexed under this heading.

Lisinopril (Electrolyte disturbances are a risk associated with this product. Concurrent use of medications that may affect electrolyte levels, such as angiotensen converting enzyme inhibitors (ACE-Is), may be associated with acute renal failure and requires caution). Products include:

Prinivil Tablets 2087
Prinzide Tablets 2092

Lithium (Electrolyte disturbances are a risk associated with this product. Concurrent use of medications that may affect electrolyte levels, such as lithium, may be associated with acute renal failure).

No products indexed under this heading.

Lithium Carbonate (Electrolyte disturbances are a risk associated with this product. Concurrent use of medications that may affect electrolyte levels, such as lithium, may be associated with acute renal failure).

No products indexed under this heading.

Lithium Citrate (Electrolyte disturbances are a risk associated with this product. Concurrent use of medications that may affect electrolyte levels, such as lithium, may be associated with acute renal failure).

No products indexed under this heading.

Losartan Potassium (Electrolyte disturbances are a risk associated with this product. Concurrent use of medications that may affect electrolyte levels, such as angiotensen receptor blockers (ARBs), may be associated with acute renal failure and requires caution). Products include:

Cozaar Tablets 1973

Meclofenamate Sodium (Electrolyte disturbances are a risk associated with this product. Concurrent use of medications that may affect electrolyte levels, such as NSAIDs, may be associated with acute renal failure).

No products indexed under this heading.

Mefenamic Acid (Electrolyte disturbances are a risk associated with this product. Concurrent use of medications that may affect electrolyte levels, such as NSAIDs, may be associated with acute renal failure).

No products indexed under this heading.

Meloxicam (Electrolyte disturbances are a risk associated with this product. Concurrent use of medications that may affect electrolyte levels, such as NSAIDs, may be associated with acute renal failure). Products include:

Mobic Oral Suspension 863
Mobic Tablets 863

Methyclothiazide (Electrolyte disturbances are a risk associated with this product. Concurrent use of medications that may affect electrolyte levels, such as diuretics, may be associated with acute renal failure and requires caution).

No products indexed under this heading.

Metolazone (Electrolyte disturbances are a risk associated with this product. Concurrent use of medications that may affect electrolyte levels, such as diuretics, may be associated with acute renal failure and requires caution).

No products indexed under this heading.

Moexipril Hydrochloride (Electrolyte disturbances are a risk associated with this product. Concurrent use of medications that may affect electrolyte levels, such as angiotensen converting enzyme inhibitors (ACE-Is), may be associated with acute renal failure and requires caution).

No products indexed under this heading.

Nabumetone (Electrolyte disturbances are a risk associated with this product. Concurrent use of medications that may affect electrolyte levels, such as NSAIDs, may be associated with acute renal failure).

No products indexed under this heading.

Naproxen (Electrolyte disturbances are a risk associated with this product. Concurrent use of medications that may affect electrolyte levels, such as NSAIDs, may be associated with acute renal failure). Products include:

EC-Naprosyn Delayed-Release Tablets... 2632
Naprosyn Suspension 2632
Naprosyn Tablets 2632

Naproxen Sodium (Electrolyte disturbances are a risk associated with this product. Concurrent use of medications that may affect electrolyte levels, such as NSAIDs, may be associated with acute renal failure). Products include:

Anaprox Tablets 2632
Anaprox DS Tablets 2632
Treximet Tablets 1616

Oxaprozin (Electrolyte disturbances are a risk associated with this product. Concurrent use of medications that may affect electrolyte levels, such as NSAIDs, may be associated with acute renal failure).

No products indexed under this heading.

Perindopril Erbumine (Electrolyte disturbances are a risk associated with this product. Concurrent use of medications that may affect electrolyte levels, such as angiotensen converting enzyme inhibitors (ACE-Is), may be associated with acute renal failure and requires caution). Products include:

Aceon Tablets (2 mg, 4 mg, 8 mg)... 3038

Phenylbutazone (Electrolyte disturbances are a risk associated with this product. Concurrent use of medications that may affect electrolyte levels, such as NSAIDs, may be associated with acute renal failure).

No products indexed under this heading.

Piroxicam (Electrolyte disturbances are a risk associated with this product. Concurrent use of medications that may affect electrolyte levels, such as NSAIDs, may be associated with acute renal failure).

No products indexed under this heading.

Polythiazide (Electrolyte disturbances are a risk associated with this product. Concurrent use of medications that may affect electrolyte levels, such as diuretics, may be associated with acute renal failure and requires caution).

No products indexed under this heading.

Potassium Phosphate (No oral phosphate supplements or other sodium phosphates preparations including sodium phosphates-based enemas or tablets should be given concomitantly). Products include:

K-Phos Neutral Tablets 813

Quinapril Hydrochloride (Electrolyte disturbances are a risk associated with this product. Concurrent use of medications that may affect electrolyte levels, such as angiotensen converting enzyme inhibitors (ACE-Is), may be associated with acute renal failure and requires caution).

No products indexed under this heading.

Ramipril (Electrolyte disturbances are a risk associated with this product. Concurrent use of medications that may affect electrolyte levels, such as angiotensen converting enzyme inhibitors (ACE-Is), may be associated with acute renal failure and requires caution).

No products indexed under this heading.

Rofecoxib (Electrolyte disturbances are a risk associated with this product. Concurrent use of medications that may affect electrolyte levels, such as NSAIDs, may be associated with acute renal failure).

No products indexed under this heading.

Spirapril Hydrochloride (Electrolyte disturbances are a risk associated with this product. Concurrent use of medications that may affect electrolyte levels, such as angiotensen converting enzyme inhibitors (ACE-Is), may be associated with acute renal failure and requires caution).

No products indexed under this heading.

Spironolactone (Electrolyte disturbances are a risk associated with this product. Concurrent use of medications that may affect electrolyte levels, such as diuretics, may be associated with acute renal failure and requires caution).

No products indexed under this heading.

Sulindac (Electrolyte disturbances are a risk associated with this product. Concurrent use of medications that may affect electrolyte levels, such as NSAIDs, may be associated with acute renal failure). Products include:

Clinoril Tablets 1962

Telmisartan (Electrolyte disturbances are a risk associated with this product. Concurrent use of medications that may affect electrolyte levels, such as angiotensen receptor blockers (ARBs), may be associated with acute renal failure and requires caution). Products include:

Micardis Tablets 852
Micardis HCT Tablets 854

Tolmetin Sodium (Electrolyte disturbances are a risk associated with this product. Concurrent use of medications that may affect electrolyte levels, such as NSAIDs, may be associated with acute renal failure).
No products indexed under this heading.

Torsemide (Electrolyte disturbances are a risk associated with this product. Concurrent use of medications that may affect electrolyte levels, such as diuretics, may be associated with acute renal failure and requires caution). Products include:
Demadex Injection 2630
Demadex Tablets 2630

Trandolapril (Electrolyte disturbances are a risk associated with this product. Concurrent use of medications that may affect electrolyte levels, such as angiotensen converting enzyme inhibitors (ACE-Is), may be associated with acute renal failure and requires caution). Products include:
Mavik Tablets 472
Tarka Tablets 511

Triamterene (Electrolyte disturbances are a risk associated with this product. Concurrent use of medications that may affect electrolyte levels, such as diuretics, may be associated with acute renal failure and requires caution). Products include:
Dyazide Capsules 1405
Dyrenium Capsules 3189

Valdecoxib (Electrolyte disturbances are a risk associated with this product. Concurrent use of medications that may affect electrolyte levels, such as NSAIDs, may be associated with acute renal failure).
No products indexed under this heading.

Valsartan (Electrolyte disturbances are a risk associated with this product. Concurrent use of medications that may affect electrolyte levels, such as angiotensen receptor blockers (ARBs), may be associated with acute renal failure and requires caution). Products include:
Diovan Tablets 2212
Diovan HCT Tablets 2216
Exforge Tablets 2238

FLEET PEDIA-LAX LIQUID STOOL SOFTENER

(Docusate Sodium) 1144
None cited in PDR database.

FLEET PEDIA-LAX LIQUID SUPPOSITORIES

(Glycerin) .... ▣605
None cited in PDR database.

FLEET PEDIA-LAX SENNA QUICK DISSOLVE STRIPS

(Sennosides) 1145
None cited in PDR database.

FLEET PEDIA-LAX SUPPOSITORIES

(Glycerin) 1142
None cited in PDR database.

FLEET PHOSPHO-SODA

(Sodium Phosphate) 1145
May interact with ACE inhibitors, oral aminoglycosides, angiotensin-II receptor antagonists, antihypertensives, diuretics, anticonvulsants, oral hypoglycemic agents, lithium preparations, non-steroidal anti-inflammatory agents, oral contraceptives, and oral phosphate supplements. Compounds in these categories include:

Acarbose (During the intake of oral sodium phosphate, the absorption of the drugs from the gastrointestinal tract may be delayed or even completely prevented. The efficacy of regularly taken oral drugs (e.g., antidiabetic) may be reduced or completely absent). Products include:
Precose Tablets 792

Acebutolol Hydrochloride (Patients that are taking hypertension medications are at a higher risk for renal failure and acute phosphate nephropathy when oral sodium phosphate products are used concomitantly).
No products indexed under this heading.

Aliskiren (Patients that are taking hypertension medications are at a higher risk for renal failure and acute phosphate nephropathy when oral sodium phosphate products are used concomitantly). Products include:
Tekturna Tablets 2321
Tekturna HCT Tablets 2324

Amiloride Hydrochloride (Patients at increased risk for acute phosphate nephropathy include those with conditions that affect renal perfusion or function or those taking medications which may decrease glomerular filtration rate or predispose to dehydration, including diuretics. Dehydration and hypovolemia from purgation may exacerbated by inadequate oral fluid intake, nausea, vomiting, loss of appetite, or use of diuretics and may be associated with acute renal failure).
No products indexed under this heading.

Amlodipine Besylate (Patients that are taking hypertension medications are at a higher risk for renal failure and acute phosphate nephropathy when oral sodium phosphate products are used concomitantly). Products include:
Azor Tablets 1005
Exforge Tablets 2238

Atenolol (Patients that are taking hypertension medications are at a higher risk for renal failure and acute phosphate nephropathy when oral sodium phosphate products are used concomitantly).
No products indexed under this heading.

Benazepril Hydrochloride (Patients that are taking hypertension medications are at a higher risk for renal failure and acute phosphate nephropathy when oral sodium phosphate products are used concomitantly).
No products indexed under this heading.

Bendroflumethiazide (Patients that are taking hypertension medications are at a higher risk for renal failure and acute phosphate nephropathy when oral sodium phosphate products are used concomitantly).
No products indexed under this heading.

Betaxolol Hydrochloride (Patients that are taking hypertension medications are at a higher risk for renal failure and acute phosphate nephropathy when oral sodium phosphate products are used concomitantly).
No products indexed under this heading.

Bisoprolol Fumarate (Patients that are taking hypertension medications are at a higher risk for renal failure and acute phosphate nephropathy when oral sodium phosphate products are used concomitantly).
No products indexed under this heading.

Bumetanide (Patients at increased risk for acute phosphate nephropathy include those with conditions that affect renal perfusion or function or those taking medications which may decrease glomerular filtration rate or predispose to dehydration, including diuretics. Dehydration and hypovolemia from purgation may exacerbated by inadequate oral fluid intake, nausea, vomiting, loss of appetite, or use of diuretics and may be associated with acute renal failure).
No products indexed under this heading.

Candesartan Cilexetil (Patients that are taking hypertension medications are at a higher risk for renal failure and acute phosphate nephropathy when oral sodium phosphate products are used concomitantly). Products include:
Atacand Tablets 639
Atacand HCT 642

Captopril (Patients that are taking hypertension medications are at a higher risk for renal failure and acute phosphate nephropathy when oral sodium phosphate products are used concomitantly). Products include:
Captopril Tablets 2182

Carbamazepine (During the intake of oral sodium phosphate, the absorption of drugs from the gastrointestinal tract may be delayed or even completely prevented. The efficacy of regularly taken oral drugs (e.g., antiepileptic drugs) may be reduced or completely absent). Products include:
Carbatrol Capsules 3019
Equetro Extended-Release Capsules 3174

Carteolol Hydrochloride (Patients that are taking hypertension medications are at a higher risk for renal failure and acute phosphate nephropathy when oral sodium phosphate products are used concomitantly).
No products indexed under this heading.

Celecoxib (Patients at increased risk for acute phosphate nephropathy include those with conditions that affect renal perfusion or function or those taking medications which may decrease glomerular filtrations rate or predispose to dehydration, including non-steroidal anti-inflammatory drugs (NSAIDs). Dehydration and hypovolemia from purgation may be exacerbated by inadequate oral fluid intake, nausea, vomiting, loss of appetite, or use of NSAIDs and may be associated with acute renal failure). Products include:
Celebrex Capsules 2979

Chlorothiazide (Patients that are taking hypertension medications are at a higher risk for renal failure and acute phosphate nephropathy when oral sodium phosphate products are used concomitantly).
No products indexed under this heading.

Chlorothiazide Sodium (Patients that are taking hypertension medications are at a higher risk for renal failure and acute phosphate nephropathy when oral sodium phosphate products are used concomitantly). Products include:
Intravenous Sodium Diuril 2490

Chlorpropamide (During the intake of oral sodium phosphate, the absorption of the drugs from the gastrointestinal tract may be delayed or even completely prevented. The efficacy of regularly taken oral drugs (e.g., antidiabetic) may be reduced or completely absent).
No products indexed under this heading.

Chlorthalidone (Patients that are taking hypertension medications are at a higher risk for renal failure and acute phosphate nephropathy when oral sodium phosphate products are used concomitantly). Products include:
Clorpres Tablets 2185

Clonidine (Patients that are taking hypertension medications are at a higher risk for renal failure and acute phosphate nephropathy when oral sodium phosphate products are used concomitantly). Products include:
Catapres-TTS 842

Clonidine Hydrochloride (Patients that are taking hypertension medications are at a higher risk for renal failure and acute phosphate nephropathy when oral sodium phosphate products are used concomitantly). Products include:
Catapres Tablets 841
Clorpres Tablets 2185

Deserpidine (Patients that are taking hypertension medications are at a higher risk for renal failure and acute phosphate nephropathy when oral sodium phosphate products are used concomitantly).
No products indexed under this heading.

Desogestrel (During the intake of oral sodium phosphate, the absorption of drugs from the gastrointestinal tract may be delayed or even completely prevented. The efficacy of regularly taken oral drugs (e.g., oral contraceptives) may be reduced or completely absent). Products include:
Mircette Tablets 1034

Diazoxide (Patients that are taking hypertension medications are at a higher risk for renal failure and acute phosphate nephropathy when oral sodium phosphate products are used concomitantly). Products include:
Proglycem Capsules 1185
Proglycem Suspension 1185

Diclofenac Epolamine (Patients at increased risk for acute phosphate nephropathy include those with conditions that affect renal perfusion or function or those taking medications which may decrease glomerular filtrations rate or predispose to dehydration, including non-steroidal anti-inflammatory drugs (NSAIDs). Dehydration and hypovolemia from purgation may be exacerbated by inadequate oral fluid intake, nausea, vomiting, loss of appetite, or use of NSAIDs and may be associated with acute renal failure). Products include:

Flector Patch 561

Diclofenac Potassium (Patients at increased risk for acute phosphate nephropathy include those with conditions that affect renal perfusion or function or those taking medications which may decrease glomerular filtrations rate or predispose to dehydration, including non-steroidal anti-inflammatory drugs (NSAIDs). Dehydration and hypovolemia from purgation may be exacerbated by inadequate oral fluid intake, nausea, vomiting, loss of appetite, or use of NSAIDs and may be associated with acute renal failure).

No products indexed under this heading.

Diclofenac Sodium (Patients at increased risk for acute phosphate nephropathy include those with conditions that affect renal perfusion or function or those taking medications which may decrease glomerular filtrations rate or predispose to dehydration, including non-steroidal anti-inflammatory drugs (NSAIDs). Dehydration and hypovolemia from purgation may be exacerbated by inadequate oral fluid intake, nausea, vomiting, loss of appetite, or use of NSAIDs and may be associated with acute renal failure). Products include:

Diclofenac Sodium Ophthalmic Solution...................................... ⊙240
Voltaren Ophthalmic Solution 2336
Voltaren Tablets 2334
Voltaren-XR Tablets 2337

Diltiazem Hydrochloride (Patients that are taking hypertension medications are at a higher risk for renal failure and acute phosphate nephropathy when oral sodium phosphate products are used concomitantly). Products include:

Cardizem LA Extended Release Tablets.. 421

Divalproex Sodium (During the intake of oral sodium phosphate, the absorption of drugs from the gastrointestinal tract may be delayed or even completely prevented. The efficacy of regularly taken oral drugs (e.g., antiepileptic drugs) may be reduced or completely absent). Products include:

Depakote ER Tablets 423

Doxazosin Mesylate (Patients that are taking hypertension medications are at a higher risk for renal failure and acute phosphate nephropathy when oral sodium phosphate products are used concomitantly).

No products indexed under this heading.

Enalapril Maleate (Patients that are taking hypertension medications are at a higher risk for renal failure and acute phosphate nephropathy when oral sodium phosphate products are used concomitantly).

No products indexed under this heading.

Enalaprilat (Patients that are taking hypertension medications are at a higher risk for renal failure and acute phosphate nephropathy when oral sodium phosphate products are used concomitantly).

No products indexed under this heading.

Eprosartan Mesylate (Patients that are taking hypertension medications are at a higher risk for renal failure and acute phosphate nephropathy when oral sodium phosphate products are used concomitantly). Products include:

Teveten Tablets 515
Teveten HCT Tablets 517

Esmolol Hydrochloride (Patients that are taking hypertension medications are at a higher risk for renal failure and acute phosphate nephropathy when oral sodium phosphate products are used concomitantly).

No products indexed under this heading.

Ethacrynic Acid (Patients at increased risk for acute phosphate nephropathy include those with conditions that affect renal perfusion or function or those taking medications which may decrease glomerular filtration rate or predispose to dehydration, including diuretics. Dehydration and hypovolemia from purgation may exacerbated by inadequate oral fluid intake, nausea, vomiting, loss of appetite, or use of diuretics and may be associated with acute renal failure). Products include:

Edecrin Tablets 698

Ethinyl Estradiol (During the intake of oral sodium phosphate, the absorption of drugs from the gastrointestinal tract may be delayed or even completely prevented. The efficacy of regularly taken oral drugs (e.g., oral contraceptives) may be reduced or completely absent). Products include:

Lybrel Tablets 3204
Mircette Tablets 1034
NuvaRing 2897
Ortho-Cyclen/Ortho Tri-Cyclen 2449
Ortho Evra Transdermal System 2437
Ortho Tri-Cyclen Lo Tablets 2458
Seasonique Tablets 1046
Yaz Tablets 805

Ethosuximide (During the intake of oral sodium phosphate, the absorption of drugs from the gastrointestinal tract may be delayed or even completely prevented. The efficacy of regularly taken oral drugs (e.g., antiepileptic drugs) may be reduced or completely absent).

No products indexed under this heading.

Ethotoin (During the intake of oral sodium phosphate, the absorption of drugs from the gastrointestinal tract may be delayed or even completely prevented. The efficacy of regularly taken oral drugs (e.g., antiepileptic drugs) may be reduced or completely absent).

No products indexed under this heading.

Ethynodiol Diacetate (During the intake of oral sodium phosphate, the absorption of drugs from the gastrointestinal tract may be delayed or even completely prevented. The efficacy of regularly taken oral drugs (e.g., oral contraceptives) may be reduced or completely absent).

No products indexed under this heading.

Etodolac (Patients at increased risk for acute phosphate nephropathy include those with conditions that affect renal perfusion or function or those taking medications which may decrease glomerular filtrations rate or predispose to dehydration, including non-steroidal anti-inflammatory drugs (NSAIDs). Dehydration and hypovolemia from purgation may be exacerbated by inadequate oral fluid intake, nausea, vomiting, loss of appetite, or use of NSAIDs and may be associated with acute renal failure).

No products indexed under this heading.

Felbamate (During the intake of oral sodium phosphate, the absorption of drugs from the gastrointestinal tract may be delayed or even completely prevented. The efficacy of regularly taken oral drugs (e.g., antiepileptic drugs) may be reduced or completely absent).

No products indexed under this heading.

Felodipine (Patients that are taking hypertension medications are at a higher risk for renal failure and acute phosphate nephropathy when oral sodium phosphate products are used concomitantly).

No products indexed under this heading.

Fenoprofen Calcium (Patients at increased risk for acute phosphate nephropathy include those with conditions that affect renal perfusion or function or those taking medications which may decrease glomerular filtrations rate or predispose to dehydration, including non-steroidal anti-inflammatory drugs (NSAIDs). Dehydration and hypovolemia from purgation may be exacerbated by inadequate oral fluid intake, nausea, vomiting, loss of appetite, or use of NSAIDs and may be associated with acute renal failure). Products include:

Nalfon Capsules 2508

Flurbiprofen (Patients at increased risk for acute phosphate nephropathy include those with conditions that affect renal perfusion or function or those taking medications which may decrease glomerular filtrations rate or predispose to dehydration, including non-steroidal anti-inflammatory drugs (NSAIDs). Dehydration and hypovolemia from purgation may be exacerbated by inadequate oral fluid intake, nausea, vomiting, loss of appetite, or use of NSAIDs and may be associated with acute renal failure).

No products indexed under this heading.

Fosinopril Sodium (Patients that are taking hypertension medications are at a higher risk for renal failure and acute phosphate nephropathy when oral sodium phosphate products are used concomitantly).

No products indexed under this heading.

Fosphenytoin (During the intake of oral sodium phosphate, the absorption of drugs from the gastrointestinal tract may be delayed or even completely prevented. The efficacy of regularly taken oral drugs (e.g., antiepileptic drugs) may be reduced or completely absent).

No products indexed under this heading.

Fosphenytoin Sodium (During the intake of oral sodium phosphate, the absorption of drugs from the gastrointestinal tract may be delayed or even completely prevented. The efficacy of regularly taken oral drugs (e.g., antiepileptic drugs) may be reduced or completely absent).

No products indexed under this heading.

Furosemide (Patients that are taking hypertension medications are at a higher risk for renal failure and acute phosphate nephropathy when oral sodium phosphate products are used concomitantly). Products include:

Furosemide Tablets 2186

Gabapentin (During the intake of oral sodium phosphate, the absorption of drugs from the gastrointestinal tract may be delayed or even completely prevented. The efficacy of regularly taken oral drugs (e.g., antiepileptic drugs) may be reduced or completely absent).

No products indexed under this heading.

Glimepiride (During the intake of oral sodium phosphate, the absorption of the drugs from the gastrointestinal tract may be delayed or even completely prevented. The efficacy of regularly taken oral drugs (e.g., antidiabetic) may be reduced or completely absent). Products include:

Avandaryl Tablets 1344
Duetact Tablets 3085

Glipizide (During the intake of oral sodium phosphate, the absorption of the drugs from the gastrointestinal tract may be delayed or even completely prevented. The efficacy of regularly taken oral drugs (e.g., antidiabetic) may be reduced or completely absent).

No products indexed under this heading.

Glyburide (During the intake of oral sodium phosphate, the absorption of the drugs from the gastrointestinal tract may be delayed or even completely prevented. The efficacy of regularly taken oral drugs (e.g., antidiabetic) may be reduced or completely absent).

No products indexed under this heading.

Guanabenz Acetate (Patients that are taking hypertension medications are at a higher risk for renal failure and acute phosphate nephropathy when oral sodium phosphate products are used concomitantly).

No products indexed under this heading.

Guanethidine Monosulfate (Patients that are taking hypertension medications are at a higher risk for renal failure and acute phosphate nephropathy when oral sodium phosphate products are used concomitantly).

No products indexed under this heading.

Hydralazine Hydrochloride (Patients that are taking hypertension medications are at a higher risk for renal failure and acute phosphate nephropathy when oral sodium phosphate products are used concomitantly).

No products indexed under this heading.

Hydrochlorothiazide (Patients that are taking hypertension medications

are at a higher risk for renal failure and acute phosphate nephropathy when oral sodium phosphate products are used concomitantly). Products include:

Atacand HCT 642
Avalide Tablets 892
Avalide Tablets 2713
Benicar HCT Tablets 1010
Diovan HCT Tablets 2216
Dyazide Capsules 1405
Micardis HCT Tablets 854
Prinzide Tablets 2092
Tekturna HCT Tablets 2324
Teveten HCT Tablets 517

Hydroflumethiazide (Patients that are taking hypertension medications are at a higher risk for renal failure and acute phosphate nephropathy when oral sodium phosphate products are used concomitantly).
No products indexed under this heading.

Ibuprofen (Patients at increased risk for acute phosphate nephropathy include those with conditions that affect renal perfusion or function or those taking medications which may decrease glomerular filtrations rate or predispose to dehydration, including non-steroidal anti-inflammatory drugs (NSAIDs). Dehydration and hypovolemia from purgation may be exacerbated by inadequate oral fluid intake, nausea, vomiting, loss of appetite, or use of NSAIDs and may be associated with acute renal failure). Products include:

Motrin IB Tablets and Caplets 1900
Children's Motrin Oral Suspension ... 1901
Children's Motrin Non-Staining Dye-Free Oral Suspension 1901
Children's Motrin Cold Oral Suspension 1899
Infants' Motrin Concentrated Drops 1901
Infants' Motrin Non-Staining Dye-Free Concentrated Drops 1901
Junior Strength Motrin Caplets and Chewable Tablets 1901
Vicoprofen Tablets 533

Indapamide (Patients that are taking hypertension medications are at a higher risk for renal failure and acute phosphate nephropathy when oral sodium phosphate products are used concomitantly). Products include:

Indapamide Tablets 2188

Indomethacin (Patients at increased risk for acute phosphate nephropathy include those with conditions that affect renal perfusion or function or those taking medications which may decrease glomerular filtrations rate or predispose to dehydration, including non-steroidal anti-inflammatory drugs (NSAIDs). Dehydration and hypovolemia from purgation may be exacerbated by inadequate oral fluid intake, nausea, vomiting, loss of appetite, or use of NSAIDs and may be associated with acute renal failure). Products include:

Indocin 2024

Indomethacin Sodium Trihydrate (Patients at increased risk for acute phosphate nephropathy include those with conditions that affect renal perfusion or function or those taking medications which may decrease glomerular filtrations rate or predispose to dehydration, including non-steroidal anti-inflammatory drugs (NSAIDs). Dehydration and hypovolemia from purgation may be exacerbated by inadequate oral fluid intake, nausea, vomiting, loss of appetite, or use of NSAIDs and may be associated with acute renal failure). Products include:

Indocin I.V. 2489

Irbesartan (Patients that are taking hypertension medications are at a higher risk for renal failure and acute phosphate nephropathy when oral sodium phosphate products are used concomitantly). Products include:

Avalide Tablets 892
Avalide Tablets 2713
Avapro Tablets 897
Avapro Tablets 2718

Isradipine (Patients that are taking hypertension medications are at a higher risk for renal failure and acute phosphate nephropathy when oral sodium phosphate products are used concomitantly). Products include:

DynaCirc CR Controlled Release Tablets 1407

Kanamycin Sulfate (During the intake of oral sodium phosphate, the absorption of drugs from the gastrointestinal tract may be delayed or even completely prevented. The efficacy of regularly taken oral antibiotics (e.g., oral aminoglycosides) may be reduced or completely absent).
No products indexed under this heading.

Ketoprofen (Patients at increased risk for acute phosphate nephropathy include those with conditions that affect renal perfusion or function or those taking medications which may decrease glomerular filtrations rate or predispose to dehydration, including non-steroidal anti-inflammatory drugs (NSAIDs). Dehydration and hypovolemia from purgation may be exacerbated by inadequate oral fluid intake, nausea, vomiting, loss of appetite, or use of NSAIDs and may be associated with acute renal failure).
No products indexed under this heading.

Ketorolac Tromethamine (Patients at increased risk for acute phosphate nephropathy include those with conditions that affect renal perfusion or function or those taking medications which may decrease glomerular filtrations rate or predispose to dehydration, including non-steroidal anti-inflammatory drugs (NSAIDs). Dehydration and hypovolemia from purgation may be exacerbated by inadequate oral fluid intake, nausea, vomiting, loss of appetite, or use of NSAIDs and may be associated with acute renal failure).
No products indexed under this heading.

Labetalol Hydrochloride (Patients that are taking hypertension medications are at a higher risk for renal failure and acute phosphate nephropathy when oral sodium phosphate products are used concomitantly).
No products indexed under this heading.

Lamotrigine (During the intake of oral sodium phosphate, the absorption of drugs from the gastrointestinal tract may be delayed or even completely prevented. The efficacy of regularly taken oral drugs (e.g., antiepileptic drugs) may be reduced or completely absent). Products include:

Lamictal 1488

Levetiracetam (During the intake of oral sodium phosphate, the absorption of drugs from the gastrointestinal tract may be delayed or even completely prevented. The efficacy of regularly taken oral drugs (e.g., antiepileptic drugs) may be reduced or completely absent). Products include:

Keppra Injection 3137
Keppra Oral Solution 3131
Keppra Tablets 3131

Levonorgestrel (During the intake of oral sodium phosphate, the absorption of drugs from the gastrointestinal tract may be delayed or even completely prevented. The efficacy of regularly taken oral drugs (e.g., oral contraceptives) may be reduced or completely absent). Products include:

Climara Pro Transdermal System 768
Lybrel Tablets 3204
Mirena Intrauterine System 779
Plan B Tablets 1044
Seasonique Tablets 1046

Lisinopril (Patients that are taking hypertension medications are at a higher risk for renal failure and acute phosphate nephropathy when oral sodium phosphate products are used concomitantly). Products include:

Prinivil Tablets 2087
Prinzide Tablets 2092

Lithium (Dehydration and hypovolemia from purgation may be exacerbated by inadequate oral fluid intake, nausea, vomiting, loss of appetite, or use of lithium or other medications that may affect electrolyte levels, and may be associated with acute renal failure).
No products indexed under this heading.

Lithium Carbonate (Dehydration and hypovolemia from purgation may be exacerbated by inadequate oral fluid intake, nausea, vomiting, loss of appetite, or use of lithium or other medications that may affect electrolyte levels, and may be associated with acute renal failure).
No products indexed under this heading.

Lithium Citrate (Dehydration and hypovolemia from purgation may be exacerbated by inadequate oral fluid intake, nausea, vomiting, loss of appetite, or use of lithium or other medications that may affect electrolyte levels, and may be associated with acute renal failure).
No products indexed under this heading.

Losartan Potassium (Patients that are taking hypertension medications are at a higher risk for renal failure and acute phosphate nephropathy when oral sodium phosphate products are used concomitantly). Products include:

Cozaar Tablets 1973

Mecamylamine Hydrochloride (Patients that are taking hypertension medications are at a higher risk for renal failure and acute phosphate nephropathy when oral sodium phosphate products are used concomitantly).
No products indexed under this heading.

Meclofenamate Sodium (Patients at increased risk for acute phosphate nephropathy include those with conditions that affect renal perfusion or function or those taking medications which may decrease glomerular filtrations rate or predispose to dehydration, including non-steroidal anti-inflammatory drugs (NSAIDs). Dehydration and hypovolemia from purgation may be exacerbated by inadequate oral fluid intake, nausea, vomiting, loss of appetite, or use of NSAIDs and may be associated with acute renal failure).
No products indexed under this heading.

Mefenamic Acid (Patients at increased risk for acute phosphate nephropathy include those with conditions that affect renal perfusion or function or those taking medications which may decrease glomerular filtrations rate or predispose to dehydration, including non-steroidal anti-inflammatory drugs (NSAIDs). Dehydration and hypovolemia from purgation may be exacerbated by inadequate oral fluid intake, nausea, vomiting, loss of appetite, or use of NSAIDs and may be associated with acute renal failure).
No products indexed under this heading.

Meloxicam (Patients at increased risk for acute phosphate nephropathy include those with conditions that affect renal perfusion or function or those taking medications which may decrease glomerular filtrations rate or predispose to dehydration, including non-steroidal anti-inflammatory drugs (NSAIDs). Dehydration and hypovolemia from purgation may be exacerbated by inadequate oral fluid intake, nausea, vomiting, loss of appetite, or use of NSAIDs and may be associated with acute renal failure). Products include:

Mobic Oral Suspension 863
Mobic Tablets 863

Mephenytoin (During the intake of oral sodium phosphate, the absorption of drugs from the gastrointestinal tract may be delayed or even completely prevented. The efficacy of regularly taken oral drugs (e.g., antiepileptic drugs) may be reduced or completely absent).
No products indexed under this heading.

Mestranol (During the intake of oral sodium phosphate, the absorption of drugs from the gastrointestinal tract may be delayed or even completely prevented. The efficacy of regularly taken oral drugs (e.g., oral contraceptives) may be reduced or completely absent).
No products indexed under this heading.

Metformin Hydrochloride (During the intake of oral sodium phosphate, the absorption of the drugs from the gastrointestinal tract may be delayed or even completely prevented. The efficacy of regularly taken oral drugs (e.g., antidiabetic) may be reduced or completely absent). Products include:

ActoPlus Met Tablets 3071
Avandamet Tablets 1336
Janumet Tablets 2041
PrandiMet Tablets 2967

Methsuximide (During the intake of oral sodium phosphate, the absorption of drugs from the gastrointestinal tract may be delayed or even completely prevented. The efficacy of regularly taken oral drugs (e.g., antiepileptic drugs) may be reduced or completely absent).
No products indexed under this heading.

Methyclothiazide (Patients that are taking hypertension medications are at a higher risk for renal failure and acute phosphate nephropathy when oral sodium phosphate products are used concomitantly).
No products indexed under this heading.

Methyldopa (Patients that are taking hypertension medications are at a higher risk for renal failure and acute phosphate nephropathy when oral sodium phosphate products are used concomitantly).
No products indexed under this heading.

Methyldopate Hydrochloride (Patients that are taking hypertension medications are at a higher risk for renal failure and acute phosphate nephropathy when oral sodium phosphate products are used concomitantly).
No products indexed under this heading.

Metolazone (Patients that are taking hypertension medications are at a higher risk for renal failure and acute phosphate nephropathy when oral sodium phosphate products are used concomitantly).
No products indexed under this heading.

Metoprolol Succinate (Patients that are taking hypertension medications are at a higher risk for renal failure and acute phosphate nephropathy when oral sodium phosphate products are used concomitantly). Products include:
Toprol-XL Tablets 666

Metoprolol Tartrate (Patients that are taking hypertension medications are at a higher risk for renal failure and acute phosphate nephropathy when oral sodium phosphate products are used concomitantly).
No products indexed under this heading.

Metyrosine (Patients that are taking hypertension medications are at a higher risk for renal failure and acute phosphate nephropathy when oral sodium phosphate products are used concomitantly). Products include:
Demser Capsules 1989

Mibefradil Dihydrochloride (Patients that are taking hypertension medications are at a higher risk for renal failure and acute phosphate nephropathy when oral sodium phosphate products are used concomitantly).
No products indexed under this heading.

Miglitol (During the intake of oral sodium phosphate, the absorption of the drugs from the gastrointestinal tract may be delayed or even completely prevented. The efficacy of regularly taken oral drugs (e.g., antidiabetic) may be reduced or completely absent).
No products indexed under this heading.

Minoxidil (Patients that are taking hypertension medications are at a higher risk for renal failure and acute phosphate nephropathy when oral sodium phosphate products are used concomitantly).
No products indexed under this heading.

Moexipril Hydrochloride (Patients that are taking hypertension medications are at a higher risk for renal failure and acute phosphate nephropathy when oral sodium phosphate products are used concomitantly).
No products indexed under this heading.

Nabumetone (Patients at increased risk for acute phosphate nephropathy include those with conditions that affect renal perfusion or function or those taking medications which may decrease glomerular filtrations rate or predispose to dehydration, including non-steroidal anti-inflammatory drugs (NSAIDs). Dehydration and hypovolemia from purgation may be exacerbated by inadequate oral fluid intake, nausea, vomiting, loss of appetite, or use of NSAIDs and may be associated with acute renal failure).
No products indexed under this heading.

Nadolol (Patients that are taking hypertension medications are at a higher risk for renal failure and acute phosphate nephropathy when oral sodium phosphate products are used concomitantly). Products include:
Nadolol Tablets 2191

Naproxen (Patients at increased risk for acute phosphate nephropathy include those with conditions that affect renal perfusion or function or those taking medications which may decrease glomerular filtrations rate or predispose to dehydration, including non-steroidal anti-inflammatory drugs (NSAIDs). Dehydration and hypovolemia from purgation may be exacerbated by inadequate oral fluid intake, nausea, vomiting, loss of appetite, or use of NSAIDs and may be associated with acute renal failure). Products include:
EC-Naprosyn Delayed-Release Tablets 2632
Naprosyn Suspension 2632
Naprosyn Tablets 2632

Naproxen Sodium (Patients at increased risk for acute phosphate nephropathy include those with conditions that affect renal perfusion or function or those taking medications which may decrease glomerular filtrations rate or predispose to dehydration, including non-steroidal anti-inflammatory drugs (NSAIDs). Dehydration and hypovolemia from purgation may be exacerbated by inadequate oral fluid intake, nausea, vomiting, loss of appetite, or use of NSAIDs and may be associated with acute renal failure). Products include:
Anaprox Tablets 2632
Anaprox DS Tablets 2632
Treximet Tablets 1616

Nateglinide (During the intake of oral sodium phosphate, the absorption of the drugs from the gastrointestinal tract may be delayed or even completely prevented. The efficacy of regularly taken oral drugs (e.g., antidiabetic) may be reduced or completely absent). Products include:
Starlix Tablets 2314

Nebivolol (Patients that are taking hypertension medications are at a higher risk for renal failure and acute phosphate nephropathy when oral sodium phosphate products are used concomitantly). Products include:
Bystolic Tablets 1155

Neomycin, oral (During the intake of oral sodium phosphate, the absorption of drugs from the gastrointestinal tract may be delayed or even completely prevented. The efficacy of regularly taken oral antibiotics (e.g., oral aminoglycosides) may be reduced or completely absent).
No products indexed under this heading.

Nicardipine Hydrochloride (Patients that are taking hypertension medications are at a higher risk for renal failure and acute phosphate nephropathy when oral sodium phosphate products are used concomitantly). Products include:
Cardene I.V. 1093

Nifedipine (Patients that are taking hypertension medications are at a higher risk for renal failure and acute phosphate nephropathy when oral sodium phosphate products are used concomitantly).
No products indexed under this heading.

Nisoldipine (Patients that are taking hypertension medications are at a higher risk for renal failure and acute phosphate nephropathy when oral sodium phosphate products are used concomitantly). Products include:
Sular Extended Release Tablets 2975

Nitroglycerin (Patients that are taking hypertension medications are at a higher risk for renal failure and acute phosphate nephropathy when oral sodium phosphate products are used concomitantly). Products include:
Nitro-Dur Transdermal Infusion System 2887
Nitrolingual Pumpspray 2965

Norethindrone (During the intake of oral sodium phosphate, the absorption of drugs from the gastrointestinal tract may be delayed or even completely prevented. The efficacy of regularly taken oral drugs (e.g., oral contraceptives) may be reduced or completely absent). Products include:
Ortho Micronor Tablets 2446

Norethynodrel (During the intake of oral sodium phosphate, the absorption of drugs from the gastrointestinal tract may be delayed or even completely prevented. The efficacy of regularly taken oral drugs (e.g., oral contraceptives) may be reduced or completely absent).
No products indexed under this heading.

Norgestimate (During the intake of oral sodium phosphate, the absorption of drugs from the gastrointestinal tract may be delayed or even completely prevented. The efficacy of regularly taken oral drugs (e.g., oral contraceptives) may be reduced or completely absent). Products include:
Ortho-Cyclen/Ortho Tri-Cyclen 2449
Ortho Tri-Cyclen Lo Tablets 2458

Norgestrel (During the intake of oral sodium phosphate, the absorption of drugs from the gastrointestinal tract may be delayed or even completely prevented. The efficacy of regularly taken oral drugs (e.g., oral contraceptives) may be reduced or completely absent).
No products indexed under this heading.

Oxaprozin (Patients at increased risk for acute phosphate nephropathy include those with conditions that affect renal perfusion or function or those taking medications which may decrease glomerular filtrations rate or predispose to dehydration, including non-steroidal anti-inflammatory drugs (NSAIDs). Dehydration and hypovolemia from purgation may be exacerbated by inadequate oral fluid intake, nausea, vomiting, loss of appetite, or use of NSAIDs and may be associated with acute renal failure).
No products indexed under this heading.

Oxcarbazepine (During the intake of oral sodium phosphate, the absorption of drugs from the gastrointestinal tract may be delayed or even completely prevented. The efficacy of regularly taken oral drugs (e.g., antiepileptic drugs) may be reduced or completely absent).
No products indexed under this heading.

Paramethadione (During the intake of oral sodium phosphate, the absorption of drugs from the gastrointestinal tract may be delayed or even completely prevented. The efficacy of regularly taken oral drugs (e.g., antiepileptic drugs) may be reduced or completely absent).
No products indexed under this heading.

Paromomycin Sulfate (During the intake of oral sodium phosphate, the absorption of drugs from the gastrointestinal tract may be delayed or even completely prevented. The efficacy of regularly taken oral antibiotics (e.g., oral aminoglycosides) may be reduced or completely absent).
No products indexed under this heading.

Penbutolol Sulfate (Patients that are taking hypertension medications are at a higher risk for renal failure and acute phosphate nephropathy when oral sodium phosphate products are used concomitantly).
No products indexed under this heading.

Perindopril Erbumine (Patients that are taking hypertension medications are at a higher risk for renal failure and acute phosphate nephropathy when oral sodium phosphate products are used concomitantly). Products include:
Aceon Tablets (2 mg, 4 mg, 8 mg) 3038

Phenacemide (During the intake of oral sodium phosphate, the absorption of drugs from the gastrointestinal tract may be delayed or even completely prevented. The efficacy of regularly taken oral drugs (e.g., antiepileptic drugs) may be reduced or completely absent).
No products indexed under this heading.

Phenobarbital (During the intake of oral sodium phosphate, the absorption of drugs from the gastrointestinal tract may be delayed or even completely prevented. The efficacy of regularly taken oral drugs (e.g., antiepileptic drugs) may be reduced or completely absent). Products include:

Donnatal Extentabs 2507

Phenoxybenzamine Hydrochloride (Patients that are taking hypertension medications are at a higher risk for renal failure and acute phosphate nephropathy when oral sodium phosphate products are used concomitantly). Products include:

Dibenzyline Capsules 3188

Phensuximide (During the intake of oral sodium phosphate, the absorption of drugs from the gastrointestinal tract may be delayed or even completely prevented. The efficacy of regularly taken oral drugs (e.g., antiepileptic drugs) may be reduced or completely absent).

No products indexed under this heading.

Phentolamine Mesylate (Patients that are taking hypertension medications are at a higher risk for renal failure and acute phosphate nephropathy when oral sodium phosphate products are used concomitantly).

No products indexed under this heading.

Phenylbutazone (Patients at increased risk for acute phosphate nephropathy include those with conditions that affect renal perfusion or function or those taking medications which may decrease glomerular filtrations rate or predispose to dehydration, including non-steroidal anti-inflammatory drugs (NSAIDs). Dehydration and hypovolemia from purgation may be exacerbated by inadequate oral fluid intake, nausea, vomiting, loss of appetite, or use of NSAIDs and may be associated with acute renal failure).

No products indexed under this heading.

Phenytoin (During the intake of oral sodium phosphate, the absorption of drugs from the gastrointestinal tract may be delayed or even completely prevented. The efficacy of regularly taken oral drugs (e.g., antiepileptic drugs) may be reduced or completely absent).

No products indexed under this heading.

Phenytoin Sodium (During the intake of oral sodium phosphate, the absorption of drugs from the gastrointestinal tract may be delayed or even completely prevented. The efficacy of regularly taken oral drugs (e.g., antiepileptic drugs) may be reduced or completely absent). Products include:

Phenytek Capsules 2192

Pindolol (Patients that are taking hypertension medications are at a higher risk for renal failure and acute phosphate nephropathy when oral sodium phosphate products are used concomitantly).

No products indexed under this heading.

Pioglitazone Hydrochloride (During the intake of oral sodium phosphate, the absorption of the drugs from the gastrointestinal tract may be delayed or even completely prevented. The efficacy of regularly taken oral drugs (e.g., antidiabetic) may be reduced or completely absent). Products include:

ActoPlus Met Tablets 3071
Actos Tablets 3077
Duetact Tablets 3085

Piroxicam (Patients at increased risk for acute phosphate nephropathy include those with conditions that affect renal perfusion or function or those taking medications which may decrease glomerular filtrations rate or predispose to dehydration, including non-steroidal anti-inflammatory drugs (NSAIDs). Dehydration and hypovolemia from purgation may be exacerbated by inadequate oral fluid intake, nausea, vomiting, loss of appetite, or use of NSAIDs and may be associated with acute renal failure).

No products indexed under this heading.

Polythiazide (Patients that are taking hypertension medications are at a higher risk for renal failure and acute phosphate nephropathy when oral sodium phosphate products are used concomitantly).

No products indexed under this heading.

Potassium Phosphate (No oral phosphate supplements or other sodium phosphates preparations including sodium phosphates-based enemas or tablets should be given concomitantly). Products include:

K-Phos Neutral Tablets 813

Prazosin Hydrochloride (Patients that are taking hypertension medications are at a higher risk for renal failure and acute phosphate nephropathy when oral sodium phosphate products are used concomitantly).

No products indexed under this heading.

Primidone (During the intake of oral sodium phosphate, the absorption of drugs from the gastrointestinal tract may be delayed or even completely prevented. The efficacy of regularly taken oral drugs (e.g., antiepileptic drugs) may be reduced or completely absent).

No products indexed under this heading.

Propranolol Hydrochloride (Patients that are taking hypertension medications are at a higher risk for renal failure and acute phosphate nephropathy when oral sodium phosphate products are used concomitantly). Products include:

InnoPran XL Extended Release Capsules 1484

Quinapril Hydrochloride (Patients that are taking hypertension medications are at a higher risk for renal failure and acute phosphate nephropathy when oral sodium phosphate products are used concomitantly).

No products indexed under this heading.

Ramipril (Patients that are taking hypertension medications are at a higher risk for renal failure and acute phosphate nephropathy when oral sodium phosphate products are used concomitantly).

No products indexed under this heading.

Rauwolfia Serpentina (Patients that are taking hypertension medications are at a higher risk for renal failure and acute phosphate nephropathy when oral sodium phosphate products are used concomitantly).

No products indexed under this heading.

Repaglinide (During the intake of oral sodium phosphate, the absorption of the drugs from the gastrointestinal tract may be delayed or even completely prevented. The efficacy of regularly taken oral drugs (e.g., antidiabetic) may be reduced or completely absent). Products include:

PrandiMet Tablets 2967
Prandin Tablets 2971

Rescinnamine (Patients that are taking hypertension medications are at a higher risk for renal failure and acute phosphate nephropathy when oral sodium phosphate products are used concomitantly).

No products indexed under this heading.

Reserpine (Patients that are taking hypertension medications are at a higher risk for renal failure and acute phosphate nephropathy when oral sodium phosphate products are used concomitantly).

No products indexed under this heading.

Rofecoxib (Patients at increased risk for acute phosphate nephropathy include those with conditions that affect renal perfusion or function or those taking medications which may decrease glomerular filtrations rate or predispose to dehydration, including non-steroidal anti-inflammatory drugs (NSAIDs). Dehydration and hypovolemia from purgation may be exacerbated by inadequate oral fluid intake, nausea, vomiting, loss of appetite, or use of NSAIDs and may be associated with acute renal failure).

No products indexed under this heading.

Rosiglitazone Maleate (During the intake of oral sodium phosphate, the absorption of the drugs from the gastrointestinal tract may be delayed or even completely prevented. The efficacy of regularly taken oral drugs (e.g., antidiabetic) may be reduced or completely absent). Products include:

Avandamet Tablets 1336
Avandaryl Tablets 1344
Avandia Tablets 1351

Sitagliptin Phosphate (During the intake of oral sodium phosphate, the absorption of the drugs from the gastrointestinal tract may be delayed or even completely prevented. The efficacy of regularly taken oral drugs (e.g., antidiabetic) may be reduced or completely absent). Products include:

Janumet Tablets 2041
Januvia Tablets 2048

Sodium Nitroprusside (Patients that are taking hypertension medications are at a higher risk for renal failure and acute phosphate nephropathy when oral sodium phosphate products are used concomitantly).

No products indexed under this heading.

Sotalol Hydrochloride (Patients that are taking hypertension medications are at a higher risk for renal failure and acute phosphate nephropathy when oral sodium phosphate products are used concomitantly).

No products indexed under this heading.

Spirapril Hydrochloride (Patients that are taking hypertension medications are at a higher risk for renal failure and acute phosphate nephropathy when oral sodium phosphate products are used concomitantly).

No products indexed under this heading.

Spironolactone (Patients at increased risk for acute phosphate nephropathy include those with conditions that affect renal perfusion or function or those taking medications which may decrease glomerular filtration rate or predispose to dehydration, including diuretics. Dehydration and hypovolemia from purgation may exacerbated by inadequate oral fluid intake, nausea, vomiting, loss of appetite, or use of diuretics and may be associated with acute renal failure).

No products indexed under this heading.

Sulindac (Patients at increased risk for acute phosphate nephropathy include those with conditions that affect renal perfusion or function or those taking medications which may decrease glomerular filtrations rate or predispose to dehydration, including non-steroidal anti-inflammatory drugs (NSAIDs). Dehydration and hypovolemia from purgation may be exacerbated by inadequate oral fluid intake, nausea, vomiting, loss of appetite, or use of NSAIDs and may be associated with acute renal failure). Products include:

Clinoril Tablets 1962

Telmisartan (Patients that are taking hypertension medications are at a higher risk for renal failure and acute phosphate nephropathy when oral sodium phosphate products are used concomitantly). Products include:

Micardis Tablets 852
Micardis HCT Tablets 854

Terazosin Hydrochloride (Patients that are taking hypertension medications are at a higher risk for renal failure and acute phosphate nephropathy when oral sodium phosphate products are used concomitantly).

No products indexed under this heading.

Tiagabine Hydrochloride (During the intake of oral sodium phosphate, the absorption of drugs from the gastrointestinal tract may be delayed or even completely prevented. The efficacy of regularly taken oral drugs (e.g., antiepileptic drugs) may be reduced or completely absent). Products include:

Gabitril Tablets 973

Timolol Maleate (Patients that are taking hypertension medications are at a higher risk for renal failure and acute phosphate nephropathy when oral sodium phosphate products are used concomitantly). Products include:

Combigan Ophthalmic Solution 553
Cosopt Sterile Ophthalmic Solution 1969
Timoptic Sterile Ophthalmic Solution 2121
Timoptic in Ocudose 2124
Timoptic-XE Sterile Ophthalmic Gel Forming Solution 2125

Tolazamide (During the intake of oral sodium phosphate, the absorption of the drugs from the gastrointestinal tract may be delayed or even completely prevented. The efficacy of regularly taken oral drugs (e.g., antidiabetic) may be reduced or completely absent).
No products indexed under this heading.

Tolbutamide (During the intake of oral sodium phosphate, the absorption of the drugs from the gastrointestinal tract may be delayed or even completely prevented. The efficacy of regularly taken oral drugs (e.g., antidiabetic) may be reduced or completely absent).
No products indexed under this heading.

Tolmetin Sodium (Patients at increased risk for acute phosphate nephropathy include those with conditions that affect renal perfusion or function or those taking medications which may decrease glomerular filtrations rate or predispose to dehydration, including non-steroidal anti-inflammatory drugs (NSAIDs). Dehydration and hypovolemia from purgation may be exacerbated by inadequate oral fluid intake, nausea, vomiting, loss of appetite, or use of NSAIDs and may be associated with acute renal failure).
No products indexed under this heading.

Topiramate (During the intake of oral sodium phosphate, the absorption of drugs from the gastrointestinal tract may be delayed or even completely prevented. The efficacy of regularly taken oral drugs (e.g., antiepileptic drugs) may be reduced or completely absent).
No products indexed under this heading.

Torsemide (Patients that are taking hypertension medications are at a higher risk for renal failure and acute phosphate nephropathy when oral sodium phosphate products are used concomitantly). Products include:
Demadex Injection 2630
Demadex Tablets 2630

Trandolapril (Patients that are taking hypertension medications are at a higher risk for renal failure and acute phosphate nephropathy when oral sodium phosphate products are used concomitantly). Products include:
Mavik Tablets 472
Tarka Tablets 511

Triamterene (Patients at increased risk for acute phosphate nephropathy include those with conditions that affect renal perfusion or function or those taking medications which may decrease glomerular filtration rate or predispose to dehydration, including diuretics. Dehydration and hypovolemia from purgation may exacerbated by inadequate oral fluid intake, nausea, vomiting, loss of appetite, or use of diuretics and may be associated with acute renal failure). Products include:
Dyazide Capsules 1405
Dyrenium Capsules 3189

Trimethadione (During the intake of oral sodium phosphate, the absorption of drugs from the gastrointestinal tract may be delayed or even completely prevented. The efficacy of regularly taken oral drugs (e.g., antiepileptic drugs) may be reduced or completely absent).
No products indexed under this heading.

Trimethaphan Camsylate (Patients that are taking hypertension medications are at a higher risk for renal failure and acute phosphate nephropathy when oral sodium phosphate products are used concomitantly).
No products indexed under this heading.

Troglitazone (During the intake of oral sodium phosphate, the absorption of the drugs from the gastrointestinal tract may be delayed or even completely prevented. The efficacy of regularly taken oral drugs (e.g., antidiabetic) may be reduced or completely absent).
No products indexed under this heading.

Valdecoxib (Patients at increased risk for acute phosphate nephropathy include those with conditions that affect renal perfusion or function or those taking medications which may decrease glomerular filtrations rate or predispose to dehydration, including non-steroidal anti-inflammatory drugs (NSAIDs). Dehydration and hypovolemia from purgation may be exacerbated by inadequate oral fluid intake, nausea, vomiting, loss of appetite, or use of NSAIDs and may be associated with acute renal failure).
No products indexed under this heading.

Valproate Sodium (During the intake of oral sodium phosphate, the absorption of drugs from the gastrointestinal tract may be delayed or even completely prevented. The efficacy of regularly taken oral drugs (e.g., antiepileptic drugs) may be reduced or completely absent).
No products indexed under this heading.

Valproic Acid (During the intake of oral sodium phosphate, the absorption of drugs from the gastrointestinal tract may be delayed or even completely prevented. The efficacy of regularly taken oral drugs (e.g., antiepileptic drugs) may be reduced or completely absent).
No products indexed under this heading.

Valsartan (Patients that are taking hypertension medications are at a higher risk for renal failure and acute phosphate nephropathy when oral sodium phosphate products are used concomitantly). Products include:
Diovan Tablets 2212
Diovan HCT Tablets 2216
Exforge Tablets 2238

Verapamil Hydrochloride (Patients that are taking hypertension medications are at a higher risk for renal failure and acute phosphate nephropathy when oral sodium phosphate products are used concomitantly). Products include:
Tarka Tablets 511

Zonisamide (During the intake of oral sodium phosphate, the absorption of drugs from the gastrointestinal tract may be delayed or even completely prevented. The efficacy of regularly taken oral drugs (e.g., antiepileptic drugs) may be reduced or completely absent). Products include:
Zonegran Capsules 1089

FLEET PHOSPHO-SODA EZ-PREP
(Sodium Phosphate) 1147
See Fleet Phospho-soda

FLEET PREP KITS
(Bisacodyl, Sodium Phosphate) 1149
May interact with ACE inhibitors, oral aminoglycosides, angiotensin-II receptor antagonists, antacids, antihypertensives, oral anticoagulants, diuretics, anticonvulsants, oral hypoglycemic agents, iron containing oral preparations, lithium preparations, non-steroidal anti-inflammatory agents, oral contraceptives, oral phosphate supplements, drugs that prolong the QT interval, oral sympathomimetics, and certain other agents. Compounds in these categories include:

Acarbose (The absorption of drugs taken concomitantly with sodium phosphate from the gastrointestinal tract may be delayed or even completely prevented). Products include:
Precose Tablets 792

Acebutolol Hydrochloride (Electrolyte disturbances area a risk associated with this product; concurrent use in patients taking agents known to disturb electrolyte balance requires caution).
No products indexed under this heading.

Albuterol Sulfate (The absorption of drugs taken concomitantly with sodium phosphate from the gastrointestinal tract may be delayed or even completely prevented). Products include:
Combivent Inhalation Aerosol 845
ProAir HFA Inhalation Aerosol 3113
Proventil HFA Inhalation Aerosol 2914
Ventolin HFA Inhalation Aerosol 1638

Aliskiren (Electrolyte disturbances area a risk associated with this product; concurrent use in patients taking agents known to disturb electrolyte balance requires caution). Products include:
Tekturna Tablets 2321
Tekturna HCT Tablets 2324

Alprazolam (Electrolyte disturbances are a risk associated with this product; concurrent use in patients taking agents known to prolong QT interval requires caution).
No products indexed under this heading.

Aluminum Carbonate (Concurrent use within one hour should be avoided).
No products indexed under this heading.

Aluminum Hydroxide (Concurrent use within one hour should be avoided).
No products indexed under this heading.

Amiloride Hydrochloride (Electrolyte disturbances are a risk associated with this product; concurrent use in patients taking agents known to disturb electrolyte balance requires caution).
No products indexed under this heading.

Amiodarone Hydrochloride (Electrolyte disturbances are a risk associated with this product; concurrent use in patients taking agents known to prolong QT interval requires caution).
No products indexed under this heading.

Amitriptyline Hydrochloride (Electrolyte disturbances are a risk associated with this product; concurrent use in patients taking agents known to prolong QT interval requires caution).
No products indexed under this heading.

Amlodipine Besylate (Electrolyte disturbances area a risk associated with this product; concurrent use in patients taking agents known to disturb electrolyte balance requires caution). Products include:
Azor Tablets 1005
Exforge Tablets 2238

Amoxapine (Electrolyte disturbances are a risk associated with this product; concurrent use in patients taking agents known to prolong QT interval requires caution).
No products indexed under this heading.

Anisindione (The absorption of drugs taken concomitantly with sodium phosphate from the gastrointestinal tract may be delayed or even completely prevented).
No products indexed under this heading.

Astemizole (Electrolyte disturbances are a risk associated with this product; concurrent use in patients taking agents known to prolong QT interval requires caution).
No products indexed under this heading.

Atenolol (Electrolyte disturbances area a risk associated with this product; concurrent use in patients taking agents known to disturb electrolyte balance requires caution).
No products indexed under this heading.

Benazepril Hydrochloride (Electrolyte disturbances are a risk associated with this product; concurrent use in patients taking agents known to disturb electrolyte balance requires caution).
No products indexed under this heading.

Bendroflumethiazide (Electrolyte disturbances are a risk associated with this product; concurrent use in patients taking agents known to disturb electrolyte balance requires caution).
No products indexed under this heading.

Betaxolol Hydrochloride (Electrolyte disturbances area a risk associated with this product; concurrent use in patients taking agents known to disturb electrolyte balance requires caution).
No products indexed under this heading.

Bisoprolol Fumarate (Electrolyte disturbances area a risk associated with this product; concurrent use in patients taking agents known to disturb electrolyte balance requires caution).
No products indexed under this heading.

Bretylium Tosylate (Electrolyte disturbances are a risk associated with this product; concurrent use in patients taking agents known to prolong QT interval requires caution).
No products indexed under this heading.

Bumetanide (Electrolyte disturbances are a risk associated with this product; concurrent use in patients taking agents known to disturb electrolyte balance requires caution).
No products indexed under this heading.

Buspirone Hydrochloride (Electrolyte disturbances are a risk associated with this product; concurrent use in patients taking agents known to prolong QT interval requires caution).
No products indexed under this heading.

Candesartan Cilexetil (Electrolyte disturbances are a risk associated with this product; concurrent use in patients taking agents known to disturb electrolyte balance requires caution). Products include:
Atacand Tablets 639
Atacand HCT 642

Captopril (Electrolyte disturbances are a risk associated with this product; concurrent use in patients taking agents known to disturb electrolyte balance requires caution). Products include:
Captopril Tablets 2182

Carbamazepine (Concomitant use may delay or even completely prevent the absorption of antiepileptic drugs. The efficacy of regularly taken antiepileptic drugs may be reduced or completely absent). Products include:
Carbatrol Capsules 3019
Equetro Extended-Release Capsules 3174

Carteolol Hydrochloride (Electrolyte disturbances area a risk associated with this product; concurrent use in patients taking agents known to disturb electrolyte balance requires caution).
No products indexed under this heading.

Celecoxib (Electrolyte disturbances are a risk associated with this product; concurrent use in patients taking agents known to disturb electrolyte balance requires caution). Products include:
Celebrex Capsules 2979

Chlordiazepoxide (Electrolyte disturbances are a risk associated with this product; concurrent use in patients taking agents known to prolong QT interval requires caution).
No products indexed under this heading.

Chlordiazepoxide Hydrochloride (Electrolyte disturbances are a risk associated with this product; concurrent use in patients taking agents known to prolong QT interval requires caution).
No products indexed under this heading.

Chlorothiazide (Electrolyte disturbances are a risk associated with this product; concurrent use in patients taking agents known to disturb electrolyte balance requires caution).
No products indexed under this heading.

Chlorothiazide Sodium (Electrolyte disturbances are a risk associated with this product; concurrent use in patients taking agents known to disturb electrolyte balance requires caution). Products include:
Intravenous Sodium Diuril 2490

Chlorpromazine (Electrolyte disturbances are a risk associated with this product; concurrent use in patients taking agents known to prolong QT interval requires caution).
No products indexed under this heading.

Chlorpromazine Hydrochloride (Electrolyte disturbances are a risk associated with this product; concurrent use in patients taking agents known to prolong QT interval requires caution).
No products indexed under this heading.

Chlorpropamide (The absorption of drugs taken concomitantly with sodium phosphate from the gastrointestinal tract may be delayed or even completely prevented).
No products indexed under this heading.

Chlorprothixene (Electrolyte disturbances are a risk associated with this product; concurrent use in patients taking agents known to prolong QT interval requires caution).
No products indexed under this heading.

Chlorprothixene Hydrochloride (Electrolyte disturbances are a risk associated with this product; concurrent use in patients taking agents known to prolong QT interval requires caution).
No products indexed under this heading.

Chlorthalidone (Electrolyte disturbances are a risk associated with this product; concurrent use in patients taking agents known to disturb electrolyte balance requires caution). Products include:
Clorpres Tablets 2185

Clomipramine Hydrochloride (Electrolyte disturbances are a risk associated with this product; concurrent use in patients taking agents known to prolong QT interval requires caution).
No products indexed under this heading.

Clonidine (Electrolyte disturbances area a risk associated with this product; concurrent use in patients taking agents known to disturb electrolyte balance requires caution). Products include:
Catapres-TTS 842

Clonidine Hydrochloride (Electrolyte disturbances area a risk associated with this product; concurrent use in patients taking agents known to disturb electrolyte balance requires caution). Products include:
Catapres Tablets 841
Clorpres Tablets 2185

Clorazepate Dipotassium (Electrolyte disturbances are a risk associated with this product; concurrent use in patients taking agents known to prolong QT interval requires caution).
No products indexed under this heading.

Clozapine (Electrolyte disturbances are a risk associated with this product; concurrent use in patients taking agents known to prolong QT interval requires caution).
No products indexed under this heading.

Deserpidine (Electrolyte disturbances area a risk associated with this product; concurrent use in patients taking agents known to disturb electrolyte balance requires caution).
No products indexed under this heading.

Desipramine Hydrochloride (Electrolyte disturbances are a risk associated with this product; concurrent use in patients taking agents known to prolong QT interval requires caution).
No products indexed under this heading.

Desogestrel (The absorption of drugs taken concomitantly with sodium phosphate from the gastrointestinal tract may be delayed or even completely prevented). Products include:
Mircette Tablets 1034

Diazepam (Electrolyte disturbances are a risk associated with this product; concurrent use in patients taking agents known to prolong QT interval requires caution). Products include:
Valium Tablets 2658

Diazoxide (Electrolyte disturbances area a risk associated with this product; concurrent use in patients taking agents known to disturb electrolyte balance requires caution). Products include:
Proglycem Capsules 1185
Proglycem Suspension 1185

Diclofenac Epolamine (Electrolyte disturbances are a risk associated with this product; concurrent use in patients taking agents known to disturb electrolyte balance requires caution). Products include:
Flector Patch 561

Diclofenac Potassium (Electrolyte disturbances are a risk associated with this product; concurrent use in patients taking agents known to disturb electrolyte balance requires caution).
No products indexed under this heading.

Diclofenac Sodium (Electrolyte disturbances are a risk associated with this product; concurrent use in patients taking agents known to disturb electrolyte balance requires caution). Products include:
Diclofenac Sodium Ophthalmic Solution .... ⊙ 240
Voltaren Ophthalmic Solution 2336
Voltaren Tablets 2334
Voltaren-XR Tablets 2337

Dicumarol (The absorption of drugs taken concomitantly with sodium phosphate from the gastrointestinal tract may be delayed or even completely prevented).
No products indexed under this heading.

Diltiazem Hydrochloride (Electrolyte disturbances area a risk associated with this product; concurrent use in patients taking agents known to disturb electrolyte balance requires caution). Products include:
Cardizem LA Extended Release Tablets 421

Disopyramide Phosphate (Electrolyte disturbances are a risk associated with this product; concurrent use in patients taking agents known to prolong QT interval requires caution).
No products indexed under this heading.

Divalproex Sodium (Concomitant use may delay or even completely prevent the absorption of antiepileptic drugs. The efficacy of regularly taken antiepileptic drugs may be reduced or completely absent). Products include:
Depakote ER Tablets 423

Dofetilide (Electrolyte disturbances are a risk associated with this product; concurrent use in patients taking agents known to prolong QT interval requires caution).
No products indexed under this heading.

Doxazosin Mesylate (Electrolyte disturbances area a risk associated with this product; concurrent use in patients taking agents known to disturb electrolyte balance requires caution).
No products indexed under this heading.

Doxepin Hydrochloride (Electrolyte disturbances are a risk associated with this product; concurrent use in patients taking agents known to prolong QT interval requires caution).
No products indexed under this heading.

Droperidol (Electrolyte disturbances are a risk associated with this product; concurrent use in patients taking agents known to prolong QT interval requires caution).
No products indexed under this heading.

Enalapril Maleate (Electrolyte disturbances are a risk associated with this product; concurrent use in patients taking agents known to disturb electrolyte balance requires caution).
No products indexed under this heading.

Enalaprilat (Electrolyte disturbances are a risk associated with this product; concurrent use in patients taking agents known to disturb electrolyte balance requires caution).
No products indexed under this heading.

Ephedrine Hydrochloride (The absorption of drugs taken concomitantly with sodium phosphate from the gastrointestinal tract may be delayed or even completely prevented).
No products indexed under this heading.

Ephedrine Sulfate (The absorption of drugs taken concomitantly with sodium phosphate from the gastrointestinal tract may be delayed or even completely prevented).
No products indexed under this heading.

Ephedrine Tannate (The absorption of drugs taken concomitantly with sodium phosphate from the gastrointestinal tract may be delayed or even completely prevented).
No products indexed under this heading.

Eprosartan Mesylate (Electrolyte disturbances are a risk associated with this product; concurrent use in patients taking agents known to disturb electrolyte balance requires caution). Products include:
Teveten Tablets 515
Teveten HCT Tablets 517

Erythromycin (Electrolyte disturbances are a risk associated with this product; concurrent use in patients taking agents known to prolong QT interval requires caution).
No products indexed under this heading.

Erythromycin Estolate (Electrolyte disturbances are a risk associated with this product; concurrent use in patients taking agents known to prolong QT interval requires caution).
No products indexed under this heading.

Erythromycin Ethylsuccinate (Electrolyte disturbances are a risk associated with this product; concurrent use in patients taking agents known to prolong QT interval requires caution). Products include:
E.E.S. 433
EryPed 431

Erythromycin Gluceptate (Electrolyte disturbances are a risk associated with this product; concurrent use in patients taking agents known to prolong QT interval requires caution).
No products indexed under this heading.

Erythromycin Lactobionate (Electrolyte disturbances are a risk associated with this product; concurrent use in patients taking agents known to prolong QT interval requires caution).
No products indexed under this heading.

Erythromycin Stearate (Electrolyte disturbances are a risk associated with this product; concurrent use in patients taking agents known to prolong QT interval requires caution).
No products indexed under this heading.

Esmolol Hydrochloride (Electrolyte disturbances area a risk associated with this product; concurrent use in patients taking agents known to disturb electrolyte balance requires caution).
No products indexed under this heading.

Ethacrynic Acid (Electrolyte disturbances are a risk associated with this product; concurrent use in patients taking agents known to disturb electrolyte balance requires caution). Products include:
Edecrin Tablets 698

Ethinyl Estradiol (The absorption of drugs taken concomitantly with sodium phosphate from the gastrointestinal tract may be delayed or even completely prevented).
Products include:
Lybrel Tablets 3204
Mircette Tablets 1034
NuvaRing 2897
Ortho-Cyclen/Ortho Tri-Cyclen 2449
Ortho Evra Transdermal System 2437
Ortho Tri-Cyclen Lo Tablets 2458
Seasonique Tablets 1046
Yaz Tablets 805

Ethosuximide (Concomitant use may delay or even completely prevent the absorption of antiepileptic drugs. The efficacy of regularly taken antiepileptic drugs may be reduced or completely absent).
No products indexed under this heading.

Ethotoin (Concomitant use may delay or even completely prevent the absorption of antiepileptic drugs. The efficacy of regularly taken antiepileptic drugs may be reduced or completely absent).
No products indexed under this heading.

Ethynodiol Diacetate (The absorption of drugs taken concomitantly with sodium phosphate from the gastrointestinal tract may be delayed or even completely prevented).
No products indexed under this heading.

Etodolac (Electrolyte disturbances are a risk associated with this product; concurrent use in patients taking agents known to disturb electrolyte balance requires caution).
No products indexed under this heading.

Felbamate (Concomitant use may delay or even completely prevent the absorption of antiepileptic drugs. The efficacy of regularly taken antiepileptic drugs may be reduced or completely absent).
No products indexed under this heading.

Felodipine (Electrolyte disturbances area a risk associated with this product; concurrent use in patients taking agents known to disturb electrolyte balance requires caution).
No products indexed under this heading.

Fenoprofen Calcium (Electrolyte disturbances are a risk associated with this product; concurrent use in patients taking agents known to disturb electrolyte balance requires caution). Products include:
Nalfon Capsules 2508

Ferrous Fumarate (The absorption of drugs taken concomitantly with sodium phosphate from the gastrointestinal tract may be delayed or even completely prevented).
No products indexed under this heading.

Ferrous Gluconate (The absorption of drugs taken concomitantly with sodium phosphate from the gastrointestinal tract may be delayed or even completely prevented).
Products include:
CitraNatal DHA Tablets 2175

Ferrous Sulfate (The absorption of drugs taken concomitantly with sodium phosphate from the gastrointestinal tract may be delayed or even completely prevented).
No products indexed under this heading.

Flecainide Acetate (Electrolyte disturbances are a risk associated with this product; concurrent use in patients taking agents known to prolong QT interval requires caution).
No products indexed under this heading.

Fluphenazine Decanoate (Electrolyte disturbances are a risk associated with this product; concurrent use in patients taking agents known to prolong QT interval requires caution).
No products indexed under this heading.

Fluphenazine Enanthate (Electrolyte disturbances are a risk associated with this product; concurrent use in patients taking agents known to prolong QT interval requires caution).
No products indexed under this heading.

Fluphenazine Hydrochloride (Electrolyte disturbances are a risk associated with this product; concurrent use in patients taking agents known to prolong QT interval requires caution).
No products indexed under this heading.

Flurbiprofen (Electrolyte disturbances are a risk associated with this product; concurrent use in patients taking agents known to disturb electrolyte balance requires caution).
No products indexed under this heading.

Fosinopril Sodium (Electrolyte disturbances are a risk associated with this product; concurrent use in patients taking agents known to disturb electrolyte balance requires caution).
No products indexed under this heading.

Fosphenytoin (Concomitant use may delay or even completely prevent the absorption of antiepileptic drugs. The efficacy of regularly taken antiepileptic drugs may be reduced or completely absent).
No products indexed under this heading.

Fosphenytoin Sodium (Concomitant use may delay or even completely prevent the absorption of antiepileptic drugs. The efficacy of regularly taken antiepileptic drugs may be reduced or completely absent).
No products indexed under this heading.

Furosemide (Electrolyte disturbances are a risk associated with this product; concurrent use in patients taking agents known to disturb electrolyte balance requires caution).
Products include:
Furosemide Tablets 2186

Gabapentin (Concomitant use may delay or even completely prevent the absorption of antiepileptic drugs. The efficacy of regularly taken antiepileptic drugs may be reduced or completely absent).
No products indexed under this heading.

Glimepiride (The absorption of drugs taken concomitantly with sodium phosphate from the gastrointestinal tract may be delayed or even completely prevented). Products include:
Avandaryl Tablets 1344
Duetact Tablets 3085

Glipizide (The absorption of drugs taken concomitantly with sodium phosphate from the gastrointestinal tract may be delayed or even completely prevented).
No products indexed under this heading.

Glyburide (The absorption of drugs taken concomitantly with sodium phosphate from the gastrointestinal tract may be delayed or even completely prevented).
No products indexed under this heading.

Guanabenz Acetate (Electrolyte disturbances area a risk associated with this product; concurrent use in patients taking agents known to disturb electrolyte balance requires caution).
No products indexed under this heading.

Guanethidine Monosulfate (Electrolyte disturbances area a risk associated with this product; concurrent use in patients taking agents known to disturb electrolyte balance requires caution).
No products indexed under this heading.

Haloperidol (Electrolyte disturbances are a risk associated with this product; concurrent use in patients taking agents known to prolong QT interval requires caution).
No products indexed under this heading.

Haloperidol Decanoate (Electrolyte disturbances are a risk associated with this product; concurrent use in patients taking agents known to prolong QT interval requires caution).
No products indexed under this heading.

Hydralazine Hydrochloride (Electrolyte disturbances area a risk associated with this product; concurrent use in patients taking agents known to disturb electrolyte balance requires caution).
No products indexed under this heading.

Hydrochlorothiazide (Electrolyte disturbances are a risk associated with this product; concurrent use in patients taking agents known to disturb electrolyte balance requires caution). Products include:
Atacand HCT 642
Avalide Tablets 892
Avalide Tablets 2713
Benicar HCT Tablets 1010
Diovan HCT Tablets 2216
Dyazide Capsules 1405
Micardis HCT Tablets 854
Prinzide Tablets 2092
Tekturna HCT Tablets 2324
Teveten HCT Tablets 517

Hydroflumethiazide (Electrolyte disturbances are a risk associated with this product; concurrent use in patients taking agents known to disturb electrolyte balance requires caution).
No products indexed under this heading.

Hydroxyzine Hydrochloride (Electrolyte disturbances are a risk associated with this product; concurrent use in patients taking agents known to prolong QT interval requires caution).
No products indexed under this heading.

Ibuprofen (Electrolyte disturbances are a risk associated with this product; concurrent use in patients taking agents known to disturb electrolyte balance requires caution).
Products include:
Motrin IB Tablets and Caplets 1900
Children's Motrin Oral Suspension 1901
Children's Motrin Non-Staining Dye-Free Oral Suspension 1901
Children's Motrin Cold Oral Suspension 1899
Infants' Motrin Concentrated Drops 1901
Infants' Motrin Non-Staining Dye-Free Concentrated Drops 1901
Junior Strength Motrin Caplets and Chewable Tablets 1901
Vicoprofen Tablets 533

Imipramine Hydrochloride (Electrolyte disturbances are a risk associated with this product; concurrent use in patients taking agents known to prolong QT interval requires caution).
No products indexed under this heading.

Imipramine Pamoate (Electrolyte disturbances are a risk associated with this product; concurrent use in patients taking agents known to prolong QT interval requires caution).
No products indexed under this heading.

Indapamide (Electrolyte disturbances are a risk associated with this product; concurrent use in patients taking agents known to disturb electrolyte balance requires caution). Products include:
Indapamide Tablets 2188

Indomethacin (Electrolyte disturbances are a risk associated with this product; concurrent use in patients taking agents known to disturb electrolyte balance requires caution). Products include:
Indocin 2024

Indomethacin Sodium Trihydrate (Electrolyte disturbances are a risk associated with this product; concurrent use in patients taking agents known to disturb electrolyte balance requires caution). Products include:
Indocin I.V. 2489

Irbesartan (Electrolyte disturbances are a risk associated with this product; concurrent use in patients taking agents known to disturb electrolyte balance requires caution). Products include:
Avalide Tablets 892
Avalide Tablets 2713
Avapro Tablets 897
Avapro Tablets 2718

Iron (The absorption of drugs taken concomitantly with sodium phosphate from the gastrointestinal tract may be delayed or even completely prevented). Products include:
Phyto-Vite Tablets .... ▣639

Isocarboxazid (Electrolyte disturbances are a risk associated with this product; concurrent use in patients taking agents known to prolong QT interval requires caution). Products include:
Marplan Tablets 3177

Isradipine (Electrolyte disturbances area a risk associated with this product; concurrent use in patients taking agents known to disturb electrolyte balance requires caution). Products include:
DynaCirc CR Controlled Release Tablets 1407

Kanamycin Sulfate (The absorption of drugs taken concomitantly with sodium phosphate from the gastrointestinal tract may be delayed or even completely prevented).
No products indexed under this heading.

Ketoprofen (Electrolyte disturbances are a risk associated with this product; concurrent use in patients taking agents known to disturb electrolyte balance requires caution).
No products indexed under this heading.

Ketorolac Tromethamine (Electrolyte disturbances are a risk associated with this product; concurrent use in patients taking agents known to disturb electrolyte balance requires caution).
No products indexed under this heading.

Labetalol Hydrochloride (Electrolyte disturbances area a risk associated with this product; concurrent use in patients taking agents known to disturb electrolyte balance requires caution).
No products indexed under this heading.

Lamotrigine (Concomitant use may delay or even completely prevent the absorption of antiepileptic drugs. The efficacy of regularly taken antiepileptic drugs may be reduced or completely absent). Products include:
Lamictal 1488

Levetiracetam (Concomitant use may delay or even completely prevent the absorption of antiepileptic drugs. The efficacy of regularly taken antiepileptic drugs may be reduced or completely absent). Products include:
Keppra Injection 3137
Keppra Oral Solution 3131
Keppra Tablets 3131

Levonorgestrel (The absorption of drugs taken concomitantly with sodium phosphate from the gastrointestinal tract may be delayed or even completely prevented). Products include:
Climara Pro Transdermal System 768
Lybrel Tablets 3204
Mirena Intrauterine System 779
Plan B Tablets 1044
Seasonique Tablets 1046

Lidocaine Hydrochloride (Electrolyte disturbances are a risk associated with this product; concurrent use in patients taking agents known to prolong QT interval requires caution).
No products indexed under this heading.

Lisinopril (Electrolyte disturbances are a risk associated with this product; concurrent use in patients taking agents known to disturb electrolyte balance requires caution). Products include:
Prinivil Tablets 2087
Prinzide Tablets 2092

Lithium (Electrolyte disturbances are a risk associated with this product; concurrent use in patients taking agents known to disturb electrolyte balance requires caution).
No products indexed under this heading.

Lithium Carbonate (Electrolyte disturbances are a risk associated with this product; concurrent use in patients taking agents known to prolong QT interval requires caution).
No products indexed under this heading.

Lithium Citrate (Electrolyte disturbances are a risk associated with this product; concurrent use in patients taking agents known to prolong QT interval requires caution).
No products indexed under this heading.

Lorazepam (Electrolyte disturbances are a risk associated with this product; concurrent use in patients taking agents known to prolong QT interval requires caution).
No products indexed under this heading.

Losartan Potassium (Electrolyte disturbances are a risk associated with this product; concurrent use in patients taking agents known to disturb electrolyte balance requires caution). Products include:
Cozaar Tablets 1973

Loxapine Hydrochloride (Electrolyte disturbances are a risk associated with this product; concurrent use in patients taking agents known to prolong QT interval requires caution).
No products indexed under this heading.

Loxapine Succinate (Electrolyte disturbances are a risk associated with this product; concurrent use in patients taking agents known to prolong QT interval requires caution).
No products indexed under this heading.

Magaldrate (Concurrent use within one hour should be avoided).
No products indexed under this heading.

Magnesium Hydroxide (Concurrent use within one hour should be avoided). Products include:
Fleet Pedia-Lax Chewable Tablets 1145
Pepcid Complete Chewable Tablets 1771
Extra Strength Rolaids Freshmint Tablets 1903
Rolaids Multi-Symptom Berry Tablets 1903
Rolaids Original Peppermint Tablets 1903

Magnesium Oxide (Concurrent use within one hour should be avoided). Products include:
Beelith Tablets 813

Maprotiline Hydrochloride (Electrolyte disturbances are a risk associated with this product; concurrent use in patients taking agents known to prolong QT interval requires caution).
No products indexed under this heading.

Mecamylamine Hydrochloride (Electrolyte disturbances area a risk associated with this product; concurrent use in patients taking agents known to disturb electrolyte balance requires caution).
No products indexed under this heading.

Meclofenamate Sodium (Electrolyte disturbances are a risk associated with this product; concurrent use in patients taking agents known to disturb electrolyte balance requires caution).
No products indexed under this heading.

Mefenamic Acid (Electrolyte disturbances are a risk associated with this product; concurrent use in patients taking agents known to disturb electrolyte balance requires caution).
No products indexed under this heading.

Meloxicam (Electrolyte disturbances are a risk associated with this product; concurrent use in patients taking agents known to disturb electrolyte balance requires caution). Products include:
Mobic Oral Suspension 863
Mobic Tablets 863

Mephenytoin (Concomitant use may delay or even completely prevent the absorption of antiepileptic drugs. The efficacy of regularly taken antiepileptic drugs may be reduced or completely absent).
No products indexed under this heading.

Meprobamate (Electrolyte disturbances are a risk associated with this product; concurrent use in patients taking agents known to prolong QT interval requires caution).
No products indexed under this heading.

Mesoridazine Besylate (Electrolyte disturbances are a risk associated with this product; concurrent use in patients taking agents known to prolong QT interval requires caution).
No products indexed under this heading.

Mestranol (The absorption of drugs taken concomitantly with sodium phosphate from the gastrointestinal tract may be delayed or even completely prevented).
No products indexed under this heading.

Metaproterenol Sulfate (The absorption of drugs taken concomitantly with sodium phosphate from the gastrointestinal tract may be delayed or even completely prevented).
No products indexed under this heading.

Metformin Hydrochloride (The absorption of drugs taken concomitantly with sodium phosphate from the gastrointestinal tract may be delayed or even completely prevented). Products include:
ActoPlus Met Tablets 3071
Avandamet Tablets 1336
Janumet Tablets 2041
PrandiMet Tablets 2967

Methsuximide (Concomitant use may delay or even completely prevent the absorption of antiepileptic drugs. The efficacy of regularly taken antiepileptic drugs may be reduced or completely absent).
No products indexed under this heading.

Methyclothiazide (Electrolyte disturbances are a risk associated with this product; concurrent use in patients taking agents known to disturb electrolyte balance requires caution).
No products indexed under this heading.

Methyldopa (Electrolyte disturbances area a risk associated with this product; concurrent use in patients taking agents known to disturb electrolyte balance requires caution).
No products indexed under this heading.

Methyldopate Hydrochloride (Electrolyte disturbances area a risk associated with this product; concurrent use in patients taking agents known to disturb electrolyte balance requires caution).
No products indexed under this heading.

Metolazone (Electrolyte disturbances are a risk associated with this product; concurrent use in patients taking agents known to disturb electrolyte balance requires caution).
No products indexed under this heading.

Metoprolol Succinate (Electrolyte disturbances area a risk associated with this product; concurrent use in patients taking agents known to disturb electrolyte balance requires caution). Products include:
Toprol-XL Tablets 666

Metoprolol Tartrate (Electrolyte disturbances area a risk associated with this product; concurrent use in patients taking agents known to disturb electrolyte balance requires caution).
No products indexed under this heading.

Metyrosine (Electrolyte disturbances area a risk associated with this product; concurrent use in patients taking agents known to disturb electrolyte balance requires caution). Products include:
Demser Capsules 1989

Mexiletine Hydrochloride (Electrolyte disturbances are a risk associated with this product; concurrent use in patients taking agents known to prolong QT interval requires caution).
No products indexed under this heading.

Mibefradil Dihydrochloride (Electrolyte disturbances area a risk associated with this product; concurrent use in patients taking agents known to disturb electrolyte balance requires caution).
No products indexed under this heading.

Midazolam Hydrochloride (Electrolyte disturbances are a risk associated with this product; concurrent use in patients taking agents known to prolong QT interval requires caution).
No products indexed under this heading.

Miglitol (The absorption of drugs taken concomitantly with sodium phosphate from the gastrointestinal tract may be delayed or even completely prevented).
No products indexed under this heading.

Minoxidil (Electrolyte disturbances area a risk associated with this product; concurrent use in patients taking agents known to disturb electrolyte balance requires caution).
No products indexed under this heading.

Moexipril Hydrochloride (Electrolyte disturbances are a risk associated with this product; concurrent use in patients taking agents known to disturb electrolyte balance requires caution).
No products indexed under this heading.

Molindone Hydrochloride (Electrolyte disturbances are a risk associated with this product; concurrent use in patients taking agents known to prolong QT interval requires caution). Products include:
Moban Tablets 1116

Nabumetone (Electrolyte disturbances are a risk associated with this product; concurrent use in patients taking agents known to disturb electrolyte balance requires caution).
No products indexed under this heading.

Nadolol (Electrolyte disturbances area a risk associated with this product; concurrent use in patients taking agents known to disturb electrolyte balance requires caution). Products include:
Nadolol Tablets 2191

Naproxen (Electrolyte disturbances are a risk associated with this product; concurrent use in patients taking agents known to disturb electrolyte balance requires caution). Products include:
EC-Naprosyn Delayed-Release Tablets 2632
Naprosyn Suspension 2632
Naprosyn Tablets 2632

Naproxen Sodium (Electrolyte disturbances are a risk associated with this product; concurrent use in patients taking agents known to disturb electrolyte balance requires caution). Products include:
Anaprox Tablets 2632
Anaprox DS Tablets 2632
Treximet Tablets 1616

Nateglinide (The absorption of drugs taken concomitantly with sodium phosphate from the gastrointestinal tract may be delayed or even completely prevented). Products include:
Starlix Tablets 2314

Nebivolol (Electrolyte disturbances area a risk associated with this product; concurrent use in patients taking agents known to disturb electrolyte balance requires caution). Products include:
Bystolic Tablets 1155

Neomycin, oral (The absorption of drugs taken concomitantly with sodium phosphate from the gastrointestinal tract may be delayed or even completely prevented).
No products indexed under this heading.

Nicardipine Hydrochloride (Electrolyte disturbances area a risk associated with this product; concurrent use in patients taking agents known to disturb electrolyte balance requires caution). Products include:
Cardene I.V. 1093

Nifedipine (Electrolyte disturbances area a risk associated with this product; concurrent use in patients taking agents known to disturb electrolyte balance requires caution).
No products indexed under this heading.

Nisoldipine (Electrolyte disturbances area a risk associated with this product; concurrent use in patients taking agents known to disturb electrolyte balance requires caution). Products include:
Sular Extended Release Tablets 2975

Nitroglycerin (Electrolyte disturbances area a risk associated with this product; concurrent use in patients taking agents known to disturb electrolyte balance requires caution). Products include:
Nitro-Dur Transdermal Infusion System.. 2887
Nitrolingual Pumpspray 2965

Norethindrone (The absorption of drugs taken concomitantly with sodium phosphate from the gastrointestinal tract may be delayed or even completely prevented). Products include:
Ortho Micronor Tablets 2446

Norethynodrel (The absorption of drugs taken concomitantly with sodium phosphate from the gastrointestinal tract may be delayed or even completely prevented).
No products indexed under this heading.

Norgestimate (The absorption of drugs taken concomitantly with sodium phosphate from the gastrointestinal tract may be delayed or even completely prevented). Products include:
Ortho-Cyclen/Ortho Tri-Cyclen 2449
Ortho Tri-Cyclen Lo Tablets 2458

Norgestrel (The absorption of drugs taken concomitantly with sodium phosphate from the gastrointestinal tract may be delayed or even completely prevented).
No products indexed under this heading.

Nortriptyline Hydrochloride (Electrolyte disturbances are a risk associated with this product; concurrent use in patients taking agents known to prolong QT interval requires caution).
No products indexed under this heading.

Olanzapine (Electrolyte disturbances are a risk associated with this product; concurrent use in patients taking agents known to prolong QT interval requires caution). Products include:
Symbyax Capsules 1871
Zyprexa Tablets 1883
Zyprexa IntraMuscular 1883
Zyprexa ZYDIS Orally Disintegrating Tablets.................. 1883

Oral Medications, unspecified (During the intake of sodium phosphate, the absorption of drugs from the gastrointestinal tract may be delayed or even completely prevented).
No products indexed under this heading.

Oxaprozin (Electrolyte disturbances are a risk associated with this product; concurrent use in patients taking agents known to disturb electrolyte balance requires caution).
No products indexed under this heading.

Oxazepam (Electrolyte disturbances are a risk associated with this product; concurrent use in patients taking agents known to prolong QT interval requires caution).
No products indexed under this heading.

Oxcarbazepine (Concomitant use may delay or even completely prevent the absorption of antiepileptic drugs. The efficacy of regularly taken antiepileptic drugs may be reduced or completely absent).
No products indexed under this heading.

Paramethadione (Concomitant use may delay or even completely prevent the absorption of antiepileptic drugs. The efficacy of regularly taken antiepileptic drugs may be reduced or completely absent).
No products indexed under this heading.

Paromomycin Sulfate (The absorption of drugs taken concomitantly with sodium phosphate from the gastrointestinal tract may be delayed or even completely prevented).
No products indexed under this heading.

Penbutolol Sulfate (Electrolyte disturbances are a risk associated with this product; concurrent use in patients taking agents known to disturb electrolyte balance requires caution).
No products indexed under this heading.

Perindopril Erbumine (Electrolyte disturbances are a risk associated with this product; concurrent use in patients taking agents known to disturb electrolyte balance requires caution). Products include:
Aceon Tablets (2 mg, 4 mg, 8 mg)... 3038

Perphenazine (Electrolyte disturbances are a risk associated with this product; concurrent use in patients taking agents known to prolong QT interval requires caution).
No products indexed under this heading.

Phenacemide (Concomitant use may delay or even completely prevent the absorption of antiepileptic drugs. The efficacy of regularly taken antiepileptic drugs may be reduced or completely absent).
No products indexed under this heading.

Phenelzine Sulfate (Electrolyte disturbances are a risk associated with this product; concurrent use in patients taking agents known to prolong QT interval requires caution).
No products indexed under this heading.

Phenobarbital (Concomitant use may delay or even completely prevent the absorption of antiepileptic drugs. The efficacy of regularly taken antiepileptic drugs may be reduced or completely absent). Products include:
Donnatal Extentabs 2507

Phenoxybenzamine Hydrochloride (Electrolyte disturbances area a risk associated with this product; concurrent use in patients taking agents known to disturb electrolyte balance requires caution). Products include:
Dibenzyline Capsules 3188

Phensuximide (Concomitant use may delay or even completely prevent the absorption of antiepileptic drugs. The efficacy of regularly taken antiepileptic drugs may be reduced or completely absent).
No products indexed under this heading.

Phentolamine Mesylate (Electrolyte disturbances area a risk associated with this product; concurrent use in patients taking agents known to disturb electrolyte balance requires caution).
No products indexed under this heading.

Phenylbutazone (Electrolyte disturbances are a risk associated with this product; concurrent use in patients taking agents known to disturb electrolyte balance requires caution).
No products indexed under this heading.

Phenylephrine Hydrochloride (The absorption of drugs taken concomitantly with sodium phosphate from the gastrointestinal tract may be delayed or even completely prevented). Products include:
Actifed Cold & Allergy Tablets 1895
Benadryl Allergy & Cold Kapgels...... 1895

Benadryl Allergy & Sinus Headache Kapgels ... **1895**
Benadryl Severe Allergy & Sinus Headache Caplets ... **1897**
Children's Benadryl-D Allergy & Sinus Liquid ... **1896**
Benadryl-D Allergy & Sinus Tablet ... **1896**
PediaCare Children's Allergy & Cold Liquid ... **1902**
PediaCare Children's Decongestant Liquid ... **1902**
PediaCare Children's Liquid Multi-Symptom Cold ... **1902**
Sinutab Non-Drying Caplets ... **1905**
Sinutab Sinus Caplets ... **1905**
Children's Sudafed PE Cold & Cough Liquid ... **1907**
Children's Sudafed PE Nasal Decongestant Liquid ... **1906**
Sudafed PE Cold & Cough Caplets ... **1907**
Sudafed PE Nasal Decongestant Tablets ... **1907**
Sudafed PE Nighttime Cold Caplets ... **1907**
Sudafed PE Non-Drying Sinus Caplets ... **1908**
Sudafed PE Severe Cold Caplets ... **1908**
Sudafed PE Sinus & Allergy Tablets ... **1908**
Sudafed PE Sinus Headache Caplets ... **1908**
Tylenol Allergy Multi-Symptom Caplets with Cool Burst and Rapid Release Gelcaps ... **1916**
Tylenol Allergy Multi-Symptom Nighttime Caplets with Cool Burst ... **1916**
Children's Tylenol Plus Cold Suspension Liquid ... **1912**
Children's Tylenol Plus Cold & Allergy Suspension Liquid ... **1914**
Children's Tylenol Plus Flu Suspension Liquid ... **1914**
Children's Tylenol Plus Multi-Symptom Cold Suspension Liquid ... **1912**
Tylenol Cold Head Congestion Daytime Caplets with Cool Burst ... **1910**
Tylenol Cold Head Congestion Nighttime Caplets with Cool Burst ... **1910**
Tylenol Cold Head Congestion Severe Daytime Caplets with Cool Burst ... **1910**
Tylenol Cold Multi-Symptom Daytime Caplets with Cool Burst and Rapid Release Gels ... **1913**
Tylenol Cold Multi-Symptom Daytime Liquid with Citrus Burst ... **1913**
Tylenol Cold Multi-Symptom Nighttime Caplets with Cool Burst ... **1913**
Tylenol Cold Multi-Symptom Nighttime Liquid with Cool Burst ... **1913**
Tylenol Cold Multi-Symptom Severe Caplets with Cool Burst ... **1913**
Tylenol Cold Multi-Symptom Severe Daytime Liquid with Citrus Burst ... **1913**
Tylenol Sinus Congestion & Pain Daytime Caplets with Cool Burst and Gelcaps ... **1917**
Tylenol Sinus Congestion & Pain Nighttime Caplets with Cool Burst ... **1917**
Tylenol Sinus Congestion & Pain Severe Caplets with Cool Burst ... **1917**
Vicks DayQuil Cold & Flu Multi-Symptom Relief ... ■**616**
Vicks DayQuil LiquiCaps ... **2567**
Vicks DayQuil Liquid ... **2567**
Vicks DayQuil Multi-Symptom Cold/Flu Relief ... **2567**

Phenylephrine Tannate (The absorption of drugs taken concomitantly with sodium phosphate from the gastrointestinal tract may be delayed or even completely prevented).
No products indexed under this heading.

Phenylpropanolamine Hydrochloride (The absorption of drugs taken concomitantly with sodium phosphate from the gastrointestinal tract may be delayed or even completely prevented).
No products indexed under this heading.

Phenytoin (Concomitant use may delay or even completely prevent the absorption of antiepileptic drugs. The efficacy of regularly taken antiepileptic drugs may be reduced or completely absent).
No products indexed under this heading.

Phenytoin Sodium (Concomitant use may delay or even completely prevent the absorption of antiepileptic drugs. The efficacy of regularly taken antiepileptic drugs may be reduced or completely absent). Products include:
Phenytek Capsules ... **2192**

Pindolol (Electrolyte disturbances area a risk associated with this product; concurrent use in patients taking agents known to disturb electrolyte balance requires caution).
No products indexed under this heading.

Pioglitazone Hydrochloride (The absorption of drugs taken concomitantly with sodium phosphate from the gastrointestinal tract may be delayed or even completely prevented). Products include:
ActoPlus Met Tablets ... **3071**
Actos Tablets ... **3077**
Duetact Tablets ... **3085**

Piroxicam (Electrolyte disturbances are a risk associated with this product; concurrent use in patients taking agents known to disturb electrolyte balance requires caution).
No products indexed under this heading.

Polysaccharide Iron Complex (The absorption of drugs taken concomitantly with sodium phosphate from the gastrointestinal tract may be delayed or even completely prevented). Products include:
Nu-Iron 150 Capsules ... **2165**

Polythiazide (Electrolyte disturbances are a risk associated with this product; concurrent use in patients taking agents known to disturb electrolyte balance requires caution).
No products indexed under this heading.

Potassium Phosphate (The absorption of drugs taken concomitantly with sodium phosphate from the gastrointestinal tract may be delayed or even completely prevented). Products include:
K-Phos Neutral Tablets ... **813**

Prazepam (Electrolyte disturbances are a risk associated with this product; concurrent use in patients taking agents known to prolong QT interval requires caution).
No products indexed under this heading.

Prazosin Hydrochloride (Electrolyte disturbances area a risk associated with this product; concurrent use in patients taking agents known to disturb electrolyte balance requires caution).
No products indexed under this heading.

Primidone (Concomitant use may delay or even completely prevent the absorption of antiepileptic drugs. The efficacy of regularly taken antiepileptic drugs may be reduced or completely absent).
No products indexed under this heading.

Procainamide Hydrochloride (Electrolyte disturbances are a risk associated with this product; concurrent use in patients taking agents known to prolong QT interval requires caution).
No products indexed under this heading.

Prochlorperazine (Electrolyte disturbances are a risk associated with this product; concurrent use in patients taking agents known to prolong QT interval requires caution).
No products indexed under this heading.

Promethazine Hydrochloride (Electrolyte disturbances are a risk associated with this product; concurrent use in patients taking agents known to prolong QT interval requires caution).
No products indexed under this heading.

Propafenone Hydrochloride (Electrolyte disturbances are a risk associated with this product; concurrent use in patients taking agents known to prolong QT interval requires caution). Products include:
Rythmol Tablets ... **1586**
Rythmol SR Capsules ... **1590**

Propranolol Hydrochloride (Electrolyte disturbances area a risk associated with this product; concurrent use in patients taking agents known to disturb electrolyte balance requires caution). Products include:
InnoPran XL Extended Release Capsules ... **1484**

Protriptyline Hydrochloride (Electrolyte disturbances are a risk associated with this product; concurrent use in patients taking agents known to prolong QT interval requires caution).
No products indexed under this heading.

Pseudoephedrine Hydrochloride (The absorption of drugs taken concomitantly with sodium phosphate from the gastrointestinal tract may be delayed or even completely prevented). Products include:
Allegra-D 12 Hour Extended-Release Tablets ... **2687**
Allegra-D 24 Hour Extended-Release Tablets ... **2690**
Children's Motrin Cold Oral Suspension ... **1899**
Sudafed 12 Hour Nasal Decongestant Non-Drowsy Caplets ... **1909**
Sudafed 24 Hour Non-Drowsy Nasal Decongestant Tablets ... **1906**
Children's Sudafed Nasal Decongestant Liquid ... **1906**
Sudafed Nasal Decongestant Tablets ... **1906**
Tylenol Cold Severe Congestion Daytime Caplets with Cool Burst ... **1912**
Tylenol Sinus Severe Congestion Caplets with Cool Burst ... **1917**
Vicks NyQuil LiquiCaps ... **2567**
Vicks NyQuil Liquid ... **2567**
Vicks NyQuil Multi-Symptom Cold/Flu Relief ... **2567**
Zyrtec-D 12 Hour Extended Release Tablets ... **1923**
Zyrtec-D Allergy & Congestion Extended-Release Tablets ... **1923**

Pseudoephedrine Sulfate (The absorption of drugs taken concomitantly with sodium phosphate from the gastrointestinal tract may be delayed or even completely prevented). Products include:
Clarinex-D 12-Hour Extended-Release Tablets ... **2831**
Clarinex-D 24-Hour Extended-Release Tablets ... **2834**

Quetiapine Fumarate (Electrolyte disturbances are a risk associated with this product; concurrent use in patients taking agents known to prolong QT interval requires caution).
No products indexed under this heading.

Quinapril Hydrochloride (Electrolyte disturbances are a risk associated with this product; concurrent use in patients taking agents known to disturb electrolyte balance requires caution).
No products indexed under this heading.

Quinidine Gluconate (Electrolyte disturbances are a risk associated with this product; concurrent use in patients taking agents known to prolong QT interval requires caution).
No products indexed under this heading.

Quinidine Polygalacturonate (Electrolyte disturbances are a risk associated with this product; concurrent use in patients taking agents known to prolong QT interval requires caution).
No products indexed under this heading.

Quinidine Sulfate (Electrolyte disturbances are a risk associated with this product; concurrent use in patients taking agents known to prolong QT interval requires caution).
No products indexed under this heading.

Ramipril (Electrolyte disturbances are a risk associated with this product; concurrent use in patients taking agents known to disturb electrolyte balance requires caution).
No products indexed under this heading.

Rauwolfia Serpentina (Electrolyte disturbances area a risk associated with this product; concurrent use in patients taking agents known to disturb electrolyte balance requires caution).
No products indexed under this heading.

Repaglinide (The absorption of drugs taken concomitantly with sodium phosphate from the gastrointestinal tract may be delayed or even completely prevented). Products include:
PrandiMet Tablets ... **2967**
Prandin Tablets ... **2971**

Rescinnamine (Electrolyte disturbances area a risk associated with this product; concurrent use in patients taking agents known to disturb electrolyte balance requires caution).
No products indexed under this heading.

Reserpine (Electrolyte disturbances area a risk associated with this product; concurrent use in patients taking agents known to disturb electrolyte balance requires caution).
No products indexed under this heading.

Risperidone (Electrolyte disturbances are a risk associated with this product; concurrent use in patients taking agents known to prolong QT interval requires caution). Products include:

Risperdal Consta Long-Acting Injection 1753

Rofecoxib (Electrolyte disturbances are a risk associated with this product; concurrent use in patients taking agents known to disturb electrolyte balance requires caution).

No products indexed under this heading.

Rosiglitazone Maleate (The absorption of drugs taken concomitantly with sodium phosphate from the gastrointestinal tract may be delayed or even completely prevented). Products include:

Avandamet Tablets 1336
Avandaryl Tablets 1344
Avandia Tablets 1351

Sitagliptin Phosphate (The absorption of drugs taken concomitantly with sodium phosphate from the gastrointestinal tract may be delayed or even completely prevented). Products include:

Janumet Tablets 2041
Januvia Tablets 2048

Sodium Bicarbonate (Concurrent use within one hour should be avoided). Products include:

Ceo-Two Laxative Suppository 815

Sodium Nitroprusside (Electrolyte disturbances area a risk associated with this product; concurrent use in patients taking agents known to disturb electrolyte balance requires caution).

No products indexed under this heading.

Sotalol Hydrochloride (Electrolyte disturbances area a risk associated with this product; concurrent use in patients taking agents known to disturb electrolyte balance requires caution).

No products indexed under this heading.

Spirapril Hydrochloride (Electrolyte disturbances are a risk associated with this product; concurrent use in patients taking agents known to disturb electrolyte balance requires caution).

No products indexed under this heading.

Spironolactone (Electrolyte disturbances are a risk associated with this product; concurrent use in patients taking agents known to disturb electrolyte balance requires caution).

No products indexed under this heading.

Sulindac (Electrolyte disturbances are a risk associated with this product; concurrent use in patients taking agents known to disturb electrolyte balance requires caution). Products include:

Clinoril Tablets 1962

Telmisartan (Electrolyte disturbances are a risk associated with this product; concurrent use in patients taking agents known to disturb electrolyte balance requires caution). Products include:

Micardis Tablets 852
Micardis HCT Tablets 854

Terazosin Hydrochloride (Electrolyte disturbances area a risk associated with this product; concurrent use in patients taking agents known to disturb electrolyte balance requires caution).

No products indexed under this heading.

Terbutaline Sulfate (The absorption of drugs taken concomitantly with sodium phosphate from the gastrointestinal tract may be delayed or even completely prevented).

No products indexed under this heading.

Thioridazine Hydrochloride (Electrolyte disturbances are a risk associated with this product; concurrent use in patients taking agents known to prolong QT interval requires caution). Products include:

Thioridazine Hydrochloride Tablets 2195

Thiothixene (Electrolyte disturbances are a risk associated with this product; concurrent use in patients taking agents known to prolong QT interval requires caution). Products include:

Thiothixene Capsules 2197

Tiagabine Hydrochloride (Concomitant use may delay or even completely prevent the absorption of antiepileptic drugs. The efficacy of regularly taken antiepileptic drugs may be reduced or completely absent). Products include:

Gabitril Tablets 973

Timolol Maleate (Electrolyte disturbances area a risk associated with this product; concurrent use in patients taking agents known to disturb electrolyte balance requires caution). Products include:

Combigan Ophthalmic Solution 553
Cosopt Sterile Ophthalmic Solution 1969
Timoptic Sterile Ophthalmic Solution 2121
Timoptic in Ocudose 2124
Timoptic-XE Sterile Ophthalmic Gel Forming Solution 2125

Tocainide Hydrochloride (Electrolyte disturbances are a risk associated with this product; concurrent use in patients taking agents known to prolong QT interval requires caution).

No products indexed under this heading.

Tolazamide (The absorption of drugs taken concomitantly with sodium phosphate from the gastrointestinal tract may be delayed or even completely prevented).

No products indexed under this heading.

Tolbutamide (The absorption of drugs taken concomitantly with sodium phosphate from the gastrointestinal tract may be delayed or even completely prevented).

No products indexed under this heading.

Tolmetin Sodium (Electrolyte disturbances are a risk associated with this product; concurrent use in patients taking agents known to disturb electrolyte balance requires caution).

No products indexed under this heading.

Topiramate (Concomitant use may delay or even completely prevent the absorption of antiepileptic drugs. The efficacy of regularly taken antiepileptic drugs may be reduced or completely absent).

No products indexed under this heading.

Torsemide (Electrolyte disturbances are a risk associated with this product; concurrent use in patients taking agents known to disturb electrolyte balance requires caution). Products include:

Demadex Injection 2630
Demadex Tablets 2630

Trandolapril (Electrolyte disturbances are a risk associated with this product; concurrent use in patients taking agents known to disturb electrolyte balance requires caution). Products include:

Mavik Tablets 472
Tarka Tablets 511

Tranylcypromine Sulfate (Electrolyte disturbances are a risk associated with this product; concurrent use in patients taking agents known to prolong QT interval requires caution). Products include:

Parnate Tablets 1532

Triamterene (Electrolyte disturbances are a risk associated with this product; concurrent use in patients taking agents known to disturb electrolyte balance requires caution). Products include:

Dyazide Capsules 1405
Dyrenium Capsules 3189

Trifluoperazine Hydrochloride (Electrolyte disturbances are a risk associated with this product; concurrent use in patients taking agents known to prolong QT interval requires caution).

No products indexed under this heading.

Trimethadione (Concomitant use may delay or even completely prevent the absorption of antiepileptic drugs. The efficacy of regularly taken antiepileptic drugs may be reduced or completely absent).

No products indexed under this heading.

Trimethaphan Camsylate (Electrolyte disturbances area a risk associated with this product; concurrent use in patients taking agents known to disturb electrolyte balance requires caution).

No products indexed under this heading.

Trimipramine Maleate (Electrolyte disturbances are a risk associated with this product; concurrent use in patients taking agents known to prolong QT interval requires caution).

No products indexed under this heading.

Troglitazone (The absorption of drugs taken concomitantly with sodium phosphate from the gastrointestinal tract may be delayed or even completely prevented).

No products indexed under this heading.

Valdecoxib (Electrolyte disturbances are a risk associated with this product; concurrent use in patients taking agents known to disturb electrolyte balance requires caution).

No products indexed under this heading.

Valproate Sodium (Concomitant use may delay or even completely prevent the absorption of antiepileptic drugs. The efficacy of regularly taken antiepileptic drugs may be reduced or completely absent).

No products indexed under this heading.

Valproic Acid (Concomitant use may delay or even completely prevent the absorption of antiepileptic drugs. The efficacy of regularly taken antiepileptic drugs may be reduced or completely absent).

No products indexed under this heading.

Valsartan (Electrolyte disturbances are a risk associated with this product; concurrent use in patients taking agents known to disturb electrolyte balance requires caution). Products include:

Diovan Tablets 2212
Diovan HCT Tablets 2216
Exforge Tablets 2238

Verapamil Hydrochloride (Electrolyte disturbances area a risk associated with this product; concurrent use in patients taking agents known to disturb electrolyte balance requires caution). Products include:

Tarka Tablets 511

Warfarin Sodium (The absorption of drugs taken concomitantly with sodium phosphate from the gastrointestinal tract may be delayed or even completely prevented).

No products indexed under this heading.

Ziprasidone Hydrochloride (Electrolyte disturbances are a risk associated with this product; concurrent use in patients taking agents known to prolong QT interval requires caution). Products include:

Geodon Capsules 2520

Zonisamide (Concomitant use may delay or even completely prevent the absorption of antiepileptic drugs. The efficacy of regularly taken antiepileptic drugs may be reduced or completely absent). Products include:

Zonegran Capsules 1089

Food Interactions

Dairy products (Concurrent use within one hour should be avoided).

FLEXBUMIN 25% I.V.

(Albumin (human)) 729
None cited in PDR database.

FLEXIBILITY CAPSULES

(Amino Acid Preparations, Hydroxypropyl Methylcellulose, Vitamins with Minerals) 637
None cited in PDR database.

FLOLAN FOR INJECTION

(Epoprostenol Sodium) 1426
May interact with antihypertensives, anticoagulants, diuretics, platelet inhibitors, vasodilators, and certain other agents. Compounds in these categories include:

Acebutolol Hydrochloride (Additional reductions in blood pressure may occur).

No products indexed under this heading.

Aliskiren (Additional reductions in blood pressure may occur). Products include:

Tekturna Tablets 2321
Tekturna HCT Tablets 2324

Amiloride Hydrochloride (Additional reductions in blood pressure may occur).
No products indexed under this heading.

Amlodipine Besylate (Additional reductions in blood pressure may occur). Products include:
Azor Tablets 1005
Exforge Tablets 2238

Amyl Nitrite (Additional reductions in blood pressure may occur).
No products indexed under this heading.

Anisindione (Potential for increased risk of bleeding).
No products indexed under this heading.

Ardeparin Sodium (Potential for increased risk of bleeding).
No products indexed under this heading.

Aspirin (Potential for increased risk of bleeding). Products include:
Aggrenox Capsules 819
Bayer Aspirin 750
Percodan Tablets 1130
St. Joseph 81 mg Aspirin Chewable and Enteric Coated Tablets 1903

Aspirin, Enteric Coated (Potential for increased risk of bleeding).
No products indexed under this heading.

Aspirin Buffered (Potential for increased risk of bleeding).
No products indexed under this heading.

Atenolol (Additional reductions in blood pressure may occur).
No products indexed under this heading.

Azlocillin Sodium (Potential for increased risk of bleeding).
No products indexed under this heading.

Benazepril Hydrochloride (Additional reductions in blood pressure may occur).
No products indexed under this heading.

Bendroflumethiazide (Additional reductions in blood pressure may occur).
No products indexed under this heading.

Betaxolol Hydrochloride (Additional reductions in blood pressure may occur).
No products indexed under this heading.

Bisoprolol Fumarate (Additional reductions in blood pressure may occur).
No products indexed under this heading.

Bumetanide (Additional reductions in blood pressure may occur).
No products indexed under this heading.

Candesartan Cilexetil (Additional reductions in blood pressure may occur). Products include:
Atacand Tablets 639
Atacand HCT 642

Captopril (Additional reductions in blood pressure may occur).
Products include:
Captopril Tablets 2182

Carbenicillin Indanyl Sodium (Potential for increased risk of bleeding).
No products indexed under this heading.

Carteolol Hydrochloride (Additional reductions in blood pressure may occur).
No products indexed under this heading.

Chlorothiazide (Additional reductions in blood pressure may occur).
No products indexed under this heading.

Chlorothiazide Sodium (Additional reductions in blood pressure may occur). Products include:
Intravenous Sodium Diuril 2490

Chlorthalidone (Additional reductions in blood pressure may occur).
Products include:
Clorpres Tablets 2185

Choline Magnesium Trisalicylate (Potential for increased risk of bleeding).
No products indexed under this heading.

Clonidine (Additional reductions in blood pressure may occur).
Products include:
Catapres-TTS 842

Clonidine Hydrochloride (Additional reductions in blood pressure may occur). Products include:
Catapres Tablets 841
Clorpres Tablets 2185

Clopidogrel Bisulfate (Potential for increased risk of bleeding).
Products include:
Plavix Tablets 926
Plavix Tablets 2767

Dalteparin Sodium (Potential for increased risk of bleeding). Products include:
Fragmin Injection 1070

Danaparoid Sodium (Potential for increased risk of bleeding).
No products indexed under this heading.

Deserpidine (Additional reductions in blood pressure may occur).
No products indexed under this heading.

Diazoxide (Additional reductions in blood pressure may occur).
Products include:
Proglycem Capsules 1185
Proglycem Suspension 1185

Diclofenac Potassium (Potential for increased risk of bleeding).
No products indexed under this heading.

Diclofenac Sodium (Potential for increased risk of bleeding). Products include:
Diclofenac Sodium Ophthalmic Solution .... ⊙ 240
Voltaren Ophthalmic Solution 2336
Voltaren Tablets 2334
Voltaren-XR Tablets 2337

Dicumarol (Potential for increased risk of bleeding).
No products indexed under this heading.

Diflunisal (Potential for increased risk of bleeding).
No products indexed under this heading.

Digoxin (Co-administration of epoprostenol with digoxin in patients with congestive heart failure has resulted in decreased apparent oral clearance values of digoxin by 15%; patients on digoxin may show elevations of digoxin concentrations after initiation of epoprostenol therapy, which may be clinically significant in patients prone to digoxin toxicity).
Products include:
Lanoxin Injection 1498
Lanoxin Injection Pediatric 1502
Lanoxin Tablets 1505

Diltiazem Hydrochloride (Additional reductions in blood pressure may occur). Products include:
Cardizem LA Extended Release Tablets 421

Dipyridamole (Potential for increased risk of bleeding). Products include:
Aggrenox Capsules 819
Persantine Tablets 869

Doxazosin Mesylate (Additional reductions in blood pressure may occur).
No products indexed under this heading.

Enalapril Maleate (Additional reductions in blood pressure may occur).
No products indexed under this heading.

Enalaprilat (Additional reductions in blood pressure may occur).
No products indexed under this heading.

Enoxaparin Sodium (Potential for increased risk of bleeding). Products include:
Lovenox Injection 2756

Eprosartan Mesylate (Additional reductions in blood pressure may occur). Products include:
Teveten Tablets 515
Teveten HCT Tablets 517

Esmolol Hydrochloride (Additional reductions in blood pressure may occur).
No products indexed under this heading.

Ethacrynic Acid (Additional reductions in blood pressure may occur).
Products include:
Edecrin Tablets 698

Ethaverine Hydrochloride (Additional reductions in blood pressure may occur).
No products indexed under this heading.

Felodipine (Additional reductions in blood pressure may occur).
No products indexed under this heading.

Fenoprofen Calcium (Potential for increased risk of bleeding). Products include:
Nalfon Capsules 2508

Flurbiprofen (Potential for increased risk of bleeding).
No products indexed under this heading.

Fondaparinux Sodium (Potential for increased risk of bleeding).
Products include:
Arixtra Injection 1313

Fosinopril Sodium (Additional reductions in blood pressure may occur).
No products indexed under this heading.

Furosemide (Co-administration in patients with congestive heart failure receiving furosemide apparent oral clearance values for furosemide were decreased by 13% on the second day of therapy and had returned to baseline values by day 87).
Products include:
Furosemide Tablets 2186

Guanabenz Acetate (Additional reductions in blood pressure may occur).
No products indexed under this heading.

Guanethidine Monosulfate (Additional reductions in blood pressure may occur).
No products indexed under this heading.

Heparin Calcium (Potential for increased risk of bleeding).
No products indexed under this heading.

Heparin Sodium (Potential for increased risk of bleeding).
No products indexed under this heading.

Hydralazine Hydrochloride (Additional reductions in blood pressure may occur).
No products indexed under this heading.

Hydrochlorothiazide (Additional reductions in blood pressure may occur). Products include:
Atacand HCT 642
Avalide Tablets 892
Avalide Tablets 2713
Benicar HCT Tablets 1010
Diovan HCT Tablets 2216
Dyazide Capsules 1405
Micardis HCT Tablets 854
Prinzide Tablets 2092
Tekturna HCT Tablets 2324
Teveten HCT Tablets 517

Hydroflumethiazide (Additional reductions in blood pressure may occur).
No products indexed under this heading.

Ibuprofen (Potential for increased risk of bleeding). Products include:
Motrin IB Tablets and Caplets 1900
Children's Motrin Oral Suspension ... 1901
Children's Motrin Non-Staining Dye-Free Oral Suspension 1901
Children's Motrin Cold Oral Suspension 1899
Infants' Motrin Concentrated Drops 1901
Infants' Motrin Non-Staining Dye-Free Concentrated Drops 1901
Junior Strength Motrin Caplets and Chewable Tablets 1901
Vicoprofen Tablets 533

Indapamide (Additional reductions in blood pressure may occur).
Products include:
Indapamide Tablets 2188

Indomethacin (Potential for increased risk of bleeding). Products include:
Indocin 2024

Indomethacin Sodium Trihydrate (Potential for increased risk of bleeding). Products include:
Indocin I.V. 2489

Irbesartan (Additional reductions in blood pressure may occur).
Products include:
Avalide Tablets 892
Avalide Tablets 2713
Avapro Tablets 897
Avapro Tablets 2718

Isosorbide Dinitrate (Additional reductions in blood pressure may occur).
No products indexed under this heading.

Isosorbide Mononitrate (Additional reductions in blood pressure may occur).
No products indexed under this heading.

Isoxsuprine Hydrochloride (Additional reductions in blood pressure may occur).
No products indexed under this heading.

Isradipine (Additional reductions in blood pressure may occur).
Products include:

DynaCirc CR Controlled Release Tablets 1407
Ketoprofen (Potential for increased risk of bleeding).
No products indexed under this heading.
Labetalol Hydrochloride (Additional reductions in blood pressure may occur).
No products indexed under this heading.
Lisinopril (Additional reductions in blood pressure may occur).
Products include:
Prinivil Tablets 2087
Prinzide Tablets 2092
Losartan Potassium (Additional reductions in blood pressure may occur). Products include:
Cozaar Tablets 1973
Low Molecular Weight Heparins (Potential for increased risk of bleeding).
No products indexed under this heading.
Magnesium Salicylate (Potential for increased risk of bleeding).
No products indexed under this heading.
Mecamylamine Hydrochloride (Additional reductions in blood pressure may occur).
No products indexed under this heading.
Meclofenamate Sodium (Potential for increased risk of bleeding).
No products indexed under this heading.
Mefenamic Acid (Potential for increased risk of bleeding).
No products indexed under this heading.
Methyclothiazide (Additional reductions in blood pressure may occur).
No products indexed under this heading.
Methyldopa (Additional reductions in blood pressure may occur).
No products indexed under this heading.
Methyldopate Hydrochloride (Additional reductions in blood pressure may occur).
No products indexed under this heading.
Metolazone (Additional reductions in blood pressure may occur).
No products indexed under this heading.
Metoprolol Succinate (Additional reductions in blood pressure may occur). Products include:
Toprol-XL Tablets 666
Metoprolol Tartrate (Additional reductions in blood pressure may occur).
No products indexed under this heading.
Metyrosine (Additional reductions in blood pressure may occur).
Products include:
Demser Capsules 1989
Mezlocillin Sodium (Potential for increased risk of bleeding).
No products indexed under this heading.
Mibefradil Dihydrochloride (Additional reductions in blood pressure may occur).
No products indexed under this heading.
Minoxidil (Additional reductions in blood pressure may occur).
No products indexed under this heading.
Moexipril Hydrochloride (Additional reductions in blood pressure may occur).
No products indexed under this heading.
Nadolol (Additional reductions in blood pressure may occur).
Products include:
Nadolol Tablets 2191
Nafcillin Sodium (Potential for increased risk of bleeding).
No products indexed under this heading.
Naproxen (Potential for increased risk of bleeding). Products include:
EC-Naprosyn Delayed-Release Tablets 2632
Naprosyn Suspension 2632
Naprosyn Tablets 2632
Naproxen Sodium (Potential for increased risk of bleeding). Products include:
Anaprox Tablets 2632
Anaprox DS Tablets 2632
Treximet Tablets 1616
Nebivolol (Additional reductions in blood pressure may occur).
Products include:
Bystolic Tablets 1155
Nicardipine Hydrochloride (Additional reductions in blood pressure may occur). Products include:
Cardene I.V. 1093
Nifedipine (Additional reductions in blood pressure may occur).
No products indexed under this heading.
Nisoldipine (Additional reductions in blood pressure may occur).
Products include:
Sular Extended Release Tablets 2975
Nitroglycerin (Additional reductions in blood pressure may occur).
Products include:
Nitro-Dur Transdermal Infusion System 2887
Nitrolingual Pumpspray 2965
Nitroglycerin, long-acting formulations (Additional reductions in blood pressure may occur).
No products indexed under this heading.
Nitroglycerin Intravenous (Additional reductions in blood pressure may occur).
No products indexed under this heading.
Papaverine (Additional reductions in blood pressure may occur).
No products indexed under this heading.
Papaverine Hydrochloride (Additional reductions in blood pressure may occur).
No products indexed under this heading.
Penbutolol Sulfate (Additional reductions in blood pressure may occur).
No products indexed under this heading.
Penicillin G Benzathine (Potential for increased risk of bleeding).
Products include:
Bicillin C-R Injectable Suspension 1775
Bicillin L-A Injection 1777
Penicillin G Procaine (Potential for increased risk of bleeding). Products include:
Bicillin C-R Injectable Suspension 1775
Bicillin L-A Injection 1777
Perindopril Erbumine (Additional reductions in blood pressure may occur). Products include:
Aceon Tablets (2 mg, 4 mg, 8 mg) 3038
Phenoxybenzamine Hydrochloride (Additional reductions in blood pressure may occur). Products include:
Dibenzyline Capsules 3188
Phentolamine Mesylate (Additional reductions in blood pressure may occur).
No products indexed under this heading.
Phenylbutazone (Potential for increased risk of bleeding).
No products indexed under this heading.
Pindolol (Additional reductions in blood pressure may occur).
No products indexed under this heading.
Piroxicam (Potential for increased risk of bleeding).
No products indexed under this heading.
Polythiazide (Additional reductions in blood pressure may occur).
No products indexed under this heading.
Prazosin Hydrochloride (Additional reductions in blood pressure may occur).
No products indexed under this heading.
Propranolol Hydrochloride (Additional reductions in blood pressure may occur). Products include:
InnoPran XL Extended Release Capsules 1484
Quinapril Hydrochloride (Additional reductions in blood pressure may occur).
No products indexed under this heading.
Ramipril (Additional reductions in blood pressure may occur).
No products indexed under this heading.
Rauwolfia Serpentina (Additional reductions in blood pressure may occur).
No products indexed under this heading.
Rescinnamine (Additional reductions in blood pressure may occur).
No products indexed under this heading.
Reserpine (Additional reductions in blood pressure may occur).
No products indexed under this heading.
Salsalate (Potential for increased risk of bleeding).
No products indexed under this heading.
Sodium Nitroprusside (Additional reductions in blood pressure may occur).
No products indexed under this heading.
Sotalol Hydrochloride (Additional reductions in blood pressure may occur).
No products indexed under this heading.
Spirapril Hydrochloride (Additional reductions in blood pressure may occur).
No products indexed under this heading.
Spironolactone (Additional reductions in blood pressure may occur).
No products indexed under this heading.
Sulindac (Potential for increased risk of bleeding). Products include:
Clinoril Tablets 1962
Telmisartan (Additional reductions in blood pressure may occur).
Products include:
Micardis Tablets 852
Micardis HCT Tablets 854
Terazosin Hydrochloride (Additional reductions in blood pressure may occur).
No products indexed under this heading.
Ticarcillin Disodium (Potential for increased risk of bleeding). Products include:
Timentin ADD-Vantage 1606
Timentin Injection Galaxy Container 1609
Timentin IV Infusion 1603
Timentin Pharmacy Bulk Package 1613
Ticlopidine Hydrochloride (Potential for increased risk of bleeding).
No products indexed under this heading.
Timolol Maleate (Additional reductions in blood pressure may occur).
Products include:
Combigan Ophthalmic Solution 553
Cosopt Sterile Ophthalmic Solution 1969
Timoptic Sterile Ophthalmic Solution 2121
Timoptic in Ocudose 2124
Timoptic-XE Sterile Ophthalmic Gel Forming Solution 2125
Tinzaparin Sodium (Potential for increased risk of bleeding).
No products indexed under this heading.
Tolazoline Hydrochloride (Additional reductions in blood pressure may occur).
No products indexed under this heading.
Tolmetin Sodium (Potential for increased risk of bleeding).
No products indexed under this heading.
Torsemide (Additional reductions in blood pressure may occur).
Products include:
Demadex Injection 2630
Demadex Tablets 2630
Trandolapril (Additional reductions in blood pressure may occur).
Products include:
Mavik Tablets 472
Tarka Tablets 511
Triamterene (Additional reductions in blood pressure may occur).
Products include:
Dyazide Capsules 1405
Dyrenium Capsules 3189
Trimethaphan Camsylate (Additional reductions in blood pressure may occur).
No products indexed under this heading.
Valsartan (Additional reductions in blood pressure may occur).
Products include:
Diovan Tablets 2212
Diovan HCT Tablets 2216
Exforge Tablets 2238
Verapamil Hydrochloride (Additional reductions in blood pressure may occur). Products include:
Tarka Tablets 511
Warfarin Sodium (Potential for increased risk of bleeding).
No products indexed under this heading.

Food Interactions

Alcohol (Additional reductions in blood pressure may occur).

FLOMAX CAPSULES
(Tamsulosin Hydrochloride) **848**
May interact with alpha adrenergic blockers, cytochrome p450 2d6 inhibitors (selected), cytochrome p450 3a4 inhibitors (selected), and certain other agents. Compounds in these categories include:

Acetazolamide (Concomitant administration of tamsulosin HCl and an inhibitor of CYP3A4 may lead to increased tamsulosin HCl plasma exposure. Tamsulosin HCl capsules should be used with caution in combination with moderate or strong inhibitors of CYP3A4 (e.g., ketoconazole), particularly at doses higher than 0.4mg).
No products indexed under this heading.

Amiodarone Hydrochloride (Concomitant administration of tamsulosin HCl and an inhibitor of CYP2D6 may lead to increased tamsulosin HCl plasma exposure. Tamsulosin HCl capsules should be used with caution in combination with moderate or strong inhibitors of CYP2D6 (e.g., fluoxetine), particularly at doses higher than 0.4mg).
No products indexed under this heading.

Amitriptyline Hydrochloride (Concomitant administration of tamsulosin HCl and an inhibitor of CYP2D6 may lead to increased tamsulosin HCl plasma exposure. Tamsulosin HCl capsules should be used with caution in combination with moderate or strong inhibitors of CYP2D6 (e.g., fluoxetine), particularly at doses higher than 0.4mg).
No products indexed under this heading.

Amoxapine (Concomitant administration of tamsulosin HCl and an inhibitor of CYP2D6 may lead to increased tamsulosin HCl plasma exposure. Tamsulosin HCl capsules should be used with caution in combination with moderate or strong inhibitors of CYP2D6 (e.g., fluoxetine), particularly at doses higher than 0.4mg).
No products indexed under this heading.

Amprenavir (Concomitant administration of tamsulosin HCl and an inhibitor of CYP3A4 may lead to increased tamsulosin HCl plasma exposure. Tamsulosin HCl capsules should be used with caution in combination with moderate or strong inhibitors of CYP3A4 (e.g., ketoconazole), particularly at doses higher than 0.4mg).
No products indexed under this heading.

Anastrozole (Concomitant administration of tamsulosin HCl and an inhibitor of CYP3A4 may lead to increased tamsulosin HCl plasma exposure. Tamsulosin HCl capsules should be used with caution in combination with moderate or strong inhibitors of CYP3A4 (e.g., ketoconazole), particularly at doses higher than 0.4mg). Products include:
Arimidex Tablets **672**

Aprepitant (Concomitant administration of tamsulosin HCl and an inhibitor of CYP3A4 may lead to increased tamsulosin HCl plasma exposure. Tamsulosin HCl capsules should be used with caution in combination with moderate or strong inhibitors of CYP3A4 (e.g., ketoconazole), particularly at doses higher than 0.4mg). Products include:
Emend Capsules **1992**

Atazanavir (Concomitant administration of tamsulosin HCl and an inhibitor of CYP3A4 may lead to increased tamsulosin HCl plasma exposure. Tamsulosin HCl capsules should be used with caution in combination with moderate or strong inhibitors of CYP3A4 (e.g., ketoconazole), particularly at doses higher than 0.4mg).
No products indexed under this heading.

Atazanavir Sulfate (Concomitant administration of tamsulosin HCl and an inhibitor of CYP3A4 may lead to increased tamsulosin HCl plasma exposure. Tamsulosin HCl capsules should be used with caution in combination with moderate or strong inhibitors of CYP3A4 (e.g., ketoconazole), particularly at doses higher than 0.4mg). Products include:
Reyataz Capsules **3299**

Bupropion Hydrochloride (Concomitant administration of tamsulosin HCl and an inhibitor of CYP2D6 may lead to increased tamsulosin HCl plasma exposure. Tamsulosin HCl capsules should be used with caution in combination with moderate or strong inhibitors of CYP2D6 (e.g., fluoxetine), particularly at doses higher than 0.4mg). Products include:
Wellbutrin Tablets **1648**
Wellbutrin SR Sustained-Release Tablets **1653**
Wellbutrin XL Extended-Release Tablets **1659**
Zyban Sustained-Release Tablets **1692**

Celecoxib (Concomitant administration of tamsulosin HCl and an inhibitor of CYP2D6 may lead to increased tamsulosin HCl plasma exposure. Tamsulosin HCl capsules should be used with caution in combination with moderate or strong inhibitors of CYP2D6 (e.g., fluoxetine), particularly at doses higher than 0.4mg). Products include:
Celebrex Capsules **2979**

Chloroquine Hydrochloride (Concomitant administration of tamsulosin HCl and an inhibitor of CYP2D6 may lead to increased tamsulosin HCl plasma exposure. Tamsulosin HCl capsules should be used with caution in combination with moderate or strong inhibitors of CYP2D6 (e.g., fluoxetine), particularly at doses higher than 0.4mg).
No products indexed under this heading.

Chloroquine Phosphate (Concomitant administration of tamsulosin HCl and an inhibitor of CYP2D6 may lead to increased tamsulosin HCl plasma exposure. Tamsulosin HCl capsules should be used with caution in combination with moderate or strong inhibitors of CYP2D6 (e.g., fluoxetine), particularly at doses higher than 0.4mg).
No products indexed under this heading.

Chlorpheniramine (Concomitant administration of tamsulosin HCl and an inhibitor of CYP2D6 may lead to increased tamsulosin HCl plasma exposure. Tamsulosin HCl capsules should be used with caution in combination with moderate or strong inhibitors of CYP2D6 (e.g., fluoxetine), particularly at doses higher than 0.4mg).
No products indexed under this heading.

Chlorpheniramine Maleate (Concomitant administration of tamsulosin HCl and an inhibitor of CYP2D6 may lead to increased tamsulosin HCl plasma exposure. Tamsulosin HCl capsules should be used with caution in combination with moderate or strong inhibitors of CYP2D6 (e.g., fluoxetine), particularly at doses higher than 0.4mg). Products include:
Actifed Cold & Allergy Tablets **1895**
Sudafed PE Sinus & Allergy Tablets **1908**
Tylenol Allergy Multi-Symptom Caplets with Cool Burst and Rapid Release Gelcaps **1916**
Children's Tylenol Plus Cold Suspension Liquid **1912**
Children's Tylenol Plus Cough & Runny Nose Suspension Liquid **1912**
Children's Tylenol Plus Flu Suspension Liquid **1914**
Children's Tylenol Plus Multi-Symptom Cold Suspension Liquid **1912**
Tylenol Cold Head Congestion Nighttime Caplets with Cool Burst **1910**
Tylenol Cold Multi-Symptom Nighttime Caplets with Cool Burst **1913**
Tylenol Sinus Congestion & Pain Nighttime Caplets with Cool Burst **1917**

Chlorpheniramine Polistirex (Concomitant administration of tamsulosin HCl and an inhibitor of CYP2D6 may lead to increased tamsulosin HCl plasma exposure. Tamsulosin HCl capsules should be used with caution in combination with moderate or strong inhibitors of CYP2D6 (e.g., fluoxetine), particularly at doses higher than 0.4mg). Products include:
Tussionex Pennkinetic Extended-Release Suspension **3154**

Chlorpheniramine Tannate (Concomitant administration of tamsulosin HCl and an inhibitor of CYP2D6 may lead to increased tamsulosin HCl plasma exposure. Tamsulosin HCl capsules should be used with caution in combination with moderate or strong inhibitors of CYP2D6 (e.g., fluoxetine), particularly at doses higher than 0.4mg).
No products indexed under this heading.

Cimetidine (Co-administration with highest recommended dose of cimetidine has resulted in a significant decrease (26%) in the clearance of tamsulosin which resulted in a moderate increase in tamsulosin AUC (44%)).
No products indexed under this heading.

Cimetidine Hydrochloride (Co-administration with highest recommended dose of cimetidine has resulted in a significant decrease (26%) in the clearance of tamsulosin which resulted in a moderate increase in tamsulosin AUC (44%)).
No products indexed under this heading.

Ciprofloxacin (Concomitant administration of tamsulosin HCl and an inhibitor of CYP3A4 may lead to increased tamsulosin HCl plasma exposure. Tamsulosin HCl capsules should be used with caution in combination with moderate or strong inhibitors of CYP3A4 (e.g., ketoconazole), particularly at doses higher than 0.4mg). Products include:
Cipro I.V. **2817**
Cipro Oral Suspension **2810**
Cipro XR Tablets **2823**
Ciprodex Otic Suspension **541**

Citalopram Hydrobromide (Concomitant administration of tamsulosin HCl and an inhibitor of CYP2D6 may lead to increased tamsulosin HCl plasma exposure. Tamsulosin HCl capsules should be used with caution in combination with moderate or strong inhibitors of CYP2D6 (e.g., fluoxetine), particularly at doses higher than 0.4mg). Products include:
Celexa **1160**

Clarithromycin (Concomitant administration of tamsulosin HCl and an inhibitor of CYP3A4 may lead to increased tamsulosin HCl plasma exposure. Tamsulosin HCl capsules should be used with caution in combination with moderate or strong inhibitors of CYP3A4 (e.g., ketoconazole), particularly at doses higher than 0.4mg). Products include:
Biaxin/Biaxin XL **411**

Clomipramine Hydrochloride (Concomitant administration of tamsulosin HCl and an inhibitor of CYP2D6 may lead to increased tamsulosin HCl plasma exposure. Tamsulosin HCl capsules should be used with caution in combination with moderate or strong inhibitors of CYP2D6 (e.g., fluoxetine), particularly at doses higher than 0.4mg).
No products indexed under this heading.

Clotrimazole (Concomitant administration of tamsulosin HCl and an inhibitor of CYP3A4 may lead to increased tamsulosin HCl plasma exposure. Tamsulosin HCl capsules should be used with caution in combination with moderate or strong inhibitors of CYP3A4 (e.g., ketoconazole), particularly at doses higher than 0.4mg). Products include:
Lotrisone **2881**

Cocaine Hydrochloride (Concomitant administration of tamsulosin HCl and an inhibitor of CYP2D6 may lead to increased tamsulosin HCl plasma exposure. Tamsulosin HCl capsules should be used with caution in combination with moderate or strong inhibitors of CYP2D6 (e.g., fluoxetine), particularly at doses higher than 0.4mg).
No products indexed under this heading.

Cyclosporine (Concomitant administration of tamsulosin HCl and an inhibitor of CYP3A4 may lead to increased tamsulosin HCl plasma exposure. Tamsulosin HCl capsules should be used with caution in combination with moderate or strong inhibitors of CYP3A4 (e.g., ketoconazole), particularly at doses higher than 0.4mg). Products include:
Gengraf Capsules **435**
Neoral Oral Solution **2280**
Neoral Soft Gelatin Capsules **2280**
Restasis Ophthalmic Emulsion **557**
Sandimmune **2296**

Dalfopristin (Concomitant administration of tamsulosin HCl and an inhibitor of CYP3A4 may lead to increased tamsulosin HCl plasma exposure. Tamsulosin HCl capsules should be used with caution in combination with moderate or strong inhibitors of CYP3A4 (e.g., ketoconazole), particularly at doses higher than 0.4mg).

No products indexed under this heading.

Danazol (Concomitant administration of tamsulosin HCl and an inhibitor of CYP3A4 may lead to increased tamsulosin HCl plasma exposure. Tamsulosin HCl capsules should be used with caution in combination with moderate or strong inhibitors of CYP3A4 (e.g., ketoconazole), particularly at doses higher than 0.4mg).

No products indexed under this heading.

Delavirdine Mesylate (Concomitant administration of tamsulosin HCl and an inhibitor of CYP3A4 may lead to increased tamsulosin HCl plasma exposure. Tamsulosin HCl capsules should be used with caution in combination with moderate or strong inhibitors of CYP3A4 (e.g., ketoconazole), particularly at doses higher than 0.4mg).

No products indexed under this heading.

Desipramine Hydrochloride (Concomitant administration of tamsulosin HCl and an inhibitor of CYP2D6 may lead to increased tamsulosin HCl plasma exposure. Tamsulosin HCl capsules should be used with caution in combination with moderate or strong inhibitors of CYP2D6 (e.g., fluoxetine), particularly at doses higher than 0.4mg).

No products indexed under this heading.

Diltiazem Hydrochloride (Concomitant administration of tamsulosin HCl and an inhibitor of CYP3A4 may lead to increased tamsulosin HCl plasma exposure. Tamsulosin HCl capsules should be used with caution in combination with moderate or strong inhibitors of CYP3A4 (e.g., ketoconazole), particularly at doses higher than 0.4mg). Products include:

Cardizem LA Extended Release Tablets **421**

Diltiazem Maleate (Concomitant administration of tamsulosin HCl and an inhibitor of CYP3A4 may lead to increased tamsulosin HCl plasma exposure. Tamsulosin HCl capsules should be used with caution in combination with moderate or strong inhibitors of CYP3A4 (e.g., ketoconazole), particularly at doses higher than 0.4mg).

No products indexed under this heading.

Diphenhydramine (Concomitant administration of tamsulosin HCl and an inhibitor of CYP2D6 may lead to increased tamsulosin HCl plasma exposure. Tamsulosin HCl capsules should be used with caution in combination with moderate or strong inhibitors of CYP2D6 (e.g., fluoxetine), particularly at doses higher than 0.4mg).

No products indexed under this heading.

Diphenhydramine Hydrochloride (Concomitant administration of tamsulosin HCl and an inhibitor of CYP2D6 may lead to increased tamsulosin HCl plasma exposure. Tamsulosin HCl capsules should be used with caution in combination with moderate or strong inhibitors of CYP2D6 (e.g., fluoxetine), particularly at doses higher than 0.4mg). Products include:

Benadryl Allergy & Cold Kapgels **1895**
Benadryl Allergy & Sinus Headache Kapgels **1895**
Benadryl Severe Allergy & Sinus Headache Caplets **1897**
Benadryl Dye-Free Allergy Liqui-gels Softgels **1897**
Benadryl Allergy Kapgels **1895**
Benadryl Allergy Quick Dissolve Strips **1896**
Benadryl Allergy Ultratab Tablets **1896**
Children's Benadryl Dye-Free Allergy Liquid **1897**
Children's Benadryl Allergy Fastmelts **1897**
Children's Benadryl Allergy Liquid **1898**
Children's Benadryl Allergy Perfect Measure **1896**
Children's Benadryl-D Allergy & Sinus Liquid **1896**
Benadryl-D Allergy & Sinus Tablet **1896**
PediaCare Children's Allergy & Cold Liquid **1902**
PediaCare Children's Allergy Liquid **1902**
Simply Sleep Caplets **1905**
Sudafed PE Nighttime Cold Caplets **1907**
Sudafed PE Severe Cold Caplets **1908**
Extra Strength Tylenol PM Caplets, Geltabs, Liquid, and Rapid Release Gels **1915**
Tylenol Allergy Multi-Symptom Nighttime Caplets with Cool Burst **1916**
Tylenol Severe Allergy Caplets **1916**
Children's Tylenol Plus Cold & Allergy Suspension Liquid **1914**
Tylenol Sore Throat Nighttime Liquid with Cool Burst **1918**

Doxazosin Mesylate (The pharmacokinetic and pharmacodynamic interactions between tamsulosin and other alpha-adrenergic blockers have not been determined; however, interactions may be expected and co-administration should be avoided).

No products indexed under this heading.

Doxepin Hydrochloride (Concomitant administration of tamsulosin HCl and an inhibitor of CYP2D6 may lead to increased tamsulosin HCl plasma exposure. Tamsulosin HCl capsules should be used with caution in combination with moderate or strong inhibitors of CYP2D6 (e.g., fluoxetine), particularly at doses higher than 0.4mg).

No products indexed under this heading.

Efavirenz (Concomitant administration of tamsulosin HCl and an inhibitor of CYP3A4 may lead to increased tamsulosin HCl plasma exposure. Tamsulosin HCl capsules should be used with caution in combination with moderate or strong inhibitors of CYP3A4 (e.g., ketoconazole), particularly at doses higher than 0.4mg). Products include:

Atripla Tablets **938**
Sustiva Capsules **930**
Sustiva Tablets **930**

Erythromycin (Concomitant administration of tamsulosin HCl and an inhibitor of CYP3A4 may lead to increased tamsulosin HCl plasma exposure. Tamsulosin HCl capsules should be used with caution in combination with moderate or strong inhibitors of CYP3A4 (e.g., ketoconazole), particularly at doses higher than 0.4mg).

No products indexed under this heading.

Erythromycin Estolate (Concomitant administration of tamsulosin HCl and an inhibitor of CYP3A4 may lead to increased tamsulosin HCl plasma exposure. Tamsulosin HCl capsules should be used with caution in combination with moderate or strong inhibitors of CYP3A4 (e.g., ketoconazole), particularly at doses higher than 0.4mg).

No products indexed under this heading.

Erythromycin Ethylsuccinate (Concomitant administration of tamsulosin HCl and an inhibitor of CYP3A4 may lead to increased tamsulosin HCl plasma exposure. Tamsulosin HCl capsules should be used with caution in combination with moderate or strong inhibitors of CYP3A4 (e.g., ketoconazole), particularly at doses higher than 0.4mg). Products include:

E.E.S. **433**
EryPed **431**

Erythromycin Gluceptate (Concomitant administration of tamsulosin HCl and an inhibitor of CYP3A4 may lead to increased tamsulosin HCl plasma exposure. Tamsulosin HCl capsules should be used with caution in combination with moderate or strong inhibitors of CYP3A4 (e.g., ketoconazole), particularly at doses higher than 0.4mg).

No products indexed under this heading.

Erythromycin Lactobionate (Concomitant administration of tamsulosin HCl and an inhibitor of CYP3A4 may lead to increased tamsulosin HCl plasma exposure. Tamsulosin HCl capsules should be used with caution in combination with moderate or strong inhibitors of CYP3A4 (e.g., ketoconazole), particularly at doses higher than 0.4mg).

No products indexed under this heading.

Erythromycin Stearate (Concomitant administration of tamsulosin HCl and an inhibitor of CYP3A4 may lead to increased tamsulosin HCl plasma exposure. Tamsulosin HCl capsules should be used with caution in combination with moderate or strong inhibitors of CYP3A4 (e.g., ketoconazole), particularly at doses higher than 0.4mg).

No products indexed under this heading.

Escitalopram Oxalate (Concomitant administration of tamsulosin HCl and an inhibitor of CYP2D6 may lead to increased tamsulosin HCl plasma exposure. Tamsulosin HCl capsules should be used with caution in combination with moderate or strong inhibitors of CYP2D6 (e.g., fluoxetine), particularly at doses higher than 0.4mg). Products include:

Lexapro Oral Suspension **1174**
Lexapro Tablets **1174**

Esomeprazole Magnesium (Concomitant administration of tamsulosin HCl and an inhibitor of CYP3A4 may lead to increased tamsulosin HCl plasma exposure. Tamsulosin HCl capsules should be used with caution in combination with moderate or strong inhibitors of CYP3A4 (e.g., ketoconazole), particularly at doses higher than 0.4mg). Products include:

Nexium Delayed-Release Capsules **645**
Nexium Delayed-Release Oral Suspension **645**

Fluconazole (Concomitant administration of tamsulosin HCl and an inhibitor of CYP3A4 may lead to increased tamsulosin HCl plasma exposure. Tamsulosin HCl capsules should be used with caution in combination with moderate or strong inhibitors of CYP3A4 (e.g., ketoconazole), particularly at doses higher than 0.4mg).

No products indexed under this heading.

Fluoxetine (Concomitant administration of tamsulosin HCl and an inhibitor of CYP2D6 may lead to increased tamsulosin HCl plasma exposure. Tamsulosin HCl capsules should be used with caution in combination with moderate or strong inhibitors of CYP2D6 (e.g., fluoxetine), particularly at doses higher than 0.4mg).

No products indexed under this heading.

Fluoxetine Hydrochloride (Concomitant administration of tamsulosin HCl and an inhibitor of CYP2D6 may lead to increased tamsulosin HCl plasma exposure. Tamsulosin HCl capsules should be used with caution in combination with moderate or strong inhibitors of CYP2D6 (e.g., fluoxetine), particularly at doses higher than 0.4mg). Products include:

Prozac Weekly Capsules **1852**
Prozac Pulvules and Liquid **1852**
Symbyax Capsules **1871**

Fluphenazine Decanoate (Concomitant administration of tamsulosin HCl and an inhibitor of CYP2D6 may lead to increased tamsulosin HCl plasma exposure. Tamsulosin HCl capsules should be used with caution in combination with moderate or strong inhibitors of CYP2D6 (e.g., fluoxetine), particularly at doses higher than 0.4mg).

No products indexed under this heading.

Fluphenazine Enanthate (Concomitant administration of tamsulosin HCl and an inhibitor of CYP2D6 may lead to increased tamsulosin HCl plasma exposure. Tamsulosin HCl capsules should be used with caution in combination with moderate or strong inhibitors of CYP2D6 (e.g., fluoxetine), particularly at doses higher than 0.4mg).

No products indexed under this heading.

Fluphenazine Hydrochloride (Concomitant administration of tamsulosin HCl and an inhibitor of CYP2D6 may lead to increased tamsulosin HCl plasma exposure. Tamsulosin HCl capsules should be used with caution in combination with moderate or strong inhibitors of CYP2D6 (e.g., fluoxetine), particularly at doses higher than 0.4mg).

No products indexed under this heading.

Fluvoxamine Maleate (Concomitant administration of tamsulosin HCl and an inhibitor of CYP2D6 may lead to increased tamsulosin HCl plasma exposure. Tamsulosin HCl capsules should be used with caution in combination with moderate or strong inhibitors of CYP2D6 (e.g., fluoxetine), particularly at doses higher than 0.4mg). Products include:
Luvox CR Extended-Release Capsules 1759

Fosamprenavir Calcium (Concomitant administration of tamsulosin HCl and an inhibitor of CYP3A4 may lead to increased tamsulosin HCl plasma exposure. Tamsulosin HCl capsules should be used with caution in combination with moderate or strong inhibitors of CYP3A4 (e.g., ketoconazole), particularly at doses higher than 0.4mg). Products include:
Lexiva Oral Suspension 1510
Lexiva Tablets 1510

Furosemide (Co-administration produces an 11% to 12% reduction in tamsulosin Cmax and AUC; these changes are expected to be clinically insignificant). Products include:
Furosemide Tablets 2186

Halofantrine Hydrochloride (Concomitant administration of tamsulosin HCl and an inhibitor of CYP2D6 may lead to increased tamsulosin HCl plasma exposure. Tamsulosin HCl capsules should be used with caution in combination with moderate or strong inhibitors of CYP2D6 (e.g., fluoxetine), particularly at doses higher than 0.4mg).
No products indexed under this heading.

Haloperidol (Concomitant administration of tamsulosin HCl and an inhibitor of CYP2D6 may lead to increased tamsulosin HCl plasma exposure. Tamsulosin HCl capsules should be used with caution in combination with moderate or strong inhibitors of CYP2D6 (e.g., fluoxetine), particularly at doses higher than 0.4mg).
No products indexed under this heading.

Haloperidol Decanoate (Concomitant administration of tamsulosin HCl and an inhibitor of CYP2D6 may lead to increased tamsulosin HCl plasma exposure. Tamsulosin HCl capsules should be used with caution in combination with moderate or strong inhibitors of CYP2D6 (e.g., fluoxetine), particularly at doses higher than 0.4mg).
No products indexed under this heading.

Hydroxychloroquine Sulfate (Concomitant administration of tamsulosin HCl and an inhibitor of CYP2D6 may lead to increased tamsulosin HCl plasma exposure. Tamsulosin HCl capsules should be used with caution in combination with moderate or strong inhibitors of CYP2D6 (e.g., fluoxetine), particularly at doses higher than 0.4mg).
No products indexed under this heading.

Imatinib Mesylate (Concomitant administration of tamsulosin HCl and an inhibitor of CYP2D6 may lead to increased tamsulosin HCl plasma exposure. Tamsulosin HCl capsules should be used with caution in combination with moderate or strong inhibitors of CYP2D6 (e.g., fluoxetine), particularly at doses higher than 0.4mg). Products include:
Gleevec Tablets 2255

Imipramine Hydrochloride (Concomitant administration of tamsulosin HCl and an inhibitor of CYP2D6 may lead to increased tamsulosin HCl plasma exposure. Tamsulosin HCl capsules should be used with caution in combination with moderate or strong inhibitors of CYP2D6 (e.g., fluoxetine), particularly at doses higher than 0.4mg).
No products indexed under this heading.

Imipramine Pamoate (Concomitant administration of tamsulosin HCl and an inhibitor of CYP2D6 may lead to increased tamsulosin HCl plasma exposure. Tamsulosin HCl capsules should be used with caution in combination with moderate or strong inhibitors of CYP2D6 (e.g., fluoxetine), particularly at doses higher than 0.4mg).
No products indexed under this heading.

Indinavir Sulfate (Concomitant administration of tamsulosin HCl and an inhibitor of CYP3A4 may lead to increased tamsulosin HCl plasma exposure. Tamsulosin HCl capsules should be used with caution in combination with moderate or strong inhibitors of CYP3A4 (e.g., ketoconazole), particularly at doses higher than 0.4mg). Products include:
Crixivan Capsules 1979

Isoniazid (Concomitant administration of tamsulosin HCl and an inhibitor of CYP3A4 may lead to increased tamsulosin HCl plasma exposure. Tamsulosin HCl capsules should be used with caution in combination with moderate or strong inhibitors of CYP3A4 (e.g., ketoconazole), particularly at doses higher than 0.4mg).
No products indexed under this heading.

Itraconazole (Concomitant administration of tamsulosin HCl and an inhibitor of CYP3A4 may lead to increased tamsulosin HCl plasma exposure. Tamsulosin HCl capsules should be used with caution in combination with moderate or strong inhibitors of CYP3A4 (e.g., ketoconazole), particularly at doses higher than 0.4mg).
No products indexed under this heading.

Ketoconazole (Concomitant administration of tamsulosin HCl and an inhibitor of CYP3A4 may lead to increased tamsulosin HCl plasma exposure. Tamsulosin HCl capsules should be used with caution in combination with moderate or strong inhibitors of CYP3A4 (e.g., ketoconazole), particularly at doses higher than 0.4mg). Products include:
Extina Foam, 2% 3057
Nizoral A-D Shampoo 1901

Lopinavir (Concomitant administration of tamsulosin HCl and an inhibitor of CYP3A4 may lead to increased tamsulosin HCl plasma exposure. Tamsulosin HCl capsules should be used with caution in combination with moderate or strong inhibitors of CYP3A4 (e.g., ketoconazole), particularly at doses higher than 0.4mg). Products include:
Kaletra 452

Loratadine (Concomitant administration of tamsulosin HCl and an inhibitor of CYP3A4 may lead to increased tamsulosin HCl plasma exposure. Tamsulosin HCl capsules should be used with caution in combination with moderate or strong inhibitors of CYP3A4 (e.g., ketoconazole), particularly at doses higher than 0.4mg).
No products indexed under this heading.

Maprotiline Hydrochloride (Concomitant administration of tamsulosin HCl and an inhibitor of CYP2D6 may lead to increased tamsulosin HCl plasma exposure. Tamsulosin HCl capsules should be used with caution in combination with moderate or strong inhibitors of CYP2D6 (e.g., fluoxetine), particularly at doses higher than 0.4mg).
No products indexed under this heading.

Methadone Hydrochloride (Concomitant administration of tamsulosin HCl and an inhibitor of CYP2D6 may lead to increased tamsulosin HCl plasma exposure. Tamsulosin HCl capsules should be used with caution in combination with moderate or strong inhibitors of CYP2D6 (e.g., fluoxetine), particularly at doses higher than 0.4mg).
No products indexed under this heading.

Metronidazole (Concomitant administration of tamsulosin HCl and an inhibitor of CYP3A4 may lead to increased tamsulosin HCl plasma exposure. Tamsulosin HCl capsules should be used with caution in combination with moderate or strong inhibitors of CYP3A4 (e.g., ketoconazole), particularly at doses higher than 0.4mg). Products include:
Pylera Capsules 714

Metronidazole Benzoate (Concomitant administration of tamsulosin HCl and an inhibitor of CYP3A4 may lead to increased tamsulosin HCl plasma exposure. Tamsulosin HCl capsules should be used with caution in combination with moderate or strong inhibitors of CYP3A4 (e.g., ketoconazole), particularly at doses higher than 0.4mg).
No products indexed under this heading.

Metronidazole Hydrochloride (Concomitant administration of tamsulosin HCl and an inhibitor of CYP3A4 may lead to increased tamsulosin HCl plasma exposure. Tamsulosin HCl capsules should be used with caution in combination with moderate or strong inhibitors of CYP3A4 (e.g., ketoconazole), particularly at doses higher than 0.4mg).
No products indexed under this heading.

Mibefradil Dihydrochloride (Concomitant administration of tamsulosin HCl and an inhibitor of CYP2D6 may lead to increased tamsulosin HCl plasma exposure. Tamsulosin HCl capsules should be used with caution in combination with moderate or strong inhibitors of CYP2D6 (e.g., fluoxetine), particularly at doses higher than 0.4mg).
No products indexed under this heading.

Miconazole (Concomitant administration of tamsulosin HCl and an inhibitor of CYP3A4 may lead to increased tamsulosin HCl plasma exposure. Tamsulosin HCl capsules should be used with caution in combination with moderate or strong inhibitors of CYP3A4 (e.g., ketoconazole), particularly at doses higher than 0.4mg).
No products indexed under this heading.

Miconazole Nitrate (Concomitant administration of tamsulosin HCl and an inhibitor of CYP3A4 may lead to increased tamsulosin HCl plasma exposure. Tamsulosin HCl capsules should be used with caution in combination with moderate or strong inhibitors of CYP3A4 (e.g., ketoconazole), particularly at doses higher than 0.4mg).
No products indexed under this heading.

Moclobemide (Concomitant administration of tamsulosin HCl and an inhibitor of CYP2D6 may lead to increased tamsulosin HCl plasma exposure. Tamsulosin HCl capsules should be used with caution in combination with moderate or strong inhibitors of CYP2D6 (e.g., fluoxetine), particularly at doses higher than 0.4mg).
No products indexed under this heading.

Nefazodone Hydrochloride (Concomitant administration of tamsulosin HCl and an inhibitor of CYP3A4 may lead to increased tamsulosin HCl plasma exposure. Tamsulosin HCl capsules should be used with caution in combination with moderate or strong inhibitors of CYP3A4 (e.g., ketoconazole), particularly at doses higher than 0.4mg).
No products indexed under this heading.

Nelfinavir Mesylate (Concomitant administration of tamsulosin HCl and an inhibitor of CYP3A4 may lead to increased tamsulosin HCl plasma exposure. Tamsulosin HCl capsules should be used with caution in combination with moderate or strong inhibitors of CYP3A4 (e.g., ketoconazole), particularly at doses higher than 0.4mg).
No products indexed under this heading.

Nevirapine (Concomitant administration of tamsulosin HCl and an inhibitor of CYP3A4 may lead to increased tamsulosin HCl plasma exposure. Tamsulosin HCl capsules should be used with caution in combination with moderate or strong inhibitors of CYP3A4 (e.g., ketoconazole), particularly at doses higher than 0.4mg). Products include:
Viramune Oral Suspension 873
Viramune Tablets 873

Niacinamide (Concomitant administration of tamsulosin HCl and an inhibitor of CYP3A4 may lead to increased tamsulosin HCl plasma exposure. Tamsulosin HCl capsules should be used with caution in combination with moderate or strong inhibitors of CYP3A4 (e.g., ketoconazole), particularly at doses higher than 0.4mg). Products include:
BioLean Free Tablets .... ▣635

Nicotinamide (Concomitant administration of tamsulosin HCl and an inhibitor of CYP3A4 may lead to increased tamsulosin HCl plasma exposure. Tamsulosin HCl capsules should be used with caution in combination with moderate or strong inhibitors of CYP3A4 (e.g., ketoconazole), particularly at doses higher than 0.4mg).
No products indexed under this heading.

Nifedipine (Concomitant administration of tamsulosin HCl and an inhibitor of CYP3A4 may lead to increased tamsulosin HCl plasma exposure. Tamsulosin HCl capsules should be used with caution in combination with moderate or strong inhibitors of CYP3A4 (e.g., ketoconazole), particularly at doses higher than 0.4mg).
No products indexed under this heading.

Norfloxacin (Concomitant administration of tamsulosin HCl and an inhibitor of CYP3A4 may lead to increased tamsulosin HCl plasma exposure. Tamsulosin HCl capsules should be used with caution in combination with moderate or strong inhibitors of CYP3A4 (e.g., ketoconazole), particularly at doses higher than 0.4mg). Products include:
Noroxin Tablets **2069**

Nortriptyline Hydrochloride (Concomitant administration of tamsulosin HCl and an inhibitor of CYP2D6 may lead to increased tamsulosin HCl plasma exposure. Tamsulosin HCl capsules should be used with caution in combination with moderate or strong inhibitors of CYP2D6 (e.g., fluoxetine), particularly at doses higher than 0.4mg).
No products indexed under this heading.

Omeprazole (Concomitant administration of tamsulosin HCl and an inhibitor of CYP3A4 may lead to increased tamsulosin HCl plasma exposure. Tamsulosin HCl capsules should be used with caution in combination with moderate or strong inhibitors of CYP3A4 (e.g., ketoconazole), particularly at doses higher than 0.4mg).
No products indexed under this heading.

Paroxetine Hydrochloride (Concomitant administration of tamsulosin HCl and an inhibitor of CYP2D6 may lead to increased tamsulosin HCl plasma exposure. Tamsulosin HCl capsules should be used with caution in combination with moderate or strong inhibitors of CYP2D6 (e.g., fluoxetine), particularly at doses higher than 0.4mg). Products include:
Paxil **1535**
Paxil CR Controlled-Release Tablets **1544**

Perphenazine (Concomitant administration of tamsulosin HCl and an inhibitor of CYP2D6 may lead to increased tamsulosin HCl plasma exposure. Tamsulosin HCl capsules should be used with caution in combination with moderate or strong inhibitors of CYP2D6 (e.g., fluoxetine), particularly at doses higher than 0.4mg).
No products indexed under this heading.

Prazosin Hydrochloride (The pharmacokinetic and pharmacodynamic interactions between tamsulosin and other alpha-adrenergic blockers have not been determined; however, interactions may be expected and co-administration should be avoided).
No products indexed under this heading.

Propafenone Hydrochloride (Concomitant administration of tamsulosin HCl and an inhibitor of CYP2D6 may lead to increased tamsulosin HCl plasma exposure. Tamsulosin HCl capsules should be used with caution in combination with moderate or strong inhibitors of CYP2D6 (e.g., fluoxetine), particularly at doses higher than 0.4mg). Products include:
Rythmol Tablets **1586**
Rythmol SR Capsules **1590**

Propoxyphene Hydrochloride (Concomitant administration of tamsulosin HCl and an inhibitor of CYP2D6 may lead to increased tamsulosin HCl plasma exposure. Tamsulosin HCl capsules should be used with caution in combination with moderate or strong inhibitors of CYP2D6 (e.g., fluoxetine), particularly at doses higher than 0.4mg).
No products indexed under this heading.

Propoxyphene Napsylate (Concomitant administration of tamsulosin HCl and an inhibitor of CYP2D6 may lead to increased tamsulosin HCl plasma exposure. Tamsulosin HCl capsules should be used with caution in combination with moderate or strong inhibitors of CYP2D6 (e.g., fluoxetine), particularly at doses higher than 0.4mg).
No products indexed under this heading.

Protriptyline Hydrochloride (Concomitant administration of tamsulosin HCl and an inhibitor of CYP2D6 may lead to increased tamsulosin HCl plasma exposure. Tamsulosin HCl capsules should be used with caution in combination with moderate or strong inhibitors of CYP2D6 (e.g., fluoxetine), particularly at doses higher than 0.4mg).
No products indexed under this heading.

Quinacrine Hydrochloride (Concomitant administration of tamsulosin HCl and an inhibitor of CYP2D6 may lead to increased tamsulosin HCl plasma exposure. Tamsulosin HCl capsules should be used with caution in combination with moderate or strong inhibitors of CYP2D6 (e.g., fluoxetine), particularly at doses higher than 0.4mg).
No products indexed under this heading.

Quinidine (Concomitant administration of tamsulosin HCl and an inhibitor of CYP3A4 may lead to increased tamsulosin HCl plasma exposure. Tamsulosin HCl capsules should be used with caution in combination with moderate or strong inhibitors of CYP3A4 (e.g., ketoconazole), particularly at doses higher than 0.4mg).
No products indexed under this heading.

Quinidine Gluconate (Concomitant administration of tamsulosin HCl and an inhibitor of CYP2D6 may lead to increased tamsulosin HCl plasma exposure. Tamsulosin HCl capsules should be used with caution in combination with moderate or strong inhibitors of CYP2D6 (e.g., fluoxetine), particularly at doses higher than 0.4mg).
No products indexed under this heading.

Quinidine Hydrochloride (Concomitant administration of tamsulosin HCl and an inhibitor of CYP2D6 may lead to increased tamsulosin HCl plasma exposure. Tamsulosin HCl capsules should be used with caution in combination with moderate or strong inhibitors of CYP2D6 (e.g., fluoxetine), particularly at doses higher than 0.4mg).
No products indexed under this heading.

Quinidine Polygalacturonate (Concomitant administration of tamsulosin HCl and an inhibitor of CYP2D6 may lead to increased tamsulosin HCl plasma exposure. Tamsulosin HCl capsules should be used with caution in combination with moderate or strong inhibitors of CYP2D6 (e.g., fluoxetine), particularly at doses higher than 0.4mg).
No products indexed under this heading.

Quinidine Sulfate (Concomitant administration of tamsulosin HCl and an inhibitor of CYP2D6 may lead to increased tamsulosin HCl plasma exposure. Tamsulosin HCl capsules should be used with caution in combination with moderate or strong inhibitors of CYP2D6 (e.g., fluoxetine), particularly at doses higher than 0.4mg).
No products indexed under this heading.

Quinine (Concomitant administration of tamsulosin HCl and an inhibitor of CYP3A4 may lead to increased tamsulosin HCl plasma exposure. Tamsulosin HCl capsules should be used with caution in combination with moderate or strong inhibitors of CYP3A4 (e.g., ketoconazole), particularly at doses higher than 0.4mg).
No products indexed under this heading.

Quinine Sulfate (Concomitant administration of tamsulosin HCl and an inhibitor of CYP3A4 may lead to increased tamsulosin HCl plasma exposure. Tamsulosin HCl capsules should be used with caution in combination with moderate or strong inhibitors of CYP3A4 (e.g., ketoconazole), particularly at doses higher than 0.4mg).
No products indexed under this heading.

Quinupristin (Concomitant administration of tamsulosin HCl and an inhibitor of CYP3A4 may lead to increased tamsulosin HCl plasma exposure. Tamsulosin HCl capsules should be used with caution in combination with moderate or strong inhibitors of CYP3A4 (e.g., ketoconazole), particularly at doses higher than 0.4mg).
No products indexed under this heading.

Ranitidine Bismuth Citrate (Concomitant administration of tamsulosin HCl and an inhibitor of CYP2D6 may lead to increased tamsulosin HCl plasma exposure. Tamsulosin HCl capsules should be used with caution in combination with moderate or strong inhibitors of CYP2D6 (e.g., fluoxetine), particularly at doses higher than 0.4mg).
No products indexed under this heading.

Ranitidine Hydrochloride (Concomitant administration of tamsulosin HCl and an inhibitor of CYP2D6 may lead to increased tamsulosin HCl plasma exposure. Tamsulosin HCl capsules should be used with caution in combination with moderate or strong inhibitors of CYP2D6 (e.g., fluoxetine), particularly at doses higher than 0.4mg). Products include:
Zantac 75 Tablets **603**
Zantac **1670**
Zantac Injection **1666**
Zantac Injection Pharmacy Bulk Package.................................... **1668**
Maximum Strength Zantac 150 Tablets.. **603**
Maximum Strength Zantac 150 Cool Mint Tablets **603**

Ritonavir (Concomitant administration of tamsulosin HCl and an inhibitor of CYP2D6 may lead to increased tamsulosin HCl plasma exposure. Tamsulosin HCl capsules should be used with caution in combination with moderate or strong inhibitors of CYP2D6 (e.g., fluoxetine), particularly at doses higher than 0.4mg). Products include:
Kaletra **452**
Norvir **489**

Saquinavir (Concomitant administration of tamsulosin HCl and an inhibitor of CYP3A4 may lead to increased tamsulosin HCl plasma exposure. Tamsulosin HCl capsules should be used with caution in combination with moderate or strong inhibitors of CYP3A4 (e.g., ketoconazole), particularly at doses higher than 0.4mg).
No products indexed under this heading.

Saquinavir Mesylate (Concomitant administration of tamsulosin HCl and an inhibitor of CYP3A4 may lead to increased tamsulosin HCl plasma exposure. Tamsulosin HCl capsules should be used with caution in combination with moderate or strong inhibitors of CYP3A4 (e.g., ketoconazole), particularly at doses higher than 0.4mg).
No products indexed under this heading.

Sertraline Hydrochloride (Concomitant administration of tamsulosin HCl and an inhibitor of CYP2D6 may lead to increased tamsulosin HCl plasma exposure. Tamsulosin HCl capsules should be used with caution in combination with moderate or strong inhibitors of CYP2D6 (e.g., fluoxetine), particularly at doses higher than 0.4mg).
No products indexed under this heading.

Sildenafil Citrate (Concomitant administration of tamsulosin HCl and an inhibitor of CYP2D6 may lead to increased tamsulosin HCl plasma exposure. Tamsulosin HCl capsules should be used with caution in combination with moderate or strong inhibitors of CYP2D6 (e.g., fluoxetine), particularly at doses higher than 0.4mg).
No products indexed under this heading.

Telithromycin (Concomitant administration of tamsulosin HCl and an inhibitor of CYP3A4 may lead to increased tamsulosin HCl plasma exposure. Tamsulosin HCl capsules should be used with caution in combination with moderate or strong inhibitors of CYP3A4 (e.g., ketoconazole), particularly at doses higher than 0.4mg). Products include:
Ketek Tablets 2744

Terazosin Hydrochloride (The pharmacokinetic and pharmacodynamic interactions between tamsulosin and other alpha-adrenergic blockers have not been determined; however, interactions may be expected and co-administration should be avoided).
No products indexed under this heading.

Terbinafine Hydrochloride (Concomitant administration of tamsulosin HCl and an inhibitor of CYP2D6 may lead to increased tamsulosin HCl plasma exposure. Tamsulosin HCl capsules should be used with caution in combination with moderate or strong inhibitors of CYP2D6 (e.g., fluoxetine), particularly at doses higher than 0.4mg). Products include:
Lamisil Oral Granules 2264
Lamisil Tablets 2266

Thioridazine Hydrochloride (Concomitant administration of tamsulosin HCl and an inhibitor of CYP2D6 may lead to increased tamsulosin HCl plasma exposure. Tamsulosin HCl capsules should be used with caution in combination with moderate or strong inhibitors of CYP2D6 (e.g., fluoxetine), particularly at doses higher than 0.4mg). Products include:
Thioridazine Hydrochloride Tablets 2195

Trimipramine Maleate (Concomitant administration of tamsulosin HCl and an inhibitor of CYP2D6 may lead to increased tamsulosin HCl plasma exposure. Tamsulosin HCl capsules should be used with caution in combination with moderate or strong inhibitors of CYP2D6 (e.g., fluoxetine), particularly at doses higher than 0.4mg).
No products indexed under this heading.

Troglitazone (Concomitant administration of tamsulosin HCl and an inhibitor of CYP3A4 may lead to increased tamsulosin HCl plasma exposure. Tamsulosin HCl capsules should be used with caution in combination with moderate or strong inhibitors of CYP3A4 (e.g., ketoconazole), particularly at doses higher than 0.4mg).
No products indexed under this heading.

Troleandomycin (Concomitant administration of tamsulosin HCl and an inhibitor of CYP3A4 may lead to increased tamsulosin HCl plasma exposure. Tamsulosin HCl capsules should be used with caution in combination with moderate or strong inhibitors of CYP3A4 (e.g., ketoconazole), particularly at doses higher than 0.4mg).
No products indexed under this heading.

Valproate Sodium (Concomitant administration of tamsulosin HCl and an inhibitor of CYP3A4 may lead to increased tamsulosin HCl plasma exposure. Tamsulosin HCl capsules should be used with caution in combination with moderate or strong inhibitors of CYP3A4 (e.g., ketoconazole), particularly at doses higher than 0.4mg).
No products indexed under this heading.

Vardenafil Hydrochloride (Concomitant administration of tamsulosin HCl and an inhibitor of CYP2D6 may lead to increased tamsulosin HCl plasma exposure. Tamsulosin HCl capsules should be used with caution in combination with moderate or strong inhibitors of CYP2D6 (e.g., fluoxetine), particularly at doses higher than 0.4mg). Products include:
Levitra Tablets 2876

Verapamil Hydrochloride (Concomitant administration of tamsulosin HCl and an inhibitor of CYP3A4 may lead to increased tamsulosin HCl plasma exposure. Tamsulosin HCl capsules should be used with caution in combination with moderate or strong inhibitors of CYP3A4 (e.g., ketoconazole), particularly at doses higher than 0.4mg). Products include:
Tarka Tablets 511

Voriconazole (Concomitant administration of tamsulosin HCl and an inhibitor of CYP3A4 may lead to increased tamsulosin HCl plasma exposure. Tamsulosin HCl capsules should be used with caution in combination with moderate or strong inhibitors of CYP3A4 (e.g., ketoconazole), particularly at doses higher than 0.4mg).
No products indexed under this heading.

Warfarin Sodium (Results from *in vitro* and *in vivo* interaction studies are inconclusive; therefore, caution should be exercised with concomitant use).
No products indexed under this heading.

Zafirlukast (Concomitant administration of tamsulosin HCl and an inhibitor of CYP3A4 may lead to increased tamsulosin HCl plasma exposure. Tamsulosin HCl capsules should be used with caution in combination with moderate or strong inhibitors of CYP3A4 (e.g., ketoconazole), particularly at doses higher than 0.4mg). Products include:
Accolate Tablets 669

Zileuton (Concomitant administration of tamsulosin HCl and an inhibitor of CYP3A4 may lead to increased tamsulosin HCl plasma exposure. Tamsulosin HCl capsules should be used with caution in combination with moderate or strong inhibitors of CYP3A4 (e.g., ketoconazole), particularly at doses higher than 0.4mg).
No products indexed under this heading.

Food Interactions

Food, unspecified (Tmax is reached by 4 to 5 hours under fasting conditions and by 6 to 7 hours when tamsulosin is administered with food; taking tamsulosin under fasted conditions results in a 30% increase in AUC and 40% to 70% increase in Cmax compared to fed conditions; Flomax should be taken approximately 30 minutes following the meal).

Grapefruit (Concomitant administration of tamsulosin HCl and an inhibitor of CYP3A4 may lead to increased tamsulosin HCl plasma exposure. Tamsulosin HCl capsules should be used with caution in combination with moderate or strong inhibitors of CYP3A4 (e.g., ketoconazole), particularly at doses higher than 0.4mg).

Grapefruit Juice (Concomitant administration of tamsulosin HCl and an inhibitor of CYP3A4 may lead to increased tamsulosin HCl plasma exposure. Tamsulosin HCl capsules should be used with caution in combination with moderate or strong inhibitors of CYP3A4 (e.g., ketoconazole), particularly at doses higher than 0.4mg).

FLONASE NASAL SPRAY

(Fluticasone Propionate) 1431
May interact with cytochrome p450 3a4 inhibitors (selected) and certain other agents. Compounds in these categories include:

Acetazolamide (Caution should be exercised when potent cytochrome P450 3A4 inhibitors are co-administered with fluticasone propionate).
No products indexed under this heading.

Amiodarone Hydrochloride (Caution should be exercised when potent cytochrome P450 3A4 inhibitors are co-administered with fluticasone propionate).
No products indexed under this heading.

Amprenavir (Caution should be exercised when potent cytochrome P450 3A4 inhibitors are co-administered with fluticasone propionate).
No products indexed under this heading.

Anastrozole (Caution should be exercised when potent cytochrome P450 3A4 inhibitors are co-administered with fluticasone propionate). Products include:
Arimidex Tablets 672

Aprepitant (Caution should be exercised when potent cytochrome P450 3A4 inhibitors are co-administered with fluticasone propionate). Products include:
Emend Capsules 1992

Atazanavir (Caution should be exercised when potent cytochrome P450 3A4 inhibitors are co-administered with fluticasone propionate).
No products indexed under this heading.

Atazanavir Sulfate (Caution should be exercised when potent cytochrome P450 3A4 inhibitors are co-administered with fluticasone propionate). Products include:
Reyataz Capsules 3299

Cimetidine (Caution should be exercised when potent cytochrome P450 3A4 inhibitors are co-administered with fluticasone propionate).
No products indexed under this heading.

Cimetidine Hydrochloride (Caution should be exercised when potent cytochrome P450 3A4 inhibitors are co-administered with fluticasone propionate).
No products indexed under this heading.

Ciprofloxacin (Caution should be exercised when potent cytochrome P450 3A4 inhibitors are co-administered with fluticasone propionate). Products include:
Cipro I.V. 2817
Cipro Oral Suspension 2810
Cipro XR Tablets 2823
Ciprodex Otic Suspension 541

Clarithromycin (Caution should be exercised when potent cytochrome P450 3A4 inhibitors are co-administered with fluticasone propionate). Products include:
Biaxin/Biaxin XL 411

Clotrimazole (Caution should be exercised when potent cytochrome P450 3A4 inhibitors are co-administered with fluticasone propionate). Products include:
Lotrisone 2881

Cyclosporine (Caution should be exercised when potent cytochrome P450 3A4 inhibitors are co-administered with fluticasone propionate). Products include:
Gengraf Capsules 435
Neoral Oral Solution 2280
Neoral Soft Gelatin Capsules 2280
Restasis Ophthalmic Emulsion 557
Sandimmune 2296

Dalfopristin (Caution should be exercised when potent cytochrome P450 3A4 inhibitors are co-administered with fluticasone propionate).
No products indexed under this heading.

Danazol (Caution should be exercised when potent cytochrome P450 3A4 inhibitors are co-administered with fluticasone propionate).
No products indexed under this heading.

Delavirdine Mesylate (Caution should be exercised when potent cytochrome P450 3A4 inhibitors are co-administered with fluticasone propionate).
No products indexed under this heading.

Diltiazem Hydrochloride (Caution should be exercised when potent cytochrome P450 3A4 inhibitors are co-administered with fluticasone propionate). Products include:
Cardizem LA Extended Release Tablets 421

Diltiazem Maleate (Caution should be exercised when potent cytochrome P450 3A4 inhibitors are co-administered with fluticasone propionate).
No products indexed under this heading.

Efavirenz (Caution should be exercised when potent cytochrome P450

3A4 inhibitors are co-administered with fluticasone propionate). Products include:

Atripla Tablets 938
Sustiva Capsules 930
Sustiva Tablets 930

Erythromycin (Caution should be exercised when potent cytochrome P450 3A4 inhibitors are co-administered with fluticasone propionate).

No products indexed under this heading.

Erythromycin Estolate (Caution should be exercised when potent cytochrome P450 3A4 inhibitors are co-administered with fluticasone propionate).

No products indexed under this heading.

Erythromycin Ethylsuccinate (Caution should be exercised when potent cytochrome P450 3A4 inhibitors are co-administered with fluticasone propionate). Products include:

E.E.S. 433
EryPed 431

Erythromycin Gluceptate (Caution should be exercised when potent cytochrome P450 3A4 inhibitors are co-administered with fluticasone propionate).

No products indexed under this heading.

Erythromycin Lactobionate (Caution should be exercised when potent cytochrome P450 3A4 inhibitors are co-administered with fluticasone propionate).

No products indexed under this heading.

Erythromycin Stearate (Caution should be exercised when potent cytochrome P450 3A4 inhibitors are co-administered with fluticasone propionate).

No products indexed under this heading.

Esomeprazole Magnesium (Caution should be exercised when potent cytochrome P450 3A4 inhibitors are co-administered with fluticasone propionate). Products include:

Nexium Delayed-Release Capsules 645
Nexium Delayed-Release Oral Suspension 645

Fluconazole (Caution should be exercised when potent cytochrome P450 3A4 inhibitors are co-administered with fluticasone propionate).

No products indexed under this heading.

Fluoxetine (Caution should be exercised when potent cytochrome P450 3A4 inhibitors are co-administered with fluticasone propionate).

No products indexed under this heading.

Fluoxetine Hydrochloride (Caution should be exercised when potent cytochrome P450 3A4 inhibitors are co-administered with fluticasone propionate). Products include:

Prozac Weekly Capsules 1852
Prozac Pulvules and Liquid 1852
Symbyax Capsules 1871

Fluvoxamine Maleate (Caution should be exercised when potent cytochrome P450 3A4 inhibitors are co-administered with fluticasone propionate). Products include:

Luvox CR Extended-Release Capsules 1759

Fosamprenavir Calcium (Caution should be exercised when potent cytochrome P450 3A4 inhibitors are co-administered with fluticasone propionate). Products include:

Lexiva Oral Suspension 1510
Lexiva Tablets 1510

Indinavir Sulfate (Caution should be exercised when potent cytochrome P450 3A4 inhibitors are co-administered with fluticasone propionate). Products include:

Crixivan Capsules 1979

Isoniazid (Caution should be exercised when potent cytochrome P450 3A4 inhibitors are co-administered with fluticasone propionate).

No products indexed under this heading.

Itraconazole (Caution should be exercised when potent cytochrome P450 3A4 inhibitors are co-administered with fluticasone propionate).

No products indexed under this heading.

Ketoconazole (Fluticasone propionate is a substrate of cytochrome P450 3A4. Co-administration with ketoconazole resulted in increased plasma fluticasone propionate exposure, a reduction in plasma cortisol AUC, and no effect on urinary excretion of cortisol. Caution should be exercised when potent cytochrome P450 3A inhibitors are co-administered with fluticasone propionate). Products include:

Extina Foam, 2% 3057
Nizoral A-D Shampoo 1901

Lopinavir (Caution should be exercised when potent cytochrome P450 3A4 inhibitors are co-administered with fluticasone propionate). Products include:

Kaletra 452

Loratadine (Caution should be exercised when potent cytochrome P450 3A4 inhibitors are co-administered with fluticasone propionate).

No products indexed under this heading.

Metronidazole (Caution should be exercised when potent cytochrome P450 3A4 inhibitors are co-administered with fluticasone propionate). Products include:

Pylera Capsules 714

Metronidazole Benzoate (Caution should be exercised when potent cytochrome P450 3A4 inhibitors are co-administered with fluticasone propionate).

No products indexed under this heading.

Metronidazole Hydrochloride (Caution should be exercised when potent cytochrome P450 3A4 inhibitors are co-administered with fluticasone propionate).

No products indexed under this heading.

Miconazole (Caution should be exercised when potent cytochrome P450 3A4 inhibitors are co-administered with fluticasone propionate).

No products indexed under this heading.

Miconazole Nitrate (Caution should be exercised when potent cytochrome P450 3A4 inhibitors are co-administered with fluticasone propionate).

No products indexed under this heading.

Nefazodone Hydrochloride (Caution should be exercised when potent cytochrome P450 3A4 inhibitors are co-administered with fluticasone propionate).

No products indexed under this heading.

Nelfinavir Mesylate (Caution should be exercised when potent cytochrome P450 3A4 inhibitors are co-administered with fluticasone propionate).

No products indexed under this heading.

Nevirapine (Caution should be exercised when potent cytochrome P450 3A4 inhibitors are co-administered with fluticasone propionate). Products include:

Viramune Oral Suspension 873
Viramune Tablets 873

Niacinamide (Caution should be exercised when potent cytochrome P450 3A4 inhibitors are co-administered with fluticasone propionate). Products include:

BioLean Free Tablets 635

Nicotinamide (Caution should be exercised when potent cytochrome P450 3A4 inhibitors are co-administered with fluticasone propionate).

No products indexed under this heading.

Nifedipine (Caution should be exercised when potent cytochrome P450 3A4 inhibitors are co-administered with fluticasone propionate).

No products indexed under this heading.

Norfloxacin (Caution should be exercised when potent cytochrome P450 3A4 inhibitors are co-administered with fluticasone propionate). Products include:

Noroxin Tablets 2069

Omeprazole (Caution should be exercised when potent cytochrome P450 3A4 inhibitors are co-administered with fluticasone propionate).

No products indexed under this heading.

Paroxetine Hydrochloride (Caution should be exercised when potent cytochrome P450 3A4 inhibitors are co-administered with fluticasone propionate). Products include:

Paxil 1535
Paxil CR Controlled-Release Tablets 1544

Propoxyphene Hydrochloride (Caution should be exercised when potent cytochrome P450 3A4 inhibitors are co-administered with fluticasone propionate).

No products indexed under this heading.

Propoxyphene Napsylate (Caution should be exercised when potent cytochrome P450 3A4 inhibitors are co-administered with fluticasone propionate).

No products indexed under this heading.

Quinidine (Caution should be exercised when potent cytochrome P450 3A4 inhibitors are co-administered with fluticasone propionate).

No products indexed under this heading.

Quinidine Hydrochloride (Caution should be exercised when potent cytochrome P450 3A4 inhibitors are co-administered with fluticasone propionate).

No products indexed under this heading.

Quinidine Polygalacturonate (Caution should be exercised when potent cytochrome P450 3A4 inhibitors are co-administered with fluticasone propionate).

No products indexed under this heading.

Quinidine Sulfate (Caution should be exercised when potent cytochrome P450 3A4 inhibitors are co-administered with fluticasone propionate).

No products indexed under this heading.

Quinine (Caution should be exercised when potent cytochrome P450 3A4 inhibitors are co-administered with fluticasone propionate).

No products indexed under this heading.

Quinine Sulfate (Caution should be exercised when potent cytochrome P450 3A4 inhibitors are co-administered with fluticasone propionate).

No products indexed under this heading.

Quinupristin (Caution should be exercised when potent cytochrome P450 3A4 inhibitors are co-administered with fluticasone propionate).

No products indexed under this heading.

Ranitidine Bismuth Citrate (Caution should be exercised when potent cytochrome P450 3A4 inhibitors are co-administered with fluticasone propionate).

No products indexed under this heading.

Ranitidine Hydrochloride (Caution should be exercised when potent cytochrome P450 3A4 inhibitors are co-administered with fluticasone propionate). Products include:

Zantac 75 Tablets 603
Zantac 1670
Zantac Injection 1666
Zantac Injection Pharmacy Bulk Package 1668
Maximum Strength Zantac 150 Tablets 603
Maximum Strength Zantac 150 Cool Mint Tablets 603

Ritonavir (Fluticasone propionate is a substrate of cytochrome P450 3A4. A drug interaction study has shown that ritonavir (a highly potent cytochrome P450 3A4 inhibitor) can significantly increase plasma fluticasone propionate exposure, resulting in significantly reduced serum cortisol concentrations. Therefore, co-administration of fluticasone propionate and ritonavir is not recommended unless the potential benefit to the patient outweighs the risk of systemic corticosteroid side effects). Products include:

Kaletra 452
Norvir 489

Saquinavir (Caution should be exercised when potent cytochrome P450 3A4 inhibitors are co-administered with fluticasone propionate).

No products indexed under this heading.

Saquinavir Mesylate (Caution should be exercised when potent cytochrome P450 3A4 inhibitors are co-administered with fluticasone propionate).
No products indexed under this heading.

Sertraline Hydrochloride (Caution should be exercised when potent cytochrome P450 3A4 inhibitors are co-administered with fluticasone propionate).
No products indexed under this heading.

Sildenafil Citrate (Caution should be exercised when potent cytochrome P450 3A4 inhibitors are co-administered with fluticasone propionate).
No products indexed under this heading.

Telithromycin (Caution should be exercised when potent cytochrome P450 3A4 inhibitors are co-administered with fluticasone propionate). Products include:
Ketek Tablets 2744

Troglitazone (Caution should be exercised when potent cytochrome P450 3A4 inhibitors are co-administered with fluticasone propionate).
No products indexed under this heading.

Troleandomycin (Caution should be exercised when potent cytochrome P450 3A4 inhibitors are co-administered with fluticasone propionate).
No products indexed under this heading.

Valproate Sodium (Caution should be exercised when potent cytochrome P450 3A4 inhibitors are co-administered with fluticasone propionate).
No products indexed under this heading.

Vardenafil Hydrochloride (Caution should be exercised when potent cytochrome P450 3A4 inhibitors are co-administered with fluticasone propionate). Products include:
Levitra Tablets 2876

Verapamil Hydrochloride (Caution should be exercised when potent cytochrome P450 3A4 inhibitors are co-administered with fluticasone propionate). Products include:
Tarka Tablets 511

Voriconazole (Caution should be exercised when potent cytochrome P450 3A4 inhibitors are co-administered with fluticasone propionate).
No products indexed under this heading.

Zafirlukast (Caution should be exercised when potent cytochrome P450 3A4 inhibitors are co-administered with fluticasone propionate). Products include:
Accolate Tablets 669

Zileuton (Caution should be exercised when potent cytochrome P450 3A4 inhibitors are co-administered with fluticasone propionate).
No products indexed under this heading.

Food Interactions

Grapefruit (Caution should be exercised when potent cytochrome P450 3A4 inhibitors are co-administered with fluticasone propionate).

Grapefruit Juice (Caution should be exercised when potent cytochrome P450 3A4 inhibitors are co-administered with fluticasone propionate).

FLOVENT DISKUS 50 MCG

(Fluticasone Propionate) 1435
May interact with cytochrome p450 3a4 inhibitors, potent and certain other agents. Compounds in these categories include:

Amprenavir (Caution should be exercised when potent cytochrome P450 3A4 inhibitors are co-administered with fluticasone. Interactions with ritonavir and ketoconazole, both potent CYP3A4 inhibitors, have resulted in increased fluticasone exposure).
No products indexed under this heading.

Atazanavir (Caution should be exercised when potent cytochrome P450 3A4 inhibitors are co-administered with fluticasone. Interactions with ritonavir and ketoconazole, both potent CYP3A4 inhibitors, have resulted in increased fluticasone exposure).
No products indexed under this heading.

Atazanavir Sulfate (Caution should be exercised when potent cytochrome P450 3A4 inhibitors are co-administered with fluticasone. Interactions with ritonavir and ketoconazole, both potent CYP3A4 inhibitors, have resulted in increased fluticasone exposure). Products include:
Reyataz Capsules 3299

Clarithromycin (Caution should be exercised when potent cytochrome P450 3A4 inhibitors are co-administered with fluticasone. Interactions with ritonavir and ketoconazole, both potent CYP3A4 inhibitors, have resulted in increased fluticasone exposure). Products include:
Biaxin/Biaxin XL 411

Delavirdine Mesylate (Caution should be exercised when potent cytochrome P450 3A4 inhibitors are co-administered with fluticasone. Interactions with ritonavir and ketoconazole, both potent CYP3A4 inhibitors, have resulted in increased fluticasone exposure).
No products indexed under this heading.

Delavirine (Caution should be exercised when potent cytochrome P450 3A4 inhibitors are co-administered with fluticasone. Interactions with ritonavir and ketoconazole, both potent CYP3A4 inhibitors, have resulted in increased fluticasone exposure).
No products indexed under this heading.

Fosamprenavir Calcium (Caution should be exercised when potent cytochrome P450 3A4 inhibitors are co-administered with fluticasone. Interactions with ritonavir and ketoconazole, both potent CYP3A4 inhibitors, have resulted in increased fluticasone exposure). Products include:
Lexiva Oral Suspension 1510
Lexiva Tablets 1510

Indinavir Sulfate (Caution should be exercised when potent cytochrome P450 3A4 inhibitors are co-administered with fluticasone. Interactions with ritonavir and ketoconazole, both potent CYP3A4 inhibitors, have resulted in increased fluticasone exposure). Products include:
Crixivan Capsules 1979

Itraconazole (Caution should be exercised when potent cytochrome P450 3A4 inhibitors are co-administered with fluticasone. Interactions with ritonavir and ketoconazole, both potent CYP3A4 inhibitors, have resulted in increased fluticasone exposure).
No products indexed under this heading.

Ketoconazole (Co-administration of a single dose of fluticasone (1000 mcg) with multiple doses of ketoconazole (200 mg) to steady state has resulted in increased mean fluticasone concentrations, a reduction in plasma cortisol AUC, and no effect on urinary excretion ofcortisol). Products include:
Extina Foam, 2% 3057
Nizoral A-D Shampoo 1901

Lopinavir (Caution should be exercised when potent cytochrome P450 3A4 inhibitors are co-administered with fluticasone. Interactions with ritonavir and ketoconazole, both potent CYP3A4 inhibitors, have resulted in increased fluticasone exposure). Products include:
Kaletra 452

Nefazodone Hydrochloride (Caution should be exercised when potent cytochrome P450 3A4 inhibitors are co-administered with fluticasone. Interactions with ritonavir and ketoconazole, both potent CYP3A4 inhibitors, have resulted in increased fluticasone exposure).
No products indexed under this heading.

Nelfinavir Mesylate (Caution should be exercised when potent cytochrome P450 3A4 inhibitors are co-administered with fluticasone. Interactions with ritonavir and ketoconazole, both potent CYP3A4 inhibitors, have resulted in increased fluticasone exposure).
No products indexed under this heading.

Ritonavir (Ritonavir can significantly increase plasma fluticasone exposure, resulting in significantly reduced serum cortisol concentrations. Cushing syndrome and adrenal suppression have been reported; therefore, co-administration is not recommended unless the potential benefit outweighs the risks). Products include:
Kaletra 452
Norvir 489

Saquinavir (Caution should be exercised when potent cytochrome P450 3A4 inhibitors are co-administered with fluticasone. Interactions with ritonavir and ketoconazole, both potent CYP3A4 inhibitors, have resulted in increased fluticasone exposure).
No products indexed under this heading.

Saquinavir Mesylate (Caution should be exercised when potent cytochrome P450 3A4 inhibitors are co-administered with fluticasone. Interactions with ritonavir and ketoconazole, both potent CYP3A4 inhibitors, have resulted in increased fluticasone exposure).
No products indexed under this heading.

Telithromycin (Caution should be exercised when potent cytochrome P450 3A4 inhibitors are co-administered with fluticasone. Interactions with ritonavir and ketoconazole, both potent CYP3A4 inhibitors, have resulted in increased fluticasone exposure). Products include:
Ketek Tablets 2744

Troleandomycin (Caution should be exercised when potent cytochrome P450 3A4 inhibitors are co-administered with fluticasone. Interactions with ritonavir and ketoconazole, both potent CYP3A4 inhibitors, have resulted in increased fluticasone exposure).
No products indexed under this heading.

Voriconazole (Caution should be exercised when potent cytochrome P450 3A4 inhibitors are co-administered with fluticasone. Interactions with ritonavir and ketoconazole, both potent CYP3A4 inhibitors, have resulted in increased fluticasone exposure).
No products indexed under this heading.

FLOVENT HFA 44 MCG INHALATION AEROSOL

(Fluticasone Propionate HFA) 1440
May interact with:

Ketoconazole (Co-administration of a single dose of fluticasone (1000 mcg) with multiple doses of ketoconazole (200 mg) to steady state has resulted in increased mean plasma fluticasone exposure, a reduction in plasma cortisol AUC, and no effect on urinary excretion of cortisol). Products include:
Extina Foam, 2% 3057
Nizoral A-D Shampoo 1901

Ritonavir (Ritonavir can significantly increase plasma fluticasone exposure, resulting in significantly reduced serum cortisol concentrations. Cushing syndrome and adrenal suppression have been reported; therefore, co-administration is not recommended unless the potential benefit outweighs the risks). Products include:
Kaletra 452
Norvir 489

FLOVENT HFA 110 MCG INHALATION AEROSOL

(Fluticasone Propionate HFA) 1440
See Flovent HFA 44 mcg Inhalation Aerosol

FLOVENT HFA 220 MCG INHALATION AEROSOL

(Fluticasone Propionate HFA) 1440
See Flovent HFA 44 mcg Inhalation Aerosol

FLUARIX VACCINE

(Influenza Virus Vaccine) 1446
May interact with alkylating agents, antimetabolites, corticosteroids, cytotoxic drugs, phenytoin, theophyllines, and certain other agents. Compounds in these categories include:

Betamethasone Acetate (Immunosuppressive therapies, corticosteroids (used in greater than physiologic doses), may reduce the immune response to vaccines).
No products indexed under this heading.

Betamethasone Sodium Phosphate (Immunosuppressive therapies, corticosteroids (used in greater than physiologic doses), may reduce the immune response to vaccines).
No products indexed under this heading.

Bleomycin Sulfate (Immunosuppressive therapies, cytotoxic drugs, may reduce the immune response to vaccines).
No products indexed under this heading.

Budesonide (Immunosuppressive therapies, corticosteroids (used in greater than physiologic doses), may reduce the immune response to vaccines). Products include:
Pulmicort Flexhaler **654**
Symbicort 80/4.5 Inhalation Aerosol **659**
Symbicort 160/4.5 Inhalation Aerosol **659**

Busulfan (Immunosuppressive therapies, alkylating agents, may reduce the immune response to vaccines). Products include:
Busulfex Injection **2477**
Myleran Tablets **1530**

Capecitabine (Immunosuppressive therapies, antimetabolites, may reduce the immune response to vaccines). Products include:
Xeloda Tablets **2662**

Carmustine (BCNU) (Immunosuppressive therapies, alkylating agents, may reduce the immune response to vaccines).
No products indexed under this heading.

Chlorambucil (Immunosuppressive therapies, alkylating agents, may reduce the immune response to vaccines). Products include:
Leukeran Tablets **1508**

Ciclesonide (Immunosuppressive therapies, corticosteroids (used in greater than physiologic doses), may reduce the immune response to vaccines). Products include:
Alvesco Inhalation Aerosol **2985**
Omnaris Nasal Spray **2998**

Cladribine (Immunosuppressive therapies, antimetabolites, may reduce the immune response to vaccines). Products include:
Leustatin Injection **2384**

Cortisone Acetate (Immunosuppressive therapies, corticosteroids (used in greater than physiologic doses), may reduce the immune response to vaccines).
No products indexed under this heading.

Cyclophosphamide (Immunosuppressive therapies, alkylating agents, may reduce the immune response to vaccines).
No products indexed under this heading.

Cytarabine (Immunosuppressive therapies, antimetabolites, may reduce the immune response to vaccines).
No products indexed under this heading.

Dacarbazine (Immunosuppressive therapies, alkylating agents, may reduce the immune response to vaccines).
No products indexed under this heading.

Daunorubicin Hydrochloride (Immunosuppressive therapies, cytotoxic drugs, may reduce the immune response to vaccines).
No products indexed under this heading.

Dexamethasone (Immunosuppressive therapies, corticosteroids (used in greater than physiologic doses), may reduce the immune response to vaccines). Products include:
Ciprodex Otic Suspension **541**

Dexamethasone Acetate (Immunosuppressive therapies, corticosteroids (used in greater than physiologic doses), may reduce the immune response to vaccines).
No products indexed under this heading.

Dexamethasone Sodium Phosphate (Immunosuppressive therapies, corticosteroids (used in greater than physiologic doses), may reduce the immune response to vaccines).
No products indexed under this heading.

Doxorubicin Hydrochloride (Immunosuppressive therapies, cytotoxic drugs, may reduce the immune response to vaccines).
No products indexed under this heading.

Epirubicin Hydrochloride (Immunosuppressive therapies, cytotoxic drugs, may reduce the immune response to vaccines).
No products indexed under this heading.

Floxuridine (Immunosuppressive therapies, antimetabolites, may reduce the immune response to vaccines).
No products indexed under this heading.

Fludarabine Phosphate (Immunosuppressive therapies, antimetabolites, may reduce the immune response to vaccines).
No products indexed under this heading.

Fludrocortisone Acetate (Immunosuppressive therapies, corticosteroids (used in greater than physiologic doses), may reduce the immune response to vaccines).
No products indexed under this heading.

Flunisolide (Immunosuppressive therapies, corticosteroids (used in greater than physiologic doses), may reduce the immune response to vaccines). Products include:
Aerobid/Aerobid-M **1153**

Fluorouracil (Immunosuppressive therapies, antimetabolites, may reduce the immune response to vaccines). Products include:
Carac Cream 0.5% **2722**

Fluticasone Propionate (Immunosuppressive therapies, corticosteroids (used in greater than physiologic doses), may reduce the immune response to vaccines). Products include:
Advair Diskus 100/50 .... **1276**
Advair Diskus 250/50 .... **1276**
Advair Diskus 500/50 .... **1276**
Advair HFA 45/21 Inhalation Aerosol **1288**
Advair HFA 115/21 Inhalation Aerosol **1288**
Advair HFA 230/21 Inhalation Aerosol **1288**
Flonase Nasal Spray **1431**
Flovent Diskus 50 mcg **1435**

Fluticasone Propionate HFA (Immunosuppressive therapies, corticosteroids (used in greater than physiologic doses), may reduce the immune response to vaccines). Products include:
Flovent HFA **1440**

Fosphenytoin Sodium (Although it has been reported that influenza vaccination may inhibit the clearance of phenytoin, controlled studies have yielded inconsistent results regarding pharmacokinetic interactions between influenza vaccine and phenytoin. Nevertheless, clinicians should consider the potential for an interaction when influenza vaccine is administered to persons receiving phenytoin).
No products indexed under this heading.

Gemcitabine Hydrochloride (Immunosuppressive therapies, antimetabolites, may reduce the immune response to vaccines). Products include:
Gemzar for Injection **1820**

Hydrocortisone (Immunosuppressive therapies, corticosteroids (used in greater than physiologic doses), may reduce the immune response to vaccines).
No products indexed under this heading.

Hydrocortisone Acetate (Immunosuppressive therapies, corticosteroids (used in greater than physiologic doses), may reduce the immune response to vaccines). Products include:
Analpram-HC **1140**
Pramosone **1141**

Hydrocortisone Sodium Phosphate (Immunosuppressive therapies, corticosteroids (used in greater than physiologic doses), may reduce the immune response to vaccines).
No products indexed under this heading.

Hydrocortisone Sodium Succinate (Immunosuppressive therapies, corticosteroids (used in greater than physiologic doses), may reduce the immune response to vaccines).
No products indexed under this heading.

Hydroxyurea (Immunosuppressive therapies, cytotoxic drugs, may reduce the immune response to vaccines).
No products indexed under this heading.

Lomustine (CCNU) (Immunosuppressive therapies, alkylating agents, may reduce the immune response to vaccines).
No products indexed under this heading.

Mechlorethamine Hydrochloride (Immunosuppressive therapies, alkylating agents, may reduce the immune response to vaccines). Products include:
Mustargen for Injection **2492**

Melphalan (Immunosuppressive therapies, alkylating agents, may reduce the immune response to vaccines).
No products indexed under this heading.

Mercaptopurine (Immunosuppressive therapies, antimetabolites, may reduce the immune response to vaccines).
No products indexed under this heading.

Methotrexate (Immunosuppressive therapies, antimetabolites, may reduce the immune response to vaccines).
No products indexed under this heading.

Methotrexate Sodium (Immunosuppressive therapies, cytotoxic drugs, may reduce the immune response to vaccines).
No products indexed under this heading.

Methylprednisolone Acetate (Immunosuppressive therapies, corticosteroids (used in greater than physiologic doses), may reduce the immune response to vaccines).
No products indexed under this heading.

Methylprednisolone Sodium Succinate (Immunosuppressive therapies, corticosteroids (used in greater than physiologic doses), may reduce the immune response to vaccines).
No products indexed under this heading.

Mitotane (Immunosuppressive therapies, cytotoxic drugs, may reduce the immune response to vaccines).
No products indexed under this heading.

Mitoxantrone Hydrochloride (Immunosuppressive therapies, cytotoxic drugs, may reduce the immune response to vaccines). Products include:
Novantrone for Injection Concentrate **1100**

Mometasone Furoate (Immunosuppressive therapies, corticosteroids (used in greater than physiologic doses), may reduce the immune response to vaccines). Products include:
Asmanex Twisthaler **2797**
Elocon Cream 0.1% **2840**
Elocon Lotion 0.1% **2841**
Elocon Ointment 0.1% **2842**

Mometasone Furoate Monohydrate (Immunosuppressive therapies, corticosteroids (used in greater than physiologic doses), may reduce the immune response to vaccines). Products include:
Nasonex Nasal Spray **2883**

Pentostatin (Immunosuppressive therapies, antimetabolites, may reduce the immune response to vaccines).
No products indexed under this heading.

Phenytoin (Although it has been reported that influenza vaccination may inhibit the clearance of phenytoin, controlled studies have yielded inconsistent results regarding pharmacokinetic interactions between influenza vaccine and phenytoin. Nevertheless, clinicians should consider the potential for an interaction when influenza vaccine is administered to persons receiving phenytoin).
No products indexed under this heading.

Phenytoin Sodium (Although it has been reported that influenza vaccination may inhibit the clearance of phenytoin, controlled studies have yielded inconsistent results regarding pharmacokinetic interactions between influenza vaccine and phenytoin. Nevertheless, clinicians should consider the potential for an interac-

tion when influenza vaccine is administered to persons receiving phenytoin). Products include:

Phenytek Capsules 2192

Prednisolone Acetate (Immunosuppressive therapies, corticosteroids (used in greater than physiologic doses), may reduce the immune response to vaccines). Products include:

Pred Forte Ophthalmic Suspension .... ⊙227
Pred Mild Ophthalmic Suspension .... ⊙230
Pred-G Ophthalmic Ointment .... ⊙229
Pred-G Ophthalmic Suspension ...... ⊙228

Prednisolone Sodium Phosphate (Immunosuppressive therapies, corticosteroids (used in greater than physiologic doses), may reduce the immune response to vaccines).

No products indexed under this heading.

Prednisolone Tebutate (Immunosuppressive therapies, corticosteroids (used in greater than physiologic doses), may reduce the immune response to vaccines).

No products indexed under this heading.

Prednisone (Immunosuppressive therapies, corticosteroids (used in greater than physiologic doses), may reduce the immune response to vaccines).

No products indexed under this heading.

Procarbazine Hydrochloride (Immunosuppressive therapies, cytotoxic drugs, may reduce the immune response to vaccines).

No products indexed under this heading.

Tamoxifen Citrate (Immunosuppressive therapies, cytotoxic drugs, may reduce the immune response to vaccines).

No products indexed under this heading.

Theophylline (Although it has been reported that influenza vaccination may inhibit the clearance of theophylline, controlled studies have yielded inconsistent results regarding pharmacokinetic interactions between influenza vaccine and theophylline. Nevertheless, clinicians should consider the potential for an interaction when influenza vaccine is administered to persons receiving theophylline).

No products indexed under this heading.

Theophylline Anhydrous (Although it has been reported that influenza vaccination may inhibit the clearance of theophylline, controlled studies have yielded inconsistent results regarding pharmacokinetic interactions between influenza vaccine and theophylline. Nevertheless, clinicians should consider the potential for an interaction when influenza vaccine is administered to persons receiving theophylline). Products include:

Uniphyl Tablets 2595

Theophylline Calcium Salicylate (Although it has been reported that influenza vaccination may inhibit the clearance of theophylline, controlled studies have yielded inconsistent results regarding pharmacokinetic interactions between influenza vaccine and theophylline. Nevertheless, clinicians should consider the potential for an interaction when influenza vaccine is administered to persons receiving theophylline).

No products indexed under this heading.

Theophylline Dihydroxypropyl (Glyceryl) (Although it has been reported that influenza vaccination may inhibit the clearance of theophylline, controlled studies have yielded inconsistent results regarding pharmacokinetic interactions between influenza vaccine and theophylline. Nevertheless, clinicians should consider the potential for an interaction when influenza vaccine is administered to persons receiving theophylline).

No products indexed under this heading.

Theophylline Ethylenediamine (Although it has been reported that influenza vaccination may inhibit the clearance of theophylline, controlled studies have yielded inconsistent results regarding pharmacokinetic interactions between influenza vaccine and theophylline. Nevertheless, clinicians should consider the potential for an interaction when influenza vaccine is administered to persons receiving theophylline).

No products indexed under this heading.

Theophylline Sodium Glycinate (Although it has been reported that influenza vaccination may inhibit the clearance of theophylline, controlled studies have yielded inconsistent results regarding pharmacokinetic interactions between influenza vaccine and theophylline. Nevertheless, clinicians should consider the potential for an interaction when influenza vaccine is administered to persons receiving theophylline).

No products indexed under this heading.

Thioguanine (Immunosuppressive therapies, antimetabolites, may reduce the immune response to vaccines). Products include:

Tabloid Tablets 1601

Thiotepa (Immunosuppressive therapies, alkylating agents, may reduce the immune response to vaccines).

No products indexed under this heading.

Triamcinolone (Immunosuppressive therapies, corticosteroids (used in greater than physiologic doses), may reduce the immune response to vaccines).

No products indexed under this heading.

Triamcinolone Acetonide (Immunosuppressive therapies, corticosteroids (used in greater than physiologic doses), may reduce the immune response to vaccines). Products include:

Azmacort Inhalation Aerosol 407
Nasacort AQ Nasal Spray 2765
Triesence Injectable Suspension .... ⊙209

Triamcinolone Diacetate (Immunosuppressive therapies, corticosteroids (used in greater than physiologic doses), may reduce the immune response to vaccines).

No products indexed under this heading.

Triamcinolone Hexacetonide (Immunosuppressive therapies, corticosteroids (used in greater than physiologic doses), may reduce the immune response to vaccines).

No products indexed under this heading.

Vincristine Sulfate (Immunosuppressive therapies, cytotoxic drugs, may reduce the immune response to vaccines).

No products indexed under this heading.

Warfarin Sodium (Although it has been reported that influenza vaccination may inhibit the clearance of warfarin, controlled studies have yielded inconsistent results regarding pharmacokinetic interactions between influenza vaccine and warfarin. Nevertheless, clinicians should consider the potential for an interaction when influenza vaccine is administered to persons receiving warfarin).

No products indexed under this heading.

FLULAVAL INJECTION VACCINE

(Influenza Virus Vaccine) 1448

May interact with immunosuppressive agents and certain other agents. Compounds in these categories include:

Azathioprine (Immunosuppressive therapies, including irradiation, antimetabolites, alkylating agents, cytotoxic drugs and corticosteroids (used in greater than physiologic doses), may reduce the immune response to influenza virus vaccine).

No products indexed under this heading.

Basiliximab (Immunosuppressive therapies, including irradiation, antimetabolites, alkylating agents, cytotoxic drugs and corticosteroids (used in greater than physiologic doses), may reduce the immune response to influenza virus vaccine). Products include:

Simulect for Injection 2306

Cyclosporine (Immunosuppressive therapies, including irradiation, antimetabolites, alkylating agents, cytotoxic drugs and corticosteroids (used in greater than physiologic doses), may reduce the immune response to influenza virus vaccine). Products include:

Gengraf Capsules 435
Neoral Oral Solution 2280
Neoral Soft Gelatin Capsules 2280
Restasis Ophthalmic Emulsion 557
Sandimmune 2296

Muromonab-CD3 (Immunosuppressive therapies, including irradiation, antimetabolites, alkylating agents, cytotoxic drugs and corticosteroids (used in greater than physiologic doses), may reduce the immune response to influenza virus vaccine). Products include:

Orthoclone OKT3 Sterile Solution 2387

Mycophenolate Mofetil (Immunosuppressive therapies, including irradiation, antimetabolites, alkylating agents, cytotoxic drugs and corticosteroids (used in greater than physiologic doses), may reduce the immune response to influenza virus vaccine). Products include:

CellCept Capsules 2622
CellCept Oral Suspension 2622
CellCept Tablets 2622

Phenytoin (Although it has been reported that influenza vaccination may inhibit the clearance of phenytoin, controlled studies have yielded inconsistent results regarding pharmacokinetic interactions between influenza vaccine and these medications. Nevertheless, clinicians should consider the potential for an interaction when influenza virus vaccine is administered to persons receiving phenytoin).

No products indexed under this heading.

Sirolimus (Immunosuppressive therapies, including irradiation, antimetabolites, alkylating agents, cytotoxic drugs and corticosteroids (used in greater than physiologic doses), may reduce the immune response to influenza virus vaccine). Products include:

Rapamune 3260

Tacrolimus (Immunosuppressive therapies, including irradiation, antimetabolites, alkylating agents, cytotoxic drugs and corticosteroids (used in greater than physiologic doses), may reduce the immune response to influenza virus vaccine). Products include:

Prograf Capsules and Injection 622
Protopic Ointment 628

Theophylline (Although it has been reported that influenza vaccination may inhibit the clearance of theophylline, controlled studies have yielded inconsistent results regarding pharmacokinetic interactions between influenza vaccine and these medications. Nevertheless, clinicians should consider the potential for an interaction when influenza virus vaccine is administered to persons receiving theophylline).

No products indexed under this heading.

Warfarin Sodium (Although it has been reported that influenza vaccination may inhibit the clearance of warfarin, controlled studies have yielded inconsistent results regarding pharmacokinetic interactions between influenza vaccine and these medications. Nevertheless, clinicians should consider the potential for an interaction when influenza virus vaccine is administered to persons receiving warfarin).

No products indexed under this heading.

FLUMADINE SYRUP

(Rimantadine Hydrochloride) 1167

See Flumadine Tablets

FLUMADINE TABLETS

(Rimantadine Hydrochloride) 1167

May interact with:

Acetaminophen (Co-administration reduces the peak concentration and AUC values for rimantadine). Products include:

Benadryl Allergy & Cold Kapgels 1895
Benadryl Allergy & Sinus Headache Kapgels 1895
Benadryl Severe Allergy & Sinus Headache Caplets 1897
Lortab 5/500 Tablets 3143
Lortab 7.5/500 Tablets 3144
Lortab 10/500 Tablets 3144
Percocet Tablets 1127
Sinutab Sinus Caplets 1905
Sudafed PE Cold & Cough Caplets 1907
Sudafed PE Nighttime Cold Caplets 1907
Sudafed PE Severe Cold Caplets 1908
Sudafed PE Sinus Headache Caplets 1908
Regular Strength Tylenol Tablets 1915
Tylenol 8 Hour Extended Release Caplets 1915
Extra Strength Tylenol Caplets, Cool Caplets, and EZ Tabs 1915
Extra Strength Tylenol Adult Rapid Blast Liquid 1915

Extra Strength Tylenol PM Caplets, Geltabs, Liquid, and Rapid Release Gels 1915
Extra Strength Tylenol Rapid Release Gels 1915
Tylenol with Codeine Tablets 2427
Tylenol Allergy Multi-Symptom Caplets with Cool Burst and Rapid Release Gelcaps 1916
Tylenol Allergy Multi-Symptom Nighttime Caplets with Cool Burst 1916
Tylenol Severe Allergy Caplets 1916
Tylenol Arthritis Pain Extended Release Geltabs/Caplets 1915
Tylenol Chest Congestion Caplets with Cool Burst 1910
Tylenol Chest Congestion Liquid with Cool Burst 1910
Children's Tylenol Plus Cold Suspension Liquid 1912
Children's Tylenol Plus Cold & Allergy Suspension Liquid 1914
Children's Tylenol Plus Cough & Runny Nose Suspension Liquid 1912
Children's Tylenol Plus Cough & Sore Throat Suspension Liquid 1912
Children's Tylenol Plus Flu Suspension Liquid 1914
Children's Tylenol Suspension Liquid 1909
Children's Tylenol Meltaways 1909
Children's Tylenol Plus Multi-Symptom Cold Suspension Liquid 1912
Tylenol Cold Severe Congestion Daytime Caplets with Cool Burst 1912
Tylenol Cold Head Congestion Daytime Caplets with Cool Burst 1910
Tylenol Cold Head Congestion Nighttime Caplets with Cool Burst 1910
Tylenol Cold Head Congestion Severe Daytime Caplets with Cool Burst 1910
Tylenol Cold Multi-Symptom Daytime Caplets with Cool Burst and Rapid Release Gels 1913
Tylenol Cold Multi-Symptom Daytime Liquid with Citrus Burst 1913
Tylenol Cold Multi-Symptom Nighttime Caplets with Cool Burst 1913
Tylenol Cold Multi-Symptom Nighttime Liquid with Cool Burst 1913
Tylenol Cold Multi-Symptom Severe Caplets with Cool Burst 1913
Tylenol Cold Multi-Symptom Severe Daytime Liquid with Citrus Burst 1913
Tylenol Cough & Sore Throat Daytime Liquid with Cool Burst 1918
Tylenol Cough & Sore Throat Nighttime Liquid with Cool Burst 1918
Concentrated Tylenol Infants' Drops 1909
Jr. Tylenol Meltaways 1909
Tylenol Sinus Congestion & Pain Daytime Caplets with Cool Burst and Gelcaps 1917
Tylenol Sinus Congestion & Pain Nighttime Caplets with Cool Burst 1917
Tylenol Sinus Congestion & Pain Severe Caplets with Cool Burst 1917
Tylenol Sinus Severe Congestion Caplets with Cool Burst 1917
Tylenol Sore Throat Daytime Liquid with Cool Burst 1918
Tylenol Sore Throat Nighttime Liquid with Cool Burst 1918
Women's Tylenol Menstrual Relief Caplets 1919
Vicks DayQuil Cold & Flu Multi-Symptom Relief 616
Vicks DayQuil LiquiCaps 2567
Vicks DayQuil Liquid 2567
Vicks DayQuil Multi-Symptom Cold/Flu Relief 2567
Vicks NyQuil Cold & Flu Multi-Symptom Relief 617
Vicks NyQuil LiquiCaps 2567
Vicks NyQuil Liquid 2567
Vicks NyQuil Multi-Symptom Cold/Flu Relief 2567
Vicodin Tablets 529
Vicodin ES Tablets 530
Vicodin HP Tablets 531
Zydone Tablets 1132

Aspirin (Co-administration reduces the peak concentration and AUC values for rimantadine). Products include:
Aggrenox Capsules 819
Bayer Aspirin 750
Percodan Tablets 1130
St. Joseph 81 mg Aspirin Chewable and Enteric Coated Tablets 1903

Cimetidine (Potential for reduced clearance of total rimantadine).
No products indexed under this heading.

Cimetidine Hydrochloride (Potential for reduced clearance of total rimantadine).
No products indexed under this heading.

Influenza Virus Vaccine Live, Intranasal (It is advisable that Influenza Virus Vaccine Live, Intranasal not be administered until 48 hours after cessation of rimantadine and that rimantadine not be administered until two weeks after the administration of Influenza Virus Vaccine Live, Intranasal unless medically indicated). Products include:
FluMist Vaccine 1945

FLUMIST VACCINE

(Influenza Virus Vaccine Live, Intranasal) 1945

May interact with alkylating agents, antivirals active against influenza, antimetabolites, aspirin-acetylsalicylic acid, corticosteroids, immunosuppressive agents, killed/inactivated vaccines, and certain other agents. Compounds in these categories include:

Amantadine Hydrochloride (The concurrent use of FluMist with antiviral agents that are active against influenza A and/or B viruses has not been evaluated. However, base upon the potential for antiviral agents to reduce the effectiveness of FluMist, do not administer FluMist until 48 hours after the cessation of antiviral therapy and antiviral agents should not be administered until two weeks after administration of FluMist unless medically indicated. If antiviral agents and Flumist are administered concomitantly, revaccination should be considered when appropriate).
No products indexed under this heading.

Arginine base (FluMist is contraindicated in individuals with history of hypersensitivity, especially anaphylactic reactions, to arginine).
No products indexed under this heading.

Arginine Hydrochloride (FluMist is contraindicated in individuals with history of hypersensitivity, especially anaphylactic reactions, to arginine).
No products indexed under this heading.

Aspirin (FluMist is contraindicated in children and adolescents (2-17 years of age) receiving aspirin therapy or aspirin-containing therapy, because of the association of Reye's syndrome with aspirin and wild-type influenza infection). Products include:
Aggrenox Capsules 819
Bayer Aspirin 750
Percodan Tablets 1130
St. Joseph 81 mg Aspirin Chewable and Enteric Coated Tablets 1903

Aspirin, Enteric Coated (FluMist is contraindicated in children and adolescents (2-17 years of age) receiving aspirin therapy or aspirin-containing therapy, because of the association of Reye's syndrome with aspirin and wild-type influenza infection).
No products indexed under this heading.

Aspirin Buffered (FluMist is contraindicated in children and adolescents (2-17 years of age) receiving aspirin therapy or aspirin-containing therapy, because of the association of Reye's syndrome with aspirin and wild-type influenza infection).
No products indexed under this heading.

Azathioprine (Administration of FluMist, a live virus vaccine, to immunocompromised persons should be based on careful consideration of potential benefits and risks).
No products indexed under this heading.

Basiliximab (Administration of FluMist, a live virus vaccine, to immunocompromised persons should be based on careful consideration of potential benefits and risks).
Products include:
Simulect for Injection 2306

Betamethasone Acetate (Administration of FluMist, a live virus vaccine, to immunocompromised persons should be based on careful consideration of potential benefits and risk).
No products indexed under this heading.

Betamethasone Sodium Phosphate (Administration of FluMist, a live virus vaccine, to immunocompromised persons should be based on careful consideration of potential benefits and risk).
No products indexed under this heading.

Budesonide (Administration of FluMist, a live virus vaccine, to immunocompromised persons should be based on careful consideration of potential benefits and risk). Products include:
Pulmicort Flexhaler 654
Symbicort 80/4.5 Inhalation Aerosol 659
Symbicort 160/4.5 Inhalation Aerosol 659

Busulfan (Adminstration of Flumist, a live virus vaccine, to immunocompromised persons should be based on careful consideration of potential benefits and risks). Products include:
Busulfex Injection 2477
Myleran Tablets 1530

Capecitabine (Adminstration of Flumist, a live virus vaccine, to immunocompromised persons should be based on careful consideration of potential benefits and risks).
Products include:
Xeloda Tablets 2662

Carmustine (BCNU) (Adminstration of Flumist, a live virus vaccine, to immunocompromised persons should be based on careful consideration of potential benefits and risks).
No products indexed under this heading.

Chlorambucil (Adminstration of Flumist, a live virus vaccine, to immunocompromised persons should be based on careful consideration of potential benefits and risks).
Products include:
Leukeran Tablets 1508

Ciclesonide (Administration of FluMist, a live virus vaccine, to immunocompromised persons should be based on careful consideration of potential benefits and risk). Products include:
Alvesco Inhalation Aerosol 2985
Omnaris Nasal Spray 2998

Cladribine (Adminstration of FluMist, a live virus vaccine, to immunocompromised persons should be based on careful consideration of potential benefits and risks).
Products include:
Leustatin Injection 2384

Cortisone Acetate (Administration of FluMist, a live virus vaccine, to immunocompromised persons should be based on careful consideration of potential benefits and risk).
No products indexed under this heading.

Cyclophosphamide (Adminstration of Flumist, a live virus vaccine, to immunocompromised persons should be based on careful consideration of potential benefits and risks).
No products indexed under this heading.

Cyclosporine (Administration of FluMist, a live virus vaccine, to immunocompromised persons should be based on careful consideration of potential benefits and risks).
Products include:
Gengraf Capsules 435
Neoral Oral Solution 2280
Neoral Soft Gelatin Capsules 2280
Restasis Ophthalmic Emulsion 557
Sandimmune 2296

Cytarabine (Adminstration of FluMist, a live virus vaccine, to immunocompromised persons should be based on careful consideration of potential benefits and risks).
No products indexed under this heading.

Dacarbazine (Adminstration of FluMist, a live virus vaccine, to immunocompromised persons should be based on careful consideration of potential benefits and risks).
No products indexed under this heading.

Dexamethasone (Administration of FluMist, a live virus vaccine, to immunocompromised persons should be based on careful consideration of potential benefits and risk). Products include:
Ciprodex Otic Suspension 541

Dexamethasone Acetate (Administration of FluMist, a live virus vaccine, to immunocompromised persons should be based on careful consideration of potential benefits and risk).
No products indexed under this heading.

Dexamethasone Sodium Phosphate (Administration of FluMist, a live virus vaccine, to immunocompromised persons should be based on careful consideration of potential benefits and risk).
No products indexed under this heading.

Diphtheria & Tetanus Toxoids and Acellular Pertussis Vaccine Adsorbed, Hepatitis B (recombinant) and Inactivated Poliovirus Vaccine Combined (The safety and immunogenicity of Flumist when

IMPORTANT NOTE: Always consult each drug listing in the patient's regimen for possible interactions.

administered concurrently with inactivated vaccines have not been determined. Studies of FluMist excluded subjects who received any inactivated or subunit vaccine within two weeks of enrollment. Therefore, healthcare providers should consider the risk and benefits of concurrent administration of Flumist with inactivated vaccines).
No products indexed under this heading.

Egg product, hyperimmune (FluMist is contraindicated in individuals with history of hypersensitivity, especially anaphylactic reactions, to eggs and egg proteins). Products include:
i26 Capsules .... ■▫629
i26 Chewable Tablets .... ■▫629

Floxuridine (Adminstration of Flumist, a live virus vaccine, to immunocompromised persons should be based on careful consideration of potential benefits and risks).
No products indexed under this heading.

Fludarabine Phosphate (Adminstration of Flumist, a live virus vaccine, to immunocompromised persons should be based on careful consideration of potential benefits and risks).
No products indexed under this heading.

Fludrocortisone Acetate (Administration of FluMist, a live virus vaccine, to immunocompromised persons should be based on careful consideration of potential benefits and risk).
No products indexed under this heading.

Flunisolide (Administration of FluMist, a live virus vaccine, to immunocompromised persons should be based on careful consideration of potential benefits and risk). Products include:
Aerobid/Aerobid-M 1153

Fluorouracil (Adminstration of Flumist, a live virus vaccine, to immunocompromised persons should be based on careful consideration of potential benefits and risks). Products include:
Carac Cream 0.5% 2722

Fluticasone Propionate (Administration of FluMist, a live virus vaccine, to immunocompromised persons should be based on careful consideration of potential benefits and risk). Products include:
Advair Diskus 100/50 1276
Advair Diskus 250/50 1276
Advair Diskus 500/50 1276
Advair HFA 45/21 Inhalation Aerosol 1288
Advair HFA 115/21 Inhalation Aerosol 1288
Advair HFA 230/21 Inhalation Aerosol 1288
Flonase Nasal Spray 1431
Flovent Diskus 50 mcg 1435

Fluticasone Propionate HFA (Administration of FluMist, a live virus vaccine, to immunocompromised persons should be based on careful consideration of potential benefits and risk). Products include:
Flovent HFA 1440

Gelatin (FluMist is contraindicated in individuals with history of hypersensitivity, especially anaphylactic reactions, to gelatin).
No products indexed under this heading.

Gelatin Preparations (FluMist is contraindicated in individuals with history of hypersensitivity, especially anaphylactic reactions, to gelatin).
No products indexed under this heading.

Gemcitabine Hydrochloride (Adminstration of Flumist, a live virus vaccine, to immunocompromised persons should be based on careful consideration of potential benefits and risks). Products include:
Gemzar for Injection 1820

Gentamicin (FluMist is contraindicated in individuals with history of hypersensitivity, especially anaphylactic reactions, to gentamicin).
No products indexed under this heading.

Gentamicin Sulfate (FluMist is contraindicated in individuals with history of hypersensitivity, especially anaphylactic reactions, to gentamicin). Products include:
Pred-G Ophthalmic Ointment .... ⊙229
Pred-G Ophthalmic Suspension .... ⊙228

Hepatitis A Vaccine, Inactivated (The safety and immunogenicity of Flumist when administered concurrently with inactivated vaccines have not been determined. Studies of FluMist excluded subjects who received any inactivated or subunit vaccine within two weeks of enrollment. Therefore, healthcare providers should consider the risk and benefits of concurrent administration of FluMist with inactivated vaccines). Products include:
Havrix Injection Vaccine 1454
Twinrix Vaccine 1628
Vaqta 2130

Hydrocortisone (Administration of FluMist, a live virus vaccine, to immunocompromised persons should be based on careful consideration of potential benefits and risk).
No products indexed under this heading.

Hydrocortisone Acetate (Administration of FluMist, a live virus vaccine, to immunocompromised persons should be based on careful consideration of potential benefits and risk). Products include:
Analpram-HC 1140
Pramosone 1141

Hydrocortisone Sodium Phosphate (Administration of FluMist, a live virus vaccine, to immunocompromised persons should be based on careful consideration of potential benefits and risk).
No products indexed under this heading.

Hydrocortisone Sodium Succinate (Administration of FluMist, a live virus vaccine, to immunocompromised persons should be based on careful consideration of potential benefits and risk).
No products indexed under this heading.

Influenza Virus Vaccine (The safety and immunogenicity of Flumist when administered concurrently with inactivated vaccines have not been determined. Studies of FluMist excluded subjects who received any inactivated or subunit vaccine within two weeks of enrollment. Therefore, healthcare providers should consider the risk and benefits of concurrent administration of Flumist with inactivated vaccines). Products include:
Fluarix Vaccine 1446
Flulaval Injection Vaccine 1448

Japanese Encephalitis Vaccine Inactivated (The safety and immunogenicity of Flumist when administered concurrently with inactivated vaccines have not been determined. Studies of FluMist excluded subjects who received any inactivated or subunit vaccine within two weeks of enrollment. Therefore, healthcare providers should consider the risk and benefits of concurrent administration of Flumist with inactivated vaccines).
No products indexed under this heading.

L-Arginine (FluMist is contraindicated in individuals with history of hypersensitivity, especially anaphylactic reactions, to arginine). Products include:
Dismutax Dietary Supplement 995
NT-Kinase Dietary Supplement 995

Lomustine (CCNU) (Adminstration of Flumist, a live virus vaccine, to immunocompromised persons should be based on careful consideration of potential benefits and risks).
No products indexed under this heading.

Mechlorethamine Hydrochloride (Adminstration of Flumist, a live virus vaccine, to immunocompromised persons should be based on careful consideration of potential benefits and risks). Products include:
Mustargen for Injection 2492

Melphalan (Adminstration of Flumist, a live virus vaccine, to immunocompromised persons should be based on careful consideration of potential benefits and risks).
No products indexed under this heading.

Mercaptopurine (Adminstration of Flumist, a live virus vaccine, to immunocompromised persons should be based on careful consideration of potential benefits and risks).
No products indexed under this heading.

Methotrexate (Adminstration of Flumist, a live virus vaccine, to immunocompromised persons should be based on careful consideration of potential benefits and risks).
No products indexed under this heading.

Methylprednisolone Acetate (Administration of FluMist, a live virus vaccine, to immunocompromised persons should be based on careful consideration of potential benefits and risk).
No products indexed under this heading.

Methylprednisolone Sodium Succinate (Administration of FluMist, a live virus vaccine, to immunocompromised persons should be based on careful consideration of potential benefits and risk).
No products indexed under this heading.

Mometasone Furoate (Administration of FluMist, a live virus vaccine, to immunocompromised persons should be based on careful consideration of potential benefits and risk). Products include:
Asmanex Twisthaler 2797
Elocon Cream 0.1% 2840
Elocon Lotion 0.1% 2841
Elocon Ointment 0.1% 2842

Mometasone Furoate Monohydrate (Administration of FluMist, a live virus vaccine, to immunocompromised persons should be based on careful consideration of potential benefits and risk). Products include:
Nasonex Nasal Spray 2883

Muromonab-CD3 (Administration of FluMist, a live virus vaccine, to immunocompromised persons should be based on careful consideration of potential benefits and risks). Products include:
Orthoclone OKT3 Sterile Solution 2387

Mycophenolate Mofetil (Administration of FluMist, a live virus vaccine, to immunocompromised persons should be based on careful consideration of potential benefits and risks). Products include:
CellCept Capsules 2622
CellCept Oral Suspension 2622
CellCept Tablets 2622

Oseltamivir Phosphate (The concurrent use of FluMist with antiviral agents that are active against influenza A and/or B viruses has not been evaluated. However, base upon the potential for antiviral agents to reduce the effectiveness of FluMist, do not administer FluMist until 48 hours after the cessation of antiviral therapy and antiviral agents should not be administered until two weeks after administration of FluMist unless medically indicated. If antiviral agents and Flumist are administered concomitantly, revaccination should be considered when appropriate). Products include:
Tamiflu Capsules 2649
Tamiflu Oral Suspension 2649

Pentostatin (Adminstration of Flumist, a live virus vaccine, to immunocompromised persons should be based on careful consideration of potential benefits and risks).
No products indexed under this heading.

Poliovirus Vaccine Inactivated (The safety and immunogenicity of Flumist when administered concurrently with inactivated vaccines have not been determined. Studies of FluMist excluded subjects who received any inactivated or subunit vaccine within two weeks of enrollment. Therefore, healthcare providers should consider the risk and benefits of concurrent administration of FluMist with inactivated vaccines). Products include:
Pediarix Vaccine 1552

Prednisolone Acetate (Administration of FluMist, a live virus vaccine, to immunocompromised persons should be based on careful consideration of potential benefits and risk). Products include:
Pred Forte Ophthalmic Suspension .... ⊙227
Pred Mild Ophthalmic Suspension .... ⊙230
Pred-G Ophthalmic Ointment .... ⊙229
Pred-G Ophthalmic Suspension .... ⊙228

Prednisolone Sodium Phosphate (Administration of FluMist, a live virus vaccine, to immunocompromised persons should be based on careful consideration of potential benefits and risk).
No products indexed under this heading.

Prednisolone Tebutate (Administration of FluMist, a live virus vaccine, to immunocompromised persons should be based on careful consideration of potential benefits and risk).
No products indexed under this heading.

Prednisone (Administration of FluMist, a live virus vaccine, to immunocompromised persons should be based on careful consideration of potential benefits and risk).
No products indexed under this heading.

Rimantadine Hydrochloride (The concurrent use of FluMist with antiviral agents that are active against influenza A and/or B viruses has not been evaluated. However, base upon the potential for antiviral agents to reduce the effectiveness of FluMist, do not administer FluMist until 48 hours after the cessation of antiviral therapy and antiviral agents should not be administered until two weeks after administration of FluMist unless medically indicated. If antiviral agents and Flumist are administered concomitantly, revaccination should be considered when appropriate).
Products include:
Flumadine 1167

Sirolimus (Administration of FluMist, a live virus vaccine, to immunocompromised persons should be based on careful consideration of potential benefits and risks).
Products include:
Rapamune 3260

Tacrolimus (Administration of FluMist, a live virus vaccine, to immunocompromised persons should be based on careful consideration of potential benefits and risks).
Products include:
Prograf Capsules and Injection 622
Protopic Ointment 628

Thioguanine (Adminstration of Flumist, a live virus vaccine, to immunocompromised persons should be based on careful consideration of potential benefits and risks).
Products include:
Tabloid Tablets 1601

Thiotepa (Adminstration of Flumist, a live virus vaccine, to immunocompromised persons should be based on careful consideration of potential benefits and risks).
No products indexed under this heading.

Triamcinolone (Administration of FluMist, a live virus vaccine, to immunocompromised persons should be based on careful consideration of potential benefits and risk).
No products indexed under this heading.

Triamcinolone Acetonide (Administration of FluMist, a live virus vaccine, to immunocompromised persons should be based on careful consideration of potential benefits and risk). Products include:
Azmacort Inhalation Aerosol 407
Nasacort AQ Nasal Spray 2765
Triesence Injectable Suspension .... ⊙209

Triamcinolone Diacetate (Administration of FluMist, a live virus vaccine, to immunocompromised persons should be based on careful consideration of potential benefits and risk).
No products indexed under this heading.

Triamcinolone Hexacetonide (Administration of FluMist, a live virus vaccine, to immunocompromised persons should be based on careful consideration of potential benefits and risk).
No products indexed under this heading.

Zanamivir (The concurrent use of FluMist with antiviral agents that are active against influenza A and/or B viruses has not been evaluated. However, base upon the potential for antiviral agents to reduce the effectiveness of FluMist, do not administer FluMist until 48 hours after the cessation of antiviral therapy and antiviral agents should not be administered until two weeks after administration of FluMist unless medically indicated. If antiviral agents and Flumist are administered concomitantly, revaccination should be considered when appropriate). Products include:
Relenza Inhalation Powder 1556

Food Interactions

Egg Product (FluMist is contraindicated in individuals with history of hypersensitivity, especially anaphylactic reactions, to eggs and egg proteins).

Eggs (FluMist is contraindicated in individuals with history of hypersensitivity, especially anaphylactic reactions, to eggs and egg proteins).

FLUORESCITE INJECTION

(Fluorescein Sodium) .... ⊙203
None cited in PDR database.

FML OPHTHALMIC OINTMENT

(Fluorometholone) .... ⊙223
None cited in PDR database.

FML OPHTHALMIC SUSPENSION

(Fluorometholone) .... ⊙224
None cited in PDR database.

FML FORTE OPHTHALMIC SUSPENSION

(Fluorometholone) .... ⊙222
None cited in PDR database.

FOCALIN XR CAPSULES

(Dexmethylphenidate Hydrochloride) 2251
May interact with antacids, antihypertensives, oral anticoagulants, histamine H_2-receptor antagonists, monoamine oxidase inhibitors, phenytoin, proton pump inhibitor, tricyclic antidepressants, vasopressors, and certain other agents. Compounds in these categories include:

Acebutolol Hydrochloride (Methylphenidate may decrease the effectiveness of antihypertensive drugs).
No products indexed under this heading.

Aliskiren (Methylphenidate may decrease the effectiveness of antihypertensive drugs). Products include:
Tekturna Tablets 2321
Tekturna HCT Tablets 2324

Aluminum Carbonate (The effects of gastrointestinal pH alterations on the absorption of dexmethylphenidate from Focalin XR have not been studied. Since the modified release characteristics of Focalin XR are pH dependent, the co-administration of antacids or acid suppressants could alter the release of dexmethylphenidate).
No products indexed under this heading.

Aluminum Hydroxide (The effects of gastrointestinal pH alterations on the absorption of dexmethylphenidate from Focalin XR have not been studied. Since the modified release characteristics of Focalin XR are pH dependent, the co-administration of antacids or acid suppressants could alter the release of dexmethylphenidate).
No products indexed under this heading.

Amitriptyline Hydrochloride (Racemic methylphenidate may inhibit the metabolism of tricyclic antidepressants).
No products indexed under this heading.

Amlodipine Besylate (Methylphenidate may decrease the effectiveness of antihypertensive drugs). Products include:
Azor Tablets 1005
Exforge Tablets 2238

Amoxapine (Racemic methylphenidate may inhibit the metabolism of tricyclic antidepressants).
No products indexed under this heading.

Anisindione (Racemic methylphenidate may inhibit the metabolism of coumarin anticoagulants).
No products indexed under this heading.

Atenolol (Methylphenidate may decrease the effectiveness of antihypertensive drugs).
No products indexed under this heading.

Benazepril Hydrochloride (Methylphenidate may decrease the effectiveness of antihypertensive drugs).
No products indexed under this heading.

Bendroflumethiazide (Methylphenidate may decrease the effectiveness of antihypertensive drugs).
No products indexed under this heading.

Betaxolol Hydrochloride (Methylphenidate may decrease the effectiveness of antihypertensive drugs).
No products indexed under this heading.

Bisoprolol Fumarate (Methylphenidate may decrease the effectiveness of antihypertensive drugs).
No products indexed under this heading.

Candesartan Cilexetil (Methylphenidate may decrease the effectiveness of antihypertensive drugs).
Products include:
Atacand Tablets 639
Atacand HCT 642

Captopril (Methylphenidate may decrease the effectiveness of antihypertensive drugs). Products include:
Captopril Tablets 2182

Carteolol Hydrochloride (Methylphenidate may decrease the effectiveness of antihypertensive drugs).
No products indexed under this heading.

Chlorothiazide (Methylphenidate may decrease the effectiveness of antihypertensive drugs).
No products indexed under this heading.

Chlorothiazide Sodium (Methylphenidate may decrease the effectiveness of antihypertensive drugs).
Products include:
Intravenous Sodium Diuril 2490

Chlorthalidone (Methylphenidate may decrease the effectiveness of antihypertensive drugs). Products include:
Clorpres Tablets 2185

Cimetidine (The effects of gastrointestinal pH alterations on the absorption of dexmethylphenidate from Focalin XR have not been studied. Since the modified release characteristics of Focalin XR are pH dependent, the co-administration of antacids or acid suppressants could alter the release of dexmethylphenidate).
No products indexed under this heading.

Cimetidine Hydrochloride (The effects of gastrointestinal pH alterations on the absorption of dexmethylphenidate from Focalin XR have not been studied. Since the modified release characteristics of Focalin XR are pH dependent, the co-administration of antacids or acid suppressants could alter the release of dexmethylphenidate).
No products indexed under this heading.

Clomipramine Hydrochloride (Racemic methylphenidate may inhibit the metabolism of tricyclic antidepressants).
No products indexed under this heading.

Clonidine (Co-administration has resulted in serious adverse events).
Products include:
Catapres-TTS 842

Clonidine Hydrochloride (Co-administration has resulted in serious adverse events). Products include:
Catapres Tablets 841
Clorpres Tablets 2185

Deserpidine (Methylphenidate may decrease the effectiveness of antihypertensive drugs).
No products indexed under this heading.

Desipramine Hydrochloride (Racemic methylphenidate may inhibit the metabolism of tricyclic antidepressants).
No products indexed under this heading.

Diazoxide (Methylphenidate may decrease the effectiveness of antihypertensive drugs). Products include:
Proglycem Capsules 1185
Proglycem Suspension 1185

Dicumarol (Racemic methylphenidate may inhibit the metabolism of coumarin anticoagulants).
No products indexed under this heading.

Diltiazem Hydrochloride (Methylphenidate may decrease the effectiveness of antihypertensive drugs).
Products include:
Cardizem LA Extended Release Tablets 421

Dobutamine (Methylphenidate has potential to increase blood pressure; concurrent use with pressor agents requires caution).
No products indexed under this heading.

Dobutamine Hydrochloride (Methylphenidate has potential to increase blood pressure; concurrent use with pressor agents requires caution).
No products indexed under this heading.

Dopamine Hydrochloride (Methylphenidate has potential to increase blood pressure; concurrent use with pressor agents requires caution).
No products indexed under this heading.

Doxazosin Mesylate (Methylphenidate may decrease the effectiveness of antihypertensive drugs).
No products indexed under this heading.

Doxepin Hydrochloride (Racemic methylphenidate may inhibit the metabolism of tricyclic antidepressants).
No products indexed under this heading.

Enalapril Maleate (Methylphenidate may decrease the effectiveness of antihypertensive drugs).
No products indexed under this heading.

Enalaprilat (Methylphenidate may decrease the effectiveness of antihypertensive drugs).
No products indexed under this heading.

Ephedrine Sulfate (Methylphenidate has potential to increase blood pressure; concurrent use with pressor agents requires caution).
No products indexed under this heading.

Epinephrine Bitartrate (Methylphenidate has potential to increase blood pressure; concurrent use with pressor agents requires caution).
No products indexed under this heading.

Epinephrine Hydrochloride (Methylphenidate has potential to increase blood pressure; concurrent use with pressor agents requires caution).
No products indexed under this heading.

Eprosartan Mesylate (Methylphenidate may decrease the effectiveness of antihypertensive drugs). Products include:
Teveten Tablets 515
Teveten HCT Tablets 517

Esmolol Hydrochloride (Methylphenidate may decrease the effectiveness of antihypertensive drugs).
No products indexed under this heading.

Esomeprazole Magnesium (The effects of gastrointestinal pH alterations on the absorption of dexmethylphenidate from Focalin XR have not been studied. Since the modified release characteristics of Focalin XR are pH dependent, the co-administration of antacids or acid suppressants could alter the release of dexmethylphenidate). Products include:
Nexium Delayed-Release Capsules 645
Nexium Delayed-Release Oral Suspension 645

Famotidine (The effects of gastrointestinal pH alterations on the absorption of dexmethylphenidate from Focalin XR have not been studied. Since the modified release characteristics of Focalin XR are pH dependent, the co-administration of antacids or acid suppressants could alter the release of dexmethylphenidate). Products include:
Pepcid Tablets 2075
Original Strength Pepcid AC Gelcaps 1771
Original Strength Pepcid AC Tablets 1771
Maximum Strength Pepcid AC Tablets 1771
Pepcid Complete Chewable Tablets 1771

Felodipine (Methylphenidate may decrease the effectiveness of antihypertensive drugs).
No products indexed under this heading.

Fosinopril Sodium (Methylphenidate may decrease the effectiveness of antihypertensive drugs).
No products indexed under this heading.

Fosphenytoin Sodium (Racemic methylphenidate may inhibit the metabolism of phenytoin).
No products indexed under this heading.

Furosemide (Methylphenidate may decrease the effectiveness of antihypertensive drugs). Products include:
Furosemide Tablets 2186

Guanabenz Acetate (Methylphenidate may decrease the effectiveness of antihypertensive drugs).
No products indexed under this heading.

Guanethidine Monosulfate (Methylphenidate may decrease the effectiveness of antihypertensive drugs).
No products indexed under this heading.

Hydralazine Hydrochloride (Methylphenidate may decrease the effectiveness of antihypertensive drugs).
No products indexed under this heading.

Hydrochlorothiazide (Methylphenidate may decrease the effectiveness of antihypertensive drugs). Products include:
Atacand HCT 642
Avalide Tablets 892
Avalide Tablets 2713
Benicar HCT Tablets 1010
Diovan HCT Tablets 2216
Dyazide Capsules 1405
Micardis HCT Tablets 854
Prinzide Tablets 2092
Tekturna HCT Tablets 2324
Teveten HCT Tablets 517

Hydroflumethiazide (Methylphenidate may decrease the effectiveness of antihypertensive drugs).
No products indexed under this heading.

Imipramine Hydrochloride (Racemic methylphenidate may inhibit the metabolism of tricyclic antidepressants).
No products indexed under this heading.

Imipramine Pamoate (Racemic methylphenidate may inhibit the metabolism of tricyclic antidepressants).
No products indexed under this heading.

Indapamide (Methylphenidate may decrease the effectiveness of antihypertensive drugs). Products include:
Indapamide Tablets 2188

Irbesartan (Methylphenidate may decrease the effectiveness of antihypertensive drugs). Products include:
Avalide Tablets 892
Avalide Tablets 2713
Avapro Tablets 897
Avapro Tablets 2718

Isocarboxazid (Co-administration with MAO inhibitor may result in hypertensive crises; concurrent and/or sequential use is contraindicated). Products include:
Marplan Tablets 3177

Isoproterenol Hydrochloride (Methylphenidate has potential to increase blood pressure; concurrent use with pressor agents requires caution).
No products indexed under this heading.

Isoproterenol Sulfate (Methylphenidate has potential to increase blood pressure; concurrent use with pressor agents requires caution).
No products indexed under this heading.

Isradipine (Methylphenidate may decrease the effectiveness of antihypertensive drugs). Products include:
DynaCirc CR Controlled Release Tablets 1407

Labetalol Hydrochloride (Methylphenidate may decrease the effectiveness of antihypertensive drugs).
No products indexed under this heading.

Lansoprazole (The effects of gastrointestinal pH alterations on the absorption of dexmethylphenidate from Focalin XR have not been studied. Since the modified release characteristics of Focalin XR are pH dependent, the co-administration of antacids or acid suppressants could alter the release of dexmethylphenidate).
No products indexed under this heading.

Lisinopril (Methylphenidate may decrease the effectiveness of antihypertensive drugs). Products include:
Prinivil Tablets 2087
Prinzide Tablets 2092

Losartan Potassium (Methylphenidate may decrease the effectiveness of antihypertensive drugs). Products include:
Cozaar Tablets 1973

Magaldrate (The effects of gastrointestinal pH alterations on the absorption of dexmethylphenidate from Focalin XR have not been studied. Since the modified release characteristics of Focalin XR are pH dependent, the co-administration of antacids or acid suppressants could alter the release of dexmethylphenidate).
No products indexed under this heading.

Magnesium Hydroxide (The effects of gastrointestinal pH alterations on the absorption of dexmethylphenidate from Focalin XR have not been studied. Since the modified release characteristics of Focalin XR are pH dependent, the co-administration of antacids or acid suppressants could alter the release of dexmethylphenidate). Products include:
Fleet Pedia-Lax Chewable Tablets 1145
Pepcid Complete Chewable Tablets 1771
Extra Strength Rolaids Freshmint Tablets 1903
Rolaids Multi-Symptom Berry Tablets 1903
Rolaids Original Peppermint Tablets 1903

Magnesium Oxide (The effects of gastrointestinal pH alterations on the absorption of dexmethylphenidate from Focalin XR have not been studied. Since the modified release characteristics of Focalin XR are pH dependent, the co-administration of antacids or acid suppressants could alter the release of dexmethylphenidate). Products include:
Beelith Tablets 813

Maprotiline Hydrochloride (Racemic methylphenidate may inhibit the metabolism of tricyclic antidepressants).
No products indexed under this heading.

Mecamylamine Hydrochloride (Methylphenidate may decrease the effectiveness of antihypertensive drugs).
No products indexed under this heading.

Mephentermine Sulfate (Methylphenidate has potential to increase blood pressure; concurrent use with pressor agents requires caution).
No products indexed under this heading.

Metaraminol Bitartrate (Methylphenidate has potential to increase blood pressure; concurrent use with pressor agents requires caution).
No products indexed under this heading.

Methoxamine Hydrochloride (Methylphenidate has potential to increase blood pressure; concurrent use with pressor agents requires caution).
No products indexed under this heading.

Methyclothiazide (Methylphenidate may decrease the effectiveness of antihypertensive drugs).
No products indexed under this heading.

Methyldopa (Methylphenidate may decrease the effectiveness of antihypertensive drugs).
No products indexed under this heading.

Methyldopate Hydrochloride (Methylphenidate may decrease the effectiveness of antihypertensive drugs).
No products indexed under this heading.

Metolazone (Methylphenidate may decrease the effectiveness of antihypertensive drugs).
No products indexed under this heading.

Metoprolol Succinate (Methylphenidate may decrease the effectiveness of antihypertensive drugs). Products include:
Toprol-XL Tablets 666

Metoprolol Tartrate (Methylphenidate may decrease the effectiveness of antihypertensive drugs).
No products indexed under this heading.

Metyrosine (Methylphenidate may decrease the effectiveness of antihypertensive drugs). Products include:
Demser Capsules 1989

Mibefradil Dihydrochloride (Methylphenidate may decrease the effectiveness of antihypertensive drugs).
No products indexed under this heading.

Minoxidil (Methylphenidate may decrease the effectiveness of antihypertensive drugs).
No products indexed under this heading.

Moclobemide (Co-administration with MAO inhibitor may result in hypertensive crises; concurrent and/or sequential use is contraindicated).
No products indexed under this heading.

Moexipril Hydrochloride (Methylphenidate may decrease the effectiveness of antihypertensive drugs).
No products indexed under this heading.

Nadolol (Methylphenidate may decrease the effectiveness of antihypertensive drugs). Products include:
Nadolol Tablets 2191

Nebivolol (Methylphenidate may decrease the effectiveness of antihypertensive drugs). Products include:
Bystolic Tablets 1155

Nicardipine Hydrochloride (Methylphenidate may decrease the effectiveness of antihypertensive drugs). Products include:
Cardene I.V. 1093

Nifedipine (Methylphenidate may decrease the effectiveness of antihypertensive drugs).
No products indexed under this heading.

Nisoldipine (Methylphenidate may decrease the effectiveness of antihypertensive drugs). Products include:
Sular Extended Release Tablets 2975

Nitroglycerin (Methylphenidate may decrease the effectiveness of antihypertensive drugs). Products include:
Nitro-Dur Transdermal Infusion System 2887
Nitrolingual Pumpspray 2965

Nizatidine (The effects of gastrointestinal pH alterations on the absorption of dexmethylphenidate from Focalin XR have not been studied. Since the modified release characteristics of Focalin XR are pH dependent, the co-administration of antacids or acid suppressants could alter the release of dexmethylphenidate). Products include:
Axid Capsules 1364

Norepinephrine Bitartrate (Methylphenidate has potential to increase blood pressure; concurrent use with pressor agents requires caution).
No products indexed under this heading.

Nortriptyline Hydrochloride (Racemic methylphenidate may inhibit the metabolism of tricyclic antidepressants).
No products indexed under this heading.

Omeprazole (The effects of gastrointestinal pH alterations on the absorption of dexmethylphenidate from Focalin XR have not been studied. Since the modified release characteristics of Focalin XR are pH dependent, the co-administration of antacids or acid suppressants could alter the release of dexmethylphenidate).
No products indexed under this heading.

Pantoprazole Sodium (The effects of gastrointestinal pH alterations on the absorption of dexmethylphenidate from Focalin XR have not been studied. Since the modified release characteristics of Focalin XR are pH dependent, the co-administration of antacids or acid suppressants could alter the release of dexmethylphenidate). Products include:
Protonix for Delayed-Release Oral Suspension 3254
Protonix Delayed-Release Tablets 3254
Protonix I.V. 3257

Pargyline Hydrochloride (Co-administration with MAO inhibitor may result in hypertensive crises; concurrent and/or sequential use is contraindicated).
No products indexed under this heading.

Penbutolol Sulfate (Methylphenidate may decrease the effectiveness of antihypertensive drugs).
No products indexed under this heading.

Perindopril Erbumine (Methylphenidate may decrease the effectiveness of antihypertensive drugs). Products include:
Aceon Tablets (2 mg, 4 mg, 8 mg) 3038

Phenelzine Sulfate (Co-administration with MAO inhibitor may result in hypertensive crises; concurrent and/or sequential use is contraindicated).
No products indexed under this heading.

Phenobarbital (Racemic methylphenidate may inhibit the metabolism of phenobarbital). Products include:
Donnatal Extentabs 2507

Phenoxybenzamine Hydrochloride (Methylphenidate may decrease the effectiveness of antihypertensive drugs). Products include:
Dibenzyline Capsules 3188

Phentolamine Mesylate (Methylphenidate may decrease the effectiveness of antihypertensive drugs).
No products indexed under this heading.

Phenylephrine Hydrochloride (Methylphenidate has potential to increase blood pressure; concurrent use with pressor agents requires caution). Products include:
Actifed Cold & Allergy Tablets 1895
Benadryl Allergy & Cold Kapgels 1895
Benadryl Allergy & Sinus Headache Kapgels 1895
Benadryl Severe Allergy & Sinus Headache Caplets 1897
Children's Benadryl-D Allergy & Sinus Liquid 1896
Benadryl-D Allergy & Sinus Tablet 1896
PediaCare Children's Allergy & Cold Liquid 1902
PediaCare Children's Decongestant Liquid 1902
PediaCare Children's Liquid Multi-Symptom Cold 1902
Sinutab Non-Drying Caplets 1905
Sinutab Sinus Caplets 1905
Children's Sudafed PE Cold & Cough Liquid 1907
Children's Sudafed PE Nasal Decongestant Liquid 1906
Sudafed PE Cold & Cough Caplets 1907
Sudafed PE Nasal Decongestant Tablets 1907
Sudafed PE Nighttime Cold Caplets 1907
Sudafed PE Non-Drying Sinus Caplets 1908
Sudafed PE Severe Cold Caplets 1908
Sudafed PE Sinus & Allergy Tablets 1908
Sudafed PE Sinus Headache Caplets 1908
Tylenol Allergy Multi-Symptom Caplets with Cool Burst and Rapid Release Gelcaps 1916
Tylenol Allergy Multi-Symptom Nighttime Caplets with Cool Burst 1916
Children's Tylenol Plus Cold Suspension Liquid 1912
Children's Tylenol Plus Cold & Allergy Suspension Liquid 1914
Children's Tylenol Plus Flu Suspension Liquid 1914
Children's Tylenol Plus Multi-Symptom Cold Suspension Liquid 1912
Tylenol Cold Head Congestion Daytime Caplets with Cool Burst 1910
Tylenol Cold Head Congestion Nighttime Caplets with Cool Burst 1910
Tylenol Cold Head Congestion Severe Daytime Caplets with Cool Burst 1910
Tylenol Cold Multi-Symptom Daytime Caplets with Cool Burst and Rapid Release Gels 1913
Tylenol Cold Multi-Symptom Daytime Liquid with Citrus Burst 1913
Tylenol Cold Multi-Symptom Nighttime Caplets with Cool Burst 1913
Tylenol Cold Multi-Symptom Nighttime Liquid with Cool Burst 1913
Tylenol Cold Multi-Symptom Severe Caplets with Cool Burst 1913
Tylenol Cold Multi-Symptom Severe Daytime Liquid with Citrus Burst 1913
Tylenol Sinus Congestion & Pain Daytime Caplets with Cool Burst and Gelcaps 1917
Tylenol Sinus Congestion & Pain Nighttime Caplets with Cool Burst 1917
Tylenol Sinus Congestion & Pain Severe Caplets with Cool Burst 1917
Vicks DayQuil Cold & Flu Multi-Symptom Relief 616
Vicks DayQuil LiquiCaps 2567
Vicks DayQuil Liquid 2567
Vicks DayQuil Multi-Symptom Cold/Flu Relief 2567

Phenytoin (Racemic methylphenidate may inhibit the metabolism of phenytoin).
No products indexed under this heading.

Phenytoin Sodium (Racemic methylphenidate may inhibit the metabolism of phenytoin). Products include:
Phenytek Capsules 2192

Pindolol (Methylphenidate may decrease the effectiveness of antihypertensive drugs).
No products indexed under this heading.

Polythiazide (Methylphenidate may decrease the effectiveness of antihypertensive drugs).
No products indexed under this heading.

Prazosin Hydrochloride (Methylphenidate may decrease the effectiveness of antihypertensive drugs).
No products indexed under this heading.

Primidone (Racemic methylphenidate may inhibit the metabolism of primidone).
No products indexed under this heading.

Procarbazine Hydrochloride (Co-administration with MAO inhibitor may result in hypertensive crises; concurrent and/or sequential use is contraindicated).
No products indexed under this heading.

Propranolol Hydrochloride (Methylphenidate may decrease the effectiveness of antihypertensive drugs). Products include:
InnoPran XL Extended Release Capsules 1484

Protriptyline Hydrochloride (Racemic methylphenidate may inhibit the metabolism of tricyclic antidepressants).
No products indexed under this heading.

Quinapril Hydrochloride (Methylphenidate may decrease the effectiveness of antihypertensive drugs).
No products indexed under this heading.

Rabeprazole Sodium (The effects of gastrointestinal pH alterations on the absorption of dexmethylphenidate from Focalin XR have not been studied. Since the modified release characteristics of Focalin XR are pH dependent, the co-administration of antacids or acid suppressants could alter the release of dexmethylphenidate). Products include:
Aciphex Tablets 1053

Ramipril (Methylphenidate may decrease the effectiveness of antihypertensive drugs).
No products indexed under this heading.

Ranitidine Bismuth Citrate (The effects of gastrointestinal pH alterations on the absorption of dexmethylphenidate from Focalin XR have not been studied. Since the modified release characteristics of Focalin XR are pH dependent, the co-administration of antacids or acid suppressants could alter the release of dexmethylphenidate).
No products indexed under this heading.

Ranitidine Hydrochloride (The effects of gastrointestinal pH alterations on the absorption of dexmethylphenidate from Focalin XR have not been studied. Since the modified release characteristics of Focalin XR are pH dependent, the co-administration of antacids or acid suppressants could alter the release of dexmethylphenidate). Products include:
Zantac 75 Tablets 603
Zantac 1670
Zantac Injection 1666
Zantac Injection Pharmacy Bulk Package 1668
Maximum Strength Zantac 150 Tablets 603
Maximum Strength Zantac 150 Cool Mint Tablets 603

Rasagiline Mesylate (Co-administration with MAO inhibitor may result in hypertensive crises; concurrent and/or sequential use is contraindicated). Products include:
Azilect Tablets 3106

Rauwolfia Serpentina (Methylphenidate may decrease the effectiveness of antihypertensive drugs).
No products indexed under this heading.

Rescinnamine (Methylphenidate may decrease the effectiveness of antihypertensive drugs).
No products indexed under this heading.

Reserpine (Methylphenidate may decrease the effectiveness of antihypertensive drugs).
No products indexed under this heading.

Selegiline (Co-administration with MAO inhibitor may result in hypertensive crises; concurrent and/or sequential use is contraindicated). Products include:
Emsam Transdermal System 905

Selegiline Hydrochloride (Co-administration with MAO inhibitor may result in hypertensive crises; concurrent and/or sequential use is contraindicated). Products include:
Eldepryl Capsules 3052

IMPORTANT NOTE: Always consult each drug listing in the patient's regimen for possible interactions.

Sodium Bicarbonate (The effects of gastrointestinal pH alterations on the absorption of dexmethylphenidate from Focalin XR have not been studied. Since the modified release characteristics of Focalin XR are pH dependent, the co-administration of antacids or acid suppressants could alter the release of dexmethylphenidate). Products include:
Ceo-Two Laxative Suppository 815

Sodium Nitroprusside (Methylphenidate may decrease the effectiveness of antihypertensive drugs).
No products indexed under this heading.

Sotalol Hydrochloride (Methylphenidate may decrease the effectiveness of antihypertensive drugs).
No products indexed under this heading.

Spirapril Hydrochloride (Methylphenidate may decrease the effectiveness of antihypertensive drugs).
No products indexed under this heading.

Telmisartan (Methylphenidate may decrease the effectiveness of antihypertensive drugs). Products include:
Micardis Tablets 852
Micardis HCT Tablets 854

Terazosin Hydrochloride (Methylphenidate may decrease the effectiveness of antihypertensive drugs).
No products indexed under this heading.

Timolol Maleate (Methylphenidate may decrease the effectiveness of antihypertensive drugs). Products include:
Combigan Ophthalmic Solution 553
Cosopt Sterile Ophthalmic Solution 1969
Timoptic Sterile Ophthalmic Solution 2121
Timoptic in Ocudose 2124
Timoptic-XE Sterile Ophthalmic Gel Forming Solution 2125

Torsemide (Methylphenidate may decrease the effectiveness of antihypertensive drugs). Products include:
Demadex Injection 2630
Demadex Tablets 2630

Trandolapril (Methylphenidate may decrease the effectiveness of antihypertensive drugs). Products include:
Mavik Tablets 472
Tarka Tablets 511

Tranylcypromine Sulfate (Co-administration with MAO inhibitor may result in hypertensive crises; concurrent and/or sequential use is contraindicated). Products include:
Parnate Tablets 1532

Trimethaphan Camsylate (Methylphenidate may decrease the effectiveness of antihypertensive drugs).
No products indexed under this heading.

Trimipramine Maleate (Racemic methylphenidate may inhibit the metabolism of tricyclic antidepressants).
No products indexed under this heading.

Valsartan (Methylphenidate may decrease the effectiveness of antihypertensive drugs). Products include:
Diovan Tablets 2212
Diovan HCT Tablets 2216
Exforge Tablets 2238

Verapamil Hydrochloride (Methylphenidate may decrease the effectiveness of antihypertensive drugs). Products include:
Tarka Tablets 511

Warfarin Sodium (Racemic methylphenidate may inhibit the metabolism of coumarin anticoagulants).
No products indexed under this heading.

FOLLISTIM AQ CARTRIDGE

(Follitropin Beta) 2844
None cited in PDR database.

FOOD FOR THOUGHT DIETARY SUPPLEMENT

(Amino Acid Preparations, Vitamins with Minerals) .... ▣637
May interact with:

Aluminum Carbonate (Concomitant use with aluminum-containing antacids should be avoided).
No products indexed under this heading.

Aluminum Hydroxide (Concomitant use with aluminum-containing antacids should be avoided).
No products indexed under this heading.

FORADIL AEROLIZER

(Formoterol Fumarate) 2849
May interact with beta blockers, diuretics, glucocorticoids, monoamine oxidase inhibitors, potassium-depleting diuretics, drugs that prolong the QT interval, sympathomimetics, tricyclic antidepressants, and xanthines. Compounds in these categories include:

Acebutolol Hydrochloride (Co-administration with beta-blockers may inhibit the effect of each other. Beta-blockers not only block the therapeutic effect of beta-agonists, such as formoterol, but may produce severe bronchospasm in patients with asthma).
No products indexed under this heading.

Albuterol (Co-administration with additional adrenergic drugs may potentiate the sympathetic effects of formoterol).
No products indexed under this heading.

Albuterol Sulfate (Co-administration with additional adrenergic drugs may potentiate the sympathetic effects of formoterol). Products include:
Combivent Inhalation Aerosol 845
ProAir HFA Inhalation Aerosol 3113
Proventil HFA Inhalation Aerosol 2914
Ventolin HFA Inhalation Aerosol 1638

Alprazolam (Co-administration with drugs known to prolong the QTc interval may lead to an increased risk of ventricular arrhythmias; co-administer with extreme caution).
No products indexed under this heading.

Amiloride Hydrochloride (Concomitant treatment with diuretics may potentiate any hypokalemic effect of adrenergic agonists).
No products indexed under this heading.

Aminophylline (Co-administration with xanthine derivatives may potentiate hypokalemic effect of adrenergic agonists).
No products indexed under this heading.

Amiodarone Hydrochloride (Co-administration with drugs known to prolong the QTc interval may lead to an increased risk of ventricular arrhythmias; co-administer with extreme caution).
No products indexed under this heading.

Amitriptyline Hydrochloride (Concurrent and/or sequential administration with tricyclic antidepressants may potentiate the action of adrenergic agonists on the cardiovascular system; co-administer with extreme caution).
No products indexed under this heading.

Amoxapine (Concurrent and/or sequential administration with tricyclic antidepressants may potentiate the action of adrenergic agonists on the cardiovascular system; co-administer with extreme caution).
No products indexed under this heading.

Astemizole (Co-administration with drugs known to prolong the QTc interval may lead to an increased risk of ventricular arrhythmias; co-administer with extreme caution).
No products indexed under this heading.

Atenolol (Co-administration with beta-blockers may inhibit the effect of each other. Beta-blockers not only block the therapeutic effect of beta-agonists, such as formoterol, but may produce severe bronchospasm in patients with asthma).
No products indexed under this heading.

Bendroflumethiazide (The ECG changes and/or hypokalemia that may result from the administration of non-potassium sparing diuretics can be acutely worsened by beta-agonists, especially when the recommended dose of beta-agonist is exceeded).
No products indexed under this heading.

Betamethasone Acetate (Co-administration with glucocorticosteroids may potentiate hypokalemic effect of adrenergic agonists).
No products indexed under this heading.

Betamethasone Sodium Phosphate (Co-administration with glucocorticosteroids may potentiate hypokalemic effect of adrenergic agonists).
No products indexed under this heading.

Betaxolol Hydrochloride (Co-administration with beta-blockers may inhibit the effect of each other. Beta-blockers not only block the therapeutic effect of beta-agonists, such as formoterol, but may produce severe bronchospasm in patients with asthma).
No products indexed under this heading.

Bisoprolol Fumarate (Co-administration with beta-blockers may inhibit the effect of each other. Beta-blockers not only block the therapeutic effect of beta-agonists, such as formoterol, but may produce severe bronchospasm in patients with asthma).
No products indexed under this heading.

Bretylium Tosylate (Co-administration with drugs known to prolong the QTc interval may lead to an increased risk of ventricular arrhythmias; co-administer with extreme caution).
No products indexed under this heading.

Bumetanide (The ECG changes and/or hypokalemia that may result from the administration of non-potassium sparing diuretics can be acutely worsened by beta-agonists, especially when the recommended dose of beta-agonist is exceeded).
No products indexed under this heading.

Buspirone Hydrochloride (Co-administration with drugs known to prolong the QTc interval may lead to an increased risk of ventricular arrhythmias; co-administer with extreme caution).
No products indexed under this heading.

Carteolol Hydrochloride (Co-administration with beta-blockers may inhibit the effect of each other. Beta-blockers not only block the therapeutic effect of beta-agonists, such as formoterol, but may produce severe bronchospasm in patients with asthma).
No products indexed under this heading.

Chlordiazepoxide (Co-administration with drugs known to prolong the QTc interval may lead to an increased risk of ventricular arrhythmias; co-administer with extreme caution).
No products indexed under this heading.

Chlordiazepoxide Hydrochloride (Co-administration with drugs known to prolong the QTc interval may lead to an increased risk of ventricular arrhythmias; co-administer with extreme caution).
No products indexed under this heading.

Chlorothiazide (The ECG changes and/or hypokalemia that may result from the administration of non-potassium sparing diuretics can be acutely worsened by beta-agonists, especially when the recommended dose of beta-agonist is exceeded).
No products indexed under this heading.

Chlorothiazide Sodium (The ECG changes and/or hypokalemia that may result from the administration of non-potassium sparing diuretics can be acutely worsened by beta-agonists, especially when the recommended dose of beta-agonist is exceeded). Products include:
Intravenous Sodium Diuril 2490

Chlorpromazine (Co-administration with drugs known to prolong the QTc interval may lead to an increased risk of ventricular arrhythmias; co-administer with extreme caution).
No products indexed under this heading.

Chlorpromazine Hydrochloride (Co-administration with drugs known to prolong the QTc interval may lead to an increased risk of ventricular arrhythmias; co-administer with extreme caution).
No products indexed under this heading.

Hydrocortisone Sodium Succinate (Co-administration with glucocorticosteroids may potentiate hypokalemic effect of adrenergic agonists).
No products indexed under this heading.

Hydroflumethiazide (The ECG changes and/or hypokalemia that may result from the administration of non-potassium sparing diuretics can be acutely worsened by beta-agonists, especially when the recommended dose of beta-agonist is exceeded).
No products indexed under this heading.

Hydroxyzine Hydrochloride (Co-administration with drugs known to prolong the QTc interval may lead to an increased risk of ventricular arrhythmias; co-administer with extreme caution).
No products indexed under this heading.

Imipramine Hydrochloride (Concurrent and/or sequential administration with tricyclic antidepressants may potentiate the action of adrenergic agonists on the cardiovascular system; co-administer with extreme caution).
No products indexed under this heading.

Imipramine Pamoate (Concurrent and/or sequential administration with tricyclic antidepressants may potentiate the action of adrenergic agonists on the cardiovascular system; co-administer with extreme caution).
No products indexed under this heading.

Indapamide (Concomitant treatment with diuretics may potentiate any hypokalemic effect of adrenergic agonists). Products include:
Indapamide Tablets 2188

Isocarboxazid (Concurrent and/or sequential administration with MAO inhibitors may potentiate the action of adrenergic agonists on the cardiovascular system; co-administer with extreme caution). Products include:
Marplan Tablets 3177

Isoproterenol Hydrochloride (Co-administration with additional adrenergic drugs may potentiate the sympathetic effects of formoterol).
No products indexed under this heading.

Isoproterenol Sulfate (Co-administration with additional adrenergic drugs may potentiate the sympathetic effects of formoterol).
No products indexed under this heading.

Labetalol Hydrochloride (Co-administration with beta-blockers may inhibit the effect of each other. Beta-blockers not only block the therapeutic effect of beta-agonists, such as formoterol, but may produce severe bronchospasm in patients with asthma).
No products indexed under this heading.

Levalbuterol Hydrochloride (Co-administration with additional adrenergic drugs may potentiate the sympathetic effects of formoterol). Products include:
Xopenex Inhalation Solution 3001
Xopenex Inhalation Solution Concentrate 3005

Levobunolol Hydrochloride (Co-administration with beta-blockers may inhibit the effect of each other. Beta-blockers not only block the therapeutic effect of beta-agonists, such as formoterol, but may produce severe bronchospasm in patients with asthma).
No products indexed under this heading.

Lidocaine Hydrochloride (Co-administration with drugs known to prolong the QTc interval may lead to an increased risk of ventricular arrhythmias; co-administer with extreme caution).
No products indexed under this heading.

Lithium Carbonate (Co-administration with drugs known to prolong the QTc interval may lead to an increased risk of ventricular arrhythmias; co-administer with extreme caution).
No products indexed under this heading.

Lithium Citrate (Co-administration with drugs known to prolong the QTc interval may lead to an increased risk of ventricular arrhythmias; co-administer with extreme caution).
No products indexed under this heading.

Lorazepam (Co-administration with drugs known to prolong the QTc interval may lead to an increased risk of ventricular arrhythmias; co-administer with extreme caution).
No products indexed under this heading.

Loxapine Hydrochloride (Co-administration with drugs known to prolong the QTc interval may lead to an increased risk of ventricular arrhythmias; co-administer with extreme caution).
No products indexed under this heading.

Loxapine Succinate (Co-administration with drugs known to prolong the QTc interval may lead to an increased risk of ventricular arrhythmias; co-administer with extreme caution).
No products indexed under this heading.

Maprotiline Hydrochloride (Concurrent and/or sequential administration with tricyclic antidepressants may potentiate the action of adrenergic agonists on the cardiovascular system; co-administer with extreme caution).
No products indexed under this heading.

Meprobamate (Co-administration with drugs known to prolong the QTc interval may lead to an increased risk of ventricular arrhythmias; co-administer with extreme caution).
No products indexed under this heading.

Mesoridazine Besylate (Co-administration with drugs known to prolong the QTc interval may lead to an increased risk of ventricular arrhythmias; co-administer with extreme caution).
No products indexed under this heading.

Metaproterenol Sulfate (Co-administration with additional adrenergic drugs may potentiate the sympathetic effects of formoterol).
No products indexed under this heading.

Metaraminol Bitartrate (Co-administration with additional adrenergic drugs may potentiate the sympathetic effects of formoterol).
No products indexed under this heading.

Methoxamine Hydrochloride (Co-administration with additional adrenergic drugs may potentiate the sympathetic effects of formoterol).
No products indexed under this heading.

Methyclothiazide (The ECG changes and/or hypokalemia that may result from the administration of non-potassium sparing diuretics can be acutely worsened by beta-agonists, especially when the recommended dose of beta-agonist is exceeded).
No products indexed under this heading.

Methylprednisolone Acetate (Co-administration with glucocorticosteroids may potentiate hypokalemic effect of adrenergic agonists).
No products indexed under this heading.

Methylprednisolone Sodium Succinate (Co-administration with glucocorticosteroids may potentiate hypokalemic effect of adrenergic agonists).
No products indexed under this heading.

Metipranolol Hydrochloride (Co-administration with beta-blockers may inhibit the effect of each other. Beta-blockers not only block the therapeutic effect of beta-agonists, such as formoterol, but may produce severe bronchospasm in patients with asthma).
No products indexed under this heading.

Metolazone (Concomitant treatment with diuretics may potentiate any hypokalemic effect of adrenergic agonists).
No products indexed under this heading.

Metoprolol Succinate (Co-administration with beta-blockers may inhibit the effect of each other. Beta-blockers not only block the therapeutic effect of beta-agonists, such as formoterol, but may produce severe bronchospasm in patients with asthma). Products include:
Toprol-XL Tablets 666

Metoprolol Tartrate (Co-administration with beta-blockers may inhibit the effect of each other. Beta-blockers not only block the therapeutic effect of beta-agonists, such as formoterol, but may produce severe bronchospasm in patients with asthma).
No products indexed under this heading.

Mexiletine Hydrochloride (Co-administration with drugs known to prolong the QTc interval may lead to an increased risk of ventricular arrhythmias; co-administer with extreme caution).
No products indexed under this heading.

Midazolam Hydrochloride (Co-administration with drugs known to prolong the QTc interval may lead to an increased risk of ventricular arrhythmias; co-administer with extreme caution).
No products indexed under this heading.

Moclobemide (Concurrent and/or sequential administration with MAO inhibitors may potentiate the action of adrenergic agonists on the cardiovascular system; co-administer with extreme caution).
No products indexed under this heading.

Molindone Hydrochloride (Co-administration with drugs known to prolong the QTc interval may lead to an increased risk of ventricular arrhythmias; co-administer with extreme caution). Products include:
Moban Tablets 1116

Nadolol (Co-administration with beta-blockers may inhibit the effect of each other. Beta-blockers not only block the therapeutic effect of beta-agonists, such as formoterol, but may produce severe bronchospasm in patients with asthma). Products include:
Nadolol Tablets 2191

Nebivolol (Co-administration with beta-blockers may inhibit the effect of each other. Beta-blockers not only block the therapeutic effect of beta-agonists, such as formoterol, but may produce severe bronchospasm in patients with asthma). Products include:
Bystolic Tablets 1155

Norepinephrine Bitartrate (Co-administration with additional adrenergic drugs may potentiate the sympathetic effects of formoterol).
No products indexed under this heading.

Nortriptyline Hydrochloride (Concurrent and/or sequential administration with tricyclic antidepressants may potentiate the action of adrenergic agonists on the cardiovascular system; co-administer with extreme caution).
No products indexed under this heading.

Olanzapine (Co-administration with drugs known to prolong the QTc interval may lead to an increased risk of ventricular arrhythmias; co-administer with extreme caution). Products include:
Symbyax Capsules 1871
Zyprexa Tablets 1883
Zyprexa IntraMuscular 1883
Zyprexa ZYDIS Orally Disintegrating Tablets 1883

Oxazepam (Co-administration with drugs known to prolong the QTc interval may lead to an increased risk of ventricular arrhythmias; co-administer with extreme caution).
No products indexed under this heading.

Pargyline Hydrochloride (Concurrent and/or sequential administration with MAO inhibitors may potentiate the action of adrenergic agonists on the cardiovascular system; co-administer with extreme caution).
No products indexed under this heading.

Penbutolol Sulfate (Co-administration with beta-blockers may inhibit the effect of each other. Beta-blockers not only block the therapeutic effect of beta-agonists, such as formoterol, but may produce severe bronchospasm in patients with asthma).
No products indexed under this heading.

vascular system; co-administer with extreme caution). Products include:
Emsam Transdermal System 905

Selegiline Hydrochloride (Concurrent and/or sequential administration with MAO inhibitors may potentiate the action of adrenergic agonists on the cardiovascular system; co-administer with extreme caution). Products include:
Eldepryl Capsules 3052

Sotalol Hydrochloride (Co-administration with beta-blockers may inhibit the effect of each other. Beta-blockers not only block the therapeutic effect of beta-agonists, such as formoterol, but may produce severe bronchospasm in patients with asthma).
No products indexed under this heading.

Spironolactone (Concomitant treatment with diuretics may potentiate any hypokalemic effect of adrenergic agonists).
No products indexed under this heading.

Terbutaline Sulfate (Co-administration with additional adrenergic drugs may potentiate the sympathetic effects of formoterol).
No products indexed under this heading.

Theophylline (Co-administration with xanthine derivatives may potentiate hypokalemic effect of adrenergic agonists).
No products indexed under this heading.

Theophylline Anhydrous (Co-administration with xanthine derivatives may potentiate hypokalemic effect of adrenergic agonists). Products include:
Uniphyl Tablets 2595

Theophylline Calcium Salicylate (Co-administration with xanthine derivatives may potentiate hypokalemic effect of adrenergic agonists).
No products indexed under this heading.

Theophylline Dihydroxypropyl (Glyceryl) (Co-administration with xanthine derivatives may potentiate hypokalemic effect of adrenergic agonists).
No products indexed under this heading.

Theophylline Ethylenediamine (Co-administration with xanthine derivatives may potentiate hypokalemic effect of adrenergic agonists).
No products indexed under this heading.

Theophylline Sodium Glycinate (Co-administration with xanthine derivatives may potentiate hypokalemic effect of adrenergic agonists).
No products indexed under this heading.

Thioridazine Hydrochloride (Co-administration with drugs known to prolong the QTc interval may lead to an increased risk of ventricular arrhythmias; co-administer with extreme caution). Products include:
Thioridazine Hydrochloride Tablets 2195

Thiothixene (Co-administration with drugs known to prolong the QTc interval may lead to an increased risk of ventricular arrhythmias; co-administer with extreme caution). Products include:
Thiothixene Capsules 2197

Timolol Hemihydrate (Co-administration with beta-blockers may inhibit the effect of each other. Beta-blockers not only block the therapeutic effect of beta-agonists, such as formoterol, but may produce severe bronchospasm in patients with asthma). Products include:
Betimol Ophthalmic Solution 3181

Timolol Maleate (Co-administration with beta-blockers may inhibit the effect of each other. Beta-blockers not only block the therapeutic effect of beta-agonists, such as formoterol, but may produce severe bronchospasm in patients with asthma). Products include:
Combigan Ophthalmic Solution 553
Cosopt Sterile Ophthalmic Solution 1969
Timoptic Sterile Ophthalmic Solution 2121
Timoptic in Ocudose 2124
Timoptic-XE Sterile Ophthalmic Gel Forming Solution 2125

Tocainide Hydrochloride (Co-administration with drugs known to prolong the QTc interval may lead to an increased risk of ventricular arrhythmias; co-administer with extreme caution).
No products indexed under this heading.

Torsemide (The ECG changes and/or hypokalemia that may result from the administration of non-potassium sparing diuretics can be acutely worsened by beta-agonists, especially when the recommended dose of beta-agonist is exceeded). Products include:
Demadex Injection 2630
Demadex Tablets 2630

Tranylcypromine Sulfate (Concurrent and/or sequential administration with MAO inhibitors may potentiate the action of adrenergic agonists on the cardiovascular system; co-administer with extreme caution). Products include:
Parnate Tablets 1532

Triamcinolone (Co-administration with glucocorticosteroids may potentiate hypokalemic effect of adrenergic agonists).
No products indexed under this heading.

Triamcinolone Acetonide (Co-administration with glucocorticosteroids may potentiate hypokalemic effect of adrenergic agonists). Products include:
Azmacort Inhalation Aerosol 407
Nasacort AQ Nasal Spray 2765
Triesence Injectable Suspension .... ⊙ 209

Triamcinolone Diacetate (Co-administration with glucocorticosteroids may potentiate hypokalemic effect of adrenergic agonists).
No products indexed under this heading.

Triamcinolone Hexacetonide (Co-administration with glucocorticosteroids may potentiate hypokalemic effect of adrenergic agonists).
No products indexed under this heading.

Triamterene (Concomitant treatment with diuretics may potentiate any hypokalemic effect of adrenergic agonists). Products include:
Dyazide Capsules 1405
Dyrenium Capsules 3189

Trifluoperazine Hydrochloride (Co-administration with drugs known to prolong the QTc interval may lead to an increased risk of ventricular arrhythmias; co-administer with extreme caution).
No products indexed under this heading.

Trimipramine Maleate (Concurrent and/or sequential administration with tricyclic antidepressants may potentiate the action of adrenergic agonists on the cardiovascular system; co-administer with extreme caution).
No products indexed under this heading.

Ziprasidone Hydrochloride (Co-administration with drugs known to prolong the QTc interval may lead to an increased risk of ventricular arrhythmias; co-administer with extreme caution). Products include:
Geodon Capsules 2520

FORMADON SOLUTION

(Formaldehyde) 1699
None cited in PDR database.

FORTAZ INJECTION

(Ceftazidime) 1450
See Fortaz for Injection

FORTAZ FOR INJECTION

(Ceftazidime) 1450
May interact with aminoglycosides, oral contraceptives, and certain other agents. Compounds in these categories include:

Amikacin Sulfate (Potential for nephrotoxicity following concomitant administration).
No products indexed under this heading.

Chloramphenicol (Possibility of antagonism *"in-vivo,"* particularly when bactericidal activity is desired; avoid this combination).
No products indexed under this heading.

Chloramphenicol Palmitate (Possibility of antagonism *"in-vivo,"* particularly when bactericidal activity is desired; avoid this combination).
No products indexed under this heading.

Chloramphenicol Sodium Succinate (Possibility of antagonism *"in-vivo,"* particularly when bactericidal activity is desired; avoid this combination).
No products indexed under this heading.

Desogestrel (In common with other antibiotics, ceftazidime may affect the gut flora, leading to lower estrogen reabsorption and reduced efficacy of combined oral estrogen/progesterone contraceptives). Products include:
Mircette Tablets 1034

Ethinyl Estradiol (In common with other antibiotics, ceftazidime may affect the gut flora, leading to lower estrogen reabsorption and reduced efficacy of combined oral estrogen/progesterone contraceptives). Products include:
Lybrel Tablets 3204
Mircette Tablets 1034
NuvaRing 2897
Ortho-Cyclen/Ortho Tri-Cyclen 2449
Ortho Evra Transdermal System 2437
Ortho Tri-Cyclen Lo Tablets 2458
Seasonique Tablets 1046
Yaz Tablets 805

Ethynodiol Diacetate (In common with other antibiotics, ceftazidime may affect the gut flora, leading to lower estrogen reabsorption and reduced efficacy of combined oral estrogen/progesterone contraceptives).
No products indexed under this heading.

Furosemide (Potential for nephrotoxicity following concomitant administration). Products include:
Furosemide Tablets 2186

Gentamicin Sulfate (Potential for nephrotoxicity following concomitant administration). Products include:
Pred-G Ophthalmic Ointment .... ⊙ 229
Pred-G Ophthalmic Suspension ...... ⊙ 228

Kanamycin Sulfate (Potential for nephrotoxicity following concomitant administration).
No products indexed under this heading.

Levonorgestrel (In common with other antibiotics, ceftazidime may affect the gut flora, leading to lower estrogen reabsorption and reduced efficacy of combined oral estrogen/progesterone contraceptives). Products include:
Climara Pro Transdermal System 768
Lybrel Tablets 3204
Mirena Intrauterine System 779
Plan B Tablets 1044
Seasonique Tablets 1046

Mestranol (In common with other antibiotics, ceftazidime may affect the gut flora, leading to lower estrogen reabsorption and reduced efficacy of combined oral estrogen/progesterone contraceptives).
No products indexed under this heading.

Norethindrone (In common with other antibiotics, ceftazidime may affect the gut flora, leading to lower estrogen reabsorption and reduced efficacy of combined oral estrogen/progesterone contraceptives). Products include:
Ortho Micronor Tablets 2446

Norethynodrel (In common with other antibiotics, ceftazidime may affect the gut flora, leading to lower estrogen reabsorption and reduced efficacy of combined oral estrogen/progesterone contraceptives).
No products indexed under this heading.

Norgestimate (In common with other antibiotics, ceftazidime may affect the gut flora, leading to lower estrogen reabsorption and reduced efficacy of combined oral estrogen/progesterone contraceptives). Products include:
Ortho-Cyclen/Ortho Tri-Cyclen 2449
Ortho Tri-Cyclen Lo Tablets 2458

Norgestrel (In common with other antibiotics, ceftazidime may affect the gut flora, leading to lower estrogen reabsorption and reduced efficacy of combined oral estrogen/progesterone contraceptives).
No products indexed under this heading.

Streptomycin Sulfate (Potential for nephrotoxicity following concomitant administration).
No products indexed under this heading.

Tobramycin (Potential for nephrotoxicity following concomitant administration). Products include:
Zylet Ophthalmic Suspension .... ⊙ 247

Tobramycin Sulfate (Potential for nephrotoxicity following concomitant administration).
No products indexed under this heading.

FORTEO FOR INJECTION

(Teriparatide) 1816
May interact with cardiac glycosides. Compounds in these categories include:

Deslanoside (Hypercalcemia may pre-dispose patients to digitalis toxicity. Because teriparatide transiently increases serum calcium, teriparatide should be used with caution in patients taking digitalis).
No products indexed under this heading.

Digitalis Glycoside Preparations (Hypercalcemia may pre-dispose patients to digitalis toxicity. Because teriparatide transiently increases serum calcium, teriparatide should be used with caution in patients taking digitalis).
No products indexed under this heading.

Digitoxin (Hypercalcemia may predispose patients to digitalis toxicity. Because teriparatide transiently increases serum calcium, teriparatide should be used with caution in patients taking digitalis).
No products indexed under this heading.

Digoxin (Hypercalcemia may predispose patients to digitalis toxicity. Because teriparatide transiently increases serum calcium, teriparatide should be used with caution in patients taking digitalis). Products include:
Lanoxin Injection 1498
Lanoxin Injection Pediatric 1502
Lanoxin Tablets 1505

FOSAMAX ORAL SOLUTION

(Alendronate Sodium) 2005
See Fosamax Tablets

FOSAMAX TABLETS

(Alendronate Sodium) 2005
May interact with antacids containing aluminum, calcium and magnesium, calcium preparations, non-steroidal anti-inflammatory agents, and certain other agents. Compounds in these categories include:

Aluminum Carbonate (May interfere with the absorption of alendronate; patient must wait at least one-half hour after taking alendronate before taking any drug).
No products indexed under this heading.

Aluminum Hydroxide (May interfere with the absorption of alendronate; patient must wait at least one-half hour after taking alendronate before taking any drug).
No products indexed under this heading.

Aspirin (Co-administration with doses of alendronate greater than 10 mg/day and aspirin-containing compounds can increase the incidence of gastrointestinal adverse events; one case of anastomotic ulcer with mild hemorrhage has been reported in a patient with history of peptic ulcer disease and gastrectomy on alendronate 10 mg/day plus aspirin). Products include:
Aggrenox Capsules 819
Bayer Aspirin 750
Percodan Tablets 1130
St. Joseph 81 mg Aspirin Chewable and Enteric Coated Tablets 1903

Aspirin, Enteric Coated (Co-administration with doses of alendronate greater than 10 mg/day and aspirin-containing compounds can increase the incidence of gastrointestinal adverse events; one case of anastomotic ulcer with mild hemorrhage has been reported in a patient with history of peptic ulcer disease and gastrectomy on alendronate 10 mg/day plus aspirin).
No products indexed under this heading.

Aspirin Buffered (Co-administration with doses of alendronate greater than 10 mg/day and aspirin-containing compounds can increase the incidence of gastrointestinal adverse events; one case of anastomotic ulcer with mild hemorrhage has been reported in a patient with history of peptic ulcer disease and gastrectomy on alendronate 10 mg/day plus aspirin).
No products indexed under this heading.

Calcium Carbonate (May interfere with the absorption of alendronate; patient must wait at least one-half hour after taking alendronate before taking any drug). Products include:
Accelerator Tablets 634
Actonel with Calcium Tablets 2574
BioLean II Tablets 635
Calcet Triple Calcium + Vitamin D Tablets 629
D-Cal Chewable Caplets 624
Elixir Capsules 636
Pepcid Complete Chewable Tablets 1771
Extra Strength Rolaids Plus Gas Relief Tropical Fruit Softchews...... 1903
Extra Strength Rolaids Softchews Vanilla Creme 1903
Extra Strength Rolaids Freshmint Tablets 1903
Rolaids Multi-Symptom Berry Tablets 1903
Rolaids Original Peppermint Tablets 1903

Calcium Chloride (May interfere with the absorption of alendronate; patient must wait at least one-half hour after taking alendronate before taking any drug).
No products indexed under this heading.

Calcium Citrate (May interfere with the absorption of alendronate; patient must wait at least one-half hour after taking alendronate before taking any drug). Products include:
Active Calcium Tablets 3173
CitraNatal DHA Tablets 2175
CitraNatal 90 DHA Tablets 2175

Calcium Glubionate (May interfere with the absorption of alendronate; patient must wait at least one-half hour after taking alendronate before taking any drug).
No products indexed under this heading.

Celecoxib (Since NSAID use is associated with gastrointestinal irritation, caution should be used during concomitant use; no increase in the incidence of gastrointestinal irritation was reported in clinical trials). Products include:
Celebrex Capsules 2979

Diclofenac Epolamine (Since NSAID use is associated with gastrointestinal irritation, caution should be used during concomitant use; no increase in the incidence of gastrointestinal irritation was reported in clinical trials). Products include:
Flector Patch 561

Diclofenac Potassium (Since NSAID use is associated with gastrointestinal irritation, caution should be used during concomitant use; no increase in the incidence of gastrointestinal irritation was reported in clinical trials).
No products indexed under this heading.

Diclofenac Sodium (Since NSAID use is associated with gastrointestinal irritation, caution should be used during concomitant use; no increase in the incidence of gastrointestinal irritation was reported in clinical trials). Products include:
Diclofenac Sodium Ophthalmic Solution.. ⊙240
Voltaren Ophthalmic Solution 2336
Voltaren Tablets 2334
Voltaren-XR Tablets 2337

Etodolac (Since NSAID use is associated with gastrointestinal irritation, caution should be used during concomitant use; no increase in the incidence of gastrointestinal irritation was reported in clinical trials).
No products indexed under this heading.

Fenoprofen Calcium (Since NSAID use is associated with gastrointestinal irritation, caution should be used during concomitant use; no increase in the incidence of gastrointestinal irritation was reported in clinical trials). Products include:
Nalfon Capsules 2508

Flurbiprofen (Since NSAID use is associated with gastrointestinal irritation, caution should be used during concomitant use; no increase in the incidence of gastrointestinal irritation was reported in clinical trials).
No products indexed under this heading.

Ibuprofen (Since NSAID use is associated with gastrointestinal irritation, caution should be used during concomitant use; no increase in the incidence of gastrointestinal irritation was reported in clinical trials).
Products include:
Motrin IB Tablets and Caplets 1900
Children's Motrin Oral Suspension ... 1901
Children's Motrin Non-Staining Dye-Free Oral Suspension............ 1901
Children's Motrin Cold Oral Suspension 1899
Infants' Motrin Concentrated Drops.. 1901
Infants' Motrin Non-Staining Dye-Free Concentrated Drops....... 1901
Junior Strength Motrin Caplets and Chewable Tablets.................. 1901
Vicoprofen Tablets 533

Indomethacin (Since NSAID use is associated with gastrointestinal irritation, caution should be used during concomitant use; no increase in the incidence of gastrointestinal irritation was reported in clinical trials).
Products include:
Indocin 2024

Indomethacin Sodium Trihydrate (Since NSAID use is associated with gastrointestinal irritation, caution should be used during concomitant use; no increase in the incidence of gastrointestinal irritation was reported in clinical trials).
Products include:
Indocin I.V. 2489

Ketoprofen (Since NSAID use is associated with gastrointestinal irritation, caution should be used during concomitant use; no increase in the incidence of gastrointestinal irritation was reported in clinical trials).
No products indexed under this heading.

Ketorolac Tromethamine (Since NSAID use is associated with gastrointestinal irritation, caution should be used during concomitant use; no increase in the incidence of gastrointestinal irritation was reported in clinical trials).
No products indexed under this heading.

Magaldrate (May interfere with the absorption of alendronate; patient must wait at least one-half hour after taking alendronate before taking any drug).
No products indexed under this heading.

Magnesium Hydroxide (May interfere with the absorption of alendronate; patient must wait at least one-half hour after taking alendronate before taking any drug). Products include:
Fleet Pedia-Lax Chewable Tablets 1145
Pepcid Complete Chewable Tablets 1771
Extra Strength Rolaids Freshmint Tablets 1903
Rolaids Multi-Symptom Berry Tablets 1903
Rolaids Original Peppermint Tablets 1903

Magnesium Oxide (May interfere with the absorption of alendronate; patient must wait at least one-half hour after taking alendronate before taking any drug). Products include:
Beelith Tablets 813

Meclofenamate Sodium (Since NSAID use is associated with gastrointestinal irritation, caution should be used during concomitant use; no increase in the incidence of gastrointestinal irritation was reported in clinical trials).
No products indexed under this heading.

Mefenamic Acid (Since NSAID use is associated with gastrointestinal irritation, caution should be used during concomitant use; no increase in the incidence of gastrointestinal irritation was reported in clinical trials).
No products indexed under this heading.

Meloxicam (Since NSAID use is associated with gastrointestinal irritation, caution should be used during concomitant use; no increase in the incidence of gastrointestinal irritation was reported in clinical trials).
Products include:
Mobic Oral Suspension 863
Mobic Tablets 863

Nabumetone (Since NSAID use is associated with gastrointestinal irritation, caution should be used during concomitant use; no increase in the incidence of gastrointestinal irritation was reported in clinical trials).
No products indexed under this heading.

Naproxen (Since NSAID use is associated with gastrointestinal irritation, caution should be used during concomitant use; no increase in the incidence of gastrointestinal irritation was reported in clinical trials).
Products include:

EC-Naprosyn Delayed-Release Tablets 2632
Naprosyn Suspension 2632
Naprosyn Tablets 2632

Naproxen Sodium (Since NSAID use is associated with gastrointestinal irritation, caution should be used during concomitant use; no increase in the incidence of gastrointestinal irritation was reported in clinical trials). Products include:
Anaprox Tablets 2632
Anaprox DS Tablets 2632
Treximet Tablets 1616

Oxaprozin (Since NSAID use is associated with gastrointestinal irritation, caution should be used during concomitant use; no increase in the incidence of gastrointestinal irritation was reported in clinical trials).
No products indexed under this heading.

Phenylbutazone (Since NSAID use is associated with gastrointestinal irritation, caution should be used during concomitant use; no increase in the incidence of gastrointestinal irritation was reported in clinical trials).
No products indexed under this heading.

Piroxicam (Since NSAID use is associated with gastrointestinal irritation, caution should be used during concomitant use; no increase in the incidence of gastrointestinal irritation was reported in clinical trials).
No products indexed under this heading.

Ranitidine Hydrochloride (Intravenous ranitidine has shown to double the bioavailability of oral alendronate; clinical significance of this increased bioavailability and whether similar increases will occur with oral ranitidine are unknown). Products include:
Zantac 75 Tablets .... ▣603
Zantac 1670
Zantac Injection 1666
Zantac Injection Pharmacy Bulk Package 1668
Maximum Strength Zantac 150 Tablets .... ▣603
Maximum Strength Zantac 150 Cool Mint Tablets .... ▣603

Rofecoxib (Since NSAID use is associated with gastrointestinal irritation, caution should be used during concomitant use; no increase in the incidence of gastrointestinal irritation was reported in clinical trials).
No products indexed under this heading.

Sulindac (Since NSAID use is associated with gastrointestinal irritation, caution should be used during concomitant use; no increase in the incidence of gastrointestinal irritation was reported in clinical trials). Products include:
Clinoril Tablets 1962

Tolmetin Sodium (Since NSAID use is associated with gastrointestinal irritation, caution should be used during concomitant use; no increase in the incidence of gastrointestinal irritation was reported in clinical trials).
No products indexed under this heading.

Valdecoxib (Since NSAID use is associated with gastrointestinal irritation, caution should be used during concomitant use; no increase in the incidence of gastrointestinal irritation was reported in clinical trials).
No products indexed under this heading.

Food Interactions

Beverages, caffeine-containing (Concomitant administration of alendronate with coffee reduces bioavailability by approximately 60%).

Meal, unspecified (Standardized breakfast decreases bioavailability by approximately 40% when alendronate is administered either one-half or 1 hour before breakfast).

Orange Juice (Concomitant administration of alendronate with orange juice reduces bioavailability by approximately 60%).

FOSAMAX PLUS D TABLETS

(Alendronate Sodium, Cholecalciferol) 2013
May interact with antacids containing aluminum, calcium and magnesium, aspirin-acetylsalicylic acid, bile acid sequestering agents, calcium preparations, anticonvulsants, nonsteroidal anti-inflammatory agents, thiazides, and certain other agents. Compounds in these categories include:

Aluminum Carbonate (Antacids may interfere with the absorption of alendronate. Therefore, patients must wait at least one-half hour after taking alendronate sodium/cholecalciferol before taking any other oral medications).
No products indexed under this heading.

Aluminum Hydroxide (Antacids may interfere with the absorption of alendronate. Therefore, patients must wait at least one-half hour after taking alendronate sodium/cholecalciferol before taking any other oral medications).
No products indexed under this heading.

Aspirin (Studies have shown an increased incidence of upper gastrointestinal adverse events in patients receiving concomitant therapy with daily doses of alendronate greater than 10 mg and aspirin-containing products). Products include:
Aggrenox Capsules 819
Bayer Aspirin 750
Percodan Tablets 1130
St. Joseph 81 mg Aspirin Chewable and Enteric Coated Tablets 1903

Aspirin, Enteric Coated (Studies have shown an increased incidence of upper gastrointestinal adverse events in patients receiving concomitant therapy with daily doses of alendronate greater than 10 mg and aspirin-containing products).
No products indexed under this heading.

Aspirin Buffered (Studies have shown an increased incidence of upper gastrointestinal adverse events in patients receiving concomitant therapy with daily doses of alendronate greater than 10 mg and aspirin-containing products).
No products indexed under this heading.

Bendroflumethiazide (Thiazides may increase the catabolism of vitamin D; consider additional vitamin D supplementation when co-administering).
No products indexed under this heading.

Calcium Carbonate (Calcium supplements may interfere with the absorption of alendronate. Therefore, patients must wait at least one-half hour after taking alendronate sodium/cholecalciferol before taking any other oral medications).
Products include:
Accelerator Tablets .... ▣634
Actonel with Calcium Tablets 2574
BioLean II Tablets .... ▣635
Calcet Triple Calcium + Vitamin D Tablets .... ▣629
D-Cal Chewable Caplets .... ▣624
Elixir Capsules .... ▣636
Pepcid Complete Chewable Tablets 1771
Extra Strength Rolaids Plus Gas Relief Tropical Fruit Softchews 1903
Extra Strength Rolaids Softchews Vanilla Creme 1903
Extra Strength Rolaids Freshmint Tablets 1903
Rolaids Multi-Symptom Berry Tablets 1903
Rolaids Original Peppermint Tablets 1903

Calcium Chloride (Calcium supplements may interfere with the absorption of alendronate. Therefore, patients must wait at least one-half hour after taking alendronate sodium/cholecalciferol before taking any other oral medications).
No products indexed under this heading.

Calcium Citrate (Calcium supplements may interfere with the absorption of alendronate. Therefore, patients must wait at least one-half hour after taking alendronate sodium/cholecalciferol before taking any other oral medications).
Products include:
Active Calcium Tablets 3173
CitraNatal DHA Tablets 2175
CitraNatal 90 DHA Tablets 2175

Calcium Glubionate (Calcium supplements may interfere with the absorption of alendronate. Therefore, patients must wait at least one-half hour after taking alendronate sodium/cholecalciferol before taking any other oral medications).
No products indexed under this heading.

Carbamazepine (Anticonvulsants may increase the catabolism of vitamin D; consider additional vitamin D supplementation when co-administering). Products include:
Carbatrol Capsules 3019
Equetro Extended-Release Capsules 3174

Celecoxib (Since NSAID use is associated with gastrointestinal irritation, caution should be used during concomitant use with alendronate sodium/cholecalciferol. No increase in the incidence of gastrointestinal irritation was reported in clinical trials). Products include:
Celebrex Capsules 2979

Chlorothiazide (Thiazides may increase the catabolism of vitamin D; consider additional vitamin D supplementation when co-administering).
No products indexed under this heading.

Chlorothiazide Sodium (Thiazides may increase the catabolism of vitamin D; consider additional vitamin D supplementation when co-administering). Products include:
Intravenous Sodium Diuril 2490

Cholestyramine (Bile-acid sequestrants may impair the absoption of vitamin D; consider additional vitamin D supplementation when co-administering).
No products indexed under this heading.

Cimetidine (Cimetidine may increase the catabolism of vitamin D; consider additional vitamin D supplementation when co-administering).
No products indexed under this heading.

Cimetidine Hydrochloride (Cimetidine may increase the catabolism of vitamin D; consider additional vitamin D supplementation when co-administering).
No products indexed under this heading.

Colesevelam Hydrochloride (Bile-acid sequestrants may impair the absoption of vitamin D; consider additional vitamin D supplementation when co-administering). Products include:
WelChol Tablets 1015

Colestipol Hydrochloride (Bile-acid sequestrants may impair the absoption of vitamin D; consider additional vitamin D supplementation when co-administering).
No products indexed under this heading.

Diclofenac Epolamine (Since NSAID use is associated with gastrointestinal irritation, caution should be used during concomitant use with alendronate sodium/cholecalciferol. No increase in the incidence of gastrointestinal irritation was reported in clinical trials). Products include:
Flector Patch 561

Diclofenac Potassium (Since NSAID use is associated with gastrointestinal irritation, caution should be used during concomitant use with alendronate sodium/cholecalciferol. No increase in the incidence of gastrointestinal irritation was reported in clinical trials).
No products indexed under this heading.

Diclofenac Sodium (Since NSAID use is associated with gastrointestinal irritation, caution should be used during concomitant use with alendronate sodium/cholecalciferol. No increase in the incidence of gastrointestinal irritation was reported in clinical trials). Products include:
Diclofenac Sodium Ophthalmic Solution .... ⊙240
Voltaren Ophthalmic Solution 2336
Voltaren Tablets 2334
Voltaren-XR Tablets 2337

Divalproex Sodium (Anticonvulsants may increase the catabolism of vitamin D; consider additional vitamin D supplementation when co-administering). Products include:
Depakote ER Tablets 423

Ethosuximide (Anticonvulsants may increase the catabolism of vitamin D; consider additional vitamin D supplementation when co-administering).
No products indexed under this heading.

Ethotoin (Anticonvulsants may increase the catabolism of vitamin D; consider additional vitamin D supplementation when co-administering).
No products indexed under this heading.

Etodolac (Since NSAID use is associated with gastrointestinal irritation, caution should be used during concomitant use with alendronate sodium/cholecalciferol. No increase in the incidence of gastrointestinal irritation was reported in clinical trials).
No products indexed under this heading.

Felbamate (Anticonvulsants may increase the catabolism of vitamin D; consider additional vitamin D supplementation when co-administering).
No products indexed under this heading.

Fenoprofen Calcium (Since NSAID use is associated with gastrointestinal irritation, caution should be used during concomitant use with alendronate sodium/cholecalciferol. No increase in the incidence of gastrointestinal irritation was reported in clinical trials). Products include:
Nalfon Capsules ... 2508

Flurbiprofen (Since NSAID use is associated with gastrointestinal irritation, caution should be used during concomitant use with alendronate sodium/cholecalciferol. No increase in the incidence of gastrointestinal irritation was reported in clinical trials).
No products indexed under this heading.

Fosphenytoin (Anticonvulsants may increase the catabolism of vitamin D; consider additional vitamin D supplementation when co-administering).
No products indexed under this heading.

Fosphenytoin Sodium (Anticonvulsants may increase the catabolism of vitamin D; consider additional vitamin D supplementation when co-administering).
No products indexed under this heading.

Gabapentin (Anticonvulsants may increase the catabolism of vitamin D; consider additional vitamin D supplementation when co-administering).
No products indexed under this heading.

Hydrochlorothiazide (Thiazides may increase the catabolism of vitamin D; consider additional vitamin D supplementation when co-administering). Products include:
Atacand HCT ... 642
Avalide Tablets ... 892
Avalide Tablets ... 2713
Benicar HCT Tablets ... 1010
Diovan HCT Tablets ... 2216
Dyazide Capsules ... 1405
Micardis HCT Tablets ... 854
Prinzide Tablets ... 2092
Tekturna HCT Tablets ... 2324
Teveten HCT Tablets ... 517

Hydroflumethiazide (Thiazides may increase the catabolism of vitamin D; consider additional vitamin D supplementation when co-administering).
No products indexed under this heading.

Ibuprofen (Since NSAID use is associated with gastrointestinal irritation, caution should be used during concomitant use with alendronate sodium/cholecalciferol. No increase in the incidence of gastrointestinal irritation was reported in clinical trials). Products include:
Motrin IB Tablets and Caplets ... 1900
Children's Motrin Oral Suspension ... 1901
Children's Motrin Non-Staining Dye-Free Oral Suspension ... 1901
Children's Motrin Cold Oral Suspension ... 1899
Infants' Motrin Concentrated Drops ... 1901
Infants' Motrin Non-Staining Dye-Free Concentrated Drops ... 1901
Junior Strength Motrin Caplets and Chewable Tablets ... 1901
Vicoprofen Tablets ... 533

Indomethacin (Since NSAID use is associated with gastrointestinal irritation, caution should be used during concomitant use with alendronate sodium/cholecalciferol. No increase in the incidence of gastrointestinal irritation was reported in clinical trials). Products include:
Indocin ... 2024

Indomethacin Sodium Trihydrate (Since NSAID use is associated with gastrointestinal irritation, caution should be used during concomitant use with alendronate sodium/cholecalciferol. No increase in the incidence of gastrointestinal irritation was reported in clinical trials). Products include:
Indocin I.V. ... 2489

Ketoprofen (Since NSAID use is associated with gastrointestinal irritation, caution should be used during concomitant use with alendronate sodium/cholecalciferol. No increase in the incidence of gastrointestinal irritation was reported in clinical trials).
No products indexed under this heading.

Ketorolac Tromethamine (Since NSAID use is associated with gastrointestinal irritation, caution should be used during concomitant use with alendronate sodium/cholecalciferol. No increase in the incidence of gastrointestinal irritation was reported in clinical trials).
No products indexed under this heading.

Lamotrigine (Anticonvulsants may increase the catabolism of vitamin D; consider additional vitamin D supplementation when co-administering). Products include:
Lamictal ... 1488

Levetiracetam (Anticonvulsants may increase the catabolism of vitamin D; consider additional vitamin D supplementation when co-administering). Products include:
Keppra Injection ... 3137
Keppra Oral Solution ... 3131
Keppra Tablets ... 3131

Magaldrate (Antacids may interfere with the absorption of alendronate. Therefore, patients must wait at least one-half hour after taking alendronate sodium/cholecalciferol before taking any other oral medications).
No products indexed under this heading.

Magnesium Hydroxide (Antacids may interfere with the absorption of alendronate. Therefore, patients must wait at least one-half hour after taking alendronate sodium/cholecalciferol before taking any other oral medications). Products include:
Fleet Pedia-Lax Chewable Tablets ... 1145
Pepcid Complete Chewable Tablets ... 1771
Extra Strength Rolaids Freshmint Tablets ... 1903
Rolaids Multi-Symptom Berry Tablets ... 1903
Rolaids Original Peppermint Tablets ... 1903

Magnesium Oxide (Antacids may interfere with the absorption of alendronate. Therefore, patients must wait at least one-half hour after taking alendronate sodium/cholecalciferol before taking any other oral medications). Products include:
Beelith Tablets ... 813

Meclofenamate Sodium (Since NSAID use is associated with gastrointestinal irritation, caution should be used during concomitant use with alendronate sodium/cholecalciferol. No increase in the incidence of gastrointestinal irritation was reported in clinical trials).
No products indexed under this heading.

Mefenamic Acid (Since NSAID use is associated with gastrointestinal irritation, caution should be used during concomitant use with alendronate sodium/cholecalciferol. No increase in the incidence of gastrointestinal irritation was reported in clinical trials).
No products indexed under this heading.

Meloxicam (Since NSAID use is associated with gastrointestinal irritation, caution should be used during concomitant use with alendronate sodium/cholecalciferol. No increase in the incidence of gastrointestinal irritation was reported in clinical trials). Products include:
Mobic Oral Suspension ... 863
Mobic Tablets ... 863

Mephenytoin (Anticonvulsants may increase the catabolism of vitamin D; consider additional vitamin D supplementation when co-administering).
No products indexed under this heading.

Methsuximide (Anticonvulsants may increase the catabolism of vitamin D; consider additional vitamin D supplementation when co-administering).
No products indexed under this heading.

Methyclothiazide (Thiazides may increase the catabolism of vitamin D; consider additional vitamin D supplementation when co-administering).
No products indexed under this heading.

Mineral Oil (Mineral oil may impair the absorption of vitamin D; consider additional vitamin D supplementation when co-administering). Products include:
Fleet Mineral Oil Enema ... 1144
Soothe XP Eye Drops ... ⊙246

Nabumetone (Since NSAID use is associated with gastrointestinal irritation, caution should be used during concomitant use with alendronate sodium/cholecalciferol. No increase in the incidence of gastrointestinal irritation was reported in clinical trials).
No products indexed under this heading.

Naproxen (Since NSAID use is associated with gastrointestinal irritation, caution should be used during concomitant use with alendronate sodium/cholecalciferol. No increase in the incidence of gastrointestinal irritation was reported in clinical trials). Products include:
EC-Naprosyn Delayed-Release Tablets ... 2632
Naprosyn Suspension ... 2632
Naprosyn Tablets ... 2632

Naproxen Sodium (Since NSAID use is associated with gastrointestinal irritation, caution should be used during concomitant use with alendronate sodium/cholecalciferol. No increase in the incidence of gastrointestinal irritation was reported in clinical trials). Products include:
Anaprox Tablets ... 2632
Anaprox DS Tablets ... 2632
Treximet Tablets ... 1616

Olestra (Olestra may impair the absorption of vitamin D; consider additional vitamin D supplementation when co-administering).
No products indexed under this heading.

Orlistat (Orlistat may impair the absorption of vitamin D; consider additional vitamin D supplementation when co-administering). Products include:
Xenical Capsules ... 2672

Oxaprozin (Since NSAID use is associated with gastrointestinal irritation, caution should be used during concomitant use with alendronate sodium/cholecalciferol. No increase in the incidence of gastrointestinal irritation was reported in clinical trials).
No products indexed under this heading.

Oxcarbazepine (Anticonvulsants may increase the catabolism of vitamin D; consider additional vitamin D supplementation when co-administering).
No products indexed under this heading.

Paramethadione (Anticonvulsants may increase the catabolism of vitamin D; consider additional vitamin D supplementation when co-administering).
No products indexed under this heading.

Phenacemide (Anticonvulsants may increase the catabolism of vitamin D; consider additional vitamin D supplementation when co-administering).
No products indexed under this heading.

Phenobarbital (Anticonvulsants may increase the catabolism of vitamin D; consider additional vitamin D supplementation when co-administering). Products include:
Donnatal Extentabs ... 2507

Phensuximide (Anticonvulsants may increase the catabolism of vitamin D; consider additional vitamin D supplementation when co-administering).
No products indexed under this heading.

Phenylbutazone (Since NSAID use is associated with gastrointestinal irritation, caution should be used during concomitant use with alendronate sodium/cholecalciferol. No increase in the incidence of gastrointestinal irritation was reported in clinical trials).
No products indexed under this heading.

Phenytoin (Anticonvulsants may increase the catabolism of vitamin D; consider additional vitamin D supplementation when co-administering).
No products indexed under this heading.

Phenytoin Sodium (Anticonvulsants may increase the catabolism of vitamin D; consider additional vitamin D supplementation when co-administering). Products include:
Phenytek Capsules 2192

Piroxicam (Since NSAID use is associated with gastrointestinal irritation, caution should be used during concomitant use with alendronate sodium/cholecalciferol. No increase in the incidence of gastrointestinal irritation was reported in clinical trials).
No products indexed under this heading.

Polythiazide (Thiazides may increase the catabolism of vitamin D; consider additional vitamin D supplementation when co-administering).
No products indexed under this heading.

Primidone (Anticonvulsants may increase the catabolism of vitamin D; consider additional vitamin D supplementation when co-administering).
No products indexed under this heading.

Ranitidine Hydrochloride (Intravenous ranitidine was shown to double the bioavailability of oral alendronate. The clinical significance of this increased bioavailability and whether similar increases will occur in patients given oral H2-antagonists is unknown). Products include:
Zantac 75 Tablets .... ◘603
Zantac 1670
Zantac Injection 1666
Zantac Injection Pharmacy Bulk Package 1668
Maximum Strength Zantac 150 Tablets .... ◘603
Maximum Strength Zantac 150 Cool Mint Tablets .... ◘603

Rofecoxib (Since NSAID use is associated with gastrointestinal irritation, caution should be used during concomitant use with alendronate sodium/cholecalciferol. No increase in the incidence of gastrointestinal irritation was reported in clinical trials).
No products indexed under this heading.

Sulindac (Since NSAID use is associated with gastrointestinal irritation, caution should be used during concomitant use with alendronate sodium/cholecalciferol. No increase in the incidence of gastrointestinal irritation was reported in clinical trials). Products include:
Clinoril Tablets 1962

Tiagabine Hydrochloride (Anticonvulsants may increase the catabolism of vitamin D; consider additional vitamin D supplementation when co-administering). Products include:
Gabitril Tablets 973

Tolmetin Sodium (Since NSAID use is associated with gastrointestinal irritation, caution should be used during concomitant use with alendronate sodium/cholecalciferol. No increase in the incidence of gastrointestinal irritation was reported in clinical trials).
No products indexed under this heading.

Topiramate (Anticonvulsants may increase the catabolism of vitamin D; consider additional vitamin D supplementation when co-administering).
No products indexed under this heading.

Trimethadione (Anticonvulsants may increase the catabolism of vitamin D; consider additional vitamin D supplementation when co-administering).
No products indexed under this heading.

Valdecoxib (Since NSAID use is associated with gastrointestinal irritation, caution should be used during concomitant use with alendronate sodium/cholecalciferol. No increase in the incidence of gastrointestinal irritation was reported in clinical trials).
No products indexed under this heading.

Valproate Sodium (Anticonvulsants may increase the catabolism of vitamin D; consider additional vitamin D supplementation when co-administering).
No products indexed under this heading.

Valproic Acid (Anticonvulsants may increase the catabolism of vitamin D; consider additional vitamin D supplementation when co-administering).
No products indexed under this heading.

Zonisamide (Anticonvulsants may increase the catabolism of vitamin D; consider additional vitamin D supplementation when co-administering). Products include:
Zonegran Capsules 1089

Food Interactions

Beverages, caffeine-containing (Concomitant administration of alendronate with coffee reduces bioavailability by approximately 60%).

Meal, unspecified (Bioavailability was decreased (by approximately 40%) when 10 mg alendronate was administered either 0.5 or 1 hour before a standardized breakfast, when compared to dosing 2 hours before eating).

Orange Juice (Concomitant administration of alendronate with orange juice reduces bioavailability by approximately 60%).

FOSRENOL CHEWABLE TABLETS

(Lanthanum Carbonate) 3027
May interact with antacids. Compounds in these categories include:

Aluminum Carbonate (Avoid administering within 2 hours of antacids).
No products indexed under this heading.

Aluminum Hydroxide (Avoid administering within 2 hours of antacids).
No products indexed under this heading.

Magaldrate (Avoid administering within 2 hours of antacids).
No products indexed under this heading.

Magnesium Hydroxide (Avoid administering within 2 hours of antacids). Products include:
Fleet Pedia-Lax Chewable Tablets 1145
Pepcid Complete Chewable Tablets 1771
Extra Strength Rolaids Freshmint Tablets 1903
Rolaids Multi-Symptom Berry Tablets 1903
Rolaids Original Peppermint Tablets 1903

Magnesium Oxide (Avoid administering within 2 hours of antacids). Products include:
Beelith Tablets 813

Sodium Bicarbonate (Avoid administering within 2 hours of antacids). Products include:
Ceo-Two Laxative Suppository 815

FOSTEUM CAPSULES

(Cholecalciferol, Genistein Aglycone, Zinc Bisglycinate) 2963
May interact with bile acid sequestering agents, anticonvulsants, thiazides, Zincs, and certain other agents. Compounds in these categories include:

Bendroflumethiazide (Thiazides may increase catabolism of vitamin D3).
No products indexed under this heading.

Carbamazepine (Anticonvulsants may increase catabolism of vitamin D3). Products include:
Carbatrol Capsules 3019
Equetro Extended-Release Capsules 3174

Chlorothiazide (Thiazides may increase catabolism of vitamin D3).
No products indexed under this heading.

Chlorothiazide Sodium (Thiazides may increase catabolism of vitamin D3). Products include:
Intravenous Sodium Diuril 2490

Cholestyramine (Cholestyramine and other bile acid sequestrants may impede absorption of vitamin D3 from the intestine).
No products indexed under this heading.

Cimetidine (Cimetidine may increase catabolism of vitamin D3).
No products indexed under this heading.

Cimetidine Hydrochloride (Cimetidine may increase catabolism of vitamin D3).
No products indexed under this heading.

Colesevelam Hydrochloride (Cholestyramine and other bile acid sequestrants may impede absorption of vitamin D3 from the intestine). Products include:
WelChol Tablets 1015

Colestipol Hydrochloride (Cholestyramine and other bile acid sequestrants may impede absorption of vitamin D3 from the intestine).
No products indexed under this heading.

Divalproex Sodium (Anticonvulsants may increase catabolism of vitamin D3). Products include:
Depakote ER Tablets 423

Ethosuximide (Anticonvulsants may increase catabolism of vitamin D3).
No products indexed under this heading.

Ethotoin (Anticonvulsants may increase catabolism of vitamin D3).
No products indexed under this heading.

Felbamate (Anticonvulsants may increase catabolism of vitamin D3).
No products indexed under this heading.

Fosphenytoin (Anticonvulsants may increase catabolism of vitamin D3).
No products indexed under this heading.

Fosphenytoin Sodium (Anticonvulsants may increase catabolism of vitamin D3).
No products indexed under this heading.

Gabapentin (Anticonvulsants may increase catabolism of vitamin D3).
No products indexed under this heading.

Hydrochlorothiazide (Thiazides may increase catabolism of vitamin D3). Products include:
Atacand HCT 642
Avalide Tablets 892
Avalide Tablets 2713
Benicar HCT Tablets 1010
Diovan HCT Tablets 2216
Dyazide Capsules 1405
Micardis HCT Tablets 854
Prinzide Tablets 2092
Tekturna HCT Tablets 2324
Teveten HCT Tablets 517

Hydroflumethiazide (Thiazides may increase catabolism of vitamin D3).
No products indexed under this heading.

Lamotrigine (Anticonvulsants may increase catabolism of vitamin D3). Products include:
Lamictal 1488

Levetiracetam (Anticonvulsants may increase catabolism of vitamin D3). Products include:
Keppra Injection 3137
Keppra Oral Solution 3131
Keppra Tablets 3131

Mephenytoin (Anticonvulsants may increase catabolism of vitamin D3).
No products indexed under this heading.

Methsuximide (Anticonvulsants may increase catabolism of vitamin D3).
No products indexed under this heading.

Methyclothiazide (Thiazides may increase catabolism of vitamin D3).
No products indexed under this heading.

Mineral Oil (Mineral oil may impede absorption of vitamin D3 from the intestine). Products include:
Fleet Mineral Oil Enema 1144
Soothe XP Eye Drops .... ⊙246

Olestra (Olestra may impede absorption of vitamin D3 from the intestine).
No products indexed under this heading.

Orlistat (Orlistat may impede absorption of vitamin D3 from the intestine). Products include:
Xenical Capsules 2672

Oxcarbazepine (Anticonvulsants may increase catabolism of vitamin D3).
No products indexed under this heading.

Paramethadione (Anticonvulsants may increase catabolism of vitamin D3).
No products indexed under this heading.

Phenacemide (Anticonvulsants may increase catabolism of vitamin D3).
No products indexed under this heading.

Phenobarbital (Anticonvulsants may increase catabolism of vitamin D3). Products include:

Donnatal Extentabs 2507

Phensuximide (Anticonvulsants may increase catabolism of vitamin D3).
No products indexed under this heading.

Phenytoin (Anticonvulsants may increase catabolism of vitamin D3).
No products indexed under this heading.

Phenytoin Sodium (Anticonvulsants may increase catabolism of vitamin D3). Products include:
Phenytek Capsules 2192

Polythiazide (Thiazides may increase catabolism of vitamin D3).
No products indexed under this heading.

Primidone (Anticonvulsants may increase catabolism of vitamin D3).
No products indexed under this heading.

Tiagabine Hydrochloride (Anticonvulsants may increase catabolism of vitamin D3). Products include:
Gabitril Tablets 973

Topiramate (Anticonvulsants may increase catabolism of vitamin D3).
No products indexed under this heading.

Trimethadione (Anticonvulsants may increase catabolism of vitamin D3).
No products indexed under this heading.

Valproate Sodium (Anticonvulsants may increase catabolism of vitamin D3).
No products indexed under this heading.

Valproic Acid (Anticonvulsants may increase catabolism of vitamin D3).
No products indexed under this heading.

Zinc (Symptoms of acute zync toxicity occur after ingestion of 2 mg or more of elemental zinc, the equivalent of 500 Fosteum Capsules at one time. Chronic zinc toxicity, resulting from induced copper deficiency, is increasingly common as the use of large doses of zinc in supplements becomes more routine. Those on long-term supplementation or high doses of zinc-containing cold medication, zinc lozenges, etc., should be monitored for zinc and copper status). Products include:
Comax Dietary Supplement 995
Glaucofit Dietary Supplement 995
Glauma Dietary Supplement 995
Tonox Dietary Supplement 995
Vibe Liquid Multi-Nutrient Supplement 626
Visutein Capsules 3159

Zinc Acetate (Symptoms of acute zync toxicity occur after ingestion of 2 mg or more of elemental zinc, the equivalent of 500 Fosteum Capsules at one time. Chronic zinc toxicity, resulting from induced copper deficiency, is increasingly common as the use of large doses of zinc in supplements becomes more routine. Those on long-term supplementation or high doses of zinc-containing cold medication, zinc lozenges, etc., should be monitored for zinc and copper status).
No products indexed under this heading.

Zinc Chloride (Symptoms of acute zync toxicity occur after ingestion of 2 mg or more of elemental zinc, the equivalent of 500 Fosteum Capsules at one time. Chronic zinc toxicity, resulting from induced copper deficiency, is increasingly common as the use of large doses of zinc in supplements becomes more routine. Those on long-term supplementation or high doses of zinc-containing cold medication, zinc lozenges, etc., should be monitored for zinc and copper status).
No products indexed under this heading.

Zinc Citrate (Symptoms of acute zync toxicity occur after ingestion of 2 mg or more of elemental zinc, the equivalent of 500 Fosteum Capsules at one time. Chronic zinc toxicity, resulting from induced copper deficiency, is increasingly common as the use of large doses of zinc in supplements becomes more routine. Those on long-term supplementation or high doses of zinc-containing cold medication, zinc lozenges, etc., should be monitored for zinc and copper status).
No products indexed under this heading.

Zinc-Containing Multivitamins (Symptoms of acute zync toxicity occur after ingestion of 2 mg or more of elemental zinc, the equivalent of 500 Fosteum Capsules at one time. Chronic zinc toxicity, resulting from induced copper deficiency, is increasingly common as the use of large doses of zinc in supplements becomes more routine. Those on long-term supplementation or high doses of zinc-containing cold medication, zinc lozenges, etc., should be monitored for zinc and copper status).
No products indexed under this heading.

Zinc Gluconate (Symptoms of acute zync toxicity occur after ingestion of 2 mg or more of elemental zinc, the equivalent of 500 Fosteum Capsules at one time. Chronic zinc toxicity, resulting from induced copper deficiency, is increasingly common as the use of large doses of zinc in supplements becomes more routine. Those on long-term supplementation or high doses of zinc-containing cold medication, zinc lozenges, etc., should be monitored for zinc and copper status).
No products indexed under this heading.

Zinc Oxide (Symptoms of acute zync toxicity occur after ingestion of 2 mg or more of elemental zinc, the equivalent of 500 Fosteum Capsules at one time. Chronic zinc toxicity, resulting from induced copper deficiency, is increasingly common as the use of large doses of zinc in supplements becomes more routine. Those on long-term supplementation or high doses of zinc-containing cold medication, zinc lozenges, etc., should be monitored for zinc and copper status). Products include:
Bausch & Lomb Ocuvite Adult 50+ Vitamin and Mineral Supplement .... ⊙ 237
CitraNatal DHA Tablets 2175
CitraNatal 90 DHA Tablets 2175

Zinc Phenosulfonate (Symptoms of acute zync toxicity occur after ingestion of 2 mg or more of elemental zinc, the equivalent of 500 Fosteum Capsules at one time. Chronic zinc toxicity, resulting from induced copper deficiency, is increasingly common as the use of large doses of zinc in supplements becomes more routine. Those on long-term supplementation or high doses of zinc-containing cold medication, zinc lozenges, etc., should be monitored for zinc and copper status).
No products indexed under this heading.

Zinc Pyrithione (Symptoms of acute zync toxicity occur after ingestion of 2 mg or more of elemental zinc, the equivalent of 500 Fosteum Capsules at one time. Chronic zinc toxicity, resulting from induced copper deficiency, is increasingly common as the use of large doses of zinc in supplements becomes more routine. Those on long-term supplementation or high doses of zinc-containing cold medication, zinc lozenges, etc., should be monitored for zinc and copper status).
No products indexed under this heading.

Zinc Sulfate (Symptoms of acute zync toxicity occur after ingestion of 2 mg or more of elemental zinc, the equivalent of 500 Fosteum Capsules at one time. Chronic zinc toxicity, resulting from induced copper deficiency, is increasingly common as the use of large doses of zinc in supplements becomes more routine. Those on long-term supplementation or high doses of zinc-containing cold medication, zinc lozenges, etc., should be monitored for zinc and copper status). Products include:
Clear Eyes Itchy Eye Relief .... ⊙ 255
Zinc-220 Capsules 564

Zinc Undecylenate (Symptoms of acute zync toxicity occur after ingestion of 2 mg or more of elemental zinc, the equivalent of 500 Fosteum Capsules at one time. Chronic zinc toxicity, resulting from induced copper deficiency, is increasingly common as the use of large doses of zinc in supplements becomes more routine. Those on long-term supplementation or high doses of zinc-containing cold medication, zinc lozenges, etc., should be monitored for zinc and copper status).
No products indexed under this heading.

Zonisamide (Anticonvulsants may increase catabolism of vitamin D3). Products include:
Zonegran Capsules 1089

FRAGMIN INJECTION

(Dalteparin Sodium) 1070
May interact with anesthetics, oral anticoagulants, platelet inhibitors, and thrombolytics. Compounds in these categories include:

Alfentanil Hydrochloride (Patients undergoing regional anesthesia should not receive dalteparin sodium for unstable angina or non-Q-wave myocardial infarction due to an increased risk of bleeding associated with the dosage of dalteparin sodium recommended for unstable angina and non-Q-wave myocardial infarction).
No products indexed under this heading.

Alteplase (Dalteparin sodium should be used with care in patients receiving oral anticoagulants, platelet inhibitors, and thrombolytic agents because of an increased risk of bleeding). Products include:
Activase I.V. 1188
Cathflo Activase 1198

Anisindione (Dalteparin sodium should be used with care in patients receiving oral anticoagulants, platelet inhibitors, and thrombolytic agents because of an increased risk of bleeding).
No products indexed under this heading.

Anistreplase (Dalteparin sodium should be used with care in patients receiving oral anticoagulants, platelet inhibitors, and thrombolytic agents because of an increased risk of bleeding).
No products indexed under this heading.

Aspirin (Dalteparin sodium should be used with care in patients receiving oral anticoagulants, platelet inhibitors, and thrombolytic agents because of an increased risk of bleeding). Products include:
Aggrenox Capsules 819
Bayer Aspirin 750
Percodan Tablets 1130
St. Joseph 81 mg Aspirin Chewable and Enteric Coated Tablets 1903

Aspirin, Enteric Coated (Dalteparin sodium should be used with care in patients receiving oral anticoagulants, platelet inhibitors, and thrombolytic agents because of an increased risk of bleeding).
No products indexed under this heading.

Aspirin Buffered (Dalteparin sodium should be used with care in patients receiving oral anticoagulants, platelet inhibitors, and thrombolytic agents because of an increased risk of bleeding).
No products indexed under this heading.

Azlocillin Sodium (Dalteparin sodium should be used with care in patients receiving oral anticoagulants, platelet inhibitors, and thrombolytic agents because of an increased risk of bleeding).
No products indexed under this heading.

Bivalirudin (Dalteparin sodium should be used with care in patients receiving oral anticoagulants, platelet inhibitors, and thrombolytic agents because of an increased risk of bleeding). Products include:
Angiomax for Injection 1933

Carbenicillin Indanyl Sodium (Dalteparin sodium should be used with care in patients receiving oral anticoagulants, platelet inhibitors, and thrombolytic agents because of an increased risk of bleeding).
No products indexed under this heading.

Choline Magnesium Trisalicylate (Dalteparin sodium should be used with care in patients receiving oral anticoagulants, platelet inhibitors, and thrombolytic agents because of an increased risk of bleeding).
No products indexed under this heading.

Clopidogrel Bisulfate (Dalteparin sodium should be used with care in patients receiving oral anticoagulants, platelet inhibitors, and thrombolytic agents because of an increased risk of bleeding). Products include:
Plavix Tablets 926
Plavix Tablets 2767

Diclofenac Potassium (Dalteparin sodium should be used with care in patients receiving oral anticoagulants, platelet inhibitors, and thrombolytic agents because of an increased risk of bleeding).
No products indexed under this heading.

Diclofenac Sodium (Dalteparin sodium should be used with care in patients receiving oral anticoagulants, platelet inhibitors, and thrombolytic agents because of an increased risk of bleeding). Products include:
Diclofenac Sodium Ophthalmic Solution .... ⊙ 240
Voltaren Ophthalmic Solution 2336
Voltaren Tablets 2334
Voltaren-XR Tablets 2337

Dicumarol (Dalteparin sodium should be used with care in patients receiving oral anticoagulants, platelet inhibitors, and thrombolytic agents because of an increased risk of bleeding).
No products indexed under this heading.

Diflunisal (Dalteparin sodium should be used with care in patients receiving oral anticoagulants, platelet inhibitors, and thrombolytic agents because of an increased risk of bleeding).
No products indexed under this heading.

Dipyridamole (Dalteparin sodium should be used with care in patients receiving oral anticoagulants, platelet inhibitors, and thrombolytic agents because of an increased risk of bleeding). Products include:
Aggrenox Capsules 819
Persantine Tablets 869

Enflurane (Patients undergoing regional anesthesia should not receive dalteparin sodium for unstable angina or non-Q-wave myocardial infarction due to an increased risk of bleeding associated with the dosage of dalteparin sodium recommended for unstable angina and non-Q-wave myocardial infarction).
No products indexed under this heading.

Fenoprofen Calcium (Dalteparin sodium should be used with care in patients receiving oral anticoagulants, platelet inhibitors, and thrombolytic agents because of an increased risk of bleeding). Products include:
Nalfon Capsules 2508

Fentanyl Citrate (Patients undergoing regional anesthesia should not receive dalteparin sodium for unstable angina or non-Q-wave myocardial infarction due to an increased risk of bleeding associated with the dosage of dalteparin sodium recommended for unstable angina and non-Q-wave myocardial infarction). Products include:
Actiq 959
Fentora Tablets 968

Flurbiprofen (Dalteparin sodium should be used with care in patients receiving oral anticoagulants, platelet inhibitors, and thrombolytic agents because of an increased risk of bleeding).
No products indexed under this heading.

Halothane (Patients undergoing regional anesthesia should not receive dalteparin sodium for unstable angina or non-Q-wave myocardial infarction due to an increased risk of bleeding associated with the dosage of dalteparin sodium recommended for unstable angina and non-Q-wave myocardial infarction).
No products indexed under this heading.

Ibuprofen (Dalteparin sodium should be used with care in patients receiving oral anticoagulants, platelet inhibitors, and thrombolytic agents because of an increased risk of bleeding). Products include:
Motrin IB Tablets and Caplets 1900
Children's Motrin Oral Suspension ... 1901
Children's Motrin Non-Staining Dye-Free Oral Suspension 1901
Children's Motrin Cold Oral Suspension 1899
Infants' Motrin Concentrated Drops 1901
Infants' Motrin Non-Staining Dye-Free Concentrated Drops 1901
Junior Strength Motrin Caplets and Chewable Tablets 1901
Vicoprofen Tablets 533

Indomethacin (Dalteparin sodium should be used with care in patients receiving oral anticoagulants, platelet inhibitors, and thrombolytic agents because of an increased risk of bleeding). Products include:
Indocin 2024

Indomethacin Sodium Trihydrate (Dalteparin sodium should be used with care in patients receiving oral anticoagulants, platelet inhibitors, and thrombolytic agents because of an increased risk of bleeding). Products include:
Indocin I.V. 2489

Isoflurane (Patients undergoing regional anesthesia should not receive dalteparin sodium for unstable angina or non-Q-wave myocardial infarction due to an increased risk of bleeding associated with the dosage of dalteparin sodium recommended for unstable angina and non-Q-wave myocardial infarction).
No products indexed under this heading.

Ketamine Hydrochloride (Patients undergoing regional anesthesia should not receive dalteparin sodium for unstable angina or non-Q-wave myocardial infarction due to an increased risk of bleeding associated with the dosage of dalteparin sodium recommended for unstable angina and non-Q-wave myocardial infarction).
No products indexed under this heading.

Ketoprofen (Dalteparin sodium should be used with care in patients receiving oral anticoagulants, platelet inhibitors, and thrombolytic agents because of an increased risk of bleeding).
No products indexed under this heading.

Magnesium Salicylate (Dalteparin sodium should be used with care in patients receiving oral anticoagulants, platelet inhibitors, and thrombolytic agents because of an increased risk of bleeding).
No products indexed under this heading.

Meclofenamate Sodium (Dalteparin sodium should be used with care in patients receiving oral anticoagulants, platelet inhibitors, and thrombolytic agents because of an increased risk of bleeding).
No products indexed under this heading.

Mefenamic Acid (Dalteparin sodium should be used with care in patients receiving oral anticoagulants, platelet inhibitors, and thrombolytic agents because of an increased risk of bleeding).
No products indexed under this heading.

Methohexital Sodium (Patients undergoing regional anesthesia should not receive dalteparin sodium for unstable angina or non-Q-wave myocardial infarction due to an increased risk of bleeding associated with the dosage of dalteparin sodium recommended for unstable angina and non-Q-wave myocardial infarction).
No products indexed under this heading.

Mezlocillin Sodium (Dalteparin sodium should be used with care in patients receiving oral anticoagulants, platelet inhibitors, and thrombolytic agents because of an increased risk of bleeding).
No products indexed under this heading.

Midazolam Hydrochloride (Patients undergoing regional anesthesia should not receive dalteparin sodium for unstable angina or non-Q-wave myocardial infarction due to an increased risk of bleeding associated with the dosage of dalteparin sodium recommended for unstable angina and non-Q-wave myocardial infarction).
No products indexed under this heading.

Nafcillin Sodium (Dalteparin sodium should be used with care in patients receiving oral anticoagulants, platelet inhibitors, and thrombolytic agents because of an increased risk of bleeding).
No products indexed under this heading.

Naproxen (Dalteparin sodium should be used with care in patients receiving oral anticoagulants, platelet inhibitors, and thrombolytic agents because of an increased risk of bleeding). Products include:
EC-Naprosyn Delayed-Release Tablets 2632
Naprosyn Suspension 2632
Naprosyn Tablets 2632

Naproxen Sodium (Dalteparin sodium should be used with care in patients receiving oral anticoagulants, platelet inhibitors, and thrombolytic agents because of an increased risk of bleeding). Products include:
Anaprox Tablets 2632
Anaprox DS Tablets 2632
Treximet Tablets 1616

Penicillin G Benzathine (Dalteparin sodium should be used with care in patients receiving oral anticoagulants, platelet inhibitors, and thrombolytic agents because of an increased risk of bleeding). Products include:
Bicillin C-R Injectable Suspension 1775
Bicillin L-A Injection 1777

Penicillin G Procaine (Dalteparin sodium should be used with care in patients receiving oral anticoagulants, platelet inhibitors, and thrombolytic agents because of an increased risk of bleeding). Products include:
Bicillin C-R Injectable Suspension 1775
Bicillin L-A Injection 1777

Phenylbutazone (Dalteparin sodium should be used with care in patients receiving oral anticoagulants, platelet inhibitors, and thrombolytic agents because of an increased risk of bleeding).
No products indexed under this heading.

Piroxicam (Dalteparin sodium should be used with care in patients receiving oral anticoagulants, platelet inhibitors, and thrombolytic agents because of an increased risk of bleeding).
No products indexed under this heading.

Propofol (Patients undergoing regional anesthesia should not receive dalteparin sodium for unstable angina or non-Q-wave myocardial infarction due to an increased risk of bleeding associated with the dosage of dalteparin sodium recommended for unstable angina and non-Q-wave myocardial infarction).
No products indexed under this heading.

Remifentanil Hydrochloride (Patients undergoing regional anesthesia should not receive dalteparin sodium for unstable angina or non-Q-wave myocardial infarction due to an increased risk of bleeding associated with the dosage of dalteparin sodium recommended for unstable angina and non-Q-wave myocardial infarction).
No products indexed under this heading.

Reteplase (Dalteparin sodium should be used with care in patients receiving oral anticoagulants, platelet inhibitors, and thrombolytic agents because of an increased risk of bleeding).
No products indexed under this heading.

Salsalate (Dalteparin sodium should be used with care in patients receiving oral anticoagulants, platelet inhibitors, and thrombolytic agents because of an increased risk of bleeding).
No products indexed under this heading.

Streptokinase (Dalteparin sodium should be used with care in patients receiving oral anticoagulants, platelet inhibitors, and thrombolytic agents because of an increased risk of bleeding).
No products indexed under this heading.

Sufentanil Citrate (Patients undergoing regional anesthesia should not receive dalteparin sodium for unstable angina or non-Q-wave myocardial infarction due to an increased risk of bleeding associated with the dosage of dalteparin sodium recommended for unstable angina and non-Q-wave myocardial infarction).
No products indexed under this heading.

Sulindac (Dalteparin sodium should be used with care in patients receiving oral anticoagulants, platelet inhibitors, and thrombolytic agents because of an increased risk of bleeding). Products include:

Clinoril Tablets **1962**

Thiamylal Sodium (Patients undergoing regional anesthesia should not receive dalteparin sodium for unstable angina or non-Q-wave myocardial infarction due to an increased risk of bleeding associated with the dosage of dalteparin sodium recommended for unstable angina and non-Q-wave myocardial infarction).

No products indexed under this heading.

Ticarcillin Disodium (Dalteparin sodium should be used with care in patients receiving oral anticoagulants, platelet inhibitors, and thrombolytic agents because of an increased risk of bleeding). Products include:

Timentin ADD-Vantage **1606**
Timentin Injection Galaxy Container **1609**
Timentin IV Infusion **1603**
Timentin Pharmacy Bulk Package **1613**

Ticlopidine Hydrochloride (Dalteparin sodium should be used with care in patients receiving oral anticoagulants, platelet inhibitors, and thrombolytic agents because of an increased risk of bleeding).

No products indexed under this heading.

Tolmetin Sodium (Dalteparin sodium should be used with care in patients receiving oral anticoagulants, platelet inhibitors, and thrombolytic agents because of an increased risk of bleeding).

No products indexed under this heading.

Urokinase (Dalteparin sodium should be used with care in patients receiving oral anticoagulants, platelet inhibitors, and thrombolytic agents because of an increased risk of bleeding).

No products indexed under this heading.

Warfarin Sodium (Dalteparin sodium should be used with care in patients receiving oral anticoagulants, platelet inhibitors, and thrombolytic agents because of an increased risk of bleeding).

No products indexed under this heading.

FRESHKOTE STERILE OPHTHALMIC SOLUTION

(Polyvinyl Alcohol, Povidone) .... ⊙**248**
None cited in PDR database.

FROVA TABLETS

(Frovatriptan Succinate) **1111**
May interact with 5HT1-receptor agonists, ergot-containing drugs, oral contraceptives, Serotonin and Norepinephrine Reuptake Inhibitors, selective serotonin reuptake inhibitors, and certain other agents. Compounds in these categories include:

Almotriptan Malate (Co-administration with other $_{max}$ agonists within 24 hours of each other is contraindicated). Products include:

Axert Tablets **2431**

Citalopram Hydrobromide (The development of a potentially life-threatening serotonin syndrome may occur with triptans, including frovatriptan succinate treatment, particularly during combined use with selective serotonin reuptake inhibitors (SSRIs) or serotonin norepinephrine reuptake inhibitors (SNRIs). If concomitant treatment with FROVA and an SSRI (eg, fluoxetine, paroxetine, sertraline, fluvoxamine, citalopram, escitalopram) or SNRI (eg, venlafaxine, duloxetine) is clinically warranted, careful observation of the patient is advised, particularly during treatment initiation and dose increases). Products include:

Celexa **1160**

Desogestrel (Retrospective analysis of pharmacokinetic data indicates that mean C_{max}x and AUC of frovatriptan are 30% higher in females taking oral contraceptives). Products include:

Mircette Tablets **1034**

Desvenlafaxine Succinate (The development of a potentially life-threatening serotonin syndrome may occur with triptans, including frovatriptan succinate treatment, particularly during combined use with selective serotonin reuptake inhibitors (SSRIs) or serotonin norepinephrine reuptake inhibitors (SNRIs). If concomitant treatment with FROVA and an SSRI (eg, fluoxetine, paroxetine, sertraline, fluvoxamine, citalopram, escitalopram) or SNRI (eg, venlafaxine, duloxetine) is clinically warranted, careful observation of the patient is advised, particularly during treatment initiation and dose increases). Products include:

Pristiq Extended-Release Tablets **3247**

Dihydroergotamine Mesylate (Ergot-containing drugs have been reported to cause prolonged vasospastic reactions; because there is a theoretical basis that these effects may be additive, use of ergot-type agents and frovatriptan within 24 hours is contraindicated).

No products indexed under this heading.

Duloxetine Hydrochloride (The development of a potentially life-threatening serotonin syndrome may occur with triptans, including frovatriptan succinate treatment, particularly during combined use with selective serotonin reuptake inhibitors (SSRIs) or serotonin norepinephrine reuptake inhibitors (SNRIs). If concomitant treatment with FROVA and an SSRI (eg, fluoxetine, paroxetine, sertraline, fluvoxamine, citalopram, escitalopram) or SNRI (eg, venlafaxine, duloxetine) is clinically warranted, careful observation of the patient is advised, particularly during treatment initiation and dose increases). Products include:

Cymbalta Delayed-Release Capsules.................................. **1801**

Eletriptan Hydrobromide (Co-administration with other $_{max}$ agonists within 24 hours of each other is contraindicated).

No products indexed under this heading.

Ergonovine Maleate (Ergot-containing drugs have been reported to cause prolonged vasospastic reactions; because there is a theoretical basis that these effects may be additive, use of ergot-type agents and frovatriptan within 24 hours is contraindicated).

No products indexed under this heading.

Ergotamine Tartrate (Ergot-containing drugs have been reported to cause prolonged vasospastic reactions; because there is a theoretical basis that these effects may be additive, use of ergot-type agents and frovatriptan within 24 hours is contraindicated).

No products indexed under this heading.

Escitalopram Oxalate (The development of a potentially life-threatening serotonin syndrome may occur with triptans, including frovatriptan succinate treatment, particularly during combined use with selective serotonin reuptake inhibitors (SSRIs) or serotonin norepinephrine reuptake inhibitors (SNRIs). If concomitant treatment with FROVA and an SSRI (eg, fluoxetine, paroxetine, sertraline, fluvoxamine, citalopram, escitalopram) or SNRI (eg, venlafaxine, duloxetine) is clinically warranted, careful observation of the patient is advised, particularly during treatment initiation and dose increases). Products include:

Lexapro Oral Suspension **1174**
Lexapro Tablets **1174**

Ethinyl Estradiol (Retrospective analysis of pharmacokinetic data indicates that mean C_{max} and AUC of frovatriptan are 30% higher in females taking oral contraceptives). Products include:

Lybrel Tablets **3204**
Mircette Tablets **1034**
NuvaRing **2897**
Ortho-Cyclen/Ortho Tri-Cyclen **2449**
Ortho Evra Transdermal System **2437**
Ortho Tri-Cyclen Lo Tablets **2458**
Seasonique Tablets **1046**
Yaz Tablets **805**

Ethynodiol Diacetate (Retrospective analysis of pharmacokinetic data indicates that mean C_{max} and AUC of frovatriptan are 30% higher in females taking oral contraceptives).

No products indexed under this heading.

Fluoxetine (The development of a potentially life-threatening serotonin syndrome may occur with triptans, including frovatriptan succinate treatment, particularly during combined use with selective serotonin reuptake inhibitors (SSRIs) or serotonin norepinephrine reuptake inhibitors (SNRIs). If concomitant treatment with FROVA and an SSRI (eg, fluoxetine, paroxetine, sertraline, fluvoxamine, citalopram, escitalopram) or SNRI (eg, venlafaxine, duloxetine) is clinically warranted, careful observation of the patient is advised, particularly during treatment initiation and dose increases).

No products indexed under this heading.

Fluoxetine Hydrochloride (The development of a potentially life-threatening serotonin syndrome may occur with triptans, including frovatriptan succinate treatment, particularly during combined use with selective serotonin reuptake inhibitors (SSRIs) or serotonin norepinephrine reuptake inhibitors (SNRIs). If concomitant treatment with FROVA and an SSRI (eg, fluoxetine, paroxetine, sertraline, fluvoxamine, citalopram, escitalopram) or SNRI (eg, venlafaxine, duloxetine) is clinically warranted, careful observation of the patient is advised, particularly during treatment initiation and dose increases). Products include:

Prozac Weekly Capsules **1852**
Prozac Pulvules and Liquid **1852**
Symbyax Capsules **1871**

Fluvoxamine Maleate (The development of a potentially life-threatening serotonin syndrome may occur with triptans, including frovatriptan succinate treatment, particularly during combined use with selective serotonin reuptake inhibitors (SSRIs) or serotonin norepinephrine reuptake inhibitors (SNRIs). If concomitant treatment with FROVA and an SSRI (eg, fluoxetine, paroxetine, sertraline, fluvoxamine, citalopram, escitalopram) or SNRI (eg, venlafaxine, duloxetine) is clinically warranted, careful observation of the patient is advised, particularly during treatment initiation and dose increases). Products include:

Luvox CR Extended-Release Capsules..................................... **1759**

Levonorgestrel (Retrospective analysis of pharmacokinetic data indicates that mean C_{max} and AUC of frovatriptan are 30% higher in females taking oral contraceptives). Products include:

Climara Pro Transdermal System **768**
Lybrel Tablets **3204**
Mirena Intrauterine System **779**
Plan B Tablets **1044**
Seasonique Tablets **1046**

Mestranol (Retrospective analysis of pharmacokinetic data indicates that mean C_{max} and AUC of frovatriptan are 30% higher in females taking oral contraceptives).

No products indexed under this heading.

Methylergonovine Maleate (Ergot-containing drugs have been reported to cause prolonged vasospastic reactions; because there is a theoretical basis that these effects may be additive, use of ergot-type agents and frovatriptan within 24 hours is contraindicated).

No products indexed under this heading.

Methysergide Maleate (Ergot-containing drugs have been reported to cause prolonged vasospastic reactions; because there is a theoretical basis that these effects may be additive, use of ergot-type agents and frovatriptan within 24 hours is contraindicated).

No products indexed under this heading.

Naratriptan Hydrochloride (Co-administration with other $_{max}$ agonists within 24 hours of each other is contraindicated). Products include:

Amerge Tablets **1301**

Nefazodone Hydrochloride (The development of a potentially life-threatening serotonin syndrome may occur with triptans, including frovatriptan succinate treatment, particularly during combined use with selective serotonin reuptake inhibitors (SSRIs) or serotonin norepinephrine reuptake inhibitors (SNRIs). If concomitant treatment with FROVA and an SSRI (eg, fluoxetine, paroxetine, sertraline, fluvoxamine, citalopram, escitalopram) or SNRI (eg, venlafaxine, duloxetine) is clinically warranted, careful observation of the patient is advised, particularly during treatment initiation and dose increases).

No products indexed under this heading.

Norethindrone (Retrospective analysis of pharmacokinetic data indicates that mean C_{max} and AUC of frovatriptan are 30% higher in females taking oral contraceptives). Products include:

Ortho Micronor Tablets **2446**

Norethynodrel (Retrospective analysis of pharmacokinetic data indicates that mean C_{max} and AUC of frovatriptan are 30% higher in females taking oral contraceptives).

No products indexed under this heading.

Norgestimate (Retrospective analysis of pharmacokinetic data indicates that mean C_{max} and AUC of frovatriptan are 30% higher in females taking oral contraceptives). Products include:

Ortho-Cyclen/Ortho Tri-Cyclen **2449**
Ortho Tri-Cyclen Lo Tablets **2458**

Norgestrel (Retrospective analysis of pharmacokinetic data indicates that mean C_{max} and AUC of frovatriptan are 30% higher in females taking oral contraceptives).

No products indexed under this heading.

Paroxetine Hydrochloride (The development of a potentially life-threatening serotonin syndrome may occur with triptans, including frovatriptan succinate treatment, particularly during combined use with selective serotonin reuptake inhibitors (SSRIs) or serotonin norepinephrine reuptake inhibitors (SNRIs). If concomitant treatment with FROVA and an SSRI (eg, fluoxetine, paroxetine, sertraline, fluvoxamine, citalopram, escitalopram) or SNRI (eg, venlafaxine, duloxetine) is clinically warranted, careful observation of the patient is advised, particularly during treatment initiation and dose increases). Products include:

Paxil **1535**
Paxil CR Controlled-Release Tablets **1544**

Propranolol Hydrochloride (Increases AUC of frovatriptan in males by 60% and in females by 29%; C_{max} was increased by 23% in males and 16% in females). Products include:

InnoPran XL Extended Release Capsules **1484**

Rizatriptan Benzoate (Co-administration with other $_{max}$ agonists within 24 hours of each other is contraindicated). Products include:

Maxalt Tablets **2056**
Maxalt-MLT Orally Disintegrating Tablets **2056**

Sertraline Hydrochloride (The development of a potentially life-threatening serotonin syndrome may occur with triptans, including frovatriptan succinate treatment, particularly during combined use with selective serotonin reuptake inhibitors (SSRIs) or serotonin norepinephrine reuptake inhibitors (SNRIs). If concomitant treatment with FROVA and an SSRI (eg, fluoxetine, paroxetine, sertraline, fluvoxamine, citalopram, escitalopram) or SNRI (eg, venlafaxine, duloxetine) is clinically warranted, careful observation of the patient is advised, particularly during treatment initiation and dose increases).

No products indexed under this heading.

Sumatriptan (Co-administration with other $_{max}$ agonists within 24 hours of each other is contraindicated). Products include:

Imitrex Nasal Spray **1470**

Sumatriptan Succinate (Co-administration with other $_{max}$ agonists within 24 hours of each other is contraindicated). Products include:

Imitrex Injection **1465**
Imitrex Tablets **1474**
Treximet Tablets **1616**

Venlafaxine Hydrochloride (The development of a potentially life-threatening serotonin syndrome may occur with triptans, including frovatriptan succinate treatment, particularly during combined use with selective serotonin reuptake inhibitors (SSRIs) or serotonin norepinephrine reuptake inhibitors (SNRIs). If concomitant treatment with FROVA and an SSRI (eg, fluoxetine, paroxetine, sertraline, fluvoxamine, citalopram, escitalopram) or SNRI (eg, venlafaxine, duloxetine) is clinically warranted, careful observation of the patient is advised, particularly during treatment initiation and dose increases). Products include:

Effexor XR Extended-Release Capsules **3195**
Venlafaxine Hydrochloride Tablets ... **2199**

Zolmitriptan (Co-administration with other $_{max}$ agonists within 24 hours of each other is contraindicated). Products include:

Zomig Tablets **694**
Zomig Nasal Spray **689**
Zomig-ZMT Tablets **694**

FUROSEMIDE TABLETS

(Furosemide) **2186**

May interact with aminoglycosides, antihypertensives, barbiturates, corticosteroids, cardiac glycosides, lithium preparations, narcotic analgesics, non-steroidal anti-inflammatory agents, salicylates, and certain other agents. Compounds in these categories include:

Acebutolol Hydrochloride (Furosemide may add to or potentiate the therapeutic effect of other antihypertensive drugs).

No products indexed under this heading.

ACTH (Co-administration with ACTH may increase the risk of hypokalemia).

No products indexed under this heading.

Alfentanil Hydrochloride (Aggravates orthostatic hypotension).

No products indexed under this heading.

Aliskiren (Furosemide may add to or potentiate the therapeutic effect of other antihypertensive drugs). Products include:

Tekturna Tablets **2321**
Tekturna HCT Tablets **2324**

Amikacin Sulfate (Potential for increased risk of ototoxicity with concomitant therapy, especially in the presence of impaired renal function; avoid concurrent use except in presence of life threatening situations).

No products indexed under this heading.

Amlodipine Besylate (Furosemide may add to or potentiate the therapeutic effect of other antihypertensive drugs). Products include:

Azor Tablets **1005**
Exforge Tablets **2238**

Aprobarbital (Aggravates orthostatic hypotension).

No products indexed under this heading.

Aspirin (Combination of furosemide and aspirin temporarily reduced creatinine clearance in patients with chronic renal insufficiency; co-administration in patients receiving high doses of salicylates may experience salicylate toxicity). Products include:

Aggrenox Capsules **819**
Bayer Aspirin **750**
Percodan Tablets **1130**
St. Joseph 81 mg Aspirin Chewable and Enteric Coated Tablets **1903**

Aspirin, Enteric Coated (Co-administration in patients receiving high doses of salicylates may experience salicylate toxicity).

No products indexed under this heading.

Aspirin Buffered (Co-administration in patients receiving high doses of salicylates may experience salicylate toxicity).

No products indexed under this heading.

Atenolol (Furosemide may add to or potentiate the therapeutic effect of other antihypertensive drugs).

No products indexed under this heading.

Benazepril Hydrochloride (Furosemide may add to or potentiate the therapeutic effect of other antihypertensive drugs).

No products indexed under this heading.

Bendroflumethiazide (Furosemide may add to or potentiate the therapeutic effect of other antihypertensive drugs).

No products indexed under this heading.

Betamethasone Acetate (Co-administration with corticosteroids may increase the risk of hypokalemia).

No products indexed under this heading.

Betamethasone Sodium Phosphate (Co-administration with corticosteroids may increase the risk of hypokalemia).

No products indexed under this heading.

Betaxolol Hydrochloride (Furosemide may add to or potentiate the therapeutic effect of other antihypertensive drugs).

No products indexed under this heading.

Bisoprolol Fumarate (Furosemide may add to or potentiate the therapeutic effect of other antihypertensive drugs).

No products indexed under this heading.

Budesonide (Co-administration with corticosteroids may increase the risk of hypokalemia). Products include:

Pulmicort Flexhaler **654**
Symbicort 80/4.5 Inhalation Aerosol **659**
Symbicort 160/4.5 Inhalation Aerosol **659**

Buprenorphine Hydrochloride (Aggravates orthostatic hypotension). Products include:

Suboxone Tablets **2601**
Subutex Tablets **2601**

Butabarbital (Aggravates orthostatic hypotension).

No products indexed under this heading.

Butalbital (Aggravates orthostatic hypotension).

No products indexed under this heading.

Candesartan Cilexetil (Furosemide may add to or potentiate the therapeutic effect of other antihypertensive drugs). Products include:

Atacand Tablets **639**
Atacand HCT **642**

Captopril (Furosemide may add to or potentiate the therapeutic effect of other antihypertensive drugs). Products include:

Captopril Tablets **2182**

Carteolol Hydrochloride (Furosemide may add to or potentiate the therapeutic effect of other antihypertensive drugs).

No products indexed under this heading.

Celecoxib (Co-administration with NSAIDs has resulted in increased BUN, serum creatinine and serum potassium levels, and weight gain). Products include:

Celebrex Capsules **2979**

Chlorothiazide (Furosemide may add to or potentiate the therapeutic effect of other antihypertensive drugs).

No products indexed under this heading.

Chlorothiazide Sodium (Furosemide may add to or potentiate the therapeutic effect of other antihypertensive drugs). Products include:

Intravenous Sodium Diuril **2490**

Chlorthalidone (Furosemide may add to or potentiate the therapeutic effect of other antihypertensive drugs). Products include:

Clorpres Tablets **2185**

Choline Magnesium Trisalicylate (Co-administration in patients receiving high doses of salicylates may experience salicylate toxicity).

No products indexed under this heading.

Ciclesonide (Co-administration with corticosteroids may increase the risk of hypokalemia). Products include:

Alvesco Inhalation Aerosol **2985**
Omnaris Nasal Spray **2998**

Clonidine (Furosemide may add to or potentiate the therapeutic effect of other antihypertensive drugs). Products include:

Catapres-TTS **842**

Clonidine Hydrochloride (Furosemide may add to or potentiate the therapeutic effect of other antihypertensive drugs). Products include:

Catapres Tablets **841**
Clorpres Tablets **2185**

Codeine Phosphate (Aggravates orthostatic hypotension). Products include:

Tylenol with Codeine Tablets **2427**

Cortisone Acetate (Co-administration with corticosteroids may increase the risk of hypokalemia).

No products indexed under this heading.

Deserpidine (Furosemide may add to or potentiate the therapeutic effect of other antihypertensive drugs).

No products indexed under this heading.

Deslanoside (Concurrent digitalis therapy may exaggerate metabolic effects of hypokalemia, especially myocardial effects).
No products indexed under this heading.

Dexamethasone (Co-administration with corticosteroids may increase the risk of hypokalemia). Products include:
Ciprodex Otic Suspension 541

Dexamethasone Acetate (Co-administration with corticosteroids may increase the risk of hypokalemia).
No products indexed under this heading.

Dexamethasone Sodium Phosphate (Co-administration with corticosteroids may increase the risk of hypokalemia).
No products indexed under this heading.

Dezocine (Aggravates orthostatic hypotension).
No products indexed under this heading.

Diazoxide (Furosemide may add to or potentiate the therapeutic effect of other antihypertensive drugs). Products include:
Proglycem Capsules 1185
Proglycem Suspension 1185

Diclofenac Epolamine (Co-administration with NSAIDs has resulted in increased BUN, serum creatinine and serum potassium levels, and weight gain). Products include:
Flector Patch 561

Diclofenac Potassium (Co-administration with NSAIDs has resulted in increased BUN, serum creatinine and serum potassium levels, and weight gain).
No products indexed under this heading.

Diclofenac Sodium (Co-administration with NSAIDs has resulted in increased BUN, serum creatinine and serum potassium levels, and weight gain). Products include:
Diclofenac Sodium Ophthalmic Solution..................................... ⊙240
Voltaren Ophthalmic Solution 2336
Voltaren Tablets 2334
Voltaren-XR Tablets 2337

Diflunisal (Co-administration in patients receiving high doses of salicylates may experience salicylate toxicity).
No products indexed under this heading.

Digitalis Glycoside Preparations (Concurrent digitalis therapy may exaggerate metabolic effects of hypokalemia, especially myocardial effects).
No products indexed under this heading.

Digitoxin (Concurrent digitalis therapy may exaggerate metabolic effects of hypokalemia, especially myocardial effects).
No products indexed under this heading.

Digoxin (Concurrent digitalis therapy may exaggerate metabolic effects of hypokalemia, especially myocardial effects). Products include:
Lanoxin Injection 1498
Lanoxin Injection Pediatric 1502
Lanoxin Tablets 1505

Diltiazem Hydrochloride (Furosemide may add to or potentiate the therapeutic effect of other antihypertensive drugs). Products include:
Cardizem LA Extended Release Tablets 421

Doxazosin Mesylate (Furosemide may add to or potentiate the therapeutic effect of other antihypertensive drugs).
No products indexed under this heading.

Enalapril Maleate (Furosemide may add to or potentiate the therapeutic effect of other antihypertensive drugs).
No products indexed under this heading.

Enalaprilat (Furosemide may add to or potentiate the therapeutic effect of other antihypertensive drugs).
No products indexed under this heading.

Eprosartan Mesylate (Furosemide may add to or potentiate the therapeutic effect of other antihypertensive drugs). Products include:
Teveten Tablets 515
Teveten HCT Tablets 517

Esmolol Hydrochloride (Furosemide may add to or potentiate the therapeutic effect of other antihypertensive drugs).
No products indexed under this heading.

Ethacrynic Acid (Potential for increased risk of ototoxicity with concomitant therapy; concurrent use should be avoided). Products include:
Edecrin Tablets 698

Etodolac (Co-administration with NSAIDs has resulted in increased BUN, serum creatinine and serum potassium levels, and weight gain).
No products indexed under this heading.

Felodipine (Furosemide may add to or potentiate the therapeutic effect of other antihypertensive drugs).
No products indexed under this heading.

Fenoprofen Calcium (Co-administration with NSAIDs has resulted in increased BUN, serum creatinine and serum potassium levels, and weight gain). Products include:
Nalfon Capsules 2508

Fentanyl (Aggravates orthostatic hypotension). Products include:
Duragesic Transdermal System 2405
Ionsys Transdermal System 2410

Fentanyl Citrate (Aggravates orthostatic hypotension). Products include:
Actiq 959
Fentora Tablets 968

Fludrocortisone Acetate (Co-administration with corticosteroids may increase the risk of hypokalemia).
No products indexed under this heading.

Flunisolide (Co-administration with corticosteroids may increase the risk of hypokalemia). Products include:
Aerobid/Aerobid-M 1153

Flurbiprofen (Co-administration with NSAIDs has resulted in increased BUN, serum creatinine and serum potassium levels, and weight gain).
No products indexed under this heading.

Fluticasone Propionate (Co-administration with corticosteroids may increase the risk of hypokalemia). Products include:
Advair Diskus 100/50 1276
Advair Diskus 250/50 1276
Advair Diskus 500/50 1276
Advair HFA 45/21 Inhalation Aerosol.. 1288
Advair HFA 115/21 Inhalation Aerosol.. 1288
Advair HFA 230/21 Inhalation Aerosol.. 1288
Flonase Nasal Spray 1431
Flovent Diskus 50 mcg 1435

Fluticasone Propionate HFA (Co-administration with corticosteroids may increase the risk of hypokalemia). Products include:
Flovent HFA 1440

Fosinopril Sodium (Furosemide may add to or potentiate the therapeutic effect of other antihypertensive drugs).
No products indexed under this heading.

Gentamicin Sulfate (Potential for increased risk of ototoxicity with concomitant therapy, especially in the presence of impaired renal function; avoid concurrent use except in presence of life threatening situations). Products include:
Pred-G Ophthalmic Ointment .... ⊙229
Pred-G Ophthalmic Suspension ...... ⊙228

Guanabenz Acetate (Furosemide may add to or potentiate the therapeutic effect of other antihypertensive drugs).
No products indexed under this heading.

Guanethidine Monosulfate (Furosemide may add to or potentiate the therapeutic effect of other antihypertensive drugs).
No products indexed under this heading.

Hydralazine Hydrochloride (Furosemide may add to or potentiate the therapeutic effect of other antihypertensive drugs).
No products indexed under this heading.

Hydrochlorothiazide (Furosemide may add to or potentiate the therapeutic effect of other antihypertensive drugs). Products include:
Atacand HCT 642
Avalide Tablets 892
Avalide Tablets 2713
Benicar HCT Tablets 1010
Diovan HCT Tablets 2216
Dyazide Capsules 1405
Micardis HCT Tablets 854
Prinzide Tablets 2092
Tekturna HCT Tablets 2324
Teveten HCT Tablets 517

Hydrocodone Bitartrate (Aggravates orthostatic hypotension). Products include:
Lortab 5/500 Tablets 3143
Lortab 7.5/500 Tablets 3144
Lortab 10/500 Tablets 3144
Vicodin Tablets 529
Vicodin ES Tablets 530
Vicodin HP Tablets 531
Vicoprofen Tablets 533
Zydone Tablets 1132

Hydrocodone Polistirex (Aggravates orthostatic hypotension). Products include:
Tussionex Pennkinetic Extended-Release Suspension 3154

Hydrocortisone (Co-administration with corticosteroids may increase the risk of hypokalemia).
No products indexed under this heading.

Hydrocortisone Acetate (Co-administration with corticosteroids may increase the risk of hypokalemia). Products include:
Analpram-HC 1140
Pramosone 1141

Hydrocortisone Sodium Phosphate (Co-administration with corticosteroids may increase the risk of hypokalemia).
No products indexed under this heading.

Hydrocortisone Sodium Succinate (Co-administration with corticosteroids may increase the risk of hypokalemia).
No products indexed under this heading.

Hydroflumethiazide (Furosemide may add to or potentiate the therapeutic effect of other antihypertensive drugs).
No products indexed under this heading.

Hydromorphone Hydrochloride (Aggravates orthostatic hypotension).
No products indexed under this heading.

Ibuprofen (Co-administration with NSAIDs has resulted in increased BUN, serum creatinine and serum potassium levels, and weight gain). Products include:
Motrin IB Tablets and Caplets 1900
Children's Motrin Oral Suspension ... 1901
Children's Motrin Non-Staining Dye-Free Oral Suspension............ 1901
Children's Motrin Cold Oral Suspension 1899
Infants' Motrin Concentrated Drops... 1901
Infants' Motrin Non-Staining Dye-Free Concentrated Drops....... 1901
Junior Strength Motrin Caplets and Chewable Tablets................. 1901
Vicoprofen Tablets 533

Indapamide (Furosemide may add to or potentiate the therapeutic effect of other antihypertensive drugs). Products include:
Indapamide Tablets 2188

Indomethacin (Co-administration may educe the natriuretic and antihypertensive effects of furosemide in some patients by inhibiting prostaglandin synthesis). Products include:
Indocin 2024

Indomethacin Sodium Trihydrate (Co-administration with NSAIDs has resulted in increased BUN, serum creatinine and serum potassium levels, and weight gain). Products include:
Indocin I.V. 2489

Irbesartan (Furosemide may add to or potentiate the therapeutic effect of other antihypertensive drugs). Products include:
Avalide Tablets 892
Avalide Tablets 2713
Avapro Tablets 897
Avapro Tablets 2718

Isradipine (Furosemide may add to or potentiate the therapeutic effect of other antihypertensive drugs). Products include:
DynaCirc CR Controlled Release Tablets 1407

IMPORTANT NOTE: Always consult each drug listing in the patient's regimen for possible interactions.

Kanamycin Sulfate (Potential for increased risk of ototoxicity with concomitant therapy, especially in the presence of impaired renal function; avoid concurrent use except in presence of life threatening situations).
No products indexed under this heading.

Ketoprofen (Co-administration with NSAIDs has resulted in increased BUN, serum creatinine and serum potassium levels, and weight gain).
No products indexed under this heading.

Ketorolac Tromethamine (Co-administration with NSAIDs has resulted in increased BUN, serum creatinine and serum potassium levels, and weight gain).
No products indexed under this heading.

Labetalol Hydrochloride (Furosemide may add to or potentiate the therapeutic effect of other antihypertensive drugs).
No products indexed under this heading.

Levorphanol Tartrate (Aggravates orthostatic hypotension).
No products indexed under this heading.

Lisinopril (Furosemide may add to or potentiate the therapeutic effect of other antihypertensive drugs). Products include:
Prinivil Tablets 2087
Prinzide Tablets 2092

Lithium (Diuretics reduce lithium's renal clearance and add a high risk of lithium toxicity).
No products indexed under this heading.

Lithium Carbonate (Diuretics reduce lithium's renal clearance and add a high risk of lithium toxicity).
No products indexed under this heading.

Lithium Citrate (Diuretics reduce lithium's renal clearance and add a high risk of lithium toxicity).
No products indexed under this heading.

Losartan Potassium (Furosemide may add to or potentiate the therapeutic effect of other antihypertensive drugs). Products include:
Cozaar Tablets 1973

Magnesium Salicylate (Co-administration in patients receiving high doses of salicylates may experience salicylate toxicity).
No products indexed under this heading.

Mecamylamine Hydrochloride (Furosemide may add to or potentiate the therapeutic effect of other antihypertensive drugs).
No products indexed under this heading.

Meclofenamate Sodium (Co-administration with NSAIDs has resulted in increased BUN, serum creatinine and serum potassium levels, and weight gain).
No products indexed under this heading.

Mefenamic Acid (Co-administration with NSAIDs has resulted in increased BUN, serum creatinine and serum potassium levels, and weight gain).
No products indexed under this heading.

Meloxicam (Co-administration with NSAIDs has resulted in increased BUN, serum creatinine and serum potassium levels, and weight gain). Products include:
Mobic Oral Suspension 863
Mobic Tablets 863

Meperidine Hydrochloride (Aggravates orthostatic hypotension).
No products indexed under this heading.

Mephobarbital (Aggravates orthostatic hypotension).
No products indexed under this heading.

Methadone Hydrochloride (Aggravates orthostatic hypotension).
No products indexed under this heading.

Methyclothiazide (Furosemide may add to or potentiate the therapeutic effect of other antihypertensive drugs).
No products indexed under this heading.

Methyldopa (Furosemide may add to or potentiate the therapeutic effect of other antihypertensive drugs).
No products indexed under this heading.

Methyldopate Hydrochloride (Furosemide may add to or potentiate the therapeutic effect of other antihypertensive drugs).
No products indexed under this heading.

Methylprednisolone Acetate (Co-administration with corticosteroids may increase the risk of hypokalemia).
No products indexed under this heading.

Methylprednisolone Sodium Succinate (Co-administration with corticosteroids may increase the risk of hypokalemia).
No products indexed under this heading.

Metolazone (Furosemide may add to or potentiate the therapeutic effect of other antihypertensive drugs).
No products indexed under this heading.

Metoprolol Succinate (Furosemide may add to or potentiate the therapeutic effect of other antihypertensive drugs). Products include:
Toprol-XL Tablets 666

Metoprolol Tartrate (Furosemide may add to or potentiate the therapeutic effect of other antihypertensive drugs).
No products indexed under this heading.

Metyrosine (Furosemide may add to or potentiate the therapeutic effect of other antihypertensive drugs). Products include:
Demser Capsules 1989

Mibefradil Dihydrochloride (Furosemide may add to or potentiate the therapeutic effect of other antihypertensive drugs).
No products indexed under this heading.

Minoxidil (Furosemide may add to or potentiate the therapeutic effect of other antihypertensive drugs).
No products indexed under this heading.

Moexipril Hydrochloride (Furosemide may add to or potentiate the therapeutic effect of other antihypertensive drugs).
No products indexed under this heading.

Mometasone Furoate (Co-administration with corticosteroids may increase the risk of hypokalemia). Products include:
Asmanex Twisthaler 2797
Elocon Cream 0.1% 2840
Elocon Lotion 0.1% 2841
Elocon Ointment 0.1% 2842

Mometasone Furoate Monohydrate (Co-administration with corticosteroids may increase the risk of hypokalemia). Products include:
Nasonex Nasal Spray 2883

Morphine Sulfate (Aggravates orthostatic hypotension). Products include:
Avinza Capsules 1772
DepoDur Injection 1095
MS Contin Tablets 2585

Nabumetone (Co-administration with NSAIDs has resulted in increased BUN, serum creatinine and serum potassium levels, and weight gain).
No products indexed under this heading.

Nadolol (Furosemide may add to or potentiate the therapeutic effect of other antihypertensive drugs). Products include:
Nadolol Tablets 2191

Naproxen (Co-administration with NSAIDs has resulted in increased BUN, serum creatinine and serum potassium levels, and weight gain). Products include:
EC-Naprosyn Delayed-Release Tablets 2632
Naprosyn Suspension 2632
Naprosyn Tablets 2632

Naproxen Sodium (Co-administration with NSAIDs has resulted in increased BUN, serum creatinine and serum potassium levels, and weight gain). Products include:
Anaprox Tablets 2632
Anaprox DS Tablets 2632
Treximet Tablets 1616

Nebivolol (Furosemide may add to or potentiate the therapeutic effect of other antihypertensive drugs). Products include:
Bystolic Tablets 1155

Nicardipine Hydrochloride (Furosemide may add to or potentiate the therapeutic effect of other antihypertensive drugs). Products include:
Cardene I.V. 1093

Nifedipine (Furosemide may add to or potentiate the therapeutic effect of other antihypertensive drugs).
No products indexed under this heading.

Nisoldipine (Furosemide may add to or potentiate the therapeutic effect of other antihypertensive drugs). Products include:
Sular Extended Release Tablets 2975

Nitroglycerin (Furosemide may add to or potentiate the therapeutic effect of other antihypertensive drugs). Products include:
Nitro-Dur Transdermal Infusion System 2887
Nitrolingual Pumpspray 2965

Norepinephrine Bitartrate (Furosemide may decrease arterial responsiveness to norepinephrine).
No products indexed under this heading.

Oxaprozin (Co-administration with NSAIDs has resulted in increased BUN, serum creatinine and serum potassium levels, and weight gain).
No products indexed under this heading.

Oxycodone Hydrochloride (Aggravates orthostatic hypotension). Products include:
OxyContin Tablets 2589
OxyIR Capsules 2593
Percocet Tablets 1127
Percodan Tablets 1130

Penbutolol Sulfate (Furosemide may add to or potentiate the therapeutic effect of other antihypertensive drugs).
No products indexed under this heading.

Pentobarbital Sodium (Aggravates orthostatic hypotension). Products include:
Nembutal Sodium Solution, USP 2494

Perindopril Erbumine (Furosemide may add to or potentiate the therapeutic effect of other antihypertensive drugs). Products include:
Aceon Tablets (2 mg, 4 mg, 8 mg) 3038

Phenobarbital (Aggravates orthostatic hypotension). Products include:
Donnatal Extentabs 2507

Phenoxybenzamine Hydrochloride (Furosemide may add to or potentiate the therapeutic effect of other antihypertensive drugs). Products include:
Dibenzyline Capsules 3188

Phentolamine Mesylate (Furosemide may add to or potentiate the therapeutic effect of other antihypertensive drugs).
No products indexed under this heading.

Phenylbutazone (Co-administration with NSAIDs has resulted in increased BUN, serum creatinine and serum potassium levels, and weight gain).
No products indexed under this heading.

Pindolol (Furosemide may add to or potentiate the therapeutic effect of other antihypertensive drugs).
No products indexed under this heading.

Piroxicam (Co-administration with NSAIDs has resulted in increased BUN, serum creatinine and serum potassium levels, and weight gain).
No products indexed under this heading.

Polythiazide (Furosemide may add to or potentiate the therapeutic effect of other antihypertensive drugs).
No products indexed under this heading.

Prazosin Hydrochloride (Furosemide may add to or potentiate the therapeutic effect of other antihypertensive drugs).
No products indexed under this heading.

Prednisolone Acetate (Co-administration with corticosteroids may increase the risk of hypokalemia). Products include:
Pred Forte Ophthalmic Suspension .... ⊙ 227
Pred Mild Ophthalmic Suspension .... ⊙ 230
Pred-G Ophthalmic Ointment .... ⊙ 229
Pred-G Ophthalmic Suspension ...... ⊙ 228

Prednisolone Sodium Phosphate (Co-administration with corticosteroids may increase the risk of hypokalemia).
No products indexed under this heading.

Prednisolone Tebutate (Co-administration with corticosteroids may increase the risk of hypokalemia).
No products indexed under this heading.

Prednisone (Co-administration with corticosteroids may increase the risk of hypokalemia).
No products indexed under this heading.

Propoxyphene Hydrochloride (Aggravates orthostatic hypotension).
No products indexed under this heading.

Propoxyphene Napsylate (Aggravates orthostatic hypotension).
No products indexed under this heading.

Propranolol Hydrochloride (Furosemide may add to or potentiate the therapeutic effect of other antihypertensive drugs). Products include:
InnoPran XL Extended Release Capsules **1484**

Quinapril Hydrochloride (Furosemide may add to or potentiate the therapeutic effect of other antihypertensive drugs).
No products indexed under this heading.

Ramipril (Furosemide may add to or potentiate the therapeutic effect of other antihypertensive drugs).
No products indexed under this heading.

Rauwolfia Serpentina (Furosemide may add to or potentiate the therapeutic effect of other antihypertensive drugs).
No products indexed under this heading.

Remifentanil Hydrochloride (Aggravates orthostatic hypotension).
No products indexed under this heading.

Rescinnamine (Furosemide may add to or potentiate the therapeutic effect of other antihypertensive drugs).
No products indexed under this heading.

Reserpine (Furosemide may add to or potentiate the therapeutic effect of other antihypertensive drugs).
No products indexed under this heading.

Rofecoxib (Co-administration with NSAIDs has resulted in increased BUN, serum creatinine and serum potassium levels, and weight gain).
No products indexed under this heading.

Salsalate (Co-administration in patients receiving high doses of salicylates may experience salicylate toxicity).
No products indexed under this heading.

Secobarbital Sodium (Aggravates orthostatic hypotension).
No products indexed under this heading.

Sodium Nitroprusside (Furosemide may add to or potentiate the therapeutic effect of other antihypertensive drugs).
No products indexed under this heading.

Sotalol Hydrochloride (Furosemide may add to or potentiate the therapeutic effect of other antihypertensive drugs).
No products indexed under this heading.

Spirapril Hydrochloride (Furosemide may add to or potentiate the therapeutic effect of other antihypertensive drugs).
No products indexed under this heading.

Streptomycin Sulfate (Potential for increased risk of ototoxicity with concomitant therapy, especially in the presence of impaired renal function; avoid concurrent use except in presence of life threatening situations).
No products indexed under this heading.

Succinylcholine Chloride (Furosemide has a tendency to potentiate the action of succinylcholine).
No products indexed under this heading.

Sucralfate (Simultaneous administration of sucralfate and furosemide may reduce the natriuretic and antihypertensive effects of furosemide; the intake of these two drugs should be separated by at least two hours). Products include:
Carafate Suspension **706**
Carafate Tablets **707**

Sufentanil Citrate (Aggravates orthostatic hypotension).
No products indexed under this heading.

Sulindac (Co-administration with NSAIDs has resulted in increased BUN, serum creatinine and serum potassium levels, and weight gain). Products include:
Clinoril Tablets **1962**

Telmisartan (Furosemide may add to or potentiate the therapeutic effect of other antihypertensive drugs). Products include:
Micardis Tablets **852**
Micardis HCT Tablets **854**

Terazosin Hydrochloride (Furosemide may add to or potentiate the therapeutic effect of other antihypertensive drugs).
No products indexed under this heading.

Thiamylal Sodium (Aggravates orthostatic hypotension).
No products indexed under this heading.

Timolol Maleate (Furosemide may add to or potentiate the therapeutic effect of other antihypertensive drugs). Products include:
Combigan Ophthalmic Solution **553**
Cosopt Sterile Ophthalmic Solution **1969**
Timoptic Sterile Ophthalmic Solution **2121**
Timoptic in Ocudose **2124**
Timoptic-XE Sterile Ophthalmic Gel Forming Solution **2125**

Tobramycin (Potential for increased risk of ototoxicity with concomitant therapy, especially in the presence of impaired renal function; avoid concurrent use except in presence of life threatening situations). Products include:
Zylet Ophthalmic Suspension .... ⊙ **247**

Tobramycin Sulfate (Potential for increased risk of ototoxicity with concomitant therapy, especially in the presence of impaired renal function; avoid concurrent use except in presence of life threatening situations).
No products indexed under this heading.

Tolmetin Sodium (Co-administration with NSAIDs has resulted in increased BUN, serum creatinine and serum potassium levels, and weight gain).
No products indexed under this heading.

Torsemide (Furosemide may add to or potentiate the therapeutic effect of other antihypertensive drugs). Products include:
Demadex Injection **2630**
Demadex Tablets **2630**

Trandolapril (Furosemide may add to or potentiate the therapeutic effect of other antihypertensive drugs). Products include:
Mavik Tablets **472**
Tarka Tablets **511**

Triamcinolone (Co-administration with corticosteroids may increase the risk of hypokalemia).
No products indexed under this heading.

Triamcinolone Acetonide (Co-administration with corticosteroids may increase the risk of hypokalemia). Products include:
Azmacort Inhalation Aerosol **407**
Nasacort AQ Nasal Spray **2765**
Triesence Injectable Suspension .... ⊙ **209**

Triamcinolone Diacetate (Co-administration with corticosteroids may increase the risk of hypokalemia).
No products indexed under this heading.

Triamcinolone Hexacetonide (Co-administration with corticosteroids may increase the risk of hypokalemia).
No products indexed under this heading.

Trimethaphan Camsylate (Furosemide may add to or potentiate the therapeutic effect of other antihypertensive drugs).
No products indexed under this heading.

Tubocurarine Chloride (Furosemide has a tendency to antagonize the skeletal muscle relaxing effects of tubocurarine).
No products indexed under this heading.

Valdecoxib (Co-administration with NSAIDs has resulted in increased BUN, serum creatinine and serum potassium levels, and weight gain).
No products indexed under this heading.

Valsartan (Furosemide may add to or potentiate the therapeutic effect of other antihypertensive drugs). Products include:
Diovan Tablets **2212**
Diovan HCT Tablets **2216**
Exforge Tablets **2238**

Verapamil Hydrochloride (Furosemide may add to or potentiate the therapeutic effect of other antihypertensive drugs). Products include:
Tarka Tablets **511**

Food Interactions

Alcohol (Aggravates orthostatic hypotension).

GABITRIL TABLETS

(Tiagabine Hydrochloride) **973**
May interact with central nervous system depressants, phenytoin, highly protein bound drugs (selected), valproate, and certain other agents. Compounds in these categories include:

Alfentanil Hydrochloride (Possible additive depressive effects).
No products indexed under this heading.

Alprazolam (Possible additive depressive effects).
No products indexed under this heading.

Amiodarone Hydrochloride (Tiagabine is 96% bound to human plasma protein and therefore has the potential to interact with other highly protein bound compounds. Such an interaction can potentially lead to higher free fractions of either tiagabine or the competing drug).
No products indexed under this heading.

Amitriptyline Hydrochloride (Tiagabine is 96% bound to human plasma protein and therefore has the potential to interact with other highly protein bound compounds. Such an interaction can potentially lead to higher free fractions of either tiagabine or the competing drug).
No products indexed under this heading.

Aprobarbital (Possible additive depressive effects).
No products indexed under this heading.

Atovaquone (Tiagabine is 96% bound to human plasma protein and therefore has the potential to interact with other highly protein bound compounds. Such an interaction can potentially lead to higher free fractions of either tiagabine or the competing drug). Products include:
Malarone Pediatric Tablets **1521**
Malarone Tablets **1521**
Mepron Suspension **1526**

Buprenorphine Hydrochloride (Possible additive depressive effects). Products include:
Suboxone Tablets **2601**
Subutex Tablets **2601**

Buspirone Hydrochloride (Possible additive depressive effects).
No products indexed under this heading.

Butabarbital (Possible additive depressive effects).
No products indexed under this heading.

Butalbital (Possible additive depressive effects).
No products indexed under this heading.

Carbamazepine (Population pharmacokinetic analyses indicate that tiagabine clearance is 60% greater in patients taking carbamazepine with or without other enzyme-inducing antiepileptic drugs; tiagabine had no effect on the steady-state plasma concentrations of carbamazepine or its epoxide metabolite in patients with epilepsy). Products include:
Carbatrol Capsules **3019**
Equetro Extended-Release Capsules **3174**

Cefonicid Sodium (Tiagabine is 96% bound to human plasma protein and therefore has the potential to interact with other highly protein bound compounds. Such an interaction can potentially lead to higher free fractions of either tiagabine or the competing drug).
No products indexed under this heading.

Celecoxib (Tiagabine is 96% bound to human plasma protein and therefore has the potential to interact with other highly protein bound compounds. Such an interaction can potentially lead to higher free fractions of either tiagabine or the competing drug). Products include:
Celebrex Capsules 2979

Chlordiazepoxide (Possible additive depressive effects).
No products indexed under this heading.

Chlordiazepoxide Hydrochloride (Possible additive depressive effects).
No products indexed under this heading.

Chlorpromazine (Possible additive depressive effects).
No products indexed under this heading.

Chlorpromazine Hydrochloride (Possible additive depressive effects).
No products indexed under this heading.

Chlorprothixene (Possible additive depressive effects).
No products indexed under this heading.

Chlorprothixene Hydrochloride (Possible additive depressive effects).
No products indexed under this heading.

Chlorprothixene Lactate (Possible additive depressive effects).
No products indexed under this heading.

Clomipramine Hydrochloride (Tiagabine is 96% bound to human plasma protein and therefore has the potential to interact with other highly protein bound compounds. Such an interaction can potentially lead to higher free fractions of either tiagabine or the competing drug).
No products indexed under this heading.

Clorazepate Dipotassium (Possible additive depressive effects).
No products indexed under this heading.

Clozapine (Possible additive depressive effects).
No products indexed under this heading.

Codeine Phosphate (Possible additive depressive effects). Products include:
Tylenol with Codeine Tablets 2427

Cyclosporine (Tiagabine is 96% bound to human plasma protein and therefore has the potential to interact with other highly protein bound compounds. Such an interaction can potentially lead to higher free fractions of either tiagabine or the competing drug). Products include:
Gengraf Capsules 435
Neoral Oral Solution 2280
Neoral Soft Gelatin Capsules 2280
Restasis Ophthalmic Emulsion 557
Sandimmune 2296

Desflurane (Possible additive depressive effects).
No products indexed under this heading.

Dezocine (Possible additive depressive effects).
No products indexed under this heading.

Diazepam (Possible additive depressive effects). Products include:
Valium Tablets 2658

Diclofenac Potassium (Tiagabine is 96% bound to human plasma protein and therefore has the potential to interact with other highly protein bound compounds. Such an interaction can potentially lead to higher free fractions of either tiagabine or the competing drug).
No products indexed under this heading.

Diclofenac Sodium (Tiagabine is 96% bound to human plasma protein and therefore has the potential to interact with other highly protein bound compounds. Such an interaction can potentially lead to higher free fractions of either tiagabine or the competing drug). Products include:
Diclofenac Sodium Ophthalmic Solution .... ⊙ 240
Voltaren Ophthalmic Solution 2336
Voltaren Tablets 2334
Voltaren-XR Tablets 2337

Dipyridamole (Tiagabine is 96% bound to human plasma protein and therefore has the potential to interact with other highly protein bound compounds. Such an interaction can potentially lead to higher free fractions of either tiagabine or the competing drug). Products include:
Aggrenox Capsules 819
Persantine Tablets 869

Divalproex Sodium (Coadministration of tiagabine in patients taking valproate chronically had no effect on tiagabine pharmacokinetics, but valproate significantly decreased tiagabine binding in vitro from 96.3% to 94.8% which resulted in an increase of approximately 40% in the tiagabine concentrations; the clinical relevance of this in vitro finding is unknown). Products include:
Depakote ER Tablets 423

Droperidol (Possible additive depressive effects).
No products indexed under this heading.

Enflurane (Possible additive depressive effects).
No products indexed under this heading.

Estazolam (Possible additive depressive effects).
No products indexed under this heading.

Ethanol (Possible additive depressive effects).
No products indexed under this heading.

Ethchlorvynol (Possible additive depressive effects).
No products indexed under this heading.

Ethinamate (Possible additive depressive effects).
No products indexed under this heading.

Ethyl Alcohol (Possible additive depressive effects).
No products indexed under this heading.

Fenoprofen Calcium (Tiagabine is 96% bound to human plasma protein and therefore has the potential to interact with other highly protein bound compounds. Such an interaction can potentially lead to higher free fractions of either tiagabine or the competing drug). Products include:
Nalfon Capsules 2508

Fentanyl (Possible additive depressive effects). Products include:
Duragesic Transdermal System 2405
Ionsys Transdermal System 2410

Fentanyl Citrate (Possible additive depressive effects). Products include:
Actiq 959
Fentora Tablets 968

Fluphenazine Decanoate (Possible additive depressive effects).
No products indexed under this heading.

Fluphenazine Enanthate (Possible additive depressive effects).
No products indexed under this heading.

Fluphenazine Hydrochloride (Possible additive depressive effects).
No products indexed under this heading.

Flurazepam Hydrochloride (Possible additive depressive effects).
No products indexed under this heading.

Flurbiprofen (Tiagabine is 96% bound to human plasma protein and therefore has the potential to interact with other highly protein bound compounds. Such an interaction can potentially lead to higher free fractions of either tiagabine or the competing drug).
No products indexed under this heading.

Fosphenytoin Sodium (Population pharmacokinetic analyses indicate that tiagabine clearance is 60% greater in patients taking phenytoin with or without other enzyme-inducing antiepileptic drugs; tiagabine had no effect on the steady-state plasma concentrations of phenytoin in patients with epilepsy).
No products indexed under this heading.

Glipizide (Tiagabine is 96% bound to human plasma protein and therefore has the potential to interact with other highly protein bound compounds. Such an interaction can potentially lead to higher free fractions of either tiagabine or the competing drug).
No products indexed under this heading.

Glutethimide (Possible additive depressive effects).
No products indexed under this heading.

Haloperidol (Possible additive depressive effects).
No products indexed under this heading.

Haloperidol Decanoate (Possible additive depressive effects).
No products indexed under this heading.

Hydrocodone Bitartrate (Possible additive depressive effects). Products include:
Lortab 5/500 Tablets 3143
Lortab 7.5/500 Tablets 3144
Lortab 10/500 Tablets 3144
Vicodin Tablets 529
Vicodin ES Tablets 530
Vicodin HP Tablets 531
Vicoprofen Tablets 533
Zydone Tablets 1132

Hydrocodone Polistirex (Possible additive depressive effects). Products include:
Tussionex Pennkinetic Extended-Release Suspension 3154

Hydromorphone Hydrochloride (Possible additive depressive effects).
No products indexed under this heading.

Hydroxyzine Hydrochloride (Possible additive depressive effects).
No products indexed under this heading.

Ibuprofen (Tiagabine is 96% bound to human plasma protein and therefore has the potential to interact with other highly protein bound compounds. Such an interaction can potentially lead to higher free fractions of either tiagabine or the competing drug). Products include:
Motrin IB Tablets and Caplets 1900
Children's Motrin Oral Suspension 1901
Children's Motrin Non-Staining Dye-Free Oral Suspension 1901
Children's Motrin Cold Oral Suspension 1899
Infants' Motrin Concentrated Drops 1901
Infants' Motrin Non-Staining Dye-Free Concentrated Drops 1901
Junior Strength Motrin Caplets and Chewable Tablets 1901
Vicoprofen Tablets 533

Imipramine Hydrochloride (Tiagabine is 96% bound to human plasma protein and therefore has the potential to interact with other highly protein bound compounds. Such an interaction can potentially lead to higher free fractions of either tiagabine or the competing drug).
No products indexed under this heading.

Imipramine Pamoate (Tiagabine is 96% bound to human plasma protein and therefore has the potential to interact with other highly protein bound compounds. Such an interaction can potentially lead to higher free fractions of either tiagabine or the competing drug).
No products indexed under this heading.

Indomethacin (Tiagabine is 96% bound to human plasma protein and therefore has the potential to interact with other highly protein bound compounds. Such an interaction can potentially lead to higher free fractions of either tiagabine or the competing drug). Products include:
Indocin 2024

Indomethacin Sodium Trihydrate (Tiagabine is 96% bound to human plasma protein and therefore has the potential to interact with other highly protein bound compounds. Such an interaction can potentially lead to higher free fractions of either tiagabine or the competing drug). Products include:
Indocin I.V. 2489

Isoflurane (Possible additive depressive effects).
No products indexed under this heading.

Ketamine Hydrochloride (Possible additive depressive effects).
No products indexed under this heading.

Ketoprofen (Tiagabine is 96% bound to human plasma protein and therefore has the potential to interact with other highly protein bound compounds. Such an interaction can potentially lead to higher free fractions of either tiagabine or the competing drug).
No products indexed under this heading.

Ketorolac Tromethamine (Tiagabine is 96% bound to human plasma protein and therefore has the potential to interact with other highly protein bound compounds. Such an interaction can potentially lead to higher free fractions of either tiagabine or the competing drug).
No products indexed under this heading.

Levomethadyl Acetate Hydrochloride (Possible additive depressive effects).
No products indexed under this heading.

Levorphanol Tartrate (Possible additive depressive effects).
No products indexed under this heading.

Lorazepam (Possible additive depressive effects).
No products indexed under this heading.

Loxapine Hydrochloride (Possible additive depressive effects).
No products indexed under this heading.

Loxapine Succinate (Possible additive depressive effects).
No products indexed under this heading.

Meclofenamate Sodium (Tiagabine is 96% bound to human plasma protein and therefore has the potential to interact with other highly protein bound compounds. Such an interaction can potentially lead to higher free fractions of either tiagabine or the competing drug).
No products indexed under this heading.

Mefenamic Acid (Tiagabine is 96% bound to human plasma protein and therefore has the potential to interact with other highly protein bound compounds. Such an interaction can potentially lead to higher free fractions of either tiagabine or the competing drug).
No products indexed under this heading.

Meperidine Hydrochloride (Possible additive depressive effects).
No products indexed under this heading.

Mephobarbital (Possible additive depressive effects).
No products indexed under this heading.

Meprobamate (Possible additive depressive effects).
No products indexed under this heading.

Mesoridazine Besylate (Possible additive depressive effects).
No products indexed under this heading.

Methadone Hydrochloride (Possible additive depressive effects).
No products indexed under this heading.

Methohexital Sodium (Possible additive depressive effects).
No products indexed under this heading.

Methotrimeprazine (Possible additive depressive effects).
No products indexed under this heading.

Methoxyflurane (Possible additive depressive effects).
No products indexed under this heading.

Midazolam Hydrochloride (Possible additive depressive effects).
No products indexed under this heading.

Molindone Hydrochloride (Possible additive depressive effects). Products include:
Moban Tablets 1116

Morphine Sulfate (Possible additive depressive effects). Products include:
Avinza Capsules 1772
DepoDur Injection 1095
MS Contin Tablets 2585

Naproxen (Tiagabine is 96% bound to human plasma protein and therefore has the potential to interact with other highly protein bound compounds. Such an interaction can potentially lead to higher free fractions of either tiagabine or the competing drug). Products include:
EC-Naprosyn Delayed-Release Tablets 2632
Naprosyn Suspension 2632
Naprosyn Tablets 2632

Naproxen Sodium (Tiagabine is 96% bound to human plasma protein and therefore has the potential to interact with other highly protein bound compounds. Such an interaction can potentially lead to higher free fractions of either tiagabine or the competing drug). Products include:
Anaprox Tablets 2632
Anaprox DS Tablets 2632
Treximet Tablets 1616

Nortriptyline Hydrochloride (Tiagabine is 96% bound to human plasma protein and therefore has the potential to interact with other highly protein bound compounds. Such an interaction can potentially lead to higher free fractions of either tiagabine or the competing drug).
No products indexed under this heading.

Olanzapine (Possible additive depressive effects). Products include:
Symbyax Capsules 1871
Zyprexa Tablets 1883
Zyprexa IntraMuscular 1883
Zyprexa ZYDIS Orally Disintegrating Tablets 1883

Oxaprozin (Tiagabine is 96% bound to human plasma protein and therefore has the potential to interact with other highly protein bound compounds. Such an interaction can potentially lead to higher free fractions of either tiagabine or the competing drug).
No products indexed under this heading.

Oxazepam (Possible additive depressive effects).
No products indexed under this heading.

Oxycodone Hydrochloride (Possible additive depressive effects). Products include:
OxyContin Tablets 2589
OxyIR Capsules 2593
Percocet Tablets 1127
Percodan Tablets 1130

Pentobarbital Sodium (Possible additive depressive effects). Products include:
Nembutal Sodium Solution, USP 2494

Perphenazine (Possible additive depressive effects).
No products indexed under this heading.

Phenobarbital (Population pharmacokinetic analyses indicate that tiagabine clearance is 60% greater in patients taking phenobarbital with or without other enzyme-inducing antiepileptic drugs; possible additive depressive effects). Products include:
Donnatal Extentabs 2507

Phenylbutazone (Tiagabine is 96% bound to human plasma protein and therefore has the potential to interact with other highly protein bound compounds. Such an interaction can potentially lead to higher free fractions of either tiagabine or the competing drug).
No products indexed under this heading.

Phenytoin (Population pharmacokinetic analyses indicate that tiagabine clearance is 60% greater in patients taking phenytoin with or without other enzyme-inducing antiepileptic drugs; tiagabine had no effect on the steady-state plasma concentrations of phenytoin in patients with epilepsy).
No products indexed under this heading.

Phenytoin Sodium (Population pharmacokinetic analyses indicate that tiagabine clearance is 60% greater in patients taking phenytoin with or without other enzyme-inducing antiepileptic drugs; tiagabine had no effect on the steady-state plasma concentrations of phenytoin in patients with epilepsy). Products include:
Phenytek Capsules 2192

Piroxicam (Tiagabine is 96% bound to human plasma protein and therefore has the potential to interact with other highly protein bound compounds. Such an interaction can potentially lead to higher free fractions of either tiagabine or the competing drug).
No products indexed under this heading.

Prazepam (Possible additive depressive effects).
No products indexed under this heading.

Prochlorperazine (Possible additive depressive effects).
No products indexed under this heading.

Promethazine Hydrochloride (Possible additive depressive effects).
No products indexed under this heading.

Propofol (Possible additive depressive effects).
No products indexed under this heading.

Propoxyphene Hydrochloride (Possible additive depressive effects).
No products indexed under this heading.

Propoxyphene Napsylate (Possible additive depressive effects).
No products indexed under this heading.

Propranolol Hydrochloride (Tiagabine is 96% bound to human plasma protein and therefore has the potential to interact with other highly protein bound compounds. Such an interaction can potentially lead to higher free fractions of either tiagabine or the competing drug). Products include:
InnoPran XL Extended Release Capsules 1484

Quazepam (Possible additive depressive effects).
No products indexed under this heading.

Quetiapine Fumarate (Possible additive depressive effects).
No products indexed under this heading.

Remifentanil Hydrochloride (Possible additive depressive effects).
No products indexed under this heading.

Risperidone (Possible additive depressive effects). Products include:
Risperdal Consta Long-Acting Injection 1753

Secobarbital Sodium (Possible additive depressive effects).
No products indexed under this heading.

Sevoflurane (Possible additive depressive effects). Products include:
Ultane Liquid for Inhalation 524

Sodium Oxybate (Possible additive depressive effects). Products include:
Xyrem Oral Solution 1766

Sufentanil Citrate (Possible additive depressive effects).
No products indexed under this heading.

Sulindac (Tiagabine is 96% bound to human plasma protein and therefore has the potential to interact with other highly protein bound compounds. Such an interaction can potentially lead to higher free fractions of either tiagabine or the competing drug). Products include:
Clinoril Tablets 1962

Temazepam (Possible additive depressive effects).
No products indexed under this heading.

Thiamylal Sodium (Possible additive depressive effects).
No products indexed under this heading.

Thioridazine Hydrochloride (Possible additive depressive effects). Products include:
Thioridazine Hydrochloride Tablets 2195

Thiothixene (Possible additive depressive effects). Products include:
Thiothixene Capsules 2197

Tolbutamide (Tiagabine is 96% bound to human plasma protein and therefore has the potential to interact with other highly protein bound compounds. Such an interaction can potentially lead to higher free fractions of either tiagabine or the competing drug).
No products indexed under this heading.

Tolmetin Sodium (Tiagabine is 96% bound to human plasma protein and therefore has the potential to interact with other highly protein bound compounds. Such an interaction can potentially lead to higher free fractions of either tiagabine or the competing drug).
No products indexed under this heading.

Triazolam (Possible additive depressive effects).
No products indexed under this heading.

Trifluoperazine Hydrochloride (Possible additive depressive effects).
No products indexed under this heading.

Trimipramine Maleate (Tiagabine is 96% bound to human plasma protein and therefore has the potential to interact with other highly protein bound compounds. Such an interaction can potentially lead to higher free fractions of either tiagabine or the competing drug).
No products indexed under this heading.

Valproate Sodium (Co-administration of tiagabine in patients taking valproate chronically had no effect on tiagabine pharmacokinetics, but valproate significantly decreased tiagabine binding in vitro from 96.3% to 94.8% which resulted in an increase of approximately 40% in the tiagabine concentrations; the clinical relevance of this in vitro finding is unknown).
No products indexed under this heading.

Valproic Acid (Co-administration of tiagabine in patients taking valproate chronically had no effect on tiagabine pharmacokinetics, but valproate significantly decreased tiagabine binding in vitro from 96.3% to 94.8% which resulted in an increase of approximately 40% in the tiagabine concentrations; the clinical relevance of this in vitro finding is unknown).
No products indexed under this heading.

Warfarin Sodium (Tiagabine is 96% bound to human plasma protein and therefore has the potential to interact with other highly protein bound compounds. Such an interaction can potentially lead to higher free fractions of either tiagabine or the competing drug).
No products indexed under this heading.

Zaleplon (Possible additive depressive effects).
No products indexed under this heading.

Ziprasidone Hydrochloride (Possible additive depressive effects). Products include:
Geodon Capsules 2520

Zolpidem Tartrate (Possible additive depressive effects). Products include:
Ambien Tablets 2692
Ambien CR Tablets 2696

Food Interactions

Alcohol (Possible additive depressive effects).

Food, unspecified (A high fat meal decreases the rate (mean Tmax was prolonged to 2.5 hours, and Cmax was reduced by about 40%) but not the extent (AUC) of tiagabine).

GAMMAGARD LIQUID

(Immune Globulin Intravenous (Human)).......................... 730
May interact with vaccines, live. Compounds in these categories include:

BCG Vaccine (Antibodies in immune globulin intravenous products may interfere with patient responses to live vaccines, such as those for measles, mumps and rubella).
No products indexed under this heading.

Influenza Vaccine, Live Attenuated (Antibodies in immune globulin intravenous products may interfere with patient responses to live vaccines, such as those for measles, mumps and rubella).
No products indexed under this heading.

Influenza Virus Vaccine Live, Intranasal (Antibodies in immune globulin intravenous products may interfere with patient responses to live vaccines, such as those for measles, mumps and rubella). Products include:
FluMist Vaccine 1945

Measles, Mumps, Rubella and Varicella Virus Vaccine Live (Antibodies in immune globulin intravenous products may interfere with patient responses to live vaccines, such as those for measles, mumps and rubella). Products include:
ProQuad 2099

Measles, Mumps & Rubella Virus Vaccine, Live (Antibodies in immune globulin intravenous products may interfere with patient responses to live vaccines, such as those for measles, mumps and rubella). Products include:
M-M-R II 2054

Measles & Rubella Virus Vaccine Live (Antibodies in immune globulin intravenous products may interfere with patient responses to live vaccines, such as those for measles, mumps and rubella).
No products indexed under this heading.

Measles Virus Vaccine Live (Antibodies in immune globulin intravenous products may interfere with patient responses to live vaccines, such as those for measles, mumps and rubella). Products include:
Attenuvax 1951

Mumps Virus Vaccine, Live (Antibodies in immune globulin intravenous products may interfere with patient responses to live vaccines, such as those for measles, mumps and rubella). Products include:
Mumpsvax 2068

Poliovirus Vaccine, Live, Oral, Trivalent, Types 1,2,3 (Sabin) (Antibodies in immune globulin intravenous products may interfere with patient responses to live vaccines, such as those for measles, mumps and rubella).
No products indexed under this heading.

Rotavirus Vaccine, Live, Oral, Tetravalent (Antibodies in immune globulin intravenous products may interfere with patient responses to live vaccines, such as those for measles, mumps and rubella).
No products indexed under this heading.

Rubella & Mumps Virus Vaccine Live (Antibodies in immune globulin intravenous products may interfere with patient responses to live vaccines, such as those for measles, mumps and rubella).
No products indexed under this heading.

Rubella Virus Vaccine Live (Antibodies in immune globulin intravenous products may interfere with patient responses to live vaccines, such as those for measles, mumps and rubella). Products include:
Meruvax II 2061

Smallpox Vaccine (Antibodies in immune globulin intravenous products may interfere with patient responses to live vaccines, such as those for measles, mumps and rubella).
No products indexed under this heading.

Typhoid Vaccine (Antibodies in immune globulin intravenous products may interfere with patient responses to live vaccines, such as those for measles, mumps and rubella).
No products indexed under this heading.

Varicella Virus Vaccine Live (Antibodies in immune globulin intravenous products may interfere with patient responses to live vaccines, such as those for measles, mumps and rubella). Products include:
Varivax 2133

Yellow Fever Vaccine (Antibodies in immune globulin intravenous products may interfere with patient responses to live vaccines, such as those for measles, mumps and rubella).
No products indexed under this heading.

Zoster Vaccine Live (Antibodies in immune globulin intravenous products may interfere with patient responses to live vaccines, such as those for measles, mumps and rubella). Products include:
Zostavax Injection 2145

GAMMAGARD S/D

(Immune Globulin Intravenous (Human)).......................... 734
May interact with vaccines, live and certain other agents. Compounds in these categories include:

BCG Vaccine (Antibodies in immune globulin intravenous products may interfere with patient responses to live vaccines, such as those for measles, mumps and rubella).
No products indexed under this heading.

Influenza Vaccine, Live Attenuated (Antibodies in immune globulin intravenous products may interfere with patient responses to live vaccines, such as those for measles, mumps and rubella).
No products indexed under this heading.

Influenza Virus Vaccine Live, Intranasal (Antibodies in immune globulin intravenous products may interfere with patient responses to live vaccines, such as those for measles, mumps and rubella). Products include:
FluMist Vaccine 1945

Measles, Mumps, Rubella and Varicella Virus Vaccine Live (Antibodies in immune globulin intravenous products may interfere with patient responses to live vaccines, such as those for measles, mumps and rubella). Products include:
ProQuad 2099

Measles, Mumps & Rubella Virus Vaccine, Live (Antibodies in immune globulin intravenous products may interfere with patient responses to live vaccines, such as those for measles, mumps and rubella). Products include:
M-M-R II 2054

Measles & Rubella Virus Vaccine Live (Antibodies in immune globulin intravenous products may interfere with patient responses to live vaccines, such as those for measles, mumps and rubella).
No products indexed under this heading.

Measles Virus Vaccine Live (Antibodies in immune globulin intravenous products may interfere with patient responses to live vaccines, such as those for measles, mumps and rubella). Products include:
Attenuvax 1951

Mumps Virus Vaccine, Live (Antibodies in immune globulin intravenous products may interfere with patient responses to live vaccines, such as those for measles, mumps and rubella). Products include:
Mumpsvax 2068

Poliovirus Vaccine, Live, Oral, Trivalent, Types 1,2,3 (Sabin) (Antibodies in immune globulin intravenous products may interfere with patient responses to live vaccines, such as those for measles, mumps and rubella).
No products indexed under this heading.

Rotavirus Vaccine, Live, Oral, Tetravalent (Antibodies in immune globulin intravenous products may interfere with patient responses to live vaccines, such as those for measles, mumps and rubella).
No products indexed under this heading.

Rubella & Mumps Virus Vaccine Live (Antibodies in immune globulin intravenous products may interfere with patient responses to live vaccines, such as those for measles, mumps and rubella).
No products indexed under this heading.

Rubella Virus Vaccine Live (Antibodies in immune globulin intravenous products may interfere with patient responses to live vaccines, such as those for measles, mumps and rubella). Products include:
Meruvax II 2061

Smallpox Vaccine (Antibodies in immune globulin intravenous products may interfere with patient responses to live vaccines, such as those for measles, mumps and rubella).
No products indexed under this heading.

Typhoid Vaccine (Antibodies in immune globulin intravenous products may interfere with patient responses to live vaccines, such as those for measles, mumps and rubella).
No products indexed under this heading.

Varicella Virus Vaccine Live (Antibodies in immune globulin intravenous products may interfere with patient responses to live vaccines, such as those for measles, mumps and rubella). Products include:

Varivax 2133

Yellow Fever Vaccine (Antibodies in immune globulin intravenous products may interfere with patient responses to live vaccines, such as those for measles, mumps and rubella).

No products indexed under this heading.

Zoster Vaccine Live (Antibodies in immune globulin intravenous products may interfere with patient responses to live vaccines, such as those for measles, mumps and rubella). Products include:

Zostavax Injection 2145

GAMUNEX

(Immune Globulin Intravenous (Human)).. 3094

May interact with:

Measles, Mumps & Rubella Virus Vaccine, Live (Co-administration may interfere with the response to live viral vaccines such as measles. Therefore, use of such vaccines should be deferred until approximately 6 months after Immune Globulin Intravenous (Human) administration). Products include:

M-M-R II 2054

Measles & Rubella Virus Vaccine Live (Co-administration may interfere with the response to live viral vaccines such as measles. Therefore, use of such vaccines should be deferred until approximately 6 months after Immune Globulin Intravenous (Human) administration).

No products indexed under this heading.

Measles Virus Vaccine Live (Co-administration may interfere with the response to live viral vaccines such as measles. Therefore, use of such vaccines should be deferred until approximately 6 months after Immune Globulin Intravenous (Human) administration). Products include:

Attenuvax 1951

Mumps Skin Test Antigen (Co-administration may interfere with the response to live viral vaccines such as mumps. Therefore, use of such vaccines should be deferred until approximately 6 months after Immune Globulin Intravenous (Human) administration).

No products indexed under this heading.

Mumps Virus Vaccine, Live (Co-administration may interfere with the response to live viral vaccines such as mumps. Therefore, use of such vaccines should be deferred until approximately 6 months after Immune Globulin Intravenous (Human) administration). Products include:

Mumpsvax 2068

Rubella & Mumps Virus Vaccine Live (Co-administration may interfere with the response to live viral vaccines such as rubella. Therefore, use of such vaccines should be deferred until approximately 6 months after Immune Globulin Intravenous (Human) administration).

No products indexed under this heading.

Rubella Virus Vaccine Live (Co-administration may interfere with the response to live viral vaccines such as rubella. Therefore, use of such vaccines should be deferred until approximately 6 months after Immune Globulin Intravenous (Human) administration). Products include:

Meruvax II 2061

GANTRISIN PEDIATRIC SUSPENSION

(Acetyl Sulfisoxazole) 2638

May interact with anticoagulants, sulfonylureas, and certain other agents. Compounds in these categories include:

Anisindione (Sulfisoxazole may prolong the prothrombin time in patients who are receiving anticoagulants, including warfarin; monitor coagulation tests closely).

No products indexed under this heading.

Ardeparin Sodium (Sulfisoxazole may prolong the prothrombin time in patients who are receiving anticoagulants, including warfarin; monitor coagulation tests closely).

No products indexed under this heading.

Chlorpropamide (Sulfisoxazole may potentiate the hypoglycemic activity of sulfonylureas, as well as cause hypoglycemia by itself).

No products indexed under this heading.

Dalteparin Sodium (Sulfisoxazole may prolong the prothrombin time in patients who are receiving anticoagulants, including warfarin; monitor coagulation tests closely). Products include:

Fragmin Injection 1070

Danaparoid Sodium (Sulfisoxazole may prolong the prothrombin time in patients who are receiving anticoagulants, including warfarin; monitor coagulation tests closely).

No products indexed under this heading.

Dicumarol (Sulfisoxazole may prolong the prothrombin time in patients who are receiving anticoagulants, including warfarin; monitor coagulation tests closely).

No products indexed under this heading.

Enoxaparin Sodium (Sulfisoxazole may prolong the prothrombin time in patients who are receiving anticoagulants, including warfarin; monitor coagulation tests closely). Products include:

Lovenox Injection 2756

Fondaparinux Sodium (Sulfisoxazole may prolong the prothrombin time in patients who are receiving anticoagulants, including warfarin; monitor coagulation tests closely). Products include:

Arixtra Injection 1313

Glimepiride (Sulfisoxazole may potentiate the hypoglycemic activity of sulfonylureas, as well as cause hypoglycemia by itself). Products include:

Avandaryl Tablets 1344

Duetact Tablets 3085

Glipizide (Sulfisoxazole may potentiate the hypoglycemic activity of sulfonylureas, as well as cause hypoglycemia by itself).

No products indexed under this heading.

Glyburide (Sulfisoxazole may potentiate the hypoglycemic activity of sulfonylureas, as well as cause hypoglycemia by itself).

No products indexed under this heading.

Heparin Calcium (Sulfisoxazole may prolong the prothrombin time in patients who are receiving anticoagulants, including warfarin; monitor coagulation tests closely).

No products indexed under this heading.

Heparin Sodium (Sulfisoxazole may prolong the prothrombin time in patients who are receiving anticoagulants, including warfarin; monitor coagulation tests closely).

No products indexed under this heading.

Low Molecular Weight Heparins (Sulfisoxazole may prolong the prothrombin time in patients who are receiving anticoagulants, including warfarin; monitor coagulation tests closely).

No products indexed under this heading.

Methotrexate (Sulfonamides can displace methotrexate from plasma protein-binding sites, thus increasing free methotrexate concentrations. Studies have shown sulfisoxazole infusions to decrease plasma protein-bound methotrexate by one-fourth).

No products indexed under this heading.

Methotrexate Sodium (Sulfonamides can displace methotrexate from plasma protein-binding sites, thus increasing free methotrexate concentrations. Studies have shown sulfisoxazole infusions to decrease plasma protein-bound methotrexate by one-fourth).

No products indexed under this heading.

Sodium Thiopental (Patients receiving sulfisoxazole may require less thiopental for anesthesia since sulfisoxazole may compete with thiopental for plasma protein-binding).

No products indexed under this heading.

Tinzaparin Sodium (Sulfisoxazole may prolong the prothrombin time in patients who are receiving anticoagulants, including warfarin; monitor coagulation tests closely).

No products indexed under this heading.

Tolazamide (Sulfisoxazole may potentiate the hypoglycemic activity of sulfonylureas, as well as cause hypoglycemia by itself).

No products indexed under this heading.

Tolbutamide (Sulfisoxazole may potentiate the hypoglycemic activity of sulfonylureas, as well as cause hypoglycemia by itself).

No products indexed under this heading.

Warfarin Sodium (Sulfisoxazole may prolong the prothrombin time in patients who are receiving anticoagulants, including warfarin; monitor coagulation tests closely).

No products indexed under this heading.

GARDASIL INJECTION

(Quadrivalent Human Papillomavirus (Types 6, 11, 16, 18) Recombinant Vaccine)............... 2019

May interact with alkylating agents, antimetabolites, corticosteroids, cytotoxic drugs, and immunosuppressive agents. Compounds in these categories include:

Azathioprine (Immunosuppressive agents may reduce the immune responses to vaccines).

No products indexed under this heading.

Basiliximab (Immunosuppressive agents may reduce the immune responses to vaccines). Products include:

Simulect for Injection 2306

Betamethasone Acetate (Corticosteroids may reduce the immune responses to vaccines).

No products indexed under this heading.

Betamethasone Sodium Phosphate (Corticosteroids may reduce the immune responses to vaccines).

No products indexed under this heading.

Bleomycin Sulfate (Cytotoxic drugs may reduce the immune responses to vaccines).

No products indexed under this heading.

Budesonide (Corticosteroids may reduce the immune responses to vaccines). Products include:

Pulmicort Flexhaler 654

Symbicort 80/4.5 Inhalation Aerosol.. 659

Symbicort 160/4.5 Inhalation Aerosol.. 659

Busulfan (Alkylating agents may reduce the immune responses to vaccines). Products include:

Busulfex Injection 2477

Myleran Tablets 1530

Capecitabine (Antimetabolites may reduce the immune responses to vaccines). Products include:

Xeloda Tablets 2662

Carmustine (BCNU) (Alkylating agents may reduce the immune responses to vaccines).

No products indexed under this heading.

Chlorambucil (Alkylating agents may reduce the immune responses to vaccines). Products include:

Leukeran Tablets 1508

Ciclesonide (Corticosteroids may reduce the immune responses to vaccines). Products include:

Alvesco Inhalation Aerosol 2985

Omnaris Nasal Spray 2998

Cladribine (Antimetabolites may reduce the immune responses to vaccines). Products include:

Leustatin Injection 2384

Cortisone Acetate (Corticosteroids may reduce the immune responses to vaccines).

No products indexed under this heading.

Cyclophosphamide (Alkylating agents may reduce the immune responses to vaccines).

No products indexed under this heading.

Cyclosporine (Immunosuppressive agents may reduce the immune responses to vaccines). Products include:

Gengraf Capsules 435

Neoral Oral Solution 2280

Neoral Soft Gelatin Capsules 2280

IMPORTANT NOTE: Always consult each drug listing in the patient's regimen for possible interactions.

Restasis Ophthalmic Emulsion 557
Sandimmune 2296

Cytarabine (Antimetabolites may reduce the immune responses to vaccines).
No products indexed under this heading.

Dacarbazine (Alkylating agents may reduce the immune responses to vaccines).
No products indexed under this heading.

Daunorubicin Hydrochloride (Cytotoxic drugs may reduce the immune responses to vaccines).
No products indexed under this heading.

Dexamethasone (Corticosteroids may reduce the immune responses to vaccines). Products include:
Ciprodex Otic Suspension 541

Dexamethasone Acetate (Corticosteroids may reduce the immune responses to vaccines).
No products indexed under this heading.

Dexamethasone Sodium Phosphate (Corticosteroids may reduce the immune responses to vaccines).
No products indexed under this heading.

Doxorubicin Hydrochloride (Cytotoxic drugs may reduce the immune responses to vaccines).
No products indexed under this heading.

Epirubicin Hydrochloride (Cytotoxic drugs may reduce the immune responses to vaccines).
No products indexed under this heading.

Floxuridine (Antimetabolites may reduce the immune responses to vaccines).
No products indexed under this heading.

Fludarabine Phosphate (Antimetabolites may reduce the immune responses to vaccines).
No products indexed under this heading.

Fludrocortisone Acetate (Corticosteroids may reduce the immune responses to vaccines).
No products indexed under this heading.

Flunisolide (Corticosteroids may reduce the immune responses to vaccines). Products include:
Aerobid/Aerobid-M 1153

Fluorouracil (Antimetabolites may reduce the immune responses to vaccines). Products include:
Carac Cream 0.5% 2722

Fluticasone Propionate (Corticosteroids may reduce the immune responses to vaccines). Products include:
Advair Diskus 100/50 1276
Advair Diskus 250/50 1276
Advair Diskus 500/50 1276
Advair HFA 45/21 Inhalation Aerosol 1288
Advair HFA 115/21 Inhalation Aerosol 1288
Advair HFA 230/21 Inhalation Aerosol 1288
Flonase Nasal Spray 1431
Flovent Diskus 50 mcg 1435

Fluticasone Propionate HFA (Corticosteroids may reduce the immune responses to vaccines). Products include:
Flovent HFA 1440

Gemcitabine Hydrochloride (Antimetabolites may reduce the immune responses to vaccines). Products include:
Gemzar for Injection 1820

Hydrocortisone (Corticosteroids may reduce the immune responses to vaccines).
No products indexed under this heading.

Hydrocortisone Acetate (Corticosteroids may reduce the immune responses to vaccines). Products include:
Analpram-HC 1140
Pramosone 1141

Hydrocortisone Sodium Phosphate (Corticosteroids may reduce the immune responses to vaccines).
No products indexed under this heading.

Hydrocortisone Sodium Succinate (Corticosteroids may reduce the immune responses to vaccines).
No products indexed under this heading.

Hydroxyurea (Cytotoxic drugs may reduce the immune responses to vaccines).
No products indexed under this heading.

Lomustine (CCNU) (Alkylating agents may reduce the immune responses to vaccines).
No products indexed under this heading.

Mechlorethamine Hydrochloride (Alkylating agents may reduce the immune responses to vaccines). Products include:
Mustargen for Injection 2492

Melphalan (Alkylating agents may reduce the immune responses to vaccines).
No products indexed under this heading.

Mercaptopurine (Antimetabolites may reduce the immune responses to vaccines).
No products indexed under this heading.

Methotrexate (Antimetabolites may reduce the immune responses to vaccines).
No products indexed under this heading.

Methotrexate Sodium (Cytotoxic drugs may reduce the immune responses to vaccines).
No products indexed under this heading.

Methylprednisolone Acetate (Corticosteroids may reduce the immune responses to vaccines).
No products indexed under this heading.

Methylprednisolone Sodium Succinate (Corticosteroids may reduce the immune responses to vaccines).
No products indexed under this heading.

Mitotane (Cytotoxic drugs may reduce the immune responses to vaccines).
No products indexed under this heading.

Mitoxantrone Hydrochloride (Cytotoxic drugs may reduce the immune responses to vaccines). Products include:
Novantrone for Injection Concentrate 1100

Mometasone Furoate (Corticosteroids may reduce the immune responses to vaccines). Products include:
Asmanex Twisthaler 2797
Elocon Cream 0.1% 2840
Elocon Lotion 0.1% 2841
Elocon Ointment 0.1% 2842

Mometasone Furoate Monohydrate (Corticosteroids may reduce the immune responses to vaccines). Products include:
Nasonex Nasal Spray 2883

Muromonab-CD3 (Immunosuppressive agents may reduce the immune responses to vaccines). Products include:
Orthoclone OKT3 Sterile Solution 2387

Mycophenolate Mofetil (Immunosuppressive agents may reduce the immune responses to vaccines). Products include:
CellCept Capsules 2622
CellCept Oral Suspension 2622
CellCept Tablets 2622

Pentostatin (Antimetabolites may reduce the immune responses to vaccines).
No products indexed under this heading.

Prednisolone Acetate (Corticosteroids may reduce the immune responses to vaccines). Products include:
Pred Forte Ophthalmic Suspension .... ⊙227
Pred Mild Ophthalmic Suspension .... ⊙230
Pred-G Ophthalmic Ointment .... ⊙229
Pred-G Ophthalmic Suspension .... ⊙228

Prednisolone Sodium Phosphate (Corticosteroids may reduce the immune responses to vaccines).
No products indexed under this heading.

Prednisolone Tebutate (Corticosteroids may reduce the immune responses to vaccines).
No products indexed under this heading.

Prednisone (Corticosteroids may reduce the immune responses to vaccines).
No products indexed under this heading.

Procarbazine Hydrochloride (Cytotoxic drugs may reduce the immune responses to vaccines).
No products indexed under this heading.

Sirolimus (Immunosuppressive agents may reduce the immune responses to vaccines). Products include:
Rapamune 3260

Tacrolimus (Immunosuppressive agents may reduce the immune responses to vaccines). Products include:
Prograf Capsules and Injection 622
Protopic Ointment 628

Tamoxifen Citrate (Cytotoxic drugs may reduce the immune responses to vaccines).
No products indexed under this heading.

Thioguanine (Antimetabolites may reduce the immune responses to vaccines). Products include:
Tabloid Tablets 1601

Thiotepa (Alkylating agents may reduce the immune responses to vaccines).
No products indexed under this heading.

Triamcinolone (Corticosteroids may reduce the immune responses to vaccines).
No products indexed under this heading.

Triamcinolone Acetonide (Corticosteroids may reduce the immune responses to vaccines). Products include:
Azmacort Inhalation Aerosol 407
Nasacort AQ Nasal Spray 2765
Triesence Injectable Suspension .... ⊙209

Triamcinolone Diacetate (Corticosteroids may reduce the immune responses to vaccines).
No products indexed under this heading.

Triamcinolone Hexacetonide (Corticosteroids may reduce the immune responses to vaccines).
No products indexed under this heading.

Vincristine Sulfate (Cytotoxic drugs may reduce the immune responses to vaccines).
No products indexed under this heading.

GEMZAR FOR INJECTION

(Gemcitabine Hydrochloride) 1820
None cited in PDR database.

GENGRAF CAPSULES

(Cyclosporine) 435
May interact with ACE inhibitors, angiotensin-II receptor antagonists, calcium channel blockers, cytochrome p450 3a inducers (selected), cytochrome p450 3a inhibitors (selected), erythromycin, HMG-CoA reductase inhibitors, immunosuppressive agents, methylprednisolone, nephrotoxic agents, non-steroidal anti-inflammatory agents, oral contraceptives, phenytoin, potassium preparations, prednisolone, protease inhibitors, potassium sparing diuretics, killed/inactivated vaccines, vaccines, live, and certain other agents. Compounds in these categories include:

Abacavir Sulfate (Care should be taken in using cyclosporine with nephrotoxic drugs). Products include:
Epzicom Tablets 1422
Trizivir Tablets 1622
Ziagen 1673

Acyclovir (Care should be taken in using cyclosporine with nephrotoxic drugs). Products include:
Zovirax 1690
Zovirax Cream 817
Zovirax Ointment 819

Acyclovir Sodium (Care should be taken in using cyclosporine with nephrotoxic drugs).
No products indexed under this heading.

Alatrofloxacin Mesylate (Care should be taken in using cyclosporine with nephrotoxic drugs).
No products indexed under this heading.

Aldesleukin (Care should be taken in using cyclosporine with nephrotoxic drugs). Products include:
Proleukin for Injection 2287

Allium sativum (Cyclosporine is extensively metabolized by CYP3A. Substances that are inducers of CYP3A could increase metabolism and decrease cyclosporine concentrations).
No products indexed under this heading.

Allopurinol (Cyclosporine is extensively metabolized by CYP450 3A. Substances that inhibit this enzyme could decrease the metabolism and increase cyclosporine concentrations).
No products indexed under this heading.

Amikacin Sulfate (Care should be taken in using cyclosporine with nephrotoxic drugs).
No products indexed under this heading.

Amiloride Hydrochloride (Cyclosporine causes hyperkalemia; concurrent use with potassium-sparing diuretics can result in increased risk of hyperkalemia; co-administration should be avoided).
No products indexed under this heading.

Amiodarone Hydrochloride (Cyclosporine is extensively metabolized by CYP450 3A. Substances that inhibit this enzyme could decrease the metabolism and increase cyclosporine concentrations).
No products indexed under this heading.

Amlodipine Besylate (While calcium antagonists can be effective agents in treating cyclosporine-associated hypertension, they can interfere with cyclosporine metabolism). Products include:
Azor Tablets 1005
Exforge Tablets 2238

Amoxicillin (Care should be taken in using cyclosporine with nephrotoxic drugs). Products include:
Amoxil Capsules 1305
Amoxil Chewable Tablets 1305
Amoxil Pediatric Drops for Oral Suspension 1305
Amoxil Powder for Oral Suspension 1305
Amoxil Tablets 1305
Augmentin 1323
Augmentin Tablets 1327
Augmentin XR Extended Release Tablets 1333
Augmentin ES-600 Powder for Oral Suspension 1329
Moxatag Tablets 2165

Amoxicillin Trihydrate (Care should be taken in using cyclosporine with nephrotoxic drugs).
No products indexed under this heading.

Amphotericin B (May potentiate renal dysfunction).
No products indexed under this heading.

Amphotericin B, liposomal (Care should be taken in using cyclosporine with nephrotoxic drugs). Products include:
AmBisome for Injection 606

Amphotericin B Cholesteryl Sulfate (Care should be taken in using cyclosporine with nephrotoxic drugs).
No products indexed under this heading.

Amphotericin B Lipid Complex (Care should be taken in using cyclosporine with nephrotoxic drugs). Products include:
Abelcet Injection 1134

Ampicillin (Care should be taken in using cyclosporine with nephrotoxic drugs).
No products indexed under this heading.

Ampicillin Sodium (Care should be taken in using cyclosporine with nephrotoxic drugs).
No products indexed under this heading.

Ampicillin Trihydrate (Care should be taken in using cyclosporine with nephrotoxic drugs).
No products indexed under this heading.

Amprenavir (the HIV protease inhibitors are known to inhibit CYP3A and thus could potentially increase the concentrations of cyclosporine; care should be exercised when these drugs are administered concomitantly).
No products indexed under this heading.

Aprepitant (Cyclosporine is extensively metabolized by CYP3A. Substances that inhibit this enzyme could decrease the metabolism and increase cyclosporine concentrations). Products include:
Emend Capsules 1992

Aspirin (Care should be taken in using cyclosporine with nephrotoxic drugs). Products include:
Aggrenox Capsules 819
Bayer Aspirin 750
Percodan Tablets 1130
St. Joseph 81 mg Aspirin Chewable and Enteric Coated Tablets 1903

Atazanavir (Care should be taken in using cyclosporine with nephrotoxic drugs).
No products indexed under this heading.

Atorvastatin Calcium (Cyclosporine may reduce the clearance of HMG-CoA reductase inhibitors. Myotoxicity, including muscle pain and weakness, myositis, and rhabdomyolysis, have been reported with concomitant administration of cyclosporine with lovastatin, simvastatin, atorvastatin, pravastatin, and, rarely, fluvastatin. Dosage of these statins should be reduced). Products include:
Lipitor Tablets 2501

Azapropazon (May potentiate renal dysfunction).
No products indexed under this heading.

Azathioprine (Psoriasis patients who are treated with cyclosporine capsules should not receive concomitant immunosuppressive agents. Co-administration with other immunosuppressive agents increases the possibility of excessive immunosuppression).
No products indexed under this heading.

Azithromycin (Cyclosporine is extensively metabolized by CYP3A. Substances that inhibit this enzyme could decrease the metabolism and increase cyclosporine concentrations). Products include:
AzaSite Ophthalmic Drops 1740

Azithromycin Dihydrate (Cyclosporine is extensively metabolized by CYP3A. Substances that inhibit this enzyme could decrease the metabolism and increase cyclosporine concentrations).
No products indexed under this heading.

Azlocillin Sodium (Care should be taken in using cyclosporine with nephrotoxic drugs).
No products indexed under this heading.

Aztreonam (Care should be taken in using cyclosporine with nephrotoxic drugs).
No products indexed under this heading.

Bacampicillin Hydrochloride (Care should be taken in using cyclosporine with nephrotoxic drugs).
No products indexed under this heading.

Balsalazide Disodium (Care should be taken in using cyclosporine with nephrotoxic drugs).
No products indexed under this heading.

Basiliximab (Psoriasis patients who are treated with cyclosporine capsules should not receive concomitant immunosuppressive agents. Co-administration with other immunosuppressive agents increases the possibility of excessive immunosuppression). Products include:
Simulect for Injection 2306

BCG Vaccine (During treatment with cyclosporine, vaccination may be less effective; and the use of live attenuated vaccines avoided).
No products indexed under this heading.

Benazepril Hydrochloride (Caution is required when co-administering cyclosporine with potassium sparing drugs, such as ACE inhibitors).
No products indexed under this heading.

Bendroflumethiazide (Care should be taken in using cyclosporine with nephrotoxic drugs).
No products indexed under this heading.

Bepridil Hydrochloride (While calcium antagonists can be effective agents in treating cyclosporine-associated hypertension, they can interfere with cyclosporine metabolism).
No products indexed under this heading.

Bezafibrate (May potentiate renal dysfunction).
No products indexed under this heading.

Bromocriptine Mesylate (Cyclosporine is extensively metabolized by CYP450 3A. Substances that inhibit this enzyme could decrease the metabolism and increase cyclosporine concentrations).
No products indexed under this heading.

Caffeine (Care should be taken in using cyclosporine with nephrotoxic drugs). Products include:
BioLean Free Tablets 635
BioLean II Tablets 635
Winrgy Dietary Supplement 642

Candesartan Cilexetil (Caution is required when co-administering cyclosporine with potassium sparing drugs, such as angiotensin II receptor antagonists). Products include:
Atacand Tablets 639
Atacand HCT 642

Captopril (Caution is required when co-administering cyclosporine with potassium sparing drugs, such as ACE inhibitors). Products include:
Captopril Tablets 2182

Carbamazepine (Co-administration with drugs that are inducers of CYP450 3A, such as carbamazepine, could increase metabolism of cyclosporine and decrease its concentrations). Products include:
Carbatrol Capsules 3019
Equetro Extended-Release Capsules 3174

Carbenicillin Disodium (Care should be taken in using cyclosporine with nephrotoxic drugs).
No products indexed under this heading.

Carbenicillin Indanyl Sodium (Care should be taken in using cyclosporine with nephrotoxic drugs).
No products indexed under this heading.

Carboplatin (Care should be taken in using cyclosporine with nephrotoxic drugs).
No products indexed under this heading.

Carmustine (BCNU) (Care should be taken in using cyclosporine with nephrotoxic drugs).
No products indexed under this heading.

Cefaclor (Care should be taken in using cyclosporine with nephrotoxic drugs).
No products indexed under this heading.

Cefadroxil (Care should be taken in using cyclosporine with nephrotoxic drugs).
No products indexed under this heading.

Cefamandole Nafate (Care should be taken in using cyclosporine with nephrotoxic drugs).
No products indexed under this heading.

Cefazolin Sodium (Care should be taken in using cyclosporine with nephrotoxic drugs).
No products indexed under this heading.

Cefdinir (Care should be taken in using cyclosporine with nephrotoxic drugs). Products include:
Omnicef Capsules 497
Omnicef for Oral Suspension 497

Cefepime Hydrochloride (Care should be taken in using cyclosporine with nephrotoxic drugs).
No products indexed under this heading.

Cefixime (Care should be taken in using cyclosporine with nephrotoxic drugs). Products include:
Suprax for Oral Suspension 1891
Suprax Tablets 1891

Cefmetazole Sodium (Care should be taken in using cyclosporine with nephrotoxic drugs).
No products indexed under this heading.

Cefonicid Sodium (Care should be taken in using cyclosporine with nephrotoxic drugs).
No products indexed under this heading.

Cefoperazone Sodium (Care should be taken in using cyclosporine with nephrotoxic drugs).
No products indexed under this heading.

Ceforanide (Care should be taken in using cyclosporine with nephrotoxic drugs).
No products indexed under this heading.

Cefotaxime Sodium (Care should be taken in using cyclosporine with nephrotoxic drugs).
No products indexed under this heading.

Cefotetan (Care should be taken in using cyclosporine with nephrotoxic drugs).
No products indexed under this heading.

Cefoxitin Sodium (Care should be taken in using cyclosporine with nephrotoxic drugs).
No products indexed under this heading.

Cefpodoxime Proxetil (Care should be taken in using cyclosporine with nephrotoxic drugs).
No products indexed under this heading.

Cefprozil (Care should be taken in using cyclosporine with nephrotoxic drugs).
No products indexed under this heading.

Ceftazidime (Care should be taken in using cyclosporine with nephrotoxic drugs). Products include:
Fortaz 1450

Ceftizoxime Sodium (Care should be taken in using cyclosporine with nephrotoxic drugs).
No products indexed under this heading.

Ceftriaxone Sodium (Care should be taken in using cyclosporine with nephrotoxic drugs). Products include:
Rocephin Injectable Vials, ADD-Vantage, Galaxy, Bulk 2642

Cefuroxime Axetil (Care should be taken in using cyclosporine with nephrotoxic drugs). Products include:
Ceftin 1380

Cefuroxime Sodium (Care should be taken in using cyclosporine with nephrotoxic drugs).
No products indexed under this heading.

Celecoxib (Cyclosporine can cause nephrotoxicity; clinical status and serum creatinine should be closely monitored when cyclosporine is used with NSAIDs in rheumatoid arthritis patients). Products include:
Celebrex Capsules 2979

Cephalexin (Care should be taken in using cyclosporine with nephrotoxic drugs).
No products indexed under this heading.

Cephalothin Sodium (Care should be taken in using cyclosporine with nephrotoxic drugs).
No products indexed under this heading.

Cephapirin Sodium (Care should be taken in using cyclosporine with nephrotoxic drugs).
No products indexed under this heading.

Cephradine (Care should be taken in using cyclosporine with nephrotoxic drugs).
No products indexed under this heading.

Cerivastatin Sodium (Cyclosporine may reduce the clearance of HMG-CoA reductase inhibitors. Myotoxicity, including muscle pain and weakness, myositis, and rhabdomyolysis, have been reported with concomitant administration of cyclosporine with lovastatin, simvastatin, atorvastatin, pravastatin, and, rarely, fluvastatin. Dosage of these statins should be reduced).
No products indexed under this heading.

Chlorothiazide (Care should be taken in using cyclosporine with nephrotoxic drugs).
No products indexed under this heading.

Chlorothiazide Sodium (Care should be taken in using cyclosporine with nephrotoxic drugs). Products include:
Intravenous Sodium Diuril 2490

Chlorpropamide (Care should be taken in using cyclosporine with nephrotoxic drugs).
No products indexed under this heading.

Cidofovir (Care should be taken in using cyclosporine with nephrotoxic drugs).
No products indexed under this heading.

Cilastatin Sodium (Care should be taken in using cyclosporine with nephrotoxic drugs). Products include:
Primaxin I.M. 2080
Primaxin I.V. 2083

Cimetidine (May potentiate renal dysfunction).
No products indexed under this heading.

Cimetidine Hydrochloride (May potentiate renal dysfunction).
No products indexed under this heading.

Ciprofloxacin (May potentiate renal dysfunction). Products include:
Cipro I.V. 2817
Cipro Oral Suspension 2810
Cipro XR Tablets 2823
Ciprodex Otic Suspension 541

Ciprofloxacin Hydrochloride (May potentiate renal dysfunction). Products include:
Cipro Tablets 2810

Cisplatin (Care should be taken in using cyclosporine with nephrotoxic drugs).
No products indexed under this heading.

Cladribine (Care should be taken in using cyclosporine with nephrotoxic drugs). Products include:
Leustatin Injection 2384

Clarithromycin (Cyclosporine is extensively metabolized by CYP450 3A. Substances that inhibit this enzyme could decrease the metabolism and increase cyclosporine concentrations). Products include:
Biaxin/Biaxin XL 411

Clozapine (Care should be taken in using cyclosporine with nephrotoxic drugs).
No products indexed under this heading.

Coal Tar (Psoriasis patients who are treated with cyclosporine capsules should not receive concomitant coal tar).
No products indexed under this heading.

Colchicine (Cyclosporine may reduce the clearance of colchicine and enhance its toxic effects, such as myopathy and neuropathy, especially in patients with renal dysfunction. Close clinical observation is required during concomitant administration).
No products indexed under this heading.

Colistimethate Sodium (Care should be taken in using cyclosporine with nephrotoxic drugs).
No products indexed under this heading.

Colistin Sulfate (Care should be taken in using cyclosporine with nephrotoxic drugs).
No products indexed under this heading.

Cyclophosphamide (Care should be taken in using cyclosporine with nephrotoxic drugs).
No products indexed under this heading.

Cytarabine (Care should be taken in using cyclosporine with nephrotoxic drugs).
No products indexed under this heading.

Cytarabine Liposome (Care should be taken in using cyclosporine with nephrotoxic drugs). Products include:
DepoCyt Injection 1136

Dalfopristin (Cyclosporine is extensively metabolized by CYP450 3A. Substances that inhibit this enzyme could decrease the metabolism and increase cyclosporine concentrations).
No products indexed under this heading.

Danazol (Cyclosporine is extensively metabolized by CYP450 3A. Substances that inhibit this enzyme could decrease the metabolism and increase cyclosporine concentrations).
No products indexed under this heading.

Darunavir (the HIV protease inhibitors are known to inhibit CYP3A and thus could potentially increase the concentrations of cyclosporine; care should be exercised when these drugs are administered concomitantly).
No products indexed under this heading.

Delavirdine Mesylate (Care should be taken in using cyclosporine with nephrotoxic drugs).
No products indexed under this heading.

Desogestrel (Cyclosporine is extensively metabolized by CYP3A. Substances that inhibit this enzyme could decrease the metabolism and increase cyclosporine concentrations). Products include:
Mircette Tablets 1034

Dexamethasone (Cyclosporine is extensively metabolized by CYP3A. Substances that are inducers of CYP3A could increase metabolism and decrease cyclosporine concentrations). Products include:
Ciprodex Otic Suspension 541

Diatrizoate Meglumine (Care should be taken in using cyclosporine with nephrotoxic drugs).
No products indexed under this heading.

Diatrizoate Sodium (Care should be taken in using cyclosporine with nephrotoxic drugs).
No products indexed under this heading.

Diclofenac Epolamine (Cyclosporine can cause nephrotoxicity; clinical status and serum creatinine should be closely monitored when cyclosporine is used with NSAIDs in rheumatoid arthritis patients). Products include:
Flector Patch 561

Diclofenac Potassium (May potentiate renal dysfunction; potential for doubling of diclofenac blood levels and occasional reports of reversible decreases in renal function have been reported with concurrent use).
No products indexed under this heading.

Diclofenac Sodium (May potentiate renal dysfunction; potential for doubling of diclofenac blood levels and occasional reports of reversible decreases in renal function have been reported with concurrent use). Products include:
Diclofenac Sodium Ophthalmic Solution .... ⊙ 240
Voltaren Ophthalmic Solution 2336
Voltaren Tablets 2334
Voltaren-XR Tablets 2337

Dicloxacillin Sodium (Care should be taken in using cyclosporine with nephrotoxic drugs).
No products indexed under this heading.

Didanosine (Care should be taken in using cyclosporine with nephrotoxic drugs).
No products indexed under this heading.

Digoxin (Cyclosporine may reduce the clearance of digoxin. Severe digitalis toxicity has been seen within days of starting cyclosporine. Close clinical observation is required during concomitant administration). Products include:
Lanoxin Injection 1498
Lanoxin Injection Pediatric 1502
Lanoxin Tablets 1505

Diltiazem Hydrochloride (Cyclosporine is extensively metabolized by CYP450 3A. Substances that inhibit this enzyme could decrease the metabolism and increase cyclosporine concentrations). Products include:
Cardizem LA Extended Release Tablets 421

Diltiazem Maleate (Cyclosporine is extensively metabolized by CYP450 3A. Substances that inhibit this enzyme could decrease the metabolism and increase cyclosporine concentrations).
No products indexed under this heading.

Diphtheria & Tetanus Toxoids and Acellular Pertussis Vaccine Adsorbed, Hepatitis B (recombinant) and Inactivated Poliovirus Vaccine Combined (During treatment with cyclosporine, vaccination may be less effective).
No products indexed under this heading.

Efavirenz (Care should be taken in using cyclosporine with nephrotoxic drugs). Products include:
Atripla Tablets 938
Sustiva Capsules 930
Sustiva Tablets 930

Emtricitabine (Care should be taken in using cyclosporine with nephrotoxic drugs). Products include:
- Atripla Tablets ... 938
- Emtriva Capsules ... 1246
- Emtriva Oral Solution ... 1246
- Truvada Tablets ... 1262

Enalapril Maleate (Caution is required when co-administering cyclosporine with potassium sparing drugs, such as ACE inhibitors).
No products indexed under this heading.

Enalaprilat (Caution is required when co-administering cyclosporine with potassium sparing drugs, such as ACE inhibitors).
No products indexed under this heading.

Enfuvirtide (Care should be taken in using cyclosporine with nephrotoxic drugs).
No products indexed under this heading.

Eprosartan Mesylate (Caution is required when co-administering cyclosporine with potassium sparing drugs, such as angiotensin II receptor antagonists). Products include:
- Teveten Tablets ... 515
- Teveten HCT Tablets ... 517

Erythromycin (Cyclosporine is extensively metabolized by CYP450 3A. Substances that inhibit this enzyme could decrease the metabolism and increase cyclosporine concentrations).
No products indexed under this heading.

Erythromycin Estolate (Cyclosporine is extensively metabolized by CYP450 3A. Substances that inhibit this enzyme could decrease the metabolism and increase cyclosporine concentrations).
No products indexed under this heading.

Erythromycin Ethylsuccinate (Cyclosporine is extensively metabolized by CYP450 3A. Substances that inhibit this enzyme could decrease the metabolism and increase cyclosporine concentrations). Products include:
- E.E.S. ... 433
- EryPed ... 431

Erythromycin Gluceptate (Cyclosporine is extensively metabolized by CYP450 3A. Substances that inhibit this enzyme could decrease the metabolism and increase cyclosporine concentrations).
No products indexed under this heading.

Erythromycin Lactobionate (Cyclosporine is extensively metabolized by CYP450 3A. Substances that inhibit this enzyme could decrease the metabolism and increase cyclosporine concentrations).
No products indexed under this heading.

Erythromycin Stearate (Cyclosporine is extensively metabolized by CYP450 3A. Substances that inhibit this enzyme could decrease the metabolism and increase cyclosporine concentrations).
No products indexed under this heading.

Ethinyl Estradiol (Cyclosporine is extensively metabolized by CYP3A. Substances that inhibit this enzyme could decrease the metabolism and increase cyclosporine concentrations). Products include:
- Lybrel Tablets ... 3204
- Mircette Tablets ... 1034
- NuvaRing ... 2897
- Ortho-Cyclen/Ortho Tri-Cyclen ... 2449
- Ortho Evra Transdermal System ... 2437
- Ortho Tri-Cyclen Lo Tablets ... 2458
- Seasonique Tablets ... 1046
- Yaz Tablets ... 805

Ethiodized Oil (Care should be taken in using cyclosporine with nephrotoxic drugs).
No products indexed under this heading.

Ethosuximide (Cyclosporine is extensively metabolized by CYP3A. Substances that are inducers of CYP3A could increase metabolism and decrease cyclosporine concentrations).
No products indexed under this heading.

Ethynodiol Diacetate (Cyclosporine is extensively metabolized by CYP3A. Substances that inhibit this enzyme could decrease the metabolism and increase cyclosporine concentrations).
No products indexed under this heading.

Etodolac (Cyclosporine can cause nephrotoxicity; clinical status and serum creatinine should be closely monitored when cyclosporine is used with NSAIDs in rheumatoid arthritis patients).
No products indexed under this heading.

Felodipine (While calcium antagonists can be effective agents in treating cyclosporine-associated hypertension, they can interfere with cyclosporine metabolism).
No products indexed under this heading.

Fenoprofen Calcium (Cyclosporine can cause nephrotoxicity; clinical status and serum creatinine should be closely monitored when cyclosporine is used with NSAIDs in rheumatoid arthritis patients). Products include:
- Nalfon Capsules ... 2508

Fibrates (May potentiate renal dysfunction).
No products indexed under this heading.

Filgrastim (Care should be taken in using cyclosporine with nephrotoxic drugs). Products include:
- Neupogen for Injection ... 589

Fluconazole (Co-administration with drugs that inhibit CYP450 3A, such as fluconazole, could decrease metabolism of cyclosporine and increase its concentrations).
No products indexed under this heading.

Fluorouracil (Care should be taken in using cyclosporine with nephrotoxic drugs). Products include:
- Carac Cream 0.5% ... 2722

Fluoxetine (Cyclosporine is extensively metabolized by CYP3A. Substances that inhibit this enzyme could decrease the metabolism and increase cyclosporine concentrations).
No products indexed under this heading.

Fluoxetine Hydrochloride (Cyclosporine is extensively metabolized by CYP3A. Substances that inhibit this enzyme could decrease the metabolism and increase cyclosporine concentrations). Products include:
- Prozac Weekly Capsules ... 1852
- Prozac Pulvules and Liquid ... 1852
- Symbyax Capsules ... 1871

Flurbiprofen (Cyclosporine can cause nephrotoxicity; clinical status and serum creatinine should be closely monitored when cyclosporine is used with NSAIDs in rheumatoid arthritis patients).
No products indexed under this heading.

Fluvastatin Sodium (Cyclosporine may reduce the clearance of HMG-CoA reductase inhibitors. Myotoxicity, including muscle pain and weakness, myositis, and rhabdomyolysis, have been reported with concomitant administration of cyclosporine with lovastatin, simvastatin, atorvastatin, pravastatin, and, rarely, fluvastatin. Dosage of these statins should be reduced). Products include:
- Lescol Capsules ... 2268
- Lescol XL Tablets ... 2268

Fluvoxamine Maleate (Cyclosporine is extensively metabolized by CYP3A. Substances that inhibit this enzyme could decrease the metabolism and increase cyclosporine concentrations). Products include:
- Luvox CR Extended-Release Capsules ... 1759

Fosamprenavir Calcium (the HIV protease inhibitors are known to inhibit CYP3A and thus could potentially increase the concentrations of cyclosporine; care should be exercised when these drugs are administered concomitantly). Products include:
- Lexiva Oral Suspension ... 1510
- Lexiva Tablets ... 1510

Foscarnet Sodium (Care should be taken in using cyclosporine with nephrotoxic drugs).
No products indexed under this heading.

Fosinopril Sodium (Caution is required when co-administering cyclosporine with potassium sparing drugs, such as ACE inhibitors).
No products indexed under this heading.

Fosphenytoin Sodium (Co-administration with drugs that are inducers of CYP450 3A, such as phenytoin, could increase metabolism of cyclosporine and decrease its concentrations).
No products indexed under this heading.

Furosemide (Care should be taken in using cyclosporine with nephrotoxic drugs). Products include:
- Furosemide Tablets ... 2186

Gadopentetate Dimeglumine (Care should be taken in using cyclosporine with nephrotoxic drugs).
No products indexed under this heading.

Gentamicin (Care should be taken in using cyclosporine with nephrotoxic drugs).
No products indexed under this heading.

Gentamicin Sulfate (May potentiate renal dysfunction). Products include:
- Pred-G Ophthalmic Ointment ... ⊙ 229
- Pred-G Ophthalmic Suspension ... ⊙ 228

Glipizide (Care should be taken in using cyclosporine with nephrotoxic drugs).
No products indexed under this heading.

Globulin, Immune (Human) (Care should be taken in using cyclosporine with nephrotoxic drugs). Products include:
- Flebogamma 5% ... 1715

Glyburide (Care should be taken in using cyclosporine with nephrotoxic drugs).
No products indexed under this heading.

Gold Therapy (Care should be taken in using cyclosporine with nephrotoxic drugs).
No products indexed under this heading.

Hepatitis A Vaccine, Inactivated (During treatment with cyclosporine, vaccination may be less effective). Products include:
- Havrix Injection Vaccine ... 1454
- Twinrix Vaccine ... 1628
- Vaqta ... 2130

HMG-CoA Reductase Inhibitors (Care should be taken in using cyclosporine with nephrotoxic drugs).
No products indexed under this heading.

Hydrochlorothiazide (Care should be taken in using cyclosporine with nephrotoxic drugs). Products include:
- Atacand HCT ... 642
- Avalide Tablets ... 892
- Avalide Tablets ... 2713
- Benicar HCT Tablets ... 1010
- Diovan HCT Tablets ... 2216
- Dyazide Capsules ... 1405
- Micardis HCT Tablets ... 854
- Prinzide Tablets ... 2092
- Tekturna HCT Tablets ... 2324
- Teveten HCT Tablets ... 517

Hydroflumethiazide (Care should be taken in using cyclosporine with nephrotoxic drugs).
No products indexed under this heading.

Hypericum (Co-administration with drugs that are inducers of CYP450 3A could increase metabolism of cyclosporine and decrease its concentrations. This interaction has been reported to produce a marked reduction in the blood concentrations of cyclosporine, resultingin subtherapeutic levels, rejection of transplant organs, and graft loss). Products include:
- Satieté Tablets ... ■ 640

Ibuprofen (Cyclosporine can cause nephrotoxicity; clinical status and serum creatinine should be closely monitored when cyclosporine is used with NSAIDs in rheumatoid arthritis patients). Products include:
- Motrin IB Tablets and Caplets ... 1900
- Children's Motrin Oral Suspension ... 1901
- Children's Motrin Non-Staining Dye-Free Oral Suspension ... 1901
- Children's Motrin Cold Oral Suspension ... 1899
- Infants' Motrin Concentrated Drops ... 1901
- Infants' Motrin Non-Staining Dye-Free Concentrated Drops ... 1901
- Junior Strength Motrin Caplets and Chewable Tablets ... 1901
- Vicoprofen Tablets ... 533

Idarubicin Hydrochloride (Care should be taken in using cyclosporine with nephrotoxic drugs).
No products indexed under this heading.

IMPORTANT NOTE: Always consult each drug listing in the patient's regimen for possible interactions.

Ifosfamide (Care should be taken in using cyclosporine with nephrotoxic drugs).
No products indexed under this heading.

Imatinib Mesylate (Cyclosporine is extensively metabolized by CYP3A. Substances that inhibit this enzyme could decrease the metabolism and increase cyclosporine concentrations). Products include:
Gleevec Tablets 2255

Imipenem (Care should be taken in using cyclosporine with nephrotoxic drugs). Products include:
Primaxin I.M. 2080
Primaxin I.V. 2083

Immune Globulin Intravenous (Human) (Care should be taken in using cyclosporine with nephrotoxic drugs). Products include:
Flebogamma 5% DIF 1718
Gammagard Liquid 730
Gammagard S/D 734
Gamunex 3094

Indinavir Sulfate (the HIV protease inhibitors are known to inhibit CYP3A and thus could potentially increase the concentrations of cyclosporine; care should be exercised when these drugs are administered concomitantly). Products include:
Crixivan Capsules 1979

Indomethacin (Cyclosporine can cause nephrotoxicity; clinical status and serum creatinine should be closely monitored when cyclosporine is used with NSAIDs in rheumatoid arthritis patients). Products include:
Indocin 2024

Indomethacin Sodium Trihydrate (Cyclosporine can cause nephrotoxicity; clinical status and serum creatinine should be closely monitored when cyclosporine is used with NSAIDs in rheumatoid arthritis patients). Products include:
Indocin I.V. 2489

Influenza Vaccine, Live Attenuated (During treatment with cyclosporine, vaccination may be less effective; and the use of live attenuated vaccines avoided).
No products indexed under this heading.

Influenza Virus Vaccine (During treatment with cyclosporine, vaccination may be less effective). Products include:
Fluarix Vaccine 1446
Flulaval Injection Vaccine 1448

Influenza Virus Vaccine Live, Intranasal (During treatment with cyclosporine, vaccination may be less effective; and the use of live attenuated vaccines avoided). Products include:
FluMist Vaccine 1945

Interferon Beta-1b (Care should be taken in using cyclosporine with nephrotoxic drugs). Products include:
Betaseron for SC Injection 756

Interleuken-2 (Care should be taken in using cyclosporine with nephrotoxic drugs).
No products indexed under this heading.

Iodamide Meglumine (Care should be taken in using cyclosporine with nephrotoxic drugs).
No products indexed under this heading.

Iohexol (Care should be taken in using cyclosporine with nephrotoxic drugs).
No products indexed under this heading.

Iopamidol (Care should be taken in using cyclosporine with nephrotoxic drugs).
No products indexed under this heading.

Iopanoic Acid (Care should be taken in using cyclosporine with nephrotoxic drugs).
No products indexed under this heading.

Iothalamate Meglumine (Care should be taken in using cyclosporine with nephrotoxic drugs).
No products indexed under this heading.

Ioxaglate Meglumine (Care should be taken in using cyclosporine with nephrotoxic drugs).
No products indexed under this heading.

Ioxaglate Sodium (Care should be taken in using cyclosporine with nephrotoxic drugs).
No products indexed under this heading.

Irbesartan (Caution is required when co-administering cyclosporine with potassium sparing drugs, such as angiotensin II receptor antagonists). Products include:
Avalide Tablets 892
Avalide Tablets 2713
Avapro Tablets 897
Avapro Tablets 2718

Isoniazid (Cyclosporine is extensively metabolized by CYP3A. Substances that inhibit this enzyme could decrease the metabolism and increase cyclosporine concentrations).
No products indexed under this heading.

Isradipine (While calcium antagonists can be effective agents in treating cyclosporine-associated hypertension, they can interfere with cyclosporine metabolism). Products include:
DynaCirc CR Controlled Release Tablets 1407

Itraconazole (Co-administration with drugs that inhibit CYP450 3A, such as itraconazole, could decrease metabolism of cyclosporine and increase its concentrations).
No products indexed under this heading.

Japanese Encephalitis Vaccine Inactivated (During treatment with cyclosporine, vaccination may be less effective).
No products indexed under this heading.

Kanamycin Sulfate (Care should be taken in using cyclosporine with nephrotoxic drugs).
No products indexed under this heading.

Ketoconazole (May potentiate renal dysfunction; co-administration with drugs that inhibit CYP4503A, such as ketoconazole, could decrease metabolism of cyclosporine and increase its concentrations). Products include:
Extina Foam, 2% 3057
Nizoral A-D Shampoo 1901

Ketoprofen (Cyclosporine can cause nephrotoxicity; clinical status and serum creatinine should be closely monitored when cyclosporine is used with NSAIDs in rheumatoid arthritis patients).
No products indexed under this heading.

Ketorolac Tromethamine (Cyclosporine can cause nephrotoxicity; clinical status and serum creatinine should be closely monitored when cyclosporine is used with NSAIDs in rheumatoid arthritis patients).
No products indexed under this heading.

Lamium album (Care should be taken in using cyclosporine with nephrotoxic drugs).
No products indexed under this heading.

Levonorgestrel (Cyclosporine is extensively metabolized by CYP3A. Substances that inhibit this enzyme could decrease the metabolism and increase cyclosporine concentrations). Products include:
Climara Pro Transdermal System 768
Lybrel Tablets 3204
Mirena Intrauterine System 779
Plan B Tablets 1044
Seasonique Tablets 1046

Lisinopril (Caution is required when co-administering cyclosporine with potassium sparing drugs, such as ACE inhibitors). Products include:
Prinivil Tablets 2087
Prinzide Tablets 2092

Lithium (Care should be taken in using cyclosporine with nephrotoxic drugs).
No products indexed under this heading.

Lithium Carbonate (Care should be taken in using cyclosporine with nephrotoxic drugs).
No products indexed under this heading.

Lithium Citrate (Care should be taken in using cyclosporine with nephrotoxic drugs).
No products indexed under this heading.

Lopinavir (the HIV protease inhibitors are known to inhibit CYP3A and thus could potentially increase the concentrations of cyclosporine; care should be exercised when these drugs are administered concomitantly). Products include:
Kaletra 452

Loracarbef (Care should be taken in using cyclosporine with nephrotoxic drugs).
No products indexed under this heading.

Losartan Potassium (Caution is required when co-administering cyclosporine with potassium sparing drugs, such as angiotensin II receptor antagonists). Products include:
Cozaar Tablets 1973

Lovastatin (Co-administration results in reduced clearance of lovastatin; myositis has been reported with concurrent use). Products include:
Advicor Tablets 402
Mevacor Tablets 2063

Measles, Mumps, Rubella and Varicella Virus Vaccine Live (During treatment with cyclosporine, vaccination may be less effective; and the use of live attenuated vaccines avoided). Products include:
ProQuad 2099

Measles, Mumps & Rubella Virus Vaccine, Live (During treatment with cyclosporine, vaccination may be less effective; and the use of live attenuated vaccines avoided). Products include:
M-M-R II 2054

Measles & Rubella Virus Vaccine Live (During treatment with cyclosporine, vaccination may be less effective; and the use of live attenuated vaccines avoided).
No products indexed under this heading.

Measles Virus Vaccine Live (During treatment with cyclosporine, vaccination may be less effective; and the use of live attenuated vaccines avoided). Products include:
Attenuvax 1951

Meclofenamate Sodium (Cyclosporine can cause nephrotoxicity; clinical status and serum creatinine should be closely monitored when cyclosporine is used with NSAIDs in rheumatoid arthritis patients).
No products indexed under this heading.

Mefenamic Acid (Cyclosporine can cause nephrotoxicity; clinical status and serum creatinine should be closely monitored when cyclosporine is used with NSAIDs in rheumatoid arthritis patients).
No products indexed under this heading.

Meloxicam (Cyclosporine can cause nephrotoxicity; clinical status and serum creatinine should be closely monitored when cyclosporine is used with NSAIDs in rheumatoid arthritis patients). Products include:
Mobic Oral Suspension 863
Mobic Tablets 863

Melphalan (May potentiate renal dysfunction).
No products indexed under this heading.

Melphalan Hydrochloride (Care should be taken in using cyclosporine with nephrotoxic drugs).
No products indexed under this heading.

Mesalamine (Care should be taken in using cyclosporine with nephrotoxic drugs). Products include:
Asacol Delayed-Release Tablets 2579
Canasa Rectal Suppositories 705
Lialda Tablets 3029
Pentasa Capsules 3030

Mestranol (Cyclosporine is extensively metabolized by CYP3A. Substances that inhibit this enzyme could decrease the metabolism and increase cyclosporine concentrations).
No products indexed under this heading.

Methimazole (Care should be taken in using cyclosporine with nephrotoxic drugs).
No products indexed under this heading.

Methotrexate (Care should be taken in using cyclosporine with nephrotoxic drugs).
No products indexed under this heading.

Methotrexate Sodium (Psoriasis patients who are treated with cyclosporine capsules should not receive concomitant methotrexate. Co-administration in rheumatoid arthritis patients has resulted in increased concentrations (AUC) of

methotrexate by approximately 30% and the concentrations of its metabolite, 7-hydromethotrexate, were decreased by approximately 80%; the clinical significance of this outcome is not known).
No products indexed under this heading.

Methyclothiazide (Care should be taken in using cyclosporine with nephrotoxic drugs).
No products indexed under this heading.

Methylprednisolone (Co-administration with drugs that inhibit CYP450 3A such as methylprednisolone, could decrease metabolism of cyclosporine and increase its concentrations; convulsions have been reported with concurrent high dose methylprednisolone).
No products indexed under this heading.

Methylprednisolone Acetate (Co-administration with drugs that inhibit CYP450 3A such as methylprednisolone, could decrease metabolism of cyclosporine and increase its concentrations; convulsions have been reported with concurrent high dose methylprednisolone).
No products indexed under this heading.

Methylprednisolone Sodium Succinate (Co-administration with drugs that inhibit CYP450 3A such as methylprednisolone, could decrease metabolism of cyclosporine and increase its concentrations; convulsions have been reported with concurrent high dose methylprednisolone).
No products indexed under this heading.

Metoclopramide Hydrochloride (Cyclosporine is extensively metabolized by CYP450 3A. Substances that inhibit this enzyme could decrease the metabolism and increase cyclosporine concentrations).
No products indexed under this heading.

Metronidazole (Cyclosporine is extensively metabolized by CYP3A. Substances that inhibit this enzyme could decrease the metabolism and increase cyclosporine concentrations). Products include:
Pylera Capsules 714

Metronidazole Benzoate (Cyclosporine is extensively metabolized by CYP3A. Substances that inhibit this enzyme could decrease the metabolism and increase cyclosporine concentrations).
No products indexed under this heading.

Metronidazole Hydrochloride (Cyclosporine is extensively metabolized by CYP3A. Substances that inhibit this enzyme could decrease the metabolism and increase cyclosporine concentrations).
No products indexed under this heading.

Mezlocillin Sodium (Care should be taken in using cyclosporine with nephrotoxic drugs).
No products indexed under this heading.

Mibefradil Dihydrochloride (While calcium antagonists can be effective agents in treating cyclosporine-associated hypertension, they can interfere with cyclosporine metabolism).
No products indexed under this heading.

Miconazole (Cyclosporine is extensively metabolized by CYP3A. Substances that inhibit this enzyme could decrease the metabolism and increase cyclosporine concentrations).
No products indexed under this heading.

Minocycline Hydrochloride (Care should be taken in using cyclosporine with nephrotoxic drugs). Products include:
Solodyn Extended Release Tablets 1938

Mitomycin (Mitomycin-C) (Care should be taken in using cyclosporine with nephrotoxic drugs).
No products indexed under this heading.

Modafinil (Cyclosporine is extensively metabolized by CYP3A. Substances that are inducers of CYP3A could increase metabolism and decrease cyclosporine concentrations). Products include:
Provigil Tablets 977

Moexipril Hydrochloride (Caution is required when co-administering cyclosporine with potassium sparing drugs, such as ACE inhibitors).
No products indexed under this heading.

Mumps Virus Vaccine, Live (During treatment with cyclosporine, vaccination may be less effective; and the use of live attenuated vaccines avoided). Products include:
Mumpsvax 2068

Muromonab-CD3 (Psoriasis patients who are treated with cyclosporine capsules should not receive concomitant immunosuppressive agents. Co-administration with other immunosuppressive agents increases the possibility of excessive immunosuppression). Products include:
Orthoclone OKT3 Sterile Solution 2387

Mycophenolate Mofetil (Psoriasis patients who are treated with cyclosporine capsules should not receive concomitant immunosuppressive agents. Co-administration with other immunosuppressive agents increases the possibility of excessive immunosuppression). Products include:
CellCept Capsules 2622
CellCept Oral Suspension 2622
CellCept Tablets 2622

Nabumetone (Cyclosporine can cause nephrotoxicity; clinical status and serum creatinine should be closely monitored when cyclosporine is used with NSAIDs in rheumatoid arthritis patients).
No products indexed under this heading.

Nafcillin Sodium (Co-administration with drugs that are inducers of CYP450 3A, such as nafcillin, could increase metabolism of cyclosporine and decrease its concentrations).
No products indexed under this heading.

Naproxen (May potentiate renal dysfunction; co-administration is associated with additive decreases in renal function). Products include:
EC-Naprosyn Delayed-Release Tablets 2632
Naprosyn Suspension 2632
Naprosyn Tablets 2632

Naproxen Sodium (May potentiate renal dysfunction; co-administration is associated with additive decreases in renal function). Products include:
Anaprox Tablets 2632
Anaprox DS Tablets 2632
Treximet Tablets 1616

Nefazodone Hydrochloride (Cyclosporine is extensively metabolized by CYP3A. Substances that inhibit this enzyme could decrease the metabolism and increase cyclosporine concentrations).
No products indexed under this heading.

Nelfinavir Mesylate (the HIV protease inhibitors are known to inhibit CYP3A and thus could potentially increase the concentrations of cyclosporine; care should be exercised when these drugs are administered concomitantly).
No products indexed under this heading.

Neomycin (Care should be taken in using cyclosporine with nephrotoxic drugs).
No products indexed under this heading.

Neomycin, oral (Care should be taken in using cyclosporine with nephrotoxic drugs).
No products indexed under this heading.

Neomycin Sulfate (Care should be taken in using cyclosporine with nephrotoxic drugs). Products include:
Neosporin Ophthalmic Solution Sterile .... ⊙252

Nevirapine (Care should be taken in using cyclosporine with nephrotoxic drugs). Products include:
Viramune Oral Suspension 873
Viramune Tablets 873

Nicardipine Hydrochloride (Cyclosporine is extensively metabolized by CYP450 3A. Substances that inhibit this enzyme could decrease the metabolism and increase cyclosporine concentrations). Products include:
Cardene I.V. 1093

Nifedipine (Co-administration results in frequent episodes of gingival hyperplasia).
No products indexed under this heading.

Nimodipine (While calcium antagonists can be effective agents in treating cyclosporine-associated hypertension, they can interfere with cyclosporine metabolism). Products include:
Nimotop Capsules 790

Nisoldipine (While calcium antagonists can be effective agents in treating cyclosporine-associated hypertension, they can interfere with cyclosporine metabolism). Products include:
Sular Extended Release Tablets 2975

Norethindrone (Cyclosporine is extensively metabolized by CYP3A. Substances that inhibit this enzyme could decrease the metabolism and increase cyclosporine concentrations). Products include:
Ortho Micronor Tablets 2446

Norethynodrel (Cyclosporine is extensively metabolized by CYP3A. Substances that inhibit this enzyme could decrease the metabolism and increase cyclosporine concentrations).
No products indexed under this heading.

Norfloxacin (Care should be taken in using cyclosporine with nephrotoxic drugs). Products include:
Noroxin Tablets 2069

Norgestimate (Cyclosporine is extensively metabolized by CYP3A. Substances that inhibit this enzyme could decrease the metabolism and increase cyclosporine concentrations). Products include:
Ortho-Cyclen/Ortho Tri-Cyclen 2449
Ortho Tri-Cyclen Lo Tablets 2458

Norgestrel (Cyclosporine is extensively metabolized by CYP3A. Substances that inhibit this enzyme could decrease the metabolism and increase cyclosporine concentrations).
No products indexed under this heading.

Octreotide Acetate (Co-administration with drugs that are inducers of CYP450 3A, such as octreotide, could increase metabolism of cyclosporine and decrease its concentrations). Products include:
Sandostatin Injection 2300
Sandostatin LAR Depot 2302

Olsalazine Sodium (Care should be taken in using cyclosporine with nephrotoxic drugs).
No products indexed under this heading.

Omeprazole (Care should be taken in using cyclosporine with nephrotoxic drugs).
No products indexed under this heading.

Orlistat (Compounds that decrease cyclosporine absorption such as orlistat should be avoided). Products include:
Xenical Capsules 2672

Oxaprozin (Cyclosporine can cause nephrotoxicity; clinical status and serum creatinine should be closely monitored when cyclosporine is used with NSAIDs in rheumatoid arthritis patients).
No products indexed under this heading.

Pamidronate Disodium (Care should be taken in using cyclosporine with nephrotoxic drugs).
No products indexed under this heading.

Paroxetine Hydrochloride (Care should be taken in using cyclosporine with nephrotoxic drugs). Products include:
Paxil 1535
Paxil CR Controlled-Release Tablets 1544

Penicillamine (Care should be taken in using cyclosporine with nephrotoxic drugs). Products include:
Cuprimine Capsules 1986

Penicillin G Benzathine (Care should be taken in using cyclosporine with nephrotoxic drugs). Products include:
Bicillin C-R Injectable Suspension 1775
Bicillin L-A Injection 1777

IMPORTANT NOTE: Always consult each drug listing in the patient's regimen for possible interactions.

Penicillin G Potassium (Care should be taken in using cyclosporine with nephrotoxic drugs).
No products indexed under this heading.

Penicillin G Procaine (Care should be taken in using cyclosporine with nephrotoxic drugs). Products include:
Bicillin C-R Injectable Suspension 1775
Bicillin L-A Injection 1777

Penicillin G Sodium (Care should be taken in using cyclosporine with nephrotoxic drugs).
No products indexed under this heading.

Penicillin V Potassium (Care should be taken in using cyclosporine with nephrotoxic drugs).
No products indexed under this heading.

Pentamidine Isethionate (Care should be taken in using cyclosporine with nephrotoxic drugs).
No products indexed under this heading.

Perindopril Erbumine (Caution is required when co-administering cyclosporine with potassium sparing drugs, such as ACE inhibitors). Products include:
Aceon Tablets (2 mg, 4 mg, 8 mg) 3038

Phenobarbital (Co-administration with drugs that are inducers of CYP450 3A, such as phenobarbital, could increase metabolism of cyclosporine and decrease its concentrations). Products include:
Donnatal Extentabs 2507

Phenylbutazone (Cyclosporine can cause nephrotoxicity; clinical status and serum creatinine should be closely monitored when cyclosporine is used with NSAIDs in rheumatoid arthritis patients).
No products indexed under this heading.

Phenytoin (Co-administration with drugs that are inducers of CYP450 3A, such as phenytoin, could increase metabolism of cyclosporine and decrease its concentrations).
No products indexed under this heading.

Phenytoin Sodium (Co-administration with drugs that are inducers of CYP450 3A, such as phenytoin, could increase metabolism of cyclosporine and decrease its concentrations). Products include:
Phenytek Capsules 2192

Piroxicam (Cyclosporine can cause nephrotoxicity; clinical status and serum creatinine should be closely monitored when cyclosporine is used with NSAIDs in rheumatoid arthritis patients).
No products indexed under this heading.

Plicamycin (Care should be taken in using cyclosporine with nephrotoxic drugs).
No products indexed under this heading.

Poliovirus Vaccine, Live, Oral, Trivalent, Types 1,2,3 (Sabin) (During treatment with cyclosporine, vaccination may be less effective; and the use of live attenuated vaccines avoided).
No products indexed under this heading.

Poliovirus Vaccine Inactivated (During treatment with cyclosporine, vaccination may be less effective). Products include:
Pediarix Vaccine 1552

Polymyxin (Care should be taken in using cyclosporine with nephrotoxic drugs).
No products indexed under this heading.

Polymyxin B Sulfate (Care should be taken in using cyclosporine with nephrotoxic drugs). Products include:
Neosporin Ophthalmic Solution Sterile ..... ⊙ 252

Polythiazide (Care should be taken in using cyclosporine with nephrotoxic drugs).
No products indexed under this heading.

Potassium Acid Phosphate (Caution is required when co-administering cyclosporine with potassium containing drugs, such as angiotensin II receptor antagonists). Products include:
K-Phos Original (Sodium Free) Tablets 814

Potassium Bicarbonate (Caution is required when co-administering cyclosporine with potassium containing drugs, such as angiotensin II receptor antagonists).
No products indexed under this heading.

Potassium Chloride (Caution is required when co-administering cyclosporine with potassium containing drugs, such as angiotensin II receptor antagonists). Products include:
MoviPrep Oral Solution 2679

Potassium Citrate (Caution is required when co-administering cyclosporine with potassium containing drugs, such as angiotensin II receptor antagonists). Products include:
BioLean Free Tablets ..... ▣ 635
Urocit-K Tablets 2176

Potassium Gluconate (Caution is required when co-administering cyclosporine with potassium containing drugs, such as angiotensin II receptor antagonists).
No products indexed under this heading.

Potassium Phosphate (Caution is required when co-administering cyclosporine with potassium containing drugs, such as angiotensin II receptor antagonists). Products include:
K-Phos Neutral Tablets 813

Pravastatin Sodium (Cyclosporine may reduce the clearance of HMG-CoA reductase inhibitors. Myotoxicity, including muscle pain and weakness, myositis, and rhabdomyolysis, have been reported with concomitant administration of cyclosporine with lovastatin, simvastatin, atorvastatin, pravastatin, and, rarely, fluvastatin. Dosage of these statins should be reduced).
No products indexed under this heading.

Prednisolone (Co-administration results in reduced clearance of prednisolone).
No products indexed under this heading.

Prednisolone Acetate (Co-administration results in reduced clearance of prednisolone). Products include:
Pred Forte Ophthalmic Suspension ..... ⊙ 227
Pred Mild Ophthalmic Suspension ..... ⊙ 230
Pred-G Ophthalmic Ointment ..... ⊙ 229
Pred-G Ophthalmic Suspension ..... ⊙ 228

Prednisolone Sodium Phosphate (Co-administration results in reduced clearance of prednisolone).
No products indexed under this heading.

Prednisolone Tebutate (Co-administration results in reduced clearance of prednisolone).
No products indexed under this heading.

Probenecid (Care should be taken in using cyclosporine with nephrotoxic drugs).
No products indexed under this heading.

Quinapril Hydrochloride (Caution is required when co-administering cyclosporine with potassium sparing drugs, such as ACE inhibitors).
No products indexed under this heading.

Quinine (Cyclosporine is extensively metabolized by CYP3A. Substances that inhibit this enzyme could decrease the metabolism and increase cyclosporine concentrations).
No products indexed under this heading.

Quinine Sulfate (Cyclosporine is extensively metabolized by CYP3A. Substances that inhibit this enzyme could decrease the metabolism and increase cyclosporine concentrations).
No products indexed under this heading.

Quinupristin (Cyclosporine is extensively metabolized by CYP450 3A. Substances that inhibit this enzyme could decrease the metabolism and increase cyclosporine concentrations).
No products indexed under this heading.

Rabeprazole Sodium (Care should be taken in using cyclosporine with nephrotoxic drugs). Products include:
Aciphex Tablets 1053

Ramipril (Caution is required when co-administering cyclosporine with potassium sparing drugs, such as ACE inhibitors).
No products indexed under this heading.

Ranitidine Hydrochloride (May potentiate renal dysfunction). Products include:
Zantac 75 Tablets ..... ▣ 603
Zantac 1670
Zantac Injection 1666
Zantac Injection Pharmacy Bulk Package 1668
Maximum Strength Zantac 150 Tablets ..... ▣ 603
Maximum Strength Zantac 150 Cool Mint Tablets ..... ▣ 603

Rifabutin (Rifabutin is known to increase the metabolism of other drugs metabolized by CYP450 system; cyclosporine is extensively metabolized by CYP450 3A system, therefore, caution should be exercised).
No products indexed under this heading.

Rifampicin (Cyclosporine is extensively metabolized by CYP3A. Substances that are inducers of CYP3A could increase metabolism and decrease cyclosporine concentrations).
No products indexed under this heading.

Rifampin (Co-administration with drugs that are inducers of CYP450 3A, such as rifampin, could increase metabolism of cyclosporine and decrease its concentrations).
No products indexed under this heading.

Rifapentine (Cyclosporine is extensively metabolized by CYP3A. Substances that are inducers of CYP3A could increase metabolism and decrease cyclosporine concentrations).
No products indexed under this heading.

Riluzole (Care should be taken in using cyclosporine with nephrotoxic drugs). Products include:
Rilutek Tablets 2771

Ritonavir (the HIV protease inhibitors are known to inhibit CYP3A and thus could potentially increase the concentrations of cyclosporine; care should be exercised when these drugs are administered concomitantly). Products include:
Kaletra 452
Norvir 489

Rofecoxib (Cyclosporine can cause nephrotoxicity; clinical status and serum creatinine should be closely monitored when cyclosporine is used with NSAIDs in rheumatoid arthritis patients).
No products indexed under this heading.

Rosuvastatin Calcium (Cyclosporine may reduce the clearance of HMG-CoA reductase inhibitors. Myotoxicity, including muscle pain and weakness, myositis, and rhabdomyolysis, have been reported with concomitant administration of cyclosporine with lovastatin, simvastatin, atorvastatin, pravastatin, and, rarely, fluvastatin. Dosage of these statins should be reduced). Products include:
Crestor Tablets 677

Rotavirus Vaccine, Live, Oral, Tetravalent (During treatment with cyclosporine, vaccination may be less effective; and the use of live attenuated vaccines avoided).
No products indexed under this heading.

Rubella & Mumps Virus Vaccine Live (During treatment with cyclosporine, vaccination may be less effective; and the use of live attenuated vaccines avoided).
No products indexed under this heading.

Rubella Virus Vaccine Live (During treatment with cyclosporine, vaccination may be less effective; and the use of live attenuated vaccines avoided). Products include:
Meruvax II 2061

Saquinavir (the HIV protease inhibitors are known to inhibit CYP3A and thus could potentially increase the concentrations of cyclosporine; care should be exercised when these drugs are administered concomitantly).
No products indexed under this heading.

Saquinavir Mesylate (the HIV protease inhibitors are known to inhibit CYP3A and thus could potentially increase the concentrations of cyclosporine; care should be exercised when these drugs are administered concomitantly).
No products indexed under this heading.

Sertraline Hydrochloride (Cyclosporine is extensively metabolized by CYP3A. Substances that inhibit this enzyme could decrease the metabolism and increase cyclosporine concentrations).
No products indexed under this heading.

Sibutramine Hydrochloride Monohydrate (Care should be taken in using cyclosporine with nephrotoxic drugs). Products include:
Meridia Capsules 475

Simvastatin (Cyclosporine may reduce the clearance of HMG-CoA reductase inhibitors. Myotoxicity, including muscle pain and weakness, myositis, and rhabdomyolysis, have been reported with concomitant administration of cyclosporine with lovastatin, simvastatin, atorvastatin, pravastatin, and, rarely, fluvastatin. Dosage of these statins should be reduced). Products include:
Simcor Tablets 502
Vytorin 10/10 Tablets 2149
Vytorin 10/10 Tablets 2939
Vytorin 10/20 Tablets 2149
Vytorin 10/20 Tablets 2939
Vytorin 10/40 Tablets 2149
Vytorin 10/40 Tablets 2939
Vytorin 10/80 Tablets 2149
Vytorin 10/80 Tablets 2939
Zocor Tablets 2136

Sirolimus (Elevations in serum creatinine were observed in studies using sirolimus in combination with full-dose cyclosporine. This effect is often reversible with cyclosporine dose reduction. Simultaneous co-administration of cyclosporine significantly increases blood levels of sirolimus; to minimize this, it is recommended that sirolimus be given 4 hours after cyclosporine administration). Products include:
Rapamune 3260

Smallpox Vaccine (During treatment with cyclosporine, vaccination may be less effective; and the use of live attenuated vaccines avoided).
No products indexed under this heading.

Spirapril Hydrochloride (Caution is required when co-administering cyclosporine with potassium sparing drugs, such as ACE inhibitors).
No products indexed under this heading.

Spironolactone (Cyclosporine causes hyperkalemia; concurrent use with potassium-sparing diuretics can result in increased risk of hyperkalemia; co-administration should be avoided).
No products indexed under this heading.

Stavudine (Care should be taken in using cyclosporine with nephrotoxic drugs).
No products indexed under this heading.

Streptomycin Sulfate (Care should be taken in using cyclosporine with nephrotoxic drugs).
No products indexed under this heading.

Streptozocin (Care should be taken in using cyclosporine with nephrotoxic drugs).
No products indexed under this heading.

Sulfacytine (Care should be taken in using cyclosporine with nephrotoxic drugs).
No products indexed under this heading.

Sulfamethizole (Care should be taken in using cyclosporine with nephrotoxic drugs).
No products indexed under this heading.

Sulfamethoxazole (May potentiate renal dysfunction).
No products indexed under this heading.

Sulfasalazine (Care should be taken in using cyclosporine with nephrotoxic drugs).
No products indexed under this heading.

Sulfinpyrazone (Cyclosporine is extensively metabolized by CYP3A. Substances that induce this enzyme could increase the metabolism and decrease cyclosporine concentrations).
No products indexed under this heading.

Sulfisoxazole Acetyl (Care should be taken in using cyclosporine with nephrotoxic drugs).
No products indexed under this heading.

Sulfisoxazole Diolamine (Care should be taken in using cyclosporine with nephrotoxic drugs).
No products indexed under this heading.

Sulindac (May potentiate renal dysfunction; co-administration is associated with additive decreases in renal function). Products include:
Clinoril Tablets 1962

Tacrolimus (May potentiate renal dysfunction; co-administration with other immunosuppressive agents increases the possibility of excessive immunosuppression). Products include:
Prograf Capsules and Injection 622
Protopic Ointment 628

Telmisartan (Caution is required when co-administering cyclosporine with potassium sparing drugs, such as angiotensin II receptor antagonists). Products include:
Micardis Tablets 852
Micardis HCT Tablets 854

Tenofovir Disoproxil Fumarate (Care should be taken in using cyclosporine with nephrotoxic drugs). Products include:
Atripla Tablets 938
Truvada Tablets 1262
Viread Tablets 1268

Terbinafine Hydrochloride (Cyclosporine is extensively metabolized by CYP3A. Substances that induce this enzyme could increase the metabolism and decrease cyclosporine concentrations). Products include:
Lamisil Oral Granules 2264
Lamisil Tablets 2266

Thioguanine (Care should be taken in using cyclosporine with nephrotoxic drugs). Products include:
Tabloid Tablets 1601

Ticarcillin Disodium (Care should be taken in using cyclosporine with nephrotoxic drugs). Products include:
Timentin ADD-Vantage 1606
Timentin Injection Galaxy Container 1609
Timentin IV Infusion 1603
Timentin Pharmacy Bulk Package 1613

Ticlopidine Hydrochloride (Co-administration with drugs that are inducers of CYP450 3A, such as ticlopidine, could increase metabolism of cyclosporine and decrease its concentrations).
No products indexed under this heading.

Tipranavir (the HIV protease inhibitors are known to inhibit CYP3A and thus could potentially increase the concentrations of cyclosporine; care should be exercised when these drugs are administered concomitantly). Products include:
Aptivus Capsules 823
Aptivus Oral Solution 823

Tobramycin (May potentiate renal dysfunction). Products include:
Zylet Ophthalmic Suspension .... ⊙ 247

Tobramycin Sulfate (May potentiate renal dysfunction).
No products indexed under this heading.

Tolazamide (Care should be taken in using cyclosporine with nephrotoxic drugs).
No products indexed under this heading.

Tolbutamide (Care should be taken in using cyclosporine with nephrotoxic drugs).
No products indexed under this heading.

Tolmetin Sodium (Cyclosporine can cause nephrotoxicity; clinical status and serum creatinine should be closely monitored when cyclosporine is used with NSAIDs in rheumatoid arthritis patients).
No products indexed under this heading.

Trandolapril (Caution is required when co-administering cyclosporine with potassium sparing drugs, such as ACE inhibitors). Products include:
Mavik Tablets 472
Tarka Tablets 511

Triamterene (Cyclosporine causes hyperkalemia; concurrent use with potassium-sparing diuretics can result in increased risk of hyperkalemia; co-administration should be avoided). Products include:
Dyazide Capsules 1405
Dyrenium Capsules 3189

Trimethadione (Care should be taken in using cyclosporine with nephrotoxic drugs).
No products indexed under this heading.

Trimethoprim (May potentiate renal dysfunction).
No products indexed under this heading.

Troleandomycin (Cyclosporine is extensively metabolized by CYP3A. Substances that inhibit this enzyme could decrease the metabolism and increase cyclosporine concentrations).
No products indexed under this heading.

Trovafloxacin Mesylate (Care should be taken in using cyclosporine with nephrotoxic drugs).
No products indexed under this heading.

Typhoid Vaccine (During treatment with cyclosporine, vaccination may be less effective; and the use of live attenuated vaccines avoided).
No products indexed under this heading.

Tyropanoate Sodium (Care should be taken in using cyclosporine with nephrotoxic drugs).
No products indexed under this heading.

Ultraviolet radiation (Psoriasis patients who are treated with cyclosporine capsules should not receive concomitant PUVA or UVB therapy).
No products indexed under this heading.

Vaccines (Live) (During treatment with cyclosporine, vaccination may be less effective and the use of live attenuated vaccines should be avoided).
No products indexed under this heading.

Valacyclovir Hydrochloride (Care should be taken in using cyclosporine with nephrotoxic drugs). Products include:
Valtrex Caplets 1635

Valdecoxib (Cyclosporine can cause nephrotoxicity; clinical status and serum creatinine should be closely monitored when cyclosporine is used with NSAIDs in rheumatoid arthritis patients).
No products indexed under this heading.

Valsartan (Caution is required when co-administering cyclosporine with potassium sparing drugs, such as angiotensin II receptor antagonists). Products include:
Diovan Tablets 2212
Diovan HCT Tablets 2216
Exforge Tablets 2238

Vancomycin Hydrochloride (May potentiate renal dysfunction).
No products indexed under this heading.

Varicella Virus Vaccine Live (During treatment with cyclosporine, vaccination may be less effective; and the use of live attenuated vaccines avoided). Products include:
Varivax 2133

Venlafaxine Hydrochloride (Cyclosporine is extensively metabolized by CYP3A. Substances that inhibit this enzyme could decrease the metabolism and increase cyclosporine concentrations). Products include:
Effexor XR Extended-Release Capsules 3195
Venlafaxine Hydrochloride Tablets 2199

Verapamil Hydrochloride (Cyclosporine is extensively metabolized by CYP450 3A. Substances that inhibit this enzyme could decrease the metabolism and increase cyclosporine concentrations). Products include:
Tarka Tablets 511

Voriconazole (Care should be taken in using cyclosporine with nephrotoxic drugs).
No products indexed under this heading.

Yellow Fever Vaccine (During treatment with cyclosporine, vaccination may be less effective; and the use of live attenuated vaccines avoided).
No products indexed under this heading.

Zafirlukast (Cyclosporine is extensively metabolized by CYP3A. Substances that inhibit this enzyme could decrease the metabolism and increase cyclosporine concentrations). Products include:
Accolate Tablets 669

Zalcitabine (Care should be taken in using cyclosporine with nephrotoxic drugs).
No products indexed under this heading.

Zidovudine (Care should be taken in using cyclosporine with nephrotoxic drugs). Products include:
Combivir Tablets 1384
Retrovir 1574
Retrovir IV Infusion 1579
Trizivir Tablets 1622

Zileuton (Cyclosporine is extensively metabolized by CYP3A. Substances that inhibit this enzyme could decrease the metabolism and increase cyclosporine concentrations).
No products indexed under this heading.

Zoledronic acid (Care should be taken in using cyclosporine with nephrotoxic drugs). Products include:
Reclast Injection 2291
Zometa for Intravenous Infusion 2341

Zoster Vaccine Live (During treatment with cyclosporine, vaccination may be less effective; and the use of live attenuated vaccines avoided). Products include:
Zostavax Injection 2145

Food Interactions

Diet, high-lipid (A high fat meal within one-half hour before cyclosporine administration decreases the AUC by 13% and Cmax by 33%).

Food, unspecified (The administration of food with Gengraf decreases the cyclosporine AUC and Cmax).

Grapefruit (Affects the metabolism of cyclosporine increasing blood concentration of cyclosporine; concurrent use should be avoided).

Grapefruit Juice (Affects the metabolism of cyclosporine increasing blood concentration of cyclosporine; concurrent use should be avoided).

GENOTROPIN LYOPHILIZED POWDER

(Somatropin) 2547
May interact with corticosteroids, anticonvulsants, estrogens, glucocorticoids, oral hypoglycemic agents, insulin, drugs which undergo biotransformation by cytochrome p-450 mixed function oxidase, sex steroids, and certain other agents. Compounds in these categories include:

Acarbose (In patients with diabetes mellitus requiring drug therapy, the dose of oral hypoglycemic agents may require adjustment when somatropin therapy is initiated). Products include:
Precose Tablets 792

Acetaminophen (Limited published data indicate that somatropin treatment increases cytochrome P450 (CYP450)-mediated antipyrine clearance in man. These data suggest that somatropin administration may alter the clearance of compounds known to be metabolized by CYP450 liver enzymes. Careful monitoring is advisable when somatropin is administered in combination with other drugs known to be metabolized by CYP450 liver enzymes. However formal drug interaction studies have not been conducted). Products include:
Benadryl Allergy & Cold Kapgels 1895
Benadryl Allergy & Sinus Headache Kapgels 1895
Benadryl Severe Allergy & Sinus Headache Caplets 1897
Lortab 5/500 Tablets 3143
Lortab 7.5/500 Tablets 3144
Lortab 10/500 Tablets 3144
Percocet Tablets 1127
Sinutab Sinus Caplets 1905
Sudafed PE Cold & Cough Caplets 1907
Sudafed PE Nighttime Cold Caplets 1907
Sudafed PE Severe Cold Caplets 1908
Sudafed PE Sinus Headache Caplets 1908
Regular Strength Tylenol Tablets 1915
Tylenol 8 Hour Extended Release Caplets 1915
Extra Strength Tylenol Caplets, Cool Caplets, and EZ Tabs 1915
Extra Strength Tylenol Adult Rapid Blast Liquid 1915
Extra Strength Tylenol PM Caplets, Geltabs, Liquid, and Rapid Release Gels 1915
Extra Strength Tylenol Rapid Release Gels 1915
Tylenol with Codeine Tablets 2427
Tylenol Allergy Multi-Symptom Caplets with Cool Burst and Rapid Release Gelcaps 1916
Tylenol Allergy Multi-Symptom Nighttime Caplets with Cool Burst 1916
Tylenol Severe Allergy Caplets 1916
Tylenol Arthritis Pain Extended Release Geltabs/Caplets 1915
Tylenol Chest Congestion Caplets with Cool Burst 1910
Tylenol Chest Congestion Liquid with Cool Burst 1910
Children's Tylenol Plus Cold Suspension Liquid 1912
Children's Tylenol Plus Cold & Allergy Suspension Liquid 1914
Children's Tylenol Plus Cough & Runny Nose Suspension Liquid 1912
Children's Tylenol Plus Cough & Sore Throat Suspension Liquid 1912
Children's Tylenol Plus Flu Suspension Liquid 1914
Children's Tylenol Suspension Liquid 1909
Children's Tylenol Meltaways 1909
Children's Tylenol Plus Multi-Symptom Cold Suspension Liquid 1912
Tylenol Cold Severe Congestion Daytime Caplets with Cool Burst 1912
Tylenol Cold Head Congestion Daytime Caplets with Cool Burst 1910
Tylenol Cold Head Congestion Nighttime Caplets with Cool Burst 1910
Tylenol Cold Head Congestion Severe Daytime Caplets with Cool Burst 1910
Tylenol Cold Multi-Symptom Daytime Caplets with Cool Burst and Rapid Release Gels 1913
Tylenol Cold Multi-Symptom Daytime Liquid with Citrus Burst 1913
Tylenol Cold Multi-Symptom Nighttime Caplets with Cool Burst 1913
Tylenol Cold Multi-Symptom Nighttime Liquid with Cool Burst 1913
Tylenol Cold Multi-Symptom Severe Caplets with Cool Burst 1913
Tylenol Cold Multi-Symptom Severe Daytime Liquid with Citrus Burst 1913
Tylenol Cough & Sore Throat Daytime Liquid with Cool Burst 1918
Tylenol Cough & Sore Throat Nighttime Liquid with Cool Burst 1918
Concentrated Tylenol Infants' Drops 1909
Jr. Tylenol Meltaways 1909
Tylenol Sinus Congestion & Pain Daytime Caplets with Cool Burst and Gelcaps 1917
Tylenol Sinus Congestion & Pain Nighttime Caplets with Cool Burst 1917
Tylenol Sinus Congestion & Pain Severe Caplets with Cool Burst 1917
Tylenol Sinus Severe Congestion Caplets with Cool Burst 1917
Tylenol Sore Throat Daytime Liquid with Cool Burst 1918
Tylenol Sore Throat Nighttime Liquid with Cool Burst 1918
Women's Tylenol Menstrual Relief Caplets 1919
Vicks DayQuil Cold & Flu Multi-Symptom Relief .... ▣ 616
Vicks DayQuil LiquiCaps 2567
Vicks DayQuil Liquid 2567
Vicks DayQuil Multi-Symptom Cold/Flu Relief 2567
Vicks NyQuil Cold & Flu Multi-Symptom Relief .... ▣ 617
Vicks NyQuil LiquiCaps 2567
Vicks NyQuil Liquid 2567
Vicks NyQuil Multi-Symptom Cold/Flu Relief 2567
Vicodin Tablets 529
Vicodin ES Tablets 530
Vicodin HP Tablets 531
Zydone Tablets 1132

Alatrofloxacin Mesylate (Limited published data indicate that somatropin treatment increases cytochrome P450 (CYP450)-mediated antipyrine clearance in man. These data suggest that somatropin administration may alter the clearance of compounds known to be metabolized by CYP450 liver enzymes. Careful monitoring is advisable when somatropin is administered in combination with other drugs known to be metabolized by CYP450 liver enzymes. However formal drug interaction studies have not been conducted).
No products indexed under this heading.

Alfentanil Hydrochloride (Limited published data indicate that somatropin treatment increases cytochrome P450 (CYP450)-mediated antipyrine clearance in man. These data suggest that somatropin administration may alter the clearance of compounds known to be metabolized by CYP450 liver enzymes. Careful monitoring is advisable when somatropin is administered in combination with other drugs known to be metabolized by CYP450 liver enzymes. However formal drug interaction studies have not been conducted).
No products indexed under this heading.

Alprazolam (Limited published data indicate that somatropin treatment increases cytochrome P450 (CYP450)-mediated antipyrine clearance in man. These data suggest that somatropin administration may alter the clearance of compounds known to be metabolized by CYP450 liver enzymes. Careful monitoring is advisable when somatropin is administered in combination with other drugs known to be metabolized by CYP450 liver enzymes. However formal drug interaction studies have not been conducted).
No products indexed under this heading.

Aminophylline (Limited published data indicate that somatropin treatment increases cytochrome P450 (CYP450)-mediated antipyrine clearance in man. These data suggest that somatropin administration may alter the clearance of compounds known to be metabolized by CYP450 liver enzymes. Careful monitoring is advisable when somatropin is administered in combination with other drugs known to be metabolized by CYP450 liver enzymes. However formal drug interaction studies have not been conducted).
No products indexed under this heading.

Amiodarone Hydrochloride (Limited published data indicate that somatropin treatment increases cytochrome P450 (CYP450)-mediated antipyrine clearance in man. These data suggest that somatropin administration may alter the clearance of compounds known to be metabolized by CYP450 liver enzymes. Careful monitoring is advisable when somatropin is administered in combination with other drugs known to be metabolized by CYP450 liver enzymes. However formal drug interaction studies have not been conducted).
No products indexed under this heading.

Amitriptyline Hydrochloride (Limited published data indicate that somatropin treatment increases cytochrome P450 (CYP450)-mediated antipyrine clearance in man. These data suggest that somatropin administration may alter the clearance of compounds known to be metabolized by CYP450 liver enzymes. Careful monitoring is advisable when somatropin is administered in combination with other drugs known to be metabolized by CYP450 liver enzymes. However formal drug interaction studies have not been conducted).
No products indexed under this heading.

Amlodipine Besylate (Limited published data indicate that somatropin treatment increases cytochrome P450 (CYP450)-mediated antipyrine clearance in man. These data suggest that somatropin administration may alter the clearance of compounds known to be metabolized by CYP450 liver enzymes. Careful monitoring is advisable when somatropin is administered in combination with other drugs known to be metabolized by CYP450 liver enzymes. However formal drug interaction studies have not been conducted). Products include:
Azor Tablets 1005
Exforge Tablets 2238

Amoxapine (Limited published data indicate that somatropin treatment increases cytochrome P450 (CYP450)-mediated antipyrine clearance in man. These data suggest that somatropin administration may alter the clearance of compounds known to be metabolized by CYP450 liver enzymes. Careful monitoring is advisable when somatropin is administered in combination with other drugs known to be metabolized by CYP450 liver enzymes. However formal drug interaction studies have not been conducted).
No products indexed under this heading.

Amphetamine Aspartate (Limited published data indicate that somatropin treatment increases cytochrome P450 (CYP450)-mediated antipyrine clearance in man. These data suggest that somatropin administration may alter the clearance of compounds known to be metabolized by

CYP450 liver enzymes. Careful monitoring is advisable when somatropin is administered in combination with other drugs known to be metabolized by CYP450 liver enzymes. However formal drug interaction studies have not been conducted). Products include:

Adderall XR Capsules 3012

Amphetamine Aspartate Monohydrate (Limited published data indicate that somatropin treatment increases cytochrome P450 (CYP450)-mediated antipyrine clearance in man. These data suggest that somatropin administration may alter the clearance of compounds known to be metabolized by CYP450 liver enzymes. Careful monitoring is advisable when somatropin is administered in combination with other drugs known to be metabolized by CYP450 liver enzymes. However formal drug interaction studies have not been conducted).

No products indexed under this heading.

Amphetamine Sulfate (Limited published data indicate that somatropin treatment increases cytochrome P450 (CYP450)-mediated antipyrine clearance in man. These data suggest that somatropin administration may alter the clearance of compounds known to be metabolized by CYP450 liver enzymes. Careful monitoring is advisable when somatropin is administered in combination with other drugs known to be metabolized by CYP450 liver enzymes. However formal drug interaction studies have not been conducted). Products include:

Adderall XR Capsules 3012

Aprepitant (Limited published data indicate that somatropin treatment increases cytochrome P450 (CYP450)-mediated antipyrine clearance in man. These data suggest that somatropin administration may alter the clearance of compounds known to be metabolized by CYP450 liver enzymes. Careful monitoring is advisable when somatropin is administered in combination with other drugs known to be metabolized by CYP450 liver enzymes. However formal drug interaction studies have not been conducted). Products include:

Emend Capsules 1992

Astemizole (Limited published data indicate that somatropin treatment increases cytochrome P450 (CYP450)-mediated antipyrine clearance in man. These data suggest that somatropin administration may alter the clearance of compounds known to be metabolized by CYP450 liver enzymes. Careful monitoring is advisable when somatropin is administered in combination with other drugs known to be metabolized by CYP450 liver enzymes. However formal drug interaction studies have not been conducted).

No products indexed under this heading.

Atomoxetine Hydrochloride (Limited published data indicate that somatropin treatment increases cytochrome P450 (CYP450)-mediated antipyrine clearance in man. These data suggest that somatropin administration may alter the clearance of compounds known to be metabolized by CYP450 liver enzymes. Careful monitoring is advisable when somatropin is administered in combination with other drugs known to be metabolized by CYP450 liver enzymes. However formal drug interaction studies have not been conducted). Products include:

Strattera Capsules 1864

Atorvastatin Calcium (Limited published data indicate that somatropin treatment increases cytochrome P450 (CYP450)-mediated antipyrine clearance in man. These data suggest that somatropin administration may alter the clearance of compounds known to be metabolized by CYP450 liver enzymes. Careful monitoring is advisable when somatropin is administered in combination with other drugs known to be metabolized by CYP450 liver enzymes. However formal drug interaction studies have not been conducted). Products include:

Lipitor Tablets 2501

Belladonna Ergotamine (Limited published data indicate that somatropin treatment increases cytochrome P450 (CYP450)-mediated antipyrine clearance in man. These data suggest that somatropin administration may alter the clearance of compounds known to be metabolized by CYP450 liver enzymes. Careful monitoring is advisable when somatropin is administered in combination with other drugs known to be metabolized by CYP450 liver enzymes. However formal drug interaction studies have not been conducted).

No products indexed under this heading.

Benzphetamine Hydrochloride (Limited published data indicate that somatropin treatment increases cytochrome P450 (CYP450)-mediated antipyrine clearance in man. These data suggest that somatropin administration may alter the clearance of compounds known to be metabolized by CYP450 liver enzymes. Careful monitoring is advisable when somatropin is administered in combination with other drugs known to be metabolized by CYP450 liver enzymes. However formal drug interaction studies have not been conducted).

No products indexed under this heading.

Betamethasone Acetate (Somatropin inhibits 11βHSD-1 in adipose/hepatic tissue and may significantly impact the metabolism of cortisone and cortisol. Patients being treated with glucocorticoid replacement therapy for hypoadrenalism may require an increase in their maintenance or stress doses; especially with cortisone acetate and prednisone, since conversion of these drugs to their biologically active metabolites is dependent on the activity of the 11μHSD-1 enzyme. Also, excessive glucocorticoid therapy may attenuate the growth-promoting effects of somatropin in children. Therefore, glucocorticoid replacement therapy should be carefully adjusted in children with concomitant GH and glucocorticoid deficiency to avoid both hypoadrenalism and an inhibitory effect on growth).

No products indexed under this heading.

Betamethasone Sodium Phosphate (Somatropin inhibits 11βHSD-1 in adipose/hepatic tissue and may significantly impact the metabolism of cortisone and cortisol. Patients being treated with glucocorticoid replacement therapy for hypoadrenalism may require an increase in their maintenance or stress doses; especially with cortisone acetate and prednisone, since conversion of these drugs to their biologically active metabolites is dependent on the activity of the 11μHSD-1 enzyme. Also, excessive glucocorticoid therapy may attenuate the growth-promoting effects of somatropin in children. Therefore, glucocorticoid replacement therapy should be carefully adjusted in children with concomitant GH and glucocorticoid deficiency to avoid both hypoadrenalism and an inhibitory effect on growth).

No products indexed under this heading.

Bisoprolol Fumarate (Limited published data indicate that somatropin treatment increases cytochrome P450 (CYP450)-mediated antipyrine clearance in man. These data suggest that somatropin administration may alter the clearance of compounds known to be metabolized by CYP450 liver enzymes. Careful monitoring is advisable when somatropin is administered in combination with other drugs known to be metabolized by CYP450 liver enzymes. However formal drug interaction studies have not been conducted).

No products indexed under this heading.

Budesonide (Limited published data indicates that somatropin treatment increases cytochrome P450 (CP450) mediated antipyrine clearance in man. This data suggests that somatropin administration may alter the clearance of compounds known to be metabolized by CP450 liver enzymes (eg, corticosteroids). Careful monitoring is advisable when somatropin is administered in combination with other drugs known to be metabolized by CP450 liver enzymes. However, formal drug interaction studies have not been conducted). Products include:

Pulmicort Flexhaler 654

Symbicort 80/4.5 Inhalation Aerosol.. 659

Symbicort 160/4.5 Inhalation Aerosol.. 659

Buspirone Hydrochloride (Limited published data indicate that somatropin treatment increases cytochrome P450 (CYP450)-mediated antipyrine clearance in man. These data suggest that somatropin administration may alter the clearance of compounds known to be metabolized by CYP450 liver enzymes. Careful monitoring is advisable when somatropin is administered in combination with other drugs known to be metabolized by CYP450 liver enzymes. However formal drug interaction studies have not been conducted).

No products indexed under this heading.

Busulfan (Limited published data indicate that somatropin treatment increases cytochrome P450 (CYP450)-mediated antipyrine clearance in man. These data suggest that somatropin administration may alter the clearance of compounds known to be metabolized by CYP450 liver enzymes. Careful monitoring is advisable when somatropin is administered in combination with other drugs known to be metabolized by CYP450 liver enzymes. However formal drug interaction studies have not been conducted). Products include:

Busulfex Injection 2477

Myleran Tablets 1530

Caffeine (Limited published data indicate that somatropin treatment increases cytochrome P450 (CYP450)-mediated antipyrine clearance in man. These data suggest that somatropin administration may alter the clearance of compounds known to be metabolized by CYP450 liver enzymes. Careful monitoring is advisable when somatropin is administered in combination with other drugs known to be metabolized by CYP450 liver enzymes. However formal drug interaction studies have not been conducted). Products include:

BioLean Free Tablets 635

BioLean II Tablets 635

Winrgy Dietary Supplement 642

Caffeine Anhydrous (Limited published data indicate that somatropin treatment increases cytochrome P450 (CYP450)-mediated antipyrine clearance in man. These data suggest that somatropin administration may alter the clearance of compounds known to be metabolized by CYP450 liver enzymes. Careful monitoring is advisable when somatropin is administered in combination with other drugs known to be metabolized by CYP450 liver enzymes. However formal drug interaction studies have not been conducted).

No products indexed under this heading.

Caffeine Citrate (Limited published data indicate that somatropin treatment increases cytochrome P450 (CYP450)-mediated antipyrine clearance in man. These data suggest that somatropin administration may alter the clearance of compounds known to be metabolized by CYP450 liver enzymes. Careful monitoring is advisable when somatropin is administered in combination with other drugs known to be metabolized by CYP450 liver enzymes. However formal drug interaction studies have not been conducted).

No products indexed under this heading.

Candesartan Cilexetil (Limited published data indicate that somatropin treatment increases cytochrome P450 (CYP450)-mediated antipyrine clearance in man. These data suggest that somatropin administration may alter the clearance of compounds known to be metabolized by CYP450 liver enzymes. Careful monitoring is advisable when somatropin is administered in combination with other drugs known to be metabolized by CYP450 liver enzymes. However formal drug interaction studies have not been conducted). Products include:

Atacand Tablets 639

Atacand HCT 642

Captopril (Limited published data indicate that somatropin treatment increases cytochrome P450 (CYP450)-mediated antipyrine clearance in man. These data suggest that somatropin administration may alter the clearance of compounds known to be metabolized by CYP450 liver enzymes. Careful monitoring is advisable when somatropin is administered in combination with other drugs known to be metabolized by CYP450 liver enzymes. However formal drug interaction studies have not been conducted). Products include:

Captopril Tablets 2182

Carbamazepine (Limited published data indicates that somatropin treatment increases cytochrome P450 (CP450) mediated antipyrine clearance in man. This data suggests that somatropin administration may alter the clearance of compounds known to be metabolized by CP450 liver enzymes (eg anticonvulsants). Careful monitoring is advisable when somatropin is administered in combination with other drugs known to be metabolized by CP450 liver enzymes. However, formal drug interaction studies have not been conducted). Products include:

Carbatrol Capsules 3019
Equetro Extended-Release Capsules 3174

Carisoprodol (Limited published data indicate that somatropin treatment increases cytochrome P450 (CYP450)-mediated antipyrine clearance in man. These data suggest that somatropin administration may alter the clearance of compounds known to be metabolized by CYP450 liver enzymes. Careful monitoring is advisable when somatropin is administered in combination with other drugs known to be metabolized by CYP450 liver enzymes. However formal drug interaction studies have not been conducted). Products include:

Soma Tablets 1931

Carvedilol (Limited published data indicate that somatropin treatment increases cytochrome P450 (CYP450)-mediated antipyrine clearance in man. These data suggest that somatropin administration may alter the clearance of compounds known to be metabolized by CYP450 liver enzymes. Careful monitoring is advisable when somatropin is administered in combination with other drugs known to be metabolized by CYP450 liver enzymes. However formal drug interaction studies have not been conducted). Products include:

Coreg Tablets 1387

Celecoxib (Limited published data indicate that somatropin treatment increases cytochrome P450 (CYP450)-mediated antipyrine clearance in man. These data suggest that somatropin administration may alter the clearance of compounds known to be metabolized by CYP450 liver enzymes. Careful monitoring is advisable when somatropin is administered in combination with other drugs known to be metabolized by CYP450 liver enzymes. However formal drug interaction studies have not been conducted). Products include:

Celebrex Capsules 2979

Cerivastatin Sodium (Limited published data indicate that somatropin treatment increases cytochrome P450 (CYP450)-mediated antipyrine clearance in man. These data suggest that somatropin administration may alter the clearance of compounds known to be metabolized by CYP450 liver enzymes. Careful monitoring is advisable when somatropin is administered in combination with other drugs known to be metabolized by CYP450 liver enzymes. However formal drug interaction studies have not been conducted).

No products indexed under this heading.

Cevimeline Hydrochloride (Limited published data indicate that somatropin treatment increases cytochrome P450 (CYP450)-mediated antipyrine clearance in man. These data suggest that somatropin administration may alter the clearance of compounds known to be metabolized by CYP450 liver enzymes. Careful monitoring is advisable when somatropin is administered in combination with other drugs known to be metabolized by CYP450 liver enzymes. However formal drug interaction studies have not been conducted). Products include:

Evoxac Capsules 1013

Chlordiazepoxide (Limited published data indicate that somatropin treatment increases cytochrome P450 (CYP450)-mediated antipyrine clearance in man. These data suggest that somatropin administration may alter the clearance of compounds known to be metabolized by CYP450 liver enzymes. Careful monitoring is advisable when somatropin is administered in combination with other drugs known to be metabolized by CYP450 liver enzymes. However formal drug interaction studies have not been conducted).

No products indexed under this heading.

Chlordiazepoxide Hydrochloride (Limited published data indicate that somatropin treatment increases cytochrome P450 (CYP450)-mediated antipyrine clearance in man. These data suggest that somatropin administration may alter the clearance of compounds known to be metabolized by CYP450 liver enzymes. Careful monitoring is advisable when somatropin is administered in combination with other drugs known to be metabolized by CYP450 liver enzymes. However formal drug interaction studies have not been conducted).

No products indexed under this heading.

Chlorotrianisene (In patients on oral estrogen replacement, a larger dose of somatropin may be required to achieve the defined treatment goal).

No products indexed under this heading.

Chlorpheniramine (Limited published data indicate that somatropin treatment increases cytochrome P450 (CYP450)-mediated antipyrine clearance in man. These data suggest that somatropin administration may alter the clearance of compounds known to be metabolized by CYP450 liver enzymes. Careful monitoring is advisable when somatropin is administered in combination with other drugs known to be metabolized by CYP450 liver enzymes. However formal drug interaction studies have not been conducted).

No products indexed under this heading.

Chlorpheniramine Maleate (Limited published data indicate that somatropin treatment increases cytochrome P450 (CYP450)-mediated antipyrine clearance in man. These data suggest that somatropin administration may alter the clearance of compounds known to be metabolized by CYP450 liver enzymes. Careful monitoring is advisable when somatropin is administered in combination with other drugs known to be metabolized by CYP450 liver enzymes. However formal drug interaction studies have not been conducted). Products include:

Actifed Cold & Allergy Tablets 1895
Sudafed PE Sinus & Allergy Tablets 1908
Tylenol Allergy Multi-Symptom Caplets with Cool Burst and Rapid Release Gelcaps 1916
Children's Tylenol Plus Cold Suspension Liquid 1912
Children's Tylenol Plus Cough & Runny Nose Suspension Liquid 1912
Children's Tylenol Plus Flu Suspension Liquid 1914
Children's Tylenol Plus Multi-Symptom Cold Suspension Liquid 1912
Tylenol Cold Head Congestion Nighttime Caplets with Cool Burst 1910
Tylenol Cold Multi-Symptom Nighttime Caplets with Cool Burst 1913
Tylenol Sinus Congestion & Pain Nighttime Caplets with Cool Burst 1917

Chlorpheniramine Polistirex (Limited published data indicate that somatropin treatment increases cytochrome P450 (CYP450)-mediated antipyrine clearance in man. These data suggest that somatropin administration may alter the clearance of compounds known to be metabolized by CYP450 liver enzymes. Careful monitoring is advisable when somatropin is administered in combination with other drugs known to be metabolized by CYP450 liver enzymes. However formal drug interaction studies have not been conducted). Products include:

Tussionex Pennkinetic Extended-Release Suspension 3154

Chlorpheniramine Tannate (Limited published data indicate that somatropin treatment increases cytochrome P450 (CYP450)-mediated antipyrine clearance in man. These data suggest that somatropin administration may alter the clearance of compounds known to be metabolized by CYP450 liver enzymes. Careful monitoring is advisable when somatropin is administered in combination with other drugs known to be metabolized by CYP450 liver enzymes. However formal drug interaction studies have not been conducted).

No products indexed under this heading.

Chlorpromazine (Limited published data indicate that somatropin treatment increases cytochrome P450 (CYP450)-mediated antipyrine clearance in man. These data suggest that somatropin administration may alter the clearance of compounds known to be metabolized by CYP450 liver enzymes. Careful monitoring is advisable when somatropin is administered in combination with other drugs known to be metabolized by CYP450 liver enzymes. However formal drug interaction studies have not been conducted).

No products indexed under this heading.

Chlorpromazine Hydrochloride (Limited published data indicate that somatropin treatment increases cytochrome P450 (CYP450)-mediated antipyrine clearance in man. These data suggest that somatropin administration may alter the clearance of compounds known to be metabolized by CYP450 liver enzymes. Careful monitoring is advisable when somatropin is administered in combination with other drugs known to be metabolized by CYP450 liver enzymes. However formal drug interaction studies have not been conducted).

No products indexed under this heading.

Chlorpropamide (In patients with diabetes mellitus requiring drug therapy, the dose of oral hypoglycemic agents may require adjustment when somatropin therapy is initiated).

No products indexed under this heading.

Ciclesonide (Limited published data indicates that somatropin treatment increases cytochrome P450 (CP450) mediated antipyrine clearance in man. This data suggests that somatropin administration may alter the clearance of compounds known to be metabolized by CP450 liver enzymes (eg, corticosteroids). Careful monitoring is advisable when somatropin is administered in combination with other drugs known to be metabolized by CP450 liver enzymes. However, formal drug interaction studies have not been conducted). Products include:

Alvesco Inhalation Aerosol 2985
Omnaris Nasal Spray 2998

Cilostazol (Limited published data indicate that somatropin treatment increases cytochrome P450 (CYP450)-mediated antipyrine clearance in man. These data suggest that somatropin administration may alter the clearance of compounds known to be metabolized by CYP450 liver enzymes. Careful monitoring is advisable when somatropin is administered in combination with other drugs known to be metabolized by CYP450 liver enzymes. However formal drug interaction studies have not been conducted). Products include:

Pletal Tablets 2481

Cimetidine Hydrochloride (Limited published data indicate that somatropin treatment increases cytochrome P450 (CYP450)-mediated antipyrine clearance in man. These data suggest that somatropin administration may alter the clearance of compounds known to be metabolized by CYP450 liver enzymes. Careful monitoring is advisable when somatropin is administered in combination with other drugs known to be metabolized by CYP450 liver enzymes. However formal drug interaction studies have not been conducted).

No products indexed under this heading.

Ciprofloxacin (Limited published data indicate that somatropin treatment increases cytochrome P450 (CYP450)-mediated antipyrine clearance in man. These data suggest that somatropin administration may alter the clearance of compounds known to be metabolized by CYP450 liver enzymes. Careful monitoring is advisable when somatropin is administered in combination with other drugs known to be metabolized by CYP450 liver enzymes. However formal drug interaction studies have not been conducted). Products include:

Cipro I.V. 2817
Cipro Oral Suspension 2810
Cipro XR Tablets 2823
Ciprodex Otic Suspension 541

Ciprofloxacin Hydrochloride (Limited published data indicate that somatropin treatment increases cytochrome P450 (CYP450)-mediated antipyrine clearance in man. These data suggest that somatropin administration may alter the clearance of compounds known to be metabolized by CYP450 liver enzymes. Careful monitoring is advisable when somatropin is administered in combination with other drugs known to be metabolized by CYP450 liver enzymes. However formal drug interaction studies have not been conducted). Products include:

Cipro Tablets 2810

Cisapride (Limited published data indicate that somatropin treatment increases cytochrome P450 (CYP450)-mediated antipyrine clearance in man. These data suggest that somatropin administration may alter the clearance of compounds known to be metabolized by CYP450 liver enzymes. Careful monitoring is advisable when somatropin is administered in combination with other drugs known to be metabolized by CYP450 liver enzymes. However formal drug interaction studies have not been conducted).

No products indexed under this heading.

Citalopram Hydrobromide (Limited published data indicate that somatropin treatment increases cytochrome P450 (CYP450)-mediated antipyrine clearance in man. These data suggest that somatropin administration may alter the clearance of compounds known to be metabolized by CYP450 liver enzymes. Careful monitoring is advisable when somatropin is administered in combination with other drugs known to be metabolized by CYP450 liver enzymes. However formal drug interaction studies have not been conducted). Products include:

Celexa 1160

Clarithromycin (Limited published data indicate that somatropin treatment increases cytochrome P450 (CYP450)-mediated antipyrine clearance in man. These data suggest that somatropin administration may alter the clearance of compounds known to be metabolized by CYP450 liver enzymes. Careful monitoring is advisable when somatropin is administered in combination with other drugs known to be metabolized by CYP450 liver enzymes. However formal drug interaction studies have not been conducted). Products include:

Biaxin/Biaxin XL 411

Clomipramine Hydrochloride (Limited published data indicate that somatropin treatment increases cytochrome P450 (CYP450)-mediated antipyrine clearance in man. These data suggest that somatropin administration may alter the clearance of compounds known to be metabolized by CYP450 liver enzymes. Careful monitoring is advisable when somatropin is administered in combination with other drugs known to be metabolized by CYP450 liver enzymes. However formal drug interaction studies have not been conducted).

No products indexed under this heading.

Clopidogrel Hydrogen Sulfate (Limited published data indicate that somatropin treatment increases cytochrome P450 (CYP450)-mediated antipyrine clearance in man. These data suggest that somatropin administration may alter the clearance of compounds known to be metabolized by CYP450 liver enzymes. Careful monitoring is advisable when somatropin is administered in combination with other drugs known to be metabolized by CYP450 liver enzymes. However formal drug interaction studies have not been conducted).

No products indexed under this heading.

Clozapine (Limited published data indicate that somatropin treatment increases cytochrome P450 (CYP450)-mediated antipyrine clearance in man. These data suggest that somatropin administration may alter the clearance of compounds known to be metabolized by CYP450 liver enzymes. Careful monitoring is advisable when somatropin is administered in combination with other drugs known to be metabolized by CYP450 liver enzymes. However formal drug interaction studies have not been conducted).

No products indexed under this heading.

Codeine Phosphate (Limited published data indicate that somatropin treatment increases cytochrome P450 (CYP450)-mediated antipyrine clearance in man. These data suggest that somatropin administration may alter the clearance of compounds known to be metabolized by CYP450 liver enzymes. Careful monitoring is advisable when somatropin is administered in combination with other drugs known to be metabolized by CYP450 liver enzymes. However formal drug interaction studies have not been conducted). Products include:

Tylenol with Codeine Tablets 2427

Codeine Sulfate (Limited published data indicate that somatropin treatment increases cytochrome P450 (CYP450)-mediated antipyrine clearance in man. These data suggest that somatropin administration may alter the clearance of compounds known to be metabolized by CYP450 liver enzymes. Careful monitoring is advisable when somatropin is administered in combination with other drugs known to be metabolized by CYP450 liver enzymes. However formal drug interaction studies have not been conducted).

No products indexed under this heading.

Cortisol (Somatropin inhibits 11β-hydroxysteroid dehydrogenase type 1 (11βHSD-1) in adipose/hepatic tissue and may significantly impact the metabolism of cortisol. Patients being treated with glucocorticoid replacement therapy for hypoadrenalism may require an increase in their maintenance or stress doses. Also excessive glucocorticoid therapy may attenuate the growth promoting effects of somatropin in children. Therefore, glucocorticoid replacement therapy should be carefully adjusted in children with concomitant GH and glucocorticoid deficiency to avoid both hypoadrenalism and an inhibitory effect on growth).

No products indexed under this heading.

Cortisone Acetate (Somatropin inhibits 11βHSD-1 in adipose/hepatic tissue and may significantly impact the metabolism of cortisone and cortisol. Patients being treated with glucocorticoid replacement therapy for hypoadrenalism may require an increase in their maintenance or stress doses; especially with cortisone acetate and prednisone, since conversion of these drugs to their biologically active metabolites is dependent on the activity of the 11μHSD-1 enzyme. Also, excessive glucocorticoid therapy may attenuate the growth-promoting effects of somatropin in children. Therefore, glucocorticoid replacement therapy should be carefully adjusted in children with concomitant GH and glucocorticoid deficiency to avoid both hypoadrenalism and an inhibitory effect on growth).

No products indexed under this heading.

Cyclobenzaprine (Limited published data indicate that somatropin treatment increases cytochrome P450 (CYP450)-mediated antipyrine clearance in man. These data suggest that somatropin administration may alter the clearance of compounds known to be metabolized by CYP450 liver enzymes. Careful monitoring is advisable when somatropin is administered in combination with other drugs known to be metabolized by CYP450 liver enzymes. However formal drug interaction studies have not been conducted).

No products indexed under this heading.

Cyclobenzaprine Hydrochloride (Limited published data indicate that somatropin treatment increases cytochrome P450 (CYP450)-mediated antipyrine clearance in man. These data suggest that somatropin administration may alter the clearance of compounds known to be metabolized by CYP450 liver enzymes. Careful monitoring is advisable when somatropin is administered in combination with other drugs known to be metabolized by CYP450 liver enzymes. However formal drug interaction studies have not been conducted). Products include:

Amrix Capsules 966

Cyclophosphamide (Limited published data indicate that somatropin treatment increases cytochrome P450 (CYP450)-mediated antipyrine clearance in man. These data suggest that somatropin administration may alter the clearance of compounds known to be metabolized by CYP450 liver enzymes. Careful monitoring is advisable when somatropin is administered in combination with other drugs known to be metabolized by CYP450 liver enzymes. However formal drug interaction studies have not been conducted).

No products indexed under this heading.

Cyclosporine (Limited published data indicate that somatropin treatment increases cytochrome P450 (CYP450) mediated antipyrine clearance in man. This data suggests that somatropin administration may alter the clearance of compounds known to be metabolized by CYP450liver enzymes (eg cyclosporine). Careful monitoring is advisable when somatropin is administered in combination with other drugs known to be metabolized by CYP450 liver enzymes. However, formal drug interaction studies have not been conducted). Products include:

Gengraf Capsules 435
Neoral Oral Solution 2280
Neoral Soft Gelatin Capsules 2280
Restasis Ophthalmic Emulsion 557
Sandimmune 2296

Desipramine Hydrochloride (Limited published data indicate that somatropin treatment increases cytochrome P450 (CYP450)-mediated antipyrine clearance in man. These data suggest that somatropin administration may alter the clearance of compounds known to be metabolized by CYP450 liver enzymes. Careful monitoring is advisable when somatropin is administered in combination with other drugs known to be metabolized by CYP450 liver enzymes. However formal drug interaction studies have not been conducted).

No products indexed under this heading.

Desogestrel (Limited published data indicates that somatropin treatment increases cytochrome P450 (CP450) mediated antipyrine clearance in man. This data suggests that somatropin administration may alter the clearance of compounds known to be metabolized by CP450 liver enzymes (eg, sex steroids). Careful monitoring is advisable when somatropin is administered in combination with other drugs known to be metabolized by CP450 liver enzymes. However, formal drug interaction studies have not been conducted). Products include:

Mircette Tablets 1034

Dexamethasone (Somatropin inhibits 11βHSD-1 in adipose/hepatic tissue and may significantly impact the metabolism of cortisone and cortisol. Patients being treated with glucocorticoid replacement therapy for hypoadrenalism may require an increase in their maintenance or stress doses; especially with cortisone acetate and prednisone, since conversion of these drugs to their biologically active metabolites is dependent on the activity of the 11μHSD-1 enzyme. Also, excessive glucocorticoid therapy may attenuate the growth-promoting effects of somatropin in children. Therefore, glucocorticoid replacement therapy should be carefully adjusted in children with concomitant GH and glucocorticoid deficiency to avoid both hypoadrenalism and an inhibitory effect on growth). Products include:

Ciprodex Otic Suspension 541

Dexamethasone Acetate (Somatropin inhibits 11βHSD-1 in adipose/hepatic tissue and may significantly impact the metabolism of cortisone and cortisol. Patients being treated with glucocorticoid replacement therapy for hypoadrenalism may require an increase in their maintenance or stress doses; especially with cortisone acetate and prednisone, since conversion of these drugs to their biologically active metabolites is dependent on the activity of the 11μHSD-1 enzyme. Also, excessive glucocorticoid therapy may attenuate the growth-promoting effects of somatropin in children. Therefore, glucocorticoid replacement therapy should be carefully adjusted in children with concomitant GH and glucocorticoid deficiency to avoid both hypoadrenalism and an inhibitory effect on growth).

No products indexed under this heading.

Dexamethasone Phosphate (Limited published data indicate that somatropin treatment increases cytochrome P450 (CYP450)-mediated antipyrine clearance in man. These data suggest that somatropin administration may alter the clearance of compounds known to be metabolized by CYP450 liver enzymes. Careful monitoring is advisable when somatropin is administered in combination with other drugs known to be metabolized by CYP450 liver enzymes. However formal drug interaction studies have not been conducted).

No products indexed under this heading.

Dexamethasone Sodium (Limited published data indicate that somatropin treatment increases cytochrome P450 (CYP450)-mediated antipyrine clearance in man. These data suggest that somatropin administration may alter the clearance of compounds known to be metabolized by CYP450 liver enzymes. Careful monitoring is advisable when somatropin is administered in combination with other drugs known to be metabolized by CYP450 liver enzymes. However formal drug interaction studies have not been conducted).

No products indexed under this heading.

Dexamethasone Sodium Phosphate (Somatropin inhibits 11βHSD-1 in adipose/hepatic tissue and may significantly impact the metabolism of cortisone and cortisol. Patients being treated with glucocorticoid replacement therapy for hypoadrenalism may require an increase in their maintenance or stress doses; especially with cortisone acetate and prednisone, since conversion of these drugs to their biologically active metabolites is dependent on the activity of the 11μHSD-1 enzyme. Also, excessive glucocorticoid therapy may attenuate the growth-promoting effects of somatropin in children. Therefore, glucocorticoid replacement therapy should be carefully adjusted in children with concomitant GH and glucocorticoid deficiency to avoid both hypoadrenalism and an inhibitory effect on growth).

No products indexed under this heading.

Dexfenfluramine Hydrochloride (Limited published data indicate that somatropin treatment increases cytochrome P450 (CYP450)-mediated antipyrine clearance in man. These data suggest that somatropin administration may alter the clearance of compounds known to be metabolized by CYP450 liver enzymes. Careful monitoring is advisable when somatropin is administered in combination with other drugs known to be metabolized by CYP450 liver enzymes. However formal drug interaction studies have not been conducted).

No products indexed under this heading.

Dextromethorphan (Limited published data indicate that somatropin treatment increases cytochrome P450 (CYP450)-mediated antipyrine clearance in man. These data suggest that somatropin administration may alter the clearance of compounds known to be metabolized by CYP450 liver enzymes. Careful monitoring is advisable when somatropin is administered in combination with other drugs known to be metabolized by CYP450 liver enzymes. However formal drug interaction studies have not been conducted).

No products indexed under this heading.

Dextromethorphan Hydrobromide (Limited published data indicate that somatropin treatment increases cytochrome P450 (CYP450)-mediated antipyrine clearance in man. These data suggest that somatropin administration may alter the clearance of compounds known to be metabolized by CYP450 liver enzymes. Careful monitoring is advisable when somatropin is administered in combination with other drugs known to be metabolized by CYP450 liver enzymes. However formal drug interaction studies have not been conducted). Products include:

PediaCare Children's Liquid Multi-Symptom Cold **1902**
PediaCare Children's Long-Acting Cough **1902**
Children's Sudafed PE Cold & Cough Liquid **1907**
Sudafed PE Cold & Cough Caplets **1907**
Children's Tylenol Plus Cough & Runny Nose Suspension Liquid **1912**
Children's Tylenol Plus Cough & Sore Throat Suspension Liquid **1912**
Children's Tylenol Plus Flu Suspension Liquid **1914**
Children's Tylenol Plus Multi-Symptom Cold Suspension Liquid **1912**
Tylenol Cold Severe Congestion Daytime Caplets with Cool Burst **1912**
Tylenol Cold Head Congestion Daytime Caplets with Cool Burst **1910**
Tylenol Cold Head Congestion Nighttime Caplets with Cool Burst **1910**
Tylenol Cold Head Congestion Severe Daytime Caplets with Cool Burst **1910**
Tylenol Cold Multi-Symptom Daytime Caplets with Cool Burst and Rapid Release Gels **1913**
Tylenol Cold Multi-Symptom Daytime Liquid with Citrus Burst **1913**
Tylenol Cold Multi-Symptom Nighttime Caplets with Cool Burst **1913**
Tylenol Cold Multi-Symptom Nighttime Liquid with Cool Burst **1913**
Tylenol Cold Multi-Symptom Severe Caplets with Cool Burst **1913**
Tylenol Cold Multi-Symptom Severe Daytime Liquid with Citrus Burst **1913**
Tylenol Cough & Sore Throat Daytime Liquid with Cool Burst **1918**
Tylenol Cough & Sore Throat Nighttime Liquid with Cool Burst **1918**
Vicks DayQuil Cold & Flu Multi-Symptom Relief .... ▣ **616**
Vicks DayQuil LiquiCaps **2567**
Vicks DayQuil Liquid **2567**
Vicks DayQuil Multi-Symptom Cold/Flu Relief **2567**
Vicks NyQuil Cold & Flu Multi-Symptom Relief .... ▣ **617**
Vicks NyQuil LiquiCaps **2567**
Vicks NyQuil Liquid **2567**
Vicks NyQuil Multi-Symptom Cold/Flu Relief **2567**

Dextromethorphan Polistirex (Limited published data indicate that somatropin treatment increases cytochrome P450 (CYP450)-mediated antipyrine clearance in man. These data suggest that somatropin administration may alter the clearance of compounds known to be metabolized by CYP450 liver enzymes. Careful monitoring is advisable when somatropin is administered in combination with other drugs known to be metabolized by CYP450 liver enzymes. However formal drug interaction studies have not been conducted).

No products indexed under this heading.

Diazepam (Limited published data indicate that somatropin treatment increases cytochrome P450 (CYP450)-mediated antipyrine clearance in man. These data suggest that somatropin administration may alter the clearance of compounds known to be metabolized by CYP450 liver enzymes. Careful monitoring is advisable when somatropin is administered in combination with other drugs known to be metabolized by CYP450 liver enzymes. However formal drug interaction studies have not been conducted). Products include:

Valium Tablets **2658**

Diclofenac Potassium (Limited published data indicate that somatropin treatment increases cytochrome P450 (CYP450)-mediated antipyrine clearance in man. These data suggest that somatropin administration may alter the clearance of compounds known to be metabolized by CYP450 liver enzymes. Careful monitoring is advisable when somatropin is administered in combination with other drugs known to be metabolized by CYP450 liver enzymes. However formal drug interaction studies have not been conducted).

No products indexed under this heading.

Diclofenac Sodium (Limited published data indicate that somatropin treatment increases cytochrome P450 (CYP450)-mediated antipyrine clearance in man. These data suggest that somatropin administration may alter the clearance of compounds known to be metabolized by CYP450 liver enzymes. Careful monitoring is advisable when somatropin is administered in combination with other drugs known to be metabolized by CYP450 liver enzymes. However formal drug interaction studies have not been conducted). Products include:

Diclofenac Sodium Ophthalmic Solution .... ⊙ **240**
Voltaren Ophthalmic Solution **2336**
Voltaren Tablets **2334**
Voltaren-XR Tablets **2337**

Dienestrol (In patients on oral estrogen replacement, a larger dose of somatropin may be required to achieve the defined treatment goal).

No products indexed under this heading.

Diethylstilbestrol (In patients on oral estrogen replacement, a larger dose of somatropin may be required to achieve the defined treatment goal).

No products indexed under this heading.

Dihydroergotamine Mesylate (Limited published data indicate that somatropin treatment increases cytochrome P450 (CYP450)-mediated antipyrine clearance in man. These data suggest that somatropin administration may alter the clearance of compounds known to be metabolized by CYP450 liver enzymes. Careful monitoring is advisable when somatropin is administered in combination with other drugs known to be metabolized by CYP450 liver enzymes. However formal drug interaction studies have not been conducted).

No products indexed under this heading.

Diltiazem Hydrochloride (Limited published data indicate that somatropin treatment increases cytochrome P450 (CYP450)-mediated antipyrine clearance in man. These data suggest that somatropin administration may alter the clearance of compounds known to be metabolized by CYP450 liver enzymes. Careful monitoring is advisable when somatropin is administered in combination with other drugs known to be metabolized by CYP450 liver enzymes. However formal drug interaction studies have not been conducted). Products include:

Cardizem LA Extended Release Tablets **421**

Diltiazem Maleate (Limited published data indicate that somatropin treatment increases cytochrome P450 (CYP450)-mediated antipyrine clearance in man. These data suggest that somatropin administration may alter the clearance of compounds known to be metabolized by CYP450 liver enzymes. Careful monitoring is advisable when somatropin is administered in combination with other drugs known to be metabolized by CYP450 liver enzymes. However formal drug interaction studies have not been conducted).

No products indexed under this heading.

Disopyramide (Limited published data indicate that somatropin treatment increases cytochrome P450 (CYP450)-mediated antipyrine clearance in man. These data suggest that somatropin administration may alter the clearance of compounds known to be metabolized by CYP450 liver enzymes. Careful monitoring is advisable when somatropin is administered in combination with other drugs known to be metabolized by CYP450 liver enzymes. However formal drug interaction studies have not been conducted).

No products indexed under this heading.

Disopyramide Phosphate (Limited published data indicate that somatropin treatment increases cytochrome P450 (CYP450)-mediated antipyrine clearance in man. These data suggest that somatropin administration may alter the clearance of compounds known to be metabolized by CYP450 liver enzymes. Careful monitoring is advisable when somatropin is administered in combination with other drugs known to be metabolized by CYP450 liver enzymes. However formal drug interaction studies have not been conducted).

No products indexed under this heading.

Divalproex Sodium (Limited published data indicates that somatropin treatment increases cytochrome P450 (CP450) mediated antipyrine clearance in man. This data suggests that somatropin administration may alter the clearance of compounds known to be metabolized by CP450 liver enzymes (eg anticonvulsants). Careful monitoring is advisable when somatropin is administered in combination with other drugs known to be metabolized by CP450 liver enzymes. However, formal drug interaction studies have not been conducted). Products include:

Depakote ER Tablets **423**

Docetaxel (Limited published data indicate that somatropin treatment increases cytochrome P450 (CYP450)-mediated antipyrine clearance in man. These data suggest that somatropin administration may alter the clearance of compounds known to be metabolized by CYP450 liver enzymes. Careful monitoring is advisable when somatropin is administered in combination with other drugs known to be metabolized by CYP450 liver enzymes. However formal drug interaction studies have not been conducted). Products include:

Taxotere Injection Concentrate **2773**

Dolasetron Mesylate (Limited published data indicate that somatropin treatment increases cytochrome P450 (CYP450)-mediated antipyrine clearance in man. These data suggest that somatropin administration may alter the clearance of compounds known to be metabolized by CYP450 liver enzymes. Careful monitoring is advisable when somatropin is administered in combination with other drugs known to be metabolized by CYP450 liver enzymes. However formal drug interaction studies have not been conducted). Products include:

Anzemet Injection **2701**
Anzemet Tablets **2704**

Donepezil Hydrochloride (Limited published data indicate that somatropin treatment increases cytochrome P450 (CYP450)-mediated antipyrine clearance in man. These data suggest that somatropin administration may alter the clearance of compounds known to be metabolized by CYP450 liver enzymes. Careful monitoring is advisable when somatropin is administered in combination with other drugs known to be metabolized by CYP450 liver enzymes. However formal drug interaction studies have not been conducted). Products include:

Aricept Tablets **1062**
Aricept ODT Tablets **1062**

Doxepin Hydrochloride (Limited published data indicate that somatropin treatment increases cytochrome P450 (CYP450)-mediated antipyrine clearance in man. These data suggest that somatropin administration may alter the clearance of compounds known to be metabolized by CYP450 liver enzymes. Careful monitoring is advisable when somatropin is administered in combination with other drugs known to be metabolized by CYP450 liver enzymes. However formal drug interaction studies have not been conducted).

No products indexed under this heading.

Doxorubicin Hydrochloride (Limited published data indicate that somatropin treatment increases cytochrome P450 (CYP450)-mediated antipyrine clearance in man. These data suggest that somatropin administration may alter the clearance of compounds known to be metabolized by CYP450 liver enzymes. Careful monitoring is advisable when somatropin is administered in combination with other drugs known to be metabolized by CYP450 liver enzymes. However formal drug interaction studies have not been conducted).

No products indexed under this heading.

Dronabinol (Limited published data indicate that somatropin treatment increases cytochrome P450 (CYP450)-mediated antipyrine clearance in man. These data suggest that somatropin administration may alter the clearance of compounds known to be metabolized by CYP450 liver enzymes. Careful monitoring is advisable when somatropin is administered in combination with other drugs known to be metabolized by CYP450 liver enzymes. However formal drug interaction studies have not been conducted). Products include:

Marinol Capsules **3163**

Drugs that Undergo Biotransformation by Cytochrome P-450 Mixed Function Oxidase (Limited published data indicate that somatropin treatment increases cytochrome P450 (CYP450)-mediated antipyrine clearance in man. These data suggest that somatropin administration may alter the clearance of compounds known to be metabolized by CYP450 liver enzymes. Careful monitoring is advisable when somatropin is administered in combination with other drugs known to be metabolized by CYP450 liver enzymes. However formal drug interaction studies have not been conducted).

No products indexed under this heading.

Dyphylline (Limited published data indicate that somatropin treatment increases cytochrome P450 (CYP450)-mediated antipyrine clearance in man. These data suggest that somatropin administration may alter the clearance of compounds known to be metabolized by CYP450 liver enzymes. Careful monitoring is advisable when somatropin is administered in combination with other drugs known to be metabolized by CYP450 liver enzymes. However formal drug interaction studies have not been conducted).

No products indexed under this heading.

Encainide Hydrochloride (Limited published data indicate that somatropin treatment increases cytochrome P450 (CYP450)-mediated antipyrine clearance in man. These data suggest that somatropin administration may alter the clearance of compounds known to be metabolized by CYP450 liver enzymes. Careful monitoring is advisable when somatropin is administered in combination with other drugs known to be metabolized by CYP450 liver enzymes. However formal drug interaction studies have not been conducted).

No products indexed under this heading.

Enoxacin (Limited published data indicate that somatropin treatment increases cytochrome P450 (CYP450)-mediated antipyrine clearance in man. These data suggest that somatropin administration may alter the clearance of compounds known to be metabolized by CYP450 liver enzymes. Careful monitoring is advisable when somatropin is administered in combination with other drugs known to be metabolized by CYP450 liver enzymes. However formal drug interaction studies have not been conducted).

No products indexed under this heading.

Eprosartan Mesylate (Limited published data indicate that somatropin treatment increases cytochrome P450 (CYP450)-mediated antipyrine clearance in man. These data suggest that somatropin administration may alter the clearance of compounds known to be metabolized by CYP450 liver enzymes. Careful monitoring is advisable when somatropin is administered in combination with other drugs known to be metabolized by CYP450 liver enzymes. However formal drug interaction studies have not been conducted). Products include:

Teveten Tablets **515**
Teveten HCT Tablets **517**

Ergotamine Tartrate (Limited published data indicate that somatropin treatment increases cytochrome P450 (CYP450)-mediated antipyrine clearance in man. These data suggest that somatropin administration may alter the clearance of compounds known to be metabolized by CYP450 liver enzymes. Careful monitoring is advisable when somatropin is administered in combination with other drugs known to be metabolized by CYP450 liver enzymes. However formal drug interaction studies have not been conducted).

No products indexed under this heading.

Erythromycin (Limited published data indicate that somatropin treatment increases cytochrome P450 (CYP450)-mediated antipyrine clearance in man. These data suggest that somatropin administration may alter the clearance of compounds known to be metabolized by CYP450 liver enzymes. Careful monitoring is advisable when somatropin is administered in combination with other drugs known to be metabolized by CYP450 liver enzymes. However formal drug interaction studies have not been conducted).

No products indexed under this heading.

Erythromycin Estolate (Limited published data indicate that somatropin treatment increases cytochrome P450 (CYP450)-mediated antipyrine clearance in man. These data suggest that somatropin administration may alter the clearance of compounds known to be metabolized by CYP450 liver enzymes. Careful monitoring is advisable when somatropin is administered in combination with other drugs known to be metabolized by CYP450 liver enzymes. However formal drug interaction studies have not been conducted).

No products indexed under this heading.

Erythromycin Ethylsuccinate (Limited published data indicate that somatropin treatment increases cytochrome P450 (CYP450)-mediated antipyrine clearance in man. These data suggest that somatropin administration may alter the clearance of compounds known to be metabolized by CYP450 liver enzymes. Careful monitoring is advisable when somatropin is administered in combination with other drugs known to be metabolized by CYP450 liver enzymes. However formal drug interaction studies have not been conducted). Products include:

E.E.S. **433**
EryPed **431**

Erythromycin Gluceptate (Limited published data indicate that somatropin treatment increases cytochrome P450 (CYP450)-mediated antipyrine clearance in man. These data suggest that somatropin administration may alter the clearance of compounds known to be metabolized by CYP450 liver enzymes. Careful monitoring is advisable when somatropin is administered in combination with other drugs known to be metabolized by CYP450 liver enzymes. However formal drug interaction studies have not been conducted).

No products indexed under this heading.

Erythromycin Lactobionate (Limited published data indicate that somatropin treatment increases cytochrome P450 (CYP450)-mediated antipyrine clearance in man. These data suggest that somatropin administration may alter the clearance of compounds known to be metabolized by CYP450 liver enzymes. Careful monitoring is advisable when somatropin is administered in combination with other drugs known to be metabolized by CYP450 liver enzymes. However formal drug interaction studies have not been conducted).

No products indexed under this heading.

Erythromycin Stearate (Limited published data indicate that somatropin treatment increases cytochrome P450 (CYP450)-mediated antipyrine clearance in man. These data suggest that somatropin administration may alter the clearance of compounds known to be metabolized by CYP450 liver enzymes. Careful monitoring is advisable when somatropin is administered in combination with other drugs known to be metabolized by CYP450 liver enzymes. However formal drug interaction studies have not been conducted).

No products indexed under this heading.

Esomeprazole Magnesium (Limited published data indicate that somatropin treatment increases cytochrome P450 (CYP450)-mediated antipyrine clearance in man. These data suggest that somatropin administration may alter the clearance of compounds known to be metabolized by CYP450 liver enzymes. Careful monitoring is advisable when somatropin is administered in combination with other drugs known to be metabolized by CYP450 liver enzymes. However formal drug interaction studies have not been conducted). Products include:

Nexium Delayed-Release Capsules 645
Nexium Delayed-Release Oral Suspension 645

Estradiol (Limited published data indicates that somatropin treatment increases cytochrome P450 (CP450) mediated antipyrine clearance in man. This data suggests that somatropin administration may alter the clearance of compounds known to be metabolized by CP450 liver enzymes (eg, sex steroids). Careful monitoring is advisable when somatropin is administered in combination with other drugs known to be metabolized by CP450 liver enzymes. However, formal drug interaction studies have not been conducted). Products include:

Activella Tablets 2347
Angeliq Tablets 751
Climara Transdermal System 763
Climara Pro Transdermal System 768
Divigel 3167
Vagifem Tablets 2375

Estradiol Benzoate (Limited published data indicate that somatropin treatment increases cytochrome P450 (CYP450)-mediated antipyrine clearance in man. These data suggest that somatropin administration may alter the clearance of compounds known to be metabolized by CYP450 liver enzymes. Careful monitoring is advisable when somatropin is administered in combination with other drugs known to be metabolized by CYP450 liver enzymes. However formal drug interaction studies have not been conducted).

No products indexed under this heading.

Estradiol Cypionate (Limited published data indicate that somatropin treatment increases cytochrome P450 (CYP450)-mediated antipyrine clearance in man. These data suggest that somatropin administration may alter the clearance of compounds known to be metabolized by CYP450 liver enzymes. Careful monitoring is advisable when somatropin is administered in combination with other drugs known to be metabolized by CYP450 liver enzymes. However formal drug interaction studies have not been conducted).

No products indexed under this heading.

Estradiol Valerate (Limited published data indicate that somatropin treatment increases cytochrome P450 (CYP450)-mediated antipyrine clearance in man. These data suggest that somatropin administration may alter the clearance of compounds known to be metabolized by CYP450 liver enzymes. Careful monitoring is advisable when somatropin is administered in combination with other drugs known to be metabolized by CYP450 liver enzymes. However formal drug interaction studies have not been conducted).

No products indexed under this heading.

Estrogen (Limited published data indicate that somatropin treatment increases cytochrome P450 (CYP450)-mediated antipyrine clearance in man. These data suggest that somatropin administration may alter the clearance of compounds known to be metabolized by CYP450 liver enzymes. Careful monitoring is advisable when somatropin is administered in combination with other drugs known to be metabolized by CYP450 liver enzymes. However formal drug interaction studies have not been conducted).

No products indexed under this heading.

Estrogens, Conjugated (Limited published data indicates that somatropin treatment increases cytochrome P450 (CP450) mediated antipyrine clearance in man. This data suggests that somatropin administration may alter the clearance of compounds known to be metabolized by CP450 liver enzymes (eg, sex steroids). Careful monitoring is advisable when somatropin is administered in combination with other drugs known to be metabolized by CP450 liver enzymes. However, formal drug interaction studies have not been conducted). Products include:

Premarin Intravenous 3217
Premarin Tablets 3221
Premarin Vaginal Cream 3228
Premphase Tablets 3232
Prempro Tablets 3232

Estrogens, Conjugated, Synthetic A (Limited published data indicate that somatropin treatment increases cytochrome P450 (CYP450)-mediated antipyrine clearance in man. These data suggest that somatropin administration may alter the clearance of compounds known to be metabolized by CYP450 liver enzymes. Careful monitoring is advisable when somatropin is administered in combination with other drugs known to be metabolized by CYP450 liver enzymes. However formal drug interaction studies have not been conducted).

No products indexed under this heading.

Estrogens, Esterified (In patients on oral estrogen replacement, a larger dose of somatropin may be required to achieve the defined treatment goal). Products include:

Estratest Tablets 3043
Estratest H.S. Tablets 3043

Estropipate (In patients on oral estrogen replacement, a larger dose of somatropin may be required to achieve the defined treatment goal).

No products indexed under this heading.

Ethinyl Estradiol (Limited published data indicates that somatropin treatment increases cytochrome P450 (CP450) mediated antipyrine clearance in man. This data suggests that somatropin administration may alter the clearance of compounds known to be metabolized by CP450 liver enzymes (eg, sex steroids). Careful monitoring is advisable when somatropin is administered in combination with other drugs known to be metabolized by CP450 liver enzymes. However, formal drug interaction studies have not been conducted). Products include:

Lybrel Tablets 3204
Mircette Tablets 1034
NuvaRing 2897
Ortho-Cyclen/Ortho Tri-Cyclen 2449
Ortho Evra Transdermal System 2437
Ortho Tri-Cyclen Lo Tablets 2458
Seasonique Tablets 1046
Yaz Tablets 805

Ethosuximide (Limited published data indicates that somatropin treatment increases cytochrome P450 (CP450) mediated antipyrine clearance in man. This data suggests that somatropin administration may alter the clearance of compounds known to be metabolized by CP450 liver enzymes (eg anticonvulsants). Careful monitoring is advisable when somatropin is administered in combination with other drugs known to be metabolized by CP450 liver enzymes. However, formal drug interaction studies have not been conducted).

No products indexed under this heading.

Ethotoin (Limited published data indicates that somatropin treatment increases cytochrome P450 (CP450) mediated antipyrine clearance in man. This data suggests that somatropin administration may alter the clearance of compounds known to be metabolized by CP450 liver enzymes (eg anticonvulsants). Careful monitoring is advisable when somatropin is administered in combination with other drugs known to be metabolized by CP450 liver enzymes. However, formal drug interaction studies have not been conducted).

No products indexed under this heading.

Ethynodiol Diacetate (Limited published data indicates that somatropin treatment increases cytochrome P450 (CP450) mediated antipyrine clearance in man. This data suggests that somatropin administration may alter the clearance of compounds known to be metabolized by CP450 liver enzymes (eg, sex steroids). Careful monitoring is advisable when somatropin is administered in combination with other drugs known to be metabolized by CP450 liver enzymes. However, formal drug interaction studies have not been conducted).

No products indexed under this heading.

Etodolac (Limited published data indicate that somatropin treatment increases cytochrome P450 (CYP450)-mediated antipyrine clearance in man. These data suggest that somatropin administration may alter the clearance of compounds known to be metabolized by CYP450 liver enzymes. Careful monitoring is advisable when somatropin is administered in combination with other drugs known to be metabolized by CYP450 liver enzymes. However formal drug interaction studies have not been conducted).

No products indexed under this heading.

Etoposide (Limited published data indicate that somatropin treatment increases cytochrome P450 (CYP450)-mediated antipyrine clearance in man. These data suggest that somatropin administration may alter the clearance of compounds known to be metabolized by CYP450 liver enzymes. Careful monitoring is advisable when somatropin is administered in combination with other drugs known to be metabolized by CYP450 liver enzymes. However formal drug interaction studies have not been conducted).

No products indexed under this heading.

Etoposide Phosphate (Limited published data indicate that somatropin treatment increases cytochrome P450 (CYP450)-mediated antipyrine clearance in man. These data suggest that somatropin administration may alter the clearance of compounds known to be metabolized by CYP450 liver enzymes. Careful monitoring is advisable when somatropin is administered in combination with other drugs known to be metabolized by CYP450 liver enzymes. However formal drug interaction studies have not been conducted).

No products indexed under this heading.

Felbamate (Limited published data indicates that somatropin treatment increases cytochrome P450 (CP450) mediated antipyrine clearance in man. This data suggests that somatropin administration may alter the clearance of compounds known to be metabolized by CP450 liver enzymes (eg anticonvulsants). Careful monitoring is advisable when somatropin is administered in combination with other drugs known to be metabolized by CP450 liver enzymes. However, formal drug interaction studies have not been conducted).

No products indexed under this heading.

Felodipine (Limited published data indicate that somatropin treatment increases cytochrome P450 (CYP450)-mediated antipyrine clearance in man. These data suggest that somatropin administration may alter the clearance of compounds known to be metabolized by CYP450 liver enzymes. Careful monitoring is advisable when somatropin is administered in combination with other drugs known to be metabolized by CYP450 liver enzymes. However formal drug interaction studies have not been conducted).

No products indexed under this heading.

Fenoprofen Calcium (Limited published data indicate that somatropin treatment increases cytochrome P450 (CYP450)-mediated antipyrine clearance in man. These data suggest that somatropin administration may alter the clearance of compounds known to be metabolized by CYP450 liver enzymes. Careful monitoring is advisable when somatropin is administered in combination with other drugs known to be metabolized by CYP450 liver enzymes. However formal drug interaction studies have not been conducted). Products include:

Nalfon Capsules 2508

Fentanyl (Limited published data indicate that somatropin treatment increases cytochrome P450 (CYP450)-mediated antipyrine clearance in man. These data suggest that somatropin administration may alter the clearance of compounds known to be metabolized by CYP450 liver enzymes. Careful monitoring is advisable when somatropin is administered in combination with other drugs known to be metabolized by CYP450 liver enzymes. However

formal drug interaction studies have not been conducted). Products include:

Duragesic Transdermal System **2405**
Ionsys Transdermal System **2410**

Fentanyl Citrate (Limited published data indicate that somatropin treatment increases cytochrome P450 (CYP450)-mediated antipyrine clearance in man. These data suggest that somatropin administration may alter the clearance of compounds known to be metabolized by CYP450 liver enzymes. Careful monitoring is advisable when somatropin is administered in combination with other drugs known to be metabolized by CYP450 liver enzymes. However formal drug interaction studies have not been conducted). Products include:

Actiq **959**
Fentora Tablets **968**

Flecainide Acetate (Limited published data indicate that somatropin treatment increases cytochrome P450 (CYP450)-mediated antipyrine clearance in man. These data suggest that somatropin administration may alter the clearance of compounds known to be metabolized by CYP450 liver enzymes. Careful monitoring is advisable when somatropin is administered in combination with other drugs known to be metabolized by CYP450 liver enzymes. However formal drug interaction studies have not been conducted).

No products indexed under this heading.

Fludrocortisone Acetate (Somatropin inhibits 11βHSD-1 in adipose/hepatic tissue and may significantly impact the metabolism of cortisone and cortisol. Patients being treated with glucocorticoid replacement therapy for hypoadrenalism may require an increase in their maintenance or stress doses; especially with cortisone acetate and prednisone, since conversion of these drugs to their biologically active metabolites is dependent on the activity of the 11μHSD-1 enzyme. Also, excessive glucocorticoid therapy may attenuate the growth-promoting effects of somatropin in children. Therefore, glucocorticoid replacement therapy should be carefully adjusted in children with concomitant GH and glucocorticoid deficiency to avoid both hypoadrenalism and an inhibitory effect on growth).

No products indexed under this heading.

Flunisolide (Limited published data indicates that somatropin treatment increases cytochrome P450 (CP450) mediated antipyrine clearance in man. This data suggests that somatropin administration may alter the clearance of compounds known to be metabolized by CP450 liver enzymes (eg, corticosteroids). Careful monitoring is advisable when somatropin is administered in combination with other drugs known to be metabolized by CP450 liver enzymes. However, formal drug interaction studies have not been conducted). Products include:

Aerobid/Aerobid-M **1153**

Fluoxetine (Limited published data indicate that somatropin treatment increases cytochrome P450 (CYP450)-mediated antipyrine clearance in man. These data suggest that somatropin administration may alter the clearance of compounds known to be metabolized by CYP450 liver enzymes. Careful monitoring is advisable when somatropin is administered in combination with other drugs known to be metabolized by CYP450 liver enzymes. However formal drug interaction studies have not been conducted).

No products indexed under this heading.

Fluoxetine Hydrochloride (Limited published data indicate that somatropin treatment increases cytochrome P450 (CYP450)-mediated antipyrine clearance in man. These data suggest that somatropin administration may alter the clearance of compounds known to be metabolized by CYP450 liver enzymes. Careful monitoring is advisable when somatropin is administered in combination with other drugs known to be metabolized by CYP450 liver enzymes. However formal drug interaction studies have not been conducted). Products include:

Prozac Weekly Capsules **1852**
Prozac Pulvules and Liquid **1852**
Symbyax Capsules **1871**

Fluoxymesterone (Limited published data indicates that somatropin treatment increases cytochrome P450 (CP450) mediated antipyrine clearance in man. This data suggests that somatropin administration may alter the clearance of compounds known to be metabolized by CP450 liver enzymes (eg, sex steroids). Careful monitoring is advisable when somatropin is administered in combination with other drugs known to be metabolized by CP450 liver enzymes. However, formal drug interaction studies have not been conducted).

No products indexed under this heading.

Fluphenazine Decanoate (Limited published data indicate that somatropin treatment increases cytochrome P450 (CYP450)-mediated antipyrine clearance in man. These data suggest that somatropin administration may alter the clearance of compounds known to be metabolized by CYP450 liver enzymes. Careful monitoring is advisable when somatropin is administered in combination with other drugs known to be metabolized by CYP450 liver enzymes. However formal drug interaction studies have not been conducted).

No products indexed under this heading.

Fluphenazine Enanthate (Limited published data indicate that somatropin treatment increases cytochrome P450 (CYP450)-mediated antipyrine clearance in man. These data suggest that somatropin administration may alter the clearance of compounds known to be metabolized by CYP450 liver enzymes. Careful monitoring is advisable when somatropin is administered in combination with other drugs known to be metabolized by CYP450 liver enzymes. However formal drug interaction studies have not been conducted).

No products indexed under this heading.

Fluphenazine Hydrochloride (Limited published data indicate that somatropin treatment increases cytochrome P450 (CYP450)-mediated antipyrine clearance in man. These data suggest that somatropin administration may alter the clearance of compounds known to be metabolized by CYP450 liver enzymes. Careful monitoring is advisable when somatropin is administered in combination with other drugs known to be metabolized by CYP450 liver enzymes. However formal drug interaction studies have not been conducted).

No products indexed under this heading.

Flurbiprofen (Limited published data indicate that somatropin treatment increases cytochrome P450 (CYP450)-mediated antipyrine clearance in man. These data suggest that somatropin administration may alter the clearance of compounds known to be metabolized by CYP450 liver enzymes. Careful monitoring is advisable when somatropin is administered in combination with other drugs known to be metabolized by CYP450 liver enzymes. However formal drug interaction studies have not been conducted).

No products indexed under this heading.

Flurbiprofen Sodium (Limited published data indicate that somatropin treatment increases cytochrome P450 (CYP450)-mediated antipyrine clearance in man. These data suggest that somatropin administration may alter the clearance of compounds known to be metabolized by CYP450 liver enzymes. Careful monitoring is advisable when somatropin is administered in combination with other drugs known to be metabolized by CYP450 liver enzymes. However formal drug interaction studies have not been conducted).

No products indexed under this heading.

Flutamide (Limited published data indicate that somatropin treatment increases cytochrome P450 (CYP450)-mediated antipyrine clearance in man. These data suggest that somatropin administration may alter the clearance of compounds known to be metabolized by CYP450 liver enzymes. Careful monitoring is advisable when somatropin is administered in combination with other drugs known to be metabolized by CYP450 liver enzymes. However formal drug interaction studies have not been conducted).

No products indexed under this heading.

Fluticasone Propionate (Limited published data indicates that somatropin treatment increases cytochrome P450 (CP450) mediated antipyrine clearance in man. This data suggests that somatropin administration may alter the clearance of compounds known to be metabolized by CP450 liver enzymes (eg, corticosteroids). Careful monitoring is advisable when somatropin is administered in combination with other drugs known to be metabolized by CP450 liver enzymes. However, formal drug interaction studies have not been conducted). Products include:

Advair Diskus 100/50 .... **1276**
Advair Diskus 250/50 .... **1276**
Advair Diskus 500/50 .... **1276**
Advair HFA 45/21 Inhalation Aerosol.. **1288**
Advair HFA 115/21 Inhalation Aerosol.. **1288**
Advair HFA 230/21 Inhalation Aerosol.. **1288**
Flonase Nasal Spray **1431**
Flovent Diskus 50 mcg **1435**

Fluticasone Propionate HFA (Limited published data indicates that somatropin treatment increases cytochrome P450 (CP450) mediated antipyrine clearance in man. This data suggests that somatropin administration may alter the clearance of compounds known to be metabolized by CP450 liver enzymes (eg, corticosteroids). Careful monitoring is advisable when somatropin is administered in combination with other drugs known to be metabolized by CP450 liver enzymes. However, formal drug interaction studies have not been conducted). Products include:

Flovent HFA **1440**

Fluvastatin Sodium (Limited published data indicate that somatropin treatment increases cytochrome P450 (CYP450)-mediated antipyrine clearance in man. These data suggest that somatropin administration may alter the clearance of compounds known to be metabolized by CYP450 liver enzymes. Careful monitoring is advisable when somatropin is administered in combination with other drugs known to be metabolized by CYP450 liver enzymes. However formal drug interaction studies have not been conducted). Products include:

Lescol Capsules **2268**
Lescol XL Tablets **2268**

Fluvoxamine Maleate (Limited published data indicate that somatropin treatment increases cytochrome P450 (CYP450)-mediated antipyrine clearance in man. These data suggest that somatropin administration may alter the clearance of compounds known to be metabolized by CYP450 liver enzymes. Careful monitoring is advisable when somatropin is administered in combination with other drugs known to be metabolized by CYP450 liver enzymes. However formal drug interaction studies have not been conducted). Products include:

Luvox CR Extended-Release Capsules....................................... **1759**

Formoterol Fumarate (Limited published data indicate that somatropin treatment increases cytochrome P450 (CYP450)-mediated antipyrine clearance in man. These data suggest that somatropin administration may alter the clearance of compounds known to be metabolized by CYP450 liver enzymes. Careful monitoring is advisable when somatropin is administered in combination with other drugs known to be metabolized by CYP450 liver enzymes. However formal drug interaction studies have not been conducted). Products include:

Foradil Aerolizer **2849**
Perforomist Inhalation Solution **1025**

Fosphenytoin (Limited published data indicates that somatropin treatment increases cytochrome P450 (CP450) mediated antipyrine clearance in man. This data suggests that somatropin administration may alter the clearance of compounds known to be metabolized by CP450 liver enzymes (eg anticonvulsants). Careful monitoring is advisable when somatropin is administered in combination with other drugs known to be

metabolized by CP450 liver enzymes. However, formal drug interaction studies have not been conducted).

No products indexed under this heading.

Fosphenytoin Sodium (Limited published data indicates that somatropin treatment increases cytochrome P450 (CP450) mediated antipyrine clearance in man. This data suggests that somatropin administration may alter the clearance of compounds known to be metabolized by CP450 liver enzymes (eg anticonvulsants). Careful monitoring is advisable when somatropin is administered in combination with other drugs known to be metabolized by CP450 liver enzymes. However, formal drug interaction studies have not been conducted).

No products indexed under this heading.

Gabapentin (Limited published data indicates that somatropin treatment increases cytochrome P450 (CP450) mediated antipyrine clearance in man. This data suggests that somatropin administration may alter the clearance of compounds known to be metabolized by CP450 liver enzymes (eg anticonvulsants). Careful monitoring is advisable when somatropin is administered in combination with other drugs known to be metabolized by CP450 liver enzymes. However, formal drug interaction studies have not been conducted).

No products indexed under this heading.

Galantamine Hydrobromide (Limited published data indicate that somatropin treatment increases cytochrome P450 (CYP450)-mediated antipyrine clearance in man. These data suggest that somatropin administration may alter the clearance of compounds known to be metabolized by CYP450 liver enzymes. Careful monitoring is advisable when somatropin is administered in combination with other drugs known to be metabolized by CYP450 liver enzymes. However formal drug interaction studies have not been conducted).

No products indexed under this heading.

Glimepiride (In patients with diabetes mellitus requiring drug therapy, the dose of oral hypoglycemic agents may require adjustment when somatropin therapy is initiated). Products include:

Avandaryl Tablets 1344
Duetact Tablets 3085

Glipizide (In patients with diabetes mellitus requiring drug therapy, the dose of oral hypoglycemic agents may require adjustment when somatropin therapy is initiated).

No products indexed under this heading.

Glyburide (In patients with diabetes mellitus requiring drug therapy, the dose of oral hypoglycemic agents may require adjustment when somatropin therapy is initiated).

No products indexed under this heading.

Grepafloxacin Hydrochloride (Limited published data indicate that somatropin treatment increases cytochrome P450 (CYP450)-mediated antipyrine clearance in man. These data suggest that somatropin administration may alter the clearance of compounds known to be metabolized by CYP450 liver enzymes. Careful monitoring is advisable when somatropin is administered in combination with other drugs known to be metabolized by CYP450 liver enzymes. However formal drug interaction studies have not been conducted).

No products indexed under this heading.

Haloperidol (Limited published data indicate that somatropin treatment increases cytochrome P450 (CYP450)-mediated antipyrine clearance in man. These data suggest that somatropin administration may alter the clearance of compounds known to be metabolized by CYP450 liver enzymes. Careful monitoring is advisable when somatropin is administered in combination with other drugs known to be metabolized by CYP450 liver enzymes. However formal drug interaction studies have not been conducted).

No products indexed under this heading.

Haloperidol Decanoate (Limited published data indicate that somatropin treatment increases cytochrome P450 (CYP450)-mediated antipyrine clearance in man. These data suggest that somatropin administration may alter the clearance of compounds known to be metabolized by CYP450 liver enzymes. Careful monitoring is advisable when somatropin is administered in combination with other drugs known to be metabolized by CYP450 liver enzymes. However formal drug interaction studies have not been conducted).

No products indexed under this heading.

Haloperidol Lactate (Limited published data indicate that somatropin treatment increases cytochrome P450 (CYP450)-mediated antipyrine clearance in man. These data suggest that somatropin administration may alter the clearance of compounds known to be metabolized by CYP450 liver enzymes. Careful monitoring is advisable when somatropin is administered in combination with other drugs known to be metabolized by CYP450 liver enzymes. However formal drug interaction studies have not been conducted).

No products indexed under this heading.

Hydrocodone Bitartrate (Limited published data indicate that somatropin treatment increases cytochrome P450 (CYP450)-mediated antipyrine clearance in man. These data suggest that somatropin administration may alter the clearance of compounds known to be metabolized by CYP450 liver enzymes. Careful monitoring is advisable when somatropin is administered in combination with other drugs known to be metabolized by CYP450 liver enzymes. However formal drug interaction studies have not been conducted). Products include:

Lortab 5/500 Tablets 3143
Lortab 7.5/500 Tablets 3144
Lortab 10/500 Tablets 3144
Vicodin Tablets 529
Vicodin ES Tablets 530
Vicodin HP Tablets 531
Vicoprofen Tablets 533
Zydone Tablets 1132

Hydrocortisone (Somatropin inhibits 11βHSD-1 in adipose/hepatic tissue and may significantly impact the metabolism of cortisone and cortisol. Patients being treated with glucocorticoid replacement therapy for hypoadrenalism may require an increase in their maintenance or stress doses; especially with cortisone acetate and prednisone, since conversion of these drugs to their biologically active metabolites is dependent on the activity of the 11μHSD-1 enzyme. Also, excessive glucocorticoid therapy may attenuate the growth-promoting effects of somatropin in children. Therefore, glucocorticoid replacement therapy should be carefully adjusted in children with concomitant GH and glucocorticoid deficiency to avoid both hypoadrenalism and an inhibitory effect on growth).

No products indexed under this heading.

Hydrocortisone Acetate (Somatropin inhibits 11βHSD-1 in adipose/hepatic tissue and may significantly impact the metabolism of cortisone and cortisol. Patients being treated with glucocorticoid replacement therapy for hypoadrenalism may require an increase in their maintenance or stress doses; especially with cortisone acetate and prednisone, since conversion of these drugs to their biologically active metabolites is dependent on the activity of the 11μHSD-1 enzyme. Also, excessive glucocorticoid therapy may attenuate the growth-promoting effects of somatropin in children. Therefore, glucocorticoid replacement therapy should be carefully adjusted in children with concomitant GH and glucocorticoid deficiency to avoid both hypoadrenalism and an inhibitory effect on growth). Products include:

Analpram-HC 1140
Pramosone 1141

Hydrocortisone Sodium Phosphate (Somatropin inhibits 11βHSD-1 in adipose/hepatic tissue and may significantly impact the metabolism of cortisone and cortisol. Patients being treated with glucocorticoid replacement therapy for hypoadrenalism may require an increase in their maintenance or stress doses; especially with cortisone acetate and prednisone, since conversion of these drugs to their biologically active metabolites is dependent on the activity of the 11μHSD-1 enzyme. Also, excessive glucocorticoid therapy may attenuate the growth-promoting effects of somatropin in children. Therefore, glucocorticoid replacement therapy should be carefully adjusted in children with concomitant GH and glucocorticoid deficiency to avoid both hypoadrenalism and an inhibitory effect on growth).

No products indexed under this heading.

Hydrocortisone Sodium Succinate (Somatropin inhibits 11βHSD-1 in adipose/hepatic tissue and may significantly impact the metabolism of cortisone and cortisol. Patients being treated with glucocorticoid replacement therapy for hypoadrenalism may require an increase in their maintenance or stress doses; especially with cortisone acetate and prednisone, since conversion of these drugs to their biologically active metabolites is dependent on the activity of the 11μHSD-1 enzyme. Also, excessive glucocorticoid therapy may attenuate the growth-promoting effects of somatropin in children. Therefore, glucocorticoid replacement therapy should be carefully adjusted in children with concomitant GH and glucocorticoid deficiency to avoid both hypoadrenalism and an inhibitory effect on growth).

No products indexed under this heading.

Ibuprofen (Limited published data indicate that somatropin treatment increases cytochrome P450 (CYP450)-mediated antipyrine clearance in man. These data suggest that somatropin administration may alter the clearance of compounds known to be metabolized by CYP450 liver enzymes. Careful monitoring is advisable when somatropin is administered in combination with other drugs known to be metabolized by CYP450 liver enzymes. However formal drug interaction studies have not been conducted). Products include:

Motrin IB Tablets and Caplets 1900
Children's Motrin Oral Suspension 1901
Children's Motrin Non-Staining Dye-Free Oral Suspension 1901
Children's Motrin Cold Oral Suspension 1899
Infants' Motrin Concentrated Drops 1901
Infants' Motrin Non-Staining Dye-Free Concentrated Drops 1901
Junior Strength Motrin Caplets and Chewable Tablets 1901
Vicoprofen Tablets 533

Imipramine Hydrochloride (Limited published data indicate that somatropin treatment increases cytochrome P450 (CYP450)-mediated antipyrine clearance in man. These data suggest that somatropin administration may alter the clearance of compounds known to be metabolized by CYP450 liver enzymes. Careful monitoring is advisable when somatropin is administered in combination with other drugs known to be metabolized by CYP450 liver enzymes. However formal drug interaction studies have not been conducted).

No products indexed under this heading.

Imipramine Pamoate (Limited published data indicate that somatropin treatment increases cytochrome P450 (CYP450)-mediated antipyrine clearance in man. These data suggest that somatropin administration may alter the clearance of compounds known to be metabolized by CYP450 liver enzymes. Careful monitoring is advisable when somatropin is administered in combination with other drugs known to be metabolized by CYP450 liver enzymes. However formal drug interaction studies have not been conducted).

No products indexed under this heading.

Indinavir Sulfate (Limited published data indicate that somatropin treatment increases cytochrome P450 (CYP450)-mediated antipyrine clearance in man. These data suggest that somatropin administration may alter the clearance of compounds known to be metabolized by CYP450 liver enzymes. Careful monitoring is advisable when somatropin

is administered in combination with other drugs known to be metabolized by CYP450 liver enzymes. However formal drug interaction studies have not been conducted). Products include:

Crixivan Capsules **1979**

Indomethacin (Limited published data indicate that somatropin treatment increases cytochrome P450 (CYP450)-mediated antipyrine clearance in man. These data suggest that somatropin administration may alter the clearance of compounds known to be metabolized by CYP450 liver enzymes. Careful monitoring is advisable when somatropin is administered in combination with other drugs known to be metabolized by CYP450 liver enzymes. However formal drug interaction studies have not been conducted). Products include:

Indocin **2024**

Indomethacin Sodium Trihydrate (Limited published data indicate that somatropin treatment increases cytochrome P450 (CYP450)-mediated antipyrine clearance in man. These data suggest that somatropin administration may alter the clearance of compounds known to be metabolized by CYP450 liver enzymes. Careful monitoring is advisable when somatropin is administered in combination with other drugs known to be metabolized by CYP450 liver enzymes. However formal drug interaction studies have not been conducted). Products include:

Indocin I.V. **2489**

Indoramin Hydrochloride (Limited published data indicate that somatropin treatment increases cytochrome P450 (CYP450)-mediated antipyrine clearance in man. These data suggest that somatropin administration may alter the clearance of compounds known to be metabolized by CYP450 liver enzymes. Careful monitoring is advisable when somatropin is administered in combination with other drugs known to be metabolized by CYP450 liver enzymes. However formal drug interaction studies have not been conducted).

No products indexed under this heading.

Insulin (In patients with diabetes mellitus requiring drug therapy, the dose of insulin may require adjustment when somatropin therapy is initiated).

No products indexed under this heading.

Insulin, Human, Zinc Suspension (In patients with diabetes mellitus requiring drug therapy, the dose of insulin may require adjustment when somatropin therapy is initiated).

No products indexed under this heading.

Insulin, Human (rDNA origin) (In patients with diabetes mellitus requiring drug therapy, the dose of insulin may require adjustment when somatropin therapy is initiated). Products include:

Exubera Inhalation Powder **2515**

Insulin, Human NPH (In patients with diabetes mellitus requiring drug therapy, the dose of insulin may require adjustment when somatropin therapy is initiated). Products include:

Humulin N Vial **1846**

Insulin, Human Regular (In patients with diabetes mellitus requiring drug therapy, the dose of insulin may require adjustment when somatropin therapy is initiated). Products include:

Humulin R **1849**
Humulin R (U-500) **1850**

Insulin, Human Regular and Human NPH Mixture (In patients with diabetes mellitus requiring drug therapy, the dose of insulin may require adjustment when somatropin therapy is initiated). Products include:

Humulin 50/50, 100 Units **1843**
Humulin 70/30 Vial **1844**

Insulin, NPH (In patients with diabetes mellitus requiring drug therapy, the dose of insulin may require adjustment when somatropin therapy is initiated).

No products indexed under this heading.

Insulin, Regular (In patients with diabetes mellitus requiring drug therapy, the dose of insulin may require adjustment when somatropin therapy is initiated).

No products indexed under this heading.

Insulin, Regular and NPH mixture (In patients with diabetes mellitus requiring drug therapy, the dose of insulin may require adjustment when somatropin therapy is initiated).

No products indexed under this heading.

Insulin, Zinc Crystals (In patients with diabetes mellitus requiring drug therapy, the dose of insulin may require adjustment when somatropin therapy is initiated).

No products indexed under this heading.

Insulin, Zinc Suspension (In patients with diabetes mellitus requiring drug therapy, the dose of insulin may require adjustment when somatropin therapy is initiated).

No products indexed under this heading.

Insulin Aspart (In patients with diabetes mellitus requiring drug therapy, the dose of insulin may require adjustment when somatropin therapy is initiated).

No products indexed under this heading.

Insulin Aspart, Human (In patients with diabetes mellitus requiring drug therapy, the dose of insulin may require adjustment when somatropin therapy is initiated). Products include:

NovoLog Mix 70/30 .... **2364**

Insulin Aspart, Human Regular (In patients with diabetes mellitus requiring drug therapy, the dose of insulin may require adjustment when somatropin therapy is initiated). Products include:

NovoLog Injection **2359**

Insulin Aspart Protamine, Human (In patients with diabetes mellitus requiring drug therapy, the dose of insulin may require adjustment when somatropin therapy is initiated). Products include:

NovoLog Mix 70/30 .... **2364**

Insulin Detemir (rDNA Origin) (In patients with diabetes mellitus requiring drug therapy, the dose of insulin may require adjustment when somatropin therapy is initiated). Products include:

Levemir Injection **2352**

Insulin glargine (In patients with diabetes mellitus requiring drug therapy, the dose of insulin may require adjustment when somatropin therapy is initiated). Products include:

Lantus Injection **2749**

Insulin Glulisine (In patients with diabetes mellitus requiring drug therapy, the dose of insulin may require adjustment when somatropin therapy is initiated). Products include:

Apidra Injection **2706**

Insulin Lispro, Human (In patients with diabetes mellitus requiring drug therapy, the dose of insulin may require adjustment when somatropin therapy is initiated). Products include:

Humalog-Pen and KwikPen **1829**
Humalog Mix 50/50-Pen and KwikPen **1833**
Humalog Mix 75/25-Pen and KwikPen **1835**

Insulin Lispro Protamine, Human (In patients with diabetes mellitus requiring drug therapy, the dose of insulin may require adjustment when somatropin therapy is initiated). Products include:

Humalog Mix 50/50-Pen and KwikPen **1833**
Humalog Mix 75/25-Pen and KwikPen **1835**

Irbesartan (Limited published data indicate that somatropin treatment increases cytochrome P450 (CYP450)-mediated antipyrine clearance in man. These data suggest that somatropin administration may alter the clearance of compounds known to be metabolized by CYP450 liver enzymes. Careful monitoring is advisable when somatropin is administered in combination with other drugs known to be metabolized by CYP450 liver enzymes. However formal drug interaction studies have not been conducted). Products include:

Avalide Tablets **892**
Avalide Tablets **2713**
Avapro Tablets **897**
Avapro Tablets **2718**

Isotretinoin (Limited published data indicate that somatropin treatment increases cytochrome P450 (CYP450)-mediated antipyrine clearance in man. These data suggest that somatropin administration may alter the clearance of compounds known to be metabolized by CYP450 liver enzymes. Careful monitoring is advisable when somatropin is administered in combination with other drugs known to be metabolized by CYP450 liver enzymes. However formal drug interaction studies have not been conducted). Products include:

Accutane Capsules **2607**

Isradipine (Limited published data indicate that somatropin treatment increases cytochrome P450 (CYP450)-mediated antipyrine clearance in man. These data suggest that somatropin administration may alter the clearance of compounds known to be metabolized by CYP450 liver enzymes. Careful monitoring is advisable when somatropin is administered in combination with other drugs known to be metabolized by CYP450 liver enzymes. However formal drug interaction studies have not been conducted). Products include:

DynaCirc CR Controlled Release Tablets **1407**

Itraconazole (Limited published data indicate that somatropin treatment increases cytochrome P450 (CYP450)-mediated antipyrine clearance in man. These data suggest that somatropin administration may alter the clearance of compounds known to be metabolized by CYP450 liver enzymes. Careful monitoring is advisable when somatropin is administered in combination with other drugs known to be metabolized by CYP450 liver enzymes. However formal drug interaction studies have not been conducted).

No products indexed under this heading.

Ketoconazole (Limited published data indicate that somatropin treatment increases cytochrome P450 (CYP450)-mediated antipyrine clearance in man. These data suggest that somatropin administration may alter the clearance of compounds known to be metabolized by CYP450 liver enzymes. Careful monitoring is advisable when somatropin is administered in combination with other drugs known to be metabolized by CYP450 liver enzymes. However formal drug interaction studies have not been conducted). Products include:

Extina Foam, 2% **3057**
Nizoral A-D Shampoo **1901**

Ketoprofen (Limited published data indicate that somatropin treatment increases cytochrome P450 (CYP450)-mediated antipyrine clearance in man. These data suggest that somatropin administration may alter the clearance of compounds known to be metabolized by CYP450 liver enzymes. Careful monitoring is advisable when somatropin is administered in combination with other drugs known to be metabolized by CYP450 liver enzymes. However formal drug interaction studies have not been conducted).

No products indexed under this heading.

Ketorolac Tromethamine (Limited published data indicate that somatropin treatment increases cytochrome P450 (CYP450)-mediated antipyrine clearance in man. These data suggest that somatropin administration may alter the clearance of compounds known to be metabolized by CYP450 liver enzymes. Careful monitoring is advisable when somatropin is administered in combination with other drugs known to be metabolized by CYP450 liver enzymes. However formal drug interaction studies have not been conducted).

No products indexed under this heading.

Labetalol Hydrochloride (Limited published data indicate that somatropin treatment increases cytochrome P450 (CYP450)-mediated antipyrine clearance in man. These data suggest that somatropin administration may alter the clearance of compounds known to be metabolized by CYP450 liver enzymes. Careful monitoring is advisable when somatropin is administered in combination with other drugs known to be metabolized by CYP450 liver enzymes. However formal drug interaction studies have not been conducted).

No products indexed under this heading.

Lamotrigine (Limited published data indicates that somatropin treatment increases cytochrome P450 (CP450) mediated antipyrine clearance in man. This data suggests that somatropin administration may alter the clearance of compounds known to be metabolized by CP450 liver enzymes (eg anticonvulsants). Careful monitoring is advisable when somatropin is administered in combination with other drugs known to be metabolized by CP450 liver enzymes. However, formal drug interaction studies have not been conducted). Products include:

Lamictal 1488

Lansoprazole (Limited published data indicate that somatropin treatment increases cytochrome P450 (CYP450)-mediated antipyrine clearance in man. These data suggest that somatropin administration may alter the clearance of compounds known to be metabolized by CYP450 liver enzymes. Careful monitoring is advisable when somatropin is administered in combination with other drugs known to be metabolized by CYP450 liver enzymes. However formal drug interaction studies have not been conducted).

No products indexed under this heading.

Levetiracetam (Limited published data indicates that somatropin treatment increases cytochrome P450 (CP450) mediated antipyrine clearance in man. This data suggests that somatropin administration may alter the clearance of compounds known to be metabolized by CP450 liver enzymes (eg anticonvulsants). Careful monitoring is advisable when somatropin is administered in combination with other drugs known to be metabolized by CP450 liver enzymes. However, formal drug interaction studies have not been conducted). Products include:

Keppra Injection 3137
Keppra Oral Solution 3131
Keppra Tablets 3131

Levobupivacaine Hydrochloride (Limited published data indicate that somatropin treatment increases cytochrome P450 (CYP450)-mediated antipyrine clearance in man. These data suggest that somatropin administration may alter the clearance of compounds known to be metabolized by CYP450 liver enzymes. Careful monitoring is advisable when somatropin is administered in combination with other drugs known to be metabolized by CYP450 liver enzymes. However formal drug interaction studies have not been conducted).

No products indexed under this heading.

Levonorgestrel (Limited published data indicates that somatropin treatment increases cytochrome P450 (CP450) mediated antipyrine clearance in man. This data suggests that somatropin administration may alter the clearance of compounds known to be metabolized by CP450 liver enzymes (eg, sex steroids). Careful monitoring is advisable when somatropin is administered in combination with other drugs known to be metabolized by CP450 liver enzymes. However, formal drug interaction studies have not been conducted). Products include:

Climara Pro Transdermal System 768
Lybrel Tablets 3204
Mirena Intrauterine System 779
Plan B Tablets 1044
Seasonique Tablets 1046

Lidocaine (Limited published data indicate that somatropin treatment increases cytochrome P450 (CYP450)-mediated antipyrine clearance in man. These data suggest that somatropin administration may alter the clearance of compounds known to be metabolized by CYP450 liver enzymes. Careful monitoring is advisable when somatropin is administered in combination with other drugs known to be metabolized by CYP450 liver enzymes. However formal drug interaction studies have not been conducted). Products include:

Lidoderm Patch 1114

Lidocaine Base (Limited published data indicate that somatropin treatment increases cytochrome P450 (CYP450)-mediated antipyrine clearance in man. These data suggest that somatropin administration may alter the clearance of compounds known to be metabolized by CYP450 liver enzymes. Careful monitoring is advisable when somatropin is administered in combination with other drugs known to be metabolized by CYP450 liver enzymes. However formal drug interaction studies have not been conducted).

No products indexed under this heading.

Lidocaine Hydrochloride (Limited published data indicate that somatropin treatment increases cytochrome P450 (CYP450)-mediated antipyrine clearance in man. These data suggest that somatropin administration may alter the clearance of compounds known to be metabolized by CYP450 liver enzymes. Careful monitoring is advisable when somatropin is administered in combination with other drugs known to be metabolized by CYP450 liver enzymes. However formal drug interaction studies have not been conducted).

No products indexed under this heading.

Lomefloxacin Hydrochloride (Limited published data indicate that somatropin treatment increases cytochrome P450 (CYP450)-mediated antipyrine clearance in man. These data suggest that somatropin administration may alter the clearance of compounds known to be metabolized by CYP450 liver enzymes. Careful monitoring is advisable when somatropin is administered in combination with other drugs known to be metabolized by CYP450 liver enzymes. However formal drug interaction studies have not been conducted).

No products indexed under this heading.

Losartan Potassium (Limited published data indicate that somatropin treatment increases cytochrome P450 (CYP450)-mediated antipyrine clearance in man. These data suggest that somatropin administration may alter the clearance of compounds known to be metabolized by CYP450 liver enzymes. Careful monitoring is advisable when somatropin is administered in combination with other drugs known to be metabolized by CYP450 liver enzymes. However formal drug interaction studies have not been conducted). Products include:

Cozaar Tablets 1973

Lovastatin (Limited published data indicate that somatropin treatment increases cytochrome P450 (CYP450)-mediated antipyrine clearance in man. These data suggest that somatropin administration may alter the clearance of compounds known to be metabolized by CYP450 liver enzymes. Careful monitoring is advisable when somatropin is administered in combination with other drugs known to be metabolized by CYP450 liver enzymes. However formal drug interaction studies have not been conducted). Products include:

Advicor Tablets 402
Mevacor Tablets 2063

Maprotiline Hydrochloride (Limited published data indicate that somatropin treatment increases cytochrome P450 (CYP450)-mediated antipyrine clearance in man. These data suggest that somatropin administration may alter the clearance of compounds known to be metabolized by CYP450 liver enzymes. Careful monitoring is advisable when somatropin is administered in combination with other drugs known to be metabolized by CYP450 liver enzymes. However formal drug interaction studies have not been conducted).

No products indexed under this heading.

Meclofenamate Sodium (Limited published data indicate that somatropin treatment increases cytochrome P450 (CYP450)-mediated antipyrine clearance in man. These data suggest that somatropin administration may alter the clearance of compounds known to be metabolized by CYP450 liver enzymes. Careful monitoring is advisable when somatropin is administered in combination with other drugs known to be metabolized by CYP450 liver enzymes. However formal drug interaction studies have not been conducted).

No products indexed under this heading.

Mefenamic Acid (Limited published data indicate that somatropin treatment increases cytochrome P450 (CYP450)-mediated antipyrine clearance in man. These data suggest that somatropin administration may alter the clearance of compounds known to be metabolized by CYP450 liver enzymes. Careful monitoring is advisable when somatropin is administered in combination with other drugs known to be metabolized by CYP450 liver enzymes. However formal drug interaction studies have not been conducted).

No products indexed under this heading.

Meloxicam (Limited published data indicate that somatropin treatment increases cytochrome P450 (CYP450)-mediated antipyrine clearance in man. These data suggest that somatropin administration may alter the clearance of compounds known to be metabolized by CYP450 liver enzymes. Careful monitoring is advisable when somatropin is administered in combination with other drugs known to be metabolized by CYP450 liver enzymes. However formal drug interaction studies have not been conducted). Products include:

Mobic Oral Suspension 863
Mobic Tablets 863

Meperidine Hydrochloride (Limited published data indicate that somatropin treatment increases cytochrome P450 (CYP450)-mediated antipyrine clearance in man. These data suggest that somatropin administration may alter the clearance of compounds known to be metabolized by CYP450 liver enzymes. Careful monitoring is advisable when somatropin is administered in combination with other drugs known to be metabolized by CYP450 liver enzymes. However formal drug interaction studies have not been conducted).

No products indexed under this heading.

Mephenytoin (Limited published data indicates that somatropin treatment increases cytochrome P450 (CP450) mediated antipyrine clearance in man. This data suggests that somatropin administration may alter the clearance of compounds known to be metabolized by CP450 liver enzymes (eg anticonvulsants). Careful monitoring is advisable when somatropin is administered in combination with other drugs known to be metabolized by CP450 liver enzymes. However, formal drug interaction studies have not been conducted).

No products indexed under this heading.

Mephobarbital (Limited published data indicate that somatropin treatment increases cytochrome P450 (CYP450)-mediated antipyrine clearance in man. These data suggest that somatropin administration may alter the clearance of compounds known to be metabolized by CYP450 liver enzymes. Careful monitoring is advisable when somatropin is administered in combination with other drugs known to be metabolized by CYP450 liver enzymes. However formal drug interaction studies have not been conducted).

No products indexed under this heading.

Meprobamate (Limited published data indicate that somatropin treatment increases cytochrome P450 (CYP450)-mediated antipyrine clearance in man. These data suggest that somatropin administration may alter the clearance of compounds known to be metabolized by CYP450 liver enzymes. Careful monitoring is advisable when somatropin is administered in combination with other drugs known to be metabolized by CYP450 liver enzymes. However formal drug interaction studies have not been conducted).

No products indexed under this heading.

Mestranol (Limited published data indicates that somatropin treatment increases cytochrome P450 (CP450) mediated antipyrine clearance in man. This data suggests that somatropin administration may alter the clearance of compounds known to be metabolized by CP450 liver enzymes (eg, sex steroids). Careful monitoring is advisable when somatropin is administered in combination with other drugs known to be metabolized by CP450 liver enzymes. How-

ever, formal drug interaction studies have not been conducted).
No products indexed under this heading.

Metformin Hydrochloride (In patients with diabetes mellitus requiring drug therapy, the dose of oral hypoglycemic agents may require adjustment when somatropin therapy is initiated). Products include:
ActoPlus Met Tablets **3071**
Avandamet Tablets **1336**
Janumet Tablets **2041**
PrandiMet Tablets **2967**

Methadone Hydrochloride (Limited published data indicate that somatropin treatment increases cytochrome P450 (CYP450)-mediated antipyrine clearance in man. These data suggest that somatropin administration may alter the clearance of compounds known to be metabolized by CYP450 liver enzymes. Careful monitoring is advisable when somatropin is administered in combination with other drugs known to be metabolized by CYP450 liver enzymes. However formal drug interaction studies have not been conducted).
No products indexed under this heading.

Methamphetamine Hydrochloride (Limited published data indicate that somatropin treatment increases cytochrome P450 (CYP450)-mediated antipyrine clearance in man. These data suggest that somatropin administration may alter the clearance of compounds known to be metabolized by CYP450 liver enzymes. Careful monitoring is advisable when somatropin is administered in combination with other drugs known to be metabolized by CYP450 liver enzymes. However formal drug interaction studies have not been conducted).
No products indexed under this heading.

Methsuximide (Limited published data indicates that somatropin treatment increases cytochrome P450 (CP450) mediated antipyrine clearance in man. This data suggests that somatropin administration may alter the clearance of compounds known to be metabolized by CP450 liver enzymes (eg anticonvulsants). Careful monitoring is advisable when somatropin is administered in combination with other drugs known to be metabolized by CP450 liver enzymes. However, formal drug interaction studies have not been conducted).
No products indexed under this heading.

Methylprednisolone Acetate (Somatropin inhibits 11βHSD-1 in adipose/hepatic tissue and may significantly impact the metabolism of cortisone and cortisol. Patients being treated with glucocorticoid replacement therapy for hypoadrenalism may require an increase in their maintenance or stress doses; especially with cortisone acetate and prednisone, since conversion of these drugs to their biologically active metabolites is dependent on the activity of the 11μHSD-1 enzyme. Also, excessive glucocorticoid therapy may attenuate the growth-promoting effects of somatropin in children. Therefore, glucocorticoid replacement therapy should be carefully adjusted in children with concomitant GH and glucocorticoid deficiency to avoid both hypoadrenalism and an inhibitory effect on growth).
No products indexed under this heading.

Methylprednisolone Sodium Succinate (Somatropin inhibits 11βHSD-1 in adipose/hepatic tissue and may significantly impact the metabolism of cortisone and cortisol. Patients being treated with glucocorticoid replacement therapy for hypoadrenalism may require an increase in their maintenance or stress doses; especially with cortisone acetate and prednisone, since conversion of these drugs to their biologically active metabolites is dependent on the activity of the 11μHSD-1 enzyme. Also, excessive glucocorticoid therapy may attenuate the growth-promoting effects of somatropin in children. Therefore, glucocorticoid replacement therapy should be carefully adjusted in children with concomitant GH and glucocorticoid deficiency to avoid both hypoadrenalism and an inhibitory effect on growth).
No products indexed under this heading.

Methyltestosterone (Limited published data indicates that somatropin treatment increases cytochrome P450 (CP450) mediated antipyrine clearance in man. This data suggests that somatropin administration may alter the clearance of compounds known to be metabolized by CP450 liver enzymes (eg, sex steroids). Careful monitoring is advisable when somatropin is administered in combination with other drugs known to be metabolized by CP450 liver enzymes. However, formal drug interaction studies have not been conducted). Products include:
Estratest Tablets **3043**
Estratest H.S. Tablets **3043**

Metoprolol Succinate (Limited published data indicate that somatropin treatment increases cytochrome P450 (CYP450)-mediated antipyrine clearance in man. These data suggest that somatropin administration may alter the clearance of compounds known to be metabolized by CYP450 liver enzymes. Careful monitoring is advisable when somatropin is administered in combination with other drugs known to be metabolized by CYP450 liver enzymes. However formal drug interaction studies have not been conducted). Products include:
Toprol-XL Tablets **666**

Metoprolol Tartrate (Limited published data indicate that somatropin treatment increases cytochrome P450 (CYP450)-mediated antipyrine clearance in man. These data suggest that somatropin administration may alter the clearance of compounds known to be metabolized by CYP450 liver enzymes. Careful monitoring is advisable when somatropin is administered in combination with other drugs known to be metabolized by CYP450 liver enzymes. However formal drug interaction studies have not been conducted).
No products indexed under this heading.

Mexiletine Hydrochloride (Limited published data indicate that somatropin treatment increases cytochrome P450 (CYP450)-mediated antipyrine clearance in man. These data suggest that somatropin administration may alter the clearance of compounds known to be metabolized by CYP450 liver enzymes. Careful monitoring is advisable when somatropin is administered in combination with other drugs known to be metabolized by CYP450 liver enzymes. However formal drug interaction studies have not been conducted).
No products indexed under this heading.

Midazolam Hydrochloride (Limited published data indicate that somatropin treatment increases cytochrome P450 (CYP450)-mediated antipyrine clearance in man. These data suggest that somatropin administration may alter the clearance of compounds known to be metabolized by CYP450 liver enzymes. Careful monitoring is advisable when somatropin is administered in combination with other drugs known to be metabolized by CYP450 liver enzymes. However formal drug interaction studies have not been conducted).
No products indexed under this heading.

Miglitol (In patients with diabetes mellitus requiring drug therapy, the dose of oral hypoglycemic agents may require adjustment when somatropin therapy is initiated).
No products indexed under this heading.

Mirtazapine (Limited published data indicate that somatropin treatment increases cytochrome P450 (CYP450)-mediated antipyrine clearance in man. These data suggest that somatropin administration may alter the clearance of compounds known to be metabolized by CYP450 liver enzymes. Careful monitoring is advisable when somatropin is administered in combination with other drugs known to be metabolized by CYP450 liver enzymes. However formal drug interaction studies have not been conducted). Products include:
Remeron Tablets **2924**
RemeronSolTab Tablets **2927**

Mometasone Furoate (Limited published data indicates that somatropin treatment increases cytochrome P450 (CP450) mediated antipyrine clearance in man. This data suggests that somatropin administration may alter the clearance of compounds known to be metabolized by CP450 liver enzymes (eg, corticosteroids). Careful monitoring is advisable when somatropin is administered in combination with other drugs known to be metabolized by CP450 liver enzymes. However, formal drug interaction studies have not been conducted). Products include:
Asmanex Twisthaler **2797**
Elocon Cream 0.1% **2840**
Elocon Lotion 0.1% **2841**
Elocon Ointment 0.1% **2842**

Mometasone Furoate Monohydrate (Limited published data indicates that somatropin treatment increases cytochrome P450 (CP450) mediated antipyrine clearance in man. This data suggests that somatropin administration may alter the clearance of compounds known to be metabolized by CP450 liver enzymes (eg, corticosteroids). Careful monitoring is advisable when somatropin is administered in combination with other drugs known to be metabolized by CP450 liver enzymes. However, formal drug interaction studies have not been conducted). Products include:
Nasonex Nasal Spray **2883**

Montelukast Sodium (Limited published data indicate that somatropin treatment increases cytochrome P450 (CYP450)-mediated antipyrine clearance in man. These data suggest that somatropin administration may alter the clearance of compounds known to be metabolized by CYP450 liver enzymes. Careful monitoring is advisable when somatropin is administered in combination with other drugs known to be metabolized by CYP450 liver enzymes. However formal drug interaction studies have not been conducted). Products include:
Singulair **2114**

Morphine Sulfate (Limited published data indicate that somatropin treatment increases cytochrome P450 (CYP450)-mediated antipyrine clearance in man. These data suggest that somatropin administration may alter the clearance of compounds known to be metabolized by CYP450 liver enzymes. Careful monitoring is advisable when somatropin is administered in combination with other drugs known to be metabolized by CYP450 liver enzymes. However formal drug interaction studies have not been conducted). Products include:
Avinza Capsules **1772**
DepoDur Injection **1095**
MS Contin Tablets **2585**

Moxifloxacin Hydrochloride (Limited published data indicate that somatropin treatment increases cytochrome P450 (CYP450)-mediated antipyrine clearance in man. These data suggest that somatropin administration may alter the clearance of compounds known to be metabolized by CYP450 liver enzymes. Careful monitoring is advisable when somatropin is administered in combination with other drugs known to be metabolized by CYP450 liver enzymes. However formal drug interaction studies have not been conducted). Products include:
Avelox **2803**
Vigamox Ophthalmic Solution **548**

Nabumetone (Limited published data indicate that somatropin treatment increases cytochrome P450 (CYP450)-mediated antipyrine clearance in man. These data suggest that somatropin administration may alter the clearance of compounds known to be metabolized by CYP450 liver enzymes. Careful monitoring is advisable when somatropin is administered in combination with other drugs known to be metabolized by CYP450 liver enzymes. However formal drug interaction studies have not been conducted).
No products indexed under this heading.

Nafcillin Sodium (Limited published data indicate that somatropin treatment increases cytochrome P450 (CYP450)-mediated antipyrine clearance in man. These data suggest that somatropin administration may alter the clearance of compounds known to be metabolized by

CYP450 liver enzymes. Careful monitoring is advisable when somatropin is administered in combination with other drugs known to be metabolized by CYP450 liver enzymes. However formal drug interaction studies have not been conducted).
No products indexed under this heading.

Naproxen (Limited published data indicate that somatropin treatment increases cytochrome P450 (CYP450)-mediated antipyrine clearance in man. These data suggest that somatropin administration may alter the clearance of compounds known to be metabolized by CYP450 liver enzymes. Careful monitoring is advisable when somatropin is administered in combination with other drugs known to be metabolized by CYP450 liver enzymes. However formal drug interaction studies have not been conducted). Products include:

EC-Naprosyn Delayed-Release Tablets 2632
Naprosyn Suspension 2632
Naprosyn Tablets 2632

Naproxen Sodium (Limited published data indicate that somatropin treatment increases cytochrome P450 (CYP450)-mediated antipyrine clearance in man. These data suggest that somatropin administration may alter the clearance of compounds known to be metabolized by CYP450 liver enzymes. Careful monitoring is advisable when somatropin is administered in combination with other drugs known to be metabolized by CYP450 liver enzymes. However formal drug interaction studies have not been conducted). Products include:

Anaprox Tablets 2632
Anaprox DS Tablets 2632
Treximet Tablets 1616

Nateglinide (In patients with diabetes mellitus requiring drug therapy, the dose of oral hypoglycemic agents may require adjustment when somatropin therapy is initiated). Products include:

Starlix Tablets 2314

Nefazodone Hydrochloride (Limited published data indicate that somatropin treatment increases cytochrome P450 (CYP450)-mediated antipyrine clearance in man. These data suggest that somatropin administration may alter the clearance of compounds known to be metabolized by CYP450 liver enzymes. Careful monitoring is advisable when somatropin is administered in combination with other drugs known to be metabolized by CYP450 liver enzymes. However formal drug interaction studies have not been conducted).
No products indexed under this heading.

Nelfinavir Mesylate (Limited published data indicate that somatropin treatment increases cytochrome P450 (CYP450)-mediated antipyrine clearance in man. These data suggest that somatropin administration may alter the clearance of compounds known to be metabolized by CYP450 liver enzymes. Careful monitoring is advisable when somatropin is administered in combination with other drugs known to be metabolized by CYP450 liver enzymes. However formal drug interaction studies have not been conducted).
No products indexed under this heading.

Nicardipine (Limited published data indicate that somatropin treatment increases cytochrome P450 (CYP450)-mediated antipyrine clearance in man. These data suggest that somatropin administration may alter the clearance of compounds known to be metabolized by CYP450 liver enzymes. Careful monitoring is advisable when somatropin is administered in combination with other drugs known to be metabolized by CYP450 liver enzymes. However formal drug interaction studies have not been conducted).
No products indexed under this heading.

Nicardipine Hydrochloride (Limited published data indicate that somatropin treatment increases cytochrome P450 (CYP450)-mediated antipyrine clearance in man. These data suggest that somatropin administration may alter the clearance of compounds known to be metabolized by CYP450 liver enzymes. Careful monitoring is advisable when somatropin is administered in combination with other drugs known to be metabolized by CYP450 liver enzymes. However formal drug interaction studies have not been conducted). Products include:

Cardene I.V. 1093

Nicotine Polacrilex (Limited published data indicate that somatropin treatment increases cytochrome P450 (CYP450)-mediated antipyrine clearance in man. These data suggest that somatropin administration may alter the clearance of compounds known to be metabolized by CYP450 liver enzymes. Careful monitoring is advisable when somatropin is administered in combination with other drugs known to be metabolized by CYP450 liver enzymes. However formal drug interaction studies have not been conducted).
No products indexed under this heading.

Nicotine Salicylate (Limited published data indicate that somatropin treatment increases cytochrome P450 (CYP450)-mediated antipyrine clearance in man. These data suggest that somatropin administration may alter the clearance of compounds known to be metabolized by CYP450 liver enzymes. Careful monitoring is advisable when somatropin is administered in combination with other drugs known to be metabolized by CYP450 liver enzymes. However formal drug interaction studies have not been conducted).
No products indexed under this heading.

Nicotine Sulfate (Limited published data indicate that somatropin treatment increases cytochrome P450 (CYP450)-mediated antipyrine clearance in man. These data suggest that somatropin administration may alter the clearance of compounds known to be metabolized by CYP450 liver enzymes. Careful monitoring is advisable when somatropin is administered in combination with other drugs known to be metabolized by CYP450 liver enzymes. However formal drug interaction studies have not been conducted).
No products indexed under this heading.

Nifedipine (Limited published data indicate that somatropin treatment increases cytochrome P450 (CYP450)-mediated antipyrine clearance in man. These data suggest that somatropin administration may alter the clearance of compounds known to be metabolized by CYP450 liver enzymes. Careful monitoring is advisable when somatropin is administered in combination with other drugs known to be metabolized by CYP450 liver enzymes. However formal drug interaction studies have not been conducted).
No products indexed under this heading.

Nilutamide (Limited published data indicate that somatropin treatment increases cytochrome P450 (CYP450)-mediated antipyrine clearance in man. These data suggest that somatropin administration may alter the clearance of compounds known to be metabolized by CYP450 liver enzymes. Careful monitoring is advisable when somatropin is administered in combination with other drugs known to be metabolized by CYP450 liver enzymes. However formal drug interaction studies have not been conducted).
No products indexed under this heading.

Nimodipine (Limited published data indicate that somatropin treatment increases cytochrome P450 (CYP450)-mediated antipyrine clearance in man. These data suggest that somatropin administration may alter the clearance of compounds known to be metabolized by CYP450 liver enzymes. Careful monitoring is advisable when somatropin is administered in combination with other drugs known to be metabolized by CYP450 liver enzymes. However formal drug interaction studies have not been conducted). Products include:

Nimotop Capsules 790

Nisoldipine (Limited published data indicate that somatropin treatment increases cytochrome P450 (CYP450)-mediated antipyrine clearance in man. These data suggest that somatropin administration may alter the clearance of compounds known to be metabolized by CYP450 liver enzymes. Careful monitoring is advisable when somatropin is administered in combination with other drugs known to be metabolized by CYP450 liver enzymes. However formal drug interaction studies have not been conducted). Products include:

Sular Extended Release Tablets 2975

Nitrendipine (Limited published data indicate that somatropin treatment increases cytochrome P450 (CYP450)-mediated antipyrine clearance in man. These data suggest that somatropin administration may alter the clearance of compounds known to be metabolized by CYP450 liver enzymes. Careful monitoring is advisable when somatropin is administered in combination with other drugs known to be metabolized by CYP450 liver enzymes. However formal drug interaction studies have not been conducted).
No products indexed under this heading.

Norethindrone (Limited published data indicates that somatropin treatment increases cytochrome P450 (CP450) mediated antipyrine clearance in man. This data suggests that somatropin administration may alter the clearance of compounds known to be metabolized by CP450 liver enzymes (eg, sex steroids). Careful monitoring is advisable when somatropin is administered in combination with other drugs known to be metabolized by CP450 liver enzymes. However, formal drug interaction studies have not been conducted). Products include:

Ortho Micronor Tablets 2446

Norethindrone Acetate (Limited published data indicates that somatropin treatment increases cytochrome P450 (CP450) mediated antipyrine clearance in man. This data suggests that somatropin administration may alter the clearance of compounds known to be metabolized by CP450 liver enzymes (eg, sex steroids). Careful monitoring is advisable when somatropin is administered in combination with other drugs known to be metabolized by CP450 liver enzymes. However, formal drug interaction studies have not been conducted). Products include:

Activella Tablets 2347

Norfloxacin (Limited published data indicate that somatropin treatment increases cytochrome P450 (CYP450)-mediated antipyrine clearance in man. These data suggest that somatropin administration may alter the clearance of compounds known to be metabolized by CYP450 liver enzymes. Careful monitoring is advisable when somatropin is administered in combination with other drugs known to be metabolized by CYP450 liver enzymes. However formal drug interaction studies have not been conducted). Products include:

Noroxin Tablets 2069

Norgestimate (Limited published data indicates that somatropin treatment increases cytochrome P450 (CP450) mediated antipyrine clearance in man. This data suggests that somatropin administration may alter the clearance of compounds known to be metabolized by CP450 liver enzymes (eg, sex steroids). Careful monitoring is advisable when somatropin is administered in combination with other drugs known to be metabolized by CP450 liver enzymes. However, formal drug interaction studies have not been conducted). Products include:

Ortho-Cyclen/Ortho Tri-Cyclen 2449
Ortho Tri-Cyclen Lo Tablets 2458

Norgestrel (Limited published data indicate that somatropin treatment increases cytochrome P450 (CYP450)-mediated antipyrine clearance in man. These data suggest that somatropin administration may alter the clearance of compounds known to be metabolized by CYP450 liver enzymes. Careful monitoring is advisable when somatropin is administered in combination with other drugs known to be metabolized by CYP450 liver enzymes. However formal drug interaction studies have not been conducted).
No products indexed under this heading.

Nortriptyline Hydrochloride (Limited published data indicate that somatropin treatment increases cytochrome P450 (CYP450)-mediated antipyrine clearance in man. These data suggest that somatropin administration may alter the clearance of compounds known to be metabolized by CYP450 liver enzymes. Careful monitoring is advisable when somatropin is administered in combination with other drugs known to be metabolized by CYP450 liver enzymes. However formal drug interaction studies have not been conducted).

No products indexed under this heading.

Ofloxacin (Limited published data indicate that somatropin treatment increases cytochrome P450 (CYP450)-mediated antipyrine clearance in man. These data suggest that somatropin administration may alter the clearance of compounds known to be metabolized by CYP450 liver enzymes. Careful monitoring is advisable when somatropin is administered in combination with other drugs known to be metabolized by CYP450 liver enzymes. However formal drug interaction studies have not been conducted). Products include:

Ofloxacin Ophthalmic Solution 0.3% ⊙ 243

Olanzapine (Limited published data indicate that somatropin treatment increases cytochrome P450 (CYP450)-mediated antipyrine clearance in man. These data suggest that somatropin administration may alter the clearance of compounds known to be metabolized by CYP450 liver enzymes. Careful monitoring is advisable when somatropin is administered in combination with other drugs known to be metabolized by CYP450 liver enzymes. However formal drug interaction studies have not been conducted). Products include:

Symbyax Capsules 1871
Zyprexa Tablets 1883
Zyprexa IntraMuscular 1883
Zyprexa ZYDIS Orally Disintegrating Tablets 1883

Omeprazole (Limited published data indicate that somatropin treatment increases cytochrome P450 (CYP450)-mediated antipyrine clearance in man. These data suggest that somatropin administration may alter the clearance of compounds known to be metabolized by CYP450 liver enzymes. Careful monitoring is advisable when somatropin is administered in combination with other drugs known to be metabolized by CYP450 liver enzymes. However formal drug interaction studies have not been conducted).

No products indexed under this heading.

Ondansetron (Limited published data indicate that somatropin treatment increases cytochrome P450 (CYP450)-mediated antipyrine clearance in man. These data suggest that somatropin administration may alter the clearance of compounds known to be metabolized by CYP450 liver enzymes. Careful monitoring is advisable when somatropin is administered in combination with other drugs known to be metabolized by CYP450 liver enzymes. However formal drug interaction studies have not been conducted). Products include:

Zofran ODT Orally Disintegrating Tablets 1687

Ondansetron Hydrochloride (Limited published data indicate that somatropin treatment increases cytochrome P450 (CYP450)-mediated antipyrine clearance in man. These data suggest that somatropin administration may alter the clearance of compounds known to be metabolized by CYP450 liver enzymes. Careful monitoring is advisable when somatropin is administered in combination with other drugs known to be metabolized by CYP450 liver enzymes. However formal drug interaction studies have not been conducted). Products include:

Zofran Injection 1682
Zofran 1687

Oxaprozin (Limited published data indicate that somatropin treatment increases cytochrome P450 (CYP450)-mediated antipyrine clearance in man. These data suggest that somatropin administration may alter the clearance of compounds known to be metabolized by CYP450 liver enzymes. Careful monitoring is advisable when somatropin is administered in combination with other drugs known to be metabolized by CYP450 liver enzymes. However formal drug interaction studies have not been conducted).

No products indexed under this heading.

Oxcarbazepine (Limited published data indicates that somatropin treatment increases cytochrome P450 (CP450) mediated antipyrine clearance in man. This data suggests that somatropin administration may alter the clearance of compounds known to be metabolized by CP450 liver enzymes (eg anticonvulsants). Careful monitoring is advisable when somatropin is administered in combination with other drugs known to be metabolized by CP450 liver enzymes. However, formal drug interaction studies have not been conducted).

No products indexed under this heading.

Oxycodone Hydrochloride (Limited published data indicate that somatropin treatment increases cytochrome P450 (CYP450)-mediated antipyrine clearance in man. These data suggest that somatropin administration may alter the clearance of compounds known to be metabolized by CYP450 liver enzymes. Careful monitoring is advisable when somatropin is administered in combination with other drugs known to be metabolized by CYP450 liver enzymes. However formal drug interaction studies have not been conducted). Products include:

OxyContin Tablets 2589
OxyIR Capsules 2593
Percocet Tablets 1127
Percodan Tablets 1130

Paclitaxel (Limited published data indicate that somatropin treatment increases cytochrome P450 (CYP450)-mediated antipyrine clearance in man. These data suggest that somatropin administration may alter the clearance of compounds known to be metabolized by CYP450 liver enzymes. Careful monitoring is advisable when somatropin is administered in combination with other drugs known to be metabolized by CYP450 liver enzymes. However formal drug interaction studies have not been conducted).

No products indexed under this heading.

Pantoprazole Sodium (Limited published data indicate that somatropin treatment increases cytochrome P450 (CYP450)-mediated antipyrine clearance in man. These data suggest that somatropin administration may alter the clearance of compounds known to be metabolized by CYP450 liver enzymes. Careful monitoring is advisable when somatropin is administered in combination with other drugs known to be metabolized by CYP450 liver enzymes. However formal drug interaction studies have not been conducted). Products include:

Protonix for Delayed-Release Oral Suspension 3254
Protonix Delayed-Release Tablets 3254
Protonix I.V. 3257

Paramethadione (Limited published data indicates that somatropin treatment increases cytochrome P450 (CP450) mediated antipyrine clearance in man. This data suggests that somatropin administration may alter the clearance of compounds known to be metabolized by CP450 liver enzymes (eg anticonvulsants). Careful monitoring is advisable when somatropin is administered in combination with other drugs known to be metabolized by CP450 liver enzymes. However, formal drug interaction studies have not been conducted).

No products indexed under this heading.

Paroxetine Hydrochloride (Limited published data indicate that somatropin treatment increases cytochrome P450 (CYP450)-mediated antipyrine clearance in man. These data suggest that somatropin administration may alter the clearance of compounds known to be metabolized by CYP450 liver enzymes. Careful monitoring is advisable when somatropin is administered in combination with other drugs known to be metabolized by CYP450 liver enzymes. However formal drug interaction studies have not been conducted). Products include:

Paxil 1535
Paxil CR Controlled-Release Tablets 1544

Pentamidine Isethionate (Limited published data indicate that somatropin treatment increases cytochrome P450 (CYP450)-mediated antipyrine clearance in man. These data suggest that somatropin administration may alter the clearance of compounds known to be metabolized by CYP450 liver enzymes. Careful monitoring is advisable when somatropin is administered in combination with other drugs known to be metabolized by CYP450 liver enzymes. However formal drug interaction studies have not been conducted).

No products indexed under this heading.

Phenacemide (Limited published data indicates that somatropin treatment increases cytochrome P450 (CP450) mediated antipyrine clearance in man. This data suggests that somatropin administration may alter the clearance of compounds known to be metabolized by CP450 liver enzymes (eg anticonvulsants). Careful monitoring is advisable when somatropin is administered in combination with other drugs known to be metabolized by CP450 liver enzymes. However, formal drug interaction studies have not been conducted).

No products indexed under this heading.

Phenobarbital (Limited published data indicates that somatropin treatment increases cytochrome P450 (CP450) mediated antipyrine clearance in man. This data suggests that somatropin administration may alter the clearance of compounds known to be metabolized by CP450 liver enzymes (eg anticonvulsants). Careful monitoring is advisable when somatropin is administered in combination with other drugs known to be metabolized by CP450 liver enzymes. However, formal drug interaction studies have not been conducted). Products include:

Donnatal Extentabs 2507

Phenobarbital Sodium (Limited published data indicate that somatropin treatment increases cytochrome P450 (CYP450)-mediated antipyrine clearance in man. These data suggest that somatropin administration may alter the clearance of compounds known to be metabolized by CYP450 liver enzymes. Careful monitoring is advisable when somatropin is administered in combination with other drugs known to be metabolized by CYP450 liver enzymes. However formal drug interaction studies have not been conducted).

No products indexed under this heading.

Phensuximide (Limited published data indicates that somatropin treatment increases cytochrome P450 (CP450) mediated antipyrine clearance in man. This data suggests that somatropin administration may alter the clearance of compounds known to be metabolized by CP450 liver enzymes (eg anticonvulsants). Careful monitoring is advisable when somatropin is administered in combination with other drugs known to be metabolized by CP450 liver enzymes. However, formal drug interaction studies have not been conducted).

No products indexed under this heading.

Phenylbutazone (Limited published data indicate that somatropin treatment increases cytochrome P450 (CYP450)-mediated antipyrine clearance in man. These data suggest that somatropin administration may alter the clearance of compounds known to be metabolized by CYP450 liver enzymes. Careful monitoring is advisable when somatropin is administered in combination with other drugs known to be metabolized by CYP450 liver enzymes. However formal drug interaction studies have not been conducted).

No products indexed under this heading.

Phenytoin (Limited published data indicates that somatropin treatment increases cytochrome P450 (CP450) mediated antipyrine clearance in man. This data suggests that

somatropin administration may alter the clearance of compounds known to be metabolized by CP450 liver enzymes (eg anticonvulsants). Careful monitoring is advisable when somatropin is administered in combination with other drugs known to be metabolized by CP450 liver enzymes. However, formal drug interaction studies have not been conducted).
No products indexed under this heading.

Phenytoin Sodium (Limited published data indicates that somatropin treatment increases cytochrome P450 (CP450) mediated antipyrine clearance in man. This data suggests that somatropin administration may alter the clearance of compounds known to be metabolized by CP450 liver enzymes (eg anticonvulsants). Careful monitoring is advisable when somatropin is administered in combination with other drugs known to be metabolized by CP450 liver enzymes. However, formal drug interaction studies have not been conducted). Products include:
Phenytek Capsules 2192

Pimozide (Limited published data indicate that somatropin treatment increases cytochrome P450 (CYP450)-mediated antipyrine clearance in man. These data suggest that somatropin administration may alter the clearance of compounds known to be metabolized by CYP450 liver enzymes. Careful monitoring is advisable when somatropin is administered in combination with other drugs known to be metabolized by CYP450 liver enzymes. However formal drug interaction studies have not been conducted).
No products indexed under this heading.

Pindolol (Limited published data indicate that somatropin treatment increases cytochrome P450 (CYP450)-mediated antipyrine clearance in man. These data suggest that somatropin administration may alter the clearance of compounds known to be metabolized by CYP450 liver enzymes. Careful monitoring is advisable when somatropin is administered in combination with other drugs known to be metabolized by CYP450 liver enzymes. However formal drug interaction studies have not been conducted).
No products indexed under this heading.

Pioglitazone Hydrochloride (In patients with diabetes mellitus requiring drug therapy, the dose of oral hypoglycemic agents may require adjustment when somatropin therapy is initiated). Products include:
ActoPlus Met Tablets 3071
Actos Tablets 3077
Duetact Tablets 3085

Piroxicam (Limited published data indicate that somatropin treatment increases cytochrome P450 (CYP450)-mediated antipyrine clearance in man. These data suggest that somatropin administration may alter the clearance of compounds known to be metabolized by CYP450 liver enzymes. Careful monitoring is advisable when somatropin is administered in combination with other drugs known to be metabolized by CYP450 liver enzymes. However formal drug interaction studies have not been conducted).
No products indexed under this heading.

Polyestradiol Phosphate (In patients on oral estrogen replacement, a larger dose of somatropin may be required to achieve the defined treatment goal).
No products indexed under this heading.

Prednisolone Acetate (Somatropin inhibits 11βHSD-1 in adipose/hepatic tissue and may significantly impact the metabolism of cortisone and cortisol. Patients being treated with glucocorticoid replacement therapy for hypoadrenalism may require an increase in their maintenance or stress doses; especially with cortisone acetate and prednisone, since conversion of these drugs to their biologically active metabolites is dependent on the activity of the 11μHSD-1 enzyme. Also, excessive glucocorticoid therapy may attenuate the growth-promoting effects of somatropin in children. Therefore, glucocorticoid replacement therapy should be carefully adjusted in children with concomitant GH and glucocorticoid deficiency to avoid both hypoadrenalism and an inhibitory effect on growth). Products include:
Pred Forte Ophthalmic Suspension .... ⊙ 227
Pred Mild Ophthalmic Suspension .... ⊙ 230
Pred-G Ophthalmic Ointment .... ⊙ 229
Pred-G Ophthalmic Suspension .... ⊙ 228

Prednisolone Sodium Phosphate (Somatropin inhibits 11βHSD-1 in adipose/hepatic tissue and may significantly impact the metabolism of cortisone and cortisol. Patients being treated with glucocorticoid replacement therapy for hypoadrenalism may require an increase in their maintenance or stress doses; especially with cortisone acetate and prednisone, since conversion of these drugs to their biologically active metabolites is dependent on the activity of the 11μHSD-1 enzyme. Also, excessive glucocorticoid therapy may attenuate the growth-promoting effects of somatropin in children. Therefore, glucocorticoid replacement therapy should be carefully adjusted in children with concomitant GH and glucocorticoid deficiency to avoid both hypoadrenalism and an inhibitory effect on growth).
No products indexed under this heading.

Prednisolone Tebutate (Somatropin inhibits 11βHSD-1 in adipose/hepatic tissue and may significantly impact the metabolism of cortisone and cortisol. Patients being treated with glucocorticoid replacement therapy for hypoadrenalism may require an increase in their maintenance or stress doses; especially with cortisone acetate and prednisone, since conversion of these drugs to their biologically active metabolites is dependent on the activity of the 11μHSD-1 enzyme. Also, excessive glucocorticoid therapy may attenuate the growth-promoting effects of somatropin in children. Therefore, glucocorticoid replacement therapy should be carefully adjusted in children with concomitant GH and glucocorticoid deficiency to avoid both hypoadrenalism and an inhibitory effect on growth).
No products indexed under this heading.

Prednisone (Somatropin inhibits 11βHSD-1 in adipose/hepatic tissue and may significantly impact the metabolism of cortisone and cortisol. Patients being treated with glucocorticoid replacement therapy for hypoadrenalism may require an increase in their maintenance or stress doses; especially with cortisone acetate and prednisone, since conversion of these drugs to their biologically active metabolites is dependent on the activity of the 11μHSD-1 enzyme. Also, excessive glucocorticoid therapy may attenuate the growth-promoting effects of somatropin in children. Therefore, glucocorticoid replacement therapy should be carefully adjusted in children with concomitant GH and glucocorticoid deficiency to avoid both hypoadrenalism and an inhibitory effect on growth).
No products indexed under this heading.

Primidone (Limited published data indicates that somatropin treatment increases cytochrome P450 (CP450) mediated antipyrine clearance in man. This data suggests that somatropin administration may alter the clearance of compounds known to be metabolized by CP450 liver enzymes (eg anticonvulsants). Careful monitoring is advisable when somatropin is administered in combination with other drugs known to be metabolized by CP450 liver enzymes. However, formal drug interaction studies have not been conducted).
No products indexed under this heading.

Progesterone (Limited published data indicate that somatropin treatment increases cytochrome P450 (CYP450)-mediated antipyrine clearance in man. These data suggest that somatropin administration may alter the clearance of compounds known to be metabolized by CYP450 liver enzymes. Careful monitoring is advisable when somatropin is administered in combination with other drugs known to be metabolized by CYP450 liver enzymes. However formal drug interaction studies have not been conducted). Products include:
Crinone 4% Gel 992
Crinone 8% Gel 992
Prometrium Capsules (100 mg, 200 mg) 3047

Proguanil Hydrochloride (Limited published data indicate that somatropin treatment increases cytochrome P450 (CYP450)-mediated antipyrine clearance in man. These data suggest that somatropin administration may alter the clearance of compounds known to be metabolized by CYP450 liver enzymes. Careful monitoring is advisable when somatropin is administered in combination with other drugs known to be metabolized by CYP450 liver enzymes. However formal drug interaction studies have not been conducted). Products include:
Malarone Pediatric Tablets 1521
Malarone Tablets 1521

Propafenone Hydrochloride (Limited published data indicate that somatropin treatment increases cytochrome P450 (CYP450)-mediated antipyrine clearance in man. These data suggest that somatropin administration may alter the clearance of compounds known to be metabolized by CYP450 liver enzymes. Careful monitoring is advisable when somatropin is administered in combination with other drugs known to be metabolized by CYP450 liver enzymes. However formal drug interaction studies have not been conducted). Products include:
Rythmol Tablets 1586
Rythmol SR Capsules 1590

Propoxyphene Hydrochloride (Limited published data indicate that somatropin treatment increases cytochrome P450 (CYP450)-mediated antipyrine clearance in man. These data suggest that somatropin administration may alter the clearance of compounds known to be metabolized by CYP450 liver enzymes. Careful monitoring is advisable when somatropin is administered in combination with other drugs known to be metabolized by CYP450 liver enzymes. However formal drug interaction studies have not been conducted).
No products indexed under this heading.

Propoxyphene Napsylate (Limited published data indicate that somatropin treatment increases cytochrome P450 (CYP450)-mediated antipyrine clearance in man. These data suggest that somatropin administration may alter the clearance of compounds known to be metabolized by CYP450 liver enzymes. Careful monitoring is advisable when somatropin is administered in combination with other drugs known to be metabolized by CYP450 liver enzymes. However formal drug interaction studies have not been conducted).
No products indexed under this heading.

Propranolol Hydrochloride (Limited published data indicate that somatropin treatment increases cytochrome P450 (CYP450)-mediated antipyrine clearance in man. These data suggest that somatropin administration may alter the clearance of compounds known to be metabolized by CYP450 liver enzymes. Careful monitoring is advisable when somatropin is administered in combination with other drugs known to be metabolized by CYP450 liver enzymes. However formal drug interaction studies have not been conducted). Products include:
InnoPran XL Extended Release Capsules 1484

Protriptyline Hydrochloride (Limited published data indicate that somatropin treatment increases cytochrome P450 (CYP450)-mediated antipyrine clearance in man. These data suggest that somatropin administration may alter the clearance of compounds known to be metabolized by CYP450 liver enzymes. Careful monitoring is advisable when somatropin is administered in combination with other drugs known to be metabolized by CYP450 liver enzymes. However formal drug interaction studies have not been conducted).
No products indexed under this heading.

Quetiapine Fumarate (Limited published data indicate that somatropin treatment increases cytochrome P450 (CYP450)-mediated antipyrine clearance in man. These data suggest that somatropin administration may alter the clearance of compounds known to be metabolized by CYP450 liver enzymes. Careful monitoring is advisable when somatropin is administered in combination with other drugs known to be metabolized by CYP450 liver enzymes. However formal drug interaction studies have not been conducted).
No products indexed under this heading.

Quinestrol (In patients on oral estrogen replacement, a larger dose of somatropin may be required to achieve the defined treatment goal).
No products indexed under this heading.

Quinidine Gluconate (Limited published data indicate that somatropin treatment increases cytochrome P450 (CYP450)-mediated antipyrine clearance in man. These data suggest that somatropin administration may alter the clearance of compounds known to be metabolized by CYP450 liver enzymes. Careful monitoring is advisable when somatropin is administered in combination with other drugs known to be metabolized by CYP450 liver enzymes. However formal drug interaction studies have not been conducted).
No products indexed under this heading.

Quinidine Hydrochloride (Limited published data indicate that somatropin treatment increases cytochrome P450 (CYP450)-mediated antipyrine clearance in man. These data suggest that somatropin administration may alter the clearance of compounds known to be metabolized by CYP450 liver enzymes. Careful monitoring is advisable when somatropin is administered in combination with other drugs known to be metabolized by CYP450 liver enzymes. However formal drug interaction studies have not been conducted).
No products indexed under this heading.

Quinidine Polygalacturonate (Limited published data indicate that somatropin treatment increases cytochrome P450 (CYP450)-mediated antipyrine clearance in man. These data suggest that somatropin administration may alter the clearance of compounds known to be metabolized by CYP450 liver enzymes. Careful monitoring is advisable when somatropin is administered in combination with other drugs known to be metabolized by CYP450 liver enzymes. However formal drug interaction studies have not been conducted).
No products indexed under this heading.

Quinidine Sulfate (Limited published data indicate that somatropin treatment increases cytochrome P450 (CYP450)-mediated antipyrine clearance in man. These data suggest that somatropin administration may alter the clearance of compounds known to be metabolized by CYP450 liver enzymes. Careful monitoring is advisable when somatropin is administered in combination with other drugs known to be metabolized by CYP450 liver enzymes. However formal drug interaction studies have not been conducted).
No products indexed under this heading.

Quinine (Limited published data indicate that somatropin treatment increases cytochrome P450 (CYP450)-mediated antipyrine clearance in man. These data suggest that somatropin administration may alter the clearance of compounds known to be metabolized by CYP450 liver enzymes. Careful monitoring is advisable when somatropin is administered in combination with other drugs known to be metabolized by CYP450 liver enzymes. However formal drug interaction studies have not been conducted).
No products indexed under this heading.

Quinine Sulfate (Limited published data indicate that somatropin treatment increases cytochrome P450 (CYP450)-mediated antipyrine clearance in man. These data suggest that somatropin administration may alter the clearance of compounds known to be metabolized by CYP450 liver enzymes. Careful monitoring is advisable when somatropin is administered in combination with other drugs known to be metabolized by CYP450 liver enzymes. However formal drug interaction studies have not been conducted).
No products indexed under this heading.

Rabeprazole Sodium (Limited published data indicate that somatropin treatment increases cytochrome P450 (CYP450)-mediated antipyrine clearance in man. These data suggest that somatropin administration may alter the clearance of compounds known to be metabolized by CYP450 liver enzymes. Careful monitoring is advisable when somatropin is administered in combination with other drugs known to be metabolized by CYP450 liver enzymes. However formal drug interaction studies have not been conducted). Products include:
Aciphex Tablets 1053

Repaglinide (In patients with diabetes mellitus requiring drug therapy, the dose of oral hypoglycemic agents may require adjustment when somatropin therapy is initiated). Products include:
PrandiMet Tablets 2967
Prandin Tablets 2971

Rifabutin (Limited published data indicate that somatropin treatment increases cytochrome P450 (CYP450)-mediated antipyrine clearance in man. These data suggest that somatropin administration may alter the clearance of compounds known to be metabolized by CYP450 liver enzymes. Careful monitoring is advisable when somatropin is administered in combination with other drugs known to be metabolized by CYP450 liver enzymes. However formal drug interaction studies have not been conducted).
No products indexed under this heading.

Riluzole (Limited published data indicate that somatropin treatment increases cytochrome P450 (CYP450)-mediated antipyrine clearance in man. These data suggest that somatropin administration may alter the clearance of compounds known to be metabolized by CYP450 liver enzymes. Careful monitoring is advisable when somatropin is administered in combination with other drugs known to be metabolized by CYP450 liver enzymes. However formal drug interaction studies have not been conducted). Products include:
Rilutek Tablets 2771

Risperidone (Limited published data indicate that somatropin treatment increases cytochrome P450 (CYP450)-mediated antipyrine clearance in man. These data suggest that somatropin administration may alter the clearance of compounds known to be metabolized by CYP450 liver enzymes. Careful monitoring is advisable when somatropin is administered in combination with other drugs known to be metabolized by CYP450 liver enzymes. However formal drug interaction studies have not been conducted). Products include:
Risperdal Consta Long-Acting Injection 1753

Ritonavir (Limited published data indicate that somatropin treatment increases cytochrome P450 (CYP450)-mediated antipyrine clearance in man. These data suggest that somatropin administration may alter the clearance of compounds known to be metabolized by CYP450 liver enzymes. Careful monitoring is advisable when somatropin is administered in combination with other drugs known to be metabolized by CYP450 liver enzymes. However formal drug interaction studies have not been conducted). Products include:
Kaletra 452
Norvir 489

Rofecoxib (Limited published data indicate that somatropin treatment increases cytochrome P450 (CYP450)-mediated antipyrine clearance in man. These data suggest that somatropin administration may alter the clearance of compounds known to be metabolized by CYP450 liver enzymes. Careful monitoring is advisable when somatropin is administered in combination with other drugs known to be metabolized by CYP450 liver enzymes. However formal drug interaction studies have not been conducted).
No products indexed under this heading.

Ropinirole Hydrochloride (Limited published data indicate that somatropin treatment increases cytochrome P450 (CYP450)-mediated antipyrine clearance in man. These data suggest that somatropin administration may alter the clearance of compounds known to be metabolized by CYP450 liver enzymes. Careful monitoring is advisable when somatropin is administered in combination with other drugs known to be metabolized by CYP450 liver enzymes. However formal drug interaction studies have not been conducted). Products include:
Requip Tablets 1561
Requip XL Tablets 1568

Ropivacaine Hydrochloride (Limited published data indicate that somatropin treatment increases cytochrome P450 (CYP450)-mediated antipyrine clearance in man. These data suggest that somatropin administration may alter the clearance of compounds known to be metabolized by CYP450 liver enzymes. Careful monitoring is advisable when somatropin is administered in combination with other drugs known to be metabolized by CYP450 liver enzymes. However formal drug interaction studies have not been conducted).
No products indexed under this heading.

Rosiglitazone Maleate (In patients with diabetes mellitus requiring drug therapy, the dose of oral hypoglycemic agents may require adjustment when somatropin therapy is initiated). Products include:
Avandamet Tablets 1336
Avandaryl Tablets 1344
Avandia Tablets 1351

Saquinavir (Limited published data indicate that somatropin treatment increases cytochrome P450 (CYP450)-mediated antipyrine clearance in man. These data suggest that somatropin administration may alter the clearance of compounds known to be metabolized by CYP450 liver enzymes. Careful monitoring is advisable when somatropin is administered in combination with other drugs known to be metabolized by CYP450 liver enzymes. However formal drug interaction studies have not been conducted).
No products indexed under this heading.

Saquinavir Mesylate (Limited published data indicate that somatropin treatment increases cytochrome P450 (CYP450)-mediated antipyrine clearance in man. These data suggest that somatropin administration may alter the clearance of compounds known to be metabolized by CYP450 liver enzymes. Careful monitoring is advisable when somatropin is administered in combination with other drugs known to be metabolized by CYP450 liver enzymes. However formal drug interaction studies have not been conducted).
No products indexed under this heading.

Sertraline Hydrochloride (Limited published data indicate that somatropin treatment increases cytochrome P450 (CYP450)-mediated antipyrine clearance in man. These data suggest that somatropin administration may alter the clearance of compounds known to be metabolized by CYP450 liver enzymes. Careful monitoring is advisable when somatropin is administered in combination with other drugs known to be metabolized by CYP450 liver enzymes. However formal drug interaction studies have not been conducted).
No products indexed under this heading.

Sildenafil Citrate (Limited published data indicate that somatropin treatment increases cytochrome P450 (CYP450)-mediated antipyrine clearance in man. These data suggest that somatropin administration may alter the clearance of compounds known to be metabolized by CYP450 liver enzymes. Careful monitoring is advisable when somatropin is administered in combination with other drugs known to be metabolized by CYP450 liver enzymes. However formal drug interaction studies have not been conducted).
No products indexed under this heading.

Simvastatin (Limited published data indicate that somatropin treatment increases cytochrome P450 (CYP450)-mediated antipyrine clearance in man. These data suggest that somatropin administration may alter the clearance of compounds known to be metabolized by CYP450 liver enzymes. Careful monitoring is advisable when somatropin is administered in combination with other drugs known to be metabolized by CYP450 liver enzymes. However formal drug interaction studies have not been conducted). Products include:

Simcor Tablets 502
Vytorin 10/10 Tablets 2149
Vytorin 10/10 Tablets 2939
Vytorin 10/20 Tablets 2149
Vytorin 10/20 Tablets 2939
Vytorin 10/40 Tablets 2149
Vytorin 10/40 Tablets 2939
Vytorin 10/80 Tablets 2149
Vytorin 10/80 Tablets 2939
Zocor Tablets 2136

Sirolimus (Limited published data indicate that somatropin treatment increases cytochrome P450 (CYP450)-mediated antipyrine clearance in man. These data suggest that somatropin administration may alter the clearance of compounds known to be metabolized by CYP450 liver enzymes. Careful monitoring is advisable when somatropin is administered in combination with other drugs known to be metabolized by CYP450 liver enzymes. However formal drug interaction studies have not been conducted). Products include:

Rapamune 3260

Sitagliptin Phosphate (In patients with diabetes mellitus requiring drug therapy, the dose of oral hypoglycemic agents may require adjustment when somatropin therapy is initiated). Products include:

Janumet Tablets 2041
Januvia Tablets 2048

Sulfamethoxazole (Limited published data indicate that somatropin treatment increases cytochrome P450 (CYP450)-mediated antipyrine clearance in man. These data suggest that somatropin administration may alter the clearance of compounds known to be metabolized by CYP450 liver enzymes. Careful monitoring is advisable when somatropin is administered in combination with other drugs known to be metabolized by CYP450 liver enzymes. However formal drug interaction studies have not been conducted).

No products indexed under this heading.

Sulindac (Limited published data indicate that somatropin treatment increases cytochrome P450 (CYP450)-mediated antipyrine clearance in man. These data suggest that somatropin administration may alter the clearance of compounds known to be metabolized by CYP450 liver enzymes. Careful monitoring is advisable when somatropin is administered in combination with other drugs known to be metabolized by CYP450 liver enzymes. However formal drug interaction studies have not been conducted). Products include:

Clinoril Tablets 1962

Suprofen (Limited published data indicate that somatropin treatment increases cytochrome P450 (CYP450)-mediated antipyrine clearance in man. These data suggest that somatropin administration may alter the clearance of compounds known to be metabolized by CYP450 liver enzymes. Careful monitoring is advisable when somatropin is administered in combination with other drugs known to be metabolized by CYP450 liver enzymes. However formal drug interaction studies have not been conducted).

No products indexed under this heading.

Tacrine Hydrochloride (Limited published data indicate that somatropin treatment increases cytochrome P450 (CYP450)-mediated antipyrine clearance in man. These data suggest that somatropin administration may alter the clearance of compounds known to be metabolized by CYP450 liver enzymes. Careful monitoring is advisable when somatropin is administered in combination with other drugs known to be metabolized by CYP450 liver enzymes. However formal drug interaction studies have not been conducted).

No products indexed under this heading.

Tacrolimus (Limited published data indicate that somatropin treatment increases cytochrome P450 (CYP450)-mediated antipyrine clearance in man. These data suggest that somatropin administration may alter the clearance of compounds known to be metabolized by CYP450 liver enzymes. Careful monitoring is advisable when somatropin is administered in combination with other drugs known to be metabolized by CYP450 liver enzymes. However formal drug interaction studies have not been conducted). Products include:

Prograf Capsules and Injection 622
Protopic Ointment 628

Tamoxifen Citrate (Limited published data indicate that somatropin treatment increases cytochrome P450 (CYP450)-mediated antipyrine clearance in man. These data suggest that somatropin administration may alter the clearance of compounds known to be metabolized by CYP450 liver enzymes. Careful monitoring is advisable when somatropin is administered in combination with other drugs known to be metabolized by CYP450 liver enzymes. However formal drug interaction studies have not been conducted).

No products indexed under this heading.

Telmisartan (Limited published data indicate that somatropin treatment increases cytochrome P450 (CYP450)-mediated antipyrine clearance in man. These data suggest that somatropin administration may alter the clearance of compounds known to be metabolized by CYP450 liver enzymes. Careful monitoring is advisable when somatropin is administered in combination with other drugs known to be metabolized by CYP450 liver enzymes. However formal drug interaction studies have not been conducted). Products include:

Micardis Tablets 852
Micardis HCT Tablets 854

Teniposide (Limited published data indicate that somatropin treatment increases cytochrome P450 (CYP450)-mediated antipyrine clearance in man. These data suggest that somatropin administration may alter the clearance of compounds known to be metabolized by CYP450 liver enzymes. Careful monitoring is advisable when somatropin is administered in combination with other drugs known to be metabolized by CYP450 liver enzymes. However formal drug interaction studies have not been conducted).

No products indexed under this heading.

Terfenadine (Limited published data indicate that somatropin treatment increases cytochrome P450 (CYP450)-mediated antipyrine clearance in man. These data suggest that somatropin administration may alter the clearance of compounds known to be metabolized by CYP450 liver enzymes. Careful monitoring is advisable when somatropin is administered in combination with other drugs known to be metabolized by CYP450 liver enzymes. However formal drug interaction studies have not been conducted).

No products indexed under this heading.

Testosterone (Limited published data indicates that somatropin treatment increases cytochrome P450 (CP450) mediated antipyrine clearance in man. This data suggests that somatropin administration may alter the clearance of compounds known to be metabolized by CP450 liver enzymes (eg, sex steroids). Careful monitoring is advisable when somatropin is administered in combination with other drugs known to be metabolized by CP450 liver enzymes. However, formal drug interaction studies have not been conducted). Products include:

AndroGel 3159
Testim 1% Gel 701

Testosterone Cypionate (Limited published data indicate that somatropin treatment increases cytochrome P450 (CYP450)-mediated antipyrine clearance in man. These data suggest that somatropin administration may alter the clearance of compounds known to be metabolized by CYP450 liver enzymes. Careful monitoring is advisable when somatropin is administered in combination with other drugs known to be metabolized by CYP450 liver enzymes. However formal drug interaction studies have not been conducted).

No products indexed under this heading.

Testosterone Enanthate (Limited published data indicate that somatropin treatment increases cytochrome P450 (CYP450)-mediated antipyrine clearance in man. These data suggest that somatropin administration may alter the clearance of compounds known to be metabolized by CYP450 liver enzymes. Careful monitoring is advisable when somatropin is administered in combination with other drugs known to be metabolized by CYP450 liver enzymes. However formal drug interaction studies have not been conducted). Products include:

Delatestryl Injection 1730

Testosterone Propionate (Limited published data indicate that somatropin treatment increases cytochrome P450 (CYP450)-mediated antipyrine clearance in man. These data suggest that somatropin administration may alter the clearance of compounds known to be metabolized by CYP450 liver enzymes. Careful monitoring is advisable when somatropin is administered in combination with other drugs known to be metabolized by CYP450 liver enzymes. However formal drug interaction studies have not been conducted).

No products indexed under this heading.

Theophylline (Limited published data indicate that somatropin treatment increases cytochrome P450 (CYP450)-mediated antipyrine clearance in man. These data suggest that somatropin administration may alter the clearance of compounds known to be metabolized by CYP450 liver enzymes. Careful monitoring is advisable when somatropin is administered in combination with other drugs known to be metabolized by CYP450 liver enzymes. However formal drug interaction studies have not been conducted).

No products indexed under this heading.

Theophylline Anhydrous (Limited published data indicate that somatropin treatment increases cytochrome P450 (CYP450)-mediated antipyrine clearance in man. These data suggest that somatropin administration may alter the clearance of compounds known to be metabolized by CYP450 liver enzymes. Careful monitoring is advisable when somatropin is administered in combination with other drugs known to be metabolized by CYP450 liver enzymes. However formal drug interaction studies have not been conducted). Products include:

Uniphyl Tablets 2595

Theophylline Sodium Glycinate (Limited published data indicate that somatropin treatment increases cytochrome P450 (CYP450)-mediated antipyrine clearance in man. These data suggest that somatropin administration may alter the clearance of compounds known to be metabolized by CYP450 liver enzymes. Careful monitoring is advisable when somatropin is administered in combination with other drugs known to be metabolized by CYP450 liver enzymes. However formal drug interaction studies have not been conducted).

No products indexed under this heading.

Thioridazine (Limited published data indicate that somatropin treatment increases cytochrome P450 (CYP450)-mediated antipyrine clearance in man. These data suggest that somatropin administration may alter the clearance of compounds known to be metabolized by CYP450 liver enzymes. Careful monitoring is advisable when somatropin is administered in combination with other drugs known to be metabolized by CYP450 liver enzymes. However formal drug interaction studies have not been conducted).

No products indexed under this heading.

Thioridazine Hydrochloride (Limited published data indicate that somatropin treatment increases cytochrome P450 (CYP450)-mediated antipyrine clearance in man. These data suggest that somatropin administration may alter the clearance of compounds known to be metabolized by CYP450

liver enzymes. Careful monitoring is advisable when somatropin is administered in combination with other drugs known to be metabolized by CYP450 liver enzymes. However formal drug interaction studies have not been conducted). Products include:

Thioridazine Hydrochloride Tablets 2195

Tiagabine Hydrochloride (Limited published data indicates that somatropin treatment increases cytochrome P450 (CP450) mediated antipyrine clearance in man. This data suggests that somatropin administration may alter the clearance of compounds known to be metabolized by CP450 liver enzymes (eg anticonvulsants). Careful monitoring is advisable when somatropin is administered in combination with other drugs known to be metabolized by CP450 liver enzymes. However, formal drug interaction studies have not been conducted). Products include:

Gabitril Tablets 973

Timolol Maleate (Limited published data indicate that somatropin treatment increases cytochrome P450 (CYP450)-mediated antipyrine clearance in man. These data suggest that somatropin administration may alter the clearance of compounds known to be metabolized by CYP450 liver enzymes. Careful monitoring is advisable when somatropin is administered in combination with other drugs known to be metabolized by CYP450 liver enzymes. However formal drug interaction studies have not been conducted). Products include:

Combigan Ophthalmic Solution 553
Cosopt Sterile Ophthalmic Solution 1969
Timoptic Sterile Ophthalmic Solution 2121
Timoptic in Ocudose 2124
Timoptic-XE Sterile Ophthalmic Gel Forming Solution 2125

Tolazamide (In patients with diabetes mellitus requiring drug therapy, the dose of oral hypoglycemic agents may require adjustment when somatropin therapy is initiated).

No products indexed under this heading.

Tolbutamide (In patients with diabetes mellitus requiring drug therapy, the dose of oral hypoglycemic agents may require adjustment when somatropin therapy is initiated).

No products indexed under this heading.

Tolbutamide Sodium (Limited published data indicate that somatropin treatment increases cytochrome P450 (CYP450)-mediated antipyrine clearance in man. These data suggest that somatropin administration may alter the clearance of compounds known to be metabolized by CYP450 liver enzymes. Careful monitoring is advisable when somatropin is administered in combination with other drugs known to be metabolized by CYP450 liver enzymes. However formal drug interaction studies have not been conducted).

No products indexed under this heading.

Tolmetin Sodium (Limited published data indicate that somatropin treatment increases cytochrome P450 (CYP450)-mediated antipyrine clearance in man. These data suggest that somatropin administration may alter the clearance of compounds known to be metabolized by CYP450 liver enzymes. Careful monitoring is advisable when somatropin is administered in combination with other drugs known to be metabolized by CYP450 liver enzymes. However formal drug interaction studies have not been conducted).

No products indexed under this heading.

Tolterodine Tartrate (Limited published data indicate that somatropin treatment increases cytochrome P450 (CYP450)-mediated antipyrine clearance in man. These data suggest that somatropin administration may alter the clearance of compounds known to be metabolized by CYP450 liver enzymes. Careful monitoring is advisable when somatropin is administered in combination with other drugs known to be metabolized by CYP450 liver enzymes. However formal drug interaction studies have not been conducted).

No products indexed under this heading.

Topiramate (Limited published data indicates that somatropin treatment increases cytochrome P450 (CP450) mediated antipyrine clearance in man. This data suggests that somatropin administration may alter the clearance of compounds known to be metabolized by CP450 liver enzymes (eg anticonvulsants). Careful monitoring is advisable when somatropin is administered in combination with other drugs known to be metabolized by CP450 liver enzymes. However, formal drug interaction studies have not been conducted).

No products indexed under this heading.

Torsemide (Limited published data indicate that somatropin treatment increases cytochrome P450 (CYP450)-mediated antipyrine clearance in man. These data suggest that somatropin administration may alter the clearance of compounds known to be metabolized by CYP450 liver enzymes. Careful monitoring is advisable when somatropin is administered in combination with other drugs known to be metabolized by CYP450 liver enzymes. However formal drug interaction studies have not been conducted). Products include:

Demadex Injection 2630
Demadex Tablets 2630

Tramadol Hydrochloride (Limited published data indicate that somatropin treatment increases cytochrome P450 (CYP450)-mediated antipyrine clearance in man. These data suggest that somatropin administration may alter the clearance of compounds known to be metabolized by CYP450 liver enzymes. Careful monitoring is advisable when somatropin is administered in combination with other drugs known to be metabolized by CYP450 liver enzymes. However formal drug interaction studies have not been conducted). Products include:

Ultram ER Extended-Release Tablets 2428

Trazodone Hydrochloride (Limited published data indicate that somatropin treatment increases cytochrome P450 (CYP450)-mediated antipyrine clearance in man. These data suggest that somatropin administration may alter the clearance of compounds known to be metabolized by CYP450 liver enzymes. Careful monitoring is advisable when somatropin is administered in combination with other drugs known to be metabolized by CYP450 liver enzymes. However formal drug interaction studies have not been conducted).

No products indexed under this heading.

Tretinoin (Limited published data indicate that somatropin treatment increases cytochrome P450 (CYP450)-mediated antipyrine clearance in man. These data suggest that somatropin administration may alter the clearance of compounds known to be metabolized by CYP450 liver enzymes. Careful monitoring is advisable when somatropin is administered in combination with other drugs known to be metabolized by CYP450 liver enzymes. However formal drug interaction studies have not been conducted). Products include:

Vesanoid Capsules 2660
Ziana Gel 1942

Triamcinolone (Somatropin inhibits 11βHSD-1 in adipose/hepatic tissue and may significantly impact the metabolism of cortisone and cortisol. Patients being treated with glucocorticoid replacement therapy for hypoadrenalism may require an increase in their maintenance or stress doses; especially with cortisone acetate and prednisone, since conversion of these drugs to their biologically active metabolites is dependent on the activity of the 11μHSD-1 enzyme. Also, excessive glucocorticoid therapy may attenuate the growth-promoting effects of somatropin in children. Therefore, glucocorticoid replacement therapy should be carefully adjusted in children with concomitant GH and glucocorticoid deficiency to avoid both hypoadrenalism and an inhibitory effect on growth).

No products indexed under this heading.

Triamcinolone Acetonide (Somatropin inhibits 11βHSD-1 in adipose/hepatic tissue and may significantly impact the metabolism of cortisone and cortisol. Patients being treated with glucocorticoid replacement therapy for hypoadrenalism may require an increase in their maintenance or stress doses; especially with cortisone acetate and prednisone, since conversion of these drugs to their biologically active metabolites is dependent on the activity of the 11μHSD-1 enzyme. Also, excessive glucocorticoid therapy may attenuate the growth-promoting effects of somatropin in children. Therefore, glucocorticoid replacement therapy should be carefully adjusted in children with concomitant GH and glucocorticoid deficiency to avoid both hypoadrenalism and an inhibitory effect on growth). Products include:

Azmacort Inhalation Aerosol 407
Nasacort AQ Nasal Spray 2765
Triesence Injectable Suspension .... ⊙209

Triamcinolone Diacetate (Somatropin inhibits 11βHSD-1 in adipose/hepatic tissue and may significantly impact the metabolism of cortisone and cortisol. Patients being treated with glucocorticoid replacement therapy for hypoadrenalism may require an increase in their maintenance or stress doses; especially with cortisone acetate and prednisone, since conversion of these drugs to their biologically active metabolites is dependent on the activity of the 11μHSD-1 enzyme. Also, excessive glucocorticoid therapy may attenuate the growth-promoting effects of somatropin in children. Therefore, glucocorticoid replacement therapy should be carefully adjusted in children with concomitant GH and glucocorticoid deficiency to avoid both hypoadrenalism and an inhibitory effect on growth).

No products indexed under this heading.

Triamcinolone Hexacetonide (Somatropin inhibits 11βHSD-1 in adipose/hepatic tissue and may significantly impact the metabolism of cortisone and cortisol. Patients being treated with glucocorticoid replacement therapy for hypoadrenalism may require an increase in their maintenance or stress doses; especially with cortisone acetate and prednisone, since conversion of these drugs to their biologically active metabolites is dependent on the activity of the 11μHSD-1 enzyme. Also, excessive glucocorticoid therapy may attenuate the growth-promoting effects of somatropin in children. Therefore, glucocorticoid replacement therapy should be carefully adjusted in children with concomitant GH and glucocorticoid deficiency to avoid both hypoadrenalism and an inhibitory effect on growth).

No products indexed under this heading.

Triazolam (Limited published data indicate that somatropin treatment increases cytochrome P450 (CYP450)-mediated antipyrine clearance in man. These data suggest that somatropin administration may alter the clearance of compounds known to be metabolized by CYP450 liver enzymes. Careful monitoring is advisable when somatropin is administered in combination with other drugs known to be metabolized by CYP450 liver enzymes. However formal drug interaction studies have not been conducted).

No products indexed under this heading.

Trimethadione (Limited published data indicates that somatropin treatment increases cytochrome P450 (CP450) mediated antipyrine clearance in man. This data suggests that somatropin administration may alter the clearance of compounds known to be metabolized by CP450 liver enzymes (eg anticonvulsants). Careful monitoring is advisable when somatropin is administered in combination with other drugs known to be metabolized by CP450 liver enzymes. However, formal drug interaction studies have not been conducted).

No products indexed under this heading.

Trimethaphan Camsylate (Limited published data indicate that somatropin treatment increases cytochrome P450 (CYP450)-mediated antipyrine clearance in man. These data suggest that somatropin administration may alter the clearance of compounds

known to be metabolized by CYP450 liver enzymes. Careful monitoring is advisable when somatropin is administered in combination with other drugs known to be metabolized by CYP450 liver enzymes. However formal drug interaction studies have not been conducted).

No products indexed under this heading.

Trimipramine Maleate (Limited published data indicate that somatropin treatment increases cytochrome P450 (CYP450)-mediated antipyrine clearance in man. These data suggest that somatropin administration may alter the clearance of compounds known to be metabolized by CYP450 liver enzymes. Careful monitoring is advisable when somatropin is administered in combination with other drugs known to be metabolized by CYP450 liver enzymes. However formal drug interaction studies have not been conducted).

No products indexed under this heading.

Troglitazone (In patients with diabetes mellitus requiring drug therapy, the dose of oral hypoglycemic agents may require adjustment when somatropin therapy is initiated).

No products indexed under this heading.

Trovafloxacin Mesylate (Limited published data indicate that somatropin treatment increases cytochrome P450 (CYP450)-mediated antipyrine clearance in man. These data suggest that somatropin administration may alter the clearance of compounds known to be metabolized by CYP450 liver enzymes. Careful monitoring is advisable when somatropin is administered in combination with other drugs known to be metabolized by CYP450 liver enzymes. However formal drug interaction studies have not been conducted).

No products indexed under this heading.

Valdecoxib (Limited published data indicate that somatropin treatment increases cytochrome P450 (CYP450)-mediated antipyrine clearance in man. These data suggest that somatropin administration may alter the clearance of compounds known to be metabolized by CYP450 liver enzymes. Careful monitoring is advisable when somatropin is administered in combination with other drugs known to be metabolized by CYP450 liver enzymes. However formal drug interaction studies have not been conducted).

No products indexed under this heading.

Valproate Sodium (Limited published data indicates that somatropin treatment increases cytochrome P450 (CP450) mediated antipyrine clearance in man. This data suggests that somatropin administration may alter the clearance of compounds known to be metabolized by CP450 liver enzymes (eg anticonvulsants). Careful monitoring is advisable when somatropin is administered in combination with other drugs known to be metabolized by CP450 liver enzymes. However, formal drug interaction studies have not been conducted).

No products indexed under this heading.

Valproic Acid (Limited published data indicates that somatropin treatment increases cytochrome P450 (CP450) mediated antipyrine clearance in man. This data suggests that somatropin administration may alter the clearance of compounds known to be metabolized by CP450 liver enzymes (eg anticonvulsants). Careful monitoring is advisable when somatropin is administered in combination with other drugs known to be metabolized by CP450 liver enzymes. However, formal drug interaction studies have not been conducted).

No products indexed under this heading.

Valsartan (Limited published data indicate that somatropin treatment increases cytochrome P450 (CYP450)-mediated antipyrine clearance in man. These data suggest that somatropin administration may alter the clearance of compounds known to be metabolized by CYP450 liver enzymes. Careful monitoring is advisable when somatropin is administered in combination with other drugs known to be metabolized by CYP450 liver enzymes. However formal drug interaction studies have not been conducted). Products include:

Diovan Tablets **2212**
Diovan HCT Tablets **2216**
Exforge Tablets **2238**

Venlafaxine Hydrochloride (Limited published data indicate that somatropin treatment increases cytochrome P450 (CYP450)-mediated antipyrine clearance in man. These data suggest that somatropin administration may alter the clearance of compounds known to be metabolized by CYP450 liver enzymes. Careful monitoring is advisable when somatropin is administered in combination with other drugs known to be metabolized by CYP450 liver enzymes. However formal drug interaction studies have not been conducted). Products include:

Effexor XR Extended-Release Capsules **3195**
Venlafaxine Hydrochloride Tablets ... **2199**

Verapamil Hydrochloride (Limited published data indicate that somatropin treatment increases cytochrome P450 (CYP450)-mediated antipyrine clearance in man. These data suggest that somatropin administration may alter the clearance of compounds known to be metabolized by CYP450 liver enzymes. Careful monitoring is advisable when somatropin is administered in combination with other drugs known to be metabolized by CYP450 liver enzymes. However formal drug interaction studies have not been conducted). Products include:

Tarka Tablets **511**

Vinblastine Sulfate (Limited published data indicate that somatropin treatment increases cytochrome P450 (CYP450)-mediated antipyrine clearance in man. These data suggest that somatropin administration may alter the clearance of compounds known to be metabolized by CYP450 liver enzymes. Careful monitoring is advisable when somatropin is administered in combination with other drugs known to be metabolized by CYP450 liver enzymes. However formal drug interaction studies have not been conducted).

No products indexed under this heading.

Vincristine Sulfate (Limited published data indicate that somatropin treatment increases cytochrome P450 (CYP450)-mediated antipyrine clearance in man. These data suggest that somatropin administration may alter the clearance of compounds known to be metabolized by CYP450 liver enzymes. Careful monitoring is advisable when somatropin is administered in combination with other drugs known to be metabolized by CYP450 liver enzymes. However formal drug interaction studies have not been conducted).

No products indexed under this heading.

Vitamin A (Limited published data indicate that somatropin treatment increases cytochrome P450 (CYP450)-mediated antipyrine clearance in man. These data suggest that somatropin administration may alter the clearance of compounds known to be metabolized by CYP450 liver enzymes. Careful monitoring is advisable when somatropin is administered in combination with other drugs known to be metabolized by CYP450 liver enzymes. However formal drug interaction studies have not been conducted). Products include:

Norwegian Cod Liver Oil **949**

Vitamin A Acetate (Limited published data indicate that somatropin treatment increases cytochrome P450 (CYP450)-mediated antipyrine clearance in man. These data suggest that somatropin administration may alter the clearance of compounds known to be metabolized by CYP450 liver enzymes. Careful monitoring is advisable when somatropin is administered in combination with other drugs known to be metabolized by CYP450 liver enzymes. However formal drug interaction studies have not been conducted).

No products indexed under this heading.

Voriconazole (Limited published data indicate that somatropin treatment increases cytochrome P450 (CYP450)-mediated antipyrine clearance in man. These data suggest that somatropin administration may alter the clearance of compounds known to be metabolized by CYP450 liver enzymes. Careful monitoring is advisable when somatropin is administered in combination with other drugs known to be metabolized by CYP450 liver enzymes. However formal drug interaction studies have not been conducted).

No products indexed under this heading.

Warfarin Sodium (Limited published data indicate that somatropin treatment increases cytochrome P450 (CYP450)-mediated antipyrine clearance in man. These data suggest that somatropin administration may alter the clearance of compounds known to be metabolized by CYP450 liver enzymes. Careful monitoring is advisable when somatropin is administered in combination with other drugs known to be metabolized by CYP450 liver enzymes. However formal drug interaction studies have not been conducted).

No products indexed under this heading.

Zafirlukast (Limited published data indicate that somatropin treatment increases cytochrome P450 (CYP450)-mediated antipyrine clearance in man. These data suggest that somatropin administration may alter the clearance of compounds known to be metabolized by CYP450 liver enzymes. Careful monitoring is advisable when somatropin is administered in combination with other drugs known to be metabolized by CYP450 liver enzymes. However formal drug interaction studies have not been conducted). Products include:

Accolate Tablets **669**

Zileuton (Limited published data indicate that somatropin treatment increases cytochrome P450 (CYP450)-mediated antipyrine clearance in man. These data suggest that somatropin administration may alter the clearance of compounds known to be metabolized by CYP450 liver enzymes. Careful monitoring is advisable when somatropin is administered in combination with other drugs known to be metabolized by CYP450 liver enzymes. However formal drug interaction studies have not been conducted).

No products indexed under this heading.

Zolmitriptan (Limited published data indicate that somatropin treatment increases cytochrome P450 (CYP450)-mediated antipyrine clearance in man. These data suggest that somatropin administration may alter the clearance of compounds known to be metabolized by CYP450 liver enzymes. Careful monitoring is advisable when somatropin is administered in combination with other drugs known to be metabolized by CYP450 liver enzymes. However formal drug interaction studies have not been conducted). Products include:

Zomig Tablets **694**
Zomig Nasal Spray **689**
Zomig-ZMT Tablets **694**

Zonisamide (Limited published data indicates that somatropin treatment increases cytochrome P450 (CP450) mediated antipyrine clearance in man. This data suggests that somatropin administration may alter the clearance of compounds known to be metabolized by CP450 liver enzymes (eg anticonvulsants). Careful monitoring is advisable when somatropin is administered in combination with other drugs known to be metabolized by CP450 liver enzymes. However, formal drug interaction studies have not been conducted). Products include:

Zonegran Capsules **1089**

Zopiclone (Limited published data indicate that somatropin treatment increases cytochrome P450 (CYP450)-mediated antipyrine clearance in man. These data suggest that somatropin administration may alter the clearance of compounds known to be metabolized by CYP450 liver enzymes. Careful monitoring is advisable when somatropin is administered in combination with other drugs known to be metabolized by CYP450 liver enzymes. However formal drug interaction studies have not been conducted).

No products indexed under this heading.

GEODON CAPSULES
(Ziprasidone Hydrochloride) 2520
May interact with antihypertensives, central nervous system depressants, dopamine agonists, erythromycin, potassium-depleting diuretics, quinidine, and certain other agents. Compounds in these categories include:

Acebutolol Hydrochloride (Ziprasidone may induce orthostatic hypotension; co-administration with certain antihypertensive drugs may enhance the hypotensive effects).
No products indexed under this heading.

Alfentanil Hydrochloride (Somnolence was a commonly reported adverse event in patients treated with ziprasidone; concurrent use with other CNS active drugs, such as depressants, should be undertaken with caution).
No products indexed under this heading.

Aliskiren (Ziprasidone may induce orthostatic hypotension; co-administration with certain antihypertensive drugs may enhance the hypotensive effects). Products include:
Tekturna Tablets 2321
Tekturna HCT Tablets 2324

Alprazolam (Somnolence was a commonly reported adverse event in patients treated with ziprasidone; concurrent use with other CNS active drugs, such as depressants, should be undertaken with caution).
No products indexed under this heading.

Amiodarone Hydrochloride (Ziprasidone produces dose-related prolongation of the QT interval; an additive effect of ziprasidone and other drugs that prolong cannot be excluded; concurrent use is not recommended).
No products indexed under this heading.

Amlodipine Besylate (Ziprasidone may induce orthostatic hypotension; co-administration with certain antihypertensive drugs may enhance the hypotensive effects). Products include:
Azor Tablets 1005
Exforge Tablets 2238

Aprobarbital (Somnolence was a commonly reported adverse event in patients treated with ziprasidone; concurrent use with other CNS active drugs, such as depressants, should be undertaken with caution).
No products indexed under this heading.

Arsenic Trioxide (Ziprasidone produces dose-related prolongation of the QT interval; an additive effect of ziprasidone and other drugs that prolong cannot be excluded; concurrent use is not recommended). Products include:
Trisenox Injection 986

Atenolol (Ziprasidone may induce orthostatic hypotension; co-administration with certain antihypertensive drugs may enhance the hypotensive effects).
No products indexed under this heading.

Benazepril Hydrochloride (Ziprasidone may induce orthostatic hypotension; co-administration with certain antihypertensive drugs may enhance the hypotensive effects).
No products indexed under this heading.

Bendroflumethiazide (Ziprasidone produces dose-related prolongation of the QT interval; hypokalemia may result from diuretic therapy and this may increase the risk of QT prolongation and arrhythmias; potential for enhanced hypotensive effect if used concurrently).
No products indexed under this heading.

Bepridil Hydrochloride (Ziprasidone produces dose-related prolongation of the QT interval; an additive effect of ziprasidone and other drugs that prolong cannot be excluded; concurrent use is not recommended).
No products indexed under this heading.

Betaxolol Hydrochloride (Ziprasidone may induce orthostatic hypotension; co-administration with certain antihypertensive drugs may enhance the hypotensive effects).
No products indexed under this heading.

Bisoprolol Fumarate (Ziprasidone may induce orthostatic hypotension; co-administration with certain antihypertensive drugs may enhance the hypotensive effects).
No products indexed under this heading.

Bromocriptine Mesylate (Ziprasidone may antagonize the effects of dopamine agonists).
No products indexed under this heading.

Bumetanide (Ziprasidone produces dose-related prolongation of the QT interval; hypokalemia may result from diuretic therapy and this may increase the risk of QT prolongation and arrhythmias; potential for enhanced hypotensive effect if used concurrently).
No products indexed under this heading.

Buprenorphine Hydrochloride (Somnolence was a commonly reported adverse event in patients treated with ziprasidone; concurrent use with other CNS active drugs, such as depressants, should be undertaken with caution). Products include:
Suboxone Tablets 2601
Subutex Tablets 2601

Buspirone Hydrochloride (Somnolence was a commonly reported adverse event in patients treated with ziprasidone; concurrent use with other CNS active drugs, such as depressants, should be undertaken with caution).
No products indexed under this heading.

Butabarbital (Somnolence was a commonly reported adverse event in patients treated with ziprasidone; concurrent use with other CNS active drugs, such as depressants, should be undertaken with caution).
No products indexed under this heading.

Butalbital (Somnolence was a commonly reported adverse event in patients treated with ziprasidone; concurrent use with other CNS active drugs, such as depressants, should be undertaken with caution).
No products indexed under this heading.

Candesartan Cilexetil (Ziprasidone may induce orthostatic hypotension; co-administration with certain antihypertensive drugs may enhance the hypotensive effects). Products include:
Atacand Tablets 639
Atacand HCT 642

Captopril (Ziprasidone may induce orthostatic hypotension; co-administration with certain antihypertensive drugs may enhance the hypotensive effects). Products include:
Captopril Tablets 2182

Carbamazepine (Co-administration with carbamazepine, an inducer of CYP3A4, has resulted in a decrease of approximately 35% in AUC of ziprasidone; this effect may be greater when higher doses of carbamazepine are administered). Products include:
Carbatrol Capsules 3019
Equetro Extended-Release Capsules 3174

Carteolol Hydrochloride (Ziprasidone may induce orthostatic hypotension; co-administration with certain antihypertensive drugs may enhance the hypotensive effects).
No products indexed under this heading.

Chlordiazepoxide (Somnolence was a commonly reported adverse event in patients treated with ziprasidone; concurrent use with other CNS active drugs, such as depressants, should be undertaken with caution).
No products indexed under this heading.

Chlordiazepoxide Hydrochloride (Somnolence was a commonly reported adverse event in patients treated with ziprasidone; concurrent use with other CNS active drugs, such as depressants, should be undertaken with caution).
No products indexed under this heading.

Chlorothiazide (Ziprasidone produces dose-related prolongation of the QT interval; hypokalemia may result from diuretic therapy and this may increase the risk of QT prolongation and arrhythmias; potential for enhanced hypotensive effect if used concurrently).
No products indexed under this heading.

Chlorothiazide Sodium (Ziprasidone produces dose-related prolongation of the QT interval; hypokalemia may result from diuretic therapy and this may increase the risk of QT prolongation and arrhythmias; potential for enhanced hypotensive effect if used concurrently). Products include:
Intravenous Sodium Diuril 2490

Chlorpromazine (Ziprasidone produces dose-related prolongation of the QT interval; an additive effect of ziprasidone and other drugs that prolong cannot be excluded; concurrent use is not recommended).
No products indexed under this heading.

Chlorpromazine Hydrochloride (Ziprasidone produces dose-related prolongation of the QT interval; an additive effect of ziprasidone and other drugs that prolong cannot be excluded; concurrent use is not recommended).
No products indexed under this heading.

Chlorprothixene (Somnolence was a commonly reported adverse event in patients treated with ziprasidone; concurrent use with other CNS active drugs, such as depressants, should be undertaken with caution).
No products indexed under this heading.

Chlorprothixene Hydrochloride (Ziprasidone produces dose-related prolongation of the QT interval; an additive effect of ziprasidone and other drugs that prolong cannot be excluded; concurrent use is not recommended).
No products indexed under this heading.

Chlorprothixene Lactate (Somnolence was a commonly reported adverse event in patients treated with ziprasidone; concurrent use with other CNS active drugs, such as depressants, should be undertaken with caution).
No products indexed under this heading.

Chlorthalidone (Ziprasidone may induce orthostatic hypotension; co-administration with certain antihypertensive drugs may enhance the hypotensive effects). Products include:
Clorpres Tablets 2185

Clonidine (Ziprasidone may induce orthostatic hypotension; co-administration with certain antihypertensive drugs may enhance the hypotensive effects). Products include:
Catapres-TTS 842

Clonidine Hydrochloride (Ziprasidone may induce orthostatic hypotension; co-administration with certain antihypertensive drugs may enhance the hypotensive effects). Products include:
Catapres Tablets 841
Clorpres Tablets 2185

Clorazepate Dipotassium (Somnolence was a commonly reported adverse event in patients treated with ziprasidone; concurrent use with other CNS active drugs, such as depressants, should be undertaken with caution).
No products indexed under this heading.

Clozapine (Somnolence was a commonly reported adverse event in patients treated with ziprasidone; concurrent use with other CNS active drugs, such as depressants, should be undertaken with caution).
No products indexed under this heading.

Codeine Phosphate (Somnolence was a commonly reported adverse event in patients treated with ziprasidone; concurrent use with other CNS active drugs, such as depressants, should be undertaken with caution). Products include:
Tylenol with Codeine Tablets 2427

Deserpidine (Ziprasidone may induce orthostatic hypotension; co-administration with certain antihypertensive drugs may enhance the hypotensive effects).
No products indexed under this heading.

Desflurane (Somnolence was a commonly reported adverse event in patients treated with ziprasidone; concurrent use with other CNS active drugs, such as depressants, should be undertaken with caution).
No products indexed under this heading.

Desipramine Hydrochloride (Ziprasidone produces dose-related prolongation of the QT interval; an additive effect of ziprasidone and other drugs that prolong cannot be excluded; concurrent use is not recommended).
No products indexed under this heading.

Dezocine (Somnolence was a commonly reported adverse event in patients treated with ziprasidone; concurrent use with other CNS active drugs, such as depressants, should be undertaken with caution).
No products indexed under this heading.

Diazepam (Somnolence was a commonly reported adverse event in patients treated with ziprasidone; concurrent use with other CNS active drugs, such as depressants, should be undertaken with caution). Products include:
Valium Tablets 2658

Diazoxide (Ziprasidone may induce orthostatic hypotension; co-administration with certain antihypertensive drugs may enhance the hypotensive effects). Products include:
Proglycem Capsules 1185
Proglycem Suspension 1185

Diltiazem Hydrochloride (Ziprasidone may induce orthostatic hypotension; co-administration with certain antihypertensive drugs may enhance the hypotensive effects). Products include:
Cardizem LA Extended Release Tablets 421

Disopyramide Phosphate (Ziprasidone produces dose-related prolongation of the QT interval; an additive effect of ziprasidone and other drugs that prolong cannot be excluded; concurrent use is not recommended).
No products indexed under this heading.

Dofetilide (Ziprasidone produces dose-related prolongation of the QT interval; an additive effect of ziprasidone and other drugs that prolong cannot be excluded; concurrent use is not recommended).
No products indexed under this heading.

Dolasetron Mesylate (Ziprasidone produces dose-related prolongation of the QT interval; an additive effect of ziprasidone and other drugs that prolong cannot be excluded; concurrent use is not recommended). Products include:
Anzemet Injection 2701
Anzemet Tablets 2704

Dopamine Hydrochloride (Ziprasidone may antagonize the effects of dopamine agonists).
No products indexed under this heading.

Doxazosin Mesylate (Ziprasidone may induce orthostatic hypotension; co-administration with certain antihypertensive drugs may enhance the hypotensive effects).
No products indexed under this heading.

Droperidol (Ziprasidone produces dose-related prolongation of the QT interval; an additive effect of ziprasidone and other drugs that prolong cannot be excluded; concurrent use is not recommended).
No products indexed under this heading.

Enalapril Maleate (Ziprasidone may induce orthostatic hypotension; co-administration with certain antihypertensive drugs may enhance the hypotensive effects).
No products indexed under this heading.

Enalaprilat (Ziprasidone may induce orthostatic hypotension; co-administration with certain antihypertensive drugs may enhance the hypotensive effects).
No products indexed under this heading.

Enflurane (Somnolence was a commonly reported adverse event in patients treated with ziprasidone; concurrent use with other CNS active drugs, such as depressants, should be undertaken with caution).
No products indexed under this heading.

Eprosartan Mesylate (Ziprasidone may induce orthostatic hypotension; co-administration with certain antihypertensive drugs may enhance the hypotensive effects). Products include:
Teveten Tablets 515
Teveten HCT Tablets 517

Erythromycin (Ziprasidone produces dose-related prolongation of the QT interval; an additive effect of ziprasidone and other drugs that prolong cannot be excluded; concurrent use is not recommended).
No products indexed under this heading.

Erythromycin Estolate (Ziprasidone produces dose-related prolongation of the QT interval; an additive effect of ziprasidone and other drugs that prolong cannot be excluded; concurrent use is not recommended).
No products indexed under this heading.

Erythromycin Ethylsuccinate (Ziprasidone produces dose-related prolongation of the QT interval; an additive effect of ziprasidone and other drugs that prolong cannot be excluded; concurrent use is not recommended). Products include:
E.E.S. 433
EryPed 431

Erythromycin Gluceptate (Ziprasidone produces dose-related prolongation of the QT interval; an additive effect of ziprasidone and other drugs that prolong cannot be excluded; concurrent use is not recommended).
No products indexed under this heading.

Erythromycin Lactobionate (Ziprasidone produces dose-related prolongation of the QT interval; an additive effect of ziprasidone and other drugs that prolong cannot be excluded; concurrent use is not recommended).
No products indexed under this heading.

Erythromycin Stearate (Ziprasidone produces dose-related prolongation of the QT interval; an additive effect of ziprasidone and other drugs that prolong cannot be excluded; concurrent use is not recommended).
No products indexed under this heading.

Esmolol Hydrochloride (Ziprasidone may induce orthostatic hypotension; co-administration with certain antihypertensive drugs may enhance the hypotensive effects).
No products indexed under this heading.

Estazolam (Somnolence was a commonly reported adverse event in patients treated with ziprasidone; concurrent use with other CNS active drugs, such as depressants, should be undertaken with caution).
No products indexed under this heading.

Ethacrynic Acid (Ziprasidone produces dose-related prolongation of the QT interval; hypokalemia may result from diuretic therapy and this may increase the risk of QT prolongation and arrhythmias; potential for enhanced hypotensive effect if used concurrently). Products include:
Edecrin Tablets 698

Ethanol (Somnolence was a commonly reported adverse event in patients treated with ziprasidone; concurrent use with other CNS active drugs, such as depressants, should be undertaken with caution).
No products indexed under this heading.

Ethchlorvynol (Somnolence was a commonly reported adverse event in patients treated with ziprasidone; concurrent use with other CNS active drugs, such as depressants, should be undertaken with caution).
No products indexed under this heading.

Ethinamate (Somnolence was a commonly reported adverse event in patients treated with ziprasidone; concurrent use with other CNS active drugs, such as depressants, should be undertaken with caution).
No products indexed under this heading.

Ethyl Alcohol (Somnolence was a commonly reported adverse event in patients treated with ziprasidone; concurrent use with other CNS active drugs, such as depressants, should be undertaken with caution).
No products indexed under this heading.

Felodipine (Ziprasidone may induce orthostatic hypotension; co-administration with certain antihypertensive drugs may enhance the hypotensive effects).
No products indexed under this heading.

Fentanyl (Somnolence was a commonly reported adverse event in patients treated with ziprasidone; concurrent use with other CNS active drugs, such as depressants, should be undertaken with caution). Products include:
Duragesic Transdermal System 2405
Ionsys Transdermal System 2410

Fentanyl Citrate (Somnolence was a commonly reported adverse event in patients treated with ziprasidone; concurrent use with other CNS active drugs, such as depressants, should be undertaken with caution). Products include:
Actiq 959
Fentora Tablets 968

Flecainide Acetate (Ziprasidone produces dose-related prolongation of the QT interval; an additive effect of ziprasidone and other drugs that prolong cannot be excluded; concurrent use is not recommended).
No products indexed under this heading.

Fluphenazine Decanoate (Somnolence was a commonly reported adverse event in patients treated with ziprasidone; concurrent use with other CNS active drugs, such as depressants, should be undertaken with caution).
No products indexed under this heading.

Fluphenazine Enanthate (Somnolence was a commonly reported adverse event in patients treated with ziprasidone; concurrent use with other CNS active drugs, such as depressants, should be undertaken with caution).
No products indexed under this heading.

Fluphenazine Hydrochloride (Somnolence was a commonly reported adverse event in patients treated with ziprasidone; concurrent use with other CNS active drugs, such as depressants, should be undertaken with caution).
No products indexed under this heading.

Flurazepam Hydrochloride (Somnolence was a commonly reported adverse event in patients treated with ziprasidone; concurrent use with other CNS active drugs, such as depressants, should be undertaken with caution).
No products indexed under this heading.

Fosinopril Sodium (Ziprasidone may induce orthostatic hypotension; co-administration with certain antihypertensive drugs may enhance the hypotensive effects).
No products indexed under this heading.

Furosemide (Ziprasidone produces dose-related prolongation of the QT interval; hypokalemia may result from diuretic therapy and this may increase the risk of QT prolongation and arrhythmias; potential for enhanced hypotensive effect if used concurrently). Products include:
Furosemide Tablets 2186

Gatifloxacin (Ziprasidone produces dose-related prolongation of the QT interval; an additive effect of ziprasidone and other drugs that prolong cannot be excluded; concurrent use is not recommended).
No products indexed under this heading.

Glutethimide (Somnolence was a commonly reported adverse event in patients treated with ziprasidone; concurrent use with other CNS active drugs, such as depressants, should be undertaken with caution).
No products indexed under this heading.

Guanabenz Acetate (Ziprasidone may induce orthostatic hypotension; co-administration with certain antihypertensive drugs may enhance the hypotensive effects).
No products indexed under this heading.

Guanethidine Monosulfate (Ziprasidone may induce orthostatic hypotension; co-administration with certain antihypertensive drugs may enhance the hypotensive effects).
No products indexed under this heading.

Halofantrine (Ziprasidone produces dose-related prolongation of the QT interval; an additive effect of ziprasidone and other drugs that prolong cannot be excluded; concurrent use is not recommended).
No products indexed under this heading.

Haloperidol (Somnolence was a commonly reported adverse event in patients treated with ziprasidone; concurrent use with other CNS active drugs, such as depressants, should be undertaken with caution).
No products indexed under this heading.

Haloperidol Decanoate (Somnolence was a commonly reported adverse event in patients treated with ziprasidone; concurrent use with other CNS active drugs, such as depressants, should be undertaken with caution).
No products indexed under this heading.

Hydralazine Hydrochloride (Ziprasidone may induce orthostatic hypotension; co-administration with certain antihypertensive drugs may enhance the hypotensive effects).
No products indexed under this heading.

Hydrochlorothiazide (Ziprasidone produces dose-related prolongation of the QT interval; hypokalemia may result from diuretic therapy and this may increase the risk of QT prolongation and arrhythmias; potential for enhanced hypotensive effect if used concurrently). Products include:
- Atacand HCT ... 642
- Avalide Tablets ... 892
- Avalide Tablets ... 2713
- Benicar HCT Tablets ... 1010
- Diovan HCT Tablets ... 2216
- Dyazide Capsules ... 1405
- Micardis HCT Tablets ... 854
- Prinzide Tablets ... 2092
- Tekturna HCT Tablets ... 2324
- Teveten HCT Tablets ... 517

Hydrocodone Bitartrate (Somnolence was a commonly reported adverse event in patients treated with ziprasidone; concurrent use with other CNS active drugs, such as depressants, should be undertaken with caution). Products include:
- Lortab 5/500 Tablets ... 3143
- Lortab 7.5/500 Tablets ... 3144
- Lortab 10/500 Tablets ... 3144
- Vicodin Tablets ... 529
- Vicodin ES Tablets ... 530
- Vicodin HP Tablets ... 531
- Vicoprofen Tablets ... 533
- Zydone Tablets ... 1132

Hydrocodone Polistirex (Somnolence was a commonly reported adverse event in patients treated with ziprasidone; concurrent use with other CNS active drugs, such as depressants, should be undertaken with caution). Products include:
- Tussionex Pennkinetic Extended-Release Suspension ... 3154

Hydroflumethiazide (Ziprasidone produces dose-related prolongation of the QT interval; hypokalemia may result from diuretic therapy and this may increase the risk of QT prolongation and arrhythmias; potential for enhanced hypotensive effect if used concurrently).
No products indexed under this heading.

Hydromorphone Hydrochloride (Somnolence was a commonly reported adverse event in patients treated with ziprasidone; concurrent use with other CNS active drugs, such as depressants, should be undertaken with caution).
No products indexed under this heading.

Hydroxyzine Hydrochloride (Somnolence was a commonly reported adverse event in patients treated with ziprasidone; concurrent use with other CNS active drugs, such as depressants, should be undertaken with caution).
No products indexed under this heading.

Ibutilide Fumarate (Ziprasidone produces dose-related prolongation of the QT interval; an additive effect of ziprasidone and other drugs that prolong cannot be excluded; concurrent use is not recommended).
No products indexed under this heading.

Indapamide (Ziprasidone may induce orthostatic hypotension; co-administration with certain antihypertensive drugs may enhance the hypotensive effects). Products include:
- Indapamide Tablets ... 2188

Irbesartan (Ziprasidone may induce orthostatic hypotension; co-administration with certain antihypertensive drugs may enhance the hypotensive effects). Products include:
- Avalide Tablets ... 892
- Avalide Tablets ... 2713
- Avapro Tablets ... 897
- Avapro Tablets ... 2718

Isoflurane (Somnolence was a commonly reported adverse event in patients treated with ziprasidone; concurrent use with other CNS active drugs, such as depressants, should be undertaken with caution).
No products indexed under this heading.

Isradipine (Ziprasidone may induce orthostatic hypotension; co-administration with certain antihypertensive drugs may enhance the hypotensive effects). Products include:
- DynaCirc CR Controlled Release Tablets ... 1407

Itraconazole (Co-administration with inhibitors of CYP3A4, such as itraconazole, may result in increased AUC and Cmax of ziprasidone).
No products indexed under this heading.

Ketamine Hydrochloride (Somnolence was a commonly reported adverse event in patients treated with ziprasidone; concurrent use with other CNS active drugs, such as depressants, should be undertaken with caution).
No products indexed under this heading.

Ketoconazole (Co-administration with ketoconazole, a potent inhibitor of CYP3A4, has resulted in increased AUC and Cmax of ziprasidone by about 35-40%). Products include:
- Extina Foam, 2% ... 3057
- Nizoral A-D Shampoo ... 1901

Labetalol Hydrochloride (Ziprasidone may induce orthostatic hypotension; co-administration with certain antihypertensive drugs may enhance the hypotensive effects).
No products indexed under this heading.

Levodopa (Ziprasidone may antagonize the effects of levodopa). Products include:
- Stalevo Tablets ... 2309

Levomethadyl Acetate Hydrochloride (Ziprasidone produces dose-related prolongation of the QT interval; an additive effect of ziprasidone and other drugs that prolong cannot be excluded; concurrent use is not recommended).
No products indexed under this heading.

Levorphanol Tartrate (Somnolence was a commonly reported adverse event in patients treated with ziprasidone; concurrent use with other CNS active drugs, such as depressants, should be undertaken with caution).
No products indexed under this heading.

Lisinopril (Ziprasidone may induce orthostatic hypotension; co-administration with certain antihypertensive drugs may enhance the hypotensive effects). Products include:
- Prinivil Tablets ... 2087
- Prinzide Tablets ... 2092

Lorazepam (Somnolence was a commonly reported adverse event in patients treated with ziprasidone; concurrent use with other CNS active drugs, such as depressants, should be undertaken with caution).
No products indexed under this heading.

Losartan Potassium (Ziprasidone may induce orthostatic hypotension; co-administration with certain antihypertensive drugs may enhance the hypotensive effects). Products include:
- Cozaar Tablets ... 1973

Loxapine Hydrochloride (Somnolence was a commonly reported adverse event in patients treated with ziprasidone; concurrent use with other CNS active drugs, such as depressants, should be undertaken with caution).
No products indexed under this heading.

Loxapine Succinate (Somnolence was a commonly reported adverse event in patients treated with ziprasidone; concurrent use with other CNS active drugs, such as depressants, should be undertaken with caution).
No products indexed under this heading.

Mecamylamine Hydrochloride (Ziprasidone may induce orthostatic hypotension; co-administration with certain antihypertensive drugs may enhance the hypotensive effects).
No products indexed under this heading.

Mefloquine Hydrochloride (Ziprasidone produces dose-related prolongation of the QT interval; an additive effect of ziprasidone and other drugs that prolong cannot be excluded; concurrent use is not recommended).
No products indexed under this heading.

Meperidine Hydrochloride (Somnolence was a commonly reported adverse event in patients treated with ziprasidone; concurrent use with other CNS active drugs, such as depressants, should be undertaken with caution).
No products indexed under this heading.

Mephobarbital (Somnolence was a commonly reported adverse event in patients treated with ziprasidone; concurrent use with other CNS active drugs, such as depressants, should be undertaken with caution).
No products indexed under this heading.

Meprobamate (Somnolence was a commonly reported adverse event in patients treated with ziprasidone; concurrent use with other CNS active drugs, such as depressants, should be undertaken with caution).
No products indexed under this heading.

Mesoridazine Besylate (Ziprasidone produces dose-related prolongation of the QT interval; an additive effect of ziprasidone and other drugs that prolong cannot be excluded; concurrent use is not recommended).
No products indexed under this heading.

Methadone Hydrochloride (Somnolence was a commonly reported adverse event in patients treated with ziprasidone; concurrent use with other CNS active drugs, such as depressants, should be undertaken with caution).
No products indexed under this heading.

Methohexital Sodium (Somnolence was a commonly reported adverse event in patients treated with ziprasidone; concurrent use with other CNS active drugs, such as depressants, should be undertaken with caution).
No products indexed under this heading.

Methotrimeprazine (Somnolence was a commonly reported adverse event in patients treated with ziprasidone; concurrent use with other CNS active drugs, such as depressants, should be undertaken with caution).
No products indexed under this heading.

Methoxyflurane (Somnolence was a commonly reported adverse event in patients treated with ziprasidone; concurrent use with other CNS active drugs, such as depressants, should be undertaken with caution).
No products indexed under this heading.

Methyclothiazide (Ziprasidone produces dose-related prolongation of the QT interval; hypokalemia may result from diuretic therapy and this may increase the risk of QT prolongation and arrhythmias; potential for enhanced hypotensive effect if used concurrently).
No products indexed under this heading.

Methyldopa (Ziprasidone may induce orthostatic hypotension; co-administration with certain antihypertensive drugs may enhance the hypotensive effects).
No products indexed under this heading.

Methyldopate Hydrochloride (Ziprasidone may induce orthostatic hypotension; co-administration with certain antihypertensive drugs may enhance the hypotensive effects).
No products indexed under this heading.

Metolazone (Ziprasidone may induce orthostatic hypotension; co-administration with certain antihypertensive drugs may enhance the hypotensive effects).
No products indexed under this heading.

Metoprolol Succinate (Ziprasidone may induce orthostatic hypotension; co-administration with certain antihypertensive drugs may enhance the hypotensive effects). Products include:
Toprol-XL Tablets ... 666

Metoprolol Tartrate (Ziprasidone may induce orthostatic hypotension; co-administration with certain antihypertensive drugs may enhance the hypotensive effects).
No products indexed under this heading.

Metyrosine (Ziprasidone may induce orthostatic hypotension; co-administration with certain antihypertensive drugs may enhance the hypotensive effects). Products include:
Demser Capsules ... 1989

Mibefradil Dihydrochloride (Ziprasidone may induce orthostatic hypotension; co-administration with certain antihypertensive drugs may enhance the hypotensive effects).
No products indexed under this heading.

Midazolam Hydrochloride (Somnolence was a commonly reported adverse event in patients treated with ziprasidone; concurrent use with other CNS active drugs, such as depressants, should be undertaken with caution).
No products indexed under this heading.

Minoxidil (Ziprasidone may induce orthostatic hypotension; co-administration with certain antihypertensive drugs may enhance the hypotensive effects).
No products indexed under this heading.

Moexipril Hydrochloride (Ziprasidone may induce orthostatic hypotension; co-administration with certain antihypertensive drugs may enhance the hypotensive effects).
No products indexed under this heading.

Molindone Hydrochloride (Somnolence was a commonly reported adverse event in patients treated with ziprasidone; concurrent use with other CNS active drugs, such as depressants, should be undertaken with caution). Products include:
Moban Tablets ... 1116

Morphine Sulfate (Somnolence was a commonly reported adverse event in patients treated with ziprasidone; concurrent use with other CNS active drugs, such as depressants, should be undertaken with caution). Products include:
Avinza Capsules ... 1772
DepoDur Injection ... 1095
MS Contin Tablets ... 2585

Moxifloxacin Hydrochloride (Ziprasidone produces dose-related prolongation of the QT interval; an additive effect of ziprasidone and other drugs that prolong cannot be excluded; concurrent use is not recommended). Products include:
Avelox ... 2803
Vigamox Ophthalmic Solution ... 548

Nadolol (Ziprasidone may induce orthostatic hypotension; co-administration with certain antihypertensive drugs may enhance the hypotensive effects). Products include:
Nadolol Tablets ... 2191

Nebivolol (Ziprasidone may induce orthostatic hypotension; co-administration with certain antihypertensive drugs may enhance the hypotensive effects). Products include:
Bystolic Tablets ... 1155

Nicardipine Hydrochloride (Ziprasidone may induce orthostatic hypotension; co-administration with certain antihypertensive drugs may enhance the hypotensive effects). Products include:
Cardene I.V. ... 1093

Nifedipine (Ziprasidone may induce orthostatic hypotension; co-administration with certain antihypertensive drugs may enhance the hypotensive effects).
No products indexed under this heading.

Nisoldipine (Ziprasidone may induce orthostatic hypotension; co-administration with certain antihypertensive drugs may enhance the hypotensive effects). Products include:
Sular Extended Release Tablets ... 2975

Nitroglycerin (Ziprasidone may induce orthostatic hypotension; co-administration with certain antihypertensive drugs may enhance the hypotensive effects). Products include:
Nitro-Dur Transdermal Infusion System ... 2887
Nitrolingual Pumpspray ... 2965

Olanzapine (Somnolence was a commonly reported adverse event in patients treated with ziprasidone; concurrent use with other CNS active drugs, such as depressants, should be undertaken with caution). Products include:
Symbyax Capsules ... 1871
Zyprexa Tablets ... 1883
Zyprexa IntraMuscular ... 1883
Zyprexa ZYDIS Orally Disintegrating Tablets ... 1883

Oxazepam (Somnolence was a commonly reported adverse event in patients treated with ziprasidone; concurrent use with other CNS active drugs, such as depressants, should be undertaken with caution).
No products indexed under this heading.

Oxycodone Hydrochloride (Somnolence was a commonly reported adverse event in patients treated with ziprasidone; concurrent use with other CNS active drugs, such as depressants, should be undertaken with caution). Products include:
OxyContin Tablets ... 2589
OxyIR Capsules ... 2593
Percocet Tablets ... 1127
Percodan Tablets ... 1130

Penbutolol Sulfate (Ziprasidone may induce orthostatic hypotension; co-administration with certain antihypertensive drugs may enhance the hypotensive effects).
No products indexed under this heading.

Pentamidine Isethionate (Ziprasidone produces dose-related prolongation of the QT interval; an additive effect of ziprasidone and other drugs that prolong cannot be excluded; concurrent use is not recommended).
No products indexed under this heading.

Pentobarbital Sodium (Somnolence was a commonly reported adverse event in patients treated with ziprasidone; concurrent use with other CNS active drugs, such as depressants, should be undertaken with caution). Products include:
Nembutal Sodium Solution, USP ... 2494

Pergolide Mesylate (Ziprasidone may antagonize the effects of dopamine agonists).
No products indexed under this heading.

Perindopril Erbumine (Ziprasidone may induce orthostatic hypotension; co-administration with certain antihypertensive drugs may enhance the hypotensive effects). Products include:
Aceon Tablets (2 mg, 4 mg, 8 mg) ... 3038

Perphenazine (Somnolence was a commonly reported adverse event in patients treated with ziprasidone; concurrent use with other CNS active drugs, such as depressants, should be undertaken with caution).
No products indexed under this heading.

Phenobarbital (Somnolence was a commonly reported adverse event in patients treated with ziprasidone; concurrent use with other CNS active drugs, such as depressants, should be undertaken with caution). Products include:
Donnatal Extentabs ... 2507

Phenoxybenzamine Hydrochloride (Ziprasidone may induce orthostatic hypotension; co-administration with certain antihypertensive drugs may enhance the hypotensive effects). Products include:
Dibenzyline Capsules ... 3188

Phentolamine Mesylate (Ziprasidone may induce orthostatic hypotension; co-administration with certain antihypertensive drugs may enhance the hypotensive effects).
No products indexed under this heading.

Pimozide (Ziprasidone produces dose-related prolongation of the QT interval; an additive effect of ziprasidone and other drugs that prolong cannot be excluded; concurrent use is not recommended).
No products indexed under this heading.

Pindolol (Ziprasidone may induce orthostatic hypotension; co-administration with certain antihypertensive drugs may enhance the hypotensive effects).
No products indexed under this heading.

Polythiazide (Ziprasidone produces dose-related prolongation of the QT interval; hypokalemia may result from diuretic therapy and this may increase the risk of QT prolongation and arrhythmias; potential for enhanced hypotensive effect if used concurrently).
No products indexed under this heading.

Pramipexole Dihydrochloride (Ziprasidone may antagonize the effects of dopamine agonists). Products include:
Mirapex Tablets ... 857

Prazepam (Somnolence was a commonly reported adverse event in patients treated with ziprasidone; concurrent use with other CNS active drugs, such as depressants, should be undertaken with caution).
No products indexed under this heading.

Prazosin Hydrochloride (Ziprasidone may induce orthostatic hypotension; co-administration with certain antihypertensive drugs may enhance the hypotensive effects).
No products indexed under this heading.

Probucol (Ziprasidone produces dose-related prolongation of the QT interval; an additive effect of ziprasidone and other drugs that prolong cannot be excluded; concurrent use is not recommended).
No products indexed under this heading.

Procainamide Hydrochloride (Ziprasidone produces dose-related prolongation of the QT interval; an additive effect of ziprasidone and other drugs that prolong cannot be excluded; concurrent use is not recommended).
No products indexed under this heading.

Prochlorperazine (Somnolence was a commonly reported adverse event in patients treated with ziprasidone; concurrent use with other CNS active drugs, such as depressants, should be undertaken with caution).
No products indexed under this heading.

Promethazine Hydrochloride (Somnolence was a commonly reported adverse event in patients treated with ziprasidone; concurrent use with other CNS active drugs, such as depressants, should be undertaken with caution).
No products indexed under this heading.

Propofol (Somnolence was a commonly reported adverse event in patients treated with ziprasidone; concurrent use with other CNS active drugs, such as depressants, should be undertaken with caution).
No products indexed under this heading.

Propoxyphene Hydrochloride (Somnolence was a commonly reported adverse event in patients treated with ziprasidone; concurrent use with other CNS active drugs, such as depressants, should be undertaken with caution).
No products indexed under this heading.

Propoxyphene Napsylate (Somnolence was a commonly reported adverse event in patients treated with ziprasidone; concurrent use with other CNS active drugs, such as depressants, should be undertaken with caution).
No products indexed under this heading.

Propranolol Hydrochloride (Ziprasidone may induce orthostatic hypotension; co-administration with certain antihypertensive drugs may enhance the hypotensive effects). Products include:
InnoPran XL Extended Release Capsules ... 1484

Quazepam (Somnolence was a commonly reported adverse event in patients treated with ziprasidone; concurrent use with other CNS active drugs, such as depressants, should be undertaken with caution).
No products indexed under this heading.

Quetiapine Fumarate (Somnolence was a commonly reported adverse event in patients treated with ziprasidone; concurrent use with other CNS active drugs, such as depressants, should be undertaken with caution).
No products indexed under this heading.

Quinapril Hydrochloride (Ziprasidone may induce orthostatic hypotension; co-administration with certain antihypertensive drugs may enhance the hypotensive effects).
No products indexed under this heading.

Quinidine (Ziprasidone produces dose-related prolongation of the QT interval; an additive effect of ziprasidone and other drugs that prolong cannot be excluded; concurrent use is not recommended).
No products indexed under this heading.

Quinidine Gluconate (Ziprasidone produces dose-related prolongation of the QT interval; an additive effect of ziprasidone and other drugs that prolong cannot be excluded; concurrent use is not recommended).
No products indexed under this heading.

Quinidine Hydrochloride (Ziprasidone produces dose-related prolongation of the QT interval; an additive effect of ziprasidone and other drugs that prolong cannot be excluded; concurrent use is not recommended).
No products indexed under this heading.

Quinidine Polygalacturonate (Ziprasidone produces dose-related prolongation of the QT interval; an additive effect of ziprasidone and other drugs that prolong cannot be excluded; concurrent use is not recommended).
No products indexed under this heading.

Quinidine Sulfate (Ziprasidone produces dose-related prolongation of the QT interval; an additive effect of ziprasidone and other drugs that prolong cannot be excluded; concurrent use is not recommended).
No products indexed under this heading.

Ramipril (Ziprasidone may induce orthostatic hypotension; co-administration with certain antihypertensive drugs may enhance the hypotensive effects).
No products indexed under this heading.

Rauwolfia Serpentina (Ziprasidone may induce orthostatic hypotension; co-administration with certain antihypertensive drugs may enhance the hypotensive effects).
No products indexed under this heading.

Remifentanil Hydrochloride (Somnolence was a commonly reported adverse event in patients treated with ziprasidone; concurrent use with other CNS active drugs, such as depressants, should be undertaken with caution).
No products indexed under this heading.

Rescinnamine (Ziprasidone may induce orthostatic hypotension; co-administration with certain antihypertensive drugs may enhance the hypotensive effects).
No products indexed under this heading.

Reserpine (Ziprasidone may induce orthostatic hypotension; co-administration with certain antihypertensive drugs may enhance the hypotensive effects).
No products indexed under this heading.

Risperidone (Somnolence was a commonly reported adverse event in patients treated with ziprasidone; concurrent use with other CNS active drugs, such as depressants, should be undertaken with caution). Products include:
Risperdal Consta Long-Acting Injection ... 1753

Ropinirole Hydrochloride (Ziprasidone may antagonize the effects of dopamine agonists). Products include:
Requip Tablets ... 1561
Requip XL Tablets ... 1568

Secobarbital Sodium (Somnolence was a commonly reported adverse event in patients treated with ziprasidone; concurrent use with other CNS active drugs, such as depressants, should be undertaken with caution).
No products indexed under this heading.

Sevoflurane (Somnolence was a commonly reported adverse event in patients treated with ziprasidone; concurrent use with other CNS active drugs, such as depressants, should be undertaken with caution). Products include:
Ultane Liquid for Inhalation ... 524

Sodium Nitroprusside (Ziprasidone may induce orthostatic hypotension; co-administration with certain antihypertensive drugs may enhance the hypotensive effects).
No products indexed under this heading.

Sodium Oxybate (Somnolence was a commonly reported adverse event in patients treated with ziprasidone; concurrent use with other CNS active drugs, such as depressants, should be undertaken with caution). Products include:
Xyrem Oral Solution ... 1766

Sotalol Hydrochloride (Ziprasidone produces dose-related prolongation of the QT interval; an additive effect of ziprasidone and other drugs that prolong cannot be excluded; concurrent use is not recommended).
No products indexed under this heading.

Sparfloxacin (Ziprasidone produces dose-related prolongation of the QT interval; an additive effect of ziprasidone and other drugs that prolong cannot be excluded; concurrent use is not recommended).
No products indexed under this heading.

Spirapril Hydrochloride (Ziprasidone may induce orthostatic hypotension; co-administration with certain antihypertensive drugs may enhance the hypotensive effects).
No products indexed under this heading.

Sufentanil Citrate (Somnolence was a commonly reported adverse event in patients treated with ziprasidone; concurrent use with other CNS active drugs, such as depressants, should be undertaken with caution).
No products indexed under this heading.

Tacrolimus (Ziprasidone produces dose-related prolongation of the QT interval; an additive effect of ziprasidone and other drugs that prolong cannot be excluded; concurrent use is not recommended). Products include:
Prograf Capsules and Injection ... 622
Protopic Ointment ... 628

Telmisartan (Ziprasidone may induce orthostatic hypotension; co-administration with certain antihypertensive drugs may enhance the hypotensive effects). Products include:
Micardis Tablets ... 852
Micardis HCT Tablets ... 854

Temazepam (Somnolence was a commonly reported adverse event in patients treated with ziprasidone; concurrent use with other CNS active drugs, such as depressants, should be undertaken with caution).
No products indexed under this heading.

Terazosin Hydrochloride (Ziprasidone may induce orthostatic hypotension; co-administration with certain antihypertensive drugs may enhance the hypotensive effects).
No products indexed under this heading.

Thiamylal Sodium (Somnolence was a commonly reported adverse event in patients treated with ziprasidone; concurrent use with other CNS active drugs, such as depressants, should be undertaken with caution).
No products indexed under this heading.

Thioridazine Hydrochloride (Ziprasidone produces dose-related prolongation of the QT interval; an additive effect of ziprasidone and other drugs that prolong cannot be excluded; concurrent use is not recommended). Products include:
Thioridazine Hydrochloride Tablets ... 2195

Thiothixene (Somnolence was a commonly reported adverse event in patients treated with ziprasidone; concurrent use with other CNS active drugs, such as depressants, should be undertaken with caution). Products include:
Thiothixene Capsules ... 2197

Timolol Maleate (Ziprasidone may induce orthostatic hypotension; co-administration with certain antihypertensive drugs may enhance the hypotensive effects). Products include:
Combigan Ophthalmic Solution ... 553
Cosopt Sterile Ophthalmic Solution ... 1969
Timoptic Sterile Ophthalmic Solution ... 2121
Timoptic in Ocudose ... 2124
Timoptic-XE Sterile Ophthalmic Gel Forming Solution ... 2125

Torsemide (Ziprasidone produces dose-related prolongation of the QT interval; hypokalemia may result from diuretic therapy and this may increase the risk of QT prolongation and arrhythmias; potential for enhanced hypotensive effect if used concurrently). Products include:
Demadex Injection ... 2630
Demadex Tablets ... 2630

Trandolapril (Ziprasidone may induce orthostatic hypotension; co-administration with certain antihypertensive drugs may enhance the hypotensive effects). Products include:
Mavik Tablets ... 472
Tarka Tablets ... 511

Triazolam (Somnolence was a commonly reported adverse event in patients treated with ziprasidone; concurrent use with other CNS active drugs, such as depressants, should be undertaken with caution).
No products indexed under this heading.

Trifluoperazine Hydrochloride (Somnolence was a commonly reported adverse event in patients treated with ziprasidone; concurrent use with other CNS active drugs, such as depressants, should be undertaken with caution).
No products indexed under this heading.

Trimethaphan Camsylate (Ziprasidone may induce orthostatic hypotension; co-administration with certain antihypertensive drugs may enhance the hypotensive effects).
No products indexed under this heading.

Valsartan (Ziprasidone may induce orthostatic hypotension; co-administration with certain antihypertensive drugs may enhance the hypotensive effects). Products include:
Diovan Tablets ... 2212
Diovan HCT Tablets ... 2216
Exforge Tablets ... 2238

Verapamil Hydrochloride (Ziprasidone may induce orthostatic hypotension; co-administration with certain antihypertensive drugs may enhance the hypotensive effects). Products include:
Tarka Tablets ... 511

Zaleplon (Somnolence was a commonly reported adverse event in patients treated with ziprasidone; concurrent use with other CNS active drugs, such as depressants, should be undertaken with caution).
No products indexed under this heading.

Zolpidem Tartrate (Somnolence was a commonly reported adverse event in patients treated with ziprasidone; concurrent use with other CNS active drugs, such as depressants, should be undertaken with caution). Products include:

Ambien Tablets 2692
Ambien CR Tablets 2696

Food Interactions

Alcohol (Somnolence was a commonly reported adverse event in patients treated with ziprasidone; concurrent use with alcohol or other CNS active drugs, such as depressants, should be undertaken with caution).

GEODON FOR INJECTION

(Ziprasidone Mesylate) 2520
See Geodon Capsules

GLAUCOFIT DIETARY SUPPLEMENT

(Alpha Lipoic Acid, Lutein, Peptidase, Rutoside, Selenium, Vitamin B_{12}, Vitamin C, Vitamin E, Zeaxanthin, Zinc) 995
None cited in PDR database.

GLAUMA DIETARY SUPPLEMENT

(Alpha Lipoic Acid, Lutein, Peptidase, Rutoside, Selenium, Vitamin B_{12}, Vitamin C, Vitamin E, Zeaxanthin, Zinc) 995
None cited in PDR database.

GLEEVEC TABLETS

(Imatinib Mesylate) 2255
May interact with calcium channel blockers that are metabolized by CYP3A4, cytochrome p450 2d6 substrates (selected), cytochrome p450 3a4 inducers (selected), cytochrome p450 3a4 inhibitors (selected), cytochrome p450 3a4 substrates (selected), HMG-CoA reductase inhibitors, triazolobenzodiazepines, and certain other agents. Compounds in these categories include:

Acetaminophen (In vitro, imatinib mesylate inhibits acetaminophen O-glucuronidation at therapeutic levels. Systemic exposure to acetaminophen is expected to be increased when co-administered with imatinib mesylate. No specific studies in humans have been performed and caution is recommended). Products include:

Benadryl Allergy & Cold Kapgels 1895
Benadryl Allergy & Sinus Headache Kapgels 1895
Benadryl Severe Allergy & Sinus Headache Caplets 1897
Lortab 5/500 Tablets 3143
Lortab 7.5/500 Tablets 3144
Lortab 10/500 Tablets 3144
Percocet Tablets 1127
Sinutab Sinus Caplets 1905
Sudafed PE Cold & Cough Caplets 1907
Sudafed PE Nighttime Cold Caplets 1907
Sudafed PE Severe Cold Caplets 1908
Sudafed PE Sinus Headache Caplets 1908
Regular Strength Tylenol Tablets 1915
Tylenol 8 Hour Extended Release Caplets 1915
Extra Strength Tylenol Caplets, Cool Caplets, and EZ Tabs 1915
Extra Strength Tylenol Adult Rapid Blast Liquid 1915
Extra Strength Tylenol PM Caplets, Geltabs, Liquid, and Rapid Release Gels 1915
Extra Strength Tylenol Rapid Release Gels 1915
Tylenol with Codeine Tablets 2427
Tylenol Allergy Multi-Symptom Caplets with Cool Burst and Rapid Release Gelcaps 1916
Tylenol Allergy Multi-Symptom Nighttime Caplets with Cool Burst 1916
Tylenol Severe Allergy Caplets 1916
Tylenol Arthritis Pain Extended Release Geltabs/Caplets 1915
Tylenol Chest Congestion Caplets with Cool Burst 1910
Tylenol Chest Congestion Liquid with Cool Burst 1910
Children's Tylenol Plus Cold Suspension Liquid 1912
Children's Tylenol Plus Cold & Allergy Suspension Liquid 1914
Children's Tylenol Plus Cough & Runny Nose Suspension Liquid 1912
Children's Tylenol Plus Cough & Sore Throat Suspension Liquid 1912
Children's Tylenol Plus Flu Suspension Liquid 1914
Children's Tylenol Suspension Liquid 1909
Children's Tylenol Meltaways 1909
Children's Tylenol Plus Multi-Symptom Cold Suspension Liquid 1912
Tylenol Cold Severe Congestion Daytime Caplets with Cool Burst 1912
Tylenol Cold Head Congestion Daytime Caplets with Cool Burst 1910
Tylenol Cold Head Congestion Nighttime Caplets with Cool Burst 1910
Tylenol Cold Head Congestion Severe Daytime Caplets with Cool Burst 1910
Tylenol Cold Multi-Symptom Daytime Caplets with Cool Burst and Rapid Release Gels 1913
Tylenol Cold Multi-Symptom Daytime Liquid with Citrus Burst 1913
Tylenol Cold Multi-Symptom Nighttime Caplets with Cool Burst 1913
Tylenol Cold Multi-Symptom Nighttime Liquid with Cool Burst 1913
Tylenol Cold Multi-Symptom Severe Caplets with Cool Burst 1913
Tylenol Cold Multi-Symptom Severe Daytime Liquid with Citrus Burst 1913
Tylenol Cough & Sore Throat Daytime Liquid with Cool Burst 1918
Tylenol Cough & Sore Throat Nighttime Liquid with Cool Burst 1918
Concentrated Tylenol Infants' Drops 1909
Jr. Tylenol Meltaways 1909
Tylenol Sinus Congestion & Pain Daytime Caplets with Cool Burst and Gelcaps 1917
Tylenol Sinus Congestion & Pain Nighttime Caplets with Cool Burst 1917
Tylenol Sinus Congestion & Pain Severe Caplets with Cool Burst 1917
Tylenol Sinus Severe Congestion Caplets with Cool Burst 1917
Tylenol Sore Throat Daytime Liquid with Cool Burst 1918
Tylenol Sore Throat Nighttime Liquid with Cool Burst 1918
Women's Tylenol Menstrual Relief Caplets 1919
Vicks DayQuil Cold & Flu Multi-Symptom Relief 616
Vicks DayQuil LiquiCaps 2567
Vicks DayQuil Liquid 2567
Vicks DayQuil Multi-Symptom Cold/Flu Relief 2567
Vicks NyQuil Cold & Flu Multi-Symptom Relief 617
Vicks NyQuil LiquiCaps 2567
Vicks NyQuil Liquid 2567
Vicks NyQuil Multi-Symptom Cold/Flu Relief 2567
Vicodin Tablets 529
Vicodin ES Tablets 530
Vicodin HP Tablets 531
Zydone Tablets 1132

Acetaminophen-containing products (In vitro, imatinib mesylate inhibits acetaminophen O-glucuronidation at therapeutic levels. Systemic exposure to acetaminophen is expected to be increased when co-administered with imatinib mesylate. No specific studies in humans have been performed and caution is recommended).
No products indexed under this heading.

Acetazolamide (CYP3A4 inhibitors may increase imatinib mesylate Cmax and AUC. There was a significant increase in exposure to imatinib (mean Cmax and AUC increased by 26% and 40% respectively) in healthy subjects when imatinib mesylate was co-administered with a singledose of ketoconazole (a CYP3A4 inhibitor). Caution is recommended when administering imatinib mesylate with strong CYP3A4 inhibitors (eg, ketoconazole, itraconazole). Grapefruit juice may also increase plasma concentrations of imatinib and should be avoided. Substances that inhibit the cytochrome P450 isoenszyme (CYP3A4) activity may decrease metabolism and increase imatinib concentrations).
No products indexed under this heading.

Alfentanil Hydrochloride (Imatinib mesylate is an inhibitor of CYP3A4 and may increase the Cmax and AUC of other drugs. Imatinib mesylate increases the mean Cmax and AUC of simvastatin (CYP3A4 substrate) 2-fold and 3.5-fold, respectively, suggesting an inhibition of the CYP3A4 byimatinib mesylate. Particular caution is recommended when administering imatinib mesylate with CYP3A4 substrates that have a narrow therapeutic window (eg, alfentanil, cyclosporine, diergotamine, ergotamine, fentanyl, pimozide, quinidine, sirolimus, or tacrolimus)).
No products indexed under this heading.

Allium sativum (CYP3A4 inducers may decrease imatinib mesylate Cmax and AUC. The use of concomitant strong CYP3A4 inducers should be avoided (eg, dexamethasone, phenytoin, carbamazepine, rifampin, rifabutin, rifampacin, phenobarbital). If patients must be co-administered a strong CYP3A4 inducer, based on pharmacokinetic studies, the dosage of imatinib mesylate should be increased by at least 50% and clinical response should be carefully monitored).
No products indexed under this heading.

Alprazolam (Imatinib mesylate is an inhibitor of CYP3A4 and may increase the Cmax and AUC of other drugs. Imatinib mesylate increases the mean Cmax and AUC of simvastatin (CYP3A4 substrate) 2-fold and 3.5-fold, suggesting an inhibition of the CYP3A4 byimatinib mesylate. Particular caution is recommended when administering imatinib mesylate with CYP3A4 substrates that have a narrow therapeutic window (eg, alfentanil, cyclosporine, diergotamine, ergotamine, fentanyl, pimozide, quinidine, sirolimus, or tacrolimus)).
No products indexed under this heading.

Amiodarone Hydrochloride (CYP3A4 inhibitors may increase imatinib mesylate Cmax and AUC. There was a significant increase in exposure to imatinib (mean Cmax and AUC increased by 26% and 40% respectively) in healthy subjects when imatinib mesylate was co-administered with a singledose of ketoconazole (a CYP3A4 inhibitor). Caution is recommended when administering imatinib mesylate with strong CYP3A4 inhibitors (eg, ketoconazole, itraconazole). Grapefruit juice may also increase plasma concentrations of imatinib and should be avoided. Substances that inhibit the cytochrome P450 isoenszyme (CYP3A4) activity may decrease metabolism and increase imatinib concentrations).
No products indexed under this heading.

Amitriptyline Hydrochloride (Imatinib mesylate is an inhibitor of CYP3A4 and may increase the Cmax and AUC of other drugs. Imatinib mesylate increases the mean Cmax and AUC of simvastatin (CYP3A4 substrate) 2-fold and 3.5-fold, respectively, suggesting an inhibition of the CYP3A4 byimatinib mesylate. Particular caution is recommended when administering imatinib mesylate with CYP3A4 substrates that have a narrow therapeutic window (eg, alfentanil, cyclosporine, diergotamine, ergotamine, fentanyl, pimozide, quinidine, sirolimus, or tacrolimus)).
No products indexed under this heading.

Amlodipine Besylate (Imatinib mesylate is an inhibitor of CYP3A4 and may increase the Cmax and AUC of other drugs. Imatinib mesylate increases the mean Cmax and AUC of simvastatin (CYP3A4 substrate) 2-fold and 3.5-fold, respectively, suggesting an inhibition of the CYP3A4 byimatinib mesylate. Particular caution is recommended when administering imatinib mesylate with CYP3A4 substrates that have a narrow therapeutic window (eg, alfentanil, cyclosporine, diergotamine, ergotamine, fentanyl, pimozide, quinidine, sirolimus, or tacrolimus)). Products include:

Azor Tablets 1005
Exforge Tablets 2238

Amphetamine Aspartate (In vitro, imatinib mesylate inhibits the cytochrome P450 isoenzyme CYP2D6 activity at similar concentrations that affect CYP3A4 activity. Systemic exposure to substrates of CYP2D6 is expected to be increased when co-administered with imatinib mesylate. No specific studies have been performed and caution is recommended). Products include:

Adderall XR Capsules 3012

Amphetamine Aspartate Monohydrate (In vitro, imatinib mesylate inhibits the cytochrome P450 isoenzyme CYP2D6 activity at similar concentrations that affect CYP3A4 activity. Systemic exposure to substrates of CYP2D6 is expected to be increased when co-administered with imatinib mesylate. No specific studies have been performed and caution is recommended).
No products indexed under this heading.

Amphetamine Sulfate (In vitro, imatinib mesylate inhibits the cytochrome P450 isoenzyme CYP2D6 activity at similar concentrations that affect CYP3A4 activity. Systemic exposure to substrates of CYP2D6 is expected to be increased when co-administered with imatinib mesylate. No specific studies have been performed and caution is recommended). Products include:

Adderall XR Capsules 3012

Amprenavir (CYP3A4 inhibitors may increase imatinib mesylate Cmax and AUC. There was a significant increase in exposure to imatinib (mean Cmax and AUC increased by 26% and 40% respectively) in healthy subjects when imatinib mesylate was co-administered with a singledose of ketoconazole (a CYP3A4 inhibitor). Caution is recommended when administering imatinib mesylate with strong CYP3A4 inhibitors (eg, ketoconazole, itraconazole). Grapefruit juice may also increase plasma concentrations of imatinib and should be avoided. Substances that inhibit the cytochrome P450 isoenszyme (CYP3A4) activity may decrease metabolism and increase imatinib concentrations).

No products indexed under this heading.

Anastrozole (CYP3A4 inhibitors may increase imatinib mesylate Cmax and AUC. There was a significant increase in exposure to imatinib (mean Cmax and AUC increased by 26% and 40% respectively) in healthy subjects when imatinib mesylate was co-administered with a singledose of ketoconazole (a CYP3A4 inhibitor). Caution is recommended when administering imatinib mesylate with strong CYP3A4 inhibitors (eg, ketoconazole, itraconazole). Grapefruit juice may also increase plasma concentrations of imatinib and should be avoided. Substances that inhibit the cytochrome P450 isoenszyme (CYP3A4) activity may decrease metabolism and increase imatinib concentrations). Products include:

Arimidex Tablets 672

Aprepitant (CYP3A4 inducers may decrease imatinib mesylate Cmax and AUC. The use of concomitant strong CYP3A4 inducers should be avoided (eg, dexamethasone, phenytoin, carbamazepine, rifampin, rifabutin, rifampacin, phenobarbital). If patients must be co-administered a strong CYP3A4 inducer, based on pharmacokinetic studies, the dosage of imatinib mesylate should be increased by at least 50% and clinical response should be carefully monitored). Products include:

Emend Capsules 1992

Astemizole (Imatinib mesylate is an inhibitor of CYP3A4 and may increase the Cmax and AUC of other drugs. Imatinib mesylate increases the mean Cmax and AUC of simvastatin (CYP3A4 substrate) 2-fold and 3.5-fold, respectively, suggesting an inhibition of the CYP3A4 byimatinib mesylate. Particular caution is recommended when administering imatinib mesylate with CYP3A4 substrates that have a narrow therapeutic window (eg, alfentanil, cyclosporine, diergotamine, ergotamine, fentanyl, pimozide, quinidine, sirolimus, or tacrolimus)).

No products indexed under this heading.

Atazanavir (CYP3A4 inhibitors may increase imatinib mesylate Cmax and AUC. There was a significant increase in exposure to imatinib (mean Cmax and AUC increased by 26% and 40% respectively) in healthy subjects when imatinib mesylate was co-administered with a singledose of ketoconazole (a CYP3A4 inhibitor). Caution is recommended when administering imatinib mesylate with strong CYP3A4 inhibitors (eg, ketoconazole, itraconazole). Grapefruit juice may also increase plasma concentrations of imatinib and should be avoided. Substances that inhibit the cytochrome P450 isoenszyme (CYP3A4) activity may decrease metabolism and increase imatinib concentrations).

No products indexed under this heading.

Atazanavir Sulfate (CYP3A4 inhibitors may increase imatinib mesylate Cmax and AUC. There was a significant increase in exposure to imatinib (mean Cmax and AUC increased by 26% and 40% respectively) in healthy subjects when imatinib mesylate was co-administered with a singledose of ketoconazole (a CYP3A4 inhibitor). Caution is recommended when administering imatinib mesylate with strong CYP3A4 inhibitors (eg, ketoconazole, itraconazole). Grapefruit juice may also increase plasma concentrations of imatinib and should be avoided. Substances that inhibit the cytochrome P450 isoenszyme (CYP3A4) activity may decrease metabolism and increase imatinib concentrations). Products include:

Reyataz Capsules 3299

Atomoxetine Hydrochloride (In vitro, imatinib mesylate inhibits the cytochrome P450 isoenzyme CYP2D6 activity at similar concentrations that affect CYP3A4 activity. Systemic exposure to substrates of CYP2D6 is expected to be increased when co-administered with imatinib mesylate. No specific studies have been performed and caution is recommended). Products include:

Strattera Capsules 1864

Atorvastatin Calcium (Imatinib will increase the plasma concentrations of certain HMG-CoA reductase inhibitors by inhibiting CYP3A4). Products include:

Lipitor Tablets 2501

Belladonna Ergotamine (Imatinib mesylate is an inhibitor of CYP3A4 and may increase the Cmax and AUC of other drugs. Imatinib mesylate increases the mean Cmax and AUC of simvastatin (CYP3A4 substrate) 2-fold and 3.5-fold, respectively, suggesting an inhibition of the CYP3A4 byimatinib mesylate. Particular caution is recommended when administering imatinib mesylate with CYP3A4 substrates that have a narrow therapeutic window (eg, alfentanil, cyclosporine, diergotamine, ergotamine, fentanyl, pimozide, quinidine, sirolimus, or tacrolimus)).

No products indexed under this heading.

Betamethasone Acetate (CYP3A4 inducers may decrease imatinib mesylate Cmax and AUC. The use of concomitant strong CYP3A4 inducers should be avoided (eg, dexamethasone, phenytoin, carbamazepine, rifampin, rifabutin, rifampacin, phenobarbital). If patients must be co-administered a strong CYP3A4 inducer, based on pharmacokinetic studies, the dosage of imatinib mesylate should be increased by at least 50% and clinical response should be carefully monitored).

No products indexed under this heading.

Betamethasone Sodium Phosphate (CYP3A4 inducers may decrease imatinib mesylate Cmax and AUC. The use of concomitant strong CYP3A4 inducers should be avoided (eg, dexamethasone, phenytoin, carbamazepine, rifampin, rifabutin, rifampacin, phenobarbital). If patients must be co-administered a strong CYP3A4 inducer, based on pharmacokinetic studies, the dosage of imatinib mesylate should be increased by at least 50% and clinical response should be carefully monitored).

No products indexed under this heading.

Bisoprolol Fumarate (In vitro, imatinib mesylate inhibits the cytochrome P450 isoenzyme CYP2D6 activity at similar concentrations that affect CYP3A4 activity. Systemic exposure to substrates of CYP2D6 is expected to be increased when co-administered with imatinib mesylate. No specific studies have been performed and caution is recommended).

No products indexed under this heading.

Buspirone Hydrochloride (Imatinib mesylate is an inhibitor of CYP3A4 and may increase the Cmax and AUC of other drugs. Imatinib mesylate increases the mean Cmax and AUC of simvastatin (CYP3A4 substrate) 2-fold and 3.5-fold, respectively, suggesting an inhibition of the CYP3A4 byimatinib mesylate. Particular caution is recommended when administering imatinib mesylate with CYP3A4 substrates that have a narrow therapeutic window (eg, alfentanil, cyclosporine, diergotamine, ergotamine, fentanyl, pimozide, quinidine, sirolimus, or tacrolimus)).

No products indexed under this heading.

Busulfan (Imatinib mesylate is an inhibitor of CYP3A4 and may increase the Cmax and AUC of other drugs. Imatinib mesylate increases the mean Cmax and AUC of simvastatin (CYP3A4 substrate) 2-fold and 3.5-fold, respectively, suggesting an inhibition of the CYP3A4 byimatinib mesylate. Particular caution is recommended when administering imatinib mesylate with CYP3A4 substrates that have a narrow therapeutic window (eg, alfentanil, cyclosporine, diergotamine, ergotamine, fentanyl, pimozide, quinidine, sirolimus, or tacrolimus)). Products include:

Busulfex Injection 2477
Myleran Tablets 1530

Captopril (In vitro, imatinib mesylate inhibits the cytochrome P450 isoenzyme CYP2D6 activity at similar concentrations that affect CYP3A4 activity. Systemic exposure to substrates of CYP2D6 is expected to be increased when co-administered with imatinib mesylate. No specific studies have been performed and caution is recommended). Products include:

Captopril Tablets 2182

Carbamazepine (Co-administration with inducers of CYP3A4, such as carbamazepine, may increase the metabolism and decrease imatinib concentrations). Products include:

Carbatrol Capsules 3019
Equetro Extended-Release Capsules 3174

Carvedilol (In vitro, imatinib mesylate inhibits the cytochrome P450 isoenzyme CYP2D6 activity at similar concentrations that affect CYP3A4 activity. Systemic exposure to substrates of CYP2D6 is expected to be increased when co-administered with imatinib mesylate. No specific studies have been performed and caution is recommended). Products include:

Coreg Tablets 1387

Cerivastatin Sodium (Imatinib will increase the plasma concentrations of certain HMG-CoA reductase inhibitors by inhibiting CYP3A4).

No products indexed under this heading.

Cevimeline Hydrochloride (In vitro, imatinib mesylate inhibits the cytochrome P450 isoenzyme CYP2D6 activity at similar concentrations that affect CYP3A4 activity. Systemic exposure to substrates of CYP2D6 is expected to be increased when co-administered with imatinib mesylate. No specific studies have been performed and caution is recommended). Products include:

Evoxac Capsules 1013

Chlorpheniramine (Imatinib mesylate is an inhibitor of CYP3A4 and may increase the Cmax and AUC of other drugs. Imatinib mesylate increases the mean Cmax and AUC of simvastatin (CYP3A4 substrate) 2-fold and 3.5-fold, respectively, suggesting an inhibition of the CYP3A4 byimatinib mesylate. Particular caution is recommended when administering imatinib mesylate with CYP3A4 substrates that have a narrow therapeutic window (eg, alfentanil, cyclosporine, diergotamine, ergotamine, fentanyl, pimozide, quinidine, sirolimus, or tacrolimus)).

No products indexed under this heading.

Chlorpheniramine Maleate (Imatinib mesylate is an inhibitor of CYP3A4 and may increase the Cmax and AUC of other drugs. Imatinib mesylate increases the mean Cmax and AUC of simvastatin (CYP3A4 substrate) 2-fold and 3.5-fold, respectively, suggesting an inhibition of the CYP3A4 byimatinib mesylate. Particular caution is recommended when administering imatinib mesylate with CYP3A4 substrates that have a narrow therapeutic window (eg, alfentanil, cyclosporine, diergotamine, ergotamine, fentanyl, pimozide, quinidine, sirolimus, or tacrolimus)). Products include:

Actifed Cold & Allergy Tablets 1895
Sudafed PE Sinus & Allergy Tablets 1908
Tylenol Allergy Multi-Symptom Caplets with Cool Burst and Rapid Release Gelcaps 1916
Children's Tylenol Plus Cold Suspension Liquid 1912
Children's Tylenol Plus Cough & Runny Nose Suspension Liquid 1912
Children's Tylenol Plus Flu Suspension Liquid 1914
Children's Tylenol Plus Multi-Symptom Cold Suspension Liquid 1912
Tylenol Cold Head Congestion Nighttime Caplets with Cool Burst 1910

IMPORTANT NOTE: Always consult each drug listing in the patient's regimen for possible interactions.

Tylenol Cold Multi-Symptom Nighttime Caplets with Cool Burst **1913**
Tylenol Sinus Congestion & Pain Nighttime Caplets with Cool Burst **1917**

Chlorpheniramine Polistirex (Imatinib mesylate is an inhibitor of CYP3A4 and may increase the Cmax and AUC of other drugs. Imatinib mesylate increases the mean Cmax and AUC of simvastatin (CYP3A4 substrate) 2-fold and 3.5-fold, respectively, suggesting an inhibition of the CYP3A4 byimatinib mesylate. Particular caution is recommended when administering imatinib mesylate with CYP3A4 substrates that have a narrow therapeutic window (eg, alfentanil, cyclosporine, diergotamine, ergotamine, fentanyl, pimozide, quinidine, sirolimus, or tacrolimus)). Products include:
Tussionex Pennkinetic Extended-Release Suspension **3154**

Chlorpheniramine Tannate (Imatinib mesylate is an inhibitor of CYP3A4 and may increase the Cmax and AUC of other drugs. Imatinib mesylate increases the mean Cmax and AUC of simvastatin (CYP3A4 substrate) 2-fold and 3.5-fold, respectively, suggesting an inhibition of the CYP3A4 byimatinib mesylate. Particular caution is recommended when administering imatinib mesylate with CYP3A4 substrates that have a narrow therapeutic window (eg, alfentanil, cyclosporine, diergotamine, ergotamine, fentanyl, pimozide, quinidine, sirolimus, or tacrolimus)).
No products indexed under this heading.

Chlorpromazine (In vitro, imatinib mesylate inhibits the cytochrome P450 isoenzyme CYP2D6 activity at similar concentrations that affect CYP3A4 activity. Systemic exposure to substrates of CYP2D6 is expected to be increased when co-administered with imatinib mesylate. No specific studies have been performed and caution is recommended).
No products indexed under this heading.

Chlorpromazine Hydrochloride (In vitro, imatinib mesylate inhibits the cytochrome P450 isoenzyme CYP2D6 activity at similar concentrations that affect CYP3A4 activity. Systemic exposure to substrates of CYP2D6 is expected to be increased when co-administered with imatinib mesylate. No specific studies have been performed and caution is recommended).
No products indexed under this heading.

Chlorpropamide (In vitro, imatinib mesylate inhibits the cytochrome P450 isoenzyme CYP2D6 activity at similar concentrations that affect CYP3A4 activity. Systemic exposure to substrates of CYP2D6 is expected to be increased when co-administered with imatinib mesylate. No specific studies have been performed and caution is recommended).
No products indexed under this heading.

Cimetidine (CYP3A4 inhibitors may increase imatinib mesylate Cmax and AUC. There was a significant increase in exposure to imatinib (mean Cmax and AUC increased by 26% and 40% respectively) in healthy subjects when imatinib mesylate was co-administered with a singledose of ketoconazole (a CYP3A4 inhibitor). Caution is recommended when administering imatinib mesylate with strong CYP3A4 inhibitors (eg, ketoconazole, itraconazole). Grapefruit juice may also increase plasma concentrations of imatinib and should be avoided. Substances that inhibit the cytochrome P450 isoenszyme (CYP3A4) activity may decrease metabolism and increase imatinib concentrations).
No products indexed under this heading.

Cimetidine Hydrochloride (CYP3A4 inhibitors may increase imatinib mesylate Cmax and AUC. There was a significant increase in exposure to imatinib (mean Cmax and AUC increased by 26% and 40% respectively) in healthy subjects when imatinib mesylate was co-administered with a singledose of ketoconazole (a CYP3A4 inhibitor). Caution is recommended when administering imatinib mesylate with strong CYP3A4 inhibitors (eg, ketoconazole, itraconazole). Grapefruit juice may also increase plasma concentrations of imatinib and should be avoided. Substances that inhibit the cytochrome P450 isoenszyme (CYP3A4) activity may decrease metabolism and increase imatinib concentrations).
No products indexed under this heading.

Ciprofloxacin (CYP3A4 inhibitors may increase imatinib mesylate Cmax and AUC. There was a significant increase in exposure to imatinib (mean Cmax and AUC increased by 26% and 40% respectively) in healthy subjects when imatinib mesylate was co-administered with a singledose of ketoconazole (a CYP3A4 inhibitor). Caution is recommended when administering imatinib mesylate with strong CYP3A4 inhibitors (eg, ketoconazole, itraconazole). Grapefruit juice may also increase plasma concentrations of imatinib and should be avoided. Substances that inhibit the cytochrome P450 isoenszyme (CYP3A4) activity may decrease metabolism and increase imatinib concentrations). Products include:
Cipro I.V. **2817**
Cipro Oral Suspension **2810**
Cipro XR Tablets **2823**
Ciprodex Otic Suspension **541**

Ciprofloxacin Hydrochloride (CYP3A4 inducers may decrease imatinib mesylate Cmax and AUC. The use of concomitant strong CYP3A4 inducers should be avoided (eg, dexamethasone, phenytoin, carbamazepine, rifampin, rifabutin, rifampacin, phenobarbital). If patients must be co-administered a strong CYP3A4 inducer, based on pharmacokinetic studies, the dosage of imatinib mesylate should be increased by at least 50% and clinical response should be carefully monitored). Products include:
Cipro Tablets **2810**

Cisapride (Imatinib mesylate is an inhibitor of CYP3A4 and may increase the Cmax and AUC of other drugs. Imatinib mesylate increases the mean Cmax and AUC of simvastatin (CYP3A4 substrate) 2-fold and 3.5-fold, respectively, suggesting an inhibition of the CYP3A4 byimatinib mesylate. Particular caution is recommended when administering imatinib mesylate with CYP3A4 substrates that have a narrow therapeutic window (eg, alfentanil, cyclosporine, diergotamine, ergotamine, fentanyl, pimozide, quinidine, sirolimus, or tacrolimus)).
No products indexed under this heading.

Cisplatin (CYP3A4 inducers may decrease imatinib mesylate Cmax and AUC. The use of concomitant strong CYP3A4 inducers should be avoided (eg, dexamethasone, phenytoin, carbamazepine, rifampin, rifabutin, rifampacin, phenobarbital). If patients must be co-administered a strong CYP3A4 inducer, based on pharmacokinetic studies, the dosage of imatinib mesylate should be increased by at least 50% and clinical response should be carefully monitored).
No products indexed under this heading.

Clarithromycin (Co-administration with CYP3A4 inhibitors, such as clarithromycin, may decrease the metabolism and increase imatinib concentrations). Products include:
Biaxin/Biaxin XL **411**

Clomipramine Hydrochloride (In vitro, imatinib mesylate inhibits the cytochrome P450 isoenzyme CYP2D6 activity at similar concentrations that affect CYP3A4 activity. Systemic exposure to substrates of CYP2D6 is expected to be increased when co-administered with imatinib mesylate. No specific studies have been performed and caution is recommended).
No products indexed under this heading.

Clotrimazole (CYP3A4 inhibitors may increase imatinib mesylate Cmax and AUC. There was a significant increase in exposure to imatinib (mean Cmax and AUC increased by 26% and 40% respectively) in healthy subjects when imatinib mesylate was co-administered with a singledose of ketoconazole (a CYP3A4 inhibitor). Caution is recommended when administering imatinib mesylate with strong CYP3A4 inhibitors (eg, ketoconazole, itraconazole). Grapefruit juice may also increase plasma concentrations of imatinib and should be avoided. Substances that inhibit the cytochrome P450 isoenszyme (CYP3A4) activity may decrease metabolism and increase imatinib concentrations). Products include:
Lotrisone **2881**

Clozapine (In vitro, imatinib mesylate inhibits the cytochrome P450 isoenzyme CYP2D6 activity at similar concentrations that affect CYP3A4 activity. Systemic exposure to substrates of CYP2D6 is expected to be increased when co-administered with imatinib mesylate. No specific studies have been performed and caution is recommended).
No products indexed under this heading.

Codeine Phosphate (In vitro, imatinib mesylate inhibits the cytochrome P450 isoenzyme CYP2D6 activity at similar concentrations that affect CYP3A4 activity. Systemic exposure to substrates of CYP2D6 is expected to be increased when co-administered with imatinib mesylate. No specific studies have been performed and caution is recommended). Products include:
Tylenol with Codeine Tablets **2427**

Codeine Sulfate (In vitro, imatinib mesylate inhibits the cytochrome P450 isoenzyme CYP2D6 activity at similar concentrations that affect CYP3A4 activity. Systemic exposure to substrates of CYP2D6 is expected to be increased when co-administered with imatinib mesylate. No specific studies have been performed and caution is recommended).
No products indexed under this heading.

Cortisone Acetate (CYP3A4 inducers may decrease imatinib mesylate Cmax and AUC. The use of concomitant strong CYP3A4 inducers should be avoided (eg, dexamethasone, phenytoin, carbamazepine, rifampin, rifabutin, rifampacin, phenobarbital). If patients must be co-administered a strong CYP3A4 inducer, based on pharmacokinetic studies, the dosage of imatinib mesylate should be increased by at least 50% and clinical response should be carefully monitored).
No products indexed under this heading.

Cyclobenzaprine Hydrochloride (In vitro, imatinib mesylate inhibits the cytochrome P450 isoenzyme CYP2D6 activity at similar concentrations that affect CYP3A4 activity. Systemic exposure to substrates of CYP2D6 is expected to be increased when co-administered with imatinib mesylate. No specific studies have been performed and caution is recommended). Products include:
Amrix Capsules **966**

Cyclosporine (Particular caution is recommended when administering imatinib with CYP3A4 substrates that have a narrow therapeutic window). Products include:
Gengraf Capsules **435**
Neoral Oral Solution **2280**
Neoral Soft Gelatin Capsules **2280**
Restasis Ophthalmic Emulsion **557**
Sandimmune **2296**

Dalfopristin (CYP3A4 inhibitors may increase imatinib mesylate Cmax and AUC. There was a significant increase in exposure to imatinib (mean Cmax and AUC increased by 26% and 40% respectively) in healthy subjects when imatinib mesylate was co-administered with a singledose of ketoconazole (a CYP3A4 inhibitor). Caution is recommended when administering imatinib mesylate with strong CYP3A4 inhibitors (eg, ketoconazole, itraconazole). Grapefruit juice may also increase plasma concentrations of imatinib and should be avoided. Substances that inhibit the cytochrome P450 isoenszyme (CYP3A4) activity may decrease metabolism and increase imatinib concentrations).
No products indexed under this heading.

Danazol (CYP3A4 inhibitors may increase imatinib mesylate Cmax and AUC. There was a significant increase in exposure to imatinib (mean Cmax and AUC increased by 26% and 40% respectively) in healthy subjects when imatinib mesylate was co-administered with a singledose of ketoconazole (a CYP3A4 inhibitor). Caution is recommended when administering imatinib mesylate with strong CYP3A4 inhibitors (eg, ketoconazole, itraconazole). Grapefruit juice may also increase plasma concentrations of imatinib and should be avoided. Substances that inhibit the cytochrome P450 isoenszyme (CYP3A4) activity may decrease metabolism and increase imatinib concentrations).

No products indexed under this heading.

Delavirdine Mesylate (CYP3A4 inhibitors may increase imatinib mesylate Cmax and AUC. There was a significant increase in exposure to imatinib (mean Cmax and AUC increased by 26% and 40% respectively) in healthy subjects when imatinib mesylate was co-administered with a singledose of ketoconazole (a CYP3A4 inhibitor). Caution is recommended when administering imatinib mesylate with strong CYP3A4 inhibitors (eg, ketoconazole, itraconazole). Grapefruit juice may also increase plasma concentrations of imatinib and should be avoided. Substances that inhibit the cytochrome P450 isoenszyme (CYP3A4) activity may decrease metabolism and increase imatinib concentrations).

No products indexed under this heading.

Desipramine Hydrochloride (In vitro, imatinib mesylate inhibits the cytochrome P450 isoenzyme CYP2D6 activity at similar concentrations that affect CYP3A4 activity. Systemic exposure to substrates of CYP2D6 is expected to be increased when co-administered with imatinib mesylate. No specific studies have been performed and caution is recommended).

No products indexed under this heading.

Desogestrel (Imatinib mesylate is an inhibitor of CYP3A4 and may increase the Cmax and AUC of other drugs. Imatinib mesylate increases the mean Cmax and AUC of simvastatin (CYP3A4 substrate) 2-fold and 3.5-fold, respectively, suggesting an inhibition of the CYP3A4 byimatinib mesylate. Particular caution is recommended when administering imatinib mesylate with CYP3A4 substrates that have a narrow therapeutic window (eg, alfentanil, cyclosporine, diergotamine, ergotamine, fentanyl, pimozide, quinidine, sirolimus, or tacrolimus)). Products include:

Mircette Tablets 1034

Dexamethasone (CYP3A4 inducers may decrease imatinib mesylate Cmax and AUC. The use of concomitant strong CYP3A4 inducers should be avoided (eg, dexamethasone, phenytoin, carbamazepine, rifampin, rifabutin, rifampacin, phenobarbital). If patients must be co-administered a strong CYP3A4 inducer, based on pharmacokinetic studies, the dosage of imatinib mesylate should be increased by at least 50% and clinical response should be carefully monitored). Products include:

Ciprodex Otic Suspension 541

Dexamethasone Acetate (CYP3A4 inducers may decrease imatinib mesylate Cmax and AUC. The use of concomitant strong CYP3A4 inducers should be avoided (eg, dexamethasone, phenytoin, carbamazepine, rifampin, rifabutin, rifampacin, phenobarbital). If patients must be co-administered a strong CYP3A4 inducer, based on pharmacokinetic studies, the dosage of imatinib mesylate should be increased by at least 50% and clinical response should be carefully monitored).

No products indexed under this heading.

Dexamethasone Sodium Phosphate (CYP3A4 inducers may decrease imatinib mesylate Cmax and AUC. The use of concomitant strong CYP3A4 inducers should be avoided (eg, dexamethasone, phenytoin, carbamazepine, rifampin, rifabutin, rifampacin, phenobarbital). If patients must be co-administered a strong CYP3A4 inducer, based on pharmacokinetic studies, the dosage of imatinib mesylate should be increased by at least 50% and clinical response should be carefully monitored).

No products indexed under this heading.

Dexfenfluramine Hydrochloride (In vitro, imatinib mesylate inhibits the cytochrome P450 isoenzyme CYP2D6 activity at similar concentrations that affect CYP3A4 activity. Systemic exposure to substrates of CYP2D6 is expected to be increased when co-administered with imatinib mesylate. No specific studies have been performed and caution is recommended).

No products indexed under this heading.

Dextromethorphan Hydrobromide (In vitro, imatinib mesylate inhibits the cytochrome P450 isoenzyme CYP2D6 activity at similar concentrations that affect CYP3A4 activity. Systemic exposure to substrates of CYP2D6 is expected to be increased when co-administered with imatinib mesylate. No specific studies have been performed and caution is recommended). Products include:

PediaCare Children's Liquid Multi-Symptom Cold..................... 1902
PediaCare Children's Long-Acting Cough 1902
Children's Sudafed PE Cold & Cough Liquid 1907
Sudafed PE Cold & Cough Caplets....................................... 1907
Children's Tylenol Plus Cough & Runny Nose Suspension Liquid..... 1912
Children's Tylenol Plus Cough & Sore Throat Suspension Liquid..... 1912
Children's Tylenol Plus Flu Suspension Liquid 1914
Children's Tylenol Plus Multi-Symptom Cold Suspension Liquid 1912
Tylenol Cold Severe Congestion Daytime Caplets with Cool Burst.. 1912
Tylenol Cold Head Congestion Daytime Caplets with Cool Burst.. 1910
Tylenol Cold Head Congestion Nighttime Caplets with Cool Burst.. 1910
Tylenol Cold Head Congestion Severe Daytime Caplets with Cool Burst............................. 1910
Tylenol Cold Multi-Symptom Daytime Caplets with Cool Burst and Rapid Release Gels....... 1913
Tylenol Cold Multi-Symptom Daytime Liquid with Citrus Burst... 1913
Tylenol Cold Multi-Symptom Nighttime Caplets with Cool Burst.. 1913
Tylenol Cold Multi-Symptom Nighttime Liquid with Cool Burst... 1913
Tylenol Cold Multi-Symptom Severe Caplets with Cool Burst..... 1913
Tylenol Cold Multi-Symptom Severe Daytime Liquid with Citrus Burst.................................. 1913
Tylenol Cough & Sore Throat Daytime Liquid with Cool Burst...... 1918
Tylenol Cough & Sore Throat Nighttime Liquid with Cool Burst... 1918
Vicks DayQuil Cold & Flu Multi-Symptom Relief 616
Vicks DayQuil LiquiCaps 2567
Vicks DayQuil Liquid 2567
Vicks DayQuil Multi-Symptom Cold/Flu Relief............................ 2567
Vicks NyQuil Cold & Flu Multi-Symptom Relief 617
Vicks NyQuil LiquiCaps 2567
Vicks NyQuil Liquid 2567
Vicks NyQuil Multi-Symptom Cold/Flu Relief............................ 2567

Dextromethorphan Polistirex (In vitro, imatinib mesylate inhibits the cytochrome P450 isoenzyme CYP2D6 activity at similar concentrations that affect CYP3A4 activity. Systemic exposure to substrates of CYP2D6 is expected to be increased when co-administered with imatinib mesylate. No specific studies have been performed and caution is recommended).

No products indexed under this heading.

Diazepam (Imatinib mesylate is an inhibitor of CYP3A4 and may increase the Cmax and AUC of other drugs. Imatinib mesylate increases the mean Cmax and AUC of simvastatin (CYP3A4 substrate) 2-fold and 3.5-fold, respectively, suggesting an inhibition of the CYP3A4 byimatinib mesylate. Particular caution is recommended when administering imatinib mesylate with CYP3A4 substrates that have a narrow therapeutic window (eg, alfentanil, cyclosporine, diergotamine, ergotamine, fentanyl, pimozide, quinidine, sirolimus, or tacrolimus)). Products include:

Valium Tablets 2658

Dihydroergotamine Mesylate (Imatinib mesylate is an inhibitor of CYP3A4 and may increase the Cmax and AUC of other drugs. Imatinib mesylate increases the mean Cmax and AUC of simvastatin (CYP3A4 substrate) 2-fold and 3.5-fold, respectively, suggesting an inhibition of the CYP3A4 byimatinib mesylate. Particular caution is recommended when administering imatinib mesylate with CYP3A4 substrates that have a narrow therapeutic window (eg, alfentanil, cyclosporine, diergotamine, ergotamine, fentanyl, pimozide, quinidine, sirolimus, or tacrolimus)).

No products indexed under this heading.

Diltiazem Hydrochloride (CYP3A4 inhibitors may increase imatinib mesylate Cmax and AUC. There was a significant increase in exposure to imatinib (mean Cmax and AUC increased by 26% and 40% respectively) in healthy subjects when imatinib mesylate was co-administered with a singledose of ketoconazole (a CYP3A4 inhibitor). Caution is recommended when administering imatinib mesylate with strong CYP3A4 inhibitors (eg, ketoconazole, itraconazole). Grapefruit juice may also increase plasma concentrations of imatinib and should be avoided. Substances that inhibit the cytochrome P450 isoenszyme (CYP3A4) activity may decrease metabolism and increase imatinib concentrations). Products include:

Cardizem LA Extended Release Tablets 421

Diltiazem Maleate (CYP3A4 inhibitors may increase imatinib mesylate Cmax and AUC. There was a significant increase in exposure to imatinib (mean Cmax and AUC increased by 26% and 40% respectively) in healthy subjects when imatinib mesylate was co-administered with a singledose of ketoconazole (a CYP3A4 inhibitor). Caution is recommended when administering imatinib mesylate with strong CYP3A4 inhibitors (eg, ketoconazole, itraconazole). Grapefruit juice may also increase plasma concentrations of imatinib and should be avoided. Substances that inhibit the cytochrome P450 isoenszyme (CYP3A4) activity may decrease metabolism and increase imatinib concentrations).

No products indexed under this heading.

Disopyramide (Imatinib mesylate is an inhibitor of CYP3A4 and may increase the Cmax and AUC of other drugs. Imatinib mesylate increases the mean Cmax and AUC of simvastatin (CYP3A4 substrate) 2-fold and 3.5-fold, respectively, suggesting an inhibition of the CYP3A4 byimatinib mesylate. Particular caution is recommended when administering imatinib mesylate with CYP3A4 substrates that have a narrow therapeutic window (eg, alfentanil, cyclosporine, diergotamine, ergotamine, fentanyl, pimozide, quinidine, sirolimus, or tacrolimus)).

No products indexed under this heading.

Disopyramide Phosphate (Imatinib mesylate is an inhibitor of CYP3A4 and may increase the Cmax and AUC of other drugs. Imatinib mesylate increases the mean Cmax and AUC of simvastatin (CYP3A4 substrate) 2-fold and 3.5-fold, respectively, suggesting an inhibition of the CYP3A4 byimatinib mesylate. Particular caution is recommended when administering imatinib mesylate with CYP3A4 substrates that have a narrow therapeutic window (eg, alfentanil, cyclosporine, diergotamine, ergotamine, fentanyl, pimozide, quinidine, sirolimus, or tacrolimus)).

No products indexed under this heading.

Disulfiram (Imatinib mesylate is an inhibitor of CYP3A4 and may increase the Cmax and AUC of other drugs. Imatinib mesylate increases the mean Cmax and AUC of simvastatin (CYP3A4 substrate) 2-fold and 3.5-fold, respectively, suggesting an inhibition of the CYP3A4 byimatinib mesylate. Particular caution is recommended when administering imatinib mesylate with CYP3A4 substrates that have a narrow therapeutic window (eg, alfentanil, cyclosporine, diergotamine, ergotamine, fentanyl, pimozide, quinidine, sirolimus, or tacrolimus)).

No products indexed under this heading.

Dolasetron Mesylate (In vitro, imatinib mesylate inhibits the cytochrome P450 isoenzyme CYP2D6 activity at similar concentrations that affect CYP3A4 activity. Systemic exposure to substrates of CYP2D6 is expected to be increased when co-administered with imatinib mesylate. No specific studies have been performed and caution is recommended). Products include:

Anzemet Injection 2701
Anzemet Tablets 2704

Donepezil Hydrochloride (In vitro, imatinib mesylate inhibits the cytochrome P450 isoenzyme CYP2D6 activity at similar concentrations that affect CYP3A4 activity. Systemic exposure to substrates of CYP2D6 is expected to be increased when co-administered with imatinib mesylate. No specific studies have been performed and caution is recommended). Products include:

Aricept Tablets 1062
Aricept ODT Tablets 1062

Doxepin Hydrochloride (In vitro, imatinib mesylate inhibits the cytochrome P450 isoenzyme CYP2D6 activity at similar concentrations that affect CYP3A4 activity. Systemic exposure to substrates of CYP2D6 is expected to be increased when co-administered with imatinib mesylate. No specific studies have been performed and caution is recommended).

No products indexed under this heading.

Doxorubicin Hydrochloride (CYP3A4 inducers may decrease imatinib mesylate Cmax and AUC. The use of concomitant strong CYP3A4 inducers should be avoided (eg, dexamethasone, phenytoin, carbamazepine, rifampin, rifabutin, rifampacin, phenobarbital). If patients must be co-administered a strong CYP3A4 inducer, based on pharmacokinetic studies, the dosage of imatinib mesylate should be increased by at least 50% and clinical response should be carefully monitored).

No products indexed under this heading.

Dronabinol (Imatinib mesylate is an inhibitor of CYP3A4 and may increase the Cmax and AUC of other drugs. Imatinib mesylate increases the mean Cmax and AUC of simvastatin (CYP3A4 substrate) 2-fold and 3.5-fold, respectively, suggesting an inhibition of the CYP3A4 byimatinib mesylate. Particular caution is recommended when administering imatinib mesylate with CYP3A4 substrates that have a narrow therapeutic window (eg, alfentanil, cyclosporine, diergotamine, ergotamine, fentanyl, pimozide, quinidine, sirolimus, or tacrolimus)). Products include:

Marinol Capsules 3163

Efavirenz (CYP3A4 inducers may decrease imatinib mesylate Cmax and AUC. The use of concomitant strong CYP3A4 inducers should be avoided (eg, dexamethasone, phenytoin, carbamazepine, rifampin, rifabutin, rifampacin, phenobarbital). If patients must be co-administered a strong CYP3A4 inducer, based on pharmacokinetic studies, the dosage of imatinib mesylate should be increased by at least 50% and clinical response should be carefully monitored). Products include:

Atripla Tablets 938
Sustiva Capsules 930
Sustiva Tablets 930

Encainide Hydrochloride (In vitro, imatinib mesylate inhibits the cytochrome P450 isoenzyme CYP2D6 activity at similar concentrations that affect CYP3A4 activity. Systemic exposure to substrates of CYP2D6 is expected to be increased when co-administered with imatinib mesylate. No specific studies have been performed and caution is recommended).

No products indexed under this heading.

Ergotamine Tartrate (Imatinib mesylate is an inhibitor of CYP3A4 and may increase the Cmax and AUC of other drugs. Imatinib mesylate increases the mean Cmax and AUC of simvastatin (CYP3A4 substrate) 2-fold and 3.5-fold, respectively, suggesting an inhibition of the CYP3A4 byimatinib mesylate. Particular caution is recommended when administering imatinib mesylate with CYP3A4 substrates that have a narrow therapeutic window (eg, alfentanil, cyclosporine, diergotamine, ergotamine, fentanyl, pimozide, quinidine, sirolimus, or tacrolimus)).

No products indexed under this heading.

Erythromycin (CYP3A4 inhibitors may increase imatinib mesylate Cmax and AUC: There was a significant increase in exposure to imatinib (mean Cmax and AUC increased by 26% and 40% respectively) in healthy subjects when imatinib mesylate was co-administered with a singledose of ketoconazole (a CYP3A4 inhibitor). Caution is recommended when administering imatinib mesylate with strong CYP3A4 inhibitors (eg, ketoconazole, itraconazole). Grapefruit juice may also increase plasma concentrations of imatinib and should be avoided. Substances that inhibit the cytochrome P450 isoenszyme (CYP3A4) activity may decrease metabolism and increase imatinib concentrations).

No products indexed under this heading.

Erythromycin Estolate (CYP3A4 inhibitors may increase imatinib mesylate Cmax and AUC. There was a significant increase in exposure to imatinib (mean Cmax and AUC increased by 26% and 40% respectively) in healthy subjects when imatinib mesylate was co-administered with a singledose of ketoconazole (a CYP3A4 inhibitor). Caution is recommended when administering imatinib mesylate with strong CYP3A4 inhibitors (eg, ketoconazole, itraconazole). Grapefruit juice may also increase plasma concentrations of imatinib and should be avoided. Substances that inhibit the cytochrome P450 isoenszyme (CYP3A4) activity may decrease metabolism and increase imatinib concentrations).

No products indexed under this heading.

Erythromycin Ethylsuccinate (CYP3A4 inhibitors may increase imatinib mesylate Cmax and AUC. There was a significant increase in exposure to imatinib (mean Cmax and AUC increased by 26% and 40% respectively) in healthy subjects when imatinib mesylate was co-administered with a singledose of ketoconazole (a CYP3A4 inhibitor). Caution is recommended when administering imatinib mesylate with strong CYP3A4 inhibitors (eg, ketoconazole, itraconazole). Grapefruit juice may also increase plasma concentrations of imatinib and should be avoided. Substances that inhibit the cytochrome P450 isoenszyme (CYP3A4) activity may decrease metabolism and increase imatinib concentrations). Products include:

E.E.S. 433
EryPed 431

Erythromycin Gluceptate (CYP3A4 inhibitors may increase imatinib mesylate Cmax and AUC. There was a significant increase in exposure to imatinib (mean Cmax and AUC increased by 26% and 40% respectively) in healthy subjects when imatinib mesylate was co-administered with a singledose of ketoconazole (a CYP3A4 inhibitor). Caution is recommended when administering imatinib mesylate with strong CYP3A4 inhibitors (eg, ketoconazole, itraconazole). Grapefruit juice may also increase plasma concentrations of imatinib and should be avoided. Substances that inhibit the cytochrome P450 isoenszyme (CYP3A4) activity may decrease metabolism and increase imatinib concentrations).

No products indexed under this heading.

Erythromycin Lactobionate (CYP3A4 inhibitors may increase imatinib mesylate Cmax and AUC. There was a significant increase in exposure to imatinib (mean Cmax and AUC increased by 26% and 40% respectively) in healthy subjects when imatinib mesylate was co-administered with a singledose of ketoconazole (a CYP3A4 inhibitor). Caution is recommended when administering imatinib mesylate with strong CYP3A4 inhibitors (eg, ketoconazole, itraconazole). Grapefruit juice may also increase plasma concentrations of imatinib and should be avoided. Substances that inhibit the cytochrome P450 isoenszyme (CYP3A4) activity may decrease metabolism and increase imatinib concentrations).

No products indexed under this heading.

Erythromycin Stearate (CYP3A4 inhibitors may increase imatinib mesylate Cmax and AUC. There was a significant increase in exposure to imatinib (mean Cmax and AUC increased by 26% and 40% respectively) in healthy subjects when imatinib mesylate was co-administered with a singledose of ketoconazole (a CYP3A4 inhibitor). Caution is recommended when administering imatinib mesylate with strong CYP3A4 inhibitors (eg, ketoconazole, itraconazole). Grapefruit juice may also increase plasma concentrations of imatinib and should be avoided. Substances that inhibit the cytochrome P450 isoenszyme (CYP3A4) activity may decrease metabolism and increase imatinib concentrations).

No products indexed under this heading.

Esomeprazole Magnesium (CYP3A4 inhibitors may increase imatinib mesylate Cmax and AUC. There was a significant increase in exposure to imatinib (mean Cmax and AUC increased by 26% and 40% respectively) in healthy subjects when imatinib mesylate was co-administered with a singledose of ketoconazole (a CYP3A4 inhibitor). Caution is recommended when administering imatinib mesylate with strong CYP3A4 inhibitors (eg, ketoconazole, itraconazole). Grapefruit juice may also increase plasma concentrations of imatinib and should be avoided. Substances that inhibit the cytochrome P450 isoenszyme (CYP3A4) activity may decrease metabolism and increase imatinib concentrations). Products include:

Nexium Delayed-Release Capsules 645
Nexium Delayed-Release Oral Suspension 645

Estradiol (Imatinib mesylate is an inhibitor of CYP3A4 and may increase the Cmax and AUC of other drugs. Imatinib mesylate increases the mean Cmax and AUC of simvastatin (CYP3A4 substrate) 2-fold and 3.5-fold, respectively, suggesting an inhibition of the CYP3A4 byimatinib mesylate. Particular caution is recommended when administering imatinib mesylate with CYP3A4 substrates that have a narrow therapeutic window (eg, alfentanil, cyclosporine, diergotamine, ergotamine, fentanyl, pimozide, quinidine, sirolimus, or tacrolimus)). Products include:

Activella Tablets 2347
Angeliq Tablets 751
Climara Transdermal System 763
Climara Pro Transdermal System 768
Divigel 3167
Vagifem Tablets 2375

Estradiol Benzoate (Imatinib mesylate is an inhibitor of CYP3A4 and may increase the Cmax and AUC of other drugs. Imatinib mesylate increases the mean Cmax and AUC of simvastatin (CYP3A4 substrate) 2-fold and 3.5-fold, respectively, suggesting an inhibition of the CYP3A4 byimatinib mesylate. Particular caution is recommended when administering imatinib mesylate with CYP3A4 substrates that have a narrow therapeutic window (eg, alfentanil, cyclosporine, diergotamine, ergotamine, fentanyl, pimozide, quinidine, sirolimus, or tacrolimus)).

No products indexed under this heading.

Estradiol Cypionate (Imatinib mesylate is an inhibitor of CYP3A4 and may increase the Cmax and AUC of other drugs. Imatinib mesylate increases the mean Cmax and AUC of simvastatin (CYP3A4 substrate) 2-fold and 3.5-fold, respectively, suggesting an inhibition of the CYP3A4 byimatinib mesylate. Particular caution is recommended when administering imatinib mesylate with CYP3A4 substrates that have a narrow therapeutic window (eg, alfentanil, cyclosporine, diergotamine, ergotamine, fentanyl, pimozide, quinidine, sirolimus, or tacrolimus)).

No products indexed under this heading.

Estradiol Valerate (Imatinib mesylate is an inhibitor of CYP3A4 and may increase the Cmax and AUC of other drugs. Imatinib mesylate increases the mean Cmax and AUC of simvastatin (CYP3A4 substrate) 2-fold and 3.5-fold, respectively, suggesting an inhibition of the CYP3A4 byimatinib mesylate. Particular caution is recommended when administering imatinib mesylate with CYP3A4 substrates that have a narrow therapeutic window (eg, alfentanil, cyclosporine, diergotamine, ergotamine, fentanyl, pimozide, quin-

idine, sirolimus, or tacrolimus)).
No products indexed under this heading.

Ethinyl Estradiol (Imatinib mesylate is an inhibitor of CYP3A4 and may increase the Cmax and AUC of other drugs. Imatinib mesylate increases the mean Cmax and AUC of simvastatin (CYP3A4 substrate) 2-fold and 3.5-fold, respectively, suggesting an inhibition of the CYP3A4 byimatinib mesylate. Particular caution is recommended when administering imatinib mesylate with CYP3A4 substrates that have a narrow therapeutic window (eg, alfentanil, cyclosporine, diergotamine, ergotamine, fentanyl, pimozide, quinidine, sirolimus, or tacrolimus)). Products include:
Lybrel Tablets **3204**
Mircette Tablets **1034**
NuvaRing **2897**
Ortho-Cyclen/Ortho Tri-Cyclen **2449**
Ortho Evra Transdermal System **2437**
Ortho Tri-Cyclen Lo Tablets **2458**
Seasonique Tablets **1046**
Yaz Tablets **805**

Ethosuximide (CYP3A4 inducers may decrease imatinib mesylate Cmax and AUC. The use of concomitant strong CYP3A4 inducers should be avoided (eg, dexamethasone, phenytoin, carbamazepine, rifampin, rifabutin, rifampacin, phenobarbital). If patients must be co-administered a strong CYP3A4 inducer, based on pharmacokinetic studies, the dosage of imatinib mesylate should be increased by at least 50% and clinical response should be carefully monitored).
No products indexed under this heading.

Ethynodiol Diacetate (Imatinib mesylate is an inhibitor of CYP3A4 and may increase the Cmax and AUC of other drugs. Imatinib mesylate increases the mean Cmax and AUC of simvastatin (CYP3A4 substrate) 2-fold and 3.5-fold, respectively, suggesting an inhibition of the CYP3A4 byimatinib mesylate. Particular caution is recommended when administering imatinib mesylate with CYP3A4 substrates that have a narrow therapeutic window (eg, alfentanil, cyclosporine, diergotamine, ergotamine, fentanyl, pimozide, quinidine, sirolimus, or tacrolimus)).
No products indexed under this heading.

Etoposide (Imatinib mesylate is an inhibitor of CYP3A4 and may increase the Cmax and AUC of other drugs. Imatinib mesylate increases the mean Cmax and AUC of simvastatin (CYP3A4 substrate) 2-fold and 3.5-fold, respectively, suggesting an inhibition of the CYP3A4 byimatinib mesylate. Particular caution is recommended when administering imatinib mesylate with CYP3A4 substrates that have a narrow therapeutic window (eg, alfentanil, cyclosporine, diergotamine, ergotamine, fentanyl, pimozide, quinidine, sirolimus, or tacrolimus)).
No products indexed under this heading.

Etoposide Phosphate (Imatinib mesylate is an inhibitor of CYP3A4 and may increase the Cmax and AUC of other drugs. Imatinib mesylate increases the mean Cmax and AUC of simvastatin (CYP3A4 substrate) 2-fold and 3.5-fold, respectively, suggesting an inhibition of the CYP3A4 byimatinib mesylate. Particular caution is recommended when administering imatinib mesylate with CYP3A4 substrates that have a narrow therapeutic window (eg, alfentanil, cyclosporine, diergotamine, ergotamine, fentanyl, pimozide, quinidine, sirolimus, or tacrolimus)).
No products indexed under this heading.

Felbamate (CYP3A4 inducers may decrease imatinib mesylate Cmax and AUC. The use of concomitant strong CYP3A4 inducers should be avoided (eg, dexamethasone, phenytoin, carbamazepine, rifampin, rifabutin, rifampacin, phenobarbital). If patients must be co-administered a strong CYP3A4 inducer, based on pharmacokinetic studies, the dosage of imatinib mesylate should be increased by at least 50% and clinical response should be carefully monitored).
No products indexed under this heading.

Felodipine (Imatinib mesylate is an inhibitor of CYP3A4 and may increase the Cmax and AUC of other drugs. Imatinib mesylate increases the mean Cmax and AUC of simvastatin (CYP3A4 substrate) 2-fold and 3.5-fold, respectively, suggesting an inhibition of the CYP3A4 byimatinib mesylate. Particular caution is recommended when administering imatinib mesylate with CYP3A4 substrates that have a narrow therapeutic window (eg, alfentanil, cyclosporine, diergotamine, ergotamine, fentanyl, pimozide, quinidine, sirolimus, or tacrolimus)).
No products indexed under this heading.

Fentanyl (Imatinib mesylate is an inhibitor of CYP3A4 and may increase the Cmax and AUC of other drugs. Imatinib mesylate increases the mean Cmax and AUC of simvastatin (CYP3A4 substrate) 2-fold and 3.5-fold, respectively, suggesting an inhibition of the CYP3A4 byimatinib mesylate. Particular caution is recommended when administering imatinib mesylate with CYP3A4 substrates that have a narrow therapeutic window (eg, alfentanil, cyclosporine, diergotamine, ergotamine, fentanyl, pimozide, quinidine, sirolimus, or tacrolimus)). Products include:
Duragesic Transdermal System **2405**
Ionsys Transdermal System **2410**

Fentanyl Citrate (Imatinib mesylate is an inhibitor of CYP3A4 and may increase the Cmax and AUC of other drugs. Imatinib mesylate increases the mean Cmax and AUC of simvastatin (CYP3A4 substrate) 2-fold and 3.5-fold, respectively, suggesting an inhibition of the CYP3A4 byimatinib mesylate. Particular caution is recommended when administering imatinib mesylate with CYP3A4 substrates that have a narrow therapeutic window (eg, alfentanil, cyclosporine, diergotamine, ergotamine, fentanyl, pimozide, quinidine, sirolimus, or tacrolimus)). Products include:
Actiq **959**
Fentora Tablets **968**

Flecainide Acetate (In vitro, imatinib mesylate inhibits the cytochrome P450 isoenzyme CYP2D6 activity at similar concentrations that affect CYP3A4 activity. Systemic exposure to substrates of CYP2D6 is expected to be increased when co-administered with imatinib mesylate. No specific studies have been performed and caution is recommended).
No products indexed under this heading.

Fluconazole (CYP3A4 inhibitors may increase imatinib mesylate Cmax and AUC. There was a significant increase in exposure to imatinib (mean Cmax and AUC increased by 26% and 40% respectively) in healthy subjects when imatinib mesylate was co-administered with a singledose of ketoconazole (a CYP3A4 inhibitor). Caution is recommended when administering imatinib mesylate with strong CYP3A4 inhibitors (eg, ketoconazole, itraconazole). Grapefruit juice may also increase plasma concentrations of imatinib and should be avoided. Substances that inhibit the cytochrome P450 isoenszyme (CYP3A4) activity may decrease metabolism and increase imatinib concentrations).
No products indexed under this heading.

Fludrocortisone Acetate (CYP3A4 inducers may decrease imatinib mesylate Cmax and AUC. The use of concomitant strong CYP3A4 inducers should be avoided (eg, dexamethasone, phenytoin, carbamazepine, rifampin, rifabutin, rifampacin, phenobarbital). If patients must be co-administered a strong CYP3A4 inducer, based on pharmacokinetic studies, the dosage of imatinib mesylate should be increased by at least 50% and clinical response should be carefully monitored).
No products indexed under this heading.

Fluoxetine (CYP3A4 inhibitors may increase imatinib mesylate Cmax and AUC. There was a significant increase in exposure to imatinib (mean Cmax and AUC increased by 26% and 40% respectively) in healthy subjects when imatinib mesylate was co-administered with a singledose of ketoconazole (a CYP3A4 inhibitor). Caution is recommended when administering imatinib mesylate with strong CYP3A4 inhibitors (eg, ketoconazole, itraconazole). Grapefruit juice may also increase plasma concentrations of imatinib and should be avoided. Substances that inhibit the cytochrome P450 isoenszyme (CYP3A4) activity may decrease metabolism and increase imatinib concentrations).
No products indexed under this heading.

Fluoxetine Hydrochloride (CYP3A4 inhibitors may increase imatinib mesylate Cmax and AUC. There was a significant increase in exposure to imatinib (mean Cmax and AUC increased by 26% and 40% respectively) in healthy subjects when imatinib mesylate was co-administered with a singledose of ketoconazole (a CYP3A4 inhibitor). Caution is recommended when administering imatinib mesylate with strong CYP3A4 inhibitors (eg, ketoconazole, itraconazole). Grapefruit juice may also increase plasma concentrations of imatinib and should be avoided. Substances that inhibit the cytochrome P450 isoenszyme (CYP3A4) activity may decrease metabolism and increase imatinib concentrations). Products include:
Prozac Weekly Capsules **1852**
Prozac Pulvules and Liquid **1852**
Symbyax Capsules **1871**

Fluphenazine Decanoate (In vitro, imatinib mesylate inhibits the cytochrome P450 isoenzyme CYP2D6 activity at similar concentrations that affect CYP3A4 activity. Systemic exposure to substrates of CYP2D6 is expected to be increased when co-administered with imatinib mesylate. No specific studies have been performed and caution is recommended).
No products indexed under this heading.

Fluphenazine Enanthate (In vitro, imatinib mesylate inhibits the cytochrome P450 isoenzyme CYP2D6 activity at similar concentrations that affect CYP3A4 activity. Systemic exposure to substrates of CYP2D6 is expected to be increased when co-administered with imatinib mesylate. No specific studies have been performed and caution is recommended).
No products indexed under this heading.

Fluphenazine Hydrochloride (In vitro, imatinib mesylate inhibits the cytochrome P450 isoenzyme CYP2D6 activity at similar concentrations that affect CYP3A4 activity. Systemic exposure to substrates of CYP2D6 is expected to be increased when co-administered with imatinib mesylate. No specific studies have been performed and caution is recommended).
No products indexed under this heading.

Fluvastatin Sodium (Imatinib mesylate will increase plasma concentration of CYP3A4 metabolized drugs (eg, certain HMG-CoA reductase inhibitors)). Products include:
Lescol Capsules **2268**
Lescol XL Tablets **2268**

Fluvoxamine Maleate (CYP3A4 inhibitors may increase imatinib mesylate Cmax and AUC. There was a significant increase in exposure to imatinib (mean Cmax and AUC increased by 26% and 40% respectively) in healthy subjects when imatinib mesylate was co-administered with a singledose of ketoconazole (a CYP3A4 inhibitor). Caution is recommended when administering imatinib mesylate with strong CYP3A4 inhibitors (eg, ketoconazole, itraconazole). Grapefruit juice may also increase plasma concentrations of imatinib and should be avoided. Substances that inhibit the cytochrome P450 isoenszyme (CYP3A4) activity may decrease metabolism and increase imatinib concentrations). Products include:
Luvox CR Extended-Release Capsules **1759**

Formoterol Fumarate (In vitro, imatinib mesylate inhibits the cytochrome P450 isoenzyme CYP2D6 activity at similar concentrations that affect CYP3A4 activity. Systemic exposure to substrates of CYP2D6 is expected to be increased when co-administered with imatinib mesyl-

ate. No specific studies have been performed and caution is recommended). Products include:
Foradil Aerolizer 2849
Perforomist Inhalation Solution 1025

Fosamprenavir Calcium (CYP3A4 inhibitors may increase imatinib mesylate Cmax and AUC. There was a significant increase in exposure to imatinib (mean Cmax and AUC increased by 26% and 40% respectively) in healthy subjects when imatinib mesylate was co-administered with a singledose of ketoconazole (a CYP3A4 inhibitor). Caution is recommended when administering imatinib mesylate with strong CYP3A4 inhibitors (eg, ketoconazole, itraconazole). Grapefruit juice may also increase plasma concentrations of imatinib and should be avoided. Substances that inhibit the cytochrome P450 isoenzyme (CYP3A4) activity may decrease metabolism and increase imatinib concentrations). Products include:
Lexiva Oral Suspension 1510
Lexiva Tablets 1510

Fosphenytoin Sodium (CYP3A4 inducers may decrease imatinib mesylate Cmax and AUC. The use of concomitant strong CYP3A4 inducers should be avoided (eg, dexamethasone, phenytoin, carbamazepine, rifampin, rifabutin, rifampacin, phenobarbital). If patients must be co-administered a strong CYP3A4 inducer, based on pharmacokinetic studies, the dosage of imatinib mesylate should be increased by at least 50% and clinical response should be carefully monitored).
No products indexed under this heading.

Galantamine Hydrobromide (In vitro, imatinib mesylate inhibits the cytochrome P450 isoenzyme CYP2D6 activity at similar concentrations that affect CYP3A4 activity. Systemic exposure to substrates of CYP2D6 is expected to be increased when co-administered with imatinib mesylate. No specific studies have been performed and caution is recommended).
No products indexed under this heading.

Garlic Extract (CYP3A4 inducers may decrease imatinib mesylate Cmax and AUC. The use of concomitant strong CYP3A4 inducers should be avoided (eg, dexamethasone, phenytoin, carbamazepine, rifampin, rifabutin, rifampacin, phenobarbital). If patients must be co-administered a strong CYP3A4 inducer, based on pharmacokinetic studies, the dosage of imatinib mesylate should be increased by at least 50% and clinical response should be carefully monitored).
No products indexed under this heading.

Garlic Oil (CYP3A4 inducers may decrease imatinib mesylate Cmax and AUC. The use of concomitant strong CYP3A4 inducers should be avoided (eg, dexamethasone, phenytoin, carbamazepine, rifampin, rifabutin, rifampacin, phenobarbital). If patients must be co-administered a strong CYP3A4 inducer, based on pharmacokinetic studies, the dosage of imatinib mesylate should be increased by at least 50% and clinical response should be carefully monitored).
No products indexed under this heading.

Haloperidol (Imatinib mesylate is an inhibitor of CYP3A4 and may increase the Cmax and AUC of other drugs. Imatinib mesylate increases the mean Cmax and AUC of simvastatin (CYP3A4 substrate) 2-fold and 3.5-fold, respectively, suggesting an inhibition of the CYP3A4 byimatinib mesylate. Particular caution is recommended when administering imatinib mesylate with CYP3A4 substrates that have a narrow therapeutic window (eg, alfentanil, cyclosporine, diergotamine, ergotamine, fentanyl, pimozide, quinidine, sirolimus, or tacrolimus)).
No products indexed under this heading.

Haloperidol Decanoate (Imatinib mesylate is an inhibitor of CYP3A4 and may increase the Cmax and AUC of other drugs. Imatinib mesylate increases the mean Cmax and AUC of simvastatin (CYP3A4 substrate) 2-fold and 3.5-fold, respectively, suggesting an inhibition of the CYP3A4 byimatinib mesylate. Particular caution is recommended when administering imatinib mesylate with CYP3A4 substrates that have a narrow therapeutic window (eg, alfentanil, cyclosporine, diergotamine, ergotamine, fentanyl, pimozide, quinidine, sirolimus, or tacrolimus)).
No products indexed under this heading.

Haloperidol Lactate (Imatinib mesylate is an inhibitor of CYP3A4 and may increase the Cmax and AUC of other drugs. Imatinib mesylate increases the mean Cmax and AUC of simvastatin (CYP3A4 substrate) 2-fold and 3.5-fold, respectively, suggesting an inhibition of the CYP3A4 byimatinib mesylate. Particular caution is recommended when administering imatinib mesylate with CYP3A4 substrates that have a narrow therapeutic window (eg, alfentanil, cyclosporine, diergotamine, ergotamine, fentanyl, pimozide, quinidine, sirolimus, or tacrolimus)).
No products indexed under this heading.

Hydrocodone Bitartrate (In vitro, imatinib mesylate inhibits the cytochrome P450 isoenzyme CYP2D6 activity at similar concentrations that affect CYP3A4 activity. Systemic exposure to substrates of CYP2D6 is expected to be increased when co-administered with imatinib mesylate. No specific studies have been performed and caution is recommended). Products include:
Lortab 5/500 Tablets 3143
Lortab 7.5/500 Tablets 3144
Lortab 10/500 Tablets 3144
Vicodin Tablets 529
Vicodin ES Tablets 530
Vicodin HP Tablets 531
Vicoprofen Tablets 533
Zydone Tablets 1132

Hydrocortisone (CYP3A4 inducers may decrease imatinib mesylate Cmax and AUC. The use of concomitant strong CYP3A4 inducers should be avoided (eg, dexamethasone, phenytoin, carbamazepine, rifampin, rifabutin, rifampacin, phenobarbital). If patients must be co-administered a strong CYP3A4 inducer, based on pharmacokinetic studies, the dosage of imatinib mesylate should be increased by at least 50% and clinical response should be carefully monitored).
No products indexed under this heading.

Hydrocortisone Acetate (CYP3A4 inducers may decrease imatinib mesylate Cmax and AUC. The use of concomitant strong CYP3A4 inducers should be avoided (eg, dexamethasone, phenytoin, carbamazepine, rifampin, rifabutin, rifampacin, phenobarbital). If patients must be co-administered a strong CYP3A4 inducer, based on pharmacokinetic studies, the dosage of imatinib mesylate should be increased by at least 50% and clinical response should be carefully monitored). Products include:
Analpram-HC 1140
Pramosone 1141

Hydrocortisone Butyrate (CYP3A4 inducers may decrease imatinib mesylate Cmax and AUC. The use of concomitant strong CYP3A4 inducers should be avoided (eg, dexamethasone, phenytoin, carbamazepine, rifampin, rifabutin, rifampacin, phenobarbital). If patients must be co-administered a strong CYP3A4 inducer, based on pharmacokinetic studies, the dosage of imatinib mesylate should be increased by at least 50% and clinical response should be carefully monitored).
No products indexed under this heading.

Hydrocortisone Cypionate (CYP3A4 inducers may decrease imatinib mesylate Cmax and AUC. The use of concomitant strong CYP3A4 inducers should be avoided (eg, dexamethasone, phenytoin, carbamazepine, rifampin, rifabutin, rifampacin, phenobarbital). If patients must be co-administered a strong CYP3A4 inducer, based on pharmacokinetic studies, the dosage of imatinib mesylate should be increased by at least 50% and clinical response should be carefully monitored).
No products indexed under this heading.

Hydrocortisone Hemisuccinate (CYP3A4 inducers may decrease imatinib mesylate Cmax and AUC. The use of concomitant strong CYP3A4 inducers should be avoided (eg, dexamethasone, phenytoin, carbamazepine, rifampin, rifabutin, rifampacin, phenobarbital). If patients must be co-administered a strong CYP3A4 inducer, based on pharmacokinetic studies, the dosage of imatinib mesylate should be increased by at least 50% and clinical response should be carefully monitored).
No products indexed under this heading.

Hydrocortisone Probutate (CYP3A4 inducers may decrease imatinib mesylate Cmax and AUC. The use of concomitant strong CYP3A4 inducers should be avoided (eg, dexamethasone, phenytoin, carbamazepine, rifampin, rifabutin, rifampacin, phenobarbital). If patients must be co-administered a strong CYP3A4 inducer, based on pharmacokinetic studies, the dosage of imatinib mesylate should be increased by at least 50% and clinical response should be carefully monitored).
No products indexed under this heading.

Hydrocortisone Sodium Phosphate (CYP3A4 inducers may decrease imatinib mesylate Cmax and AUC. The use of concomitant strong CYP3A4 inducers should be avoided (eg, dexamethasone, phenytoin, carbamazepine, rifampin, rifabutin, rifampacin, phenobarbital). If patients must be co-administered a strong CYP3A4 inducer, based on pharmacokinetic studies, the dosage of imatinib mesylate should be increased by at least 50% and clinical response should be carefully monitored).
No products indexed under this heading.

Hydrocortisone Sodium Succinate (CYP3A4 inducers may decrease imatinib mesylate Cmax and AUC. The use of concomitant strong CYP3A4 inducers should be avoided (eg, dexamethasone, phenytoin, carbamazepine, rifampin, rifabutin, rifampacin, phenobarbital). If patients must be co-administered a strong CYP3A4 inducer, based on pharmacokinetic studies, the dosage of imatinib mesylate should be increased by at least 50% and clinical response should be carefully monitored).
No products indexed under this heading.

Hydrocortisone Valerate (CYP3A4 inducers may decrease imatinib mesylate Cmax and AUC. The use of concomitant strong CYP3A4 inducers should be avoided (eg, dexamethasone, phenytoin, carbamazepine, rifampin, rifabutin, rifampacin, phenobarbital). If patients must be co-administered a strong CYP3A4 inducer, based on pharmacokinetic studies, the dosage of imatinib mesylate should be increased by at least 50% and clinical response should be carefully monitored).
No products indexed under this heading.

Hypericum (Co-administration with inducers of CYP3A4, such as St. John's Wort, may increase the metabolism and decrease imatinib concentrations). Products include:
Satieté Tablets .... ▣ 640

Hypericum Perforatum (CYP3A4 inducers may decrease imatinib mesylate Cmax and AUC. The use of concomitant strong CYP3A4 inducers should be avoided (eg, dexamethasone, phenytoin, carbamazepine, rifampin, rifabutin, rifampacin, phenobarbital). If patients must be co-administered a strong CYP3A4 inducer, based on pharmacokinetic studies, the dosage of imatinib mesylate should be increased by at least 50% and clinical response should be carefully monitored).
No products indexed under this heading.

Imipramine Hydrochloride (In vitro, imatinib mesylate inhibits the cytochrome P450 isoenzyme CYP2D6 activity at similar concentrations that affect CYP3A4 activity. Systemic exposure to substrates of CYP2D6 is expected to be increased when co-administered with imatinib mesylate. No specific studies have been performed and caution is recommended).
No products indexed under this heading.

Imipramine Pamoate (In vitro, imatinib mesylate inhibits the cytochrome P450 isoenzyme CYP2D6 activity at similar concentrations that affect CYP3A4 activity. Systemic exposure to substrates of CYP2D6 is expected to be increased when co-administered with imatinib mesylate. No specific studies have been performed and caution is recommended).
No products indexed under this heading.

Indinavir Sulfate (CYP3A4 inhibitors may increase imatinib mesylate Cmax and AUC. There was a significant increase in exposure to imatinib (mean Cmax and AUC increased by 26% and 40% respectively) in healthy subjects when imatinib mesylate was co-administered with a singledose of ketoconazole (a CYP3A4 inhibitor). Caution is recommended when administering imatinib mesylate with strong CYP3A4 inhibitors (eg, ketoconazole, itraconazole). Grapefruit juice may also increase plasma concentrations of imatinib and should be avoided. Substances that inhibit the cytochrome P450 isoenzyme (CYP3A4) activity may decrease metabolism and increase imatinib concentrations). Products include:
Crixivan Capsules 1979

Indoramin Hydrochloride (In vitro, imatinib mesylate inhibits the cytochrome P450 isoenzyme CYP2D6 activity at similar concentrations that affect CYP3A4 activity. Systemic exposure to substrates of CYP2D6 is expected to be increased when co-administered with imatinib mesylate. No specific studies have been performed and caution is recommended).
No products indexed under this heading.

Isoniazid (CYP3A4 inhibitors may increase imatinib mesylate Cmax and AUC. There was a significant increase in exposure to imatinib (mean Cmax and AUC increased by 26% and 40% respectively) in healthy subjects when imatinib mesylate was co-administered with a singledose of ketoconazole (a CYP3A4 inhibitor). Caution is recommended when administering imatinib mesylate with strong CYP3A4 inhibitors (eg, ketoconazole, itraconazole). Grapefruit juice may also increase plasma concentrations of imatinib and should be avoided. Substances that inhibit the cytochrome P450 isoenzyme (CYP3A4) activity may decrease metabolism and increase imatinib concentrations).
No products indexed under this heading.

Isradipine (Imatinib mesylate is an inhibitor of CYP3A4 and may increase the Cmax and AUC of other drugs. Imatinib mesylate increases the mean Cmax and AUC of simvastatin (CYP3A4 substrate) 2-fold and 3.5-fold, respectively, suggesting an inhibition of the CYP3A4 byimatinib mesylate. Particular caution is recommended when administering imatinib mesylate with CYP3A4 substrates that have a narrow therapeutic window (eg, alfentanil, cyclosporine, diergotamine, ergotamine, fentanyl, pimozide, quinidine, sirolimus, or tacrolimus)). Products include:
DynaCirc CR Controlled Release Tablets 1407

Itraconazole (Co-administration with CYP3A4 inhibitors, such as itraconazole, may decrease the metabolism and increase imatinib concentrations).
No products indexed under this heading.

Ixabepilone (Imatinib mesylate is an inhibitor of CYP3A4 and may increase the Cmax and AUC of other drugs. Imatinib mesylate increases the mean Cmax and AUC of simvastatin (CYP3A4 substrate) 2-fold and 3.5-fold, respectively, suggesting an inhibition of the CYP3A4 byimatinib mesylate. Particular caution is recommended when administering imatinib mesylate with CYP3A4 substrates that have a narrow therapeutic window (eg, alfentanil, cyclosporine, diergotamine, ergotamine, fentanyl, pimozide, quinidine, sirolimus, or tacrolimus)). Products include:
Ixempra Kit for Injection 915

Ketoconazole (Co-administration with inhibitors of CYP3A4, such as ketoconazole, may decrease the metabolism and increase imatinib concentrations; there is a significant increase in exposure to imatinib when co-administered with ketoconazole). Products include:
Extina Foam, 2% 3057
Nizoral A-D Shampoo 1901

Labetalol Hydrochloride (In vitro, imatinib mesylate inhibits the cytochrome P450 isoenzyme CYP2D6 activity at similar concentrations that affect CYP3A4 activity. Systemic exposure to substrates of CYP2D6 is expected to be increased when co-administered with imatinib mesylate. No specific studies have been performed and caution is recommended).
No products indexed under this heading.

Levonorgestrel (Imatinib mesylate is an inhibitor of CYP3A4 and may increase the Cmax and AUC of other drugs. Imatinib mesylate increases the mean Cmax and AUC of simvastatin (CYP3A4 substrate) 2-fold and 3.5-fold, respectively, suggesting an inhibition of the CYP3A4 byimatinib mesylate. Particular caution is recommended when administering imatinib mesylate with CYP3A4 substrates that have a narrow therapeutic window (eg, alfentanil, cyclosporine, diergotamine, ergotamine, fentanyl, pimozide, quinidine, sirolimus, or tacrolimus)). Products include:
Climara Pro Transdermal System 768
Lybrel Tablets 3204
Mirena Intrauterine System 779
Plan B Tablets 1044
Seasonique Tablets 1046

Lidocaine (Imatinib mesylate is an inhibitor of CYP3A4 and may increase the Cmax and AUC of other drugs. Imatinib mesylate increases the mean Cmax and AUC of simvastatin (CYP3A4 substrate) 2-fold and 3.5-fold, respectively, suggesting an inhibition of the CYP3A4 byimatinib mesylate. Particular caution is recommended when administering imatinib mesylate with CYP3A4 substrates that have a narrow therapeutic window (eg, alfentanil, cyclosporine, diergotamine, ergotamine, fentanyl, pimozide, quinidine, sirolimus, or tacrolimus)). Products include:
Lidoderm Patch 1114

Lidocaine Hydrochloride (Imatinib mesylate is an inhibitor of CYP3A4 and may increase the Cmax and AUC of other drugs. Imatinib mesylate increases the mean Cmax and AUC of simvastatin (CYP3A4 substrate) 2-fold and 3.5-fold, respectively, suggesting an inhibition of the CYP3A4 byimatinib mesylate. Particular caution is recommended when administering imatinib mesylate with CYP3A4 substrates that have a narrow therapeutic window (eg, alfentanil, cyclosporine, diergotamine, ergotamine, fentanyl, pimozide, quinidine, sirolimus, or tacrolimus)).
No products indexed under this heading.

Lopinavir (CYP3A4 inhibitors may increase imatinib mesylate Cmax and AUC. There was a significant increase in exposure to imatinib (mean Cmax and AUC increased by 26% and 40% respectively) in healthy subjects when imatinib mesylate was co-administered with a singledose of ketoconazole (a CYP3A4 inhibitor). Caution is recommended when administering imatinib mesylate with strong CYP3A4 inhibitors (eg, ketoconazole, itraconazole). Grapefruit juice may also increase plasma concentrations of imatinib and should be avoided. Substances that inhibit the cytochrome P450 isoenzyme (CYP3A4) activity may decrease metabolism and increase imatinib concentrations). Products include:
Kaletra 452

Loratadine (CYP3A4 inhibitors may increase imatinib mesylate Cmax and AUC. There was a significant increase in exposure to imatinib (mean Cmax and AUC increased by 26% and 40% respectively) in healthy subjects when imatinib mesylate was co-administered with a singledose of ketoconazole (a CYP3A4 inhibitor). Caution is recommended when administering imatinib mesylate with strong CYP3A4 inhibitors (eg, ketoconazole, itraconazole). Grapefruit juice may also increase plasma concentrations of imatinib and should be avoided. Substances that inhibit the cytochrome P450 isoenzyme (CYP3A4) activity may decrease metabolism and increase imatinib concentrations).
No products indexed under this heading.

Lovastatin (Imatinib will increase the plasma concentrations of certain HMG-CoA reductase inhibitors by inhibiting CYP3A4). Products include:
Advicor Tablets 402
Mevacor Tablets 2063

Maprotiline Hydrochloride (In vitro, imatinib mesylate inhibits the cytochrome P450 isoenzyme CYP2D6 activity at similar concentrations that affect CYP3A4 activity. Systemic exposure to substrates of CYP2D6 is expected to be increased when co-administered with imatinib mesylate. No specific studies have been performed and caution is recommended).
No products indexed under this heading.

Meperidine Hydrochloride (In vitro, imatinib mesylate inhibits the cytochrome P450 isoenzyme CYP2D6 activity at similar concentrations that affect CYP3A4 activity. Systemic exposure to substrates of CYP2D6 is expected to be increased when co-administered with imatinib mesylate. No specific studies have been performed and caution is recommended).
No products indexed under this heading.

Mephenytoin (CYP3A4 inducers may decrease imatinib mesylate Cmax and AUC. The use of concomitant strong CYP3A4 inducers should be avoided (eg, dexamethasone, phenytoin, carbamazepine, rifampin, rifabutin, rifampacin, phenobarbital). If patients must be co-administered a strong CYP3A4 inducer, based on pharmacokinetic studies, the dosage of imatinib mesylate should be increased by at least 50% and clinical response should be carefully monitored).
No products indexed under this heading.

Mestranol (Imatinib mesylate is an inhibitor of CYP3A4 and may increase the Cmax and AUC of other drugs. Imatinib mesylate increases the mean Cmax and AUC of simvastatin (CYP3A4 substrate) 2-fold and 3.5-fold, respectively, suggesting an inhibition of the CYP3A4 byimatinib mesylate. Particular caution is recommended when administering imatinib mesylate with CYP3A4 substrates that have a narrow therapeutic window (eg, alfentanil, cyclosporine, diergotamine, ergotamine, fentanyl, pimozide, quinidine, sirolimus, or tacrolimus)).
No products indexed under this heading.

Methadone Hydrochloride (Imatinib mesylate is an inhibitor of CYP3A4 and may increase the Cmax and AUC of other drugs. Imatinib mesylate increases the mean Cmax and AUC of simvastatin (CYP3A4 substrate) 2-fold and 3.5-fold, respectively, suggesting an inhibition of the CYP3A4 byimatinib mesylate. Particular caution is recommended when administering imatinib mesylate with CYP3A4 substrates that have a narrow therapeutic window (eg, alfentanil, cyclosporine, diergotamine, ergotamine, fentanyl, pimozide, quinidine, sirolimus, or tacrolimus)).
No products indexed under this heading.

Methamphetamine Hydrochloride (In vitro, imatinib mesylate inhibits the cytochrome P450 isoenzyme CYP2D6 activity at similar concentrations that affect CYP3A4 activity. Systemic exposure to substrates of CYP2D6 is expected to be increased when co-administered with imatinib mesylate. No specific studies have been performed and caution is recommended).
No products indexed under this heading.

Methsuximide (CYP3A4 inducers may decrease imatinib mesylate Cmax and AUC. The use of concomitant strong CYP3A4 inducers should be avoided (eg, dexamethasone, phenytoin, carbamazepine, rifampin, rifabutin, rifampacin, phenobarbital). If patients must be co-administered a strong CYP3A4 inducer, based on pharmacokinetic studies, the dosage of imatinib mesylate should be increased by at least 50% and clinical response should be carefully monitored).

No products indexed under this heading.

Methylprednisolone (CYP3A4 inducers may decrease imatinib mesylate Cmax and AUC. The use of concomitant strong CYP3A4 inducers should be avoided (eg, dexamethasone, phenytoin, carbamazepine, rifampin, rifabutin, rifampacin, phenobarbital). If patients must be co-administered a strong CYP3A4 inducer, based on pharmacokinetic studies, the dosage of imatinib mesylate should be increased by at least 50% and clinical response should be carefully monitored).

No products indexed under this heading.

Methylprednisolone Acetate (CYP3A4 inducers may decrease imatinib mesylate Cmax and AUC. The use of concomitant strong CYP3A4 inducers should be avoided (eg, dexamethasone, phenytoin, carbamazepine, rifampin, rifabutin, rifampacin, phenobarbital). If patients must be co-administered a strong CYP3A4 inducer, based on pharmacokinetic studies, the dosage of imatinib mesylate should be increased by at least 50% and clinical response should be carefully monitored).

No products indexed under this heading.

Methylprednisolone Sodium Succinate (CYP3A4 inducers may decrease imatinib mesylate Cmax and AUC. The use of concomitant strong CYP3A4 inducers should be avoided (eg, dexamethasone, phenytoin, carbamazepine, rifampin, rifabutin, rifampacin, phenobarbital). If patients must be co-administered a strong CYP3A4 inducer, based on pharmacokinetic studies, the dosage of imatinib mesylate should be increased by at least 50% and clinical response should be carefully monitored).

No products indexed under this heading.

Metoprolol Succinate (In vitro, imatinib mesylate inhibits the cytochrome P450 isoenzyme CYP2D6 activity at similar concentrations that affect CYP3A4 activity. Systemic exposure to substrates of CYP2D6 is expected to be increased when co-administered with imatinib mesylate. No specific studies have been performed and caution is recommended). Products include:

Toprol-XL Tablets 666

Metoprolol Tartrate (In vitro, imatinib mesylate inhibits the cytochrome P450 isoenzyme CYP2D6 activity at similar concentrations that affect CYP3A4 activity. Systemic exposure to substrates of CYP2D6 is expected to be increased when co-administered with imatinib mesylate. No specific studies have been performed and caution is recommended).

No products indexed under this heading.

Metronidazole (CYP3A4 inhibitors may increase imatinib mesylate Cmax and AUC. There was a significant increase in exposure to imatinib (mean Cmax and AUC increased by 26% and 40% respectively) in healthy subjects when imatinib mesylate was co-administered with a singledose of ketoconazole (a CYP3A4 inhibitor). Caution is recommended when administering imatinib mesylate with strong CYP3A4 inhibitors (eg, ketoconazole, itraconazole). Grapefruit juice may also increase plasma concentrations of imatinib and should be avoided. Substances that inhibit the cytochrome P450 isoenzyme (CYP3A4) activity may decrease metabolism and increase imatinib concentrations). Products include:

Pylera Capsules 714

Metronidazole Benzoate (CYP3A4 inhibitors may increase imatinib mesylate Cmax and AUC. There was a significant increase in exposure to imatinib (mean Cmax and AUC increased by 26% and 40% respectively) in healthy subjects when imatinib mesylate was co-administered with a singledose of ketoconazole (a CYP3A4 inhibitor). Caution is recommended when administering imatinib mesylate with strong CYP3A4 inhibitors (eg, ketoconazole, itraconazole). Grapefruit juice may also increase plasma concentrations of imatinib and should be avoided. Substances that inhibit the cytochrome P450 isoenzyme (CYP3A4) activity may decrease metabolism and increase imatinib concentrations).

No products indexed under this heading.

Metronidazole Hydrochloride (CYP3A4 inhibitors may increase imatinib mesylate Cmax and AUC. There was a significant increase in exposure to imatinib (mean Cmax and AUC increased by 26% and 40% respectively) in healthy subjects when imatinib mesylate was co-administered with a singledose of ketoconazole (a CYP3A4 inhibitor). Caution is recommended when administering imatinib mesylate with strong CYP3A4 inhibitors (eg, ketoconazole, itraconazole). Grapefruit juice may also increase plasma concentrations of imatinib and should be avoided. Substances that inhibit the cytochrome P450 isoenzyme (CYP3A4) activity may decrease metabolism and increase imatinib concentrations).

No products indexed under this heading.

Mexiletine Hydrochloride (In vitro, imatinib mesylate inhibits the cytochrome P450 isoenzyme CYP2D6 activity at similar concentrations that affect CYP3A4 activity. Systemic exposure to substrates of CYP2D6 is expected to be increased when co-administered with imatinib mesylate. No specific studies have been performed and caution is recommended).

No products indexed under this heading.

Miconazole (CYP3A4 inhibitors may increase imatinib mesylate Cmax and AUC. There was a significant increase in exposure to imatinib (mean Cmax and AUC increased by 26% and 40% respectively) in healthy subjects when imatinib mesylate was co-administered with a singledose of ketoconazole (a CYP3A4 inhibitor). Caution is recommended when administering imatinib mesylate with strong CYP3A4 inhibitors (eg, ketoconazole, itraconazole). Grapefruit juice may also increase plasma concentrations of imatinib and should be avoided. Substances that inhibit the cytochrome P450 isoenzyme (CYP3A4) activity may decrease metabolism and increase imatinib concentrations).

No products indexed under this heading.

Miconazole Nitrate (CYP3A4 inhibitors may increase imatinib mesylate Cmax and AUC. There was a significant increase in exposure to imatinib (mean Cmax and AUC increased by 26% and 40% respectively) in healthy subjects when imatinib mesylate was co-administered with a singledose of ketoconazole (a CYP3A4 inhibitor). Caution is recommended when administering imatinib mesylate with strong CYP3A4 inhibitors (eg, ketoconazole, itraconazole). Grapefruit juice may also increase plasma concentrations of imatinib and should be avoided. Substances that inhibit the cytochrome P450 isoenzyme (CYP3A4) activity may decrease metabolism and increase imatinib concentrations).

No products indexed under this heading.

Midazolam Hydrochloride (Imatinib mesylate is an inhibitor of CYP3A4 and may increase the Cmax and AUC of other drugs. Imatinib mesylate increases the mean Cmax and AUC of simvastatin (CYP3A4 substrate) 2-fold and 3.5-fold, respectively, suggesting an inhibition of the CYP3A4 byimatinib mesylate. Particular caution is recommended when administering imatinib mesylate with CYP3A4 substrates that have a narrow therapeutic window (eg, alfentanil, cyclosporine, dihergotamine, ergotamine, fentanyl, pimozide, quinidine, sirolimus, or tacrolimus)).

No products indexed under this heading.

Mirtazapine (In vitro, imatinib mesylate inhibits the cytochrome P450 isoenzyme CYP2D6 activity at similar concentrations that affect CYP3A4 activity. Systemic exposure to substrates of CYP2D6 is expected to be increased when co-administered with imatinib mesylate. No specific studies have been performed and caution is recommended). Products include:

Remeron Tablets 2924
RemeronSolTab Tablets 2927

Modafinil (CYP3A4 inducers may decrease imatinib mesylate Cmax and AUC. The use of concomitant strong CYP3A4 inducers should be avoided (eg, dexamethasone, phenytoin, carbamazepine, rifampin, rifabutin, rifampacin, phenobarbital). If patients must be co-administered a strong CYP3A4 inducer, based on pharmacokinetic studies, the dosage of imatinib mesylate should be increased by at least 50% and clinical response should be carefully monitored). Products include:

Provigil Tablets 977

Morphine Sulfate (In vitro, imatinib mesylate inhibits the cytochrome P450 isoenzyme CYP2D6 activity at similar concentrations that affect CYP3A4 activity. Systemic exposure to substrates of CYP2D6 is expected to be increased when co-administered with imatinib mesylate. No specific studies have been performed and caution is recommended). Products include:

Avinza Capsules 1772
DepoDur Injection 1095
MS Contin Tablets 2585

Nefazodone Hydrochloride (CYP3A4 inhibitors may increase imatinib mesylate Cmax and AUC. There was a significant increase in exposure to imatinib (mean Cmax and AUC increased by 26% and 40% respectively) in healthy subjects when imatinib mesylate was co-administered with a singledose of ketoconazole (a CYP3A4 inhibitor). Caution is recommended when administering imatinib mesylate with strong CYP3A4 inhibitors (eg, ketoconazole, itraconazole). Grapefruit juice may also increase plasma concentrations of imatinib and should be avoided. Substances that inhibit the cytochrome P450 isoenzyme (CYP3A4) activity may decrease metabolism and increase imatinib concentrations).

No products indexed under this heading.

Nelfinavir Mesylate (CYP3A4 inhibitors may increase imatinib mesylate Cmax and AUC. There was a significant increase in exposure to imatinib (mean Cmax and AUC increased by 26% and 40% respectively) in healthy subjects when imatinib mesylate was co-administered with a singledose of ketoconazole (a CYP3A4 inhibitor). Caution is recommended when administering imatinib mesylate with strong CYP3A4 inhibitors (eg, ketoconazole, itraconazole). Grapefruit juice may also increase plasma concentrations of imatinib and should be avoided. Substances that inhibit the cytochrome P450 isoenzyme (CYP3A4) activity may decrease metabolism and increase imatinib concentrations).

No products indexed under this heading.

Nevirapine (CYP3A4 inducers may decrease imatinib mesylate Cmax and AUC. The use of concomitant strong CYP3A4 inducers should be avoided (eg, dexamethasone, phenytoin, carbamazepine, rifampin, rifabutin, rifampacin, phenobarbital). If patients must be co-administered a strong CYP3A4 inducer, based on pharmacokinetic studies, the dosage of imatinib mesylate should be increased by at least 50% and clinical response should be carefully monitored). Products include:

Viramune Oral Suspension 873
Viramune Tablets 873

Niacinamide (CYP3A4 inhibitors may increase imatinib mesylate Cmax and AUC. There was a significant increase in exposure to imatinib (mean Cmax and AUC increased by 26% and 40% respectively) in healthy subjects when imatinib mesylate was co-administered with a singledose of ketoconazole (a CYP3A4 inhibitor). Caution is recommended when administering imatinib mesylate with strong CYP3A4 inhibitors (eg, ketoconazole, itraconazole). Grapefruit juice may also increase plasma concentrations of imatinib and should be avoided. Substances that inhibit the cytochrome P450 isoenzyme (CYP3A4) activity may decrease metabolism and increase imatinib concentrations). Products include:

BioLean Free Tablets 635

Nicardipine Hydrochloride (Imatinib mesylate is an inhibitor of CYP3A4 and may increase the Cmax and AUC of other drugs. Imatinib mesylate increases the mean Cmax and AUC of simvastatin (CYP3A4 substrate) 2-fold and 3.5-fold, respectively, suggesting an inhibition of the CYP3A4 byimatinib mesylate. Particular caution is recommended when administering imatinib mesylate with CYP3A4 substrates that have a narrow therapeutic window (eg, alfentanil, cyclosporine, diergotamine, ergotamine, fentanyl, pimozide, quinidine, sirolimus, or tacrolimus)). Products include:

Cardene I.V. **1093**

Nicotinamide (CYP3A4 inhibitors may increase imatinib mesylate Cmax and AUC. There was a significant increase in exposure to imatinib (mean Cmax and AUC increased by 26% and 40% respectively) in healthy subjects when imatinib mesylate was co-administered with a singledose of ketoconazole (a CYP3A4 inhibitor). Caution is recommended when administering imatinib mesylate with strong CYP3A4 inhibitors (eg, ketoconazole, itraconazole). Grapefruit juice may also increase plasma concentrations of imatinib and should be avoided. Substances that inhibit the cytochrome P450 isoenszyme (CYP3A4) activity may decrease metabolism and increase imatinib concentrations).

No products indexed under this heading.

Nifedipine (CYP3A4 inhibitors may increase imatinib mesylate Cmax and AUC. There was a significant increase in exposure to imatinib (mean Cmax and AUC increased by 26% and 40% respectively) in healthy subjects when imatinib mesylate was co-administered with a singledose of ketoconazole (a CYP3A4 inhibitor). Caution is recommended when administering imatinib mesylate with strong CYP3A4 inhibitors (eg, ketoconazole, itraconazole). Grapefruit juice may also increase plasma concentrations of imatinib and should be avoided. Substances that inhibit the cytochrome P450 isoenszyme (CYP3A4) activity may decrease metabolism and increase imatinib concentrations).

No products indexed under this heading.

Nimodipine (Imatinib mesylate is an inhibitor of CYP3A4 and may increase the Cmax and AUC of other drugs. Imatinib mesylate increases the mean Cmax and AUC of simvastatin (CYP3A4 substrate) 2-fold and 3.5-fold, respectively, suggesting an inhibition of the CYP3A4 byimatinib mesylate. Particular caution is recommended when administering imatinib mesylate with CYP3A4 substrates that have a narrow therapeutic window (eg, alfentanil, cyclosporine, diergotamine, ergotamine, fentanyl, pimozide, quinidine, sirolimus, or tacrolimus)). Products include:

Nimotop Capsules **790**

Nisoldipine (Imatinib mesylate is an inhibitor of CYP3A4 and may increase the Cmax and AUC of other drugs. Imatinib mesylate increases the mean Cmax and AUC of simvastatin (CYP3A4 substrate) 2-fold and 3.5-fold, respectively, suggesting an inhibition of the CYP3A4 byimatinib mesylate. Particular caution is recommended when administering imatinib mesylate with CYP3A4 substrates that have a narrow therapeutic window (eg, alfentanil, cyclosporine, diergotamine, ergotamine, fentanyl, pimozide, quinidine, sirolimus, or tacrolimus)). Products include:

Sular Extended Release Tablets **2975**

Nitrendipine (Imatinib mesylate is an inhibitor of CYP3A4 and may increase the Cmax and AUC of other drugs. Imatinib mesylate increases the mean Cmax and AUC of simvastatin (CYP3A4 substrate) 2-fold and 3.5-fold, respectively, suggesting an inhibition of the CYP3A4 byimatinib mesylate. Particular caution is recommended when administering imatinib mesylate with CYP3A4 substrates that have a narrow therapeutic window (eg, alfentanil, cyclosporine, diergotamine, ergotamine, fentanyl, pimozide, quinidine, sirolimus, or tacrolimus)).

No products indexed under this heading.

Norethindrone (Imatinib mesylate is an inhibitor of CYP3A4 and may increase the Cmax and AUC of other drugs. Imatinib mesylate increases the mean Cmax and AUC of simvastatin (CYP3A4 substrate) 2-fold and 3.5-fold, respectively, suggesting an inhibition of the CYP3A4 byimatinib mesylate. Particular caution is recommended when administering imatinib mesylate with CYP3A4 substrates that have a narrow therapeutic window (eg, alfentanil, cyclosporine, diergotamine, ergotamine, fentanyl, pimozide, quinidine, sirolimus, or tacrolimus)). Products include:

Ortho Micronor Tablets **2446**

Norethindrone Acetate (Imatinib mesylate is an inhibitor of CYP3A4 and may increase the Cmax and AUC of other drugs. Imatinib mesylate increases the mean Cmax and AUC of simvastatin (CYP3A4 substrate) 2-fold and 3.5-fold, respectively, suggesting an inhibition of the CYP3A4 byimatinib mesylate. Particular caution is recommended when administering imatinib mesylate with CYP3A4 substrates that have a narrow therapeutic window (eg, alfentanil, cyclosporine, diergotamine, ergotamine, fentanyl, pimozide, quinidine, sirolimus, or tacrolimus)). Products include:

Activella Tablets **2347**

Norfloxacin (CYP3A4 inhibitors may increase imatinib mesylate Cmax and AUC. There was a significant increase in exposure to imatinib (mean Cmax and AUC increased by 26% and 40% respectively) in healthy subjects when imatinib mesylate was co-administered with a singledose of ketoconazole (a CYP3A4 inhibitor). Caution is recommended when administering imatinib mesylate with strong CYP3A4 inhibitors (eg, ketoconazole, itraconazole). Grapefruit juice may also increase plasma concentrations of imatinib and should be avoided. Substances that inhibit the cytochrome P450 isoenszyme (CYP3A4) activity may decrease metabolism and increase imatinib concentrations). Products include:

Noroxin Tablets **2069**

Norgestrel (Imatinib mesylate is an inhibitor of CYP3A4 and may increase the Cmax and AUC of other drugs. Imatinib mesylate increases the mean Cmax and AUC of simvastatin (CYP3A4 substrate) 2-fold and 3.5-fold, respectively, suggesting an inhibition of the CYP3A4 byimatinib mesylate. Particular caution is recommended when administering imatinib mesylate with CYP3A4 substrates that have a narrow therapeutic window (eg, alfentanil, cyclosporine, diergotamine, ergotamine, fentanyl, pimozide, quinidine, sirolimus, or tacrolimus)).

No products indexed under this heading.

Nortriptyline Hydrochloride (In vitro, imatinib mesylate inhibits the cytochrome P450 isoenzyme CYP2D6 activity at similar concentrations that affect CYP3A4 activity. Systemic exposure to substrates of CYP2D6 is expected to be increased when co-administered with imatinib mesylate. No specific studies have been performed and caution is recommended).

No products indexed under this heading.

Olanzapine (In vitro, imatinib mesylate inhibits the cytochrome P450 isoenzyme CYP2D6 activity at similar concentrations that affect CYP3A4 activity. Systemic exposure to substrates of CYP2D6 is expected to be increased when co-administered with imatinib mesylate. No specific studies have been performed and caution is recommended). Products include:

Symbyax Capsules **1871**
Zyprexa Tablets **1883**
Zyprexa IntraMuscular **1883**
Zyprexa ZYDIS Orally Disintegrating Tablets **1883**

Omeprazole (CYP3A4 inhibitors may increase imatinib mesylate Cmax and AUC. There was a significant increase in exposure to imatinib (mean Cmax and AUC increased by 26% and 40% respectively) in healthy subjects when imatinib mesylate was co-administered with a singledose of ketoconazole (a CYP3A4 inhibitor). Caution is recommended when administering imatinib mesylate with strong CYP3A4 inhibitors (eg, ketoconazole, itraconazole). Grapefruit juice may also increase plasma concentrations of imatinib and should be avoided. Substances that inhibit the cytochrome P450 isoenszyme (CYP3A4) activity may decrease metabolism and increase imatinib concentrations).

No products indexed under this heading.

Ondansetron (Imatinib mesylate is an inhibitor of CYP3A4 and may increase the Cmax and AUC of other drugs. Imatinib mesylate increases the mean Cmax and AUC of simvastatin (CYP3A4 substrate) 2-fold and 3.5-fold, respectively, suggesting an inhibition of the CYP3A4 byimatinib mesylate. Particular caution is recommended when administering imatinib mesylate with CYP3A4 substrates that have a narrow therapeutic window (eg, alfentanil, cyclosporine, diergotamine, ergotamine, fentanyl, pimozide, quinidine, sirolimus, or tacrolimus)). Products include:

Zofran ODT Orally Disintegrating Tablets **1687**

Ondansetron Hydrochloride (Imatinib mesylate is an inhibitor of CYP3A4 and may increase the Cmax and AUC of other drugs. Imatinib mesylate increases the mean Cmax and AUC of simvastatin (CYP3A4 substrate) 2-fold and 3.5-fold, respectively, suggesting an inhibition of the CYP3A4 byimatinib mesylate. Particular caution is recommended when administering imatinib mesylate with CYP3A4 substrates that have a narrow therapeutic window (eg, alfentanil, cyclosporine, diergotamine, ergotamine, fentanyl, pimozide, quinidine, sirolimus, or tacrolimus)). Products include:

Zofran Injection **1682**
Zofran **1687**

Oxcarbazepine (CYP3A4 inducers may decrease imatinib mesylate Cmax and AUC. The use of concomitant strong CYP3A4 inducers should be avoided (eg, dexamethasone, phenytoin, carbamazepine, rifampin, rifabutin, rifampacin, phenobarbital). If patients must be co-administered a strong CYP3A4 inducer, based on pharmacokinetic studies, the dosage of imatinib mesylate should be increased by at least 50% and clinical response should be carefully monitored).

No products indexed under this heading.

Oxycodone Hydrochloride (In vitro, imatinib mesylate inhibits the cytochrome P450 isoenzyme CYP2D6 activity at similar concentrations that affect CYP3A4 activity. Systemic exposure to substrates of CYP2D6 is expected to be increased when co-administered with imatinib mesylate. No specific studies have been performed and caution is recommended). Products include:

OxyContin Tablets **2589**
OxyIR Capsules **2593**
Percocet Tablets **1127**
Percodan Tablets **1130**

Paclitaxel (Imatinib mesylate is an inhibitor of CYP3A4 and may increase the Cmax and AUC of other drugs. Imatinib mesylate increases the mean Cmax and AUC of simvastatin (CYP3A4 substrate) 2-fold and 3.5-fold, respectively, suggesting an inhibition of the CYP3A4 byimatinib mesylate. Particular caution is recommended when administering imatinib mesylate with CYP3A4 substrates that have a narrow therapeutic window (eg, alfentanil, cyclosporine, diergotamine, ergotamine, fentanyl, pimozide, quinidine, sirolimus, or tacrolimus)).

No products indexed under this heading.

Paroxetine Hydrochloride (CYP3A4 inhibitors may increase imatinib mesylate Cmax and AUC. There was a significant increase in exposure to imatinib (mean Cmax and AUC increased by 26% and 40% respectively) in healthy subjects when imatinib mesylate was co-administered with a singledose of ketoconazole (a CYP3A4 inhibitor). Caution is recommended when administering imatinib mesylate with strong CYP3A4 inhibitors (eg, ketoconazole, itraconazole). Grapefruit juice may also increase plasma concentrations of imatinib and should be avoided. Substances that inhibit the cytochrome P450 isoenszyme

(CYP3A4) activity may decrease metabolism and increase imatinib concentrations). Products include:

Paxil 1535

Paxil CR Controlled-Release Tablets 1544

Phenobarbital (Co-administration with inducers of CYP3A4, such as phenobarbital, may increase the metabolism and decrease imatinib concentrations). Products include:

Donnatal Extentabs 2507

Phenobarbital Sodium (CYP3A4 inducers may decrease imatinib mesylate Cmax and AUC. The use of concomitant strong CYP3A4 inducers should be avoided (eg, dexamethasone, phenytoin, carbamazepine, rifampin, rifabutin, rifampacin, phenobarbital). If patients must be co-administered a strong CYP3A4 inducer, based on pharmacokinetic studies, the dosage of imatinib mesylate should be increased by at least 50% and clinical response should be carefully monitored).

No products indexed under this heading.

Phenytoin (CYP3A4 inducers may decrease imatinib mesylate Cmax and AUC. The use of concomitant strong CYP3A4 inducers should be avoided (eg, dexamethasone, phenytoin, carbamazepine, rifampin, rifabutin, rifampacin, phenobarbital). If patients must be co-administered a strong CYP3A4 inducer, based on pharmacokinetic studies, the dosage of imatinib mesylate should be increased by at least 50% and clinical response should be carefully monitored).

No products indexed under this heading.

Phenytoin Sodium (CYP3A4 inducers may decrease imatinib mesylate Cmax and AUC. The use of concomitant strong CYP3A4 inducers should be avoided (eg, dexamethasone, phenytoin, carbamazepine, rifampin, rifabutin, rifampacin, phenobarbital). If patients must be co-administered a strong CYP3A4 inducer, based on pharmacokinetic studies, the dosage of imatinib mesylate should be increased by at least 50% and clinical response should be carefully monitored). Products include:

Phenytek Capsules 2192

Pimozide (Particular caution is recommended when administering imatinib with CYP3A4 substrates that have a narrow therapeutic window).

No products indexed under this heading.

Pindolol (In vitro, imatinib mesylate inhibits the cytochrome P450 isoenzyme CYP2D6 activity at similar concentrations that affect CYP3A4 activity. Systemic exposure to substrates of CYP2D6 is expected to be increased when co-administered with imatinib mesylate. No specific studies have been performed and caution is recommended).

No products indexed under this heading.

Polyestradiol Phosphate (Imatinib mesylate is an inhibitor of CYP3A4 and may increase the Cmax and AUC of other drugs. Imatinib mesylate increases the mean Cmax and AUC of simvastatin (CYP3A4 substrate) 2-fold and 3.5-fold, respectively, suggesting an inhibition of the CYP3A4 byimatinib mesylate. Particular caution is recommended when administering imatinib mesylate with CYP3A4 substrates that have a narrow therapeutic window (eg, alfentanil, cyclosporine, diergotamine, ergotamine, fentanyl, pimozide, quinidine, sirolimus, or tacrolimus)).

No products indexed under this heading.

Pravastatin Sodium (Imatinib mesylate will increase plasma concentration of CYP3A4 metabolized drugs (eg, certain HMG-CoA reductase inhibitors)).

No products indexed under this heading.

Prednisolone Acetate (CYP3A4 inducers may decrease imatinib mesylate Cmax and AUC. The use of concomitant strong CYP3A4 inducers should be avoided (eg, dexamethasone, phenytoin, carbamazepine, rifampin, rifabutin, rifampacin, phenobarbital). If patients must be co-administered a strong CYP3A4 inducer, based on pharmacokinetic studies, the dosage of imatinib mesylate should be increased by at least 50% and clinical response should be carefully monitored). Products include:

Pred Forte Ophthalmic Suspension .... ⊙227

Pred Mild Ophthalmic Suspension .... ⊙230

Pred-G Ophthalmic Ointment .... ⊙229

Pred-G Ophthalmic Suspension ...... ⊙228

Prednisolone Sodium Phosphate (CYP3A4 inducers may decrease imatinib mesylate Cmax and AUC. The use of concomitant strong CYP3A4 inducers should be avoided (eg, dexamethasone, phenytoin, carbamazepine, rifampin, rifabutin, rifampacin, phenobarbital). If patients must be co-administered a strong CYP3A4 inducer, based on pharmacokinetic studies, the dosage of imatinib mesylate should be increased by at least 50% and clinical response should be carefully monitored).

No products indexed under this heading.

Prednisolone Tebutate (CYP3A4 inducers may decrease imatinib mesylate Cmax and AUC. The use of concomitant strong CYP3A4 inducers should be avoided (eg, dexamethasone, phenytoin, carbamazepine, rifampin, rifabutin, rifampacin, phenobarbital). If patients must be co-administered a strong CYP3A4 inducer, based on pharmacokinetic studies, the dosage of imatinib mesylate should be increased by at least 50% and clinical response should be carefully monitored).

No products indexed under this heading.

Prednisone (CYP3A4 inducers may decrease imatinib mesylate Cmax and AUC. The use of concomitant strong CYP3A4 inducers should be avoided (eg, dexamethasone, phenytoin, carbamazepine, rifampin, rifabutin, rifampacin, phenobarbital). If patients must be co-administered a strong CYP3A4 inducer, based on pharmacokinetic studies, the dosage of imatinib mesylate should be increased by at least 50% and clinical response should be carefully monitored).

No products indexed under this heading.

Primidone (CYP3A4 inducers may decrease imatinib mesylate Cmax and AUC. The use of concomitant strong CYP3A4 inducers should be avoided (eg, dexamethasone, phenytoin, carbamazepine, rifampin, rifabutin, rifampacin, phenobarbital). If patients must be co-administered a strong CYP3A4 inducer, based on pharmacokinetic studies, the dosage of imatinib mesylate should be increased by at least 50% and clinical response should be carefully monitored).

No products indexed under this heading.

Propafenone Hydrochloride (In vitro, imatinib mesylate inhibits the cytochrome P450 isoenzyme CYP2D6 activity at similar concentrations that affect CYP3A4 activity. Systemic exposure to substrates of CYP2D6 is expected to be increased when co-administered with imatinib mesylate. No specific studies have been performed and caution is recommended). Products include:

Rythmol Tablets 1586

Rythmol SR Capsules 1590

Propoxyphene Hydrochloride (CYP3A4 inhibitors may increase imatinib mesylate Cmax and AUC. There was a significant increase in exposure to imatinib (mean Cmax and AUC increased by 26% and 40% respectively) in healthy subjects when imatinib mesylate was co-administered with a singledose of ketoconazole (a CYP3A4 inhibitor). Caution is recommended when administering imatinib mesylate with strong CYP3A4 inhibitors (eg, ketoconazole, itraconazole). Grapefruit juice may also increase plasma concentrations of imatinib and should be avoided. Substances that inhibit the cytochrome P450 isoenszyme (CYP3A4) activity may decrease metabolism and increase imatinib concentrations).

No products indexed under this heading.

Propoxyphene Napsylate (CYP3A4 inhibitors may increase imatinib mesylate Cmax and AUC. There was a significant increase in exposure to imatinib (mean Cmax and AUC increased by 26% and 40% respectively) in healthy subjects when imatinib mesylate was co-administered with a singledose of ketoconazole (a CYP3A4 inhibitor). Caution is recommended when administering imatinib mesylate with strong CYP3A4 inhibitors (eg, ketoconazole, itraconazole). Grapefruit juice may also increase plasma concentrations of imatinib and should be avoided. Substances that inhibit the cytochrome P450 isoenszyme (CYP3A4) activity may decrease metabolism and increase imatinib concentrations).

No products indexed under this heading.

Propranolol Hydrochloride (In vitro, imatinib mesylate inhibits the cytochrome P450 isoenzyme CYP2D6 activity at similar concentrations that affect CYP3A4 activity. Systemic exposure to substrates of CYP2D6 is expected to be increased when co-administered with imatinib mesylate. No specific studies have been performed and caution is recommended). Products include:

InnoPran XL Extended Release Capsules 1484

Quetiapine Fumarate (In vitro, imatinib mesylate inhibits the cytochrome P450 isoenzyme CYP2D6 activity at similar concentrations that affect CYP3A4 activity. Systemic exposure to substrates of CYP2D6 is expected to be increased when co-administered with imatinib mesylate. No specific studies have been performed and caution is recommended).

No products indexed under this heading.

Quinidine (CYP3A4 inhibitors may increase imatinib mesylate Cmax and AUC. There was a significant increase in exposure to imatinib (mean Cmax and AUC increased by 26% and 40% respectively) in healthy subjects when imatinib mesylate was co-administered with a singledose of ketoconazole (a CYP3A4 inhibitor). Caution is recommended when administering imatinib mesylate with strong CYP3A4 inhibitors (eg, ketoconazole, itraconazole). Grapefruit juice may also increase plasma concentrations of imatinib and should be avoided. Substances that inhibit the cytochrome P450 isoenszyme (CYP3A4) activity may decrease metabolism and increase imatinib concentrations).

No products indexed under this heading.

Quinidine Gluconate (Imatinib mesylate is an inhibitor of CYP3A4 and may increase the Cmax and AUC of other drugs. Imatinib mesylate increases the mean Cmax and AUC of simvastatin (CYP3A4 substrate) 2-fold and 3.5-fold, respectively, suggesting an inhibition of the CYP3A4 byimatinib mesylate. Particular caution is recommended when administering imatinib mesylate with CYP3A4 substrates that have a narrow therapeutic window (eg, alfentanil, cyclosporine, diergotamine, ergotamine, fentanyl, pimozide, quinidine, sirolimus, or tacrolimus)).

No products indexed under this heading.

Quinidine Hydrochloride (CYP3A4 inhibitors may increase imatinib mesylate Cmax and AUC. There was a significant increase in exposure to imatinib (mean Cmax and AUC increased by 26% and 40% respectively) in healthy subjects when imatinib mesylate was co-administered with a singledose of ketoconazole (a CYP3A4 inhibitor). Caution is recommended when administering imatinib mesylate with strong CYP3A4 inhibitors (eg, ketoconazole, itraconazole). Grapefruit juice may also increase plasma concentrations of imatinib and should be avoided. Substances that inhibit the cytochrome P450 isoenszyme (CYP3A4) activity may decrease metabolism and increase imatinib concentrations).

No products indexed under this heading.

Quinidine Polygalacturonate (CYP3A4 inhibitors may increase imatinib mesylate Cmax and AUC. There was a significant increase in exposure to imatinib (mean Cmax and AUC increased by 26% and 40% respectively) in healthy subjects when imatinib mesylate was co-administered with a singledose of ketoconazole (a CYP3A4 inhibitor). Caution is recommended when administering imatinib mesylate with strong CYP3A4 inhibitors (eg, ketoconazole, itraconazole). Grapefruit juice may also increase plasma concentrations of imatinib and should be avoided. Substances that inhibit the cytochrome P450 isoenszyme (CYP3A4) activity may decrease metabolism and increase imatinib concentrations).

No products indexed under this heading.

Quinidine Sulfate (CYP3A4 inhibitors may increase imatinib mesylate Cmax and AUC. There was a significant increase in exposure to imatinib (mean Cmax and AUC increased by 26% and 40% respectively) in healthy subjects when imatinib mesylate was co-administered with a singledose of ketoconazole (a CYP3A4 inhibitor). Caution is recommended when administering imatinib mesylate with strong CYP3A4 inhibitors (eg, ketoconazole, itraconazole). Grapefruit juice may also increase plasma concentrations of imatinib and should be avoided. Substances that inhibit the cytochrome P450 isoenszyme (CYP3A4) activity may decrease metabolism and increase imatinib concentrations).

No products indexed under this heading.

Quinine (CYP3A4 inhibitors may increase imatinib mesylate Cmax and AUC. There was a significant increase in exposure to imatinib (mean Cmax and AUC increased by 26% and 40% respectively) in healthy subjects when imatinib mesylate was co-administered with a singledose of ketoconazole (a CYP3A4 inhibitor). Caution is recommended when administering imatinib mesylate with strong CYP3A4 inhibitors (eg, ketoconazole, itraconazole). Grapefruit juice may also increase plasma concentrations of imatinib and should be avoided. Substances that inhibit the cytochrome P450 isoenszyme (CYP3A4) activity may decrease metabolism and increase imatinib concentrations).

No products indexed under this heading.

Quinine Sulfate (CYP3A4 inhibitors may increase imatinib mesylate Cmax and AUC. There was a significant increase in exposure to imatinib (mean Cmax and AUC increased by 26% and 40% respectively) in healthy subjects when imatinib mesylate was co-administered with a singledose of ketoconazole (a CYP3A4 inhibitor). Caution is recommended when administering imatinib mesylate with strong CYP3A4 inhibitors (eg, ketoconazole, itraconazole). Grapefruit juice may also increase plasma concentrations of imatinib and should be avoided. Substances that inhibit the cytochrome P450 isoenszyme (CYP3A4) activity may decrease metabolism and increase imatinib concentrations).

No products indexed under this heading.

Quinupristin (CYP3A4 inhibitors may increase imatinib mesylate Cmax and AUC. There was a significant increase in exposure to imatinib (mean Cmax and AUC increased by 26% and 40% respectively) in healthy subjects when imatinib mesylate was co-administered with a singledose of ketoconazole (a CYP3A4 inhibitor). Caution is recommended when administering imatinib mesylate with strong CYP3A4 inhibitors (eg, ketoconazole, itraconazole). Grapefruit juice may also increase plasma concentrations of imatinib and should be avoided. Substances that inhibit the cytochrome P450 isoenszyme (CYP3A4) activity may decrease metabolism and increase imatinib concentrations).

No products indexed under this heading.

Ranitidine Bismuth Citrate (CYP3A4 inhibitors may increase imatinib mesylate Cmax and AUC. There was a significant increase in exposure to imatinib (mean Cmax and AUC increased by 26% and 40% respectively) in healthy subjects when imatinib mesylate was co-administered with a singledose of ketoconazole (a CYP3A4 inhibitor). Caution is recommended when administering imatinib mesylate with strong CYP3A4 inhibitors (eg, ketoconazole, itraconazole). Grapefruit juice may also increase plasma concentrations of imatinib and should be avoided. Substances that inhibit the cytochrome P450 isoenszyme (CYP3A4) activity may decrease metabolism and increase imatinib concentrations).

No products indexed under this heading.

Ranitidine Hydrochloride (CYP3A4 inhibitors may increase imatinib mesylate Cmax and AUC. There was a significant increase in exposure to imatinib (mean Cmax and AUC increased by 26% and 40% respectively) in healthy subjects when imatinib mesylate was co-administered with a singledose of ketoconazole (a CYP3A4 inhibitor). Caution is recommended when administering imatinib mesylate with strong CYP3A4 inhibitors (eg, ketoconazole, itraconazole). Grapefruit juice may also increase plasma concentrations of imatinib and should be avoided. Substances that inhibit the cytochrome P450 isoenszyme (CYP3A4) activity may decrease metabolism and increase imatinib concentrations). Products include:

Zantac 75 Tablets 603
Zantac 1670
Zantac Injection 1666
Zantac Injection Pharmacy Bulk Package 1668
Maximum Strength Zantac 150 Tablets 603
Maximum Strength Zantac 150 Cool Mint Tablets 603

Rifabutin (CYP3A4 inducers may decrease imatinib mesylate Cmax and AUC. The use of concomitant strong CYP3A4 inducers should be avoided (eg, dexamethasone, phenytoin, carbamazepine, rifampin, rifabutin, rifampacin, phenobarbital). If patients must be co-administered a strong CYP3A4 inducer, based on pharmacokinetic studies, the dosage of imatinib mesylate should be increased by at least 50% and clinical response should be carefully monitored).

No products indexed under this heading.

Rifampicin (CYP3A4 inducers may decrease imatinib mesylate Cmax and AUC. The use of concomitant strong CYP3A4 inducers should be avoided (eg, dexamethasone, phenytoin, carbamazepine, rifampin, rifabutin, rifampacin, phenobarbital). If patients must be co-administered a strong CYP3A4 inducer, based on pharmacokinetic studies, the dosage of imatinib mesylate should be increased by at least 50% and clinical response should be carefully monitored).

No products indexed under this heading.

Rifampin (Pretreatment of healthy volunteers with multiple doses of rifampin followed by a single dose of imatinib mesylate, increased imatinib mesylate oral-dose clearance by 3.8 fold, which significantly ($p<0.05$) decreased mean Cmax and AUC. If alternative treatment cannot be administered, a dose adjustment should be considered).

No products indexed under this heading.

Rifapentine (CYP3A4 inducers may decrease imatinib mesylate Cmax and AUC. The use of concomitant strong CYP3A4 inducers should be avoided (eg, dexamethasone, phenytoin, carbamazepine, rifampin, rifabutin, rifampacin, phenobarbital). If patients must be co-administered a strong CYP3A4 inducer, based on pharmacokinetic studies, the dosage of imatinib mesylate should be increased by at least 50% and clinical response should be carefully monitored).

No products indexed under this heading.

Risperidone (In vitro, imatinib mesylate inhibits the cytochrome P450 isoenzyme CYP2D6 activity at similar concentrations that affect CYP3A4 activity. Systemic exposure to substrates of CYP2D6 is expected to be increased when co-administered with imatinib mesylate. No specific studies have been performed and caution is recommended). Products include:

Risperdal Consta Long-Acting Injection 1753

Ritonavir (CYP3A4 inhibitors may increase imatinib mesylate Cmax and AUC. There was a significant increase in exposure to imatinib (mean Cmax and AUC increased by 26% and 40% respectively) in healthy subjects when imatinib mesylate was co-administered with a singledose of ketoconazole (a CYP3A4 inhibitor). Caution is recommended when administering imatinib mesylate with strong CYP3A4 inhibitors (eg, ketoconazole, itraconazole). Grapefruit juice may also increase plasma concentrations of imatinib and should be avoided. Substances that inhibit the cytochrome P450 isoenszyme (CYP3A4) activity may decrease metabolism and increase imatinib concentrations). Products include:

Kaletra 452
Norvir 489

Rosuvastatin Calcium (Imatinib mesylate will increase plasma concentration of CYP3A4 metabolized drugs (eg, certain HMG-CoA reductase inhibitors)). Products include:

Crestor Tablets 677

Saquinavir (CYP3A4 inhibitors may increase imatinib mesylate Cmax and AUC. There was a significant increase in exposure to imatinib (mean Cmax and AUC increased by 26% and 40% respectively) in healthy subjects when imatinib mesylate was co-administered with a singledose of ketoconazole (a CYP3A4 inhibitor). Caution is recommended when administering imatinib mesylate with strong CYP3A4 inhibitors (eg, ketoconazole, itraconazole). Grapefruit juice may also increase plasma concentrations of imatinib and should be avoided. Substances that inhibit the cytochrome P450 isoenszyme (CYP3A4) activity may decrease metabolism and increase imatinib concentrations).

No products indexed under this heading.

Saquinavir Mesylate (CYP3A4 inhibitors may increase imatinib mesylate Cmax and AUC. There was a significant increase in exposure to imatinib (mean Cmax and AUC increased by 26% and 40% respectively) in healthy subjects when imatinib mesylate was co-administered with a singledose of ketoconazole (a CYP3A4 inhibitor). Caution is recommended when administering imatinib mesylate with strong CYP3A4 inhibitors (eg, ketoconazole, itraconazole). Grapefruit juice may also increase plasma concentrations of imatinib and should be avoided. Substances that inhibit the cytochrome P450 isoenszyme (CYP3A4) activity may decrease metabolism and increase imatinib concentrations).

No products indexed under this heading.

Sertraline Hydrochloride (CYP3A4 inhibitors may increase imatinib mesylate Cmax and AUC. There was a significant increase in exposure to imatinib (mean Cmax and AUC increased by 26% and 40% respectively) in healthy subjects when imatinib mesylate was co-administered with a singledose of ketoconazole (a CYP3A4 inhibitor). Caution is recommended when administering imatinib mesylate with strong CYP3A4 inhibitors (eg, ketoconazole, itraconazole). Grapefruit juice may also increase plasma concentrations of imatinib and should be avoided. Substances that inhibit the cytochrome P450 isoenszyme (CYP3A4) activity may decrease metabolism and increase imatinib concentrations).

No products indexed under this heading.

Sildenafil Citrate (CYP3A4 inhibitors may increase imatinib mesylate Cmax and AUC. There was a significant increase in exposure to imatinib (mean Cmax and AUC increased by 26% and 40% respectively) in healthy subjects when imatinib mesylate was co-administered with a singledose of ketoconazole (a CYP3A4 inhibitor). Caution is recommended when administering imatinib mesylate with strong CYP3A4 inhibitors (eg, ketoconazole, itraconazole). Grapefruit juice may also increase plasma concentrations of imatinib and should be avoided. Substances that inhibit the cytochrome P450 isoenszyme (CYP3A4) activity may decrease metabolism and increase imatinib concentrations).

No products indexed under this heading.

Simvastatin (Imatinib increases the mean Cmax and AUC of simvastatin 2-fold and 3.5-fold, respectively by inhibiting CYP3A4). Products include:

Simcor Tablets 502
Vytorin 10/10 Tablets 2149
Vytorin 10/10 Tablets 2939
Vytorin 10/20 Tablets 2149
Vytorin 10/20 Tablets 2939
Vytorin 10/40 Tablets 2149
Vytorin 10/40 Tablets 2939

Vytorin 10/80 Tablets **2149**
Vytorin 10/80 Tablets **2939**
Zocor Tablets **2136**

Sirolimus (Imatinib mesylate is an inhibitor of CYP3A4 and may increase the Cmax and AUC of other drugs. Imatinib mesylate increases the mean Cmax and AUC of simvastatin (CYP3A4 substrate) 2-fold and 3.5-fold, respectively, suggesting an inhibition of the CYP3A4 byimatinib mesylate. Particular caution is recommended when administering imatinib mesylate with CYP3A4 substrates that have a narrow therapeutic window (eg, alfentanil, cyclosporine, diergotamine, ergotamine, fentanyl, pimozide, quinidine, sirolimus, or tacrolimus)). Products include:

Rapamune **3260**

Sulfinpyrazone (CYP3A4 inducers may decrease imatinib mesylate Cmax and AUC. The use of concomitant strong CYP3A4 inducers should be avoided (eg, dexamethasone, phenytoin, carbamazepine, rifampin, rifabutin, rifampacin, phenobarbital). If patients must be co-administered a strong CYP3A4 inducer, based on pharmacokinetic studies, the dosage of imatinib mesylate should be increased by at least 50% and clinical response should be carefully monitored).

No products indexed under this heading.

Tacrolimus (Imatinib mesylate is an inhibitor of CYP3A4 and may increase the Cmax and AUC of other drugs. Imatinib mesylate increases the mean Cmax and AUC of simvastatin (CYP3A4 substrate) 2-fold and 3.5-fold, respectively, suggesting an inhibition of the CYP3A4 byimatinib mesylate. Particular caution is recommended when administering imatinib mesylate with CYP3A4 substrates that have a narrow therapeutic window (eg, alfentanil, cyclosporine, diergotamine, ergotamine, fentanyl, pimozide, quinidine, sirolimus, or tacrolimus)). Products include:

Prograf Capsules and Injection **622**
Protopic Ointment **628**

Tadalafil (Imatinib mesylate is an inhibitor of CYP3A4 and may increase the Cmax and AUC of other drugs. Imatinib mesylate increases the mean Cmax and AUC of simvastatin (CYP3A4 substrate) 2-fold and 3.5-fold, respectively, suggesting an inhibition of the CYP3A4 byimatinib mesylate. Particular caution is recommended when administering imatinib mesylate with CYP3A4 substrates that have a narrow therapeutic window (eg, alfentanil, cyclosporine, diergotamine, ergotamine, fentanyl, pimozide, quinidine, sirolimus, or tacrolimus)). Products include:

Cialis Tablets **1792**

Tamoxifen Citrate (Imatinib mesylate is an inhibitor of CYP3A4 and may increase the Cmax and AUC of other drugs. Imatinib mesylate increases the mean Cmax and AUC of simvastatin (CYP3A4 substrate) 2-fold and 3.5-fold, respectively, suggesting an inhibition of the CYP3A4 byimatinib mesylate. Particular caution is recommended when administering imatinib mesylate with CYP3A4 substrates that have a narrow therapeutic window (eg, alfentanil, cyclosporine, diergotamine, ergotamine, fentanyl, pimozide, quinidine, sirolimus, or tacrolimus)).

No products indexed under this heading.

Telithromycin (CYP3A4 inhibitors may increase imatinib mesylate Cmax and AUC. There was a significant increase in exposure to imatinib (mean Cmax and AUC increased by 26% and 40% respectively) in healthy subjects when imatinib mesylate was co-administered with a singledose of ketoconazole (a CYP3A4 inhibitor). Caution is recommended when administering imatinib mesylate with strong CYP3A4 inhibitors (eg, ketoconazole, itraconazole). Grapefruit juice may also increase plasma concentrations of imatinib and should be avoided. Substances that inhibit the cytochrome P450 isoenszyme (CYP3A4) activity may decrease metabolism and increase imatinib concentrations). Products include:

Ketek Tablets **2744**

Teniposide (*in vitro*, imatinib mesylate inhibits the cytochrome P450 isoenzyme CYP2D6 activity at similar concentrations that affect CYP3A4 activity. Systemic exposure to substrates of CYP2D6 is expected to be increased when co-administered with imatinib mesylate. No specific studies have been performed and caution is recommended).

No products indexed under this heading.

Testosterone (In vitro, imatinib mesylate inhibits the cytochrome P450 isoenzyme CYP2D6 activity at similar concentrations that affect CYP3A4 activity. Systemic exposure to substrates of CYP2D6 is expected to be increased when co-administered with imatinib mesylate. No specific studies have been performed and caution is recommended). Products include:

AndroGel **3159**
Testim 1% Gel **701**

Testosterone Cypionate (In vitro, imatinib mesylate inhibits the cytochrome P450 isoenzyme CYP2D6 activity at similar concentrations that affect CYP3A4 activity. Systemic exposure to substrates of CYP2D6 is expected to be increased when co-administered with imatinib mesylate. No specific studies have been performed and caution is recommended).

No products indexed under this heading.

Testosterone Enanthate (In vitro, imatinib mesylate inhibits the cytochrome P450 isoenzyme CYP2D6 activity at similar concentrations that affect CYP3A4 activity. Systemic exposure to substrates of CYP2D6 is expected to be increased when co-administered with imatinib mesylate. No specific studies have been performed and caution is recommended). Products include:

Delatestryl Injection **1730**

Testosterone Propionate (In vitro, imatinib mesylate inhibits the cytochrome P450 isoenzyme CYP2D6 activity at similar concentrations that affect CYP3A4 activity. Systemic exposure to substrates of CYP2D6 is expected to be increased when co-administered with imatinib mesylate. No specific studies have been performed and caution is recommended).

No products indexed under this heading.

Theophylline (CYP3A4 inducers may decrease imatinib mesylate Cmax and AUC. The use of concomitant strong CYP3A4 inducers should be avoided (eg, dexamethasone, phenytoin, carbamazepine, rifampin, rifabutin, rifampacin, phenobarbital). If patients must be co-administered a strong CYP3A4 inducer, based on pharmacokinetic studies, the dosage of imatinib mesylate should be increased by at least 50% and clinical response should be carefully monitored).

No products indexed under this heading.

Theophylline Anhydrous (CYP3A4 inducers may decrease imatinib mesylate Cmax and AUC. The use of concomitant strong CYP3A4 inducers should be avoided (eg, dexamethasone, phenytoin, carbamazepine, rifampin, rifabutin, rifampacin, phenobarbital). If patients must be co-administered a strong CYP3A4 inducer, based on pharmacokinetic studies, the dosage of imatinib mesylate should be increased by at least 50% and clinical response should be carefully monitored). Products include:

Uniphyl Tablets **2595**

Theophylline Calcium Salicylate (CYP3A4 inducers may decrease imatinib mesylate Cmax and AUC. The use of concomitant strong CYP3A4 inducers should be avoided (eg, dexamethasone, phenytoin, carbamazepine, rifampin, rifabutin, rifampacin, phenobarbital). If patients must be co-administered a strong CYP3A4 inducer, based on pharmacokinetic studies, the dosage of imatinib mesylate should be increased by at least 50% and clinical response should be carefully monitored).

No products indexed under this heading.

Theophylline Dihydroxypropyl (Glyceryl) (CYP3A4 inducers may decrease imatinib mesylate Cmax and AUC. The use of concomitant strong CYP3A4 inducers should be avoided (eg, dexamethasone, phenytoin, carbamazepine, rifampin, rifabutin, rifampacin, phenobarbital). If patients must be co-administered a strong CYP3A4 inducer, based on pharmacokinetic studies, the dosage of imatinib mesylate should be increased by at least 50% and clinical response should be carefully monitored).

No products indexed under this heading.

Theophylline Ethylenediamine (CYP3A4 inducers may decrease imatinib mesylate Cmax and AUC. The use of concomitant strong CYP3A4 inducers should be avoided (eg, dexamethasone, phenytoin, carbamazepine, rifampin, rifabutin, rifampacin, phenobarbital). If patients must be co-administered a strong CYP3A4 inducer, based on pharmacokinetic studies, the dosage of imatinib mesylate should be increased by at least 50% and clinical response should be carefully monitored).

No products indexed under this heading.

Thioridazine (In vitro, imatinib mesylate inhibits the cytochrome P450 isoenzyme CYP2D6 activity at similar concentrations that affect CYP3A4 activity. Systemic exposure to substrates of CYP2D6 is expected to be increased when co-administered with imatinib mesylate. No specific studies have been performed and caution is recommended).

No products indexed under this heading.

Thioridazine Hydrochloride (In vitro, imatinib mesylate inhibits the cytochrome P450 isoenzyme CYP2D6 activity at similar concentrations that affect CYP3A4 activity. Systemic exposure to substrates of CYP2D6 is expected to be increased when co-administered with imatinib mesylate. No specific studies have been performed and caution is recommended). Products include:

Thioridazine Hydrochloride Tablets **2195**

Tiagabine Hydrochloride (Imatinib mesylate is an inhibitor of CYP3A4 and may increase the Cmax and AUC of other drugs. Imatinib mesylate increases the mean Cmax and AUC of simvastatin (CYP3A4 substrate) 2-fold and 3.5-fold, respectively, suggesting an inhibition of the CYP3A4 byimatinib mesylate. Particular caution is recommended when administering imatinib mesylate with CYP3A4 substrates that have a narrow therapeutic window (eg, alfentanil, cyclosporine, diergotamine, ergotamine, fentanyl, pimozide, quinidine, sirolimus, or tacrolimus)). Products include:

Gabitril Tablets **973**

Timolol Maleate (In vitro, imatinib mesylate inhibits the cytochrome P450 isoenzyme CYP2D6 activity at similar concentrations that affect CYP3A4 activity. Systemic exposure to substrates of CYP2D6 is expected to be increased when co-administered with imatinib mesylate. No specific studies have been performed and caution is recommended). Products include:

Combigan Ophthalmic Solution **553**
Cosopt Sterile Ophthalmic Solution **1969**
Timoptic Sterile Ophthalmic Solution **2121**
Timoptic in Ocudose **2124**
Timoptic-XE Sterile Ophthalmic Gel Forming Solution **2125**

Tolterodine Tartrate (Imatinib mesylate is an inhibitor of CYP3A4 and may increase the Cmax and AUC of other drugs. Imatinib mesylate increases the mean Cmax and AUC of simvastatin (CYP3A4 substrate) 2-fold and 3.5-fold, respectively, suggesting an inhibition of the CYP3A4 byimatinib mesylate. Particular caution is recommended when administering imatinib mesylate with CYP3A4 substrates that have a narrow therapeutic window (eg, alfentanil, cyclosporine, diergotamine, ergotamine, fentanyl, pimozide, quinidine, sirolimus, or tacrolimus)).

No products indexed under this heading.

Tramadol Hydrochloride (In vitro, imatinib mesylate inhibits the cytochrome P450 isoenzyme CYP2D6 activity at similar concentrations that affect CYP3A4 activity. Systemic exposure to substrates of CYP2D6 is expected to be increased when co-administered with imatinib mesylate. No specific studies have been performed and caution is recommended). Products include:

Ultram ER Extended-Release Tablets **2428**

Trazodone Hydrochloride (Imatinib mesylate is an inhibitor of CYP3A4 and may increase the Cmax and AUC of other drugs. Imatinib mesylate increases the mean Cmax and AUC of simvastatin (CYP3A4 substrate) 2-fold and 3.5-fold, respectively, suggesting an inhibition of the CYP3A4 byimatinib mesylate. Particular caution is recommended when administering imatinib mesylate with CYP3A4 substrates that have a narrow therapeutic window (eg, alfentanil, cyclosporine, diergotamine, ergotamine, fentanyl, pimozide, quinidine, sirolimus, or tacrolimus)).
No products indexed under this heading.

Triamcinolone (CYP3A4 inducers may decrease imatinib mesylate Cmax and AUC. The use of concomitant strong CYP3A4 inducers should be avoided (eg, dexamethasone, phenytoin, carbamazepine, rifampin, rifabutin, rifampacin, phenobarbital). If patients must be co-administered a strong CYP3A4 inducer, based on pharmacokinetic studies, the dosage of imatinib mesylate should be increased by at least 50% and clinical response should be carefully monitored).
No products indexed under this heading.

Triamcinolone Acetonide (CYP3A4 inducers may decrease imatinib mesylate Cmax and AUC. The use of concomitant strong CYP3A4 inducers should be avoided (eg, dexamethasone, phenytoin, carbamazepine, rifampin, rifabutin, rifampacin, phenobarbital). If patients must be co-administered a strong CYP3A4 inducer, based on pharmacokinetic studies, the dosage of imatinib mesylate should be increased by at least 50% and clinical response should be carefully monitored). Products include:
Azmacort Inhalation Aerosol 407
Nasacort AQ Nasal Spray 2765
Triesence Injectable Suspension .... ⊙209

Triamcinolone Diacetate (CYP3A4 inducers may decrease imatinib mesylate Cmax and AUC. The use of concomitant strong CYP3A4 inducers should be avoided (eg, dexamethasone, phenytoin, carbamazepine, rifampin, rifabutin, rifampacin, phenobarbital). If patients must be co-administered a strong CYP3A4 inducer, based on pharmacokinetic studies, the dosage of imatinib mesylate should be increased by at least 50% and clinical response should be carefully monitored).
No products indexed under this heading.

Triamcinolone Hexacetonide (CYP3A4 inducers may decrease imatinib mesylate Cmax and AUC. The use of concomitant strong CYP3A4 inducers should be avoided (eg, dexamethasone, phenytoin, carbamazepine, rifampin, rifabutin, rifampacin, phenobarbital). If patients must be co-administered a strong CYP3A4 inducer, based on pharmacokinetic studies, the dosage of imatinib mesylate should be increased by at least 50% and clinical response should be carefully monitored).
No products indexed under this heading.

Triazolam (Imatinib mesylate is an inhibitor of CYP3A4 and may increase the Cmax and AUC of other drugs. Imatinib mesylate increases the mean Cmax and AUC of simvastatin (CYP3A4 substrate) 2-fold and 3.5-fold, respectively, suggesting an inhibition of the CYP3A4 byimatinib mesylate. Particular caution is recommended when administering imatinib mesylate with CYP3A4 substrates that have a narrow therapeutic window (eg, alfentanil, cyclosporine, diergotamine, ergotamine, fentanyl, pimozide, quinidine, sirolimus, or tacrolimus)).
No products indexed under this heading.

Trimipramine Maleate (In vitro, imatinib mesylate inhibits the cytochrome P450 isoenzyme CYP2D6 activity at similar concentrations that affect CYP3A4 activity. Systemic exposure to substrates of CYP2D6 is expected to be increased when co-administered with imatinib mesylate. No specific studies have been performed and caution is recommended).
No products indexed under this heading.

Troglitazone (CYP3A4 inducers may decrease imatinib mesylate Cmax and AUC. The use of concomitant strong CYP3A4 inducers should be avoided (eg, dexamethasone, phenytoin, carbamazepine, rifampin, rifabutin, rifampacin, phenobarbital). If patients must be co-administered a strong CYP3A4 inducer, based on pharmacokinetic studies, the dosage of imatinib mesylate should be increased by at least 50% and clinical response should be carefully monitored).
No products indexed under this heading.

Troleandomycin (CYP3A4 inhibitors may increase imatinib mesylate Cmax and AUC. There was a significant increase in exposure to imatinib (mean Cmax and AUC increased by 26% and 40% respectively) in healthy subjects when imatinib mesylate was co-administered with a singledose of ketoconazole (a CYP3A4 inhibitor). Caution is recommended when administering imatinib mesylate with strong CYP3A4 inhibitors (eg, ketoconazole, itraconazole). Grapefruit juice may also increase plasma concentrations of imatinib and should be avoided. Substances that inhibit the cytochrome P450 isoenszyme (CYP3A4) activity may decrease metabolism and increase imatinib concentrations).
No products indexed under this heading.

Valproate Sodium (CYP3A4 inhibitors may increase imatinib mesylate Cmax and AUC. There was a significant increase in exposure to imatinib (mean Cmax and AUC increased by 26% and 40% respectively) in healthy subjects when imatinib mesylate was co-administered with a singledose of ketoconazole (a CYP3A4 inhibitor). Caution is recommended when administering imatinib mesylate with strong CYP3A4 inhibitors (eg, ketoconazole, itraconazole). Grapefruit juice may also increase plasma concentrations of imatinib and should be avoided. Substances that inhibit the cytochrome P450 isoenszyme (CYP3A4) activity may decrease metabolism and increase imatinib concentrations).
No products indexed under this heading.

Vardenafil Hydrochloride (CYP3A4 inhibitors may increase imatinib mesylate Cmax and AUC. There was a significant increase in exposure to imatinib (mean Cmax and AUC increased by 26% and 40% respectively) in healthy subjects when imatinib mesylate was co-administered with a singledose of ketoconazole (a CYP3A4 inhibitor). Caution is recommended when administering imatinib mesylate with strong CYP3A4 inhibitors (eg, ketoconazole, itraconazole). Grapefruit juice may also increase plasma concentrations of imatinib and should be avoided. Substances that inhibit the cytochrome P450 isoenszyme (CYP3A4) activity may decrease metabolism and increase imatinib concentrations). Products include:
Levitra Tablets 2876

Venlafaxine Hydrochloride (In vitro, imatinib mesylate inhibits the cytochrome P450 isoenzyme CYP2D6 activity at similar concentrations that affect CYP3A4 activity. Systemic exposure to substrates of CYP2D6 is expected to be increased when co-administered with imatinib mesylate. No specific studies have been performed and caution is recommended). Products include:
Effexor XR Extended-Release Capsules 3195
Venlafaxine Hydrochloride Tablets ... 2199

Verapamil Hydrochloride (CYP3A4 inhibitors may increase imatinib mesylate Cmax and AUC. There was a significant increase in exposure to imatinib (mean Cmax and AUC increased by 26% and 40% respectively) in healthy subjects when imatinib mesylate was co-administered with a singledose of ketoconazole (a CYP3A4 inhibitor). Caution is recommended when administering imatinib mesylate with strong CYP3A4 inhibitors (eg, ketoconazole, itraconazole). Grapefruit juice may also increase plasma concentrations of imatinib and should be avoided. Substances that inhibit the cytochrome P450 isoenszyme (CYP3A4) activity may decrease metabolism and increase imatinib concentrations). Products include:
Tarka Tablets 511

Vinblastine Sulfate (Imatinib mesylate is an inhibitor of CYP3A4 and may increase the Cmax and AUC of other drugs. Imatinib mesylate increases the mean Cmax and AUC of simvastatin (CYP3A4 substrate) 2-fold and 3.5-fold, respectively, suggesting an inhibition of the CYP3A4 byimatinib mesylate. Particular caution is recommended when administering imatinib mesylate with CYP3A4 substrates that have a narrow therapeutic window (eg, alfentanil, cyclosporine, diergotamine, ergotamine, fentanyl, pimozide, quinidine, sirolimus, or tacrolimus)).
No products indexed under this heading.

Vincristine Sulfate (Imatinib mesylate is an inhibitor of CYP3A4 and may increase the Cmax and AUC of other drugs. Imatinib mesylate increases the mean Cmax and AUC of simvastatin (CYP3A4 substrate) 2-fold and 3.5-fold, respectively, suggesting an inhibition of the CYP3A4 byimatinib mesylate. Particular caution is recommended when administering imatinib mesylate with CYP3A4 substrates that have a narrow therapeutic window (eg, alfentanil, cyclosporine, diergotamine, ergotamine, fentanyl, pimozide, quinidine, sirolimus, or tacrolimus)).
No products indexed under this heading.

Voriconazole (CYP3A4 inhibitors may increase imatinib mesylate Cmax and AUC. There was a significant increase in exposure to imatinib (mean Cmax and AUC increased by 26% and 40% respectively) in healthy subjects when imatinib mesylate was co-administered with a singledose of ketoconazole (a CYP3A4 inhibitor). Caution is recommended when administering imatinib mesylate with strong CYP3A4 inhibitors (eg, ketoconazole, itraconazole). Grapefruit juice may also increase plasma concentrations of imatinib and should be avoided. Substances that inhibit the cytochrome P450 isoenszyme (CYP3A4) activity may decrease metabolism and increase imatinib concentrations).
No products indexed under this heading.

Warfarin Sodium (Because warfarin is metabolized by CYP2C9 and CYP3A4, patients who require anticoagulation should receive low-molecular weight or standard heparin instead of warfarin).
No products indexed under this heading.

Zafirlukast (CYP3A4 inhibitors may increase imatinib mesylate Cmax and AUC. There was a significant increase in exposure to imatinib (mean Cmax and AUC increased by 26% and 40% respectively) in healthy subjects when imatinib mesylate was co-administered with a singledose of ketoconazole (a CYP3A4 inhibitor). Caution is recommended when administering imatinib mesylate with strong CYP3A4 inhibitors (eg, ketoconazole, itraconazole). Grapefruit juice may also increase plasma concentrations of imatinib and should be avoided. Substances that inhibit the cytochrome P450 isoenszyme (CYP3A4) activity may decrease metabolism and increase imatinib concentrations). Products include:
Accolate Tablets 669

Zileuton (CYP3A4 inhibitors may increase imatinib mesylate Cmax and AUC. There was a significant increase in exposure to imatinib (mean Cmax and AUC increased by 26% and 40% respectively) in healthy subjects when imatinib mesylate was co-administered with a singledose of ketoconazole (a CYP3A4 inhibitor). Caution is recommended when administering imatinib mesylate with strong CYP3A4 inhibitors (eg, ketoconazole, itraconazole). Grapefruit juice may also increase plasma concentrations of imatinib and should be avoided. Substances that inhibit the cytochrome P450 isoenszyme (CYP3A4) activity may decrease metabolism and increase imatinib concentrations).
No products indexed under this heading.

Zonisamide (In vitro, imatinib mesylate inhibits the cytochrome P450 isoenzyme CYP2D6 activity at similar concentrations that affect CYP3A4 activity. Systemic exposure

to substrates of CYP2D6 is expected to be increased when co-administered with imatinib mesylate. No specific studies have been performed and caution is recommended). Products include:
Zonegran Capsules 1089

Food Interactions

Grapefruit (There was a significant increase in exposure to imatinib (mean Cmax and AUC increased by 26% and 40% respectively) in healthy subjects when imatinib mesylate was co-administered with a single dose of ketoconazole (a CYP3A4 inhibitor). Caution is recommended when administering imatinib mesylate with strong CYP3A4 inhibitors (eg, ketoconazole, itraconazole, clarithromycin, atazanavir, indinavir, nefazodone, nelfinavir, ritonavir, saquinavir, telithromycin, and voriconazole). Grapefruit juice may also increase plasma concentrations of imatinib and should be avoided. Substances that inhibit the cytochrome P450 isoenzyme (CPY3A4) activity may decrease metabolism and increase imatinib concentrations).

Grapefruit Juice (There was a significant increase in exposure to imatinib (mean Cmax and AUC increased by 26% and 40% respectively) in healthy subjects when imatinib mesylate was co-administered with a single dose of ketoconazole (a CYP3A4 inhibitor). Caution is recommended when administering imatinib mesylate with strong CYP3A4 inhibitors (eg, ketoconazole, itraconazole, clarithromycin, atazanavir, indinavir, nefazodone, nelfinavir, ritonavir, saquinavir, telithromycin, and voriconazole). Grapefruit juice may also increase plasma concentrations of imatinib and should be avoided. Substances that inhibit the cytochrome P450 isoenzyme (CPY3A4) activity may decrease metabolism and increase imatinib concentrations).

GLIADEL WAFER
(Polifeprosan 20 with Carmustine) 1076
None cited in PDR database.

GLUCAGON FOR INJECTION VIALS AND EMERGENCY KIT
(Glucagon) 1827
None cited in PDR database.

GORDOCHOM SOLUTION
(Chloroxylenol, Undecylenic Acid) 1699
None cited in PDR database.

GRIS-PEG TABLETS
(Griseofulvin) 2507
May interact with barbiturates, oral contraceptives, and certain other agents. Compounds in these categories include:

Aprobarbital (Barbiturates usually depress griseofulvin activity and co-administration requires a dosage adjustment of the antifungal agent).
No products indexed under this heading.

Butabarbital (Barbiturates usually depress griseofulvin activity and co-administration requires a dosage adjustment of the antifungal agent).
No products indexed under this heading.

Butalbital (Barbiturates usually depress griseofulvin activity and co-administration requires a dosage adjustment of the antifungal agent).
No products indexed under this heading.

Desogestrel (There have been reports in the literature of possible interactions between griseofulvin and oral contraceptives). Products include:
Mircette Tablets 1034

Ethinyl Estradiol (There have been reports in the literature of possible interactions between griseofulvin and oral contraceptives). Products include:
Lybrel Tablets 3204
Mircette Tablets 1034
NuvaRing 2897
Ortho-Cyclen/Ortho Tri-Cyclen 2449
Ortho Evra Transdermal System 2437
Ortho Tri-Cyclen Lo Tablets 2458
Seasonique Tablets 1046
Yaz Tablets 805

Ethynodiol Diacetate (There have been reports in the literature of possible interactions between griseofulvin and oral contraceptives).
No products indexed under this heading.

Levonorgestrel (There have been reports in the literature of possible interactions between griseofulvin and oral contraceptives). Products include:
Climara Pro Transdermal System 768
Lybrel Tablets 3204
Mirena Intrauterine System 779
Plan B Tablets 1044
Seasonique Tablets 1046

Mephobarbital (Barbiturates usually depress griseofulvin activity and co-administration requires a dosage adjustment of the antifungal agent).
No products indexed under this heading.

Mestranol (There have been reports in the literature of possible interactions between griseofulvin and oral contraceptives).
No products indexed under this heading.

Norethindrone (There have been reports in the literature of possible interactions between griseofulvin and oral contraceptives). Products include:
Ortho Micronor Tablets 2446

Norethynodrel (There have been reports in the literature of possible interactions between griseofulvin and oral contraceptives).
No products indexed under this heading.

Norgestimate (There have been reports in the literature of possible interactions between griseofulvin and oral contraceptives). Products include:
Ortho-Cyclen/Ortho Tri-Cyclen 2449
Ortho Tri-Cyclen Lo Tablets 2458

Norgestrel (There have been reports in the literature of possible interactions between griseofulvin and oral contraceptives).
No products indexed under this heading.

Pentobarbital Sodium (Barbiturates usually depress griseofulvin activity and co-administration requires a dosage adjustment of the antifungal agent). Products include:
Nembutal Sodium Solution, USP 2494

Phenobarbital (Barbiturates usually depress griseofulvin activity and co-administration requires a dosage adjustment of the antifungal agent). Products include:
Donnatal Extentabs 2507

Secobarbital Sodium (Barbiturates usually depress griseofulvin activity and co-administration requires a dosage adjustment of the antifungal agent).
No products indexed under this heading.

Thiamylal Sodium (Barbiturates usually depress griseofulvin activity and co-administration requires a dosage adjustment of the antifungal agent).
No products indexed under this heading.

Warfarin Sodium (Griseofulvin decreases the activity of warfarin-type anticoagulants).
No products indexed under this heading.

Food Interactions

Alcohol (The effects of alcohol may be potentiated by griseofulvin, producing such effects as tachycardia and flushing).

HAVRIX INJECTION VACCINE
(Hepatitis A Vaccine, Inactivated) 1454
None cited in PDR database.

HEMOFIL M
(Antihemophilic Factor (Human)) 737
None cited in PDR database.

HEP-FORTE CAPSULES
(Vitamins with Minerals) 1894
None cited in PDR database.

HEPSERA TABLETS
(Adefovir dipivoxil) 1253
May interact with aminoglycosides, nephrotoxic agents, inhibitors of renal tubular secretion or resorption, and certain other agents. Compounds in these categories include:

Abacavir Sulfate (Since adefovir is eliminated by the kidney, co-administration of adefovir with drugs that reduce renal function may increase serum concentrations of either adefovir and/or these co-administered drugs). Products include:
Epzicom Tablets 1422
Trizivir Tablets 1622
Ziagen 1673

Acyclovir (Since adefovir is eliminated by the kidney, co-administration of adefovir with drugs that reduce renal function may increase serum concentrations of either adefovir and/or these co-administered drugs). Products include:
Zovirax 1690
Zovirax Cream 817
Zovirax Ointment 819

Acyclovir Sodium (Since adefovir is eliminated by the kidney, co-administration of adefovir with drugs that reduce renal function may increase serum concentrations of either adefovir and/or these co-administered drugs).
No products indexed under this heading.

Alatrofloxacin Mesylate (Since adefovir is eliminated by the kidney, co-administration of adefovir with drugs that reduce renal function may increase serum concentrations of either adefovir and/or these co-administered drugs).
No products indexed under this heading.

Aldesleukin (Since adefovir is eliminated by the kidney, co-administration of adefovir with drugs that reduce renal function may increase serum concentrations of either adefovir and/or these co-administered drugs). Products include:
Proleukin for Injection 2287

Amikacin Sulfate (Patients should be monitored closely for adverse events when adefovir dipivoxil is co-administered with other drugs that are known to affect renal function).
No products indexed under this heading.

Amoxicillin (Since adefovir is eliminated by the kidney, co-administration of adefovir with drugs that reduce renal function may increase serum concentrations of either adefovir and/or these co-administered drugs). Products include:
Amoxil Capsules 1305
Amoxil Chewable Tablets 1305
Amoxil Pediatric Drops for Oral Suspension 1305
Amoxil Powder for Oral Suspension 1305
Amoxil Tablets 1305
Augmentin 1323
Augmentin Tablets 1327
Augmentin XR Extended Release Tablets 1333
Augmentin ES-600 Powder for Oral Suspension 1329
Moxatag Tablets 2165

Amoxicillin Trihydrate (Since adefovir is eliminated by the kidney, co-administration of adefovir with drugs that reduce renal function may increase serum concentrations of either adefovir and/or these co-administered drugs).
No products indexed under this heading.

Amphotericin B (Since adefovir is eliminated by the kidney, co-administration of adefovir with drugs that reduce renal function may increase serum concentrations of either adefovir and/or these co-administered drugs).
No products indexed under this heading.

Amphotericin B, liposomal (Since adefovir is eliminated by the kidney, co-administration of adefovir with drugs that reduce renal function may increase serum concentrations of either adefovir and/or these co-administered drugs). Products include:
AmBisome for Injection 606

Amphotericin B Cholesteryl Sulfate (Since adefovir is eliminated by the kidney, co-administration of adefovir with drugs that reduce renal function may increase serum concentrations of either adefovir and/or these co-administered drugs).
No products indexed under this heading.

Amphotericin B Lipid Complex (Since adefovir is eliminated by the kidney, co-administration of adefovir with drugs that reduce renal function may increase serum concentrations of either adefovir and/or these co-administered drugs). Products include:
Abelcet Injection 1134

Ampicillin (Since adefovir is eliminated by the kidney, co-administration of adefovir with drugs that reduce renal function may increase serum concentrations of either adefovir and/or these co-administered drugs).
No products indexed under this heading.

Ampicillin Sodium (Since adefovir is eliminated by the kidney, co-administration of adefovir with drugs that reduce renal function may increase serum concentrations of either adefovir and/or these co-administered drugs).
No products indexed under this heading.

Ampicillin Trihydrate (Since adefovir is eliminated by the kidney, co-administration of adefovir with drugs that reduce renal function may increase serum concentrations of either adefovir and/or these co-administered drugs).
No products indexed under this heading.

Amprenavir (Since adefovir is eliminated by the kidney, co-administration of adefovir with drugs that reduce renal function may increase serum concentrations of either adefovir and/or these co-administered drugs).
No products indexed under this heading.

Aspirin (Since adefovir is eliminated by the kidney, co-administration of adefovir with drugs that reduce renal function may increase serum concentrations of either adefovir and/or these co-administered drugs).
Products include:
- Aggrenox Capsules 819
- Bayer Aspirin 750
- Percodan Tablets 1130
- St. Joseph 81 mg Aspirin Chewable and Enteric Coated Tablets 1903

Atazanavir (Since adefovir is eliminated by the kidney, co-administration of adefovir with drugs that reduce renal function may increase serum concentrations of either adefovir and/or these co-administered drugs).
No products indexed under this heading.

Atorvastatin Calcium (Since adefovir is eliminated by the kidney, co-administration of adefovir with drugs that reduce renal function may increase serum concentrations of either adefovir and/or these co-administered drugs). Products include:
- Lipitor Tablets 2501

Azithromycin Dihydrate (Since adefovir is eliminated by the kidney, co-administration of adefovir with drugs that reduce renal function may increase serum concentrations of either adefovir and/or these co-administered drugs).
No products indexed under this heading.

Azlocillin Sodium (Since adefovir is eliminated by the kidney, co-administration of adefovir with drugs that reduce renal function may increase serum concentrations of either adefovir and/or these co-administered drugs).
No products indexed under this heading.

Aztreonam (Since adefovir is eliminated by the kidney, co-administration of adefovir with drugs that reduce renal function may increase serum concentrations of either adefovir and/or these co-administered drugs).
No products indexed under this heading.

Bacampicillin Hydrochloride (Since adefovir is eliminated by the kidney, co-administration of adefovir with drugs that reduce renal function may increase serum concentrations of either adefovir and/or these co-administered drugs).
No products indexed under this heading.

Balsalazide Disodium (Since adefovir is eliminated by the kidney, co-administration of adefovir with drugs that reduce renal function may increase serum concentrations of either adefovir and/or these co-administered drugs).
No products indexed under this heading.

Benazepril Hydrochloride (Since adefovir is eliminated by the kidney, co-administration of adefovir with drugs that reduce renal function may increase serum concentrations of either adefovir and/or these co-administered drugs).
No products indexed under this heading.

Bendroflumethiazide (Since adefovir is eliminated by the kidney, co-administration of adefovir with drugs that reduce renal function may increase serum concentrations of either adefovir and/or these co-administered drugs).
No products indexed under this heading.

Caffeine (Since adefovir is eliminated by the kidney, co-administration of adefovir with drugs that reduce renal function may increase serum concentrations of either adefovir and/or these co-administered drugs). Products include:
- BioLean Free Tablets 635
- BioLean II Tablets 635
- Winrgy Dietary Supplement 642

Captopril (Since adefovir is eliminated by the kidney, co-administration of adefovir with drugs that reduce renal function may increase serum concentrations of either adefovir and/or these co-administered drugs). Products include:
- Captopril Tablets 2182

Carbenicillin Disodium (Since adefovir is eliminated by the kidney, co-administration of adefovir with drugs that reduce renal function may increase serum concentrations of either adefovir and/or these co-administered drugs).
No products indexed under this heading.

Carbenicillin Indanyl Sodium (Since adefovir is eliminated by the kidney, co-administration of adefovir with drugs that reduce renal function may increase serum concentrations of either adefovir and/or these co-administered drugs).
No products indexed under this heading.

Carboplatin (Since adefovir is eliminated by the kidney, co-administration of adefovir with drugs that reduce renal function may increase serum concentrations of either adefovir and/or these co-administered drugs).
No products indexed under this heading.

Carmustine (BCNU) (Since adefovir is eliminated by the kidney, co-administration of adefovir with drugs that reduce renal function may increase serum concentrations of either adefovir and/or these co-administered drugs).
No products indexed under this heading.

Cefaclor (Since adefovir is eliminated by the kidney, co-administration of adefovir with drugs that reduce renal function may increase serum concentrations of either adefovir and/or these co-administered drugs).
No products indexed under this heading.

Cefadroxil (Since adefovir is eliminated by the kidney, co-administration of adefovir with drugs that reduce renal function may increase serum concentrations of either adefovir and/or these co-administered drugs).
No products indexed under this heading.

Cefamandole Nafate (Since adefovir is eliminated by the kidney, co-administration of adefovir with drugs that reduce renal function may increase serum concentrations of either adefovir and/or these co-administered drugs).
No products indexed under this heading.

Cefazolin Sodium (Since adefovir is eliminated by the kidney, co-administration of adefovir with drugs that reduce renal function may increase serum concentrations of either adefovir and/or these co-administered drugs).
No products indexed under this heading.

Cefdinir (Since adefovir is eliminated by the kidney, co-administration of adefovir with drugs that reduce renal function may increase serum concentrations of either adefovir and/or these co-administered drugs). Products include:
- Omnicef Capsules 497
- Omnicef for Oral Suspension 497

Cefepime Hydrochloride (Since adefovir is eliminated by the kidney, co-administration of adefovir with drugs that reduce renal function may increase serum concentrations of either adefovir and/or these co-administered drugs).
No products indexed under this heading.

Cefixime (Since adefovir is eliminated by the kidney, co-administration of adefovir with drugs that reduce renal function may increase serum concentrations of either adefovir and/or these co-administered drugs). Products include:
- Suprax for Oral Suspension 1891
- Suprax Tablets 1891

Cefmetazole Sodium (Since adefovir is eliminated by the kidney, co-administration of adefovir with drugs that reduce renal function may increase serum concentrations of either adefovir and/or these co-administered drugs).
No products indexed under this heading.

Cefonicid Sodium (Since adefovir is eliminated by the kidney, co-administration of adefovir with drugs that reduce renal function may increase serum concentrations of either adefovir and/or these co-administered drugs).
No products indexed under this heading.

Cefoperazone Sodium (Since adefovir is eliminated by the kidney, co-administration of adefovir with drugs that reduce renal function may increase serum concentrations of either adefovir and/or these co-administered drugs).
No products indexed under this heading.

Cefoxanide (Since adefovir is eliminated by the kidney, co-administration of adefovir with drugs that reduce renal function may increase serum concentrations of either adefovir and/or these co-administered drugs).
No products indexed under this heading.

Cefotaxime Sodium (Since adefovir is eliminated by the kidney, co-administration of adefovir with drugs that reduce renal function may increase serum concentrations of either adefovir and/or these co-administered drugs).
No products indexed under this heading.

Cefotetan (Since adefovir is eliminated by the kidney, co-administration of adefovir with drugs that reduce renal function may increase serum concentrations of either adefovir and/or these co-administered drugs).
No products indexed under this heading.

Cefoxitin Sodium (Since adefovir is eliminated by the kidney, co-administration of adefovir with drugs that reduce renal function may increase serum concentrations of either adefovir and/or these co-administered drugs).
No products indexed under this heading.

Cefpodoxime Proxetil (Since adefovir is eliminated by the kidney, co-administration of adefovir with drugs that reduce renal function may increase serum concentrations of either adefovir and/or these co-administered drugs).
No products indexed under this heading.

Cefprozil (Since adefovir is eliminated by the kidney, co-administration of adefovir with drugs that reduce renal function may increase serum concentrations of either adefovir and/or these co-administered drugs).
No products indexed under this heading.

Ceftazidime (Since adefovir is eliminated by the kidney, co-administration of adefovir with drugs that reduce renal function may increase serum concentrations of

either adefovir and/or these co-administered drugs). Products include:
Fortaz 1450

Ceftizoxime Sodium (Since adefovir is eliminated by the kidney, co-administration of adefovir with drugs that reduce renal function may increase serum concentrations of either adefovir and/or these co-administered drugs).
No products indexed under this heading.

Ceftriaxone Sodium (Since adefovir is eliminated by the kidney, co-administration of adefovir with drugs that reduce renal function may increase serum concentrations of either adefovir and/or these co-administered drugs). Products include:
Rocephin Injectable Vials, ADD-Vantage, Galaxy, Bulk 2642

Cefuroxime Axetil (Since adefovir is eliminated by the kidney, co-administration of adefovir with drugs that reduce renal function may increase serum concentrations of either adefovir and/or these co-administered drugs). Products include:
Ceftin 1380

Cefuroxime Sodium (Since adefovir is eliminated by the kidney, co-administration of adefovir with drugs that reduce renal function may increase serum concentrations of either adefovir and/or these co-administered drugs).
No products indexed under this heading.

Celecoxib (Since adefovir is eliminated by the kidney, co-administration of adefovir with drugs that reduce renal function may increase serum concentrations of either adefovir and/or these co-administered drugs). Products include:
Celebrex Capsules 2979

Cephalexin (Since adefovir is eliminated by the kidney, co-administration of adefovir with drugs that reduce renal function may increase serum concentrations of either adefovir and/or these co-administered drugs).
No products indexed under this heading.

Cephalothin Sodium (Since adefovir is eliminated by the kidney, co-administration of adefovir with drugs that reduce renal function may increase serum concentrations of either adefovir and/or these co-administered drugs).
No products indexed under this heading.

Cephapirin Sodium (Since adefovir is eliminated by the kidney, co-administration of adefovir with drugs that reduce renal function may increase serum concentrations of either adefovir and/or these co-administered drugs).
No products indexed under this heading.

Cephradine (Since adefovir is eliminated by the kidney, co-administration of adefovir with drugs that reduce renal function may increase serum concentrations of either adefovir and/or these co-administered drugs).
No products indexed under this heading.

Cerivastatin Sodium (Since adefovir is eliminated by the kidney, co-administration of adefovir with drugs that reduce renal function may increase serum concentrations of either adefovir and/or these co-administered drugs).
No products indexed under this heading.

Chlorothiazide (Since adefovir is eliminated by the kidney, co-administration of adefovir with drugs that reduce renal function may increase serum concentrations of either adefovir and/or these co-administered drugs).
No products indexed under this heading.

Chlorothiazide Sodium (Since adefovir is eliminated by the kidney, co-administration of adefovir with drugs that reduce renal function may increase serum concentrations of either adefovir and/or these co-administered drugs). Products include:
Intravenous Sodium Diuril 2490

Chlorpropamide (Since adefovir is eliminated by the kidney, co-administration of adefovir with drugs that reduce renal function may increase serum concentrations of either adefovir and/or these co-administered drugs).
No products indexed under this heading.

Cidofovir (Since adefovir is eliminated by the kidney, co-administration of adefovir with drugs that reduce renal function may increase serum concentrations of either adefovir and/or these co-administered drugs).
No products indexed under this heading.

Cilastatin Sodium (Since adefovir is eliminated by the kidney, co-administration of adefovir with drugs that reduce renal function may increase serum concentrations of either adefovir and/or these co-administered drugs). Products include:
Primaxin I.M. 2080
Primaxin I.V. 2083

Cimetidine (Since adefovir is eliminated by the kidney, co-administration of adefovir with drugs that reduce renal function may increase serum concentrations of either adefovir and/or these co-administered drugs).
No products indexed under this heading.

Cimetidine Hydrochloride (Since adefovir is eliminated by the kidney, co-administration of adefovir with drugs that reduce renal function may increase serum concentrations of either adefovir and/or these co-administered drugs).
No products indexed under this heading.

Cisplatin (Since adefovir is eliminated by the kidney, co-administration of adefovir with drugs that reduce renal function may increase serum concentrations of either adefovir and/or these co-administered drugs).
No products indexed under this heading.

Cladribine (Since adefovir is eliminated by the kidney, co-administration of adefovir with drugs that reduce renal function may increase serum concentrations of either adefovir and/or these co-administered drugs). Products include:
Leustatin Injection 2384

Clozapine (Since adefovir is eliminated by the kidney, co-administration of adefovir with drugs that reduce renal function may increase serum concentrations of either adefovir and/or these co-administered drugs).
No products indexed under this heading.

Colistimethate Sodium (Since adefovir is eliminated by the kidney, co-administration of adefovir with drugs that reduce renal function may increase serum concentrations of either adefovir and/or these co-administered drugs).
No products indexed under this heading.

Colistin Sulfate (Since adefovir is eliminated by the kidney, co-administration of adefovir with drugs that reduce renal function may increase serum concentrations of either adefovir and/or these co-administered drugs).
No products indexed under this heading.

Cyclophosphamide (Since adefovir is eliminated by the kidney, co-administration of adefovir with drugs that reduce renal function may increase serum concentrations of either adefovir and/or these co-administered drugs).
No products indexed under this heading.

Cyclosporine (Since adefovir is eliminated by the kidney, co-administration of adefovir with drugs that reduce renal function may increase serum concentrations of either adefovir and/or these co-administered drugs). Products include:
Gengraf Capsules 435
Neoral Oral Solution 2280
Neoral Soft Gelatin Capsules 2280
Restasis Ophthalmic Emulsion 557
Sandimmune 2296

Cytarabine (Since adefovir is eliminated by the kidney, co-administration of adefovir with drugs that reduce renal function may increase serum concentrations of either adefovir and/or these co-administered drugs).
No products indexed under this heading.

Cytarabine Liposome (Since adefovir is eliminated by the kidney, co-administration of adefovir with drugs that reduce renal function may increase serum concentrations of either adefovir and/or these co-administered drugs). Products include:
DepoCyt Injection 1136

Delavirdine Mesylate (Since adefovir is eliminated by the kidney, co-administration of adefovir with drugs that reduce renal function may increase serum concentrations of either adefovir and/or these co-administered drugs).
No products indexed under this heading.

Diatrizoate Meglumine (Since adefovir is eliminated by the kidney, co-administration of adefovir with drugs that reduce renal function may increase serum concentrations of either adefovir and/or these co-administered drugs).
No products indexed under this heading.

Diatrizoate Sodium (Since adefovir is eliminated by the kidney, co-administration of adefovir with drugs that reduce renal function may increase serum concentrations of either adefovir and/or these co-administered drugs).
No products indexed under this heading.

Diclofenac Potassium (Since adefovir is eliminated by the kidney, co-administration of adefovir with drugs that reduce renal function may increase serum concentrations of either adefovir and/or these co-administered drugs).
No products indexed under this heading.

Diclofenac Sodium (Since adefovir is eliminated by the kidney, co-administration of adefovir with drugs that reduce renal function may increase serum concentrations of either adefovir and/or these co-administered drugs). Products include:
Diclofenac Sodium Ophthalmic Solution .... ⊙240
Voltaren Ophthalmic Solution 2336
Voltaren Tablets 2334
Voltaren-XR Tablets 2337

Dicloxacillin Sodium (Since adefovir is eliminated by the kidney, co-administration of adefovir with drugs that reduce renal function may increase serum concentrations of either adefovir and/or these co-administered drugs).
No products indexed under this heading.

Didanosine (Since adefovir is eliminated by the kidney, co-administration of adefovir with drugs that reduce renal function may increase serum concentrations of either adefovir and/or these co-administered drugs).
No products indexed under this heading.

Efavirenz (Since adefovir is eliminated by the kidney, co-administration of adefovir with drugs that reduce renal function may increase serum concentrations of either adefovir and/or these co-administered drugs). Products include:
Atripla Tablets 938
Sustiva Capsules 930
Sustiva Tablets 930

Emtricitabine (Since adefovir is eliminated by the kidney, co-administration of adefovir with drugs that reduce renal function may increase serum concentrations of either adefovir and/or these co-administered drugs). Products include:
Atripla Tablets 938
Emtriva Capsules 1246
Emtriva Oral Solution 1246
Truvada Tablets 1262

Enalapril Maleate (Since adefovir is eliminated by the kidney, co-administration of adefovir with drugs that reduce renal function may increase serum concentrations of either adefovir and/or these co-administered drugs).
No products indexed under this heading.

Enalaprilat (Since adefovir is eliminated by the kidney, co-administration of adefovir with drugs that reduce renal function may increase serum concentrations of either adefovir and/or these co-administered drugs).
No products indexed under this heading.

Enfuvirtide (Since adefovir is eliminated by the kidney, co-administration of adefovir with drugs that reduce renal function may increase serum concentrations of either adefovir and/or these co-administered drugs).
No products indexed under this heading.

Ethiodized Oil (Since adefovir is eliminated by the kidney, co-administration of adefovir with drugs that reduce renal function may increase serum concentrations of either adefovir and/or these co-administered drugs).
No products indexed under this heading.

Etodolac (Since adefovir is eliminated by the kidney, co-administration of adefovir with drugs that reduce renal function may increase serum concentrations of either adefovir and/or these co-administered drugs).
No products indexed under this heading.

Fenoprofen Calcium (Since adefovir is eliminated by the kidney, co-administration of adefovir with drugs that reduce renal function may increase serum concentrations of either adefovir and/or these co-administered drugs). Products include:
Nalfon Capsules 2508

Filgrastim (Since adefovir is eliminated by the kidney, co-administration of adefovir with drugs that reduce renal function may increase serum concentrations of either adefovir and/or these co-administered drugs). Products include:
Neupogen for Injection 589

Fluorouracil (Since adefovir is eliminated by the kidney, co-administration of adefovir with drugs that reduce renal function may increase serum concentrations of either adefovir and/or these co-administered drugs). Products include:
Carac Cream 0.5% 2722

Flurbiprofen (Since adefovir is eliminated by the kidney, co-administration of adefovir with drugs that reduce renal function may increase serum concentrations of either adefovir and/or these co-administered drugs).
No products indexed under this heading.

Fluvastatin Sodium (Since adefovir is eliminated by the kidney, co-administration of adefovir with drugs that reduce renal function may increase serum concentrations of either adefovir and/or these co-administered drugs). Products include:
Lescol Capsules 2268
Lescol XL Tablets 2268

Foscarnet Sodium (Since adefovir is eliminated by the kidney, co-administration of adefovir with drugs that reduce renal function may increase serum concentrations of either adefovir and/or these co-administered drugs).
No products indexed under this heading.

Fosinopril Sodium (Since adefovir is eliminated by the kidney, co-administration of adefovir with drugs that reduce renal function may increase serum concentrations of either adefovir and/or these co-administered drugs).
No products indexed under this heading.

Furosemide (Since adefovir is eliminated by the kidney, co-administration of adefovir with drugs that reduce renal function may increase serum concentrations of either adefovir and/or these co-administered drugs). Products include:
Furosemide Tablets 2186

Gadopentetate Dimeglumine (Since adefovir is eliminated by the kidney, co-administration of adefovir with drugs that reduce renal function may increase serum concentrations of either adefovir and/or these co-administered drugs).
No products indexed under this heading.

Gentamicin (Since adefovir is eliminated by the kidney, co-administration of adefovir with drugs that reduce renal function may increase serum concentrations of either adefovir and/or these co-administered drugs).
No products indexed under this heading.

Gentamicin Sulfate (Patients should be monitored closely for adverse events when adefovir dipivoxil is co-administered with other drugs that are known to affect renal function). Products include:
Pred-G Ophthalmic Ointment .... ⊙ 229
Pred-G Ophthalmic Suspension .... ⊙ 228

Glipizide (Since adefovir is eliminated by the kidney, co-administration of adefovir with drugs that reduce renal function may increase serum concentrations of either adefovir and/or these co-administered drugs).
No products indexed under this heading.

Globulin, Immune (Human) (Since adefovir is eliminated by the kidney, co-administration of adefovir with drugs that reduce renal function may increase serum concentrations of either adefovir and/or these co-administered drugs). Products include:
Flebogamma 5% 1715

Glyburide (Since adefovir is eliminated by the kidney, co-administration of adefovir with drugs that reduce renal function may increase serum concentrations of either adefovir and/or these co-administered drugs).
No products indexed under this heading.

Gold Therapy (Since adefovir is eliminated by the kidney, co-administration of adefovir with drugs that reduce renal function may increase serum concentrations of either adefovir and/or these co-administered drugs).
No products indexed under this heading.

HMG-CoA Reductase Inhibitors (Since adefovir is eliminated by the kidney, co-administration of adefovir with drugs that reduce renal function may increase serum concentrations of either adefovir and/or these co-administered drugs).
No products indexed under this heading.

Hydrochlorothiazide (Since adefovir is eliminated by the kidney, co-administration of adefovir with drugs that reduce renal function may increase serum concentrations of either adefovir and/or these co-administered drugs). Products include:
Atacand HCT 642
Avalide Tablets 892
Avalide Tablets 2713
Benicar HCT Tablets 1010
Diovan HCT Tablets 2216
Dyazide Capsules 1405
Micardis HCT Tablets 854
Prinzide Tablets 2092
Tekturna HCT Tablets 2324
Teveten HCT Tablets 517

Hydroflumethiazide (Since adefovir is eliminated by the kidney, co-administration of adefovir with drugs that reduce renal function may increase serum concentrations of either adefovir and/or these co-administered drugs).
No products indexed under this heading.

Ibuprofen (When adefovir was co-administered with ibuprofen, increases in adefovir Cmax (33%), AUC (23%) and urinary recovery were observed. These increases appear to be due to higher oral bioavailability, not a reduction in renal clearance of adefovir). Products include:
Motrin IB Tablets and Caplets 1900
Children's Motrin Oral Suspension 1901
Children's Motrin Non-Staining Dye-Free Oral Suspension 1901
Children's Motrin Cold Oral Suspension 1899
Infants' Motrin Concentrated Drops 1901
Infants' Motrin Non-Staining Dye-Free Concentrated Drops 1901
Junior Strength Motrin Caplets and Chewable Tablets 1901
Vicoprofen Tablets 533

Idarubicin Hydrochloride (Since adefovir is eliminated by the kidney, co-administration of adefovir with drugs that reduce renal function may increase serum concentrations of either adefovir and/or these co-administered drugs).
No products indexed under this heading.

Ifosfamide (Since adefovir is eliminated by the kidney, co-administration of adefovir with drugs that reduce renal function may increase serum concentrations of either adefovir and/or these co-administered drugs).
No products indexed under this heading.

Imipenem (Since adefovir is eliminated by the kidney, co-administration of adefovir with drugs that reduce renal function may increase serum concentrations of either adefovir and/or these co-administered drugs). Products include:
Primaxin I.M. 2080
Primaxin I.V. 2083

Immune Globulin Intravenous (Human) (Since adefovir is eliminated by the kidney, co-administration of adefovir with drugs that reduce renal function may increase serum concentrations of either adefovir and/or these co-administered drugs). Products include:
Flebogamma 5% DIF 1718
Gammagard Liquid 730
Gammagard S/D 734
Gamunex 3094

Indinavir Sulfate (Since adefovir is eliminated by the kidney, co-administration of adefovir with drugs that reduce renal function may increase serum concentrations of either adefovir and/or these co-administered drugs). Products include:
Crixivan Capsules 1979

Indomethacin (Since adefovir is eliminated by the kidney, co-administration of adefovir with drugs that reduce renal function may increase serum concentrations of either adefovir and/or these co-administered drugs). Products include:
Indocin 2024

Indomethacin Sodium Trihydrate (Since adefovir is eliminated by the kidney, co-administration of adefovir with drugs that reduce renal function may increase serum concentrations of either adefovir and/or these co-administered drugs). Products include:
Indocin I.V. 2489

Interferon Beta-1b (Since adefovir is eliminated by the kidney, co-administration of adefovir with drugs that reduce renal function may increase serum concentrations of either adefovir and/or these co-administered drugs). Products include:
Betaseron for SC Injection 756

Interleuken-2 (Since adefovir is eliminated by the kidney, co-administration of adefovir with drugs that reduce renal function may increase serum concentrations of either adefovir and/or these co-administered drugs).
No products indexed under this heading.

Iodamide Meglumine (Since adefovir is eliminated by the kidney, co-administration of adefovir with drugs that reduce renal function may increase serum concentrations of either adefovir and/or these co-administered drugs).
No products indexed under this heading.

Iohexol (Since adefovir is eliminated by the kidney, co-administration of adefovir with drugs that reduce renal function may increase serum concentrations of either adefovir and/or these co-administered drugs).
No products indexed under this heading.

Iopamidol (Since adefovir is eliminated by the kidney, co-administration of adefovir with drugs that reduce renal function may increase serum concentrations of either adefovir and/or these co-administered drugs).
No products indexed under this heading.

Iopanoic Acid (Since adefovir is eliminated by the kidney, co-administration of adefovir with drugs that reduce renal function may increase serum concentrations of either adefovir and/or these co-administered drugs).
No products indexed under this heading.

Iothalamate Meglumine (Since adefovir is eliminated by the kidney, co-administration of adefovir with drugs that reduce renal function may increase serum concentrations of either adefovir and/or these co-administered drugs).
No products indexed under this heading.

Ioxaglate Meglumine (Since adefovir is eliminated by the kidney, co-administration of adefovir with drugs that reduce renal function may increase serum concentrations of either adefovir and/or these co-administered drugs).
No products indexed under this heading.

Ioxaglate Sodium (Since adefovir is eliminated by the kidney, co-administration of adefovir with drugs that reduce renal function may increase serum concentrations of either adefovir and/or these co-administered drugs).
No products indexed under this heading.

Kanamycin Sulfate (Patients should be monitored closely for adverse events when adefovir dipivoxil is co-administered with other drugs that are known to affect renal function).
No products indexed under this heading.

Ketoprofen (Since adefovir is eliminated by the kidney, co-administration of adefovir with drugs that reduce renal function may increase serum concentrations of either adefovir and/or these co-administered drugs).
No products indexed under this heading.

Ketorolac Tromethamine (Since adefovir is eliminated by the kidney, co-administration of adefovir with drugs that reduce renal function may increase serum concentrations of either adefovir and/or these co-administered drugs).
No products indexed under this heading.

Lamium album (Since adefovir is eliminated by the kidney, co-administration of adefovir with drugs that reduce renal function may increase serum concentrations of either adefovir and/or these co-administered drugs).
No products indexed under this heading.

Lisinopril (Since adefovir is eliminated by the kidney, co-administration of adefovir with drugs that reduce renal function may increase serum concentrations of either adefovir and/or these co-administered drugs). Products include:
Prinivil Tablets 2087
Prinzide Tablets 2092

Lithium (Since adefovir is eliminated by the kidney, co-administration of adefovir with drugs that reduce renal function may increase serum concentrations of either adefovir and/or these co-administered drugs).
No products indexed under this heading.

Lithium Carbonate (Since adefovir is eliminated by the kidney, co-administration of adefovir with drugs that reduce renal function may increase serum concentrations of either adefovir and/or these co-administered drugs).
No products indexed under this heading.

Lithium Citrate (Since adefovir is eliminated by the kidney, co-administration of adefovir with drugs that reduce renal function may increase serum concentrations of either adefovir and/or these co-administered drugs).
No products indexed under this heading.

Lopinavir (Since adefovir is eliminated by the kidney, co-administration of adefovir with drugs that reduce renal function may increase serum concentrations of either adefovir and/or these co-administered drugs). Products include:
Kaletra 452

Loracarbef (Since adefovir is eliminated by the kidney, co-administration of adefovir with drugs that reduce renal function may increase serum concentrations of either adefovir and/or these co-administered drugs).
No products indexed under this heading.

Lovastatin (Since adefovir is eliminated by the kidney, co-administration of adefovir with drugs that reduce renal function may increase serum concentrations of either adefovir and/or these co-administered drugs). Products include:
Advicor Tablets 402
Mevacor Tablets 2063

Meclofenamate Sodium (Since adefovir is eliminated by the kidney, co-administration of adefovir with drugs that reduce renal function may increase serum concentrations of either adefovir and/or these co-administered drugs).
No products indexed under this heading.

Mefenamic Acid (Since adefovir is eliminated by the kidney, co-administration of adefovir with drugs that reduce renal function may increase serum concentrations of either adefovir and/or these co-administered drugs).
No products indexed under this heading.

Meloxicam (Since adefovir is eliminated by the kidney, co-administration of adefovir with drugs that reduce renal function may increase serum concentrations of either adefovir and/or these co-administered drugs). Products include:
Mobic Oral Suspension 863
Mobic Tablets 863

Melphalan Hydrochloride (Since adefovir is eliminated by the kidney, co-administration of adefovir with drugs that reduce renal function may increase serum concentrations of either adefovir and/or these co-administered drugs).
No products indexed under this heading.

Mesalamine (Since adefovir is eliminated by the kidney, co-administration of adefovir with drugs that reduce renal function may increase serum concentrations of either adefovir and/or these co-administered drugs). Products include:
Asacol Delayed-Release Tablets 2579
Canasa Rectal Suppositories 705
Lialda Tablets 3029
Pentasa Capsules 3030

Methimazole (Since adefovir is eliminated by the kidney, co-administration of adefovir with drugs that reduce renal function may increase serum concentrations of either adefovir and/or these co-administered drugs).
No products indexed under this heading.

Methotrexate (Since adefovir is eliminated by the kidney, co-administration of adefovir with drugs that reduce renal function may increase serum concentrations of either adefovir and/or these co-administered drugs).
No products indexed under this heading.

Methotrexate Sodium (Since adefovir is eliminated by the kidney, co-administration of adefovir with drugs that reduce renal function may increase serum concentrations of either adefovir and/or these co-administered drugs).
No products indexed under this heading.

Methyclothiazide (Since adefovir is eliminated by the kidney, co-administration of adefovir with drugs that reduce renal function may increase serum concentrations of either adefovir and/or these co-administered drugs).
No products indexed under this heading.

Mezlocillin Sodium (Since adefovir is eliminated by the kidney, co-administration of adefovir with drugs that reduce renal function may increase serum concentrations of either adefovir and/or these co-administered drugs).
No products indexed under this heading.

Minocycline Hydrochloride (Since adefovir is eliminated by the kidney, co-administration of adefovir with drugs that reduce renal function may increase serum concentrations of either adefovir and/or these co-administered drugs). Products include:
Solodyn Extended Release Tablets 1938

Mitomycin (Mitomycin-C) (Since adefovir is eliminated by the kidney, co-administration of adefovir with drugs that reduce renal function may increase serum concentrations of either adefovir and/or these co-administered drugs).
No products indexed under this heading.

Moexipril Hydrochloride (Since adefovir is eliminated by the kidney, co-administration of adefovir with drugs that reduce renal function may increase serum concentrations of either adefovir and/or these co-administered drugs).
No products indexed under this heading.

Muromonab-CD3 (Since adefovir is eliminated by the kidney, co-administration of adefovir with drugs that reduce renal function may increase serum concentrations of either adefovir and/or these co-administered drugs). Products include:
Orthoclone OKT3 Sterile Solution 2387

Nabumetone (Since adefovir is eliminated by the kidney, co-administration of adefovir with drugs that reduce renal function may increase serum concentrations of either adefovir and/or these co-administered drugs).
No products indexed under this heading.

Nafcillin Sodium (Since adefovir is eliminated by the kidney, co-administration of adefovir with drugs that reduce renal function may increase serum concentrations of either adefovir and/or these co-administered drugs).
No products indexed under this heading.

Naproxen (Since adefovir is eliminated by the kidney, co-administration of adefovir with drugs that reduce renal function may increase serum concentrations of either adefovir and/or these co-administered drugs). Products include:
EC-Naprosyn Delayed-Release Tablets 2632
Naprosyn Suspension 2632
Naprosyn Tablets 2632

Naproxen Sodium (Since adefovir is eliminated by the kidney, co-administration of adefovir with drugs that reduce renal function may increase serum concentrations of either adefovir and/or these co-administered drugs). Products include:
Anaprox Tablets 2632
Anaprox DS Tablets 2632
Treximet Tablets 1616

Nelfinavir Mesylate (Since adefovir is eliminated by the kidney, co-administration of adefovir with drugs that reduce renal function may increase serum concentrations of either adefovir and/or these co-administered drugs).
No products indexed under this heading.

Neomycin (Since adefovir is eliminated by the kidney, co-administration of adefovir with drugs that reduce renal function may increase serum concentrations of either adefovir and/or these co-administered drugs).
No products indexed under this heading.

Neomycin, oral (Since adefovir is eliminated by the kidney, co-administration of adefovir with drugs that reduce renal function may increase serum concentrations of either adefovir and/or these co-administered drugs).
No products indexed under this heading.

Neomycin Sulfate (Since adefovir is eliminated by the kidney, co-administration of adefovir with drugs that reduce renal function may increase serum concentrations of either adefovir and/or these co-administered drugs). Products include:

Neosporin Ophthalmic Solution Sterile ⊙ 252

Nevirapine (Since adefovir is eliminated by the kidney, co-administration of adefovir with drugs that reduce renal function may increase serum concentrations of either adefovir and/or these co-administered drugs). Products include:

Viramune Oral Suspension 873
Viramune Tablets 873

Norfloxacin (Since adefovir is eliminated by the kidney, co-administration of adefovir with drugs that reduce renal function may increase serum concentrations of either adefovir and/or these co-administered drugs). Products include:

Noroxin Tablets 2069

Olsalazine Sodium (Since adefovir is eliminated by the kidney, co-administration of adefovir with drugs that reduce renal function may increase serum concentrations of either adefovir and/or these co-administered drugs).

No products indexed under this heading.

Omeprazole (Since adefovir is eliminated by the kidney, co-administration of adefovir with drugs that reduce renal function may increase serum concentrations of either adefovir and/or these co-administered drugs).

No products indexed under this heading.

Oxaprozin (Since adefovir is eliminated by the kidney, co-administration of adefovir with drugs that reduce renal function may increase serum concentrations of either adefovir and/or these co-administered drugs).

No products indexed under this heading.

Pamidronate Disodium (Since adefovir is eliminated by the kidney, co-administration of adefovir with drugs that reduce renal function may increase serum concentrations of either adefovir and/or these co-administered drugs).

No products indexed under this heading.

Paroxetine Hydrochloride (Since adefovir is eliminated by the kidney, co-administration of adefovir with drugs that reduce renal function may increase serum concentrations of either adefovir and/or these co-administered drugs). Products include:

Paxil 1535
Paxil CR Controlled-Release Tablets 1544

Penicillamine (Since adefovir is eliminated by the kidney, co-administration of adefovir with drugs that reduce renal function may increase serum concentrations of either adefovir and/or these co-administered drugs). Products include:

Cuprimine Capsules 1986

Penicillin G Benzathine (Since adefovir is eliminated by the kidney, co-administration of adefovir with drugs that reduce renal function may increase serum concentrations of either adefovir and/or these co-administered drugs). Products include:

Bicillin C-R Injectable Suspension 1775
Bicillin L-A Injection 1777

Penicillin G Potassium (Since adefovir is eliminated by the kidney, co-administration of adefovir with drugs that reduce renal function may increase serum concentrations of either adefovir and/or these co-administered drugs).

No products indexed under this heading.

Penicillin G Procaine (Since adefovir is eliminated by the kidney, co-administration of adefovir with drugs that reduce renal function may increase serum concentrations of either adefovir and/or these co-administered drugs). Products include:

Bicillin C-R Injectable Suspension 1775
Bicillin L-A Injection 1777

Penicillin G Sodium (Since adefovir is eliminated by the kidney, co-administration of adefovir with drugs that reduce renal function may increase serum concentrations of either adefovir and/or these co-administered drugs).

No products indexed under this heading.

Penicillin V Potassium (Since adefovir is eliminated by the kidney, co-administration of adefovir with drugs that reduce renal function may increase serum concentrations of either adefovir and/or these co-administered drugs).

No products indexed under this heading.

Pentamidine Isethionate (Since adefovir is eliminated by the kidney, co-administration of adefovir with drugs that reduce renal function may increase serum concentrations of either adefovir and/or these co-administered drugs).

No products indexed under this heading.

Perindopril Erbumine (Since adefovir is eliminated by the kidney, co-administration of adefovir with drugs that reduce renal function may increase serum concentrations of either adefovir and/or these co-administered drugs). Products include:

Aceon Tablets (2 mg, 4 mg, 8 mg) 3038

Phenylbutazone (Since adefovir is eliminated by the kidney, co-administration of adefovir with drugs that reduce renal function may increase serum concentrations of either adefovir and/or these co-administered drugs).

No products indexed under this heading.

Piroxicam (Since adefovir is eliminated by the kidney, co-administration of adefovir with drugs that reduce renal function may increase serum concentrations of either adefovir and/or these co-administered drugs).

No products indexed under this heading.

Plicamycin (Since adefovir is eliminated by the kidney, co-administration of adefovir with drugs that reduce renal function may increase serum concentrations of either adefovir and/or these co-administered drugs).

No products indexed under this heading.

Polymyxin (Since adefovir is eliminated by the kidney, co-administration of adefovir with drugs that reduce renal function may increase serum concentrations of either adefovir and/or these co-administered drugs).

No products indexed under this heading.

Polymyxin B Sulfate (Since adefovir is eliminated by the kidney, co-administration of adefovir with drugs that reduce renal function may increase serum concentrations of either adefovir and/or these co-administered drugs). Products include:

Neosporin Ophthalmic Solution Sterile ⊙ 252

Polythiazide (Since adefovir is eliminated by the kidney, co-administration of adefovir with drugs that reduce renal function may increase serum concentrations of either adefovir and/or these co-administered drugs).

No products indexed under this heading.

Pravastatin Sodium (Since adefovir is eliminated by the kidney, co-administration of adefovir with drugs that reduce renal function may increase serum concentrations of either adefovir and/or these co-administered drugs).

No products indexed under this heading.

Probenecid (Since adefovir is eliminated by the kidney, co-administration of adefovir with drugs that reduce renal function may increase serum concentrations of either adefovir and/or these co-administered drugs).

No products indexed under this heading.

Quinapril Hydrochloride (Since adefovir is eliminated by the kidney, co-administration of adefovir with drugs that reduce renal function may increase serum concentrations of either adefovir and/or these co-administered drugs).

No products indexed under this heading.

Rabeprazole Sodium (Since adefovir is eliminated by the kidney, co-administration of adefovir with drugs that reduce renal function may increase serum concentrations of either adefovir and/or these co-administered drugs). Products include:

Aciphex Tablets 1053

Ramipril (Since adefovir is eliminated by the kidney, co-administration of adefovir with drugs that reduce renal function may increase serum concentrations of either adefovir and/or these co-administered drugs).

No products indexed under this heading.

Rifampin (Since adefovir is eliminated by the kidney, co-administration of adefovir with drugs that reduce renal function may increase serum concentrations of either adefovir and/or these co-administered drugs).

No products indexed under this heading.

Riluzole (Since adefovir is eliminated by the kidney, co-administration of adefovir with drugs that reduce renal function may increase serum concentrations of either adefovir and/or these co-administered drugs). Products include:

Rilutek Tablets 2771

Ritonavir (Since adefovir is eliminated by the kidney, co-administration of adefovir with drugs that reduce renal function may increase serum concentrations of either adefovir and/or these co-administered drugs). Products include:

Kaletra 452
Norvir 489

Rofecoxib (Since adefovir is eliminated by the kidney, co-administration of adefovir with drugs that reduce renal function may increase serum concentrations of either adefovir and/or these co-administered drugs).

No products indexed under this heading.

Saquinavir (Since adefovir is eliminated by the kidney, co-administration of adefovir with drugs that reduce renal function may increase serum concentrations of either adefovir and/or these co-administered drugs).

No products indexed under this heading.

Sibutramine Hydrochloride Monohydrate (Since adefovir is eliminated by the kidney, co-administration of adefovir with drugs that reduce renal function may increase serum concentrations of either adefovir and/or these co-administered drugs). Products include:

Meridia Capsules 475

Simvastatin (Since adefovir is eliminated by the kidney, co-administration of adefovir with drugs that reduce renal function may increase serum concentrations of either adefovir and/or these co-administered drugs). Products include:

Simcor Tablets 502
Vytorin 10/10 Tablets 2149
Vytorin 10/10 Tablets 2939
Vytorin 10/20 Tablets 2149
Vytorin 10/20 Tablets 2939
Vytorin 10/40 Tablets 2149
Vytorin 10/40 Tablets 2939
Vytorin 10/80 Tablets 2149
Vytorin 10/80 Tablets 2939
Zocor Tablets 2136

Spirapril Hydrochloride (Since adefovir is eliminated by the kidney, co-administration of adefovir with drugs that reduce renal function may increase serum concentrations of either adefovir and/or these co-administered drugs).

No products indexed under this heading.

Stavudine (Since adefovir is eliminated by the kidney, co-administration of adefovir with drugs that reduce renal function may increase serum concentrations of either adefovir and/or these co-administered drugs).
No products indexed under this heading.

Streptomycin Sulfate (Patients should be monitored closely for adverse events when adefovir dipivoxil is co-administered with other drugs that are known to affect renal function).
No products indexed under this heading.

Streptozocin (Since adefovir is eliminated by the kidney, co-administration of adefovir with drugs that reduce renal function may increase serum concentrations of either adefovir and/or these co-administered drugs).
No products indexed under this heading.

Sulfacytine (Since adefovir is eliminated by the kidney, co-administration of adefovir with drugs that reduce renal function may increase serum concentrations of either adefovir and/or these co-administered drugs).
No products indexed under this heading.

Sulfamethizole (Since adefovir is eliminated by the kidney, co-administration of adefovir with drugs that reduce renal function may increase serum concentrations of either adefovir and/or these co-administered drugs).
No products indexed under this heading.

Sulfamethoxazole (Since adefovir is eliminated by the kidney, co-administration of adefovir with drugs that reduce renal function may increase serum concentrations of either adefovir and/or these co-administered drugs).
No products indexed under this heading.

Sulfasalazine (Since adefovir is eliminated by the kidney, co-administration of adefovir with drugs that reduce renal function may increase serum concentrations of either adefovir and/or these co-administered drugs).
No products indexed under this heading.

Sulfinpyrazone (Since adefovir is eliminated by the kidney, co-administration of adefovir with drugs that reduce renal function may increase serum concentrations of either adefovir and/or these co-administered drugs).
No products indexed under this heading.

Sulfisoxazole Acetyl (Since adefovir is eliminated by the kidney, co-administration of adefovir with drugs that reduce renal function may increase serum concentrations of either adefovir and/or these co-administered drugs).
No products indexed under this heading.

Sulfisoxazole Diolamine (Since adefovir is eliminated by the kidney, co-administration of adefovir with drugs that reduce renal function may increase serum concentrations of either adefovir and/or these co-administered drugs).
No products indexed under this heading.

Sulindac (Since adefovir is eliminated by the kidney, co-administration of adefovir with drugs that reduce renal function may increase serum concentrations of either adefovir and/or these co-administered drugs). Products include:
Clinoril Tablets **1962**

Tacrolimus (Since adefovir is eliminated by the kidney, co-administration of adefovir with drugs that reduce renal function may increase serum concentrations of either adefovir and/or these co-administered drugs). Products include:
Prograf Capsules and Injection **622**
Protopic Ointment **628**

Tenofovir Disoproxil Fumarate (Since adefovir is eliminated by the kidney, co-administration of adefovir with drugs that reduce renal function may increase serum concentrations of either adefovir and/or these co-administered drugs). Products include:
Atripla Tablets **938**
Truvada Tablets **1262**
Viread Tablets **1268**

Thioguanine (Since adefovir is eliminated by the kidney, co-administration of adefovir with drugs that reduce renal function may increase serum concentrations of either adefovir and/or these co-administered drugs). Products include:
Tabloid Tablets **1601**

Ticarcillin Disodium (Since adefovir is eliminated by the kidney, co-administration of adefovir with drugs that reduce renal function may increase serum concentrations of either adefovir and/or these co-administered drugs). Products include:
Timentin ADD-Vantage **1606**
Timentin Injection Galaxy Container **1609**
Timentin IV Infusion **1603**
Timentin Pharmacy Bulk Package **1613**

Tobramycin (Patients should be monitored closely for adverse events when adefovir dipivoxil is co-administered with other drugs that are known to affect renal function). Products include:
Zylet Ophthalmic Suspension .... ⊙**247**

Tobramycin Sulfate (Patients should be monitored closely for adverse events when adefovir dipivoxil is co-administered with other drugs that are known to affect renal function).
No products indexed under this heading.

Tolazamide (Since adefovir is eliminated by the kidney, co-administration of adefovir with drugs that reduce renal function may increase serum concentrations of either adefovir and/or these co-administered drugs).
No products indexed under this heading.

Tolbutamide (Since adefovir is eliminated by the kidney, co-administration of adefovir with drugs that reduce renal function may increase serum concentrations of either adefovir and/or these co-administered drugs).
No products indexed under this heading.

Tolmetin Sodium (Since adefovir is eliminated by the kidney, co-administration of adefovir with drugs that reduce renal function may increase serum concentrations of either adefovir and/or these co-administered drugs).
No products indexed under this heading.

Trandolapril (Since adefovir is eliminated by the kidney, co-administration of adefovir with drugs that reduce renal function may increase serum concentrations of either adefovir and/or these co-administered drugs). Products include:
Mavik Tablets **472**
Tarka Tablets **511**

Triamterene (Since adefovir is eliminated by the kidney, co-administration of adefovir with drugs that reduce renal function may increase serum concentrations of either adefovir and/or these co-administered drugs). Products include:
Dyazide Capsules **1405**
Dyrenium Capsules **3189**

Trimethadione (Since adefovir is eliminated by the kidney, co-administration of adefovir with drugs that reduce renal function may increase serum concentrations of either adefovir and/or these co-administered drugs).
No products indexed under this heading.

Trovafloxacin Mesylate (Since adefovir is eliminated by the kidney, co-administration of adefovir with drugs that reduce renal function may increase serum concentrations of either adefovir and/or these co-administered drugs).
No products indexed under this heading.

Tyropanoate Sodium (Since adefovir is eliminated by the kidney, co-administration of adefovir with drugs that reduce renal function may increase serum concentrations of either adefovir and/or these co-administered drugs).
No products indexed under this heading.

Valacyclovir Hydrochloride (Since adefovir is eliminated by the kidney, co-administration of adefovir with drugs that reduce renal function may increase serum concentrations of either adefovir and/or these co-administered drugs). Products include:
Valtrex Caplets **1635**

Valdecoxib (Since adefovir is eliminated by the kidney, co-administration of adefovir with drugs that reduce renal function may increase serum concentrations of either adefovir and/or these co-administered drugs).
No products indexed under this heading.

Vancomycin Hydrochloride (Since adefovir is eliminated by the kidney, co-administration of adefovir with drugs that reduce renal function may increase serum concentrations of either adefovir and/or these co-administered drugs).
No products indexed under this heading.

Voriconazole (Since adefovir is eliminated by the kidney, co-administration of adefovir with drugs that reduce renal function may increase serum concentrations of either adefovir and/or these co-administered drugs).
No products indexed under this heading.

Zalcitabine (Since adefovir is eliminated by the kidney, co-administration of adefovir with drugs that reduce renal function may increase serum concentrations of either adefovir and/or these co-administered drugs).
No products indexed under this heading.

Zidovudine (Since adefovir is eliminated by the kidney, co-administration of adefovir with drugs that reduce renal function may increase serum concentrations of either adefovir and/or these co-administered drugs). Products include:
Combivir Tablets **1384**
Retrovir **1574**
Retrovir IV Infusion **1579**
Trizivir Tablets **1622**

Zoledronic acid (Since adefovir is eliminated by the kidney, co-administration of adefovir with drugs that reduce renal function may increase serum concentrations of either adefovir and/or these co-administered drugs). Products include:
Reclast Injection **2291**
Zometa for Intravenous Infusion **2341**

HERCEPTIN I.V.

(Trastuzumab) **1199**
May interact with anthracycline antibiotics and their derivatives and certain other agents. Compounds in these categories include:

Cyclophosphamide (The increase and severity of cardiac dysfunction is particularly high in patients who receive trastuzumab in combination with cyclophosphamide).
No products indexed under this heading.

Daunorubicin Hydrochloride (Co-administration may cause cardiomyopathy. Concurrent use of trastuzumab with anthracyclines have a greater risk of sub-clinical and clinical cardiac failure manifesting as CHF, and decreased LVEF. Evaluate cardiac function prior to and during treatment. Discontinue trastuzumab for cardiomyopathy).
No products indexed under this heading.

Doxorubicin Hydrochloride (Co-administration may cause cardiomyopathy. Concurrent use of trastuzumab with anthracyclines have a greater risk of sub-clinical and clinical cardiac failure manifesting as CHF, and decreased LVEF. Evaluate cardiac function prior to and during treatment. Discontinue trastuzumab for cardiomyopathy).
No products indexed under this heading.

Epirubicin Hydrochloride (Co-administration may cause cardiomyopathy. Concurrent use of trastuzumab with anthracyclines have a greater risk of sub-clinical and clinical cardiac failure manifesting as CHF, and decreased LVEF. Evaluate cardiac function prior to and during treatment. Discontinue trastuzumab for cardiomyopathy).
No products indexed under this heading.

Idarubicin Hydrochloride (Co-administration may cause cardiomyopathy. Concurrent use of trastuzumab with anthracyclines have a greater risk of sub-clinical and clinical cardiac failure manifesting as CHF, and decreased LVEF. Evaluate cardiac function prior to and during treatment. Discontinue trastuzumab for cardiomyopathy).
No products indexed under this heading.

Paclitaxel (Co-administration has resulted in a 1.5-fold increase in trastuzumab serum levels in clinical studies).
No products indexed under this heading.

HEXALEN CAPSULES

(Altretamine) 1078
May interact with monoamine oxidase inhibitors and certain other agents. Compounds in these categories include:

Isocarboxazid (Concurrent administration of altretamine capsules and antidepressants of the MAO inhibitor class may cause severe orthostatic hypotensions). Products include:
Marplan Tablets 3177

Moclobemide (Concurrent administration of altretamine capsules and antidepressants of the MAO inhibitor class may cause severe orthostatic hypotensions).
No products indexed under this heading.

Pargyline Hydrochloride (Concurrent administration of altretamine capsules and antidepressants of the MAO inhibitor class may cause severe orthostatic hypotensions).
No products indexed under this heading.

Phenelzine Sulfate (Concurrent administration of altretamine capsules and antidepressants of the MAO inhibitor class may cause severe orthostatic hypotensions).
No products indexed under this heading.

Procarbazine Hydrochloride (Concurrent administration of altretamine capsules and antidepressants of the MAO inhibitor class may cause severe orthostatic hypotensions).
No products indexed under this heading.

Pyridoxine (Concomitant adminstration of pyridoxine with altrelamine should be avoided. There are possible adverse response duration effects).
No products indexed under this heading.

Rasagiline Mesylate (Concurrent administration of altretamine capsules and antidepressants of the MAO inhibitor class may cause severe orthostatic hypotensions). Products include:
Azilect Tablets 3106

Selegiline (Concurrent administration of altretamine capsules and antidepressants of the MAO inhibitor class may cause severe orthostatic hypotensions). Products include:
Emsam Transdermal System 905

Selegiline Hydrochloride (Concurrent administration of altretamine capsules and antidepressants of the MAO inhibitor class may cause severe orthostatic hypotensions). Products include:
Eldepryl Capsules 3052

Tranylcypromine Sulfate (Concurrent administration of altretamine capsules and antidepressants of the MAO inhibitor class may cause severe orthostatic hypotensions). Products include:
Parnate Tablets 1532

HUMALOG-PEN AND KWIKPEN

(Insulin Lispro, Human) 1829
May interact with ACE inhibitors, angiotensin-II receptor antagonists, beta blockers, corticosteroids, estrogens, oral hypoglycemic agents, oral contraceptives, phenothiazines, salicylates, thyroid preparations, and certain other agents. Compounds in these categories include:

Acarbose (Co-administration with drugs with hypoglycemic activity, such as oral hypoglycemic agents, may result in decreased insulin requirements). Products include:
Precose Tablets 792

Acebutolol Hydrochloride (Co-administration with drugs with hypoglycemic activity, such as beta blockers, may result in decreased insulin requirements; beta blockers may mask the symptoms of hypoglycemia in some patients).
No products indexed under this heading.

Aspirin (Co-administration with drugs with hypoglycemic activity, such as salicylates, may result in decreased insulin requirements). Products include:
Aggrenox Capsules 819
Bayer Aspirin 750
Percodan Tablets 1130
St. Joseph 81 mg Aspirin Chewable and Enteric Coated Tablets 1903

Aspirin, Enteric Coated (Co-administration with drugs with hypoglycemic activity, such as salicylates, may result in decreased insulin requirements).
No products indexed under this heading.

Aspirin Buffered (Co-administration with drugs with hypoglycemic activity, such as salicylates, may result in decreased insulin requirements).
No products indexed under this heading.

Atenolol (Co-administration with drugs with hypoglycemic activity, such as beta blockers, may result in decreased insulin requirements; beta blockers may mask the symptoms of hypoglycemia in some patients).
No products indexed under this heading.

Benazepril Hydrochloride (Co-administration with drugs with hypoglycemic activity, such as certain ACE inhibitors, may result in decreased insulin requirements).
No products indexed under this heading.

Betamethasone Acetate (Co-administration may result in increased insulin requirements).
No products indexed under this heading.

Betamethasone Sodium Phosphate (Co-administration may result in increased insulin requirements).
No products indexed under this heading.

Betaxolol Hydrochloride (Co-administration with drugs with hypoglycemic activity, such as beta blockers, may result in decreased insulin requirements; beta blockers may mask the symptoms of hypoglycemia in some patients).
No products indexed under this heading.

Bisoprolol Fumarate (Co-administration with drugs with hypoglycemic activity, such as beta blockers, may result in decreased insulin requirements; beta blockers may mask the symptoms of hypoglycemia in some patients).
No products indexed under this heading.

Budesonide (Co-administration may result in increased insulin requirements). Products include:
Pulmicort Flexhaler 654
Symbicort 80/4.5 Inhalation Aerosol 659
Symbicort 160/4.5 Inhalation Aerosol 659

Candesartan Cilexetil (Insulin requirements may be decreased in the presence of drugs with hypoglycemicartivity, such as angiotension II receptor blocking agents). Products include:
Atacand Tablets 639
Atacand HCT 642

Captopril (Co-administration with drugs with hypoglycemic activity, such as certain ACE inhibitors, may result in decreased insulin requirements). Products include:
Captopril Tablets 2182

Carteolol Hydrochloride (Co-administration with drugs with hypoglycemic activity, such as beta blockers, may result in decreased insulin requirements; beta blockers may mask the symptoms of hypoglycemia in some patients).
No products indexed under this heading.

Chlorotrianisene (Co-administration may result in increased insulin requirements).
No products indexed under this heading.

Chlorpromazine (Co-administration with phenothiazines may result in increased insulin requirements).
No products indexed under this heading.

Chlorpromazine Hydrochloride (Co-administration with phenothiazines may result in increased insulin requirements).
No products indexed under this heading.

Chlorpropamide (Co-administration with drugs with hypoglycemic activity, such as oral hypoglycemic agents, may result in decreased insulin requirements).
No products indexed under this heading.

Choline Magnesium Trisalicylate (Co-administration with drugs with hypoglycemic activity, such as salicylates, may result in decreased insulin requirements).
No products indexed under this heading.

Ciclesonide (Co-administration may result in increased insulin requirements). Products include:
Alvesco Inhalation Aerosol 2985
Omnaris Nasal Spray 2998

Cortisone Acetate (Co-administration may result in increased insulin requirements).
No products indexed under this heading.

Desogestrel (Co-admininstration with oral contraceptives may result in increased insulin requirements). Products include:
Mircette Tablets 1034

Dexamethasone (Co-administration may result in increased insulin requirements). Products include:
Ciprodex Otic Suspension 541

Dexamethasone Acetate (Co-administration may result in increased insulin requirements).
No products indexed under this heading.

Dexamethasone Sodium Phosphate (Co-administration may result in increased insulin requirements).
No products indexed under this heading.

Dienestrol (Co-administration may result in increased insulin requirements).
No products indexed under this heading.

Diethylstilbestrol (Co-administration may result in increased insulin requirements).
No products indexed under this heading.

Diflunisal (Co-administration with drugs with hypoglycemic activity, such as salicylates, may result in decreased insulin requirements).
No products indexed under this heading.

Enalapril Maleate (Co-administration with drugs with hypoglycemic activity, such as certain ACE inhibitors, may result in decreased insulin requirements).
No products indexed under this heading.

Enalaprilat (Co-administration with drugs with hypoglycemic activity, such as certain ACE inhibitors, may result in decreased insulin requirements).
No products indexed under this heading.

Eprosartan Mesylate (Insulin requirements may be decreased in the presence of drugs with hypoglycemicartivity, such as angiotension II receptor blocking agents). Products include:
Teveten Tablets 515
Teveten HCT Tablets 517

Esmolol Hydrochloride (Co-administration with drugs with hypoglycemic activity, such as beta blockers, may result in decreased insulin requirements; beta blockers may mask the symptoms of hypoglycemia in some patients).
No products indexed under this heading.

Estradiol (Co-administration may result in increased insulin requirements). Products include:
Activella Tablets 2347
Angeliq Tablets 751
Climara Transdermal System 763
Climara Pro Transdermal System 768
Divigel 3167
Vagifem Tablets 2375

Estrogens, Conjugated (Co-administration may result in increased insulin requirements). Products include:
Premarin Intravenous 3217
Premarin Tablets 3221
Premarin Vaginal Cream 3228
Premphase Tablets 3232
Prempro Tablets 3232

Estrogens, Esterified (Co-administration may result in increased insulin requirements). Products include:
Estratest Tablets 3043
Estratest H.S. Tablets 3043

Estropipate (Co-administration may result in increased insulin requirements).
No products indexed under this heading.

Ethinyl Estradiol (Co-administration may result in increased insulin requirements). Products include:
Lybrel Tablets 3204
Mircette Tablets 1034
NuvaRing 2897
Ortho-Cyclen/Ortho Tri-Cyclen 2449
Ortho Evra Transdermal System 2437
Ortho Tri-Cyclen Lo Tablets 2458
Seasonique Tablets 1046
Yaz Tablets 805

Ethynodiol Diacetate (Co-admininstration with oral contraceptives may result in increased insulin requirements).
No products indexed under this heading.

Fludrocortisone Acetate (Co-administration may result in increased insulin requirements).
No products indexed under this heading.

Flunisolide (Co-administration may result in increased insulin requirements). Products include:
Aerobid/Aerobid-M 1153

Fluphenazine Decanoate (Co-administration with phenothiazines may result in increased insulin requirements).
No products indexed under this heading.

Fluphenazine Enanthate (Co-administration with phenothiazines may result in increased insulin requirements).
No products indexed under this heading.

Fluphenazine Hydrochloride (Co-administration with phenothiazines may result in increased insulin requirements).
No products indexed under this heading.

Fluticasone Propionate (Co-administration may result in increased insulin requirements). Products include:
Advair Diskus 100/50 1276
Advair Diskus 250/50 1276
Advair Diskus 500/50 1276
Advair HFA 45/21 Inhalation Aerosol 1288
Advair HFA 115/21 Inhalation Aerosol 1288
Advair HFA 230/21 Inhalation Aerosol 1288
Flonase Nasal Spray 1431
Flovent Diskus 50 mcg 1435

Fluticasone Propionate HFA (Co-administration may result in increased insulin requirements). Products include:
Flovent HFA 1440

Fosinopril Sodium (Co-administration with drugs with hypoglycemic activity, such as certain ACE inhibitors, may result in decreased insulin requirements).
No products indexed under this heading.

Glimepiride (Co-administration with drugs with hypoglycemic activity, such as oral hypoglycemic agents, may result in decreased insulin requirements). Products include:
Avandaryl Tablets 1344
Duetact Tablets 3085

Glipizide (Co-administration with drugs with hypoglycemic activity, such as oral hypoglycemic agents, may result in decreased insulin requirements).
No products indexed under this heading.

Glyburide (Co-administration with drugs with hypoglycemic activity, such as oral hypoglycemic agents, may result in decreased insulin requirements).
No products indexed under this heading.

Hydrocortisone (Co-administration may result in increased insulin requirements).
No products indexed under this heading.

Hydrocortisone Acetate (Co-administration may result in increased insulin requirements). Products include:
Analpram-HC 1140
Pramosone 1141

Hydrocortisone Sodium Phosphate (Co-administration may result in increased insulin requirements).
No products indexed under this heading.

Hydrocortisone Sodium Succinate (Co-administration may result in increased insulin requirements).
No products indexed under this heading.

Irbesartan (Insulin requirements may be decreased in the presence of drugs with hypoglycemicartivity, such as angiotension II receptor blocking agents). Products include:
Avalide Tablets 892
Avalide Tablets 2713
Avapro Tablets 897
Avapro Tablets 2718

Isoniazid (Co-administration may result in increased insulin requirements).
No products indexed under this heading.

Labetalol Hydrochloride (Co-administration with drugs with hypoglycemic activity, such as beta blockers, may result in decreased insulin requirements; beta blockers may mask the symptoms of hypoglycemia in some patients).
No products indexed under this heading.

Levobunolol Hydrochloride (Co-administration with drugs with hypoglycemic activity, such as beta blockers, may result in decreased insulin requirements; beta blockers may mask the symptoms of hypoglycemia in some patients).
No products indexed under this heading.

Levonorgestrel (Co-admininstration with oral contraceptives may result in increased insulin requirements). Products include:
Climara Pro Transdermal System 768
Lybrel Tablets 3204
Mirena Intrauterine System 779
Plan B Tablets 1044
Seasonique Tablets 1046

Levothyroxine Sodium (Co-administration with thyroid replacement therapy may result in increased insulin requirements). Products include:
Levothroid Tablets 1170
Levoxyl Tablets 1780
Synthroid Tablets 507

Liothyronine Sodium (Co-administration with thyroid replacement therapy may result in increased insulin requirements). Products include:
Cytomel Tablets 1778

Liotrix (Co-administration with thyroid replacement therapy may result in increased insulin requirements).
No products indexed under this heading.

Lisinopril (Co-administration with drugs with hypoglycemic activity, such as certain ACE inhibitors, may result in decreased insulin requirements). Products include:
Prinivil Tablets 2087
Prinzide Tablets 2092

Losartan Potassium (Insulin requirements may be decreased in the presence of drugs with hypoglycemicartivity, such as angiotension II receptor blocking agents). Products include:
Cozaar Tablets 1973

Magnesium Salicylate (Co-administration with drugs with hypoglycemic activity, such as salicylates, may result in decreased insulin requirements).
No products indexed under this heading.

Mesoridazine Besylate (Co-administration with phenothiazines may result in increased insulin requirements).
No products indexed under this heading.

Mestranol (Co-admininstration with oral contraceptives may result in increased insulin requirements).
No products indexed under this heading.

Metformin Hydrochloride (Co-administration with drugs with hypoglycemic activity, such as oral hypoglycemic agents, may result in decreased insulin requirements). Products include:
ActoPlus Met Tablets 3071
Avandamet Tablets 1336
Janumet Tablets 2041
PrandiMet Tablets 2967

Methotrimeprazine (Co-administration with phenothiazines may result in increased insulin requirements).
No products indexed under this heading.

Methylprednisolone Acetate (Co-administration may result in increased insulin requirements).
No products indexed under this heading.

Methylprednisolone Sodium Succinate (Co-administration may result in increased insulin requirements).
No products indexed under this heading.

Metipranolol Hydrochloride (Co-administration with drugs with hypoglycemic activity, such as beta blockers, may result in decreased insulin requirements; beta blockers may mask the symptoms of hypoglycemia in some patients).
No products indexed under this heading.

Metoprolol Succinate (Co-administration with drugs with hypoglycemic activity, such as beta blockers, may result in decreased insulin requirements; beta blockers may mask the symptoms of hypoglycemia in some patients). Products include:
Toprol-XL Tablets 666

Metoprolol Tartrate (Co-administration with drugs with hypoglycemic activity, such as beta blockers, may result in decreased insulin requirements; beta blockers may mask the symptoms of hypoglycemia in some patients).
No products indexed under this heading.

Miglitol (Co-administration with drugs with hypoglycemic activity, such as oral hypoglycemic agents, may result in decreased insulin requirements).
No products indexed under this heading.

Moexipril Hydrochloride (Co-administration with drugs with hypoglycemic activity, such as certain ACE inhibitors, may result in decreased insulin requirements).
No products indexed under this heading.

Mometasone Furoate (Co-administration may result in increased insulin requirements). Products include:
Asmanex Twisthaler 2797
Elocon Cream 0.1% 2840
Elocon Lotion 0.1% 2841
Elocon Ointment 0.1% 2842

Mometasone Furoate Monohydrate (Co-administration may result in increased insulin requirements). Products include:
Nasonex Nasal Spray 2883

Nadolol (Co-administration with drugs with hypoglycemic activity, such as beta blockers, may result in decreased insulin requirements; beta blockers may mask the symptoms of hypoglycemia in some patients). Products include:
Nadolol Tablets 2191

Nateglinide (Co-administration with drugs with hypoglycemic activity, such as oral hypoglycemic agents, may result in decreased insulin requirements). Products include:
Starlix Tablets 2314

Nebivolol (Co-administration with drugs with hypoglycemic activity, such as beta blockers, may result in decreased insulin requirements; beta blockers may mask the symptoms of hypoglycemia in some patients). Products include:
Bystolic Tablets 1155

Niacin (Co-administration may result in increased insulin requirements). Products include:
Advicor Tablets 402
Bausch & Lomb Ocuvite DF Vitamin Supplement .... ⊙238
Dismutax Dietary Supplement 995
Niaspan Extended-Release Tablets 480
NT-Kinase Dietary Supplement 995
Simcor Tablets 502

Norethindrone (Co-admininstration with oral contraceptives may result in increased insulin requirements). Products include:
Ortho Micronor Tablets ... 2446

Norethynodrel (Co-admininstration with oral contraceptives may result in increased insulin requirements).
No products indexed under this heading.

Norgestimate (Co-admininstration with oral contraceptives may result in increased insulin requirements). Products include:
Ortho-Cyclen/Ortho Tri-Cyclen ... 2449
Ortho Tri-Cyclen Lo Tablets ... 2458

Norgestrel (Co-admininstration with oral contraceptives may result in increased insulin requirements).
No products indexed under this heading.

Octreotide Acetate (Co-administration with drugs with hypoglycemic activity, such as inhibitors of pancreatic function, may result in decreased insulin requirements). Products include:
Sandostatin Injection ... 2300
Sandostatin LAR Depot ... 2302

Penbutolol Sulfate (Co-administration with drugs with hypoglycemic activity, such as beta blockers, may result in decreased insulin requirements; beta blockers may mask the symptoms of hypoglycemia in some patients).
No products indexed under this heading.

Perindopril Erbumine (Co-administration with drugs with hypoglycemic activity, such as certain ACE inhibitors, may result in decreased insulin requirements). Products include:
Aceon Tablets (2 mg, 4 mg, 8 mg) ... 3038

Perphenazine (Co-administration with phenothiazines may result in increased insulin requirements).
No products indexed under this heading.

Phenelzine Sulfate (Co-administration with drugs with hypoglycemic activity, such as certain MAO inhibitor antidepressants, may result in decreased insulin requirements).
No products indexed under this heading.

Pindolol (Co-administration with drugs with hypoglycemic activity, such as beta blockers, may result in decreased insulin requirements; beta blockers may mask the symptoms of hypoglycemia in some patients).
No products indexed under this heading.

Pioglitazone Hydrochloride (Co-administration with drugs with hypoglycemic activity, such as oral hypoglycemic agents, may result in decreased insulin requirements). Products include:
ActoPlus Met Tablets ... 3071
Actos Tablets ... 3077
Duetact Tablets ... 3085

Polyestradiol Phosphate (Co-administration may result in increased insulin requirements).
No products indexed under this heading.

Prednisolone Acetate (Co-administration may result in increased insulin requirements). Products include:
Pred Forte Ophthalmic Suspension ... ⊙ 227
Pred Mild Ophthalmic Suspension ... ⊙ 230
Pred-G Ophthalmic Ointment ... ⊙ 229
Pred-G Ophthalmic Suspension ... ⊙ 228

Prednisolone Sodium Phosphate (Co-administration may result in increased insulin requirements).
No products indexed under this heading.

Prednisolone Tebutate (Co-administration may result in increased insulin requirements).
No products indexed under this heading.

Prednisone (Co-administration may result in increased insulin requirements).
No products indexed under this heading.

Prochlorperazine (Co-administration with phenothiazines may result in increased insulin requirements).
No products indexed under this heading.

Promethazine Hydrochloride (Co-administration with phenothiazines may result in increased insulin requirements).
No products indexed under this heading.

Propranolol Hydrochloride (Co-administration with drugs with hypoglycemic activity, such as beta blockers, may result in decreased insulin requirements; beta blockers may mask the symptoms of hypoglycemia in some patients). Products include:
InnoPran XL Extended Release Capsules ... 1484

Quinapril Hydrochloride (Co-administration with drugs with hypoglycemic activity, such as certain ACE inhibitors, may result in decreased insulin requirements).
No products indexed under this heading.

Quinestrol (Co-administration may result in increased insulin requirements).
No products indexed under this heading.

Ramipril (Co-administration with drugs with hypoglycemic activity, such as certain ACE inhibitors, may result in decreased insulin requirements).
No products indexed under this heading.

Repaglinide (Co-administration with drugs with hypoglycemic activity, such as oral hypoglycemic agents, may result in decreased insulin requirements). Products include:
PrandiMet Tablets ... 2967
Prandin Tablets ... 2971

Rosiglitazone Maleate (Co-administration with drugs with hypoglycemic activity, such as oral hypoglycemic agents, may result in decreased insulin requirements). Products include:
Avandamet Tablets ... 1336
Avandaryl Tablets ... 1344
Avandia Tablets ... 1351

Salsalate (Co-administration with drugs with hypoglycemic activity, such as salicylates, may result in decreased insulin requirements).
No products indexed under this heading.

Sitagliptin Phosphate (Co-administration with drugs with hypoglycemic activity, such as oral hypoglycemic agents, may result in decreased insulin requirements). Products include:
Janumet Tablets ... 2041
Januvia Tablets ... 2048

Sotalol Hydrochloride (Co-administration with drugs with hypoglycemic activity, such as beta blockers, may result in decreased insulin requirements; beta blockers may mask the symptoms of hypoglycemia in some patients).
No products indexed under this heading.

Spirapril Hydrochloride (Co-administration with drugs with hypoglycemic activity, such as certain ACE inhibitors, may result in decreased insulin requirements).
No products indexed under this heading.

Sulfacytine (Co-administration with drugs with hypoglycemic activity, such as sulfa antibiotics, may result in decreased insulin requirements).
No products indexed under this heading.

Sulfamethizole (Co-administration with drugs with hypoglycemic activity, such as sulfa antibiotics, may result in decreased insulin requirements).
No products indexed under this heading.

Sulfamethoxazole (Co-administration with drugs with hypoglycemic activity, such as sulfa antibiotics, may result in decreased insulin requirements).
No products indexed under this heading.

Sulfasalazine (Co-administration with drugs with hypoglycemic activity, such as sulfa antibiotics, may result in decreased insulin requirements).
No products indexed under this heading.

Telmisartan (Insulin requirements may be decreased in the presence of drugs with hypoglycemicartivity, such as angiotension II receptor blocking agents). Products include:
Micardis Tablets ... 852
Micardis HCT Tablets ... 854

Thioridazine Hydrochloride (Co-administration with phenothiazines may result in increased insulin requirements). Products include:
Thioridazine Hydrochloride Tablets ... 2195

Thyroglobulin (Co-administration with thyroid replacement therapy may result in increased insulin requirements).
No products indexed under this heading.

Thyroid (Co-administration with thyroid replacement therapy may result in increased insulin requirements). Products include:
Naturethroid Tablets ... 2605

Thyroxine (Co-administration with thyroid replacement therapy may result in increased insulin requirements).
No products indexed under this heading.

Thyroxine Sodium (Co-administration with thyroid replacement therapy may result in increased insulin requirements).
No products indexed under this heading.

Timolol Hemihydrate (Co-administration with drugs with hypoglycemic activity, such as beta blockers, may result in decreased insulin requirements; beta blockers may mask the symptoms of hypoglycemia in some patients). Products include:
Betimol Ophthalmic Solution ... 3181

Timolol Maleate (Co-administration with drugs with hypoglycemic activity, such as beta blockers, may result in decreased insulin requirements; beta blockers may mask the symptoms of hypoglycemia in some patients). Products include:
Combigan Ophthalmic Solution ... 553
Cosopt Sterile Ophthalmic Solution ... 1969
Timoptic Sterile Ophthalmic Solution ... 2121
Timoptic in Ocudose ... 2124
Timoptic-XE Sterile Ophthalmic Gel Forming Solution ... 2125

Tolazamide (Co-administration with drugs with hypoglycemic activity, such as oral hypoglycemic agents, may result in decreased insulin requirements).
No products indexed under this heading.

Tolbutamide (Co-administration with drugs with hypoglycemic activity, such as oral hypoglycemic agents, may result in decreased insulin requirements).
No products indexed under this heading.

Trandolapril (Co-administration with drugs with hypoglycemic activity, such as certain ACE inhibitors, may result in decreased insulin requirements). Products include:
Mavik Tablets ... 472
Tarka Tablets ... 511

Tranylcypromine Sulfate (Co-administration with drugs with hypoglycemic activity, such as certain MAO inhibitor antidepressants, may result in decreased insulin requirements). Products include:
Parnate Tablets ... 1532

Triamcinolone (Co-administration may result in increased insulin requirements).
No products indexed under this heading.

Triamcinolone Acetonide (Co-administration may result in increased insulin requirements). Products include:
Azmacort Inhalation Aerosol ... 407
Nasacort AQ Nasal Spray ... 2765
Triesence Injectable Suspension ... ⊙ 209

Triamcinolone Diacetate (Co-administration may result in increased insulin requirements).
No products indexed under this heading.

Triamcinolone Hexacetonide (Co-administration may result in increased insulin requirements).
No products indexed under this heading.

Trifluoperazine Hydrochloride (Co-administration with phenothiazines may result in increased insulin requirements).
No products indexed under this heading.

Troglitazone (Co-administration with drugs with hypoglycemic activity, such as oral hypoglycemic agents, may result in decreased insulin requirements).
No products indexed under this heading.

Valsartan (Insulin requirements may be decreased in the presence of

drugs with hypoglycemicartivity, such as angiotension II receptor blocking agents). Products include:
Diovan Tablets 2212
Diovan HCT Tablets 2216
Exforge Tablets 2238

Food Interactions

Alcohol (Co-administration with drugs with hypoglycemic activity may result in decreased insulin requirements).

HUMALOG MIX 50/50-PEN AND KWIKPEN
(Insulin Lispro, Human, Insulin Lispro Protamine, Human) 1833
May interact with ACE inhibitors, beta blockers, corticosteroids, estrogens, oral hypoglycemic agents, monoamine oxidase inhibitors, oral contraceptives, phenothiazines, salicylates, thyroid preparations, and certain other agents. Compounds in these categories include:

Acarbose (Insulin requirements may be decreased in the presence of drugs with with hypoglycemic activity, such as oral antidiabetic agents). Products include:
Precose Tablets 792

Acebutolol Hydrochloride (Beta-adrenergic blockers may mask the symptoms of hypoglycemia in some patients).
No products indexed under this heading.

Aspirin (Insulin requirements may be decreased in the presence of drugs with hypoglycemic activity, such as salicylates). Products include:
Aggrenox Capsules 819
Bayer Aspirin 750
Percodan Tablets 1130
St. Joseph 81 mg Aspirin Chewable and Enteric Coated Tablets 1903

Aspirin, Enteric Coated (Insulin requirements may be decreased in the presence of drugs with hypoglycemic activity, such as salicylates).
No products indexed under this heading.

Aspirin Buffered (Insulin requirements may be decreased in the presence of drugs with hypoglycemic activity, such as salicylates).
No products indexed under this heading.

Atenolol (Beta-adrenergic blockers may mask the symptoms of hypoglycemia in some patients).
No products indexed under this heading.

Benazepril Hydrochloride (Insulin requirements may be decreased in the presence of drugs with hypoglycemic activity, such as certain angiotensin converting enzyme inhibitors).
No products indexed under this heading.

Betamethasone Acetate (Insulin requirements may be increased by medications with hypoglycemic activity, such as corticosteroids).
No products indexed under this heading.

Betamethasone Sodium Phosphate (Insulin requirements may be increased by medications with hypoglycemic activity, such as corticosteroids).
No products indexed under this heading.

Betaxolol Hydrochloride (Beta-adrenergic blockers may mask the symptoms of hypoglycemia in some patients).
No products indexed under this heading.

Bisoprolol Fumarate (Beta-adrenergic blockers may mask the symptoms of hypoglycemia in some patients).
No products indexed under this heading.

Budesonide (Insulin requirements may be increased by medications with hypoglycemic activity, such as corticosteroids). Products include:
Pulmicort Flexhaler 654
Symbicort 80/4.5 Inhalation Aerosol 659
Symbicort 160/4.5 Inhalation Aerosol 659

Captopril (Insulin requirements may be decreased in the presence of drugs with hypoglycemic activity, such as certain angiotensin converting enzyme inhibitors). Products include:
Captopril Tablets 2182

Carteolol Hydrochloride (Beta-adrenergic blockers may mask the symptoms of hypoglycemia in some patients).
No products indexed under this heading.

Chlorotrianisene (Insulin requirements may be increased by medications with hypoglycemic activity, such as estrogens).
No products indexed under this heading.

Chlorpromazine (Insulin requirements may be increased by medications with hypoglycemic activity, such as phenothiazines).
No products indexed under this heading.

Chlorpromazine Hydrochloride (Insulin requirements may be increased by medications with hypoglycemic activity, such as phenothiazines).
No products indexed under this heading.

Chlorpropamide (Insulin requirements may be decreased in the presence of drugs with with hypoglycemic activity, such as oral antidiabetic agents).
No products indexed under this heading.

Choline Magnesium Trisalicylate (Insulin requirements may be decreased in the presence of drugs with hypoglycemic activity, such as salicylates).
No products indexed under this heading.

Ciclesonide (Insulin requirements may be increased by medications with hypoglycemic activity, such as corticosteroids). Products include:
Alvesco Inhalation Aerosol 2985
Omnaris Nasal Spray 2998

Cortisone Acetate (Insulin requirements may be increased by medications with hypoglycemic activity, such as corticosteroids).
No products indexed under this heading.

Desogestrel (Insulin requirements may be increased by medications with hypoglycemic activity, such as oral contraceptives). Products include:
Mircette Tablets 1034

Dexamethasone (Insulin requirements may be increased by medications with hypoglycemic activity, such as corticosteroids). Products include:
Ciprodex Otic Suspension 541

Dexamethasone Acetate (Insulin requirements may be increased by medications with hypoglycemic activity, such as corticosteroids).
No products indexed under this heading.

Dexamethasone Sodium Phosphate (Insulin requirements may be increased by medications with hypoglycemic activity, such as corticosteroids).
No products indexed under this heading.

Dienestrol (Insulin requirements may be increased by medications with hypoglycemic activity, such as estrogens).
No products indexed under this heading.

Diethylstilbestrol (Insulin requirements may be increased by medications with hypoglycemic activity, such as estrogens).
No products indexed under this heading.

Diflunisal (Insulin requirements may be decreased in the presence of drugs with hypoglycemic activity, such as salicylates).
No products indexed under this heading.

Enalapril Maleate (Insulin requirements may be decreased in the presence of drugs with hypoglycemic activity, such as certain angiotensin converting enzyme inhibitors).
No products indexed under this heading.

Enalaprilat (Insulin requirements may be decreased in the presence of drugs with hypoglycemic activity, such as certain angiotensin converting enzyme inhibitors).
No products indexed under this heading.

Esmolol Hydrochloride (Beta-adrenergic blockers may mask the symptoms of hypoglycemia in some patients).
No products indexed under this heading.

Estradiol (Insulin requirements may be increased by medications with hypoglycemic activity, such as estrogens). Products include:
Activella Tablets 2347
Angeliq Tablets 751
Climara Transdermal System 763
Climara Pro Transdermal System 768
Divigel 3167
Vagifem Tablets 2375

Estrogens, Conjugated (Insulin requirements may be increased by medications with hypoglycemic activity, such as estrogens). Products include:
Premarin Intravenous 3217
Premarin Tablets 3221
Premarin Vaginal Cream 3228
Premphase Tablets 3232
Prempro Tablets 3232

Estrogens, Esterified (Insulin requirements may be increased by medications with hypoglycemic activity, such as estrogens). Products include:
Estratest Tablets 3043
Estratest H.S. Tablets 3043

Estropipate (Insulin requirements may be increased by medications with hypoglycemic activity, such as estrogens).
No products indexed under this heading.

Ethanol (Insulin requirements may be decreased in the presence of drugs with hypoglycemic activity, such as ethanol).
No products indexed under this heading.

Ethinyl Estradiol (Insulin requirements may be increased by medications with hypoglycemic activity, such as oral contraceptives). Products include:
Lybrel Tablets 3204
Mircette Tablets 1034
NuvaRing 2897
Ortho-Cyclen/Ortho Tri-Cyclen 2449
Ortho Evra Transdermal System 2437
Ortho Tri-Cyclen Lo Tablets 2458
Seasonique Tablets 1046
Yaz Tablets 805

Ethyl Alcohol (Insulin requirements may be decreased in the presence of drugs with hypoglycemic activity, such as alcohol).
No products indexed under this heading.

Ethynodiol Diacetate (Insulin requirements may be increased by medications with hypoglycemic activity, such as oral contraceptives).
No products indexed under this heading.

Fludrocortisone Acetate (Insulin requirements may be increased by medications with hypoglycemic activity, such as corticosteroids).
No products indexed under this heading.

Flunisolide (Insulin requirements may be increased by medications with hypoglycemic activity, such as corticosteroids). Products include:
Aerobid/Aerobid-M 1153

Fluphenazine Decanoate (Insulin requirements may be increased by medications with hypoglycemic activity, such as phenothiazines).
No products indexed under this heading.

Fluphenazine Enanthate (Insulin requirements may be increased by medications with hypoglycemic activity, such as phenothiazines).
No products indexed under this heading.

Fluphenazine Hydrochloride (Insulin requirements may be increased by medications with hypoglycemic activity, such as phenothiazines).
No products indexed under this heading.

Fluticasone Propionate (Insulin requirements may be increased by medications with hypoglycemic activity, such as corticosteroids). Products include:
Advair Diskus 100/50 1276
Advair Diskus 250/50 1276
Advair Diskus 500/50 1276
Advair HFA 45/21 Inhalation Aerosol 1288
Advair HFA 115/21 Inhalation Aerosol 1288
Advair HFA 230/21 Inhalation Aerosol 1288
Flonase Nasal Spray 1431
Flovent Diskus 50 mcg 1435

Fluticasone Propionate HFA (Insulin requirements may be

increased by medications with hypoglycemic activity, such as corticosteroids). Products include:
Flovent HFA ... 1440

Fosinopril Sodium (Insulin requirements may be decreased in the presence of drugs with hypoglycemic activity, such as certain angiotensin converting enzyme inhibitors).
No products indexed under this heading.

Glimepiride (Insulin requirements may be decreased in the presence of drugs with with hypoglycemic activity, such as oral antidiabetic agents). Products include:
Avandaryl Tablets ... 1344
Duetact Tablets ... 3085

Glipizide (Insulin requirements may be decreased in the presence of drugs with with hypoglycemic activity, such as oral antidiabetic agents).
No products indexed under this heading.

Glyburide (Insulin requirements may be decreased in the presence of drugs with with hypoglycemic activity, such as oral antidiabetic agents).
No products indexed under this heading.

Hydrocortisone (Insulin requirements may be increased by medications with hypoglycemic activity, such as corticosteroids).
No products indexed under this heading.

Hydrocortisone Acetate (Insulin requirements may be increased by medications with hypoglycemic activity, such as corticosteroids). Products include:
Analpram-HC ... 1140
Pramosone ... 1141

Hydrocortisone Sodium Phosphate (Insulin requirements may be increased by medications with hypoglycemic activity, such as corticosteroids).
No products indexed under this heading.

Hydrocortisone Sodium Succinate (Insulin requirements may be increased by medications with hypoglycemic activity, such as corticosteroids).
No products indexed under this heading.

Isocarboxazid (Insulin requirements may be decreased in the presence of drugs with hypoglycemic activity, such as monoamine oxidase inhibitors). Products include:
Marplan Tablets ... 3177

Isoniazid (Insulin requirements may be increased by medications with hypoglycemic activity, such as isoniazid).
No products indexed under this heading.

Labetalol Hydrochloride (Beta-adrenergic blockers may mask the symptoms of hypoglycemia in some patients).
No products indexed under this heading.

Levobunolol Hydrochloride (Beta-adrenergic blockers may mask the symptoms of hypoglycemia in some patients).
No products indexed under this heading.

Levonorgestrel (Insulin requirements may be increased by medications with hypoglycemic activity, such as oral contraceptives). Products include:
Climara Pro Transdermal System ... 768
Lybrel Tablets ... 3204
Mirena Intrauterine System ... 779
Plan B Tablets ... 1044
Seasonique Tablets ... 1046

Levothyroxine Sodium (Insulin requirements may be increased by medications with hypoglycemic activity, such as thyroid replacement therapy). Products include:
Levothroid Tablets ... 1170
Levoxyl Tablets ... 1780
Synthroid Tablets ... 507

Liothyronine Sodium (Insulin requirements may be increased by medications with hypoglycemic activity, such as thyroid replacement therapy). Products include:
Cytomel Tablets ... 1778

Liotrix (Insulin requirements may be increased by medications with hypoglycemic activity, such as thyroid replacement therapy).
No products indexed under this heading.

Lisinopril (Insulin requirements may be decreased in the presence of drugs with hypoglycemic activity, such as certain angiotensin converting enzyme inhibitors). Products include:
Prinivil Tablets ... 2087
Prinzide Tablets ... 2092

Magnesium Salicylate (Insulin requirements may be decreased in the presence of drugs with hypoglycemic activity, such as salicylates).
No products indexed under this heading.

Mesoridazine Besylate (Insulin requirements may be increased by medications with hypoglycemic activity, such as phenothiazines).
No products indexed under this heading.

Mestranol (Insulin requirements may be increased by medications with hypoglycemic activity, such as oral contraceptives).
No products indexed under this heading.

Metformin Hydrochloride (Insulin requirements may be decreased in the presence of drugs with with hypoglycemic activity, such as oral antidiabetic agents). Products include:
ActoPlus Met Tablets ... 3071
Avandamet Tablets ... 1336
Janumet Tablets ... 2041
PrandiMet Tablets ... 2967

Methotrimeprazine (Insulin requirements may be increased by medications with hypoglycemic activity, such as phenothiazines).
No products indexed under this heading.

Methylprednisolone Acetate (Insulin requirements may be increased by medications with hypoglycemic activity, such as corticosteroids).
No products indexed under this heading.

Methylprednisolone Sodium Succinate (Insulin requirements may be increased by medications with hypoglycemic activity, such as corticosteroids).
No products indexed under this heading.

Metipranolol Hydrochloride (Beta-adrenergic blockers may mask the symptoms of hypoglycemia in some patients).
No products indexed under this heading.

Metoprolol Succinate (Beta-adrenergic blockers may mask the symptoms of hypoglycemia in some patients). Products include:
Toprol-XL Tablets ... 666

Metoprolol Tartrate (Beta-adrenergic blockers may mask the symptoms of hypoglycemia in some patients).
No products indexed under this heading.

Miglitol (Insulin requirements may be decreased in the presence of drugs with with hypoglycemic activity, such as oral antidiabetic agents).
No products indexed under this heading.

Moclobemide (Insulin requirements may be decreased in the presence of drugs with hypoglycemic activity, such as monoamine oxidase inhibitors).
No products indexed under this heading.

Moexipril Hydrochloride (Insulin requirements may be decreased in the presence of drugs with hypoglycemic activity, such as certain angiotensin converting enzyme inhibitors).
No products indexed under this heading.

Mometasone Furoate (Insulin requirements may be increased by medications with hypoglycemic activity, such as corticosteroids). Products include:
Asmanex Twisthaler ... 2797
Elocon Cream 0.1% ... 2840
Elocon Lotion 0.1% ... 2841
Elocon Ointment 0.1% ... 2842

Mometasone Furoate Monohydrate (Insulin requirements may be increased by medications with hypoglycemic activity, such as corticosteroids). Products include:
Nasonex Nasal Spray ... 2883

Nadolol (Beta-adrenergic blockers may mask the symptoms of hypoglycemia in some patients). Products include:
Nadolol Tablets ... 2191

Nateglinide (Insulin requirements may be decreased in the presence of drugs with with hypoglycemic activity, such as oral antidiabetic agents). Products include:
Starlix Tablets ... 2314

Nebivolol (Beta-adrenergic blockers may mask the symptoms of hypoglycemia in some patients). Products include:
Bystolic Tablets ... 1155

Niacin (Insulin requirements may be increased by medications with hypoglycemic activity such as certain lipid-lowering drugs (niacin)). Products include:
Advicor Tablets ... 402
Bausch & Lomb Ocuvite DF Vitamin Supplement ... ⊙ 238
Dismutax Dietary Supplement ... 995
Niaspan Extended-Release Tablets ... 480
NT-Kinase Dietary Supplement ... 995
Simcor Tablets ... 502

Niacinamide (Insulin requirements may be increased by medications with hypoglycemic activity such as certain lipid-lowering drugs (niacin)). Products include:
BioLean Free Tablets ... 635

Norethindrone (Insulin requirements may be increased by medications with hypoglycemic activity, such as oral contraceptives). Products include:
Ortho Micronor Tablets ... 2446

Norethynodrel (Insulin requirements may be increased by medications with hypoglycemic activity, such as oral contraceptives).
No products indexed under this heading.

Norgestimate (Insulin requirements may be increased by medications with hypoglycemic activity, such as oral contraceptives). Products include:
Ortho-Cyclen/Ortho Tri-Cyclen ... 2449
Ortho Tri-Cyclen Lo Tablets ... 2458

Norgestrel (Insulin requirements may be increased by medications with hypoglycemic activity, such as oral contraceptives).
No products indexed under this heading.

Octreotide Acetate (Insulin requirements may be decreased in the presence of drugs with hypoglycemic activity, such as inhibitors of pancreatic function (octreotide)). Products include:
Sandostatin Injection ... 2300
Sandostatin LAR Depot ... 2302

Pargyline Hydrochloride (Insulin requirements may be decreased in the presence of drugs with hypoglycemic activity, such as monoamine oxidase inhibitors).
No products indexed under this heading.

Penbutolol Sulfate (Beta-adrenergic blockers may mask the symptoms of hypoglycemia in some patients).
No products indexed under this heading.

Perindopril Erbumine (Insulin requirements may be decreased in the presence of drugs with hypoglycemic activity, such as certain angiotensin converting enzyme inhibitors). Products include:
Aceon Tablets (2 mg, 4 mg, 8 mg) ... 3038

Perphenazine (Insulin requirements may be increased by medications with hypoglycemic activity, such as phenothiazines).
No products indexed under this heading.

Phenelzine Sulfate (Insulin requirements may be decreased in the presence of drugs with hypoglycemic activity, such as monoamine oxidase inhibitors).
No products indexed under this heading.

Pindolol (Beta-adrenergic blockers may mask the symptoms of hypoglycemia in some patients).
No products indexed under this heading.

Pioglitazone Hydrochloride (Insulin requirements may be decreased in the presence of drugs with with hypoglycemic activity, such as oral antidiabetic agents). Products include:
ActoPlus Met Tablets ... 3071
Actos Tablets ... 3077
Duetact Tablets ... 3085

Polyestradiol Phosphate (Insulin requirements may be increased by medications with hypoglycemic activity, such as estrogens).
No products indexed under this heading.

Prednisolone Acetate (Insulin requirements may be increased by medications with hypoglycemic activity, such as corticosteroids). Products include:

Pred Forte Ophthalmic Suspension .... ⊙227
Pred Mild Ophthalmic Suspension .... ⊙230
Pred-G Ophthalmic Ointment .... ⊙229
Pred-G Ophthalmic Suspension .... ⊙228

Prednisolone Sodium Phosphate (Insulin requirements may be increased by medications with hypoglycemic activity, such as corticosteroids).
No products indexed under this heading.

Prednisolone Tebutate (Insulin requirements may be increased by medications with hypoglycemic activity, such as corticosteroids).
No products indexed under this heading.

Prednisone (Insulin requirements may be increased by medications with hypoglycemic activity, such as corticosteroids).
No products indexed under this heading.

Procarbazine Hydrochloride (Insulin requirements may be decreased in the presence of drugs with hypoglycemic activity, such as monoamine oxidase inhibitors).
No products indexed under this heading.

Prochlorperazine (Insulin requirements may be increased by medications with hypoglycemic activity, such as phenothiazines).
No products indexed under this heading.

Promethazine Hydrochloride (Insulin requirements may be increased by medications with hypoglycemic activity, such as phenothiazines).
No products indexed under this heading.

Propranolol Hydrochloride (Beta-adrenergic blockers may mask the symptoms of hypoglycemia in some patients). Products include:
InnoPran XL Extended Release Capsules 1484

Quinapril Hydrochloride (Insulin requirements may be decreased in the presence of drugs with hypoglycemic activity, such as certain angiotensin converting enzyme inhibitors).
No products indexed under this heading.

Quinestrol (Insulin requirements may be increased by medications with hypoglycemic activity, such as estrogens).
No products indexed under this heading.

Ramipril (Insulin requirements may be decreased in the presence of drugs with hypoglycemic activity, such as certain angiotensin converting enzyme inhibitors).
No products indexed under this heading.

Rasagiline Mesylate (Insulin requirements may be decreased in the presence of drugs with hypoglycemic activity, such as monoamine oxidase inhibitors). Products include:
Azilect Tablets 3106

Repaglinide (Insulin requirements may be decreased in the presence of drugs with with hypoglycemic activity, such as oral antidiabetic agents). Products include:
PrandiMet Tablets 2967
Prandin Tablets 2971

Rosiglitazone Maleate (Insulin requirements may be decreased in the presence of drugs with with hypoglycemic activity, such as oral antidiabetic agents). Products include:
Avandamet Tablets 1336
Avandaryl Tablets 1344
Avandia Tablets 1351

Salsalate (Insulin requirements may be decreased in the presence of drugs with hypoglycemic activity, such as salicylates).
No products indexed under this heading.

Selegiline (Insulin requirements may be decreased in the presence of drugs with hypoglycemic activity, such as monoamine oxidase inhibitors). Products include:
Emsam Transdermal System 905

Selegiline Hydrochloride (Insulin requirements may be decreased in the presence of drugs with hypoglycemic activity, such as monoamine oxidase inhibitors). Products include:
Eldepryl Capsules 3052

Sitagliptin Phosphate (Insulin requirements may be decreased in the presence of drugs with with hypoglycemic activity, such as oral antidiabetic agents). Products include:
Janumet Tablets 2041
Januvia Tablets 2048

Sotalol Hydrochloride (Beta-adrenergic blockers may mask the symptoms of hypoglycemia in some patients).
No products indexed under this heading.

Spirapril Hydrochloride (Insulin requirements may be decreased in the presence of drugs with hypoglycemic activity, such as certain angiotensin converting enzyme inhibitors).
No products indexed under this heading.

Thioridazine Hydrochloride (Insulin requirements may be increased by medications with hypoglycemic activity, such as phenothiazines). Products include:
Thioridazine Hydrochloride Tablets 2195

Thyroglobulin (Insulin requirements may be increased by medications with hypoglycemic activity, such as thyroid replacement therapy).
No products indexed under this heading.

Thyroid (Insulin requirements may be increased by medications with hypoglycemic activity, such as thyroid replacement therapy). Products include:
Naturethroid Tablets 2605

Thyroxine (Insulin requirements may be increased by medications with hypoglycemic activity, such as thyroid replacement therapy).
No products indexed under this heading.

Thyroxine Sodium (Insulin requirements may be increased by medications with hypoglycemic activity, such as thyroid replacement therapy).
No products indexed under this heading.

Timolol Hemihydrate (Beta-adrenergic blockers may mask the symptoms of hypoglycemia in some patients). Products include:
Betimol Ophthalmic Solution 3181

Timolol Maleate (Beta-adrenergic blockers may mask the symptoms of hypoglycemia in some patients). Products include:
Combigan Ophthalmic Solution 553
Cosopt Sterile Ophthalmic Solution 1969
Timoptic Sterile Ophthalmic Solution 2121
Timoptic in Ocudose 2124
Timoptic-XE Sterile Ophthalmic Gel Forming Solution 2125

Tolazamide (Insulin requirements may be decreased in the presence of drugs with with hypoglycemic activity, such as oral antidiabetic agents).
No products indexed under this heading.

Tolbutamide (Insulin requirements may be decreased in the presence of drugs with with hypoglycemic activity, such as oral antidiabetic agents).
No products indexed under this heading.

Trandolapril (Insulin requirements may be decreased in the presence of drugs with hypoglycemic activity, such as certain angiotensin converting enzyme inhibitors). Products include:
Mavik Tablets 472
Tarka Tablets 511

Tranylcypromine Sulfate (Insulin requirements may be decreased in the presence of drugs with hypoglycemic activity, such as monoamine oxidase inhibitors). Products include:
Parnate Tablets 1532

Triamcinolone (Insulin requirements may be increased by medications with hypoglycemic activity, such as corticosteroids).
No products indexed under this heading.

Triamcinolone Acetonide (Insulin requirements may be increased by medications with hypoglycemic activity, such as corticosteroids). Products include:
Azmacort Inhalation Aerosol 407
Nasacort AQ Nasal Spray 2765
Triesence Injectable Suspension .... ⊙209

Triamcinolone Diacetate (Insulin requirements may be increased by medications with hypoglycemic activity, such as corticosteroids).
No products indexed under this heading.

Triamcinolone Hexacetonide (Insulin requirements may be increased by medications with hypoglycemic activity, such as corticosteroids).
No products indexed under this heading.

Trifluoperazine Hydrochloride (Insulin requirements may be increased by medications with hypoglycemic activity, such as phenothiazines).
No products indexed under this heading.

Troglitazone (Insulin requirements may be decreased in the presence of drugs with with hypoglycemic activity, such as oral antidiabetic agents).
No products indexed under this heading.

Food Interactions

Alcohol (Insulin requirements may be decreased in the presence of drugs with hypoglycemic activity, such as alcohol).

HUMALOG MIX 75/25-PEN AND KWIKPEN

(Insulin Lispro, Human, Insulin Lispro Protamine, Human) 1835
See Humalog-Pen and KwikPen

HUMAN ALBUMIN GRIFOLS 25%

(Albumin (human)) 1706
None cited in PDR database.

HUMATROPE VIALS AND CARTRIDGES

(Somatropin) 1838
May interact with corticosteroids, anticonvulsants, estrogens, glucocorticoids, oral hypoglycemic agents, insulin, drugs which undergo biotransformation by cytochrome p-450 mixed function oxidase, sex steroids, and certain other agents. Compounds in these categories include:

Acarbose (For diabetes, oral hypoglycemics may require dose adjustment when somatropin therapy is instituted). Products include:
Precose Tablets 792

Acetaminophen (Somatropin administration may alter the clearance of compounds known to be metabolized by CYP450 liver enzymes: monitor carefully). Products include:
Benadryl Allergy & Cold Kapgels 1895
Benadryl Allergy & Sinus Headache Kapgels 1895
Benadryl Severe Allergy & Sinus Headache Caplets 1897
Lortab 5/500 Tablets 3143
Lortab 7.5/500 Tablets 3144
Lortab 10/500 Tablets 3144
Percocet Tablets 1127
Sinutab Sinus Caplets 1905
Sudafed PE Cold & Cough Caplets 1907
Sudafed PE Nighttime Cold Caplets 1907
Sudafed PE Severe Cold Caplets 1908
Sudafed PE Sinus Headache Caplets 1908
Regular Strength Tylenol Tablets 1915
Tylenol 8 Hour Extended Release Caplets 1915
Extra Strength Tylenol Caplets, Cool Caplets, and EZ Tabs 1915
Extra Strength Tylenol Adult Rapid Blast Liquid 1915
Extra Strength Tylenol PM Caplets, Geltabs, Liquid, and Rapid Release Gels 1915
Extra Strength Tylenol Rapid Release Gels 1915
Tylenol with Codeine Tablets 2427
Tylenol Allergy Multi-Symptom Caplets with Cool Burst and Rapid Release Gelcaps 1916
Tylenol Allergy Multi-Symptom Nighttime Caplets with Cool Burst 1916
Tylenol Severe Allergy Caplets 1916
Tylenol Arthritis Pain Extended Release Geltabs/Caplets 1915
Tylenol Chest Congestion Caplets with Cool Burst 1910
Tylenol Chest Congestion Liquid with Cool Burst 1910
Children's Tylenol Plus Cold Suspension Liquid 1912
Children's Tylenol Plus Cold & Allergy Suspension Liquid 1914
Children's Tylenol Plus Cough & Runny Nose Suspension Liquid 1912
Children's Tylenol Plus Cough & Sore Throat Suspension Liquid 1912
Children's Tylenol Plus Flu Suspension Liquid 1914
Children's Tylenol Suspension Liquid 1909
Children's Tylenol Meltaways 1909
Children's Tylenol Plus Multi-Symptom Cold Suspension Liquid 1912
Tylenol Cold Severe Congestion Daytime Caplets with Cool Burst 1912
Tylenol Cold Head Congestion Daytime Caplets with Cool Burst 1910

Tylenol Cold Head Congestion Nighttime Caplets with Cool Burst 1910
Tylenol Cold Head Congestion Severe Daytime Caplets with Cool Burst 1910
Tylenol Cold Multi-Symptom Daytime Caplets with Cool Burst and Rapid Release Gels 1913
Tylenol Cold Multi-Symptom Daytime Liquid with Citrus Burst ... 1913
Tylenol Cold Multi-Symptom Nighttime Caplets with Cool Burst 1913
Tylenol Cold Multi-Symptom Nighttime Liquid with Cool Burst ... 1913
Tylenol Cold Multi-Symptom Severe Caplets with Cool Burst 1913
Tylenol Cold Multi-Symptom Severe Daytime Liquid with Citrus Burst 1913
Tylenol Cough & Sore Throat Daytime Liquid with Cool Burst 1918
Tylenol Cough & Sore Throat Nighttime Liquid with Cool Burst ... 1918
Concentrated Tylenol Infants' Drops 1909
Jr. Tylenol Meltaways 1909
Tylenol Sinus Congestion & Pain Daytime Caplets with Cool Burst and Gelcaps 1917
Tylenol Sinus Congestion & Pain Nighttime Caplets with Cool Burst 1917
Tylenol Sinus Congestion & Pain Severe Caplets with Cool Burst 1917
Tylenol Sinus Severe Congestion Caplets with Cool Burst 1917
Tylenol Sore Throat Daytime Liquid with Cool Burst 1918
Tylenol Sore Throat Nighttime Liquid with Cool Burst 1918
Women's Tylenol Menstrual Relief Caplets 1919
Vicks DayQuil Cold & Flu Multi-Symptom Relief 616
Vicks DayQuil LiquiCaps 2567
Vicks DayQuil Liquid 2567
Vicks DayQuil Multi-Symptom Cold/Flu Relief 2567
Vicks NyQuil Cold & Flu Multi-Symptom Relief 617
Vicks NyQuil LiquiCaps 2567
Vicks NyQuil Liquid 2567
Vicks NyQuil Multi-Symptom Cold/Flu Relief 2567
Vicodin Tablets 529
Vicodin ES Tablets 530
Vicodin HP Tablets 531
Zydone Tablets 1132

ACTH (Excessive glucocorticoid therapy will inhibit the growth promoting effect of somatropin; growth hormone administration may alter the clearance of compounds known to be metabolized by cytochrome P450 liver enzymes; such as corticosteroids).
No products indexed under this heading.

Alatrofloxacin Mesylate (Somatropin administration may alter the clearance of compounds known to be metabolized by CYP450 liver enzymes: monitor carefully).
No products indexed under this heading.

Alfentanil Hydrochloride (Somatropin administration may alter the clearance of compounds known to be metabolized by CYP450 liver enzymes: monitor carefully).
No products indexed under this heading.

Alprazolam (Somatropin administration may alter the clearance of compounds known to be metabolized by CYP450 liver enzymes: monitor carefully).
No products indexed under this heading.

Aminophylline (Somatropin administration may alter the clearance of compounds known to be metabolized by CYP450 liver enzymes: monitor carefully).
No products indexed under this heading.

Amiodarone Hydrochloride (Somatropin administration may alter the clearance of compounds known to be metabolized by CYP450 liver enzymes: monitor carefully).
No products indexed under this heading.

Amitriptyline Hydrochloride (Somatropin administration may alter the clearance of compounds known to be metabolized by CYP450 liver enzymes: monitor carefully).
No products indexed under this heading.

Amlodipine Besylate (Somatropin administration may alter the clearance of compounds known to be metabolized by CYP450 liver enzymes: monitor carefully).
Products include:
Azor Tablets 1005
Exforge Tablets 2238

Amoxapine (Somatropin administration may alter the clearance of compounds known to be metabolized by CYP450 liver enzymes: monitor carefully).
No products indexed under this heading.

Amphetamine Aspartate (Somatropin administration may alter the clearance of compounds known to be metabolized by CYP450 liver enzymes: monitor carefully).
Products include:
Adderall XR Capsules 3012

Amphetamine Aspartate Monohydrate (Somatropin administration may alter the clearance of compounds known to be metabolized by CYP450 liver enzymes: monitor carefully).
No products indexed under this heading.

Amphetamine Sulfate (Somatropin administration may alter the clearance of compounds known to be metabolized by CYP450 liver enzymes: monitor carefully).
Products include:
Adderall XR Capsules 3012

Aprepitant (Somatropin administration may alter the clearance of compounds known to be metabolized by CYP450 liver enzymes: monitor carefully). Products include:
Emend Capsules 1992

Astemizole (Somatropin administration may alter the clearance of compounds known to be metabolized by CYP450 liver enzymes: monitor carefully).
No products indexed under this heading.

Atomoxetine Hydrochloride (Somatropin administration may alter the clearance of compounds known to be metabolized by CYP450 liver enzymes: monitor carefully).
Products include:
Strattera Capsules 1864

Atorvastatin Calcium (Somatropin administration may alter the clearance of compounds known to be metabolized by CYP450 liver enzymes: monitor carefully).
Products include:
Lipitor Tablets 2501

Belladonna Ergotamine (Somatropin administration may alter the clearance of compounds known to be metabolized by CYP450 liver enzymes: monitor carefully).
No products indexed under this heading.

Benzphetamine Hydrochloride (Somatropin administration may alter the clearance of compounds known to be metabolized by CYP450 liver enzymes: monitor carefully).
No products indexed under this heading.

Betamethasone Acetate (Excessive glucocorticoid therapy will inhibit the growth promoting effect of somatropin; growth hormone administration may alter the clearance of compounds known to be metabolized by cytochrome P450 liver enzymes; such as corticosteroids).
No products indexed under this heading.

Betamethasone Sodium Phosphate (Excessive glucocorticoid therapy will inhibit the growth promoting effect of somatropin; growth hormone administration may alter the clearance of compounds known to be metabolized by cytochrome P450 liver enzymes; such as corticosteroids).
No products indexed under this heading.

Bisoprolol Fumarate (Somatropin administration may alter the clearance of compounds known to be metabolized by CYP450 liver enzymes: monitor carefully).
No products indexed under this heading.

Budesonide (Growth hormone administration may alter the clearance of compounds known to be metabolized by CYP450 liver enzymes, such as corticosteroids).
Products include:
Pulmicort Flexhaler 654
Symbicort 80/4.5 Inhalation Aerosol 659
Symbicort 160/4.5 Inhalation Aerosol 659

Buspirone Hydrochloride (Somatropin administration may alter the clearance of compounds known to be metabolized by CYP450 liver enzymes: monitor carefully).
No products indexed under this heading.

Busulfan (Somatropin administration may alter the clearance of compounds known to be metabolized by CYP450 liver enzymes: monitor carefully). Products include:
Busulfex Injection 2477
Myleran Tablets 1530

Caffeine (Somatropin administration may alter the clearance of compounds known to be metabolized by CYP450 liver enzymes: monitor carefully). Products include:
BioLean Free Tablets 635
BioLean II Tablets 635
Winrgy Dietary Supplement 642

Caffeine Anhydrous (Somatropin administration may alter the clearance of compounds known to be metabolized by CYP450 liver enzymes: monitor carefully).
No products indexed under this heading.

Caffeine Citrate (Somatropin administration may alter the clearance of compounds known to be metabolized by CYP450 liver enzymes: monitor carefully).
No products indexed under this heading.

Candesartan Cilexetil (Somatropin administration may alter the clearance of compounds known to be metabolized by CYP450 liver enzymes: monitor carefully).
Products include:
Atacand Tablets 639
Atacand HCT 642

Captopril (Somatropin administration may alter the clearance of compounds known to be metabolized by CYP450 liver enzymes: monitor carefully). Products include:
Captopril Tablets 2182

Carbamazepine (Growth hormone adminstration may alter the clearance of compounds known to be metabolized by CYP450 liver enzymes, such as anticonvulsants).
Products include:
Carbatrol Capsules 3019
Equetro Extended-Release Capsules 3174

Carisoprodol (Somatropin administration may alter the clearance of compounds known to be metabolized by CYP450 liver enzymes: monitor carefully). Products include:
Soma Tablets 1931

Carvedilol (Somatropin administration may alter the clearance of compounds known to be metabolized by CYP450 liver enzymes: monitor carefully). Products include:
Coreg Tablets 1387

Celecoxib (Somatropin administration may alter the clearance of compounds known to be metabolized by CYP450 liver enzymes: monitor carefully). Products include:
Celebrex Capsules 2979

Cerivastatin Sodium (Somatropin administration may alter the clearance of compounds known to be metabolized by CYP450 liver enzymes: monitor carefully).
No products indexed under this heading.

Cevimeline Hydrochloride (Somatropin administration may alter the clearance of compounds known to be metabolized by CYP450 liver enzymes: monitor carefully).
Products include:
Evoxac Capsules 1013

Chlordiazepoxide (Somatropin administration may alter the clearance of compounds known to be metabolized by CYP450 liver enzymes: monitor carefully).
No products indexed under this heading.

Chlordiazepoxide Hydrochloride (Somatropin administration may alter the clearance of compounds known to be metabolized by CYP450 liver enzymes: monitor carefully).
No products indexed under this heading.

Chlorotrianisene (A larger dose of somatropin may be required to achieve the defined treatment goal in adult women on oral estrogen replacement).
No products indexed under this heading.

IMPORTANT NOTE: Always consult each drug listing in the patient's regimen for possible interactions.

Chlorpheniramine (Somatropin administration may alter the clearance of compounds known to be metabolized by CYP450 liver enzymes: monitor carefully).
No products indexed under this heading.

Chlorpheniramine Maleate (Somatropin administration may alter the clearance of compounds known to be metabolized by CYP450 liver enzymes: monitor carefully). Products include:
Actifed Cold & Allergy Tablets 1895
Sudafed PE Sinus & Allergy Tablets 1908
Tylenol Allergy Multi-Symptom Caplets with Cool Burst and Rapid Release Gelcaps 1916
Children's Tylenol Plus Cold Suspension Liquid 1912
Children's Tylenol Plus Cough & Runny Nose Suspension Liquid 1912
Children's Tylenol Plus Flu Suspension Liquid 1914
Children's Tylenol Plus Multi-Symptom Cold Suspension Liquid 1912
Tylenol Cold Head Congestion Nighttime Caplets with Cool Burst 1910
Tylenol Cold Multi-Symptom Nighttime Caplets with Cool Burst 1913
Tylenol Sinus Congestion & Pain Nighttime Caplets with Cool Burst 1917

Chlorpheniramine Polistirex (Somatropin administration may alter the clearance of compounds known to be metabolized by CYP450 liver enzymes: monitor carefully). Products include:
Tussionex Pennkinetic Extended-Release Suspension 3154

Chlorpheniramine Tannate (Somatropin administration may alter the clearance of compounds known to be metabolized by CYP450 liver enzymes: monitor carefully).
No products indexed under this heading.

Chlorpromazine (Somatropin administration may alter the clearance of compounds known to be metabolized by CYP450 liver enzymes: monitor carefully).
No products indexed under this heading.

Chlorpromazine Hydrochloride (Somatropin administration may alter the clearance of compounds known to be metabolized by CYP450 liver enzymes: monitor carefully).
No products indexed under this heading.

Chlorpropamide (For diabetes, oral hypoglycemics may require dose adjustment when somatropin therapy is instituted).
No products indexed under this heading.

Ciclesonide (Growth hormone administration may alter the clearance of compounds known to be metabolized by CYP450 liver enzymes, such as corticosteroids). Products include:
Alvesco Inhalation Aerosol 2985
Omnaris Nasal Spray 2998

Cilostazol (Somatropin administration may alter the clearance of compounds known to be metabolized by CYP450 liver enzymes: monitor carefully). Products include:
Pletal Tablets 2481

Cimetidine Hydrochloride (Somatropin administration may alter the clearance of compounds known to be metabolized by CYP450 liver enzymes: monitor carefully).
No products indexed under this heading.

Ciprofloxacin (Somatropin administration may alter the clearance of compounds known to be metabolized by CYP450 liver enzymes: monitor carefully). Products include:
Cipro I.V. 2817
Cipro Oral Suspension 2810
Cipro XR Tablets 2823
Ciprodex Otic Suspension 541

Ciprofloxacin Hydrochloride (Somatropin administration may alter the clearance of compounds known to be metabolized by CYP450 liver enzymes: monitor carefully). Products include:
Cipro Tablets 2810

Cisapride (Somatropin administration may alter the clearance of compounds known to be metabolized by CYP450 liver enzymes: monitor carefully).
No products indexed under this heading.

Citalopram Hydrobromide (Somatropin administration may alter the clearance of compounds known to be metabolized by CYP450 liver enzymes: monitor carefully). Products include:
Celexa 1160

Clarithromycin (Somatropin administration may alter the clearance of compounds known to be metabolized by CYP450 liver enzymes: monitor carefully). Products include:
Biaxin/Biaxin XL 411

Clomipramine Hydrochloride (Somatropin administration may alter the clearance of compounds known to be metabolized by CYP450 liver enzymes: monitor carefully).
No products indexed under this heading.

Clopidogrel Hydrogen Sulfate (Somatropin administration may alter the clearance of compounds known to be metabolized by CYP450 liver enzymes: monitor carefully).
No products indexed under this heading.

Clozapine (Somatropin administration may alter the clearance of compounds known to be metabolized by CYP450 liver enzymes: monitor carefully).
No products indexed under this heading.

Codeine Phosphate (Somatropin administration may alter the clearance of compounds known to be metabolized by CYP450 liver enzymes: monitor carefully). Products include:
Tylenol with Codeine Tablets 2427

Codeine Sulfate (Somatropin administration may alter the clearance of compounds known to be metabolized by CYP450 liver enzymes: monitor carefully).
No products indexed under this heading.

Cortisone Acetate (Excessive glucocorticoid therapy will inhibit the growth promoting effect of somatropin; growth hormone administration may alter the clearance of compounds known to be metabolized by cytochrome P450 liver enzymes; such as corticosteroids).
No products indexed under this heading.

Cyclobenzaprine (Somatropin administration may alter the clearance of compounds known to be metabolized by CYP450 liver enzymes: monitor carefully).
No products indexed under this heading.

Cyclobenzaprine Hydrochloride (Somatropin administration may alter the clearance of compounds known to be metabolized by CYP450 liver enzymes: monitor carefully). Products include:
Amrix Capsules 966

Cyclophosphamide (Somatropin administration may alter the clearance of compounds known to be metabolized by CYP450 liver enzymes: monitor carefully).
No products indexed under this heading.

Cyclosporine (Growth hormone administration may alter the clearance of compounds known to be metabolized by cytochrome P450 liver enzymes, such as cyclosporine). Products include:
Gengraf Capsules 435
Neoral Oral Solution 2280
Neoral Soft Gelatin Capsules 2280
Restasis Ophthalmic Emulsion 557
Sandimmune 2296

Desipramine Hydrochloride (Somatropin administration may alter the clearance of compounds known to be metabolized by CYP450 liver enzymes: monitor carefully).
No products indexed under this heading.

Desogestrel (Growth hormone administration may alter the clearance of compounds known to be metabolized by cytochrome P450 liver enzymes, such as sex steroids). Products include:
Mircette Tablets 1034

Dexamethasone (Excessive glucocorticoid therapy will inhibit the growth promoting effect of somatropin; growth hormone administration may alter the clearance of compounds known to be metabolized by cytochrome P450 liver enzymes; such as corticosteroids). Products include:
Ciprodex Otic Suspension 541

Dexamethasone Acetate (Excessive glucocorticoid therapy will inhibit the growth promoting effect of somatropin; growth hormone administration may alter the clearance of compounds known to be metabolized by cytochrome P450 liver enzymes; such as corticosteroids).
No products indexed under this heading.

Dexamethasone Phosphate (Somatropin administration may alter the clearance of compounds known to be metabolized by CYP450 liver enzymes: monitor carefully).
No products indexed under this heading.

Dexamethasone Sodium (Somatropin administration may alter the clearance of compounds known to be metabolized by CYP450 liver enzymes: monitor carefully).
No products indexed under this heading.

Dexamethasone Sodium Phosphate (Excessive glucocorticoid therapy will inhibit the growth promoting effect of somatropin; growth hormone administration may alter the clearance of compounds known to be metabolized by cytochrome P450 liver enzymes; such as corticosteroids).
No products indexed under this heading.

Dexfenfluramine Hydrochloride (Somatropin administration may alter the clearance of compounds known to be metabolized by CYP450 liver enzymes: monitor carefully).
No products indexed under this heading.

Dextromethorphan (Somatropin administration may alter the clearance of compounds known to be metabolized by CYP450 liver enzymes: monitor carefully).
No products indexed under this heading.

Dextromethorphan Hydrobromide (Somatropin administration may alter the clearance of compounds known to be metabolized by CYP450 liver enzymes: monitor carefully). Products include:
PediaCare Children's Liquid Multi-Symptom Cold 1902
PediaCare Children's Long-Acting Cough 1902
Children's Sudafed PE Cold & Cough Liquid 1907
Sudafed PE Cold & Cough Caplets 1907
Children's Tylenol Plus Cough & Runny Nose Suspension Liquid 1912
Children's Tylenol Plus Cough & Sore Throat Suspension Liquid 1912
Children's Tylenol Plus Flu Suspension Liquid 1914
Children's Tylenol Plus Multi-Symptom Cold Suspension Liquid 1912
Tylenol Cold Severe Congestion Daytime Caplets with Cool Burst 1912
Tylenol Cold Head Congestion Daytime Caplets with Cool Burst 1910
Tylenol Cold Head Congestion Nighttime Caplets with Cool Burst 1910
Tylenol Cold Head Congestion Severe Daytime Caplets with Cool Burst 1910
Tylenol Cold Multi-Symptom Daytime Caplets with Cool Burst and Rapid Release Gels 1913
Tylenol Cold Multi-Symptom Daytime Liquid with Citrus Burst 1913
Tylenol Cold Multi-Symptom Nighttime Caplets with Cool Burst 1913
Tylenol Cold Multi-Symptom Nighttime Liquid with Cool Burst 1913
Tylenol Cold Multi-Symptom Severe Caplets with Cool Burst 1913
Tylenol Cold Multi-Symptom Severe Daytime Liquid with Citrus Burst 1913
Tylenol Cough & Sore Throat Daytime Liquid with Cool Burst 1918
Tylenol Cough & Sore Throat Nighttime Liquid with Cool Burst 1918
Vicks DayQuil Cold & Flu Multi-Symptom Relief .... ◘616
Vicks DayQuil LiquiCaps 2567
Vicks DayQuil Liquid 2567
Vicks DayQuil Multi-Symptom Cold/Flu Relief 2567

Vicks NyQuil Cold & Flu Multi-Symptom Relief 617
Vicks NyQuil LiquiCaps 2567
Vicks NyQuil Liquid 2567
Vicks NyQuil Multi-Symptom Cold/Flu Relief 2567

Dextromethorphan Polistirex (Somatropin administration may alter the clearance of compounds known to be metabolized by CYP450 liver enzymes: monitor carefully).
No products indexed under this heading.

Diazepam (Somatropin administration may alter the clearance of compounds known to be metabolized by CYP450 liver enzymes: monitor carefully). Products include:
Valium Tablets 2658

Diclofenac Potassium (Somatropin administration may alter the clearance of compounds known to be metabolized by CYP450 liver enzymes: monitor carefully).
No products indexed under this heading.

Diclofenac Sodium (Somatropin administration may alter the clearance of compounds known to be metabolized by CYP450 liver enzymes: monitor carefully). Products include:
Diclofenac Sodium Ophthalmic Solution .... ⊙ 240
Voltaren Ophthalmic Solution 2336
Voltaren Tablets 2334
Voltaren-XR Tablets 2337

Dienestrol (A larger dose of somatropin may be required to achieve the defined treatment goal in adult women on oral estrogen replacement).
No products indexed under this heading.

Diethylstilbestrol (A larger dose of somatropin may be required to achieve the defined treatment goal in adult women on oral estrogen replacement).
No products indexed under this heading.

Dihydroergotamine Mesylate (Somatropin administration may alter the clearance of compounds known to be metabolized by CYP450 liver enzymes: monitor carefully).
No products indexed under this heading.

Diltiazem Hydrochloride (Somatropin administration may alter the clearance of compounds known to be metabolized by CYP450 liver enzymes: monitor carefully). Products include:
Cardizem LA Extended Release Tablets 421

Diltiazem Maleate (Somatropin administration may alter the clearance of compounds known to be metabolized by CYP450 liver enzymes: monitor carefully).
No products indexed under this heading.

Disopyramide (Somatropin administration may alter the clearance of compounds known to be metabolized by CYP450 liver enzymes: monitor carefully).
No products indexed under this heading.

Disopyramide Phosphate (Somatropin administration may alter the clearance of compounds known to be metabolized by CYP450 liver enzymes: monitor carefully).
No products indexed under this heading.

Divalproex Sodium (Growth hormone adminstration may alter the clearance of compounds known to be metabolized by CYP450 liver enzymes, such as anticonvulsants). Products include:
Depakote ER Tablets 423

Docetaxel (Somatropin administration may alter the clearance of compounds known to be metabolized by CYP450 liver enzymes: monitor carefully). Products include:
Taxotere Injection Concentrate 2773

Dolasetron Mesylate (Somatropin administration may alter the clearance of compounds known to be metabolized by CYP450 liver enzymes: monitor carefully). Products include:
Anzemet Injection 2701
Anzemet Tablets 2704

Donepezil Hydrochloride (Somatropin administration may alter the clearance of compounds known to be metabolized by CYP450 liver enzymes: monitor carefully). Products include:
Aricept Tablets 1062
Aricept ODT Tablets 1062

Doxepin Hydrochloride (Somatropin administration may alter the clearance of compounds known to be metabolized by CYP450 liver enzymes: monitor carefully).
No products indexed under this heading.

Doxorubicin Hydrochloride (Somatropin administration may alter the clearance of compounds known to be metabolized by CYP450 liver enzymes: monitor carefully).
No products indexed under this heading.

Dronabinol (Somatropin administration may alter the clearance of compounds known to be metabolized by CYP450 liver enzymes: monitor carefully). Products include:
Marinol Capsules 3163

Drugs that Undergo Biotransformation by Cytochrome P-450 Mixed Function Oxidase (Somatropin administration may alter the clearance of compounds known to be metabolized by CYP450 liver enzymes: monitor carefully).
No products indexed under this heading.

Dyphylline (Somatropin administration may alter the clearance of compounds known to be metabolized by CYP450 liver enzymes: monitor carefully).
No products indexed under this heading.

Encainide Hydrochloride (Somatropin administration may alter the clearance of compounds known to be metabolized by CYP450 liver enzymes: monitor carefully).
No products indexed under this heading.

Enoxacin (Somatropin administration may alter the clearance of compounds known to be metabolized by CYP450 liver enzymes: monitor carefully).
No products indexed under this heading.

Eprosartan Mesylate (Somatropin administration may alter the clearance of compounds known to be metabolized by CYP450 liver enzymes: monitor carefully). Products include:
Teveten Tablets 515
Teveten HCT Tablets 517

Ergotamine Tartrate (Somatropin administration may alter the clearance of compounds known to be metabolized by CYP450 liver enzymes: monitor carefully).
No products indexed under this heading.

Erythromycin (Somatropin administration may alter the clearance of compounds known to be metabolized by CYP450 liver enzymes: monitor carefully).
No products indexed under this heading.

Erythromycin Estolate (Somatropin administration may alter the clearance of compounds known to be metabolized by CYP450 liver enzymes: monitor carefully).
No products indexed under this heading.

Erythromycin Ethylsuccinate (Somatropin administration may alter the clearance of compounds known to be metabolized by CYP450 liver enzymes: monitor carefully). Products include:
E.E.S. 433
EryPed 431

Erythromycin Gluceptate (Somatropin administration may alter the clearance of compounds known to be metabolized by CYP450 liver enzymes: monitor carefully).
No products indexed under this heading.

Erythromycin Lactobionate (Somatropin administration may alter the clearance of compounds known to be metabolized by CYP450 liver enzymes: monitor carefully).
No products indexed under this heading.

Erythromycin Stearate (Somatropin administration may alter the clearance of compounds known to be metabolized by CYP450 liver enzymes: monitor carefully).
No products indexed under this heading.

Esomeprazole Magnesium (Somatropin administration may alter the clearance of compounds known to be metabolized by CYP450 liver enzymes: monitor carefully). Products include:
Nexium Delayed-Release Capsules 645
Nexium Delayed-Release Oral Suspension 645

Estradiol (Growth hormone administration may alter the clearance of compounds known to be metabolized by cytochrome P450 liver enzymes, such as sex steroids). Products include:
Activella Tablets 2347
Angeliq Tablets 751
Climara Transdermal System 763
Climara Pro Transdermal System 768
Divigel 3167
Vagifem Tablets 2375

Estradiol Benzoate (Somatropin administration may alter the clearance of compounds known to be metabolized by CYP450 liver enzymes: monitor carefully).
No products indexed under this heading.

Estradiol Cypionate (Somatropin administration may alter the clearance of compounds known to be metabolized by CYP450 liver enzymes: monitor carefully).
No products indexed under this heading.

Estradiol Valerate (Somatropin administration may alter the clearance of compounds known to be metabolized by CYP450 liver enzymes: monitor carefully).
No products indexed under this heading.

Estrogen (Somatropin administration may alter the clearance of compounds known to be metabolized by CYP450 liver enzymes: monitor carefully).
No products indexed under this heading.

Estrogens, Conjugated (Growth hormone administration may alter the clearance of compounds known to be metabolized by cytochrome P450 liver enzymes, such as sex steroids). Products include:
Premarin Intravenous 3217
Premarin Tablets 3221
Premarin Vaginal Cream 3228
Premphase Tablets 3232
Prempro Tablets 3232

Estrogens, Conjugated, Synthetic A (Somatropin administration may alter the clearance of compounds known to be metabolized by CYP450 liver enzymes: monitor carefully).
No products indexed under this heading.

Estrogens, Esterified (A larger dose of somatropin may be required to achieve the defined treatment goal in adult women on oral estrogen replacement). Products include:
Estratest Tablets 3043
Estratest H.S. Tablets 3043

Estropipate (A larger dose of somatropin may be required to achieve the defined treatment goal in adult women on oral estrogen replacement).
No products indexed under this heading.

Ethinyl Estradiol (Growth hormone administration may alter the clearance of compounds known to be metabolized by cytochrome P450 liver enzymes, such as sex steroids). Products include:
Lybrel Tablets 3204
Mircette Tablets 1034
NuvaRing 2897
Ortho-Cyclen/Ortho Tri-Cyclen 2449
Ortho Evra Transdermal System 2437
Ortho Tri-Cyclen Lo Tablets 2458
Seasonique Tablets 1046
Yaz Tablets 805

Ethosuximide (Growth hormone adminstration may alter the clearance of compounds known to be metabolized by CYP450 liver enzymes, such as anticonvulsants).
No products indexed under this heading.

Ethotoin (Growth hormone adminstration may alter the clearance of compounds known to be metabolized by CYP450 liver enzymes, such as anticonvulsants).
No products indexed under this heading.

Ethynodiol Diacetate (Growth hormone administration may alter the clearance of compounds known to be metabolized by cytochrome P450 liver enzymes, such as sex steroids).
No products indexed under this heading.

Etodolac (Somatropin administration may alter the clearance of compounds known to be metabolized by CYP450 liver enzymes: monitor carefully).
No products indexed under this heading.

Etoposide (Somatropin administration may alter the clearance of compounds known to be metabolized by CYP450 liver enzymes: monitor carefully).
No products indexed under this heading.

Etoposide Phosphate (Somatropin administration may alter the clearance of compounds known to be metabolized by CYP450 liver enzymes: monitor carefully).
No products indexed under this heading.

Felbamate (Growth hormone adminstration may alter the clearance of compounds known to be metabolized by CYP450 liver enzymes, such as anticonvulsants).
No products indexed under this heading.

Felodipine (Somatropin administration may alter the clearance of compounds known to be metabolized by CYP450 liver enzymes: monitor carefully).
No products indexed under this heading.

Fenoprofen Calcium (Somatropin administration may alter the clearance of compounds known to be metabolized by CYP450 liver enzymes: monitor carefully).
Products include:
Nalfon Capsules **2508**

Fentanyl (Somatropin administration may alter the clearance of compounds known to be metabolized by CYP450 liver enzymes: monitor carefully). Products include:
Duragesic Transdermal System **2405**
Ionsys Transdermal System **2410**

Fentanyl Citrate (Somatropin administration may alter the clearance of compounds known to be metabolized by CYP450 liver enzymes: monitor carefully).
Products include:
Actiq **959**
Fentora Tablets **968**

Flecainide Acetate (Somatropin administration may alter the clearance of compounds known to be metabolized by CYP450 liver enzymes: monitor carefully).
No products indexed under this heading.

Fludrocortisone Acetate (Excessive glucocorticoid therapy will inhibit the growth promoting effect of somatropin; growth hormone administration may alter the clearance of compounds known to be metabolized by cytochrome P450 liver enzymes; such as corticosteroids).
No products indexed under this heading.

Flunisolide (Growth hormone administration may alter the clearance of compounds known to be metabolized by CYP450 liver enzymes, such as corticosteroids).
Products include:
Aerobid/Aerobid-M **1153**

Fluoxetine (Somatropin administration may alter the clearance of compounds known to be metabolized by CYP450 liver enzymes: monitor carefully).
No products indexed under this heading.

Fluoxetine Hydrochloride (Somatropin administration may alter the clearance of compounds known to be metabolized by CYP450 liver enzymes: monitor carefully).
Products include:
Prozac Weekly Capsules **1852**
Prozac Pulvules and Liquid **1852**
Symbyax Capsules **1871**

Fluoxymesterone (Growth hormone administration may alter the clearance of compounds known to be metabolized by cytochrome P450 liver enzymes, such as sex steroids).
No products indexed under this heading.

Fluphenazine Decanoate (Somatropin administration may alter the clearance of compounds known to be metabolized by CYP450 liver enzymes: monitor carefully).
No products indexed under this heading.

Fluphenazine Enanthate (Somatropin administration may alter the clearance of compounds known to be metabolized by CYP450 liver enzymes: monitor carefully).
No products indexed under this heading.

Fluphenazine Hydrochloride (Somatropin administration may alter the clearance of compounds known to be metabolized by CYP450 liver enzymes: monitor carefully).
No products indexed under this heading.

Flurbiprofen (Somatropin administration may alter the clearance of compounds known to be metabolized by CYP450 liver enzymes: monitor carefully).
No products indexed under this heading.

Flurbiprofen Sodium (Somatropin administration may alter the clearance of compounds known to be metabolized by CYP450 liver enzymes: monitor carefully).
No products indexed under this heading.

Flutamide (Somatropin administration may alter the clearance of compounds known to be metabolized by CYP450 liver enzymes: monitor carefully).
No products indexed under this heading.

Fluticasone Propionate (Growth hormone administration may alter the clearance of compounds known to be metabolized by CYP450 liver enzymes, such as corticosteroids).
Products include:
Advair Diskus 100/50 .... **1276**
Advair Diskus 250/50 .... **1276**
Advair Diskus 500/50 .... **1276**
Advair HFA 45/21 Inhalation Aerosol **1288**
Advair HFA 115/21 Inhalation Aerosol **1288**
Advair HFA 230/21 Inhalation Aerosol **1288**
Flonase Nasal Spray **1431**
Flovent Diskus 50 mcg **1435**

Fluticasone Propionate HFA (Growth hormone administration may alter the clearance of compounds known to be metabolized by CYP450 liver enzymes, such as corticosteroids). Products include:
Flovent HFA **1440**

Fluvastatin Sodium (Somatropin administration may alter the clearance of compounds known to be metabolized by CYP450 liver enzymes: monitor carefully).
Products include:
Lescol Capsules **2268**
Lescol XL Tablets **2268**

Fluvoxamine Maleate (Somatropin administration may alter the clearance of compounds known to be metabolized by CYP450 liver enzymes: monitor carefully).
Products include:
Luvox CR Extended-Release Capsules **1759**

Formoterol Fumarate (Somatropin administration may alter the clearance of compounds known to be metabolized by CYP450 liver enzymes: monitor carefully).
Products include:
Foradil Aerolizer **2849**
Perforomist Inhalation Solution **1025**

Fosphenytoin (Growth hormone adminstration may alter the clearance of compounds known to be metabolized by CYP450 liver enzymes, such as anticonvulsants).
No products indexed under this heading.

Fosphenytoin Sodium (Growth hormone adminstration may alter the clearance of compounds known to be metabolized by CYP450 liver enzymes, such as anticonvulsants).
No products indexed under this heading.

Gabapentin (Growth hormone adminstration may alter the clearance of compounds known to be metabolized by CYP450 liver enzymes, such as anticonvulsants).
No products indexed under this heading.

Galantamine Hydrobromide (Somatropin administration may alter the clearance of compounds known to be metabolized by CYP450 liver enzymes: monitor carefully).
No products indexed under this heading.

Glimepiride (For diabetes, oral hypoglycemics may require dose adjustment when somatropin therapy is instituted). Products include:
Avandaryl Tablets **1344**
Duetact Tablets **3085**

Glipizide (For diabetes, oral hypoglycemics may require dose adjustment when somatropin therapy is instituted).
No products indexed under this heading.

Glyburide (For diabetes, oral hypoglycemics may require dose adjustment when somatropin therapy is instituted).
No products indexed under this heading.

Grepafloxacin Hydrochloride (Somatropin administration may alter the clearance of compounds known to be metabolized by CYP450 liver enzymes: monitor carefully).
No products indexed under this heading.

Haloperidol (Somatropin administration may alter the clearance of compounds known to be metabolized by CYP450 liver enzymes: monitor carefully).
No products indexed under this heading.

Haloperidol Decanoate (Somatropin administration may alter the clearance of compounds known to be metabolized by CYP450 liver enzymes: monitor carefully).
No products indexed under this heading.

Haloperidol Lactate (Somatropin administration may alter the clearance of compounds known to be metabolized by CYP450 liver enzymes: monitor carefully).
No products indexed under this heading.

Hydrocodone Bitartrate (Somatropin administration may alter the clearance of compounds known to be metabolized by CYP450 liver enzymes: monitor carefully).
Products include:
Lortab 5/500 Tablets **3143**
Lortab 7.5/500 Tablets **3144**
Lortab 10/500 Tablets **3144**
Vicodin Tablets **529**
Vicodin ES Tablets **530**
Vicodin HP Tablets **531**
Vicoprofen Tablets **533**
Zydone Tablets **1132**

Hydrocortisone (Excessive glucocorticoid therapy will inhibit the growth promoting effect of somatropin; growth hormone administration may alter the clearance of compounds known to be metabolized by cytochrome P450 liver enzymes; such as corticosteroids).
No products indexed under this heading.

Hydrocortisone Acetate (Excessive glucocorticoid therapy will inhibit the growth promoting effect of somatropin; growth hormone administration may alter the clearance of compounds known to be metabolized by cytochrome P450 liver enzymes; such as corticosteroids).
Products include:
Analpram-HC **1140**
Pramosone **1141**

Hydrocortisone Sodium Phosphate (Excessive glucocorticoid therapy will inhibit the growth promoting effect of somatropin; growth hormone administration may alter the clearance of compounds known to be metabolized by cytochrome P450 liver enzymes; such as corticosteroids).
No products indexed under this heading.

Hydrocortisone Sodium Succinate (Excessive glucocorticoid therapy will inhibit the growth promoting effect of somatropin; growth hormone administration may alter the clearance of compounds known to be metabolized by cytochrome P450 liver enzymes; such as corticosteroids).
No products indexed under this heading.

Ibuprofen (Somatropin administration may alter the clearance of compounds known to be metabolized by CYP450 liver enzymes: monitor carefully). Products include:
Motrin IB Tablets and Caplets **1900**
Children's Motrin Oral Suspension ... **1901**
Children's Motrin Non-Staining Dye-Free Oral Suspension **1901**

Children's Motrin Cold Oral Suspension 1899
Infants' Motrin Concentrated Drops 1901
Infants' Motrin Non-Staining Dye-Free Concentrated Drops 1901
Junior Strength Motrin Caplets and Chewable Tablets 1901
Vicoprofen Tablets 533

Imipramine Hydrochloride (Somatropin administration may alter the clearance of compounds known to be metabolized by CYP450 liver enzymes: monitor carefully).
No products indexed under this heading.

Imipramine Pamoate (Somatropin administration may alter the clearance of compounds known to be metabolized by CYP450 liver enzymes: monitor carefully).
No products indexed under this heading.

Indinavir Sulfate (Somatropin administration may alter the clearance of compounds known to be metabolized by CYP450 liver enzymes: monitor carefully).
Products include:
Crixivan Capsules 1979

Indomethacin (Somatropin administration may alter the clearance of compounds known to be metabolized by CYP450 liver enzymes: monitor carefully). Products include:
Indocin 2024

Indomethacin Sodium Trihydrate (Somatropin administration may alter the clearance of compounds known to be metabolized by CYP450 liver enzymes: monitor carefully). Products include:
Indocin I.V. 2489

Indoramin Hydrochloride (Somatropin administration may alter the clearance of compounds known to be metabolized by CYP450 liver enzymes: monitor carefully).
No products indexed under this heading.

Insulin (For diabetes, the insulin dose may require adjustment when somatropin therapy is instituted; growth hormone may induce a state of insulin resistance; patients should be observed for evidence of glucose intolerance).
No products indexed under this heading.

Insulin, Human, Zinc Suspension (For diabetes, the insulin dose may require adjustment when somatropin therapy is instituted; growth hormone may induce a state of insulin resistance; patients should be observed for evidence of glucose intolerance).
No products indexed under this heading.

Insulin, Human (rDNA origin) (For diabetes, the insulin dose may require adjustment when somatropin therapy is instituted; growth hormone may induce a state of insulin resistance; patients should be observed for evidence of glucose intolerance). Products include:
Exubera Inhalation Powder 2515

Insulin, Human NPH (For diabetes, the insulin dose may require adjustment when somatropin therapy is instituted; growth hormone may induce a state of insulin resistance; patients should be observed for evidence of glucose intolerance).
Products include:
Humulin N Vial 1846

Insulin, Human Regular (For diabetes, the insulin dose may require adjustment when somatropin therapy is instituted; growth hormone may induce a state of insulin resistance; patients should be observed for evidence of glucose intolerance).
Products include:
Humulin R 1849
Humulin R (U-500) 1850

Insulin, Human Regular and Human NPH Mixture (For diabetes, the insulin dose may require adjustment when somatropin therapy is instituted; growth hormone may induce a state of insulin resistance; patients should be observed for evidence of glucose intolerance).
Products include:
Humulin 50/50, 100 Units 1843
Humulin 70/30 Vial 1844

Insulin, NPH (For diabetes, the insulin dose may require adjustment when somatropin therapy is instituted; growth hormone may induce a state of insulin resistance; patients should be observed for evidence of glucose intolerance).
No products indexed under this heading.

Insulin, Regular (For diabetes, the insulin dose may require adjustment when somatropin therapy is instituted; growth hormone may induce a state of insulin resistance; patients should be observed for evidence of glucose intolerance).
No products indexed under this heading.

Insulin, Regular and NPH mixture (For diabetes, the insulin dose may require adjustment when somatropin therapy is instituted; growth hormone may induce a state of insulin resistance; patients should be observed for evidence of glucose intolerance).
No products indexed under this heading.

Insulin, Zinc Crystals (For diabetes, the insulin dose may require adjustment when somatropin therapy is instituted; growth hormone may induce a state of insulin resistance; patients should be observed for evidence of glucose intolerance).
No products indexed under this heading.

Insulin, Zinc Suspension (For diabetes, the insulin dose may require adjustment when somatropin therapy is instituted; growth hormone may induce a state of insulin resistance; patients should be observed for evidence of glucose intolerance).
No products indexed under this heading.

Insulin Aspart (For diabetes, the insulin dose may require adjustment when somatropin therapy is instituted; growth hormone may induce a state of insulin resistance; patients should be observed for evidence of glucose intolerance).
No products indexed under this heading.

Insulin Aspart, Human (For diabetes, the insulin dose may require adjustment when somatropin therapy is instituted; growth hormone may induce a state of insulin resistance; patients should be observed for evidence of glucose intolerance).
Products include:
NovoLog Mix 70/30 2364

Insulin Aspart, Human Regular (For diabetes, the insulin dose may require adjustment when somatropin therapy is instituted; growth hormone may induce a state of insulin resistance; patients should be observed for evidence of glucose intolerance). Products include:
NovoLog Injection 2359

Insulin Aspart Protamine, Human (For diabetes, the insulin dose may require adjustment when somatropin therapy is instituted; growth hormone may induce a state of insulin resistance; patients should be observed for evidence of glucose intolerance). Products include:
NovoLog Mix 70/30 2364

Insulin Detemir (rDNA Origin) (For diabetes, the insulin dose may require adjustment when somatropin therapy is instituted; growth hormone may induce a state of insulin resistance; patients should be observed for evidence of glucose intolerance). Products include:
Levemir Injection 2352

Insulin glargine (For diabetes, the insulin dose may require adjustment when somatropin therapy is instituted; growth hormone may induce a state of insulin resistance; patients should be observed for evidence of glucose intolerance). Products include:
Lantus Injection 2749

Insulin Glulisine (For diabetes, the insulin dose may require adjustment when somatropin therapy is instituted; growth hormone may induce a state of insulin resistance; patients should be observed for evidence of glucose intolerance). Products include:
Apidra Injection 2706

Insulin Lispro, Human (For diabetes, the insulin dose may require adjustment when somatropin therapy is instituted; growth hormone may induce a state of insulin resistance; patients should be observed for evidence of glucose intolerance).
Products include:
Humalog-Pen and KwikPen 1829
Humalog Mix 50/50-Pen and KwikPen 1833
Humalog Mix 75/25-Pen and KwikPen 1835

Insulin Lispro Protamine, Human (For diabetes, the insulin dose may require adjustment when somatropin therapy is instituted; growth hormone may induce a state of insulin resistance; patients should be observed for evidence of glucose intolerance). Products include:
Humalog Mix 50/50-Pen and KwikPen 1833
Humalog Mix 75/25-Pen and KwikPen 1835

Irbesartan (Somatropin administration may alter the clearance of compounds known to be metabolized by CYP450 liver enzymes: monitor carefully). Products include:
Avalide Tablets 892
Avalide Tablets 2713
Avapro Tablets 897
Avapro Tablets 2718

Isotretinoin (Somatropin administration may alter the clearance of compounds known to be metabolized by CYP450 liver enzymes: monitor carefully). Products include:
Accutane Capsules 2607

Isradipine (Somatropin administration may alter the clearance of compounds known to be metabolized by CYP450 liver enzymes: monitor carefully). Products include:
DynaCirc CR Controlled Release Tablets 1407

Itraconazole (Somatropin administration may alter the clearance of compounds known to be metabolized by CYP450 liver enzymes: monitor carefully).
No products indexed under this heading.

Ketoconazole (Somatropin administration may alter the clearance of compounds known to be metabolized by CYP450 liver enzymes: monitor carefully). Products include:
Extina Foam, 2% 3057
Nizoral A-D Shampoo 1901

Ketoprofen (Somatropin administration may alter the clearance of compounds known to be metabolized by CYP450 liver enzymes: monitor carefully).
No products indexed under this heading.

Ketorolac Tromethamine (Somatropin administration may alter the clearance of compounds known to be metabolized by CYP450 liver enzymes: monitor carefully).
No products indexed under this heading.

Labetalol Hydrochloride (Somatropin administration may alter the clearance of compounds known to be metabolized by CYP450 liver enzymes: monitor carefully).
No products indexed under this heading.

Lamotrigine (Growth hormone adminstration may alter the clearance of compounds known to be metabolized by CYP450 liver enzymes, such as anticonvulsants).
Products include:
Lamictal 1488

Lansoprazole (Somatropin administration may alter the clearance of compounds known to be metabolized by CYP450 liver enzymes: monitor carefully).
No products indexed under this heading.

Levetiracetam (Growth hormone adminstration may alter the clearance of compounds known to be metabolized by CYP450 liver enzymes, such as anticonvulsants).
Products include:
Keppra Injection 3137
Keppra Oral Solution 3131
Keppra Tablets 3131

Levobupivacaine Hydrochloride (Somatropin administration may alter the clearance of compounds known to be metabolized by CYP450 liver enzymes: monitor carefully).
No products indexed under this heading.

Levonorgestrel (Growth hormone administration may alter the clearance of compounds known to be metabolized by cytochrome P450 liver enzymes, such as sex steroids).
Products include:
Climara Pro Transdermal System 768
Lybrel Tablets 3204
Mirena Intrauterine System 779
Plan B Tablets 1044
Seasonique Tablets 1046

Lidocaine (Somatropin administration may alter the clearance of compounds known to be metabolized by CYP450 liver enzymes: monitor carefully). Products include:
Lidoderm Patch 1114

Lidocaine Base (Somatropin administration may alter the clearance of compounds known to be metabolized by CYP450 liver enzymes: monitor carefully).
No products indexed under this heading.

Lidocaine Hydrochloride (Somatropin administration may alter the clearance of compounds known to be metabolized by CYP450 liver enzymes: monitor carefully).
No products indexed under this heading.

Lomefloxacin Hydrochloride (Somatropin administration may alter the clearance of compounds known to be metabolized by CYP450 liver enzymes: monitor carefully).
No products indexed under this heading.

Losartan Potassium (Somatropin administration may alter the clearance of compounds known to be metabolized by CYP450 liver enzymes: monitor carefully). Products include:
Cozaar Tablets ... **1973**

Lovastatin (Somatropin administration may alter the clearance of compounds known to be metabolized by CYP450 liver enzymes: monitor carefully). Products include:
Advicor Tablets ... **402**
Mevacor Tablets ... **2063**

Maprotiline Hydrochloride (Somatropin administration may alter the clearance of compounds known to be metabolized by CYP450 liver enzymes: monitor carefully).
No products indexed under this heading.

Meclofenamate Sodium (Somatropin administration may alter the clearance of compounds known to be metabolized by CYP450 liver enzymes: monitor carefully).
No products indexed under this heading.

Mefenamic Acid (Somatropin administration may alter the clearance of compounds known to be metabolized by CYP450 liver enzymes: monitor carefully).
No products indexed under this heading.

Meloxicam (Somatropin administration may alter the clearance of compounds known to be metabolized by CYP450 liver enzymes: monitor carefully). Products include:
Mobic Oral Suspension ... **863**
Mobic Tablets ... **863**

Meperidine Hydrochloride (Somatropin administration may alter the clearance of compounds known to be metabolized by CYP450 liver enzymes: monitor carefully).
No products indexed under this heading.

Mephenytoin (Growth hormone adminstration may alter the clearance of compounds known to be metabolized by CYP450 liver enzymes, such as anticonvulsants).
No products indexed under this heading.

Mephobarbital (Somatropin administration may alter the clearance of compounds known to be metabolized by CYP450 liver enzymes: monitor carefully).
No products indexed under this heading.

Meprobamate (Somatropin administration may alter the clearance of compounds known to be metabolized by CYP450 liver enzymes: monitor carefully).
No products indexed under this heading.

Mestranol (Growth hormone administration may alter the clearance of compounds known to be metabolized by cytochrome P450 liver enzymes, such as sex steroids).
No products indexed under this heading.

Metformin Hydrochloride (For diabetes, oral hypoglycemics may require dose adjustment when somatropin therapy is instituted). Products include:
ActoPlus Met Tablets ... **3071**
Avandamet Tablets ... **1336**
Janumet Tablets ... **2041**
PrandiMet Tablets ... **2967**

Methadone Hydrochloride (Somatropin administration may alter the clearance of compounds known to be metabolized by CYP450 liver enzymes: monitor carefully).
No products indexed under this heading.

Methamphetamine Hydrochloride (Somatropin administration may alter the clearance of compounds known to be metabolized by CYP450 liver enzymes: monitor carefully).
No products indexed under this heading.

Methsuximide (Growth hormone adminstration may alter the clearance of compounds known to be metabolized by CYP450 liver enzymes, such as anticonvulsants).
No products indexed under this heading.

Methylprednisolone Acetate (Excessive glucocorticoid therapy will inhibit the growth promoting effect of somatropin; growth hormone administration may alter the clearance of compounds known to be metabolized by cytochrome P450 liver enzymes; such as corticosteroids).
No products indexed under this heading.

Methylprednisolone Sodium Succinate (Excessive glucocorticoid therapy will inhibit the growth promoting effect of somatropin; growth hormone administration may alter the clearance of compounds known to be metabolized by cytochrome P450 liver enzymes; such as corticosteroids).
No products indexed under this heading.

Methyltestosterone (Growth hormone administration may alter the clearance of compounds known to be metabolized by cytochrome P450 liver enzymes, such as sex steroids). Products include:
Estratest Tablets ... **3043**
Estratest H.S. Tablets ... **3043**

Metoprolol Succinate (Somatropin administration may alter the clearance of compounds known to be metabolized by CYP450 liver enzymes: monitor carefully). Products include:
Toprol-XL Tablets ... **666**

Metoprolol Tartrate (Somatropin administration may alter the clearance of compounds known to be metabolized by CYP450 liver enzymes: monitor carefully).
No products indexed under this heading.

Mexiletine Hydrochloride (Somatropin administration may alter the clearance of compounds known to be metabolized by CYP450 liver enzymes: monitor carefully).
No products indexed under this heading.

Midazolam Hydrochloride (Somatropin administration may alter the clearance of compounds known to be metabolized by CYP450 liver enzymes: monitor carefully).
No products indexed under this heading.

Miglitol (For diabetes, oral hypoglycemics may require dose adjustment when somatropin therapy is instituted).
No products indexed under this heading.

Mirtazapine (Somatropin administration may alter the clearance of compounds known to be metabolized by CYP450 liver enzymes: monitor carefully). Products include:
Remeron Tablets ... **2924**
RemeronSolTab Tablets ... **2927**

Mometasone Furoate (Growth hormone administration may alter the clearance of compounds known to be metabolized by CYP450 liver enzymes, such as corticosteroids). Products include:
Asmanex Twisthaler ... **2797**
Elocon Cream 0.1% ... **2840**
Elocon Lotion 0.1% ... **2841**
Elocon Ointment 0.1% ... **2842**

Mometasone Furoate Monohydrate (Growth hormone administration may alter the clearance of compounds known to be metabolized by CYP450 liver enzymes, such as corticosteroids). Products include:
Nasonex Nasal Spray ... **2883**

Montelukast Sodium (Somatropin administration may alter the clearance of compounds known to be metabolized by CYP450 liver enzymes: monitor carefully). Products include:
Singulair ... **2114**

Morphine Sulfate (Somatropin administration may alter the clearance of compounds known to be metabolized by CYP450 liver enzymes: monitor carefully). Products include:
Avinza Capsules ... **1772**
DepoDur Injection ... **1095**
MS Contin Tablets ... **2585**

Moxifloxacin Hydrochloride (Somatropin administration may alter the clearance of compounds known to be metabolized by CYP450 liver enzymes: monitor carefully). Products include:
Avelox ... **2803**
Vigamox Ophthalmic Solution ... **548**

Nabumetone (Somatropin administration may alter the clearance of compounds known to be metabolized by CYP450 liver enzymes: monitor carefully).
No products indexed under this heading.

Nafcillin Sodium (Somatropin administration may alter the clearance of compounds known to be metabolized by CYP450 liver enzymes: monitor carefully).
No products indexed under this heading.

Naproxen (Somatropin administration may alter the clearance of compounds known to be metabolized by CYP450 liver enzymes: monitor carefully). Products include:
EC-Naprosyn Delayed-Release Tablets ... **2632**
Naprosyn Suspension ... **2632**
Naprosyn Tablets ... **2632**

Naproxen Sodium (Somatropin administration may alter the clearance of compounds known to be metabolized by CYP450 liver enzymes: monitor carefully). Products include:
Anaprox Tablets ... **2632**
Anaprox DS Tablets ... **2632**
Treximet Tablets ... **1616**

Nateglinide (For diabetes, oral hypoglycemics may require dose adjustment when somatropin therapy is instituted). Products include:
Starlix Tablets ... **2314**

Nefazodone Hydrochloride (Somatropin administration may alter the clearance of compounds known to be metabolized by CYP450 liver enzymes: monitor carefully).
No products indexed under this heading.

Nelfinavir Mesylate (Somatropin administration may alter the clearance of compounds known to be metabolized by CYP450 liver enzymes: monitor carefully).
No products indexed under this heading.

Nicardipine (Somatropin administration may alter the clearance of compounds known to be metabolized by CYP450 liver enzymes: monitor carefully).
No products indexed under this heading.

Nicardipine Hydrochloride (Somatropin administration may alter the clearance of compounds known to be metabolized by CYP450 liver enzymes: monitor carefully). Products include:
Cardene I.V. ... **1093**

Nicotine Polacrilex (Somatropin administration may alter the clearance of compounds known to be metabolized by CYP450 liver enzymes: monitor carefully).
No products indexed under this heading.

Nicotine Salicylate (Somatropin administration may alter the clearance of compounds known to be metabolized by CYP450 liver enzymes: monitor carefully).
No products indexed under this heading.

Nicotine Sulfate (Somatropin administration may alter the clearance of compounds known to be metabolized by CYP450 liver enzymes: monitor carefully).
No products indexed under this heading.

Nifedipine (Somatropin administration may alter the clearance of compounds known to be metabolized by CYP450 liver enzymes: monitor carefully).
No products indexed under this heading.

Nilutamide (Somatropin administration may alter the clearance of compounds known to be metabolized by CYP450 liver enzymes: monitor carefully).
No products indexed under this heading.

Nimodipine (Somatropin administration may alter the clearance of compounds known to be metabolized by CYP450 liver enzymes: monitor carefully). Products include:
Nimotop Capsules 790

Nisoldipine (Somatropin administration may alter the clearance of compounds known to be metabolized by CYP450 liver enzymes: monitor carefully). Products include:
Sular Extended Release Tablets 2975

Nitrendipine (Somatropin administration may alter the clearance of compounds known to be metabolized by CYP450 liver enzymes: monitor carefully).
No products indexed under this heading.

Norethindrone (Growth hormone administration may alter the clearance of compounds known to be metabolized by cytochrome P450 liver enzymes, such as sex steroids). Products include:
Ortho Micronor Tablets 2446

Norethindrone Acetate (Growth hormone administration may alter the clearance of compounds known to be metabolized by cytochrome P450 liver enzymes, such as sex steroids). Products include:
Activella Tablets 2347

Norfloxacin (Somatropin administration may alter the clearance of compounds known to be metabolized by CYP450 liver enzymes: monitor carefully). Products include:
Noroxin Tablets 2069

Norgestimate (Growth hormone administration may alter the clearance of compounds known to be metabolized by cytochrome P450 liver enzymes, such as sex steroids). Products include:
Ortho-Cyclen/Ortho Tri-Cyclen 2449
Ortho Tri-Cyclen Lo Tablets 2458

Norgestrel (Somatropin administration may alter the clearance of compounds known to be metabolized by CYP450 liver enzymes: monitor carefully).
No products indexed under this heading.

Nortriptyline Hydrochloride (Somatropin administration may alter the clearance of compounds known to be metabolized by CYP450 liver enzymes: monitor carefully).
No products indexed under this heading.

Ofloxacin (Somatropin administration may alter the clearance of compounds known to be metabolized by CYP450 liver enzymes: monitor carefully). Products include:
Ofloxacin Ophthalmic Solution 0.3% .... ⊙ 243

Olanzapine (Somatropin administration may alter the clearance of compounds known to be metabolized by CYP450 liver enzymes: monitor carefully). Products include:
Symbyax Capsules 1871
Zyprexa Tablets 1883
Zyprexa IntraMuscular 1883
Zyprexa ZYDIS Orally Disintegrating Tablets 1883

Omeprazole (Somatropin administration may alter the clearance of compounds known to be metabolized by CYP450 liver enzymes: monitor carefully).
No products indexed under this heading.

Ondansetron (Somatropin administration may alter the clearance of compounds known to be metabolized by CYP450 liver enzymes: monitor carefully). Products include:
Zofran ODT Orally Disintegrating Tablets 1687

Ondansetron Hydrochloride (Somatropin administration may alter the clearance of compounds known to be metabolized by CYP450 liver enzymes: monitor carefully). Products include:
Zofran Injection 1682
Zofran 1687

Oxaprozin (Somatropin administration may alter the clearance of compounds known to be metabolized by CYP450 liver enzymes: monitor carefully).
No products indexed under this heading.

Oxcarbazepine (Growth hormone adminstration may alter the clearance of compounds known to be metabolized by CYP450 liver enzymes, such as anticonvulsants).
No products indexed under this heading.

Oxycodone Hydrochloride (Somatropin administration may alter the clearance of compounds known to be metabolized by CYP450 liver enzymes: monitor carefully). Products include:
OxyContin Tablets 2589
OxyIR Capsules 2593
Percocet Tablets 1127
Percodan Tablets 1130

Paclitaxel (Somatropin administration may alter the clearance of compounds known to be metabolized by CYP450 liver enzymes: monitor carefully).
No products indexed under this heading.

Pantoprazole Sodium (Somatropin administration may alter the clearance of compounds known to be metabolized by CYP450 liver enzymes: monitor carefully). Products include:
Protonix for Delayed-Release Oral Suspension 3254
Protonix Delayed-Release Tablets 3254
Protonix I.V. 3257

Paramethadione (Growth hormone adminstration may alter the clearance of compounds known to be metabolized by CYP450 liver enzymes, such as anticonvulsants).
No products indexed under this heading.

Paroxetine Hydrochloride (Somatropin administration may alter the clearance of compounds known to be metabolized by CYP450 liver enzymes: monitor carefully). Products include:
Paxil 1535
Paxil CR Controlled-Release Tablets 1544

Pentamidine Isethionate (Somatropin administration may alter the clearance of compounds known to be metabolized by CYP450 liver enzymes: monitor carefully).
No products indexed under this heading.

Phenacemide (Growth hormone adminstration may alter the clearance of compounds known to be metabolized by CYP450 liver enzymes, such as anticonvulsants).
No products indexed under this heading.

Phenobarbital (Growth hormone adminstration may alter the clearance of compounds known to be metabolized by CYP450 liver enzymes, such as anticonvulsants). Products include:
Donnatal Extentabs 2507

Phenobarbital Sodium (Somatropin administration may alter the clearance of compounds known to be metabolized by CYP450 liver enzymes: monitor carefully).
No products indexed under this heading.

Phensuximide (Growth hormone adminstration may alter the clearance of compounds known to be metabolized by CYP450 liver enzymes, such as anticonvulsants).
No products indexed under this heading.

Phenylbutazone (Somatropin administration may alter the clearance of compounds known to be metabolized by CYP450 liver enzymes: monitor carefully).
No products indexed under this heading.

Phenytoin (Growth hormone adminstration may alter the clearance of compounds known to be metabolized by CYP450 liver enzymes, such as anticonvulsants).
No products indexed under this heading.

Phenytoin Sodium (Growth hormone adminstration may alter the clearance of compounds known to be metabolized by CYP450 liver enzymes, such as anticonvulsants). Products include:
Phenytek Capsules 2192

Pimozide (Somatropin administration may alter the clearance of compounds known to be metabolized by CYP450 liver enzymes: monitor carefully).
No products indexed under this heading.

Pindolol (Somatropin administration may alter the clearance of compounds known to be metabolized by CYP450 liver enzymes: monitor carefully).
No products indexed under this heading.

Pioglitazone Hydrochloride (For diabetes, oral hypoglycemics may require dose adjustment when somatropin therapy is instituted). Products include:
ActoPlus Met Tablets 3071
Actos Tablets 3077
Duetact Tablets 3085

Piroxicam (Somatropin administration may alter the clearance of compounds known to be metabolized by CYP450 liver enzymes: monitor carefully).
No products indexed under this heading.

Polyestradiol Phosphate (A larger dose of somatropin may be required to achieve the defined treatment goal in adult women on oral estrogen replacement).
No products indexed under this heading.

Prednisolone Acetate (Excessive glucocorticoid therapy will inhibit the growth promoting effect of somatropin; growth hormone administration may alter the clearance of compounds known to be metabolized by cytochrome P450 liver enzymes; such as corticosteroids). Products include:
Pred Forte Ophthalmic Suspension .... ⊙ 227
Pred Mild Ophthalmic Suspension .... ⊙ 230
Pred-G Ophthalmic Ointment .... ⊙ 229
Pred-G Ophthalmic Suspension .... ⊙ 228

Prednisolone Sodium Phosphate (Excessive glucocorticoid therapy will inhibit the growth promoting effect of somatropin; growth hormone administration may alter the clearance of compounds known to be metabolized by cytochrome P450 liver enzymes; such as corticosteroids).
No products indexed under this heading.

Prednisolone Tebutate (Excessive glucocorticoid therapy will inhibit the growth promoting effect of somatropin; growth hormone administration may alter the clearance of compounds known to be metabolized by cytochrome P450 liver enzymes; such as corticosteroids).
No products indexed under this heading.

Prednisone (Excessive glucocorticoid therapy will inhibit the growth promoting effect of somatropin; growth hormone administration may alter the clearance of compounds known to be metabolized by cytochrome P450 liver enzymes; such as corticosteroids).
No products indexed under this heading.

Primidone (Growth hormone adminstration may alter the clearance of compounds known to be metabolized by CYP450 liver enzymes, such as anticonvulsants).
No products indexed under this heading.

Progesterone (Somatropin administration may alter the clearance of compounds known to be metabolized by CYP450 liver enzymes: monitor carefully). Products include:
Crinone 4% Gel 992
Crinone 8% Gel 992
Prometrium Capsules (100 mg, 200 mg) 3047

Proguanil Hydrochloride (Somatropin administration may alter the clearance of compounds known to be metabolized by CYP450 liver enzymes: monitor carefully). Products include:
Malarone Pediatric Tablets 1521
Malarone Tablets 1521

Propafenone Hydrochloride (Somatropin administration may alter the clearance of compounds known to be metabolized by CYP450 liver enzymes: monitor carefully). Products include:
Rythmol Tablets 1586
Rythmol SR Capsules 1590

Propoxyphene Hydrochloride (Somatropin administration may alter the clearance of compounds known to be metabolized by CYP450 liver enzymes: monitor carefully).
No products indexed under this heading.

Propoxyphene Napsylate (Somatropin administration may alter the clearance of compounds known to be metabolized by CYP450 liver enzymes: monitor carefully).
No products indexed under this heading.

Propranolol Hydrochloride (Somatropin administration may alter the clearance of compounds known to be metabolized by CYP450 liver enzymes: monitor carefully).
Products include:
InnoPran XL Extended Release Capsules 1484

Protriptyline Hydrochloride (Somatropin administration may alter the clearance of compounds known to be metabolized by CYP450 liver enzymes: monitor carefully).
No products indexed under this heading.

Quetiapine Fumarate (Somatropin administration may alter the clearance of compounds known to be metabolized by CYP450 liver enzymes: monitor carefully).
No products indexed under this heading.

Quinestrol (A larger dose of somatropin may be required to achieve the defined treatment goal in adult women on oral estrogen replacement).
No products indexed under this heading.

Quinidine Gluconate (Somatropin administration may alter the clearance of compounds known to be metabolized by CYP450 liver enzymes: monitor carefully).
No products indexed under this heading.

Quinidine Hydrochloride (Somatropin administration may alter the clearance of compounds known to be metabolized by CYP450 liver enzymes: monitor carefully).
No products indexed under this heading.

Quinidine Polygalacturonate (Somatropin administration may alter the clearance of compounds known to be metabolized by CYP450 liver enzymes: monitor carefully).
No products indexed under this heading.

Quinidine Sulfate (Somatropin administration may alter the clearance of compounds known to be metabolized by CYP450 liver enzymes: monitor carefully).
No products indexed under this heading.

Quinine (Somatropin administration may alter the clearance of compounds known to be metabolized by CYP450 liver enzymes: monitor carefully).
No products indexed under this heading.

Quinine Sulfate (Somatropin administration may alter the clearance of compounds known to be metabolized by CYP450 liver enzymes: monitor carefully).
No products indexed under this heading.

Rabeprazole Sodium (Somatropin administration may alter the clearance of compounds known to be metabolized by CYP450 liver enzymes: monitor carefully).
Products include:
Aciphex Tablets 1053

Repaglinide (For diabetes, oral hypoglycemics may require dose adjustment when somatropin therapy is instituted). Products include:
PrandiMet Tablets 2967
Prandin Tablets 2971

Rifabutin (Somatropin administration may alter the clearance of compounds known to be metabolized by CYP450 liver enzymes: monitor carefully).
No products indexed under this heading.

Riluzole (Somatropin administration may alter the clearance of compounds known to be metabolized by CYP450 liver enzymes: monitor carefully). Products include:
Rilutek Tablets 2771

Risperidone (Somatropin administration may alter the clearance of compounds known to be metabolized by CYP450 liver enzymes: monitor carefully). Products include:
Risperdal Consta Long-Acting Injection 1753

Ritonavir (Somatropin administration may alter the clearance of compounds known to be metabolized by CYP450 liver enzymes: monitor carefully). Products include:
Kaletra 452
Norvir 489

Rofecoxib (Somatropin administration may alter the clearance of compounds known to be metabolized by CYP450 liver enzymes: monitor carefully).
No products indexed under this heading.

Ropinirole Hydrochloride (Somatropin administration may alter the clearance of compounds known to be metabolized by CYP450 liver enzymes: monitor carefully).
Products include:
Requip Tablets 1561
Requip XL Tablets 1568

Ropivacaine Hydrochloride (Somatropin administration may alter the clearance of compounds known to be metabolized by CYP450 liver enzymes: monitor carefully).
No products indexed under this heading.

Rosiglitazone Maleate (For diabetes, oral hypoglycemics may require dose adjustment when somatropin therapy is instituted). Products include:
Avandamet Tablets 1336
Avandaryl Tablets 1344
Avandia Tablets 1351

Saquinavir (Somatropin administration may alter the clearance of compounds known to be metabolized by CYP450 liver enzymes: monitor carefully).
No products indexed under this heading.

Saquinavir Mesylate (Somatropin administration may alter the clearance of compounds known to be metabolized by CYP450 liver enzymes: monitor carefully).
No products indexed under this heading.

Sertraline Hydrochloride (Somatropin administration may alter the clearance of compounds known to be metabolized by CYP450 liver enzymes: monitor carefully).
No products indexed under this heading.

Sildenafil Citrate (Somatropin administration may alter the clearance of compounds known to be metabolized by CYP450 liver enzymes: monitor carefully).
No products indexed under this heading.

Simvastatin (Somatropin administration may alter the clearance of compounds known to be metabolized by CYP450 liver enzymes: monitor carefully). Products include:
Simcor Tablets 502
Vytorin 10/10 Tablets 2149
Vytorin 10/10 Tablets 2939
Vytorin 10/20 Tablets 2149
Vytorin 10/20 Tablets 2939
Vytorin 10/40 Tablets 2149
Vytorin 10/40 Tablets 2939
Vytorin 10/80 Tablets 2149
Vytorin 10/80 Tablets 2939
Zocor Tablets 2136

Sirolimus (Somatropin administration may alter the clearance of compounds known to be metabolized by CYP450 liver enzymes: monitor carefully). Products include:
Rapamune 3260

Sitagliptin Phosphate (For diabetes, oral hypoglycemics may require dose adjustment when somatropin therapy is instituted). Products include:
Janumet Tablets 2041
Januvia Tablets 2048

Sulfamethoxazole (Somatropin administration may alter the clearance of compounds known to be metabolized by CYP450 liver enzymes: monitor carefully).
No products indexed under this heading.

Sulindac (Somatropin administration may alter the clearance of compounds known to be metabolized by CYP450 liver enzymes: monitor carefully). Products include:
Clinoril Tablets 1962

Suprofen (Somatropin administration may alter the clearance of compounds known to be metabolized by CYP450 liver enzymes: monitor carefully).
No products indexed under this heading.

Tacrine Hydrochloride (Somatropin administration may alter the clearance of compounds known to be metabolized by CYP450 liver enzymes: monitor carefully).
No products indexed under this heading.

Tacrolimus (Somatropin administration may alter the clearance of compounds known to be metabolized by CYP450 liver enzymes: monitor carefully). Products include:
Prograf Capsules and Injection 622
Protopic Ointment 628

Tamoxifen Citrate (Somatropin administration may alter the clearance of compounds known to be metabolized by CYP450 liver enzymes: monitor carefully).
No products indexed under this heading.

Telmisartan (Somatropin administration may alter the clearance of compounds known to be metabolized by CYP450 liver enzymes: monitor carefully). Products include:
Micardis Tablets 852
Micardis HCT Tablets 854

Teniposide (Somatropin administration may alter the clearance of compounds known to be metabolized by CYP450 liver enzymes: monitor carefully).
No products indexed under this heading.

Terfenadine (Somatropin administration may alter the clearance of compounds known to be metabolized by CYP450 liver enzymes: monitor carefully).
No products indexed under this heading.

Testosterone (Growth hormone administration may alter the clearance of compounds known to be metabolized by cytochrome P450 liver enzymes, such as sex steroids).
Products include:
AndroGel 3159
Testim 1% Gel 701

Testosterone Cypionate (Somatropin administration may alter the clearance of compounds known to be metabolized by CYP450 liver enzymes: monitor carefully).
No products indexed under this heading.

Testosterone Enanthate (Somatropin administration may alter the clearance of compounds known to be metabolized by CYP450 liver enzymes: monitor carefully).
Products include:
Delatestryl Injection 1730

Testosterone Propionate (Somatropin administration may alter the clearance of compounds known to be metabolized by CYP450 liver enzymes: monitor carefully).
No products indexed under this heading.

Theophylline (Somatropin administration may alter the clearance of compounds known to be metabolized by CYP450 liver enzymes: monitor carefully).
No products indexed under this heading.

Theophylline Anhydrous (Somatropin administration may alter the clearance of compounds known to be metabolized by CYP450 liver enzymes: monitor carefully).
Products include:
Uniphyl Tablets 2595

Theophylline Sodium Glycinate (Somatropin administration may alter the clearance of compounds known to be metabolized by CYP450 liver enzymes: monitor carefully).
No products indexed under this heading.

Thioridazine (Somatropin administration may alter the clearance of compounds known to be metabolized by CYP450 liver enzymes: monitor carefully).
No products indexed under this heading.

Thioridazine Hydrochloride (Somatropin administration may alter the clearance of compounds known to be metabolized by CYP450 liver enzymes: monitor carefully).
Products include:
Thioridazine Hydrochloride Tablets 2195

Tiagabine Hydrochloride (Growth hormone adminstration may alter the clearance of compounds known to be metabolized by CYP450 liver enzymes, such as anticonvulsants).
Products include:
Gabitril Tablets 973

Timolol Maleate (Somatropin administration may alter the clearance of compounds known to be metabolized by CYP450 liver enzymes: monitor carefully). Products include:
Combigan Ophthalmic Solution 553
Cosopt Sterile Ophthalmic Solution 1969
Timoptic Sterile Ophthalmic Solution 2121
Timoptic in Ocudose 2124
Timoptic-XE Sterile Ophthalmic Gel Forming Solution 2125

Tolazamide (For diabetes, oral hypoglycemics may require dose adjustment when somatropin therapy is instituted).
No products indexed under this heading.

Tolbutamide (For diabetes, oral hypoglycemics may require dose adjustment when somatropin therapy is instituted).
No products indexed under this heading.

Tolbutamide Sodium (Somatropin administration may alter the clearance of compounds known to be metabolized by CYP450 liver enzymes: monitor carefully).
No products indexed under this heading.

Tolmetin Sodium (Somatropin administration may alter the clearance of compounds known to be metabolized by CYP450 liver enzymes: monitor carefully).
No products indexed under this heading.

Tolterodine Tartrate (Somatropin administration may alter the clearance of compounds known to be metabolized by CYP450 liver enzymes: monitor carefully).
No products indexed under this heading.

Topiramate (Growth hormone adminstration may alter the clearance of compounds known to be metabolized by CYP450 liver enzymes, such as anticonvulsants).
No products indexed under this heading.

Torsemide (Somatropin administration may alter the clearance of compounds known to be metabolized by CYP450 liver enzymes: monitor carefully). Products include:
Demadex Injection 2630
Demadex Tablets 2630

Tramadol Hydrochloride (Somatropin administration may alter the clearance of compounds known to be metabolized by CYP450 liver enzymes: monitor carefully). Products include:
Ultram ER Extended-Release Tablets 2428

Trazodone Hydrochloride (Somatropin administration may alter the clearance of compounds known to be metabolized by CYP450 liver enzymes: monitor carefully).
No products indexed under this heading.

Tretinoin (Somatropin administration may alter the clearance of compounds known to be metabolized by CYP450 liver enzymes: monitor carefully). Products include:
Vesanoid Capsules 2660
Ziana Gel 1942

Triamcinolone (Excessive glucocorticoid therapy will inhibit the growth promoting effect of somatropin; growth hormone administration may alter the clearance of compounds known to be metabolized by cytochrome P450 liver enzymes; such as corticosteroids).
No products indexed under this heading.

Triamcinolone Acetonide (Excessive glucocorticoid therapy will inhibit the growth promoting effect of somatropin; growth hormone administration may alter the clearance of compounds known to be metabolized by cytochrome P450 liver enzymes; such as corticosteroids). Products include:
Azmacort Inhalation Aerosol 407
Nasacort AQ Nasal Spray 2765
Triesence Injectable Suspension .... ⊙ 209

Triamcinolone Diacetate (Excessive glucocorticoid therapy will inhibit the growth promoting effect of somatropin; growth hormone administration may alter the clearance of compounds known to be metabolized by cytochrome P450 liver enzymes; such as corticosteroids).
No products indexed under this heading.

Triamcinolone Hexacetonide (Excessive glucocorticoid therapy will inhibit the growth promoting effect of somatropin; growth hormone administration may alter the clearance of compounds known to be metabolized by cytochrome P450 liver enzymes; such as corticosteroids).
No products indexed under this heading.

Triazolam (Somatropin administration may alter the clearance of compounds known to be metabolized by CYP450 liver enzymes: monitor carefully).
No products indexed under this heading.

Trimethadione (Growth hormone adminstration may alter the clearance of compounds known to be metabolized by CYP450 liver enzymes, such as anticonvulsants).
No products indexed under this heading.

Trimethaphan Camsylate (Somatropin administration may alter the clearance of compounds known to be metabolized by CYP450 liver enzymes: monitor carefully).
No products indexed under this heading.

Trimipramine Maleate (Somatropin administration may alter the clearance of compounds known to be metabolized by CYP450 liver enzymes: monitor carefully).
No products indexed under this heading.

Troglitazone (For diabetes, oral hypoglycemics may require dose adjustment when somatropin therapy is instituted).
No products indexed under this heading.

Trovafloxacin Mesylate (Somatropin administration may alter the clearance of compounds known to be metabolized by CYP450 liver enzymes: monitor carefully).
No products indexed under this heading.

Valdecoxib (Somatropin administration may alter the clearance of compounds known to be metabolized by CYP450 liver enzymes: monitor carefully).
No products indexed under this heading.

Valproate Sodium (Growth hormone adminstration may alter the clearance of compounds known to be metabolized by CYP450 liver enzymes, such as anticonvulsants).
No products indexed under this heading.

Valproic Acid (Growth hormone adminstration may alter the clearance of compounds known to be metabolized by CYP450 liver enzymes, such as anticonvulsants).
No products indexed under this heading.

Valsartan (Somatropin administration may alter the clearance of compounds known to be metabolized by CYP450 liver enzymes: monitor carefully). Products include:
Diovan Tablets 2212
Diovan HCT Tablets 2216
Exforge Tablets 2238

Venlafaxine Hydrochloride (Somatropin administration may alter the clearance of compounds known to be metabolized by CYP450 liver enzymes: monitor carefully). Products include:
Effexor XR Extended-Release Capsules 3195
Venlafaxine Hydrochloride Tablets ... 2199

Verapamil Hydrochloride (Somatropin administration may alter the clearance of compounds known to be metabolized by CYP450 liver enzymes: monitor carefully). Products include:
Tarka Tablets 511

Vinblastine Sulfate (Somatropin administration may alter the clearance of compounds known to be metabolized by CYP450 liver enzymes: monitor carefully).
No products indexed under this heading.

Vincristine Sulfate (Somatropin administration may alter the clearance of compounds known to be metabolized by CYP450 liver enzymes: monitor carefully).
No products indexed under this heading.

Vitamin A (Somatropin administration may alter the clearance of compounds known to be metabolized by CYP450 liver enzymes: monitor carefully). Products include:
Norwegian Cod Liver Oil 949

Vitamin A Acetate (Somatropin administration may alter the clearance of compounds known to be metabolized by CYP450 liver enzymes: monitor carefully).
No products indexed under this heading.

Voriconazole (Somatropin administration may alter the clearance of compounds known to be metabolized by CYP450 liver enzymes: monitor carefully).
No products indexed under this heading.

Warfarin Sodium (Somatropin administration may alter the clearance of compounds known to be metabolized by CYP450 liver enzymes: monitor carefully).
No products indexed under this heading.

Zafirlukast (Somatropin administration may alter the clearance of compounds known to be metabolized by CYP450 liver enzymes: monitor carefully). Products include:
Accolate Tablets 669

Zileuton (Somatropin administration may alter the clearance of compounds known to be metabolized by CYP450 liver enzymes: monitor carefully).
No products indexed under this heading.

Zolmitriptan (Somatropin administration may alter the clearance of compounds known to be metabolized by CYP450 liver enzymes: monitor carefully). Products include:
Zomig Tablets 694
Zomig Nasal Spray 689
Zomig-ZMT Tablets 694

Zonisamide (Growth hormone adminstration may alter the clearance of compounds known to be metabolized by CYP450 liver enzymes, such as anticonvulsants). Products include:
Zonegran Capsules 1089

Zopiclone (Somatropin administration may alter the clearance of compounds known to be metabolized by CYP450 liver enzymes: monitor carefully).
No products indexed under this heading.

HUMIRA INJECTION
(Adalimumab) 442
May interact with:

Anakinra (Concurrent administration of anakinra (an interleukin-1 antagonist) and another TNF-blocking agent has been associated with an increased risk of serious infections, an increased risk of neutropenia and no additional benefit compared to these medicinal agents alone. Therefore, the combination of anakinra with other TNF-blocking agents, including adalimumab, may also result in similar toxicities). Products include:
Kineret Injection 585

Methotrexate (Methotrexate reduced adalimumab apparent clearance after single and multiple dosing by 29% and 44% respectively).
No products indexed under this heading.

Vaccines (Live) (Live vaccines should not be given concurrently with Humira).
No products indexed under this heading.

HUMULIN 50/50, 100 UNITS
(Insulin, Human Regular and Human NPH Mixture) 1843
See Humulin N Vial

HUMULIN 70/30 VIAL
(Insulin, Human Regular and Human NPH Mixture) 1844
See Humulin N Vial

HUMULIN N VIAL
(Insulin, Human NPH) 1846
May interact with antihypertensives, corticosteroids, oral hypoglycemic agents, oral contraceptives, salicylates, sulfonamides, thyroid preparations, and certain other agents. Compounds in these categories include:

Acarbose (Co-administration with drugs with hypoglycemic activity,

such as oral hypoglycemic agents, may result in decreased insulin requirements). Products include:

Precose Tablets ... 792

Acebutolol Hydrochloride (Insulin requirements may be reduced in the presence of drugs that lower blood glucose or affect how the body responds to insulin).

No products indexed under this heading.

Aliskiren (Insulin requirements may be reduced in the presence of drugs that lower blood glucose or affect how the body responds to insulin). Products include:

Tekturna Tablets ... 2321
Tekturna HCT Tablets ... 2324

Amlodipine Besylate (Insulin requirements may be reduced in the presence of drugs that lower blood glucose or affect how the body responds to insulin). Products include:

Azor Tablets ... 1005
Exforge Tablets ... 2238

Aspirin (Co-administration with drugs with hypoglycemic activity, such as salicylates, may result in decreased insulin requirements). Products include:

Aggrenox Capsules ... 819
Bayer Aspirin ... 750
Percodan Tablets ... 1130
St. Joseph 81 mg Aspirin Chewable and Enteric Coated Tablets ... 1903

Aspirin, Enteric Coated (Co-administration with drugs with hypoglycemic activity, such as salicylates, may result in decreased insulin requirements).

No products indexed under this heading.

Aspirin Buffered (Co-administration with drugs with hypoglycemic activity, such as salicylates, may result in decreased insulin requirements).

No products indexed under this heading.

Atenolol (Insulin requirements may be reduced in the presence of drugs that lower blood glucose or affect how the body responds to insulin).

No products indexed under this heading.

Benazepril Hydrochloride (Insulin requirements may be reduced in the presence of drugs that lower blood glucose or affect how the body responds to insulin).

No products indexed under this heading.

Bendroflumethiazide (Insulin requirements may be reduced in the presence of drugs that lower blood glucose or affect how the body responds to insulin).

No products indexed under this heading.

Betamethasone Acetate (Co-administration may result in increased insulin requirements).

No products indexed under this heading.

Betamethasone Sodium Phosphate (Co-administration may result in increased insulin requirements).

No products indexed under this heading.

Betaxolol Hydrochloride (Insulin requirements may be reduced in the presence of drugs that lower blood glucose or affect how the body responds to insulin).

No products indexed under this heading.

Bisoprolol Fumarate (Insulin requirements may be reduced in the presence of drugs that lower blood glucose or affect how the body responds to insulin).

No products indexed under this heading.

Budesonide (Co-administration may result in increased insulin requirements). Products include:

Pulmicort Flexhaler ... 654
Symbicort 80/4.5 Inhalation Aerosol ... 659
Symbicort 160/4.5 Inhalation Aerosol ... 659

Candesartan Cilexetil (Insulin requirements may be reduced in the presence of drugs that lower blood glucose or affect how the body responds to insulin). Products include:

Atacand Tablets ... 639
Atacand HCT ... 642

Captopril (Insulin requirements may be reduced in the presence of drugs that lower blood glucose or affect how the body responds to insulin). Products include:

Captopril Tablets ... 2182

Carteolol Hydrochloride (Insulin requirements may be reduced in the presence of drugs that lower blood glucose or affect how the body responds to insulin).

No products indexed under this heading.

Chlorothiazide (Insulin requirements may be reduced in the presence of drugs that lower blood glucose or affect how the body responds to insulin).

No products indexed under this heading.

Chlorothiazide Sodium (Insulin requirements may be reduced in the presence of drugs that lower blood glucose or affect how the body responds to insulin). Products include:

Intravenous Sodium Diuril ... 2490

Chlorpropamide (Co-administration with drugs with hypoglycemic activity, such as oral hypoglycemic agents, may result in decreased insulin requirements).

No products indexed under this heading.

Chlorthalidone (Insulin requirements may be reduced in the presence of drugs that lower blood glucose or affect how the body responds to insulin). Products include:

Clorpres Tablets ... 2185

Choline Magnesium Trisalicylate (Co-administration with drugs with hypoglycemic activity, such as salicylates, may result in decreased insulin requirements).

No products indexed under this heading.

Ciclesonide (Co-administration may result in increased insulin requirements). Products include:

Alvesco Inhalation Aerosol ... 2985
Omnaris Nasal Spray ... 2998

Clonidine (Insulin requirements may be reduced in the presence of drugs that lower blood glucose or affect how the body responds to insulin). Products include:

Catapres-TTS ... 842

Clonidine Hydrochloride (Insulin requirements may be reduced in the presence of drugs that lower blood glucose or affect how the body responds to insulin). Products include:

Catapres Tablets ... 841
Clorpres Tablets ... 2185

Cortisone Acetate (Co-administration may result in increased insulin requirements).

No products indexed under this heading.

Deserpidine (Insulin requirements may be reduced in the presence of drugs that lower blood glucose or affect how the body responds to insulin).

No products indexed under this heading.

Desogestrel (Co-administration with oral contraceptives may result in increased insulin requirements). Products include:

Mircette Tablets ... 1034

Dexamethasone (Co-administration may result in increased insulin requirements). Products include:

Ciprodex Otic Suspension ... 541

Dexamethasone Acetate (Co-administration may result in increased insulin requirements).

No products indexed under this heading.

Dexamethasone Sodium Phosphate (Co-administration may result in increased insulin requirements).

No products indexed under this heading.

Diazoxide (Insulin requirements may be reduced in the presence of drugs that lower blood glucose or affect how the body responds to insulin). Products include:

Proglycem Capsules ... 1185
Proglycem Suspension ... 1185

Diflunisal (Co-administration with drugs with hypoglycemic activity, such as salicylates, may result in decreased insulin requirements).

No products indexed under this heading.

Diltiazem Hydrochloride (Insulin requirements may be reduced in the presence of drugs that lower blood glucose or affect how the body responds to insulin). Products include:

Cardizem LA Extended Release Tablets ... 421

Doxazosin Mesylate (Insulin requirements may be reduced in the presence of drugs that lower blood glucose or affect how the body responds to insulin).

No products indexed under this heading.

Enalapril Maleate (Insulin requirements may be reduced in the presence of drugs that lower blood glucose or affect how the body responds to insulin).

No products indexed under this heading.

Enalaprilat (Insulin requirements may be reduced in the presence of drugs that lower blood glucose or affect how the body responds to insulin).

No products indexed under this heading.

Eprosartan Mesylate (Insulin requirements may be reduced in the presence of drugs that lower blood glucose or affect how the body responds to insulin). Products include:

Teveten Tablets ... 515
Teveten HCT Tablets ... 517

Esmolol Hydrochloride (Insulin requirements may be reduced in the presence of drugs that lower blood glucose or affect how the body responds to insulin).

No products indexed under this heading.

Ethinyl Estradiol (Co-administration with oral contraceptives may result in increased insulin requirements). Products include:

Lybrel Tablets ... 3204
Mircette Tablets ... 1034
NuvaRing ... 2897
Ortho-Cyclen/Ortho Tri-Cyclen ... 2449
Ortho Evra Transdermal System ... 2437
Ortho Tri-Cyclen Lo Tablets ... 2458
Seasonique Tablets ... 1046
Yaz Tablets ... 805

Ethynodiol Diacetate (Co-administration with oral contraceptives may result in increased insulin requirements).

No products indexed under this heading.

Felodipine (Insulin requirements may be reduced in the presence of drugs that lower blood glucose or affect how the body responds to insulin).

No products indexed under this heading.

Fludrocortisone Acetate (Co-administration may result in increased insulin requirements).

No products indexed under this heading.

Flunisolide (Co-administration may result in increased insulin requirements). Products include:

Aerobid/Aerobid-M ... 1153

Fluticasone Propionate (Co-administration may result in increased insulin requirements). Products include:

Advair Diskus 100/50 ... 1276
Advair Diskus 250/50 ... 1276
Advair Diskus 500/50 ... 1276
Advair HFA 45/21 Inhalation Aerosol ... 1288
Advair HFA 115/21 Inhalation Aerosol ... 1288
Advair HFA 230/21 Inhalation Aerosol ... 1288
Flonase Nasal Spray ... 1431
Flovent Diskus 50 mcg ... 1435

Fluticasone Propionate HFA (Co-administration may result in increased insulin requirements). Products include:

Flovent HFA ... 1440

Fosinopril Sodium (Insulin requirements may be reduced in the presence of drugs that lower blood glucose or affect how the body responds to insulin).

No products indexed under this heading.

Furosemide (Insulin requirements may be reduced in the presence of drugs that lower blood glucose or affect how the body responds to insulin). Products include:

Furosemide Tablets ... 2186

Glimepiride (Co-administration with drugs with hypoglycemic activity, such as oral hypoglycemic agents, may result in decreased insulin requirements). Products include:

Avandaryl Tablets ... 1344
Duetact Tablets ... 3085

Glipizide (Co-administration with drugs with hypoglycemic activity, such as oral hypoglycemic agents, may result in decreased insulin requirements).
No products indexed under this heading.

Glyburide (Co-administration with drugs with hypoglycemic activity, such as oral hypoglycemic agents, may result in decreased insulin requirements).
No products indexed under this heading.

Guanabenz Acetate (Insulin requirements may be reduced in the presence of drugs that lower blood glucose or affect how the body responds to insulin).
No products indexed under this heading.

Guanethidine Monosulfate (Insulin requirements may be reduced in the presence of drugs that lower blood glucose or affect how the body responds to insulin).
No products indexed under this heading.

Hydralazine Hydrochloride (Insulin requirements may be reduced in the presence of drugs that lower blood glucose or affect how the body responds to insulin).
No products indexed under this heading.

Hydrochlorothiazide (Insulin requirements may be reduced in the presence of drugs that lower blood glucose or affect how the body responds to insulin). Products include:
- Atacand HCT 642
- Avalide Tablets 892
- Avalide Tablets 2713
- Benicar HCT Tablets 1010
- Diovan HCT Tablets 2216
- Dyazide Capsules 1405
- Micardis HCT Tablets 854
- Prinzide Tablets 2092
- Tekturna HCT Tablets 2324
- Teveten HCT Tablets 517

Hydrocortisone (Co-administration may result in increased insulin requirements).
No products indexed under this heading.

Hydrocortisone Acetate (Co-administration may result in increased insulin requirements). Products include:
- Analpram-HC 1140
- Pramosone 1141

Hydrocortisone Sodium Phosphate (Co-administration may result in increased insulin requirements).
No products indexed under this heading.

Hydrocortisone Sodium Succinate (Co-administration may result in increased insulin requirements).
No products indexed under this heading.

Hydroflumethiazide (Insulin requirements may be reduced in the presence of drugs that lower blood glucose or affect how the body responds to insulin).
No products indexed under this heading.

Indapamide (Insulin requirements may be reduced in the presence of drugs that lower blood glucose or affect how the body responds to insulin). Products include:
- Indapamide Tablets 2188

Irbesartan (Insulin requirements may be reduced in the presence of drugs that lower blood glucose or affect how the body responds to insulin). Products include:
- Avalide Tablets 892
- Avalide Tablets 2713
- Avapro Tablets 897
- Avapro Tablets 2718

Isradipine (Insulin requirements may be reduced in the presence of drugs that lower blood glucose or affect how the body responds to insulin). Products include:
- DynaCirc CR Controlled Release Tablets 1407

Labetalol Hydrochloride (Insulin requirements may be reduced in the presence of drugs that lower blood glucose or affect how the body responds to insulin).
No products indexed under this heading.

Levonorgestrel (Co-administration with oral contraceptives may result in increased insulin requirements). Products include:
- Climara Pro Transdermal System 768
- Lybrel Tablets 3204
- Mirena Intrauterine System 779
- Plan B Tablets 1044
- Seasonique Tablets 1046

Levothyroxine Sodium (Co-administration with thyroid replacement therapy may result in increased insulin requirements). Products include:
- Levothroid Tablets 1170
- Levoxyl Tablets 1780
- Synthroid Tablets 507

Liothyronine Sodium (Co-administration with thyroid replacement therapy may result in increased insulin requirements). Products include:
- Cytomel Tablets 1778

Liotrix (Co-administration with thyroid replacement therapy may result in increased insulin requirements).
No products indexed under this heading.

Lisinopril (Insulin requirements may be reduced in the presence of drugs that lower blood glucose or affect how the body responds to insulin). Products include:
- Prinivil Tablets 2087
- Prinzide Tablets 2092

Losartan Potassium (Insulin requirements may be reduced in the presence of drugs that lower blood glucose or affect how the body responds to insulin). Products include:
- Cozaar Tablets 1973

Magnesium Salicylate (Co-administration with drugs with hypoglycemic activity, such as salicylates, may result in decreased insulin requirements).
No products indexed under this heading.

Mecamylamine Hydrochloride (Insulin requirements may be reduced in the presence of drugs that lower blood glucose or affect how the body responds to insulin).
No products indexed under this heading.

Mestranol (Co-administration with oral contraceptives may result in increased insulin requirements).
No products indexed under this heading.

Metformin Hydrochloride (Co-administration with drugs with hypoglycemic activity, such as oral hypoglycemic agents, may result in decreased insulin requirements). Products include:
- ActoPlus Met Tablets 3071
- Avandamet Tablets 1336
- Janumet Tablets 2041
- PrandiMet Tablets 2967

Methyclothiazide (Insulin requirements may be reduced in the presence of drugs that lower blood glucose or affect how the body responds to insulin).
No products indexed under this heading.

Methyldopa (Insulin requirements may be reduced in the presence of drugs that lower blood glucose or affect how the body responds to insulin).
No products indexed under this heading.

Methyldopate Hydrochloride (Insulin requirements may be reduced in the presence of drugs that lower blood glucose or affect how the body responds to insulin).
No products indexed under this heading.

Methylprednisolone Acetate (Co-administration may result in increased insulin requirements).
No products indexed under this heading.

Methylprednisolone Sodium Succinate (Co-administration may result in increased insulin requirements).
No products indexed under this heading.

Metolazone (Insulin requirements may be reduced in the presence of drugs that lower blood glucose or affect how the body responds to insulin).
No products indexed under this heading.

Metoprolol Succinate (Insulin requirements may be reduced in the presence of drugs that lower blood glucose or affect how the body responds to insulin). Products include:
- Toprol-XL Tablets 666

Metoprolol Tartrate (Insulin requirements may be reduced in the presence of drugs that lower blood glucose or affect how the body responds to insulin).
No products indexed under this heading.

Metyrosine (Insulin requirements may be reduced in the presence of drugs that lower blood glucose or affect how the body responds to insulin). Products include:
- Demser Capsules 1989

Mibefradil Dihydrochloride (Insulin requirements may be reduced in the presence of drugs that lower blood glucose or affect how the body responds to insulin).
No products indexed under this heading.

Miglitol (Co-administration with drugs with hypoglycemic activity, such as oral hypoglycemic agents, may result in decreased insulin requirements).
No products indexed under this heading.

Minoxidil (Insulin requirements may be reduced in the presence of drugs that lower blood glucose or affect how the body responds to insulin).
No products indexed under this heading.

Moexipril Hydrochloride (Insulin requirements may be reduced in the presence of drugs that lower blood glucose or affect how the body responds to insulin).
No products indexed under this heading.

Mometasone Furoate (Co-administration may result in increased insulin requirements). Products include:
- Asmanex Twisthaler 2797
- Elocon Cream 0.1% 2840
- Elocon Lotion 0.1% 2841
- Elocon Ointment 0.1% 2842

Mometasone Furoate Monohydrate (Co-administration may result in increased insulin requirements). Products include:
- Nasonex Nasal Spray 2883

Nadolol (Insulin requirements may be reduced in the presence of drugs that lower blood glucose or affect how the body responds to insulin). Products include:
- Nadolol Tablets 2191

Nateglinide (Co-administration with drugs with hypoglycemic activity, such as oral hypoglycemic agents, may result in decreased insulin requirements). Products include:
- Starlix Tablets 2314

Nebivolol (Insulin requirements may be reduced in the presence of drugs that lower blood glucose or affect how the body responds to insulin). Products include:
- Bystolic Tablets 1155

Nicardipine Hydrochloride (Insulin requirements may be reduced in the presence of drugs that lower blood glucose or affect how the body responds to insulin). Products include:
- Cardene I.V. 1093

Nifedipine (Insulin requirements may be reduced in the presence of drugs that lower blood glucose or affect how the body responds to insulin).
No products indexed under this heading.

Nisoldipine (Insulin requirements may be reduced in the presence of drugs that lower blood glucose or affect how the body responds to insulin). Products include:
- Sular Extended Release Tablets 2975

Nitroglycerin (Insulin requirements may be reduced in the presence of drugs that lower blood glucose or affect how the body responds to insulin). Products include:
- Nitro-Dur Transdermal Infusion System 2887
- Nitrolingual Pumpspray 2965

Norethindrone (Co-administration with oral contraceptives may result in increased insulin requirements). Products include:
- Ortho Micronor Tablets 2446

Norethynodrel (Co-administration with oral contraceptives may result in increased insulin requirements).
No products indexed under this heading.

Norgestimate (Co-administration with oral contraceptives may result in increased insulin requirements). Products include:
- Ortho-Cyclen/Ortho Tri-Cyclen 2449
- Ortho Tri-Cyclen Lo Tablets 2458

Norgestrel (Co-administration with oral contraceptives may result in increased insulin requirements).
No products indexed under this heading.

IMPORTANT NOTE: Always consult each drug listing in the patient's regimen for possible interactions.

Penbutolol Sulfate (Insulin requirements may be reduced in the presence of drugs that lower blood glucose or affect how the body responds to insulin).
No products indexed under this heading.

Perindopril Erbumine (Insulin requirements may be reduced in the presence of drugs that lower blood glucose or affect how the body responds to insulin). Products include:
Aceon Tablets (2 mg, 4 mg, 8 mg) **3038**

Phenelzine Sulfate (Co-administration with drugs with hypoglycemic activity, such as certain MAO inhibitor antidepressants, may result in decreased insulin requirements).
No products indexed under this heading.

Phenoxybenzamine Hydrochloride (Insulin requirements may be reduced in the presence of drugs that lower blood glucose or affect how the body responds to insulin). Products include:
Dibenzyline Capsules **3188**

Phentolamine Mesylate (Insulin requirements may be reduced in the presence of drugs that lower blood glucose or affect how the body responds to insulin).
No products indexed under this heading.

Pindolol (Insulin requirements may be reduced in the presence of drugs that lower blood glucose or affect how the body responds to insulin).
No products indexed under this heading.

Pioglitazone Hydrochloride (Co-administration with drugs with hypoglycemic activity, such as oral hypoglycemic agents, may result in decreased insulin requirements). Products include:
ActoPlus Met Tablets **3071**
Actos Tablets **3077**
Duetact Tablets **3085**

Polythiazide (Insulin requirements may be reduced in the presence of drugs that lower blood glucose or affect how the body responds to insulin).
No products indexed under this heading.

Prazosin Hydrochloride (Insulin requirements may be reduced in the presence of drugs that lower blood glucose or affect how the body responds to insulin).
No products indexed under this heading.

Prednisolone Acetate (Co-administration may result in increased insulin requirements). Products include:
Pred Forte Ophthalmic Suspension .... ⊙**227**
Pred Mild Ophthalmic Suspension .... ⊙**230**
Pred-G Ophthalmic Ointment .... ⊙**229**
Pred-G Ophthalmic Suspension .... ⊙**228**

Prednisolone Sodium Phosphate (Co-administration may result in increased insulin requirements).
No products indexed under this heading.

Prednisolone Tebutate (Co-administration may result in increased insulin requirements).
No products indexed under this heading.

Prednisone (Co-administration may result in increased insulin requirements).
No products indexed under this heading.

Propranolol Hydrochloride (Insulin requirements may be reduced in the presence of drugs that lower blood glucose or affect how the body responds to insulin). Products include:
InnoPran XL Extended Release Capsules **1484**

Quinapril Hydrochloride (Insulin requirements may be reduced in the presence of drugs that lower blood glucose or affect how the body responds to insulin).
No products indexed under this heading.

Ramipril (Insulin requirements may be reduced in the presence of drugs that lower blood glucose or affect how the body responds to insulin).
No products indexed under this heading.

Rauwolfia Serpentina (Insulin requirements may be reduced in the presence of drugs that lower blood glucose or affect how the body responds to insulin).
No products indexed under this heading.

Repaglinide (Co-administration with drugs with hypoglycemic activity, such as oral hypoglycemic agents, may result in decreased insulin requirements). Products include:
PrandiMet Tablets **2967**
Prandin Tablets **2971**

Rescinnamine (Insulin requirements may be reduced in the presence of drugs that lower blood glucose or affect how the body responds to insulin).
No products indexed under this heading.

Reserpine (Insulin requirements may be reduced in the presence of drugs that lower blood glucose or affect how the body responds to insulin).
No products indexed under this heading.

Rosiglitazone Maleate (Co-administration with drugs with hypoglycemic activity, such as oral hypoglycemic agents, may result in decreased insulin requirements). Products include:
Avandamet Tablets **1336**
Avandaryl Tablets **1344**
Avandia Tablets **1351**

Salsalate (Co-administration with drugs with hypoglycemic activity, such as salicylates, may result in decreased insulin requirements).
No products indexed under this heading.

Sitagliptin Phosphate (Co-administration with drugs with hypoglycemic activity, such as oral hypoglycemic agents, may result in decreased insulin requirements). Products include:
Janumet Tablets **2041**
Januvia Tablets **2048**

Sodium Nitroprusside (Insulin requirements may be reduced in the presence of drugs that lower blood glucose or affect how the body responds to insulin).
No products indexed under this heading.

Sotalol Hydrochloride (Insulin requirements may be reduced in the presence of drugs that lower blood glucose or affect how the body responds to insulin).
No products indexed under this heading.

Spirapril Hydrochloride (Insulin requirements may be reduced in the presence of drugs that lower blood glucose or affect how the body responds to insulin).
No products indexed under this heading.

Sulfacytine (Co-administration with drugs with hypoglycemic activity, such as sulfa antibiotics, may result in decreased insulin requirements).
No products indexed under this heading.

Sulfamethizole (Co-administration with drugs with hypoglycemic activity, such as sulfa antibiotics, may result in decreased insulin requirements).
No products indexed under this heading.

Sulfamethoxazole (Co-administration with drugs with hypoglycemic activity, such as sulfa antibiotics, may result in decreased insulin requirements).
No products indexed under this heading.

Sulfasalazine (Co-administration with drugs with hypoglycemic activity, such as sulfa antibiotics, may result in decreased insulin requirements).
No products indexed under this heading.

Sulfinpyrazone (Insulin requirements may be reduced in the presence of drugs that lower blood glucose or affect how the body responds to insulin).
No products indexed under this heading.

Sulfisoxazole Acetyl (Insulin requirements may be reduced in the presence of drugs that lower blood glucose or affect how the body responds to insulin).
No products indexed under this heading.

Sulfisoxazole Diolamine (Insulin requirements may be reduced in the presence of drugs that lower blood glucose or affect how the body responds to insulin).
No products indexed under this heading.

Telmisartan (Insulin requirements may be reduced in the presence of drugs that lower blood glucose or affect how the body responds to insulin). Products include:
Micardis Tablets **852**
Micardis HCT Tablets **854**

Terazosin Hydrochloride (Insulin requirements may be reduced in the presence of drugs that lower blood glucose or affect how the body responds to insulin).
No products indexed under this heading.

Thyroglobulin (Co-administration with thyroid replacement therapy may result in increased insulin requirements).
No products indexed under this heading.

Thyroid (Co-administration with thyroid replacement therapy may result in increased insulin requirements). Products include:
Naturethroid Tablets **2605**

Thyroxine (Co-administration with thyroid replacement therapy may result in increased insulin requirements).
No products indexed under this heading.

Thyroxine Sodium (Co-administration with thyroid replacement therapy may result in increased insulin requirements).
No products indexed under this heading.

Timolol Maleate (Insulin requirements may be reduced in the presence of drugs that lower blood glucose or affect how the body responds to insulin). Products include:
Combigan Ophthalmic Solution **553**
Cosopt Sterile Ophthalmic Solution **1969**
Timoptic Sterile Ophthalmic Solution **2121**
Timoptic in Ocudose **2124**
Timoptic-XE Sterile Ophthalmic Gel Forming Solution **2125**

Tolazamide (Co-administration with drugs with hypoglycemic activity, such as oral hypoglycemic agents, may result in decreased insulin requirements).
No products indexed under this heading.

Tolbutamide (Co-administration with drugs with hypoglycemic activity, such as oral hypoglycemic agents, may result in decreased insulin requirements).
No products indexed under this heading.

Torsemide (Insulin requirements may be reduced in the presence of drugs that lower blood glucose or affect how the body responds to insulin). Products include:
Demadex Injection **2630**
Demadex Tablets **2630**

Trandolapril (Insulin requirements may be reduced in the presence of drugs that lower blood glucose or affect how the body responds to insulin). Products include:
Mavik Tablets **472**
Tarka Tablets **511**

Tranylcypromine Sulfate (Co-administration with drugs with hypoglycemic activity, such as certain MAO inhibitor antidepressants, may result in decreased insulin requirements). Products include:
Parnate Tablets **1532**

Triamcinolone (Co-administration may result in increased insulin requirements).
No products indexed under this heading.

Triamcinolone Acetonide (Co-administration may result in increased insulin requirements). Products include:
Azmacort Inhalation Aerosol **407**
Nasacort AQ Nasal Spray **2765**
Triesence Injectable Suspension .... ⊙**209**

Triamcinolone Diacetate (Co-administration may result in increased insulin requirements).
No products indexed under this heading.

Triamcinolone Hexacetonide (Co-administration may result in increased insulin requirements).
No products indexed under this heading.

Trimethaphan Camsylate (Insulin requirements may be reduced in the presence of drugs that lower blood glucose or affect how the body responds to insulin).
No products indexed under this heading.

Troglitazone (Co-administration with drugs with hypoglycemic activity, such as oral hypoglycemic agents, may result in decreased insulin requirements).
No products indexed under this heading.

Valsartan (Insulin requirements may be reduced in the presence of drugs that lower blood glucose or affect how the body responds to insulin). Products include:
Diovan Tablets 2212
Diovan HCT Tablets 2216
Exforge Tablets 2238

Verapamil Hydrochloride (Insulin requirements may be reduced in the presence of drugs that lower blood glucose or affect how the body responds to insulin). Products include:
Tarka Tablets 511

Food Interactions

Alcohol (Insulin requirements may be reduced in the presence of drugs that lower blood glucose or affect how the body responds to insulin).

HUMULIN R

(Insulin, Human Regular) 1849
May interact with oral hypoglycemic agents. Compounds in these categories include:

Acarbose (The concurrent use of oral hypoglycemic agents with regular human insulin is not recommended). Products include:
Precose Tablets 792

Chlorpropamide (The concurrent use of oral hypoglycemic agents with regular human insulin is not recommended).
No products indexed under this heading.

Glimepiride (The concurrent use of oral hypoglycemic agents with regular human insulin is not recommended). Products include:
Avandaryl Tablets 1344
Duetact Tablets 3085

Glipizide (The concurrent use of oral hypoglycemic agents with regular human insulin is not recommended).
No products indexed under this heading.

Glyburide (The concurrent use of oral hypoglycemic agents with regular human insulin is not recommended).
No products indexed under this heading.

Metformin Hydrochloride (The concurrent use of oral hypoglycemic agents with regular human insulin is not recommended). Products include:
ActoPlus Met Tablets 3071
Avandamet Tablets 1336
Janumet Tablets 2041
PrandiMet Tablets 2967

Miglitol (The concurrent use of oral hypoglycemic agents with regular human insulin is not recommended).
No products indexed under this heading.

Nateglinide (The concurrent use of oral hypoglycemic agents with regular human insulin is not recommended). Products include:
Starlix Tablets 2314

Pioglitazone Hydrochloride (The concurrent use of oral hypoglycemic agents with regular human insulin is not recommended). Products include:
ActoPlus Met Tablets 3071
Actos Tablets 3077
Duetact Tablets 3085

Repaglinide (The concurrent use of oral hypoglycemic agents with regular human insulin is not recommended). Products include:
PrandiMet Tablets 2967
Prandin Tablets 2971

Rosiglitazone Maleate (The concurrent use of oral hypoglycemic agents with regular human insulin is not recommended). Products include:
Avandamet Tablets 1336
Avandaryl Tablets 1344
Avandia Tablets 1351

Sitagliptin Phosphate (The concurrent use of oral hypoglycemic agents with regular human insulin is not recommended). Products include:
Janumet Tablets 2041
Januvia Tablets 2048

Tolazamide (The concurrent use of oral hypoglycemic agents with regular human insulin is not recommended).
No products indexed under this heading.

Tolbutamide (The concurrent use of oral hypoglycemic agents with regular human insulin is not recommended).
No products indexed under this heading.

Troglitazone (The concurrent use of oral hypoglycemic agents with regular human insulin is not recommended).
No products indexed under this heading.

HUMULIN R (U-500)

(Insulin, Human Regular) 1850
May interact with ACE inhibitors, angiotensin-II receptor antagonists, beta blockers, corticosteroids, estrogens, oral hypoglycemic agents, monoamine oxidase inhibitors, oral contraceptives, phenothiazines, salicylates, sulfonamides, thyroid preparations, and certain other agents. Compounds in these categories include:

Acarbose (Insulin requirements may be decreased in the presence of drugs that increase insulin sensitivity or have hypoglycemic activity, such as oral hypoglycemic agents). Products include:
Precose Tablets 792

Acebutolol Hydrochloride (Insulin requirements may be decreased in the presence of drugs that increase insulin sensitivity or have hypoglycemic activity, such as beta-adrenergic blockers. Beta-adrenergic blockers may mask the symptoms of hypoglycemia in some patients).
No products indexed under this heading.

Aspirin (Insulin requirements may be decreased in the presence of drugs that increase insulin sensitivity or have hypoglycemic activity, such as salicylates). Products include:
Aggrenox Capsules 819
Bayer Aspirin 750
Percodan Tablets 1130
St. Joseph 81 mg Aspirin Chewable and Enteric Coated Tablets 1903

Aspirin, Enteric Coated (Insulin requirements may be decreased in the presence of drugs that increase insulin sensitivity or have hypoglycemic activity, such as salicylates).
No products indexed under this heading.

Aspirin Buffered (Insulin requirements may be decreased in the presence of drugs that increase insulin sensitivity or have hypoglycemic activity, such as salicylates).
No products indexed under this heading.

Atenolol (Insulin requirements may be decreased in the presence of drugs that increase insulin sensitivity or have hypoglycemic activity, such as beta-adrenergic blockers. Beta-adrenergic blockers may mask the symptoms of hypoglycemia in some patients).
No products indexed under this heading.

Benazepril Hydrochloride (Insulin requirements may be decreased in the presence of drugs that increase insulin sensitivity or have hypoglycemic activity, such as ACE inhibitors).
No products indexed under this heading.

Bendroflumethiazide (Insulin requirements may be decreased in the presence of drugs that increase insulin sensitivity or have hypoglycemic activity, such as sulfa antibiotics).
No products indexed under this heading.

Betamethasone Acetate (Insulin requirements may be increased by medications with hyperglycemic activity such as corticosteroids).
No products indexed under this heading.

Betamethasone Sodium Phosphate (Insulin requirements may be increased by medications with hyperglycemic activity such as corticosteroids).
No products indexed under this heading.

Betaxolol Hydrochloride (Insulin requirements may be decreased in the presence of drugs that increase insulin sensitivity or have hypoglycemic activity, such as beta-adrenergic blockers. Beta-adrenergic blockers may mask the symptoms of hypoglycemia in some patients).
No products indexed under this heading.

Bisoprolol Fumarate (Insulin requirements may be decreased in the presence of drugs that increase insulin sensitivity or have hypoglycemic activity, such as beta-adrenergic blockers. Beta-adrenergic blockers may mask the symptoms of hypoglycemia in some patients).
No products indexed under this heading.

Budesonide (Insulin requirements may be increased by medications with hyperglycemic activity such as corticosteroids). Products include:
Pulmicort Flexhaler 654
Symbicort 80/4.5 Inhalation Aerosol 659
Symbicort 160/4.5 Inhalation Aerosol 659

Candesartan Cilexetil (Insulin requirements may be decreased in the presence of drugs that increase insulin sensitivity or have hypoglycemic activity, such as angiotensin-II receptor antagonists). Products include:
Atacand Tablets 639
Atacand HCT 642

Captopril (Insulin requirements may be decreased in the presence of drugs that increase insulin sensitivity or have hypoglycemic activity, such as ACE inhibitors). Products include:
Captopril Tablets 2182

Carteolol Hydrochloride (Insulin requirements may be decreased in the presence of drugs that increase insulin sensitivity or have hypoglycemic activity, such as beta-adrenergic blockers. Beta-adrenergic blockers may mask the symptoms of hypoglycemia in some patients).
No products indexed under this heading.

Chlorothiazide (Insulin requirements may be decreased in the presence of drugs that increase insulin sensitivity or have hypoglycemic activity, such as sulfa antibiotics).
No products indexed under this heading.

Chlorothiazide Sodium (Insulin requirements may be decreased in the presence of drugs that increase insulin sensitivity or have hypoglycemic activity, such as sulfa antibiotics). Products include:
Intravenous Sodium Diuril 2490

Chlorotrianisene (Insulin requirements may increase by estrogens).
No products indexed under this heading.

Chlorpromazine (Insulin requirements may be increased by phenothiazines).
No products indexed under this heading.

Chlorpromazine Hydrochloride (Insulin requirements may be increased by phenothiazines).
No products indexed under this heading.

Chlorpropamide (Insulin requirements may be decreased in the presence of drugs that increase insulin sensitivity or have hypoglycemic activity, such as oral hypoglycemic agents).
No products indexed under this heading.

Choline Magnesium Trisalicylate (Insulin requirements may be decreased in the presence of drugs that increase insulin sensitivity or have hypoglycemic activity, such as salicylates).
No products indexed under this heading.

Ciclesonide (Insulin requirements may be increased by medications with hyperglycemic activity such as corticosteroids). Products include:
Alvesco Inhalation Aerosol 2985
Omnaris Nasal Spray 2998

Cortisone Acetate (Insulin requirements may be increased by medications with hyperglycemic activity such as corticosteroids).
No products indexed under this heading.

Desogestrel (Insulin requirements may be increased by oral contraceptives). Products include:
Mircette Tablets 1034

Dexamethasone (Insulin requirements may be increased by medica-

tions with hyperglycemic activity such as corticosteroids). Products include:
Ciprodex Otic Suspension 541

Dexamethasone Acetate (Insulin requirements may be increased by medications with hyperglycemic activity such as corticosteroids).
No products indexed under this heading.

Dexamethasone Sodium Phosphate (Insulin requirements may be increased by medications with hyperglycemic activity such as corticosteroids).
No products indexed under this heading.

Dienestrol (Insulin requirements may increase by estrogens).
No products indexed under this heading.

Diethylstilbestrol (Insulin requirements may increase by estrogens).
No products indexed under this heading.

Diflunisal (Insulin requirements may be decreased in the presence of drugs that increase insulin sensitivity or have hypoglycemic activity, such as salicylates).
No products indexed under this heading.

Enalapril Maleate (Insulin requirements may be decreased in the presence of drugs that increase insulin sensitivity or have hypoglycemic activity, such as ACE inhibitors).
No products indexed under this heading.

Enalaprilat (Insulin requirements may be decreased in the presence of drugs that increase insulin sensitivity or have hypoglycemic activity, such as ACE inhibitors).
No products indexed under this heading.

Eprosartan Mesylate (Insulin requirements may be decreased in the presence of drugs that increase insulin sensitivity or have hypoglycemic activity, such as angiotensin-II receptor antagonists). Products include:
Teveten Tablets 515
Teveten HCT Tablets 517

Esmolol Hydrochloride (Insulin requirements may be decreased in the presence of drugs that increase insulin sensitivity or have hypoglycemic activity, such as beta-adrenergic blockers. Beta-adrenergic blockers may mask the symptoms of hypoglycemia in some patients).
No products indexed under this heading.

Estradiol (Insulin requirements may increase by estrogens). Products include:
Activella Tablets 2347
Angeliq Tablets 751
Climara Transdermal System 763
Climara Pro Transdermal System 768
Divigel 3167
Vagifem Tablets 2375

Estrogens, Conjugated (Insulin requirements may increase by estrogens). Products include:
Premarin Intravenous 3217
Premarin Tablets 3221
Premarin Vaginal Cream 3228
Premphase Tablets 3232
Prempro Tablets 3232

Estrogens, Esterified (Insulin requirements may increase by estrogens). Products include:
Estratest Tablets 3043
Estratest H.S. Tablets 3043

Estropipate (Insulin requirements may increase by estrogens).
No products indexed under this heading.

Ethinyl Estradiol (Insulin requirements may be increased by oral contraceptives). Products include:
Lybrel Tablets 3204
Mircette Tablets 1034
NuvaRing 2897
Ortho-Cyclen/Ortho Tri-Cyclen 2449
Ortho Evra Transdermal System 2437
Ortho Tri-Cyclen Lo Tablets 2458
Seasonique Tablets 1046
Yaz Tablets 805

Ethyl Alcohol (Insulin requirements may be decreased in the presence of drugs that increase insulin sensitivity or have hypoglycemic activity, such as alcohol).
No products indexed under this heading.

Ethynodiol Diacetate (Insulin requirements may be increased by oral contraceptives).
No products indexed under this heading.

Fludrocortisone Acetate (Insulin requirements may be increased by medications with hyperglycemic activity such as corticosteroids).
No products indexed under this heading.

Flunisolide (Insulin requirements may be increased by medications with hyperglycemic activity such as corticosteroids). Products include:
Aerobid/Aerobid-M 1153

Fluphenazine Decanoate (Insulin requirements may be increased by phenothiazines).
No products indexed under this heading.

Fluphenazine Enanthate (Insulin requirements may be increased by phenothiazines).
No products indexed under this heading.

Fluphenazine Hydrochloride (Insulin requirements may be increased by phenothiazines).
No products indexed under this heading.

Fluticasone Propionate (Insulin requirements may be increased by medications with hyperglycemic activity such as corticosteroids). Products include:
Advair Diskus 100/50 1276
Advair Diskus 250/50 1276
Advair Diskus 500/50 1276
Advair HFA 45/21 Inhalation Aerosol 1288
Advair HFA 115/21 Inhalation Aerosol 1288
Advair HFA 230/21 Inhalation Aerosol 1288
Flonase Nasal Spray 1431
Flovent Diskus 50 mcg 1435

Fluticasone Propionate HFA (Insulin requirements may be increased by medications with hyperglycemic activity such as corticosteroids). Products include:
Flovent HFA 1440

Fosinopril Sodium (Insulin requirements may be decreased in the presence of drugs that increase insulin sensitivity or have hypoglycemic activity, such as ACE inhibitors).
No products indexed under this heading.

Glimepiride (Insulin requirements may be decreased in the presence of drugs that increase insulin sensitivity or have hypoglycemic activity, such as oral hypoglycemic agents). Products include:
Avandaryl Tablets 1344
Duetact Tablets 3085

Glipizide (Insulin requirements may be decreased in the presence of drugs that increase insulin sensitivity or have hypoglycemic activity, such as oral hypoglycemic agents).
No products indexed under this heading.

Glyburide (Insulin requirements may be decreased in the presence of drugs that increase insulin sensitivity or have hypoglycemic activity, such as oral hypoglycemic agents).
No products indexed under this heading.

Hydrochlorothiazide (Insulin requirements may be decreased in the presence of drugs that increase insulin sensitivity or have hypoglycemic activity, such as sulfa antibiotics). Products include:
Atacand HCT 642
Avalide Tablets 892
Avalide Tablets 2713
Benicar HCT Tablets 1010
Diovan HCT Tablets 2216
Dyazide Capsules 1405
Micardis HCT Tablets 854
Prinzide Tablets 2092
Tekturna HCT Tablets 2324
Teveten HCT Tablets 517

Hydrocortisone (Insulin requirements may be increased by medications with hyperglycemic activity such as corticosteroids).
No products indexed under this heading.

Hydrocortisone Acetate (Insulin requirements may be increased by medications with hyperglycemic activity such as corticosteroids). Products include:
Analpram-HC 1140
Pramosone 1141

Hydrocortisone Sodium Phosphate (Insulin requirements may be increased by medications with hyperglycemic activity such as corticosteroids).
No products indexed under this heading.

Hydrocortisone Sodium Succinate (Insulin requirements may be increased by medications with hyperglycemic activity such as corticosteroids).
No products indexed under this heading.

Hydroflumethiazide (Insulin requirements may be decreased in the presence of drugs that increase insulin sensitivity or have hypoglycemic activity, such as sulfa antibiotics).
No products indexed under this heading.

Irbesartan (Insulin requirements may be decreased in the presence of drugs that increase insulin sensitivity or have hypoglycemic activity, such as angiotensin-II receptor antagonists). Products include:
Avalide Tablets 892
Avalide Tablets 2713
Avapro Tablets 897
Avapro Tablets 2718

Isocarboxazid (Insulin requirements may be decreased in the presence of drugs that increase insulin sensitivity or have hypoglycemic activity, such as monoamine oxidase inhibitors). Products include:
Marplan Tablets 3177

Isoniazid (Insulin requirements may be increased by isoniazid).
No products indexed under this heading.

Isopropyl Alcohol (Insulin requirements may be decreased in the presence of drugs that increase insulin sensitivity or have hypoglycemic activity, such as alcohol).
No products indexed under this heading.

Labetalol Hydrochloride (Insulin requirements may be decreased in the presence of drugs that increase insulin sensitivity or have hypoglycemic activity, such as beta-adrenergic blockers. Beta-adrenergic blockers may mask the symptoms of hypoglycemia in some patients).
No products indexed under this heading.

Levobunolol Hydrochloride (Insulin requirements may be decreased in the presence of drugs that increase insulin sensitivity or have hypoglycemic activity, such as beta-adrenergic blockers. Beta-adrenergic blockers may mask the symptoms of hypoglycemia in some patients).
No products indexed under this heading.

Levonorgestrel (Insulin requirements may be increased by oral contraceptives). Products include:
Climara Pro Transdermal System 768
Lybrel Tablets 3204
Mirena Intrauterine System 779
Plan B Tablets 1044
Seasonique Tablets 1046

Levothyroxine Sodium (Insulin requirements may increase by thyroid replacement therapy/thyroid preparations). Products include:
Levothroid Tablets 1170
Levoxyl Tablets 1780
Synthroid Tablets 507

Liothyronine Sodium (Insulin requirements may increase by thyroid replacement therapy/thyroid preparations). Products include:
Cytomel Tablets 1778

Liotrix (Insulin requirements may increase by thyroid replacement therapy/thyroid preparations).
No products indexed under this heading.

Lisinopril (Insulin requirements may be decreased in the presence of drugs that increase insulin sensitivity or have hypoglycemic activity, such as ACE inhibitors). Products include:
Prinivil Tablets 2087
Prinzide Tablets 2092

Losartan Potassium (Insulin requirements may be decreased in the presence of drugs that increase insulin sensitivity or have hypoglycemic activity, such as angiotensin-II receptor antagonists). Products include:
Cozaar Tablets 1973

Magnesium Salicylate (Insulin requirements may be decreased in the presence of drugs that increase insulin sensitivity or have hypoglycemic activity, such as salicylates).
No products indexed under this heading.

Mesoridazine Besylate (Insulin requirements may be increased by phenothiazines).
No products indexed under this heading.

Mestranol (Insulin requirements may be increased by oral contraceptives).
No products indexed under this heading.

Metformin Hydrochloride (Insulin requirements may be decreased in the presence of drugs that increase insulin sensitivity or have hypoglycemic activity, such as oral hypoglycemic agents). Products include:
ActoPlus Met Tablets 3071
Avandamet Tablets 1336
Janumet Tablets 2041
PrandiMet Tablets 2967

Methotrimeprazine (Insulin requirements may be increased by phenothiazines).
No products indexed under this heading.

Methyclothiazide (Insulin requirements may be decreased in the presence of drugs that increase insulin sensitivity or have hypoglycemic activity, such as sulfa antibiotics).
No products indexed under this heading.

Methylprednisolone Acetate (Insulin requirements may be increased by medications with hyperglycemic activity such as corticosteroids).
No products indexed under this heading.

Methylprednisolone Sodium Succinate (Insulin requirements may be increased by medications with hyperglycemic activity such as corticosteroids).
No products indexed under this heading.

Metipranolol Hydrochloride (Insulin requirements may be decreased in the presence of drugs that increase insulin sensitivity or have hypoglycemic activity, such as beta-adrenergic blockers. Beta-adrenergic blockers may mask the symptoms of hypoglycemia in some patients).
No products indexed under this heading.

Metoprolol Succinate (Insulin requirements may be decreased in the presence of drugs that increase insulin sensitivity or have hypoglycemic activity, such as beta-adrenergic blockers. Beta-adrenergic blockers may mask the symptoms of hypoglycemia in some patients). Products include:
Toprol-XL Tablets 666

Metoprolol Tartrate (Insulin requirements may be decreased in the presence of drugs that increase insulin sensitivity or have hypoglycemic activity, such as beta-adrenergic blockers. Beta-adrenergic blockers may mask the symptoms of hypoglycemia in some patients).
No products indexed under this heading.

Miglitol (Insulin requirements may be decreased in the presence of drugs that increase insulin sensitivity or have hypoglycemic activity, such as oral hypoglycemic agents).
No products indexed under this heading.

Moclobemide (Insulin requirements may be decreased in the presence of drugs that increase insulin sensitivity or have hypoglycemic activity, such as monoamine oxidase inhibitors).
No products indexed under this heading.

Moexipril Hydrochloride (Insulin requirements may be decreased in the presence of drugs that increase insulin sensitivity or have hypoglycemic activity, such as ACE inhibitors).
No products indexed under this heading.

Mometasone Furoate (Insulin requirements may be increased by medications with hyperglycemic activity such as corticosteroids). Products include:
Asmanex Twisthaler 2797
Elocon Cream 0.1% 2840
Elocon Lotion 0.1% 2841
Elocon Ointment 0.1% 2842

Mometasone Furoate Monohydrate (Insulin requirements may be increased by medications with hyperglycemic activity such as corticosteroids). Products include:
Nasonex Nasal Spray 2883

Nadolol (Insulin requirements may be decreased in the presence of drugs that increase insulin sensitivity or have hypoglycemic activity, such as beta-adrenergic blockers. Beta-adrenergic blockers may mask the symptoms of hypoglycemia in some patients). Products include:
Nadolol Tablets 2191

Nateglinide (Insulin requirements may be decreased in the presence of drugs that increase insulin sensitivity or have hypoglycemic activity, such as oral hypoglycemic agents). Products include:
Starlix Tablets 2314

Nebivolol (Insulin requirements may be decreased in the presence of drugs that increase insulin sensitivity or have hypoglycemic activity, such as beta-adrenergic blockers. Beta-adrenergic blockers may mask the symptoms of hypoglycemia in some patients). Products include:
Bystolic Tablets 1155

Niacin (Insulin requirements may be increased by certain lipid-lowering drugs (e.g., niacin)). Products include:
Advicor Tablets 402
Bausch & Lomb Ocuvite DF Vitamin Supplement.......... ⊙238
Dismutax Dietary Supplement 995
Niaspan Extended-Release Tablets 480
NT-Kinase Dietary Supplement 995
Simcor Tablets 502

Norethindrone (Insulin requirements may be increased by oral contraceptives). Products include:
Ortho Micronor Tablets 2446

Norethynodrel (Insulin requirements may be increased by oral contraceptives).
No products indexed under this heading.

Norgestimate (Insulin requirements may be increased by oral contraceptives). Products include:
Ortho-Cyclen/Ortho Tri-Cyclen 2449
Ortho Tri-Cyclen Lo Tablets 2458

Norgestrel (Insulin requirements may be increased by oral contraceptives).
No products indexed under this heading.

Octreotide Acetate (Insulin requirements may be decreased in the presence of drugs that increase insulin sensitivity or have hypoglycemic activity, such as inhibitors of pancreatic function (e.g., octreotide)). Products include:
Sandostatin Injection 2300
Sandostatin LAR Depot 2302

Pargyline Hydrochloride (Insulin requirements may be decreased in the presence of drugs that increase insulin sensitivity or have hypoglycemic activity, such as monoamine oxidase inhibitors).
No products indexed under this heading.

Penbutolol Sulfate (Insulin requirements may be decreased in the presence of drugs that increase insulin sensitivity or have hypoglycemic activity, such as beta-adrenergic blockers. Beta-adrenergic blockers may mask the symptoms of hypoglycemia in some patients).
No products indexed under this heading.

Perindopril Erbumine (Insulin requirements may be decreased in the presence of drugs that increase insulin sensitivity or have hypoglycemic activity, such as ACE inhibitors). Products include:
Aceon Tablets (2 mg, 4 mg, 8 mg).......... 3038

Perphenazine (Insulin requirements may be increased by phenothiazines).
No products indexed under this heading.

Phenelzine Sulfate (Insulin requirements may be decreased in the presence of drugs that increase insulin sensitivity or have hypoglycemic activity, such as monoamine oxidase inhibitors).
No products indexed under this heading.

Pindolol (Insulin requirements may be decreased in the presence of drugs that increase insulin sensitivity or have hypoglycemic activity, such as beta-adrenergic blockers. Beta-adrenergic blockers may mask the symptoms of hypoglycemia in some patients).
No products indexed under this heading.

Pioglitazone Hydrochloride (Insulin requirements may be decreased in the presence of drugs that increase insulin sensitivity or have hypoglycemic activity, such as oral hypoglycemic agents). Products include:
ActoPlus Met Tablets 3071
Actos Tablets 3077
Duetact Tablets 3085

Polyestradiol Phosphate (Insulin requirements may increase by estrogens).
No products indexed under this heading.

Polythiazide (Insulin requirements may be decreased in the presence of drugs that increase insulin sensitivity or have hypoglycemic activity, such as sulfa antibiotics).
No products indexed under this heading.

Prednisolone Acetate (Insulin requirements may be increased by medications with hyperglycemic activity such as corticosteroids). Products include:
Pred Forte Ophthalmic Suspension .... ⊙227
Pred Mild Ophthalmic Suspension .... ⊙230
Pred-G Ophthalmic Ointment .... ⊙229
Pred-G Ophthalmic Suspension .... ⊙228

Prednisolone Sodium Phosphate (Insulin requirements may be increased by medications with hyperglycemic activity such as corticosteroids).
No products indexed under this heading.

Prednisolone Tebutate (Insulin requirements may be increased by medications with hyperglycemic activity such as corticosteroids).
No products indexed under this heading.

Prednisone (Insulin requirements may be increased by medications with hyperglycemic activity such as corticosteroids).
No products indexed under this heading.

Procarbazine Hydrochloride (Insulin requirements may be decreased in the presence of drugs that increase insulin sensitivity or have hypoglycemic activity, such as monoamine oxidase inhibitors).
No products indexed under this heading.

Prochlorperazine (Insulin requirements may be increased by phenothiazines).
No products indexed under this heading.

Promethazine Hydrochloride (Insulin requirements may be increased by phenothiazines).
No products indexed under this heading.

Propranolol Hydrochloride (Insulin requirements may be decreased in the presence of drugs that increase insulin sensitivity or have hypoglycemic activity, such as beta-adrenergic blockers. Beta-adrenergic blockers may mask the symptoms of hypoglycemia in some patients). Products include:
InnoPran XL Extended Release Capsules 1484

Quinapril Hydrochloride (Insulin requirements may be decreased in the presence of drugs that increase insulin sensitivity or have hypoglycemic activity, such as ACE inhibitors).
No products indexed under this heading.

Quinestrol (Insulin requirements may increase by estrogens).
No products indexed under this heading.

Ramipril (Insulin requirements may be decreased in the presence of drugs that increase insulin sensitivity or have hypoglycemic activity, such as ACE inhibitors).
No products indexed under this heading.

Rasagiline Mesylate (Insulin requirements may be decreased in the presence of drugs that increase insulin sensitivity or have hypoglycemic activity, such as monoamine oxidase inhibitors). Products include:
Azilect Tablets 3106

Repaglinide (Insulin requirements may be decreased in the presence of drugs that increase insulin sensitivity or have hypoglycemic activity, such as oral hypoglycemic agents). Products include:
PrandiMet Tablets 2967
Prandin Tablets 2971

Rosiglitazone Maleate (Insulin requirements may be decreased in the presence of drugs that increase insulin sensitivity or have hypoglycemic activity, such as oral hypoglycemic agents). Products include:

Avandamet Tablets 1336
Avandaryl Tablets 1344
Avandia Tablets 1351

Salsalate (Insulin requirements may be decreased in the presence of drugs that increase insulin sensitivity or have hypoglycemic activity, such as salicylates).
No products indexed under this heading.

Selegiline (Insulin requirements may be decreased in the presence of drugs that increase insulin sensitivity or have hypoglycemic activity, such as monoamine oxidase inhibitors). Products include:
Emsam Transdermal System 905

Selegiline Hydrochloride (Insulin requirements may be decreased in the presence of drugs that increase insulin sensitivity or have hypoglycemic activity, such as monoamine oxidase inhibitors). Products include:
Eldepryl Capsules 3052

Sitagliptin Phosphate (Insulin requirements may be decreased in the presence of drugs that increase insulin sensitivity or have hypoglycemic activity, such as oral hypoglycemic agents). Products include:
Janumet Tablets 2041
Januvia Tablets 2048

Sotalol Hydrochloride (Insulin requirements may be decreased in the presence of drugs that increase insulin sensitivity or have hypoglycemic activity, such as beta-adrenergic blockers. Beta-adrenergic blockers may mask the symptoms of hypoglycemia in some patients).
No products indexed under this heading.

Spirapril Hydrochloride (Insulin requirements may be decreased in the presence of drugs that increase insulin sensitivity or have hypoglycemic activity, such as ACE inhibitors).
No products indexed under this heading.

Sulfacytine (Insulin requirements may be decreased in the presence of drugs that increase insulin sensitivity or have hypoglycemic activity, such as sulfa antibiotics).
No products indexed under this heading.

Sulfamethizole (Insulin requirements may be decreased in the presence of drugs that increase insulin sensitivity or have hypoglycemic activity, such as sulfa antibiotics).
No products indexed under this heading.

Sulfamethoxazole (Insulin requirements may be decreased in the presence of drugs that increase insulin sensitivity or have hypoglycemic activity, such as sulfa antibiotics).
No products indexed under this heading.

Sulfasalazine (Insulin requirements may be decreased in the presence of drugs that increase insulin sensitivity or have hypoglycemic activity, such as sulfa antibiotics).
No products indexed under this heading.

Sulfinpyrazone (Insulin requirements may be decreased in the presence of drugs that increase insulin sensitivity or have hypoglycemic activity, such as sulfa antibiotics).
No products indexed under this heading.

Sulfisoxazole Acetyl (Insulin requirements may be decreased in the presence of drugs that increase insulin sensitivity or have hypoglycemic activity, such as sulfa antibiotics).
No products indexed under this heading.

Sulfisoxazole Diolamine (Insulin requirements may be decreased in the presence of drugs that increase insulin sensitivity or have hypoglycemic activity, such as sulfa antibiotics).
No products indexed under this heading.

Telmisartan (Insulin requirements may be decreased in the presence of drugs that increase insulin sensitivity or have hypoglycemic activity, such as angiotensin-II receptor antagonists). Products include:
Micardis Tablets 852
Micardis HCT Tablets 854

Thioridazine Hydrochloride (Insulin requirements may be increased by phenothiazines). Products include:
Thioridazine Hydrochloride Tablets 2195

Thyroglobulin (Insulin requirements may increase by thyroid replacement therapy/thyroid preparations).
No products indexed under this heading.

Thyroid (Insulin requirements may increase by thyroid replacement therapy/thyroid preparations). Products include:
Naturethroid Tablets 2605

Thyroxine (Insulin requirements may increase by thyroid replacement therapy/thyroid preparations).
No products indexed under this heading.

Thyroxine Sodium (Insulin requirements may increase by thyroid replacement therapy/thyroid preparations).
No products indexed under this heading.

Timolol Hemihydrate (Insulin requirements may be decreased in the presence of drugs that increase insulin sensitivity or have hypoglycemic activity, such as beta-adrenergic blockers. Beta-adrenergic blockers may mask the symptoms of hypoglycemia in some patients). Products include:
Betimol Ophthalmic Solution 3181

Timolol Maleate (Insulin requirements may be decreased in the presence of drugs that increase insulin sensitivity or have hypoglycemic activity, such as beta-adrenergic blockers. Beta-adrenergic blockers may mask the symptoms of hypoglycemia in some patients). Products include:
Combigan Ophthalmic Solution 553
Cosopt Sterile Ophthalmic Solution 1969
Timoptic Sterile Ophthalmic Solution 2121
Timoptic in Ocudose 2124
Timoptic-XE Sterile Ophthalmic Gel Forming Solution 2125

Tolazamide (Insulin requirements may be decreased in the presence of drugs that increase insulin sensitivity or have hypoglycemic activity, such as oral hypoglycemic agents).
No products indexed under this heading.

Tolbutamide (Insulin requirements may be decreased in the presence of drugs that increase insulin sensitivity or have hypoglycemic activity, such as oral hypoglycemic agents).
No products indexed under this heading.

Trandolapril (Insulin requirements may be decreased in the presence of drugs that increase insulin sensitivity or have hypoglycemic activity, such as ACE inhibitors). Products include:
Mavik Tablets 472
Tarka Tablets 511

Tranylcypromine Sulfate (Insulin requirements may be decreased in the presence of drugs that increase insulin sensitivity or have hypoglycemic activity, such as monoamine oxidase inhibitors). Products include:
Parnate Tablets 1532

Triamcinolone (Insulin requirements may be increased by medications with hyperglycemic activity such as corticosteroids).
No products indexed under this heading.

Triamcinolone Acetonide (Insulin requirements may be increased by medications with hyperglycemic activity such as corticosteroids). Products include:
Azmacort Inhalation Aerosol 407
Nasacort AQ Nasal Spray 2765
Triesence Injectable Suspension .... ⊙209

Triamcinolone Diacetate (Insulin requirements may be increased by medications with hyperglycemic activity such as corticosteroids).
No products indexed under this heading.

Triamcinolone Hexacetonide (Insulin requirements may be increased by medications with hyperglycemic activity such as corticosteroids).
No products indexed under this heading.

Trifluoperazine Hydrochloride (Insulin requirements may be increased by phenothiazines).
No products indexed under this heading.

Troglitazone (Insulin requirements may be decreased in the presence of drugs that increase insulin sensitivity or have hypoglycemic activity, such as oral hypoglycemic agents).
No products indexed under this heading.

Valsartan (Insulin requirements may be decreased in the presence of drugs that increase insulin sensitivity or have hypoglycemic activity, such as angiotensin-II receptor antagonists). Products include:
Diovan Tablets 2212
Diovan HCT Tablets 2216
Exforge Tablets 2238

Food Interactions

Alcohol (Insulin requirements may be decreased in the presence of drugs that increase insulin sensitivity or have hypoglycemic activity, such as alcohol).

HURRICAINE TOPICAL ANESTHETIC

(Benzocaine) 815
None cited in PDR database.

HYALGAN SOLUTION

(Sodium Hyaluronate) 2742
None cited in PDR database.

HYCAMTIN FOR INJECTION

(Topotecan Hydrochloride) 1459
May interact with cytotoxic drugs and certain other agents. Compounds in these categories include:

Bleomycin Sulfate (Greater myelosuppression is also likely to be seen when Hycamtin is used in combination with other cytotoxic agents, thereby necessitating a dose reduction).
No products indexed under this heading.

Carboplatin (Greater myelosuppression is likely to be seen when topotecan hydrochloride is used in combination with other cytotoxic agents, thereby necessitating a dose reduction. However, when combining topotecan hydrochloride with platinum agents (e.g., carboplatin), a distinct sequence dependent interaction on myelosuppression has been reported).
No products indexed under this heading.

Cisplatin (Co-administration has resulted in severe myelosuppression; a case of neutropenia and fatal neutropenic sepsis has been reported).
No products indexed under this heading.

Cyclophosphamide (Greater myelosuppression is also likely to be seen when Hycamtin is used in combination with other cytotoxic agents, thereby necessitating a dose reduction).
No products indexed under this heading.

Daunorubicin Hydrochloride (Greater myelosuppression is also likely to be seen when Hycamtin is used in combination with other cytotoxic agents, thereby necessitating a dose reduction).
No products indexed under this heading.

Doxorubicin Hydrochloride (Greater myelosuppression is also likely to be seen when Hycamtin is used in combination with other cytotoxic agents, thereby necessitating a dose reduction).
No products indexed under this heading.

Epirubicin Hydrochloride (Greater myelosuppression is also likely to be seen when Hycamtin is used in combination with other cytotoxic agents, thereby necessitating a dose reduction).
No products indexed under this heading.

Filgrastim (Concomitant administration of granulocyte colony stimulating factor (G-CSF) can prolong the duration of neutropenia, so if G-CSF is to be used, it should not be initiated until day 6 of the course of therapy, 24 hours after completion of treatment with topotecan hydrochloride). Products include:
Neupogen for Injection 589

Fluorouracil (Greater myelosuppression is also likely to be seen when Hycamtin is used in combination with other cytotoxic agents, thereby necessitating a dose reduction). Products include:
Carac Cream 0.5% 2722

Hydroxyurea (Greater myelosuppression is also likely to be seen when Hycamtin is used in combination with other cytotoxic agents, thereby necessitating a dose reduction).
No products indexed under this heading.

Methotrexate Sodium (Greater myelosuppression is also likely to be seen when Hycamtin is used in combination with other cytotoxic agents, thereby necessitating a dose reduction).
No products indexed under this heading.

Mitotane (Greater myelosuppression is also likely to be seen when Hycamtin is used in combination with other cytotoxic agents, thereby necessitating a dose reduction).
No products indexed under this heading.

Mitoxantrone Hydrochloride (Greater myelosuppression is also likely to be seen when Hycamtin is used in combination with other cytotoxic agents, thereby necessitating a dose reduction). Products include:
Novantrone for Injection Concentrate 1100

Procarbazine Hydrochloride (Greater myelosuppression is also likely to be seen when Hycamtin is used in combination with other cytotoxic agents, thereby necessitating a dose reduction).
No products indexed under this heading.

Tamoxifen Citrate (Greater myelosuppression is also likely to be seen when Hycamtin is used in combination with other cytotoxic agents, thereby necessitating a dose reduction).
No products indexed under this heading.

Vincristine Sulfate (Greater myelosuppression is also likely to be seen when Hycamtin is used in combination with other cytotoxic agents, thereby necessitating a dose reduction).
No products indexed under this heading.

HYCAMTIN CAPSULES

(Topotecan Hydrochloride) 1456
May interact with quinidine and certain other agents. Compounds in these categories include:

Cyclosporine (Topotecan is a substrate for both ABCB1 [P-glycoprotein (P-gp)] and ABCG2 (BCRP). Elacridar (inhibitor of ABCB1 and ABCG2) administered with topotecan capsules increased topotecan exposure to approximately 2.5-fold of control. Cyclosporine A (inhibitor of ABCB1, ABCC1 [MRP-1], and CYP3A4) with topotecan capsules increased topotecan exposure to 2- to 3-fold of control. Patients should be carefully monitored for adverse reactions when topotecan capsules are administered with a drug known to inhibit these transporters). Products include:
Gengraf Capsules 435
Neoral Oral Solution 2280
Neoral Soft Gelatin Capsules 2280
Restasis Ophthalmic Emulsion 557
Sandimmune 2296

Elacridar (Topotecan is a substrate for both ABCB1 [P-glycoprotein (P-gp)] and ABCG2 (BCRP). Elacridar (inhibitor of ABCB1 and ABCG2) administered with topotecan capsules increased topotecan exposure to approximately 2.5-fold of control. Cyclosporine A (inhibitor of ABCB1, ABCC1 [MRP-1], and CYP3A4) with topotecan capsules increased topotecan exposure to 2- to 3-fold of control. Patients should be carefully monitored for adverse reactions when topotecan capsules are administered with a drug known to inhibit these transporters).
No products indexed under this heading.

Quinidine (Topotecan is a substrate for both ABCB1 [P-glycoprotein (P-gp)] and ABCG2 (BCRP). Elacridar (inhibitor of ABCB1 and ABCG2) administered with topotecan capsules increased topotecan exposure to approximately 2.5-fold of control. Cyclosporine A (inhibitor of ABCB1, ABCC1 [MRP-1], and CYP3A4) with topotecan capsules increased topotecan exposure to 2- to 3-fold of control. Patients should be carefully monitored for adverse reactions when topotecan capsules are administered with a drug known to inhibit these transporters).
No products indexed under this heading.

Quinidine Gluconate (Topotecan is a substrate for both ABCB1 [P-glycoprotein (P-gp)] and ABCG2 (BCRP). Elacridar (inhibitor of ABCB1 and ABCG2) administered with topotecan capsules increased topotecan exposure to approximately 2.5-fold of control. Cyclosporine A (inhibitor of ABCB1, ABCC1 [MRP-1], and CYP3A4) with topotecan capsules increased topotecan exposure to 2- to 3-fold of control. Patients should be carefully monitored for adverse reactions when topotecan capsules are administered with a drug known to inhibit these transporters).
No products indexed under this heading.

Quinidine Hydrochloride (Topotecan is a substrate for both ABCB1 [P-glycoprotein (P-gp)] and ABCG2 (BCRP). Elacridar (inhibitor of ABCB1 and ABCG2) administered with topotecan capsules increased topotecan exposure to approximately 2.5-fold of control. Cyclosporine A (inhibitor of ABCB1, ABCC1 [MRP-1], and CYP3A4) with topotecan capsules increased topotecan exposure to 2- to 3-fold of control. Patients should be carefully monitored for adverse reactions when topotecan capsules are administered with a drug known to inhibit these transporters).
No products indexed under this heading.

Quinidine Polygalacturonate (Topotecan is a substrate for both ABCB1 [P-glycoprotein (P-gp)] and ABCG2 (BCRP). Elacridar (inhibitor of ABCB1 and ABCG2) administered with topotecan capsules increased topotecan exposure to approximately 2.5-fold of control. Cyclosporine A (inhibitor of ABCB1, ABCC1 [MRP-1], and CYP3A4) with topotecan capsules increased topotecan exposure to 2- to 3-fold of control. Patients should be carefully monitored for adverse reactions when topotecan capsules are administered with a drug known to inhibit these transporters).
No products indexed under this heading.

Quinidine Sulfate (Topotecan is a substrate for both ABCB1 [P-glycoprotein (P-gp)] and ABCG2 (BCRP). Elacridar (inhibitor of ABCB1 and ABCG2) administered with topotecan capsules increased topotecan exposure to approximately 2.5-fold of control. Cyclosporine A (inhibitor of ABCB1, ABCC1 [MRP-1], and CYP3A4) with topotecan capsules increased topotecan exposure to 2- to 3-fold of control. Patients should be carefully monitored for adverse reactions when topotecan capsules are administered with a drug known to inhibit these transporters).
No products indexed under this heading.

Verapamil Hydrochloride (Topotecan is a substrate for both ABCB1 [P-glycoprotein (P-gp)] and ABCG2 (BCRP). Elacridar (inhibitor of ABCB1 and ABCG2) administered with topotecan capsules increased topotecan exposure to approximately 2.5-fold of control. Cyclosporine A (inhibitor of ABCB1, ABCC1 [MRP-1], and CYP3A4) with topotecan capsules increased topotecan exposure to 2- to 3-fold of control. Patients should be carefully monitored for adverse reactions when topotecan capsules are administered with a drug known to inhibit these transporters). Products include:
Tarka Tablets 511

HYLAND'S BACKACHE WITH ARNICA CAPLETS

(Homeopathic Formulations) 618
None cited in PDR database.

HYLAND'S CALMS FORTE TABLETS AND CAPLETS

(Homeopathic Formulations) 618
None cited in PDR database.

HYLAND'S CALMS FORTE 4 KIDS TABLETS

(Homeopathic Formulations, Sulfur).. 619
None cited in PDR database.

HYLAND'S COLIC TABLETS

(Chamomilla, Colocynthis, Disocorea, Homeopathic Formulations).. 619
None cited in PDR database.

HYLAND'S COUGH SYRUP WITH HONEY

(Homeopathic Formulations) 619
None cited in PDR database.

HYLAND'S EARACHE DROPS

(Herbals, Multiple) 619
None cited in PDR database.

HYLAND'S EARACHE TABLETS

(Homeopathic Formulations) 620
None cited in PDR database.

HYLAND'S LEG CRAMPS WITH QUININE TABLETS AND CAPLETS

(Homeopathic Formulations) 620
None cited in PDR database.

HYLAND'S NERVE TONIC TABLETS AND CAPLETS

(Homeopathic Formulations) 620
None cited in PDR database.

HYLAND'S RESTFUL LEGS TABLETS

(Homeopathic Formulations) 620
None cited in PDR database.

HYLAND'S SNIFFLES 'N SNEEZES 4 KIDS TABLETS

(Dietary Supplement) 621
None cited in PDR database.

HYLAND'S TEETHING GEL

(Homeopathic Formulations) 621
None cited in PDR database.

HYLAND'S TEETHING TABLETS

(Belladonna Alkaloids, Homeopathic Formulations).............. 621
None cited in PDR database.

I26 CAPSULES

(Egg product, hyperimmune) 629
None cited in PDR database.

I26 CHEWABLE TABLETS

(Egg product, hyperimmune) 629
None cited in PDR database.

IMITREX INJECTION

(Sumatriptan Succinate) 1465
See Imitrex Tablets

IMITREX NASAL SPRAY

(Sumatriptan) 1470
See Imitrex Tablets

IMITREX TABLETS

(Sumatriptan Succinate) 1474
May interact with 5HT1-receptor agonists, ergot-containing drugs, nonselective MAO inhibitors, Serotonin and Norepinephrine Reuptake Inhibitors, selective serotonin reuptake inhibitors, and certain other agents. Compounds in these categories include:

Almotriptan Malate (Co-administration with other $_{max}$ agonists within 24 hours of each other is contraindicated because the vasospastic effects may be additive). Products include:
Axert Tablets 2431

Citalopram Hydrobromide (The development of a potentially life-threatening serotonin syndrome may occur with triptans, including sumatriptan treatment, particularly during combined use with selective serotonin reuptake inhibitors (SSRIs) or serotonin norepinephrine reuptake inhibitors (SNRIs). If concomitant treatment with sumatriptan and an SSRI (eg, fluoxetine, paroxetine, sertraline, fluvoxamine, citalopram, escitalopram) or SNRI (eg, venlafaxine, duloxetine) is clinically warranted, careful observation of the patient is advised, particularly during treatment initiation and dose increases). Products include:
Celexa 1160

Desvenlafaxine Succinate (The development of a potentially life-threatening serotonin syndrome may occur with triptans, including sumatriptan treatment, particularly during combined use with selective serotonin reuptake inhibitors (SSRIs) or serotonin norepinephrine reuptake inhibitors (SNRIs). If concomitant treatment with sumatriptan and an SSRI (eg, fluoxetine, paroxetine, sertraline, fluvoxamine, citalopram, escitalopram) or SNRI (eg, venlafaxine, duloxetine) is clinically warranted, careful observation of the patient is advised, particularly during treatment initiation and dose increases). Products include:

Pristiq Extended-Release Tablets 3247

Dihydroergotamine Mesylate (Ergot-containing drugs have been reported to cause prolonged vasospastic reactions; because there is a theoretical basis that these effects may be additive, use of ergot-type agents and sumatriptan within 24 hours is contraindicated).

No products indexed under this heading.

Duloxetine Hydrochloride (Cases of life-threatening serotonin syndrome have been reported during combined use of serotonin and norepinephrine reuptake inhibitors (SNRIs) and triptans. If concomitant treatment with sumatriptan succinate is clinically warranted, careful observation of the patient is advised, particularly during treatment initiation and dose increases. Serotonin syndrome symptoms may include mental status changes, autonomic instability, neuromuscular aberrations and/or gastrointestinal symptoms). Products include:

Cymbalta Delayed-Release Capsules 1801

Eletriptan Hydrobromide (Co-administration with other ${}_{max}$ agonists within 24 hours of each other is contraindicated because the vasospastic effects may be additive).

No products indexed under this heading.

Ergonovine Maleate (Ergot-containing drugs have been reported to cause prolonged vasospastic reactions; because there is a theoretical basis that these effects may be additive, use of ergot-type agents and sumatriptan within 24 hours is contraindicated).

No products indexed under this heading.

Ergotamine Tartrate (Ergot-containing drugs have been reported to cause prolonged vasospastic reactions; because there is a theoretical basis that these effects may be additive, use of ergot-type agents and sumatriptan within 24 hours is contraindicated).

No products indexed under this heading.

Escitalopram Oxalate (The development of a potentially life-threatening serotonin syndrome may occur with triptans, including sumatriptan treatment, particularly during combined use with selective serotonin reuptake inhibitors (SSRIs) or serotonin norepinephrine reuptake inhibitors (SNRIs). If concomitant treatment with sumatriptan and an SSRI (eg, fluoxetine, paroxetine, sertraline, fluvoxamine, citalopram, escitalopram) or SNRI (eg, venlafaxine, duloxetine) is clinically warranted, careful observation of the patient is advised, particularly during treatment initiation and dose increases). Products include:

Lexapro Oral Suspension 1174
Lexapro Tablets 1174

Fluoxetine (The development of a potentially life-threatening serotonin syndrome may occur with triptans, including sumatriptan treatment, particularly during combined use with selective serotonin reuptake inhibitors (SSRIs) or serotonin norepinephrine reuptake inhibitors (SNRIs). If concomitant treatment with sumatriptan and an SSRI (eg, fluoxetine, paroxetine, sertraline, fluvoxamine, citalopram, escitalopram) or SNRI (eg, venlafaxine, duloxetine) is clinically warranted, careful observation of the patient is advised, particularly during treatment initiation and dose increases).

No products indexed under this heading.

Fluoxetine Hydrochloride (The development of a potentially life-threatening serotonin syndrome may occur with triptans, including sumatriptan treatment, particularly during combined use with selective serotonin reuptake inhibitors (SSRIs) or serotonin norepinephrine reuptake inhibitors (SNRIs). If concomitant treatment with sumatriptan and an SSRI (eg, fluoxetine, paroxetine, sertraline, fluvoxamine, citalopram, escitalopram) or SNRI (eg, venlafaxine, duloxetine) is clinically warranted, careful observation of the patient is advised, particularly during treatment initiation and dose increases). Products include:

Prozac Weekly Capsules 1852
Prozac Pulvules and Liquid 1852
Symbyax Capsules 1871

Fluvoxamine Maleate (The development of a potentially life-threatening serotonin syndrome may occur with triptans, including sumatriptan treatment, particularly during combined use with selective serotonin reuptake inhibitors (SSRIs) or serotonin norepinephrine reuptake inhibitors (SNRIs). If concomitant treatment with sumatriptan and an SSRI (eg, fluoxetine, paroxetine, sertraline, fluvoxamine, citalopram, escitalopram) or SNRI (eg, venlafaxine, duloxetine) is clinically warranted, careful observation of the patient is advised, particularly during treatment initiation and dose increases). Products include:

Luvox CR Extended-Release Capsules 1759

Frovatriptan Succinate (Co-administration with other ${}_{max}$ agonists within 24 hours of each other is contraindicated because the vasospastic effects may be additive). Products include:

Frova Tablets 1111

Isocarboxazid (MAO-A inhibitors reduce sumatriptan clearance and significantly increasing systemic exposure; concurrent and/or sequential use is contraindicated). Products include:

Marplan Tablets 3177

Methylergonovine Maleate (Ergot-containing drugs have been reported to cause prolonged vasospastic reactions; because there is a theoretical basis that these effects may be additive, use of ergot-type agents and sumatriptan within 24 hours is contraindicated).

No products indexed under this heading.

Methysergide Maleate (Ergot-containing drugs have been reported to cause prolonged vasospastic reactions; because there is a theoretical basis that these effects may be additive, use of ergot-type agents and sumatriptan within 24 hours is contraindicated).

No products indexed under this heading.

Naratriptan Hydrochloride (Co-administration with other ${}_{max}$ agonists within 24 hours of each other is contraindicated because the vasospastic effects may be additive). Products include:

Amerge Tablets 1301

Nefazodone Hydrochloride (Cases of life-threatening serotonin syndrome have been reported during combined use of serotonin and norepinephrine reuptake inhibitors (SNRIs) and triptans. If concomitant treatment with sumatriptan succinate is clinically warranted, careful observation of the patient is advised, particularly during treatment initiation and dose increases. Serotonin syndrome symptoms may include mental status changes, autonomic instability, neuromuscular aberrations and/or gastrointestinal symptoms).

No products indexed under this heading.

Pargyline Hydrochloride (MAO-A inhibitors reduce sumatriptan clearance and significantly increasing systemic exposure; concurrent and/or sequential use is contraindicated).

No products indexed under this heading.

Paroxetine Hydrochloride (The development of a potentially life-threatening serotonin syndrome may occur with triptans, including sumatriptan treatment, particularly during combined use with selective serotonin reuptake inhibitors (SSRIs) or serotonin norepinephrine reuptake inhibitors (SNRIs). If concomitant treatment with sumatriptan and an SSRI (eg, fluoxetine, paroxetine, sertraline, fluvoxamine, citalopram, escitalopram) or SNRI (eg, venlafaxine, duloxetine) is clinically warranted, careful observation of the patient is advised, particularly during treatment initiation and dose increases). Products include:

Paxil 1535
Paxil CR Controlled-Release Tablets 1544

Phenelzine Sulfate (MAO-A inhibitors reduce sumatriptan clearance and significantly increasing systemic exposure; concurrent and/or sequential use is contraindicated).

No products indexed under this heading.

Procarbazine Hydrochloride (MAO-A inhibitors reduce sumatriptan clearance and significantly increasing systemic exposure; concurrent and/or sequential use is contraindicated).

No products indexed under this heading.

Rizatriptan Benzoate (Co-administration with other ${}_{max}$ agonists within 24 hours of each other is contraindicated because the vasospastic effects may be additive). Products include:

Maxalt Tablets 2056
Maxalt-MLT Orally Disintegrating Tablets 2056

Sertraline Hydrochloride (The development of a potentially life-threatening serotonin syndrome may occur with triptans, including sumatriptan treatment, particularly during combined use with selective serotonin reuptake inhibitors (SSRIs) or serotonin norepinephrine reuptake inhibitors (SNRIs). If concomitant treatment with sumatriptan and an SSRI (eg, fluoxetine, paroxetine, sertraline, fluvoxamine, citalopram, escitalopram) or SNRI (eg, venlafaxine, duloxetine) is clinically warranted, careful observation of the patient is advised, particularly during treatment initiation and dose increases).

No products indexed under this heading.

Sumatriptan (Co-administration with other ${}_{max}$ agonists within 24 hours of each other is contraindicated because the vasospastic effects may be additive). Products include:

Imitrex Nasal Spray 1470

Tranylcypromine Sulfate (MAO-A inhibitors reduce sumatriptan clearance and significantly increasing systemic exposure; concurrent and/or sequential use is contraindicated). Products include:

Parnate Tablets 1532

Venlafaxine Hydrochloride (Cases of life-threatening serotonin syndrome have been reported during combined use of serotonin and norepinephrine reuptake inhibitors (SNRIs) and triptans. If concomitant treatment with sumatriptan succinate is clinically warranted, careful observation of the patient is advised, particularly during treatment initiation and dose increases. Serotonin syndrome symptoms may include mental status changes, autonomic instability, neuromuscular aberrations and/or gastrointestinal symptoms). Products include:

Effexor XR Extended-Release Capsules 3195
Venlafaxine Hydrochloride Tablets ... 2199

Zolmitriptan (Co-administration with other ${}_{max}$ agonists within 24 hours of each other is contraindicated because the vasospastic effects may be additive). Products include:

Zomig Tablets 694
Zomig Nasal Spray 689
Zomig-ZMT Tablets 694

Food Interactions

Food, unspecified (Delays the Tmax slightly by about 0.5 hour with no significant effect on the bioavailability).

IMMUNE FORMULATION 200

(Amino Acid Preparations, L-Cysteine, L-Glutamine, Glycine, L-Glutamic Acid, Selenomethionine).... 2585
None cited in PDR database.

IMMUNOCAL POWDER SACHETS

(Whey Protein Isolate) 1729
None cited in PDR database.

IMODIUM A-D LIQUID, CAPLETS, AND EZ CHEWS

(Loperamide Hydrochloride) 1898
None cited in PDR database.

IMODIUM MULTI-SYMPTOM RELIEF CAPLETS AND CHEWABLE TABLETS

(Loperamide Hydrochloride, Simethicone)....................................... 1899
None cited in PDR database.

INCRELEX INJECTION

(Mecasermin [rDNA origin]) 3100
None cited in PDR database.

INDAPAMIDE TABLETS

(Indapamide) 2188

May interact with antihypertensives, barbiturates, corticosteroids, cardiac glycosides, insulin, lithium preparations, narcotic analgesics, and certain other agents. Compounds in these categories include:

Acebutolol Hydrochloride (Indapamide may add to or potentiate the therapeutic effect of other antihypertensive drugs).
No products indexed under this heading.

ACTH (Co-administration with ACTH may increase the risk of hypokalemia).
No products indexed under this heading.

Alfentanil Hydrochloride (Aggravates orthostatic hypotension).
No products indexed under this heading.

Aliskiren (Indapamide may add to or potentiate the therapeutic effect of other antihypertensive drugs). Products include:
Tekturna Tablets 2321
Tekturna HCT Tablets 2324

Amlodipine Besylate (Indapamide may add to or potentiate the therapeutic effect of other antihypertensive drugs). Products include:
Azor Tablets 1005
Exforge Tablets 2238

Aprobarbital (Aggravates orthostatic hypotension).
No products indexed under this heading.

Atenolol (Indapamide may add to or potentiate the therapeutic effect of other antihypertensive drugs).
No products indexed under this heading.

Benazepril Hydrochloride (Indapamide may add to or potentiate the therapeutic effect of other antihypertensive drugs).
No products indexed under this heading.

Bendroflumethiazide (Indapamide may add to or potentiate the therapeutic effect of other antihypertensive drugs).
No products indexed under this heading.

Betamethasone Acetate (Co-administration with corticosteroids may increase the risk of hypokalemia).
No products indexed under this heading.

Betamethasone Sodium Phosphate (Co-administration with corticosteroids may increase the risk of hypokalemia).
No products indexed under this heading.

Betaxolol Hydrochloride (Indapamide may add to or potentiate the therapeutic effect of other antihypertensive drugs).
No products indexed under this heading.

Bisoprolol Fumarate (Indapamide may add to or potentiate the therapeutic effect of other antihypertensive drugs).
No products indexed under this heading.

Budesonide (Co-administration with corticosteroids may increase the risk of hypokalemia). Products include:
Pulmicort Flexhaler 654
Symbicort 80/4.5 Inhalation Aerosol... 659
Symbicort 160/4.5 Inhalation Aerosol... 659

Buprenorphine Hydrochloride (Aggravates orthostatic hypotension). Products include:
Suboxone Tablets 2601
Subutex Tablets 2601

Butabarbital (Aggravates orthostatic hypotension).
No products indexed under this heading.

Butalbital (Aggravates orthostatic hypotension).
No products indexed under this heading.

Candesartan Cilexetil (Indapamide may add to or potentiate the therapeutic effect of other antihypertensive drugs). Products include:
Atacand Tablets 639
Atacand HCT 642

Captopril (Indapamide may add to or potentiate the therapeutic effect of other antihypertensive drugs). Products include:
Captopril Tablets 2182

Carteolol Hydrochloride (Indapamide may add to or potentiate the therapeutic effect of other antihypertensive drugs).
No products indexed under this heading.

Chlorothiazide (Indapamide may add to or potentiate the therapeutic effect of other antihypertensive drugs).
No products indexed under this heading.

Chlorothiazide Sodium (Indapamide may add to or potentiate the therapeutic effect of other antihypertensive drugs). Products include:
Intravenous Sodium Diuril 2490

Chlorthalidone (Indapamide may add to or potentiate the therapeutic effect of other antihypertensive drugs). Products include:
Clorpres Tablets 2185

Ciclesonide (Co-administration with corticosteroids may increase the risk of hypokalemia). Products include:
Alvesco Inhalation Aerosol 2985
Omnaris Nasal Spray 2998

Clonidine (Indapamide may add to or potentiate the therapeutic effect of other antihypertensive drugs). Products include:
Catapres-TTS 842

Clonidine Hydrochloride (Indapamide may add to or potentiate the therapeutic effect of other antihypertensive drugs). Products include:
Catapres Tablets 841
Clorpres Tablets 2185

Codeine Phosphate (Aggravates orthostatic hypotension). Products include:
Tylenol with Codeine Tablets 2427

Cortisone Acetate (Co-administration with corticosteroids may increase the risk of hypokalemia).
No products indexed under this heading.

Deserpidine (Indapamide may add to or potentiate the therapeutic effect of other antihypertensive drugs).
No products indexed under this heading.

Deslanoside (Concurrent digitalis therapy may exaggerate metabolic effects of hypokalemia; especially myocardial effects such as increase ventricular irritability).
No products indexed under this heading.

Dexamethasone (Co-administration with corticosteroids may increase the risk of hypokalemia). Products include:
Ciprodex Otic Suspension 541

Dexamethasone Acetate (Co-administration with corticosteroids may increase the risk of hypokalemia).
No products indexed under this heading.

Dexamethasone Sodium Phosphate (Co-administration with corticosteroids may increase the risk of hypokalemia).
No products indexed under this heading.

Dezocine (Aggravates orthostatic hypotension).
No products indexed under this heading.

Diazoxide (Indapamide may add to or potentiate the therapeutic effect of other antihypertensive drugs). Products include:
Proglycem Capsules 1185
Proglycem Suspension 1185

Digitalis Glycoside Preparations (Concurrent digitalis therapy may exaggerate metabolic effects of hypokalemia; especially myocardial effects such as increase ventricular irritability).
No products indexed under this heading.

Digitoxin (Concurrent digitalis therapy may exaggerate metabolic effects of hypokalemia; especially myocardial effects such as increase ventricular irritability).
No products indexed under this heading.

Digoxin (Concurrent digitalis therapy may exaggerate metabolic effects of hypokalemia; especially myocardial effects such as increase ventricular irritability). Products include:
Lanoxin Injection 1498
Lanoxin Injection Pediatric 1502
Lanoxin Tablets 1505

Diltiazem Hydrochloride (Indapamide may add to or potentiate the therapeutic effect of other antihypertensive drugs). Products include:
Cardizem LA Extended Release Tablets 421

Doxazosin Mesylate (Indapamide may add to or potentiate the therapeutic effect of other antihypertensive drugs).
No products indexed under this heading.

Enalapril Maleate (Indapamide may add to or potentiate the therapeutic effect of other antihypertensive drugs).
No products indexed under this heading.

Enalaprilat (Indapamide may add to or potentiate the therapeutic effect of other antihypertensive drugs).
No products indexed under this heading.

Eprosartan Mesylate (Indapamide may add to or potentiate the therapeutic effect of other antihypertensive drugs). Products include:
Teveten Tablets 515
Teveten HCT Tablets 517

Esmolol Hydrochloride (Indapamide may add to or potentiate the therapeutic effect of other antihypertensive drugs).
No products indexed under this heading.

Felodipine (Indapamide may add to or potentiate the therapeutic effect of other antihypertensive drugs).
No products indexed under this heading.

Fentanyl (Aggravates orthostatic hypotension). Products include:
Duragesic Transdermal System 2405
Ionsys Transdermal System 2410

Fentanyl Citrate (Aggravates orthostatic hypotension). Products include:
Actiq 959
Fentora Tablets 968

Fludrocortisone Acetate (Co-administration with corticosteroids may increase the risk of hypokalemia).
No products indexed under this heading.

Flunisolide (Co-administration with corticosteroids may increase the risk of hypokalemia). Products include:
Aerobid/Aerobid-M 1153

Fluticasone Propionate (Co-administration with corticosteroids may increase the risk of hypokalemia). Products include:
Advair Diskus 100/50 1276
Advair Diskus 250/50 1276
Advair Diskus 500/50 1276
Advair HFA 45/21 Inhalation Aerosol... 1288
Advair HFA 115/21 Inhalation Aerosol... 1288
Advair HFA 230/21 Inhalation Aerosol... 1288
Flonase Nasal Spray 1431
Flovent Diskus 50 mcg 1435

Fluticasone Propionate HFA (Co-administration with corticosteroids may increase the risk of hypokalemia). Products include:
Flovent HFA 1440

Fosinopril Sodium (Indapamide may add to or potentiate the therapeutic effect of other antihypertensive drugs).
No products indexed under this heading.

Furosemide (Indapamide may add to or potentiate the therapeutic effect of other antihypertensive drugs). Products include:
Furosemide Tablets 2186

Guanabenz Acetate (Indapamide may add to or potentiate the therapeutic effect of other antihypertensive drugs).
No products indexed under this heading.

Guanethidine Monosulfate (Indapamide may add to or potentiate the therapeutic effect of other antihypertensive drugs).
No products indexed under this heading.

Hydralazine Hydrochloride (Indapamide may add to or potentiate the therapeutic effect of other antihypertensive drugs).
No products indexed under this heading.

Hydrochlorothiazide (Indapamide may add to or potentiate the therapeutic effect of other antihypertensive drugs). Products include:
Atacand HCT 642
Avalide Tablets 892

Avalide Tablets ... 2713
Benicar HCT Tablets ... 1010
Diovan HCT Tablets ... 2216
Dyazide Capsules ... 1405
Micardis HCT Tablets ... 854
Prinzide Tablets ... 2092
Tekturna HCT Tablets ... 2324
Teveten HCT Tablets ... 517

Hydrocodone Bitartrate (Aggravates orthostatic hypotension). Products include:
Lortab 5/500 Tablets ... 3143
Lortab 7.5/500 Tablets ... 3144
Lortab 10/500 Tablets ... 3144
Vicodin Tablets ... 529
Vicodin ES Tablets ... 530
Vicodin HP Tablets ... 531
Vicoprofen Tablets ... 533
Zydone Tablets ... 1132

Hydrocodone Polistirex (Aggravates orthostatic hypotension). Products include:
Tussionex Pennkinetic Extended-Release Suspension ... 3154

Hydrocortisone (Co-administration with corticosteroids may increase the risk of hypokalemia).
No products indexed under this heading.

Hydrocortisone Acetate (Co-administration with corticosteroids may increase the risk of hypokalemia). Products include:
Analpram-HC ... 1140
Pramosone ... 1141

Hydrocortisone Sodium Phosphate (Co-administration with corticosteroids may increase the risk of hypokalemia).
No products indexed under this heading.

Hydrocortisone Sodium Succinate (Co-administration with corticosteroids may increase the risk of hypokalemia).
No products indexed under this heading.

Hydroflumethiazide (Indapamide may add to or potentiate the therapeutic effect of other antihypertensive drugs).
No products indexed under this heading.

Hydromorphone Hydrochloride (Aggravates orthostatic hypotension).
No products indexed under this heading.

Insulin (Hyperglycemia has been reported with the use of indapamide; co-administration may require adjustment in insulin dosage in diabetic patients).
No products indexed under this heading.

Insulin, Human, Zinc Suspension (Hyperglycemia has been reported with the use of indapamide; co-administration may require adjustment in insulin dosage in diabetic patients).
No products indexed under this heading.

Insulin, Human (rDNA origin) (Hyperglycemia has been reported with the use of indapamide; co-administration may require adjustment in insulin dosage in diabetic patients). Products include:
Exubera Inhalation Powder ... 2515

Insulin, Human NPH (Hyperglycemia has been reported with the use of indapamide; co-administration may require adjustment in insulin dosage in diabetic patients). Products include:
Humulin N Vial ... 1846

Insulin, Human Regular (Hyperglycemia has been reported with the use of indapamide; co-administration may require adjustment in insulin dosage in diabetic patients). Products include:
Humulin R ... 1849
Humulin R (U-500) ... 1850

Insulin, Human Regular and Human NPH Mixture (Hyperglycemia has been reported with the use of indapamide; co-administration may require adjustment in insulin dosage in diabetic patients). Products include:
Humulin 50/50, 100 Units ... 1843
Humulin 70/30 Vial ... 1844

Insulin, NPH (Hyperglycemia has been reported with the use of indapamide; co-administration may require adjustment in insulin dosage in diabetic patients).
No products indexed under this heading.

Insulin, Regular (Hyperglycemia has been reported with the use of indapamide; co-administration may require adjustment in insulin dosage in diabetic patients).
No products indexed under this heading.

Insulin, Regular and NPH mixture (Hyperglycemia has been reported with the use of indapamide; co-administration may require adjustment in insulin dosage in diabetic patients).
No products indexed under this heading.

Insulin, Zinc Crystals (Hyperglycemia has been reported with the use of indapamide; co-administration may require adjustment in insulin dosage in diabetic patients).
No products indexed under this heading.

Insulin, Zinc Suspension (Hyperglycemia has been reported with the use of indapamide; co-administration may require adjustment in insulin dosage in diabetic patients).
No products indexed under this heading.

Insulin Aspart (Hyperglycemia has been reported with the use of indapamide; co-administration may require adjustment in insulin dosage in diabetic patients).
No products indexed under this heading.

Insulin Aspart, Human (Hyperglycemia has been reported with the use of indapamide; co-administration may require adjustment in insulin dosage in diabetic patients). Products include:
NovoLog Mix 70/30 ... 2364

Insulin Aspart, Human Regular (Hyperglycemia has been reported with the use of indapamide; co-administration may require adjustment in insulin dosage in diabetic patients). Products include:
NovoLog Injection ... 2359

Insulin Aspart Protamine, Human (Hyperglycemia has been reported with the use of indapamide; co-administration may require adjustment in insulin dosage in diabetic patients). Products include:
NovoLog Mix 70/30 ... 2364

Insulin Detemir (rDNA Origin) (Hyperglycemia has been reported with the use of indapamide; co-administration may require adjustment in insulin dosage in diabetic patients). Products include:
Levemir Injection ... 2352

Insulin glargine (Hyperglycemia has been reported with the use of indapamide; co-administration may require adjustment in insulin dosage in diabetic patients). Products include:
Lantus Injection ... 2749

Insulin Glulisine (Hyperglycemia has been reported with the use of indapamide; co-administration may require adjustment in insulin dosage in diabetic patients). Products include:
Apidra Injection ... 2706

Insulin Lispro, Human (Hyperglycemia has been reported with the use of indapamide; co-administration may require adjustment in insulin dosage in diabetic patients). Products include:
Humalog-Pen and KwikPen ... 1829
Humalog Mix 50/50-Pen and KwikPen ... 1833
Humalog Mix 75/25-Pen and KwikPen ... 1835

Insulin Lispro Protamine, Human (Hyperglycemia has been reported with the use of indapamide; co-administration may require adjustment in insulin dosage in diabetic patients). Products include:
Humalog Mix 50/50-Pen and KwikPen ... 1833
Humalog Mix 75/25-Pen and KwikPen ... 1835

Irbesartan (Indapamide may add to or potentiate the therapeutic effect of other antihypertensive drugs). Products include:
Avalide Tablets ... 892
Avalide Tablets ... 2713
Avapro Tablets ... 897
Avapro Tablets ... 2718

Isradipine (Indapamide may add to or potentiate the therapeutic effect of other antihypertensive drugs). Products include:
DynaCirc CR Controlled Release Tablets ... 1407

Labetalol Hydrochloride (Indapamide may add to or potentiate the therapeutic effect of other antihypertensive drugs).
No products indexed under this heading.

Levorphanol Tartrate (Aggravates orthostatic hypotension).
No products indexed under this heading.

Lisinopril (Indapamide may add to or potentiate the therapeutic effect of other antihypertensive drugs). Products include:
Prinivil Tablets ... 2087
Prinzide Tablets ... 2092

Lithium (Diuretics reduce lithium's renal clearance and add a high risk of lithium toxicity).
No products indexed under this heading.

Lithium Carbonate (Diuretics reduce lithium's renal clearance and add a high risk of lithium toxicity).
No products indexed under this heading.

Lithium Citrate (Diuretics reduce lithium's renal clearance and add a high risk of lithium toxicity).
No products indexed under this heading.

Losartan Potassium (Indapamide may add to or potentiate the therapeutic effect of other antihypertensive drugs). Products include:
Cozaar Tablets ... 1973

Mecamylamine Hydrochloride (Indapamide may add to or potentiate the therapeutic effect of other antihypertensive drugs).
No products indexed under this heading.

Meperidine Hydrochloride (Aggravates orthostatic hypotension).
No products indexed under this heading.

Mephobarbital (Aggravates orthostatic hypotension).
No products indexed under this heading.

Methadone Hydrochloride (Aggravates orthostatic hypotension).
No products indexed under this heading.

Methyclothiazide (Indapamide may add to or potentiate the therapeutic effect of other antihypertensive drugs).
No products indexed under this heading.

Methyldopa (Indapamide may add to or potentiate the therapeutic effect of other antihypertensive drugs).
No products indexed under this heading.

Methyldopate Hydrochloride (Indapamide may add to or potentiate the therapeutic effect of other antihypertensive drugs).
No products indexed under this heading.

Methylprednisolone Acetate (Co-administration with corticosteroids may increase the risk of hypokalemia).
No products indexed under this heading.

Methylprednisolone Sodium Succinate (Co-administration with corticosteroids may increase the risk of hypokalemia).
No products indexed under this heading.

Metolazone (Indapamide may add to or potentiate the therapeutic effect of other antihypertensive drugs).
No products indexed under this heading.

Metoprolol Succinate (Indapamide may add to or potentiate the therapeutic effect of other antihypertensive drugs). Products include:
Toprol-XL Tablets ... 666

Metoprolol Tartrate (Indapamide may add to or potentiate the therapeutic effect of other antihypertensive drugs).
No products indexed under this heading.

Metyrosine (Indapamide may add to or potentiate the therapeutic effect of other antihypertensive drugs). Products include:
Demser Capsules ... 1989

Mibefradil Dihydrochloride (Indapamide may add to or potentiate the therapeutic effect of other antihypertensive drugs).
No products indexed under this heading.

Minoxidil (Indapamide may add to or potentiate the therapeutic effect of other antihypertensive drugs).
No products indexed under this heading.

Moexipril Hydrochloride (Indapamide may add to or potentiate the therapeutic effect of other antihypertensive drugs).
No products indexed under this heading.

Mometasone Furoate (Co-administration with corticosteroids may increase the risk of hypokalemia). Products include:
Asmanex Twisthaler 2797
Elocon Cream 0.1% 2840
Elocon Lotion 0.1% 2841
Elocon Ointment 0.1% 2842

Mometasone Furoate Monohydrate (Co-administration with corticosteroids may increase the risk of hypokalemia). Products include:
Nasonex Nasal Spray 2883

Morphine Sulfate (Aggravates orthostatic hypotension). Products include:
Avinza Capsules 1772
DepoDur Injection 1095
MS Contin Tablets 2585

Nadolol (Indapamide may add to or potentiate the therapeutic effect of other antihypertensive drugs). Products include:
Nadolol Tablets 2191

Nebivolol (Indapamide may add to or potentiate the therapeutic effect of other antihypertensive drugs). Products include:
Bystolic Tablets 1155

Nicardipine Hydrochloride (Indapamide may add to or potentiate the therapeutic effect of other antihypertensive drugs). Products include:
Cardene I.V. 1093

Nifedipine (Indapamide may add to or potentiate the therapeutic effect of other antihypertensive drugs).
No products indexed under this heading.

Nisoldipine (Indapamide may add to or potentiate the therapeutic effect of other antihypertensive drugs). Products include:
Sular Extended Release Tablets 2975

Nitroglycerin (Indapamide may add to or potentiate the therapeutic effect of other antihypertensive drugs). Products include:
Nitro-Dur Transdermal Infusion System 2887
Nitrolingual Pumpspray 2965

Norepinephrine Bitartrate (Indapamide may decrease arterial responsiveness to norepinephrine).
No products indexed under this heading.

Oxycodone Hydrochloride (Aggravates orthostatic hypotension). Products include:
OxyContin Tablets 2589
OxyIR Capsules 2593
Percocet Tablets 1127
Percodan Tablets 1130

Penbutolol Sulfate (Indapamide may add to or potentiate the therapeutic effect of other antihypertensive drugs).
No products indexed under this heading.

Pentobarbital Sodium (Aggravates orthostatic hypotension). Products include:
Nembutal Sodium Solution, USP 2494

Perindopril Erbumine (Indapamide may add to or potentiate the therapeutic effect of other antihypertensive drugs). Products include:
Aceon Tablets (2 mg, 4 mg, 8 mg) 3038

Phenobarbital (Aggravates orthostatic hypotension). Products include:
Donnatal Extentabs 2507

Phenoxybenzamine Hydrochloride (Indapamide may add to or potentiate the therapeutic effect of other antihypertensive drugs). Products include:
Dibenzyline Capsules 3188

Phentolamine Mesylate (Indapamide may add to or potentiate the therapeutic effect of other antihypertensive drugs).
No products indexed under this heading.

Pindolol (Indapamide may add to or potentiate the therapeutic effect of other antihypertensive drugs).
No products indexed under this heading.

Polythiazide (Indapamide may add to or potentiate the therapeutic effect of other antihypertensive drugs).
No products indexed under this heading.

Prazosin Hydrochloride (Indapamide may add to or potentiate the therapeutic effect of other antihypertensive drugs).
No products indexed under this heading.

Prednisolone Acetate (Co-administration with corticosteroids may increase the risk of hypokalemia). Products include:
Pred Forte Ophthalmic Suspension .... ⊙ 227
Pred Mild Ophthalmic Suspension .... ⊙ 230
Pred-G Ophthalmic Ointment .... ⊙ 229
Pred-G Ophthalmic Suspension .... ⊙ 228

Prednisolone Sodium Phosphate (Co-administration with corticosteroids may increase the risk of hypokalemia).
No products indexed under this heading.

Prednisolone Tebutate (Co-administration with corticosteroids may increase the risk of hypokalemia).
No products indexed under this heading.

Prednisone (Co-administration with corticosteroids may increase the risk of hypokalemia).
No products indexed under this heading.

Propoxyphene Hydrochloride (Aggravates orthostatic hypotension).
No products indexed under this heading.

Propoxyphene Napsylate (Aggravates orthostatic hypotension).
No products indexed under this heading.

Propranolol Hydrochloride (Indapamide may add to or potentiate the therapeutic effect of other antihypertensive drugs). Products include:
InnoPran XL Extended Release Capsules 1484

Quinapril Hydrochloride (Indapamide may add to or potentiate the therapeutic effect of other antihypertensive drugs).
No products indexed under this heading.

Ramipril (Indapamide may add to or potentiate the therapeutic effect of other antihypertensive drugs).
No products indexed under this heading.

Rauwolfia Serpentina (Indapamide may add to or potentiate the therapeutic effect of other antihypertensive drugs).
No products indexed under this heading.

Remifentanil Hydrochloride (Aggravates orthostatic hypotension).
No products indexed under this heading.

Rescinnamine (Indapamide may add to or potentiate the therapeutic effect of other antihypertensive drugs).
No products indexed under this heading.

Reserpine (Indapamide may add to or potentiate the therapeutic effect of other antihypertensive drugs).
No products indexed under this heading.

Secobarbital Sodium (Aggravates orthostatic hypotension).
No products indexed under this heading.

Sodium Nitroprusside (Indapamide may add to or potentiate the therapeutic effect of other antihypertensive drugs).
No products indexed under this heading.

Sotalol Hydrochloride (Indapamide may add to or potentiate the therapeutic effect of other antihypertensive drugs).
No products indexed under this heading.

Spirapril Hydrochloride (Indapamide may add to or potentiate the therapeutic effect of other antihypertensive drugs).
No products indexed under this heading.

Sufentanil Citrate (Aggravates orthostatic hypotension).
No products indexed under this heading.

Telmisartan (Indapamide may add to or potentiate the therapeutic effect of other antihypertensive drugs). Products include:
Micardis Tablets 852
Micardis HCT Tablets 854

Terazosin Hydrochloride (Indapamide may add to or potentiate the therapeutic effect of other antihypertensive drugs).
No products indexed under this heading.

Thiamylal Sodium (Aggravates orthostatic hypotension).
No products indexed under this heading.

Timolol Maleate (Indapamide may add to or potentiate the therapeutic effect of other antihypertensive drugs). Products include:
Combigan Ophthalmic Solution 553
Cosopt Sterile Ophthalmic Solution 1969
Timoptic Sterile Ophthalmic Solution 2121
Timoptic in Ocudose 2124
Timoptic-XE Sterile Ophthalmic Gel Forming Solution 2125

Torsemide (Indapamide may add to or potentiate the therapeutic effect of other antihypertensive drugs). Products include:
Demadex Injection 2630
Demadex Tablets 2630

Trandolapril (Indapamide may add to or potentiate the therapeutic effect of other antihypertensive drugs). Products include:
Mavik Tablets 472
Tarka Tablets 511

Triamcinolone (Co-administration with corticosteroids may increase the risk of hypokalemia).
No products indexed under this heading.

Triamcinolone Acetonide (Co-administration with corticosteroids may increase the risk of hypokalemia). Products include:
Azmacort Inhalation Aerosol 407
Nasacort AQ Nasal Spray 2765
Triesence Injectable Suspension .... ⊙ 209

Triamcinolone Diacetate (Co-administration with corticosteroids may increase the risk of hypokalemia).
No products indexed under this heading.

Triamcinolone Hexacetonide (Co-administration with corticosteroids may increase the risk of hypokalemia).
No products indexed under this heading.

Trimethaphan Camsylate (Indapamide may add to or potentiate the therapeutic effect of other antihypertensive drugs).
No products indexed under this heading.

Valsartan (Indapamide may add to or potentiate the therapeutic effect of other antihypertensive drugs). Products include:
Diovan Tablets 2212
Diovan HCT Tablets 2216
Exforge Tablets 2238

Verapamil Hydrochloride (Indapamide may add to or potentiate the therapeutic effect of other antihypertensive drugs). Products include:
Tarka Tablets 511

Food Interactions

Alcohol (Aggravates orthostatic hypotension).

INDOCIN CAPSULES

(Indomethacin) 2024

May interact with ACE inhibitors, angiotensin-II receptor antagonists, beta blockers, anticoagulants, lithium preparations, loop diuretics, non-steroidal anti-inflammatory agents, potassium sparing diuretics, thiazides, and certain other agents. Compounds in these categories include:

Acebutolol Hydrochloride (Blunting of antihypertensive effect of beta blockers).
No products indexed under this heading.

Amiloride Hydrochloride (Reduced diuretic, natriuretic and antihypertensive effects of increased serum potassium levels).
No products indexed under this heading.

Anisindione (Bleeding has been reported in patients on concomitant treatment with anticoagulants and indomethacin. Caution should be exercised when indomethacin and anticoagulants are administered concomitantly).
No products indexed under this heading.

Ardeparin Sodium (Bleeding has been reported in patients on concomitant treatment with anticoagulants and indomethacin. Caution should be exercised when indomethacin and anticoagulants are administered concomitantly).
No products indexed under this heading.

IMPORTANT NOTE: Always consult each drug listing in the patient's regimen for possible interactions.

Aspirin (When indomethacin is administered with aspirin, its protein binding is reduced, although the clearance of free indomethacin is not altered. The clinical significance of this interaction is not known; however, as with other NSAIDs, concomitant administration of indomethacin and aspirin is not generally recommended because of the potential of increased adverse effects). Products include:
Aggrenox Capsules 819
Bayer Aspirin 750
Percodan Tablets 1130
St. Joseph 81 mg Aspirin Chewable and Enteric Coated Tablets 1903

Atenolol (Blunting of antihypertensive effect of beta blockers).
No products indexed under this heading.

Benazepril Hydrochloride (Reports suggest that NSAIDs may diminish the antihypertensive effect of ACE-inhibitors and angiotensin II antagonists. These interactions should be given consideration in patients taking NSAIDs concomitantly with ACE-inhibitors or angiotensin II antagonists. In some patients with compromised renal function, the co-administration of an NSAID and an ACE-inhibitor or an angiotensin II antagonist may result in further deterioration of renal funchtion, including possible acute renal failure, which is usually reversible).
No products indexed under this heading.

Bendroflumethiazide (Reduced diuretic, natriuretic, and antihypertensive effects of thiazide diuretics).
No products indexed under this heading.

Betaxolol Hydrochloride (Blunting of antihypertensive effect of beta blockers).
No products indexed under this heading.

Bisoprolol Fumarate (Blunting of antihypertensive effect of beta blockers).
No products indexed under this heading.

Bumetanide (Reduced diuretic, natriuretic, and antihypertensive effects of loop diuretics).
No products indexed under this heading.

Candesartan Cilexetil (Reports suggest that NSAIDs may diminish the antihypertensive effect of ACE-inhibitors and angiotensin II antagonists. These interactions should be given consideration in patients taking NSAIDs concomitantly with ACE-inhibitors or angiotensin II antagonists. In some patients with compromised renal function, the co-administration of an NSAID and an ACE-inhibitor or an angiotensin II antagonist may result in further deterioration of renal funchtion, including possible acute renal failure, which is usually reversible). Products include:
Atacand Tablets 639
Atacand HCT 642

Captopril (Reduced antihypertensive effect of captopril). Products include:
Captopril Tablets 2182

Carteolol Hydrochloride (Blunting of antihypertensive effect of beta blockers).
No products indexed under this heading.

Celecoxib (Concomitant use is not recommended due to the increased possibility of gastrointestinal toxicity, with little or no increase in efficacy). Products include:
Celebrex Capsules 2979

Chlorothiazide (Reduced diuretic, natriuretic, and antihypertensive effects of thiazide diuretics).
No products indexed under this heading.

Chlorothiazide Sodium (Reduced diuretic, natriuretic, and antihypertensive effects of thiazide diuretics). Products include:
Intravenous Sodium Diuril 2490

Cyclosporine (Increase in cyclosporine-induced toxicity). Products include:
Gengraf Capsules 435
Neoral Oral Solution 2280
Neoral Soft Gelatin Capsules 2280
Restasis Ophthalmic Emulsion 557
Sandimmune 2296

Dalteparin Sodium (Bleeding has been reported in patients on concomitant treatment with anticoagulants and indomethacin. Caution should be exercised when indomethacin and anticoagulants are administered concomitantly). Products include:
Fragmin Injection 1070

Danaparoid Sodium (Bleeding has been reported in patients on concomitant treatment with anticoagulants and indomethacin. Caution should be exercised when indomethacin and anticoagulants are administered concomitantly).
No products indexed under this heading.

Dexamethasone (False-negative results in dexamethasone suppression test). Products include:
Ciprodex Otic Suspension 541

Dexamethasone Acetate (False-negative results in dexamethasone suppression test).
No products indexed under this heading.

Dexamethasone Sodium Phosphate (False-negative results in dexamethasone suppression test).
No products indexed under this heading.

Diclofenac Epolamine (Concomitant use is not recommended due to the increased possibility of gastrointestinal toxicity, with little or no increase in efficacy). Products include:
Flector Patch 561

Diclofenac Potassium (Concomitant use is not recommended due to the increased possibility of gastrointestinal toxicity, with little or no increase in efficacy).
No products indexed under this heading.

Diclofenac Sodium (Concomitant use is not recommended due to the increased possibility of gastrointestinal toxicity, with little or no increase in efficacy). Products include:
Diclofenac Sodium Ophthalmic Solution .... ⊙240
Voltaren Ophthalmic Solution 2336
Voltaren Tablets 2334
Voltaren-XR Tablets 2337

Dicumarol (Bleeding has been reported in patients on concomitant treatment with anticoagulants and indomethacin. Caution should be exercised when indomethacin and anticoagulants are administered concomitantly).
No products indexed under this heading.

Diflunisal (Co-administration results in decreased renal clearance and significant increase in the plasma levels of indomethacin; in some patients combined therapy has been associated with fatal gastrointestinal hemorrhage; concurrent use is not recommended).
No products indexed under this heading.

Digoxin (Increased serum digoxin concentration and prolonged half-life). Products include:
Lanoxin Injection 1498
Lanoxin Injection Pediatric 1502
Lanoxin Tablets 1505

Enalapril Maleate (Reports suggest that NSAIDs may diminish the antihypertensive effect of ACE-inhibitors and angiotensin II antagonists. These interactions should be given consideration in patients taking NSAIDs concomitantly with ACE-inhibitors or angiotensin II antagonists. In some patients with compromised renal function, the co-administration of an NSAID and an ACE-inhibitor or an angiotensin II antagonist may result in further deterioration of renal funchtion, including possible acute renal failure, which is usually reversible).
No products indexed under this heading.

Enalaprilat (Reports suggest that NSAIDs may diminish the antihypertensive effect of ACE-inhibitors and angiotensin II antagonists. These interactions should be given consideration in patients taking NSAIDs concomitantly with ACE-inhibitors or angiotensin II antagonists. In some patients with compromised renal function, the co-administration of an NSAID and an ACE-inhibitor or an angiotensin II antagonist may result in further deterioration of renal funchtion, including possible acute renal failure, which is usually reversible).
No products indexed under this heading.

Enoxaparin Sodium (Bleeding has been reported in patients on concomitant treatment with anticoagulants and indomethacin. Caution should be exercised when indomethacin and anticoagulants are administered concomitantly). Products include:
Lovenox Injection 2756

Eprosartan Mesylate (Reports suggest that NSAIDs may diminish the antihypertensive effect of ACE-inhibitors and angiotensin II antagonists. These interactions should be given consideration in patients taking NSAIDs concomitantly with ACE-inhibitors or angiotensin II antagonists. In some patients with compromised renal function, the co-administration of an NSAID and an ACE-inhibitor or an angiotensin II antagonist may result in further deterioration of renal funchtion, including possible acute renal failure, which is usually reversible). Products include:
Teveten Tablets 515
Teveten HCT Tablets 517

Esmolol Hydrochloride (Blunting of antihypertensive effect of beta blockers).
No products indexed under this heading.

Ethacrynic Acid (Reduced diuretic, natriuretic, and antihypertensive effects of loop diuretics). Products include:
Edecrin Tablets 698

Etodolac (Concomitant use is not recommended due to the increased possibility of gastrointestinal toxicity, with little or no increase in efficacy).
No products indexed under this heading.

Fenoprofen Calcium (Concomitant use is not recommended due to the increased possibility of gastrointestinal toxicity, with little or no increase in efficacy). Products include:
Nalfon Capsules 2508

Flurbiprofen (Concomitant use is not recommended due to the increased possibility of gastrointestinal toxicity, with little or no increase in efficacy).
No products indexed under this heading.

Fondaparinux Sodium (Bleeding has been reported in patients on concomitant treatment with anticoagulants and indomethacin. Caution should be exercised when indomethacin and anticoagulants are administered concomitantly). Products include:
Arixtra Injection 1313

Fosinopril Sodium (Reports suggest that NSAIDs may diminish the antihypertensive effect of ACE-inhibitors and angiotensin II antagonists. These interactions should be given consideration in patients taking NSAIDs concomitantly with ACE-inhibitors or angiotensin II antagonists. In some patients with compromised renal function, the co-administration of an NSAID and an ACE-inhibitor or an angiotensin II antagonist may result in further deterioration of renal funchtion, including possible acute renal failure, which is usually reversible).
No products indexed under this heading.

Furosemide (Indomethacin reduces basal plasma renin activity (PRA) induced by furosemide; reduced diuretic, natriuretic, and antihypertensive effects of loop diuretics). Products include:
Furosemide Tablets 2186

Heparin Calcium (Bleeding has been reported in patients on concomitant treatment with anticoagulants and indomethacin. Caution should be exercised when indomethacin and anticoagulants are administered concomitantly).
No products indexed under this heading.

Heparin Sodium (Bleeding has been reported in patients on concomitant treatment with anticoagulants and indomethacin. Caution should be exercised when indomethacin and anticoagulants are administered concomitantly).
No products indexed under this heading.

Hydrochlorothiazide (Reduced diuretic, natriuretic, and antihypertensive effects of thiazide diuretics). Products include:

Atacand HCT 642
Avalide Tablets 892
Avalide Tablets 2713
Benicar HCT Tablets 1010
Diovan HCT Tablets 2216
Dyazide Capsules 1405
Micardis HCT Tablets 854
Prinzide Tablets 2092
Tekturna HCT Tablets 2324
Teveten HCT Tablets 517

Hydroflumethiazide (Reduced diuretic, natriuretic, and antihypertensive effects of thiazide diuretics).
No products indexed under this heading.

Ibuprofen (Concomitant use is not recommended due to the increased possibility of gastrointestinal toxicity, with little or no increase in efficacy). Products include:
Motrin IB Tablets and Caplets 1900
Children's Motrin Oral Suspension ... 1901
Children's Motrin Non-Staining Dye-Free Oral Suspension 1901
Children's Motrin Cold Oral Suspension 1899
Infants' Motrin Concentrated Drops 1901
Infants' Motrin Non-Staining Dye-Free Concentrated Drops 1901
Junior Strength Motrin Caplets and Chewable Tablets 1901
Vicoprofen Tablets 533

Indomethacin Sodium Trihydrate (Concomitant use is not recommended due to the increased possibility of gastrointestinal toxicity, with little or no increase in efficacy). Products include:
Indocin I.V. 2489

Irbesartan (Reports suggest that NSAIDs may diminish the antihypertensive effect of ACE-inhibitors and angiotensin II antagonists. These interactions should be given consideration in patients taking NSAIDs concomitantly with ACE-inhibitors or angiotensin II antagonists. In some patients with compromised renal function, the co-administration of an NSAID and an ACE-inhibitor or an angiotensin II antagonist may result in further deterioration of renal funchtion, including possible acute renal failure, which is usually reversible). Products include:
Avalide Tablets 892
Avalide Tablets 2713
Avapro Tablets 897
Avapro Tablets 2718

Ketoprofen (Concomitant use is not recommended due to the increased possibility of gastrointestinal toxicity, with little or no increase in efficacy).
No products indexed under this heading.

Ketorolac Tromethamine (Concomitant use is not recommended due to the increased possibility of gastrointestinal toxicity, with little or no increase in efficacy).
No products indexed under this heading.

Labetalol Hydrochloride (Blunting of antihypertensive effect of beta blockers).
No products indexed under this heading.

Levobunolol Hydrochloride (Blunting of antihypertensive effect of beta blockers).
No products indexed under this heading.

Lisinopril (Reports suggest that NSAIDs may diminish the antihypertensive effect of ACE-inhibitors and angiotensin II antagonists. These interactions should be given consideration in patients taking NSAIDs concomitantly with ACE-inhibitors or angiotensin II antagonists. In some patients with compromised renal function, the co-administration of an NSAID and an ACE-inhibitor or an angiotensin II antagonist may result in further deterioration of renal funchtion, including possible acute renal failure, which is usually reversible). Products include:
Prinivil Tablets 2087
Prinzide Tablets 2092

Lithium (Co-administration produces a clinically relevant elevation of plasma lithium and reduction in renal lithium clearance with a potential for lithium toxicity).
No products indexed under this heading.

Lithium Carbonate (Co-administration produces a clinically relevant elevation of plasma lithium and reduction in renal lithium clearance with a potential for lithium toxicity).
No products indexed under this heading.

Lithium Citrate (Co-administration produces a clinically relevant elevation of plasma lithium and reduction in renal lithium clearance with a potential for lithium toxicity).
No products indexed under this heading.

Losartan Potassium (Reports suggest that NSAIDs may diminish the antihypertensive effect of ACE-inhibitors and angiotensin II antagonists. These interactions should be given consideration in patients taking NSAIDs concomitantly with ACE-inhibitors or angiotensin II antagonists. In some patients with compromised renal function, the co-administration of an NSAID and an ACE-inhibitor or an angiotensin II antagonist may result in further deterioration of renal funchtion, including possible acute renal failure, which is usually reversible). Products include:
Cozaar Tablets 1973

Low Molecular Weight Heparins (Bleeding has been reported in patients on concomitant treatment with anticoagulants and indomethacin. Caution should be exercised when indomethacin and anticoagulants are administered concomitantly).
No products indexed under this heading.

Meclofenamate Sodium (Concomitant use is not recommended due to the increased possibility of gastrointestinal toxicity, with little or no increase in efficacy).
No products indexed under this heading.

Mefenamic Acid (Concomitant use is not recommended due to the increased possibility of gastrointestinal toxicity, with little or no increase in efficacy).
No products indexed under this heading.

Meloxicam (Concomitant use is not recommended due to the increased possibility of gastrointestinal toxicity, with little or no increase in efficacy). Products include:
Mobic Oral Suspension 863
Mobic Tablets 863

Methotrexate Sodium (Potentiation of methotrexate toxicity).
No products indexed under this heading.

Methyclothiazide (Reduced diuretic, natriuretic, and antihypertensive effects of thiazide diuretics).
No products indexed under this heading.

Metipranolol Hydrochloride (Blunting of antihypertensive effect of beta blockers).
No products indexed under this heading.

Metoprolol Succinate (Blunting of antihypertensive effect of beta blockers). Products include:
Toprol-XL Tablets 666

Metoprolol Tartrate (Blunting of antihypertensive effect of beta blockers).
No products indexed under this heading.

Moexipril Hydrochloride (Reports suggest that NSAIDs may diminish the antihypertensive effect of ACE-inhibitors and angiotensin II antagonists. These interactions should be given consideration in patients taking NSAIDs concomitantly with ACE-inhibitors or angiotensin II antagonists. In some patients with compromised renal function, the co-administration of an NSAID and an ACE-inhibitor or an angiotensin II antagonist may result in further deterioration of renal funchtion, including possible acute renal failure, which is usually reversible).
No products indexed under this heading.

Nabumetone (Concomitant use is not recommended due to the increased possibility of gastrointestinal toxicity, with little or no increase in efficacy).
No products indexed under this heading.

Nadolol (Blunting of antihypertensive effect of beta blockers). Products include:
Nadolol Tablets 2191

Naproxen (Concomitant use is not recommended due to the increased possibility of gastrointestinal toxicity, with little or no increase in efficacy). Products include:
EC-Naprosyn Delayed-Release Tablets 2632
Naprosyn Suspension 2632
Naprosyn Tablets 2632

Naproxen Sodium (Concomitant use is not recommended due to the increased possibility of gastrointestinal toxicity, with little or no increase in efficacy). Products include:
Anaprox Tablets 2632
Anaprox DS Tablets 2632
Treximet Tablets 1616

Nebivolol (Blunting of antihypertensive effect of beta blockers). Products include:
Bystolic Tablets 1155

Nephrotoxic Drugs (Overt renal decompensation).
No products indexed under this heading.

Oxaprozin (Concomitant use is not recommended due to the increased possibility of gastrointestinal toxicity, with little or no increase in efficacy).
No products indexed under this heading.

Penbutolol Sulfate (Blunting of antihypertensive effect of beta blockers).
No products indexed under this heading.

Perindopril Erbumine (Reports suggest that NSAIDs may diminish the antihypertensive effect of ACE-inhibitors and angiotensin II antagonists. These interactions should be given consideration in patients taking NSAIDs concomitantly with ACE-inhibitors or angiotensin II antagonists. In some patients with compromised renal function, the co-administration of an NSAID and an ACE-inhibitor or an angiotensin II antagonist may result in further deterioration of renal funchtion, including possible acute renal failure, which is usually reversible). Products include:
Aceon Tablets (2 mg, 4 mg, 8 mg) 3038

Phenylbutazone (Concomitant use is not recommended due to the increased possibility of gastrointestinal toxicity, with little or no increase in efficacy).
No products indexed under this heading.

Pindolol (Blunting of antihypertensive effect of beta blockers).
No products indexed under this heading.

Piroxicam (Concomitant use is not recommended due to the increased possibility of gastrointestinal toxicity, with little or no increase in efficacy).
No products indexed under this heading.

Polythiazide (Reduced diuretic, natriuretic, and antihypertensive effects of thiazide diuretics).
No products indexed under this heading.

Probenecid (Increased plasma levels of indomethacin).
No products indexed under this heading.

Propranolol Hydrochloride (Blunting of antihypertensive effect of beta blockers). Products include:
InnoPran XL Extended Release Capsules 1484

Quinapril Hydrochloride (Reports suggest that NSAIDs may diminish the antihypertensive effect of ACE-inhibitors and angiotensin II antagonists. These interactions should be given consideration in patients taking NSAIDs concomitantly with ACE-inhibitors or angiotensin II antagonists. In some patients with compromised renal function, the co-administration of an NSAID and an ACE-inhibitor or an angiotensin II antagonist may result in further deterioration of renal funchtion, including possible acute renal failure, which is usually reversible).
No products indexed under this heading.

Ramipril (Reports suggest that NSAIDs may diminish the antihypertensive effect of ACE-inhibitors and angiotensin II antagonists. These interactions should be given consideration in patients taking NSAIDs concomitantly with ACE-inhibitors or angiotensin II antagonists. In some patients with compromised renal function, the co-administration of an NSAID and an ACE-inhibitor or an angiotensin II antagonist may result in further deterioration of renal funchtion, including possible acute renal failure, which is usually reversible).
No products indexed under this heading.

Rofecoxib (Concomitant use is not recommended due to the increased possibility of gastrointestinal toxicity, with little or no increase in efficacy).
No products indexed under this heading.

Sotalol Hydrochloride (Blunting of antihypertensive effect of beta blockers).
No products indexed under this heading.

Spirapril Hydrochloride (Reports suggest that NSAIDs may diminish the antihypertensive effect of ACE-inhibitors and angiotensin II antagonists. These interactions should be given consideration in patients taking NSAIDs concomitantly with ACE-inhibitors or angiotensin II antagonists. In some patients with compromised renal function, the co-administration of an NSAID and an ACE-inhibitor or an angiotensin II antagonist may result in further deterioration of renal funchtion, including possible acute renal failure, which is usually reversible).
No products indexed under this heading.

Spironolactone (Reduced diuretic, natriuretic and antihypertensive effects of increased serum potassium levels).
No products indexed under this heading.

Sulindac (Concomitant use is not recommended due to the increased possibility of gastrointestinal toxicity, with little or no increase in efficacy). Products include:
Clinoril Tablets ... 1962

Telmisartan (Reports suggest that NSAIDs may diminish the antihypertensive effect of ACE-inhibitors and angiotensin II antagonists. These interactions should be given consideration in patients taking NSAIDs concomitantly with ACE-inhibitors or angiotensin II antagonists. In some patients with compromised renal function, the co-administration of an NSAID and an ACE-inhibitor or an angiotensin II antagonist may result in further deterioration of renal funchtion, including possible acute renal failure, which is usually reversible). Products include:
Micardis Tablets ... 852
Micardis HCT Tablets ... 854

Timolol Hemihydrate (Blunting of antihypertensive effect of beta blockers). Products include:
Betimol Ophthalmic Solution ... 3181

Timolol Maleate (Blunting of antihypertensive effect of beta blockers). Products include:
Combigan Ophthalmic Solution ... 553
Cosopt Sterile Ophthalmic Solution ... 1969
Timoptic Sterile Ophthalmic Solution ... 2121
Timoptic in Ocudose ... 2124
Timoptic-XE Sterile Ophthalmic Gel Forming Solution ... 2125

Tinzaparin Sodium (Bleeding has been reported in patients on concomitant treatment with anticoagulants and indomethacin. Caution should be exercised when indomethacin and anticoagulants are administered concomitantly).
No products indexed under this heading.

Tolmetin Sodium (Concomitant use is not recommended due to the increased possibility of gastrointestinal toxicity, with little or no increase in efficacy).
No products indexed under this heading.

Torsemide (Reduced diuretic, natriuretic, and antihypertensive effects of loop diuretics). Products include:
Demadex Injection ... 2630
Demadex Tablets ... 2630

Trandolapril (Reports suggest that NSAIDs may diminish the antihypertensive effect of ACE-inhibitors and angiotensin II antagonists. These interactions should be given consideration in patients taking NSAIDs concomitantly with ACE-inhibitors or angiotensin II antagonists. In some patients with compromised renal function, the co-administration of an NSAID and an ACE-inhibitor or an angiotensin II antagonist may result in further deterioration of renal funchtion, including possible acute renal failure, which is usually reversible). Products include:
Mavik Tablets ... 472
Tarka Tablets ... 511

Triamterene (The addition of triamterene to maintenance schedule of indomethacin has resulted in reversible acute renal failure; potential for increased hyperkalemia; concurrent therapy should be avoided). Products include:
Dyazide Capsules ... 1405
Dyrenium Capsules ... 3189

Valdecoxib (Concomitant use is not recommended due to the increased possibility of gastrointestinal toxicity, with little or no increase in efficacy).
No products indexed under this heading.

Valsartan (Reports suggest that NSAIDs may diminish the antihypertensive effect of ACE-inhibitors and angiotensin II antagonists. These interactions should be given consideration in patients taking NSAIDs concomitantly with ACE-inhibitors or angiotensin II antagonists. In some patients with compromised renal function, the co-administration of an NSAID and an ACE-inhibitor or an angiotensin II antagonist may result in further deterioration of renal funchtion, including possible acute renal failure, which is usually reversible). Products include:
Diovan Tablets ... 2212
Diovan HCT Tablets ... 2216
Exforge Tablets ... 2238

Warfarin Sodium (Bleeding has been reported in patients on concomitant treatment with anticoagulants and indomethacin. Caution should be exercised when indomethacin and anticoagulants are administered concomitantly).
No products indexed under this heading.

INDOCIN I.V.

(Indomethacin Sodium Trihydrate) ... 2489
May interact with ACE inhibitors, angiotensin-II receptor antagonists, anticoagulants, cardiac glycosides, and certain other agents. Compounds in these categories include:

Amikacin Sulfate (Serum levels of amikacin significantly elevated).
No products indexed under this heading.

Anisindione (Bleeding has been reported in patients on concomitant treatment with anticoagulants and indomethacin, therefore they should be co-administered with caution).
No products indexed under this heading.

Ardeparin Sodium (Bleeding has been reported in patients on concomitant treatment with anticoagulants and indomethacin, therefore they should be co-administered with caution).
No products indexed under this heading.

Benazepril Hydrochloride (In patients with compromised renal function, the co-administration of an NSAID and an ACE inhibitor may result in further deterioration of renal function, including possible acute renal failure, which is usually reversible).
No products indexed under this heading.

Candesartan Cilexetil (In patients with compromised renal function, the co-administration of an NSAID and an angiotensin II antagonist may result in further deterioration of renal function, including possible acute renal failure, which is usually reversible). Products include:
Atacand Tablets ... 639
Atacand HCT ... 642

Captopril (In patients with compromised renal function, the co-administration of an NSAID and an ACE inhibitor may result in further deterioration of renal function, including possible acute renal failure, which is usually reversible). Products include:
Captopril Tablets ... 2182

Dalteparin Sodium (Bleeding has been reported in patients on concomitant treatment with anticoagulants and indomethacin, therefore they should be co-administered with caution). Products include:
Fragmin Injection ... 1070

Danaparoid Sodium (Bleeding has been reported in patients on concomitant treatment with anticoagulants and indomethacin, therefore they should be co-administered with caution).
No products indexed under this heading.

Deslanoside (Half-life of digitalis may be prolonged when given concomitantly).
No products indexed under this heading.

Dicumarol (Bleeding has been reported in patients on concomitant treatment with anticoagulants and indomethacin, therefore they should be co-administered with caution).
No products indexed under this heading.

Digitalis Glycoside Preparations (Half-life of digitalis may be prolonged when given concomitantly).
No products indexed under this heading.

Digitoxin (Half-life of digitalis may be prolonged when given concomitantly).
No products indexed under this heading.

Digoxin (Half-life of digitalis may be prolonged when given concomitantly). Products include:
Lanoxin Injection ... 1498
Lanoxin Injection Pediatric ... 1502
Lanoxin Tablets ... 1505

Enalapril Maleate (In patients with compromised renal function, the co-administration of an NSAID and an ACE inhibitor may result in further deterioration of renal function, including possible acute renal failure, which is usually reversible).
No products indexed under this heading.

Enalaprilat (In patients with compromised renal function, the co-administration of an NSAID and an ACE inhibitor may result in further deterioration of renal function, including possible acute renal failure, which is usually reversible).
No products indexed under this heading.

Enoxaparin Sodium (Bleeding has been reported in patients on concomitant treatment with anticoagulants and indomethacin, therefore they should be co-administered with caution). Products include:
Lovenox Injection ... 2756

Eprosartan Mesylate (In patients with compromised renal function, the co-administration of an NSAID and an angiotensin II antagonist may result in further deterioration of renal function, including possible acute renal failure, which is usually reversible). Products include:
Teveten Tablets ... 515
Teveten HCT Tablets ... 517

Fondaparinux Sodium (Bleeding has been reported in patients on concomitant treatment with anticoagulants and indomethacin, therefore they should be co-administered with caution). Products include:
Arixtra Injection ... 1313

Fosinopril Sodium (In patients with compromised renal function, the co-administration of an NSAID and an ACE inhibitor may result in further deterioration of renal function, including possible acute renal failure, which is usually reversible).
No products indexed under this heading.

Furosemide (Blunted natriuretic effect of furosemide). Products include:
Furosemide Tablets ... 2186

Gentamicin Sulfate (Serum levels of gentamicin significantly elevated). Products include:
Pred-G Ophthalmic Ointment ... ⊙229
Pred-G Ophthalmic Suspension ... ⊙228

Heparin Calcium (Bleeding has been reported in patients on concomitant treatment with anticoagulants and indomethacin, therefore they should be co-administered with caution).
No products indexed under this heading.

Heparin Sodium (Bleeding has been reported in patients on concomitant treatment with anticoagulants and indomethacin, therefore they should be co-administered with caution).
No products indexed under this heading.

Irbesartan (In patients with compromised renal function, the co-administration of an NSAID and an angiotensin II antagonist may result in further deterioration of renal function, including possible acute renal failure, which is usually reversible). Products include:
Avalide Tablets ... 892

Avalide Tablets 2713
Avapro Tablets 897
Avapro Tablets 2718

Lisinopril (In patients with compromised renal function, the co-administration of an NSAID and an ACE inhibitor may result in further deterioration of renal function, including possible acute renal failure, which is usually reversible). Products include:
Prinivil Tablets 2087
Prinzide Tablets 2092

Losartan Potassium (In patients with compromised renal function, the co-administration of an NSAID and an angiotensin II antagonist may result in further deterioration of renal function, including possible acute renal failure, which is usually reversible). Products include:
Cozaar Tablets 1973

Low Molecular Weight Heparins (Bleeding has been reported in patients on concomitant treatment with anticoagulants and indomethacin, therefore they should be co-administered with caution).
No products indexed under this heading.

Moexipril Hydrochloride (In patients with compromised renal function, the co-administration of an NSAID and an ACE inhibitor may result in further deterioration of renal function, including possible acute renal failure, which is usually reversible).
No products indexed under this heading.

Perindopril Erbumine (In patients with compromised renal function, the co-administration of an NSAID and an ACE inhibitor may result in further deterioration of renal function, including possible acute renal failure, which is usually reversible). Products include:
Aceon Tablets (2 mg, 4 mg, 8 mg) 3038

Quinapril Hydrochloride (In patients with compromised renal function, the co-administration of an NSAID and an ACE inhibitor may result in further deterioration of renal function, including possible acute renal failure, which is usually reversible).
No products indexed under this heading.

Ramipril (In patients with compromised renal function, the co-administration of an NSAID and an ACE inhibitor may result in further deterioration of renal function, including possible acute renal failure, which is usually reversible).
No products indexed under this heading.

Spirapril Hydrochloride (In patients with compromised renal function, the co-administration of an NSAID and an ACE inhibitor may result in further deterioration of renal function, including possible acute renal failure, which is usually reversible).
No products indexed under this heading.

Telmisartan (In patients with compromised renal function, the co-administration of an NSAID and an angiotensin II antagonist may result in further deterioration of renal function, including possible acute renal failure, which is usually reversible). Products include:
Micardis Tablets 852
Micardis HCT Tablets 854

Tinzaparin Sodium (Bleeding has been reported in patients on concomitant treatment with anticoagulants and indomethacin, therefore they should be co-administered with caution).
No products indexed under this heading.

Trandolapril (In patients with compromised renal function, the co-administration of an NSAID and an ACE inhibitor may result in further deterioration of renal function, including possible acute renal failure, which is usually reversible). Products include:
Mavik Tablets 472
Tarka Tablets 511

Valsartan (In patients with compromised renal function, the co-administration of an NSAID and an angiotensin II antagonist may result in further deterioration of renal function, including possible acute renal failure, which is usually reversible). Products include:
Diovan Tablets 2212
Diovan HCT Tablets 2216
Exforge Tablets 2238

Warfarin Sodium (Bleeding has been reported in patients on concomitant treatment with anticoagulants and indomethacin, therefore they should be co-administered with caution).
No products indexed under this heading.

INDOCIN ORAL SUSPENSION

(Indomethacin) 2024
See Indocin Capsules

INDOCIN SUPPOSITORIES

(Indomethacin) 2024
See Indocin Capsules

INFANRIX VACCINE

(Diphtheria & Tetanus Toxoids and Acellular Pertussis Vaccine Adsorbed) 1479
May interact with alkylating agents, antimetabolites, corticosteroids, cytotoxic drugs, and immunosuppressive agents. Compounds in these categories include:

Azathioprine (Concurrent immunosuppressive therapy may reduce the immune response to vaccine).
No products indexed under this heading.

Basiliximab (Concurrent immunosuppressive therapy may reduce the immune response to vaccine). Products include:
Simulect for Injection 2306

Betamethasone Acetate (Concurrent immunosuppressive therapy with greater than physiologic doses of corticosteroids may reduce the immune response to vaccine).
No products indexed under this heading.

Betamethasone Sodium Phosphate (Concurrent immunosuppressive therapy with greater than physiologic doses of corticosteroids may reduce the immune response to vaccine).
No products indexed under this heading.

Bleomycin Sulfate (Cytotoxic drugs may reduce the immune response to vaccine).
No products indexed under this heading.

Budesonide (Concurrent immunosuppressive therapy with greater than physiologic doses of corticosteroids may reduce the immune response to vaccine). Products include:
Pulmicort Flexhaler 654
Symbicort 80/4.5 Inhalation Aerosol 659
Symbicort 160/4.5 Inhalation Aerosol 659

Busulfan (Alkylating drugs may reduce the immune response to vaccine). Products include:
Busulfex Injection 2477
Myleran Tablets 1530

Capecitabine (Immunosuppressive therapies may reduce the immune response to vaccines). Products include:
Xeloda Tablets 2662

Carmustine (BCNU) (Alkylating drugs may reduce the immune response to vaccine).
No products indexed under this heading.

Chlorambucil (Alkylating drugs may reduce the immune response to vaccine). Products include:
Leukeran Tablets 1508

Ciclesonide (Concurrent immunosuppressive therapy with greater than physiologic doses of corticosteroids may reduce the immune response to vaccine). Products include:
Alvesco Inhalation Aerosol 2985
Omnaris Nasal Spray 2998

Cladribine (Immunosuppressive therapies may reduce the immune response to vaccines). Products include:
Leustatin Injection 2384

Cortisone Acetate (Concurrent immunosuppressive therapy with greater than physiologic doses of corticosteroids may reduce the immune response to vaccine).
No products indexed under this heading.

Cyclophosphamide (Alkylating drugs may reduce the immune response to vaccine).
No products indexed under this heading.

Cyclosporine (Concurrent immunosuppressive therapy may reduce the immune response to vaccine). Products include:
Gengraf Capsules 435
Neoral Oral Solution 2280
Neoral Soft Gelatin Capsules 2280
Restasis Ophthalmic Emulsion 557
Sandimmune 2296

Cytarabine (Immunosuppressive therapies may reduce the immune response to vaccines).
No products indexed under this heading.

Dacarbazine (Alkylating drugs may reduce the immune response to vaccine).
No products indexed under this heading.

Daunorubicin Hydrochloride (Cytotoxic drugs may reduce the immune response to vaccine).
No products indexed under this heading.

Dexamethasone (Concurrent immunosuppressive therapy with greater than physiologic doses of corticosteroids may reduce the immune response to vaccine). Products include:
Ciprodex Otic Suspension 541

Dexamethasone Acetate (Concurrent immunosuppressive therapy with greater than physiologic doses of corticosteroids may reduce the immune response to vaccine).
No products indexed under this heading.

Dexamethasone Sodium Phosphate (Concurrent immunosuppressive therapy with greater than physiologic doses of corticosteroids may reduce the immune response to vaccine).
No products indexed under this heading.

Doxorubicin Hydrochloride (Cytotoxic drugs may reduce the immune response to vaccine).
No products indexed under this heading.

Epirubicin Hydrochloride (Cytotoxic drugs may reduce the immune response to vaccine).
No products indexed under this heading.

Floxuridine (Immunosuppressive therapies may reduce the immune response to vaccines).
No products indexed under this heading.

Fludarabine Phosphate (Immunosuppressive therapies may reduce the immune response to vaccines).
No products indexed under this heading.

Fludrocortisone Acetate (Concurrent immunosuppressive therapy with greater than physiologic doses of corticosteroids may reduce the immune response to vaccine).
No products indexed under this heading.

Flunisolide (Concurrent immunosuppressive therapy with greater than physiologic doses of corticosteroids may reduce the immune response to vaccine). Products include:
Aerobid/Aerobid-M 1153

Fluorouracil (Immunosuppressive therapies may reduce the immune response to vaccines). Products include:
Carac Cream 0.5% 2722

Fluticasone Propionate (Concurrent immunosuppressive therapy with greater than physiologic doses of corticosteroids may reduce the immune response to vaccine). Products include:
Advair Diskus 100/50 1276
Advair Diskus 250/50 1276
Advair Diskus 500/50 1276
Advair HFA 45/21 Inhalation Aerosol 1288
Advair HFA 115/21 Inhalation Aerosol 1288
Advair HFA 230/21 Inhalation Aerosol 1288
Flonase Nasal Spray 1431
Flovent Diskus 50 mcg 1435

Fluticasone Propionate HFA (Concurrent immunosuppressive therapy with greater than physiologic doses of corticosteroids may reduce the immune response to vaccine). Products include:
Flovent HFA 1440

Gemcitabine Hydrochloride (Immunosuppressive therapies may reduce the immune response to vaccines). Products include:
Gemzar for Injection 1820

Hydrocortisone (Concurrent immunosuppressive therapy with greater than physiologic doses of corticosteroids may reduce the immune response to vaccine).
No products indexed under this heading.

Hydrocortisone Acetate (Concurrent immunosuppressive therapy with greater than physiologic doses of corticosteroids may reduce the immune response to vaccine). Products include:
Analpram-HC 1140
Pramosone 1141

Hydrocortisone Sodium Phosphate (Concurrent immunosuppressive therapy with greater than physiologic doses of corticosteroids may reduce the immune response to vaccine).
No products indexed under this heading.

Hydrocortisone Sodium Succinate (Concurrent immunosuppressive therapy with greater than physiologic doses of corticosteroids may reduce the immune response to vaccine).
No products indexed under this heading.

Hydroxyurea (Cytotoxic drugs may reduce the immune response to vaccine).
No products indexed under this heading.

Lomustine (CCNU) (Alkylating drugs may reduce the immune response to vaccine).
No products indexed under this heading.

Mechlorethamine Hydrochloride (Alkylating drugs may reduce the immune response to vaccine). Products include:
Mustargen for Injection 2492

Melphalan (Alkylating drugs may reduce the immune response to vaccine).
No products indexed under this heading.

Mercaptopurine (Immunosuppressive therapies may reduce the immune response to vaccines).
No products indexed under this heading.

Methotrexate (Immunosuppressive therapies may reduce the immune response to vaccines).
No products indexed under this heading.

Methotrexate Sodium (Cytotoxic drugs may reduce the immune response to vaccine).
No products indexed under this heading.

Methylprednisolone Acetate (Concurrent immunosuppressive therapy with greater than physiologic doses of corticosteroids may reduce the immune response to vaccine).
No products indexed under this heading.

Methylprednisolone Sodium Succinate (Concurrent immunosuppressive therapy with greater than physiologic doses of corticosteroids may reduce the immune response to vaccine).
No products indexed under this heading.

Mitotane (Cytotoxic drugs may reduce the immune response to vaccine).
No products indexed under this heading.

Mitoxantrone Hydrochloride (Cytotoxic drugs may reduce the immune response to vaccine). Products include:
Novantrone for Injection Concentrate 1100

Mometasone Furoate (Concurrent immunosuppressive therapy with greater than physiologic doses of corticosteroids may reduce the immune response to vaccine). Products include:
Asmanex Twisthaler 2797
Elocon Cream 0.1% 2840
Elocon Lotion 0.1% 2841
Elocon Ointment 0.1% 2842

Mometasone Furoate Monohydrate (Concurrent immunosuppressive therapy with greater than physiologic doses of corticosteroids may reduce the immune response to vaccine). Products include:
Nasonex Nasal Spray 2883

Muromonab-CD3 (Concurrent immunosuppressive therapy may reduce the immune response to vaccine). Products include:
Orthoclone OKT3 Sterile Solution 2387

Mycophenolate Mofetil (Concurrent immunosuppressive therapy may reduce the immune response to vaccine). Products include:
CellCept Capsules 2622
CellCept Oral Suspension 2622
CellCept Tablets 2622

Pentostatin (Immunosuppressive therapies may reduce the immune response to vaccines).
No products indexed under this heading.

Prednisolone Acetate (Concurrent immunosuppressive therapy with greater than physiologic doses of corticosteroids may reduce the immune response to vaccine). Products include:
Pred Forte Ophthalmic Suspension .... ⊙227
Pred Mild Ophthalmic Suspension .... ⊙230
Pred-G Ophthalmic Ointment .... ⊙229
Pred-G Ophthalmic Suspension .... ⊙228

Prednisolone Sodium Phosphate (Concurrent immunosuppressive therapy with greater than physiologic doses of corticosteroids may reduce the immune response to vaccine).
No products indexed under this heading.

Prednisolone Tebutate (Concurrent immunosuppressive therapy with greater than physiologic doses of corticosteroids may reduce the immune response to vaccine).
No products indexed under this heading.

Prednisone (Concurrent immunosuppressive therapy with greater than physiologic doses of corticosteroids may reduce the immune response to vaccine).
No products indexed under this heading.

Procarbazine Hydrochloride (Cytotoxic drugs may reduce the immune response to vaccine).
No products indexed under this heading.

Sirolimus (Concurrent immunosuppressive therapy may reduce the immune response to vaccine). Products include:
Rapamune 3260

Tacrolimus (Concurrent immunosuppressive therapy may reduce the immune response to vaccine). Products include:
Prograf Capsules and Injection 622
Protopic Ointment 628

Tamoxifen Citrate (Cytotoxic drugs may reduce the immune response to vaccine).
No products indexed under this heading.

Thioguanine (Immunosuppressive therapies may reduce the immune response to vaccines). Products include:
Tabloid Tablets 1601

Thiotepa (Alkylating drugs may reduce the immune response to vaccine).
No products indexed under this heading.

Triamcinolone (Concurrent immunosuppressive therapy with greater than physiologic doses of corticosteroids may reduce the immune response to vaccine).
No products indexed under this heading.

Triamcinolone Acetonide (Concurrent immunosuppressive therapy with greater than physiologic doses of corticosteroids may reduce the immune response to vaccine). Products include:
Azmacort Inhalation Aerosol 407
Nasacort AQ Nasal Spray 2765
Triesence Injectable Suspension .... ⊙209

Triamcinolone Diacetate (Concurrent immunosuppressive therapy with greater than physiologic doses of corticosteroids may reduce the immune response to vaccine).
No products indexed under this heading.

Triamcinolone Hexacetonide (Concurrent immunosuppressive therapy with greater than physiologic doses of corticosteroids may reduce the immune response to vaccine).
No products indexed under this heading.

Vincristine Sulfate (Cytotoxic drugs may reduce the immune response to vaccine).
No products indexed under this heading.

INFASURF INTRATRACHEAL SUSPENSION

(Calfactant) 1168
None cited in PDR database.

INNOPRAN XL EXTENDED RELEASE CAPSULES

(Propranolol Hydrochloride) 1484
May interact with ACE inhibitors, catecholamine depleting drugs, calcium channel blockers, cytochrome p450 1a2 inhibitors (selected), cytochrome p450 1a2 substrates (selected), cytochrome p450 2c19 inhibitors (selected), cytochrome p450 2c19 substrates (selected), cytochrome p450 2d6 inhibitors (selected), cytochrome p450 2d6 substrates (selected), epinephrine-containing products, cardiac glycosides, hepatic microsomal enzyme inducers, insulin, monoamine oxidase inhibitors, non-steroidal anti-inflammatory agents, quinidine, theophyllines, tricyclic antidepressants, and certain other agents. Compounds in these categories include:

Acetaminophen (Blood levels and/or toxicity of propranolol may be increased by administration of propranolol extended-release capsules with substrates of CYP1A2). Products include:
Benadryl Allergy & Cold Kapgels 1895
Benadryl Allergy & Sinus Headache Kapgels 1895
Benadryl Severe Allergy & Sinus Headache Caplets 1897
Lortab 5/500 Tablets 3143
Lortab 7.5/500 Tablets 3144
Lortab 10/500 Tablets 3144
Percocet Tablets 1127
Sinutab Sinus Caplets 1905
Sudafed PE Cold & Cough Caplets 1907
Sudafed PE Nighttime Cold Caplets 1907
Sudafed PE Severe Cold Caplets 1908
Sudafed PE Sinus Headache Caplets 1908
Regular Strength Tylenol Tablets 1915
Tylenol 8 Hour Extended Release Caplets 1915
Extra Strength Tylenol Caplets, Cool Caplets, and EZ Tabs 1915
Extra Strength Tylenol Adult Rapid Blast Liquid 1915
Extra Strength Tylenol PM Caplets, Geltabs, Liquid, and Rapid Release Gels 1915
Extra Strength Tylenol Rapid Release Gels 1915
Tylenol with Codeine Tablets 2427
Tylenol Allergy Multi-Symptom Caplets with Cool Burst and Rapid Release Gelcaps 1916
Tylenol Allergy Multi-Symptom Nighttime Caplets with Cool Burst 1916
Tylenol Severe Allergy Caplets 1916
Tylenol Arthritis Pain Extended Release Geltabs/Caplets 1915
Tylenol Chest Congestion Caplets with Cool Burst 1910
Tylenol Chest Congestion Liquid with Cool Burst 1910
Children's Tylenol Plus Cold Suspension Liquid 1912
Children's Tylenol Plus Cold & Allergy Suspension Liquid 1914
Children's Tylenol Plus Cough & Runny Nose Suspension Liquid 1912
Children's Tylenol Plus Cough & Sore Throat Suspension Liquid 1912
Children's Tylenol Plus Flu Suspension Liquid 1914
Children's Tylenol Suspension Liquid 1909
Children's Tylenol Meltaways 1909
Children's Tylenol Plus Multi-Symptom Cold Suspension Liquid 1912
Tylenol Cold Severe Congestion Daytime Caplets with Cool Burst 1912
Tylenol Cold Head Congestion Daytime Caplets with Cool Burst 1910
Tylenol Cold Head Congestion Nighttime Caplets with Cool Burst 1910
Tylenol Cold Head Congestion Severe Daytime Caplets with Cool Burst 1910
Tylenol Cold Multi-Symptom Daytime Caplets with Cool Burst and Rapid Release Gels 1913
Tylenol Cold Multi-Symptom Daytime Liquid with Citrus Burst 1913
Tylenol Cold Multi-Symptom Nighttime Caplets with Cool Burst 1913
Tylenol Cold Multi-Symptom Nighttime Liquid with Cool Burst 1913
Tylenol Cold Multi-Symptom Severe Caplets with Cool Burst 1913
Tylenol Cold Multi-Symptom Severe Daytime Liquid with Citrus Burst 1913
Tylenol Cough & Sore Throat Daytime Liquid with Cool Burst 1918
Tylenol Cough & Sore Throat Nighttime Liquid with Cool Burst 1918
Concentrated Tylenol Infants' Drops 1909
Jr. Tylenol Meltaways 1909
Tylenol Sinus Congestion & Pain Daytime Caplets with Cool Burst and Gelcaps 1917
Tylenol Sinus Congestion & Pain Nighttime Caplets with Cool Burst 1917

Tylenol Sinus Congestion & Pain Severe Caplets with Cool Burst..... 1917
Tylenol Sinus Severe Congestion Caplets with Cool Burst............... 1917
Tylenol Sore Throat Daytime Liquid with Cool Burst.................. 1918
Tylenol Sore Throat Nighttime Liquid with Cool Burst.................. 1918
Women's Tylenol Menstrual Relief Caplets.................................... 1919
Vicks DayQuil Cold & Flu Multi-Symptom Relief.................. 616
Vicks DayQuil LiquiCaps.................. 2567
Vicks DayQuil Liquid...................... 2567
Vicks DayQuil Multi-Symptom Cold/Flu Relief............................ 2567
Vicks NyQuil Cold & Flu Multi-Symptom Relief.................. 617
Vicks NyQuil LiquiCaps.................. 2567
Vicks NyQuil Liquid........................ 2567
Vicks NyQuil Multi-Symptom Cold/Flu Relief............................ 2567
Vicodin Tablets.............................. 529
Vicodin ES Tablets.......................... 530
Vicodin HP Tablets.......................... 531
Zydone Tablets.............................. 1132

Alatrofloxacin Mesylate (Blood levels and/or toxicity of propranolol may be increased by administration of propranolol extended-release capsules with substrates of CYP1A2).
No products indexed under this heading.

Aluminum Hydroxide (Co-administration of propranolol with aluminum hydroxide gel (1,200 mg) resulted in a 50% decrease in propranolol concentrations).
No products indexed under this heading.

Amiodarone Hydrochloride (Amiodarone is an antiarrhythmic agent with negative chronotropic properties that may be additive to those seen with propranolol).
No products indexed under this heading.

Amitriptyline Hydrochloride (The hypotensive effects of tricyclic antidepressants may be exacerbated when administered with beta-blockers by interfering with the beta-blocking activity of propranolol).
No products indexed under this heading.

Amlodipine Besylate (Caution should be exercised when patients receiving a beta-blocker are administered a calcium-channel-blocking drug with negative inotropic and/or chronotropic effects. Both agents may depress myocardial contractility or atrioventricular conduction). Products include:
Azor Tablets.................................. 1005
Exforge Tablets.............................. 2238

Amoxapine (The hypotensive effects of tricyclic antidepressants may be exacerbated when administered with beta-blockers by interfering with the beta-blocking activity of propranolol).
No products indexed under this heading.

Amphetamine Aspartate (Blood levels and/or toxicity of propranolol may be increased by administration of propranolol extended-release capsules with substrates of CYP2D6). Products include:
Adderall XR Capsules..................... 3012

Amphetamine Aspartate Monohydrate (Blood levels and/or toxicity of propranolol may be increased by administration of propranolol extended-release capsules with substrates of CYP2D6).
No products indexed under this heading.

Amphetamine Sulfate (Blood levels and/or toxicity of propranolol may be increased by administration of propranolol extended-release capsules with substrates of CYP2D6). Products include:
Adderall XR Capsules..................... 3012

Anagrelide Hydrochloride (Blood levels and/or toxicity of propranolol may be increased by administration of propranolol extended-release capsules with substrates of CYP1A2). Products include:
Agrylin Capsules............................ 3017

Anastrozole (Blood levels and/or toxicity of propranolol may be increased by administration of propranolol hydrochloride extended-release capsules with inhibitors of CYP1A2). Products include:
Arimidex Tablets............................ 672

Atomoxetine Hydrochloride (Blood levels and/or toxicity of propranolol may be increased by administration of propranolol extended-release capsules with substrates of CYP2D6). Products include:
Strattera Capsules......................... 1864

Benazepril Hydrochloride (When combined with beta-blockers, ACE inhibitors can cause hypotension, particularly in the setting of acute myocardial infarction. Certain ACE inhibitors have been reported to increase bronchial hyper-reactivity when administered with propranolol).
No products indexed under this heading.

Bepridil Hydrochloride (Caution should be exercised when patients receiving a beta-blocker are administered a calcium-channel-blocking drug with negative inotropic and/or chronotropic effects. Both agents may depress myocardial contractility or atrioventricular conduction).
No products indexed under this heading.

Bisoprolol Fumarate (Blood levels and/or toxicity of propranolol may be increased by administration of propranolol extended-release capsules with substrates of CYP2D6).
No products indexed under this heading.

Bupropion Hydrochloride (Blood levels and/or toxicity of propranolol may be increased by administration of propranolol extended-release capsules with inhibitors of CYP2D6). Products include:
Wellbutrin Tablets.......................... 1648
Wellbutrin SR Sustained-Release Tablets.................................... 1653
Wellbutrin XL Extended-Release Tablets.................................... 1659
Zyban Sustained-Release Tablets..... 1692

Caffeine (Blood levels and/or toxicity of propranolol may be increased by administration of propranolol extended-release capsules with substrates of CYP1A2). Products include:
BioLean Free Tablets.................... 635
BioLean II Tablets......................... 635
Winrgy Dietary Supplement........... 642

Caffeine Anhydrous (Blood levels and/or toxicity of propranolol may be increased by administration of propranolol extended-release capsules with substrates of CYP1A2).
No products indexed under this heading.

Captopril (When combined with beta-blockers, ACE inhibitors can cause hypotension, particularly in the setting of acute myocardial infarction. Certain ACE inhibitors have been reported to increase bronchial hyper-reactivity when administered with propranolol). Products include:
Captopril Tablets........................... 2182

Carbamazepine (Blood levels of propranolol may be decreased by administration of propranolol extended-release capsules with inducers of hepatic drug metabolism). Products include:
Carbatrol Capsules........................ 3019
Equetro Extended-Release Capsules.................................... 3174

Carisoprodol (Blood levels and/or toxicity of propranolol may be increased by administration of propranolol extended-release capsules with substrates of CYP2C19). Products include:
Soma Tablets................................ 1931

Carvedilol (Blood levels and/or toxicity of propranolol may be increased by administration of propranolol extended-release capsules with substrates of CYP2D6). Products include:
Coreg Tablets............................... 1387

Celecoxib (Non-steroidal anti-inflammatory drugs (NSAIDs) have been reported to blunt the antihypertensive effects of beta-adreno receptor blocking agents). Products include:
Celebrex Capsules........................ 2979

Cevimeline Hydrochloride (Blood levels and/or toxicity of propranolol may be increased by administration of propranolol extended-release capsules with substrates of CYP2D6). Products include:
Evoxac Capsules........................... 1013

Chlordiazepoxide (Blood levels and/or toxicity of propranolol may be increased by administration of propranolol extended-release capsules with substrates of CYP1A2).
No products indexed under this heading.

Chlordiazepoxide Hydrochloride (Blood levels and/or toxicity of propranolol may be increased by administration of propranolol extended-release capsules with substrates of CYP1A2).
No products indexed under this heading.

Chloroquine Hydrochloride (Blood levels and/or toxicity of propranolol may be increased by administration of propranolol extended-release capsules with inhibitors of CYP2D6).
No products indexed under this heading.

Chloroquine Phosphate (Blood levels and/or toxicity of propranolol may be increased by administration of propranolol extended-release capsules with inhibitors of CYP2D6).
No products indexed under this heading.

Chlorpheniramine (Blood levels and/or toxicity of propranolol may be increased by administration of propranolol extended-release capsules with inhibitors of CYP2D6).
No products indexed under this heading.

Chlorpheniramine Maleate (Blood levels and/or toxicity of propranolol may be increased by administration of propranolol extended-release capsules with inhibitors of CYP2D6). Products include:
Actifed Cold & Allergy Tablets.......... 1895
Sudafed PE Sinus & Allergy Tablets....................................... 1908
Tylenol Allergy Multi-Symptom Caplets with Cool Burst and Rapid Release Gelcaps................ 1916
Children's Tylenol Plus Cold Suspension Liquid........................ 1912
Children's Tylenol Plus Cough & Runny Nose Suspension Liquid..... 1912
Children's Tylenol Plus Flu Suspension Liquid........................ 1914
Children's Tylenol Plus Multi-Symptom Cold Suspension Liquid........................ 1912
Tylenol Cold Head Congestion Nighttime Caplets with Cool Burst... 1910
Tylenol Cold Multi-Symptom Nighttime Caplets with Cool Burst... 1913
Tylenol Sinus Congestion & Pain Nighttime Caplets with Cool Burst... 1917

Chlorpheniramine Polistirex (Blood levels and/or toxicity of propranolol may be increased by administration of propranolol extended-release capsules with inhibitors of CYP2D6). Products include:
Tussionex Pennkinetic Extended-Release Suspension...... 3154

Chlorpheniramine Tannate (Blood levels and/or toxicity of propranolol may be increased by administration of propranolol extended-release capsules with inhibitors of CYP2D6).
No products indexed under this heading.

Chlorpromazine (Co-administration of chlorpromazine with propranolol resulted in increased plasma levels of both drugs (70% increase in propranolol concentrations)).
No products indexed under this heading.

Chlorpromazine Hydrochloride (Co-administration of chlorpromazine with propranolol resulted in increased plasma levels of both drugs (70% increase in propranolol concentrations)).
No products indexed under this heading.

Chlorpropamide (Blood levels of propranolol may be decreased by administration of propranolol extended-release capsules with inducers of hepatic drug metabolism).
No products indexed under this heading.

Cilostazol (Blood levels and/or toxicity of propranolol may be increased by administration of propranolol extended-release capsules with substrates of CYP2C19). Products include:
Pletal Tablets................................ 2481

Cimetidine (Co-administration of propranolol with cimetidine, a non-specific CYP450 inhibitor, increased propranolol concentrations by about 40%).
No products indexed under this heading.

Cimetidine Hydrochloride (Co-administration of propranolol with cimetidine, a non-specific CYP450 inhibitor, increased propranolol concentrations by about 40%).
No products indexed under this heading.

Ciprofloxacin (Blood levels and/or toxicity of propranolol may be increased by administration of propranolol extended-release capsules with substrates of CYP1A2). Products include:
Cipro I.V...................................... 2817
Cipro Oral Suspension.................... 2810

Cipro XR Tablets ... **2823**
Ciprodex Otic Suspension ... **541**

Ciprofloxacin Hydrochloride (Blood levels and/or toxicity of propranolol may be increased by administration of propranolol extended-release capsules with substrates of CYP1A2). Products include:
Cipro Tablets ... **2810**

Citalopram Hydrobromide (Blood levels and/or toxicity of propranolol may be increased by administration of propranolol extended-release capsules with inhibitors of CYP2D6). Products include:
Celexa ... **1160**

Clarithromycin (Blood levels and/or toxicity of propranolol may be increased by administration of propranolol hydrochloride extended-release capsules with inhibitors of CYP1A2). Products include:
Biaxin/Biaxin XL ... **411**

Clomipramine Hydrochloride (The hypotensive effects of tricyclic antidepressants may be exacerbated when administered with beta-blockers by interfering with the beta-blocking activity of propranolol).
No products indexed under this heading.

Clonidine (The antihypertensive effects of clonidine may be antagonized by beta-blockers. Propranolol extended-release capsules should be administered cautiously to patients withdrawing from clonidine). Products include:
Catapres-TTS ... **842**

Clonidine Hydrochloride (The antihypertensive effects of clonidine may be antagonized by beta-blockers. Propranolol extended-release capsules should be administered cautiously to patients withdrawing from clonidine). Products include:
Catapres Tablets ... **841**
Clorpres Tablets ... **2185**

Clopidogrel Bisulfate (Blood levels and/or toxicity of propranolol may be increased by administration of propranolol extended-release capsules with substrates of CYP1A2). Products include:
Plavix Tablets ... **926**
Plavix Tablets ... **2767**

Clozapine (Blood levels and/or toxicity of propranolol may be increased by administration of propranolol extended-release capsules with substrates of CYP2D6).
No products indexed under this heading.

Cocaine Hydrochloride (Blood levels and/or toxicity of propranolol may be increased by administration of propranolol extended-release capsules with inhibitors of CYP2D6).
No products indexed under this heading.

Codeine Phosphate (Blood levels and/or toxicity of propranolol may be increased by administration of propranolol extended-release capsules with substrates of CYP2D6). Products include:
Tylenol with Codeine Tablets ... **2427**

Codeine Sulfate (Blood levels and/or toxicity of propranolol may be increased by administration of propranolol extended-release capsules with substrates of CYP2D6).
No products indexed under this heading.

Colestipol (Co-administration of colestipol with propranolol resulted in up to 50% decrease in propranolol concentrations).
No products indexed under this heading.

Colestipol Hydrochloride (Co-administration of colestipol with propranolol resulted in up to 50% decrease in propranolol concentrations).
No products indexed under this heading.

Cyclobenzaprine (Blood levels and/or toxicity of propranolol may be increased by administration of propranolol extended-release capsules with substrates of CYP1A2).
No products indexed under this heading.

Cyclobenzaprine Hydrochloride (Blood levels and/or toxicity of propranolol may be increased by administration of propranolol extended-release capsules with substrates of CYP2D6). Products include:
Amrix Capsules ... **966**

Cyclophosphamide (Blood levels and/or toxicity of propranolol may be increased by administration of propranolol extended-release capsules with substrates of CYP2C19).
No products indexed under this heading.

Delavirdine Mesylate (Blood levels and/or toxicity of propranolol may be increased by administration of propranolol extended-release capsules with inhibitors of CYP2C19).
No products indexed under this heading.

Deserpidine (Patients receiving catecholamine-depleting drugs, (e.g. reserpine) and propranolol extended release capsules, should be closely observed for excessive reduction of resting sympathetic nervous activity, which may result in hypotension, marked bradycardia,vertigo, syncopal attacks, or orthostatic hypotension).
No products indexed under this heading.

Desipramine Hydrochloride (The hypotensive effects of tricyclic antidepressants may be exacerbated when administered with beta-blockers by interfering with the beta-blocking activity of propranolol).
No products indexed under this heading.

Deslanoside (Both digitalis glycosides and beta-blockers slow atrioventricular conduction and decrease heart rate. Concomitant use can increase the risk of bradycardia).
No products indexed under this heading.

Desogestrel (Blood levels and/or toxicity of propranolol may be increased by administration of propranolol hydrochloride extended-release capsules with inhibitors of CYP1A2). Products include:
Mircette Tablets ... **1034**

Dexfenfluramine Hydrochloride (Blood levels and/or toxicity of propranolol may be increased by administration of propranolol extended-release capsules with substrates of CYP2D6).
No products indexed under this heading.

Dextromethorphan (Blood levels and/or toxicity of propranolol may be increased by administration of propranolol extended-release capsules with substrates of CYP2C19).
No products indexed under this heading.

Dextromethorphan Hydrobromide (Blood levels and/or toxicity of propranolol may be increased by administration of propranolol extended-release capsules with substrates of CYP2D6). Products include:
PediaCare Children's Liquid Multi-Symptom Cold ... **1902**
PediaCare Children's Long-Acting Cough ... **1902**
Children's Sudafed PE Cold & Cough Liquid ... **1907**
Sudafed PE Cold & Cough Caplets ... **1907**
Children's Tylenol Plus Cough & Runny Nose Suspension Liquid ... **1912**
Children's Tylenol Plus Cough & Sore Throat Suspension Liquid ... **1912**
Children's Tylenol Plus Flu Suspension Liquid ... **1914**
Children's Tylenol Plus Multi-Symptom Cold Suspension Liquid ... **1912**
Tylenol Cold Severe Congestion Daytime Caplets with Cool Burst ... **1912**
Tylenol Cold Head Congestion Daytime Caplets with Cool Burst ... **1910**
Tylenol Cold Head Congestion Nighttime Caplets with Cool Burst ... **1910**
Tylenol Cold Head Congestion Severe Daytime Caplets with Cool Burst ... **1910**
Tylenol Cold Multi-Symptom Daytime Caplets with Cool Burst and Rapid Release Gels ... **1913**
Tylenol Cold Multi-Symptom Daytime Liquid with Citrus Burst ... **1913**
Tylenol Cold Multi-Symptom Nighttime Caplets with Cool Burst ... **1913**
Tylenol Cold Multi-Symptom Nighttime Liquid with Cool Burst ... **1913**
Tylenol Cold Multi-Symptom Severe Caplets with Cool Burst ... **1913**
Tylenol Cold Multi-Symptom Severe Daytime Liquid with Citrus Burst ... **1913**
Tylenol Cough & Sore Throat Daytime Liquid with Cool Burst ... **1918**
Tylenol Cough & Sore Throat Nighttime Liquid with Cool Burst ... **1918**
Vicks DayQuil Cold & Flu Multi-Symptom Relief ... ▣**616**
Vicks DayQuil LiquiCaps ... **2567**
Vicks DayQuil Liquid ... **2567**
Vicks DayQuil Multi-Symptom Cold/Flu Relief ... **2567**
Vicks NyQuil Cold & Flu Multi-Symptom Relief ... ▣**617**
Vicks NyQuil LiquiCaps ... **2567**
Vicks NyQuil Liquid ... **2567**
Vicks NyQuil Multi-Symptom Cold/Flu Relief ... **2567**

Dextromethorphan Polistirex (Blood levels and/or toxicity of propranolol may be increased by administration of propranolol extended-release capsules with substrates of CYP2D6).
No products indexed under this heading.

Diazepam (Propranolol can inhibit the metabolism of diazepam, resulting in increased concentrations of diazepam and its metabolites. Diazepam does not alter the pharmacokinetics of propranolol). Products include:
Valium Tablets ... **2658**

Diclofenac Epolamine (Non-steroidal anti-inflammatory drugs (NSAIDs) have been reported to blunt the antihypertensive effects of beta-adreno receptor blocking agents). Products include:
Flector Patch ... **561**

Diclofenac Potassium (Non-steroidal anti-inflammatory drugs (NSAIDs) have been reported to blunt the antihypertensive effects of beta-adreno receptor blocking agents).
No products indexed under this heading.

Diclofenac Sodium (Non-steroidal anti-inflammatory drugs (NSAIDs) have been reported to blunt the antihypertensive effects of beta-adreno receptor blocking agents). Products include:
Diclofenac Sodium Ophthalmic Solution ... ⊙**240**
Voltaren Ophthalmic Solution ... **2336**
Voltaren Tablets ... **2334**
Voltaren-XR Tablets ... **2337**

Digitalis Glycoside Preparations (Both digitalis glycosides and beta-blockers slow atrioventricular conduction and decrease heart rate. Concomitant use can increase the risk of bradycardia).
No products indexed under this heading.

Digitoxin (Both digitalis glycosides and beta-blockers slow atrioventricular conduction and decrease heart rate. Concomitant use can increase the risk of bradycardia).
No products indexed under this heading.

Digoxin (Both digitalis glycosides and beta-blockers slow atrioventricular conduction and decrease heart rate. Concomitant use can increase the risk of bradycardia). Products include:
Lanoxin Injection ... **1498**
Lanoxin Injection Pediatric ... **1502**
Lanoxin Tablets ... **1505**

Diltiazem Hydrochloride (Caution should be exercised when patients receiving a beta-blocker are administered a calcium-channel-blocking drug with negative inotropic and/or chronotropic effects. Both agents may depress myocardial contractility or atrioventricular conduction). Products include:
Cardizem LA Extended Release Tablets ... **421**

Diltiazem Maleate (Blood levels and/or toxicity of propranolol may be increased by administration of propranolol extended-release capsules with substrates of CYP1A2).
No products indexed under this heading.

Diphenhydramine (Blood levels and/or toxicity of propranolol may be increased by administration of propranolol extended-release capsules with inhibitors of CYP2D6).
No products indexed under this heading.

Diphenhydramine Hydrochloride (Blood levels and/or toxicity of propranolol may be increased by administration of propranolol extended-release capsules with inhibitors of CYP2D6). Products include:
Benadryl Allergy & Cold Kapgels ... **1895**
Benadryl Allergy & Sinus Headache Kapgels ... **1895**
Benadryl Severe Allergy & Sinus Headache Caplets ... **1897**
Benadryl Dye-Free Allergy Liqui-gels Softgels ... **1897**
Benadryl Allergy Kapgels ... **1895**
Benadryl Allergy Quick Dissolve Strips ... **1896**

Benadryl Allergy Ultratab Tablets **1896**
Children's Benadryl Dye-Free Allergy Liquid **1897**
Children's Benadryl Allergy Fastmelts **1897**
Children's Benadryl Allergy Liquid **1898**
Children's Benadryl Allergy Perfect Measure **1896**
Children's Benadryl-D Allergy & Sinus Liquid **1896**
Benadryl-D Allergy & Sinus Tablet **1896**
PediaCare Children's Allergy & Cold Liquid **1902**
PediaCare Children's Allergy Liquid **1902**
Simply Sleep Caplets **1905**
Sudafed PE Nighttime Cold Caplets **1907**
Sudafed PE Severe Cold Caplets **1908**
Extra Strength Tylenol PM Caplets, Geltabs, Liquid, and Rapid Release Gels **1915**
Tylenol Allergy Multi-Symptom Nighttime Caplets with Cool Burst **1916**
Tylenol Severe Allergy Caplets **1916**
Children's Tylenol Plus Cold & Allergy Suspension Liquid **1914**
Tylenol Sore Throat Nighttime Liquid with Cool Burst **1918**

Disopyramide (Disopyramide is a Type I antiarrhythmic drug with potent negative inotropic and chronotropic effects and has been associated with severe bradycardia, asystole, and heart failure when administered with propranolol).
No products indexed under this heading.

Disopyramide Phosphate (Disopyramide is a Type I antiarrhythmic drug with potent negative inotropic and chronotropic effects and has been associated with severe bradycardia, asystole, and heart failure when administered with propranolol).
No products indexed under this heading.

Divalproex Sodium (Blood levels and/or toxicity of propranolol may be increased by administration of propranolol extended-release capsules with substrates of CYP2C19). Products include:
Depakote ER Tablets **423**

Dobutamine (Propranolol is a competitive inhibitor of beta-receptor agonists, and its effects can be reversed by administration of such agents, eg, dobutamine. Also propranolol may reduce sensitivity to dobutamine stress echocardiography in patients undergoing evaluation for myocardial ischemia).
No products indexed under this heading.

Dobutamine Hydrochloride (Propranolol is a competitive inhibitor of beta-receptor agonists, and its effects can be reversed by administration of such agents, eg, dobutamine. Also propranolol may reduce sensitivity to dobutamine stress echocardiography in patients undergoing evaluation for myocardial ischemia).
No products indexed under this heading.

Dolasetron Mesylate (Blood levels and/or toxicity of propranolol may be increased by administration of propranolol extended-release capsules with substrates of CYP2D6). Products include:
Anzemet Injection **2701**
Anzemet Tablets **2704**

Donepezil Hydrochloride (Blood levels and/or toxicity of propranolol may be increased by administration of propranolol extended-release capsules with substrates of CYP2D6). Products include:
Aricept Tablets **1062**
Aricept ODT Tablets **1062**

Doxazosin Mesylate (Postural hypotension has been reported in patients taking both beta-blockers and doxazosin).
No products indexed under this heading.

Doxepin Hydrochloride (The hypotensive effects of tricyclic antidepressants may be exacerbated when administered with beta-blockers by interfering with the beta-blocking activity of propranolol).
No products indexed under this heading.

Efavirenz (Blood levels and/or toxicity of propranolol may be increased by administration of propranolol extended-release capsules with inhibitors of CYP2C19). Products include:
Atripla Tablets **938**
Sustiva Capsules **930**
Sustiva Tablets **930**

Enalapril Maleate (When combined with beta-blockers, ACE inhibitors can cause hypotension, particularly in the setting of acute myocardial infarction. Certain ACE inhibitors have been reported to increase bronchial hyper-reactivity when administered with propranolol).
No products indexed under this heading.

Enalaprilat (When combined with beta-blockers, ACE inhibitors can cause hypotension, particularly in the setting of acute myocardial infarction. Certain ACE inhibitors have been reported to increase bronchial hyper-reactivity when administered with propranolol).
No products indexed under this heading.

Encainide Hydrochloride (Blood levels and/or toxicity of propranolol may be increased by administration of propranolol extended-release capsules with substrates of CYP2D6).
No products indexed under this heading.

Enoxacin (Blood levels and/or toxicity of propranolol may be increased by administration of propranolol extended-release capsules with substrates of CYP1A2).
No products indexed under this heading.

Epinephrine (Patients on long term therapy with propranolol may experience uncontrolled hypertension if administered epinephrine as a consequence of unopposed alpha-receptor stimulation. Epinephrine is therefore not indicated in the treatment of propranolol overdose). Products include:
EpiPen **1024**

Epinephrine Bitartrate (Patients on long term therapy with propranolol may experience uncontrolled hypertension if administered epinephrine as a consequence of unopposed alpha-receptor stimulation. Epinephrine is therefore not indicated in the treatment of propranolol overdose).
No products indexed under this heading.

Epinephrine Hydrochloride (Patients on long term therapy with propranolol may experience uncontrolled hypertension if administered epinephrine as a consequence of unopposed alpha-receptor stimulation. Epinephrine is therefore not indicated in the treatment of propranolol overdose).
No products indexed under this heading.

Erythromycin (Blood levels and/or toxicity of propranolol may be increased by administration of propranolol extended-release capsules with substrates of CYP1A2).
No products indexed under this heading.

Erythromycin Estolate (Blood levels and/or toxicity of propranolol may be increased by administration of propranolol extended-release capsules with substrates of CYP1A2).
No products indexed under this heading.

Erythromycin Ethylsuccinate (Blood levels and/or toxicity of propranolol may be increased by administration of propranolol extended-release capsules with substrates of CYP1A2). Products include:
E.E.S. **433**
EryPed **431**

Erythromycin Gluceptate (Blood levels and/or toxicity of propranolol may be increased by administration of propranolol extended-release capsules with substrates of CYP1A2).
No products indexed under this heading.

Erythromycin Lactobionate (Blood levels and/or toxicity of propranolol may be increased by administration of propranolol extended-release capsules with substrates of CYP1A2).
No products indexed under this heading.

Erythromycin Stearate (Blood levels and/or toxicity of propranolol may be increased by administration of propranolol extended-release capsules with substrates of CYP1A2).
No products indexed under this heading.

Escitalopram Oxalate (Blood levels and/or toxicity of propranolol may be increased by administration of propranolol extended-release capsules with inhibitors of CYP2D6). Products include:
Lexapro Oral Suspension **1174**
Lexapro Tablets **1174**

Esomeprazole Magnesium (Blood levels and/or toxicity of propranolol may be increased by administration of propranolol extended-release capsules with substrates of CYP2C19). Products include:
Nexium Delayed-Release Capsules **645**
Nexium Delayed-Release Oral Suspension **645**

Estradiol (Blood levels and/or toxicity of propranolol may be increased by administration of propranolol extended-release capsules with substrates of CYP1A2). Products include:
Activella Tablets **2347**
Angeliq Tablets **751**
Climara Transdermal System **763**
Climara Pro Transdermal System **768**
Divigel **3167**
Vagifem Tablets **2375**

Estradiol Benzoate (Blood levels and/or toxicity of propranolol may be increased by administration of propranolol extended-release capsules with substrates of CYP1A2).
No products indexed under this heading.

Estradiol Cypionate (Blood levels and/or toxicity of propranolol may be increased by administration of propranolol extended-release capsules with substrates of CYP1A2).
No products indexed under this heading.

Ethanol (Blood levels of propranolol may be decreased by administration of propranolol extended-release capsules with inducers of hepatic drug metabolism).
No products indexed under this heading.

Ethinyl Estradiol (Blood levels and/or toxicity of propranolol may be increased by administration of propranolol hydrochloride extended-release capsules with inhibitors of CYP1A2). Products include:
Lybrel Tablets **3204**
Mircette Tablets **1034**
NuvaRing **2897**
Ortho-Cyclen/Ortho Tri-Cyclen **2449**
Ortho Evra Transdermal System **2437**
Ortho Tri-Cyclen Lo Tablets **2458**
Seasonique Tablets **1046**
Yaz Tablets **805**

Ethosuximide (Blood levels and/or toxicity of propranolol may be increased by administration of propranolol extended-release capsules with substrates of CYP2C19).
No products indexed under this heading.

Ethotoin (Blood levels and/or toxicity of propranolol may be increased by administration of propranolol extended-release capsules with substrates of CYP2C19).
No products indexed under this heading.

Ethynodiol Diacetate (Blood levels and/or toxicity of propranolol may be increased by administration of propranolol extended-release capsules with inhibitors of CYP2C19).
No products indexed under this heading.

Etodolac (Non-steroidal anti-inflammatory drugs (NSAIDs) have been reported to blunt the antihypertensive effects of beta-adreno receptor blocking agents).
No products indexed under this heading.

Felbamate (Blood levels and/or toxicity of propranolol may be increased by administration of propranolol extended-release capsules with substrates of CYP2C19).
No products indexed under this heading.

Felodipine (Caution should be exercised when patients receiving a beta-blocker are administered a calcium-channel-blocking drug with negative inotropic and/or chronotropic effects. Both agents may depress myocardial contractility or atrioventricular conduction).
No products indexed under this heading.

Fenoprofen Calcium (Non-steroidal anti-inflammatory drugs (NSAIDs) have been reported to blunt the antihypertensive effects of beta-adreno receptor blocking agents). Products include:
Nalfon Capsules **2508**

Fentanyl (Blood levels and/or toxicity of propranolol may be increased by administration of propranolol extended-release capsules with substrates of CYP2D6). Products include:
Duragesic Transdermal System 2405
Ionsys Transdermal System 2410

Fentanyl Citrate (Blood levels and/or toxicity of propranolol may be increased by administration of propranolol extended-release capsules with substrates of CYP2D6). Products include:
Actiq 959
Fentora Tablets 968

Flecainide Acetate (Blood levels and/or toxicity of propranolol may be increased by administration of propranolol extended-release capsules with substrates of CYP2D6).
No products indexed under this heading.

Fluconazole (Blood levels and/or toxicity of propranolol may be increased by administration of propranolol extended release capsules with inhibitors of CYP2C19 such as fluconazole).
No products indexed under this heading.

Fluoxetine (Blood levels and/or toxicity of propranolol may be increased by administration of propranolol extended-release capsules with substrates of CYP2D6).
No products indexed under this heading.

Fluoxetine Hydrochloride (Blood levels and/or toxicity of propranolol may be increased by administration of propranolol extended-release capsules with substrates of CYP2D6). Products include:
Prozac Weekly Capsules 1852
Prozac Pulvules and Liquid 1852
Symbyax Capsules 1871

Fluphenazine Decanoate (Blood levels and/or toxicity of propranolol may be increased by administration of propranolol extended-release capsules with substrates of CYP2D6).
No products indexed under this heading.

Fluphenazine Enanthate (Blood levels and/or toxicity of propranolol may be increased by administration of propranolol extended-release capsules with substrates of CYP2D6).
No products indexed under this heading.

Fluphenazine Hydrochloride (Blood levels and/or toxicity of propranolol may be increased by administration of propranolol extended-release capsules with substrates of CYP2D6).
No products indexed under this heading.

Flurbiprofen (Non-steroidal anti-inflammatory drugs (NSAIDs) have been reported to blunt the antihypertensive effects of beta-adreno receptor blocking agents).
No products indexed under this heading.

Flutamide (Blood levels and/or toxicity of propranolol may be increased by administration of propranolol extended-release capsules with substrates of CYP1A2).
No products indexed under this heading.

Fluticasone Propionate (Blood levels and/or toxicity of propranolol may be increased by administration of propranolol extended-release capsules with substrates of CYP1A2). Products include:
Advair Diskus 100/50 1276
Advair Diskus 250/50 1276
Advair Diskus 500/50 1276
Advair HFA 45/21 Inhalation Aerosol 1288
Advair HFA 115/21 Inhalation Aerosol 1288
Advair HFA 230/21 Inhalation Aerosol 1288
Flonase Nasal Spray 1431
Flovent Diskus 50 mcg 1435

Fluvastatin Sodium (Blood levels and/or toxicity of propranolol may be increased by administration of propranolol extended-release capsules with inhibitors of CYP2C19). Products include:
Lescol Capsules 2268
Lescol XL Tablets 2268

Fluvoxamine (Blood levels and/or toxicity of propranolol may be increased by administration of propranolol hydrochloride extended-release capsules with inhibitors of CYP1A2).
No products indexed under this heading.

Fluvoxamine Maleate (Blood levels and/or toxicity of propranolol may be increased by administration of propranolol extended-release capsules with substrates of CYP2D6). Products include:
Luvox CR Extended-Release Capsules 1759

Formoterol Fumarate (Blood levels and/or toxicity of propranolol may be increased by administration of propranolol extended-release capsules with substrates of CYP2D6). Products include:
Foradil Aerolizer 2849
Perforomist Inhalation Solution 1025

Fosinopril Sodium (When combined with beta-blockers, ACE inhibitors can cause hypotension, particularly in the setting of acute myocardial infarction. Certain ACE inhibitors have been reported to increase bronchial hyper-reactivity when administered with propranolol).
No products indexed under this heading.

Fosphenytoin (Blood levels and/or toxicity of propranolol may be increased by administration of propranolol extended-release capsules with substrates of CYP2C19).
No products indexed under this heading.

Fosphenytoin Sodium (Blood levels of propranolol may be decreased by administration of propranolol extended-release capsules with inducers of hepatic drug metabolism).
No products indexed under this heading.

Gabapentin (Blood levels and/or toxicity of propranolol may be increased by administration of propranolol extended-release capsules with substrates of CYP2C19).
No products indexed under this heading.

Galantamine Hydrobromide (Blood levels and/or toxicity of propranolol may be increased by administration of propranolol extended-release capsules with substrates of CYP2D6).
No products indexed under this heading.

Gatifloxacin (Blood levels and/or toxicity of propranolol may be increased by administration of propranolol hydrochloride extended-release capsules with inhibitors of CYP1A2).
No products indexed under this heading.

Gemifloxacin Mesylate (Blood levels and/or toxicity of propranolol may be increased by administration of propranolol hydrochloride extended-release capsules with inhibitors of CYP1A2).
No products indexed under this heading.

Glipizide (Blood levels of propranolol may be decreased by administration of propranolol extended-release capsules with inducers of hepatic drug metabolism).
No products indexed under this heading.

Glyburide (Blood levels of propranolol may be decreased by administration of propranolol extended-release capsules with inducers of hepatic drug metabolism).
No products indexed under this heading.

Grepafloxacin Hydrochloride (Blood levels and/or toxicity of propranolol may be increased by administration of propranolol extended-release capsules with substrates of CYP1A2).
No products indexed under this heading.

Guanethidine Monosulfate (Patients receiving catecholamine-depleting drugs, (e.g. reserpine) and propranolol extended release capsules, should be closely observed for excessive reduction of resting sympathetic nervous activity, which may result in hypotension, marked bradycardia,vertigo, syncopal attacks, or orthostatic hypotension).
No products indexed under this heading.

Halofantrine Hydrochloride (Blood levels and/or toxicity of propranolol may be increased by administration of propranolol extended-release capsules with inhibitors of CYP2D6).
No products indexed under this heading.

Haloperidol (Hypotension and cardiac arrest have been reported with the concomitant use of propranolol and haloperidol).
No products indexed under this heading.

Haloperidol Decanoate (Hypotension and cardiac arrest have been reported with the concomitant use of propranolol and haloperidol).
No products indexed under this heading.

Haloperidol Lactate (Hypotension and cardiac arrest have been reported with the concomitant use of propranolol and haloperidol).
No products indexed under this heading.

Hydrocodone Bitartrate (Blood levels and/or toxicity of propranolol may be increased by administration of propranolol extended-release capsules with substrates of CYP2D6). Products include:
Lortab 5/500 Tablets 3143
Lortab 7.5/500 Tablets 3144
Lortab 10/500 Tablets 3144
Vicodin Tablets 529
Vicodin ES Tablets 530
Vicodin HP Tablets 531
Vicoprofen Tablets 533
Zydone Tablets 1132

Hydroxychloroquine Sulfate (Blood levels and/or toxicity of propranolol may be increased by administration of propranolol extended-release capsules with inhibitors of CYP2D6).
No products indexed under this heading.

Ibuprofen (Non-steroidal anti-inflammatory drugs (NSAIDs) have been reported to blunt the antihypertensive effects of beta-adreno receptor blocking agents). Products include:
Motrin IB Tablets and Caplets 1900
Children's Motrin Oral Suspension ... 1901
Children's Motrin Non-Staining Dye-Free Oral Suspension 1901
Children's Motrin Cold Oral Suspension 1899
Infants' Motrin Concentrated Drops 1901
Infants' Motrin Non-Staining Dye-Free Concentrated Drops 1901
Junior Strength Motrin Caplets and Chewable Tablets 1901
Vicoprofen Tablets 533

Imatinib Mesylate (Blood levels and/or toxicity of propranolol may be increased by administration of propranolol extended-release capsules with inhibitors of CYP2D6). Products include:
Gleevec Tablets 2255

Imipramine Hydrochloride (The hypotensive effects of tricyclic antidepressants may be exacerbated when administered with beta-blockers by interfering with the beta-blocking activity of propranolol).
No products indexed under this heading.

Imipramine Pamoate (The hypotensive effects of tricyclic antidepressants may be exacerbated when administered with beta-blockers by interfering with the beta-blocking activity of propranolol).
No products indexed under this heading.

Indomethacin (Administration of indomethacin with propranolol may reduce the efficacy of propranolol in reducing blood pressure and heart rate). Products include:
Indocin 2024

Indomethacin Sodium Trihydrate (Administration of indomethacin with propranolol may reduce the efficacy of propranolol in reducing blood pressure and heart rate). Products include:
Indocin I.V. 2489

Indoramin Hydrochloride (Blood levels and/or toxicity of propranolol may be increased by administration of propranolol extended-release capsules with substrates of CYP2D6).
No products indexed under this heading.

Insulin (Beta-adrenergic blockade may prevent the appearance of certain premonitory signs and symptoms (pulse rate and blood pressure changes) of acute hypoglycemia, especially in labile insulin-dependent diabetics. In these patients, it may be more difficult to adjust the dosage of insulin).
No products indexed under this heading.

Insulin, Human, Zinc Suspension (Beta-adrenergic blockade may prevent the appearance of certain premonitory signs and symptoms (pulse rate and blood pressure changes) of acute hypoglycemia, especially in labile insulin-dependent diabetics. In these patients, it may be more difficult to adjust the dosage of insulin).
No products indexed under this heading.

Insulin, Human (rDNA origin) (Beta-adrenergic blockade may prevent the appearance of certain premonitory signs and symptoms (pulse rate and blood pressure changes) of acute hypoglycemia, especially in labile insulin-dependent diabetics. In these patients, it may be more difficult to adjust the dosage of insulin). Products include:
Exubera Inhalation Powder 2515

Insulin, Human NPH (Beta-adrenergic blockade may prevent the appearance of certain premonitory signs and symptoms (pulse rate and blood pressure changes) of acute hypoglycemia, especially in labile insulin-dependent diabetics. In these patients, it may be more difficult to adjust the dosage of insulin).
Products include:
Humulin N Vial 1846

Insulin, Human Regular (Beta-adrenergic blockade may prevent the appearance of certain premonitory signs and symptoms (pulse rate and blood pressure changes) of acute hypoglycemia, especially in labile insulin-dependent diabetics. In these patients, it may be more difficult to adjust the dosage of insulin).
Products include:
Humulin R 1849
Humulin R (U-500) 1850

Insulin, Human Regular and Human NPH Mixture (Beta-adrenergic blockade may prevent the appearance of certain premonitory signs and symptoms (pulse rate and blood pressure changes) of acute hypoglycemia, especially in labile insulin-dependent diabetics. In these patients, it may be more difficult to adjust the dosage of insulin).
Products include:
Humulin 50/50, 100 Units 1843
Humulin 70/30 Vial 1844

Insulin, NPH (Beta-adrenergic blockade may prevent the appearance of certain premonitory signs and symptoms (pulse rate and blood pressure changes) of acute hypoglycemia, especially in labile insulin-dependent diabetics. In these patients, it may be more difficult to adjust the dosage of insulin).
No products indexed under this heading.

Insulin, Regular (Beta-adrenergic blockade may prevent the appearance of certain premonitory signs and symptoms (pulse rate and blood pressure changes) of acute hypoglycemia, especially in labile insulin-dependent diabetics. In these patients, it may be more difficult to adjust the dosage of insulin).
No products indexed under this heading.

Insulin, Regular and NPH mixture (Beta-adrenergic blockade may prevent the appearance of certain premonitory signs and symptoms (pulse rate and blood pressure changes) of acute hypoglycemia, especially in labile insulin-dependent diabetics. In these patients, it may be more difficult to adjust the dosage of insulin).
No products indexed under this heading.

Insulin, Zinc Crystals (Beta-adrenergic blockade may prevent the appearance of certain premonitory signs and symptoms (pulse rate and blood pressure changes) of acute hypoglycemia, especially in labile insulin-dependent diabetics. In these patients, it may be more difficult to adjust the dosage of insulin).
No products indexed under this heading.

Insulin, Zinc Suspension (Beta-adrenergic blockade may prevent the appearance of certain premonitory signs and symptoms (pulse rate and blood pressure changes) of acute hypoglycemia, especially in labile insulin-dependent diabetics. In these patients, it may be more difficult to adjust the dosage of insulin).
No products indexed under this heading.

Insulin Aspart (Beta-adrenergic blockade may prevent the appearance of certain premonitory signs and symptoms (pulse rate and blood pressure changes) of acute hypoglycemia, especially in labile insulin-dependent diabetics. In these patients, it may be more difficult to adjust the dosage of insulin).
No products indexed under this heading.

Insulin Aspart, Human (Beta-adrenergic blockade may prevent the appearance of certain premonitory signs and symptoms (pulse rate and blood pressure changes) of acute hypoglycemia, especially in labile insulin-dependent diabetics. In these patients, it may be more difficult to adjust the dosage of insulin).
Products include:
NovoLog Mix 70/30 2364

Insulin Aspart, Human Regular (Beta-adrenergic blockade may prevent the appearance of certain premonitory signs and symptoms (pulse rate and blood pressure changes) of acute hypoglycemia, especially in labile insulin-dependent diabetics. In these patients, it may be more difficult to adjust the dosage of insulin).
Products include:
NovoLog Injection 2359

Insulin Aspart Protamine, Human (Beta-adrenergic blockade may prevent the appearance of certain premonitory signs and symptoms (pulse rate and blood pressure changes) of acute hypoglycemia, especially in labile insulin-dependent diabetics. In these patients, it may be more difficult to adjust the dosage of insulin). Products include:
NovoLog Mix 70/30 2364

Insulin Detemir (rDNA Origin) (Beta-adrenergic blockade may prevent the appearance of certain premonitory signs and symptoms (pulse rate and blood pressure changes) of acute hypoglycemia, especially in labile insulin-dependent diabetics. In these patients, it may be more difficult to adjust the dosage of insulin).
Products include:
Levemir Injection 2352

Insulin glargine (Beta-adrenergic blockade may prevent the appearance of certain premonitory signs and symptoms (pulse rate and blood pressure changes) of acute hypoglycemia, especially in labile insulin-dependent diabetics. In these patients, it may be more difficult to adjust the dosage of insulin).
Products include:
Lantus Injection 2749

Insulin Glulisine (Beta-adrenergic blockade may prevent the appearance of certain premonitory signs and symptoms (pulse rate and blood pressure changes) of acute hypoglycemia, especially in labile insulin-dependent diabetics. In these patients, it may be more difficult to adjust the dosage of insulin).
Products include:
Apidra Injection 2706

Insulin Lispro, Human (Beta-adrenergic blockade may prevent the appearance of certain premonitory signs and symptoms (pulse rate and blood pressure changes) of acute hypoglycemia, especially in labile insulin-dependent diabetics. In these patients, it may be more difficult to adjust the dosage of insulin).
Products include:
Humalog-Pen and KwikPen 1829
Humalog Mix 50/50-Pen and KwikPen 1833
Humalog Mix 75/25-Pen and KwikPen 1835

Insulin Lispro Protamine, Human (Beta-adrenergic blockade may prevent the appearance of certain premonitory signs and symptoms (pulse rate and blood pressure changes) of acute hypoglycemia, especially in labile insulin-dependent diabetics. In these patients, it may be more difficult to adjust the dosage of insulin).
Products include:
Humalog Mix 50/50-Pen and KwikPen 1833
Humalog Mix 75/25-Pen and KwikPen 1835

Isocarboxazid (The hypotensive effects of MAO inhibitors may be exacerbated when administered with beta-blockers by interfering with the beta-blocking activity of propranolol).
Products include:
Marplan Tablets 3177

Isoniazid (Blood levels and/or toxicity of propranolol may be increased by administration of propranolol hydrochloride extended-release capsules with inhibitors of CYP1A2).
No products indexed under this heading.

Isoproterenol Hydrochloride (Propranolol is a competitive inhibitor of beta-receptor agonists, and its effects can be reversed by administration of such agents, eg, isoproterenol).
No products indexed under this heading.

Isoproterenol Sulfate (Propranolol is a competitive inhibitor of beta-receptor agonists, and its effects can be reversed by administration of such agents, eg, isoproterenol).
No products indexed under this heading.

Isradipine (Caution should be exercised when patients receiving a beta-blocker are administered a calcium-channel-blocking drug with negative inotropic and/or chronotropic effects. Both agents may depress myocardial contractility or atrioventricular conduction). Products include:
DynaCirc CR Controlled Release Tablets 1407

Ketoconazole (Blood levels and/or toxicity of propranolol may be increased by administration of propranolol hydrochloride extended-release capsules with inhibitors of CYP1A2). Products include:
Extina Foam, 2% 3057
Nizoral A-D Shampoo 1901

Ketoprofen (Non-steroidal anti-inflammatory drugs (NSAIDs) have been reported to blunt the antihypertensive effects of beta-adreno receptor blocking agents).
No products indexed under this heading.

Ketorolac Tromethamine (Non-steroidal anti-inflammatory drugs (NSAIDs) have been reported to blunt the antihypertensive effects of beta-adreno receptor blocking agents).
No products indexed under this heading.

Labetalol Hydrochloride (Blood levels and/or toxicity of propranolol may be increased by administration of propranolol extended-release capsules with substrates of CYP2D6).
No products indexed under this heading.

Lamotrigine (Blood levels and/or toxicity of propranolol may be increased by administration of propranolol extended-release capsules with substrates of CYP2C19).
Products include:
Lamictal 1488

Lansoprazole (Blood levels and/or toxicity of propranolol may be increased by administration of propranolol extended-release capsules with substrates of CYP2C19).
No products indexed under this heading.

Letrozole (Blood levels and/or toxicity of propranolol may be increased by administration of propranolol extended-release capsules with inhibitors of CYP2C19). Products include:
Femara Tablets 2246

Levetiracetam (Blood levels and/or toxicity of propranolol may be increased by administration of propranolol extended-release capsules with substrates of CYP2C19).
Products include:
Keppra Injection 3137
Keppra Oral Solution 3131
Keppra Tablets 3131

Levobupivacaine Hydrochloride (Blood levels and/or toxicity of propranolol may be increased by administration of propranolol extended-release capsules with substrates of CYP1A2).
No products indexed under this heading.

Levofloxacin (Blood levels and/or toxicity of propranolol may be increased by administration of propranolol hydrochloride extended-release capsules with inhibitors of CYP1A2). Products include:
Iquix Ophthalmic Solution 3183
Levaquin 2416
Levaquin in 5% Dextrose Injection 2416
Quixin Ophthalmic Solution 3184

Levonorgestrel (Blood levels and/or toxicity of propranolol may be

increased by administration of propranolol hydrochloride extended-release capsules with inhibitors of CYP1A2). Products include:
Climara Pro Transdermal System 768
Lybrel Tablets 3204
Mirena Intrauterine System 779
Plan B Tablets 1044
Seasonique Tablets 1046

Lidocaine (The metabolism of lidocaine is inhibited by co-administration of propranolol, resulting in a 25% increase in lidocaine concentrations. Lidocaine toxicity has been reported following co-administration with propranolol. Caution should be exercised when administering propranolol extended release capsules with drugs that slow A-V nodal conduction eg, lidocaine). Products include:
Lidoderm Patch 1114

Lidocaine Base (The metabolism of lidocaine is inhibited by co-administration of propranolol, resulting in a 25% increase in lidocaine concentrations. Lidocaine toxicity has been reported following co-administration with propranolol. Caution should be exercised when administering propranolol extended release capsules with drugs that slow A-V nodal conduction eg, lidocaine).
No products indexed under this heading.

Lidocaine Hydrochloride (The metabolism of lidocaine is inhibited by co-administration of propranolol, resulting in a 25% increase in lidocaine concentrations. Lidocaine toxicity has been reported following co-administration with propranolol. Caution should be exercised when administering propranolol extended release capsules with drugs that slow A-V nodal conduction eg, lidocaine).
No products indexed under this heading.

Lisinopril (When combined with beta-blockers, ACE inhibitors can cause hypotension, particularly in the setting of acute myocardial infarction. Certain ACE inhibitors have been reported to increase bronchial hyper-reactivity when administered with propranolol). Products include:
Prinivil Tablets 2087
Prinzide Tablets 2092

Lomefloxacin Hydrochloride (Blood levels and/or toxicity of propranolol may be increased by administration of propranolol extended-release capsules with substrates of CYP1A2).
No products indexed under this heading.

Lovastatin (Co-administration of propranolol with lovastatin decreased the AUC of lovastatin by 20% to 25% but did not alter its pharmacodynamics). Products include:
Advicor Tablets 402
Mevacor Tablets 2063

Maprotiline Hydrochloride (The hypotensive effects of tricyclic antidepressants may be exacerbated when administered with beta-blockers by interfering with the beta-blocking activity of propranolol).
No products indexed under this heading.

Meclofenamate Sodium (Non-steroidal anti-inflammatory drugs (NSAIDs) have been reported to blunt the antihypertensive effects of beta-adreno receptor blocking agents).
No products indexed under this heading.

Mefenamic Acid (Non-steroidal anti-inflammatory drugs (NSAIDs) have been reported to blunt the antihypertensive effects of beta-adreno receptor blocking agents).
No products indexed under this heading.

Meloxicam (Non-steroidal anti-inflammatory drugs (NSAIDs) have been reported to blunt the antihypertensive effects of beta-adreno receptor blocking agents). Products include:
Mobic Oral Suspension 863
Mobic Tablets 863

Meperidine Hydrochloride (Blood levels and/or toxicity of propranolol may be increased by administration of propranolol extended-release capsules with substrates of CYP2D6).
No products indexed under this heading.

Mephenytoin (Blood levels and/or toxicity of propranolol may be increased by administration of propranolol extended-release capsules with substrates of CYP2C19).
No products indexed under this heading.

Mephobarbital (Blood levels and/or toxicity of propranolol may be increased by administration of propranolol extended-release capsules with substrates of CYP2C19).
No products indexed under this heading.

Meprobamate (Blood levels and/or toxicity of propranolol may be increased by administration of propranolol extended-release capsules with substrates of CYP2C19).
No products indexed under this heading.

Mestranol (Blood levels and/or toxicity of propranolol may be increased by administration of propranolol hydrochloride extended-release capsules with inhibitors of CYP1A2).
No products indexed under this heading.

Methadone Hydrochloride (Blood levels and/or toxicity of propranolol may be increased by administration of propranolol extended-release capsules with substrates of CYP2D6).
No products indexed under this heading.

Methamphetamine Hydrochloride (Blood levels and/or toxicity of propranolol may be increased by administration of propranolol extended-release capsules with substrates of CYP2D6).
No products indexed under this heading.

Methoxsalen (Blood levels and/or toxicity of propranolol may be increased by administration of propranolol hydrochloride extended-release capsules with inhibitors of CYP1A2).
No products indexed under this heading.

Methoxyflurane (Methoxyflurane may depress myocardial contractility when administered with propranolol).
No products indexed under this heading.

Methsuximide (Blood levels and/or toxicity of propranolol may be increased by administration of propranolol extended-release capsules with substrates of CYP2C19).
No products indexed under this heading.

Metoprolol Succinate (Blood levels and/or toxicity of propranolol may be increased by administration of propranolol extended-release capsules with substrates of CYP2D6). Products include:
Toprol-XL Tablets 666

Metoprolol Tartrate (Blood levels and/or toxicity of propranolol may be increased by administration of propranolol extended-release capsules with substrates of CYP2D6).
No products indexed under this heading.

Mexiletine Hydrochloride (Blood levels and/or toxicity of propranolol may be increased by administration of propranolol extended-release capsules with substrates of CYP2D6).
No products indexed under this heading.

Mibefradil Dihydrochloride (Caution should be exercised when patients receiving a beta-blocker are administered a calcium-channel-blocking drug with negative inotropic and/or chronotropic effects. Both agents may depress myocardial contractility or atrioventricular conduction).
No products indexed under this heading.

Midazolam Hydrochloride (Blood levels and/or toxicity of propranolol may be increased by administration of propranolol extended-release capsules with substrates of CYP2C19).
No products indexed under this heading.

Mirtazapine (Blood levels and/or toxicity of propranolol may be increased by administration of propranolol extended-release capsules with substrates of CYP2D6). Products include:
Remeron Tablets 2924
RemeronSolTab Tablets 2927

Moclobemide (The hypotensive effects of MAO inhibitors may be exacerbated when administered with beta-blockers by interfering with the beta-blocking activity of propranolol).
No products indexed under this heading.

Modafinil (Blood levels and/or toxicity of propranolol may be increased by administration of propranolol extended-release capsules with inhibitors of CYP2C19). Products include:
Provigil Tablets 977

Moexipril Hydrochloride (When combined with beta-blockers, ACE inhibitors can cause hypotension, particularly in the setting of acute myocardial infarction. Certain ACE inhibitors have been reported to increase bronchial hyper-reactivity when administered with propranolol).
No products indexed under this heading.

Morphine Sulfate (Blood levels and/or toxicity of propranolol may be increased by administration of propranolol extended-release capsules with substrates of CYP2D6). Products include:
Avinza Capsules 1772
DepoDur Injection 1095
MS Contin Tablets 2585

Moxifloxacin Hydrochloride (Blood levels and/or toxicity of propranolol may be increased by administration of propranolol extended-release capsules with substrates of CYP1A2). Products include:
Avelox 2803
Vigamox Ophthalmic Solution 548

Nabumetone (Non-steroidal anti-inflammatory drugs (NSAIDs) have been reported to blunt the antihypertensive effects of beta-adreno receptor blocking agents).
No products indexed under this heading.

Nafcillin Sodium (Blood levels and/or toxicity of propranolol may be increased by administration of propranolol extended-release capsules with substrates of CYP1A2).
No products indexed under this heading.

Nalidixic Acid (Blood levels and/or toxicity of propranolol may be increased by administration of propranolol hydrochloride extended-release capsules with inhibitors of CYP1A2).
No products indexed under this heading.

Naproxen (Non-steroidal anti-inflammatory drugs (NSAIDs) have been reported to blunt the antihypertensive effects of beta-adreno receptor blocking agents). Products include:
EC-Naprosyn Delayed-Release Tablets 2632
Naprosyn Suspension 2632
Naprosyn Tablets 2632

Naproxen Sodium (Non-steroidal anti-inflammatory drugs (NSAIDs) have been reported to blunt the antihypertensive effects of beta-adreno receptor blocking agents). Products include:
Anaprox Tablets 2632
Anaprox DS Tablets 2632
Treximet Tablets 1616

Nelfinavir Mesylate (Blood levels and/or toxicity of propranolol may be increased by administration of propranolol extended-release capsules with substrates of CYP2D6).
No products indexed under this heading.

Nicardipine (The mean Cmax and AUC of propranolol are increased respectively, by 80% and 47% by co-administration of nicardipine).
No products indexed under this heading.

Nicardipine Hydrochloride (The mean Cmax and AUC of propranolol are increased respectively, by 80% and 47% by co-administration of nicardipine). Products include:
Cardene I.V. 1093

Nicotine Polacrilex (Blood levels and/or toxicity of propranolol may be increased by administration of propranolol extended-release capsules with substrates of CYP1A2).
No products indexed under this heading.

Nicotine Salicylate (Blood levels and/or toxicity of propranolol may be increased by administration of propranolol extended-release capsules with substrates of CYP1A2).
No products indexed under this heading.

Nicotine Sulfate (Blood levels and/or toxicity of propranolol may be increased by administration of propranolol extended-release capsules with substrates of CYP1A2).
No products indexed under this heading.

Nifedipine (The mean Cmax and AUC of nifedipine are increased by 64% and 79% respectively, by co-administration of propranolol).
No products indexed under this heading.

Nilutamide (Blood levels and/or toxicity of propranolol may be increased by administration of propranolol extended-release capsules with substrates of CYP2C19).
No products indexed under this heading.

Nimodipine (Caution should be exercised when patients receiving a beta-blocker are administered a calcium-channel-blocking drug with negative inotropic and/or chronotropic effects. Both agents may depress myocardial contractility or atrioventricular conduction).
Products include:
Nimotop Capsules 790

Nisoldipine (The mean Cmax and AUC of propranolol are increased by respectively, by 50% and 30% by co-administration of nisoldipine).
Products include:
Sular Extended Release Tablets 2975

Norethindrone (Blood levels and/or toxicity of propranolol may be increased by administration of propranolol hydrochloride extended-release capsules with inhibitors of CYP1A2). Products include:
Ortho Micronor Tablets 2446

Norethindrone Acetate (Blood levels and/or toxicity of propranolol may be increased by administration of propranolol extended-release capsules with substrates of CYP1A2).
Products include:
Activella Tablets 2347

Norethynodrel (Blood levels and/or toxicity of propranolol may be increased by administration of propranolol extended-release capsules with inhibitors of CYP2C19).
No products indexed under this heading.

Norfloxacin (Blood levels and/or toxicity of propranolol may be increased by administration of propranolol extended-release capsules with substrates of CYP1A2).
Products include:
Noroxin Tablets 2069

Norgestimate (Blood levels and/or toxicity of propranolol may be increased by administration of propranolol extended-release capsules with inhibitors of CYP2C19).
Products include:
Ortho-Cyclen/Ortho Tri-Cyclen 2449
Ortho Tri-Cyclen Lo Tablets 2458

Norgestrel (Blood levels and/or toxicity of propranolol may be increased by administration of propranolol hydrochloride extended-release capsules with inhibitors of CYP1A2).
No products indexed under this heading.

Nortriptyline Hydrochloride (The hypotensive effects of tricyclic antidepressants may be exacerbated when administered with beta-blockers by interfering with the beta-blocking activity of propranolol).
No products indexed under this heading.

Ofloxacin (Blood levels and/or toxicity of propranolol may be increased by administration of propranolol extended-release capsules with substrates of CYP1A2). Products include:
Ofloxacin Ophthalmic Solution 0.3% .... ⊙ 243

Olanzapine (Blood levels and/or toxicity of propranolol may be increased by administration of propranolol extended-release capsules with substrates of CYP2D6).
Products include:
Symbyax Capsules 1871
Zyprexa Tablets 1883
Zyprexa IntraMuscular 1883
Zyprexa ZYDIS Orally Disintegrating Tablets 1883

Omeprazole (Blood levels and/or toxicity of propranolol may be increased by administration of propranolol extended-release capsules with substrates of CYP2D6).
No products indexed under this heading.

Ondansetron (Blood levels and/or toxicity of propranolol may be increased by administration of propranolol extended-release capsules with substrates of CYP2D6).
Products include:
Zofran ODT Orally Disintegrating Tablets 1687

Ondansetron Hydrochloride (Blood levels and/or toxicity of propranolol may be increased by administration of propranolol extended-release capsules with substrates of CYP2D6). Products include:
Zofran Injection 1682
Zofran 1687

Oxaprozin (Non-steroidal anti-inflammatory drugs (NSAIDs) have been reported to blunt the antihypertensive effects of beta-adreno receptor blocking agents).
No products indexed under this heading.

Oxcarbazepine (Blood levels and/or toxicity of propranolol may be increased by administration of propranolol extended-release capsules with substrates of CYP2C19).
No products indexed under this heading.

Oxycodone Hydrochloride (Blood levels and/or toxicity of propranolol may be increased by administration of propranolol extended-release capsules with substrates of CYP2D6).
Products include:
OxyContin Tablets 2589
OxyIR Capsules 2593
Percocet Tablets 1127
Percodan Tablets 1130

Paclitaxel (Blood levels and/or toxicity of propranolol may be increased by administration of propranolol extended-release capsules with substrates of CYP2D6).
No products indexed under this heading.

Pantoprazole Sodium (Blood levels and/or toxicity of propranolol may be increased by administration of propranolol extended-release capsules with substrates of CYP2C19).
Products include:
Protonix for Delayed-Release Oral Suspension 3254
Protonix Delayed-Release Tablets 3254
Protonix I.V. 3257

Paramethadione (Blood levels and/or toxicity of propranolol may be increased by administration of propranolol extended-release capsules with substrates of CYP2C19).
No products indexed under this heading.

Pargyline Hydrochloride (The hypotensive effects of MAO inhibitors may be exacerbated when administered with beta-blockers by interfering with the beta-blocking activity of propranolol).
No products indexed under this heading.

Paroxetine Hydrochloride (Blood levels and/or toxicity of propranolol may be increased by administration of propranolol extended-release capsules with substrates of CYP2D6).
Products include:
Paxil 1535
Paxil CR Controlled-Release Tablets 1544

Pentamidine Isethionate (Blood levels and/or toxicity of propranolol may be increased by administration of propranolol extended-release capsules with substrates of CYP2C19).
No products indexed under this heading.

Perindopril Erbumine (When combined with beta-blockers, ACE inhibitors can cause hypotension, particularly in the setting of acute myocardial infarction. Certain ACE inhibitors have been reported to increase bronchial hyper-reactivity when administered with propranolol).
Products include:
Aceon Tablets (2 mg, 4 mg, 8 mg) 3038

Perphenazine (Blood levels and/or toxicity of propranolol may be increased by administration of propranolol extended-release capsules with inhibitors of CYP2D6).
No products indexed under this heading.

Phenacemide (Blood levels and/or toxicity of propranolol may be increased by administration of propranolol extended-release capsules with substrates of CYP2C19).
No products indexed under this heading.

Phenelzine Sulfate (The hypotensive effects of MAO inhibitors may be exacerbated when administered with beta-blockers by interfering with the beta-blocking activity of propranolol).
No products indexed under this heading.

Phenobarbital (Blood levels of propranolol may be decreased by administration of propranolol extended-release capsules with inducers of hepatic drug metabolism). Products include:
Donnatal Extentabs 2507

Phenobarbital Sodium (Blood levels and/or toxicity of propranolol may be increased by administration of propranolol extended-release capsules with substrates of CYP1A2).
No products indexed under this heading.

Phensuximide (Blood levels and/or toxicity of propranolol may be increased by administration of propranolol extended-release capsules with substrates of CYP2C19).
No products indexed under this heading.

Phenylbutazone (Blood levels of propranolol may be decreased by administration of propranolol extended-release capsules with inducers of hepatic drug metabolism).
No products indexed under this heading.

Phenytoin (Blood levels of propranolol may be decreased by administration of propranolol extended-release capsules with inducers of hepatic drug metabolism).
No products indexed under this heading.

Phenytoin Sodium (Blood levels of propranolol may be decreased by administration of propranolol extended-release capsules with inducers of hepatic drug metabolism). Products include:
Phenytek Capsules 2192

Pindolol (Blood levels and/or toxicity of propranolol may be increased by administration of propranolol extended-release capsules with substrates of CYP2D6).
No products indexed under this heading.

Piroxicam (Non-steroidal anti-inflammatory drugs (NSAIDs) have been reported to blunt the antihypertensive effects of beta-adreno receptor blocking agents).
No products indexed under this heading.

Pravastatin Sodium (Co-administration of propranolol with pravastatin decreased the AUC of pravastatin by 20% to 25% but did not alter its pharmacodynamics).
No products indexed under this heading.

Prazosin Hydrochloride (Prazosin has been associated with prolongation of first dose hypotension in the presence of beta-blockers).
No products indexed under this heading.

Primidone (Blood levels and/or toxicity of propranolol may be increased by administration of propranolol extended-release capsules with substrates of CYP2C19).
No products indexed under this heading.

Procarbazine Hydrochloride (The hypotensive effects of MAO inhibitors may be exacerbated when administered with beta-blockers by interfering with the beta-blocking activity of propranolol).
No products indexed under this heading.

Progesterone (Blood levels and/or toxicity of propranolol may be increased by administration of propranolol extended-release capsules with substrates of CYP2C19).
Products include:
Crinone 4% Gel 992
Crinone 8% Gel 992
Prometrium Capsules (100 mg, 200 mg) 3047

Proguanil Hydrochloride (Blood levels and/or toxicity of propranolol may be increased by administration of propranolol extended-release capsules with substrates of CYP2C19).
Products include:

IMPORTANT NOTE: Always consult each drug listing in the patient's regimen for possible interactions.

Malarone Pediatric Tablets 1521
Malarone Tablets 1521

Propafenone Hydrochloride (Propafenone has negative inotropic and beta-blocking properties that can be additive to those of propranolol. The concomitant administration of propranolol and propafenone increased propranolol average steady-state plasma concentrations (213%), AUC (113%), Cmax (83%), Tmax (55%), and T1/2 (30%), and significantly decreased plasma levels of 4-hydroxy-propranolol. Co-administration of propranolol and propafenone did not produce any significant change in propafenone pharmacokinetics. While the therapeuticrange for propranolol is wide, a reduction in dosage may be necessary during concomitant administration with propafenone). Products include:

Rythmol Tablets 1586
Rythmol SR Capsules 1590

Propoxyphene Hydrochloride (Blood levels and/or toxicity of propranolol may be increased by administration of propranolol extended-release capsules with substrates of CYP2D6).
No products indexed under this heading.

Propoxyphene Napsylate (Blood levels and/or toxicity of propranolol may be increased by administration of propranolol extended-release capsules with substrates of CYP2D6).
No products indexed under this heading.

Protriptyline Hydrochloride (The hypotensive effects of tricyclic antidepressants may be exacerbated when administered with beta-blockers by interfering with the beta-blocking activity of propranolol).
No products indexed under this heading.

Quetiapine Fumarate (Blood levels and/or toxicity of propranolol may be increased by administration of propranolol extended-release capsules with substrates of CYP2D6).
No products indexed under this heading.

Quinacrine Hydrochloride (Blood levels and/or toxicity of propranolol may be increased by administration of propranolol extended-release capsules with inhibitors of CYP2D6).
No products indexed under this heading.

Quinapril Hydrochloride (When combined with beta-blockers, ACE inhibitors can cause hypotension, particularly in the setting of acute myocardial infarction. Certain ACE inhibitors have been reported to increase bronchial hyper-reactivity when administered with propranolol).
No products indexed under this heading.

Quinidine (The metabolism of propranolol is reduced by co-administration of quinidine, leading to a 2- to 3-fold increase in blood concentrations and greater degrees of clinical beta-blockade. Concurrent use my cause postural hypotension).
No products indexed under this heading.

Quinidine Gluconate (The metabolism of propranolol is reduced by co-administration of quinidine, leading to a 2- to 3-fold increase in blood concentrations and greater degrees of clinical beta-blockade. Concurrent use my cause postural hypotension).
No products indexed under this heading.

Quinidine Hydrochloride (The metabolism of propranolol is reduced by co-administration of quinidine, leading to a 2- to 3-fold increase in blood concentrations and greater degrees of clinical beta-blockade. Concurrent use my cause postural hypotension).
No products indexed under this heading.

Quinidine Polygalacturonate (The metabolism of propranolol is reduced by co-administration of quinidine, leading to a 2- to 3-fold increase in blood concentrations and greater degrees of clinical beta-blockade. Concurrent use my cause postural hypotension).
No products indexed under this heading.

Quinidine Sulfate (The metabolism of propranolol is reduced by co-administration of quinidine, leading to a 2- to 3-fold increase in blood concentrations and greater degrees of clinical beta-blockade. Concurrent use my cause postural hypotension).
No products indexed under this heading.

Rabeprazole Sodium (Blood levels and/or toxicity of propranolol may be increased by administration of propranolol extended-release capsules with substrates of CYP2C19). Products include:

Aciphex Tablets 1053

Ramipril (When combined with beta-blockers, ACE inhibitors can cause hypotension, particularly in the setting of acute myocardial infarction. Certain ACE inhibitors have been reported to increase bronchial hyper-reactivity when administered with propranolol).
No products indexed under this heading.

Ranitidine Bismuth Citrate (Blood levels and/or toxicity of propranolol may be increased by administration of propranolol extended-release capsules with inhibitors of CYP2D6).
No products indexed under this heading.

Ranitidine Hydrochloride (Blood levels and/or toxicity of propranolol may be increased by administration of propranolol extended-release capsules with inhibitors of CYP2D6). Products include:

Zantac 75 Tablets .... ▣ 603
Zantac 1670
Zantac Injection 1666
Zantac Injection Pharmacy Bulk Package 1668
Maximum Strength Zantac 150 Tablets .... ▣ 603
Maximum Strength Zantac 150 Cool Mint Tablets .... ▣ 603

Rasagiline Mesylate (The hypotensive effects of MAO inhibitors may be exacerbated when administered with beta-blockers by interfering with the beta-blocking activity of propranolol). Products include:

Azilect Tablets 3106

Rauwolfia Serpentina (Patients receiving catecholamine-depleting drugs, (e.g. reserpine) and propranolol extended release capsules, should be closely observed for excessive reduction of resting sympathetic nervous activity, which may result in hypotension, marked bradycardia,vertigo, syncopal attacks, or orthostatic hypotension).
No products indexed under this heading.

Rescinnamine (Patients receiving catecholamine-depleting drugs, (e.g. reserpine) and propranolol extended release capsules, should be closely observed for excessive reduction of resting sympathetic nervous activity, which may result in hypotension, marked bradycardia, vertigo, syncopal attacks, or orthostatic hypotension).
No products indexed under this heading.

Reserpine (Patients receiving catecholamine-depleting drugs such as reserpine and propranolol hydrochloride extended-release capsules should be observed closely for excessive reduction of resting sympathetic nervous activity, which may result in hypotension, marked bradycardia, vertigo, syncopal attacks, or orthostatic hypotension. Administration of reserpine with propranolol may also potentiate depression).
No products indexed under this heading.

Rifampin (Blood levels of propranolol may be decreased by administration of propranolol extended-release capsules with inducers of hepatic drug metabolism).
No products indexed under this heading.

Rifapentine (Blood levels of propranolol may be decreased by administration of propranolol extended-release capsules with inducers of hepatic drug metabolism).
No products indexed under this heading.

Riluzole (Blood levels and/or toxicity of propranolol may be increased by administration of propranolol extended-release capsules with substrates of CYP1A2). Products include:

Rilutek Tablets 2771

Risperidone (Blood levels and/or toxicity of propranolol may be increased by administration of propranolol extended-release capsules with substrates of CYP2D6). Products include:

Risperdal Consta Long-Acting Injection 1753

Ritonavir (Blood levels and/or toxicity of propranolol may be increased by administration of propranolol extended-release capsules with substrates of CYP2D6). Products include:

Kaletra 452
Norvir 489

Rizatriptan Benzoate (Administration of rizatriptan with propranolol resulted in increased concentrations of rizatriptan (the AUC and Cmax were increased by 67% and 75%, respectively)). Products include:

Maxalt Tablets 2056
Maxalt-MLT Orally Disintegrating Tablets 2056

Rofecoxib (Non-steroidal anti-inflammatory drugs (NSAIDs) have been reported to blunt the antihypertensive effects of beta-adreno receptor blocking agents).
No products indexed under this heading.

Ropinirole Hydrochloride (Blood levels and/or toxicity of propranolol may be increased by administration of propranolol extended-release capsules with substrates of CYP1A2). Products include:

Requip Tablets 1561
Requip XL Tablets 1568

Ropivacaine Hydrochloride (Blood levels and/or toxicity of propranolol may be increased by administration of propranolol extended-release capsules with substrates of CYP1A2).
No products indexed under this heading.

Selegiline (The hypotensive effects of MAO inhibitors may be exacerbated when administered with beta-blockers by interfering with the beta-blocking activity of propranolol). Products include:

Emsam Transdermal System 905

Selegiline Hydrochloride (The hypotensive effects of MAO inhibitors may be exacerbated when administered with beta-blockers by interfering with the beta-blocking activity of propranolol). Products include:

Eldepryl Capsules 3052

Sertraline Hydrochloride (Blood levels and/or toxicity of propranolol may be increased by administration of propranolol extended-release capsules with inhibitors of CYP2D6).
No products indexed under this heading.

Sildenafil Citrate (Blood levels and/or toxicity of propranolol may be increased by administration of propranolol extended-release capsules with inhibitors of CYP2D6).
No products indexed under this heading.

Sparfloxacin (Blood levels and/or toxicity of propranolol may be increased by administration of propranolol hydrochloride extended-release capsules with inhibitors of CYP1A2).
No products indexed under this heading.

Spirapril Hydrochloride (When combined with beta-blockers, ACE inhibitors can cause hypotension, particularly in the setting of acute myocardial infarction. Certain ACE inhibitors have been reported to increase bronchial hyper-reactivity when administered with propranolol).
No products indexed under this heading.

Sulfaphenazole (Blood levels and/or toxicity of propranolol may be increased by administration of propranolol extended-release capsules with inhibitors of CYP2C19).
No products indexed under this heading.

Sulindac (Non-steroidal anti-inflammatory drugs (NSAIDs) have been reported to blunt the antihypertensive effects of beta-adreno receptor blocking agents). Products include:

Clinoril Tablets 1962

Tacrine Hydrochloride (Blood levels and/or toxicity of propranolol may be increased by administration of propranolol extended-release capsules with substrates of CYP1A2).
No products indexed under this heading.

Tamoxifen Citrate (Blood levels and/or toxicity of propranolol may be increased by administration of propranolol extended-release capsules with substrates of CYP2D6).
No products indexed under this heading.

Telmisartan (Blood levels and/or toxicity of propranolol may be increased by administration of propranolol extended-release capsules with inhibitors of CYP2C19).
Products include:
Micardis Tablets **852**
Micardis HCT Tablets **854**

Teniposide (Blood levels and/or toxicity of propranolol may be increased by administration of propranolol extended-release capsules with substrates of CYP2D6).
No products indexed under this heading.

Terazosin Hydrochloride (Postural hypotension has been reported in patients taking both beta-blockers and terazosin).
No products indexed under this heading.

Terbinafine Hydrochloride (Blood levels and/or toxicity of propranolol may be increased by administration of propranolol extended-release capsules with inhibitors of CYP2D6).
Products include:
Lamisil Oral Granules **2264**
Lamisil Tablets **2266**

Testosterone (Blood levels and/or toxicity of propranolol may be increased by administration of propranolol extended-release capsules with substrates of CYP2D6).
Products include:
AndroGel **3159**
Testim 1% Gel **701**

Testosterone Cypionate (Blood levels and/or toxicity of propranolol may be increased by administration of propranolol extended-release capsules with substrates of CYP2D6).
No products indexed under this heading.

Testosterone Enanthate (Blood levels and/or toxicity of propranolol may be increased by administration of propranolol extended-release capsules with substrates of CYP2D6).
Products include:
Delatestryl Injection **1730**

Testosterone Propionate (Blood levels and/or toxicity of propranolol may be increased by administration of propranolol extended-release capsules with substrates of CYP2D6).
No products indexed under this heading.

Theophylline (Co-administration of theophylline with propranolol decreases theophylline oral clearance by 33% to 52%).
No products indexed under this heading.

Theophylline Anhydrous (Co-administration of theophylline with propranolol decreases theophylline oral clearance by 33% to 52%).
Products include:
Uniphyl Tablets **2595**

Theophylline Calcium Salicylate (Co-administration of theophylline with propranolol decreases theophylline oral clearance by 33% to 52%).
No products indexed under this heading.

Theophylline Dihydroxypropyl (Glyceryl) (Co-administration of theophylline with propranolol decreases theophylline oral clearance by 33% to 52%).
No products indexed under this heading.

Theophylline Ethylenediamine (Co-administration of theophylline with propranolol decreases theophylline oral clearance by 33% to 52%).
No products indexed under this heading.

Theophylline Sodium Glycinate (Co-administration of theophylline with propranolol decreases theophylline oral clearance by 33% to 52%).
No products indexed under this heading.

Thioridazine (Co-administration of propranolol at doses greater than or equal to 160 mg/day resulted in increased thioridazine plasma concentrations, ranging from 50% to 370% and increased thioridazine metabolite concentrations ranging from 33% to 210%).
No products indexed under this heading.

Thioridazine Hydrochloride (Co-administration of propranolol at doses greater than or equal to 160 mg/day resulted in increased thioridazine plasma concentrations, ranging from 50% to 370% and increased thioridazine metabolite concentrations ranging from 33% to 210%). Products include:
Thioridazine Hydrochloride Tablets **2195**

Thyroxine (Thyroxine may result in a lower than expected T3 concentration when used concomitantly with propranolol).
No products indexed under this heading.

Thyroxine Sodium (Thyroxine may result in a lower than expected T3 concentration when used concomitantly with propranolol).
No products indexed under this heading.

Tiagabine Hydrochloride (Blood levels and/or toxicity of propranolol may be increased by administration of propranolol extended-release capsules with substrates of CYP2C19).
Products include:
Gabitril Tablets **973**

Ticlopidine Hydrochloride (Blood levels and/or toxicity of propranolol may be increased by administration of propranolol hydrochloride extended-release capsules with inhibitors of CYP1A2).
No products indexed under this heading.

Timolol Maleate (Blood levels and/or toxicity of propranolol may be increased by administration of propranolol extended-release capsules with substrates of CYP2D6).
Products include:
Combigan Ophthalmic Solution **553**
Cosopt Sterile Ophthalmic Solution **1969**
Timoptic Sterile Ophthalmic Solution **2121**
Timoptic in Ocudose **2124**
Timoptic-XE Sterile Ophthalmic Gel Forming Solution **2125**

Tolazamide (Blood levels of propranolol may be decreased by administration of propranolol extended-release capsules with inducers of hepatic drug metabolism).
No products indexed under this heading.

Tolbutamide (Blood levels of propranolol may be decreased by administration of propranolol extended-release capsules with inducers of hepatic drug metabolism).
No products indexed under this heading.

Tolbutamide Sodium (Blood levels and/or toxicity of propranolol may be increased by administration of propranolol extended-release capsules with substrates of CYP2C19).
No products indexed under this heading.

Tolmetin Sodium (Non-steroidal anti-inflammatory drugs (NSAIDs) have been reported to blunt the antihypertensive effects of beta-adreno receptor blocking agents).
No products indexed under this heading.

Tolterodine Tartrate (Blood levels and/or toxicity of propranolol may be increased by administration of propranolol extended-release capsules with substrates of CYP2D6).
No products indexed under this heading.

Topiramate (Blood levels and/or toxicity of propranolol may be increased by administration of propranolol extended-release capsules with substrates of CYP2C19).
No products indexed under this heading.

Tramadol Hydrochloride (Blood levels and/or toxicity of propranolol may be increased by administration of propranolol extended-release capsules with substrates of CYP2D6).
Products include:
Ultram ER Extended-Release Tablets **2428**

Trandolapril (When combined with beta-blockers, ACE inhibitors can cause hypotension, particularly in the setting of acute myocardial infarction. Certain ACE inhibitors have been reported to increase bronchial hyper-reactivity when administered with propranolol). Products include:
Mavik Tablets **472**
Tarka Tablets **511**

Tranylcypromine Sulfate (The hypotensive effects of MAO inhibitors may be exacerbated when administered with beta-blockers by interfering with the beta-blocking activity of propranolol). Products include:
Parnate Tablets **1532**

Trazodone Hydrochloride (Blood levels and/or toxicity of propranolol may be increased by administration of propranolol extended-release capsules with substrates of CYP2D6).
No products indexed under this heading.

Triazolam (Blood levels and/or toxicity of propranolol may be increased by administration of propranolol extended-release capsules with substrates of CYP2D6).
No products indexed under this heading.

Trichloroethylene (Trichloroethylene may depress myocardial contractility when administered with propranolol).
No products indexed under this heading.

Trimethadione (Blood levels and/or toxicity of propranolol may be increased by administration of propranolol extended-release capsules with substrates of CYP2C19).
No products indexed under this heading.

Trimethaphan Camsylate (Blood levels and/or toxicity of propranolol may be increased by administration of propranolol extended-release capsules with substrates of CYP1A2).
No products indexed under this heading.

Trimipramine Maleate (The hypotensive effects of tricyclic antidepressants may be exacerbated when administered with beta-blockers by interfering with the beta-blocking activity of propranolol).
No products indexed under this heading.

Troleandomycin (Blood levels and/or toxicity of propranolol may be increased by administration of propranolol hydrochloride extended-release capsules with inhibitors of CYP1A2).
No products indexed under this heading.

Trovafloxacin Mesylate (Blood levels and/or toxicity of propranolol may be increased by administration of propranolol extended-release capsules with substrates of CYP1A2).
No products indexed under this heading.

Valdecoxib (Non-steroidal anti-inflammatory drugs (NSAIDs) have been reported to blunt the antihypertensive effects of beta-adreno receptor blocking agents).
No products indexed under this heading.

Valproate Sodium (Blood levels and/or toxicity of propranolol may be increased by administration of propranolol extended-release capsules with substrates of CYP2C19).
No products indexed under this heading.

Valproic Acid (Blood levels and/or toxicity of propranolol may be increased by administration of propranolol extended-release capsules with substrates of CYP2C19).
No products indexed under this heading.

Vardenafil Hydrochloride (Blood levels and/or toxicity of propranolol may be increased by administration of propranolol extended-release capsules with inhibitors of CYP2D6).
Products include:
Levitra Tablets **2876**

Venlafaxine Hydrochloride (Blood levels and/or toxicity of propranolol may be increased by administration of propranolol extended-release capsules with substrates of CYP2D6).
Products include:
Effexor XR Extended-Release Capsules **3195**
Venlafaxine Hydrochloride Tablets ... **2199**

Verapamil Hydrochloride (There have been reports of significant bradycardia, heart failure, and cardiovascular collapse with concurrent use of verapamil and beta-blockers).
Products include:

Tarka Tablets 511

Vinblastine Sulfate (Blood levels and/or toxicity of propranolol may be increased by administration of propranolol extended-release capsules with substrates of CYP2D6).

No products indexed under this heading.

Voriconazole (Blood levels and/or toxicity of propranolol may be increased by administration of propranolol extended-release capsules with substrates of CYP2C19).

No products indexed under this heading.

Warfarin Sodium (Propranolol when administered with warfarin increases the concentration of warfarin. Prothrombin time, therefore, should be monitored).

No products indexed under this heading.

Zileuton (Blood levels and/or toxicity of propranolol may be increased by administration of propranolol extended-release capsules with substrates of CYP1A2).

No products indexed under this heading.

Zolmitriptan (Administration of zolmitriptan with propranolol resulted in increased concentrations of zolmitriptan (AUC increased by 56% and Cmax by 37%)). Products include:

Zomig Tablets 694
Zomig Nasal Spray 689
Zomig-ZMT Tablets 694

Zonisamide (Blood levels and/or toxicity of propranolol may be increased by administration of propranolol extended-release capsules with substrates of CYP2D6). Products include:

Zonegran Capsules 1089

Food Interactions

Grapefruit Juice (Blood levels and/or toxicity of propranolol may be increased by administration of propranolol hydrochloride extended-release capsules with inhibitors of CYP1A2).

INTEGRILIN INJECTION

(Eptifibatide) 2855

May interact with oral anticoagulants, glycoprotein (GP) IIb/IIIa inhibitors, non-steroidal anti-inflammatory agents, and certain other agents. Compounds in these categories include:

Abciximab (Current or planned administration of another parenteral GP IIb/IIIa inhibitor is contraindicated). Products include:

ReoPro Vials 1860

Anisindione (Potential for additive pharmacologic effects because eptifibatide inhibits platelet aggregation; concurrent use requires caution).

No products indexed under this heading.

Aspirin (Co-administration of eptifibatide with heparin and aspirin has resulted in cerebral, GI and pulmonary hemorrhage). Products include:

Aggrenox Capsules 819
Bayer Aspirin 750
Percodan Tablets 1130
St. Joseph 81 mg Aspirin Chewable and Enteric Coated Tablets 1903

Celecoxib (Potential for additive pharmacologic effects because eptifibatide inhibits platelet aggregation; concurrent use requires caution). Products include:

Celebrex Capsules 2979

Clopidogrel Bisulfate (Potential for additive pharmacologic effects because eptifibatide inhibits platelet aggregation; concurrent use requires caution). Products include:

Plavix Tablets 926
Plavix Tablets 2767

Diclofenac Epolamine (Potential for additive pharmacologic effects because eptifibatide inhibits platelet aggregation; concurrent use requires caution). Products include:

Flector Patch 561

Diclofenac Potassium (Potential for additive pharmacologic effects because eptifibatide inhibits platelet aggregation; concurrent use requires caution).

No products indexed under this heading.

Diclofenac Sodium (Potential for additive pharmacologic effects because eptifibatide inhibits platelet aggregation; concurrent use requires caution). Products include:

Diclofenac Sodium Ophthalmic Solution .... ⊙240
Voltaren Ophthalmic Solution 2336
Voltaren Tablets 2334
Voltaren-XR Tablets 2337

Dicumarol (Potential for additive pharmacologic effects because eptifibatide inhibits platelet aggregation; concurrent use requires caution).

No products indexed under this heading.

Dipyridamole (Potential for additive pharmacologic effects because eptifibatide inhibits platelet aggregation; concurrent use requires caution). Products include:

Aggrenox Capsules 819
Persantine Tablets 869

Etodolac (Potential for additive pharmacologic effects because eptifibatide inhibits platelet aggregation; concurrent use requires caution).

No products indexed under this heading.

Fenoprofen Calcium (Potential for additive pharmacologic effects because eptifibatide inhibits platelet aggregation; concurrent use requires caution). Products include:

Nalfon Capsules 2508

Flurbiprofen (Potential for additive pharmacologic effects because eptifibatide inhibits platelet aggregation; concurrent use requires caution).

No products indexed under this heading.

Heparin Sodium (Co-administration of eptifibatide with heparin and aspirin has resulted in cerebral, GI and pulmonary hemorrhage).

No products indexed under this heading.

Ibuprofen (Potential for additive pharmacologic effects because eptifibatide inhibits platelet aggregation; concurrent use requires caution). Products include:

Motrin IB Tablets and Caplets 1900
Children's Motrin Oral Suspension ... 1901
Children's Motrin Non-Staining Dye-Free Oral Suspension 1901
Children's Motrin Cold Oral Suspension 1899
Infants' Motrin Concentrated Drops 1901
Infants' Motrin Non-Staining Dye-Free Concentrated Drops....... 1901
Junior Strength Motrin Caplets and Chewable Tablets.................. 1901
Vicoprofen Tablets 533

Indomethacin (Potential for additive pharmacologic effects because eptifibatide inhibits platelet aggregation; concurrent use requires caution). Products include:

Indocin 2024

Indomethacin Sodium Trihydrate (Potential for additive pharmacologic effects because eptifibatide inhibits platelet aggregation; concurrent use requires caution). Products include:

Indocin I.V. 2489

Ketoprofen (Potential for additive pharmacologic effects because eptifibatide inhibits platelet aggregation; concurrent use requires caution).

No products indexed under this heading.

Ketorolac Tromethamine (Potential for additive pharmacologic effects because eptifibatide inhibits platelet aggregation; concurrent use requires caution).

No products indexed under this heading.

Meclofenamate Sodium (Potential for additive pharmacologic effects because eptifibatide inhibits platelet aggregation; concurrent use requires caution).

No products indexed under this heading.

Mefenamic Acid (Potential for additive pharmacologic effects because eptifibatide inhibits platelet aggregation; concurrent use requires caution).

No products indexed under this heading.

Meloxicam (Potential for additive pharmacologic effects because eptifibatide inhibits platelet aggregation; concurrent use requires caution). Products include:

Mobic Oral Suspension 863
Mobic Tablets 863

Nabumetone (Potential for additive pharmacologic effects because eptifibatide inhibits platelet aggregation; concurrent use requires caution).

No products indexed under this heading.

Naproxen (Potential for additive pharmacologic effects because eptifibatide inhibits platelet aggregation; concurrent use requires caution). Products include:

EC-Naprosyn Delayed-Release Tablets 2632
Naprosyn Suspension 2632
Naprosyn Tablets 2632

Naproxen Sodium (Potential for additive pharmacologic effects because eptifibatide inhibits platelet aggregation; concurrent use requires caution). Products include:

Anaprox Tablets 2632
Anaprox DS Tablets 2632
Treximet Tablets 1616

Oxaprozin (Potential for additive pharmacologic effects because eptifibatide inhibits platelet aggregation; concurrent use requires caution).

No products indexed under this heading.

Phenylbutazone (Potential for additive pharmacologic effects because eptifibatide inhibits platelet aggregation; concurrent use requires caution).

No products indexed under this heading.

Piroxicam (Potential for additive pharmacologic effects because eptifibatide inhibits platelet aggregation; concurrent use requires caution).

No products indexed under this heading.

Rofecoxib (Potential for additive pharmacologic effects because eptifibatide inhibits platelet aggregation; concurrent use requires caution).

No products indexed under this heading.

Sulindac (Potential for additive pharmacologic effects because eptifibatide inhibits platelet aggregation; concurrent use requires caution). Products include:

Clinoril Tablets 1962

Ticlopidine Hydrochloride (Potential for additive pharmacologic effects because eptifibatide inhibits platelet aggregation; concurrent use requires caution).

No products indexed under this heading.

Tirofiban Hydrochloride (Current or planned administration of another parenteral GP IIb/IIIa inhibitor is contraindicated).

No products indexed under this heading.

Tolmetin Sodium (Potential for additive pharmacologic effects because eptifibatide inhibits platelet aggregation; concurrent use requires caution).

No products indexed under this heading.

Valdecoxib (Potential for additive pharmacologic effects because eptifibatide inhibits platelet aggregation; concurrent use requires caution).

No products indexed under this heading.

Warfarin Sodium (Potential for additive pharmacologic effects because eptifibatide inhibits platelet aggregation; concurrent use requires caution).

No products indexed under this heading.

INTELECTOL TABLETS

(Vinpocetine) .... ■629

None cited in PDR database.

INTELENCE TABLETS

(Etravirine) 3119

May interact with antiarrhythmics, cytochrome p450 2c19 inducers (selected), cytochrome p450 2c19 inhibitors (selected), cytochrome p450 2c19 substrates (selected), cytochrome p450 2c9 inducers (selected), cytochrome p450 2c9 inhibitors (selected), cytochrome p450 2c9 substrates (selected), cytochrome p450 3a4 inducers (selected), cytochrome p450 3a4 inhibitors (selected), cytochrome p450 3a4 substrates (selected), Non-nucleoside reverse transcriptase inhibitors, phenytoin, and protease inhibitors. Compounds in these categories include:

Acarbose (Etravirine is an inducer of CYP3A4 and inhibitor of CYP2C9 and CYP2C19. Therefore, co-administration of drugs that are substrates of CYP3A4, CYP2C9 and CYP2C19 with etravirine may alter the therapeutic effect or adverse reaction profile of the co-administered drug(s)). Products include:

Precose Tablets 792

Acebutolol Hydrochloride (Concentrations of these antiarrhythmics may be decreased when co-administered with etravirine. Etravirine and antiarrhythmics should be co-administered with caution. Drug concentration monitoring is recommended, if available).
No products indexed under this heading.

Acetazolamide (Etravirine is a substrate of CYP3A4, CYP2C9, and CYP2C19. Therefore, co-administration of etravirine with drugs that induce or inhibit CYP3A4, CYP2C9, and CYP2C19 may alter the therapeutic effect or adverse reaction profile of etravirine).
No products indexed under this heading.

Adenosine (Concentrations of these antiarrhythmics may be decreased when co-administered with etravirine. Etravirine and antiarrhythmics should be co-administered with caution. Drug concentration monitoring is recommended, if available). Products include:
Adenocard IV Injection 603
Adenoscan 605

Alfentanil Hydrochloride (Etravirine is an inducer of CYP3A4 and inhibitor of CYP2C9 and CYP2C19. Therefore, co-administration of drugs that are substrates of CYP3A4, CYP2C9 and CYP2C19 with etravirine may alter the therapeutic effect or adverse reaction profile of the co-administered drug(s)).
No products indexed under this heading.

Allium sativum (Etravirine is a substrate of CYP3A4, CYP2C9, and CYP2C19. Therefore, co-administration of etravirine with drugs that induce or inhibit CYP3A4, CYP2C9, and CYP2C19 may alter the therapeutic effect or adverse reaction profile of etravirine).
No products indexed under this heading.

Alprazolam (Etravirine is an inducer of CYP3A4 and inhibitor of CYP2C9 and CYP2C19. Therefore, co-administration of drugs that are substrates of CYP3A4, CYP2C9 and CYP2C19 with etravirine may alter the therapeutic effect or adverse reaction profile of the co-administered drug(s)).
No products indexed under this heading.

Amiodarone Hydrochloride (Concentrations of these antiarrhythmics may be decreased when co-administered with etravirine. Etravirine and antiarrhythmics should be co-administered with caution. Drug concentration monitoring is recommended, if available).
No products indexed under this heading.

Amitriptyline Hydrochloride (Etravirine is an inducer of CYP3A4 and inhibitor of CYP2C9 and CYP2C19. Therefore, co-administration of drugs that are substrates of CYP3A4, CYP2C9 and CYP2C19 with etravirine may alter the therapeutic effect or adverse reaction profile of the co-administered drug(s)).
No products indexed under this heading.

Amlodipine Besylate (Etravirine is an inducer of CYP3A4 and inhibitor of CYP2C9 and CYP2C19. Therefore, co-administration of drugs that are substrates of CYP3A4, CYP2C9 and CYP2C19 with etravirine may alter the therapeutic effect or adverse reaction profile of the co-administered drug(s)). Products include:
Azor Tablets 1005
Exforge Tablets 2238

Amoxapine (Etravirine is an inducer of CYP3A4 and inhibitor of CYP2C9 and CYP2C19. Therefore, co-administration of drugs that are substrates of CYP3A4, CYP2C9 and CYP2C19 with etravirine may alter the therapeutic effect or adverse reaction profile of the co-administered drug(s)).
No products indexed under this heading.

Amprenavir (Concomitant use of etravirine with protease inhibitors (PIs) without co-administration of low-dose ritonavir may cause a significant alteration in the plasma concentrations of the PI. Etravirine should not be co-administered with PIs without low-dose ritonavir).
No products indexed under this heading.

Anastrozole (Etravirine is a substrate of CYP3A4, CYP2C9, and CYP2C19. Therefore, co-administration of etravirine with drugs that induce or inhibit CYP3A4, CYP2C9, and CYP2C19 may alter the therapeutic effect or adverse reaction profile of etravirine). Products include:
Arimidex Tablets 672

Aprepitant (Etravirine is a substrate of CYP3A4, CYP2C9, and CYP2C19. Therefore, co-administration of etravirine with drugs that induce or inhibit CYP3A4, CYP2C9, and CYP2C19 may alter the therapeutic effect or adverse reaction profile of etravirine). Products include:
Emend Capsules 1992

Astemizole (Etravirine is an inducer of CYP3A4 and inhibitor of CYP2C9 and CYP2C19. Therefore, co-administration of drugs that are substrates of CYP3A4, CYP2C9 and CYP2C19 with etravirine may alter the therapeutic effect or adverse reaction profile of the co-administered drug(s)).
No products indexed under this heading.

Atazanavir (Concomitant use of etravirine with protease inhibitors (PIs) without co-administration of low-dose ritonavir may cause a significant alteration in the plasma concentrations of the PI. Etravirine should not be co-administered with PIs without low-dose ritonavir. Concomitant use of etravirine with atazanavir/ritonavir may cause a significant decrease in atazanavir Cmin by about 38% and loss of therapeutic effect of atazanavir. In addition, the mean systemic exposure (AUC) of etravirine after co-administration of etravirine with atazanavir/ritonavir is anticipated to be about 100% higher than the mean systemic exposure of etravirine observed in the Phase 3 trials. Etravirine and atazanavir/ritonavir should not be co-administered).
No products indexed under this heading.

Atazanavir Sulfate (Concomitant use of etravirine with protease inhibitors (PIs) without co-administration of low-dose ritonavir may cause a significant alteration in the plasma concentrations of the PI. Etravirine should not be co-administered with PIs without low-dose ritonavir. Concomitant use of etravirine with atazanavir/ritonavir may cause a significant decrease in atazanavir Cmin by about 38% and loss of therapeutic effect of atazanavir. In addition, the mean systemic exposure (AUC) of etravirine after co-administration of etravirine with atazanavir/ritonavir is anticipated to be about 100% higher than the mean systemic exposure of etravirine observed in the Phase 3 trials. Etravirine and atazanavir/ritonavir should not be co-administered). Products include:
Reyataz Capsules 3299

Atorvastatin Calcium (The combination of etravirine and atorvastatin can be given without any dose adjustments, however, the dose of atorvastatin may need to be altered based on clinical response). Products include:
Lipitor Tablets 2501

Belladonna Ergotamine (Etravirine is an inducer of CYP3A4 and inhibitor of CYP2C9 and CYP2C19. Therefore, co-administration of drugs that are substrates of CYP3A4, CYP2C9 and CYP2C19 with etravirine may alter the therapeutic effect or adverse reaction profile of the co-administered drug(s)).
No products indexed under this heading.

Bendroflumethiazide (Etravirine is a substrate of CYP3A4, CYP2C9, and CYP2C19. Therefore, co-administration of etravirine with drugs that induce or inhibit CYP3A4, CYP2C9, and CYP2C19 may alter the therapeutic effect or adverse reaction profile of etravirine).
No products indexed under this heading.

Betamethasone Acetate (Etravirine is a substrate of CYP3A4, CYP2C9, and CYP2C19. Therefore, co-administration of etravirine with drugs that induce or inhibit CYP3A4, CYP2C9, and CYP2C19 may alter the therapeutic effect or adverse reaction profile of etravirine).
No products indexed under this heading.

Betamethasone Sodium Phosphate (Etravirine is a substrate of CYP3A4, CYP2C9, and CYP2C19. Therefore, co-administration of etravirine with drugs that induce or inhibit CYP3A4, CYP2C9, and CYP2C19 may alter the therapeutic effect or adverse reaction profile of etravirine).
No products indexed under this heading.

Bretylium Tosylate (Concentrations of these antiarrhythmics may be decreased when co-administered with etravirine. Etravirine and antiarrhythmics should be co-administered with caution. Drug concentration monitoring is recommended, if available).
No products indexed under this heading.

Buspirone Hydrochloride (Etravirine is an inducer of CYP3A4 and inhibitor of CYP2C9 and CYP2C19. Therefore, co-administration of drugs that are substrates of CYP3A4, CYP2C9 and CYP2C19 with etravirine may alter the therapeutic effect or adverse reaction profile of the co-administered drug(s)).
No products indexed under this heading.

Busulfan (Etravirine is an inducer of CYP3A4 and inhibitor of CYP2C9 and CYP2C19. Therefore, co-administration of drugs that are substrates of CYP3A4, CYP2C9 and CYP2C19 with etravirine may alter the therapeutic effect or adverse reaction profile of the co-administered drug(s)). Products include:
Busulfex Injection 2477
Myleran Tablets 1530

Candesartan Cilexetil (Etravirine is an inducer of CYP3A4 and inhibitor of CYP2C9 and CYP2C19. Therefore, co-administration of drugs that are substrates of CYP3A4, CYP2C9 and CYP2C19 with etravirine may alter the therapeutic effect or adverse reaction profile of the co-administered drug(s)). Products include:
Atacand Tablets 639
Atacand HCT 642

Carbamazepine (Carbamazepine, phenobarbital and phenyoin are inducers of CYP450 enzymes. Etravirine should not be used in combination with carbamazepine, phenobarbital, or phenytoin as co-administration may cause significant decreases in etravirine plasma concentrations and loss of therapeutic effect of etravirine). Products include:
Carbatrol Capsules 3019
Equetro Extended-Release Capsules 3174

Carisoprodol (Etravirine is an inducer of CYP3A4 and inhibitor of CYP2C9 and CYP2C19. Therefore, co-administration of drugs that are substrates of CYP3A4, CYP2C9 and CYP2C19 with etravirine may alter the therapeutic effect or adverse reaction profile of the co-administered drug(s)). Products include:
Soma Tablets 1931

Carvedilol (Etravirine is an inducer of CYP3A4 and inhibitor of CYP2C9 and CYP2C19. Therefore, co-administration of drugs that are substrates of CYP3A4, CYP2C9 and CYP2C19 with etravirine may alter the therapeutic effect or adverse reaction profile of the co-administered drug(s)). Products include:
Coreg Tablets 1387

Celecoxib (Etravirine is an inducer of CYP3A4 and inhibitor of CYP2C9 and CYP2C19. Therefore, co-administration of drugs that are substrates of CYP3A4, CYP2C9 and CYP2C19 with etravirine may alter the therapeutic effect or adverse reaction profile of the co-administered drug(s)). Products include:
Celebrex Capsules 2979

Cerivastatin Sodium (Etravirine is an inducer of CYP3A4 and inhibitor of CYP2C9 and CYP2C19. Therefore, co-administration of drugs that are substrates of CYP3A4, CYP2C9 and CYP2C19 with etravirine may alter the therapeutic effect or adverse reaction profile of the co-administered drug(s)).
No products indexed under this heading.

Chloramphenicol (Etravirine is a substrate of CYP3A4, CYP2C9, and CYP2C19. Therefore, co-administration of etravirine with drugs that induce or inhibit CYP3A4, CYP2C9, and CYP2C19 may alter the therapeutic effect or adverse reaction profile of etravirine).
No products indexed under this heading.

Chlorothiazide (Etravirine is a substrate of CYP3A4, CYP2C9, and CYP2C19. Therefore, co-administration of etravirine with drugs that induce or inhibit CYP3A4, CYP2C9, and CYP2C19 may alter the therapeutic effect or adverse reaction profile of etravirine).
No products indexed under this heading.

Chlorothiazide Sodium (Etravirine is a substrate of CYP3A4, CYP2C9, and CYP2C19. Therefore, co-administration of etravirine with drugs that induce or inhibit CYP3A4, CYP2C9, and CYP2C19 may alter the therapeutic effect or adverse reaction profile of etravirine). Products include:
Intravenous Sodium Diuril 2490

Chlorpheniramine (Etravirine is an inducer of CYP3A4 and inhibitor of CYP2C9 and CYP2C19. Therefore, co-administration of drugs that are substrates of CYP3A4, CYP2C9 and CYP2C19 with etravirine may alter the therapeutic effect or adverse reaction profile of the co-administered drug(s)).
No products indexed under this heading.

Chlorpheniramine Maleate (Etravirine is an inducer of CYP3A4 and inhibitor of CYP2C9 and CYP2C19. Therefore, co-administration of drugs that are substrates of CYP3A4, CYP2C9 and CYP2C19 with etravirine may alter the therapeutic effect or adverse reaction profile of the co-administered drug(s)). Products include:
Actifed Cold & Allergy Tablets 1895
Sudafed PE Sinus & Allergy Tablets 1908
Tylenol Allergy Multi-Symptom Caplets with Cool Burst and Rapid Release Gelcaps 1916
Children's Tylenol Plus Cold Suspension Liquid 1912
Children's Tylenol Plus Cough & Runny Nose Suspension Liquid 1912
Children's Tylenol Plus Flu Suspension Liquid 1914
Children's Tylenol Plus Multi-Symptom Cold Suspension Liquid 1912
Tylenol Cold Head Congestion Nighttime Caplets with Cool Burst 1910
Tylenol Cold Multi-Symptom Nighttime Caplets with Cool Burst 1913
Tylenol Sinus Congestion & Pain Nighttime Caplets with Cool Burst 1917

Chlorpheniramine Polistirex (Etravirine is an inducer of CYP3A4 and inhibitor of CYP2C9 and CYP2C19. Therefore, co-administration of drugs that are substrates of CYP3A4, CYP2C9 and CYP2C19 with etravirine may alter the therapeutic effect or adverse reaction profile of the co-administered drug(s)). Products include:
Tussionex Pennkinetic Extended-Release Suspension 3154

Chlorpheniramine Tannate (Etravirine is an inducer of CYP3A4 and inhibitor of CYP2C9 and CYP2C19. Therefore, co-administration of drugs that are substrates of CYP3A4, CYP2C9 and CYP2C19 with etravirine may alter the therapeutic effect or adverse reaction profile of the co-administered drug(s)).
No products indexed under this heading.

Chlorpropamide (Etravirine is a substrate of CYP3A4, CYP2C9, and CYP2C19. Therefore, co-administration of etravirine with drugs that induce or inhibit CYP3A4, CYP2C9, and CYP2C19 may alter the therapeutic effect or adverse reaction profile of etravirine).
No products indexed under this heading.

Cilostazol (Etravirine is an inducer of CYP3A4 and inhibitor of CYP2C9 and CYP2C19. Therefore, co-administration of drugs that are substrates of CYP3A4, CYP2C9 and CYP2C19 with etravirine may alter the therapeutic effect or adverse reaction profile of the co-administered drug(s)). Products include:
Pletal Tablets 2481

Cimetidine (Etravirine is a substrate of CYP3A4, CYP2C9, and CYP2C19. Therefore, co-administration of etravirine with drugs that induce or inhibit CYP3A4, CYP2C9, and CYP2C19 may alter the therapeutic effect or adverse reaction profile of etravirine).
No products indexed under this heading.

Cimetidine Hydrochloride (Etravirine is a substrate of CYP3A4, CYP2C9, and CYP2C19. Therefore, co-administration of etravirine with drugs that induce or inhibit CYP3A4, CYP2C9, and CYP2C19 may alter the therapeutic effect or adverse reaction profile of etravirine).
No products indexed under this heading.

Ciprofloxacin (Etravirine is a substrate of CYP3A4, CYP2C9, and CYP2C19. Therefore, co-administration of etravirine with drugs that induce or inhibit CYP3A4, CYP2C9, and CYP2C19 may alter the therapeutic effect or adverse reaction profile of etravirine). Products include:
Cipro I.V. 2817
Cipro Oral Suspension 2810
Cipro XR Tablets 2823
Ciprodex Otic Suspension 541

Ciprofloxacin Hydrochloride (Etravirine is a substrate of CYP3A4, CYP2C9, and CYP2C19. Therefore, co-administration of etravirine with drugs that induce or inhibit CYP3A4, CYP2C9, and CYP2C19 may alter the therapeutic effect or adverse reaction profile of etravirine). Products include:
Cipro Tablets 2810

Cisapride (Etravirine is an inducer of CYP3A4 and inhibitor of CYP2C9 and CYP2C19. Therefore, co-administration of drugs that are substrates of CYP3A4, CYP2C9 and CYP2C19 with etravirine may alter the therapeutic effect or adverse reaction profile of the co-administered drug(s)).
No products indexed under this heading.

Cisplatin (Etravirine is a substrate of CYP3A4, CYP2C9, and CYP2C19. Therefore, co-administration of etravirine with drugs that induce or inhibit CYP3A4, CYP2C9, and CYP2C19 may alter the therapeutic effect or adverse reaction profile of etravirine).
No products indexed under this heading.

Citalopram Hydrobromide (Etravirine is a substrate of CYP3A4, CYP2C9, and CYP2C19. Therefore, co-administration of etravirine with drugs that induce or inhibit CYP3A4, CYP2C9, and CYP2C19 may alter the therapeutic effect or adverse reaction profile of etravirine). Products include:
Celexa 1160

Clarithromycin (Clarithromycin exposure was decreased by etravirine; however, concentrations of the active metabolite, 14-hydroxy-clarithromycin has reduced activity against Mycobacterium avium complex (MAC), overall activity against this pathogen may be altered. Alternatives to clarithromycin, such as azithromycin, should be considered for the treatment of MAC). Products include:
Biaxin/Biaxin XL 411

Clomipramine Hydrochloride (Etravirine is an inducer of CYP3A4 and inhibitor of CYP2C9 and CYP2C19. Therefore, co-administration of drugs that are substrates of CYP3A4, CYP2C9 and CYP2C19 with etravirine may alter the therapeutic effect or adverse reaction profile of the co-administered drug(s)).
No products indexed under this heading.

Clopidogrel Hydrogen Sulfate (Etravirine is a substrate of CYP3A4, CYP2C9, and CYP2C19. Therefore, co-administration of etravirine with drugs that induce or inhibit CYP3A4, CYP2C9, and CYP2C19 may alter the therapeutic effect or adverse reaction profile of etravirine).
No products indexed under this heading.

Clotrimazole (Etravirine is a substrate of CYP3A4, CYP2C9, and CYP2C19. Therefore, co-administration of etravirine with drugs that induce or inhibit CYP3A4, CYP2C9, and CYP2C19 may alter the therapeutic effect or adverse reaction profile of etravirine). Products include:
Lotrisone 2881

Cortisone Acetate (Etravirine is a substrate of CYP3A4, CYP2C9, and CYP2C19. Therefore, co-administration of etravirine with drugs that induce or inhibit CYP3A4, CYP2C9, and CYP2C19 may alter the therapeutic effect or adverse reaction profile of etravirine).
No products indexed under this heading.

Cyclophosphamide (Etravirine is an inducer of CYP3A4 and inhibitor of CYP2C9 and CYP2C19. Therefore, co-administration of drugs that are substrates of CYP3A4, CYP2C9 and CYP2C19 with etravirine may alter the therapeutic effect or adverse reaction profile of the co-administered drug(s)).
No products indexed under this heading.

Cyclosporine (Etravirine and systemic immunosuppressants should be co-administered with caution because plasma concentrations of cyclosporine, sirolimus, or tacrolimus may be affected). Products include:
Gengraf Capsules 435
Neoral Oral Solution 2280
Neoral Soft Gelatin Capsules 2280
Restasis Ophthalmic Emulsion 557
Sandimmune 2296

Dalfopristin (Etravirine is a substrate of CYP3A4, CYP2C9, and CYP2C19. Therefore, co-administration of etravirine with drugs that induce or inhibit CYP3A4, CYP2C9, and CYP2C19 may alter the therapeutic effect or adverse reaction profile of etravirine).
No products indexed under this heading.

Danazol (Etravirine is a substrate of CYP3A4, CYP2C9, and CYP2C19. Therefore, co-administration of etravirine with drugs that induce or inhibit CYP3A4, CYP2C9, and CYP2C19 may alter the therapeutic effect or adverse reaction profile of etravirine).
No products indexed under this heading.

Darunavir (Concomitant use of etravirine with protease inhibitors (PIs) without co-administration of low-dose ritonavir may cause a significant alteration in the plasma concentrations of the PI. Etravirine should not be co-administered with PIs without low-dose ritonavir. The mean systemic exposure (AUC) of etravirine was reduced by about 37% when etravirine was co-administered with darunavir/ritonavir. Because all subjects in the Phase 3 trials received darunavir/ritonavir as part of the background regimen and etravirine exposures from these trials were determined to be safe and effective, etravirine and darunavir/ritonavir can be co-administered without any dose adjustments).
No products indexed under this heading.

Delavirdine Mesylate (Combining two NNRTIs has not been shown to be beneficial. Intelence and delavirdine should not be co-administered).
No products indexed under this heading.

Desipramine Hydrochloride (Etravirine is an inducer of CYP3A4 and inhibitor of CYP2C9 and CYP2C19. Therefore, co-administration of drugs that are substrates of CYP3A4, CYP2C9 and CYP2C19 with etravirine may alter the therapeutic effect or adverse reaction profile of the co-administered drug(s)).
No products indexed under this heading.

Desogestrel (Etravirine is a substrate of CYP3A4, CYP2C9, and CYP2C19. Therefore, co-administration of etravirine with

drugs that induce or inhibit CYP3A4, CYP2C9, and CYP2C19 may alter the therapeutic effect or adverse reaction profile of etravirine). Products include:

Mircette Tablets **1034**

Dexamethasone (Systemic dexamethasone induces CYP3A4 and can decrease etravirine plasma concentrations. This may result in loss of therapeutic effect of etravirine. Systemic dexamethasone should be used with caution or alternatives should be considered, particularly for long-term use). Products include:

Ciprodex Otic Suspension **541**

Dexamethasone Acetate (Systemic dexamethasone induces CYP3A4 and can decrease etravirine plasma concentrations. This may result in loss of therapeutic effect of etravirine. Systemic dexamethasone should be used with caution or alternatives should be considered, particularly for long-term use).

No products indexed under this heading.

Dexamethasone Phosphate (Systemic dexamethasone induces CYP3A4 and can decrease etravirine plasma concentrations. This may result in loss of therapeutic effect of etravirine. Systemic dexamethasone should be used with caution or alternatives should be considered, particularly for long-term use).

No products indexed under this heading.

Dexamethasone Sodium (Systemic dexamethasone induces CYP3A4 and can decrease etravirine plasma concentrations. This may result in loss of therapeutic effect of etravirine. Systemic dexamethasone should be used with caution or alternatives should be considered, particularly for long-term use).

No products indexed under this heading.

Dexamethasone Sodium Phosphate (Systemic dexamethasone induces CYP3A4 and can decrease etravirine plasma concentrations. This may result in loss of therapeutic effect of etravirine. Systemic dexamethasone should be used with caution or alternatives should be considered, particularly for long-term use).

No products indexed under this heading.

Dexamethasone Sodium Phosphate Injection (Systemic dexamethasone induces CYP3A4 and can decrease etravirine plasma concentrations. This may result in loss of therapeutic effect of etravirine. Systemic dexamethasone should be used with caution or alternatives should be considered, particularly for long-term use).

No products indexed under this heading.

Dextromethorphan (Etravirine is an inducer of CYP3A4 and inhibitor of CYP2C9 and CYP2C19. Therefore, co-administration of drugs that are substrates of CYP3A4, CYP2C9 and CYP2C19 with etravirine may alter the therapeutic effect or adverse reaction profile of the co-administered drug(s)).

No products indexed under this heading.

Dextromethorphan Hydrobromide (Etravirine is an inducer of CYP3A4 and inhibitor of CYP2C9 and CYP2C19. Therefore, co-administration of drugs that are substrates of CYP3A4, CYP2C9 and CYP2C19 with etravirine may alter the therapeutic effect or adverse reaction profile of the co-administered drug(s)). Products include:

PediaCare Children's Liquid Multi-Symptom Cold..................... **1902**
PediaCare Children's Long-Acting Cough.. **1902**
Children's Sudafed PE Cold & Cough Liquid.............................. **1907**
Sudafed PE Cold & Cough Caplets.. **1907**
Children's Tylenol Plus Cough & Runny Nose Suspension Liquid..... **1912**
Children's Tylenol Plus Cough & Sore Throat Suspension Liquid..... **1912**
Children's Tylenol Plus Flu Suspension Liquid **1914**
Children's Tylenol Plus Multi-Symptom Cold Suspension Liquid **1912**
Tylenol Cold Severe Congestion Daytime Caplets with Cool Burst... **1912**
Tylenol Cold Head Congestion Daytime Caplets with Cool Burst.. **1910**
Tylenol Cold Head Congestion Nighttime Caplets with Cool Burst.. **1910**
Tylenol Cold Head Congestion Severe Daytime Caplets with Cool Burst.................................. **1910**
Tylenol Cold Multi-Symptom Daytime Caplets with Cool Burst and Rapid Release Gels....... **1913**
Tylenol Cold Multi-Symptom Daytime Liquid with Citrus Burst... **1913**
Tylenol Cold Multi-Symptom Nighttime Caplets with Cool Burst.. **1913**
Tylenol Cold Multi-Symptom Nighttime Liquid with Cool Burst... **1913**
Tylenol Cold Multi-Symptom Severe Caplets with Cool Burst..... **1913**
Tylenol Cold Multi-Symptom Severe Daytime Liquid with Citrus Burst................................ **1913**
Tylenol Cough & Sore Throat Daytime Liquid with Cool Burst...... **1918**
Tylenol Cough & Sore Throat Nighttime Liquid with Cool Burst... **1918**
Vicks DayQuil Cold & Flu Multi-Symptom Relief................. ▣**616**
Vicks DayQuil LiquiCaps **2567**
Vicks DayQuil Liquid **2567**
Vicks DayQuil Multi-Symptom Cold/Flu Relief............................ **2567**
Vicks NyQuil Cold & Flu Multi-Symptom Relief................. ▣**617**
Vicks NyQuil LiquiCaps **2567**
Vicks NyQuil Liquid **2567**
Vicks NyQuil Multi-Symptom Cold/Flu Relief............................ **2567**

Diazepam (Concomitant use of etravirine with diazepam may increase plasma concentrations of diazepam. A decrease in diazepam dose may be needed). Products include:

Valium Tablets **2658**

Diclofenac Potassium (Etravirine is a substrate of CYP3A4, CYP2C9, and CYP2C19. Therefore, co-administration of etravirine with drugs that induce or inhibit CYP3A4, CYP2C9, and CYP2C19 may alter the therapeutic effect or adverse reaction profile of etravirine).

No products indexed under this heading.

Diclofenac Sodium (Etravirine is a substrate of CYP3A4, CYP2C9, and CYP2C19. Therefore, co-administration of etravirine with drugs that induce or inhibit CYP3A4, CYP2C9, and CYP2C19 may alter the therapeutic effect or adverse reaction profile of etravirine). Products include:

Diclofenac Sodium Ophthalmic Solution.. ⊙**240**
Voltaren Ophthalmic Solution **2336**
Voltaren Tablets **2334**
Voltaren-XR Tablets **2337**

Dihydroergotamine Mesylate (Etravirine is an inducer of CYP3A4 and inhibitor of CYP2C9 and CYP2C19. Therefore, co-administration of drugs that are substrates of CYP3A4, CYP2C9 and CYP2C19 with etravirine may alter the therapeutic effect or adverse reaction profile of the co-administered drug(s)).

No products indexed under this heading.

Diltiazem Hydrochloride (Etravirine is a substrate of CYP3A4, CYP2C9, and CYP2C19. Therefore, co-administration of etravirine with drugs that induce or inhibit CYP3A4, CYP2C9, and CYP2C19 may alter the therapeutic effect or adverse reaction profile of etravirine). Products include:

Cardizem LA Extended Release Tablets.. **421**

Diltiazem Maleate (Etravirine is a substrate of CYP3A4, CYP2C9, and CYP2C19. Therefore, co-administration of etravirine with drugs that induce or inhibit CYP3A4, CYP2C9, and CYP2C19 may alter the therapeutic effect or adverse reaction profile of etravirine).

No products indexed under this heading.

Disopyramide (Etravirine is an inducer of CYP3A4 and inhibitor of CYP2C9 and CYP2C19. Therefore, co-administration of drugs that are substrates of CYP3A4, CYP2C9 and CYP2C19 with etravirine may alter the therapeutic effect or adverse reaction profile of the co-administered drug(s)).

No products indexed under this heading.

Disopyramide Phosphate (Concentrations of these antiarrhythmics may be decreased when co-administered with etravirine. Etravirine and antiarrhythmics should be co-administered with caution. Drug concentration monitoring is recommended, if available).

No products indexed under this heading.

Disulfiram (Etravirine is a substrate of CYP3A4, CYP2C9, and CYP2C19. Therefore, co-administration of etravirine with drugs that induce or inhibit CYP3A4, CYP2C9, and CYP2C19 may alter the therapeutic effect or adverse reaction profile of etravirine).

No products indexed under this heading.

Divalproex Sodium (Etravirine is an inducer of CYP3A4 and inhibitor of CYP2C9 and CYP2C19. Therefore, co-administration of drugs that are substrates of CYP3A4, CYP2C9 and CYP2C19 with etravirine may alter the therapeutic effect or adverse reaction profile of the co-administered drug(s)). Products include:

Depakote ER Tablets **423**

Dofetilide (Concentrations of these antiarrhythmics may be decreased when co-administered with etravirine. Etravirine and antiarrhythmics should be co-administered with caution. Drug concentration monitoring is recommended, if available).

No products indexed under this heading.

Doxepin Hydrochloride (Etravirine is an inducer of CYP3A4 and inhibitor of CYP2C9 and CYP2C19. Therefore, co-administration of drugs that are substrates of CYP3A4, CYP2C9 and CYP2C19 with etravirine may alter the therapeutic effect or adverse reaction profile of the co-administered drug(s)).

No products indexed under this heading.

Doxorubicin Hydrochloride (Etravirine is a substrate of CYP3A4, CYP2C9, and CYP2C19. Therefore, co-administration of etravirine with drugs that induce or inhibit CYP3A4, CYP2C9, and CYP2C19 may alter the therapeutic effect or adverse reaction profile of etravirine).

No products indexed under this heading.

Dronabinol (Etravirine is an inducer of CYP3A4 and inhibitor of CYP2C9 and CYP2C19. Therefore, co-administration of drugs that are substrates of CYP3A4, CYP2C9 and CYP2C19 with etravirine may alter the therapeutic effect or adverse reaction profile of the co-administered drug(s)). Products include:

Marinol Capsules **3163**

Efavirenz (Combining two NNRTIs has not been shown to be beneficial. Concomitant use of etravirine with efavirenz or nevirapine may cause a significant decrease in the plasma concentrations of etravirine and loss of therapeutic effect of etravirine. Etravirine and other NNRTIs should no be co-administered). Products include:

Atripla Tablets **938**
Sustiva Capsules **930**
Sustiva Tablets **930**

Eprosartan Mesylate (Etravirine is an inducer of CYP3A4 and inhibitor of CYP2C9 and CYP2C19. Therefore, co-administration of drugs that are substrates of CYP3A4, CYP2C9 and CYP2C19 with etravirine may alter the therapeutic effect or adverse reaction profile of the co-administered drug(s)). Products include:

Teveten Tablets **515**
Teveten HCT Tablets **517**

Ergotamine Tartrate (Etravirine is an inducer of CYP3A4 and inhibitor of CYP2C9 and CYP2C19. Therefore, co-administration of drugs that are substrates of CYP3A4, CYP2C9 and CYP2C19 with etravirine may alter the therapeutic effect or adverse reaction profile of the co-administered drug(s)).

No products indexed under this heading.

Erythromycin (Etravirine is a substrate of CYP3A4, CYP2C9, and CYP2C19. Therefore, co-administration of etravirine with drugs that induce or inhibit CYP3A4, CYP2C9, and CYP2C19 may alter the therapeutic effect or adverse reaction profile of etravirine).

No products indexed under this heading.

Erythromycin Estolate (Etravirine is a substrate of CYP3A4, CYP2C9, and CYP2C19. Therefore, co-administration of etravirine with drugs that induce or inhibit CYP3A4, CYP2C9, and CYP2C19 may alter the therapeutic effect or adverse reaction profile of etravirine).

No products indexed under this heading.

Erythromycin Ethylsuccinate (Etravirine is a substrate of CYP3A4, CYP2C9, and CYP2C19. Therefore, co-administration of etravirine with drugs that induce or inhibit CYP3A4, CYP2C9, and CYP2C19 may alter the therapeutic effect or adverse reaction profile of etravirine).
Products include:
E.E.S. ... 433
EryPed ... 431

Erythromycin Gluceptate (Etravirine is a substrate of CYP3A4, CYP2C9, and CYP2C19. Therefore, co-administration of etravirine with drugs that induce or inhibit CYP3A4, CYP2C9, and CYP2C19 may alter the therapeutic effect or adverse reaction profile of etravirine).
No products indexed under this heading.

Erythromycin Lactobionate (Etravirine is a substrate of CYP3A4, CYP2C9, and CYP2C19. Therefore, co-administration of etravirine with drugs that induce or inhibit CYP3A4, CYP2C9, and CYP2C19 may alter the therapeutic effect or adverse reaction profile of etravirine).
No products indexed under this heading.

Erythromycin Stearate (Etravirine is a substrate of CYP3A4, CYP2C9, and CYP2C19. Therefore, co-administration of etravirine with drugs that induce or inhibit CYP3A4, CYP2C9, and CYP2C19 may alter the therapeutic effect or adverse reaction profile of etravirine).
No products indexed under this heading.

Esomeprazole Magnesium (Etravirine is a substrate of CYP3A4, CYP2C9, and CYP2C19. Therefore, co-administration of etravirine with drugs that induce or inhibit CYP3A4, CYP2C9, and CYP2C19 may alter the therapeutic effect or adverse reaction profile of etravirine).
Products include:
Nexium Delayed-Release Capsules ... 645
Nexium Delayed-Release Oral Suspension ... 645

Estradiol (Etravirine is an inducer of CYP3A4 and inhibitor of CYP2C9 and CYP2C19. Therefore, co-administration of drugs that are substrates of CYP3A4, CYP2C9 and CYP2C19 with etravirine may alter the therapeutic effect or adverse reaction profile of the co-administered drug(s)). Products include:
Activella Tablets ... 2347
Angeliq Tablets ... 751
Climara Transdermal System ... 763
Climara Pro Transdermal System ... 768
Divigel ... 3167
Vagifem Tablets ... 2375

Estradiol Benzoate (Etravirine is an inducer of CYP3A4 and inhibitor of CYP2C9 and CYP2C19. Therefore, co-administration of drugs that are substrates of CYP3A4, CYP2C9 and CYP2C19 with etravirine may alter the therapeutic effect or adverse reaction profile of the co-administered drug(s)).
No products indexed under this heading.

Estradiol Cypionate (Etravirine is an inducer of CYP3A4 and inhibitor of CYP2C9 and CYP2C19. Therefore, co-administration of drugs that are substrates of CYP3A4, CYP2C9 and CYP2C19 with etravirine may alter the therapeutic effect or adverse reaction profile of the co-administered drug(s)).
No products indexed under this heading.

Estradiol Valerate (Etravirine is an inducer of CYP3A4 and inhibitor of CYP2C9 and CYP2C19. Therefore, co-administration of drugs that are substrates of CYP3A4, CYP2C9 and CYP2C19 with etravirine may alter the therapeutic effect or adverse reaction profile of the co-administered drug(s)).
No products indexed under this heading.

Ethinyl Estradiol (Etravirine is a substrate of CYP3A4, CYP2C9, and CYP2C19. Therefore, co-administration of etravirine with drugs that induce or inhibit CYP3A4, CYP2C9, and CYP2C19 may alter the therapeutic effect or adverse reaction profile of etravirine).
Products include:
Lybrel Tablets ... 3204
Mircette Tablets ... 1034
NuvaRing ... 2897
Ortho-Cyclen/Ortho Tri-Cyclen ... 2449
Ortho Evra Transdermal System ... 2437
Ortho Tri-Cyclen Lo Tablets ... 2458
Seasonique Tablets ... 1046
Yaz Tablets ... 805

Ethosuximide (Etravirine is a substrate of CYP3A4, CYP2C9, and CYP2C19. Therefore, co-administration of etravirine with drugs that induce or inhibit CYP3A4, CYP2C9, and CYP2C19 may alter the therapeutic effect or adverse reaction profile of etravirine).
No products indexed under this heading.

Ethotoin (Etravirine is an inducer of CYP3A4 and inhibitor of CYP2C9 and CYP2C19. Therefore, co-administration of drugs that are substrates of CYP3A4, CYP2C9 and CYP2C19 with etravirine may alter the therapeutic effect or adverse reaction profile of the co-administered drug(s)).
No products indexed under this heading.

Ethynodiol Diacetate (Etravirine is a substrate of CYP3A4, CYP2C9, and CYP2C19. Therefore, co-administration of etravirine with drugs that induce or inhibit CYP3A4, CYP2C9, and CYP2C19 may alter the therapeutic effect or adverse reaction profile of etravirine).
No products indexed under this heading.

Etodolac (Etravirine is an inducer of CYP3A4 and inhibitor of CYP2C9 and CYP2C19. Therefore, co-administration of drugs that are substrates of CYP3A4, CYP2C9 and CYP2C19 with etravirine may alter the therapeutic effect or adverse reaction profile of the co-administered drug(s)).
No products indexed under this heading.

Etoposide (Etravirine is an inducer of CYP3A4 and inhibitor of CYP2C9 and CYP2C19. Therefore, co-administration of drugs that are substrates of CYP3A4, CYP2C9 and CYP2C19 with etravirine may alter the therapeutic effect or adverse reaction profile of the co-administered drug(s)).
No products indexed under this heading.

Etoposide Phosphate (Etravirine is an inducer of CYP3A4 and inhibitor of CYP2C9 and CYP2C19. Therefore, co-administration of drugs that are substrates of CYP3A4, CYP2C9 and CYP2C19 with etravirine may alter the therapeutic effect or adverse reaction profile of the co-administered drug(s)).
No products indexed under this heading.

Felbamate (Etravirine is a substrate of CYP3A4, CYP2C9, and CYP2C19. Therefore, co-administration of etravirine with drugs that induce or inhibit CYP3A4, CYP2C9, and CYP2C19 may alter the therapeutic effect or adverse reaction profile of etravirine).
No products indexed under this heading.

Felodipine (Etravirine is an inducer of CYP3A4 and inhibitor of CYP2C9 and CYP2C19. Therefore, co-administration of drugs that are substrates of CYP3A4, CYP2C9 and CYP2C19 with etravirine may alter the therapeutic effect or adverse reaction profile of the co-administered drug(s)).
No products indexed under this heading.

Fenofibrate (Etravirine is a substrate of CYP3A4, CYP2C9, and CYP2C19. Therefore, co-administration of etravirine with drugs that induce or inhibit CYP3A4, CYP2C9, and CYP2C19 may alter the therapeutic effect or adverse reaction profile of etravirine).
Products include:
Fenoglide Tablets ... 2960
Tricor Tablets ... 520

Fenoprofen Calcium (Etravirine is an inducer of CYP3A4 and inhibitor of CYP2C9 and CYP2C19. Therefore, co-administration of drugs that are substrates of CYP3A4, CYP2C9 and CYP2C19 with etravirine may alter the therapeutic effect or adverse reaction profile of the co-administered drug(s)). Products include:
Nalfon Capsules ... 2508

Fentanyl (Etravirine is an inducer of CYP3A4 and inhibitor of CYP2C9 and CYP2C19. Therefore, co-administration of drugs that are substrates of CYP3A4, CYP2C9 and CYP2C19 with etravirine may alter the therapeutic effect or adverse reaction profile of the co-administered drug(s)). Products include:
Duragesic Transdermal System ... 2405
Ionsys Transdermal System ... 2410

Fentanyl Citrate (Etravirine is an inducer of CYP3A4 and inhibitor of CYP2C9 and CYP2C19. Therefore, co-administration of drugs that are substrates of CYP3A4, CYP2C9 and CYP2C19 with etravirine may alter the therapeutic effect or adverse reaction profile of the co-administered drug(s)). Products include:
Actiq ... 959
Fentora Tablets ... 968

Flecainide Acetate (Concentrations of these antiarrhythmics may be decreased when co-administered with etravirine. Etravirine and antiarrhythmics should be co-administered with caution. Drug concentration monitoring is recommended, if available).
No products indexed under this heading.

Fluconazole (Posaconazole is a potent inhibitor of CYP3A4 and fluconazole is a potent inhibitor of CYP2C9; both may increase plasma concentrations of etravirine. Itraconazole and ketoconazole are potent inhibitors as well as substrates of CYP3A4. Concomitant systemic use of itraconazole or ketoconazole and etravirine may increase plasma concentrations of etravirine. Simultaneously, plasma concentrations of itraconazole or ketoconazole may be decreased by etravirine. Voriconazole is a CYP2C19 substrate and CYP3A4, CYP2C9 and CYP2C19 inhibitor. Concomitant use of voriconazole and etravirine may increase plasma concentrations of both drugs. Dose adjustments for itraconazole, ketoconazole or voriconazole may be necessary depending on other co-administered drugs).
No products indexed under this heading.

Fludrocortisone Acetate (Etravirine is a substrate of CYP3A4, CYP2C9, and CYP2C19. Therefore, co-administration of etravirine with drugs that induce or inhibit CYP3A4, CYP2C9, and CYP2C19 may alter the therapeutic effect or adverse reaction profile of etravirine).
No products indexed under this heading.

Fluorouracil (Etravirine is a substrate of CYP3A4, CYP2C9, and CYP2C19. Therefore, co-administration of etravirine with drugs that induce or inhibit CYP3A4, CYP2C9, and CYP2C19 may alter the therapeutic effect or adverse reaction profile of etravirine).
Products include:
Carac Cream 0.5% ... 2722

Fluoxetine (Etravirine is a substrate of CYP3A4, CYP2C9, and CYP2C19. Therefore, co-administration of etravirine with drugs that induce or inhibit CYP3A4, CYP2C9, and CYP2C19 may alter the therapeutic effect or adverse reaction profile of etravirine).
No products indexed under this heading.

Fluoxetine Hydrochloride (Etravirine is a substrate of CYP3A4, CYP2C9, and CYP2C19. Therefore, co-administration of etravirine with drugs that induce or inhibit CYP3A4, CYP2C9, and CYP2C19 may alter the therapeutic effect or adverse reaction profile of etravirine).
Products include:
Prozac Weekly Capsules ... 1852
Prozac Pulvules and Liquid ... 1852
Symbyax Capsules ... 1871

Flurbiprofen (Etravirine is a substrate of CYP3A4, CYP2C9, and CYP2C19. Therefore, co-administration of etravirine with drugs that induce or inhibit CYP3A4, CYP2C9, and CYP2C19 may alter the therapeutic effect or adverse reaction profile of etravirine).
No products indexed under this heading.

Flurbiprofen Sodium (Etravirine is a substrate of CYP3A4, CYP2C9, and CYP2C19. Therefore, co-administration of etravirine with drugs that induce or inhibit CYP3A4, CYP2C9, and CYP2C19 may alter the therapeutic effect or adverse reaction profile of etravirine).
No products indexed under this heading.

Fluvastatin Sodium (Lovastatin and simvastatin are CYP3A4 substrates and co-administration with etravirine may result in lower plasma concentrations of the HMG-CoA reductase inhibitor. Fluvastatin is metabolized by CYP2C9 and co-administration with etravirine may result in higher plasma concentrations of the HMG-CoA reductase inhibitor. Dose adjustments for these HMG-CoA reductase inhibitors may be necessary). Products include:
Lescol Capsules 2268
Lescol XL Tablets 2268

Fluvoxamine (Etravirine is a substrate of CYP3A4, CYP2C9, and CYP2C19. Therefore, co-administration of etravirine with drugs that induce or inhibit CYP3A4, CYP2C9, and CYP2C19 may alter the therapeutic effect or adverse reaction profile of etravirine).
No products indexed under this heading.

Fluvoxamine Maleate (Etravirine is a substrate of CYP3A4, CYP2C9, and CYP2C19. Therefore, co-administration of etravirine with drugs that induce or inhibit CYP3A4, CYP2C9, and CYP2C19 may alter the therapeutic effect or adverse reaction profile of etravirine). Products include:
Luvox CR Extended-Release Capsules 1759

Formoterol Fumarate (Etravirine is an inducer of CYP3A4 and inhibitor of CYP2C9 and CYP2C19. Therefore, co-administration of drugs that are substrates of CYP3A4, CYP2C9 and CYP2C19 with etravirine may alter the therapeutic effect or adverse reaction profile of the co-administered drug(s)). Products include:
Foradil Aerolizer 2849
Perforomist Inhalation Solution 1025

Fosamprenavir Calcium (Concomitant use of etravirine with protease inhibitors (PIs) without co-administration of low-dose ritonavir may cause a significant alteration in the plasma concentrations of the PI. Etravirine should not be co-administered with PIs without low-dose ritonavir. Due to a significant increase in the systemic exposure of amprenavir, the appropriate doses of the cobination of etravirine and fosamprenavir/ritonavir have not been established. Etravirine and fosamprenavir/ritonavir should not be co-administered). Products include:
Lexiva Oral Suspension 1510
Lexiva Tablets 1510

Fosphenytoin (Etravirine is an inducer of CYP3A4 and inhibitor of CYP2C9 and CYP2C19. Therefore, co-administration of drugs that are substrates of CYP3A4, CYP2C9 and CYP2C19 with etravirine may alter the therapeutic effect or adverse reaction profile of the co-administered drug(s)).
No products indexed under this heading.

Fosphenytoin Sodium (Carbamazepine, phenobarbital and phenytoin are inducers of CYP450 enzymes. Etravirine should not be used in combination with carbamazepine, phenobarbital, or phenytoin as co-administration may cause significant decreases with etravirine plasma concentrations and loss of therapeutic effect of etravirine).
No products indexed under this heading.

Gabapentin (Etravirine is an inducer of CYP3A4 and inhibitor of CYP2C9 and CYP2C19. Therefore, co-administration of drugs that are substrates of CYP3A4, CYP2C9 and CYP2C19 with etravirine may alter the therapeutic effect or adverse reaction profile of the co-administered drug(s)).
No products indexed under this heading.

Garlic Extract (Etravirine is a substrate of CYP3A4, CYP2C9, and CYP2C19. Therefore, co-administration of etravirine with drugs that induce or inhibit CYP3A4, CYP2C9, and CYP2C19 may alter the therapeutic effect or adverse reaction profile of etravirine).
No products indexed under this heading.

Garlic Oil (Etravirine is a substrate of CYP3A4, CYP2C9, and CYP2C19. Therefore, co-administration of etravirine with drugs that induce or inhibit CYP3A4, CYP2C9, and CYP2C19 may alter the therapeutic effect or adverse reaction profile of etravirine).
No products indexed under this heading.

Gemfibrozil (Etravirine is a substrate of CYP3A4, CYP2C9, and CYP2C19. Therefore, co-administration of etravirine with drugs that induce or inhibit CYP3A4, CYP2C9, and CYP2C19 may alter the therapeutic effect or adverse reaction profile of etravirine).
No products indexed under this heading.

Glimepiride (Etravirine is an inducer of CYP3A4 and inhibitor of CYP2C9 and CYP2C19. Therefore, co-administration of drugs that are substrates of CYP3A4, CYP2C9 and CYP2C19 with etravirine may alter the therapeutic effect or adverse reaction profile of the co-administered drug(s)). Products include:
Avandaryl Tablets 1344
Duetact Tablets 3085

Glipizide (Etravirine is a substrate of CYP3A4, CYP2C9, and CYP2C19. Therefore, co-administration of etravirine with drugs that induce or inhibit CYP3A4, CYP2C9, and CYP2C19 may alter the therapeutic effect or adverse reaction profile of etravirine).
No products indexed under this heading.

Glyburide (Etravirine is a substrate of CYP3A4, CYP2C9, and CYP2C19. Therefore, co-administration of etravirine with drugs that induce or inhibit CYP3A4, CYP2C9, and CYP2C19 may alter the therapeutic effect or adverse reaction profile of etravirine).
No products indexed under this heading.

Haloperidol (Etravirine is an inducer of CYP3A4 and inhibitor of CYP2C9 and CYP2C19. Therefore, co-administration of drugs that are substrates of CYP3A4, CYP2C9 and CYP2C19 with etravirine may alter the therapeutic effect or adverse reaction profile of the co-administered drug(s)).
No products indexed under this heading.

Haloperidol Decanoate (Etravirine is an inducer of CYP3A4 and inhibitor of CYP2C9 and CYP2C19. Therefore, co-administration of drugs that are substrates of CYP3A4, CYP2C9 and CYP2C19 with etravirine may alter the therapeutic effect or adverse reaction profile of the co-administered drug(s)).
No products indexed under this heading.

Haloperidol Lactate (Etravirine is an inducer of CYP3A4 and inhibitor of CYP2C9 and CYP2C19. Therefore, co-administration of drugs that are substrates of CYP3A4, CYP2C9 and CYP2C19 with etravirine may alter the therapeutic effect or adverse reaction profile of the co-administered drug(s)).
No products indexed under this heading.

Hydrochlorothiazide (Etravirine is a substrate of CYP3A4, CYP2C9, and CYP2C19. Therefore, co-administration of etravirine with drugs that induce or inhibit CYP3A4, CYP2C9, and CYP2C19 may alter the therapeutic effect or adverse reaction profile of etravirine). Products include:
Atacand HCT 642
Avalide Tablets 892
Avalide Tablets 2713
Benicar HCT Tablets 1010
Diovan HCT Tablets 2216
Dyazide Capsules 1405
Micardis HCT Tablets 854
Prinzide Tablets 2092
Tekturna HCT Tablets 2324
Teveten HCT Tablets 517

Hydrocortisone (Etravirine is a substrate of CYP3A4, CYP2C9, and CYP2C19. Therefore, co-administration of etravirine with drugs that induce or inhibit CYP3A4, CYP2C9, and CYP2C19 may alter the therapeutic effect or adverse reaction profile of etravirine).
No products indexed under this heading.

Hydrocortisone Acetate (Etravirine is a substrate of CYP3A4, CYP2C9, and CYP2C19. Therefore, co-administration of etravirine with drugs that induce or inhibit CYP3A4, CYP2C9, and CYP2C19 may alter the therapeutic effect or adverse reaction profile of etravirine). Products include:
Analpram-HC 1140
Pramosone 1141

Hydrocortisone Butyrate (Etravirine is a substrate of CYP3A4, CYP2C9, and CYP2C19. Therefore, co-administration of etravirine with drugs that induce or inhibit CYP3A4, CYP2C9, and CYP2C19 may alter the therapeutic effect or adverse reaction profile of etravirine).
No products indexed under this heading.

Hydrocortisone Cypionate (Etravirine is a substrate of CYP3A4, CYP2C9, and CYP2C19. Therefore, co-administration of etravirine with drugs that induce or inhibit CYP3A4, CYP2C9, and CYP2C19 may alter the therapeutic effect or adverse reaction profile of etravirine).
No products indexed under this heading.

Hydrocortisone Hemisuccinate (Etravirine is a substrate of CYP3A4, CYP2C9, and CYP2C19. Therefore, co-administration of etravirine with drugs that induce or inhibit CYP3A4, CYP2C9, and CYP2C19 may alter the therapeutic effect or adverse reaction profile of etravirine).
No products indexed under this heading.

Hydrocortisone Probutate (Etravirine is a substrate of CYP3A4, CYP2C9, and CYP2C19. Therefore, co-administration of etravirine with drugs that induce or inhibit CYP3A4, CYP2C9, and CYP2C19 may alter the therapeutic effect or adverse reaction profile of etravirine).
No products indexed under this heading.

Hydrocortisone Sodium Phosphate (Etravirine is a substrate of CYP3A4, CYP2C9, and CYP2C19. Therefore, co-administration of etravirine with drugs that induce or inhibit CYP3A4, CYP2C9, and CYP2C19 may alter the therapeutic effect or adverse reaction profile of etravirine).
No products indexed under this heading.

Hydrocortisone Sodium Succinate (Etravirine is a substrate of CYP3A4, CYP2C9, and CYP2C19. Therefore, co-administration of etravirine with drugs that induce or inhibit CYP3A4, CYP2C9, and CYP2C19 may alter the therapeutic effect or adverse reaction profile of etravirine).
No products indexed under this heading.

Hydrocortisone Valerate (Etravirine is a substrate of CYP3A4, CYP2C9, and CYP2C19. Therefore, co-administration of etravirine with drugs that induce or inhibit CYP3A4, CYP2C9, and CYP2C19 may alter the therapeutic effect or adverse reaction profile of etravirine).
No products indexed under this heading.

Hydroflumethiazide (Etravirine is a substrate of CYP3A4, CYP2C9, and CYP2C19. Therefore, co-administration of etravirine with drugs that induce or inhibit CYP3A4, CYP2C9, and CYP2C19 may alter the therapeutic effect or adverse reaction profile of etravirine).
No products indexed under this heading.

Hypericum (Concomitant use of etravirine with products containing St. John's wort may cause significant decreases in etravirine plasma concentrations and loss of therapeu-

tic effect of etravirine. Etravirine and products containing St. John's wort should not be co-administered). Products include:

Satieté Tablets .... ■ 640

Hypericum Perforatum (Concomitant use of etravirine with products containing St. John's wort may cause significant decreases in etravirine plasma concentrations and loss of therapeutic effect of etravirine. Etravirine and products containing St. John's wort should not be co-administered).

No products indexed under this heading.

Ibuprofen (Etravirine is an inducer of CYP3A4 and inhibitor of CYP2C9 and CYP2C19. Therefore, co-administration of drugs that are substrates of CYP3A4, CYP2C9 and CYP2C19 with etravirine may alter the therapeutic effect or adverse reaction profile of the co-administered drug(s)). Products include:

Motrin IB Tablets and Caplets 1900
Children's Motrin Oral Suspension ... 1901
Children's Motrin Non-Staining Dye-Free Oral Suspension............ 1901
Children's Motrin Cold Oral Suspension 1899
Infants' Motrin Concentrated Drops.. 1901
Infants' Motrin Non-Staining Dye-Free Concentrated Drops....... 1901
Junior Strength Motrin Caplets and Chewable Tablets.................. 1901
Vicoprofen Tablets 533

Imatinib Mesylate (Etravirine is a substrate of CYP3A4, CYP2C9, and CYP2C19. Therefore, co-administration of etravirine with drugs that induce or inhibit CYP3A4, CYP2C9, and CYP2C19 may alter the therapeutic effect or adverse reaction profile of etravirine). Products include:

Gleevec Tablets 2255

Imipramine Hydrochloride (Etravirine is an inducer of CYP3A4 and inhibitor of CYP2C9 and CYP2C19. Therefore, co-administration of drugs that are substrates of CYP3A4, CYP2C9 and CYP2C19 with etravirine may alter the therapeutic effect or adverse reaction profile of the co-administered drug(s)).

No products indexed under this heading.

Imipramine Pamoate (Etravirine is an inducer of CYP3A4 and inhibitor of CYP2C9 and CYP2C19. Therefore, co-administration of drugs that are substrates of CYP3A4, CYP2C9 and CYP2C19 with etravirine may alter the therapeutic effect or adverse reaction profile of the co-administered drug(s)).

No products indexed under this heading.

Indinavir Sulfate (Concomitant use of etravirine with protease inhibitors (PIs) without co-administration of low-dose ritonavir may cause a significant alteration in the plasma concentrations of the PI. Etravirine should not be co-administered with PIs without low-dose ritonavir). Products include:

Crixivan Capsules 1979

Indomethacin (Etravirine is a substrate of CYP3A4, CYP2C9, and CYP2C19. Therefore, co-administration of etravirine with drugs that induce or inhibit CYP3A4, CYP2C9, and CYP2C19 may alter the therapeutic effect or adverse reaction profile of etravirine). Products include:

Indocin 2024

Indomethacin Sodium Trihydrate (Etravirine is a substrate of CYP3A4, CYP2C9, and CYP2C19. Therefore, co-administration of etravirine with drugs that induce or inhibit CYP3A4, CYP2C9, and CYP2C19 may alter the therapeutic effect or adverse reaction profile of etravirine). Products include:

Indocin I.V. 2489

Irbesartan (Etravirine is an inducer of CYP3A4 and inhibitor of CYP2C9 and CYP2C19. Therefore, co-administration of drugs that are substrates of CYP3A4, CYP2C9 and CYP2C19 with etravirine may alter the therapeutic effect or adverse reaction profile of the co-administered drug(s)). Products include:

Avalide Tablets 892
Avalide Tablets 2713
Avapro Tablets 897
Avapro Tablets 2718

Isoniazid (Etravirine is a substrate of CYP3A4, CYP2C9, and CYP2C19. Therefore, co-administration of etravirine with drugs that induce or inhibit CYP3A4, CYP2C9, and CYP2C19 may alter the therapeutic effect or adverse reaction profile of etravirine).

No products indexed under this heading.

Isradipine (Etravirine is an inducer of CYP3A4 and inhibitor of CYP2C9 and CYP2C19. Therefore, co-administration of drugs that are substrates of CYP3A4, CYP2C9 and CYP2C19 with etravirine may alter the therapeutic effect or adverse reaction profile of the co-administered drug(s)). Products include:

DynaCirc CR Controlled Release Tablets 1407

Itraconazole (Etravirine is a substrate of CYP3A4, CYP2C9, and CYP2C19. Therefore, co-administration of etravirine with drugs that induce or inhibit CYP3A4, CYP2C9, and CYP2C19 may alter the therapeutic effect or adverse reaction profile of etravirine).

No products indexed under this heading.

Ixabepilone (Etravirine is an inducer of CYP3A4 and inhibitor of CYP2C9 and CYP2C19. Therefore, co-administration of drugs that are substrates of CYP3A4, CYP2C9 and CYP2C19 with etravirine may alter the therapeutic effect or adverse reaction profile of the co-administered drug(s)). Products include:

Ixempra Kit for Injection 915

Ketoconazole (Posaconazole is a potent inhibitor of CYP3A4 and fluconazole is a potent inhibitor of CYP2C9; both may increase plasma concentrations of etravirine. Itraconazole and ketoconazole are potent inhibitors as well as substrates of CYP3A4. Concomitant systemic use of itraconazole or ketoconazole and etravirine may increase plasma concentrations of etravirine. Simultaneously, plasma concentrations of itraconazole or ketoconazole may be decreased by etravirine. Voriconazole is a CYP2C19 substrate and CYP3A4, CYP2C9 and CYP2C19 inhibitor. Concomitant use of voriconazole and etravirine may increase plasma concentrations of both drugs. Dose adjustments for itraconazole, ketoconazole or voriconazole may be necessary depending on other co-administered drugs). Products include:

Extina Foam, 2% 3057
Nizoral A-D Shampoo 1901

Ketoprofen (Etravirine is a substrate of CYP3A4, CYP2C9, and CYP2C19. Therefore, co-administration of etravirine with drugs that induce or inhibit CYP3A4, CYP2C9, and CYP2C19 may alter the therapeutic effect or adverse reaction profile of etravirine).

No products indexed under this heading.

Ketorolac Tromethamine (Etravirine is an inducer of CYP3A4 and inhibitor of CYP2C9 and CYP2C19. Therefore, co-administration of drugs that are substrates of CYP3A4, CYP2C9 and CYP2C19 with etravirine may alter the therapeutic effect or adverse reaction profile of the co-administered drug(s)).

No products indexed under this heading.

Lamotrigine (Etravirine is an inducer of CYP3A4 and inhibitor of CYP2C9 and CYP2C19. Therefore, co-administration of drugs that are substrates of CYP3A4, CYP2C9 and CYP2C19 with etravirine may alter the therapeutic effect or adverse reaction profile of the co-administered drug(s)). Products include:

Lamictal 1488

Lansoprazole (Etravirine is a substrate of CYP3A4, CYP2C9, and CYP2C19. Therefore, co-administration of etravirine with drugs that induce or inhibit CYP3A4, CYP2C9, and CYP2C19 may alter the therapeutic effect or adverse reaction profile of etravirine).

No products indexed under this heading.

Leflunomide (Etravirine is a substrate of CYP3A4, CYP2C9, and CYP2C19. Therefore, co-administration of etravirine with drugs that induce or inhibit CYP3A4, CYP2C9, and CYP2C19 may alter the therapeutic effect or adverse reaction profile of etravirine).

No products indexed under this heading.

Letrozole (Etravirine is a substrate of CYP3A4, CYP2C9, and CYP2C19. Therefore, co-administration of etravirine with drugs that induce or inhibit CYP3A4, CYP2C9, and CYP2C19 may alter the therapeutic effect or adverse reaction profile of etravirine). Products include:

Femara Tablets 2246

Levetiracetam (Etravirine is an inducer of CYP3A4 and inhibitor of CYP2C9 and CYP2C19. Therefore, co-administration of drugs that are substrates of CYP3A4, CYP2C9 and CYP2C19 with etravirine may alter the therapeutic effect or adverse reaction profile of the co-administered drug(s)). Products include:

Keppra Injection 3137
Keppra Oral Solution 3131
Keppra Tablets 3131

Levonorgestrel (Etravirine is a substrate of CYP3A4, CYP2C9, and CYP2C19. Therefore, co-administration of etravirine with drugs that induce or inhibit CYP3A4, CYP2C9, and CYP2C19 may alter the therapeutic effect or adverse reaction profile of etravirine). Products include:

Climara Pro Transdermal System 768
Lybrel Tablets 3204
Mirena Intrauterine System 779
Plan B Tablets 1044
Seasonique Tablets 1046

Lidocaine (Etravirine is an inducer of CYP3A4 and inhibitor of CYP2C9 and CYP2C19. Therefore, co-administration of drugs that are substrates of CYP3A4, CYP2C9 and CYP2C19 with etravirine may alter the therapeutic effect or adverse reaction profile of the co-administered drug(s)). Products include:

Lidoderm Patch 1114

Lidocaine Hydrochloride (Concentrations of these antiarrhythmics may be decreased when co-administered with etravirine. Etravirine and antiarrhythmics should be co-administered with caution. Drug concentration monitoring is recommended, if available).

No products indexed under this heading.

Lopinavir (Concomitant use of etravirine with protease inhibitors (PIs) without co-administration of low-dose ritonavir may cause a significant alteration in the plasma concentrations of the PI. Etravirine should not be co-administered with PIs without low-dose ritonavir. The mean system exposure (AUC) of etravirine after co-administration of etravirine with lopinavir/ritonavir is anticipated to be about 85% higher than the mean systemic exposure of etravirine observed in the Phase 3 trials. The amount of safetydata at these increased etravirine exposures is limited, therefore, etravirine and lopinavir/ritonavir should be co-administered with caution). Products include:

Kaletra 452

Loratadine (Etravirine is a substrate of CYP3A4, CYP2C9, and CYP2C19. Therefore, co-administration of etravirine with drugs that induce or inhibit CYP3A4, CYP2C9, and CYP2C19 may alter the therapeutic effect or adverse reaction profile of etravirine).

No products indexed under this heading.

Losartan Potassium (Etravirine is an inducer of CYP3A4 and inhibitor of CYP2C9 and CYP2C19. Therefore, co-administration of drugs that are substrates of CYP3A4, CYP2C9 and CYP2C19 with etravirine may alter the therapeutic effect or adverse reaction profile of the co-administered drug(s)). Products include:

Cozaar Tablets 1973

Lovastatin (Lovastatin and simvastatin are CYP3A4 substrates and co-administration with etravirine may result in lower plasma concentrations of the HMG-CoA reductase inhibitor. Fluvastatin is metabolized by CYP2C9 and co-administration with etravirine may result in higher plasma concentrations of the HMG-CoA reductase inhibitor. Dose adjustments for these HMG-CoA reductase inhibitors may be necessary). Products include:

Advicor Tablets 402
Mevacor Tablets 2063

Maprotiline Hydrochloride (Etravirine is an inducer of CYP3A4 and inhibitor of CYP2C9 and CYP2C19. Therefore, co-administration of drugs that are substrates of CYP3A4, CYP2C9 and CYP2C19 with etravirine may alter the therapeutic effect or adverse reaction profile of the co-administered drug(s)).
No products indexed under this heading.

Meclofenamate Sodium (Etravirine is an inducer of CYP3A4 and inhibitor of CYP2C9 and CYP2C19. Therefore, co-administration of drugs that are substrates of CYP3A4, CYP2C9 and CYP2C19 with etravirine may alter the therapeutic effect or adverse reaction profile of the co-administered drug(s)).
No products indexed under this heading.

Mefenamic Acid (Etravirine is an inducer of CYP3A4 and inhibitor of CYP2C9 and CYP2C19. Therefore, co-administration of drugs that are substrates of CYP3A4, CYP2C9 and CYP2C19 with etravirine may alter the therapeutic effect or adverse reaction profile of the co-administered drug(s)).
No products indexed under this heading.

Meloxicam (Etravirine is an inducer of CYP3A4 and inhibitor of CYP2C9 and CYP2C19. Therefore, co-administration of drugs that are substrates of CYP3A4, CYP2C9 and CYP2C19 with etravirine may alter the therapeutic effect or adverse reaction profile of the co-administered drug(s)). Products include:
Mobic Oral Suspension 863
Mobic Tablets 863

Mephenytoin (Etravirine is a substrate of CYP3A4, CYP2C9, and CYP2C19. Therefore, co-administration of etravirine with drugs that induce or inhibit CYP3A4, CYP2C9, and CYP2C19 may alter the therapeutic effect or adverse reaction profile of etravirine).
No products indexed under this heading.

Mephobarbital (Etravirine is an inducer of CYP3A4 and inhibitor of CYP2C9 and CYP2C19. Therefore, co-administration of drugs that are substrates of CYP3A4, CYP2C9 and CYP2C19 with etravirine may alter the therapeutic effect or adverse reaction profile of the co-administered drug(s)).
No products indexed under this heading.

Meprobamate (Etravirine is an inducer of CYP3A4 and inhibitor of CYP2C9 and CYP2C19. Therefore, co-administration of drugs that are substrates of CYP3A4, CYP2C9 and CYP2C19 with etravirine may alter the therapeutic effect or adverse reaction profile of the co-administered drug(s)).
No products indexed under this heading.

Mestranol (Etravirine is a substrate of CYP3A4, CYP2C9, and CYP2C19. Therefore, co-administration of etravirine with drugs that induce or inhibit CYP3A4, CYP2C9, and CYP2C19 may alter the therapeutic effect or adverse reaction profile of etravirine).
No products indexed under this heading.

Metformin Hydrochloride (Etravirine is an inducer of CYP3A4 and inhibitor of CYP2C9 and CYP2C19. Therefore, co-administration of drugs that are substrates of CYP3A4, CYP2C9 and CYP2C19 with etravirine may alter the therapeutic effect or adverse reaction profile of the co-administered drug(s)). Products include:
ActoPlus Met Tablets 3071
Avandamet Tablets 1336
Janumet Tablets 2041
PrandiMet Tablets 2967

Methadone Hydrochloride (Etravirine and methadone can be co-administered without dose adjustments, however, clinical monitoring for withdrawal symptoms is recommended as methadone maintenance therapy may need to be adjusted in some patients).
No products indexed under this heading.

Methsuximide (Etravirine is a substrate of CYP3A4, CYP2C9, and CYP2C19. Therefore, co-administration of etravirine with drugs that induce or inhibit CYP3A4, CYP2C9, and CYP2C19 may alter the therapeutic effect or adverse reaction profile of etravirine).
No products indexed under this heading.

Methyclothiazide (Etravirine is a substrate of CYP3A4, CYP2C9, and CYP2C19. Therefore, co-administration of etravirine with drugs that induce or inhibit CYP3A4, CYP2C9, and CYP2C19 may alter the therapeutic effect or adverse reaction profile of etravirine).
No products indexed under this heading.

Methylprednisolone (Etravirine is a substrate of CYP3A4, CYP2C9, and CYP2C19. Therefore, co-administration of etravirine with drugs that induce or inhibit CYP3A4, CYP2C9, and CYP2C19 may alter the therapeutic effect or adverse reaction profile of etravirine).
No products indexed under this heading.

Methylprednisolone Acetate (Etravirine is a substrate of CYP3A4, CYP2C9, and CYP2C19. Therefore, co-administration of etravirine with drugs that induce or inhibit CYP3A4, CYP2C9, and CYP2C19 may alter the therapeutic effect or adverse reaction profile of etravirine).
No products indexed under this heading.

Methylprednisolone Sodium Succinate (Etravirine is a substrate of CYP3A4, CYP2C9, and CYP2C19. Therefore, co-administration of etravirine with drugs that induce or inhibit CYP3A4, CYP2C9, and CYP2C19 may alter the therapeutic effect or adverse reaction profile of etravirine).
No products indexed under this heading.

Metronidazole (Etravirine is a substrate of CYP3A4, CYP2C9, and CYP2C19. Therefore, co-administration of etravirine with drugs that induce or inhibit CYP3A4, CYP2C9, and CYP2C19 may alter the therapeutic effect or adverse reaction profile of etravirine). Products include:
Pylera Capsules 714

Metronidazole Benzoate (Etravirine is a substrate of CYP3A4, CYP2C9, and CYP2C19. Therefore, co-administration of etravirine with drugs that induce or inhibit CYP3A4, CYP2C9, and CYP2C19 may alter the therapeutic effect or adverse reaction profile of etravirine).
No products indexed under this heading.

Metronidazole Hydrochloride (Etravirine is a substrate of CYP3A4, CYP2C9, and CYP2C19. Therefore, co-administration of etravirine with drugs that induce or inhibit CYP3A4, CYP2C9, and CYP2C19 may alter the therapeutic effect or adverse reaction profile of etravirine).
No products indexed under this heading.

Metronidazole Sodium (Etravirine is a substrate of CYP3A4, CYP2C9, and CYP2C19. Therefore, co-administration of etravirine with drugs that induce or inhibit CYP3A4, CYP2C9, and CYP2C19 may alter the therapeutic effect or adverse reaction profile of etravirine).
No products indexed under this heading.

Mexiletine Hydrochloride (Concentrations of these antiarrhythmics may be decreased when co-administered with etravirine. Etravirine and antiarrhythmics should be co-administered with caution. Drug concentration monitoring is recommended, if available).
No products indexed under this heading.

Miconazole (Etravirine is a substrate of CYP3A4, CYP2C9, and CYP2C19. Therefore, co-administration of etravirine with drugs that induce or inhibit CYP3A4, CYP2C9, and CYP2C19 may alter the therapeutic effect or adverse reaction profile of etravirine).
No products indexed under this heading.

Miconazole Nitrate (Etravirine is a substrate of CYP3A4, CYP2C9, and CYP2C19. Therefore, co-administration of etravirine with drugs that induce or inhibit CYP3A4, CYP2C9, and CYP2C19 may alter the therapeutic effect or adverse reaction profile of etravirine).
No products indexed under this heading.

Midazolam Hydrochloride (Etravirine is an inducer of CYP3A4 and inhibitor of CYP2C9 and CYP2C19. Therefore, co-administration of drugs that are substrates of CYP3A4, CYP2C9 and CYP2C19 with etravirine may alter the therapeutic effect or adverse reaction profile of the co-administered drug(s)).
No products indexed under this heading.

Miglitol (Etravirine is an inducer of CYP3A4 and inhibitor of CYP2C9 and CYP2C19. Therefore, co-administration of drugs that are substrates of CYP3A4, CYP2C9 and CYP2C19 with etravirine may alter the therapeutic effect or adverse reaction profile of the co-administered drug(s)).
No products indexed under this heading.

Mirtazapine (Etravirine is an inducer of CYP3A4 and inhibitor of CYP2C9 and CYP2C19. Therefore, co-administration of drugs that are substrates of CYP3A4, CYP2C9 and CYP2C19 with etravirine may alter the therapeutic effect or adverse reaction profile of the co-administered drug(s)). Products include:
Remeron Tablets 2924
RemeronSolTab Tablets 2927

Modafinil (Etravirine is a substrate of CYP3A4, CYP2C9, and CYP2C19. Therefore, co-administration of etravirine with drugs that induce or inhibit CYP3A4, CYP2C9, and CYP2C19 may alter the therapeutic effect or adverse reaction profile of etravirine). Products include:
Provigil Tablets 977

Montelukast Sodium (Etravirine is an inducer of CYP3A4 and inhibitor of CYP2C9 and CYP2C19. Therefore, co-administration of drugs that are substrates of CYP3A4, CYP2C9 and CYP2C19 with etravirine may alter the therapeutic effect or adverse reaction profile of the co-administered drug(s)). Products include:
Singulair 2114

Moricizine Hydrochloride (Concentrations of these antiarrhythmics may be decreased when co-administered with etravirine. Etravirine and antiarrhythmics should be co-administered with caution. Drug concentration monitoring is recommended, if available).
No products indexed under this heading.

Nabumetone (Etravirine is an inducer of CYP3A4 and inhibitor of CYP2C9 and CYP2C19. Therefore, co-administration of drugs that are substrates of CYP3A4, CYP2C9 and CYP2C19 with etravirine may alter the therapeutic effect or adverse reaction profile of the co-administered drug(s)).
No products indexed under this heading.

Naproxen (Etravirine is an inducer of CYP3A4 and inhibitor of CYP2C9 and CYP2C19. Therefore, co-administration of drugs that are substrates of CYP3A4, CYP2C9 and CYP2C19 with etravirine may alter the therapeutic effect or adverse reaction profile of the co-administered drug(s)). Products include:
EC-Naprosyn Delayed-Release Tablets 2632
Naprosyn Suspension 2632
Naprosyn Tablets 2632

Naproxen Sodium (Etravirine is an inducer of CYP3A4 and inhibitor of CYP2C9 and CYP2C19. Therefore, co-administration of drugs that are substrates of CYP3A4, CYP2C9 and CYP2C19 with etravirine may alter the therapeutic effect or adverse reaction profile of the co-administered drug(s)). Products include:

Anaprox Tablets **2632**
Anaprox DS Tablets **2632**
Treximet Tablets **1616**

Nateglinide (Etravirine is an inducer of CYP3A4 and inhibitor of CYP2C9 and CYP2C19. Therefore, co-administration of drugs that are substrates of CYP3A4, CYP2C9 and CYP2C19 with etravirine may alter the therapeutic effect or adverse reaction profile of the co-administered drug(s)). Products include:

Starlix Tablets **2314**

Nefazodone Hydrochloride (Etravirine is a substrate of CYP3A4, CYP2C9, and CYP2C19. Therefore, co-administration of etravirine with drugs that induce or inhibit CYP3A4, CYP2C9, and CYP2C19 may alter the therapeutic effect or adverse reaction profile of etravirine).

No products indexed under this heading.

Nelfinavir Mesylate (Concomitant use of etravirine with protease inhibitors (PIs) without co-administration of low-dose ritonavir may cause a significant alteration in the plasma concentrations of the PI. Etravirine should not be co-administered with PIs without low-dose ritonavir).

No products indexed under this heading.

Nevirapine (Combining two NNRTIs has not been shown to be beneficial. Concomitant use of etravirine with efavirenz or nevirapine may cause a significant decrease in the plasma concentrations of etravirine and loss of therapeutic effect of etravirine. Etravirine and other NNRTIs should no be co-administered). Products include:

Viramune Oral Suspension **873**
Viramune Tablets **873**

Niacinamide (Etravirine is a substrate of CYP3A4, CYP2C9, and CYP2C19. Therefore, co-administration of etravirine with drugs that induce or inhibit CYP3A4, CYP2C9, and CYP2C19 may alter the therapeutic effect or adverse reaction profile of etravirine). Products include:

BioLean Free Tablets .... ▣**635**

Nicardipine Hydrochloride (Etravirine is an inducer of CYP3A4 and inhibitor of CYP2C9 and CYP2C19. Therefore, co-administration of drugs that are substrates of CYP3A4, CYP2C9 and CYP2C19 with etravirine may alter the therapeutic effect or adverse reaction profile of the co-administered drug(s)). Products include:

Cardene I.V. **1093**

Nicotinamide (Etravirine is a substrate of CYP3A4, CYP2C9, and CYP2C19. Therefore, co-administration of etravirine with drugs that induce or inhibit CYP3A4, CYP2C9, and CYP2C19 may alter the therapeutic effect or adverse reaction profile of etravirine).

No products indexed under this heading.

Nifedipine (Etravirine is a substrate of CYP3A4, CYP2C9, and CYP2C19. Therefore, co-administration of etravirine with drugs that induce or inhibit CYP3A4, CYP2C9, and CYP2C19 may alter the therapeutic effect or adverse reaction profile of etravirine).

No products indexed under this heading.

Nilutamide (Etravirine is an inducer of CYP3A4 and inhibitor of CYP2C9 and CYP2C19. Therefore, co-administration of drugs that are substrates of CYP3A4, CYP2C9 and CYP2C19 with etravirine may alter the therapeutic effect or adverse reaction profile of the co-administered drug(s)).

No products indexed under this heading.

Nimodipine (Etravirine is an inducer of CYP3A4 and inhibitor of CYP2C9 and CYP2C19. Therefore, co-administration of drugs that are substrates of CYP3A4, CYP2C9 and CYP2C19 with etravirine may alter the therapeutic effect or adverse reaction profile of the co-administered drug(s)). Products include:

Nimotop Capsules **790**

Nisoldipine (Etravirine is an inducer of CYP3A4 and inhibitor of CYP2C9 and CYP2C19. Therefore, co-administration of drugs that are substrates of CYP3A4, CYP2C9 and CYP2C19 with etravirine may alter the therapeutic effect or adverse reaction profile of the co-administered drug(s)). Products include:

Sular Extended Release Tablets **2975**

Nitrendipine (Etravirine is an inducer of CYP3A4 and inhibitor of CYP2C9 and CYP2C19. Therefore, co-administration of drugs that are substrates of CYP3A4, CYP2C9 and CYP2C19 with etravirine may alter the therapeutic effect or adverse reaction profile of the co-administered drug(s)).

No products indexed under this heading.

Norethindrone (Etravirine is a substrate of CYP3A4, CYP2C9, and CYP2C19. Therefore, co-administration of etravirine with drugs that induce or inhibit CYP3A4, CYP2C9, and CYP2C19 may alter the therapeutic effect or adverse reaction profile of etravirine). Products include:

Ortho Micronor Tablets **2446**

Norethindrone Acetate (Etravirine is a substrate of CYP3A4, CYP2C9, and CYP2C19. Therefore, co-administration of etravirine with drugs that induce or inhibit CYP3A4, CYP2C9, and CYP2C19 may alter the therapeutic effect or adverse reaction profile of etravirine). Products include:

Activella Tablets **2347**

Norethynodrel (Etravirine is a substrate of CYP3A4, CYP2C9, and CYP2C19. Therefore, co-administration of etravirine with drugs that induce or inhibit CYP3A4, CYP2C9, and CYP2C19 may alter the therapeutic effect or adverse reaction profile of etravirine).

No products indexed under this heading.

Norfloxacin (Etravirine is a substrate of CYP3A4, CYP2C9, and CYP2C19. Therefore, co-administration of etravirine with drugs that induce or inhibit CYP3A4, CYP2C9, and CYP2C19 may alter the therapeutic effect or adverse reaction profile of etravirine). Products include:

Noroxin Tablets **2069**

Norgestimate (Etravirine is a substrate of CYP3A4, CYP2C9, and CYP2C19. Therefore, co-administration of etravirine with drugs that induce or inhibit CYP3A4, CYP2C9, and CYP2C19 may alter the therapeutic effect or adverse reaction profile of etravirine). Products include:

Ortho-Cyclen/Ortho Tri-Cyclen **2449**
Ortho Tri-Cyclen Lo Tablets **2458**

Norgestrel (Etravirine is a substrate of CYP3A4, CYP2C9, and CYP2C19. Therefore, co-administration of etravirine with drugs that induce or inhibit CYP3A4, CYP2C9, and CYP2C19 may alter the therapeutic effect or adverse reaction profile of etravirine).

No products indexed under this heading.

Nortriptyline Hydrochloride (Etravirine is an inducer of CYP3A4 and inhibitor of CYP2C9 and CYP2C19. Therefore, co-administration of drugs that are substrates of CYP3A4, CYP2C9 and CYP2C19 with etravirine may alter the therapeutic effect or adverse reaction profile of the co-administered drug(s)).

No products indexed under this heading.

Omeprazole (Etravirine is a substrate of CYP3A4, CYP2C9, and CYP2C19. Therefore, co-administration of etravirine with drugs that induce or inhibit CYP3A4, CYP2C9, and CYP2C19 may alter the therapeutic effect or adverse reaction profile of etravirine).

No products indexed under this heading.

Ondansetron (Etravirine is an inducer of CYP3A4 and inhibitor of CYP2C9 and CYP2C19. Therefore, co-administration of drugs that are substrates of CYP3A4, CYP2C9 and CYP2C19 with etravirine may alter the therapeutic effect or adverse reaction profile of the co-administered drug(s)). Products include:

Zofran ODT Orally Disintegrating Tablets **1687**

Ondansetron Hydrochloride (Etravirine is an inducer of CYP3A4 and inhibitor of CYP2C9 and CYP2C19. Therefore, co-administration of drugs that are substrates of CYP3A4, CYP2C9 and CYP2C19 with etravirine may alter the therapeutic effect or adverse reaction profile of the co-administered drug(s)). Products include:

Zofran Injection **1682**
Zofran **1687**

Oxaprozin (Etravirine is an inducer of CYP3A4 and inhibitor of CYP2C9 and CYP2C19. Therefore, co-administration of drugs that are substrates of CYP3A4, CYP2C9 and CYP2C19 with etravirine may alter the therapeutic effect or adverse reaction profile of the co-administered drug(s)).

No products indexed under this heading.

Oxcarbazepine (Etravirine is a substrate of CYP3A4, CYP2C9, and CYP2C19. Therefore, co-administration of etravirine with drugs that induce or inhibit CYP3A4, CYP2C9, and CYP2C19 may alter the therapeutic effect or adverse reaction profile of etravirine).

No products indexed under this heading.

Oxiconazole Nitrate (Etravirine is a substrate of CYP3A4, CYP2C9, and CYP2C19. Therefore, co-administration of etravirine with drugs that induce or inhibit CYP3A4, CYP2C9, and CYP2C19 may alter the therapeutic effect or adverse reaction profile of etravirine).

No products indexed under this heading.

Paclitaxel (Etravirine is an inducer of CYP3A4 and inhibitor of CYP2C9 and CYP2C19. Therefore, co-administration of drugs that are substrates of CYP3A4, CYP2C9 and CYP2C19 with etravirine may alter the therapeutic effect or adverse reaction profile of the co-administered drug(s)).

No products indexed under this heading.

Pantoprazole Sodium (Etravirine is an inducer of CYP3A4 and inhibitor of CYP2C9 and CYP2C19. Therefore, co-administration of drugs that are substrates of CYP3A4, CYP2C9 and CYP2C19 with etravirine may alter the therapeutic effect or adverse reaction profile of the co-administered drug(s)). Products include:

Protonix for Delayed-Release Oral Suspension **3254**
Protonix Delayed-Release Tablets **3254**
Protonix I.V. **3257**

Paramethadione (Etravirine is an inducer of CYP3A4 and inhibitor of CYP2C9 and CYP2C19. Therefore, co-administration of drugs that are substrates of CYP3A4, CYP2C9 and CYP2C19 with etravirine may alter the therapeutic effect or adverse reaction profile of the co-administered drug(s)).

No products indexed under this heading.

Paroxetine Hydrochloride (Etravirine is a substrate of CYP3A4, CYP2C9, and CYP2C19. Therefore, co-administration of etravirine with drugs that induce or inhibit CYP3A4, CYP2C9, and CYP2C19 may alter the therapeutic effect or adverse reaction profile of etravirine). Products include:

Paxil **1535**
Paxil CR Controlled-Release Tablets **1544**

Pentamidine Isethionate (Etravirine is an inducer of CYP3A4 and inhibitor of CYP2C9 and CYP2C19. Therefore, co-administration of drugs that are substrates of CYP3A4, CYP2C9 and CYP2C19 with etravirine may alter the therapeutic effect or adverse reaction profile of the co-administered drug(s)).

No products indexed under this heading.

Phenacemide (Etravirine is an inducer of CYP3A4 and inhibitor of CYP2C9 and CYP2C19. Therefore, co-administration of drugs that are substrates of CYP3A4, CYP2C9 and CYP2C19 with etravirine may alter the therapeutic effect or adverse reaction profile of the co-administered drug(s)).

No products indexed under this heading.

Phenobarbital (Carbamazepine, phenobarbital and phenytoin are inducers of CYP450 enzymes. Etravirine should not be used in combination with carbamazepine, phenobarbital, or phenytoin as co-administration may cause significant decreases in etravirine plasma concentrations and loss of therapeutic effect of etravirine). Products include:

Donnatal Extentabs **2507**

Phenobarbital Sodium (Carbamazepine, phenobarbital and phenytoin are inducers of CYP450 enzymes. Etravirine should not be used in combination with carbamazepine, phenobarbital, or phenytoin as co-administration may cause significant decreases in etravirine plasma concentrations and loss of therapeutic effect of etravirine).

No products indexed under this heading.

Phensuximide (Etravirine is an inducer of CYP3A4 and inhibitor of CYP2C9 and CYP2C19. Therefore, co-administration of drugs that are substrates of CYP3A4, CYP2C9 and CYP2C19 with etravirine may alter the therapeutic effect or adverse reaction profile of the co-administered drug(s)).

No products indexed under this heading.

Phenylbutazone (Etravirine is a substrate of CYP3A4, CYP2C9, and CYP2C19. Therefore, co-administration of etravirine with drugs that induce or inhibit CYP3A4, CYP2C9, and CYP2C19 may alter the therapeutic effect or adverse reaction profile of etravirine).

No products indexed under this heading.

Phenytoin (Carbamazepine, phenobarbital and phenytoin are inducers of CYP450 enzymes. Etravirine should not be used in combination with carbamazepine, phenobarbital, or phenytoin as co-administration may cause significant decreases with etravirine plasma concentrations and loss of therapeutic effect of etravirine).

No products indexed under this heading.

Phenytoin Sodium (Carbamazepine, phenobarbital and phenytoin are inducers of CYP450 enzymes. Etravirine should not be used in combination with carbamazepine, phenobarbital, or phenytoin as co-administration may cause significant decreases with etravirine plasma concentrations and loss of therapeutic effect of etravirine). Products include:

Phenytek Capsules **2192**

Pimozide (Etravirine is an inducer of CYP3A4 and inhibitor of CYP2C9 and CYP2C19. Therefore, co-administration of drugs that are substrates of CYP3A4, CYP2C9 and CYP2C19 with etravirine may alter the therapeutic effect or adverse reaction profile of the co-administered drug(s)).

No products indexed under this heading.

Pioglitazone Hydrochloride (Etravirine is an inducer of CYP3A4 and inhibitor of CYP2C9 and CYP2C19. Therefore, co-administration of drugs that are substrates of CYP3A4, CYP2C9 and CYP2C19 with etravirine may alter the therapeutic effect or adverse reaction profile of the co-administered drug(s)). Products include:

ActoPlus Met Tablets **3071**
Actos Tablets **3077**
Duetact Tablets **3085**

Piroxicam (Etravirine is an inducer of CYP3A4 and inhibitor of CYP2C9 and CYP2C19. Therefore, co-administration of drugs that are substrates of CYP3A4, CYP2C9 and CYP2C19 with etravirine may alter the therapeutic effect or adverse reaction profile of the co-administered drug(s)).

No products indexed under this heading.

Polyestradiol Phosphate (Etravirine is an inducer of CYP3A4 and inhibitor of CYP2C9 and CYP2C19. Therefore, co-administration of drugs that are substrates of CYP3A4, CYP2C9 and CYP2C19 with etravirine may alter the therapeutic effect or adverse reaction profile of the co-administered drug(s)).

No products indexed under this heading.

Polythiazide (Etravirine is a substrate of CYP3A4, CYP2C9, and CYP2C19. Therefore, co-administration of etravirine with drugs that induce or inhibit CYP3A4, CYP2C9, and CYP2C19 may alter the therapeutic effect or adverse reaction profile of etravirine).

No products indexed under this heading.

Posaconazole (Posaconazole is a potent inhibitor of CYP3A4 and fluconazole is a potent inhibitor of CYP2C9; both may increase plasma concentrations of etravirine. Itraconazole and ketoconazole are potent inhibitors as well as substrates of CYP3A4. Concomitant systemic use of itraconazole or ketoconazole and etravirine may increase plasma concentrations of etravirine. Simultaneously, plasma concentrations of itraconazole or ketoconazole may be decreased by etravirine. Voriconazole is a CYP2C19 substrate and CYP3A4, CYP2C9 and CYP2C19 inhibitor. Concomitant use of voriconazole and etravirine may increase plasma concentrations of both drugs. Dose adjustments for itraconazole, ketoconazole or voriconazole may be necessary depending on other co-administered drugs). Products include:

Noxafil Oral Suspension **2889**

Prednisolone Acetate (Etravirine is a substrate of CYP3A4, CYP2C9, and CYP2C19. Therefore, co-administration of etravirine with drugs that induce or inhibit CYP3A4, CYP2C9, and CYP2C19 may alter the therapeutic effect or adverse reaction profile of etravirine). Products include:

Pred Forte Ophthalmic Suspension .... ⊙**227**
Pred Mild Ophthalmic Suspension .... ⊙**230**
Pred-G Ophthalmic Ointment .... ⊙**229**
Pred-G Ophthalmic Suspension ...... ⊙**228**

Prednisolone Sodium Phosphate (Etravirine is a substrate of CYP3A4, CYP2C9, and CYP2C19. Therefore, co-administration of etravirine with drugs that induce or inhibit CYP3A4, CYP2C9, and CYP2C19 may alter the therapeutic effect or adverse reaction profile of etravirine).

No products indexed under this heading.

Prednisolone Tebutate (Etravirine is a substrate of CYP3A4, CYP2C9, and CYP2C19. Therefore, co-administration of etravirine with drugs that induce or inhibit CYP3A4, CYP2C9, and CYP2C19 may alter the therapeutic effect or adverse reaction profile of etravirine).

No products indexed under this heading.

Prednisone (Etravirine is a substrate of CYP3A4, CYP2C9, and CYP2C19. Therefore, co-administration of etravirine with drugs that induce or inhibit CYP3A4, CYP2C9, and CYP2C19 may alter the therapeutic effect or adverse reaction profile of etravirine).

No products indexed under this heading.

Primidone (Etravirine is a substrate of CYP3A4, CYP2C9, and CYP2C19. Therefore, co-administration of etravirine with drugs that induce or inhibit CYP3A4, CYP2C9, and CYP2C19 may alter the therapeutic effect or adverse reaction profile of etravirine).

No products indexed under this heading.

Procainamide Hydrochloride (Concentrations of these antiarrhythmics may be decreased when co-administered with etravirine. Etravirine and antiarrhythmics should be co-administered with caution. Drug concentration monitoring is recommended, if available).

No products indexed under this heading.

Progesterone (Etravirine is an inducer of CYP3A4 and inhibitor of CYP2C9 and CYP2C19. Therefore, co-administration of drugs that are substrates of CYP3A4, CYP2C9 and CYP2C19 with etravirine may alter the therapeutic effect or adverse reaction profile of the co-administered drug(s)). Products include:

Crinone 4% Gel **992**
Crinone 8% Gel **992**
Prometrium Capsules (100 mg, 200 mg) **3047**

Proguanil Hydrochloride (Etravirine is an inducer of CYP3A4 and inhibitor of CYP2C9 and CYP2C19. Therefore, co-administration of drugs that are substrates of CYP3A4, CYP2C9 and CYP2C19 with etravirine may alter the therapeutic effect or adverse reaction profile of the co-administered drug(s)). Products include:

Malarone Pediatric Tablets **1521**
Malarone Tablets **1521**

Propafenone Hydrochloride (Concentrations of these antiarrhythmics may be decreased when co-administered with etravirine. Etravirine and antiarrhythmics should be co-administered with caution. Drug concentration monitoring is recommended, if available). Products include:

Rythmol Tablets **1586**
Rythmol SR Capsules **1590**

Propoxyphene Hydrochloride (Etravirine is a substrate of CYP3A4, CYP2C9, and CYP2C19. Therefore, co-administration of etravirine with drugs that induce or inhibit CYP3A4, CYP2C9, and CYP2C19 may alter the therapeutic effect or adverse reaction profile of etravirine).

No products indexed under this heading.

Propoxyphene Napsylate (Etravirine is a substrate of CYP3A4, CYP2C9, and CYP2C19. Therefore, co-administration of etravirine with drugs that induce or inhibit CYP3A4, CYP2C9, and CYP2C19 may alter the therapeutic effect or adverse reaction profile of etravirine).

No products indexed under this heading.

Propranolol Hydrochloride (Concentrations of these antiarrhythmics may be decreased when co-administered with etravirine. Etravirine and antiarrhythmics should be co-administered with caution. Drug concentration monitoring is recommended, if available). Products include:

InnoPran XL Extended Release Capsules.................................... **1484**

Protriptyline Hydrochloride (Etravirine is an inducer of CYP3A4 and inhibitor of CYP2C9 and CYP2C19. Therefore, co-administration of drugs that are substrates of CYP3A4, CYP2C9 and CYP2C19 with etravirine may alter the therapeutic effect or adverse reaction profile of the co-administered drug(s)).

No products indexed under this heading.

Quinidine (Etravirine is a substrate of CYP3A4, CYP2C9, and CYP2C19. Therefore, co-administration of etravirine with drugs that induce or inhibit CYP3A4, CYP2C9, and CYP2C19 may alter the therapeutic effect or adverse reaction profile of etravirine).

No products indexed under this heading.

Quinidine Gluconate (Concentrations of these antiarrhythmics may be decreased when co-administered with etravirine. Etravirine and antiarrhythmics should be co-administered with caution. Drug concentration monitoring is recommended, if available).

No products indexed under this heading.

Quinidine Hydrochloride (Etravirine is a substrate of CYP3A4, CYP2C9, and CYP2C19. Therefore, co-administration of etravirine with drugs that induce or inhibit CYP3A4, CYP2C9, and CYP2C19 may alter the therapeutic effect or adverse reaction profile of etravirine).

No products indexed under this heading.

Quinidine Polygalacturonate (Concentrations of these antiarrhythmics may be decreased when co-administered with etravirine. Etravirine and antiarrhythmics should be co-administered with caution. Drug concentration monitoring is recommended, if available).

No products indexed under this heading.

Quinidine Sulfate (Concentrations of these antiarrhythmics may be decreased when co-administered with etravirine. Etravirine and antiarrhythmics should be co-administered with caution. Drug concentration monitoring is recommended, if available).

No products indexed under this heading.

Quinine (Etravirine is a substrate of CYP3A4, CYP2C9, and CYP2C19. Therefore, co-administration of etravirine with drugs that induce or inhibit CYP3A4, CYP2C9, and CYP2C19 may alter the therapeutic effect or adverse reaction profile of etravirine).
No products indexed under this heading.

Quinine Sulfate (Etravirine is a substrate of CYP3A4, CYP2C9, and CYP2C19. Therefore, co-administration of etravirine with drugs that induce or inhibit CYP3A4, CYP2C9, and CYP2C19 may alter the therapeutic effect or adverse reaction profile of etravirine).
No products indexed under this heading.

Quinupristin (Etravirine is a substrate of CYP3A4, CYP2C9, and CYP2C19. Therefore, co-administration of etravirine with drugs that induce or inhibit CYP3A4, CYP2C9, and CYP2C19 may alter the therapeutic effect or adverse reaction profile of etravirine).
No products indexed under this heading.

Rabeprazole Sodium (Etravirine is an inducer of CYP3A4 and inhibitor of CYP2C9 and CYP2C19. Therefore, co-administration of drugs that are substrates of CYP3A4, CYP2C9 and CYP2C19 with etravirine may alter the therapeutic effect or adverse reaction profile of the co-administered drug(s)). Products include:
Aciphex Tablets 1053

Ranitidine Bismuth Citrate (Etravirine is a substrate of CYP3A4, CYP2C9, and CYP2C19. Therefore, co-administration of etravirine with drugs that induce or inhibit CYP3A4, CYP2C9, and CYP2C19 may alter the therapeutic effect or adverse reaction profile of etravirine).
No products indexed under this heading.

Ranitidine Hydrochloride (Etravirine is a substrate of CYP3A4, CYP2C9, and CYP2C19. Therefore, co-administration of etravirine with drugs that induce or inhibit CYP3A4, CYP2C9, and CYP2C19 may alter the therapeutic effect or adverse reaction profile of etravirine). Products include:
Zantac 75 Tablets .... ▣603
Zantac 1670
Zantac Injection 1666
Zantac Injection Pharmacy Bulk Package 1668
Maximum Strength Zantac 150 Tablets .... ▣603
Maximum Strength Zantac 150 Cool Mint Tablets .... ▣603

Repaglinide (Etravirine is an inducer of CYP3A4 and inhibitor of CYP2C9 and CYP2C19. Therefore, co-administration of drugs that are substrates of CYP3A4, CYP2C9 and CYP2C19 with etravirine may alter the therapeutic effect or adverse reaction profile of the co-administered drug(s)). Products include:
PrandiMet Tablets 2967
Prandin Tablets 2971

Rifabutin (If etravirine is NOT co-adminsitered with a protease inhibitor/ritonavir, then rifabutin at a dose of 300 mg qd is recommended. If etravirine is co-administered with darunavir/ritonavir or saquinavir/ritonavir, then rifabutin should not be co-administered with due to the potential for significant reductions in etravirine exposure).
No products indexed under this heading.

Rifampicin (Etravirine is a substrate of CYP3A4, CYP2C9, and CYP2C19. Therefore, co-administration of etravirine with drugs that induce or inhibit CYP3A4, CYP2C9, and CYP2C19 may alter the therapeutic effect or adverse reaction profile of etravirine).
No products indexed under this heading.

Rifampin (Rifampin and rifapentine are potent inducers of CYP450 enzymes. Etravirine should not be used with rifampin or rifapentine as co-administration may cause significant decreases in etravirine plasma concentrations and loss of therapeutic effect of etravirine).
No products indexed under this heading.

Rifapentine (Rifampin and rifapentine are potent inducers of CYP450 enzymes. Etravirine should not be used with rifampin or rifapentine as co-administration may cause significant decreases in etravirine plasma concentrations and loss of therapeutic effect of etravirine).
No products indexed under this heading.

Ritonavir (Concomitant use of etravirine with ritonavir 600 mg b.i.d. may cause a significant decrease in the plasma concentration of etravirine and loss of therapeutic effect of etravirine. Etravirine and ritonavir 600 mg b.i.d. should not be co-administered). Products include:
Kaletra 452
Norvir 489

Rofecoxib (Etravirine is an inducer of CYP3A4 and inhibitor of CYP2C9 and CYP2C19. Therefore, co-administration of drugs that are substrates of CYP3A4, CYP2C9 and CYP2C19 with etravirine may alter the therapeutic effect or adverse reaction profile of the co-administered drug(s)).
No products indexed under this heading.

Rosiglitazone Maleate (Etravirine is an inducer of CYP3A4 and inhibitor of CYP2C9 and CYP2C19. Therefore, co-administration of drugs that are substrates of CYP3A4, CYP2C9 and CYP2C19 with etravirine may alter the therapeutic effect or adverse reaction profile of the co-administered drug(s)). Products include:
Avandamet Tablets 1336
Avandaryl Tablets 1344
Avandia Tablets 1351

Saquinavir (Concomitant use of etravirine with protease inhibitors (PIs) without co-administration of low-dose ritonavir may cause a significant alteration in the plasma concentrations of the PI. Etravirine should not be co-administered with PIs without low-dose ritonavir. The mean systemic exposure (AUC) of etravirine was reduced by about 33% when etravirine was co-administered with saquinavir/ritonavir. Because the reduction in the systemic exposures of etravirine in the presence of saquinavir/ritonavir is similar to the reduction in mean systemic exposures of etravirine in the presence of darunavir/ritonavir, etravirine and saquinavir/ritonavir can be co-administered without any dose adjustments).
No products indexed under this heading.

Saquinavir Mesylate (Concomitant use of etravirine with protease inhibitors (PIs) without co-administration of low-dose ritonavir may cause a significant alteration in the plasma concentrations of the PI. Etravirine should not be co-administered with PIs without low-dose ritonavir. The mean systemic exposure (AUC) of etravirine was reduced by about 33% when etravirine was co-administered with saquinavir/ritonavir. Because the reduction in the systemic exposures of etravirine in the presence of saquinavir/ritonavir is similar to the reduction in mean systemic exposures of etravirine in the presence of darunavir/ritonavir, etravirine and saquinavir/ritonavir can be co-administered without any dose adjustments).
No products indexed under this heading.

Secobarbital Sodium (Etravirine is a substrate of CYP3A4, CYP2C9, and CYP2C19. Therefore, co-administration of etravirine with drugs that induce or inhibit CYP3A4, CYP2C9, and CYP2C19 may alter the therapeutic effect or adverse reaction profile of etravirine).
No products indexed under this heading.

Sertraline Hydrochloride (Etravirine is a substrate of CYP3A4, CYP2C9, and CYP2C19. Therefore, co-administration of etravirine with drugs that induce or inhibit CYP3A4, CYP2C9, and CYP2C19 may alter the therapeutic effect or adverse reaction profile of etravirine).
No products indexed under this heading.

Sildenafil Citrate (Etravirine and sildenafil can be co-administered without dose adjustments, however, the dose of sildenafil may need to be altered based on clinical effect).
No products indexed under this heading.

Simvastatin (Lovastatin and simvastatin are CYP3A4 substrates and co-administration with etravirine may result in lower plasma concentrations of the HMG-CoA reductase inhibitor. Fluvastatin is metabolized by CYP2C9 and co-administration with etravirine may result in higher plasma concentrations of the HMG-CoA reductase inhibitor. Dose adjustments for these HMG-CoA reductase inhibitors may be necessary). Products include:
Simcor Tablets 502
Vytorin 10/10 Tablets 2149
Vytorin 10/10 Tablets 2939
Vytorin 10/20 Tablets 2149
Vytorin 10/20 Tablets 2939
Vytorin 10/40 Tablets 2149
Vytorin 10/40 Tablets 2939
Vytorin 10/80 Tablets 2149
Vytorin 10/80 Tablets 2939
Zocor Tablets 2136

Sirolimus (Etravirine and systemic immunosuppressants should be co-administered with caution because plasma concentrations of cyclosporine, sirolimus, or tacrolimus may be affected). Products include:
Rapamune 3260

Sotalol Hydrochloride (Concentrations of these antiarrhythmics may be decreased when co-administered with etravirine. Etravirine and antiarrhythmics should be co-administered with caution. Drug concentration monitoring is recommended, if available).
No products indexed under this heading.

Sulfacytine (Etravirine is a substrate of CYP3A4, CYP2C9, and CYP2C19. Therefore, co-administration of etravirine with drugs that induce or inhibit CYP3A4, CYP2C9, and CYP2C19 may alter the therapeutic effect or adverse reaction profile of etravirine).
No products indexed under this heading.

Sulfamethizole (Etravirine is a substrate of CYP3A4, CYP2C9, and CYP2C19. Therefore, co-administration of etravirine with drugs that induce or inhibit CYP3A4, CYP2C9, and CYP2C19 may alter the therapeutic effect or adverse reaction profile of etravirine).
No products indexed under this heading.

Sulfamethoxazole (Etravirine is a substrate of CYP3A4, CYP2C9, and CYP2C19. Therefore, co-administration of etravirine with drugs that induce or inhibit CYP3A4, CYP2C9, and CYP2C19 may alter the therapeutic effect or adverse reaction profile of etravirine).
No products indexed under this heading.

Sulfaphenazole (Etravirine is a substrate of CYP3A4, CYP2C9, and CYP2C19. Therefore, co-administration of etravirine with drugs that induce or inhibit CYP3A4, CYP2C9, and CYP2C19 may alter the therapeutic effect or adverse reaction profile of etravirine).
No products indexed under this heading.

Sulfasalazine (Etravirine is a substrate of CYP3A4, CYP2C9, and CYP2C19. Therefore, co-administration of etravirine with drugs that induce or inhibit CYP3A4, CYP2C9, and CYP2C19 may alter the therapeutic effect or adverse reaction profile of etravirine).
No products indexed under this heading.

Sulfinpyrazone (Etravirine is a substrate of CYP3A4, CYP2C9, and CYP2C19. Therefore, co-administration of etravirine with drugs that induce or inhibit CYP3A4, CYP2C9, and CYP2C19 may alter the therapeutic effect or adverse reaction profile of etravirine).
No products indexed under this heading.

Sulfisoxazole Acetyl (Etravirine is a substrate of CYP3A4, CYP2C9, and CYP2C19. Therefore, co-administration of etravirine with drugs that induce or inhibit CYP3A4, CYP2C9, and CYP2C19 may alter the therapeutic effect or adverse reaction profile of etravirine).
No products indexed under this heading.

Sulfisoxazole Diolamine (Etravirine is a substrate of CYP3A4, CYP2C9, and CYP2C19. Therefore, co-administration of etravirine with drugs that induce or inhibit CYP3A4, CYP2C9, and CYP2C19 may alter the therapeutic effect or adverse reaction profile of etravirine).
No products indexed under this heading.

Sulindac (Etravirine is an inducer of CYP3A4 and inhibitor of CYP2C9 and CYP2C19. Therefore, co-administration of drugs that are substrates of CYP3A4, CYP2C9 and CYP2C19 with etravirine may alter the therapeutic effect or adverse reaction profile of the co-administered drug(s)). Products include:
Clinoril Tablets **1962**

Suprofen (Etravirine is an inducer of CYP3A4 and inhibitor of CYP2C9 and CYP2C19. Therefore, co-administration of drugs that are substrates of CYP3A4, CYP2C9 and CYP2C19 with etravirine may alter the therapeutic effect or adverse reaction profile of the co-administered drug(s)).
No products indexed under this heading.

Tacrolimus (Etravirine and systemic immunosuppressants should be co-administered with caution because plasma concentrations of cyclosporine, sirolimus, or tacrolimus may be affected). Products include:
Prograf Capsules and Injection **622**
Protopic Ointment **628**

Tadalafil (Etravirine is an inducer of CYP3A4 and inhibitor of CYP2C9 and CYP2C19. Therefore, co-administration of drugs that are substrates of CYP3A4, CYP2C9 and CYP2C19 with etravirine may alter the therapeutic effect or adverse reaction profile of the co-administered drug(s)). Products include:
Cialis Tablets **1792**

Tamoxifen Citrate (Etravirine is an inducer of CYP3A4 and inhibitor of CYP2C9 and CYP2C19. Therefore, co-administration of drugs that are substrates of CYP3A4, CYP2C9 and CYP2C19 with etravirine may alter the therapeutic effect or adverse reaction profile of the co-administered drug(s)).
No products indexed under this heading.

Telithromycin (Etravirine is a substrate of CYP3A4, CYP2C9, and CYP2C19. Therefore, co-administration of etravirine with drugs that induce or inhibit CYP3A4, CYP2C9, and CYP2C19 may alter the therapeutic effect or adverse reaction profile of etravirine). Products include:
Ketek Tablets **2744**

Telmisartan (Etravirine is a substrate of CYP3A4, CYP2C9, and CYP2C19. Therefore, co-administration of etravirine with drugs that induce or inhibit CYP3A4, CYP2C9, and CYP2C19 may alter the therapeutic effect or adverse reaction profile of etravirine). Products include:
Micardis Tablets **852**
Micardis HCT Tablets **854**

Teniposide (Etravirine is an inducer of CYP3A4 and inhibitor of CYP2C9 and CYP2C19. Therefore, co-administration of drugs that are substrates of CYP3A4, CYP2C9 and CYP2C19 with etravirine may alter the therapeutic effect or adverse reaction profile of the co-administered drug(s)).
No products indexed under this heading.

Terconazole (Etravirine is a substrate of CYP3A4, CYP2C9, and CYP2C19. Therefore, co-administration of etravirine with drugs that induce or inhibit CYP3A4, CYP2C9, and CYP2C19 may alter the therapeutic effect or adverse reaction profile of etravirine).
No products indexed under this heading.

Theophylline (Etravirine is a substrate of CYP3A4, CYP2C9, and CYP2C19. Therefore, co-administration of etravirine with drugs that induce or inhibit CYP3A4, CYP2C9, and CYP2C19 may alter the therapeutic effect or adverse reaction profile of etravirine).
No products indexed under this heading.

Theophylline Anhydrous (Etravirine is a substrate of CYP3A4, CYP2C9, and CYP2C19. Therefore, co-administration of etravirine with drugs that induce or inhibit CYP3A4, CYP2C9, and CYP2C19 may alter the therapeutic effect or adverse reaction profile of etravirine). Products include:
Uniphyl Tablets **2595**

Theophylline Calcium Salicylate (Etravirine is a substrate of CYP3A4, CYP2C9, and CYP2C19. Therefore, co-administration of etravirine with drugs that induce or inhibit CYP3A4, CYP2C9, and CYP2C19 may alter the therapeutic effect or adverse reaction profile of etravirine).
No products indexed under this heading.

Theophylline Dihydroxypropyl (Glyceryl) (Etravirine is a substrate of CYP3A4, CYP2C9, and CYP2C19. Therefore, co-administration of etravirine with drugs that induce or inhibit CYP3A4, CYP2C9, and CYP2C19 may alter the therapeutic effect or adverse reaction profile of etravirine).
No products indexed under this heading.

Theophylline Ethylenediamine (Etravirine is a substrate of CYP3A4, CYP2C9, and CYP2C19. Therefore, co-administration of etravirine with drugs that induce or inhibit CYP3A4, CYP2C9, and CYP2C19 may alter the therapeutic effect or adverse reaction profile of etravirine).
No products indexed under this heading.

Thioridazine (Etravirine is an inducer of CYP3A4 and inhibitor of CYP2C9 and CYP2C19. Therefore, co-administration of drugs that are substrates of CYP3A4, CYP2C9 and CYP2C19 with etravirine may alter the therapeutic effect or adverse reaction profile of the co-administered drug(s)).
No products indexed under this heading.

Thioridazine Hydrochloride (Etravirine is an inducer of CYP3A4 and inhibitor of CYP2C9 and CYP2C19. Therefore, co-administration of drugs that are substrates of CYP3A4, CYP2C9 and CYP2C19 with etravirine may alter the therapeutic effect or adverse reaction profile of the co-administered drug(s)). Products include:
Thioridazine Hydrochloride Tablets **2195**

Tiagabine Hydrochloride (Etravirine is an inducer of CYP3A4 and inhibitor of CYP2C9 and CYP2C19. Therefore, co-administration of drugs that are substrates of CYP3A4, CYP2C9 and CYP2C19 with etravirine may alter the therapeutic effect or adverse reaction profile of the co-administered drug(s)). Products include:
Gabitril Tablets **973**

Ticlopidine Hydrochloride (Etravirine is a substrate of CYP3A4, CYP2C9, and CYP2C19. Therefore, co-administration of etravirine with drugs that induce or inhibit CYP3A4, CYP2C9, and CYP2C19 may alter the therapeutic effect or adverse reaction profile of etravirine).
No products indexed under this heading.

Tipranavir (Concomitant use of etravirine with protease inhibitors (PIs) without co-administration of low-dose ritonavir may cause a significant alteration in the plasma concentrations of the PI. Etravirine should not be co-administered with PIs without low-dose ritonavir. Concomitant use of etravirine with tipranavir/ritonavir may cause a significant decrease in the plasma concentrations of etravirine and loss of therapeutic effect of etravirine. Etravirine and tipranavir/ritonavir should not be co-administered). Products include:
Aptivus Capsules **823**
Aptivus Oral Solution **823**

Tocainide Hydrochloride (Concentrations of these antiarrhythmics may be decreased when co-administered with etravirine. Etravirine and antiarrhythmics should be co-administered with caution. Drug concentration monitoring is recommended, if available).
No products indexed under this heading.

Tolazamide (Etravirine is a substrate of CYP3A4, CYP2C9, and CYP2C19. Therefore, co-administration of etravirine with drugs that induce or inhibit CYP3A4, CYP2C9, and CYP2C19 may alter the therapeutic effect or adverse reaction profile of etravirine).
No products indexed under this heading.

Tolbutamide (Etravirine is a substrate of CYP3A4, CYP2C9, and CYP2C19. Therefore, co-administration of etravirine with drugs that induce or inhibit CYP3A4, CYP2C9, and CYP2C19 may alter the therapeutic effect or adverse reaction profile of etravirine).
No products indexed under this heading.

Tolbutamide Sodium (Etravirine is a substrate of CYP3A4, CYP2C9, and CYP2C19. Therefore, co-administration of etravirine with drugs that induce or inhibit CYP3A4, CYP2C9, and CYP2C19 may alter the therapeutic effect or adverse reaction profile of etravirine).
No products indexed under this heading.

Tolmetin Sodium (Etravirine is an inducer of CYP3A4 and inhibitor of CYP2C9 and CYP2C19. Therefore, co-administration of drugs that are substrates of CYP3A4, CYP2C9 and CYP2C19 with etravirine may alter the therapeutic effect or adverse reaction profile of the co-administered drug(s)).
No products indexed under this heading.

Tolterodine Tartrate (Etravirine is an inducer of CYP3A4 and inhibitor of CYP2C9 and CYP2C19. Therefore, co-administration of drugs that are substrates of CYP3A4, CYP2C9 and CYP2C19 with etravirine may alter the therapeutic effect or adverse reaction profile of the co-administered drug(s)).
No products indexed under this heading.

Topiramate (Etravirine is a substrate of CYP3A4, CYP2C9, and CYP2C19. Therefore, co-administration of etravirine with drugs that induce or inhibit CYP3A4, CYP2C9, and CYP2C19 may alter the therapeutic effect or adverse reaction profile of etravirine).
No products indexed under this heading.

Torsemide (Etravirine is an inducer of CYP3A4 and inhibitor of CYP2C9 and CYP2C19. Therefore, co-administration of drugs that are substrates of CYP3A4, CYP2C9 and CYP2C19 with etravirine may alter the therapeutic effect or adverse reaction profile of the co-administered drug(s)). Products include:
Demadex Injection **2630**
Demadex Tablets **2630**

Trazodone Hydrochloride (Etravirine is an inducer of CYP3A4 and inhibitor of CYP2C9 and CYP2C19. Therefore, co-administration of drugs that are substrates of CYP3A4, CYP2C9 and CYP2C19 with etravirine may alter the therapeutic effect or adverse reaction profile of the co-administered drug(s)).
No products indexed under this heading.

Triamcinolone (Etravirine is a substrate of CYP3A4, CYP2C9, and CYP2C19. Therefore, co-administration of etravirine with drugs that induce or inhibit CYP3A4, CYP2C9, and CYP2C19 may alter the therapeutic effect or adverse reaction profile of etravirine).
No products indexed under this heading.

Triamcinolone Acetonide (Etravirine is a substrate of CYP3A4, CYP2C9, and CYP2C19. Therefore, co-administration of etravirine with drugs that induce or inhibit CYP3A4, CYP2C9, and CYP2C19 may alter the therapeutic effect or adverse reaction profile of etravirine). Products include:
Azmacort Inhalation Aerosol **407**
Nasacort AQ Nasal Spray **2765**
Triesence Injectable Suspension .... ⊙ **209**

Triamcinolone Diacetate (Etravirine is a substrate of CYP3A4, CYP2C9, and CYP2C19. Therefore, co-administration of etravirine with drugs that induce or inhibit CYP3A4, CYP2C9, and CYP2C19 may alter the therapeutic effect or adverse reaction profile of etravirine).
No products indexed under this heading.

Triamcinolone Hexacetonide (Etravirine is a substrate of CYP3A4, CYP2C9, and CYP2C19. Therefore, co-administration of etravirine with drugs that induce or inhibit CYP3A4, CYP2C9, and CYP2C19 may alter the therapeutic effect or adverse reaction profile of etravirine).
No products indexed under this heading.

Triazolam (Etravirine is an inducer of CYP3A4 and inhibitor of CYP2C9 and CYP2C19. Therefore, co-administration of drugs that are substrates of CYP3A4, CYP2C9 and CYP2C19 with etravirine may alter the therapeutic effect or adverse reaction profile of the co-administered drug(s)).
No products indexed under this heading.

Trimethadione (Etravirine is an inducer of CYP3A4 and inhibitor of CYP2C9 and CYP2C19. Therefore, co-administration of drugs that are substrates of CYP3A4, CYP2C9 and CYP2C19 with etravirine may alter the therapeutic effect or adverse reaction profile of the co-administered drug(s)).
No products indexed under this heading.

Trimipramine Maleate (Etravirine is an inducer of CYP3A4 and inhibitor of CYP2C9 and CYP2C19. Therefore, co-administration of drugs that are substrates of CYP3A4, CYP2C9 and CYP2C19 with etravirine may alter the therapeutic effect or adverse reaction profile of the co-administered drug(s)).
No products indexed under this heading.

Troglitazone (Etravirine is a substrate of CYP3A4, CYP2C9, and CYP2C19. Therefore, co-administration of etravirine with drugs that induce or inhibit CYP3A4, CYP2C9, and CYP2C19 may alter the therapeutic effect or adverse reaction profile of etravirine).
No products indexed under this heading.

Troleandomycin (Etravirine is a substrate of CYP3A4, CYP2C9, and CYP2C19. Therefore, co-administration of etravirine with drugs that induce or inhibit CYP3A4, CYP2C9, and CYP2C19 may alter the therapeutic effect or adverse reaction profile of etravirine).
No products indexed under this heading.

Valdecoxib (Etravirine is an inducer of CYP3A4 and inhibitor of CYP2C9 and CYP2C19. Therefore, co-administration of drugs that are substrates of CYP3A4, CYP2C9 and CYP2C19 with etravirine may alter the therapeutic effect or adverse reaction profile of the co-administered drug(s)).
No products indexed under this heading.

Valproate Sodium (Etravirine is a substrate of CYP3A4, CYP2C9, and CYP2C19. Therefore, co-administration of etravirine with drugs that induce or inhibit CYP3A4, CYP2C9, and CYP2C19 may alter the therapeutic effect or adverse reaction profile of etravirine).
No products indexed under this heading.

Valproic Acid (Etravirine is an inducer of CYP3A4 and inhibitor of CYP2C9 and CYP2C19. Therefore, co-administration of drugs that are substrates of CYP3A4, CYP2C9 and CYP2C19 with etravirine may alter the therapeutic effect or adverse reaction profile of the co-administered drug(s)).
No products indexed under this heading.

Valsartan (Etravirine is an inducer of CYP3A4 and inhibitor of CYP2C9 and CYP2C19. Therefore, co-administration of drugs that are substrates of CYP3A4, CYP2C9 and CYP2C19 with etravirine may alter the therapeutic effect or adverse reaction profile of the co-administered drug(s)). Products include:
Diovan Tablets 2212
Diovan HCT Tablets 2216
Exforge Tablets 2238

Vardenafil Hydrochloride (Etravirine is a substrate of CYP3A4, CYP2C9, and CYP2C19. Therefore, co-administration of etravirine with drugs that induce or inhibit CYP3A4, CYP2C9, and CYP2C19 may alter the therapeutic effect or adverse reaction profile of etravirine). Products include:
Levitra Tablets 2876

Verapamil Hydrochloride (Concentrations of these antiarrhythmics may be decreased when co-administered with etravirine. Etravirine and antiarrhythmics should be co-administered with caution. Drug concentration monitoring is recommended, if available). Products include:
Tarka Tablets 511

Vinblastine Sulfate (Etravirine is an inducer of CYP3A4 and inhibitor of CYP2C9 and CYP2C19. Therefore, co-administration of drugs that are substrates of CYP3A4, CYP2C9 and CYP2C19 with etravirine may alter the therapeutic effect or adverse reaction profile of the co-administered drug(s)).
No products indexed under this heading.

Vincristine Sulfate (Etravirine is an inducer of CYP3A4 and inhibitor of CYP2C9 and CYP2C19. Therefore, co-administration of drugs that are substrates of CYP3A4, CYP2C9 and CYP2C19 with etravirine may alter the therapeutic effect or adverse reaction profile of the co-administered drug(s)).
No products indexed under this heading.

Voriconazole (Posaconazole is a potent inhibitor of CYP3A4 and fluconazole is a potent inhibitor of CYP2C9; both may increase plasma concentrations of etravirine. Itraconazole and ketoconazole are potent inhibitors as well as substrates of CYP3A4. Concomitant systemic use of itraconazole or ketoconazole and etravirine may increase plasma concentrations of etravirine. Simultaneously, plasma concentrations of itraconazole or ketoconazole may be decreased by etravirine. Voriconazole is a CYP2C19 substrate and CYP3A4, CYP2C9 and CYP2C19 inhibitor. Concomitant use of voriconazole and etravirine may increase plasma concentrations of both drugs. Dose adjustments for itraconazole, ketoconazole or voriconazole may be necessary depending on other co-administered drugs).
No products indexed under this heading.

Warfarin Sodium (Warfarin concentrations may be increased when co-administered with etravirine. The international normalized ratio (INR) should be monitored when warfarin is combined with etravirine).
No products indexed under this heading.

Zafirlukast (Etravirine is a substrate of CYP3A4, CYP2C9, and CYP2C19. Therefore, co-administration of etravirine with drugs that induce or inhibit CYP3A4, CYP2C9, and CYP2C19 may alter the therapeutic effect or adverse reaction profile of etravirine). Products include:
Accolate Tablets 669

Zileuton (Etravirine is a substrate of CYP3A4, CYP2C9, and CYP2C19. Therefore, co-administration of etravirine with drugs that induce or inhibit CYP3A4, CYP2C9, and CYP2C19 may alter the therapeutic effect or adverse reaction profile of etravirine).
No products indexed under this heading.

Zonisamide (Etravirine is an inducer of CYP3A4 and inhibitor of CYP2C9 and CYP2C19. Therefore, co-administration of drugs that are substrates of CYP3A4, CYP2C9 and CYP2C19 with etravirine may alter the therapeutic effect or adverse reaction profile of the co-administered drug(s)). Products include:
Zonegran Capsules 1089

Food Interactions

Grapefruit (Etravirine is a substrate of CYP3A4, CYP2C9, and CYP2C19. Therefore, co-administration of etravirine with drugs that induce or inhibit CYP3A4, CYP2C9, and CYP2C19 may alter the therapeutic effect or adverse reaction profile of etravirine).

Grapefruit Juice (Etravirine is a substrate of CYP3A4, CYP2C9, and CYP2C19. Therefore, co-administration of etravirine with drugs that induce or inhibit CYP3A4, CYP2C9, and CYP2C19 may alter the therapeutic effect or adverse reaction profile of etravirine).

INTRAVENOUS SODIUM DIURIL

(Chlorothiazide Sodium) 2490
May interact with antihypertensives, barbiturates, corticosteroids, cardiac glycosides, oral hypoglycemic agents, insulin, lithium preparations, narcotic analgesics, nondepolarizing neuromuscular blocking agents, nonsteroidal anti-inflammatory agents, and certain other agents. Compounds in these categories include:

Acarbose (Thiazide-induced hyperglycemia may require dosage adjustment of hypoglycemic agents). Products include:
Precose Tablets 792

Acebutolol Hydrochloride (Concurrent use with other antihypertensive agents may result in additive effect or potentiation).
No products indexed under this heading.

ACTH (Intensified electrolyte depletion particularly hypokalemia).
No products indexed under this heading.

Alfentanil Hydrochloride (Potentiation of orthostatic hypotension may occur).
No products indexed under this heading.

Aliskiren (Concurrent use with other antihypertensive agents may result in additive effect or potentiation). Products include:
Tekturna Tablets 2321
Tekturna HCT Tablets 2324

Amlodipine Besylate (Concurrent use with other antihypertensive agents may result in additive effect or potentiation). Products include:
Azor Tablets 1005
Exforge Tablets 2238

Aprobarbital (Potentiation of orthostatic hypotension may occur).
No products indexed under this heading.

Atenolol (Concurrent use with other antihypertensive agents may result in additive effect or potentiation).
No products indexed under this heading.

Atracurium Besylate (Possible increased responsiveness to the muscle relaxants).
No products indexed under this heading.

Benazepril Hydrochloride (Concurrent use with other antihypertensive agents may result in additive effect or potentiation).
No products indexed under this heading.

Bendroflumethiazide (Concurrent use with other antihypertensive agents may result in additive effect or potentiation).
No products indexed under this heading.

Betamethasone Acetate (Intensified electrolyte depletion particularly hypokalemia).
No products indexed under this heading.

Betamethasone Sodium Phosphate (Intensified electrolyte depletion particularly hypokalemia).
No products indexed under this heading.

Betaxolol Hydrochloride (Concurrent use with other antihypertensive agents may result in additive effect or potentiation).
No products indexed under this heading.

Bisoprolol Fumarate (Concurrent use with other antihypertensive agents may result in additive effect or potentiation).
No products indexed under this heading.

Budesonide (Intensified electrolyte depletion particularly hypokalemia). Products include:
Pulmicort Flexhaler 654
Symbicort 80/4.5 Inhalation Aerosol 659
Symbicort 160/4.5 Inhalation Aerosol 659

Buprenorphine Hydrochloride (Potentiation of orthostatic hypotension may occur). Products include:
Suboxone Tablets 2601
Subutex Tablets 2601

Butabarbital (Potentiation of orthostatic hypotension may occur).
No products indexed under this heading.

Butalbital (Potentiation of orthostatic hypotension may occur).
No products indexed under this heading.

Candesartan Cilexetil (Concurrent use with other antihypertensive agents may result in additive effect or potentiation). Products include:
Atacand Tablets 639
Atacand HCT 642

Captopril (Concurrent use with other antihypertensive agents may result in additive effect or potentiation). Products include:
Captopril Tablets 2182

Carteolol Hydrochloride (Concurrent use with other antihypertensive agents may result in additive effect or potentiation).
No products indexed under this heading.

Celecoxib (Reduces diuretic, natriuretiç, and antihypertensive effects). Products include:
Celebrex Capsules 2979

Chlorothiazide (Concurrent use with other antihypertensive agents may result in additive effect or potentiation).
No products indexed under this heading.

Chlorpropamide (Thiazide-induced hyperglycemia may require dosage adjustment of hypoglycemic agents).
No products indexed under this heading.

Chlorthalidone (Concurrent use with other antihypertensive agents may result in additive effect or potentiation). Products include:
Clorpres Tablets 2185

Ciclesonide (Intensified electrolyte depletion particularly hypokalemia). Products include:
Alvesco Inhalation Aerosol 2985
Omnaris Nasal Spray 2998

Cisatracurium Besylate (Possible increased responsiveness to the muscle relaxants). Products include:
Nimbex Injection 484

Clonidine (Concurrent use with other antihypertensive agents may result in additive effect or potentiation). Products include:
Catapres-TTS 842

Clonidine Hydrochloride (Concurrent use with other antihypertensive agents may result in additive effect or potentiation). Products include:
Catapres Tablets 841
Clorpres Tablets 2185

Codeine Phosphate (Potentiation of orthostatic hypotension may occur). Products include:
Tylenol with Codeine Tablets 2427

Cortisone Acetate (Intensified electrolyte depletion particularly hypokalemia).
No products indexed under this heading.

Deserpidine (Concurrent use with other antihypertensive agents may result in additive effect or potentiation).
No products indexed under this heading.

Deslanoside (Thiazide-induced hypokalemia may sensitize or exaggerate the response of the heart to the toxic effects of digitalis).
No products indexed under this heading.

Dexamethasone (Intensified electrolyte depletion particularly hypokalemia). Products include:
Ciprodex Otic Suspension 541

Dexamethasone Acetate (Intensified electrolyte depletion particularly hypokalemia).
No products indexed under this heading.

Dexamethasone Sodium Phosphate (Intensified electrolyte depletion particularly hypokalemia).
No products indexed under this heading.

Dezocine (Potentiation of orthostatic hypotension may occur).
No products indexed under this heading.

Diazoxide (Concurrent use with other antihypertensive agents may result in additive effect or potentiation). Products include:
Proglycem Capsules 1185
Proglycem Suspension 1185

Diclofenac Epolamine (Reduces diuretic, natriuretic, and antihypertensive effects). Products include:
Flector Patch 561

Diclofenac Potassium (Reduces diuretic, natriuretic, and antihypertensive effects).
No products indexed under this heading.

Diclofenac Sodium (Reduces diuretic, natriuretic, and antihypertensive effects). Products include:
Diclofenac Sodium Ophthalmic Solution .... ⊙ 240
Voltaren Ophthalmic Solution 2336
Voltaren Tablets 2334
Voltaren-XR Tablets 2337

Digitalis Glycoside Preparations (Thiazide-induced hypokalemia may sensitize or exaggerate the response of the heart to the toxic effects of digitalis).
No products indexed under this heading.

Digitoxin (Thiazide-induced hypokalemia may sensitize or exaggerate the response of the heart to the toxic effects of digitalis).
No products indexed under this heading.

Digoxin (Thiazide-induced hypokalemia may sensitize or exaggerate the response of the heart to the toxic effects of digitalis). Products include:
Lanoxin Injection 1498
Lanoxin Injection Pediatric 1502
Lanoxin Tablets 1505

Diltiazem Hydrochloride (Concurrent use with other antihypertensive agents may result in additive effect or potentiation). Products include:
Cardizem LA Extended Release Tablets 421

Doxazosin Mesylate (Concurrent use with other antihypertensive agents may result in additive effect or potentiation).
No products indexed under this heading.

Enalapril Maleate (Concurrent use with other antihypertensive agents may result in additive effect or potentiation).
No products indexed under this heading.

Enalaprilat (Concurrent use with other antihypertensive agents may result in additive effect or potentiation).
No products indexed under this heading.

Eprosartan Mesylate (Concurrent use with other antihypertensive agents may result in additive effect or potentiation). Products include:
Teveten Tablets 515
Teveten HCT Tablets 517

Esmolol Hydrochloride (Concurrent use with other antihypertensive agents may result in additive effect or potentiation).
No products indexed under this heading.

Etodolac (Reduces diuretic, natriuretic, and antihypertensive effects).
No products indexed under this heading.

Felodipine (Concurrent use with other antihypertensive agents may result in additive effect or potentiation).
No products indexed under this heading.

Fenoprofen Calcium (Reduces diuretic, natriuretic, and antihypertensive effects). Products include:
Nalfon Capsules 2508

Fentanyl (Potentiation of orthostatic hypotension may occur). Products include:
Duragesic Transdermal System 2405
Ionsys Transdermal System 2410

Fentanyl Citrate (Potentiation of orthostatic hypotension may occur). Products include:
Actiq 959
Fentora Tablets 968

Fludrocortisone Acetate (Intensified electrolyte depletion particularly hypokalemia).
No products indexed under this heading.

Flunisolide (Intensified electrolyte depletion particularly hypokalemia). Products include:
Aerobid/Aerobid-M 1153

Flurbiprofen (Reduces diuretic, natriuretic, and antihypertensive effects).
No products indexed under this heading.

Fluticasone Propionate (Intensified electrolyte depletion particularly hypokalemia). Products include:
Advair Diskus 100/50 1276
Advair Diskus 250/50 1276
Advair Diskus 500/50 1276
Advair HFA 45/21 Inhalation Aerosol 1288
Advair HFA 115/21 Inhalation Aerosol 1288
Advair HFA 230/21 Inhalation Aerosol 1288
Flonase Nasal Spray 1431
Flovent Diskus 50 mcg 1435

Fluticasone Propionate HFA (Intensified electrolyte depletion particularly hypokalemia). Products include:
Flovent HFA 1440

Fosinopril Sodium (Concurrent use with other antihypertensive agents may result in additive effect or potentiation).
No products indexed under this heading.

Furosemide (Concurrent use with other antihypertensive agents may result in additive effect or potentiation). Products include:
Furosemide Tablets 2186

Glimepiride (Thiazide-induced hyperglycemia may require dosage adjustment of hypoglycemic agents). Products include:
Avandaryl Tablets 1344
Duetact Tablets 3085

Glipizide (Thiazide-induced hyperglycemia may require dosage adjustment of hypoglycemic agents).
No products indexed under this heading.

Glyburide (Thiazide-induced hyperglycemia may require dosage adjustment of hypoglycemic agents).
No products indexed under this heading.

Guanabenz Acetate (Concurrent use with other antihypertensive agents may result in additive effect or potentiation).
No products indexed under this heading.

Guanethidine Monosulfate (Concurrent use with other antihypertensive agents may result in additive effect or potentiation).
No products indexed under this heading.

Hydralazine Hydrochloride (Concurrent use with other antihypertensive agents may result in additive effect or potentiation).
No products indexed under this heading.

Hydrochlorothiazide (Concurrent use with other antihypertensive agents may result in additive effect or potentiation). Products include:
Atacand HCT 642
Avalide Tablets 892
Avalide Tablets 2713
Benicar HCT Tablets 1010
Diovan HCT Tablets 2216
Dyazide Capsules 1405
Micardis HCT Tablets 854
Prinzide Tablets 2092
Tekturna HCT Tablets 2324
Teveten HCT Tablets 517

Hydrocodone Bitartrate (Potentiation of orthostatic hypotension may occur). Products include:
Lortab 5/500 Tablets 3143
Lortab 7.5/500 Tablets 3144
Lortab 10/500 Tablets 3144
Vicodin Tablets 529
Vicodin ES Tablets 530
Vicodin HP Tablets 531
Vicoprofen Tablets 533
Zydone Tablets 1132

Hydrocodone Polistirex (Potentiation of orthostatic hypotension may occur). Products include:
Tussionex Pennkinetic Extended-Release Suspension 3154

Hydrocortisone (Intensified electrolyte depletion particularly hypokalemia).
No products indexed under this heading.

Hydrocortisone Acetate (Intensified electrolyte depletion particularly hypokalemia). Products include:
Analpram-HC 1140
Pramosone 1141

Hydrocortisone Sodium Phosphate (Intensified electrolyte depletion particularly hypokalemia).
No products indexed under this heading.

Hydrocortisone Sodium Succinate (Intensified electrolyte depletion particularly hypokalemia).
No products indexed under this heading.

Hydroflumethiazide (Concurrent use with other antihypertensive agents may result in additive effect or potentiation).
No products indexed under this heading.

Hydromorphone Hydrochloride (Potentiation of orthostatic hypotension may occur).
No products indexed under this heading.

Ibuprofen (Reduces diuretic, natriuretic, and antihypertensive effects). Products include:

Motrin IB Tablets and Caplets 1900
Children's Motrin Oral Suspension ... 1901
Children's Motrin Non-Staining Dye-Free Oral Suspension............ 1901
Children's Motrin Cold Oral Suspension................................ 1899
Infants' Motrin Concentrated Drops.. 1901
Infants' Motrin Non-Staining Dye-Free Concentrated Drops....... 1901
Junior Strength Motrin Caplets and Chewable Tablets.................. 1901
Vicoprofen Tablets 533

Indapamide (Concurrent use with other antihypertensive agents may result in additive effect or potentiation). Products include:
Indapamide Tablets 2188

Indomethacin (Reduces diuretic, natriuretic, and antihypertensive effects). Products include:
Indocin 2024

Indomethacin Sodium Trihydrate (Reduces diuretic, natriuretic, and antihypertensive effects). Products include:
Indocin I.V. 2489

Insulin (Thiazide-induced hyperglycemia may require dosage adjustment of hypoglycemic agents).
No products indexed under this heading.

Insulin, Human, Zinc Suspension (Thiazide-induced hyperglycemia may require dosage adjustment of hypoglycemic agents).
No products indexed under this heading.

Insulin, Human (rDNA origin) (Thiazide-induced hyperglycemia may require dosage adjustment of hypoglycemic agents). Products include:
Exubera Inhalation Powder 2515

Insulin, Human NPH (Thiazide-induced hyperglycemia may require dosage adjustment of hypoglycemic agents). Products include:
Humulin N Vial 1846

Insulin, Human Regular (Thiazide-induced hyperglycemia may require dosage adjustment of hypoglycemic agents). Products include:
Humulin R 1849
Humulin R (U-500) 1850

Insulin, Human Regular and Human NPH Mixture (Thiazide-induced hyperglycemia may require dosage adjustment of hypoglycemic agents). Products include:
Humulin 50/50, 100 Units 1843
Humulin 70/30 Vial 1844

Insulin, NPH (Thiazide-induced hyperglycemia may require dosage adjustment of hypoglycemic agents).
No products indexed under this heading.

Insulin, Regular (Thiazide-induced hyperglycemia may require dosage adjustment of hypoglycemic agents).
No products indexed under this heading.

Insulin, Regular and NPH mixture (Thiazide-induced hyperglycemia may require dosage adjustment of hypoglycemic agents).
No products indexed under this heading.

Insulin, Zinc Crystals (Thiazide-induced hyperglycemia may require dosage adjustment of hypoglycemic agents).
No products indexed under this heading.

Insulin, Zinc Suspension (Thiazide-induced hyperglycemia may require dosage adjustment of hypoglycemic agents).
No products indexed under this heading.

Insulin Aspart (Thiazide-induced hyperglycemia may require dosage adjustment of hypoglycemic agents).
No products indexed under this heading.

Insulin Aspart, Human (Thiazide-induced hyperglycemia may require dosage adjustment of hypoglycemic agents). Products include:
NovoLog Mix 70/30 2364

Insulin Aspart, Human Regular (Thiazide-induced hyperglycemia may require dosage adjustment of hypoglycemic agents). Products include:
NovoLog Injection 2359

Insulin Aspart Protamine, Human (Thiazide-induced hyperglycemia may require dosage adjustment of hypoglycemic agents). Products include:
NovoLog Mix 70/30 2364

Insulin Detemir (rDNA Origin) (Thiazide-induced hyperglycemia may require dosage adjustment of hypoglycemic agents). Products include:
Levemir Injection 2352

Insulin glargine (Thiazide-induced hyperglycemia may require dosage adjustment of hypoglycemic agents). Products include:
Lantus Injection 2749

Insulin Glulisine (Thiazide-induced hyperglycemia may require dosage adjustment of hypoglycemic agents). Products include:
Apidra Injection 2706

Insulin Lispro, Human (Thiazide-induced hyperglycemia may require dosage adjustment of hypoglycemic agents). Products include:
Humalog-Pen and KwikPen 1829
Humalog Mix 50/50-Pen and KwikPen.. 1833
Humalog Mix 75/25-Pen and KwikPen.. 1835

Insulin Lispro Protamine, Human (Thiazide-induced hyperglycemia may require dosage adjustment of hypoglycemic agents). Products include:
Humalog Mix 50/50-Pen and KwikPen.. 1833
Humalog Mix 75/25-Pen and KwikPen.. 1835

Irbesartan (Concurrent use with other antihypertensive agents may result in additive effect or potentiation). Products include:
Avalide Tablets 892
Avalide Tablets 2713
Avapro Tablets 897
Avapro Tablets 2718

Isradipine (Concurrent use with other antihypertensive agents may result in additive effect or potentiation). Products include:
DynaCirc CR Controlled Release Tablets... 1407

Ketoprofen (Reduces diuretic, natriuretic, and antihypertensive effects).
No products indexed under this heading.

Ketorolac Tromethamine (Reduces diuretic, natriuretic, and antihypertensive effects).
No products indexed under this heading.

Labetalol Hydrochloride (Concurrent use with other antihypertensive agents may result in additive effect or potentiation).
No products indexed under this heading.

Levobunolol Hydrochloride (Concurrent use with other antihypertensive agents may result in additive effect or potentiation).
No products indexed under this heading.

Levorphanol Tartrate (Potentiation of orthostatic hypotension may occur).
No products indexed under this heading.

Lisinopril (Concurrent use with other antihypertensive agents may result in additive effect or potentiation). Products include:
Prinivil Tablets................................. 2087
Prinzide Tablets 2092

Lithium (Diuretics reduce the renal clearance of lithium and this may lead to lithium toxicity).
No products indexed under this heading.

Lithium Carbonate (Diuretics reduce the renal clearance of lithium and this may lead to lithium toxicity).
No products indexed under this heading.

Lithium Citrate (Diuretics reduce the renal clearance of lithium and this may lead to lithium toxicity).
No products indexed under this heading.

Losartan Potassium (Concurrent use with other antihypertensive agents may result in additive effect or potentiation). Products include:
Cozaar Tablets 1973

Mecamylamine Hydrochloride (Concurrent use with other antihypertensive agents may result in additive effect or potentiation).
No products indexed under this heading.

Meclofenamate Sodium (Reduces diuretic, natriuretic, and antihypertensive effects).
No products indexed under this heading.

Mefenamic Acid (Reduces diuretic, natriuretic, and antihypertensive effects).
No products indexed under this heading.

Meloxicam (Reduces diuretic, natriuretic, and antihypertensive effects). Products include:
Mobic Oral Suspension 863
Mobic Tablets 863

Meperidine Hydrochloride (Potentiation of orthostatic hypotension may occur).
No products indexed under this heading.

Mephobarbital (Potentiation of orthostatic hypotension may occur).
No products indexed under this heading.

Metformin Hydrochloride (Thiazide-induced hyperglycemia may require dosage adjustment of hypoglycemic agents). Products include:
ActoPlus Met Tablets 3071
Avandamet Tablets 1336
Janumet Tablets 2041
PrandiMet Tablets 2967

Methadone Hydrochloride (Potentiation of orthostatic hypotension may occur).
No products indexed under this heading.

Methyclothiazide (Concurrent use with other antihypertensive agents may result in additive effect or potentiation).
No products indexed under this heading.

Methyldopa (Concurrent use with other antihypertensive agents may result in additive effect or potentiation).
No products indexed under this heading.

Methyldopate Hydrochloride (Concurrent use with other antihypertensive agents may result in additive effect or potentiation).
No products indexed under this heading.

Methylprednisolone Acetate (Intensified electrolyte depletion particularly hypokalemia).
No products indexed under this heading.

Methylprednisolone Sodium Succinate (Intensified electrolyte depletion particularly hypokalemia).
No products indexed under this heading.

Metipranolol Hydrochloride (Concurrent use with other antihypertensive agents may result in additive effect or potentiation).
No products indexed under this heading.

Metocurine Iodide (Possible increased responsiveness to the muscle relaxants).
No products indexed under this heading.

Metolazone (Concurrent use with other antihypertensive agents may result in additive effect or potentiation).
No products indexed under this heading.

Metoprolol Succinate (Concurrent use with other antihypertensive agents may result in additive effect or potentiation). Products include:
Toprol-XL Tablets 666

Metoprolol Tartrate (Concurrent use with other antihypertensive agents may result in additive effect or potentiation).
No products indexed under this heading.

Metyrosine (Concurrent use with other antihypertensive agents may result in additive effect or potentiation). Products include:
Demser Capsules 1989

Mibefradil Dihydrochloride (Concurrent use with other antihypertensive agents may result in additive effect or potentiation).
No products indexed under this heading.

Miglitol (Thiazide-induced hyperglycemia may require dosage adjustment of hypoglycemic agents).
No products indexed under this heading.

Minoxidil (Concurrent use with other antihypertensive agents may result in additive effect or potentiation).
No products indexed under this heading.

Mivacurium Chloride (Possible increased responsiveness to the muscle relaxants).
No products indexed under this heading.

Moexipril Hydrochloride (Concurrent use with other antihypertensive agents may result in additive effect or potentiation).
No products indexed under this heading.

Mometasone Furoate (Intensified electrolyte depletion particularly hypokalemia). Products include:
- Asmanex Twisthaler **2797**
- Elocon Cream 0.1% **2840**
- Elocon Lotion 0.1% **2841**
- Elocon Ointment 0.1% **2842**

Mometasone Furoate Monohydrate (Intensified electrolyte depletion particularly hypokalemia). Products include:
- Nasonex Nasal Spray **2883**

Morphine Sulfate (Potentiation of orthostatic hypotension may occur). Products include:
- Avinza Capsules **1772**
- DepoDur Injection **1095**
- MS Contin Tablets **2585**

Nabumetone (Reduces diuretic, natriuretic, and antihypertensive effects).
No products indexed under this heading.

Nadolol (Concurrent use with other antihypertensive agents may result in additive effect or potentiation). Products include:
- Nadolol Tablets **2191**

Naproxen (Reduces diuretic, natriuretic, and antihypertensive effects). Products include:
- EC-Naprosyn Delayed-Release Tablets **2632**
- Naprosyn Suspension **2632**
- Naprosyn Tablets **2632**

Naproxen Sodium (Reduces diuretic, natriuretic, and antihypertensive effects). Products include:
- Anaprox Tablets **2632**
- Anaprox DS Tablets **2632**
- Treximet Tablets **1616**

Nateglinide (Thiazide-induced hyperglycemia may require dosage adjustment of hypoglycemic agents). Products include:
- Starlix Tablets **2314**

Nebivolol (Concurrent use with other antihypertensive agents may result in additive effect or potentiation). Products include:
- Bystolic Tablets **1155**

Nicardipine Hydrochloride (Concurrent use with other antihypertensive agents may result in additive effect or potentiation). Products include:
- Cardene I.V. **1093**

Nifedipine (Concurrent use with other antihypertensive agents may result in additive effect or potentiation).
No products indexed under this heading.

Nisoldipine (Concurrent use with other antihypertensive agents may result in additive effect or potentiation). Products include:
- Sular Extended Release Tablets **2975**

Nitroglycerin (Concurrent use with other antihypertensive agents may result in additive effect or potentiation). Products include:
- Nitro-Dur Transdermal Infusion System **2887**
- Nitrolingual Pumpspray **2965**

Norepinephrine Hydrochloride (Decreased arterial responsiveness to pressor amine).
No products indexed under this heading.

Oxaprozin (Reduces diuretic, natriuretic, and antihypertensive effects).
No products indexed under this heading.

Oxycodone Hydrochloride (Potentiation of orthostatic hypotension may occur). Products include:
- OxyContin Tablets **2589**
- OxyIR Capsules **2593**
- Percocet Tablets **1127**
- Percodan Tablets **1130**

Pancuronium Bromide (Possible increased responsiveness to the muscle relaxants).
No products indexed under this heading.

Penbutolol Sulfate (Concurrent use with other antihypertensive agents may result in additive effect or potentiation).
No products indexed under this heading.

Pentobarbital Sodium (Potentiation of orthostatic hypotension may occur). Products include:
- Nembutal Sodium Solution, USP **2494**

Perindopril Erbumine (Concurrent use with other antihypertensive agents may result in additive effect or potentiation). Products include:
- Aceon Tablets (2 mg, 4 mg, 8 mg) **3038**

Phenobarbital (Potentiation of orthostatic hypotension may occur). Products include:
- Donnatal Extentabs **2507**

Phenoxybenzamine Hydrochloride (Concurrent use with other antihypertensive agents may result in additive effect or potentiation). Products include:
- Dibenzyline Capsules **3188**

Phentolamine Mesylate (Concurrent use with other antihypertensive agents may result in additive effect or potentiation).
No products indexed under this heading.

Phenylbutazone (Reduces diuretic, natriuretic, and antihypertensive effects).
No products indexed under this heading.

Pindolol (Concurrent use with other antihypertensive agents may result in additive effect or potentiation).
No products indexed under this heading.

Pioglitazone Hydrochloride (Thiazide-induced hyperglycemia may require dosage adjustment of hypoglycemic agents). Products include:
- ActoPlus Met Tablets **3071**
- Actos Tablets **3077**
- Duetact Tablets **3085**

Piroxicam (Reduces diuretic, natriuretic, and antihypertensive effects).
No products indexed under this heading.

Polythiazide (Concurrent use with other antihypertensive agents may result in additive effect or potentiation).
No products indexed under this heading.

Prazosin Hydrochloride (Concurrent use with other antihypertensive agents may result in additive effect or potentiation).
No products indexed under this heading.

Prednisolone Acetate (Intensified electrolyte depletion particularly hypokalemia). Products include:
- Pred Forte Ophthalmic Suspension .... ⊙**227**
- Pred Mild Ophthalmic Suspension .... ⊙**230**
- Pred-G Ophthalmic Ointment .... ⊙**229**
- Pred-G Ophthalmic Suspension .... ⊙**228**

Prednisolone Sodium Phosphate (Intensified electrolyte depletion particularly hypokalemia).
No products indexed under this heading.

Prednisolone Tebutate (Intensified electrolyte depletion particularly hypokalemia).
No products indexed under this heading.

Prednisone (Intensified electrolyte depletion particularly hypokalemia).
No products indexed under this heading.

Propoxyphene Hydrochloride (Potentiation of orthostatic hypotension may occur).
No products indexed under this heading.

Propoxyphene Napsylate (Potentiation of orthostatic hypotension may occur).
No products indexed under this heading.

Propranolol Hydrochloride (Concurrent use with other antihypertensive agents may result in additive effect or potentiation). Products include:
- InnoPran XL Extended Release Capsules **1484**

Quinapril Hydrochloride (Concurrent use with other antihypertensive agents may result in additive effect or potentiation).
No products indexed under this heading.

Ramipril (Concurrent use with other antihypertensive agents may result in additive effect or potentiation).
No products indexed under this heading.

Rapacuronium Bromide (Possible increased responsiveness to the muscle relaxants).
No products indexed under this heading.

Rauwolfia Serpentina (Concurrent use with other antihypertensive agents may result in additive effect or potentiation).
No products indexed under this heading.

Remifentanil Hydrochloride (Potentiation of orthostatic hypotension may occur).
No products indexed under this heading.

Repaglinide (Thiazide-induced hyperglycemia may require dosage adjustment of hypoglycemic agents). Products include:
- PrandiMet Tablets **2967**
- Prandin Tablets **2971**

Rescinnamine (Concurrent use with other antihypertensive agents may result in additive effect or potentiation).
No products indexed under this heading.

Reserpine (Concurrent use with other antihypertensive agents may result in additive effect or potentiation).
No products indexed under this heading.

Rocuronium Bromide (Possible increased responsiveness to the muscle relaxants). Products include:
- Zemuron Injection **2947**

Rofecoxib (Reduces diuretic, natriuretic, and antihypertensive effects).
No products indexed under this heading.

Rosiglitazone Maleate (Thiazide-induced hyperglycemia may require dosage adjustment of hypoglycemic agents). Products include:
- Avandamet Tablets **1336**
- Avandaryl Tablets **1344**
- Avandia Tablets **1351**

Secobarbital Sodium (Potentiation of orthostatic hypotension may occur).
No products indexed under this heading.

Sitagliptin Phosphate (Thiazide-induced hyperglycemia may require dosage adjustment of hypoglycemic agents). Products include:
- Janumet Tablets **2041**
- Januvia Tablets **2048**

Sodium Nitroprusside (Concurrent use with other antihypertensive agents may result in additive effect or potentiation).
No products indexed under this heading.

Sotalol Hydrochloride (Concurrent use with other antihypertensive agents may result in additive effect or potentiation).
No products indexed under this heading.

Spirapril Hydrochloride (Concurrent use with other antihypertensive agents may result in additive effect or potentiation).
No products indexed under this heading.

Sufentanil Citrate (Potentiation of orthostatic hypotension may occur).
No products indexed under this heading.

Sulindac (Reduces diuretic, natriuretic, and antihypertensive effects). Products include:
- Clinoril Tablets **1962**

Telmisartan (Concurrent use with other antihypertensive agents may result in additive effect or potentiation). Products include:
- Micardis Tablets **852**
- Micardis HCT Tablets **854**

Terazosin Hydrochloride (Concurrent use with other antihypertensive agents may result in additive effect or potentiation).
No products indexed under this heading.

Thiamylal Sodium (Potentiation of orthostatic hypotension may occur).
No products indexed under this heading.

Timolol Maleate (Concurrent use with other antihypertensive agents may result in additive effect or potentiation). Products include:
- Combigan Ophthalmic Solution **553**
- Cosopt Sterile Ophthalmic Solution **1969**
- Timoptic Sterile Ophthalmic Solution **2121**
- Timoptic in Ocudose **2124**
- Timoptic-XE Sterile Ophthalmic Gel Forming Solution **2125**

Tolazamide (Thiazide-induced hyperglycemia may require dosage adjustment of hypoglycemic agents).
No products indexed under this heading.

IMPORTANT NOTE: Always consult each drug listing in the patient's regimen for possible interactions.

Tolbutamide (Thiazide-induced hyperglycemia may require dosage adjustment of hypoglycemic agents).
No products indexed under this heading.

Tolmetin Sodium (Reduces diuretic, natriuretic, and antihypertensive effects).
No products indexed under this heading.

Torsemide (Concurrent use with other antihypertensive agents may result in additive effect or potentiation). Products include:
Demadex Injection 2630
Demadex Tablets 2630

Trandolapril (Concurrent use with other antihypertensive agents may result in additive effect or potentiation). Products include:
Mavik Tablets 472
Tarka Tablets 511

Triamcinolone (Intensified electrolyte depletion particularly hypokalemia).
No products indexed under this heading.

Triamcinolone Acetonide (Intensified electrolyte depletion particularly hypokalemia). Products include:
Azmacort Inhalation Aerosol 407
Nasacort AQ Nasal Spray 2765
Triesence Injectable Suspension .... ⊙ 209

Triamcinolone Diacetate (Intensified electrolyte depletion particularly hypokalemia).
No products indexed under this heading.

Triamcinolone Hexacetonide (Intensified electrolyte depletion particularly hypokalemia).
No products indexed under this heading.

Trimethaphan Camsylate (Concurrent use with other antihypertensive agents may result in additive effect or potentiation).
No products indexed under this heading.

Troglitazone (Thiazide-induced hyperglycemia may require dosage adjustment of hypoglycemic agents).
No products indexed under this heading.

Tubocurarine Chloride (Possible increased responsiveness to the muscle relaxants).
No products indexed under this heading.

Valdecoxib (Reduces diuretic, natriuretic, and antihypertensive effects).
No products indexed under this heading.

Valsartan (Concurrent use with other antihypertensive agents may result in additive effect or potentiation). Products include:
Diovan Tablets 2212
Diovan HCT Tablets 2216
Exforge Tablets 2238

Vecuronium Bromide (Possible increased responsiveness to the muscle relaxants).
No products indexed under this heading.

Verapamil Hydrochloride (Concurrent use with other antihypertensive agents may result in additive effect or potentiation). Products include:
Tarka Tablets 511

Food Interactions

Alcohol (Potentiation of orthostatic hypotension may occur).

INTRON A FOR INJECTION

(Interferon alfa-2b, Recombinant) 2859
May interact with xanthines and certain other agents. Compounds in these categories include:

Aminophylline (Co-administration results in decreased theophylline clearance resulting in a 100% increase in serum theophylline levels).
No products indexed under this heading.

Bone Marrow Depressants, unspecified (Careful monitoring of the WBC count is indicated).
No products indexed under this heading.

Dyphylline (Co-administration results in decreased theophylline clearance resulting in a 100% increase in serum theophylline levels).
No products indexed under this heading.

Theophylline (Co-administration results in decreased theophylline clearance resulting in a 100% increase in serum theophylline levels).
No products indexed under this heading.

Theophylline Anhydrous (Co-administration results in decreased theophylline clearance resulting in a 100% increase in serum theophylline levels). Products include:
Uniphyl Tablets 2595

Theophylline Calcium Salicylate (Co-administration results in decreased theophylline clearance resulting in a 100% increase in serum theophylline levels).
No products indexed under this heading.

Theophylline Dihydroxypropyl (Glyceryl) (Co-administration results in decreased theophylline clearance resulting in a 100% increase in serum theophylline levels).
No products indexed under this heading.

Theophylline Ethylenediamine (Co-administration results in decreased theophylline clearance resulting in a 100% increase in serum theophylline levels).
No products indexed under this heading.

Theophylline Sodium Glycinate (Co-administration results in decreased theophylline clearance resulting in a 100% increase in serum theophylline levels).
No products indexed under this heading.

Zidovudine (Concomitant administration may result in a higher incidence of neutropenia). Products include:
Combivir Tablets 1384
Retrovir 1574
Retrovir IV Infusion 1579
Trizivir Tablets 1622

INVANZ FOR INJECTION

(Ertapenem) 2029
May interact with valproate and certain other agents. Compounds in these categories include:

Divalproex Sodium (Carbapenems, including ertapenem, may reduce serum valproic acid concentrations to subtherapeutic levels, resulting in loss of seizure control. Serum valproic acid concentrations should be monitored frequently after initiating carbapenem therapy. Alternative antibacterial or anticonvulsant therapy should be considered if serum valproic acid concentrations drop below the therapeutic range or seizure occurs). Products include:
Depakote ER Tablets 423

Probenecid (Competes for active tubular secretion and reduces the renal clearance of ertapenem).
No products indexed under this heading.

Valproate Sodium (Carbapenems, including ertapenem, may reduce serum valproic acid concentrations to subtherapeutic levels, resulting in loss of seizure control. Serum valproic acid concentrations should be monitored frequently after initiating carbapenem therapy. Alternative antibacterial or anticonvulsant therapy should be considered if serum valproic acid concentrations drop below the therapeutic range or seizure occurs).
No products indexed under this heading.

Valproic Acid (Carbapenems, including ertapenem, may reduce serum valproic acid concentrations to subtherapeutic levels, resulting in loss of seizure control. Serum valproic acid concentrations should be monitored frequently after initiating carbapenem therapy. Alternative antibacterial or anticonvulsant therapy should be considered if serum valproic acid concentrations drop below the therapeutic range or seizure occurs).
No products indexed under this heading.

INVEGA EXTENDED-RELEASE TABLETS

(Paliperidone) 1748
May interact with class 1A antiarrhythmics, class III antiarrhythmics, antihypertensives, central nervous system depressants, central nervous system stimulants, dopamine agonists, and certain other agents. Compounds in these categories include:

Acebutolol Hydrochloride (Because of its potential for inducing hypotension, paliperidone may enhance the hypotensive effects of other therapeutic agents with this potential).
No products indexed under this heading.

Alfentanil Hydrochloride (Given the primary CNS effects of paliperidone, caution should be used if taken with other centrally-acting drugs).
No products indexed under this heading.

Aliskiren (Because of its potential for inducing hypotension, paliperidone may enhance the hypotensive effects of other therapeutic agents with this potential). Products include:
Tekturna Tablets 2321
Tekturna HCT Tablets 2324

Alprazolam (Given the primary CNS effects of paliperidone, caution should be used if taken with other centrally-acting drugs).
No products indexed under this heading.

Amiodarone Hydrochloride (Paliperidone causes a modest increase in the corrected QT (QTc) interval. The use of paliperidone should be avoided in combination with other drugs that are known to prolong QTc including Class III antiarrhythmic medications).
No products indexed under this heading.

Amlodipine Besylate (Because of its potential for inducing hypotension, paliperidone may enhance the hypotensive effects of other therapeutic agents with this potential). Products include:
Azor Tablets 1005
Exforge Tablets 2238

Amphetamine Resins (Given the primary CNS effects of paliperidone, caution should be used if taken with other centrally-acting drugs).
No products indexed under this heading.

Aprobarbital (Given the primary CNS effects of paliperidone, caution should be used if taken with other centrally-acting drugs).
No products indexed under this heading.

Atenolol (Because of its potential for inducing hypotension, paliperidone may enhance the hypotensive effects of other therapeutic agents with this potential).
No products indexed under this heading.

Benazepril Hydrochloride (Because of its potential for inducing hypotension, paliperidone may enhance the hypotensive effects of other therapeutic agents with this potential).
No products indexed under this heading.

Bendroflumethiazide (Because of its potential for inducing hypotension, paliperidone may enhance the hypotensive effects of other therapeutic agents with this potential).
No products indexed under this heading.

Betaxolol Hydrochloride (Because of its potential for inducing hypotension, paliperidone may enhance the hypotensive effects of other therapeutic agents with this potential).
No products indexed under this heading.

Bisoprolol Fumarate (Because of its potential for inducing hypotension, paliperidone may enhance the hypotensive effects of other therapeutic agents with this potential).
No products indexed under this heading.

Bretylium Tosylate (Paliperidone causes a modest increase in the corrected QT (QTc) interval. The use of paliperidone should be avoided in combination with other drugs that are known to prolong QTc including Class III antiarrhythmic medications).
No products indexed under this heading.

Bromocriptine Mesylate (Paliperidone may antagonize the effect of dopamine agonists).
No products indexed under this heading.

Buprenorphine Hydrochloride (Given the primary CNS effects of paliperidone, caution should be used if taken with other centrally-acting drugs). Products include:

Suboxone Tablets 2601
Subutex Tablets 2601

Buspirone Hydrochloride (Given the primary CNS effects of paliperidone, caution should be used if taken with other centrally-acting drugs).
No products indexed under this heading.

Butabarbital (Given the primary CNS effects of paliperidone, caution should be used if taken with other centrally-acting drugs).
No products indexed under this heading.

Butalbital (Given the primary CNS effects of paliperidone, caution should be used if taken with other centrally-acting drugs).
No products indexed under this heading.

Candesartan Cilexetil (Because of its potential for inducing hypotension, paliperidone may enhance the hypotensive effects of other therapeutic agents with this potential). Products include:
Atacand Tablets 639
Atacand HCT 642

Captopril (Because of its potential for inducing hypotension, paliperidone may enhance the hypotensive effects of other therapeutic agents with this potential). Products include:
Captopril Tablets 2182

Carteolol Hydrochloride (Because of its potential for inducing hypotension, paliperidone may enhance the hypotensive effects of other therapeutic agents with this potential).
No products indexed under this heading.

Chlordiazepoxide (Given the primary CNS effects of paliperidone, caution should be used if taken with other centrally-acting drugs).
No products indexed under this heading.

Chlordiazepoxide Hydrochloride (Given the primary CNS effects of paliperidone, caution should be used if taken with other centrally-acting drugs).
No products indexed under this heading.

Chlorothiazide (Because of its potential for inducing hypotension, paliperidone may enhance the hypotensive effects of other therapeutic agents with this potential).
No products indexed under this heading.

Chlorothiazide Sodium (Because of its potential for inducing hypotension, paliperidone may enhance the hypotensive effects of other therapeutic agents with this potential). Products include:
Intravenous Sodium Diuril 2490

Chlorpromazine (Paliperidone causes a modest increase in the corrected QT (QTc) interval. The use of paliperidone should be avoided in combination with other drugs that are known to prolong QTc such as chlorpromazine).
No products indexed under this heading.

Chlorpromazine Hydrochloride (Paliperidone causes a modest increase in the corrected QT (QTc) interval. The use of paliperidone should be avoided in combination with other drugs that are known to prolong QTc such as chlorpromazine).
No products indexed under this heading.

Chlorprothixene (Given the primary CNS effects of paliperidone, caution should be used if taken with other centrally-acting drugs).
No products indexed under this heading.

Chlorprothixene Hydrochloride (Given the primary CNS effects of paliperidone, caution should be used if taken with other centrally-acting drugs).
No products indexed under this heading.

Chlorprothixene Lactate (Given the primary CNS effects of paliperidone, caution should be used if taken with other centrally-acting drugs).
No products indexed under this heading.

Chlorthalidone (Because of its potential for inducing hypotension, paliperidone may enhance the hypotensive effects of other therapeutic agents with this potential). Products include:
Clorpres Tablets 2185

Clonidine (Because of its potential for inducing hypotension, paliperidone may enhance the hypotensive effects of other therapeutic agents with this potential). Products include:
Catapres-TTS 842

Clonidine Hydrochloride (Because of its potential for inducing hypotension, paliperidone may enhance the hypotensive effects of other therapeutic agents with this potential). Products include:
Catapres Tablets 841
Clorpres Tablets 2185

Clorazepate Dipotassium (Given the primary CNS effects of paliperidone, caution should be used if taken with other centrally-acting drugs).
No products indexed under this heading.

Clozapine (Given the primary CNS effects of paliperidone, caution should be used if taken with other centrally-acting drugs).
No products indexed under this heading.

Codeine Phosphate (Given the primary CNS effects of paliperidone, caution should be used if taken with other centrally-acting drugs). Products include:
Tylenol with Codeine Tablets 2427

Deserpidine (Because of its potential for inducing hypotension, paliperidone may enhance the hypotensive effects of other therapeutic agents with this potential).
No products indexed under this heading.

Desflurane (Given the primary CNS effects of paliperidone, caution should be used if taken with other centrally-acting drugs).
No products indexed under this heading.

Dextroamphetamine Sulfate (Given the primary CNS effects of paliperidone, caution should be used if taken with other centrally-acting drugs). Products include:
Adderall XR Capsules 3012
Dexedrine 1401

Dezocine (Given the primary CNS effects of paliperidone, caution should be used if taken with other centrally-acting drugs).
No products indexed under this heading.

Diazepam (Given the primary CNS effects of paliperidone, caution should be used if taken with other centrally-acting drugs). Products include:
Valium Tablets 2658

Diazoxide (Because of its potential for inducing hypotension, paliperidone may enhance the hypotensive effects of other therapeutic agents with this potential). Products include:
Proglycem Capsules 1185
Proglycem Suspension 1185

Diltiazem Hydrochloride (Because of its potential for inducing hypotension, paliperidone may enhance the hypotensive effects of other therapeutic agents with this potential). Products include:
Cardizem LA Extended Release Tablets 421

Disopyramide (Paliperidone causes a modest increase in the corrected QT (QTc) interval. The use of paliperidone should be avoided in combination with other drugs that are known to prolong QTc including Class 1A antiarrhythmic medications).
No products indexed under this heading.

Dopamine Hydrochloride (Paliperidone may antagonize the effect of dopamine agonists).
No products indexed under this heading.

Doxazosin Mesylate (Because of its potential for inducing hypotension, paliperidone may enhance the hypotensive effects of other therapeutic agents with this potential).
No products indexed under this heading.

Droperidol (Given the primary CNS effects of paliperidone, caution should be used if taken with other centrally-acting drugs).
No products indexed under this heading.

Enalapril Maleate (Because of its potential for inducing hypotension, paliperidone may enhance the hypotensive effects of other therapeutic agents with this potential).
No products indexed under this heading.

Enalaprilat (Because of its potential for inducing hypotension, paliperidone may enhance the hypotensive effects of other therapeutic agents with this potential).
No products indexed under this heading.

Enflurane (Given the primary CNS effects of paliperidone, caution should be used if taken with other centrally-acting drugs).
No products indexed under this heading.

Eprosartan Mesylate (Because of its potential for inducing hypotension, paliperidone may enhance the hypotensive effects of other therapeutic agents with this potential). Products include:
Teveten Tablets 515
Teveten HCT Tablets 517

Esmolol Hydrochloride (Because of its potential for inducing hypotension, paliperidone may enhance the hypotensive effects of other therapeutic agents with this potential).
No products indexed under this heading.

Estazolam (Given the primary CNS effects of paliperidone, caution should be used if taken with other centrally-acting drugs).
No products indexed under this heading.

Ethanol (Given the primary CNS effects of paliperidone, caution should be used if taken with other centrally-acting drugs).
No products indexed under this heading.

Ethchlorvynol (Given the primary CNS effects of paliperidone, caution should be used if taken with other centrally-acting drugs).
No products indexed under this heading.

Ethinamate (Given the primary CNS effects of paliperidone, caution should be used if taken with other centrally-acting drugs).
No products indexed under this heading.

Ethyl Alcohol (Given the primary CNS effects of paliperidone, caution should be used if taken with other centrally-acting drugs).
No products indexed under this heading.

Felodipine (Because of its potential for inducing hypotension, paliperidone may enhance the hypotensive effects of other therapeutic agents with this potential).
No products indexed under this heading.

Fentanyl (Given the primary CNS effects of paliperidone, caution should be used if taken with other centrally-acting drugs). Products include:
Duragesic Transdermal System 2405
Ionsys Transdermal System 2410

Fentanyl Citrate (Given the primary CNS effects of paliperidone, caution should be used if taken with other centrally-acting drugs). Products include:
Actiq 959
Fentora Tablets 968

Fluphenazine Decanoate (Given the primary CNS effects of paliperidone, caution should be used if taken with other centrally-acting drugs).
No products indexed under this heading.

Fluphenazine Enanthate (Given the primary CNS effects of paliperidone, caution should be used if taken with other centrally-acting drugs).
No products indexed under this heading.

Fluphenazine Hydrochloride (Given the primary CNS effects of paliperidone, caution should be used if taken with other centrally-acting drugs).
No products indexed under this heading.

IMPORTANT NOTE: Always consult each drug listing in the patient's regimen for possible interactions.

Flurazepam Hydrochloride (Given the primary CNS effects of paliperidone, caution should be used if taken with other centrally-acting drugs).
No products indexed under this heading.

Fosinopril Sodium (Because of its potential for inducing hypotension, paliperidone may enhance the hypotensive effects of other therapeutic agents with this potential).
No products indexed under this heading.

Furosemide (Because of its potential for inducing hypotension, paliperidone may enhance the hypotensive effects of other therapeutic agents with this potential). Products include:
Furosemide Tablets **2186**

Gatifloxacin (Paliperidone causes a modest increase in the corrected QT (QTc) interval. The use of paliperidone should be avoided in combination with other drugs that are unknown to prolong QTc such as gatifloxacin).
No products indexed under this heading.

Glutethimide (Given the primary CNS effects of paliperidone, caution should be used if taken with other centrally-acting drugs).
No products indexed under this heading.

Guanabenz Acetate (Because of its potential for inducing hypotension, paliperidone may enhance the hypotensive effects of other therapeutic agents with this potential).
No products indexed under this heading.

Guanethidine Monosulfate (Because of its potential for inducing hypotension, paliperidone may enhance the hypotensive effects of other therapeutic agents with this potential).
No products indexed under this heading.

Haloperidol (Given the primary CNS effects of paliperidone, caution should be used if taken with other centrally-acting drugs).
No products indexed under this heading.

Haloperidol Decanoate (Given the primary CNS effects of paliperidone, caution should be used if taken with other centrally-acting drugs).
No products indexed under this heading.

Hydralazine Hydrochloride (Because of its potential for inducing hypotension, paliperidone may enhance the hypotensive effects of other therapeutic agents with this potential).
No products indexed under this heading.

Hydrochlorothiazide (Because of its potential for inducing hypotension, paliperidone may enhance the hypotensive effects of other therapeutic agents with this potential). Products include:
Atacand HCT **642**
Avalide Tablets **892**
Avalide Tablets **2713**
Benicar HCT Tablets **1010**
Diovan HCT Tablets **2216**
Dyazide Capsules **1405**
Micardis HCT Tablets **854**
Prinzide Tablets **2092**
Tekturna HCT Tablets **2324**
Teveten HCT Tablets **517**

Hydrocodone Bitartrate (Given the primary CNS effects of paliperidone, caution should be used if taken with other centrally-acting drugs). Products include:
Lortab 5/500 Tablets **3143**
Lortab 7.5/500 Tablets **3144**
Lortab 10/500 Tablets **3144**
Vicodin Tablets **529**
Vicodin ES Tablets **530**
Vicodin HP Tablets **531**
Vicoprofen Tablets **533**
Zydone Tablets **1132**

Hydrocodone Polistirex (Given the primary CNS effects of paliperidone, caution should be used if taken with other centrally-acting drugs). Products include:
Tussionex Pennkinetic Extended-Release Suspension **3154**

Hydroflumethiazide (Because of its potential for inducing hypotension, paliperidone may enhance the hypotensive effects of other therapeutic agents with this potential).
No products indexed under this heading.

Hydromorphone Hydrochloride (Given the primary CNS effects of paliperidone, caution should be used if taken with other centrally-acting drugs).
No products indexed under this heading.

Hydroxyzine Hydrochloride (Given the primary CNS effects of paliperidone, caution should be used if taken with other centrally-acting drugs).
No products indexed under this heading.

Indapamide (Because of its potential for inducing hypotension, paliperidone may enhance the hypotensive effects of other therapeutic agents with this potential). Products include:
Indapamide Tablets **2188**

Irbesartan (Because of its potential for inducing hypotension, paliperidone may enhance the hypotensive effects of other therapeutic agents with this potential). Products include:
Avalide Tablets **892**
Avalide Tablets **2713**
Avapro Tablets **897**
Avapro Tablets **2718**

Isoflurane (Given the primary CNS effects of paliperidone, caution should be used if taken with other centrally-acting drugs).
No products indexed under this heading.

Isradipine (Because of its potential for inducing hypotension, paliperidone may enhance the hypotensive effects of other therapeutic agents with this potential). Products include:
DynaCirc CR Controlled Release Tablets **1407**

Ketamine Hydrochloride (Given the primary CNS effects of paliperidone, caution should be used if taken with other centrally-acting drugs).
No products indexed under this heading.

Labetalol Hydrochloride (Because of its potential for inducing hypotension, paliperidone may enhance the hypotensive effects of other therapeutic agents with this potential).
No products indexed under this heading.

Levodopa (Paliperidone may antagonize the effect of dopamine agonists). Products include:
Stalevo Tablets **2309**

Levomethadyl Acetate Hydrochloride (Given the primary CNS effects of paliperidone, caution should be used if taken with other centrally-acting drugs).
No products indexed under this heading.

Levorphanol Tartrate (Given the primary CNS effects of paliperidone, caution should be used if taken with other centrally-acting drugs).
No products indexed under this heading.

Lisinopril (Because of its potential for inducing hypotension, paliperidone may enhance the hypotensive effects of other therapeutic agents with this potential). Products include:
Prinivil Tablets **2087**
Prinzide Tablets **2092**

Lorazepam (Given the primary CNS effects of paliperidone, caution should be used if taken with other centrally-acting drugs).
No products indexed under this heading.

Losartan Potassium (Because of its potential for inducing hypotension, paliperidone may enhance the hypotensive effects of other therapeutic agents with this potential). Products include:
Cozaar Tablets **1973**

Loxapine Hydrochloride (Given the primary CNS effects of paliperidone, caution should be used if taken with other centrally-acting drugs).
No products indexed under this heading.

Loxapine Succinate (Given the primary CNS effects of paliperidone, caution should be used if taken with other centrally-acting drugs).
No products indexed under this heading.

Mecamylamine Hydrochloride (Because of its potential for inducing hypotension, paliperidone may enhance the hypotensive effects of other therapeutic agents with this potential).
No products indexed under this heading.

Meperidine Hydrochloride (Given the primary CNS effects of paliperidone, caution should be used if taken with other centrally-acting drugs).
No products indexed under this heading.

Mephobarbital (Given the primary CNS effects of paliperidone, caution should be used if taken with other centrally-acting drugs).
No products indexed under this heading.

Meprobamate (Given the primary CNS effects of paliperidone, caution should be used if taken with other centrally-acting drugs).
No products indexed under this heading.

Mesoridazine Besylate (Given the primary CNS effects of paliperidone, caution should be used if taken with other centrally-acting drugs).
No products indexed under this heading.

Methadone Hydrochloride (Given the primary CNS effects of paliperidone, caution should be used if taken with other centrally-acting drugs).
No products indexed under this heading.

Methamphetamine Hydrochloride (Given the primary CNS effects of paliperidone, caution should be used if taken with other centrally-acting drugs).
No products indexed under this heading.

Methohexital Sodium (Given the primary CNS effects of paliperidone, caution should be used if taken with other centrally-acting drugs).
No products indexed under this heading.

Methotrimeprazine (Given the primary CNS effects of paliperidone, caution should be used if taken with other centrally-acting drugs).
No products indexed under this heading.

Methoxyflurane (Given the primary CNS effects of paliperidone, caution should be used if taken with other centrally-acting drugs).
No products indexed under this heading.

Methyclothiazide (Because of its potential for inducing hypotension, paliperidone may enhance the hypotensive effects of other therapeutic agents with this potential).
No products indexed under this heading.

Methyldopa (Because of its potential for inducing hypotension, paliperidone may enhance the hypotensive effects of other therapeutic agents with this potential).
No products indexed under this heading.

Methyldopate Hydrochloride (Because of its potential for inducing hypotension, paliperidone may enhance the hypotensive effects of other therapeutic agents with this potential).
No products indexed under this heading.

Methylphenidate (Given the primary CNS effects of paliperidone, caution should be used if taken with other centrally-acting drugs). Products include:
Daytrana Transdermal Patch **3022**

Methylphenidate Hydrochloride (Given the primary CNS effects of paliperidone, caution should be used if taken with other centrally-acting drugs). Products include:
Concerta Extended-Release Tablets **1925**
Metadate CD Capsules **3146**

Metolazone (Because of its potential for inducing hypotension, paliperidone may enhance the hypotensive effects of other therapeutic agents with this potential).
No products indexed under this heading.

Metoprolol Succinate (Because of its potential for inducing hypotension, paliperidone may enhance the hypotensive effects of other therapeutic agents with this potential). Products include:
Toprol-XL Tablets **666**

Metoprolol Tartrate (Because of its potential for inducing hypotension, paliperidone may enhance the hypotensive effects of other therapeutic agents with this potential).
No products indexed under this heading.

Metyrosine (Because of its potential for inducing hypotension, paliperidone may enhance the hypoten-

sive effects of other therapeutic agents with this potential). Products include:
Demser Capsules 1989

Mibefradil Dihydrochloride (Because of its potential for inducing hypotension, paliperidone may enhance the hypotensive effects of other therapeutic agents with this potential).
No products indexed under this heading.

Midazolam Hydrochloride (Given the primary CNS effects of paliperidone, caution should be used if taken with other centrally-acting drugs).
No products indexed under this heading.

Minoxidil (Because of its potential for inducing hypotension, paliperidone may enhance the hypotensive effects of other therapeutic agents with this potential).
No products indexed under this heading.

Moexipril Hydrochloride (Because of its potential for inducing hypotension, paliperidone may enhance the hypotensive effects of other therapeutic agents with this potential).
No products indexed under this heading.

Molindone Hydrochloride (Given the primary CNS effects of paliperidone, caution should be used if taken with other centrally-acting drugs). Products include:
Moban Tablets 1116

Moricizine Hydrochloride (Paliperidone causes a modest increase in the corrected QT (QTc) interval. The use of paliperidone should be avoided in combination with other drugs that are known to prolong QTc including Class 1A antiarrhythmic medications).
No products indexed under this heading.

Morphine Sulfate (Given the primary CNS effects of paliperidone, caution should be used if taken with other centrally-acting drugs). Products include:
Avinza Capsules 1772
DepoDur Injection 1095
MS Contin Tablets 2585

Moxifloxacin Hydrochloride (Paliperidone causes a modest increase in the corrected QT (QTc) interval. The use of paliperidone should be avoided in combination with other drugs that are known to prolong QTc such as moxifloxacin). Products include:
Avelox 2803
Vigamox Ophthalmic Solution 548

Nadolol (Because of its potential for inducing hypotension, paliperidone may enhance the hypotensive effects of other therapeutic agents with this potential). Products include:
Nadolol Tablets 2191

Nebivolol (Because of its potential for inducing hypotension, paliperidone may enhance the hypotensive effects of other therapeutic agents with this potential). Products include:
Bystolic Tablets 1155

Nicardipine Hydrochloride (Because of its potential for inducing hypotension, paliperidone may enhance the hypotensive effects of other therapeutic agents with this potential). Products include:
Cardene I.V. 1093

Nifedipine (Because of its potential for inducing hypotension, paliperidone may enhance the hypotensive effects of other therapeutic agents with this potential).
No products indexed under this heading.

Nisoldipine (Because of its potential for inducing hypotension, paliperidone may enhance the hypotensive effects of other therapeutic agents with this potential). Products include:
Sular Extended Release Tablets 2975

Nitroglycerin (Because of its potential for inducing hypotension, paliperidone may enhance the hypotensive effects of other therapeutic agents with this potential). Products include:
Nitro-Dur Transdermal Infusion System....................................... 2887
Nitrolingual Pumpspray 2965

Olanzapine (Given the primary CNS effects of paliperidone, caution should be used if taken with other centrally-acting drugs). Products include:
Symbyax Capsules 1871
Zyprexa Tablets 1883
Zyprexa IntraMuscular 1883
Zyprexa ZYDIS Orally Disintegrating Tablets.................. 1883

Oxazepam (Given the primary CNS effects of paliperidone, caution should be used if taken with other centrally-acting drugs).
No products indexed under this heading.

Oxycodone Hydrochloride (Given the primary CNS effects of paliperidone, caution should be used if taken with other centrally-acting drugs). Products include:
OxyContin Tablets 2589
OxyIR Capsules 2593
Percocet Tablets 1127
Percodan Tablets 1130

Paroxetine (Paliperidone is metabolized to a limited extent by CYP2D6. In an interaction study in healthy subjects in which a single 3 mg dose of paliperidone was administered concomitantly with 20 mg per day of paroxetine (a potent CYP2D6 inhibitor), paliperidone exposures were on average 16% higher in CYP2D6 extensive metabolizers. Higher doses of paroxetine have not been studied. The clinical relevance is unknown).
No products indexed under this heading.

Paroxetine Hydrochloride (Paliperidone is metabolized to a limited extent by CYP2D6. In an interaction study in healthy subjects in which a single 3 mg dose of paliperidone was administered concomitantly with 20 mg per day of paroxetine (a potent CYP2D6 inhibitor), paliperidone exposures were on average 16% higher in CYP2D6 extensive metabolizers. Higher doses of paroxetine have not been studied. The clinical relevance is unknown). Products include:
Paxil 1535
Paxil CR Controlled-Release Tablets...................................... 1544

Paroxetine Mesylate (Paliperidone is metabolized to a limited extent by CYP2D6. In an interaction study in healthy subjects in which a single 3 mg dose of paliperidone was administered concomitantly with 20 mg per day of paroxetine (a potent CYP2D6 inhibitor), paliperidone exposures were on average 16% higher in CYP2D6 extensive metabolizers. Higher doses of paroxetine have not been studied. The clinical relevance is unknown).
No products indexed under this heading.

Pemoline (Given the primary CNS effects of paliperidone, caution should be used if taken with other centrally-acting drugs).
No products indexed under this heading.

Penbutolol Sulfate (Because of its potential for inducing hypotension, paliperidone may enhance the hypotensive effects of other therapeutic agents with this potential).
No products indexed under this heading.

Pentobarbital Sodium (Given the primary CNS effects of paliperidone, caution should be used if taken with other centrally-acting drugs). Products include:
Nembutal Sodium Solution, USP 2494

Pergolide Mesylate (Paliperidone may antagonize the effect of dopamine agonists).
No products indexed under this heading.

Perindopril Erbumine (Because of its potential for inducing hypotension, paliperidone may enhance the hypotensive effects of other therapeutic agents with this potential). Products include:
Aceon Tablets (2 mg, 4 mg, 8 mg)... 3038

Perphenazine (Given the primary CNS effects of paliperidone, caution should be used if taken with other centrally-acting drugs).
No products indexed under this heading.

Phenobarbital (Given the primary CNS effects of paliperidone, caution should be used if taken with other centrally-acting drugs). Products include:
Donnatal Extentabs 2507

Phenoxybenzamine Hydrochloride (Because of its potential for inducing hypotension, paliperidone may enhance the hypotensive effects of other therapeutic agents with this potential). Products include:
Dibenzyline Capsules 3188

Phentolamine Mesylate (Because of its potential for inducing hypotension, paliperidone may enhance the hypotensive effects of other therapeutic agents with this potential).
No products indexed under this heading.

Pindolol (Because of its potential for inducing hypotension, paliperidone may enhance the hypotensive effects of other therapeutic agents with this potential).
No products indexed under this heading.

Polythiazide (Because of its potential for inducing hypotension, paliperidone may enhance the hypotensive effects of other therapeutic agents with this potential).
No products indexed under this heading.

Pramipexole Dihydrochloride (Paliperidone may antagonize the effect of dopamine agonists). Products include:
Mirapex Tablets 857

Prazepam (Given the primary CNS effects of paliperidone, caution should be used if taken with other centrally-acting drugs).
No products indexed under this heading.

Prazosin Hydrochloride (Because of its potential for inducing hypotension, paliperidone may enhance the hypotensive effects of other therapeutic agents with this potential).
No products indexed under this heading.

Procainamide (Paliperidone causes a modest increase in the corrected QT (QTc) interval. The use of paliperidone should be avoided in combination with other drugs that are known to prolong QTc including Class 1A antiarrhythmic medications).
No products indexed under this heading.

Prochlorperazine (Given the primary CNS effects of paliperidone, caution should be used if taken with other centrally-acting drugs).
No products indexed under this heading.

Promethazine Hydrochloride (Given the primary CNS effects of paliperidone, caution should be used if taken with other centrally-acting drugs).
No products indexed under this heading.

Propofol (Given the primary CNS effects of paliperidone, caution should be used if taken with other centrally-acting drugs).
No products indexed under this heading.

Propoxyphene Hydrochloride (Given the primary CNS effects of paliperidone, caution should be used if taken with other centrally-acting drugs).
No products indexed under this heading.

Propoxyphene Napsylate (Given the primary CNS effects of paliperidone, caution should be used if taken with other centrally-acting drugs).
No products indexed under this heading.

Propranolol Hydrochloride (Because of its potential for inducing hypotension, paliperidone may enhance the hypotensive effects of other therapeutic agents with this potential). Products include:
InnoPran XL Extended Release Capsules.................................... 1484

Quazepam (Given the primary CNS effects of paliperidone, caution should be used if taken with other centrally-acting drugs).
No products indexed under this heading.

Quetiapine Fumarate (Given the primary CNS effects of paliperidone, caution should be used if taken with other centrally-acting drugs).
No products indexed under this heading.

Quinapril Hydrochloride (Because of its potential for inducing hypotension, paliperidone may enhance the hypotensive effects of other therapeutic agents with this potential).
No products indexed under this heading.

Quinidine (Paliperidone causes a modest increase in the corrected QT (QTc) interval. The use of paliperidone should be avoided in combination with other drugs that are known to prolong QTc including Class 1A antiarrhythmic medications).
No products indexed under this heading.

Quinidine Gluconate (Paliperidone causes a modest increase in the corrected QT (QTc) interval. The use of paliperidone should be avoided in combination with other drugs that are known to prolong QTc including Class 1A antiarrhythmic medications).
No products indexed under this heading.

Quinidine Hydrochloride (Paliperidone causes a modest increase in the corrected QT (QTc) interval. The use of paliperidone should be avoided in combination with other drugs that are known to prolong QTc including Class 1A antiarrhythmic medications).
No products indexed under this heading.

Quinidine Polygalacturonate (Paliperidone causes a modest increase in the corrected QT (QTc) interval. The use of paliperidone should be avoided in combination with other drugs that are known to prolong QTc including Class 1A antiarrhythmic medications).
No products indexed under this heading.

Quinidine Sulfate (Paliperidone causes a modest increase in the corrected QT (QTc) interval. The use of paliperidone should be avoided in combination with other drugs that are known to prolong QTc including Class 1A antiarrhythmic medications).
No products indexed under this heading.

Ramipril (Because of its potential for inducing hypotension, paliperidone may enhance the hypotensive effects of other therapeutic agents with this potential).
No products indexed under this heading.

Rauwolfia Serpentina (Because of its potential for inducing hypotension, paliperidone may enhance the hypotensive effects of other therapeutic agents with this potential).
No products indexed under this heading.

Remifentanil Hydrochloride (Given the primary CNS effects of paliperidone, caution should be used if taken with other centrally-acting drugs).
No products indexed under this heading.

Rescinnamine (Because of its potential for inducing hypotension, paliperidone may enhance the hypotensive effects of other therapeutic agents with this potential).
No products indexed under this heading.

Reserpine (Because of its potential for inducing hypotension, paliperidone may enhance the hypotensive effects of other therapeutic agents with this potential).
No products indexed under this heading.

Risperidone (Given the primary CNS effects of paliperidone, caution should be used if taken with other centrally-acting drugs). Products include:
Risperdal Consta Long-Acting Injection **1753**

Ropinirole Hydrochloride (Paliperidone may antagonize the effect of dopamine agonists). Products include:
Requip Tablets **1561**
Requip XL Tablets **1568**

Secobarbital Sodium (Given the primary CNS effects of paliperidone, caution should be used if taken with other centrally-acting drugs).
No products indexed under this heading.

Sevoflurane (Given the primary CNS effects of paliperidone, caution should be used if taken with other centrally-acting drugs). Products include:
Ultane Liquid for Inhalation **524**

Sodium Nitroprusside (Because of its potential for inducing hypotension, paliperidone may enhance the hypotensive effects of other therapeutic agents with this potential).
No products indexed under this heading.

Sodium Oxybate (Given the primary CNS effects of paliperidone, caution should be used if taken with other centrally-acting drugs). Products include:
Xyrem Oral Solution **1766**

Sotalol Hydrochloride (Because of its potential for inducing hypotension, paliperidone may enhance the hypotensive effects of other therapeutic agents with this potential).
No products indexed under this heading.

Spirapril Hydrochloride (Because of its potential for inducing hypotension, paliperidone may enhance the hypotensive effects of other therapeutic agents with this potential).
No products indexed under this heading.

Sufentanil Citrate (Given the primary CNS effects of paliperidone, caution should be used if taken with other centrally-acting drugs).
No products indexed under this heading.

Telmisartan (Because of its potential for inducing hypotension, paliperidone may enhance the hypotensive effects of other therapeutic agents with this potential). Products include:
Micardis Tablets **852**
Micardis HCT Tablets **854**

Temazepam (Given the primary CNS effects of paliperidone, caution should be used if taken with other centrally-acting drugs).
No products indexed under this heading.

Terazosin Hydrochloride (Because of its potential for inducing hypotension, paliperidone may enhance the hypotensive effects of other therapeutic agents with this potential).
No products indexed under this heading.

Thiamylal Sodium (Given the primary CNS effects of paliperidone, caution should be used if taken with other centrally-acting drugs).
No products indexed under this heading.

Thioridazine (Paliperidone causes a modest increase in the corrected QT (QTc) interval. The use of paliperidone should be avoided in combination with other drugs that are known to prolong QTc such as thioridazine).
No products indexed under this heading.

Thioridazine Hydrochloride (Paliperidone causes a modest increase in the corrected QT (QTc) interval. The use of paliperidone should be avoided in combination with other drugs that are known to prolong QTc such as thioridazine). Products include:
Thioridazine Hydrochloride Tablets **2195**

Thiothixene (Given the primary CNS effects of paliperidone, caution should be used if taken with other centrally-acting drugs). Products include:
Thiothixene Capsules **2197**

Timolol Maleate (Because of its potential for inducing hypotension, paliperidone may enhance the hypotensive effects of other therapeutic agents with this potential). Products include:
Combigan Ophthalmic Solution **553**
Cosopt Sterile Ophthalmic Solution **1969**
Timoptic Sterile Ophthalmic Solution **2121**
Timoptic in Ocudose **2124**
Timoptic-XE Sterile Ophthalmic Gel Forming Solution **2125**

Torsemide (Because of its potential for inducing hypotension, paliperidone may enhance the hypotensive effects of other therapeutic agents with this potential). Products include:
Demadex Injection **2630**
Demadex Tablets **2630**

Trandolapril (Because of its potential for inducing hypotension, paliperidone may enhance the hypotensive effects of other therapeutic agents with this potential). Products include:
Mavik Tablets **472**
Tarka Tablets **511**

Triazolam (Given the primary CNS effects of paliperidone, caution should be used if taken with other centrally-acting drugs).
No products indexed under this heading.

Trifluoperazine Hydrochloride (Given the primary CNS effects of paliperidone, caution should be used if taken with other centrally-acting drugs).
No products indexed under this heading.

Trimethaphan Camsylate (Because of its potential for inducing hypotension, paliperidone may enhance the hypotensive effects of other therapeutic agents with this potential).
No products indexed under this heading.

Valsartan (Because of its potential for inducing hypotension, paliperidone may enhance the hypotensive effects of other therapeutic agents with this potential). Products include:
Diovan Tablets **2212**
Diovan HCT Tablets **2216**
Exforge Tablets **2238**

Verapamil Hydrochloride (Because of its potential for inducing hypotension, paliperidone may enhance the hypotensive effects of other therapeutic agents with this potential). Products include:
Tarka Tablets **511**

Zaleplon (Given the primary CNS effects of paliperidone, caution should be used if taken with other centrally-acting drugs).
No products indexed under this heading.

Ziprasidone Hydrochloride (Given the primary CNS effects of paliperidone, caution should be used if taken with other centrally-acting drugs). Products include:
Geodon Capsules **2520**

Zolpidem Tartrate (Given the primary CNS effects of paliperidone, caution should be used if taken with other centrally-acting drugs). Products include:
Ambien Tablets **2692**
Ambien CR Tablets **2696**

Food Interactions

Alcohol (Given the primary CNS effects of paliperidone, caution should be used if taken with other centrally-acting drugs).

IONSYS TRANSDERMAL SYSTEM

(Fentanyl) **2410**

May interact with anesthetics, cytochrome p450 3a4 inducers (selected), cytochrome p450 3a4 inhibitors (selected), hypnotics and sedatives, narcotic analgesics, phenothiazines, sedating antihistamines, skeletal muscle relaxants, tranquilizers, and certain other agents. Compounds in these categories include:

Acetazolamide (The concomitant use of fentanyl with CYP3A4 inhibitors may result in a decrease in fentanyl clearance, which could increase or prolong adverse drug effects including serious respiratory depression. In this situation, special patient care and observation is appropriate).
No products indexed under this heading.

Acrivastine (The concomitant use of other central nervous system depressants, such as sedating antihistamines, may produce additive depressant effects. Hypoventilation, hypotension, profound sedation, and coma may occur. Therefore, use of concomitant CNS depressants requires individual adjustment of dosage of the concomitant medication and observation of a given patient).
No products indexed under this heading.

Alfentanil Hydrochloride (The concomitant use of other central nervous system depressants, such as opiods, may produce additive depressant effects. Hypoventilation, hypotension, profound sedation, and coma may occur. Therefore, use of concomitant CNS depressants requires individual adjustment of dosage of the concomitant medication and observation of a given patient).

No products indexed under this heading.

Allium sativum (Co-administration with agents that induce CYP3A4 activity may cause increased clearance of fentanyl and reduce its efficacy).

No products indexed under this heading.

Alprazolam (The concomitant use of other central nervous system depressants, such as tranquilizers, may produce additive depressant effects. Hypoventilation, hypotension, profound sedation, and coma may occur. Therefore, use of concomitant CNS depressants requires individual adjustment of dosage of the concomitant medication and observation of a given patient).

No products indexed under this heading.

Amiodarone Hydrochloride (The concomitant use of fentanyl with CYP3A4 inhibitors may result in a decrease in fentanyl clearance, which could increase or prolong adverse drug effects including serious respiratory depression. In this situation, special patient care and observation is appropriate).

No products indexed under this heading.

Amprenavir (The concomitant use of fentanyl with CYP3A4 inhibitors may result in a decrease in fentanyl clearance, which could increase or prolong adverse drug effects including serious respiratory depression. In this situation, special patient care and observation is appropriate).

No products indexed under this heading.

Anastrozole (The concomitant use of fentanyl with CYP3A4 inhibitors may result in a decrease in fentanyl clearance, which could increase or prolong adverse drug effects including serious respiratory depression. In this situation, special patient care and observation is appropriate). Products include:

Arimidex Tablets 672

Aprepitant (The concomitant use of fentanyl with CYP3A4 inhibitors may result in a decrease in fentanyl clearance, which could increase or prolong adverse drug effects including serious respiratory depression. In this situation, special patient care and observation is appropriate). Products include:

Emend Capsules 1992

Atazanavir (The concomitant use of fentanyl with CYP3A4 inhibitors may result in a decrease in fentanyl clearance, which could increase or prolong adverse drug effects including serious respiratory depression. In this situation, special patient care and observation is appropriate).

No products indexed under this heading.

Atazanavir Sulfate (The concomitant use of fentanyl with CYP3A4 inhibitors may result in a decrease in fentanyl clearance, which could increase or prolong adverse drug effects including serious respiratory depression. In this situation, special patient care and observation is appropriate). Products include:

Reyataz Capsules 3299

Azatadine Maleate (The concomitant use of other central nervous system depressants, such as sedating antihistamines, may produce additive depressant effects. Hypoventilation, hypotension, profound sedation, and coma may occur. Therefore, use of concomitant CNS depressants requires individual adjustment of dosage of the concomitant medication and observation of a given patient).

No products indexed under this heading.

Baclofen (The concomitant use of other central nervous system depressants, such as skeletal muscle relaxants, may produce additive depressant effects. Hypoventilation, hypotension, profound sedation, and coma may occur. Therefore, use of concomitant CNS depressants requires individual adjustment of dosage of the concomitant medication and observation of a given patient).

No products indexed under this heading.

Betamethasone Acetate (Co-administration with agents that induce CYP3A4 activity may cause increased clearance of fentanyl and reduce its efficacy).

No products indexed under this heading.

Betamethasone Sodium Phosphate (Co-administration with agents that induce CYP3A4 activity may cause increased clearance of fentanyl and reduce its efficacy).

No products indexed under this heading.

Bromodiphenhydramine Hydrochloride (The concomitant use of other central nervous system depressants, such as sedating antihistamines, may produce additive depressant effects. Hypoventilation, hypotension, profound sedation, and coma may occur. Therefore, use of concomitant CNS depressants requires individual adjustment of dosage of the concomitant medication and observation of a given patient).

No products indexed under this heading.

Brompheniramine Maleate (The concomitant use of other central nervous system depressants, such as sedating antihistamines, may produce additive depressant effects. Hypoventilation, hypotension, profound sedation, and coma may occur. Therefore, use of concomitant CNS depressants requires individual adjustment of dosage of the concomitant medication and observation of a given patient).

No products indexed under this heading.

Buprenorphine Hydrochloride (The concomitant use of other central nervous system depressants, such as opiods, may produce additive depressant effects. Hypoventilation, hypotension, profound sedation, and coma may occur. Therefore, use of concomitant CNS depressants requires individual adjustment of dosage of the concomitant medication and observation of a given patient). Products include:

Suboxone Tablets 2601
Subutex Tablets 2601

Buspirone Hydrochloride (The concomitant use of other central nervous system depressants, such as tranquilizers, may produce additive depressant effects. Hypoventilation, hypotension, profound sedation, and coma may occur. Therefore, use of concomitant CNS depressants requires individual adjustment of dosage of the concomitant medication and observation of a given patient).

No products indexed under this heading.

Butabarbital (The concomitant use of other central nervous system depressants, such as sedatives and hypnotics, may produce additive depressant effects. Hypoventilation, hypotension, profound sedation, and coma may occur. Therefore, use of concomitant CNS depressants requires individual adjustment of dosage of the concomitant medication and observation of a given patient).

No products indexed under this heading.

Butabarbital Sodium (The concomitant use of other central nervous system depressants, such as sedatives and hypnotics, may produce additive depressant effects. Hypoventilation, hypotension, profound sedation, and coma may occur. Therefore, use of concomitant CNS depressants requires individual adjustment of dosage of the concomitant medication and observation of a given patient).

No products indexed under this heading.

Carbamazepine (Co-administration with agents that induce CYP3A4 activity may cause increased clearance of fentanyl and reduce its efficacy). Products include:

Carbatrol Capsules 3019
Equetro Extended-Release Capsules 3174

Carisoprodol (The concomitant use of other central nervous system depressants, such as skeletal muscle relaxants, may produce additive depressant effects. Hypoventilation, hypotension, profound sedation, and coma may occur. Therefore, use of concomitant CNS depressants requires individual adjustment of dosage of the concomitant medication and observation of a given patient). Products include:

Soma Tablets 1931

Chloral Hydrate (The concomitant use of other central nervous system depressants, such as sedatives and hypnotics, may produce additive depressant effects. Hypoventilation, hypotension, profound sedation, and coma may occur. Therefore, use of concomitant CNS depressants requires individual adjustment of dosage of the concomitant medication and observation of a given patient).

No products indexed under this heading.

Chlordiazepoxide (The concomitant use of other central nervous system depressants, such as tranquilizers, may produce additive depressant effects. Hypoventilation, hypotension, profound sedation, and coma may occur. Therefore, use of concomitant CNS depressants requires individual adjustment of dosage of the concomitant medication and observation of a given patient).

No products indexed under this heading.

Chlordiazepoxide Hydrochloride (The concomitant use of other central nervous system depressants, such as tranquilizers, may produce additive depressant effects. Hypoventilation, hypotension, profound sedation, and coma may occur. Therefore, use of concomitant CNS depressants requires individual adjustment of dosage of the concomitant medication and observation of a given patient).

No products indexed under this heading.

Chlorpheniramine Maleate (The concomitant use of other central nervous system depressants, such as sedating antihistamines, may produce additive depressant effects. Hypoventilation, hypotension, profound sedation, and coma may occur. Therefore, use of concomitant CNS depressants requires individual adjustment of dosage of the concomitant medication and observation of a given patient). Products include:

Actifed Cold & Allergy Tablets 1895
Sudafed PE Sinus & Allergy Tablets 1908
Tylenol Allergy Multi-Symptom Caplets with Cool Burst and Rapid Release Gelcaps 1916
Children's Tylenol Plus Cold Suspension Liquid 1912
Children's Tylenol Plus Cough & Runny Nose Suspension Liquid 1912
Children's Tylenol Plus Flu Suspension Liquid 1914
Children's Tylenol Plus Multi-Symptom Cold Suspension Liquid 1912
Tylenol Cold Head Congestion Nighttime Caplets with Cool Burst 1910
Tylenol Cold Multi-Symptom Nighttime Caplets with Cool Burst 1913
Tylenol Sinus Congestion & Pain Nighttime Caplets with Cool Burst 1917

Chlorpheniramine Polistirex (The concomitant use of other central nervous system depressants, such as sedating antihistamines, may produce additive depressant effects. Hypoventilation, hypotension, profound sedation, and coma may occur. Therefore, use of concomitant CNS depressants requires individual adjustment of dosage of the concomitant medication and observation of a given patient). Products include:

Tussionex Pennkinetic Extended-Release Suspension 3154

Chlorpheniramine Tannate (The concomitant use of other central nervous system depressants, such as sedating antihistamines, may produce additive depressant effects. Hypoventilation, hypotension, profound sedation, and coma may occur. Therefore, use of concomitant CNS depressants requires individual adjustment of dosage of the concomitant medication and observation of a given patient).

No products indexed under this heading.

Chlorpromazine (The concomitant use of other central nervous system depressants, such as phenothiazines, may produce additive depressant effects. Hypoventilation, hypotension, profound sedation, and coma may occur. Therefore, use of concomitant CNS depressants requires individual adjustment of dosage of the concomitant medication and observation of a given patient).

No products indexed under this heading.

Chlorpromazine Hydrochloride (The concomitant use of other central nervous system depressants, such as phenothiazines, may produce additive depressant effects. Hypoventilation, hypotension, profound sedation, and coma may occur. Therefore, use of concomitant CNS depressants requires individual adjustment of dosage of the concomitant medication and observation of a given patient).

No products indexed under this heading.

Chlorprothixene (The concomitant use of other central nervous system depressants, such as tranquilizers, may produce additive depressant effects. Hypoventilation, hypotension, profound sedation, and coma may occur. Therefore, use of concomitant CNS depressants requires individual adjustment of dosage of the concomitant medication and observation of a given patient).

No products indexed under this heading.

Chlorprothixene Hydrochloride (The concomitant use of other central nervous system depressants, such as tranquilizers, may produce additive depressant effects. Hypoventilation, hypotension, profound sedation, and coma may occur. Therefore, use of concomitant CNS depressants requires individual adjustment of dosage of the concomitant medication and observation of a given patient).

No products indexed under this heading.

Chlorzoxazone (The concomitant use of other central nervous system depressants, such as skeletal muscle relaxants, may produce additive depressant effects. Hypoventilation, hypotension, profound sedation, and coma may occur. Therefore, use of concomitant CNS depressants requires individual adjustment of dosage of the concomitant medication and observation of a given patient).

No products indexed under this heading.

Cimetidine (The concomitant use of fentanyl with CYP3A4 inhibitors may result in a decrease in fentanyl clearance, which could increase or prolong adverse drug effects including serious respiratory depression. In this situation, special patient care and observation is appropriate).

No products indexed under this heading.

Cimetidine Hydrochloride (The concomitant use of fentanyl with CYP3A4 inhibitors may result in a decrease in fentanyl clearance, which could increase or prolong adverse drug effects including serious respiratory depression. In this situation, special patient care and observation is appropriate).

No products indexed under this heading.

Ciprofloxacin (The concomitant use of fentanyl with CYP3A4 inhibitors may result in a decrease in fentanyl clearance, which could increase or prolong adverse drug effects including serious respiratory depression. In this situation, special patient care and observation is appropriate). Products include:

Cipro I.V. **2817**
Cipro Oral Suspension **2810**
Cipro XR Tablets **2823**
Ciprodex Otic Suspension **541**

Ciprofloxacin Hydrochloride (Co-administration with agents that induce CYP3A4 activity may cause increased clearance of fentanyl and reduce its efficacy). Products include:

Cipro Tablets **2810**

Cisplatin (Co-administration with agents that induce CYP3A4 activity may cause increased clearance of fentanyl and reduce its efficacy).

No products indexed under this heading.

Clarithromycin (The concomitant use of fentanyl with CYP3A4 inhibitors may result in a decrease in fentanyl clearance, which could increase or prolong adverse drug effects including serious respiratory depression. In this situation, special patient care and observation is appropriate). Products include:

Biaxin/Biaxin XL **411**

Clemastine Fumarate (The concomitant use of other central nervous system depressants, such as sedating antihistamines, may produce additive depressant effects. Hypoventilation, hypotension, profound sedation, and coma may occur. Therefore, use of concomitant CNS depressants requires individual adjustment of dosage of the concomitant medication and observation of a given patient).

No products indexed under this heading.

Clorazepate Dipotassium (The concomitant use of other central nervous system depressants, such as tranquilizers, may produce additive depressant effects. Hypoventilation, hypotension, profound sedation, and coma may occur. Therefore, use of concomitant CNS depressants requires individual adjustment of dosage of the concomitant medication and observation of a given patient).

No products indexed under this heading.

Clotrimazole (The concomitant use of fentanyl with CYP3A4 inhibitors may result in a decrease in fentanyl clearance, which could increase or prolong adverse drug effects including serious respiratory depression. In this situation, special patient care and observation is appropriate). Products include:

Lotrisone **2881**

Codeine Phosphate (The concomitant use of other central nervous system depressants, such as opioids, may produce additive depressant effects. Hypoventilation, hypotension, profound sedation, and coma may occur. Therefore, use of concomitant CNS depressants requires individual adjustment of dosage of the concomitant medication and observation of a given patient). Products include:

Tylenol with Codeine Tablets **2427**

Cortisone Acetate (Co-administration with agents that induce CYP3A4 activity may cause increased clearance of fentanyl and reduce its efficacy).

No products indexed under this heading.

Cyclobenzaprine Hydrochloride (The concomitant use of other central nervous system depressants, such as skeletal muscle relaxants, may produce additive depressant effects. Hypoventilation, hypotension, profound sedation, and coma may occur. Therefore, use of concomitant CNS depressants requires individual adjustment of dosage of the concomitant medication and observation of a given patient). Products include:

Amrix Capsules **966**

Cyclosporine (The concomitant use of fentanyl with CYP3A4 inhibitors may result in a decrease in fentanyl clearance, which could increase or prolong adverse drug effects including serious respiratory depression. In this situation, special patient care and observation is appropriate). Products include:

Gengraf Capsules **435**
Neoral Oral Solution **2280**
Neoral Soft Gelatin Capsules **2280**
Restasis Ophthalmic Emulsion **557**
Sandimmune **2296**

Cyproheptadine Hydrochloride (The concomitant use of other central nervous system depressants, such as sedating antihistamines, may produce additive depressant effects. Hypoventilation, hypotension, profound sedation, and coma may occur. Therefore, use of concomitant CNS depressants requires individual adjustment of dosage of the concomitant medication and observation of a given patient).

No products indexed under this heading.

Dalfopristin (The concomitant use of fentanyl with CYP3A4 inhibitors may result in a decrease in fentanyl clearance, which could increase or prolong adverse drug effects including serious respiratory depression. In this situation, special patient care and observation is appropriate).

No products indexed under this heading.

Danazol (The concomitant use of fentanyl with CYP3A4 inhibitors may result in a decrease in fentanyl clearance, which could increase or prolong adverse drug effects including serious respiratory depression. In this situation, special patient care and observation is appropriate).

No products indexed under this heading.

Dantrolene Sodium (The concomitant use of other central nervous system depressants, such as skeletal muscle relaxants, may produce additive depressant effects. Hypoventilation, hypotension, profound sedation, and coma may occur. Therefore, use of concomitant CNS depressants requires individual adjustment of dosage of the concomitant medication and observation of a given patient). Products include:

Dantrium Capsules **2580**
Dantrium Intravenous **2582**

Delavirdine Mesylate (The concomitant use of fentanyl with CYP3A4 inhibitors may result in a decrease in fentanyl clearance, which could increase or prolong adverse drug effects including serious respiratory depression. In this situation, special patient care and observation is appropriate).

No products indexed under this heading.

Dexamethasone (Co-administration with agents that induce CYP3A4 activity may cause increased clearance of fentanyl and reduce its efficacy). Products include:

Ciprodex Otic Suspension **541**

Dexamethasone Acetate (Co-administration with agents that induce CYP3A4 activity may cause increased clearance of fentanyl and reduce its efficacy).

No products indexed under this heading.

Dexamethasone Sodium Phosphate (Co-administration with agents that induce CYP3A4 activity may cause increased clearance of fentanyl and reduce its efficacy).

No products indexed under this heading.

Dexchlorpheniramine Maleate (The concomitant use of other central nervous system depressants, such as sedating antihistamines, may produce additive depressant effects. Hypoventilation, hypotension, profound sedation, and coma may occur. Therefore, use of concomitant CNS depressants requires individual adjustment of dosage of the concomitant medication and observation of a given patient).

No products indexed under this heading.

Dezocine (The concomitant use of other central nervous system depressants, such as opioids, may produce additive depressant effects. Hypoventilation, hypotension, profound sedation, and coma may occur. Therefore, use of concomitant CNS depressants requires individual adjustment of dosage of the concomitant medication and observation of a given patient).

No products indexed under this heading.

Diazepam (The concomitant use of other central nervous system depressants, such as tranquilizers, may produce additive depressant effects. Hypoventilation, hypotension, profound sedation, and coma may occur. Therefore, use of concomitant CNS depressants requires individual adjustment of dosage of the concomitant medication and observation of a given patient). Products include:

Valium Tablets **2658**

Diltiazem Hydrochloride (The concomitant use of fentanyl with CYP3A4 inhibitors may result in a decrease in fentanyl clearance, which could increase or prolong adverse drug effects including serious respiratory depression. In this situation, special patient care and observation is appropriate). Products include:

Cardizem LA Extended Release Tablets **421**

Diltiazem Maleate (The concomitant use of fentanyl with CYP3A4 inhibitors may result in a decrease in fentanyl clearance, which could increase or prolong adverse drug effects including serious respiratory depression. In this situation, special patient care and observation is appropriate).
No products indexed under this heading.

Diphenhydramine Citrate (The concomitant use of other central nervous system depressants, such as sedating antihistamines, may produce additive depressant effects. Hypoventilation, hypotension, profound sedation, and coma may occur. Therefore, use of concomitant CNS depressants requires individual adjustment of dosage of the concomitant medication and observation of a given patient).
No products indexed under this heading.

Diphenhydramine Hydrochloride (The concomitant use of other central nervous system depressants, such as sedating antihistamines, may produce additive depressant effects. Hypoventilation, hypotension, profound sedation, and coma may occur. Therefore, use of concomitant CNS depressants requires individual adjustment of dosage of the concomitant medication and observation of a given patient). Products include:
Benadryl Allergy & Cold Kapgels **1895**
Benadryl Allergy & Sinus Headache Kapgels **1895**
Benadryl Severe Allergy & Sinus Headache Caplets **1897**
Benadryl Dye-Free Allergy Liqui-gels Softgels **1897**
Benadryl Allergy Kapgels **1895**
Benadryl Allergy Quick Dissolve Strips **1896**
Benadryl Allergy Ultratab Tablets **1896**
Children's Benadryl Dye-Free Allergy Liquid **1897**
Children's Benadryl Allergy Fastmelts **1897**
Children's Benadryl Allergy Liquid **1898**
Children's Benadryl Allergy Perfect Measure **1896**
Children's Benadryl-D Allergy & Sinus Liquid **1896**
Benadryl-D Allergy & Sinus Tablet **1896**
PediaCare Children's Allergy & Cold Liquid **1902**
PediaCare Children's Allergy Liquid **1902**
Simply Sleep Caplets **1905**
Sudafed PE Nighttime Cold Caplets **1907**
Sudafed PE Severe Cold Caplets **1908**
Extra Strength Tylenol PM Caplets, Geltabs, Liquid, and Rapid Release Gels **1915**
Tylenol Allergy Multi-Symptom Nighttime Caplets with Cool Burst **1916**
Tylenol Severe Allergy Caplets **1916**
Children's Tylenol Plus Cold & Allergy Suspension Liquid **1914**
Tylenol Sore Throat Nighttime Liquid with Cool Burst **1918**

Diphenylpyraline Hydrochloride (The concomitant use of other central nervous system depressants, such as sedating antihistamines, may produce additive depressant effects. Hypoventilation, hypotension, profound sedation, and coma may occur. Therefore, use of concomitant CNS depressants requires individual adjustment of dosage of the concomitant medication and observation of a given patient).
No products indexed under this heading.

Doxorubicin Hydrochloride (Co-administration with agents that induce CYP3A4 activity may cause increased clearance of fentanyl and reduce its efficacy).
No products indexed under this heading.

Droperidol (The concomitant use of other central nervous system depressants, such as tranquilizers, may produce additive depressant effects. Hypoventilation, hypotension, profound sedation, and coma may occur. Therefore, use of concomitant CNS depressants requires individual adjustment of dosage of the concomitant medication and observation of a given patient).
No products indexed under this heading.

Efavirenz (The concomitant use of fentanyl with CYP3A4 inhibitors may result in a decrease in fentanyl clearance, which could increase or prolong adverse drug effects including serious respiratory depression. In this situation, special patient care and observation is appropriate). Products include:
Atripla Tablets **938**
Sustiva Capsules **930**
Sustiva Tablets **930**

Enflurane (The concomitant use of other central nervous system depressants, such as general anesthetics, may produce additive depressant effects. Hypoventilation, hypotension, profound sedation, and coma may occur. Therefore, use of concomitant CNS depressants requires individual adjustment of dosage of the concomitant medication and observation of a given patient).
No products indexed under this heading.

Erythromycin (The concomitant use of fentanyl with CYP3A4 inhibitors may result in a decrease in fentanyl clearance, which could increase or prolong adverse drug effects including serious respiratory depression. In this situation, special patient care and observation is appropriate).
No products indexed under this heading.

Erythromycin Estolate (The concomitant use of fentanyl with CYP3A4 inhibitors may result in a decrease in fentanyl clearance, which could increase or prolong adverse drug effects including serious respiratory depression. In this situation, special patient care and observation is appropriate).
No products indexed under this heading.

Erythromycin Ethylsuccinate (The concomitant use of fentanyl with CYP3A4 inhibitors may result in a decrease in fentanyl clearance, which could increase or prolong adverse drug effects including serious respiratory depression. In this situation, special patient care and observation is appropriate). Products include:
E.E.S. **433**
EryPed **431**

Erythromycin Gluceptate (The concomitant use of fentanyl with CYP3A4 inhibitors may result in a decrease in fentanyl clearance, which could increase or prolong adverse drug effects including serious respiratory depression. In this situation, special patient care and observation is appropriate).
No products indexed under this heading.

Erythromycin Lactobionate (The concomitant use of fentanyl with CYP3A4 inhibitors may result in a decrease in fentanyl clearance, which could increase or prolong adverse drug effects including serious respiratory depression. In this situation, special patient care and observation is appropriate).
No products indexed under this heading.

Erythromycin Stearate (The concomitant use of fentanyl with CYP3A4 inhibitors may result in a decrease in fentanyl clearance, which could increase or prolong adverse drug effects including serious respiratory depression. In this situation, special patient care and observation is appropriate).
No products indexed under this heading.

Esomeprazole Magnesium (The concomitant use of fentanyl with CYP3A4 inhibitors may result in a decrease in fentanyl clearance, which could increase or prolong adverse drug effects including serious respiratory depression. In this situation, special patient care and observation is appropriate). Products include:
Nexium Delayed-Release Capsules **645**
Nexium Delayed-Release Oral Suspension **645**

Estazolam (The concomitant use of other central nervous system depressants, such as sedatives and hypnotics, may produce additive depressant effects. Hypoventilation, hypotension, profound sedation, and coma may occur. Therefore, use of concomitant CNS depressants requires individual adjustment of dosage of the concomitant medication and observation of a given patient).
No products indexed under this heading.

Ethchlorvynol (The concomitant use of other central nervous system depressants, such as sedatives and hypnotics, may produce additive depressant effects. Hypoventilation, hypotension, profound sedation, and coma may occur. Therefore, use of concomitant CNS depressants requires individual adjustment of dosage of the concomitant medication and observation of a given patient).
No products indexed under this heading.

Ethinamate (The concomitant use of other central nervous system depressants, such as sedatives and hypnotics, may produce additive depressant effects. Hypoventilation, hypotension, profound sedation, and coma may occur. Therefore, use of concomitant CNS depressants requires individual adjustment of dosage of the concomitant medication and observation of a given patient).
No products indexed under this heading.

Ethosuximide (Co-administration with agents that induce CYP3A4 activity may cause increased clearance of fentanyl and reduce its efficacy).
No products indexed under this heading.

Felbamate (Co-administration with agents that induce CYP3A4 activity may cause increased clearance of fentanyl and reduce its efficacy).
No products indexed under this heading.

Fentanyl Citrate (The concomitant use of other central nervous system depressants, such as opiods, may produce additive depressant effects. Hypoventilation, hypotension, profound sedation, and coma may occur. Therefore, use of concomitant CNS depressants requires individual adjustment of dosage of the concomitant medication and observation of a given patient). Products include:
Actiq **959**
Fentora Tablets **968**

Fluconazole (The concomitant use of fentanyl with CYP3A4 inhibitors may result in a decrease in fentanyl clearance, which could increase or prolong adverse drug effects including serious respiratory depression. In this situation, special patient care and observation is appropriate).
No products indexed under this heading.

Fludrocortisone Acetate (Co-administration with agents that induce CYP3A4 activity may cause increased clearance of fentanyl and reduce its efficacy).
No products indexed under this heading.

Fluoxetine (The concomitant use of fentanyl with CYP3A4 inhibitors may result in a decrease in fentanyl clearance, which could increase or prolong adverse drug effects including serious respiratory depression. In this situation, special patient care and observation is appropriate).
No products indexed under this heading.

Fluoxetine Hydrochloride (The concomitant use of fentanyl with CYP3A4 inhibitors may result in a decrease in fentanyl clearance, which could increase or prolong adverse drug effects including serious respiratory depression. In this situation, special patient care and observation is appropriate). Products include:
Prozac Weekly Capsules **1852**
Prozac Pulvules and Liquid **1852**
Symbyax Capsules **1871**

Fluphenazine Decanoate (The concomitant use of other central nervous system depressants, such as phenothiazines, may produce additive depressant effects. Hypoventilation, hypotension, profound sedation, and coma may occur. Therefore, use of concomitant CNS depressants requires individual adjustment of dosage of the concomitant medication and observation of a given patient).
No products indexed under this heading.

Fluphenazine Enanthate (The concomitant use of other central nervous system depressants, such as phenothiazines, may produce additive depressant effects. Hypoventilation, hypotension, profound sedation, and coma may occur. Therefore, use of concomitant CNS depressants requires individual adjustment of dosage of the concomitant medication and observation of a given patient).
No products indexed under this heading.

Fluphenazine Hydrochloride (The concomitant use of other central nervous system depressants, such as phenothiazines, may produce additive depressant effects. Hypoventilation, hypotension, profound sedation, and coma may occur. Therefore, use of concomitant CNS depressants requires individual adjustment of dosage of the concomitant medication and observation of a given patient).
No products indexed under this heading.

Flurazepam Hydrochloride (The concomitant use of other central nervous system depressants, such as sedatives and hypnotics, may produce additive depressant effects. Hypoventilation, hypotension, profound sedation, and coma may occur. Therefore, use of concomitant CNS depressants requires individual adjustment of dosage of the concomitant medication and observation of a given patient).
No products indexed under this heading.

Fluvoxamine Maleate (The concomitant use of fentanyl with CYP3A4 inhibitors may result in a decrease in fentanyl clearance, which could increase or prolong adverse drug effects including serious respiratory depression. In this situation, special patient care and observation is appropriate). Products include:
Luvox CR Extended-Release Capsules 1759

Fosamprenavir Calcium (The concomitant use of fentanyl with CYP3A4 inhibitors may result in a decrease in fentanyl clearance, which could increase or prolong adverse drug effects including serious respiratory depression. In this situation, special patient care and observation is appropriate). Products include:
Lexiva Oral Suspension 1510
Lexiva Tablets 1510

Fosphenytoin Sodium (Co-administration with agents that induce CYP3A4 activity may cause increased clearance of fentanyl and reduce its efficacy).
No products indexed under this heading.

Garlic Extract (Co-administration with agents that induce CYP3A4 activity may cause increased clearance of fentanyl and reduce its efficacy).
No products indexed under this heading.

Garlic Oil (Co-administration with agents that induce CYP3A4 activity may cause increased clearance of fentanyl and reduce its efficacy).
No products indexed under this heading.

Glutethimide (The concomitant use of other central nervous system depressants, such as sedatives and hypnotics, may produce additive depressant effects. Hypoventilation, hypotension, profound sedation, and coma may occur. Therefore, use of concomitant CNS depressants requires individual adjustment of dosage of the concomitant medication and observation of a given patient).
No products indexed under this heading.

Haloperidol (The concomitant use of other central nervous system depressants, such as tranquilizers, may produce additive depressant effects. Hypoventilation, hypotension, profound sedation, and coma may occur. Therefore, use of concomitant CNS depressants requires individual adjustment of dosage of the concomitant medication and observation of a given patient).
No products indexed under this heading.

Haloperidol Decanoate (The concomitant use of other central nervous system depressants, such as tranquilizers, may produce additive depressant effects. Hypoventilation, hypotension, profound sedation, and coma may occur. Therefore, use of concomitant CNS depressants requires individual adjustment of dosage of the concomitant medication and observation of a given patient).
No products indexed under this heading.

Halothane (The concomitant use of other central nervous system depressants, such as general anesthetics, may produce additive depressant effects. Hypoventilation, hypotension, profound sedation, and coma may occur. Therefore, use of concomitant CNS depressants requires individual adjustment of dosage of the concomitant medication and observation of a given patient).
No products indexed under this heading.

Hydrocodone Bitartrate (The concomitant use of other central nervous system depressants, such as opiods, may produce additive depressant effects. Hypoventilation, hypotension, profound sedation, and coma may occur. Therefore, use of concomitant CNS depressants requires individual adjustment of dosage of the concomitant medication and observation of a given patient). Products include:
Lortab 5/500 Tablets 3143
Lortab 7.5/500 Tablets 3144
Lortab 10/500 Tablets 3144
Vicodin Tablets 529
Vicodin ES Tablets 530
Vicodin HP Tablets 531
Vicoprofen Tablets 533
Zydone Tablets 1132

Hydrocodone Polistirex (The concomitant use of other central nervous system depressants, such as opiods, may produce additive depressant effects. Hypoventilation, hypotension, profound sedation, and coma may occur. Therefore, use of concomitant CNS depressants requires individual adjustment of dosage of the concomitant medication and observation of a given patient). Products include:
Tussionex Pennkinetic Extended-Release Suspension...... 3154

Hydrocortisone (Co-administration with agents that induce CYP3A4 activity may cause increased clearance of fentanyl and reduce its efficacy).
No products indexed under this heading.

Hydrocortisone Acetate (Co-administration with agents that induce CYP3A4 activity may cause increased clearance of fentanyl and reduce its efficacy). Products include:
Analpram-HC 1140
Pramosone 1141

Hydrocortisone Butyrate (Co-administration with agents that induce CYP3A4 activity may cause increased clearance of fentanyl and reduce its efficacy).
No products indexed under this heading.

Hydrocortisone Cypionate (Co-administration with agents that induce CYP3A4 activity may cause increased clearance of fentanyl and reduce its efficacy).
No products indexed under this heading.

Hydrocortisone Hemisuccinate (Co-administration with agents that induce CYP3A4 activity may cause increased clearance of fentanyl and reduce its efficacy).
No products indexed under this heading.

Hydrocortisone Probutate (Co-administration with agents that induce CYP3A4 activity may cause increased clearance of fentanyl and reduce its efficacy).
No products indexed under this heading.

Hydrocortisone Sodium Phosphate (Co-administration with agents that induce CYP3A4 activity may cause increased clearance of fentanyl and reduce its efficacy).
No products indexed under this heading.

Hydrocortisone Sodium Succinate (Co-administration with agents that induce CYP3A4 activity may cause increased clearance of fentanyl and reduce its efficacy).
No products indexed under this heading.

Hydrocortisone Valerate (Co-administration with agents that induce CYP3A4 activity may cause increased clearance of fentanyl and reduce its efficacy).
No products indexed under this heading.

Hydromorphone Hydrochloride (The concomitant use of other central nervous system depressants, such as opiods, may produce additive depressant effects. Hypoventilation, hypotension, profound sedation, and coma may occur. Therefore, use of concomitant CNS depressants requires individual adjustment of dosage of the concomitant medication and observation of a given patient).
No products indexed under this heading.

Hydroxyzine Hydrochloride (The concomitant use of other central nervous system depressants, such as tranquilizers, may produce additive depressant effects. Hypoventilation, hypotension, profound sedation, and coma may occur. Therefore, use of concomitant CNS depressants requires individual adjustment of dosage of the concomitant medication and observation of a given patient).
No products indexed under this heading.

Hypericum (Co-administration with agents that induce CYP3A4 activity may cause increased clearance of fentanyl and reduce its efficacy). Products include:
Satieté Tablets .... ▣ 640

Hypericum Perforatum (Co-administration with agents that induce CYP3A4 activity may cause increased clearance of fentanyl and reduce its efficacy).
No products indexed under this heading.

Indinavir Sulfate (The concomitant use of fentanyl with CYP3A4 inhibitors may result in a decrease in fentanyl clearance, which could increase or prolong adverse drug effects including serious respiratory depression. In this situation, special patient care and observation is appropriate). Products include:
Crixivan Capsules 1979

Isoflurane (The concomitant use of other central nervous system depressants, such as general anesthetics, may produce additive depressant effects. Hypoventilation, hypotension, profound sedation, and coma may occur. Therefore, use of concomitant CNS depressants requires individual adjustment of dosage of the concomitant medication and observation of a given patient).
No products indexed under this heading.

Isoniazid (The concomitant use of fentanyl with CYP3A4 inhibitors may result in a decrease in fentanyl clearance, which could increase or prolong adverse drug effects including serious respiratory depression. In this situation, special patient care and observation is appropriate).
No products indexed under this heading.

Itraconazole (The concomitant use of fentanyl with CYP3A4 inhibitors may result in a decrease in fentanyl clearance, which could increase or prolong adverse drug effects including serious respiratory depression. In this situation, special patient care and observation is appropriate).
No products indexed under this heading.

Ketamine Hydrochloride (The concomitant use of other central nervous system depressants, such as general anesthetics, may produce additive depressant effects. Hypoventilation, hypotension, profound sedation, and coma may occur. Therefore, use of concomitant CNS depressants requires individual adjustment of dosage of the concomitant medication and observation of a given patient).
No products indexed under this heading.

Ketoconazole (The concomitant use of fentanyl with CYP3A4 inhibitors may result in a decrease in fentanyl clearance, which could increase or prolong adverse drug effects including serious respiratory depression. In this situation, special patient care and observation is appropriate). Products include:

Extina Foam, 2% 3057
Nizoral A-D Shampoo 1901

Levorphanol Tartrate (The concomitant use of other central nervous system depressants, such as opiods, may produce additive depressant effects. Hypoventilation, hypotension, profound sedation, and coma may occur. Therefore, use of concomitant CNS depressants requires individual adjustment of dosage of the concomitant medication and observation of a given patient).
No products indexed under this heading.

Lopinavir (The concomitant use of fentanyl with CYP3A4 inhibitors may result in a decrease in fentanyl clearance, which could increase or prolong adverse drug effects including serious respiratory depression. In this situation, special patient care and observation is appropriate). Products include:

Kaletra 452

Loratadine (The concomitant use of fentanyl with CYP3A4 inhibitors may result in a decrease in fentanyl clearance, which could increase or prolong adverse drug effects including serious respiratory depression. In this situation, special patient care and observation is appropriate).
No products indexed under this heading.

Lorazepam (The concomitant use of other central nervous system depressants, such as sedatives and hypnotics, may produce additive depressant effects. Hypoventilation, hypotension, profound sedation, and coma may occur. Therefore, use of concomitant CNS depressants requires individual adjustment of dosage of the concomitant medication and observation of a given patient).
No products indexed under this heading.

Loxapine Hydrochloride (The concomitant use of other central nervous system depressants, such as tranquilizers, may produce additive depressant effects. Hypoventilation, hypotension, profound sedation, and coma may occur. Therefore, use of concomitant CNS depressants requires individual adjustment of dosage of the concomitant medication and observation of a given patient).
No products indexed under this heading.

Loxapine Succinate (The concomitant use of other central nervous system depressants, such as tranquilizers, may produce additive depressant effects. Hypoventilation, hypotension, profound sedation, and coma may occur. Therefore, use of concomitant CNS depressants requires individual adjustment of dosage of the concomitant medication and observation of a given patient).
No products indexed under this heading.

Meperidine Hydrochloride (The concomitant use of other central nervous system depressants, such as opiods, may produce additive depressant effects. Hypoventilation, hypotension, profound sedation, and coma may occur. Therefore, use of concomitant CNS depressants requires individual adjustment of dosage of the concomitant medication and observation of a given patient).
No products indexed under this heading.

Mephenytoin (Co-administration with agents that induce CYP3A4 activity may cause increased clearance of fentanyl and reduce its efficacy).
No products indexed under this heading.

Meprobamate (The concomitant use of other central nervous system depressants, such as tranquilizers, may produce additive depressant effects. Hypoventilation, hypotension, profound sedation, and coma may occur. Therefore, use of concomitant CNS depressants requires individual adjustment of dosage of the concomitant medication and observation of a given patient).
No products indexed under this heading.

Mesoridazine Besylate (The concomitant use of other central nervous system depressants, such as phenothiazines, may produce additive depressant effects. Hypoventilation, hypotension, profound sedation, and coma may occur. Therefore, use of concomitant CNS depressants requires individual adjustment of dosage of the concomitant medication and observation of a given patient).
No products indexed under this heading.

Metaxalone (The concomitant use of other central nervous system depressants, such as skeletal muscle relaxants, may produce additive depressant effects. Hypoventilation, hypotension, profound sedation, and coma may occur. Therefore, use of concomitant CNS depressants requires individual adjustment of dosage of the concomitant medication and observation of a given patient). Products include:

Skelaxin Tablets 1784

Methadone Hydrochloride (The concomitant use of other central nervous system depressants, such as opiods, may produce additive depressant effects. Hypoventilation, hypotension, profound sedation, and coma may occur. Therefore, use of concomitant CNS depressants requires individual adjustment of dosage of the concomitant medication and observation of a given patient).
No products indexed under this heading.

Methdilazine Hydrochloride (The concomitant use of other central nervous system depressants, such as sedating antihistamines, may produce additive depressant effects. Hypoventilation, hypotension, profound sedation, and coma may occur. Therefore, use of concomitant CNS depressants requires individual adjustment of dosage of the concomitant medication and observation of a given patient).
No products indexed under this heading.

Methocarbamol (The concomitant use of other central nervous system depressants, such as skeletal muscle relaxants, may produce additive depressant effects. Hypoventilation, hypotension, profound sedation, and coma may occur. Therefore, use of concomitant CNS depressants requires individual adjustment of dosage of the concomitant medication and observation of a given patient).
No products indexed under this heading.

Methohexital Sodium (The concomitant use of other central nervous system depressants, such as general anesthetics, may produce additive depressant effects. Hypoventilation, hypotension, profound sedation, and coma may occur. Therefore, use of concomitant CNS depressants requires individual adjustment of dosage of the concomitant medication and observation of a given patient).
No products indexed under this heading.

Methotrimeprazine (The concomitant use of other central nervous system depressants, such as phenothiazines, may produce additive depressant effects. Hypoventilation, hypotension, profound sedation, and coma may occur. Therefore, use of concomitant CNS depressants requires individual adjustment of dosage of the concomitant medication and observation of a given patient).
No products indexed under this heading.

Methsuximide (Co-administration with agents that induce CYP3A4 activity may cause increased clearance of fentanyl and reduce its efficacy).
No products indexed under this heading.

Methylprednisolone (Co-administration with agents that induce CYP3A4 activity may cause increased clearance of fentanyl and reduce its efficacy).
No products indexed under this heading.

Methylprednisolone Acetate (Co-administration with agents that induce CYP3A4 activity may cause increased clearance of fentanyl and reduce its efficacy).
No products indexed under this heading.

Methylprednisolone Sodium Succinate (Co-administration with agents that induce CYP3A4 activity may cause increased clearance of fentanyl and reduce its efficacy).
No products indexed under this heading.

Metronidazole (The concomitant use of fentanyl with CYP3A4 inhibitors may result in a decrease in fentanyl clearance, which could increase or prolong adverse drug effects including serious respiratory depression. In this situation, special patient care and observation is appropriate). Products include:

Pylera Capsules 714

Metronidazole Benzoate (The concomitant use of fentanyl with CYP3A4 inhibitors may result in a decrease in fentanyl clearance, which could increase or prolong adverse drug effects including serious respiratory depression. In this situation, special patient care and observation is appropriate).
No products indexed under this heading.

Metronidazole Hydrochloride (The concomitant use of fentanyl with CYP3A4 inhibitors may result in a decrease in fentanyl clearance, which could increase or prolong adverse drug effects including serious respiratory depression. In this situation, special patient care and observation is appropriate).
No products indexed under this heading.

Metronidazole Sodium (The concomitant use of fentanyl with CYP3A4 inhibitors may result in a decrease in fentanyl clearance, which could increase or prolong adverse drug effects including serious respiratory depression. In this situation, special patient care and observation is appropriate).
No products indexed under this heading.

Miconazole (The concomitant use of fentanyl with CYP3A4 inhibitors may result in a decrease in fentanyl clearance, which could increase or prolong adverse drug effects including serious respiratory depression. In this situation, special patient care and observation is appropriate).
No products indexed under this heading.

Miconazole Nitrate (The concomitant use of fentanyl with CYP3A4 inhibitors may result in a decrease in fentanyl clearance, which could increase or prolong adverse drug effects including serious respiratory depression. In this situation, special patient care and observation is appropriate).
No products indexed under this heading.

Midazolam Hydrochloride (The concomitant use of other central nervous system depressants, such as sedatives and hypnotics, may produce additive depressant effects. Hypoventilation, hypotension, profound sedation, and coma may occur. Therefore, use of concomitant CNS depressants requires individual adjustment of dosage of the concomitant medication and observation of a given patient).
No products indexed under this heading.

Modafinil (Co-administration with agents that induce CYP3A4 activity may cause increased clearance of fentanyl and reduce its efficacy). Products include:

Provigil Tablets 977

Molindone Hydrochloride (The concomitant use of other central nervous system depressants, such as tranquilizers, may produce additive depressant effects. Hypoventilation, hypotension, profound sedation, and coma may occur. Therefore, use of concomitant CNS depressants requires individual adjustment of dosage of the concomitant medication and observation of a given patient). Products include:

Moban Tablets 1116

Morphine Sulfate (The concomitant use of other central nervous system depressants, such as opiods, may produce additive depressant effects. Hypoventilation, hypotension, profound sedation, and coma may occur. Therefore, use of concomitant CNS depressants requires individual adjustment of dosage of the concomitant medication and observation of a given patient). Products include:

Avinza Capsules 1772
DepoDur Injection 1095
MS Contin Tablets 2585

Nefazodone Hydrochloride (The concomitant use of fentanyl with CYP3A4 inhibitors may result in a decrease in fentanyl clearance, which could increase or prolong adverse drug effects including serious respiratory depression. In this situation, special patient care and observation is appropriate).

No products indexed under this heading.

Nelfinavir Mesylate (The concomitant use of fentanyl with CYP3A4 inhibitors may result in a decrease in fentanyl clearance, which could increase or prolong adverse drug effects including serious respiratory depression. In this situation, special patient care and observation is appropriate).

No products indexed under this heading.

Nevirapine (The concomitant use of fentanyl with CYP3A4 inhibitors may result in a decrease in fentanyl clearance, which could increase or prolong adverse drug effects including serious respiratory depression. In this situation, special patient care and observation is appropriate). Products include:

Viramune Oral Suspension 873
Viramune Tablets 873

Niacinamide (The concomitant use of fentanyl with CYP3A4 inhibitors may result in a decrease in fentanyl clearance, which could increase or prolong adverse drug effects including serious respiratory depression. In this situation, special patient care and observation is appropriate). Products include:

BioLean Free Tablets .... ▣635

Nicotinamide (The concomitant use of fentanyl with CYP3A4 inhibitors may result in a decrease in fentanyl clearance, which could increase or prolong adverse drug effects including serious respiratory depression. In this situation, special patient care and observation is appropriate).

No products indexed under this heading.

Nifedipine (The concomitant use of fentanyl with CYP3A4 inhibitors may result in a decrease in fentanyl clearance, which could increase or prolong adverse drug effects including serious respiratory depression. In this situation, special patient care and observation is appropriate).

No products indexed under this heading.

Norfloxacin (The concomitant use of fentanyl with CYP3A4 inhibitors may result in a decrease in fentanyl clearance, which could increase or prolong adverse drug effects including serious respiratory depression. In this situation, special patient care and observation is appropriate). Products include:

Noroxin Tablets 2069

Omeprazole (The concomitant use of fentanyl with CYP3A4 inhibitors may result in a decrease in fentanyl clearance, which could increase or prolong adverse drug effects including serious respiratory depression. In this situation, special patient care and observation is appropriate).

No products indexed under this heading.

Orphenadrine Citrate (The concomitant use of other central nervous system depressants, such as skeletal muscle relaxants, may produce additive depressant effects. Hypoventilation, hypotension, profound sedation, and coma may occur. Therefore, use of concomitant CNS depressants requires individual adjustment of dosage of the concomitant medication and observation of a given patient).

No products indexed under this heading.

Oxazepam (The concomitant use of other central nervous system depressants, such as tranquilizers, may produce additive depressant effects. Hypoventilation, hypotension, profound sedation, and coma may occur. Therefore, use of concomitant CNS depressants requires individual adjustment of dosage of the concomitant medication and observation of a given patient).

No products indexed under this heading.

Oxcarbazepine (Co-administration with agents that induce CYP3A4 activity may cause increased clearance of fentanyl and reduce its efficacy).

No products indexed under this heading.

Oxycodone Hydrochloride (The concomitant use of other central nervous system depressants, such as opiods, may produce additive depressant effects. Hypoventilation, hypotension, profound sedation, and coma may occur. Therefore, use of concomitant CNS depressants requires individual adjustment of dosage of the concomitant medication and observation of a given patient). Products include:

OxyContin Tablets 2589
OxyIR Capsules 2593
Percocet Tablets 1127
Percodan Tablets 1130

Paroxetine Hydrochloride (The concomitant use of fentanyl with CYP3A4 inhibitors may result in a decrease in fentanyl clearance, which could increase or prolong adverse drug effects including serious respiratory depression. In this situation, special patient care and observation is appropriate). Products include:

Paxil 1535
Paxil CR Controlled-Release Tablets 1544

Perphenazine (The concomitant use of other central nervous system depressants, such as phenothiazines, may produce additive depressant effects. Hypoventilation, hypotension, profound sedation, and coma may occur. Therefore, use of concomitant CNS depressants requires individual adjustment of dosage of the concomitant medication and observation of a given patient).

No products indexed under this heading.

Phenobarbital (Co-administration with agents that induce CYP3A4 activity may cause increased clearance of fentanyl and reduce its efficacy). Products include:

Donnatal Extentabs 2507

Phenobarbital Sodium (Co-administration with agents that induce CYP3A4 activity may cause increased clearance of fentanyl and reduce its efficacy).

No products indexed under this heading.

Phenytoin (Co-administration with agents that induce CYP3A4 activity may cause increased clearance of fentanyl and reduce its efficacy).

No products indexed under this heading.

Phenytoin Sodium (Co-administration with agents that induce CYP3A4 activity may cause increased clearance of fentanyl and reduce its efficacy). Products include:

Phenytek Capsules 2192

Prazepam (The concomitant use of other central nervous system depressants, such as tranquilizers, may produce additive depressant effects. Hypoventilation, hypotension, profound sedation, and coma may occur. Therefore, use of concomitant CNS depressants requires individual adjustment of dosage of the concomitant medication and observation of a given patient).

No products indexed under this heading.

Prednisolone Acetate (Co-administration with agents that induce CYP3A4 activity may cause increased clearance of fentanyl and reduce its efficacy). Products include:

Pred Forte Ophthalmic Suspension .... ⊙227
Pred Mild Ophthalmic Suspension .... ⊙230
Pred-G Ophthalmic Ointment .... ⊙229
Pred-G Ophthalmic Suspension .... ⊙228

Prednisolone Sodium Phosphate (Co-administration with agents that induce CYP3A4 activity may cause increased clearance of fentanyl and reduce its efficacy).

No products indexed under this heading.

Prednisolone Tebutate (Co-administration with agents that induce CYP3A4 activity may cause increased clearance of fentanyl and reduce its efficacy).

No products indexed under this heading.

Prednisone (Co-administration with agents that induce CYP3A4 activity may cause increased clearance of fentanyl and reduce its efficacy).

No products indexed under this heading.

Primidone (Co-administration with agents that induce CYP3A4 activity may cause increased clearance of fentanyl and reduce its efficacy).

No products indexed under this heading.

Prochlorperazine (The concomitant use of other central nervous system depressants, such as phenothiazines, may produce additive depressant effects. Hypoventilation, hypotension, profound sedation, and coma may occur. Therefore, use of concomitant CNS depressants requires individual adjustment of dosage of the concomitant medication and observation of a given patient).

No products indexed under this heading.

Promethazine Hydrochloride (The concomitant use of other central nervous system depressants, such as phenothiazines, may produce additive depressant effects. Hypoventilation, hypotension, profound sedation, and coma may occur. Therefore, use of concomitant CNS depressants requires individual adjustment of dosage of the concomitant medication and observation of a given patient).

No products indexed under this heading.

Propofol (The concomitant use of other central nervous system depressants, such as sedatives and hypnotics, may produce additive depressant effects. Hypoventilation, hypotension, profound sedation, and coma may occur. Therefore, use of concomitant CNS depressants requires individual adjustment of dosage of the concomitant medication and observation of a given patient).

No products indexed under this heading.

Propoxyphene Hydrochloride (The concomitant use of other central nervous system depressants, such as opiods, may produce additive depressant effects. Hypoventilation, hypotension, profound sedation, and coma may occur. Therefore, use of concomitant CNS depressants requires individual adjustment of dosage of the concomitant medication and observation of a given patient).

No products indexed under this heading.

Propoxyphene Napsylate (The concomitant use of other central nervous system depressants, such as opiods, may produce additive depressant effects. Hypoventilation, hypotension, profound sedation, and coma may occur. Therefore, use of concomitant CNS depressants requires individual adjustment of dosage of the concomitant medication and observation of a given patient).

No products indexed under this heading.

Pyrilamine Maleate (The concomitant use of other central nervous system depressants, such as sedating antihistamines, may produce additive depressant effects. Hypoventilation, hypotension, profound sedation, and coma may occur. Therefore, use of concomitant CNS depressants requires individual adjustment of dosage of the concomitant medication and observation of a given patient).

No products indexed under this heading.

Pyrilamine Tannate (The concomitant use of other central nervous system depressants, such as sedating antihistamines, may produce additive depressant effects. Hypoventilation, hypotension, profound sedation, and coma may occur. Therefore, use of concomitant CNS depressants requires individual adjustment of dosage of the concomitant medication and observation of a given patient).

No products indexed under this heading.

Quazepam (The concomitant use of other central nervous system depressants, such as sedatives and hypnotics, may produce additive depressant effects. Hypoventilation, hypotension, profound sedation, and coma may occur. Therefore, use of concomitant CNS depressants requires individual adjustment of dosage of the concomitant medication and observation of a given patient).
No products indexed under this heading.

Quinidine (The concomitant use of fentanyl with CYP3A4 inhibitors may result in a decrease in fentanyl clearance, which could increase or prolong adverse drug effects including serious respiratory depression. In this situation, special patient care and observation is appropriate).
No products indexed under this heading.

Quinidine Hydrochloride (The concomitant use of fentanyl with CYP3A4 inhibitors may result in a decrease in fentanyl clearance, which could increase or prolong adverse drug effects including serious respiratory depression. In this situation, special patient care and observation is appropriate).
No products indexed under this heading.

Quinidine Polygalacturonate (The concomitant use of fentanyl with CYP3A4 inhibitors may result in a decrease in fentanyl clearance, which could increase or prolong adverse drug effects including serious respiratory depression. In this situation, special patient care and observation is appropriate).
No products indexed under this heading.

Quinidine Sulfate (The concomitant use of fentanyl with CYP3A4 inhibitors may result in a decrease in fentanyl clearance, which could increase or prolong adverse drug effects including serious respiratory depression. In this situation, special patient care and observation is appropriate).
No products indexed under this heading.

Quinine (The concomitant use of fentanyl with CYP3A4 inhibitors may result in a decrease in fentanyl clearance, which could increase or prolong adverse drug effects including serious respiratory depression. In this situation, special patient care and observation is appropriate).
No products indexed under this heading.

Quinine Sulfate (The concomitant use of fentanyl with CYP3A4 inhibitors may result in a decrease in fentanyl clearance, which could increase or prolong adverse drug effects including serious respiratory depression. In this situation, special patient care and observation is appropriate).
No products indexed under this heading.

Quinupristin (The concomitant use of fentanyl with CYP3A4 inhibitors may result in a decrease in fentanyl clearance, which could increase or prolong adverse drug effects including serious respiratory depression. In this situation, special patient care and observation is appropriate).
No products indexed under this heading.

Ramelteon (The concomitant use of other central nervous system depressants, such as sedatives and hypnotics, may produce additive depressant effects. Hypoventilation, hypotension, profound sedation, and coma may occur. Therefore, use of concomitant CNS depressants requires individual adjustment of dosage of the concomitant medication and observation of a given patient). Products include:
Rozerem Tablets 3091

Ranitidine Bismuth Citrate (The concomitant use of fentanyl with CYP3A4 inhibitors may result in a decrease in fentanyl clearance, which could increase or prolong adverse drug effects including serious respiratory depression. In this situation, special patient care and observation is appropriate).
No products indexed under this heading.

Ranitidine Hydrochloride (The concomitant use of fentanyl with CYP3A4 inhibitors may result in a decrease in fentanyl clearance, which could increase or prolong adverse drug effects including serious respiratory depression. In this situation, special patient care and observation is appropriate).
Products include:
Zantac 75 Tablets 603
Zantac 1670
Zantac Injection 1666
Zantac Injection Pharmacy Bulk Package 1668
Maximum Strength Zantac 150 Tablets 603
Maximum Strength Zantac 150 Cool Mint Tablets 603

Remifentanil Hydrochloride (The concomitant use of other central nervous system depressants, such as opiods, may produce additive depressant effects. Hypoventilation, hypotension, profound sedation, and coma may occur. Therefore, use of concomitant CNS depressants requires individual adjustment of dosage of the concomitant medication and observation of a given patient).
No products indexed under this heading.

Rifabutin (Co-administration with agents that induce CYP3A4 activity may cause increased clearance of fentanyl and reduce its efficacy).
No products indexed under this heading.

Rifampicin (Co-administration with agents that induce CYP3A4 activity may cause increased clearance of fentanyl and reduce its efficacy).
No products indexed under this heading.

Rifampin (Co-administration with agents that induce CYP3A4 activity may cause increased clearance of fentanyl and reduce its efficacy).
No products indexed under this heading.

Rifapentine (Co-administration with agents that induce CYP3A4 activity may cause increased clearance of fentanyl and reduce its efficacy).
No products indexed under this heading.

Ritonavir (The concomitant use of fentanyl with CYP3A4 inhibitors may result in a decrease in fentanyl clearance, which could increase or prolong adverse drug effects including serious respiratory depression. In this situation, special patient care and observation is appropriate).
Products include:
Kaletra 452
Norvir 489

Saquinavir (The concomitant use of fentanyl with CYP3A4 inhibitors may result in a decrease in fentanyl clearance, which could increase or prolong adverse drug effects including serious respiratory depression. In this situation, special patient care and observation is appropriate).
No products indexed under this heading.

Saquinavir Mesylate (The concomitant use of fentanyl with CYP3A4 inhibitors may result in a decrease in fentanyl clearance, which could increase or prolong adverse drug effects including serious respiratory depression. In this situation, special patient care and observation is appropriate).
No products indexed under this heading.

Secobarbital Sodium (The concomitant use of other central nervous system depressants, such as sedatives and hypnotics, may produce additive depressant effects. Hypoventilation, hypotension, profound sedation, and coma may occur. Therefore, use of concomitant CNS depressants requires individual adjustment of dosage of the concomitant medication and observation of a given patient).
No products indexed under this heading.

Sertraline Hydrochloride (The concomitant use of fentanyl with CYP3A4 inhibitors may result in a decrease in fentanyl clearance, which could increase or prolong adverse drug effects including serious respiratory depression. In this situation, special patient care and observation is appropriate).
No products indexed under this heading.

Sildenafil Citrate (The concomitant use of fentanyl with CYP3A4 inhibitors may result in a decrease in fentanyl clearance, which could increase or prolong adverse drug effects including serious respiratory depression. In this situation, special patient care and observation is appropriate).
No products indexed under this heading.

Sodium Butabarbital (The concomitant use of other central nervous system depressants, such as sedatives and hypnotics, may produce additive depressant effects. Hypoventilation, hypotension, profound sedation, and coma may occur. Therefore, use of concomitant CNS depressants requires individual adjustment of dosage of the concomitant medication and observation of a given patient).
No products indexed under this heading.

Sufentanil Citrate (The concomitant use of other central nervous system depressants, such as opiods, may produce additive depressant effects. Hypoventilation, hypotension, profound sedation, and coma may occur. Therefore, use of concomitant CNS depressants requires individual adjustment of dosage of the concomitant medication and observation of a given patient).
No products indexed under this heading.

Sulfinpyrazone (Co-administration with agents that induce CYP3A4 activity may cause increased clearance of fentanyl and reduce its efficacy).
No products indexed under this heading.

Telithromycin (The concomitant use of fentanyl with CYP3A4 inhibitors may result in a decrease in fentanyl clearance, which could increase or prolong adverse drug effects including serious respiratory depression. In this situation, special patient care and observation is appropriate). Products include:
Ketek Tablets 2744

Temazepam (The concomitant use of other central nervous system depressants, such as sedatives and hypnotics, may produce additive depressant effects. Hypoventilation, hypotension, profound sedation, and coma may occur. Therefore, use of concomitant CNS depressants requires individual adjustment of dosage of the concomitant medication and observation of a given patient).
No products indexed under this heading.

Theophylline (Co-administration with agents that induce CYP3A4 activity may cause increased clearance of fentanyl and reduce its efficacy).
No products indexed under this heading.

Theophylline Anhydrous (Co-administration with agents that induce CYP3A4 activity may cause increased clearance of fentanyl and reduce its efficacy). Products include:
Uniphyl Tablets 2595

Theophylline Calcium Salicylate (Co-administration with agents that induce CYP3A4 activity may cause increased clearance of fentanyl and reduce its efficacy).
No products indexed under this heading.

Theophylline Dihydroxypropyl (Glyceryl) (Co-administration with agents that induce CYP3A4 activity may cause increased clearance of fentanyl and reduce its efficacy).
No products indexed under this heading.

Theophylline Ethylenediamine (Co-administration with agents that induce CYP3A4 activity may cause increased clearance of fentanyl and reduce its efficacy).
No products indexed under this heading.

Thiamylal Sodium (The concomitant use of other central nervous system depressants, such as general anesthetics, may produce additive depressant effects. Hypoventilation, hypotension, profound sedation, and coma may occur. Therefore, use of concomitant CNS depressants requires individual adjustment of dosage of the concomitant medication and observation of a given patient).
No products indexed under this heading.

Thioridazine Hydrochloride (The concomitant use of other central nervous system depressants, such as phenothiazines, may produce additive depressant effects. Hypoventilation, hypotension, profound sedation, and coma may occur. Therefore, use of concomitant CNS depressants requires individual

adjustment of dosage of the concomitant medication and observation of a given patient). Products include:
Thioridazine Hydrochloride Tablets 2195

Thiothixene (The concomitant use of other central nervous system depressants, such as tranquilizers, may produce additive depressant effects. Hypoventilation, hypotension, profound sedation, and coma may occur. Therefore, use of concomitant CNS depressants requires individual adjustment of dosage of the concomitant medication and observation of a given patient). Products include:
Thiothixene Capsules 2197

Triamcinolone (Co-administration with agents that induce CYP3A4 activity may cause increased clearance of fentanyl and reduce its efficacy).
No products indexed under this heading.

Triamcinolone Acetonide (Co-administration with agents that induce CYP3A4 activity may cause increased clearance of fentanyl and reduce its efficacy). Products include:
Azmacort Inhalation Aerosol 407
Nasacort AQ Nasal Spray 2765
Triesence Injectable Suspension .... ⊙209

Triamcinolone Diacetate (Co-administration with agents that induce CYP3A4 activity may cause increased clearance of fentanyl and reduce its efficacy).
No products indexed under this heading.

Triamcinolone Hexacetonide (Co-administration with agents that induce CYP3A4 activity may cause increased clearance of fentanyl and reduce its efficacy).
No products indexed under this heading.

Triazolam (The concomitant use of other central nervous system depressants, such as sedatives and hypnotics, may produce additive depressant effects. Hypoventilation, hypotension, profound sedation, and coma may occur. Therefore, use of concomitant CNS depressants requires individual adjustment of dosage of the concomitant medication and observation of a given patient).
No products indexed under this heading.

Trifluoperazine Hydrochloride (The concomitant use of other central nervous system depressants, such as phenothiazines, may produce additive depressant effects. Hypoventilation, hypotension, profound sedation, and coma may occur. Therefore, use of concomitant CNS depressants requires individual adjustment of dosage of the concomitant medication and observation of a given patient).
No products indexed under this heading.

Trimeprazine Tartrate (The concomitant use of other central nervous system depressants, such as sedating antihistamines, may produce additive depressant effects. Hypoventilation, hypotension, profound sedation, and coma may occur. Therefore, use of concomitant CNS depressants requires individual adjustment of dosage of the concomitant medication and observation of a given patient).
No products indexed under this heading.

Tripelennamine Hydrochloride (The concomitant use of other central nervous system depressants, such as sedating antihistamines, may produce additive depressant effects. Hypoventilation, hypotension, profound sedation, and coma may occur. Therefore, use of concomitant CNS depressants requires individual adjustment of dosage of the concomitant medication and observation of a given patient).
No products indexed under this heading.

Triprolidine Hydrochloride (The concomitant use of other central nervous system depressants, such as sedating antihistamines, may produce additive depressant effects. Hypoventilation, hypotension, profound sedation, and coma may occur. Therefore, use of concomitant CNS depressants requires individual adjustment of dosage of the concomitant medication and observation of a given patient).
No products indexed under this heading.

Troglitazone (The concomitant use of fentanyl with CYP3A4 inhibitors may result in a decrease in fentanyl clearance, which could increase or prolong adverse drug effects including serious respiratory depression. In this situation, special patient care and observation is appropriate).
No products indexed under this heading.

Troleandomycin (The concomitant use of fentanyl with CYP3A4 inhibitors may result in a decrease in fentanyl clearance, which could increase or prolong adverse drug effects including serious respiratory depression. In this situation, special patient care and observation is appropriate).
No products indexed under this heading.

Valproate Sodium (The concomitant use of fentanyl with CYP3A4 inhibitors may result in a decrease in fentanyl clearance, which could increase or prolong adverse drug effects including serious respiratory depression. In this situation, special patient care and observation is appropriate).
No products indexed under this heading.

Vardenafil Hydrochloride (The concomitant use of fentanyl with CYP3A4 inhibitors may result in a decrease in fentanyl clearance, which could increase or prolong adverse drug effects including serious respiratory depression. In this situation, special patient care and observation is appropriate). Products include:
Levitra Tablets 2876

Verapamil Hydrochloride (The concomitant use of fentanyl with CYP3A4 inhibitors may result in a decrease in fentanyl clearance, which could increase or prolong adverse drug effects including serious respiratory depression. In this situation, special patient care and observation is appropriate). Products include:
Tarka Tablets 511

Voriconazole (The concomitant use of fentanyl with CYP3A4 inhibitors may result in a decrease in fentanyl clearance, which could increase or prolong adverse drug effects including serious respiratory depression. In this situation, special patient care and observation is appropriate).
No products indexed under this heading.

Zafirlukast (The concomitant use of fentanyl with CYP3A4 inhibitors may result in a decrease in fentanyl clearance, which could increase or prolong adverse drug effects including serious respiratory depression. In this situation, special patient care and observation is appropriate). Products include:
Accolate Tablets 669

Zaleplon (The concomitant use of other central nervous system depressants, such as sedatives and hypnotics, may produce additive depressant effects. Hypoventilation, hypotension, profound sedation, and coma may occur. Therefore, use of concomitant CNS depressants requires individual adjustment of dosage of the concomitant medication and observation of a given patient).
No products indexed under this heading.

Zileuton (The concomitant use of fentanyl with CYP3A4 inhibitors may result in a decrease in fentanyl clearance, which could increase or prolong adverse drug effects including serious respiratory depression. In this situation, special patient care and observation is appropriate).
No products indexed under this heading.

Zolpidem Tartrate (The concomitant use of other central nervous system depressants, such as sedatives and hypnotics, may produce additive depressant effects. Hypoventilation, hypotension, profound sedation, and coma may occur. Therefore, use of concomitant CNS depressants requires individual adjustment of dosage of the concomitant medication and observation of a given patient). Products include:
Ambien Tablets 2692
Ambien CR Tablets 2696

Food Interactions

Alcohol (The concomitant use of other central nervous system depressants, such as alcoholic beverages, may produce additive depressant effects. Hypoventilation, hypotension, profound sedation, and coma may occur. Therefore, use of concomitant CNS depressants requires individual adjustment of dosage of the concomitant medication and observation of a given patient).

Grapefruit (The concomitant use of fentanyl with CYP3A4 inhibitors may result in a decrease in fentanyl clearance, which could increase or prolong adverse drug effects including serious respiratory depression. In this situation, special patient care and observation is appropriate).

Grapefruit Juice (The concomitant use of fentanyl with CYP3A4 inhibitors may result in a decrease in fentanyl clearance, which could increase or prolong adverse drug effects including serious respiratory depression. In this situation, special patient care and observation is appropriate).

IQUIX OPHTHALMIC SOLUTION

(Levofloxacin) 3183
May interact with xanthines and certain other agents. Compounds in these categories include:

Aminophylline (Systemic administration of some quinolones has been shown to elevate plasma concentrations of theophylline).
No products indexed under this heading.

Caffeine (Systemic administration of some quinolones has been shown to interfere with the metabolism of caffeine). Products include:
BioLean Free Tablets .... ▣635
BioLean II Tablets .... ▣635
Winrgy Dietary Supplement .... ▣642

Caffeine Anhydrous (Systemic administration of some quinolones has been shown to interfere with the metabolism of caffeine).
No products indexed under this heading.

Caffeine Citrate (Systemic administration of some quinolones has been shown to interfere with the metabolism of caffeine).
No products indexed under this heading.

Caffeine-containing medications (Systemic administration of some quinolones has been shown to interfere with the metabolism of caffeine).
No products indexed under this heading.

Caffeine Sodium Benzoate (Systemic administration of some quinolones has been shown to interfere with the metabolism of caffeine).
No products indexed under this heading.

Cyclosporine (Systemic administration of some quinolones has been associated with transient elevations in serum creatinine in patients receiving systemic cyclosporine concomitantly). Products include:
Gengraf Capsules 435
Neoral Oral Solution 2280
Neoral Soft Gelatin Capsules 2280
Restasis Ophthalmic Emulsion 557
Sandimmune 2296

Dyphylline (Systemic administration of some quinolones has been shown to elevate plasma concentrations of theophylline).
No products indexed under this heading.

Theophylline (Systemic administration of some quinolones has been shown to elevate plasma concentrations of theophylline).
No products indexed under this heading.

Theophylline Anhydrous (Systemic administration of some quinolones has been shown to elevate plasma concentrations of theophylline). Products include:
Uniphyl Tablets 2595

Theophylline Calcium Salicylate (Systemic administration of some quinolones has been shown to elevate plasma concentrations of theophylline).
No products indexed under this heading.

Theophylline Dihydroxypropyl (Glyceryl) (Systemic administration of some quinolones has been shown to elevate plasma concentrations of theophylline).

No products indexed under this heading.

Theophylline Ethylenediamine (Systemic administration of some quinolones has been shown to elevate plasma concentrations of theophylline).

No products indexed under this heading.

Theophylline Sodium Glycinate (Systemic administration of some quinolones has been shown to elevate plasma concentrations of theophylline).

No products indexed under this heading.

Warfarin Sodium (Systemic administration of some quinolones has been shown to enhance the effects of warfarin).

No products indexed under this heading.

Food Interactions

Beverages, caffeine-containing (Systemic administration of some quinolones has been shown to interfere with the metabolism of caffeine).

Food, caffeine-containing (Systemic administration of some quinolones has been shown to interfere with the metabolism of caffeine).

ISENTRESS TABLETS

(Raltegravir) 2036

May interact with HMG-CoA reductase inhibitors and certain other agents. Compounds in these categories include:

Atazanavir (Co-administration of raltegravir with other drugs that inhibit UGT1A1 may increase plasma levels of raltegravir. However, studies have shown that concomitant use of raltegravir and atazanavir/ritonavir did not result in a unique safety signal. Based on these data, atazanavir/ritonavir may be co-administered with raltegravir without dose adjustments of raltegravir).

No products indexed under this heading.

Atazanavir Sulfate (Co-administration of raltegravir with other drugs that inhibit UGT1A1 may increase plasma levels of raltegravir. However, studies have shown that concomitant use of raltegravir and atazanavir/ritonavir did not result in a unique safety signal. Based on these data, atazanavir/ritonavir may be co-administered with raltegravir without dose adjustments of raltegravir). Products include:

Reyataz Capsules 3299

Atorvastatin Calcium (Use with caution in patients at increased risk of myopathy or rhabdomyolysis, such as patients receiving concomitant medications known to cause these conditions). Products include:

Lipitor Tablets 2501

Cerivastatin Sodium (Use with caution in patients at increased risk of myopathy or rhabdomyolysis, such as patients receiving concomitant medications known to cause these conditions).

No products indexed under this heading.

Fluvastatin Sodium (Use with caution in patients at increased risk of myopathy or rhabdomyolysis, such as patients receiving concomitant medications known to cause these conditions). Products include:

Lescol Capsules 2268
Lescol XL Tablets 2268

Lovastatin (Use with caution in patients at increased risk of myopathy or rhabdomyolysis, such as patients receiving concomitant medications known to cause these conditions). Products include:

Advicor Tablets 402
Mevacor Tablets 2063

Pravastatin Sodium (Use with caution in patients at increased risk of myopathy or rhabdomyolysis, such as patients receiving concomitant medications known to cause these conditions).

No products indexed under this heading.

Rifampin (Rifampin, a strong inducer of UGT1A1, reduces plasma concentrations of raltegravir. Therefore, caution should be used when co-administering raltegravir with rifampin or other strong inducers of UGT1A1).

No products indexed under this heading.

Rosuvastatin Calcium (Use with caution in patients at increased risk of myopathy or rhabdomyolysis, such as patients receiving concomitant medications known to cause these conditions). Products include:

Crestor Tablets 677

Simvastatin (Use with caution in patients at increased risk of myopathy or rhabdomyolysis, such as patients receiving concomitant medications known to cause these conditions). Products include:

Simcor Tablets 502
Vytorin 10/10 Tablets 2149
Vytorin 10/10 Tablets 2939
Vytorin 10/20 Tablets 2149
Vytorin 10/20 Tablets 2939
Vytorin 10/40 Tablets 2149
Vytorin 10/40 Tablets 2939
Vytorin 10/80 Tablets 2149
Vytorin 10/80 Tablets 2939
Zocor Tablets 2136

Tenofovir Disoproxil Fumarate (Co-administration of raltegravir with other drugs that inhibit UGT1A1 may increase plasma levels of raltegravir). Products include:

Atripla Tablets 938
Truvada Tablets 1262
Viread Tablets 1268

IVY BLOCK

(Bentoquatam) 621

None cited in PDR database.

IXEMPRA KIT FOR INJECTION

(Ixabepilone) 915

May interact with cytochrome p450 3a4 inducers (selected), cytochrome p450 3a4 inhibitors (selected), cytochrome p450 3a4 inhibitors, potent, and certain other agents. Compounds in these categories include:

Acetazolamide (The effect of mild or moderate CYP3A4 inhibitors (e.g., erythromycin, fluconazole, or verapamil) on exposure to ixabepilone has not been studied. Therefore, caution should be used when administering mild or moderate CYP3A4 inhibitors during treatment with ixabepilone, and alternative therapeutic agents that do not inhibit CYP3A4 should be considered. Patients receiving CYP3A4 inhibitors during treatment with ixabepilone should be monitored closely for acute toxicities (e.g., frequent monitoring of peripheral blood counts between cycles of ixabepilone)).

No products indexed under this heading.

Allium sativum (Ixabepiloneis a CYP3A4 substrate. Strong CYP3A4 inducers (e.g., dexamethasone, phenytoin, carbamazepine, rifampin, rifampicin, rifabutin, and phenobarbital) may decrease ixabepilone concentrations leading to subtherapeutic levels. Therefore, therapeutic agents with low enzyme induction potential should be considered for co-administration with ixabepilone).

No products indexed under this heading.

Amiodarone Hydrochloride (The effect of mild or moderate CYP3A4 inhibitors (e.g., erythromycin, fluconazole, or verapamil) on exposure to ixabepilone has not been studied. Therefore, caution should be used when administering mild or moderate CYP3A4 inhibitors during treatment with ixabepilone, and alternative therapeutic agents that do not inhibit CYP3A4 should be considered. Patients receiving CYP3A4 inhibitors during treatment with ixabepilone should be monitored closely for acute toxicities (e.g., frequent monitoring of peripheral blood counts between cycles of ixabepilone)).

No products indexed under this heading.

Amprenavir (The use of concomitant strong CYP3A4 inhibitors should be avoided (e.g., ketocnazole, itraconazole, clarithromycin, atazanavir, nefazodone, saquinavir, telithromycin, ritonavir, amprenavir, indinavir, nelfinavir, delavirdine, or voriconazole). Based on pharmacokinetic studies, if a strong CYP3A4 inhibitor must be co-administered, a dose reduction to 20 mg/m^2 is predicted to adjust the ixabepilone AUC to the range observed without inhibitors and should be considered. If the strong inhibitor is discontinued, a washout period of approximately 1 week should be allowed before the ixabepilone dose is adjusted upward to the indicated dose).

No products indexed under this heading.

Anastrozole (The effect of mild or moderate CYP3A4 inhibitors (e.g., erythromycin, fluconazole, or verapamil) on exposure to ixabepilone has not been studied. Therefore, caution should be used when administering mild or moderate CYP3A4 inhibitors during treatment with ixabepilone, and alternative therapeutic agents that do not inhibit CYP3A4 should be considered. Patients receiving CYP3A4 inhibitors during treatment with ixabepilone should be monitored closely for acute toxicities (e.g., frequent monitoring of peripheral blood counts between cycles of ixabepilone)). Products include:

Arimidex Tablets 672

Aprepitant (The effect of mild or moderate CYP3A4 inhibitors (e.g., erythromycin, fluconazole, or verapamil) on exposure to ixabepilone has not been studied. Therefore, caution should be used when administering mild or moderate CYP3A4 inhibitors during treatment with ixabepilone, and alternative therapeutic agents that do not inhibit CYP3A4 should be considered. Patients receiving CYP3A4 inhibitors during treatment with ixabepilone should be monitored closely for acute toxicities (e.g., frequent monitoring of peripheral blood counts between cycles of ixabepilone)). Products include:

Emend Capsules 1992

Atazanavir (The use of concomitant strong CYP3A4 inhibitors should be avoided (e.g., ketocnazole, itraconazole, clarithromycin, atazanavir, nefazodone, saquinavir, telithromycin, ritonavir, amprenavir, indinavir, nelfinavir, delavirdine, or voriconazole). Based on pharmacokinetic studies, if a strong CYP3A4 inhibitor must be co-administered, a dose reduction to 20 mg/m^2 is predicted to adjust the ixabepilone AUC to the range observed without inhibitors and should be considered. If the strong inhibitor is discontinued, a washout period of approximately 1 week should be allowed before the ixabepilone dose is adjusted upward to the indicated dose).

No products indexed under this heading.

Atazanavir Sulfate (The use of concomitant strong CYP3A4 inhibitors should be avoided (e.g., ketocnazole, itraconazole, clarithromycin, atazanavir, nefazodone, saquinavir, telithromycin, ritonavir, amprenavir, indinavir, nelfinavir, delavirdine, or voriconazole). Based on pharmacokinetic studies, if a strong CYP3A4 inhibitor must be co-administered, a dose reduction to 20 mg/m^2 is predicted to adjust the ixabepilone AUC to the range observed without inhibitors and should be considered. If the strong inhibitor is discontinued, a washout period of approximately 1 week should be allowed before the ixabepilone dose is adjusted upward to the indicated dose). Products include:

Reyataz Capsules 3299

Betamethasone Acetate (Ixabepiloneis a CYP3A4 substrate. Strong CYP3A4 inducers (e.g., dexamethasone, phenytoin, carbamazepine, rifampin, rifampicin, rifabutin, and phenobarbital) may decrease ixabepilone concentrations leading to subtherapeutic levels. Therefore, therapeutic agents with low enzyme induction potential should be considered for co-administration with ixabepilone).

No products indexed under this heading.

Betamethasone Sodium Phosphate (Ixabepiloneis a CYP3A4 substrate. Strong CYP3A4 inducers (e.g., dexamethasone, phenytoin, carbamazepine, rifampin, rifampicin, rifabutin, and phenobarbital) may decrease ixabepilone concentrations leading to subtherapeutic levels. Therefore, therapeutic agents with low enzyme induction potential should be considered for co-administration with ixabepilone).

No products indexed under this heading.

Carbamazepine (Ixabepiloneis a CYP3A4 substrate. Strong CYP3A4 inducers (e.g., dexamethasone, phenytoin, carbamazepine, rifampin, rifampicin, rifabutin, and phenobarbital) may decrease ixabepilone concentrations leading to subtherapeutic levels. Therefore, therapeutic

erythromycin, fluconazole, or verapamil) on exposure to ixabepilone has not been studied. Therefore, caution should be used when administering mild or moderate CYP3A4 inhibitors during treatment with ixabepilone, and alternative therapeutic agents that do not inhibit CYP3A4 should be considered. Patients receiving CYP3A4 inhibitors during treatment with ixabepilone should be monitored closely for acute toxicities (e.g., frequent monitoring of peripheral blood counts between cycles of ixabepilone)). Products include:

Atripla Tablets **938**
Sustiva Capsules **930**
Sustiva Tablets **930**

Erythromycin (The effect of mild or moderate CYP3A4 inhibitors (e.g., erythromycin, fluconazole, or verapamil) on exposure to ixabepilone has not been studied. Therefore, caution should be used when administering mild or moderate CYP3A4 inhibitors during treatment with ixabepilone, and alternative therapeutic agents that do not inhibit CYP3A4 should be considered. Patients receiving CYP3A4 inhibitors during treatment with ixabepilone should be monitored closely for acute toxicities (e.g., frequent monitoring of peripheral blood counts between cycles of ixabepilone)).

No products indexed under this heading.

Erythromycin Estolate (The effect of mild or moderate CYP3A4 inhibitors (e.g., erythromycin, fluconazole, or verapamil) on exposure to ixabepilone has not been studied. Therefore, caution should be used when administering mild or moderate CYP3A4 inhibitors during treatment with ixabepilone, and alternative therapeutic agents that do not inhibit CYP3A4 should be considered. Patients receiving CYP3A4 inhibitors during treatment with ixabepilone should be monitored closely for acute toxicities (e.g., frequent monitoring of peripheral blood counts between cycles of ixabepilone)).

No products indexed under this heading.

Erythromycin Ethylsuccinate (The effect of mild or moderate CYP3A4 inhibitors (e.g., erythromycin, fluconazole, or verapamil) on exposure to ixabepilone has not been studied. Therefore, caution should be used when administering mild or moderate CYP3A4 inhibitors during treatment with ixabepilone, and alternative therapeutic agents that do not inhibit CYP3A4 should be considered. Patients receiving CYP3A4 inhibitors during treatment with ixabepilone should be monitored closely for acute toxicities (e.g., frequent monitoring of peripheral blood counts between cycles of ixabepilone)). Products include:

E.E.S. **433**
EryPed **431**

Erythromycin Gluceptate (The effect of mild or moderate CYP3A4 inhibitors (e.g., erythromycin, fluconazole, or verapamil) on exposure to ixabepilone has not been studied. Therefore, caution should be used when administering mild or moderate CYP3A4 inhibitors during treatment with ixabepilone, and alternative therapeutic agents that do not inhibit CYP3A4 should be considered. Patients receiving CYP3A4 inhibitors during treatment with ixabepilone should be monitored closely for acute toxicities (e.g., frequent monitoring of peripheral blood counts between cycles of ixabepilone)).

No products indexed under this heading.

Erythromycin Lactobionate (The effect of mild or moderate CYP3A4 inhibitors (e.g., erythromycin, fluconazole, or verapamil) on exposure to ixabepilone has not been studied. Therefore, caution should be used when administering mild or moderate CYP3A4 inhibitors during treatment with ixabepilone, and alternative therapeutic agents that do not inhibit CYP3A4 should be considered. Patients receiving CYP3A4 inhibitors during treatment with ixabepilone should be monitored closely for acute toxicities (e.g., frequent monitoring of peripheral blood counts between cycles of ixabepilone)).

No products indexed under this heading.

Erythromycin Stearate (The effect of mild or moderate CYP3A4 inhibitors (e.g., erythromycin, fluconazole, or verapamil) on exposure to ixabepilone has not been studied. Therefore, caution should be used when administering mild or moderate CYP3A4 inhibitors during treatment with ixabepilone, and alternative therapeutic agents that do not inhibit CYP3A4 should be considered. Patients receiving CYP3A4 inhibitors during treatment with ixabepilone should be monitored closely for acute toxicities (e.g., frequent monitoring of peripheral blood counts between cycles of ixabepilone)).

No products indexed under this heading.

Esomeprazole Magnesium (The effect of mild or moderate CYP3A4 inhibitors (e.g., erythromycin, fluconazole, or verapamil) on exposure to ixabepilone has not been studied. Therefore, caution should be used when administering mild or moderate CYP3A4 inhibitors during treatment with ixabepilone, and alternative therapeutic agents that do not inhibit CYP3A4 should be considered. Patients receiving CYP3A4 inhibitors during treatment with ixabepilone should be monitored closely for acute toxicities (e.g., frequent monitoring of peripheral blood counts between cycles of ixabepilone)). Products include:

Nexium Delayed-Release Capsules **645**
Nexium Delayed-Release Oral Suspension................................. **645**

Ethosuximide (Ixabepiloneis a CYP3A4 substrate. Strong CYP3A4 inducers (e.g., dexamethasone, phenytoin, carbamazepine, rifampin, rifampicin, rifabutin, and phenobarbital) may decrease ixabepilone concentrations leading to subtherapeutic levels. Therefore, therapeutic agents with low enzyme induction potential should be considered for co-administration with ixabepilone).

No products indexed under this heading.

Felbamate (Ixabepiloneis a CYP3A4 substrate. Strong CYP3A4 inducers (e.g., dexamethasone, phenytoin, carbamazepine, rifampin, rifampicin, rifabutin, and phenobarbital) may decrease ixabepilone concentrations leading to subtherapeutic levels. Therefore, therapeutic agents with low enzyme induction potential should be considered for co-administration with ixabepilone).

No products indexed under this heading.

Fluconazole (The effect of mild or moderate CYP3A4 inhibitors (e.g., erythromycin, fluconazole, or verapamil) on exposure to ixabepilone has not been studied. Therefore, caution should be used when administering mild or moderate CYP3A4 inhibitors during treatment with ixabepilone, and alternative therapeutic agents that do not inhibit CYP3A4 should be considered. Patients receiving CYP3A4 inhibitors during treatment with ixabepilone should be monitored closely for acute toxicities (e.g., frequent monitoring of peripheral blood counts between cycles of ixabepilone)).

No products indexed under this heading.

Fludrocortisone Acetate (Ixabepiloneis a CYP3A4 substrate. Strong CYP3A4 inducers (e.g., dexamethasone, phenytoin, carbamazepine, rifampin, rifampicin, rifabutin, and phenobarbital) may decrease ixabepilone concentrations leading to subtherapeutic levels. Therefore, therapeutic agents with low enzyme induction potential should be considered for co-administration with ixabepilone).

No products indexed under this heading.

Fluoxetine (The effect of mild or moderate CYP3A4 inhibitors (e.g., erythromycin, fluconazole, or verapamil) on exposure to ixabepilone has not been studied. Therefore, caution should be used when administering mild or moderate CYP3A4 inhibitors during treatment with ixabepilone, and alternative therapeutic agents that do not inhibit CYP3A4 should be considered. Patients receiving CYP3A4 inhibitors during treatment with ixabepilone should be monitored closely for acute toxicities (e.g., frequent monitoring of peripheral blood counts between cycles of ixabepilone)).

No products indexed under this heading.

Fluoxetine Hydrochloride (The effect of mild or moderate CYP3A4 inhibitors (e.g., erythromycin, fluconazole, or verapamil) on exposure to ixabepilone has not been studied. Therefore, caution should be used when administering mild or moderate CYP3A4 inhibitors during treatment with ixabepilone, and alternative therapeutic agents that do not inhibit CYP3A4 should be considered. Patients receiving CYP3A4 inhibitors during treatment with ixabepilone should be monitored closely for acute toxicities (e.g., frequent monitoring of peripheral blood counts between cycles of ixabepilone)). Products include:

Prozac Weekly Capsules **1852**
Prozac Pulvules and Liquid **1852**
Symbyax Capsules **1871**

Fluvoxamine Maleate (The effect of mild or moderate CYP3A4 inhibitors (e.g., erythromycin, fluconazole, or verapamil) on exposure to ixabepilone has not been studied. Therefore, caution should be used when administering mild or moderate CYP3A4 inhibitors during treatment with ixabepilone, and alternative therapeutic agents that do not inhibit CYP3A4 should be considered. Patients receiving CYP3A4 inhibitors during treatment with ixabepilone should be monitored closely for acute toxicities (e.g., frequent monitoring of peripheral blood counts between cycles of ixabepilone)). Products include:

Luvox CR Extended-Release Capsules.................................... **1759**

Fosamprenavir Calcium (The use of concomitant strong CYP3A4 inhibitors should be avoided (e.g., ketocnazole, itraconazole, clarithromycin, atazanavir, nefazodone, saquinavir, telithromycin, ritonavir, amprenavir, indinavir, nelfinavir, delavirdine, or voriconazole). Based on pharmacokinetic studies, if a strong CYP3A4 inhibitor must be co-administered, a dose reduction to 20 mg/m^2 is predicted to adjust the ixabepilone AUC to the range observed without inhibitors and should be considered. If the strong inhibitor is discontinued, a washout period of approximately 1 week should be allowed before the ixabepilone dose is adjusted upward to the indicated dose). Products include:

Lexiva Oral Suspension **1510**
Lexiva Tablets **1510**

Fosphenytoin Sodium (Ixabepiloneis a CYP3A4 substrate. Strong CYP3A4 inducers (e.g., dexamethasone, phenytoin, carbamazepine, rifampin, rifampicin, rifabutin, and phenobarbital) may decrease ixabepilone concentrations leading to subtherapeutic levels. Therefore, therapeutic agents with low enzyme induction potential should be considered for co-administration with ixabepilone).

No products indexed under this heading.

Garlic Extract (Ixabepiloneis a CYP3A4 substrate. Strong CYP3A4 inducers (e.g., dexamethasone, phenytoin, carbamazepine, rifampin, rifampicin, rifabutin, and phenobarbital) may decrease ixabepilone concentrations leading to subtherapeutic levels. Therefore, therapeutic agents with low enzyme induction potential should be considered for co-administration with ixabepilone).

No products indexed under this heading.

Garlic Oil (Ixabepiloneis a CYP3A4 substrate. Strong CYP3A4 inducers (e.g., dexamethasone, phenytoin, carbamazepine, rifampin, rifampicin, rifabutin, and phenobarbital) may decrease ixabepilone concentrations leading to subtherapeutic levels. Therefore, therapeutic agents with low enzyme induction potential should be considered for co-administration with ixabepilone).

No products indexed under this heading.

Hydrocortisone (Ixabepiloneis a CYP3A4 substrate. Strong CYP3A4 inducers (e.g., dexamethasone, phenytoin, carbamazepine, rifampin, rifampicin, rifabutin, and phenobarbital) may decrease ixabepilone concentrations leading to subtherapeutic levels. Therefore, therapeutic agents with low enzyme induction potential should be considered for co-administration with ixabepilone).
No products indexed under this heading.

Hydrocortisone Acetate (Ixabepiloneis a CYP3A4 substrate. Strong CYP3A4 inducers (e.g., dexamethasone, phenytoin, carbamazepine, rifampin, rifampicin, rifabutin, and phenobarbital) may decrease ixabepilone concentrations leading to subtherapeutic levels. Therefore, therapeutic agents with low enzyme induction potential should be considered for co-administration with ixabepilone). Products include:
Analpram-HC **1140**
Pramosone **1141**

Hydrocortisone Butyrate (Ixabepiloneis a CYP3A4 substrate. Strong CYP3A4 inducers (e.g., dexamethasone, phenytoin, carbamazepine, rifampin, rifampicin, rifabutin, and phenobarbital) may decrease ixabepilone concentrations leading to subtherapeutic levels. Therefore, therapeutic agents with low enzyme induction potential should be considered for co-administration with ixabepilone).
No products indexed under this heading.

Hydrocortisone Cypionate (Ixabepiloneis a CYP3A4 substrate. Strong CYP3A4 inducers (e.g., dexamethasone, phenytoin, carbamazepine, rifampin, rifampicin, rifabutin, and phenobarbital) may decrease ixabepilone concentrations leading to subtherapeutic levels. Therefore, therapeutic agents with low enzyme induction potential should be considered for co-administration with ixabepilone).
No products indexed under this heading.

Hydrocortisone Hemisuccinate (Ixabepiloneis a CYP3A4 substrate. Strong CYP3A4 inducers (e.g., dexamethasone, phenytoin, carbamazepine, rifampin, rifampicin, rifabutin, and phenobarbital) may decrease ixabepilone concentrations leading to subtherapeutic levels. Therefore, therapeutic agents with low enzyme induction potential should be considered for co-administration with ixabepilone).
No products indexed under this heading.

Hydrocortisone Probutate (Ixabepiloneis a CYP3A4 substrate. Strong CYP3A4 inducers (e.g., dexamethasone, phenytoin, carbamazepine, rifampin, rifampicin, rifabutin, and phenobarbital) may decrease ixabepilone concentrations leading to subtherapeutic levels. Therefore, therapeutic agents with low enzyme induction potential should be considered for co-administration with ixabepilone).
No products indexed under this heading.

Hydrocortisone Sodium Phosphate (Ixabepiloneis a CYP3A4 substrate. Strong CYP3A4 inducers (e.g., dexamethasone, phenytoin, carbamazepine, rifampin, rifampicin, rifabutin, and phenobarbital) may decrease ixabepilone concentrations leading to subtherapeutic levels. Therefore, therapeutic agents with low enzyme induction potential should be considered for co-administration with ixabepilone).
No products indexed under this heading.

Hydrocortisone Sodium Succinate (Ixabepiloneis a CYP3A4 substrate. Strong CYP3A4 inducers (e.g., dexamethasone, phenytoin, carbamazepine, rifampin, rifampicin, rifabutin, and phenobarbital) may decrease ixabepilone concentrations leading to subtherapeutic levels. Therefore, therapeutic agents with low enzyme induction potential should be considered for co-administration with ixabepilone).
No products indexed under this heading.

Hydrocortisone Valerate (Ixabepiloneis a CYP3A4 substrate. Strong CYP3A4 inducers (e.g., dexamethasone, phenytoin, carbamazepine, rifampin, rifampicin, rifabutin, and phenobarbital) may decrease ixabepilone concentrations leading to subtherapeutic levels. Therefore, therapeutic agents with low enzyme induction potential should be considered for co-administration with ixabepilone).
No products indexed under this heading.

Hypericum (St. John's wort may decrease ixabepilone plasma concentrations unpredictably and should be avoided). Products include:
Satieté Tablets .... ▣ **640**

Hypericum Perforatum (St. John's wort may decrease ixabepilone plasma concentrations unpredictably and should be avoided).
No products indexed under this heading.

Indinavir Sulfate (The use of concomitant strong CYP3A4 inhibitors should be avoided (e.g., ketocnazole, itraconazole, clarithromycin, atazanavir, nefazodone, saquinavir, telithromycin, ritonavir, amprenavir, indinavir, nelfinavir, delavirdine, or voriconazole). Based on pharmacokinetic studies, if a strong CYP3A4 inhibitor must be co-administered, a dose reduction to 20 mg/m^2 is predicted to adjust the ixabepilone AUC to the range observed without inhibitors and should be considered. If the strong inhibitor is discontinued, a washout period of approximately 1 week should be allowed before the ixabepilone dose is adjusted upward to the indicated dose). Products include:
Crixivan Capsules **1979**

Isoniazid (The effect of mild or moderate CYP3A4 inhibitors (e.g., erythromycin, fluconazole, or verapamil) on exposure to ixabepilone has not been studied. Therefore, caution should be used when administering mild or moderate CYP3A4 inhibitors during treatment with ixabepilone, and alternative therapeutic agents that do not inhibit CYP3A4 should be considered. Patients receiving CYP3A4 inhibitors during treatment with ixabepilone should be monitored closely for acute toxicities (e.g., frequent monitoring of peripheral blood counts between cycles of ixabepilone)).
No products indexed under this heading.

Itraconazole (The use of concomitant strong CYP3A4 inhibitors should be avoided (e.g., ketocnazole, itraconazole, clarithromycin, atazanavir, nefazodone, saquinavir, telithromycin, ritonavir, amprenavir, indinavir, nelfinavir, delavirdine, or voriconazole). Based on pharmacokinetic studies, if a strong CYP3A4 inhibitor must be co-administered, a dose reduction to 20 mg/m^2 is predicted to adjust the ixabepilone AUC to the range observed without inhibitors and should be considered. If the strong inhibitor is discontinued, a washout period of approximately 1 week should be allowed before the ixabepilone dose is adjusted upward to the indicated dose).
No products indexed under this heading.

Ketoconazole (The use of concomitant strong CYP3A4 inhibitors should be avoided (e.g., ketocnazole, itraconazole, clarithromycin, atazanavir, nefazodone, saquinavir, telithromycin, ritonavir, amprenavir, indinavir, nelfinavir, delavirdine, or voriconazole). Based on pharmacokinetic studies, if a strong CYP3A4 inhibitor must be co-administered, a dose reduction to 20 mg/m^2 is predicted to adjust the ixabepilone AUC to the range observed without inhibitors and should be considered. If the strong inhibitor is discontinued, a washout period of approximately 1 week should be allowed before the ixabepilone dose is adjusted upward to the indicated dose). Products include:
Extina Foam, 2% **3057**
Nizoral A-D Shampoo **1901**

Lopinavir (The use of concomitant strong CYP3A4 inhibitors should be avoided (e.g., ketocnazole, itraconazole, clarithromycin, atazanavir, nefazodone, saquinavir, telithromycin, ritonavir, amprenavir, indinavir, nelfinavir, delavirdine, or voriconazole). Based on pharmacokinetic studies, if a strong CYP3A4 inhibitor must be co-administered, a dose reduction to 20 mg/m^2 is predicted to adjust the ixabepilone AUC to the range observed without inhibitors and should be considered. If the strong inhibitor is discontinued, a washout period of approximately 1 week should be allowed before the ixabepilone dose is adjusted upward to the indicated dose). Products include:
Kaletra **452**

Loratadine (The effect of mild or moderate CYP3A4 inhibitors (e.g., erythromycin, fluconazole, or verapamil) on exposure to ixabepilone has not been studied. Therefore, caution should be used when administering mild or moderate CYP3A4 inhibitors during treatment with ixabepilone, and alternative therapeutic agents that do not inhibit CYP3A4 should be considered. Patients receiving CYP3A4 inhibitors during treatment with ixabepilone should be monitored closely for acute toxicities (e.g., frequent monitoring of peripheral blood counts between cycles of ixabepilone)).
No products indexed under this heading.

Mephenytoin (Ixabepiloneis a CYP3A4 substrate. Strong CYP3A4 inducers (e.g., dexamethasone, phenytoin, carbamazepine, rifampin, rifampicin, rifabutin, and phenobarbital) may decrease ixabepilone concentrations leading to subtherapeutic levels. Therefore, therapeutic agents with low enzyme induction potential should be considered for co-administration with ixabepilone).
No products indexed under this heading.

Methsuximide (Ixabepiloneis a CYP3A4 substrate. Strong CYP3A4 inducers (e.g., dexamethasone, phenytoin, carbamazepine, rifampin, rifampicin, rifabutin, and phenobarbital) may decrease ixabepilone concentrations leading to subtherapeutic levels. Therefore, therapeutic agents with low enzyme induction potential should be considered for co-administration with ixabepilone).
No products indexed under this heading.

Methylprednisolone (Ixabepiloneis a CYP3A4 substrate. Strong CYP3A4 inducers (e.g., dexamethasone, phenytoin, carbamazepine, rifampin, rifampicin, rifabutin, and phenobarbital) may decrease ixabepilone concentrations leading to subtherapeutic levels. Therefore, therapeutic agents with low enzyme induction potential should be considered for co-administration with ixabepilone).
No products indexed under this heading.

Methylprednisolone Acetate (Ixabepiloneis a CYP3A4 substrate. Strong CYP3A4 inducers (e.g., dexamethasone, phenytoin, carbamazepine, rifampin, rifampicin, rifabutin, and phenobarbital) may decrease ixabepilone concentrations leading to subtherapeutic levels. Therefore, therapeutic agents with low enzyme induction potential should be considered for co-administration with ixabepilone).
No products indexed under this heading.

Methylprednisolone Sodium Succinate (Ixabepiloneis a CYP3A4 substrate. Strong CYP3A4 inducers (e.g., dexamethasone, phenytoin, carbamazepine, rifampin, rifampicin, rifabutin, and phenobarbital) may decrease ixabepilone concentrations leading to subtherapeutic levels. Therefore, therapeutic agents with low enzyme induction potential should be considered for co-administration with ixabepilone).
No products indexed under this heading.

Metronidazole (The effect of mild or moderate CYP3A4 inhibitors (e.g., erythromycin, fluconazole, or verapamil) on exposure to ixabepilone has not been studied. Therefore, caution should be used when administering mild or moderate CYP3A4 inhibitors during treatment with ixabepilone, and alternative therapeutic agents that do not inhibit CYP3A4 should be considered. Patients receiving CYP3A4 inhibitors during treatment with ixabepilone should be monitored closely for acute toxicities (e.g., frequent monitoring of peripheral blood counts between cycles of ixabepilone)). Products include:
Pylera Capsules **714**

Metronidazole Benzoate (The effect of mild or moderate CYP3A4 inhibitors (e.g., erythromycin, fluconazole, or verapamil) on exposure to ixabepilone has not been studied. Therefore, caution should be used when administering mild or moderate CYP3A4 inhibitors during treatment with ixabepilone, and alternative therapeutic agents that do not inhibit CYP3A4 should be considered. Patients receiving CYP3A4 inhibitors during treatment with ixabepilone should be monitored closely for acute toxicities (e.g., frequent monitoring of peripheral blood counts between cycles of ixabepilone)).

No products indexed under this heading.

Metronidazole Hydrochloride (The effect of mild or moderate CYP3A4 inhibitors (e.g., erythromycin, fluconazole, or verapamil) on exposure to ixabepilone has not been studied. Therefore, caution should be used when administering mild or moderate CYP3A4 inhibitors during treatment with ixabepilone, and alternative therapeutic agents that do not inhibit CYP3A4 should be considered. Patients receiving CYP3A4 inhibitors during treatment with ixabepilone should be monitored closely for acute toxicities (e.g., frequent monitoring of peripheral blood counts between cycles of ixabepilone)).

No products indexed under this heading.

Metronidazole Sodium (The effect of mild or moderate CYP3A4 inhibitors (e.g., erythromycin, fluconazole, or verapamil) on exposure to ixabepilone has not been studied. Therefore, caution should be used when administering mild or moderate CYP3A4 inhibitors during treatment with ixabepilone, and alternative therapeutic agents that do not inhibit CYP3A4 should be considered. Patients receiving CYP3A4 inhibitors during treatment with ixabepilone should be monitored closely for acute toxicities (e.g., frequent monitoring of peripheral blood counts between cycles of ixabepilone)).

No products indexed under this heading.

Miconazole (The effect of mild or moderate CYP3A4 inhibitors (e.g., erythromycin, fluconazole, or verapamil) on exposure to ixabepilone has not been studied. Therefore, caution should be used when administering mild or moderate CYP3A4 inhibitors during treatment with ixabepilone, and alternative therapeutic agents that do not inhibit CYP3A4 should be considered. Patients receiving CYP3A4 inhibitors during treatment with ixabepilone should be monitored closely for acute toxicities (e.g., frequent monitoring of peripheral blood counts between cycles of ixabepilone)).

No products indexed under this heading.

Miconazole Nitrate (The effect of mild or moderate CYP3A4 inhibitors (e.g., erythromycin, fluconazole, or verapamil) on exposure to ixabepilone has not been studied. Therefore, caution should be used when administering mild or moderate CYP3A4 inhibitors during treatment with ixabepilone, and alternative therapeutic agents that do not inhibit CYP3A4 should be considered. Patients receiving CYP3A4 inhibitors during treatment with ixabepilone should be monitored closely for acute toxicities (e.g., frequent monitoring of peripheral blood counts between cycles of ixabepilone)).

No products indexed under this heading.

Modafinil (Ixabepiloneis a CYP3A4 substrate. Strong CYP3A4 inducers (e.g., dexamethasone, phenytoin, carbamazepine, rifampin, rifampicin, rifabutin, and phenobarbital) may decrease ixabepilone concentrations leading to subtherapeutic levels. Therefore, therapeutic agents with low enzyme induction potential should be considered for co-administration with ixabepilone). Products include:

Provigil Tablets 977

Nefazodone Hydrochloride (The use of concomitant strong CYP3A4 inhibitors should be avoided (e.g., ketoconazole, itraconazole, clarithromycin, atazanavir, nefazodone, saquinavir, telithromycin, ritonavir, amprenavir, indinavir, nelfinavir, delavirdine, or voriconazole). Based on pharmacokinetic studies, if a strong CYP3A4 inhibitor must be co-administered, a dose reduction to 20 mg/m^2 is predicted to adjust the ixabepilone AUC to the range observed without inhibitors and should be considered. If the strong inhibitor is discontinued, a washout period of approximately 1 week should be allowed before the ixabepilone dose is adjusted upward to the indicated dose).

No products indexed under this heading.

Nelfinavir Mesylate (The use of concomitant strong CYP3A4 inhibitors should be avoided (e.g., ketoconazole, itraconazole, clarithromycin, atazanavir, nefazodone, saquinavir, telithromycin, ritonavir, amprenavir, indinavir, nelfinavir, delavirdine, or voriconazole). Based on pharmacokinetic studies, if a strong CYP3A4 inhibitor must be co-administered, a dose reduction to 20 mg/m^2 is predicted to adjust the ixabepilone AUC to the range observed without inhibitors and should be considered. If the strong inhibitor is discontinued, a washout period of approximately 1 week should be allowed before the ixabepilone dose is adjusted upward to the indicated dose).

No products indexed under this heading.

Nevirapine (The effect of mild or moderate CYP3A4 inhibitors (e.g., erythromycin, fluconazole, or verapamil) on exposure to ixabepilone has not been studied. Therefore, caution should be used when administering mild or moderate CYP3A4 inhibitors during treatment with ixabepilone, and alternative therapeutic agents that do not inhibit CYP3A4 should be considered. Patients receiving CYP3A4 inhibitors during treatment with ixabepilone should be monitored closely for acute toxicities (e.g., frequent monitoring of peripheral blood counts between cycles of ixabepilone)). Products include:

Viramune Oral Suspension 873
Viramune Tablets 873

Niacinamide (The effect of mild or moderate CYP3A4 inhibitors (e.g., erythromycin, fluconazole, or verapamil) on exposure to ixabepilone has not been studied. Therefore, caution should be used when administering mild or moderate CYP3A4 inhibitors during treatment with ixabepilone, and alternative therapeutic agents that do not inhibit CYP3A4 should be considered. Patients receiving CYP3A4 inhibitors during treatment with ixabepilone should be monitored closely for acute toxicities (e.g., frequent monitoring of peripheral blood counts between cycles of ixabepilone)). Products include:

BioLean Free Tablets .... ▣635

Nicotinamide (The effect of mild or moderate CYP3A4 inhibitors (e.g., erythromycin, fluconazole, or verapamil) on exposure to ixabepilone has not been studied. Therefore, caution should be used when administering mild or moderate CYP3A4 inhibitors during treatment with ixabepilone, and alternative therapeutic agents that do not inhibit CYP3A4 should be considered. Patients receiving CYP3A4 inhibitors during treatment with ixabepilone should be monitored closely for acute toxicities (e.g., frequent monitoring of peripheral blood counts between cycles of ixabepilone)).

No products indexed under this heading.

Nifedipine (The effect of mild or moderate CYP3A4 inhibitors (e.g., erythromycin, fluconazole, or verapamil) on exposure to ixabepilone has not been studied. Therefore, caution should be used when administering mild or moderate CYP3A4 inhibitors during treatment with ixabepilone, and alternative therapeutic agents that do not inhibit CYP3A4 should be considered. Patients receiving CYP3A4 inhibitors during treatment with ixabepilone should be monitored closely for acute toxicities (e.g., frequent monitoring of peripheral blood counts between cycles of ixabepilone)).

No products indexed under this heading.

Norfloxacin (The effect of mild or moderate CYP3A4 inhibitors (e.g., erythromycin, fluconazole, or verapamil) on exposure to ixabepilone has not been studied. Therefore, caution should be used when administering mild or moderate CYP3A4 inhibitors during treatment with ixabepilone, and alternative therapeutic agents that do not inhibit CYP3A4 should be considered. Patients receiving CYP3A4 inhibitors during treatment with ixabepilone should be monitored closely for acute toxicities (e.g., frequent monitoring of peripheral blood counts between cycles of ixabepilone)). Products include:

Noroxin Tablets 2069

Omeprazole (The effect of mild or moderate CYP3A4 inhibitors (e.g., erythromycin, fluconazole, or verapamil) on exposure to ixabepilone has not been studied. Therefore, caution should be used when administering mild or moderate CYP3A4 inhibitors during treatment with ixabepilone, and alternative therapeutic agents that do not inhibit CYP3A4 should be considered. Patients receiving CYP3A4 inhibitors during treatment with ixabepilone should be monitored closely for acute toxicities (e.g., frequent monitoring of peripheral blood counts between cycles of ixabepilone)).

No products indexed under this heading.

Oxcarbazepine (Ixabepiloneis a CYP3A4 substrate. Strong CYP3A4 inducers (e.g., dexamethasone, phenytoin, carbamazepine, rifampin, rifampicin, rifabutin, and phenobarbital) may decrease ixabepilone concentrations leading to subtherapeutic levels. Therefore, therapeutic agents with low enzyme induction potential should be considered for co-administration with ixabepilone).

No products indexed under this heading.

Paroxetine Hydrochloride (The effect of mild or moderate CYP3A4 inhibitors (e.g., erythromycin, fluconazole, or verapamil) on exposure to ixabepilone has not been studied. Therefore, caution should be used when administering mild or moderate CYP3A4 inhibitors during treatment with ixabepilone, and alternative therapeutic agents that do not inhibit CYP3A4 should be considered. Patients receiving CYP3A4 inhibitors during treatment with ixabepilone should be monitored closely for acute toxicities (e.g., frequent monitoring of peripheral blood counts between cycles of ixabepilone)). Products include:

Paxil 1535
Paxil CR Controlled-Release Tablets 1544

Phenobarbital (Ixabepiloneis a CYP3A4 substrate. Strong CYP3A4 inducers (e.g., dexamethasone, phenytoin, carbamazepine, rifampin, rifampicin, rifabutin, and phenobarbital) may decrease ixabepilone concentrations leading to subtherapeutic levels. Therefore, therapeutic agents with low enzyme induction potential should be considered for co-administration with ixabepilone). Products include:

Donnatal Extentabs 2507

Phenobarbital Sodium (Ixabepiloneis a CYP3A4 substrate. Strong CYP3A4 inducers (e.g., dexamethasone, phenytoin, carbamazepine, rifampin, rifampicin, rifabutin, and phenobarbital) may decrease ixabepilone concentrations leading to subtherapeutic levels. Therefore, therapeutic agents with low enzyme induction potential should be considered for co-administration with ixabepilone).

No products indexed under this heading.

Phenytoin (Ixabepiloneis a CYP3A4 substrate. Strong CYP3A4 inducers (e.g., dexamethasone, phenytoin, carbamazepine, rifampin, rifampicin, rifabutin, and phenobarbital) may decrease ixabepilone concentrations leading to subtherapeutic levels. Therefore, therapeutic agents with low enzyme induction potential should be considered for co-administration with ixabepilone).

No products indexed under this heading.

Phenytoin Sodium (Ixabepiloneis a CYP3A4 substrate. Strong CYP3A4 inducers (e.g., dexamethasone, phenytoin, carbamazepine, rifampin, rifampicin, rifabutin, and phenobarbital) may decrease ixabepilone concentrations leading to subtherapeutic levels. Therefore, therapeutic agents with low enzyme induction potential should be considered for co-administration with ixabepilone). Products include:

Phenytek Capsules 2192

Prednisolone Acetate (Ixabepiloneis a CYP3A4 substrate. Strong CYP3A4 inducers (e.g., dexamethasone, phenytoin, carbamazepine, rifampin, rifampicin, rifabutin, and phenobarbital) may decrease ixabepilone concentrations leading to subtherapeutic levels. Therefore, therapeutic agents with low enzyme induction potential should be considered for co-administration with ixabepilone). Products include:

Pred Forte Ophthalmic Suspension .... ⊙ **227**
Pred Mild Ophthalmic Suspension .... ⊙ **230**
Pred-G Ophthalmic Ointment .... ⊙ **229**
Pred-G Ophthalmic Suspension ...... ⊙ **228**

Prednisolone Sodium Phosphate (Ixabepiloneis a CYP3A4 substrate. Strong CYP3A4 inducers (e.g., dexamethasone, phenytoin, carbamazepine, rifampin, rifampicin, rifabutin, and phenobarbital) may decrease ixabepilone concentrations leading to subtherapeutic levels. Therefore, therapeutic agents with low enzyme induction potential should be considered for co-administration with ixabepilone).

No products indexed under this heading.

Prednisolone Tebutate (Ixabepiloneis a CYP3A4 substrate. Strong CYP3A4 inducers (e.g., dexamethasone, phenytoin, carbamazepine, rifampin, rifampicin, rifabutin, and phenobarbital) may decrease ixabepilone concentrations leading to subtherapeutic levels. Therefore, therapeutic agents with low enzyme induction potential should be considered for co-administration with ixabepilone).

No products indexed under this heading.

Prednisone (Ixabepiloneis a CYP3A4 substrate. Strong CYP3A4 inducers (e.g., dexamethasone, phenytoin, carbamazepine, rifampin, rifampicin, rifabutin, and phenobarbital) may decrease ixabepilone concentrations leading to subtherapeutic levels. Therefore, therapeutic agents with low enzyme induction potential should be considered for co-administration with ixabepilone).

No products indexed under this heading.

Primidone (Ixabepiloneis a CYP3A4 substrate. Strong CYP3A4 inducers (e.g., dexamethasone, phenytoin, carbamazepine, rifampin, rifampicin, rifabutin, and phenobarbital) may decrease ixabepilone concentrations leading to subtherapeutic levels. Therefore, therapeutic agents with low enzyme induction potential should be considered for co-administration with ixabepilone).

No products indexed under this heading.

Propoxyphene Hydrochloride (The effect of mild or moderate CYP3A4 inhibitors (e.g., erythromycin, fluconazole, or verapamil) on exposure to ixabepilone has not been studied. Therefore, caution should be used when administering mild or moderate CYP3A4 inhibitors during treatment with ixabepilone, and alternative therapeutic agents that do not inhibit CYP3A4 should be considered. Patients receiving CYP3A4 inhibitors during treatment with ixabepilone should be monitored closely for acute toxicities (e.g., frequent monitoring of peripheral blood counts between cycles of ixabepilone)).

No products indexed under this heading.

Propoxyphene Napsylate (The effect of mild or moderate CYP3A4 inhibitors (e.g., erythromycin, fluconazole, or verapamil) on exposure to ixabepilone has not been studied. Therefore, caution should be used when administering mild or moderate CYP3A4 inhibitors during treatment with ixabepilone, and alternative therapeutic agents that do not inhibit CYP3A4 should be considered. Patients receiving CYP3A4 inhibitors during treatment with ixabepilone should be monitored closely for acute toxicities (e.g., frequent monitoring of peripheral blood counts between cycles of ixabepilone)).

No products indexed under this heading.

Quinidine (The effect of mild or moderate CYP3A4 inhibitors (e.g., erythromycin, fluconazole, or verapamil) on exposure to ixabepilone has not been studied. Therefore, caution should be used when administering mild or moderate CYP3A4 inhibitors during treatment with ixabepilone, and alternative therapeutic agents that do not inhibit CYP3A4 should be considered. Patients receiving CYP3A4 inhibitors during treatment with ixabepilone should be monitored closely for acute toxicities (e.g., frequent monitoring of peripheral blood counts between cycles of ixabepilone)).

No products indexed under this heading.

Quinidine Hydrochloride (The effect of mild or moderate CYP3A4 inhibitors (e.g., erythromycin, fluconazole, or verapamil) on exposure to ixabepilone has not been studied. Therefore, caution should be used when administering mild or moderate CYP3A4 inhibitors during treatment with ixabepilone, and alternative therapeutic agents that do not inhibit CYP3A4 should be considered. Patients receiving CYP3A4 inhibitors during treatment with ixabepilone should be monitored closely for acute toxicities (e.g., frequent monitoring of peripheral blood counts between cycles of ixabepilone)).

No products indexed under this heading.

Quinidine Polygalacturonate (The effect of mild or moderate CYP3A4 inhibitors (e.g., erythromycin, fluconazole, or verapamil) on exposure to ixabepilone has not been studied. Therefore, caution should be used when administering mild or moderate CYP3A4 inhibitors during treatment with ixabepilone, and alternative therapeutic agents that do not inhibit CYP3A4 should be considered. Patients receiving CYP3A4 inhibitors during treatment with ixabepilone should be monitored closely for acute toxicities (e.g., frequent monitoring of peripheral blood counts between cycles of ixabepilone)).

No products indexed under this heading.

Quinidine Sulfate (The effect of mild or moderate CYP3A4 inhibitors (e.g., erythromycin, fluconazole, or verapamil) on exposure to ixabepilone has not been studied. Therefore, caution should be used when administering mild or moderate CYP3A4 inhibitors during treatment with ixabepilone, and alternative therapeutic agents that do not inhibit CYP3A4 should be considered. Patients receiving CYP3A4 inhibitors during treatment with ixabepilone should be monitored closely for acute toxicities (e.g., frequent monitoring of peripheral blood counts between cycles of ixabepilone)).

No products indexed under this heading.

Quinine (The effect of mild or moderate CYP3A4 inhibitors (e.g., erythromycin, fluconazole, or verapamil) on exposure to ixabepilone has not been studied. Therefore, caution should be used when administering mild or moderate CYP3A4 inhibitors during treatment with ixabepilone, and alternative therapeutic agents that do not inhibit CYP3A4 should be considered. Patients receiving CYP3A4 inhibitors during treatment with ixabepilone should be monitored closely for acute toxicities (e.g., frequent monitoring of peripheral blood counts between cycles of ixabepilone)).

No products indexed under this heading.

Quinine Sulfate (The effect of mild or moderate CYP3A4 inhibitors (e.g., erythromycin, fluconazole, or verapamil) on exposure to ixabepilone has not been studied. Therefore, caution should be used when administering mild or moderate CYP3A4 inhibitors during treatment with ixabepilone, and alternative therapeutic agents that do not inhibit CYP3A4 should be considered. Patients receiving CYP3A4 inhibitors during treatment with ixabepilone should be monitored closely for acute toxicities (e.g., frequent monitoring of peripheral blood counts between cycles of ixabepilone)).

No products indexed under this heading.

Quinupristin (The effect of mild or moderate CYP3A4 inhibitors (e.g., erythromycin, fluconazole, or verapamil) on exposure to ixabepilone has not been studied. Therefore, caution should be used when administering mild or moderate CYP3A4 inhibitors during treatment with ixabepilone, and alternative therapeutic agents that do not inhibit CYP3A4 should be considered. Patients receiving CYP3A4 inhibitors during treatment with ixabepilone should be monitored closely for acute toxicities (e.g., frequent monitoring of peripheral blood counts between cycles of ixabepilone)).

No products indexed under this heading.

Ranitidine Bismuth Citrate (The effect of mild or moderate CYP3A4 inhibitors (e.g., erythromycin, fluconazole, or verapamil) on exposure to ixabepilone has not been studied. Therefore, caution should be used when administering mild or moderate CYP3A4 inhibitors during treatment with ixabepilone, and alternative therapeutic agents that do not inhibit CYP3A4 should be considered. Patients receiving CYP3A4 inhibitors during treatment with ixabepilone should be monitored closely for acute toxicities (e.g., frequent monitoring of peripheral blood counts between cycles of ixabepilone)).

No products indexed under this heading.

Ranitidine Hydrochloride (The effect of mild or moderate CYP3A4 inhibitors (e.g., erythromycin, fluconazole, or verapamil) on exposure to ixabepilone has not been studied. Therefore, caution should be used when administering mild or moderate CYP3A4 inhibitors during treatment with ixabepilone, and alternative therapeutic agents that do not inhibit CYP3A4 should be considered. Patients receiving CYP3A4 inhibitors during treatment with ixabepilone should be monitored closely for acute toxicities (e.g., frequent monitoring of peripheral blood counts between cycles of ixabepilone)). Products include:

Zantac 75 Tablets .... ▣ **603**
Zantac **1670**
Zantac Injection **1666**
Zantac Injection Pharmacy Bulk Package **1668**
Maximum Strength Zantac 150 Tablets .... ▣ **603**
Maximum Strength Zantac 150 Cool Mint Tablets .... ▣ **603**

Rifabutin (Ixabepiloneis a CYP3A4 substrate. Strong CYP3A4 inducers (e.g., dexamethasone, phenytoin, carbamazepine, rifampin, rifampicin, rifabutin, and phenobarbital) may decrease ixabepilone concentrations leading to subtherapeutic levels. Therefore, therapeutic agents with low enzyme induction potential should be considered for co-administration with ixabepilone).

No products indexed under this heading.

Rifampicin (Ixabepiloneis a CYP3A4 substrate. Strong CYP3A4 inducers (e.g., dexamethasone, phenytoin, carbamazepine, rifampin, rifampicin, rifabutin, and phenobarbital) may decrease ixabepilone concentrations leading to subtherapeutic levels. Therefore, therapeutic agents with low enzyme induction potential should be considered for co-administration with ixabepilone).

No products indexed under this heading.

Rifampin (Ixabepiloneis a CYP3A4 substrate. Strong CYP3A4 inducers (e.g., dexamethasone, phenytoin, carbamazepine, rifampin, rifampicin, rifabutin, and phenobarbital) may decrease ixabepilone concentrations leading to subtherapeutic levels. Therefore, therapeutic agents with low enzyme induction potential should be considered for co-administration with ixabepilone).

No products indexed under this heading.

Rifapentine (Ixabepiloneis a CYP3A4 substrate. Strong CYP3A4 inducers (e.g., dexamethasone, phenytoin, carbamazepine, rifampin, rifampicin, rifabutin, and phenobarbital) may decrease ixabepilone concentrations leading to subtherapeutic levels. Therefore, therapeutic agents with low enzyme induction potential should be considered for co-administration with ixabepilone).

No products indexed under this heading.

Ritonavir (The use of concomitant strong CYP3A4 inhibitors should be avoided (e.g., ketocnazole, itraconazole, clarithromycin, atazanavir, nefazodone, saquinavir, telithromycin, ritonavir, amprenavir, indinavir, nelfinavir, delavirdine, or voriconazole). Based on pharmacokinetic studies, if a strong CYP3A4 inhibitor must be co-administered, a dose reduction to 20 mg/m^2 is predicted to adjust the ixabepilone AUC to the range observed without inhibitors and should be considered. If the strong inhibitor is discontinued, a washout period of approximately 1 week should be allowed before the ixabepilone dose is adjusted upward to the indicated dose). Products include:

Kaletra **452**
Norvir **489**

Saquinavir (The use of concomitant strong CYP3A4 inhibitors should be avoided (e.g., ketocnazole, itraconazole, clarithromycin, atazanavir, nefazodone, saquinavir, telithromycin, ritonavir, amprenavir, indinavir, nelfinavir, delavirdine, or voriconazole). Based on pharmacokinetic studies, if a strong CYP3A4 inhibitor must be co-administered, a dose reduction to 20 mg/m^2 is predicted to adjust the ixabepilone AUC to the range observed without inhibitors and should be considered. If the strong inhibitor is discontinued, a washout period of approximately 1 week should be allowed before the ixabepilone dose is adjusted upward to the indicated dose).
No products indexed under this heading.

Saquinavir Mesylate (The use of concomitant strong CYP3A4 inhibitors should be avoided (e.g., ketocnazole, itraconazole, clarithromycin, atazanavir, nefazodone, saquinavir, telithromycin, ritonavir, amprenavir, indinavir, nelfinavir, delavirdine, or voriconazole). Based on pharmacokinetic studies, if a strong CYP3A4 inhibitor must be co-administered, a dose reduction to 20 mg/m^2 is predicted to adjust the ixabepilone AUC to the range observed without inhibitors and should be considered. If the strong inhibitor is discontinued, a washout period of approximately 1 week should be allowed before the ixabepilone dose is adjusted upward to the indicated dose).
No products indexed under this heading.

Sertraline Hydrochloride (The effect of mild or moderate CYP3A4 inhibitors (e.g., erythromycin, fluconazole, or verapamil) on exposure to ixabepilone has not been studied. Therefore, caution should be used when administering mild or moderate CYP3A4 inhibitors during treatment with ixabepilone, and alternative therapeutic agents that do not inhibit CYP3A4 should be considered. Patients receiving CYP3A4 inhibitors during treatment with ixabepilone should be monitored closely for acute toxicities (e.g., frequent monitoring of peripheral blood counts between cycles of ixabepilone)).
No products indexed under this heading.

Sildenafil Citrate (The effect of mild or moderate CYP3A4 inhibitors (e.g., erythromycin, fluconazole, or verapamil) on exposure to ixabepilone has not been studied. Therefore, caution should be used when administering mild or moderate CYP3A4 inhibitors during treatment with ixabepilone, and alternative therapeutic agents that do not inhibit CYP3A4 should be considered. Patients receiving CYP3A4 inhibitors during treatment with ixabepilone should be monitored closely for acute toxicities (e.g., frequent monitoring of peripheral blood counts between cycles of ixabepilone)).
No products indexed under this heading.

Sulfinpyrazone (Ixabepiloneis a CYP3A4 substrate. Strong CYP3A4 inducers (e.g., dexamethasone, phenytoin, carbamazepine, rifampin, rifampicin, rifabutin, and phenobarbital) may decrease ixabepilone concentrations leading to subtherapeutic levels. Therefore, therapeutic agents with low enzyme induction potential should be considered for co-administration with ixabepilone).
No products indexed under this heading.

Telithromycin (The use of concomitant strong CYP3A4 inhibitors should be avoided (e.g., ketocnazole, itraconazole, clarithromycin, atazanavir, nefazodone, saquinavir, telithromycin, ritonavir, amprenavir, indinavir, nelfinavir, delavirdine, or voriconazole). Based on pharmacokinetic studies, if a strong CYP3A4 inhibitor must be co-administered, a dose reduction to 20 mg/m^2 is predicted to adjust the ixabepilone AUC to the range observed without inhibitors and should be considered. If the strong inhibitor is discontinued, a washout period of approximately 1 week should be allowed before the ixabepilone dose is adjusted upward to the indicated dose). Products include:

Ketek Tablets **2744**

Theophylline (Ixabepiloneis a CYP3A4 substrate. Strong CYP3A4 inducers (e.g., dexamethasone, phenytoin, carbamazepine, rifampin, rifampicin, rifabutin, and phenobarbital) may decrease ixabepilone concentrations leading to subtherapeutic levels. Therefore, therapeutic agents with low enzyme induction potential should be considered for co-administration with ixabepilone).
No products indexed under this heading.

Theophylline Anhydrous (Ixabepiloneis a CYP3A4 substrate. Strong CYP3A4 inducers (e.g., dexamethasone, phenytoin, carbamazepine, rifampin, rifampicin, rifabutin, and phenobarbital) may decrease ixabepilone concentrations leading to subtherapeutic levels. Therefore, therapeutic agents with low enzyme induction potential should be considered for co-administration with ixabepilone). Products include:

Uniphyl Tablets **2595**

Theophylline Calcium Salicylate (Ixabepiloneis a CYP3A4 substrate. Strong CYP3A4 inducers (e.g., dexamethasone, phenytoin, carbamazepine, rifampin, rifampicin, rifabutin, and phenobarbital) may decrease ixabepilone concentrations leading to subtherapeutic levels. Therefore, therapeutic agents with low enzyme induction potential should be considered for co-administration with ixabepilone).
No products indexed under this heading.

Theophylline Dihydroxypropyl (Glyceryl) (Ixabepiloneis a CYP3A4 substrate. Strong CYP3A4 inducers (e.g., dexamethasone, phenytoin, carbamazepine, rifampin, rifampicin, rifabutin, and phenobarbital) may decrease ixabepilone concentrations leading to subtherapeutic levels. Therefore, therapeutic agents with low enzyme induction potential should be considered for co-administration with ixabepilone).
No products indexed under this heading.

Theophylline Ethylenediamine (Ixabepiloneis a CYP3A4 substrate. Strong CYP3A4 inducers (e.g., dexamethasone, phenytoin, carbamazepine, rifampin, rifampicin, rifabutin, and phenobarbital) may decrease ixabepilone concentrations leading to subtherapeutic levels. Therefore, therapeutic agents with low enzyme induction potential should be considered for co-administration with ixabepilone).
No products indexed under this heading.

Triamcinolone (Ixabepiloneis a CYP3A4 substrate. Strong CYP3A4 inducers (e.g., dexamethasone, phenytoin, carbamazepine, rifampin, rifampicin, rifabutin, and phenobarbital) may decrease ixabepilone concentrations leading to subtherapeutic levels. Therefore, therapeutic agents with low enzyme induction potential should be considered for co-administration with ixabepilone).
No products indexed under this heading.

Triamcinolone Acetonide (Ixabepiloneis a CYP3A4 substrate. Strong CYP3A4 inducers (e.g., dexamethasone, phenytoin, carbamazepine, rifampin, rifampicin, rifabutin, and phenobarbital) may decrease ixabepilone concentrations leading to subtherapeutic levels. Therefore, therapeutic agents with low enzyme induction potential should be considered for co-administration with ixabepilone). Products include:

Azmacort Inhalation Aerosol **407**
Nasacort AQ Nasal Spray **2765**
Triesence Injectable Suspension .... ⊙ **209**

Triamcinolone Diacetate (Ixabepiloneis a CYP3A4 substrate. Strong CYP3A4 inducers (e.g., dexamethasone, phenytoin, carbamazepine, rifampin, rifampicin, rifabutin, and phenobarbital) may decrease ixabepilone concentrations leading to subtherapeutic levels. Therefore, therapeutic agents with low enzyme induction potential should be considered for co-administration with ixabepilone).
No products indexed under this heading.

Triamcinolone Hexacetonide (Ixabepiloneis a CYP3A4 substrate. Strong CYP3A4 inducers (e.g., dexamethasone, phenytoin, carbamazepine, rifampin, rifampicin, rifabutin, and phenobarbital) may decrease ixabepilone concentrations leading to subtherapeutic levels. Therefore, therapeutic agents with low enzyme induction potential should be considered for co-administration with ixabepilone).
No products indexed under this heading.

Troglitazone (The effect of mild or moderate CYP3A4 inhibitors (e.g., erythromycin, fluconazole, or verapamil) on exposure to ixabepilone has not been studied. Therefore, caution should be used when administering mild or moderate CYP3A4 inhibitors during treatment with ixabepilone, and alternative therapeutic agents that do not inhibit CYP3A4 should be considered. Patients receiving CYP3A4 inhibitors during treatment with ixabepilone should be monitored closely for acute toxicities (e.g., frequent monitoring of peripheral blood counts between cycles of ixabepilone)).
No products indexed under this heading.

Troleandomycin (The use of concomitant strong CYP3A4 inhibitors should be avoided (e.g., ketocnazole, itraconazole, clarithromycin, atazanavir, nefazodone, saquinavir, telithromycin, ritonavir, amprenavir, indinavir, nelfinavir, delavirdine, or voriconazole). Based on pharmacokinetic studies, if a strong CYP3A4 inhibitor must be co-administered, a dose reduction to 20 mg/m^2 is predicted to adjust the ixabepilone AUC to the range observed without inhibitors and should be considered. If the strong inhibitor is discontinued, a washout period of approximately 1 week should be allowed before the ixabepilone dose is adjusted upward to the indicated dose).
No products indexed under this heading.

Valproate Sodium (The effect of mild or moderate CYP3A4 inhibitors (e.g., erythromycin, fluconazole, or verapamil) on exposure to ixabepilone has not been studied. Therefore, caution should be used when administering mild or moderate CYP3A4 inhibitors during treatment with ixabepilone, and alternative therapeutic agents that do not inhibit CYP3A4 should be considered. Patients receiving CYP3A4 inhibitors during treatment with ixabepilone should be monitored closely for acute toxicities (e.g., frequent monitoring of peripheral blood counts between cycles of ixabepilone)).
No products indexed under this heading.

Vardenafil Hydrochloride (The effect of mild or moderate CYP3A4 inhibitors (e.g., erythromycin, fluconazole, or verapamil) on exposure to ixabepilone has not been studied. Therefore, caution should be used when administering mild or moderate CYP3A4 inhibitors during treatment with ixabepilone, and alternative therapeutic agents that do not inhibit CYP3A4 should be considered. Patients receiving CYP3A4 inhibitors during treatment with ixabepilone should be monitored closely for acute toxicities (e.g., frequent monitoring of peripheral blood counts between cycles of ixabepilone)). Products include:

Levitra Tablets **2876**

Verapamil Hydrochloride (The effect of mild or moderate CYP3A4 inhibitors (e.g., erythromycin, fluconazole, or verapamil) on exposure to ixabepilone has not been studied. Therefore, caution should be used when administering mild or moderate CYP3A4 inhibitors during treatment with ixabepilone, and alternative therapeutic agents that do not inhibit CYP3A4 should be considered. Patients receiving CYP3A4 inhibitors during treatment with ixabepilone should be monitored closely for acute toxicities (e.g., frequent monitoring of peripheral blood counts between cycles of ixabepilone)). Products include:

Tarka Tablets **511**

Voriconazole (The use of concomitant strong CYP3A4 inhibitors should be avoided (e.g., ketocnazole, itraconazole, clarithromycin, atazanavir, nefazodone, saquinavir, telithromycin, ritonavir, amprenavir, indinavir, nelfinavir, delavirdine, or voriconazole). Based on pharmacokinetic studies, if a strong CYP3A4 inhibitor must be co-administered, a dose reduction to 20 mg/m^2 is predicted to adjust the ixabepilone AUC to the range observed without inhibitors and should be considered. If the strong inhibitor is discontinued, a washout period of approximately 1 week should be allowed before the ixabepilone dose is adjusted upward to the indicated dose).

No products indexed under this heading.

Zafirlukast (The effect of mild or moderate CYP3A4 inhibitors (e.g., erythromycin, fluconazole, or verapamil) on exposure to ixabepilone has not been studied. Therefore, caution should be used when administering mild or moderate CYP3A4 inhibitors during treatment with ixabepilone, and alternative therapeutic agents that do not inhibit CYP3A4 should be considered. Patients receiving CYP3A4 inhibitors during treatment with ixabepilone should be monitored closely for acute toxicities (e.g., frequent monitoring of peripheral blood counts between cycles of ixabepilone)). Products include:

Accolate Tablets 669

Zileuton (The effect of mild or moderate CYP3A4 inhibitors (e.g., erythromycin, fluconazole, or verapamil) on exposure to ixabepilone has not been studied. Therefore, caution should be used when administering mild or moderate CYP3A4 inhibitors during treatment with ixabepilone, and alternative therapeutic agents that do not inhibit CYP3A4 should be considered. Patients receiving CYP3A4 inhibitors during treatment with ixabepilone should be monitored closely for acute toxicities (e.g., frequent monitoring of peripheral blood counts between cycles of ixabepilone)).

No products indexed under this heading.

Food Interactions

Grapefruit (Grapefruit juice may increase plasma concentrations of ixabepilone and should be avoided).

Grapefruit Juice (Grapefruit juice may increase plasma concentrations of ixabepilone and should be avoided).

JANUMET TABLETS

(Metformin Hydrochloride, Sitagliptin Phosphate) 2041

May interact with cationic drugs that are eliminated by renal tubular, calcium channel blockers, corticosteroids, diuretics, estrogens, oral hypoglycemic agents, oral contraceptives, phenothiazines, phenytoin, sympathomimetics, thiazides, thyroid preparations, and certain other agents. Compounds in these categories include:

Acarbose (Patients also receiving an insulin secretagogue (e.g., sulfonylurea, meglitinide) may require a lower dose of the insulin secretagogue to reduce the risk of hypoglycemia). Products include:

Precose Tablets 792

Albuterol (Sympathomimetics tend to produce hyperglycemia and may lead to loss of glycemic control. When sympathomimetics are administered to a patient receiving Janumet, the patient should be closely observed to maintain adequate glycemic control).

No products indexed under this heading.

Albuterol Sulfate (Sympathomimetics tend to produce hyperglycemia and may lead to loss of glycemic control. When sympathomimetics are administered to a patient receiving Janumet, the patient should be closely observed to maintain adequate glycemic control). Products include:

Combivent Inhalation Aerosol 845
ProAir HFA Inhalation Aerosol 3113
Proventil HFA Inhalation Aerosol 2914
Ventolin HFA Inhalation Aerosol 1638

Amiloride Hydrochloride (Diuretics tend to produce hyperglycemia and may lead to loss of glycemic control. When diuretics are administered to a patient receiving Janumet, the patient should be closely observed to maintain adequate glycemic control).

No products indexed under this heading.

Amlodipine Besylate (Calcium channel blocking agents tend to produce hyperglycemia and may lead to loss of glycemic control. When calcium channel blocking agents are administered to a patient receiving Janumet, the patient should be closely observed to maintain adequate glycemic control). Products include:

Azor Tablets 1005
Exforge Tablets 2238

Bendroflumethiazide (Thiazides tend to produce hyperglycemia and may lead to loss of glycemic control. When thiazides are administered to a patient receiving Janumet, the patient should be closely observed to maintain adequate glycemic control).

No products indexed under this heading.

Bepridil Hydrochloride (Calcium channel blocking agents tend to produce hyperglycemia and may lead to loss of glycemic control. When calcium channel blocking agents are administered to a patient receiving Janumet, the patient should be closely observed to maintain adequate glycemic control).

No products indexed under this heading.

Betamethasone Acetate (Corticosteroids tend to produce hyperglycemia and may lead to loss of glycemic control. When corticosteroids are administered to a patient receiving Janumet, the patient should be closely observed to maintain adequate glycemic control).

No products indexed under this heading.

Betamethasone Sodium Phosphate (Corticosteroids tend to produce hyperglycemia and may lead to loss of glycemic control. When corticosteroids are administered to a patient receiving Janumet, the patient should be closely observed to maintain adequate glycemic control).

No products indexed under this heading.

Budesonide (Corticosteroids tend to produce hyperglycemia and may lead to loss of glycemic control. When corticosteroids are administered to a patient receiving Janumet, the patient should be closely observed to maintain adequate glycemic control). Products include:

Pulmicort Flexhaler 654
Symbicort 80/4.5 Inhalation Aerosol 659
Symbicort 160/4.5 Inhalation Aerosol 659

Bumetanide (Diuretics tend to produce hyperglycemia and may lead to loss of glycemic control. When diuretics are administered to a patient receiving Janumet, the patient should be closely observed to maintain adequate glycemic control).

No products indexed under this heading.

Chlorothiazide (Thiazides tend to produce hyperglycemia and may lead to loss of glycemic control. When thiazides are administered to a patient receiving Janumet, the patient should be closely observed to maintain adequate glycemic control).

No products indexed under this heading.

Chlorothiazide Sodium (Thiazides tend to produce hyperglycemia and may lead to loss of glycemic control. When thiazides are administered to a patient receiving Janumet, the patient should be closely observed to maintain adequate glycemic control). Products include:

Intravenous Sodium Diuril 2490

Chlorotrianisene (Estrogens tend to produce hyperglycemia and may lead to loss of glycemic control. When estrogens are administered to a patient receiving Janumet, the patient should be closely observed to maintain adequate glycemic control).

No products indexed under this heading.

Chlorpromazine (Phenothiazines tend to produce hyperglycemia and may lead to loss of glycemic control. When phenothiazines are administered to a patient receiving Janumet, the patient should be closely observed to maintain adequate glycemic control).

No products indexed under this heading.

Chlorpromazine Hydrochloride (Phenothiazines tend to produce hyperglycemia and may lead to loss of glycemic control. When phenothiazines are administered to a patient receiving Janumet, the patient should be closely observed to maintain adequate glycemic control).

No products indexed under this heading.

Chlorpropamide (Patients also receiving an insulin secretagogue (e.g., sulfonylurea, meglitinide) may require a lower dose of the insulin secretagogue to reduce the risk of hypoglycemia).

No products indexed under this heading.

Chlorthalidone (Diuretics tend to produce hyperglycemia and may lead to loss of glycemic control. When diuretics are administered to a patient receiving Janumet, the patient should be closely observed to maintain adequate glycemic control). Products include:

Clorpres Tablets 2185

Ciclesonide (Corticosteroids tend to produce hyperglycemia and may lead to loss of glycemic control. When corticosteroids are administered to a patient receiving Janumet, the patient should be closely observed to maintain adequate glycemic control). Products include:

Alvesco Inhalation Aerosol 2985
Omnaris Nasal Spray 2998

Cortisone Acetate (Corticosteroids tend to produce hyperglycemia and may lead to loss of glycemic control. When corticosteroids are administered to a patient receiving Janumet, the patient should be closely observed to maintain adequate glycemic control).

No products indexed under this heading.

Cyclosporine (Cyclosporine is a potent inhibitor of p-glycoprotein. Co-administration of 600 mg oral dose of cyclosprone with 100 mg of sitagliptin shows an increase in area under the curve (AUC) and maximum concentration (Cmax) of sitagliptin). Products include:

Gengraf Capsules 435
Neoral Oral Solution 2280
Neoral Soft Gelatin Capsules 2280
Restasis Ophthalmic Emulsion 557
Sandimmune 2296

Desogestrel (Oral contraceptives tend to produce hyperglycemia and may lead to loss of glycemic control. When oral contraceptives are administered to a patient receiving Janumet, the patient should be closely observed to maintain adequate glycemic control). Products include:

Mircette Tablets 1034

Dexamethasone (Corticosteroids tend to produce hyperglycemia and may lead to loss of glycemic control. When corticosteroids are administered to a patient receiving Janumet, the patient should be closely observed to maintain adequate glycemic control). Products include:

Ciprodex Otic Suspension 541

Dexamethasone Acetate (Corticosteroids tend to produce hyperglycemia and may lead to loss of glycemic control. When corticosteroids are administered to a patient receiving Janumet, the patient should be closely observed to maintain adequate glycemic control).

No products indexed under this heading.

Dexamethasone Sodium Phosphate (Corticosteroids tend to produce hyperglycemia and may lead to loss of glycemic control. When corticosteroids are administered to a patient receiving Janumet, the patient should be closely observed to maintain adequate glycemic control).

No products indexed under this heading.

Dienestrol (Estrogens tend to produce hyperglycemia and may lead to loss of glycemic control. When estrogens are administered to a patient receiving Janumet, the patient should be closely observed to maintain adequate glycemic control).

No products indexed under this heading.

Diethylstilbestrol (Estrogens tend to produce hyperglycemia and may lead to loss of glycemic control. When estrogens are administered to a patient receiving Janumet, the patient should be closely observed to maintain adequate glycemic control).
No products indexed under this heading.

Digoxin (Digoxin, a cationic drug, has the potential to compete with metformin for common renal tubular transport systems, thus affecting the serum concentrations of either digoxin, metformin or both. Patients receiving digoxin should be monitored appropriately. No dosage adjustment if digoxin or Janumet is recommended. There was a slight increase in the area under the curve (AUC, 11%) and mean peak drug concentration (Cmax, 18%) of digoxin with the co-administration of 100 mg sitagliptin for 10 days). Products include:
Lanoxin Injection **1498**
Lanoxin Injection Pediatric **1502**
Lanoxin Tablets **1505**

Diltiazem Hydrochloride (Calcium channel blocking agents tend to produce hyperglycemia and may lead to loss of glycemic control. When calcium channel blocking agents are administered to a patient receiving Janumet, the patient should be closely observed to maintain adequate glycemic control). Products include:
Cardizem LA Extended Release Tablets **421**

Dobutamine Hydrochloride (Sympathomimetics tend to produce hyperglycemia and may lead to loss of glycemic control. When sympathomimetics are administered to a patient receiving Janumet, the patient should be closely observed to maintain adequate glycemic control).
No products indexed under this heading.

Dopamine Hydrochloride (Sympathomimetics tend to produce hyperglycemia and may lead to loss of glycemic control. When sympathomimetics are administered to a patient receiving Janumet, the patient should be closely observed to maintain adequate glycemic control).
No products indexed under this heading.

Ephedrine Hydrochloride (Sympathomimetics tend to produce hyperglycemia and may lead to loss of glycemic control. When sympathomimetics are administered to a patient receiving Janumet, the patient should be closely observed to maintain adequate glycemic control).
No products indexed under this heading.

Ephedrine Sulfate (Sympathomimetics tend to produce hyperglycemia and may lead to loss of glycemic control. When sympathomimetics are administered to a patient receiving Janumet, the patient should be closely observed to maintain adequate glycemic control).
No products indexed under this heading.

Ephedrine Tannate (Sympathomimetics tend to produce hyperglycemia and may lead to loss of glycemic control. When sympathomimetics are administered to a patient receiving Janumet, the patient should be closely observed to maintain adequate glycemic control).
No products indexed under this heading.

Epinephrine (Sympathomimetics tend to produce hyperglycemia and may lead to loss of glycemic control. When sympathomimetics are administered to a patient receiving Janumet, the patient should be closely observed to maintain adequate glycemic control). Products include:
EpiPen **1024**

Epinephrine Bitartrate (Sympathomimetics tend to produce hyperglycemia and may lead to loss of glycemic control. When sympathomimetics are administered to a patient receiving Janumet, the patient should be closely observed to maintain adequate glycemic control).
No products indexed under this heading.

Epinephrine Hydrochloride (Sympathomimetics tend to produce hyperglycemia and may lead to loss of glycemic control. When sympathomimetics are administered to a patient receiving Janumet, the patient should be closely observed to maintain adequate glycemic control).
No products indexed under this heading.

Estradiol (Estrogens tend to produce hyperglycemia and may lead to loss of glycemic control. When estrogens are administered to a patient receiving Janumet, the patient should be closely observed to maintain adequate glycemic control). Products include:
Activella Tablets **2347**
Angeliq Tablets **751**
Climara Transdermal System **763**
Climara Pro Transdermal System **768**
Divigel **3167**
Vagifem Tablets **2375**

Estrogens, Conjugated (Estrogens tend to produce hyperglycemia and may lead to loss of glycemic control. When estrogens are administered to a patient receiving Janumet, the patient should be closely observed to maintain adequate glycemic control). Products include:
Premarin Intravenous **3217**
Premarin Tablets **3221**
Premarin Vaginal Cream **3228**
Premphase Tablets **3232**
Prempro Tablets **3232**

Estrogens, Esterified (Estrogens tend to produce hyperglycemia and may lead to loss of glycemic control. When estrogens are administered to a patient receiving Janumet, the patient should be closely observed to maintain adequate glycemic control). Products include:
Estratest Tablets **3043**
Estratest H.S. Tablets **3043**

Estropipate (Estrogens tend to produce hyperglycemia and may lead to loss of glycemic control. When estrogens are administered to a patient receiving Janumet, the patient should be closely observed to maintain adequate glycemic control).
No products indexed under this heading.

Ethacrynic Acid (Diuretics tend to produce hyperglycemia and may lead to loss of glycemic control. When diuretics are administered to a patient receiving Janumet, the patient should be closely observed to maintain adequate glycemic control). Products include:
Edecrin Tablets **698**

Ethinyl Estradiol (Estrogens tend to produce hyperglycemia and may lead to loss of glycemic control. When estrogens are administered to a patient receiving Janumet, the patient should be closely observed to maintain adequate glycemic control). Products include:
Lybrel Tablets **3204**
Mircette Tablets **1034**
NuvaRing **2897**
Ortho-Cyclen/Ortho Tri-Cyclen **2449**
Ortho Evra Transdermal System **2437**
Ortho Tri-Cyclen Lo Tablets **2458**
Seasonique Tablets **1046**
Yaz Tablets **805**

Ethynodiol Diacetate (Oral contraceptives tend to produce hyperglycemia and may lead to loss of glycemic control. When oral contraceptives are administered to a patient receiving Janumet, the patient should be closely observed to maintain adequate glycemic control).
No products indexed under this heading.

Felodipine (Calcium channel blocking agents tend to produce hyperglycemia and may lead to loss of glycemic control. When calcium channel blocking agents are administered to a patient receiving Janumet, the patient should be closely observed to maintain adequate glycemic control).
No products indexed under this heading.

Fludrocortisone Acetate (Corticosteroids tend to produce hyperglycemia and may lead to loss of glycemic control. When corticosteroids are administered to a patient receiving Janumet, the patient should be closely observed to maintain adequate glycemic control).
No products indexed under this heading.

Flunisolide (Corticosteroids tend to produce hyperglycemia and may lead to loss of glycemic control. When corticosteroids are administered to a patient receiving Janumet, the patient should be closely observed to maintain adequate glycemic control). Products include:
Aerobid/Aerobid-M **1153**

Fluphenazine Decanoate (Phenothiazines tend to produce hyperglycemia and may lead to loss of glycemic control. When phenothiazines are administered to a patient receiving Janumet, the patient should be closely observed to maintain adequate glycemic control).
No products indexed under this heading.

Fluphenazine Enanthate (Phenothiazines tend to produce hyperglycemia and may lead to loss of glycemic control. When phenothiazines are administered to a patient receiving Janumet, the patient should be closely observed to maintain adequate glycemic control).
No products indexed under this heading.

Fluphenazine Hydrochloride (Phenothiazines tend to produce hyperglycemia and may lead to loss of glycemic control. When phenothiazines are administered to a patient receiving Janumet, the patient should be closely observed to maintain adequate glycemic control).
No products indexed under this heading.

Fluticasone Propionate (Corticosteroids tend to produce hyperglycemia and may lead to loss of glycemic control. When corticosteroids are administered to a patient receiving Janumet, the patient should be closely observed to maintain adequate glycemic control). Products include:
Advair Diskus 100/50 .... **1276**
Advair Diskus 250/50 .... **1276**
Advair Diskus 500/50 .... **1276**
Advair HFA 45/21 Inhalation Aerosol **1288**
Advair HFA 115/21 Inhalation Aerosol **1288**
Advair HFA 230/21 Inhalation Aerosol **1288**
Flonase Nasal Spray **1431**
Flovent Diskus 50 mcg **1435**

Fluticasone Propionate HFA (Corticosteroids tend to produce hyperglycemia and may lead to loss of glycemic control. When corticosteroids are administered to a patient receiving Janumet, the patient should be closely observed to maintain adequate glycemic control). Products include:
Flovent HFA **1440**

Fosphenytoin Sodium (Phenytoin tends to produce hyperglycemia and may lead to loss of glycemic control. When phenytoin is administered to a patient receiving Janumet, the patient should be closely observed to maintain adequate glycemic control).
No products indexed under this heading.

Furosemide (Furosemide has been shown to increase the metformin plasma and blood Cmax by 22% and blood AUC by 15%, without any significant change in metformin renal clearance. When administered with metformin, there may be a decrease in Cmax and AUC of furosemide than when administered alone, and the terminal half-life of metformin may be decreased without any significant change in furosemide renal clearance. Diuretics tend to produce hyperglycemia and may lead to loss of glycemic control. When diuretics are administered to a patient receiving sitagliptin/metformin HCL, the patient should be closely observed to maintain adequate glycemic control). Products include:
Furosemide Tablets **2186**

Glimepiride (Patients also receiving an insulin secretagogue (e.g., sulfonylurea, meglitinide) may require a lower dose of the insulin secretagogue to reduce the risk of hypoglycemia). Products include:
Avandaryl Tablets **1344**
Duetact Tablets **3085**

Glipizide (Patients also receiving an insulin secretagogue (e.g., sulfonylurea, meglitinide) may require a lower dose of the insulin secretagogue to reduce the risk of hypoglycemia).
No products indexed under this heading.

Glyburide (A decrease in glyburide area under the curve (AUC) and mean peak drug concentration (Cmax) were observed but were highly variable in a single-dose interaction study in type 2 diabetes patients when co-administering metforming with glyburide).
No products indexed under this heading.

Hydrochlorothiazide (Thiazides tend to produce hyperglycemia and may lead to loss of glycemic control. When thiazides are administered to a patient receiving Janumet, the patient should be closely observed to maintain adequate glycemic control). Products include:
Atacand HCT 642
Avalide Tablets 892
Avalide Tablets 2713
Benicar HCT Tablets 1010
Diovan HCT Tablets 2216
Dyazide Capsules 1405
Micardis HCT Tablets 854
Prinzide Tablets 2092
Tekturna HCT Tablets 2324
Teveten HCT Tablets 517

Hydrocortisone (Corticosteroids tend to produce hyperglycemia and may lead to loss of glycemic control. When corticosteroids are administered to a patient receiving Janumet, the patient should be closely observed to maintain adequate glycemic control).
No products indexed under this heading.

Hydrocortisone Acetate (Corticosteroids tend to produce hyperglycemia and may lead to loss of glycemic control. When corticosteroids are administered to a patient receiving Janumet, the patient should be closely observed to maintain adequate glycemic control). Products include:
Analpram-HC 1140
Pramosone 1141

Hydrocortisone Sodium Phosphate (Corticosteroids tend to produce hyperglycemia and may lead to loss of glycemic control. When corticosteroids are administered to a patient receiving Janumet, the patient should be closely observed to maintain adequate glycemic control).
No products indexed under this heading.

Hydrocortisone Sodium Succinate (Corticosteroids tend to produce hyperglycemia and may lead to loss of glycemic control. When corticosteroids are administered to a patient receiving Janumet, the patient should be closely observed to maintain adequate glycemic control).
No products indexed under this heading.

Hydroflumethiazide (Thiazides tend to produce hyperglycemia and may lead to loss of glycemic control. When thiazides are administered to a patient receiving Janumet, the patient should be closely observed to maintain adequate glycemic control).
No products indexed under this heading.

Indapamide (Diuretics tend to produce hyperglycemia and may lead to loss of glycemic control. When diuretics are administered to a patient receiving Janumet, the patient should be closely observed to maintain adequate glycemic control). Products include:
Indapamide Tablets 2188

Isoniazid (Isoniazides tend to produce hyperglycemia and may lead to loss of glycemic control. When isoniazides are administered to a patient receiving Janumet, the patient should be closely observed to maintain adequate glycemic control).
No products indexed under this heading.

Isoproterenol Hydrochloride (Sympathomimetics tend to produce hyperglycemia and may lead to loss of glycemic control. When sympathomimetics are administered to a patient receiving Janumet, the patient should be closely observed to maintain adequate glycemic control).
No products indexed under this heading.

Isoproterenol Sulfate (Sympathomimetics tend to produce hyperglycemia and may lead to loss of glycemic control. When sympathomimetics are administered to a patient receiving Janumet, the patient should be closely observed to maintain adequate glycemic control).
No products indexed under this heading.

Isradipine (Calcium channel blocking agents tend to produce hyperglycemia and may lead to loss of glycemic control. When calcium channel blocking agents are administered to a patient receiving Janumet, the patient should be closely observed to maintain adequate glycemic control). Products include:
DynaCirc CR Controlled Release Tablets 1407

Levalbuterol Hydrochloride (Sympathomimetics tend to produce hyperglycemia and may lead to loss of glycemic control. When sympathomimetics are administered to a patient receiving Janumet, the patient should be closely observed to maintain adequate glycemic control). Products include:
Xopenex Inhalation Solution 3001
Xopenex Inhalation Solution Concentrate 3005

Levonorgestrel (Oral contraceptives tend to produce hyperglycemia and may lead to loss of glycemic control. When oral contraceptives are administered to a patient receiving Janumet, the patient should be closely observed to maintain adequate glycemic control). Products include:
Climara Pro Transdermal System 768
Lybrel Tablets 3204
Mirena Intrauterine System 779
Plan B Tablets 1044
Seasonique Tablets 1046

Levothyroxine Sodium (Thyroid products tend to produce hyperglycemia and may lead to loss of glycemic control. When thyroid products are administered to a patient receiving Janumet, the patient should be closely observed to maintain adequate glycemic control). Products include:
Levothroid Tablets 1170
Levoxyl Tablets 1780
Synthroid Tablets 507

Liothyronine Sodium (Thyroid products tend to produce hyperglycemia and may lead to loss of glycemic control. When thyroid products are administered to a patient receiving Janumet, the patient should be closely observed to maintain adequate glycemic control). Products include:
Cytomel Tablets 1778

Liotrix (Thyroid products tend to produce hyperglycemia and may lead to loss of glycemic control. When thyroid products are administered to a patient receiving Janumet, the patient should be closely observed to maintain adequate glycemic control).
No products indexed under this heading.

Mesoridazine Besylate (Phenothiazines tend to produce hyperglycemia and may lead to loss of glycemic control. When phenothiazines are administered to a patient receiving Janumet, the patient should be closely observed to maintain adequate glycemic control).
No products indexed under this heading.

Mestranol (Oral contraceptives tend to produce hyperglycemia and may lead to loss of glycemic control. When oral contraceptives are administered to a patient receiving Janumet, the patient should be closely observed to maintain adequate glycemic control).
No products indexed under this heading.

Metaproterenol Sulfate (Sympathomimetics tend to produce hyperglycemia and may lead to loss of glycemic control. When sympathomimetics are administered to a patient receiving Janumet, the patient should be closely observed to maintain adequate glycemic control).
No products indexed under this heading.

Metaraminol Bitartrate (Sympathomimetics tend to produce hyperglycemia and may lead to loss of glycemic control. When sympathomimetics are administered to a patient receiving Janumet, the patient should be closely observed to maintain adequate glycemic control).
No products indexed under this heading.

Methotrimeprazine (Phenothiazines tend to produce hyperglycemia and may lead to loss of glycemic control. When phenothiazines are administered to a patient receiving Janumet, the patient should be closely observed to maintain adequate glycemic control).
No products indexed under this heading.

Methoxamine Hydrochloride (Sympathomimetics tend to produce hyperglycemia and may lead to loss of glycemic control. When sympathomimetics are administered to a patient receiving Janumet, the patient should be closely observed to maintain adequate glycemic control).
No products indexed under this heading.

Methyclothiazide (Thiazides tend to produce hyperglycemia and may lead to loss of glycemic control. When thiazides are administered to a patient receiving Janumet, the patient should be closely observed to maintain adequate glycemic control).
No products indexed under this heading.

Methylprednisolone Acetate (Corticosteroids tend to produce hyperglycemia and may lead to loss of glycemic control. When corticosteroids are administered to a patient receiving Janumet, the patient should be closely observed to maintain adequate glycemic control).
No products indexed under this heading.

Methylprednisolone Sodium Succinate (Corticosteroids tend to produce hyperglycemia and may lead to loss of glycemic control. When corticosteroids are administered to a patient receiving Janumet, the patient should be closely observed to maintain adequate glycemic control).
No products indexed under this heading.

Metolazone (Diuretics tend to produce hyperglycemia and may lead to loss of glycemic control. When diuretics are administered to a patient receiving Janumet, the patient should be closely observed to maintain adequate glycemic control).
No products indexed under this heading.

Mibefradil Dihydrochloride (Calcium channel blocking agents tend to produce hyperglycemia and may lead to loss of glycemic control. When calcium channel blocking agents are administered to a patient receiving Janumet, the patient should be closely observed to maintain adequate glycemic control).
No products indexed under this heading.

Miglitol (Patients also receiving an insulin secretagogue (e.g., sulfonylurea, meglitinide) may require a lower dose of the insulin secretagogue to reduce the risk of hypoglycemia).
No products indexed under this heading.

Mometasone Furoate (Corticosteroids tend to produce hyperglycemia and may lead to loss of glycemic control. When corticosteroids are administered to a patient receiving Janumet, the patient should be closely observed to maintain adequate glycemic control). Products include:
Asmanex Twisthaler 2797
Elocon Cream 0.1% 2840
Elocon Lotion 0.1% 2841
Elocon Ointment 0.1% 2842

Mometasone Furoate Monohydrate (Corticosteroids tend to produce hyperglycemia and may lead to loss of glycemic control. When corticosteroids are administered to a patient receiving Janumet, the patient should be closely observed to maintain adequate glycemic control). Products include:
Nasonex Nasal Spray 2883

Morphine Sulfate (Cationic drugs that are eliminated by renal tubular secretion theoretically have the potential for interaction with metformin by competing for common renal tubular transport systems. Careful patient monitoring and dose adjustment of Janumet and/or interfering drug is recommended in patients taking cationic medications that are excreted via the proximal renal tubular secretory system). Products include:
Avinza Capsules 1772
DepoDur Injection 1095

MS Contin Tablets 2585

Nateglinide (Patients also receiving an insulin secretagogue (e.g., sulfonylurea, meglitinide) may require a lower dose of the insulin secretagogue to reduce the risk of hypoglycemia). Products include:

Starlix Tablets 2314

Nicardipine Hydrochloride (Calcium channel blocking agents tend to produce hyperglycemia and may lead to loss of glycemic control. When calcium channel blocking agents are administered to a patient receiving Janumet, the patient should be closely observed to maintain adequate glycemic control). Products include:

Cardene I.V. 1093

Nicotinic Acid (Nicotinic acid tends to produce hyperglycemia and may lead to loss of glycemic control. When nicotinic acid is administered to a patient receiving Janumet, the patient should be closely observed to maintain adequate glycemic control).

No products indexed under this heading.

Nifedipine (A single-dose, metformin-nifedipine drug interaction study in normal healthy volunteers demonstrated an increase in plasma metformin Cmax and AUC by 10% to 9%, respectively in co-administering metformin with nifedipine and increased the amount excreted in the urine. Nifedipine appears to enhance the absorption of metforming. Metformin had minimal effects on nifedipine).

No products indexed under this heading.

Nimodipine (Calcium channel blocking agents tend to produce hyperglycemia and may lead to loss of glycemic control. When calcium channel blocking agents are administered to a patient receiving Janumet, the patient should be closely observed to maintain adequate glycemic control). Products include:

Nimotop Capsules 790

Nisoldipine (Calcium channel blocking agents tend to produce hyperglycemia and may lead to loss of glycemic control. When calcium channel blocking agents are administered to a patient receiving Janumet, the patient should be closely observed to maintain adequate glycemic control). Products include:

Sular Extended Release Tablets 2975

Norepinephrine Bitartrate (Sympathomimetics tend to produce hyperglycemia and may lead to loss of glycemic control. When sympathomimetics are administered to a patient receiving Janumet, the patient should be closely observed to maintain adequate glycemic control).

No products indexed under this heading.

Norethindrone (Oral contraceptives tend to produce hyperglycemia and may lead to loss of glycemic control. When oral contraceptives are administered to a patient receiving Janumet, the patient should be closely observed to maintain adequate glycemic control). Products include:

Ortho Micronor Tablets 2446

Norethynodrel (Oral contraceptives tend to produce hyperglycemia and may lead to loss of glycemic control. When oral contraceptives are administered to a patient receiving Janumet, the patient should be closely observed to maintain adequate glycemic control).

No products indexed under this heading.

Norgestimate (Oral contraceptives tend to produce hyperglycemia and may lead to loss of glycemic control. When oral contraceptives are administered to a patient receiving Janumet, the patient should be closely observed to maintain adequate glycemic control). Products include:

Ortho-Cyclen/Ortho Tri-Cyclen 2449
Ortho Tri-Cyclen Lo Tablets 2458

Norgestrel (Oral contraceptives tend to produce hyperglycemia and may lead to loss of glycemic control. When oral contraceptives are administered to a patient receiving Janumet, the patient should be closely observed to maintain adequate glycemic control).

No products indexed under this heading.

Perphenazine (Phenothiazines tend to produce hyperglycemia and may lead to loss of glycemic control. When phenothiazines are administered to a patient receiving Janumet, the patient should be closely observed to maintain adequate glycemic control).

No products indexed under this heading.

Phenylephrine Bitartrate (Sympathomimetics tend to produce hyperglycemia and may lead to loss of glycemic control. When sympathomimetics are administered to a patient receiving Janumet, the patient should be closely observed to maintain adequate glycemic control).

No products indexed under this heading.

Phenylephrine Hydrochloride (Sympathomimetics tend to produce hyperglycemia and may lead to loss of glycemic control. When sympathomimetics are administered to a patient receiving Janumet, the patient should be closely observed to maintain adequate glycemic control). Products include:

Actifed Cold & Allergy Tablets 1895
Benadryl Allergy & Cold Kapgels 1895
Benadryl Allergy & Sinus Headache Kapgels 1895
Benadryl Severe Allergy & Sinus Headache Caplets 1897
Children's Benadryl-D Allergy & Sinus Liquid 1896
Benadryl-D Allergy & Sinus Tablet 1896
PediaCare Children's Allergy & Cold Liquid 1902
PediaCare Children's Decongestant Liquid 1902
PediaCare Children's Liquid Multi-Symptom Cold 1902
Sinutab Non-Drying Caplets 1905
Sinutab Sinus Caplets 1905
Children's Sudafed PE Cold & Cough Liquid 1907
Children's Sudafed PE Nasal Decongestant Liquid 1906
Sudafed PE Cold & Cough Caplets 1907
Sudafed PE Nasal Decongestant Tablets 1907
Sudafed PE Nighttime Cold Caplets 1907
Sudafed PE Non-Drying Sinus Caplets 1908
Sudafed PE Severe Cold Caplets 1908
Sudafed PE Sinus & Allergy Tablets 1908
Sudafed PE Sinus Headache Caplets 1908
Tylenol Allergy Multi-Symptom Caplets with Cool Burst and Rapid Release Gelcaps 1916
Tylenol Allergy Multi-Symptom Nighttime Caplets with Cool Burst 1916
Children's Tylenol Plus Cold Suspension Liquid 1912
Children's Tylenol Plus Cold & Allergy Suspension Liquid 1914
Children's Tylenol Plus Flu Suspension Liquid 1914
Children's Tylenol Plus Multi-Symptom Cold Suspension Liquid 1912
Tylenol Cold Head Congestion Daytime Caplets with Cool Burst 1910
Tylenol Cold Head Congestion Nighttime Caplets with Cool Burst 1910
Tylenol Cold Head Congestion Severe Daytime Caplets with Cool Burst 1910
Tylenol Cold Multi-Symptom Daytime Caplets with Cool Burst and Rapid Release Gels 1913
Tylenol Cold Multi-Symptom Daytime Liquid with Citrus Burst ... 1913
Tylenol Cold Multi-Symptom Nighttime Caplets with Cool Burst 1913
Tylenol Cold Multi-Symptom Nighttime Liquid with Cool Burst ... 1913
Tylenol Cold Multi-Symptom Severe Caplets with Cool Burst..... 1913
Tylenol Cold Multi-Symptom Severe Daytime Liquid with Citrus Burst 1913
Tylenol Sinus Congestion & Pain Daytime Caplets with Cool Burst and Gelcaps 1917
Tylenol Sinus Congestion & Pain Nighttime Caplets with Cool Burst 1917
Tylenol Sinus Congestion & Pain Severe Caplets with Cool Burst..... 1917
Vicks DayQuil Cold & Flu Multi-Symptom Relief 616
Vicks DayQuil LiquiCaps 2567
Vicks DayQuil Liquid 2567
Vicks DayQuil Multi-Symptom Cold/Flu Relief 2567

Phenylephrine Tannate (Sympathomimetics tend to produce hyperglycemia and may lead to loss of glycemic control. When sympathomimetics are administered to a patient receiving Janumet, the patient should be closely observed to maintain adequate glycemic control).

No products indexed under this heading.

Phenylpropanolamine Hydrochloride (Sympathomimetics tend to produce hyperglycemia and may lead to loss of glycemic control. When sympathomimetics are administered to a patient receiving Janumet, the patient should be closely observed to maintain adequate glycemic control).

No products indexed under this heading.

Phenytoin (Phenytoin tends to produce hyperglycemia and may lead to loss of glycemic control. When phenytoin is administered to a patient receiving Janumet, the patient should be closely observed to maintain adequate glycemic control).

No products indexed under this heading.

Phenytoin Sodium (Phenytoin tends to produce hyperglycemia and may lead to loss of glycemic control. When phenytoin is administered to a patient receiving Janumet, the patient should be closely observed to maintain adequate glycemic control). Products include:

Phenytek Capsules 2192

Pioglitazone Hydrochloride (Patients also receiving an insulin secretagogue (e.g., sulfonylurea, meglitinide) may require a lower dose of the insulin secretagogue to reduce the risk of hypoglycemia). Products include:

ActoPlus Met Tablets 3071
Actos Tablets 3077
Duetact Tablets 3085

Pirbuterol Acetate (Sympathomimetics tend to produce hyperglycemia and may lead to loss of glycemic control. When sympathomimetics are administered to a patient receiving Janumet, the patient should be closely observed to maintain adequate glycemic control). Products include:

Maxair Autohaler 1705

Polyestradiol Phosphate (Estrogens tend to produce hyperglycemia and may lead to loss of glycemic control. When estrogens are administered to a patient receiving Janumet, the patient should be closely observed to maintain adequate glycemic control).

No products indexed under this heading.

Polythiazide (Thiazides tend to produce hyperglycemia and may lead to loss of glycemic control. When thiazides are administered to a patient receiving Janumet, the patient should be closely observed to maintain adequate glycemic control).

No products indexed under this heading.

Prednisolone Acetate (Corticosteroids tend to produce hyperglycemia and may lead to loss of glycemic control. When corticosteroids are administered to a patient receiving Janumet, the patient should be closely observed to maintain adequate glycemic control). Products include:

Pred Forte Ophthalmic Suspension .... ⊙227
Pred Mild Ophthalmic Suspension .... ⊙230
Pred-G Ophthalmic Ointment .... ⊙229
Pred-G Ophthalmic Suspension ...... ⊙228

Prednisolone Sodium Phosphate (Corticosteroids tend to produce hyperglycemia and may lead to loss of glycemic control. When corticosteroids are administered to a patient receiving Janumet, the patient should be closely observed to maintain adequate glycemic control).

No products indexed under this heading.

Prednisolone Tebutate (Corticosteroids tend to produce hyperglycemia and may lead to loss of glycemic control. When corticosteroids are administered to a patient receiving Janumet, the patient should be closely observed to maintain adequate glycemic control).

No products indexed under this heading.

Prednisone (Corticosteroids tend to produce hyperglycemia and may lead to loss of glycemic control. When corticosteroids are administered to a patient receiving Janumet, the patient should be closely observed to maintain adequate glycemic control).

No products indexed under this heading.

Procainamide Hydrochloride (Cationic drugs that are eliminated by renal tubular secretion theoretically have the potential for interaction with metformin by competing for common renal tubular transport systems. Careful patient monitoring and dose adjustment of Janumet and/or interfering drug is recommended in patients taking cationic medications that are excreted via the proximal renal tubular secretory system).
No products indexed under this heading.

Prochlorperazine (Phenothiazines tend to produce hyperglycemia and may lead to loss of glycemic control. When phenothiazines are administered to a patient receiving Janumet, the patient should be closely observed to maintain adequate glycemic control).
No products indexed under this heading.

Promethazine Hydrochloride (Phenothiazines tend to produce hyperglycemia and may lead to loss of glycemic control. When phenothiazines are administered to a patient receiving Janumet, the patient should be closely observed to maintain adequate glycemic control).
No products indexed under this heading.

Pseudoephedrine Hydrochloride (Sympathomimetics tend to produce hyperglycemia and may lead to loss of glycemic control. When sympathomimetics are administered to a patient receiving Janumet, the patient should be closely observed to maintain adequate glycemic control). Products include:

- Allegra-D 12 Hour Extended-Release Tablets 2687
- Allegra-D 24 Hour Extended-Release Tablets 2690
- Children's Motrin Cold Oral Suspension 1899
- Sudafed 12 Hour Nasal Decongestant Non-Drowsy Caplets 1909
- Sudafed 24 Hour Non-Drowsy Nasal Decongestant Tablets 1906
- Children's Sudafed Nasal Decongestant Liquid 1906
- Sudafed Nasal Decongestant Tablets 1906
- Tylenol Cold Severe Congestion Daytime Caplets with Cool Burst 1912
- Tylenol Sinus Severe Congestion Caplets with Cool Burst 1917
- Vicks NyQuil LiquiCaps 2567
- Vicks NyQuil Liquid 2567
- Vicks NyQuil Multi-Symptom Cold/Flu Relief 2567
- Zyrtec-D 12 Hour Extended Release Tablets 1923
- Zyrtec-D Allergy & Congestion Extended-Release Tablets 1923

Pseudoephedrine Sulfate (Sympathomimetics tend to produce hyperglycemia and may lead to loss of glycemic control. When sympathomimetics are administered to a patient receiving Janumet, the patient should be closely observed to maintain adequate glycemic control). Products include:

- Clarinex-D 12-Hour Extended-Release Tablets 2831
- Clarinex-D 24-Hour Extended-Release Tablets 2834

Quinestrol (Estrogens tend to produce hyperglycemia and may lead to loss of glycemic control. When estrogens are administered to a patient receiving Janumet, the patient should be closely observed to maintain adequate glycemic control).
No products indexed under this heading.

Quinidine Gluconate (Cationic drugs that are eliminated by renal tubular secretion theoretically have the potential for interaction with metformin by competing for common renal tubular transport systems. Careful patient monitoring and dose adjustment of Janumet and/or interfering drug is recommended in patients taking cationic medications that are excreted via the proximal renal tubular secretory system).
No products indexed under this heading.

Quinidine Polygalacturonate (Cationic drugs that are eliminated by renal tubular secretion theoretically have the potential for interaction with metformin by competing for common renal tubular transport systems. Careful patient monitoring and dose adjustment of Janumet and/or interfering drug is recommended in patients taking cationic medications that are excreted via the proximal renal tubular secretory system).
No products indexed under this heading.

Quinidine Sulfate (Cationic drugs that are eliminated by renal tubular secretion theoretically have the potential for interaction with metformin by competing for common renal tubular transport systems. Careful patient monitoring and dose adjustment of Janumet and/or interfering drug is recommended in patients taking cationic medications that are excreted via the proximal renal tubular secretory system).
No products indexed under this heading.

Quinine Sulfate (Cationic drugs that are eliminated by renal tubular secretion theoretically have the potential for interaction with metformin by competing for common renal tubular transport systems. Careful patient monitoring and dose adjustment of Janumet and/or interfering drug is recommended in patients taking cationic medications that are excreted via the proximal renal tubular secretory system).
No products indexed under this heading.

Ranitidine Hydrochloride (Cationic drugs that are eliminated by renal tubular secretion theoretically have the potential for interaction with metformin by competing for common renal tubular transport systems. Careful patient monitoring and dose adjustment of Janumet and/or interfering drug is recommended in patients taking cationic medications that are excreted via the proximal renal tubular secretory system). Products include:

- Zantac 75 Tablets .... ▣603
- Zantac 1670
- Zantac Injection 1666
- Zantac Injection Pharmacy Bulk Package 1668
- Maximum Strength Zantac 150 Tablets .... ▣603
- Maximum Strength Zantac 150 Cool Mint Tablets .... ▣603

Repaglinide (Patients also receiving an insulin secretagogue (e.g., sulfonylurea, meglitinide) may require a lower dose of the insulin secretagogue to reduce the risk of hypoglycemia). Products include:

- PrandiMet Tablets 2967
- Prandin Tablets 2971

Rosiglitazone Maleate (Patients also receiving an insulin secretagogue (e.g., sulfonylurea, meglitinide) may require a lower dose of the insulin secretagogue to reduce the risk of hypoglycemia). Products include:

- Avandamet Tablets 1336
- Avandaryl Tablets 1344
- Avandia Tablets 1351

Salmeterol Xinafoate (Sympathomimetics tend to produce hyperglycemia and may lead to loss of glycemic control. When sympathomimetics are administered to a patient receiving Janumet, the patient should be closely observed to maintain adequate glycemic control). Products include:

- Advair Diskus 100/50 1276
- Advair Diskus 250/50 1276
- Advair Diskus 500/50 1276
- Advair HFA 45/21 Inhalation Aerosol 1288
- Advair HFA 115/21 Inhalation Aerosol 1288
- Advair HFA 230/21 Inhalation Aerosol 1288
- Serevent Diskus 1594

Spironolactone (Diuretics tend to produce hyperglycemia and may lead to loss of glycemic control. When diuretics are administered to a patient receiving Janumet, the patient should be closely observed to maintain adequate glycemic control).
No products indexed under this heading.

Terbutaline Sulfate (Sympathomimetics tend to produce hyperglycemia and may lead to loss of glycemic control. When sympathomimetics are administered to a patient receiving Janumet, the patient should be closely observed to maintain adequate glycemic control).
No products indexed under this heading.

Thioridazine Hydrochloride (Phenothiazines tend to produce hyperglycemia and may lead to loss of glycemic control. When phenothiazines are administered to a patient receiving Janumet, the patient should be closely observed to maintain adequate glycemic control). Products include:

- Thioridazine Hydrochloride Tablets 2195

Thyroglobulin (Thyroid products tend to produce hyperglycemia and may lead to loss of glycemic control. When thyroid products are administered to a patient receiving Janumet, the patient should be closely observed to maintain adequate glycemic control).
No products indexed under this heading.

Thyroid (Thyroid products tend to produce hyperglycemia and may lead to loss of glycemic control. When thyroid products are administered to a patient receiving Janumet, the patient should be closely observed to maintain adequate glycemic control). Products include:

- Naturethroid Tablets 2605

Thyroxine (Thyroid products tend to produce hyperglycemia and may lead to loss of glycemic control. When thyroid products are administered to a patient receiving Janumet, the patient should be closely observed to maintain adequate glycemic control).
No products indexed under this heading.

Thyroxine Sodium (Thyroid products tend to produce hyperglycemia and may lead to loss of glycemic control. When thyroid products are administered to a patient receiving Janumet, the patient should be closely observed to maintain adequate glycemic control).
No products indexed under this heading.

Tolazamide (Patients also receiving an insulin secretagogue (e.g., sulfonylurea, meglitinide) may require a lower dose of the insulin secretagogue to reduce the risk of hypoglycemia).
No products indexed under this heading.

Tolbutamide (Patients also receiving an insulin secretagogue (e.g., sulfonylurea, meglitinide) may require a lower dose of the insulin secretagogue to reduce the risk of hypoglycemia).
No products indexed under this heading.

Torsemide (Diuretics tend to produce hyperglycemia and may lead to loss of glycemic control. When diuretics are administered to a patient receiving Janumet, the patient should be closely observed to maintain adequate glycemic control). Products include:

- Demadex Injection 2630
- Demadex Tablets 2630

Triamcinolone (Corticosteroids tend to produce hyperglycemia and may lead to loss of glycemic control. When corticosteroids are administered to a patient receiving Janumet, the patient should be closely observed to maintain adequate glycemic control).
No products indexed under this heading.

Triamcinolone Acetonide (Corticosteroids tend to produce hyperglycemia and may lead to loss of glycemic control. When corticosteroids are administered to a patient receiving Janumet, the patient should be closely observed to maintain adequate glycemic control). Products include:

- Azmacort Inhalation Aerosol 407
- Nasacort AQ Nasal Spray 2765
- Triesence Injectable Suspension .... ⊙209

Triamcinolone Diacetate (Corticosteroids tend to produce hyperglycemia and may lead to loss of glycemic control. When corticosteroids are administered to a patient receiving Janumet, the patient should be closely observed to maintain adequate glycemic control).
No products indexed under this heading.

Triamcinolone Hexacetonide (Corticosteroids tend to produce hyperglycemia and may lead to loss of glycemic control. When corticosteroids are administered to a patient receiving Janumet, the patient should be closely observed to maintain adequate glycemic control).
No products indexed under this heading.

Triamterene (Diuretics tend to produce hyperglycemia and may lead to loss of glycemic control. When diuretics are administered to a patient receiving Janumet, the patient should be closely observed to maintain adequate glycemic control). Products include:
Dyazide Capsules 1405
Dyrenium Capsules 3189

Trifluoperazine Hydrochloride (Phenothiazines tend to produce hyperglycemia and may lead to loss of glycemic control. When phenothiazines are administered to a patient receiving Janumet, the patient should be closely observed to maintain adequate glycemic control).
No products indexed under this heading.

Trimethoprim (Cationic drugs that are eliminated by renal tubular secretion theoretically have the potential for interaction with metformin by competing for common renal tubular transport systems. Careful patient monitoring and dose adjustment of Janumet and/or interfering drug is recommended in patients taking cationic medications that are excreted via the proximal renal tubular secretory system).
No products indexed under this heading.

Trimethoprim Sulfate (Cationic drugs that are eliminated by renal tubular secretion theoretically have the potential for interaction with metformin by competing for common renal tubular transport systems. Careful patient monitoring and dose adjustment of Janumet and/or interfering drug is recommended in patients taking cationic medications that are excreted via the proximal renal tubular secretory system).
No products indexed under this heading.

Troglitazone (Patients also receiving an insulin secretagogue (e.g., sulfonylurea, meglitinide) may require a lower dose of the insulin secretagogue to reduce the risk of hypoglycemia).
No products indexed under this heading.

Vancomycin Hydrochloride (Cationic drugs that are eliminated by renal tubular secretion theoretically have the potential for interaction with metformin by competing for common renal tubular transport systems. Careful patient monitoring and dose adjustment of Janumet and/or interfering drug is recommended in patients taking cationic medications that are excreted via the proximal renal tubular secretory system).
No products indexed under this heading.

Verapamil Hydrochloride (Calcium channel blocking agents tend to produce hyperglycemia and may lead to loss of glycemic control. When calcium channel blocking agents are administered to a patient receiving Janumet, the patient should be closely observed to maintain adequate glycemic control). Products include:
Tarka Tablets 511

JANUVIA TABLETS

(Sitagliptin Phosphate) 2048
May interact with:

Digoxin (Co-administration may increase digoxin levels. Patients receiving digoxin should be monitored appropriately. No dosage adjustment of digoxin or sitagliptin phosphate is recommended). Products include:
Lanoxin Injection 1498
Lanoxin Injection Pediatric 1502
Lanoxin Tablets 1505

KALETRA ORAL SOLUTION

(Lopinavir, Ritonavir) 452
See Kaletra Tablets

KALETRA TABLETS

(Lopinavir, Ritonavir) 452
May interact with cytochrome p450 3a inducers (selected), dexamethasone, dihydropyridine calcium channel blockers, ergot-containing drugs, phenytoin, quinidine, and certain other agents. Compounds in these categories include:

Abacavir Sulfate (Kaletra induces glucuronidation; therefore, Kaletra has the potential to reduce abacavir plasma concentrations; the clinical significance is unknown). Products include:
Epzicom Tablets 1422
Trizivir Tablets 1622
Ziagen 1673

Allium sativum (Co-administration is contraindicated with potent CYP3A4 inducers where significantly reduced lopinavir plasma concentrations may be associated with the potential for loss of virologic response and possible resistance and cross-resistance).
No products indexed under this heading.

Amiodarone Hydrochloride (Co-administration can result in increased amiodarone plasma concentrations; caution and monitoring is recommended).
No products indexed under this heading.

Amlodipine Besylate (Increased plasma concentrations of dihydropyridine calcium channel blockers; caution is warranted and clinical monitoring of patients is recommended). Products include:
Azor Tablets 1005
Exforge Tablets 2238

Amprenavir (Co-administration may result in increased amprenavir plasma concentration. Kaletra should not be administered once-daily in combination with amprenavir).
No products indexed under this heading.

Aprepitant (Co-administration is contraindicated with potent CYP3A4 inducers where significantly reduced lopinavir plasma concentrations may be associated with the potential for loss of virologic response and possible resistance and cross-resistance). Products include:
Emend Capsules 1992

Astemizole (Kaletra is an inhibitor of the CYP450 3A. Co-administration with drugs that are highly dependent on CYP450 3A for clearance and for which elevated plasma concentrations are associated with serious and/or life threatening events, such as astemizole, is contraindicated).
No products indexed under this heading.

Atorvastatin Calcium (Co-administration with HMG-CoA reductase inhibitors that are metabolized by the CYP3A pathway, such as atorvastatin, increases the risk of myopathy including rhabdomyolysis; caution is recommended). Products include:
Lipitor Tablets 2501

Atovaquone (Co-administration can result in decreased atovaquone plasma concentrations; clinical significance is unknown; however, increase in atovaquone doses may be needed). Products include:
Malarone Pediatric Tablets 1521
Malarone Tablets 1521
Mepron Suspension 1526

Bepridil Hydrochloride (Co-administration can result in increased bepridil plasma concentrations; caution and monitoring is recommended).
No products indexed under this heading.

Carbamazepine (Co-administration can result in decreased lopinavir plasma concentrations; Kaletra may be less effective due to decreased lopinavir plasma concentrations; use with caution). Products include:
Carbatrol Capsules 3019
Equetro Extended-Release Capsules 3174

Cisapride (Kaletra is an inhibitor of the CYP450 3A. Co-administration with drugs that are highly dependent on CYP450 3A for clearance and for which elevated plasma concentrations are associated with serious and/or life threatening events, such as cisapride, is contraindicated).
No products indexed under this heading.

Clarithromycin (Co-administration can result in increased clarithromycin plasma concentrations; for patients with renal impairment, the dosage may need to be adjusted). Products include:
Biaxin/Biaxin XL 411

Cyclosporine (Co-administration results in increased plasma concentrations of immunosuppressants; monitoring is recommended). Products include:
Gengraf Capsules 435
Neoral Oral Solution 2280
Neoral Soft Gelatin Capsules 2280
Restasis Ophthalmic Emulsion 557
Sandimmune 2296

Delavirdine Mesylate (Co-administration has a potential to increase lopinavir plasma concentrations).
No products indexed under this heading.

Dexamethasone (Co-administration can result in decreased lopinavir plasma concentrations; Kaletra may be less effective due to decreased lopinavir plasma concentrations in patients taking these agents concomitantly. Co-administer with caution). Products include:
Ciprodex Otic Suspension 541

Dexamethasone Acetate (Co-administration can result in decreased lopinavir plasma concentrations; Kaletra may be less effective due to decreased lopinavir plasma concentrations in patients taking these agents concomitantly. Co-administer with caution).
No products indexed under this heading.

Dexamethasone Sodium Phosphate (Co-administration can result in decreased lopinavir plasma concentrations; Kaletra may be less effective due to decreased lopinavir plasma concentrations in patients taking these agents concomitantly. Co-administer with caution).
No products indexed under this heading.

Didanosine (Kaletra tablets can be administered simultaneously with didanosine without food. For Kaletra oral solution, it is recommended that didanosine be administered on an empty stomach, therefore, didanosine should be given one hour before or two hours after Kaletra oral solution (given with food)).
No products indexed under this heading.

Dihydroergotamine Mesylate (Co-administration of Kaletra is contraindicated with potent CYP3A4 inducers where significantly reduced lopinavir plasma concentrations may be associated with the potential for loss of virologic response and possible resistance and cross-resistance. Co-administration may lead to the potential for causing acute ergot toxicity characterized by peripheral vasospasm and ischemia of the extremities and other tissues).
No products indexed under this heading.

Disulfiram (Kaletra oral solution contains alcohol which can produce disulfiram-like reactions when co-administered with disulfiram).
No products indexed under this heading.

Efavirenz (Efavirenz may decrease concentration of lopinavir. Kaletra should not be administered once-daily in combination with enfavirenz). Products include:
Atripla Tablets 938
Sustiva Capsules 930
Sustiva Tablets 930

Ergonovine Maleate (Co-administration of Kaletra is contraindicated with potent CYP3A4 inducers where significantly reduced lopinavir plasma concentrations may be associated with the potential for loss of virologic response and possible resistance and cross-resistance. Co-administration may lead to the potential for causing acute ergot toxicity characterized by peripheral vasospam and ischemia of the extremities and other tissues).
No products indexed under this heading.

Ergotamine Tartrate (Co-administration of Kaletra is contraindicated with potent CYP3A4 inducers where significantly reduced lopinavir plasma concentrations may be associated with the potential for loss of virologic response and possible resistance and cross-resistance. Co-administration may lead to the potential for causing acute ergot toxicity characterized by peripheral vasospam and ischemia of the extremities and other tissues).
No products indexed under this heading.

Ethinyl Estradiol (Co-administration results in decreased plasma concentrations of ethinyl estradiol; alternative methods of non-hormonal contraception should be used when estrogen-based oral contraceptives and Kaletra are co-administered). Products include:

Lybrel Tablets 3204
Mircette Tablets 1034
NuvaRing 2897
Ortho-Cyclen/Ortho Tri-Cyclen 2449
Ortho Evra Transdermal System 2437
Ortho Tri-Cyclen Lo Tablets 2458
Seasonique Tablets 1046
Yaz Tablets 805

Ethosuximide (Co-administration is contraindicated with potent CYP3A4 inducers where significantly reduced lopinavir plasma concentrations may be associated with the potential for loss of virologic response and possible resistance and cross-resistance).
No products indexed under this heading.

Felodipine (Increased plasma concentrations of dihydropyridine calcium channel blockers; caution is warranted and clinical monitoring of patients is recommended).
No products indexed under this heading.

Flecainide Acetate (Kaletra is an in vitro inhibitor of the CYP450 3A and inhibits CYP2D6 to a lesser extent; co-administration with drugs that are highly dependent on these isoforms for clearance and for which elevated plasma concentrations are associated with serious and/or life threatening events, such as flecainide, is contraindicated).
No products indexed under this heading.

Fluticasone Propionate (Concomitant use of fluticasone propionate and Kaletra may increase plasma concentrations of fluticasone propionate, resulting in significantly reduced serum cortisol concentrations. Co-administration of fluticasone propionate and Kaletra is not recommended unless the potential benefit to the patient outweighs the risk of system corticosteroid side effect). Products include:
Advair Diskus 100/50 1276
Advair Diskus 250/50 1276
Advair Diskus 500/50 1276
Advair HFA 45/21 Inhalation Aerosol 1288
Advair HFA 115/21 Inhalation Aerosol 1288
Advair HFA 230/21 Inhalation Aerosol 1288
Flonase Nasal Spray 1431
Flovent Diskus 50 mcg 1435

Fluticasone Propionate HFA (Concomitant use of fluticasone propionate and Kaletra may increase plasma concentrations of fluticasone propionate, resulting in significantly reduced serum cortisol concentrations. Co-administration of fluticasone propionate and Kaletra is not recommended unless the potential benefit to the patient outweighs the risk of system corticosteroid side effect). Products include:
Flovent HFA 1440

Fosamprenavir Calcium (Co-administration may result in decreased levels of amprenavir and/or lopinavir. An increased rate of adverse effects has also been observed with co-administration of these medications). Products include:
Lexiva Oral Suspension 1510
Lexiva Tablets 1510

Fosphenytoin Sodium (Co-administration can result in decreased lopinavir plasma concentrations; Kaletra may be less effective due to decreased lopinavir plasma concentrations. Co-administer with caution).
No products indexed under this heading.

Hypericum (Co-administration of Kaletra is contraindicated with potent CYP3A4 inducers where significantly reduced lopinavir plasma concentrations may be associated with the potential for loss of virologic response and possible resistance and cross-resistance. Co-administration may lead to loss of virologic response and possible resistance to Kaletra or to the class of protease inhibitors). Products include:
Satieté Tablets .... ▣640

Hypericum Perforatum (Co-administration of Kaletra is contraindicated with potent CYP3A4 inducers where significantly reduced lopinavir plasma concentrations may be associated with the potential for loss of virologic response and possible resistance and cross-resistance. Co-administration may lead to loss of virologic response and possible resistance to Kaletra or to the class of protease inhibitors).
No products indexed under this heading.

Indinavir Sulfate (Co-administration may result in increased indinavir concentrations, decreased Cmax and increased Cmin. Decreased indinavir dose to 600mg BID, when co-administered with Kaletra 400/100mg BID. Kaletra once-daily has not been studied in combination with indinavir). Products include:
Crixivan Capsules 1979

Isradipine (Increased plasma concentrations of dihydropyridine calcium channel blockers; caution is warranted and clinical monitoring of patients is recommended). Products include:
DynaCirc CR Controlled Release Tablets 1407

Itraconazole (Co-administration can result in increased itraconazole plasma concentrations; high doses of itraconazole (>200 mg/day) are not recommended).
No products indexed under this heading.

Ketoconazole (Co-administration can result in increased ketoconazole plasma concentrations; high doses of ketoconazole (>200 mg/day) are not recommended). Products include:
Extina Foam, 2% 3057
Nizoral A-D Shampoo 1901

Lidocaine Hydrochloride (Co-administration with systemic lidocaine can result in increased lidocaine plasma concentrations; caution and monitoring is recommended).
No products indexed under this heading.

Lovastatin (Co-administration of Kaletra is contraindicated with potent CYP3A4 inducers where significantly reduced lopinavir plasma concentrations may be associated with the potential for loss of virologic response and possible resistance and cross-resistance. Co-administration may lead to the potential for myopathy including rhabdomyolysis). Products include:
Advicor Tablets 402
Mevacor Tablets 2063

Methadone Hydrochloride (Co-administration results in decreased plasma concentrations of methadone; dosage of methadone may need to be increased when co-administered).
No products indexed under this heading.

Methylergonovine Maleate (Co-administration of Kaletra is contraindicated with potent CYP3A4 inducers where significantly reduced lopinavir plasma concentrations may be associated with the potential for loss of virologic response and possible resistance and cross-resistance. Co-administration may lead to the potential for causing acute ergot toxicity characterized by peripheral vasospam and ischemia of the extremities and other tissues).
No products indexed under this heading.

Methysergide Maleate (Kaletra is an inhibitor of CYP450 3A. Co-administration is contraindicated due to potential for serious and/or life threatening reactions such as acute ergot toxiety).
No products indexed under this heading.

Metronidazole (Kaletra oral solution contains alcohol, which can produce disulfiram-like reactions when co-administered with disulfiram or other drugs that produce this reaction, such as metronidazole). Products include:
Pylera Capsules 714

Metronidazole Hydrochloride (Kaletra oral solution contains alcohol, which can produce disulfiram-like reactions when co-administered with disulfiram or other drugs that produce this reaction, such as metronidazole).
No products indexed under this heading.

Midazolam Hydrochloride (Co-administration of Kaletra is contraindicated with potent CYP3A4 inducers where significantly reduced lopinavir plasma concentrations may be associated with the potential for loss of virologic response and possible resistance and cross-resistance. Co-administration may lead to prolonged or increased sedation or respiratory depression).
No products indexed under this heading.

Modafinil (Co-administration is contraindicated with potent CYP3A4 inducers where significantly reduced lopinavir plasma concentrations may be associated with the potential for loss of virologic response and possible resistance and cross-resistance). Products include:
Provigil Tablets 977

Nelfinavir Mesylate (Co-administration may result in increased nelfinavir plasma concentration. Kaletra should not be administered once-daily in combination with nelfinavir).
No products indexed under this heading.

Nevirapine (Nevirapine may decrease concentration of lopinavir. Kaletra should not be administered once-daily in combination with nevirapine). Products include:
Viramune Oral Suspension 873
Viramune Tablets 873

Nicardipine Hydrochloride (Increased plasma concentrations of dihydropyridine calcium channel blockers; caution is warranted and clinical monitoring of patients is recommended). Products include:
Cardene I.V. 1093

Nifedipine (Increased plasma concentrations of dihydropyridine calcium channel blockers; caution is warranted and clinical monitoring of patients is recommended).
No products indexed under this heading.

Nimodipine (Increased plasma concentrations of dihydropyridine calcium channel blockers; caution is warranted and clinical monitoring of patients is recommended). Products include:
Nimotop Capsules 790

Phenobarbital (Co-administration can result in decreased lopinavir plasma concentrations; Kaletra may be less effective due to decreased lopinavir plasma concentrations. Co-administer with caution). Products include:
Donnatal Extentabs 2507

Phenytoin (Co-administration can result in decreased lopinavir plasma concentrations; Kaletra may be less effective due to decreased lopinavir plasma concentrations. Co-administer with caution).
No products indexed under this heading.

Phenytoin Sodium (Co-administration can result in decreased lopinavir plasma concentrations; Kaletra may be less effective due to decreased lopinavir plasma concentrations. Co-administer with caution). Products include:
Phenytek Capsules 2192

Pimozide (Co-administration of Kaletra is contraindicated with potent CYP3A4 inducers where significantly reduced lopinavir plasma concentrations may be associated with the potential for loss of virologic response and possible resistance and cross-resistance. Co-administration may lead to the potential for cardiac arrhythmias).
No products indexed under this heading.

Propafenone Hydrochloride (Kaletra is an inhibitor of CYP450 3A. Co-administration with drugs that are highly dependent on CYP450 3A for clearance and for which elevated plasma concentrations are associated with serious and/or life threatening events, such as propafenone, is contraindicated). Products include:
Rythmol Tablets 1586
Rythmol SR Capsules 1590

Quinidine (Co-administration can result in increased quinidine plasma concentrations; caution and monitoring is recommended).
No products indexed under this heading.

Quinidine Gluconate (Co-administration can result in increased quinidine plasma concentrations; caution and monitoring is recommended).
No products indexed under this heading.

Quinidine Hydrochloride (Co-administration can result in increased quinidine plasma concentrations; caution and monitoring is recommended).
No products indexed under this heading.

Quinidine Polygalacturonate (Co-administration can result in increased quinidine plasma concentrations; caution and monitoring is recommended).
No products indexed under this heading.

Quinidine Sulfate (Co-administration can result in increased quinidine plasma concentrations; caution and monitoring is recommended).
No products indexed under this heading.

Rapamycin (Co-administration results in increased plasma concentrations of immunosuppressants; monitoring is recommended).
No products indexed under this heading.

Rifabutin (Co-administration can result in increased rifabutin and rifabutin metabolite plasma concentrations; dosage reduction of rifabutin by at least 75% of the usual dose of 300 mg/day is recommended; increased monitoring for adverse reactions is warranted).
No products indexed under this heading.

Rifampicin (Co-administration is contraindicated with potent CYP3A4 inducers where significantly reduced lopinavir plasma concentrations may be associated with the potential for loss of virologic response and possible resistance and cross-resistance).
No products indexed under this heading.

Rifampin (Co-administration of Kaletra is contraindicated with potent CYP3A4 inducers where significantly reduced lopinavir plasma concentrations may be associated with the potential for loss of virologic response and possible resistance and cross-resistance. Co-administration may lead to loss of virologic response and possible resistance to Kaletra or to the class of protease inhibitors or other co-administered antiretroviral agents).
No products indexed under this heading.

Rifapentine (Co-administration is contraindicated with potent CYP3A4 inducers where significantly reduced lopinavir plasma concentrations may be associated with the potential for loss of virologic response and possible resistance and cross-resistance).
No products indexed under this heading.

Saquinavir (Co-administration may increase saquinavir concentrations. The saquinavir dose is 1000mg BID, when co-administered with Kaletra 400/100mg. Kaletra once-daily has not been studied in combination with saquinavir).
No products indexed under this heading.

Saquinavir Mesylate (Co-administration may increase saquinavir concentrations. The saquinavir dose is 1000mg BID, when co-administered with Kaletra 400/100mg. Kaletra once-daily has not been studied in combination with saquinavir).
No products indexed under this heading.

Sildenafil Citrate (Co-administration is expected to substantially increase sildenafil concentrations and may result in an increase in sildenafil-associated adverse events including hypotension, syncope, visual changes and prolonged erection; Dosage reductions of 25 mg every 48 hours with increased monitoring for adverse events).
No products indexed under this heading.

Simvastatin (Co-administration of Kaletra is contraindicated with potent CYP3A4 inducers where significantly reduced lopinavir plasma concentrations may be associated with the potential for loss of virologic response and possible resistance and cross-resistance. Co-administration may lead to the potential for myopathy including rhabdomyolysis). Products include:
Simcor Tablets ... 502
Vytorin 10/10 Tablets ... 2149
Vytorin 10/10 Tablets ... 2939
Vytorin 10/20 Tablets ... 2149
Vytorin 10/20 Tablets ... 2939
Vytorin 10/40 Tablets ... 2149
Vytorin 10/40 Tablets ... 2939
Vytorin 10/80 Tablets ... 2149
Vytorin 10/80 Tablets ... 2939
Zocor Tablets ... 2136

Tacrolimus (Co-administration results in increased plasma concentrations of immunosuppressants; monitoring is recommended). Products include:
Prograf Capsules and Injection ... 622
Protopic Ointment ... 628

Tadalafil (Co-administration is expected to substantially increase tadalafil concentrations and may result in an increase in tadalafil associated adverse drug events including hypotension, syncope, visual changes and prolonged erection; Dosage reduction recommended10 mg every 72 hours with increased monitoring for adverse events). Products include:
Cialis Tablets ... 1792

Tenofovir Disoproxil Fumarate (Co-administration results in increased plasma concentrations of nucleoside reverse transcriptase inhibitors; Co-administer with caution. Patients receiving Kaletra and tenofovir should be monitored for adverse reactions associated with tenofovir). Products include:
Atripla Tablets ... 938
Truvada Tablets ... 1262
Viread Tablets ... 1268

Terfenadine (Kaletra is an inhibitor of CYP450 3A. Co-administration with drugs that are highly dependent on CYP450 3A for clearance and for which elevated plasma concentrations are associated with serious and/or life threatening events, such as terfenadine, is contraindicated).
No products indexed under this heading.

Tipranavir (Co-administration may result in a decrease in lopinavir AUC and Cmin. Kaletra should not be administered with tipranavir (500 mg twice-daily) or co-administered with ritonavir (200 mg twice-daily)). Products include:
Aptivus Capsules ... 823
Aptivus Oral Solution ... 823

Trazodone Hydrochloride (Concomitant use of trazodone and Kaletra may increase concentrations of trazodone. Adverse events of nausea, dizziness, hypotension and syncope have been observed following co-administration of trazodone and ritonavir. If trazodone is used with a CYP3A4 inhibitor such as ritonavir, the combination should be used with caution and a lower dose of trazodone should be considered).
No products indexed under this heading.

Triazolam (Co-administration of Kaletra is contraindicated with potent CYP3A4 inducers where significantly reduced lopinavir plasma concentrations may be associated with the potential for loss of virologic response and possible resistance and cross-resistance. Co-administration may lead to prolonged or increased sedation or respiratory depression).
No products indexed under this heading.

Vardenafil Hydrochloride (Co-administration is expected to substantially increase vardenafil concentrations and may result in an increase in vardenafil associated adverse drug events including hypotension, syncope, visual changes and prolonged erection; Dosage reduction of 2.5 mg every 72 hours with increased monitoring for adverse effects). Products include:
Levitra Tablets ... 2876

Voriconazole (Co-administration of voriconazole with Kaletra has not been studied. However, administration of voriconazole with ritonavir 400 mg every 12 hours decreased voriconazole steady-state AUC by an average of 82%. The effect of lower ritonavir doses on voriconazole is not known at this time. Until data is available, voriconazole should not be administered to patients receiving Kaletra).
No products indexed under this heading.

Warfarin Sodium (Co-administration can affect concentrations of warfarin; it is recommended that INR be monitored).
No products indexed under this heading.

Zidovudine (Kaletra induces glucuronidation; therefore, Kaletra has the potential to reduce zidovudine plasma concentrations; the clinical significance is unknown). Products include:
Combivir Tablets ... 1384
Retrovir ... 1574
Retrovir IV Infusion ... 1579
Trizivir Tablets ... 1622

Food Interactions

Food, unspecified (Co-administration with moderate fat meal was associated with a mean increase in AUC and Cmax; to enhance bioavailability Kaletra should be taken with food).

KEPIVANCE

(Palifermin) ... 583
May interact with:

Heparin Calcium (Palifermin has been shown to bind to heparin in vitro. Therefore, if heparin is used to maintain an IV line, saline should be used to rinse the line prior to and after palifermin administration).
No products indexed under this heading.

Heparin Sodium (Palifermin has been shown to bind to heparin in vitro. Therefore, if heparin is used to maintain an IV line, saline should be used to rinse the line prior to and after palifermin administration).
No products indexed under this heading.

KEPPRA INJECTION

(Levetiracetam) ... 3137
May interact with:

Probenecid (Probenecid, a renal tubular secretion blocking agent, administered at a dose of 500mg four times a day, did not change the pharmacokinetics of levetiracetam 1000mg twice daily. Cmax of the metabolite, ucb L057, was approximately doubled in the presence of probenecid while the fraction of drug excreted unchanged in the urine remained the same. Renal clearance of ucb L057 in the presence of probenecid decreased 60%, probably related to competitive inhibition of tubular secretion of ucb L057).
No products indexed under this heading.

KEPPRA ORAL SOLUTION

(Levetiracetam) ... 3131
See Keppra Tablets

KEPPRA TABLETS

(Levetiracetam) ... 3131
May interact with:

Probenecid (Probenecid, a renal tubular secretion blocking agent, administered at a dose of 500 mg four times a day, did not change the pharmacokinetics of levetiracetam 1000 mg twice daily. Css max of the metabolite ucb L057 was approximately doubled in the presence of probenecid, while the fraction of drug excreted unchanged in the urine remained the same. Renal clearance of ucb L057 in the presence of probenecid decreased 60%; probably related to competitive inhibition of tubular secretion of ucb L057. The effect of levetiracetam on probenecid was not studied).
No products indexed under this heading.

Food Interactions

Food, unspecified (Food does not affect the extent of absorption of levetiracetam but it decreases Cmax by 20% and delays Tmax by 1.5 hours).

KETEK TABLETS

(Telithromycin) ... 2744
May interact with benzodiazepine that are metabolized by CYP3A4, cytochrome p450 3a4 inducers (selected), cytochrome p450 3a4 substrates (selected), ergot-containing drugs, drugs which undergo biotransformation by cytochrome p-450 mixed function oxidase, and certain other agents. Compounds in these categories include:

Acarbose (Elevated levels of drugs metabolized by the CYP450 system

may be observed when co-administered with telithromycin; therefore, increases or prolongation of the therapeutic and/or adverse effects of the concomitant drug may be observed). Products include:
Precose Tablets 792

Acetaminophen (Elevated levels of drugs metabolized by the CYP450 system may be observed when co-administered with telithromycin; therefore, increases or prolongation of the therapeutic and/or adverse effects of the concomitant drug may be observed). Products include:
Benadryl Allergy & Cold Kapgels 1895
Benadryl Allergy & Sinus Headache Kapgels 1895
Benadryl Severe Allergy & Sinus Headache Caplets 1897
Lortab 5/500 Tablets 3143
Lortab 7.5/500 Tablets 3144
Lortab 10/500 Tablets 3144
Percocet Tablets 1127
Sinutab Sinus Caplets 1905
Sudafed PE Cold & Cough Caplets 1907
Sudafed PE Nighttime Cold Caplets 1907
Sudafed PE Severe Cold Caplets 1908
Sudafed PE Sinus Headache Caplets 1908
Regular Strength Tylenol Tablets 1915
Tylenol 8 Hour Extended Release Caplets 1915
Extra Strength Tylenol Caplets, Cool Caplets, and EZ Tabs 1915
Extra Strength Tylenol Adult Rapid Blast Liquid 1915
Extra Strength Tylenol PM Caplets, Geltabs, Liquid, and Rapid Release Gels 1915
Extra Strength Tylenol Rapid Release Gels 1915
Tylenol with Codeine Tablets 2427
Tylenol Allergy Multi-Symptom Caplets with Cool Burst and Rapid Release Gelcaps 1916
Tylenol Allergy Multi-Symptom Nighttime Caplets with Cool Burst 1916
Tylenol Severe Allergy Caplets 1916
Tylenol Arthritis Pain Extended Release Geltabs/Caplets 1915
Tylenol Chest Congestion Caplets with Cool Burst 1910
Tylenol Chest Congestion Liquid with Cool Burst 1910
Children's Tylenol Plus Cold Suspension Liquid 1912
Children's Tylenol Plus Cold & Allergy Suspension Liquid 1914
Children's Tylenol Plus Cough & Runny Nose Suspension Liquid 1912
Children's Tylenol Plus Cough & Sore Throat Suspension Liquid 1912
Children's Tylenol Plus Flu Suspension Liquid 1914
Children's Tylenol Suspension Liquid 1909
Children's Tylenol Meltaways 1909
Children's Tylenol Plus Multi-Symptom Cold Suspension Liquid 1912
Tylenol Cold Severe Congestion Daytime Caplets with Cool Burst 1912
Tylenol Cold Head Congestion Daytime Caplets with Cool Burst 1910
Tylenol Cold Head Congestion Nighttime Caplets with Cool Burst 1910
Tylenol Cold Head Congestion Severe Daytime Caplets with Cool Burst 1910
Tylenol Cold Multi-Symptom Daytime Caplets with Cool Burst and Rapid Release Gels 1913
Tylenol Cold Multi-Symptom Daytime Liquid with Citrus Burst ... 1913
Tylenol Cold Multi-Symptom Nighttime Caplets with Cool Burst 1913
Tylenol Cold Multi-Symptom Nighttime Liquid with Cool Burst ... 1913
Tylenol Cold Multi-Symptom Severe Caplets with Cool Burst 1913
Tylenol Cold Multi-Symptom Severe Daytime Liquid with Citrus Burst 1913
Tylenol Cough & Sore Throat Daytime Liquid with Cool Burst 1918
Tylenol Cough & Sore Throat Nighttime Liquid with Cool Burst ... 1918
Concentrated Tylenol Infants' Drops 1909
Jr. Tylenol Meltaways 1909
Tylenol Sinus Congestion & Pain Daytime Caplets with Cool Burst and Gelcaps 1917
Tylenol Sinus Congestion & Pain Nighttime Caplets with Cool Burst 1917
Tylenol Sinus Congestion & Pain Severe Caplets with Cool Burst 1917
Tylenol Sinus Severe Congestion Caplets with Cool Burst 1917
Tylenol Sore Throat Daytime Liquid with Cool Burst 1918
Tylenol Sore Throat Nighttime Liquid with Cool Burst 1918
Women's Tylenol Menstrual Relief Caplets 1919
Vicks DayQuil Cold & Flu Multi-Symptom Relief .... ▣616
Vicks DayQuil LiquiCaps 2567
Vicks DayQuil Liquid 2567
Vicks DayQuil Multi-Symptom Cold/Flu Relief 2567
Vicks NyQuil Cold & Flu Multi-Symptom Relief .... ▣617
Vicks NyQuil LiquiCaps 2567
Vicks NyQuil Liquid 2567
Vicks NyQuil Multi-Symptom Cold/Flu Relief 2567
Vicodin Tablets 529
Vicodin ES Tablets 530
Vicodin HP Tablets 531
Zydone Tablets 1132

Alatrofloxacin Mesylate (Elevated levels of drugs metabolized by the CYP450 system may be observed when co-administered with telithromycin; therefore, increases or prolongation of the therapeutic and/or adverse effects of the concomitant drug may be observed).
No products indexed under this heading.

Alfentanil Hydrochloride (Co-administration of telithromycin with a drug primarily metabolized by the CYP 3A4 enzyme system may result in increased plasma concentrations of the drug co-administered with telithromycin that could increase or prolong both the therapeutic and adverse effects).
No products indexed under this heading.

Allium sativum (Concomitant administration of CYP 3A4 inducers is likely to result in subtherapeutic levels of telithromycin and loss of effect).
No products indexed under this heading.

Alprazolam (Co-administration of telithromycin with a drug primarily metabolized by the CYP 3A4 enzyme system may result in increased plasma concentrations of the drug co-administered with telithromycin that could increase or prolong both the therapeutic and adverse effects).
No products indexed under this heading.

Aminophylline (Elevated levels of drugs metabolized by the CYP450 system may be observed when co-administered with telithromycin; therefore, increases or prolongation of the therapeutic and/or adverse effects of the concomitant drug may be observed).
No products indexed under this heading.

Amiodarone Hydrochloride (Co-administration of telithromycin with a drug primarily metabolized by the CYP 3A4 enzyme system may result in increased plasma concentrations of the drug co-administered with telithromycin that could increase or prolong both the therapeutic and adverse effects).
No products indexed under this heading.

Amitriptyline Hydrochloride (Co-administration of telithromycin with a drug primarily metabolized by the CYP 3A4 enzyme system may result in increased plasma concentrations of the drug co-administered with telithromycin that could increase or prolong both the therapeutic and adverse effects).
No products indexed under this heading.

Amlodipine Besylate (Co-administration of telithromycin with a drug primarily metabolized by the CYP 3A4 enzyme system may result in increased plasma concentrations of the drug co-administered with telithromycin that could increase or prolong both the therapeutic and adverse effects). Products include:
Azor Tablets 1005
Exforge Tablets 2238

Amoxapine (Elevated levels of drugs metabolized by the CYP450 system may be observed when co-administered with telithromycin; therefore, increases or prolongation of the therapeutic and/or adverse effects of the concomitant drug may be observed).
No products indexed under this heading.

Amphetamine Aspartate (Elevated levels of drugs metabolized by the CYP450 system may be observed when co-administered with telithromycin; therefore, increases or prolongation of the therapeutic and/or adverse effects of the concomitant drug may be observed).
Products include:
Adderall XR Capsules 3012

Amphetamine Aspartate Monohydrate (Elevated levels of drugs metabolized by the CYP450 system may be observed when co-administered with telithromycin; therefore, increases or prolongation of the therapeutic and/or adverse effects of the concomitant drug may be observed).
No products indexed under this heading.

Amphetamine Sulfate (Elevated levels of drugs metabolized by the CYP450 system may be observed when co-administered with telithromycin; therefore, increases or prolongation of the therapeutic and/or adverse effects of the concomitant drug may be observed). Products include:
Adderall XR Capsules 3012

Aprepitant (Co-administration of telithromycin with a drug primarily metabolized by the CYP 3A4 enzyme system may result in increased plasma concentrations of the drug co-administered with telithromycin that could increase or prolong both the therapeutic and adverse effects).
Products include:
Emend Capsules 1992

Astemizole (Co-administration of telithromycin with a drug primarily metabolized by the CYP 3A4 enzyme system may result in increased plasma concentrations of the drug co-administered with telithromycin that could increase or prolong both the therapeutic and adverse effects).
No products indexed under this heading.

Atomoxetine Hydrochloride (Elevated levels of drugs metabolized by the CYP450 system may be observed when co-administered with telithromycin; therefore, increases or prolongation of the therapeutic and/or adverse effects of the concomitant drug may be observed).
Products include:
Strattera Capsules 1864

Atorvastatin Calcium (Atorvastatin levels were increased due to CYP 3A4 inhibition by telithromycin, thereby increasing the risk of myopathy. Co-administration should be avoided). Products include:
Lipitor Tablets 2501

Belladonna Ergotamine (Co-administration of telithromycin with a drug primarily metabolized by the CYP 3A4 enzyme system may result in increased plasma concentrations of the drug co-administered with telithromycin that could increase or prolong both the therapeutic and adverse effects).
No products indexed under this heading.

Benzphetamine Hydrochloride (Elevated levels of drugs metabolized by the CYP450 system may be observed when co-administered with telithromycin; therefore, increases or prolongation of the therapeutic and/or adverse effects of the concomitant drug may be observed).
No products indexed under this heading.

Betamethasone Acetate (Concomitant administration of CYP 3A4 inducers is likely to result in subtherapeutic levels of telithromycin and loss of effect).
No products indexed under this heading.

Betamethasone Sodium Phosphate (Concomitant administration of CYP 3A4 inducers is likely to result in subtherapeutic levels of telithromycin and loss of effect).
No products indexed under this heading.

Bisoprolol Fumarate (Elevated levels of drugs metabolized by the CYP450 system may be observed when co-administered with telithromycin; therefore, increases or prolongation of the therapeutic and/or adverse effects of the concomitant drug may be observed).
No products indexed under this heading.

Buspirone Hydrochloride (Co-administration of telithromycin with a drug primarily metabolized by the CYP 3A4 enzyme system may result in increased plasma concentrations of the drug co-administered with telithromycin that could increase or prolong both the therapeutic and adverse effects).
No products indexed under this heading.

Busulfan (Co-administration of telithromycin with a drug primarily metabolized by the CYP 3A4 enzyme system may result in increased plas-

ma concentrations of the drug co-administered with telithromycin that could increase or prolong both the therapeutic and adverse effects). Products include:
Busulfex Injection 2477
Myleran Tablets 1530

Caffeine (Elevated levels of drugs metabolized by the CYP450 system may be observed when co-administered with telithromycin; therefore, increases or prolongation of the therapeutic and/or adverse effects of the concomitant drug may be observed). Products include:
BioLean Free Tablets 635
BioLean II Tablets 635
Winrgy Dietary Supplement 642

Caffeine Anhydrous (Elevated levels of drugs metabolized by the CYP450 system may be observed when co-administered with telithromycin; therefore, increases or prolongation of the therapeutic and/or adverse effects of the concomitant drug may be observed).
No products indexed under this heading.

Caffeine Citrate (Elevated levels of drugs metabolized by the CYP450 system may be observed when co-administered with telithromycin; therefore, increases or prolongation of the therapeutic and/or adverse effects of the concomitant drug may be observed).
No products indexed under this heading.

Candesartan Cilexetil (Elevated levels of drugs metabolized by the CYP450 system may be observed when co-administered with telithromycin; therefore, increases or prolongation of the therapeutic and/or adverse effects of the concomitant drug may be observed). Products include:
Atacand Tablets 639
Atacand HCT 642

Captopril (Elevated levels of drugs metabolized by the CYP450 system may be observed when co-administered with telithromycin; therefore, increases or prolongation of the therapeutic and/or adverse effects of the concomitant drug may be observed). Products include:
Captopril Tablets 2182

Carbamazepine (Co-administration of telithromycin with a drug primarily metabolized by the CYP 3A4 enzyme system may result in increased plasma concentrations of the drug co-administered with telithromycin that could increase or prolong both the therapeutic and adverse effects). Products include:
Carbatrol Capsules 3019
Equetro Extended-Release Capsules 3174

Carisoprodol (Elevated levels of drugs metabolized by the CYP450 system may be observed when co-administered with telithromycin; therefore, increases or prolongation of the therapeutic and/or adverse effects of the concomitant drug may be observed). Products include:
Soma Tablets 1931

Carvedilol (Elevated levels of drugs metabolized by the CYP450 system may be observed when co-administered with telithromycin; therefore, increases or prolongation of the therapeutic and/or adverse effects of the concomitant drug may be observed). Products include:
Coreg Tablets 1387

Celecoxib (Elevated levels of drugs metabolized by the CYP450 system may be observed when co-administered with telithromycin; therefore, increases or prolongation of the therapeutic and/or adverse effects of the concomitant drug may be observed). Products include:
Celebrex Capsules 2979

Cerivastatin Sodium (Co-administration of telithromycin with a drug primarily metabolized by the CYP 3A4 enzyme system may result in increased plasma concentrations of the drug co-administered with telithromycin that could increase or prolong both the therapeutic and adverse effects).
No products indexed under this heading.

Cevimeline Hydrochloride (Elevated levels of drugs metabolized by the CYP450 system may be observed when co-administered with telithromycin; therefore, increases or prolongation of the therapeutic and/or adverse effects of the concomitant drug may be observed). Products include:
Evoxac Capsules 1013

Chlordiazepoxide (Elevated levels of drugs metabolized by the CYP450 system may be observed when co-administered with telithromycin; therefore, increases or prolongation of the therapeutic and/or adverse effects of the concomitant drug may be observed).
No products indexed under this heading.

Chlordiazepoxide Hydrochloride (Elevated levels of drugs metabolized by the CYP450 system may be observed when co-administered with telithromycin; therefore, increases or prolongation of the therapeutic and/or adverse effects of the concomitant drug may be observed).
No products indexed under this heading.

Chlorpheniramine (Co-administration of telithromycin with a drug primarily metabolized by the CYP 3A4 enzyme system may result in increased plasma concentrations of the drug co-administered with telithromycin that could increase or prolong both the therapeutic and adverse effects).
No products indexed under this heading.

Chlorpheniramine Maleate (Co-administration of telithromycin with a drug primarily metabolized by the CYP 3A4 enzyme system may result in increased plasma concentrations of the drug co-administered with telithromycin that could increase or prolong both the therapeutic and adverse effects). Products include:
Actifed Cold & Allergy Tablets 1895
Sudafed PE Sinus & Allergy Tablets 1908
Tylenol Allergy Multi-Symptom Caplets with Cool Burst and Rapid Release Gelcaps 1916
Children's Tylenol Plus Cold Suspension Liquid 1912
Children's Tylenol Plus Cough & Runny Nose Suspension Liquid 1912
Children's Tylenol Plus Flu Suspension Liquid 1914
Children's Tylenol Plus Multi-Symptom Cold Suspension Liquid 1912
Tylenol Cold Head Congestion Nighttime Caplets with Cool Burst 1910
Tylenol Cold Multi-Symptom Nighttime Caplets with Cool Burst 1913
Tylenol Sinus Congestion & Pain Nighttime Caplets with Cool Burst 1917

Chlorpheniramine Polistirex (Co-administration of telithromycin with a drug primarily metabolized by the CYP 3A4 enzyme system may result in increased plasma concentrations of the drug co-administered with telithromycin that could increase or prolong both the therapeutic and adverse effects). Products include:
Tussionex Pennkinetic Extended-Release Suspension...... 3154

Chlorpheniramine Tannate (Co-administration of telithromycin with a drug primarily metabolized by the CYP 3A4 enzyme system may result in increased plasma concentrations of the drug co-administered with telithromycin that could increase or prolong both the therapeutic and adverse effects).
No products indexed under this heading.

Chlorpromazine (Elevated levels of drugs metabolized by the CYP450 system may be observed when co-administered with telithromycin; therefore, increases or prolongation of the therapeutic and/or adverse effects of the concomitant drug may be observed).
No products indexed under this heading.

Chlorpromazine Hydrochloride (Elevated levels of drugs metabolized by the CYP450 system may be observed when co-administered with telithromycin; therefore, increases or prolongation of the therapeutic and/or adverse effects of the concomitant drug may be observed).
No products indexed under this heading.

Chlorpropamide (Elevated levels of drugs metabolized by the CYP450 system may be observed when co-administered with telithromycin; therefore, increases or prolongation of the therapeutic and/or adverse effects of the concomitant drug may be observed).
No products indexed under this heading.

Cilostazol (Elevated levels of drugs metabolized by the CYP450 system may be observed when co-administered with telithromycin; therefore, increases or prolongation of the therapeutic and/or adverse effects of the concomitant drug may be observed). Products include:
Pletal Tablets 2481

Cimetidine Hydrochloride (Elevated levels of drugs metabolized by the CYP450 system may be observed when co-administered with telithromycin; therefore, increases or prolongation of the therapeutic and/or adverse effects of the concomitant drug may be observed).
No products indexed under this heading.

Ciprofloxacin (Elevated levels of drugs metabolized by the CYP450 system may be observed when co-administered with telithromycin; therefore, increases or prolongation of the therapeutic and/or adverse effects of the concomitant drug may be observed). Products include:
Cipro I.V. 2817
Cipro Oral Suspension 2810
Cipro XR Tablets 2823
Ciprodex Otic Suspension 541

Ciprofloxacin Hydrochloride (Concomitant administration of CYP 3A4 inducers is likely to result in subtherapeutic levels of telithromycin and loss of effect). Products include:
Cipro Tablets 2810

Cisapride (Steady-state peak plasma concentrations of cisapride were increased when co-administered with repeated doses of telithromycin, resulting in significant increases in QTc. Co-administration is contraindicated).
No products indexed under this heading.

Cisplatin (Concomitant administration of CYP 3A4 inducers is likely to result in subtherapeutic levels of telithromycin and loss of effect).
No products indexed under this heading.

Citalopram Hydrobromide (Elevated levels of drugs metabolized by the CYP450 system may be observed when co-administered with telithromycin; therefore, increases or prolongation of the therapeutic and/or adverse effects of the concomitant drug may be observed). Products include:
Celexa 1160

Clarithromycin (Co-administration of telithromycin with a drug primarily metabolized by the CYP 3A4 enzyme system may result in increased plasma concentrations of the drug co-administered with telithromycin that could increase or prolong both the therapeutic and adverse effects). Products include:
Biaxin/Biaxin XL 411

Clomipramine Hydrochloride (Elevated levels of drugs metabolized by the CYP450 system may be observed when co-administered with telithromycin; therefore, increases or prolongation of the therapeutic and/or adverse effects of the concomitant drug may be observed).
No products indexed under this heading.

Clopidogrel Hydrogen Sulfate (Elevated levels of drugs metabolized by the CYP450 system may be observed when co-administered with telithromycin; therefore, increases or prolongation of the therapeutic and/or adverse effects of the concomitant drug may be observed).
No products indexed under this heading.

Clozapine (Elevated levels of drugs metabolized by the CYP450 system may be observed when co-administered with telithromycin; therefore, increases or prolongation of the therapeutic and/or adverse effects of the concomitant drug may be observed).
No products indexed under this heading.

Codeine Phosphate (Elevated levels of drugs metabolized by the CYP450 system may be observed when co-administered with telithromycin; therefore, increases or prolongation of the therapeutic and/or adverse effects of the concomitant drug may be observed). Products include:
Tylenol with Codeine Tablets 2427

Codeine Sulfate (Elevated levels of drugs metabolized by the CYP450 system may be observed when co-administered with telithromycin; therefore, increases or prolongation of the therapeutic and/or adverse effects of the concomitant drug may be observed).
No products indexed under this heading.

Cortisone Acetate (Concomitant administration of CYP 3A4 inducers is likely to result in subtherapeutic levels of telithromycin and loss of effect).
No products indexed under this heading.

Cyclobenzaprine (Elevated levels of drugs metabolized by the CYP450 system may be observed when co-administered with telithromycin; therefore, increases or prolongation of the therapeutic and/or adverse effects of the concomitant drug may be observed).
No products indexed under this heading.

Cyclobenzaprine Hydrochloride (Elevated levels of drugs metabolized by the CYP450 system may be observed when co-administered with telithromycin; therefore, increases or prolongation of the therapeutic and/or adverse effects of the concomitant drug may be observed).
Products include:
Amrix Capsules 966

Cyclophosphamide (Elevated levels of drugs metabolized by the CYP450 system may be observed when co-administered with telithromycin; therefore, increases or prolongation of the therapeutic and/or adverse effects of the concomitant drug may be observed).
No products indexed under this heading.

Cyclosporine (Co-administration of telithromycin with a drug primarily metabolized by the CYP 3A4 enzyme system may result in increased plasma concentrations of the drug co-administered with telithromycin that could increase or prolong both the therapeutic and adverse effects).
Products include:
Gengraf Capsules 435
Neoral Oral Solution 2280
Neoral Soft Gelatin Capsules 2280
Restasis Ophthalmic Emulsion 557
Sandimmune 2296

Desipramine Hydrochloride (Elevated levels of drugs metabolized by the CYP450 system may be observed when co-administered with telithromycin; therefore, increases or prolongation of the therapeutic and/or adverse effects of the concomitant drug may be observed).
No products indexed under this heading.

Desogestrel (Co-administration of telithromycin with a drug primarily metabolized by the CYP 3A4 enzyme system may result in increased plasma concentrations of the drug co-administered with telithromycin that could increase or prolong both the therapeutic and adverse effects).
Products include:
Mircette Tablets 1034

Dexamethasone (Concomitant administration of CYP 3A4 inducers is likely to result in subtherapeutic levels of telithromycin and loss of effect). Products include:
Ciprodex Otic Suspension 541

Dexamethasone Acetate (Concomitant administration of CYP 3A4 inducers is likely to result in subtherapeutic levels of telithromycin and loss of effect).
No products indexed under this heading.

Dexamethasone Phosphate (Elevated levels of drugs metabolized by the CYP450 system may be observed when co-administered with telithromycin; therefore, increases or prolongation of the therapeutic and/or adverse effects of the concomitant drug may be observed).
No products indexed under this heading.

Dexamethasone Sodium (Elevated levels of drugs metabolized by the CYP450 system may be observed when co-administered with telithromycin; therefore, increases or prolongation of the therapeutic and/or adverse effects of the concomitant drug may be observed).
No products indexed under this heading.

Dexamethasone Sodium Phosphate (Concomitant administration of CYP 3A4 inducers is likely to result in subtherapeutic levels of telithromycin and loss of effect).
No products indexed under this heading.

Dexfenfluramine Hydrochloride (Elevated levels of drugs metabolized by the CYP450 system may be observed when co-administered with telithromycin; therefore, increases or prolongation of the therapeutic and/or adverse effects of the concomitant drug may be observed).
No products indexed under this heading.

Dextromethorphan (Elevated levels of drugs metabolized by the CYP450 system may be observed when co-administered with telithromycin; therefore, increases or prolongation of the therapeutic and/or adverse effects of the concomitant drug may be observed).
No products indexed under this heading.

Dextromethorphan Hydrobromide (Elevated levels of drugs metabolized by the CYP450 system may be observed when co-administered with telithromycin; therefore, increases or prolongation of the therapeutic and/or adverse effects of the concomitant drug may be observed). Products include:
PediaCare Children's Liquid Multi-Symptom Cold 1902
PediaCare Children's Long-Acting Cough 1902
Children's Sudafed PE Cold & Cough Liquid 1907
Sudafed PE Cold & Cough Caplets 1907
Children's Tylenol Plus Cough & Runny Nose Suspension Liquid 1912
Children's Tylenol Plus Cough & Sore Throat Suspension Liquid 1912
Children's Tylenol Plus Flu Suspension Liquid 1914
Children's Tylenol Plus Multi-Symptom Cold Suspension Liquid 1912
Tylenol Cold Severe Congestion Daytime Caplets with Cool Burst 1912
Tylenol Cold Head Congestion Daytime Caplets with Cool Burst 1910
Tylenol Cold Head Congestion Nighttime Caplets with Cool Burst 1910
Tylenol Cold Head Congestion Severe Daytime Caplets with Cool Burst 1910
Tylenol Cold Multi-Symptom Daytime Caplets with Cool Burst and Rapid Release Gels 1913
Tylenol Cold Multi-Symptom Daytime Liquid with Citrus Burst 1913
Tylenol Cold Multi-Symptom Nighttime Caplets with Cool Burst 1913
Tylenol Cold Multi-Symptom Nighttime Liquid with Cool Burst 1913
Tylenol Cold Multi-Symptom Severe Caplets with Cool Burst 1913
Tylenol Cold Multi-Symptom Severe Daytime Liquid with Citrus Burst 1913
Tylenol Cough & Sore Throat Daytime Liquid with Cool Burst 1918
Tylenol Cough & Sore Throat Nighttime Liquid with Cool Burst 1918
Vicks DayQuil Cold & Flu Multi-Symptom Relief .... ▣616
Vicks DayQuil LiquiCaps 2567
Vicks DayQuil Liquid 2567
Vicks DayQuil Multi-Symptom Cold/Flu Relief 2567
Vicks NyQuil Cold & Flu Multi-Symptom Relief .... ▣617
Vicks NyQuil LiquiCaps 2567
Vicks NyQuil Liquid 2567
Vicks NyQuil Multi-Symptom Cold/Flu Relief 2567

Dextromethorphan Polistirex (Elevated levels of drugs metabolized by the CYP450 system may be observed when co-administered with telithromycin; therefore, increases or prolongation of the therapeutic and/or adverse effects of the concomitant drug may be observed).
No products indexed under this heading.

Diazepam (Co-administration of telithromycin with a drug primarily metabolized by the CYP 3A4 enzyme system may result in increased plasma concentrations of the drug co-administered with telithromycin that could increase or prolong both the therapeutic and adverse effects).
Products include:
Valium Tablets 2658

Diclofenac Potassium (Elevated levels of drugs metabolized by the CYP450 system may be observed when co-administered with telithromycin; therefore, increases or prolongation of the therapeutic and/or adverse effects of the concomitant drug may be observed).
No products indexed under this heading.

Diclofenac Sodium (Elevated levels of drugs metabolized by the CYP450 system may be observed when co-administered with telithromycin; therefore, increases or prolongation of the therapeutic and/or adverse effects of the concomitant drug may be observed). Products include:
Diclofenac Sodium Ophthalmic Solution .... ⊙240
Voltaren Ophthalmic Solution 2336
Voltaren Tablets 2334
Voltaren-XR Tablets 2337

Digoxin (Plasma peak and trough levels of digoxin were increased when co-administered with telithromycin; however, trough concentrations of digoxin ranged from 0.74 to 2.17 ng/mL). Products include:
Lanoxin Injection 1498
Lanoxin Injection Pediatric 1502
Lanoxin Tablets 1505

Dihydroergotamine Mesylate (Co-administration is not recommended because acute ergot toxicity characterized by severe peripheral vasospasm and dyesthesia have been reported with macrolide antibiotics).
No products indexed under this heading.

Diltiazem Hydrochloride (Co-administration of telithromycin with a drug primarily metabolized by the CYP 3A4 enzyme system may result in increased plasma concentrations of the drug co-administered with telithromycin that could increase or prolong both the therapeutic and adverse effects). Products include:
Cardizem LA Extended Release Tablets 421

Diltiazem Maleate (Co-administration of telithromycin with a drug primarily metabolized by the CYP 3A4 enzyme system may result in increased plasma concentrations of the drug co-administered with telithromycin that could increase or prolong both the therapeutic and adverse effects).
No products indexed under this heading.

Disopyramide (Co-administration of telithromycin with a drug primarily metabolized by the CYP 3A4 enzyme system may result in increased plasma concentrations of the drug co-administered with telithromycin that could increase or prolong both the therapeutic and adverse effects).
No products indexed under this heading.

Disopyramide Phosphate (Co-administration of telithromycin with a drug primarily metabolized by the CYP 3A4 enzyme system may result in increased plasma concentrations of the drug co-administered with telithromycin that could increase or prolong both the therapeutic and adverse effects).
No products indexed under this heading.

Disulfiram (Co-administration of telithromycin with a drug primarily metabolized by the CYP 3A4 enzyme system may result in increased plasma concentrations of the drug co-administered with telithromycin that could increase or prolong both the therapeutic and adverse effects).
No products indexed under this heading.

Divalproex Sodium (Elevated levels of drugs metabolized by the CYP450 system may be observed when co-administered with telithromycin; therefore, increases or prolongation of the therapeutic and/or adverse effects of the concomitant drug may be observed). Products include:
Depakote ER Tablets 423

Docetaxel (Elevated levels of drugs metabolized by the CYP450 system may be observed when co-administered with telithromycin; therefore, increases or prolongation of the therapeutic and/or adverse effects of the concomitant drug may be observed). Products include:
Taxotere Injection Concentrate 2773

Dolasetron Mesylate (Elevated levels of drugs metabolized by the CYP450 system may be observed when co-administered with telithromycin; therefore, increases or prolongation of the therapeutic and/or

adverse effects of the concomitant drug may be observed). Products include:

Anzemet Injection 2701
Anzemet Tablets 2704

Donepezil Hydrochloride (Elevated levels of drugs metabolized by the CYP450 system may be observed when co-administered with telithromycin; therefore, increases or prolongation of the therapeutic and/or adverse effects of the concomitant drug may be observed). Products include:

Aricept Tablets 1062
Aricept ODT Tablets 1062

Doxepin Hydrochloride (Elevated levels of drugs metabolized by the CYP450 system may be observed when co-administered with telithromycin; therefore, increases or prolongation of the therapeutic and/or adverse effects of the concomitant drug may be observed).

No products indexed under this heading.

Doxorubicin Hydrochloride (Co-administration of telithromycin with a drug primarily metabolized by the CYP 3A4 enzyme system may result in increased plasma concentrations of the drug co-administered with telithromycin that could increase or prolong both the therapeutic and adverse effects).

No products indexed under this heading.

Dronabinol (Co-administration of telithromycin with a drug primarily metabolized by the CYP 3A4 enzyme system may result in increased plasma concentrations of the drug co-administered with telithromycin that could increase or prolong both the therapeutic and adverse effects). Products include:

Marinol Capsules 3163

Drugs that Undergo Biotransformation by Cytochrome P-450 Mixed Function Oxidase (Elevated levels of drugs metabolized by the CYP450 system may be observed when co-administered with telithromycin; therefore, increases or prolongation of the therapeutic and/or adverse effects of the concomitant drug may be observed).

No products indexed under this heading.

Dyphylline (Elevated levels of drugs metabolized by the CYP450 system may be observed when co-administered with telithromycin; therefore, increases or prolongation of the therapeutic and/or adverse effects of the concomitant drug may be observed).

No products indexed under this heading.

Efavirenz (Concomitant administration of CYP 3A4 inducers is likely to result in subtherapeutic levels of telithromycin and loss of effect). Products include:

Atripla Tablets 938
Sustiva Capsules 930
Sustiva Tablets 930

Encainide Hydrochloride (Elevated levels of drugs metabolized by the CYP450 system may be observed when co-administered with telithromycin; therefore, increases or prolongation of the therapeutic and/or adverse effects of the concomitant drug may be observed).

No products indexed under this heading.

Enoxacin (Elevated levels of drugs metabolized by the CYP450 system may be observed when co-administered with telithromycin; therefore, increases or prolongation of the therapeutic and/or adverse effects of the concomitant drug may be observed).

No products indexed under this heading.

Eprosartan Mesylate (Elevated levels of drugs metabolized by the CYP450 system may be observed when co-administered with telithromycin; therefore, increases or prolongation of the therapeutic and/or adverse effects of the concomitant drug may be observed). Products include:

Teveten Tablets 515
Teveten HCT Tablets 517

Ergonovine Maleate (Co-administration is not recommended because acute ergot toxicity characterized by severe peripheral vasospasm and dyesthesia have been reported with macrolide antibiotics).

No products indexed under this heading.

Ergotamine Tartrate (Co-administration is not recommended because acute ergot toxicity characterized by severe peripheral vasospasm and dyesthesia have been reported with macrolide antibiotics).

No products indexed under this heading.

Erythromycin (Co-administration of telithromycin with a drug primarily metabolized by the CYP 3A4 enzyme system may result in increased plasma concentrations of the drug co-administered with telithromycin that could increase or prolong both the therapeutic and adverse effects).

No products indexed under this heading.

Erythromycin Estolate (Co-administration of telithromycin with a drug primarily metabolized by the CYP 3A4 enzyme system may result in increased plasma concentrations of the drug co-administered with telithromycin that could increase or prolong both the therapeutic and adverse effects).

No products indexed under this heading.

Erythromycin Ethylsuccinate (Co-administration of telithromycin with a drug primarily metabolized by the CYP 3A4 enzyme system may result in increased plasma concentrations of the drug co-administered with telithromycin that could increase or prolong both the therapeutic and adverse effects). Products include:

E.E.S. 433
EryPed 431

Erythromycin Gluceptate (Co-administration of telithromycin with a drug primarily metabolized by the CYP 3A4 enzyme system may result in increased plasma concentrations of the drug co-administered with telithromycin that could increase or prolong both the therapeutic and adverse effects).

No products indexed under this heading.

Erythromycin Lactobionate (Co-administration of telithromycin with a drug primarily metabolized by the CYP 3A4 enzyme system may result in increased plasma concentrations of the drug co-administered with telithromycin that could increase or prolong both the therapeutic and adverse effects).

No products indexed under this heading.

Erythromycin Stearate (Co-administration of telithromycin with a drug primarily metabolized by the CYP 3A4 enzyme system may result in increased plasma concentrations of the drug co-administered with telithromycin that could increase or prolong both the therapeutic and adverse effects).

No products indexed under this heading.

Esomeprazole Magnesium (Elevated levels of drugs metabolized by the CYP450 system may be observed when co-administered with telithromycin; therefore, increases or prolongation of the therapeutic and/or adverse effects of the concomitant drug may be observed). Products include:

Nexium Delayed-Release Capsules 645
Nexium Delayed-Release Oral Suspension 645

Estradiol (Co-administration of telithromycin with a drug primarily metabolized by the CYP 3A4 enzyme system may result in increased plasma concentrations of the drug co-administered with telithromycin that could increase or prolong both the therapeutic and adverse effects). Products include:

Activella Tablets 2347
Angeliq Tablets 751
Climara Transdermal System 763
Climara Pro Transdermal System 768
Divigel 3167
Vagifem Tablets 2375

Estradiol Benzoate (Co-administration of telithromycin with a drug primarily metabolized by the CYP 3A4 enzyme system may result in increased plasma concentrations of the drug co-administered with telithromycin that could increase or prolong both the therapeutic and adverse effects).

No products indexed under this heading.

Estradiol Cypionate (Co-administration of telithromycin with a drug primarily metabolized by the CYP 3A4 enzyme system may result in increased plasma concentrations of the drug co-administered with telithromycin that could increase or prolong both the therapeutic and adverse effects).

No products indexed under this heading.

Estradiol Valerate (Co-administration of telithromycin with a drug primarily metabolized by the CYP 3A4 enzyme system may result in increased plasma concentrations of the drug co-administered with telithromycin that could increase or prolong both the therapeutic and adverse effects).

No products indexed under this heading.

Estrogen (Elevated levels of drugs metabolized by the CYP450 system may be observed when co-administered with telithromycin; therefore, increases or prolongation of the therapeutic and/or adverse effects of the concomitant drug may be observed).

No products indexed under this heading.

Estrogens, Conjugated (Elevated levels of drugs metabolized by the CYP450 system may be observed when co-administered with telithromycin; therefore, increases or prolongation of the therapeutic and/or adverse effects of the concomitant drug may be observed). Products include:

Premarin Intravenous 3217
Premarin Tablets 3221
Premarin Vaginal Cream 3228
Premphase Tablets 3232
Prempro Tablets 3232

Estrogens, Conjugated, Synthetic A (Elevated levels of drugs metabolized by the CYP450 system may be observed when co-administered with telithromycin; therefore, increases or prolongation of the therapeutic and/or adverse effects of the concomitant drug may be observed).

No products indexed under this heading.

Estrogens, Esterified (Elevated levels of drugs metabolized by the CYP450 system may be observed when co-administered with telithromycin; therefore, increases or prolongation of the therapeutic and/or adverse effects of the concomitant drug may be observed). Products include:

Estratest Tablets 3043
Estratest H.S. Tablets 3043

Ethinyl Estradiol (Co-administration of telithromycin with a drug primarily metabolized by the CYP 3A4 enzyme system may result in increased plasma concentrations of the drug co-administered with telithromycin that could increase or prolong both the therapeutic and adverse effects). Products include:

Lybrel Tablets 3204
Mircette Tablets 1034
NuvaRing 2897
Ortho-Cyclen/Ortho Tri-Cyclen 2449
Ortho Evra Transdermal System 2437
Ortho Tri-Cyclen Lo Tablets 2458
Seasonique Tablets 1046
Yaz Tablets 805

Ethosuximide (Co-administration of telithromycin with a drug primarily metabolized by the CYP 3A4 enzyme system may result in increased plasma concentrations of the drug co-administered with telithromycin that could increase or prolong both the therapeutic and adverse effects).

No products indexed under this heading.

Ethotoin (Elevated levels of drugs metabolized by the CYP450 system may be observed when co-administered with telithromycin; therefore, increases or prolongation of the therapeutic and/or adverse effects of the concomitant drug may be observed).

No products indexed under this heading.

Ethynodiol Diacetate (Co-administration of telithromycin with a drug primarily metabolized by the CYP 3A4 enzyme system may result in increased plasma concentrations of the drug co-administered with telithromycin that could increase or prolong both the therapeutic and adverse effects).
No products indexed under this heading.

Etodolac (Elevated levels of drugs metabolized by the CYP450 system may be observed when co-administered with telithromycin; therefore, increases or prolongation of the therapeutic and/or adverse effects of the concomitant drug may be observed).
No products indexed under this heading.

Etoposide (Co-administration of telithromycin with a drug primarily metabolized by the CYP 3A4 enzyme system may result in increased plasma concentrations of the drug co-administered with telithromycin that could increase or prolong both the therapeutic and adverse effects).
No products indexed under this heading.

Etoposide Phosphate (Co-administration of telithromycin with a drug primarily metabolized by the CYP 3A4 enzyme system may result in increased plasma concentrations of the drug co-administered with telithromycin that could increase or prolong both the therapeutic and adverse effects).
No products indexed under this heading.

Felbamate (Concomitant administration of CYP 3A4 inducers is likely to result in subtherapeutic levels of telithromycin and loss of effect).
No products indexed under this heading.

Felodipine (Co-administration of telithromycin with a drug primarily metabolized by the CYP 3A4 enzyme system may result in increased plasma concentrations of the drug co-administered with telithromycin that could increase or prolong both the therapeutic and adverse effects).
No products indexed under this heading.

Fenoprofen Calcium (Elevated levels of drugs metabolized by the CYP450 system may be observed when co-administered with telithromycin; therefore, increases or prolongation of the therapeutic and/or adverse effects of the concomitant drug may be observed). Products include:
Nalfon Capsules 2508

Fentanyl (Co-administration of telithromycin with a drug primarily metabolized by the CYP 3A4 enzyme system may result in increased plasma concentrations of the drug co-administered with telithromycin that could increase or prolong both the therapeutic and adverse effects).
Products include:
Duragesic Transdermal System 2405
Ionsys Transdermal System 2410

Fentanyl Citrate (Co-administration of telithromycin with a drug primarily metabolized by the CYP 3A4 enzyme system may result in increased plasma concentrations of the drug co-administered with telithromycin that could increase or prolong both the therapeutic and adverse effects).
Products include:
Actiq 959
Fentora Tablets 968

Flecainide Acetate (Elevated levels of drugs metabolized by the CYP450 system may be observed when co-administered with telithromycin; therefore, increases or prolongation of the therapeutic and/or adverse effects of the concomitant drug may be observed).
No products indexed under this heading.

Fludrocortisone Acetate (Concomitant administration of CYP 3A4 inducers is likely to result in subtherapeutic levels of telithromycin and loss of effect).
No products indexed under this heading.

Fluoxetine (Elevated levels of drugs metabolized by the CYP450 system may be observed when co-administered with telithromycin; therefore, increases or prolongation of the therapeutic and/or adverse effects of the concomitant drug may be observed).
No products indexed under this heading.

Fluoxetine Hydrochloride (Elevated levels of drugs metabolized by the CYP450 system may be observed when co-administered with telithromycin; therefore, increases or prolongation of the therapeutic and/ or adverse effects of the concomitant drug may be observed).
Products include:
Prozac Weekly Capsules 1852
Prozac Pulvules and Liquid 1852
Symbyax Capsules 1871

Fluphenazine Decanoate (Elevated levels of drugs metabolized by the CYP450 system may be observed when co-administered with telithromycin; therefore, increases or prolongation of the therapeutic and/ or adverse effects of the concomitant drug may be observed).
No products indexed under this heading.

Fluphenazine Enanthate (Elevated levels of drugs metabolized by the CYP450 system may be observed when co-administered with telithromycin; therefore, increases or prolongation of the therapeutic and/ or adverse effects of the concomitant drug may be observed).
No products indexed under this heading.

Fluphenazine Hydrochloride (Elevated levels of drugs metabolized by the CYP450 system may be observed when co-administered with telithromycin; therefore, increases or prolongation of the therapeutic and/ or adverse effects of the concomitant drug may be observed).
No products indexed under this heading.

Flurbiprofen (Elevated levels of drugs metabolized by the CYP450 system may be observed when co-administered with telithromycin; therefore, increases or prolongation of the therapeutic and/or adverse effects of the concomitant drug may be observed).
No products indexed under this heading.

Flurbiprofen Sodium (Elevated levels of drugs metabolized by the CYP450 system may be observed when co-administered with telithromycin; therefore, increases or prolongation of the therapeutic and/or adverse effects of the concomitant drug may be observed).
No products indexed under this heading.

Flutamide (Elevated levels of drugs metabolized by the CYP450 system may be observed when co-administered with telithromycin; therefore, increases or prolongation of the therapeutic and/or adverse effects of the concomitant drug may be observed).
No products indexed under this heading.

Fluticasone Propionate (Elevated levels of drugs metabolized by the CYP450 system may be observed when co-administered with telithromycin; therefore, increases or prolongation of the therapeutic and/or adverse effects of the concomitant drug may be observed). Products include:
Advair Diskus 100/50 1276
Advair Diskus 250/50 1276
Advair Diskus 500/50 1276
Advair HFA 45/21 Inhalation Aerosol 1288
Advair HFA 115/21 Inhalation Aerosol 1288
Advair HFA 230/21 Inhalation Aerosol 1288
Flonase Nasal Spray 1431
Flovent Diskus 50 mcg 1435

Fluvastatin Sodium (Elevated levels of drugs metabolized by the CYP450 system may be observed when co-administered with telithromycin; therefore, increases or prolongation of the therapeutic and/or adverse effects of the concomitant drug may be observed). Products include:
Lescol Capsules 2268
Lescol XL Tablets 2268

Fluvoxamine Maleate (Elevated levels of drugs metabolized by the CYP450 system may be observed when co-administered with telithromycin; therefore, increases or prolongation of the therapeutic and/or adverse effects of the concomitant drug may be observed). Products include:
Luvox CR Extended-Release Capsules 1759

Formoterol Fumarate (Elevated levels of drugs metabolized by the CYP450 system may be observed when co-administered with telithromycin; therefore, increases or prolongation of the therapeutic and/or adverse effects of the concomitant drug may be observed). Products include:
Foradil Aerolizer 2849
Perforomist Inhalation Solution 1025

Fosphenytoin (Elevated levels of drugs metabolized by the CYP450 system may be observed when co-administered with telithromycin; therefore, increases or prolongation of the therapeutic and/or adverse effects of the concomitant drug may be observed).
No products indexed under this heading.

Fosphenytoin Sodium (Concomitant administration of CYP 3A4 inducers is likely to result in subtherapeutic levels of telithromycin and loss of effect).
No products indexed under this heading.

Gabapentin (Elevated levels of drugs metabolized by the CYP450 system may be observed when co-administered with telithromycin; therefore, increases or prolongation of the therapeutic and/or adverse effects of the concomitant drug may be observed).
No products indexed under this heading.

Galantamine Hydrobromide (Elevated levels of drugs metabolized by the CYP450 system may be observed when co-administered with telithromycin; therefore, increases or prolongation of the therapeutic and/ or adverse effects of the concomitant drug may be observed).
No products indexed under this heading.

Garlic Extract (Concomitant administration of CYP 3A4 inducers is likely to result in subtherapeutic levels of telithromycin and loss of effect).
No products indexed under this heading.

Garlic Oil (Concomitant administration of CYP 3A4 inducers is likely to result in subtherapeutic levels of telithromycin and loss of effect).
No products indexed under this heading.

Glimepiride (Elevated levels of drugs metabolized by the CYP450 system may be observed when co-administered with telithromycin; therefore, increases or prolongation of the therapeutic and/or adverse effects of the concomitant drug may be observed). Products include:
Avandaryl Tablets 1344
Duetact Tablets 3085

Glipizide (Elevated levels of drugs metabolized by the CYP450 system may be observed when co-administered with telithromycin; therefore, increases or prolongation of the therapeutic and/or adverse effects of the concomitant drug may be observed).
No products indexed under this heading.

Glyburide (Elevated levels of drugs metabolized by the CYP450 system may be observed when co-administered with telithromycin; therefore, increases or prolongation of the therapeutic and/or adverse effects of the concomitant drug may be observed).
No products indexed under this heading.

Grepafloxacin Hydrochloride (Elevated levels of drugs metabolized by the CYP450 system may be observed when co-administered with telithromycin; therefore, increases or prolongation of the therapeutic and/ or adverse effects of the concomitant drug may be observed).
No products indexed under this heading.

Haloperidol (Co-administration of telithromycin with a drug primarily metabolized by the CYP 3A4 enzyme system may result in increased plasma concentrations of the drug co-administered with telithromycin that could increase or prolong both the therapeutic and adverse effects).
No products indexed under this heading.

Haloperidol Decanoate (Co-administration of telithromycin with a drug primarily metabolized by the CYP 3A4 enzyme system may result in increased plasma concentrations of the drug co-administered with telithromycin that could increase or prolong both the therapeutic and adverse effects).
No products indexed under this heading.

Haloperidol Lactate (Co-administration of telithromycin with a drug primarily metabolized by the CYP 3A4 enzyme system may result in increased plasma concentrations of the drug co-administered with telithromycin that could increase or prolong both the therapeutic and adverse effects).
No products indexed under this heading.

Hydrocodone Bitartrate (Elevated levels of drugs metabolized by the CYP450 system may be observed when co-administered with telithromycin; therefore, increases or prolongation of the therapeutic and/or adverse effects of the concomitant drug may be observed). Products include:
Lortab 5/500 Tablets 3143
Lortab 7.5/500 Tablets 3144
Lortab 10/500 Tablets 3144
Vicodin Tablets 529
Vicodin ES Tablets 530
Vicodin HP Tablets 531
Vicoprofen Tablets 533
Zydone Tablets 1132

Hydrocortisone (Concomitant administration of CYP 3A4 inducers is likely to result in subtherapeutic levels of telithromycin and loss of effect).
No products indexed under this heading.

Hydrocortisone Acetate (Concomitant administration of CYP 3A4 inducers is likely to result in subtherapeutic levels of telithromycin and loss of effect). Products include:
Analpram-HC 1140
Pramosone 1141

Hydrocortisone Butyrate (Concomitant administration of CYP 3A4 inducers is likely to result in subtherapeutic levels of telithromycin and loss of effect).
No products indexed under this heading.

Hydrocortisone Cypionate (Concomitant administration of CYP 3A4 inducers is likely to result in subtherapeutic levels of telithromycin and loss of effect).
No products indexed under this heading.

Hydrocortisone Hemisuccinate (Concomitant administration of CYP 3A4 inducers is likely to result in subtherapeutic levels of telithromycin and loss of effect).
No products indexed under this heading.

Hydrocortisone Probutate (Concomitant administration of CYP 3A4 inducers is likely to result in subtherapeutic levels of telithromycin and loss of effect).
No products indexed under this heading.

Hydrocortisone Sodium Phosphate (Concomitant administration of CYP 3A4 inducers is likely to result in subtherapeutic levels of telithromycin and loss of effect).
No products indexed under this heading.

Hydrocortisone Sodium Succinate (Concomitant administration of CYP 3A4 inducers is likely to result in subtherapeutic levels of telithromycin and loss of effect).
No products indexed under this heading.

Hydrocortisone Valerate (Concomitant administration of CYP 3A4 inducers is likely to result in subtherapeutic levels of telithromycin and loss of effect).
No products indexed under this heading.

Hypericum (Concomitant administration of CYP 3A4 inducers is likely to result in subtherapeutic levels of telithromycin and loss of effect). Products include:
Satieté Tablets 640

Hypericum Perforatum (Concomitant administration of CYP 3A4 inducers is likely to result in subtherapeutic levels of telithromycin and loss of effect).
No products indexed under this heading.

Ibuprofen (Elevated levels of drugs metabolized by the CYP450 system may be observed when co-administered with telithromycin; therefore, increases or prolongation of the therapeutic and/or adverse effects of the concomitant drug may be observed). Products include:
Motrin IB Tablets and Caplets 1900
Children's Motrin Oral Suspension ... 1901
Children's Motrin Non-Staining Dye-Free Oral Suspension 1901
Children's Motrin Cold Oral Suspension 1899
Infants' Motrin Concentrated Drops 1901
Infants' Motrin Non-Staining Dye-Free Concentrated Drops 1901
Junior Strength Motrin Caplets and Chewable Tablets 1901
Vicoprofen Tablets 533

Imipramine Hydrochloride (Elevated levels of drugs metabolized by the CYP450 system may be observed when co-administered with telithromycin; therefore, increases or prolongation of the therapeutic and/or adverse effects of the concomitant drug may be observed).
No products indexed under this heading.

Imipramine Pamoate (Elevated levels of drugs metabolized by the CYP450 system may be observed when co-administered with telithromycin; therefore, increases or prolongation of the therapeutic and/or adverse effects of the concomitant drug may be observed).
No products indexed under this heading.

Indinavir Sulfate (Co-administration of telithromycin with a drug primarily metabolized by the CYP 3A4 enzyme system may result in increased plasma concentrations of the drug co-administered with telithromycin that could increase or prolong both the therapeutic and adverse effects). Products include:
Crixivan Capsules 1979

Indomethacin (Elevated levels of drugs metabolized by the CYP450 system may be observed when co-administered with telithromycin; therefore, increases or prolongation of the therapeutic and/or adverse effects of the concomitant drug may be observed). Products include:
Indocin 2024

Indomethacin Sodium Trihydrate (Elevated levels of drugs metabolized by the CYP450 system may be observed when co-administered with telithromycin; therefore, increases or prolongation of the therapeutic and/or adverse effects of the concomitant drug may be observed). Products include:
Indocin I.V. 2489

Indoramin Hydrochloride (Elevated levels of drugs metabolized by the CYP450 system may be observed when co-administered with telithromycin; therefore, increases or prolongation of the therapeutic and/or adverse effects of the concomitant drug may be observed).
No products indexed under this heading.

Irbesartan (Elevated levels of drugs metabolized by the CYP450 system may be observed when co-administered with telithromycin; therefore, increases or prolongation of the therapeutic and/or adverse effects of the concomitant drug may be observed). Products include:
Avalide Tablets 892
Avalide Tablets 2713
Avapro Tablets 897
Avapro Tablets 2718

Isotretinoin (Elevated levels of drugs metabolized by the CYP450 system may be observed when co-administered with telithromycin; therefore, increases or prolongation of the therapeutic and/or adverse effects of the concomitant drug may be observed). Products include:
Accutane Capsules 2607

Isradipine (Co-administration of telithromycin with a drug primarily metabolized by the CYP 3A4 enzyme system may result in increased plasma concentrations of the drug co-administered with telithromycin that could increase or prolong both the therapeutic and adverse effects). Products include:
DynaCirc CR Controlled Release Tablets 1407

Itraconazole (A study with itraconazole showed the Cmax and AUC of telithromycin were increased).
No products indexed under this heading.

Ixabepilone (Co-administration of telithromycin with a drug primarily metabolized by the CYP 3A4 enzyme system may result in increased plasma concentrations of the drug co-administered with telithromycin that could increase or prolong both the therapeutic and adverse effects). Products include:
Ixempra Kit for Injection 915

Ketoconazole (A study with ketoconazole showed the Cmax and AUC of telithromycin were increased). Products include:
Extina Foam, 2% 3057
Nizoral A-D Shampoo 1901

Ketoprofen (Elevated levels of drugs metabolized by the CYP450 system may be observed when co-administered with telithromycin; therefore, increases or prolongation of the therapeutic and/or adverse effects of the concomitant drug may be observed).
No products indexed under this heading.

Ketorolac Tromethamine (Elevated levels of drugs metabolized by the CYP450 system may be observed when co-administered with telithromycin; therefore, increases or prolongation of the therapeutic and/or adverse effects of the concomitant drug may be observed).
No products indexed under this heading.

Labetalol Hydrochloride (Elevated levels of drugs metabolized by the CYP450 system may be observed when co-administered with telithromycin; therefore, increases or prolongation of the therapeutic and/or adverse effects of the concomitant drug may be observed).
No products indexed under this heading.

Lamotrigine (Elevated levels of drugs metabolized by the CYP450 system may be observed when co-administered with telithromycin; therefore, increases or prolongation of the therapeutic and/or adverse effects of the concomitant drug may be observed). Products include:
Lamictal 1488

Lansoprazole (Elevated levels of drugs metabolized by the CYP450 system may be observed when co-administered with telithromycin; therefore, increases or prolongation of the therapeutic and/or adverse effects of the concomitant drug may be observed).
No products indexed under this heading.

Levetiracetam (Elevated levels of drugs metabolized by the CYP450 system may be observed when co-administered with telithromycin; therefore, increases or prolongation of the therapeutic and/or adverse effects of the concomitant drug may be observed). Products include:
Keppra Injection 3137
Keppra Oral Solution 3131
Keppra Tablets 3131

Levobupivacaine Hydrochloride (Elevated levels of drugs metabolized by the CYP450 system may be observed when co-administered with telithromycin; therefore, increases or prolongation of the therapeutic and/or adverse effects of the concomitant drug may be observed).
No products indexed under this heading.

Levonorgestrel (When oral contraceptives containing ethinyl estradiol and levonorgestrel were co-administered with telithromycin, the steady-state AUC of ethinyl estradiol did not change but the AUC of levonorgestrel increased. However, telithromycin did not interfere with the antiovulatory effect of the oral contraceptives). Products include:
Climara Pro Transdermal System 768
Lybrel Tablets 3204
Mirena Intrauterine System 779
Plan B Tablets 1044
Seasonique Tablets 1046

Lidocaine (Co-administration of telithromycin with a drug primarily

metabolized by the CYP 3A4 enzyme system may result in increased plasma concentrations of the drug co-administered with telithromycin that could increase or prolong both the therapeutic and adverse effects). Products include:
Lidoderm Patch 1114

Lidocaine Base (Elevated levels of drugs metabolized by the CYP450 system may be observed when co-administered with telithromycin; therefore, increases or prolongation of the therapeutic and/or adverse effects of the concomitant drug may be observed).
No products indexed under this heading.

Lidocaine Hydrochloride (Co-administration of telithromycin with a drug primarily metabolized by the CYP 3A4 enzyme system may result in increased plasma concentrations of the drug co-administered with telithromycin that could increase or prolong both the therapeutic and adverse effects).
No products indexed under this heading.

Lomefloxacin Hydrochloride (Elevated levels of drugs metabolized by the CYP450 system may be observed when co-administered with telithromycin; therefore, increases or prolongation of the therapeutic and/or adverse effects of the concomitant drug may be observed).
No products indexed under this heading.

Losartan Potassium (Elevated levels of drugs metabolized by the CYP450 system may be observed when co-administered with telithromycin; therefore, increases or prolongation of the therapeutic and/or adverse effects of the concomitant drug may be observed). Products include:
Cozaar Tablets 1973

Lovastatin (Lovastatin levels were increased due to CYP 3A4 inhibition by telithromycin, thereby increasing the risk of myopathy. Co-administration should be avoided). Products include:
Advicor Tablets 402
Mevacor Tablets 2063

Maprotiline Hydrochloride (Elevated levels of drugs metabolized by the CYP450 system may be observed when co-administered with telithromycin; therefore, increases or prolongation of the therapeutic and/or adverse effects of the concomitant drug may be observed).
No products indexed under this heading.

Meclofenamate Sodium (Elevated levels of drugs metabolized by the CYP450 system may be observed when co-administered with telithromycin; therefore, increases or prolongation of the therapeutic and/or adverse effects of the concomitant drug may be observed).
No products indexed under this heading.

Mefenamic Acid (Elevated levels of drugs metabolized by the CYP450 system may be observed when co-administered with telithromycin; therefore, increases or prolongation of the therapeutic and/or adverse effects of the concomitant drug may be observed).
No products indexed under this heading.

Meloxicam (Elevated levels of drugs metabolized by the CYP450 system may be observed when co-administered with telithromycin; therefore, increases or prolongation of the therapeutic and/or adverse effects of the concomitant drug may be observed). Products include:
Mobic Oral Suspension 863
Mobic Tablets 863

Meperidine Hydrochloride (Elevated levels of drugs metabolized by the CYP450 system may be observed when co-administered with telithromycin; therefore, increases or prolongation of the therapeutic and/or adverse effects of the concomitant drug may be observed).
No products indexed under this heading.

Mephenytoin (Concomitant administration of CYP 3A4 inducers is likely to result in subtherapeutic levels of telithromycin and loss of effect).
No products indexed under this heading.

Mephobarbital (Elevated levels of drugs metabolized by the CYP450 system may be observed when co-administered with telithromycin; therefore, increases or prolongation of the therapeutic and/or adverse effects of the concomitant drug may be observed).
No products indexed under this heading.

Meprobamate (Elevated levels of drugs metabolized by the CYP450 system may be observed when co-administered with telithromycin; therefore, increases or prolongation of the therapeutic and/or adverse effects of the concomitant drug may be observed).
No products indexed under this heading.

Mestranol (Co-administration of telithromycin with a drug primarily metabolized by the CYP 3A4 enzyme system may result in increased plasma concentrations of the drug co-administered with telithromycin that could increase or prolong both the therapeutic and adverse effects).
No products indexed under this heading.

Metformin Hydrochloride (Elevated levels of drugs metabolized by the CYP450 system may be observed when co-administered with telithromycin; therefore, increases or prolongation of the therapeutic and/or adverse effects of the concomitant drug may be observed). Products include:
ActoPlus Met Tablets 3071
Avandamet Tablets 1336
Janumet Tablets 2041
PrandiMet Tablets 2967

Methadone Hydrochloride (Co-administration of telithromycin with a drug primarily metabolized by the CYP 3A4 enzyme system may result in increased plasma concentrations of the drug co-administered with telithromycin that could increase or prolong both the therapeutic and adverse effects).
No products indexed under this heading.

Methamphetamine Hydrochloride (Elevated levels of drugs metabolized by the CYP450 system may be observed when co-administered with telithromycin; therefore, increases or prolongation of the therapeutic and/or adverse effects of the concomitant drug may be observed).
No products indexed under this heading.

Methsuximide (Concomitant administration of CYP 3A4 inducers is likely to result in subtherapeutic levels of telithromycin and loss of effect).
No products indexed under this heading.

Methylergonovine Maleate (Co-administration is not recommended because acute ergot toxicity characterized by severe peripheral vasospasm and dyesthesia have been reported with macrolide antibiotics).
No products indexed under this heading.

Methylprednisolone (Concomitant administration of CYP 3A4 inducers is likely to result in subtherapeutic levels of telithromycin and loss of effect).
No products indexed under this heading.

Methylprednisolone Acetate (Concomitant administration of CYP 3A4 inducers is likely to result in subtherapeutic levels of telithromycin and loss of effect).
No products indexed under this heading.

Methylprednisolone Sodium Succinate (Concomitant administration of CYP 3A4 inducers is likely to result in subtherapeutic levels of telithromycin and loss of effect).
No products indexed under this heading.

Methysergide Maleate (Co-administration is not recommended because acute ergot toxicity characterized by severe peripheral vasospasm and dyesthesia have been reported with macrolide antibiotics).
No products indexed under this heading.

Metoprolol Succinate (Co-administration increased the Cmax and AUC of metoprolol; however, there was no effect on the elimination half-life. The increased exposure to metoprolol may be of clinical importance). Products include:
Toprol-XL Tablets 666

Metoprolol Tartrate (Co-administration increased the Cmax and AUC of metoprolol; however, there was no effect on the elimination half-life. The increased exposure to metoprolol may be of clinical importance).
No products indexed under this heading.

Mexiletine Hydrochloride (Elevated levels of drugs metabolized by the CYP450 system may be observed when co-administered with telithromycin; therefore, increases or prolongation of the therapeutic and/or adverse effects of the concomitant drug may be observed).
No products indexed under this heading.

Midazolam Hydrochloride (Concomitant administration of telithromycin with midazolam increased the AUC of midazolam. Dosage adjustment of midazolam should be considered if necessary).
No products indexed under this heading.

Miglitol (Elevated levels of drugs metabolized by the CYP450 system may be observed when co-administered with telithromycin; therefore, increases or prolongation of the therapeutic and/or adverse effects of the concomitant drug may be observed).
No products indexed under this heading.

Mirtazapine (Elevated levels of drugs metabolized by the CYP450 system may be observed when co-administered with telithromycin; therefore, increases or prolongation of the therapeutic and/or adverse effects of the concomitant drug may be observed). Products include:
Remeron Tablets 2924
RemeronSolTab Tablets 2927

Modafinil (Concomitant administration of CYP 3A4 inducers is likely to result in subtherapeutic levels of telithromycin and loss of effect). Products include:
Provigil Tablets 977

Montelukast Sodium (Elevated levels of drugs metabolized by the CYP450 system may be observed when co-administered with telithromycin; therefore, increases or prolongation of the therapeutic and/or adverse effects of the concomitant drug may be observed). Products include:
Singulair 2114

Morphine Sulfate (Elevated levels of drugs metabolized by the CYP450 system may be observed when co-administered with telithromycin; therefore, increases or prolongation of the therapeutic and/or adverse effects of the concomitant drug may be observed). Products include:
Avinza Capsules 1772
DepoDur Injection 1095
MS Contin Tablets 2585

Moxifloxacin Hydrochloride (Elevated levels of drugs metabolized by the CYP450 system may be observed when co-administered with telithromycin; therefore, increases or prolongation of the therapeutic and/or adverse effects of the concomitant drug may be observed). Products include:
Avelox 2803
Vigamox Ophthalmic Solution 548

Nabumetone (Elevated levels of drugs metabolized by the CYP450 system may be observed when co-administered with telithromycin; therefore, increases or prolongation of the therapeutic and/or adverse effects of the concomitant drug may be observed).
No products indexed under this heading.

Nafcillin Sodium (Elevated levels of drugs metabolized by the CYP450 system may be observed when co-administered with telithromycin; therefore, increases or prolongation of the therapeutic and/or adverse effects of the concomitant drug may be observed).
No products indexed under this heading.

Naproxen (Elevated levels of drugs metabolized by the CYP450 system

may be observed when co-administered with telithromycin; therefore, increases or prolongation of the therapeutic and/or adverse effects of the concomitant drug may be observed). Products include:

EC-Naprosyn Delayed-Release Tablets ... 2632
Naprosyn Suspension ... 2632
Naprosyn Tablets ... 2632

Naproxen Sodium (Elevated levels of drugs metabolized by the CYP450 system may be observed when co-administered with telithromycin; therefore, increases or prolongation of the therapeutic and/or adverse effects of the concomitant drug may be observed). Products include:

Anaprox Tablets ... 2632
Anaprox DS Tablets ... 2632
Treximet Tablets ... 1616

Nateglinide (Elevated levels of drugs metabolized by the CYP450 system may be observed when co-administered with telithromycin; therefore, increases or prolongation of the therapeutic and/or adverse effects of the concomitant drug may be observed). Products include:

Starlix Tablets ... 2314

Nefazodone Hydrochloride (Co-administration of telithromycin with a drug primarily metabolized by the CYP 3A4 enzyme system may result in increased plasma concentrations of the drug co-administered with telithromycin that could increase or prolong both the therapeutic and adverse effects).

No products indexed under this heading.

Nelfinavir Mesylate (Co-administration of telithromycin with a drug primarily metabolized by the CYP 3A4 enzyme system may result in increased plasma concentrations of the drug co-administered with telithromycin that could increase or prolong both the therapeutic and adverse effects).

No products indexed under this heading.

Nevirapine (Concomitant administration of CYP 3A4 inducers is likely to result in subtherapeutic levels of telithromycin and loss of effect). Products include:

Viramune Oral Suspension ... 873
Viramune Tablets ... 873

Nicardipine (Elevated levels of drugs metabolized by the CYP450 system may be observed when co-administered with telithromycin; therefore, increases or prolongation of the therapeutic and/or adverse effects of the concomitant drug may be observed).

No products indexed under this heading.

Nicardipine Hydrochloride (Co-administration of telithromycin with a drug primarily metabolized by the CYP 3A4 enzyme system may result in increased plasma concentrations of the drug co-administered with telithromycin that could increase or prolong both the therapeutic and adverse effects). Products include:

Cardene I.V. ... 1093

Nicotine Polacrilex (Elevated levels of drugs metabolized by the CYP450 system may be observed when co-administered with telithromycin; therefore, increases or prolongation of the therapeutic and/or adverse effects of the concomitant drug may be observed).

No products indexed under this heading.

Nicotine Salicylate (Elevated levels of drugs metabolized by the CYP450 system may be observed when co-administered with telithromycin; therefore, increases or prolongation of the therapeutic and/or adverse effects of the concomitant drug may be observed).

No products indexed under this heading.

Nicotine Sulfate (Elevated levels of drugs metabolized by the CYP450 system may be observed when co-administered with telithromycin; therefore, increases or prolongation of the therapeutic and/or adverse effects of the concomitant drug may be observed).

No products indexed under this heading.

Nifedipine (Co-administration of telithromycin with a drug primarily metabolized by the CYP 3A4 enzyme system may result in increased plasma concentrations of the drug co-administered with telithromycin that could increase or prolong both the therapeutic and adverse effects).

No products indexed under this heading.

Nilutamide (Elevated levels of drugs metabolized by the CYP450 system may be observed when co-administered with telithromycin; therefore, increases or prolongation of the therapeutic and/or adverse effects of the concomitant drug may be observed).

No products indexed under this heading.

Nimodipine (Co-administration of telithromycin with a drug primarily metabolized by the CYP 3A4 enzyme system may result in increased plasma concentrations of the drug co-administered with telithromycin that could increase or prolong both the therapeutic and adverse effects). Products include:

Nimotop Capsules ... 790

Nisoldipine (Co-administration of telithromycin with a drug primarily metabolized by the CYP 3A4 enzyme system may result in increased plasma concentrations of the drug co-administered with telithromycin that could increase or prolong both the therapeutic and adverse effects). Products include:

Sular Extended Release Tablets ... 2975

Nitrendipine (Co-administration of telithromycin with a drug primarily metabolized by the CYP 3A4 enzyme system may result in increased plasma concentrations of the drug co-administered with telithromycin that could increase or prolong both the therapeutic and adverse effects).

No products indexed under this heading.

Norethindrone (Co-administration of telithromycin with a drug primarily metabolized by the CYP 3A4 enzyme system may result in increased plasma concentrations of the drug co-administered with telithromycin that could increase or prolong both the therapeutic and adverse effects). Products include:

Ortho Micronor Tablets ... 2446

Norethindrone Acetate (Co-administration of telithromycin with a drug primarily metabolized by the CYP 3A4 enzyme system may result in increased plasma concentrations of the drug co-administered with telithromycin that could increase or prolong both the therapeutic and adverse effects). Products include:

Activella Tablets ... 2347

Norfloxacin (Elevated levels of drugs metabolized by the CYP450 system may be observed when co-administered with telithromycin; therefore, increases or prolongation of the therapeutic and/or adverse effects of the concomitant drug may be observed). Products include:

Noroxin Tablets ... 2069

Norgestrel (Co-administration of telithromycin with a drug primarily metabolized by the CYP 3A4 enzyme system may result in increased plasma concentrations of the drug co-administered with telithromycin that could increase or prolong both the therapeutic and adverse effects).

No products indexed under this heading.

Nortriptyline Hydrochloride (Elevated levels of drugs metabolized by the CYP450 system may be observed when co-administered with telithromycin; therefore, increases or prolongation of the therapeutic and/or adverse effects of the concomitant drug may be observed).

No products indexed under this heading.

Ofloxacin (Elevated levels of drugs metabolized by the CYP450 system may be observed when co-administered with telithromycin; therefore, increases or prolongation of the therapeutic and/or adverse effects of the concomitant drug may be observed). Products include:

Ofloxacin Ophthalmic Solution 0.3% ... ⊙ 243

Olanzapine (Elevated levels of drugs metabolized by the CYP450 system may be observed when co-administered with telithromycin; therefore, increases or prolongation of the therapeutic and/or adverse effects of the concomitant drug may be observed). Products include:

Symbyax Capsules ... 1871
Zyprexa Tablets ... 1883
Zyprexa IntraMuscular ... 1883
Zyprexa ZYDIS Orally Disintegrating Tablets ... 1883

Omeprazole (Elevated levels of drugs metabolized by the CYP450 system may be observed when co-administered with telithromycin; therefore, increases or prolongation of the therapeutic and/or adverse effects of the concomitant drug may be observed).

No products indexed under this heading.

Ondansetron (Co-administration of telithromycin with a drug primarily metabolized by the CYP 3A4 enzyme system may result in increased plasma concentrations of the drug co-administered with telithromycin that could increase or prolong both the therapeutic and adverse effects). Products include:

Zofran ODT Orally Disintegrating Tablets ... 1687

Ondansetron Hydrochloride (Co-administration of telithromycin with a drug primarily metabolized by the CYP 3A4 enzyme system may result in increased plasma concentrations of the drug co-administered with telithromycin that could increase or prolong both the therapeutic and adverse effects). Products include:

Zofran Injection ... 1682
Zofran ... 1687

Oxaprozin (Elevated levels of drugs metabolized by the CYP450 system may be observed when co-administered with telithromycin; therefore, increases or prolongation of the therapeutic and/or adverse effects of the concomitant drug may be observed).

No products indexed under this heading.

Oxcarbazepine (Concomitant administration of CYP 3A4 inducers is likely to result in subtherapeutic levels of telithromycin and loss of effect).

No products indexed under this heading.

Oxycodone Hydrochloride (Elevated levels of drugs metabolized by the CYP450 system may be observed when co-administered with telithromycin; therefore, increases or prolongation of the therapeutic and/or adverse effects of the concomitant drug may be observed). Products include:

OxyContin Tablets ... 2589
OxyIR Capsules ... 2593
Percocet Tablets ... 1127
Percodan Tablets ... 1130

Paclitaxel (Co-administration of telithromycin with a drug primarily metabolized by the CYP 3A4 enzyme system may result in increased plasma concentrations of the drug co-administered with telithromycin that could increase or prolong both the therapeutic and adverse effects).

No products indexed under this heading.

Pantoprazole Sodium (Elevated levels of drugs metabolized by the CYP450 system may be observed when co-administered with telithromycin; therefore, increases or prolongation of the therapeutic and/or adverse effects of the concomitant drug may be observed). Products include:

Protonix for Delayed-Release Oral Suspension ... 3254
Protonix Delayed-Release Tablets ... 3254
Protonix I.V. ... 3257

Paramethadione (Elevated levels of drugs metabolized by the CYP450 system may be observed when co-administered with telithromycin; therefore, increases or prolongation of the therapeutic and/or adverse effects of the concomitant drug may be observed).

No products indexed under this heading.

Paroxetine Hydrochloride (Elevated levels of drugs metabolized by the CYP450 system may be observed when co-administered with telithromycin; therefore, increases or prolongation of the therapeutic and/or adverse effects of the concomitant drug may be observed). Products include:

Paxil ... 1535
Paxil CR Controlled-Release Tablets ... 1544

Pentamidine Isethionate (Elevated levels of drugs metabolized by the CYP450 system may be observed when co-administered with telithromycin; therefore, increases or prolongation of the therapeutic and/or adverse effects of the concomitant drug may be observed).

No products indexed under this heading.

Phenacemide (Elevated levels of drugs metabolized by the CYP450 system may be observed when co-administered with telithromycin; therefore, increases or prolongation of the therapeutic and/or adverse effects of the concomitant drug may be observed).
No products indexed under this heading.

Phenobarbital (Concomitant administration of CYP 3A4 inducers is likely to result in subtherapeutic levels of telithromycin and loss of effect). Products include:
Donnatal Extentabs 2507

Phenobarbital Sodium (Concomitant administration of CYP 3A4 inducers is likely to result in subtherapeutic levels of telithromycin and loss of effect).
No products indexed under this heading.

Phensuximide (Elevated levels of drugs metabolized by the CYP450 system may be observed when co-administered with telithromycin; therefore, increases or prolongation of the therapeutic and/or adverse effects of the concomitant drug may be observed).
No products indexed under this heading.

Phenylbutazone (Elevated levels of drugs metabolized by the CYP450 system may be observed when co-administered with telithromycin; therefore, increases or prolongation of the therapeutic and/or adverse effects of the concomitant drug may be observed).
No products indexed under this heading.

Phenytoin (Concomitant administration of CYP 3A4 inducers is likely to result in subtherapeutic levels of telithromycin and loss of effect).
No products indexed under this heading.

Phenytoin Sodium (Concomitant administration of CYP 3A4 inducers is likely to result in subtherapeutic levels of telithromycin and loss of effect). Products include:
Phenytek Capsules 2192

Pimozide (There is a potential risk of increased pimozide plasma levels by inhibition of CYP 3A4 pathways by telithromycin. Co-administration is contraindicated).
No products indexed under this heading.

Pindolol (Elevated levels of drugs metabolized by the CYP450 system may be observed when co-administered with telithromycin; therefore, increases or prolongation of the therapeutic and/or adverse effects of the concomitant drug may be observed).
No products indexed under this heading.

Pioglitazone Hydrochloride (Elevated levels of drugs metabolized by the CYP450 system may be observed when co-administered with telithromycin; therefore, increases or prolongation of the therapeutic and/or adverse effects of the concomitant drug may be observed).
Products include:
ActoPlus Met Tablets 3071
Actos Tablets 3077
Duetact Tablets 3085

Piroxicam (Elevated levels of drugs metabolized by the CYP450 system may be observed when co-administered with telithromycin; therefore, increases or prolongation of the therapeutic and/or adverse effects of the concomitant drug may be observed).
No products indexed under this heading.

Polyestradiol Phosphate (Co-administration of telithromycin with a drug primarily metabolized by the CYP 3A4 enzyme system may result in increased plasma concentrations of the drug co-administered with telithromycin that could increase or prolong both the therapeutic and adverse effects).
No products indexed under this heading.

Prednisolone Acetate (Concomitant administration of CYP 3A4 inducers is likely to result in subtherapeutic levels of telithromycin and loss of effect). Products include:
Pred Forte Ophthalmic Suspension .... ⊙ 227
Pred Mild Ophthalmic Suspension .... ⊙ 230
Pred-G Ophthalmic Ointment .... ⊙ 229
Pred-G Ophthalmic Suspension .... ⊙ 228

Prednisolone Sodium Phosphate (Concomitant administration of CYP 3A4 inducers is likely to result in subtherapeutic levels of telithromycin and loss of effect).
No products indexed under this heading.

Prednisolone Tebutate (Concomitant administration of CYP 3A4 inducers is likely to result in subtherapeutic levels of telithromycin and loss of effect).
No products indexed under this heading.

Prednisone (Concomitant administration of CYP 3A4 inducers is likely to result in subtherapeutic levels of telithromycin and loss of effect).
No products indexed under this heading.

Primidone (Concomitant administration of CYP 3A4 inducers is likely to result in subtherapeutic levels of telithromycin and loss of effect).
No products indexed under this heading.

Progesterone (Elevated levels of drugs metabolized by the CYP450 system may be observed when co-administered with telithromycin; therefore, increases or prolongation of the therapeutic and/or adverse effects of the concomitant drug may be observed). Products include:
Crinone 4% Gel 992
Crinone 8% Gel 992
Prometrium Capsules (100 mg, 200 mg) 3047

Proguanil Hydrochloride (Elevated levels of drugs metabolized by the CYP450 system may be observed when co-administered with telithromycin; therefore, increases or prolongation of the therapeutic and/or adverse effects of the concomitant drug may be observed).
Products include:
Malarone Pediatric Tablets 1521
Malarone Tablets 1521

Propafenone Hydrochloride (Elevated levels of drugs metabolized by the CYP450 system may be observed when co-administered with telithromycin; therefore, increases or prolongation of the therapeutic and/or adverse effects of the concomitant drug may be observed).
Products include:
Rythmol Tablets 1586
Rythmol SR Capsules 1590

Propoxyphene Hydrochloride (Elevated levels of drugs metabolized by the CYP450 system may be observed when co-administered with telithromycin; therefore, increases or prolongation of the therapeutic and/or adverse effects of the concomitant drug may be observed).
No products indexed under this heading.

Propoxyphene Napsylate (Elevated levels of drugs metabolized by the CYP450 system may be observed when co-administered with telithromycin; therefore, increases or prolongation of the therapeutic and/or adverse effects of the concomitant drug may be observed).
No products indexed under this heading.

Propranolol Hydrochloride (Elevated levels of drugs metabolized by the CYP450 system may be observed when co-administered with telithromycin; therefore, increases or prolongation of the therapeutic and/or adverse effects of the concomitant drug may be observed).
Products include:
InnoPran XL Extended Release Capsules 1484

Protriptyline Hydrochloride (Elevated levels of drugs metabolized by the CYP450 system may be observed when co-administered with telithromycin; therefore, increases or prolongation of the therapeutic and/or adverse effects of the concomitant drug may be observed).
No products indexed under this heading.

Quetiapine Fumarate (Elevated levels of drugs metabolized by the CYP450 system may be observed when co-administered with telithromycin; therefore, increases or prolongation of the therapeutic and/or adverse effects of the concomitant drug may be observed).
No products indexed under this heading.

Quinidine Gluconate (Co-administration of telithromycin with a drug primarily metabolized by the CYP 3A4 enzyme system may result in increased plasma concentrations of the drug co-administered with telithromycin that could increase or prolong both the therapeutic and adverse effects).
No products indexed under this heading.

Quinidine Hydrochloride (Elevated levels of drugs metabolized by the CYP450 system may be observed when co-administered with telithromycin; therefore, increases or prolongation of the therapeutic and/or adverse effects of the concomitant drug may be observed).
No products indexed under this heading.

Quinidine Polygalacturonate (Co-administration of telithromycin with a drug primarily metabolized by the CYP 3A4 enzyme system may result in increased plasma concentrations of the drug co-administered with telithromycin that could increase or prolong both the therapeutic and adverse effects).
No products indexed under this heading.

Quinidine Sulfate (Co-administration of telithromycin with a drug primarily metabolized by the CYP 3A4 enzyme system may result in increased plasma concentrations of the drug co-administered with telithromycin that could increase or prolong both the therapeutic and adverse effects).
No products indexed under this heading.

Quinine (Elevated levels of drugs metabolized by the CYP450 system may be observed when co-administered with telithromycin; therefore, increases or prolongation of the therapeutic and/or adverse effects of the concomitant drug may be observed).
No products indexed under this heading.

Quinine Sulfate (Elevated levels of drugs metabolized by the CYP450 system may be observed when co-administered with telithromycin; therefore, increases or prolongation of the therapeutic and/or adverse effects of the concomitant drug may be observed).
No products indexed under this heading.

Rabeprazole Sodium (Elevated levels of drugs metabolized by the CYP450 system may be observed when co-administered with telithromycin; therefore, increases or prolongation of the therapeutic and/or adverse effects of the concomitant drug may be observed). Products include:
Aciphex Tablets 1053

Repaglinide (Elevated levels of drugs metabolized by the CYP450 system may be observed when co-administered with telithromycin; therefore, increases or prolongation of the therapeutic and/or adverse effects of the concomitant drug may be observed). Products include:
PrandiMet Tablets 2967
Prandin Tablets 2971

Rifabutin (Co-administration of telithromycin with a drug primarily metabolized by the CYP 3A4 enzyme system may result in increased plasma concentrations of the drug co-administered with telithromycin that could increase or prolong both the therapeutic and adverse effects).
No products indexed under this heading.

Rifampicin (Concomitant administration of CYP 3A4 inducers is likely to result in subtherapeutic levels of telithromycin and loss of effect).
No products indexed under this heading.

Rifampin (Co-administration of rifampin, a CYP 3A4 inducer, with telithromycin in repeated doses decreased the Cmax and AUC of telithromycin. Avoid concomitant treatment).
No products indexed under this heading.

Rifapentine (Concomitant administration of CYP 3A4 inducers is likely to result in subtherapeutic levels of telithromycin and loss of effect).
No products indexed under this heading.

Riluzole (Elevated levels of drugs metabolized by the CYP450 system may be observed when co-administered with telithromycin; therefore, increases or prolongation

of the therapeutic and/or adverse effects of the concomitant drug may be observed). Products include:
Rilutek Tablets 2771

Risperidone (Elevated levels of drugs metabolized by the CYP450 system may be observed when co-administered with telithromycin; therefore, increases or prolongation of the therapeutic and/or adverse effects of the concomitant drug may be observed). Products include:
Risperdal Consta Long-Acting Injection 1753

Ritonavir (Co-administration of telithromycin with a drug primarily metabolized by the CYP 3A4 enzyme system may result in increased plasma concentrations of the drug co-administered with telithromycin that could increase or prolong both the therapeutic and adverse effects). Products include:
Kaletra 452
Norvir 489

Rofecoxib (Elevated levels of drugs metabolized by the CYP450 system may be observed when co-administered with telithromycin; therefore, increases or prolongation of the therapeutic and/or adverse effects of the concomitant drug may be observed).
No products indexed under this heading.

Ropinirole Hydrochloride (Elevated levels of drugs metabolized by the CYP450 system may be observed when co-administered with telithromycin; therefore, increases or prolongation of the therapeutic and/or adverse effects of the concomitant drug may be observed). Products include:
Requip Tablets 1561
Requip XL Tablets 1568

Ropivacaine Hydrochloride (Elevated levels of drugs metabolized by the CYP450 system may be observed when co-administered with telithromycin; therefore, increases or prolongation of the therapeutic and/or adverse effects of the concomitant drug may be observed).
No products indexed under this heading.

Rosiglitazone Maleate (Elevated levels of drugs metabolized by the CYP450 system may be observed when co-administered with telithromycin; therefore, increases or prolongation of the therapeutic and/or adverse effects of the concomitant drug may be observed). Products include:
Avandamet Tablets 1336
Avandaryl Tablets 1344
Avandia Tablets 1351

Saquinavir (Co-administration of telithromycin with a drug primarily metabolized by the CYP 3A4 enzyme system may result in increased plasma concentrations of the drug co-administered with telithromycin that could increase or prolong both the therapeutic and adverse effects).
No products indexed under this heading.

Saquinavir Mesylate (Co-administration of telithromycin with a drug primarily metabolized by the CYP 3A4 enzyme system may result in increased plasma concentrations of the drug co-administered with telithromycin that could increase or prolong both the therapeutic and adverse effects).
No products indexed under this heading.

Sertraline Hydrochloride (Co-administration of telithromycin with a drug primarily metabolized by the CYP 3A4 enzyme system may result in increased plasma concentrations of the drug co-administered with telithromycin that could increase or prolong both the therapeutic and adverse effects).
No products indexed under this heading.

Sildenafil Citrate (Co-administration of telithromycin with a drug primarily metabolized by the CYP 3A4 enzyme system may result in increased plasma concentrations of the drug co-administered with telithromycin that could increase or prolong both the therapeutic and adverse effects).
No products indexed under this heading.

Simvastatin (Simvastatin levels were increased due to CYP 3A4 inhibition by telithromycin, thereby increasing the risk of myopathy. Co-administration should be avoided). Products include:
Simcor Tablets 502
Vytorin 10/10 Tablets 2149
Vytorin 10/10 Tablets 2939
Vytorin 10/20 Tablets 2149
Vytorin 10/20 Tablets 2939
Vytorin 10/40 Tablets 2149
Vytorin 10/40 Tablets 2939
Vytorin 10/80 Tablets 2149
Vytorin 10/80 Tablets 2939
Zocor Tablets 2136

Sirolimus (Co-administration of telithromycin with a drug primarily metabolized by the CYP 3A4 enzyme system may result in increased plasma concentrations of the drug co-administered with telithromycin that could increase or prolong both the therapeutic and adverse effects). Products include:
Rapamune 3260

Sotalol Hydrochloride (Telithromycin has been shown to decrease the Cmax and AUC of sotalol due to decreased absorption).
No products indexed under this heading.

Sulfamethoxazole (Elevated levels of drugs metabolized by the CYP450 system may be observed when co-administered with telithromycin; therefore, increases or prolongation of the therapeutic and/or adverse effects of the concomitant drug may be observed).
No products indexed under this heading.

Sulfinpyrazone (Concomitant administration of CYP 3A4 inducers is likely to result in subtherapeutic levels of telithromycin and loss of effect).
No products indexed under this heading.

Sulindac (Elevated levels of drugs metabolized by the CYP450 system may be observed when co-administered with telithromycin; therefore, increases or prolongation of the therapeutic and/or adverse effects of the concomitant drug may be observed). Products include:
Clinoril Tablets 1962

Suprofen (Elevated levels of drugs metabolized by the CYP450 system may be observed when co-administered with telithromycin; therefore, increases or prolongation of the therapeutic and/or adverse effects of the concomitant drug may be observed).
No products indexed under this heading.

Tacrine Hydrochloride (Elevated levels of drugs metabolized by the CYP450 system may be observed when co-administered with telithromycin; therefore, increases or prolongation of the therapeutic and/or adverse effects of the concomitant drug may be observed).
No products indexed under this heading.

Tacrolimus (Co-administration of telithromycin with a drug primarily metabolized by the CYP 3A4 enzyme system may result in increased plasma concentrations of the drug co-administered with telithromycin that could increase or prolong both the therapeutic and adverse effects). Products include:
Prograf Capsules and Injection 622
Protopic Ointment 628

Tadalafil (Co-administration of telithromycin with a drug primarily metabolized by the CYP 3A4 enzyme system may result in increased plasma concentrations of the drug co-administered with telithromycin that could increase or prolong both the therapeutic and adverse effects). Products include:
Cialis Tablets 1792

Tamoxifen Citrate (Co-administration of telithromycin with a drug primarily metabolized by the CYP 3A4 enzyme system may result in increased plasma concentrations of the drug co-administered with telithromycin that could increase or prolong both the therapeutic and adverse effects).
No products indexed under this heading.

Telmisartan (Elevated levels of drugs metabolized by the CYP450 system may be observed when co-administered with telithromycin; therefore, increases or prolongation of the therapeutic and/or adverse effects of the concomitant drug may be observed). Products include:
Micardis Tablets 852
Micardis HCT Tablets 854

Teniposide (Elevated levels of drugs metabolized by the CYP450 system may be observed when co-administered with telithromycin; therefore, increases or prolongation of the therapeutic and/or adverse effects of the concomitant drug may be observed).
No products indexed under this heading.

Terfenadine (Elevated levels of drugs metabolized by the CYP450 system may be observed when co-administered with telithromycin; therefore, increases or prolongation of the therapeutic and/or adverse effects of the concomitant drug may be observed).
No products indexed under this heading.

Testosterone (Elevated levels of drugs metabolized by the CYP450 system may be observed when co-administered with telithromycin; therefore, increases or prolongation of the therapeutic and/or adverse effects of the concomitant drug may be observed). Products include:
AndroGel 3159
Testim 1% Gel 701

Testosterone Cypionate (Elevated levels of drugs metabolized by the CYP450 system may be observed when co-administered with telithromycin; therefore, increases or prolongation of the therapeutic and/or adverse effects of the concomitant drug may be observed).
No products indexed under this heading.

Testosterone Enanthate (Elevated levels of drugs metabolized by the CYP450 system may be observed when co-administered with telithromycin; therefore, increases or prolongation of the therapeutic and/or adverse effects of the concomitant drug may be observed). Products include:
Delatestryl Injection 1730

Testosterone Propionate (Elevated levels of drugs metabolized by the CYP450 system may be observed when co-administered with telithromycin; therefore, increases or prolongation of the therapeutic and/or adverse effects of the concomitant drug may be observed).
No products indexed under this heading.

Theophylline (Co-administration increased steady state Cmax and AUC of theophylline and may worsen GI side effects, especially in female patients. Theophylline and telithromycin should be taken 1 hour apart).
No products indexed under this heading.

Theophylline Anhydrous (Co-administration increased steady state Cmax and AUC of theophylline and may worsen GI side effects, especially in female patients. Theophylline and telithromycin should be taken 1 hour apart). Products include:
Uniphyl Tablets 2595

Theophylline Calcium Salicylate (Co-administration increased steady state Cmax and AUC of theophylline and may worsen GI side effects, especially in female patients. Theophylline and telithromycin should be taken 1 hour apart).
No products indexed under this heading.

Theophylline Dihydroxypropyl (Glyceryl) (Co-administration increased steady state Cmax and AUC of theophylline and may worsen GI side effects, especially in female patients. Theophylline and telithromycin should be taken 1 hour apart).
No products indexed under this heading.

Theophylline Ethylenediamine (Co-administration increased steady state Cmax and AUC of theophylline and may worsen GI side effects, especially in female patients. Theophylline and telithromycin should be taken 1 hour apart).
No products indexed under this heading.

Theophylline Sodium Glycinate (Co-administration increased steady state Cmax and AUC of theophylline and may worsen GI side effects, especially in female patients. Theophylline and telithromycin should be taken 1 hour apart).
No products indexed under this heading.

Thioridazine (Elevated levels of drugs metabolized by the CYP450 system may be observed when co-administered with telithromycin; therefore, increases or prolongation of the therapeutic and/or adverse effects of the concomitant drug may be observed).
No products indexed under this heading.

Thioridazine Hydrochloride (Elevated levels of drugs metabolized by the CYP450 system may be observed when co-administered with telithromycin; therefore, increases or prolongation of the therapeutic and/or adverse effects of the concomitant drug may be observed). Products include:
Thioridazine Hydrochloride Tablets 2195

Tiagabine Hydrochloride (Co-administration of telithromycin with a drug primarily metabolized by the CYP 3A4 enzyme system may result in increased plasma concentrations of the drug co-administered with telithromycin that could increase or prolong both the therapeutic and adverse effects). Products include:
Gabitril Tablets 973

Timolol Maleate (Elevated levels of drugs metabolized by the CYP450 system may be observed when co-administered with telithromycin; therefore, increases or prolongation of the therapeutic and/or adverse effects of the concomitant drug may be observed). Products include:
Combigan Ophthalmic Solution 553
Cosopt Sterile Ophthalmic Solution 1969
Timoptic Sterile Ophthalmic Solution 2121
Timoptic in Ocudose 2124
Timoptic-XE Sterile Ophthalmic Gel Forming Solution 2125

Tolazamide (Elevated levels of drugs metabolized by the CYP450 system may be observed when co-administered with telithromycin; therefore, increases or prolongation of the therapeutic and/or adverse effects of the concomitant drug may be observed).
No products indexed under this heading.

Tolbutamide (Elevated levels of drugs metabolized by the CYP450 system may be observed when co-administered with telithromycin; therefore, increases or prolongation of the therapeutic and/or adverse effects of the concomitant drug may be observed).
No products indexed under this heading.

Tolbutamide Sodium (Elevated levels of drugs metabolized by the CYP450 system may be observed when co-administered with telithromycin; therefore, increases or prolongation of the therapeutic and/or adverse effects of the concomitant drug may be observed).
No products indexed under this heading.

Tolmetin Sodium (Elevated levels of drugs metabolized by the CYP450 system may be observed when co-administered with telithromycin; therefore, increases or prolongation of the therapeutic and/or adverse effects of the concomitant drug may be observed).
No products indexed under this heading.

Tolterodine Tartrate (Co-administration of telithromycin with a drug primarily metabolized by the CYP 3A4 enzyme system may result in increased plasma concentrations of the drug co-administered with telithromycin that could increase or prolong both the therapeutic and adverse effects).
No products indexed under this heading.

Topiramate (Elevated levels of drugs metabolized by the CYP450 system may be observed when co-administered with telithromycin; therefore, increases or prolongation of the therapeutic and/or adverse effects of the concomitant drug may be observed).
No products indexed under this heading.

Torsemide (Elevated levels of drugs metabolized by the CYP450 system may be observed when co-administered with telithromycin; therefore, increases or prolongation of the therapeutic and/or adverse effects of the concomitant drug may be observed). Products include:
Demadex Injection 2630
Demadex Tablets 2630

Tramadol Hydrochloride (Elevated levels of drugs metabolized by the CYP450 system may be observed when co-administered with telithromycin; therefore, increases or prolongation of the therapeutic and/or adverse effects of the concomitant drug may be observed). Products include:
Ultram ER Extended-Release Tablets 2428

Trazodone Hydrochloride (Co-administration of telithromycin with a drug primarily metabolized by the CYP 3A4 enzyme system may result in increased plasma concentrations of the drug co-administered with telithromycin that could increase or prolong both the therapeutic and adverse effects).
No products indexed under this heading.

Tretinoin (Elevated levels of drugs metabolized by the CYP450 system may be observed when co-administered with telithromycin; therefore, increases or prolongation of the therapeutic and/or adverse effects of the concomitant drug may be observed). Products include:
Vesanoid Capsules 2660
Ziana Gel 1942

Triamcinolone (Concomitant administration of CYP 3A4 inducers is likely to result in subtherapeutic levels of telithromycin and loss of effect).
No products indexed under this heading.

Triamcinolone Acetonide (Concomitant administration of CYP 3A4 inducers is likely to result in subtherapeutic levels of telithromycin and loss of effect). Products include:
Azmacort Inhalation Aerosol 407
Nasacort AQ Nasal Spray 2765
Triesence Injectable Suspension .... ⊙209

Triamcinolone Diacetate (Concomitant administration of CYP 3A4 inducers is likely to result in subtherapeutic levels of telithromycin and loss of effect).
No products indexed under this heading.

Triamcinolone Hexacetonide (Concomitant administration of CYP 3A4 inducers is likely to result in subtherapeutic levels of telithromycin and loss of effect).
No products indexed under this heading.

Triazolam (Co-administration of telithromycin with a drug primarily metabolized by the CYP 3A4 enzyme system may result in increased plasma concentrations of the drug co-administered with telithromycin that could increase or prolong both the therapeutic and adverse effects).
No products indexed under this heading.

Trimethadione (Elevated levels of drugs metabolized by the CYP450 system may be observed when co-administered with telithromycin; therefore, increases or prolongation of the therapeutic and/or adverse effects of the concomitant drug may be observed).
No products indexed under this heading.

Trimethaphan Camsylate (Elevated levels of drugs metabolized by the CYP450 system may be observed when co-administered with telithromycin; therefore, increases or prolongation of the therapeutic and/or adverse effects of the concomitant drug may be observed).
No products indexed under this heading.

Trimipramine Maleate (Elevated levels of drugs metabolized by the CYP450 system may be observed when co-administered with telithromycin; therefore, increases or prolongation of the therapeutic and/or adverse effects of the concomitant drug may be observed).
No products indexed under this heading.

Troglitazone (Concomitant administration of CYP 3A4 inducers is likely to result in subtherapeutic levels of telithromycin and loss of effect).
No products indexed under this heading.

Trovafloxacin Mesylate (Elevated levels of drugs metabolized by the CYP450 system may be observed when co-administered with telithromycin; therefore, increases or prolongation of the therapeutic and/or adverse effects of the concomitant drug may be observed).
No products indexed under this heading.

Valdecoxib (Elevated levels of drugs metabolized by the CYP450 system may be observed when co-administered with telithromycin; therefore, increases or prolongation of the therapeutic and/or adverse effects of the concomitant drug may be observed).
No products indexed under this heading.

Valproate Sodium (Elevated levels of drugs metabolized by the CYP450 system may be observed when co-administered with telithromycin; therefore, increases or prolongation of the therapeutic and/or adverse effects of the concomitant drug may be observed).
No products indexed under this heading.

Valproic Acid (Elevated levels of drugs metabolized by the CYP450 system may be observed when co-administered with telithromycin; therefore, increases or prolongation of the therapeutic and/or adverse effects of the concomitant drug may be observed).
No products indexed under this heading.

Valsartan (Elevated levels of drugs metabolized by the CYP450 system may be observed when co-administered with telithromycin; therefore, increases or prolongation of the therapeutic and/or adverse effects of the concomitant drug may be observed). Products include:
Diovan Tablets 2212
Diovan HCT Tablets 2216
Exforge Tablets 2238

Vardenafil Hydrochloride (Co-administration of telithromycin with a drug primarily metabolized by the CYP 3A4 enzyme system may result in increased plasma concentrations of the drug co-administered with telithromycin that could increase or prolong both the therapeutic and adverse effects). Products include:
Levitra Tablets 2876

Venlafaxine Hydrochloride (Elevated levels of drugs metabolized by the CYP450 system may be observed when co-administered with telithromycin; therefore, increases or prolongation of the therapeutic and/or adverse effects of the concomitant drug may be observed). Products include:
Effexor XR Extended-Release Capsules 3195
Venlafaxine Hydrochloride Tablets ... 2199

Verapamil Hydrochloride (Co-administration of telithromycin with a drug primarily metabolized by the CYP 3A4 enzyme system may result in increased plasma concentrations of the drug co-administered with telithromycin that could increase or prolong both the therapeutic and adverse effects). Products include:
Tarka Tablets 511

Vinblastine Sulfate (Co-administration of telithromycin with a drug primarily metabolized by the CYP 3A4 enzyme system may result in increased plasma concentrations of the drug co-administered with telithromycin that could increase or prolong both the therapeutic and adverse effects).
No products indexed under this heading.

Vincristine Sulfate (Co-administration of telithromycin with a drug primarily metabolized by the CYP 3A4 enzyme system may result in increased plasma concentrations of the drug co-administered with telithromycin that could increase or prolong both the therapeutic and adverse effects).
No products indexed under this heading.

Vitamin A (Elevated levels of drugs metabolized by the CYP450 system may be observed when co-

administered with telithromycin; therefore, increases or prolongation of the therapeutic and/or adverse effects of the concomitant drug may be observed). Products include:

Norwegian Cod Liver Oil 949

Vitamin A Acetate (Elevated levels of drugs metabolized by the CYP450 system may be observed when co-administered with telithromycin; therefore, increases or prolongation of the therapeutic and/or adverse effects of the concomitant drug may be observed).

No products indexed under this heading.

Voriconazole (Elevated levels of drugs metabolized by the CYP450 system may be observed when co-administered with telithromycin; therefore, increases or prolongation of the therapeutic and/or adverse effects of the concomitant drug may be observed).

No products indexed under this heading.

Warfarin Sodium (Co-administration of telithromycin with a drug primarily metabolized by the CYP 3A4 enzyme system may result in increased plasma concentrations of the drug co-administered with telithromycin that could increase or prolong both the therapeutic and adverse effects).

No products indexed under this heading.

Zafirlukast (Elevated levels of drugs metabolized by the CYP450 system may be observed when co-administered with telithromycin; therefore, increases or prolongation of the therapeutic and/or adverse effects of the concomitant drug may be observed). Products include:

Accolate Tablets 669

Zileuton (Elevated levels of drugs metabolized by the CYP450 system may be observed when co-administered with telithromycin; therefore, increases or prolongation of the therapeutic and/or adverse effects of the concomitant drug may be observed).

No products indexed under this heading.

Zolmitriptan (Elevated levels of drugs metabolized by the CYP450 system may be observed when co-administered with telithromycin; therefore, increases or prolongation of the therapeutic and/or adverse effects of the concomitant drug may be observed). Products include:

Zomig Tablets 694
Zomig Nasal Spray 689
Zomig-ZMT Tablets 694

Zonisamide (Elevated levels of drugs metabolized by the CYP450 system may be observed when co-administered with telithromycin; therefore, increases or prolongation of the therapeutic and/or adverse effects of the concomitant drug may be observed). Products include:

Zonegran Capsules 1089

Zopiclone (Elevated levels of drugs metabolized by the CYP450 system may be observed when co-administered with telithromycin; therefore, increases or prolongation of the therapeutic and/or adverse effects of the concomitant drug may be observed).

No products indexed under this heading.

KINERET INJECTION

(Anakinra) 585
May interact with vaccines, live and certain other agents. Compounds in these categories include:

Adalimumab (Use of anakinra in combination with TNF-blocking agents is not recommended). Products include:

Humira Injection 442

BCG Vaccine (Live vaccines should not be given concurently with anakinra due to lack of data on either the effects or the secondary transmission of infection by live vaccination).

No products indexed under this heading.

Diphtheria & Tetanus Toxoids and Acellular Pertussis Vaccine Adsorbed, Hepatitis B (recombinant) and Inactivated Poliovirus Vaccine Combined (Vaccination may not be effective in patients receiving anakinra).

No products indexed under this heading.

Etanercept (In a study in which patients with active RA were treated for up to 24 weeks with concurrent anakinra and etanercept therapy, a 7% rate of serious infections was observed, which was higher than that observed with etanercept alone (0%). Two percent of patients treated concurrently with anakinra and etanercept developed neutropenia. Use of anakinra in combination with TNF-blocking agents is not recommended). Products include:

Enbrel for Injection 569

Hepatitis A Vaccine, Inactivated (Vaccination may not be effective in patients receiving anakinra). Products include:

Havrix Injection Vaccine 1454
Twinrix Vaccine 1628
Vaqta 2130

Infliximab (Use of anakinra in combination with TNF-blocking agents is not recommended). Products include:

Remicade for IV Injection 950

Influenza Vaccine, Live Attenuated (Live vaccines should not be given concurently with anakinra due to lack of data on either the effects or the secondary transmission of infection by live vaccination).

No products indexed under this heading.

Influenza Virus Vaccine (Vaccination may not be effective in patients receiving anakinra). Products include:

Fluarix Vaccine 1446
Flulaval Injection Vaccine 1448

Influenza Virus Vaccine Live, Intranasal (Live vaccines should not be given concurently with anakinra due to lack of data on either the effects or the secondary transmission of infection by live vaccination). Products include:

FluMist Vaccine 1945

Japanese Encephalitis Vaccine Inactivated (Vaccination may not be effective in patients receiving anakinra).

No products indexed under this heading.

Measles, Mumps, Rubella and Varicella Virus Vaccine Live (Live vaccines should not be given concurently with anakinra due to lack of data on either the effects or the secondary transmission of infection by live vaccination). Products include:

ProQuad 2099

Measles, Mumps & Rubella Virus Vaccine, Live (Live vaccines should not be given concurently with anakinra due to lack of data on either the effects or the secondary transmission of infection by live vaccination). Products include:

M-M-R II 2054

Measles & Rubella Virus Vaccine Live (Live vaccines should not be given concurently with anakinra due to lack of data on either the effects or the secondary transmission of infection by live vaccination).

No products indexed under this heading.

Measles Virus Vaccine Live (Live vaccines should not be given concurently with anakinra due to lack of data on either the effects or the secondary transmission of infection by live vaccination). Products include:

Attenuvax 1951

Mumps Virus Vaccine, Live (Live vaccines should not be given concurently with anakinra due to lack of data on either the effects or the secondary transmission of infection by live vaccination). Products include:

Mumpsvax 2068

Poliovirus Vaccine, Live, Oral, Trivalent, Types 1,2,3 (Sabin) (Live vaccines should not be given concurently with anakinra due to lack of data on either the effects or the secondary transmission of infection by live vaccination).

No products indexed under this heading.

Poliovirus Vaccine Inactivated (Vaccination may not be effective in patients receiving anakinra). Products include:

Pediarix Vaccine 1552

Rotavirus Vaccine, Live, Oral, Tetravalent (Live vaccines should not be given concurently with anakinra due to lack of data on either the effects or the secondary transmission of infection by live vaccination).

No products indexed under this heading.

Rubella & Mumps Virus Vaccine Live (Live vaccines should not be given concurently with anakinra due to lack of data on either the effects or the secondary transmission of infection by live vaccination).

No products indexed under this heading.

Rubella Virus Vaccine Live (Live vaccines should not be given concurently with anakinra due to lack of data on either the effects or the secondary transmission of infection by live vaccination). Products include:

Meruvax II 2061

Smallpox Vaccine (Live vaccines should not be given concurently with anakinra due to lack of data on either the effects or the secondary transmission of infection by live vaccination).

No products indexed under this heading.

Typhoid Vaccine (Live vaccines should not be given concurently with anakinra due to lack of data on either the effects or the secondary transmission of infection by live vaccination).

No products indexed under this heading.

Varicella Virus Vaccine Live (Live vaccines should not be given concurently with anakinra due to lack of data on either the effects or the secondary transmission of infection by live vaccination). Products include:

Varivax 2133

Yellow Fever Vaccine (Live vaccines should not be given concurently with anakinra due to lack of data on either the effects or the secondary transmission of infection by live vaccination).

No products indexed under this heading.

Zoster Vaccine Live (Live vaccines should not be given concurently with anakinra due to lack of data on either the effects or the secondary transmission of infection by live vaccination). Products include:

Zostavax Injection 2145

KINRIX INJECTION VACCINE

(Diphtheria and Tetanus Toxoids and Acellular Pertussis Adsorbed and Inactivated Poliovirus Vaccine)...... 1486
May interact with alkylating agents, antimetabolites, corticosteroids, cytotoxic drugs, immunosuppressive agents, killed/inactivated vaccines, vaccines, live, and certain other agents. Compounds in these categories include:

Azathioprine (Immunosuppressive therapies may reduce the immune response to Kinrix).

No products indexed under this heading.

Basiliximab (Immunosuppressive therapies may reduce the immune response to Kinrix). Products include:

Simulect for Injection 2306

BCG Vaccine (When Kinrix is administered concomitantly with other injectable vaccines, they should be given with separate syringes. Kinrix should not be mixed with any other vaccine in the same syringe or vial).

No products indexed under this heading.

Betamethasone Acetate (Immunosuppressive therapies, including corticosteroids, may reduce the immune response to Kinrix).

No products indexed under this heading.

Betamethasone Sodium Phosphate (Immunosuppressive therapies, including corticosteroids, may reduce the immune response to Kinrix).

No products indexed under this heading.

Bleomycin Sulfate (Immunosuppressive therapies, including cytotoxic drugs, may reduce the immune response to Kinrix).

No products indexed under this heading.

Budesonide (Immunosuppressive therapies, including corticosteroids, may reduce the immune response to Kinrix). Products include:

Pulmicort Flexhaler 654
Symbicort 80/4.5 Inhalation Aerosol.. 659
Symbicort 160/4.5 Inhalation Aerosol.. 659

Busulfan (Immunosuppressive therapies, including alkylating agents, may reduce the immune response to Kinrix). Products include:

Busulfex Injection 2477
Myleran Tablets 1530

Capecitabine (Immunosuppressive therapies, including antimetabolites, may reduce the immune response to Kinrix). Products include:
Xeloda Tablets 2662
Carmustine (BCNU) (Immunosuppressive therapies, including alkylating agents, may reduce the immune response to Kinrix).
No products indexed under this heading.
Chlorambucil (Immunosuppressive therapies, including alkylating agents, may reduce the immune response to Kinrix). Products include:
Leukeran Tablets 1508
Ciclesonide (Immunosuppressive therapies, including corticosteroids, may reduce the immune response to Kinrix). Products include:
Alvesco Inhalation Aerosol 2985
Omnaris Nasal Spray 2998
Cladribine (Immunosuppressive therapies, including antimetabolites, may reduce the immune response to Kinrix). Products include:
Leustatin Injection 2384
Cortisone Acetate (Immunosuppressive therapies, including corticosteroids, may reduce the immune response to Kinrix).
No products indexed under this heading.
Cyclophosphamide (Immunosuppressive therapies, including alkylating agents, may reduce the immune response to Kinrix).
No products indexed under this heading.
Cyclosporine (Immunosuppressive therapies may reduce the immune response to Kinrix). Products include:
Gengraf Capsules 435
Neoral Oral Solution 2280
Neoral Soft Gelatin Capsules 2280
Restasis Ophthalmic Emulsion 557
Sandimmune 2296
Cytarabine (Immunosuppressive therapies, including antimetabolites, may reduce the immune response to Kinrix).
No products indexed under this heading.
Dacarbazine (Immunosuppressive therapies, including alkylating agents, may reduce the immune response to Kinrix).
No products indexed under this heading.
Daunorubicin Hydrochloride (Immunosuppressive therapies, including cytotoxic drugs, may reduce the immune response to Kinrix).
No products indexed under this heading.
Dexamethasone (Immunosuppressive therapies, including corticosteroids, may reduce the immune response to Kinrix). Products include:
Ciprodex Otic Suspension 541
Dexamethasone Acetate (Immunosuppressive therapies, including corticosteroids, may reduce the immune response to Kinrix).
No products indexed under this heading.
Dexamethasone Sodium Phosphate (Immunosuppressive therapies, including corticosteroids, may reduce the immune response to Kinrix).
No products indexed under this heading.
Diphtheria & Tetanus Toxoids and Acellular Pertussis Vaccine Adsorbed, Hepatitis B (recombinant) and Inactivated Poliovirus Vaccine Combined (When Kinrix is administered concomitantly with other injectable vaccines, they should be given with separate syringes. Kinrix should not be mixed with any other vaccine in the same syringe or vial).
No products indexed under this heading.
Doxorubicin Hydrochloride (Immunosuppressive therapies, including cytotoxic drugs, may reduce the immune response to Kinrix).
No products indexed under this heading.
Epirubicin Hydrochloride (Immunosuppressive therapies, including cytotoxic drugs, may reduce the immune response to Kinrix).
No products indexed under this heading.
Floxuridine (Immunosuppressive therapies, including antimetabolites, may reduce the immune response to Kinrix).
No products indexed under this heading.
Fludarabine Phosphate (Immunosuppressive therapies, including antimetabolites, may reduce the immune response to Kinrix).
No products indexed under this heading.
Fludrocortisone Acetate (Immunosuppressive therapies, including corticosteroids, may reduce the immune response to Kinrix).
No products indexed under this heading.
Flunisolide (Immunosuppressive therapies, including corticosteroids, may reduce the immune response to Kinrix). Products include:
Aerobid/Aerobid-M 1153
Fluorouracil (Immunosuppressive therapies, including antimetabolites, may reduce the immune response to Kinrix). Products include:
Carac Cream 0.5% 2722
Fluticasone Propionate (Immunosuppressive therapies, including corticosteroids, may reduce the immune response to Kinrix). Products include:
Advair Diskus 100/50 1276
Advair Diskus 250/50 1276
Advair Diskus 500/50 1276
Advair HFA 45/21 Inhalation Aerosol 1288
Advair HFA 115/21 Inhalation Aerosol 1288
Advair HFA 230/21 Inhalation Aerosol 1288
Flonase Nasal Spray 1431
Flovent Diskus 50 mcg 1435
Fluticasone Propionate HFA (Immunosuppressive therapies, including corticosteroids, may reduce the immune response to Kinrix). Products include:
Flovent HFA 1440
Gemcitabine Hydrochloride (Immunosuppressive therapies, including antimetabolites, may reduce the immune response to Kinrix). Products include:
Gemzar for Injection 1820
Hepatitis A Vaccine, Inactivated (When Kinrix is administered concomitantly with other injectable vaccines, they should be given with separate syringes. Kinrix should not be mixed with any other vaccine in the same syringe or vial). Products include:
Havrix Injection Vaccine 1454
Twinrix Vaccine 1628
Vaqta 2130
Hydrocortisone (Immunosuppressive therapies, including corticosteroids, may reduce the immune response to Kinrix).
No products indexed under this heading.
Hydrocortisone Acetate (Immunosuppressive therapies, including corticosteroids, may reduce the immune response to Kinrix). Products include:
Analpram-HC 1140
Pramosone 1141
Hydrocortisone Sodium Phosphate (Immunosuppressive therapies, including corticosteroids, may reduce the immune response to Kinrix).
No products indexed under this heading.
Hydrocortisone Sodium Succinate (Immunosuppressive therapies, including corticosteroids, may reduce the immune response to Kinrix).
No products indexed under this heading.
Hydroxyurea (Immunosuppressive therapies, including cytotoxic drugs, may reduce the immune response to Kinrix).
No products indexed under this heading.
Influenza Vaccine, Live Attenuated (When Kinrix is administered concomitantly with other injectable vaccines, they should be given with separate syringes. Kinrix should not be mixed with any other vaccine in the same syringe or vial).
No products indexed under this heading.
Influenza Virus Vaccine (When Kinrix is administered concomitantly with other injectable vaccines, they should be given with separate syringes. Kinrix should not be mixed with any other vaccine in the same syringe or vial). Products include:
Fluarix Vaccine 1446
Flulaval Injection Vaccine 1448
Influenza Virus Vaccine Live, Intranasal (When Kinrix is administered concomitantly with other injectable vaccines, they should be given with separate syringes. Kinrix should not be mixed with any other vaccine in the same syringe or vial). Products include:
FluMist Vaccine 1945
Japanese Encephalitis Vaccine Inactivated (When Kinrix is administered concomitantly with other injectable vaccines, they should be given with separate syringes. Kinrix should not be mixed with any other vaccine in the same syringe or vial).
No products indexed under this heading.
Lomustine (CCNU) (Immunosuppressive therapies, including alkylating agents, may reduce the immune response to Kinrix).
No products indexed under this heading.
Measles, Mumps, Rubella and Varicella Virus Vaccine Live (When Kinrix is administered concomitantly with other injectable vaccines, they should be given with separate syringes. Kinrix should not be mixed with any other vaccine in the same syringe or vial). Products include:
ProQuad 2099
Measles, Mumps & Rubella Virus Vaccine, Live (When Kinrix is administered concomitantly with other injectable vaccines, they should be given with separate syringes. Kinrix should not be mixed with any other vaccine in the same syringe or vial). Products include:
M-M-R II 2054
Measles & Rubella Virus Vaccine Live (When Kinrix is administered concomitantly with other injectable vaccines, they should be given with separate syringes. Kinrix should not be mixed with any other vaccine in the same syringe or vial).
No products indexed under this heading.
Measles Virus Vaccine Live (When Kinrix is administered concomitantly with other injectable vaccines, they should be given with separate syringes. Kinrix should not be mixed with any other vaccine in the same syringe or vial). Products include:
Attenuvax 1951
Mechlorethamine Hydrochloride (Immunosuppressive therapies, including alkylating agents, may reduce the immune response to Kinrix). Products include:
Mustargen for Injection 2492
Melphalan (Immunosuppressive therapies, including alkylating agents, may reduce the immune response to Kinrix).
No products indexed under this heading.
Mercaptopurine (Immunosuppressive therapies, including antimetabolites, may reduce the immune response to Kinrix).
No products indexed under this heading.
Methotrexate (Immunosuppressive therapies, including antimetabolites, may reduce the immune response to Kinrix).
No products indexed under this heading.
Methotrexate Sodium (Immunosuppressive therapies, including cytotoxic drugs, may reduce the immune response to Kinrix).
No products indexed under this heading.
Methylprednisolone Acetate (Immunosuppressive therapies, including corticosteroids, may reduce the immune response to Kinrix).
No products indexed under this heading.
Methylprednisolone Sodium Succinate (Immunosuppressive therapies, including corticosteroids, may reduce the immune response to Kinrix).
No products indexed under this heading.
Mitotane (Immunosuppressive therapies, including cytotoxic drugs, may reduce the immune response to Kinrix).
No products indexed under this heading.
Mitoxantrone Hydrochloride (Immunosuppressive therapies, including cytotoxic drugs, may reduce the immune response to Kinrix). Products include:

Novantrone for Injection Concentrate 1100

Mometasone Furoate (Immunosuppressive therapies, including corticosteroids, may reduce the immune response to Kinrix). Products include:
Asmanex Twisthaler 2797
Elocon Cream 0.1% 2840
Elocon Lotion 0.1% 2841
Elocon Ointment 0.1% 2842

Mometasone Furoate Monohydrate (Immunosuppressive therapies, including corticosteroids, may reduce the immune response to Kinrix). Products include:
Nasonex Nasal Spray 2883

Mumps Virus Vaccine, Live (When Kinrix is administered concomitantly with other injectable vaccines, they should be given with separate syringes. Kinrix should not be mixed with any other vaccine in the same syringe or vial). Products include:
Mumpsvax 2068

Muromonab-CD3 (Immunosuppressive therapies may reduce the immune response to Kinrix). Products include:
Orthoclone OKT3 Sterile Solution 2387

Mycophenolate Mofetil (Immunosuppressive therapies may reduce the immune response to Kinrix). Products include:
CellCept Capsules 2622
CellCept Oral Suspension 2622
CellCept Tablets 2622

Pentostatin (Immunosuppressive therapies, including antimetabolites, may reduce the immune response to Kinrix).
No products indexed under this heading.

Poliovirus Vaccine, Live, Oral, Trivalent, Types 1,2,3 (Sabin) (When Kinrix is administered concomitantly with other injectable vaccines, they should be given with separate syringes. Kinrix should not be mixed with any other vaccine in the same syringe or vial).
No products indexed under this heading.

Poliovirus Vaccine Inactivated (When Kinrix is administered concomitantly with other injectable vaccines, they should be given with separate syringes. Kinrix should not be mixed with any other vaccine in the same syringe or vial). Products include:
Pediarix Vaccine 1552

Prednisolone Acetate (Immunosuppressive therapies, including corticosteroids, may reduce the immune response to Kinrix). Products include:
Pred Forte Ophthalmic Suspension .... ⊙227
Pred Mild Ophthalmic Suspension .... ⊙230
Pred-G Ophthalmic Ointment .... ⊙229
Pred-G Ophthalmic Suspension .... ⊙228

Prednisolone Sodium Phosphate (Immunosuppressive therapies, including corticosteroids, may reduce the immune response to Kinrix).
No products indexed under this heading.

Prednisolone Tebutate (Immunosuppressive therapies, including corticosteroids, may reduce the immune response to Kinrix).
No products indexed under this heading.

Prednisone (Immunosuppressive therapies, including corticosteroids, may reduce the immune response to Kinrix).
No products indexed under this heading.

Procarbazine Hydrochloride (Immunosuppressive therapies, including cytotoxic drugs, may reduce the immune response to Kinrix).
No products indexed under this heading.

Radiation (Immunosuppressive therapies, including irradiation, may reduce the immune response to Kinrix).
No products indexed under this heading.

Rotavirus Vaccine, Live, Oral, Tetravalent (When Kinrix is administered concomitantly with other injectable vaccines, they should be given with separate syringes. Kinrix should not be mixed with any other vaccine in the same syringe or vial).
No products indexed under this heading.

Rubella & Mumps Virus Vaccine Live (When Kinrix is administered concomitantly with other injectable vaccines, they should be given with separate syringes. Kinrix should not be mixed with any other vaccine in the same syringe or vial).
No products indexed under this heading.

Rubella Virus Vaccine Live (When Kinrix is administered concomitantly with other injectable vaccines, they should be given with separate syringes. Kinrix should not be mixed with any other vaccine in the same syringe or vial). Products include:
Meruvax II 2061

Sirolimus (Immunosuppressive therapies may reduce the immune response to Kinrix). Products include:
Rapamune 3260

Smallpox Vaccine (When Kinrix is administered concomitantly with other injectable vaccines, they should be given with separate syringes. Kinrix should not be mixed with any other vaccine in the same syringe or vial).
No products indexed under this heading.

Tacrolimus (Immunosuppressive therapies may reduce the immune response to Kinrix). Products include:
Prograf Capsules and Injection 622
Protopic Ointment 628

Tamoxifen Citrate (Immunosuppressive therapies, including cytotoxic drugs, may reduce the immune response to Kinrix).
No products indexed under this heading.

Thioguanine (Immunosuppressive therapies, including antimetabolites, may reduce the immune response to Kinrix). Products include:
Tabloid Tablets 1601

Thiotepa (Immunosuppressive therapies, including alkylating agents, may reduce the immune response to Kinrix).
No products indexed under this heading.

Triamcinolone (Immunosuppressive therapies, including corticosteroids, may reduce the immune response to Kinrix).
No products indexed under this heading.

Triamcinolone Acetonide (Immunosuppressive therapies, including corticosteroids, may reduce the immune response to Kinrix). Products include:
Azmacort Inhalation Aerosol 407
Nasacort AQ Nasal Spray 2765
Triesence Injectable Suspension .... ⊙209

Triamcinolone Diacetate (Immunosuppressive therapies, including corticosteroids, may reduce the immune response to Kinrix).
No products indexed under this heading.

Triamcinolone Hexacetonide (Immunosuppressive therapies, including corticosteroids, may reduce the immune response to Kinrix).
No products indexed under this heading.

Typhoid Vaccine (When Kinrix is administered concomitantly with other injectable vaccines, they should be given with separate syringes. Kinrix should not be mixed with any other vaccine in the same syringe or vial).
No products indexed under this heading.

Varicella Virus Vaccine Live (When Kinrix is administered concomitantly with other injectable vaccines, they should be given with separate syringes. Kinrix should not be mixed with any other vaccine in the same syringe or vial). Products include:
Varivax 2133

Vincristine Sulfate (Immunosuppressive therapies, including cytotoxic drugs, may reduce the immune response to Kinrix).
No products indexed under this heading.

Yellow Fever Vaccine (When Kinrix is administered concomitantly with other injectable vaccines, they should be given with separate syringes. Kinrix should not be mixed with any other vaccine in the same syringe or vial).
No products indexed under this heading.

Zoster Vaccine Live (When Kinrix is administered concomitantly with other injectable vaccines, they should be given with separate syringes. Kinrix should not be mixed with any other vaccine in the same syringe or vial). Products include:
Zostavax Injection 2145

KLONOPIN TABLETS

(Clonazepam) 2639

May interact with central nervous system depressants, anticonvulsants, monoamine oxidase inhibitors, phenytoin, tricyclic antidepressants, and certain other agents. Compounds in these categories include:

Alfentanil Hydrochloride (Potentiates CNS-depressant action).
No products indexed under this heading.

Alprazolam (Potentiates CNS-depressant action).
No products indexed under this heading.

Amitriptyline Hydrochloride (Potentiates CNS-depressant action).
No products indexed under this heading.

Amoxapine (Potentiates CNS-depressant action).
No products indexed under this heading.

Aprobarbital (Potentiates CNS-depressant action).
No products indexed under this heading.

Buprenorphine Hydrochloride (Potentiates CNS-depressant action). Products include:
Suboxone Tablets 2601
Subutex Tablets 2601

Buspirone Hydrochloride (Potentiates CNS-depressant action).
No products indexed under this heading.

Butabarbital (Potentiates CNS-depressant action).
No products indexed under this heading.

Butalbital (Potentiates CNS-depressant action).
No products indexed under this heading.

Carbamazepine (Induces clonazepam metabolism causing an approximately 30% decrease in plasma clonazepam levels). Products include:
Carbatrol Capsules 3019
Equetro Extended-Release Capsules 3174

Chlordiazepoxide (Potentiates CNS-depressant action).
No products indexed under this heading.

Chlordiazepoxide Hydrochloride (Potentiates CNS-depressant action).
No products indexed under this heading.

Chlorpromazine (Potentiates CNS-depressant action).
No products indexed under this heading.

Chlorpromazine Hydrochloride (Potentiates CNS-depressant action).
No products indexed under this heading.

Chlorprothixene (Potentiates CNS-depressant action).
No products indexed under this heading.

Chlorprothixene Hydrochloride (Potentiates CNS-depressant action).
No products indexed under this heading.

Chlorprothixene Lactate (Potentiates CNS-depressant action).
No products indexed under this heading.

Clomipramine Hydrochloride (Potentiates CNS-depressant action).
No products indexed under this heading.

Clorazepate Dipotassium (Potentiates CNS-depressant action).
No products indexed under this heading.

Clozapine (Potentiates CNS-depressant action).
No products indexed under this heading.

Codeine Phosphate (Potentiates CNS-depressant action). Products include:
Tylenol with Codeine Tablets 2427

Desflurane (Potentiates CNS-depressant action).
No products indexed under this heading.

IMPORTANT NOTE: Always consult each drug listing in the patient's regimen for possible interactions.

Desipramine Hydrochloride (Potentiates CNS-depressant action).
No products indexed under this heading.

Dezocine (Potentiates CNS-depressant action).
No products indexed under this heading.

Diazepam (Potentiates CNS-depressant action). Products include:
Valium Tablets 2658

Divalproex Sodium (Potentiates CNS-depressant action). Products include:
Depakote ER Tablets 423

Doxepin Hydrochloride (Potentiates CNS-depressant action).
No products indexed under this heading.

Droperidol (Potentiates CNS-depressant action).
No products indexed under this heading.

Enflurane (Potentiates CNS-depressant action).
No products indexed under this heading.

Estazolam (Potentiates CNS-depressant action).
No products indexed under this heading.

Ethanol (Potentiates CNS-depressant action).
No products indexed under this heading.

Ethchlorvynol (Potentiates CNS-depressant action).
No products indexed under this heading.

Ethinamate (Potentiates CNS-depressant action).
No products indexed under this heading.

Ethosuximide (Potentiates CNS-depressant action).
No products indexed under this heading.

Ethotoin (Potentiates CNS-depressant action).
No products indexed under this heading.

Ethyl Alcohol (Potentiates CNS-depressant action).
No products indexed under this heading.

Felbamate (Potentiates CNS-depressant action).
No products indexed under this heading.

Fentanyl (Potentiates CNS-depressant action). Products include:
Duragesic Transdermal System 2405
Ionsys Transdermal System 2410

Fentanyl Citrate (Potentiates CNS-depressant action). Products include:
Actiq 959
Fentora Tablets 968

Fluphenazine Decanoate (Potentiates CNS-depressant action).
No products indexed under this heading.

Fluphenazine Enanthate (Potentiates CNS-depressant action).
No products indexed under this heading.

Fluphenazine Hydrochloride (Potentiates CNS-depressant action).
No products indexed under this heading.

Flurazepam Hydrochloride (Potentiates CNS-depressant action).
No products indexed under this heading.

Fosphenytoin (Potentiates CNS-depressant action).
No products indexed under this heading.

Fosphenytoin Sodium (Induces clonazepam metabolism causing an approximately 30% decrease in plasma clonazepam levels).
No products indexed under this heading.

Gabapentin (Potentiates CNS-depressant action).
No products indexed under this heading.

Glutethimide (Potentiates CNS-depressant action).
No products indexed under this heading.

Haloperidol (Potentiates CNS-depressant action).
No products indexed under this heading.

Haloperidol Decanoate (Potentiates CNS-depressant action).
No products indexed under this heading.

Hydrocodone Bitartrate (Potentiates CNS-depressant action). Products include:
Lortab 5/500 Tablets 3143
Lortab 7.5/500 Tablets 3144
Lortab 10/500 Tablets 3144
Vicodin Tablets 529
Vicodin ES Tablets 530
Vicodin HP Tablets 531
Vicoprofen Tablets 533
Zydone Tablets 1132

Hydrocodone Polistirex (Potentiates CNS-depressant action). Products include:
Tussionex Pennkinetic Extended-Release Suspension 3154

Hydromorphone Hydrochloride (Potentiates CNS-depressant action).
No products indexed under this heading.

Hydroxyzine Hydrochloride (Potentiates CNS-depressant action).
No products indexed under this heading.

Imipramine Hydrochloride (Potentiates CNS-depressant action).
No products indexed under this heading.

Imipramine Pamoate (Potentiates CNS-depressant action).
No products indexed under this heading.

Isocarboxazid (Potentiates CNS-depressant action). Products include:
Marplan Tablets 3177

Isoflurane (Potentiates CNS-depressant action).
No products indexed under this heading.

Itraconazole (Co-administration with CYP450 3A inhibitors should be undertaken with caution).
No products indexed under this heading.

Ketamine Hydrochloride (Potentiates CNS-depressant action).
No products indexed under this heading.

Ketoconazole (Co-administration with CYP450 3A inhibitors should be undertaken with caution). Products include:
Extina Foam, 2% 3057
Nizoral A-D Shampoo 1901

Lamotrigine (Potentiates CNS-depressant action). Products include:
Lamictal 1488

Levetiracetam (Potentiates CNS-depressant action). Products include:
Keppra Injection 3137
Keppra Oral Solution 3131
Keppra Tablets 3131

Levomethadyl Acetate Hydrochloride (Potentiates CNS-depressant action).
No products indexed under this heading.

Levorphanol Tartrate (Potentiates CNS-depressant action).
No products indexed under this heading.

Lorazepam (Potentiates CNS-depressant action).
No products indexed under this heading.

Loxapine Hydrochloride (Potentiates CNS-depressant action).
No products indexed under this heading.

Loxapine Succinate (Potentiates CNS-depressant action).
No products indexed under this heading.

Maprotiline Hydrochloride (Potentiates CNS-depressant action).
No products indexed under this heading.

Meperidine Hydrochloride (Potentiates CNS-depressant action).
No products indexed under this heading.

Mephenytoin (Potentiates CNS-depressant action).
No products indexed under this heading.

Mephobarbital (Potentiates CNS-depressant action).
No products indexed under this heading.

Meprobamate (Potentiates CNS-depressant action).
No products indexed under this heading.

Mesoridazine Besylate (Potentiates CNS-depressant action).
No products indexed under this heading.

Methadone Hydrochloride (Potentiates CNS-depressant action).
No products indexed under this heading.

Methohexital Sodium (Potentiates CNS-depressant action).
No products indexed under this heading.

Methotrimeprazine (Potentiates CNS-depressant action).
No products indexed under this heading.

Methoxyflurane (Potentiates CNS-depressant action).
No products indexed under this heading.

Methsuximide (Potentiates CNS-depressant action).
No products indexed under this heading.

Midazolam Hydrochloride (Potentiates CNS-depressant action).
No products indexed under this heading.

Moclobemide (Potentiates CNS-depressant action).
No products indexed under this heading.

Molindone Hydrochloride (Potentiates CNS-depressant action). Products include:
Moban Tablets 1116

Morphine Sulfate (Potentiates CNS-depressant action). Products include:
Avinza Capsules 1772
DepoDur Injection 1095
MS Contin Tablets 2585

Nortriptyline Hydrochloride (Potentiates CNS-depressant action).
No products indexed under this heading.

Olanzapine (Potentiates CNS-depressant action). Products include:
Symbyax Capsules 1871
Zyprexa Tablets 1883
Zyprexa IntraMuscular 1883
Zyprexa ZYDIS Orally Disintegrating Tablets 1883

Oxazepam (Potentiates CNS-depressant action).
No products indexed under this heading.

Oxcarbazepine (Potentiates CNS-depressant action).
No products indexed under this heading.

Oxycodone Hydrochloride (Potentiates CNS-depressant action). Products include:
OxyContin Tablets 2589
OxyIR Capsules 2593
Percocet Tablets 1127
Percodan Tablets 1130

Paramethadione (Potentiates CNS-depressant action).
No products indexed under this heading.

Pargyline Hydrochloride (Potentiates CNS-depressant action).
No products indexed under this heading.

Pentobarbital Sodium (Potentiates CNS-depressant action). Products include:
Nembutal Sodium Solution, USP 2494

Perphenazine (Potentiates CNS-depressant action).
No products indexed under this heading.

Phenacemide (Potentiates CNS-depressant action).
No products indexed under this heading.

Phenelzine Sulfate (Potentiates CNS-depressant action).
No products indexed under this heading.

Phenobarbital (Induces clonazepam metabolism causing an approximately 30% decrease in plasma clonazepam levels; CNS depressant action may be potentiated). Products include:
Donnatal Extentabs 2507

Phensuximide (Potentiates CNS-depressant action).
No products indexed under this heading.

Phenytoin (Induces clonazepam metabolism causing an approximately 30% decrease in plasma clonazepam levels).
No products indexed under this heading.

Phenytoin Sodium (Induces clonazepam metabolism causing an approximately 30% decrease in plasma clonazepam levels). Products include:
Phenytek Capsules 2192

Prazepam (Potentiates CNS-depressant action).
No products indexed under this heading.

Primidone (Potentiates CNS-depressant action).
No products indexed under this heading.

Procarbazine Hydrochloride (Potentiates CNS-depressant action).
No products indexed under this heading.

Prochlorperazine (Potentiates CNS-depressant action).
No products indexed under this heading.

Promethazine Hydrochloride (Potentiates CNS-depressant action).
No products indexed under this heading.

Propofol (Potentiates CNS-depressant action).
No products indexed under this heading.

Propoxyphene Hydrochloride (Potentiates CNS-depressant action).
No products indexed under this heading.

Propoxyphene Napsylate (Potentiates CNS-depressant action).
No products indexed under this heading.

Protriptyline Hydrochloride (Potentiates CNS-depressant action).
No products indexed under this heading.

Quazepam (Potentiates CNS-depressant action).
No products indexed under this heading.

Quetiapine Fumarate (Potentiates CNS-depressant action).
No products indexed under this heading.

Rasagiline Mesylate (Potentiates CNS-depressant action). Products include:
Azilect Tablets 3106

Remifentanil Hydrochloride (Potentiates CNS-depressant action).
No products indexed under this heading.

Risperidone (Potentiates CNS-depressant action). Products include:
Risperdal Consta Long-Acting Injection 1753

Secobarbital Sodium (Potentiates CNS-depressant action).
No products indexed under this heading.

Selegiline (Potentiates CNS-depressant action). Products include:
Emsam Transdermal System 905

Selegiline Hydrochloride (Potentiates CNS-depressant action). Products include:
Eldepryl Capsules 3052

Sevoflurane (Potentiates CNS-depressant action). Products include:
Ultane Liquid for Inhalation 524

Sufentanil Citrate (Potentiates CNS-depressant action).
No products indexed under this heading.

Temazepam (Potentiates CNS-depressant action).
No products indexed under this heading.

Thiamylal Sodium (Potentiates CNS-depressant action).
No products indexed under this heading.

Thioridazine Hydrochloride (Potentiates CNS-depressant action). Products include:
Thioridazine Hydrochloride Tablets 2195

Thiothixene (Potentiates CNS-depressant action). Products include:
Thiothixene Capsules 2197

Tiagabine Hydrochloride (Potentiates CNS-depressant action). Products include:
Gabitril Tablets 973

Topiramate (Potentiates CNS-depressant action).
No products indexed under this heading.

Tranylcypromine Sulfate (Potentiates CNS-depressant action). Products include:
Parnate Tablets 1532

Triazolam (Potentiates CNS-depressant action).
No products indexed under this heading.

Trifluoperazine Hydrochloride (Potentiates CNS-depressant action).
No products indexed under this heading.

Trimethadione (Potentiates CNS-depressant action).
No products indexed under this heading.

Trimipramine Maleate (Potentiates CNS-depressant action).
No products indexed under this heading.

Valproate Sodium (Potentiates CNS-depressant action).
No products indexed under this heading.

Valproic Acid (Potentiates CNS-depressant action).
No products indexed under this heading.

Zaleplon (Potentiates CNS-depressant action).
No products indexed under this heading.

Ziprasidone Hydrochloride (Potentiates CNS-depressant action). Products include:
Geodon Capsules 2520

Zolpidem Tartrate (Potentiates CNS-depressant action). Products include:
Ambien Tablets 2692
Ambien CR Tablets 2696

Zonisamide (Potentiates CNS-depressant action). Products include:
Zonegran Capsules 1089

Food Interactions

Alcohol (Potentiates CNS-depressant action).

KLONOPIN WAFERS

(Clonazepam) 2639
See Klonopin Tablets

KOGENATE FS

(Antihemophilic Factor (Recombinant)) 746
None cited in PDR database.

KOGENATE FS WITH BIO-SET

(Antihemophilic Factor (Recombinant)) 748
None cited in PDR database.

K-PHOS ORIGINAL (SODIUM FREE) TABLETS

(Potassium Acid Phosphate) 814
May interact with antacids, potassium preparations, potassium sparing diuretics, salicylates, and certain other agents. Compounds in these categories include:

Aluminum Carbonate (May bind phosphate and prevent its absorption).
No products indexed under this heading.

Aluminum Hydroxide (May bind phosphate and prevent its absorption).
No products indexed under this heading.

Amiloride Hydrochloride (Hyperkalemia).
No products indexed under this heading.

Aspirin (Increased serum salicylate levels; possible toxicity). Products include:
Aggrenox Capsules 819
Bayer Aspirin 750
Percodan Tablets 1130
St. Joseph 81 mg Aspirin Chewable and Enteric Coated Tablets 1903

Aspirin, Enteric Coated (Increased serum salicylate levels; possible toxicity).
No products indexed under this heading.

Aspirin Buffered (Increased serum salicylate levels; possible toxicity).
No products indexed under this heading.

Choline Magnesium Trisalicylate (Increased serum salicylate levels; possible toxicity).
No products indexed under this heading.

Diflunisal (Increased serum salicylate levels; possible toxicity).
No products indexed under this heading.

Magaldrate (May bind phosphate and prevent its absorption).
No products indexed under this heading.

Magnesium Hydroxide (May bind phosphate and prevent its absorption). Products include:
Fleet Pedia-Lax Chewable Tablets 1145
Pepcid Complete Chewable Tablets 1771
Extra Strength Rolaids Freshmint Tablets 1903
Rolaids Multi-Symptom Berry Tablets 1903
Rolaids Original Peppermint Tablets 1903

Magnesium Oxide (May bind phosphate and prevent its absorption). Products include:
Beelith Tablets 813

Magnesium Salicylate (Increased serum salicylate levels; possible toxicity).
No products indexed under this heading.

Potassium Bicarbonate (Potential for hyperkalemia).
No products indexed under this heading.

Potassium Chloride (Potential for hyperkalemia). Products include:
MoviPrep Oral Solution 2679

Potassium Citrate (Potential for hyperkalemia). Products include:
BioLean Free Tablets 635
Urocit-K Tablets 2176

Potassium Gluconate (Potential for hyperkalemia).
No products indexed under this heading.

Potassium Phosphate (Potential for hyperkalemia). Products include:
K-Phos Neutral Tablets 813

Salsalate (Increased serum salicylate levels; possible toxicity).
No products indexed under this heading.

Sodium Bicarbonate (May bind phosphate and prevent its absorption). Products include:
Ceo-Two Laxative Suppository 815

Spironolactone (Hyperkalemia).
No products indexed under this heading.

Triamterene (Hyperkalemia). Products include:
Dyazide Capsules 1405
Dyrenium Capsules 3189

K-PHOS NEUTRAL TABLETS

(Potassium Phosphate, Sodium Phosphate) 813
May interact with antacids containing aluminum, calcium and magnesium, calcium preparations, potassium preparations, potassium sparing diuretics, and certain other agents. Compounds in these categories include:

ACTH (Concurrent use with corticotropin may result in hypernatremia).
No products indexed under this heading.

Aluminum Carbonate (Coadministration with antacids may bind the phosphate and prevent its absorption).
No products indexed under this heading.

Aluminum Hydroxide (Coadministration with antacids may bind the phosphate and prevent its absorption).
No products indexed under this heading.

Amiloride Hydrochloride (Concurrent use with potassium-sparing diuretics may cause hyperkalemia).
No products indexed under this heading.

Calcium Carbonate (Concurrent use with calcium-containing preparations may antagonize the effects of phosphates in the treatment of hypercalcemia). Products include:
Accelerator Tablets 634
Actonel with Calcium Tablets 2574
BioLean II Tablets 635
Calcet Triple Calcium + Vitamin D Tablets 629
D-Cal Chewable Caplets 624
Elixir Capsules 636
Pepcid Complete Chewable Tablets 1771
Extra Strength Rolaids Plus Gas Relief Tropical Fruit Softchews...... 1903
Extra Strength Rolaids Softchews Vanilla Creme 1903
Extra Strength Rolaids Freshmint Tablets 1903
Rolaids Multi-Symptom Berry Tablets 1903
Rolaids Original Peppermint Tablets 1903

Calcium Chloride (Concurrent use with calcium-containing preparations may antagonize the effects of phosphates in the treatment of hypercalcemia).
No products indexed under this heading.

Calcium Citrate (Concurrent use with calcium-containing preparations may antagonize the effects of phosphates in the treatment of hypercalcemia). Products include:

- Active Calcium Tablets ... 3173
- CitraNatal DHA Tablets ... 2175
- CitraNatal 90 DHA Tablets ... 2175

Calcium Glubionate (Concurrent use with calcium-containing preparations may antagonize the effects of phosphates in the treatment of hypercalcemia).

No products indexed under this heading.

Deserpidine (Concurrent use with antihypertensives, such as rauwolfia alkaloids, may result in hypernatremia).

No products indexed under this heading.

Diazoxide (Concurrent use with antihypertensives, such as diazoxide, may result in hypernatremia). Products include:

- Proglycem Capsules ... 1185
- Proglycem Suspension ... 1185

Fludrocortisone Acetate (Concurrent use with mineralocorticoids may result in hypernatremia).

No products indexed under this heading.

Guanethidine Monosulfate (Concurrent use with antihypertensives, such as guanethidine, may result in hypernatremia).

No products indexed under this heading.

Hydralazine Hydrochloride (Concurrent use with antihypertensives, such as hydralazine, may result in hypernatremia).

No products indexed under this heading.

Magaldrate (Co-administration with antacids may bind the phosphate and prevent its absorption).

No products indexed under this heading.

Magnesium Hydroxide (Co-administration with antacids may bind the phosphate and prevent its absorption). Products include:

- Fleet Pedia-Lax Chewable Tablets ... 1145
- Pepcid Complete Chewable Tablets ... 1771
- Extra Strength Rolaids Freshmint Tablets ... 1903
- Rolaids Multi-Symptom Berry Tablets ... 1903
- Rolaids Original Peppermint Tablets ... 1903

Magnesium Oxide (Co-administration with antacids may bind the phosphate and prevent its absorption). Products include:

- Beelith Tablets ... 813

Methyldopa (Concurrent use with antihypertensives, such as methyldopa, may result in hypernatremia).

No products indexed under this heading.

Potassium Acid Phosphate (Concurrent use with potassium-containing medications may cause hyperkalemia). Products include:

- K-Phos Original (Sodium Free) Tablets ... 814

Potassium Bicarbonate (Concurrent use with potassium-containing medications may cause hyperkalemia).

No products indexed under this heading.

Potassium Chloride (Concurrent use with potassium-containing medications may cause hyperkalemia). Products include:

- MoviPrep Oral Solution ... 2679

Potassium Citrate (Concurrent use with potassium-containing medications may cause hyperkalemia). Products include:

- BioLean Free Tablets ... ▣635
- Urocit-K Tablets ... 2176

Potassium Gluconate (Concurrent use with potassium-containing medications may cause hyperkalemia).

No products indexed under this heading.

Rauwolfia Serpentina (Concurrent use with antihypertensives, such as rauwolfia alkaloids, may result in hypernatremia).

No products indexed under this heading.

Rescinnamine (Concurrent use with antihypertensives, such as rauwolfia alkaloids, may result in hypernatremia).

No products indexed under this heading.

Reserpine (Concurrent use with antihypertensives, such as rauwolfia alkaloids, may result in hypernatremia).

No products indexed under this heading.

Spironolactone (Concurrent use with potassium-sparing diuretics may cause hyperkalemia).

No products indexed under this heading.

Triamterene (Concurrent use with potassium-sparing diuretics may cause hyperkalemia). Products include:

- Dyazide Capsules ... 1405
- Dyrenium Capsules ... 3189

Vitamin D (Concurrent use with vitamin D may antagonize the effects of phosphates in the treatment of hypercalcemia). Products include:

- Active Calcium Tablets ... 3173
- D-Cal Chewable Caplets ... ▣624
- Norwegian Cod Liver Oil ... 949

KRISTALOSE FOR ORAL SOLUTION

(Lactulose) ... 1004

May interact with nonabsorbable antacids. Compounds in these categories include:

Aluminum Carbonate (Results of preliminary studies suggests that nonabsorbable antacids given concurrently with lactulose may inhibit the desired lactulose-induced drop in colonic pH).

No products indexed under this heading.

Aluminum Hydroxide (Results of preliminary studies suggests that nonabsorbable antacids given concurrently with lactulose may inhibit the desired lactulose-induced drop in colonic pH).

No products indexed under this heading.

Calcium Carbonate (Results of preliminary studies suggests that nonabsorbable antacids given concurrently with lactulose may inhibit the desired lactulose-induced drop in colonic pH). Products include:

- Accelerator Tablets ... ▣634
- Actonel with Calcium Tablets ... 2574
- BioLean II Tablets ... ▣635
- Calcet Triple Calcium + Vitamin D Tablets ... ▣629
- D-Cal Chewable Caplets ... ▣624
- Elixir Capsules ... ▣636
- Pepcid Complete Chewable Tablets ... 1771
- Extra Strength Rolaids Plus Gas Relief Tropical Fruit Softchews ... 1903
- Extra Strength Rolaids Softchews Vanilla Creme ... 1903
- Extra Strength Rolaids Freshmint Tablets ... 1903
- Rolaids Multi-Symptom Berry Tablets ... 1903
- Rolaids Original Peppermint Tablets ... 1903

Magnesium Carbonate (Results of preliminary studies suggests that nonabsorbable antacids given concurrently with lactulose may inhibit the desired lactulose-induced drop in colonic pH).

No products indexed under this heading.

Magnesium Hydroxide (Results of preliminary studies suggests that nonabsorbable antacids given concurrently with lactulose may inhibit the desired lactulose-induced drop in colonic pH). Products include:

- Fleet Pedia-Lax Chewable Tablets ... 1145
- Pepcid Complete Chewable Tablets ... 1771
- Extra Strength Rolaids Freshmint Tablets ... 1903
- Rolaids Multi-Symptom Berry Tablets ... 1903
- Rolaids Original Peppermint Tablets ... 1903

LACRISERT STERILE OPHTHALMIC INSERT

(Hydroxypropyl Cellulose) ... ⊙233

None cited in PDR database.

LAMICTAL CHEWABLE DISPERSIBLE TABLETS

(Lamotrigine) ... 1488

See Lamictal Tablets

LAMICTAL TABLETS

(Lamotrigine) ... 1488

May interact with dihydrofolate reductase inhibitors, lithium preparations, oral contraceptives, phenytoin, valproate, and certain other agents. Compounds in these categories include:

Carbamazepine (Potential for higher incidence of dizziness, diplopia, ataxia, and blurred vision; decreases lamotrigine steady-state concentrations by approximately 40%; lamotrigine has no appreciable effect on steady-state carbamazepine plasma concentration). Products include:

- Carbatrol Capsules ... 3019
- Equetro Extended-Release Capsules ... 3174

Desogestrel (Some estrogen-containing oral contraceptives have been shown to decrease serum concentrations of lamotrigine. Dosage adjustments will be necessary in most patients who start or stop estrogen-containing oral contraceptives while taking lamotrigine. Duringthe week of inactive hormone preparation ("pill-free" week) of oral contraceptive therapy, plasma levels are expected to rise, as much as doubling by the end of the week. Adverse events consistent with elevated levels of lamotrigine, such as dizziness, ataxia and diplopia, could occur). Products include:

- Mircette Tablets ... 1034

Divalproex Sodium (Co-administration in healthy volunteers resulted in decreased trough steady-state VPA concentrations; the addition of VPA increases lamotrigine steady-state concentrations in normal volunteers by slightly more than two-fold). Products include:

- Depakote ER Tablets ... 423

Ethinyl Estradiol (Some estrogen-containing oral contraceptives have been shown to decrease serum concentrations of lamotrigine. Dosage adjustments will be necessary in most patients who start or stop estrogen-containing oral contraceptives while taking lamotrigine. Duringthe week of inactive hormone preparation ("pill-free" week) of oral contraceptive therapy, plasma levels are expected to rise, as much as doubling by the end of the week. Adverse events consistent with elevated levels of lamotrigine, such as dizziness, ataxia and diplopia, could occur). Products include:

- Lybrel Tablets ... 3204
- Mircette Tablets ... 1034
- NuvaRing ... 2897
- Ortho-Cyclen/Ortho Tri-Cyclen ... 2449
- Ortho Evra Transdermal System ... 2437
- Ortho Tri-Cyclen Lo Tablets ... 2458
- Seasonique Tablets ... 1046
- Yaz Tablets ... 805

Ethynodiol Diacetate (Some estrogen-containing oral contraceptives have been shown to decrease serum concentrations of lamotrigine. Dosage adjustments will be necessary in most patients who start or stop estrogen-containing oral contraceptives while taking lamotrigine. Duringthe week of inactive hormone preparation ("pill-free" week) of oral contraceptive therapy, plasma levels are expected to rise, as much as doubling by the end of the week. Adverse events consistent with elevated levels of lamotrigine, such as dizziness, ataxia and diplopia, could occur).

No products indexed under this heading.

Fosphenytoin Sodium (Decreases lamotrigine steady-state concentrations by approximately 40%).

No products indexed under this heading.

Levetiracetam (Potential drug interactions between levetiracetam and lamotrigene were assessed by evaluating serum concentrations of both agents during placebo-controlled clinical trials. These data indicate that lamotrigene does not influence the pharmacokinetics of levetiracetam). Products include:

- Keppra Injection ... 3137
- Keppra Oral Solution ... 3131
- Keppra Tablets ... 3131

Levonorgestrel (Some estrogen-containing oral contraceptives have been shown to decrease serum concentrations of lamotrigine. Dosage adjustments will be necessary in most patients who start or stop estrogen-containing oral contraceptives while taking lamotrigine. Duringthe week of inactive hormone preparation ("pill-free" week) of oral contraceptive therapy, plasma levels are expected to rise, as much as doubling by the end of the week. Adverse events consistent with elevated levels of lamotrigine, such as dizziness, ataxia and diplopia, could occur). Products include:

- Climara Pro Transdermal System ... 768
- Lybrel Tablets ... 3204
- Mirena Intrauterine System ... 779
- Plan B Tablets ... 1044
- Seasonique Tablets ... 1046

Lithium (The pharmacokinetics of lithium were not altered in healthy subjects by co-administration of 100 m/day lamotrigene for six days).
No products indexed under this heading.

Lithium Carbonate (The pharmacokinetics of lithium were not altered in healthy subjects by co-administration of 100 m/day lamotrigene for six days).
No products indexed under this heading.

Lithium Citrate (The pharmacokinetics of lithium were not altered in healthy subjects by co-administration of 100 m/day lamotrigene for six days).
No products indexed under this heading.

Mestranol (Some estrogen-containing oral contraceptives have been shown to decrease serum concentrations of lamotrigine. Dosage adjustments will be necessary in most patients who start or stop estrogen-containing oral contraceptives while taking lamotrigine. Duringthe week of inactive hormone preparation ("pill-free" week) of oral contraceptive therapy, plasma levels are expected to rise, as much as doubling by the end of the week. Adverse events consistent with elevated levels of lamotrigine, such as dizziness, ataxia and diplopia, could occur).
No products indexed under this heading.

Methotrexate Sodium (Lamotrigine is an inhibitor of dihydrofolate reductase; use caution when prescribing other medications that inhibit folate metabolism).
No products indexed under this heading.

Norethindrone (Some estrogen-containing oral contraceptives have been shown to decrease serum concentrations of lamotrigine. Dosage adjustments will be necessary in most patients who start or stop estrogen-containing oral contraceptives while taking lamotrigine. Duringthe week of inactive hormone preparation ("pill-free" week) of oral contraceptive therapy, plasma levels are expected to rise, as much as doubling by the end of the week. Adverse events consistent with elevated levels of lamotrigine, such as dizziness, ataxia and diplopia, could occur). Products include:
Ortho Micronor Tablets 2446

Norethynodrel (Some estrogen-containing oral contraceptives have been shown to decrease serum concentrations of lamotrigine. Dosage adjustments will be necessary in most patients who start or stop estrogen-containing oral contraceptives while taking lamotrigine. Duringthe week of inactive hormone preparation ("pill-free" week) of oral contraceptive therapy, plasma levels are expected to rise, as much as doubling by the end of the week. Adverse events consistent with elevated levels of lamotrigine, such as dizziness, ataxia and diplopia, could occur).
No products indexed under this heading.

Norgestimate (Some estrogen-containing oral contraceptives have been shown to decrease serum concentrations of lamotrigine. Dosage adjustments will be necessary in most patients who start or stop estrogen-containing oral contraceptives while taking lamotrigine. Duringthe week of inactive hormone preparation ("pill-free" week) of oral contraceptive therapy, plasma levels are expected to rise, as much as doubling by the end of the week. Adverse events consistent with elevated levels of lamotrigine, such as dizziness, ataxia and diplopia, could occur). Products include:
Ortho-Cyclen/Ortho Tri-Cyclen 2449
Ortho Tri-Cyclen Lo Tablets 2458

Norgestrel (Some estrogen-containing oral contraceptives have been shown to decrease serum concentrations of lamotrigine. Dosage adjustments will be necessary in most patients who start or stop estrogen-containing oral contraceptives while taking lamotrigine. Duringthe week of inactive hormone preparation ("pill-free" week) of oral contraceptive therapy, plasma levels are expected to rise, as much as doubling by the end of the week. Adverse events consistent with elevated levels of lamotrigine, such as dizziness, ataxia and diplopia, could occur).
No products indexed under this heading.

Olanzapine (The AUC and Cmax of lamotrigine was reduced on average by 24% and 20%, respectively, following the addition of olanzapine (15 mg once daily) to lamotrigine (200 mg once daily) in healthy male volunteers (n=16) compared to healthy male volunteers receiving lamotrigine alone (n=12). This reduction in lamotrigine plasma concentration is not expected to be clinically relevant). Products include:
Symbyax Capsules 1871
Zyprexa Tablets 1883
Zyprexa IntraMuscular 1883
Zyprexa ZYDIS Orally Disintegrating Tablets.................. 1883

Oral Contraceptives (There have been reports of decreased lamotrigine concentrations following introduction of oral contraceptives and reports of increased lamotrigine concentrations following withdrawal of oral contraceptives).
No products indexed under this heading.

Oxcarbazepine (The AUC and Cmax of oxcarbazepine and its active 10-monohydroxy oxcarbazepine metabolite were not significantly different following the addition of oxcarbazepine (600 mg twice daily) to lamotrigene (200 mg once daily) in healthy male volunteers compared to healthy male volunteers receiving oxcarbazepine alone. Limited clinical data suggests a higher incidence of headache, dizziness, nausea and somnolence with co-administration of lamotrigene and oxcarbazepine compared to lamotrigene alone or oxcarbazepine alone).
No products indexed under this heading.

Phenobarbital (Decreases lamotrigine steady-state concentrations by approximately 40%). Products include:
Donnatal Extentabs 2507

Phenytoin (Decreases lamotrigine steady-state concentrations by approximately 40%).
No products indexed under this heading.

Phenytoin Sodium (Decreases lamotrigine steady-state concentrations by approximately 40%). Products include:
Phenytek Capsules 2192

Primidone (Decreases lamotrigine steady-state concentrations by approximately 40%).
No products indexed under this heading.

Rifampin (Co-administration of rifampin has been shown to increase the apparent clearance of lamotrigine).
No products indexed under this heading.

Trimethoprim (Lamotrigine is an inhibitor of dihydrofolate reductase; use caution when prescribing other medications that inhibit folate metabolism).
No products indexed under this heading.

Trimetrexate Glucuronate (Lamotrigine is an inhibitor of dihydrofolate reductase; use caution when prescribing other medications that inhibit folate metabolism).
No products indexed under this heading.

Valproate Sodium (Co-administration in healthy volunteers resulted in decreased trough steady-state VPA concentrations; the addition of VPA increases lamotrigine steady-state concentrations in normal volunteers by slightly more than two-fold).
No products indexed under this heading.

Valproic Acid (Co-administration in healthy volunteers resulted in decreased trough steady-state VPA concentrations; the addition of VPA increases lamotrigine steady-state concentrations in normal volunteers by slightly more than two-fold).
No products indexed under this heading.

LAMISIL ORAL GRANULES

(Terbinafine Hydrochloride) 2264
May interact with cytochrome p450 2c9 inhibitors (selected), cytochrome p450 2d6 substrates (selected), cytochrome p450 3a4 inhibitors (selected), monoamine oxidase inhibitors, selective serotonin reuptake inhibitors, tricyclic antidepressants, and certain other agents. Compounds in these categories include:

Acetazolamide (It is likely that inhibitors of both CYP2C9 and CYP3A4 may lead to substantial increase in the systemic exposure (Cmax and AUC) of terbinafine).
No products indexed under this heading.

Amiodarone Hydrochloride (Concurrent use with amiodarone, an inhibitor of both CYP2C9 and CYP3A4 may lead to a substantial increase in the systemic exposure (Cmax and AUC) of terbinafine).
No products indexed under this heading.

Amitriptyline Hydrochloride (Studies have shown that terbinafine is an inhibitor of the CYP450 2D6 isozyme. Co-administration of terbinafine hydrochloride oral granules should be done with careful monitoring and may require a reduction in dose of the 2D6-metabolized drug).
No products indexed under this heading.

Amoxapine (Studies have shown that terbinafine is an inhibitor of the CYP450 2D6 isozyme. Co-administration of terbinafine hydrochloride oral granules should be done with careful monitoring and may require a reduction in dose of the 2D6-metabolized drug).
No products indexed under this heading.

Amphetamine Aspartate (Studies have shown that terbinafine is an inhibitor of the CYP450 2D6 isozyme. Co-administration of terbinafine hydrochloride oral granules should be done with careful monitoring and may require a reduction in dose of the 2D6-metabolized drug). Products include:
Adderall XR Capsules 3012

Amphetamine Aspartate Monohydrate (Studies have shown that terbinafine is an inhibitor of the CYP450 2D6 isozyme. Co-administration of terbinafine hydrochloride oral granules should be done with careful monitoring and may require a reduction in dose of the 2D6-metabolized drug).
No products indexed under this heading.

Amphetamine Sulfate (Studies have shown that terbinafine is an inhibitor of the CYP450 2D6 isozyme. Co-administration of terbinafine hydrochloride oral granules should be done with careful monitoring and may require a reduction in dose of the 2D6-metabolized drug). Products include:
Adderall XR Capsules 3012

Amprenavir (It is likely that inhibitors of both CYP2C9 and CYP3A4 may lead to substantial increase in the systemic exposure (Cmax and AUC) of terbinafine).
No products indexed under this heading.

Anastrozole (It is likely that inhibitors of both CYP2C9 and CYP3A4 may lead to substantial increase in the systemic exposure (Cmax and AUC) of terbinafine). Products include:
Arimidex Tablets 672

Aprepitant (It is likely that inhibitors of both CYP2C9 and CYP3A4 may lead to substantial increase in the systemic exposure (Cmax and AUC) of terbinafine). Products include:
Emend Capsules 1992

Atazanavir (It is likely that inhibitors of both CYP2C9 and CYP3A4 may lead to substantial increase in the systemic exposure (Cmax and AUC) of terbinafine).
No products indexed under this heading.

Atazanavir Sulfate (It is likely that inhibitors of both CYP2C9 and CYP3A4 may lead to substantial increase in the systemic exposure (Cmax and AUC) of terbinafine). Products include:
Reyataz Capsules 3299

Atomoxetine Hydrochloride (Studies have shown that terbinafine is an inhibitor of the CYP450 2D6 isozyme. Co-administration of terbinafine hydrochloride oral granules should be done with careful monitoring and may require a reduction in dose of the 2D6-metabolized drug). Products include:
Strattera Capsules 1864

Bendroflumethiazide (It is likely that inhibitors of both CYP2C9 and CYP3A4 may lead to substantial increase in the systemic exposure (Cmax and AUC) of terbinafine).
No products indexed under this heading.

Bisoprolol Fumarate (Studies have shown that terbinafine is an inhibitor of the CYP450 2D6 isozyme. Co-administration of terbinafine hydrochloride oral granules should be done with careful monitoring and may require a reduction in dose of the 2D6-metabolized drug).
No products indexed under this heading.

Caffeine (Terbinafine decreases the clearance of caffeine by 19%).
Products include:
BioLean Free Tablets .... ■635
BioLean II Tablets .... ■635
Winrgy Dietary Supplement .... ■642

Caffeine Citrate (Terbinafine decreases the clearance of caffeine by 19%).
No products indexed under this heading.

Captopril (Studies have shown that terbinafine is an inhibitor of the CYP450 2D6 isozyme. Co-administration of terbinafine hydrochloride oral granules should be done with careful monitoring and may require a reduction in dose of the 2D6-metabolized drug). Products include:
Captopril Tablets 2182

Carvedilol (Studies have shown that terbinafine is an inhibitor of the CYP450 2D6 isozyme. Co-administration of terbinafine hydrochloride oral granules should be done with careful monitoring and may require a reduction in dose of the 2D6-metabolized drug). Products include:
Coreg Tablets 1387

Cevimeline Hydrochloride (Studies have shown that terbinafine is an inhibitor of the CYP450 2D6 isozyme. Co-administration of terbinafine hydrochloride oral granules should be done with careful monitoring and may require a reduction in dose of the 2D6-metabolized drug).
Products include:
Evoxac Capsules 1013

Chloramphenicol (It is likely that inhibitors of both CYP2C9 and CYP3A4 may lead to substantial increase in the systemic exposure (Cmax and AUC) of terbinafine).
No products indexed under this heading.

Chlorothiazide (It is likely that inhibitors of both CYP2C9 and CYP3A4 may lead to substantial increase in the systemic exposure (Cmax and AUC) of terbinafine).
No products indexed under this heading.

Chlorothiazide Sodium (It is likely that inhibitors of both CYP2C9 and CYP3A4 may lead to substantial increase in the systemic exposure (Cmax and AUC) of terbinafine).
Products include:
Intravenous Sodium Diuril 2490

Chlorpromazine (Studies have shown that terbinafine is an inhibitor of the CYP450 2D6 isozyme. Co-administration of terbinafine hydrochloride oral granules should be done with careful monitoring and may require a reduction in dose of the 2D6-metabolized drug).
No products indexed under this heading.

Chlorpromazine Hydrochloride (Studies have shown that terbinafine is an inhibitor of the CYP450 2D6 isozyme. Co-administration of terbinafine hydrochloride oral granules should be done with careful monitoring and may require a reduction in dose of the 2D6-metabolized drug).
No products indexed under this heading.

Chlorpropamide (Studies have shown that terbinafine is an inhibitor of the CYP450 2D6 isozyme. Co-administration of terbinafine hydrochloride oral granules should be done with careful monitoring and may require a reduction in dose of the 2D6-metabolized drug).
No products indexed under this heading.

Cimetidine (Terbinafine is decreased 33% by cimetidine, a CYP450 enzyme inhibitor).
No products indexed under this heading.

Cimetidine Hydrochloride (Terbinafine is decreased 33% by cimetidine, a CYP450 enzyme inhibitor).
No products indexed under this heading.

Ciprofloxacin (It is likely that inhibitors of both CYP2C9 and CYP3A4 may lead to substantial increase in the systemic exposure (Cmax and AUC) of terbinafine). Products include:
Cipro I.V. 2817
Cipro Oral Suspension 2810
Cipro XR Tablets 2823
Ciprodex Otic Suspension 541

Citalopram Hydrobromide (Studies have shown that terbinafine is an inhibitor of the CYP450 2D6 isozyme. Co-administration of terbinafine hydrochloride oral granules should be done with careful monitoring and may require a reduction in dose of the 2D6-metabolized drug).
Products include:
Celexa 1160

Clarithromycin (It is likely that inhibitors of both CYP2C9 and CYP3A4 may lead to substantial increase in the systemic exposure (Cmax and AUC) of terbinafine).
Products include:
Biaxin/Biaxin XL 411

Clomipramine Hydrochloride (Studies have shown that terbinafine is an inhibitor of the CYP450 2D6 isozyme. Co-administration of terbinafine hydrochloride oral granules should be done with careful monitoring and may require a reduction in dose of the 2D6-metabolized drug).
No products indexed under this heading.

Clopidogrel Hydrogen Sulfate (It is likely that inhibitors of both CYP2C9 and CYP3A4 may lead to substantial increase in the systemic exposure (Cmax and AUC) of terbinafine).
No products indexed under this heading.

Clotrimazole (It is likely that inhibitors of both CYP2C9 and CYP3A4 may lead to substantial increase in the systemic exposure (Cmax and AUC) of terbinafine). Products include:
Lotrisone 2881

Clozapine (Studies have shown that terbinafine is an inhibitor of the CYP450 2D6 isozyme. Co-administration of terbinafine hydrochloride oral granules should be done with careful monitoring and may require a reduction in dose of the 2D6-metabolized drug).
No products indexed under this heading.

Codeine Phosphate (Studies have shown that terbinafine is an inhibitor of the CYP450 2D6 isozyme. Co-administration of terbinafine hydrochloride oral granules should be done with careful monitoring and may require a reduction in dose of the 2D6-metabolized drug). Products include:
Tylenol with Codeine Tablets 2427

Codeine Sulfate (Studies have shown that terbinafine is an inhibitor of the CYP450 2D6 isozyme. Co-administration of terbinafine hydrochloride oral granules should be done with careful monitoring and may require a reduction in dose of the 2D6-metabolized drug).
No products indexed under this heading.

Cyclobenzaprine Hydrochloride (Studies have shown that terbinafine is an inhibitor of the CYP450 2D6 isozyme. Co-administration of terbinafine hydrochloride oral granules should be done with careful monitoring and may require a reduction in dose of the 2D6-metabolized drug).
Products include:
Amrix Capsules 966

Cyclosporine (Terbinafine increases the clearance of cyclosporine by 15%; terbinafine clearance is unaffected by cyclosporine).
Products include:
Gengraf Capsules 435
Neoral Oral Solution 2280
Neoral Soft Gelatin Capsules 2280
Restasis Ophthalmic Emulsion 557
Sandimmune 2296

Dalfopristin (It is likely that inhibitors of both CYP2C9 and CYP3A4 may lead to substantial increase in the systemic exposure (Cmax and AUC) of terbinafine).
No products indexed under this heading.

Danazol (It is likely that inhibitors of both CYP2C9 and CYP3A4 may lead to substantial increase in the systemic exposure (Cmax and AUC) of terbinafine).
No products indexed under this heading.

Delavirdine Mesylate (It is likely that inhibitors of both CYP2C9 and CYP3A4 may lead to substantial increase in the systemic exposure (Cmax and AUC) of terbinafine).
No products indexed under this heading.

Desipramine Hydrochloride (In a study to assess the effects of terbinafine on desipramine in healthy volunteers characterized as normal metabolizers, the administration of terbinafine resulted in a 2-fold increase in Cmax and a 5-fold increase in AUC. In this study, these effects were shown to persist at the last observation at 4 weeks after discontinuation of terbinafine).
No products indexed under this heading.

Dexfenfluramine Hydrochloride (Studies have shown that terbinafine is an inhibitor of the CYP450 2D6 isozyme. Co-administration of terbinafine hydrochloride oral granules should be done with careful monitoring and may require a reduction in dose of the 2D6-metabolized drug).
No products indexed under this heading.

Dextromethorphan (In studies in healthy subjects characterized as extensive metabolizers of dextromethorphan, terbinafine increases the dextromethorphan/dextrorphan metabolite ratio in urine by 16- to 97-fold, on average).
No products indexed under this heading.

Dextromethorphan Hydrobromide (In studies in healthy subjects characterized as extensive metabolizers of dextromethorphan, terbinafine increases the dextromethorphan/dextrorphan metabolite ratio in urine by 16- to 97-fold, on average). Products include:
PediaCare Children's Liquid Multi-Symptom Cold 1902
PediaCare Children's Long-Acting Cough 1902
Children's Sudafed PE Cold & Cough Liquid 1907
Sudafed PE Cold & Cough Caplets 1907
Children's Tylenol Plus Cough & Runny Nose Suspension Liquid 1912
Children's Tylenol Plus Cough & Sore Throat Suspension Liquid 1912
Children's Tylenol Plus Flu Suspension Liquid 1914
Children's Tylenol Plus Multi-Symptom Cold Suspension Liquid 1912
Tylenol Cold Severe Congestion Daytime Caplets with Cool Burst 1912
Tylenol Cold Head Congestion Daytime Caplets with Cool Burst 1910
Tylenol Cold Head Congestion Nighttime Caplets with Cool Burst 1910
Tylenol Cold Head Congestion Severe Daytime Caplets with Cool Burst 1910
Tylenol Cold Multi-Symptom Daytime Caplets with Cool Burst and Rapid Release Gels 1913
Tylenol Cold Multi-Symptom Daytime Liquid with Citrus Burst ... 1913
Tylenol Cold Multi-Symptom Nighttime Caplets with Cool Burst 1913
Tylenol Cold Multi-Symptom Nighttime Liquid with Cool Burst ... 1913
Tylenol Cold Multi-Symptom Severe Caplets with Cool Burst 1913
Tylenol Cold Multi-Symptom Severe Daytime Liquid with Citrus Burst 1913
Tylenol Cough & Sore Throat Daytime Liquid with Cool Burst 1918
Tylenol Cough & Sore Throat Nighttime Liquid with Cool Burst ... 1918
Vicks DayQuil Cold & Flu Multi-Symptom Relief .... ■616
Vicks DayQuil LiquiCaps 2567
Vicks DayQuil Liquid 2567
Vicks DayQuil Multi-Symptom Cold/Flu Relief 2567
Vicks NyQuil Cold & Flu Multi-Symptom Relief .... ■617
Vicks NyQuil LiquiCaps 2567
Vicks NyQuil Liquid 2567
Vicks NyQuil Multi-Symptom Cold/Flu Relief 2567

Dextromethorphan Polistirex (In studies in healthy subjects characterized as extensive metabolizers of dextromethorphan, terbinafine increases the dextromethorphan/ dextrorphan metabolite ratio in urine by 16- to 97-fold, on average).
No products indexed under this heading.

Dextromethorphan tannate (In studies in healthy subjects characterized as extensive metabolizers of dextromethorphan, terbinafine increases the dextromethorphan/ dextrorphan metabolite ratio in urine by 16- to 97-fold, on average).
No products indexed under this heading.

Diclofenac Potassium (It is likely that inhibitors of both CYP2C9 and CYP3A4 may lead to substantial increase in the systemic exposure (Cmax and AUC) of terbinafine).
No products indexed under this heading.

Diclofenac Sodium (It is likely that inhibitors of both CYP2C9 and CYP3A4 may lead to substantial increase in the systemic exposure (Cmax and AUC) of terbinafine). Products include:
Diclofenac Sodium Ophthalmic Solution.......... ⊙ 240
Voltaren Ophthalmic Solution 2336
Voltaren Tablets 2334
Voltaren-XR Tablets 2337

Diltiazem Hydrochloride (It is likely that inhibitors of both CYP2C9 and CYP3A4 may lead to substantial increase in the systemic exposure (Cmax and AUC) of terbinafine). Products include:
Cardizem LA Extended Release Tablets 421

Diltiazem Maleate (It is likely that inhibitors of both CYP2C9 and CYP3A4 may lead to substantial increase in the systemic exposure (Cmax and AUC) of terbinafine).
No products indexed under this heading.

Disulfiram (It is likely that inhibitors of both CYP2C9 and CYP3A4 may lead to substantial increase in the systemic exposure (Cmax and AUC) of terbinafine).
No products indexed under this heading.

Dolasetron Mesylate (Studies have shown that terbinafine is an inhibitor of the CYP450 2D6 isozyme. Co-administration of terbinafine hydrochloride oral granules should be done with careful monitoring and may require a reduction in dose of the 2D6-metabolized drug). Products include:
Anzemet Injection 2701
Anzemet Tablets 2704

Donepezil Hydrochloride (Studies have shown that terbinafine is an inhibitor of the CYP450 2D6 isozyme. Co-administration of terbinafine hydrochloride oral granules should be done with careful monitoring and may require a reduction in dose of the 2D6-metabolized drug). Products include:
Aricept Tablets 1062
Aricept ODT Tablets 1062

Doxepin Hydrochloride (Studies have shown that terbinafine is an inhibitor of the CYP450 2D6 isozyme. Co-administration of terbinafine hydrochloride oral granules should be done with careful monitoring and may require a reduction in dose of the 2D6-metabolized drug).
No products indexed under this heading.

Efavirenz (It is likely that inhibitors of both CYP2C9 and CYP3A4 may lead to substantial increase in the systemic exposure (Cmax and AUC) of terbinafine). Products include:
Atripla Tablets 938
Sustiva Capsules 930
Sustiva Tablets 930

Encainide Hydrochloride (Studies have shown that terbinafine is an inhibitor of the CYP450 2D6 isozyme. Co-administration of terbinafine hydrochloride oral granules should be done with careful monitoring and may require a reduction in dose of the 2D6-metabolized drug).
No products indexed under this heading.

Erythromycin (It is likely that inhibitors of both CYP2C9 and CYP3A4 may lead to substantial increase in the systemic exposure (Cmax and AUC) of terbinafine).
No products indexed under this heading.

Erythromycin Estolate (It is likely that inhibitors of both CYP2C9 and CYP3A4 may lead to substantial increase in the systemic exposure (Cmax and AUC) of terbinafine).
No products indexed under this heading.

Erythromycin Ethylsuccinate (It is likely that inhibitors of both CYP2C9 and CYP3A4 may lead to substantial increase in the systemic exposure (Cmax and AUC) of terbinafine). Products include:
E.E.S. 433
EryPed 431

Erythromycin Gluceptate (It is likely that inhibitors of both CYP2C9 and CYP3A4 may lead to substantial increase in the systemic exposure (Cmax and AUC) of terbinafine).
No products indexed under this heading.

Erythromycin Lactobionate (It is likely that inhibitors of both CYP2C9 and CYP3A4 may lead to substantial increase in the systemic exposure (Cmax and AUC) of terbinafine).
No products indexed under this heading.

Erythromycin Stearate (It is likely that inhibitors of both CYP2C9 and CYP3A4 may lead to substantial increase in the systemic exposure (Cmax and AUC) of terbinafine).
No products indexed under this heading.

Escitalopram Oxalate (Studies have shown that terbinafine is an inhibitor of the CYP450 2D6 isozyme. Co-administration of terbinafine hydrochloride oral granules should be done with careful monitoring and may require a reduction in dose of the 2D6-metabolized drug). Products include:
Lexapro Oral Suspension 1174
Lexapro Tablets 1174

Esomeprazole Magnesium (It is likely that inhibitors of both CYP2C9 and CYP3A4 may lead to substantial increase in the systemic exposure (Cmax and AUC) of terbinafine). Products include:
Nexium Delayed-Release Capsules 645
Nexium Delayed-Release Oral Suspension 645

Fenofibrate (It is likely that inhibitors of both CYP2C9 and CYP3A4 may lead to substantial increase in the systemic exposure (Cmax and AUC) of terbinafine). Products include:
Fenoglide Tablets 2960
Tricor Tablets 520

Fentanyl (Studies have shown that terbinafine is an inhibitor of the CYP450 2D6 isozyme. Co-administration of terbinafine hydrochloride oral granules should be done with careful monitoring and may require a reduction in dose of the 2D6-metabolized drug). Products include:
Duragesic Transdermal System 2405
Ionsys Transdermal System 2410

Fentanyl Citrate (Studies have shown that terbinafine is an inhibitor of the CYP450 2D6 isozyme. Co-administration of terbinafine hydrochloride oral granules should be done with careful monitoring and may require a reduction in dose of the 2D6-metabolized drug). Products include:
Actiq 959
Fentora Tablets 968

Flecainide Acetate (Studies have shown that terbinafine is an inhibitor of the CYP450 2D6 isozyme. Co-administration of terbinafine hydrochloride oral granules should be done with careful monitoring and may require a reduction in dose of the 2D6-metabolized drug).
No products indexed under this heading.

Fluconazole (Fluconazole is an inhibitor of CYP2C9 and CYP3A enzymes. Co-administration of a single dose of fluconazole (100 mg) with a single dose of terbinafine resulted in a 52% and 69% increase in terbinafine Cmax and AUC, respectively).
No products indexed under this heading.

Fluorouracil (It is likely that inhibitors of both CYP2C9 and CYP3A4 may lead to substantial increase in the systemic exposure (Cmax and AUC) of terbinafine). Products include:
Carac Cream 0.5% 2722

Fluoxetine (Studies have shown that terbinafine is an inhibitor of the CYP450 2D6 isozyme. Co-administration of terbinafine hydrochloride oral granules should be done with careful monitoring and may require a reduction in dose of the 2D6-metabolized drug).
No products indexed under this heading.

Fluoxetine Hydrochloride (Studies have shown that terbinafine is an inhibitor of the CYP450 2D6 isozyme. Co-administration of terbinafine hydrochloride oral granules should be done with careful monitoring and may require a reduction in dose of the 2D6-metabolized drug). Products include:
Prozac Weekly Capsules 1852
Prozac Pulvules and Liquid 1852
Symbyax Capsules 1871

Fluphenazine Decanoate (Studies have shown that terbinafine is an inhibitor of the CYP450 2D6 isozyme. Co-administration of terbinafine hydrochloride oral granules should be done with careful monitoring and may require a reduction in dose of the 2D6-metabolized drug).
No products indexed under this heading.

Fluphenazine Enanthate (Studies have shown that terbinafine is an inhibitor of the CYP450 2D6 isozyme. Co-administration of terbinafine hydrochloride oral granules should be done with careful monitoring and may require a reduction in dose of the 2D6-metabolized drug).
No products indexed under this heading.

Fluphenazine Hydrochloride (Studies have shown that terbinafine is an inhibitor of the CYP450 2D6 isozyme. Co-administration of terbinafine hydrochloride oral granules should be done with careful monitoring and may require a reduction in dose of the 2D6-metabolized drug).
No products indexed under this heading.

Flurbiprofen (It is likely that inhibitors of both CYP2C9 and CYP3A4 may lead to substantial increase in the systemic exposure (Cmax and AUC) of terbinafine).
No products indexed under this heading.

Flurbiprofen Sodium (It is likely that inhibitors of both CYP2C9 and CYP3A4 may lead to substantial increase in the systemic exposure (Cmax and AUC) of terbinafine).
No products indexed under this heading.

Fluvastatin Sodium (It is likely that inhibitors of both CYP2C9 and CYP3A4 may lead to substantial increase in the systemic exposure (Cmax and AUC) of terbinafine). Products include:
Lescol Capsules 2268
Lescol XL Tablets 2268

Fluvoxamine Maleate (Studies have shown that terbinafine is an inhibitor of the CYP450 2D6 isozyme. Co-administration of terbinafine hydrochloride oral granules should be done with careful monitoring and may require a reduction in dose of the 2D6-metabolized drug). Products include:
Luvox CR Extended-Release Capsules 1759

Formoterol Fumarate (Studies have shown that terbinafine is an inhibitor of the CYP450 2D6 isozyme. Co-administration of terbinafine hydrochloride oral granules should be done with careful monitoring and may require a reduction in dose of the 2D6-metabolized drug). Products include:
Foradil Aerolizer 2849
Perforomist Inhalation Solution 1025

Fosamprenavir Calcium (It is likely that inhibitors of both CYP2C9 and CYP3A4 may lead to substantial increase in the systemic exposure (Cmax and AUC) of terbinafine). Products include:
Lexiva Oral Suspension 1510
Lexiva Tablets 1510

Galantamine Hydrobromide (Studies have shown that terbinafine is an inhibitor of the CYP450 2D6 isozyme. Co-administration of terbinafine hydrochloride oral granules should be done with careful monitoring and may require a reduction in dose of the 2D6-metabolized drug).
No products indexed under this heading.

Gemfibrozil (It is likely that inhibitors of both CYP2C9 and CYP3A4 may lead to substantial increase in the systemic exposure (Cmax and AUC) of terbinafine).
No products indexed under this heading.

Glipizide (It is likely that inhibitors of both CYP2C9 and CYP3A4 may lead to substantial increase in the systemic exposure (Cmax and AUC) of terbinafine).
No products indexed under this heading.

Glyburide (It is likely that inhibitors of both CYP2C9 and CYP3A4 may lead to substantial increase in the systemic exposure (Cmax and AUC) of terbinafine).
No products indexed under this heading.

Haloperidol (Studies have shown that terbinafine is an inhibitor of the CYP450 2D6 isozyme. Co-administration of terbinafine hydrochloride oral granules should be done with careful monitoring and may require a reduction in dose of the 2D6-metabolized drug).
No products indexed under this heading.

Haloperidol Decanoate (Studies have shown that terbinafine is an inhibitor of the CYP450 2D6 isozyme. Co-administration of terbinafine hydrochloride oral granules should be done with careful monitoring and may require a reduction in dose of the 2D6-metabolized drug).
No products indexed under this heading.

Hydrochlorothiazide (It is likely that inhibitors of both CYP2C9 and CYP3A4 may lead to substantial increase in the systemic exposure (Cmax and AUC) of terbinafine).
Products include:
Atacand HCT 642
Avalide Tablets 892
Avalide Tablets 2713
Benicar HCT Tablets 1010
Diovan HCT Tablets 2216
Dyazide Capsules 1405
Micardis HCT Tablets 854
Prinzide Tablets 2092
Tekturna HCT Tablets 2324
Teveten HCT Tablets 517

Hydrocodone Bitartrate (Studies have shown that terbinafine is an inhibitor of the CYP450 2D6 isozyme. Co-administration of terbinafine hydrochloride oral granules should be done with careful monitoring and may require a reduction in dose of the 2D6-metabolized drug).
Products include:
Lortab 5/500 Tablets 3143
Lortab 7.5/500 Tablets 3144
Lortab 10/500 Tablets 3144
Vicodin Tablets 529
Vicodin ES Tablets 530
Vicodin HP Tablets 531
Vicoprofen Tablets 533
Zydone Tablets 1132

Hydroflumethiazide (It is likely that inhibitors of both CYP2C9 and CYP3A4 may lead to substantial increase in the systemic exposure (Cmax and AUC) of terbinafine).
No products indexed under this heading.

Imatinib Mesylate (It is likely that inhibitors of both CYP2C9 and CYP3A4 may lead to substantial increase in the systemic exposure (Cmax and AUC) of terbinafine).
Products include:
Gleevec Tablets 2255

Imipramine Hydrochloride (Studies have shown that terbinafine is an inhibitor of the CYP450 2D6 isozyme. Co-administration of terbinafine hydrochloride oral granules should be done with careful monitoring and may require a reduction in dose of the 2D6-metabolized drug).
No products indexed under this heading.

Imipramine Pamoate (Studies have shown that terbinafine is an inhibitor of the CYP450 2D6 isozyme. Co-administration of terbinafine hydrochloride oral granules should be done with careful monitoring and may require a reduction in dose of the 2D6-metabolized drug).
No products indexed under this heading.

Indinavir Sulfate (It is likely that inhibitors of both CYP2C9 and CYP3A4 may lead to substantial increase in the systemic exposure (Cmax and AUC) of terbinafine).
Products include:
Crixivan Capsules 1979

Indoramin Hydrochloride (Studies have shown that terbinafine is an inhibitor of the CYP450 2D6 isozyme. Co-administration of terbinafine hydrochloride oral granules should be done with careful monitoring and may require a reduction in dose of the 2D6-metabolized drug).
No products indexed under this heading.

Isocarboxazid (Studies have shown that terbinafine is an inhibitor of the CYP450 2D6 isozyme. Co-administration of terbinafine hydrochloride oral granules should be done with careful monitoring and may require a reduction in dose of the 2D6-metabolized drug). Products include:
Marplan Tablets 3177

Isoniazid (It is likely that inhibitors of both CYP2C9 and CYP3A4 may lead to substantial increase in the systemic exposure (Cmax and AUC) of terbinafine).
No products indexed under this heading.

Itraconazole (It is likely that inhibitors of both CYP2C9 and CYP3A4 may lead to substantial increase in the systemic exposure (Cmax and AUC) of terbinafine).
No products indexed under this heading.

Ketoconazole (Concurrent use with ketoconazole, an inhibitor of both CYP2C9 and CYP3A4 may lead to a substantial increase in the systemic exposure (Cmax and AUC) of terbinafine). Products include:
Extina Foam, 2% 3057
Nizoral A-D Shampoo 1901

Ketoprofen (It is likely that inhibitors of both CYP2C9 and CYP3A4 may lead to substantial increase in the systemic exposure (Cmax and AUC) of terbinafine).
No products indexed under this heading.

Labetalol Hydrochloride (Studies have shown that terbinafine is an inhibitor of the CYP450 2D6 isozyme. Co-administration of terbinafine hydrochloride oral granules should be done with careful monitoring and may require a reduction in dose of the 2D6-metabolized drug).
No products indexed under this heading.

Leflunomide (It is likely that inhibitors of both CYP2C9 and CYP3A4 may lead to substantial increase in the systemic exposure (Cmax and AUC) of terbinafine).
No products indexed under this heading.

Lidocaine (Studies have shown that terbinafine is an inhibitor of the CYP450 2D6 isozyme. Co-administration of terbinafine hydrochloride oral granules should be done with careful monitoring and may require a reduction in dose of the 2D6-metabolized drug). Products include:
Lidoderm Patch 1114

Lidocaine Hydrochloride (Studies have shown that terbinafine is an inhibitor of the CYP450 2D6 isozyme. Co-administration of terbinafine hydrochloride oral granules should be done with careful monitoring and may require a reduction in dose of the 2D6-metabolized drug).
No products indexed under this heading.

Lopinavir (It is likely that inhibitors of both CYP2C9 and CYP3A4 may lead to substantial increase in the systemic exposure (Cmax and AUC) of terbinafine). Products include:
Kaletra 452

Loratadine (It is likely that inhibitors of both CYP2C9 and CYP3A4 may lead to substantial increase in the systemic exposure (Cmax and AUC) of terbinafine).
No products indexed under this heading.

Lovastatin (It is likely that inhibitors of both CYP2C9 and CYP3A4 may lead to substantial increase in the systemic exposure (Cmax and AUC) of terbinafine). Products include:
Advicor Tablets 402
Mevacor Tablets 2063

Maprotiline Hydrochloride (Studies have shown that terbinafine is an inhibitor of the CYP450 2D6 isozyme. Co-administration of terbinafine hydrochloride oral granules should be done with careful monitoring and may require a reduction in dose of the 2D6-metabolized drug).
No products indexed under this heading.

Meperidine Hydrochloride (Studies have shown that terbinafine is an inhibitor of the CYP450 2D6 isozyme. Co-administration of terbinafine hydrochloride oral granules should be done with careful monitoring and may require a reduction in dose of the 2D6-metabolized drug).
No products indexed under this heading.

Methadone Hydrochloride (Studies have shown that terbinafine is an inhibitor of the CYP450 2D6 isozyme. Co-administration of terbinafine hydrochloride oral granules should be done with careful monitoring and may require a reduction in dose of the 2D6-metabolized drug).
No products indexed under this heading.

Methamphetamine Hydrochloride (Studies have shown that terbinafine is an inhibitor of the CYP450 2D6 isozyme. Co-administration of terbinafine hydrochloride oral granules should be done with careful monitoring and may require a reduction in dose of the 2D6-metabolized drug).
No products indexed under this heading.

Methyclothiazide (It is likely that inhibitors of both CYP2C9 and CYP3A4 may lead to substantial increase in the systemic exposure (Cmax and AUC) of terbinafine).
No products indexed under this heading.

Metoprolol Succinate (Studies have shown that terbinafine is an inhibitor of the CYP450 2D6 isozyme. Co-administration of terbinafine hydrochloride oral granules should be done with careful monitoring and may require a reduction in dose of the 2D6-metabolized drug).
Products include:
Toprol-XL Tablets 666

Metoprolol Tartrate (Studies have shown that terbinafine is an inhibitor of the CYP450 2D6 isozyme. Co-administration of terbinafine hydrochloride oral granules should be done with careful monitoring and may require a reduction in dose of the 2D6-metabolized drug).
No products indexed under this heading.

Metronidazole (It is likely that inhibitors of both CYP2C9 and CYP3A4 may lead to substantial increase in the systemic exposure (Cmax and AUC) of terbinafine).
Products include:
Pylera Capsules 714

Metronidazole Benzoate (It is likely that inhibitors of both CYP2C9 and CYP3A4 may lead to substantial increase in the systemic exposure (Cmax and AUC) of terbinafine).
No products indexed under this heading.

Metronidazole Hydrochloride (It is likely that inhibitors of both CYP2C9 and CYP3A4 may lead to substantial increase in the systemic exposure (Cmax and AUC) of terbinafine).
No products indexed under this heading.

Metronidazole Sodium (It is likely that inhibitors of both CYP2C9 and CYP3A4 may lead to substantial increase in the systemic exposure (Cmax and AUC) of terbinafine).
No products indexed under this heading.

Mexiletine Hydrochloride (Studies have shown that terbinafine is an inhibitor of the CYP450 2D6 isozyme. Co-administration of terbinafine hydrochloride oral granules should be done with careful monitoring and may require a reduction in dose of the 2D6-metabolized drug).
No products indexed under this heading.

Miconazole (It is likely that inhibitors of both CYP2C9 and CYP3A4 may lead to substantial increase in the systemic exposure (Cmax and AUC) of terbinafine).
No products indexed under this heading.

Miconazole Nitrate (It is likely that inhibitors of both CYP2C9 and CYP3A4 may lead to substantial increase in the systemic exposure (Cmax and AUC) of terbinafine).
No products indexed under this heading.

Mirtazapine (Studies have shown that terbinafine is an inhibitor of the CYP450 2D6 isozyme. Co-administration of terbinafine hydrochloride oral granules should be done with careful monitoring and may require a reduction in dose of the 2D6-metabolized drug). Products include:
Remeron Tablets 2924
RemeronSolTab Tablets 2927

Moclobemide (Studies have shown that terbinafine is an inhibitor of the CYP450 2D6 isozyme. Co-administration of terbinafine hydrochloride oral granules should be done with careful monitoring and may require a reduction in dose of the 2D6-metabolized drug).
No products indexed under this heading.

Modafinil (It is likely that inhibitors of both CYP2C9 and CYP3A4 may lead to substantial increase in the systemic exposure (Cmax and AUC) of terbinafine). Products include:
Provigil Tablets 977

Morphine Sulfate (Studies have shown that terbinafine is an inhibitor of the CYP450 2D6 isozyme. Co-administration of terbinafine hydrochloride oral granules should be done with careful monitoring and may require a reduction in dose of the 2D6-metabolized drug). Products include:
Avinza Capsules 1772
DepoDur Injection 1095
MS Contin Tablets 2585

Nefazodone Hydrochloride (It is likely that inhibitors of both CYP2C9 and CYP3A4 may lead to substantial increase in the systemic exposure (Cmax and AUC) of terbinafine).
No products indexed under this heading.

Nelfinavir Mesylate (Studies have shown that terbinafine is an inhibitor of the CYP450 2D6 isozyme. Co-administration of terbinafine hydrochloride oral granules should be done with careful monitoring and may require a reduction in dose of the 2D6-metabolized drug).
No products indexed under this heading.

Nevirapine (It is likely that inhibitors of both CYP2C9 and CYP3A4 may lead to substantial increase in the systemic exposure (Cmax and AUC) of terbinafine). Products include:
Viramune Oral Suspension 873
Viramune Tablets 873

Niacinamide (It is likely that inhibitors of both CYP2C9 and CYP3A4 may lead to substantial increase in the systemic exposure (Cmax and AUC) of terbinafine). Products include:
BioLean Free Tablets 635

Nicotinamide (It is likely that inhibitors of both CYP2C9 and CYP3A4 may lead to substantial increase in the systemic exposure (Cmax and AUC) of terbinafine).
No products indexed under this heading.

Nifedipine (It is likely that inhibitors of both CYP2C9 and CYP3A4 may lead to substantial increase in the systemic exposure (Cmax and AUC) of terbinafine).
No products indexed under this heading.

Norfloxacin (It is likely that inhibitors of both CYP2C9 and CYP3A4 may lead to substantial increase in the systemic exposure (Cmax and AUC) of terbinafine). Products include:
Noroxin Tablets 2069

Nortriptyline Hydrochloride (Studies have shown that terbinafine is an inhibitor of the CYP450 2D6 isozyme. Co-administration of terbinafine hydrochloride oral granules should be done with careful monitoring and may require a reduction in dose of the 2D6-metabolized drug).
No products indexed under this heading.

Olanzapine (Studies have shown that terbinafine is an inhibitor of the CYP450 2D6 isozyme. Co-administration of terbinafine hydrochloride oral granules should be done with careful monitoring and may require a reduction in dose of the 2D6-metabolized drug). Products include:
Symbyax Capsules 1871
Zyprexa Tablets 1883
Zyprexa IntraMuscular 1883
Zyprexa ZYDIS Orally Disintegrating Tablets 1883

Omeprazole (Studies have shown that terbinafine is an inhibitor of the CYP450 2D6 isozyme. Co-administration of terbinafine hydrochloride oral granules should be done with careful monitoring and may require a reduction in dose of the 2D6-metabolized drug).
No products indexed under this heading.

Ondansetron (Studies have shown that terbinafine is an inhibitor of the CYP450 2D6 isozyme. Co-administration of terbinafine hydrochloride oral granules should be done with careful monitoring and may require a reduction in dose of the 2D6-metabolized drug). Products include:
Zofran ODT Orally Disintegrating Tablets 1687

Ondansetron Hydrochloride (Studies have shown that terbinafine is an inhibitor of the CYP450 2D6 isozyme. Co-administration of terbinafine hydrochloride oral granules should be done with careful monitoring and may require a reduction in dose of the 2D6-metabolized drug). Products include:
Zofran Injection 1682
Zofran 1687

Oxiconazole Nitrate (It is likely that inhibitors of both CYP2C9 and CYP3A4 may lead to substantial increase in the systemic exposure (Cmax and AUC) of terbinafine).
No products indexed under this heading.

Oxycodone Hydrochloride (Studies have shown that terbinafine is an inhibitor of the CYP450 2D6 isozyme. Co-administration of terbinafine hydrochloride oral granules should be done with careful monitoring and may require a reduction in dose of the 2D6-metabolized drug). Products include:
OxyContin Tablets 2589
OxyIR Capsules 2593
Percocet Tablets 1127
Percodan Tablets 1130

Paclitaxel (Studies have shown that terbinafine is an inhibitor of the CYP450 2D6 isozyme. Co-administration of terbinafine hydrochloride oral granules should be done with careful monitoring and may require a reduction in dose of the 2D6-metabolized drug).
No products indexed under this heading.

Pargyline Hydrochloride (Studies have shown that terbinafine is an inhibitor of the CYP450 2D6 isozyme. Co-administration of terbinafine hydrochloride oral granules should be done with careful monitoring and may require a reduction in dose of the 2D6-metabolized drug).
No products indexed under this heading.

Paroxetine Hydrochloride (Studies have shown that terbinafine is an inhibitor of the CYP450 2D6 isozyme. Co-administration of terbinafine hydrochloride oral granules should be done with careful monitoring and may require a reduction in dose of the 2D6-metabolized drug). Products include:
Paxil 1535
Paxil CR Controlled-Release Tablets 1544

Phenelzine Sulfate (Studies have shown that terbinafine is an inhibitor of the CYP450 2D6 isozyme. Co-administration of terbinafine hydrochloride oral granules should be done with careful monitoring and may require a reduction in dose of the 2D6-metabolized drug).
No products indexed under this heading.

Phenylbutazone (It is likely that inhibitors of both CYP2C9 and CYP3A4 may lead to substantial increase in the systemic exposure (Cmax and AUC) of terbinafine).
No products indexed under this heading.

Pindolol (Studies have shown that terbinafine is an inhibitor of the CYP450 2D6 isozyme. Co-administration of terbinafine hydrochloride oral granules should be done with careful monitoring and may require a reduction in dose of the 2D6-metabolized drug).
No products indexed under this heading.

Polythiazide (It is likely that inhibitors of both CYP2C9 and CYP3A4 may lead to substantial increase in the systemic exposure (Cmax and AUC) of terbinafine).
No products indexed under this heading.

Procarbazine Hydrochloride (Studies have shown that terbinafine is an inhibitor of the CYP450 2D6 isozyme. Co-administration of terbinafine hydrochloride oral granules should be done with careful monitoring and may require a reduction in dose of the 2D6-metabolized drug).
No products indexed under this heading.

Propafenone Hydrochloride (Studies have shown that terbinafine is an inhibitor of the CYP450 2D6 isozyme. Co-administration of terbinafine hydrochloride oral granules should be done with careful monitoring and may require a reduction in dose of the 2D6-metabolized drug). Products include:
Rythmol Tablets 1586
Rythmol SR Capsules 1590

Propoxyphene Hydrochloride (Studies have shown that terbinafine is an inhibitor of the CYP450 2D6 isozyme. Co-administration of terbinafine hydrochloride oral granules should be done with careful monitoring and may require a reduction in dose of the 2D6-metabolized drug).
No products indexed under this heading.

Propoxyphene Napsylate (Studies have shown that terbinafine is an inhibitor of the CYP450 2D6 isozyme. Co-administration of terbinafine hydrochloride oral granules should be done with careful monitoring and may require a reduction in dose of the 2D6-metabolized drug).
No products indexed under this heading.

Propranolol Hydrochloride (Studies have shown that terbinafine is an inhibitor of the CYP450 2D6 isozyme. Co-administration of terbinafine hydrochloride oral granules should be done with careful monitoring and may require a reduction in dose of the 2D6-metabolized drug). Products include:
InnoPran XL Extended Release Capsules 1484

Protriptyline Hydrochloride (Studies have shown that terbinafine is an inhibitor of the CYP450 2D6 isozyme. Co-administration of terbinafine hydrochloride oral granules should be done with careful monitoring and may require a reduction in dose of the 2D6-metabolized drug).
No products indexed under this heading.

Quetiapine Fumarate (Studies have shown that terbinafine is an inhibitor of the CYP450 2D6 isozyme. Co-administration of terbinafine hydrochloride oral granules should be done with careful monitoring and may require a reduction in dose of the 2D6-metabolized drug).
No products indexed under this heading.

Quinidine (It is likely that inhibitors of both CYP2C9 and CYP3A4 may lead to substantial increase in the systemic exposure (Cmax and AUC) of terbinafine).
No products indexed under this heading.

Quinidine Gluconate (Studies have shown that terbinafine is an inhibitor of the CYP450 2D6 isozyme. Co-administration of terbinafine hydrochloride oral granules should be done with careful monitoring and may require a reduction in dose of the 2D6-metabolized drug).
No products indexed under this heading.

Quinidine Hydrochloride (Studies have shown that terbinafine is an inhibitor of the CYP450 2D6 isozyme. Co-administration of terbinafine hydrochloride oral granules should be done with careful monitoring and may require a reduction in dose of the 2D6-metabolized drug).
No products indexed under this heading.

Quinidine Polygalacturonate (Studies have shown that terbinafine is an inhibitor of the CYP450 2D6 isozyme. Co-administration of terbinafine hydrochloride oral granules should be done with careful monitoring and may require a reduction in dose of the 2D6-metabolized drug).
No products indexed under this heading.

Quinidine Sulfate (Studies have shown that terbinafine is an inhibitor of the CYP450 2D6 isozyme. Co-administration of terbinafine hydrochloride oral granules should be done with careful monitoring and may require a reduction in dose of the 2D6-metabolized drug).
No products indexed under this heading.

Quinine (It is likely that inhibitors of both CYP2C9 and CYP3A4 may lead to substantial increase in the systemic exposure (Cmax and AUC) of terbinafine).
No products indexed under this heading.

Quinine Sulfate (It is likely that inhibitors of both CYP2C9 and CYP3A4 may lead to substantial increase in the systemic exposure (Cmax and AUC) of terbinafine).
No products indexed under this heading.

Quinupristin (It is likely that inhibitors of both CYP2C9 and CYP3A4 may lead to substantial increase in the systemic exposure (Cmax and AUC) of terbinafine).
No products indexed under this heading.

Ranitidine Bismuth Citrate (It is likely that inhibitors of both CYP2C9 and CYP3A4 may lead to substantial increase in the systemic exposure (Cmax and AUC) of terbinafine).
No products indexed under this heading.

Ranitidine Hydrochloride (It is likely that inhibitors of both CYP2C9 and CYP3A4 may lead to substantial increase in the systemic exposure (Cmax and AUC) of terbinafine). Products include:
Zantac 75 Tablets .... ▣603
Zantac 1670
Zantac Injection 1666
Zantac Injection Pharmacy Bulk Package 1668
Maximum Strength Zantac 150 Tablets .... ▣603
Maximum Strength Zantac 150 Cool Mint Tablets .... ▣603

Rasagiline Mesylate (Studies have shown that terbinafine is an inhibitor of the CYP450 2D6 isozyme. Co-administration of terbinafine hydrochloride oral granules should be done with careful monitoring and may require a reduction in dose of the 2D6-metabolized drug). Products include:
Azilect Tablets 3106

Rifampin (Terbinafine clearance is increased 100% by rifampin, a CYP450 enzyme inducer).
No products indexed under this heading.

Risperidone (Studies have shown that terbinafine is an inhibitor of the CYP450 2D6 isozyme. Co-administration of terbinafine hydrochloride oral granules should be done with careful monitoring and may require a reduction in dose of the 2D6-metabolized drug). Products include:
Risperdal Consta Long-Acting Injection 1753

Ritonavir (Studies have shown that terbinafine is an inhibitor of the CYP450 2D6 isozyme. Co-administration of terbinafine hydrochloride oral granules should be done with careful monitoring and may require a reduction in dose of the 2D6-metabolized drug). Products include:
Kaletra 452
Norvir 489

Saquinavir (It is likely that inhibitors of both CYP2C9 and CYP3A4 may lead to substantial increase in the systemic exposure (Cmax and AUC) of terbinafine).
No products indexed under this heading.

Saquinavir Mesylate (It is likely that inhibitors of both CYP2C9 and CYP3A4 may lead to substantial increase in the systemic exposure (Cmax and AUC) of terbinafine).
No products indexed under this heading.

Selegiline (Studies have shown that terbinafine is an inhibitor of the CYP450 2D6 isozyme. Co-administration of terbinafine hydrochloride oral granules should be done with careful monitoring and may require a reduction in dose of the 2D6-metabolized drug). Products include:
Emsam Transdermal System 905

Selegiline Hydrochloride (Studies have shown that terbinafine is an inhibitor of the CYP450 2D6 isozyme. Co-administration of terbinafine hydrochloride oral granules should be done with careful monitoring and may require a reduction in dose of the 2D6-metabolized drug). Products include:
Eldepryl Capsules 3052

Sertraline Hydrochloride (Studies have shown that terbinafine is an inhibitor of the CYP450 2D6 isozyme. Co-administration of terbinafine hydrochloride oral granules should be done with careful monitoring and may require a reduction in dose of the 2D6-metabolized drug).
No products indexed under this heading.

Sildenafil Citrate (It is likely that inhibitors of both CYP2C9 and CYP3A4 may lead to substantial increase in the systemic exposure (Cmax and AUC) of terbinafine).
No products indexed under this heading.

Sulfacytine (It is likely that inhibitors of both CYP2C9 and CYP3A4 may lead to substantial increase in the systemic exposure (Cmax and AUC) of terbinafine).
No products indexed under this heading.

Sulfamethizole (It is likely that inhibitors of both CYP2C9 and CYP3A4 may lead to substantial increase in the systemic exposure (Cmax and AUC) of terbinafine).
No products indexed under this heading.

Sulfamethoxazole (It is likely that inhibitors of both CYP2C9 and CYP3A4 may lead to substantial increase in the systemic exposure (Cmax and AUC) of terbinafine).
No products indexed under this heading.

Sulfasalazine (It is likely that inhibitors of both CYP2C9 and CYP3A4 may lead to substantial increase in the systemic exposure (Cmax and AUC) of terbinafine).
No products indexed under this heading.

Sulfinpyrazone (It is likely that inhibitors of both CYP2C9 and CYP3A4 may lead to substantial increase in the systemic exposure (Cmax and AUC) of terbinafine).
No products indexed under this heading.

Sulfisoxazole Acetyl (It is likely that inhibitors of both CYP2C9 and CYP3A4 may lead to substantial increase in the systemic exposure (Cmax and AUC) of terbinafine).
No products indexed under this heading.

Sulfisoxazole Diolamine (It is likely that inhibitors of both CYP2C9 and CYP3A4 may lead to substantial increase in the systemic exposure (Cmax and AUC) of terbinafine).
No products indexed under this heading.

Tamoxifen Citrate (Studies have shown that terbinafine is an inhibitor of the CYP450 2D6 isozyme. Co-administration of terbinafine hydrochloride oral granules should be done with careful monitoring and may require a reduction in dose of the 2D6-metabolized drug).
No products indexed under this heading.

Telithromycin (It is likely that inhibitors of both CYP2C9 and CYP3A4 may lead to substantial increase in the systemic exposure (Cmax and AUC) of terbinafine). Products include:
Ketek Tablets 2744

Teniposide (Studies have shown that terbinafine is an inhibitor of the CYP450 2D6 isozyme. Co-administration of terbinafine hydrochloride oral granules should be done with careful monitoring and may require a reduction in dose of the 2D6-metabolized drug).
No products indexed under this heading.

Terconazole (It is likely that inhibitors of both CYP2C9 and CYP3A4 may lead to substantial increase in the systemic exposure (Cmax and AUC) of terbinafine).
No products indexed under this heading.

Testosterone (Studies have shown that terbinafine is an inhibitor of the CYP450 2D6 isozyme. Co-administration of terbinafine hydrochloride oral granules should be done with careful monitoring and may require a reduction in dose of the 2D6-metabolized drug). Products include:
AndroGel 3159
Testim 1% Gel 701

Testosterone Cypionate (Studies have shown that terbinafine is an inhibitor of the CYP450 2D6 isozyme. Co-administration of terbinafine hydrochloride oral granules should be done with careful monitoring and may require a reduction in dose of the 2D6-metabolized drug).
No products indexed under this heading.

Testosterone Enanthate (Studies have shown that terbinafine is an inhibitor of the CYP450 2D6 isozyme. Co-administration of terbinafine hydrochloride oral granules should be done with careful monitoring and may require a reduction in dose of the 2D6-metabolized drug). Products include:
Delatestryl Injection 1730

Testosterone Propionate (Studies have shown that terbinafine is an inhibitor of the CYP450 2D6 isozyme. Co-administration of terbinafine hydrochloride oral granules should be done with careful monitoring and may require a reduction in dose of the 2D6-metabolized drug).
No products indexed under this heading.

Thioridazine (Studies have shown that terbinafine is an inhibitor of the CYP450 2D6 isozyme. Co-administration of terbinafine hydrochloride oral granules should be done with careful monitoring and may require a reduction in dose of the 2D6-metabolized drug).
No products indexed under this heading.

Thioridazine Hydrochloride (Studies have shown that terbinafine is an inhibitor of the CYP450 2D6 isozyme. Co-administration of terbinafine hydrochloride oral granules should be done with careful monitoring and may require a reduction in dose of the 2D6-metabolized drug). Products include:
Thioridazine Hydrochloride Tablets 2195

Ticlopidine Hydrochloride (It is likely that inhibitors of both CYP2C9 and CYP3A4 may lead to substantial increase in the systemic exposure (Cmax and AUC) of terbinafine).
No products indexed under this heading.

Timolol Maleate (Studies have shown that terbinafine is an inhibitor of the CYP450 2D6 isozyme. Co-administration of terbinafine hydrochloride oral granules should be done with careful monitoring and may require a reduction in dose of the 2D6-metabolized drug). Products include:
Combigan Ophthalmic Solution 553
Cosopt Sterile Ophthalmic Solution 1969
Timoptic Sterile Ophthalmic Solution 2121
Timoptic in Ocudose 2124
Timoptic-XE Sterile Ophthalmic Gel Forming Solution 2125

Tolazamide (It is likely that inhibitors of both CYP2C9 and CYP3A4 may lead to substantial increase in the systemic exposure (Cmax and AUC) of terbinafine).
No products indexed under this heading.

Tolbutamide (It is likely that inhibitors of both CYP2C9 and CYP3A4 may lead to substantial increase in the systemic exposure (Cmax and AUC) of terbinafine).
No products indexed under this heading.

Tolbutamide Sodium (It is likely that inhibitors of both CYP2C9 and CYP3A4 may lead to substantial increase in the systemic exposure (Cmax and AUC) of terbinafine).
No products indexed under this heading.

Tolterodine Tartrate (Studies have shown that terbinafine is an inhibitor of the CYP450 2D6 isozyme. Co-administration of terbinafine hydrochloride oral granules should be done with careful monitoring and may require a reduction in dose of the 2D6-metabolized drug).
No products indexed under this heading.

Tramadol Hydrochloride (Studies have shown that terbinafine is an inhibitor of the CYP450 2D6 isozyme. Co-administration of terbinafine hydrochloride oral granules should be done with careful monitoring and may require a reduction in dose of the 2D6-metabolized drug). Products include:
Ultram ER Extended-Release Tablets 2428

Tranylcypromine Sulfate (Studies have shown that terbinafine is an inhibitor of the CYP450 2D6 isozyme. Co-administration of terbinafine hydrochloride oral granules should be done with careful monitoring and may require a reduction in dose of the 2D6-metabolized drug). Products include:
Parnate Tablets 1532

Trazodone Hydrochloride (Studies have shown that terbinafine is an inhibitor of the CYP450 2D6 isozyme. Co-administration of terbinafine hydrochloride oral granules should be done with careful monitoring and may require a reduction in dose of the 2D6-metabolized drug).
No products indexed under this heading.

Triazolam (Studies have shown that terbinafine is an inhibitor of the CYP450 2D6 isozyme. Co-administration of terbinafine hydrochloride oral granules should be done with careful monitoring and may require a reduction in dose of the 2D6-metabolized drug).
No products indexed under this heading.

Trimipramine Maleate (Studies have shown that terbinafine is an inhibitor of the CYP450 2D6 isozyme. Co-administration of terbinafine hydrochloride oral granules should be done with careful monitoring and may require a reduction in dose of the 2D6-metabolized drug).
No products indexed under this heading.

Troglitazone (It is likely that inhibitors of both CYP2C9 and CYP3A4 may lead to substantial increase in the systemic exposure (Cmax and AUC) of terbinafine).
No products indexed under this heading.

Troleandomycin (It is likely that inhibitors of both CYP2C9 and CYP3A4 may lead to substantial increase in the systemic exposure (Cmax and AUC) of terbinafine).
No products indexed under this heading.

Valproate Sodium (It is likely that inhibitors of both CYP2C9 and CYP3A4 may lead to substantial increase in the systemic exposure (Cmax and AUC) of terbinafine).
No products indexed under this heading.

Vardenafil Hydrochloride (It is likely that inhibitors of both CYP2C9 and CYP3A4 may lead to substantial increase in the systemic exposure (Cmax and AUC) of terbinafine). Products include:
Levitra Tablets 2876

Venlafaxine Hydrochloride (Studies have shown that terbinafine is an inhibitor of the CYP450 2D6 isozyme. Co-administration of terbinafine hydrochloride oral granules should be done with careful monitoring and may require a reduction in dose of the 2D6-metabolized drug). Products include:
Effexor XR Extended-Release Capsules 3195
Venlafaxine Hydrochloride Tablets ... 2199

Verapamil Hydrochloride (It is likely that inhibitors of both CYP2C9 and CYP3A4 may lead to substantial increase in the systemic exposure (Cmax and AUC) of terbinafine). Products include:
Tarka Tablets 511

Vinblastine Sulfate (Studies have shown that terbinafine is an inhibitor of the CYP450 2D6 isozyme. Co-administration of terbinafine hydrochloride oral granules should be done with careful monitoring and may require a reduction in dose of the 2D6-metabolized drug).
No products indexed under this heading.

Voriconazole (It is likely that inhibitors of both CYP2C9 and CYP3A4 may lead to substantial increase in the systemic exposure (Cmax and AUC) of terbinafine).
No products indexed under this heading.

Warfarin Sodium (There have been spontaneous reports of increase or decrease in prothrombin times in patients concomitantly taking oral terbinafine and warfarin).
No products indexed under this heading.

Zafirlukast (It is likely that inhibitors of both CYP2C9 and CYP3A4 may lead to substantial increase in the systemic exposure (Cmax and AUC) of terbinafine). Products include:
Accolate Tablets 669

Zileuton (It is likely that inhibitors of both CYP2C9 and CYP3A4 may lead to substantial increase in the systemic exposure (Cmax and AUC) of terbinafine).
No products indexed under this heading.

Zonisamide (Studies have shown that terbinafine is an inhibitor of the CYP450 2D6 isozyme. Co-administration of terbinafine hydrochloride oral granules should be done with careful monitoring and may require a reduction in dose of the 2D6-metabolized drug). Products include:
Zonegran Capsules 1089

Food Interactions

Grapefruit (It is likely that inhibitors of both CYP2C9 and CYP3A4 may lead to substantial increase in the systemic exposure (Cmax and AUC) of terbinafine).

Grapefruit Juice (It is likely that inhibitors of both CYP2C9 and CYP3A4 may lead to substantial increase in the systemic exposure (Cmax and AUC) of terbinafine).

LAMISIL TABLETS

(Terbinafine Hydrochloride) 2266
May interact with beta blockers, cytochrome p450 2d6 substrates (selected), monoamine oxidase inhibitors, selective serotonin reuptake inhibitors, tricyclic antidepressants, and certain other agents. Compounds in these categories include:

Acebutolol Hydrochloride (Studies have shown that terbinafine is an inhibitor of the CYP450 2D6 isoenzyme. Co-administration of terbinafine with drugs predominantly metabolized by the CYP450 2D6 isoenzyme should be done with careful monitoring and may require a reduction in dose of the 2D6-metabolized drug).
No products indexed under this heading.

Amitriptyline Hydrochloride (Studies have shown that terbinafine is an inhibitor of the CYP450 2D6 isoenzyme. Co-administration of terbinafine with drugs predominantly metabolized by the CYP450 2D6 isoenzyme should be done with careful monitoring and may require a reduction in dose of the 2D6-metabolized drug).
No products indexed under this heading.

Amoxapine (Studies have shown that terbinafine is an inhibitor of the CYP450 2D6 isoenzyme. Co-administration of terbinafine with drugs predominantly metabolized by the CYP450 2D6 isoenzyme should be done with careful monitoring and may require a reduction in dose of the 2D6-metabolized drug).
No products indexed under this heading.

Amphetamine Aspartate (Studies have shown that terbinafine is an inhibitor of the CYP450 2D6 isoenzyme. Co-administration of terbinafine with drugs predominantly metabolized by the CYP450 2D6 isoenzyme should be done with careful monitoring and may require a reduction in dose of the 2D6-metabolized drug). Products include:
Adderall XR Capsules 3012

Amphetamine Aspartate Monohydrate (Studies have shown that terbinafine is an inhibitor of the CYP450 2D6 isoenzyme. Co-administration of terbinafine with drugs predominantly metabolized by the CYP450 2D6 isoenzyme should be done with careful monitoring and may require a reduction in dose of the 2D6-metabolized drug).
No products indexed under this heading.

Amphetamine Sulfate (Studies have shown that terbinafine is an inhibitor of the CYP450 2D6 isoenzyme. Co-administration of terbinafine with drugs predominantly metabolized by the CYP450 2D6 isoenzyme should be done with careful monitoring and may require a reduction in dose of the 2D6-metabolized drug). Products include:
Adderall XR Capsules 3012

Atenolol (Studies have shown that terbinafine is an inhibitor of the CYP450 2D6 isoenzyme. Co-administration of terbinafine with drugs predominantly metabolized by the CYP450 2D6 isoenzyme should be done with careful monitoring and may require a reduction in dose of the 2D6-metabolized drug).
No products indexed under this heading.

Atomoxetine Hydrochloride (Studies have shown that terbinafine is an inhibitor of the CYP450 2D6 isoenzyme. Co-administration of terbinafine with drugs predominantly metabolized by the CYP450 2D6 isoenzyme should be done with careful monitoring and may require a reduction in dose of the 2D6-metabolized drug). Products include:
Strattera Capsules 1864

Betaxolol Hydrochloride (Studies have shown that terbinafine is an inhibitor of the CYP450 2D6 isoenzyme. Co-administration of terbinafine with drugs predominantly metabolized by the CYP450 2D6 isoenzyme should be done with careful monitoring and may require a reduction in dose of the 2D6-metabolized drug).
No products indexed under this heading.

Bisoprolol Fumarate (Studies have shown that terbinafine is an inhibitor of the CYP450 2D6 isoenzyme. Co-administration of terbinafine with drugs predominantly metabolized by the CYP450 2D6 isoenzyme should be done with careful monitoring and may require a reduction in dose of the 2D6-metabolized drug).
No products indexed under this heading.

Caffeine (Terbinafine decreases the clearance of intravenously administered caffeine by 19%). Products include:
BioLean Free Tablets 635
BioLean II Tablets 635
Winrgy Dietary Supplement 642

Caffeine Citrate (Terbinafine decreases the clearance of intravenously administered caffeine by 19%).
No products indexed under this heading.

Captopril (Studies have shown that terbinafine is an inhibitor of the CYP450 2D6 isoenzyme. Co-administration of terbinafine with drugs predominantly metabolized by the CYP450 2D6 isoenzyme should be done with careful monitoring and may require a reduction in dose of the 2D6-metabolized drug). Products include:
Captopril Tablets 2182

Carteolol Hydrochloride (Studies have shown that terbinafine is an inhibitor of the CYP450 2D6 isoenzyme. Co-administration of terbinafine with drugs predominantly metabolized by the CYP450 2D6 isoenzyme should be done with careful monitoring and may require a reduction in dose of the 2D6-metabolized drug).
No products indexed under this heading.

Carvedilol (Studies have shown that terbinafine is an inhibitor of the CYP450 2D6 isoenzyme. Co-administration of terbinafine with

drugs predominantly metabolized by the CYP450 2D6 isoenzyme should be done with careful monitoring and may require a reduction in dose of the 2D6-metabolized drug). Products include:

Coreg Tablets 1387

Cevimeline Hydrochloride (Studies have shown that terbinafine is an inhibitor of the CYP450 2D6 isoenzyme. Co-administration of terbinafine with drugs predominantly metabolized by the CYP450 2D6 isoenzyme should be done with careful monitoring and may require a reduction in dose of the 2D6-metabolized drug). Products include:

Evoxac Capsules 1013

Chlorpromazine (Studies have shown that terbinafine is an inhibitor of the CYP450 2D6 isoenzyme. Co-administration of terbinafine with drugs predominantly metabolized by the CYP450 2D6 isoenzyme should be done with careful monitoring and may require a reduction in dose of the 2D6-metabolized drug).

No products indexed under this heading.

Chlorpromazine Hydrochloride (Studies have shown that terbinafine is an inhibitor of the CYP450 2D6 isoenzyme. Co-administration of terbinafine with drugs predominantly metabolized by the CYP450 2D6 isoenzyme should be done with careful monitoring and may require a reduction in dose of the 2D6-metabolized drug).

No products indexed under this heading.

Chlorpropamide (Studies have shown that terbinafine is an inhibitor of the CYP450 2D6 isoenzyme. Co-administration of terbinafine with drugs predominantly metabolized by the CYP450 2D6 isoenzyme should be done with careful monitoring and may require a reduction in dose of the 2D6-metabolized drug).

No products indexed under this heading.

Cimetidine (Terbinafine clearance is decreased 33% by cimetidine, a CYP450 enzyme inhibitor).

No products indexed under this heading.

Cimetidine Hydrochloride (Terbinafine clearance is decreased 33% by cimetidine, a CYP450 enzyme inhibitor).

No products indexed under this heading.

Citalopram Hydrobromide (Studies have shown that terbinafine is an inhibitor of the CYP450 2D6 isoenzyme. Co-administration of terbinafine with drugs predominantly metabolized by the CYP450 2D6 isoenzyme should be done with careful monitoring and may require a reduction in dose of the 2D6-metabolized drug). Products include:

Celexa 1160

Clomipramine Hydrochloride (Studies have shown that terbinafine is an inhibitor of the CYP450 2D6 isoenzyme. Co-administration of terbinafine with drugs predominantly metabolized by the CYP450 2D6 isoenzyme should be done with careful monitoring and may require a reduction in dose of the 2D6-metabolized drug).

No products indexed under this heading.

Clozapine (Studies have shown that terbinafine is an inhibitor of the CYP450 2D6 isoenzyme. Co-administration of terbinafine with drugs predominantly metabolized by the CYP450 2D6 isoenzyme should be done with careful monitoring and may require a reduction in dose of the 2D6-metabolized drug).

No products indexed under this heading.

Codeine Phosphate (Studies have shown that terbinafine is an inhibitor of the CYP450 2D6 isoenzyme. Co-administration of terbinafine with drugs predominantly metabolized by the CYP450 2D6 isoenzyme should be done with careful monitoring and may require a reduction in dose of the 2D6-metabolized drug). Products include:

Tylenol with Codeine Tablets 2427

Codeine Sulfate (Studies have shown that terbinafine is an inhibitor of the CYP450 2D6 isoenzyme. Co-administration of terbinafine with drugs predominantly metabolized by the CYP450 2D6 isoenzyme should be done with careful monitoring and may require a reduction in dose of the 2D6-metabolized drug).

No products indexed under this heading.

Cyclobenzaprine Hydrochloride (Studies have shown that terbinafine is an inhibitor of the CYP450 2D6 isoenzyme. Co-administration of terbinafine with drugs predominantly metabolized by the CYP450 2D6 isoenzyme should be done with careful monitoring and may require a reduction in dose of the 2D6-metabolized drug). Products include:

Amrix Capsules 966

Cyclosporine (Terbinafine increases the clearance of cyclosporine by 15%; terbinafine clearance is unaffected by cyclosporine). Products include:

Gengraf Capsules 435
Neoral Oral Solution 2280
Neoral Soft Gelatin Capsules 2280
Restasis Ophthalmic Emulsion 557
Sandimmune 2296

Desipramine Hydrochloride (Studies have shown that terbinafine is an inhibitor of the CYP450 2D6 isoenzyme. Co-administration of terbinafine with drugs predominantly metabolized by the CYP450 2D6 isoenzyme should be done with careful monitoring and may require a reduction in dose of the 2D6-metabolized drug).

No products indexed under this heading.

Dexfenfluramine Hydrochloride (Studies have shown that terbinafine is an inhibitor of the CYP450 2D6 isoenzyme. Co-administration of terbinafine with drugs predominantly metabolized by the CYP450 2D6 isoenzyme should be done with careful monitoring and may require a reduction in dose of the 2D6-metabolized drug).

No products indexed under this heading.

Dextromethorphan Hydrobromide (Studies have shown that terbinafine is an inhibitor of the CYP450 2D6 isoenzyme. Co-administration of terbinafine with drugs predominantly metabolized by the CYP450 2D6 isoenzyme should be done with careful monitoring and may require a reduction in dose of the 2D6-metabolized drug). Products include:

PediaCare Children's Liquid Multi-Symptom Cold.................. 1902
PediaCare Children's Long-Acting Cough.. 1902
Children's Sudafed PE Cold & Cough Liquid.............................. 1907
Sudafed PE Cold & Cough Caplets... 1907
Children's Tylenol Plus Cough & Runny Nose Suspension Liquid..... 1912
Children's Tylenol Plus Cough & Sore Throat Suspension Liquid..... 1912
Children's Tylenol Plus Flu Suspension Liquid........................ 1914
Children's Tylenol Plus Multi-Symptom Cold Suspension Liquid....................... 1912
Tylenol Cold Severe Congestion Daytime Caplets with Cool Burst.. 1912
Tylenol Cold Head Congestion Daytime Caplets with Cool Burst.. 1910
Tylenol Cold Head Congestion Nighttime Caplets with Cool Burst.. 1910
Tylenol Cold Head Congestion Severe Daytime Caplets with Cool Burst.................................. 1910
Tylenol Cold Multi-Symptom Daytime Caplets with Cool, Burst and Rapid Release Gels....... 1913
Tylenol Cold Multi-Symptom Daytime Liquid with Citrus Burst... 1913
Tylenol Cold Multi-Symptom Nighttime Caplets with Cool Burst.. 1913
Tylenol Cold Multi-Symptom Nighttime Liquid with Cool Burst... 1913
Tylenol Cold Multi-Symptom Severe Caplets with Cool Burst..... 1913
Tylenol Cold Multi-Symptom Severe Daytime Liquid with Citrus Burst.................................. 1913
Tylenol Cough & Sore Throat Daytime Liquid with Cool Burst...... 1918
Tylenol Cough & Sore Throat Nighttime Liquid with Cool Burst... 1918
Vicks DayQuil Cold & Flu Multi-Symptom Relief................. ■616
Vicks DayQuil LiquiCaps 2567
Vicks DayQuil Liquid 2567
Vicks DayQuil Multi-Symptom Cold/Flu Relief.......................... 2567
Vicks NyQuil Cold & Flu Multi-Symptom Relief................. ■617
Vicks NyQuil LiquiCaps 2567
Vicks NyQuil Liquid 2567
Vicks NyQuil Multi-Symptom Cold/Flu Relief.......................... 2567

Dextromethorphan Polistirex (Studies have shown that terbinafine is an inhibitor of the CYP450 2D6 isoenzyme. Co-administration of terbinafine with drugs predominantly metabolized by the CYP450 2D6 isoenzyme should be done with careful monitoring and may require a reduction in dose of the 2D6-metabolized drug).

No products indexed under this heading.

Dolasetron Mesylate (Studies have shown that terbinafine is an inhibitor of the CYP450 2D6 isoenzyme. Co-administration of terbinafine with drugs predominantly metabolized by the CYP450 2D6 isoenzyme should be done with careful monitoring and may require a reduction in dose of the 2D6-metabolized drug). Products include:

Anzemet Injection 2701
Anzemet Tablets 2704

Donepezil Hydrochloride (Studies have shown that terbinafine is an inhibitor of the CYP450 2D6 isoenzyme. Co-administration of terbinafine with drugs predominantly metabolized by the CYP450 2D6 isoenzyme should be done with careful monitoring and may require a reduction in dose of the 2D6-metabolized drug). Products include:

Aricept Tablets 1062
Aricept ODT Tablets 1062

Doxepin Hydrochloride (Studies have shown that terbinafine is an inhibitor of the CYP450 2D6 isoenzyme. Co-administration of terbinafine with drugs predominantly metabolized by the CYP450 2D6 isoenzyme should be done with careful monitoring and may require a reduction in dose of the 2D6-metabolized drug).

No products indexed under this heading.

Encainide Hydrochloride (Studies have shown that terbinafine is an inhibitor of the CYP450 2D6 isoenzyme. Co-administration of terbinafine with drugs predominantly metabolized by the CYP450 2D6 isoenzyme should be done with careful monitoring and may require a reduction in dose of the 2D6-metabolized drug).

No products indexed under this heading.

Escitalopram Oxalate (Studies have shown that terbinafine is an inhibitor of the CYP450 2D6 isoenzyme. Co-administration of terbinafine with drugs predominantly metabolized by the CYP450 2D6 isoenzyme should be done with careful monitoring and may require a reduction in dose of the 2D6-metabolized drug). Products include:

Lexapro Oral Suspension 1174
Lexapro Tablets 1174

Esmolol Hydrochloride (Studies have shown that terbinafine is an inhibitor of the CYP450 2D6 isoenzyme. Co-administration of terbinafine with drugs predominantly metabolized by the CYP450 2D6 isoenzyme should be done with careful monitoring and may require a reduction in dose of the 2D6-metabolized drug).

No products indexed under this heading.

Fentanyl (Studies have shown that terbinafine is an inhibitor of the CYP450 2D6 isoenzyme. Co-administration of terbinafine with drugs predominantly metabolized by the CYP450 2D6 isoenzyme should be done with careful monitoring and may require a reduction in dose of the 2D6-metabolized drug). Products include:

Duragesic Transdermal System 2405
Ionsys Transdermal System 2410

Fentanyl Citrate (Studies have shown that terbinafine is an inhibitor of the CYP450 2D6 isoenzyme. Co-administration of terbinafine with drugs predominantly metabolized by the CYP450 2D6 isoenzyme should be done with careful monitoring and may require a reduction in dose of the 2D6-metabolized drug). Products include:

Actiq 959
Fentora Tablets 968

Flecainide Acetate (Studies have shown that terbinafine is an inhibitor of the CYP450 2D6 isoenzyme. Co-administration of terbinafine with drugs predominantly metabolized by the CYP450 2D6 isoenzyme should be done with careful monitoring and may require a reduction in dose of the 2D6-metabolized drug).
No products indexed under this heading.

Fluoxetine (Studies have shown that terbinafine is an inhibitor of the CYP450 2D6 isoenzyme. Co-administration of terbinafine with drugs predominantly metabolized by the CYP450 2D6 isoenzyme should be done with careful monitoring and may require a reduction in dose of the 2D6-metabolized drug).
No products indexed under this heading.

Fluoxetine Hydrochloride (Studies have shown that terbinafine is an inhibitor of the CYP450 2D6 isoenzyme. Co-administration of terbinafine with drugs predominantly metabolized by the CYP450 2D6 isoenzyme should be done with careful monitoring and may require a reduction in dose of the 2D6-metabolized drug). Products include:
Prozac Weekly Capsules **1852**
Prozac Pulvules and Liquid **1852**
Symbyax Capsules **1871**

Fluphenazine Decanoate (Studies have shown that terbinafine is an inhibitor of the CYP450 2D6 isoenzyme. Co-administration of terbinafine with drugs predominantly metabolized by the CYP450 2D6 isoenzyme should be done with careful monitoring and may require a reduction in dose of the 2D6-metabolized drug).
No products indexed under this heading.

Fluphenazine Enanthate (Studies have shown that terbinafine is an inhibitor of the CYP450 2D6 isoenzyme. Co-administration of terbinafine with drugs predominantly metabolized by the CYP450 2D6 isoenzyme should be done with careful monitoring and may require a reduction in dose of the 2D6-metabolized drug).
No products indexed under this heading.

Fluphenazine Hydrochloride (Studies have shown that terbinafine is an inhibitor of the CYP450 2D6 isoenzyme. Co-administration of terbinafine with drugs predominantly metabolized by the CYP450 2D6 isoenzyme should be done with careful monitoring and may require a reduction in dose of the 2D6-metabolized drug).
No products indexed under this heading.

Fluvoxamine Maleate (Studies have shown that terbinafine is an inhibitor of the CYP450 2D6 isoenzyme. Co-administration of terbinafine with drugs predominantly metabolized by the CYP450 2D6 isoenzyme should be done with careful monitoring and may require a reduction in dose of the 2D6-metabolized drug). Products include:
Luvox CR Extended-Release Capsules **1759**

Formoterol Fumarate (Studies have shown that terbinafine is an inhibitor of the CYP450 2D6 isoenzyme. Co-administration of terbinafine with drugs predominantly metabolized by the CYP450 2D6 isoenzyme should be done with careful monitoring and may require a reduction in dose of the 2D6-metabolized drug). Products include:
Foradil Aerolizer **2849**
Perforomist Inhalation Solution **1025**

Galantamine Hydrobromide (Studies have shown that terbinafine is an inhibitor of the CYP450 2D6 isoenzyme. Co-administration of terbinafine with drugs predominantly metabolized by the CYP450 2D6 isoenzyme should be done with careful monitoring and may require a reduction in dose of the 2D6-metabolized drug).
No products indexed under this heading.

Haloperidol (Studies have shown that terbinafine is an inhibitor of the CYP450 2D6 isoenzyme. Co-administration of terbinafine with drugs predominantly metabolized by the CYP450 2D6 isoenzyme should be done with careful monitoring and may require a reduction in dose of the 2D6-metabolized drug).
No products indexed under this heading.

Haloperidol Decanoate (Studies have shown that terbinafine is an inhibitor of the CYP450 2D6 isoenzyme. Co-administration of terbinafine with drugs predominantly metabolized by the CYP450 2D6 isoenzyme should be done with careful monitoring and may require a reduction in dose of the 2D6-metabolized drug).
No products indexed under this heading.

Hydrocodone Bitartrate (Studies have shown that terbinafine is an inhibitor of the CYP450 2D6 isoenzyme. Co-administration of terbinafine with drugs predominantly metabolized by the CYP450 2D6 isoenzyme should be done with careful monitoring and may require a reduction in dose of the 2D6-metabolized drug). Products include:
Lortab 5/500 Tablets **3143**
Lortab 7.5/500 Tablets **3144**
Lortab 10/500 Tablets **3144**
Vicodin Tablets **529**
Vicodin ES Tablets **530**
Vicodin HP Tablets **531**
Vicoprofen Tablets **533**
Zydone Tablets **1132**

Imipramine Hydrochloride (Studies have shown that terbinafine is an inhibitor of the CYP450 2D6 isoenzyme. Co-administration of terbinafine with drugs predominantly metabolized by the CYP450 2D6 isoenzyme should be done with careful monitoring and may require a reduction in dose of the 2D6-metabolized drug).
No products indexed under this heading.

Imipramine Pamoate (Studies have shown that terbinafine is an inhibitor of the CYP450 2D6 isoenzyme. Co-administration of terbinafine with drugs predominantly metabolized by the CYP450 2D6 isoenzyme should be done with careful monitoring and may require a reduction in dose of the 2D6-metabolized drug).
No products indexed under this heading.

Indoramin Hydrochloride (Studies have shown that terbinafine is an inhibitor of the CYP450 2D6 isoenzyme. Co-administration of terbinafine with drugs predominantly metabolized by the CYP450 2D6 isoenzyme should be done with careful monitoring and may require a reduction in dose of the 2D6-metabolized drug).
No products indexed under this heading.

Isocarboxazid (Studies have shown that terbinafine is an inhibitor of the CYP450 2D6 isoenzyme. Co-administration of terbinafine with drugs predominantly metabolized by the CYP450 2D6 isoenzyme should be done with careful monitoring and may require a reduction in dose of the 2D6-metabolized drug). Products include:
Marplan Tablets **3177**

Labetalol Hydrochloride (Studies have shown that terbinafine is an inhibitor of the CYP450 2D6 isoenzyme. Co-administration of terbinafine with drugs predominantly metabolized by the CYP450 2D6 isoenzyme should be done with careful monitoring and may require a reduction in dose of the 2D6-metabolized drug).
No products indexed under this heading.

Levobunolol Hydrochloride (Studies have shown that terbinafine is an inhibitor of the CYP450 2D6 isoenzyme. Co-administration of terbinafine with drugs predominantly metabolized by the CYP450 2D6 isoenzyme should be done with careful monitoring and may require a reduction in dose of the 2D6-metabolized drug).
No products indexed under this heading.

Lidocaine (Studies have shown that terbinafine is an inhibitor of the CYP450 2D6 isoenzyme. Co-administration of terbinafine with drugs predominantly metabolized by the CYP450 2D6 isoenzyme should be done with careful monitoring and may require a reduction in dose of the 2D6-metabolized drug). Products include:
Lidoderm Patch **1114**

Lidocaine Hydrochloride (Studies have shown that terbinafine is an inhibitor of the CYP450 2D6 isoenzyme. Co-administration of terbinafine with drugs predominantly metabolized by the CYP450 2D6 isoenzyme should be done with careful monitoring and may require a reduction in dose of the 2D6-metabolized drug).
No products indexed under this heading.

Maprotiline Hydrochloride (Studies have shown that terbinafine is an inhibitor of the CYP450 2D6 isoenzyme. Co-administration of terbinafine with drugs predominantly metabolized by the CYP450 2D6 isoenzyme should be done with careful monitoring and may require a reduction in dose of the 2D6-metabolized drug).
No products indexed under this heading.

Meperidine Hydrochloride (Studies have shown that terbinafine is an inhibitor of the CYP450 2D6 isoenzyme. Co-administration of terbinafine with drugs predominantly metabolized by the CYP450 2D6 isoenzyme should be done with careful monitoring and may require a reduction in dose of the 2D6-metabolized drug).
No products indexed under this heading.

Methadone Hydrochloride (Studies have shown that terbinafine is an inhibitor of the CYP450 2D6 isoenzyme. Co-administration of terbinafine with drugs predominantly metabolized by the CYP450 2D6 isoenzyme should be done with careful monitoring and may require a reduction in dose of the 2D6-metabolized drug).
No products indexed under this heading.

Methamphetamine Hydrochloride (Studies have shown that terbinafine is an inhibitor of the CYP450 2D6 isoenzyme. Co-administration of terbinafine with drugs predominantly metabolized by the CYP450 2D6 isoenzyme should be done with careful monitoring and may require a reduction in dose of the 2D6-metabolized drug).
No products indexed under this heading.

Metipranolol Hydrochloride (Studies have shown that terbinafine is an inhibitor of the CYP450 2D6 isoenzyme. Co-administration of terbinafine with drugs predominantly metabolized by the CYP450 2D6 isoenzyme should be done with careful monitoring and may require a reduction in dose of the 2D6-metabolized drug).
No products indexed under this heading.

Metoprolol Succinate (Studies have shown that terbinafine is an inhibitor of the CYP450 2D6 isoenzyme. Co-administration of terbinafine with drugs predominantly metabolized by the CYP450 2D6 isoenzyme should be done with careful monitoring and may require a reduction in dose of the 2D6-metabolized drug). Products include:
Toprol-XL Tablets **666**

Metoprolol Tartrate (Studies have shown that terbinafine is an inhibitor of the CYP450 2D6 isoenzyme. Co-administration of terbinafine with drugs predominantly metabolized by the CYP450 2D6 isoenzyme should be done with careful monitoring and may require a reduction in dose of the 2D6-metabolized drug).
No products indexed under this heading.

Mexiletine Hydrochloride (Studies have shown that terbinafine is an inhibitor of the CYP450 2D6 isoenzyme. Co-administration of terbinafine with drugs predominantly metabolized by the CYP450 2D6 isoenzyme should be done with careful monitoring and may require a reduction in dose of the 2D6-metabolized drug).
No products indexed under this heading.

Mirtazapine (Studies have shown that terbinafine is an inhibitor of the CYP450 2D6 isoenzyme. Co-administration of terbinafine with

drugs predominantly metabolized by the CYP450 2D6 isoenzyme should be done with careful monitoring and may require a reduction in dose of the 2D6-metabolized drug). Products include:

Remeron Tablets ... 2924
RemeronSolTab Tablets ... 2927

Moclobemide (Studies have shown that terbinafine is an inhibitor of the CYP450 2D6 isoenzyme. Co-administration of terbinafine with drugs predominantly metabolized by the CYP450 2D6 isoenzyme should be done with careful monitoring and may require a reduction in dose of the 2D6-metabolized drug).

No products indexed under this heading.

Morphine Sulfate (Studies have shown that terbinafine is an inhibitor of the CYP450 2D6 isoenzyme. Co-administration of terbinafine with drugs predominantly metabolized by the CYP450 2D6 isoenzyme should be done with careful monitoring and may require a reduction in dose of the 2D6-metabolized drug). Products include:

Avinza Capsules ... 1772
DepoDur Injection ... 1095
MS Contin Tablets ... 2585

Nadolol (Studies have shown that terbinafine is an inhibitor of the CYP450 2D6 isoenzyme. Co-administration of terbinafine with drugs predominantly metabolized by the CYP450 2D6 isoenzyme should be done with careful monitoring and may require a reduction in dose of the 2D6-metabolized drug). Products include:

Nadolol Tablets ... 2191

Nebivolol (Studies have shown that terbinafine is an inhibitor of the CYP450 2D6 isoenzyme. Co-administration of terbinafine with drugs predominantly metabolized by the CYP450 2D6 isoenzyme should be done with careful monitoring and may require a reduction in dose of the 2D6-metabolized drug). Products include:

Bystolic Tablets ... 1155

Nelfinavir Mesylate (Studies have shown that terbinafine is an inhibitor of the CYP450 2D6 isoenzyme. Co-administration of terbinafine with drugs predominantly metabolized by the CYP450 2D6 isoenzyme should be done with careful monitoring and may require a reduction in dose of the 2D6-metabolized drug).

No products indexed under this heading.

Nortriptyline Hydrochloride (Studies have shown that terbinafine is an inhibitor of the CYP450 2D6 isoenzyme. Co-administration of terbinafine with drugs predominantly metabolized by the CYP450 2D6 isoenzyme should be done with careful monitoring and may require a reduction in dose of the 2D6-metabolized drug).

No products indexed under this heading.

Olanzapine (Studies have shown that terbinafine is an inhibitor of the CYP450 2D6 isoenzyme. Co-administration of terbinafine with drugs predominantly metabolized by the CYP450 2D6 isoenzyme should be done with careful monitoring and may require a reduction in dose of the 2D6-metabolized drug). Products include:

Symbyax Capsules ... 1871
Zyprexa Tablets ... 1883
Zyprexa IntraMuscular ... 1883
Zyprexa ZYDIS Orally Disintegrating Tablets ... 1883

Omeprazole (Studies have shown that terbinafine is an inhibitor of the CYP450 2D6 isoenzyme. Co-administration of terbinafine with drugs predominantly metabolized by the CYP450 2D6 isoenzyme should be done with careful monitoring and may require a reduction in dose of the 2D6-metabolized drug).

No products indexed under this heading.

Ondansetron (Studies have shown that terbinafine is an inhibitor of the CYP450 2D6 isoenzyme. Co-administration of terbinafine with drugs predominantly metabolized by the CYP450 2D6 isoenzyme should be done with careful monitoring and may require a reduction in dose of the 2D6-metabolized drug). Products include:

Zofran ODT Orally Disintegrating Tablets ... 1687

Ondansetron Hydrochloride (Studies have shown that terbinafine is an inhibitor of the CYP450 2D6 isoenzyme. Co-administration of terbinafine with drugs predominantly metabolized by the CYP450 2D6 isoenzyme should be done with careful monitoring and may require a reduction in dose of the 2D6-metabolized drug). Products include:

Zofran Injection ... 1682
Zofran ... 1687

Oxycodone Hydrochloride (Studies have shown that terbinafine is an inhibitor of the CYP450 2D6 isoenzyme. Co-administration of terbinafine with drugs predominantly metabolized by the CYP450 2D6 isoenzyme should be done with careful monitoring and may require a reduction in dose of the 2D6-metabolized drug). Products include:

OxyContin Tablets ... 2589
OxyIR Capsules ... 2593
Percocet Tablets ... 1127
Percodan Tablets ... 1130

Paclitaxel (Studies have shown that terbinafine is an inhibitor of the CYP450 2D6 isoenzyme. Co-administration of terbinafine with drugs predominantly metabolized by the CYP450 2D6 isoenzyme should be done with careful monitoring and may require a reduction in dose of the 2D6-metabolized drug).

No products indexed under this heading.

Pargyline Hydrochloride (Studies have shown that terbinafine is an inhibitor of the CYP450 2D6 isoenzyme. Co-administration of terbinafine with drugs predominantly metabolized by the CYP450 2D6 isoenzyme should be done with careful monitoring and may require a reduction in dose of the 2D6-metabolized drug).

No products indexed under this heading.

Paroxetine Hydrochloride (Studies have shown that terbinafine is an inhibitor of the CYP450 2D6 isoenzyme. Co-administration of terbinafine with drugs predominantly metabolized by the CYP450 2D6 isoenzyme should be done with careful monitoring and may require a reduction in dose of the 2D6-metabolized drug). Products include:

Paxil ... 1535
Paxil CR Controlled-Release Tablets ... 1544

Penbutolol Sulfate (Studies have shown that terbinafine is an inhibitor of the CYP450 2D6 isoenzyme. Co-administration of terbinafine with drugs predominantly metabolized by the CYP450 2D6 isoenzyme should be done with careful monitoring and may require a reduction in dose of the 2D6-metabolized drug).

No products indexed under this heading.

Phenelzine Sulfate (Studies have shown that terbinafine is an inhibitor of the CYP450 2D6 isoenzyme. Co-administration of terbinafine with drugs predominantly metabolized by the CYP450 2D6 isoenzyme should be done with careful monitoring and may require a reduction in dose of the 2D6-metabolized drug).

No products indexed under this heading.

Pindolol (Studies have shown that terbinafine is an inhibitor of the CYP450 2D6 isoenzyme. Co-administration of terbinafine with drugs predominantly metabolized by the CYP450 2D6 isoenzyme should be done with careful monitoring and may require a reduction in dose of the 2D6-metabolized drug).

No products indexed under this heading.

Procarbazine Hydrochloride (Studies have shown that terbinafine is an inhibitor of the CYP450 2D6 isoenzyme. Co-administration of terbinafine with drugs predominantly metabolized by the CYP450 2D6 isoenzyme should be done with careful monitoring and may require a reduction in dose of the 2D6-metabolized drug).

No products indexed under this heading.

Propafenone Hydrochloride (Studies have shown that terbinafine is an inhibitor of the CYP450 2D6 isoenzyme. Co-administration of terbinafine with drugs predominantly metabolized by the CYP450 2D6 isoenzyme should be done with careful monitoring and may require a reduction in dose of the 2D6-metabolized drug). Products include:

Rythmol Tablets ... 1586
Rythmol SR Capsules ... 1590

Propoxyphene Hydrochloride (Studies have shown that terbinafine is an inhibitor of the CYP450 2D6 isoenzyme. Co-administration of terbinafine with drugs predominantly metabolized by the CYP450 2D6 isoenzyme should be done with careful monitoring and may require a reduction in dose of the 2D6-metabolized drug).

No products indexed under this heading.

Propoxyphene Napsylate (Studies have shown that terbinafine is an inhibitor of the CYP450 2D6 isoenzyme. Co-administration of terbinafine with drugs predominantly metabolized by the CYP450 2D6 isoenzyme should be done with careful monitoring and may require a reduction in dose of the 2D6-metabolized drug).

No products indexed under this heading.

Propranolol Hydrochloride (Studies have shown that terbinafine is an inhibitor of the CYP450 2D6 isoenzyme. Co-administration of terbinafine with drugs predominantly metabolized by the CYP450 2D6 isoenzyme should be done with careful monitoring and may require a reduction in dose of the 2D6-metabolized drug). Products include:

InnoPran XL Extended Release Capsules ... 1484

Protriptyline Hydrochloride (Studies have shown that terbinafine is an inhibitor of the CYP450 2D6 isoenzyme. Co-administration of terbinafine with drugs predominantly metabolized by the CYP450 2D6 isoenzyme should be done with careful monitoring and may require a reduction in dose of the 2D6-metabolized drug).

No products indexed under this heading.

Quetiapine Fumarate (Studies have shown that terbinafine is an inhibitor of the CYP450 2D6 isoenzyme. Co-administration of terbinafine with drugs predominantly metabolized by the CYP450 2D6 isoenzyme should be done with careful monitoring and may require a reduction in dose of the 2D6-metabolized drug).

No products indexed under this heading.

Quinidine Gluconate (Studies have shown that terbinafine is an inhibitor of the CYP450 2D6 isoenzyme. Co-administration of terbinafine with drugs predominantly metabolized by the CYP450 2D6 isoenzyme should be done with careful monitoring and may require a reduction in dose of the 2D6-metabolized drug).

No products indexed under this heading.

Quinidine Hydrochloride (Studies have shown that terbinafine is an inhibitor of the CYP450 2D6 isoenzyme. Co-administration of terbinafine with drugs predominantly metabolized by the CYP450 2D6 isoenzyme should be done with careful monitoring and may require a reduction in dose of the 2D6-metabolized drug).

No products indexed under this heading.

Quinidine Polygalacturonate (Studies have shown that terbinafine is an inhibitor of the CYP450 2D6 isoenzyme. Co-administration of terbinafine with drugs predominantly metabolized by the CYP450 2D6 isoenzyme should be done with careful monitoring and may require a reduction in dose of the 2D6-metabolized drug).

No products indexed under this heading.

Quinidine Sulfate (Studies have shown that terbinafine is an inhibitor of the CYP450 2D6 isoenzyme. Co-administration of terbinafine with drugs predominantly metabolized by the CYP450 2D6 isoenzyme should be done with careful monitoring and may require a reduction in dose of the 2D6-metabolized drug).

No products indexed under this heading.

Rasagiline Mesylate (Studies have shown that terbinafine is an inhibitor of the CYP450 2D6 isoenzyme. Co-administration of terbinafine with

drugs predominantly metabolized by the CYP450 2D6 isoenzyme should be done with careful monitoring and may require a reduction in dose of the 2D6-metabolized drug). Products include:

Azilect Tablets 3106

Rifampin (Terbinafine clearance is increased 100% by rifampin, a CYP450 enzyme inducer).

No products indexed under this heading.

Risperidone (Studies have shown that terbinafine is an inhibitor of the CYP450 2D6 isoenzyme. Co-administration of terbinafine with drugs predominantly metabolized by the CYP450 2D6 isoenzyme should be done with careful monitoring and may require a reduction in dose of the 2D6-metabolized drug). Products include:

Risperdal Consta Long-Acting Injection 1753

Ritonavir (Studies have shown that terbinafine is an inhibitor of the CYP450 2D6 isoenzyme. Co-administration of terbinafine with drugs predominantly metabolized by the CYP450 2D6 isoenzyme should be done with careful monitoring and may require a reduction in dose of the 2D6-metabolized drug). Products include:

Kaletra 452
Norvir 489

Selegiline (Studies have shown that terbinafine is an inhibitor of the CYP450 2D6 isoenzyme. Co-administration of terbinafine with drugs predominantly metabolized by the CYP450 2D6 isoenzyme should be done with careful monitoring and may require a reduction in dose of the 2D6-metabolized drug). Products include:

Emsam Transdermal System 905

Selegiline Hydrochloride (In vitro studies show that terbinafine inhibits CYP2D6 mediated metabolism; this may be of clinical relevance for compounds predominantly metabolized by this enzyme, such as type B MAO inhibitor, if they have a narrow therapeutic window). Products include:

Eldepryl Capsules 3052

Sertraline Hydrochloride (Studies have shown that terbinafine is an inhibitor of the CYP450 2D6 isoenzyme. Co-administration of terbinafine with drugs predominantly metabolized by the CYP450 2D6 isoenzyme should be done with careful monitoring and may require a reduction in dose of the 2D6-metabolized drug).

No products indexed under this heading.

Sotalol Hydrochloride (Studies have shown that terbinafine is an inhibitor of the CYP450 2D6 isoenzyme. Co-administration of terbinafine with drugs predominantly metabolized by the CYP450 2D6 isoenzyme should be done with careful monitoring and may require a reduction in dose of the 2D6-metabolized drug).

No products indexed under this heading.

Tamoxifen Citrate (Studies have shown that terbinafine is an inhibitor of the CYP450 2D6 isoenzyme. Co-administration of terbinafine with drugs predominantly metabolized by the CYP450 2D6 isoenzyme should be done with careful monitoring and may require a reduction in dose of the 2D6-metabolized drug).

No products indexed under this heading.

Teniposide (Studies have shown that terbinafine is an inhibitor of the CYP450 2D6 isoenzyme. Co-administration of terbinafine with drugs predominantly metabolized by the CYP450 2D6 isoenzyme should be done with careful monitoring and may require a reduction in dose of the 2D6-metabolized drug).

No products indexed under this heading.

Terfenadine (Terbinafine clearance is decreased 16% by terfenadine).

No products indexed under this heading.

Testosterone (Studies have shown that terbinafine is an inhibitor of the CYP450 2D6 isoenzyme. Co-administration of terbinafine with drugs predominantly metabolized by the CYP450 2D6 isoenzyme should be done with careful monitoring and may require a reduction in dose of the 2D6-metabolized drug). Products include:

AndroGel 3159
Testim 1% Gel 701

Testosterone Cypionate (Studies have shown that terbinafine is an inhibitor of the CYP450 2D6 isoenzyme. Co-administration of terbinafine with drugs predominantly metabolized by the CYP450 2D6 isoenzyme should be done with careful monitoring and may require a reduction in dose of the 2D6-metabolized drug).

No products indexed under this heading.

Testosterone Enanthate (Studies have shown that terbinafine is an inhibitor of the CYP450 2D6 isoenzyme. Co-administration of terbinafine with drugs predominantly metabolized by the CYP450 2D6 isoenzyme should be done with careful monitoring and may require a reduction in dose of the 2D6-metabolized drug). Products include:

Delatestryl Injection 1730

Testosterone Propionate (Studies have shown that terbinafine is an inhibitor of the CYP450 2D6 isoenzyme. Co-administration of terbinafine with drugs predominantly metabolized by the CYP450 2D6 isoenzyme should be done with careful monitoring and may require a reduction in dose of the 2D6-metabolized drug).

No products indexed under this heading.

Thioridazine (Studies have shown that terbinafine is an inhibitor of the CYP450 2D6 isoenzyme. Co-administration of terbinafine with drugs predominantly metabolized by the CYP450 2D6 isoenzyme should be done with careful monitoring and may require a reduction in dose of the 2D6-metabolized drug).

No products indexed under this heading.

Thioridazine Hydrochloride (Studies have shown that terbinafine is an inhibitor of the CYP450 2D6 isoenzyme. Co-administration of terbinafine with drugs predominantly metabolized by the CYP450 2D6 isoenzyme should be done with careful monitoring and may require a reduction in dose of the 2D6-metabolized drug). Products include:

Thioridazine Hydrochloride Tablets 2195

Timolol Hemihydrate (Studies have shown that terbinafine is an inhibitor of the CYP450 2D6 isoenzyme. Co-administration of terbinafine with drugs predominantly metabolized by the CYP450 2D6 isoenzyme should be done with careful monitoring and may require a reduction in dose of the 2D6-metabolized drug). Products include:

Betimol Ophthalmic Solution 3181

Timolol Maleate (Studies have shown that terbinafine is an inhibitor of the CYP450 2D6 isoenzyme. Co-administration of terbinafine with drugs predominantly metabolized by the CYP450 2D6 isoenzyme should be done with careful monitoring and may require a reduction in dose of the 2D6-metabolized drug). Products include:

Combigan Ophthalmic Solution 553
Cosopt Sterile Ophthalmic Solution...................................... 1969
Timoptic Sterile Ophthalmic Solution.. 2121
Timoptic in Ocudose 2124
Timoptic-XE Sterile Ophthalmic Gel Forming Solution.................. 2125

Tolterodine Tartrate (Studies have shown that terbinafine is an inhibitor of the CYP450 2D6 isoenzyme. Co-administration of terbinafine with drugs predominantly metabolized by the CYP450 2D6 isoenzyme should be done with careful monitoring and may require a reduction in dose of the 2D6-metabolized drug).

No products indexed under this heading.

Tramadol Hydrochloride (Studies have shown that terbinafine is an inhibitor of the CYP450 2D6 isoenzyme. Co-administration of terbinafine with drugs predominantly metabolized by the CYP450 2D6 isoenzyme should be done with careful monitoring and may require a reduction in dose of the 2D6-metabolized drug). Products include:

Ultram ER Extended-Release Tablets 2428

Tranylcypromine Sulfate (Studies have shown that terbinafine is an inhibitor of the CYP450 2D6 isoenzyme. Co-administration of terbinafine with drugs predominantly metabolized by the CYP450 2D6 isoenzyme should be done with careful monitoring and may require a reduction in dose of the 2D6-metabolized drug). Products include:

Parnate Tablets 1532

Trazodone Hydrochloride (Studies have shown that terbinafine is an inhibitor of the CYP450 2D6 isoenzyme. Co-administration of terbinafine with drugs predominantly metabolized by the CYP450 2D6 isoenzyme should be done with careful monitoring and may require a reduction in dose of the 2D6-metabolized drug).

No products indexed under this heading.

Triazolam (Studies have shown that terbinafine is an inhibitor of the CYP450 2D6 isoenzyme. Co-administration of terbinafine with drugs predominantly metabolized by the CYP450 2D6 isoenzyme should be done with careful monitoring and may require a reduction in dose of the 2D6-metabolized drug).

No products indexed under this heading.

Trimipramine Maleate (Studies have shown that terbinafine is an inhibitor of the CYP450 2D6 isoenzyme. Co-administration of terbinafine with drugs predominantly metabolized by the CYP450 2D6 isoenzyme should be done with careful monitoring and may require a reduction in dose of the 2D6-metabolized drug).

No products indexed under this heading.

Venlafaxine Hydrochloride (Studies have shown that terbinafine is an inhibitor of the CYP450 2D6 isoenzyme. Co-administration of terbinafine with drugs predominantly metabolized by the CYP450 2D6 isoenzyme should be done with careful monitoring and may require a reduction in dose of the 2D6-metabolized drug). Products include:

Effexor XR Extended-Release Capsules...................................... 3195
Venlafaxine Hydrochloride Tablets ... 2199

Vinblastine Sulfate (Studies have shown that terbinafine is an inhibitor of the CYP450 2D6 isoenzyme. Co-administration of terbinafine with drugs predominantly metabolized by the CYP450 2D6 isoenzyme should be done with careful monitoring and may require a reduction in dose of the 2D6-metabolized drug).

No products indexed under this heading.

Warfarin Sodium (Co-administration has resulted in altered prothrombin time (prolongation and reduction)).

No products indexed under this heading.

Zonisamide (Studies have shown that terbinafine is an inhibitor of the CYP450 2D6 isoenzyme. Co-administration of terbinafine with drugs predominantly metabolized by the CYP450 2D6 isoenzyme should be done with careful monitoring and may require a reduction in dose of the 2D6-metabolized drug). Products include:

Zonegran Capsules 1089

Food Interactions

Food, unspecified (Co-administration has resulted in an increase in the AUC of terbinafine of less than 20%).

LANOXIN INJECTION

(Digoxin) 1498
See Lanoxin Tablets

LANOXIN INJECTION PEDIATRIC

(Digoxin) 1502
See Lanoxin Tablets

IMPORTANT NOTE: Always consult each drug listing in the patient's regimen for possible interactions.

LANOXIN TABLETS

(Digoxin) 1505

May interact with antacids, beta blockers, calcium channel blockers, corticosteroids, erythromycin, macrolide antibiotics, potassium-depleting diuretics, quinidine, sympathomimetics, tetracyclines, thyroid preparations, and certain other agents. Compounds in these categories include:

Acebutolol Hydrochloride (Concomitant use of digoxin and beta-andrenergic blockers may result in the additive effects on AV node conduction).
No products indexed under this heading.

Albuterol (Concomitant use of digoxin and sympathomimetics increases the risk of cardiac arrhythmias).
No products indexed under this heading.

Albuterol Sulfate (Concomitant use of digoxin and sympathomimetics increases the risk of cardiac arrhythmias). Products include:
Combivent Inhalation Aerosol 845
ProAir HFA Inhalation Aerosol 3113
Proventil HFA Inhalation Aerosol 2914
Ventolin HFA Inhalation Aerosol 1638

Alprazolam (Raises the serum digoxin concentration due to reduction in clearance and/or volume of distribution of the drug, with the implication that digitalis intoxication may result).
No products indexed under this heading.

Aluminum Carbonate (Antacids may interfere with intestinal digoxin absorption, resulting in unexpectedly low serum concentrations; antacids may cause hypokalemia or hypomagnesemia and co-administration can cause digitalis toxicity).
No products indexed under this heading.

Aluminum Hydroxide (Antacids may interfere with intestinal digoxin absorption, resulting in unexpectedly low serum concentrations; antacids may cause hypokalemia or hypomagnesemia and co-administration can cause digitalis toxicity).
No products indexed under this heading.

Amiodarone Hydrochloride (Raises the serum digoxin concentration due to reduction in clearance and/or volume of distribution of the drug, with the implication that digitalis intoxication may result).
No products indexed under this heading.

Amlodipine Besylate (Concomitant use of digoxin and calcium channel blockers may result in the additive effects on AV node conduction). Products include:
Azor Tablets 1005
Exforge Tablets 2238

Amphotericin B (Can cause hypokalemia or hypomagnesemia and potassium or magnesium depletion can sensitize the myocardium to digoxin resulting in digitails toxicity).
No products indexed under this heading.

Anticancer Drugs, unspecified (May interfere with intestinal digoxin absorption, resulting in unexpectedly low serum concentrations).
No products indexed under this heading.

Atenolol (Concomitant use of digoxin and beta-andrenergic blockers may result in the additive effects on AV node conduction).
No products indexed under this heading.

Azithromycin Dihydrate (Macrolide antibiotics may possibly increase digoxin absorption in patients who inactivate digoxin by bacterial metabolism in the lower intestine, so that digitalis intoxication may result).
No products indexed under this heading.

Bendroflumethiazide (Potassium-depleting diuretics can cause hypokalemia and co-administration can result in digitalis toxicity).
No products indexed under this heading.

Bepridil Hydrochloride (Concomitant use of digoxin and calcium channel blockers may result in the additive effects on AV node conduction).
No products indexed under this heading.

Betamethasone Acetate (Corticosteroids can cause hypokalemia or hypomagnesemia and potassium or magnesium depletion can sensitize the myocardium to digoxin resulting in digitalis toxicity).
No products indexed under this heading.

Betamethasone Sodium Phosphate (Corticosteroids can cause hypokalemia or hypomagnesemia and potassium or magnesium depletion can sensitize the myocardium to digoxin resulting in digitalis toxicity).
No products indexed under this heading.

Betaxolol Hydrochloride (Concomitant use of digoxin and beta-andrenergic blockers may result in the additive effects on AV node conduction).
No products indexed under this heading.

Bisoprolol Fumarate (Concomitant use of digoxin and beta-andrenergic blockers may result in the additive effects on AV node conduction).
No products indexed under this heading.

Budesonide (Corticosteroids can cause hypokalemia or hypomagnesemia and potassium or magnesium depletion can sensitize the myocardium to digoxin resulting in digitalis toxicity). Products include:
Pulmicort Flexhaler 654
Symbicort 80/4.5 Inhalation Aerosol.. 659
Symbicort 160/4.5 Inhalation Aerosol.. 659

Bumetanide (Potassium-depleting diuretics can cause hypokalemia and co-administration can result in digitalis toxicity).
No products indexed under this heading.

Calcium, intravenous (Co-administration with calcium, particularly if administered rapidly by the intravenous route may produce serious arrhythmias in digitalized patients).
No products indexed under this heading.

Carteolol Hydrochloride (Concomitant use of digoxin and beta-andrenergic blockers may result in the additive effects on AV node conduction).
No products indexed under this heading.

Chlorothiazide (Potassium-depleting diuretics can cause hypokalemia and co-administration can result in digitalis toxicity).
No products indexed under this heading.

Chlorothiazide Sodium (Potassium-depleting diuretics can cause hypokalemia and co-administration can result in digitalis toxicity). Products include:
Intravenous Sodium Diuril 2490

Cholestyramine (May interfere with intestinal digoxin absorption, resulting in unexpectedly low serum concentrations).
No products indexed under this heading.

Ciclesonide (Corticosteroids can cause hypokalemia or hypomagnesemia and potassium or magnesium depletion can sensitize the myocardium to digoxin resulting in digitalis toxicity). Products include:
Alvesco Inhalation Aerosol 2985
Omnaris Nasal Spray 2998

Clarithromycin (May increase digoxin absorption in patients who inactivate digoxin by bacterial metabolism in the lower intestine, so that digitalis intoxication may result). Products include:
Biaxin/Biaxin XL 411

Cortisone Acetate (Corticosteroids can cause hypokalemia or hypomagnesemia and potassium or magnesium depletion can sensitize the myocardium to digoxin resulting in digitalis toxicity).
No products indexed under this heading.

Demeclocycline Hydrochloride (May increase digoxin absorption in patients who inactivate digoxin by bacterial metabolism in the lower intestine, so that digitalis intoxication may result).
No products indexed under this heading.

Dexamethasone (Corticosteroids can cause hypokalemia or hypomagnesemia and potassium or magnesium depletion can sensitize the myocardium to digoxin resulting in digitalis toxicity). Products include:
Ciprodex Otic Suspension 541

Dexamethasone Acetate (Corticosteroids can cause hypokalemia or hypomagnesemia and potassium or magnesium depletion can sensitize the myocardium to digoxin resulting in digitalis toxicity).
No products indexed under this heading.

Dexamethasone Sodium Phosphate (Corticosteroids can cause hypokalemia or hypomagnesemia and potassium or magnesium depletion can sensitize the myocardium to digoxin resulting in digitalis toxicity).
No products indexed under this heading.

Diltiazem Hydrochloride (Concomitant use of digoxin and calcium channel blockers may result in the additive effects on AV node conduction). Products include:
Cardizem LA Extended Release Tablets....................................... 421

Diphenoxylate Hydrochloride (Decreases gut motility and may increase digoxin absorption).
No products indexed under this heading.

Dirithromycin (Macrolide antibiotics may possibly increase digoxin absorption in patients who inactivate digoxin by bacterial metabolism in the lower intestine, so that digitalis intoxication may result).
No products indexed under this heading.

Dobutamine Hydrochloride (Concomitant use of digoxin and sympathomimetics increases the risk of cardiac arrhythmias).
No products indexed under this heading.

Dopamine Hydrochloride (Concomitant use of digoxin and sympathomimetics increases the risk of cardiac arrhythmias).
No products indexed under this heading.

Doxycycline Calcium (May increase digoxin absorption in patients who inactivate digoxin by bacterial metabolism in the lower intestine, so that digitalis intoxication may result).
No products indexed under this heading.

Doxycycline Hyclate (May increase digoxin absorption in patients who inactivate digoxin by bacterial metabolism in the lower intestine, so that digitalis intoxication may result).
No products indexed under this heading.

Doxycycline Monohydrate (May increase digoxin absorption in patients who inactivate digoxin by bacterial metabolism in the lower intestine, so that digitalis intoxication may result).
No products indexed under this heading.

Ephedrine Hydrochloride (Concomitant use of digoxin and sympathomimetics increases the risk of cardiac arrhythmias).
No products indexed under this heading.

Ephedrine Sulfate (Concomitant use of digoxin and sympathomimetics increases the risk of cardiac arrhythmias).
No products indexed under this heading.

Ephedrine Tannate (Concomitant use of digoxin and sympathomimetics increases the risk of cardiac arrhythmias).
No products indexed under this heading.

Epinephrine (Concomitant use of digoxin and sympathomimetics increases the risk of cardiac arrhythmias). Products include:
EpiPen 1024

Epinephrine Bitartrate (Concomitant use of digoxin and sympathomimetics increases the risk of cardiac arrhythmias).
No products indexed under this heading.

Epinephrine Hydrochloride (Concomitant use of digoxin and sympathomimetics increases the risk of cardiac arrhythmias).
No products indexed under this heading.

Erythromycin (May increase digoxin absorption in patients who inactivate digoxin by bacterial metabolism in the lower intestine, so that digitalis intoxication may result).
No products indexed under this heading.

Erythromycin Estolate (May increase digoxin absorption in patients who inactivate digoxin by bacterial metabolism in the lower intestine, so that digitalis intoxication may result).
No products indexed under this heading.

Erythromycin Ethylsuccinate (May increase digoxin absorption in patients who inactivate digoxin by bacterial metabolism in the lower intestine, so that digitalis intoxication may result). Products include:
- E.E.S. 433
- EryPed 431

Erythromycin Gluceptate (May increase digoxin absorption in patients who inactivate digoxin by bacterial metabolism in the lower intestine, so that digitalis intoxication may result).
No products indexed under this heading.

Erythromycin Lactobionate (May increase digoxin absorption in patients who inactivate digoxin by bacterial metabolism in the lower intestine, so that digitalis intoxication may result).
No products indexed under this heading.

Erythromycin Stearate (May increase digoxin absorption in patients who inactivate digoxin by bacterial metabolism in the lower intestine, so that digitalis intoxication may result).
No products indexed under this heading.

Esmolol Hydrochloride (Concomitant use of digoxin and beta-andrenergic blockers may result in the additive effects on AV node conduction).
No products indexed under this heading.

Ethacrynic Acid (Potassium-depleting diuretics can cause hypokalemia and co-administration can result in digitalis toxicity). Products include:
- Edecrin Tablets 698

Felodipine (Concomitant use of digoxin and calcium channel blockers may result in the additive effects on AV node conduction).
No products indexed under this heading.

Fludrocortisone Acetate (Corticosteroids can cause hypokalemia or hypomagnesemia and potassium or magnesium depletion can sensitize the myocardium to digoxin resulting in digitalis toxicity).
No products indexed under this heading.

Flunisolide (Corticosteroids can cause hypokalemia or hypomagnesemia and potassium or magnesium depletion can sensitize the myocardium to digoxin resulting in digitalis toxicity). Products include:
- Aerobid/Aerobid-M 1153

Fluticasone Propionate (Corticosteroids can cause hypokalemia or hypomagnesemia and potassium or magnesium depletion can sensitize the myocardium to digoxin resulting in digitalis toxicity). Products include:
- Advair Diskus 100/50 1276
- Advair Diskus 250/50 1276
- Advair Diskus 500/50 1276
- Advair HFA 45/21 Inhalation Aerosol 1288
- Advair HFA 115/21 Inhalation Aerosol 1288
- Advair HFA 230/21 Inhalation Aerosol 1288
- Flonase Nasal Spray 1431
- Flovent Diskus 50 mcg 1435

Fluticasone Propionate HFA (Corticosteroids can cause hypokalemia or hypomagnesemia and potassium or magnesium depletion can sensitize the myocardium to digoxin resulting in digitalis toxicity).
Products include:
- Flovent HFA 1440

Furosemide (Potassium-depleting diuretics can cause hypokalemia and co-administration can result in digitalis toxicity). Products include:
- Furosemide Tablets 2186

Hydrochlorothiazide (Potassium-depleting diuretics can cause hypokalemia and co-administration can result in digitalis toxicity). Products include:
- Atacand HCT 642
- Avalide Tablets 892
- Avalide Tablets 2713
- Benicar HCT Tablets 1010
- Diovan HCT Tablets 2216
- Dyazide Capsules 1405
- Micardis HCT Tablets 854
- Prinzide Tablets 2092
- Tekturna HCT Tablets 2324
- Teveten HCT Tablets 517

Hydrocortisone (Corticosteroids can cause hypokalemia or hypomagnesemia and potassium or magnesium depletion can sensitize the myocardium to digoxin resulting in digitalis toxicity).
No products indexed under this heading.

Hydrocortisone Acetate (Corticosteroids can cause hypokalemia or hypomagnesemia and potassium or magnesium depletion can sensitize the myocardium to digoxin resulting in digitalis toxicity).
Products include:
- Analpram-HC 1140
- Pramosone 1141

Hydrocortisone Sodium Phosphate (Corticosteroids can cause hypokalemia or hypomagnesemia and potassium or magnesium depletion can sensitize the myocardium to digoxin resulting in digitalis toxicity).
No products indexed under this heading.

Hydrocortisone Sodium Succinate (Corticosteroids can cause hypokalemia or hypomagnesemia and potassium or magnesium depletion can sensitize the myocardium to digoxin resulting in digitalis toxicity).
No products indexed under this heading.

Hydroflumethiazide (Potassium-depleting diuretics can cause hypokalemia and co-administration can result in digitalis toxicity).
No products indexed under this heading.

Indomethacin (Raises the serum digoxin concentration due to reduction in clearance and/or volume of distribution of the drug, with the implication that digitalis intoxication may result). Products include:
- Indocin 2024

Indomethacin Sodium Trihydrate (Raises the serum digoxin concentration due to reduction in clearance and/or volume of distribution of the drug, with the implication that digitalis intoxication may result).
Products include:
- Indocin I.V. 2489

Isoproterenol Hydrochloride (Concomitant use of digoxin and sympathomimetics increases the risk of cardiac arrhythmias).
No products indexed under this heading.

Isoproterenol Sulfate (Concomitant use of digoxin and sympathomimetics increases the risk of cardiac arrhythmias).
No products indexed under this heading.

Isradipine (Concomitant use of digoxin and calcium channel blockers may result in the additive effects on AV node conduction). Products include:
- DynaCirc CR Controlled Release Tablets 1407

Itraconazole (Raises the serum digoxin concentration due to reduction in clearance and/or volume of distribution of the drug, with the implication that digitalis intoxication may result).
No products indexed under this heading.

Kaolin (May interfere with intestinal digoxin absorption, resulting in unexpectedly low serum concentrations).
No products indexed under this heading.

Labetalol Hydrochloride (Concomitant use of digoxin and beta-andrenergic blockers may result in the additive effects on AV node conduction).
No products indexed under this heading.

Levalbuterol Hydrochloride (Concomitant use of digoxin and sympathomimetics increases the risk of cardiac arrhythmias). Products include:
- Xopenex Inhalation Solution 3001
- Xopenex Inhalation Solution Concentrate 3005

Levobunolol Hydrochloride (Concomitant use of digoxin and beta-andrenergic blockers may result in the additive effects on AV node conduction).
No products indexed under this heading.

Levothyroxine Sodium (Thyroid administration to a digitalized, hypothyroid patient may increase the dose requirement of digoxin).
Products include:
- Levothroid Tablets 1170
- Levoxyl Tablets 1780
- Synthroid Tablets 507

Liothyronine Sodium (Thyroid administration to a digitalized, hypothyroid patient may increase the dose requirement of digoxin).
Products include:
- Cytomel Tablets 1778

Liotrix (Thyroid administration to a digitalized, hypothyroid patient may increase the dose requirement of digoxin).
No products indexed under this heading.

Magaldrate (Antacids may interfere with intestinal digoxin absorption, resulting in unexpectedly low serum concentrations; antacids may cause hypokalemia or hypomagnesemia and co-administration can cause digitalis toxicity).
No products indexed under this heading.

Magnesium Hydroxide (Antacids may interfere with intestinal digoxin absorption, resulting in unexpectedly low serum concentrations; antacids may cause hypokalemia or hypomagnesemia and co-administration can cause digitalis toxicity).
Products include:
- Fleet Pedia-Lax Chewable Tablets 1145
- Pepcid Complete Chewable Tablets 1771
- Extra Strength Rolaids Freshmint Tablets 1903
- Rolaids Multi-Symptom Berry Tablets 1903
- Rolaids Original Peppermint Tablets 1903

Magnesium Oxide (Antacids may interfere with intestinal digoxin absorption, resulting in unexpectedly low serum concentrations; antacids may cause hypokalemia or hypomagnesemia and co-administration can cause digitalis toxicity).
Products include:
- Beelith Tablets 813

Metaproterenol Sulfate (Concomitant use of digoxin and sympathomimetics increases the risk of cardiac arrhythmias).
No products indexed under this heading.

Metaraminol Bitartrate (Concomitant use of digoxin and sympathomimetics increases the risk of cardiac arrhythmias).
No products indexed under this heading.

Methacycline Hydrochloride (May increase digoxin absorption in patients who inactivate digoxin by bacterial metabolism in the lower intestine, so that digitalis intoxication may result).
No products indexed under this heading.

Methoxamine Hydrochloride (Concomitant use of digoxin and sympathomimetics increases the risk of cardiac arrhythmias).
No products indexed under this heading.

Methyclothiazide (Potassium-depleting diuretics can cause hypokalemia and co-administration can result in digitalis toxicity).
No products indexed under this heading.

Methylprednisolone Acetate (Corticosteroids can cause hypokalemia or hypomagnesemia and potassium or magnesium depletion can sensitize the myocardium to digoxin resulting in digitalis toxicity).
No products indexed under this heading.

Methylprednisolone Sodium Succinate (Corticosteroids can cause hypokalemia or hypomagnesemia and potassium or magnesium depletion can sensitize the myocardium to digoxin resulting in digitalis toxicity).
No products indexed under this heading.

Metipranolol Hydrochloride (Concomitant use of digoxin and beta-andrenergic blockers may result in the additive effects on AV node conduction).
No products indexed under this heading.

Metoclopramide Hydrochloride (May interfere with intestinal digoxin absorption, resulting in unexpectedly low serum concentrations).
No products indexed under this heading.

Metoprolol Succinate (Concomitant use of digoxin and beta-andrenergic blockers may result in the additive effects on AV node conduction). Products include:
Toprol-XL Tablets 666

Metoprolol Tartrate (Concomitant use of digoxin and beta-andrenergic blockers may result in the additive effects on AV node conduction).
No products indexed under this heading.

Mibefradil Dihydrochloride (Concomitant use of digoxin and calcium channel blockers may result in the additive effects on AV node conduction).
No products indexed under this heading.

Minocycline Hydrochloride (May increase digoxin absorption in patients who inactivate digoxin by bacterial metabolism in the lower intestine, so that digitalis intoxication may result). Products include:
Solodyn Extended Release Tablets 1938

Mometasone Furoate (Corticosteroids can cause hypokalemia or hypomagnesemia and potassium or magnesium depletion can sensitize the myocardium to digoxin resulting in digitalis toxicity). Products include:
Asmanex Twisthaler 2797
Elocon Cream 0.1% 2840
Elocon Lotion 0.1% 2841
Elocon Ointment 0.1% 2842

Mometasone Furoate Monohydrate (Corticosteroids can cause hypokalemia or hypomagnesemia and potassium or magnesium depletion can sensitize the myocardium to digoxin resulting in digitalis toxicity). Products include:
Nasonex Nasal Spray 2883

Nadolol (Concomitant use of digoxin and beta-andrenergic blockers may result in the additive effects on AV node conduction). Products include:
Nadolol Tablets 2191

Nebivolol (Concomitant use of digoxin and beta-andrenergic blockers may result in the additive effects on AV node conduction). Products include:
Bystolic Tablets 1155

Neomycin, oral (May interfere with intestinal digoxin absorption, resulting in unexpectedly low serum concentrations).
No products indexed under this heading.

Nicardipine Hydrochloride (Concomitant use of digoxin and calcium channel blockers may result in the additive effects on AV node conduction). Products include:
Cardene I.V. 1093

Nifedipine (Concomitant use of digoxin and calcium channel blockers may result in the additive effects on AV node conduction).
No products indexed under this heading.

Nimodipine (Concomitant use of digoxin and calcium channel blockers may result in the additive effects on AV node conduction). Products include:
Nimotop Capsules 790

Nisoldipine (Concomitant use of digoxin and calcium channel blockers may result in the additive effects on AV node conduction). Products include:
Sular Extended Release Tablets 2975

Norepinephrine Bitartrate (Concomitant use of digoxin and sympathomimetics increases the risk of cardiac arrhythmias).
No products indexed under this heading.

Oxytetracycline Hydrochloride (May increase digoxin absorption in patients who inactivate digoxin by bacterial metabolism in the lower intestine, so that digitalis intoxication may result).
No products indexed under this heading.

Pectin (May interfere with intestinal digoxin absorption, resulting in unexpectedly low serum concentrations).
No products indexed under this heading.

Penbutolol Sulfate (Concomitant use of digoxin and beta-andrenergic blockers may result in the additive effects on AV node conduction).
No products indexed under this heading.

Penicillamine (Co-administration has resulted in inconsistent reports regarding the effects of penicillamine on serum digoxin concentration). Products include:
Cuprimine Capsules 1986

Phenylephrine Bitartrate (Concomitant use of digoxin and sympathomimetics increases the risk of cardiac arrhythmias).
No products indexed under this heading.

Phenylephrine Hydrochloride (Concomitant use of digoxin and sympathomimetics increases the risk of cardiac arrhythmias). Products include:
Actifed Cold & Allergy Tablets 1895
Benadryl Allergy & Cold Kapgels 1895
Benadryl Allergy & Sinus Headache Kapgels 1895
Benadryl Severe Allergy & Sinus Headache Caplets 1897
Children's Benadryl-D Allergy & Sinus Liquid 1896
Benadryl-D Allergy & Sinus Tablet 1896
PediaCare Children's Allergy & Cold Liquid 1902
PediaCare Children's Decongestant Liquid 1902
PediaCare Children's Liquid Multi-Symptom Cold 1902
Sinutab Non-Drying Caplets 1905
Sinutab Sinus Caplets 1905
Children's Sudafed PE Cold & Cough Liquid 1907
Children's Sudafed PE Nasal Decongestant Liquid 1906
Sudafed PE Cold & Cough Caplets 1907
Sudafed PE Nasal Decongestant Tablets 1907
Sudafed PE Nighttime Cold Caplets 1907
Sudafed PE Non-Drying Sinus Caplets 1908
Sudafed PE Severe Cold Caplets 1908
Sudafed PE Sinus & Allergy Tablets 1908
Sudafed PE Sinus Headache Caplets 1908
Tylenol Allergy Multi-Symptom Caplets with Cool Burst and Rapid Release Gelcaps 1916
Tylenol Allergy Multi-Symptom Nighttime Caplets with Cool Burst 1916
Children's Tylenol Plus Cold Suspension Liquid 1912
Children's Tylenol Plus Cold & Allergy Suspension Liquid 1914
Children's Tylenol Plus Flu Suspension Liquid 1914
Children's Tylenol Plus Multi-Symptom Cold Suspension Liquid 1912
Tylenol Cold Head Congestion Daytime Caplets with Cool Burst 1910
Tylenol Cold Head Congestion Nighttime Caplets with Cool Burst 1910
Tylenol Cold Head Congestion Severe Daytime Caplets with Cool Burst 1910
Tylenol Cold Multi-Symptom Daytime Caplets with Cool Burst and Rapid Release Gels 1913
Tylenol Cold Multi-Symptom Daytime Liquid with Citrus Burst ... 1913
Tylenol Cold Multi-Symptom Nighttime Caplets with Cool Burst 1913
Tylenol Cold Multi-Symptom Nighttime Liquid with Cool Burst ... 1913
Tylenol Cold Multi-Symptom Severe Caplets with Cool Burst 1913
Tylenol Cold Multi-Symptom Severe Daytime Liquid with Citrus Burst 1913
Tylenol Sinus Congestion & Pain Daytime Caplets with Cool Burst and Gelcaps 1917
Tylenol Sinus Congestion & Pain Nighttime Caplets with Cool Burst 1917
Tylenol Sinus Congestion & Pain Severe Caplets with Cool Burst 1917
Vicks DayQuil Cold & Flu Multi-Symptom Relief .... ■■616
Vicks DayQuil LiquiCaps 2567
Vicks DayQuil Liquid 2567
Vicks DayQuil Multi-Symptom Cold/Flu Relief 2567

Phenylephrine Tannate (Concomitant use of digoxin and sympathomimetics increases the risk of cardiac arrhythmias).
No products indexed under this heading.

Phenylpropanolamine Hydrochloride (Concomitant use of digoxin and sympathomimetics increases the risk of cardiac arrhythmias).
No products indexed under this heading.

Pindolol (Concomitant use of digoxin and beta-andrenergic blockers may result in the additive effects on AV node conduction).
No products indexed under this heading.

Pirbuterol Acetate (Concomitant use of digoxin and sympathomimetics increases the risk of cardiac arrhythmias). Products include:
Maxair Autohaler 1705

Polythiazide (Potassium-depleting diuretics can cause hypokalemia and co-administration can result in digitalis toxicity).
No products indexed under this heading.

Prednisolone Acetate (Corticosteroids can cause hypokalemia or hypomagnesemia and potassium or magnesium depletion can sensitize the myocardium to digoxin resulting in digitalis toxicity). Products include:
Pred Forte Ophthalmic Suspension .... ⊙227
Pred Mild Ophthalmic Suspension .... ⊙230
Pred-G Ophthalmic Ointment .... ⊙229
Pred-G Ophthalmic Suspension .... ⊙228

Prednisolone Sodium Phosphate (Corticosteroids can cause hypokalemia or hypomagnesemia and potassium or magnesium depletion can sensitize the myocardium to digoxin resulting in digitalis toxicity).
No products indexed under this heading.

Prednisolone Tebutate (Corticosteroids can cause hypokalemia or hypomagnesemia and potassium or magnesium depletion can sensitize the myocardium to digoxin resulting in digitalis toxicity).
No products indexed under this heading.

Prednisone (Corticosteroids can cause hypokalemia or hypomagnesemia and potassium or magnesium depletion can sensitize the myocardium to digoxin resulting in digitalis toxicity).
No products indexed under this heading.

Propafenone Hydrochloride (Raises the serum digoxin concentration due to reduction in clearance and/or volume of distribution of the drug, with the implication that digitalis intoxication may result). Products include:
Rythmol Tablets 1586
Rythmol SR Capsules 1590

Propantheline Bromide (Decreases gut motility and may increase digoxin absorption).
No products indexed under this heading.

Propranolol Hydrochloride (Concomitant use of digoxin and beta-andrenergic blockers may result in the additive effects on AV node conduction). Products include:
InnoPran XL Extended Release Capsules 1484

Pseudoephedrine Hydrochloride (Concomitant use of digoxin and sympathomimetics increases the risk of cardiac arrhythmias). Products include:
Allegra-D 12 Hour Extended-Release Tablets 2687
Allegra-D 24 Hour Extended-Release Tablets 2690
Children's Motrin Cold Oral Suspension 1899
Sudafed 12 Hour Nasal Decongestant Non-Drowsy Caplets 1909
Sudafed 24 Hour Non-Drowsy Nasal Decongestant Tablets 1906
Children's Sudafed Nasal Decongestant Liquid 1906
Sudafed Nasal Decongestant Tablets 1906
Tylenol Cold Severe Congestion Daytime Caplets with Cool Burst 1912
Tylenol Sinus Severe Congestion Caplets with Cool Burst 1917
Vicks NyQuil LiquiCaps 2567
Vicks NyQuil Liquid 2567
Vicks NyQuil Multi-Symptom Cold/Flu Relief 2567
Zyrtec-D 12 Hour Extended Release Tablets 1923
Zyrtec-D Allergy & Congestion Extended-Release Tablets 1923

Pseudoephedrine Sulfate (Concomitant use of digoxin and sympathomimetics increases the risk of cardiac arrhythmias). Products include:

Clarinex-D 12-Hour Extended-Release Tablets 2831
Clarinex-D 24-Hour Extended-Release Tablets 2834

Quinidine (Raises the serum digoxin concentration due to reduction in clearance and/or volume of distribution of the drug, with the implication that digitalis intoxication may result).
No products indexed under this heading.

Quinidine Gluconate (Raises the serum digoxin concentration due to reduction in clearance and/or volume of distribution of the drug, with the implication that digitalis intoxication may result).
No products indexed under this heading.

Quinidine Hydrochloride (Raises the serum digoxin concentration due to reduction in clearance and/or volume of distribution of the drug, with the implication that digitalis intoxication may result).
No products indexed under this heading.

Quinidine Polygalacturonate (Raises the serum digoxin concentration due to reduction in clearance and/or volume of distribution of the drug, with the implication that digitalis intoxication may result).
No products indexed under this heading.

Quinidine Sulfate (Raises the serum digoxin concentration due to reduction in clearance and/or volume of distribution of the drug, with the implication that digitalis intoxication may result).
No products indexed under this heading.

Quinine (Co-administration has resulted in inconsistent reports regarding the effects of quinine on serum digoxin concentration).
No products indexed under this heading.

Rifampin (May decrease serum digoxin concentration, especially in patients with renal dysfunction, by increasing the non-renal clearance of digoxin).
No products indexed under this heading.

Salmeterol Xinafoate (Concomitant use of digoxin and sympathomimetics increases the risk of cardiac arrhythmias). Products include:
Advair Diskus 100/50 1276
Advair Diskus 250/50 1276
Advair Diskus 500/50 1276
Advair HFA 45/21 Inhalation Aerosol 1288
Advair HFA 115/21 Inhalation Aerosol 1288
Advair HFA 230/21 Inhalation Aerosol 1288
Serevent Diskus 1594

Sodium Bicarbonate (Antacids may interfere with intestinal digoxin absorption, resulting in unexpectedly low serum concentrations; antacids may cause hypokalemia or hypomagnesemia and co-administration can cause digitalis toxicity). Products include:
Ceo-Two Laxative Suppository 815

Sotalol Hydrochloride (Concomitant use of digoxin and beta-andrenergic blockers may result in the additive effects on AV node conduction).
No products indexed under this heading.

Spironolactone (Raises the serum digoxin concentration due to reduction in clearance and/or volume of distribution of the drug, with the implication that digitalis intoxication may result).
No products indexed under this heading.

Succinylcholine Chloride (May cause a sudden extrusion of potassium from muscle cells, and may thereby cause arrhythmias in digitalized patients).
No products indexed under this heading.

Sulfasalazine (May interfere with intestinal digoxin absorption, resulting in unexpectedly low serum concentrations).
No products indexed under this heading.

Terbutaline Sulfate (Concomitant use of digoxin and sympathomimetics increases the risk of cardiac arrhythmias).
No products indexed under this heading.

Tetracycline Hydrochloride (May increase digoxin absorption in patients who inactivate digoxin by bacterial metabolism in the lower intestine, so that digitalis intoxication may result). Products include:
Pylera Capsules 714

Thyroglobulin (Thyroid administration to a digitalized, hypothyroid patient may increase the dose requirement of digoxin).
No products indexed under this heading.

Thyroid (Thyroid administration to a digitalized, hypothyroid patient may increase the dose requirement of digoxin). Products include:
Naturethroid Tablets 2605

Thyroxine (Thyroid administration to a digitalized, hypothyroid patient may increase the dose requirement of digoxin).
No products indexed under this heading.

Thyroxine Sodium (Thyroid administration to a digitalized, hypothyroid patient may increase the dose requirement of digoxin).
No products indexed under this heading.

Timolol Hemihydrate (Concomitant use of digoxin and beta-andrenergic blockers may result in the additive effects on AV node conduction). Products include:
Betimol Ophthalmic Solution 3181

Timolol Maleate (Concomitant use of digoxin and beta-andrenergic blockers may result in the additive effects on AV node conduction). Products include:
Combigan Ophthalmic Solution 553
Cosopt Sterile Ophthalmic Solution 1969
Timoptic Sterile Ophthalmic Solution 2121
Timoptic in Ocudose 2124
Timoptic-XE Sterile Ophthalmic Gel Forming Solution 2125

Torsemide (Potassium-depleting diuretics can cause hypokalemia and co-administration can result in digitalis toxicity). Products include:
Demadex Injection 2630
Demadex Tablets 2630

Triamcinolone (Corticosteroids can cause hypokalemia or hypomagnesemia and potassium or magnesium depletion can sensitize the myocardium to digoxin resulting in digitalis toxicity).
No products indexed under this heading.

Triamcinolone Acetonide (Corticosteroids can cause hypokalemia or hypomagnesemia and potassium or magnesium depletion can sensitize the myocardium to digoxin resulting in digitalis toxicity). Products include:
Azmacort Inhalation Aerosol 407
Nasacort AQ Nasal Spray 2765
Triesence Injectable Suspension .... ⊙ 209

Triamcinolone Diacetate (Corticosteroids can cause hypokalemia or hypomagnesemia and potassium or magnesium depletion can sensitize the myocardium to digoxin resulting in digitalis toxicity).
No products indexed under this heading.

Triamcinolone Hexacetonide (Corticosteroids can cause hypokalemia or hypomagnesemia and potassium or magnesium depletion can sensitize the myocardium to digoxin resulting in digitalis toxicity).
No products indexed under this heading.

Troleandomycin (Macrolide antibiotics may possibly increase digoxin absorption in patients who inactivate digoxin by bacterial metabolism in the lower intestine, so that digitalis intoxication may result).
No products indexed under this heading.

Verapamil Hydrochloride (Raises the serum digoxin concentration due to reduction in clearance and/or volume of distribution of the drug, with the implication that digitalis intoxication may result). Products include:
Tarka Tablets 511

Food Interactions

Meal, high in bran fiber (The amount of digoxin from an oral dose may be reduced).

Meal, unspecified (Slows the rate of absorption).

LANTUS INJECTION

(Insulin glargine) 2749
May interact with ACE inhibitors, beta blockers, corticosteroids, diuretics, fibrates, oral hypoglycemic agents, lithium preparations, monoamine oxidase inhibitors, oral contraceptives, phenothiazines, protease inhibitors, salicylates, sympathomimetics, thyroid preparations, and certain other agents. Compounds in these categories include:

Acarbose (May increase the blood-glucose-lowering effect and susceptibility to hypoglycemia). Products include:
Precose Tablets 792

Acebutolol Hydrochloride (Beta-blockers may either potentiate or weaken the blood-glucose-lowering effect of insulin; signs of hypoglycemia may be reduced or absent with co-administration).
No products indexed under this heading.

Albuterol (Sympathomimetic agents may reduce the blood-glucose-lowering effect of insulin).
No products indexed under this heading.

Albuterol Sulfate (Sympathomimetic agents may reduce the blood-glucose-lowering effect of insulin). Products include:
Combivent Inhalation Aerosol 845
ProAir HFA Inhalation Aerosol 3113
Proventil HFA Inhalation Aerosol 2914
Ventolin HFA Inhalation Aerosol 1638

Amiloride Hydrochloride (Diuretics may reduce the blood-glucose-lowering effect of insulin).
No products indexed under this heading.

Amprenavir (May reduce the blood-glucose lowering effect of insulin).
No products indexed under this heading.

Aspirin (May increase the blood-glucose-lowering effect and susceptibility to hypoglycemia). Products include:
Aggrenox Capsules 819
Bayer Aspirin 750
Percodan Tablets 1130
St. Joseph 81 mg Aspirin Chewable and Enteric Coated Tablets 1903

Aspirin, Enteric Coated (May increase the blood-glucose-lowering effect and susceptibility to hypoglycemia).
No products indexed under this heading.

Aspirin Buffered (May increase the blood-glucose-lowering effect and susceptibility to hypoglycemia).
No products indexed under this heading.

Atenolol (Beta-blockers may either potentiate or weaken the blood-glucose-lowering effect of insulin; signs of hypoglycemia may be reduced or absent with co-administration).
No products indexed under this heading.

Benazepril Hydrochloride (May increase the blood-glucose-lowering effect and susceptibility to hypoglycemia).
No products indexed under this heading.

Bendroflumethiazide (Diuretics may reduce the blood-glucose-lowering effect of insulin).
No products indexed under this heading.

Betamethasone Acetate (Co-administration with corticosteroids may reduce the blood-glucose-lowering effect of insulin).
No products indexed under this heading.

Betamethasone Sodium Phosphate (Co-administration with corticosteroids may reduce the blood-glucose-lowering effect of insulin).
No products indexed under this heading.

Betaxolol Hydrochloride (Beta-blockers may either potentiate or weaken the blood-glucose-lowering effect of insulin; signs of hypoglycemia may be reduced or absent with co-administration).
No products indexed under this heading.

Bisoprolol Fumarate (Beta-blockers may either potentiate or weaken the blood-glucose-lowering effect of insulin; signs of hypoglycemia may be reduced or absent with co-administration).
No products indexed under this heading.

Budesonide (Co-administration with corticosteroids may reduce the blood-glucose-lowering effect of insulin). Products include:
Pulmicort Flexhaler 654
Symbicort 80/4.5 Inhalation Aerosol........................ 659
Symbicort 160/4.5 Inhalation Aerosol........................ 659

Bumetanide (Diuretics may reduce the blood-glucose-lowering effect of insulin).
No products indexed under this heading.

Captopril (May increase the blood-glucose-lowering effect and susceptibility to hypoglycemia). Products include:
Captopril Tablets 2182

Carteolol Hydrochloride (Beta-blockers may either potentiate or weaken the blood-glucose-lowering effect of insulin; signs of hypoglycemia may be reduced or absent with co-administration).
No products indexed under this heading.

Chlorothiazide (Diuretics may reduce the blood-glucose-lowering effect of insulin).
No products indexed under this heading.

Chlorothiazide Sodium (Diuretics may reduce the blood-glucose-lowering effect of insulin). Products include:
Intravenous Sodium Diuril 2490

Chlorpromazine (Phenothiazine derivatives may reduce the blood-glucose-lowering effect of insulin).
No products indexed under this heading.

Chlorpromazine Hydrochloride (Phenothiazine derivatives may reduce the blood-glucose-lowering effect of insulin).
No products indexed under this heading.

Chlorpropamide (May increase the blood-glucose-lowering effect and susceptibility to hypoglycemia).
No products indexed under this heading.

Chlorthalidone (Diuretics may reduce the blood-glucose-lowering effect of insulin). Products include:
Clorpres Tablets 2185

Choline Magnesium Trisalicylate (May increase the blood-glucose-lowering effect and susceptibility to hypoglycemia).
No products indexed under this heading.

Ciclesonide (Co-administration with corticosteroids may reduce the blood-glucose-lowering effect of insulin). Products include:
Alvesco Inhalation Aerosol 2985
Omnaris Nasal Spray 2998

Clofibrate (May increase the blood-glucose-lowering effect and susceptibility to hypoglycemia).
No products indexed under this heading.

Clonidine (Signs of hypoglycemia may be reduced or absent with co-administration). Products include:
Catapres-TTS 842

Clonidine Hydrochloride (Signs of hypoglycemia may be reduced or absent with co-administration). Products include:
Catapres Tablets 841
Clorpres Tablets 2185

Cortisone Acetate (Co-administration with corticosteroids may reduce the blood-glucose-lowering effect of insulin).
No products indexed under this heading.

Danazol (May reduce the blood-glucose-lowering effect of insulin).
No products indexed under this heading.

Darunavir (May reduce the blood-glucose lowering effect of insulin).
No products indexed under this heading.

Desogestrel (Oral contraceptives may reduce the blood-glucose-lowering effect of insulin). Products include:
Mircette Tablets 1034

Dexamethasone (Co-administration with corticosteroids may reduce the blood-glucose-lowering effect of insulin). Products include:
Ciprodex Otic Suspension 541

Dexamethasone Acetate (Co-administration with corticosteroids may reduce the blood-glucose-lowering effect of insulin).
No products indexed under this heading.

Dexamethasone Sodium Phosphate (Co-administration with corticosteroids may reduce the blood-glucose-lowering effect of insulin).
No products indexed under this heading.

Diflunisal (May increase the blood-glucose-lowering effect and susceptibility to hypoglycemia).
No products indexed under this heading.

Disopyramide Phosphate (May increase the blood-glucose-lowering effect and susceptibility to hypoglycemia).
No products indexed under this heading.

Dobutamine Hydrochloride (Sympathomimetic agents may reduce the blood-glucose-lowering effect of insulin).
No products indexed under this heading.

Dopamine Hydrochloride (Sympathomimetic agents may reduce the blood-glucose-lowering effect of insulin).
No products indexed under this heading.

Enalapril Maleate (May increase the blood-glucose-lowering effect and susceptibility to hypoglycemia).
No products indexed under this heading.

Enalaprilat (May increase the blood-glucose-lowering effect and susceptibility to hypoglycemia).
No products indexed under this heading.

Ephedrine Hydrochloride (Sympathomimetic agents may reduce the blood-glucose-lowering effect of insulin).
No products indexed under this heading.

Ephedrine Sulfate (Sympathomimetic agents may reduce the blood-glucose-lowering effect of insulin).
No products indexed under this heading.

Ephedrine Tannate (Sympathomimetic agents may reduce the blood-glucose-lowering effect of insulin).
No products indexed under this heading.

Epinephrine (Sympathomimetic agents may reduce the blood-glucose-lowering effect of insulin). Products include:
EpiPen 1024

Epinephrine Bitartrate (Sympathomimetic agents may reduce the blood-glucose-lowering effect of insulin).
No products indexed under this heading.

Epinephrine Hydrochloride (Sympathomimetic agents may reduce the blood-glucose-lowering effect of insulin).
No products indexed under this heading.

Esmolol Hydrochloride (Beta-blockers may either potentiate or weaken the blood-glucose-lowering effect of insulin; signs of hypoglycemia may be reduced or absent with co-administration).
No products indexed under this heading.

Ethacrynic Acid (Diuretics may reduce the blood-glucose-lowering effect of insulin). Products include:
Edecrin Tablets 698

Ethinyl Estradiol (Oral contraceptives may reduce the blood-glucose-lowering effect of insulin). Products include:
Lybrel Tablets 3204
Mircette Tablets 1034
NuvaRing 2897
Ortho-Cyclen/Ortho Tri-Cyclen 2449
Ortho Evra Transdermal System 2437
Ortho Tri-Cyclen Lo Tablets 2458
Seasonique Tablets 1046
Yaz Tablets 805

Ethynodiol Diacetate (Oral contraceptives may reduce the blood-glucose-lowering effect of insulin).
No products indexed under this heading.

Fenofibrate (May increase the blood-glucose-lowering effect and susceptibility to hypoglycemia). Products include:
Fenoglide Tablets 2960
Tricor Tablets 520

Fludrocortisone Acetate (Co-administration with corticosteroids may reduce the blood-glucose-lowering effect of insulin).
No products indexed under this heading.

Flunisolide (Co-administration with corticosteroids may reduce the blood-glucose-lowering effect of insulin). Products include:
Aerobid/Aerobid-M 1153

Fluoxetine Hydrochloride (May increase the blood-glucose-lowering effect and susceptibility to hypoglycemia). Products include:
Prozac Weekly Capsules 1852
Prozac Pulvules and Liquid 1852
Symbyax Capsules 1871

Fluphenazine Decanoate (Phenothiazine derivatives may reduce the blood-glucose-lowering effect of insulin).
No products indexed under this heading.

Fluphenazine Enanthate (Phenothiazine derivatives may reduce the blood-glucose-lowering effect of insulin).
No products indexed under this heading.

Fluphenazine Hydrochloride (Phenothiazine derivatives may reduce the blood-glucose-lowering effect of insulin).
No products indexed under this heading.

Fluticasone Propionate (Co-administration with corticosteroids may reduce the blood-glucose-lowering effect of insulin). Products include:
Advair Diskus 100/50 1276
Advair Diskus 250/50 1276
Advair Diskus 500/50 1276
Advair HFA 45/21 Inhalation Aerosol........................ 1288
Advair HFA 115/21 Inhalation Aerosol........................ 1288
Advair HFA 230/21 Inhalation Aerosol........................ 1288
Flonase Nasal Spray 1431
Flovent Diskus 50 mcg 1435

Fluticasone Propionate HFA (Co-administration with corticosteroids may reduce the blood-glucose-lowering effect of insulin). Products include:
Flovent HFA 1440

Fosamprenavir Calcium (May reduce the blood-glucose lowering effect of insulin). Products include:
Lexiva Oral Suspension 1510
Lexiva Tablets 1510

Fosinopril Sodium (May increase the blood-glucose-lowering effect and susceptibility to hypoglycemia).
No products indexed under this heading.

Furosemide (Diuretics may reduce the blood-glucose-lowering effect of insulin). Products include:
Furosemide Tablets 2186

Gemfibrozil (May increase the blood-glucose-lowering effect and susceptibility to hypoglycemia).
No products indexed under this heading.

Glimepiride (May increase the blood-glucose-lowering effect and susceptibility to hypoglycemia). Products include:
Avandaryl Tablets 1344
Duetact Tablets 3085

Glipizide (May increase the blood-glucose-lowering effect and susceptibility to hypoglycemia).
No products indexed under this heading.

Glyburide (May increase the blood-glucose-lowering effect and susceptibility to hypoglycemia).
No products indexed under this heading.

Guanethidine Monosulfate (Signs of hypoglycemia may be reduced or absent with co-administration).
No products indexed under this heading.

Hydrochlorothiazide (Diuretics may reduce the blood-glucose-lowering effect of insulin). Products include:
Atacand HCT 642
Avalide Tablets 892
Avalide Tablets 2713
Benicar HCT Tablets 1010
Diovan HCT Tablets 2216
Dyazide Capsules 1405
Micardis HCT Tablets 854
Prinzide Tablets 2092
Tekturna HCT Tablets 2324
Teveten HCT Tablets 517

Hydrocortisone (Co-administration with corticosteroids may reduce the blood-glucose-lowering effect of insulin).
No products indexed under this heading.

Hydrocortisone Acetate (Co-administration with corticosteroids may reduce the blood-glucose-lowering effect of insulin). Products include:
Analpram-HC 1140
Pramosone 1141

Hydrocortisone Sodium Phosphate (Co-administration with corticosteroids may reduce the blood-glucose-lowering effect of insulin).
No products indexed under this heading.

Hydrocortisone Sodium Succinate (Co-administration with corticosteroids may reduce the blood-glucose-lowering effect of insulin).
No products indexed under this heading.

Hydroflumethiazide (Diuretics may reduce the blood-glucose-lowering effect of insulin).
No products indexed under this heading.

Indapamide (Diuretics may reduce the blood-glucose-lowering effect of insulin). Products include:
Indapamide Tablets 2188

Indinavir Sulfate (May reduce the blood-glucose lowering effect of insulin). Products include:
Crixivan Capsules 1979

Isocarboxazid (May increase the blood-glucose-lowering effect and susceptibility to hypoglycemia). Products include:
Marplan Tablets 3177

Isoniazid (May reduce the blood-glucose-lowering effect of insulin).
No products indexed under this heading.

Isoproterenol Hydrochloride (Sympathomimetic agents may reduce the blood-glucose-lowering effect of insulin).
No products indexed under this heading.

Isoproterenol Sulfate (Sympathomimetic agents may reduce the blood-glucose-lowering effect of insulin).
No products indexed under this heading.

Labetalol Hydrochloride (Beta-blockers may either potentiate or weaken the blood-glucose-lowering effect of insulin; signs of hypoglycemia may be reduced or absent with co-administration).
No products indexed under this heading.

Levalbuterol Hydrochloride (Sympathomimetic agents may reduce the blood-glucose-lowering effect of insulin). Products include:
Xopenex Inhalation Solution 3001
Xopenex Inhalation Solution Concentrate 3005

Levobunolol Hydrochloride (Beta-blockers may either potentiate or weaken the blood-glucose-lowering effect of insulin; signs of hypoglycemia may be reduced or absent with co-administration).
No products indexed under this heading.

Levonorgestrel (Oral contraceptives may reduce the blood-glucose-lowering effect of insulin). Products include:
Climara Pro Transdermal System 768
Lybrel Tablets 3204
Mirena Intrauterine System 779
Plan B Tablets 1044
Seasonique Tablets 1046

Levothyroxine Sodium (May reduce the blood-glucose-lowering effect of insulin). Products include:
Levothroid Tablets 1170
Levoxyl Tablets 1780
Synthroid Tablets 507

Liothyronine Sodium (May reduce the blood-glucose-lowering effect of insulin). Products include:
Cytomel Tablets 1778

Liotrix (May reduce the blood-glucose-lowering effect of insulin).
No products indexed under this heading.

Lisinopril (May increase the blood-glucose-lowering effect and susceptibility to hypoglycemia). Products include:
Prinivil Tablets 2087
Prinzide Tablets 2092

Lithium (May either potentiate or weaken the blood-glucose-lowering effect of insulin).
No products indexed under this heading.

Lithium Carbonate (May either potentiate or weaken the blood-glucose-lowering effect of insulin).
No products indexed under this heading.

Lithium Citrate (May either potentiate or weaken the blood-glucose-lowering effect of insulin).
No products indexed under this heading.

Lopinavir (May reduce the blood-glucose lowering effect of insulin). Products include:
Kaletra 452

Magnesium Salicylate (May increase the blood-glucose-lowering effect and susceptibility to hypoglycemia).
No products indexed under this heading.

Mesoridazine Besylate (Phenothiazine derivatives may reduce the blood-glucose-lowering effect of insulin).
No products indexed under this heading.

Mestranol (Oral contraceptives may reduce the blood-glucose-lowering effect of insulin).
No products indexed under this heading.

Metaproterenol Sulfate (Sympathomimetic agents may reduce the blood-glucose-lowering effect of insulin).
No products indexed under this heading.

Metaraminol Bitartrate (Sympathomimetic agents may reduce the blood-glucose-lowering effect of insulin).
No products indexed under this heading.

Metformin Hydrochloride (May increase the blood-glucose-lowering effect and susceptibility to hypoglycemia). Products include:
ActoPlus Met Tablets 3071
Avandamet Tablets 1336
Janumet Tablets 2041
PrandiMet Tablets 2967

Methotrimeprazine (Phenothiazine derivatives may reduce the blood-glucose-lowering effect of insulin).
No products indexed under this heading.

Methoxamine Hydrochloride (Sympathomimetic agents may reduce the blood-glucose-lowering effect of insulin).
No products indexed under this heading.

Methyclothiazide (Diuretics may reduce the blood-glucose-lowering effect of insulin).
No products indexed under this heading.

Methylprednisolone Acetate (Co-administration with corticosteroids may reduce the blood-glucose-lowering effect of insulin).
No products indexed under this heading.

Methylprednisolone Sodium Succinate (Co-administration with corticosteroids may reduce the blood-glucose-lowering effect of insulin).
No products indexed under this heading.

Metipranolol Hydrochloride (Beta-blockers may either potentiate or weaken the blood-glucose-lowering effect of insulin; signs of hypoglycemia may be reduced or absent with co-administration).
No products indexed under this heading.

Metolazone (Diuretics may reduce the blood-glucose-lowering effect of insulin).
No products indexed under this heading.

Metoprolol Succinate (Beta-blockers may either potentiate or weaken the blood-glucose-lowering effect of insulin; signs of hypoglycemia may be reduced or absent with co-administration). Products include:
Toprol-XL Tablets 666

Metoprolol Tartrate (Beta-blockers may either potentiate or weaken the blood-glucose-lowering effect of insulin; signs of hypoglycemia may be reduced or absent with co-administration).
No products indexed under this heading.

Miglitol (May increase the blood-glucose-lowering effect and susceptibility to hypoglycemia).
No products indexed under this heading.

Moclobemide (May increase the blood-glucose-lowering effect and susceptibility to hypoglycemia).
No products indexed under this heading.

Moexipril Hydrochloride (May increase the blood-glucose-lowering effect and susceptibility to hypoglycemia).
No products indexed under this heading.

Mometasone Furoate (Co-administration with corticosteroids may reduce the blood-glucose-lowering effect of insulin). Products include:
Asmanex Twisthaler 2797
Elocon Cream 0.1% 2840
Elocon Lotion 0.1% 2841
Elocon Ointment 0.1% 2842

Mometasone Furoate Monohydrate (Co-administration with corticosteroids may reduce the blood-glucose-lowering effect of insulin). Products include:
Nasonex Nasal Spray 2883

Nadolol (Beta-blockers may either potentiate or weaken the blood-glucose-lowering effect of insulin; signs of hypoglycemia may be reduced or absent with co-administration). Products include:
Nadolol Tablets 2191

Nateglinide (May increase the blood-glucose-lowering effect and susceptibility to hypoglycemia). Products include:
Starlix Tablets 2314

Nebivolol (Beta-blockers may either potentiate or weaken the blood-glucose-lowering effect of insulin; signs of hypoglycemia may be reduced or absent with co-administration). Products include:
Bystolic Tablets 1155

Nelfinavir Mesylate (May reduce the blood-glucose lowering effect of insulin).
No products indexed under this heading.

Norepinephrine Bitartrate (Sympathomimetic agents may reduce the blood-glucose-lowering effect of insulin).
No products indexed under this heading.

Norethindrone (Oral contraceptives may reduce the blood-glucose-lowering effect of insulin). Products include:
Ortho Micronor Tablets 2446

Norethynodrel (Oral contraceptives may reduce the blood-glucose-lowering effect of insulin).
No products indexed under this heading.

Norgestimate (Oral contraceptives may reduce the blood-glucose-lowering effect of insulin). Products include:
Ortho-Cyclen/Ortho Tri-Cyclen 2449
Ortho Tri-Cyclen Lo Tablets 2458

Norgestrel (Oral contraceptives may reduce the blood-glucose-lowering effect of insulin).
No products indexed under this heading.

Octreotide Acetate (May increase the blood-glucose-lowering effect and susceptibility to hypoglycemia). Products include:
Sandostatin Injection 2300
Sandostatin LAR Depot 2302

Pargyline Hydrochloride (May increase the blood-glucose-lowering effect and susceptibility to hypoglycemia).
No products indexed under this heading.

Penbutolol Sulfate (Beta-blockers may either potentiate or weaken the blood-glucose-lowering effect of insulin; signs of hypoglycemia may be reduced or absent with co-administration).
No products indexed under this heading.

Pentamidine Isethionate (May cause hypoglycemia, which may sometimes be followed by hyperglycemia).
No products indexed under this heading.

Perindopril Erbumine (May increase the blood-glucose-lowering effect and susceptibility to hypoglycemia). Products include:
Aceon Tablets (2 mg, 4 mg, 8 mg) 3038

Perphenazine (Phenothiazine derivatives may reduce the blood-glucose-lowering effect of insulin).
No products indexed under this heading.

Phenelzine Sulfate (May increase the blood-glucose-lowering effect and susceptibility to hypoglycemia).
No products indexed under this heading.

IMPORTANT NOTE: Always consult each drug listing in the patient's regimen for possible interactions.

Phenylephrine Bitartrate (Sympathomimetic agents may reduce the blood-glucose-lowering effect of insulin).
No products indexed under this heading.

Phenylephrine Hydrochloride (Sympathomimetic agents may reduce the blood-glucose-lowering effect of insulin). Products include:
Actifed Cold & Allergy Tablets 1895
Benadryl Allergy & Cold Kapgels 1895
Benadryl Allergy & Sinus Headache Kapgels 1895
Benadryl Severe Allergy & Sinus Headache Caplets 1897
Children's Benadryl-D Allergy & Sinus Liquid................................ 1896
Benadryl-D Allergy & Sinus Tablet 1896
PediaCare Children's Allergy & Cold Liquid 1902
PediaCare Children's Decongestant Liquid.................... 1902
PediaCare Children's Liquid Multi-Symptom Cold..................... 1902
Sinutab Non-Drying Caplets 1905
Sinutab Sinus Caplets 1905
Children's Sudafed PE Cold & Cough Liquid 1907
Children's Sudafed PE Nasal Decongestant Liquid.................... 1906
Sudafed PE Cold & Cough Caplets.. 1907
Sudafed PE Nasal Decongestant Tablets.. 1907
Sudafed PE Nighttime Cold Caplets.. 1907
Sudafed PE Non-Drying Sinus Caplets.. 1908
Sudafed PE Severe Cold Caplets 1908
Sudafed PE Sinus & Allergy Tablets 1908
Sudafed PE Sinus Headache Caplets.. 1908
Tylenol Allergy Multi-Symptom Caplets with Cool Burst and Rapid Release Gelcaps................ 1916
Tylenol Allergy Multi-Symptom Nighttime Caplets with Cool Burst.. 1916
Children's Tylenol Plus Cold Suspension Liquid 1912
Children's Tylenol Plus Cold & Allergy Suspension Liquid............ 1914
Children's Tylenol Plus Flu Suspension Liquid 1914
Children's Tylenol Plus Multi-Symptom Cold Suspension Liquid 1912
Tylenol Cold Head Congestion Daytime Caplets with Cool Burst.. 1910
Tylenol Cold Head Congestion Nighttime Caplets with Cool Burst.. 1910
Tylenol Cold Head Congestion Severe Daytime Caplets with Cool Burst.................................. 1910
Tylenol Cold Multi-Symptom Daytime Caplets with Cool Burst and Rapid Release Gels....... 1913
Tylenol Cold Multi-Symptom Daytime Liquid with Citrus Burst ... 1913
Tylenol Cold Multi-Symptom Nighttime Caplets with Cool Burst.. 1913
Tylenol Cold Multi-Symptom Nighttime Liquid with Cool Burst... 1913
Tylenol Cold Multi-Symptom Severe Caplets with Cool Burst..... 1913
Tylenol Cold Multi-Symptom Severe Daytime Liquid with Citrus Burst................................ 1913
Tylenol Sinus Congestion & Pain Daytime Caplets with Cool Burst and Gelcaps...................... 1917
Tylenol Sinus Congestion & Pain Nighttime Caplets with Cool Burst.. 1917
Tylenol Sinus Congestion & Pain Severe Caplets with Cool Burst..... 1917
Vicks DayQuil Cold & Flu Multi-Symptom Relief .... ▣616
Vicks DayQuil LiquiCaps 2567
Vicks DayQuil Liquid 2567
Vicks DayQuil Multi-Symptom Cold/Flu Relief.............................. 2567

Phenylephrine Tannate (Sympathomimetic agents may reduce the blood-glucose-lowering effect of insulin).
No products indexed under this heading.

Phenylpropanolamine Hydrochloride (Sympathomimetic agents may reduce the blood-glucose-lowering effect of insulin).
No products indexed under this heading.

Pindolol (Beta-blockers may either potentiate or weaken the blood-glucose-lowering effect of insulin; signs of hypoglycemia may be reduced or absent with co-administration).
No products indexed under this heading.

Pioglitazone Hydrochloride (May increase the blood-glucose-lowering effect and susceptibility to hypoglycemia). Products include:
ActoPlus Met Tablets 3071
Actos Tablets 3077
Duetact Tablets 3085

Pirbuterol Acetate (Sympathomimetic agents may reduce the blood-glucose-lowering effect of insulin). Products include:
Maxair Autohaler 1705

Polythiazide (Diuretics may reduce the blood-glucose-lowering effect of insulin).
No products indexed under this heading.

Prednisolone Acetate (Co-administration with corticosteroids may reduce the blood-glucose-lowering effect of insulin). Products include:
Pred Forte Ophthalmic Suspension .... ⊙227
Pred Mild Ophthalmic Suspension .... ⊙230
Pred-G Ophthalmic Ointment .... ⊙229
Pred-G Ophthalmic Suspension ...... ⊙228

Prednisolone Sodium Phosphate (Co-administration with corticosteroids may reduce the blood-glucose-lowering effect of insulin).
No products indexed under this heading.

Prednisolone Tebutate (Co-administration with corticosteroids may reduce the blood-glucose-lowering effect of insulin).
No products indexed under this heading.

Prednisone (Co-administration with corticosteroids may reduce the blood-glucose-lowering effect of insulin).
No products indexed under this heading.

Procarbazine Hydrochloride (May increase the blood-glucose-lowering effect and susceptibility to hypoglycemia).
No products indexed under this heading.

Prochlorperazine (Phenothiazine derivatives may reduce the blood-glucose-lowering effect of insulin).
No products indexed under this heading.

Promethazine Hydrochloride (Phenothiazine derivatives may reduce the blood-glucose-lowering effect of insulin).
No products indexed under this heading.

Propoxyphene Hydrochloride (May increase the blood-glucose-lowering effect and susceptibility to hypoglycemia).
No products indexed under this heading.

Propoxyphene Napsylate (May increase the blood-glucose-lowering effect and susceptibility to hypoglycemia).
No products indexed under this heading.

Propranolol Hydrochloride (Beta-blockers may either potentiate or weaken the blood-glucose-lowering effect of insulin; signs of hypoglycemia may be reduced or absent with co-administration). Products include:
InnoPran XL Extended Release Capsules...................................... 1484

Pseudoephedrine Hydrochloride (Sympathomimetic agents may reduce the blood-glucose-lowering effect of insulin). Products include:
Allegra-D 12 Hour Extended-Release Tablets............ 2687
Allegra-D 24 Hour Extended-Release Tablets............ 2690
Children's Motrin Cold Oral Suspension 1899
Sudafed 12 Hour Nasal Decongestant Non-Drowsy Caplets.................................... 1909
Sudafed 24 Hour Non-Drowsy Nasal Decongestant Tablets........ 1906
Children's Sudafed Nasal Decongestant Liquid.................... 1906
Sudafed Nasal Decongestant Tablets 1906
Tylenol Cold Severe Congestion Daytime Caplets with Cool Burst.. 1912
Tylenol Sinus Severe Congestion Caplets with Cool Burst 1917
Vicks NyQuil LiquiCaps 2567
Vicks NyQuil Liquid 2567
Vicks NyQuil Multi-Symptom Cold/Flu Relief............................ 2567
Zyrtec-D 12 Hour Extended Release Tablets.............................. 1923
Zyrtec-D Allergy & Congestion Extended-Release Tablets............ 1923

Pseudoephedrine Sulfate (Sympathomimetic agents may reduce the blood-glucose-lowering effect of insulin). Products include:
Clarinex-D 12-Hour Extended-Release Tablets............ 2831
Clarinex-D 24-Hour Extended-Release Tablets............ 2834

Quinapril Hydrochloride (May increase the blood-glucose-lowering effect and susceptibility to hypoglycemia).
No products indexed under this heading.

Ramipril (May increase the blood-glucose-lowering effect and susceptibility to hypoglycemia).
No products indexed under this heading.

Rasagiline Mesylate (May increase the blood-glucose-lowering effect and susceptibility to hypoglycemia). Products include:
Azilect Tablets 3106

Repaglinide (May increase the blood-glucose-lowering effect and susceptibility to hypoglycemia). Products include:
PrandiMet Tablets 2967
Prandin Tablets 2971

Reserpine (Signs of hypoglycemia may be reduced or absent with co-administration).
No products indexed under this heading.

Ritonavir (May reduce the blood-glucose lowering effect of insulin). Products include:
Kaletra 452
Norvir 489

Rosiglitazone Maleate (May increase the blood-glucose-lowering effect and susceptibility to hypoglycemia). Products include:
Avandamet Tablets 1336
Avandaryl Tablets 1344
Avandia Tablets 1351

Salmeterol Xinafoate (Sympathomimetic agents may reduce the blood-glucose-lowering effect of insulin). Products include:
Advair Diskus 100/50 1276
Advair Diskus 250/50 1276
Advair Diskus 500/50 1276
Advair HFA 45/21 Inhalation Aerosol.. 1288
Advair HFA 115/21 Inhalation Aerosol.. 1288
Advair HFA 230/21 Inhalation Aerosol.. 1288
Serevent Diskus 1594

Salsalate (May increase the blood-glucose-lowering effect and susceptibility to hypoglycemia).
No products indexed under this heading.

Saquinavir (May reduce the blood-glucose lowering effect of insulin).
No products indexed under this heading.

Saquinavir Mesylate (May reduce the blood-glucose lowering effect of insulin).
No products indexed under this heading.

Selegiline (May increase the blood-glucose-lowering effect and susceptibility to hypoglycemia). Products include:
Emsam Transdermal System 905

Selegiline Hydrochloride (May increase the blood-glucose-lowering effect and susceptibility to hypoglycemia). Products include:
Eldepryl Capsules 3052

Sitagliptin Phosphate (May increase the blood-glucose-lowering effect and susceptibility to hypoglycemia). Products include:
Janumet Tablets 2041
Januvia Tablets 2048

Somatropin (May reduce the blood-glucose-lowering effect of insulin). Products include:
Genotropin Lyophilized Powder 2547
Humatrope Vials and Cartridges 1838
Nutropin for Injection 1208
Nutropin AQ Injection 1212
Nutropin AQ NuSpin Injection 1212
Nutropin AQ Pen 1212
Nutropin AQ Pen Cartridge 1212

Sotalol Hydrochloride (Beta-blockers may either potentiate or weaken the blood-glucose-lowering effect of insulin; signs of hypoglycemia may be reduced or absent with co-administration).
No products indexed under this heading.

Spirapril Hydrochloride (May increase the blood-glucose-lowering effect and susceptibility to hypoglycemia).
No products indexed under this heading.

Spironolactone (Diuretics may reduce the blood-glucose-lowering effect of insulin).
No products indexed under this heading.

Sulfamethoxazole (Co-administration with sulfonamide antibiotics may increase the blood-glucose-lowering effect and susceptibility to hypoglycemia).
No products indexed under this heading.

Sulfisoxazole Acetyl (Co-administration with sulfonamide antibiotics may increase the blood-glucose-lowering effect and susceptibility to hypoglycemia).
No products indexed under this heading.

Terbutaline Sulfate (Sympathomimetic agents may reduce the blood-glucose-lowering effect of insulin).
No products indexed under this heading.

Thioridazine Hydrochloride (Phenothiazine derivatives may reduce the blood-glucose-lowering effect of insulin). Products include:
Thioridazine Hydrochloride Tablets 2195

Thyroglobulin (May reduce the blood-glucose-lowering effect of insulin).
No products indexed under this heading.

Thyroid (May reduce the blood-glucose-lowering effect of insulin). Products include:
Naturethroid Tablets 2605

Thyroxine (May reduce the blood-glucose-lowering effect of insulin).
No products indexed under this heading.

Thyroxine Sodium (May reduce the blood-glucose-lowering effect of insulin).
No products indexed under this heading.

Timolol Hemihydrate (Beta-blockers may either potentiate or weaken the blood-glucose-lowering effect of insulin; signs of hypoglycemia may be reduced or absent with co-administration). Products include:
Betimol Ophthalmic Solution 3181

Timolol Maleate (Beta-blockers may either potentiate or weaken the blood-glucose-lowering effect of insulin; signs of hypoglycemia may be reduced or absent with co-administration). Products include:
Combigan Ophthalmic Solution 553
Cosopt Sterile Ophthalmic Solution 1969
Timoptic Sterile Ophthalmic Solution 2121
Timoptic in Ocudose 2124
Timoptic-XE Sterile Ophthalmic Gel Forming Solution 2125

Tipranavir (May reduce the blood-glucose lowering effect of insulin). Products include:
Aptivus Capsules 823
Aptivus Oral Solution 823

Tolazamide (May increase the blood-glucose-lowering effect and susceptibility to hypoglycemia).
No products indexed under this heading.

Tolbutamide (May increase the blood-glucose-lowering effect and susceptibility to hypoglycemia).
No products indexed under this heading.

Torsemide (Diuretics may reduce the blood-glucose-lowering effect of insulin). Products include:
Demadex Injection 2630
Demadex Tablets 2630

Trandolapril (May increase the blood-glucose-lowering effect and susceptibility to hypoglycemia). Products include:
Mavik Tablets 472
Tarka Tablets 511

Tranylcypromine Sulfate (May increase the blood-glucose-lowering effect and susceptibility to hypoglycemia). Products include:
Parnate Tablets 1532

Triamcinolone (Co-administration with corticosteroids may reduce the blood-glucose-lowering effect of insulin).
No products indexed under this heading.

Triamcinolone Acetonide (Co-administration with corticosteroids may reduce the blood-glucose-lowering effect of insulin). Products include:
Azmacort Inhalation Aerosol 407
Nasacort AQ Nasal Spray 2765
Triesence Injectable Suspension .... ⊙209

Triamcinolone Diacetate (Co-administration with corticosteroids may reduce the blood-glucose-lowering effect of insulin).
No products indexed under this heading.

Triamcinolone Hexacetonide (Co-administration with corticosteroids may reduce the blood-glucose-lowering effect of insulin).
No products indexed under this heading.

Triamterene (Diuretics may reduce the blood-glucose-lowering effect of insulin). Products include:
Dyazide Capsules 1405
Dyrenium Capsules 3189

Trifluoperazine Hydrochloride (Phenothiazine derivatives may reduce the blood-glucose-lowering effect of insulin).
No products indexed under this heading.

Troglitazone (May increase the blood-glucose-lowering effect and susceptibility to hypoglycemia).
No products indexed under this heading.

Food Interactions

Alcohol (May either potentiate or weaken the blood-glucose-lowering effect of insulin).

LESCOL CAPSULES

(Fluvastatin Sodium) 2268
May interact with erythromycin, fibrates, and certain other agents. Compounds in these categories include:

Cholestyramine (Administration of fluvastatin with, or up to 4 hours after cholestyramine results in significant reductions in AUC and Cmax of fluvastatin; however, use of fluvastatin 4 hours after resin results in clinically significant additive effect).
No products indexed under this heading.

Cimetidine (Co-administration results in a significant increase in the fluvastatin Cmax and AUC and a decrease in plasma clearance).
No products indexed under this heading.

Cimetidine Hydrochloride (Co-administration results in a significant increase in the fluvastatin Cmax and AUC and a decrease in plasma clearance).
No products indexed under this heading.

Clofibrate (Myopathy has occasionally been associated with fibrates; combined use should generally be avoided).
No products indexed under this heading.

Cyclosporine (The risk of myopathy and/or rhabdomyolysis during treatment with HMG-CoA reductase inhibitor has been reported to be increased with concurrent cyclosporine; caution should be exercised). Products include:
Gengraf Capsules 435
Neoral Oral Solution 2280
Neoral Soft Gelatin Capsules 2280
Restasis Ophthalmic Emulsion 557
Sandimmune 2296

Diclofenac Potassium (Co-administration increases the mean Cmax and AUC of diclofenac by 60% and 25% respectively).
No products indexed under this heading.

Diclofenac Sodium (Co-administration increases the mean Cmax and AUC of diclofenac by 60% and 25% respectively). Products include:
Diclofenac Sodium Ophthalmic Solution .... ⊙240
Voltaren Ophthalmic Solution 2336
Voltaren Tablets 2334
Voltaren-XR Tablets 2337

Digoxin (Co-administration in patients on chronic digoxin may result in a small increase in digoxin Cmax (11%) and urinary clearance). Products include:
Lanoxin Injection 1498
Lanoxin Injection Pediatric 1502
Lanoxin Tablets 1505

Erythromycin (The risk of myopathy and/or rhabdomyolysis during treatment with HMG-CoA reductase inhibitor has been reported to be increased with concurrent erythromycin; caution should be exercised).
No products indexed under this heading.

Erythromycin Estolate (The risk of myopathy and/or rhabdomyolysis during treatment with HMG-CoA reductase inhibitor has been reported to be increased with concurrent erythromycin; caution should be exercised).
No products indexed under this heading.

Erythromycin Ethylsuccinate (The risk of myopathy and/or rhabdomyolysis during treatment with HMG-CoA reductase inhibitor has been reported to be increased with concurrent erythromycin; caution should be exercised). Products include:
E.E.S. 433
EryPed 431

Erythromycin Gluceptate (The risk of myopathy and/or rhabdomyolysis during treatment with HMG-CoA reductase inhibitor has been reported to be increased with concurrent erythromycin; caution should be exercised).
No products indexed under this heading.

Erythromycin Lactobionate (The risk of myopathy and/or rhabdomyolysis during treatment with HMG-CoA reductase inhibitor has been reported to be increased with concurrent erythromycin; caution should be exercised).
No products indexed under this heading.

Erythromycin Stearate (The risk of myopathy and/or rhabdomyolysis during treatment with HMG-CoA reductase inhibitor has been reported to be increased with concurrent erythromycin; caution should be exercised).
No products indexed under this heading.

Fenofibrate (Myopathy has occasionally been associated with fibrates; combined use should generally be avoided). Products include:
Fenoglide Tablets 2960
Tricor Tablets 520

Fluconazole (Administration of fluvastatin to volunteers pre-treated with fluconazole for 4 days results in an increase of fluvastatin Cmax and AUC by 44% and 84% respectively; caution should be exercised when fluvastatin is co-administered with fluconazole).
No products indexed under this heading.

Gemfibrozil (The risk of myopathy and/or rhabdomyolysis during treatment with HMG-CoA reductase inhibitor has been reported to be increased with concurrent gemfibrozil; combined use should generally be avoided).
No products indexed under this heading.

Glyburide (Co-administration results in increased mean Cmax, AUC, and t1/2 of glyburide approximately 50%, 69% and 121% respectively; glyburide increased the mean Cmax and AUC of fluvastatin by 44% and 51% respectively).
No products indexed under this heading.

Ketoconazole (Caution should be exercised if used concurrently with drugs that may decrease the levels of endogenous steroid hormones; increased potential for endocrine dysfunction). Products include:
Extina Foam, 2% 3057
Nizoral A-D Shampoo 1901

Nicotinic Acid (The risk of myopathy and/or rhabdomyolysis during treatment with HMG-CoA reductase inhibitor has been reported to be increased with concurrent niacin; caution should be exercised).
No products indexed under this heading.

Omeprazole (Co-administration results in a significant increase in the fluvastatin Cmax and AUC and a decrease in plasma clearance).
No products indexed under this heading.

Ranitidine Hydrochloride (Co-administration results in a significant increase in the fluvastatin Cmax and AUC and a decrease in plasma clearance). Products include:
Zantac 75 Tablets 603
Zantac 1670
Zantac Injection 1666
Zantac Injection Pharmacy Bulk Package 1668
Maximum Strength Zantac 150 Tablets 603
Maximum Strength Zantac 150 Cool Mint Tablets 603

Rifampicin (Co-administration in patients pretreated with rifampin results in significant reduction in Cmax (59%) and AUC (51%) with a large increase (95%) in plasma clearance).
No products indexed under this heading.

Spironolactone (Caution should be exercised if used concurrently with drugs that may decrease the levels of endogenous steroid hormones; increased potential for endocrine dysfunction).
No products indexed under this heading.

Warfarin Sodium (Bleeding and/or increased prothrombin time has been reported with other HMG-CoA reductase inhibitors when used concurrently; no interactions at therapeutic concentrations have been demonstrated with fluvastatin and warfarin).
No products indexed under this heading.

Food Interactions

Food, unspecified (Administration of regular formulation of fluvastatin with food reduces the rate but not the extent of absorption; administration with evening meal results in a two-fold decrease in Cmax and more than a two-fold increase in tmax as compared to administration 4 hours after the evening meal; administration of Lescol XL with a high fat meal delayed the absorption and increased the bioavailability by 50%).

LESCOL XL TABLETS

(Fluvastatin Sodium) 2268
See Lescol Capsules

LETAIRIS TABLETS

(Ambrisentan) 1258
May interact with cytochrome p450 1a2 inducers (selected), cytochrome p450 2c19 inducers (selected), cytochrome p450 2c19 inhibitors (selected), cytochrome p450 2c8 inducers (selected), cytochrome p450 2c9 inducers (selected), cytochrome p450 2d6 inducers (selected), cytochrome p450 3a4 inducers (selected), cytochrome p450 3a inducers (selected), cytochrome p450 3a inhibitors (selected), and certain other agents. Compounds in these categories include:

Allium sativum (Use caution when ambrisentan is co-administered with inducers of CYP).
No products indexed under this heading.

Amiodarone Hydrochloride (Use caution when ambrisentan is co-administered with strong CYP3A inhibitors).
No products indexed under this heading.

Amprenavir (Use caution when ambrisentan is co-administered with strong CYP3A inhibitors).
No products indexed under this heading.

Aprepitant (Use caution when ambrisentan is co-administered with strong CYP3A inhibitors). Products include:
Emend Capsules 1992

Betamethasone Acetate (Use caution when ambrisentan is co-administered with inducers of CYP).
No products indexed under this heading.

Betamethasone Sodium Phosphate (Use caution when ambrisentan is co-administered with inducers of CYP).
No products indexed under this heading.

Carbamazepine (Use caution when ambrisentan is co-administered with inducers of CYP). Products include:
Carbatrol Capsules 3019
Equetro Extended-Release Capsules 3174

Cimetidine (Use caution when ambrisentan is co-administered with strong CYP2C19 inhibitors).
No products indexed under this heading.

Cimetidine Hydrochloride (Use caution when ambrisentan is co-administered with strong CYP2C19 inhibitors).
No products indexed under this heading.

Ciprofloxacin (Use caution when ambrisentan is co-administered with strong CYP3A inhibitors). Products include:
Cipro I.V. 2817
Cipro Oral Suspension 2810
Cipro XR Tablets 2823
Ciprodex Otic Suspension 541

Ciprofloxacin Hydrochloride (Use caution when ambrisentan is co-administered with strong CYP3A inhibitors). Products include:
Cipro Tablets 2810

Cisplatin (Use caution when ambrisentan is co-administered with inducers of CYP).
No products indexed under this heading.

Citalopram Hydrobromide (Use caution when ambrisentan is co-administered with strong CYP2C19 inhibitors). Products include:
Celexa 1160

Clarithromycin (Use caution when ambrisentan is co-administered with strong CYP3A inhibitors). Products include:
Biaxin/Biaxin XL 411

Cortisone Acetate (Use caution when ambrisentan is co-administered with inducers of CYP).
No products indexed under this heading.

Cyclosporine (Use caution when ambrisentan is co-administered with cyclosporine A because cyclosporine A may cause increased exposure to ambrisentan). Products include:
Gengraf Capsules 435
Neoral Oral Solution 2280
Neoral Soft Gelatin Capsules 2280
Restasis Ophthalmic Emulsion 557
Sandimmune 2296

Delavirdine Mesylate (Use caution when ambrisentan is co-administered with strong CYP2C19 inhibitors).
No products indexed under this heading.

Desogestrel (Use caution when ambrisentan is co-administered with strong CYP2C19 inhibitors). Products include:
Mircette Tablets 1034

Dexamethasone (Use caution when ambrisentan is co-administered with inducers of CYP). Products include:
Ciprodex Otic Suspension 541

Dexamethasone Acetate (Use caution when ambrisentan is co-administered with inducers of CYP).
No products indexed under this heading.

Dexamethasone Sodium Phosphate (Use caution when ambrisentan is co-administered with inducers of CYP).
No products indexed under this heading.

Diltiazem Hydrochloride (Use caution when ambrisentan is co-administered with strong CYP3A inhibitors). Products include:
Cardizem LA Extended Release Tablets 421

Diltiazem Maleate (Use caution when ambrisentan is co-administered with strong CYP3A inhibitors).
No products indexed under this heading.

Doxorubicin Hydrochloride (Use caution when ambrisentan is co-administered with inducers of CYP).
No products indexed under this heading.

Efavirenz (Use caution when ambrisentan is co-administered with strong CYP2C19 inhibitors). Products include:
Atripla Tablets 938
Sustiva Capsules 930
Sustiva Tablets 930

Erythromycin (Use caution when ambrisentan is co-administered with strong CYP3A inhibitors).
No products indexed under this heading.

Erythromycin Estolate (Use caution when ambrisentan is co-administered with inducers of CYP).
No products indexed under this heading.

Erythromycin Ethylsuccinate (Use caution when ambrisentan is co-administered with inducers of CYP). Products include:
E.E.S. 433
EryPed 431

Erythromycin Gluceptate (Use caution when ambrisentan is co-administered with inducers of CYP).
No products indexed under this heading.

Erythromycin Lactobionate (Use caution when ambrisentan is co-administered with inducers of CYP).
No products indexed under this heading.

Erythromycin Stearate (Use caution when ambrisentan is co-administered with inducers of CYP).
No products indexed under this heading.

Ethanol (Use caution when ambrisentan is co-administered with inducers of CYP).
No products indexed under this heading.

Ethinyl Estradiol (Use caution when ambrisentan is co-administered with strong CYP2C19 inhibitors). Products include:
Lybrel Tablets 3204
Mircette Tablets 1034
NuvaRing 2897
Ortho-Cyclen/Ortho Tri-Cyclen 2449
Ortho Evra Transdermal System 2437
Ortho Tri-Cyclen Lo Tablets 2458
Seasonique Tablets 1046
Yaz Tablets 805

Ethosuximide (Use caution when ambrisentan is co-administered with inducers of CYP).
No products indexed under this heading.

Ethynodiol Diacetate (Use caution when ambrisentan is co-administered with strong CYP2C19 inhibitors).
No products indexed under this heading.

Felbamate (Use caution when ambrisentan is co-administered with strong CYP2C19 inhibitors).
No products indexed under this heading.

Flavonoids (Use caution when ambrisentan is co-administered with inducers of UGTs (uridine 5'-diphophate glucuronosyltransferases)).
No products indexed under this heading.

Fluconazole (Use caution when ambrisentan is co-administered with strong CYP3A inhibitors).
No products indexed under this heading.

Fludrocortisone Acetate (Use caution when ambrisentan is co-administered with inducers of CYP).
No products indexed under this heading.

Fluoxetine (Use caution when ambrisentan is co-administered with strong CYP2C19 inhibitors).
No products indexed under this heading.

Fluoxetine Hydrochloride (Use caution when ambrisentan is co-administered with strong CYP2C19 inhibitors). Products include:
Prozac Weekly Capsules 1852
Prozac Pulvules and Liquid 1852
Symbyax Capsules 1871

Fluvastatin Sodium (Use caution when ambrisentan is co-administered with strong CYP2C19 inhibitors). Products include:
Lescol Capsules 2268
Lescol XL Tablets 2268

Fluvoxamine (Use caution when ambrisentan is co-administered with strong CYP2C19 inhibitors).
No products indexed under this heading.

Fluvoxamine Maleate (Use caution when ambrisentan is co-administered with strong CYP2C19 inhibitors). Products include:
Luvox CR Extended-Release Capsules 1759

Fosphenytoin Sodium (Use caution when ambrisentan is co-administered with inducers of CYP).
No products indexed under this heading.

Garlic Extract (Use caution when ambrisentan is co-administered with inducers of CYP).
No products indexed under this heading.

Garlic Oil (Use caution when ambrisentan is co-administered with inducers of CYP).
No products indexed under this heading.

Hydrocortisone (Use caution when ambrisentan is co-administered with inducers of CYP).
No products indexed under this heading.

Hydrocortisone Acetate (Use caution when ambrisentan is co-administered with inducers of CYP). Products include:
Analpram-HC 1140
Pramosone 1141

Hydrocortisone Butyrate (Use caution when ambrisentan is co-administered with inducers of CYP).
No products indexed under this heading.

Hydrocortisone Cypionate (Use caution when ambrisentan is co-administered with inducers of CYP).
No products indexed under this heading.

Hydrocortisone Hemisuccinate (Use caution when ambrisentan is co-administered with inducers of CYP).
No products indexed under this heading.

Hydrocortisone Probutate (Use caution when ambrisentan is co-administered with inducers of CYP).
No products indexed under this heading.

Hydrocortisone Sodium Phosphate (Use caution when ambrisentan is co-administered with inducers of CYP).
No products indexed under this heading.

Hydrocortisone Sodium Succinate (Use caution when ambrisentan is co-administered with inducers of CYP).
No products indexed under this heading.

Hydrocortisone Valerate (Use caution when ambrisentan is co-administered with inducers of CYP).
No products indexed under this heading.

Hypericum (Use caution when ambrisentan is co-administered with inducers of CYP). Products include:
Satieté Tablets 640

Hypericum Perforatum (Use caution when ambrisentan is co-administered with inducers of CYP).
No products indexed under this heading.

Indinavir Sulfate (Use caution when ambrisentan is co-administered with strong CYP3A inhibitors).
Products include:
Crixivan Capsules 1979

Indomethacin (Use caution when ambrisentan is co-administered with strong CYP2C19 inhibitors).
Products include:
Indocin 2024

Indomethacin Sodium Trihydrate (Use caution when ambrisentan is co-administered with strong CYP2C19 inhibitors). Products include:
Indocin I.V. 2489

Insulin (Use caution when ambrisentan is co-administered with inducers of CYP).
No products indexed under this heading.

Isoniazid (Use caution when ambrisentan is co-administered with strong CYP2C19 inhibitors).
No products indexed under this heading.

Itraconazole (Use caution when ambrisentan is co-administered with strong CYP3A inhibitors).
No products indexed under this heading.

Ketoconazole (Use caution when ambrisentan is co-administered with strong CYP2C19 inhibitors).
Products include:
Extina Foam, 2% 3057
Nizoral A-D Shampoo 1901

Lansoprazole (Use caution when ambrisentan is co-administered with strong CYP2C19 inhibitors).
No products indexed under this heading.

Letrozole (Use caution when ambrisentan is co-administered with strong CYP2C19 inhibitors).
Products include:
Femara Tablets 2246

Levonorgestrel (Use caution when ambrisentan is co-administered with strong CYP2C19 inhibitors).
Products include:
Climara Pro Transdermal System 768
Lybrel Tablets 3204
Mirena Intrauterine System 779
Plan B Tablets 1044
Seasonique Tablets 1046

Lopinavir (Use caution when ambrisentan is co-administered with strong CYP3A inhibitors). Products include:
Kaletra 452

Mephenytoin (Use caution when ambrisentan is co-administered with inducers of CYP).
No products indexed under this heading.

Mestranol (Use caution when ambrisentan is co-administered with strong CYP2C19 inhibitors).
No products indexed under this heading.

Methsuximide (Use caution when ambrisentan is co-administered with inducers of CYP).
No products indexed under this heading.

Methylprednisolone (Use caution when ambrisentan is co-administered with inducers of CYP).
No products indexed under this heading.

Methylprednisolone Acetate (Use caution when ambrisentan is co-administered with inducers of CYP).
No products indexed under this heading.

Methylprednisolone Sodium Succinate (Use caution when ambrisentan is co-administered with inducers of CYP).
No products indexed under this heading.

Metronidazole (Use caution when ambrisentan is co-administered with strong CYP3A inhibitors). Products include:
Pylera Capsules 714

Metronidazole Benzoate (Use caution when ambrisentan is co-administered with strong CYP3A inhibitors).
No products indexed under this heading.

Metronidazole Hydrochloride (Use caution when ambrisentan is co-administered with strong CYP3A inhibitors).
No products indexed under this heading.

Miconazole (Use caution when ambrisentan is co-administered with strong CYP3A inhibitors).
No products indexed under this heading.

Modafinil (Use caution when ambrisentan is co-administered with strong CYP2C19 inhibitors).
Products include:
Provigil Tablets 977

Nafcillin Sodium (Use caution when ambrisentan is co-administered with inducers of CYP).
No products indexed under this heading.

Nefazodone Hydrochloride (Use caution when ambrisentan is co-administered with strong CYP3A inhibitors).
No products indexed under this heading.

Nelfinavir Mesylate (Use caution when ambrisentan is co-administered with strong CYP3A inhibitors).
No products indexed under this heading.

Nevirapine (Use caution when ambrisentan is co-administered with inducers of CYP). Products include:
Viramune Oral Suspension 873
Viramune Tablets 873

Nicotine (Use caution when ambrisentan is co-administered with inducers of CYP).
No products indexed under this heading.

Nicotine Polacrilex (Use caution when ambrisentan is co-administered with inducers of CYP).
No products indexed under this heading.

Nicotine Salicylate (Use caution when ambrisentan is co-administered with inducers of CYP).
No products indexed under this heading.

Nicotine Sulfate (Use caution when ambrisentan is co-administered with inducers of CYP).
No products indexed under this heading.

Nifedipine (Use caution when ambrisentan is co-administered with strong CYP3A inhibitors).
No products indexed under this heading.

Norethindrone (Use caution when ambrisentan is co-administered with strong CYP2C19 inhibitors).
Products include:
Ortho Micronor Tablets 2446

Norethindrone Acetate (Use caution when ambrisentan is co-administered with inducers of CYP).
Products include:
Activella Tablets 2347

Norethynodrel (Use caution when ambrisentan is co-administered with strong CYP2C19 inhibitors).
No products indexed under this heading.

Norfloxacin (Use caution when ambrisentan is co-administered with strong CYP3A inhibitors). Products include:
Noroxin Tablets 2069

Norgestimate (Use caution when ambrisentan is co-administered with strong CYP2C19 inhibitors).
Products include:
Ortho-Cyclen/Ortho Tri-Cyclen 2449
Ortho Tri-Cyclen Lo Tablets 2458

Norgestrel (Use caution when ambrisentan is co-administered with strong CYP2C19 inhibitors).
No products indexed under this heading.

Omeprazole (Use caution when ambrisentan is co-administered with strong CYP2C19 inhibitors).
No products indexed under this heading.

Oxcarbazepine (Use caution when ambrisentan is co-administered with strong CYP2C19 inhibitors).
No products indexed under this heading.

Paroxetine Hydrochloride (Use caution when ambrisentan is co-administered with strong CYP2C19 inhibitors). Products include:
Paxil 1535
Paxil CR Controlled-Release Tablets 1544

Phenobarbital (Use caution when ambrisentan is co-administered with inducers of UGTs (uridine 5'-diphophate glucuronosyltransferases)). Products include:
Donnatal Extentabs 2507

Phenobarbital Sodium (Use caution when ambrisentan is co-administered with inducers of UGTs (uridine 5'-diphophate glucuronosyltransferases)).
No products indexed under this heading.

Phenytoin (Use caution when ambrisentan is co-administered with inducers of CYP).
No products indexed under this heading.

Phenytoin Sodium (Use caution when ambrisentan is co-administered with inducers of CYP). Products include:
Phenytek Capsules 2192

Prednisolone Acetate (Use caution when ambrisentan is co-administered with inducers of CYP).
Products include:
Pred Forte Ophthalmic Suspension .... ⊙ 227
Pred Mild Ophthalmic Suspension .... ⊙ 230
Pred-G Ophthalmic Ointment .... ⊙ 229
Pred-G Ophthalmic Suspension ...... ⊙ 228

Prednisolone Sodium Phosphate (Use caution when ambrisentan is co-administered with inducers of CYP).
No products indexed under this heading.

Prednisolone Tebutate (Use caution when ambrisentan is co-administered with inducers of CYP).
No products indexed under this heading.

Prednisone (Use caution when ambrisentan is co-administered with inducers of CYP).
No products indexed under this heading.

Primidone (Use caution when ambrisentan is co-administered with inducers of CYP).
No products indexed under this heading.

Quinine (Use caution when ambrisentan is co-administered with strong CYP3A inhibitors).
No products indexed under this heading.

Quinine Sulfate (Use caution when ambrisentan is co-administered with strong CYP3A inhibitors).
No products indexed under this heading.

Rifabutin (Use caution when ambrisentan is co-administered with inducers of CYP).
No products indexed under this heading.

Rifampicin (Use caution when ambrisentan is co-administered with inducers of CYP).
No products indexed under this heading.

Rifampin (Use caution when ambrisentan is co-administered with inducers of P-gp and UGTs (uridine 5'-diphophate glucuronosyltransferases)).
No products indexed under this heading.

Rifapentine (Use caution when ambrisentan is co-administered with inducers of CYP).
No products indexed under this heading.

Ritonavir (Use caution when ambrisentan is co-administered with strong CYP2C19 inhibitors). Products include:
- Kaletra 452
- Norvir 489

Saquinavir (Use caution when ambrisentan is co-administered with strong CYP3A inhibitors).
No products indexed under this heading.

Saquinavir Mesylate (Use caution when ambrisentan is co-administered with strong CYP3A inhibitors).
No products indexed under this heading.

Secobarbital Sodium (Use caution when ambrisentan is co-administered with inducers of CYP).
No products indexed under this heading.

Sertraline Hydrochloride (Use caution when ambrisentan is co-administered with strong CYP2C19 inhibitors).
No products indexed under this heading.

Sildenafil Citrate (Use caution when ambrisentan is co-administered with strong CYP2C19 inhibitors).
No products indexed under this heading.

Sulfaphenazole (Use caution when ambrisentan is co-administered with strong CYP2C19 inhibitors).
No products indexed under this heading.

Sulfinpyrazone (Use caution when ambrisentan is co-administered with inducers of CYP).
No products indexed under this heading.

Telmisartan (Use caution when ambrisentan is co-administered with strong CYP2C19 inhibitors). Products include:
- Micardis Tablets 852
- Micardis HCT Tablets 854

Theophylline (Use caution when ambrisentan is co-administered with inducers of CYP).
No products indexed under this heading.

Theophylline Anhydrous (Use caution when ambrisentan is co-administered with inducers of CYP). Products include:
- Uniphyl Tablets 2595

Theophylline Calcium Salicylate (Use caution when ambrisentan is co-administered with inducers of CYP).
No products indexed under this heading.

Theophylline Dihydroxypropyl (Glyceryl) (Use caution when ambrisentan is co-administered with inducers of CYP).
No products indexed under this heading.

Theophylline Ethylenediamine (Use caution when ambrisentan is co-administered with inducers of CYP).
No products indexed under this heading.

Ticlopidine Hydrochloride (Use caution when ambrisentan is co-administered with strong CYP2C19 inhibitors).
No products indexed under this heading.

Tobacco (Use caution when ambrisentan is co-administered with inducers of CYP).
No products indexed under this heading.

Tolbutamide (Use caution when ambrisentan is co-administered with strong CYP2C19 inhibitors).
No products indexed under this heading.

Tolbutamide Sodium (Use caution when ambrisentan is co-administered with strong CYP2C19 inhibitors).
No products indexed under this heading.

Topiramate (Use caution when ambrisentan is co-administered with strong CYP2C19 inhibitors).
No products indexed under this heading.

Triamcinolone (Use caution when ambrisentan is co-administered with inducers of CYP).
No products indexed under this heading.

Triamcinolone Acetonide (Use caution when ambrisentan is co-administered with inducers of CYP). Products include:
- Azmacort Inhalation Aerosol 407
- Nasacort AQ Nasal Spray 2765
- Triesence Injectable Suspension .... ⊙ 209

Triamcinolone Diacetate (Use caution when ambrisentan is co-administered with inducers of CYP).
No products indexed under this heading.

Triamcinolone Hexacetonide (Use caution when ambrisentan is co-administered with inducers of CYP).
No products indexed under this heading.

Troglitazone (Use caution when ambrisentan is co-administered with inducers of CYP).
No products indexed under this heading.

Troleandomycin (Use caution when ambrisentan is co-administered with strong CYP3A inhibitors).
No products indexed under this heading.

Vardenafil Hydrochloride (Use caution when ambrisentan is co-administered with strong CYP2C19 inhibitors). Products include:
- Levitra Tablets 2876

Venlafaxine Hydrochloride (Use caution when ambrisentan is co-administered with strong CYP3A inhibitors). Products include:
- Effexor XR Extended-Release Capsules 3195
- Venlafaxine Hydrochloride Tablets ... 2199

Verapamil Hydrochloride (Use caution when ambrisentan is co-administered with strong CYP3A inhibitors). Products include:
- Tarka Tablets 511

Voriconazole (Use caution when ambrisentan is co-administered with strong CYP2C19 inhibitors).
No products indexed under this heading.

Zafirlukast (Use caution when ambrisentan is co-administered with strong CYP3A inhibitors). Products include:
- Accolate Tablets 669

Zileuton (Use caution when ambrisentan is co-administered with strong CYP3A inhibitors).
No products indexed under this heading.

Food Interactions

Broccoli (Use caution when ambrisentan is co-administered with inducers of CYP).

Brussel Sprouts (Use caution when ambrisentan is co-administered with inducers of CYP).

Charbroiled Food (Use caution when ambrisentan is co-administered with inducers of CYP).

Grapefruit (Use caution when ambrisentan is co-administered with strong CYP3A inhibitors).

LEUKERAN TABLETS

(Chlorambucil) 1508

May interact with vaccines, live. Compounds in these categories include:

BCG Vaccine (Administration of live vaccines to immunocompromised patients should be avoided).
No products indexed under this heading.

Influenza Vaccine, Live Attenuated (Administration of live vaccines to immunocompromised patients should be avoided).
No products indexed under this heading.

Influenza Virus Vaccine Live, Intranasal (Administration of live vaccines to immunocompromised patients should be avoided). Products include:
- FluMist Vaccine 1945

Measles, Mumps, Rubella and Varicella Virus Vaccine Live (Administration of live vaccines to immunocompromised patients should be avoided). Products include:
- ProQuad 2099

Measles, Mumps & Rubella Virus Vaccine, Live (Administration of live vaccines to immunocompromised patients should be avoided). Products include:
- M-M-R II 2054

Measles & Rubella Virus Vaccine Live (Administration of live vaccines to immunocompromised patients should be avoided).
No products indexed under this heading.

Measles Virus Vaccine Live (Administration of live vaccines to immunocompromised patients should be avoided). Products include:
- Attenuvax 1951

Mumps Virus Vaccine, Live (Administration of live vaccines to immunocompromised patients should be avoided). Products include:
- Mumpsvax 2068

Poliovirus Vaccine, Live, Oral, Trivalent, Types 1,2,3 (Sabin) (Administration of live vaccines to immunocompromised patients should be avoided).
No products indexed under this heading.

Rotavirus Vaccine, Live, Oral, Tetravalent (Administration of live vaccines to immunocompromised patients should be avoided).
No products indexed under this heading.

Rubella & Mumps Virus Vaccine Live (Administration of live vaccines to immunocompromised patients should be avoided).
No products indexed under this heading.

Rubella Virus Vaccine Live (Administration of live vaccines to immunocompromised patients should be avoided). Products include:
- Meruvax II 2061

Smallpox Vaccine (Administration of live vaccines to immunocompromised patients should be avoided).
No products indexed under this heading.

Typhoid Vaccine (Administration of live vaccines to immunocompromised patients should be avoided).
No products indexed under this heading.

Varicella Virus Vaccine Live (Administration of live vaccines to immunocompromised patients should be avoided). Products include:
- Varivax 2133

Yellow Fever Vaccine (Administration of live vaccines to immunocompromised patients should be avoided).
No products indexed under this heading.

Zoster Vaccine Live (Administration of live vaccines to immunocompromised patients should be avoided). Products include:
- Zostavax Injection 2145

LEUKINE

(Sargramostim) 774

May interact with antimetabolites, cytotoxic drugs, drugs with myeloproliferative effects, and certain other agents. Compounds in these categories include:

Betamethasone Acetate (May potentiate the myeloproliferative effect).
No products indexed under this heading.

Betamethasone Sodium Phosphate (May potentiate the myeloproliferative effect).
No products indexed under this heading.

Bleomycin Sulfate (Co-administration within 24 hours preceding or following chemotherapy is not recommended because of potential sensitivity of rapidly dividing hematopoietic progenitor cells to cytotoxic therapy).
No products indexed under this heading.

Capecitabine (In patients who have been exposed to multiple myelotoxic agents, the effect of Leukine on myeloid reconstitution may be limited). Products include:
- Xeloda Tablets 2662

Cladribine (In patients who have been exposed to multiple myelotoxic agents, the effect of Leukine on myeloid reconstitution may be limited). Products include:
- Leustatin Injection 2384

Cortisone Acetate (May potentiate the myeloproliferative effect).
No products indexed under this heading.

Cyclophosphamide (Co-administration within 24 hours preceding or following chemotherapy is not recommended because of potential sensitivity of rapidly dividing hematopoietic progenitor cells to cytotoxic therapy).
No products indexed under this heading.

Cytarabine (In patients who have been exposed to multiple myelotoxic agents, the effect of Leukine on myeloid reconstitution may be limited).
No products indexed under this heading.

Daunorubicin Hydrochloride (Co-administration within 24 hours preceding or following chemotherapy is not recommended because of potential sensitivity of rapidly dividing hematopoietic progenitor cells to cytotoxic therapy).
No products indexed under this heading.

Dexamethasone (May potentiate the myeloproliferative effect). Products include:
Ciprodex Otic Suspension 541

Dexamethasone Acetate (May potentiate the myeloproliferative effect).
No products indexed under this heading.

Dexamethasone Sodium Phosphate (May potentiate the myeloproliferative effect).
No products indexed under this heading.

Doxorubicin Hydrochloride (Co-administration within 24 hours preceding or following chemotherapy is not recommended because of potential sensitivity of rapidly dividing hematopoietic progenitor cells to cytotoxic therapy).
No products indexed under this heading.

Epirubicin Hydrochloride (Co-administration within 24 hours preceding or following chemotherapy is not recommended because of potential sensitivity of rapidly dividing hematopoietic progenitor cells to cytotoxic therapy).
No products indexed under this heading.

Floxuridine (In patients who have been exposed to multiple myelotoxic agents, the effect of Leukine on myeloid reconstitution may be limited).
No products indexed under this heading.

Fludarabine Phosphate (In patients who have been exposed to multiple myelotoxic agents, the effect of Leukine on myeloid reconstitution may be limited).
No products indexed under this heading.

Fluorouracil (Co-administration within 24 hours preceding or following chemotherapy is not recommended because of potential sensitivity of rapidly dividing hematopoietic progenitor cells to cytotoxic therapy). Products include:
Carac Cream 0.5% 2722

Gemcitabine Hydrochloride (In patients who have been exposed to multiple myelotoxic agents, the effect of Leukine on myeloid reconstitution may be limited). Products include:
Gemzar for Injection 1820

Hydrocortisone (May potentiate the myeloproliferative effect).
No products indexed under this heading.

Hydrocortisone Acetate (May potentiate the myeloproliferative effect). Products include:
Analpram-HC 1140
Pramosone 1141

Hydrocortisone Sodium Phosphate (May potentiate the myeloproliferative effect).
No products indexed under this heading.

Hydrocortisone Sodium Succinate (May potentiate the myeloproliferative effect).
No products indexed under this heading.

Hydroxyurea (Co-administration within 24 hours preceding or following chemotherapy is not recommended because of potential sensitivity of rapidly dividing hematopoietic progenitor cells to cytotoxic therapy).
No products indexed under this heading.

Lithium Carbonate (May potentiate the myeloproliferative effect).
No products indexed under this heading.

Lithium Citrate (May potentiate the myeloproliferative effect).
No products indexed under this heading.

Mercaptopurine (In patients who have been exposed to multiple myelotoxic agents, the effect of Leukine on myeloid reconstitution may be limited).
No products indexed under this heading.

Methotrexate (In patients who have been exposed to multiple myelotoxic agents, the effect of Leukine on myeloid reconstitution may be limited).
No products indexed under this heading.

Methotrexate Sodium (Co-administration within 24 hours preceding or following chemotherapy is not recommended because of potential sensitivity of rapidly dividing hematopoietic progenitor cells to cytotoxic therapy).
No products indexed under this heading.

Methylprednisolone Acetate (May potentiate the myeloproliferative effect).
No products indexed under this heading.

Methylprednisolone Sodium Succinate (May potentiate the myeloproliferative effect).
No products indexed under this heading.

Mitotane (Co-administration within 24 hours preceding or following chemotherapy is not recommended because of potential sensitivity of rapidly dividing hematopoietic progenitor cells to cytotoxic therapy).
No products indexed under this heading.

Mitoxantrone Hydrochloride (Co-administration within 24 hours preceding or following chemotherapy is not recommended because of potential sensitivity of rapidly dividing hematopoietic progenitor cells to cytotoxic therapy). Products include:
Novantrone for Injection Concentrate 1100

Pentostatin (In patients who have been exposed to multiple myelotoxic agents, the effect of Leukine on myeloid reconstitution may be limited).
No products indexed under this heading.

Prednisolone Acetate (May potentiate the myeloproliferative effect). Products include:
Pred Forte Ophthalmic Suspension .... ⊙227
Pred Mild Ophthalmic Suspension .... ⊙230
Pred-G Ophthalmic Ointment .... ⊙229
Pred-G Ophthalmic Suspension ...... ⊙228

Prednisolone Sodium Phosphate (May potentiate the myeloproliferative effect).
No products indexed under this heading.

Prednisolone Tebutate (May potentiate the myeloproliferative effect).
No products indexed under this heading.

Prednisone (May potentiate the myeloproliferative effect).
No products indexed under this heading.

Procarbazine Hydrochloride (Co-administration within 24 hours preceding or following chemotherapy is not recommended because of potential sensitivity of rapidly dividing hematopoietic progenitor cells to cytotoxic therapy).
No products indexed under this heading.

Tamoxifen Citrate (Co-administration within 24 hours preceding or following chemotherapy is not recommended because of potential sensitivity of rapidly dividing hematopoietic progenitor cells to cytotoxic therapy).
No products indexed under this heading.

Thioguanine (In patients who have been exposed to multiple myelotoxic agents, the effect of Leukine on myeloid reconstitution may be limited). Products include:
Tabloid Tablets 1601

Triamcinolone (May potentiate the myeloproliferative effect).
No products indexed under this heading.

Triamcinolone Acetonide (May potentiate the myeloproliferative effect). Products include:
Azmacort Inhalation Aerosol 407
Nasacort AQ Nasal Spray 2765
Triesence Injectable Suspension .... ⊙209

Triamcinolone Diacetate (May potentiate the myeloproliferative effect).
No products indexed under this heading.

Triamcinolone Hexacetonide (May potentiate the myeloproliferative effect).
No products indexed under this heading.

Vincristine Sulfate (Co-administration within 24 hours preceding or following chemotherapy is not recommended because of potential sensitivity of rapidly dividing hematopoietic progenitor cells to cytotoxic therapy).
No products indexed under this heading.

LEUSTATIN INJECTION

(Cladribine) 2384
May interact with immunosuppressive agents, agents associated with myelosuppression, and certain other agents. Compounds in these categories include:

Altretamine (Caution should be exercised if co-administered with other drugs known to cause immunosuppression). Products include:
Hexalen Capsules 1078

Azathioprine (Caution should be exercised if co-administered with other drugs known to cause immunosuppression).
No products indexed under this heading.

Basiliximab (Caution should be exercised if co-administered with other drugs known to cause immunosuppression). Products include:
Simulect for Injection 2306

Bone Marrow Depressants, unspecified (Caution should be exercised if co-administered with other drugs known to cause myelosuppression).
No products indexed under this heading.

Busulfan (Caution should be exercised if co-administered with other drugs known to cause immunosuppression). Products include:
Busulfex Injection 2477
Myleran Tablets 1530

Chlorambucil (Caution should be exercised if co-administered with other drugs known to cause immunosuppression). Products include:
Leukeran Tablets 1508

Cyclosporine (Caution should be exercised if co-administered with other drugs known to cause immunosuppression). Products include:
Gengraf Capsules 435
Neoral Oral Solution 2280
Neoral Soft Gelatin Capsules 2280
Restasis Ophthalmic Emulsion 557
Sandimmune 2296

Daunorubicin Citrate Liposome (Caution should be exercised if co-administered with other drugs known to cause immunosuppression).
No products indexed under this heading.

Daunorubicin Hydrochloride (Caution should be exercised if co-administered with other drugs known to cause immunosuppression).
No products indexed under this heading.

Dexrazoxane (Caution should be exercised if co-administered with other drugs known to cause immunosuppression).
No products indexed under this heading.

Doxorubicin Hydrochloride (Caution should be exercised if co-administered with other drugs known to cause immunosuppression).
No products indexed under this heading.

Doxorubicin Hydrochloride Liposome (Caution should be exercised if co-administered with other drugs known to cause immunosuppression). Products include:
Doxil Injection 2378

Fludarabine Phosphate (Caution should be exercised if co-administered with other drugs known to cause immunosuppression).
No products indexed under this heading.

Gemcitabine Hydrochloride (Caution should be exercised if co-administered with other drugs known to cause immunosuppression). Products include:
Gemzar for Injection 1820

Gemtuzumab Ozogamicin (Caution should be exercised if co-administered with other drugs known to cause immunosuppression). Products include:

Mylotarg for Injection 3212

Idarubicin Hydrochloride (Caution should be exercised if co-administered with other drugs known to cause immunosuppression).
No products indexed under this heading.

Immunosuppressants (Caution should be exercised if co-administered with other drugs known to cause immunosuppression).
No products indexed under this heading.

Interferon alfa-2a, Recombinant (Caution should be exercised if co-administered with other drugs known to cause immunosuppression).
No products indexed under this heading.

Irinotecan Hydrochloride (Caution should be exercised if co-administered with other drugs known to cause immunosuppression).
No products indexed under this heading.

Melphalan Hydrochloride (Caution should be exercised if co-administered with other drugs known to cause immunosuppression).
No products indexed under this heading.

Mercaptopurine (Caution should be exercised if co-administered with other drugs known to cause immunosuppression).
No products indexed under this heading.

Mitoxantrone Hydrochloride (Caution should be exercised if co-administered with other drugs known to cause immunosuppression). Products include:
Novantrone for Injection Concentrate 1100

Muromonab-CD3 (Caution should be exercised if co-administered with other drugs known to cause immunosuppression). Products include:
Orthoclone OKT3 Sterile Solution 2387

Mycophenolate Mofetil (Caution should be exercised if co-administered with other drugs known to cause immunosuppression). Products include:
CellCept Capsules 2622
CellCept Oral Suspension 2622
CellCept Tablets 2622

Sirolimus (Caution should be exercised if co-administered with other drugs known to cause immunosuppression). Products include:
Rapamune 3260

Tacrolimus (Caution should be exercised if co-administered with other drugs known to cause immunosuppression). Products include:
Prograf Capsules and Injection 622
Protopic Ointment 628

Temozolomide (Caution should be exercised if co-administered with other drugs known to cause immunosuppression). Products include:
Temodar Capsules 2931

Thioguanine (Caution should be exercised if co-administered with other drugs known to cause immunosuppression). Products include:
Tabloid Tablets 1601

Vinorelbine Tartrate (Caution should be exercised if co-administered with other drugs known to cause immunosuppression).
No products indexed under this heading.

LEVAQUIN INJECTION

(Levofloxacin) 2416
May interact with class 1A antiarrhythmics, class III antiarrhythmics, corticosteroids, erythromycin, oral hypoglycemic agents, insulin, nonsteroidal anti-inflammatory agents, psychotropics, drugs that prolong the QT interval, quinidine, tricyclic antidepressants, xanthines, and certain other agents. Compounds in these categories include:

Acarbose (Disturbances of blood glucose, including hyper- and hypoglycemia, have been reported in patients treated concomitantly with quinolones and an antidiabetic agent; careful monitoring of blood glucose levels is recommended). Products include:
Precose Tablets 792

Alprazolam (Prolongation of the QT interval and isolated cases of torsade de pointes have been reported. Avoid concurrent use with other drugs that prolong the QT interval).
No products indexed under this heading.

Aminophylline (Co-administration of other quinolones with theophylline has resulted in prolonged elimination half-life, elevated serum theophylline levels, and increased risk of theophylline related toxicity; no significant effect of levofloxacin on theophylline pharmacokinetic parameters has been detected; however, caution should be exercised and theophylline levels monitored closely).
No products indexed under this heading.

Amiodarone Hydrochloride (Levofloxacin has been associated with prolongation of the QTc interval; co-administration with drugs known to prolong QT interval should be avoided).
No products indexed under this heading.

Amitriptyline Hydrochloride (Prolongation of the QT interval and isolated cases of torsade de pointes have been reported. Avoid concurrent use with other drugs that prolong the QT interval).
No products indexed under this heading.

Amoxapine (Prolongation of the QT interval and isolated cases of torsade de pointes have been reported. Avoid concurrent use with other drugs that prolong the QT interval).
No products indexed under this heading.

Arsenic Trioxide (Levofloxacin has been associated with prolongation of the QTc interval; co-administration with drugs known to prolong QT interval should be avoided). Products include:
Trisenox Injection 986

Astemizole (Prolongation of the QT interval and isolated cases of torsade de pointes have been reported. Avoid concurrent use with other drugs that prolong the QT interval).
No products indexed under this heading.

Betamethasone Acetate (Achilles and other tendon ruptures have been reported with quinolones, post-market surveillance reports indicate that the risk may be increased in patients on concomitant corticosteroids).
No products indexed under this heading.

Betamethasone Sodium Phosphate (Achilles and other tendon ruptures have been reported with quinolones, post-market surveillance reports indicate that the risk may be increased in patients on concomitant corticosteroids).
No products indexed under this heading.

Bretylium Tosylate (Levofloxacin has been associated with prolongation of the QT interval and infrequent cases of arrhythmia. Rare cases of torsades de pointes have been spontaneously reported during post-marketing surveillance in patients receiving levofloxacin. Levofloxacin should be avoided in patients receiving class III antiarrhythmic agents).
No products indexed under this heading.

Budesonide (Achilles and other tendon ruptures have been reported with quinolones, post-market surveillance reports indicate that the risk may be increased in patients on concomitant corticosteroids). Products include:
Pulmicort Flexhaler 654
Symbicort 80/4.5 Inhalation Aerosol....................................... 659
Symbicort 160/4.5 Inhalation Aerosol....................................... 659

Buspirone Hydrochloride (Prolongation of the QT interval and isolated cases of torsade de pointes have been reported. Avoid concurrent use with other drugs that prolong the QT interval).
No products indexed under this heading.

Celecoxib (Co-administration may increase the risk of CNS stimulation and convulsive seizures). Products include:
Celebrex Capsules 2979

Chlordiazepoxide (Prolongation of the QT interval and isolated cases of torsade de pointes have been reported. Avoid concurrent use with other drugs that prolong the QT interval).
No products indexed under this heading.

Chlordiazepoxide Hydrochloride (Prolongation of the QT interval and isolated cases of torsade de pointes have been reported. Avoid concurrent use with other drugs that prolong the QT interval).
No products indexed under this heading.

Chlorpromazine (Prolongation of the QT interval and isolated cases of torsade de pointes have been reported. Avoid concurrent use with other drugs that prolong the QT interval).
No products indexed under this heading.

Chlorpromazine Hydrochloride (Prolongation of the QT interval and isolated cases of torsade de pointes have been reported. Avoid concurrent use with other drugs that prolong the QT interval).
No products indexed under this heading.

Chlorpropamide (Disturbances of blood glucose, including hyper- and hypoglycemia, have been reported in patients treated concomitantly with quinolones and an antidiabetic agent; careful monitoring of blood glucose levels is recommended).
No products indexed under this heading.

Chlorprothixene (Prolongation of the QT interval and isolated cases of torsade de pointes have been reported. Avoid concurrent use with other drugs that prolong the QT interval).
No products indexed under this heading.

Chlorprothixene Hydrochloride (Prolongation of the QT interval and isolated cases of torsade de pointes have been reported. Avoid concurrent use with other drugs that prolong the QT interval).
No products indexed under this heading.

Ciclesonide (Achilles and other tendon ruptures have been reported with quinolones, post-market surveillance reports indicate that the risk may be increased in patients on concomitant corticosteroids). Products include:
Alvesco Inhalation Aerosol 2985
Omnaris Nasal Spray 2998

Cimetidine (Co-administration has resulted in higher levofloxacin AUC and t1/2, while CL/F and CLr were lower during concomitant treatment with cimetidine).
No products indexed under this heading.

Cimetidine Hydrochloride (Co-administration has resulted in higher levofloxacin AUC and t1/2, while CL/F and CLr were lower during concomitant treatment with cimetidine).
No products indexed under this heading.

Cisapride (Levofloxacin has been associated with prolongation of the QTc interval; co-administration with drugs known to prolong QT interval should be avoided).
No products indexed under this heading.

Clomipramine Hydrochloride (Prolongation of the QT interval and isolated cases of torsade de pointes have been reported. Avoid concurrent use with other drugs that prolong the QT interval).
No products indexed under this heading.

Clorazepate Dipotassium (Prolongation of the QT interval and isolated cases of torsade de pointes have been reported. Avoid concurrent use with other drugs that prolong the QT interval).
No products indexed under this heading.

Clozapine (Prolongation of the QT interval and isolated cases of torsade de pointes have been reported. Avoid concurrent use with other drugs that prolong the QT interval).
No products indexed under this heading.

Cortisone Acetate (Achilles and other tendon ruptures have been reported with quinolones, post-market surveillance reports indicate that the risk may be increased in patients on concomitant corticosteroids).
No products indexed under this heading.

Cyclosporine (Levofloxacin Cmax and Ke were slightly lower while Tmax and t1/2 were slightly longer in the presence of cyclosporine.These differences, however, are not clinically significant, therefore, no dosage adjustment is required). Products include:
Gengraf Capsules 435

Neoral Oral Solution **2280**
Neoral Soft Gelatin Capsules **2280**
Restasis Ophthalmic Emulsion **557**
Sandimmune **2296**

Desipramine Hydrochloride (Prolongation of the QT interval and isolated cases of torsade de pointes have been reported. Avoid concurrent use with other drugs that prolong the QT interval).
No products indexed under this heading.

Dexamethasone (Achilles and other tendon ruptures have been reported with quinolones, post-market surveillance reports indicate that the risk may be increased in patients on concomitant corticosteroids). Products include:
Ciprodex Otic Suspension **541**

Dexamethasone Acetate (Achilles and other tendon ruptures have been reported with quinolones, post-market surveillance reports indicate that the risk may be increased in patients on concomitant corticosteroids).
No products indexed under this heading.

Dexamethasone Sodium Phosphate (Achilles and other tendon ruptures have been reported with quinolones, post-market surveillance reports indicate that the risk may be increased in patients on concomitant corticosteroids).
No products indexed under this heading.

Diazepam (Prolongation of the QT interval and isolated cases of torsade de pointes have been reported. Avoid concurrent use with other drugs that prolong the QT interval). Products include:
Valium Tablets **2658**

Diclofenac Epolamine (Co-administration may increase the risk of CNS stimulation and convulsive seizures). Products include:
Flector Patch **561**

Diclofenac Potassium (Co-administration may increase the risk of CNS stimulation and convulsive seizures).
No products indexed under this heading.

Diclofenac Sodium (Co-administration may increase the risk of CNS stimulation and convulsive seizures). Products include:
Diclofenac Sodium Ophthalmic Solution.................................. ⊙ **240**
Voltaren Ophthalmic Solution **2336**
Voltaren Tablets **2334**
Voltaren-XR Tablets **2337**

Disopyramide (Levofloxacin has been associated with prolongation of the QT interval and infrequent cases of arrhythmia. Rare cases of torsades de pointes have been spontaneously reported during post-marketing surveillance in patients receiving levofloxacin. Levofloxacin should be avoided in patients receiving class IA antiarrhythmic agents).
No products indexed under this heading.

Disopyramide Phosphate (Prolongation of the QT interval and isolated cases of torsade de pointes have been reported. Avoid concurrent use with other drugs that prolong the QT interval).
No products indexed under this heading.

Dofetilide (Prolongation of the QT interval and isolated cases of torsade de pointes have been reported. Avoid concurrent use with other drugs that prolong the QT interval).
No products indexed under this heading.

Doxepin Hydrochloride (Prolongation of the QT interval and isolated cases of torsade de pointes have been reported. Avoid concurrent use with other drugs that prolong the QT interval).
No products indexed under this heading.

Droperidol (Prolongation of the QT interval and isolated cases of torsade de pointes have been reported. Avoid concurrent use with other drugs that prolong the QT interval).
No products indexed under this heading.

Dyphylline (Co-administration of other quinolones with theophylline has resulted in prolonged elimination half-life, elevated serum theophylline levels, and increased risk of theophylline related toxicity; no significant effect of levofloxacin on theophylline pharmacokinetic parameters has been detected; however, caution should be exercised and theophylline levels monitored closely).
No products indexed under this heading.

Erythromycin (Prolongation of the QT interval and isolated cases of torsade de pointes have been reported. Avoid concurrent use with other drugs that prolong the QT interval).
No products indexed under this heading.

Erythromycin Estolate (Prolongation of the QT interval and isolated cases of torsade de pointes have been reported. Avoid concurrent use with other drugs that prolong the QT interval).
No products indexed under this heading.

Erythromycin Ethylsuccinate (Prolongation of the QT interval and isolated cases of torsade de pointes have been reported. Avoid concurrent use with other drugs that prolong the QT interval). Products include:
E.E.S. **433**
EryPed **431**

Erythromycin Gluceptate (Prolongation of the QT interval and isolated cases of torsade de pointes have been reported. Avoid concurrent use with other drugs that prolong the QT interval).
No products indexed under this heading.

Erythromycin Lactobionate (Prolongation of the QT interval and isolated cases of torsade de pointes have been reported. Avoid concurrent use with other drugs that prolong the QT interval).
No products indexed under this heading.

Erythromycin Stearate (Prolongation of the QT interval and isolated cases of torsade de pointes have been reported. Avoid concurrent use with other drugs that prolong the QT interval).
No products indexed under this heading.

Etodolac (Co-administration may increase the risk of CNS stimulation and convulsive seizures).
No products indexed under this heading.

Fenoprofen Calcium (Co-administration may increase the risk of CNS stimulation and convulsive seizures). Products include:
Nalfon Capsules **2508**

Flecainide Acetate (Prolongation of the QT interval and isolated cases of torsade de pointes have been reported. Avoid concurrent use with other drugs that prolong the QT interval).
No products indexed under this heading.

Fludrocortisone Acetate (Achilles and other tendon ruptures have been reported with quinolones, post-market surveillance reports indicate that the risk may be increased in patients on concomitant corticosteroids).
No products indexed under this heading.

Flunisolide (Achilles and other tendon ruptures have been reported with quinolones, post-market surveillance reports indicate that the risk may be increased in patients on concomitant corticosteroids). Products include:
Aerobid/Aerobid-M **1153**

Fluphenazine Decanoate (Prolongation of the QT interval and isolated cases of torsade de pointes have been reported. Avoid concurrent use with other drugs that prolong the QT interval).
No products indexed under this heading.

Fluphenazine Enanthate (Prolongation of the QT interval and isolated cases of torsade de pointes have been reported. Avoid concurrent use with other drugs that prolong the QT interval).
No products indexed under this heading.

Fluphenazine Hydrochloride (Prolongation of the QT interval and isolated cases of torsade de pointes have been reported. Avoid concurrent use with other drugs that prolong the QT interval).
No products indexed under this heading.

Flurbiprofen (Co-administration may increase the risk of CNS stimulation and convulsive seizures).
No products indexed under this heading.

Fluticasone Propionate (Achilles and other tendon ruptures have been reported with quinolones, post-market surveillance reports indicate that the risk may be increased in patients on concomitant corticosteroids). Products include:
Advair Diskus 100/50 .... **1276**
Advair Diskus 250/50 .... **1276**
Advair Diskus 500/50 .... **1276**
Advair HFA 45/21 Inhalation Aerosol.. **1288**
Advair HFA 115/21 Inhalation Aerosol.. **1288**
Advair HFA 230/21 Inhalation Aerosol.. **1288**
Flonase Nasal Spray **1431**
Flovent Diskus 50 mcg **1435**

Fluticasone Propionate HFA (Achilles and other tendon ruptures have been reported with quinolones, post-market surveillance reports indicate that the risk may be increased in patients on concomitant corticosteroids). Products include:
Flovent HFA **1440**

Glimepiride (Disturbances of blood glucose, including hyper- and hypoglycemia, have been reported in patients treated concomitantly with quinolones and an antidiabetic agent; careful monitoring of blood glucose levels is recommended). Products include:
Avandaryl Tablets **1344**
Duetact Tablets **3085**

Glipizide (Disturbances of blood glucose, including hyper- and hypoglycemia, have been reported in patients treated concomitantly with quinolones and an antidiabetic agent; careful monitoring of blood glucose levels is recommended).
No products indexed under this heading.

Glyburide (Disturbances of blood glucose, including hyper- and hypoglycemia, have been reported in patients treated concomitantly with quinolones and an antidiabetic agent; careful monitoring of blood glucose levels is recommended).
No products indexed under this heading.

Haloperidol (Prolongation of the QT interval and isolated cases of torsade de pointes have been reported. Avoid concurrent use with other drugs that prolong the QT interval).
No products indexed under this heading.

Haloperidol Decanoate (Prolongation of the QT interval and isolated cases of torsade de pointes have been reported. Avoid concurrent use with other drugs that prolong the QT interval).
No products indexed under this heading.

Hydrocortisone (Achilles and other tendon ruptures have been reported with quinolones, post-market surveillance reports indicate that the risk may be increased in patients on concomitant corticosteroids).
No products indexed under this heading.

Hydrocortisone Acetate (Achilles and other tendon ruptures have been reported with quinolones, post-market surveillance reports indicate that the risk may be increased in patients on concomitant corticosteroids). Products include:
Analpram-HC **1140**
Pramosone **1141**

Hydrocortisone Sodium Phosphate (Achilles and other tendon ruptures have been reported with quinolones, post-market surveillance reports indicate that the risk may be increased in patients on concomitant corticosteroids).
No products indexed under this heading.

Hydrocortisone Sodium Succinate (Achilles and other tendon ruptures have been reported with quinolones, post-market surveillance reports indicate that the risk may be increased in patients on concomitant corticosteroids).
No products indexed under this heading.

Hydroxyzine Hydrochloride (Prolongation of the QT interval and isolated cases of torsade de pointes have been reported. Avoid concurrent use with other drugs that prolong the QT interval).
No products indexed under this heading.

Ibuprofen (Co-administration may increase the risk of CNS stimulation and convulsive seizures). Products include:
Motrin IB Tablets and Caplets 1900
Children's Motrin Oral Suspension ... 1901
Children's Motrin Non-Staining Dye-Free Oral Suspension............ 1901
Children's Motrin Cold Oral Suspension.............................. 1899
Infants' Motrin Concentrated Drops.. 1901
Infants' Motrin Non-Staining Dye-Free Concentrated Drops...... 1901
Junior Strength Motrin Caplets and Chewable Tablets.................. 1901
Vicoprofen Tablets 533

Imipramine Hydrochloride (Prolongation of the QT interval and isolated cases of torsade de pointes have been reported. Avoid concurrent use with other drugs that prolong the QT interval).
No products indexed under this heading.

Imipramine Pamoate (Prolongation of the QT interval and isolated cases of torsade de pointes have been reported. Avoid concurrent use with other drugs that prolong the QT interval).
No products indexed under this heading.

Indomethacin (Co-administration may increase the risk of CNS stimulation and convulsive seizures). Products include:
Indocin 2024

Indomethacin Sodium Trihydrate (Co-administration may increase the risk of CNS stimulation and convulsive seizures). Products include:
Indocin I.V. 2489

Insulin (Disturbances of blood glucose, including hyper- and hypoglycemia, have been reported in patients treated concomitantly with quinolones and an antidiabetic agent; careful monitoring of blood glucose levels is recommended).
No products indexed under this heading.

Insulin, Human, Zinc Suspension (Disturbances of blood glucose, including hyper- and hypoglycemia, have been reported in patients treated concomitantly with quinolones and an antidiabetic agent; careful monitoring of blood glucose levels is recommended).
No products indexed under this heading.

Insulin, Human (rDNA origin) (Disturbances of blood glucose, including hyper- and hypoglycemia, have been reported in patients treated concomitantly with quinolones and an antidiabetic agent; careful monitoring of blood glucose levels is recommended). Products include:
Exubera Inhalation Powder 2515

Insulin, Human NPH (Disturbances of blood glucose, including hyper- and hypoglycemia, have been reported in patients treated concomitantly with quinolones and an antidiabetic agent; careful monitoring of blood glucose levels is recommended). Products include:
Humulin N Vial 1846

Insulin, Human Regular (Disturbances of blood glucose, including hyper- and hypoglycemia, have been reported in patients treated concomitantly with quinolones and an antidiabetic agent; careful monitoring of blood glucose levels is recommended). Products include:
Humulin R.. 1849
Humulin R (U-500) 1850

Insulin, Human Regular and Human NPH Mixture (Disturbances of blood glucose, including hyper- and hypoglycemia, have been reported in patients treated concomitantly with quinolones and an antidiabetic agent; careful monitoring of blood glucose levels is recommended). Products include:
Humulin 50/50, 100 Units 1843
Humulin 70/30 Vial 1844

Insulin, NPH (Disturbances of blood glucose, including hyper- and hypoglycemia, have been reported in patients treated concomitantly with quinolones and an antidiabetic agent; careful monitoring of blood glucose levels is recommended).
No products indexed under this heading.

Insulin, Regular (Disturbances of blood glucose, including hyper- and hypoglycemia, have been reported in patients treated concomitantly with quinolones and an antidiabetic agent; careful monitoring of blood glucose levels is recommended).
No products indexed under this heading.

Insulin, Regular and NPH mixture (Disturbances of blood glucose, including hyper- and hypoglycemia, have been reported in patients treated concomitantly with quinolones and an antidiabetic agent; careful monitoring of blood glucose levels is recommended).
No products indexed under this heading.

Insulin, Zinc Crystals (Disturbances of blood glucose, including hyper- and hypoglycemia, have been reported in patients treated concomitantly with quinolones and an antidiabetic agent; careful monitoring of blood glucose levels is recommended).
No products indexed under this heading.

Insulin, Zinc Suspension (Disturbances of blood glucose, including hyper- and hypoglycemia, have been reported in patients treated concomitantly with quinolones and an antidiabetic agent; careful monitoring of blood glucose levels is recommended).
No products indexed under this heading.

Insulin Aspart (Disturbances of blood glucose, including hyper- and hypoglycemia, have been reported in patients treated concomitantly with quinolones and an antidiabetic agent; careful monitoring of blood glucose levels is recommended).
No products indexed under this heading.

Insulin Aspart, Human (Disturbances of blood glucose, including hyper- and hypoglycemia, have been reported in patients treated concomitantly with quinolones and an antidiabetic agent; careful monitoring of blood glucose levels is recommended). Products include:
NovoLog Mix 70/30 2364

Insulin Aspart, Human Regular (Disturbances of blood glucose, including hyper- and hypoglycemia, have been reported in patients treated concomitantly with quinolones and an antidiabetic agent; careful monitoring of blood glucose levels is recommended). Products include:
NovoLog Injection 2359

Insulin Aspart Protamine, Human (Disturbances of blood glucose, including hyper- and hypoglycemia, have been reported in patients treated concomitantly with quinolones and an antidiabetic agent; careful monitoring of blood glucose levels is recommended). Products include:
NovoLog Mix 70/30 2364

Insulin Detemir (rDNA Origin) (Disturbances of blood glucose, including hyper- and hypoglycemia, have been reported in patients treated concomitantly with quinolones and an antidiabetic agent; careful monitoring of blood glucose levels is recommended). Products include:
Levemir Injection 2352

Insulin glargine (Disturbances of blood glucose, including hyper- and hypoglycemia, have been reported in patients treated concomitantly with quinolones and an antidiabetic agent; careful monitoring of blood glucose levels is recommended). Products include:
Lantus Injection 2749

Insulin Glulisine (Disturbances of blood glucose, including hyper- and hypoglycemia, have been reported in patients treated concomitantly with quinolones and an antidiabetic agent; careful monitoring of blood glucose levels is recommended). Products include:
Apidra Injection 2706

Insulin Lispro, Human (Disturbances of blood glucose, including hyper- and hypoglycemia, have been reported in patients treated concomitantly with quinolones and an antidiabetic agent; careful monitoring of blood glucose levels is recommended). Products include:
Humalog-Pen and KwikPen 1829
Humalog Mix 50/50-Pen and KwikPen.. 1833
Humalog Mix 75/25-Pen and KwikPen.. 1835

Insulin Lispro Protamine, Human (Disturbances of blood glucose, including hyper- and hypoglycemia, have been reported in patients treated concomitantly with quinolones and an antidiabetic agent; careful monitoring of blood glucose levels is recommended). Products include:
Humalog Mix 50/50-Pen and KwikPen.. 1833
Humalog Mix 75/25-Pen and KwikPen.. 1835

Isocarboxazid (Prolongation of the QT interval and isolated cases of torsade de pointes have been reported. Avoid concurrent use with other drugs that prolong the QT interval). Products include:
Marplan Tablets 3177

Ketoprofen (Co-administration may increase the risk of CNS stimulation and convulsive seizures).
No products indexed under this heading.

Ketorolac Tromethamine (Co-administration may increase the risk of CNS stimulation and convulsive seizures).
No products indexed under this heading.

Lidocaine Hydrochloride (Prolongation of the QT interval and isolated cases of torsade de pointes have been reported. Avoid concurrent use with other drugs that prolong the QT interval).
No products indexed under this heading.

Lithium Carbonate (Prolongation of the QT interval and isolated cases of torsade de pointes have been reported. Avoid concurrent use with other drugs that prolong the QT interval).
No products indexed under this heading.

Lithium Citrate (Prolongation of the QT interval and isolated cases of torsade de pointes have been reported. Avoid concurrent use with other drugs that prolong the QT interval).
No products indexed under this heading.

Lorazepam (Prolongation of the QT interval and isolated cases of torsade de pointes have been reported. Avoid concurrent use with other drugs that prolong the QT interval).
No products indexed under this heading.

Loxapine Hydrochloride (Prolongation of the QT interval and isolated cases of torsade de pointes have been reported. Avoid concurrent use with other drugs that prolong the QT interval).
No products indexed under this heading.

Loxapine Succinate (Prolongation of the QT interval and isolated cases of torsade de pointes have been reported. Avoid concurrent use with other drugs that prolong the QT interval).
No products indexed under this heading.

Maprotiline Hydrochloride (Prolongation of the QT interval and isolated cases of torsade de pointes have been reported. Avoid concurrent use with other drugs that prolong the QT interval).
No products indexed under this heading.

Meclofenamate Sodium (Co-administration may increase the risk of CNS stimulation and convulsive seizures).
No products indexed under this heading.

Mefenamic Acid (Co-administration may increase the risk of CNS stimulation and convulsive seizures).
No products indexed under this heading.

Meloxicam (Co-administration may increase the risk of CNS stimulation and convulsive seizures). Products include:
Mobic Oral Suspension 863
Mobic Tablets 863

Meprobamate (Prolongation of the QT interval and isolated cases of torsade de pointes have been reported. Avoid concurrent use with other drugs that prolong the QT interval).
No products indexed under this heading.

Mesoridazine Besylate (Prolongation of the QT interval and isolated cases of torsade de pointes have been reported. Avoid concurrent use with other drugs that prolong the QT interval).
No products indexed under this heading.

Metformin Hydrochloride (Disturbances of blood glucose, including hyper- and hypoglycemia, have been reported in patients treated concomitantly with quinolones and an antidiabetic agent; careful monitoring of blood glucose levels is recommended). Products include:
ActoPlus Met Tablets **3071**
Avandamet Tablets **1336**
Janumet Tablets **2041**
PrandiMet Tablets **2967**

Methylprednisolone Acetate (Achilles and other tendon ruptures have been reported with quinolones, post-market surveillance reports indicate that the risk may be increased in patients on concomitant corticosteroids).
No products indexed under this heading.

Methylprednisolone Sodium Succinate (Achilles and other tendon ruptures have been reported with quinolones, post-market surveillance reports indicate that the risk may be increased in patients on concomitant corticosteroids).
No products indexed under this heading.

Mexiletine Hydrochloride (Prolongation of the QT interval and isolated cases of torsade de pointes have been reported. Avoid concurrent use with other drugs that prolong the QT interval).
No products indexed under this heading.

Midazolam Hydrochloride (Prolongation of the QT interval and isolated cases of torsade de pointes have been reported. Avoid concurrent use with other drugs that prolong the QT interval).
No products indexed under this heading.

Miglitol (Disturbances of blood glucose, including hyper- and hypoglycemia, have been reported in patients treated concomitantly with quinolones and an antidiabetic agent; careful monitoring of blood glucose levels is recommended).
No products indexed under this heading.

Molindone Hydrochloride (Prolongation of the QT interval and isolated cases of torsade de pointes have been reported. Avoid concurrent use with other drugs that prolong the QT interval). Products include:
Moban Tablets **1116**

Mometasone Furoate (Achilles and other tendon ruptures have been reported with quinolones, post-market surveillance reports indicate that the risk may be increased in patients on concomitant corticosteroids). Products include:
Asmanex Twisthaler **2797**
Elocon Cream 0.1% **2840**
Elocon Lotion 0.1% **2841**
Elocon Ointment 0.1% **2842**

Mometasone Furoate Monohydrate (Achilles and other tendon ruptures have been reported with quinolones, post-market surveillance reports indicate that the risk may be increased in patients on concomitant corticosteroids). Products include:
Nasonex Nasal Spray **2883**

Moricizine Hydrochloride (Levofloxacin has been associated with prolongation of the QT interval and infrequent cases of arrhythmia. Rare cases of torsades de pointes have been spontaneously reported during post-marketing surveillance in patients receiving levofloxacin. Levofloxacin should be avoided in patients receiving class IA antiarrhythmic agents).
No products indexed under this heading.

Nabumetone (Co-administration may increase the risk of CNS stimulation and convulsive seizures).
No products indexed under this heading.

Naproxen (Co-administration may increase the risk of CNS stimulation and convulsive seizures). Products include:
EC-Naprosyn Delayed-Release Tablets **2632**
Naprosyn Suspension **2632**
Naprosyn Tablets **2632**

Naproxen Sodium (Co-administration may increase the risk of CNS stimulation and convulsive seizures). Products include:
Anaprox Tablets **2632**
Anaprox DS Tablets **2632**
Treximet Tablets **1616**

Nateglinide (Disturbances of blood glucose, including hyper- and hypoglycemia, have been reported in patients treated concomitantly with quinolones and an antidiabetic agent; careful monitoring of blood glucose levels is recommended). Products include:
Starlix Tablets **2314**

Nortriptyline Hydrochloride (Prolongation of the QT interval and isolated cases of torsade de pointes have been reported. Avoid concurrent use with other drugs that prolong the QT interval).
No products indexed under this heading.

Olanzapine (Prolongation of the QT interval and isolated cases of torsade de pointes have been reported. Avoid concurrent use with other drugs that prolong the QT interval). Products include:
Symbyax Capsules **1871**
Zyprexa Tablets **1883**
Zyprexa IntraMuscular **1883**
Zyprexa ZYDIS Orally Disintegrating Tablets **1883**

Oxaprozin (Co-administration may increase the risk of CNS stimulation and convulsive seizures).
No products indexed under this heading.

Oxazepam (Prolongation of the QT interval and isolated cases of torsade de pointes have been reported. Avoid concurrent use with other drugs that prolong the QT interval).
No products indexed under this heading.

Paliperidone (Prolongation of the QT interval and isolated cases of torsade de pointes have been reported. Avoid concurrent use with other drugs that prolong the QT interval). Products include:
Invega Extended-Release Tablets **1748**

Perphenazine (Prolongation of the QT interval and isolated cases of torsade de pointes have been reported. Avoid concurrent use with other drugs that prolong the QT interval).
No products indexed under this heading.

Phenelzine Sulfate (Prolongation of the QT interval and isolated cases of torsade de pointes have been reported. Avoid concurrent use with other drugs that prolong the QT interval).
No products indexed under this heading.

Phenylbutazone (Co-administration may increase the risk of CNS stimulation and convulsive seizures).
No products indexed under this heading.

Pioglitazone Hydrochloride (Disturbances of blood glucose, including hyper- and hypoglycemia, have been reported in patients treated concomitantly with quinolones and an antidiabetic agent; careful monitoring of blood glucose levels is recommended). Products include:
ActoPlus Met Tablets **3071**
Actos Tablets **3077**
Duetact Tablets **3085**

Piroxicam (Co-administration may increase the risk of CNS stimulation and convulsive seizures).
No products indexed under this heading.

Prazepam (Prolongation of the QT interval and isolated cases of torsade de pointes have been reported. Avoid concurrent use with other drugs that prolong the QT interval).
No products indexed under this heading.

Prednisolone Acetate (Achilles and other tendon ruptures have been reported with quinolones, post-market surveillance reports indicate that the risk may be increased in patients on concomitant corticosteroids). Products include:
Pred Forte Ophthalmic Suspension .... ⊙**227**
Pred Mild Ophthalmic Suspension .... ⊙**230**
Pred-G Ophthalmic Ointment .... ⊙**229**
Pred-G Ophthalmic Suspension .... ⊙**228**

Prednisolone Sodium Phosphate (Achilles and other tendon ruptures have been reported with quinolones, post-market surveillance reports indicate that the risk may be increased in patients on concomitant corticosteroids).
No products indexed under this heading.

Prednisolone Tebutate (Achilles and other tendon ruptures have been reported with quinolones, post-market surveillance reports indicate that the risk may be increased in patients on concomitant corticosteroids).
No products indexed under this heading.

Prednisone (Achilles and other tendon ruptures have been reported with quinolones, post-market surveillance reports indicate that the risk may be increased in patients on concomitant corticosteroids).
No products indexed under this heading.

Probenecid (Co-administration has resulted in higher levofloxacin AUC and T1/2, while CL/F and CLr were lower during concomitant treatment with probenecid).
No products indexed under this heading.

Procainamide (Levofloxacin has been associated with prolongation of the QT interval and infrequent cases of arrhythmia. Rare cases of torsades de pointes have been spontaneously reported during post-marketing surveillance in patients receiving levofloxacin. Levofloxacin should be avoided in patients receiving class IA antiarrhythmic agents).
No products indexed under this heading.

Procainamide Hydrochloride (Levofloxacin has been associated with prolongation of the QTc interval; co-administration with drugs known to prolong QT interval should be avoided).
No products indexed under this heading.

Prochlorperazine (Prolongation of the QT interval and isolated cases of torsade de pointes have been reported. Avoid concurrent use with other drugs that prolong the QT interval).
No products indexed under this heading.

Promethazine Hydrochloride (Prolongation of the QT interval and isolated cases of torsade de pointes have been reported. Avoid concurrent use with other drugs that prolong the QT interval).
No products indexed under this heading.

Propafenone Hydrochloride (Prolongation of the QT interval and isolated cases of torsade de pointes have been reported. Avoid concurrent use with other drugs that prolong the QT interval). Products include:
Rythmol Tablets **1586**
Rythmol SR Capsules **1590**

Protriptyline Hydrochloride (Prolongation of the QT interval and isolated cases of torsade de pointes have been reported. Avoid concurrent use with other drugs that prolong the QT interval).
No products indexed under this heading.

Quetiapine Fumarate (Prolongation of the QT interval and isolated cases of torsade de pointes have been reported. Avoid concurrent use with other drugs that prolong the QT interval).
No products indexed under this heading.

Quinidine (Levofloxacin has been associated with prolongation of the QTc interval; co-administration with drugs known to prolong QT interval should be avoided).
No products indexed under this heading.

Quinidine Gluconate (Levofloxacin has been associated with prolongation of the QTc interval; co-administration with drugs known to prolong QT interval should be avoided).
No products indexed under this heading.

Quinidine Hydrochloride (Levofloxacin has been associated with prolongation of the QTc interval; co-administration with drugs known to prolong QT interval should be avoided).
No products indexed under this heading.

Quinidine Polygalacturonate (Levofloxacin has been associated with prolongation of the QTc interval; co-administration with drugs known to prolong QT interval should be avoided).
No products indexed under this heading.

Quinidine Sulfate (Levofloxacin has been associated with prolongation of the QTc interval; co-administration with drugs known to prolong QT interval should be avoided).
No products indexed under this heading.

Repaglinide (Disturbances of blood glucose, including hyper- and hypoglycemia, have been reported in patients treated concomitantly with quinolones and an antidiabetic agent; careful monitoring of blood glucose levels is recommended). Products include:
PrandiMet Tablets 2967
Prandin Tablets 2971

Risperidone (Prolongation of the QT interval and isolated cases of torsade de pointes have been reported. Avoid concurrent use with other drugs that prolong the QT interval). Products include:
Risperdal Consta Long-Acting Injection 1753

Rofecoxib (Co-administration may increase the risk of CNS stimulation and convulsive seizures).
No products indexed under this heading.

Rosiglitazone Maleate (Disturbances of blood glucose, including hyper- and hypoglycemia, have been reported in patients treated concomitantly with quinolones and an antidiabetic agent; careful monitoring of blood glucose levels is recommended). Products include:
Avandamet Tablets 1336
Avandaryl Tablets 1344
Avandia Tablets 1351

Sitagliptin Phosphate (Disturbances of blood glucose, including hyper- and hypoglycemia, have been reported in patients treated concomitantly with quinolones and an antidiabetic agent; careful monitoring of blood glucose levels is recommended). Products include:
Janumet Tablets 2041
Januvia Tablets 2048

Sotalol Hydrochloride (Levofloxacin has been associated with prolongation of the QTc interval; co-administration with drugs known to prolong QT interval should be avoided).
No products indexed under this heading.

Sulindac (Co-administration may increase the risk of CNS stimulation and convulsive seizures). Products include:
Clinoril Tablets 1962

Theophylline (Co-administration of other quinolones with theophylline has resulted in prolonged elimination half-life, elevated serum theophylline levels, and increased risk of theophylline related toxicity; no significant effect of levofloxacin on theophylline pharmacokinetic parameters has been detected; however, caution should be exercised and theophylline levels monitored closely).
No products indexed under this heading.

Theophylline Anhydrous (Co-administration of other quinolones with theophylline has resulted in prolonged elimination half-life, elevated serum theophylline levels, and increased risk of theophylline related toxicity; no significant effect of levofloxacin on theophylline pharmacokinetic parameters has been detected; however, caution should be exercised and theophylline levels monitored closely). Products include:
Uniphyl Tablets 2595

Theophylline Calcium Salicylate (Co-administration of other quinolones with theophylline has resulted in prolonged elimination half-life, elevated serum theophylline levels, and increased risk of theophylline related toxicity; no significant effect of levofloxacin on theophylline pharmacokinetic parameters has been detected; however, caution should be exercised and theophylline levels monitored closely).
No products indexed under this heading.

Theophylline Dihydroxypropyl (Glyceryl) (Co-administration of other quinolones with theophylline has resulted in prolonged elimination half-life, elevated serum theophylline levels, and increased risk of theophylline related toxicity; no significant effect of levofloxacin on theophylline pharmacokinetic parameters has been detected; however, caution should be exercised and theophylline levels monitored closely).
No products indexed under this heading.

Theophylline Ethylenediamine (Co-administration of other quinolones with theophylline has resulted in prolonged elimination half-life, elevated serum theophylline levels, and increased risk of theophylline related toxicity; no significant effect of levofloxacin on theophylline pharmacokinetic parameters has been detected; however, caution should be exercised and theophylline levels monitored closely).
No products indexed under this heading.

Theophylline Sodium Glycinate (Co-administration of other quinolones with theophylline has resulted in prolonged elimination half-life, elevated serum theophylline levels, and increased risk of theophylline related toxicity; no significant effect of levofloxacin on theophylline pharmacokinetic parameters has been detected; however, caution should be exercised and theophylline levels monitored closely).
No products indexed under this heading.

Thioridazine Hydrochloride (Prolongation of the QT interval and isolated cases of torsade de pointes have been reported. Avoid concurrent use with other drugs that prolong the QT interval). Products include:
Thioridazine Hydrochloride Tablets 2195

Thiothixene (Prolongation of the QT interval and isolated cases of torsade de pointes have been reported. Avoid concurrent use with other drugs that prolong the QT interval). Products include:
Thiothixene Capsules 2197

Tocainide Hydrochloride (Prolongation of the QT interval and isolated cases of torsade de pointes have been reported. Avoid concurrent use with other drugs that prolong the QT interval).
No products indexed under this heading.

Tolazamide (Disturbances of blood glucose, including hyper- and hypoglycemia, have been reported in patients treated concomitantly with quinolones and an antidiabetic agent; careful monitoring of blood glucose levels is recommended).
No products indexed under this heading.

Tolbutamide (Disturbances of blood glucose, including hyper- and hypoglycemia, have been reported in patients treated concomitantly with quinolones and an antidiabetic agent; careful monitoring of blood glucose levels is recommended).
No products indexed under this heading.

Tolmetin Sodium (Co-administration may increase the risk of CNS stimulation and convulsive seizures).
No products indexed under this heading.

Tranylcypromine Sulfate (Prolongation of the QT interval and isolated cases of torsade de pointes have been reported. Avoid concurrent use with other drugs that prolong the QT interval). Products include:
Parnate Tablets 1532

Triamcinolone (Achilles and other tendon ruptures have been reported with quinolones, post-market surveillance reports indicate that the risk may be increased in patients on concomitant corticosteroids).
No products indexed under this heading.

Triamcinolone Acetonide (Achilles and other tendon ruptures have been reported with quinolones, post-market surveillance reports indicate that the risk may be increased in patients on concomitant corticosteroids). Products include:
Azmacort Inhalation Aerosol 407
Nasacort AQ Nasal Spray 2765
Triesence Injectable Suspension .... ⊙209

Triamcinolone Diacetate (Achilles and other tendon ruptures have been reported with quinolones, post-market surveillance reports indicate that the risk may be increased in patients on concomitant corticosteroids).
No products indexed under this heading.

Triamcinolone Hexacetonide (Achilles and other tendon ruptures have been reported with quinolones, post-market surveillance reports indicate that the risk may be increased in patients on concomitant corticosteroids).
No products indexed under this heading.

Trifluoperazine Hydrochloride (Prolongation of the QT interval and isolated cases of torsade de pointes have been reported. Avoid concurrent use with other drugs that prolong the QT interval).
No products indexed under this heading.

Trimipramine Maleate (Prolongation of the QT interval and isolated cases of torsade de pointes have been reported. Avoid concurrent use with other drugs that prolong the QT interval).
No products indexed under this heading.

Troglitazone (Disturbances of blood glucose, including hyper- and hypoglycemia, have been reported in patients treated concomitantly with quinolones and an antidiabetic agent; careful monitoring of blood glucose levels is recommended).
No products indexed under this heading.

Valdecoxib (Co-administration may increase the risk of CNS stimulation and convulsive seizures).
No products indexed under this heading.

Warfarin Sodium (Co-administration of other quinolones with warfarin has resulted in enhanced effects of warfarin; no significant effect of levofloxacin on warfarin pharmacokinetic parameters has been detected in clinical studies, however, caution should be exercised and coagulation test should be closely monitored).
No products indexed under this heading.

Ziprasidone Hydrochloride (Prolongation of the QT interval and isolated cases of torsade de pointes have been reported. Avoid concurrent use with other drugs that prolong the QT interval). Products include:
Geodon Capsules 2520

Food Interactions

Food, unspecified (Co-administration slightly prolongs the time to peak concentration by approximately 1 hour and slightly decreases the peak concentration by approximately 14%; levofloxacin can be administered without regard to food).

LEVAQUIN ORAL SOLUTION

(Levofloxacin) 2416
See Levaquin Tablets

LEVAQUIN TABLETS

(Levofloxacin) 2416
May interact with antacids containing aluminum, calcium and magnesium, class 1A antiarrhythmics, class III antiarrhythmics, cations, corticosteroids, erythromycin, oral hypoglycemic agents, insulin, iron containing oral preparations, nonsteroidal anti-inflammatory agents, psychotropics, drugs that prolong the QT interval, quinidine, tricyclic antidepressants, xanthines, and certain other agents. Compounds in these categories include:

Acarbose (Disturbances of blood glucose, including hyper- and hypoglycemia, have been reported in patients treated concomitantly with quinolones and an antidiabetic agent; careful monitoring of blood glucose levels is recommended). Products include:

Precose Tablets ... 792

Alprazolam (Prolongation of the QT interval and isolated cases of torsade de pointes have been reported. Avoid concurrent use with other drugs that prolong the QT interval).
No products indexed under this heading.

Aluminum Carbonate (Antacids containing aluminum or magnesium may interfere with the gastrointestinal absorption of levofloxacin resulting in systemic levels considerably lower than desired; these agents should be taken at least 2 hours before or after levofloxacin administration).
No products indexed under this heading.

Aluminum-containing Compounds, unspecified (Concurrent administration of levofloxacin with metal cations may interfere with the GI absorption of levofloxacin, resulting in systemic levels considerably lower than desired; these agents containing metal cations should be taken at least 2 hours before or 2 hours after levofloxacin administration).
No products indexed under this heading.

Aluminum Hydroxide (Antacids containing aluminum or magnesium may interfere with the gastrointestinal absorption of levofloxacin resulting in systemic levels considerably lower than desired; these agents should be taken at least 2 hours before or after levofloxacin administration).
No products indexed under this heading.

Aminophylline (Co-administration of other quinolones with theophylline has resulted in prolonged elimination half-life, elevated serum theophylline levels, and increased risk of theophylline related toxicity; no significant effect of levofloxacin on theophylline pharmacokinetic parameters has been detected, however, caution should be exercised and theophylline levels monitored closely).
No products indexed under this heading.

Amiodarone Hydrochloride (Levofloxacin has been associated with prolongation of the QTc interval; co-administration with drugs known to prolong QT interval should be avoided).
No products indexed under this heading.

Amitriptyline Hydrochloride (Prolongation of the QT interval and isolated cases of torsade de pointes have been reported. Avoid concurrent use with other drugs that prolong the QT interval).
No products indexed under this heading.

Amoxapine (Prolongation of the QT interval and isolated cases of torsade de pointes have been reported. Avoid concurrent use with other drugs that prolong the QT interval).
No products indexed under this heading.

Arsenic Trioxide (Levofloxacin has been associated with prolongation of the QTc interval; co-administration with drugs known to prolong QT interval should be avoided). Products include:
Trisenox Injection ... 986

Astemizole (Prolongation of the QT interval and isolated cases of torsade de pointes have been reported. Avoid concurrent use with other drugs that prolong the QT interval).
No products indexed under this heading.

Betamethasone Acetate (Achilles and other tendon ruptures have been reported with quinolones; post-market surveillance reports indicate that the risk may be increased in patients on concomitant corticosteroids).[1]
No products indexed under this heading.

Betamethasone Sodium Phosphate (Achilles and other tendon ruptures have been reported with quinolones; post-market surveillance reports indicate that the risk may be increased in patients on concomitant corticosteroids).
No products indexed under this heading.

Bretylium Tosylate (Levofloxacin has been associated with prolongation of the QT interval and infrequent cases of arrhythmia. Rare cases of torsades de pointes have been spontaneously reported during post-marketing surveillance in patients receiving levofloxacin. Levofloxacin should be avoided in patients receiving class III antiarrhythmic agents).
No products indexed under this heading.

Budesonide (Achilles and other tendon ruptures have been reported with quinolones; post-market surveillance reports indicate that the risk may be increased in patients on concomitant corticosteroids). Products include:
Pulmicort Flexhaler ... 654
Symbicort 80/4.5 Inhalation Aerosol ... 659
Symbicort 160/4.5 Inhalation Aerosol ... 659

Buspirone Hydrochloride (Prolongation of the QT interval and isolated cases of torsade de pointes have been reported. Avoid concurrent use with other drugs that prolong the QT interval).
No products indexed under this heading.

Calcium (Concurrent administration of levofloxacin with metal cations may interfere with the GI absorption of levofloxacin, resulting in systemic levels considerably lower than desired; these agents containing metal cations should be taken at least 2 hours before or 2 hours after levofloxacin administration).
Products include:
Phyto-Vite Tablets ... 639
Vibe Liquid Multi-Nutrient Supplement ... 626

Celecoxib (Co-administration may increase the risk of CNS stimulation and convulsive seizures). Products include:
Celebrex Capsules ... 2979

Chlordiazepoxide (Prolongation of the QT interval and isolated cases of torsade de pointes have been reported. Avoid concurrent use with other drugs that prolong the QT interval).
No products indexed under this heading.

Chlordiazepoxide Hydrochloride (Prolongation of the QT interval and isolated cases of torsade de pointes have been reported. Avoid concurrent use with other drugs that prolong the QT interval).
No products indexed under this heading.

Chlorpromazine (Prolongation of the QT interval and isolated cases of torsade de pointes have been reported. Avoid concurrent use with other drugs that prolong the QT interval).
No products indexed under this heading.

Chlorpromazine Hydrochloride (Prolongation of the QT interval and isolated cases of torsade de pointes have been reported. Avoid concurrent use with other drugs that prolong the QT interval).
No products indexed under this heading.

Chlorpropamide (Disturbances of blood glucose, including hyper- and hypoglycemia, have been reported in patients treated concomitantly with quinolones and an antidiabetic agent; careful monitoring of blood glucose levels is recommended).
No products indexed under this heading.

Chlorprothixene (Prolongation of the QT interval and isolated cases of torsade de pointes have been reported. Avoid concurrent use with other drugs that prolong the QT interval).
No products indexed under this heading.

Chlorprothixene Hydrochloride (Prolongation of the QT interval and isolated cases of torsade de pointes have been reported. Avoid concurrent use with other drugs that prolong the QT interval).
No products indexed under this heading.

Ciclesonide (Achilles and other tendon ruptures have been reported with quinolones; post-market surveillance reports indicate that the risk may be increased in patients on concomitant corticosteroids). Products include:
Alvesco Inhalation Aerosol ... 2985
Omnaris Nasal Spray ... 2998

Cimetidine (Co-administration has resulted in higher levofloxacin AUC and t1/2, while CL/F and CLr were lower during concomitant treatment with cimetidine).
No products indexed under this heading.

Cimetidine Hydrochloride (Co-administration has resulted in higher levofloxacin AUC and t1/2, while CL/F and CLr were lower during concomitant treatment with cimetidine).
No products indexed under this heading.

Cisapride (Levofloxacin has been associated with prolongation of the QTc interval; co-administration with drugs known to prolong QT interval should be avoided).
No products indexed under this heading.

Clomipramine Hydrochloride (Prolongation of the QT interval and isolated cases of torsade de pointes have been reported. Avoid concurrent use with other drugs that prolong the QT interval).
No products indexed under this heading.

Clorazepate Dipotassium (Prolongation of the QT interval and isolated cases of torsade de pointes have been reported. Avoid concurrent use with other drugs that prolong the QT interval).
No products indexed under this heading.

Clozapine (Prolongation of the QT interval and isolated cases of torsade de pointes have been reported. Avoid concurrent use with other drugs that prolong the QT interval).
No products indexed under this heading.

Cortisone Acetate (Achilles and other tendon ruptures have been reported with quinolones; post-market surveillance reports indicate that the risk may be increased in patients on concomitant corticosteroids).
No products indexed under this heading.

Cyclosporine (Levofloxacin Cmax and Ke were slightly lower while Tmax and t1/2 were slightly longer in the presence of cyclosporine; these differences, however, are not clinically significant, therefore, no dosage adjustment is required).
Products include:
Gengraf Capsules ... 435
Neoral Oral Solution ... 2280
Neoral Soft Gelatin Capsules ... 2280
Restasis Ophthalmic Emulsion ... 557
Sandimmune ... 2296

Desipramine Hydrochloride (Prolongation of the QT interval and isolated cases of torsade de pointes have been reported. Avoid concurrent use with other drugs that prolong the QT interval).
No products indexed under this heading.

Dexamethasone (Achilles and other tendon ruptures have been reported with quinolones; post-market surveillance reports indicate that the risk may be increased in patients on concomitant corticosteroids).
Products include:
Ciprodex Otic Suspension ... 541

Dexamethasone Acetate (Achilles and other tendon ruptures have been reported with quinolones; post-market surveillance reports indicate that the risk may be increased in patients on concomitant corticosteroids).
No products indexed under this heading.

Dexamethasone Sodium Phosphate (Achilles and other tendon ruptures have been reported with quinolones; post-market surveillance reports indicate that the risk may be increased in patients on concomitant corticosteroids).
No products indexed under this heading.

Diazepam (Prolongation of the QT interval and isolated cases of torsade de pointes have been reported. Avoid concurrent use with other drugs that prolong the QT interval).
Products include:
Valium Tablets ... 2658

Diclofenac Epolamine (Co-administration may increase the risk of CNS stimulation and convulsive seizures). Products include:
Flector Patch ... 561

IMPORTANT NOTE: Always consult each drug listing in the patient's regimen for possible interactions.

Diclofenac Potassium (Co-administration may increase the risk of CNS stimulation and convulsive seizures).
No products indexed under this heading.

Diclofenac Sodium (Co-administration may increase the risk of CNS stimulation and convulsive seizures). Products include:
Diclofenac Sodium Ophthalmic Solution ⊙ 240
Voltaren Ophthalmic Solution 2336
Voltaren Tablets 2334
Voltaren-XR Tablets 2337

Didanosine (Antacids contained in Videx chewable/buffered tablets or pediatric powder for oral solution may substantially interfere with the gastrointestinal absorption of levofloxacin, resulting in systemic levels considerably lower than desired).
No products indexed under this heading.

Disopyramide (Levofloxacin has been associated with prolongation of the QT interval and infrequent cases of arrhythmia. Rare cases of torsades de pointes have been spontaneously reported during post-marketing surveillance in patients receiving levofloxacin. Levofloxacin should be avoided in patients receiving class IA antiarrhythmic agents).
No products indexed under this heading.

Disopyramide Phosphate (Prolongation of the QT interval and isolated cases of torsade de pointes have been reported. Avoid concurrent use with other drugs that prolong the QT interval).
No products indexed under this heading.

Dofetilide (Prolongation of the QT interval and isolated cases of torsade de pointes have been reported. Avoid concurrent use with other drugs that prolong the QT interval).
No products indexed under this heading.

Doxepin Hydrochloride (Prolongation of the QT interval and isolated cases of torsade de pointes have been reported. Avoid concurrent use with other drugs that prolong the QT interval).
No products indexed under this heading.

Droperidol (Prolongation of the QT interval and isolated cases of torsade de pointes have been reported. Avoid concurrent use with other drugs that prolong the QT interval).
No products indexed under this heading.

Dyphylline (Co-administration of other quinolones with theophylline has resulted in prolonged elimination half-life, elevated serum theophylline levels, and increased risk of theophylline related toxicity; no significant effect of levofloxacin on theophylline pharmacokinetic parameters has been detected, however, caution should be exercised and theophylline levels monitored closely).
No products indexed under this heading.

Erythromycin (Prolongation of the QT interval and isolated cases of torsade de pointes have been reported. Avoid concurrent use with other drugs that prolong the QT interval).
No products indexed under this heading.

Erythromycin Estolate (Prolongation of the QT interval and isolated cases of torsade de pointes have been reported. Avoid concurrent use with other drugs that prolong the QT interval).
No products indexed under this heading.

Erythromycin Ethylsuccinate (Prolongation of the QT interval and isolated cases of torsade de pointes have been reported. Avoid concurrent use with other drugs that prolong the QT interval). Products include:
E.E.S. 433
EryPed 431

Erythromycin Gluceptate (Prolongation of the QT interval and isolated cases of torsade de pointes have been reported. Avoid concurrent use with other drugs that prolong the QT interval).
No products indexed under this heading.

Erythromycin Lactobionate (Prolongation of the QT interval and isolated cases of torsade de pointes have been reported. Avoid concurrent use with other drugs that prolong the QT interval).
No products indexed under this heading.

Erythromycin Stearate (Prolongation of the QT interval and isolated cases of torsade de pointes have been reported. Avoid concurrent use with other drugs that prolong the QT interval).
No products indexed under this heading.

Etodolac (Co-administration may increase the risk of CNS stimulation and convulsive seizures).
No products indexed under this heading.

Fenoprofen Calcium (Co-administration may increase the risk of CNS stimulation and convulsive seizures). Products include:
Nalfon Capsules 2508

Ferrous Fumarate (Iron-containing preparations may interfere with the gastrointestinal absorption of levofloxacin resulting in systemic levels considerably lower than desired; these agents should be taken at least 2 hours before or after levofloxacin administration).
No products indexed under this heading.

Ferrous Gluconate (Iron-containing preparations may interfere with the gastrointestinal absorption of levofloxacin resulting in systemic levels considerably lower than desired; these agents should be taken at least 2 hours before or after levofloxacin administration). Products include:
CitraNatal DHA Tablets 2175

Ferrous Sulfate (Iron-containing preparations may interfere with the gastrointestinal absorption of levofloxacin resulting in systemic levels considerably lower than desired; these agents should be taken at least 2 hours before or after levofloxacin administration).
No products indexed under this heading.

Flecainide Acetate (Prolongation of the QT interval and isolated cases of torsade de pointes have been reported. Avoid concurrent use with other drugs that prolong the QT interval).
No products indexed under this heading.

Fludrocortisone Acetate (Achilles and other tendon ruptures have been reported with quinolones; post-market surveillance reports indicate that the risk may be increased in patients on concomitant corticosteroids).
No products indexed under this heading.

Flunisolide (Achilles and other tendon ruptures have been reported with quinolones; post-market surveillance reports indicate that the risk may be increased in patients on concomitant corticosteroids). Products include:
Aerobid/Aerobid-M 1153

Fluphenazine Decanoate (Prolongation of the QT interval and isolated cases of torsade de pointes have been reported. Avoid concurrent use with other drugs that prolong the QT interval).
No products indexed under this heading.

Fluphenazine Enanthate (Prolongation of the QT interval and isolated cases of torsade de pointes have been reported. Avoid concurrent use with other drugs that prolong the QT interval).
No products indexed under this heading.

Fluphenazine Hydrochloride (Prolongation of the QT interval and isolated cases of torsade de pointes have been reported. Avoid concurrent use with other drugs that prolong the QT interval).
No products indexed under this heading.

Flurbiprofen (Co-administration may increase the risk of CNS stimulation and convulsive seizures).
No products indexed under this heading.

Fluticasone Propionate (Achilles and other tendon ruptures have been reported with quinolones; post-market surveillance reports indicate that the risk may be increased in patients on concomitant corticosteroids). Products include:
Advair Diskus 100/50 1276
Advair Diskus 250/50 1276
Advair Diskus 500/50 1276
Advair HFA 45/21 Inhalation Aerosol 1288
Advair HFA 115/21 Inhalation Aerosol 1288
Advair HFA 230/21 Inhalation Aerosol 1288
Flonase Nasal Spray 1431
Flovent Diskus 50 mcg 1435

Fluticasone Propionate HFA (Achilles and other tendon ruptures have been reported with quinolones; post-market surveillance reports indicate that the risk may be increased in patients on concomitant corticosteroids). Products include:
Flovent HFA 1440

Glimepiride (Disturbances of blood glucose, including hyper- and hypoglycemia, have been reported in patients treated concomitantly with quinolones and an antidiabetic agent; careful monitoring of blood glucose levels is recommended). Products include:
Avandaryl Tablets 1344
Duetact Tablets 3085

Glipizide (Disturbances of blood glucose, including hyper- and hypoglycemia, have been reported in patients treated concomitantly with quinolones and an antidiabetic agent; careful monitoring of blood glucose levels is recommended).
No products indexed under this heading.

Glyburide (Disturbances of blood glucose, including hyper- and hypoglycemia, have been reported in patients treated concomitantly with quinolones and an antidiabetic agent; careful monitoring of blood glucose levels is recommended).
No products indexed under this heading.

Haloperidol (Prolongation of the QT interval and isolated cases of torsade de pointes have been reported. Avoid concurrent use with other drugs that prolong the QT interval).
No products indexed under this heading.

Haloperidol Decanoate (Prolongation of the QT interval and isolated cases of torsade de pointes have been reported. Avoid concurrent use with other drugs that prolong the QT interval).
No products indexed under this heading.

Hydrocortisone (Achilles and other tendon ruptures have been reported with quinolones; post-market surveillance reports indicate that the risk may be increased in patients on concomitant corticosteroids).
No products indexed under this heading.

Hydrocortisone Acetate (Achilles and other tendon ruptures have been reported with quinolones; post-market surveillance reports indicate that the risk may be increased in patients on concomitant corticosteroids). Products include:
Analpram-HC 1140
Pramosone 1141

Hydrocortisone Sodium Phosphate (Achilles and other tendon ruptures have been reported with quinolones; post-market surveillance reports indicate that the risk may be increased in patients on concomitant corticosteroids).
No products indexed under this heading.

Hydrocortisone Sodium Succinate (Achilles and other tendon ruptures have been reported with quinolones; post-market surveillance reports indicate that the risk may be increased in patients on concomitant corticosteroids).
No products indexed under this heading.

Hydroxyzine Hydrochloride (Prolongation of the QT interval and isolated cases of torsade de pointes have been reported. Avoid concurrent use with other drugs that prolong the QT interval).
No products indexed under this heading.

Ibuprofen (Co-administration may increase the risk of CNS stimulation and convulsive seizures). Products include:
Motrin IB Tablets and Caplets 1900

Children's Motrin Oral Suspension ... 1901
Children's Motrin Non-Staining Dye-Free Oral Suspension............ 1901
Children's Motrin Cold Oral Suspension.............................. 1899
Infants' Motrin Concentrated Drops.. 1901
Infants' Motrin Non-Staining Dye-Free Concentrated Drops....... 1901
Junior Strength Motrin Caplets and Chewable Tablets.................. 1901
Vicoprofen Tablets 533

Imipramine Hydrochloride (Prolongation of the QT interval and isolated cases of torsade de pointes have been reported. Avoid concurrent use with other drugs that prolong the QT interval).
No products indexed under this heading.

Imipramine Pamoate (Prolongation of the QT interval and isolated cases of torsade de pointes have been reported. Avoid concurrent use with other drugs that prolong the QT interval).
No products indexed under this heading.

Indomethacin (Co-administration may increase the risk of CNS stimulation and convulsive seizures). Products include:
Indocin 2024

Indomethacin Sodium Trihydrate (Co-administration may increase the risk of CNS stimulation and convulsive seizures). Products include:
Indocin I.V. 2489

Insulin (Disturbances of blood glucose, including hyper- and hypoglycemia, have been reported in patients treated concomitantly with quinolones and an antidiabetic agent; careful monitoring of blood glucose levels is recommended).
No products indexed under this heading.

Insulin, Human, Zinc Suspension (Disturbances of blood glucose, including hyper- and hypoglycemia, have been reported in patients treated concomitantly with quinolones and an antidiabetic agent; careful monitoring of blood glucose levels is recommended).
No products indexed under this heading.

Insulin, Human (rDNA origin) (Disturbances of blood glucose, including hyper- and hypoglycemia, have been reported in patients treated concomitantly with quinolones and an antidiabetic agent; careful monitoring of blood glucose levels is recommended). Products include:
Exubera Inhalation Powder 2515

Insulin, Human NPH (Disturbances of blood glucose, including hyper- and hypoglycemia, have been reported in patients treated concomitantly with quinolones and an antidiabetic agent; careful monitoring of blood glucose levels is recommended). Products include:
Humulin N Vial 1846

Insulin, Human Regular (Disturbances of blood glucose, including hyper- and hypoglycemia, have been reported in patients treated concomitantly with quinolones and an antidiabetic agent; careful monitoring of blood glucose levels is recommended). Products include:
Humulin R.. 1849
Humulin R (U-500) 1850

Insulin, Human Regular and Human NPH Mixture (Disturbances of blood glucose, including hyper- and hypoglycemia, have been reported in patients treated concomitantly with quinolones and an antidiabetic agent; careful monitoring of blood glucose levels is recommended). Products include:
Humulin 50/50, 100 Units 1843
Humulin 70/30 Vial 1844

Insulin, NPH (Disturbances of blood glucose, including hyper- and hypoglycemia, have been reported in patients treated concomitantly with quinolones and an antidiabetic agent; careful monitoring of blood glucose levels is recommended).
No products indexed under this heading.

Insulin, Regular (Disturbances of blood glucose, including hyper- and hypoglycemia, have been reported in patients treated concomitantly with quinolones and an antidiabetic agent; careful monitoring of blood glucose levels is recommended).
No products indexed under this heading.

Insulin, Regular and NPH mixture (Disturbances of blood glucose, including hyper- and hypoglycemia, have been reported in patients treated concomitantly with quinolones and an antidiabetic agent; careful monitoring of blood glucose levels is recommended).
No products indexed under this heading.

Insulin, Zinc Crystals (Disturbances of blood glucose, including hyper- and hypoglycemia, have been reported in patients treated concomitantly with quinolones and an antidiabetic agent; careful monitoring of blood glucose levels is recommended).
No products indexed under this heading.

Insulin, Zinc Suspension (Disturbances of blood glucose, including hyper- and hypoglycemia, have been reported in patients treated concomitantly with quinolones and an antidiabetic agent; careful monitoring of blood glucose levels is recommended).
No products indexed under this heading.

Insulin Aspart (Disturbances of blood glucose, including hyper- and hypoglycemia, have been reported in patients treated concomitantly with quinolones and an antidiabetic agent; careful monitoring of blood glucose levels is recommended).
No products indexed under this heading.

Insulin Aspart, Human (Disturbances of blood glucose, including hyper- and hypoglycemia, have been reported in patients treated concomitantly with quinolones and an antidiabetic agent; careful monitoring of blood glucose levels is recommended). Products include:
NovoLog Mix 70/30 2364

Insulin Aspart, Human Regular (Disturbances of blood glucose, including hyper- and hypoglycemia, have been reported in patients treated concomitantly with quinolones and an antidiabetic agent; careful monitoring of blood glucose levels is recommended). Products include:
NovoLog Injection 2359

Insulin Aspart Protamine, Human (Disturbances of blood glucose, including hyper- and hypoglycemia, have been reported in patients treated concomitantly with quinolones and an antidiabetic agent; careful monitoring of blood glucose levels is recommended). Products include:
NovoLog Mix 70/30 2364

Insulin Detemir (rDNA Origin) (Disturbances of blood glucose, including hyper- and hypoglycemia, have been reported in patients treated concomitantly with quinolones and an antidiabetic agent; careful monitoring of blood glucose levels is recommended). Products include:
Levemir Injection 2352

Insulin glargine (Disturbances of blood glucose, including hyper- and hypoglycemia, have been reported in patients treated concomitantly with quinolones and an antidiabetic agent; careful monitoring of blood glucose levels is recommended). Products include:
Lantus Injection 2749

Insulin Glulisine (Disturbances of blood glucose, including hyper- and hypoglycemia, have been reported in patients treated concomitantly with quinolones and an antidiabetic agent; careful monitoring of blood glucose levels is recommended). Products include:
Apidra Injection 2706

Insulin Lispro, Human (Disturbances of blood glucose, including hyper- and hypoglycemia, have been reported in patients treated concomitantly with quinolones and an antidiabetic agent; careful monitoring of blood glucose levels is recommended). Products include:
Humalog-Pen and KwikPen 1829
Humalog Mix 50/50-Pen and KwikPen.. 1833
Humalog Mix 75/25-Pen and KwikPen.. 1835

Insulin Lispro Protamine, Human (Disturbances of blood glucose, including hyper- and hypoglycemia, have been reported in patients treated concomitantly with quinolones and an antidiabetic agent; careful monitoring of blood glucose levels is recommended). Products include:
Humalog Mix 50/50-Pen and KwikPen.. 1833
Humalog Mix 75/25-Pen and KwikPen.. 1835

Iron (Iron-containing preparations may interfere with the gastrointestinal absorption of levofloxacin resulting in systemic levels considerably lower than desired; these agents should be taken at least 2 hours before or after levofloxacin administration). Products include:
Phyto-Vite Tablets 639

Isocarboxazid (Prolongation of the QT interval and isolated cases of torsade de pointes have been reported. Avoid concurrent use with other drugs that prolong the QT interval). Products include:
Marplan Tablets 3177

Ketoprofen (Co-administration may increase the risk of CNS stimulation and convulsive seizures).
No products indexed under this heading.

Ketorolac Tromethamine (Co-administration may increase the risk of CNS stimulation and convulsive seizures).
No products indexed under this heading.

Lidocaine Hydrochloride (Prolongation of the QT interval and isolated cases of torsade de pointes have been reported. Avoid concurrent use with other drugs that prolong the QT interval).
No products indexed under this heading.

Lithium Carbonate (Prolongation of the QT interval and isolated cases of torsade de pointes have been reported. Avoid concurrent use with other drugs that prolong the QT interval).
No products indexed under this heading.

Lithium Citrate (Prolongation of the QT interval and isolated cases of torsade de pointes have been reported. Avoid concurrent use with other drugs that prolong the QT interval).
No products indexed under this heading.

Lorazepam (Prolongation of the QT interval and isolated cases of torsade de pointes have been reported. Avoid concurrent use with other drugs that prolong the QT interval).
No products indexed under this heading.

Loxapine Hydrochloride (Prolongation of the QT interval and isolated cases of torsade de pointes have been reported. Avoid concurrent use with other drugs that prolong the QT interval).
No products indexed under this heading.

Loxapine Succinate (Prolongation of the QT interval and isolated cases of torsade de pointes have been reported. Avoid concurrent use with other drugs that prolong the QT interval).
No products indexed under this heading.

Magaldrate (Antacids containing aluminum or magnesium may interfere with the gastrointestinal absorption of levofloxacin resulting in systemic levels considerably lower than desired; these agents should be taken at least 2 hours before or after levofloxacin administration).
No products indexed under this heading.

Magnesium (Concurrent administration of levofloxacin with metal cations may interfere with the GI absorption of levofloxacin, resulting in systemic levels considerably lower than desired; these agents containing metal cations should be taken at least 2 hours before or 2 hours after levofloxacin administration). Products include:
Protector Capsules 639
Vibe Liquid Multi-Nutrient Supplement.................................. 626

Magnesium Hydroxide (Antacids containing aluminum or magnesium may interfere with the gastrointestinal absorption of levofloxacin resulting in systemic levels considerably lower than desired; these agents should be taken at least 2 hours before or after levofloxacin administration). Products include:
Fleet Pedia-Lax Chewable Tablets 1145
Pepcid Complete Chewable Tablets.. 1771
Extra Strength Rolaids Freshmint Tablets.. 1903
Rolaids Multi-Symptom Berry Tablets.. 1903
Rolaids Original Peppermint Tablets.. 1903

Magnesium Oxide (Antacids containing aluminum or magnesium may interfere with the gastrointestinal absorption of levofloxacin resulting in systemic levels considerably lower than desired; these agents should be taken at least 2 hours before or after levofloxacin administration). Products include:

Beelith Tablets 813

Maprotiline Hydrochloride (Prolongation of the QT interval and isolated cases of torsade de pointes have been reported. Avoid concurrent use with other drugs that prolong the QT interval).

No products indexed under this heading.

Meclofenamate Sodium (Co-administration may increase the risk of CNS stimulation and convulsive seizures).

No products indexed under this heading.

Mefenamic Acid (Co-administration may increase the risk of CNS stimulation and convulsive seizures).

No products indexed under this heading.

Meloxicam (Co-administration may increase the risk of CNS stimulation and convulsive seizures). Products include:

Mobic Oral Suspension 863
Mobic Tablets 863

Meprobamate (Prolongation of the QT interval and isolated cases of torsade de pointes have been reported. Avoid concurrent use with other drugs that prolong the QT interval).

No products indexed under this heading.

Mesoridazine Besylate (Prolongation of the QT interval and isolated cases of torsade de pointes have been reported. Avoid concurrent use with other drugs that prolong the QT interval).

No products indexed under this heading.

Metformin Hydrochloride (Disturbances of blood glucose, including hyper- and hypoglycemia, have been reported in patients treated concomitantly with quinolones and an antidiabetic agent; careful monitoring of blood glucose levels is recommended). Products include:

ActoPlus Met Tablets 3071
Avandamet Tablets 1336
Janumet Tablets 2041
PrandiMet Tablets 2967

Methylprednisolone Acetate (Achilles and other tendon ruptures have been reported with quinolones; post-market surveillance reports indicate that the risk may be increased in patients on concomitant corticosteroids).

No products indexed under this heading.

Methylprednisolone Sodium Succinate (Achilles and other tendon ruptures have been reported with quinolones; post-market surveillance reports indicate that the risk may be increased in patients on concomitant corticosteroids).

No products indexed under this heading.

Mexiletine Hydrochloride (Prolongation of the QT interval and isolated cases of torsade de pointes have been reported. Avoid concurrent use with other drugs that prolong the QT interval).

No products indexed under this heading.

Midazolam Hydrochloride (Prolongation of the QT interval and isolated cases of torsade de pointes have been reported. Avoid concurrent use with other drugs that prolong the QT interval).

No products indexed under this heading.

Miglitol (Disturbances of blood glucose, including hyper- and hypoglycemia, have been reported in patients treated concomitantly with quinolones and an antidiabetic agent; careful monitoring of blood glucose levels is recommended).

No products indexed under this heading.

Molindone Hydrochloride (Prolongation of the QT interval and isolated cases of torsade de pointes have been reported. Avoid concurrent use with other drugs that prolong the QT interval). Products include:

Moban Tablets 1116

Mometasone Furoate (Achilles and other tendon ruptures have been reported with quinolones; post-market surveillance reports indicate that the risk may be increased in patients on concomitant corticosteroids). Products include:

Asmanex Twisthaler 2797
Elocon Cream 0.1% 2840
Elocon Lotion 0.1% 2841
Elocon Ointment 0.1% 2842

Mometasone Furoate Monohydrate (Achilles and other tendon ruptures have been reported with quinolones; post-market surveillance reports indicate that the risk may be increased in patients on concomitant corticosteroids). Products include:

Nasonex Nasal Spray 2883

Moricizine Hydrochloride (Levofloxacin has been associated with prolongation of the QT interval and infrequent cases of arrhythmia. Rare cases of torsades de pointes have been spontaneously reported during post-marketing surveillance in patients receiving levofloxacin. Levofloxacin should be avoided in patients receiving class IA antiarrhythmic agents).

No products indexed under this heading.

Nabumetone (Co-administration may increase the risk of CNS stimulation and convulsive seizures).

No products indexed under this heading.

Naproxen (Co-administration may increase the risk of CNS stimulation and convulsive seizures). Products include:

EC-Naprosyn Delayed-Release Tablets 2632
Naprosyn Suspension 2632
Naprosyn Tablets 2632

Naproxen Sodium (Co-administration may increase the risk of CNS stimulation and convulsive seizures). Products include:

Anaprox Tablets 2632
Anaprox DS Tablets 2632
Treximet Tablets 1616

Nateglinide (Disturbances of blood glucose, including hyper- and hypoglycemia, have been reported in patients treated concomitantly with quinolones and an antidiabetic agent; careful monitoring of blood glucose levels is recommended). Products include:

Starlix Tablets 2314

Nortriptyline Hydrochloride (Prolongation of the QT interval and isolated cases of torsade de pointes have been reported. Avoid concurrent use with other drugs that prolong the QT interval).

No products indexed under this heading.

Olanzapine (Prolongation of the QT interval and isolated cases of torsade de pointes have been reported. Avoid concurrent use with other drugs that prolong the QT interval). Products include:

Symbyax Capsules 1871
Zyprexa Tablets 1883
Zyprexa IntraMuscular 1883
Zyprexa ZYDIS Orally Disintegrating Tablets 1883

Oxaprozin (Co-administration may increase the risk of CNS stimulation and convulsive seizures).

No products indexed under this heading.

Oxazepam (Prolongation of the QT interval and isolated cases of torsade de pointes have been reported. Avoid concurrent use with other drugs that prolong the QT interval).

No products indexed under this heading.

Paliperidone (Prolongation of the QT interval and isolated cases of torsade de pointes have been reported. Avoid concurrent use with other drugs that prolong the QT interval). Products include:

Invega Extended-Release Tablets 1748

Perphenazine (Prolongation of the QT interval and isolated cases of torsade de pointes have been reported. Avoid concurrent use with other drugs that prolong the QT interval).

No products indexed under this heading.

Phenelzine Sulfate (Prolongation of the QT interval and isolated cases of torsade de pointes have been reported. Avoid concurrent use with other drugs that prolong the QT interval).

No products indexed under this heading.

Phenylbutazone (Co-administration may increase the risk of CNS stimulation and convulsive seizures).

No products indexed under this heading.

Pimozide (Levofloxacin has been associated with prolongation of the QTc interval; co-administration with drugs known to prolong QT interval should be avoided).

No products indexed under this heading.

Pioglitazone Hydrochloride (Disturbances of blood glucose, including hyper- and hypoglycemia, have been reported in patients treated concomitantly with quinolones and an antidiabetic agent; careful monitoring of blood glucose levels is recommended). Products include:

ActoPlus Met Tablets 3071
Actos Tablets 3077
Duetact Tablets 3085

Piroxicam (Co-administration may increase the risk of CNS stimulation and convulsive seizures).

No products indexed under this heading.

Polysaccharide Iron Complex (Iron-containing preparations may interfere with the gastrointestinal absorption of levofloxacin resulting in systemic levels considerably lower than desired; these agents should be taken at least 2 hours before or after levofloxacin administration). Products include:

Nu-Iron 150 Capsules 2165

Prazepam (Prolongation of the QT interval and isolated cases of torsade de pointes have been reported. Avoid concurrent use with other drugs that prolong the QT interval).

No products indexed under this heading.

Prednisolone Acetate (Achilles and other tendon ruptures have been reported with quinolones; post-market surveillance reports indicate that the risk may be increased in patients on concomitant corticosteroids). Products include:

Pred Forte Ophthalmic Suspension .... ⊙227
Pred Mild Ophthalmic Suspension .... ⊙230
Pred-G Ophthalmic Ointment .... ⊙229
Pred-G Ophthalmic Suspension .... ⊙228

Prednisolone Sodium Phosphate (Achilles and other tendon ruptures have been reported with quinolones; post-market surveillance reports indicate that the risk may be increased in patients on concomitant corticosteroids).

No products indexed under this heading.

Prednisolone Tebutate (Achilles and other tendon ruptures have been reported with quinolones; post-market surveillance reports indicate that the risk may be increased in patients on concomitant corticosteroids).

No products indexed under this heading.

Prednisone (Achilles and other tendon ruptures have been reported with quinolones; post-market surveillance reports indicate that the risk may be increased in patients on concomitant corticosteroids).

No products indexed under this heading.

Probenecid (Co-administration has resulted in higher levofloxacin AUC and t1/2, while CL/F and CLr were lower during concomitant treatment with probenecid).

No products indexed under this heading.

Procainamide (Levofloxacin has been associated with prolongation of the QT interval and infrequent cases of arrhythmia. Rare cases of torsades de pointes have been spontaneously reported during post-marketing surveillance in patients receiving levofloxacin. Levofloxacin should be avoided in patients receiving class IA antiarrhythmic agents).

No products indexed under this heading.

Procainamide Hydrochloride (Levofloxacin has been associated with prolongation of the QTc interval; co-administration with drugs known to prolong QT interval should be avoided).

No products indexed under this heading.

Prochlorperazine (Prolongation of the QT interval and isolated cases of torsade de pointes have been reported. Avoid concurrent use with other drugs that prolong the QT interval).
No products indexed under this heading.

Promethazine Hydrochloride (Prolongation of the QT interval and isolated cases of torsade de pointes have been reported. Avoid concurrent use with other drugs that prolong the QT interval).
No products indexed under this heading.

Propafenone Hydrochloride (Prolongation of the QT interval and isolated cases of torsade de pointes have been reported. Avoid concurrent use with other drugs that prolong the QT interval). Products include:
Rythmol Tablets **1586**
Rythmol SR Capsules **1590**

Protriptyline Hydrochloride (Prolongation of the QT interval and isolated cases of torsade de pointes have been reported. Avoid concurrent use with other drugs that prolong the QT interval).
No products indexed under this heading.

Quetiapine Fumarate (Prolongation of the QT interval and isolated cases of torsade de pointes have been reported. Avoid concurrent use with other drugs that prolong the QT interval).
No products indexed under this heading.

Quinidine (Levofloxacin has been associated with prolongation of the QTc interval; co-administration with drugs known to prolong QT interval should be avoided).
No products indexed under this heading.

Quinidine Gluconate (Levofloxacin has been associated with prolongation of the QTc interval; co-administration with drugs known to prolong QT interval should be avoided).
No products indexed under this heading.

Quinidine Hydrochloride (Levofloxacin has been associated with prolongation of the QTc interval; co-administration with drugs known to prolong QT interval should be avoided).
No products indexed under this heading.

Quinidine Polygalacturonate (Levofloxacin has been associated with prolongation of the QTc interval; co-administration with drugs known to prolong QT interval should be avoided).
No products indexed under this heading.

Quinidine Sulfate (Levofloxacin has been associated with prolongation of the QTc interval; co-administration with drugs known to prolong QT interval should be avoided).
No products indexed under this heading.

Repaglinide (Disturbances of blood glucose, including hyper- and hypoglycemia, have been reported in patients treated concomitantly with quinolones and an antidiabetic agent; careful monitoring of blood glucose levels is recommended). Products include:
PrandiMet Tablets **2967**
Prandin Tablets **2971**

Risperidone (Prolongation of the QT interval and isolated cases of torsade de pointes have been reported. Avoid concurrent use with other drugs that prolong the QT interval). Products include:
Risperdal Consta Long-Acting Injection **1753**

Rofecoxib (Co-administration may increase the risk of CNS stimulation and convulsive seizures).
No products indexed under this heading.

Rosiglitazone Maleate (Disturbances of blood glucose, including hyper- and hypoglycemia, have been reported in patients treated concomitantly with quinolones and an antidiabetic agent; careful monitoring of blood glucose levels is recommended). Products include:
Avandamet Tablets **1336**
Avandaryl Tablets **1344**
Avandia Tablets **1351**

Sitagliptin Phosphate (Disturbances of blood glucose, including hyper- and hypoglycemia, have been reported in patients treated concomitantly with quinolones and an antidiabetic agent; careful monitoring of blood glucose levels is recommended). Products include:
Janumet Tablets **2041**
Januvia Tablets **2048**

Sotalol Hydrochloride (Levofloxacin has been associated with prolongation of the QTc interval; co-administration with drugs known to prolong QT interval should be avoided).
No products indexed under this heading.

Sucralfate (May interfere with the gastrointestinal absorption of levofloxacin resulting in systemic levels considerably lower than desired; sucralfate should be taken at least 2 hours before or after levofloxacin administration). Products include:
Carafate Suspension **706**
Carafate Tablets **707**

Sulindac (Co-administration may increase the risk of CNS stimulation and convulsive seizures). Products include:
Clinoril Tablets **1962**

Theophylline (Co-administration of other quinolones with theophylline has resulted in prolonged elimination half-life, elevated serum theophylline levels, and increased risk of theophylline related toxicity; no significant effect of levofloxacin on theophylline pharmacokinetic parameters has been detected, however, caution should be exercised and theophylline levels monitored closely).
No products indexed under this heading.

Theophylline Anhydrous (Co-administration of other quinolones with theophylline has resulted in prolonged elimination half-life, elevated serum theophylline levels, and increased risk of theophylline related toxicity; no significant effect of levofloxacin on theophylline pharmacokinetic parameters has been detected, however, caution should be exercised and theophylline levels monitored closely). Products include:
Uniphyl Tablets **2595**

Theophylline Calcium Salicylate (Co-administration of other quinolones with theophylline has resulted in prolonged elimination half-life, elevated serum theophylline levels, and increased risk of theophylline related toxicity; no significant effect of levofloxacin on theophylline pharmacokinetic parameters has been detected, however, caution should be exercised and theophylline levels monitored closely).
No products indexed under this heading.

Theophylline Dihydroxypropyl (Glyceryl) (Co-administration of other quinolones with theophylline has resulted in prolonged elimination half-life, elevated serum theophylline levels, and increased risk of theophylline related toxicity; no significant effect of levofloxacin on theophylline pharmacokinetic parameters has been detected, however, caution should be exercised and theophylline levels monitored closely).
No products indexed under this heading.

Theophylline Ethylenediamine (Co-administration of other quinolones with theophylline has resulted in prolonged elimination half-life, elevated serum theophylline levels, and increased risk of theophylline related toxicity; no significant effect of levofloxacin on theophylline pharmacokinetic parameters has been detected, however, caution should be exercised and theophylline levels monitored closely).
No products indexed under this heading.

Theophylline Sodium Glycinate (Co-administration of other quinolones with theophylline has resulted in prolonged elimination half-life, elevated serum theophylline levels, and increased risk of theophylline related toxicity; no significant effect of levofloxacin on theophylline pharmacokinetic parameters has been detected, however, caution should be exercised and theophylline levels monitored closely).
No products indexed under this heading.

Thioridazine Hydrochloride (Prolongation of the QT interval and isolated cases of torsade de pointes have been reported. Avoid concurrent use with other drugs that prolong the QT interval). Products include:
Thioridazine Hydrochloride Tablets **2195**

Thiothixene (Prolongation of the QT interval and isolated cases of torsade de pointes have been reported. Avoid concurrent use with other drugs that prolong the QT interval). Products include:
Thiothixene Capsules **2197**

Tocainide Hydrochloride (Prolongation of the QT interval and isolated cases of torsade de pointes have been reported. Avoid concurrent use with other drugs that prolong the QT interval).
No products indexed under this heading.

Tolazamide (Disturbances of blood glucose, including hyper- and hypoglycemia, have been reported in patients treated concomitantly with quinolones and an antidiabetic agent; careful monitoring of blood glucose levels is recommended).
No products indexed under this heading.

Tolbutamide (Disturbances of blood glucose, including hyper- and hypoglycemia, have been reported in patients treated concomitantly with quinolones and an antidiabetic agent; careful monitoring of blood glucose levels is recommended).
No products indexed under this heading.

Tolmetin Sodium (Co-administration may increase the risk of CNS stimulation and convulsive seizures).
No products indexed under this heading.

Tranylcypromine Sulfate (Prolongation of the QT interval and isolated cases of torsade de pointes have been reported. Avoid concurrent use with other drugs that prolong the QT interval). Products include:
Parnate Tablets **1532**

Triamcinolone (Achilles and other tendon ruptures have been reported with quinolones; post-market surveillance reports indicate that the risk may be increased in patients on concomitant corticosteroids).
No products indexed under this heading.

Triamcinolone Acetonide (Achilles and other tendon ruptures have been reported with quinolones; post-market surveillance reports indicate that the risk may be increased in patients on concomitant corticosteroids). Products include:
Azmacort Inhalation Aerosol **407**
Nasacort AQ Nasal Spray **2765**
Triesence Injectable Suspension .... ⊙ **209**

Triamcinolone Diacetate (Achilles and other tendon ruptures have been reported with quinolones; post-market surveillance reports indicate that the risk may be increased in patients on concomitant corticosteroids).
No products indexed under this heading.

Triamcinolone Hexacetonide (Achilles and other tendon ruptures have been reported with quinolones; post-market surveillance reports indicate that the risk may be increased in patients on concomitant corticosteroids).
No products indexed under this heading.

Trifluoperazine Hydrochloride (Prolongation of the QT interval and isolated cases of torsade de pointes have been reported. Avoid concurrent use with other drugs that prolong the QT interval).
No products indexed under this heading.

Trimipramine Maleate (Prolongation of the QT interval and isolated cases of torsade de pointes have been reported. Avoid concurrent use with other drugs that prolong the QT interval).
No products indexed under this heading.

Troglitazone (Disturbances of blood glucose, including hyper- and hypoglycemia, have been reported in patients treated concomitantly with quinolones and an antidiabetic agent; careful monitoring of blood glucose levels is recommended).
No products indexed under this heading.

Valdecoxib (Co-administration may increase the risk of CNS stimulation and convulsive seizures).
No products indexed under this heading.

Warfarin Sodium (Co-administration of other quinolones with warfarin has resulted in enhanced effects of warfarin; no significant effect of levofloxacin on warfarin pharmacokinetic parameters has been detected in clinical studies, however, caution should be exercised and coagulation test should be closely monitored).
No products indexed under this heading.

Zinc (Concurrent administration of levofloxacin with metal cations may interfere with the GI absorption of levofloxacin, resulting in systemic levels considerably lower than desired; these agents containing metal cations should be taken at least 2 hours before or 2 hours after levofloxacin administration). Products include:
Comax Dietary Supplement 995
Glaucofit Dietary Supplement 995
Glauma Dietary Supplement 995
Tonox Dietary Supplement 995
Vibe Liquid Multi-Nutrient Supplement .... ▣626
Visutein Capsules 3159

Ziprasidone Hydrochloride (Levofloxacin has been associated with prolongation of the QTc interval; co-administration with drugs known to prolong QT interval should be avoided). Products include:
Geodon Capsules 2520

Food Interactions

Food, unspecified (Co-administration slightly prolongs the time to peak concentration by approximately 1 hour and slightly decreases the peak concentration by approximately 14%; levofloxacin can be administered without regard to food).

LEVAQUIN IN 5% DEXTROSE INJECTION

(Levofloxacin) 2416
See Levaquin Injection

LEVEMIR INJECTION

(Insulin Detemir (rDNA Origin)) 2352
May interact with ACE inhibitors, beta blockers, corticosteroids, diuretics, estrogens, fibrates, oral hypoglycemic agents, lithium preparations, monoamine oxidase inhibitors, phenothiazines, progestins, salicylates, sulfonamides, sympathomimetics, thyroid preparations, and certain other agents. Compounds in these categories include:

Acarbose (Co-administration may reduce the blood-glucose-lowering effect of insulin and susceptibility to hypoglycemia). Products include:
Precose Tablets 792

Acebutolol Hydrochloride (Co-administration may either potentiate or weaken the blood-glucose-lowering effect of insulin. Signs of hypoglycemia may be reduced or absent).
No products indexed under this heading.

Albuterol (Co-administration may reduce the blood-glucose-lowering effect of insulin).
No products indexed under this heading.

Albuterol Sulfate (Co-administration may reduce the blood-glucose-lowering effect of insulin). Products include:
Combivent Inhalation Aerosol 845
ProAir HFA Inhalation Aerosol 3113
Proventil HFA Inhalation Aerosol 2914
Ventolin HFA Inhalation Aerosol 1638

Amiloride Hydrochloride (Co-administration may reduce the blood-glucose-lowering effect of insulin).
No products indexed under this heading.

Aspirin (Co-administration may reduce the blood-glucose-lowering effect of insulin and susceptibility to hypoglycemia). Products include:
Aggrenox Capsules 819
Bayer Aspirin 750
Percodan Tablets 1130
St. Joseph 81 mg Aspirin Chewable and Enteric Coated Tablets 1903

Aspirin, Enteric Coated (Co-administration may reduce the blood-glucose-lowering effect of insulin and susceptibility to hypoglycemia).
No products indexed under this heading.

Aspirin Buffered (Co-administration may reduce the blood-glucose-lowering effect of insulin and susceptibility to hypoglycemia).
No products indexed under this heading.

Atenolol (Co-administration may either potentiate or weaken the blood-glucose-lowering effect of insulin. Signs of hypoglycemia may be reduced or absent).
No products indexed under this heading.

Benazepril Hydrochloride (Co-administration may reduce the blood-glucose-lowering effect of insulin and susceptibility to hypoglycemia).
No products indexed under this heading.

Bendroflumethiazide (Co-administration may reduce the blood-glucose-lowering effect of insulin).
No products indexed under this heading.

Betamethasone Acetate (Co-administration may reduce the blood-glucose-lowering effect of insulin).
No products indexed under this heading.

Betamethasone Sodium Phosphate (Co-administration may reduce the blood-glucose-lowering effect of insulin).
No products indexed under this heading.

Betaxolol Hydrochloride (Co-administration may either potentiate or weaken the blood-glucose-lowering effect of insulin. Signs of hypoglycemia may be reduced or absent).
No products indexed under this heading.

Bisoprolol Fumarate (Co-administration may either potentiate or weaken the blood-glucose-lowering effect of insulin. Signs of hypoglycemia may be reduced or absent).
No products indexed under this heading.

Budesonide (Co-administration may reduce the blood-glucose-lowering effect of insulin). Products include:
Pulmicort Flexhaler 654
Symbicort 80/4.5 Inhalation Aerosol.. 659
Symbicort 160/4.5 Inhalation Aerosol.. 659

Bumetanide (Co-administration may reduce the blood-glucose-lowering effect of insulin).
No products indexed under this heading.

Captopril (Co-administration may reduce the blood-glucose-lowering effect of insulin and susceptibility to hypoglycemia). Products include:
Captopril Tablets 2182

Carteolol Hydrochloride (Co-administration may either potentiate or weaken the blood-glucose-lowering effect of insulin. Signs of hypoglycemia may be reduced or absent).
No products indexed under this heading.

Chlorothiazide (Co-administration may reduce the blood-glucose-lowering effect of insulin).
No products indexed under this heading.

Chlorothiazide Sodium (Co-administration may reduce the blood-glucose-lowering effect of insulin). Products include:
Intravenous Sodium Diuril 2490

Chlorotrianisene (Co-administration may reduce the blood-glucose-lowering effect of insulin).
No products indexed under this heading.

Chlorpromazine (Co-administration may reduce the blood-glucose-lowering effect of insulin).
No products indexed under this heading.

Chlorpromazine Hydrochloride (Co-administration may reduce the blood-glucose-lowering effect of insulin).
No products indexed under this heading.

Chlorpropamide (Co-administration may reduce the blood-glucose-lowering effect of insulin and susceptibility to hypoglycemia).
No products indexed under this heading.

Chlorthalidone (Co-administration may reduce the blood-glucose-lowering effect of insulin). Products include:
Clorpres Tablets 2185

Choline Magnesium Trisalicylate (Co-administration may reduce the blood-glucose-lowering effect of insulin and susceptibility to hypoglycemia).
No products indexed under this heading.

Ciclesonide (Co-administration may reduce the blood-glucose-lowering effect of insulin). Products include:
Alvesco Inhalation Aerosol 2985
Omnaris Nasal Spray 2998

Clofibrate (Co-administration may reduce the blood-glucose-lowering effect of insulin and susceptibility to hypoglycemia).
No products indexed under this heading.

Clonidine (Co-administration may either potentiate or weaken the blood-glucose lowering effect of insulin. Signs of hypoglycemia may be reduced or absent). Products include:
Catapres-TTS 842

Cortisone Acetate (Co-administration may reduce the blood-glucose-lowering effect of insulin).
No products indexed under this heading.

Danazol (Co-administration may reduce the blood-glucose-lowering effect of insulin).
No products indexed under this heading.

Desogestrel (Co-administration may reduce the blood-glucose-lowering effect of insulin). Products include:
Mircette Tablets 1034

Dexamethasone (Co-administration may reduce the blood-glucose-lowering effect of insulin). Products include:
Ciprodex Otic Suspension 541

Dexamethasone Acetate (Co-administration may reduce the blood-glucose-lowering effect of insulin).
No products indexed under this heading.

Dexamethasone Sodium Phosphate (Co-administration may reduce the blood-glucose-lowering effect of insulin).
No products indexed under this heading.

Dienestrol (Co-administration may reduce the blood-glucose-lowering effect of insulin).
No products indexed under this heading.

Diethylstilbestrol (Co-administration may reduce the blood-glucose-lowering effect of insulin).
No products indexed under this heading.

Diflunisal (Co-administration may reduce the blood-glucose-lowering effect of insulin and susceptibility to hypoglycemia).
No products indexed under this heading.

Disopyramide (Co-administration may reduce the blood-glucose-lowering effect of insulin and susceptibility to hypoglycemia).
No products indexed under this heading.

Dobutamine Hydrochloride (Co-administration may reduce the blood-glucose-lowering effect of insulin).
No products indexed under this heading.

Dopamine Hydrochloride (Co-administration may reduce the blood-glucose-lowering effect of insulin).
No products indexed under this heading.

Enalapril Maleate (Co-administration may reduce the blood-glucose-lowering effect of insulin and susceptibility to hypoglycemia).
No products indexed under this heading.

Enalaprilat (Co-administration may reduce the blood-glucose-lowering effect of insulin and susceptibility to hypoglycemia).
No products indexed under this heading.

Ephedrine Hydrochloride (Co-administration may reduce the blood-glucose-lowering effect of insulin).
No products indexed under this heading.

Ephedrine Sulfate (Co-administration may reduce the blood-glucose-lowering effect of insulin).
No products indexed under this heading.

Ephedrine Tannate (Co-administration may reduce the blood-glucose-lowering effect of insulin).
No products indexed under this heading.

Epinephrine (Co-administration may reduce the blood-glucose-lowering effect of insulin). Products include:
EpiPen 1024

Epinephrine Bitartrate (Co-administration may reduce the blood-glucose-lowering effect of insulin).
No products indexed under this heading.

Epinephrine Hydrochloride (Co-administration may reduce the blood-glucose-lowering effect of insulin).
No products indexed under this heading.

Esmolol Hydrochloride (Co-administration may either potentiate or weaken the blood-glucose-lowering effect of insulin. Signs of hypoglycemia may be reduced or absent).
No products indexed under this heading.

Estradiol (Co-administration may reduce the blood-glucose-lowering effect of insulin). Products include:
Activella Tablets 2347
Angeliq Tablets 751
Climara Transdermal System 763
Climara Pro Transdermal System 768
Divigel 3167
Vagifem Tablets 2375

Estrogens, Conjugated (Co-administration may reduce the blood-glucose-lowering effect of insulin). Products include:
Premarin Intravenous 3217
Premarin Tablets 3221
Premarin Vaginal Cream 3228
Premphase Tablets 3232
Prempro Tablets 3232

Estrogens, Esterified (Co-administration may reduce the blood-glucose-lowering effect of insulin). Products include:
Estratest Tablets 3043
Estratest H.S. Tablets 3043

Estropipate (Co-administration may reduce the blood-glucose-lowering effect of insulin).
No products indexed under this heading.

Ethacrynic Acid (Co-administration may reduce the blood-glucose-lowering effect of insulin). Products include:
Edecrin Tablets 698

Ethinyl Estradiol (Co-administration may reduce the blood-glucose-lowering effect of insulin). Products include:
Lybrel Tablets 3204
Mircette Tablets 1034
NuvaRing 2897
Ortho-Cyclen/Ortho Tri-Cyclen 2449
Ortho Evra Transdermal System 2437
Ortho Tri-Cyclen Lo Tablets 2458
Seasonique Tablets 1046
Yaz Tablets 805

Fenofibrate (Co-administration may reduce the blood-glucose-lowering effect of insulin and susceptibility to hypoglycemia). Products include:
Fenoglide Tablets 2960
Tricor Tablets 520

Fludrocortisone Acetate (Co-administration may reduce the blood-glucose-lowering effect of insulin).
No products indexed under this heading.

Flunisolide (Co-administration may reduce the blood-glucose-lowering effect of insulin). Products include:
Aerobid/Aerobid-M 1153

Fluoxetine (Co-administration may reduce the blood-glucose-lowering effect of insulin and susceptibility to hypoglycemia).
No products indexed under this heading.

Fluphenazine Decanoate (Co-administration may reduce the blood-glucose-lowering effect of insulin).
No products indexed under this heading.

Fluphenazine Enanthate (Co-administration may reduce the blood-glucose-lowering effect of insulin).
No products indexed under this heading.

Fluphenazine Hydrochloride (Co-administration may reduce the blood-glucose-lowering effect of insulin).
No products indexed under this heading.

Fluticasone Propionate (Co-administration may reduce the blood-glucose-lowering effect of insulin). Products include:
Advair Diskus 100/50 1276
Advair Diskus 250/50 1276
Advair Diskus 500/50 1276
Advair HFA 45/21 Inhalation Aerosol 1288
Advair HFA 115/21 Inhalation Aerosol 1288
Advair HFA 230/21 Inhalation Aerosol 1288
Flonase Nasal Spray 1431
Flovent Diskus 50 mcg 1435

Fluticasone Propionate HFA (Co-administration may reduce the blood-glucose-lowering effect of insulin). Products include:
Flovent HFA 1440

Fosinopril Sodium (Co-administration may reduce the blood-glucose-lowering effect of insulin and susceptibility to hypoglycemia).
No products indexed under this heading.

Furosemide (Co-administration may reduce the blood-glucose-lowering effect of insulin). Products include:
Furosemide Tablets 2186

Gemfibrozil (Co-administration may reduce the blood-glucose-lowering effect of insulin and susceptibility to hypoglycemia).
No products indexed under this heading.

Glimepiride (Co-administration may reduce the blood-glucose-lowering effect of insulin and susceptibility to hypoglycemia). Products include:
Avandaryl Tablets 1344
Duetact Tablets 3085

Glipizide (Co-administration may reduce the blood-glucose-lowering effect of insulin and susceptibility to hypoglycemia).
No products indexed under this heading.

Glyburide (Co-administration may reduce the blood-glucose-lowering effect of insulin and susceptibility to hypoglycemia).
No products indexed under this heading.

Guanethidine (Signs of hypoglycemia may be reduced or absent).
No products indexed under this heading.

Hydrochlorothiazide (Co-administration may reduce the blood-glucose-lowering effect of insulin). Products include:
Atacand HCT 642
Avalide Tablets 892
Avalide Tablets 2713
Benicar HCT Tablets 1010
Diovan HCT Tablets 2216
Dyazide Capsules 1405
Micardis HCT Tablets 854
Prinzide Tablets 2092
Tekturna HCT Tablets 2324
Teveten HCT Tablets 517

Hydrocortisone (Co-administration may reduce the blood-glucose-lowering effect of insulin).
No products indexed under this heading.

Hydrocortisone Acetate (Co-administration may reduce the blood-glucose-lowering effect of insulin). Products include:
Analpram-HC 1140
Pramosone 1141

Hydrocortisone Sodium Phosphate (Co-administration may reduce the blood-glucose-lowering effect of insulin).
No products indexed under this heading.

Hydrocortisone Sodium Succinate (Co-administration may reduce the blood-glucose-lowering effect of insulin).
No products indexed under this heading.

Hydroflumethiazide (Co-administration may reduce the blood-glucose-lowering effect of insulin).
No products indexed under this heading.

Indapamide (Co-administration may reduce the blood-glucose-lowering effect of insulin). Products include:
Indapamide Tablets 2188

Isocarboxazid (Co-administration may reduce the blood-glucose-lowering effect of insulin and susceptibility to hypoglycemia). Products include:
Marplan Tablets 3177

Isoniazid (Co-administration may reduce the blood-glucose-lowering effect of insulin).
No products indexed under this heading.

Isoproterenol Hydrochloride (Co-administration may reduce the blood-glucose-lowering effect of insulin).
No products indexed under this heading.

Isoproterenol Sulfate (Co-administration may reduce the blood-glucose-lowering effect of insulin).
No products indexed under this heading.

Labetalol Hydrochloride (Co-administration may either potentiate or weaken the blood-glucose-lowering effect of insulin. Signs of hypoglycemia may be reduced or absent).
No products indexed under this heading.

Levalbuterol Hydrochloride (Co-administration may reduce the blood-glucose-lowering effect of insulin). Products include:
Xopenex Inhalation Solution 3001
Xopenex Inhalation Solution Concentrate 3005

Levobunolol Hydrochloride (Co-administration may either potentiate or weaken the blood-glucose-lowering effect of insulin. Signs of hypoglycemia may be reduced or absent).
No products indexed under this heading.

Levothyroxine Sodium (Co-administration may reduce the blood-glucose-lowering effect of insulin). Products include:
Levothroid Tablets 1170
Levoxyl Tablets 1780
Synthroid Tablets 507

Liothyronine Sodium (Co-administration may reduce the blood-glucose-lowering effect of insulin). Products include:
Cytomel Tablets 1778

Liotrix (Co-administration may reduce the blood-glucose-lowering effect of insulin).
No products indexed under this heading.

Lisinopril (Co-administration may reduce the blood-glucose-lowering effect of insulin and susceptibility to hypoglycemia). Products include:
Prinivil Tablets 2087
Prinzide Tablets 2092

Lithium (Co-administration may either potentiate or weaken the blood-glucose-lowering effect of insulin).
No products indexed under this heading.

Lithium Carbonate (Co-administration may either potentiate or weaken the blood-glucose-lowering effect of insulin).
No products indexed under this heading.

Lithium Citrate (Co-administration may either potentiate or weaken the blood-glucose-lowering effect of insulin).
No products indexed under this heading.

Magnesium Salicylate (Co-administration may reduce the blood-glucose-lowering effect of insulin and susceptibility to hypoglycemia).
No products indexed under this heading.

Medroxyprogesterone Acetate (Co-administration may reduce the blood-glucose-lowering effect of insulin). Products include:
Premphase Tablets 3232
Prempro Tablets 3232

Megestrol Acetate (Co-administration may reduce the blood-glucose-lowering effect of insulin). Products include:
Megace ES Oral Suspension 2499

Mesoridazine Besylate (Co-administration may reduce the blood-glucose-lowering effect of insulin).
No products indexed under this heading.

Metaproterenol Sulfate (Co-administration may reduce the blood-glucose-lowering effect of insulin).
No products indexed under this heading.

Metaraminol Bitartrate (Co-administration may reduce the blood-glucose-lowering effect of insulin).
No products indexed under this heading.

Metformin Hydrochloride (Co-administration may reduce the blood-glucose-lowering effect of insulin and susceptibility to hypoglycemia). Products include:
ActoPlus Met Tablets 3071
Avandamet Tablets 1336
Janumet Tablets 2041
PrandiMet Tablets 2967

Methotrimeprazine (Co-administration may reduce the blood-glucose-lowering effect of insulin).
No products indexed under this heading.

Methoxamine Hydrochloride (Co-administration may reduce the blood-glucose-lowering effect of insulin).
No products indexed under this heading.

Methyclothiazide (Co-administration may reduce the blood-glucose-lowering effect of insulin).
No products indexed under this heading.

Methylprednisolone Acetate (Co-administration may reduce the blood-glucose-lowering effect of insulin).
No products indexed under this heading.

Methylprednisolone Sodium Succinate (Co-administration may reduce the blood-glucose-lowering effect of insulin).
No products indexed under this heading.

Metipranolol Hydrochloride (Co-administration may either potentiate or weaken the blood-glucose-lowering effect of insulin. Signs of hypoglycemia may be reduced or absent).
No products indexed under this heading.

Metolazone (Co-administration may reduce the blood-glucose-lowering effect of insulin).
No products indexed under this heading.

Metoprolol Succinate (Co-administration may either potentiate or weaken the blood-glucose-lowering effect of insulin. Signs of hypoglycemia may be reduced or absent). Products include:
Toprol-XL Tablets **666**

Metoprolol Tartrate (Co-administration may either potentiate or weaken the blood-glucose-lowering effect of insulin. Signs of hypoglycemia may be reduced or absent).
No products indexed under this heading.

Miglitol (Co-administration may reduce the blood-glucose-lowering effect of insulin and susceptibility to hypoglycemia).
No products indexed under this heading.

Moclobemide (Co-administration may reduce the blood-glucose-lowering effect of insulin and susceptibility to hypoglycemia).
No products indexed under this heading.

Moexipril Hydrochloride (Co-administration may reduce the blood-glucose-lowering effect of insulin and susceptibility to hypoglycemia).
No products indexed under this heading.

Mometasone Furoate (Co-administration may reduce the blood-glucose-lowering effect of insulin). Products include:
Asmanex Twisthaler **2797**
Elocon Cream 0.1% **2840**
Elocon Lotion 0.1% **2841**
Elocon Ointment 0.1% **2842**

Mometasone Furoate Monohydrate (Co-administration may reduce the blood-glucose-lowering effect of insulin). Products include:
Nasonex Nasal Spray **2883**

Nadolol (Co-administration may either potentiate or weaken the blood-glucose-lowering effect of insulin. Signs of hypoglycemia may be reduced or absent). Products include:
Nadolol Tablets **2191**

Nateglinide (Co-administration may reduce the blood-glucose-lowering effect of insulin and susceptibility to hypoglycemia). Products include:
Starlix Tablets **2314**

Nebivolol (Co-administration may either potentiate or weaken the blood-glucose-lowering effect of insulin. Signs of hypoglycemia may be reduced or absent). Products include:
Bystolic Tablets **1155**

Norepinephrine Bitartrate (Co-administration may reduce the blood-glucose-lowering effect of insulin).
No products indexed under this heading.

Norgestimate (Co-administration may reduce the blood-glucose-lowering effect of insulin). Products include:
Ortho-Cyclen/Ortho Tri-Cyclen **2449**
Ortho Tri-Cyclen Lo Tablets **2458**

Octreotide Acetate (Co-administration may increase the blood-glucose-lowering effect of insulin and susceptibility to hypoglycemia). Products include:
Sandostatin Injection **2300**
Sandostatin LAR Depot **2302**

Pargyline Hydrochloride (Co-administration may reduce the blood-glucose-lowering effect of insulin and susceptibility to hypoglycemia).
No products indexed under this heading.

Penbutolol Sulfate (Co-administration may either potentiate or weaken the blood-glucose-lowering effect of insulin. Signs of hypoglycemia may be reduced or absent).
No products indexed under this heading.

Pentamidine Isethionate (Co-administration may cause hypoglycemia, which may sometimes be followed by hyperglycemia).
No products indexed under this heading.

Perindopril Erbumine (Co-administration may reduce the blood-glucose-lowering effect of insulin and susceptibility to hypoglycemia). Products include:
Aceon Tablets (2 mg, 4 mg, 8 mg) **3038**

Perphenazine (Co-administration may reduce the blood-glucose-lowering effect of insulin).
No products indexed under this heading.

Phenelzine Sulfate (Co-administration may reduce the blood-glucose-lowering effect of insulin and susceptibility to hypoglycemia).
No products indexed under this heading.

Phenylephrine Bitartrate (Co-administration may reduce the blood-glucose-lowering effect of insulin).
No products indexed under this heading.

Phenylephrine Hydrochloride (Co-administration may reduce the blood-glucose-lowering effect of insulin). Products include:
Actifed Cold & Allergy Tablets **1895**
Benadryl Allergy & Cold Kapgels **1895**
Benadryl Allergy & Sinus Headache Kapgels **1895**
Benadryl Severe Allergy & Sinus Headache Caplets **1897**
Children's Benadryl-D Allergy & Sinus Liquid **1896**
Benadryl-D Allergy & Sinus Tablet **1896**
PediaCare Children's Allergy & Cold Liquid **1902**
PediaCare Children's Decongestant Liquid **1902**
PediaCare Children's Liquid Multi-Symptom Cold **1902**
Sinutab Non-Drying Caplets **1905**
Sinutab Sinus Caplets **1905**
Children's Sudafed PE Cold & Cough Liquid **1907**
Children's Sudafed PE Nasal Decongestant Liquid **1906**
Sudafed PE Cold & Cough Caplets **1907**
Sudafed PE Nasal Decongestant Tablets **1907**
Sudafed PE Nighttime Cold Caplets **1907**
Sudafed PE Non-Drying Sinus Caplets **1908**
Sudafed PE Severe Cold Caplets **1908**
Sudafed PE Sinus & Allergy Tablets **1908**
Sudafed PE Sinus Headache Caplets **1908**
Tylenol Allergy Multi-Symptom Caplets with Cool Burst and Rapid Release Gelcaps **1916**
Tylenol Allergy Multi-Symptom Nighttime Caplets with Cool Burst **1916**
Children's Tylenol Plus Cold Suspension Liquid **1912**
Children's Tylenol Plus Cold & Allergy Suspension Liquid **1914**
Children's Tylenol Plus Flu Suspension Liquid **1914**
Children's Tylenol Plus Multi-Symptom Cold Suspension Liquid **1912**
Tylenol Cold Head Congestion Daytime Caplets with Cool Burst **1910**
Tylenol Cold Head Congestion Nighttime Caplets with Cool Burst **1910**
Tylenol Cold Head Congestion Severe Daytime Caplets with Cool Burst **1910**
Tylenol Cold Multi-Symptom Daytime Caplets with Cool Burst and Rapid Release Gels **1913**
Tylenol Cold Multi-Symptom Daytime Liquid with Citrus Burst **1913**
Tylenol Cold Multi-Symptom Nighttime Caplets with Cool Burst **1913**
Tylenol Cold Multi-Symptom Nighttime Liquid with Cool Burst **1913**
Tylenol Cold Multi-Symptom Severe Caplets with Cool Burst **1913**
Tylenol Cold Multi-Symptom Severe Daytime Liquid with Citrus Burst **1913**
Tylenol Sinus Congestion & Pain Daytime Caplets with Cool Burst and Gelcaps **1917**
Tylenol Sinus Congestion & Pain Nighttime Caplets with Cool Burst **1917**
Tylenol Sinus Congestion & Pain Severe Caplets with Cool Burst **1917**
Vicks DayQuil Cold & Flu Multi-Symptom Relief ..... ▣**616**
Vicks DayQuil LiquiCaps **2567**
Vicks DayQuil Liquid **2567**
Vicks DayQuil Multi-Symptom Cold/Flu Relief **2567**

Phenylephrine Tannate (Co-administration may reduce the blood-glucose-lowering effect of insulin).
No products indexed under this heading.

Phenylpropanolamine Hydrochloride (Co-administration may reduce the blood-glucose-lowering effect of insulin).
No products indexed under this heading.

Pindolol (Co-administration may either potentiate or weaken the blood-glucose-lowering effect of insulin. Signs of hypoglycemia may be reduced or absent).
No products indexed under this heading.

Pioglitazone Hydrochloride (Co-administration may reduce the blood-glucose-lowering effect of insulin and susceptibility to hypoglycemia). Products include:
ActoPlus Met Tablets **3071**
Actos Tablets **3077**
Duetact Tablets **3085**

Pirbuterol Acetate (Co-administration may reduce the blood-glucose-lowering effect of insulin). Products include:
Maxair Autohaler **1705**

Polyestradiol Phosphate (Co-administration may reduce the blood-glucose-lowering effect of insulin).
No products indexed under this heading.

Polythiazide (Co-administration may reduce the blood-glucose-lowering effect of insulin).
No products indexed under this heading.

Prednisolone Acetate (Co-administration may reduce the blood-glucose-lowering effect of insulin). Products include:
Pred Forte Ophthalmic Suspension ..... ⊙**227**
Pred Mild Ophthalmic Suspension ..... ⊙**230**
Pred-G Ophthalmic Ointment ..... ⊙**229**
Pred-G Ophthalmic Suspension ..... ⊙**228**

Prednisolone Sodium Phosphate (Co-administration may reduce the blood-glucose-lowering effect of insulin).
No products indexed under this heading.

Prednisolone Tebutate (Co-administration may reduce the blood-glucose-lowering effect of insulin).
No products indexed under this heading.

Prednisone (Co-administration may reduce the blood-glucose-lowering effect of insulin).
No products indexed under this heading.

Procarbazine Hydrochloride (Co-administration may reduce the blood-glucose-lowering effect of insulin and susceptibility to hypoglycemia).
No products indexed under this heading.

Prochlorperazine (Co-administration may reduce the blood-glucose-lowering effect of insulin).
No products indexed under this heading.

Promethazine Hydrochloride (Co-administration may reduce the blood-glucose-lowering effect of insulin).
No products indexed under this heading.

Propoxyphene Hydrochloride (Co-administration may increase the blood-glucose-lowering effect of insulin and susceptibility to hypoglycemia).
No products indexed under this heading.

Propoxyphene Napsylate (Co-administration may increase the blood-glucose-lowering effect of insulin and susceptibility to hypoglycemia).
No products indexed under this heading.

Propranolol Hydrochloride (Co-administration may either potentiate or weaken the blood-glucose-lowering effect of insulin. Signs of hypoglycemia may be reduced or absent). Products include:
InnoPran XL Extended Release Capsules 1484

Pseudoephedrine Hydrochloride (Co-administration may reduce the blood-glucose-lowering effect of insulin). Products include:
Allegra-D 12 Hour Extended-Release Tablets 2687
Allegra-D 24 Hour Extended-Release Tablets 2690
Children's Motrin Cold Oral Suspension 1899
Sudafed 12 Hour Nasal Decongestant Non-Drowsy Caplets 1909
Sudafed 24 Hour Non-Drowsy Nasal Decongestant Tablets 1906
Children's Sudafed Nasal Decongestant Liquid 1906
Sudafed Nasal Decongestant Tablets 1906
Tylenol Cold Severe Congestion Daytime Caplets with Cool Burst 1912
Tylenol Sinus Severe Congestion Caplets with Cool Burst 1917
Vicks NyQuil LiquiCaps 2567
Vicks NyQuil Liquid 2567
Vicks NyQuil Multi-Symptom Cold/Flu Relief 2567
Zyrtec-D 12 Hour Extended Release Tablets 1923
Zyrtec-D Allergy & Congestion Extended-Release Tablets 1923

Pseudoephedrine Sulfate (Co-administration may reduce the blood-glucose-lowering effect of insulin). Products include:
Clarinex-D 12-Hour Extended-Release Tablets 2831
Clarinex-D 24-Hour Extended-Release Tablets 2834

Quinapril Hydrochloride (Co-administration may reduce the blood-glucose-lowering effect of insulin and susceptibility to hypoglycemia).
No products indexed under this heading.

Quinestrol (Co-administration may reduce the blood-glucose-lowering effect of insulin).
No products indexed under this heading.

Ramipril (Co-administration may reduce the blood-glucose-lowering effect of insulin and susceptibility to hypoglycemia).
No products indexed under this heading.

Rasagiline Mesylate (Co-administration may reduce the blood-glucose-lowering effect of insulin and susceptibility to hypoglycemia). Products include:
Azilect Tablets 3106

Repaglinide (Co-administration may reduce the blood-glucose-lowering effect of insulin and susceptibility to hypoglycemia). Products include:
PrandiMet Tablets 2967
Prandin Tablets 2971

Reserpine (Signs of hypoglycemia may be reduced or absent).
No products indexed under this heading.

Rosiglitazone Maleate (Co-administration may reduce the blood-glucose-lowering effect of insulin and susceptibility to hypoglycemia). Products include:
Avandamet Tablets 1336
Avandaryl Tablets 1344
Avandia Tablets 1351

Salmeterol Xinafoate (Co-administration may reduce the blood-glucose-lowering effect of insulin). Products include:
Advair Diskus 100/50 1276
Advair Diskus 250/50 1276
Advair Diskus 500/50 1276
Advair HFA 45/21 Inhalation Aerosol 1288
Advair HFA 115/21 Inhalation Aerosol 1288
Advair HFA 230/21 Inhalation Aerosol 1288
Serevent Diskus 1594

Salsalate (Co-administration may reduce the blood-glucose-lowering effect of insulin and susceptibility to hypoglycemia).
No products indexed under this heading.

Selegiline (Co-administration may reduce the blood-glucose-lowering effect of insulin and susceptibility to hypoglycemia). Products include:
Emsam Transdermal System 905

Selegiline Hydrochloride (Co-administration may reduce the blood-glucose-lowering effect of insulin and susceptibility to hypoglycemia). Products include:
Eldepryl Capsules 3052

Sitagliptin Phosphate (Co-administration may reduce the blood-glucose-lowering effect of insulin and susceptibility to hypoglycemia). Products include:
Janumet Tablets 2041
Januvia Tablets 2048

Somatropin (Co-administration may reduce the blood-glucose-lowering effect of insulin). Products include:
Genotropin Lyophilized Powder 2547
Humatrope Vials and Cartridges 1838
Nutropin for Injection 1208
Nutropin AQ Injection 1212
Nutropin AQ NuSpin Injection 1212
Nutropin AQ Pen 1212
Nutropin AQ Pen Cartridge 1212

Sotalol Hydrochloride (Co-administration may either potentiate or weaken the blood-glucose-lowering effect of insulin. Signs of hypoglycemia may be reduced or absent).
No products indexed under this heading.

Spirapril Hydrochloride (Co-administration may reduce the blood-glucose-lowering effect of insulin and susceptibility to hypoglycemia).
No products indexed under this heading.

Spironolactone (Co-administration may reduce the blood-glucose-lowering effect of insulin).
No products indexed under this heading.

Sulfacytine (Co-administration may reduce the blood-glucose-lowering effect of insulin and susceptibility to hypoglycemia).
No products indexed under this heading.

Sulfamethizole (Co-administration may reduce the blood-glucose-lowering effect of insulin and susceptibility to hypoglycemia).
No products indexed under this heading.

Sulfamethoxazole (Co-administration may reduce the blood-glucose-lowering effect of insulin and susceptibility to hypoglycemia).
No products indexed under this heading.

Sulfasalazine (Co-administration may reduce the blood-glucose-lowering effect of insulin and susceptibility to hypoglycemia).
No products indexed under this heading.

Sulfinpyrazone (Co-administration may reduce the blood-glucose-lowering effect of insulin and susceptibility to hypoglycemia).
No products indexed under this heading.

Sulfisoxazole Acetyl (Co-administration may reduce the blood-glucose-lowering effect of insulin and susceptibility to hypoglycemia).
No products indexed under this heading.

Sulfisoxazole Diolamine (Co-administration may reduce the blood-glucose-lowering effect of insulin and susceptibility to hypoglycemia).
No products indexed under this heading.

Terbutaline Sulfate (Co-administration may reduce the blood-glucose-lowering effect of insulin).
No products indexed under this heading.

Thioridazine Hydrochloride (Co-administration may reduce the blood-glucose-lowering effect of insulin). Products include:
Thioridazine Hydrochloride Tablets 2195

Thyroglobulin (Co-administration may reduce the blood-glucose-lowering effect of insulin).
No products indexed under this heading.

Thyroid (Co-administration may reduce the blood-glucose-lowering effect of insulin). Products include:
Naturethroid Tablets 2605

Thyroxine (Co-administration may reduce the blood-glucose-lowering effect of insulin).
No products indexed under this heading.

Thyroxine Sodium (Co-administration may reduce the blood-glucose-lowering effect of insulin).
No products indexed under this heading.

Timolol Hemihydrate (Co-administration may either potentiate or weaken the blood-glucose-lowering effect of insulin. Signs of hypoglycemia may be reduced or absent). Products include:
Betimol Ophthalmic Solution 3181

Timolol Maleate (Co-administration may either potentiate or weaken the blood-glucose-lowering effect of insulin. Signs of hypoglycemia may be reduced or absent). Products include:
Combigan Ophthalmic Solution 553
Cosopt Sterile Ophthalmic Solution 1969
Timoptic Sterile Ophthalmic Solution 2121
Timoptic in Ocudose 2124
Timoptic-XE Sterile Ophthalmic Gel Forming Solution 2125

Tolazamide (Co-administration may reduce the blood-glucose-lowering effect of insulin and susceptibility to hypoglycemia).
No products indexed under this heading.

Tolbutamide (Co-administration may reduce the blood-glucose-lowering effect of insulin and susceptibility to hypoglycemia).
No products indexed under this heading.

Torsemide (Co-administration may reduce the blood-glucose-lowering effect of insulin). Products include:
Demadex Injection 2630
Demadex Tablets 2630

Trandolapril (Co-administration may reduce the blood-glucose-lowering effect of insulin and susceptibility to hypoglycemia). Products include:
Mavik Tablets 472
Tarka Tablets 511

Tranylcypromine Sulfate (Co-administration may reduce the blood-glucose-lowering effect of insulin and susceptibility to hypoglycemia). Products include:
Parnate Tablets 1532

Triamcinolone (Co-administration may reduce the blood-glucose-lowering effect of insulin).
No products indexed under this heading.

Triamcinolone Acetonide (Co-administration may reduce the blood-glucose-lowering effect of insulin). Products include:
Azmacort Inhalation Aerosol 407
Nasacort AQ Nasal Spray 2765
Triesence Injectable Suspension .... ⊙209

Triamcinolone Diacetate (Co-administration may reduce the blood-glucose-lowering effect of insulin).
No products indexed under this heading.

Triamcinolone Hexacetonide (Co-administration may reduce the blood-glucose-lowering effect of insulin).
No products indexed under this heading.

Triamterene (Co-administration may reduce the blood-glucose-lowering effect of insulin). Products include:
Dyazide Capsules 1405
Dyrenium Capsules 3189

Trifluoperazine Hydrochloride (Co-administration may reduce the blood-glucose-lowering effect of insulin).
No products indexed under this heading.

Troglitazone (Co-administration may reduce the blood-glucose-lowering effect of insulin and susceptibility to hypoglycemia).
No products indexed under this heading.

Food Interactions

Alcohol (Co-administration may either potentiate or weaken the blood-glucose lowering effect of insulin).

LEVITRA TABLETS

(Vardenafil Hydrochloride) 2876
May interact with alpha adrenergic blockers, class 1A antiarrhythmics, class III antiarrhythmics, cytochrome p450 2c9 inhibitors (selected), cytochrome p450 3a4 inhibitors (selected), cytochrome p450 3a4 inhibitors, potent, erythromycin, nitrates and nitrites, protease inhibitors, drugs that prolong the QT interval, and certain other agents. Compounds in these categories include:

Acetazolamide (Studies in human liver microsomes showed that vardenafil is metabolized primarily by cytochrome P450 (CYP) isoforms 3A4/5, and to a lesser degree, by CYP2C9. Therefore, inhibitors of CYP3A4 are expected to reduce vardenafil clearance).
No products indexed under this heading.

Alprazolam (In a study of the effect of vardenafil on QT interval in 59 healthy males, therapeutic (10 mg) and supratherapeutic (80 mg) doses of vardenafil and the active control moxifloxacin (400 mg) produced similar increases in QTc interval. A postmarketing study evaluating the effect of combining vardenafil with another drug of comparable QT effect showed an additive QT effect when compared with either drug alone. These observations should be considered in clinical decisions when prescribing vardenafil to patients taking medications known to prolong the QT interval).
No products indexed under this heading.

Amiodarone Hydrochloride (Patients taking Class III antiarrhythmic medications should avoid using vardenafil).
No products indexed under this heading.

Amitriptyline Hydrochloride (In a study of the effect of vardenafil on QT interval in 59 healthy males, therapeutic (10 mg) and supratherapeutic (80 mg) doses of vardenafil and the active control moxifloxacin (400 mg) produced similar increases in QTc interval. A postmarketing study evaluating the effect of combining vardenafil with another drug of comparable QT effect showed an additive QT effect when compared with either drug alone. These observations should be considered in clinical decisions when prescribing vardenafil to patients taking medications known to prolong the QT interval).
No products indexed under this heading.

Amoxapine (In a study of the effect of vardenafil on QT interval in 59 healthy males, therapeutic (10 mg) and supratherapeutic (80 mg) doses of vardenafil and the active control moxifloxacin (400 mg) produced similar increases in QTc interval. A postmarketing study evaluating the effect of combining vardenafil with another drug of comparable QT effect showed an additive QT effect when compared with either drug alone. These observations should be considered in clinical decisions when prescribing vardenafil to patients taking medications known to prolong the QT interval).
No products indexed under this heading.

Amprenavir (Studies in human liver microsomes showed that vardenafil is metabolized primarily by cytochrome P450 (CYP) isoforms 3A4/5, and to a lesser degree, by CYP2C9. Therefore, inhibitors of CYP3A4 are expected to reduce vardenafil clearance. Patients taking potent CYP3A4 inhibitors should not exceed a dose of vardenafil 2.5 mg once daily).
No products indexed under this heading.

Amyl Nitrite (The blood pressure lowering effects of sublingual nitrates (0.4 mg) taken 1 and 4 hours after vardenafil and increases in heart rate were taken at 1, 4, and 8 hours were potentiated by a 20 mg dose of vardenafil in healthy middle-aged subjects. These effects were not observed when vardenafil 20 mg was taken 24 hours before the NTG. Potentiation of the hypotensive effects of nitrates for patients with ischemic heart disease has not been evaluated, and concomitant use of vardenafil and nitrates is contraindicated).
No products indexed under this heading.

Anastrozole (Studies in human liver microsomes showed that vardenafil is metabolized primarily by cytochrome P450 (CYP) isoforms 3A4/5, and to a lesser degree, by CYP2C9. Therefore, inhibitors of CYP3A4 are expected to reduce vardenafil clearance). Products include:
Arimidex Tablets 672

Aprepitant (Studies in human liver microsomes showed that vardenafil is metabolized primarily by cytochrome P450 (CYP) isoforms 3A4/5, and to a lesser degree, by CYP2C9. Therefore, inhibitors of CYP3A4 are expected to reduce vardenafil clearance). Products include:
Emend Capsules 1992

Astemizole (In a study of the effect of vardenafil on QT interval in 59 healthy males, therapeutic (10 mg) and supratherapeutic (80 mg) doses of vardenafil and the active control moxifloxacin (400 mg) produced similar increases in QTc interval. A postmarketing study evaluating the effect of combining vardenafil with another drug of comparable QT effect showed an additive QT effect when compared with either drug alone. These observations should be considered in clinical decisions when prescribing vardenafil to patients taking medications known to prolong the QT interval).
No products indexed under this heading.

Atazanavir (Patients taking atazanavir, a potent CYP3A4 inhibitor should not exceed a dose of vardenafil 2.5 mg once daily. Long-term safety information is not available on the concomitant administration of vardenafil with HIV protease inhibitors).
No products indexed under this heading.

Atazanavir Sulfate (Patients taking atazanavir, a potent CYP3A4 inhibitor should not exceed a dose of vardenafil 2.5 mg once daily. Long-term safety information is not available on the concomitant administration of vardenafil with HIV protease inhibitors). Products include:
Reyataz Capsules 3299

Bendroflumethiazide (Studies in human liver microsomes showed that vardenafil is metabolized primarily by cytochrome P450 (CYP) isoforms 3A4/5, and to a lesser degree, by CYP2C9. Therefore, inhibitors of CYP2C9 are expected to reduce vardenafil clearance).
No products indexed under this heading.

Bretylium Tosylate (Patients taking Class III antiarrhythmic medications should avoid using vardenafil).
No products indexed under this heading.

Buspirone Hydrochloride (In a study of the effect of vardenafil on QT interval in 59 healthy males, therapeutic (10 mg) and supratherapeutic (80 mg) doses of vardenafil and the active control moxifloxacin (400 mg) produced similar increases in QTc interval. A postmarketing study evaluating the effect of combining vardenafil with another drug of comparable QT effect showed an additive QT effect when compared with either drug alone. These observations should be considered in clinical decisions when prescribing vardenafil to patients taking medications known to prolong the QT interval).
No products indexed under this heading.

Chloramphenicol (Studies in human liver microsomes showed that vardenafil is metabolized primarily by cytochrome P450 (CYP) isoforms 3A4/5, and to a lesser degree, by CYP2C9. Therefore, inhibitors of CYP2C9 are expected to reduce vardenafil clearance).
No products indexed under this heading.

Chlordiazepoxide (In a study of the effect of vardenafil on QT interval in 59 healthy males, therapeutic (10 mg) and supratherapeutic (80 mg) doses of vardenafil and the active control moxifloxacin (400 mg) produced similar increases in QTc interval. A postmarketing study evaluating the effect of combining vardenafil with another drug of comparable QT effect showed an additive QT effect when compared with either drug alone. These observations should be considered in clinical decisions when prescribing vardenafil to patients taking medications known to prolong the QT interval).
No products indexed under this heading.

Chlordiazepoxide Hydrochloride (In a study of the effect of vardenafil on QT interval in 59 healthy males, therapeutic (10 mg) and supratherapeutic (80 mg) doses of vardenafil and the active control moxifloxacin (400 mg) produced similar increases in QTc interval. A postmarketing study evaluating the effect of combining vardenafil with another drug of comparable QT effect showed an additive QT effect when compared with either drug alone. These observations should be considered in clinical decisions when prescribing vardenafil to patients taking medications known to prolong the QT interval).
No products indexed under this heading.

Chlorothiazide (Studies in human liver microsomes showed that vardenafil is metabolized primarily by cytochrome P450 (CYP) isoforms 3A4/5, and to a lesser degree, by CYP2C9. Therefore, inhibitors of CYP2C9 are expected to reduce vardenafil clearance).
No products indexed under this heading.

Chlorothiazide Sodium (Studies in human liver microsomes showed that vardenafil is metabolized primarily by cytochrome P450 (CYP) isoforms 3A4/5, and to a lesser degree, by CYP2C9. Therefore, inhibitors of CYP2C9 are expected to reduce vardenafil clearance). Products include:
Intravenous Sodium Diuril 2490

Chlorpromazine (In a study of the effect of vardenafil on QT interval in 59 healthy males, therapeutic (10 mg) and supratherapeutic (80 mg) doses of vardenafil and the active control moxifloxacin (400 mg) produced similar increases in QTc interval. A postmarketing study evaluating the effect of combining vardenafil with another drug of comparable QT effect showed an additive QT effect when compared with either drug alone. These observations should be considered in clinical decisions when prescribing vardenafil to patients taking medications known to prolong the QT interval).
No products indexed under this heading.

Chlorpromazine Hydrochloride (In a study of the effect of vardenafil on QT interval in 59 healthy males, therapeutic (10 mg) and supratherapeutic (80 mg) doses of vardenafil and the active control moxifloxacin (400 mg) produced similar increases in QTc interval. A postmarketing study evaluating the effect of combining vardenafil with another drug of comparable QT effect showed an additive QT effect when compared with either drug alone. These observations should be considered in clinical decisions when prescribing vardenafil to patients taking medications known to prolong the QT interval).
No products indexed under this heading.

Chlorpropamide (Studies in human liver microsomes showed that vardenafil is metabolized primarily by cytochrome P450 (CYP) isoforms 3A4/5, and to a lesser degree, by CYP2C9. Therefore, inhibitors of CYP2C9 are expected to reduce vardenafil clearance).
No products indexed under this heading.

Chlorprothixene (In a study of the effect of vardenafil on QT interval in 59 healthy males, therapeutic (10 mg) and supratherapeutic (80 mg) doses of vardenafil and the active control moxifloxacin (400 mg) produced similar increases in QTc interval. A postmarketing study evaluating the effect of combining vardenafil with another drug of comparable QT effect showed an additive QT effect when compared with either drug alone. These observations should be considered in clinical decisions when prescribing vardenafil to patients taking medications known to prolong the QT interval).
No products indexed under this heading.

Chlorprothixene Hydrochloride (In a study of the effect of vardenafil on QT interval in 59 healthy males, therapeutic (10 mg) and supratherapeutic (80 mg) doses of vardenafil and the active control moxifloxacin (400 mg) produced similar increases in QTc interval. A postmarketing study evaluating the effect of combining vardenafil with another drug of comparable QT effect showed an additive QT effect when compared with either drug alone. These observations should be considered in clinical decisions when prescribing vardenafil to patients taking medications known to prolong the QT interval).
No products indexed under this heading.

Cimetidine (Studies in human liver microsomes showed that vardenafil is metabolized primarily by cytochrome P450 (CYP) isoforms 3A4/5, and to a lesser degree, by CYP2C9. Therefore, inhibitors of CYP3A4 are expected to reduce vardenafil clearance).
No products indexed under this heading.

Cimetidine Hydrochloride (Studies in human liver microsomes showed that vardenafil is metabolized primarily by cytochrome P450 (CYP) isoforms 3A4/5, and to a lesser degree, by CYP2C9. Therefore, inhibitors of CYP3A4 are expected to reduce vardenafil clearance).
No products indexed under this heading.

Ciprofloxacin (Studies in human liver microsomes showed that vardenafil is metabolized primarily by cytochrome P450 (CYP) isoforms 3A4/5, and to a lesser degree, by CYP2C9. Therefore, inhibitors of CYP3A4 are expected to reduce vardenafil clearance). Products include:
Cipro I.V. 2817
Cipro Oral Suspension 2810
Cipro XR Tablets 2823
Ciprodex Otic Suspension 541

Clarithromycin (Patients taking clarithromycin, a potent CYP3A4 inhibitor, should not exceed a dose of vardenafil 2.5 mg once daily). Products include:
Biaxin/Biaxin XL 411

Clomipramine Hydrochloride (In a study of the effect of vardenafil on QT interval in 59 healthy males, therapeutic (10 mg) and supratherapeutic (80 mg) doses of vardenafil and the active control moxifloxacin (400 mg) produced similar increases in QTc interval. A postmarketing study evaluating the effect of combining vardenafil with another drug of comparable QT effect showed an additive QT effect when compared with either drug alone. These observations should be considered in clinical decisions when prescribing vardenafil to patients taking medications known to prolong the QT interval).
No products indexed under this heading.

Clopidogrel Hydrogen Sulfate (Studies in human liver microsomes showed that vardenafil is metabolized primarily by cytochrome P450 (CYP) isoforms 3A4/5, and to a lesser degree, by CYP2C9. Therefore, inhibitors of CYP2C9 are expected to reduce vardenafil clearance).
No products indexed under this heading.

Clorazepate Dipotassium (In a study of the effect of vardenafil on QT interval in 59 healthy males, therapeutic (10 mg) and supratherapeutic (80 mg) doses of vardenafil and the active control moxifloxacin (400 mg) produced similar increases in QTc interval. A postmarketing study evaluating the effect of combining vardenafil with another drug of comparable QT effect showed an additive QT effect when compared with either drug alone. These observations should be considered in clinical decisions when prescribing vardenafil to patients taking medications known to prolong the QT interval).
No products indexed under this heading.

Clotrimazole (Studies in human liver microsomes showed that vardenafil is metabolized primarily by cytochrome P450 (CYP) isoforms 3A4/5, and to a lesser degree, by CYP2C9. Therefore, inhibitors of CYP3A4 are expected to reduce vardenafil clearance). Products include:
Lotrisone 2881

Clozapine (In a study of the effect of vardenafil on QT interval in 59 healthy males, therapeutic (10 mg) and supratherapeutic (80 mg) doses of vardenafil and the active control moxifloxacin (400 mg) produced similar increases in QTc interval. A postmarketing study evaluating the effect of combining vardenafil with another drug of comparable QT effect showed an additive QT effect when compared with either drug alone. These observations should be considered in clinical decisions when prescribing vardenafil to patients taking medications known to prolong the QT interval).
No products indexed under this heading.

Cyclosporine (Studies in human liver microsomes showed that vardenafil is metabolized primarily by cytochrome P450 (CYP) isoforms 3A4/5, and to a lesser degree, by CYP2C9. Therefore, inhibitors of CYP3A4 are expected to reduce vardenafil clearance). Products include:
Gengraf Capsules 435
Neoral Oral Solution 2280
Neoral Soft Gelatin Capsules 2280
Restasis Ophthalmic Emulsion 557
Sandimmune 2296

Dalfopristin (Studies in human liver microsomes showed that vardenafil is metabolized primarily by cytochrome P450 (CYP) isoforms 3A4/5, and to a lesser degree, by CYP2C9. Therefore, inhibitors of CYP3A4 are expected to reduce vardenafil clearance).
No products indexed under this heading.

Danazol (Studies in human liver microsomes showed that vardenafil is metabolized primarily by cytochrome P450 (CYP) isoforms 3A4/5, and to a lesser degree, by CYP2C9. Therefore, inhibitors of CYP3A4 are expected to reduce vardenafil clearance).
No products indexed under this heading.

Darunavir (Long-term safety information is not available on the concomitant administration of vardenafil with HIV protease inhibitors).
No products indexed under this heading.

Delavirdine Mesylate (Studies in human liver microsomes showed that vardenafil is metabolized primarily by cytochrome P450 (CYP) isoforms 3A4/5, and to a lesser degree, by CYP2C9. Therefore, inhibitors of CYP3A4 are expected to reduce vardenafil clearance. Patients taking potent CYP3A4 inhibitors should not exceed a dose of vardenafil 2.5 mg once daily).
No products indexed under this heading.

Delavirine (Studies in human liver microsomes showed that vardenafil is metabolized primarily by cytochrome P450 (CYP) isoforms 3A4/5, and to a lesser degree, by CYP2C9. Therefore, inhibitors of CYP3A4 are expected to reduce vardenafil clearance. Patients taking potent CYP3A4 inhibitors should not exceed a dose of vardenafil 2.5 mg once daily).
No products indexed under this heading.

Desipramine Hydrochloride (In a study of the effect of vardenafil on QT interval in 59 healthy males, therapeutic (10 mg) and supratherapeutic (80 mg) doses of vardenafil and the active control moxifloxacin (400 mg) produced similar increases in QTc interval. A postmarketing study evaluating the effect of combining vardenafil with another drug of comparable QT effect showed an additive QT effect when compared with either drug alone. These observations should be considered in clinical decisions when prescribing vardenafil to patients taking medications known to prolong the QT interval).
No products indexed under this heading.

Diazepam (In a study of the effect of vardenafil on QT interval in 59 healthy males, therapeutic (10 mg) and supratherapeutic (80 mg) doses of vardenafil and the active control moxifloxacin (400 mg) produced similar increases in QTc interval. A postmarketing study evaluating the effect of combining vardenafil with another drug of comparable QT effect showed an additive QT effect when compared with either drug alone. These observations should be considered in clinical decisions when prescribing vardenafil to patients taking medications known to prolong the QT interval). Products include:
Valium Tablets 2658

Diclofenac Potassium (Studies in human liver microsomes showed that vardenafil is metabolized primarily by cytochrome P450 (CYP) isoforms 3A4/5, and to a lesser degree, by CYP2C9. Therefore, inhibitors of CYP2C9 are expected to reduce vardenafil clearance).
No products indexed under this heading.

Diclofenac Sodium (Studies in human liver microsomes showed that vardenafil is metabolized primarily by cytochrome P450 (CYP) isoforms 3A4/5, and to a lesser degree, by CYP2C9. Therefore, inhibitors of CYP2C9 are expected to reduce vardenafil clearance). Products include:
Diclofenac Sodium Ophthalmic Solution .... ⊙ 240
Voltaren Ophthalmic Solution 2336
Voltaren Tablets 2334
Voltaren-XR Tablets 2337

Diltiazem Hydrochloride (Studies in human liver microsomes showed that vardenafil is metabolized primarily by cytochrome P450 (CYP) isoforms 3A4/5, and to a lesser degree, by CYP2C9. Therefore, inhibitors of CYP3A4 are expected to reduce vardenafil clearance). Products include:
Cardizem LA Extended Release Tablets 421

Diltiazem Maleate (Studies in human liver microsomes showed that vardenafil is metabolized primarily by cytochrome P450 (CYP) isoforms 3A4/5, and to a lesser degree, by CYP2C9. Therefore, inhibitors of CYP3A4 are expected to reduce vardenafil clearance).
No products indexed under this heading.

Disopyramide (Patients taking Class 1A antiarrhythmic medications should avoid using vardenafil).
No products indexed under this heading.

Disopyramide Phosphate (In a study of the effect of vardenafil on QT interval in 59 healthy males, therapeutic (10 mg) and supratherapeutic (80 mg) doses of vardenafil and the active control moxifloxacin (400 mg) produced similar increases in QTc interval. A postmarketing study evaluating the effect of combining vardenafil with another drug of comparable QT effect showed an additive QT effect when compared with either drug alone. These observations should be considered in clinical decisions when prescribing vardenafil to patients taking medications known to prolong the QT interval).
No products indexed under this heading.

Disulfiram (Studies in human liver microsomes showed that vardenafil is metabolized primarily by cytochrome P450 (CYP) isoforms 3A4/5, and to a lesser degree, by CYP2C9. Therefore, inhibitors of CYP2C9 are expected to reduce vardenafil clearance).
No products indexed under this heading.

Dofetilide (In a study of the effect of vardenafil on QT interval in 59 healthy males, therapeutic (10 mg) and supratherapeutic (80 mg) doses of vardenafil and the active control moxifloxacin (400 mg) produced similar increases in QTc interval. A postmarketing study evaluating the effect of combining vardenafil with another drug of comparable QT effect showed an additive QT effect when compared with either drug alone. These observations should be considered in clinical decisions when prescribing vardenafil to patients taking medications known to prolong the QT interval).
No products indexed under this heading.

Doxazosin Mesylate (Caution is advised when phosphodiesterase type 5 (PDE5) inhibitors are co-administered with alpha-blockers. PDE5 inhibitors, including vardenafil, and alpha-adrenergic blocking agents are both vasodilators with blood pressure lowering effects. When vasodilators are used in combination, an additive effect on blood pressure may be anticipated. In some patients, concomitant use of these two drug classes can lower blood pressure significantly, leading to symptomatic hypotension (e.g., fainting). Concomitant treatment with vardenafil and alpha-blockers should be initiated only if the patient is stable on his alpha-blocker therapy. Vardenafil should be initiated at the lowest recommended starting dose).
No products indexed under this heading.

Doxepin Hydrochloride (In a study of the effect of vardenafil on QT interval in 59 healthy males, therapeutic (10 mg) and supratherapeutic (80 mg) doses of vardenafil and the active control moxifloxacin (400 mg) produced similar increases in QTc interval. A postmarketing study evaluating the effect of combining vardenafil with another drug of comparable QT effect showed an additive QT effect when compared with either drug alone. These observations should be considered in clinical decisions when prescribing vardenafil to patients taking medications known to prolong the QT interval).
No products indexed under this heading.

Droperidol (In a study of the effect of vardenafil on QT interval in 59 healthy males, therapeutic (10 mg) and supratherapeutic (80 mg) doses of vardenafil and the active control moxifloxacin (400 mg) produced similar increases in QTc interval. A postmarketing study evaluating the effect of combining vardenafil with another drug of comparable QT effect showed an additive QT effect when compared with either drug alone. These observations should be considered in clinical decisions when prescribing vardenafil to patients taking medications known to prolong the QT interval).

No products indexed under this heading.

Efavirenz (Studies in human liver microsomes showed that vardenafil is metabolized primarily by cytochrome P450 (CYP) isoforms 3A4/5, and to a lesser degree, by CYP2C9. Therefore, inhibitors of CYP3A4 are expected to reduce vardenafil clearance). Products include:

Atripla Tablets **938**
Sustiva Capsules **930**
Sustiva Tablets **930**

Erythrityl Tetranitrate (The blood pressure lowering effects of sublingual nitrates (0.4 mg) taken 1 and 4 hours after vardenafil and increases in heart rate were taken at 1, 4, and 8 hours were potentiated by a 20 mg dose of vardenafil in healthy middle-aged subjects. These effects were not observed when vardenafil 20 mg was taken 24 hours before the NTG. Potentiation of the hypotensive effects of nitrates for patients with ischemic heart disease has not been evaluated, and concomitant use of vardenafil and nitrates is contraindicated).

No products indexed under this heading.

Erythromycin (Erythromycin (500 mg t.i.d.) produced a 4-fold increase in vardenafil AUC and a 3-fold increase in Cmax when co-administered with vardenafil 5 mg in healthy volunteers. It is recommended not to exceed a single 5 mg dose of vardenafil in a 24 hour period when used in combination with erythromycin).

No products indexed under this heading.

Erythromycin Estolate (Erythromycin (500 mg t.i.d.) produced a 4-fold increase in vardenafil AUC and a 3-fold increase in Cmax when co-administered with vardenafil 5 mg in healthy volunteers. It is recommended not to exceed a single 5 mg dose of vardenafil in a 24 hour period when used in combination with erythromycin).

No products indexed under this heading.

Erythromycin Ethylsuccinate (Erythromycin (500 mg t.i.d.) produced a 4-fold increase in vardenafil AUC and a 3-fold increase in Cmax when co-administered with vardenafil 5 mg in healthy volunteers. It is recommended not to exceed a single 5 mg dose of vardenafil in a 24 hour period when used in combination with erythromycin). Products include:

E.E.S. **433**
EryPed **431**

Erythromycin Gluceptate (Erythromycin (500 mg t.i.d.) produced a 4-fold increase in vardenafil AUC and a 3-fold increase in Cmax when co-administered with vardenafil 5 mg in healthy volunteers. It is recommended not to exceed a single 5 mg dose of vardenafil in a 24 hour period when used in combination with erythromycin).

No products indexed under this heading.

Erythromycin Lactobionate (Erythromycin (500 mg t.i.d.) produced a 4-fold increase in vardenafil AUC and a 3-fold increase in Cmax when co-administered with vardenafil 5 mg in healthy volunteers. It is recommended not to exceed a single 5 mg dose of vardenafil in a 24 hour period when used in combination with erythromycin).

No products indexed under this heading.

Erythromycin Stearate (Erythromycin (500 mg t.i.d.) produced a 4-fold increase in vardenafil AUC and a 3-fold increase in Cmax when co-administered with vardenafil 5 mg in healthy volunteers. It is recommended not to exceed a single 5 mg dose of vardenafil in a 24 hour period when used in combination with erythromycin).

No products indexed under this heading.

Esomeprazole Magnesium (Studies in human liver microsomes showed that vardenafil is metabolized primarily by cytochrome P450 (CYP) isoforms 3A4/5, and to a lesser degree, by CYP2C9. Therefore, inhibitors of CYP3A4 are expected to reduce vardenafil clearance). Products include:

Nexium Delayed-Release Capsules.................................... **645**
Nexium Delayed-Release Oral Suspension.................................. **645**

Fenofibrate (Studies in human liver microsomes showed that vardenafil is metabolized primarily by cytochrome P450 (CYP) isoforms 3A4/5, and to a lesser degree, by CYP2C9. Therefore, inhibitors of CYP2C9 are expected to reduce vardenafil clearance). Products include:

Fenoglide Tablets **2960**
Tricor Tablets **520**

Flecainide Acetate (In a study of the effect of vardenafil on QT interval in 59 healthy males, therapeutic (10 mg) and supratherapeutic (80 mg) doses of vardenafil and the active control moxifloxacin (400 mg) produced similar increases in QTc interval. A postmarketing study evaluating the effect of combining vardenafil with another drug of comparable QT effect showed an additive QT effect when compared with either drug alone. These observations should be considered in clinical decisions when prescribing vardenafil to patients taking medications known to prolong the QT interval).

No products indexed under this heading.

Fluconazole (Studies in human liver microsomes showed that vardenafil is metabolized primarily by cytochrome P450 (CYP) isoforms 3A4/5, and to a lesser degree, by CYP2C9. Therefore, inhibitors of CYP3A4 are expected to reduce vardenafil clearance).

No products indexed under this heading.

Fluorouracil (Studies in human liver microsomes showed that vardenafil is metabolized primarily by cytochrome P450 (CYP) isoforms 3A4/5, and to a lesser degree, by CYP2C9. Therefore, inhibitors of CYP2C9 are expected to reduce vardenafil clearance). Products include:

Carac Cream 0.5% **2722**

Fluoxetine (Studies in human liver microsomes showed that vardenafil is metabolized primarily by cytochrome P450 (CYP) isoforms 3A4/5, and to a lesser degree, by CYP2C9. Therefore, inhibitors of CYP3A4 are expected to reduce vardenafil clearance).

No products indexed under this heading.

Fluoxetine Hydrochloride (Studies in human liver microsomes showed that vardenafil is metabolized primarily by cytochrome P450 (CYP) isoforms 3A4/5, and to a lesser degree, by CYP2C9. Therefore, inhibitors of CYP3A4 are expected to reduce vardenafil clearance). Products include:

Prozac Weekly Capsules **1852**
Prozac Pulvules and Liquid **1852**
Symbyax Capsules **1871**

Fluphenazine Decanoate (In a study of the effect of vardenafil on QT interval in 59 healthy males, therapeutic (10 mg) and supratherapeutic (80 mg) doses of vardenafil and the active control moxifloxacin (400 mg) produced similar increases in QTc interval. A postmarketing study evaluating the effect of combining vardenafil with another drug of comparable QT effect showed an additive QT effect when compared with either drug alone. These observations should be considered in clinical decisions when prescribing vardenafil to patients taking medications known to prolong the QT interval).

No products indexed under this heading.

Fluphenazine Enanthate (In a study of the effect of vardenafil on QT interval in 59 healthy males, therapeutic (10 mg) and supratherapeutic (80 mg) doses of vardenafil and the active control moxifloxacin (400 mg) produced similar increases in QTc interval. A postmarketing study evaluating the effect of combining vardenafil with another drug of comparable QT effect showed an additive QT effect when compared with either drug alone. These observations should be considered in clinical decisions when prescribing vardenafil to patients taking medications known to prolong the QT interval).

No products indexed under this heading.

Fluphenazine Hydrochloride (In a study of the effect of vardenafil on QT interval in 59 healthy males, therapeutic (10 mg) and supratherapeutic (80 mg) doses of vardenafil and the active control moxifloxacin (400 mg) produced similar increases in QTc interval. A postmarketing study evaluating the effect of combining vardenafil with another drug of comparable QT effect showed an additive QT effect when compared with either drug alone. These observations should be considered in clinical decisions when prescribing vardenafil to patients taking medications known to prolong the QT interval).

No products indexed under this heading.

Flurbiprofen (Studies in human liver microsomes showed that vardenafil is metabolized primarily by cytochrome P450 (CYP) isoforms 3A4/5, and to a lesser degree, by CYP2C9. Therefore, inhibitors of CYP2C9 are expected to reduce vardenafil clearance).

No products indexed under this heading.

Flurbiprofen Sodium (Studies in human liver microsomes showed that vardenafil is metabolized primarily by cytochrome P450 (CYP) isoforms 3A4/5, and to a lesser degree, by CYP2C9. Therefore, inhibitors of CYP2C9 are expected to reduce vardenafil clearance).

No products indexed under this heading.

Fluvastatin Sodium (Studies in human liver microsomes showed that vardenafil is metabolized primarily by cytochrome P450 (CYP) isoforms 3A4/5, and to a lesser degree, by CYP2C9. Therefore, inhibitors of CYP2C9 are expected to reduce vardenafil clearance). Products include:

Lescol Capsules **2268**
Lescol XL Tablets **2268**

Fluvoxamine Maleate (Studies in human liver microsomes showed that vardenafil is metabolized primarily by cytochrome P450 (CYP) isoforms 3A4/5, and to a lesser degree, by CYP2C9. Therefore, inhibitors of CYP3A4 are expected to reduce vardenafil clearance). Products include:

Luvox CR Extended-Release Capsules.. **1759**

Fosamprenavir Calcium (Studies in human liver microsomes showed that vardenafil is metabolized primarily by cytochrome P450 (CYP) isoforms 3A4/5, and to a lesser degree, by CYP2C9. Therefore, inhibitors of CYP3A4 are expected to reduce vardenafil clearance. Patients taking potent CYP3A4 inhibitors should not exceed a dose of vardenafil 2.5 mg once daily). Products include:

Lexiva Oral Suspension **1510**
Lexiva Tablets **1510**

Gemfibrozil (Studies in human liver microsomes showed that vardenafil is metabolized primarily by cytochrome P450 (CYP) isoforms 3A4/5, and to a lesser degree, by CYP2C9. Therefore, inhibitors of CYP2C9 are expected to reduce vardenafil clearance).

No products indexed under this heading.

Glipizide (Studies in human liver microsomes showed that vardenafil is metabolized primarily by cytochrome P450 (CYP) isoforms 3A4/5, and to a lesser degree, by CYP2C9. Therefore, inhibitors of CYP2C9 are expected to reduce vardenafil clearance).

No products indexed under this heading.

Glyburide (Studies in human liver microsomes showed that vardenafil is metabolized primarily by cytochrome P450 (CYP) isoforms 3A4/5, and to a lesser degree, by CYP2C9. Therefore, inhibitors of CYP2C9 are expected to reduce vardenafil clearance).

No products indexed under this heading.

Haloperidol (In a study of the effect of vardenafil on QT interval in 59 healthy males, therapeutic (10 mg) and supratherapeutic (80 mg) doses of vardenafil and the active control moxifloxacin (400 mg) produced similar increases in QTc interval. A postmarketing study evaluating the effect of combining vardenafil with another drug of comparable QT effect showed an additive QT effect when compared with either drug alone. These observations should be considered in clinical decisions when prescribing vardenafil to patients taking medications known to prolong the QT interval).
No products indexed under this heading.

Haloperidol Decanoate (In a study of the effect of vardenafil on QT interval in 59 healthy males, therapeutic (10 mg) and supratherapeutic (80 mg) doses of vardenafil and the active control moxifloxacin (400 mg) produced similar increases in QTc interval. A postmarketing study evaluating the effect of combining vardenafil with another drug of comparable QT effect showed an additive QT effect when compared with either drug alone. These observations should be considered in clinical decisions when prescribing vardenafil to patients taking medications known to prolong the QT interval).
No products indexed under this heading.

Hydrochlorothiazide (Studies in human liver microsomes showed that vardenafil is metabolized primarily by cytochrome P450 (CYP) isoforms 3A4/5, and to a lesser degree, by CYP2C9. Therefore, inhibitors of CYP2C9 are expected to reduce vardenafil clearance). Products include:
Atacand HCT **642**
Avalide Tablets **892**
Avalide Tablets **2713**
Benicar HCT Tablets **1010**
Diovan HCT Tablets **2216**
Dyazide Capsules **1405**
Micardis HCT Tablets **854**
Prinzide Tablets **2092**
Tekturna HCT Tablets **2324**
Teveten HCT Tablets **517**

Hydroflumethiazide (Studies in human liver microsomes showed that vardenafil is metabolized primarily by cytochrome P450 (CYP) isoforms 3A4/5, and to a lesser degree, by CYP2C9. Therefore, inhibitors of CYP2C9 are expected to reduce vardenafil clearance).
No products indexed under this heading.

Hydroxyzine Hydrochloride (In a study of the effect of vardenafil on QT interval in 59 healthy males, therapeutic (10 mg) and supratherapeutic (80 mg) doses of vardenafil and the active control moxifloxacin (400 mg) produced similar increases in QTc interval. A postmarketing study evaluating the effect of combining vardenafil with another drug of comparable QT effect showed an additive QT effect when compared with either drug alone. These observations should be considered in clinical decisions when prescribing vardenafil to patients taking medications known to prolong the QT interval).
No products indexed under this heading.

Imatinib Mesylate (Studies in human liver microsomes showed that vardenafil is metabolized primarily by cytochrome P450 (CYP) isoforms 3A4/5, and to a lesser degree, by CYP2C9. Therefore, inhibitors of CYP2C9 are expected to reduce vardenafil clearance). Products include:
Gleevec Tablets **2255**

Imipramine Hydrochloride (In a study of the effect of vardenafil on QT interval in 59 healthy males, therapeutic (10 mg) and supratherapeutic (80 mg) doses of vardenafil and the active control moxifloxacin (400 mg) produced similar increases in QTc interval. A postmarketing study evaluating the effect of combining vardenafil with another drug of comparable QT effect showed an additive QT effect when compared with either drug alone. These observations should be considered in clinical decisions when prescribing vardenafil to patients taking medications known to prolong the QT interval).
No products indexed under this heading.

Imipramine Pamoate (In a study of the effect of vardenafil on QT interval in 59 healthy males, therapeutic (10 mg) and supratherapeutic (80 mg) doses of vardenafil and the active control moxifloxacin (400 mg) produced similar increases in QTc interval. A postmarketing study evaluating the effect of combining vardenafil with another drug of comparable QT effect showed an additive QT effect when compared with either drug alone. These observations should be considered in clinical decisions when prescribing vardenafil to patients taking medications known to prolong the QT interval).
No products indexed under this heading.

Indinavir Sulfate (Indinavir (800 mg b.i.d.) co-administered with vardenafil 10 mg resulted in a 16-fold increase in vardenafil AUC a 7-fold increase in vardenafil Cmax and a 2-fold increase in vardenafil half-life. It is recommended not to exceed a single 2.5 mg vardenafil dose in a 24 hour period when used in combination with indinavir. Long-term safety information is not available on the concomitant administration of vardenafil with HIV protease inhibitors). Products include:
Crixivan Capsules **1979**

Isocarboxazid (In a study of the effect of vardenafil on QT interval in 59 healthy males, therapeutic (10 mg) and supratherapeutic (80 mg) doses of vardenafil and the active control moxifloxacin (400 mg) produced similar increases in QTc interval. A postmarketing study evaluating the effect of combining vardenafil with another drug of comparable QT effect showed an additive QT effect when compared with either drug alone. These observations should be considered in clinical decisions when prescribing vardenafil to patients taking medications known to prolong the QT interval). Products include:
Marplan Tablets **3177**

Isoniazid (Studies in human liver microsomes showed that vardenafil is metabolized primarily by cytochrome P450 (CYP) isoforms 3A4/5, and to a lesser degree, by CYP2C9. Therefore, inhibitors of CYP3A4 are expected to reduce vardenafil clearance).
No products indexed under this heading.

Isosorbide Dinitrate (The blood pressure lowering effects of sublingual nitrates (0.4 mg) taken 1 and 4 hours after vardenafil and increases in heart rate were taken at 1, 4, and 8 hours were potentiated by a 20 mg dose of vardenafil in healthy middle-aged subjects. These effects were not observed when vardenafil 20 mg was taken 24 hours before the NTG. Potentiation of the hypotensive effects of nitrates for patients with ischemic heart disease has not been evaluated, and concomitant use of vardenafil and nitrates is contraindicated).
No products indexed under this heading.

Isosorbide Mononitrate (The blood pressure lowering effects of sublingual nitrates (0.4 mg) taken 1 and 4 hours after vardenafil and increases in heart rate were taken at 1, 4, and 8 hours were potentiated by a 20 mg dose of vardenafil in healthy middle-aged subjects. These effects were not observed when vardenafil 20 mg was taken 24 hours before the NTG. Potentiation of the hypotensive effects of nitrates for patients with ischemic heart disease has not been evaluated, and concomitant use of vardenafil and nitrates is contraindicated).
No products indexed under this heading.

Itraconazole (Patients taking itraconazole 400 mg daily should not exceed a dose of vardenafil 2.5 mg once daily. For patients taking itraconazole 200 mg daily, a single dose of 5 mg of vardenafil should not be exceeded in a 24 hour period).
No products indexed under this heading.

Ketoconazole (Ketoconazole (200 mg once daily), produced a 10-fold increase in vardenafil AUC and a 4-fold increase in Cmax when co-administered with vardenafil (5 mg) in healthy volunteers. A 5 mg vardenafil dose should not be exceeded when used in combination with 200 mg once daily ketoconazole. Since higher doses of ketoconazole (400 mg daily) may result in higher increases in Cmax and AUC, a single 2.5 mg dose of vardenafil should not be exceeded in a 24 hour period when used in combination with ketoconazole 400 mg daily). Products include:
Extina Foam, 2% **3057**
Nizoral A-D Shampoo **1901**

Ketoprofen (Studies in human liver microsomes showed that vardenafil is metabolized primarily by cytochrome P450 (CYP) isoforms 3A4/5, and to a lesser degree, by CYP2C9. Therefore, inhibitors of CYP2C9 are expected to reduce vardenafil clearance).
No products indexed under this heading.

Leflunomide (Studies in human liver microsomes showed that vardenafil is metabolized primarily by cytochrome P450 (CYP) isoforms 3A4/5, and to a lesser degree, by CYP2C9. Therefore, inhibitors of CYP2C9 are expected to reduce vardenafil clearance).
No products indexed under this heading.

Lidocaine Hydrochloride (In a study of the effect of vardenafil on QT interval in 59 healthy males, therapeutic (10 mg) and supratherapeutic (80 mg) doses of vardenafil and the active control moxifloxacin (400 mg) produced similar increases in QTc interval. A postmarketing study evaluating the effect of combining vardenafil with another drug of comparable QT effect showed an additive QT effect when compared with either drug alone. These observations should be considered in clinical decisions when prescribing vardenafil to patients taking medications known to prolong the QT interval).
No products indexed under this heading.

Lithium Carbonate (In a study of the effect of vardenafil on QT interval in 59 healthy males, therapeutic (10 mg) and supratherapeutic (80 mg) doses of vardenafil and the active control moxifloxacin (400 mg) produced similar increases in QTc interval. A postmarketing study evaluating the effect of combining vardenafil with another drug of comparable QT effect showed an additive QT effect when compared with either drug alone. These observations should be considered in clinical decisions when prescribing vardenafil to patients taking medications known to prolong the QT interval).
No products indexed under this heading.

Lithium Citrate (In a study of the effect of vardenafil on QT interval in 59 healthy males, therapeutic (10 mg) and supratherapeutic (80 mg) doses of vardenafil and the active control moxifloxacin (400 mg) produced similar increases in QTc interval. A postmarketing study evaluating the effect of combining vardenafil with another drug of comparable QT effect showed an additive QT effect when compared with either drug alone. These observations should be considered in clinical decisions when prescribing vardenafil to patients taking medications known to prolong the QT interval).
No products indexed under this heading.

Lopinavir (Studies in human liver microsomes showed that vardenafil is metabolized primarily by cytochrome P450 (CYP) isoforms 3A4/5, and to a lesser degree, by CYP2C9. Therefore, inhibitors of CYP3A4 are expected to reduce vardenafil clearance. Patients taking potent CYP3A4 inhibitors should not exceed a dose of vardenafil 2.5 mg once daily). Products include:
Kaletra **452**

Loratadine (Studies in human liver microsomes showed that vardenafil is metabolized primarily by cytochrome P450 (CYP) isoforms 3A4/5, and to a lesser degree, by CYP2C9. Therefore, inhibitors of CYP3A4 are expected to reduce vardenafil clearance).
No products indexed under this heading.

Lorazepam (In a study of the effect of vardenafil on QT interval in 59 healthy males, therapeutic (10 mg) and supratherapeutic (80 mg) doses of vardenafil and the active control moxifloxacin (400 mg) produced similar increases in QTc interval. A postmarketing study evaluating the effect of combining vardenafil with another drug of comparable QT effect showed an additive QT effect when compared with either drug alone. These observations should be considered in clinical decisions when prescribing vardenafil to patients taking medications known to prolong the QT interval).
No products indexed under this heading.

Lovastatin (Studies in human liver microsomes showed that vardenafil is metabolized primarily by cytochrome P450 (CYP) isoforms 3A4/5, and to a lesser degree, by CYP2C9. Therefore, inhibitors of CYP2C9 are expected to reduce vardenafil clearance). Products include:
Advicor Tablets 402
Mevacor Tablets 2063

Loxapine Hydrochloride (In a study of the effect of vardenafil on QT interval in 59 healthy males, therapeutic (10 mg) and supratherapeutic (80 mg) doses of vardenafil and the active control moxifloxacin (400 mg) produced similar increases in QTc interval. A postmarketing study evaluating the effect of combining vardenafil with another drug of comparable QT effect showed an additive QT effect when compared with either drug alone. These observations should be considered in clinical decisions when prescribing vardenafil to patients taking medications known to prolong the QT interval).
No products indexed under this heading.

Loxapine Succinate (In a study of the effect of vardenafil on QT interval in 59 healthy males, therapeutic (10 mg) and supratherapeutic (80 mg) doses of vardenafil and the active control moxifloxacin (400 mg) produced similar increases in QTc interval. A postmarketing study evaluating the effect of combining vardenafil with another drug of comparable QT effect showed an additive QT effect when compared with either drug alone. These observations should be considered in clinical decisions when prescribing vardenafil to patients taking medications known to prolong the QT interval).
No products indexed under this heading.

Maprotiline Hydrochloride (In a study of the effect of vardenafil on QT interval in 59 healthy males, therapeutic (10 mg) and supratherapeutic (80 mg) doses of vardenafil and the active control moxifloxacin (400 mg) produced similar increases in QTc interval. A postmarketing study evaluating the effect of combining vardenafil with another drug of comparable QT effect showed an additive QT effect when compared with either drug alone. These observations should be considered in clinical decisions when prescribing vardenafil to patients taking medications known to prolong the QT interval).
No products indexed under this heading.

Meprobamate (In a study of the effect of vardenafil on QT interval in 59 healthy males, therapeutic (10 mg) and supratherapeutic (80 mg) doses of vardenafil and the active control moxifloxacin (400 mg) produced similar increases in QTc interval. A postmarketing study evaluating the effect of combining vardenafil with another drug of comparable QT effect showed an additive QT effect when compared with either drug alone. These observations should be considered in clinical decisions when prescribing vardenafil to patients taking medications known to prolong the QT interval).
No products indexed under this heading.

Mesoridazine Besylate (In a study of the effect of vardenafil on QT interval in 59 healthy males, therapeutic (10 mg) and supratherapeutic (80 mg) doses of vardenafil and the active control moxifloxacin (400 mg) produced similar increases in QTc interval. A postmarketing study evaluating the effect of combining vardenafil with another drug of comparable QT effect showed an additive QT effect when compared with either drug alone. These observations should be considered in clinical decisions when prescribing vardenafil to patients taking medications known to prolong the QT interval).
No products indexed under this heading.

Methyclothiazide (Studies in human liver microsomes showed that vardenafil is metabolized primarily by cytochrome P450 (CYP) isoforms 3A4/5, and to a lesser degree, by CYP2C9. Therefore, inhibitors of CYP2C9 are expected to reduce vardenafil clearance).
No products indexed under this heading.

Metronidazole (Studies in human liver microsomes showed that vardenafil is metabolized primarily by cytochrome P450 (CYP) isoforms 3A4/5, and to a lesser degree, by CYP2C9. Therefore, inhibitors of CYP3A4 are expected to reduce vardenafil clearance). Products include:
Pylera Capsules 714

Metronidazole Benzoate (Studies in human liver microsomes showed that vardenafil is metabolized primarily by cytochrome P450 (CYP) isoforms 3A4/5, and to a lesser degree, by CYP2C9. Therefore, inhibitors of CYP3A4 are expected to reduce vardenafil clearance).
No products indexed under this heading.

Metronidazole Hydrochloride (Studies in human liver microsomes showed that vardenafil is metabolized primarily by cytochrome P450 (CYP) isoforms 3A4/5, and to a lesser degree, by CYP2C9. Therefore, inhibitors of CYP3A4 are expected to reduce vardenafil clearance).
No products indexed under this heading.

Metronidazole Sodium (Studies in human liver microsomes showed that vardenafil is metabolized primarily by cytochrome P450 (CYP) isoforms 3A4/5, and to a lesser degree, by CYP2C9. Therefore, inhibitors of CYP3A4 are expected to reduce vardenafil clearance).
No products indexed under this heading.

Mexiletine Hydrochloride (In a study of the effect of vardenafil on QT interval in 59 healthy males, therapeutic (10 mg) and supratherapeutic (80 mg) doses of vardenafil and the active control moxifloxacin (400 mg) produced similar increases in QTc interval. A postmarketing study evaluating the effect of combining vardenafil with another drug of comparable QT effect showed an additive QT effect when compared with either drug alone. These observations should be considered in clinical decisions when prescribing vardenafil to patients taking medications known to prolong the QT interval).
No products indexed under this heading.

Miconazole (Studies in human liver microsomes showed that vardenafil is metabolized primarily by cytochrome P450 (CYP) isoforms 3A4/5, and to a lesser degree, by CYP2C9. Therefore, inhibitors of CYP3A4 are expected to reduce vardenafil clearance).
No products indexed under this heading.

Miconazole Nitrate (Studies in human liver microsomes showed that vardenafil is metabolized primarily by cytochrome P450 (CYP) isoforms 3A4/5, and to a lesser degree, by CYP2C9. Therefore, inhibitors of CYP3A4 are expected to reduce vardenafil clearance).
No products indexed under this heading.

Midazolam Hydrochloride (In a study of the effect of vardenafil on QT interval in 59 healthy males, therapeutic (10 mg) and supratherapeutic (80 mg) doses of vardenafil and the active control moxifloxacin (400 mg) produced similar increases in QTc interval. A postmarketing study evaluating the effect of combining vardenafil with another drug of comparable QT effect showed an additive QT effect when compared with either drug alone. These observations should be considered in clinical decisions when prescribing vardenafil to patients taking medications known to prolong the QT interval).
No products indexed under this heading.

Modafinil (Studies in human liver microsomes showed that vardenafil is metabolized primarily by cytochrome P450 (CYP) isoforms 3A4/5, and to a lesser degree, by CYP2C9. Therefore, inhibitors of CYP2C9 are expected to reduce vardenafil clearance). Products include:
Provigil Tablets 977

Molindone Hydrochloride (In a study of the effect of vardenafil on QT interval in 59 healthy males, therapeutic (10 mg) and supratherapeutic (80 mg) doses of vardenafil and the active control moxifloxacin (400 mg) produced similar increases in QTc interval. A postmarketing study evaluating the effect of combining vardenafil with another drug of comparable QT effect showed an additive QT effect when compared with either drug alone. These observations should be considered in clinical decisions when prescribing vardenafil to patients taking medications known to prolong the QT interval). Products include:
Moban Tablets 1116

Moricizine Hydrochloride (Patients taking Class 1A antiarrhythmic medications should avoid using vardenafil).
No products indexed under this heading.

Nefazodone Hydrochloride (Studies in human liver microsomes showed that vardenafil is metabolized primarily by cytochrome P450 (CYP) isoforms 3A4/5, and to a lesser degree, by CYP2C9. Therefore, inhibitors of CYP3A4 are expected to reduce vardenafil clearance. Patients taking potent CYP3A4 inhibitors should not exceed a dose of vardenafil 2.5 mg once daily).
No products indexed under this heading.

Nelfinavir Mesylate (Studies in human liver microsomes showed that vardenafil is metabolized primarily by cytochrome P450 (CYP) isoforms 3A4/5, and to a lesser degree, by CYP2C9. Therefore, inhibitors of CYP3A4 are expected to reduce vardenafil clearance. Patients taking potent CYP3A4 inhibitors should not exceed a dose of vardenafil 2.5 mg once daily).
No products indexed under this heading.

Nevirapine (Studies in human liver microsomes showed that vardenafil is metabolized primarily by cytochrome P450 (CYP) isoforms 3A4/5, and to a lesser degree, by CYP2C9. Therefore, inhibitors of CYP3A4 are expected to reduce vardenafil clearance). Products include:
Viramune Oral Suspension 873
Viramune Tablets 873

Niacinamide (Studies in human liver microsomes showed that vardenafil is metabolized primarily by cytochrome P450 (CYP) isoforms 3A4/5, and to a lesser degree, by CYP2C9. Therefore, inhibitors of CYP3A4 are expected to reduce vardenafil clearance). Products include:
BioLean Free Tablets .... ▣635

Nicotinamide (Studies in human liver microsomes showed that vardenafil is metabolized primarily by cytochrome P450 (CYP) isoforms 3A4/5, and to a lesser degree, by CYP2C9. Therefore, inhibitors of CYP3A4 are expected to reduce vardenafil clearance).
No products indexed under this heading.

Nifedipine (In patients whose hypertension was controlled with nifedipine, vardenafil 20 mg produced mean additional supine systolic/diastolic blood pressure reductions of 6/5 mmHg compared to placebo).
No products indexed under this heading.

Nitroglycerin (The blood pressure lowering effects of sublingual nitrates (0.4 mg) taken 1 and 4 hours after vardenafil and increases in heart rate were taken at 1, 4, and 8 hours were potentiated by a 20 mg dose of vardenafil in healthy middle-aged subjects. These effects were not observed when vardenafil 20 mg was taken 24 hours before the NTG. Potentiation of the hypotensive effects of nitrates for patients with ischemic heart disease has not been evaluated, and concomitant use of vardenafil and nitrates is contraindicated). Products include:

Nitro-Dur Transdermal Infusion System **2887**
Nitrolingual Pumpspray **2965**

Norfloxacin (Studies in human liver microsomes showed that vardenafil is metabolized primarily by cytochrome P450 (CYP) isoforms 3A4/5, and to a lesser degree, by CYP2C9. Therefore, inhibitors of CYP3A4 are expected to reduce vardenafil clearance). Products include:
Noroxin Tablets **2069**

Nortriptyline Hydrochloride (In a study of the effect of vardenafil on QT interval in 59 healthy males, therapeutic (10 mg) and supratherapeutic (80 mg) doses of vardenafil and the active control moxifloxacin (400 mg) produced similar increases in QTc interval. A postmarketing study evaluating the effect of combining vardenafil with another drug of comparable QT effect showed an additive QT effect when compared with either drug alone. These observations should be considered in clinical decisions when prescribing vardenafil to patients taking medications known to prolong the QT interval).
No products indexed under this heading.

Olanzapine (In a study of the effect of vardenafil on QT interval in 59 healthy males, therapeutic (10 mg) and supratherapeutic (80 mg) doses of vardenafil and the active control moxifloxacin (400 mg) produced similar increases in QTc interval. A postmarketing study evaluating the effect of combining vardenafil with another drug of comparable QT effect showed an additive QT effect when compared with either drug alone. These observations should be considered in clinical decisions when prescribing vardenafil to patients taking medications known to prolong the QT interval). Products include:
Symbyax Capsules **1871**
Zyprexa Tablets **1883**
Zyprexa IntraMuscular **1883**
Zyprexa ZYDIS Orally Disintegrating Tablets **1883**

Omeprazole (Studies in human liver microsomes showed that vardenafil is metabolized primarily by cytochrome P450 (CYP) isoforms 3A4/5, and to a lesser degree, by CYP2C9. Therefore, inhibitors of CYP3A4 are expected to reduce vardenafil clearance).
No products indexed under this heading.

Oxazepam (In a study of the effect of vardenafil on QT interval in 59 healthy males, therapeutic (10 mg) and supratherapeutic (80 mg) doses of vardenafil and the active control moxifloxacin (400 mg) produced similar increases in QTc interval. A postmarketing study evaluating the effect of combining vardenafil with another drug of comparable QT effect showed an additive QT effect when compared with either drug alone. These observations should be considered in clinical decisions when prescribing vardenafil to patients taking medications known to prolong the QT interval).
No products indexed under this heading.

Oxiconazole Nitrate (Studies in human liver microsomes showed that vardenafil is metabolized primarily by cytochrome P450 (CYP) isoforms 3A4/5, and to a lesser degree, by CYP2C9. Therefore, inhibitors of CYP2C9 are expected to reduce vardenafil clearance).
No products indexed under this heading.

Paroxetine Hydrochloride (Studies in human liver microsomes showed that vardenafil is metabolized primarily by cytochrome P450 (CYP) isoforms 3A4/5, and to a lesser degree, by CYP2C9. Therefore, inhibitors of CYP3A4 are expected to reduce vardenafil clearance). Products include:
Paxil **1535**
Paxil CR Controlled-Release Tablets **1544**

Pentaerythritol Tetranitrate (The blood pressure lowering effects of sublingual nitrates (0.4 mg) taken 1 and 4 hours after vardenafil and increases in heart rate were taken at 1, 4, and 8 hours were potentiated by a 20 mg dose of vardenafil in healthy middle-aged subjects. These effects were not observed when vardenafil 20 mg was taken 24 hours before the NTG. Potentiation of the hypotensive effects of nitrates for patients with ischemic heart disease has not been evaluated, and concomitant use of vardenafil and nitrates is contraindicated).
No products indexed under this heading.

Perphenazine (In a study of the effect of vardenafil on QT interval in 59 healthy males, therapeutic (10 mg) and supratherapeutic (80 mg) doses of vardenafil and the active control moxifloxacin (400 mg) produced similar increases in QTc interval. A postmarketing study evaluating the effect of combining vardenafil with another drug of comparable QT effect showed an additive QT effect when compared with either drug alone. These observations should be considered in clinical decisions when prescribing vardenafil to patients taking medications known to prolong the QT interval).
No products indexed under this heading.

Phenelzine Sulfate (In a study of the effect of vardenafil on QT interval in 59 healthy males, therapeutic (10 mg) and supratherapeutic (80 mg) doses of vardenafil and the active control moxifloxacin (400 mg) produced similar increases in QTc interval. A postmarketing study evaluating the effect of combining vardenafil with another drug of comparable QT effect showed an additive QT effect when compared with either drug alone. These observations should be considered in clinical decisions when prescribing vardenafil to patients taking medications known to prolong the QT interval).
No products indexed under this heading.

Phenylbutazone (Studies in human liver microsomes showed that vardenafil is metabolized primarily by cytochrome P450 (CYP) isoforms 3A4/5, and to a lesser degree, by CYP2C9. Therefore, inhibitors of CYP2C9 are expected to reduce vardenafil clearance).
No products indexed under this heading.

Polythiazide (Studies in human liver microsomes showed that vardenafil is metabolized primarily by cytochrome P450 (CYP) isoforms 3A4/5, and to a lesser degree, by CYP2C9. Therefore, inhibitors of CYP2C9 are expected to reduce vardenafil clearance).
No products indexed under this heading.

Prazepam (In a study of the effect of vardenafil on QT interval in 59 healthy males, therapeutic (10 mg) and supratherapeutic (80 mg) doses of vardenafil and the active control moxifloxacin (400 mg) produced similar increases in QTc interval. A postmarketing study evaluating the effect of combining vardenafil with another drug of comparable QT effect showed an additive QT effect when compared with either drug alone. These observations should be considered in clinical decisions when prescribing vardenafil to patients taking medications known to prolong the QT interval).
No products indexed under this heading.

Prazosin Hydrochloride (Caution is advised when phosphodiesterase type 5 (PDE5) inhibitors are co-administered with alpha-blockers. PDE5 inhibitors, including vardenafil, and alpha-adrenergic blocking agents are both vasodilators with blood pressure lowering effects. When vasodilators are used in combination, an additive effect on blood pressure may be anticipated. In some patients, concomitant use of these two drug classes can lower blood pressure significantly, leading to symptomatic hypotension (e.g., fainting). Concomitant treatment with vardenafil and alpha-blockers should be initiated only if the patient is stable on his alpha-blocker therapy. Vardenafil should be initiated at the lowest recommended starting dose).
No products indexed under this heading.

Procainamide (Patients taking Class 1A antiarrhythmic medications should avoid using vardenafil).
No products indexed under this heading.

Procainamide Hydrochloride (In a study of the effect of vardenafil on QT interval in 59 healthy males, therapeutic (10 mg) and supratherapeutic (80 mg) doses of vardenafil and the active control moxifloxacin (400 mg) produced similar increases in QTc interval. A postmarketing study evaluating the effect of combining vardenafil with another drug of comparable QT effect showed an additive QT effect when compared with either drug alone. These observations should be considered in clinical decisions when prescribing vardenafil to patients taking medications known to prolong the QT interval).
No products indexed under this heading.

Prochlorperazine (In a study of the effect of vardenafil on QT interval in 59 healthy males, therapeutic (10 mg) and supratherapeutic (80 mg) doses of vardenafil and the active control moxifloxacin (400 mg) produced similar increases in QTc interval. A postmarketing study evaluating the effect of combining vardenafil with another drug of comparable QT effect showed an additive QT effect when compared with either drug alone. These observations should be considered in clinical decisions when prescribing vardenafil to patients taking medications known to prolong the QT interval).
No products indexed under this heading.

Promethazine Hydrochloride (In a study of the effect of vardenafil on QT interval in 59 healthy males, therapeutic (10 mg) and supratherapeutic (80 mg) doses of vardenafil and the active control moxifloxacin (400 mg) produced similar increases in QTc interval. A postmarketing study evaluating the effect of combining vardenafil with another drug of comparable QT effect showed an additive QT effect when compared with either drug alone. These observations should be considered in clinical decisions when prescribing vardenafil to patients taking medications known to prolong the QT interval).
No products indexed under this heading.

Propafenone Hydrochloride (In a study of the effect of vardenafil on QT interval in 59 healthy males, therapeutic (10 mg) and supratherapeutic (80 mg) doses of vardenafil and the active control moxifloxacin (400 mg) produced similar increases in QTc interval. A postmarketing study evaluating the effect of combining vardenafil with another drug of comparable QT effect showed an additive QT effect when compared with either drug alone. These observations should be considered in clinical decisions when prescribing vardenafil to patients taking medications known to prolong the QT interval). Products include:
Rythmol Tablets **1586**
Rythmol SR Capsules **1590**

Propoxyphene Hydrochloride (Studies in human liver microsomes showed that vardenafil is metabolized primarily by cytochrome P450 (CYP) isoforms 3A4/5, and to a lesser degree, by CYP2C9. Therefore, inhibitors of CYP3A4 are expected to reduce vardenafil clearance).
No products indexed under this heading.

Propoxyphene Napsylate (Studies in human liver microsomes showed that vardenafil is metabolized primarily by cytochrome P450 (CYP) isoforms 3A4/5, and to a lesser degree, by CYP2C9. Therefore, inhibitors of CYP3A4 are expected to reduce vardenafil clearance).
No products indexed under this heading.

Protriptyline Hydrochloride (In a study of the effect of vardenafil on QT interval in 59 healthy males, therapeutic (10 mg) and supratherapeutic (80 mg) doses of vardenafil and the active control moxifloxacin (400 mg) produced similar increases in QTc interval. A postmarketing study evaluating the effect of combining vardenafil with another drug of comparable QT effect showed an additive QT effect when compared with either drug alone. These observations should be considered in clinical decisions when prescribing vardenafil to patients taking medications known to prolong the QT interval).
No products indexed under this heading.

Quetiapine Fumarate (In a study of the effect of vardenafil on QT interval in 59 healthy males, thera-

peutic (10 mg) and supratherapeutic (80 mg) doses of vardenafil and the active control moxifloxacin (400 mg) produced similar increases in QTc interval. A postmarketing study evaluating the effect of combining vardenafil with another drug of comparable QT effect showed an additive QT effect when compared with either drug alone. These observations should be considered in clinical decisions when prescribing vardenafil to patients taking medications known to prolong the QT interval).
No products indexed under this heading.

Quinidine (Patients taking Class 1A antiarrhythmic medications should avoid using vardenafil).
No products indexed under this heading.

Quinidine Gluconate (In a study of the effect of vardenafil on QT interval in 59 healthy males, therapeutic (10 mg) and supratherapeutic (80 mg) doses of vardenafil and the active control moxifloxacin (400 mg) produced similar increases in QTc interval. A postmarketing study evaluating the effect of combining vardenafil with another drug of comparable QT effect showed an additive QT effect when compared with either drug alone. These observations should be considered in clinical decisions when prescribing vardenafil to patients taking medications known to prolong the QT interval).
No products indexed under this heading.

Quinidine Hydrochloride (Patients taking Class 1A antiarrhythmic medications should avoid using vardenafil).
No products indexed under this heading.

Quinidine Polygalacturonate (In a study of the effect of vardenafil on QT interval in 59 healthy males, therapeutic (10 mg) and supratherapeutic (80 mg) doses of vardenafil and the active control moxifloxacin (400 mg) produced similar increases in QTc interval. A postmarketing study evaluating the effect of combining vardenafil with another drug of comparable QT effect showed an additive QT effect when compared with either drug alone. These observations should be considered in clinical decisions when prescribing vardenafil to patients taking medications known to prolong the QT interval).
No products indexed under this heading.

Quinidine Sulfate (In a study of the effect of vardenafil on QT interval in 59 healthy males, therapeutic (10 mg) and supratherapeutic (80 mg) doses of vardenafil and the active control moxifloxacin (400 mg) produced similar increases in QTc interval. A postmarketing study evaluating the effect of combining vardenafil with another drug of comparable QT effect showed an additive QT effect when compared with either drug alone. These observations should be considered in clinical decisions when prescribing vardenafil to patients taking medications known to prolong the QT interval).
No products indexed under this heading.

Quinine (Studies in human liver microsomes showed that vardenafil is metabolized primarily by cytochrome P450 (CYP) isoforms 3A4/5, and to a lesser degree, by CYP2C9. Therefore, inhibitors of CYP3A4 are expected to reduce vardenafil clearance).
No products indexed under this heading.

Quinine Sulfate (Studies in human liver microsomes showed that vardenafil is metabolized primarily by cytochrome P450 (CYP) isoforms 3A4/5, and to a lesser degree, by CYP2C9. Therefore, inhibitors of CYP3A4 are expected to reduce vardenafil clearance).
No products indexed under this heading.

Quinupristin (Studies in human liver microsomes showed that vardenafil is metabolized primarily by cytochrome P450 (CYP) isoforms 3A4/5, and to a lesser degree, by CYP2C9. Therefore, inhibitors of CYP3A4 are expected to reduce vardenafil clearance).
No products indexed under this heading.

Ranitidine Bismuth Citrate (Studies in human liver microsomes showed that vardenafil is metabolized primarily by cytochrome P450 (CYP) isoforms 3A4/5, and to a lesser degree, by CYP2C9. Therefore, inhibitors of CYP3A4 are expected to reduce vardenafil clearance).
No products indexed under this heading.

Ranitidine Hydrochloride (Studies in human liver microsomes showed that vardenafil is metabolized primarily by cytochrome P450 (CYP) isoforms 3A4/5, and to a lesser degree, by CYP2C9. Therefore, inhibitors of CYP3A4 are expected to reduce vardenafil clearance).
Products include:
Zantac 75 Tablets .... ▣ 603
Zantac 1670
Zantac Injection 1666
Zantac Injection Pharmacy Bulk Package 1668
Maximum Strength Zantac 150 Tablets .... ▣ 603
Maximum Strength Zantac 150 Cool Mint Tablets .... ▣ 603

Risperidone (In a study of the effect of vardenafil on QT interval in 59 healthy males, therapeutic (10 mg) and supratherapeutic (80 mg) doses of vardenafil and the active control moxifloxacin (400 mg) produced similar increases in QTc interval. A postmarketing study evaluating the effect of combining vardenafil with another drug of comparable QT effect showed an additive QT effect when compared with either drug alone. These observations should be considered in clinical decisions when prescribing vardenafil to patients taking medications known to prolong the QT interval). Products include:
Risperdal Consta Long-Acting Injection 1753

Ritonavir (Ritonavir (600 mg b.i.d.) co-administered with vardenafil 5 mg resulted in a 49-fold increase in vardenafil AUC and a 13-fold increase in vardenafil Cmax. The interaction is a consequence of blocking hepatic metabolism of vardenafil by ritonavir, a highly potent CYP3A4 inhibitor, which also inhibits CYP2C9. Ritonavir significantly prolonged the half-life of vardenafil to 26 hours. Consequently, it is recommended not to exceed a single 2.5 mg vardenafil dose in a 72 hour period when used in combination with ritonavir. Long-term safety information is not available on the concomitant administration of vardenafil with HIV protease inhibitors).
Products include:
Kaletra 452
Norvir 489

Saquinavir (Patients taking saquinavir, a potent CYP3A4 inhibitor should not exceed a dose of vardenafil 2.5 mg once daily. Long-term safety information is not available on the concomitant administration of vardenafil with HIV protease inhibitors).
No products indexed under this heading.

Saquinavir Mesylate (Patients taking saquinavir, a potent CYP3A4 inhibitor should not exceed a dose of vardenafil 2.5 mg once daily. Long-term safety information is not available on the concomitant administration of vardenafil with HIV protease inhibitors).
No products indexed under this heading.

Sertraline Hydrochloride (Studies in human liver microsomes showed that vardenafil is metabolized primarily by cytochrome P450 (CYP) isoforms 3A4/5, and to a lesser degree, by CYP2C9. Therefore, inhibitors of CYP3A4 are expected to reduce vardenafil clearance).
No products indexed under this heading.

Sildenafil Citrate (The safety and efficacy of vardenafil used in combination with other treatments for erectile dysfunction have not been studied. Therefore the use of such combinations is not recommended).
No products indexed under this heading.

Sotalol Hydrochloride (Patients taking Class III antiarrhythmic medications should avoid using vardenafil).
No products indexed under this heading.

Sulfacytine (Studies in human liver microsomes showed that vardenafil is metabolized primarily by cytochrome P450 (CYP) isoforms 3A4/5, and to a lesser degree, by CYP2C9. Therefore, inhibitors of CYP2C9 are expected to reduce vardenafil clearance).
No products indexed under this heading.

Sulfamethizole (Studies in human liver microsomes showed that vardenafil is metabolized primarily by cytochrome P450 (CYP) isoforms 3A4/5, and to a lesser degree, by CYP2C9. Therefore, inhibitors of CYP2C9 are expected to reduce vardenafil clearance).
No products indexed under this heading.

Sulfamethoxazole (Studies in human liver microsomes showed that vardenafil is metabolized primarily by cytochrome P450 (CYP) isoforms 3A4/5, and to a lesser degree, by CYP2C9. Therefore, inhibitors of CYP2C9 are expected to reduce vardenafil clearance).
No products indexed under this heading.

Sulfasalazine (Studies in human liver microsomes showed that vardenafil is metabolized primarily by cytochrome P450 (CYP) isoforms 3A4/5, and to a lesser degree, by CYP2C9. Therefore, inhibitors of CYP2C9 are expected to reduce vardenafil clearance).
No products indexed under this heading.

Sulfinpyrazone (Studies in human liver microsomes showed that vardenafil is metabolized primarily by cytochrome P450 (CYP) isoforms 3A4/5, and to a lesser degree, by CYP2C9. Therefore, inhibitors of CYP2C9 are expected to reduce vardenafil clearance).
No products indexed under this heading.

Sulfisoxazole Acetyl (Studies in human liver microsomes showed that vardenafil is metabolized primarily by cytochrome P450 (CYP) isoforms 3A4/5, and to a lesser degree, by CYP2C9. Therefore, inhibitors of CYP2C9 are expected to reduce vardenafil clearance).
No products indexed under this heading.

Sulfisoxazole Diolamine (Studies in human liver microsomes showed that vardenafil is metabolized primarily by cytochrome P450 (CYP) isoforms 3A4/5, and to a lesser degree, by CYP2C9. Therefore, inhibitors of CYP2C9 are expected to reduce vardenafil clearance).
No products indexed under this heading.

Tamsulosin Hydrochloride (Caution is advised when phosphodiesterase type 5 (PDE5) inhibitors are co-administered with alpha-blockers. PDE5 inhibitors, including vardenafil, and alpha-adrenergic blocking agents are both vasodilators with blood pressure lowering effects. When vasodilators are used in combination, an additive effect on blood pressure may be anticipated. In some patients, concomitant use of these two drug classes can lower blood pressure significantly, leading to symptomatic hypotension (e.g., fainting). Concomitant treatment with vardenafil and alpha-blockers should be initiated only if the patient is stable on his alpha-blocker therapy. Vardenafil should be initiated at the lowest recommended starting dose). Products include:
Flomax Capsules 848

Telithromycin (Studies in human liver microsomes showed that vardenafil is metabolized primarily by cytochrome P450 (CYP) isoforms 3A4/5, and to a lesser degree, by CYP2C9. Therefore, inhibitors of CYP3A4 are expected to reduce vardenafil clearance. Patients taking potent CYP3A4 inhibitors should not exceed a dose of vardenafil 2.5 mg once daily). Products include:
Ketek Tablets 2744

Terazosin Hydrochloride (Caution is advised when phosphodiesterase type 5 (PDE5) inhibitors are co-administered with alpha-blockers. PDE5 inhibitors, including vardenafil, and alpha-adrenergic blocking agents are both vasodilators with blood pressure lowering effects. When vasodilators are used in combination, an additive effect on blood pressure may be anticipated. In some patients, concomitant use of these two drug classes can lower

blood pressure significantly, leading to symptomatic hypotension (e.g., fainting). Concomitant treatment with vardenafil and alpha-blockers should be initiated only if the patient is stable on his alpha-blocker therapy. Vardenafil should be initiated at the lowest recommended starting dose).
No products indexed under this heading.

Terconazole (Studies in human liver microsomes showed that vardenafil is metabolized primarily by cytochrome P450 (CYP) isoforms 3A4/5, and to a lesser degree, by CYP2C9. Therefore, inhibitors of CYP2C9 are expected to reduce vardenafil clearance).
No products indexed under this heading.

Thioridazine Hydrochloride (In a study of the effect of vardenafil on QT interval in 59 healthy males, therapeutic (10 mg) and supratherapeutic (80 mg) doses of vardenafil and the active control moxifloxacin (400 mg) produced similar increases in QTc interval. A postmarketing study evaluating the effect of combining vardenafil with another drug of comparable QT effect showed an additive QT effect when compared with either drug alone. These observations should be considered in clinical decisions when prescribing vardenafil to patients taking medications known to prolong the QT interval). Products include:
Thioridazine Hydrochloride Tablets 2195

Thiothixene (In a study of the effect of vardenafil on QT interval in 59 healthy males, therapeutic (10 mg) and supratherapeutic (80 mg) doses of vardenafil and the active control moxifloxacin (400 mg) produced similar increases in QTc interval. A postmarketing study evaluating the effect of combining vardenafil with another drug of comparable QT effect showed an additive QT effect when compared with either drug alone. These observations should be considered in clinical decisions when prescribing vardenafil to patients taking medications known to prolong the QT interval). Products include:
Thiothixene Capsules 2197

Ticlopidine Hydrochloride (Studies in human liver microsomes showed that vardenafil is metabolized primarily by cytochrome P450 (CYP) isoforms 3A4/5, and to a lesser degree, by CYP2C9. Therefore, inhibitors of CYP2C9 are expected to reduce vardenafil clearance).
No products indexed under this heading.

Tipranavir (Long-term safety information is not available on the concomitant administration of vardenafil with HIV protease inhibitors).
Products include:
Aptivus Capsules 823
Aptivus Oral Solution 823

Tocainide Hydrochloride (In a study of the effect of vardenafil on QT interval in 59 healthy males, therapeutic (10 mg) and supratherapeutic (80 mg) doses of vardenafil and the active control moxifloxacin (400 mg) produced similar increases in QTc interval. A postmarketing study evaluating the effect of combining vardenafil with another drug of comparable QT effect showed an additive QT effect when compared with either drug alone. These observations should be considered in clinical decisions when prescribing vardenafil to patients taking medications known to prolong the QT interval).
No products indexed under this heading.

Tolazamide (Studies in human liver microsomes showed that vardenafil is metabolized primarily by cytochrome P450 (CYP) isoforms 3A4/5, and to a lesser degree, by CYP2C9. Therefore, inhibitors of CYP2C9 are expected to reduce vardenafil clearance).
No products indexed under this heading.

Tolbutamide (Studies in human liver microsomes showed that vardenafil is metabolized primarily by cytochrome P450 (CYP) isoforms 3A4/5, and to a lesser degree, by CYP2C9. Therefore, inhibitors of CYP2C9 are expected to reduce vardenafil clearance).
No products indexed under this heading.

Tolbutamide Sodium (Studies in human liver microsomes showed that vardenafil is metabolized primarily by cytochrome P450 (CYP) isoforms 3A4/5, and to a lesser degree, by CYP2C9. Therefore, inhibitors of CYP2C9 are expected to reduce vardenafil clearance).
No products indexed under this heading.

Tranylcypromine Sulfate (In a study of the effect of vardenafil on QT interval in 59 healthy males, therapeutic (10 mg) and supratherapeutic (80 mg) doses of vardenafil and the active control moxifloxacin (400 mg) produced similar increases in QTc interval. A postmarketing study evaluating the effect of combining vardenafil with another drug of comparable QT effect showed an additive QT effect when compared with either drug alone. These observations should be considered in clinical decisions when prescribing vardenafil to patients taking medications known to prolong the QT interval).
Products include:
Parnate Tablets 1532

Trifluoperazine Hydrochloride (In a study of the effect of vardenafil on QT interval in 59 healthy males, therapeutic (10 mg) and supratherapeutic (80 mg) doses of vardenafil and the active control moxifloxacin (400 mg) produced similar increases in QTc interval. A postmarketing study evaluating the effect of combining vardenafil with another drug of comparable QT effect showed an additive QT effect when compared with either drug alone. These observations should be considered in clinical decisions when prescribing vardenafil to patients taking medications known to prolong the QT interval).
No products indexed under this heading.

Trimipramine Maleate (In a study of the effect of vardenafil on QT interval in 59 healthy males, therapeutic (10 mg) and supratherapeutic (80 mg) doses of vardenafil and the active control moxifloxacin (400 mg) produced similar increases in QTc interval. A postmarketing study evaluating the effect of combining vardenafil with another drug of comparable QT effect showed an additive QT effect when compared with either drug alone. These observations should be considered in clinical decisions when prescribing vardenafil to patients taking medications known to prolong the QT interval).
No products indexed under this heading.

Troglitazone (Studies in human liver microsomes showed that vardenafil is metabolized primarily by cytochrome P450 (CYP) isoforms 3A4/5, and to a lesser degree, by CYP2C9. Therefore, inhibitors of CYP3A4 are expected to reduce vardenafil clearance).
No products indexed under this heading.

Troleandomycin (Studies in human liver microsomes showed that vardenafil is metabolized primarily by cytochrome P450 (CYP) isoforms 3A4/5, and to a lesser degree, by CYP2C9. Therefore, inhibitors of CYP3A4 are expected to reduce vardenafil clearance. Patients taking potent CYP3A4 inhibitors should not exceed a dose of vardenafil 2.5 mg once daily).
No products indexed under this heading.

Valproate Sodium (Studies in human liver microsomes showed that vardenafil is metabolized primarily by cytochrome P450 (CYP) isoforms 3A4/5, and to a lesser degree, by CYP2C9. Therefore, inhibitors of CYP3A4 are expected to reduce vardenafil clearance).
No products indexed under this heading.

Verapamil Hydrochloride (Studies in human liver microsomes showed that vardenafil is metabolized primarily by cytochrome P450 (CYP) isoforms 3A4/5, and to a lesser degree, by CYP2C9. Therefore, inhibitors of CYP3A4 are expected to reduce vardenafil clearance).
Products include:
Tarka Tablets 511

Voriconazole (Studies in human liver microsomes showed that vardenafil is metabolized primarily by cytochrome P450 (CYP) isoforms 3A4/5, and to a lesser degree, by CYP2C9. Therefore, inhibitors of CYP3A4 are expected to reduce vardenafil clearance. Patients taking potent CYP3A4 inhibitors should not exceed a dose of vardenafil 2.5 mg once daily).
No products indexed under this heading.

Zafirlukast (Studies in human liver microsomes showed that vardenafil is metabolized primarily by cytochrome P450 (CYP) isoforms 3A4/5, and to a lesser degree, by CYP2C9. Therefore, inhibitors of CYP3A4 are expected to reduce vardenafil clearance). Products include:
Accolate Tablets 669

Zileuton (Studies in human liver microsomes showed that vardenafil is metabolized primarily by cytochrome P450 (CYP) isoforms 3A4/5, and to a lesser degree, by CYP2C9. Therefore, inhibitors of CYP3A4 are expected to reduce vardenafil clearance).
No products indexed under this heading.

Ziprasidone Hydrochloride (In a study of the effect of vardenafil on QT interval in 59 healthy males, therapeutic (10 mg) and supratherapeutic (80 mg) doses of vardenafil and the active control moxifloxacin (400 mg) produced similar increases in QTc interval. A postmarketing study evaluating the effect of combining vardenafil with another drug of comparable QT effect showed an additive QT effect when compared with either drug alone. These observations should be considered in clinical decisions when prescribing vardenafil to patients taking medications known to prolong the QT interval).
Products include:
Geodon Capsules 2520

Food Interactions

Grapefruit (Although specific interactions have not been studied, other CYP3A4 inhibitors, including grapefruit juice, would likely increase vardenafil exposure).

Grapefruit Juice (Although specific interactions have not been studied, other CYP3A4 inhibitors, including grapefruit juice, would likely increase vardenafil exposure).

LEVOTHROID TABLETS

(Levothyroxine Sodium) 1170
May interact with androgens, antacids, beta blockers, oral anticoagulants, dopamine agonists, estrogens, glucocorticoids, cardiac glycosides, hydantoin anticonvulsants, oral hypoglycemic agents, insulin, oral contraceptives, radiographic iodinated contrast media, salicylates, sympathomimetics, thiazides, tricyclic antidepressants, xanthines, and certain other agents. Compounds in these categories include:

Acarbose (Addition of levothyroxine to antidiabetic therapy may result in increased antidiabetic agent requirements. Careful monitoring of diabetic control is recommended, especially when thyroid therapy is started, changed, or discontinued). Products include:
Precose Tablets 792

Acebutolol Hydrochloride (Actions of particular beta-adrenergic antagonists may be impaired when the hypothyroid patient is converted to the euthroid state).
No products indexed under this heading.

Albuterol (Concurrent use may increase the effects of sympathomimetics or thyroid hormone. Thyroid hormones may increase the risk of coronary insufficiency when sympathomimetic agents are administered to patients with coronary artery disease).
No products indexed under this heading.

Albuterol Sulfate (Concurrent use may increase the effects of sympathomimetics or thyroid hormone. Thyroid hormones may increase the risk of coronary insufficiency when sympathomimetic agents are administered to patients with coronary artery disease). Products include:
Combivent Inhalation Aerosol 845
ProAir HFA Inhalation Aerosol 3113
Proventil HFA Inhalation Aerosol 2914
Ventolin HFA Inhalation Aerosol 1638

Aluminum Carbonate (Concurrent use with antacids may reduce the efficacy of levothyroxine by binding and delaying or preventing the absorption, potentially resulting in hypothyroidism. Administer levothyroxine at least four hours apart from these agents).
No products indexed under this heading.

Aluminum Hydroxide (Concurrent use with antacids may reduce the efficacy of levothyroxine by binding and delaying or preventing the absorption, potentially resulting in hypothyroidism. Administer levothyroxine at least four hours apart from these agents).
No products indexed under this heading.

Aminoglutethimide (Long-term aminoglutethimide therapy may minimally decrease T4 and T3 levels and increase TSH, although all values remain within normal limits in most patients).
No products indexed under this heading.

Aminophylline (Decreased theophylline clearance may occur in hypothyroid patients; clearance returns to normal when the euthroid state is achieved).
No products indexed under this heading.

Amiodarone Hydrochloride (Administration may decrease the peripheral conversion of T4 to T3, leading to decreased T3 levels. However, serum T4 levels are usually normal but may occasionally be slightly increased. Amiodarone may also induce hyperthyroidism by causing thyroiditis).
No products indexed under this heading.

Amitriptyline Hydrochloride (Concurrent use of tricyclic antidepressants and levothyroxine may increase the therapeutic and toxic effects of both drugs, possibly due to increased receptor sensitivity to catecholamines. Onset of action of tricyclics may be accelerated).
No products indexed under this heading.

Amoxapine (Concurrent use of tricyclic antidepressants and levothyroxine may increase the therapeutic and toxic effects of both drugs, possibly due to increased receptor sensitivity to catecholamines. Onset of action of tricyclics may be accelerated).
No products indexed under this heading.

Anisindione (Thyroid hormones appear to increase the catabolism of vitamin-K dependent clotting factors, thereby increasing the anticoagulant activity of oral anticoagulants. Concomitant use of these agents impairs the compensatory increases in clotting factor synthesis. Prothrombin time should be carefully monitored in patients taking levothyroxine and oral anticoagulants and the dose of anticoagulant therapy adjusted accordingly).
No products indexed under this heading.

Asparaginase (Asparaginase may decrease serum TBG concentration). Products include:
Elspar for Injection 1990
Elspar for Injection 2488

Aspirin (Salicylates inhibit binding of T4 and T3 to TBG and transthyretin. An initial increase in FT4 is followed by return of FT4 to normal levels with sustained therapeutic serum salicylate concentrations, although total T4 levels may decrease by as much as 30%). Products include:
Aggrenox Capsules 819
Bayer Aspirin 750
Percodan Tablets 1130
St. Joseph 81 mg Aspirin Chewable and Enteric Coated Tablets 1903

Aspirin, Enteric Coated (Salicylates inhibit binding of T4 and T3 to TBG and transthyretin. An initial increase in FT4 is followed by return of FT4 to normal levels with sustained therapeutic serum salicylate concentrations, although total T4 levels may decrease by as much as 30%).
No products indexed under this heading.

Aspirin Buffered (Salicylates inhibit binding of T4 and T3 to TBG and transthyretin. An initial increase in FT4 is followed by return of FT4 to normal levels with sustained therapeutic serum salicylate concentrations, although total T4 levels may decrease by as much as 30%).
No products indexed under this heading.

Atenolol (Actions of particular beta-adrenergic antagonists may be impaired when the hypothyroid patient is converted to the euthroid state).
No products indexed under this heading.

Bendroflumethiazide (Thiazide diuretics are associated with thyroid hormone and/or TSH level alterations).
No products indexed under this heading.

Betamethasone Acetate (Glucocorticoids may result in a transient reduction in TSH secretion when administered at doses greater than 100mg/day of hydrocortisone or equivalent. Short-term administration of large doses of glucocorticoids may decrease serum T3 concentrations by 30% with minimal change in serum T4 levels. However, long-term glucocorticoid therapy may result in slightly decreased T3 and T4 levels due to decreased TBG production).
No products indexed under this heading.

Betamethasone Sodium Phosphate (Glucocorticoids may result in a transient reduction in TSH secretion when administered at doses greater than 100mg/day of hydrocortisone or equivalent. Short-term administration of large doses of glucocorticoids may decrease serum T3 concentrations by 30% with minimal change in serum T4 levels. However, long-term glucocorticoid therapy may result in slightly decreased T3 and T4 levels due to decreased TBG production).
No products indexed under this heading.

Betaxolol Hydrochloride (Actions of particular beta-adrenergic antagonists may be impaired when the hypothyroid patient is converted to the euthroid state).
No products indexed under this heading.

Bisoprolol Fumarate (Actions of particular beta-adrenergic antagonists may be impaired when the hypothyroid patient is converted to the euthroid state).
No products indexed under this heading.

Bromocriptine Mesylate (Dopamine and dopamine agonists may result in a transient reduction in TSH secretion when administered at dopamine doses greater than or equal to 1 mcg/kg/min).
No products indexed under this heading.

Calcium Carbonate (Calcium carbonate may form an insoluble chelate with levothyroxine. Concurrent use may reduce the efficacy of levothyroxine by binding and delaying or preventing the absorption, potentially resulting in hypothyroidism. Administer levothyroxine at least four hours apart from calcium carbonate-containing products). Products include:
Accelerator Tablets .... ■ 634
Actonel with Calcium Tablets 2574
BioLean II Tablets .... ■ 635
Calcet Triple Calcium + Vitamin D Tablets .... ■ 629
D-Cal Chewable Caplets .... ■ 624
Elixir Capsules .... ■ 636
Pepcid Complete Chewable Tablets 1771
Extra Strength Rolaids Plus Gas Relief Tropical Fruit Softchews 1903
Extra Strength Rolaids Softchews Vanilla Creme 1903
Extra Strength Rolaids Freshmint Tablets 1903
Rolaids Multi-Symptom Berry Tablets 1903
Rolaids Original Peppermint Tablets 1903

Carbamazepine (Stimulation of hepatic microsomal drug-metabolizing activity may cause increased hepatic degradation of levothyroxine, resulting in increased levothyroxine requirements). Products include:
Carbatrol Capsules 3019
Equetro Extended-Release Capsules 3174

Carteolol Hydrochloride (Actions of particular beta-adrenergic antagonists may be impaired when the hypothyroid patient is converted to the euthroid state).
No products indexed under this heading.

Chloral Hydrate (Chloral Hydrate has been associated with thyroid hormone and/or TSH level alterations).
No products indexed under this heading.

Chlorothiazide (Thiazide diuretics are associated with thyroid hormone and/or TSH level alterations).
No products indexed under this heading.

Chlorothiazide Sodium (Thiazide diuretics are associated with thyroid hormone and/or TSH level alterations). Products include:
Intravenous Sodium Diuril 2490

Chlorotrianisene (Estrogen may increase serum TBG concentration).
No products indexed under this heading.

Chlorpropamide (Addition of levothyroxine to antidiabetic therapy may result in increased antidiabetic agent requirements. Careful monitoring of diabetic control is recommended, especially when thyroid therapy is started, changed, or discontinued).
No products indexed under this heading.

Cholestyramine (Concurrent use with cholestyramine may reduce the efficacy of levothyroxine by binding and delaying or preventing the absorption, potentially resulting in hypothyroidism. Administer levothyroxine at least four hours apart from cholestyramine).
No products indexed under this heading.

Choline Magnesium Trisalicylate (Salicylates inhibit binding of T4 and T3 to TBG and transthyretin. An initial increase in FT4 is followed by return of FT4 to normal levels with sustained therapeutic serum salicylate concentrations, although total T4 levels may decrease by as much as 30%).
No products indexed under this heading.

Clofibrate (Clofibrate may increase serum TBG concentration).
No products indexed under this heading.

Clomipramine Hydrochloride (Concurrent use of tricyclic antidepressants and levothyroxine may increase the therapeutic and toxic effects of both drugs, possibly due to increased receptor sensitivity to catecholamines. Onset of action of tricyclics may be accelerated).
No products indexed under this heading.

Colestipol (Concurrent use with colestipol may reduce the efficacy of levothyroxine by binding and delaying or preventing the absorption, potentially resulting in hypothyroidism. Administer levothyroxine at least four hours apart from colestipol).
No products indexed under this heading.

Colestipol Hydrochloride (Concurrent use with colestipol may reduce the efficacy of levothyroxine by binding and delaying or preventing the absorption, potentially resulting in hypothyroidism. Administer levothyroxine at least four hours apart from colestipol).
No products indexed under this heading.

Cortisone Acetate (Glucocorticoids may result in a transient reduction in TSH secretion when administered at doses greater than 100mg/day of hydrocortisone or equivalent. Short-term administration of large doses of glucocorticoids may decrease serum T3 concentrations by 30% with minimal change in serum T4 levels. However, long-term glucocorticoid therapy may result in slightly decreased T3 and T4 levels due to decreased TBG production).
No products indexed under this heading.

Desipramine Hydrochloride (Concurrent use of tricyclic antidepressants and levothyroxine may increase the therapeutic and toxic effects of both drugs, possibly due to increased receptor sensitivity to catecholamines. Onset of action of tricyclics may be accelerated).
No products indexed under this heading.

Deslanoside (Serum digitalis glycoside levels may be reduced in hyperthyroidism or when the hypothyroid patient is converted to the euthroid state. Therapeutic effect of digitalis glycosides may be reduced).
No products indexed under this heading.

Desogestrel (Estrogen-containing oral contraceptives may increase serum TBG concentration). Products include:

Mircette Tablets 1034

Dexamethasone (Glucocorticoids may result in a transient reduction in TSH secretion when administered at doses greater than 100mg/day of hydrocortisone or equivalent. Short-term administration of large doses of glucocorticoids may decrease serum T3 concentrations by 30% with minimal change in serum T4 levels. However, long-term glucocorticoid therapy may result in slightly decreased T3 and T4 levels due to decreased TBG production). Products include:

Ciprodex Otic Suspension 541

Dexamethasone Acetate (Glucocorticoids may result in a transient reduction in TSH secretion when administered at doses greater than 100mg/day of hydrocortisone or equivalent. Short-term administration of large doses of glucocorticoids may decrease serum T3 concentrations by 30% with minimal change in serum T4 levels. However, long-term glucocorticoid therapy may result in slightly decreased T3 and T4 levels due to decreased TBG production).

No products indexed under this heading.

Dexamethasone Sodium Phosphate (Glucocorticoids may result in a transient reduction in TSH secretion when administered at doses greater than 100mg/day of hydrocortisone or equivalent. Short-term administration of large doses of glucocorticoids may decrease serum T3 concentrations by 30% with minimal change in serum T4 levels. However, long-term glucocorticoid therapy may result in slightly decreased T3 and T4 levels due to decreased TBG production).

No products indexed under this heading.

Diatrizoate Meglumine (Iodide and drugs that contain pharmacologic amounts of iodide may cause hyperthyroidism in euthroid patients with Grave's disease previously treated with antithyroid drugs or in euthroid patients with thyroid autonomy. Hyperthyroidism may develop over several weeks and may persist for several months after therapy discontinuation. Thyroid hormones may also reduce the uptake of I-123 and I-131).

No products indexed under this heading.

Diatrizoate Sodium (Iodide and drugs that contain pharmacologic amounts of iodide may cause hyperthyroidism in euthroid patients with Grave's disease previously treated with antithyroid drugs or in euthroid patients with thyroid autonomy. Hyperthyroidism may develop over several weeks and may persist for several months after therapy discontinuation. Thyroid hormones may also reduce the uptake of I-123 and I-131).

No products indexed under this heading.

Diazepam (Diazepam is associated with thyroid hormone and/or TSH level alterations). Products include:

Valium Tablets 2658

Dicumarol (Thyroid hormones appear to increase the catabolism of vitamin-K dependent clotting factors, thereby increasing the anticoagulant activity of oral anticoagulants. Concomitant use of these agents impairs the compensatory increases in clotting factor synthesis. Prothrombin time should be carefully monitored in patients taking levothyroxine and oral anticoagulants and the dose of anticoagulant therapy adjusted accordingly).

No products indexed under this heading.

Dienestrol (Estrogen may increase serum TBG concentration).

No products indexed under this heading.

Diethylstilbestrol (Estrogen may increase serum TBG concentration).

No products indexed under this heading.

Diflunisal (Salicylates inhibit binding of T4 and T3 to TBG and transthyretin. An initial increase in FT4 is followed by return of FT4 to normal levels with sustained therapeutic serum salicylate concentrations, although total T4 levels may decrease by as much as 30%).

No products indexed under this heading.

Digitalis Glycoside Preparations (Serum digitalis glycoside levels may be reduced in hyperthyroidism or when the hypothyroid patient is converted to the euthroid state. Therapeutic effect of digitalis glycosides may be reduced).

No products indexed under this heading.

Digitoxin (Serum digitalis glycoside levels may be reduced in hyperthyroidism or when the hypothyroid patient is converted to the euthroid state. Therapeutic effect of digitalis glycosides may be reduced).

No products indexed under this heading.

Digoxin (Serum digitalis glycoside levels may be reduced in hyperthyroidism or when the hypothyroid patient is converted to the euthroid state. Therapeutic effect of digitalis glycosides may be reduced). Products include:

Lanoxin Injection 1498
Lanoxin Injection Pediatric 1502
Lanoxin Tablets 1505

Dobutamine Hydrochloride (Concurrent use may increase the effects of sympathomimetics or thyroid hormone. Thyroid hormones may increase the risk of coronary insufficiency when sympathomimetic agents are administered to patients with coronary artery disease).

No products indexed under this heading.

Dopamine Hydrochloride (Concurrent use may increase the effects of sympathomimetics or thyroid hormone. Thyroid hormones may increase the risk of coronary insufficiency when sympathomimetic agents are administered to patients with coronary artery disease).

No products indexed under this heading.

Doxepin Hydrochloride (Concurrent use of tricyclic antidepressants and levothyroxine may increase the therapeutic and toxic effects of both drugs, possibly due to increased receptor sensitivity to catecholamines. Onset of action of tricyclics may be accelerated).

No products indexed under this heading.

Dyphylline (Decreased theophylline clearance may occur in hypothyroid patients; clearance returns to normal when the euthroid state is achieved).

No products indexed under this heading.

Ephedrine Hydrochloride (Concurrent use may increase the effects of sympathomimetics or thyroid hormone. Thyroid hormones may increase the risk of coronary insufficiency when sympathomimetic agents are administered to patients with coronary artery disease).

No products indexed under this heading.

Ephedrine Sulfate (Concurrent use may increase the effects of sympathomimetics or thyroid hormone. Thyroid hormones may increase the risk of coronary insufficiency when sympathomimetic agents are administered to patients with coronary artery disease).

No products indexed under this heading.

Ephedrine Tannate (Concurrent use may increase the effects of sympathomimetics or thyroid hormone. Thyroid hormones may increase the risk of coronary insufficiency when sympathomimetic agents are administered to patients with coronary artery disease).

No products indexed under this heading.

Epinephrine (Concurrent use may increase the effects of sympathomimetics or thyroid hormone. Thyroid hormones may increase the risk of coronary insufficiency when sympathomimetic agents are administered to patients with coronary artery disease). Products include:

EpiPen 1024

Epinephrine Bitartrate (Concurrent use may increase the effects of sympathomimetics or thyroid hormone. Thyroid hormones may increase the risk of coronary insufficiency when sympathomimetic agents are administered to patients with coronary artery disease).

No products indexed under this heading.

Epinephrine Hydrochloride (Concurrent use may increase the effects of sympathomimetics or thyroid hormone. Thyroid hormones may increase the risk of coronary insufficiency when sympathomimetic agents are administered to patients with coronary artery disease).

No products indexed under this heading.

Esmolol Hydrochloride (Actions of particular beta-adrenergic antagonists may be impaired when the hypothyroid patient is converted to the euthroid state).

No products indexed under this heading.

Estradiol (Estrogen may increase serum TBG concentration). Products include:

Activella Tablets 2347
Angeliq Tablets 751
Climara Transdermal System 763
Climara Pro Transdermal System 768
Divigel 3167
Vagifem Tablets 2375

Estrogens, Conjugated (Estrogen may increase serum TBG concentration). Products include:

Premarin Intravenous 3217
Premarin Tablets 3221
Premarin Vaginal Cream 3228
Premphase Tablets 3232
Prempro Tablets 3232

Estrogens, Esterified (Estrogen may increase serum TBG concentration). Products include:

Estratest Tablets 3043
Estratest H.S. Tablets 3043

Estropipate (Estrogen may increase serum TBG concentration).

No products indexed under this heading.

Ethinyl Estradiol (Estrogen-containing oral contraceptives may increase serum TBG concentration). Products include:

Lybrel Tablets 3204
Mircette Tablets 1034
NuvaRing 2897
Ortho-Cyclen/Ortho Tri-Cyclen 2449
Ortho Evra Transdermal System 2437
Ortho Tri-Cyclen Lo Tablets 2458
Seasonique Tablets 1046
Yaz Tablets 805

Ethiodized Oil (Iodide and drugs that contain pharmacologic amounts of iodide may cause hyperthyroidism in euthroid patients with Grave's disease previously treated with antithyroid drugs or in euthroid patients with thyroid autonomy. Hyperthyroidism may develop over several weeks and may persist for several months after therapy discontinuation. Thyroid hormones may also reduce the uptake of I-123 and I-131).

No products indexed under this heading.

Ethionamide (Ethionamide is associated with thyroid hormone and/or TSH level alterations).

No products indexed under this heading.

Ethotoin (Stimulation of hepatic microsomal drug-metabolizing activity may cause increased hepatic degradation of levothyroxine, resulting in increased levothyroxine requirements).

No products indexed under this heading.

Ethynodiol Diacetate (Estrogen-containing oral contraceptives may increase serum TBG concentration).

No products indexed under this heading.

Ferrous Sulfate (Ferrous sulfate likely forms a ferric-thyroxine complex. Concurrent use may reduce the efficacy of levothyroxine by binding and delaying or preventing the absorption, potentially resulting in hypothyroidism. Administer levothyroxine at least four hours apart from ferrous sulfate-containing products).

No products indexed under this heading.

Fludrocortisone Acetate (Glucocorticoids may result in a transient reduction in TSH secretion when administered at doses greater than 100mg/day of hydrocortisone or equivalent. Short-term administration of large doses of glucocorticoids may decrease serum T3 concentrations by 30% with minimal change in serum T4 levels. However, long-term glucocorticoid therapy may result in slightly decreased T3 and T4 levels due to decreased TBG production).

No products indexed under this heading.

Fluorouracil (Fluorouracil may increase serum TBG concentration). Products include:

Carac Cream 0.5% 2722

Fluoxymesterone (Androgens/anabolic steroids may decrease serum TBG concentration).
No products indexed under this heading.

Fosphenytoin Sodium (Stimulation of hepatic microsomal drug-metabolizing activity may cause increased hepatic degradation of levothyroxine, resulting in increased levothyroxine requirements).
No products indexed under this heading.

Furosemide (Co-administration of furosemide (greater than 80mg IV) with levothyroxine results in an initial transient increase in FT4. Continued administration results in a decrease in serum T4 and normal FT4 and TSH concentrations and, therefore, patients are clinically euthroid).
Products include:
Furosemide Tablets **2186**

Gadopentetate Dimeglumine (Iodide and drugs that contain pharmacologic amounts of iodide may cause hyperthyroidism in euthroid patients with Grave's disease previously treated with antithyroid drugs or in euthroid patients with thyroid autonomy. Hyperthyroidism may develop over several weeks and may persist for several months after therapy discontinuation. Thyroid hormones may also reduce the uptake of I-123 and I-131).
No products indexed under this heading.

Glimepiride (Addition of levothyroxine to antidiabetic therapy may result in increased antidiabetic agent requirements. Careful monitoring of diabetic control is recommended, especially when thyroid therapy is started, changed, or discontinued).
Products include:
Avandaryl Tablets **1344**
Duetact Tablets **3085**

Glipizide (Addition of levothyroxine to antidiabetic therapy may result in increased antidiabetic agent requirements. Careful monitoring of diabetic control is recommended, especially when thyroid therapy is started, changed, or discontinued).
No products indexed under this heading.

Glyburide (Addition of levothyroxine to antidiabetic therapy may result in increased antidiabetic agent requirements. Careful monitoring of diabetic control is recommended, especially when thyroid therapy is started, changed, or discontinued).
No products indexed under this heading.

Heparin Calcium (Co-administration of heparin with levothyroxine results in an initial transient increase in FT4. Continued administration results in a decrease in serum T4 and normal FT4 and TSH concentrations and, therefore, patients are clinically euthroid).
No products indexed under this heading.

Heparin Sodium (Co-administration of heparin with levothyroxine results in an initial transient increase in FT4. Continued administration results in a decrease in serum T4 and normal FT4 and TSH concentrations and, therefore, patients are clinically euthroid).
No products indexed under this heading.

Heroin (Heroin may increase serum TBG concentration).
No products indexed under this heading.

Hydrochlorothiazide (Thiazide diuretics are associated with thyroid hormone and/or TSH level alterations). Products include:
Atacand HCT **642**
Avalide Tablets **892**
Avalide Tablets **2713**
Benicar HCT Tablets **1010**
Diovan HCT Tablets **2216**
Dyazide Capsules **1405**
Micardis HCT Tablets **854**
Prinzide Tablets **2092**
Tekturna HCT Tablets **2324**
Teveten HCT Tablets **517**

Hydrocortisone (Glucocorticoids may result in a transient reduction in TSH secretion when administered at doses greater than 100mg/day of hydrocortisone or equivalent. Short-term administration of large doses of glucocorticoids may decrease serum T3 concentrations by 30% with minimal change in serum T4 levels. However, long-term glucocorticoid therapy may result in slightly decreased T3 and T4 levels due to decreased TBG production).
No products indexed under this heading.

Hydrocortisone Acetate (Glucocorticoids may result in a transient reduction in TSH secretion when administered at doses greater than 100mg/day of hydrocortisone or equivalent. Short-term administration of large doses of glucocorticoids may decrease serum T3 concentrations by 30% with minimal change in serum T4 levels. However, long-term glucocorticoid therapy may result in slightly decreased T3 and T4 levels due to decreased TBG production).
Products include:
Analpram-HC **1140**
Pramosone **1141**

Hydrocortisone Sodium Phosphate (Glucocorticoids may result in a transient reduction in TSH secretion when administered at doses greater than 100mg/day of hydrocortisone or equivalent. Short-term administration of large doses of glucocorticoids may decrease serum T3 concentrations by 30% with minimal change in serum T4 levels. However, long-term glucocorticoid therapy may result in slightly decreased T3 and T4 levels due to decreased TBG production).
No products indexed under this heading.

Hydrocortisone Sodium Succinate (Glucocorticoids may result in a transient reduction in TSH secretion when administered at doses greater than 100mg/day of hydrocortisone or equivalent. Short-term administration of large doses of glucocorticoids may decrease serum T3 concentrations by 30% with minimal change in serum T4 levels. However, long-term glucocorticoid therapy may result in slightly decreased T3 and T4 levels due to decreased TBG production).
No products indexed under this heading.

Hydroflumethiazide (Thiazide diuretics are associated with thyroid hormone and/or TSH level alterations).
No products indexed under this heading.

Imipramine Hydrochloride (Concurrent use of tricyclic antidepressants and levothyroxine may increase the therapeutic and toxic effects of both drugs, possibly due to increased receptor sensitivity to catecholamines. Onset of action of tricyclics may be accelerated).
No products indexed under this heading.

Imipramine Pamoate (Concurrent use of tricyclic antidepressants and levothyroxine may increase the therapeutic and toxic effects of both drugs, possibly due to increased receptor sensitivity to catecholamines. Onset of action of tricyclics may be accelerated).
No products indexed under this heading.

Insulin (Addition of levothyroxine to insulin therapy may result in increased insulin requirements. Careful monitoring of diabetic control is recommended, especially when thyroid therapy is started, changed, or discontinued).
No products indexed under this heading.

Insulin, Human, Zinc Suspension (Addition of levothyroxine to insulin therapy may result in increased insulin requirements. Careful monitoring of diabetic control is recommended, especially when thyroid therapy is started, changed, or discontinued).
No products indexed under this heading.

Insulin, Human (rDNA origin) (Addition of levothyroxine to insulin therapy may result in increased insulin requirements. Careful monitoring of diabetic control is recommended, especially when thyroid therapy is started, changed, or discontinued).
Products include:
Exubera Inhalation Powder **2515**

Insulin, Human NPH (Addition of levothyroxine to insulin therapy may result in increased insulin requirements. Careful monitoring of diabetic control is recommended, especially when thyroid therapy is started, changed, or discontinued). Products include:
Humulin N Vial **1846**

Insulin, Human Regular (Addition of levothyroxine to insulin therapy may result in increased insulin requirements. Careful monitoring of diabetic control is recommended, especially when thyroid therapy is started, changed, or discontinued).
Products include:
Humulin R **1849**
Humulin R (U-500) **1850**

Insulin, Human Regular and Human NPH Mixture (Addition of levothyroxine to insulin therapy may result in increased insulin requirements. Careful monitoring of diabetic control is recommended, especially when thyroid therapy is started, changed, or discontinued). Products include:
Humulin 50/50, 100 Units **1843**
Humulin 70/30 Vial **1844**

Insulin, NPH (Addition of levothyroxine to insulin therapy may result in increased insulin requirements. Careful monitoring of diabetic control is recommended, especially when thyroid therapy is started, changed, or discontinued).
No products indexed under this heading.

Insulin, Regular (Addition of levothyroxine to insulin therapy may result in increased insulin requirements. Careful monitoring of diabetic control is recommended, especially when thyroid therapy is started, changed, or discontinued).
No products indexed under this heading.

Insulin, Regular and NPH mixture (Addition of levothyroxine to insulin therapy may result in increased insulin requirements. Careful monitoring of diabetic control is recommended, especially when thyroid therapy is started, changed, or discontinued).
No products indexed under this heading.

Insulin, Zinc Crystals (Addition of levothyroxine to insulin therapy may result in increased insulin requirements. Careful monitoring of diabetic control is recommended, especially when thyroid therapy is started, changed, or discontinued).
No products indexed under this heading.

Insulin, Zinc Suspension (Addition of levothyroxine to insulin therapy may result in increased insulin requirements. Careful monitoring of diabetic control is recommended, especially when thyroid therapy is started, changed, or discontinued).
No products indexed under this heading.

Insulin Aspart (Addition of levothyroxine to insulin therapy may result in increased insulin requirements. Careful monitoring of diabetic control is recommended, especially when thyroid therapy is started, changed, or discontinued).
No products indexed under this heading.

Insulin Aspart, Human (Addition of levothyroxine to insulin therapy may result in increased insulin requirements. Careful monitoring of diabetic control is recommended, especially when thyroid therapy is started, changed, or discontinued). Products include:
NovoLog Mix 70/30 .... **2364**

Insulin Aspart, Human Regular (Addition of levothyroxine to insulin therapy may result in increased insulin requirements. Careful monitoring of diabetic control is recommended, especially when thyroid therapy is started, changed, or discontinued).
Products include:
NovoLog Injection **2359**

Insulin Aspart Protamine, Human (Addition of levothyroxine to insulin therapy may result in increased insulin requirements. Careful monitoring of diabetic control is recommended, especially when thyroid therapy is started, changed, or discontinued). Products include:
NovoLog Mix 70/30 .... **2364**

Insulin Detemir (rDNA Origin) (Addition of levothyroxine to insulin therapy may result in increased insulin requirements. Careful monitoring of diabetic control is recommended, especially when thyroid therapy is started, changed, or discontinued).
Products include:
Levemir Injection **2352**

Insulin glargine (Addition of levothyroxine to insulin therapy may result in increased insulin requirements. Careful monitoring of diabetic control is recommended, especially when thyroid therapy is started, changed, or discontinued). Products include:

Lantus Injection **2749**

Insulin Glulisine (Addition of levothyroxine to insulin therapy may result in increased insulin requirements. Careful monitoring of diabetic control is recommended, especially when thyroid therapy is started, changed, or discontinued). Products include:

Apidra Injection **2706**

Insulin Lispro, Human (Addition of levothyroxine to insulin therapy may result in increased insulin requirements. Careful monitoring of diabetic control is recommended, especially when thyroid therapy is started, changed, or discontinued). Products include:

Humalog-Pen and KwikPen **1829**
Humalog Mix 50/50-Pen and KwikPen **1833**
Humalog Mix 75/25-Pen and KwikPen **1835**

Insulin Lispro Protamine, Human (Addition of levothyroxine to insulin therapy may result in increased insulin requirements. Careful monitoring of diabetic control is recommended, especially when thyroid therapy is started, changed, or discontinued). Products include:

Humalog Mix 50/50-Pen and KwikPen **1833**
Humalog Mix 75/25-Pen and KwikPen **1835**

Interferon alfa-2a, Recombinant (Therapy with interferon-alpha has been associated with the development of antithyroid microsomal antibodies in 20% of patients and some have transient hypothyroidism, hyperthyroidism, or both).

No products indexed under this heading.

Interferon alfa-2b, Recombinant (Therapy with interferon-alpha has been associated with the development of antithyroid microsomal antibodies in 20% of patients and some have transient hypothyroidism, hyperthyroidism, or both). Products include:

Intron A for Injection **2859**

Iodamide Meglumine (Iodide and drugs that contain pharmacologic amounts of iodide may cause hyperthyroidism in euthroid patients with Grave's disease previously treated with antithyroid drugs or in euthroid patients with thyroid autonomy. Hyperthyroidism may develop over several weeks and may persist for several months after therapy discontinuation. Thyroid hormones may also reduce the uptake of I-123 and I-131).

No products indexed under this heading.

Iohexol (Iodide and drugs that contain pharmacologic amounts of iodide may cause hyperthyroidism in euthroid patients with Grave's disease previously treated with antithyroid drugs or in euthroid patients with thyroid autonomy. Hyperthyroidism may develop over several weeks and may persist for several months after therapy discontinuation. Thyroid hormones may also reduce the uptake of I-123 and I-131).

No products indexed under this heading.

Iopamidol (Iodide and drugs that contain pharmacologic amounts of iodide may cause hyperthyroidism in euthroid patients with Grave's disease previously treated with antithyroid drugs or in euthroid patients with thyroid autonomy. Hyperthyroidism may develop over several weeks and may persist for several months after therapy discontinuation. Thyroid hormones may also reduce the uptake of I-123 and I-131).

No products indexed under this heading.

Iopanoic Acid (Iodide and drugs that contain pharmacologic amounts of iodide may cause hyperthyroidism in euthroid patients with Grave's disease previously treated with antithyroid drugs or in euthroid patients with thyroid autonomy. Hyperthyroidism may develop over several weeks and may persist for several months after therapy discontinuation. Thyroid hormones may also reduce the uptake of I-123 and I-131).

No products indexed under this heading.

Iothalamate Meglumine (Iodide and drugs that contain pharmacologic amounts of iodide may cause hyperthyroidism in euthroid patients with Grave's disease previously treated with antithyroid drugs or in euthroid patients with thyroid autonomy. Hyperthyroidism may develop over several weeks and may persist for several months after therapy discontinuation. Thyroid hormones may also reduce the uptake of I-123 and I-131).

No products indexed under this heading.

Ioxaglate Meglumine (Iodide and drugs that contain pharmacologic amounts of iodide may cause hyperthyroidism in euthroid patients with Grave's disease previously treated with antithyroid drugs or in euthroid patients with thyroid autonomy. Hyperthyroidism may develop over several weeks and may persist for several months after therapy discontinuation. Thyroid hormones may also reduce the uptake of I-123 and I-131).

No products indexed under this heading.

Ioxaglate Sodium (Iodide and drugs that contain pharmacologic amounts of iodide may cause hyperthyroidism in euthroid patients with Grave's disease previously treated with antithyroid drugs or in euthroid patients with thyroid autonomy. Hyperthyroidism may develop over several weeks and may persist for several months after therapy discontinuation. Thyroid hormones may also reduce the uptake of I-123 and I-131).

No products indexed under this heading.

Isoproterenol Hydrochloride (Concurrent use may increase the effects of sympathomimetics or thyroid hormone. Thyroid hormones may increase the risk of coronary insufficiency when sympathomimetic agents are administered to patients with coronary artery disease).

No products indexed under this heading.

Isoproterenol Sulfate (Concurrent use may increase the effects of sympathomimetics or thyroid hormone. Thyroid hormones may increase the risk of coronary insufficiency when sympathomimetic agents are administered to patients with coronary artery disease).

No products indexed under this heading.

Ketamine (Concurrent use may produce marked hypertension and tachycardia; cautious administration to patients receiving thyroid therapy is recommended).

No products indexed under this heading.

Ketamine Hydrochloride (Concurrent use may produce marked hypertension and tachycardia; cautious administration to patients receiving thyroid therapy is recommended).

No products indexed under this heading.

Labetalol Hydrochloride (Actions of particular beta-adrenergic antagonists may be impaired when the hypothyroid patient is converted to the euthroid state).

No products indexed under this heading.

Levalbuterol Hydrochloride (Concurrent use may increase the effects of sympathomimetics or thyroid hormone. Thyroid hormones may increase the risk of coronary insufficiency when sympathomimetic agents are administered to patients with coronary artery disease). Products include:

Xopenex Inhalation Solution **3001**
Xopenex Inhalation Solution Concentrate **3005**

Levobunolol Hydrochloride (Actions of particular beta-adrenergic antagonists may be impaired when the hypothyroid patient is converted to the euthroid state).

No products indexed under this heading.

Levodopa (Dopamine and dopamine agonists may result in a transient reduction in TSH secretion when administered at dopamine doses greater than or equal to 1 mcg/kg/min). Products include:

Stalevo Tablets **2309**

Levonorgestrel (Estrogen-containing oral contraceptives may increase serum TBG concentration). Products include:

Climara Pro Transdermal System **768**
Lybrel Tablets **3204**
Mirena Intrauterine System **779**
Plan B Tablets **1044**
Seasonique Tablets **1046**

Lithium (Long-term lithium therapy can result in goiter in up to 50% of patients, and either subclinical or overt hypothyroidism, each in up to 20% of patients).

No products indexed under this heading.

Lithium Carbonate (Long-term lithium therapy can result in goiter in up to 50% of patients, and either subclinical or overt hypothyroidism, each in up to 20% of patients).

No products indexed under this heading.

Lithium Citrate (Long-term lithium therapy can result in goiter in up to 50% of patients, and either subclinical or overt hypothyroidism, each in up to 20% of patients).

No products indexed under this heading.

Lovastatin (Lovastatin is associated with thyroid hormone and/or TSH level alterations). Products include:

Advicor Tablets **402**
Mevacor Tablets **2063**

Magaldrate (Concurrent use with antacids may reduce the efficacy of levothyroxine by binding and delaying or preventing the absorption, potentially resulting in hypothyroidism. Administer levothyroxine at least four hours apart from these agents).

No products indexed under this heading.

Magnesium Hydroxide (Concurrent use with antacids may reduce the efficacy of levothyroxine by binding and delaying or preventing the absorption, potentially resulting in hypothyroidism. Administer levothyroxine at least four hours apart from these agents). Products include:

Fleet Pedia-Lax Chewable Tablets **1145**
Pepcid Complete Chewable Tablets **1771**
Extra Strength Rolaids Freshmint Tablets **1903**
Rolaids Multi-Symptom Berry Tablets **1903**
Rolaids Original Peppermint Tablets **1903**

Magnesium Oxide (Concurrent use with antacids may reduce the efficacy of levothyroxine by binding and delaying or preventing the absorption, potentially resulting in hypothyroidism. Administer levothyroxine at least four hours apart from these agents). Products include:

Beelith Tablets **813**

Magnesium Salicylate (Salicylates inhibit binding of T4 and T3 to TBG and transthyretin. An initial increase in FT4 is followed by return of FT4 to normal levels with sustained therapeutic serum salicylate concentrations, although total T4 levels may decrease by as much as 30%).

No products indexed under this heading.

Maprotiline Hydrochloride (Concurrent use of tetracyclic antidepressants and levothyroxine may increase the therapeutic and toxic effects of both drugs, possibly due to increased receptor sensitivity to catecholamines).

No products indexed under this heading.

Meclofenamate Sodium (Co-administration of fenamates with levothyroxine results in an initial transient increase in FT4. Continued administration results in a decrease in serum T4 and normal FT4 and TSH concentrations and, therefore, patients are clinically euthroid).

No products indexed under this heading.

Mephenytoin (Stimulation of hepatic microsomal drug-metabolizing activity may cause increased hepatic degradation of levothyroxine, resulting in increased levothyroxine requirements).

No products indexed under this heading.

Mercaptopurine (Mercaptopurine is associated with thyroid hormone and/or TSH level alterations).

No products indexed under this heading.

Mestranol (Estrogen-containing oral contraceptives may increase serum TBG concentration).

No products indexed under this heading.

IMPORTANT NOTE: Always consult each drug listing in the patient's regimen for possible interactions.

Metaproterenol Sulfate (Concurrent use may increase the effects of sympathomimetics or thyroid hormone. Thyroid hormones may increase the risk of coronary insufficiency when sympathomimetic agents are administered to patients with coronary artery disease).
No products indexed under this heading.

Metaraminol Bitartrate (Concurrent use may increase the effects of sympathomimetics or thyroid hormone. Thyroid hormones may increase the risk of coronary insufficiency when sympathomimetic agents are administered to patients with coronary artery disease).
No products indexed under this heading.

Metformin Hydrochloride (Addition of levothyroxine to antidiabetic therapy may result in increased antidiabetic agent requirements. Careful monitoring of diabetic control is recommended, especially when thyroid therapy is started, changed, or discontinued). Products include:
ActoPlus Met Tablets 3071
Avandamet Tablets 1336
Janumet Tablets 2041
PrandiMet Tablets 2967

Methadone Hydrochloride (Methadone may increase serum TBG concentration).
No products indexed under this heading.

Methoxamine Hydrochloride (Concurrent use may increase the effects of sympathomimetics or thyroid hormone. Thyroid hormones may increase the risk of coronary insufficiency when sympathomimetic agents are administered to patients with coronary artery disease).
No products indexed under this heading.

Methyclothiazide (Thiazide diuretics are associated with thyroid hormone and/or TSH level alterations).
No products indexed under this heading.

Methylprednisolone Acetate (Glucocorticoids may result in a transient reduction in TSH secretion when administered at doses greater than 100mg/day of hydrocortisone or equivalent. Short-term administration of large doses of glucocorticoids may decrease serum T3 concentrations by 30% with minimal change in serum T4 levels. However, long-term glucocorticoid therapy may result in slightly decreased T3 and T4 levels due to decreased TBG production).
No products indexed under this heading.

Methylprednisolone Sodium Succinate (Glucocorticoids may result in a transient reduction in TSH secretion when administered at doses greater than 100mg/day of hydrocortisone or equivalent. Short-term administration of large doses of glucocorticoids may decrease serum T3 concentrations by 30% with minimal change in serum T4 levels. However, long-term glucocorticoid therapy may result in slightly decreased T3 and T4 levels due to decreased TBG production).
No products indexed under this heading.

Methyltestosterone (Androgens/anabolic steroids may decrease serum TBG concentration). Products include:
Estratest Tablets 3043
Estratest H.S. Tablets 3043

Metipranolol Hydrochloride (Actions of particular beta-adrenergic antagonists may be impaired when the hypothyroid patient is converted to the euthroid state).
No products indexed under this heading.

Metoclopramide Hydrochloride (Metoclopramide is associated with thyroid hormone and/or TSH level alterations).
No products indexed under this heading.

Metoprolol Succinate (Actions of particular beta-adrenergic antagonists may be impaired when the hypothyroid patient is converted to the euthroid state). Products include:
Toprol-XL Tablets 666

Metoprolol Tartrate (Actions of particular beta-adrenergic antagonists may be impaired when the hypothyroid patient is converted to the euthroid state).
No products indexed under this heading.

Miglitol (Addition of levothyroxine to antidiabetic therapy may result in increased antidiabetic agent requirements. Careful monitoring of diabetic control is recommended, especially when thyroid therapy is started, changed, or discontinued).
No products indexed under this heading.

Mirtazapine (Concurrent use of tetracyclic antidepressants and levothyroxine may increase the therapeutic and toxic effects of both drugs, possibly due to increased receptor sensitivity to catecholamines). Products include:
Remeron Tablets 2924
RemeronSolTab Tablets 2927

Mitotane (Mitotane may increase serum TBG concentration).
No products indexed under this heading.

Nadolol (Actions of particular beta-adrenergic antagonists may be impaired when the hypothyroid patient is converted to the euthroid state). Products include:
Nadolol Tablets 2191

Nateglinide (Addition of levothyroxine to antidiabetic therapy may result in increased antidiabetic agent requirements. Careful monitoring of diabetic control is recommended, especially when thyroid therapy is started, changed, or discontinued). Products include:
Starlix Tablets 2314

Nebivolol (Actions of particular beta-adrenergic antagonists may be impaired when the hypothyroid patient is converted to the euthroid state). Products include:
Bystolic Tablets 1155

Nicotinic Acid (Slow-release nicotinic acid may decrease TBG concentration).
No products indexed under this heading.

Norepinephrine Bitartrate (Concurrent use may increase the effects of sympathomimetics or thyroid hormone. Thyroid hormones may increase the risk of coronary insufficiency when sympathomimetic agents are administered to patients with coronary artery disease).
No products indexed under this heading.

Norethindrone (Estrogen-containing oral contraceptives may increase serum TBG concentration). Products include:
Ortho Micronor Tablets 2446

Norethynodrel (Estrogen-containing oral contraceptives may increase serum TBG concentration).
No products indexed under this heading.

Norgestimate (Estrogen-containing oral contraceptives may increase serum TBG concentration). Products include:
Ortho-Cyclen/Ortho Tri-Cyclen 2449
Ortho Tri-Cyclen Lo Tablets 2458

Norgestrel (Estrogen-containing oral contraceptives may increase serum TBG concentration).
No products indexed under this heading.

Nortriptyline Hydrochloride (Concurrent use of tricyclic antidepressants and levothyroxine may increase the therapeutic and toxic effects of both drugs, possibly due to increased receptor sensitivity to catecholamines. Onset of action of tricyclics may be accelerated).
No products indexed under this heading.

Octreotide Acetate (Octreotide may result in a transient reduction in TSH secretion when administered at doses greater than 100 mcg/day). Products include:
Sandostatin Injection 2300
Sandostatin LAR Depot 2302

Oxandrolone (Androgens/anabolic steroids may decrease serum TBG concentration).
No products indexed under this heading.

Oxymetholone (Androgens/anabolic steroids may decrease serum TBG concentration).
No products indexed under this heading.

Para-Aminosalicylate Sodium (Para-aminosalicylate sodium is associated with thyroid hormone and/or TSH level alterations).
No products indexed under this heading.

Penbutolol Sulfate (Actions of particular beta-adrenergic antagonists may be impaired when the hypothyroid patient is converted to the euthroid state).
No products indexed under this heading.

Pergolide Mesylate (Dopamine and dopamine agonists may result in a transient reduction in TSH secretion when administered at dopamine doses greater than or equal to 1 mcg/kg/min).
No products indexed under this heading.

Perphenazine (Perphenazine is associated with thyroid hormone and/or TSH level alterations).
No products indexed under this heading.

Phenobarbital (Stimulation of hepatic microsomal drug-metabolizing activity may cause increased hepatic degradation of levothyroxine, resulting in increased levothyroxine requirements). Products include:
Donnatal Extentabs 2507

Phenobarbital Sodium (Stimulation of hepatic microsomal drug-metabolizing activity may cause increased hepatic degradation of levothyroxine, resulting in increased levothyroxine requirements).
No products indexed under this heading.

Phenylbutazone (Co-administration of phenylbutazone with levothyroxine results in an initial transient increase in FT4. Continued administration results in a decrease in serum T4 and normal FT4 and TSH concentrations and, therefore, patients are clinically euthroid).
No products indexed under this heading.

Phenylephrine Bitartrate (Concurrent use may increase the effects of sympathomimetics or thyroid hormone. Thyroid hormones may increase the risk of coronary insufficiency when sympathomimetic agents are administered to patients with coronary artery disease).
No products indexed under this heading.

Phenylephrine Hydrochloride (Concurrent use may increase the effects of sympathomimetics or thyroid hormone. Thyroid hormones may increase the risk of coronary insufficiency when sympathomimetic agents are administered to patients with coronary artery disease). Products include:
Actifed Cold & Allergy Tablets 1895
Benadryl Allergy & Cold Kapgels 1895
Benadryl Allergy & Sinus Headache Kapgels 1895
Benadryl Severe Allergy & Sinus Headache Caplets 1897
Children's Benadryl-D Allergy & Sinus Liquid 1896
Benadryl-D Allergy & Sinus Tablet 1896
PediaCare Children's Allergy & Cold Liquid 1902
PediaCare Children's Decongestant Liquid 1902
PediaCare Children's Liquid Multi-Symptom Cold 1902
Sinutab Non-Drying Caplets 1905
Sinutab Sinus Caplets 1905
Children's Sudafed PE Cold & Cough Liquid 1907
Children's Sudafed PE Nasal Decongestant Liquid 1906
Sudafed PE Cold & Cough Caplets 1907
Sudafed PE Nasal Decongestant Tablets 1907
Sudafed PE Nighttime Cold Caplets 1907
Sudafed PE Non-Drying Sinus Caplets 1908
Sudafed PE Severe Cold Caplets 1908
Sudafed PE Sinus & Allergy Tablets 1908
Sudafed PE Sinus Headache Caplets 1908
Tylenol Allergy Multi-Symptom Caplets with Cool Burst and Rapid Release Gelcaps 1916
Tylenol Allergy Multi-Symptom Nighttime Caplets with Cool Burst 1916
Children's Tylenol Plus Cold Suspension Liquid 1912
Children's Tylenol Plus Cold & Allergy Suspension Liquid 1914
Children's Tylenol Plus Flu Suspension Liquid 1914
Children's Tylenol Plus Multi-Symptom Cold Suspension Liquid 1912
Tylenol Cold Head Congestion Daytime Caplets with Cool Burst 1910
Tylenol Cold Head Congestion Nighttime Caplets with Cool Burst 1910

Tylenol Cold Head Congestion Severe Daytime Caplets with Cool Burst 1910
Tylenol Cold Multi-Symptom Daytime Caplets with Cool Burst and Rapid Release Gels 1913
Tylenol Cold Multi-Symptom Daytime Liquid with Citrus Burst 1913
Tylenol Cold Multi-Symptom Nighttime Caplets with Cool Burst 1913
Tylenol Cold Multi-Symptom Nighttime Liquid with Cool Burst 1913
Tylenol Cold Multi-Symptom Severe Caplets with Cool Burst 1913
Tylenol Cold Multi-Symptom Severe Daytime Liquid with Citrus Burst 1913
Tylenol Sinus Congestion & Pain Daytime Caplets with Cool Burst and Gelcaps 1917
Tylenol Sinus Congestion & Pain Nighttime Caplets with Cool Burst 1917
Tylenol Sinus Congestion & Pain Severe Caplets with Cool Burst 1917
Vicks DayQuil Cold & Flu Multi-Symptom Relief 616
Vicks DayQuil LiquiCaps 2567
Vicks DayQuil Liquid 2567
Vicks DayQuil Multi-Symptom Cold/Flu Relief 2567

Phenylephrine Tannate (Concurrent use may increase the effects of sympathomimetics or thyroid hormone. Thyroid hormones may increase the risk of coronary insufficiency when sympathomimetic agents are administered to patients with coronary artery disease).
No products indexed under this heading.

Phenylpropanolamine Hydrochloride (Concurrent use may increase the effects of sympathomimetics or thyroid hormone. Thyroid hormones may increase the risk of coronary insufficiency when sympathomimetic agents are administered to patients with coronary artery disease).
No products indexed under this heading.

Phenytoin (Stimulation of hepatic microsomal drug-metabolizing activity may cause increased hepatic degradation of levothyroxine, resulting in increased levothyroxine requirements).
No products indexed under this heading.

Phenytoin Sodium (Stimulation of hepatic microsomal drug-metabolizing activity may cause increased hepatic degradation of levothyroxine, resulting in increased levothyroxine requirements).
Products include:
Phenytek Capsules 2192

Pindolol (Actions of particular beta-adrenergic antagonists may be impaired when the hypothyroid patient is converted to the euthroid state).
No products indexed under this heading.

Pioglitazone Hydrochloride (Addition of levothyroxine to antidiabetic therapy may result in increased antidiabetic agent requirements. Careful monitoring of diabetic control is recommended, especially when thyroid therapy is started, changed, or discontinued). Products include:
ActoPlus Met Tablets 3071
Actos Tablets 3077
Duetact Tablets 3085

Pirbuterol Acetate (Concurrent use may increase the effects of sympathomimetics or thyroid hormone. Thyroid hormones may increase the risk of coronary insufficiency when sympathomimetic agents are administered to patients with coronary artery disease). Products include:
Maxair Autohaler 1705

Polyestradiol Phosphate (Estrogen may increase serum TBG concentration).
No products indexed under this heading.

Polythiazide (Thiazide diuretics are associated with thyroid hormone and/or TSH level alterations).
No products indexed under this heading.

Pramipexole Dihydrochloride (Dopamine and dopamine agonists may result in a transient reduction in TSH secretion when administered at dopamine doses greater than or equal to 1 mcg/kg/min). Products include:
Mirapex Tablets 857

Prednisolone Acetate (Glucocorticoids may result in a transient reduction in TSH secretion when administered at doses greater than 100mg/day of hydrocortisone or equivalent. Short-term administration of large doses of glucocorticoids may decrease serum T3 concentrations by 30% with minimal change in serum T4 levels. However, long-term glucocorticoid therapy may result in slightly decreased T3 and T4 levels due to decreased TBG production). Products include:
Pred Forte Ophthalmic Suspension .... ⊙ 227
Pred Mild Ophthalmic Suspension .... ⊙ 230
Pred-G Ophthalmic Ointment .... ⊙ 229
Pred-G Ophthalmic Suspension .... ⊙ 228

Prednisolone Sodium Phosphate (Glucocorticoids may result in a transient reduction in TSH secretion when administered at doses greater than 100mg/day of hydrocortisone or equivalent. Short-term administration of large doses of glucocorticoids may decrease serum T3 concentrations by 30% with minimal change in serum T4 levels. However, long-term glucocorticoid therapy may result in slightly decreased T3 and T4 levels due to decreased TBG production).
No products indexed under this heading.

Prednisolone Tebutate (Glucocorticoids may result in a transient reduction in TSH secretion when administered at doses greater than 100mg/day of hydrocortisone or equivalent. Short-term administration of large doses of glucocorticoids may decrease serum T3 concentrations by 30% with minimal change in serum T4 levels. However, long-term glucocorticoid therapy may result in slightly decreased T3 and T4 levels due to decreased TBG production).
No products indexed under this heading.

Prednisone (Glucocorticoids may result in a transient reduction in TSH secretion when administered at doses greater than 100mg/day of hydrocortisone or equivalent. Short-term administration of large doses of glucocorticoids may decrease serum T3 concentrations by 30% with minimal change in serum T4 levels. However, long-term glucocorticoid therapy may result in slightly decreased T3 and T4 levels due to decreased TBG production).
No products indexed under this heading.

Propranolol Hydrochloride (In patients treated with large doses of propranolol (greater than 160mg/day), T3 and T4 levels change slightly, TSH levels remain normal, and patients are clinically euthroid). Products include:
InnoPran XL Extended Release Capsules 1484

Protriptyline Hydrochloride (Concurrent use of tricyclic antidepressants and levothyroxine may increase the therapeutic and toxic effects of both drugs, possibly due to increased receptor sensitivity to catecholamines. Onset of action of tricyclics may be accelerated).
No products indexed under this heading.

Pseudoephedrine Hydrochloride (Concurrent use may increase the effects of sympathomimetics or thyroid hormone. Thyroid hormones may increase the risk of coronary insufficiency when sympathomimetic agents are administered to patients with coronary artery disease).
Products include:
Allegra-D 12 Hour Extended-Release Tablets 2687
Allegra-D 24 Hour Extended-Release Tablets 2690
Children's Motrin Cold Oral Suspension 1899
Sudafed 12 Hour Nasal Decongestant Non-Drowsy Caplets 1909
Sudafed 24 Hour Non-Drowsy Nasal Decongestant Tablets 1906
Children's Sudafed Nasal Decongestant Liquid 1906
Sudafed Nasal Decongestant Tablets 1906
Tylenol Cold Severe Congestion Daytime Caplets with Cool Burst 1912
Tylenol Sinus Severe Congestion Caplets with Cool Burst 1917
Vicks NyQuil LiquiCaps 2567
Vicks NyQuil Liquid 2567
Vicks NyQuil Multi-Symptom Cold/Flu Relief 2567
Zyrtec-D 12 Hour Extended Release Tablets 1923
Zyrtec-D Allergy & Congestion Extended-Release Tablets 1923

Pseudoephedrine Sulfate (Concurrent use may increase the effects of sympathomimetics or thyroid hormone. Thyroid hormones may increase the risk of coronary insufficiency when sympathomimetic agents are administered to patients with coronary artery disease).
Products include:
Clarinex-D 12-Hour Extended-Release Tablets 2831
Clarinex-D 24-Hour Extended-Release Tablets 2834

Quinestrol (Estrogen may increase serum TBG concentration).
No products indexed under this heading.

Repaglinide (Addition of levothyroxine to antidiabetic therapy may result in increased antidiabetic agent requirements. Careful monitoring of diabetic control is recommended, especially when thyroid therapy is started, changed, or discontinued).
Products include:
PrandiMet Tablets 2967
Prandin Tablets 2971

Resorcinol (Excessive topical use of resorcinol has been associated with thyroid hormone and/or TSH level alterations).
No products indexed under this heading.

Rifampin (Stimulation of hepatic microsomal drug-metabolizing activity may cause increased hepatic degradation of levothyroxine, resulting in increased levothyroxine requirements).
No products indexed under this heading.

Ropinirole Hydrochloride (Dopamine and dopamine agonists may result in a transient reduction in TSH secretion when administered at dopamine doses greater than or equal to 1 mcg/kg/min). Products include:
Requip Tablets 1561
Requip XL Tablets 1568

Rosiglitazone Maleate (Addition of levothyroxine to antidiabetic therapy may result in increased antidiabetic agent requirements. Careful monitoring of diabetic control is recommended, especially when thyroid therapy is started, changed, or discontinued). Products include:
Avandamet Tablets 1336
Avandaryl Tablets 1344
Avandia Tablets 1351

Salmeterol Xinafoate (Concurrent use may increase the effects of sympathomimetics or thyroid hormone. Thyroid hormones may increase the risk of coronary insufficiency when sympathomimetic agents are administered to patients with coronary artery disease). Products include:
Advair Diskus 100/50 1276
Advair Diskus 250/50 1276
Advair Diskus 500/50 1276
Advair HFA 45/21 Inhalation Aerosol 1288
Advair HFA 115/21 Inhalation Aerosol 1288
Advair HFA 230/21 Inhalation Aerosol 1288
Serevent Diskus 1594

Salsalate (Salicylates inhibit binding of T4 and T3 to TBG and transthyretin. An initial increase in FT4 is followed by return of FT4 to normal levels with sustained therapeutic serum salicylate concentrations, although total T4 levels may decrease by as much as 30%).
No products indexed under this heading.

Sertraline Hydrochloride (Administration of sertraline in patients stabilized on levothyroxine may result in increased levothyroxine requirements).
No products indexed under this heading.

Simethicone (Concurrent use with simethicone may reduce the efficacy of levothyroxine by binding and delaying or preventing the absorption, potentially resulting in hypothyroidism. Administer levothyroxine at least 4 hours apart from simethicone). Products include:
Imodium Multi-Symptom Relief Caplets and Chewable Tablets 1899
Extra Strength Rolaids Plus Gas Relief Tropical Fruit Softchews 1903
Rolaids Multi-Symptom Berry Tablets 1903

Sitagliptin Phosphate (Addition of levothyroxine to antidiabetic therapy may result in increased antidiabetic agent requirements. Careful monitoring of diabetic control is recommended, especially when thyroid therapy is started, changed, or discontinued). Products include:

Janumet Tablets 2041
Januvia Tablets 2048

Sodium Bicarbonate (Concurrent use with antacids may reduce the efficacy of levothyroxine by binding and delaying or preventing the absorption, potentially resulting in hypothyroidism. Administer levothyroxine at least four hours apart from these agents). Products include:

Ceo-Two Laxative Suppository 815

Sodium Nitroprusside (Nitroprusside is associated with thyroid hormone and/or TSH level alterations).

No products indexed under this heading.

Sodium Polystyrene Sulfonate (Concurrent use with sodium polystyrene sulfonate may reduce the efficacy of levothyroxine by binding and delaying or preventing the absorption, potentially resulting in hypothyroidism. Administer levothyroxine at least 4 hours apart from sodium polystyrene sodium).

No products indexed under this heading.

Somatrem (Excessive use of thyroid hormones with growth hormones may accelerate epiphyseal closure. However, untreated hypothyroidism may interfere with growth response to growth hormone).

No products indexed under this heading.

Somatropin (Excessive use of thyroid hormones with growth hormones may accelerate epiphyseal closure. However, untreated hypothyroidism may interfere with growth response to growth hormone).

Products include:

Genotropin Lyophilized Powder 2547
Humatrope Vials and Cartridges 1838
Nutropin for Injection 1208
Nutropin AQ Injection 1212
Nutropin AQ NuSpin Injection 1212
Nutropin AQ Pen 1212
Nutropin AQ Pen Cartridge 1212

Sotalol Hydrochloride (Actions of particular beta-adrenergic antagonists may be impaired when the hypothyroid patient is converted to the euthroid state).

No products indexed under this heading.

Stanozolol (Androgens/anabolic steroids may decrease serum TBG concentration).

No products indexed under this heading.

Sucralfate (Concurrent use with sucralfate may reduce the efficacy of levothyroxine by binding and delaying or preventing the absorption, potentially resulting in hypothyroidism. Administer levothyroxine at least four hours apart from sucralfate). Products include:

Carafate Suspension 706
Carafate Tablets 707

Tamoxifen Citrate (Tamoxifen may increase serum TBG concentration).

No products indexed under this heading.

Terbutaline Sulfate (Concurrent use may increase the effects of sympathomimetics or thyroid hormone. Thyroid hormones may increase the risk of coronary insufficiency when sympathomimetic agents are administered to patients with coronary artery disease).

No products indexed under this heading.

Theophylline (Decreased theophylline clearance may occur in hypothyroid patients; clearance returns to normal when the euthroid state is achieved).

No products indexed under this heading.

Theophylline Anhydrous (Decreased theophylline clearance may occur in hypothyroid patients; clearance returns to normal when the euthroid state is achieved). Products include:

Uniphyl Tablets 2595

Theophylline Calcium Salicylate (Decreased theophylline clearance may occur in hypothyroid patients; clearance returns to normal when the euthroid state is achieved).

No products indexed under this heading.

Theophylline Dihydroxypropyl (Glyceryl) (Decreased theophylline clearance may occur in hypothyroid patients; clearance returns to normal when the euthroid state is achieved).

No products indexed under this heading.

Theophylline Ethylenediamine (Decreased theophylline clearance may occur in hypothyroid patients; clearance returns to normal when the euthroid state is achieved).

No products indexed under this heading.

Theophylline Sodium Glycinate (Decreased theophylline clearance may occur in hypothyroid patients; clearance returns to normal when the euthroid state is achieved).

No products indexed under this heading.

Timolol Hemihydrate (Actions of particular beta-adrenergic antagonists may be impaired when the hypothyroid patient is converted to the euthroid state). Products include:

Betimol Ophthalmic Solution 3181

Timolol Maleate (Actions of particular beta-adrenergic antagonists may be impaired when the hypothyroid patient is converted to the euthroid state). Products include:

Combigan Ophthalmic Solution 553
Cosopt Sterile Ophthalmic Solution 1969
Timoptic Sterile Ophthalmic Solution 2121
Timoptic in Ocudose 2124
Timoptic-XE Sterile Ophthalmic Gel Forming Solution 2125

Tolazamide (Addition of levothyroxine to antidiabetic therapy may result in increased antidiabetic agent requirements. Careful monitoring of diabetic control is recommended, especially when thyroid therapy is started, changed, or discontinued).

No products indexed under this heading.

Tolbutamide (Addition of levothyroxine to antidiabetic therapy may result in increased antidiabetic agent requirements. Careful monitoring of diabetic control is recommended, especially when thyroid therapy is started, changed, or discontinued).

No products indexed under this heading.

Triamcinolone (Glucocorticoids may result in a transient reduction in TSH secretion when administered at doses greater than 100mg/day of hydrocortisone or equivalent. Short-term administration of large doses of glucocorticoids may decrease serum T3 concentrations by 30% with minimal change in serum T4 levels. However, long-term glucocorticoid therapy may result in slightly decreased T3 and T4 levels due to decreased TBG production).

No products indexed under this heading.

Triamcinolone Acetonide (Glucocorticoids may result in a transient reduction in TSH secretion when administered at doses greater than 100mg/day of hydrocortisone or equivalent. Short-term administration of large doses of glucocorticoids may decrease serum T3 concentrations by 30% with minimal change in serum T4 levels. However, long-term glucocorticoid therapy may result in slightly decreased T3 and T4 levels due to decreased TBG production). Products include:

Azmacort Inhalation Aerosol 407
Nasacort AQ Nasal Spray 2765
Triesence Injectable Suspension .... ⊙209

Triamcinolone Diacetate (Glucocorticoids may result in a transient reduction in TSH secretion when administered at doses greater than 100mg/day of hydrocortisone or equivalent. Short-term administration of large doses of glucocorticoids may decrease serum T3 concentrations by 30% with minimal change in serum T4 levels. However, long-term glucocorticoid therapy may result in slightly decreased T3 and T4 levels due to decreased TBG production).

No products indexed under this heading.

Triamcinolone Hexacetonide (Glucocorticoids may result in a transient reduction in TSH secretion when administered at doses greater than 100mg/day of hydrocortisone or equivalent. Short-term administration of large doses of glucocorticoids may decrease serum T3 concentrations by 30% with minimal change in serum T4 levels. However, long-term glucocorticoid therapy may result in slightly decreased T3 and T4 levels due to decreased TBG production).

No products indexed under this heading.

Trimipramine Maleate (Concurrent use of tricyclic antidepressants and levothyroxine may increase the therapeutic and toxic effects of both drugs, possibly due to increased receptor sensitivity to catecholamines. Onset of action of tricyclics may be accelerated).

No products indexed under this heading.

Troglitazone (Addition of levothyroxine to antidiabetic therapy may result in increased antidiabetic agent requirements. Careful monitoring of diabetic control is recommended, especially when thyroid therapy is started, changed, or discontinued).

No products indexed under this heading.

Tyropanoate Sodium (Iodide and drugs that contain pharmacologic amounts of iodide may cause hyperthyroidism in euthroid patients with Grave's disease previously treated with antithyroid drugs or in euthroid patients with thyroid autonomy. Hyperthyroidism may develop over several weeks and may persist for several months after therapy discontinuation. Thyroid hormones may also reduce the uptake of I-123 and I-131).

No products indexed under this heading.

Warfarin Sodium (Thyroid hormones appear to increase the catabolism of vitamin-K dependent clotting factors, thereby increasing the anticoagulant activity of oral anticoagulants. Concomitant use of these agents impairs the compensatory increases in clotting factor synthesis. Prothrombin time should be carefully monitored in patients taking levothyroxine and oral anticoagulants and the dose of anticoagulant therapy adjusted accordingly).

No products indexed under this heading.

LEVOXYL TABLETS

(Levothyroxine Sodium) 1780

May interact with androgens, antacids containing aluminum, calcium and magnesium, beta blockers, oral anticoagulants, dopamine agonists, estrogens, glucocorticoids, cardiac glycosides, hydantoin anticonvulsants, oral hypoglycemic agents, insulin, lithium preparations, phenytoin, radiographic iodinated contrast media, salicylates, sympathomimetics, thiazides, tricyclic antidepressants, and xanthines. Compounds in these categories include:

Acarbose (Addition of levothyroxine to antidiabetic therapy may result in increased antidiabetic agent requirements). Products include:

Precose Tablets 792

Acebutolol Hydrochloride (Co-administration with beta-blockers may decrease T_4 5'-deiodinase activity; action of beta-blocker may be impaired when the hypothyroid patient is converted to euthyroid).

No products indexed under this heading.

Albuterol (Co-administration of sympathomimetic agents may increase the effects of sympathomimetics or thyroid hormone; thyroid hormones may increase risk of coronary insufficiency when sympathomimetic agents are administered to patients with coronary disease).

No products indexed under this heading.

Albuterol Sulfate (Co-administration of sympathomimetic agents may increase the effects of sympathomimetics or thyroid hormone; thyroid hormones may increase risk of coronary insufficiency when sympathomimetic agents are administered to patients with coronary disease). Products include:

Combivent Inhalation Aerosol 845
ProAir HFA Inhalation Aerosol 3113
Proventil HFA Inhalation Aerosol 2914
Ventolin HFA Inhalation Aerosol 1638

Aldesleukin (Co-administration has been associated with transient painless thyroiditis in 20% of patients). Products include:
Proleukin for Injection 2287

Aluminum Carbonate (Co-administration with antacids may reduce the efficacy of levothyroxine by binding and delaying or preventing absorption, potentially resulting in hypothyroidism; administer levothyroxine at least 4 hours apart from these agents).
No products indexed under this heading.

Aluminum Hydroxide (Co-administration with antacids may reduce the efficacy of levothyroxine by binding and delaying or preventing absorption, potentially resulting in hypothyroidism; administer levothyroxine at least 4 hours apart from these agents).
No products indexed under this heading.

Aminoglutethimide (May decrease thyroid hormone secretion, which may result in hypothyrodism).
No products indexed under this heading.

Aminophylline (Decreased theophylline clearance may occur in hypothyroid patients; clearance returns to normal when euthyroid state is achieved).
No products indexed under this heading.

p-Aminosalicylic Acid (Co-administration has been associated with thyroid hormone and/or TSH level alterations by various mechanisms).
No products indexed under this heading.

Amiodarone Hydrochloride (May decrease thyroid hormone secretion, which may result in hypothyrodism; amiodarone is slowly excreted, producing more prolonged hypothyroidism; amiodarone may induce hyperthyroidism by causing thyroiditis).
No products indexed under this heading.

Amitriptyline Hydrochloride (Co-administration may increase the therapeutic and toxic effects of both drugs possibly due to increased receptor sensitivity to catecholamines; toxic effects may include increased risk of arrhythmias and CNS stimulation; onset of tricyclics may be accelerated).
No products indexed under this heading.

Amoxapine (Co-administration may increase the therapeutic and toxic effects of both drugs possibly due to increased receptor sensitivity to catecholamines; toxic effects may include increased risk of arrhythmias and CNS stimulation; onset of tricyclics may be accelerated).
No products indexed under this heading.

Anisindione (Thyroid hormones appear to increase the catabolism of vitamin K-dependent clotting factors, thereby increasing the anticoagulant activity of oral anticoagulants).
No products indexed under this heading.

Asparaginase (Co-administration may result in decreased serum TBG concentration). Products include:
Elspar for Injection 1990
Elspar for Injection 2488

Aspirin (Co-administration with salicylates at greater than 2 gm inhibit binding of T_4 and T_3 to TBG and transthyrelin; an initial increase in serum FT_4 is followed by return of FT_4 to normal levels with sustained therapeutic salicylate concentrations, although total T_4 levels may decrease by as much as 30%). Products include:
Aggrenox Capsules 819
Bayer Aspirin 750
Percodan Tablets 1130
St. Joseph 81 mg Aspirin Chewable and Enteric Coated Tablets 1903

Aspirin, Enteric Coated (Co-administration with salicylates at greater than 2 gm inhibit binding of T_4 and T_3 to TBG and transthyrelin; an initial increase in serum FT_4 is followed by return of FT_4 to normal levels with sustained therapeutic salicylate concentrations, although total T_4 levels may decrease by as much as 30%).
No products indexed under this heading.

Aspirin Buffered (Co-administration with salicylates at greater than 2 gm inhibit binding of T_4 and T_3 to TBG and transthyrelin; an initial increase in serum FT_4 is followed by return of FT_4 to normal levels with sustained therapeutic salicylate concentrations, although total T_4 levels may decrease by as much as 30%).
No products indexed under this heading.

Atenolol (Co-administration with beta-blockers may decrease T_4 5'-deiodinase activity; action of beta-blocker may be impaired when the hypothyroid patient is converted to euthyroid).
No products indexed under this heading.

Bendroflumethiazide (Co-administration has been associated with thyroid hormone and/or TSH level alterations by various mechanisms).
No products indexed under this heading.

Betamethasone Acetate (Co-administration with glucocorticoids may result in a transient reduction in TSH secretion; the reduction is not sustained, therefore, hypothyroidism does not occur; glucocorticoids may decrease serum TBG concentration).
No products indexed under this heading.

Betamethasone Sodium Phosphate (Co-administration with glucocorticoids may result in a transient reduction in TSH secretion; the reduction is not sustained, therefore, hypothyroidism does not occur; glucocorticoids may decrease serum TBG concentration).
No products indexed under this heading.

Betaxolol Hydrochloride (Co-administration with beta-blockers may decrease T_4 5'-deiodinase activity; action of beta-blocker may be impaired when the hypothyroid patient is converted to euthyroid).
No products indexed under this heading.

Bisoprolol Fumarate (Co-administration with beta-blockers may decrease T_4 5'-deiodinase activity; action of beta-blocker may be impaired when the hypothyroid patient is converted to euthyroid).
No products indexed under this heading.

Bromocriptine Mesylate (Co-administration with dopamine agonists may result in a transient reduction in TSH secretion; the reduction is not sustained, therefore, hypothyroidism does not occur).
No products indexed under this heading.

Calcium Carbonate (Co-administration with calcium carbonate may form insoluble chelate with levothyroxine, which may result in hypothyroidism; administer levothyroxine at least 4 hours apart from these agents). Products include:
Accelerator Tablets 634
Actonel with Calcium Tablets 2574
BioLean II Tablets 635
Calcet Triple Calcium + Vitamin D Tablets 629
D-Cal Chewable Caplets 624
Elixir Capsules 636
Pepcid Complete Chewable Tablets 1771
Extra Strength Rolaids Plus Gas Relief Tropical Fruit Softchews...... 1903
Extra Strength Rolaids Softchews Vanilla Creme 1903
Extra Strength Rolaids Freshmint Tablets 1903
Rolaids Multi-Symptom Berry Tablets 1903
Rolaids Original Peppermint Tablets 1903

Carbamazepine (Co-administration may increase hepatic metabolism, which may result in hypothyroidism, resulting in increased levothyroxine requirements; carbamazepine reduces serum protein binding of levothyroxine, and total- and free-T_4 may be reduced by 20% to 40%, but most patients have normal serum TSH levels and are clinically euthyroid). Products include:
Carbatrol Capsules 3019
Equetro Extended-Release Capsules 3174

Carteolol Hydrochloride (Co-administration with beta-blockers may decrease T_4 5'-deiodinase activity; action of beta-blocker may be impaired when the hypothyroid patient is converted to euthyroid).
No products indexed under this heading.

Chloral Hydrate (Co-administration has been associated with thyroid hormone and/or TSH level alterations by various mechanisms).
No products indexed under this heading.

Chlorothiazide (Co-administration has been associated with thyroid hormone and/or TSH level alterations by various mechanisms).
No products indexed under this heading.

Chlorothiazide Sodium (Co-administration has been associated with thyroid hormone and/or TSH level alterations by various mechanisms). Products include:
Intravenous Sodium Diuril 2490

Chlorotrianisene (Co-administration with oral estrogens may result in increased serum TBG concentrations).
No products indexed under this heading.

Chlorpropamide (Addition of levothyroxine to antidiabetic therapy may result in increased antidiabetic agent requirements).
No products indexed under this heading.

Cholestyramine (Co-administration may result in decreased T_4 absorption, which may result in hypothyroidism; administer levothyroxine at least 4 hours apart from these agents).
No products indexed under this heading.

Choline Magnesium Trisalicylate (Co-administration with salicylates at greater than 2 gm inhibit binding of T_4 and T_3 to TBG and transthyrelin; an initial increase in serum FT_4 is followed by return of FT_4 to normal levels with sustained therapeutic salicylate concentrations, although total T_4 levels may decrease by as much as 30%).
No products indexed under this heading.

Clofibrate (Co-administration may result in increased serum TBG concentrations).
No products indexed under this heading.

Clomipramine Hydrochloride (Co-administration may increase the therapeutic and toxic effects of both drugs possibly due to increased receptor sensitivity to catecholamines; toxic effects may include increased risk of arrhythmias and CNS stimulation; onset of tricyclics may be accelerated).
No products indexed under this heading.

Colestipol Hydrochloride (Co-administration may result in decreased T_4 absorption, which may result in hypothyroidism; administer levothyroxine at least 4 hours apart from these agents).
No products indexed under this heading.

Cortisone Acetate (Co-administration with glucocorticoids may result in a transient reduction in TSH secretion; the reduction is not sustained, therefore, hypothyroidism does not occur; glucocorticoids may decrease serum TBG concentration).
No products indexed under this heading.

Desipramine Hydrochloride (Co-administration may increase the therapeutic and toxic effects of both drugs possibly due to increased receptor sensitivity to catecholamines; toxic effects may include increased risk of arrhythmias and CNS stimulation; onset of tricyclics may be accelerated).
No products indexed under this heading.

Deslanoside (Co-administration may result in reduced serum digitalis glycosides in hyperthyroidism or when the hypothyroid patient is converted to euthyroid state; therapeutic effect of digitalis glycoside may be reduced).
No products indexed under this heading.

Dexamethasone (Co-administration with glucocorticoids may result in a transient reduction in TSH secretion; the reduction is not sustained, therefore, hypothyroidism does not occur; glucocorticoids may decrease serum TBG concentration). Products include:

Ciprodex Otic Suspension 541

Dexamethasone Acetate (Co-administration with glucocorticoids may result in a transient reduction in TSH secretion; the reduction is not sustained, therefore, hypothyroidism does not occur; glucocorticoids may decrease serum TBG concentration).
No products indexed under this heading.

Dexamethasone Sodium Phosphate (Co-administration with glucocorticoids may result in a transient reduction in TSH secretion; the reduction is not sustained, therefore, hypothyroidism does not occur; glucocorticoids may decrease serum TBG concentration).
No products indexed under this heading.

Diatrizoate Meglumine (May decrease thyroid hormone secretion, which may result in hypothyrodism; the fetus, elderly, and euthyroid patients with underlying thyroid disease are among those individuals who are susceptible to iodine-induced hypothyroidism; oral cholecytographic agents slowly excreted, producing more prolonged hypothyroidism; iodide drugs that contain pharmacologic amounts of iodide may cause hypothyroidism in euthyroid patients with Grave's disease previously treated with thyroid autonomy; hyperthyroidism may develop over several weeks and may persist for several months after therapy discontinuation).
No products indexed under this heading.

Diatrizoate Sodium (May decrease thyroid hormone secretion, which may result in hypothyrodism; the fetus, elderly, and euthyroid patients with underlying thyroid disease are among those individuals who are susceptible to iodine-induced hypothyroidism; oral cholecytographic agents slowly excreted, producing more prolonged hypothyroidism; iodide drugs that contain pharmacologic amounts of iodide may cause hypothyroidism in euthyroid patients with Grave's disease previously treated with thyroid autonomy; hyperthyroidism may develop over several weeks and may persist for several months after therapy discontinuation).
No products indexed under this heading.

Diazepam (Co-administration has been associated with thyroid hormone and/or TSH level alterations by various mechanisms). Products include:
Valium Tablets 2658

Dicumarol (Thyroid hormones appear to increase the catabolism of vitamin K-dependent clotting factors, thereby increasing the anticoagulant activity of oral anticoagulants).
No products indexed under this heading.

Dienestrol (Co-administration with oral estrogens may result in increased serum TBG concentrations).
No products indexed under this heading.

Diethylstilbestrol (Co-administration with oral estrogens may result in increased serum TBG concentrations).
No products indexed under this heading.

Diflunisal (Co-administration with salicylates at greater than 2 gm inhibit binding of T_4 and T_3 to TBG and transthyretin; an initial increase in serum FT_4 is followed by return of FT_4 to normal levels with sustained therapeutic salicylate concentrations, although total T_4 levels may decrease by as much as 30%).
No products indexed under this heading.

Digitalis Glycoside Preparations (Co-administration may result in reduced serum digitalis glycosides in hyperthyroidism or when the hypothyroid patient is converted to euthyroid state; therapeutic effect of digitalis glycoside may be reduced).
No products indexed under this heading.

Digitoxin (Co-administration may result in reduced serum digitalis glycosides in hyperthyroidism or when the hypothyroid patient is converted to euthyroid state; therapeutic effect of digitalis glycoside may be reduced).
No products indexed under this heading.

Digoxin (Co-administration may result in reduced serum digitalis glycosides in hyperthyroidism or when the hypothyroid patient is converted to euthyroid state; therapeutic effect of digitalis glycoside may be reduced). Products include:
Lanoxin Injection 1498
Lanoxin Injection Pediatric 1502
Lanoxin Tablets 1505

Dobutamine Hydrochloride (Co-administration of sympathomimetic agents may increase the effects of sympathomimetics or thyroid hormone; thyroid hormones may increase risk of coronary insufficiency when sympathomimetic agents are administered to patients with coronary disease).
No products indexed under this heading.

Dopamine Hydrochloride (Co-administration with dopamine may result in a transient reduction in TSH secretion; the reduction is not sustained, therefore, hypothyroidism does not occur).
No products indexed under this heading.

Doxepin Hydrochloride (Co-administration may increase the therapeutic and toxic effects of both drugs possibly due to increased receptor sensitivity to catecholamines; toxic effects may include increased risk of arrhythmias and CNS stimulation; onset of tricyclics may be accelerated).
No products indexed under this heading.

Dyphylline (Decreased theophylline clearance may occur in hypothyroid patients; clearance returns to normal when euthyroid state is achieved).
No products indexed under this heading.

Ephedrine Hydrochloride (Co-administration of sympathomimetic agents may increase the effects of sympathomimetics or thyroid hormone; thyroid hormones may increase risk of coronary insufficiency when sympathomimetic agents are administered to patients with coronary disease).
No products indexed under this heading.

Ephedrine Sulfate (Co-administration of sympathomimetic agents may increase the effects of sympathomimetics or thyroid hormone; thyroid hormones may increase risk of coronary insufficiency when sympathomimetic agents are administered to patients with coronary disease).
No products indexed under this heading.

Ephedrine Tannate (Co-administration of sympathomimetic agents may increase the effects of sympathomimetics or thyroid hormone; thyroid hormones may increase risk of coronary insufficiency when sympathomimetic agents are administered to patients with coronary disease).
No products indexed under this heading.

Epinephrine (Co-administration of sympathomimetic agents may increase the effects of sympathomimetics or thyroid hormone; thyroid hormones may increase risk of coronary insufficiency when sympathomimetic agents are administered to patients with coronary disease). Products include:
EpiPen 1024

Epinephrine Bitartrate (Co-administration of sympathomimetic agents may increase the effects of sympathomimetics or thyroid hormone; thyroid hormones may increase risk of coronary insufficiency when sympathomimetic agents are administered to patients with coronary disease).
No products indexed under this heading.

Epinephrine Hydrochloride (Co-administration of sympathomimetic agents may increase the effects of sympathomimetics or thyroid hormone; thyroid hormones may increase risk of coronary insufficiency when sympathomimetic agents are administered to patients with coronary disease).
No products indexed under this heading.

Esmolol Hydrochloride (Co-administration with beta-blockers may decrease T_4 5'-deiodinase activity; action of beta-blocker may be impaired when the hypothyroid patient is converted to euthyroid).
No products indexed under this heading.

Estradiol (Co-administration with oral estrogens may result in increased serum TBG concentrations). Products include:
Activella Tablets 2347
Angeliq Tablets 751
Climara Transdermal System 763
Climara Pro Transdermal System 768
Divigel 3167
Vagifem Tablets 2375

Estrogens, Conjugated (Co-administration with oral estrogens may result in increased serum TBG concentrations). Products include:
Premarin Intravenous 3217
Premarin Tablets 3221
Premarin Vaginal Cream 3228
Premphase Tablets 3232
Prempro Tablets 3232

Estrogens, Esterified (Co-administration with oral estrogens may result in increased serum TBG concentrations). Products include:
Estratest Tablets 3043
Estratest H.S. Tablets 3043

Estropipate (Co-administration with oral estrogens may result in increased serum TBG concentrations).
No products indexed under this heading.

Ethinyl Estradiol (Co-administration with estrogen containing oral contraceptives may result in increased serum TBG concentrations). Products include:
Lybrel Tablets 3204
Mircette Tablets 1034
NuvaRing 2897
Ortho-Cyclen/Ortho Tri-Cyclen 2449
Ortho Evra Transdermal System 2437
Ortho Tri-Cyclen Lo Tablets 2458
Seasonique Tablets 1046
Yaz Tablets 805

Ethiodized Oil (May decrease thyroid hormone secretion, which may result in hypothyrodism; the fetus, elderly, and euthyroid patients with underlying thyroid disease are among those individuals who are susceptible to iodine-induced hypothyroidism; oral cholecytographic agents slowly excreted, producing more prolonged hypothyroidism; iodide drugs that contain pharmacologic amounts of iodide may cause hypothyroidism in euthyroid patients with Grave's disease previously treated with thyroid autonomy; hyperthyroidism may develop over several weeks and may persist for several months after therapy discontinuation).
No products indexed under this heading.

Ethionamide (Co-administration has been associated with thyroid hormone and/or TSH level alterations by various mechanisms).
No products indexed under this heading.

Ethotoin (Hydantoins may cause protein-binding site displacement; co-administration results in an initial transient increase in FT_4; continued administration results in a decrease in serum T_4 and normal FT_4 and TSH concentrations and, therefore, patients are clinically euthyroid).
No products indexed under this heading.

Ferrous Sulfate (Co-administration may result in decreased T_4 absorption, which may result in hypothyroidism; ferrous sulfate may form a ferric-thyroxine complex; administer levothyroxine at least 4 hours apart from these agents).
No products indexed under this heading.

Fiber Supplement (Concurrent use of dietary fiber may bind and decrease the absorption of levothyroxine sodium from GI tract).
No products indexed under this heading.

Fludrocortisone Acetate (Co-administration with glucocorticoids may result in a transient reduction in TSH secretion; the reduction is not sustained, therefore, hypothyroidism does not occur; glucocorticoids may decrease serum TBG concentration).
No products indexed under this heading.

Fluorouracil (Co-administration with 5-FU may result in increased serum TBG concentrations). Products include:
Carac Cream 0.5% 2722

Fluoxymesterone (Co-administration with androgens/anabolic steroids may result in decreased serum TBG concentration).
No products indexed under this heading.

Fosphenytoin Sodium (Hydantoins may cause protein-binding site displacement; co-administration results in an initial transient increase in FT_4; co-administration may increase hepatic metabolism, which may result in hypothyroidism, resulting in increased levothyroxine requirements; phenytoin reduces serum protein binding of levothyroxine, and total- and free-T_4 may be reduced by 20% to 40%, but most patients have normal serum TSH levels and are clinicly euthyroid).
No products indexed under this heading.

Furosemide (May cause protein-binding site displacement at greater than 80 mg IV; co-administration results in an initial transient increase in FT_4; continued administration results in a decrease in serum T_4 and normal FT_4 and TSH concentrations and, therefore, patients are clinically euthyroid). Products include:
Furosemide Tablets 2186

Gadopentetate Dimeglumine (May decrease thyroid hormone secretion, which may result in hypothyrodism; the fetus, elderly, and euthyroid patients with underlying thyroid disease are among those individuals who are susceptible to iodine-induced hypothyroidism; oral cholecytographic agents slowly excreted, producing more prolonged hypothyroidism; iodide drugs that contain pharmacologic amounts of iodide may cause hypothyroidism in euthyroid patients with Grave's disease previously treated with thyroid autonomy; hyperthyroidism may develop over several weeks and may persist for several months after therapy discontinuation).
No products indexed under this heading.

Glimepiride (Addition of levothyroxine to antidiabetic therapy may result in increased antidiabetic agent requirements). Products include:
Avandaryl Tablets 1344
Duetact Tablets 3085

Glipizide (Addition of levothyroxine to antidiabetic therapy may result in increased antidiabetic agent requirements).
No products indexed under this heading.

Glyburide (Addition of levothyroxine to antidiabetic therapy may result in increased antidiabetic agent requirements).
No products indexed under this heading.

Heparin Sodium (May cause protein-binding site displacement; co-administration results in an initial transient increase in FT_4; continued administration results in a decrease in serum T_4 and normal FT_4 and TSH concentrations and, therefore, patients are clinically euthyroid).
No products indexed under this heading.

Heroin (Co-administration may result in increased serum TBG concentrations).
No products indexed under this heading.

Hydrochlorothiazide (Co-administration has been associated with thyroid hormone and/or TSH level alterations by various mechanisms). Products include:
Atacand HCT 642
Avalide Tablets 892
Avalide Tablets 2713
Benicar HCT Tablets 1010
Diovan HCT Tablets 2216
Dyazide Capsules 1405
Micardis HCT Tablets 854
Prinzide Tablets 2092
Tekturna HCT Tablets 2324
Teveten HCT Tablets 517

Hydrocortisone (Co-administration with glucocorticoids may result in a transient reduction in TSH secretion; the reduction is not sustained, therefore, hypothyroidism does not occur; glucocorticoids may decrease serum TBG concentration).
No products indexed under this heading.

Hydrocortisone Acetate (Co-administration with glucocorticoids may result in a transient reduction in TSH secretion; the reduction is not sustained, therefore, hypothyroidism does not occur; glucocorticoids may decrease serum TBG concentration). Products include:
Analpram-HC 1140
Pramosone 1141

Hydrocortisone Sodium Phosphate (Co-administration with glucocorticoids may result in a transient reduction in TSH secretion; the reduction is not sustained, therefore, hypothyroidism does not occur; glucocorticoids may decrease serum TBG concentration).
No products indexed under this heading.

Hydrocortisone Sodium Succinate (Co-administration with glucocorticoids may result in a transient reduction in TSH secretion; the reduction is not sustained, therefore, hypothyroidism does not occur; glucocorticoids may decrease serum TBG concentration).
No products indexed under this heading.

Hydroflumethiazide (Co-administration has been associated with thyroid hormone and/or TSH level alterations by various mechanisms).
No products indexed under this heading.

Imipramine Hydrochloride (Co-administration may increase the therapeutic and toxic effects of both drugs possibly due to increased receptor sensitivity to catecholamines; toxic effects may include increased risk of arrhythmias and CNS stimulation; onset of tricyclics may be accelerated).
No products indexed under this heading.

Imipramine Pamoate (Co-administration may increase the therapeutic and toxic effects of both drugs possibly due to increased receptor sensitivity to catecholamines; toxic effects may include increased risk of arrhythmias and CNS stimulation; onset of tricyclics may be accelerated).
No products indexed under this heading.

Infant Formula (Concurrent use of soybean flour may bind and decrease the absorption of levothyroxine sodium from GI tract).
No products indexed under this heading.

Insulin (Addition of levothyroxine to insulin therapy may result in increased insulin requirements).
No products indexed under this heading.

Insulin, Human, Zinc Suspension (Addition of levothyroxine to insulin therapy may result in increased insulin requirements).
No products indexed under this heading.

Insulin, Human (rDNA origin) (Addition of levothyroxine to insulin therapy may result in increased insulin requirements). Products include:
Exubera Inhalation Powder 2515

Insulin, Human NPH (Addition of levothyroxine to insulin therapy may result in increased insulin requirements). Products include:
Humulin N Vial 1846

Insulin, Human Regular (Addition of levothyroxine to insulin therapy may result in increased insulin requirements). Products include:
Humulin R 1849
Humulin R (U-500) 1850

Insulin, Human Regular and Human NPH Mixture (Addition of levothyroxine to insulin therapy may result in increased insulin requirements). Products include:
Humulin 50/50, 100 Units 1843
Humulin 70/30 Vial 1844

Insulin, NPH (Addition of levothyroxine to insulin therapy may result in increased insulin requirements).
No products indexed under this heading.

Insulin, Regular (Addition of levothyroxine to insulin therapy may result in increased insulin requirements).
No products indexed under this heading.

Insulin, Regular and NPH mixture (Addition of levothyroxine to insulin therapy may result in increased insulin requirements).
No products indexed under this heading.

Insulin, Zinc Crystals (Addition of levothyroxine to insulin therapy may result in increased insulin requirements).
No products indexed under this heading.

Insulin, Zinc Suspension (Addition of levothyroxine to insulin therapy may result in increased insulin requirements).
No products indexed under this heading.

Insulin Aspart (Addition of levothyroxine to insulin therapy may result in increased insulin requirements).
No products indexed under this heading.

Insulin Aspart, Human (Addition of levothyroxine to insulin therapy may result in increased insulin requirements). Products include:
NovoLog Mix 70/30 2364

Insulin Aspart, Human Regular (Addition of levothyroxine to insulin therapy may result in increased insulin requirements). Products include:
NovoLog Injection 2359

Insulin Aspart Protamine, Human (Addition of levothyroxine to insulin therapy may result in increased insulin requirements). Products include:
NovoLog Mix 70/30 2364

Insulin Detemir (rDNA Origin) (Addition of levothyroxine to insulin therapy may result in increased insulin requirements). Products include:
Levemir Injection 2352

Insulin glargine (Addition of levothyroxine to insulin therapy may result in increased insulin requirements). Products include:
Lantus Injection 2749

Insulin Glulisine (Addition of levothyroxine to insulin therapy may result in increased insulin requirements). Products include:
Apidra Injection 2706

Insulin Lispro, Human (Addition of levothyroxine to insulin therapy may result in increased insulin requirements). Products include:
Humalog-Pen and KwikPen 1829
Humalog Mix 50/50-Pen and KwikPen 1833
Humalog Mix 75/25-Pen and KwikPen 1835

Insulin Lispro Protamine, Human (Addition of levothyroxine to insulin therapy may result in increased insulin requirements). Products include:
Humalog Mix 50/50-Pen and KwikPen 1833
Humalog Mix 75/25-Pen and KwikPen 1835

Interferon alfa-2a, Recombinant (Co-administration with interferon alpha has been associated with the development of antithyroid microsomal antibodies in 20% of patients and some have transient hypothyroidism, hyperthyroidism, or both; patients who have antithyroid antibodies before treatment are at higher risk for thyroid dysfunction).
No products indexed under this heading.

Interferon alfa-2b, Recombinant (Co-administration with interferon alpha has been associated with the development of antithyroid microsomal antibodies in 20% of patients and some have transient hypothyroidism, hyperthyroidism, or both; patients who have antithyroid antibodies before treatment are at higher risk for thyroid dysfunction). Products include:
Intron A for Injection 2859

Interferon alfa-N3 (Human Leukocyte Derived) (Co-administration with interferon alpha has been associated with the development of antithyroid microsomal antibodies in 20% of patients and some have transient hypothyroidism, hyperthyroidism, or both; patients who have antithyroid antibodies before treatment are at higher risk for thyroid dysfunction). Products include:
Alferon N Injection 1726

Iodamide Meglumine (May decrease thyroid hormone secretion, which may result in hypothyrodism; the fetus, elderly, and euthyroid patients with underlying thyroid disease are among those individuals who are susceptible to iodine-induced hypothyroidism; oral cholecytographic agents slowly excreted, producing more prolonged hypothyroidism; iodide drugs that contain pharmacologic amounts of iodide may cause hypothyroidism in euthyroid patients with Grave's disease previously treated with thyroid autonomy; hyperthyroidism may develop

over several weeks and may persist for several months after therapy discontinuation).
No products indexed under this heading.

Iohexol (May decrease thyroid hormone secretion, which may result in hypothyrodism; the fetus, elderly, and euthyroid patients with underlying thyroid disease are among those individuals who are susceptible to iodine-induced hypothyroidism; oral cholecytographic agents slowly excreted, producing more prolonged hypothyroidism; iodide drugs that contain pharmacologic amounts of iodide may cause hypothyroidism in euthyroid patients with Grave's disease previously treated with thyroid autonomy; hyperthyroidism may develop over several weeks and may persist for several months after therapy discontinuation).
No products indexed under this heading.

Iopamidol (May decrease thyroid hormone secretion, which may result in hypothyrodism; the fetus, elderly, and euthyroid patients with underlying thyroid disease are among those individuals who are susceptible to iodine-induced hypothyroidism; oral cholecytographic agents slowly excreted, producing more prolonged hypothyroidism; iodide drugs that contain pharmacologic amounts of iodide may cause hypothyroidism in euthyroid patients with Grave's disease previously treated with thyroid autonomy; hyperthyroidism may develop over several weeks and may persist for several months after therapy discontinuation).
No products indexed under this heading.

Iopanoic Acid (May decrease thyroid hormone secretion, which may result in hypothyrodism; the fetus, elderly, and euthyroid patients with underlying thyroid disease are among those individuals who are susceptible to iodine-induced hypothyroidism; oral cholecytographic agents slowly excreted, producing more prolonged hypothyroidism; iodide drugs that contain pharmacologic amounts of iodide may cause hypothyroidism in euthyroid patients with Grave's disease previously treated with thyroid autonomy; hyperthyroidism may develop over several weeks and may persist for several months after therapy discontinuation).
No products indexed under this heading.

Iothalamate Meglumine (May decrease thyroid hormone secretion, which may result in hypothyrodism; the fetus, elderly, and euthyroid patients with underlying thyroid disease are among those individuals who are susceptible to iodine-induced hypothyroidism; oral cholecytographic agents slowly excreted, producing more prolonged hypothyroidism; iodide drugs that contain pharmacologic amounts of iodide may cause hypothyroidism in euthyroid patients with Grave's disease previously treated with thyroid autonomy; hyperthyroidism may develop over several weeks and may persist for several months after therapy discontinuation).
No products indexed under this heading.

Ioxaglate Meglumine (May decrease thyroid hormone secretion, which may result in hypothyrodism; the fetus, elderly, and euthyroid patients with underlying thyroid disease are among those individuals who are susceptible to iodine-induced hypothyroidism; oral cholecytographic agents slowly excreted, producing more prolonged hypothyroidism; iodide drugs that contain pharmacologic amounts of iodide may cause hypothyroidism in euthyroid patients with Grave's disease previously treated with thyroid autonomy; hyperthyroidism may develop over several weeks and may persist for several months after therapy discontinuation).
No products indexed under this heading.

Ioxaglate Sodium (May decrease thyroid hormone secretion, which may result in hypothyrodism; the fetus, elderly, and euthyroid patients with underlying thyroid disease are among those individuals who are susceptible to iodine-induced hypothyroidism; oral cholecytographic agents slowly excreted, producing more prolonged hypothyroidism; iodide drugs that contain pharmacologic amounts of iodide may cause hypothyroidism in euthyroid patients with Grave's disease previously treated with thyroid autonomy; hyperthyroidism may develop over several weeks and may persist for several months after therapy discontinuation).
No products indexed under this heading.

Isoproterenol Hydrochloride (Co-administration of sympathomimetic agents may increase the effects of sympathomimetics or thyroid hormone; thyroid hormones may increase risk of coronary insufficiency when sympathomimetic agents are administered to patients with coronary disease).
No products indexed under this heading.

Isoproterenol Sulfate (Co-administration of sympathomimetic agents may increase the effects of sympathomimetics or thyroid hormone; thyroid hormones may increase risk of coronary insufficiency when sympathomimetic agents are administered to patients with coronary disease).
No products indexed under this heading.

Ketamine Hydrochloride (Co-administration may produce marked hypertension and tachycardia).
No products indexed under this heading.

Labetalol Hydrochloride (Co-administration with beta-blockers may decrease T_4 5'-deiodinase activity; action of beta-blocker may be impaired when the hypothyroid patient is converted to euthyroid).
No products indexed under this heading.

Levalbuterol Hydrochloride (Co-administration of sympathomimetic agents may increase the effects of sympathomimetics or thyroid hormone; thyroid hormones may increase risk of coronary insufficiency when sympathomimetic agents are administered to patients with coronary disease). Products include:

Xopenex Inhalation Solution 3001
Xopenex Inhalation Solution Concentrate 3005

Levobunolol Hydrochloride (Co-administration with beta-blockers may decrease T_4 5'-deiodinase activity; action of beta-blocker may be impaired when the hypothyroid patient is converted to euthyroid).
No products indexed under this heading.

Levodopa (Co-administration with dopamine agonists may result in a transient reduction in TSH secretion; the reduction is not sustained, therefore, hypothyroidism does not occur). Products include:

Stalevo Tablets 2309

Lithium (May decrease thyroid hormone secretion, which may result in hypothyrodism; long-term lithium therapy can result in goiter in up to 50% of patients, and either subclinical or overt hypothyroidism, each in up to 20% of patients).
No products indexed under this heading.

Lithium Carbonate (May decrease thyroid hormone secretion, which may result in hypothyrodism; long-term lithium therapy can result in goiter in up to 50% of patients, and either subclinical or overt hypothyroidism, each in up to 20% of patients).
No products indexed under this heading.

Lithium Citrate (May decrease thyroid hormone secretion, which may result in hypothyrodism; long-term lithium therapy can result in goiter in up to 50% of patients, and either subclinical or overt hypothyroidism, each in up to 20% of patients).
No products indexed under this heading.

Lovastatin (Co-administration has been associated with thyroid hormone and/or TSH level alterations by various mechanisms). Products include:

Advicor Tablets 402
Mevacor Tablets 2063

Magaldrate (Co-administration with antacids may reduce the efficacy of levothyroxine by binding and delaying or preventing absorption, potentially resulting in hypothyroidism; administer levothyroxine at least 4 hours apart from these agents).
No products indexed under this heading.

Magnesium Hydroxide (Co-administration with antacids may reduce the efficacy of levothyroxine by binding and delaying or preventing absorption, potentially resulting in hypothyroidism; administer levothyroxine at least 4 hours apart from these agents). Products include:

Fleet Pedia-Lax Chewable Tablets 1145
Pepcid Complete Chewable Tablets 1771
Extra Strength Rolaids Freshmint Tablets 1903
Rolaids Multi-Symptom Berry Tablets 1903
Rolaids Original Peppermint Tablets 1903

Magnesium Oxide (Co-administration with antacids may reduce the efficacy of levothyroxine by binding and delaying or preventing absorption, potentially resulting in hypothyroidism; administer levothyroxine at least 4 hours apart from these agents). Products include:

Beelith Tablets 813

Magnesium Salicylate (Co-administration with salicylates at greater than 2 gm inhibit binding of T_4 and T_3 to TBG and transthyrelin; an initial increase in serum FT_4 is followed by return of FT_4 to normal levels with sustained therapeutic salicylate concentrations, although total T_4 levels may decrease by as much as 30%).
No products indexed under this heading.

Maprotiline Hydrochloride (Co-administration may increase the therapeutic and toxic effects of both drugs possibly due to increased receptor sensitivity to catecholamines; toxic effects may include increased risk of arrhythmias and CNS stimulation; onset of tricyclics may be accelerated).
No products indexed under this heading.

Meclofenamate Sodium (Co-administration with fenamate NSAID may result in decreased serum TBG concentration).
No products indexed under this heading.

Mefenamic Acid (Co-administration with fenamate NSAID may result in decreased serum TBG concentration).
No products indexed under this heading.

Mephenytoin (Hydantoins may cause protein-binding site displacement; co-administration results in an initial transient increase in FT_4; continued administration results in a decrease in serum T_4 and normal FT_4 and TSH concentrations and, therefore, patients are clinically euthyroid).
No products indexed under this heading.

Mercaptopurine (Co-administration has been associated with thyroid hormone and/or TSH level alterations by various mechanisms).
No products indexed under this heading.

Mestranol (Co-administration with estrogen containing oral contraceptives may result in increased serum TBG concentrations).
No products indexed under this heading.

Metaproterenol Sulfate (Co-administration of sympathomimetic agents may increase the effects of sympathomimetics or thyroid hormone; thyroid hormones may increase risk of coronary insufficiency when sympathomimetic agents are administered to patients with coronary disease).
No products indexed under this heading.

Metaraminol Bitartrate (Co-administration of sympathomimetic agents may increase the effects of sympathomimetics or thyroid hormone; thyroid hormones may increase risk of coronary insufficiency when sympathomimetic agents are administered to patients with coronary disease).
No products indexed under this heading.

Metformin Hydrochloride (Addition of levothyroxine to antidiabetic therapy may result in increased antidiabetic agent requirements). Products include:

ActoPlus Met Tablets 3071
Avandamet Tablets 1336
Janumet Tablets 2041
PrandiMet Tablets 2967

Methadone Hydrochloride (Co-administration may result in increased serum TBG concentrations).
No products indexed under this heading.

Methimazole (May decrease thyroid hormone secretion, which may result in hypothyrodism).
No products indexed under this heading.

Methoxamine Hydrochloride (Co-administration of sympathomimetic agents may increase the effects of sympathomimetics or thyroid hormone; thyroid hormones may increase risk of coronary insufficiency when sympathomimetic agents are administered to patients with coronary disease).
No products indexed under this heading.

Methyclothiazide (Co-administration has been associated with thyroid hormone and/or TSH level alterations by various mechanisms).
No products indexed under this heading.

Methylprednisolone Acetate (Co-administration with glucocorticoids may result in a transient reduction in TSH secretion; the reduction is not sustained, therefore, hypothyroidism does not occur; glucocorticoids may decrease serum TBG concentration).
No products indexed under this heading.

Methylprednisolone Sodium Succinate (Co-administration with glucocorticoids may result in a transient reduction in TSH secretion; the reduction is not sustained, therefore, hypothyroidism does not occur; glucocorticoids may decrease serum TBG concentration).
No products indexed under this heading.

Methyltestosterone (Co-administration with androgens/anabolic steroids may result in decreased serum TBG concentration). Products include:
Estratest Tablets 3043
Estratest H.S. Tablets 3043

Metipranolol Hydrochloride (Co-administration with beta-blockers may decrease T_4 5'-deiodinase activity; action of beta-blocker may be impaired when the hypothyroid patient is converted to euthyroid).
No products indexed under this heading.

Metoclopramide Hydrochloride (Co-administration has been associated with thyroid hormone and/or TSH level alterations by various mechanisms).
No products indexed under this heading.

Metoprolol Succinate (Co-administration with beta-blockers may decrease T_4 5'-deiodinase activity; action of beta-blocker may be impaired when the hypothyroid patient is converted to euthyroid). Products include:
Toprol-XL Tablets 666

Metoprolol Tartrate (Co-administration with beta-blockers may decrease T_4 5'-deiodinase activity; action of beta-blocker may be impaired when the hypothyroid patient is converted to euthyroid).
No products indexed under this heading.

Miglitol (Addition of levothyroxine to antidiabetic therapy may result in increased antidiabetic agent requirements).
No products indexed under this heading.

Mitotane (Co-administration may result in increased serum TBG concentrations).
No products indexed under this heading.

Nadolol (Co-administration with beta-blockers may decrease T_4 5'-deiodinase activity; action of beta-blocker may be impaired when the hypothyroid patient is converted to euthyroid). Products include:
Nadolol Tablets 2191

Nateglinide (Addition of levothyroxine to antidiabetic therapy may result in increased antidiabetic agent requirements). Products include:
Starlix Tablets 2314

Nebivolol (Co-administration with beta-blockers may decrease T_4 5'-deiodinase activity; action of beta-blocker may be impaired when the hypothyroid patient is converted to euthyroid). Products include:
Bystolic Tablets 1155

Niacin (Co-administration with slow-release nicotinic acid may result in decreased serum TBG concentration). Products include:
Advicor Tablets 402
Bausch & Lomb Ocuvite DF Vitamin Supplement .... ⊙238
Dismutax Dietary Supplement 995
Niaspan Extended-Release Tablets 480
NT-Kinase Dietary Supplement 995
Simcor Tablets 502

Norepinephrine Bitartrate (Co-administration of sympathomimetic agents may increase the effects of sympathomimetics or thyroid hormone; thyroid hormones may increase risk of coronary insufficiency when sympathomimetic agents are administered to patients with coronary disease).
No products indexed under this heading.

Nortriptyline Hydrochloride (Co-administration may increase the therapeutic and toxic effects of both drugs possibly due to increased receptor sensitivity to catecholamines; toxic effects may include increased risk of arrhythmias and CNS stimulation; onset of tricyclics may be accelerated).
No products indexed under this heading.

Octreotide Acetate (Co-administration with octreotide may result in a transient reduction in TSH secretion; the reduction is not sustained, therefore, hypothyroidism does not occur). Products include:
Sandostatin Injection 2300
Sandostatin LAR Depot 2302

Orlistat (Concurrent use may reduce the efficacy of levothyroxine by binding and delaying or preventing absorption, potentially resulting in hypothyroidism. Patients treated concomitantly with orlistat and levothyroxine should be monitored for change in thyroid function). Products include:
Xenical Capsules 2672

Oxandrolone (Co-administration with androgens/anabolic steroids may result in decreased serum TBG concentration).
No products indexed under this heading.

Oxymetholone (Co-administration with androgens/anabolic steroids may result in decreased serum TBG concentration).
No products indexed under this heading.

Penbutolol Sulfate (Co-administration with beta-blockers may decrease T_4 5'-deiodinase activity; action of beta-blocker may be impaired when the hypothyroid patient is converted to euthyroid).
No products indexed under this heading.

Pergolide Mesylate (Co-administration with dopamine agonists may result in a transient reduction in TSH secretion; the reduction is not sustained, therefore, hypothyroidism does not occur).
No products indexed under this heading.

Perphenazine (Co-administration has been associated with thyroid hormone and/or TSH level alterations by various mechanisms).
No products indexed under this heading.

Phenobarbital (Co-administration may increase hepatic metabolism, which may result in hypothyroidism, resulting in increased levothyroxine requirements). Products include:
Donnatal Extentabs 2507

Phenylbutazone (Co-administration may cause protein-binding site displacement).
No products indexed under this heading.

Phenylephrine Bitartrate (Co-administration of sympathomimetic agents may increase the effects of sympathomimetics or thyroid hormone; thyroid hormones may increase risk of coronary insufficiency when sympathomimetic agents are administered to patients with coronary disease).
No products indexed under this heading.

Phenylephrine Hydrochloride (Co-administration of sympathomimetic agents may increase the effects of sympathomimetics or thyroid hormone; thyroid hormones may increase risk of coronary insufficiency when sympathomimetic agents are administered to patients with coronary disease). Products include:
Actifed Cold & Allergy Tablets 1895
Benadryl Allergy & Cold Kapgels 1895
Benadryl Allergy & Sinus Headache Kapgels 1895
Benadryl Severe Allergy & Sinus Headache Caplets 1897
Children's Benadryl-D Allergy & Sinus Liquid 1896
Benadryl-D Allergy & Sinus Tablet 1896
PediaCare Children's Allergy & Cold Liquid 1902
PediaCare Children's Decongestant Liquid 1902
PediaCare Children's Liquid Multi-Symptom Cold..................... 1902
Sinutab Non-Drying Caplets 1905
Sinutab Sinus Caplets 1905
Children's Sudafed PE Cold & Cough Liquid 1907
Children's Sudafed PE Nasal Decongestant Liquid 1906
Sudafed PE Cold & Cough Caplets 1907
Sudafed PE Nasal Decongestant Tablets 1907
Sudafed PE Nighttime Cold Caplets 1907
Sudafed PE Non-Drying Sinus Caplets 1908
Sudafed PE Severe Cold Caplets 1908
Sudafed PE Sinus & Allergy Tablets 1908
Sudafed PE Sinus Headache Caplets 1908
Tylenol Allergy Multi-Symptom Caplets with Cool Burst and Rapid Release Gelcaps 1916
Tylenol Allergy Multi-Symptom Nighttime Caplets with Cool Burst 1916
Children's Tylenol Plus Cold Suspension Liquid 1912
Children's Tylenol Plus Cold & Allergy Suspension Liquid 1914
Children's Tylenol Plus Flu Suspension Liquid 1914
Children's Tylenol Plus Multi-Symptom Cold Suspension Liquid 1912
Tylenol Cold Head Congestion Daytime Caplets with Cool Burst 1910
Tylenol Cold Head Congestion Nighttime Caplets with Cool Burst 1910
Tylenol Cold Head Congestion Severe Daytime Caplets with Cool Burst 1910
Tylenol Cold Multi-Symptom Daytime Caplets with Cool Burst and Rapid Release Gels 1913
Tylenol Cold Multi-Symptom Daytime Liquid with Citrus Burst ... 1913
Tylenol Cold Multi-Symptom Nighttime Caplets with Cool Burst 1913
Tylenol Cold Multi-Symptom Nighttime Liquid with Cool Burst ... 1913
Tylenol Cold Multi-Symptom Severe Caplets with Cool Burst 1913
Tylenol Cold Multi-Symptom Severe Daytime Liquid with Citrus Burst 1913
Tylenol Sinus Congestion & Pain Daytime Caplets with Cool Burst and Gelcaps 1917
Tylenol Sinus Congestion & Pain Nighttime Caplets with Cool Burst 1917
Tylenol Sinus Congestion & Pain Severe Caplets with Cool Burst 1917
Vicks DayQuil Cold & Flu Multi-Symptom Relief .... ■616
Vicks DayQuil LiquiCaps 2567
Vicks DayQuil Liquid 2567
Vicks DayQuil Multi-Symptom Cold/Flu Relief 2567

Phenylephrine Tannate (Co-administration of sympathomimetic agents may increase the effects of sympathomimetics or thyroid hormone; thyroid hormones may increase risk of coronary insufficiency when sympathomimetic agents are administered to patients with coronary disease).
No products indexed under this heading.

Phenylpropanolamine Hydrochloride (Co-administration of sympathomimetic agents may increase the effects of sympathomimetics or thyroid hormone; thyroid hormones may increase risk of coronary insufficiency when sympathomimetic agents are administered to patients with coronary disease).
No products indexed under this heading.

Phenytoin (Hydantoins may cause protein-binding site displacement; co-administration results in an initial

transient increase in FT_4; co-administration may increase hepatic metabolism, which may result in hypothyroidism, resulting in increased levothyroxine requirements; phenytoin reduces serum protein binding of levothyroxine, and total- and free-T_4 may be reduced by 20% to 40%, but most patients have normal serum TSH levels and are clinicly euthyroid).
No products indexed under this heading.

Phenytoin Sodium (Hydantoins may cause protein-binding site displacement; co-administration results in an initial transient increase in FT_4; co-administration may increase hepatic metabolism, which may result in hypothyroidism, resulting in increased levothyroxine requirements; phenytoin reduces serum protein binding of levothyroxine, and total- and free-T_4 may be reduced by 20% to 40%, but most patients have normal serum TSH levels and are clinicly euthyroid). Products include:
Phenytek Capsules 2192

Pindolol (Co-administration with beta-blockers may decrease T_4 5'-deiodinase activity; action of beta-blocker may be impaired when the hypothyroid patient is converted to euthyroid).
No products indexed under this heading.

Pioglitazone Hydrochloride (Addition of levothyroxine to antidiabetic therapy may result in increased antidiabetic agent requirements). Products include:
ActoPlus Met Tablets 3071
Actos Tablets 3077
Duetact Tablets 3085

Pirbuterol Acetate (Co-administration of sympathomimetic agents may increase the effects of sympathomimetics or thyroid hormone; thyroid hormones may increase risk of coronary insufficiency when sympathomimetic agents are administered to patients with coronary disease). Products include:
Maxair Autohaler 1705

Polyestradiol Phosphate (Co-administration with oral estrogens may result in increased serum TBG concentrations).
No products indexed under this heading.

Polythiazide (Co-administration has been associated with thyroid hormone and/or TSH level alterations by various mechanisms).
No products indexed under this heading.

Potassium Iodide (May decrease thyroid hormone secretion, which may result in hypothyrodism; iodide drugs that contain pharmacologic amounts of iodide may cause hypothyroidism in euthyroid patients with Grave's disease previously treated with thyroid autonomy; hyperthyroidism may develop over several weeks and may persist for several months after therapy discontinuation). Products include:
CitraNatal DHA Tablets 2175
CitraNatal 90 DHA Tablets 2175

Pramipexole Dihydrochloride (Co-administration with dopamine agonists may result in a transient reduction in TSH secretion; the reduction is not sustained, therefore, hypothyroidism does not occur). Products include:
Mirapex Tablets 857

Prednisolone Acetate (Co-administration with glucocorticoids may result in a transient reduction in TSH secretion; the reduction is not sustained, therefore, hypothyroidism does not occur; glucocorticoids may decrease serum TBG concentration). Products include:
Pred Forte Ophthalmic Suspension .... ⊙227
Pred Mild Ophthalmic Suspension .... ⊙230
Pred-G Ophthalmic Ointment .... ⊙229
Pred-G Ophthalmic Suspension ...... ⊙228

Prednisolone Sodium Phosphate (Co-administration with glucocorticoids may result in a transient reduction in TSH secretion; the reduction is not sustained, therefore, hypothyroidism does not occur; glucocorticoids may decrease serum TBG concentration).
No products indexed under this heading.

Prednisolone Tebutate (Co-administration with glucocorticoids may result in a transient reduction in TSH secretion; the reduction is not sustained, therefore, hypothyroidism does not occur; glucocorticoids may decrease serum TBG concentration).
No products indexed under this heading.

Prednisone (Co-administration with glucocorticoids may result in a transient reduction in TSH secretion; the reduction is not sustained, therefore, hypothyroidism does not occur; glucocorticoids may decrease serum TBG concentration).
No products indexed under this heading.

Propranolol Hydrochloride (Co-administration with beta-blockers may decrease T_4 5'-deiodinase activity; in patients treated with large doses of propranolol, greater than 160 mg/day, T_3 and T_4 levels change slightly, TSH levels remain normal, and patients are clinically euthyroid; action of beta-blocker may be impaired when the hypothyroid patient is converted to euthyroid). Products include:
InnoPran XL Extended Release Capsules 1484

Propylthiouracil (May decrease thyroid hormone secretion, which may result in hypothyrodism).
No products indexed under this heading.

Protriptyline Hydrochloride (Co-administration may increase the therapeutic and toxic effects of both drugs possibly due to increased receptor sensitivity to catecholamines; toxic effects may include increased risk of arrhythmias and CNS stimulation; onset of tricyclics may be accelerated).
No products indexed under this heading.

Pseudoephedrine Hydrochloride (Co-administration of sympathomimetic agents may increase the effects of sympathomimetics or thyroid hormone; thyroid hormones may increase risk of coronary insufficiency when sympathomimetic agents are administered to patients with coronary disease). Products include:
Allegra-D 12 Hour Extended-Release Tablets 2687
Allegra-D 24 Hour Extended-Release Tablets 2690
Children's Motrin Cold Oral Suspension 1899
Sudafed 12 Hour Nasal Decongestant Non-Drowsy Caplets 1909
Sudafed 24 Hour Non-Drowsy Nasal Decongestant Tablets 1906
Children's Sudafed Nasal Decongestant Liquid 1906
Sudafed Nasal Decongestant Tablets 1906
Tylenol Cold Severe Congestion Daytime Caplets with Cool Burst 1912
Tylenol Sinus Severe Congestion Caplets with Cool Burst 1917
Vicks NyQuil LiquiCaps 2567
Vicks NyQuil Liquid 2567
Vicks NyQuil Multi-Symptom Cold/Flu Relief 2567
Zyrtec-D 12 Hour Extended Release Tablets 1923
Zyrtec-D Allergy & Congestion Extended-Release Tablets 1923

Pseudoephedrine Sulfate (Co-administration of sympathomimetic agents may increase the effects of sympathomimetics or thyroid hormone; thyroid hormones may increase risk of coronary insufficiency when sympathomimetic agents are administered to patients with coronary disease). Products include:
Clarinex-D 12-Hour Extended-Release Tablets 2831
Clarinex-D 24-Hour Extended-Release Tablets 2834

Quinestrol (Co-administration with oral estrogens may result in increased serum TBG concentrations).
No products indexed under this heading.

Repaglinide (Addition of levothyroxine to antidiabetic therapy may result in increased antidiabetic agent requirements). Products include:
PrandiMet Tablets 2967
Prandin Tablets 2971

Resorcinol (Co-administration of excessive topical use of resorcinol has been associated with thyroid hormone and/or TSH level alterations by various mechanisms).
No products indexed under this heading.

Rifampin (Co-administration may increase hepatic metabolism, which may result in hypothyroidism, resulting in increased levothyroxine requirements).
No products indexed under this heading.

Ropinirole Hydrochloride (Co-administration with dopamine agonists may result in a transient reduction in TSH secretion; the reduction is not sustained, therefore, hypothyroidism does not occur). Products include:
Requip Tablets 1561
Requip XL Tablets 1568

Rosiglitazone Maleate (Addition of levothyroxine to antidiabetic therapy may result in increased antidiabetic agent requirements). Products include:
Avandamet Tablets 1336
Avandaryl Tablets 1344
Avandia Tablets 1351

Salmeterol Xinafoate (Co-administration of sympathomimetic agents may increase the effects of sympathomimetics or thyroid hormone; thyroid hormones may increase risk of coronary insufficiency when sympathomimetic agents are administered to patients with coronary disease). Products include:
Advair Diskus 100/50 1276
Advair Diskus 250/50 1276
Advair Diskus 500/50 1276
Advair HFA 45/21 Inhalation Aerosol 1288
Advair HFA 115/21 Inhalation Aerosol 1288
Advair HFA 230/21 Inhalation Aerosol 1288
Serevent Diskus 1594

Salsalate (Co-administration with salicylates at greater than 2 gm inhibit binding of T_4 and T_3 to TBG and transthyrelin; an initial increase in serum FT_4 is followed by return of FT_4 to normal levels with sustained therapeutic salicylate concentrations, although total T_4 levels may decrease by as much as 30%).
No products indexed under this heading.

Sertraline Hydrochloride (Co-administration of sertraline in patients stabilized on levothyroxine may result in increased levothyroxine requirements).
No products indexed under this heading.

Sitagliptin Phosphate (Addition of levothyroxine to antidiabetic therapy may result in increased antidiabetic agent requirements). Products include:
Janumet Tablets 2041
Januvia Tablets 2048

Sodium Nitroprusside (Co-administration has been associated with thyroid hormone and/or TSH level alterations by various mechanisms).
No products indexed under this heading.

Sodium Polystyrene Sulfonate (Co-administration may result in decreased T_4 absorption, which may result in hypothyroidism; administer levothyroxine at least 4 hours apart from these agents).
No products indexed under this heading.

Somatrem (Excessive use of thyroid hormone with growth hormones may accelerate epiphyseal closure; however, untreated hypothyroidism may interfere with growth response to growth hormone).
No products indexed under this heading.

Somatropin (Excessive use of thyroid hormone with growth hormones may accelerate epiphyseal closure; however, untreated hypothyroidism may interfere with growth response to growth hormone). Products include:
Genotropin Lyophilized Powder 2547
Humatrope Vials and Cartridges 1838
Nutropin for Injection 1208
Nutropin AQ Injection 1212
Nutropin AQ NuSpin Injection 1212
Nutropin AQ Pen 1212
Nutropin AQ Pen Cartridge 1212

Sotalol Hydrochloride (Co-administration with beta-blockers may decrease T_4 5'-deiodinase activity; action of beta-blocker may be impaired when the hypothyroid patient is converted to euthyroid).
No products indexed under this heading.

Soybean Preparations (Concurrent use of soybean flour may bind and decrease the absorption of levothyroxine sodium from GI tract).
No products indexed under this heading.

Stanozolol (Co-administration with androgens/anabolic steroids may result in decreased serum TBG concentration).
No products indexed under this heading.

Sucralfate (Co-administration may result in decreased T_4 absorption, which may result in hypothyroidism; administer levothyroxine at least 4 hours apart from these agents).
Products include:
Carafate Suspension 706
Carafate Tablets 707

Sulfamethoxazole (May decrease thyroid hormone secretion, which may result in hypothyrodism).
No products indexed under this heading.

Sulfisoxazole Acetyl (May decrease thyroid hormone secretion, which may result in hypothyrodism).
No products indexed under this heading.

Tamoxifen Citrate (Co-administration may result in increased serum TBG concentrations).
No products indexed under this heading.

Terbutaline Sulfate (Co-administration of sympathomimetic agents may increase the effects of sympathomimetics or thyroid hormone; thyroid hormones may increase risk of coronary insufficiency when sympathomimetic agents are administered to patients with coronary disease).
No products indexed under this heading.

Theophylline (Decreased theophylline clearance may occur in hypothyroid patients; clearance returns to normal when euthyroid state is achieved).
No products indexed under this heading.

Theophylline Anhydrous (Decreased theophylline clearance may occur in hypothyroid patients; clearance returns to normal when euthyroid state is achieved).
Products include:
Uniphyl Tablets 2595

Theophylline Calcium Salicylate (Decreased theophylline clearance may occur in hypothyroid patients; clearance returns to normal when euthyroid state is achieved).
No products indexed under this heading.

Theophylline Dihydroxypropyl (Glyceryl) (Decreased theophylline clearance may occur in hypothyroid patients; clearance returns to normal when euthyroid state is achieved).
No products indexed under this heading.

Theophylline Ethylenediamine (Decreased theophylline clearance may occur in hypothyroid patients; clearance returns to normal when euthyroid state is achieved).
No products indexed under this heading.

Theophylline Sodium Glycinate (Decreased theophylline clearance may occur in hypothyroid patients; clearance returns to normal when euthyroid state is achieved).
No products indexed under this heading.

Timolol Hemihydrate (Co-administration with beta-blockers may decrease T_4 5'-deiodinase activity; action of beta-blocker may be impaired when the hypothyroid patient is converted to euthyroid).
Products include:
Betimol Ophthalmic Solution 3181

Timolol Maleate (Co-administration with beta-blockers may decrease T_4 5'-deiodinase activity; action of beta-blocker may be impaired when the hypothyroid patient is converted to euthyroid). Products include:
Combigan Ophthalmic Solution 553
Cosopt Sterile Ophthalmic Solution 1969
Timoptic Sterile Ophthalmic Solution 2121
Timoptic in Ocudose 2124
Timoptic-XE Sterile Ophthalmic Gel Forming Solution 2125

Tolazamide (Addition of levothyroxine to antidiabetic therapy may result in increased antidiabetic agent requirements).
No products indexed under this heading.

Tolbutamide (May decrease thyroid hormone secretion, which may result in hypothyrodism).
No products indexed under this heading.

Triamcinolone (Co-administration with glucocorticoids may result in a transient reduction in TSH secretion; the reduction is not sustained, therefore, hypothyroidism does not occur; glucocorticoids may decrease serum TBG concentration).
No products indexed under this heading.

Triamcinolone Acetonide (Co-administration with glucocorticoids may result in a transient reduction in TSH secretion; the reduction is not sustained, therefore, hypothyroidism does not occur; glucocorticoids may decrease serum TBG concentration).
Products include:
Azmacort Inhalation Aerosol 407
Nasacort AQ Nasal Spray 2765
Triesence Injectable Suspension .... ⊙209

Triamcinolone Diacetate (Co-administration with glucocorticoids may result in a transient reduction in TSH secretion; the reduction is not sustained, therefore, hypothyroidism does not occur; glucocorticoids may decrease serum TBG concentration).
No products indexed under this heading.

Triamcinolone Hexacetonide (Co-administration with glucocorticoids may result in a transient reduction in TSH secretion; the reduction is not sustained, therefore, hypothyroidism does not occur; glucocorticoids may decrease serum TBG concentration).
No products indexed under this heading.

Trimipramine Maleate (Co-administration may increase the therapeutic and toxic effects of both drugs possibly due to increased receptor sensitivity to catecholamines; toxic effects may include increased risk of arrhythmias and CNS stimulation; onset of tricyclics may be accelerated).
No products indexed under this heading.

Troglitazone (Addition of levothyroxine to antidiabetic therapy may result in increased antidiabetic agent requirements).
No products indexed under this heading.

Tyropanoate Sodium (May decrease thyroid hormone secretion, which may result in hypothyrodism; the fetus, elderly, and euthyroid patients with underlying thyroid disease are among those individuals who are susceptible to iodine-induced hypothyroidism; oral cholecytographic agents slowly excreted, producing more prolonged hypothyroidism; iodide drugs that contain pharmacologic amounts of iodide may cause hypothyroidism in euthyroid patients with Grave's disease previously treated with thyroid autonomy; hyperthyroidism may develop over several weeks and may persist for several months after therapy discontinuation).
No products indexed under this heading.

Warfarin Sodium (Thyroid hormones appear to increase the catabolism of vitamin K-dependent clotting factors, thereby increasing the anticoagulant activity of oral anticoagulants).
No products indexed under this heading.

Food Interactions

Cotton seed meal (Concurrent use of cotton seed meal may bind and decrease the absorption of levothyroxine sodium from GI tract).

Dietary Fiber (Concurrent use of dietary fiber may bind and decrease the absorption of levothyroxine sodium from GI tract).

Soybean Formula, Children's (Concurrent use of soybean flour may bind and decrease the absorption of levothyroxine sodium from GI tract).

Walnuts (Concurrent use of walnuts may bind and decrease the absorption of levothyroxine sodium from GI tract).

LEXAPRO ORAL SUSPENSION

(Escitalopram Oxalate) 1174
See Lexapro Tablets

LEXAPRO TABLETS

(Escitalopram Oxalate) 1174
May interact with anticoagulants, cytochrome p450 2c19 inhibitors (selected), cytochrome p450 2d6 substrates (selected), cytochrome p450 3a4 inhibitors (selected), lithium preparations, monoamine oxidase inhibitors, non-steroidal anti-inflammatory agents, serotoninergic agents, triptans, and certain other agents. Compounds in these categories include:

Acetazolamide (In vitro studies indicated that CYP3A4 and -2C19 are the primary enzymes involved in the metabolism of escitalopram. However, co-administration of escitalopram oxalate (20 mg) and ritonavir (600 mg), a potent inhibitor of CYP3A4, did not significantly affect the pharmacokinetics of escitalopram oxalate. Because escitalopram oxalate is metabolized by multiple enzyme systems, inhibition of a single enzyme may not appreciably decrease escitalopram clearance).
No products indexed under this heading.

Almotriptan Malate (There have been rare post-marketing reports of serotonin syndrome with use of a SSRI and a triptan. If concomitant treatment of escitalopram oxalate with a triptan is clinically warranted, careful observation of the patient is advised, particularly during treatment initiation and dose increases).
Products include:
Axert Tablets 2431

Amiodarone Hydrochloride (In vitro studies indicated that CYP3A4 and -2C19 are the primary enzymes involved in the metabolism of escitalopram. However, co-administration of escitalopram oxalate (20 mg) and ritonavir (600 mg), a potent inhibitor of CYP3A4, did not significantly affect the pharmacokinetics of escitalopram oxalate. Because escitalopram oxalate is metabolized by multiple enzyme systems, inhibition of a single enzyme may not appreciably decrease escitalopram clearance).
No products indexed under this heading.

Amitriptyline Hydrochloride (In vitro studies did not reveal an inhibitory effect of escitalopram on CYP2D6. In addition, steady state levels of racemic citalopram were not significantly different in poor metabolizers and extensive CYP2D6 metabolizers after multi-dose administration of citalopram, suggesting that co-administration, with escitalopram, of a drug that inhibits CYP2D6, is unlikely to have clinically significant effects on escitalopram metabolism. However, there are limited in vivo data suggesting a modest CYP2D6 inhibitory effect for escitalopram. Caution is indicated in the co-administration of escitalopram and drugs metabolized by CYP2D6).
No products indexed under this heading.

Amphetamine Aspartate (In vitro studies did not reveal an inhibitory effect of escitalopram on CYP2D6. In addition, steady state levels of racemic citalopram were not significantly different in poor metabolizers and extensive CYP2D6 metabolizers after multi-dose administration of citalopram, suggesting that co-administration, with escitalopram, of a drug that inhibits CYP2D6, is unlikely to have clinically significant effects on escitalopram metabolism. However, there are limited in vivo data suggesting a modest CYP2D6 inhibitory effect for escitalopram. Caution is indicated in the co-administration of escitalopram and drugs metabolized by CYP2D6).
Products include:
Adderall XR Capsules 3012

Amphetamine Aspartate Monohydrate (In vitro studies did not reveal an inhibitory effect of escitalopram on CYP2D6. In addition, steady state levels of racemic citalopram were not significantly different in poor metabolizers and extensive CYP2D6 metabolizers after multi-dose administration of citalopram,

suggesting that co-administration, with escitalopram, of a drug that inhibits CYP2D6, is unlikely to have clinically significant effects on escitalopram metabolism. However, there are limited in vivo data suggesting a modest CYP2D6 inhibitory effect for escitalopram. Caution is indicated in the co-administration of escitalopram and drugs metabolized by CYP2D6).

No products indexed under this heading.

Amphetamine Sulfate (In vitro studies did not reveal an inhibitory effect of escitalopram on CYP2D6. In addition, steady state levels of racemic citalopram were not significantly different in poor metabolizers and extensive CYP2D6 metabolizers after multi-dose administration of citalopram, suggesting that co-administration, with escitalopram, of a drug that inhibits CYP2D6, is unlikely to have clinically significant effects on escitalopram metabolism. However, there are limited in vivo data suggesting a modest CYP2D6 inhibitory effect for escitalopram. Caution is indicated in the co-administration of escitalopram and drugs metabolized by CYP2D6). Products include:

Adderall XR Capsules 3012

Amprenavir (In vitro studies indicated that CYP3A4 and -2C19 are the primary enzymes involved in the metabolism of escitalopram. However, co-administration of escitalopram oxalate (20 mg) and ritonavir (600 mg), a potent inhibitor of CYP3A4, did not significantly affect the pharmacokinetics of escitalopram oxalate. Because escitalopram oxalate is metabolized by multiple enzyme systems, inhibition of a single enzyme may not appreciably decrease escitalopram clearance).

No products indexed under this heading.

Anastrozole (In vitro studies indicated that CYP3A4 and -2C19 are the primary enzymes involved in the metabolism of escitalopram. However, co-administration of escitalopram oxalate (20 mg) and ritonavir (600 mg), a potent inhibitor of CYP3A4, did not significantly affect the pharmacokinetics of escitalopram oxalate. Because escitalopram oxalate is metabolized by multiple enzyme systems, inhibition of a single enzyme may not appreciably decrease escitalopram clearance). Products include:

Arimidex Tablets 672

Anisindione (The combined use of psychotropic drugs that interfere with serotonin reuptake and drugs that affect coagulation has been associated with an increased risk of bleeding).

No products indexed under this heading.

Aprepitant (In vitro studies indicated that CYP3A4 and -2C19 are the primary enzymes involved in the metabolism of escitalopram. However, co-administration of escitalopram oxalate (20 mg) and ritonavir (600 mg), a potent inhibitor of CYP3A4, did not significantly affect the pharmacokinetics of escitalopram oxalate. Because escitalopram oxalate is metabolized by multiple enzyme systems, inhibition of a single enzyme may not appreciably decrease escitalopram clearance). Products include:

Emend Capsules 1992

Ardeparin Sodium (The combined use of psychotropic drugs that interfere with serotonin reuptake and drugs that affect coagulation has been associated with an increased risk of bleeding).

No products indexed under this heading.

Aspirin (The combined use of psychotropic drugs that interfere with serotonin reuptake and drugs that affect coagulation has been associated with an increased risk of bleeding. Use caution when co-administering). Products include:

Aggrenox Capsules 819
Bayer Aspirin 750
Percodan Tablets 1130
St. Joseph 81 mg Aspirin Chewable and Enteric Coated Tablets 1903

Aspirin, Enteric Coated (The combined use of psychotropic drugs that interfere with serotonin reuptake and drugs that affect coagulation has been associated with an increased risk of bleeding. Use caution when co-administering).

No products indexed under this heading.

Aspirin Buffered (The combined use of psychotropic drugs that interfere with serotonin reuptake and drugs that affect coagulation has been associated with an increased risk of bleeding. Use caution when co-administering).

No products indexed under this heading.

Atazanavir (In vitro studies indicated that CYP3A4 and -2C19 are the primary enzymes involved in the metabolism of escitalopram. However, co-administration of escitalopram oxalate (20 mg) and ritonavir (600 mg), a potent inhibitor of CYP3A4, did not significantly affect the pharmacokinetics of escitalopram oxalate. Because escitalopram oxalate is metabolized by multiple enzyme systems, inhibition of a single enzyme may not appreciably decrease escitalopram clearance).

No products indexed under this heading.

Atazanavir Sulfate (In vitro studies indicated that CYP3A4 and -2C19 are the primary enzymes involved in the metabolism of escitalopram. However, co-administration of escitalopram oxalate (20 mg) and ritonavir (600 mg), a potent inhibitor of CYP3A4, did not significantly affect the pharmacokinetics of escitalopram oxalate. Because escitalopram oxalate is metabolized by multiple enzyme systems, inhibition of a single enzyme may not appreciably decrease escitalopram clearance). Products include:

Reyataz Capsules 3299

Atomoxetine Hydrochloride (In vitro studies did not reveal an inhibitory effect of escitalopram on CYP2D6. In addition, steady state levels of racemic citalopram were not significantly different in poor metabolizers and extensive CYP2D6 metabolizers after multi-dose administration of citalopram, suggesting that co-administration, with escitalopram, of a drug that inhibits CYP2D6, is unlikely to have clinically significant effects on escitalopram metabolism. However, there are limited in vivo data suggesting a modest CYP2D6 inhibitory effect for escitalopram. Caution is indicated in the co-administration of escitalopram and drugs metabolized by CYP2D6). Products include:

Strattera Capsules 1864

Bisoprolol Fumarate (In vitro studies did not reveal an inhibitory effect of escitalopram on CYP2D6. In addition, steady state levels of racemic citalopram were not significantly different in poor metabolizers and extensive CYP2D6 metabolizers after multi-dose administration of citalopram, suggesting that co-administration, with escitalopram, of a drug that inhibits CYP2D6, is unlikely to have clinically significant effects on escitalopram metabolism. However, there are limited in vivo data suggesting a modest CYP2D6 inhibitory effect for escitalopram. Caution is indicated in the co-administration of escitalopram and drugs metabolized by CYP2D6).

No products indexed under this heading.

Captopril (In vitro studies did not reveal an inhibitory effect of escitalopram on CYP2D6. In addition, steady state levels of racemic citalopram were not significantly different in poor metabolizers and extensive CYP2D6 metabolizers after multi-dose administration of citalopram, suggesting that co-administration, with escitalopram, of a drug that inhibits CYP2D6, is unlikely to have clinically significant effects on escitalopram metabolism. However, there are limited in vivo data suggesting a modest CYP2D6 inhibitory effect for escitalopram. Caution is indicated in the co-administration of escitalopram and drugs metabolized by CYP2D6). Products include:

Captopril Tablets 2182

Carbamazepine (Potential for increased clearance of escitalopram, although trough citalopram plasma levels were unaffected during co-administration. The possibility that carbamazepine might increase the clearance of escitalopram should be considered if the two drugs are co-administered). Products include:

Carbatrol Capsules 3019
Equetro Extended-Release Capsules 3174

Carvedilol (In vitro studies did not reveal an inhibitory effect of escitalopram on CYP2D6. In addition, steady state levels of racemic citalopram were not significantly different in poor metabolizers and extensive CYP2D6 metabolizers after multi-dose administration of citalopram, suggesting that co-administration, with escitalopram, of a drug that inhibits CYP2D6, is unlikely to have clinically significant effects on escitalopram metabolism. However, there are limited in vivo data suggesting a modest CYP2D6 inhibitory effect for escitalopram. Caution is indicated in the co-administration of escitalopram and drugs metabolized by CYP2D6). Products include:

Coreg Tablets 1387

Celecoxib (The combined use of psychotropic drugs that interfere with serotonin reuptake and drugs that affect coagulation has been associated with an increased risk of bleeding; use caution when co-administering). Products include:

Celebrex Capsules 2979

Cevimeline Hydrochloride (In vitro studies did not reveal an inhibitory effect of escitalopram on CYP2D6. In addition, steady state levels of racemic citalopram were not significantly different in poor metabolizers and extensive CYP2D6 metabolizers after multi-dose administration of citalopram, suggesting that co-administration, with escitalopram, of a drug that inhibits CYP2D6, is unlikely to have clinically significant effects on escitalopram metabolism. However, there are limited in vivo data suggesting a modest CYP2D6 inhibitory effect for escitalopram. Caution is indicated in the co-administration of escitalopram and drugs metabolized by CYP2D6). Products include:

Evoxac Capsules 1013

Chlorpromazine (In vitro studies did not reveal an inhibitory effect of escitalopram on CYP2D6. In addition, steady state levels of racemic citalopram were not significantly different in poor metabolizers and extensive CYP2D6 metabolizers after multi-dose administration of citalopram, suggesting that co-administration, with escitalopram, of a drug that inhibits CYP2D6, is unlikely to have clinically significant effects on escitalopram metabolism. However, there are limited in vivo data suggesting a modest CYP2D6 inhibitory effect for escitalopram. Caution is indicated in the co-administration of escitalopram and drugs metabolized by CYP2D6).

No products indexed under this heading.

Chlorpromazine Hydrochloride (In vitro studies did not reveal an inhibitory effect of escitalopram on CYP2D6. In addition, steady state levels of racemic citalopram were not significantly different in poor metabolizers and extensive CYP2D6 metabolizers after multi-dose administration of citalopram, suggesting that co-administration, with escitalopram, of a drug that inhibits CYP2D6, is unlikely to have clinically significant effects on escitalopram metabolism. However, there are limited in vivo data suggesting a modest CYP2D6 inhibitory effect for escitalopram. Caution is indicated in the co-administration of escitalopram and drugs metabolized by CYP2D6).

No products indexed under this heading.

Chlorpropamide (In vitro studies did not reveal an inhibitory effect of escitalopram on CYP2D6. In addition, steady state levels of racemic citalopram were not significantly different in poor metabolizers and extensive CYP2D6 metabolizers after multi-dose administration of citalopram, suggesting that co-administration, with escitalopram, of a drug that inhibits CYP2D6, is unlikely to have clinically significant effects on escitalopram metabolism. However, there are limited in vivo data suggesting a modest CYP2D6 inhibitory effect for escitalopram. Caution is indicated in the co-administration of escitalopram and drugs metabolized by CYP2D6).

No products indexed under this heading.

Cimetidine (Co-administration of racemic citalopram with cimetidine has resulted in an increase in citalopram AUC and Cmax).

No products indexed under this heading.

Cimetidine Hydrochloride (Co-administration of racemic citalopram with cimetidine has resulted in an increase in citalopram AUC and Cmax).

No products indexed under this heading.

Ciprofloxacin (In vitro studies indicated that CYP3A4 and -2C19 are the primary enzymes involved in the metabolism of escitalopram. However, co-administration of escitalopram oxalate (20 mg) and ritonavir (600 mg), a potent inhibitor of CYP3A4, did not significantly affect the pharmacokinetics of escitalopram oxalate. Because escitalopram oxalate is metabolized by multiple enzyme systems, inhibition of a single enzyme may not appreciably decrease escitalopram clearance). Products include:

Cipro I.V. 2817
Cipro Oral Suspension 2810
Cipro XR Tablets 2823
Ciprodex Otic Suspension 541

Citalopram Hydrobromide (Since escitalopram is the active isomer of racemic citalopram, the two agents should not be co-administered). Products include:

Celexa 1160

Clarithromycin (In vitro studies indicated that CYP3A4 and -2C19 are the primary enzymes involved in the metabolism of escitalopram. However, co-administration of escitalopram oxalate (20 mg) and ritonavir (600 mg), a potent inhibitor of CYP3A4, did not significantly affect the pharmacokinetics of escitalopram oxalate. Because escitalopram oxalate is metabolized by multiple enzyme systems, inhibition of a single enzyme may not appreciably decrease escitalopram clearance). Products include:

Biaxin/Biaxin XL 411

Clomipramine Hydrochloride (In vitro studies did not reveal an inhibitory effect of escitalopram on CYP2D6. In addition, steady state levels of racemic citalopram were not significantly different in poor metabolizers and extensive CYP2D6 metabolizers after multi-dose administration of citalopram, suggesting that co-administration, with escitalopram, of a drug that inhibits CYP2D6, is unlikely to have clinically significant effects on escitalopram metabolism. However, there are limited in vivo data suggesting a modest CYP2D6 inhibitory effect for escitalopram. Caution is indicated in the co-administration of escitalopram and drugs metabolized by CYP2D6).

No products indexed under this heading.

Clotrimazole (In vitro studies indicated that CYP3A4 and -2C19 are the primary enzymes involved in the metabolism of escitalopram. However, co-administration of escitalopram oxalate (20 mg) and ritonavir (600 mg), a potent inhibitor of CYP3A4, did not significantly affect the pharmacokinetics of escitalopram oxalate. Because escitalopram oxalate is metabolized by multiple enzyme systems, inhibition of a single enzyme may not appreciably decrease escitalopram clearance). Products include:

Lotrisone 2881

Clozapine (In vitro studies did not reveal an inhibitory effect of escitalopram on CYP2D6. In addition, steady state levels of racemic citalopram were not significantly different in poor metabolizers and extensive CYP2D6 metabolizers after multi-dose administration of citalopram, suggesting that co-administration, with escitalopram, of a drug that inhibits CYP2D6, is unlikely to have clinically significant effects on escitalopram metabolism. However, there are limited in vivo data suggesting a modest CYP2D6 inhibitory effect for escitalopram. Caution is indicated in the co-administration of escitalopram and drugs metabolized by CYP2D6).

No products indexed under this heading.

Codeine Phosphate (In vitro studies did not reveal an inhibitory effect of escitalopram on CYP2D6. In addition, steady state levels of racemic citalopram were not significantly different in poor metabolizers and extensive CYP2D6 metabolizers after multi-dose administration of citalopram, suggesting that co-administration, with escitalopram, of a drug that inhibits CYP2D6, is unlikely to have clinically significant effects on escitalopram metabolism. However, there are limited in vivo data suggesting a modest CYP2D6 inhibitory effect for escitalopram. Caution is indicated in the co-administration of escitalopram and drugs metabolized by CYP2D6). Products include:

Tylenol with Codeine Tablets 2427

Codeine Sulfate (In vitro studies did not reveal an inhibitory effect of escitalopram on CYP2D6. In addition, steady state levels of racemic citalopram were not significantly different in poor metabolizers and extensive CYP2D6 metabolizers after multi-dose administration of citalopram, suggesting that co-administration, with escitalopram, of a drug that inhibits CYP2D6, is unlikely to have clinically significant effects on escitalopram metabolism. However, there are limited in vivo data suggesting a modest CYP2D6 inhibitory effect for escitalopram. Caution is indicated in the co-administration of escitalopram and drugs metabolized by CYP2D6).

No products indexed under this heading.

Cyclobenzaprine Hydrochloride (In vitro studies did not reveal an inhibitory effect of escitalopram on CYP2D6. In addition, steady state levels of racemic citalopram were not significantly different in poor metabolizers and extensive CYP2D6 metabolizers after multi-dose administration of citalopram, suggesting that co-administration, with escitalopram, of a drug that inhibits CYP2D6, is unlikely to have clinically significant effects on escitalopram metabolism. However, there are limited in vivo data suggesting a modest CYP2D6 inhibitory effect for escitalopram. Caution is indicated in the co-administration of escitalopram and drugs metabolized by CYP2D6). Products include:

Amrix Capsules 966

Cyclosporine (In vitro studies indicated that CYP3A4 and -2C19 are the primary enzymes involved in the metabolism of escitalopram. However, co-administration of escitalopram oxalate (20 mg) and ritonavir (600 mg), a potent inhibitor of CYP3A4, did not significantly affect the pharmacokinetics of escitalopram oxalate. Because escitalopram oxalate is metabolized by multiple enzyme systems, inhibition of a single enzyme may not appreciably decrease escitalopram clearance). Products include:

Gengraf Capsules 435
Neoral Oral Solution 2280
Neoral Soft Gelatin Capsules 2280
Restasis Ophthalmic Emulsion 557
Sandimmune 2296

Dalfopristin (In vitro studies indicated that CYP3A4 and -2C19 are the primary enzymes involved in the metabolism of escitalopram. However, co-administration of escitalopram oxalate (20 mg) and ritonavir (600 mg), a potent inhibitor of CYP3A4, did not significantly affect the pharmacokinetics of escitalopram oxalate. Because escitalopram oxalate is metabolized by multiple enzyme systems, inhibition of a single enzyme may not appreciably decrease escitalopram clearance).

No products indexed under this heading.

Dalteparin Sodium (The combined use of psychotropic drugs that interfere with serotonin reuptake and drugs that affect coagulation has been associated with an increased risk of bleeding). Products include:

Fragmin Injection 1070

Danaparoid Sodium (The combined use of psychotropic drugs that interfere with serotonin reuptake and drugs that affect coagulation has been associated with an increased risk of bleeding).

No products indexed under this heading.

Danazol (In vitro studies indicated that CYP3A4 and -2C19 are the primary enzymes involved in the metabolism of escitalopram. However, co-administration of escitalopram oxalate (20 mg) and ritonavir (600 mg), a potent inhibitor of CYP3A4, did not significantly affect the pharmacokinetics of escitalopram oxalate. Because escitalopram oxalate is metabolized by multiple enzyme systems, inhibition of a single enzyme may not appreciably decrease escitalopram clearance).

No products indexed under this heading.

Delavirdine Mesylate (In vitro studies indicated that CYP3A4 and -2C19 are the primary enzymes involved in the metabolism of escitalopram. However, co-administration of escitalopram oxalate (20 mg) and ritonavir (600 mg), a potent inhibitor of CYP3A4, did not significantly affect the pharmacokinetics of escitalopram oxalate. Because escitalopram oxalate is metabolized by multiple enzyme systems, inhibition of a single enzyme may not appreciably decrease escitalopram clearance).

No products indexed under this heading.

Desipramine Hydrochloride (Co-administration has resulted in an increase in Cmax and AUC of desipramine; the clinical significance of this finding is unknown).

No products indexed under this heading.

Desogestrel (In vitro studies indicated that CYP3A4 and -2C19 are the primary enzymes involved in the metabolism of escitalopram. However, co-administration of escitalopram oxalate (20 mg) and ritonavir (600 mg), a potent inhibitor of CYP3A4, did not significantly affect the pharmacokinetics of escitalopram oxalate. Because escitalopram oxalate is metabolized by multiple enzyme systems, inhibition of a single enzyme may not appreciably decrease escitalopram clearance). Products include:

Mircette Tablets 1034

Dexfenfluramine Hydrochloride (In vitro studies did not reveal an inhibitory effect of escitalopram on CYP2D6. In addition, steady state levels of racemic citalopram were not significantly different in poor metabolizers and extensive CYP2D6 metabolizers after multi-dose administration of citalopram, suggesting that co-administration, with escitalopram, of a drug that inhibits CYP2D6, is unlikely to have clinically significant effects on escitalopram metabolism. However, there are limited in vivo data suggesting a modest CYP2D6 inhibitory effect for escitalopram. Caution is indicated in the co-administration of escitalopram and drugs metabolized by CYP2D6).

No products indexed under this heading.

Dextromethorphan Hydrobromide (In vitro studies did not reveal an inhibitory effect of escitalopram on CYP2D6. In addition, steady state levels of racemic citalopram were not significantly different in poor metabolizers and extensive CYP2D6 metabolizers after multi-dose administration of citalopram, suggesting that co-administration, with escitalopram, of a drug that inhibits CYP2D6, is unlikely to have clinically significant effects on escitalopram metabolism. However, there are limited in vivo data suggesting a modest CYP2D6 inhibitory effect for escitalopram. Caution is indicated in the co-administration of escitalopram and drugs metabolized by CYP2D6). Products include:

PediaCare Children's Liquid Multi-Symptom Cold 1902
PediaCare Children's Long-Acting Cough 1902
Children's Sudafed PE Cold & Cough Liquid 1907
Sudafed PE Cold & Cough Caplets 1907
Children's Tylenol Plus Cough & Runny Nose Suspension Liquid 1912
Children's Tylenol Plus Cough & Sore Throat Suspension Liquid 1912
Children's Tylenol Plus Flu Suspension Liquid 1914
Children's Tylenol Plus Multi-Symptom Cold Suspension Liquid 1912
Tylenol Cold Severe Congestion Daytime Caplets with Cool Burst 1912
Tylenol Cold Head Congestion Daytime Caplets with Cool Burst 1910
Tylenol Cold Head Congestion Nighttime Caplets with Cool Burst 1910

Tylenol Cold Head Congestion Severe Daytime Caplets with Cool Burst **1910**
Tylenol Cold Multi-Symptom Daytime Caplets with Cool Burst and Rapid Release Gels **1913**
Tylenol Cold Multi-Symptom Daytime Liquid with Citrus Burst **1913**
Tylenol Cold Multi-Symptom Nighttime Caplets with Cool Burst **1913**
Tylenol Cold Multi-Symptom Nighttime Liquid with Cool Burst **1913**
Tylenol Cold Multi-Symptom Severe Caplets with Cool Burst **1913**
Tylenol Cold Multi-Symptom Severe Daytime Liquid with Citrus Burst **1913**
Tylenol Cough & Sore Throat Daytime Liquid with Cool Burst **1918**
Tylenol Cough & Sore Throat Nighttime Liquid with Cool Burst **1918**
Vicks DayQuil Cold & Flu Multi-Symptom Relief .... ▣**616**
Vicks DayQuil LiquiCaps **2567**
Vicks DayQuil Liquid **2567**
Vicks DayQuil Multi-Symptom Cold/Flu Relief **2567**
Vicks NyQuil Cold & Flu Multi-Symptom Relief .... ▣**617**
Vicks NyQuil LiquiCaps **2567**
Vicks NyQuil Liquid **2567**
Vicks NyQuil Multi-Symptom Cold/Flu Relief **2567**

Dextromethorphan Polistirex (In vitro studies did not reveal an inhibitory effect of escitalopram on CYP2D6. In addition, steady state levels of racemic citalopram were not significantly different in poor metabolizers and extensive CYP2D6 metabolizers after multi-dose administration of citalopram, suggesting that co-administration, with escitalopram, of a drug that inhibits CYP2D6, is unlikely to have clinically significant effects on escitalopram metabolism. However, there are limited in vivo data suggesting a modest CYP2D6 inhibitory effect for escitalopram. Caution is indicated in the co-administration of escitalopram and drugs metabolized by CYP2D6).
No products indexed under this heading.

Diclofenac Epolamine (The combined use of psychotropic drugs that interfere with serotonin reuptake and drugs that affect coagulation has been associated with an increased risk of bleeding; use caution when co-administering). Products include:
Flector Patch **561**

Diclofenac Potassium (The combined use of psychotropic drugs that interfere with serotonin reuptake and drugs that affect coagulation has been associated with an increased risk of bleeding; use caution when co-administering).
No products indexed under this heading.

Diclofenac Sodium (The combined use of psychotropic drugs that interfere with serotonin reuptake and drugs that affect coagulation has been associated with an increased risk of bleeding; use caution when co-administering). Products include:
Diclofenac Sodium Ophthalmic Solution .... ⊙**240**
Voltaren Ophthalmic Solution **2336**
Voltaren Tablets **2334**
Voltaren-XR Tablets **2337**

Dicumarol (The combined use of psychotropic drugs that interfere with serotonin reuptake and drugs that affect coagulation has been associated with an increased risk of bleeding).
No products indexed under this heading.

Diltiazem Hydrochloride (In vitro studies indicated that CYP3A4 and -2C19 are the primary enzymes involved in the metabolism of escitalopram. However, co-administration of escitalopram oxalate (20 mg) and ritonavir (600 mg), a potent inhibitor of CYP3A4, did not significantly affect the pharmacokinetics of escitalopram oxalate. Because escitalopram oxalate is metabolized by multiple enzyme systems, inhibition of a single enzyme may not appreciably decrease escitalopram clearance). Products include:
Cardizem LA Extended Release Tablets **421**

Diltiazem Maleate (In vitro studies indicated that CYP3A4 and -2C19 are the primary enzymes involved in the metabolism of escitalopram. However, co-administration of escitalopram oxalate (20 mg) and ritonavir (600 mg), a potent inhibitor of CYP3A4, did not significantly affect the pharmacokinetics of escitalopram oxalate. Because escitalopram oxalate is metabolized by multiple enzyme systems, inhibition of a single enzyme may not appreciably decrease escitalopram clearance).
No products indexed under this heading.

Dolasetron Mesylate (In vitro studies did not reveal an inhibitory effect of escitalopram on CYP2D6. In addition, steady state levels of racemic citalopram were not significantly different in poor metabolizers and extensive CYP2D6 metabolizers after multi-dose administration of citalopram, suggesting that co-administration, with escitalopram, of a drug that inhibits CYP2D6, is unlikely to have clinically significant effects on escitalopram metabolism. However, there are limited in vivo data suggesting a modest CYP2D6 inhibitory effect for escitalopram. Caution is indicated in the co-administration of escitalopram and drugs metabolized by CYP2D6). Products include:
Anzemet Injection **2701**
Anzemet Tablets **2704**

Donepezil Hydrochloride (In vitro studies did not reveal an inhibitory effect of escitalopram on CYP2D6. In addition, steady state levels of racemic citalopram were not significantly different in poor metabolizers and extensive CYP2D6 metabolizers after multi-dose administration of citalopram, suggesting that co-administration, with escitalopram, of a drug that inhibits CYP2D6, is unlikely to have clinically significant effects on escitalopram metabolism. However, there are limited in vivo data suggesting a modest CYP2D6 inhibitory effect for escitalopram. Caution is indicated in the co-administration of escitalopram and drugs metabolized by CYP2D6). Products include:
Aricept Tablets **1062**
Aricept ODT Tablets **1062**

Doxepin Hydrochloride (In vitro studies did not reveal an inhibitory effect of escitalopram on CYP2D6. In addition, steady state levels of racemic citalopram were not significantly different in poor metabolizers and extensive CYP2D6 metabolizers after multi-dose administration of citalopram, suggesting that co-administration, with escitalopram, of a drug that inhibits CYP2D6, is unlikely to have clinically significant effects on escitalopram metabolism. However, there are limited in vivo data suggesting a modest CYP2D6 inhibitory effect for escitalopram. Caution is indicated in the co-administration of escitalopram and drugs metabolized by CYP2D6).
No products indexed under this heading.

Efavirenz (In vitro studies indicated that CYP3A4 and -2C19 are the primary enzymes involved in the metabolism of escitalopram. However, co-administration of escitalopram oxalate (20 mg) and ritonavir (600 mg), a potent inhibitor of CYP3A4, did not significantly affect the pharmacokinetics of escitalopram oxalate. Because escitalopram oxalate is metabolized by multiple enzyme systems, inhibition of a single enzyme may not appreciably decrease escitalopram clearance). Products include:
Atripla Tablets **938**
Sustiva Capsules **930**
Sustiva Tablets **930**

Eletriptan Hydrobromide (There have been rare post-marketing reports of serotonin syndrome with use of a SSRI and a triptan. If concomitant treatment of escitalopram oxalate with a triptan is clinically warranted, careful observation of the patient is advised, particularly during treatment initiation and dose increases).
No products indexed under this heading.

Encainide Hydrochloride (In vitro studies did not reveal an inhibitory effect of escitalopram on CYP2D6. In addition, steady state levels of racemic citalopram were not significantly different in poor metabolizers and extensive CYP2D6 metabolizers after multi-dose administration of citalopram, suggesting that co-administration, with escitalopram, of a drug that inhibits CYP2D6, is unlikely to have clinically significant effects on escitalopram metabolism. However, there are limited in vivo data suggesting a modest CYP2D6 inhibitory effect for escitalopram. Caution is indicated in the co-administration of escitalopram and drugs metabolized by CYP2D6).
No products indexed under this heading.

Enoxaparin Sodium (The combined use of psychotropic drugs that interfere with serotonin reuptake and drugs that affect coagulation has been associated with an increased risk of bleeding). Products include:
Lovenox Injection **2756**

Erythromycin (In vitro studies indicated that CYP3A4 and -2C19 are the primary enzymes involved in the metabolism of escitalopram. However, co-administration of escitalopram oxalate (20 mg) and ritonavir (600 mg), a potent inhibitor of CYP3A4, did not significantly affect the pharmacokinetics of escitalopram oxalate. Because escitalopram oxalate is metabolized by multiple enzyme systems, inhibition of a single enzyme may not appreciably decrease escitalopram clearance).
No products indexed under this heading.

Erythromycin Estolate (In vitro studies indicated that CYP3A4 and -2C19 are the primary enzymes involved in the metabolism of escitalopram. However, co-administration of escitalopram oxalate (20 mg) and ritonavir (600 mg), a potent inhibitor of CYP3A4, did not significantly affect the pharmacokinetics of escitalopram oxalate. Because escitalopram oxalate is metabolized by multiple enzyme systems, inhibition of a single enzyme may not appreciably decrease escitalopram clearance).
No products indexed under this heading.

Erythromycin Ethylsuccinate (In vitro studies indicated that CYP3A4 and -2C19 are the primary enzymes involved in the metabolism of escitalopram. However, co-administration of escitalopram oxalate (20 mg) and ritonavir (600 mg), a potent inhibitor of CYP3A4, did not significantly affect the pharmacokinetics of escitalopram oxalate. Because escitalopram oxalate is metabolized by multiple enzyme systems, inhibition of a single enzyme may not appreciably decrease escitalopram clearance). Products include:
E.E.S. **433**
EryPed **431**

Erythromycin Gluceptate (In vitro studies indicated that CYP3A4 and -2C19 are the primary enzymes involved in the metabolism of escitalopram. However, co-administration of escitalopram oxalate (20 mg) and ritonavir (600 mg), a potent inhibitor of CYP3A4, did not significantly affect the pharmacokinetics of escitalopram oxalate. Because escitalopram oxalate is metabolized by multiple enzyme systems, inhibition of a single enzyme may not appreciably decrease escitalopram clearance).
No products indexed under this heading.

Erythromycin Lactobionate (In vitro studies indicated that CYP3A4 and -2C19 are the primary enzymes involved in the metabolism of escitalopram. However, co-administration of escitalopram oxalate (20 mg) and ritonavir (600 mg), a potent inhibitor of CYP3A4, did not significantly affect the pharmacokinetics of escitalopram oxalate. Because escitalopram oxalate is metabolized by multiple enzyme systems, inhibition of a single enzyme may not appreciably decrease escitalopram clearance).
No products indexed under this heading.

Erythromycin Stearate (In vitro studies indicated that CYP3A4 and -2C19 are the primary enzymes involved in the metabolism of escitalopram. However, co-administration of escitalopram oxalate (20 mg) and ritonavir (600 mg), a potent inhibitor of CYP3A4, did not significantly affect the pharmacokinetics of escitalopram oxalate. Because escitalopram oxalate is metabolized by multiple enzyme systems, inhibition of a single enzyme may not appreciably decrease escitalopram clearance).
No products indexed under this heading.

Esomeprazole Magnesium (In vitro studies indicated that CYP3A4 and -2C19 are the primary enzymes involved in the metabolism of escitalopram. However, co-administration of escitalopram oxalate (20 mg) and ritonavir (600 mg), a potent inhibitor of CYP3A4, did not significantly affect the pharmacokinetics of escitalopram oxalate. Because escitalopram oxalate is metabolized by multiple enzyme systems, inhibition of a single enzyme may not appreciably decrease escitalopram clearance). Products include:

Nexium Delayed-Release Capsules 645
Nexium Delayed-Release Oral Suspension 645

Ethinyl Estradiol (In vitro studies indicated that CYP3A4 and -2C19 are the primary enzymes involved in the metabolism of escitalopram. However, co-administration of escitalopram oxalate (20 mg) and ritonavir (600 mg), a potent inhibitor of CYP3A4, did not significantly affect the pharmacokinetics of escitalopram oxalate. Because escitalopram oxalate is metabolized by multiple enzyme systems, inhibition of a single enzyme may not appreciably decrease escitalopram clearance). Products include:

Lybrel Tablets 3204
Mircette Tablets 1034
NuvaRing 2897
Ortho-Cyclen/Ortho Tri-Cyclen 2449
Ortho Evra Transdermal System 2437
Ortho Tri-Cyclen Lo Tablets 2458
Seasonique Tablets 1046
Yaz Tablets 805

Ethynodiol Diacetate (In vitro studies indicated that CYP3A4 and -2C19 are the primary enzymes involved in the metabolism of escitalopram. However, co-administration of escitalopram oxalate (20 mg) and ritonavir (600 mg), a potent inhibitor of CYP3A4, did not significantly affect the pharmacokinetics of escitalopram oxalate. Because escitalopram oxalate is metabolized by multiple enzyme systems, inhibition of a single enzyme may not appreciably decrease escitalopram clearance).

No products indexed under this heading.

Etodolac (The combined use of psychotropic drugs that interfere with serotonin reuptake and drugs that affect coagulation has been associated with an increased risk of bleeding; use caution when co-administering).

No products indexed under this heading.

Felbamate (In vitro studies indicated that CYP3A4 and -2C19 are the primary enzymes involved in the metabolism of escitalopram. However, co-administration of escitalopram oxalate (20 mg) and ritonavir (600 mg), a potent inhibitor of CYP3A4, did not significantly affect the pharmacokinetics of escitalopram oxalate. Because escitalopram oxalate is metabolized by multiple enzyme systems, inhibition of a single enzyme may not appreciably decrease escitalopram clearance).

No products indexed under this heading.

Fenoprofen Calcium (The combined use of psychotropic drugs that interfere with serotonin reuptake and drugs that affect coagulation has been associated with an increased risk of bleeding; use caution when co-administering). Products include:

Nalfon Capsules 2508

Fentanyl (In vitro studies did not reveal an inhibitory effect of escitalopram on CYP2D6. In addition, steady state levels of racemic citalopram were not significantly different in poor metabolizers and extensive CYP2D6 metabolizers after multi-dose administration of citalopram, suggesting that co-administration, with escitalopram, of a drug that inhibits CYP2D6, is unlikely to have clinically significant effects on escitalopram metabolism. However, there are limited in vivo data suggesting a modest CYP2D6 inhibitory effect for escitalopram. Caution is indicated in the co-administration of escitalopram and drugs metabolized by CYP2D6). Products include:

Duragesic Transdermal System 2405
Ionsys Transdermal System 2410

Fentanyl Citrate (In vitro studies did not reveal an inhibitory effect of escitalopram on CYP2D6. In addition, steady state levels of racemic citalopram were not significantly different in poor metabolizers and extensive CYP2D6 metabolizers after multi-dose administration of citalopram, suggesting that co-administration, with escitalopram, of a drug that inhibits CYP2D6, is unlikely to have clinically significant effects on escitalopram metabolism. However, there are limited in vivo data suggesting a modest CYP2D6 inhibitory effect for escitalopram. Caution is indicated in the co-administration of escitalopram and drugs metabolized by CYP2D6). Products include:

Actiq 959
Fentora Tablets 968

Flecainide Acetate (In vitro studies did not reveal an inhibitory effect of escitalopram on CYP2D6. In addition, steady state levels of racemic citalopram were not significantly different in poor metabolizers and extensive CYP2D6 metabolizers after multi-dose administration of citalopram, suggesting that co-administration, with escitalopram, of a drug that inhibits CYP2D6, is unlikely to have clinically significant effects on escitalopram metabolism. However, there are limited in vivo data suggesting a modest CYP2D6 inhibitory effect for escitalopram. Caution is indicated in the co-administration of escitalopram and drugs metabolized by CYP2D6).

No products indexed under this heading.

Fluconazole (In vitro studies indicated that CYP3A4 and -2C19 are the primary enzymes involved in the metabolism of escitalopram. However, co-administration of escitalopram oxalate (20 mg) and ritonavir (600 mg), a potent inhibitor of CYP3A4, did not significantly affect the pharmacokinetics of escitalopram oxalate. Because escitalopram oxalate is metabolized by multiple enzyme systems, inhibition of a single enzyme may not appreciably decrease escitalopram clearance).

No products indexed under this heading.

Fluoxetine (In vitro studies did not reveal an inhibitory effect of escitalopram on CYP2D6. In addition, steady state levels of racemic citalopram were not significantly different in poor metabolizers and extensive CYP2D6 metabolizers after multi-dose administration of citalopram, suggesting that co-administration, with escitalopram, of a drug that inhibits CYP2D6, is unlikely to have clinically significant effects on escitalopram metabolism. However, there are limited in vivo data suggesting a modest CYP2D6 inhibitory effect for escitalopram. Caution is indicated in the co-administration of escitalopram and drugs metabolized by CYP2D6).

No products indexed under this heading.

Fluoxetine Hydrochloride (Development of a potentially life-threatening serotonin syndrome may occur with SSRIs, particularly with concomitant use of serotinergic drugs, including triptans. Caution is advised when escitalopram oxalate is co-administered with other drugs that may affect the serotinergic neurotransmitter systems). Products include:

Prozac Weekly Capsules 1852
Prozac Pulvules and Liquid 1852
Symbyax Capsules 1871

Fluphenazine Decanoate (In vitro studies did not reveal an inhibitory effect of escitalopram on CYP2D6. In addition, steady state levels of racemic citalopram were not significantly different in poor metabolizers and extensive CYP2D6 metabolizers after multi-dose administration of citalopram, suggesting that co-administration, with escitalopram, of a drug that inhibits CYP2D6, is unlikely to have clinically significant effects on escitalopram metabolism. However, there are limited in vivo data suggesting a modest CYP2D6 inhibitory effect for escitalopram. Caution is indicated in the co-administration of escitalopram and drugs metabolized by CYP2D6).

No products indexed under this heading.

Fluphenazine Enanthate (In vitro studies did not reveal an inhibitory effect of escitalopram on CYP2D6. In addition, steady state levels of racemic citalopram were not significantly different in poor metabolizers and extensive CYP2D6 metabolizers after multi-dose administration of citalopram, suggesting that co-administration, with escitalopram, of a drug that inhibits CYP2D6, is unlikely to have clinically significant effects on escitalopram metabolism. However, there are limited in vivo data suggesting a modest CYP2D6 inhibitory effect for escitalopram. Caution is indicated in the co-administration of escitalopram and drugs metabolized by CYP2D6).

No products indexed under this heading.

Fluphenazine Hydrochloride (In vitro studies did not reveal an inhibitory effect of escitalopram on CYP2D6. In addition, steady state levels of racemic citalopram were not significantly different in poor metabolizers and extensive CYP2D6 metabolizers after multi-dose administration of citalopram, suggesting that co-administration, with escitalopram, of a drug that inhibits CYP2D6, is unlikely to have clinically significant effects on escitalopram metabolism. However, there are limited in vivo data suggesting a modest CYP2D6 inhibitory effect for escitalopram. Caution is indicated in the co-administration of escitalopram and drugs metabolized by CYP2D6).

No products indexed under this heading.

Flurbiprofen (The combined use of psychotropic drugs that interfere with serotonin reuptake and drugs that affect coagulation has been associated with an increased risk of bleeding; use caution when co-administering).

No products indexed under this heading.

Fluvastatin Sodium (In vitro studies indicated that CYP3A4 and -2C19 are the primary enzymes involved in the metabolism of escitalopram. However, co-administration of escitalopram oxalate (20 mg) and ritonavir (600 mg), a potent inhibitor of CYP3A4, did not significantly affect the pharmacokinetics of escitalopram oxalate. Because escitalopram oxalate is metabolized by multiple enzyme systems, inhibition of a single enzyme may not appreciably decrease escitalopram clearance). Products include:

Lescol Capsules 2268
Lescol XL Tablets 2268

Fluvoxamine (In vitro studies indicated that CYP3A4 and -2C19 are the primary enzymes involved in the metabolism of escitalopram. However, co-administration of escitalopram oxalate (20 mg) and ritonavir (600 mg), a potent inhibitor of CYP3A4, did not significantly affect the pharmacokinetics of escitalopram oxalate. Because escitalopram oxalate is metabolized by multiple enzyme systems, inhibition of a single enzyme may not appreciably decrease escitalopram clearance).

No products indexed under this heading.

Fluvoxamine Maleate (Development of a potentially life-threatening serotonin syndrome may occur with SSRIs, particularly with concomitant use of serotinergic drugs, including triptans. Caution is advised when escitalopram oxalate is co-administered with other drugs that may affect the serotinergic neurotransmitter systems). Products include:

Luvox CR Extended-Release Capsules 1759

Fondaparinux Sodium (The combined use of psychotropic drugs that interfere with serotonin reuptake and drugs that affect coagulation has been associated with an increased risk of bleeding). Products include:

Arixtra Injection 1313

Formoterol Fumarate (In vitro studies did not reveal an inhibitory effect of escitalopram on CYP2D6. In addition, steady state levels of racemic citalopram were not significantly different in poor metabolizers and extensive CYP2D6 metabolizers after multi-dose administration of citalopram, suggesting that co-administration, with escitalopram, of a drug that inhibits CYP2D6, is unlikely to have clinically significant effects on escitalopram metabolism. However, there are limited in vivo data suggesting a modest CYP2D6 inhibitory effect for escitalopram. Caution is indicated in the co-administration of escitalopram and drugs metabolized by CYP2D6). Products include:

Foradil Aerolizer 2849
Perforomist Inhalation Solution 1025

Fosamprenavir Calcium (In vitro studies indicated that CYP3A4 and -2C19 are the primary enzymes involved in the metabolism of escitalopram. However, co-administration of escitalopram oxalate (20 mg) and ritonavir (600 mg), a potent inhibitor of CYP3A4, did not significantly affect the pharmacokinetics of escitalopram oxalate. Because escitalopram oxalate is metabolized by multiple enzyme systems, inhibition of a single enzyme may not appreciably decrease escitalopram clearance). Products include:

Lexiva Oral Suspension **1510**
Lexiva Tablets **1510**

Frovatriptan Succinate (There have been rare post-marketing reports of serotonin syndrome with use of a SSRI and a triptan. If concomitant treatment of escitalopram oxalate with a triptan is clinically warranted, careful observation of the patient is advised, particularly during treatment initiation and dose increases). Products include:

Frova Tablets **1111**

Galantamine Hydrobromide (In vitro studies did not reveal an inhibitory effect of escitalopram on CYP2D6. In addition, steady state levels of racemic citalopram were not significantly different in poor metabolizers and extensive CYP2D6 metabolizers after multi-dose administration of citalopram, suggesting that co-administration, with escitalopram, of a drug that inhibits CYP2D6, is unlikely to have clinically significant effects on escitalopram metabolism. However, there are limited in vivo data suggesting a modest CYP2D6 inhibitory effect for escitalopram. Caution is indicated in the co-administration of escitalopram and drugs metabolized by CYP2D6).

No products indexed under this heading.

Haloperidol (In vitro studies did not reveal an inhibitory effect of escitalopram on CYP2D6. In addition, steady state levels of racemic citalopram were not significantly different in poor metabolizers and extensive CYP2D6 metabolizers after multi-dose administration of citalopram, suggesting that co-administration, with escitalopram, of a drug that inhibits CYP2D6, is unlikely to have clinically significant effects on escitalopram metabolism. However, there are limited in vivo data suggesting a modest CYP2D6 inhibitory effect for escitalopram. Caution is indicated in the co-administration of escitalopram and drugs metabolized by CYP2D6).

No products indexed under this heading.

Haloperidol Decanoate (In vitro studies did not reveal an inhibitory effect of escitalopram on CYP2D6. In addition, steady state levels of racemic citalopram were not significantly different in poor metabolizers and extensive CYP2D6 metabolizers after multi-dose administration of citalopram, suggesting that co-administration, with escitalopram, of a drug that inhibits CYP2D6, is unlikely to have clinically significant effects on escitalopram metabolism. However, there are limited in vivo data suggesting a modest CYP2D6 inhibitory effect for escitalopram. Caution is indicated in the co-administration of escitalopram and drugs metabolized by CYP2D6).

No products indexed under this heading.

Heparin Calcium (The combined use of psychotropic drugs that interfere with serotonin reuptake and drugs that affect coagulation has been associated with an increased risk of bleeding).

No products indexed under this heading.

Heparin Sodium (The combined use of psychotropic drugs that interfere with serotonin reuptake and drugs that affect coagulation has been associated with an increased risk of bleeding).

No products indexed under this heading.

Hydrocodone Bitartrate (In vitro studies did not reveal an inhibitory effect of escitalopram on CYP2D6. In addition, steady state levels of racemic citalopram were not significantly different in poor metabolizers and extensive CYP2D6 metabolizers after multi-dose administration of citalopram, suggesting that co-administration, with escitalopram, of a drug that inhibits CYP2D6, is unlikely to have clinically significant effects on escitalopram metabolism. However, there are limited in vivo data suggesting a modest CYP2D6 inhibitory effect for escitalopram. Caution is indicated in the co-administration of escitalopram and drugs metabolized by CYP2D6). Products include:

Lortab 5/500 Tablets **3143**
Lortab 7.5/500 Tablets **3144**
Lortab 10/500 Tablets **3144**
Vicodin Tablets **529**
Vicodin ES Tablets **530**
Vicodin HP Tablets **531**
Vicoprofen Tablets **533**
Zydone Tablets **1132**

Hypericum (There is a risk of serotonin syndrome with concomitant use of escitalopram oxalate and tramadol. Caution is advised when escitalopram oxalate is co-administered with other drugs that may affect the serotinergic neurotransmitter systems, such as St. John's Wort). Products include:

Satieté Tablets .... ▣**640**

Ibuprofen (The combined use of psychotropic drugs that interfere with serotonin reuptake and drugs that affect coagulation has been associated with an increased risk of bleeding; use caution when co-administering). Products include:

Motrin IB Tablets and Caplets **1900**
Children's Motrin Oral Suspension ... **1901**
Children's Motrin Non-Staining Dye-Free Oral Suspension............ **1901**
Children's Motrin Cold Oral Suspension **1899**
Infants' Motrin Concentrated Drops.. **1901**
Infants' Motrin Non-Staining Dye-Free Concentrated Drops....... **1901**
Junior Strength Motrin Caplets and Chewable Tablets.................. **1901**
Vicoprofen Tablets **533**

Imipramine Hydrochloride (In vitro studies did not reveal an inhibitory effect of escitalopram on CYP2D6. In addition, steady state levels of racemic citalopram were not significantly different in poor metabolizers and extensive CYP2D6 metabolizers after multi-dose administration of citalopram, suggesting that co-administration, with escitalopram, of a drug that inhibits CYP2D6, is unlikely to have clinically significant effects on escitalopram metabolism. However, there are limited in vivo data suggesting a modest CYP2D6 inhibitory effect for escitalopram. Caution is indicated in the co-administration of escitalopram and drugs metabolized by CYP2D6).

No products indexed under this heading.

Imipramine Pamoate (In vitro studies did not reveal an inhibitory effect of escitalopram on CYP2D6. In addition, steady state levels of racemic citalopram were not significantly different in poor metabolizers and extensive CYP2D6 metabolizers after multi-dose administration of citalopram, suggesting that co-administration, with escitalopram, of a drug that inhibits CYP2D6, is unlikely to have clinically significant effects on escitalopram metabolism. However, there are limited in vivo data suggesting a modest CYP2D6 inhibitory effect for escitalopram. Caution is indicated in the co-administration of escitalopram and drugs metabolized by CYP2D6).

No products indexed under this heading.

Indinavir Sulfate (In vitro studies indicated that CYP3A4 and -2C19 are the primary enzymes involved in the metabolism of escitalopram. However, co-administration of escitalopram oxalate (20 mg) and ritonavir (600 mg), a potent inhibitor of CYP3A4, did not significantly affect the pharmacokinetics of escitalopram oxalate. Because escitalopram oxalate is metabolized by multiple enzyme systems, inhibition of a single enzyme may not appreciably decrease escitalopram clearance). Products include:

Crixivan Capsules **1979**

Indomethacin (The combined use of psychotropic drugs that interfere with serotonin reuptake and drugs that affect coagulation has been associated with an increased risk of bleeding; use caution when co-administering). Products include:

Indocin **2024**

Indomethacin Sodium Trihydrate (The combined use of psychotropic drugs that interfere with serotonin reuptake and drugs that affect coagulation has been associated with an increased risk of bleeding; use caution when co-administering). Products include:

Indocin I.V. **2489**

Indoramin Hydrochloride (In vitro studies did not reveal an inhibitory effect of escitalopram on CYP2D6. In addition, steady state levels of racemic citalopram were not significantly different in poor metabolizers and extensive CYP2D6 metabolizers after multi-dose administration of citalopram, suggesting that co-administration, with escitalopram, of a drug that inhibits CYP2D6, is unlikely to have clinically significant effects on escitalopram metabolism. However, there are limited in vivo data suggesting a modest CYP2D6 inhibitory effect for escitalopram. Caution is indicated in the co-administration of escitalopram and drugs metabolized by CYP2D6).

No products indexed under this heading.

Isocarboxazid (Co-administration of SSRIs and MAO inhibitors has resulted in serious, sometimes fatal, reactions including hyperthermia, rigidity, myoclonus, autonomic instability, agitation progressing to delirium serotonin syndrome and coma; concurrent and/or sequential use is contraindicated). Products include:

Marplan Tablets **3177**

Isoniazid (In vitro studies indicated that CYP3A4 and -2C19 are the primary enzymes involved in the metabolism of escitalopram. However, co-administration of escitalopram oxalate (20 mg) and ritonavir (600 mg), a potent inhibitor of CYP3A4, did not significantly affect the pharmacokinetics of escitalopram oxalate. Because escitalopram oxalate is metabolized by multiple enzyme systems, inhibition of a single enzyme may not appreciably decrease escitalopram clearance).

No products indexed under this heading.

Itraconazole (In vitro studies indicated that CYP3A4 and -2C19 are the primary enzymes involved in the metabolism of escitalopram. However, co-administration of escitalopram oxalate (20 mg) and ritonavir (600 mg), a potent inhibitor of CYP3A4, did not significantly affect the pharmacokinetics of escitalopram oxalate. Because escitalopram oxalate is metabolized by multiple enzyme systems, inhibition of a single enzyme may not appreciably decrease escitalopram clearance).

No products indexed under this heading.

Ketoconazole (Co-administration of racemic citalopram and ketoconazole resulted in decrease in Cmax and AUC of ketoconazole). Products include:

Extina Foam, 2% **3057**
Nizoral A-D Shampoo **1901**

Ketoprofen (The combined use of psychotropic drugs that interfere with serotonin reuptake and drugs that affect coagulation has been associated with an increased risk of bleeding; use caution when co-administering).

No products indexed under this heading.

Ketorolac Tromethamine (The combined use of psychotropic drugs that interfere with serotonin reuptake and drugs that affect coagulation has been associated with an increased risk of bleeding; use caution when co-administering).

No products indexed under this heading.

Labetalol Hydrochloride (In vitro studies did not reveal an inhibitory effect of escitalopram on CYP2D6. In addition, steady state levels of racemic citalopram were not significantly different in poor metabolizers and extensive CYP2D6 metabolizers after multi-dose administration of citalopram, suggesting that co-administration, with escitalopram, of a drug that inhibits CYP2D6, is unlikely to have clinically significant effects on escitalopram metabolism. However, there are limited in vivo data suggesting a modest CYP2D6 inhibitory effect for escitalopram. Caution is indicated in the co-administration of escitalopram and drugs metabolized by CYP2D6).

No products indexed under this heading.

Lansoprazole (In vitro studies indicated that CYP3A4 and -2C19 are the primary enzymes involved in the metabolism of escitalopram. However, co-administration of escitalopram oxalate (20 mg) and ritonavir

(600 mg), a potent inhibitor of CYP3A4, did not significantly affect the pharmacokinetics of escitalopram oxalate. Because escitalopram oxalate is metabolized by multiple enzyme systems, inhibition of a single enzyme may not appreciably decrease escitalopram clearance).

No products indexed under this heading.

Letrozole (In vitro studies indicated that CYP3A4 and -2C19 are the primary enzymes involved in the metabolism of escitalopram. However, co-administration of escitalopram oxalate (20 mg) and ritonavir (600 mg), a potent inhibitor of CYP3A4, did not significantly affect the pharmacokinetics of escitalopram oxalate. Because escitalopram oxalate is metabolized by multiple enzyme systems, inhibition of a single enzyme may not appreciably decrease escitalopram clearance). Products include:

Femara Tablets 2246

Levonorgestrel (In vitro studies indicated that CYP3A4 and -2C19 are the primary enzymes involved in the metabolism of escitalopram. However, co-administration of escitalopram oxalate (20 mg) and ritonavir (600 mg), a potent inhibitor of CYP3A4, did not significantly affect the pharmacokinetics of escitalopram oxalate. Because escitalopram oxalate is metabolized by multiple enzyme systems, inhibition of a single enzyme may not appreciably decrease escitalopram clearance). Products include:

Climara Pro Transdermal System 768
Lybrel Tablets 3204
Mirena Intrauterine System 779
Plan B Tablets 1044
Seasonique Tablets 1046

Lidocaine (In vitro studies did not reveal an inhibitory effect of escitalopram on CYP2D6. In addition, steady state levels of racemic citalopram were not significantly different in poor metabolizers and extensive CYP2D6 metabolizers after multi-dose administration of citalopram, suggesting that co-administration, with escitalopram, of a drug that inhibits CYP2D6, is unlikely to have clinically significant effects on escitalopram metabolism. However, there are limited in vivo data suggesting a modest CYP2D6 inhibitory effect for escitalopram. Caution is indicated in the co-administration of escitalopram and drugs metabolized by CYP2D6). Products include:

Lidoderm Patch 1114

Lidocaine Hydrochloride (In vitro studies did not reveal an inhibitory effect of escitalopram on CYP2D6. In addition, steady state levels of racemic citalopram were not significantly different in poor metabolizers and extensive CYP2D6 metabolizers after multi-dose administration of citalopram, suggesting that co-administration, with escitalopram, of a drug that inhibits CYP2D6, is unlikely to have clinically significant effects on escitalopram metabolism. However, there are limited in vivo data suggesting a modest CYP2D6 inhibitory effect for escitalopram. Caution is indicated in the co-administration of escitalopram and drugs metabolized by CYP2D6).

No products indexed under this heading.

Linezolid (There is a risk of serotonin syndrome with concomitant use of escitalopram oxalate and tramadol. Caution is advised when escitalopram oxalate is co-administered with other drugs that may affect the serotinergic neurotransmitter systems, such as linezolid). Products include:

Zyvox 2552

Lithium (There is a risk of serotonin syndrome with concomitant use of escitalopram oxalate and tramadol. Caution is advised when escitalopram oxalate is co-administration with other drugs that may affect the serotinergic neurotransmitter systems, such as lithium as it may enhance serotinergic effects of escitalopram).

No products indexed under this heading.

Lithium Carbonate (There is a risk of serotonin syndrome with concomitant use of escitalopram oxalate and tramadol. Caution is advised when escitalopram oxalate is co-administration with other drugs that may affect the serotinergic neurotransmitter systems, such as lithium as it may enhance serotinergic effects of escitalopram).

No products indexed under this heading.

Lithium Citrate (There is a risk of serotonin syndrome with concomitant use of escitalopram oxalate and tramadol. Caution is advised when escitalopram oxalate is co-administration with other drugs that may affect the serotinergic neurotransmitter systems, such as lithium as it may enhance serotinergic effects of escitalopram).

No products indexed under this heading.

Lopinavir (In vitro studies indicated that CYP3A4 and -2C19 are the primary enzymes involved in the metabolism of escitalopram. However, co-administration of escitalopram oxalate (20 mg) and ritonavir (600 mg), a potent inhibitor of CYP3A4, did not significantly affect the pharmacokinetics of escitalopram oxalate. Because escitalopram oxalate is metabolized by multiple enzyme systems, inhibition of a single enzyme may not appreciably decrease escitalopram clearance). Products include:

Kaletra 452

Loratadine (In vitro studies indicated that CYP3A4 and -2C19 are the primary enzymes involved in the metabolism of escitalopram. However, co-administration of escitalopram oxalate (20 mg) and ritonavir (600 mg), a potent inhibitor of CYP3A4, did not significantly affect the pharmacokinetics of escitalopram oxalate. Because escitalopram oxalate is metabolized by multiple enzyme systems, inhibition of a single enzyme may not appreciably decrease escitalopram clearance).

No products indexed under this heading.

Low Molecular Weight Heparins (The combined use of psychotropic drugs that interfere with serotonin reuptake and drugs that affect coagulation has been associated with an increased risk of bleeding).

No products indexed under this heading.

Maprotiline Hydrochloride (In vitro studies did not reveal an inhibitory effect of escitalopram on CYP2D6. In addition, steady state levels of racemic citalopram were not significantly different in poor metabolizers and extensive CYP2D6 metabolizers after multi-dose administration of citalopram, suggesting that co-administration, with escitalopram, of a drug that inhibits CYP2D6, is unlikely to have clinically significant effects on escitalopram metabolism. However, there are limited in vivo data suggesting a modest CYP2D6 inhibitory effect for escitalopram. Caution is indicated in the co-administration of escitalopram and drugs metabolized by CYP2D6).

No products indexed under this heading.

Meclofenamate Sodium (The combined use of psychotropic drugs that interfere with serotonin reuptake and drugs that affect coagulation has been associated with an increased risk of bleeding; use caution when co-administering).

No products indexed under this heading.

Mefenamic Acid (The combined use of psychotropic drugs that interfere with serotonin reuptake and drugs that affect coagulation has been associated with an increased risk of bleeding; use caution when co-administering).

No products indexed under this heading.

Meloxicam (The combined use of psychotropic drugs that interfere with serotonin reuptake and drugs that affect coagulation has been associated with an increased risk of bleeding; use caution when co-administering). Products include:

Mobic Oral Suspension 863
Mobic Tablets 863

Meperidine Hydrochloride (In vitro studies did not reveal an inhibitory effect of escitalopram on CYP2D6. In addition, steady state levels of racemic citalopram were not significantly different in poor metabolizers and extensive CYP2D6 metabolizers after multi-dose administration of citalopram, suggesting that co-administration, with escitalopram, of a drug that inhibits CYP2D6, is unlikely to have clinically significant effects on escitalopram metabolism. However, there are limited in vivo data suggesting a modest CYP2D6 inhibitory effect for escitalopram. Caution is indicated in the co-administration of escitalopram and drugs metabolized by CYP2D6).

No products indexed under this heading.

Mestranol (In vitro studies indicated that CYP3A4 and -2C19 are the primary enzymes involved in the metabolism of escitalopram. However, co-administration of escitalopram oxalate (20 mg) and ritonavir (600 mg), a potent inhibitor of CYP3A4, did not significantly affect the pharmacokinetics of escitalopram oxalate. Because escitalopram oxalate is metabolized by multiple enzyme systems, inhibition of a single enzyme may not appreciably decrease escitalopram clearance).

No products indexed under this heading.

Methadone Hydrochloride (In vitro studies did not reveal an inhibitory effect of escitalopram on CYP2D6. In addition, steady state levels of racemic citalopram were not significantly different in poor metabolizers and extensive CYP2D6 metabolizers after multi-dose administration of citalopram, suggesting that co-administration, with escitalopram, of a drug that inhibits CYP2D6, is unlikely to have clinically significant effects on escitalopram metabolism. However, there are limited in vivo data suggesting a modest CYP2D6 inhibitory effect for escitalopram. Caution is indicated in the co-administration of escitalopram and drugs metabolized by CYP2D6).

No products indexed under this heading.

Methamphetamine Hydrochloride (In vitro studies did not reveal an inhibitory effect of escitalopram on CYP2D6. In addition, steady state levels of racemic citalopram were not significantly different in poor metabolizers and extensive CYP2D6 metabolizers after multi-dose administration of citalopram, suggesting that co-administration, with escitalopram, of a drug that inhibits CYP2D6, is unlikely to have clinically significant effects on escitalopram metabolism. However, there are limited in vivo data suggesting a modest CYP2D6 inhibitory effect for escitalopram. Caution is indicated in the co-administration of escitalopram and drugs metabolized by CYP2D6).

No products indexed under this heading.

Metoprolol Succinate (Co-administration has resulted in an increase in Cmax and AUC of metoprolol; increased metoprolol plasma levels have been associated with decreased cardioselectivity). Products include:

Toprol-XL Tablets 666

Metoprolol Tartrate (Co-administration has resulted in an increase in Cmax and AUC of metoprolol; increased metoprolol plasma levels have been associated with decreased cardioselectivity).

No products indexed under this heading.

Metronidazole (In vitro studies indicated that CYP3A4 and -2C19 are the primary enzymes involved in the metabolism of escitalopram. However, co-administration of escitalopram oxalate (20 mg) and ritonavir (600 mg), a potent inhibitor of CYP3A4, did not significantly affect the pharmacokinetics of escitalopram oxalate. Because escitalopram oxalate is metabolized by multiple enzyme systems, inhibition of a single enzyme may not appreciably decrease escitalopram clearance). Products include:

Pylera Capsules 714

Metronidazole Benzoate (In vitro studies indicated that CYP3A4 and -2C19 are the primary enzymes involved in the metabolism of escitalopram. However, co-administration of escitalopram oxalate (20 mg) and ritonavir (600 mg), a potent inhibitor of CYP3A4, did not significantly affect the pharmacokinetics of escitalopram oxalate. Because escitalopram oxalate is metabolized by multiple enzyme systems, inhibition of a single enzyme may not appreciably decrease escitalopram clearance).

No products indexed under this heading.

Metronidazole Hydrochloride (In vitro studies indicated that CYP3A4 and -2C19 are the primary enzymes involved in the metabolism of escitalopram. However, co-administration of escitalopram oxalate (20 mg) and ritonavir (600 mg), a potent inhibitor of CYP3A4, did not significantly affect the pharmacokinetics of escitalopram oxalate. Because escitalopram oxalate is metabolized by multiple enzyme systems, inhibition of a single enzyme may not appreciably decrease escitalopram clearance).

No products indexed under this heading.

Metronidazole Sodium (In vitro studies indicated that CYP3A4 and -2C19 are the primary enzymes involved in the metabolism of escitalopram. However, co-administration of escitalopram oxalate (20 mg) and ritonavir (600 mg), a potent inhibitor of CYP3A4, did not significantly affect the pharmacokinetics of escitalopram oxalate. Because escitalopram oxalate is metabolized by multiple enzyme systems, inhibition of a single enzyme may not appreciably decrease escitalopram clearance).

No products indexed under this heading.

Mexiletine Hydrochloride (In vitro studies did not reveal an inhibitory effect of escitalopram on CYP2D6. In addition, steady state levels of racemic citalopram were not significantly different in poor metabolizers and extensive CYP2D6 metabolizers after multi-dose administration of citalopram, suggesting that co-administration, with escitalopram, of a drug that inhibits CYP2D6, is unlikely to have clinically significant effects on escitalopram metabolism. However, there are limited in vivo data suggesting a modest CYP2D6 inhibitory effect for escitalopram. Caution is indicated in the co-administration of escitalopram and drugs metabolized by CYP2D6).

No products indexed under this heading.

Miconazole (In vitro studies indicated that CYP3A4 and -2C19 are the primary enzymes involved in the metabolism of escitalopram. However, co-administration of escitalopram oxalate (20 mg) and ritonavir (600 mg), a potent inhibitor of CYP3A4, did not significantly affect the pharmacokinetics of escitalopram oxalate. Because escitalopram oxalate is metabolized by multiple enzyme systems, inhibition of a single enzyme may not appreciably decrease escitalopram clearance).

No products indexed under this heading.

Miconazole Nitrate (In vitro studies indicated that CYP3A4 and -2C19 are the primary enzymes involved in the metabolism of escitalopram. However, co-administration of escitalopram oxalate (20 mg) and ritonavir (600 mg), a potent inhibitor of CYP3A4, did not significantly affect the pharmacokinetics of escitalopram oxalate. Because escitalopram oxalate is metabolized by multiple enzyme systems, inhibition of a single enzyme may not appreciably decrease escitalopram clearance).

No products indexed under this heading.

Mirtazapine (In vitro studies did not reveal an inhibitory effect of escitalopram on CYP2D6. In addition, steady state levels of racemic citalopram were not significantly different in poor metabolizers and extensive CYP2D6 metabolizers after multi-dose administration of citalopram, suggesting that co-administration, with escitalopram, of a drug that inhibits CYP2D6, is unlikely to have clinically significant effects on escitalopram metabolism. However, there are limited in vivo data suggesting a modest CYP2D6 inhibitory effect for escitalopram. Caution is indicated in the co-administration of escitalopram and drugs metabolized by CYP2D6). Products include:

Remeron Tablets **2924**
RemeronSolTab Tablets **2927**

Moclobemide (Co-administration of SSRIs and MAO inhibitors has resulted in serious, sometimes fatal, reactions including hyperthermia, rigidity, myoclonus, autonomic instability, agitation progressing to delirium serotonin syndrome and coma; concurrent and/or sequential use is contraindicated).

No products indexed under this heading.

Modafinil (In vitro studies indicated that CYP3A4 and -2C19 are the primary enzymes involved in the metabolism of escitalopram. However, co-administration of escitalopram oxalate (20 mg) and ritonavir (600 mg), a potent inhibitor of CYP3A4, did not significantly affect the pharmacokinetics of escitalopram oxalate. Because escitalopram oxalate is metabolized by multiple enzyme systems, inhibition of a single enzyme may not appreciably decrease escitalopram clearance). Products include:

Provigil Tablets **977**

Morphine Sulfate (In vitro studies did not reveal an inhibitory effect of escitalopram on CYP2D6. In addition, steady state levels of racemic citalopram were not significantly different in poor metabolizers and extensive CYP2D6 metabolizers after multi-dose administration of citalopram, suggesting that co-administration, with escitalopram, of a drug that inhibits CYP2D6, is unlikely to have clinically significant effects on escitalopram metabolism. However, there are limited in vivo data suggesting a modest CYP2D6 inhibitory effect for escitalopram. Caution is indicated in the co-administration of escitalopram and drugs metabolized by CYP2D6). Products include:

Avinza Capsules **1772**
DepoDur Injection **1095**
MS Contin Tablets **2585**

Nabumetone (The combined use of psychotropic drugs that interfere with serotonin reuptake and drugs that affect coagulation has been associated with an increased risk of bleeding; use caution when co-administering).

No products indexed under this heading.

Naproxen (The combined use of psychotropic drugs that interfere with serotonin reuptake and drugs that affect coagulation has been associated with an increased risk of bleeding; use caution when co-administering). Products include:

EC-Naprosyn Delayed-Release Tablets **2632**
Naprosyn Suspension **2632**
Naprosyn Tablets **2632**

Naproxen Sodium (The combined use of psychotropic drugs that interfere with serotonin reuptake and drugs that affect coagulation has been associated with an increased risk of bleeding; use caution when co-administering). Products include:

Anaprox Tablets **2632**
Anaprox DS Tablets **2632**
Treximet Tablets **1616**

Naratriptan Hydrochloride (There have been rare post-marketing reports of serotonin syndrome with use of a SSRI and a triptan. If concomitant treatment of escitalopram oxalate with a triptan is clinically warranted, careful observation of the patient is advised, particularly during treatment initiation and dose increases). Products include:

Amerge Tablets **1301**

Nefazodone Hydrochloride (In vitro studies indicated that CYP3A4 and -2C19 are the primary enzymes involved in the metabolism of escitalopram. However, co-administration of escitalopram oxalate (20 mg) and ritonavir (600 mg), a potent inhibitor of CYP3A4, did not significantly affect the pharmacokinetics of escitalopram oxalate. Because escitalopram oxalate is metabolized by multiple enzyme systems, inhibition of a single enzyme may not appreciably decrease escitalopram clearance).

No products indexed under this heading.

Nelfinavir Mesylate (In vitro studies did not reveal an inhibitory effect of escitalopram on CYP2D6. In addition, steady state levels of racemic citalopram were not significantly different in poor metabolizers and extensive CYP2D6 metabolizers after multi-dose administration of citalopram, suggesting that co-administration, with escitalopram, of a drug that inhibits CYP2D6, is unlikely to have clinically significant effects on escitalopram metabolism. However, there are limited in vivo data suggesting a modest CYP2D6 inhibitory effect for escitalopram. Caution is indicated in the co-administration of escitalopram and drugs metabolized by CYP2D6).

No products indexed under this heading.

Nevirapine (In vitro studies indicated that CYP3A4 and -2C19 are the primary enzymes involved in the metabolism of escitalopram. However, co-administration of escitalopram oxalate (20 mg) and ritonavir (600 mg), a potent inhibitor of CYP3A4, did not significantly affect the pharmacokinetics of escitalopram oxalate. Because escitalopram oxalate is metabolized by multiple enzyme systems, inhibition of a single enzyme may not appreciably decrease escitalopram clearance). Products include:

Viramune Oral Suspension **873**
Viramune Tablets **873**

Niacinamide (In vitro studies indicated that CYP3A4 and -2C19 are the primary enzymes involved in the metabolism of escitalopram. However, co-administration of escitalopram oxalate (20 mg) and ritonavir (600 mg), a potent inhibitor of CYP3A4, did not significantly affect the pharmacokinetics of escitalopram oxalate. Because escitalopram oxalate is metabolized by multiple enzyme systems, inhibition of a single enzyme may not appreciably decrease escitalopram clearance). Products include:

BioLean Free Tablets .... ▣ **635**

Nicotinamide (In vitro studies indicated that CYP3A4 and -2C19 are the primary enzymes involved in the metabolism of escitalopram. However, co-administration of escitalopram oxalate (20 mg) and ritonavir (600 mg), a potent inhibitor of CYP3A4, did not significantly affect the pharmacokinetics of escitalopram oxalate. Because escitalopram oxalate is metabolized by multiple enzyme systems, inhibition of a single enzyme may not appreciably decrease escitalopram clearance).

No products indexed under this heading.

Nifedipine (In vitro studies indicated that CYP3A4 and -2C19 are the primary enzymes involved in the metabolism of escitalopram. However, co-administration of escitalopram oxalate (20 mg) and ritonavir (600 mg), a potent inhibitor of CYP3A4, did not significantly affect the pharmacokinetics of escitalopram oxalate. Because escitalopram oxalate is metabolized by multiple enzyme systems, inhibition of a single enzyme may not appreciably decrease escitalopram clearance).

No products indexed under this heading.

Norethindrone (In vitro studies indicated that CYP3A4 and -2C19 are the primary enzymes involved in the metabolism of escitalopram. However, co-administration of escitalopram oxalate (20 mg) and ritonavir (600 mg), a potent inhibitor of CYP3A4, did not significantly affect the pharmacokinetics of escitalopram oxalate. Because escitalopram oxalate is metabolized by multiple enzyme systems, inhibition of a single enzyme may not appreciably decrease escitalopram clearance). Products include:

Ortho Micronor Tablets **2446**

Norethynodrel (In vitro studies indicated that CYP3A4 and -2C19 are the primary enzymes involved in the metabolism of escitalopram. However, co-administration of escitalopram oxalate (20 mg) and ritonavir (600 mg), a potent inhibitor of CYP3A4, did not significantly affect the pharmacokinetics of escitalopram oxalate. Because escitalopram oxalate is metabolized by multiple enzyme systems, inhibition of a single enzyme may not appreciably decrease escitalopram clearance).

No products indexed under this heading.

Norfloxacin (In vitro studies indicated that CYP3A4 and -2C19 are the primary enzymes involved in the metabolism of escitalopram. However, co-administration of escitalopram oxalate (20 mg) and ritonavir (600 mg), a potent inhibitor of CYP3A4, did not significantly affect the pharmacokinetics of escitalopram oxalate. Because escitalopram oxalate is metabolized by multiple enzyme systems, inhibition of a single enzyme may not appreciably decrease escitalopram clearance). Products include:

Noroxin Tablets **2069**

Norgestimate (In vitro studies indicated that CYP3A4 and -2C19 are the primary enzymes involved in the metabolism of escitalopram. However, co-administration of escitalopram oxalate (20 mg) and ritonavir (600 mg), a potent inhibitor of CYP3A4, did not significantly affect the pharmacokinetics of escitalopram oxalate. Because escitalopram oxalate is metabolized by multiple enzyme systems, inhibition of a single enzyme may not appreciably decrease escitalopram clearance). Products include:

Ortho-Cyclen/Ortho Tri-Cyclen **2449**
Ortho Tri-Cyclen Lo Tablets **2458**

Norgestrel (In vitro studies indicated that CYP3A4 and -2C19 are the primary enzymes involved in the metabolism of escitalopram. However, co-administration of escitalopram oxalate (20 mg) and ritonavir (600 mg), a potent inhibitor of CYP3A4, did not significantly affect the pharmacokinetics of escitalopram oxalate. Because escitalopram oxalate is metabolized by multiple enzyme systems, inhibition of a single enzyme may not appreciably decrease escitalopram clearance).

No products indexed under this heading.

Nortriptyline Hydrochloride (In vitro studies did not reveal an inhibitory effect of escitalopram on CYP2D6. In addition, steady state levels of racemic citalopram were not significantly different in poor metabolizers and extensive CYP2D6 metabolizers after multi-dose administration of citalopram, suggesting that co-administration, with escitalopram, of a drug that inhibits CYP2D6, is unlikely to have clinically significant effects on escitalopram metabolism. However, there are limited in vivo data suggesting a modest CYP2D6 inhibitory effect for escitalopram. Caution is indicated in the co-administration of escitalopram and drugs metabolized by CYP2D6).

No products indexed under this heading.

Olanzapine (In vitro studies did not reveal an inhibitory effect of escitalopram on CYP2D6. In addition, steady state levels of racemic citalopram were not significantly different in poor metabolizers and extensive CYP2D6 metabolizers after multi-dose administration of citalopram, suggesting that co-administration, with escitalopram, of a drug that inhibits CYP2D6, is unlikely to have clinically significant effects on escitalopram metabolism. However, there are limited in vivo data suggesting a modest CYP2D6 inhibitory effect for escitalopram. Caution is indicated in the co-administration of escitalopram and drugs metabolized by CYP2D6). Products include:

Symbyax Capsules **1871**
Zyprexa Tablets **1883**
Zyprexa IntraMuscular **1883**
Zyprexa ZYDIS Orally Disintegrating Tablets................... **1883**

Omeprazole (In vitro studies did not reveal an inhibitory effect of escitalopram on CYP2D6. In addition, steady state levels of racemic citalopram were not significantly different in poor metabolizers and extensive CYP2D6 metabolizers after multi-dose administration of citalopram, suggesting that co-administration, with escitalopram, of a drug that inhibits CYP2D6, is unlikely to have clinically significant effects on escitalopram metabolism. However, there are limited in vivo data suggesting a modest CYP2D6 inhibitory effect for escitalopram. Caution is indicated in the co-administration of escitalopram and drugs metabolized by CYP2D6).

No products indexed under this heading.

Ondansetron (In vitro studies did not reveal an inhibitory effect of escitalopram on CYP2D6. In addition, steady state levels of racemic citalopram were not significantly different in poor metabolizers and extensive CYP2D6 metabolizers after multi-dose administration of citalopram, suggesting that co-administration, with escitalopram, of a drug that inhibits CYP2D6, is unlikely to have clinically significant effects on escitalopram metabolism. However, there are limited in vivo data suggesting a modest CYP2D6 inhibitory effect for escitalopram. Caution is indicated in the co-administration of escitalopram and drugs metabolized by CYP2D6). Products include:

Zofran ODT Orally Disintegrating Tablets... **1687**

Ondansetron Hydrochloride (In vitro studies did not reveal an inhibitory effect of escitalopram on CYP2D6. In addition, steady state levels of racemic citalopram were not significantly different in poor metabolizers and extensive CYP2D6 metabolizers after multi-dose administration of citalopram, suggesting that co-administration, with escitalopram, of a drug that inhibits CYP2D6, is unlikely to have clinically significant effects on escitalopram metabolism. However, there are limited in vivo data suggesting a modest CYP2D6 inhibitory effect for escitalopram. Caution is indicated in the co-administration of escitalopram and drugs metabolized by CYP2D6). Products include:

Zofran Injection **1682**
Zofran **1687**

Oxaprozin (The combined use of psychotropic drugs that interfere with serotonin reuptake and drugs that affect coagulation has been associated with an increased risk of bleeding; use caution when co-administering).

No products indexed under this heading.

Oxcarbazepine (In vitro studies indicated that CYP3A4 and -2C19 are the primary enzymes involved in the metabolism of escitalopram. However, co-administration of escitalopram oxalate (20 mg) and ritonavir (600 mg), a potent inhibitor of CYP3A4, did not significantly affect the pharmacokinetics of escitalopram oxalate. Because escitalopram oxalate is metabolized by multiple enzyme systems, inhibition of a single enzyme may not appreciably decrease escitalopram clearance).

No products indexed under this heading.

Oxycodone Hydrochloride (In vitro studies did not reveal an inhibitory effect of escitalopram on CYP2D6. In addition, steady state levels of racemic citalopram were not significantly different in poor metabolizers and extensive CYP2D6 metabolizers after multi-dose administration of citalopram, suggesting that co-administration, with escitalopram, of a drug that inhibits CYP2D6, is unlikely to have clinically significant effects on escitalopram metabolism. However, there are limited in vivo data suggesting a modest CYP2D6 inhibitory effect for escitalopram. Caution is indicated in the co-administration of escitalopram and drugs metabolized by CYP2D6). Products include:

OxyContin Tablets **2589**
OxyIR Capsules **2593**
Percocet Tablets **1127**
Percodan Tablets **1130**

Paclitaxel (In vitro studies did not reveal an inhibitory effect of escitalopram on CYP2D6. In addition, steady state levels of racemic citalopram were not significantly different in poor metabolizers and extensive CYP2D6 metabolizers after multi-dose administration of citalopram, suggesting that co-administration, with escitalopram, of a drug that inhibits CYP2D6, is unlikely to have clinically significant effects on escitalopram metabolism. However, there are limited in vivo data suggesting a modest CYP2D6 inhibitory effect for escitalopram. Caution is indicated in the co-administration of escitalopram and drugs metabolized by CYP2D6).

No products indexed under this heading.

Pargyline Hydrochloride (Co-administration of SSRIs and MAO inhibitors has resulted in serious, sometimes fatal, reactions including hyperthermia, rigidity, myoclonus, autonomic instability, agitation progressing to delirium serotonin syndrome and coma; concurrent and/or sequential use is contraindicated).

No products indexed under this heading.

Paroxetine Hydrochloride (Development of a potentially life-threatening serotonin syndrome may occur with SSRIs, particularly with concomitant use of serotinergic drugs, including triptans. Caution is advised when escitalopram oxalate is co-administered with other drugs that may affect the serotinergic neurotransmitter systems). Products include:

Paxil **1535**
Paxil CR Controlled-Release Tablets **1544**

Phenelzine Sulfate (Co-administration of SSRIs and MAO inhibitors has resulted in serious, sometimes fatal, reactions including hyperthermia, rigidity, myoclonus, autonomic instability, agitation progressing to delirium serotonin syndrome and coma; concurrent and/or sequential use is contraindicated).

No products indexed under this heading.

Phenylbutazone (The combined use of psychotropic drugs that interfere with serotonin reuptake and drugs that affect coagulation has been associated with an increased risk of bleeding; use caution when co-administering).

No products indexed under this heading.

Pimozide (In a controlled study, a single dose of pimozide 2 mg co-administered with citalopram 40 mg given once daily for 11 days was associated with a mean increase in QTc values of approximately 10 msec. compared to pimozide given alone).

No products indexed under this heading.

Pindolol (In vitro studies did not reveal an inhibitory effect of escitalopram on CYP2D6. In addition, steady state levels of racemic citalopram were not significantly different in poor metabolizers and extensive CYP2D6 metabolizers after multi-dose administration of citalopram, suggesting that co-administration, with escitalopram, of a drug that inhibits CYP2D6, is unlikely to have clinically significant effects on escitalopram metabolism. However, there are limited in vivo data suggesting a modest CYP2D6 inhibitory effect for escitalopram. Caution is indicated in the co-administration of escitalopram and drugs metabolized by CYP2D6).

No products indexed under this heading.

Piroxicam (The combined use of psychotropic drugs that interfere with serotonin reuptake and drugs that affect coagulation has been associated with an increased risk of bleeding; use caution when co-administering).

No products indexed under this heading.

Procarbazine Hydrochloride (Co-administration of SSRIs and MAO inhibitors has resulted in serious, sometimes fatal, reactions including hyperthermia, rigidity, myoclonus, autonomic instability, agitation progressing to delirium serotonin syndrome and coma; concurrent and/or sequential use is contraindicated).

No products indexed under this heading.

Propafenone Hydrochloride (In vitro studies did not reveal an inhibitory effect of escitalopram on CYP2D6. In addition, steady state levels of racemic citalopram were not significantly different in poor metabolizers and extensive CYP2D6 metabolizers after multi-dose administration of citalopram, suggesting that co-administration, with escitalopram, of a drug that inhibits CYP2D6, is unlikely to have clinically significant effects on escitalopram metabolism. However, there are limited in vivo data suggesting a modest CYP2D6 inhibitory effect for escitalopram. Caution is indicated in the co-administration of escitalopram and drugs metabolized by CYP2D6). Products include:

Rythmol Tablets **1586**
Rythmol SR Capsules **1590**

Propoxyphene Hydrochloride (In vitro studies did not reveal an inhibitory effect of escitalopram on CYP2D6. In addition, steady state levels of racemic citalopram were not significantly different in poor metabolizers and extensive CYP2D6 metabolizers after multi-dose administration of citalopram, suggesting that co-administration, with escitalopram, of a drug that inhibits CYP2D6, is unlikely to have clinically significant effects on escitalopram metabolism. However, there are limited in vivo data suggesting a modest CYP2D6 inhibitory effect for escitalopram. Caution is indicated in the co-administration of escitalopram and drugs metabolized by CYP2D6).

No products indexed under this heading.

Propoxyphene Napsylate (In vitro studies did not reveal an inhibitory effect of escitalopram on CYP2D6. In addition, steady state levels of racemic citalopram were not significantly different in poor metabolizers and extensive CYP2D6 metabolizers after multi-dose administration of citalopram, suggesting that co-administration, with escitalopram, of a drug that inhibits CYP2D6, is unlikely to have clinically significant effects on escitalopram metabolism. However, there are limited in vivo data suggesting a modest CYP2D6 inhibitory effect for escitalopram. Caution is indicated in the co-administration of escitalopram and drugs metabolized by CYP2D6).

No products indexed under this heading.

Propranolol Hydrochloride (In vitro studies did not reveal an inhibitory effect of escitalopram on CYP2D6. In addition, steady state levels of racemic citalopram were not significantly different in poor metabolizers and extensive CYP2D6 metabolizers after multi-dose administration of citalopram, suggesting that co-administration, with escitalopram, of a drug that inhibits CYP2D6, is unlikely to have clinically significant effects on escitalopram metabolism. However, there are limited in vivo data suggesting a modest CYP2D6 inhibitory effect for escitalopram. Caution is indicated in the co-administration of escitalopram and drugs metabolized by CYP2D6). Products include:

InnoPran XL Extended Release Capsules 1484

Quetiapine Fumarate (In vitro studies did not reveal an inhibitory effect of escitalopram on CYP2D6. In addition, steady state levels of racemic citalopram were not significantly different in poor metabolizers and extensive CYP2D6 metabolizers after multi-dose administration of citalopram, suggesting that co-administration, with escitalopram, of a drug that inhibits CYP2D6, is unlikely to have clinically significant effects on escitalopram metabolism. However, there are limited in vivo data suggesting a modest CYP2D6 inhibitory effect for escitalopram. Caution is indicated in the co-administration of escitalopram and drugs metabolized by CYP2D6).

No products indexed under this heading.

Quinidine (In vitro studies indicated that CYP3A4 and -2C19 are the primary enzymes involved in the metabolism of escitalopram. However, co-administration of escitalopram oxalate (20 mg) and ritonavir (600 mg), a potent inhibitor of CYP3A4, did not significantly affect the pharmacokinetics of escitalopram oxalate. Because escitalopram oxalate is metabolized by multiple enzyme systems, inhibition of a single enzyme may not appreciably decrease escitalopram clearance).

No products indexed under this heading.

Quinidine Gluconate (In vitro studies did not reveal an inhibitory effect of escitalopram on CYP2D6. In addition, steady state levels of racemic citalopram were not significantly different in poor metabolizers and extensive CYP2D6 metabolizers after multi-dose administration of citalopram, suggesting that co-administration, with escitalopram, of a drug that inhibits CYP2D6, is unlikely to have clinically significant effects on escitalopram metabolism. However, there are limited in vivo data suggesting a modest CYP2D6 inhibitory effect for escitalopram. Caution is indicated in the co-administration of escitalopram and drugs metabolized by CYP2D6).

No products indexed under this heading.

Quinidine Hydrochloride (In vitro studies did not reveal an inhibitory effect of escitalopram on CYP2D6. In addition, steady state levels of racemic citalopram were not significantly different in poor metabolizers and extensive CYP2D6 metabolizers after multi-dose administration of citalopram, suggesting that co-administration, with escitalopram, of a drug that inhibits CYP2D6, is unlikely to have clinically significant effects on escitalopram metabolism. However, there are limited in vivo data suggesting a modest CYP2D6 inhibitory effect for escitalopram. Caution is indicated in the co-administration of escitalopram and drugs metabolized by CYP2D6).

No products indexed under this heading.

Quinidine Polygalacturonate (In vitro studies did not reveal an inhibitory effect of escitalopram on CYP2D6. In addition, steady state levels of racemic citalopram were not significantly different in poor metabolizers and extensive CYP2D6 metabolizers after multi-dose administration of citalopram, suggesting that co-administration, with escitalopram, of a drug that inhibits CYP2D6, is unlikely to have clinically significant effects on escitalopram metabolism. However, there are limited in vivo data suggesting a modest CYP2D6 inhibitory effect for escitalopram. Caution is indicated in the co-administration of escitalopram and drugs metabolized by CYP2D6).

No products indexed under this heading.

Quinidine Sulfate (In vitro studies did not reveal an inhibitory effect of escitalopram on CYP2D6. In addition, steady state levels of racemic citalopram were not significantly different in poor metabolizers and extensive CYP2D6 metabolizers after multi-dose administration of citalopram, suggesting that co-administration, with escitalopram, of a drug that inhibits CYP2D6, is unlikely to have clinically significant effects on escitalopram metabolism. However, there are limited in vivo data suggesting a modest CYP2D6 inhibitory effect for escitalopram. Caution is indicated in the co-administration of escitalopram and drugs metabolized by CYP2D6).

No products indexed under this heading.

Quinine (In vitro studies indicated that CYP3A4 and -2C19 are the primary enzymes involved in the metabolism of escitalopram. However, co-administration of escitalopram oxalate (20 mg) and ritonavir (600 mg), a potent inhibitor of CYP3A4, did not significantly affect the pharmacokinetics of escitalopram oxalate. Because escitalopram oxalate is metabolized by multiple enzyme systems, inhibition of a single enzyme may not appreciably decrease escitalopram clearance).

No products indexed under this heading.

Quinine Sulfate (In vitro studies indicated that CYP3A4 and -2C19 are the primary enzymes involved in the metabolism of escitalopram. However, co-administration of escitalopram oxalate (20 mg) and ritonavir (600 mg), a potent inhibitor of CYP3A4, did not significantly affect the pharmacokinetics of escitalopram oxalate. Because escitalopram oxalate is metabolized by multiple enzyme systems, inhibition of a single enzyme may not appreciably decrease escitalopram clearance).

No products indexed under this heading.

Quinupristin (In vitro studies indicated that CYP3A4 and -2C19 are the primary enzymes involved in the metabolism of escitalopram. However, co-administration of escitalopram oxalate (20 mg) and ritonavir (600 mg), a potent inhibitor of CYP3A4, did not significantly affect the pharmacokinetics of escitalopram oxalate. Because escitalopram oxalate is metabolized by multiple enzyme systems, inhibition of a single enzyme may not appreciably decrease escitalopram clearance).

No products indexed under this heading.

Ranitidine Bismuth Citrate (In vitro studies indicated that CYP3A4 and -2C19 are the primary enzymes involved in the metabolism of escitalopram. However, co-administration of escitalopram oxalate (20 mg) and ritonavir (600 mg), a potent inhibitor of CYP3A4, did not significantly affect the pharmacokinetics of escitalopram oxalate. Because escitalopram oxalate is metabolized by multiple enzyme systems, inhibition of a single enzyme may not appreciably decrease escitalopram clearance).

No products indexed under this heading.

Ranitidine Hydrochloride (In vitro studies indicated that CYP3A4 and -2C19 are the primary enzymes involved in the metabolism of escitalopram. However, co-administration of escitalopram oxalate (20 mg) and ritonavir (600 mg), a potent inhibitor of CYP3A4, did not significantly affect the pharmacokinetics of escitalopram oxalate. Because escitalopram oxalate is metabolized by multiple enzyme systems, inhibition of a single enzyme may not appreciably decrease escitalopram clearance). Products include:

Zantac 75 Tablets .... ▣ 603
Zantac 1670
Zantac Injection 1666
Zantac Injection Pharmacy Bulk Package 1668
Maximum Strength Zantac 150 Tablets .... ▣ 603
Maximum Strength Zantac 150 Cool Mint Tablets .... ▣ 603

Rasagiline Mesylate (Co-administration of SSRIs and MAO inhibitors has resulted in serious, sometimes fatal, reactions including hyperthermia, rigidity, myoclonus, autonomic instability, agitation progressing to delirium serotonin syndrome and coma; concurrent and/or sequential use is contraindicated). Products include:

Azilect Tablets 3106

Risperidone (In vitro studies did not reveal an inhibitory effect of escitalopram on CYP2D6. In addition, steady state levels of racemic citalopram were not significantly different in poor metabolizers and extensive CYP2D6 metabolizers after multi-dose administration of citalopram, suggesting that co-administration, with escitalopram, of a drug that inhibits CYP2D6, is unlikely to have clinically significant effects on escitalopram metabolism. However, there are limited in vivo data suggesting a modest CYP2D6 inhibitory effect for escitalopram. Caution is indicated in the co-administration of escitalopram and drugs metabolized by CYP2D6). Products include:

Risperdal Consta Long-Acting Injection 1753

Ritonavir (In vitro studies did not reveal an inhibitory effect of escitalopram on CYP2D6. In addition, steady state levels of racemic citalopram were not significantly different in poor metabolizers and extensive CYP2D6 metabolizers after multi-dose administration of citalopram, suggesting that co-administration, with escitalopram, of a drug that inhibits CYP2D6, is unlikely to have clinically significant effects on escitalopram metabolism. However, there are limited in vivo data suggesting a modest CYP2D6 inhibitory effect for escitalopram. Caution is indicated in the co-administration of escitalopram and drugs metabolized by CYP2D6). Products include:

Kaletra 452
Norvir 489

Rizatriptan Benzoate (There have been rare post-marketing reports of serotonin syndrome with use of a SSRI and a triptan. If concomitant treatment of escitalopram oxalate with a triptan is clinically warranted, careful observation of the patient is advised, particularly during treatment initiation and dose increases). Products include:

Maxalt Tablets 2056
Maxalt-MLT Orally Disintegrating Tablets 2056

Rofecoxib (The combined use of psychotropic drugs that interfere with serotonin reuptake and drugs that affect coagulation has been associated with an increased risk of bleeding; use caution when co-administering).

No products indexed under this heading.

Saquinavir (In vitro studies indicated that CYP3A4 and -2C19 are the primary enzymes involved in the metabolism of escitalopram. However, co-administration of escitalopram oxalate (20 mg) and ritonavir (600 mg), a potent inhibitor of CYP3A4, did not significantly affect the pharmacokinetics of escitalopram oxalate. Because escitalopram oxalate is metabolized by multiple enzyme systems, inhibition of a single enzyme may not appreciably decrease escitalopram clearance).

No products indexed under this heading.

Saquinavir Mesylate (In vitro studies indicated that CYP3A4 and -2C19 are the primary enzymes involved in the metabolism of escitalopram. However, co-administration of escitalopram oxalate (20 mg) and ritonavir (600 mg), a potent inhibitor of CYP3A4, did not significantly affect the pharmacokinetics of escitalopram oxalate. Because escitalopram oxalate is metabolized by multiple enzyme systems, inhibition of a single enzyme may not appreciably decrease escitalopram clearance).

No products indexed under this heading.

Selegiline (Co-administration of SSRIs and MAO inhibitors has resulted in serious, sometimes fatal, reactions including hyperthermia, rigidity, myoclonus, autonomic instability, agitation progressing to delirium serotonin syndrome and coma; concurrent and/or sequential use is contraindicated). Products include:

Emsam Transdermal System 905

Selegiline Hydrochloride (Co-administration of SSRIs and MAO inhibitors has resulted in serious, sometimes fatal, reactions including hyperthermia, rigidity, myoclonus, autonomic instability, agitation progressing to delirium serotonin syndrome and coma; concurrent and/or sequential use is contraindicated). Products include:

Eldepryl Capsules 3052

Sertraline Hydrochloride (Development of a potentially life-threatening serotonin syndrome may occur with SSRIs, particularly with concomitant use of serotinergic drugs, including triptans. Caution is advised when escitalopram oxalate is co-administered with other drugs that may affect the serotinergic neurotransmitter systems).

No products indexed under this heading.

Sildenafil Citrate (In vitro studies indicated that CYP3A4 and -2C19 are the primary enzymes involved in the metabolism of escitalopram. However, co-administration of escitalopram oxalate (20 mg) and ritonavir (600 mg), a potent inhibitor of CYP3A4, did not significantly affect the pharmacokinetics of escitalopram oxalate. Because escitalopram oxalate is metabolized by multiple enzyme systems, inhibition of a single enzyme may not appreciably decrease escitalopram clearance).

No products indexed under this heading.

Sulfaphenazole (In vitro studies indicated that CYP3A4 and -2C19 are the primary enzymes involved in the metabolism of escitalopram. However, co-administration of escitalopram oxalate (20 mg) and ritonavir (600 mg), a potent inhibitor of CYP3A4, did not significantly affect the pharmacokinetics of escitalopram oxalate. Because escitalopram oxalate is metabolized by multiple enzyme systems, inhibition of a single enzyme may not appreciably decrease escitalopram clearance).

No products indexed under this heading.

Sulindac (The combined use of psychotropic drugs that interfere with serotonin reuptake and drugs that affect coagulation has been associated with an increased risk of bleeding; use caution when co-administering). Products include:

Clinoril Tablets 1962

Sumatriptan (Co-administration of SSRIs and sumatriptan has resulted in weakness, hyperreflexia, and incoordination). Products include:

Imitrex Nasal Spray 1470

Sumatriptan Succinate (Co-administration of SSRIs and sumatriptan has resulted in weakness, hyperreflexia, and incoordination). Products include:

Imitrex Injection 1465
Imitrex Tablets 1474
Treximet Tablets 1616

Tamoxifen Citrate (In vitro studies did not reveal an inhibitory effect of escitalopram on CYP2D6. In addition, steady state levels of racemic citalopram were not significantly different in poor metabolizers and extensive CYP2D6 metabolizers after multi-dose administration of citalopram, suggesting that co-administration, with escitalopram, of a drug that inhibits CYP2D6, is unlikely to have clinically significant effects on escitalopram metabolism. However, there are limited in vivo data suggesting a modest CYP2D6 inhibitory effect for escitalopram. Caution is indicated in the co-administration of escitalopram and drugs metabolized by CYP2D6).

No products indexed under this heading.

Telithromycin (In vitro studies indicated that CYP3A4 and -2C19 are the primary enzymes involved in the metabolism of escitalopram. However, co-administration of escitalopram oxalate (20 mg) and ritonavir (600 mg), a potent inhibitor of CYP3A4, did not significantly affect the pharmacokinetics of escitalopram oxalate. Because escitalopram oxalate is metabolized by multiple enzyme systems, inhibition of a single enzyme may not appreciably decrease escitalopram clearance). Products include:

Ketek Tablets 2744

Telmisartan (In vitro studies indicated that CYP3A4 and -2C19 are the primary enzymes involved in the metabolism of escitalopram. However, co-administration of escitalopram oxalate (20 mg) and ritonavir (600 mg), a potent inhibitor of CYP3A4, did not significantly affect the pharmacokinetics of escitalopram oxalate. Because escitalopram oxalate is metabolized by multiple enzyme systems, inhibition of a single enzyme may not appreciably decrease escitalopram clearance). Products include:

Micardis Tablets 852
Micardis HCT Tablets 854

Teniposide (In vitro studies did not reveal an inhibitory effect of escitalopram on CYP2D6. In addition, steady state levels of racemic citalopram were not significantly different in poor metabolizers and extensive CYP2D6 metabolizers after multi-dose administration of citalopram, suggesting that co-administration, with escitalopram, of a drug that inhibits CYP2D6, is unlikely to have clinically significant effects on escitalopram metabolism. However, there are limited in vivo data suggesting a modest CYP2D6 inhibitory effect for escitalopram. Caution is indicated in the co-administration of escitalopram and drugs metabolized by CYP2D6).

No products indexed under this heading.

Testosterone (In vitro studies did not reveal an inhibitory effect of escitalopram on CYP2D6. In addition, steady state levels of racemic citalopram were not significantly different in poor metabolizers and extensive CYP2D6 metabolizers after multi-dose administration of citalopram, suggesting that co-administration, with escitalopram, of a drug that inhibits CYP2D6, is unlikely to have clinically significant effects on escitalopram metabolism. However, there are limited in vivo data suggesting a modest CYP2D6 inhibitory effect for escitalopram. Caution is indicated in the co-administration of escitalopram and drugs metabolized by CYP2D6). Products include:

AndroGel 3159
Testim 1% Gel 701

Testosterone Cypionate (In vitro studies did not reveal an inhibitory effect of escitalopram on CYP2D6. In addition, steady state levels of racemic citalopram were not significantly different in poor metabolizers and extensive CYP2D6 metabolizers after multi-dose administration of citalopram, suggesting that co-administration, with escitalopram, of a drug that inhibits CYP2D6, is unlikely to have clinically significant effects on escitalopram metabolism. However, there are limited in vivo data suggesting a modest CYP2D6 inhibitory effect for escitalopram. Caution is indicated in the co-administration of escitalopram and drugs metabolized by CYP2D6).

No products indexed under this heading.

Testosterone Enanthate (In vitro studies did not reveal an inhibitory effect of escitalopram on CYP2D6. In addition, steady state levels of racemic citalopram were not significantly different in poor metabolizers and extensive CYP2D6 metabolizers after multi-dose administration of citalopram, suggesting that co-administration, with escitalopram, of a drug that inhibits CYP2D6, is unlikely to have clinically significant effects on escitalopram metabolism. However, there are limited in vivo data suggesting a modest CYP2D6 inhibitory effect for escitalopram. Caution is indicated in the co-administration of escitalopram and drugs metabolized by CYP2D6). Products include:

Delatestryl Injection 1730

Testosterone Propionate (In vitro studies did not reveal an inhibitory effect of escitalopram on CYP2D6. In addition, steady state levels of racemic citalopram were not significantly different in poor metabolizers and extensive CYP2D6 metabolizers after multi-dose administration of citalopram, suggesting that co-administration, with escitalopram, of a drug that inhibits CYP2D6, is unlikely to have clinically significant effects on escitalopram metabolism. However, there are limited in vivo data suggesting a modest CYP2D6 inhibitory effect for escitalopram. Caution is indicated in the co-administration of escitalopram and drugs metabolized by CYP2D6).

No products indexed under this heading.

Theophylline (Combined administration of racemic escitalopram oxalate (40 mg/day for 21 days) and the CYP1A2 substrate theophylline (single dose of 300 mg) did not affect the pharmacokinetics of theophylline. The effect of theophylline of the pharmacokinetics of escitalopram oxalate was not evaluated).

No products indexed under this heading.

Thioridazine (In vitro studies did not reveal an inhibitory effect of escitalopram on CYP2D6. In addition, steady state levels of racemic citalopram were not significantly different in poor metabolizers and extensive CYP2D6 metabolizers after multi-dose administration of citalopram, suggesting that co-administration, with escitalopram, of a drug that inhibits CYP2D6, is unlikely to have clinically significant effects on escitalopram metabolism. However, there are limited in vivo data suggesting a modest CYP2D6 inhibitory effect for escitalopram. Caution is indicated in the co-administration of escitalopram and drugs metabolized by CYP2D6).

No products indexed under this heading.

Thioridazine Hydrochloride (In vitro studies did not reveal an inhibitory effect of escitalopram on CYP2D6. In addition, steady state levels of racemic citalopram were not significantly different in poor metabolizers and extensive CYP2D6 metabolizers after multi-dose administration of citalopram, suggesting that co-administration, with escitalopram, of a drug that inhibits CYP2D6, is unlikely to have clinically significant effects on escitalopram metabolism. However, there are limited in vivo data suggesting a modest CYP2D6 inhibitory effect for escitalopram. Caution is indicated in the co-administration of escitalopram and drugs metabolized by CYP2D6). Products include:

Thioridazine Hydrochloride Tablets 2195

Ticlopidine Hydrochloride (In vitro studies indicated that CYP3A4 and -2C19 are the primary enzymes involved in the metabolism of escitalopram. However, co-administration of escitalopram oxalate (20 mg) and ritonavir (600 mg), a potent inhibitor of CYP3A4, did not significantly affect the pharmacokinetics of escitalopram oxalate. Because escitalopram oxalate is metabolized by multiple enzyme systems, inhibition of a single enzyme may not appreciably decrease escitalopram clearance).

No products indexed under this heading.

Timolol Maleate (In vitro studies did not reveal an inhibitory effect of escitalopram on CYP2D6. In addition, steady state levels of racemic citalopram were not significantly different in poor metabolizers and extensive CYP2D6 metabolizers after multi-dose administration of citalopram, suggesting that co-administration, with escitalopram, of a drug that inhibits CYP2D6, is unlikely to have clinically significant effects on escitalopram metabolism. However, there are limited in vivo data suggesting a modest CYP2D6 inhibitory effect for escitalopram. Caution is indicated in the co-administration of escitalopram and drugs metabolized by CYP2D6). Products include:

Combigan Ophthalmic Solution 553
Cosopt Sterile Ophthalmic Solution 1969
Timoptic Sterile Ophthalmic Solution 2121
Timoptic in Ocudose 2124
Timoptic-XE Sterile Ophthalmic Gel Forming Solution 2125

Tinzaparin Sodium (The combined use of psychotropic drugs that interfere with serotonin reuptake and drugs that affect coagulation has been associated with an increased risk of bleeding).

No products indexed under this heading.

Tolbutamide (In vitro studies indicated that CYP3A4 and -2C19 are the primary enzymes involved in the metabolism of escitalopram. However, co-administration of escitalopram oxalate (20 mg) and ritonavir (600 mg), a potent inhibitor of CYP3A4, did not significantly affect the pharmacokinetics of escitalopram oxalate. Because escitalopram oxalate is metabolized by multiple enzyme systems, inhibition of a single enzyme may not appreciably decrease escitalopram clearance).

No products indexed under this heading.

Tolbutamide Sodium (In vitro studies indicated that CYP3A4 and -2C19 are the primary enzymes involved in the metabolism of escitalopram. However, co-administration of escitalopram oxalate (20 mg) and ritonavir (600 mg), a potent inhibitor of CYP3A4, did not significantly affect the pharmacokinetics of escitalopram oxalate. Because escitalopram oxalate is metabolized by multiple enzyme systems, inhibition of a single enzyme may not appreciably decrease escitalopram clearance).

No products indexed under this heading.

Tolmetin Sodium (The combined use of psychotropic drugs that interfere with serotonin reuptake and drugs that affect coagulation has been associated with an increased risk of bleeding; use caution when co-administering).

No products indexed under this heading.

Tolterodine Tartrate (In vitro studies did not reveal an inhibitory effect of escitalopram on CYP2D6. In addition, steady state levels of racemic citalopram were not significantly different in poor metabolizers and extensive CYP2D6 metabolizers after multi-dose administration of citalopram, suggesting that co-administration, with escitalopram, of a drug that inhibits CYP2D6, is unlikely to have clinically significant effects on escitalopram metabolism. However, there are limited in vivo data suggesting a modest CYP2D6 inhibitory effect for escitalopram. Caution is indicated in the co-administration of escitalopram and drugs metabolized by CYP2D6).

No products indexed under this heading.

Topiramate (In vitro studies indicated that CYP3A4 and -2C19 are the primary enzymes involved in the metabolism of escitalopram. However, co-administration of escitalopram oxalate (20 mg) and ritonavir (600 mg), a potent inhibitor of CYP3A4, did not significantly affect the pharmacokinetics of escitalopram oxalate. Because escitalopram oxalate is metabolized by multiple enzyme systems, inhibition of a single enzyme may not appreciably decrease escitalopram clearance).

No products indexed under this heading.

Tramadol Hydrochloride (There is a risk of serotonin sydrome with concomitant use of escitalopram oxalate and tramadol. Caution is advised when escitalopram oxalate is co-administered with other drugs that may affect the seroinergic neurotransmitter systems, such as tramadol). Products include:

Ultram ER Extended-Release Tablets 2428

Tranylcypromine Sulfate (Co-administration of SSRIs and MAO inhibitors has resulted in serious, sometimes fatal, reactions including hyperthermia, rigidity, myoclonus, autonomic instability, agitation progressing to delirium serotonin syndrome and coma; concurrent and/or sequential use is contraindicated). Products include:

Parnate Tablets 1532

Trazodone Hydrochloride (In vitro studies did not reveal an inhibitory effect of escitalopram on CYP2D6. In addition, steady state levels of racemic citalopram were not significantly different in poor metabolizers and extensive CYP2D6 metabolizers after multi-dose administration of citalopram, suggesting that co-administration, with escitalopram, of a drug that inhibits CYP2D6, is unlikely to have clinically significant effects on escitalopram metabolism. However, there are limited in vivo data suggesting a modest CYP2D6 inhibitory effect for escitalopram. Caution is indicated in the co-administration of escitalopram and drugs metabolized by CYP2D6).

No products indexed under this heading.

Triazolam (In vitro studies did not reveal an inhibitory effect of escitalopram on CYP2D6. In addition, steady state levels of racemic citalopram were not significantly different in poor metabolizers and extensive CYP2D6 metabolizers after multi-dose administration of citalopram, suggesting that co-administration, with escitalopram, of a drug that inhibits CYP2D6, is unlikely to have clinically significant effects on escitalopram metabolism. However, there are limited in vivo data suggesting a modest CYP2D6 inhibitory effect for escitalopram. Caution is indicated in the co-administration of escitalopram and drugs metabolized by CYP2D6).

No products indexed under this heading.

Trimipramine Maleate (In vitro studies did not reveal an inhibitory effect of escitalopram on CYP2D6. In addition, steady state levels of racemic citalopram were not significantly different in poor metabolizers and extensive CYP2D6 metabolizers after multi-dose administration of citalopram, suggesting that co-administration, with escitalopram, of a drug that inhibits CYP2D6, is unlikely to have clinically significant effects on escitalopram metabolism. However, there are limited in vivo data suggesting a modest CYP2D6 inhibitory effect for escitalopram. Caution is indicated in the co-administration of escitalopram and drugs metabolized by CYP2D6).

No products indexed under this heading.

Troglitazone (In vitro studies indicated that CYP3A4 and -2C19 are the primary enzymes involved in the metabolism of escitalopram. However, co-administration of escitalopram oxalate (20 mg) and ritonavir (600 mg), a potent inhibitor of CYP3A4, did not significantly affect the pharmacokinetics of escitalopram oxalate. Because escitalopram oxalate is metabolized by multiple enzyme systems, inhibition of a single enzyme may not appreciably decrease escitalopram clearance).

No products indexed under this heading.

Troleandomycin (In vitro studies indicated that CYP3A4 and -2C19 are the primary enzymes involved in the metabolism of escitalopram. However, co-administration of escitalopram oxalate (20 mg) and ritonavir (600 mg), a potent inhibitor of CYP3A4, did not significantly affect the pharmacokinetics of escitalopram oxalate. Because escitalopram oxalate is metabolized by multiple enzyme systems, inhibition of a single enzyme may not appreciably decrease escitalopram clearance).

No products indexed under this heading.

Valdecoxib (The combined use of psychotropic drugs that interfere with serotonin reuptake and drugs that affect coagulation has been associated with an increased risk of bleeding; use caution when co-administering).

No products indexed under this heading.

Valproate Sodium (In vitro studies indicated that CYP3A4 and -2C19 are the primary enzymes involved in the metabolism of escitalopram. However, co-administration of escitalopram oxalate (20 mg) and ritonavir (600 mg), a potent inhibitor of CYP3A4, did not significantly affect the pharmacokinetics of escitalopram oxalate. Because escitalopram oxalate is metabolized by multiple enzyme systems, inhibition of a single enzyme may not appreciably decrease escitalopram clearance).

No products indexed under this heading.

Vardenafil Hydrochloride (In vitro studies indicated that CYP3A4 and -2C19 are the primary enzymes involved in the metabolism of escitalopram. However, co-administration of escitalopram oxalate (20 mg) and ritonavir (600 mg), a potent inhibitor of CYP3A4, did not significantly affect the pharmacokinetics of escitalopram oxalate. Because escitalopram oxalate is metabolized by multiple enzyme systems, inhibition of a single enzyme may not appreciably decrease escitalopram clearance). Products include:

Levitra Tablets 2876

Venlafaxine Hydrochloride (Development of a potentially life-threatening serotonin syndrome may occur with SSRIs, particularly with concomitant use of serotinergic drugs, including triptans. Caution is advised when escitalopram oxalate is co-administered with other drugs that may affect the serotinergic neurotransmitter systems). Products include:

Effexor XR Extended-Release Capsules 3195

Venlafaxine Hydrochloride Tablets ... 2199

Verapamil Hydrochloride (In vitro studies indicated that CYP3A4 and -2C19 are the primary enzymes involved in the metabolism of escitalopram. However, co-administration of escitalopram oxalate (20 mg) and ritonavir (600 mg), a potent inhibitor of CYP3A4, did not significantly affect the pharmacokinetics of escitalopram oxalate. Because escitalopram oxalate is metabolized by multiple enzyme systems, inhibition of a single enzyme may not appreciably decrease escitalopram clearance). Products include:

Tarka Tablets 511

Vinblastine Sulfate (In vitro studies did not reveal an inhibitory effect of escitalopram on CYP2D6. In addition, steady state levels of racemic citalopram were not significantly different in poor metabolizers and extensive CYP2D6 metabolizers after multi-dose administration of citalopram, suggesting that co-administration, with escitalopram, of a drug that inhibits CYP2D6, is unlikely to have clinically significant effects on escitalopram metabolism. However, there are limited in vivo data suggesting a modest CYP2D6 inhibitory effect for escitalopram. Caution is indicated in the co-administration of escitalopram and drugs metabolized by CYP2D6).

No products indexed under this heading.

Voriconazole (In vitro studies indicated that CYP3A4 and -2C19 are the primary enzymes involved in the metabolism of escitalopram. However, co-administration of escitalopram oxalate (20 mg) and ritonavir (600 mg), a potent inhibitor of CYP3A4, did not significantly affect the pharmacokinetics of escitalopram oxalate. Because escitalopram oxalate is metabolized by multiple enzyme systems, inhibition of a single enzyme may not appreciably decrease escitalopram clearance).

No products indexed under this heading.

Warfarin Sodium (The combined use of psychotropic drugs that interfere with serotonin reuptake and drugs that affect coagulation has been associated with an increased risk of bleeding).

No products indexed under this heading.

Zafirlukast (In vitro studies indicated that CYP3A4 and -2C19 are the primary enzymes involved in the metabolism of escitalopram. However, co-administration of escitalopram oxalate (20 mg) and ritonavir (600 mg), a potent inhibitor of CYP3A4, did not significantly affect the pharmacokinetics of escitalopram oxalate. Because escitalopram oxalate is metabolized by multiple enzyme systems, inhibition of a single enzyme may not appreciably decrease escitalopram clearance). Products include:

Accolate Tablets 669

Zileuton (In vitro studies indicated that CYP3A4 and -2C19 are the primary enzymes involved in the metabolism of escitalopram. However, co-administration of escitalopram oxalate (20 mg) and ritonavir (600 mg), a potent inhibitor of CYP3A4, did not significantly affect the pharmacokinetics of escitalopram oxalate. Because escitalopram oxalate is metabolized by multiple enzyme systems, inhibition of a single enzyme may not appreciably decrease escitalopram clearance).

No products indexed under this heading.

Zolmitriptan (There have been rare post-marketing reports of serotonin syndrome with use of a SSRI and a triptan. If concomitant treatment of escitalopram oxalate with a triptan is clinically warranted, careful observation of the patient is advised, particularly during treatment initiation and dose increases). Products include:

Zomig Tablets 694

Zomig Nasal Spray 689
Zomig-ZMT Tablets 694

Zonisamide (In vitro studies did not reveal an inhibitory effect of escitalopram on CYP2D6. In addition, steady state levels of racemic citalopram were not significantly different in poor metabolizers and extensive CYP2D6 metabolizers after multi-dose administration of citalopram, suggesting that co-administration, with escitalopram, of a drug that inhibits CYP2D6, is unlikely to have clinically significant effects on escitalopram metabolism. However, there are limited in vivo data suggesting a modest CYP2D6 inhibitory effect for escitalopram. Caution is indicated in the co-administration of escitalopram and drugs metabolized by CYP2D6). Products include:

Zonegran Capsules 1089

Food Interactions

Alcohol (Although escitalopram did not potentiate the cognitive and motor effects of alcohol in a clinical trial, as with other psychotropic medications, the use of alcohol by patients taking escitalopram is not recommended).

Grapefruit (In vitro studies indicated that CYP3A4 and -2C19 are the primary enzymes involved in the metabolism of escitalopram. However, co-administration of escitalopram oxalate (20 mg) and ritonavir (600 mg), a potent inhibitor of CYP3A4, did not significantly affect the pharmacokinetics of escitalopram oxalate. Because escitalopram oxalate is metabolized by multiple enzyme systems, inhibition of a single enzyme may not appreciably decrease escitalopram clearance).

Grapefruit Juice (In vitro studies indicated that CYP3A4 and -2C19 are the primary enzymes involved in the metabolism of escitalopram. However, co-administration of escitalopram oxalate (20 mg) and ritonavir (600 mg), a potent inhibitor of CYP3A4, did not significantly affect the pharmacokinetics of escitalopram oxalate. Because escitalopram oxalate is metabolized by multiple enzyme systems, inhibition of a single enzyme may not appreciably decrease escitalopram clearance).

LEXISCAN INJECTION

(Regadenoson) 614

May interact with theophyllines and certain other agents. Compounds in these categories include:

Caffeine (Methylxanthines (e.g., caffeine) are non-specific adenosine receptor antagonists and may interfere with the vasodilation activity of regadenoson. Patients should avoid consumption of any products containing methylxanthines as well as any drugs containing theophylline for at least 12 hours before regadenoson administration). Products include:

BioLean Free Tablets 635
BioLean II Tablets 635
Winrgy Dietary Supplement 642

Dipyridamole (Dipyridamole may change the effects of regadenoson. When possible, withhold dipyridamole for at least two days prior to regadenoson administration). Products include:

Aggrenox Capsules 819
Persantine Tablets 869

Theophylline (Methylxanthines (e.g., theophylline) are non-specific adenosine receptor antagonists and may interfere with the vasodilation activity of regadenoson. Patients should avoid consumption of any products containing methylxanthines as well as any drugs containing theophylline for at least 12 hour before regadenoson administration).

No products indexed under this heading.

Theophylline Anhydrous (Methylxanthines (e.g., theophylline) are non-specific adenosine receptor antagonists and may interfere with the vasodilation activity of regadenoson. Patients should avoid consumption of any products containing methylxanthines as well as any drugs containing theophylline for at least 12 hour before regadenoson administration). Products include:

Uniphyl Tablets 2595

Theophylline Calcium Salicylate (Methylxanthines (e.g., theophylline) are non-specific adenosine receptor antagonists and may interfere with the vasodilation activity of regadenoson. Patients should avoid consumption of any products containing methylxanthines as well as any drugs containing theophylline for at least 12 hour before regadenoson administration).

No products indexed under this heading.

Theophylline Dihydroxypropyl (Glyceryl) (Methylxanthines (e.g., theophylline) are non-specific adenosine receptor antagonists and may interfere with the vasodilation activity of regadenoson. Patients should avoid consumption of any products containing methylxanthines as well as any drugs containing theophylline for at least 12 hour before regadenoson administration).

No products indexed under this heading.

Theophylline Ethylenediamine (Methylxanthines (e.g., theophylline) are non-specific adenosine receptor antagonists and may interfere with the vasodilation activity of regadenoson. Patients should avoid consumption of any products containing methylxanthines as well as any drugs containing theophylline for at least 12 hour before regadenoson administration).

No products indexed under this heading.

Theophylline Sodium Glycinate (Methylxanthines (e.g., theophylline) are non-specific adenosine receptor antagonists and may interfere with the vasodilation activity of regadenoson. Patients should avoid consumption of any products containing methylxanthines as well as any drugs containing theophylline for at least 12 hour before regadenoson administration).

No products indexed under this heading.

LEXIVA ORAL SUSPENSION

(Fosamprenavir Calcium) 1510

See Lexiva Tablets

LEXIVA TABLETS

(Fosamprenavir Calcium) 1510

May interact with cytochrome p450 3a4 inducers (selected), cytochrome p450 3a4 inhibitors (selected), cytochrome p450 3a4 substrates (selected), histamine H_2-receptor antagonists, phenytoin, and certain other agents. Compounds in these categories include:

Acetazolamide (Amprenavir is metabolized by CYP 3A4. Co-administration of fosamprenavir calcium and drugs that inhibit CYP3A4 may increase amprenavir concentrations and increase the incidence of adverse effects).

No products indexed under this heading.

Alfentanil Hydrochloride (Amprenavir, the active metabolite of fosamprenavir, is an inhibitor of cytochrome P450 3A4 metabolism and therefore should not be administered concurrently with medications with narrow therapeutic windows that are substrates of CYP3A4. Data also suggests that amprenavir induces CYP3A4).

No products indexed under this heading.

Allium sativum (Amprenavir is metabolized by CYP3A4. Co-administration of fosamprenavir calcium and drugs that induce CYP3A4 may decrease amprenavir concentrations and reduce its therapeutic effect).

No products indexed under this heading.

Alprazolam (Co-administration may increase alprazolam levels; may need to decrease alprazolam dose).

No products indexed under this heading.

Amiodarone Hydrochloride (Co-administration may lead to increased levels of amiodarone. Caution is warranted and therapeutic concentration monitoring is recommended for antiarrhythmics when co-administered with fosamprenavir).

No products indexed under this heading.

Amitriptyline Hydrochloride (Co-administration may lead to increased levels of amitriptyline. Therapeutic concentration monitoring is recommended for tricyclic antidepressants when co-administered with fosamprenavir).

No products indexed under this heading.

Amlodipine Besylate (Co-administration may increase levels of amlodipine; caution is warranted and clinical monitoring is recommended). Products include:

Azor Tablets 1005
Exforge Tablets 2238

Amprenavir (Amprenavir is metabolized by CYP 3A4. Co-administration of fosamprenavir calcium and drugs that inhibit CYP3A4 may increase amprenavir concentrations and increase the incidence of adverse effects).

No products indexed under this heading.

Anastrozole (Amprenavir is metabolized by CYP 3A4. Co-administration of fosamprenavir calcium and drugs that inhibit CYP3A4 may increase amprenavir concentrations and increase the incidence of adverse effects). Products include:

Arimidex Tablets 672

Aprepitant (Amprenavir, the active metabolite of fosamprenavir, is an inhibitor of cytochrome P450 3A4 metabolism and therefore should not be administered concurrently with medications with narrow therapeutic windows that are substrates of CYP3A4. Data also suggests that amprenavir induces CYP3A4). Products include:

Emend Capsules 1992

Astemizole (Amprenavir, the active metabolite of fosamprenavir, is an inhibitor of cytochrome P450 3A4 metabolism and therefore should not be administered concurrently with medications with narrow therapeutic windows that are substrates of CYP3A4. Data also suggests that amprenavir induces CYP3A4).

No products indexed under this heading.

Atazanavir (Co-administration with fosamprenavir/ritonavir combination may lead to decreased levels of atazanavir).

No products indexed under this heading.

Atazanavir Sulfate (Co-administration with fosamprenavir/ritonavir combination may lead to decreased levels of atazanavir). Products include:

Reyataz Capsules 3299

Atorvastatin Calcium (Co-administration may lead to increased atorvastatin levels. Use less than or equal to 20mg/day of atorvastatin with careful monitoring or consider other HMG-CoA reductase inhibitors in combination with fosamprenavir). Products include:

Lipitor Tablets 2501

Belladonna Ergotamine (Amprenavir, the active metabolite of fosamprenavir, is an inhibitor of cytochrome P450 3A4 metabolism and therefore should not be administered concurrently with medications with narrow therapeutic windows that are substrates of CYP3A4. Data also suggests that amprenavir induces CYP3A4).

No products indexed under this heading.

Bepridil Hydrochloride (Co-administration may lead to increased levels of bepridil. Use with caution; increased levels of bepridil may be associated with life-threatening reactions such as cardiac arrhythmias).

No products indexed under this heading.

Betamethasone Acetate (Amprenavir is metabolized by CYP3A4. Co-administration of fosamprenavir calcium and drugs that induce CYP3A4 may decrease amprenavir concentrations and reduce its therapeutic effect).

No products indexed under this heading.

Betamethasone Sodium Phosphate (Amprenavir is metabolized by CYP3A4. Co-administration of fosamprenavir calcium and drugs that induce CYP3A4 may decrease amprenavir concentrations and reduce its therapeutic effect).

No products indexed under this heading.

Disopyramide (Amprenavir, the active metabolite of fosamprenavir, is an inhibitor of cytochrome P450 3A4 metabolism and therefore should not be administered concurrently with medications with narrow therapeutic windows that are substrates of CYP3A4. Data also suggests that amprenavir induces CYP3A4).
No products indexed under this heading.

Disopyramide Phosphate (Amprenavir, the active metabolite of fosamprenavir, is an inhibitor of cytochrome P450 3A4 metabolism and therefore should not be administered concurrently with medications with narrow therapeutic windows that are substrates of CYP3A4. Data also suggests that amprenavir induces CYP3A4).
No products indexed under this heading.

Disulfiram (Amprenavir, the active metabolite of fosamprenavir, is an inhibitor of cytochrome P450 3A4 metabolism and therefore should not be administered concurrently with medications with narrow therapeutic windows that are substrates of CYP3A4. Data also suggests that amprenavir induces CYP3A4).
No products indexed under this heading.

Doxorubicin Hydrochloride (Amprenavir, the active metabolite of fosamprenavir, is an inhibitor of cytochrome P450 3A4 metabolism and therefore should not be administered concurrently with medications with narrow therapeutic windows that are substrates of CYP3A4. Data also suggests that amprenavir induces CYP3A4).
No products indexed under this heading.

Dronabinol (Amprenavir, the active metabolite of fosamprenavir, is an inhibitor of cytochrome P450 3A4 metabolism and therefore should not be administered concurrently with medications with narrow therapeutic windows that are substrates of CYP3A4. Data also suggests that amprenavir induces CYP3A4). Products include:
Marinol Capsules **3163**

Efavirenz (Co-administration may lead to decreased amprenavir levels. An additional 100mg/day (300mg total) of ritonavir is recommended when efavirenz is administered with fosamprenavjr/ritonavir once daily. No change in the ritonavir dose is required when efavirenz is administered with fosamprenavir plus ritonavir twice daily). Products include:
Atripla Tablets **938**
Sustiva Capsules **930**
Sustiva Tablets **930**

Ergonovine Maleate (Co-administration with ergonovine is contraindicated due to the potential for serious and/or life-threatening reactions such as acute ergot toxicity characterized by peripheral vasospasm and ischemia of the extremities and other tissues).
No products indexed under this heading.

Ergotamine Tartrate (Co-administration with ergotamine is contraindicated due to the potential for serious and/or life-threatening reactions such as acute ergot toxicity characterized by peripheral vasospasm and ischemia of the extremities and other tissues).
No products indexed under this heading.

Erythromycin (Amprenavir, the active metabolite of fosamprenavir, is an inhibitor of cytochrome P450 3A4 metabolism and therefore should not be administered concurrently with medications with narrow therapeutic windows that are substrates of CYP3A4. Data also suggests that amprenavir induces CYP3A4).
No products indexed under this heading.

Erythromycin Estolate (Amprenavir, the active metabolite of fosamprenavir, is an inhibitor of cytochrome P450 3A4 metabolism and therefore should not be administered concurrently with medications with narrow therapeutic windows that are substrates of CYP3A4. Data also suggests that amprenavir induces CYP3A4).
No products indexed under this heading.

Erythromycin Ethylsuccinate (Amprenavir, the active metabolite of fosamprenavir, is an inhibitor of cytochrome P450 3A4 metabolism and therefore should not be administered concurrently with medications with narrow therapeutic windows that are substrates of CYP3A4. Data also suggests that amprenavir induces CYP3A4). Products include:
E.E.S. **433**
EryPed **431**

Erythromycin Gluceptate (Amprenavir, the active metabolite of fosamprenavir, is an inhibitor of cytochrome P450 3A4 metabolism and therefore should not be administered concurrently with medications with narrow therapeutic windows that are substrates of CYP3A4. Data also suggests that amprenavir induces CYP3A4).
No products indexed under this heading.

Erythromycin Lactobionate (Amprenavir, the active metabolite of fosamprenavir, is an inhibitor of cytochrome P450 3A4 metabolism and therefore should not be administered concurrently with medications with narrow therapeutic windows that are substrates of CYP3A4. Data also suggests that amprenavir induces CYP3A4).
No products indexed under this heading.

Erythromycin Stearate (Amprenavir, the active metabolite of fosamprenavir, is an inhibitor of cytochrome P450 3A4 metabolism and therefore should not be administered concurrently with medications with narrow therapeutic windows that are substrates of CYP3A4. Data also suggests that amprenavir induces CYP3A4).
No products indexed under this heading.

Esomeprazole Magnesium (Concurrent administration may lead to increased levels of esomeprazole). Products include:
Nexium Delayed-Release Capsules **645**
Nexium Delayed-Release Oral Suspension **645**

Estradiol (Amprenavir, the active metabolite of fosamprenavir, is an inhibitor of cytochrome P450 3A4 metabolism and therefore should not be administered concurrently with medications with narrow therapeutic windows that are substrates of CYP3A4. Data also suggests that amprenavir induces CYP3A4). Products include:
Activella Tablets **2347**
Angeliq Tablets **751**
Climara Transdermal System **763**
Climara Pro Transdermal System **768**
Divigel **3167**
Vagifem Tablets **2375**

Estradiol Benzoate (Amprenavir, the active metabolite of fosamprenavir, is an inhibitor of cytochrome P450 3A4 metabolism and therefore should not be administered concurrently with medications with narrow therapeutic windows that are substrates of CYP3A4. Data also suggests that amprenavir induces CYP3A4).
No products indexed under this heading.

Estradiol Cypionate (Amprenavir, the active metabolite of fosamprenavir, is an inhibitor of cytochrome P450 3A4 metabolism and therefore should not be administered concurrently with medications with narrow therapeutic windows that are substrates of CYP3A4. Data also suggests that amprenavir induces CYP3A4).
No products indexed under this heading.

Estradiol Valerate (Amprenavir, the active metabolite of fosamprenavir, is an inhibitor of cytochrome P450 3A4 metabolism and therefore should not be administered concurrently with medications with narrow therapeutic windows that are substrates of CYP3A4. Data also suggests that amprenavir induces CYP3A4).
No products indexed under this heading.

Ethinyl Estradiol (Co-administration of fosamprenavir alone with oral contraceptives containing the combination ethinyl estradiol/norethindrone may lead to increased levels of ethinyl estradiol/norethindrone. Because these hormonal levels may be altered, alternative methods of non-hormonal contraception are recommended). Products include:
Lybrel Tablets **3204**
Mircette Tablets **1034**
NuvaRing **2897**
Ortho-Cyclen/Ortho Tri-Cyclen **2449**
Ortho Evra Transdermal System **2437**
Ortho Tri-Cyclen Lo Tablets **2458**
Seasonique Tablets **1046**
Yaz Tablets **805**

Ethosuximide (Amprenavir, the active metabolite of fosamprenavir, is an inhibitor of cytochrome P450 3A4 metabolism and therefore should not be administered concurrently with medications with narrow therapeutic windows that are substrates of CYP3A4. Data also suggests that amprenavir induces CYP3A4).
No products indexed under this heading.

Ethynodiol Diacetate (Amprenavir, the active metabolite of fosamprenavir, is an inhibitor of cytochrome P450 3A4 metabolism and therefore should not be administered concurrently with medications with narrow therapeutic windows that are substrates of CYP3A4. Data also suggests that amprenavir induces CYP3A4).
No products indexed under this heading.

Etoposide (Amprenavir, the active metabolite of fosamprenavir, is an inhibitor of cytochrome P450 3A4 metabolism and therefore should not be administered concurrently with medications with narrow therapeutic windows that are substrates of CYP3A4. Data also suggests that amprenavir induces CYP3A4).
No products indexed under this heading.

Etoposide Phosphate (Amprenavir, the active metabolite of fosamprenavir, is an inhibitor of cytochrome P450 3A4 metabolism and therefore should not be administered concurrently with medications with narrow therapeutic windows that are substrates of CYP3A4. Data also suggests that amprenavir induces CYP3A4).
No products indexed under this heading.

Famotidine (Co-administration of fosamprenavir alone and histamine H2-receptor antagonists may lead to decreased levels of fosamprenavir. Use with caution since fosamprenavir may be less effective due to decreased amprenavir plasma concentrations in patients taking these agents concomitantly). Products include:
Pepcid Tablets **2075**
Original Strength Pepcid AC Gelcaps **1771**
Original Strength Pepcid AC Tablets **1771**
Maximum Strength Pepcid AC Tablets **1771**
Pepcid Complete Chewable Tablets **1771**

Felbamate (Amprenavir is metabolized by CYP3A4. Co-administration of fosamprenavir calcium and drugs that induce CYP3A4 may decrease amprenavir concentrations and reduce its therapeutic effect).
No products indexed under this heading.

Felodipine (Co-administration may increase levels of felodipine; caution is warranted and clinical monitoring is recommended).
No products indexed under this heading.

Fentanyl (Amprenavir, the active metabolite of fosamprenavir, is an inhibitor of cytochrome P450 3A4 metabolism and therefore should not be administered concurrently with medications with narrow therapeutic windows that are substrates of CYP3A4. Data also suggests that amprenavir induces CYP3A4). Products include:
Duragesic Transdermal System **2405**
Ionsys Transdermal System **2410**

Fentanyl Citrate (Amprenavir, the active metabolite of fosamprenavir, is an inhibitor of cytochrome P450 3A4 metabolism and therefore should not be administered concurrently with medications with narrow therapeutic windows that are sub-

strates of CYP3A4. Data also suggests that amprenavir induces CYP3A4). Products include:

Actiq ... 959
Fentora Tablets ... 968

Flecainide Acetate (If fosamprenavir is co-administered with ritonavir, the antiarrhythmic agent flecainide is contraindicated due to the potential for serious and/or life-threatening reactions such as cardiac arrhythmias secondary to increases in plasma concentrations of flecainide).

No products indexed under this heading.

Fluconazole (Amprenavir is metabolized by CYP 3A4. Co-administration of fosamprenavir calcium and drugs that inhibit CYP3A4 may increase amprenavir concentrations and increase the incidence of adverse effects).

No products indexed under this heading.

Fludrocortisone Acetate (Amprenavir is metabolized by CYP3A4. Co-administration of fosamprenavir calcium and drugs that induce CYP3A4 may decrease amprenavir concentrations and reduce its therapeutic effect).

No products indexed under this heading.

Fluoxetine (Amprenavir is metabolized by CYP 3A4. Co-administration of fosamprenavir calcium and drugs that inhibit CYP3A4 may increase amprenavir concentrations and increase the incidence of adverse effects).

No products indexed under this heading.

Fluoxetine Hydrochloride (Amprenavir is metabolized by CYP 3A4. Co-administration of fosamprenavir calcium and drugs that inhibit CYP3A4 may increase amprenavir concentrations and increase the incidence of adverse effects). Products include:

Prozac Weekly Capsules ... 1852
Prozac Pulvules and Liquid ... 1852
Symbyax Capsules ... 1871

Flurazepam Hydrochloride (Co-administration may increase flurazepam levels; may need to decrease flurazepam dose).

No products indexed under this heading.

Fluticasone Propionate (Co-administration may lead to increased fluticasone levels. Concomitant use of fluticasone propionate and fosamprenavir calcium (without ritonavir) may increase plasma concentrations of fluticasone propionate; use with caution and consider alternatives to fluticasone propionate, particularly for long-term use. Concomitant use of fluticasone propionate and fosamprenavir calcium/ritonavir may increase plasma concentrations of fluticasone propionate, resulting in significantly reduced serum cortisol concentrations. Co-administration of fluticasone propionate and fosamprenavir calcium/ritonavir is not recommended unless the potential benefit to the patient outweighs the risk of systemic corticosteroid side effects). Products include:

Advair Diskus 100/50 ... 1276
Advair Diskus 250/50 ... 1276
Advair Diskus 500/50 ... 1276
Advair HFA 45/21 Inhalation Aerosol ... 1288
Advair HFA 115/21 Inhalation Aerosol ... 1288
Advair HFA 230/21 Inhalation Aerosol ... 1288
Flonase Nasal Spray ... 1431
Flovent Diskus 50 mcg ... 1435

Fluticasone Propionate HFA (Co-administration may lead to increased fluticasone levels. Concomitant use of fluticasone propionate and fosamprenavir calcium (without ritonavir) may increase plasma concentrations of fluticasone propionate; use with caution and consider alternatives to fluticasone propionate, particularly for long-term use. Concomitant use of fluticasone propionate and fosamprenavir calcium/ritonavir may increase plasma concentrations of fluticasone propionate, resulting in significantly reduced serum cortisol concentrations. Co-administration of fluticasone propionate and fosamprenavir calcium/ritonavir is not recommended unless the potential benefit to the patient outweighs the risk of systemic corticosteroid side effects). Products include:

Flovent HFA ... 1440

Fluvoxamine Maleate (Amprenavir is metabolized by CYP 3A4. Co-administration of fosamprenavir calcium and drugs that inhibit CYP3A4 may increase amprenavir concentrations and increase the incidence of adverse effects). Products include:

Luvox CR Extended-Release Capsules ... 1759

Fosphenytoin Sodium (Co-administration may lead to decreased amprenavir levels. Use with caution; fosamprenavir may be less effective due to decreased plasma concentrations in patients taking these agents concomitantly).

No products indexed under this heading.

Garlic Extract (Amprenavir is metabolized by CYP3A4. Co-administration of fosamprenavir calcium and drugs that induce CYP3A4 may decrease amprenavir concentrations and reduce its therapeutic effect).

No products indexed under this heading.

Garlic Oil (Amprenavir is metabolized by CYP3A4. Co-administration of fosamprenavir calcium and drugs that induce CYP3A4 may decrease amprenavir concentrations and reduce its therapeutic effect).

No products indexed under this heading.

Haloperidol (Amprenavir, the active metabolite of fosamprenavir, is an inhibitor of cytochrome P450 3A4 metabolism and therefore should not be administered concurrently with medications with narrow therapeutic windows that are substrates of CYP3A4. Data also suggests that amprenavir induces CYP3A4).

No products indexed under this heading.

Haloperidol Decanoate (Amprenavir, the active metabolite of fosamprenavir, is an inhibitor of cytochrome P450 3A4 metabolism and therefore should not be administered concurrently with medications with narrow therapeutic windows that are substrates of CYP3A4. Data also suggests that amprenavir induces CYP3A4).

No products indexed under this heading.

Haloperidol Lactate (Amprenavir, the active metabolite of fosamprenavir, is an inhibitor of cytochrome P450 3A4 metabolism and therefore should not be administered concurrently with medications with narrow therapeutic windows that are substrates of CYP3A4. Data also suggests that amprenavir induces CYP3A4).

No products indexed under this heading.

Hydrocortisone (Amprenavir is metabolized by CYP3A4. Co-administration of fosamprenavir calcium and drugs that induce CYP3A4 may decrease amprenavir concentrations and reduce its therapeutic effect).

No products indexed under this heading.

Hydrocortisone Acetate (Amprenavir is metabolized by CYP3A4. Co-administration of fosamprenavir calcium and drugs that induce CYP3A4 may decrease amprenavir concentrations and reduce its therapeutic effect). Products include:

Analpram-HC ... 1140
Pramosone ... 1141

Hydrocortisone Butyrate (Amprenavir is metabolized by CYP3A4. Co-administration of fosamprenavir calcium and drugs that induce CYP3A4 may decrease amprenavir concentrations and reduce its therapeutic effect).

No products indexed under this heading.

Hydrocortisone Cypionate (Amprenavir is metabolized by CYP3A4. Co-administration of fosamprenavir calcium and drugs that induce CYP3A4 may decrease amprenavir concentrations and reduce its therapeutic effect).

No products indexed under this heading.

Hydrocortisone Hemisuccinate (Amprenavir is metabolized by CYP3A4. Co-administration of fosamprenavir calcium and drugs that induce CYP3A4 may decrease amprenavir concentrations and reduce its therapeutic effect).

No products indexed under this heading.

Hydrocortisone Probutate (Amprenavir is metabolized by CYP3A4. Co-administration of fosamprenavir calcium and drugs that induce CYP3A4 may decrease amprenavir concentrations and reduce its therapeutic effect).

No products indexed under this heading.

Hydrocortisone Sodium Phosphate (Amprenavir is metabolized by CYP3A4. Co-administration of fosamprenavir calcium and drugs that induce CYP3A4 may decrease amprenavir concentrations and reduce its therapeutic effect).

No products indexed under this heading.

Hydrocortisone Sodium Succinate (Amprenavir is metabolized by CYP3A4. Co-administration of fosamprenavir calcium and drugs that induce CYP3A4 may decrease amprenavir concentrations and reduce its therapeutic effect).

No products indexed under this heading.

Hydrocortisone Valerate (Amprenavir is metabolized by CYP3A4. Co-administration of fosamprenavir calcium and drugs that induce CYP3A4 may decrease amprenavir concentrations and reduce its therapeutic effect).

No products indexed under this heading.

Hypericum (Co-administration may lead to loss of virologic response and possible resistance to fosamprenavir or other protease inhibitors). Products include:

Satieté Tablets ... ▣ 640

Hypericum Perforatum (Co-administration may lead to loss of virologic response and possible resistance to fosamprenavir or other protease inhibitors).

No products indexed under this heading.

Imipramine Hydrochloride (Co-administration may lead to increased levels of imipramine. Therapeutic concentration monitoring is recommended for tricyclic antidepressants when co-administered with fosamprenavir).

No products indexed under this heading.

Imipramine Pamoate (Co-administration may lead to increased levels of imipramine. Therapeutic concentration monitoring is recommended for tricyclic antidepressants when co-administered with fosamprenavir).

No products indexed under this heading.

Indinavir Sulfate (Co-administration with fosamprenavir alone may lead to increased amprenavir levels). Products include:

Crixivan Capsules ... 1979

Isoniazid (Amprenavir is metabolized by CYP 3A4. Co-administration of fosamprenavir calcium and drugs that inhibit CYP3A4 may increase amprenavir concentrations and increase the incidence of adverse effects).

No products indexed under this heading.

Isradipine (Co-administration may increase levels of isradipine; caution is warranted and clinical monitoring is recommended). Products include:

DynaCirc CR Controlled Release Tablets ... 1407

Itraconazole (Co-administration may increase itraconazole levels; increase monitoring for adverse events due to itraconazole. When co-administered with fosamprenavir alone, itraconazole dose reduction may be needed for patients receiving more than 400mg of itraconazole per day. If patient is receiving fosamprenavir/ritonavir combination, co-administration of high doses of itraconazole (>200mg/day) are not recommended).

No products indexed under this heading.

Ixabepilone (Amprenavir, the active metabolite of fosamprenavir, is an inhibitor of cytochrome P450 3A4 metabolism and therefore should not be administered concurrently with medications with narrow therapeutic windows that are substrates of CYP3A4. Data also suggests that amprenavir induces CYP3A4). Products include:

Ixempra Kit for Injection ... 915

Ketoconazole (Co-administration may increase ketoconazole levels; increase monitoring for adverse events due to ketoconazole. When co-administered with fosamprenavir alone, ketoconazole dose reduction may be needed for patients receiving more than 400mg of ketoconazole per day. If patient is receiving fosamprenavir/ritonavir combination, co-administration of high doses of ketoconazole (>200mg/day) are not recommended). Products include:

Extina Foam, 2% 3057
Nizoral A-D Shampoo 1901

Levonorgestrel (Amprenavir, the active metabolite of fosamprenavir, is an inhibitor of cytochrome P450 3A4 metabolism and therefore should not be administered concurrently with medications with narrow therapeutic windows that are substrates of CYP3A4. Data also suggests that amprenavir induces CYP3A4). Products include:

Climara Pro Transdermal System 768
Lybrel Tablets 3204
Mirena Intrauterine System 779
Plan B Tablets 1044
Seasonique Tablets 1046

Lidocaine (Co-administration may lead to increased levels of lidocaine. Caution is warranted and therapeutic concentration monitoring is recommended for antiarrhythmics when co-administered with fosamprenavir). Products include:

Lidoderm Patch 1114

Lidocaine Hydrochloride (Co-administration may lead to increased levels of lidocaine. Caution is warranted and therapeutic concentration monitoring is recommended for antiarrhythmics when co-administered with fosamprenavir).

No products indexed under this heading.

Lopinavir (Co-administration of lopinavir/ritonavir and fosamprenavir may lead to decreased levels of amprenavir and lopinavir. An increased rate of adverse events has also been observed with co-administration of these medications). Products include:

Kaletra 452

Loratadine (Amprenavir is metabolized by CYP 3A4. Co-administration of fosamprenavir calcium and drugs that inhibit CYP3A4 may increase amprenavir concentrations and increase the incidence of adverse effects).

No products indexed under this heading.

Lovastatin (Co-administration may lead to the potential for serious reactions such as risk of myopathy including rhabdomyolysis). Products include:

Advicor Tablets 402
Mevacor Tablets 2063

Mephenytoin (Amprenavir is metabolized by CYP3A4. Co-administration of fosamprenavir calcium and drugs that induce CYP3A4 may decrease amprenavir concentrations and reduce its therapeutic effect).

No products indexed under this heading.

Mestranol (Amprenavir, the active metabolite of fosamprenavir, is an inhibitor of cytochrome P450 3A4 metabolism and therefore should not be administered concurrently with medications with narrow therapeutic windows that are substrates of CYP3A4. Data also suggests that amprenavir induces CYP3A4).

No products indexed under this heading.

Methadone Hydrochloride (Co-administration may lead to decreased levels of methadone; dosage of methadone may need to be increased when co-administered with fosamprenavir).

No products indexed under this heading.

Methsuximide (Amprenavir is metabolized by CYP3A4. Co-administration of fosamprenavir calcium and drugs that induce CYP3A4 may decrease amprenavir concentrations and reduce its therapeutic effect).

No products indexed under this heading.

Methylergonovine Maleate (Co-administration with methylergonovine is contraindicated due to the potential for serious and/or life-threatening reactions such as acute ergot toxicity characterized by peripheral vasospasm and ischemia of the extremities and other tissues).

No products indexed under this heading.

Methylprednisolone (Amprenavir is metabolized by CYP3A4. Co-administration of fosamprenavir calcium and drugs that induce CYP3A4 may decrease amprenavir concentrations and reduce its therapeutic effect).

No products indexed under this heading.

Methylprednisolone Acetate (Amprenavir is metabolized by CYP3A4. Co-administration of fosamprenavir calcium and drugs that induce CYP3A4 may decrease amprenavir concentrations and reduce its therapeutic effect).

No products indexed under this heading.

Methylprednisolone Sodium Succinate (Amprenavir is metabolized by CYP3A4. Co-administration of fosamprenavir calcium and drugs that induce CYP3A4 may decrease amprenavir concentrations and reduce its therapeutic effect).

No products indexed under this heading.

Metronidazole (Amprenavir is metabolized by CYP 3A4. Co-administration of fosamprenavir calcium and drugs that inhibit CYP3A4 may increase amprenavir concentrations and increase the incidence of adverse effects). Products include:

Pylera Capsules 714

Metronidazole Benzoate (Amprenavir is metabolized by CYP 3A4. Co-administration of fosamprenavir calcium and drugs that inhibit CYP3A4 may increase amprenavir concentrations and increase the incidence of adverse effects).

No products indexed under this heading.

Metronidazole Hydrochloride (Amprenavir is metabolized by CYP 3A4. Co-administration of fosamprenavir calcium and drugs that inhibit CYP3A4 may increase amprenavir concentrations and increase the incidence of adverse effects).

No products indexed under this heading.

Metronidazole Sodium (Amprenavir is metabolized by CYP 3A4. Co-administration of fosamprenavir calcium and drugs that inhibit CYP3A4 may increase amprenavir concentrations and increase the incidence of adverse effects).

No products indexed under this heading.

Miconazole (Amprenavir is metabolized by CYP 3A4. Co-administration of fosamprenavir calcium and drugs that inhibit CYP3A4 may increase amprenavir concentrations and increase the incidence of adverse effects).

No products indexed under this heading.

Miconazole Nitrate (Amprenavir is metabolized by CYP 3A4. Co-administration of fosamprenavir calcium and drugs that inhibit CYP3A4 may increase amprenavir concentrations and increase the incidence of adverse effects).

No products indexed under this heading.

Midazolam Hydrochloride (Co-administration with midazolam is contraindicated due to potential for serious and/or life-threatening reactions such as prolonged or increased sedation or respiratory depression).

No products indexed under this heading.

Modafinil (Amprenavir is metabolized by CYP3A4. Co-administration of fosamprenavir calcium and drugs that induce CYP3A4 may decrease amprenavir concentrations and reduce its therapeutic effect). Products include:

Provigil Tablets 977

Nefazodone Hydrochloride (Amprenavir, the active metabolite of fosamprenavir, is an inhibitor of cytochrome P450 3A4 metabolism and therefore should not be administered concurrently with medications with narrow therapeutic windows that are substrates of CYP3A4. Data also suggests that amprenavir induces CYP3A4).

No products indexed under this heading.

Nelfinavir Mesylate (Co-administration with fosamprenavir alone may lead to increased amprenavir levels).

No products indexed under this heading.

Nevirapine (Co-administration may lead to decreased amprenavir levels and increased nevirapine levels. Co-administration of nevirapine and fosamprenavir calcium without ritonavir is not recommended). Products include:

Viramune Oral Suspension 873
Viramune Tablets 873

Niacinamide (Amprenavir is metabolized by CYP 3A4. Co-administration of fosamprenavir calcium and drugs that inhibit CYP3A4 may increase amprenavir concentrations and increase the incidence of adverse effects). Products include:

BioLean Free Tablets .... ▣635

Nicardipine (Co-administration may increase levels of nicardipine; caution is warranted and clinical monitoring is recommended).

No products indexed under this heading.

Nicardipine Hydrochloride (Co-administration may increase levels of nicardipine; caution is warranted and clinical monitoring is recommended). Products include:

Cardene I.V. 1093

Nicotinamide (Amprenavir is metabolized by CYP 3A4. Co-administration of fosamprenavir calcium and drugs that inhibit CYP3A4 may increase amprenavir concentrations and increase the incidence of adverse effects).

No products indexed under this heading.

Nifedipine (Co-administration may increase levels of nifedipine, caution is warranted and clinical monitoring is recommended).

No products indexed under this heading.

Nimodipine (Co-administration may increase levels of nimodipine; caution is warranted and clinical monitoring is recommended). Products include:

Nimotop Capsules 790

Nisoldipine (Co-administration may increase levels of nisoldipine; caution is warranted and clinical monitoring is recommended). Products include:

Sular Extended Release Tablets 2975

Nitrendipine (Amprenavir, the active metabolite of fosamprenavir, is an inhibitor of cytochrome P450 3A4 metabolism and therefore should not be administered concurrently with medications with narrow therapeutic windows that are substrates of CYP3A4. Data also suggests that amprenavir induces CYP3A4).

No products indexed under this heading.

Nizatidine (Co-administration of fosamprenavir alone and histamine H2-receptor antagonists may lead to decreased levels of fosamprenavir. Use with caution since fosamprenavir may be less effective due to decreased amprenavir plasma concentrations in patients taking these agents concomitantly). Products include:

Axid Capsules 1364

Norethindrone (Co-administration of fosamprenavir alone with oral contraceptives containing the combination ethinyl estradiol/norethindrone may lead to increased levels of ethinyl estradiol/norethindrone. Because these hormonal levels may be altered, alternative methods of non-hormonal contraception are recommended). Products include:

Ortho Micronor Tablets 2446

Norethindrone Acetate (Co-administration of fosamprenavir alone with oral contraceptives containing the combination ethinyl estradiol/norethindrone may lead to increased levels of ethinyl estradiol/norethindrone. Because these hormonal levels may be altered, alterna-

tive methods of non-hormonal contraception are recommended). Products include:
Activella Tablets 2347

Norfloxacin (Amprenavir is metabolized by CYP 3A4. Co-administration of fosamprenavir calcium and drugs that inhibit CYP3A4 may increase amprenavir concentrations and increase the incidence of adverse effects). Products include:
Noroxin Tablets 2069

Norgestrel (Amprenavir, the active metabolite of fosamprenavir, is an inhibitor of cytochrome P450 3A4 metabolism and therefore should not be administered concurrently with medications with narrow therapeutic windows that are substrates of CYP3A4. Data also suggests that amprenavir induces CYP3A4).
No products indexed under this heading.

Omeprazole (Amprenavir is metabolized by CYP 3A4. Co-administration of fosamprenavir calcium and drugs that inhibit CYP3A4 may increase amprenavir concentrations and increase the incidence of adverse effects).
No products indexed under this heading.

Ondansetron (Amprenavir, the active metabolite of fosamprenavir, is an inhibitor of cytochrome P450 3A4 metabolism and therefore should not be administered concurrently with medications with narrow therapeutic windows that are substrates of CYP3A4. Data also suggests that amprenavir induces CYP3A4). Products include:
Zofran ODT Orally Disintegrating Tablets 1687

Ondansetron Hydrochloride (Amprenavir, the active metabolite of fosamprenavir, is an inhibitor of cytochrome P450 3A4 metabolism and therefore should not be administered concurrently with medications with narrow therapeutic windows that are substrates of CYP3A4. Data also suggests that amprenavir induces CYP3A4). Products include:
Zofran Injection 1682
Zofran 1687

Oxcarbazepine (Amprenavir is metabolized by CYP3A4. Co-administration of fosamprenavir calcium and drugs that induce CYP3A4 may decrease amprenavir concentrations and reduce its therapeutic effect).
No products indexed under this heading.

Paclitaxel (Amprenavir, the active metabolite of fosamprenavir, is an inhibitor of cytochrome P450 3A4 metabolism and therefore should not be administered concurrently with medications with narrow therapeutic windows that are substrates of CYP3A4. Data also suggests that amprenavir induces CYP3A4).
No products indexed under this heading.

Paroxetine Hydrochloride (Amprenavir is metabolized by CYP 3A4. Co-administration of fosamprenavir calcium and drugs that inhibit CYP3A4 may increase amprenavir concentrations and increase the incidence of adverse effects). Products include:
Paxil 1535
Paxil CR Controlled-Release Tablets 1544

Phenobarbital (Co-administration may lead to decreased amprenavir levels. Use with caution; fosamprenavir may be less effective due to decreased plasma concentrations in patients taking these agents concomitantly). Products include:
Donnatal Extentabs 2507

Phenobarbital Sodium (Co-administration may lead to decreased amprenavir levels. Use with caution; fosamprenavir may be less effective due to decreased plasma concentrations in patients taking these agents concomitantly).
No products indexed under this heading.

Phenytoin (Co-administration may lead to decreased amprenavir levels. Use with caution; fosamprenavir may be less effective due to decreased plasma concentrations in patients taking these agents concomitantly).
No products indexed under this heading.

Phenytoin Sodium (Co-administration may lead to decreased amprenavir levels. Use with caution; fosamprenavir may be less effective due to decreased plasma concentrations in patients taking these agents concomitantly). Products include:
Phenytek Capsules 2192

Pimozide (Co-administration with pimozide is contraindicated due to potential for serious and/or life-threatening reactions such as cardiac arrhythmias).
No products indexed under this heading.

Polyestradiol Phosphate (Amprenavir, the active metabolite of fosamprenavir, is an inhibitor of cytochrome P450 3A4 metabolism and therefore should not be administered concurrently with medications with narrow therapeutic windows that are substrates of CYP3A4. Data also suggests that amprenavir induces CYP3A4).
No products indexed under this heading.

Prednisolone Acetate (Amprenavir is metabolized by CYP3A4. Co-administration of fosamprenavir calcium and drugs that induce CYP3A4 may decrease amprenavir concentrations and reduce its therapeutic effect). Products include:
Pred Forte Ophthalmic Suspension .... ⊙227
Pred Mild Ophthalmic Suspension .... ⊙230
Pred-G Ophthalmic Ointment .... ⊙229
Pred-G Ophthalmic Suspension .... ⊙228

Prednisolone Sodium Phosphate (Amprenavir is metabolized by CYP3A4. Co-administration of fosamprenavir calcium and drugs that induce CYP3A4 may decrease amprenavir concentrations and reduce its therapeutic effect).
No products indexed under this heading.

Prednisolone Tebutate (Amprenavir is metabolized by CYP3A4. Co-administration of fosamprenavir calcium and drugs that induce CYP3A4 may decrease amprenavir concentrations and reduce its therapeutic effect).
No products indexed under this heading.

Prednisone (Amprenavir is metabolized by CYP3A4. Co-administration of fosamprenavir calcium and drugs that induce CYP3A4 may decrease amprenavir concentrations and reduce its therapeutic effect).
No products indexed under this heading.

Primidone (Amprenavir is metabolized by CYP3A4. Co-administration of fosamprenavir calcium and drugs that induce CYP3A4 may decrease amprenavir concentrations and reduce its therapeutic effect).
No products indexed under this heading.

Propafenone Hydrochloride (If fosamprenavir is co-administered with ritonavir, the antiarrhythmic agent propafenone is contraindicated due to the potential for serious and/or life-threatening reactions such as cardiac arrhythmias secondary to increases in plasma concentrations of propafenone). Products include:
Rythmol Tablets 1586
Rythmol SR Capsules 1590

Propoxyphene Hydrochloride (Amprenavir is metabolized by CYP 3A4. Co-administration of fosamprenavir calcium and drugs that inhibit CYP3A4 may increase amprenavir concentrations and increase the incidence of adverse effects).
No products indexed under this heading.

Propoxyphene Napsylate (Amprenavir is metabolized by CYP 3A4. Co-administration of fosamprenavir calcium and drugs that inhibit CYP3A4 may increase amprenavir concentrations and increase the incidence of adverse effects).
No products indexed under this heading.

Quinidine (Co-administration may lead to increased levels of quinidine. Caution is warranted and therapeutic concentration monitoring is recommended for antiarrhythmics when co-administered with fosamprenavir).
No products indexed under this heading.

Quinidine Gluconate (Co-administration may lead to increased levels of quinidine. Caution is warranted and therapeutic concentration monitoring is recommended for antiarrhythmics when co-administered with fosamprenavir).
No products indexed under this heading.

Quinidine Hydrochloride (Co-administration may lead to increased levels of quinidine. Caution is warranted and therapeutic concentration monitoring is recommended for antiarrhythmics when co-administered with fosamprenavir).
No products indexed under this heading.

Quinidine Polygalacturonate (Co-administration may lead to increased levels of quinidine. Caution is warranted and therapeutic concentration monitoring is recommended for antiarrhythmics when co-administered with fosamprenavir).
No products indexed under this heading.

Quinidine Sulfate (Co-administration may lead to increased levels of quinidine. Caution is warranted and therapeutic concentration monitoring is recommended for antiarrhythmics when co-administered with fosamprenavir).
No products indexed under this heading.

Quinine (Amprenavir is metabolized by CYP 3A4. Co-administration of fosamprenavir calcium and drugs that inhibit CYP3A4 may increase amprenavir concentrations and increase the incidence of adverse effects).
No products indexed under this heading.

Quinine Sulfate (Amprenavir is metabolized by CYP 3A4. Co-administration of fosamprenavir calcium and drugs that inhibit CYP3A4 may increase amprenavir concentrations and increase the incidence of adverse effects).
No products indexed under this heading.

Quinupristin (Amprenavir is metabolized by CYP 3A4. Co-administration of fosamprenavir calcium and drugs that inhibit CYP3A4 may increase amprenavir concentrations and increase the incidence of adverse effects).
No products indexed under this heading.

Ranitidine Bismuth Citrate (Co-administration of fosamprenavir alone and histamine H2-receptor antagonists may lead to decreased levels of fosamprenavir. Use with caution since fosamprenavir may be less effective due to decreased amprenavir plasma concentrations in patients taking these agents concomitantly).
No products indexed under this heading.

Ranitidine Hydrochloride (Co-administration of fosamprenavir alone and histamine H2-receptor antagonists may lead to decreased levels of fosamprenavir. Use with caution since fosamprenavir may be less effective due to decreased amprenavir plasma concentrations in patients taking these agents concomitantly). Products include:
Zantac 75 Tablets .... ▣603
Zantac 1670
Zantac Injection 1666
Zantac Injection Pharmacy Bulk Package 1668
Maximum Strength Zantac 150 Tablets .... ▣603
Maximum Strength Zantac 150 Cool Mint Tablets .... ▣603

Rapamycin (Co-administration may lead to increased levels of rapamycin. Therapeutic concentration monitoring is recommended for immunosuppressant agents when co-administered with fosamprenavir).
No products indexed under this heading.

Rifabutin (Co-administration may cause increased levels of rifabutin and its metabolite; perform CBC weekly and as clinically indicated in order to monitor for neutropenia in patients receiving concurrent administration. In patients receiving fosamprenavir alone, a dosage reduction of rifabutin by at least half the recommended dose is required. In patients receiving fosamprenavir/ritonavir combination, dosage reduction of rifabutin by at least 75% of the usual dose of 300mg/day is recommended (maximum dose of 150mg every other day or three times weekly)).

No products indexed under this heading.

Rifampicin (Amprenavir is metabolized by CYP3A4. Co-administration of fosamprenavir calcium and drugs that induce CYP3A4 may decrease amprenavir concentrations and reduce its therapeutic effect).

No products indexed under this heading.

Rifampin (Co-administration may lead to loss of virologic response and possible resistance to fosamprenavir or other protease inhibitors. Co-administration with rifampin is contraindicated).

No products indexed under this heading.

Rifapentine (Amprenavir is metabolized by CYP3A4. Co-administration of fosamprenavir calcium and drugs that induce CYP3A4 may decrease amprenavir concentrations and reduce its therapeutic effect).

No products indexed under this heading.

Ritonavir (Co-administration of lopinavir/ritonavir and fosamprenavir may lead to decreased levels of amprenavir and lopinavir (when given in combination with ritonavir). An increased rate of adverse events has also been observed with co-administration of these medications. Concomitant use of fosamprenavir calcium and ritonavir is not recommended since the combination may result in clinically significant hepatic transaminase elevations). Products include:

Kaletra 452
Norvir 489

Saquinavir (Co-administration with fosamprenavir alone may lead to decreased levels of amprenavir).

No products indexed under this heading.

Saquinavir Mesylate (Amprenavir, the active metabolite of fosamprenavir, is an inhibitor of cytochrome P450 3A4 metabolism and therefore should not be administered concurrently with medications with narrow therapeutic windows that are substrates of CYP3A4. Data also suggests that amprenavir induces CYP3A4).

No products indexed under this heading.

Sertraline Hydrochloride (Amprenavir, the active metabolite of fosamprenavir, is an inhibitor of cytochrome P450 3A4 metabolism and therefore should not be administered concurrently with medications with narrow therapeutic windows that are substrates of CYP3A4. Data also suggests that amprenavir induces CYP3A4).

No products indexed under this heading.

Sildenafil Citrate (Co-administration may lead to increased levels of sildenafil; use sildenafil with caution at reduced doses of 25mg every 48 hours with increased monitoring for adverse events).

No products indexed under this heading.

Simvastatin (Co-administration may lead to the potential for serious reactions such as risk of myopathy including rhabdomyolysis). Products include:

Simcor Tablets 502
Vytorin 10/10 Tablets 2149
Vytorin 10/10 Tablets 2939
Vytorin 10/20 Tablets 2149
Vytorin 10/20 Tablets 2939
Vytorin 10/40 Tablets 2149
Vytorin 10/40 Tablets 2939
Vytorin 10/80 Tablets 2149
Vytorin 10/80 Tablets 2939
Zocor Tablets 2136

Sirolimus (Amprenavir, the active metabolite of fosamprenavir, is an inhibitor of cytochrome P450 3A4 metabolism and therefore should not be administered concurrently with medications with narrow therapeutic windows that are substrates of CYP3A4. Data also suggests that amprenavir induces CYP3A4). Products include:

Rapamune 3260

Sulfinpyrazone (Amprenavir is metabolized by CYP3A4. Co-administration of fosamprenavir calcium and drugs that induce CYP3A4 may decrease amprenavir concentrations and reduce its therapeutic effect).

No products indexed under this heading.

Tacrolimus (Co-administration may lead to increased levels of tacrolimus. Therapeutic concentration monitoring is recommended for immunosuppressant agents when co-administered with fosamprenavir). Products include:

Prograf Capsules and Injection 622
Protopic Ointment 628

Tadalafil (Amprenavir, the active metabolite of fosamprenavir, is an inhibitor of cytochrome P450 3A4 metabolism and therefore should not be administered concurrently with medications with narrow therapeutic windows that are substrates of CYP3A4. Data also suggests that amprenavir induces CYP3A4). Products include:

Cialis Tablets 1792

Tamoxifen Citrate (Amprenavir, the active metabolite of fosamprenavir, is an inhibitor of cytochrome P450 3A4 metabolism and therefore should not be administered concurrently with medications with narrow therapeutic windows that are substrates of CYP3A4. Data also suggests that amprenavir induces CYP3A4).

No products indexed under this heading.

Telithromycin (Amprenavir is metabolized by CYP 3A4. Co-administration of fosamprenavir calcium and drugs that inhibit CYP3A4 may increase amprenavir concentrations and increase the incidence of adverse effects). Products include:

Ketek Tablets 2744

Theophylline (Amprenavir is metabolized by CYP3A4. Co-administration of fosamprenavir calcium and drugs that induce CYP3A4 may decrease amprenavir concentrations and reduce its therapeutic effect).

No products indexed under this heading.

Theophylline Anhydrous (Amprenavir is metabolized by CYP3A4. Co-administration of fosamprenavir calcium and drugs that induce CYP3A4 may decrease amprenavir concentrations and reduce its therapeutic effect). Products include:

Uniphyl Tablets 2595

Theophylline Calcium Salicylate (Amprenavir is metabolized by CYP3A4. Co-administration of fosamprenavir calcium and drugs that induce CYP3A4 may decrease amprenavir concentrations and reduce its therapeutic effect).

No products indexed under this heading.

Theophylline Dihydroxypropyl (Glyceryl) (Amprenavir is metabolized by CYP3A4. Co-administration of fosamprenavir calcium and drugs that induce CYP3A4 may decrease amprenavir concentrations and reduce its therapeutic effect).

No products indexed under this heading.

Theophylline Ethylenediamine (Amprenavir is metabolized by CYP3A4. Co-administration of fosamprenavir calcium and drugs that induce CYP3A4 may decrease amprenavir concentrations and reduce its therapeutic effect).

No products indexed under this heading.

Tiagabine Hydrochloride (Amprenavir, the active metabolite of fosamprenavir, is an inhibitor of cytochrome P450 3A4 metabolism and therefore should not be administered concurrently with medications with narrow therapeutic windows that are substrates of CYP3A4. Data also suggests that amprenavir induces CYP3A4). Products include:

Gabitril Tablets 973

Tolterodine Tartrate (Amprenavir, the active metabolite of fosamprenavir, is an inhibitor of cytochrome P450 3A4 metabolism and therefore should not be administered concurrently with medications with narrow therapeutic windows that are substrates of CYP3A4. Data also suggests that amprenavir induces CYP3A4).

No products indexed under this heading.

Trazodone Hydrochloride (Concomitant use of trazodone and fosamprenavir calcium with or without ritonavir may increase plasma concentrations of trazodone. Adverse events have been observed during co-administration. If trazodone is used with a CYP3A4 inhibitor such as fosamaprenavir calcium, the combination should be used with caution and a lower dose of trazodone should be considered).

No products indexed under this heading.

Triamcinolone (Amprenavir is metabolized by CYP3A4. Co-administration of fosamprenavir calcium and drugs that induce CYP3A4 may decrease amprenavir concentrations and reduce its therapeutic effect).

No products indexed under this heading.

Triamcinolone Acetonide (Amprenavir is metabolized by CYP3A4. Co-administration of fosamprenavir calcium and drugs that induce CYP3A4 may decrease amprenavir concentrations and reduce its therapeutic effect). Products include:

Azmacort Inhalation Aerosol 407
Nasacort AQ Nasal Spray 2765
Triesence Injectable Suspension .... ⊙ 209

Triamcinolone Diacetate (Amprenavir is metabolized by CYP3A4. Co-administration of fosamprenavir calcium and drugs that induce CYP3A4 may decrease amprenavir concentrations and reduce its therapeutic effect).

No products indexed under this heading.

Triamcinolone Hexacetonide (Amprenavir is metabolized by CYP3A4. Co-administration of fosamprenavir calcium and drugs that induce CYP3A4 may decrease amprenavir concentrations and reduce its therapeutic effect).

No products indexed under this heading.

Triazolam (Co-administration with triazolam is contraindicated due to potential for serious and/or life-threatening reactions such as prolonged or increased sedation or respiratory depression).

No products indexed under this heading.

Troglitazone (Amprenavir is metabolized by CYP3A4. Co-administration of fosamprenavir calcium and drugs that induce CYP3A4 may decrease amprenavir concentrations and reduce its therapeutic effect).

No products indexed under this heading.

Troleandomycin (Amprenavir is metabolized by CYP 3A4. Co-administration of fosamprenavir calcium and drugs that inhibit CYP3A4 may increase amprenavir concentrations and increase the incidence of adverse effects).

No products indexed under this heading.

Valproate Sodium (Amprenavir is metabolized by CYP 3A4. Co-administration of fosamprenavir calcium and drugs that inhibit CYP3A4 may increase amprenavir concentrations and increase the incidence of adverse effects).

No products indexed under this heading.

Vardenafil Hydrochloride (Co-administration may lead to increased levels of vardenafil. When co-administered with fosamprenavir alone, use vardenafil with caution at reduced doses of no more than 2.5mg every 24 hours with increased monitoring for adverse events. When co-administered with fosamprenavir/ritonavir combination, use vardenafil with caution at reduced doses of no more than 2.5mg every 72 hours with increased monitoring for adverse events). Products include:

Levitra Tablets 2876

Verapamil Hydrochloride (Co-administration may increase levels of verapamil; caution is warranted and clinical monitoring is recommended). Products include:

Tarka Tablets 511

Vinblastine Sulfate (Amprenavir, the active metabolite of fosamprenavir, is an inhibitor of cytochrome P450 3A4 metabolism and therefore should not be administered concurrently with medications with narrow therapeutic windows that are substrates of CYP3A4. Data also suggests that amprenavir induces CYP3A4).

No products indexed under this heading.

Vincristine Sulfate (Amprenavir, the active metabolite of fosamprenavir, is an inhibitor of cytochrome P450 3A4 metabolism and therefore should not be administered concurrently with medications with narrow therapeutic windows that are substrates of CYP3A4. Data also suggests that amprenavir induces CYP3A4).
No products indexed under this heading.

Voriconazole (Amprenavir is metabolized by CYP 3A4. Co-administration of fosamprenavir calcium and drugs that inhibit CYP3A4 may increase amprenavir concentrations and increase the incidence of adverse effects).
No products indexed under this heading.

Warfarin Sodium (Concentrations of warfarin may be affected. It is recommended that INR be monitored).
No products indexed under this heading.

Zafirlukast (Amprenavir is metabolized by CYP 3A4. Co-administration of fosamprenavir calcium and drugs that inhibit CYP3A4 may increase amprenavir concentrations and increase the incidence of adverse effects). Products include:
Accolate Tablets 669

Zileuton (Amprenavir is metabolized by CYP 3A4. Co-administration of fosamprenavir calcium and drugs that inhibit CYP3A4 may increase amprenavir concentrations and increase the incidence of adverse effects).
No products indexed under this heading.

Food Interactions

Grapefruit (Amprenavir is metabolized by CYP 3A4. Co-administration of fosamprenavir calcium and drugs that inhibit CYP3A4 may increase amprenavir concentrations and increase the incidence of adverse effects).

Grapefruit Juice (Amprenavir is metabolized by CYP 3A4. Co-administration of fosamprenavir calcium and drugs that inhibit CYP3A4 may increase amprenavir concentrations and increase the incidence of adverse effects).

LIALDA TABLETS

(Mesalamine) 3029

May interact with nephrotoxic agents and certain other agents. Compounds in these categories include:

Abacavir Sulfate (The concurrent use of mesalimine with known nephrotoxic agents, including non-steroidal anti-inflammatory drugs (NSAIDs) may increase the risk of renal reactions). Products include:
Epzicom Tablets 1422
Trizivir Tablets 1622
Ziagen 1673

Acyclovir (The concurrent use of mesalimine with known nephrotoxic agents, including non-steroidal anti-inflammatory drugs (NSAIDs) may increase the risk of renal reactions). Products include:
Zovirax 1690
Zovirax Cream 817
Zovirax Ointment 819

Acyclovir Sodium (The concurrent use of mesalimine with known nephrotoxic agents, including non-steroidal anti-inflammatory drugs (NSAIDs) may increase the risk of renal reactions).
No products indexed under this heading.

Alatrofloxacin Mesylate (The concurrent use of mesalimine with known nephrotoxic agents, including non-steroidal anti-inflammatory drugs (NSAIDs) may increase the risk of renal reactions).
No products indexed under this heading.

Aldesleukin (The concurrent use of mesalimine with known nephrotoxic agents, including non-steroidal anti-inflammatory drugs (NSAIDs) may increase the risk of renal reactions). Products include:
Proleukin for Injection 2287

Amikacin Sulfate (The concurrent use of mesalimine with known nephrotoxic agents, including non-steroidal anti-inflammatory drugs (NSAIDs) may increase the risk of renal reactions).
No products indexed under this heading.

Amoxicillin (The concurrent use of mesalimine with known nephrotoxic agents, including non-steroidal anti-inflammatory drugs (NSAIDs) may increase the risk of renal reactions). Products include:
Amoxil Capsules 1305
Amoxil Chewable Tablets 1305
Amoxil Pediatric Drops for Oral Suspension 1305
Amoxil Powder for Oral Suspension 1305
Amoxil Tablets 1305
Augmentin 1323
Augmentin Tablets 1327
Augmentin XR Extended Release Tablets 1333
Augmentin ES-600 Powder for Oral Suspension 1329
Moxatag Tablets 2165

Amoxicillin Trihydrate (The concurrent use of mesalimine with known nephrotoxic agents, including non-steroidal anti-inflammatory drugs (NSAIDs) may increase the risk of renal reactions).
No products indexed under this heading.

Amphotericin B (The concurrent use of mesalimine with known nephrotoxic agents, including non-steroidal anti-inflammatory drugs (NSAIDs) may increase the risk of renal reactions).
No products indexed under this heading.

Amphotericin B, liposomal (The concurrent use of mesalimine with known nephrotoxic agents, including non-steroidal anti-inflammatory drugs (NSAIDs) may increase the risk of renal reactions). Products include:
AmBisome for Injection 606

Amphotericin B Cholesteryl Sulfate (The concurrent use of mesalimine with known nephrotoxic agents, including non-steroidal anti-inflammatory drugs (NSAIDs) may increase the risk of renal reactions).
No products indexed under this heading.

Amphotericin B Lipid Complex (The concurrent use of mesalimine with known nephrotoxic agents, including non-steroidal anti-inflammatory drugs (NSAIDs) may increase the risk of renal reactions). Products include:
Abelcet Injection 1134

Ampicillin (The concurrent use of mesalimine with known nephrotoxic agents, including non-steroidal anti-inflammatory drugs (NSAIDs) may increase the risk of renal reactions).
No products indexed under this heading.

Ampicillin Sodium (The concurrent use of mesalimine with known nephrotoxic agents, including non-steroidal anti-inflammatory drugs (NSAIDs) may increase the risk of renal reactions).
No products indexed under this heading.

Ampicillin Trihydrate (The concurrent use of mesalimine with known nephrotoxic agents, including non-steroidal anti-inflammatory drugs (NSAIDs) may increase the risk of renal reactions).
No products indexed under this heading.

Amprenavir (The concurrent use of mesalimine with known nephrotoxic agents, including non-steroidal anti-inflammatory drugs (NSAIDs) may increase the risk of renal reactions).
No products indexed under this heading.

Aspirin (The concurrent use of mesalimine with known nephrotoxic agents, including non-steroidal anti-inflammatory drugs (NSAIDs) may increase the risk of renal reactions). Products include:
Aggrenox Capsules 819
Bayer Aspirin 750
Percodan Tablets 1130
St. Joseph 81 mg Aspirin Chewable and Enteric Coated Tablets 1903

Atazanavir (The concurrent use of mesalimine with known nephrotoxic agents, including non-steroidal anti-inflammatory drugs (NSAIDs) may increase the risk of renal reactions).
No products indexed under this heading.

Atorvastatin Calcium (The concurrent use of mesalimine with known nephrotoxic agents, including non-steroidal anti-inflammatory drugs (NSAIDs) may increase the risk of renal reactions). Products include:
Lipitor Tablets 2501

Azathioprine (The concurrent use of mesalamine with azathioprine can increase the potential for blood disorders).
No products indexed under this heading.

Azithromycin Dihydrate (The concurrent use of mesalimine with known nephrotoxic agents, including non-steroidal anti-inflammatory drugs (NSAIDs) may increase the risk of renal reactions).
No products indexed under this heading.

Azlocillin Sodium (The concurrent use of mesalimine with known nephrotoxic agents, including non-steroidal anti-inflammatory drugs (NSAIDs) may increase the risk of renal reactions).
No products indexed under this heading.

Aztreonam (The concurrent use of mesalimine with known nephrotoxic agents, including non-steroidal anti-inflammatory drugs (NSAIDs) may increase the risk of renal reactions).
No products indexed under this heading.

Bacampicillin Hydrochloride (The concurrent use of mesalimine with known nephrotoxic agents, including non-steroidal anti-inflammatory drugs (NSAIDs) may increase the risk of renal reactions).
No products indexed under this heading.

Balsalazide Disodium (The concurrent use of mesalimine with known nephrotoxic agents, including non-steroidal anti-inflammatory drugs (NSAIDs) may increase the risk of renal reactions).
No products indexed under this heading.

Benazepril Hydrochloride (The concurrent use of mesalimine with known nephrotoxic agents, including non-steroidal anti-inflammatory drugs (NSAIDs) may increase the risk of renal reactions).
No products indexed under this heading.

Bendroflumethiazide (The concurrent use of mesalimine with known nephrotoxic agents, including non-steroidal anti-inflammatory drugs (NSAIDs) may increase the risk of renal reactions).
No products indexed under this heading.

Caffeine (The concurrent use of mesalimine with known nephrotoxic agents, including non-steroidal anti-inflammatory drugs (NSAIDs) may increase the risk of renal reactions). Products include:
BioLean Free Tablets .... ▣ 635
BioLean II Tablets .... ▣ 635
Winrgy Dietary Supplement .... ▣ 642

Captopril (The concurrent use of mesalimine with known nephrotoxic agents, including non-steroidal anti-inflammatory drugs (NSAIDs) may increase the risk of renal reactions). Products include:
Captopril Tablets 2182

Carbenicillin Disodium (The concurrent use of mesalimine with known nephrotoxic agents, including non-steroidal anti-inflammatory drugs (NSAIDs) may increase the risk of renal reactions).
No products indexed under this heading.

Carbenicillin Indanyl Sodium (The concurrent use of mesalimine with known nephrotoxic agents, including non-steroidal anti-inflammatory drugs (NSAIDs) may increase the risk of renal reactions).
No products indexed under this heading.

Carboplatin (The concurrent use of mesalimine with known nephrotoxic agents, including non-steroidal anti-inflammatory drugs (NSAIDs) may increase the risk of renal reactions).
No products indexed under this heading.

Carmustine (BCNU) (The concurrent use of mesalimine with known nephrotoxic agents, including non-steroidal anti-inflammatory drugs (NSAIDs) may increase the risk of renal reactions).
No products indexed under this heading.

Cefaclor (The concurrent use of mesalimine with known nephrotoxic agents, including non-steroidal anti-inflammatory drugs (NSAIDs) may increase the risk of renal reactions).
No products indexed under this heading.

Cefadroxil (The concurrent use of mesalimine with known nephrotoxic agents, including non-steroidal anti-inflammatory drugs (NSAIDs) may increase the risk of renal reactions).
No products indexed under this heading.

Cefamandole Nafate (The concurrent use of mesalimine with known nephrotoxic agents, including non-steroidal anti-inflammatory drugs (NSAIDs) may increase the risk of renal reactions).
No products indexed under this heading.

Cefazolin Sodium (The concurrent use of mesalimine with known nephrotoxic agents, including non-steroidal anti-inflammatory drugs (NSAIDs) may increase the risk of renal reactions).
No products indexed under this heading.

Cefdinir (The concurrent use of mesalimine with known nephrotoxic agents, including non-steroidal anti-inflammatory drugs (NSAIDs) may increase the risk of renal reactions). Products include:
Omnicef Capsules 497
Omnicef for Oral Suspension 497

Cefepime Hydrochloride (The concurrent use of mesalimine with known nephrotoxic agents, including non-steroidal anti-inflammatory drugs (NSAIDs) may increase the risk of renal reactions).
No products indexed under this heading.

Cefixime (The concurrent use of mesalimine with known nephrotoxic agents, including non-steroidal anti-inflammatory drugs (NSAIDs) may increase the risk of renal reactions). Products include:
Suprax for Oral Suspension 1891
Suprax Tablets 1891

Cefmetazole Sodium (The concurrent use of mesalimine with known nephrotoxic agents, including non-steroidal anti-inflammatory drugs (NSAIDs) may increase the risk of renal reactions).
No products indexed under this heading.

Cefonicid Sodium (The concurrent use of mesalimine with known nephrotoxic agents, including non-steroidal anti-inflammatory drugs (NSAIDs) may increase the risk of renal reactions).
No products indexed under this heading.

Cefoperazone Sodium (The concurrent use of mesalimine with known nephrotoxic agents, including non-steroidal anti-inflammatory drugs (NSAIDs) may increase the risk of renal reactions).
No products indexed under this heading.

Ceforanide (The concurrent use of mesalimine with known nephrotoxic agents, including non-steroidal anti-inflammatory drugs (NSAIDs) may increase the risk of renal reactions).
No products indexed under this heading.

Cefotaxime Sodium (The concurrent use of mesalimine with known nephrotoxic agents, including non-steroidal anti-inflammatory drugs (NSAIDs) may increase the risk of renal reactions).
No products indexed under this heading.

Cefotetan (The concurrent use of mesalimine with known nephrotoxic agents, including non-steroidal anti-inflammatory drugs (NSAIDs) may increase the risk of renal reactions).
No products indexed under this heading.

Cefoxitin Sodium (The concurrent use of mesalimine with known nephrotoxic agents, including non-steroidal anti-inflammatory drugs (NSAIDs) may increase the risk of renal reactions).
No products indexed under this heading.

Cefpodoxime Proxetil (The concurrent use of mesalimine with known nephrotoxic agents, including non-steroidal anti-inflammatory drugs (NSAIDs) may increase the risk of renal reactions).
No products indexed under this heading.

Cefprozil (The concurrent use of mesalimine with known nephrotoxic agents, including non-steroidal anti-inflammatory drugs (NSAIDs) may increase the risk of renal reactions).
No products indexed under this heading.

Ceftazidime (The concurrent use of mesalimine with known nephrotoxic agents, including non-steroidal anti-inflammatory drugs (NSAIDs) may increase the risk of renal reactions). Products include:
Fortaz 1450

Ceftizoxime Sodium (The concurrent use of mesalimine with known nephrotoxic agents, including non-steroidal anti-inflammatory drugs (NSAIDs) may increase the risk of renal reactions).
No products indexed under this heading.

Ceftriaxone Sodium (The concurrent use of mesalimine with known nephrotoxic agents, including non-steroidal anti-inflammatory drugs (NSAIDs) may increase the risk of renal reactions). Products include:
Rocephin Injectable Vials, ADD-Vantage, Galaxy, Bulk 2642

Cefuroxime Axetil (The concurrent use of mesalimine with known nephrotoxic agents, including non-steroidal anti-inflammatory drugs (NSAIDs) may increase the risk of renal reactions). Products include:
Ceftin 1380

Cefuroxime Sodium (The concurrent use of mesalimine with known nephrotoxic agents, including non-steroidal anti-inflammatory drugs (NSAIDs) may increase the risk of renal reactions).
No products indexed under this heading.

Celecoxib (The concurrent use of mesalimine with known nephrotoxic agents, including non-steroidal anti-inflammatory drugs (NSAIDs) may increase the risk of renal reactions). Products include:
Celebrex Capsules 2979

Cephalexin (The concurrent use of mesalimine with known nephrotoxic agents, including non-steroidal anti-inflammatory drugs (NSAIDs) may increase the risk of renal reactions).
No products indexed under this heading.

Cephalothin Sodium (The concurrent use of mesalimine with known nephrotoxic agents, including non-steroidal anti-inflammatory drugs (NSAIDs) may increase the risk of renal reactions).
No products indexed under this heading.

Cephapirin Sodium (The concurrent use of mesalimine with known nephrotoxic agents, including non-steroidal anti-inflammatory drugs (NSAIDs) may increase the risk of renal reactions).
No products indexed under this heading.

Cephradine (The concurrent use of mesalimine with known nephrotoxic agents, including non-steroidal anti-inflammatory drugs (NSAIDs) may increase the risk of renal reactions).
No products indexed under this heading.

Cerivastatin Sodium (The concurrent use of mesalimine with known nephrotoxic agents, including non-steroidal anti-inflammatory drugs (NSAIDs) may increase the risk of renal reactions).
No products indexed under this heading.

Chlorothiazide (The concurrent use of mesalimine with known nephrotoxic agents, including non-steroidal anti-inflammatory drugs (NSAIDs) may increase the risk of renal reactions).
No products indexed under this heading.

Chlorothiazide Sodium (The concurrent use of mesalimine with known nephrotoxic agents, including non-steroidal anti-inflammatory drugs (NSAIDs) may increase the risk of renal reactions). Products include:
Intravenous Sodium Diuril 2490

Chlorpropamide (The concurrent use of mesalimine with known nephrotoxic agents, including non-steroidal anti-inflammatory drugs (NSAIDs) may increase the risk of renal reactions).
No products indexed under this heading.

Cidofovir (The concurrent use of mesalimine with known nephrotoxic agents, including non-steroidal anti-inflammatory drugs (NSAIDs) may increase the risk of renal reactions).
No products indexed under this heading.

Cilastatin Sodium (The concurrent use of mesalimine with known nephrotoxic agents, including non-steroidal anti-inflammatory drugs (NSAIDs) may increase the risk of renal reactions). Products include:
Primaxin I.M. 2080
Primaxin I.V. 2083

Cimetidine (The concurrent use of mesalimine with known nephrotoxic agents, including non-steroidal anti-inflammatory drugs (NSAIDs) may increase the risk of renal reactions).
No products indexed under this heading.

Cimetidine Hydrochloride (The concurrent use of mesalimine with known nephrotoxic agents, including non-steroidal anti-inflammatory drugs (NSAIDs) may increase the risk of renal reactions).
No products indexed under this heading.

Cisplatin (The concurrent use of mesalimine with known nephrotoxic agents, including non-steroidal anti-inflammatory drugs (NSAIDs) may increase the risk of renal reactions).
No products indexed under this heading.

Cladribine (The concurrent use of mesalimine with known nephrotoxic agents, including non-steroidal anti-inflammatory drugs (NSAIDs) may increase the risk of renal reactions). Products include:
Leustatin Injection 2384

Clozapine (The concurrent use of mesalimine with known nephrotoxic agents, including non-steroidal anti-inflammatory drugs (NSAIDs) may increase the risk of renal reactions).
No products indexed under this heading.

Colistimethate Sodium (The concurrent use of mesalimine with known nephrotoxic agents, including non-steroidal anti-inflammatory drugs (NSAIDs) may increase the risk of renal reactions).
No products indexed under this heading.

Colistin Sulfate (The concurrent use of mesalimine with known nephrotoxic agents, including non-steroidal anti-inflammatory drugs (NSAIDs) may increase the risk of renal reactions).
No products indexed under this heading.

Cyclophosphamide (The concurrent use of mesalimine with known nephrotoxic agents, including non-steroidal anti-inflammatory drugs (NSAIDs) may increase the risk of renal reactions).
No products indexed under this heading.

Cyclosporine (The concurrent use of mesalimine with known nephrotoxic agents, including non-steroidal anti-inflammatory drugs (NSAIDs) may increase the risk of renal reactions). Products include:
Gengraf Capsules 435
Neoral Oral Solution 2280
Neoral Soft Gelatin Capsules 2280
Restasis Ophthalmic Emulsion 557
Sandimmune 2296

IMPORTANT NOTE: Always consult each drug listing in the patient's regimen for possible interactions.

Cytarabine (The concurrent use of mesalimine with known nephrotoxic agents, including non-steroidal anti-inflammatory drugs (NSAIDs) may increase the risk of renal reactions).
No products indexed under this heading.

Cytarabine Liposome (The concurrent use of mesalimine with known nephrotoxic agents, including non-steroidal anti-inflammatory drugs (NSAIDs) may increase the risk of renal reactions). Products include:
DepoCyt Injection 1136

Delavirdine Mesylate (The concurrent use of mesalimine with known nephrotoxic agents, including non-steroidal anti-inflammatory drugs (NSAIDs) may increase the risk of renal reactions).
No products indexed under this heading.

Diatrizoate Meglumine (The concurrent use of mesalimine with known nephrotoxic agents, including non-steroidal anti-inflammatory drugs (NSAIDs) may increase the risk of renal reactions).
No products indexed under this heading.

Diatrizoate Sodium (The concurrent use of mesalimine with known nephrotoxic agents, including non-steroidal anti-inflammatory drugs (NSAIDs) may increase the risk of renal reactions).
No products indexed under this heading.

Diclofenac Potassium (The concurrent use of mesalimine with known nephrotoxic agents, including non-steroidal anti-inflammatory drugs (NSAIDs) may increase the risk of renal reactions).
No products indexed under this heading.

Diclofenac Sodium (The concurrent use of mesalimine with known nephrotoxic agents, including non-steroidal anti-inflammatory drugs (NSAIDs) may increase the risk of renal reactions). Products include:
Diclofenac Sodium Ophthalmic Solution........ ⊙240
Voltaren Ophthalmic Solution 2336
Voltaren Tablets 2334
Voltaren-XR Tablets 2337

Dicloxacillin Sodium (The concurrent use of mesalimine with known nephrotoxic agents, including non-steroidal anti-inflammatory drugs (NSAIDs) may increase the risk of renal reactions).
No products indexed under this heading.

Didanosine (The concurrent use of mesalimine with known nephrotoxic agents, including non-steroidal anti-inflammatory drugs (NSAIDs) may increase the risk of renal reactions).
No products indexed under this heading.

Efavirenz (The concurrent use of mesalimine with known nephrotoxic agents, including non-steroidal anti-inflammatory drugs (NSAIDs) may increase the risk of renal reactions). Products include:
Atripla Tablets 938
Sustiva Capsules 930
Sustiva Tablets 930

Emtricitabine (The concurrent use of mesalimine with known nephrotoxic agents, including non-steroidal anti-inflammatory drugs (NSAIDs) may increase the risk of renal reactions). Products include:
Atripla Tablets 938
Emtriva Capsules 1246
Emtriva Oral Solution 1246
Truvada Tablets 1262

Enalapril Maleate (The concurrent use of mesalimine with known nephrotoxic agents, including non-steroidal anti-inflammatory drugs (NSAIDs) may increase the risk of renal reactions).
No products indexed under this heading.

Enalaprilat (The concurrent use of mesalimine with known nephrotoxic agents, including non-steroidal anti-inflammatory drugs (NSAIDs) may increase the risk of renal reactions).
No products indexed under this heading.

Enfuvirtide (The concurrent use of mesalimine with known nephrotoxic agents, including non-steroidal anti-inflammatory drugs (NSAIDs) may increase the risk of renal reactions).
No products indexed under this heading.

Ethiodized Oil (The concurrent use of mesalimine with known nephrotoxic agents, including non-steroidal anti-inflammatory drugs (NSAIDs) may increase the risk of renal reactions).
No products indexed under this heading.

Etodolac (The concurrent use of mesalimine with known nephrotoxic agents, including non-steroidal anti-inflammatory drugs (NSAIDs) may increase the risk of renal reactions).
No products indexed under this heading.

Fenoprofen Calcium (The concurrent use of mesalimine with known nephrotoxic agents, including non-steroidal anti-inflammatory drugs (NSAIDs) may increase the risk of renal reactions). Products include:
Nalfon Capsules 2508

Filgrastim (The concurrent use of mesalimine with known nephrotoxic agents, including non-steroidal anti-inflammatory drugs (NSAIDs) may increase the risk of renal reactions). Products include:
Neupogen for Injection 589

Fluorouracil (The concurrent use of mesalimine with known nephrotoxic agents, including non-steroidal anti-inflammatory drugs (NSAIDs) may increase the risk of renal reactions). Products include:
Carac Cream 0.5% 2722

Flurbiprofen (The concurrent use of mesalimine with known nephrotoxic agents, including non-steroidal anti-inflammatory drugs (NSAIDs) may increase the risk of renal reactions).
No products indexed under this heading.

Fluvastatin Sodium (The concurrent use of mesalimine with known nephrotoxic agents, including non-steroidal anti-inflammatory drugs (NSAIDs) may increase the risk of renal reactions). Products include:
Lescol Capsules 2268
Lescol XL Tablets 2268

Foscarnet Sodium (The concurrent use of mesalimine with known nephrotoxic agents, including non-steroidal anti-inflammatory drugs (NSAIDs) may increase the risk of renal reactions).
No products indexed under this heading.

Fosinopril Sodium (The concurrent use of mesalimine with known nephrotoxic agents, including non-steroidal anti-inflammatory drugs (NSAIDs) may increase the risk of renal reactions).
No products indexed under this heading.

Furosemide (The concurrent use of mesalimine with known nephrotoxic agents, including non-steroidal anti-inflammatory drugs (NSAIDs) may increase the risk of renal reactions). Products include:
Furosemide Tablets 2186

Gadopentetate Dimeglumine (The concurrent use of mesalimine with known nephrotoxic agents, including non-steroidal anti-inflammatory drugs (NSAIDs) may increase the risk of renal reactions).
No products indexed under this heading.

Gentamicin (The concurrent use of mesalimine with known nephrotoxic agents, including non-steroidal anti-inflammatory drugs (NSAIDs) may increase the risk of renal reactions).
No products indexed under this heading.

Gentamicin Sulfate (The concurrent use of mesalimine with known nephrotoxic agents, including non-steroidal anti-inflammatory drugs (NSAIDs) may increase the risk of renal reactions). Products include:
Pred-G Ophthalmic Ointment .... ⊙229
Pred-G Ophthalmic Suspension .... ⊙228

Glipizide (The concurrent use of mesalimine with known nephrotoxic agents, including non-steroidal anti-inflammatory drugs (NSAIDs) may increase the risk of renal reactions).
No products indexed under this heading.

Globulin, Immune (Human) (The concurrent use of mesalimine with known nephrotoxic agents, including non-steroidal anti-inflammatory drugs (NSAIDs) may increase the risk of renal reactions). Products include:
Flebogamma 5% 1715

Glyburide (The concurrent use of mesalimine with known nephrotoxic agents, including non-steroidal anti-inflammatory drugs (NSAIDs) may increase the risk of renal reactions).
No products indexed under this heading.

Gold Therapy (The concurrent use of mesalimine with known nephrotoxic agents, including non-steroidal anti-inflammatory drugs (NSAIDs) may increase the risk of renal reactions).
No products indexed under this heading.

HMG-CoA Reductase Inhibitors (The concurrent use of mesalimine with known nephrotoxic agents, including non-steroidal anti-inflammatory drugs (NSAIDs) may increase the risk of renal reactions).
No products indexed under this heading.

Hydrochlorothiazide (The concurrent use of mesalimine with known nephrotoxic agents, including non-steroidal anti-inflammatory drugs (NSAIDs) may increase the risk of renal reactions). Products include:
Atacand HCT 642
Avalide Tablets 892
Avalide Tablets 2713
Benicar HCT Tablets 1010
Diovan HCT Tablets 2216
Dyazide Capsules 1405
Micardis HCT Tablets 854
Prinzide Tablets 2092
Tekturna HCT Tablets 2324
Teveten HCT Tablets 517

Hydroflumethiazide (The concurrent use of mesalimine with known nephrotoxic agents, including non-steroidal anti-inflammatory drugs (NSAIDs) may increase the risk of renal reactions).
No products indexed under this heading.

Ibuprofen (The concurrent use of mesalimine with known nephrotoxic agents, including non-steroidal anti-inflammatory drugs (NSAIDs) may increase the risk of renal reactions). Products include:
Motrin IB Tablets and Caplets 1900
Children's Motrin Oral Suspension ... 1901
Children's Motrin Non-Staining Dye-Free Oral Suspension........ 1901
Children's Motrin Cold Oral Suspension 1899
Infants' Motrin Concentrated Drops........ 1901
Infants' Motrin Non-Staining Dye-Free Concentrated Drops....... 1901
Junior Strength Motrin Caplets and Chewable Tablets........ 1901
Vicoprofen Tablets 533

Idarubicin Hydrochloride (The concurrent use of mesalimine with known nephrotoxic agents, including non-steroidal anti-inflammatory drugs (NSAIDs) may increase the risk of renal reactions).
No products indexed under this heading.

Ifosfamide (The concurrent use of mesalimine with known nephrotoxic agents, including non-steroidal anti-inflammatory drugs (NSAIDs) may increase the risk of renal reactions).
No products indexed under this heading.

Imipenem (The concurrent use of mesalimine with known nephrotoxic agents, including non-steroidal anti-inflammatory drugs (NSAIDs) may increase the risk of renal reactions). Products include:
Primaxin I.M. 2080
Primaxin I.V. 2083

Immune Globulin Intravenous (Human) (The concurrent use of mesalimine with known nephrotoxic agents, including non-steroidal anti-inflammatory drugs (NSAIDs) may increase the risk of renal reactions). Products include:
Flebogamma 5% DIF 1718
Gammagard Liquid 730
Gammagard S/D 734
Gamunex 3094

Indinavir Sulfate (The concurrent use of mesalimine with known nephrotoxic agents, including non-steroidal anti-inflammatory drugs (NSAIDs) may increase the risk of renal reactions). Products include:
Crixivan Capsules 1979

Indomethacin (The concurrent use of mesalimine with known nephrotoxic agents, including non-steroidal

anti-inflammatory drugs (NSAIDs) may increase the risk of renal reactions). Products include:
Indocin 2024

Indomethacin Sodium Trihydrate (The concurrent use of mesalimine with known nephrotoxic agents, including non-steroidal anti-inflammatory drugs (NSAIDs) may increase the risk of renal reactions). Products include:
Indocin I.V. 2489

Interferon Beta-1b (The concurrent use of mesalimine with known nephrotoxic agents, including non-steroidal anti-inflammatory drugs (NSAIDs) may increase the risk of renal reactions). Products include:
Betaseron for SC Injection 756

Interleuken-2 (The concurrent use of mesalimine with known nephrotoxic agents, including non-steroidal anti-inflammatory drugs (NSAIDs) may increase the risk of renal reactions).
No products indexed under this heading.

Iodamide Meglumine (The concurrent use of mesalimine with known nephrotoxic agents, including non-steroidal anti-inflammatory drugs (NSAIDs) may increase the risk of renal reactions).
No products indexed under this heading.

Iohexol (The concurrent use of mesalimine with known nephrotoxic agents, including non-steroidal anti-inflammatory drugs (NSAIDs) may increase the risk of renal reactions).
No products indexed under this heading.

Iopamidol (The concurrent use of mesalimine with known nephrotoxic agents, including non-steroidal anti-inflammatory drugs (NSAIDs) may increase the risk of renal reactions).
No products indexed under this heading.

Iopanoic Acid (The concurrent use of mesalimine with known nephrotoxic agents, including non-steroidal anti-inflammatory drugs (NSAIDs) may increase the risk of renal reactions).
No products indexed under this heading.

Iothalamate Meglumine (The concurrent use of mesalimine with known nephrotoxic agents, including non-steroidal anti-inflammatory drugs (NSAIDs) may increase the risk of renal reactions).
No products indexed under this heading.

Ioxaglate Meglumine (The concurrent use of mesalimine with known nephrotoxic agents, including non-steroidal anti-inflammatory drugs (NSAIDs) may increase the risk of renal reactions).
No products indexed under this heading.

Ioxaglate Sodium (The concurrent use of mesalimine with known nephrotoxic agents, including non-steroidal anti-inflammatory drugs (NSAIDs) may increase the risk of renal reactions).
No products indexed under this heading.

Kanamycin Sulfate (The concurrent use of mesalimine with known nephrotoxic agents, including non-steroidal anti-inflammatory drugs (NSAIDs) may increase the risk of renal reactions).
No products indexed under this heading.

Ketoprofen (The concurrent use of mesalimine with known nephrotoxic agents, including non-steroidal anti-inflammatory drugs (NSAIDs) may increase the risk of renal reactions).
No products indexed under this heading.

Ketorolac Tromethamine (The concurrent use of mesalimine with known nephrotoxic agents, including non-steroidal anti-inflammatory drugs (NSAIDs) may increase the risk of renal reactions).
No products indexed under this heading.

Lamium album (The concurrent use of mesalimine with known nephrotoxic agents, including non-steroidal anti-inflammatory drugs (NSAIDs) may increase the risk of renal reactions).
No products indexed under this heading.

Lisinopril (The concurrent use of mesalimine with known nephrotoxic agents, including non-steroidal anti-inflammatory drugs (NSAIDs) may increase the risk of renal reactions). Products include:
Prinivil Tablets 2087
Prinzide Tablets 2092

Lithium (The concurrent use of mesalimine with known nephrotoxic agents, including non-steroidal anti-inflammatory drugs (NSAIDs) may increase the risk of renal reactions).
No products indexed under this heading.

Lithium Carbonate (The concurrent use of mesalimine with known nephrotoxic agents, including non-steroidal anti-inflammatory drugs (NSAIDs) may increase the risk of renal reactions).
No products indexed under this heading.

Lithium Citrate (The concurrent use of mesalimine with known nephrotoxic agents, including non-steroidal anti-inflammatory drugs (NSAIDs) may increase the risk of renal reactions).
No products indexed under this heading.

Lopinavir (The concurrent use of mesalimine with known nephrotoxic agents, including non-steroidal anti-inflammatory drugs (NSAIDs) may increase the risk of renal reactions). Products include:
Kaletra 452

Loracarbef (The concurrent use of mesalimine with known nephrotoxic agents, including non-steroidal anti-inflammatory drugs (NSAIDs) may increase the risk of renal reactions).
No products indexed under this heading.

Lovastatin (The concurrent use of mesalimine with known nephrotoxic agents, including non-steroidal anti-inflammatory drugs (NSAIDs) may increase the risk of renal reactions). Products include:
Advicor Tablets 402
Mevacor Tablets 2063

Meclofenamate Sodium (The concurrent use of mesalimine with known nephrotoxic agents, including non-steroidal anti-inflammatory drugs (NSAIDs) may increase the risk of renal reactions).
No products indexed under this heading.

Mefenamic Acid (The concurrent use of mesalimine with known nephrotoxic agents, including non-steroidal anti-inflammatory drugs (NSAIDs) may increase the risk of renal reactions).
No products indexed under this heading.

Meloxicam (The concurrent use of mesalimine with known nephrotoxic agents, including non-steroidal anti-inflammatory drugs (NSAIDs) may increase the risk of renal reactions). Products include:
Mobic Oral Suspension 863
Mobic Tablets 863

Melphalan Hydrochloride (The concurrent use of mesalimine with known nephrotoxic agents, including non-steroidal anti-inflammatory drugs (NSAIDs) may increase the risk of renal reactions).
No products indexed under this heading.

Mercaptopurine (The concurrent use of mesalamine with 6-mercaptopurine can increase the potential for blood disorders).
No products indexed under this heading.

Methimazole (The concurrent use of mesalimine with known nephrotoxic agents, including non-steroidal anti-inflammatory drugs (NSAIDs) may increase the risk of renal reactions).
No products indexed under this heading.

Methotrexate (The concurrent use of mesalimine with known nephrotoxic agents, including non-steroidal anti-inflammatory drugs (NSAIDs) may increase the risk of renal reactions).
No products indexed under this heading.

Methotrexate Sodium (The concurrent use of mesalimine with known nephrotoxic agents, including non-steroidal anti-inflammatory drugs (NSAIDs) may increase the risk of renal reactions).
No products indexed under this heading.

Methyclothiazide (The concurrent use of mesalimine with known nephrotoxic agents, including non-steroidal anti-inflammatory drugs (NSAIDs) may increase the risk of renal reactions).
No products indexed under this heading.

Mezlocillin Sodium (The concurrent use of mesalimine with known nephrotoxic agents, including non-steroidal anti-inflammatory drugs (NSAIDs) may increase the risk of renal reactions).
No products indexed under this heading.

Minocycline Hydrochloride (The concurrent use of mesalimine with known nephrotoxic agents, including non-steroidal anti-inflammatory drugs (NSAIDs) may increase the risk of renal reactions). Products include:
Solodyn Extended Release Tablets 1938

Mitomycin (Mitomycin-C) (The concurrent use of mesalimine with known nephrotoxic agents, including non-steroidal anti-inflammatory drugs (NSAIDs) may increase the risk of renal reactions).
No products indexed under this heading.

Moexipril Hydrochloride (The concurrent use of mesalimine with known nephrotoxic agents, including non-steroidal anti-inflammatory drugs (NSAIDs) may increase the risk of renal reactions).
No products indexed under this heading.

Muromonab-CD3 (The concurrent use of mesalimine with known nephrotoxic agents, including non-steroidal anti-inflammatory drugs (NSAIDs) may increase the risk of renal reactions). Products include:
Orthoclone OKT3 Sterile Solution 2387

Nabumetone (The concurrent use of mesalimine with known nephrotoxic agents, including non-steroidal anti-inflammatory drugs (NSAIDs) may increase the risk of renal reactions).
No products indexed under this heading.

Nafcillin Sodium (The concurrent use of mesalimine with known nephrotoxic agents, including non-steroidal anti-inflammatory drugs (NSAIDs) may increase the risk of renal reactions).
No products indexed under this heading.

Naproxen (The concurrent use of mesalimine with known nephrotoxic agents, including non-steroidal anti-inflammatory drugs (NSAIDs) may increase the risk of renal reactions). Products include:
EC-Naprosyn Delayed-Release Tablets 2632
Naprosyn Suspension 2632
Naprosyn Tablets 2632

Naproxen Sodium (The concurrent use of mesalimine with known nephrotoxic agents, including non-steroidal anti-inflammatory drugs (NSAIDs) may increase the risk of renal reactions). Products include:
Anaprox Tablets 2632
Anaprox DS Tablets 2632
Treximet Tablets 1616

Nelfinavir Mesylate (The concurrent use of mesalimine with known nephrotoxic agents, including non-steroidal anti-inflammatory drugs (NSAIDs) may increase the risk of renal reactions).
No products indexed under this heading.

Neomycin (The concurrent use of mesalimine with known nephrotoxic agents, including non-steroidal anti-inflammatory drugs (NSAIDs) may increase the risk of renal reactions).
No products indexed under this heading.

Neomycin, oral (The concurrent use of mesalimine with known nephrotoxic agents, including non-steroidal anti-inflammatory drugs (NSAIDs) may increase the risk of renal reactions).
No products indexed under this heading.

Neomycin Sulfate (The concurrent use of mesalimine with known nephrotoxic agents, including non-

steroidal anti-inflammatory drugs (NSAIDs) may increase the risk of renal reactions). Products include:
Neosporin Ophthalmic Solution Sterile .... ⊙252

Nevirapine (The concurrent use of mesalimine with known nephrotoxic agents, including non-steroidal anti-inflammatory drugs (NSAIDs) may increase the risk of renal reactions). Products include:
Viramune Oral Suspension 873
Viramune Tablets 873

Norfloxacin (The concurrent use of mesalimine with known nephrotoxic agents, including non-steroidal anti-inflammatory drugs (NSAIDs) may increase the risk of renal reactions). Products include:
Noroxin Tablets 2069

Olsalazine Sodium (The concurrent use of mesalimine with known nephrotoxic agents, including non-steroidal anti-inflammatory drugs (NSAIDs) may increase the risk of renal reactions).
No products indexed under this heading.

Omeprazole (The concurrent use of mesalimine with known nephrotoxic agents, including non-steroidal anti-inflammatory drugs (NSAIDs) may increase the risk of renal reactions).
No products indexed under this heading.

Oxaprozin (The concurrent use of mesalimine with known nephrotoxic agents, including non-steroidal anti-inflammatory drugs (NSAIDs) may increase the risk of renal reactions).
No products indexed under this heading.

Pamidronate Disodium (The concurrent use of mesalimine with known nephrotoxic agents, including non-steroidal anti-inflammatory drugs (NSAIDs) may increase the risk of renal reactions).
No products indexed under this heading.

Paroxetine Hydrochloride (The concurrent use of mesalimine with known nephrotoxic agents, including non-steroidal anti-inflammatory drugs (NSAIDs) may increase the risk of renal reactions). Products include:
Paxil 1535
Paxil CR Controlled-Release Tablets 1544

Penicillamine (The concurrent use of mesalimine with known nephrotoxic agents, including non-steroidal anti-inflammatory drugs (NSAIDs) may increase the risk of renal reactions). Products include:
Cuprimine Capsules 1986

Penicillin G Benzathine (The concurrent use of mesalimine with known nephrotoxic agents, including non-steroidal anti-inflammatory drugs (NSAIDs) may increase the risk of renal reactions). Products include:
Bicillin C-R Injectable Suspension 1775
Bicillin L-A Injection 1777

Penicillin G Potassium (The concurrent use of mesalimine with known nephrotoxic agents, including non-steroidal anti-inflammatory drugs (NSAIDs) may increase the risk of renal reactions).
No products indexed under this heading.

Penicillin G Procaine (The concurrent use of mesalimine with known nephrotoxic agents, including non-steroidal anti-inflammatory drugs (NSAIDs) may increase the risk of renal reactions). Products include:
Bicillin C-R Injectable Suspension 1775
Bicillin L-A Injection 1777

Penicillin G Sodium (The concurrent use of mesalimine with known nephrotoxic agents, including non-steroidal anti-inflammatory drugs (NSAIDs) may increase the risk of renal reactions).
No products indexed under this heading.

Penicillin V Potassium (The concurrent use of mesalimine with known nephrotoxic agents, including non-steroidal anti-inflammatory drugs (NSAIDs) may increase the risk of renal reactions).
No products indexed under this heading.

Pentamidine Isethionate (The concurrent use of mesalimine with known nephrotoxic agents, including non-steroidal anti-inflammatory drugs (NSAIDs) may increase the risk of renal reactions).
No products indexed under this heading.

Perindopril Erbumine (The concurrent use of mesalimine with known nephrotoxic agents, including non-steroidal anti-inflammatory drugs (NSAIDs) may increase the risk of renal reactions). Products include:
Aceon Tablets (2 mg, 4 mg, 8 mg) 3038

Phenylbutazone (The concurrent use of mesalimine with known nephrotoxic agents, including non-steroidal anti-inflammatory drugs (NSAIDs) may increase the risk of renal reactions).
No products indexed under this heading.

Piroxicam (The concurrent use of mesalimine with known nephrotoxic agents, including non-steroidal anti-inflammatory drugs (NSAIDs) may increase the risk of renal reactions).
No products indexed under this heading.

Plicamycin (The concurrent use of mesalimine with known nephrotoxic agents, including non-steroidal anti-inflammatory drugs (NSAIDs) may increase the risk of renal reactions).
No products indexed under this heading.

Polymyxin (The concurrent use of mesalimine with known nephrotoxic agents, including non-steroidal anti-inflammatory drugs (NSAIDs) may increase the risk of renal reactions).
No products indexed under this heading.

Polymyxin B Sulfate (The concurrent use of mesalimine with known nephrotoxic agents, including non-steroidal anti-inflammatory drugs (NSAIDs) may increase the risk of renal reactions). Products include:
Neosporin Ophthalmic Solution Sterile .... ⊙252

Polythiazide (The concurrent use of mesalimine with known nephrotoxic agents, including non-steroidal anti-inflammatory drugs (NSAIDs) may increase the risk of renal reactions).
No products indexed under this heading.

Pravastatin Sodium (The concurrent use of mesalimine with known nephrotoxic agents, including non-steroidal anti-inflammatory drugs (NSAIDs) may increase the risk of renal reactions).
No products indexed under this heading.

Probenecid (The concurrent use of mesalimine with known nephrotoxic agents, including non-steroidal anti-inflammatory drugs (NSAIDs) may increase the risk of renal reactions).
No products indexed under this heading.

Quinapril Hydrochloride (The concurrent use of mesalimine with known nephrotoxic agents, including non-steroidal anti-inflammatory drugs (NSAIDs) may increase the risk of renal reactions).
No products indexed under this heading.

Rabeprazole Sodium (The concurrent use of mesalimine with known nephrotoxic agents, including non-steroidal anti-inflammatory drugs (NSAIDs) may increase the risk of renal reactions). Products include:
Aciphex Tablets 1053

Ramipril (The concurrent use of mesalimine with known nephrotoxic agents, including non-steroidal anti-inflammatory drugs (NSAIDs) may increase the risk of renal reactions).
No products indexed under this heading.

Rifampin (The concurrent use of mesalimine with known nephrotoxic agents, including non-steroidal anti-inflammatory drugs (NSAIDs) may increase the risk of renal reactions).
No products indexed under this heading.

Riluzole (The concurrent use of mesalimine with known nephrotoxic agents, including non-steroidal anti-inflammatory drugs (NSAIDs) may increase the risk of renal reactions). Products include:
Rilutek Tablets 2771

Ritonavir (The concurrent use of mesalimine with known nephrotoxic agents, including non-steroidal anti-inflammatory drugs (NSAIDs) may increase the risk of renal reactions). Products include:
Kaletra 452
Norvir 489

Rofecoxib (The concurrent use of mesalimine with known nephrotoxic agents, including non-steroidal anti-inflammatory drugs (NSAIDs) may increase the risk of renal reactions).
No products indexed under this heading.

Saquinavir (The concurrent use of mesalimine with known nephrotoxic agents, including non-steroidal anti-inflammatory drugs (NSAIDs) may increase the risk of renal reactions).
No products indexed under this heading.

Sibutramine Hydrochloride Monohydrate (The concurrent use of mesalimine with known nephrotoxic agents, including non-steroidal anti-inflammatory drugs (NSAIDs) may increase the risk of renal reactions). Products include:
Meridia Capsules 475

Simvastatin (The concurrent use of mesalimine with known nephrotoxic agents, including non-steroidal anti-inflammatory drugs (NSAIDs) may increase the risk of renal reactions). Products include:
Simcor Tablets 502
Vytorin 10/10 Tablets 2149
Vytorin 10/10 Tablets 2939
Vytorin 10/20 Tablets 2149
Vytorin 10/20 Tablets 2939
Vytorin 10/40 Tablets 2149
Vytorin 10/40 Tablets 2939
Vytorin 10/80 Tablets 2149
Vytorin 10/80 Tablets 2939
Zocor Tablets 2136

Spirapril Hydrochloride (The concurrent use of mesalimine with known nephrotoxic agents, including non-steroidal anti-inflammatory drugs (NSAIDs) may increase the risk of renal reactions).
No products indexed under this heading.

Stavudine (The concurrent use of mesalimine with known nephrotoxic agents, including non-steroidal anti-inflammatory drugs (NSAIDs) may increase the risk of renal reactions).
No products indexed under this heading.

Streptomycin Sulfate (The concurrent use of mesalimine with known nephrotoxic agents, including non-steroidal anti-inflammatory drugs (NSAIDs) may increase the risk of renal reactions).
No products indexed under this heading.

Streptozocin (The concurrent use of mesalimine with known nephrotoxic agents, including non-steroidal anti-inflammatory drugs (NSAIDs) may increase the risk of renal reactions).
No products indexed under this heading.

Sulfacytine (The concurrent use of mesalimine with known nephrotoxic agents, including non-steroidal anti-inflammatory drugs (NSAIDs) may increase the risk of renal reactions).
No products indexed under this heading.

Sulfamethizole (The concurrent use of mesalimine with known nephrotoxic agents, including non-steroidal anti-inflammatory drugs (NSAIDs) may increase the risk of renal reactions).
No products indexed under this heading.

Sulfamethoxazole (The concurrent use of mesalimine with known nephrotoxic agents, including non-steroidal anti-inflammatory drugs (NSAIDs) may increase the risk of renal reactions).
No products indexed under this heading.

Sulfasalazine (The concurrent use of mesalimine with known nephrotoxic agents, including non-steroidal anti-inflammatory drugs (NSAIDs) may increase the risk of renal reactions).
No products indexed under this heading.

Sulfinpyrazone (The concurrent use of mesalimine with known nephrotoxic agents, including non-steroidal anti-inflammatory drugs (NSAIDs) may increase the risk of renal reactions).
No products indexed under this heading.

Sulfisoxazole Acetyl (The concurrent use of mesalamine with known nephrotoxic agents, including non-steroidal anti-inflammatory drugs (NSAIDs) may increase the risk of renal reactions).
No products indexed under this heading.

Sulfisoxazole Diolamine (The concurrent use of mesalamine with known nephrotoxic agents, including non-steroidal anti-inflammatory drugs (NSAIDs) may increase the risk of renal reactions).
No products indexed under this heading.

Sulindac (The concurrent use of mesalamine with known nephrotoxic agents, including non-steroidal anti-inflammatory drugs (NSAIDs) may increase the risk of renal reactions). Products include:
Clinoril Tablets ... 1962

Tacrolimus (The concurrent use of mesalamine with known nephrotoxic agents, including non-steroidal anti-inflammatory drugs (NSAIDs) may increase the risk of renal reactions). Products include:
Prograf Capsules and Injection ... 622
Protopic Ointment ... 628

Tenofovir Disoproxil Fumarate (The concurrent use of mesalamine with known nephrotoxic agents, including non-steroidal anti-inflammatory drugs (NSAIDs) may increase the risk of renal reactions). Products include:
Atripla Tablets ... 938
Truvada Tablets ... 1262
Viread Tablets ... 1268

Thioguanine (The concurrent use of mesalamine with known nephrotoxic agents, including non-steroidal anti-inflammatory drugs (NSAIDs) may increase the risk of renal reactions). Products include:
Tabloid Tablets ... 1601

Ticarcillin Disodium (The concurrent use of mesalamine with known nephrotoxic agents, including non-steroidal anti-inflammatory drugs (NSAIDs) may increase the risk of renal reactions). Products include:
Timentin ADD-Vantage ... 1606
Timentin Injection Galaxy Container ... 1609
Timentin IV Infusion ... 1603
Timentin Pharmacy Bulk Package ... 1613

Tobramycin (The concurrent use of mesalamine with known nephrotoxic agents, including non-steroidal anti-inflammatory drugs (NSAIDs) may increase the risk of renal reactions). Products include:
Zylet Ophthalmic Suspension ... ⊙247

Tobramycin Sulfate (The concurrent use of mesalamine with known nephrotoxic agents, including non-steroidal anti-inflammatory drugs (NSAIDs) may increase the risk of renal reactions).
No products indexed under this heading.

Tolazamide (The concurrent use of mesalamine with known nephrotoxic agents, including non-steroidal anti-inflammatory drugs (NSAIDs) may increase the risk of renal reactions).
No products indexed under this heading.

Tolbutamide (The concurrent use of mesalamine with known nephrotoxic agents, including non-steroidal anti-inflammatory drugs (NSAIDs) may increase the risk of renal reactions).
No products indexed under this heading.

Tolmetin Sodium (The concurrent use of mesalamine with known nephrotoxic agents, including non-steroidal anti-inflammatory drugs (NSAIDs) may increase the risk of renal reactions).
No products indexed under this heading.

Trandolapril (The concurrent use of mesalamine with known nephrotoxic agents, including non-steroidal anti-inflammatory drugs (NSAIDs) may increase the risk of renal reactions). Products include:
Mavik Tablets ... 472
Tarka Tablets ... 511

Triamterene (The concurrent use of mesalamine with known nephrotoxic agents, including non-steroidal anti-inflammatory drugs (NSAIDs) may increase the risk of renal reactions). Products include:
Dyazide Capsules ... 1405
Dyrenium Capsules ... 3189

Trimethadione (The concurrent use of mesalamine with known nephrotoxic agents, including non-steroidal anti-inflammatory drugs (NSAIDs) may increase the risk of renal reactions).
No products indexed under this heading.

Trovafloxacin Mesylate (The concurrent use of mesalamine with known nephrotoxic agents, including non-steroidal anti-inflammatory drugs (NSAIDs) may increase the risk of renal reactions).
No products indexed under this heading.

Tyropanoate Sodium (The concurrent use of mesalamine with known nephrotoxic agents, including non-steroidal anti-inflammatory drugs (NSAIDs) may increase the risk of renal reactions).
No products indexed under this heading.

Valacyclovir Hydrochloride (The concurrent use of mesalamine with known nephrotoxic agents, including non-steroidal anti-inflammatory drugs (NSAIDs) may increase the risk of renal reactions). Products include:
Valtrex Caplets ... 1635

Valdecoxib (The concurrent use of mesalamine with known nephrotoxic agents, including non-steroidal anti-inflammatory drugs (NSAIDs) may increase the risk of renal reactions).
No products indexed under this heading.

Vancomycin Hydrochloride (The concurrent use of mesalamine with known nephrotoxic agents, including non-steroidal anti-inflammatory drugs (NSAIDs) may increase the risk of renal reactions).
No products indexed under this heading.

Voriconazole (The concurrent use of mesalamine with known nephrotoxic agents, including non-steroidal anti-inflammatory drugs (NSAIDs) may increase the risk of renal reactions).
No products indexed under this heading.

Zalcitabine (The concurrent use of mesalamine with known nephrotoxic agents, including non-steroidal anti-inflammatory drugs (NSAIDs) may increase the risk of renal reactions).
No products indexed under this heading.

Zidovudine (The concurrent use of mesalamine with known nephrotoxic agents, including non-steroidal anti-inflammatory drugs (NSAIDs) may increase the risk of renal reactions). Products include:
Combivir Tablets ... 1384
Retrovir ... 1574
Retrovir IV Infusion ... 1579
Trizivir Tablets ... 1622

Zoledronic acid (The concurrent use of mesalamine with known nephrotoxic agents, including non-steroidal anti-inflammatory drugs (NSAIDs) may increase the risk of renal reactions). Products include:
Reclast Injection ... 2291
Zometa for Intravenous Infusion ... 2341

LIDODERM PATCH

(Lidocaine) ... 1114
May interact with class 1A antiarrhythmics, local anesthetics, and certain other agents. Compounds in these categories include:

Bupivacaine Hydrochloride (When used concomitantly with other products containing local anesthetic agents, the amount absorbed from all formulations must be considered).
No products indexed under this heading.

Chloroprocaine Hydrochloride (When used concomitantly with other products containing local anesthetic agents, the amount absorbed from all formulations must be considered).
No products indexed under this heading.

Disopyramide (Should be used with caution in patients receiving Class I antiarrhythmic drugs since the toxic effects are additive and potentially synergistic).
No products indexed under this heading.

Etidocaine Hydrochloride (When used concomitantly with other products containing local anesthetic agents, the amount absorbed from all formulations must be considered).
No products indexed under this heading.

Levobupivacaine Hydrochloride (When used concomitantly with other products containing local anesthetic agents, the amount absorbed from all formulations must be considered).
No products indexed under this heading.

Lidocaine Hydrochloride (When used concomitantly with other products containing local anesthetic agents, the amount absorbed from all formulations must be considered).
No products indexed under this heading.

Mepivacaine Hydrochloride (When used concomitantly with other products containing local anesthetic agents, the amount absorbed from all formulations must be considered).
No products indexed under this heading.

Mexiletine Hydrochloride (Co-administration in patients receiving Class-1 antiarrhythmic drugs, such as mexiletine, may result in additive toxic effects).
No products indexed under this heading.

Moricizine Hydrochloride (Should be used with caution in patients receiving Class I antiarrhythmic drugs since the toxic effects are additive and potentially synergistic).
No products indexed under this heading.

Procainamide (Should be used with caution in patients receiving Class I antiarrhythmic drugs since the toxic effects are additive and potentially synergistic).
No products indexed under this heading.

Procaine Hydrochloride (When used concomitantly with other products containing local anesthetic agents, the amount absorbed from all formulations must be considered).
No products indexed under this heading.

Quinidine (Should be used with caution in patients receiving Class I antiarrhythmic drugs since the toxic effects are additive and potentially synergistic).
No products indexed under this heading.

Quinidine Gluconate (Should be used with caution in patients receiving Class I antiarrhythmic drugs since the toxic effects are additive and potentially synergistic).
No products indexed under this heading.

Quinidine Hydrochloride (Should be used with caution in patients receiving Class I antiarrhythmic drugs since the toxic effects are additive and potentially synergistic).
No products indexed under this heading.

Quinidine Polygalacturonate (Should be used with caution in patients receiving Class I antiarrhythmic drugs since the toxic effects are additive and potentially synergistic).
No products indexed under this heading.

Quinidine Sulfate (Should be used with caution in patients receiving Class I antiarrhythmic drugs since the toxic effects are additive and potentially synergistic).
No products indexed under this heading.

Tetracaine Hydrochloride (When used concomitantly with other products containing local anesthetic agents, the amount absorbed from all formulations must be considered).
No products indexed under this heading.

Tocainide Hydrochloride (Co-administration in patients receiving Class-1 antiarrhythmic drugs, such as tocainide, may result in additive toxic effects).
No products indexed under this heading.

LIFEGENES SPRAY

(Thymus polypeptide) ... 564
None cited in PDR database.

LIFEPAK CAPSULES

(Vitamins with Minerals) ... 2560
None cited in PDR database.

LIMBREL CAPSULES
(Flavocoxid) 2561
May interact with:

Warfarin Sodium (Flavocoxid was administered to 59 patients who were taking warfarin chronically. Prothrombin times measured 2 weeks after the addition of flavocoxid were unchanged in the majority of patients. In 2 patients the prothrombin time was lengthened, and in 2patients it was shortened beyond 2 standard deviations. It is not known whether these represented variation in laboratory testing or reflect a CYP450 polymorphism affecting warfarin metabolism. Because of this, physicians are advised to check prothrombin time one to two weeks after initiating flavocoxid in patients anticoagulated with warfarin).
No products indexed under this heading.

LIPITOR TABLETS
(Atorvastatin Calcium) 2501
May interact with antacids, azole antifungals, cytochrome p450 3a4 inducers (selected), cytochrome p450 3a4 inhibitors (selected), erythromycin, fibrates, immunosuppressive agents, oral contraceptives, and certain other agents. Compounds in these categories include:

Acetazolamide (Atorvastatin is metabolized by cytochrome P450 3A4. Concomitant administration of atorvastatin with inhibitors of cytochrome P450 3A4 can lead to increases in plasma concentrations of atorvastatin. The extent of interaction and potentiation of effects depends on the variability of effect on cytochrome P450 3A4).
No products indexed under this heading.

Allium sativum (Concomitant administration of atorvastatin with inducers of cytochrome P450 3A4 can lead to variable reductions in plasma concentrations of atorvastatin).
No products indexed under this heading.

Aluminum Carbonate (When atorvastatin and Maalox TC suspension were co-administered, plasma concentrations of atorvastatin decreased approximately 35%. However, LDL-C reduction was not altered).
No products indexed under this heading.

Aluminum Hydroxide (When atorvastatin and Maalox TC suspension were co-administered, plasma concentrations of atorvastatin decreased approximately 35%. However, LDL-C reduction was not altered).
No products indexed under this heading.

Amiodarone Hydrochloride (Atorvastatin is metabolized by cytochrome P450 3A4. Concomitant administration of atorvastatin with inhibitors of cytochrome P450 3A4 can lead to increases in plasma concentrations of atorvastatin. The extent of interaction and potentiation of effects depends on the variability of effect on cytochrome P450 3A4).
No products indexed under this heading.

Amlodipine Besylate (In a drug-drug interaction study in healthy subjects, co-administration of atorvastatin 80 mg and amlodipine 10 mg resulted in an 18% increase in exposure to atorvastatin which was not clinically meaningful). Products include:
Azor Tablets 1005
Exforge Tablets 2238

Amprenavir (Atorvastatin is metabolized by cytochrome P450 3A4. Concomitant administration of atorvastatin with inhibitors of cytochrome P450 3A4 can lead to increases in plasma concentrations of atorvastatin. The extent of interaction and potentiation of effects depends on the variability of effect on cytochrome P450 3A4).
No products indexed under this heading.

Anastrozole (Atorvastatin is metabolized by cytochrome P450 3A4. Concomitant administration of atorvastatin with inhibitors of cytochrome P450 3A4 can lead to increases in plasma concentrations of atorvastatin. The extent of interaction and potentiation of effects depends on the variability of effect on cytochrome P450 3A4). Products include:
Arimidex Tablets 672

Aprepitant (Atorvastatin is metabolized by cytochrome P450 3A4. Concomitant administration of atorvastatin with inhibitors of cytochrome P450 3A4 can lead to increases in plasma concentrations of atorvastatin. The extent of interaction and potentiation of effects depends on the variability of effect on cytochrome P450 3A4). Products include:
Emend Capsules 1992

Atazanavir (Atorvastatin is metabolized by cytochrome P450 3A4. Concomitant administration of atorvastatin with inhibitors of cytochrome P450 3A4 can lead to increases in plasma concentrations of atorvastatin. The extent of interaction and potentiation of effects depends on the variability of effect on cytochrome P450 3A4).
No products indexed under this heading.

Atazanavir Sulfate (Atorvastatin is metabolized by cytochrome P450 3A4. Concomitant administration of atorvastatin with inhibitors of cytochrome P450 3A4 can lead to increases in plasma concentrations of atorvastatin. The extent of interaction and potentiation of effects depends on the variability of effect on cytochrome P450 3A4). Products include:
Reyataz Capsules 3299

Azathioprine (Physicians considering combined therapy with immunosuppressive drugs should carefully weigh the potential benefits and risks, and should carefully monitor patients for any signs or symptoms of muscle pain, tenderness, or weakness, particularly during theintial months of therapy and during any upward dosage titration of either drug. Lower starting and maintenance doses of atorvastatin should be considered when taken concomitantly with immunosuppressive drugs. Periodic creatine phosphokinase (CPK) determinations may be considered in such situations, but there is no assurance that such monitoring will prevent the occurrence of severe myopathy).
No products indexed under this heading.

Basiliximab (Physicians considering combined therapy with immunosuppressive drugs should carefully weigh the potential benefits and risks, and should carefully monitor patients for any signs or symptoms of muscle pain, tenderness, or weakness, particularly during theintial months of therapy and during any upward dosage titration of either drug. Lower starting and maintenance doses of atorvastatin should be considered when taken concomitantly with immunosuppressive drugs. Periodic creatine phosphokinase (CPK) determinations may be considered in such situations, but there is no assurance that such monitoring will prevent the occurrence of severe myopathy). Products include:
Simulect for Injection 2306

Betamethasone Acetate (Concomitant administration of atorvastatin with inducers of cytochrome P450 3A4 can lead to variable reductions in plasma concentrations of atorvastatin).
No products indexed under this heading.

Betamethasone Sodium Phosphate (Concomitant administration of atorvastatin with inducers of cytochrome P450 3A4 can lead to variable reductions in plasma concentrations of atorvastatin).
No products indexed under this heading.

Carbamazepine (Concomitant administration of atorvastatin with inducers of cytochrome P450 3A4 can lead to variable reductions in plasma concentrations of atorvastatin). Products include:
Carbatrol Capsules 3019
Equetro Extended-Release Capsules 3174

Cimetidine (HMG-CoA reductase inhibitors interfere with cholesterol synthesis and theoretically might blunt adrenal and/or gonadal steroid production. Clinical studies have shown that atorvastatin does not reduce basal plasma cortisol concentration or impair adrenal reserve. Caution should be exercised if an HMG-CoA reductase inhibitor is administered concomitantly with drugs that may decrease levels or activity of endogenous steroid hormones, such as cimetidine).
No products indexed under this heading.

Cimetidine Hydrochloride (HMG-CoA reductase inhibitors interfere with cholesterol synthesis and theoretically might blunt adrenal and/or gonadal steroid production. Clinical studies have shown that atorvastatin does not reduce basal plasma cortisol concentration or impair adrenal reserve. Caution should be exercised if an HMG-CoA reductase inhibitor is administered concomitantly with drugs that may decrease levels or activity of endogenous steroid hormones, such as cimetidine).
No products indexed under this heading.

Ciprofloxacin (Atorvastatin is metabolized by cytochrome P450 3A4. Concomitant administration of atorvastatin with inhibitors of cytochrome P450 3A4 can lead to increases in plasma concentrations of atorvastatin. The extent of interaction and potentiation of effects depends on the variability of effect on cytochrome P450 3A4). Products include:
Cipro I.V. 2817
Cipro Oral Suspension 2810
Cipro XR Tablets 2823
Ciprodex Otic Suspension 541

Ciprofloxacin Hydrochloride (Concomitant administration of atorvastatin with inducers of cytochrome P450 3A4 can lead to variable reductions in plasma concentrations of atorvastatin). Products include:
Cipro Tablets 2810

Cisplatin (Concomitant administration of atorvastatin with inducers of cytochrome P450 3A4 can lead to variable reductions in plasma concentrations of atorvastatin).
No products indexed under this heading.

Clarithromycin (Concomitant administration of atorvastatin 80 mg with clarithromycin (500 mg b.i.d.) resulted in a 4.4-fold increase in atorvastatin AUC. The risk of myopathy during treatment with atorvastatin is increased with concurrent administration of clarithromycin. Physicians considering concurrent use of atorvastatin and clarithromycin should weigh the benefits and risks, and should monitor patients for any signs or symptoms of muscle pain, tenderness, or weakness, particularly during the initial months of therapy and during periods of upward dosage titration of either drug. Lower starting and maintenance doses of atorvastatin should be considered when taken concomitantly with clarithromycin. Periodic CPK determinations may be considered in such situations). Products include:
Biaxin/Biaxin XL 411

Clofibrate (The risk of myopathy during treatment with atorvastatin is increased with concurrent administration of fibric acid derivatives. Physicians considered combined therapy with atorvastatin and fibric derivatives should be carefully weigh the potential benefits and risks, and should carefully monitor patients for any signs or symptoms of muscle pain, tenderness, or weakness, particularly during the initial months of therapy and during any periods of upward dosage titration of either drug. Lower starting and maintenance doses of atorvastatin should be considered when taken concomitantly with fibric acid derivatives. Periodic CPK determinations may be considered in such situations. The combination of atorvastatin and fibrates should generally be avoided).
No products indexed under this heading.

Clotrimazole (The risk of myopathy during treatment with atorvastatin is increased with concurrent administration of azole antifungals. Physicians considering combined therapy with atorvastatin and azole antifungals should carefully weigh the potential benefits and risks, and should carefully monitor patients for any signs or symptoms of muscle pain, tenderness, or weakness, particularly during the initial months of therapy and during any periods of upward dosage titration of either drug. Lower starting and maintenance doses of atorvastatin should be considered when taken concomi-

tantly with azole antifungals. Periodic creatine phosphokinase (CPK) determinations may be considered in such situations). Products include:

Lotrisone 2881

Colestipol (Plasma concentrations of atorvastatin decreased approximately 25% when colestipol and atorvastatin were co-administered. However, LDL-C reduction was greater when atorvastatin and colestipol were co-administered than when either drug was given alone).

No products indexed under this heading.

Colestipol Hydrochloride (Plasma concentrations of atorvastatin decreased approximately 25% when colestipol and atorvastatin were co-administered. However, LDL-C reduction was greater when atorvastatin and colestipol were co-administered than when either drug was given alone).

No products indexed under this heading.

Cortisone Acetate (Concomitant administration of atorvastatin with inducers of cytochrome P450 3A4 can lead to variable reductions in plasma concentrations of atorvastatin).

No products indexed under this heading.

Cyclosporine (Atorvastatin and atorvastatin-metabolites are substrates of the OATP1B1 transporter. Inhibitors of the OATP1B1 such as cyclosporine can increase the bioavailability of atorvastatin. Concomitant administration of atorvastatin 10 mg and cyclosporine 5.2 mg/kg/day resulted in an 8.7-fold increase in atorvastatin AUC. In cases where co-administration of atorvastatin with cyclosporine is necessary, the dose of atorvastatin should not exceed 10 mg. The risk of myopathy during treatment with atorvastatin may increase with concurrent administration of cyclosporine). Products include:

Gengraf Capsules 435
Neoral Oral Solution 2280
Neoral Soft Gelatin Capsules 2280
Restasis Ophthalmic Emulsion 557
Sandimmune 2296

Dalfopristin (Atorvastatin is metabolized by cytochrome P450 3A4. Concomitant administration of atorvastatin with inhibitors of cytochrome P450 3A4 can lead to increases in plasma concentrations of atorvastatin. The extent of interaction and potentiation of effects depends on the variability of effect on cytochrome P450 3A4).

No products indexed under this heading.

Danazol (Atorvastatin is metabolized by cytochrome P450 3A4. Concomitant administration of atorvastatin with inhibitors of cytochrome P450 3A4 can lead to increases in plasma concentrations of atorvastatin. The extent of interaction and potentiation of effects depends on the variability of effect on cytochrome P450 3A4).

No products indexed under this heading.

Delavirdine Mesylate (Atorvastatin is metabolized by cytochrome P450 3A4. Concomitant administration of atorvastatin with inhibitors of cytochrome P450 3A4 can lead to increases in plasma concentrations of atorvastatin. The extent of interaction and potentiation of effects depends on the variability of effect on cytochrome P450 3A4).

No products indexed under this heading.

Desogestrel (Co-administration of atorvastatin and an oral contraceptive increased AUC values for norethindrone and ethinyl estradiol by approximately 30% and 20%. These increases should be considered when selecting an oral contraceptive for a woman taking atorvastatin). Products include:

Mircette Tablets 1034

Dexamethasone (Concomitant administration of atorvastatin with inducers of cytochrome P450 3A4 can lead to variable reductions in plasma concentrations of atorvastatin). Products include:

Ciprodex Otic Suspension 541

Dexamethasone Acetate (Concomitant administration of atorvastatin with inducers of cytochrome P450 3A4 can lead to variable reductions in plasma concentrations of atorvastatin).

No products indexed under this heading.

Dexamethasone Sodium Phosphate (Concomitant administration of atorvastatin with inducers of cytochrome P450 3A4 can lead to variable reductions in plasma concentrations of atorvastatin).

No products indexed under this heading.

Digoxin (When multiple doses of atorvastatin and digoxin were co-administered, steady state plasma digoxin concentrations increased by approximately 20%. Patients taking digoxin should be monitored appropriately). Products include:

Lanoxin Injection 1498
Lanoxin Injection Pediatric 1502
Lanoxin Tablets 1505

Diltiazem Hydrochloride (Co-administration of atorvastatin (40 mg) with diltiazem (240 mg) was associated with higher plasma concentrations of atorvastatin). Products include:

Cardizem LA Extended Release Tablets 421

Diltiazem Maleate (Atorvastatin is metabolized by cytochrome P450 3A4. Concomitant administration of atorvastatin with inhibitors of cytochrome P450 3A4 can lead to increases in plasma concentrations of atorvastatin. The extent of interaction and potentiation of effects depends on the variability of effect on cytochrome P450 3A4).

No products indexed under this heading.

Doxorubicin Hydrochloride (Concomitant administration of atorvastatin with inducers of cytochrome P450 3A4 can lead to variable reductions in plasma concentrations of atorvastatin).

No products indexed under this heading.

Efavirenz (Atorvastatin is metabolized by cytochrome P450 3A4. Concomitant administration of atorvastatin with inhibitors of cytochrome P450 3A4 can lead to increases in plasma concentrations of atorvastatin. The extent of interaction and potentiation of effects depends on the variability of effect on cytochrome P450 3A4). Products include:

Atripla Tablets 938
Sustiva Capsules 930
Sustiva Tablets 930

Erythromycin (Plasma concentrations of atorvastatin increased approximately 40% with co-administration of atorvastatin and erythromycin. The risk of myopathy during treatment with atorvastatin is increased with concurrent administration of erythromycin. Physicians considering combined therapy with atorvastatin and erythromycin should carefully weight the potential benefits and risk, and should monitor patients for any signs or symptoms of muscle pain, tenderness, or weakness, particularly during the initial months of therapy and during any periods of upward dosage titration of either drug. Lower starting and maintenance doses of atorvastatin should be considered when taken concomitantly with erythromycin. Periodic CPK determinations may be considered in such situations).

No products indexed under this heading.

Erythromycin Estolate (Plasma concentrations of atorvastatin increased approximately 40% with co-administration of atorvastatin and erythromycin. The risk of myopathy during treatment with atorvastatin is increased with concurrent administration of erythromycin. Physicians considering combined therapy with atorvastatin and erythromycin should carefully weight the potential benefits and risk, and should monitor patients for any signs or symptoms of muscle pain, tenderness, or weakness, particularly during the initial months of therapy and during any periods of upward dosage titration of either drug. Lower starting and maintenance doses of atorvastatin should be considered when taken concomitantly with erythromycin. Periodic CPK determinations may be considered in such situations).

No products indexed under this heading.

Erythromycin Ethylsuccinate (Plasma concentrations of atorvastatin increased approximately 40% with co-administration of atorvastatin and erythromycin. The risk of myopathy during treatment with atorvastatin is increased with concurrent administration of erythromycin. Physicians considering combined therapy with atorvastatin and erythromycin should carefully weight the potential benefits and risk, and should monitor patients for any signs or symptoms of muscle pain, tenderness, or weakness, particularly during the initial months of therapy and during any periods of upward dosage titration of either drug. Lower starting and maintenance doses of atorvastatin should be considered when taken concomitantly with erythromycin. Periodic CPK determinations may be considered in such situations). Products include:

E.E.S. 433
EryPed 431

Erythromycin Gluceptate (Plasma concentrations of atorvastatin increased approximately 40% with co-administration of atorvastatin and erythromycin. The risk of myopathy during treatment with atorvastatin is increased with concurrent administration of erythromycin. Physicians considering combined therapy with atorvastatin and erythromycin should carefully weight the potential benefits and risk, and should monitor patients for any signs or symptoms of muscle pain, tenderness, or weakness, particularly during the initial months of therapy and during any periods of upward dosage titration of either drug. Lower starting and maintenance doses of atorvastatin should be considered when taken concomitantly with erythromycin. Periodic CPK determinations may be considered in such situations).

No products indexed under this heading.

Erythromycin Lactobionate (Plasma concentrations of atorvastatin increased approximately 40% with co-administration of atorvastatin and erythromycin. The risk of myopathy during treatment with atorvastatin is increased with concurrent administration of erythromycin. Physicians considering combined therapy with atorvastatin and erythromycin should carefully weight the potential benefits and risk, and should monitor patients for any signs or symptoms of muscle pain, tenderness, or weakness, particularly during the initial months of therapy and during any periods of upward dosage titration of either drug. Lower starting and maintenance doses of atorvastatin should be considered when taken concomitantly with erythromycin. Periodic CPK determinations may be considered in such situations).

No products indexed under this heading.

Erythromycin Stearate (Plasma concentrations of atorvastatin increased approximately 40% with co-administration of atorvastatin and erythromycin. The risk of myopathy during treatment with atorvastatin is increased with concurrent administration of erythromycin. Physicians considering combined therapy with atorvastatin and erythromycin should carefully weight the potential benefits and risk, and should monitor patients for any signs or symptoms of muscle pain, tenderness, or weakness, particularly during the initial months of therapy and during any periods of upward dosage titration of either drug. Lower starting and maintenance doses of atorvastatin should be considered when taken concomitantly with erythromycin. Periodic CPK determinations may be considered in such situations).

No products indexed under this heading.

Esomeprazole Magnesium (Atorvastatin is metabolized by cytochrome P450 3A4. Concomitant administration of atorvastatin with inhibitors of cytochrome P450 3A4 can lead to increases in plasma concentrations of atorvastatin. The extent of interaction and potentiation of effects depends on the variability of effect on cytochrome P450 3A4). Products include:

Nexium Delayed-Release Capsules 645
Nexium Delayed-Release Oral Suspension 645

Ethinyl Estradiol (Co-administration of atorvastatin and an oral contraceptive increased AUC values for norethindrone and ethinyl estradiol by approximately 30% and 20%. These increases should be considered when selecting an oral contraceptive for a woman taking atorvastatin). Products include:

Lybrel Tablets ... 3204
Mircette Tablets ... 1034
NuvaRing ... 2897
Ortho-Cyclen/Ortho Tri-Cyclen ... 2449
Ortho Evra Transdermal System ... 2437
Ortho Tri-Cyclen Lo Tablets ... 2458
Seasonique Tablets ... 1046
Yaz Tablets ... 805

Ethosuximide (Concomitant administration of atorvastatin with inducers of cytochrome P450 3A4 can lead to variable reductions in plasma concentrations of atorvastatin).
No products indexed under this heading.

Ethynodiol Diacetate (Co-administration of atorvastatin and an oral contraceptive increased AUC values for norethindrone and ethinyl estradiol by approximately 30% and 20%. These increases should be considered when selecting an oral contraceptive for a woman taking atorvastatin).
No products indexed under this heading.

Felbamate (Concomitant administration of atorvastatin with inducers of cytochrome P450 3A4 can lead to variable reductions in plasma concentrations of atorvastatin).
No products indexed under this heading.

Fenofibrate (The risk of myopathy during treatment with atorvastatin is increased with concurrent administration of fibric acid derivatives. Physicians considered combined therapy with atorvastatin and fibric derivatives should be carefully weigh the potential benefits and risks, and should carefully monitor patients for any signs or symptoms of muscle pain, tenderness, or weakness, particularly during the initial months of therapy and during any periods of upward dosage titration of either drug. Lower starting and maintenance doses of atorvastatin should be considered when taken concomitantly with fibric acid derivatives. Periodic CPK determinations may be considered in such situations. The combination of atorvastatin and fibrates should generally be avoided). Products include:

Fenoglide Tablets ... 2960
Tricor Tablets ... 520

Fluconazole (The risk of myopathy during treatment with atorvastatin is increased with concurrent administration of azole antifungals. Physicians considering combined therapy with atorvastatin and azole antifungals should carefully weigh the potential benefits and risks, and should carefully monitor patients for any signs or symptoms of muscle pain, tenderness, or weakness, particularly during the initial months of therapy and during any periods of upward dosage titration of either drug. Lower starting and maintenance doses of atorvastatin should be considered when taken concomitantly with azole antifungals. Periodic creatine phosphokinase (CPK) determinations may be considered in such situations).
No products indexed under this heading.

Fludrocortisone Acetate (Concomitant administration of atorvastatin with inducers of cytochrome P450 3A4 can lead to variable reductions in plasma concentrations of atorvastatin).
No products indexed under this heading.

Fluoxetine (Atorvastatin is metabolized by cytochrome P450 3A4. Concomitant administration of atorvastatin with inhibitors of cytochrome P450 3A4 can lead to increases in plasma concentrations of atorvastatin. The extent of interaction and potentiation of effects depends on the variability of effect on cytochrome P450 3A4).
No products indexed under this heading.

Fluoxetine Hydrochloride (Atorvastatin is metabolized by cytochrome P450 3A4. Concomitant administration of atorvastatin with inhibitors of cytochrome P450 3A4 can lead to increases in plasma concentrations of atorvastatin. The extent of interaction and potentiation of effects depends on the variability of effect on cytochrome P450 3A4). Products include:

Prozac Weekly Capsules ... 1852
Prozac Pulvules and Liquid ... 1852
Symbyax Capsules ... 1871

Fluvoxamine Maleate (Atorvastatin is metabolized by cytochrome P450 3A4. Concomitant administration of atorvastatin with inhibitors of cytochrome P450 3A4 can lead to increases in plasma concentrations of atorvastatin. The extent of interaction and potentiation of effects depends on the variability of effect on cytochrome P450 3A4). Products include:

Luvox CR Extended-Release Capsules ... 1759

Fosamprenavir Calcium (Atorvastatin is metabolized by cytochrome P450 3A4. Concomitant administration of atorvastatin with inhibitors of cytochrome P450 3A4 can lead to increases in plasma concentrations of atorvastatin. The extent of interaction and potentiation of effects depends on the variability of effect on cytochrome P450 3A4). Products include:

Lexiva Oral Suspension ... 1510
Lexiva Tablets ... 1510

Fosphenytoin Sodium (Concomitant administration of atorvastatin with inducers of cytochrome P450 3A4 can lead to variable reductions in plasma concentrations of atorvastatin).
No products indexed under this heading.

Garlic Extract (Concomitant administration of atorvastatin with inducers of cytochrome P450 3A4 can lead to variable reductions in plasma concentrations of atorvastatin).
No products indexed under this heading.

Garlic Oil (Concomitant administration of atorvastatin with inducers of cytochrome P450 3A4 can lead to variable reductions in plasma concentrations of atorvastatin).
No products indexed under this heading.

Gemfibrozil (The risk of myopathy during treatment with atorvastatin is increased with concurrent administration of fibric acid derivatives. Physicians considered combined therapy with atorvastatin and fibric derivatives should be carefully weigh the potential benefits and risks, and should carefully monitor patients for any signs or symptoms of muscle pain, tenderness, or weakness, particularly during the initial months of therapy and during any periods of upward dosage titration of either drug. Lower starting and maintenance doses of atorvastatin should be considered when taken concomitantly with fibric acid derivatives. Periodic CPK determinations may be considered in such situations. The combination of atorvastatin and fibrates should generally be avoided).
No products indexed under this heading.

Hydrocortisone (Concomitant administration of atorvastatin with inducers of cytochrome P450 3A4 can lead to variable reductions in plasma concentrations of atorvastatin).
No products indexed under this heading.

Hydrocortisone Acetate (Concomitant administration of atorvastatin with inducers of cytochrome P450 3A4 can lead to variable reductions in plasma concentrations of atorvastatin). Products include:

Analpram-HC ... 1140
Pramosone ... 1141

Hydrocortisone Butyrate (Concomitant administration of atorvastatin with inducers of cytochrome P450 3A4 can lead to variable reductions in plasma concentrations of atorvastatin).
No products indexed under this heading.

Hydrocortisone Cypionate (Concomitant administration of atorvastatin with inducers of cytochrome P450 3A4 can lead to variable reductions in plasma concentrations of atorvastatin).
No products indexed under this heading.

Hydrocortisone Hemisuccinate (Concomitant administration of atorvastatin with inducers of cytochrome P450 3A4 can lead to variable reductions in plasma concentrations of atorvastatin).
No products indexed under this heading.

Hydrocortisone Probutate (Concomitant administration of atorvastatin with inducers of cytochrome P450 3A4 can lead to variable reductions in plasma concentrations of atorvastatin).
No products indexed under this heading.

Hydrocortisone Sodium Phosphate (Concomitant administration of atorvastatin with inducers of cytochrome P450 3A4 can lead to variable reductions in plasma concentrations of atorvastatin).
No products indexed under this heading.

Hydrocortisone Sodium Succinate (Concomitant administration of atorvastatin with inducers of cytochrome P450 3A4 can lead to variable reductions in plasma concentrations of atorvastatin).
No products indexed under this heading.

Hydrocortisone Valerate (Concomitant administration of atorvastatin with inducers of cytochrome P450 3A4 can lead to variable reductions in plasma concentrations of atorvastatin).
No products indexed under this heading.

Hypericum (Concomitant administration of atorvastatin with inducers of cytochrome P450 3A4 can lead to variable reductions in plasma concentrations of atorvastatin). Products include:

Satieté Tablets ... ▣640

Hypericum Perforatum (Concomitant administration of atorvastatin with inducers of cytochrome P450 3A4 can lead to variable reductions in plasma concentrations of atorvastatin).
No products indexed under this heading.

Indinavir Sulfate (Atorvastatin is metabolized by cytochrome P450 3A4. Concomitant administration of atorvastatin with inhibitors of cytochrome P450 3A4 can lead to increases in plasma concentrations of atorvastatin. The extent of interaction and potentiation of effects depends on the variability of effect on cytochrome P450 3A4). Products include:

Crixivan Capsules ... 1979

Isoniazid (Atorvastatin is metabolized by cytochrome P450 3A4. Concomitant administration of atorvastatin with inhibitors of cytochrome P450 3A4 can lead to increases in plasma concentrations of atorvastatin. The extent of interaction and potentiation of effects depends on the variability of effect on cytochrome P450 3A4).
No products indexed under this heading.

Itraconazole (Concomitant administration of atorvastatin and itraconazole was associated with a 2.5-3.3-fold increase in atorvastatin AUC. The risk of myopathy during treatment with atorvastatin is increased with concurrent administration of itraconazole. Physicians considering combined therapy with atorvastatin and itraconazole should carefully weigh the potential benefits and risks, and should monitor for any signs or symptoms of muscle pain, tenderness, or weakness, particularly during the intitial months of therapy and during any periods of upward dosage titration of either drug. Lower starting and maintenance doses of atorvastatin should be considered when taken concomitantly with itraconazole. Periodic CPK determinations may be considered in such situations).
No products indexed under this heading.

Ketoconazole (The risk of myopathy during treatment with atorvastatin is increased with concurrent administration of azole antifungals. Physicians considering combined therapy with atorvastatin and azole antifungals should carefully weigh the potential benefits and risks, and should carefully monitor patients for any signs or symptoms of muscle pain, tenderness, or weakness, particularly during the initial months of therapy and during any periods of upward dosage titration of either drug. Lower starting and maintenance doses of atorvastatin should be considered when taken concomitantly with azole antifungals. Periodic creatine phosphokinase (CPK) determinations may be considered in such situations). Products include:

Extina Foam, 2% 3057
Nizoral A-D Shampoo 1901

Levonorgestrel (Co-administration of atorvastatin and an oral contraceptive increased AUC values for norethindrone and ethinyl estradiol by approximately 30% and 20%. These increases should be considered when selecting an oral contraceptive for a woman taking atorvastatin). Products include:

Climara Pro Transdermal System 768
Lybrel Tablets 3204
Mirena Intrauterine System 779
Plan B Tablets 1044
Seasonique Tablets 1046

Lopinavir (The risk of myopathy during treatment with atorvastatin is increased with concurrent administration of combination of lopinavir plus ritonavir. Physicians considering combined therpay with atorvastatin and combination of lopinavir plus ritonavir, should carefully weigh the potential benefits and risks, and should carefully monitor patients for any signs or symptoms of muscle pain, tenderness, or weakness, particularly during the initial months of therapy and during any periods of upward dosage titration of either drug. Lower starting and maintenance doses of atorvastatin should be considered when taken concomitantly with a combination of lopinavir plus ritonavir. Periodic creatine phosphokinase (CPK) determinations may be considered in such situations). Products include:

Kaletra 452

Loratadine (Atorvastatin is metabolized by cytochrome P450 3A4. Concomitant administration of atorvastatin with inhibitors of cytochrome P450 3A4 can lead to increases in plasma concentrations of atorvastatin. The extent of interaction and potentiation of effects depends on the variability of effect on cytochrome P450 3A4).

No products indexed under this heading.

Magaldrate (When atorvastatin and Maalox TC suspension were co-administered, plasma concentrations of atorvastatin decreased approximately 35%. However, LDL-C reduction was not altered).

No products indexed under this heading.

Magnesium Hydroxide (When atorvastatin and Maalox TC suspension were co-administered, plasma concentrations of atorvastatin decreased approximately 35%. However, LDL-C reduction was not altered). Products include:

Fleet Pedia-Lax Chewable Tablets 1145
Pepcid Complete Chewable Tablets 1771
Extra Strength Rolaids Freshmint Tablets 1903
Rolaids Multi-Symptom Berry Tablets 1903
Rolaids Original Peppermint Tablets 1903

Magnesium Oxide (When atorvastatin and Maalox TC suspension were co-administered, plasma concentrations of atorvastatin decreased approximately 35%. However, LDL-C reduction was not altered). Products include:

Beelith Tablets 813

Mephenytoin (Concomitant administration of atorvastatin with inducers of cytochrome P450 3A4 can lead to variable reductions in plasma concentrations of atorvastatin).

No products indexed under this heading.

Mestranol (Co-administration of atorvastatin and an oral contraceptive increased AUC values for norethindrone and ethinyl estradiol by approximately 30% and 20%. These increases should be considered when selecting an oral contraceptive for a woman taking atorvastatin).

No products indexed under this heading.

Methsuximide (Concomitant administration of atorvastatin with inducers of cytochrome P450 3A4 can lead to variable reductions in plasma concentrations of atorvastatin).

No products indexed under this heading.

Methylprednisolone (Concomitant administration of atorvastatin with inducers of cytochrome P450 3A4 can lead to variable reductions in plasma concentrations of atorvastatin).

No products indexed under this heading.

Methylprednisolone Acetate (Concomitant administration of atorvastatin with inducers of cytochrome P450 3A4 can lead to variable reductions in plasma concentrations of atorvastatin).

No products indexed under this heading.

Methylprednisolone Sodium Succinate (Concomitant administration of atorvastatin with inducers of cytochrome P450 3A4 can lead to variable reductions in plasma concentrations of atorvastatin).

No products indexed under this heading.

Metronidazole (Atorvastatin is metabolized by cytochrome P450 3A4. Concomitant administration of atorvastatin with inhibitors of cytochrome P450 3A4 can lead to increases in plasma concentrations of atorvastatin. The extent of interaction and potentiation of effects depends on the variability of effect on cytochrome P450 3A4). Products include:

Pylera Capsules 714

Metronidazole Benzoate (Atorvastatin is metabolized by cytochrome P450 3A4. Concomitant administration of atorvastatin with inhibitors of cytochrome P450 3A4 can lead to increases in plasma concentrations of atorvastatin. The extent of interaction and potentiation of effects depends on the variability of effect on cytochrome P450 3A4).

No products indexed under this heading.

Metronidazole Hydrochloride (Atorvastatin is metabolized by cytochrome P450 3A4. Concomitant administration of atorvastatin with inhibitors of cytochrome P450 3A4 can lead to increases in plasma concentrations of atorvastatin. The extent of interaction and potentiation of effects depends on the variability of effect on cytochrome P450 3A4).

No products indexed under this heading.

Metronidazole Sodium (Atorvastatin is metabolized by cytochrome P450 3A4. Concomitant administration of atorvastatin with inhibitors of cytochrome P450 3A4 can lead to increases in plasma concentrations of atorvastatin. The extent of interaction and potentiation of effects depends on the variability of effect on cytochrome P450 3A4).

No products indexed under this heading.

Miconazole (The risk of myopathy during treatment with atorvastatin is increased with concurrent administration of azole antifungals. Physicians considering combined therapy with atorvastatin and azole antifungals should carefully weigh the potential benefits and risks, and should carefully monitor patients for any signs or symptoms of muscle pain, tenderness, or weakness, particularly during the initial months of therapy and during any periods of upward dosage titration of either drug. Lower starting and maintenance doses of atorvastatin should be considered when taken concomitantly with azole antifungals. Periodic creatine phosphokinase (CPK) determinations may be considered in such situations).

No products indexed under this heading.

Miconazole Nitrate (Atorvastatin is metabolized by cytochrome P450 3A4. Concomitant administration of atorvastatin with inhibitors of cytochrome P450 3A4 can lead to increases in plasma concentrations of atorvastatin. The extent of interaction and potentiation of effects depends on the variability of effect on cytochrome P450 3A4).

No products indexed under this heading.

Modafinil (Concomitant administration of atorvastatin with inducers of cytochrome P450 3A4 can lead to variable reductions in plasma concentrations of atorvastatin). Products include:

Provigil Tablets 977

Muromonab-CD3 (Physicians considering combined therapy with immunosuspressive drugs should carefully weigh the potential benefits and risks, and should carefully monitor patients for any signs or symptoms of muscle pain, tenderness, or weakness, particularly during theinitial months of therapy and during any upward dosage titration of either drug. Lower starting and maintenance doses of atorvastatin should be considered when taken concomitantly with immunosuppressive drugs. Periodic creatine phosphokinase (CPK) determinations may be considered in such situations, but there is no assurance that such monitoring will prevent the occurrence of severe myopathy). Products include:

Orthoclone OKT3 Sterile Solution 2387

Mycophenolate Mofetil (Physicians considering combined therapy with immunosuspressive drugs should carefully weigh the potential benefits and risks, and should carefully monitor patients for any signs or symptoms of muscle pain, tenderness, or weakness, particularly during theintial months of therapy and during any upward dosage titration of either drug. Lower starting and maintenance doses of atorvastatin should be considered when taken concomitantly with immunosuppressive drugs. Periodic creatine phosphokinase (CPK) determinations may be considered in such situations, but there is no assurance that such monitoring will prevent the occurrence of severe myopathy). Products include:

CellCept Capsules 2622
CellCept Oral Suspension 2622
CellCept Tablets 2622

Nefazodone Hydrochloride (Atorvastatin is metabolized by cytochrome P450 3A4. Concomitant administration of atorvastatin with inhibitors of cytochrome P450 3A4 can lead to increases in plasma concentrations of atorvastatin. The extent of interaction and potentiation of effects depends on the variability of effect on cytochrome P450 3A4).

No products indexed under this heading.

Nelfinavir Mesylate (Atorvastatin is metabolized by cytochrome P450 3A4. Concomitant administration of atorvastatin with inhibitors of cytochrome P450 3A4 can lead to increases in plasma concentrations of atorvastatin. The extent of interaction and potentiation of effects depends on the variability of effect on cytochrome P450 3A4).

No products indexed under this heading.

Nevirapine (Atorvastatin is metabolized by cytochrome P450 3A4. Concomitant administration of atorvastatin with inhibitors of cytochrome P450 3A4 can lead to increases in plasma concentrations of atorvastatin. The extent of interaction and potentiation of effects depends on the variability of effect on cytochrome P450 3A4). Products include:

Viramune Oral Suspension 873
Viramune Tablets 873

Niacin (The risk of myopathy during treatment with atorvastatin is increased with concurrent administration of niacin. Physicians considering combined therapy with atorvastatin and lipid-modifying doses of niacin should carefully weigh the potential benefits and risks, and should carefully monitor patients for any signs or symptoms of muscle pain, tenderness, or weaknes, particularly during the initial months of therapy and during any periods of upward dosage titration of either drug. Lower starting and maintenance doses of atorvastatin should be considered when taken concomitantly with lipid modifying doses of niacin. Periodic CPK determinations may be considered in such situations). Products include:

Advicor Tablets 402
Bausch & Lomb Ocuvite DF Vitamin Supplement .... ⊙238
Dismutax Dietary Supplement 995
Niaspan Extended-Release Tablets 480
NT-Kinase Dietary Supplement 995
Simcor Tablets 502

Niacinamide (The risk of myopathy during treatment with atorvastatin is increased with concurrent administration of niacin. Physicians considering combined therapy with atorvastatin and lipid-modifying doses of niacin should carefully weigh the potential benefits and risks, and should carefully monitor patients for any signs or symptoms of muscle pain, tenderness, or weaknes, particularly during the initial months of therapy and during any periods of upward dosage titration of either drug. Lower starting and maintenance doses of atorvastatin should be considered when taken concomitantly with lipid modifying doses of niacin. Periodic CPK determinations may be considered in such situations). Products include:

BioLean Free Tablets .... ▣635

Niacinamide Hydroiodide (The risk of myopathy during treatment with atorvastatin is increased with concurrent administration of niacin. Physicians considering combined therapy with atorvastatin and lipid-modifying doses of niacin should carefully weigh the potential benefits and risks, and should carefully monitor patients for any signs or symptoms of muscle pain, tenderness, or weaknes, particularly during the initial months of therapy and during any periods of upward dosage titration of either drug. Lower starting and maintenance doses of atorvastatin should be considered when taken concomitantly with lipid modifying doses of niacin. Periodic CPK determinations may be considered in such situations).

No products indexed under this heading.

Nicotinamide (Atorvastatin is metabolized by cytochrome P450 3A4. Concomitant administration of atorvastatin with inhibitors of cytochrome P450 3A4 can lead to increases in plasma concentrations of atorvastatin. The extent of interaction and potentiation of effects depends on the variability of effect on cytochrome P450 3A4).

No products indexed under this heading.

Nifedipine (Atorvastatin is metabolized by cytochrome P450 3A4. Concomitant administration of atorvastatin with inhibitors of cytochrome P450 3A4 can lead to increases in plasma concentrations of atorvastatin. The extent of interaction and potentiation of effects depends on the variability of effect on cytochrome P450 3A4).

No products indexed under this heading.

Norethindrone (Co-administration of atorvastatin and an oral contraceptive increased AUC values for norethindrone and ethinyl estradiol by approximately 30% and 20%. These increases should be considered when selecting an oral contraceptive for a woman taking atorvastatin). Products include:

Ortho Micronor Tablets 2446

Norethynodrel (Co-administration of atorvastatin and an oral contraceptive increased AUC values for norethindrone and ethinyl estradiol by approximately 30% and 20%. These increases should be considered when selecting an oral contraceptive for a woman taking atorvastatin).

No products indexed under this heading.

Norfloxacin (Atorvastatin is metabolized by cytochrome P450 3A4. Concomitant administration of atorvastatin with inhibitors of cytochrome P450 3A4 can lead to increases in plasma concentrations of atorvastatin. The extent of interaction and potentiation of effects depends on the variability of effect on cytochrome P450 3A4). Products include:

Noroxin Tablets 2069

Norgestimate (Co-administration of atorvastatin and an oral contraceptive increased AUC values for norethindrone and ethinyl estradiol by approximately 30% and 20%. These increases should be considered when selecting an oral contraceptive for a woman taking atorvastatin). Products include:

Ortho-Cyclen/Ortho Tri-Cyclen 2449
Ortho Tri-Cyclen Lo Tablets 2458

Norgestrel (Co-administration of atorvastatin and an oral contraceptive increased AUC values for norethindrone and ethinyl estradiol by approximately 30% and 20%. These increases should be considered when selecting an oral contraceptive for a woman taking atorvastatin).

No products indexed under this heading.

Omeprazole (Atorvastatin is metabolized by cytochrome P450 3A4. Concomitant administration of atorvastatin with inhibitors of cytochrome P450 3A4 can lead to increases in plasma concentrations of atorvastatin. The extent of interaction and potentiation of effects depends on the variability of effect on cytochrome P450 3A4).

No products indexed under this heading.

Oxcarbazepine (Concomitant administration of atorvastatin with inducers of cytochrome P450 3A4 can lead to variable reductions in plasma concentrations of atorvastatin).

No products indexed under this heading.

Oxiconazole Nitrate (The risk of myopathy during treatment with atorvastatin is increased with concurrent administration of azole antifungals. Physicians considering combined therapy with atorvastatin and azole antifungals should carefully weigh the potential benefits and risks, and should carefully monitor patients for any signs or symptoms of muscle pain, tenderness, or weakness, particularly during the initial months of therapy and during any periods of upward dosage titration of either drug. Lower starting and maintenance doses of atorvastatin should be considered when taken concomitantly with azole antifungals. Periodic creatine phosphokinase (CPK) determinations may be considered in such situations).

No products indexed under this heading.

Paroxetine Hydrochloride (Atorvastatin is metabolized by cytochrome P450 3A4. Concomitant administration of atorvastatin with inhibitors of cytochrome P450 3A4 can lead to increases in plasma concentrations of atorvastatin. The extent of interaction and potentiation of effects depends on the variability of effect on cytochrome P450 3A4). Products include:

Paxil 1535
Paxil CR Controlled-Release Tablets 1544

Phenobarbital (Concomitant administration of atorvastatin with inducers of cytochrome P450 3A4 can lead to variable reductions in plasma concentrations of atorvastatin). Products include:

Donnatal Extentabs 2507

Phenobarbital Sodium (Concomitant administration of atorvastatin with inducers of cytochrome P450 3A4 can lead to variable reductions in plasma concentrations of atorvastatin).

No products indexed under this heading.

Phenytoin (Concomitant administration of atorvastatin with inducers of cytochrome P450 3A4 can lead to variable reductions in plasma concentrations of atorvastatin).

No products indexed under this heading.

Phenytoin Sodium (Concomitant administration of atorvastatin with inducers of cytochrome P450 3A4 can lead to variable reductions in plasma concentrations of atorvastatin). Products include:

Phenytek Capsules 2192

Posaconazole (The risk of myopathy during treatment with atorvastatin is increased with concurrent administration of azole antifungals. Physicians considering combined therapy with atorvastatin and azole antifungals should carefully weigh the potential benefits and risks, and should carefully monitor patients for any signs or symptoms of muscle pain, tenderness, or weakness, particularly during the initial months of therapy and during any periods of upward dosage titration of either drug. Lower starting and maintenance doses of atorvastatin should be considered when taken concomitantly with azole antifungals. Periodic creatine phosphokinase (CPK) determinations may be considered in such situations). Products include:

Noxafil Oral Suspension 2889

Prednisolone Acetate (Concomitant administration of atorvastatin with inducers of cytochrome P450 3A4 can lead to variable reductions in plasma concentrations of atorvastatin). Products include:

Pred Forte Ophthalmic Suspension .... ⊙227
Pred Mild Ophthalmic Suspension .... ⊙230
Pred-G Ophthalmic Ointment .... ⊙229
Pred-G Ophthalmic Suspension ...... ⊙228

Prednisolone Sodium Phosphate (Concomitant administration of atorvastatin with inducers of cytochrome P450 3A4 can lead to variable reductions in plasma concentrations of atorvastatin).

No products indexed under this heading.

Prednisolone Tebutate (Concomitant administration of atorvastatin with inducers of cytochrome P450 3A4 can lead to variable reductions in plasma concentrations of atorvastatin).

No products indexed under this heading.

Prednisone (Concomitant administration of atorvastatin with inducers of cytochrome P450 3A4 can lead to variable reductions in plasma concentrations of atorvastatin).

No products indexed under this heading.

Primidone (Concomitant administration of atorvastatin with inducers of cytochrome P450 3A4 can lead to variable reductions in plasma concentrations of atorvastatin).

No products indexed under this heading.

Propoxyphene Hydrochloride (Atorvastatin is metabolized by cytochrome P450 3A4. Concomitant administration of atorvastatin with inhibitors of cytochrome P450 3A4 can lead to increases in plasma concentrations of atorvastatin. The extent of interaction and potentiation of effects depends on the variability of effect on cytochrome P450 3A4).

No products indexed under this heading.

Propoxyphene Napsylate (Atorvastatin is metabolized by cytochrome P450 3A4. Concomitant administration of atorvastatin with inhibitors of cytochrome P450 3A4 can lead to increases in plasma concentrations of atorvastatin. The extent of interaction and potentiation of effects depends on the variability of effect on cytochrome P450 3A4).

No products indexed under this heading.

Quinidine (Atorvastatin is metabolized by cytochrome P450 3A4. Concomitant administration of atorvastatin with inhibitors of cytochrome P450 3A4 can lead to increases in plasma concentrations of atorvastatin. The extent of interaction and potentiation of effects depends on the variability of effect on cytochrome P450 3A4).

No products indexed under this heading.

Quinidine Hydrochloride (Atorvastatin is metabolized by cytochrome P450 3A4. Concomitant administration of atorvastatin with inhibitors of cytochrome P450 3A4 can lead to increases in plasma concentrations of atorvastatin. The extent of interaction and potentiation of effects depends on the variability of effect on cytochrome P450 3A4).

No products indexed under this heading.

Quinidine Polygalacturonate (Atorvastatin is metabolized by cytochrome P450 3A4. Concomitant administration of atorvastatin with inhibitors of cytochrome P450 3A4 can lead to increases in plasma concentrations of atorvastatin. The extent of interaction and potentiation of effects depends on the variability of effect on cytochrome P450 3A4).

No products indexed under this heading.

Quinidine Sulfate (Atorvastatin is metabolized by cytochrome P450 3A4. Concomitant administration of atorvastatin with inhibitors of cytochrome P450 3A4 can lead to increases in plasma concentrations of atorvastatin. The extent of interaction and potentiation of effects depends on the variability of effect on cytochrome P450 3A4).

No products indexed under this heading.

Quinine (Atorvastatin is metabolized by cytochrome P450 3A4. Concomitant administration of atorvastatin with inhibitors of cytochrome P450 3A4 can lead to increases in plasma concentrations of atorvastatin. The extent of interaction and potentiation of effects depends on the variability of effect on cytochrome P450 3A4).

No products indexed under this heading.

Quinine Sulfate (Atorvastatin is metabolized by cytochrome P450 3A4. Concomitant administration of atorvastatin with inhibitors of cytochrome P450 3A4 can lead to increases in plasma concentrations of atorvastatin. The extent of interaction and potentiation of effects depends on the variability of effect on cytochrome P450 3A4).
No products indexed under this heading.

Quinupristin (Atorvastatin is metabolized by cytochrome P450 3A4. Concomitant administration of atorvastatin with inhibitors of cytochrome P450 3A4 can lead to increases in plasma concentrations of atorvastatin. The extent of interaction and potentiation of effects depends on the variability of effect on cytochrome P450 3A4).
No products indexed under this heading.

Ranitidine Bismuth Citrate (Atorvastatin is metabolized by cytochrome P450 3A4. Concomitant administration of atorvastatin with inhibitors of cytochrome P450 3A4 can lead to increases in plasma concentrations of atorvastatin. The extent of interaction and potentiation of effects depends on the variability of effect on cytochrome P450 3A4).
No products indexed under this heading.

Ranitidine Hydrochloride (Atorvastatin is metabolized by cytochrome P450 3A4. Concomitant administration of atorvastatin with inhibitors of cytochrome P450 3A4 can lead to increases in plasma concentrations of atorvastatin. The extent of interaction and potentiation of effects depends on the variability of effect on cytochrome P450 3A4). Products include:
- Zantac 75 Tablets 603
- Zantac 1670
- Zantac Injection 1666
- Zantac Injection Pharmacy Bulk Package 1668
- Maximum Strength Zantac 150 Tablets 603
- Maximum Strength Zantac 150 Cool Mint Tablets 603

Rifabutin (Concomitant administration of atorvastatin with inducers of cytochrome P450 3A4 can lead to variable reductions in plasma concentrations of atorvastatin).
No products indexed under this heading.

Rifampicin (Concomitant administration of atorvastatin with inducers of cytochrome P450 3A4 can lead to variable reductions in plasma concentrations of atorvastatin).
No products indexed under this heading.

Rifampin (Concomitant administration of atorvastatin with inducers of cytochrome P450 3A4 (e.g., rifampin) can lead to variable reductions in plasma concentrations of atorvastatin. Due to the dual interaction mechanism of rifampin, simultaneous co-administration of atorvastatin with rifampin is recommended, as delayed administration of atorvastatin after administration of rifampin has been associated with a significant reduction in atorvastatin plasma concentrations).
No products indexed under this heading.

Rifapentine (Concomitant administration of atorvastatin with inducers of cytochrome P450 3A4 can lead to variable reductions in plasma concentrations of atorvastatin).
No products indexed under this heading.

Ritonavir (The risk of myopathy during treatment with atorvastatin is increased with concurrent administration of combination of ritonavir plus saquinavir or lopinavir plus ritonavir. Physicians considering combined therapy with atorvastatin and a combination of ritonavir plus saquinavir or lopinavir plus ritonavir, should carefully weigh the potential benefits and risks, and should carefully monitor for any signs or symptoms of muscle pain, tenderness, or weakness, particularly during initial months of therapy and during any periods of upward dosage titration of either drug. Lower starting and maintenence doses of atorvastatin should be considered when taken concomitantly with such agents. Periodic CPK determinations may be considered in such situations). Products include:
- Kaletra 452
- Norvir 489

Saquinavir (The risk of myopathy during treatment with atorvastatin is increased with concurrent administration of combination of ritonavir plus saquinavir. Physicians considering combined therapy with atorvastatin and a combination of ritonavir plus saquinavir should carefully weigh the potential benefits and risk, and should carefully monitor patients for any signs or symptoms of muscl pain, tenderness, or weakness, particularly during the initial months of therapy and during any periods of upward dosage titration of either drug. Lower starting and maintenance doses of atorvastatin should be considered when taken concomitantly with a combination of ritonavir and saquinavir. Periodic CPK determinations may be considered in such situations).
No products indexed under this heading.

Saquinavir Mesylate (The risk of myopathy during treatment with atorvastatin is increased with concurrent administration of combination of ritonavir plus saquinavir. Physicians considering combined therapy with atorvastatin and a combination of ritonavir plus saquinavir should carefully weigh the potential benefits and risk, and should carefully monitor patients for any signs or symptoms of muscl pain, tenderness, or weakness, particularly during the initial months of therapy and during any periods of upward dosage titration of either drug. Lower starting and maintenance doses of atorvastatin should be considered when taken concomitantly with a combination of ritonavir and saquinavir. Periodic CPK determinations may be considered in such situations).
No products indexed under this heading.

Sertraline Hydrochloride (Atorvastatin is metabolized by cytochrome P450 3A4. Concomitant administration of atorvastatin with inhibitors of cytochrome P450 3A4 can lead to increases in plasma concentrations of atorvastatin. The extent of interaction and potentiation of effects depends on the variability of effect on cytochrome P450 3A4).
No products indexed under this heading.

Sildenafil Citrate (Atorvastatin is metabolized by cytochrome P450 3A4. Concomitant administration of atorvastatin with inhibitors of cytochrome P450 3A4 can lead to increases in plasma concentrations of atorvastatin. The extent of interaction and potentiation of effects depends on the variability of effect on cytochrome P450 3A4).
No products indexed under this heading.

Sirolimus (Physicians considering combined therapy with immunosuspressive drugs should carefully weigh the potential benefits and risks, and should carefully monitor patients for any signs or symptoms of muscle pain, tenderness, or weakness, particularly during theintial months of therapy and during any upward dosage titration of either drug. Lower starting and maintenance doses of atorvastatin should be considered when taken concomitantly with immunosuppressive drugs. Periodic creatine phosphokinase (CPK) determinations may be considered in such situations, but there is no assurance that such monitoring will prevent the occurrence of severe myopathy). Products include:
- Rapamune 3260

Sodium Bicarbonate (When atorvastatin and Maalox TC suspension were co-administered, plasma concentrations of atorvastatin decreased approximately 35%. However, LDL-C reduction was not altered). Products include:
- Ceo-Two Laxative Suppository 815

Spironolactone (HMG-CoA reductase inhibitors interfere with cholesterol synthesis and theoretically might blunt adrenal and/or gonadal steroid production. Clinical studies have shown that atorvastatin does not reduce basal plasma cortisol concentration or impair adrenal reserve. Caution should be exercised if an HMG-CoA reductase inhibitor is administered concomitantly with drugs that may decrease levels or activity of endogenous steroid hormones, such as cimetidine).
No products indexed under this heading.

Sulfinpyrazone (Concomitant administration of atorvastatin with inducers of cytochrome P450 3A4 can lead to variable reductions in plasma concentrations of atorvastatin).
No products indexed under this heading.

Tacrolimus (Physicians considering combined therapy with immunosuspressive drugs should carefully weigh the potential benefits and risks, and should carefully monitor patients for any signs or symptoms of muscle pain, tenderness, or weakness, particularly during theintial months of therapy and during any upward dosage titration of either drug. Lower starting and maintenance doses of atorvastatin should be considered when taken concomitantly with immunosuppressive drugs. Periodic creatine phosphokinase (CPK) determinations may be considered in such situations, but there is no assurance that such monitoring will prevent the occurrence of severe myopathy). Products include:
- Prograf Capsules and Injection 622
- Protopic Ointment 628

Telithromycin (Atorvastatin is metabolized by cytochrome P450 3A4. Concomitant administration of atorvastatin with inhibitors of cytochrome P450 3A4 can lead to increases in plasma concentrations of atorvastatin. The extent of interaction and potentiation of effects depends on the variability of effect on cytochrome P450 3A4). Products include:
- Ketek Tablets 2744

Terconazole (The risk of myopathy during treatment with atorvastatin is increased with concurrent administration of azole antifungals. Physicians considering combined therapy with atorvastatin and azole antifungals should carefully weigh the potential benefits and risks, and should carefully monitor patients for any signs or symptoms of muscle pain, tenderness, or weakness, particularly during the initial months of therapy and during any periods of upward dosage titration of either drug. Lower starting and maintenance doses of atorvastatin should be considered when taken concomitantly with azole antifungals. Periodic creatine phosphokinase (CPK) determinations may be considered in such situations).
No products indexed under this heading.

Theophylline (Concomitant administration of atorvastatin with inducers of cytochrome P450 3A4 can lead to variable reductions in plasma concentrations of atorvastatin).
No products indexed under this heading.

Theophylline Anhydrous (Concomitant administration of atorvastatin with inducers of cytochrome P450 3A4 can lead to variable reductions in plasma concentrations of atorvastatin). Products include:
- Uniphyl Tablets 2595

Theophylline Calcium Salicylate (Concomitant administration of atorvastatin with inducers of cytochrome P450 3A4 can lead to variable reductions in plasma concentrations of atorvastatin).
No products indexed under this heading.

Theophylline Dihydroxypropyl (Glyceryl) (Concomitant administration of atorvastatin with inducers of cytochrome P450 3A4 can lead to variable reductions in plasma concentrations of atorvastatin).
No products indexed under this heading.

Theophylline Ethylenediamine (Concomitant administration of atorvastatin with inducers of cytochrome P450 3A4 can lead to variable reductions in plasma concentrations of atorvastatin).
No products indexed under this heading.

Triamcinolone (Concomitant administration of atorvastatin with inducers of cytochrome P450 3A4 can lead to variable reductions in plasma concentrations of atorvastatin).
No products indexed under this heading.

Triamcinolone Acetonide (Concomitant administration of atorvastatin with inducers of cytochrome P450 3A4 can lead to variable reductions in plasma concentrations of atorvastatin). Products include:

Azmacort Inhalation Aerosol 407
Nasacort AQ Nasal Spray 2765
Triesence Injectable Suspension .... ⊙ 209

Triamcinolone Diacetate (Concomitant administration of atorvastatin with inducers of cytochrome P450 3A4 can lead to variable reductions in plasma concentrations of atorvastatin).

No products indexed under this heading.

Triamcinolone Hexacetonide (Concomitant administration of atorvastatin with inducers of cytochrome P450 3A4 can lead to variable reductions in plasma concentrations of atorvastatin).

No products indexed under this heading.

Troglitazone (Atorvastatin is metabolized by cytochrome P450 3A4. Concomitant administration of atorvastatin with inhibitors of cytochrome P450 3A4 can lead to increases in plasma concentrations of atorvastatin. The extent of interaction and potentiation of effects depends on the variability of effect on cytochrome P450 3A4).

No products indexed under this heading.

Troleandomycin (Atorvastatin is metabolized by cytochrome P450 3A4. Concomitant administration of atorvastatin with inhibitors of cytochrome P450 3A4 can lead to increases in plasma concentrations of atorvastatin. The extent of interaction and potentiation of effects depends on the variability of effect on cytochrome P450 3A4).

No products indexed under this heading.

Valproate Sodium (Atorvastatin is metabolized by cytochrome P450 3A4. Concomitant administration of atorvastatin with inhibitors of cytochrome P450 3A4 can lead to increases in plasma concentrations of atorvastatin. The extent of interaction and potentiation of effects depends on the variability of effect on cytochrome P450 3A4).

No products indexed under this heading.

Vardenafil Hydrochloride (Atorvastatin is metabolized by cytochrome P450 3A4. Concomitant administration of atorvastatin with inhibitors of cytochrome P450 3A4 can lead to increases in plasma concentrations of atorvastatin. The extent of interaction and potentiation of effects depends on the variability of effect on cytochrome P450 3A4). Products include:

Levitra Tablets 2876

Verapamil Hydrochloride (Atorvastatin is metabolized by cytochrome P450 3A4. Concomitant administration of atorvastatin with inhibitors of cytochrome P450 3A4 can lead to increases in plasma concentrations of atorvastatin. The extent of interaction and potentiation of effects depends on the variability of effect on cytochrome P450 3A4). Products include:

Tarka Tablets 511

Voriconazole (The risk of myopathy during treatment with atorvastatin is increased with concurrent administration of azole antifungals. Physicians considering combined therapy with atorvastatin and azole antifungals should carefully weigh the potential benefits and risks, and should carefully monitor patients for any signs or symptoms of muscle pain, tenderness, or weakness, particularly during the initial months of therapy and during any periods of upward dosage titration of either drug. Lower starting and maintenance doses of atorvastatin should be considered when taken concomitantly with azole antifungals. Periodic creatine phosphokinase (CPK) determinations may be considered in such situations).

No products indexed under this heading.

Zafirlukast (Atorvastatin is metabolized by cytochrome P450 3A4. Concomitant administration of atorvastatin with inhibitors of cytochrome P450 3A4 can lead to increases in plasma concentrations of atorvastatin. The extent of interaction and potentiation of effects depends on the variability of effect on cytochrome P450 3A4). Products include:

Accolate Tablets 669

Zileuton (Atorvastatin is metabolized by cytochrome P450 3A4. Concomitant administration of atorvastatin with inhibitors of cytochrome P450 3A4 can lead to increases in plasma concentrations of atorvastatin. The extent of interaction and potentiation of effects depends on the variability of effect on cytochrome P450 3A4).

No products indexed under this heading.

Food Interactions

Grapefruit (Contains one or more components that inhibit CYP 3A4 and can increase plasma concentrations of atorvastatin, especially with excessive grapefruit consumption (greater than 1.2 liters per day)).

Grapefruit Juice (Contains one or more components that inhibit CYP 3A4 and can increase plasma concentrations of atorvastatin, especially with excessive grapefruit consumption (greater than 1.2 liters per day)).

LIPOTRIM CAPSULES

(Herbals with Minerals) .... ▣638
None cited in PDR database.

L-O-M MUS SOFTGEL CAPSULES

(Carotenoids, Phytoene, Phytofluene, Soy oil, Soy-containing dietary supplements)................................... 2499
None cited in PDR database.

LORTAB 5/500 TABLETS

(Acetaminophen, Hydrocodone Bitartrate)... 3143

May interact with antihistamines, central nervous system depressants, hypnotics and sedatives, monoamine oxidase inhibitors, narcotic analgesics, psychotropics, tranquilizers, tricyclic antidepressants, and certain other agents. Compounds in these categories include:

Acrivastine (Concomitant use may cause additive CNS depression. When combined therapy is contemplated, the dose of one or both agents should be reduced).

No products indexed under this heading.

Alfentanil Hydrochloride (Concomitant use may cause additive CNS depression. When combined therapy is contemplated, the dose of one or both agents should be reudced).

No products indexed under this heading.

Alprazolam (Concomitant use may cause additive CNS depression. When combined therapy is contemplated, the dose of one or both agents should be reduced).

No products indexed under this heading.

Amitriptyline Hydrochloride (The use of tricyclic antidepressants with hydrocodone preparations may increase the effect of either the antidepressant or hydrocodone).

No products indexed under this heading.

Amoxapine (The use of tricyclic antidepressants with hydrocodone preparations may increase the effect of either the antidepressant or hydrocodone).

No products indexed under this heading.

Astemizole (Concomitant use may cause additive CNS depression. When combined therapy is contemplated, the dose of one or both agents should be reduced).

No products indexed under this heading.

Azatadine Maleate (Concomitant use may cause additive CNS depression. When combined therapy is contemplated, the dose of one or both agents should be reduced).

No products indexed under this heading.

Bromodiphenhydramine Hydrochloride (Concomitant use may cause additive CNS depression. When combined therapy is contemplated, the dose of one or both agents should be reduced).

No products indexed under this heading.

Brompheniramine Maleate (Concomitant use may cause additive CNS depression. When combined therapy is contemplated, the dose of one or both agents should be reduced).

No products indexed under this heading.

Buprenorphine Hydrochloride (Concomitant use may cause additive CNS depression. When combined therapy is contemplated, the dose of one or both agents should be reudced). Products include:

Suboxone Tablets 2601
Subutex Tablets 2601

Buspirone Hydrochloride (Concomitant use may cause additive CNS depression. When combined therapy is contemplated, the dose of one or both agents should be reduced).

No products indexed under this heading.

Butabarbital (Concomitant use may cause additive CNS depression. When combined therapy is contemplated, the dose of one or both agents should be reduced).

No products indexed under this heading.

Butabarbital Sodium (Concomitant use may cause additive CNS depression. When combined therapy is contemplated, the dose of one or both agents should be reduced).

No products indexed under this heading.

Cetirizine Hydrochloride (Concomitant use may cause additive CNS depression. When combined therapy is contemplated, the dose of one or both agents should be reduced). Products include:

Zyrtec Allergy Tablets 1919
Zyrtec Chewable Tablets 1920
Children's Zyrtec Allergy Chewable Tablets 1922
Children's Zyrtec Allergy Syrup 1920
Children's Zyrtec Hives Relief Syrup 1920
Zyrtec Syrup 1920
Zyrtec Tablets 1920
Zyrtec-D 12 Hour Extended Release Tablets 1923
Zyrtec-D Allergy & Congestion Extended-Release Tablets 1923

Chloral Hydrate (Concomitant use may cause additive CNS depression. When combined therapy is contemplated, the dose of one or both agents should be reduced).

No products indexed under this heading.

Chlordiazepoxide (Concomitant use may cause additive CNS depression. When combined therapy is contemplated, the dose of one or both agents should be reduced).

No products indexed under this heading.

Chlordiazepoxide Hydrochloride (Concomitant use may cause additive CNS depression. When combined therapy is contemplated, the dose of one or both agents should be reduced).

No products indexed under this heading.

Chlorpheniramine Maleate (Concomitant use may cause additive CNS depression. When combined therapy is contemplated, the dose of one or both agents should be reduced). Products include:

Actifed Cold & Allergy Tablets 1895
Sudafed PE Sinus & Allergy Tablets 1908
Tylenol Allergy Multi-Symptom Caplets with Cool Burst and Rapid Release Gelcaps 1916
Children's Tylenol Plus Cold Suspension Liquid 1912
Children's Tylenol Plus Cough & Runny Nose Suspension Liquid..... 1912
Children's Tylenol Plus Flu Suspension Liquid 1914
Children's Tylenol Plus Multi-Symptom Cold Suspension Liquid 1912
Tylenol Cold Head Congestion Nighttime Caplets with Cool Burst 1910
Tylenol Cold Multi-Symptom Nighttime Caplets with Cool Burst 1913
Tylenol Sinus Congestion & Pain Nighttime Caplets with Cool Burst 1917

Chlorpheniramine Polistirex (Concomitant use may cause additive CNS depression. When combined therapy is contemplated, the dose of one or both agents should be reduced). Products include:

Tussionex Pennkinetic Extended-Release Suspension 3154

Chlorpheniramine Tannate (Concomitant use may cause additive CNS depression. When combined therapy is contemplated, the dose of one or both agents should be reduced).
No products indexed under this heading.

Chlorpromazine (Concomitant use may cause additive CNS depression. When combined therapy is contemplated, the dose of one or both agents should be reduced).
No products indexed under this heading.

Chlorpromazine Hydrochloride (Concomitant use may cause additive CNS depression. When combined therapy is contemplated, the dose of one or both agents should be reduced).
No products indexed under this heading.

Chlorprothixene (Concomitant use may cause additive CNS depression. When combined therapy is contemplated, the dose of one or both agents should be reduced).
No products indexed under this heading.

Chlorprothixene Hydrochloride (Concomitant use may cause additive CNS depression. When combined therapy is contemplated, the dose of one or both agents should be reduced).
No products indexed under this heading.

Clemastine Fumarate (Concomitant use may cause additive CNS depression. When combined therapy is contemplated, the dose of one or both agents should be reduced).
No products indexed under this heading.

Clomipramine Hydrochloride (The use of tricyclic antidepressants with hydrocodone preparations may increase the effect of either the antidepressant or hydrocodone).
No products indexed under this heading.

Clorazepate Dipotassium (Concomitant use may cause additive CNS depression. When combined therapy is contemplated, the dose of one or both agents should be reduced).
No products indexed under this heading.

Clozapine (Concomitant use may cause additive CNS depression. When combined therapy is contemplated, the dose of one or both agents should be reduced).
No products indexed under this heading.

Codeine Phosphate (Concomitant use may cause additive CNS depression. When combined therapy is contemplated, the dose of one or both agents should be reudced). Products include:
Tylenol with Codeine Tablets **2427**

Cyproheptadine Hydrochloride (Concomitant use may cause additive CNS depression. When combined therapy is contemplated, the dose of one or both agents should be reduced).
No products indexed under this heading.

Desipramine Hydrochloride (The use of tricyclic antidepressants with hydrocodone preparations may increase the effect of either the antidepressant or hydrocodone).
No products indexed under this heading.

Dexchlorpheniramine Maleate (Concomitant use may cause additive CNS depression. When combined therapy is contemplated, the dose of one or both agents should be reduced).
No products indexed under this heading.

Dezocine (Concomitant use may cause additive CNS depression. When combined therapy is contemplated, the dose of one or both agents should be reudced).
No products indexed under this heading.

Diazepam (Concomitant use may cause additive CNS depression. When combined therapy is contemplated, the dose of one or both agents should be reduced). Products include:
Valium Tablets **2658**

Diphenhydramine Citrate (Concomitant use may cause additive CNS depression. When combined therapy is contemplated, the dose of one or both agents should be reduced).
No products indexed under this heading.

Diphenhydramine Hydrochloride (Concomitant use may cause additive CNS depression. When combined therapy is contemplated, the dose of one or both agents should be reduced). Products include:
Benadryl Allergy & Cold Kapgels **1895**
Benadryl Allergy & Sinus Headache Kapgels **1895**
Benadryl Severe Allergy & Sinus Headache Caplets **1897**
Benadryl Dye-Free Allergy Liqui-gels Softgels **1897**
Benadryl Allergy Kapgels **1895**
Benadryl Allergy Quick Dissolve Strips **1896**
Benadryl Allergy Ultratab Tablets **1896**
Children's Benadryl Dye-Free Allergy Liquid **1897**
Children's Benadryl Allergy Fastmelts **1897**
Children's Benadryl Allergy Liquid **1898**
Children's Benadryl Allergy Perfect Measure **1896**
Children's Benadryl-D Allergy & Sinus Liquid **1896**
Benadryl-D Allergy & Sinus Tablet **1896**
PediaCare Children's Allergy & Cold Liquid **1902**
PediaCare Children's Allergy Liquid **1902**
Simply Sleep Caplets **1905**
Sudafed PE Nighttime Cold Caplets **1907**
Sudafed PE Severe Cold Caplets **1908**
Extra Strength Tylenol PM Caplets, Geltabs, Liquid, and Rapid Release Gels **1915**
Tylenol Allergy Multi-Symptom Nighttime Caplets with Cool Burst **1916**
Tylenol Severe Allergy Caplets **1916**
Children's Tylenol Plus Cold & Allergy Suspension Liquid **1914**
Tylenol Sore Throat Nighttime Liquid with Cool Burst **1918**

Diphenylpyraline Hydrochloride (Concomitant use may cause additive CNS depression. When combined therapy is contemplated, the dose of one or both agents should be reduced).
No products indexed under this heading.

Doxepin Hydrochloride (The use of tricyclic antidepressants with hydrocodone preparations may increase the effect of either the antidepressant or hydrocodone).
No products indexed under this heading.

Droperidol (Concomitant use may cause additive CNS depression. When combined therapy is contemplated, the dose of one or both agents should be reduced).
No products indexed under this heading.

Estazolam (Concomitant use may cause additive CNS depression. When combined therapy is contemplated, the dose of one or both agents should be reduced).
No products indexed under this heading.

Ethanol (Concomitant use may cause additive CNS depression. When combined therapy is contemplated, the dose of one or both agents should be reduced).
No products indexed under this heading.

Ethchlorvynol (Concomitant use may cause additive CNS depression. When combined therapy is contemplated, the dose of one or both agents should be reduced).
No products indexed under this heading.

Ethinamate (Concomitant use may cause additive CNS depression. When combined therapy is contemplated, the dose of one or both agents should be reduced).
No products indexed under this heading.

Ethyl Alcohol (Concomitant use may cause additive CNS depression. When combined therapy is contemplated, the dose of one or both agents should be reduced).
No products indexed under this heading.

Fentanyl (Concomitant use may cause additive CNS depression. When combined therapy is contemplated, the dose of one or both agents should be reudced). Products include:
Duragesic Transdermal System **2405**
Ionsys Transdermal System **2410**

Fentanyl Citrate (Concomitant use may cause additive CNS depression. When combined therapy is contemplated, the dose of one or both agents should be reudced). Products include:
Actiq **959**
Fentora Tablets **968**

Fexofenadine Hydrochloride (Concomitant use may cause additive CNS depression. When combined therapy is contemplated, the dose of one or both agents should be reduced). Products include:
Allegra Oral Solution **2684**
Allegra Tablets **2684**
Allegra-D 12 Hour Extended-Release Tablets **2687**
Allegra-D 24 Hour Extended-Release Tablets **2690**

Fluphenazine Decanoate (Concomitant use may cause additive CNS depression. When combined therapy is contemplated, the dose of one or both agents should be reduced).
No products indexed under this heading.

Fluphenazine Enanthate (Concomitant use may cause additive CNS depression. When combined therapy is contemplated, the dose of one or both agents should be reduced).
No products indexed under this heading.

Fluphenazine Hydrochloride (Concomitant use may cause additive CNS depression. When combined therapy is contemplated, the dose of one or both agents should be reduced).
No products indexed under this heading.

Flurazepam Hydrochloride (Concomitant use may cause additive CNS depression. When combined therapy is contemplated, the dose of one or both agents should be reduced).
No products indexed under this heading.

Glutethimide (Concomitant use may cause additive CNS depression. When combined therapy is contemplated, the dose of one or both agents should be reduced).
No products indexed under this heading.

Haloperidol (Concomitant use may cause additive CNS depression. When combined therapy is contemplated, the dose of one or both agents should be reduced).
No products indexed under this heading.

Haloperidol Decanoate (Concomitant use may cause additive CNS depression. When combined therapy is contemplated, the dose of one or both agents should be reduced).
No products indexed under this heading.

Hydrocodone Polistirex (Concomitant use may cause additive CNS depression. When combined therapy is contemplated, the dose of one or both agents should be reudced). Products include:
Tussionex Pennkinetic Extended-Release Suspension **3154**

Hydromorphone Hydrochloride (Concomitant use may cause additive CNS depression. When combined therapy is contemplated, the dose of one or both agents should be reudced).
No products indexed under this heading.

Hydroxyzine Hydrochloride (Concomitant use may cause additive CNS depression. When combined therapy is contemplated, the dose of one or both agents should be reduced).
No products indexed under this heading.

Imipramine Hydrochloride (The use of tricyclic antidepressants with hydrocodone preparations may increase the effect of either the antidepressant or hydrocodone).
No products indexed under this heading.

Imipramine Pamoate (The use of tricyclic antidepressants with hydrocodone preparations may increase the effect of either the antidepressant or hydrocodone).
No products indexed under this heading.

Isocarboxazid (The use of MAO inhibitors with hydrocodone prepara-

tions may increase the effect of either the antidepressant or hydrocodone). Products include:
Marplan Tablets 3177

Levorphanol Tartrate (Concomitant use may cause additive CNS depression. When combined therapy is contemplated, the dose of one or both agents should be reudced).
No products indexed under this heading.

Lithium Carbonate (Concomitant use may cause additive CNS depression. When combined therapy is contemplated, the dose of one or both agents should be reduced).
No products indexed under this heading.

Lithium Citrate (Concomitant use may cause additive CNS depression. When combined therapy is contemplated, the dose of one or both agents should be reduced).
No products indexed under this heading.

Loratadine (Concomitant use may cause additive CNS depression. When combined therapy is contemplated, the dose of one or both agents should be reduced).
No products indexed under this heading.

Lorazepam (Concomitant use may cause additive CNS depression. When combined therapy is contemplated, the dose of one or both agents should be reduced).
No products indexed under this heading.

Loxapine Hydrochloride (Concomitant use may cause additive CNS depression. When combined therapy is contemplated, the dose of one or both agents should be reduced).
No products indexed under this heading.

Loxapine Succinate (Concomitant use may cause additive CNS depression. When combined therapy is contemplated, the dose of one or both agents should be reduced).
No products indexed under this heading.

Maprotiline Hydrochloride (The use of tricyclic antidepressants with hydrocodone preparations may increase the effect of either the antidepressant or hydrocodone).
No products indexed under this heading.

Meperidine Hydrochloride (Concomitant use may cause additive CNS depression. When combined therapy is contemplated, the dose of one or both agents should be reudced).
No products indexed under this heading.

Meprobamate (Concomitant use may cause additive CNS depression. When combined therapy is contemplated, the dose of one or both agents should be reduced).
No products indexed under this heading.

Mesoridazine Besylate (Concomitant use may cause additive CNS depression. When combined therapy is contemplated, the dose of one or both agents should be reduced).
No products indexed under this heading.

Methadone Hydrochloride (Concomitant use may cause additive CNS depression. When combined therapy is contemplated, the dose of one or both agents should be reudced).
No products indexed under this heading.

Methdilazine Hydrochloride (Concomitant use may cause additive CNS depression. When combined therapy is contemplated, the dose of one or both agents should be reduced).
No products indexed under this heading.

Midazolam Hydrochloride (Concomitant use may cause additive CNS depression. When combined therapy is contemplated, the dose of one or both agents should be reduced).
No products indexed under this heading.

Moclobemide (The use of MAO inhibitors with hydrocodone preparations may increase the effect of either the antidepressant or hydrocodone).
No products indexed under this heading.

Molindone Hydrochloride (Concomitant use may cause additive CNS depression. When combined therapy is contemplated, the dose of one or both agents should be reduced). Products include:
Moban Tablets 1116

Morphine Sulfate (Concomitant use may cause additive CNS depression. When combined therapy is contemplated, the dose of one or both agents should be reudced). Products include:
Avinza Capsules 1772
DepoDur Injection 1095
MS Contin Tablets 2585

Nortriptyline Hydrochloride (The use of tricyclic antidepressants with hydrocodone preparations may increase the effect of either the antidepressant or hydrocodone).
No products indexed under this heading.

Olanzapine (Concomitant use may cause additive CNS depression. When combined therapy is contemplated, the dose of one or both agents should be reduced). Products include:
Symbyax Capsules 1871
Zyprexa Tablets 1883
Zyprexa IntraMuscular 1883
Zyprexa ZYDIS Orally Disintegrating Tablets 1883

Oxazepam (Concomitant use may cause additive CNS depression. When combined therapy is contemplated, the dose of one or both agents should be reduced).
No products indexed under this heading.

Oxycodone Hydrochloride (Concomitant use may cause additive CNS depression. When combined therapy is contemplated, the dose of one or both agents should be reudced). Products include:
OxyContin Tablets 2589
OxyIR Capsules 2593
Percocet Tablets 1127
Percodan Tablets 1130

Paliperidone (Concomitant use may cause additive CNS depression. When combined therapy is contemplated, the dose of one or both agents should be reduced). Products include:
Invega Extended-Release Tablets 1748

Pargyline Hydrochloride (The use of MAO inhibitors with hydrocodone preparations may increase the effect of either the antidepressant or hydrocodone).
No products indexed under this heading.

Perphenazine (Concomitant use may cause additive CNS depression. When combined therapy is contemplated, the dose of one or both agents should be reduced).
No products indexed under this heading.

Phenelzine Sulfate (The use of MAO inhibitors with hydrocodone preparations may increase the effect of either the antidepressant or hydrocodone).
No products indexed under this heading.

Prazepam (Concomitant use may cause additive CNS depression. When combined therapy is contemplated, the dose of one or both agents should be reduced).
No products indexed under this heading.

Procarbazine Hydrochloride (The use of MAO inhibitors with hydrocodone preparations may increase the effect of either the antidepressant or hydrocodone).
No products indexed under this heading.

Prochlorperazine (Concomitant use may cause additive CNS depression. When combined therapy is contemplated, the dose of one or both agents should be reduced).
No products indexed under this heading.

Promethazine Hydrochloride (Concomitant use may cause additive CNS depression. When combined therapy is contemplated, the dose of one or both agents should be reduced).
No products indexed under this heading.

Propoxyphene Hydrochloride (Concomitant use may cause additive CNS depression. When combined therapy is contemplated, the dose of one or both agents should be reudced).
No products indexed under this heading.

Propoxyphene Napsylate (Concomitant use may cause additive CNS depression. When combined therapy is contemplated, the dose of one or both agents should be reudced).
No products indexed under this heading.

Protriptyline Hydrochloride (The use of tricyclic antidepressants with hydrocodone preparations may increase the effect of either the antidepressant or hydrocodone).
No products indexed under this heading.

Pyrilamine Maleate (Concomitant use may cause additive CNS depression. When combined therapy is contemplated, the dose of one or both agents should be reduced).
No products indexed under this heading.

Pyrilamine Tannate (Concomitant use may cause additive CNS depression. When combined therapy is contemplated, the dose of one or both agents should be reduced).
No products indexed under this heading.

Quetiapine Fumarate (Concomitant use may cause additive CNS depression. When combined therapy is contemplated, the dose of one or both agents should be reduced).
No products indexed under this heading.

Ramelteon (Concomitant use may cause additive CNS depression. When combined therapy is contemplated, the dose of one or both agents should be reduced). Products include:
Rozerem Tablets 3091

Rasagiline Mesylate (The use of MAO inhibitors with hydrocodone preparations may increase the effect of either the antidepressant or hydrocodone). Products include:
Azilect Tablets 3106

Remifentanil Hydrochloride (Concomitant use may cause additive CNS depression. When combined therapy is contemplated, the dose of one or both agents should be reudced).
No products indexed under this heading.

Risperidone (Concomitant use may cause additive CNS depression. When combined therapy is contemplated, the dose of one or both agents should be reduced). Products include:
Risperdal Consta Long-Acting Injection 1753

Selegiline (The use of MAO inhibitors with hydrocodone preparations may increase the effect of either the antidepressant or hydrocodone). Products include:
Emsam Transdermal System 905

Selegiline Hydrochloride (The use of MAO inhibitors with hydrocodone preparations may increase the effect of either the antidepressant or hydrocodone). Products include:
Eldepryl Capsules 3052

Sufentanil Citrate (Concomitant use may cause additive CNS depression. When combined therapy is contemplated, the dose of one or both agents should be reudced).
No products indexed under this heading.

Terfenadine (Concomitant use may cause additive CNS depression. When combined therapy is contemplated, the dose of one or both agents should be reduced).
No products indexed under this heading.

Thioridazine Hydrochloride (Concomitant use may cause additive CNS depression. When combined therapy is contemplated, the dose of one or both agents should be reduced). Products include:
Thioridazine Hydrochloride Tablets 2195

Thiothixene (Concomitant use may cause additive CNS depression. When combined therapy is contemplated, the dose of one or both agents should be reduced). Products include:
Thiothixene Capsules 2197

Tranylcypromine Sulfate (The use of MAO inhibitors with hydrocodone

preparations may increase the effect of either the antidepressant or hydrocodone). Products include:
Parnate Tablets 1532

Trifluoperazine Hydrochloride (Concomitant use may cause additive CNS depression. When combined therapy is contemplated, the dose of one or both agents should be reduced).
No products indexed under this heading.

Trimeprazine Tartrate (Concomitant use may cause additive CNS depression. When combined therapy is contemplated, the dose of one or both agents should be reduced).
No products indexed under this heading.

Trimipramine Maleate (The use of tricyclic antidepressants with hydrocodone preparations may increase the effect of either the antidepressant or hydrocodone).
No products indexed under this heading.

Tripelennamine Hydrochloride (Concomitant use may cause additive CNS depression. When combined therapy is contemplated, the dose of one or both agents should be reduced).
No products indexed under this heading.

Triprolidine Hydrochloride (Concomitant use may cause additive CNS depression. When combined therapy is contemplated, the dose of one or both agents should be reduced).
No products indexed under this heading.

Ziprasidone Hydrochloride (Concomitant use may cause additive CNS depression. When combined therapy is contemplated, the dose of one or both agents should be reduced). Products include:
Geodon Capsules 2520

Food Interactions

Alcohol (Concomitant use may cause additive CBS depression. When combined therapy is contemplated, the dose of one or both agents should be reduced).

LORTAB 7.5/500 TABLETS

(Acetaminophen, Hydrocodone Bitartrate) 3144

May interact with antihistamines, central nervous system depressants, monoamine oxidase inhibitors, narcotic analgesics, drugs which undergo biotransformation by cytochrome p-450 mixed function oxidase, tranquilizers, tricyclic antidepressants, and certain other agents. Compounds in these categories include:

Acarbose (Co-administration may exhibit additive CNS-depression). Products include:
Precose Tablets 792

Acrivastine (Co-administration may exhibit additive CNS-depression).
No products indexed under this heading.

Alatrofloxacin Mesylate (Co-administration may exhibit additive CNS-depression).
No products indexed under this heading.

Alfentanil Hydrochloride (Co-administration may exhibit additive CNS-depression).
No products indexed under this heading.

Alprazolam (Co-administration may exhibit additive CNS-depression).
No products indexed under this heading.

Aminophylline (Co-administration may exhibit additive CNS-depression).
No products indexed under this heading.

Amiodarone Hydrochloride (Co-administration may exhibit additive CNS-depression).
No products indexed under this heading.

Amitriptyline Hydrochloride (Co-administration may increase the effect of either the antidepressant or hydrocodone).
No products indexed under this heading.

Amlodipine Besylate (Co-administration may exhibit additive CNS-depression). Products include:
Azor Tablets 1005
Exforge Tablets 2238

Amoxapine (Co-administration may increase the effect of either the antidepressant or hydrocodone).
No products indexed under this heading.

Amphetamine Aspartate (Co-administration may exhibit additive CNS-depression). Products include:
Adderall XR Capsules 3012

Amphetamine Aspartate Monohydrate (Co-administration may exhibit additive CNS-depression).
No products indexed under this heading.

Amphetamine Sulfate (Co-administration may exhibit additive CNS-depression). Products include:
Adderall XR Capsules 3012

Aprepitant (Co-administration may exhibit additive CNS-depression). Products include:
Emend Capsules 1992

Aprobarbital (Co-administration may exhibit additive CNS-depression).
No products indexed under this heading.

Astemizole (Co-administration may exhibit additive CNS-depression).
No products indexed under this heading.

Atomoxetine Hydrochloride (Co-administration may exhibit additive CNS-depression). Products include:
Strattera Capsules 1864

Atorvastatin Calcium (Co-administration may exhibit additive CNS-depression). Products include:
Lipitor Tablets 2501

Azatadine Maleate (Co-administration may exhibit additive CNS-depression).
No products indexed under this heading.

Belladonna Ergotamine (Co-administration may exhibit additive CNS-depression).
No products indexed under this heading.

Benzphetamine Hydrochloride (Co-administration may exhibit additive CNS-depression).
No products indexed under this heading.

Bisoprolol Fumarate (Co-administration may exhibit additive CNS-depression).
No products indexed under this heading.

Bromodiphenhydramine Hydrochloride (Co-administration may exhibit additive CNS-depression).
No products indexed under this heading.

Brompheniramine Maleate (Co-administration may exhibit additive CNS-depression).
No products indexed under this heading.

Buprenorphine Hydrochloride (Co-administration may exhibit additive CNS-depression). Products include:
Suboxone Tablets 2601
Subutex Tablets 2601

Buspirone Hydrochloride (Co-administration may exhibit additive CNS-depression).
No products indexed under this heading.

Busulfan (Co-administration may exhibit additive CNS-depression). Products include:
Busulfex Injection 2477
Myleran Tablets 1530

Butabarbital (Co-administration may exhibit additive CNS-depression).
No products indexed under this heading.

Butalbital (Co-administration may exhibit additive CNS-depression).
No products indexed under this heading.

Caffeine (Co-administration may exhibit additive CNS-depression). Products include:
BioLean Free Tablets 635
BioLean II Tablets 635
Winrgy Dietary Supplement 642

Caffeine Anhydrous (Co-administration may exhibit additive CNS-depression).
No products indexed under this heading.

Caffeine Citrate (Co-administration may exhibit additive CNS-depression).
No products indexed under this heading.

Candesartan Cilexetil (Co-administration may exhibit additive CNS-depression). Products include:
Atacand Tablets 639
Atacand HCT 642

Captopril (Co-administration may exhibit additive CNS-depression). Products include:
Captopril Tablets 2182

Carbamazepine (Co-administration may exhibit additive CNS-depression). Products include:
Carbatrol Capsules 3019
Equetro Extended-Release Capsules 3174

Carisoprodol (Co-administration may exhibit additive CNS-depression). Products include:
Soma Tablets 1931

Carvedilol (Co-administration may exhibit additive CNS-depression). Products include:
Coreg Tablets 1387

Celecoxib (Co-administration may exhibit additive CNS-depression). Products include:
Celebrex Capsules 2979

Cerivastatin Sodium (Co-administration may exhibit additive CNS-depression).
No products indexed under this heading.

Cetirizine Hydrochloride (Co-administration may exhibit additive CNS-depression). Products include:
Zyrtec Allergy Tablets 1919
Zyrtec Chewable Tablets 1920
Children's Zyrtec Allergy Chewable Tablets 1922
Children's Zyrtec Allergy Syrup 1920
Children's Zyrtec Hives Relief Syrup 1920
Zyrtec Syrup 1920
Zyrtec Tablets 1920
Zyrtec-D 12 Hour Extended Release Tablets 1923
Zyrtec-D Allergy & Congestion Extended-Release Tablets 1923

Cevimeline Hydrochloride (Co-administration may exhibit additive CNS-depression). Products include:
Evoxac Capsules 1013

Chlordiazepoxide (Co-administration may exhibit additive CNS-depression).
No products indexed under this heading.

Chlordiazepoxide Hydrochloride (Co-administration may exhibit additive CNS-depression).
No products indexed under this heading.

Chlorpheniramine (Co-administration may exhibit additive CNS-depression).
No products indexed under this heading.

Chlorpheniramine Maleate (Co-administration may exhibit additive CNS-depression). Products include:
Actifed Cold & Allergy Tablets 1895
Sudafed PE Sinus & Allergy Tablets 1908
Tylenol Allergy Multi-Symptom Caplets with Cool Burst and Rapid Release Gelcaps 1916
Children's Tylenol Plus Cold Suspension Liquid 1912
Children's Tylenol Plus Cough & Runny Nose Suspension Liquid 1912
Children's Tylenol Plus Flu Suspension Liquid 1914
Children's Tylenol Plus Multi-Symptom Cold Suspension Liquid 1912
Tylenol Cold Head Congestion Nighttime Caplets with Cool Burst 1910
Tylenol Cold Multi-Symptom Nighttime Caplets with Cool Burst 1913
Tylenol Sinus Congestion & Pain Nighttime Caplets with Cool Burst 1917

Chlorpheniramine Polistirex (Co-administration may exhibit additive CNS-depression). Products include:
Tussionex Pennkinetic Extended-Release Suspension 3154

Chlorpheniramine Tannate (Co-administration may exhibit additive CNS-depression).
No products indexed under this heading.

Chlorpromazine (Co-administration may exhibit additive CNS-depression).
No products indexed under this heading.

Chlorpromazine Hydrochloride (Co-administration may exhibit additive CNS-depression).
No products indexed under this heading.

Chlorpropamide (Co-administration may exhibit additive CNS-depression).
No products indexed under this heading.

Chlorprothixene (Co-administration may exhibit additive CNS-depression).
No products indexed under this heading.

IMPORTANT NOTE: Always consult each drug listing in the patient's regimen for possible interactions.

Chlorprothixene Hydrochloride (Co-administration may exhibit additive CNS-depression).
No products indexed under this heading.

Chlorprothixene Lactate (Co-administration may exhibit additive CNS-depression).
No products indexed under this heading.

Cilostazol (Co-administration may exhibit additive CNS-depression). Products include:
Pletal Tablets 2481

Cimetidine Hydrochloride (Co-administration may exhibit additive CNS-depression).
No products indexed under this heading.

Ciprofloxacin (Co-administration may exhibit additive CNS-depression). Products include:
Cipro I.V. 2817
Cipro Oral Suspension 2810
Cipro XR Tablets 2823
Ciprodex Otic Suspension 541

Ciprofloxacin Hydrochloride (Co-administration may exhibit additive CNS-depression). Products include:
Cipro Tablets 2810

Cisapride (Co-administration may exhibit additive CNS-depression).
No products indexed under this heading.

Citalopram Hydrobromide (Co-administration may exhibit additive CNS-depression). Products include:
Celexa 1160

Clarithromycin (Co-administration may exhibit additive CNS-depression). Products include:
Biaxin/Biaxin XL 411

Clemastine Fumarate (Co-administration may exhibit additive CNS-depression).
No products indexed under this heading.

Clomipramine Hydrochloride (Co-administration may increase the effect of either the antidepressant or hydrocodone).
No products indexed under this heading.

Clopidogrel Hydrogen Sulfate (Co-administration may exhibit additive CNS-depression).
No products indexed under this heading.

Clorazepate Dipotassium (Co-administration may exhibit additive CNS-depression).
No products indexed under this heading.

Clozapine (Co-administration may exhibit additive CNS-depression).
No products indexed under this heading.

Codeine Phosphate (Co-administration may exhibit additive CNS-depression). Products include:
Tylenol with Codeine Tablets 2427

Codeine Sulfate (Co-administration may exhibit additive CNS-depression).
No products indexed under this heading.

Cyclobenzaprine (Co-administration may exhibit additive CNS-depression).
No products indexed under this heading.

Cyclobenzaprine Hydrochloride (Co-administration may exhibit additive CNS-depression). Products include:
Amrix Capsules 966

Cyclophosphamide (Co-administration may exhibit additive CNS-depression).
No products indexed under this heading.

Cyclosporine (Co-administration may exhibit additive CNS-depression). Products include:
Gengraf Capsules 435
Neoral Oral Solution 2280
Neoral Soft Gelatin Capsules 2280
Restasis Ophthalmic Emulsion 557
Sandimmune 2296

Cyproheptadine Hydrochloride (Co-administration may exhibit additive CNS-depression).
No products indexed under this heading.

Desflurane (Co-administration may exhibit additive CNS-depression).
No products indexed under this heading.

Desipramine Hydrochloride (Co-administration may increase the effect of either the antidepressant or hydrocodone).
No products indexed under this heading.

Desogestrel (Co-administration may exhibit additive CNS-depression). Products include:
Mircette Tablets 1034

Dexamethasone (Co-administration may exhibit additive CNS-depression). Products include:
Ciprodex Otic Suspension 541

Dexamethasone Acetate (Co-administration may exhibit additive CNS-depression).
No products indexed under this heading.

Dexamethasone Phosphate (Co-administration may exhibit additive CNS-depression).
No products indexed under this heading.

Dexamethasone Sodium (Co-administration may exhibit additive CNS-depression).
No products indexed under this heading.

Dexamethasone Sodium Phosphate (Co-administration may exhibit additive CNS-depression).
No products indexed under this heading.

Dexchlorpheniramine Maleate (Co-administration may exhibit additive CNS-depression).
No products indexed under this heading.

Dexfenfluramine Hydrochloride (Co-administration may exhibit additive CNS-depression).
No products indexed under this heading.

Dextromethorphan (Co-administration may exhibit additive CNS-depression).
No products indexed under this heading.

Dextromethorphan Hydrobromide (Co-administration may exhibit additive CNS-depression). Products include:
PediaCare Children's Liquid Multi-Symptom Cold 1902
PediaCare Children's Long-Acting Cough 1902
Children's Sudafed PE Cold & Cough Liquid 1907
Sudafed PE Cold & Cough Caplets 1907
Children's Tylenol Plus Cough & Runny Nose Suspension Liquid 1912
Children's Tylenol Plus Cough & Sore Throat Suspension Liquid 1912
Children's Tylenol Plus Flu Suspension Liquid 1914
Children's Tylenol Plus Multi-Symptom Cold Suspension Liquid 1912
Tylenol Cold Severe Congestion Daytime Caplets with Cool Burst 1912
Tylenol Cold Head Congestion Daytime Caplets with Cool Burst 1910
Tylenol Cold Head Congestion Nighttime Caplets with Cool Burst 1910
Tylenol Cold Head Congestion Severe Daytime Caplets with Cool Burst 1910
Tylenol Cold Multi-Symptom Daytime Caplets with Cool Burst and Rapid Release Gels 1913
Tylenol Cold Multi-Symptom Daytime Liquid with Citrus Burst 1913
Tylenol Cold Multi-Symptom Nighttime Caplets with Cool Burst 1913
Tylenol Cold Multi-Symptom Nighttime Liquid with Cool Burst 1913
Tylenol Cold Multi-Symptom Severe Caplets with Cool Burst 1913
Tylenol Cold Multi-Symptom Severe Daytime Liquid with Citrus Burst 1913
Tylenol Cough & Sore Throat Daytime Liquid with Cool Burst 1918
Tylenol Cough & Sore Throat Nighttime Liquid with Cool Burst 1918
Vicks DayQuil Cold & Flu Multi-Symptom Relief .... ▣616
Vicks DayQuil LiquiCaps 2567
Vicks DayQuil Liquid 2567
Vicks DayQuil Multi-Symptom Cold/Flu Relief 2567
Vicks NyQuil Cold & Flu Multi-Symptom Relief .... ▣617
Vicks NyQuil LiquiCaps 2567
Vicks NyQuil Liquid 2567
Vicks NyQuil Multi-Symptom Cold/Flu Relief 2567

Dextromethorphan Polistirex (Co-administration may exhibit additive CNS-depression).
No products indexed under this heading.

Dezocine (Co-administration may exhibit additive CNS-depression).
No products indexed under this heading.

Diazepam (Co-administration may exhibit additive CNS-depression). Products include:
Valium Tablets 2658

Diclofenac Potassium (Co-administration may exhibit additive CNS-depression).
No products indexed under this heading.

Diclofenac Sodium (Co-administration may exhibit additive CNS-depression). Products include:
Diclofenac Sodium Ophthalmic Solution .... ⊙240
Voltaren Ophthalmic Solution 2336
Voltaren Tablets 2334
Voltaren-XR Tablets 2337

Dihydroergotamine Mesylate (Co-administration may exhibit additive CNS-depression).
No products indexed under this heading.

Diltiazem Hydrochloride (Co-administration may exhibit additive CNS-depression). Products include:
Cardizem LA Extended Release Tablets 421

Diltiazem Maleate (Co-administration may exhibit additive CNS-depression).
No products indexed under this heading.

Diphenhydramine Citrate (Co-administration may exhibit additive CNS-depression).
No products indexed under this heading.

Diphenhydramine Hydrochloride (Co-administration may exhibit additive CNS-depression). Products include:
Benadryl Allergy & Cold Kapgels 1895
Benadryl Allergy & Sinus Headache Kapgels 1895
Benadryl Severe Allergy & Sinus Headache Caplets 1897
Benadryl Dye-Free Allergy Liqui-gels Softgels 1897
Benadryl Allergy Kapgels 1895
Benadryl Allergy Quick Dissolve Strips 1896
Benadryl Allergy Ultratab Tablets 1896
Children's Benadryl Dye-Free Allergy Liquid 1897
Children's Benadryl Allergy Fastmelts 1897
Children's Benadryl Allergy Liquid 1898
Children's Benadryl Allergy Perfect Measure 1896
Children's Benadryl-D Allergy & Sinus Liquid 1896
Benadryl-D Allergy & Sinus Tablet 1896
PediaCare Children's Allergy & Cold Liquid 1902
PediaCare Children's Allergy Liquid 1902
Simply Sleep Caplets 1905
Sudafed PE Nighttime Cold Caplets 1907
Sudafed PE Severe Cold Caplets 1908
Extra Strength Tylenol PM Caplets, Geltabs, Liquid, and Rapid Release Gels 1915
Tylenol Allergy Multi-Symptom Nighttime Caplets with Cool Burst 1916
Tylenol Severe Allergy Caplets 1916
Children's Tylenol Plus Cold & Allergy Suspension Liquid 1914
Tylenol Sore Throat Nighttime Liquid with Cool Burst 1918

Diphenylpyraline Hydrochloride (Co-administration may exhibit additive CNS-depression).
No products indexed under this heading.

Disopyramide (Co-administration may exhibit additive CNS-depression).
No products indexed under this heading.

Disopyramide Phosphate (Co-administration may exhibit additive CNS-depression).
No products indexed under this heading.

Divalproex Sodium (Co-administration may exhibit additive CNS-depression). Products include:
Depakote ER Tablets 423

Docetaxel (Co-administration may exhibit additive CNS-depression). Products include:
Taxotere Injection Concentrate 2773

Dolasetron Mesylate (Co-administration may exhibit additive CNS-depression). Products include:
Anzemet Injection 2701
Anzemet Tablets 2704

Donepezil Hydrochloride (Co-administration may exhibit additive CNS-depression). Products include:
Aricept Tablets 1062
Aricept ODT Tablets 1062

Doxepin Hydrochloride (Co-administration may increase the effect of either the antidepressant or hydrocodone).
No products indexed under this heading.

Doxorubicin Hydrochloride (Co-administration may exhibit additive CNS-depression).
No products indexed under this heading.

Dronabinol (Co-administration may exhibit additive CNS-depression). Products include:
Marinol Capsules 3163

Droperidol (Co-administration may exhibit additive CNS-depression).
No products indexed under this heading.

Drugs that Undergo Biotransformation by Cytochrome P-450 Mixed Function Oxidase (Co-administration may exhibit additive CNS-depression).
No products indexed under this heading.

Dyphylline (Co-administration may exhibit additive CNS-depression).
No products indexed under this heading.

Encainide Hydrochloride (Co-administration may exhibit additive CNS-depression).
No products indexed under this heading.

Enflurane (Co-administration may exhibit additive CNS-depression).
No products indexed under this heading.

Enoxacin (Co-administration may exhibit additive CNS-depression).
No products indexed under this heading.

Eprosartan Mesylate (Co-administration may exhibit additive CNS-depression). Products include:
Teveten Tablets 515
Teveten HCT Tablets 517

Ergotamine Tartrate (Co-administration may exhibit additive CNS-depression).
No products indexed under this heading.

Erythromycin (Co-administration may exhibit additive CNS-depression).
No products indexed under this heading.

Erythromycin Estolate (Co-administration may exhibit additive CNS-depression).
No products indexed under this heading.

Erythromycin Ethylsuccinate (Co-administration may exhibit additive CNS-depression). Products include:
E.E.S. 433
EryPed 431

Erythromycin Gluceptate (Co-administration may exhibit additive CNS-depression).
No products indexed under this heading.

Erythromycin Lactobionate (Co-administration may exhibit additive CNS-depression).
No products indexed under this heading.

Erythromycin Stearate (Co-administration may exhibit additive CNS-depression).
No products indexed under this heading.

Esomeprazole Magnesium (Co-administration may exhibit additive CNS-depression). Products include:
Nexium Delayed-Release Capsules 645
Nexium Delayed-Release Oral Suspension 645

Estazolam (Co-administration may exhibit additive CNS-depression).
No products indexed under this heading.

Estradiol (Co-administration may exhibit additive CNS-depression). Products include:
Activella Tablets 2347
Angeliq Tablets 751
Climara Transdermal System 763
Climara Pro Transdermal System 768
Divigel 3167
Vagifem Tablets 2375

Estradiol Benzoate (Co-administration may exhibit additive CNS-depression).
No products indexed under this heading.

Estradiol Cypionate (Co-administration may exhibit additive CNS-depression).
No products indexed under this heading.

Estradiol Valerate (Co-administration may exhibit additive CNS-depression).
No products indexed under this heading.

Estrogen (Co-administration may exhibit additive CNS-depression).
No products indexed under this heading.

Estrogens, Conjugated (Co-administration may exhibit additive CNS-depression). Products include:
Premarin Intravenous 3217
Premarin Tablets 3221
Premarin Vaginal Cream 3228
Premphase Tablets 3232
Prempro Tablets 3232

Estrogens, Conjugated, Synthetic A (Co-administration may exhibit additive CNS-depression).
No products indexed under this heading.

Estrogens, Esterified (Co-administration may exhibit additive CNS-depression). Products include:
Estratest Tablets 3043
Estratest H.S. Tablets 3043

Ethanol (Co-administration may exhibit additive CNS-depression).
No products indexed under this heading.

Ethchlorvynol (Co-administration may exhibit additive CNS-depression).
No products indexed under this heading.

Ethinamate (Co-administration may exhibit additive CNS-depression).
No products indexed under this heading.

Ethinyl Estradiol (Co-administration may exhibit additive CNS-depression). Products include:
Lybrel Tablets 3204
Mircette Tablets 1034
NuvaRing 2897
Ortho-Cyclen/Ortho Tri-Cyclen 2449
Ortho Evra Transdermal System 2437
Ortho Tri-Cyclen Lo Tablets 2458
Seasonique Tablets 1046
Yaz Tablets 805

Ethosuximide (Co-administration may exhibit additive CNS-depression).
No products indexed under this heading.

Ethotoin (Co-administration may exhibit additive CNS-depression).
No products indexed under this heading.

Ethyl Alcohol (Co-administration may exhibit additive CNS-depression).
No products indexed under this heading.

Ethynodiol Diacetate (Co-administration may exhibit additive CNS-depression).
No products indexed under this heading.

Etodolac (Co-administration may exhibit additive CNS-depression).
No products indexed under this heading.

Etoposide (Co-administration may exhibit additive CNS-depression).
No products indexed under this heading.

Etoposide Phosphate (Co-administration may exhibit additive CNS-depression).
No products indexed under this heading.

Felbamate (Co-administration may exhibit additive CNS-depression).
No products indexed under this heading.

Felodipine (Co-administration may exhibit additive CNS-depression).
No products indexed under this heading.

Fenoprofen Calcium (Co-administration may exhibit additive CNS-depression). Products include:
Nalfon Capsules 2508

Fentanyl (Co-administration may exhibit additive CNS-depression). Products include:
Duragesic Transdermal System 2405
Ionsys Transdermal System 2410

Fentanyl Citrate (Co-administration may exhibit additive CNS-depression). Products include:
Actiq 959
Fentora Tablets 968

Fexofenadine Hydrochloride (Co-administration may exhibit additive CNS-depression). Products include:
Allegra Oral Solution 2684
Allegra Tablets 2684
Allegra-D 12 Hour Extended-Release Tablets 2687
Allegra-D 24 Hour Extended-Release Tablets 2690

Flecainide Acetate (Co-administration may exhibit additive CNS-depression).
No products indexed under this heading.

Fluoxetine (Co-administration may exhibit additive CNS-depression).
No products indexed under this heading.

Fluoxetine Hydrochloride (Co-administration may exhibit additive CNS-depression). Products include:
Prozac Weekly Capsules 1852
Prozac Pulvules and Liquid 1852
Symbyax Capsules 1871

Fluphenazine Decanoate (Co-administration may exhibit additive CNS-depression).
No products indexed under this heading.

Fluphenazine Enanthate (Co-administration may exhibit additive CNS-depression).
No products indexed under this heading.

Fluphenazine Hydrochloride (Co-administration may exhibit additive CNS-depression).
No products indexed under this heading.

Flurazepam Hydrochloride (Co-administration may exhibit additive CNS-depression).
No products indexed under this heading.

Flurbiprofen (Co-administration may exhibit additive CNS-depression).
No products indexed under this heading.

Flurbiprofen Sodium (Co-administration may exhibit additive CNS-depression).
No products indexed under this heading.

Flutamide (Co-administration may exhibit additive CNS-depression).
No products indexed under this heading.

Fluticasone Propionate (Co-administration may exhibit additive CNS-depression). Products include:
Advair Diskus 100/50 1276
Advair Diskus 250/50 1276
Advair Diskus 500/50 1276
Advair HFA 45/21 Inhalation Aerosol 1288
Advair HFA 115/21 Inhalation Aerosol 1288
Advair HFA 230/21 Inhalation Aerosol 1288
Flonase Nasal Spray 1431
Flovent Diskus 50 mcg 1435

Fluvastatin Sodium (Co-administration may exhibit additive CNS-depression). Products include:
Lescol Capsules 2268
Lescol XL Tablets 2268

Fluvoxamine Maleate (Co-administration may exhibit additive CNS-depression). Products include:
Luvox CR Extended-Release Capsules 1759

Formoterol Fumarate (Co-administration may exhibit additive CNS-depression). Products include:
Foradil Aerolizer 2849
Perforomist Inhalation Solution 1025

Fosphenytoin (Co-administration may exhibit additive CNS-depression).
No products indexed under this heading.

Fosphenytoin Sodium (Co-administration may exhibit additive CNS-depression).
No products indexed under this heading.

Gabapentin (Co-administration may exhibit additive CNS-depression).
No products indexed under this heading.

Galantamine Hydrobromide (Co-administration may exhibit additive CNS-depression).
No products indexed under this heading.

Glimepiride (Co-administration may exhibit additive CNS-depression). Products include:
Avandaryl Tablets 1344
Duetact Tablets 3085

Glipizide (Co-administration may exhibit additive CNS-depression).
No products indexed under this heading.

Glutethimide (Co-administration may exhibit additive CNS-depression).
No products indexed under this heading.

Glyburide (Co-administration may exhibit additive CNS-depression).
No products indexed under this heading.

IMPORTANT NOTE: Always consult each drug listing in the patient's regimen for possible interactions.

Moclobemide (Co-administration may increase the effect of either the MAO inhibitor or hydrocodone).
No products indexed under this heading.

Molindone Hydrochloride (Co-administration may exhibit additive CNS-depression). Products include:
Moban Tablets ... 1116

Montelukast Sodium (Co-administration may exhibit additive CNS-depression). Products include:
Singulair ... 2114

Morphine Sulfate (Co-administration may exhibit additive CNS-depression). Products include:
Avinza Capsules ... 1772
DepoDur Injection ... 1095
MS Contin Tablets ... 2585

Moxifloxacin Hydrochloride (Co-administration may exhibit additive CNS-depression). Products include:
Avelox ... 2803
Vigamox Ophthalmic Solution ... 548

Nabumetone (Co-administration may exhibit additive CNS-depression).
No products indexed under this heading.

Nafcillin Sodium (Co-administration may exhibit additive CNS-depression).
No products indexed under this heading.

Naproxen (Co-administration may exhibit additive CNS-depression). Products include:
EC-Naprosyn Delayed-Release Tablets ... 2632
Naprosyn Suspension ... 2632
Naprosyn Tablets ... 2632

Naproxen Sodium (Co-administration may exhibit additive CNS-depression). Products include:
Anaprox Tablets ... 2632
Anaprox DS Tablets ... 2632
Treximet Tablets ... 1616

Nateglinide (Co-administration may exhibit additive CNS-depression). Products include:
Starlix Tablets ... 2314

Nefazodone Hydrochloride (Co-administration may exhibit additive CNS-depression).
No products indexed under this heading.

Nelfinavir Mesylate (Co-administration may exhibit additive CNS-depression).
No products indexed under this heading.

Nicardipine (Co-administration may exhibit additive CNS-depression).
No products indexed under this heading.

Nicardipine Hydrochloride (Co-administration may exhibit additive CNS-depression). Products include:
Cardene I.V. ... 1093

Nicotine Polacrilex (Co-administration may exhibit additive CNS-depression).
No products indexed under this heading.

Nicotine Salicylate (Co-administration may exhibit additive CNS-depression).
No products indexed under this heading.

Nicotine Sulfate (Co-administration may exhibit additive CNS-depression).
No products indexed under this heading.

Nifedipine (Co-administration may exhibit additive CNS-depression).
No products indexed under this heading.

Nilutamide (Co-administration may exhibit additive CNS-depression).
No products indexed under this heading.

Nimodipine (Co-administration may exhibit additive CNS-depression). Products include:
Nimotop Capsules ... 790

Nisoldipine (Co-administration may exhibit additive CNS-depression). Products include:
Sular Extended Release Tablets ... 2975

Nitrendipine (Co-administration may exhibit additive CNS-depression).
No products indexed under this heading.

Norethindrone (Co-administration may exhibit additive CNS-depression). Products include:
Ortho Micronor Tablets ... 2446

Norethindrone Acetate (Co-administration may exhibit additive CNS-depression). Products include:
Activella Tablets ... 2347

Norfloxacin (Co-administration may exhibit additive CNS-depression). Products include:
Noroxin Tablets ... 2069

Norgestrel (Co-administration may exhibit additive CNS-depression).
No products indexed under this heading.

Nortriptyline Hydrochloride (Co-administration may increase the effect of either the antidepressant or hydrocodone).
No products indexed under this heading.

Ofloxacin (Co-administration may exhibit additive CNS-depression). Products include:
Ofloxacin Ophthalmic Solution 0.3% ... ⊙243

Olanzapine (Co-administration may exhibit additive CNS-depression). Products include:
Symbyax Capsules ... 1871
Zyprexa Tablets ... 1883
Zyprexa IntraMuscular ... 1883
Zyprexa ZYDIS Orally Disintegrating Tablets ... 1883

Omeprazole (Co-administration may exhibit additive CNS-depression).
No products indexed under this heading.

Ondansetron (Co-administration may exhibit additive CNS-depression). Products include:
Zofran ODT Orally Disintegrating Tablets ... 1687

Ondansetron Hydrochloride (Co-administration may exhibit additive CNS-depression). Products include:
Zofran Injection ... 1682
Zofran ... 1687

Oxaprozin (Co-administration may exhibit additive CNS-depression).
No products indexed under this heading.

Oxazepam (Co-administration may exhibit additive CNS-depression).
No products indexed under this heading.

Oxcarbazepine (Co-administration may exhibit additive CNS-depression).
No products indexed under this heading.

Oxycodone Hydrochloride (Co-administration may exhibit additive CNS-depression). Products include:
OxyContin Tablets ... 2589
OxyIR Capsules ... 2593
Percocet Tablets ... 1127
Percodan Tablets ... 1130

Paclitaxel (Co-administration may exhibit additive CNS-depression).
No products indexed under this heading.

Pantoprazole Sodium (Co-administration may exhibit additive CNS-depression). Products include:
Protonix for Delayed-Release Oral Suspension ... 3254
Protonix Delayed-Release Tablets ... 3254
Protonix I.V. ... 3257

Paramethadione (Co-administration may exhibit additive CNS-depression).
No products indexed under this heading.

Pargyline Hydrochloride (Co-administration may increase the effect of either the MAO inhibitor or hydrocodone).
No products indexed under this heading.

Paroxetine Hydrochloride (Co-administration may exhibit additive CNS-depression). Products include:
Paxil ... 1535
Paxil CR Controlled-Release Tablets ... 1544

Pentamidine Isethionate (Co-administration may exhibit additive CNS-depression).
No products indexed under this heading.

Pentobarbital Sodium (Co-administration may exhibit additive CNS-depression). Products include:
Nembutal Sodium Solution, USP ... 2494

Perphenazine (Co-administration may exhibit additive CNS-depression).
No products indexed under this heading.

Phenacemide (Co-administration may exhibit additive CNS-depression).
No products indexed under this heading.

Phenelzine Sulfate (Co-administration may increase the effect of either the MAO inhibitor or hydrocodone).
No products indexed under this heading.

Phenobarbital (Co-administration may exhibit additive CNS-depression). Products include:
Donnatal Extentabs ... 2507

Phenobarbital Sodium (Co-administration may exhibit additive CNS-depression).
No products indexed under this heading.

Phensuximide (Co-administration may exhibit additive CNS-depression).
No products indexed under this heading.

Phenylbutazone (Co-administration may exhibit additive CNS-depression).
No products indexed under this heading.

Phenytoin (Co-administration may exhibit additive CNS-depression).
No products indexed under this heading.

Phenytoin Sodium (Co-administration may exhibit additive CNS-depression). Products include:
Phenytek Capsules ... 2192

Pimozide (Co-administration may exhibit additive CNS-depression).
No products indexed under this heading.

Pindolol (Co-administration may exhibit additive CNS-depression).
No products indexed under this heading.

Pioglitazone Hydrochloride (Co-administration may exhibit additive CNS-depression). Products include:
ActoPlus Met Tablets ... 3071
Actos Tablets ... 3077
Duetact Tablets ... 3085

Piroxicam (Co-administration may exhibit additive CNS-depression).
No products indexed under this heading.

Polyestradiol Phosphate (Co-administration may exhibit additive CNS-depression).
No products indexed under this heading.

Prazepam (Co-administration may exhibit additive CNS-depression).
No products indexed under this heading.

Primidone (Co-administration may exhibit additive CNS-depression).
No products indexed under this heading.

Procarbazine Hydrochloride (Co-administration may increase the effect of either the MAO inhibitor or hydrocodone).
No products indexed under this heading.

Prochlorperazine (Co-administration may exhibit additive CNS-depression).
No products indexed under this heading.

Progesterone (Co-administration may exhibit additive CNS-depression). Products include:
Crinone 4% Gel ... 992
Crinone 8% Gel ... 992
Prometrium Capsules (100 mg, 200 mg) ... 3047

Proguanil Hydrochloride (Co-administration may exhibit additive CNS-depression). Products include:
Malarone Pediatric Tablets ... 1521
Malarone Tablets ... 1521

Promethazine Hydrochloride (Co-administration may exhibit additive CNS-depression).
No products indexed under this heading.

Propafenone Hydrochloride (Co-administration may exhibit additive CNS-depression). Products include:
Rythmol Tablets ... 1586
Rythmol SR Capsules ... 1590

Propofol (Co-administration may exhibit additive CNS-depression).
No products indexed under this heading.

Propoxyphene Hydrochloride (Co-administration may exhibit additive CNS-depression).
No products indexed under this heading.

Propoxyphene Napsylate (Co-administration may exhibit additive CNS-depression).
No products indexed under this heading.

Propranolol Hydrochloride (Co-administration may exhibit additive CNS-depression). Products include:
InnoPran XL Extended Release Capsules ... 1484

IMPORTANT NOTE: Always consult each drug listing in the patient's regimen for possible interactions.

Ziana Gel 1942

Triazolam (Co-administration may exhibit additive CNS-depression).
No products indexed under this heading.

Trifluoperazine Hydrochloride (Co-administration may exhibit additive CNS-depression).
No products indexed under this heading.

Trimeprazine Tartrate (Co-administration may exhibit additive CNS-depression).
No products indexed under this heading.

Trimethadione (Co-administration may exhibit additive CNS-depression).
No products indexed under this heading.

Trimethaphan Camsylate (Co-administration may exhibit additive CNS-depression).
No products indexed under this heading.

Trimipramine Maleate (Co-administration may increase the effect of either the antidepressant or hydrocodone).
No products indexed under this heading.

Tripelennamine Hydrochloride (Co-administration may exhibit additive CNS-depression).
No products indexed under this heading.

Triprolidine Hydrochloride (Co-administration may exhibit additive CNS-depression).
No products indexed under this heading.

Troglitazone (Co-administration may exhibit additive CNS-depression).
No products indexed under this heading.

Trovafloxacin Mesylate (Co-administration may exhibit additive CNS-depression).
No products indexed under this heading.

Valdecoxib (Co-administration may exhibit additive CNS-depression).
No products indexed under this heading.

Valproate Sodium (Co-administration may exhibit additive CNS-depression).
No products indexed under this heading.

Valproic Acid (Co-administration may exhibit additive CNS-depression).
No products indexed under this heading.

Valsartan (Co-administration may exhibit additive CNS-depression). Products include:
Diovan Tablets 2212
Diovan HCT Tablets 2216
Exforge Tablets 2238

Venlafaxine Hydrochloride (Co-administration may exhibit additive CNS-depression). Products include:
Effexor XR Extended-Release Capsules 3195
Venlafaxine Hydrochloride Tablets ... 2199

Verapamil Hydrochloride (Co-administration may exhibit additive CNS-depression). Products include:
Tarka Tablets 511

Vinblastine Sulfate (Co-administration may exhibit additive CNS-depression).
No products indexed under this heading.

Vincristine Sulfate (Co-administration may exhibit additive CNS-depression).
No products indexed under this heading.

Vitamin A (Co-administration may exhibit additive CNS-depression). Products include:
Norwegian Cod Liver Oil 949

Vitamin A Acetate (Co-administration may exhibit additive CNS-depression).
No products indexed under this heading.

Voriconazole (Co-administration may exhibit additive CNS-depression).
No products indexed under this heading.

Warfarin Sodium (Co-administration may exhibit additive CNS-depression).
No products indexed under this heading.

Zafirlukast (Co-administration may exhibit additive CNS-depression). Products include:
Accolate Tablets 669

Zaleplon (Co-administration may exhibit additive CNS-depression).
No products indexed under this heading.

Zileuton (Co-administration may exhibit additive CNS-depression).
No products indexed under this heading.

Ziprasidone Hydrochloride (Co-administration may exhibit additive CNS-depression). Products include:
Geodon Capsules 2520

Zolmitriptan (Co-administration may exhibit additive CNS-depression). Products include:
Zomig Tablets 694
Zomig Nasal Spray 689
Zomig-ZMT Tablets 694

Zolpidem Tartrate (Co-administration may exhibit additive CNS-depression). Products include:
Ambien Tablets 2692
Ambien CR Tablets 2696

Zonisamide (Co-administration may exhibit additive CNS-depression). Products include:
Zonegran Capsules 1089

Zopiclone (Co-administration may exhibit additive CNS-depression).
No products indexed under this heading.

Food Interactions

Alcohol (Co-administration may exhibit additive CNS-depression; concurrent use should be avoided).

LORTAB 10/500 TABLETS
(Acetaminophen, Hydrocodone Bitartrate)... 3144
See Lortab 7.5/500 Tablets

LOTEMAX OPHTHALMIC SUSPENSION 0.5%
(Loteprednol Etabonate) .... ⊙241
None cited in PDR database.

LOTRISONE CREAM
(Betamethasone Dipropionate, Clotrimazole)....................................... 2881
None cited in PDR database.

LOTRISONE LOTION
(Betamethasone Dipropionate, Clotrimazole)....................................... 2881
None cited in PDR database.

LOVAZA CAPSULES
(Omega-3-acid ethyl esters) 1520
May interact with anticoagulants. Compounds in these categories include:

Anisindione (Possible prolongation of bleeding time with concomitant anticoagulants administration).
No products indexed under this heading.

Ardeparin Sodium (Possible prolongation of bleeding time with concomitant anticoagulants administration).
No products indexed under this heading.

Dalteparin Sodium (Possible prolongation of bleeding time with concomitant anticoagulants administration). Products include:
Fragmin Injection 1070

Danaparoid Sodium (Possible prolongation of bleeding time with concomitant anticoagulants administration).
No products indexed under this heading.

Dicumarol (Possible prolongation of bleeding time with concomitant anticoagulants administration).
No products indexed under this heading.

Enoxaparin Sodium (Possible prolongation of bleeding time with concomitant anticoagulants administration). Products include:
Lovenox Injection 2756

Fondaparinux Sodium (Possible prolongation of bleeding time with concomitant anticoagulants administration). Products include:
Arixtra Injection 1313

Heparin Calcium (Possible prolongation of bleeding time with concomitant anticoagulants administration).
No products indexed under this heading.

Heparin Sodium (Possible prolongation of bleeding time with concomitant anticoagulants administration).
No products indexed under this heading.

Low Molecular Weight Heparins (Possible prolongation of bleeding time with concomitant anticoagulants administration).
No products indexed under this heading.

Tinzaparin Sodium (Possible prolongation of bleeding time with concomitant anticoagulants administration).
No products indexed under this heading.

Warfarin Sodium (Possible prolongation of bleeding time with concomitant anticoagulants administration).
No products indexed under this heading.

LOVENOX INJECTION
(Enoxaparin Sodium) 2756
May interact with anticoagulants, non-steroidal anti-inflammatory agents, salicylates, and certain other agents. Compounds in these categories include:

Anisindione (Agents which may enhance the risk of hemorrhage, such as other anticoagulants, should be discontinued prior to initiation of Lovenox therapy; the risk of developing epidural or spinal hematoma which can result in long-term or permanent paralysis is increased by the concomitant use of drugs affecting hemostasis).
No products indexed under this heading.

Ardeparin Sodium (Agents which may enhance the risk of hemorrhage, such as other anticoagulants, should be discontinued prior to initiation of Lovenox therapy; the risk of developing epidural or spinal hematoma which can result in long-term or permanent paralysis is increased by the concomitant use of drugs affecting hemostasis).
No products indexed under this heading.

Aspirin (Agents which may enhance the risk of hemorrhage, such as platelet inhibitors, should be discontinued prior to initiation of Lovenox therapy; the risk of developing epidural or spinal hematoma which can result in long-term or permanent paralysis is increased by the concomitant use of drugs affecting hemostasis). Products include:
Aggrenox Capsules 819
Bayer Aspirin 750
Percodan Tablets 1130
St. Joseph 81 mg Aspirin Chewable and Enteric Coated Tablets 1903

Aspirin, Enteric Coated (Agents which may enhance the risk of hemorrhage, such as platelet inhibitors, should be discontinued prior to initiation of Lovenox therapy; the risk of developing epidural or spinal hematoma which can result in long-term or permanent paralysis is increased by the concomitant use of drugs affecting hemostasis).
No products indexed under this heading.

Aspirin Buffered (Agents which may enhance the risk of hemorrhage, such as platelet inhibitors, should be discontinued prior to initiation of Lovenox therapy; the risk of developing epidural or spinal hematoma which can result in long-term or permanent paralysis is increased by the concomitant use of drugs affecting hemostasis).
No products indexed under this heading.

Celecoxib (Agents which may enhance the risk of hemorrhage, such as platelet inhibitors, should be discontinued prior to initiation of Lovenox therapy; the risk of developing epidural or spinal hematoma which can result in long-term or permanent paralysis is increased by the concomitant use of drugs affecting hemostasis). Products include:
Celebrex Capsules 2979

Choline Magnesium Trisalicylate (Agents which may enhance the risk of hemorrhage, such as platelet inhibitors, should be discontinued prior to initiation of Lovenox therapy; the risk of developing epidural or spinal hematoma which can result in long-term or permanent paralysis is increased by the concomitant use of drugs affecting hemostasis).
No products indexed under this heading.

Clopidogrel Bisulfate (Agents which may enhance the risk of hemorrhage, such as platelet aggregation inhibitors, should be discontinued prior to initiation of Lovenox therapy; the risk of developing epidural or spinal hematoma which can result in long-term or permanent paralysis is increased by the concomitant use of drugs affecting hemostasis). Products include:
Plavix Tablets 926
Plavix Tablets 2767

Dalteparin Sodium (Agents which may enhance the risk of hemorrhage, such as other anticoagulants, should be discontinued prior to initiation of Lovenox therapy; the risk of developing epidural or spinal hematoma which can result in long-term or permanent paralysis is increased by the concomitant use of drugs affecting hemostasis). Products include:
Fragmin Injection 1070

Danaparoid Sodium (Agents which may enhance the risk of hemorrhage, such as other anticoagulants, should be discontinued prior to initiation of Lovenox therapy; the risk of developing epidural or spinal hematoma which can result in long-term or permanent paralysis is increased by the concomitant use of drugs affecting hemostasis).
No products indexed under this heading.

Diclofenac Epolamine (Agents which may enhance the risk of hemorrhage, such as platelet inhibitors, should be discontinued prior to initiation of Lovenox therapy; the risk of developing epidural or spinal hematoma which can result in long-term or permanent paralysis is increased by the concomitant use of drugs affecting hemostasis). Products include:
Flector Patch 561

Diclofenac Potassium (Agents which may enhance the risk of hemorrhage, such as platelet inhibitors, should be discontinued prior to initiation of Lovenox therapy; the risk of developing epidural or spinal hematoma which can result in long-term or permanent paralysis is increased by the concomitant use of drugs affecting hemostasis).
No products indexed under this heading.

Diclofenac Sodium (Agents which may enhance the risk of hemorrhage, such as platelet inhibitors, should be discontinued prior to initiation of Lovenox therapy; the risk of developing epidural or spinal hematoma which can result in long-term or permanent paralysis is increased by the concomitant use of drugs affecting hemostasis). Products include:
Diclofenac Sodium Ophthalmic Solution .... ⊙ 240
Voltaren Ophthalmic Solution 2336
Voltaren Tablets 2334
Voltaren-XR Tablets 2337

Dicumarol (Agents which may enhance the risk of hemorrhage, such as other anticoagulants, should be discontinued prior to initiation of Lovenox therapy; the risk of developing epidural or spinal hematoma which can result in long-term or permanent paralysis is increased by the concomitant use of drugs affecting hemostasis).
No products indexed under this heading.

Diflunisal (Agents which may enhance the risk of hemorrhage, such as platelet inhibitors, should be discontinued prior to initiation of Lovenox therapy; the risk of developing epidural or spinal hematoma which can result in long-term or permanent paralysis is increased by the concomitant use of drugs affecting hemostasis).
No products indexed under this heading.

Dipyridamole (Agents which may enhance the risk of hemorrhage, such as dipyridamole, should be discontinued prior to initiation of Lovenox therapy). Products include:
Aggrenox Capsules 819
Persantine Tablets 869

Eptifibatide (Agents which may enhance the risk of hemorrhage, such as platelet aggregation inhibitors, should be discontinued prior to initiation of Lovenox therapy; the risk of developing epidural or spinal hematoma which can result in long-term or permanent paralysis is increased by the concomitant use of drugs affecting hemostasis).
Products include:
Integrilin Injection 2855

Etodolac (Agents which may enhance the risk of hemorrhage, such as platelet inhibitors, should be discontinued prior to initiation of Lovenox therapy; the risk of developing epidural or spinal hematoma which can result in long-term or permanent paralysis is increased by the concomitant use of drugs affecting hemostasis).
No products indexed under this heading.

Fenoprofen Calcium (Agents which may enhance the risk of hemorrhage, such as platelet inhibitors, should be discontinued prior to initiation of Lovenox therapy; the risk of developing epidural or spinal hematoma which can result in long-term or permanent paralysis is increased by the concomitant use of drugs affecting hemostasis). Products include:
Nalfon Capsules 2508

Flurbiprofen (Agents which may enhance the risk of hemorrhage, such as platelet inhibitors, should be discontinued prior to initiation of Lovenox therapy; the risk of developing epidural or spinal hematoma which can result in long-term or permanent paralysis is increased by the concomitant use of drugs affecting hemostasis).
No products indexed under this heading.

Fondaparinux Sodium (Agents which may enhance the risk of hemorrhage, such as other anticoagulants, should be discontinued prior to initiation of Lovenox therapy; the risk of developing epidural or spinal hematoma which can result in long-term or permanent paralysis is increased by the concomitant use of drugs affecting hemostasis).
Products include:
Arixtra Injection 1313

Heparin Calcium (Agents which may enhance the risk of hemorrhage, such as other anticoagulants, should be discontinued prior to initiation of Lovenox therapy; the risk of developing epidural or spinal hematoma which can result in long-term or permanent paralysis is increased by the concomitant use of drugs affecting hemostasis).
No products indexed under this heading.

Heparin Sodium (Agents which may enhance the risk of hemorrhage, such as other anticoagulants, should be discontinued prior to initiation of Lovenox therapy; the risk of developing epidural or spinal hematoma which can result in long-term or permanent paralysis is increased by the concomitant use of drugs affecting hemostasis).
No products indexed under this heading.

Ibuprofen (Agents which may enhance the risk of hemorrhage, such as platelet inhibitors, should be discontinued prior to initiation of Lovenox therapy; the risk of developing epidural or spinal hematoma which can result in long-term or permanent paralysis is increased by the concomitant use of drugs affecting hemostasis). Products include:
Motrin IB Tablets and Caplets 1900
Children's Motrin Oral Suspension ... 1901
Children's Motrin Non-Staining Dye-Free Oral Suspension........ 1901
Children's Motrin Cold Oral Suspension 1899
Infants' Motrin Concentrated Drops........ 1901
Infants' Motrin Non-Staining Dye-Free Concentrated Drops........ 1901
Junior Strength Motrin Caplets and Chewable Tablets........ 1901
Vicoprofen Tablets 533

Indomethacin (Agents which may enhance the risk of hemorrhage, such as platelet inhibitors, should be discontinued prior to initiation of Lovenox therapy; the risk of developing epidural or spinal hematoma which can result in long-term or permanent paralysis is increased by the concomitant use of drugs affecting hemostasis). Products include:
Indocin 2024

Indomethacin Sodium Trihydrate (Agents which may enhance the risk of hemorrhage, such as platelet inhibitors, should be discontinued prior to initiation of Lovenox therapy; the risk of developing epidural or spinal hematoma which can result in long-term or permanent paralysis is increased by the concomitant use of drugs affecting hemostasis). Products include:
Indocin I.V. 2489

Ketoprofen (Agents which may enhance the risk of hemorrhage, such as platelet inhibitors, should be discontinued prior to initiation of Lovenox therapy; the risk of developing epidural or spinal hematoma which can result in long-term or permanent paralysis is increased by the concomitant use of drugs affecting hemostasis).
No products indexed under this heading.

Ketorolac Tromethamine (Agents which may enhance the risk of hemorrhage, such as platelet inhibitors, should be discontinued prior to initiation of Lovenox therapy; the risk of developing epidural or spinal hematoma which can result in long-term or permanent paralysis is increased by the concomitant use of drugs affecting hemostasis).
No products indexed under this heading.

Low Molecular Weight Heparins (Agents which may enhance the risk of hemorrhage, such as other anticoagulants, should be discontinued prior to initiation of Lovenox therapy; the risk of developing epidural or spinal hematoma which can result in long-term or permanent paralysis is increased by the concomitant use of drugs affecting hemostasis).
No products indexed under this heading.

Magnesium Salicylate (Agents which may enhance the risk of hemorrhage, such as platelet inhibitors, should be discontinued prior to initiation of Lovenox therapy; the risk of developing epidural or spinal hematoma which can result in long-term or permanent paralysis is increased by the concomitant use of drugs affecting hemostasis).
No products indexed under this heading.

Meclofenamate Sodium (Agents which may enhance the risk of hemorrhage, such as platelet inhibitors, should be discontinued prior to initiation of Lovenox therapy; the risk of developing epidural or spinal hematoma which can result in long-term or permanent paralysis is increased by the concomitant use of drugs affecting hemostasis).
No products indexed under this heading.

Mefenamic Acid (Agents which may enhance the risk of hemorrhage, such as platelet inhibitors, should be discontinued prior to initiation of Lovenox therapy; the risk of developing epidural or spinal hematoma which can result in long-term or permanent paralysis is increased by the concomitant use of drugs affecting hemostasis).
No products indexed under this heading.

Meloxicam (Agents which may enhance the risk of hemorrhage, such as platelet inhibitors, should be discontinued prior to initiation of Lovenox therapy; the risk of developing epidural or spinal hematoma which can result in long-term or permanent paralysis is increased by the concomitant use of drugs affecting hemostasis). Products include:
Mobic Oral Suspension 863
Mobic Tablets 863

Nabumetone (Agents which may enhance the risk of hemorrhage, such as platelet inhibitors, should be discontinued prior to initiation of Lovenox therapy; the risk of developing epidural or spinal hematoma which can result in long-term or permanent paralysis is increased by the concomitant use of drugs affecting hemostasis).
No products indexed under this heading.

Naproxen (Agents which may enhance the risk of hemorrhage, such as platelet inhibitors, should be

discontinued prior to initiation of Lovenox therapy; the risk of developing epidural or spinal hematoma which can result in long-term or permanent paralysis is increased by the concomitant use of drugs affecting hemostasis). Products include:
EC-Naprosyn Delayed-Release Tablets 2632
Naprosyn Suspension 2632
Naprosyn Tablets 2632

Naproxen Sodium (Agents which may enhance the risk of hemorrhage, such as platelet inhibitors, should be discontinued prior to initiation of Lovenox therapy; the risk of developing epidural or spinal hematoma which can result in long-term or permanent paralysis is increased by the concomitant use of drugs affecting hemostasis). Products include:
Anaprox Tablets 2632
Anaprox DS Tablets 2632
Treximet Tablets 1616

Oxaprozin (Agents which may enhance the risk of hemorrhage, such as platelet inhibitors, should be discontinued prior to initiation of Lovenox therapy; the risk of developing epidural or spinal hematoma which can result in long-term or permanent paralysis is increased by the concomitant use of drugs affecting hemostasis).
No products indexed under this heading.

Phenylbutazone (Agents which may enhance the risk of hemorrhage, such as platelet inhibitors, should be discontinued prior to initiation of Lovenox therapy; the risk of developing epidural or spinal hematoma which can result in long-term or permanent paralysis is increased by the concomitant use of drugs affecting hemostasis).
No products indexed under this heading.

Piroxicam (Agents which may enhance the risk of hemorrhage, such as platelet inhibitors, should be discontinued prior to initiation of Lovenox therapy; the risk of developing epidural or spinal hematoma which can result in long-term or permanent paralysis is increased by the concomitant use of drugs affecting hemostasis).
No products indexed under this heading.

Rofecoxib (Agents which may enhance the risk of hemorrhage, such as platelet inhibitors, should be discontinued prior to initiation of Lovenox therapy; the risk of developing epidural or spinal hematoma which can result in long-term or permanent paralysis is increased by the concomitant use of drugs affecting hemostasis).
No products indexed under this heading.

Salsalate (Agents which may enhance the risk of hemorrhage, such as platelet inhibitors, should be discontinued prior to initiation of Lovenox therapy; the risk of developing epidural or spinal hematoma which can result in long-term or permanent paralysis is increased by the concomitant use of drugs affecting hemostasis).
No products indexed under this heading.

Sulfinpyrazone (Agents which may enhance the risk of hemorrhage, such as sulfinpyrazone, should be discontinued prior to initiation of Lovenox therapy).
No products indexed under this heading.

Sulindac (Agents which may enhance the risk of hemorrhage, such as platelet inhibitors, should be discontinued prior to initiation of Lovenox therapy; the risk of developing epidural or spinal hematoma which can result in long-term or permanent paralysis is increased by the concomitant use of drugs affecting hemostasis). Products include:
Clinoril Tablets 1962

Tinzaparin Sodium (Agents which may enhance the risk of hemorrhage, such as other anticoagulants, should be discontinued prior to initiation of Lovenox therapy; the risk of developing epidural or spinal hematoma which can result in long-term or permanent paralysis is increased by the concomitant use of drugs affecting hemostasis).
No products indexed under this heading.

Tirofiban Hydrochloride (Agents which may enhance the risk of hemorrhage, such as platelet aggregation inhibitors, should be discontinued prior to initiation of Lovenox therapy; the risk of developing epidural or spinal hematoma which can result in long-term or permanent paralysis is increased by the concomitant use of drugs affecting hemostasis).
No products indexed under this heading.

Tolmetin Sodium (Agents which may enhance the risk of hemorrhage, such as platelet inhibitors, should be discontinued prior to initiation of Lovenox therapy; the risk of developing epidural or spinal hematoma which can result in long-term or permanent paralysis is increased by the concomitant use of drugs affecting hemostasis).
No products indexed under this heading.

Valdecoxib (Agents which may enhance the risk of hemorrhage, such as platelet inhibitors, should be discontinued prior to initiation of Lovenox therapy; the risk of developing epidural or spinal hematoma which can result in long-term or permanent paralysis is increased by the concomitant use of drugs affecting hemostasis).
No products indexed under this heading.

Warfarin Sodium (Agents which may enhance the risk of hemorrhage, such as other anticoagulants, should be discontinued prior to initiation of Lovenox therapy; the risk of developing epidural or spinal hematoma which can result in long-term or permanent paralysis is increased by the concomitant use of drugs affecting hemostasis).
No products indexed under this heading.

LOVPIL CAPSULES
(Amino Acid Preparations, Herbals with Vitamins & Minerals, Soy-containing dietary supplements) 638
None cited in PDR database.

LUCENTIS INJECTION
(Ranibizumab) 1205
May interact with:

Verteporfin (11% of patients developed serious intraocular inflammation when ranibizumab was used concomitantly with verteporfin). Products include:
Visudyne for Injection 2332

LUMIGAN OPHTHALMIC SOLUTION
(Bimatoprost) 556
None cited in PDR database.

LUNESTA TABLETS
(Eszopiclone) 2994
May interact with cytochrome p450 3a4 inhibitors, potent and certain other agents. Compounds in these categories include:

Amprenavir (CYP3A4 is a major metabolic pathway for elimination of eszopiclone. The AUC of eszopiclone was increased 2.2-fold by co-administration of ketoconazole, a potent inhibitor of CYP3A4, 400 mg daily for 5 days. Cmax and T1/2 were increased 1.4-fold and 1.3-fold, respectively. Other strong inhibitors of CYP3A4 (e.g., itraconazole, clarithromycin, nefazodone, troleandomycin, ritonavir, nelfinavir) would be expected to behave similarly).
No products indexed under this heading.

Atazanavir (CYP3A4 is a major metabolic pathway for elimination of eszopiclone. The AUC of eszopiclone was increased 2.2-fold by co-administration of ketoconazole, a potent inhibitor of CYP3A4, 400 mg daily for 5 days. Cmax and T1/2 were increased 1.4-fold and 1.3-fold, respectively. Other strong inhibitors of CYP3A4 (e.g., itraconazole, clarithromycin, nefazodone, troleandomycin, ritonavir, nelfinavir) would be expected to behave similarly).
No products indexed under this heading.

Atazanavir Sulfate (CYP3A4 is a major metabolic pathway for elimination of eszopiclone. The AUC of eszopiclone was increased 2.2-fold by co-administration of ketoconazole, a potent inhibitor of CYP3A4, 400 mg daily for 5 days. Cmax and T1/2 were increased 1.4-fold and 1.3-fold, respectively. Other strong inhibitors of CYP3A4 (e.g., itraconazole, clarithromycin, nefazodone, troleandomycin, ritonavir, nelfinavir) would be expected to behave similarly). Products include:
Reyataz Capsules 3299

Clarithromycin (CYP3A4 is a major metabolic pathway for elimination of eszopiclone. The AUC of eszopiclone was increased 2.2-fold by co-administration of ketoconazole, a potent inhibitor of CYP3A4, 400 mg daily for 5 days. Cmax and T1/2 were increased 1.4-fold and 1.3-fold, respectively. Other strong inhibitors of CYP3A4 (e.g., itraconazole, clarithromycin, nefazodone, troleandomycin, ritonavir, nelfinavir) would be expected to behave similarly).
Products include:
Biaxin/Biaxin XL 411

Delavirdine Mesylate (CYP3A4 is a major metabolic pathway for elimination of eszopiclone. The AUC of eszopiclone was increased 2.2-fold by co-administration of ketoconazole, a potent inhibitor of CYP3A4, 400 mg daily for 5 days. Cmax and T1/2 were increased 1.4-fold and 1.3-fold, respectively. Other strong inhibitors of CYP3A4 (e.g., itraconazole, clarithromycin, nefazodone, troleandomycin, ritonavir, nelfinavir) would be expected to behave similarly).
No products indexed under this heading.

Delavirine (CYP3A4 is a major metabolic pathway for elimination of eszopiclone. The AUC of eszopiclone was increased 2.2-fold by co-administration of ketoconazole, a potent inhibitor of CYP3A4, 400 mg daily for 5 days. Cmax and T1/2 were increased 1.4-fold and 1.3-fold, respectively. Other strong inhibitors of CYP3A4 (e.g., itraconazole, clarithromycin, nefazodone, troleandomycin, ritonavir, nelfinavir) would be expected to behave similarly).
No products indexed under this heading.

Ethanol (An additive effect on psychomotor performance was seen with co-administration of eszopiclone and ethanol 0.70 g/kg for up to 4 hours after ethanol administration).
No products indexed under this heading.

Fosamprenavir Calcium (CYP3A4 is a major metabolic pathway for elimination of eszopiclone. The AUC of eszopiclone was increased 2.2-fold by co-administration of ketoconazole, a potent inhibitor of CYP3A4, 400 mg daily for 5 days. Cmax and T1/2 were increased 1.4-fold and 1.3-fold, respectively. Other strong inhibitors of CYP3A4 (e.g., itraconazole, clarithromycin, nefazodone, troleandomycin, ritonavir, nelfinavir) would be expected to behave similarly).
Products include:
Lexiva Oral Suspension 1510
Lexiva Tablets 1510

Indinavir Sulfate (CYP3A4 is a major metabolic pathway for elimination of eszopiclone. The AUC of eszopiclone was increased 2.2-fold by co-administration of ketoconazole, a potent inhibitor of CYP3A4, 400 mg daily for 5 days. Cmax and T1/2 were increased 1.4-fold and 1.3-fold, respectively. Other strong inhibitors of CYP3A4 (e.g., itraconazole, clarithromycin, nefazodone, troleandomycin, ritonavir, nelfinavir) would be expected to behave similarly). Products include:
Crixivan Capsules 1979

Itraconazole (CYP3A4 is a major metabolic pathway for elimination of eszopiclone. The AUC of eszopiclone was increased 2.2-fold by co-administration of ketoconazole, a potent inhibitor of CYP3A4, 400 mg daily for 5 days. Cmax and T1/2 were increased 1.4-fold and 1.3-fold, respectively. Other strong inhibitors of CYP3A4 (e.g., itraconazole, clarithromycin, nefazodone, troleandomycin, ritonavir, nelfinavir) would be expected to behave similarly).
No products indexed under this heading.

Ketoconazole (CYP3A4 is a major metabolic pathway for elimination of eszopiclone. The AUC of eszopiclone was increased 2.2-fold by co-administration of ketoconazole, a potent inhibitor of CYP3A4, 400 mg daily for 5 days. Cmax and T1/2 were increased 1.4-fold and 1.3-fold,

respectively. Other strong inhibitors of CYP3A4 (e.g., itraconazole, clarithromycin, nefazodone, troleandomycin, ritonavir, nelfinavir) would be expected to behave similarly). Products include:

Extina Foam, 2% 3057
Nizoral A-D Shampoo 1901

Lopinavir (CYP3A4 is a major metabolic pathway for elimination of eszopiclone. The AUC of eszopiclone was increased 2.2-fold by co-administration of ketoconazole, a potent inhibitor of CYP3A4, 400 mg daily for 5 days. Cmax and T1/2 were increased 1.4-fold and 1.3-fold, respectively. Other strong inhibitors of CYP3A4 (e.g., itraconazole, clarithromycin, nefazodone, troleandomycin, ritonavir, nelfinavir) would be expected to behave similarly). Products include:

Kaletra 452

Lorazepam (Co-administration of Eszopiclone and lorazepam decreased the Cmax of both drugs by 22%).

No products indexed under this heading.

Nefazodone Hydrochloride (CYP3A4 is a major metabolic pathway for elimination of eszopiclone. The AUC of eszopiclone was increased 2.2-fold by co-administration of ketoconazole, a potent inhibitor of CYP3A4, 400 mg daily for 5 days. Cmax and T1/2 were increased 1.4-fold and 1.3-fold, respectively. Other strong inhibitors of CYP3A4 (e.g., itraconazole, clarithromycin, nefazodone, troleandomycin, ritonavir, nelfinavir) would be expected to behave similarly).

No products indexed under this heading.

Nelfinavir Mesylate (CYP3A4 is a major metabolic pathway for elimination of eszopiclone. The AUC of eszopiclone was increased 2.2-fold by co-administration of ketoconazole, a potent inhibitor of CYP3A4, 400 mg daily for 5 days. Cmax and T1/2 were increased 1.4-fold and 1.3-fold, respectively. Other strong inhibitors of CYP3A4 (e.g., itraconazole, clarithromycin, nefazodone, troleandomycin, ritonavir, nelfinavir) would be expected to behave similarly).

No products indexed under this heading.

Olanzapine (Co-administration of eszopiclone 3 mg and olanzapine 10 mg produced a decrease in DSST scores. The interaction was pharmacodynamic; there was no alteration in the pharmacokinetics of either drug). Products include:

Symbyax Capsules 1871
Zyprexa Tablets 1883
Zyprexa IntraMuscular 1883
Zyprexa ZYDIS Orally Disintegrating Tablets 1883

Rifampicin (Racemic zopiclone exposure was decreased 80% by concomitant use of rifampicin, a potent inducer of CYP3A4. A similar effect would be expected with eszopiclone).

No products indexed under this heading.

Ritonavir (CYP3A4 is a major metabolic pathway for elimination of eszopiclone. The AUC of eszopiclone was increased 2.2-fold by co-administration of ketoconazole, a potent inhibitor of CYP3A4, 400 mg daily for 5 days. Cmax and T1/2 were increased 1.4-fold and 1.3-fold, respectively. Other strong inhibitors of CYP3A4 (e.g., itraconazole, clarithromycin, nefazodone, troleandomycin, ritonavir, nelfinavir) would be expected to behave similarly). Products include:

Kaletra 452
Norvir 489

Saquinavir (CYP3A4 is a major metabolic pathway for elimination of eszopiclone. The AUC of eszopiclone was increased 2.2-fold by co-administration of ketoconazole, a potent inhibitor of CYP3A4, 400 mg daily for 5 days. Cmax and T1/2 were increased 1.4-fold and 1.3-fold, respectively. Other strong inhibitors of CYP3A4 (e.g., itraconazole, clarithromycin, nefazodone, troleandomycin, ritonavir, nelfinavir) would be expected to behave similarly).

No products indexed under this heading.

Saquinavir Mesylate (CYP3A4 is a major metabolic pathway for elimination of eszopiclone. The AUC of eszopiclone was increased 2.2-fold by co-administration of ketoconazole, a potent inhibitor of CYP3A4, 400 mg daily for 5 days. Cmax and T1/2 were increased 1.4-fold and 1.3-fold, respectively. Other strong inhibitors of CYP3A4 (e.g., itraconazole, clarithromycin, nefazodone, troleandomycin, ritonavir, nelfinavir) would be expected to behave similarly).

No products indexed under this heading.

Telithromycin (CYP3A4 is a major metabolic pathway for elimination of eszopiclone. The AUC of eszopiclone was increased 2.2-fold by co-administration of ketoconazole, a potent inhibitor of CYP3A4, 400 mg daily for 5 days. Cmax and T1/2 were increased 1.4-fold and 1.3-fold, respectively. Other strong inhibitors of CYP3A4 (e.g., itraconazole, clarithromycin, nefazodone, troleandomycin, ritonavir, nelfinavir) would be expected to behave similarly). Products include:

Ketek Tablets 2744

Troleandomycin (CYP3A4 is a major metabolic pathway for elimination of eszopiclone. The AUC of eszopiclone was increased 2.2-fold by co-administration of ketoconazole, a potent inhibitor of CYP3A4, 400 mg daily for 5 days. Cmax and T1/2 were increased 1.4-fold and 1.3-fold, respectively. Other strong inhibitors of CYP3A4 (e.g., itraconazole, clarithromycin, nefazodone, troleandomycin, ritonavir, nelfinavir) would be expected to behave similarly).

No products indexed under this heading.

Voriconazole (CYP3A4 is a major metabolic pathway for elimination of eszopiclone. The AUC of eszopiclone was increased 2.2-fold by co-administration of ketoconazole, a potent inhibitor of CYP3A4, 400 mg daily for 5 days. Cmax and T1/2 were increased 1.4-fold and 1.3-fold, respectively. Other strong inhibitors of CYP3A4 (e.g., itraconazole, clarithromycin, nefazodone, troleandomycin, ritonavir, nelfinavir) would be expected to behave similarly).

No products indexed under this heading.

Food Interactions

Alcohol (An additive effect on psychomotor performance was seen with co-administration of eszopiclone and alcohol 0.70 g/kg for up to 4 hours after alcohol consumption).

LUPRON DEPOT 3.75 MG

(Leuprolide Acetate) 462
None cited in PDR database.

LUPRON DEPOT 7.5 MG

(Leuprolide Acetate) 469
None cited in PDR database.

LUPRON DEPOT--3 MONTH 11.25 MG

(Leuprolide Acetate) 462
None cited in PDR database.

LUPRON DEPOT-PED 7.5 MG, 11.25 MG AND 15 MG

(Leuprolide Acetate) 471
None cited in PDR database.

LUVOX CR EXTENDED-RELEASE CAPSULES

(Fluvoxamine Maleate) 1759

May interact with aspirin-acetylsalicylic acid, benzodiazepines, oral anticoagulants, cytochrome p450 1a2 substrates (selected), cytochrome p450 3a4 inhibitors (selected), lithium preparations, monoamine oxidase inhibitors, non-steroidal anti-inflammatory agents, serotoninergic agents, theophyllines, tricyclic antidepressants, triptans, and certain other agents. Compounds in these categories include:

Acetaminophen (Fluvoxamine is a known potent inhibitor of CYP1A2 and also inhibits CYP3A4, CYP2C9, and CYP2C19). Products include:

Benadryl Allergy & Cold Kapgels 1895
Benadryl Allergy & Sinus Headache Kapgels 1895
Benadryl Severe Allergy & Sinus Headache Caplets 1897
Lortab 5/500 Tablets 3143
Lortab 7.5/500 Tablets 3144
Lortab 10/500 Tablets 3144
Percocet Tablets 1127
Sinutab Sinus Caplets 1905
Sudafed PE Cold & Cough Caplets 1907
Sudafed PE Nighttime Cold Caplets 1907
Sudafed PE Severe Cold Caplets 1908
Sudafed PE Sinus Headache Caplets 1908
Regular Strength Tylenol Tablets 1915
Tylenol 8 Hour Extended Release Caplets 1915
Extra Strength Tylenol Caplets, Cool Caplets, and EZ Tabs 1915
Extra Strength Tylenol Adult Rapid Blast Liquid 1915
Extra Strength Tylenol PM Caplets, Geltabs, Liquid, and Rapid Release Gels 1915
Extra Strength Tylenol Rapid Release Gels 1915
Tylenol with Codeine Tablets 2427
Tylenol Allergy Multi-Symptom Caplets with Cool Burst and Rapid Release Gelcaps 1916
Tylenol Allergy Multi-Symptom Nighttime Caplets with Cool Burst 1916
Tylenol Severe Allergy Caplets 1916
Tylenol Arthritis Pain Extended Release Geltabs/Caplets 1915
Tylenol Chest Congestion Caplets with Cool Burst 1910
Tylenol Chest Congestion Liquid with Cool Burst 1910
Children's Tylenol Plus Cold Suspension Liquid 1912
Children's Tylenol Plus Cold & Allergy Suspension Liquid 1914
Children's Tylenol Plus Cough & Runny Nose Suspension Liquid 1912
Children's Tylenol Plus Cough & Sore Throat Suspension Liquid 1912
Children's Tylenol Plus Flu Suspension Liquid 1914
Children's Tylenol Suspension Liquid 1909
Children's Tylenol Meltaways 1909
Children's Tylenol Plus Multi-Symptom Cold Suspension Liquid 1912
Tylenol Cold Severe Congestion Daytime Caplets with Cool Burst 1912
Tylenol Cold Head Congestion Daytime Caplets with Cool Burst 1910
Tylenol Cold Head Congestion Nighttime Caplets with Cool Burst 1910
Tylenol Cold Head Congestion Severe Daytime Caplets with Cool Burst 1910
Tylenol Cold Multi-Symptom Daytime Caplets with Cool Burst and Rapid Release Gels 1913
Tylenol Cold Multi-Symptom Daytime Liquid with Citrus Burst 1913
Tylenol Cold Multi-Symptom Nighttime Caplets with Cool Burst 1913
Tylenol Cold Multi-Symptom Nighttime Liquid with Cool Burst 1913
Tylenol Cold Multi-Symptom Severe Caplets with Cool Burst 1913
Tylenol Cold Multi-Symptom Severe Daytime Liquid with Citrus Burst 1913
Tylenol Cough & Sore Throat Daytime Liquid with Cool Burst 1918
Tylenol Cough & Sore Throat Nighttime Liquid with Cool Burst 1918
Concentrated Tylenol Infants' Drops 1909
Jr. Tylenol Meltaways 1909
Tylenol Sinus Congestion & Pain Daytime Caplets with Cool Burst and Gelcaps 1917
Tylenol Sinus Congestion & Pain Nighttime Caplets with Cool Burst 1917
Tylenol Sinus Congestion & Pain Severe Caplets with Cool Burst 1917
Tylenol Sinus Severe Congestion Caplets with Cool Burst 1917
Tylenol Sore Throat Daytime Liquid with Cool Burst 1918
Tylenol Sore Throat Nighttime Liquid with Cool Burst 1918
Women's Tylenol Menstrual Relief Caplets 1919
Vicks DayQuil Cold & Flu Multi-Symptom Relief .... ■616
Vicks DayQuil LiquiCaps 2567
Vicks DayQuil Liquid 2567
Vicks DayQuil Multi-Symptom Cold/Flu Relief 2567
Vicks NyQuil Cold & Flu Multi-Symptom Relief .... ■617
Vicks NyQuil LiquiCaps 2567
Vicks NyQuil Liquid 2567
Vicks NyQuil Multi-Symptom Cold/Flu Relief 2567
Vicodin Tablets 529
Vicodin ES Tablets 530
Vicodin HP Tablets 531
Zydone Tablets 1132

Acetazolamide (Fluvoxamine is a known potent inhibitor of CYP1A2 and also inhibits CYP3A4, CYP2C9, and CYP2C19).

No products indexed under this heading.

Alatrofloxacin Mesylate (Fluvoxamine is a known potent inhibitor of CYP1A2 and also inhibits CYP3A4, CYP2C9, and CYP2C19).

No products indexed under this heading.

Almotriptan Malate (The development of a potentially life-threatening serotonin syndrome may occur with Luvox CR capsules treatment, particularly with concomitant use of serotonergic drugs (including triptans) and with drugs that impair metabolism of serotonin (including MAOIs). Serotonin syndrome symptoms may include mental status changes (eg, agitation, hallucinations, coma), autonomic instability (eg, tachycardia, labile BP, hyperthermia), neuromuscular aberrations (eg, hyperreflexia, incoordination) and/or GI symptoms (eg, nausea, vomiting, diarrhea)). Products include:

Axert Tablets 2431

Alosetron Hydrochloride (Fluvoxamine, an inhibitor of several CYP isozymes, has been shown to increase alosetrone plasma concentrations (AUC) approximately 6-fold and prolonged the half-life by approximately 3-fold. Co-administration of alosterone with Luvox CR capsules is contraindicated).

No products indexed under this heading.

Alprazolam (When immediate-release fluvoxamine maleate tablets (100 mg given once daily) and alprazolam (1 mg given q.i.d.) were co-administered to steady state, plasma concentrations and other pharmacokinetic parameters (AUC, Cmax, T1/2) of alprazolam were approximately twice those observed when alprazolam concentrations resulted in decreased psychomotor performance and memory. If alprazolam is co-administered with Luvox CR capsules, the initial alprazolam dosage should be at least halved and titration to the lowest effective dose is recommended. No dosage adjustment is required for Luvox CR capsules).

No products indexed under this heading.

Amiodarone Hydrochloride (Fluvoxamine is a known potent inhibitor of CYP1A2 and also inhibits CYP3A4, CYP2C9, and CYP2C19).

No products indexed under this heading.

Amitriptyline Hydrochloride (Significantly increased plasma TCA levels have been reported with the co-administration of immediate-release fluvoxamine maleate tablets and amitriptyline, clomipramine, or imipramine. Caution is indicated with the co-administration of Luvox CR capsules and TCAs; plasma TCA concentrations may need to be monitored, and the dose of TCA may be reduced).

No products indexed under this heading.

Amoxapine (Significantly increased plasma TCA levels have been reported with the co-administration of immediate-release fluvoxamine maleate tablets and amitriptyline, clomipramine, or imipramine. Caution is indicated with the co-administration of Luvox CR capsules and TCAs; plasma TCA concentrations may need to be monitored, and the dose of TCA may be reduced).

No products indexed under this heading.

Amprenavir (Fluvoxamine is a known potent inhibitor of CYP1A2 and also inhibits CYP3A4, CYP2C9, and CYP2C19).

No products indexed under this heading.

Anagrelide Hydrochloride (Fluvoxamine is a known potent inhibitor of CYP1A2 and also inhibits CYP3A4, CYP2C9, and CYP2C19). Products include:

Agrylin Capsules 3017

Anastrozole (Fluvoxamine is a known potent inhibitor of CYP1A2 and also inhibits CYP3A4, CYP2C9, and CYP2C19). Products include:

Arimidex Tablets 672

Anisindione (When immediate-release fluvoxamine maleate tablets (50 mg given t.i.d.) were administered concomitantly with warfarin for two weeks, warfarin plasma concentrations increased by 98% and prothrombin times were prolonged. Thus patients receiving oral anticoagulants and Luvox CR capsules should have their prothrombin time monitored and their anticoagulant dose adjusted accordingly. No dosage adjustment is required for Luvox CR capsules).

No products indexed under this heading.

Aprepitant (Fluvoxamine is a known potent inhibitor of CYP1A2 and also inhibits CYP3A4, CYP2C9, and CYP2C19). Products include:

Emend Capsules 1992

Aspirin (Serotonin release by platelets plays an important role in hemostasis. Epidemiological studies of the case-control and cohort design that have demonstrated an association between use of psychotropic drugs that interfere with serotonin reuptake and the occurrence of upper GI bleeding. These studies have also shown that concurrent use of an NSAID or aspirin may potentiate this risk of bleeding). Products include:

Aggrenox Capsules 819
Bayer Aspirin 750
Percodan Tablets 1130
St. Joseph 81 mg Aspirin Chewable and Enteric Coated Tablets 1903

Aspirin, Enteric Coated (Serotonin release by platelets plays an important role in hemostasis. Epidemiological studies of the case-control and cohort design that have demonstrated an association between use of psychotropic drugs that interfere with serotonin reuptake and the occurrence of upper GI bleeding. These studies have also shown that concurrent use of an NSAID or aspirin may potentiate this risk of bleeding).

No products indexed under this heading.

Aspirin Buffered (Serotonin release by platelets plays an important role in hemostasis. Epidemiological studies of the case-control and cohort design that have demonstrated an association between use of psychotropic drugs that interfere with serotonin reuptake and the occurrence of upper GI bleeding. These studies have also shown that concurrent use of an NSAID or aspirin may potentiate this risk of bleeding).

No products indexed under this heading.

Atazanavir (Fluvoxamine is a known potent inhibitor of CYP1A2 and also inhibits CYP3A4, CYP2C9, and CYP2C19).

No products indexed under this heading.

Atazanavir Sulfate (Fluvoxamine is a known potent inhibitor of CYP1A2 and also inhibits CYP3A4, CYP2C9, and CYP2C19). Products include:

Reyataz Capsules 3299

Caffeine (Fluvoxamine is a known potent inhibitor of CYP1A2 and also inhibits CYP3A4, CYP2C9, and CYP2C19). Products include:

BioLean Free Tablets 635
BioLean II Tablets 635
Winrgy Dietary Supplement 642

Caffeine Anhydrous (Fluvoxamine is a known potent inhibitor of CYP1A2 and also inhibits CYP3A4, CYP2C9, and CYP2C19).

No products indexed under this heading.

Carbamazepine (Elevated carbamazepine levels and symptoms of toxicity have been reported with the co-administration of immediate-release fluvoxamine maleate tablets and carbamazepine). Products include:

Carbatrol Capsules 3019
Equetro Extended-Release Capsules 3174

Celecoxib (Serotonin release by platelets plays an important role in hemostasis. Epidemiological studies of the case-control and cohort design that have demonstrated an association between use of psychotropic drugs that interfere with serotonin reuptake and the occurrence of upper GI bleeding. These studies have also shown that concurrent use of an NSAID or aspirin may potentiate this risk of bleeding). Products include:

Celebrex Capsules 2979

Chlordiazepoxide (Benzodiazepines metabolized by hepatic oxidation (eg, alprazolam, midazolam, triazolam) should be used with caution because the clearance of these drugs is likely to be reduced by fluvoxamine. The clearance of benzodiazepines metabolized by glucuronidation (eg, lorazepam, oxazepam, temazepam) is unlikely to be affected by fluvoxamine).

No products indexed under this heading.

Chlordiazepoxide Hydrochloride (Benzodiazepines metabolized by hepatic oxidation (eg, alprazolam, midazolam, triazolam) should be used with caution because the clearance of these drugs is likely to be reduced by fluvoxamine. The clearance of benzodiazepines metabolized by glucuronidation (eg, lorazepam, oxazepam, temazepam) is unlikely to be affected by fluvoxamine).

No products indexed under this heading.

Cimetidine (Fluvoxamine is a known potent inhibitor of CYP1A2 and also inhibits CYP3A4, CYP2C9, and CYP2C19).

No products indexed under this heading.

Cimetidine Hydrochloride (Fluvoxamine is a known potent inhibitor of CYP1A2 and also inhibits CYP3A4, CYP2C9, and CYP2C19).

No products indexed under this heading.

Ciprofloxacin (Fluvoxamine is a known potent inhibitor of CYP1A2 and also inhibits CYP3A4, CYP2C9, and CYP2C19). Products include:

Cipro I.V. 2817
Cipro Oral Suspension 2810
Cipro XR Tablets 2823
Ciprodex Otic Suspension 541

Ciprofloxacin Hydrochloride (Fluvoxamine is a known potent inhibitor of CYP1A2 and also inhibits CYP3A4, CYP2C9, and CYP2C19). Products include:

Cipro Tablets 2810

Citalopram Hydrobromide (The development of a potentially life-threatening serotonin syndrome may occur with Luvox CR capsules treatment, particularly with concomitant use of serotonergic drugs (including triptans) and with drugs that impair metabolism of serotonin (including MAOIs). Serotonin syndrome symptoms may include mental status changes (eg, agitation, hallucinations, coma), autonomic instability (eg, tachycardia, labile BP, hyperthermia), neuromuscular aberrations (eg, hyperreflexia, incoordination) and/or GI symptoms (eg, nausea, vomiting, diarrhea)). Products include:

Celexa 1160

Clarithromycin (Fluvoxamine is a known potent inhibitor of CYP1A2 and also inhibits CYP3A4, CYP2C9, and CYP2C19). Products include:

Biaxin/Biaxin XL 411

Clomipramine Hydrochloride (Significantly increased plasma TCA levels have been reported with the co-administration of immediate-release fluvoxamine maleate tablets and amitriptyline, clomipramine, or imipramine. Caution is indicated with the co-administration of Luvox CR capsules and TCAs; plasma TCA concentrations may need to be monitored, and the dose of TCA may be reduced).

No products indexed under this heading.

Clopidogrel Bisulfate (Fluvoxamine is a known potent inhibitor of CYP1A2 and also inhibits CYP3A4, CYP2C9, and CYP2C19). Products include:

Plavix Tablets 926
Plavix Tablets 2767

Clorazepate Dipotassium (Benzodiazepines metabolized by hepatic oxidation (eg, alprazolam, midazolam, triazolam) should be used with caution because the clearance of these drugs is likely to be reduced by fluvoxamine. The clearance of benzodiazepines metabolized by glucuronidation (eg, lorazepam, oxazepam, temazepam) is unlikely to be affected by fluvoxamine).

No products indexed under this heading.

Clotrimazole (Fluvoxamine is a known potent inhibitor of CYP1A2 and also inhibits CYP3A4, CYP2C9, and CYP2C19). Products include:

Lotrisone 2881

Clozapine (Elevated serum levels of clozapine have been reported in patients taking immediate-release fluvoxamine maleate tablets and clozapine. Since clozapine-related seizures and orthostatic hypotension appear to be closely related, the risk of these adverse events may be higher when fluvoxamine and clozapine are co-administered. Patients should be closely monitored when Luvox CR capsules and clozapine are used concurrently).

No products indexed under this heading.

Cyclobenzaprine (Fluvoxamine is a known potent inhibitor of CYP1A2 and also inhibits CYP3A4, CYP2C9, and CYP2C19).
No products indexed under this heading.

Cyclobenzaprine Hydrochloride (Fluvoxamine is a known potent inhibitor of CYP1A2 and also inhibits CYP3A4, CYP2C9, and CYP2C19). Products include:
Amrix Capsules ... 966

Cyclosporine (Fluvoxamine is a known potent inhibitor of CYP1A2 and also inhibits CYP3A4, CYP2C9, and CYP2C19). Products include:
Gengraf Capsules ... 435
Neoral Oral Solution ... 2280
Neoral Soft Gelatin Capsules ... 2280
Restasis Ophthalmic Emulsion ... 557
Sandimmune ... 2296

Dalfopristin (Fluvoxamine is a known potent inhibitor of CYP1A2 and also inhibits CYP3A4, CYP2C9, and CYP2C19).
No products indexed under this heading.

Danazol (Fluvoxamine is a known potent inhibitor of CYP1A2 and also inhibits CYP3A4, CYP2C9, and CYP2C19).
No products indexed under this heading.

Delavirdine Mesylate (Fluvoxamine is a known potent inhibitor of CYP1A2 and also inhibits CYP3A4, CYP2C9, and CYP2C19).
No products indexed under this heading.

Desipramine Hydrochloride (Significantly increased plasma TCA levels have been reported with the co-administration of immediate-release fluvoxamine maleate tablets and amitriptyline, clomipramine, or imipramine. Caution is indicated with the co-administration of Luvox CR capsules and TCAs; plasma TCA concentrations may need to be monitored, and the dose of TCA may be reduced).
No products indexed under this heading.

Diazepam (The co-administration of Luvox CR capsules and diazepam is generally not advisable. Because fluvoxamine reduces the clearance of both diazepam and its active metabolite, N-desmethyldiazepam, there is a strong likelihood of substantial accumulation of both species during chronic co-administration). Products include:
Valium Tablets ... 2658

Diclofenac Epolamine (Serotonin release by platelets plays an important role in hemostasis. Epidemiological studies of the case-control and cohort design that have demonstrated an association between use of psychotropic drugs that interfere with serotonin reuptake and the occurrence of upper GI bleeding. These studies have also shown that concurrent use of an NSAID or aspirin may potentiate this risk of bleeding). Products include:
Flector Patch ... 561

Diclofenac Potassium (Serotonin release by platelets plays an important role in hemostasis. Epidemiological studies of the case-control and cohort design that have demonstrated an association between use of psychotropic drugs that interfere with serotonin reuptake and the occurrence of upper GI bleeding. These studies have also shown that concurrent use of an NSAID or aspirin may potentiate this risk of bleeding).
No products indexed under this heading.

Diclofenac Sodium (Serotonin release by platelets plays an important role in hemostasis. Epidemiological studies of the case-control and cohort design that have demonstrated an association between use of psychotropic drugs that interfere with serotonin reuptake and the occurrence of upper GI bleeding. These studies have also shown that concurrent use of an NSAID or aspirin may potentiate this risk of bleeding). Products include:
Diclofenac Sodium Ophthalmic Solution ... ⊙240
Voltaren Ophthalmic Solution ... 2336
Voltaren Tablets ... 2334
Voltaren-XR Tablets ... 2337

Dicumarol (When immediate-release fluvoxamine maleate tablets (50 mg given t.i.d.) were administered concomitantly with warfarin for two weeks, warfarin plasma concentrations increased by 98% and prothrombin times were prolonged. Thus patients receiving oral anticoagulants and Luvox CR capsules should have their prothrombin time monitored and their anticoagulant dose adjusted accordingly. No dosage adjustment is required for Luvox CR capsules).
No products indexed under this heading.

Diltiazem Hydrochloride (Bradycardia has been reported with the co-administration of immediate-release fluvoxamine maleate tablets and diltiazem). Products include:
Cardizem LA Extended Release Tablets ... 421

Diltiazem Maleate (Bradycardia has been reported with the co-administration of immediate-release fluvoxamine maleate tablets and diltiazem).
No products indexed under this heading.

Doxepin Hydrochloride (Significantly increased plasma TCA levels have been reported with the co-administration of immediate-release fluvoxamine maleate tablets and amitriptyline, clomipramine, or imipramine. Caution is indicated with the co-administration of Luvox CR capsules and TCAs; plasma TCA concentrations may need to be monitored, and the dose of TCA may be reduced).
No products indexed under this heading.

Efavirenz (Fluvoxamine is a known potent inhibitor of CYP1A2 and also inhibits CYP3A4, CYP2C9, and CYP2C19). Products include:
Atripla Tablets ... 938
Sustiva Capsules ... 930
Sustiva Tablets ... 930

Eletriptan Hydrobromide (The development of a potentially life-threatening serotonin syndrome may occur with Luvox CR capsules treatment, particularly with concomitant use of serotonergic drugs (including triptans) and with drugs that impair metabolism of serotonin (including MAOIs). Serotonin syndrome symptoms may include mental status changes (eg, agitation, hallucinations, coma), autonomic instability (eg, tachycardia, labile BP, hyperthermia), neuromuscular aberrations (eg, hyperreflexia, incoordination) and/or GI symptoms (eg, nausea, vomiting, diarrhea)).
No products indexed under this heading.

Enoxacin (Fluvoxamine is a known potent inhibitor of CYP1A2 and also inhibits CYP3A4, CYP2C9, and CYP2C19).
No products indexed under this heading.

Erythromycin (Fluvoxamine is a known potent inhibitor of CYP1A2 and also inhibits CYP3A4, CYP2C9, and CYP2C19).
No products indexed under this heading.

Erythromycin Estolate (Fluvoxamine is a known potent inhibitor of CYP1A2 and also inhibits CYP3A4, CYP2C9, and CYP2C19).
No products indexed under this heading.

Erythromycin Ethylsuccinate (Fluvoxamine is a known potent inhibitor of CYP1A2 and also inhibits CYP3A4, CYP2C9, and CYP2C19). Products include:
E.E.S. ... 433
EryPed ... 431

Erythromycin Gluceptate (Fluvoxamine is a known potent inhibitor of CYP1A2 and also inhibits CYP3A4, CYP2C9, and CYP2C19).
No products indexed under this heading.

Erythromycin Lactobionate (Fluvoxamine is a known potent inhibitor of CYP1A2 and also inhibits CYP3A4, CYP2C9, and CYP2C19).
No products indexed under this heading.

Erythromycin Stearate (Fluvoxamine is a known potent inhibitor of CYP1A2 and also inhibits CYP3A4, CYP2C9, and CYP2C19).
No products indexed under this heading.

Escitalopram Oxalate (The development of a potentially life-threatening serotonin syndrome may occur with Luvox CR capsules treatment, particularly with concomitant use of serotonergic drugs (including triptans) and with drugs that impair metabolism of serotonin (including MAOIs). Serotonin syndrome symptoms may include mental status changes (eg, agitation, hallucinations, coma), autonomic instability (eg, tachycardia, labile BP, hyperthermia), neuromuscular aberrations (eg, hyperreflexia, incoordination) and/or GI symptoms (eg, nausea, vomiting, diarrhea)). Products include:
Lexapro Oral Suspension ... 1174
Lexapro Tablets ... 1174

Esomeprazole Magnesium (Fluvoxamine is a known potent inhibitor of CYP1A2 and also inhibits CYP3A4, CYP2C9, and CYP2C19). Products include:
Nexium Delayed-Release Capsules ... 645
Nexium Delayed-Release Oral Suspension ... 645

Estazolam (Benzodiazepines metabolized by hepatic oxidation (eg, alprazolam, midazolam, triazolam) should be used with caution because the clearance of these drugs is likely to be reduced by fluvoxamine. The clearance of benzodiazepines metabolized by glucuronidation (eg, lorazepam, oxazepam, temazepam) is unlikely to be affected by fluvoxamine).
No products indexed under this heading.

Estradiol (Fluvoxamine is a known potent inhibitor of CYP1A2 and also inhibits CYP3A4, CYP2C9, and CYP2C19). Products include:
Activella Tablets ... 2347
Angeliq Tablets ... 751
Climara Transdermal System ... 763
Climara Pro Transdermal System ... 768
Divigel ... 3167
Vagifem Tablets ... 2375

Estradiol Benzoate (Fluvoxamine is a known potent inhibitor of CYP1A2 and also inhibits CYP3A4, CYP2C9, and CYP2C19).
No products indexed under this heading.

Estradiol Cypionate (Fluvoxamine is a known potent inhibitor of CYP1A2 and also inhibits CYP3A4, CYP2C9, and CYP2C19).
No products indexed under this heading.

Ethanol (Patients should be advised to avoid taking alcohol while taking Luvox CR capsules).
No products indexed under this heading.

Ethyl Alcohol (Patients should be advised to avoid taking alcohol while taking Luvox CR capsules).
No products indexed under this heading.

Etodolac (Serotonin release by platelets plays an important role in hemostasis. Epidemiological studies of the case-control and cohort design that have demonstrated an association between use of psychotropic drugs that interfere with serotonin reuptake and the occurrence of upper GI bleeding. These studies have also shown that concurrent use of an NSAID or aspirin may potentiate this risk of bleeding).
No products indexed under this heading.

Fenoprofen Calcium (Serotonin release by platelets plays an important role in hemostasis. Epidemiological studies of the case-control and cohort design that have demonstrated an association between use of psychotropic drugs that interfere with serotonin reuptake and the occurrence of upper GI bleeding. These studies have also shown that concurrent use of an NSAID or aspirin may potentiate this risk of bleeding). Products include:
Nalfon Capsules ... 2508

Fluconazole (Fluvoxamine is a known potent inhibitor of CYP1A2 and also inhibits CYP3A4, CYP2C9, and CYP2C19).
No products indexed under this heading.

Fluoxetine (Fluvoxamine is a known potent inhibitor of CYP1A2 and also inhibits CYP3A4, CYP2C9, and CYP2C19).
No products indexed under this heading.

Fluoxetine Hydrochloride (The development of a potentially life-

threatening serotonin syndrome may occur with Luvox CR capsules treatment, particularly with concomitant use of serotonergic drugs (including triptans) and with drugs that impair metabolism of serotonin (including MAOIs). Serotonin syndrome symptoms may include mental status changes (eg, agitation, hallucinations, coma), autonomic instability (eg, tachycardia, labile BP, hyperthermia), neuromuscular aberrations (eg, hyperreflexia, incoordination) and/or GI symptoms (eg, nausea, vomiting, diarrhea)). Products include:

Prozac Weekly Capsules **1852**
Prozac Pulvules and Liquid **1852**
Symbyax Capsules **1871**

Flurazepam Hydrochloride (Benzodiazepines metabolized by hepatic oxidation (eg, alprazolam, midazolam, triazolam) should be used with caution because the clearance of these drugs is likely to be reduced by fluvoxamine. The clearance of benzodiazepines metabolized by glucuronidation (eg, lorazepam, oxazepam, temazepam) is unlikely to be affected by fluvoxamine).

No products indexed under this heading.

Flurbiprofen (Serotonin release by platelets plays an important role in hemostasis. Epidemiological studies of the case-control and cohort design that have demonstrated an association between use of psychotropic drugs that interfere with serotonin reuptake and the occurrence of upper GI bleeding. These studies have also shown that concurrent use of an NSAID or aspirin may potentiate this risk of bleeding).

No products indexed under this heading.

Flutamide (Fluvoxamine is a known potent inhibitor of CYP1A2 and also inhibits CYP3A4, CYP2C9, and CYP2C19).

No products indexed under this heading.

Fluticasone Propionate (Fluvoxamine is a known potent inhibitor of CYP1A2 and also inhibits CYP3A4, CYP2C9, and CYP2C19). Products include:

Advair Diskus 100/50 .... **1276**
Advair Diskus 250/50 .... **1276**
Advair Diskus 500/50 .... **1276**
Advair HFA 45/21 Inhalation Aerosol.. **1288**
Advair HFA 115/21 Inhalation Aerosol.. **1288**
Advair HFA 230/21 Inhalation Aerosol.. **1288**
Flonase Nasal Spray **1431**
Flovent Diskus 50 mcg **1435**

Fosamprenavir Calcium (Fluvoxamine is a known potent inhibitor of CYP1A2 and also inhibits CYP3A4, CYP2C9, and CYP2C19). Products include:

Lexiva Oral Suspension **1510**
Lexiva Tablets **1510**

Frovatriptan Succinate (The development of a potentially life-threatening serotonin syndrome may occur with Luvox CR capsules treatment, particularly with concomitant use of serotonergic drugs (including triptans) and with drugs that impair metabolism of serotonin (including MAOIs). Serotonin syndrome symptoms may include mental status changes (eg, agitation, hallucinations, coma), autonomic instability (eg, tachycardia, labile BP, hyperthermia), neuromuscular aberrations (eg, hyperreflexia, incoordination) and/or GI symptoms (eg, nausea, vomiting, diarrhea)). Products include:

Frova Tablets **1111**

Grepafloxacin Hydrochloride (Fluvoxamine is a known potent inhibitor of CYP1A2 and also inhibits CYP3A4, CYP2C9, and CYP2C19).

No products indexed under this heading.

Halazepam (Benzodiazepines metabolized by hepatic oxidation (eg, alprazolam, midazolam, triazolam) should be used with caution because the clearance of these drugs is likely to be reduced by fluvoxamine. The clearance of benzodiazepines metabolized by glucuronidation (eg, lorazepam, oxazepam, temazepam) is unlikely to be affected by fluvoxamine).

No products indexed under this heading.

Haloperidol (Fluvoxamine is a known potent inhibitor of CYP1A2 and also inhibits CYP3A4, CYP2C9, and CYP2C19).

No products indexed under this heading.

Haloperidol Decanoate (Fluvoxamine is a known potent inhibitor of CYP1A2 and also inhibits CYP3A4, CYP2C9, and CYP2C19).

No products indexed under this heading.

Haloperidol Lactate (Fluvoxamine is a known potent inhibitor of CYP1A2 and also inhibits CYP3A4, CYP2C9, and CYP2C19).

No products indexed under this heading.

Ibuprofen (Serotonin release by platelets plays an important role in hemostasis. Epidemiological studies of the case-control and cohort design that have demonstrated an association between use of psychotropic drugs that interfere with serotonin reuptake and the occurrence of upper GI bleeding. These studies have also shown that concurrent use of an NSAID or aspirin may potentiate this risk of bleeding). Products include:

Motrin IB Tablets and Caplets **1900**
Children's Motrin Oral Suspension ... **1901**
Children's Motrin Non-Staining Dye-Free Oral Suspension............ **1901**
Children's Motrin Cold Oral Suspension **1899**
Infants' Motrin Concentrated Drops.. **1901**
Infants' Motrin Non-Staining Dye-Free Concentrated Drops....... **1901**
Junior Strength Motrin Caplets and Chewable Tablets................. **1901**
Vicoprofen Tablets **533**

Imipramine Hydrochloride (Significantly increased plasma TCA levels have been reported with the co-administration of immediate-release fluvoxamine maleate tablets and amitriptyline, clomipramine, or imipramine. Caution is indicated with the co-administration of Luvox CR capsules and TCAs; plasma TCA concentrations may need to be monitored, and the dose of TCA may be reduced).

No products indexed under this heading.

Imipramine Pamoate (Significantly increased plasma TCA levels have been reported with the co-administration of immediate-release fluvoxamine maleate tablets and amitriptyline, clomipramine, or imipramine. Caution is indicated with the co-administration of Luvox CR capsules and TCAs; plasma TCA concentrations may need to be monitored, and the dose of TCA may be reduced).

No products indexed under this heading.

Indinavir Sulfate (Fluvoxamine is a known potent inhibitor of CYP1A2 and also inhibits CYP3A4, CYP2C9, and CYP2C19). Products include:

Crixivan Capsules **1979**

Indomethacin (Serotonin release by platelets plays an important role in hemostasis. Epidemiological studies of the case-control and cohort design that have demonstrated an association between use of psychotropic drugs that interfere with serotonin reuptake and the occurrence of upper GI bleeding. These studies have also shown that concurrent use of an NSAID or aspirin may potentiate this risk of bleeding). Products include:

Indocin **2024**

Indomethacin Sodium Trihydrate (Serotonin release by platelets plays an important role in hemostasis. Epidemiological studies of the case-control and cohort design that have demonstrated an association between use of psychotropic drugs that interfere with serotonin reuptake and the occurrence of upper GI bleeding. These studies have also shown that concurrent use of an NSAID or aspirin may potentiate this risk of bleeding). Products include:

Indocin I.V. **2489**

Isocarboxazid (In patients receiving another serotonin reuptake inhibitor drug in combination with monoamine oxidase inhibitors (MAOIs), there have been reports of serious, sometimes fatal reactions including hyperthermia, rigidity, myoclonus, autonomic instability with possible rapid fluctuations of vital signs, and mental status changes that include extreme agitation progressing to delirium and coma. These reactions have also been reported in patients who have discontinued the drug and have started on an MAOI. Some cases presented with features resembling a serotonin syndrome or neuroleptic malignant syndrome. Therefore, concomitant administration with MAOI, or within 14 days of discontinuing treatment with an MAOI, is contraindicated). Products include:

Marplan Tablets **3177**

Isoniazid (Fluvoxamine is a known potent inhibitor of CYP1A2 and also inhibits CYP3A4, CYP2C9, and CYP2C19).

No products indexed under this heading.

Itraconazole (Fluvoxamine is a known potent inhibitor of CYP1A2 and also inhibits CYP3A4, CYP2C9, and CYP2C19).

No products indexed under this heading.

Ketoconazole (Fluvoxamine is a known potent inhibitor of CYP1A2 and also inhibits CYP3A4, CYP2C9, and CYP2C19). Products include:

Extina Foam, 2% **3057**
Nizoral A-D Shampoo **1901**

Ketoprofen (Serotonin release by platelets plays an important role in hemostasis. Epidemiological studies of the case-control and cohort design that have demonstrated an association between use of psychotropic drugs that interfere with serotonin reuptake and the occurrence of upper GI bleeding. These studies have also shown that concurrent use of an NSAID or aspirin may potentiate this risk of bleeding).

No products indexed under this heading.

Ketorolac Tromethamine (Serotonin release by platelets plays an important role in hemostasis. Epidemiological studies of the case-control and cohort design that have demonstrated an association between use of psychotropic drugs that interfere with serotonin reuptake and the occurrence of upper GI bleeding. These studies have also shown that concurrent use of an NSAID or aspirin may potentiate this risk of bleeding).

No products indexed under this heading.

Levobupivacaine Hydrochloride (Fluvoxamine is a known potent inhibitor of CYP1A2 and also inhibits CYP3A4, CYP2C9, and CYP2C19).

No products indexed under this heading.

Lithium (As with other serotonergic drugs, lithium may enhance the serotonergic effects of fluvoxamine and therefore the combination should be used with caution. Seizures have been reported with the co-administration of immediate-release fluvoxamine maleate tablets and lithium).

No products indexed under this heading.

Lithium Carbonate (As with other serotonergic drugs, lithium may enhance the serotonergic effects of fluvoxamine and therefore the combination should be used with caution. Seizures have been reported with the co-administration of immediate-release fluvoxamine maleate tablets and lithium).

No products indexed under this heading.

Lithium Citrate (As with other serotonergic drugs, lithium may enhance the serotonergic effects of fluvoxamine and therefore the combination should be used with caution. Seizures have been reported with the co-administration of immediate-release fluvoxamine maleate tablets and lithium).

No products indexed under this heading.

Lomefloxacin Hydrochloride (Fluvoxamine is a known potent inhibitor of CYP1A2 and also inhibits CYP3A4, CYP2C9, and CYP2C19).

No products indexed under this heading.

Lopinavir (Fluvoxamine is a known potent inhibitor of CYP1A2 and also inhibits CYP3A4, CYP2C9, and CYP2C19). Products include:

Kaletra **452**

Loratadine (Fluvoxamine is a known potent inhibitor of CYP1A2 and also inhibits CYP3A4, CYP2C9, and CYP2C19).

No products indexed under this heading.

Lorazepam (A study of multiple doses of immediate-release fluvoxamine tablets (50 mg given b.i.d.) in healthy male volunteers (N = 12) and a single dose of lorazepam (4 mg single dose) indicated no significant pharmacokinetic interaction. On average, both lorazepam alone and lorazepam with fluvoxamine produced substantial decrements in cognitive functioning; however, the co-administration of fluvoxamine and lorazepam did not produce larger mean decrements compared to lorazepam alone).
No products indexed under this heading.

Maprotiline Hydrochloride (Significantly increased plasma TCA levels have been reported with the co-administration of immediate-release fluvoxamine maleate tablets and amitriptyline, clomipramine, or imipramine. Caution is indicated with the co-administration of Luvox CR capsules and TCAs; plasma TCA concentrations may need to be monitored, and the dose of TCA may be reduced).
No products indexed under this heading.

Meclofenamate Sodium (Serotonin release by platelets plays an important role in hemostasis. Epidemiological studies of the case-control and cohort design that have demonstrated an association between use of psychotropic drugs that interfere with serotonin reuptake and the occurrence of upper GI bleeding. These studies have also shown that concurrent use of an NSAID or aspirin may potentiate this risk of bleeding).
No products indexed under this heading.

Mefenamic Acid (Serotonin release by platelets plays an important role in hemostasis. Epidemiological studies of the case-control and cohort design that have demonstrated an association between use of psychotropic drugs that interfere with serotonin reuptake and the occurrence of upper GI bleeding. These studies have also shown that concurrent use of an NSAID or aspirin may potentiate this risk of bleeding).
No products indexed under this heading.

Meloxicam (Serotonin release by platelets plays an important role in hemostasis. Epidemiological studies of the case-control and cohort design that have demonstrated an association between use of psychotropic drugs that interfere with serotonin reuptake and the occurrence of upper GI bleeding. These studies have also shown that concurrent use of an NSAID or aspirin may potentiate this risk of bleeding). Products include:
Mobic Oral Suspension 863
Mobic Tablets 863

Methacycline Hydrochloride (Significantly increased methadone (plasma level:dose) ratios have been reported when immediate-release fluvoxamine maleate tablets were administered to patients receiving maintenance methadone treatment, with symptoms of opioid intoxication in one patient. Opiod withdrawl symptoms were reported following fluvoxamine maleate discontinuation in another patient).
No products indexed under this heading.

Methadone Hydrochloride (Significantly increased methadone (plasma level:dose) ratios have been reported when immediate-release fluvoxamine maleate tablets were administered to patients receiving maintenance methadone treatment, with symptoms of opioid intoxication in one patient. Opioid withdrawal symptoms were reported following fluvoxamine maleate discontinuation in another patient).
No products indexed under this heading.

Metoprolol Succinate (One case of bradycardia and hypotension and a second case of orthostatic hypotension have been reported with the co-administration of immediate-release fluvoxamine maleate tablets and metoprolol. If metoprolol is co-administered with Luvox CR capsules, a reduction in the initial beta-blocker dose and more caution dose titration are recommended. No dosage adjustment is required for Luvox CR capsules). Products include:
Toprol-XL Tablets 666

Metoprolol Tartrate (One case of bradycardia and hypotension and a second case of orthostatic hypotension have been reported with the co-administration of immediate-release fluvoxamine maleate tablets and metoprolol. If metoprolol is co-administered with Luvox CR capsules, a reduction in the initial beta-blocker dose and more caution dose titration are recommended. No dosage adjustment is required for Luvox CR capsules).
No products indexed under this heading.

Metronidazole (Fluvoxamine is a known potent inhibitor of CYP1A2 and also inhibits CYP3A4, CYP2C9, and CYP2C19). Products include:
Pylera Capsules 714

Metronidazole Benzoate (Fluvoxamine is a known potent inhibitor of CYP1A2 and also inhibits CYP3A4, CYP2C9, and CYP2C19).
No products indexed under this heading.

Metronidazole Hydrochloride (Fluvoxamine is a known potent inhibitor of CYP1A2 and also inhibits CYP3A4, CYP2C9, and CYP2C19).
No products indexed under this heading.

Metronidazole Sodium (Fluvoxamine is a known potent inhibitor of CYP1A2 and also inhibits CYP3A4, CYP2C9, and CYP2C19).
No products indexed under this heading.

Mexiletine Hydrochloride (The effect of steady-state immediate release fluvoxamine maleate tablets (50 mg tablets given b.i.d. for 7 days) on the single-dose pharmacokinetics of mexiletine (200 mg) was evaluated in 6 healthy Japanese males. The clearance of mexiletine was reduced by 38% following co-administration with fluvoxamine compared to mexiletine alone. If fluvoxamine and mexiletine are co-administered, serum mexiletine levels should be monitored).
No products indexed under this heading.

Miconazole (Fluvoxamine is a known potent inhibitor of CYP1A2 and also inhibits CYP3A4, CYP2C9, and CYP2C19).
No products indexed under this heading.

Miconazole Nitrate (Fluvoxamine is a known potent inhibitor of CYP1A2 and also inhibits CYP3A4, CYP2C9, and CYP2C19).
No products indexed under this heading.

Midazolam Hydrochloride (Benzodiazepines metabolized by hepatic oxidation (eg, alprazolam, midazolam, triazolam) should be used with caution because the clearance of these drugs is likely to be reduced by fluvoxamine. The clearance of benzodiazepines metabolized by glucuronidation (eg, lorazepam, oxazepam, temazepam) is unlikely to be affected by fluvoxamine).
No products indexed under this heading.

Mirtazapine (Fluvoxamine is a known potent inhibitor of CYP1A2 and also inhibits CYP3A4, CYP2C9, and CYP2C19). Products include:
Remeron Tablets 2924
RemeronSolTab Tablets 2927

Moclobemide (In patients receiving another serotonin reuptake inhibitor drug in combination with monoamine oxidase inhibitors (MAOIs), there have been reports of serious, sometimes fatal reactions including hyperthermia, rigidity, myoclonus, autonomic instability with possible rapid fluctuations of vital signs, and mental status changes that include extreme agitation progressing to delirium and coma. These reactions have also been reported in patients who have discontinued the drug and have started on an MAOI. Some cases presented with features resembling a serotonin syndrome or neuroleptic malignant syndrome. Therefore, concomitant administration with MAOI, or within 14 days of discontinuing treatment with an MAOI, is contraindicated).
No products indexed under this heading.

Moxifloxacin Hydrochloride (Fluvoxamine is a known potent inhibitor of CYP1A2 and also inhibits CYP3A4, CYP2C9, and CYP2C19). Products include:
Avelox 2803
Vigamox Ophthalmic Solution .... ⊙ 548

Nabumetone (Serotonin release by platelets plays an important role in hemostasis. Epidemiological studies of the case-control and cohort design that have demonstrated an association between use of psychotropic drugs that interfere with serotonin reuptake and the occurrence of upper GI bleeding. These studies have also shown that concurrent use of an NSAID or aspirin may potentiate this risk of bleeding).
No products indexed under this heading.

Nafcillin Sodium (Fluvoxamine is a known potent inhibitor of CYP1A2 and also inhibits CYP3A4, CYP2C9, and CYP2C19).
No products indexed under this heading.

Naproxen (Serotonin release by platelets plays an important role in hemostasis. Epidemiological studies of the case-control and cohort design that have demonstrated an association between use of psychotropic drugs that interfere with serotonin reuptake and the occurrence of upper GI bleeding. These studies have also shown that concurrent use of an NSAID or aspirin may potentiate this risk of bleeding). Products include:
EC-Naprosyn Delayed-Release Tablets 2632
Naprosyn Suspension 2632
Naprosyn Tablets 2632

Naproxen Sodium (Serotonin release by platelets plays an important role in hemostasis. Epidemiological studies of the case-control and cohort design that have demonstrated an association between use of psychotropic drugs that interfere with serotonin reuptake and the occurrence of upper GI bleeding. These studies have also shown that concurrent use of an NSAID or aspirin may potentiate this risk of bleeding). Products include:
Anaprox Tablets 2632
Anaprox DS Tablets 2632
Treximet Tablets 1616

Naratriptan Hydrochloride (The development of a potentially life-threatening serotonin syndrome may occur with Luvox CR capsules treatment, particularly with concomitant use of serotonergic drugs (including triptans) and with drugs that impair metabolism of serotonin (including MAOIs). Serotonin syndrome symptoms may include mental status changes (eg, agitation, hallucinations, coma), autonomic instability (eg, tachycardia, labile BP, hyperthermia), neuromuscular aberrations (eg, hyperreflexia, incoordination) and/or GI symptoms (eg, nausea, vomiting, diarrhea)). Products include:
Amerge Tablets 1301

Nefazodone Hydrochloride (Fluvoxamine is a known potent inhibitor of CYP1A2 and also inhibits CYP3A4, CYP2C9, and CYP2C19).
No products indexed under this heading.

Nelfinavir Mesylate (Fluvoxamine is a known potent inhibitor of CYP1A2 and also inhibits CYP3A4, CYP2C9, and CYP2C19).
No products indexed under this heading.

Nevirapine (Fluvoxamine is a known potent inhibitor of CYP1A2 and also inhibits CYP3A4, CYP2C9, and CYP2C19). Products include:
Viramune Oral Suspension 873
Viramune Tablets 873

Niacinamide (Fluvoxamine is a known potent inhibitor of CYP1A2 and also inhibits CYP3A4, CYP2C9, and CYP2C19). Products include:
BioLean Free Tablets .... ■ 635

Nicotinamide (Fluvoxamine is a known potent inhibitor of CYP1A2 and also inhibits CYP3A4, CYP2C9, and CYP2C19).
No products indexed under this heading.

Nicotine Polacrilex (Fluvoxamine is a known potent inhibitor of CYP1A2 and also inhibits CYP3A4, CYP2C9, and CYP2C19).
No products indexed under this heading.

Nicotine Salicylate (Fluvoxamine is a known potent inhibitor of CYP1A2 and also inhibits CYP3A4, CYP2C9, and CYP2C19).
No products indexed under this heading.

Nicotine Sulfate (Fluvoxamine is a known potent inhibitor of CYP1A2 and also inhibits CYP3A4, CYP2C9, and CYP2C19).
No products indexed under this heading.

Nifedipine (Fluvoxamine is a known potent inhibitor of CYP1A2 and also inhibits CYP3A4, CYP2C9, and CYP2C19).
No products indexed under this heading.

Norethindrone Acetate (Fluvoxamine is a known potent inhibitor of CYP1A2 and also inhibits CYP3A4, CYP2C9, and CYP2C19). Products include:
Activella Tablets 2347

Norfloxacin (Fluvoxamine is a known potent inhibitor of CYP1A2 and also inhibits CYP3A4, CYP2C9, and CYP2C19). Products include:
Noroxin Tablets 2069

Nortriptyline Hydrochloride (Significantly increased plasma TCA levels have been reported with the co-administration of immediate-release fluvoxamine maleate tablets and amitriptyline, clomipramine, or imipramine. Caution is indicated with the co-administration of Luvox CR capsules and TCAs; plasma TCA concentrations may need to be monitored, and the dose of TCA may be reduced).
No products indexed under this heading.

Ofloxacin (Fluvoxamine is a known potent inhibitor of CYP1A2 and also inhibits CYP3A4, CYP2C9, and CYP2C19). Products include:
Ofloxacin Ophthalmic Solution 0.3% .... ⊙ 243

Olanzapine (Fluvoxamine is a known potent inhibitor of CYP1A2 and also inhibits CYP3A4, CYP2C9, and CYP2C19). Products include:
Symbyax Capsules 1871
Zyprexa Tablets 1883
Zyprexa IntraMuscular 1883
Zyprexa ZYDIS Orally Disintegrating Tablets 1883

Omeprazole (Fluvoxamine is a known potent inhibitor of CYP1A2 and also inhibits CYP3A4, CYP2C9, and CYP2C19).
No products indexed under this heading.

Ondansetron (Fluvoxamine is a known potent inhibitor of CYP1A2 and also inhibits CYP3A4, CYP2C9, and CYP2C19). Products include:
Zofran ODT Orally Disintegrating Tablets 1687

Ondansetron Hydrochloride (Fluvoxamine is a known potent inhibitor of CYP1A2 and also inhibits CYP3A4, CYP2C9, and CYP2C19). Products include:
Zofran Injection 1682
Zofran 1687

Oxaprozin (Serotonin release by platelets plays an important role in hemostasis. Epidemiological studies of the case-control and cohort design that have demonstrated an association between use of psychotropic drugs that interfere with serotonin reuptake and the occurrence of upper GI bleeding. These studies have also shown that concurrent use of an NSAID or aspirin may potentiate this risk of bleeding).
No products indexed under this heading.

Oxazepam (Benzodiazepines metabolized by hepatic oxidation (eg, alprazolam, midazolam, triazolam) should be used with caution because the clearance of these drugs is likely to be reduced by fluvoxamine. The clearance of benzodiazepines metabolized by glucuronidation (eg, lorazepam, oxazepam, temazepam) is unlikely to be affected by fluvoxamine).
No products indexed under this heading.

Pargyline Hydrochloride (In patients receiving another serotonin reuptake inhibitor drug in combination with monoamine oxidase inhibitors (MAOIs), there have been reports of serious, sometimes fatal reactions including hyperthermia, rigidity, myoclonus, autonomic instability with possible rapid fluctuations of vital signs, and mental status changes that include extreme agitation progressing to delirium and coma. These reactions have also been reported in patients who have discontinued the drug and have started on an MAOI. Some cases presented with features resembling a serotonin syndrome or neuroleptic malignant syndrome. Therefore, concomitant administration with MAOI, or within 14 days of discontinuing treatment with an MAOI, is contraindicated).
No products indexed under this heading.

Paroxetine Hydrochloride (The development of a potentially life-threatening serotonin syndrome may occur with Luvox CR capsules treatment, particularly with concomitant use of serotonergic drugs (including triptans) and with drugs that impair metabolism of serotonin (including MAOIs). Serotonin syndrome symptoms may include mental status changes (eg, agitation, hallucinations, coma), autonomic instability (eg, tachycardia, labile BP, hyperthermia), neuromuscular aberrations (eg, hyperreflexia, incoordination) and/or GI symptoms (eg, nausea, vomiting, diarrhea)). Products include:
Paxil 1535
Paxil CR Controlled-Release Tablets 1544

Phenelzine Sulfate (In patients receiving another serotonin reuptake inhibitor drug in combination with monoamine oxidase inhibitors (MAOIs), there have been reports of serious, sometimes fatal reactions including hyperthermia, rigidity, myoclonus, autonomic instability with possible rapid fluctuations of vital signs, and mental status changes that include extreme agitation progressing to delirium and coma. These reactions have also been reported in patients who have discontinued the drug and have started on an MAOI. Some cases presented with features resembling a serotonin syndrome or neuroleptic malignant syndrome. Therefore, concomitant administration with MAOI, or within 14 days of discontinuing treatment with an MAOI, is contraindicated).
No products indexed under this heading.

Phenobarbital Sodium (Fluvoxamine is a known potent inhibitor of CYP1A2 and also inhibits CYP3A4, CYP2C9, and CYP2C19).
No products indexed under this heading.

Phenylbutazone (Serotonin release by platelets plays an important role in hemostasis. Epidemiological studies of the case-control and cohort design that have demonstrated an association between use of psychotropic drugs that interfere with serotonin reuptake and the occurrence of upper GI bleeding. These studies have also shown that concurrent use of an NSAID or aspirin may potentiate this risk of bleeding).
No products indexed under this heading.

Phenytoin Sodium (Fluvoxamine is a known potent inhibitor of CYP1A2 and also inhibits CYP3A4, CYP2C9, and CYP2C19). Products include:
Phenytek Capsules 2192

Pimozide (Pimozide is metabolized by the CYP3A4 isozyme, and it has been demonstrated that ketoconazole, a potent inhibitor of CYP3A4, blocks the metabolism of this drug, resulting in increased plasma concentrations of parent drug. Increased plasma concentration of pimozide causes QT prolongation and has been associated with torsade de pointes-type ventricular tachycardia, sometimes fatal. A substantial pharmacokinetic interaction has been observed for fluvoxamine in combination with alprazolam, a drug known to be metabolized by the CYP3A4 isozyme. Therefore, co-administration of pimozide with Luvox CR capsules is contraindicated).
No products indexed under this heading.

Piroxicam (Serotonin release by platelets plays an important role in hemostasis. Epidemiological studies of the case-control and cohort design that have demonstrated an association between use of psychotropic drugs that interfere with serotonin reuptake and the occurrence of upper GI bleeding. These studies have also shown that concurrent use of an NSAID or aspirin may potentiate this risk of bleeding).
No products indexed under this heading.

Prazepam (Benzodiazepines metabolized by hepatic oxidation (eg, alprazolam, midazolam, triazolam) should be used with caution because the clearance of these drugs is likely to be reduced by fluvoxamine. The clearance of benzodiazepines metabolized by glucuronidation (eg, lorazepam, oxazepam, temazepam) is unlikely to be affected by fluvoxamine).
No products indexed under this heading.

Procarbazine Hydrochloride (In patients receiving another serotonin reuptake inhibitor drug in combination with monoamine oxidase inhibitors (MAOIs), there have been reports of serious, sometimes fatal reactions including hyperthermia, rigidity, myoclonus, autonomic instability with possible rapid fluctuations of vital signs, and mental status changes that include extreme agitation progressing to delirium and coma. These reactions have also been reported in patients who have discontinued the drug and have started on an MAOI. Some cases presented with features resembling a serotonin syndrome or neuroleptic malignant syndrome. Therefore, concomitant administration with MAOI, or within 14 days of discontinuing treatment with an MAOI, is contraindicated).
No products indexed under this heading.

Propafenone Hydrochloride (Fluvoxamine is a known potent inhibitor of CYP1A2 and also inhibits CYP3A4, CYP2C9, and CYP2C19). Products include:
Rythmol Tablets 1586
Rythmol SR Capsules 1590

Propoxyphene Hydrochloride (Fluvoxamine is a known potent inhibitor of CYP1A2 and also inhibits CYP3A4, CYP2C9, and CYP2C19).
No products indexed under this heading.

Propoxyphene Napsylate (Fluvoxamine is a known potent inhibitor of CYP1A2 and also inhibits CYP3A4, CYP2C9, and CYP2C19).
No products indexed under this heading.

Propranolol (Co-administration of immediate-release fluvoxamine maleate tablets 100 mg per day and propranolol 160 mg per day in normal volunteers resulted in a mean 5-fold increase (range 2-fold to 17-fold) in minimum propranolol plasma concentrations. In this study, there was a slight potentiation of the propranolol-induced reduction in heart rate and reduction in the exercise diastolic pressure. If propranolol is co-administered with Luvox CR caps, a reduction in the initial beta-blocker dose and more cautious dose titration are recommended. No dosage adjustment is required for Luvox CR caps).
No products indexed under this heading.

Propranolol Hydrochloride (Co-administration of immediate-release fluvoxamine maleate tablets 100 mg per day and propranolol 160 mg per day in normal volunteers resulted in a mean 5-fold increase (range 2-fold to 17-fold) in minimum propranolol plasma concentrations. In this study, there was a slight potentiation of the propranolol-induced reduction in heart rate and reduction in the exercise diastolic pressure. If propranolol is co-administered with Luvox CR caps, a reduction in the initial beta-blocker dose and more cautious dose titration are recommended. No dosage adjustment is required for Luvox CR caps). Products include:
InnoPran XL Extended Release Capsules 1484

Protriptyline Hydrochloride (Significantly increased plasma TCA levels have been reported with the co-administration of immediate-release fluvoxamine maleate tablets and amitriptyline, clomipramine, or imipramine. Caution is indicated with the co-administration of Luvox CR capsules and TCAs; plasma TCA concentrations may need to be monitored, and the dose of TCA may be reduced).
No products indexed under this heading.

Quazepam (Benzodiazepines metabolized by hepatic oxidation (eg, alprazolam, midazolam, triazolam) should be used with caution because the clearance of these drugs is likely to be reduced by fluvoxamine. The clearance of benzodiazepines metabolized by glucuronidation (eg, lorazepam, oxazepam, temazepam) is unlikely to be affected by fluvoxamine).
No products indexed under this heading.

Quinidine (Fluvoxamine is a known potent inhibitor of CYP1A2 and also inhibits CYP3A4, CYP2C9, and CYP2C19).
No products indexed under this heading.

Quinidine Hydrochloride (Fluvoxamine is a known potent inhibitor of CYP1A2 and also inhibits CYP3A4, CYP2C9, and CYP2C19).
No products indexed under this heading.

Quinidine Polygalacturonate (Fluvoxamine is a known potent inhibitor of CYP1A2 and also inhibits CYP3A4, CYP2C9, and CYP2C19).
No products indexed under this heading.

Quinidine Sulfate (Fluvoxamine is a known potent inhibitor of CYP1A2 and also inhibits CYP3A4, CYP2C9, and CYP2C19).
No products indexed under this heading.

Quinine (Fluvoxamine is a known potent inhibitor of CYP1A2 and also inhibits CYP3A4, CYP2C9, and CYP2C19).
No products indexed under this heading.

Quinine Sulfate (Fluvoxamine is a known potent inhibitor of CYP1A2 and also inhibits CYP3A4, CYP2C9, and CYP2C19).
No products indexed under this heading.

Quinupristin (Fluvoxamine is a known potent inhibitor of CYP1A2 and also inhibits CYP3A4, CYP2C9, and CYP2C19).
No products indexed under this heading.

Ramelteon (When immediate-release fluvoxamine maleate tablets 100 mg twice daily was administered for 3 days prior to single-dose co-administration of ramelteon 16 mg and immediate-release fluvoxamine maleate tablets, the AUC for ramelteon increased approximately 190-fold and the Cmax increased approximately 70-fold compared to ramelteon administered alone. Ramelteon should not be used in combination with Luvox CR capsules). Products include:
Rozerem Tablets 3091

Ranitidine Bismuth Citrate (Fluvoxamine is a known potent inhibitor of CYP1A2 and also inhibits CYP3A4, CYP2C9, and CYP2C19).
No products indexed under this heading.

Ranitidine Hydrochloride (Fluvoxamine is a known potent inhibitor of CYP1A2 and also inhibits CYP3A4, CYP2C9, and CYP2C19). Products include:
Zantac 75 Tablets .... ▣ 603
Zantac 1670
Zantac Injection 1666
Zantac Injection Pharmacy Bulk Package 1668
Maximum Strength Zantac 150 Tablets .... ▣ 603
Maximum Strength Zantac 150 Cool Mint Tablets .... ▣ 603

Rasagiline Mesylate (In patients receiving another serotonin reuptake inhibitor drug in combination with monoamine oxidase inhibitors (MAOIs), there have been reports of serious, sometimes fatal reactions including hyperthermia, rigidity, myoclonus, autonomic instability with possible rapid fluctuations of vital signs, and mental status changes that include extreme agitation progressing to delirium and coma. These reactions have also been reported in patients who have discontinued the drug and have started on an MAOI. Some cases presented with features resembling a serotonin syndrome or neuroleptic malignant syndrome. Therefore, concomitant administration with MAOI, or within 14 days of discontinuing treatment with an MAOI, is contraindicated). Products include:
Azilect Tablets 3106

Riluzole (Fluvoxamine is a known potent inhibitor of CYP1A2 and also inhibits CYP3A4, CYP2C9, and CYP2C19). Products include:
Rilutek Tablets 2771

Ritonavir (Fluvoxamine is a known potent inhibitor of CYP1A2 and also inhibits CYP3A4, CYP2C9, and CYP2C19). Products include:
Kaletra 452
Norvir 489

Rizatriptan Benzoate (The development of a potentially life-threatening serotonin syndrome may occur with Luvox CR capsules treatment, particularly with concomitant use of serotonergic drugs (including triptans) and with drugs that impair metabolism of serotonin (including MAOIs). Serotonin syndrome symptoms may include mental status changes (eg, agitation, hallucinations, coma), autonomic instability (eg, tachycardia, labile BP, hyperthermia), neuromuscular aberrations (eg, hyperreflexia, incoordination) and/or GI symptoms (eg, nausea, vomiting, diarrhea)). Products include:
Maxalt Tablets 2056
Maxalt-MLT Orally Disintegrating Tablets 2056

Rofecoxib (Serotonin release by platelets plays an important role in hemostasis. Epidemiological studies of the case-control and cohort design that have demonstrated an association between use of psychotropic drugs that interfere with serotonin reuptake and the occurrence of upper GI bleeding. These studies have also shown that concurrent use of an NSAID or aspirin may potentiate this risk of bleeding).
No products indexed under this heading.

Ropinirole Hydrochloride (Fluvoxamine is a known potent inhibitor of CYP1A2 and also inhibits CYP3A4, CYP2C9, and CYP2C19). Products include:
Requip Tablets 1561
Requip XL Tablets 1568

Ropivacaine Hydrochloride (Fluvoxamine is a known potent inhibitor of CYP1A2 and also inhibits CYP3A4, CYP2C9, and CYP2C19).
No products indexed under this heading.

Saquinavir (Fluvoxamine is a known potent inhibitor of CYP1A2 and also inhibits CYP3A4, CYP2C9, and CYP2C19).
No products indexed under this heading.

Saquinavir Mesylate (Fluvoxamine is a known potent inhibitor of CYP1A2 and also inhibits CYP3A4, CYP2C9, and CYP2C19).
No products indexed under this heading.

Selegiline (In patients receiving another serotonin reuptake inhibitor drug in combination with monoamine oxidase inhibitors (MAOIs), there have been reports of serious, sometimes fatal reactions including hyperthermia, rigidity, myoclonus, autonomic instability with possible rapid fluctuations of vital signs, and mental status changes that include extreme agitation progressing to delirium and coma. These reactions have also been reported in patients who have discontinued the drug and have started on an MAOI. Some cases presented with features resembling a serotonin syndrome or neuroleptic malignant syndrome. Therefore, concomitant administration with MAOI, or within 14 days of discontinuing treatment with an MAOI, is contraindicated). Products include:
Emsam Transdermal System 905

Selegiline Hydrochloride (In patients receiving another serotonin reuptake inhibitor drug in combination with monoamine oxidase inhibitors (MAOIs), there have been reports of serious, sometimes fatal reactions including hyperthermia, rigidity, myoclonus, autonomic instability with possible rapid fluctuations of vital signs, and mental status changes that include extreme agitation progressing to delirium and coma. These reactions have also been reported in patients who have discontinued the drug and have started on an MAOI. Some cases presented with features resembling a serotonin syndrome or neuroleptic malignant syndrome. Therefore, concomitant administration with MAOI, or within 14 days of discontinuing treatment with an MAOI, is contraindicated). Products include:
Eldepryl Capsules 3052

Sertraline Hydrochloride (The development of a potentially life-threatening serotonin syndrome may occur with Luvox CR capsules treatment, particularly with concomitant use of serotonergic drugs (including triptans) and with drugs that impair metabolism of serotonin (including MAOIs). Serotonin syndrome symptoms may include mental status changes (eg, agitation, hallucinations, coma), autonomic instability (eg, tachycardia, labile BP, hyperthermia), neuromuscular aberrations (eg, hyperreflexia, incoordination) and/or GI symptoms (eg, nausea, vomiting, diarrhea)).
No products indexed under this heading.

Sildenafil Citrate (Fluvoxamine is a known potent inhibitor of CYP1A2 and also inhibits CYP3A4, CYP2C9, and CYP2C19).
No products indexed under this heading.

Sulindac (Serotonin release by platelets plays an important role in hemostasis. Epidemiological studies of the case-control and cohort design that have demonstrated an association between use of psychotropic drugs that interfere with serotonin reuptake and the occurrence of upper GI bleeding. These studies have also shown that concurrent use of an NSAID or aspirin may potentiate this risk of bleeding). Products include:
Clinoril Tablets 1962

Sumatriptan (There have been rare postmarketing reports describing patients with weakness, hyperreflexia, and incoordination following the use of a selective serotonin reuptake inhibitor (SSRI) and sumatriptan. If concomitant treatment with sumatriptan and an SSRI (eg, fluoxetine, fluvoxamine, paroxetine, sertraline) is clinically warranted, appropriate observation of the patient is advised). Products include:
Imitrex Nasal Spray 1470

Sumatriptan Succinate (The development of a potentially life-threatening serotonin syndrome may occur with Luvox CR capsules treatment, particularly with concomitant use of serotonergic drugs (including triptans) and with drugs that impair metabolism of serotonin (including MAOIs). Serotonin syndrome symptoms may include mental status changes (eg, agitation, hallucinations, coma), autonomic instability (eg, tachycardia, labile BP, hyperthermia), neuromuscular aberrations (eg, hyperreflexia, incoordination) and/or GI symptoms (eg, nausea, vomiting, diarrhea)). Products include:
Imitrex Injection 1465
Imitrex Tablets 1474
Treximet Tablets 1616

Tacrine Hydrochloride (In a study of 13 healthy, male volunteers, a single 40 mg dose of tacrine added to immediate-release fluvoxamine maleate tablets 100 mg/day administered at steady state was associated with 5-fold and 8-fold increases in tacrine Cmax and AUC, respectively, compared to the administration of tacrine alone. Five subjects experienced nausea, vomiting, sweating, and diarrhea following co-administration, consistent with cholinergic effects of tacrine).
No products indexed under this heading.

Tamoxifen Citrate (Fluvoxamine is a known potent inhibitor of CYP1A2 and also inhibits CYP3A4, CYP2C9, and CYP2C19).
No products indexed under this heading.

Telithromycin (Fluvoxamine is a known potent inhibitor of CYP1A2 and also inhibits CYP3A4, CYP2C9, and CYP2C19). Products include:
Ketek Tablets 2744

Temazepam (Benzodiazepines metabolized by hepatic oxidation (eg, alprazolam, midazolam, triazolam) should be used with caution because the clearance of these drugs is likely to be reduced by fluvoxamine. The clearance of benzodiazepines metabolized by glucuronidation (eg, lorazepam, oxazepam, temazepam) is unlikely to be affected by fluvoxamine).
No products indexed under this heading.

Theophylline (The effect of steady-state immediate-release fluvoxamine maleate tablets (50 mg tablets given b.i.d.) on the pharmacokinetics of a single dose of theophylline (375 mg as 442 mg aminophylline) was evaluated in 12 healthy non-smoking male volunteers. The clearance of theophylline was decreased approximately 3-fold. Therefore if theophylline is co-administered with fluvoxamine maleate, its dose should be reduced to one third of the usual daily maintenance dose and plasma concentrations of theophylline should be monitored. No dosage is required for Luvox CR capsules).

No products indexed under this heading.

Theophylline Anhydrous (The effect of steady-state immediate-release fluvoxamine maleate tablets (50 mg tablets given b.i.d.) on the pharmacokinetics of a single dose of theophylline (375 mg as 442 mg aminophylline) was evaluated in 12 healthy non-smoking male volunteers. The clearance of theophylline was decreased approximately 3-fold. Therefore if theophylline is co-administered with fluvoxamine maleate, its dose should be reduced to one third of the usual daily maintenance dose and plasma concentrations of theophylline should be monitored. No dosage is required for Luvox CR capsules). Products include:

Uniphyl Tablets 2595

Theophylline Calcium Salicylate (The effect of steady-state immediate-release fluvoxamine maleate tablets (50 mg tablets given b.i.d.) on the pharmacokinetics of a single dose of theophylline (375 mg as 442 mg aminophylline) was evaluated in 12 healthy non-smoking male volunteers. The clearance of theophylline was decreased approximately 3-fold. Therefore if theophylline is co-administered with fluvoxamine maleate, its dose should be reduced to one third of the usual daily maintenance dose and plasma concentrations of theophylline should be monitored. No dosage is required for Luvox CR capsules).

No products indexed under this heading.

Theophylline Dihydroxypropyl (Glyceryl) (The effect of steady-state immediate-release fluvoxamine maleate tablets (50 mg tablets given b.i.d.) on the pharmacokinetics of a single dose of theophylline (375 mg as 442 mg aminophylline) was evaluated in 12 healthy non-smoking male volunteers. The clearance of theophylline was decreased approximately 3-fold. Therefore if theophylline is co-administered with fluvoxamine maleate, its dose should be reduced to one third of the usual daily maintenance dose and plasma concentrations of theophylline should be monitored. No dosage is required for Luvox CR capsules).

No products indexed under this heading.

Theophylline Ethylenediamine (The effect of steady-state immediate-release fluvoxamine maleate tablets (50 mg tablets given b.i.d.) on the pharmacokinetics of a single dose of theophylline (375 mg as 442 mg aminophylline) was evaluated in 12 healthy non-smoking male volunteers. The clearance of theophylline was decreased approximately 3-fold. Therefore if theophylline is co-administered with fluvoxamine maleate, its dose should be reduced to one third of the usual daily maintenance dose and plasma concentrations of theophylline should be monitored. No dosage is required for Luvox CR capsules).

No products indexed under this heading.

Theophylline Sodium Glycinate (The effect of steady-state immediate-release fluvoxamine maleate tablets (50 mg tablets given b.i.d.) on the pharmacokinetics of a single dose of theophylline (375 mg as 442 mg aminophylline) was evaluated in 12 healthy non-smoking male volunteers. The clearance of theophylline was decreased approximately 3-fold. Therefore if theophylline is co-administered with fluvoxamine maleate, its dose should be reduced to one third of the usual daily maintenance dose and plasma concentrations of theophylline should be monitored. No dosage is required for Luvox CR capsules).

No products indexed under this heading.

Thioridazine (Concentrations of thioridazine and its two active metabolites, mesoridazine and sulforidazine, increased 3-fold following co-administration of fluvoxamine. Thioridazine administration produces a dose related prolongation of the QTc interval, which is associated with serious ventricular arrhythmias, such as torsades de pointes-type arrhythmias, and sudden death. It is likely that this experience underestimates the degree of risk that might occur with higher doses of thioridazine. Moreover, the effect of fluvoxamine may be even more pronounced when it is administered at higher doses. Therefore, co-administration of thioridazine with Luvox CR capsules is contraindicated).

No products indexed under this heading.

Tizanidine (Fluvoxamine, an inhibitor of CYP1A2, and tizandine is a CYP1A2 substrate. Co-administration may increase tizanidine Cmax, AUC, and elimination half-life. Because of the potential for the increased risk of serious adverse reactions, including severe lowering of BP and sedation, co-administration of tizanidine with Luvox CR capsules is contraindicated).

No products indexed under this heading.

Tolmetin Sodium (Serotonin release by platelets plays an important role in hemostasis. Epidemiological studies of the case-control and cohort design that have demonstrated an association between use of psychotropic drugs that interfere with serotonin reuptake and the occurrence of upper GI bleeding. These studies have also shown that concurrent use of an NSAID or aspirin may potentiate this risk of bleeding).

No products indexed under this heading.

Tranylcypromine Sulfate (In patients receiving another serotonin reuptake inhibitor drug in combination with monoamine oxidase inhibitors (MAOIs), there have been reports of serious, sometimes fatal reactions including hyperthermia, rigidity, myoclonus, autonomic instability with possible rapid fluctuations of vital signs, and mental status changes that include extreme agitation progressing to delirium and coma. These reactions have also been reported in patients who have discontinued the drug and have started on an MAOI. Some cases presented with features resembling a serotonin syndrome or neuroleptic malignant syndrome. Therefore, concomitant administration with MAOI, or within 14 days of discontinuing treatment with an MAOI, is contraindicated). Products include:

Parnate Tablets 1532

Triazolam (Benzodiazepines metabolized by hepatic oxidation (eg, alprazolam, midazolam, triazolam) should be used with caution because the clearance of these drugs is likely to be reduced by fluvoxamine. The clearance of benzodiazepines metabolized by glucuronidation (eg, lorazepam, oxazepam, temazepam) is unlikely to be affected by fluvoxamine).

No products indexed under this heading.

Trimethaphan Camsylate (Fluvoxamine is a known potent inhibitor of CYP1A2 and also inhibits CYP3A4, CYP2C9, and CYP2C19).

No products indexed under this heading.

Trimipramine Maleate (Significantly increased plasma TCA levels have been reported with the co-administration of immediate-release fluvoxamine maleate tablets and amitriptyline, clomipramine, or imipramine. Caution is indicated with the co-administration of Luvox CR capsules and TCAs; plasma TCA concentrations may need to be monitored, and the dose of TCA may be reduced).

No products indexed under this heading.

Troglitazone (Fluvoxamine is a known potent inhibitor of CYP1A2 and also inhibits CYP3A4, CYP2C9, and CYP2C19).

No products indexed under this heading.

Troleandomycin (Fluvoxamine is a known potent inhibitor of CYP1A2 and also inhibits CYP3A4, CYP2C9, and CYP2C19).

No products indexed under this heading.

Trovafloxacin Mesylate (Fluvoxamine is a known potent inhibitor of CYP1A2 and also inhibits CYP3A4, CYP2C9, and CYP2C19).

No products indexed under this heading.

Tryptophan (Tryptophan may enhance the serotonergic effects of fluvoxamine, and therefore, the combination should be used with caution. Severe vomiting has been reported with the co-administration of immediate-release fluvoxamine maleate tablets and tryptophan).

No products indexed under this heading.

L-Tryptophan (Tryptophan may enhance the serotonergic effects of fluvoxamine, and therefore, the combination should be used with caution. Severe vomiting has been reported with the co-administration of immediate-release fluvoxamine maleate tablets and tryptophan).

No products indexed under this heading.

Valdecoxib (Serotonin release by platelets plays an important role in hemostasis. Epidemiological studies of the case-control and cohort design that have demonstrated an association between use of psychotropic drugs that interfere with serotonin reuptake and the occurrence of upper GI bleeding. These studies have also shown that concurrent use of an NSAID or aspirin may potentiate this risk of bleeding).

No products indexed under this heading.

Valproate Sodium (Fluvoxamine is a known potent inhibitor of CYP1A2 and also inhibits CYP3A4, CYP2C9, and CYP2C19).

No products indexed under this heading.

Vardenafil Hydrochloride (Fluvoxamine is a known potent inhibitor of CYP1A2 and also inhibits CYP3A4, CYP2C9, and CYP2C19). Products include:

Levitra Tablets 2876

Venlafaxine Hydrochloride (The development of a potentially life-threatening serotonin syndrome may occur with Luvox CR capsules treatment, particularly with concomitant use of serotonergic drugs (including triptans) and with drugs that impair metabolism of serotonin (including MAOIs). Serotonin syndrome symptoms may include mental status changes (eg, agitation, hallucinations, coma), autonomic instability (eg, tachycardia, labile BP, hyperthermia), neuromuscular aberrations (eg, hyperreflexia, incoordination) and/or GI symptoms (eg, nausea, vomiting, diarrhea)). Products include:

Effexor XR Extended-Release Capsules 3195
Venlafaxine Hydrochloride Tablets ... 2199

Verapamil Hydrochloride (Fluvoxamine is a known potent inhibitor of CYP1A2 and also inhibits CYP3A4, CYP2C9, and CYP2C19). Products include:

Tarka Tablets 511

Voriconazole (Fluvoxamine is a known potent inhibitor of CYP1A2 and also inhibits CYP3A4, CYP2C9, and CYP2C19).

No products indexed under this heading.

Warfarin Sodium (When immediate-release fluvoxamine maleate tablets (50 mg given t.i.d.) were administered concomitantly with warfarin for two weeks, warfarin plasma concentrations increased by 98% and prothrombin times were prolonged. Thus patients receiving oral anticoagulants and Luvox CR capsules should have their prothrombin time monitored and their anticoagulant dose adjusted accordingly. No dosage adjustment is required for Luvox CR capsules).

No products indexed under this heading.

Zafirlukast (Fluvoxamine is a known potent inhibitor of CYP1A2 and also inhibits CYP3A4, CYP2C9, and CYP2C19). Products include:

Accolate Tablets 669

Zileuton (Fluvoxamine is a known potent inhibitor of CYP1A2 and also inhibits CYP3A4, CYP2C9, and CYP2C19).

No products indexed under this heading.

Zolmitriptan (The development of a potentially life-threatening serotonin syndrome may occur with Luvox CR capsules treatment, particularly with concomitant use of serotonergic drugs (including triptans) and with drugs that impair metabolism of serotonin (including MAOIs). Serotonin syndrome symptoms may include mental status changes (eg, agitation, hallucinations, coma), autonomic instability (eg, tachycardia, labile BP, hyperthermia), neuromuscular aberrations (eg, hyperreflexia, incoordination) and/or GI symptoms (eg, nausea, vomiting, diarrhea)).
Products include:
Zomig Tablets 694
Zomig Nasal Spray 689
Zomig-ZMT Tablets 694

Food Interactions

Alcohol (Patients should be advised to avoid taking alcohol while taking Luvox CR capsules).

Grapefruit (Fluvoxamine is a known potent inhibitor of CYP1A2 and also inhibits CYP3A4, CYP2C9, and CYP2C19).

Grapefruit Juice (Fluvoxamine is a known potent inhibitor of CYP1A2 and also inhibits CYP3A4, CYP2C9, and CYP2C19).

LUXIQ FOAM

(Betamethasone Valerate) 3058
None cited in PDR database.

LYBREL TABLETS

(Ethinyl Estradiol, Levonorgestrel) 3204
May interact with barbiturates, corticosteroids, cytochrome p450 3a4 inducers (selected), cytochrome p450 3a4 inhibitors (selected), anticonvulsants, estrogens, drugs affecting gastrointestinal motility, drugs which undergo biotransformation by cytochrome p-450 mixed function oxidase, penicillins, protease inhibitors, tetracyclines, and certain other agents. Compounds in these categories include:

Acarbose (Contraceptive effectiveness may be reduced when hormonal contraceptives are co-administered with antibiotics, anticonvulsants, and other drugs that increase the metabolism of contraceptive steroids. This could result in unintended pregnancy or unscheduled bleeding. In such cases a nonhormonal back-up method of birth control should be considered).
Products include:
Precose Tablets 792

Acetaminophen (Acetaminophen increases the bioavailability of ethinyl estradiol since these drugs act as competitive inhibitors for sulfation of ethinyl estradiol in the gastrointestinal wall, a known pathway of elimination for ethinyl estradiol. Decreased plasma concentrations of acetaminophen due to induction of conjugation (particularly glucuronidation) have been noted when this drug is administered with oral contraceptives).
Products include:
Benadryl Allergy & Cold Kapgels 1895
Benadryl Allergy & Sinus Headache Kapgels 1895
Benadryl Severe Allergy & Sinus Headache Caplets 1897
Lortab 5/500 Tablets 3143
Lortab 7.5/500 Tablets 3144
Lortab 10/500 Tablets 3144
Percocet Tablets 1127
Sinutab Sinus Caplets 1905
Sudafed PE Cold & Cough Caplets 1907
Sudafed PE Nighttime Cold Caplets 1907
Sudafed PE Severe Cold Caplets 1908
Sudafed PE Sinus Headache Caplets 1908
Regular Strength Tylenol Tablets 1915
Tylenol 8 Hour Extended Release Caplets 1915
Extra Strength Tylenol Caplets, Cool Caplets, and EZ Tabs 1915
Extra Strength Tylenol Adult Rapid Blast Liquid 1915
Extra Strength Tylenol PM Caplets, Geltabs, Liquid, and Rapid Release Gels 1915
Extra Strength Tylenol Rapid Release Gels 1915
Tylenol with Codeine Tablets 2427
Tylenol Allergy Multi-Symptom Caplets with Cool Burst and Rapid Release Gelcaps 1916
Tylenol Allergy Multi-Symptom Nighttime Caplets with Cool Burst 1916
Tylenol Severe Allergy Caplets 1916
Tylenol Arthritis Pain Extended Release Geltabs/Caplets 1915
Tylenol Chest Congestion Caplets with Cool Burst 1910
Tylenol Chest Congestion Liquid with Cool Burst 1910
Children's Tylenol Plus Cold Suspension Liquid 1912
Children's Tylenol Plus Cold & Allergy Suspension Liquid 1914
Children's Tylenol Plus Cough & Runny Nose Suspension Liquid 1912
Children's Tylenol Plus Cough & Sore Throat Suspension Liquid 1912
Children's Tylenol Plus Flu Suspension Liquid 1914
Children's Tylenol Suspension Liquid 1909
Children's Tylenol Meltaways 1909
Children's Tylenol Plus Multi-Symptom Cold Suspension Liquid 1912
Tylenol Cold Severe Congestion Daytime Caplets with Cool Burst 1912
Tylenol Cold Head Congestion Daytime Caplets with Cool Burst 1910
Tylenol Cold Head Congestion Nighttime Caplets with Cool Burst 1910
Tylenol Cold Head Congestion Severe Daytime Caplets with Cool Burst 1910
Tylenol Cold Multi-Symptom Daytime Caplets with Cool Burst and Rapid Release Gels 1913
Tylenol Cold Multi-Symptom Daytime Liquid with Citrus Burst ... 1913
Tylenol Cold Multi-Symptom Nighttime Caplets with Cool Burst 1913
Tylenol Cold Multi-Symptom Nighttime Liquid with Cool Burst ... 1913
Tylenol Cold Multi-Symptom Severe Caplets with Cool Burst 1913
Tylenol Cold Multi-Symptom Severe Daytime Liquid with Citrus Burst 1913
Tylenol Cough & Sore Throat Daytime Liquid with Cool Burst 1918
Tylenol Cough & Sore Throat Nighttime Liquid with Cool Burst ... 1918
Concentrated Tylenol Infants' Drops 1909
Jr. Tylenol Meltaways 1909
Tylenol Sinus Congestion & Pain Daytime Caplets with Cool Burst and Gelcaps 1917
Tylenol Sinus Congestion & Pain Nighttime Caplets with Cool Burst 1917
Tylenol Sinus Congestion & Pain Severe Caplets with Cool Burst 1917
Tylenol Sinus Severe Congestion Caplets with Cool Burst 1917
Tylenol Sore Throat Daytime Liquid with Cool Burst 1918
Tylenol Sore Throat Nighttime Liquid with Cool Burst 1918
Women's Tylenol Menstrual Relief Caplets 1919
Vicks DayQuil Cold & Flu Multi-Symptom Relief .... ■616
Vicks DayQuil LiquiCaps 2567
Vicks DayQuil Liquid 2567
Vicks DayQuil Multi-Symptom Cold/Flu Relief 2567
Vicks NyQuil Cold & Flu Multi-Symptom Relief .... ■617
Vicks NyQuil LiquiCaps 2567
Vicks NyQuil Liquid 2567
Vicks NyQuil Multi-Symptom Cold/Flu Relief 2567
Vicodin Tablets 529
Vicodin ES Tablets 530
Vicodin HP Tablets 531
Zydone Tablets 1132

Acetazolamide (CYP 3A4 inhibitors such as indinavir, itraconazole, ketoconazole, fluconazole, and troleandomycin may increase plasma hormone levels. Troleandomycin may also increase the risk of intrahepatic cholestasis during co-administration with combination oral contraceptives).
No products indexed under this heading.

Alatrofloxacin Mesylate (Contraceptive effectiveness may be reduced when hormonal contraceptives are co-administered with antibiotics, anticonvulsants, and other drugs that increase the metabolism of contraceptive steroids. This could result in unintended pregnancy or unscheduled bleeding. In such cases a nonhormonal back-up method of birth control should be considered).
No products indexed under this heading.

Albuterol (Enterohepatic recirculation of estrogens may also be decreased by substances that reduce gut transit time).
No products indexed under this heading.

Albuterol Sulfate (Enterohepatic recirculation of estrogens may also be decreased by substances that reduce gut transit time). Products include:
Combivent Inhalation Aerosol 845
ProAir HFA Inhalation Aerosol 3113
Proventil HFA Inhalation Aerosol 2914
Ventolin HFA Inhalation Aerosol 1638

Alfentanil Hydrochloride (Contraceptive effectiveness may be reduced when hormonal contraceptives are co-administered with antibiotics, anticonvulsants, and other drugs that increase the metabolism of contraceptive steroids. This could result in unintended pregnancy or unscheduled bleeding. In such cases a nonhormonal back-up method of birth control should be considered).
No products indexed under this heading.

Allium sativum (Contraceptive effectiveness may be reduced when hormonal contraceptives are co-administered with antibiotics, anticonvulsants, and other drugs that increase the metabolism of contraceptive steroids. This could result in unintended pregnancy or unscheduled bleeding. In such cases a nonhormonal back-up method of birth control should be considered).
No products indexed under this heading.

Alprazolam (Contraceptive effectiveness may be reduced when hormonal contraceptives are co-administered with antibiotics, anticonvulsants, and other drugs that increase the metabolism of contraceptive steroids. This could result in unintended pregnancy or unscheduled bleeding. In such cases a nonhormonal back-up method of birth control should be considered).
No products indexed under this heading.

5-Amino-Salicylic Acid (Several cases of contraceptive failure and unscheduled bleeding have been reported in the literature with concomitant administration of antibiotics such as ampicillin and other penicillins, and tetracyclines. However, clinical pharmacology studies investigating drug interactions between combined oral contraceptives and these antibiotics have reported inconsistent results).
No products indexed under this heading.

Aminophylline (Contraceptive effectiveness may be reduced when hormonal contraceptives are co-administered with antibiotics, anticonvulsants, and other drugs that increase the metabolism of contraceptive steroids. This could result in unintended pregnancy or unscheduled bleeding. In such cases a nonhormonal back-up method of birth control should be considered).
No products indexed under this heading.

Amiodarone Hydrochloride (Contraceptive effectiveness may be reduced when hormonal contraceptives are co-administered with antibiotics, anticonvulsants, and other drugs that increase the metabolism of contraceptive steroids. This could result in unintended pregnancy or unscheduled bleeding. In such cases a nonhormonal back-up method of birth control should be considered).
No products indexed under this heading.

Amitriptyline Hydrochloride (Contraceptive effectiveness may be reduced when hormonal contraceptives are co-administered with antibiotics, anticonvulsants, and other drugs that increase the metabolism of contraceptive steroids. This could result in unintended pregnancy or unscheduled bleeding. In such cases a nonhormonal back-up method of birth control should be considered).
No products indexed under this heading.

Amlodipine Besylate (Contraceptive effectiveness may be reduced when hormonal contraceptives are co-administered with antibiotics, anticonvulsants, and other drugs that increase the metabolism of contraceptive steroids. This could result in unintended pregnancy or unscheduled bleeding. In such cases a nonhormonal back-up method of birth control should be considered).
Products include:
Azor Tablets 1005
Exforge Tablets 2238

Amoxapine (Contraceptive effectiveness may be reduced when hormonal contraceptives are co-administered with antibiotics, anticonvulsants, and other drugs that increase the metabolism of contraceptive steroids. This could result in unintended pregnancy or unscheduled bleeding. In such cases a nonhormonal back-up method of birth control should be considered).
No products indexed under this heading.

Amoxicillin (Several cases of contraceptive failure and unscheduled bleeding have been reported in the literature with concomitant administration of antibiotics such as ampicillin and other penicillins, and tetracyclines. However, clinical pharmacology studies investigating drug interactions between combined oral contraceptives and these antibiotics have reported inconsistent results). Products include:
Amoxil Capsules **1305**
Amoxil Chewable Tablets **1305**
Amoxil Pediatric Drops for Oral Suspension **1305**
Amoxil Powder for Oral Suspension **1305**
Amoxil Tablets **1305**
Augmentin **1323**
Augmentin Tablets **1327**
Augmentin XR Extended Release Tablets **1333**
Augmentin ES-600 Powder for Oral Suspension **1329**
Moxatag Tablets **2165**

Amoxicillin Trihydrate (Several cases of contraceptive failure and unscheduled bleeding have been reported in the literature with concomitant administration of antibiotics such as ampicillin and other penicillins, and tetracyclines. However, clinical pharmacology studies investigating drug interactions between combined oral contraceptives and these antibiotics have reported inconsistent results).
No products indexed under this heading.

Amphetamine Aspartate (Contraceptive effectiveness may be reduced when hormonal contraceptives are co-administered with antibiotics, anticonvulsants, and other drugs that increase the metabolism of contraceptive steroids. This could result in unintended pregnancy or unscheduled bleeding. In such cases a nonhormonal back-up method of birth control should be considered). Products include:
Adderall XR Capsules **3012**

Amphetamine Aspartate Monohydrate (Contraceptive effectiveness may be reduced when hormonal contraceptives are co-administered with antibiotics, anticonvulsants, and other drugs that increase the metabolism of contraceptive steroids. This could result in unintended pregnancy or unscheduled bleeding. In such cases a nonhormonal back-up method of birth control should be considered).
No products indexed under this heading.

Amphetamine Sulfate (Contraceptive effectiveness may be reduced when hormonal contraceptives are co-administered with antibiotics, anticonvulsants, and other drugs that increase the metabolism of contraceptive steroids. This could result in unintended pregnancy or unscheduled bleeding. In such cases a nonhormonal back-up method of birth control should be considered). Products include:
Adderall XR Capsules **3012**

Ampicillin (Several cases of contraceptive failure and unscheduled bleeding have been reported in the literature with concomitant administration of antibiotics such as ampicillin and other penicillins, and tetracyclines. However, clinical pharmacology studies investigating drug interactions between combined oral contraceptives and these antibiotics have reported inconsistent results).
No products indexed under this heading.

Ampicillin Sodium (Several cases of contraceptive failure and unscheduled bleeding have been reported in the literature with concomitant administration of antibiotics such as ampicillin and other penicillins, and tetracyclines. However, clinical pharmacology studies investigating drug interactions between combined oral contraceptives and these antibiotics have reported inconsistent results).
No products indexed under this heading.

Ampicillin Trihydrate (Several cases of contraceptive failure and unscheduled bleeding have been reported in the literature with concomitant administration of antibiotics such as ampicillin and other penicillins, and tetracyclines. However, clinical pharmacology studies investigating drug interactions between combined oral contraceptives and these antibiotics have reported inconsistent results).
No products indexed under this heading.

Amprenavir (Several of the anti-HIV protease inhibitors have been studied with co-administration of oral combination hormonal contraceptives; significant changes (increase and decrease) in the plasma levels of the estrogen and progestin have been noted in some cases. The safety and efficacy of oral contraceptive products may be affected with co-administration of anti-HIV protease inhibitors. Health care professionals should refer to the label of the individual anti-HIV protease inhibitors for further drug-drug interaction information).
No products indexed under this heading.

Anastrozole (CYP 3A4 inhibitors such as indinavir, itraconazole, ketoconazole, fluconazole, and troleandomycin may increase plasma hormone levels. Troleandomycin may also increase the risk of intrahepatic cholestasis during co-administration with combination oral contraceptives). Products include:
Arimidex Tablets **672**

Aprepitant (Contraceptive effectiveness may be reduced when hormonal contraceptives are co-administered with antibiotics, anticonvulsants, and other drugs that increase the metabolism of contraceptive steroids. This could result in unintended pregnancy or unscheduled bleeding. In such cases a nonhormonal back-up method of birth control should be considered). Products include:
Emend Capsules **1992**

Aprobarbital (Contraceptive effectiveness may be reduced when hormonal contraceptives are co-administered with antibiotics, anticonvulsants, and other drugs that increase the metabolism of contraceptive steroids. This could result in unintended pregnancy or unscheduled bleeding. In such cases a nonhormonal back-up method of birth control should be considered).
No products indexed under this heading.

Astemizole (Contraceptive effectiveness may be reduced when hormonal contraceptives are co-administered with antibiotics, anticonvulsants, and other drugs that increase the metabolism of contraceptive steroids. This could result in unintended pregnancy or unscheduled bleeding. In such cases a nonhormonal back-up method of birth control should be considered).
No products indexed under this heading.

Atazanavir (CYP 3A4 inhibitors such as indinavir, itraconazole, ketoconazole, fluconazole, and troleandomycin may increase plasma hormone levels. Troleandomycin may also increase the risk of intrahepatic cholestasis during co-administration with combination oral contraceptives).
No products indexed under this heading.

Atazanavir Sulfate (CYP 3A4 inhibitors such as indinavir, itraconazole, ketoconazole, fluconazole, and troleandomycin may increase plasma hormone levels. Troleandomycin may also increase the risk of intrahepatic cholestasis during co-administration with combination oral contraceptives). Products include:
Reyataz Capsules **3299**

Atomoxetine Hydrochloride (Contraceptive effectiveness may be reduced when hormonal contraceptives are co-administered with antibiotics, anticonvulsants, and other drugs that increase the metabolism of contraceptive steroids. This could result in unintended pregnancy or unscheduled bleeding. In such cases a nonhormonal back-up method of birth control should be considered). Products include:
Strattera Capsules **1864**

Atorvastatin Calcium (Co-administration of atorvastatin increases AUC values for ethinyl estradiol by approximately 20%). Products include:
Lipitor Tablets **2501**

Atropine Sulfate (Enterohepatic recirculation of estrogens may also be decreased by substances that reduce gut transit time). Products include:
Donnatal Extentabs **2507**

Azatadine Maleate (Enterohepatic recirculation of estrogens may also be decreased by substances that reduce gut transit time).
No products indexed under this heading.

Azlocillin Sodium (Several cases of contraceptive failure and unscheduled bleeding have been reported in the literature with concomitant administration of antibiotics such as ampicillin and other penicillins, and tetracyclines. However, clinical pharmacology studies investigating drug interactions between combined oral contraceptives and these antibiotics have reported inconsistent results).
No products indexed under this heading.

Bacampicillin Hydrochloride (Several cases of contraceptive failure and unscheduled bleeding have been reported in the literature with concomitant administration of antibiotics such as ampicillin and other penicillins, and tetracyclines. However, clinical pharmacology studies investigating drug interactions between combined oral contraceptives and these antibiotics have reported inconsistent results).
No products indexed under this heading.

Belladonna Alkaloids (Enterohepatic recirculation of estrogens may also be decreased by substances that reduce gut transit time). Products include:
Hyland's Teething Tablets **621**

Belladonna Ergotamine (Contraceptive effectiveness may be reduced when hormonal contraceptives are co-administered with antibiotics, anticonvulsants, and other drugs that increase the metabolism of contraceptive steroids. This could result in unintended pregnancy or unscheduled bleeding. In such cases a nonhormonal back-up method of birth control should be considered).
No products indexed under this heading.

Benzphetamine Hydrochloride (Contraceptive effectiveness may be reduced when hormonal contraceptives are co-administered with antibiotics, anticonvulsants, and other drugs that increase the metabolism of contraceptive steroids. This could result in unintended pregnancy or unscheduled bleeding. In such cases a nonhormonal back-up method of birth control should be considered).
No products indexed under this heading.

Benztropine Mesylate (Enterohepatic recirculation of estrogens may also be decreased by substances that reduce gut transit time).
No products indexed under this heading.

Bepridil Hydrochloride (Enterohepatic recirculation of estrogens may also be decreased by substances that reduce gut transit time).
No products indexed under this heading.

Betamethasone Acetate (Contraceptive effectiveness may be reduced when hormonal contraceptives are co-administered with antibiotics, anticonvulsants, and other drugs that increase the metabolism of contraceptive steroids. This could result in unintended pregnancy or unscheduled bleeding. In such cases a nonhormonal back-up method of birth control should be considered).
No products indexed under this heading.

Betamethasone Sodium Phosphate (Contraceptive effectiveness may be reduced when hormonal contraceptives are co-administered with antibiotics, anticonvulsants, and other drugs that increase the metabolism of contraceptive steroids. This could result in unintended pregnancy or unscheduled bleeding. In such cases a nonhormonal back-up method of birth control should be considered).
No products indexed under this heading.

Bethanechol Chloride (Enterohepatic recirculation of estrogens may also be decreased by substances that reduce gut transit time).
No products indexed under this heading.

Biperiden Hydrochloride (Enterohepatic recirculation of estrogens may also be decreased by substances that reduce gut transit time).
No products indexed under this heading.

Bisoprolol Fumarate (Contraceptive effectiveness may be reduced when hormonal contraceptives are co-administered with antibiotics, anticonvulsants, and other drugs that increase the metabolism of contraceptive steroids. This could result in unintended pregnancy or unscheduled bleeding. In such cases a nonhormonal back-up method of birth control should be considered).
No products indexed under this heading.

Bitolterol Mesylate (Enterohepatic recirculation of estrogens may also be decreased by substances that reduce gut transit time).
No products indexed under this heading.

Bromocriptine Mesylate (Enterohepatic recirculation of estrogens may also be decreased by substances that reduce gut transit time).
No products indexed under this heading.

Bromodiphenhydramine Hydrochloride (Enterohepatic recirculation of estrogens may also be decreased by substances that reduce gut transit time).
No products indexed under this heading.

Brompheniramine Maleate (Enterohepatic recirculation of estrogens may also be decreased by substances that reduce gut transit time).
No products indexed under this heading.

Budesonide (Increased plasma concentrations of cyclosporine, prednisolone and other corticosteroids, have been reported with concomitant administration of oral contraceptives). Products include:
Pulmicort Flexhaler 654
Symbicort 80/4.5 Inhalation Aerosol 659
Symbicort 160/4.5 Inhalation Aerosol 659

Buprenorphine Hydrochloride (Enterohepatic recirculation of estrogens may also be decreased by substances that reduce gut transit time).
Products include:
Suboxone Tablets 2601
Subutex Tablets 2601

Buspirone Hydrochloride (Contraceptive effectiveness may be reduced when hormonal contraceptives are co-administered with antibiotics, anticonvulsants, and other drugs that increase the metabolism of contraceptive steroids. This could result in unintended pregnancy or unscheduled bleeding. In such cases a nonhormonal back-up method of birth control should be considered).
No products indexed under this heading.

Busulfan (Contraceptive effectiveness may be reduced when hormonal contraceptives are co-administered with antibiotics, anticonvulsants, and other drugs that increase the metabolism of contraceptive steroids. This could result in unintended pregnancy or unscheduled bleeding. In such cases a nonhormonal back-up method of birth control should be considered).
Products include:
Busulfex Injection 2477
Myleran Tablets 1530

Butabarbital (Contraceptive effectiveness may be reduced when hormonal contraceptives are co-administered with antibiotics, anticonvulsants, and other drugs that increase the metabolism of contraceptive steroids. This could result in unintended pregnancy or unscheduled bleeding. In such cases a nonhormonal back-up method of birth control should be considered).
No products indexed under this heading.

Butalbital (Contraceptive effectiveness may be reduced when hormonal contraceptives are co-administered with antibiotics, anticonvulsants, and other drugs that increase the metabolism of contraceptive steroids. This could result in unintended pregnancy or unscheduled bleeding. In such cases a nonhormonal back-up method of birth control should be considered).
No products indexed under this heading.

Caffeine (Contraceptive effectiveness may be reduced when hormonal contraceptives are co-administered with antibiotics, anticonvulsants, and other drugs that increase the metabolism of contraceptive steroids. This could result in unintended pregnancy or unscheduled bleeding. In such cases a nonhormonal back-up method of birth control should be considered).
Products include:
BioLean Free Tablets .... ▣635
BioLean II Tablets .... ▣635
Winrgy Dietary Supplement .... ▣642

Caffeine Anhydrous (Contraceptive effectiveness may be reduced when hormonal contraceptives are co-administered with antibiotics, anticonvulsants, and other drugs that increase the metabolism of contraceptive steroids. This could result in unintended pregnancy or unscheduled bleeding. In such cases a nonhormonal back-up method of birth control should be considered).
No products indexed under this heading.

Caffeine Citrate (Contraceptive effectiveness may be reduced when hormonal contraceptives are co-administered with antibiotics, anticonvulsants, and other drugs that increase the metabolism of contraceptive steroids. This could result in unintended pregnancy or unscheduled bleeding. In such cases a nonhormonal back-up method of birth control should be considered).
No products indexed under this heading.

Candesartan Cilexetil (Contraceptive effectiveness may be reduced when hormonal contraceptives are co-administered with antibiotics, anticonvulsants, and other drugs that increase the metabolism of contraceptive steroids. This could result in unintended pregnancy or unscheduled bleeding. In such cases a nonhormonal back-up method of birth control should be considered).
Products include:
Atacand Tablets 639
Atacand HCT 642

Captopril (Contraceptive effectiveness may be reduced when hormonal contraceptives are co-administered with antibiotics, anticonvulsants, and other drugs that increase the metabolism of contraceptive steroids. This could result in unintended pregnancy or unscheduled bleeding. In such cases a nonhormonal back-up method of birth control should be considered).
Products include:
Captopril Tablets 2182

Carbamazepine (Contraceptive effectiveness may be reduced when hormonal contraceptives are co-administered with antibiotics, anticonvulsants, and other drugs that increase the metabolism of contraceptive steroids. This could result in unintended pregnancy or unscheduled bleeding. In such cases a nonhormonal back-up method of birth control should be considered).
Products include:
Carbatrol Capsules 3019
Equetro Extended-Release Capsules 3174

Carbenicillin Disodium (Several cases of contraceptive failure and unscheduled bleeding have been reported in the literature with concomitant administration of antibiotics such as ampicillin and other penicillins, and tetracyclines. However, clinical pharmacology studies investigating drug interactions between combined oral contraceptives and these antibiotics have reported inconsistent results).
No products indexed under this heading.

Carbenicillin Indanyl Sodium (Several cases of contraceptive failure and unscheduled bleeding have been reported in the literature with concomitant administration of antibiotics such as ampicillin and other penicillins, and tetracyclines. However, clinical pharmacology studies investigating drug interactions between combined oral contraceptives and these antibiotics have reported inconsistent results).
No products indexed under this heading.

Carisoprodol (Contraceptive effectiveness may be reduced when hormonal contraceptives are co-administered with antibiotics, anticonvulsants, and other drugs that increase the metabolism of contraceptive steroids. This could result in unintended pregnancy or unscheduled bleeding. In such cases a nonhormonal back-up method of birth control should be considered).
Products include:
Soma Tablets 1931

Carvedilol (Contraceptive effectiveness may be reduced when hormonal contraceptives are co-administered with antibiotics, anticonvulsants, and other drugs that increase the metabolism of contraceptive steroids. This could result in unintended pregnancy or unscheduled bleeding. In such cases a nonhormonal back-up method of birth control should be considered).
Products include:
Coreg Tablets 1387

Celecoxib (Contraceptive effectiveness may be reduced when hormonal contraceptives are co-administered with antibiotics, anticonvulsants, and other drugs that increase the metabolism of contraceptive steroids. This could result in unintended pregnancy or unscheduled bleeding. In such cases a nonhormonal back-up method of birth control should be considered).
Products include:
Celebrex Capsules 2979

Cerivastatin Sodium (Contraceptive effectiveness may be reduced when hormonal contraceptives are co-administered with antibiotics, anticonvulsants, and other drugs that increase the metabolism of contraceptive steroids. This could result in unintended pregnancy or unscheduled bleeding. In such cases a nonhormonal back-up method of birth control should be considered).
No products indexed under this heading.

Cevimeline Hydrochloride (Contraceptive effectiveness may be reduced when hormonal contraceptives are co-administered with antibiotics, anticonvulsants, and other drugs that increase the metabolism of contraceptive steroids. This could result in unintended pregnancy or unscheduled bleeding. In such cases a nonhormonal back-up method of birth control should be considered).
Products include:
Evoxac Capsules 1013

Chlordiazepoxide (Contraceptive effectiveness may be reduced when hormonal contraceptives are co-administered with antibiotics, anticonvulsants, and other drugs that increase the metabolism of contraceptive steroids. This could result in unintended pregnancy or unscheduled bleeding. In such cases a nonhormonal back-up method of birth control should be considered).
No products indexed under this heading.

Chlordiazepoxide Hydrochloride (Contraceptive effectiveness may be reduced when hormonal contraceptives are co-administered with antibiotics, anticonvulsants, and other drugs that increase the metabolism of contraceptive steroids. This could result in unintended pregnancy or unscheduled bleeding. In such cases a nonhormonal back-up method of birth control should be considered).
No products indexed under this heading.

Chlorotrianisene (Co-administration of certain oral contraceptives containing ethinyl estradiol increases AUC values for ethinyl estradiol by approximately 20%).
No products indexed under this heading.

Chlorpheniramine (Contraceptive effectiveness may be reduced when hormonal contraceptives are co-administered with antibiotics, anticonvulsants, and other drugs that increase the metabolism of contraceptive steroids. This could result in unintended pregnancy or unscheduled bleeding. In such cases a nonhormonal back-up method of birth control should be considered).
No products indexed under this heading.

Chlorpheniramine Maleate (Contraceptive effectiveness may be reduced when hormonal contraceptives are co-administered with antibiotics, anticonvulsants, and other drugs that increase the metabolism of contraceptive steroids. This could result in unintended pregnancy or unscheduled bleeding. In such cases a nonhormonal back-up method of birth control should be considered). Products include:

Actifed Cold & Allergy Tablets **1895**
Sudafed PE Sinus & Allergy Tablets **1908**
Tylenol Allergy Multi-Symptom Caplets with Cool Burst and Rapid Release Gelcaps **1916**
Children's Tylenol Plus Cold Suspension Liquid **1912**
Children's Tylenol Plus Cough & Runny Nose Suspension Liquid **1912**
Children's Tylenol Plus Flu Suspension Liquid **1914**
Children's Tylenol Plus Multi-Symptom Cold Suspension Liquid **1912**
Tylenol Cold Head Congestion Nighttime Caplets with Cool Burst **1910**
Tylenol Cold Multi-Symptom Nighttime Caplets with Cool Burst **1913**
Tylenol Sinus Congestion & Pain Nighttime Caplets with Cool Burst **1917**

Chlorpheniramine Polistirex (Contraceptive effectiveness may be reduced when hormonal contraceptives are co-administered with antibiotics, anticonvulsants, and other drugs that increase the metabolism of contraceptive steroids. This could result in unintended pregnancy or unscheduled bleeding. In such cases a nonhormonal back-up method of birth control should be considered). Products include:

Tussionex Pennkinetic Extended-Release Suspension **3154**

Chlorpheniramine Tannate (Contraceptive effectiveness may be reduced when hormonal contraceptives are co-administered with antibiotics, anticonvulsants, and other drugs that increase the metabolism of contraceptive steroids. This could result in unintended pregnancy or unscheduled bleeding. In such cases a nonhormonal back-up method of birth control should be considered).

No products indexed under this heading.

Chlorpromazine (Contraceptive effectiveness may be reduced when hormonal contraceptives are co-administered with antibiotics, anticonvulsants, and other drugs that increase the metabolism of contraceptive steroids. This could result in unintended pregnancy or unscheduled bleeding. In such cases a nonhormonal back-up method of birth control should be considered).

No products indexed under this heading.

Chlorpromazine Hydrochloride (Contraceptive effectiveness may be reduced when hormonal contraceptives are co-administered with antibiotics, anticonvulsants, and other drugs that increase the metabolism of contraceptive steroids. This could result in unintended pregnancy or unscheduled bleeding. In such cases a nonhormonal back-up method of birth control should be considered).

No products indexed under this heading.

Chlorpropamide (Contraceptive effectiveness may be reduced when hormonal contraceptives are co-administered with antibiotics, anticonvulsants, and other drugs that increase the metabolism of contraceptive steroids. This could result in unintended pregnancy or unscheduled bleeding. In such cases a nonhormonal back-up method of birth control should be considered).

No products indexed under this heading.

Ciclesonide (Increased plasma concentrations of cyclosporine, prednisolone and other corticosteroids, have been reported with concomitant administration of oral contraceptives). Products include:

Alvesco Inhalation Aerosol **2985**
Omnaris Nasal Spray **2998**

Cilostazol (Contraceptive effectiveness may be reduced when hormonal contraceptives are co-administered with antibiotics, anticonvulsants, and other drugs that increase the metabolism of contraceptive steroids. This could result in unintended pregnancy or unscheduled bleeding. In such cases a nonhormonal back-up method of birth control should be considered). Products include:

Pletal Tablets **2481**

Cimetidine (CYP 3A4 inhibitors such as indinavir, itraconazole, ketoconazole, fluconazole, and troleandomycin may increase plasma hormone levels. Troleandomycin may also increase the risk of intrahepatic cholestasis during co-administration with combination oral contraceptives).

No products indexed under this heading.

Cimetidine Hydrochloride (Contraceptive effectiveness may be reduced when hormonal contraceptives are co-administered with antibiotics, anticonvulsants, and other drugs that increase the metabolism of contraceptive steroids. This could result in unintended pregnancy or unscheduled bleeding. In such cases a nonhormonal back-up method of birth control should be considered).

No products indexed under this heading.

Ciprofloxacin (Contraceptive effectiveness may be reduced when hormonal contraceptives are co-administered with antibiotics, anticonvulsants, and other drugs that increase the metabolism of contraceptive steroids. This could result in unintended pregnancy or unscheduled bleeding. In such cases a nonhormonal back-up method of birth control should be considered). Products include:

Cipro I.V. **2817**
Cipro Oral Suspension **2810**
Cipro XR Tablets **2823**
Ciprodex Otic Suspension **541**

Ciprofloxacin Hydrochloride (Contraceptive effectiveness may be reduced when hormonal contraceptives are co-administered with antibiotics, anticonvulsants, and other drugs that increase the metabolism of contraceptive steroids. This could result in unintended pregnancy or unscheduled bleeding. In such cases a nonhormonal back-up method of birth control should be considered). Products include:

Cipro Tablets **2810**

Cisapride (Contraceptive effectiveness may be reduced when hormonal contraceptives are co-administered with antibiotics, anticonvulsants, and other drugs that increase the metabolism of contraceptive steroids. This could result in unintended pregnancy or unscheduled bleeding. In such cases a nonhormonal back-up method of birth control should be considered).

No products indexed under this heading.

Cisplatin (Contraceptive effectiveness may be reduced when hormonal contraceptives are co-administered with antibiotics, anticonvulsants, and other drugs that increase the metabolism of contraceptive steroids. This could result in unintended pregnancy or unscheduled bleeding. In such cases a nonhormonal back-up method of birth control should be considered).

No products indexed under this heading.

Citalopram Hydrobromide (Contraceptive effectiveness may be reduced when hormonal contraceptives are co-administered with antibiotics, anticonvulsants, and other drugs that increase the metabolism of contraceptive steroids. This could result in unintended pregnancy or unscheduled bleeding. In such cases a nonhormonal back-up method of birth control should be considered). Products include:

Celexa **1160**

Clarithromycin (Contraceptive effectiveness may be reduced when hormonal contraceptives are co-administered with antibiotics, anticonvulsants, and other drugs that increase the metabolism of contraceptive steroids. This could result in unintended pregnancy or unscheduled bleeding. In such cases a nonhormonal back-up method of birth control should be considered). Products include:

Biaxin/Biaxin XL **411**

Clemastine Fumarate (Enterohepatic recirculation of estrogens may also be decreased by substances that reduce gut transit time).

No products indexed under this heading.

Clidinium Bromide (Enterohepatic recirculation of estrogens may also be decreased by substances that reduce gut transit time).

No products indexed under this heading.

Clofibric Acid (Increased clearance of clofibric acid, due to induction of conjugation (particularly glucuronidation), have been noted when this drug is administered with oral contraceptives).

No products indexed under this heading.

Clomipramine Hydrochloride (Contraceptive effectiveness may be reduced when hormonal contraceptives are co-administered with antibiotics, anticonvulsants, and other drugs that increase the metabolism of contraceptive steroids. This could result in unintended pregnancy or unscheduled bleeding. In such cases a nonhormonal back-up method of birth control should be considered).

No products indexed under this heading.

Clopidogrel Hydrogen Sulfate (Contraceptive effectiveness may be reduced when hormonal contraceptives are co-administered with antibiotics, anticonvulsants, and other drugs that increase the metabolism of contraceptive steroids. This could result in unintended pregnancy or unscheduled bleeding. In such cases a nonhormonal back-up method of birth control should be considered).

No products indexed under this heading.

Clotrimazole (CYP 3A4 inhibitors such as indinavir, itraconazole, ketoconazole, fluconazole, and troleandomycin may increase plasma hormone levels. Troleandomycin may also increase the risk of intrahepatic cholestasis during co-administration with combination oral contraceptives). Products include:

Lotrisone **2881**

Clozapine (Contraceptive effectiveness may be reduced when hormonal contraceptives are co-administered with antibiotics, anticonvulsants, and other drugs that increase the metabolism of contraceptive steroids. This could result in unintended pregnancy or unscheduled bleeding. In such cases a nonhormonal back-up method of birth control should be considered).

No products indexed under this heading.

Codeine Phosphate (Contraceptive effectiveness may be reduced when hormonal contraceptives are co-administered with antibiotics, anticonvulsants, and other drugs that increase the metabolism of contraceptive steroids. This could result in unintended pregnancy or unscheduled bleeding. In such cases a nonhormonal back-up method of birth control should be considered). Products include:

Tylenol with Codeine Tablets **2427**

Codeine Sulfate (Contraceptive effectiveness may be reduced when hormonal contraceptives are co-administered with antibiotics, anticonvulsants, and other drugs that increase the metabolism of contraceptive steroids. This could result in unintended pregnancy or unscheduled bleeding. In such cases a nonhormonal back-up method of birth control should be considered).

No products indexed under this heading.

Cortisone Acetate (Contraceptive effectiveness may be reduced when hormonal contraceptives are co-administered with antibiotics, anticonvulsants, and other drugs that increase the metabolism of contraceptive steroids. This could result in unintended pregnancy or unscheduled bleeding. In such cases a nonhormonal back-up method of birth control should be considered).

No products indexed under this heading.

Cyclobenzaprine (Contraceptive effectiveness may be reduced when hormonal contraceptives are co-administered with antibiotics, anticonvulsants, and other drugs that increase the metabolism of contraceptive steroids. This could result in unintended pregnancy or unscheduled bleeding. In such cases a nonhormonal back-up method of birth control should be considered).

No products indexed under this heading.

Cyclobenzaprine Hydrochloride (Contraceptive effectiveness may be reduced when hormonal contraceptives are co-administered with antibiotics, anticonvulsants, and other drugs that increase the metabolism of contraceptive steroids. This could result in unintended pregnancy or unscheduled bleeding. In such cases a nonhormonal back-up method of birth control should be considered). Products include:

Amrix Capsules **966**

Cyclophosphamide (Contraceptive effectiveness may be reduced when hormonal contraceptives are co-administered with antibiotics, anticonvulsants, and other drugs that increase the metabolism of contraceptive steroids. This could result in unintended pregnancy or unscheduled bleeding. In such cases a nonhormonal back-up method of birth control should be considered).

No products indexed under this heading.

Cyclosporine (Contraceptive effectiveness may be reduced when hormonal contraceptives are co-administered with antibiotics, anticonvulsants, and other drugs that increase the metabolism of contraceptive steroids. This could result in unintended pregnancy or unscheduled bleeding. In such cases a nonhormonal back-up method of birth control should be considered). Products include:

Gengraf Capsules **435**
Neoral Oral Solution **2280**
Neoral Soft Gelatin Capsules **2280**
Restasis Ophthalmic Emulsion **557**
Sandimmune **2296**

Cyproheptadine Hydrochloride (Enterohepatic recirculation of estrogens may also be decreased by substances that reduce gut transit time).

No products indexed under this heading.

Dalfopristin (CYP 3A4 inhibitors such as indinavir, itraconazole, ketoconazole, fluconazole, and troleandomycin may increase plasma hormone levels. Troleandomycin may also increase the risk of intrahepatic cholestasis during co-administration with combination oral contraceptives).

No products indexed under this heading.

Danazol (CYP 3A4 inhibitors such as indinavir, itraconazole, ketoconazole, fluconazole, and troleandomycin may increase plasma hormone levels. Troleandomycin may also increase the risk of intrahepatic cholestasis during co-administration with combination oral contraceptives).

No products indexed under this heading.

Darunavir (Several of the anti-HIV protease inhibitors have been studied with co-administration of oral combination hormonal contraceptives; significant changes (increase and decrease) in the plasma levels of the estrogen and progestin have been noted in some cases. The safety and efficacy of oral contraceptive products may be affected with co-administration of anti-HIV protease inhibitors. Health care professionals should refer to the label of the individual anti-HIV protease inhibitors for further drug-drug interaction information).

No products indexed under this heading.

Delavirdine Mesylate (CYP 3A4 inhibitors such as indinavir, itraconazole, ketoconazole, fluconazole, and troleandomycin may increase plasma hormone levels. Troleandomycin may also increase the risk of intrahepatic cholestasis during co-administration with combination oral contraceptives).

No products indexed under this heading.

Demeclocycline Hydrochloride (Several cases of contraceptive failure and unscheduled bleeding have been reported in the literature with concomitant administration of antibiotics such as ampicillin and other penicillins, and tetracyclines. However, clinical pharmacology studies investigating drug interactions between combined oral contraceptives and these antibiotics have reported inconsistent results).

No products indexed under this heading.

Desipramine Hydrochloride (Contraceptive effectiveness may be reduced when hormonal contraceptives are co-administered with antibiotics, anticonvulsants, and other drugs that increase the metabolism of contraceptive steroids. This could result in unintended pregnancy or unscheduled bleeding. In such cases a nonhormonal back-up method of birth control should be considered).

No products indexed under this heading.

Desogestrel (Contraceptive effectiveness may be reduced when hormonal contraceptives are co-administered with antibiotics, anticonvulsants, and other drugs that increase the metabolism of contraceptive steroids. This could result in unintended pregnancy or unscheduled bleeding. In such cases a nonhormonal back-up method of birth control should be considered). Products include:

Mircette Tablets **1034**

Dexamethasone (Contraceptive effectiveness may be reduced when hormonal contraceptives are co-administered with antibiotics, anticonvulsants, and other drugs that increase the metabolism of contraceptive steroids. This could result in unintended pregnancy or unscheduled bleeding. In such cases a nonhormonal back-up method of birth control should be considered). Products include:

Ciprodex Otic Suspension **541**

Dexamethasone Acetate (Contraceptive effectiveness may be reduced when hormonal contraceptives are co-administered with antibiotics, anticonvulsants, and other drugs that increase the metabolism of contraceptive steroids. This could result in unintended pregnancy or unscheduled bleeding. In such cases a nonhormonal back-up method of birth control should be considered).

No products indexed under this heading.

Dexamethasone Phosphate (Contraceptive effectiveness may be reduced when hormonal contraceptives are co-administered with antibiotics, anticonvulsants, and other drugs that increase the metabolism of contraceptive steroids. This could result in unintended pregnancy or unscheduled bleeding. In such cases a nonhormonal back-up method of birth control should be considered).

No products indexed under this heading.

Dexamethasone Sodium (Contraceptive effectiveness may be reduced when hormonal contraceptives are co-administered with antibiotics, anticonvulsants, and other drugs that increase the metabolism of contraceptive steroids. This could result in unintended pregnancy or unscheduled bleeding. In such cases a nonhormonal back-up method of birth control should be considered).

No products indexed under this heading.

Dexamethasone Sodium Phosphate (Contraceptive effectiveness may be reduced when hormonal contraceptives are co-administered with antibiotics, anticonvulsants, and other drugs that increase the metabolism of contraceptive steroids. This could result in unintended pregnancy or unscheduled bleeding. In such cases a nonhormonal back-up method of birth control should be considered).

No products indexed under this heading.

Dexchlorpheniramine Maleate (Enterohepatic recirculation of estrogens may also be decreased by substances that reduce gut transit time).

No products indexed under this heading.

Dexfenfluramine Hydrochloride (Contraceptive effectiveness may be reduced when hormonal contraceptives are co-administered with antibiotics, anticonvulsants, and other drugs that increase the metabolism of contraceptive steroids. This could result in unintended pregnancy or unscheduled bleeding. In such cases a nonhormonal back-up method of birth control should be considered).

No products indexed under this heading.

Dextromethorphan (Contraceptive effectiveness may be reduced when hormonal contraceptives are co-administered with antibiotics, anticonvulsants, and other drugs that increase the metabolism of contraceptive steroids. This could result in unintended pregnancy or unscheduled bleeding. In such cases a nonhormonal back-up method of birth control should be considered).

No products indexed under this heading.

Dextromethorphan Hydrobromide (Contraceptive effectiveness may be reduced when hormonal contraceptives are co-administered with antibiotics, anticonvulsants, and other drugs that increase the metabolism of contraceptive steroids. This could result in unintended pregnancy or unscheduled bleeding. In such cases a nonhormonal back-up method of birth control should be considered). Products include:

PediaCare Children's Liquid Multi-Symptom Cold **1902**
PediaCare Children's Long-Acting Cough **1902**
Children's Sudafed PE Cold & Cough Liquid **1907**
Sudafed PE Cold & Cough Caplets **1907**
Children's Tylenol Plus Cough & Runny Nose Suspension Liquid **1912**
Children's Tylenol Plus Cough & Sore Throat Suspension Liquid **1912**
Children's Tylenol Plus Flu Suspension Liquid **1914**
Children's Tylenol Plus Multi-Symptom Cold Suspension Liquid **1912**
Tylenol Cold Severe Congestion Daytime Caplets with Cool Burst **1912**
Tylenol Cold Head Congestion Daytime Caplets with Cool Burst **1910**
Tylenol Cold Head Congestion Nighttime Caplets with Cool Burst **1910**
Tylenol Cold Head Congestion Severe Daytime Caplets with Cool Burst **1910**
Tylenol Cold Multi-Symptom Daytime Caplets with Cool Burst and Rapid Release Gels **1913**
Tylenol Cold Multi-Symptom Daytime Liquid with Citrus Burst **1913**
Tylenol Cold Multi-Symptom Nighttime Caplets with Cool Burst **1913**
Tylenol Cold Multi-Symptom Nighttime Liquid with Cool Burst **1913**
Tylenol Cold Multi-Symptom Severe Caplets with Cool Burst **1913**
Tylenol Cold Multi-Symptom Severe Daytime Liquid with Citrus Burst **1913**
Tylenol Cough & Sore Throat Daytime Liquid with Cool Burst **1918**
Tylenol Cough & Sore Throat Nighttime Liquid with Cool Burst **1918**
Vicks DayQuil Cold & Flu Multi-Symptom Relief .... ▣**616**
Vicks DayQuil LiquiCaps **2567**
Vicks DayQuil Liquid **2567**
Vicks DayQuil Multi-Symptom Cold/Flu Relief **2567**
Vicks NyQuil Cold & Flu Multi-Symptom Relief .... ▣**617**
Vicks NyQuil LiquiCaps **2567**
Vicks NyQuil Liquid **2567**
Vicks NyQuil Multi-Symptom Cold/Flu Relief **2567**

Dextromethorphan Polistirex (Contraceptive effectiveness may be reduced when hormonal contraceptives are co-administered with antibiotics, anticonvulsants, and other drugs that increase the metabolism of contraceptive steroids. This could result in unintended pregnancy or unscheduled bleeding. In such cases a nonhormonal back-up method of birth control should be considered).

No products indexed under this heading.

Dezocine (Enterohepatic recirculation of estrogens may also be decreased by substances that reduce gut transit time).

No products indexed under this heading.

Diazepam (Contraceptive effectiveness may be reduced when hormonal contraceptives are co-administered with antibiotics, anticonvulsants, and other drugs that increase the metabolism of contraceptive steroids. This could result in unintended pregnancy or unscheduled bleeding. In such cases a nonhormonal back-up method of birth control should be considered). Products include:

Valium Tablets **2658**

Diclofenac Potassium (Contraceptive effectiveness may be reduced when hormonal contraceptives are co-administered with antibiotics, anticonvulsants, and other drugs that increase the metabolism of contraceptive steroids. This could result in unintended pregnancy or unscheduled bleeding. In such cases a nonhormonal back-up method of birth control should be considered).

No products indexed under this heading.

Diclofenac Sodium (Contraceptive effectiveness may be reduced when hormonal contraceptives are co-administered with antibiotics, anticonvulsants, and other drugs that increase the metabolism of contraceptive steroids. This could result in unintended pregnancy or unscheduled bleeding. In such cases a nonhormonal back-up method of birth control should be considered).
Products include:
Diclofenac Sodium Ophthalmic Solution ⊙ 240
Voltaren Ophthalmic Solution 2336
Voltaren Tablets 2334
Voltaren-XR Tablets 2337

Dicloxacillin Sodium (Several cases of contraceptive failure and unscheduled bleeding have been reported in the literature with concomitant administration of antibiotics such as ampicillin and other penicillins, and tetracyclines. However, clinical pharmacology studies investigating drug interactions between combined oral contraceptives and these antibiotics have reported inconsistent results).
No products indexed under this heading.

Dicyclomine Hydrochloride (Enterohepatic recirculation of estrogens may also be decreased by substances that reduce gut transit time).
Products include:
Bentyl Capsules 703
Bentyl Injection 703
Bentyl Syrup 703
Bentyl Tablets 703

Dienestrol (Co-administration of certain oral contraceptives containing ethinyl estradiol increases AUC values for ethinyl estradiol by approximately 20%).
No products indexed under this heading.

Diethylstilbestrol (Co-administration of certain oral contraceptives containing ethinyl estradiol increases AUC values for ethinyl estradiol by approximately 20%).
No products indexed under this heading.

Dihydroergotamine Mesylate (Contraceptive effectiveness may be reduced when hormonal contraceptives are co-administered with antibiotics, anticonvulsants, and other drugs that increase the metabolism of contraceptive steroids. This could result in unintended pregnancy or unscheduled bleeding. In such cases a nonhormonal back-up method of birth control should be considered).
No products indexed under this heading.

Diltiazem Hydrochloride (Contraceptive effectiveness may be reduced when hormonal contraceptives are co-administered with antibiotics, anticonvulsants, and other drugs that increase the metabolism of contraceptive steroids. This could result in unintended pregnancy or unscheduled bleeding. In such cases a nonhormonal back-up method of birth control should be considered).
Products include:
Cardizem LA Extended Release Tablets 421

Diltiazem Maleate (Contraceptive effectiveness may be reduced when hormonal contraceptives are co-administered with antibiotics, anticonvulsants, and other drugs that increase the metabolism of contraceptive steroids. This could result in unintended pregnancy or unscheduled bleeding. In such cases a nonhormonal back-up method of birth control should be considered).
No products indexed under this heading.

Diphenhydramine Citrate (Enterohepatic recirculation of estrogens may also be decreased by substances that reduce gut transit time).
No products indexed under this heading.

Diphenhydramine Hydrochloride (Enterohepatic recirculation of estrogens may also be decreased by substances that reduce gut transit time).
Products include:
Benadryl Allergy & Cold Kapgels 1895
Benadryl Allergy & Sinus Headache Kapgels 1895
Benadryl Severe Allergy & Sinus Headache Caplets 1897
Benadryl Dye-Free Allergy Liqui-gels Softgels 1897
Benadryl Allergy Kapgels 1895
Benadryl Allergy Quick Dissolve Strips 1896
Benadryl Allergy Ultratab Tablets 1896
Children's Benadryl Dye-Free Allergy Liquid 1897
Children's Benadryl Allergy Fastmelts 1897
Children's Benadryl Allergy Liquid 1898
Children's Benadryl Allergy Perfect Measure 1896
Children's Benadryl-D Allergy & Sinus Liquid 1896
Benadryl-D Allergy & Sinus Tablet 1896
PediaCare Children's Allergy & Cold Liquid 1902
PediaCare Children's Allergy Liquid 1902
Simply Sleep Caplets 1905
Sudafed PE Nighttime Cold Caplets 1907
Sudafed PE Severe Cold Caplets 1908
Extra Strength Tylenol PM Caplets, Geltabs, Liquid, and Rapid Release Gels 1915
Tylenol Allergy Multi-Symptom Nighttime Caplets with Cool Burst 1916
Tylenol Severe Allergy Caplets 1916
Children's Tylenol Plus Cold & Allergy Suspension Liquid 1914
Tylenol Sore Throat Nighttime Liquid with Cool Burst 1918

Diphenylpyraline Hydrochloride (Enterohepatic recirculation of estrogens may also be decreased by substances that reduce gut transit time).
No products indexed under this heading.

Disopyramide (Contraceptive effectiveness may be reduced when hormonal contraceptives are co-administered with antibiotics, anticonvulsants, and other drugs that increase the metabolism of contraceptive steroids. This could result in unintended pregnancy or unscheduled bleeding. In such cases a nonhormonal back-up method of birth control should be considered).
No products indexed under this heading.

Disopyramide Phosphate (Contraceptive effectiveness may be reduced when hormonal contraceptives are co-administered with antibiotics, anticonvulsants, and other drugs that increase the metabolism of contraceptive steroids. This could result in unintended pregnancy or unscheduled bleeding. In such cases a nonhormonal back-up method of birth control should be considered).
No products indexed under this heading.

Divalproex Sodium (Contraceptive effectiveness may be reduced when hormonal contraceptives are co-administered with antibiotics, anticonvulsants, and other drugs that increase the metabolism of contraceptive steroids. This could result in unintended pregnancy or unscheduled bleeding. In such cases a nonhormonal back-up method of birth control should be considered).
Products include:
Depakote ER Tablets 423

Dobutamine (Enterohepatic recirculation of estrogens may also be decreased by substances that reduce gut transit time).
No products indexed under this heading.

Dobutamine Hydrochloride (Enterohepatic recirculation of estrogens may also be decreased by substances that reduce gut transit time).
No products indexed under this heading.

Docetaxel (Contraceptive effectiveness may be reduced when hormonal contraceptives are co-administered with antibiotics, anticonvulsants, and other drugs that increase the metabolism of contraceptive steroids. This could result in unintended pregnancy or unscheduled bleeding. In such cases a nonhormonal back-up method of birth control should be considered).
Products include:
Taxotere Injection Concentrate 2773

Dolasetron Mesylate (Contraceptive effectiveness may be reduced when hormonal contraceptives are co-administered with antibiotics, anticonvulsants, and other drugs that increase the metabolism of contraceptive steroids. This could result in unintended pregnancy or unscheduled bleeding. In such cases a nonhormonal back-up method of birth control should be considered).
Products include:
Anzemet Injection 2701
Anzemet Tablets 2704

Domperidone (Enterohepatic recirculation of estrogens may also be decreased by substances that reduce gut transit time).
No products indexed under this heading.

Donepezil Hydrochloride (Contraceptive effectiveness may be reduced when hormonal contraceptives are co-administered with antibiotics, anticonvulsants, and other drugs that increase the metabolism of contraceptive steroids. This could result in unintended pregnancy or unscheduled bleeding. In such cases a nonhormonal back-up method of birth control should be considered).
Products include:
Aricept Tablets 1062
Aricept ODT Tablets 1062

Dopamine Hydrochloride (Enterohepatic recirculation of estrogens may also be decreased by substances that reduce gut transit time).
No products indexed under this heading.

Doxepin Hydrochloride (Contraceptive effectiveness may be reduced when hormonal contraceptives are co-administered with antibiotics, anticonvulsants, and other drugs that increase the metabolism of contraceptive steroids. This could result in unintended pregnancy or unscheduled bleeding. In such cases a nonhormonal back-up method of birth control should be considered).
No products indexed under this heading.

Doxorubicin Hydrochloride (Contraceptive effectiveness may be reduced when hormonal contraceptives are co-administered with antibiotics, anticonvulsants, and other drugs that increase the metabolism of contraceptive steroids. This could result in unintended pregnancy or unscheduled bleeding. In such cases a nonhormonal back-up method of birth control should be considered).
No products indexed under this heading.

Doxycycline Calcium (Several cases of contraceptive failure and unscheduled bleeding have been reported in the literature with concomitant administration of antibiotics such as ampicillin and other penicillins, and tetracyclines. However, clinical pharmacology studies investigating drug interactions between combined oral contraceptives and these antibiotics have reported inconsistent results).
No products indexed under this heading.

Doxycycline Hyclate (Several cases of contraceptive failure and unscheduled bleeding have been reported in the literature with concomitant administration of antibiotics such as ampicillin and other penicillins, and tetracyclines. However, clinical pharmacology studies investigating drug interactions between combined oral contraceptives and these antibiotics have reported inconsistent results).
No products indexed under this heading.

Doxycycline Monohydrate (Several cases of contraceptive failure and unscheduled bleeding have been reported in the literature with concomitant administration of antibiotics such as ampicillin and other penicillins, and tetracyclines. However, clinical pharmacology studies investigating drug interactions between combined oral contraceptives and these antibiotics have reported inconsistent results).
No products indexed under this heading.

Dronabinol (Contraceptive effectiveness may be reduced when hormonal contraceptives are co-administered with antibiotics, anticonvulsants, and other drugs that increase the metabolism of contraceptive steroids. This could result in unintended pregnancy or unscheduled bleeding. In such cases a nonhormonal back-up method of birth control should be considered).
Products include:
Marinol Capsules 3163

Drugs that Undergo Biotransformation by Cytochrome P-450 Mixed Function Oxidase (Contraceptive effectiveness may be reduced when hormonal contraceptives are co-administered with antibiotics, anticonvulsants, and other drugs that increase the metabolism of contraceptive steroids. This could result in unintended pregnancy or unscheduled bleeding. In such cases a nonhormonal back-up method of birth control should be considered).
No products indexed under this heading.

Dyphylline (Contraceptive effectiveness may be reduced when hormonal contraceptives are co-administered with antibiotics, anticonvulsants, and other drugs that increase the metabolism of contraceptive steroids. This could result in unintended pregnancy or unscheduled bleeding. In such cases a nonhormonal back-up method of birth control should be considered).
No products indexed under this heading.

Edrophonium Chloride (Enterohepatic recirculation of estrogens may also be decreased by substances that reduce gut transit time).
No products indexed under this heading.

Efavirenz (Contraceptive effectiveness may be reduced when hormonal contraceptives are co-administered with antibiotics, anticonvulsants, and other drugs that increase the metabolism of contraceptive steroids. This could result in unintended pregnancy or unscheduled bleeding. In such cases a nonhormonal back-up method of birth control should be considered).
Products include:
Atripla Tablets **938**
Sustiva Capsules **930**
Sustiva Tablets **930**

Encainide Hydrochloride (Contraceptive effectiveness may be reduced when hormonal contraceptives are co-administered with antibiotics, anticonvulsants, and other drugs that increase the metabolism of contraceptive steroids. This could result in unintended pregnancy or unscheduled bleeding. In such cases a nonhormonal back-up method of birth control should be considered).
No products indexed under this heading.

Enoxacin (Contraceptive effectiveness may be reduced when hormonal contraceptives are co-administered with antibiotics, anticonvulsants, and other drugs that increase the metabolism of contraceptive steroids. This could result in unintended pregnancy or unscheduled bleeding. In such cases a nonhormonal back-up method of birth control should be considered).
No products indexed under this heading.

Ephedrine Hydrochloride (Enterohepatic recirculation of estrogens may also be decreased by substances that reduce gut transit time).
No products indexed under this heading.

Ephedrine Sulfate (Enterohepatic recirculation of estrogens may also be decreased by substances that reduce gut transit time).
No products indexed under this heading.

Ephedrine Tannate (Enterohepatic recirculation of estrogens may also be decreased by substances that reduce gut transit time).
No products indexed under this heading.

Epinephrine (Enterohepatic recirculation of estrogens may also be decreased by substances that reduce gut transit time). Products include:
EpiPen **1024**

Epinephrine Hydrochloride (Enterohepatic recirculation of estrogens may also be decreased by substances that reduce gut transit time).
No products indexed under this heading.

Eprosartan Mesylate (Contraceptive effectiveness may be reduced when hormonal contraceptives are co-administered with antibiotics, anticonvulsants, and other drugs that increase the metabolism of contraceptive steroids. This could result in unintended pregnancy or unscheduled bleeding. In such cases a nonhormonal back-up method of birth control should be considered).
Products include:
Teveten Tablets **515**
Teveten HCT Tablets **517**

Ergotamine Tartrate (Contraceptive effectiveness may be reduced when hormonal contraceptives are co-administered with antibiotics, anticonvulsants, and other drugs that increase the metabolism of contraceptive steroids. This could result in unintended pregnancy or unscheduled bleeding. In such cases a nonhormonal back-up method of birth control should be considered).
No products indexed under this heading.

Erythromycin (Contraceptive effectiveness may be reduced when hormonal contraceptives are co-administered with antibiotics, anticonvulsants, and other drugs that increase the metabolism of contraceptive steroids. This could result in unintended pregnancy or unscheduled bleeding. In such cases a nonhormonal back-up method of birth control should be considered).
No products indexed under this heading.

Erythromycin Estolate (Contraceptive effectiveness may be reduced when hormonal contraceptives are co-administered with antibiotics, anticonvulsants, and other drugs that increase the metabolism of contraceptive steroids. This could result in unintended pregnancy or unscheduled bleeding. In such cases a nonhormonal back-up method of birth control should be considered).
No products indexed under this heading.

Erythromycin Ethylsuccinate (Contraceptive effectiveness may be reduced when hormonal contraceptives are co-administered with antibiotics, anticonvulsants, and other drugs that increase the metabolism of contraceptive steroids. This could result in unintended pregnancy or unscheduled bleeding. In such cases a nonhormonal back-up method of birth control should be considered).
Products include:
E.E.S. **433**
EryPed **431**

Erythromycin Gluceptate (Contraceptive effectiveness may be reduced when hormonal contraceptives are co-administered with antibiotics, anticonvulsants, and other drugs that increase the metabolism of contraceptive steroids. This could result in unintended pregnancy or unscheduled bleeding. In such cases a nonhormonal back-up method of birth control should be considered).
No products indexed under this heading.

Erythromycin Lactobionate (Contraceptive effectiveness may be reduced when hormonal contraceptives are co-administered with antibiotics, anticonvulsants, and other drugs that increase the metabolism of contraceptive steroids. This could result in unintended pregnancy or unscheduled bleeding. In such cases a nonhormonal back-up method of birth control should be considered).
No products indexed under this heading.

Erythromycin Stearate (Contraceptive effectiveness may be reduced when hormonal contraceptives are co-administered with antibiotics, anticonvulsants, and other drugs that increase the metabolism of contraceptive steroids. This could result in unintended pregnancy or unscheduled bleeding. In such cases a nonhormonal back-up method of birth control should be considered).
No products indexed under this heading.

Esomeprazole Magnesium (Contraceptive effectiveness may be reduced when hormonal contraceptives are co-administered with antibiotics, anticonvulsants, and other drugs that increase the metabolism of contraceptive steroids. This could result in unintended pregnancy or unscheduled bleeding. In such cases a nonhormonal back-up method of birth control should be considered).
Products include:
Nexium Delayed-Release Capsules **645**
Nexium Delayed-Release Oral Suspension **645**

Estradiol (Contraceptive effectiveness may be reduced when hormonal contraceptives are co-administered with antibiotics, anticonvulsants, and other drugs that increase the metabolism of contraceptive steroids. This could result in unintended pregnancy or unscheduled bleeding. In such cases a nonhormonal back-up method of birth control should be considered).
Products include:
Activella Tablets **2347**
Angeliq Tablets **751**
Climara Transdermal System **763**
Climara Pro Transdermal System **768**
Divigel **3167**
Vagifem Tablets **2375**

Estradiol Benzoate (Contraceptive effectiveness may be reduced when hormonal contraceptives are co-administered with antibiotics, anticonvulsants, and other drugs that increase the metabolism of contraceptive steroids. This could result in unintended pregnancy or unscheduled bleeding. In such cases a nonhormonal back-up method of birth control should be considered).
No products indexed under this heading.

Estradiol Cypionate (Contraceptive effectiveness may be reduced when hormonal contraceptives are co-administered with antibiotics, anticonvulsants, and other drugs that increase the metabolism of contraceptive steroids. This could result in unintended pregnancy or unscheduled bleeding. In such cases a nonhormonal back-up method of birth control should be considered).
No products indexed under this heading.

Estradiol Valerate (Contraceptive effectiveness may be reduced when hormonal contraceptives are co-administered with antibiotics, anticonvulsants, and other drugs that increase the metabolism of contraceptive steroids. This could result in unintended pregnancy or unscheduled bleeding. In such cases a nonhormonal back-up method of birth control should be considered).
No products indexed under this heading.

Estrogen (Contraceptive effectiveness may be reduced when hormonal contraceptives are co-administered with antibiotics, anticonvulsants, and other drugs that increase the metabolism of contraceptive steroids. This could result in unintended pregnancy or unscheduled bleeding. In such cases a nonhormonal back-up method of birth control should be considered).
No products indexed under this heading.

Estrogens, Conjugated (Contraceptive effectiveness may be reduced when hormonal contraceptives are co-administered with antibiotics, anticonvulsants, and other drugs that increase the metabolism of contraceptive steroids. This could result in unintended pregnancy or unscheduled bleeding. In such cases a nonhormonal back-up method of birth control should be considered).
Products include:
Premarin Intravenous **3217**
Premarin Tablets **3221**
Premarin Vaginal Cream **3228**
Premphase Tablets **3232**
Prempro Tablets **3232**

Estrogens, Conjugated, Synthetic A (Contraceptive effectiveness may be reduced when hormonal contraceptives are co-administered with antibiotics, anticonvulsants, and other drugs that increase the metabolism of contraceptive steroids. This could result in unintended pregnancy or unscheduled bleeding. In such cases a nonhormonal back-up method of birth control should be considered).
No products indexed under this heading.

Estrogens, Esterified (Contraceptive effectiveness may be reduced when hormonal contraceptives are co-administered with antibiotics, anticonvulsants, and other drugs that increase the metabolism of contraceptive steroids. This could result in unintended pregnancy or unscheduled bleeding. In such cases a nonhormonal back-up method of birth control should be considered).
Products include:
Estratest Tablets **3043**
Estratest H.S. Tablets **3043**

Estropipate (Co-administration of certain oral contraceptives containing ethinyl estradiol increases AUC values for ethinyl estradiol by approximately 20%).
No products indexed under this heading.

Ethosuximide (Contraceptive effectiveness may be reduced when hormonal contraceptives are co-administered with antibiotics, anticonvulsants, and other drugs that increase the metabolism of contraceptive steroids. This could result in unintended pregnancy or unscheduled bleeding. In such cases a nonhormonal back-up method of birth control should be considered).
No products indexed under this heading.

Ethotoin (Contraceptive effectiveness may be reduced when hormonal contraceptives are co-administered with antibiotics, anticonvulsants, and other drugs that increase the metabolism of contraceptive steroids. This could result in unintended pregnancy or unscheduled bleeding. In such cases a non-hormonal back-up method of birth control should be considered).
No products indexed under this heading.

Ethynodiol Diacetate (Contraceptive effectiveness may be reduced when hormonal contraceptives are co-administered with antibiotics, anticonvulsants, and other drugs that increase the metabolism of contraceptive steroids. This could result in unintended pregnancy or unscheduled bleeding. In such cases a non-hormonal back-up method of birth control should be considered).
No products indexed under this heading.

Etodolac (Contraceptive effectiveness may be reduced when hormonal contraceptives are co-administered with antibiotics, anticonvulsants, and other drugs that increase the metabolism of contraceptive steroids. This could result in unintended pregnancy or unscheduled bleeding. In such cases a non-hormonal back-up method of birth control should be considered).
No products indexed under this heading.

Etoposide (Contraceptive effectiveness may be reduced when hormonal contraceptives are co-administered with antibiotics, anticonvulsants, and other drugs that increase the metabolism of contraceptive steroids. This could result in unintended pregnancy or unscheduled bleeding. In such cases a non-hormonal back-up method of birth control should be considered).
No products indexed under this heading.

Etoposide Phosphate (Contraceptive effectiveness may be reduced when hormonal contraceptives are co-administered with antibiotics, anticonvulsants, and other drugs that increase the metabolism of contraceptive steroids. This could result in unintended pregnancy or unscheduled bleeding. In such cases a non-hormonal back-up method of birth control should be considered).
No products indexed under this heading.

Felbamate (Contraceptive effectiveness may be reduced when hormonal contraceptives are co-administered with antibiotics, anticonvulsants, and other drugs that increase the metabolism of contraceptive steroids. This could result in unintended pregnancy or unscheduled bleeding. In such cases a non-hormonal back-up method of birth control should be considered).
No products indexed under this heading.

Felodipine (Contraceptive effectiveness may be reduced when hormonal contraceptives are co-administered with antibiotics, anticonvulsants, and other drugs that increase the metabolism of contraceptive steroids. This could result in unintended pregnancy or unscheduled bleeding. In such cases a non-hormonal back-up method of birth control should be considered).
No products indexed under this heading.

Fenoprofen Calcium (Contraceptive effectiveness may be reduced when hormonal contraceptives are co-administered with antibiotics, anticonvulsants, and other drugs that increase the metabolism of contraceptive steroids. This could result in unintended pregnancy or unscheduled bleeding. In such cases a non-hormonal back-up method of birth control should be considered). Products include:
Nalfon Capsules **2508**

Fentanyl (Contraceptive effectiveness may be reduced when hormonal contraceptives are co-administered with antibiotics, anticonvulsants, and other drugs that increase the metabolism of contraceptive steroids. This could result in unintended pregnancy or unscheduled bleeding. In such cases a non-hormonal back-up method of birth control should be considered). Products include:
Duragesic Transdermal System **2405**
Ionsys Transdermal System **2410**

Fentanyl Citrate (Contraceptive effectiveness may be reduced when hormonal contraceptives are co-administered with antibiotics, anticonvulsants, and other drugs that increase the metabolism of contraceptive steroids. This could result in unintended pregnancy or unscheduled bleeding. In such cases a non-hormonal back-up method of birth control should be considered). Products include:
Actiq **959**
Fentora Tablets **968**

Flecainide Acetate (Contraceptive effectiveness may be reduced when hormonal contraceptives are co-administered with antibiotics, anticonvulsants, and other drugs that increase the metabolism of contraceptive steroids. This could result in unintended pregnancy or unscheduled bleeding. In such cases a non-hormonal back-up method of birth control should be considered).
No products indexed under this heading.

Fluconazole (CYP 3A4 inhibitors such as indinavir, itraconazole, ketoconazole, fluconazole, and troleandomycin may increase plasma hormone levels. Troleandomycin may also increase the risk of intrahepatic cholestasis during co-administration with combination oral contraceptives).
No products indexed under this heading.

Fludrocortisone Acetate (Contraceptive effectiveness may be reduced when hormonal contraceptives are co-administered with antibiotics, anticonvulsants, and other drugs that increase the metabolism of contraceptive steroids. This could result in unintended pregnancy or unscheduled bleeding. In such cases a nonhormonal back-up method of birth control should be considered).
No products indexed under this heading.

Flunisolide (Increased plasma concentrations of cyclosporine, prednisolone and other corticosteroids, have been reported with concomitant administration of oral contraceptives). Products include:
Aerobid/Aerobid-M **1153**

Fluoxetine (Contraceptive effectiveness may be reduced when hormonal contraceptives are co-administered with antibiotics, anticonvulsants, and other drugs that increase the metabolism of contraceptive steroids. This could result in unintended pregnancy or unscheduled bleeding. In such cases a non-hormonal back-up method of birth control should be considered).
No products indexed under this heading.

Fluoxetine Hydrochloride (Contraceptive effectiveness may be reduced when hormonal contraceptives are co-administered with antibiotics, anticonvulsants, and other drugs that increase the metabolism of contraceptive steroids. This could result in unintended pregnancy or unscheduled bleeding. In such cases a nonhormonal back-up method of birth control should be considered). Products include:
Prozac Weekly Capsules **1852**
Prozac Pulvules and Liquid **1852**
Symbyax Capsules **1871**

Fluphenazine Decanoate (Contraceptive effectiveness may be reduced when hormonal contraceptives are co-administered with antibiotics, anticonvulsants, and other drugs that increase the metabolism of contraceptive steroids. This could result in unintended pregnancy or unscheduled bleeding. In such cases a nonhormonal back-up method of birth control should be considered).
No products indexed under this heading.

Fluphenazine Enanthate (Contraceptive effectiveness may be reduced when hormonal contraceptives are co-administered with antibiotics, anticonvulsants, and other drugs that increase the metabolism of contraceptive steroids. This could result in unintended pregnancy or unscheduled bleeding. In such cases a nonhormonal back-up method of birth control should be considered).
No products indexed under this heading.

Fluphenazine Hydrochloride (Contraceptive effectiveness may be reduced when hormonal contraceptives are co-administered with antibiotics, anticonvulsants, and other drugs that increase the metabolism of contraceptive steroids. This could result in unintended pregnancy or unscheduled bleeding. In such cases a nonhormonal back-up method of birth control should be considered).
No products indexed under this heading.

Flurbiprofen (Contraceptive effectiveness may be reduced when hormonal contraceptives are co-administered with antibiotics, anticonvulsants, and other drugs that increase the metabolism of contraceptive steroids. This could result in unintended pregnancy or unscheduled bleeding. In such cases a non-hormonal back-up method of birth control should be considered).
No products indexed under this heading.

Flurbiprofen Sodium (Contraceptive effectiveness may be reduced when hormonal contraceptives are co-administered with antibiotics, anticonvulsants, and other drugs that increase the metabolism of contraceptive steroids. This could result in unintended pregnancy or unscheduled bleeding. In such cases a non-hormonal back-up method of birth control should be considered).
No products indexed under this heading.

Flutamide (Contraceptive effectiveness may be reduced when hormonal contraceptives are co-administered with antibiotics, anticonvulsants, and other drugs that increase the metabolism of contraceptive steroids. This could result in unintended pregnancy or unscheduled bleeding. In such cases a non-hormonal back-up method of birth control should be considered).
No products indexed under this heading.

Fluticasone Propionate (Contraceptive effectiveness may be reduced when hormonal contraceptives are co-administered with antibiotics, anticonvulsants, and other drugs that increase the metabolism of contraceptive steroids. This could result in unintended pregnancy or unscheduled bleeding. In such cases a nonhormonal back-up method of birth control should be considered). Products include:
Advair Diskus 100/50 .... **1276**
Advair Diskus 250/50 .... **1276**
Advair Diskus 500/50 .... **1276**
Advair HFA 45/21 Inhalation Aerosol **1288**
Advair HFA 115/21 Inhalation Aerosol **1288**
Advair HFA 230/21 Inhalation Aerosol **1288**
Flonase Nasal Spray **1431**
Flovent Diskus 50 mcg **1435**

Fluticasone Propionate HFA (Increased plasma concentrations of cyclosporine, prednisolone and other corticosteroids, have been reported with concomitant administration of oral contraceptives). Products include:
Flovent HFA **1440**

Fluvastatin Sodium (Contraceptive effectiveness may be reduced when hormonal contraceptives are co-administered with antibiotics, anticonvulsants, and other drugs that increase the metabolism of contraceptive steroids. This could result in unintended pregnancy or unscheduled bleeding. In such cases a non-hormonal back-up method of birth control should be considered). Products include:
Lescol Capsules **2268**
Lescol XL Tablets **2268**

Fluvoxamine Maleate (Contraceptive effectiveness may be reduced when hormonal contraceptives are co-administered with antibiotics, anti-

convulsants, and other drugs that increase the metabolism of contraceptive steroids. This could result in unintended pregnancy or unscheduled bleeding. In such cases a nonhormonal back-up method of birth control should be considered).
Products include:
Luvox CR Extended-Release Capsules 1759

Formoterol Fumarate (Contraceptive effectiveness may be reduced when hormonal contraceptives are co-administered with antibiotics, anticonvulsants, and other drugs that increase the metabolism of contraceptive steroids. This could result in unintended pregnancy or unscheduled bleeding. In such cases a nonhormonal back-up method of birth control should be considered).
Products include:
Foradil Aerolizer 2849
Perforomist Inhalation Solution 1025

Fosamprenavir Calcium (Several of the anti-HIV protease inhibitors have been studied with co-administration of oral combination hormonal contraceptives; significant changes (increase and decrease) in the plasma levels of the estrogen and progestin have been noted in some cases. The safety and efficacy of oral contraceptive products may be affected with co-administration of anti-HIV protease inhibitors. Health care professionals should refer to the label of the individual anti-HIV protease inhibitors for further drug-drug interaction information).
Products include:
Lexiva Oral Suspension 1510
Lexiva Tablets 1510

Fosphenytoin (Contraceptive effectiveness may be reduced when hormonal contraceptives are co-administered with antibiotics, anticonvulsants, and other drugs that increase the metabolism of contraceptive steroids. This could result in unintended pregnancy or unscheduled bleeding. In such cases a nonhormonal back-up method of birth control should be considered).
No products indexed under this heading.

Fosphenytoin Sodium (Contraceptive effectiveness may be reduced when hormonal contraceptives are co-administered with antibiotics, anticonvulsants, and other drugs that increase the metabolism of contraceptive steroids. This could result in unintended pregnancy or unscheduled bleeding. In such cases a nonhormonal back-up method of birth control should be considered).
No products indexed under this heading.

Gabapentin (Contraceptive effectiveness may be reduced when hormonal contraceptives are co-administered with antibiotics, anticonvulsants, and other drugs that increase the metabolism of contraceptive steroids. This could result in unintended pregnancy or unscheduled bleeding. In such cases a nonhormonal back-up method of birth control should be considered).
No products indexed under this heading.

Galantamine Hydrobromide (Contraceptive effectiveness may be reduced when hormonal contraceptives are co-administered with antibiotics, anticonvulsants, and other drugs that increase the metabolism of contraceptive steroids. This could result in unintended pregnancy or unscheduled bleeding. In such cases a nonhormonal back-up method of birth control should be considered).
No products indexed under this heading.

Garlic Extract (Contraceptive effectiveness may be reduced when hormonal contraceptives are co-administered with antibiotics, anticonvulsants, and other drugs that increase the metabolism of contraceptive steroids. This could result in unintended pregnancy or unscheduled bleeding. In such cases a nonhormonal back-up method of birth control should be considered).
No products indexed under this heading.

Garlic Oil (Contraceptive effectiveness may be reduced when hormonal contraceptives are co-administered with antibiotics, anticonvulsants, and other drugs that increase the metabolism of contraceptive steroids. This could result in unintended pregnancy or unscheduled bleeding. In such cases a nonhormonal back-up method of birth control should be considered).
No products indexed under this heading.

Glimepiride (Contraceptive effectiveness may be reduced when hormonal contraceptives are co-administered with antibiotics, anticonvulsants, and other drugs that increase the metabolism of contraceptive steroids. This could result in unintended pregnancy or unscheduled bleeding. In such cases a nonhormonal back-up method of birth control should be considered).
Products include:
Avandaryl Tablets 1344
Duetact Tablets 3085

Glipizide (Contraceptive effectiveness may be reduced when hormonal contraceptives are co-administered with antibiotics, anticonvulsants, and other drugs that increase the metabolism of contraceptive steroids. This could result in unintended pregnancy or unscheduled bleeding. In such cases a nonhormonal back-up method of birth control should be considered).
No products indexed under this heading.

Glyburide (Contraceptive effectiveness may be reduced when hormonal contraceptives are co-administered with antibiotics, anticonvulsants, and other drugs that increase the metabolism of contraceptive steroids. This could result in unintended pregnancy or unscheduled bleeding. In such cases a nonhormonal back-up method of birth control should be considered).
No products indexed under this heading.

Glycopyrrolate (Enterohepatic recirculation of estrogens may also be decreased by substances that reduce gut transit time).
No products indexed under this heading.

Grepafloxacin Hydrochloride (Contraceptive effectiveness may be reduced when hormonal contraceptives are co-administered with antibiotics, anticonvulsants, and other drugs that increase the metabolism of contraceptive steroids. This could result in unintended pregnancy or unscheduled bleeding. In such cases a nonhormonal back-up method of birth control should be considered).
No products indexed under this heading.

Griseofulvin (Contraceptive effectiveness may be reduced when hormonal contraceptives are co-administered with antibiotics, anticonvulsants, and other drugs that increase the metabolism of contraceptive steroids. This could result in unintended pregnancy or unscheduled bleeding. In such cases a nonhormonal back-up method of birth control should be considered).
Products include:
Gris-PEG Tablets 2507

Haloperidol (Contraceptive effectiveness may be reduced when hormonal contraceptives are co-administered with antibiotics, anticonvulsants, and other drugs that increase the metabolism of contraceptive steroids. This could result in unintended pregnancy or unscheduled bleeding. In such cases a nonhormonal back-up method of birth control should be considered).
No products indexed under this heading.

Haloperidol Decanoate (Contraceptive effectiveness may be reduced when hormonal contraceptives are co-administered with antibiotics, anticonvulsants, and other drugs that increase the metabolism of contraceptive steroids. This could result in unintended pregnancy or unscheduled bleeding. In such cases a nonhormonal back-up method of birth control should be considered).
No products indexed under this heading.

Haloperidol Lactate (Contraceptive effectiveness may be reduced when hormonal contraceptives are co-administered with antibiotics, anticonvulsants, and other drugs that increase the metabolism of contraceptive steroids. This could result in unintended pregnancy or unscheduled bleeding. In such cases a nonhormonal back-up method of birth control should be considered).
No products indexed under this heading.

Hydrocodone Bitartrate (Contraceptive effectiveness may be reduced when hormonal contraceptives are co-administered with antibiotics, anticonvulsants, and other drugs that increase the metabolism of contraceptive steroids. This could result in unintended pregnancy or unscheduled bleeding. In such cases a nonhormonal back-up method of birth control should be considered).
Products include:
Lortab 5/500 Tablets 3143
Lortab 7.5/500 Tablets 3144
Lortab 10/500 Tablets 3144
Vicodin Tablets 529
Vicodin ES Tablets 530
Vicodin HP Tablets 531
Vicoprofen Tablets 533
Zydone Tablets 1132

Hydrocodone Polistirex (Enterohepatic recirculation of estrogens may also be decreased by substances that reduce gut transit time).
Products include:
Tussionex Pennkinetic Extended-Release Suspension 3154

Hydrocortisone (Contraceptive effectiveness may be reduced when hormonal contraceptives are co-administered with antibiotics, anticonvulsants, and other drugs that increase the metabolism of contraceptive steroids. This could result in unintended pregnancy or unscheduled bleeding. In such cases a nonhormonal back-up method of birth control should be considered).
No products indexed under this heading.

Hydrocortisone Acetate (Contraceptive effectiveness may be reduced when hormonal contraceptives are co-administered with antibiotics, anticonvulsants, and other drugs that increase the metabolism of contraceptive steroids. This could result in unintended pregnancy or unscheduled bleeding. In such cases a nonhormonal back-up method of birth control should be considered).
Products include:
Analpram-HC 1140
Pramosone 1141

Hydrocortisone Butyrate (Contraceptive effectiveness may be reduced when hormonal contraceptives are co-administered with antibiotics, anticonvulsants, and other drugs that increase the metabolism of contraceptive steroids. This could result in unintended pregnancy or unscheduled bleeding. In such cases a nonhormonal back-up method of birth control should be considered).
No products indexed under this heading.

Hydrocortisone Cypionate (Contraceptive effectiveness may be reduced when hormonal contraceptives are co-administered with antibiotics, anticonvulsants, and other drugs that increase the metabolism of contraceptive steroids. This could result in unintended pregnancy or unscheduled bleeding. In such cases a nonhormonal back-up method of birth control should be considered).
No products indexed under this heading.

Hydrocortisone Hemisuccinate (Contraceptive effectiveness may be reduced when hormonal contraceptives are co-administered with antibiotics, anticonvulsants, and other drugs that increase the metabolism of contraceptive steroids. This could result in unintended pregnancy or unscheduled bleeding. In such cases a nonhormonal back-up method of birth control should be considered).
No products indexed under this heading.

Hydrocortisone Probutate (Contraceptive effectiveness may be reduced when hormonal contraceptives are co-administered with antibiotics, anticonvulsants, and other drugs that increase the metabolism of contraceptive steroids. This could result in unintended pregnancy or unscheduled bleeding. In such cases a nonhormonal back-up method of birth control should be considered).
No products indexed under this heading.

Hydrocortisone Sodium Phosphate (Contraceptive effectiveness may be reduced when hormonal contraceptives are co-administered with antibiotics, anticonvulsants, and other drugs that increase the metabolism of contraceptive steroids. This could result in unintended pregnancy or unscheduled bleeding. In such cases a nonhormonal back-up method of birth control should be considered).
No products indexed under this heading.

Hydrocortisone Sodium Succinate (Contraceptive effectiveness may be reduced when hormonal contraceptives are co-administered with antibiotics, anticonvulsants, and other drugs that increase the metabolism of contraceptive steroids. This could result in unintended pregnancy or unscheduled bleeding. In such cases a nonhormonal back-up method of birth control should be considered).
No products indexed under this heading.

Hydrocortisone Valerate (Contraceptive effectiveness may be reduced when hormonal contraceptives are co-administered with antibiotics, anticonvulsants, and other drugs that increase the metabolism of contraceptive steroids. This could result in unintended pregnancy or unscheduled bleeding. In such cases a nonhormonal back-up method of birth control should be considered).
No products indexed under this heading.

Hydromorphone Hydrochloride (Enterohepatic recirculation of estrogens may also be decreased by substances that reduce gut transit time).
No products indexed under this heading.

Hyoscyamine (Enterohepatic recirculation of estrogens may also be decreased by substances that reduce gut transit time).
No products indexed under this heading.

Hyoscyamine Sulfate (Enterohepatic recirculation of estrogens may also be decreased by substances that reduce gut transit time).
Products include:
Donnatal Extentabs 2507

Hypericum (Contraceptive effectiveness may be reduced when hormonal contraceptives are co-administered with antibiotics, anticonvulsants, and other drugs that increase the metabolism of contraceptive steroids. This could result in unintended pregnancy or unscheduled bleeding. In such cases a nonhormonal back-up method of birth control should be considered).
Products include:
Satieté Tablets 640

Hypericum Perforatum (Contraceptive effectiveness may be reduced when hormonal contraceptives are co-administered with antibiotics, anticonvulsants, and other drugs that increase the metabolism of contraceptive steroids. This could result in unintended pregnancy or unscheduled bleeding. In such cases a nonhormonal back-up method of birth control should be considered).
No products indexed under this heading.

Ibuprofen (Contraceptive effectiveness may be reduced when hormonal contraceptives are co-administered with antibiotics, anticonvulsants, and other drugs that increase the metabolism of contraceptive steroids. This could result in unintended pregnancy or unscheduled bleeding. In such cases a nonhormonal back-up method of birth control should be considered).
Products include:
Motrin IB Tablets and Caplets 1900
Children's Motrin Oral Suspension ... 1901
Children's Motrin Non-Staining Dye-Free Oral Suspension 1901
Children's Motrin Cold Oral Suspension 1899
Infants' Motrin Concentrated Drops 1901
Infants' Motrin Non-Staining Dye-Free Concentrated Drops 1901
Junior Strength Motrin Caplets and Chewable Tablets 1901
Vicoprofen Tablets 533

Imipramine Hydrochloride (Contraceptive effectiveness may be reduced when hormonal contraceptives are co-administered with antibiotics, anticonvulsants, and other drugs that increase the metabolism of contraceptive steroids. This could result in unintended pregnancy or unscheduled bleeding. In such cases a nonhormonal back-up method of birth control should be considered).
No products indexed under this heading.

Imipramine Pamoate (Contraceptive effectiveness may be reduced when hormonal contraceptives are co-administered with antibiotics, anticonvulsants, and other drugs that increase the metabolism of contraceptive steroids. This could result in unintended pregnancy or unscheduled bleeding. In such cases a nonhormonal back-up method of birth control should be considered).
No products indexed under this heading.

Indinavir Sulfate (Contraceptive effectiveness may be reduced when hormonal contraceptives are co-administered with antibiotics, anticonvulsants, and other drugs that increase the metabolism of contraceptive steroids. This could result in unintended pregnancy or unscheduled bleeding. In such cases a nonhormonal back-up method of birth control should be considered).
Products include:
Crixivan Capsules 1979

Indomethacin (Contraceptive effectiveness may be reduced when hormonal contraceptives are co-administered with antibiotics, anticonvulsants, and other drugs that increase the metabolism of contraceptive steroids. This could result in unintended pregnancy or unscheduled bleeding. In such cases a nonhormonal back-up method of birth control should be considered).
Products include:
Indocin 2024

Indomethacin Sodium Trihydrate (Contraceptive effectiveness may be reduced when hormonal contraceptives are co-administered with antibiotics, anticonvulsants, and other drugs that increase the metabolism of contraceptive steroids. This could result in unintended pregnancy or unscheduled bleeding. In such cases a nonhormonal back-up method of birth control should be considered). Products include:
Indocin I.V. 2489

Indoramin Hydrochloride (Contraceptive effectiveness may be reduced when hormonal contraceptives are co-administered with antibiotics, anticonvulsants, and other drugs that increase the metabolism of contraceptive steroids. This could result in unintended pregnancy or unscheduled bleeding. In such cases a nonhormonal back-up method of birth control should be considered).
No products indexed under this heading.

Ipratropium Bromide (Enterohepatic recirculation of estrogens may also be decreased by substances that reduce gut transit time).
Products include:
Atrovent HFA Inhalation Aerosol 839
Atrovent Nasal Spray 0.03% 834
Atrovent Nasal Spray 0.06% 836
Combivent Inhalation Aerosol 845

Irbesartan (Contraceptive effectiveness may be reduced when hormonal contraceptives are co-administered with antibiotics, anticonvulsants, and other drugs that increase the metabolism of contraceptive steroids. This could result in unintended pregnancy or unscheduled bleeding. In such cases a nonhormonal back-up method of birth control should be considered).
Products include:
Avalide Tablets 892
Avalide Tablets 2713
Avapro Tablets 897
Avapro Tablets 2718

Isoetharine (Enterohepatic recirculation of estrogens may also be decreased by substances that reduce gut transit time).
No products indexed under this heading.

Isoniazid (CYP 3A4 inhibitors such as indinavir, itraconazole, ketoconazole, fluconazole, and troleandomycin may increase plasma hormone levels. Troleandomycin may also increase the risk of intrahepatic cholestasis during co-administration with combination oral contraceptives).
No products indexed under this heading.

Isoproterenol Hydrochloride (Enterohepatic recirculation of estrogens may also be decreased by substances that reduce gut transit time).
No products indexed under this heading.

Isoproterenol Sulfate (Enterohepatic recirculation of estrogens may also be decreased by substances that reduce gut transit time).
No products indexed under this heading.

Isotretinoin (Contraceptive effectiveness may be reduced when hormonal contraceptives are co-administered with antibiotics, anticonvulsants, and other drugs that increase the metabolism of contraceptive steroids. This could result in unintended pregnancy or unscheduled bleeding. In such cases a nonhormonal back-up method of birth control should be considered).
Products include:
Accutane Capsules 2607

Isradipine (Contraceptive effectiveness may be reduced when hormonal contraceptives are co-administered with antibiotics, anticonvulsants, and other drugs that increase the metabolism of contraceptive steroids. This could result in unintended pregnancy or unscheduled bleeding. In such cases a nonhormonal back-up method of birth control should be considered).
Products include:
DynaCirc CR Controlled Release Tablets 1407

Itraconazole (Contraceptive effectiveness may be reduced when hormonal contraceptives are co-administered with antibiotics, anticonvulsants, and other drugs that increase the metabolism of contraceptive steroids. This could result in unintended pregnancy or unscheduled bleeding. In such cases a nonhormonal back-up method of birth control should be considered).
No products indexed under this heading.

Ketoconazole (Contraceptive effectiveness may be reduced when hormonal contraceptives are co-administered with antibiotics, anticonvulsants, and other drugs that increase the metabolism of contraceptive steroids. This could result in unintended pregnancy or unscheduled bleeding. In such cases a nonhormonal back-up method of birth control should be considered).
Products include:
Extina Foam, 2% 3057
Nizoral A-D Shampoo 1901

Ketoprofen (Contraceptive effectiveness may be reduced when hormonal contraceptives are co-administered with antibiotics, anticonvulsants, and other drugs that increase the metabolism of contraceptive steroids. This could result in unintended pregnancy or unscheduled bleeding. In such cases a nonhormonal back-up method of birth control should be considered).
No products indexed under this heading.

Ketorolac Tromethamine (Contraceptive effectiveness may be reduced when hormonal contraceptives are co-administered with antibiotics, anticonvulsants, and other drugs that increase the metabolism of contraceptive steroids. This could result in unintended pregnancy or unscheduled bleeding. In such cases a nonhormonal back-up method of birth control should be considered).
No products indexed under this heading.

Labetalol Hydrochloride (Contraceptive effectiveness may be reduced when hormonal contraceptives are co-administered with antibiotics, anticonvulsants, and other drugs that increase the metabolism of contraceptive steroids. This could result in unintended pregnancy or unscheduled bleeding. In such cases a nonhormonal back-up method of birth control should be considered).
No products indexed under this heading.

Lamotrigine (Decreased plasma concentrations of lamotrigine due to induction of conjugation (particularly glucuronidation), have been noted when this drug is administered with oral contraceptives). Products include:
Lamictal 1488

Lansoprazole (Contraceptive effectiveness may be reduced when hormonal contraceptives are co-administered with antibiotics, anticonvulsants, and other drugs that increase the metabolism of contraceptive steroids. This could result in unintended pregnancy or unscheduled bleeding. In such cases a nonhormonal back-up method of birth control should be considered).
No products indexed under this heading.

Levalbuterol Hydrochloride (Enterohepatic recirculation of estrogens may also be decreased by substances that reduce gut transit time). Products include:
Xopenex Inhalation Solution 3001
Xopenex Inhalation Solution Concentrate 3005

Levetiracetam (Contraceptive effectiveness may be reduced when hormonal contraceptives are co-administered with antibiotics, anticonvulsants, and other drugs that increase the metabolism of contraceptive steroids. This could result in unintended pregnancy or unscheduled bleeding. In such cases a nonhormonal back-up method of birth control should be considered). Products include:
Keppra Injection 3137
Keppra Oral Solution 3131
Keppra Tablets 3131

Levobupivacaine Hydrochloride (Contraceptive effectiveness may be reduced when hormonal contraceptives are co-administered with antibiotics, anticonvulsants, and other drugs that increase the metabolism of contraceptive steroids. This could result in unintended pregnancy or unscheduled bleeding. In such cases a nonhormonal back-up method of birth control should be considered).
No products indexed under this heading.

Levorphanol Tartrate (Enterohepatic recirculation of estrogens may also be decreased by substances that reduce gut transit time).
No products indexed under this heading.

Lidocaine (Contraceptive effectiveness may be reduced when hormonal contraceptives are co-administered with antibiotics, anticonvulsants, and other drugs that increase the metabolism of contraceptive steroids. This could result in unintended pregnancy or unscheduled bleeding. In such cases a nonhormonal back-up method of birth control should be considered). Products include:
Lidoderm Patch 1114

Lidocaine Base (Contraceptive effectiveness may be reduced when hormonal contraceptives are co-administered with antibiotics, anticonvulsants, and other drugs that increase the metabolism of contraceptive steroids. This could result in unintended pregnancy or unscheduled bleeding. In such cases a nonhormonal back-up method of birth control should be considered).
No products indexed under this heading.

Lidocaine Hydrochloride (Contraceptive effectiveness may be reduced when hormonal contraceptives are co-administered with antibiotics, anticonvulsants, and other drugs that increase the metabolism of contraceptive steroids. This could result in unintended pregnancy or unscheduled bleeding. In such cases a nonhormonal back-up method of birth control should be considered).
No products indexed under this heading.

Lomefloxacin Hydrochloride (Contraceptive effectiveness may be reduced when hormonal contraceptives are co-administered with antibiotics, anticonvulsants, and other drugs that increase the metabolism of contraceptive steroids. This could result in unintended pregnancy or unscheduled bleeding. In such cases a nonhormonal back-up method of birth control should be considered).
No products indexed under this heading.

Lopinavir (Several of the anti-HIV protease inhibitors have been studied with co-administration of oral combination hormonal contraceptives; significant changes (increase and decrease) in the plasma levels of the estrogen and progestin have been noted in some cases. The safety and efficacy of oral contraceptive products may be affected with co-administration of anti-HIV protease inhibitors. Health care professionals should refer to the label of the individual anti-HIV protease inhibitors for further drug-drug interaction information). Products include:
Kaletra 452

Loratadine (CYP 3A4 inhibitors such as indinavir, itraconazole, ketoconazole, fluconazole, and troleandomycin may increase plasma hormone levels. Troleandomycin may also increase the risk of intrahepatic cholestasis during co-administration with combination oral contraceptives).
No products indexed under this heading.

Losartan Potassium (Contraceptive effectiveness may be reduced when hormonal contraceptives are co-administered with antibiotics, anticonvulsants, and other drugs that increase the metabolism of contraceptive steroids. This could result in unintended pregnancy or unscheduled bleeding. In such cases a nonhormonal back-up method of birth control should be considered). Products include:
Cozaar Tablets 1973

Lovastatin (Contraceptive effectiveness may be reduced when hormonal contraceptives are co-administered with antibiotics, anticonvulsants, and other drugs that increase the metabolism of contraceptive steroids. This could result in unintended pregnancy or unscheduled bleeding. In such cases a nonhormonal back-up method of birth control should be considered). Products include:
Advicor Tablets 402
Mevacor Tablets 2063

Maprotiline Hydrochloride (Contraceptive effectiveness may be reduced when hormonal contraceptives are co-administered with antibiotics, anticonvulsants, and other drugs that increase the metabolism of contraceptive steroids. This could result in unintended pregnancy or unscheduled bleeding. In such cases a nonhormonal back-up method of birth control should be considered).
No products indexed under this heading.

Meclofenamate Sodium (Contraceptive effectiveness may be reduced when hormonal contraceptives are co-administered with antibiotics, anticonvulsants, and other drugs that increase the metabolism of contraceptive steroids. This could result in unintended pregnancy or unscheduled bleeding. In such cases a nonhormonal back-up method of birth control should be considered).
No products indexed under this heading.

Mefenamic Acid (Contraceptive effectiveness may be reduced when hormonal contraceptives are co-administered with antibiotics, anticonvulsants, and other drugs that increase the metabolism of contraceptive steroids. This could result in unintended pregnancy or unscheduled bleeding. In such cases a nonhormonal back-up method of birth control should be considered).
No products indexed under this heading.

Meloxicam (Contraceptive effectiveness may be reduced when hormonal contraceptives are co-administered with antibiotics, anticonvulsants, and other drugs that increase the metabolism of contraceptive steroids. This could result in unintended pregnancy or unscheduled bleeding. In such cases a nonhormonal back-up method of birth control should be considered). Products include:
Mobic Oral Suspension 863
Mobic Tablets 863

Mepenzolate Bromide (Enterohepatic recirculation of estrogens may also be decreased by substances that reduce gut transit time).
No products indexed under this heading.

Meperidine Hydrochloride (Contraceptive effectiveness may be reduced when hormonal contraceptives are co-administered with antibiotics, anticonvulsants, and other drugs that increase the metabolism of contraceptive steroids. This could result in unintended pregnancy or unscheduled bleeding. In such cases a nonhormonal back-up method of birth control should be considered).
No products indexed under this heading.

Mephenytoin (Contraceptive effectiveness may be reduced when hormonal contraceptives are co-administered with antibiotics, anticonvulsants, and other drugs that increase the metabolism of contraceptive steroids. This could result in unintended pregnancy or unscheduled bleeding. In such cases a nonhormonal back-up method of birth control should be considered).
No products indexed under this heading.

Mephobarbital (Contraceptive effectiveness may be reduced when hormonal contraceptives are co-administered with antibiotics, anticonvulsants, and other drugs that increase the metabolism of contraceptive steroids. This could result in unintended pregnancy or unscheduled bleeding. In such cases a nonhormonal back-up method of birth control should be considered).
No products indexed under this heading.

Meprobamate (Contraceptive effectiveness may be reduced when hormonal contraceptives are co-administered with antibiotics, anticonvulsants, and other drugs that increase the metabolism of contraceptive steroids. This could result in unintended pregnancy or unscheduled bleeding. In such cases a nonhormonal back-up method of birth control should be considered).
No products indexed under this heading.

Mestranol (Contraceptive effectiveness may be reduced when hormonal contraceptives are co-administered with antibiotics, anticonvulsants, and other drugs that increase the metabolism of contraceptive steroids. This could result in unintended pregnancy or unscheduled bleeding. In such cases a nonhormonal back-up method of birth control should be considered).
No products indexed under this heading.

Metaproterenol Sulfate (Enterohepatic recirculation of estrogens may also be decreased by substances that reduce gut transit time).
No products indexed under this heading.

Metformin Hydrochloride (Contraceptive effectiveness may be reduced when hormonal contraceptives are co-administered with antibiotics, anticonvulsants, and other drugs that increase the metabolism of contraceptive steroids. This could result in unintended pregnancy or unscheduled bleeding. In such cases a nonhormonal back-up method of birth control should be considered). Products include:
ActoPlus Met Tablets 3071
Avandamet Tablets 1336
Janumet Tablets 2041
PrandiMet Tablets 2967

Methacycline Hydrochloride (Several cases of contraceptive failure and unscheduled bleeding have been reported in the literature with concomitant administration of antibiotics such as ampicillin and other penicillins, and tetracyclines. However, clinical pharmacology studies investigating drug interactions between combined oral contraceptives and these antibiotics have reported inconsistent results).
No products indexed under this heading.

Methadone Hydrochloride (Contraceptive effectiveness may be reduced when hormonal contraceptives are co-administered with antibiotics, anticonvulsants, and other drugs that increase the metabolism of contraceptive steroids. This could result in unintended pregnancy or unscheduled bleeding. In such cases a nonhormonal back-up method of birth control should be considered).
No products indexed under this heading.

Methamphetamine Hydrochloride (Contraceptive effectiveness may be reduced when hormonal contraceptives are co-administered with antibiotics, anticonvulsants, and other drugs that increase the metabolism of contraceptive steroids. This could result in unintended pregnancy or unscheduled bleeding. In such cases a nonhormonal back-up method of birth control should be considered).
No products indexed under this heading.

Methdilazine Hydrochloride (Enterohepatic recirculation of estrogens may also be decreased by substances that reduce gut transit time).
No products indexed under this heading.

Methsuximide (Contraceptive effectiveness may be reduced when hormonal contraceptives are co-administered with antibiotics, anticonvulsants, and other drugs that increase the metabolism of contraceptive steroids. This could result in unintended pregnancy or unscheduled bleeding. In such cases a nonhormonal back-up method of birth control should be considered).
No products indexed under this heading.

Methylprednisolone (Contraceptive effectiveness may be reduced when hormonal contraceptives are co-administered with antibiotics, anticonvulsants, and other drugs that increase the metabolism of contraceptive steroids. This could result in unintended pregnancy or unscheduled bleeding. In such cases a nonhormonal back-up method of birth control should be considered).
No products indexed under this heading.

Methylprednisolone Acetate (Contraceptive effectiveness may be reduced when hormonal contraceptives are co-administered with antibiotics, anticonvulsants, and other drugs that increase the metabolism of contraceptive steroids. This could result in unintended pregnancy or unscheduled bleeding. In such cases a nonhormonal back-up method of birth control should be considered).
No products indexed under this heading.

Methylprednisolone Sodium Succinate (Contraceptive effectiveness may be reduced when hormonal contraceptives are co-administered with antibiotics, anticonvulsants, and other drugs that increase the metabolism of contraceptive steroids. This could result in unintended pregnancy or unscheduled bleeding. In such cases a nonhormonal back-up method of birth control should be considered).
No products indexed under this heading.

Metoclopramide Hydrochloride (Enterohepatic recirculation of estrogens may also be decreased by substances that reduce gut transit time).
No products indexed under this heading.

Metoprolol Succinate (Contraceptive effectiveness may be reduced when hormonal contraceptives are co-administered with antibiotics, anticonvulsants, and other drugs that increase the metabolism of contraceptive steroids. This could result in unintended pregnancy or unscheduled bleeding. In such cases a nonhormonal back-up method of birth control should be considered). Products include:
Toprol-XL Tablets 666

Metoprolol Tartrate (Contraceptive effectiveness may be reduced when hormonal contraceptives are co-administered with antibiotics, anticonvulsants, and other drugs that increase the metabolism of contraceptive steroids. This could result in unintended pregnancy or unscheduled bleeding. In such cases a nonhormonal back-up method of birth control should be considered).
No products indexed under this heading.

Metronidazole (CYP 3A4 inhibitors such as indinavir, itraconazole, ketoconazole, fluconazole, and troleandomycin may increase plasma hormone levels. Troleandomycin may also increase the risk of intrahepatic cholestasis during co-administration with combination oral contraceptives). Products include:
Pylera Capsules 714

Metronidazole Benzoate (CYP 3A4 inhibitors such as indinavir, itraconazole, ketoconazole, fluconazole, and troleandomycin may increase plasma hormone levels. Troleandomycin may also increase the risk of intrahepatic cholestasis during co-administration with combination oral contraceptives).
No products indexed under this heading.

Metronidazole Hydrochloride (CYP 3A4 inhibitors such as indinavir, itraconazole, ketoconazole, fluconazole, and troleandomycin may increase plasma hormone levels. Troleandomycin may also increase the risk of intrahepatic cholestasis during co-administration with combination oral contraceptives).
No products indexed under this heading.

Mexiletine Hydrochloride (Contraceptive effectiveness may be reduced when hormonal contraceptives are co-administered with antibiotics, anticonvulsants, and other drugs that increase the metabolism of contraceptive steroids. This could result in unintended pregnancy or unscheduled bleeding. In such cases a nonhormonal back-up method of birth control should be considered).
No products indexed under this heading.

Mezlocillin Sodium (Several cases of contraceptive failure and unscheduled bleeding have been reported in the literature with concomitant administration of antibiotics such as ampicillin and other penicillins, and tetracyclines. However, clinical pharmacology studies investigating drug interactions between combined oral contraceptives and these antibiotics have reported inconsistent results).
No products indexed under this heading.

Mibefradil Dihydrochloride (Enterohepatic recirculation of estrogens may also be decreased by substances that reduce gut transit time).
No products indexed under this heading.

Miconazole (CYP 3A4 inhibitors such as indinavir, itraconazole, ketoconazole, fluconazole, and troleandomycin may increase plasma hormone levels. Troleandomycin may also increase the risk of intrahepatic cholestasis during co-administration with combination oral contraceptives).
No products indexed under this heading.

Miconazole Nitrate (CYP 3A4 inhibitors such as indinavir, itraconazole, ketoconazole, fluconazole, and troleandomycin may increase plasma hormone levels. Troleandomycin may also increase the risk of intrahepatic cholestasis during co-administration with combination oral contraceptives).
No products indexed under this heading.

Midazolam Hydrochloride (Contraceptive effectiveness may be reduced when hormonal contraceptives are co-administered with antibiotics, anticonvulsants, and other drugs that increase the metabolism of contraceptive steroids. This could result in unintended pregnancy or unscheduled bleeding. In such cases a nonhormonal back-up method of birth control should be considered).
No products indexed under this heading.

Miglitol (Contraceptive effectiveness may be reduced when hormonal contraceptives are co-administered with antibiotics, anticonvulsants, and other drugs that increase the metabolism of contraceptive steroids. This could result in unintended pregnancy or unscheduled bleeding. In such cases a nonhormonal back-up method of birth control should be considered).
No products indexed under this heading.

Minocycline Hydrochloride (Several cases of contraceptive failure and unscheduled bleeding have been reported in the literature with concomitant administration of antibiotics such as ampicillin and other penicillins, and tetracyclines. However, clinical pharmacology studies investigating drug interactions between combined oral contraceptives and these antibiotics have reported inconsistent results). Products include:
Solodyn Extended Release Tablets 1938

Mirtazapine (Contraceptive effectiveness may be reduced when hormonal contraceptives are co-administered with antibiotics, anticonvulsants, and other drugs that increase the metabolism of contraceptive steroids. This could result in unintended pregnancy or unscheduled bleeding. In such cases a nonhormonal back-up method of birth control should be considered). Products include:
Remeron Tablets 2924
RemeronSolTab Tablets 2927

Modafinil (Contraceptive effectiveness may be reduced when hormonal contraceptives are co-administered with antibiotics, anticonvulsants, and other drugs that increase the metabolism of contraceptive steroids. This could result in unintended pregnancy or unscheduled bleeding. In such cases a nonhormonal back-up method of birth control should be considered). Products include:
Provigil Tablets 977

Mometasone Furoate (Increased plasma concentrations of cyclosporine, prednisolone and other corticosteroids, have been reported with concomitant administration of oral contraceptives). Products include:
Asmanex Twisthaler 2797
Elocon Cream 0.1% 2840
Elocon Lotion 0.1% 2841
Elocon Ointment 0.1% 2842

Mometasone Furoate Monohydrate (Increased plasma concentrations of cyclosporine, prednisolone and other corticosteroids, have been reported with concomitant administration of oral contraceptives). Products include:
Nasonex Nasal Spray 2883

Montelukast Sodium (Contraceptive effectiveness may be reduced when hormonal contraceptives are co-administered with antibiotics, anticonvulsants, and other drugs that increase the metabolism of contraceptive steroids. This could result in unintended pregnancy or unscheduled bleeding. In such cases a nonhormonal back-up method of birth control should be considered). Products include:
Singulair 2114

Morphine Sulfate (Increased clearance of morphine, due to induction of conjugation (particularly glucuronidation), have been noted when this drug is administered with oral contraceptives). Products include:
Avinza Capsules 1772
DepoDur Injection 1095
MS Contin Tablets 2585

Morphine sulfate, liposomal (Increased clearance of morphine, due to induction of conjugation (particularly glucuronidation), have been noted when this drug is administered with oral contraceptives).
No products indexed under this heading.

Moxifloxacin Hydrochloride (Contraceptive effectiveness may be reduced when hormonal contraceptives are co-administered with antibiotics, anticonvulsants, and other drugs that increase the metabolism of contraceptive steroids. This could result in unintended pregnancy or unscheduled bleeding. In such cases a nonhormonal back-up method of birth control should be considered). Products include:
Avelox 2803
Vigamox Ophthalmic Solution 548

Nabumetone (Contraceptive effectiveness may be reduced when hormonal contraceptives are co-administered with antibiotics, anticonvulsants, and other drugs that increase the metabolism of contraceptive steroids. This could result in unintended pregnancy or unscheduled bleeding. In such cases a nonhormonal back-up method of birth control should be considered).
No products indexed under this heading.

Nafcillin Sodium (Contraceptive effectiveness may be reduced when hormonal contraceptives are co-administered with antibiotics, anticonvulsants, and other drugs that increase the metabolism of contraceptive steroids. This could result in unintended pregnancy or unscheduled bleeding. In such cases a nonhormonal back-up method of birth control should be considered).
No products indexed under this heading.

Naproxen (Contraceptive effectiveness may be reduced when hormonal contraceptives are co-administered with antibiotics, anticonvulsants, and other drugs that increase the metabolism of contraceptive steroids. This could result in unintended pregnancy or unscheduled bleeding. In such cases a nonhormonal back-up method of birth control should be considered).
Products include:
EC-Naprosyn Delayed-Release Tablets 2632
Naprosyn Suspension 2632
Naprosyn Tablets 2632

Naproxen Sodium (Contraceptive effectiveness may be reduced when hormonal contraceptives are co-administered with antibiotics, anticonvulsants, and other drugs that increase the metabolism of contraceptive steroids. This could result in unintended pregnancy or unscheduled bleeding. In such cases a nonhormonal back-up method of birth control should be considered).
Products include:
Anaprox Tablets 2632
Anaprox DS Tablets 2632
Treximet Tablets 1616

Nateglinide (Contraceptive effectiveness may be reduced when hormonal contraceptives are co-administered with antibiotics, anticonvulsants, and other drugs that increase the metabolism of contraceptive steroids. This could result in unintended pregnancy or unscheduled bleeding. In such cases a nonhormonal back-up method of birth control should be considered).
Products include:
Starlix Tablets 2314

Nefazodone Hydrochloride (Contraceptive effectiveness may be reduced when hormonal contraceptives are co-administered with antibiotics, anticonvulsants, and other drugs that increase the metabolism of contraceptive steroids. This could result in unintended pregnancy or unscheduled bleeding. In such cases a nonhormonal back-up method of birth control should be considered).
No products indexed under this heading.

Nelfinavir Mesylate (Contraceptive effectiveness may be reduced when hormonal contraceptives are co-administered with antibiotics, anticonvulsants, and other drugs that increase the metabolism of contraceptive steroids. This could result in unintended pregnancy or unscheduled bleeding. In such cases a nonhormonal back-up method of birth control should be considered).
No products indexed under this heading.

Neostigmine Bromide (Enterohepatic recirculation of estrogens may also be decreased by substances that reduce gut transit time).
No products indexed under this heading.

Neostigmine Methylsulfate (Enterohepatic recirculation of estrogens may also be decreased by substances that reduce gut transit time).
No products indexed under this heading.

Nevirapine (Contraceptive effectiveness may be reduced when hormonal contraceptives are co-administered with antibiotics, anticonvulsants, and other drugs that increase the metabolism of contraceptive steroids. This could result in unintended pregnancy or unscheduled bleeding. In such cases a nonhormonal back-up method of birth control should be considered).
Products include:
Viramune Oral Suspension 873
Viramune Tablets 873

Niacinamide (CYP 3A4 inhibitors such as indinavir, itraconazole, ketoconazole, fluconazole, and troleandomycin may increase plasma hormone levels. Troleandomycin may also increase the risk of intrahepatic cholestasis during co-administration with combination oral contraceptives). Products include:
BioLean Free Tablets .... ▣635

Nicardipine (Contraceptive effectiveness may be reduced when hormonal contraceptives are co-administered with antibiotics, anticonvulsants, and other drugs that increase the metabolism of contraceptive steroids. This could result in unintended pregnancy or unscheduled bleeding. In such cases a nonhormonal back-up method of birth control should be considered).
No products indexed under this heading.

Nicardipine Hydrochloride (Contraceptive effectiveness may be reduced when hormonal contraceptives are co-administered with antibiotics, anticonvulsants, and other drugs that increase the metabolism of contraceptive steroids. This could result in unintended pregnancy or unscheduled bleeding. In such cases a nonhormonal back-up method of birth control should be considered).
Products include:
Cardene I.V. 1093

Nicotinamide (CYP 3A4 inhibitors such as indinavir, itraconazole, ketoconazole, fluconazole, and troleandomycin may increase plasma hormone levels. Troleandomycin may also increase the risk of intrahepatic cholestasis during co-administration with combination oral contraceptives).
No products indexed under this heading.

Nicotine Polacrilex (Contraceptive effectiveness may be reduced when hormonal contraceptives are co-administered with antibiotics, anticonvulsants, and other drugs that increase the metabolism of contraceptive steroids. This could result in unintended pregnancy or unscheduled bleeding. In such cases a nonhormonal back-up method of birth control should be considered).
No products indexed under this heading.

Nicotine Salicylate (Contraceptive effectiveness may be reduced when hormonal contraceptives are co-administered with antibiotics, anticonvulsants, and other drugs that increase the metabolism of contraceptive steroids. This could result in unintended pregnancy or unscheduled bleeding. In such cases a nonhormonal back-up method of birth control should be considered).
No products indexed under this heading.

Nicotine Sulfate (Contraceptive effectiveness may be reduced when hormonal contraceptives are co-administered with antibiotics, anticonvulsants, and other drugs that increase the metabolism of contraceptive steroids. This could result in unintended pregnancy or unscheduled bleeding. In such cases a nonhormonal back-up method of birth control should be considered).
No products indexed under this heading.

Nifedipine (Contraceptive effectiveness may be reduced when hormonal contraceptives are co-administered with antibiotics, anticonvulsants, and other drugs that increase the metabolism of contraceptive steroids. This could result in unintended pregnancy or unscheduled bleeding. In such cases a nonhormonal back-up method of birth control should be considered).
No products indexed under this heading.

Nilutamide (Contraceptive effectiveness may be reduced when hormonal contraceptives are co-administered with antibiotics, anticonvulsants, and other drugs that increase the metabolism of contraceptive steroids. This could result in unintended pregnancy or unscheduled bleeding. In such cases a nonhormonal back-up method of birth control should be considered).
No products indexed under this heading.

Nimodipine (Contraceptive effectiveness may be reduced when hormonal contraceptives are co-administered with antibiotics, anticonvulsants, and other drugs that increase the metabolism of contraceptive steroids. This could result in unintended pregnancy or unscheduled bleeding. In such cases a nonhormonal back-up method of birth control should be considered).
Products include:
Nimotop Capsules 790

Nisoldipine (Contraceptive effectiveness may be reduced when hormonal contraceptives are co-administered with antibiotics, anticonvulsants, and other drugs that increase the metabolism of contraceptive steroids. This could result in unintended pregnancy or unscheduled bleeding. In such cases a nonhormonal back-up method of birth control should be considered).
Products include:
Sular Extended Release Tablets 2975

Nitrendipine (Contraceptive effectiveness may be reduced when hormonal contraceptives are co-administered with antibiotics, anticonvulsants, and other drugs that increase the metabolism of contraceptive steroids. This could result in unintended pregnancy or unscheduled bleeding. In such cases a nonhormonal back-up method of birth control should be considered).
No products indexed under this heading.

Norethindrone (Contraceptive effectiveness may be reduced when hormonal contraceptives are co-administered with antibiotics, anticonvulsants, and other drugs that increase the metabolism of contraceptive steroids. This could result in unintended pregnancy or unscheduled bleeding. In such cases a nonhormonal back-up method of birth control should be considered).
Products include:
Ortho Micronor Tablets 2446

Norethindrone Acetate (Contraceptive effectiveness may be reduced when hormonal contraceptives are co-administered with antibiotics, anticonvulsants, and other drugs that increase the metabolism of contraceptive steroids. This could result in unintended pregnancy or unscheduled bleeding. In such cases a nonhormonal back-up method of birth control should be considered).
Products include:
Activella Tablets 2347

Norfloxacin (Contraceptive effectiveness may be reduced when hormonal contraceptives are co-administered with antibiotics, anticonvulsants, and other drugs that increase the metabolism of contraceptive steroids. This could result in unintended pregnancy or unscheduled bleeding. In such cases a nonhormonal back-up method of birth control should be considered).
Products include:
Noroxin Tablets 2069

Norgestrel (Contraceptive effectiveness may be reduced when hormonal contraceptives are co-administered with antibiotics, anticonvulsants, and other drugs that increase the metabolism of contraceptive steroids. This could result in unintended pregnancy or unscheduled bleeding. In such cases a nonhormonal back-up method of birth control should be considered).
No products indexed under this heading.

Nortriptyline Hydrochloride (Contraceptive effectiveness may be reduced when hormonal contraceptives are co-administered with antibiotics, anticonvulsants, and other drugs that increase the metabolism of contraceptive steroids. This could result in unintended pregnancy or unscheduled bleeding. In such cases a nonhormonal back-up method of birth control should be considered).
No products indexed under this heading.

Octreotide Acetate (Enterohepatic recirculation of estrogens may also be decreased by substances that reduce gut transit time). Products include:
Sandostatin Injection 2300
Sandostatin LAR Depot 2302

Ofloxacin (Contraceptive effectiveness may be reduced when hormon-

al contraceptives are co-administered with antibiotics, anticonvulsants, and other drugs that increase the metabolism of contraceptive steroids. This could result in unintended pregnancy or unscheduled bleeding. In such cases a non-hormonal back-up method of birth control should be considered).
Products include:
Ofloxacin Ophthalmic Solution 0.3% .... ⊙243

Olanzapine (Contraceptive effectiveness may be reduced when hormonal contraceptives are co-administered with antibiotics, anticonvulsants, and other drugs that increase the metabolism of contraceptive steroids. This could result in unintended pregnancy or unscheduled bleeding. In such cases a non-hormonal back-up method of birth control should be considered).
Products include:
Symbyax Capsules 1871
Zyprexa Tablets 1883
Zyprexa IntraMuscular 1883
Zyprexa ZYDIS Orally Disintegrating Tablets 1883

Omeprazole (Contraceptive effectiveness may be reduced when hormonal contraceptives are co-administered with antibiotics, anticonvulsants, and other drugs that increase the metabolism of contraceptive steroids. This could result in unintended pregnancy or unscheduled bleeding. In such cases a non-hormonal back-up method of birth control should be considered).
No products indexed under this heading.

Ondansetron (Contraceptive effectiveness may be reduced when hormonal contraceptives are co-administered with antibiotics, anticonvulsants, and other drugs that increase the metabolism of contraceptive steroids. This could result in unintended pregnancy or unscheduled bleeding. In such cases a non-hormonal back-up method of birth control should be considered).
Products include:
Zofran ODT Orally Disintegrating Tablets 1687

Ondansetron Hydrochloride (Contraceptive effectiveness may be reduced when hormonal contraceptives are co-administered with antibiotics, anticonvulsants, and other drugs that increase the metabolism of contraceptive steroids. This could result in unintended pregnancy or unscheduled bleeding. In such cases a nonhormonal back-up method of birth control should be considered).
Products include:
Zofran Injection 1682
Zofran 1687

Oxaprozin (Contraceptive effectiveness may be reduced when hormonal contraceptives are co-administered with antibiotics, anticonvulsants, and other drugs that increase the metabolism of contraceptive steroids. This could result in unintended pregnancy or unscheduled bleeding. In such cases a non-hormonal back-up method of birth control should be considered).
No products indexed under this heading.

Oxcarbazepine (Contraceptive effectiveness may be reduced when hormonal contraceptives are co-administered with antibiotics, anticonvulsants, and other drugs that increase the metabolism of contraceptive steroids. This could result in unintended pregnancy or unscheduled bleeding. In such cases a non-hormonal back-up method of birth control should be considered).
No products indexed under this heading.

Oxybutynin Chloride (Enterohepatic recirculation of estrogens may also be decreased by substances that reduce gut transit time).
No products indexed under this heading.

Oxycodone Hydrochloride (Contraceptive effectiveness may be reduced when hormonal contraceptives are co-administered with antibiotics, anticonvulsants, and other drugs that increase the metabolism of contraceptive steroids. This could result in unintended pregnancy or unscheduled bleeding. In such cases a nonhormonal back-up method of birth control should be considered).
Products include:
OxyContin Tablets 2589
OxyIR Capsules 2593
Percocet Tablets 1127
Percodan Tablets 1130

Oxyphenonium Bromide (Enterohepatic recirculation of estrogens may also be decreased by substances that reduce gut transit time).
No products indexed under this heading.

Oxytetracycline Hydrochloride (Several cases of contraceptive failure and unscheduled bleeding have been reported in the literature with concomitant administration of antibiotics such as ampicillin and other penicillins, and tetracyclines. However, clinical pharmacology studies investigating drug interactions between combined oral contraceptives and these antibiotics have reported inconsistent results).
No products indexed under this heading.

Paclitaxel (Contraceptive effectiveness may be reduced when hormonal contraceptives are co-administered with antibiotics, anticonvulsants, and other drugs that increase the metabolism of contraceptive steroids. This could result in unintended pregnancy or unscheduled bleeding. In such cases a non-hormonal back-up method of birth control should be considered).
No products indexed under this heading.

Pantoprazole Sodium (Contraceptive effectiveness may be reduced when hormonal contraceptives are co-administered with antibiotics, anticonvulsants, and other drugs that increase the metabolism of contraceptive steroids. This could result in unintended pregnancy or unscheduled bleeding. In such cases a non-hormonal back-up method of birth control should be considered).
Products include:
Protonix for Delayed-Release Oral Suspension 3254
Protonix Delayed-Release Tablets 3254
Protonix I.V. 3257

Paramethadione (Contraceptive effectiveness may be reduced when hormonal contraceptives are co-administered with antibiotics, anticonvulsants, and other drugs that increase the metabolism of contraceptive steroids. This could result in unintended pregnancy or unscheduled bleeding. In such cases a non-hormonal back-up method of birth control should be considered).
No products indexed under this heading.

Paroxetine Hydrochloride (Contraceptive effectiveness may be reduced when hormonal contraceptives are co-administered with antibiotics, anticonvulsants, and other drugs that increase the metabolism of contraceptive steroids. This could result in unintended pregnancy or unscheduled bleeding. In such cases a nonhormonal back-up method of birth control should be considered).
Products include:
Paxil 1535
Paxil CR Controlled-Release Tablets 1544

Penicillin G Benzathine (Several cases of contraceptive failure and unscheduled bleeding have been reported in the literature with concomitant administration of antibiotics such as ampicillin and other penicillins, and tetracyclines. However, clinical pharmacology studies investigating drug interactions between combined oral contraceptives and these antibiotics have reported inconsistent results). Products include:
Bicillin C-R Injectable Suspension 1775
Bicillin L-A Injection 1777

Penicillin G Potassium (Several cases of contraceptive failure and unscheduled bleeding have been reported in the literature with concomitant administration of antibiotics such as ampicillin and other penicillins, and tetracyclines. However, clinical pharmacology studies investigating drug interactions between combined oral contraceptives and these antibiotics have reported inconsistent results).
No products indexed under this heading.

Penicillin G Procaine (Several cases of contraceptive failure and unscheduled bleeding have been reported in the literature with concomitant administration of antibiotics such as ampicillin and other penicillins, and tetracyclines. However, clinical pharmacology studies investigating drug interactions between combined oral contraceptives and these antibiotics have reported inconsistent results). Products include:
Bicillin C-R Injectable Suspension 1775
Bicillin L-A Injection 1777

Penicillin G Sodium (Several cases of contraceptive failure and unscheduled bleeding have been reported in the literature with concomitant administration of antibiotics such as ampicillin and other penicillins, and tetracyclines. However, clinical pharmacology studies investigating drug interactions between combined oral contraceptives and these antibiotics have reported inconsistent results).
No products indexed under this heading.

Penicillin V Potassium (Several cases of contraceptive failure and unscheduled bleeding have been reported in the literature with concomitant administration of antibiotics such as ampicillin and other penicillins, and tetracyclines. However, clinical pharmacology studies investigating drug interactions between combined oral contraceptives and these antibiotics have reported inconsistent results).
No products indexed under this heading.

Pentamidine Isethionate (Contraceptive effectiveness may be reduced when hormonal contraceptives are co-administered with antibiotics, anticonvulsants, and other drugs that increase the metabolism of contraceptive steroids. This could result in unintended pregnancy or unscheduled bleeding. In such cases a nonhormonal back-up method of birth control should be considered).
No products indexed under this heading.

Pentobarbital Sodium (Contraceptive effectiveness may be reduced when hormonal contraceptives are co-administered with antibiotics, anticonvulsants, and other drugs that increase the metabolism of contraceptive steroids. This could result in unintended pregnancy or unscheduled bleeding. In such cases a non-hormonal back-up method of birth control should be considered).
Products include:
Nembutal Sodium Solution, USP 2494

Pergolide Mesylate (Enterohepatic recirculation of estrogens may also be decreased by substances that reduce gut transit time).
No products indexed under this heading.

Phenacemide (Contraceptive effectiveness may be reduced when hormonal contraceptives are co-administered with antibiotics, anticonvulsants, and other drugs that increase the metabolism of contraceptive steroids. This could result in unintended pregnancy or unscheduled bleeding. In such cases a non-hormonal back-up method of birth control should be considered).
No products indexed under this heading.

Phenobarbital (Contraceptive effectiveness may be reduced when hormonal contraceptives are co-administered with antibiotics, anticonvulsants, and other drugs that increase the metabolism of contraceptive steroids. This could result in unintended pregnancy or unscheduled bleeding. In such cases a non-hormonal back-up method of birth control should be considered).
Products include:
Donnatal Extentabs 2507

Phenobarbital Sodium (Contraceptive effectiveness may be reduced when hormonal contraceptives are co-administered with antibiotics, anticonvulsants, and other drugs that increase the metabolism of contraceptive steroids. This could result in unintended pregnancy or unscheduled bleeding. In such cases a nonhormonal back-up method of birth control should be considered).
No products indexed under this heading.

Phensuximide (Contraceptive effectiveness may be reduced when hormonal contraceptives are co-administered with antibiotics, anticonvulsants, and other drugs that increase the metabolism of contraceptive steroids. This could result in unintended pregnancy or unscheduled bleeding. In such cases a nonhormonal back-up method of birth control should be considered).
No products indexed under this heading.

Phenylbutazone (Contraceptive effectiveness may be reduced when hormonal contraceptives are co-administered with antibiotics, anticonvulsants, and other drugs that increase the metabolism of contraceptive steroids. This could result in unintended pregnancy or unscheduled bleeding. In such cases a nonhormonal back-up method of birth control should be considered).
No products indexed under this heading.

Phenytoin (Contraceptive effectiveness may be reduced when hormonal contraceptives are co-administered with antibiotics, anticonvulsants, and other drugs that increase the metabolism of contraceptive steroids. This could result in unintended pregnancy or unscheduled bleeding. In such cases a nonhormonal back-up method of birth control should be considered).
No products indexed under this heading.

Phenytoin Sodium (Contraceptive effectiveness may be reduced when hormonal contraceptives are co-administered with antibiotics, anticonvulsants, and other drugs that increase the metabolism of contraceptive steroids. This could result in unintended pregnancy or unscheduled bleeding. In such cases a nonhormonal back-up method of birth control should be considered).
Products include:
Phenytek Capsules **2192**

Pimozide (Contraceptive effectiveness may be reduced when hormonal contraceptives are co-administered with antibiotics, anticonvulsants, and other drugs that increase the metabolism of contraceptive steroids. This could result in unintended pregnancy or unscheduled bleeding. In such cases a nonhormonal back-up method of birth control should be considered).
No products indexed under this heading.

Pindolol (Contraceptive effectiveness may be reduced when hormonal contraceptives are co-administered with antibiotics, anticonvulsants, and other drugs that increase the metabolism of contraceptive steroids. This could result in unintended pregnancy or unscheduled bleeding. In such cases a nonhormonal back-up method of birth control should be considered).
No products indexed under this heading.

Pioglitazone Hydrochloride (Contraceptive effectiveness may be reduced when hormonal contraceptives are co-administered with antibiotics, anticonvulsants, and other drugs that increase the metabolism of contraceptive steroids. This could result in unintended pregnancy or unscheduled bleeding. In such cases a nonhormonal back-up method of birth control should be considered).
Products include:
ActoPlus Met Tablets **3071**
Actos Tablets **3077**
Duetact Tablets **3085**

Pirbuterol Acetate (Enterohepatic recirculation of estrogens may also be decreased by substances that reduce gut transit time). Products include:
Maxair Autohaler **1705**

Piroxicam (Contraceptive effectiveness may be reduced when hormonal contraceptives are co-administered with antibiotics, anticonvulsants, and other drugs that increase the metabolism of contraceptive steroids. This could result in unintended pregnancy or unscheduled bleeding. In such cases a nonhormonal back-up method of birth control should be considered).
No products indexed under this heading.

Polyestradiol Phosphate (Contraceptive effectiveness may be reduced when hormonal contraceptives are co-administered with antibiotics, anticonvulsants, and other drugs that increase the metabolism of contraceptive steroids. This could result in unintended pregnancy or unscheduled bleeding. In such cases a nonhormonal back-up method of birth control should be considered).
No products indexed under this heading.

Pramipexole Dihydrochloride (Enterohepatic recirculation of estrogens may also be decreased by substances that reduce gut transit time). Products include:
Mirapex Tablets **857**

Prednisolone Acetate (Contraceptive effectiveness may be reduced when hormonal contraceptives are co-administered with antibiotics, anticonvulsants, and other drugs that increase the metabolism of contraceptive steroids. This could result in unintended pregnancy or unscheduled bleeding. In such cases a nonhormonal back-up method of birth control should be considered).
Products include:
Pred Forte Ophthalmic Suspension .... ⊙ **227**
Pred Mild Ophthalmic Suspension .... ⊙ **230**
Pred-G Ophthalmic Ointment .... ⊙ **229**
Pred-G Ophthalmic Suspension ...... ⊙ **228**

Prednisolone Sodium Phosphate (Contraceptive effectiveness may be reduced when hormonal contraceptives are co-administered with antibiotics, anticonvulsants, and other drugs that increase the metabolism of contraceptive steroids. This could result in unintended pregnancy or unscheduled bleeding. In such cases a nonhormonal back-up method of birth control should be considered).
No products indexed under this heading.

Prednisolone Tebutate (Contraceptive effectiveness may be reduced when hormonal contraceptives are co-administered with antibiotics, anticonvulsants, and other drugs that increase the metabolism of contraceptive steroids. This could result in unintended pregnancy or unscheduled bleeding. In such cases a nonhormonal back-up method of birth control should be considered).
No products indexed under this heading.

Prednisone (Contraceptive effectiveness may be reduced when hormonal contraceptives are co-administered with antibiotics, anticonvulsants, and other drugs that increase the metabolism of contraceptive steroids. This could result in unintended pregnancy or unscheduled bleeding. In such cases a nonhormonal back-up method of birth control should be considered).
No products indexed under this heading.

Primidone (Contraceptive effectiveness may be reduced when hormonal contraceptives are co-administered with antibiotics, anticonvulsants, and other drugs that increase the metabolism of contraceptive steroids. This could result in unintended pregnancy or unscheduled bleeding. In such cases a nonhormonal back-up method of birth control should be considered).
No products indexed under this heading.

Procainamide Hydrochloride (Enterohepatic recirculation of estrogens may also be decreased by substances that reduce gut transit time).
No products indexed under this heading.

Procyclidine Hydrochloride (Enterohepatic recirculation of estrogens may also be decreased by substances that reduce gut transit time).
No products indexed under this heading.

Progesterone (Contraceptive effectiveness may be reduced when hormonal contraceptives are co-administered with antibiotics, anticonvulsants, and other drugs that increase the metabolism of contraceptive steroids. This could result in unintended pregnancy or unscheduled bleeding. In such cases a nonhormonal back-up method of birth control should be considered).
Products include:
Crinone 4% Gel **992**
Crinone 8% Gel **992**
Prometrium Capsules (100 mg, 200 mg)...................................... **3047**

Proguanil Hydrochloride (Contraceptive effectiveness may be reduced when hormonal contraceptives are co-administered with antibiotics, anticonvulsants, and other drugs that increase the metabolism of contraceptive steroids. This could result in unintended pregnancy or unscheduled bleeding. In such cases a nonhormonal back-up method of birth control should be considered).
Products include:
Malarone Pediatric Tablets **1521**
Malarone Tablets **1521**

Promethazine Hydrochloride (Enterohepatic recirculation of estrogens may also be decreased by substances that reduce gut transit time).
No products indexed under this heading.

Propafenone Hydrochloride (Contraceptive effectiveness may be reduced when hormonal contraceptives are co-administered with antibiotics, anticonvulsants, and other drugs that increase the metabolism of contraceptive steroids. This could result in unintended pregnancy or unscheduled bleeding. In such cases a nonhormonal back-up method of birth control should be considered).
Products include:
Rythmol Tablets **1586**
Rythmol SR Capsules **1590**

Propantheline Bromide (Enterohepatic recirculation of estrogens may also be decreased by substances that reduce gut transit time).
No products indexed under this heading.

Propoxyphene Hydrochloride (Contraceptive effectiveness may be reduced when hormonal contraceptives are co-administered with antibiotics, anticonvulsants, and other drugs that increase the metabolism of contraceptive steroids. This could result in unintended pregnancy or unscheduled bleeding. In such cases a nonhormonal back-up method of birth control should be considered).
No products indexed under this heading.

Propoxyphene Napsylate (Contraceptive effectiveness may be reduced when hormonal contraceptives are co-administered with antibiotics, anticonvulsants, and other drugs that increase the metabolism of contraceptive steroids. This could result in unintended pregnancy or unscheduled bleeding. In such cases a nonhormonal back-up method of birth control should be considered).
No products indexed under this heading.

Propranolol Hydrochloride (Contraceptive effectiveness may be reduced when hormonal contraceptives are co-administered with antibiotics, anticonvulsants, and other drugs that increase the metabolism of contraceptive steroids. This could result in unintended pregnancy or unscheduled bleeding. In such cases a nonhormonal back-up method of birth control should be considered).
Products include:
InnoPran XL Extended Release Capsules.................................... **1484**

Protriptyline Hydrochloride (Contraceptive effectiveness may be reduced when hormonal contraceptives are co-administered with antibiotics, anticonvulsants, and other drugs that increase the metabolism of contraceptive steroids. This could result in unintended pregnancy or unscheduled bleeding. In such cases a nonhormonal back-up method of birth control should be considered).
No products indexed under this heading.

Pyridostigmine Bromide (Enterohepatic recirculation of estrogens may also be decreased by substances that reduce gut transit time).
No products indexed under this heading.

Pyrilamine Maleate (Enterohepatic recirculation of estrogens may also be decreased by substances that reduce gut transit time).
No products indexed under this heading.

Pyrilamine Tannate (Enterohepatic recirculation of estrogens may also be decreased by substances that reduce gut transit time).
No products indexed under this heading.

Quetiapine Fumarate (Contraceptive effectiveness may be reduced when hormonal contraceptives are co-administered with antibiotics, anticonvulsants, and other drugs that increase the metabolism of contraceptive steroids. This could result in unintended pregnancy or unscheduled bleeding. In such cases a nonhormonal back-up method of birth control should be considered).
No products indexed under this heading.

Quinestrol (Co-administration of certain oral contraceptives containing ethinyl estradiol increases AUC values for ethinyl estradiol by approximately 20%).
No products indexed under this heading.

Quinidine (CYP 3A4 inhibitors such as indinavir, itraconazole, ketoconazole, fluconazole, and troleandomycin may increase plasma hormone levels. Troleandomycin may also increase the risk of intrahepatic cholestasis during co-administration with combination oral contraceptives).
No products indexed under this heading.

Quinidine Gluconate (Contraceptive effectiveness may be reduced when hormonal contraceptives are co-administered with antibiotics, anticonvulsants, and other drugs that increase the metabolism of contraceptive steroids. This could result in unintended pregnancy or unscheduled bleeding. In such cases a nonhormonal back-up method of birth control should be considered).
No products indexed under this heading.

Quinidine Hydrochloride (Contraceptive effectiveness may be reduced when hormonal contraceptives are co-administered with antibiotics, anticonvulsants, and other drugs that increase the metabolism of contraceptive steroids. This could result in unintended pregnancy or unscheduled bleeding. In such cases a nonhormonal back-up method of birth control should be considered).
No products indexed under this heading.

Quinidine Polygalacturonate (Contraceptive effectiveness may be reduced when hormonal contraceptives are co-administered with antibiotics, anticonvulsants, and other drugs that increase the metabolism of contraceptive steroids. This could result in unintended pregnancy or unscheduled bleeding. In such cases a nonhormonal back-up method of birth control should be considered).
No products indexed under this heading.

Quinidine Sulfate (Contraceptive effectiveness may be reduced when hormonal contraceptives are co-administered with antibiotics, anticonvulsants, and other drugs that increase the metabolism of contraceptive steroids. This could result in unintended pregnancy or unscheduled bleeding. In such cases a nonhormonal back-up method of birth control should be considered).
No products indexed under this heading.

Quinine (Contraceptive effectiveness may be reduced when hormonal contraceptives are co-administered with antibiotics, anticonvulsants, and other drugs that increase the metabolism of contraceptive steroids. This could result in unintended pregnancy or unscheduled bleeding. In such cases a nonhormonal back-up method of birth control should be considered).
No products indexed under this heading.

Quinine Sulfate (Contraceptive effectiveness may be reduced when hormonal contraceptives are co-administered with antibiotics, anticonvulsants, and other drugs that increase the metabolism of contraceptive steroids. This could result in unintended pregnancy or unscheduled bleeding. In such cases a nonhormonal back-up method of birth control should be considered).
No products indexed under this heading.

Quinupristin (CYP 3A4 inhibitors such as indinavir, itraconazole, ketoconazole, fluconazole, and troleandomycin may increase plasma hormone levels. Troleandomycin may also increase the risk of intrahepatic cholestasis during co-administration with combination oral contraceptives).
No products indexed under this heading.

Rabeprazole Sodium (Contraceptive effectiveness may be reduced when hormonal contraceptives are co-administered with antibiotics, anticonvulsants, and other drugs that increase the metabolism of contraceptive steroids. This could result in unintended pregnancy or unscheduled bleeding. In such cases a nonhormonal back-up method of birth control should be considered).
Products include:
Aciphex Tablets 1053

Ranitidine Bismuth Citrate (CYP 3A4 inhibitors such as indinavir, itraconazole, ketoconazole, fluconazole, and troleandomycin may increase plasma hormone levels. Troleandomycin may also increase the risk of intrahepatic cholestasis during co-administration with combination oral contraceptives).
No products indexed under this heading.

Ranitidine Hydrochloride (CYP 3A4 inhibitors such as indinavir, itraconazole, ketoconazole, fluconazole, and troleandomycin may increase plasma hormone levels. Troleandomycin may also increase the risk of intrahepatic cholestasis during co-administration with combination oral contraceptives). Products include:
Zantac 75 Tablets 603
Zantac 1670
Zantac Injection 1666
Zantac Injection Pharmacy Bulk Package 1668
Maximum Strength Zantac 150 Tablets 603
Maximum Strength Zantac 150 Cool Mint Tablets 603

Remifentanil Hydrochloride (Enterohepatic recirculation of estrogens may also be decreased by substances that reduce gut transit time).
No products indexed under this heading.

Repaglinide (Contraceptive effectiveness may be reduced when hormonal contraceptives are co-administered with antibiotics, anticonvulsants, and other drugs that increase the metabolism of contraceptive steroids. This could result in unintended pregnancy or unscheduled bleeding. In such cases a nonhormonal back-up method of birth control should be considered).
Products include:
PrandiMet Tablets 2967
Prandin Tablets 2971

Rifabutin (Contraceptive effectiveness may be reduced when hormonal contraceptives are co-administered with antibiotics, anticonvulsants, and other drugs that increase the metabolism of contraceptive steroids. This could result in unintended pregnancy or unscheduled bleeding. In such cases a nonhormonal back-up method of birth control should be considered).
No products indexed under this heading.

Rifampicin (Contraceptive effectiveness may be reduced when hormonal contraceptives are co-administered with antibiotics, anticonvulsants, and other drugs that increase the metabolism of contraceptive steroids. This could result in unintended pregnancy or unscheduled bleeding. In such cases a nonhormonal back-up method of birth control should be considered).
No products indexed under this heading.

Rifampin (Contraceptive effectiveness may be reduced when hormonal contraceptives are co-administered with antibiotics, anticonvulsants, and other drugs that increase the metabolism of contraceptive steroids. This could result in unintended pregnancy or unscheduled bleeding. In such cases a nonhormonal back-up method of birth control should be considered).
No products indexed under this heading.

Rifapentine (Contraceptive effectiveness may be reduced when hormonal contraceptives are co-administered with antibiotics, anticonvulsants, and other drugs that increase the metabolism of contraceptive steroids. This could result in unintended pregnancy or unscheduled bleeding. In such cases a nonhormonal back-up method of birth control should be considered).
No products indexed under this heading.

Riluzole (Contraceptive effectiveness may be reduced when hormonal contraceptives are co-administered with antibiotics, anticonvulsants, and other drugs that increase the metabolism of contraceptive steroids. This could result in unintended pregnancy or unscheduled bleeding. In such cases a nonhormonal back-up method of birth control should be considered).
Products include:
Rilutek Tablets 2771

Risperidone (Contraceptive effectiveness may be reduced when hormonal contraceptives are co-administered with antibiotics, anticonvulsants, and other drugs that increase the metabolism of contraceptive steroids. This could result in unintended pregnancy or unscheduled bleeding. In such cases a nonhormonal back-up method of birth control should be considered).
Products include:
Risperdal Consta Long-Acting Injection 1753

Ritonavir (Contraceptive effectiveness may be reduced when hormonal contraceptives are co-administered with antibiotics, anticonvulsants, and other drugs that increase the metabolism of contraceptive steroids. This could result in unintended pregnancy or unscheduled bleeding. In such cases a nonhormonal back-up method of birth control should be considered).
Products include:
Kaletra 452
Norvir 489

Rivastigmine Tartrate (Enterohepatic recirculation of estrogens may also be decreased by substances that reduce gut transit time).
Products include:
Exelon Capsules 2229
Exelon Oral Solution 2229
Exelon Patch 2233

Rofecoxib (Contraceptive effectiveness may be reduced when hormonal contraceptives are co-administered with antibiotics, anticonvulsants, and other drugs that increase the metabolism of contraceptive steroids. This could result in unintended pregnancy or unscheduled bleeding. In such cases a nonhormonal back-up method of birth control should be considered).
No products indexed under this heading.

Ropinirole Hydrochloride (Contraceptive effectiveness may be reduced when hormonal contraceptives are co-administered with antibiotics, anticonvulsants, and other drugs that increase the metabolism of contraceptive steroids. This could result in unintended pregnancy or unscheduled bleeding. In such cases a nonhormonal back-up method of birth control should be considered).
Products include:
Requip Tablets 1561
Requip XL Tablets 1568

Ropivacaine Hydrochloride (Contraceptive effectiveness may be reduced when hormonal contraceptives are co-administered with antibiotics, anticonvulsants, and other drugs that increase the metabolism of contraceptive steroids. This could result in unintended pregnancy or unscheduled bleeding. In such cases a nonhormonal back-up method of birth control should be considered).
No products indexed under this heading.

Rosiglitazone Maleate (Contraceptive effectiveness may be reduced when hormonal contraceptives are co-administered with antibiotics, anticonvulsants, and other drugs that increase the metabolism of contraceptive steroids. This could result in unintended pregnancy or unscheduled bleeding. In such cases a nonhormonal back-up method of birth control should be considered).
Products include:
Avandamet Tablets 1336
Avandaryl Tablets 1344
Avandia Tablets 1351

Salicylic Acid (Increased clearance of salicylic adid, due to induction of conjugation (particularly glucuronidation), have been noted when this drug is administered with oral contraceptives).

No products indexed under this heading.

Salmeterol Xinafoate (Enterohepatic recirculation of estrogens may also be decreased by substances that reduce gut transit time). Products include:

Advair Diskus 100/50 1276
Advair Diskus 250/50 1276
Advair Diskus 500/50 1276
Advair HFA 45/21 Inhalation Aerosol.................... 1288
Advair HFA 115/21 Inhalation Aerosol.................... 1288
Advair HFA 230/21 Inhalation Aerosol.................... 1288
Serevent Diskus 1594

Saquinavir (Contraceptive effectiveness may be reduced when hormonal contraceptives are co-administered with antibiotics, anticonvulsants, and other drugs that increase the metabolism of contraceptive steroids. This could result in unintended pregnancy or unscheduled bleeding. In such cases a nonhormonal back-up method of birth control should be considered).

No products indexed under this heading.

Saquinavir Mesylate (Contraceptive effectiveness may be reduced when hormonal contraceptives are co-administered with antibiotics, anticonvulsants, and other drugs that increase the metabolism of contraceptive steroids. This could result in unintended pregnancy or unscheduled bleeding. In such cases a nonhormonal back-up method of birth control should be considered).

No products indexed under this heading.

Scopolamine (Enterohepatic recirculation of estrogens may also be decreased by substances that reduce gut transit time). Products include:

Transderm Scōp Transdermal Therapeutic System 2206

Scopolamine Hydrobromide (Enterohepatic recirculation of estrogens may also be decreased by substances that reduce gut transit time). Products include:

Donnatal Extentabs 2507

Secobarbital Sodium (Contraceptive effectiveness may be reduced when hormonal contraceptives are co-administered with antibiotics, anticonvulsants, and other drugs that increase the metabolism of contraceptive steroids. This could result in unintended pregnancy or unscheduled bleeding. In such cases a nonhormonal back-up method of birth control should be considered).

No products indexed under this heading.

Sertraline Hydrochloride (Contraceptive effectiveness may be reduced when hormonal contraceptives are co-administered with antibiotics, anticonvulsants, and other drugs that increase the metabolism of contraceptive steroids. This could result in unintended pregnancy or unscheduled bleeding. In such cases a nonhormonal back-up method of birth control should be considered).

No products indexed under this heading.

Sildenafil Citrate (Contraceptive effectiveness may be reduced when hormonal contraceptives are co-administered with antibiotics, anticonvulsants, and other drugs that increase the metabolism of contraceptive steroids. This could result in unintended pregnancy or unscheduled bleeding. In such cases a nonhormonal back-up method of birth control should be considered).

No products indexed under this heading.

Simvastatin (Contraceptive effectiveness may be reduced when hormonal contraceptives are co-administered with antibiotics, anticonvulsants, and other drugs that increase the metabolism of contraceptive steroids. This could result in unintended pregnancy or unscheduled bleeding. In such cases a nonhormonal back-up method of birth control should be considered). Products include:

Simcor Tablets 502
Vytorin 10/10 Tablets 2149
Vytorin 10/10 Tablets 2939
Vytorin 10/20 Tablets 2149
Vytorin 10/20 Tablets 2939
Vytorin 10/40 Tablets 2149
Vytorin 10/40 Tablets 2939
Vytorin 10/80 Tablets 2149
Vytorin 10/80 Tablets 2939
Zocor Tablets 2136

Sirolimus (Contraceptive effectiveness may be reduced when hormonal contraceptives are co-administered with antibiotics, anticonvulsants, and other drugs that increase the metabolism of contraceptive steroids. This could result in unintended pregnancy or unscheduled bleeding. In such cases a nonhormonal back-up method of birth control should be considered). Products include:

Rapamune 3260

Sucralfate (Enterohepatic recirculation of estrogens may also be decreased by substances that reduce gut transit time). Products include:

Carafate Suspension 706
Carafate Tablets 707

Sufentanil Citrate (Enterohepatic recirculation of estrogens may also be decreased by substances that reduce gut transit time).

No products indexed under this heading.

Sulfamethoxazole (Contraceptive effectiveness may be reduced when hormonal contraceptives are co-administered with antibiotics, anticonvulsants, and other drugs that increase the metabolism of contraceptive steroids. This could result in unintended pregnancy or unscheduled bleeding. In such cases a nonhormonal back-up method of birth control should be considered).

No products indexed under this heading.

Sulfinpyrazone (Contraceptive effectiveness may be reduced when hormonal contraceptives are co-administered with antibiotics, anticonvulsants, and other drugs that increase the metabolism of contraceptive steroids. This could result in unintended pregnancy or unscheduled bleeding. In such cases a nonhormonal back-up method of birth control should be considered).

No products indexed under this heading.

Sulindac (Contraceptive effectiveness may be reduced when hormonal contraceptives are co-administered with antibiotics, anticonvulsants, and other drugs that increase the metabolism of contraceptive steroids. This could result in unintended pregnancy or unscheduled bleeding. In such cases a nonhormonal back-up method of birth control should be considered). Products include:

Clinoril Tablets 1962

Suprofen (Contraceptive effectiveness may be reduced when hormonal contraceptives are co-administered with antibiotics, anticonvulsants, and other drugs that increase the metabolism of contraceptive steroids. This could result in unintended pregnancy or unscheduled bleeding. In such cases a nonhormonal back-up method of birth control should be considered).

No products indexed under this heading.

Tacrine Hydrochloride (Contraceptive effectiveness may be reduced when hormonal contraceptives are co-administered with antibiotics, anticonvulsants, and other drugs that increase the metabolism of contraceptive steroids. This could result in unintended pregnancy or unscheduled bleeding. In such cases a nonhormonal back-up method of birth control should be considered).

No products indexed under this heading.

Tacrolimus (Contraceptive effectiveness may be reduced when hormonal contraceptives are co-administered with antibiotics, anticonvulsants, and other drugs that increase the metabolism of contraceptive steroids. This could result in unintended pregnancy or unscheduled bleeding. In such cases a nonhormonal back-up method of birth control should be considered). Products include:

Prograf Capsules and Injection 622
Protopic Ointment 628

Tamoxifen Citrate (Contraceptive effectiveness may be reduced when hormonal contraceptives are co-administered with antibiotics, anticonvulsants, and other drugs that increase the metabolism of contraceptive steroids. This could result in unintended pregnancy or unscheduled bleeding. In such cases a nonhormonal back-up method of birth control should be considered).

No products indexed under this heading.

Telithromycin (CYP 3A4 inhibitors such as indinavir, itraconazole, ketoconazole, fluconazole, and troleandomycin may increase plasma hormone levels. Troleandomycin may also increase the risk of intrahepatic cholestasis during co-administration with combination oral contraceptives). Products include:

Ketek Tablets 2744

Telmisartan (Contraceptive effectiveness may be reduced when hormonal contraceptives are co-administered with antibiotics, anticonvulsants, and other drugs that increase the metabolism of contraceptive steroids. This could result in unintended pregnancy or unscheduled bleeding. In such cases a nonhormonal back-up method of birth control should be considered). Products include:

Micardis Tablets 852
Micardis HCT Tablets 854

Temazepam (Increased clearance of temazepam, due to induction of conjugation (particularly glucuronidation), have been noted when this drug is administered with oral contraceptives).

No products indexed under this heading.

Teniposide (Contraceptive effectiveness may be reduced when hormonal contraceptives are co-administered with antibiotics, anticonvulsants, and other drugs that increase the metabolism of contraceptive steroids. This could result in unintended pregnancy or unscheduled bleeding. In such cases a nonhormonal back-up method of birth control should be considered).

No products indexed under this heading.

Terbutaline Sulfate (Enterohepatic recirculation of estrogens may also be decreased by substances that reduce gut transit time).

No products indexed under this heading.

Terfenadine (Contraceptive effectiveness may be reduced when hormonal contraceptives are co-administered with antibiotics, anticonvulsants, and other drugs that increase the metabolism of contraceptive steroids. This could result in unintended pregnancy or unscheduled bleeding. In such cases a nonhormonal back-up method of birth control should be considered).

No products indexed under this heading.

Testosterone (Contraceptive effectiveness may be reduced when hormonal contraceptives are co-administered with antibiotics, anticonvulsants, and other drugs that increase the metabolism of contraceptive steroids. This could result in unintended pregnancy or unscheduled bleeding. In such cases a nonhormonal back-up method of birth control should be considered). Products include:

AndroGel 3159
Testim 1% Gel 701

Testosterone Cypionate (Contraceptive effectiveness may be reduced when hormonal contraceptives are co-administered with antibiotics, anticonvulsants, and other drugs that increase the metabolism of contraceptive steroids. This could result in unintended pregnancy or unscheduled bleeding. In such cases a nonhormonal back-up method of birth control should be considered).

No products indexed under this heading.

Testosterone Enanthate (Contraceptive effectiveness may be reduced when hormonal contraceptives are co-administered with antibiotics, anticonvulsants, and other drugs that increase the metabolism of contraceptive steroids. This could result in unintended pregnancy or unscheduled bleeding. In such cases a nonhormonal back-up method of birth control should be considered). Products include:

Delatestryl Injection 1730

Testosterone Propionate (Contraceptive effectiveness may be reduced when hormonal contraceptives are co-administered with antibiotics, anticonvulsants, and other drugs that increase the metabolism of contraceptive steroids. This could result in unintended pregnancy or unscheduled bleeding. In such cases a nonhormonal back-up method of birth control should be considered).

No products indexed under this heading.

Tetracycline Hydrochloride (Several cases of contraceptive failure and unscheduled bleeding have been reported in the literature with concomitant administration of antibiotics such as ampicillin and other penicillins, and tetracyclines. However, clinical pharmacology studies investigating drug interactions between combined oral contraceptives and these antibiotics have reported inconsistent results). Products include:

Pylera Capsules 714

Theophylline (Increased plasma concentrations of theophylline have been reported with concomitant administration of oral contraceptives).

No products indexed under this heading.

Theophylline Anhydrous (Contraceptive effectiveness may be reduced when hormonal contraceptives are co-administered with antibiotics, anticonvulsants, and other drugs that increase the metabolism of contraceptive steroids. This could result in unintended pregnancy or unscheduled bleeding. In such cases a nonhormonal back-up method of birth control should be considered). Products include:

Uniphyl Tablets 2595

Theophylline Calcium Salicylate (Contraceptive effectiveness may be reduced when hormonal contraceptives are co-administered with antibiotics, anticonvulsants, and other drugs that increase the metabolism of contraceptive steroids. This could result in unintended pregnancy or unscheduled bleeding. In such cases a nonhormonal back-up method of birth control should be considered).

No products indexed under this heading.

Theophylline Dihydroxypropyl (Glyceryl) (Contraceptive effectiveness may be reduced when hormonal contraceptives are co-administered with antibiotics, anticonvulsants, and other drugs that increase the metabolism of contraceptive steroids. This could result in unintended pregnancy or unscheduled bleeding. In such cases a nonhormonal back-up method of birth control should be considered).

No products indexed under this heading.

Theophylline Ethylenediamine (Contraceptive effectiveness may be reduced when hormonal contraceptives are co-administered with antibiotics, anticonvulsants, and other drugs that increase the metabolism of contraceptive steroids. This could result in unintended pregnancy or unscheduled bleeding. In such cases a nonhormonal back-up method of birth control should be considered).

No products indexed under this heading.

Theophylline Sodium Glycinate (Contraceptive effectiveness may be reduced when hormonal contraceptives are co-administered with antibiotics, anticonvulsants, and other drugs that increase the metabolism of contraceptive steroids. This could result in unintended pregnancy or unscheduled bleeding. In such cases a nonhormonal back-up method of birth control should be considered).

No products indexed under this heading.

Thiamylal Sodium (Contraceptive effectiveness may be reduced when hormonal contraceptives are co-administered with antibiotics, anticonvulsants, and other drugs that increase the metabolism of contraceptive steroids. This could result in unintended pregnancy or unscheduled bleeding. In such cases a nonhormonal back-up method of birth control should be considered).

No products indexed under this heading.

Thioridazine (Contraceptive effectiveness may be reduced when hormonal contraceptives are co-administered with antibiotics, anticonvulsants, and other drugs that increase the metabolism of contraceptive steroids. This could result in unintended pregnancy or unscheduled bleeding. In such cases a nonhormonal back-up method of birth control should be considered).

No products indexed under this heading.

Thioridazine Hydrochloride (Contraceptive effectiveness may be reduced when hormonal contraceptives are co-administered with antibiotics, anticonvulsants, and other drugs that increase the metabolism of contraceptive steroids. This could result in unintended pregnancy or unscheduled bleeding. In such cases a nonhormonal back-up method of birth control should be considered). Products include:

Thioridazine Hydrochloride Tablets 2195

Tiagabine Hydrochloride (Contraceptive effectiveness may be reduced when hormonal contraceptives are co-administered with antibiotics, anticonvulsants, and other drugs that increase the metabolism of contraceptive steroids. This could result in unintended pregnancy or unscheduled bleeding. In such cases a nonhormonal back-up method of birth control should be considered). Products include:

Gabitril Tablets 973

Ticarcillin Disodium (Several cases of contraceptive failure and unscheduled bleeding have been reported in the literature with concomitant administration of antibiotics such as ampicillin and other penicillins, and tetracyclines. However, clinical pharmacology studies investigating drug interactions between combined oral contraceptives and these antibiotics have reported inconsistent results). Products include:

Timentin ADD-Vantage 1606
Timentin Injection Galaxy Container 1609
Timentin IV Infusion 1603
Timentin Pharmacy Bulk Package 1613

Timolol Maleate (Contraceptive effectiveness may be reduced when hormonal contraceptives are co-administered with antibiotics, anticonvulsants, and other drugs that increase the metabolism of contraceptive steroids. This could result in unintended pregnancy or unscheduled bleeding. In such cases a nonhormonal back-up method of birth control should be considered). Products include:

Combigan Ophthalmic Solution 553
Cosopt Sterile Ophthalmic Solution 1969
Timoptic Sterile Ophthalmic Solution 2121
Timoptic in Ocudose 2124
Timoptic-XE Sterile Ophthalmic Gel Forming Solution 2125

Tipranavir (Several of the anti-HIV protease inhibitors have been studied with co-administration of oral combination hormonal contraceptives; significant changes (increase and decrease) in the plasma levels of the estrogen and progestin have been noted in some cases. The safety and efficacy of oral contraceptive products may be affected with co-administration of anti-HIV protease inhibitors. Health care professionals should refer to the label of the individual anti-HIV protease inhibitors for further drug-drug interaction information). Products include:

Aptivus Capsules 823
Aptivus Oral Solution 823

Tolazamide (Contraceptive effectiveness may be reduced when hormonal contraceptives are co-administered with antibiotics, anticonvulsants, and other drugs that increase the metabolism of contraceptive steroids. This could result in unintended pregnancy or unscheduled bleeding. In such cases a nonhormonal back-up method of birth control should be considered).

No products indexed under this heading.

Tolbutamide (Contraceptive effectiveness may be reduced when hormonal contraceptives are co-administered with antibiotics, anticonvulsants, and other drugs that increase the metabolism of contraceptive steroids. This could result in unintended pregnancy or unscheduled bleeding. In such cases a nonhormonal back-up method of birth control should be considered).

No products indexed under this heading.

Tolbutamide Sodium (Contraceptive effectiveness may be reduced when hormonal contraceptives are co-administered with antibiotics, anticonvulsants, and other drugs that increase the metabolism of contraceptive steroids. This could result in unintended pregnancy or unscheduled bleeding. In such cases a nonhormonal back-up method of birth control should be considered).

No products indexed under this heading.

Tolmetin Sodium (Contraceptive effectiveness may be reduced when hormonal contraceptives are co-administered with antibiotics, anticonvulsants, and other drugs that increase the metabolism of contraceptive steroids. This could result in unintended pregnancy or unscheduled bleeding. In such cases a nonhormonal back-up method of birth control should be considered).

No products indexed under this heading.

Tolterodine Tartrate (Contraceptive effectiveness may be reduced when hormonal contraceptives are co-administered with antibiotics, anticonvulsants, and other drugs that increase the metabolism of contraceptive steroids. This could result in unintended pregnancy or unscheduled bleeding. In such cases a nonhormonal back-up method of birth control should be considered).

No products indexed under this heading.

Topiramate (Contraceptive effectiveness may be reduced when hormonal contraceptives are co-administered with antibiotics, anticonvulsants, and other drugs that increase the metabolism of contraceptive steroids. This could result in unintended pregnancy or unscheduled bleeding. In such cases a nonhormonal back-up method of birth control should be considered).

No products indexed under this heading.

Torsemide (Contraceptive effectiveness may be reduced when hormonal contraceptives are co-administered with antibiotics, anticonvulsants, and other drugs that increase the metabolism of contraceptive steroids. This could result in unintended pregnancy or unscheduled bleeding. In such cases a nonhormonal back-up method of birth control should be considered). Products include:

Demadex Injection 2630
Demadex Tablets 2630

Tramadol Hydrochloride (Contraceptive effectiveness may be reduced when hormonal contraceptives are co-administered with antibiotics, anticonvulsants, and other drugs that increase the metabolism of contraceptive steroids. This could result in unintended pregnancy or unscheduled bleeding. In such cases a nonhormonal back-up method of birth control should be considered). Products include:

Ultram ER Extended-Release Tablets 2428

Trazodone Hydrochloride (Contraceptive effectiveness may be reduced when hormonal contraceptives are co-administered with antibiotics, anticonvulsants, and other drugs that increase the metabolism of contraceptive steroids. This could result in unintended pregnancy or unscheduled bleeding. In such cases a nonhormonal back-up method of birth control should be considered).

No products indexed under this heading.

Tretinoin (Contraceptive effectiveness may be reduced when hormonal contraceptives are co-administered with antibiotics, anticonvulsants, and other drugs that increase the metabolism of contraceptive steroids. This could result in unintended pregnancy or unscheduled bleeding. In such cases a nonhormonal back-up method of birth control should be considered). Products include:

Vesanoid Capsules 2660
Ziana Gel 1942

Triamcinolone (Contraceptive effectiveness may be reduced when hormonal contraceptives are co-administered with antibiotics, anticonvulsants, and other drugs that increase the metabolism of contraceptive steroids. This could result in unintended pregnancy or unscheduled bleeding. In such cases a nonhormonal back-up method of birth control should be considered).
No products indexed under this heading.

Triamcinolone Acetonide (Contraceptive effectiveness may be reduced when hormonal contraceptives are co-administered with antibiotics, anticonvulsants, and other drugs that increase the metabolism of contraceptive steroids. This could result in unintended pregnancy or unscheduled bleeding. In such cases a nonhormonal back-up method of birth control should be considered).
Products include:
Azmacort Inhalation Aerosol **407**
Nasacort AQ Nasal Spray **2765**
Triesence Injectable Suspension .... **⊙209**

Triamcinolone Diacetate (Contraceptive effectiveness may be reduced when hormonal contraceptives are co-administered with antibiotics, anticonvulsants, and other drugs that increase the metabolism of contraceptive steroids. This could result in unintended pregnancy or unscheduled bleeding. In such cases a nonhormonal back-up method of birth control should be considered).
No products indexed under this heading.

Triamcinolone Hexacetonide (Contraceptive effectiveness may be reduced when hormonal contraceptives are co-administered with antibiotics, anticonvulsants, and other drugs that increase the metabolism of contraceptive steroids. This could result in unintended pregnancy or unscheduled bleeding. In such cases a nonhormonal back-up method of birth control should be considered).
No products indexed under this heading.

Triazolam (Contraceptive effectiveness may be reduced when hormonal contraceptives are co-administered with antibiotics, anticonvulsants, and other drugs that increase the metabolism of contraceptive steroids. This could result in unintended pregnancy or unscheduled bleeding. In such cases a nonhormonal back-up method of birth control should be considered).
No products indexed under this heading.

Tridihexethyl Chloride (Enterohepatic recirculation of estrogens may also be decreased by substances that reduce gut transit time).
No products indexed under this heading.

Trihexyphenidyl Hydrochloride (Enterohepatic recirculation of estrogens may also be decreased by substances that reduce gut transit time).
No products indexed under this heading.

Trimeprazine Tartrate (Enterohepatic recirculation of estrogens may also be decreased by substances that reduce gut transit time).
No products indexed under this heading.

Trimethadione (Contraceptive effectiveness may be reduced when hormonal contraceptives are co-administered with antibiotics, anticonvulsants, and other drugs that increase the metabolism of contraceptive steroids. This could result in unintended pregnancy or unscheduled bleeding. In such cases a nonhormonal back-up method of birth control should be considered).
No products indexed under this heading.

Trimethaphan Camsylate (Contraceptive effectiveness may be reduced when hormonal contraceptives are co-administered with antibiotics, anticonvulsants, and other drugs that increase the metabolism of contraceptive steroids. This could result in unintended pregnancy or unscheduled bleeding. In such cases a nonhormonal back-up method of birth control should be considered).
No products indexed under this heading.

Trimipramine Maleate (Contraceptive effectiveness may be reduced when hormonal contraceptives are co-administered with antibiotics, anticonvulsants, and other drugs that increase the metabolism of contraceptive steroids. This could result in unintended pregnancy or unscheduled bleeding. In such cases a nonhormonal back-up method of birth control should be considered).
No products indexed under this heading.

Tripelennamine Hydrochloride (Enterohepatic recirculation of estrogens may also be decreased by substances that reduce gut transit time).
No products indexed under this heading.

Triprolidine Hydrochloride (Enterohepatic recirculation of estrogens may also be decreased by substances that reduce gut transit time).
No products indexed under this heading.

Troglitazone (Contraceptive effectiveness may be reduced when hormonal contraceptives are co-administered with antibiotics, anticonvulsants, and other drugs that increase the metabolism of contraceptive steroids. This could result in unintended pregnancy or unscheduled bleeding. In such cases a nonhormonal back-up method of birth control should be considered).
No products indexed under this heading.

Troleandomycin (CYP 3A4 inhibitors such as indinavir, itraconazole, ketoconazole, fluconazole, and troleandomycin may increase plasma hormone levels. Troleandomycin may also increase the risk of intrahepatic cholestasis during co-administration with combination oral contraceptives).
No products indexed under this heading.

Trovafloxacin Mesylate (Contraceptive effectiveness may be reduced when hormonal contraceptives are co-administered with antibiotics, anticonvulsants, and other drugs that increase the metabolism of contraceptive steroids. This could result in unintended pregnancy or unscheduled bleeding. In such cases a nonhormonal back-up method of birth control should be considered).
No products indexed under this heading.

Valdecoxib (Contraceptive effectiveness may be reduced when hormonal contraceptives are co-administered with antibiotics, anticonvulsants, and other drugs that increase the metabolism of contraceptive steroids. This could result in unintended pregnancy or unscheduled bleeding. In such cases a nonhormonal back-up method of birth control should be considered).
No products indexed under this heading.

Valproate Sodium (Contraceptive effectiveness may be reduced when hormonal contraceptives are co-administered with antibiotics, anticonvulsants, and other drugs that increase the metabolism of contraceptive steroids. This could result in unintended pregnancy or unscheduled bleeding. In such cases a nonhormonal back-up method of birth control should be considered).
No products indexed under this heading.

Valproic Acid (Contraceptive effectiveness may be reduced when hormonal contraceptives are co-administered with antibiotics, anticonvulsants, and other drugs that increase the metabolism of contraceptive steroids. This could result in unintended pregnancy or unscheduled bleeding. In such cases a nonhormonal back-up method of birth control should be considered).
No products indexed under this heading.

Valsartan (Contraceptive effectiveness may be reduced when hormonal contraceptives are co-administered with antibiotics, anticonvulsants, and other drugs that increase the metabolism of contraceptive steroids. This could result in unintended pregnancy or unscheduled bleeding. In such cases a nonhormonal back-up method of birth control should be considered).
Products include:
Diovan Tablets **2212**
Diovan HCT Tablets **2216**
Exforge Tablets **2238**

Vardenafil Hydrochloride (CYP 3A4 inhibitors such as indinavir, itraconazole, ketoconazole, fluconazole, and troleandomycin may increase plasma hormone levels. Troleandomycin may also increase the risk of intrahepatic cholestasis during co-administration with combination oral contraceptives). Products include:
Levitra Tablets **2876**

Venlafaxine Hydrochloride (Contraceptive effectiveness may be reduced when hormonal contraceptives are co-administered with antibiotics, anticonvulsants, and other drugs that increase the metabolism of contraceptive steroids. This could result in unintended pregnancy or unscheduled bleeding. In such cases a nonhormonal back-up method of birth control should be considered).
Products include:
Effexor XR Extended-Release Capsules.................................... **3195**
Venlafaxine Hydrochloride Tablets ... **2199**

Verapamil Hydrochloride (Contraceptive effectiveness may be reduced when hormonal contraceptives are co-administered with antibiotics, anticonvulsants, and other drugs that increase the metabolism of contraceptive steroids. This could result in unintended pregnancy or unscheduled bleeding. In such cases a nonhormonal back-up method of birth control should be considered).
Products include:
Tarka Tablets **511**

Vinblastine Sulfate (Contraceptive effectiveness may be reduced when hormonal contraceptives are co-administered with antibiotics, anticonvulsants, and other drugs that increase the metabolism of contraceptive steroids. This could result in unintended pregnancy or unscheduled bleeding. In such cases a nonhormonal back-up method of birth control should be considered).
No products indexed under this heading.

Vincristine Sulfate (Contraceptive effectiveness may be reduced when hormonal contraceptives are co-administered with antibiotics, anticonvulsants, and other drugs that increase the metabolism of contraceptive steroids. This could result in unintended pregnancy or unscheduled bleeding. In such cases a nonhormonal back-up method of birth control should be considered).
No products indexed under this heading.

Vitamin A (Contraceptive effectiveness may be reduced when hormonal contraceptives are co-administered with antibiotics, anticonvulsants, and other drugs that increase the metabolism of contraceptive steroids. This could result in unintended pregnancy or unscheduled bleeding. In such cases a nonhormonal back-up method of birth control should be considered).
Products include:
Norwegian Cod Liver Oil **949**

Vitamin A Acetate (Contraceptive effectiveness may be reduced when hormonal contraceptives are co-administered with antibiotics, anticonvulsants, and other drugs that increase the metabolism of contraceptive steroids. This could result in unintended pregnancy or unscheduled bleeding. In such cases a nonhormonal back-up method of birth control should be considered).
No products indexed under this heading.

Vitamin C (Ascorbic acid increases the bioavailability of ethinyl estradiol since these drugs act as competitive inhibitors for sulfation of ethinyl estradiol in the gastrointestinal wall, a known pathway of elimination for ethinyl estradiol). Products include:
Bausch & Lomb Ocuvite Adult 50+ Vitamin and Mineral Supplement.................................. **⊙237**
Comax Dietary Supplement **995**
Ferralet 90 Tablets **2175**
Glaucofit Dietary Supplement **995**
Glauma Dietary Supplement **995**
MoviPrep Oral Solution **2679**
Procosa II Tablets **3174**
Proflavanol 90 Tablets **3174**
Tonox Dietary Supplement **995**
Vibe Liquid Multi-Nutrient Supplement.................................. **■626**

Voriconazole (Contraceptive effectiveness may be reduced when hormonal contraceptives are co-administered with antibiotics, anticonvulsants, and other drugs that increase the metabolism of contraceptive steroids. This could result in unintended pregnancy or unscheduled bleeding. In such cases a nonhormonal back-up method of birth control should be considered).
No products indexed under this heading.

Warfarin Sodium (Contraceptive effectiveness may be reduced when hormonal contraceptives are co-administered with antibiotics, anticonvulsants, and other drugs that increase the metabolism of contraceptive steroids. This could result in unintended pregnancy or unscheduled bleeding. In such cases a non-hormonal back-up method of birth control should be considered).
No products indexed under this heading.

Zafirlukast (Contraceptive effectiveness may be reduced when hormonal contraceptives are co-administered with antibiotics, anticonvulsants, and other drugs that increase the metabolism of contraceptive steroids. This could result in unintended pregnancy or unscheduled bleeding. In such cases a non-hormonal back-up method of birth control should be considered). Products include:
Accolate Tablets 669

Zileuton (Contraceptive effectiveness may be reduced when hormonal contraceptives are co-administered with antibiotics, anticonvulsants, and other drugs that increase the metabolism of contraceptive steroids. This could result in unintended pregnancy or unscheduled bleeding. In such cases a non-hormonal back-up method of birth control should be considered).
No products indexed under this heading.

Zolmitriptan (Contraceptive effectiveness may be reduced when hormonal contraceptives are co-administered with antibiotics, anticonvulsants, and other drugs that increase the metabolism of contraceptive steroids. This could result in unintended pregnancy or unscheduled bleeding. In such cases a non-hormonal back-up method of birth control should be considered). Products include:
Zomig Tablets 694
Zomig Nasal Spray 689
Zomig-ZMT Tablets 694

Zonisamide (Contraceptive effectiveness may be reduced when hormonal contraceptives are co-administered with antibiotics, anticonvulsants, and other drugs that increase the metabolism of contraceptive steroids. This could result in unintended pregnancy or unscheduled bleeding. In such cases a non-hormonal back-up method of birth control should be considered). Products include:
Zonegran Capsules 1089

Zopiclone (Contraceptive effectiveness may be reduced when hormonal contraceptives are co-administered with antibiotics, anticonvulsants, and other drugs that increase the metabolism of contraceptive steroids. This could result in unintended pregnancy or unscheduled bleeding. In such cases a non-hormonal back-up method of birth control should be considered).
No products indexed under this heading.

Food Interactions

Grapefruit (CYP 3A4 inhibitors such as indinavir, itraconazole, ketoconazole, fluconazole, and troleandomycin may increase plasma hormone levels. Troleandomycin may also increase the risk of intrahepatic cholestasis during co-administration with combination oral contraceptives).

Grapefruit Juice (CYP 3A4 inhibitors such as indinavir, itraconazole, ketoconazole, fluconazole, and troleandomycin may increase plasma hormone levels. Troleandomycin may also increase the risk of intrahepatic cholestasis during co-administration with combination oral contraceptives).

LYRICA CAPSULES

(Pregabalin) 2527
May interact with ACE inhibitors, central nervous system depressants, and certain other agents. Compounds in these categories include:

Alfentanil Hydrochloride (Patients who require concomitant treatment with CNS depressants (eg, opiates or benzodiazepines) should be informed that they may experience additive CNS side effects, such as somnolence).
No products indexed under this heading.

Alprazolam (Patients who require concomitant treatment with CNS depressants (eg, opiates or benzodiazepines) should be informed that they may experience additive CNS side effects, such as somnolence).
No products indexed under this heading.

Aprobarbital (Patients who require concomitant treatment with CNS depressants (eg, opiates or benzodiazepines) should be informed that they may experience additive CNS side effects, such as somnolence).
No products indexed under this heading.

Benazepril Hydrochloride (Concomitant use with drugs associated with angioedema increases the risk of angioedema occuring).
No products indexed under this heading.

Buprenorphine Hydrochloride (Patients who require concomitant treatment with CNS depressants (eg, opiates or benzodiazepines) should be informed that they may experience additive CNS side effects, such as somnolence). Products include:
Suboxone Tablets 2601
Subutex Tablets 2601

Buspirone Hydrochloride (Patients who require concomitant treatment with CNS depressants (eg, opiates or benzodiazepines) should be informed that they may experience additive CNS side effects, such as somnolence).
No products indexed under this heading.

Butabarbital (Patients who require concomitant treatment with CNS depressants (eg, opiates or benzodiazepines) should be informed that they may experience additive CNS side effects, such as somnolence).
No products indexed under this heading.

Butalbital (Patients who require concomitant treatment with CNS depressants (eg, opiates or benzodiazepines) should be informed that they may experience additive CNS side effects, such as somnolence).
No products indexed under this heading.

Captopril (Concomitant use with drugs associated with angioedema increases the risk of angioedema occuring). Products include:
Captopril Tablets 2182

Chlordiazepoxide (Patients who require concomitant treatment with CNS depressants (eg, opiates or benzodiazepines) should be informed that they may experience additive CNS side effects, such as somnolence).
No products indexed under this heading.

Chlordiazepoxide Hydrochloride (Patients who require concomitant treatment with CNS depressants (eg, opiates or benzodiazepines) should be informed that they may experience additive CNS side effects, such as somnolence).
No products indexed under this heading.

Chlorpromazine (Patients who require concomitant treatment with CNS depressants (eg, opiates or benzodiazepines) should be informed that they may experience additive CNS side effects, such as somnolence).
No products indexed under this heading.

Chlorpromazine Hydrochloride (Patients who require concomitant treatment with CNS depressants (eg, opiates or benzodiazepines) should be informed that they may experience additive CNS side effects, such as somnolence).
No products indexed under this heading.

Chlorprothixene (Patients who require concomitant treatment with CNS depressants (eg, opiates or benzodiazepines) should be informed that they may experience additive CNS side effects, such as somnolence).
No products indexed under this heading.

Chlorprothixene Hydrochloride (Patients who require concomitant treatment with CNS depressants (eg, opiates or benzodiazepines) should be informed that they may experience additive CNS side effects, such as somnolence).
No products indexed under this heading.

Chlorprothixene Lactate (Patients who require concomitant treatment with CNS depressants (eg, opiates or benzodiazepines) should be informed that they may experience additive CNS side effects, such as somnolence).
No products indexed under this heading.

Clorazepate Dipotassium (Patients who require concomitant treatment with CNS depressants (eg, opiates or benzodiazepines) should be informed that they may experience additive CNS side effects, such as somnolence).
No products indexed under this heading.

Clozapine (Patients who require concomitant treatment with CNS depressants (eg, opiates or benzodiazepines) should be informed that they may experience additive CNS side effects, such as somnolence).
No products indexed under this heading.

Codeine Phosphate (Patients who require concomitant treatment with CNS depressants (eg, opiates or benzodiazepines) should be informed that they may experience additive CNS side effects, such as somnolence). Products include:
Tylenol with Codeine Tablets 2427

Desflurane (Patients who require concomitant treatment with CNS depressants (eg, opiates or benzodiazepines) should be informed that they may experience additive CNS side effects, such as somnolence).
No products indexed under this heading.

Dezocine (Patients who require concomitant treatment with CNS depressants (eg, opiates or benzodiazepines) should be informed that they may experience additive CNS side effects, such as somnolence).
No products indexed under this heading.

Diazepam (Patients who require concomitant treatment with CNS depressants (eg, opiates or benzodiazepines) should be informed that they may experience additive CNS side effects, such as somnolence). Products include:
Valium Tablets 2658

Droperidol (Patients who require concomitant treatment with CNS depressants (eg, opiates or benzodiazepines) should be informed that they may experience additive CNS side effects, such as somnolence).
No products indexed under this heading.

Enalapril Maleate (Concomitant use with drugs associated with angioedema increases the risk of angioedema occuring).
No products indexed under this heading.

Enalaprilat (Concomitant use with drugs associated with angioedema increases the risk of angioedema occuring).
No products indexed under this heading.

Enflurane (Patients who require concomitant treatment with CNS depressants (eg, opiates or benzodiazepines) should be informed that they may experience additive CNS side effects, such as somnolence).
No products indexed under this heading.

Estazolam (Patients who require concomitant treatment with CNS depressants (eg, opiates or benzodiazepines) should be informed that they may experience additive CNS side effects, such as somnolence).
No products indexed under this heading.

Ethanol (Alcohol consumption should be avoided while taking pregabalin, as pregabalin may potentiate the impairment of motor skills and sedation of alcohol).
No products indexed under this heading.

Ethchlorvynol (Patients who require concomitant treatment with CNS depressants (eg, opiates or benzodiazepines) should be informed that they may experience additive CNS side effects, such as somnolence).
No products indexed under this heading.

Ethinamate (Patients who require concomitant treatment with CNS depressants (eg, opiates or benzodiazepines) should be informed that they may experience additive CNS side effects, such as somnolence).
No products indexed under this heading.

Ethyl Alcohol (Alcohol consumption should be avoided while taking pregabalin, as pregabalin may potentiate the impairment of motor skills and sedation of alcohol).
No products indexed under this heading.

Fentanyl (Patients who require concomitant treatment with CNS depressants (eg, opiates or benzodiazepines) should be informed that they may experience additive CNS side effects, such as somnolence). Products include:
Duragesic Transdermal System 2405
Ionsys Transdermal System 2410

Fentanyl Citrate (Patients who require concomitant treatment with CNS depressants (eg, opiates or benzodiazepines) should be informed that they may experience additive CNS side effects, such as somnolence). Products include:
Actiq 959
Fentora Tablets 968

Fluphenazine Decanoate (Patients who require concomitant treatment with CNS depressants (eg, opiates or benzodiazepines) should be informed that they may experience additive CNS side effects, such as somnolence).
No products indexed under this heading.

Fluphenazine Enanthate (Patients who require concomitant treatment with CNS depressants (eg, opiates or benzodiazepines) should be informed that they may experience additive CNS side effects, such as somnolence).
No products indexed under this heading.

Fluphenazine Hydrochloride (Patients who require concomitant treatment with CNS depressants (eg, opiates or benzodiazepines) should be informed that they may experience additive CNS side effects, such as somnolence).
No products indexed under this heading.

Flurazepam Hydrochloride (Patients who require concomitant treatment with CNS depressants (eg, opiates or benzodiazepines) should be informed that they may experience additive CNS side effects, such as somnolence).
No products indexed under this heading.

Fosinopril Sodium (Concomitant use with drugs associated with angioedema increases the risk of angioedema occuring).
No products indexed under this heading.

Glutethimide (Patients who require concomitant treatment with CNS depressants (eg, opiates or benzodiazepines) should be informed that they may experience additive CNS side effects, such as somnolence).
No products indexed under this heading.

Haloperidol (Patients who require concomitant treatment with CNS depressants (eg, opiates or benzodiazepines) should be informed that they may experience additive CNS side effects, such as somnolence).
No products indexed under this heading.

Haloperidol Decanoate (Patients who require concomitant treatment with CNS depressants (eg, opiates or benzodiazepines) should be informed that they may experience additive CNS side effects, such as somnolence).
No products indexed under this heading.

Hydrocodone Bitartrate (Patients who require concomitant treatment with CNS depressants (eg, opiates or benzodiazepines) should be informed that they may experience additive CNS side effects, such as somnolence). Products include:
Lortab 5/500 Tablets 3143
Lortab 7.5/500 Tablets 3144
Lortab 10/500 Tablets 3144
Vicodin Tablets 529
Vicodin ES Tablets 530
Vicodin HP Tablets 531
Vicoprofen Tablets 533
Zydone Tablets 1132

Hydrocodone Polistirex (Patients who require concomitant treatment with CNS depressants (eg, opiates or benzodiazepines) should be informed that they may experience additive CNS side effects, such as somnolence). Products include:
Tussionex Pennkinetic Extended-Release Suspension 3154

Hydromorphone Hydrochloride (Patients who require concomitant treatment with CNS depressants (eg, opiates or benzodiazepines) should be informed that they may experience additive CNS side effects, such as somnolence).
No products indexed under this heading.

Hydroxyzine Hydrochloride (Patients who require concomitant treatment with CNS depressants (eg, opiates or benzodiazepines) should be informed that they may experience additive CNS side effects, such as somnolence).
No products indexed under this heading.

Isoflurane (Patients who require concomitant treatment with CNS depressants (eg, opiates or benzodiazepines) should be informed that they may experience additive CNS side effects, such as somnolence).
No products indexed under this heading.

Ketamine Hydrochloride (Patients who require concomitant treatment with CNS depressants (eg, opiates or benzodiazepines) should be informed that they may experience additive CNS side effects, such as somnolence).
No products indexed under this heading.

Levomethadyl Acetate Hydrochloride (Patients who require concomitant treatment with CNS depressants (eg, opiates or benzodiazepines) should be informed that they may experience additive CNS side effects, such as somnolence).
No products indexed under this heading.

Levorphanol Tartrate (Patients who require concomitant treatment with CNS depressants (eg, opiates or benzodiazepines) should be informed that they may experience additive CNS side effects, such as somnolence).
No products indexed under this heading.

Lisinopril (Concomitant use with drugs associated with angioedema increases the risk of angioedema occuring). Products include:
Prinivil Tablets 2087
Prinzide Tablets 2092

Lorazepam (Patients who require concomitant treatment with CNS depressants (eg, opiates or benzodiazepines) should be informed that they may experience additive CNS side effects, such as somnolence).
No products indexed under this heading.

Loxapine Hydrochloride (Patients who require concomitant treatment with CNS depressants (eg, opiates or benzodiazepines) should be informed that they may experience additive CNS side effects, such as somnolence).
No products indexed under this heading.

Loxapine Succinate (Patients who require concomitant treatment with CNS depressants (eg, opiates or benzodiazepines) should be informed that they may experience additive CNS side effects, such as somnolence).
No products indexed under this heading.

Meperidine Hydrochloride (Patients who require concomitant treatment with CNS depressants (eg, opiates or benzodiazepines) should be informed that they may experience additive CNS side effects, such as somnolence).
No products indexed under this heading.

Mephobarbital (Patients who require concomitant treatment with CNS depressants (eg, opiates or benzodiazepines) should be informed that they may experience additive CNS side effects, such as somnolence).
No products indexed under this heading.

Meprobamate (Patients who require concomitant treatment with CNS depressants (eg, opiates or benzodiazepines) should be informed that they may experience additive CNS side effects, such as somnolence).
No products indexed under this heading.

Mesoridazine Besylate (Patients who require concomitant treatment with CNS depressants (eg, opiates or benzodiazepines) should be informed that they may experience additive CNS side effects, such as somnolence).
No products indexed under this heading.

Methadone Hydrochloride (Patients who require concomitant treatment with CNS depressants (eg, opiates or benzodiazepines) should be informed that they may experience additive CNS side effects, such as somnolence).
No products indexed under this heading.

Methohexital Sodium (Patients who require concomitant treatment with CNS depressants (eg, opiates or benzodiazepines) should be informed that they may experience additive CNS side effects, such as somnolence).
No products indexed under this heading.

Methotrimeprazine (Patients who require concomitant treatment with CNS depressants (eg, opiates or benzodiazepines) should be informed that they may experience additive CNS side effects, such as somnolence).
No products indexed under this heading.

Methoxyflurane (Patients who require concomitant treatment with CNS depressants (eg, opiates or benzodiazepines) should be informed that they may experience additive CNS side effects, such as somnolence).
No products indexed under this heading.

Midazolam Hydrochloride (Patients who require concomitant treatment with CNS depressants (eg, opiates or benzodiazepines) should be informed that they may experience additive CNS side effects, such as somnolence).
No products indexed under this heading.

Moexipril Hydrochloride (Concomitant use with drugs associated with angioedema increases the risk of angioedema occuring).
No products indexed under this heading.

Molindone Hydrochloride (Patients who require concomitant treatment with CNS depressants (eg, opiates or benzodiazepines) should be informed that they may experience additive CNS side effects, such as somnolence). Products include:
Moban Tablets 1116

Morphine Sulfate (Patients who require concomitant treatment with CNS depressants (eg, opiates or benzodiazepines) should be informed that they may experience additive CNS side effects, such as somnolence). Products include:
Avinza Capsules 1772
DepoDur Injection 1095
MS Contin Tablets 2585

Olanzapine (Patients who require concomitant treatment with CNS depressants (eg, opiates or benzodiazepines) should be informed that they may experience additive CNS side effects, such as somnolence). Products include:
Symbyax Capsules 1871
Zyprexa Tablets 1883
Zyprexa IntraMuscular 1883
Zyprexa ZYDIS Orally Disintegrating Tablets 1883

Oxazepam (Patients who require concomitant treatment with CNS depressants (eg, opiates or benzodiazepines) should be informed that they may experience additive CNS side effects, such as somnolence).
No products indexed under this heading.

Oxycodone Hydrochloride (Patients who require concomitant treatment with CNS depressants (eg, opiates or benzodiazepines) should be informed that they may experience additive CNS side effects, such as somnolence). Products include:

OxyContin Tablets 2589
OxyIR Capsules 2593
Percocet Tablets 1127
Percodan Tablets 1130

Pentobarbital Sodium (Patients who require concomitant treatment with CNS depressants (eg, opiates or benzodiazepines) should be informed that they may experience additive CNS side effects, such as somnolence). Products include:
Nembutal Sodium Solution, USP 2494

Perindopril Erbumine (Concomitant use with drugs associated with angioedema increases the risk of angioedema occuring). Products include:
Aceon Tablets (2 mg, 4 mg, 8 mg)... 3038

Perphenazine (Patients who require concomitant treatment with CNS depressants (eg, opiates or benzodiazepines) should be informed that they may experience additive CNS side effects, such as somnolence).
No products indexed under this heading.

Phenobarbital (Patients who require concomitant treatment with CNS depressants (eg, opiates or benzodiazepines) should be informed that they may experience additive CNS side effects, such as somnolence). Products include:
Donnatal Extentabs 2507

Prazepam (Patients who require concomitant treatment with CNS depressants (eg, opiates or benzodiazepines) should be informed that they may experience additive CNS side effects, such as somnolence).
No products indexed under this heading.

Prochlorperazine (Patients who require concomitant treatment with CNS depressants (eg, opiates or benzodiazepines) should be informed that they may experience additive CNS side effects, such as somnolence).
No products indexed under this heading.

Promethazine Hydrochloride (Patients who require concomitant treatment with CNS depressants (eg, opiates or benzodiazepines) should be informed that they may experience additive CNS side effects, such as somnolence).
No products indexed under this heading.

Propofol (Patients who require concomitant treatment with CNS depressants (eg, opiates or benzodiazepines) should be informed that they may experience additive CNS side effects, such as somnolence).
No products indexed under this heading.

Propoxyphene Hydrochloride (Patients who require concomitant treatment with CNS depressants (eg, opiates or benzodiazepines) should be informed that they may experience additive CNS side effects, such as somnolence).
No products indexed under this heading.

Propoxyphene Napsylate (Patients who require concomitant treatment with CNS depressants (eg, opiates or benzodiazepines) should be informed that they may experience additive CNS side effects, such as somnolence).
No products indexed under this heading.

Quazepam (Patients who require concomitant treatment with CNS depressants (eg, opiates or benzodiazepines) should be informed that they may experience additive CNS side effects, such as somnolence).
No products indexed under this heading.

Quetiapine Fumarate (Patients who require concomitant treatment with CNS depressants (eg, opiates or benzodiazepines) should be informed that they may experience additive CNS side effects, such as somnolence).
No products indexed under this heading.

Quinapril Hydrochloride (Concomitant use with drugs associated with angioedema increases the risk of angioedema occuring).
No products indexed under this heading.

Ramipril (Concomitant use with drugs associated with angioedema increases the risk of angioedema occuring).
No products indexed under this heading.

Remifentanil Hydrochloride (Patients who require concomitant treatment with CNS depressants (eg, opiates or benzodiazepines) should be informed that they may experience additive CNS side effects, such as somnolence).
No products indexed under this heading.

Risperidone (Patients who require concomitant treatment with CNS depressants (eg, opiates or benzodiazepines) should be informed that they may experience additive CNS side effects, such as somnolence). Products include:
Risperdal Consta Long-Acting Injection 1753

Secobarbital Sodium (Patients who require concomitant treatment with CNS depressants (eg, opiates or benzodiazepines) should be informed that they may experience additive CNS side effects, such as somnolence).
No products indexed under this heading.

Sevoflurane (Patients who require concomitant treatment with CNS depressants (eg, opiates or benzodiazepines) should be informed that they may experience additive CNS side effects, such as somnolence). Products include:
Ultane Liquid for Inhalation 524

Sodium Oxybate (Patients who require concomitant treatment with CNS depressants (eg, opiates or benzodiazepines) should be informed that they may experience additive CNS side effects, such as somnolence). Products include:
Xyrem Oral Solution 1766

Spirapril Hydrochloride (Concomitant use with drugs associated with angioedema increases the risk of angioedema occuring).
No products indexed under this heading.

Sufentanil Citrate (Patients who require concomitant treatment with CNS depressants (eg, opiates or benzodiazepines) should be informed that they may experience additive CNS side effects, such as somnolence).
No products indexed under this heading.

Temazepam (Patients who require concomitant treatment with CNS depressants (eg, opiates or benzodiazepines) should be informed that they may experience additive CNS side effects, such as somnolence).
No products indexed under this heading.

Thiamylal Sodium (Patients who require concomitant treatment with CNS depressants (eg, opiates or benzodiazepines) should be informed that they may experience additive CNS side effects, such as somnolence).
No products indexed under this heading.

Thioridazine Hydrochloride (Patients who require concomitant treatment with CNS depressants (eg, opiates or benzodiazepines) should be informed that they may experience additive CNS side effects, such as somnolence). Products include:
Thioridazine Hydrochloride Tablets.. 2195

Thiothixene (Patients who require concomitant treatment with CNS depressants (eg, opiates or benzodiazepines) should be informed that they may experience additive CNS side effects, such as somnolence). Products include:
Thiothixene Capsules 2197

Trandolapril (Concomitant use with drugs associated with angioedema increases the risk of angioedema occuring). Products include:
Mavik Tablets 472
Tarka Tablets 511

Triazolam (Patients who require concomitant treatment with CNS depressants (eg, opiates or benzodiazepines) should be informed that they may experience additive CNS side effects, such as somnolence).
No products indexed under this heading.

Trifluoperazine Hydrochloride (Patients who require concomitant treatment with CNS depressants (eg, opiates or benzodiazepines) should be informed that they may experience additive CNS side effects, such as somnolence).
No products indexed under this heading.

Zaleplon (Patients who require concomitant treatment with CNS depressants (eg, opiates or benzodiazepines) should be informed that they may experience additive CNS side effects, such as somnolence).
No products indexed under this heading.

Ziprasidone Hydrochloride (Patients who require concomitant treatment with CNS depressants (eg, opiates or benzodiazepines) should be informed that they may experience additive CNS side effects, such as somnolence). Products include:
Geodon Capsules 2520

Zolpidem Tartrate (Patients who require concomitant treatment with CNS depressants (eg, opiates or benzodiazepines) should be informed that they may experience additive CNS side effects, such as somnolence). Products include:
Ambien Tablets 2692
Ambien CR Tablets 2696

Food Interactions

Alcohol (Alcohol consumption should be avoided while taking pregabalin, as pregabalin may potentiate the impairment of motor skills and sedation of alcohol).

MACUTEIN MEGA-30 MG PLUS MCT DIETARY SUPPLEMENT

(Lutein, Medium-Chain Triglycerides, Vitamins with Minerals, Zeaxanthin)......................... 995
None cited in PDR database.

MALARONE PEDIATRIC TABLETS

(Atovaquone, Proguanil Hydrochloride)................................... 1521
See Malarone Tablets

MALARONE TABLETS

(Atovaquone, Proguanil Hydrochloride)................................... 1521
May interact with oral anticoagulants, tetracyclines, and certain other agents. Compounds in these categories include:

Anisindione (Proguanil may potentiate the anti-coagulant effect of warfarin and similar anti-coagulants through possible interference with metabolic pathways. Caution is advised when initiating or withdrawing malaria prophylaxis with Malarone in patients on continuous treatment with anti-coagulants metabolized by CYP2C9).
No products indexed under this heading.

Demeclocycline Hydrochloride (Co-administration with tetracyclines has been associated with approximately a 40% reduction in plasma concentrations of atovaquone).
No products indexed under this heading.

Dicumarol (Proguanil may potentiate the anti-coagulant effect of warfarin and similar anti-coagulants through possible interference with metabolic pathways. Caution is advised when initiating or withdrawing malaria prophylaxis with Malarone in patients on continuous treatment with anti-coagulants metabolized by CYP2C9).
No products indexed under this heading.

Doxycycline Calcium (Co-administration with tetracyclines has been associated with approximately a 40% reduction in plasma concentrations of atovaquone).
No products indexed under this heading.

Doxycycline Hyclate (Co-administration with tetracyclines has been associated with approximately a 40% reduction in plasma concentrations of atovaquone).
No products indexed under this heading.

Doxycycline Monohydrate (Co-administration with tetracyclines has been associated with approximately a 40% reduction in plasma concentrations of atovaquone).
No products indexed under this heading.

Indinavir Sulfate (Concomitant administration of atovaquone and indinavir results in a decrease in the Ctrough of indinavir. Caution should be exercised when prescribing atovaquione with indinavir due to the decrease in trough levels of indinavir). Products include:
Crixivan Capsules 1979

Methacycline Hydrochloride (Co-administration with tetracyclines has been associated with approximately a 40% reduction in plasma concentrations of atovaquone).
No products indexed under this heading.

Metoclopramide Hydrochloride (May reduce the bioavailability of atovaquone and should be used only if other antiemetics are not available).
No products indexed under this heading.

Minocycline Hydrochloride (Co-administration with tetracyclines has been associated with approximately a 40% reduction in plasma concentrations of atovaquone). Products include:
Solodyn Extended Release Tablets 1938

Oxytetracycline Hydrochloride (Co-administration with tetracyclines has been associated with approximately a 40% reduction in plasma concentrations of atovaquone).
No products indexed under this heading.

Rifabutin (Co-administration of rifabutin is known to reduce atovaquone levels by approximately 34%; concomitant therapy is not recommended).
No products indexed under this heading.

Rifampin (Co-administration of rifampin is known to reduce atovaquone levels by approximately 50%; concomitant therapy is not recommended).
No products indexed under this heading.

Tetracycline Hydrochloride (Co-administration with tetracyclines has been associated with approximately a 40% reduction in plasma concentrations of atovaquone). Products include:
Pylera Capsules 714

Warfarin Sodium (Proguanil may potentiate the anti-coagulant effect of warfarin and similar anti-coagulants through possible interference with metabolic pathways. Caution is advised when initiating or withdrawing malaria prophylaxis with Malarone in patients on continuous treatment with anti-coagulants metabolized by CYP2C9).
No products indexed under this heading.

Food Interactions

Food, unspecified (Dietary fat intake with atovaquone increases the rate and extent of absorption; Malarone should be taken with food or milky drink).

MARINEOMEGA SOFTGEL CAPSULES

(Fatty Acids, Vitamin E) 2560
None cited in PDR database.

MARINOL CAPSULES

(Dronabinol) 3163
May interact with anticholinergics, antihistamines, barbiturates, benzodiazepines, central nervous system depressants, lithium preparations, muscle relaxants, narcotic analgesics, sympathomimetics, tricyclic antidepressants, xanthines, and certain other agents. Compounds in these categories include:

Acrivastine (Co-administration results in additive CNS depression or super-additive tachycardia and drowsiness).
No products indexed under this heading.

Albuterol (Co-administration with sympathomimetics may result in additive hypertension, tachycardia, and possibly cardiotoxicity).
No products indexed under this heading.

Albuterol Sulfate (Co-administration with sympathomimetics may result in additive hypertension, tachycardia, and possibly cardiotoxicity). Products include:
Combivent Inhalation Aerosol 845
ProAir HFA Inhalation Aerosol 3113
Proventil HFA Inhalation Aerosol 2914
Ventolin HFA Inhalation Aerosol 1638

Alfentanil Hydrochloride (Co-administration results in additive drowsiness and CNS depression).
No products indexed under this heading.

Alprazolam (Co-administration results in additive drowsiness and CNS depression).
No products indexed under this heading.

Aminophylline (Increased theophylline metabolism has resulted with smoking marijuana).
No products indexed under this heading.

Amitriptyline Hydrochloride (Co-administration results in additive tachycardia, hypertension, and drowsiness).
No products indexed under this heading.

Amoxapine (Co-administration results in additive tachycardia, hypertension, and drowsiness).
No products indexed under this heading.

Amphetamine Sulfate (Co-administration with amphetamine may result in additive hypertension, tachycardia, and possibly cardiotoxicity). Products include:
Adderall XR Capsules 3012

Antipyrine (Co-administration results in decreased clearance of barbiturates via competitive inhibition of metabolism; additive drowsiness and CNS depression).
No products indexed under this heading.

Aprobarbital (Co-administration results in decreased clearance of barbiturates via competitive inhibition of metabolism; additive drowsiness and CNS depression).
No products indexed under this heading.

Astemizole (Co-administration results in additive CNS depression or super-additive tachycardia and drowsiness).
No products indexed under this heading.

Atracurium Besylate (Co-administration results in additive drowsiness and CNS depression).
No products indexed under this heading.

Atropine Sulfate (Co-administration with anticholinergic agents may result in additive or super-additive tachycardia and drowsiness). Products include:
Donnatal Extentabs 2507

Azatadine Maleate (Co-administration results in additive CNS depression or super-additive tachycardia and drowsiness).
No products indexed under this heading.

Baclofen (Co-administration results in additive drowsiness and CNS depression).
No products indexed under this heading.

Belladonna Alkaloids (Co-administration with anticholinergic agents may result in additive or super-additive tachycardia and drowsiness). Products include:
Hyland's Teething Tablets .... ▣621

Benztropine Mesylate (Co-administration with anticholinergic agents may result in additive or super-additive tachycardia and drowsiness).
No products indexed under this heading.

Biperiden Hydrochloride (Co-administration with anticholinergic agents may result in additive or super-additive tachycardia and drowsiness).
No products indexed under this heading.

Bromodiphenhydramine Hydrochloride (Co-administration results in additive CNS depression or super-additive tachycardia and drowsiness).
No products indexed under this heading.

Brompheniramine Maleate (Co-administration results in additive CNS depression or super-additive tachycardia and drowsiness).
No products indexed under this heading.

Buprenorphine Hydrochloride (Co-administration results in additive drowsiness and CNS depression). Products include:
Suboxone Tablets 2601
Subutex Tablets 2601

Buspirone Hydrochloride (Co-administration results in additive drowsiness and CNS depression).
No products indexed under this heading.

Butabarbital (Co-administration results in decreased clearance of barbiturates via competitive inhibition of metabolism; additive drowsiness and CNS depression).
No products indexed under this heading.

Butalbital (Co-administration results in decreased clearance of barbiturates via competitive inhibition of metabolism; additive drowsiness and CNS depression).
No products indexed under this heading.

Carisoprodol (Co-administration with muscle relaxants may result in additive drowsiness and CNS depression). Products include:
Soma Tablets 1931

Cetirizine Hydrochloride (Co-administration results in additive CNS depression or super-additive tachycardia and drowsiness). Products include:
Zyrtec Allergy Tablets 1919
Zyrtec Chewable Tablets 1920
Children's Zyrtec Allergy Chewable Tablets 1922
Children's Zyrtec Allergy Syrup 1920
Children's Zyrtec Hives Relief Syrup 1920
Zyrtec Syrup 1920
Zyrtec Tablets 1920
Zyrtec-D 12 Hour Extended Release Tablets 1923
Zyrtec-D Allergy & Congestion Extended-Release Tablets 1923

Chlordiazepoxide (Co-administration results in additive drowsiness and CNS depression).
No products indexed under this heading.

Chlordiazepoxide Hydrochloride (Co-administration results in additive drowsiness and CNS depression).
No products indexed under this heading.

Chlorpheniramine Maleate (Co-administration results in additive CNS depression or super-additive tachycardia and drowsiness). Products include:
Actifed Cold & Allergy Tablets 1895
Sudafed PE Sinus & Allergy Tablets 1908
Tylenol Allergy Multi-Symptom Caplets with Cool Burst and Rapid Release Gelcaps 1916
Children's Tylenol Plus Cold Suspension Liquid 1912
Children's Tylenol Plus Cough & Runny Nose Suspension Liquid 1912
Children's Tylenol Plus Flu Suspension Liquid 1914
Children's Tylenol Plus Multi-Symptom Cold Suspension Liquid 1912
Tylenol Cold Head Congestion Nighttime Caplets with Cool Burst 1910
Tylenol Cold Multi-Symptom Nighttime Caplets with Cool Burst 1913
Tylenol Sinus Congestion & Pain Nighttime Caplets with Cool Burst 1917

Chlorpheniramine Polistirex (Co-administration results in additive CNS depression or super-additive tachycardia and drowsiness). Products include:
Tussionex Pennkinetic Extended-Release Suspension 3154

Chlorpheniramine Tannate (Co-administration results in additive CNS depression or super-additive tachycardia and drowsiness).
No products indexed under this heading.

Chlorpromazine (Co-administration results in additive drowsiness and CNS depression).
No products indexed under this heading.

Chlorpromazine Hydrochloride (Co-administration results in additive drowsiness and CNS depression).
No products indexed under this heading.

Chlorprothixene (Co-administration results in additive drowsiness and CNS depression).
No products indexed under this heading.

Chlorprothixene Hydrochloride (Co-administration results in additive drowsiness and CNS depression).
No products indexed under this heading.

Chlorprothixene Lactate (Co-administration results in additive drowsiness and CNS depression).
No products indexed under this heading.

Chlorzoxazone (Co-administration with muscle relaxants may result in additive drowsiness and CNS depression).
No products indexed under this heading.

Cisatracurium Besylate (Co-administration results in additive drowsiness and CNS depression). Products include:
Nimbex Injection 484

Clemastine Fumarate (Co-administration results in additive CNS depression or super-additive tachycardia and drowsiness).
No products indexed under this heading.

Clidinium Bromide (Co-administration with anticholinergic agents may result in additive or super-additive tachycardia and drowsiness).
No products indexed under this heading.

Clomipramine Hydrochloride (Co-administration results in additive tachycardia, hypertension, and drowsiness).
No products indexed under this heading.

Clorazepate Dipotassium (Co-administration results in additive drowsiness and CNS depression).
No products indexed under this heading.

Clozapine (Co-administration results in additive drowsiness and CNS depression).
No products indexed under this heading.

Cocaine Hydrochloride (Co-administration with cocaine may result in additive hypertension, tachycardia, and possibly cardiotoxicity).
No products indexed under this heading.

Codeine Phosphate (Co-administration results in additive drowsiness and CNS depression). Products include:
Tylenol with Codeine Tablets 2427

Cyclobenzaprine Hydrochloride (Co-administration with muscle relaxants may result in additive drowsiness and CNS depression). Products include:
Amrix Capsules 966

Cyproheptadine Hydrochloride (Co-administration results in additive CNS depression or super-additive tachycardia and drowsiness).
No products indexed under this heading.

Dantrolene Sodium (Co-administration results in additive drowsiness and CNS depression). Products include:
Dantrium Capsules 2580
Dantrium Intravenous 2582

Desflurane (Co-administration results in additive drowsiness and CNS depression).
No products indexed under this heading.

Desipramine Hydrochloride (Co-administration results in additive tachycardia, hypertension, and drowsiness).
No products indexed under this heading.

Dexchlorpheniramine Maleate (Co-administration results in additive CNS depression or super-additive tachycardia and drowsiness).
No products indexed under this heading.

Dextroamphetamine Sulfate (Co-administration with amphetamine may result in additive hypertension, tachycardia, and possibly cardiotoxicity). Products include:
Adderall XR Capsules 3012
Dexedrine 1401

Dezocine (Co-administration results in additive drowsiness and CNS depression).
No products indexed under this heading.

Diazepam (Co-administration results in additive drowsiness and CNS depression). Products include:
Valium Tablets 2658

Dicyclomine Hydrochloride (Co-administration with anticholinergic agents may result in additive or super-additive tachycardia and drowsiness). Products include:
Bentyl Capsules 703
Bentyl Injection 703
Bentyl Syrup 703
Bentyl Tablets 703

Diphenhydramine Citrate (Co-administration results in additive CNS depression or super-additive tachycardia and drowsiness).
No products indexed under this heading.

Diphenhydramine Hydrochloride (Co-administration results in additive CNS depression or super-additive tachycardia and drowsiness). Products include:
Benadryl Allergy & Cold Kapgels 1895
Benadryl Allergy & Sinus Headache Kapgels 1895
Benadryl Severe Allergy & Sinus Headache Caplets 1897
Benadryl Dye-Free Allergy Liqui-gels Softgels 1897
Benadryl Allergy Kapgels 1895
Benadryl Allergy Quick Dissolve Strips 1896
Benadryl Allergy Ultratab Tablets 1896
Children's Benadryl Dye-Free Allergy Liquid 1897
Children's Benadryl Allergy Fastmelts 1897
Children's Benadryl Allergy Liquid 1898
Children's Benadryl Allergy Perfect Measure 1896
Children's Benadryl-D Allergy & Sinus Liquid 1896
Benadryl-D Allergy & Sinus Tablet 1896
PediaCare Children's Allergy & Cold Liquid 1902
PediaCare Children's Allergy Liquid 1902
Simply Sleep Caplets 1905
Sudafed PE Nighttime Cold Caplets 1907
Sudafed PE Severe Cold Caplets 1908
Extra Strength Tylenol PM Caplets, Geltabs, Liquid, and Rapid Release Gels 1915
Tylenol Allergy Multi-Symptom Nighttime Caplets with Cool Burst 1916
Tylenol Severe Allergy Caplets 1916
Children's Tylenol Plus Cold & Allergy Suspension Liquid 1914
Tylenol Sore Throat Nighttime Liquid with Cool Burst 1918

Diphenylpyraline Hydrochloride (Co-administration results in additive CNS depression or super-additive tachycardia and drowsiness).
No products indexed under this heading.

Disulfiram (Co-administration of disulfiram in a patient who smoked marijuana has resulted in a reversible hypomanic reaction).
No products indexed under this heading.

Dobutamine Hydrochloride (Co-administration with sympathomimetics may result in additive hypertension, tachycardia, and possibly cardiotoxicity).
No products indexed under this heading.

Dopamine Hydrochloride (Co-administration with sympathomimetics may result in additive hypertension, tachycardia, and possibly cardiotoxicity).
No products indexed under this heading.

Doxacurium Chloride (Co-administration results in additive drowsiness and CNS depression).
No products indexed under this heading.

Doxepin Hydrochloride (Co-administration results in additive tachycardia, hypertension, and drowsiness).
No products indexed under this heading.

Droperidol (Co-administration results in additive drowsiness and CNS depression).
No products indexed under this heading.

Dyphylline (Increased theophylline metabolism has resulted with smoking marijuana).
No products indexed under this heading.

Enflurane (Co-administration results in additive drowsiness and CNS depression).
No products indexed under this heading.

Ephedrine Hydrochloride (Co-administration with sympathomimetics may result in additive hypertension, tachycardia, and possibly cardiotoxicity).
No products indexed under this heading.

Ephedrine Sulfate (Co-administration with sympathomimetics may result in additive hypertension, tachycardia, and possibly cardiotoxicity).
No products indexed under this heading.

Ephedrine Tannate (Co-administration with sympathomimetics may result in additive hypertension, tachycardia, and possibly cardiotoxicity).
No products indexed under this heading.

Epinephrine (Co-administration with sympathomimetics may result in additive hypertension, tachycardia, and possibly cardiotoxicity). Products include:
EpiPen 1024

Epinephrine Bitartrate (Co-administration with sympathomimetics may result in additive hypertension, tachycardia, and possibly cardiotoxicity).
No products indexed under this heading.

Epinephrine Hydrochloride (Co-administration with sympathomimetics may result in additive hypertension, tachycardia, and possibly cardiotoxicity).
No products indexed under this heading.

Estazolam (Co-administration results in additive drowsiness and CNS depression).
No products indexed under this heading.

Ethanol (Co-administration results in additive drowsiness and CNS depression).
No products indexed under this heading.

Ethchlorvynol (Co-administration results in additive drowsiness and CNS depression).
No products indexed under this heading.

Ethinamate (Co-administration results in additive drowsiness and CNS depression).
No products indexed under this heading.

Ethyl Alcohol (Co-administration results in additive drowsiness and CNS depression).
No products indexed under this heading.

Fentanyl (Co-administration results in additive drowsiness and CNS depression). Products include:
Duragesic Transdermal System 2405
Ionsys Transdermal System 2410

Fentanyl Citrate (Co-administration results in additive drowsiness and CNS depression). Products include:
Actiq 959
Fentora Tablets 968

Fexofenadine Hydrochloride (Co-administration results in additive CNS depression or super-additive tachycardia and drowsiness). Products include:
Allegra Oral Solution 2684
Allegra Tablets 2684
Allegra-D 12 Hour Extended-Release Tablets 2687
Allegra-D 24 Hour Extended-Release Tablets 2690

Fluoxetine Hydrochloride (Co-administration of fluoxetine in a patient who smoked marijuana has resulted in a hypomanic reaction). Products include:
Prozac Weekly Capsules 1852
Prozac Pulvules and Liquid 1852
Symbyax Capsules 1871

Fluphenazine Decanoate (Co-administration results in additive drowsiness and CNS depression).
No products indexed under this heading.

Fluphenazine Enanthate (Co-administration results in additive drowsiness and CNS depression).
No products indexed under this heading.

Fluphenazine Hydrochloride (Co-administration results in additive drowsiness and CNS depression).
No products indexed under this heading.

Flurazepam Hydrochloride (Co-administration results in additive drowsiness and CNS depression).
No products indexed under this heading.

Glutethimide (Co-administration results in additive drowsiness and CNS depression).
No products indexed under this heading.

Glycopyrrolate (Co-administration with anticholinergic agents may result in additive or super-additive tachycardia and drowsiness).
No products indexed under this heading.

Halazepam (Co-administration results in additive drowsiness and CNS depression).
No products indexed under this heading.

Haloperidol (Co-administration results in additive drowsiness and CNS depression).
No products indexed under this heading.

Haloperidol Decanoate (Co-administration results in additive drowsiness and CNS depression).
No products indexed under this heading.

Hydrocodone Bitartrate (Co-administration results in additive drowsiness and CNS depression). Products include:
Lortab 5/500 Tablets 3143
Lortab 7.5/500 Tablets 3144
Lortab 10/500 Tablets 3144
Vicodin Tablets 529
Vicodin ES Tablets 530
Vicodin HP Tablets 531
Vicoprofen Tablets 533
Zydone Tablets 1132

Hydrocodone Polistirex (Co-administration results in additive drowsiness and CNS depression). Products include:
Tussionex Pennkinetic Extended-Release Suspension 3154

Hydromorphone Hydrochloride (Co-administration results in additive drowsiness and CNS depression).
No products indexed under this heading.

Hydroxyzine Hydrochloride (Co-administration results in additive drowsiness and CNS depression).
No products indexed under this heading.

Hyoscyamine (Co-administration with anticholinergic agents may result in additive or super-additive tachycardia and drowsiness).
No products indexed under this heading.

Hyoscyamine Sulfate (Co-administration with anticholinergic agents may result in additive or super-additive tachycardia and drowsiness). Products include:
Donnatal Extentabs 2507

Imipramine Hydrochloride (Co-administration results in additive tachycardia, hypertension, and drowsiness).
No products indexed under this heading.

Imipramine Pamoate (Co-administration results in additive tachycardia, hypertension, and drowsiness).
No products indexed under this heading.

Ipratropium Bromide (Co-administration with anticholinergic agents may result in additive or super-additive tachycardia and drowsiness). Products include:
Atrovent HFA Inhalation Aerosol 839
Atrovent Nasal Spray 0.03% 834
Atrovent Nasal Spray 0.06% 836
Combivent Inhalation Aerosol 845

Isoflurane (Co-administration results in additive drowsiness and CNS depression).
No products indexed under this heading.

Isoproterenol Hydrochloride (Co-administration with sympathomimetics may result in additive hypertension, tachycardia, and possibly cardiotoxicity).
No products indexed under this heading.

Isoproterenol Sulfate (Co-administration with sympathomimetics may result in additive hypertension, tachycardia, and possibly cardiotoxicity).
No products indexed under this heading.

Ketamine Hydrochloride (Co-administration results in additive drowsiness and CNS depression).
No products indexed under this heading.

Levalbuterol Hydrochloride (Co-administration with sympathomimetics may result in additive hypertension, tachycardia, and possibly cardiotoxicity). Products include:
Xopenex Inhalation Solution 3001
Xopenex Inhalation Solution Concentrate 3005

Levomethadyl Acetate Hydrochloride (Co-administration results in additive drowsiness and CNS depression).
No products indexed under this heading.

Levorphanol Tartrate (Co-administration results in additive drowsiness and CNS depression).
No products indexed under this heading.

Lithium (Co-administration results in additive drowsiness and CNS depression).
No products indexed under this heading.

Lithium Carbonate (Co-administration results in additive drowsiness and CNS depression).
No products indexed under this heading.

Lithium Citrate (Co-administration results in additive drowsiness and CNS depression).
No products indexed under this heading.

Loratadine (Co-administration results in additive CNS depression or super-additive tachycardia and drowsiness).
No products indexed under this heading.

Lorazepam (Co-administration results in additive drowsiness and CNS depression).
No products indexed under this heading.

Loxapine Hydrochloride (Co-administration results in additive drowsiness and CNS depression).
No products indexed under this heading.

Loxapine Succinate (Co-administration results in additive drowsiness and CNS depression).
No products indexed under this heading.

Maprotiline Hydrochloride (Co-administration results in additive tachycardia, hypertension, and drowsiness).
No products indexed under this heading.

Mepenzolate Bromide (Co-administration with anticholinergic agents may result in additive or super-additive tachycardia and drowsiness).
No products indexed under this heading.

Meperidine Hydrochloride (Co-administration results in additive drowsiness and CNS depression).
No products indexed under this heading.

Mephobarbital (Co-administration results in decreased clearance of barbiturates via competitive inhibition of metabolism; additive drowsiness and CNS depression).
No products indexed under this heading.

Meprobamate (Co-administration results in additive drowsiness and CNS depression).
No products indexed under this heading.

Mesoridazine Besylate (Co-administration results in additive drowsiness and CNS depression).
No products indexed under this heading.

Metaproterenol Sulfate (Co-administration with sympathomimetics may result in additive hypertension, tachycardia, and possibly cardiotoxicity).
No products indexed under this heading.

Metaraminol Bitartrate (Co-administration with sympathomimetics may result in additive hypertension, tachycardia, and possibly cardiotoxicity).
No products indexed under this heading.

Metaxalone (Co-administration results in additive drowsiness and CNS depression). Products include:
Skelaxin Tablets 1784

Methadone Hydrochloride (Co-administration results in additive drowsiness and CNS depression).
No products indexed under this heading.

Methamphetamine Hydrochloride (Co-administration with amphetamine may result in additive hypertension, tachycardia, and possibly cardiotoxicity).
No products indexed under this heading.

Methdilazine Hydrochloride (Co-administration results in additive CNS depression or super-additive tachycardia and drowsiness).
No products indexed under this heading.

Methocarbamol (Co-administration with muscle relaxants may result in additive drowsiness and CNS depression).
No products indexed under this heading.

Methohexital Sodium (Co-administration results in additive drowsiness and CNS depression).
No products indexed under this heading.

Methotrimeprazine (Co-administration results in additive drowsiness and CNS depression).
No products indexed under this heading.

Methoxamine Hydrochloride (Co-administration with sympathomimetics may result in additive hypertension, tachycardia, and possibly cardiotoxicity).
No products indexed under this heading.

Methoxyflurane (Co-administration results in additive drowsiness and CNS depression).
No products indexed under this heading.

Metocurine Iodide (Co-administration results in additive drowsiness and CNS depression).
No products indexed under this heading.

Midazolam Hydrochloride (Co-administration results in additive drowsiness and CNS depression).
No products indexed under this heading.

Mivacurium Chloride (Co-administration results in additive drowsiness and CNS depression).
No products indexed under this heading.

Molindone Hydrochloride (Co-administration results in additive drowsiness and CNS depression). Products include:
Moban Tablets 1116

Morphine Sulfate (Co-administration results in additive drowsiness and CNS depression). Products include:
Avinza Capsules 1772
DepoDur Injection 1095
MS Contin Tablets 2585

Norepinephrine Bitartrate (Co-administration with sympathomimetics may result in additive hypertension, tachycardia, and possibly cardiotoxicity).
No products indexed under this heading.

Nortriptyline Hydrochloride (Co-administration results in additive tachycardia, hypertension, and drowsiness).
No products indexed under this heading.

Olanzapine (Co-administration results in additive drowsiness and CNS depression). Products include:
Symbyax Capsules 1871
Zyprexa Tablets 1883
Zyprexa IntraMuscular 1883
Zyprexa ZYDIS Orally Disintegrating Tablets 1883

Orphenadrine Citrate (Co-administration with muscle relaxants may result in additive drowsiness and CNS depression).
No products indexed under this heading.

Oxazepam (Co-administration results in additive drowsiness and CNS depression).
No products indexed under this heading.

Oxybutynin Chloride (Co-administration with anticholinergic agents may result in additive or super-additive tachycardia and drowsiness).
No products indexed under this heading.

Oxycodone Hydrochloride (Co-administration results in additive drowsiness and CNS depression). Products include:
OxyContin Tablets 2589
OxyIR Capsules 2593
Percocet Tablets 1127
Percodan Tablets 1130

Pancuronium Bromide (Co-administration results in additive drowsiness and CNS depression).
No products indexed under this heading.

Pentobarbital Sodium (Co-administration results in decreased clearance of barbiturates via competitive inhibition of metabolism; additive drowsiness and CNS depression). Products include:
Nembutal Sodium Solution, USP 2494

Perphenazine (Co-administration results in additive drowsiness and CNS depression).
No products indexed under this heading.

Phenobarbital (Co-administration results in decreased clearance of barbiturates via competitive inhibition of metabolism; additive drowsiness and CNS depression). Products include:
Donnatal Extentabs 2507

Phenylephrine Bitartrate (Co-administration with sympathomimetics may result in additive hypertension, tachycardia, and possibly cardiotoxicity).
No products indexed under this heading.

Phenylephrine Hydrochloride (Co-administration with sympathomimetics may result in additive hypertension, tachycardia, and possibly cardiotoxicity). Products include:
Actifed Cold & Allergy Tablets 1895
Benadryl Allergy & Cold Kapgels 1895
Benadryl Allergy & Sinus Headache Kapgels 1895
Benadryl Severe Allergy & Sinus Headache Caplets 1897
Children's Benadryl-D Allergy & Sinus Liquid 1896
Benadryl-D Allergy & Sinus Tablet 1896
PediaCare Children's Allergy & Cold Liquid 1902
PediaCare Children's Decongestant Liquid 1902
PediaCare Children's Liquid Multi-Symptom Cold 1902
Sinutab Non-Drying Caplets 1905
Sinutab Sinus Caplets 1905
Children's Sudafed PE Cold & Cough Liquid 1907
Children's Sudafed PE Nasal Decongestant Liquid 1906
Sudafed PE Cold & Cough Caplets 1907
Sudafed PE Nasal Decongestant Tablets 1907
Sudafed PE Nighttime Cold Caplets 1907
Sudafed PE Non-Drying Sinus Caplets 1908
Sudafed PE Severe Cold Caplets 1908
Sudafed PE Sinus & Allergy Tablets 1908
Sudafed PE Sinus Headache Caplets 1908
Tylenol Allergy Multi-Symptom Caplets with Cool Burst and Rapid Release Gelcaps 1916
Tylenol Allergy Multi-Symptom Nighttime Caplets with Cool Burst 1916
Children's Tylenol Plus Cold Suspension Liquid 1912
Children's Tylenol Plus Cold & Allergy Suspension Liquid 1914
Children's Tylenol Plus Flu Suspension Liquid 1914
Children's Tylenol Plus Multi-Symptom Cold Suspension Liquid 1912
Tylenol Cold Head Congestion Daytime Caplets with Cool Burst 1910
Tylenol Cold Head Congestion Nighttime Caplets with Cool Burst 1910
Tylenol Cold Head Congestion Severe Daytime Caplets with Cool Burst 1910
Tylenol Cold Multi-Symptom Daytime Caplets with Cool Burst and Rapid Release Gels 1913
Tylenol Cold Multi-Symptom Daytime Liquid with Citrus Burst 1913
Tylenol Cold Multi-Symptom Nighttime Caplets with Cool Burst 1913
Tylenol Cold Multi-Symptom Nighttime Liquid with Cool Burst 1913
Tylenol Cold Multi-Symptom Severe Caplets with Cool Burst 1913
Tylenol Cold Multi-Symptom Severe Daytime Liquid with Citrus Burst 1913
Tylenol Sinus Congestion & Pain Daytime Caplets with Cool Burst and Gelcaps 1917
Tylenol Sinus Congestion & Pain Nighttime Caplets with Cool Burst 1917
Tylenol Sinus Congestion & Pain Severe Caplets with Cool Burst 1917
Vicks DayQuil Cold & Flu Multi-Symptom Relief .... ◙616
Vicks DayQuil LiquiCaps 2567
Vicks DayQuil Liquid 2567
Vicks DayQuil Multi-Symptom Cold/Flu Relief 2567

Phenylephrine Tannate (Co-administration with sympathomimetics may result in additive hypertension, tachycardia, and possibly cardiotoxicity).
No products indexed under this heading.

Phenylpropanolamine Hydrochloride (Co-administration with sympathomimetics may result in additive hypertension, tachycardia, and possibly cardiotoxicity).
No products indexed under this heading.

Pirbuterol Acetate (Co-administration with sympathomimetics may result in additive hypertension, tachycardia, and possibly cardiotoxicity). Products include:
Maxair Autohaler 1705

Prazepam (Co-administration results in additive drowsiness and CNS depression).
No products indexed under this heading.

Prochlorperazine (Co-administration results in additive drowsiness and CNS depression).
No products indexed under this heading.

Procyclidine Hydrochloride (Co-administration with anticholinergic agents may result in additive or super-additive tachycardia and drowsiness).
No products indexed under this heading.

Promethazine Hydrochloride (Co-administration results in additive drowsiness and CNS depression).
No products indexed under this heading.

Propantheline Bromide (Co-administration with anticholinergic agents may result in additive or super-additive tachycardia and drowsiness).
No products indexed under this heading.

Propofol (Co-administration results in additive drowsiness and CNS depression).
No products indexed under this heading.

Propoxyphene Hydrochloride (Co-administration results in additive drowsiness and CNS depression).
No products indexed under this heading.

Propoxyphene Napsylate (Co-administration results in additive drowsiness and CNS depression).
No products indexed under this heading.

Protriptyline Hydrochloride (Co-administration results in additive tachycardia, hypertension, and drowsiness).
No products indexed under this heading.

Pseudoephedrine Hydrochloride (Co-administration with sympathomimetics may result in additive hypertension, tachycardia, and possibly cardiotoxicity). Products include:
Allegra-D 12 Hour Extended-Release Tablets 2687
Allegra-D 24 Hour Extended-Release Tablets 2690
Children's Motrin Cold Oral Suspension 1899
Sudafed 12 Hour Nasal Decongestant Non-Drowsy Caplets 1909
Sudafed 24 Hour Non-Drowsy Nasal Decongestant Tablets 1906
Children's Sudafed Nasal Decongestant Liquid 1906
Sudafed Nasal Decongestant Tablets 1906
Tylenol Cold Severe Congestion Daytime Caplets with Cool Burst 1912
Tylenol Sinus Severe Congestion Caplets with Cool Burst 1917
Vicks NyQuil LiquiCaps 2567
Vicks NyQuil Liquid 2567
Vicks NyQuil Multi-Symptom Cold/Flu Relief 2567
Zyrtec-D 12 Hour Extended Release Tablets 1923
Zyrtec-D Allergy & Congestion Extended-Release Tablets 1923

Pseudoephedrine Sulfate (Co-administration with sympathomimetics may result in additive hypertension, tachycardia, and possibly cardiotoxicity). Products include:
Clarinex-D 12-Hour Extended-Release Tablets 2831
Clarinex-D 24-Hour Extended-Release Tablets 2834

Pyrilamine Maleate (Co-administration results in additive CNS depression or super-additive tachycardia and drowsiness).
No products indexed under this heading.

Pyrilamine Tannate (Co-administration results in additive CNS depression or super-additive tachycardia and drowsiness).
No products indexed under this heading.

Quazepam (Co-administration results in additive drowsiness and CNS depression).
No products indexed under this heading.

Quetiapine Fumarate (Co-administration results in additive drowsiness and CNS depression).
No products indexed under this heading.

Rapacuronium Bromide (Co-administration results in additive drowsiness and CNS depression).
No products indexed under this heading.

Remifentanil Hydrochloride (Co-administration results in additive drowsiness and CNS depression).
No products indexed under this heading.

Risperidone (Co-administration results in additive drowsiness and CNS depression). Products include:
Risperdal Consta Long-Acting Injection 1753

Rocuronium Bromide (Co-administration results in additive drowsiness and CNS depression). Products include:
Zemuron Injection 2947

Salmeterol Xinafoate (Co-administration with sympathomimetics may result in additive hypertension, tachycardia, and possibly cardiotoxicity). Products include:
Advair Diskus 100/50 1276
Advair Diskus 250/50 1276
Advair Diskus 500/50 1276
Advair HFA 45/21 Inhalation Aerosol 1288
Advair HFA 115/21 Inhalation Aerosol 1288
Advair HFA 230/21 Inhalation Aerosol 1288
Serevent Diskus 1594

Scopolamine (Co-administration with anticholinergic agents may result in additive or super-additive tachycardia and drowsiness). Products include:
Transderm Scōp Transdermal Therapeutic System 2206

Scopolamine Hydrobromide (Co-administration with anticholinergic agents may result in additive or super-additive tachycardia and drowsiness). Products include:
Donnatal Extentabs 2507

Secobarbital Sodium (Co-administration results in decreased clearance of barbiturates via competitive inhibition of metabolism; additive drowsiness and CNS depression).
No products indexed under this heading.

Sevoflurane (Co-administration results in additive drowsiness and CNS depression). Products include:
Ultane Liquid for Inhalation 524

Sodium Oxybate (Co-administration results in additive drowsiness and CNS depression). Products include:
Xyrem Oral Solution 1766

Succinylcholine Chloride (Co-administration results in additive drowsiness and CNS depression).
No products indexed under this heading.

Sufentanil Citrate (Co-administration results in additive drowsiness and CNS depression).
No products indexed under this heading.

Temazepam (Co-administration results in additive drowsiness and CNS depression).
No products indexed under this heading.

Terbutaline Sulfate (Co-administration with sympathomimetics may result in additive hypertension, tachycardia, and possibly cardiotoxicity).
No products indexed under this heading.

Terfenadine (Co-administration results in additive CNS depression or super-additive tachycardia and drowsiness).
No products indexed under this heading.

Theophylline (Increased theophylline metabolism has resulted with smoking marijuana).
No products indexed under this heading.

Theophylline Anhydrous (Increased theophylline metabolism has resulted with smoking marijuana). Products include:
Uniphyl Tablets 2595

Theophylline Calcium Salicylate (Increased theophylline metabolism has resulted with smoking marijuana).
No products indexed under this heading.

Theophylline Dihydroxypropyl (Glyceryl) (Increased theophylline metabolism has resulted with smoking marijuana).
No products indexed under this heading.

Theophylline Ethylenediamine (Increased theophylline metabolism has resulted with smoking marijuana).
No products indexed under this heading.

Theophylline Sodium Glycinate (Increased theophylline metabolism has resulted with smoking marijuana).
No products indexed under this heading.

Thiamylal Sodium (Co-administration results in decreased clearance of barbiturates via competitive inhibition of metabolism; additive drowsiness and CNS depression).
No products indexed under this heading.

Thioridazine Hydrochloride (Co-administration results in additive drowsiness and CNS depression). Products include:
Thioridazine Hydrochloride Tablets **2195**

Thiothixene (Co-administration results in additive drowsiness and CNS depression). Products include:
Thiothixene Capsules **2197**

Tolterodine Tartrate (Co-administration with anticholinergic agents may result in additive or super-additive tachycardia and drowsiness).
No products indexed under this heading.

Triazolam (Co-administration results in additive drowsiness and CNS depression).
No products indexed under this heading.

Tridihexethyl Chloride (Co-administration with anticholinergic agents may result in additive or super-additive tachycardia and drowsiness).
No products indexed under this heading.

Trifluoperazine Hydrochloride (Co-administration results in additive drowsiness and CNS depression).
No products indexed under this heading.

Trihexyphenidyl Hydrochloride (Co-administration with anticholinergic agents may result in additive or super-additive tachycardia and drowsiness).
No products indexed under this heading.

Trimeprazine Tartrate (Co-administration results in additive CNS depression or super-additive tachycardia and drowsiness).
No products indexed under this heading.

Trimipramine Maleate (Co-administration results in additive tachycardia, hypertension, and drowsiness).
No products indexed under this heading.

Tripelennamine Hydrochloride (Co-administration results in additive CNS depression or super-additive tachycardia and drowsiness).
No products indexed under this heading.

Triprolidine Hydrochloride (Co-administration results in additive CNS depression or super-additive tachycardia and drowsiness).
No products indexed under this heading.

Vecuronium Bromide (Co-administration results in additive drowsiness and CNS depression).
No products indexed under this heading.

Zaleplon (Co-administration results in additive drowsiness and CNS depression).
No products indexed under this heading.

Ziprasidone Hydrochloride (Co-administration results in additive drowsiness and CNS depression). Products include:
Geodon Capsules **2520**

Zolpidem Tartrate (Co-administration results in additive drowsiness and CNS depression). Products include:
Ambien Tablets **2692**
Ambien CR Tablets **2696**

Food Interactions

Alcohol (Co-administration results in additive drowsiness and CNS depression).

MARLYN FORMULA 50 CAPSULES

(Amino Acid Preparations, Vitamin B_6) **1894**
None cited in PDR database.

MARPLAN TABLETS

(Isocarboxazid) **3177**
May interact with amphetamines, anesthetics, antihistamines, antihypertensives, central nervous system depressants, dibenzazepines, diuretics, hypnotics and sedatives, monoamine oxidase inhibitors, narcotic analgesics, selective serotonin reuptake inhibitors, sympathomimetics, and certain other agents. Compounds in these categories include:

Acebutolol Hydrochloride (Isocarboxazid should not be used in combination with anti-hypertensive agents, including thiazide diuretics. A marked potentiating effect on these drugs has been reported, resulting in hypotension).
No products indexed under this heading.

Acrivastine (Isocarboxazid should not be administered in combination with antihistamines).
No products indexed under this heading.

Albuterol (Isocarboxazid should not be administered in combination with sympathomimetics, including amphetamines, or with over-the-counter drugs such as cold, hay fever, or weight-reducing preparations that contain vasoconstrictors).
No products indexed under this heading.

Albuterol Sulfate (Isocarboxazid should not be administered in combination with sympathomimetics, including amphetamines, or with over-the-counter drugs such as cold, hay fever, or weight-reducing preparations that contain vasoconstrictors). Products include:
Combivent Inhalation Aerosol **845**
ProAir HFA Inhalation Aerosol **3113**
Proventil HFA Inhalation Aerosol **2914**
Ventolin HFA Inhalation Aerosol **1638**

Alfentanil Hydrochloride (Isocarboxazid should not be administered in combination with some central nervous system depressants including narcotic analgesics).
No products indexed under this heading.

Aliskiren (Isocarboxazid should not be used in combination with anti-hypertensive agents, including thiazide diuretics. A marked potentiating effect on these drugs has been reported, resulting in hypotension). Products include:
Tekturna Tablets **2321**
Tekturna HCT Tablets **2324**

Alprazolam (Isocarboxazid should not be administered in combination with central nervous system depressants).
No products indexed under this heading.

Amiloride Hydrochloride (Isocarboxazid should not be used in combination with anti-hypertensive agents, including thiazide diuretics. A marked potentiating effect on these drugs has been reported, resulting in hypotension).
No products indexed under this heading.

Amitriptyline Hydrochloride (Isocarboxazid should not be administered in combination with dibenzazepines. In patients being transferred to isocarboxazid from dibenzazepine-related entities, a medication-free interval of at least 1 week should be allowed, after which isocarboxazid therapy should be started using half the normal starting dosage for at least the first week of therapy. Similarly, at least 1 week should elapse between the discontinuation of isocarboxazid and initiation of other dibenzazepine-related entities, or the re-administration of isocarboxazid).
No products indexed under this heading.

Amlodipine Besylate (Isocarboxazid should not be used in combination with anti-hypertensive agents, including thiazide diuretics. A marked potentiating effect on these drugs has been reported, resulting in hypotension). Products include:
Azor Tablets **1005**
Exforge Tablets **2238**

Amoxapine (Isocarboxazid should not be administered in combination with dibenzazepines. In patients being transferred to isocarboxazid from dibenzazepine-related entities, a medication-free interval of at least 1 week should be allowed, after which isocarboxazid therapy should be started using half the normal starting dosage for at least the first week of therapy. Similarly, at least 1 week should elapse between the discontinuation of isocarboxazid and initiation of other dibenzazepine-related entities, or the re-administration of isocarboxazid).
No products indexed under this heading.

Amphetamine Resins (Isocarboxazid should not be administered in combination with sympathomimetics including amphetamines).
No products indexed under this heading.

Amphetamine Sulfate (Isocarboxazid should not be administered in combination with sympathomimetics including amphetamines). Products include:
Adderall XR Capsules **3012**

Aprobarbital (Isocarboxazid should not be administered in combination with central nervous system depressants).
No products indexed under this heading.

Astemizole (Isocarboxazid should not be administered in combination with antihistamines).
No products indexed under this heading.

Atenolol (Isocarboxazid should not be used in combination with anti-hypertensive agents, including thiazide diuretics. A marked potentiating effect on these drugs has been reported, resulting in hypotension).
No products indexed under this heading.

Azatadine Maleate (Isocarboxazid should not be administered in combination with antihistamines).
No products indexed under this heading.

Benazepril Hydrochloride (Isocarboxazid should not be used in combination with anti-hypertensive agents, including thiazide diuretics. A marked potentiating effect on these drugs has been reported, resulting in hypotension).
No products indexed under this heading.

Bendroflumethiazide (Isocarboxazid should not be used in combination with anti-hypertensive agents, including thiazide diuretics. A marked potentiating effect on these drugs has been reported, resulting in hypotension).
No products indexed under this heading.

Betaxolol Hydrochloride (Isocarboxazid should not be used in combination with anti-hypertensive agents, including thiazide diuretics. A marked potentiating effect on these drugs has been reported, resulting in hypotension).
No products indexed under this heading.

Bisoprolol Fumarate (Isocarboxazid should not be used in combination with anti-hypertensive agents, including thiazide diuretics. A marked potentiating effect on these drugs has been reported, resulting in hypotension).
No products indexed under this heading.

Bromodiphenhydramine Hydrochloride (Isocarboxazid should not be administered in combination with antihistamines).
No products indexed under this heading.

Brompheniramine Maleate (Isocarboxazid should not be administered in combination with antihistamines).
No products indexed under this heading.

Bumetanide (Isocarboxazid should not be used in combination with anti-hypertensive agents, including thiazide diuretics. A marked potentiating effect on these drugs has been reported, resulting in hypotension).
No products indexed under this heading.

Buprenorphine Hydrochloride (Isocarboxazid should not be admin-

istered in combination with some central nervous system depressants including narcotic analgesics). Products include:
- Suboxone Tablets 2601
- Subutex Tablets 2601

Bupropion Hydrochloride (Isocarboxazid should not be administered in combination with bupropion hydrochloride. The concurrent administration of a MAOI and bupropion hydrochloride is contraindicated. At least 14 days should elapse between discontinuation of an MAOI and initiationof treatment with bupropion hydrochloride). Products include:
- Wellbutrin Tablets 1648
- Wellbutrin SR Sustained-Release Tablets 1653
- Wellbutrin XL Extended-Release Tablets 1659
- Zyban Sustained-Release Tablets 1692

Buspirone Hydrochloride (Isocarboxazid should not be administered in combination with buspirone hydrochloride. At least 10 days should elapse between the discontinuation of isocarboxazid and the institution of buspirone hydrochloride).
No products indexed under this heading.

Butabarbital (Isocarboxazid should not be administered in combination with hypnotics and sedatives).
No products indexed under this heading.

Butabarbital Sodium (Isocarboxazid should not be administered in combination with hypnotics and sedatives).
No products indexed under this heading.

Butalbital (Isocarboxazid should not be administered in combination with central nervous system depressants).
No products indexed under this heading.

Caffeine (Isocarboxazid should not be administered in combination with excessive quantities of caffeine). Products include:
- BioLean Free Tablets 635
- BioLean II Tablets 635
- Winrgy Dietary Supplement 642

Candesartan Cilexetil (Isocarboxazid should not be used in combination with anti-hypertensive agents, including thiazide diuretics. A marked potentiating effect on these drugs has been reported, resulting in hypotension). Products include:
- Atacand Tablets 639
- Atacand HCT 642

Captopril (Isocarboxazid should not be used in combination with anti-hypertensive agents, including thiazide diuretics. A marked potentiating effect on these drugs has been reported, resulting in hypotension). Products include:
- Captopril Tablets 2182

Carbamazepine (Isocarboxazid should not be administered in combination with dibenzazepines. In patients being transferred to isocarboxazid from dibenzazepine-related entities, a medication-free interval of at least 1 week should be allowed, after which isocarboxazid therapy should be started using half the normal starting dosage for at least the first week of therapy. Similarly, at least 1 week should elapse between the discontinuation of isocarboxazid and initiation of other dibenzazepine-related entities, or the re-administration of isocarboxazid). Products include:
- Carbatrol Capsules 3019
- Equetro Extended-Release Capsules 3174

Carteolol Hydrochloride (Isocarboxazid should not be used in combination with anti-hypertensive agents, including thiazide diuretics. A marked potentiating effect on these drugs has been reported, resulting in hypotension).
No products indexed under this heading.

Cetirizine Hydrochloride (Isocarboxazid should not be administered in combination with antihistamines). Products include:
- Zyrtec Allergy Tablets 1919
- Zyrtec Chewable Tablets 1920
- Children's Zyrtec Allergy Chewable Tablets 1922
- Children's Zyrtec Allergy Syrup 1920
- Children's Zyrtec Hives Relief Syrup 1920
- Zyrtec Syrup 1920
- Zyrtec Tablets 1920
- Zyrtec-D 12 Hour Extended Release Tablets 1923
- Zyrtec-D Allergy & Congestion Extended-Release Tablets 1923

Chloral Hydrate (Isocarboxazid should not be administered in combination with hypnotics and sedatives).
No products indexed under this heading.

Chlordiazepoxide (Isocarboxazid should not be administered in combination with central nervous system depressants).
No products indexed under this heading.

Chlordiazepoxide Hydrochloride (Isocarboxazid should not be administered in combination with central nervous system depressants).
No products indexed under this heading.

Chlorothiazide (Isocarboxazid should not be used in combination with anti-hypertensive agents, including thiazide diuretics. A marked potentiating effect on these drugs has been reported, resulting in hypotension).
No products indexed under this heading.

Chlorothiazide Sodium (Isocarboxazid should not be used in combination with anti-hypertensive agents, including thiazide diuretics. A marked potentiating effect on these drugs has been reported, resulting in hypotension). Products include:
- Intravenous Sodium Diuril 2490

Chlorpheniramine Maleate (Isocarboxazid should not be administered in combination with antihistamines). Products include:
- Actifed Cold & Allergy Tablets 1895
- Sudafed PE Sinus & Allergy Tablets 1908
- Tylenol Allergy Multi-Symptom Caplets with Cool Burst and Rapid Release Gelcaps 1916
- Children's Tylenol Plus Cold Suspension Liquid 1912
- Children's Tylenol Plus Cough & Runny Nose Suspension Liquid 1912
- Children's Tylenol Plus Flu Suspension Liquid 1914
- Children's Tylenol Plus Multi-Symptom Cold Suspension Liquid 1912
- Tylenol Cold Head Congestion Nighttime Caplets with Cool Burst 1910
- Tylenol Cold Multi-Symptom Nighttime Caplets with Cool Burst 1913
- Tylenol Sinus Congestion & Pain Nighttime Caplets with Cool Burst 1917

Chlorpheniramine Polistirex (Isocarboxazid should not be administered in combination with antihistamines). Products include:
- Tussionex Pennkinetic Extended-Release Suspension 3154

Chlorpheniramine Tannate (Isocarboxazid should not be administered in combination with antihistamines).
No products indexed under this heading.

Chlorpromazine (Isocarboxazid should not be administered in combination with central nervous system depressants).
No products indexed under this heading.

Chlorpromazine Hydrochloride (Isocarboxazid should not be administered in combination with central nervous system depressants).
No products indexed under this heading.

Chlorprothixene (Isocarboxazid should not be administered in combination with central nervous system depressants).
No products indexed under this heading.

Chlorprothixene Hydrochloride (Isocarboxazid should not be administered in combination with central nervous system depressants).
No products indexed under this heading.

Chlorprothixene Lactate (Isocarboxazid should not be administered in combination with central nervous system depressants).
No products indexed under this heading.

Chlorthalidone (Isocarboxazid should not be used in combination with anti-hypertensive agents, including thiazide diuretics. A marked potentiating effect on these drugs has been reported, resulting in hypotension). Products include:
- Clorpres Tablets 2185

Citalopram Hydrobromide (Isocarboxazid should not be administered in combination with any selective serotonin reuptake inhibitors. At least 2 weeks should be allowed after stopping sertraline or paroxetine before starting isocarboxazid. In addition, there should be an interval of at least 10 days between discontinuation of isocarboxazid and initiation of SSRIs). Products include:
- Celexa 1160

Clemastine Fumarate (Isocarboxazid should not be administered in combination with antihistamines).
No products indexed under this heading.

Clomipramine Hydrochloride (Isocarboxazid should not be administered in combination with dibenzazepines. In patients being transferred to isocarboxazid from dibenzazepine-related entities, a medication-free interval of at least 1 week should be allowed, after which isocarboxazid therapy should be started using half the normal starting dosage for at least the first week of therapy. Similarly, at least 1 week should elapse between the discontinuation of isocarboxazid and initiation of other dibenzazepine-related entities, or the re-administration of isocarboxazid).
No products indexed under this heading.

Clonidine (Isocarboxazid should not be used in combination with anti-hypertensive agents, including thiazide diuretics. A marked potentiating effect on these drugs has been reported, resulting in hypotension). Products include:
- Catapres-TTS 842

Clonidine Hydrochloride (Isocarboxazid should not be used in combination with anti-hypertensive agents, including thiazide diuretics. A marked potentiating effect on these drugs has been reported, resulting in hypotension). Products include:
- Catapres Tablets 841
- Clorpres Tablets 2185

Clorazepate Dipotassium (Isocarboxazid should not be administered in combination with central nervous system depressants).
No products indexed under this heading.

Clozapine (Isocarboxazid should not be administered in combination with dibenzazepines. In patients being transferred to isocarboxazid from dibenzazepine-related entities, a medication-free interval of at least 1 week should be allowed, after which isocarboxazid therapy should be started using half the normal starting dosage for at least the first week of therapy. Similarly, at least 1 week should elapse between the discontinuation of isocarboxazid and initiation of other dibenzazepine-related entities, or the re-administration of isocarboxazid).
No products indexed under this heading.

Codeine Phosphate (Isocarboxazid should not be administered in combination with some central nervous system depressants including narcotic analgesics). Products include:
- Tylenol with Codeine Tablets 2427

Cyclobenzaprine Hydrochloride (Isocarboxazid should not be administered in combination with dibenzazepines. In patients being transferred to isocarboxazid from dibenzazepine-related entities, a medication-free interval of at least 1 week should be allowed, after which isocarboxazid therapy should be started using half the normal starting dosage for at least the first week of therapy. Similarly, at least 1 week should elapse between the discontinuation of isocarboxazid and initiation of other dibenzazepine-related entities, or the re-administration of isocarboxazid). Products include:
- Amrix Capsules 966

Cyproheptadine Hydrochloride (Isocarboxazid should not be administered in combination with antihistamines).
No products indexed under this heading.

Deserpidine (Isocarboxazid should not be used in combination with anti-hypertensive agents, including thiazide diuretics. A marked potentiating effect on these drugs has been reported, resulting in hypotension).
No products indexed under this heading.

Desflurane (Isocarboxazid should not be administered in combination with central nervous system depressants).
No products indexed under this heading.

Desipramine Hydrochloride (Isocarboxazid should not be administered in combination with dibenzazepines. In patients being transferred to isocarboxazid from dibenzazepine-related entities, a medication-free interval of at least 1 week should be allowed, after which isocarboxazid therapy should be started using half the normal starting dosage for at least the first week of therapy. Similarly, at least 1 week should elapse between the discontinuation of isocarboxazid and initiation of other dibenzazepine-related entities, or the re-administration of isocarboxazid).
No products indexed under this heading.

Dexchlorpheniramine Maleate (Isocarboxazid should not be administered in combination with antihistamines).
No products indexed under this heading.

Dextroamphetamine Sulfate (Isocarboxazid should not be administered in combination with sympathomimetics including amphetamines). Products include:
Adderall XR Capsules ... 3012
Dexedrine ... 1401

Dextromethorphan (Isocarboxazid should not be administered in combination with dextromethorphan. The combination of MAO inhibitors and dextromethorphan has been reported to cause brief episodes of psychosis or bizarre behavior).
No products indexed under this heading.

Dezocine (Isocarboxazid should not be administered in combination with some central nervous system depressants including narcotic analgesics).
No products indexed under this heading.

Diazepam (Isocarboxazid should not be administered in combination with central nervous system depressants). Products include:
Valium Tablets ... 2658

Diazoxide (Isocarboxazid should not be used in combination with antihypertensive agents, including thiazide diuretics. A marked potentiating effect on these drugs has been reported, resulting in hypotension). Products include:
Proglycem Capsules ... 1185
Proglycem Suspension ... 1185

Diltiazem Hydrochloride (Isocarboxazid should not be used in combination with anti-hypertensive agents, including thiazide diuretics. A marked potentiating effect on these drugs has been reported, resulting in hypotension). Products include:
Cardizem LA Extended Release Tablets ... 421

Diphenhydramine Citrate (Isocarboxazid should not be administered in combination with antihistamines).
No products indexed under this heading.

Diphenhydramine Hydrochloride (Isocarboxazid should not be administered in combination with antihistamines). Products include:
Benadryl Allergy & Cold Kapgels ... 1895
Benadryl Allergy & Sinus Headache Kapgels ... 1895
Benadryl Severe Allergy & Sinus Headache Caplets ... 1897
Benadryl Dye-Free Allergy Liqui-gels Softgels ... 1897
Benadryl Allergy Kapgels ... 1895
Benadryl Allergy Quick Dissolve Strips ... 1896
Benadryl Allergy Ultratab Tablets ... 1896
Children's Benadryl Dye-Free Allergy Liquid ... 1897
Children's Benadryl Allergy Fastmelts ... 1897
Children's Benadryl Allergy Liquid ... 1898
Children's Benadryl Allergy Perfect Measure ... 1896
Children's Benadryl-D Allergy & Sinus Liquid ... 1896
Benadryl-D Allergy & Sinus Tablet ... 1896
PediaCare Children's Allergy & Cold Liquid ... 1902
PediaCare Children's Allergy Liquid ... 1902
Simply Sleep Caplets ... 1905
Sudafed PE Nighttime Cold Caplets ... 1907
Sudafed PE Severe Cold Caplets ... 1908
Extra Strength Tylenol PM Caplets, Geltabs, Liquid, and Rapid Release Gels ... 1915
Tylenol Allergy Multi-Symptom Nighttime Caplets with Cool Burst ... 1916
Tylenol Severe Allergy Caplets ... 1916
Children's Tylenol Plus Cold & Allergy Suspension Liquid ... 1914
Tylenol Sore Throat Nighttime Liquid with Cool Burst ... 1918

Diphenylpyraline Hydrochloride (Isocarboxazid should not be administered in combination with antihistamines).
No products indexed under this heading.

Dobutamine Hydrochloride (Isocarboxazid should not be administered in combination with sympathomimetics, including amphetamines, or with over-the-counter drugs such as cold, hay fever, or weight-reducing preparations that contain vasoconstrictors).
No products indexed under this heading.

Dopamine Hydrochloride (Isocarboxazid should not be administered in combination with sympathomimetics, including amphetamines, or with over-the-counter drugs such as cold, hay fever, or weight-reducing preparations that contain vasoconstrictors).
No products indexed under this heading.

Doxazosin Mesylate (Isocarboxazid should not be used in combination with anti-hypertensive agents, including thiazide diuretics. A marked potentiating effect on these drugs has been reported, resulting in hypotension).
No products indexed under this heading.

Doxepin Hydrochloride (Isocarboxazid should not be administered in combination with dibenzazepines. In patients being transferred to isocarboxazid from dibenzazepine-related entities, a medication-free interval of at least 1 week should be allowed, after which isocarboxazid therapy should be started using half the normal starting dosage for at least the first week of therapy. Similarly, at least 1 week should elapse between the discontinuation of isocarboxazid and initiation of other dibenzazepine-related entities, or the re-administration of isocarboxazid).
No products indexed under this heading.

Droperidol (Isocarboxazid should not be administered in combination with central nervous system depressants).
No products indexed under this heading.

Enalapril Maleate (Isocarboxazid should not be used in combination with anti-hypertensive agents, including thiazide diuretics. A marked potentiating effect on these drugs has been reported, resulting in hypotension).
No products indexed under this heading.

Enalaprilat (Isocarboxazid should not be used in combination with antihypertensive agents, including thiazide diuretics. A marked potentiating effect on these drugs has been reported, resulting in hypotension).
No products indexed under this heading.

Enflurane (Isocarboxazid should not be administered in combination with anesthetic drugs. Patients taking isocarboxazid should not undergo elective surgery requiring general anesthesia. Also, they should not be given cocaine or local anesthesia containing sympathomimetic vasoconstrictors. The possible combined hypotensive effects of isocarboxazid and spinal anesthesia should be kept in mind. Isocarboxazid should be discontinued at least 10 days before elective surgery).
No products indexed under this heading.

Ephedrine Hydrochloride (Isocarboxazid should not be administered in combination with sympathomimetics, including amphetamines, or with over-the-counter drugs such as cold, hay fever, or weight-reducing preparations that contain vasoconstrictors).
No products indexed under this heading.

Ephedrine Sulfate (Isocarboxazid should not be administered in combination with sympathomimetics, including amphetamines, or with over-the-counter drugs such as cold, hay fever, or weight-reducing preparations that contain vasoconstrictors).
No products indexed under this heading.

Ephedrine Tannate (Isocarboxazid should not be administered in combination with sympathomimetics, including amphetamines, or with over-the-counter drugs such as cold, hay fever, or weight-reducing preparations that contain vasoconstrictors).
No products indexed under this heading.

Epinephrine (Isocarboxazid should not be administered in combination with sympathomimetics, including amphetamines, or with over-the-counter drugs such as cold, hay fever, or weight-reducing preparations that contain vasoconstrictors). Products include:
EpiPen ... 1024

Epinephrine Bitartrate (Isocarboxazid should not be administered in combination with sympathomimetics, including amphetamines, or with over-the-counter drugs such as cold, hay fever, or weight-reducing preparations that contain vasoconstrictors).
No products indexed under this heading.

Epinephrine Hydrochloride (Isocarboxazid should not be administered in combination with sympathomimetics, including amphetamines, or with over-the-counter drugs such as cold, hay fever, or weight-reducing preparations that contain vasoconstrictors).
No products indexed under this heading.

Eprosartan Mesylate (Isocarboxazid should not be used in combination with anti-hypertensive agents, including thiazide diuretics. A marked potentiating effect on these drugs has been reported, resulting in hypotension). Products include:
Teveten Tablets ... 515
Teveten HCT Tablets ... 517

Escitalopram Oxalate (Isocarboxazid should not be administered in combination with any selective serotonin reuptake inhibitors. At least 2 weeks should be allowed after stopping sertraline or paroxetine before starting isocarboxazid. In addition, there should be an interval of at least 10 days between discontinuation of isocarboxazid and initiation of SSRIs). Products include:
Lexapro Oral Suspension ... 1174
Lexapro Tablets ... 1174

Esmolol Hydrochloride (Isocarboxazid should not be used in combination with anti-hypertensive agents, including thiazide diuretics. A marked potentiating effect on these drugs has been reported, resulting in hypotension).
No products indexed under this heading.

Estazolam (Isocarboxazid should not be administered in combination with hypnotics and sedatives).
No products indexed under this heading.

Ethacrynic Acid (Isocarboxazid should not be used in combination with anti-hypertensive agents, including thiazide diuretics. A marked potentiating effect on these drugs has been reported, resulting in hypotension). Products include:
Edecrin Tablets ... 698

Ethanol (Isocarboxazid should not be administered in combination with central nervous system depressants).
No products indexed under this heading.

Ethchlorvynol (Isocarboxazid should not be administered in combination with hypnotics and sedatives).
No products indexed under this heading.

Ethinamate (Isocarboxazid should not be administered in combination with hypnotics and sedatives).
No products indexed under this heading.

Ethyl Alcohol (Isocarboxazid should not be administered in combination with central nervous system depressants).
No products indexed under this heading.

Felodipine (Isocarboxazid should not be used in combination with anti-hypertensive agents, including thiazide diuretics. A marked potentiating effect on these drugs has been reported, resulting in hypotension).
No products indexed under this heading.

Fentanyl (Isocarboxazid should not be administered in combination with some central nervous system depressants including narcotic analgesics). Products include:
Duragesic Transdermal System **2405**
Ionsys Transdermal System **2410**

Fentanyl Citrate (Isocarboxazid should not be administered in combination with some central nervous system depressants including narcotic analgesics). Products include:
Actiq **959**
Fentora Tablets **968**

Fexofenadine Hydrochloride (Isocarboxazid should not be administered in combination with antihistamines). Products include:
Allegra Oral Solution **2684**
Allegra Tablets **2684**
Allegra-D 12 Hour Extended-Release Tablets **2687**
Allegra-D 24 Hour Extended-Release Tablets **2690**

Fluoxetine (Isocarboxazid should not be administered in combination with any SSRI. There have been reports of serious, sometimes fatal, reactions in patients receiving fluoxetine in combination with a MAOI, and in patients who have recently discontinued fluoxetine and are then started on a MAOI. Fluoxetine and other SSRIs should not be used in combination with isocarboxazid, or within 14 days of discontinuing therapy with isocarboxazid. As fluoxetine and its major metabolite have very long elimination half-lives, at least 5 weeks should be allowed after stopping fluoxetine before starting isocarboxazid).
No products indexed under this heading.

Fluoxetine Hydrochloride (Isocarboxazid should not be administered in combination with any selective serotonin reuptake inhibitors. At least 2 weeks should be allowed after stopping sertraline or paroxetine before starting isocarboxazid. In addition, there should be an interval of at least 10 days between discontinuation of isocarboxazid and initiation of SSRIs). Products include:
Prozac Weekly Capsules **1852**
Prozac Pulvules and Liquid **1852**
Symbyax Capsules **1871**

Fluphenazine Decanoate (Isocarboxazid should not be administered in combination with central nervous system depressants).
No products indexed under this heading.

Fluphenazine Enanthate (Isocarboxazid should not be administered in combination with central nervous system depressants).
No products indexed under this heading.

Fluphenazine Hydrochloride (Isocarboxazid should not be administered in combination with central nervous system depressants).
No products indexed under this heading.

Flurazepam Hydrochloride (Isocarboxazid should not be administered in combination with hypnotics and sedatives).
No products indexed under this heading.

Fluvoxamine Maleate (Isocarboxazid should not be administered in combination with any selective serotonin reuptake inhibitors. At least 2 weeks should be allowed after stopping sertraline or paroxetine before starting isocarboxazid. In addition, there should be an interval of at least 10 days between discontinuation of isocarboxazid and initiation of SSRIs). Products include:
Luvox CR Extended-Release Capsules **1759**

Fosinopril Sodium (Isocarboxazid should not be used in combination with anti-hypertensive agents, including thiazide diuretics. A marked potentiating effect on these drugs has been reported, resulting in hypotension).
No products indexed under this heading.

Furosemide (Isocarboxazid should not be used in combination with anti-hypertensive agents, including thiazide diuretics. A marked potentiating effect on these drugs has been reported, resulting in hypotension). Products include:
Furosemide Tablets **2186**

Glutethimide (Isocarboxazid should not be administered in combination with hypnotics and sedatives).
No products indexed under this heading.

Guanabenz Acetate (Isocarboxazid should not be used in combination with anti-hypertensive agents, including thiazide diuretics. A marked potentiating effect on these drugs has been reported, resulting in hypotension).
No products indexed under this heading.

Guanethidine Monosulfate (Isocarboxazid should not be used in combination with anti-hypertensive agents, including thiazide diuretics. A marked potentiating effect on these drugs has been reported, resulting in hypotension).
No products indexed under this heading.

Haloperidol (Isocarboxazid should not be administered in combination with central nervous system depressants).
No products indexed under this heading.

Haloperidol Decanoate (Isocarboxazid should not be administered in combination with central nervous system depressants).
No products indexed under this heading.

Halothane (Isocarboxazid should not be administered in combination with anesthetic drugs. Patients taking isocarboxazid should not undergo elective surgery requiring general anesthesia. Also, they should not be given cocaine or local anesthesia containing sympathomimetic vasoconstrictors. The possible combined hypotensive effects of isocarboxazid and spinal anesthesia should be kept in mind. Isocarboxazid should be discontinued at least 10 days before elective surgery).
No products indexed under this heading.

Hydralazine Hydrochloride (Isocarboxazid should not be used in combination with anti-hypertensive agents, including thiazide diuretics. A marked potentiating effect on these drugs has been reported, resulting in hypotension).
No products indexed under this heading.

Hydrochlorothiazide (Isocarboxazid should not be used in combination with anti-hypertensive agents, including thiazide diuretics. A marked potentiating effect on these drugs has been reported, resulting in hypotension). Products include:
Atacand HCT **642**
Avalide Tablets **892**
Avalide Tablets **2713**
Benicar HCT Tablets **1010**
Diovan HCT Tablets **2216**
Dyazide Capsules **1405**
Micardis HCT Tablets **854**
Prinzide Tablets **2092**
Tekturna HCT Tablets **2324**
Teveten HCT Tablets **517**

Hydrocodone Bitartrate (Isocarboxazid should not be administered in combination with some central nervous system depressants including narcotic analgesics). Products include:
Lortab 5/500 Tablets **3143**
Lortab 7.5/500 Tablets **3144**
Lortab 10/500 Tablets **3144**
Vicodin Tablets **529**
Vicodin ES Tablets **530**
Vicodin HP Tablets **531**
Vicoprofen Tablets **533**
Zydone Tablets **1132**

Hydrocodone Polistirex (Isocarboxazid should not be administered in combination with some central nervous system depressants including narcotic analgesics). Products include:
Tussionex Pennkinetic Extended-Release Suspension **3154**

Hydroflumethiazide (Isocarboxazid should not be used in combination with anti-hypertensive agents, including thiazide diuretics. A marked potentiating effect on these drugs has been reported, resulting in hypotension).
No products indexed under this heading.

Hydromorphone Hydrochloride (Isocarboxazid should not be administered in combination with some central nervous system depressants including narcotic analgesics).
No products indexed under this heading.

Hydroxyzine Hydrochloride (Isocarboxazid should not be administered in combination with central nervous system depressants).
No products indexed under this heading.

Imipramine Hydrochloride (Isocarboxazid should not be administered in combination with dibenzazepines. In patients being transferred to isocarboxazid from dibenzazepine-related entities, a medication-free interval of at least 1 week should be allowed, after which isocarboxazid therapy should be started using half the normal starting dosage for at least the first week of therapy. Similarly, at least 1 week should elapse between the discontinuation of isocarboxazid and initiation of other dibenzazepine-related entities, or the re-administration of isocarboxazid).
No products indexed under this heading.

Imipramine Pamoate (Isocarboxazid should not be administered in combination with dibenzazepines. In patients being transferred to isocarboxazid from dibenzazepine-related entities, a medication-free interval of at least 1 week should be allowed, after which isocarboxazid therapy should be started using half the normal starting dosage for at least the first week of therapy. Similarly, at least 1 week should elapse between the discontinuation of isocarboxazid and initiation of other dibenzazepine-related entities, or the re-administration of isocarboxazid).
No products indexed under this heading.

Indapamide (Isocarboxazid should not be used in combination with anti-hypertensive agents, including thiazide diuretics. A marked potentiating effect on these drugs has been reported, resulting in hypotension). Products include:
Indapamide Tablets **2188**

Irbesartan (Isocarboxazid should not be used in combination with anti-hypertensive agents, including thiazide diuretics. A marked potentiating effect on these drugs has been reported, resulting in hypotension). Products include:
Avalide Tablets **892**
Avalide Tablets **2713**
Avapro Tablets **897**
Avapro Tablets **2718**

Isoflurane (Isocarboxazid should not be administered in combination with anesthetic drugs. Patients taking isocarboxazid should not undergo elective surgery requiring general anesthesia. Also, they should not be given cocaine or local anesthesia containing sympathomimetic vasoconstrictors. The possible combined hypotensive effects of isocarboxazid and spinal anesthesia should be kept in mind. Isocarboxazid should be discontinued at least 10 days before elective surgery).
No products indexed under this heading.

Isoproterenol Hydrochloride (Isocarboxazid should not be administered in combination with sympathomimetics, including amphetamines, or with over-the-counter drugs such as cold, hay fever, or weight-reducing preparations that contain vasoconstrictors).
No products indexed under this heading.

Isoproterenol Sulfate (Isocarboxazid should not be administered in combination with sympathomimetics, including amphetamines, or with over-the-counter drugs such as cold, hay fever, or weight-reducing preparations that contain vasoconstrictors).
No products indexed under this heading.

Isradipine (Isocarboxazid should not be used in combination with anti-hypertensive agents, including thiazide diuretics. A marked potentiating effect on these drugs has been reported, resulting in hypotension). Products include:
DynaCirc CR Controlled Release Tablets **1407**

Ketamine Hydrochloride (Isocarboxazid should not be administered in combination with anesthetic drugs. Patients taking isocarboxazid should not undergo elective surgery requiring general anesthesia. Also,

they should not be given cocaine or local anesthesia containing sympathomimetic vasoconstrictors. The possible combined hypotensive effects of isocarboxazid and spinal anesthesia should be kept in mind. Isocarboxazid should be discontinued at least 10 days before elective surgery).

No products indexed under this heading.

Labetalol Hydrochloride (Isocarboxazid should not be used in combination with anti-hypertensive agents, including thiazide diuretics. A marked potentiating effect on these drugs has been reported, resulting in hypotension).

No products indexed under this heading.

Levalbuterol Hydrochloride (Isocarboxazid should not be administered in combination with sympathomimetics, including amphetamines, or with over-the-counter drugs such as cold, hay fever, or weight-reducing preparations that contain vasoconstrictors). Products include:

Xopenex Inhalation Solution 3001
Xopenex Inhalation Solution Concentrate 3005

Levomethadyl Acetate Hydrochloride (Isocarboxazid should not be administered in combination with central nervous system depressants).

No products indexed under this heading.

Levorphanol Tartrate (Isocarboxazid should not be administered in combination with some central nervous system depressants including narcotic analgesics).

No products indexed under this heading.

Lisinopril (Isocarboxazid should not be used in combination with anti-hypertensive agents, including thiazide diuretics. A marked potentiating effect on these drugs has been reported, resulting in hypotension). Products include:

Prinivil Tablets 2087
Prinzide Tablets 2092

Loratadine (Isocarboxazid should not be administered in combination with antihistamines).

No products indexed under this heading.

Lorazepam (Isocarboxazid should not be administered in combination with hypnotics and sedatives).

No products indexed under this heading.

Losartan Potassium (Isocarboxazid should not be used in combination with anti-hypertensive agents, including thiazide diuretics. A marked potentiating effect on these drugs has been reported, resulting in hypotension). Products include:

Cozaar Tablets 1973

Loxapine Hydrochloride (Isocarboxazid should not be administered in combination with central nervous system depressants).

No products indexed under this heading.

Loxapine Succinate (Isocarboxazid should not be administered in combination with central nervous system depressants).

No products indexed under this heading.

Maprotiline Hydrochloride (Isocarboxazid should not be administered in combination with dibenzazepines. In patients being transferred to isocarboxazid from dibenzazepine-related entities, a medication-free interval of at least 1 week should be allowed, after which isocarboxazid therapy should be started using half the normal starting dosage for at least the first week of therapy. Similarly, at least 1 week should elapse between the discontinuation of isocarboxazid and initiation of other dibenzazepine-related entities, or the re-administration of isocarboxazid).

No products indexed under this heading.

Mecamylamine Hydrochloride (Isocarboxazid should not be used in combination with anti-hypertensive agents, including thiazide diuretics. A marked potentiating effect on these drugs has been reported, resulting in hypotension).

No products indexed under this heading.

Meperidine Hydrochloride (Meperidine should not be used concomitantly with MAOI or within 2 or 3 weeks following MAO therapy. Serious reactions have been precipitated with concomitant use).

No products indexed under this heading.

Mephobarbital (Isocarboxazid should not be administered in combination with central nervous system depressants).

No products indexed under this heading.

Meprobamate (Isocarboxazid should not be administered in combination with central nervous system depressants).

No products indexed under this heading.

Mesoridazine Besylate (Isocarboxazid should not be administered in combination with central nervous system depressants).

No products indexed under this heading.

Metaproterenol Sulfate (Isocarboxazid should not be administered in combination with sympathomimetics, including amphetamines, or with over-the-counter drugs such as cold, hay fever, or weight-reducing preparations that contain vasoconstrictors).

No products indexed under this heading.

Metaraminol Bitartrate (Isocarboxazid should not be administered in combination with sympathomimetics, including amphetamines, or with over-the-counter drugs such as cold, hay fever, or weight-reducing preparations that contain vasoconstrictors).

No products indexed under this heading.

Methadone Hydrochloride (Isocarboxazid should not be administered in combination with some central nervous system depressants including narcotic analgesics).

No products indexed under this heading.

Methamphetamine Hydrochloride (Isocarboxazid should not be administered in combination with sympathomimetics including amphetamines).

No products indexed under this heading.

Methdilazine Hydrochloride (Isocarboxazid should not be administered in combination with antihistamines).

No products indexed under this heading.

Methohexital Sodium (Isocarboxazid should not be administered in combination with anesthetic drugs. Patients taking isocarboxazid should not undergo elective surgery requiring general anesthesia. Also, they should not be given cocaine or local anesthesia containing sympathomimetic vasoconstrictors. The possible combined hypotensive effects of isocarboxazid and spinal anesthesia should be kept in mind. Isocarboxazid should be discontinued at least 10 days before elective surgery).

No products indexed under this heading.

Methotrimeprazine (Isocarboxazid should not be administered in combination with central nervous system depressants).

No products indexed under this heading.

Methoxamine Hydrochloride (Isocarboxazid should not be administered in combination with sympathomimetics, including amphetamines, or with over-the-counter drugs such as cold, hay fever, or weight-reducing preparations that contain vasoconstrictors).

No products indexed under this heading.

Methoxyflurane (Isocarboxazid should not be administered in combination with central nervous system depressants).

No products indexed under this heading.

Methyclothiazide (Isocarboxazid should not be used in combination with anti-hypertensive agents, including thiazide diuretics. A marked potentiating effect on these drugs has been reported, resulting in hypotension).

No products indexed under this heading.

Methyldopa (Isocarboxazid should not be used in combination with anti-hypertensive agents, including thiazide diuretics. A marked potentiating effect on these drugs has been reported, resulting in hypotension).

No products indexed under this heading.

Methyldopate Hydrochloride (Isocarboxazid should not be used in combination with anti-hypertensive agents, including thiazide diuretics. A marked potentiating effect on these drugs has been reported, resulting in hypotension).

No products indexed under this heading.

Metolazone (Isocarboxazid should not be used in combination with anti-hypertensive agents, including thiazide diuretics. A marked potentiating effect on these drugs has been reported, resulting in hypotension).

No products indexed under this heading.

Metoprolol Succinate (Isocarboxazid should not be used in combination with anti-hypertensive agents, including thiazide diuretics. A marked potentiating effect on these drugs has been reported, resulting in hypotension). Products include:

Toprol-XL Tablets 666

Metoprolol Tartrate (Isocarboxazid should not be used in combination with anti-hypertensive agents, including thiazide diuretics. A marked potentiating effect on these drugs has been reported, resulting in hypotension).

No products indexed under this heading.

Metyrosine (Isocarboxazid should not be used in combination with anti-hypertensive agents, including thiazide diuretics. A marked potentiating effect on these drugs has been reported, resulting in hypotension). Products include:

Demser Capsules 1989

Mibefradil Dihydrochloride (Isocarboxazid should not be used in combination with anti-hypertensive agents, including thiazide diuretics. A marked potentiating effect on these drugs has been reported, resulting in hypotension).

No products indexed under this heading.

Midazolam Hydrochloride (Isocarboxazid should not be administered in combination with anesthetic drugs. Patients taking isocarboxazid should not undergo elective surgery requiring general anesthesia. Also, they should not be given cocaine or local anesthesia containing sympathomimetic vasoconstrictors. The possible combined hypotensive effects of isocarboxazid and spinal anesthesia should be kept in mind. Isocarboxazid should be discontinued at least 10 days before elective surgery).

No products indexed under this heading.

Minoxidil (Isocarboxazid should not be used in combination with anti-hypertensive agents, including thiazide diuretics. A marked potentiating effect on these drugs has been reported, resulting in hypotension).

No products indexed under this heading.

Moclobemide (Isocarboxazid should not be administered in combination with monoamine oxidase inhibitors. In patients being transferred to isocarboxazid from other MAOI, a medication-free interval of at least 1 week should be allowed, after which isocarboxazid therapy should be started using half the normal starting dosage for at least the first week of therapy. Similarly, at least 1 week should elapse between the discontinuation of isocarboxazid and initiation of another MAOI, or the re-administration of isocarboxazid).

No products indexed under this heading.

Moexipril Hydrochloride (Isocarboxazid should not be used in combination with anti-hypertensive agents, including thiazide diuretics. A marked potentiating effect on these drugs has been reported, resulting in hypotension).

No products indexed under this heading.

Molindone Hydrochloride (Isocarboxazid should not be administered in combination with central nervous system depressants). Products include:

Moban Tablets 1116

Morphine Sulfate (Isocarboxazid should not be administered in combination with some central nervous

system depressants including narcotic analgesics). Products include:
Avinza Capsules 1772
DepoDur Injection 1095
MS Contin Tablets 2585

Nadolol (Isocarboxazid should not be used in combination with anti-hypertensive agents, including thiazide diuretics. A marked potentiating effect on these drugs has been reported, resulting in hypotension). Products include:
Nadolol Tablets 2191

Nebivolol (Isocarboxazid should not be used in combination with anti-hypertensive agents, including thiazide diuretics. A marked potentiating effect on these drugs has been reported, resulting in hypotension). Products include:
Bystolic Tablets 1155

Nicardipine Hydrochloride (Isocarboxazid should not be used in combination with anti-hypertensive agents, including thiazide diuretics. A marked potentiating effect on these drugs has been reported, resulting in hypotension). Products include:
Cardene I.V. 1093

Nifedipine (Isocarboxazid should not be used in combination with anti-hypertensive agents, including thiazide diuretics. A marked potentiating effect on these drugs has been reported, resulting in hypotension).
No products indexed under this heading.

Nisoldipine (Isocarboxazid should not be used in combination with anti-hypertensive agents, including thiazide diuretics. A marked potentiating effect on these drugs has been reported, resulting in hypotension). Products include:
Sular Extended Release Tablets 2975

Nitroglycerin (Isocarboxazid should not be used in combination with anti-hypertensive agents, including thiazide diuretics. A marked potentiating effect on these drugs has been reported, resulting in hypotension). Products include:
Nitro-Dur Transdermal Infusion System.. 2887
Nitrolingual Pumpspray 2965

Norepinephrine Bitartrate (Isocarboxazid should not be administered in combination with sympathomimetics, including amphetamines, or with over-the-counter drugs such as cold, hay fever, or weight-reducing preparations that contain vasoconstrictors).
No products indexed under this heading.

Nortriptyline Hydrochloride (Isocarboxazid should not be administered in combination with dibenzazepines. In patients being transferred to isocarboxazid from dibenzazepine-related entities, a medication-free interval of at least 1 week should be allowed, after which isocarboxazid therapy should be started using half the normal starting dosage for at least the first week of therapy. Similarly, at least 1 week should elapse between the discontinuation of isocarboxazid and initiation of other dibenzazepine-related entities, or the re-administration of isocarboxazid).
No products indexed under this heading.

Olanzapine (Isocarboxazid should not be administered in combination with central nervous system depressants). Products include:
Symbyax Capsules 1871
Zyprexa Tablets 1883
Zyprexa IntraMuscular 1883
Zyprexa ZYDIS Orally Disintegrating Tablets.................. 1883

Oxazepam (Isocarboxazid should not be administered in combination with central nervous system depressants).
No products indexed under this heading.

Oxycodone Hydrochloride (Isocarboxazid should not be administered in combination with some central nervous system depressants including narcotic analgesics). Products include:
OxyContin Tablets 2589
OxyIR Capsules 2593
Percocet Tablets 1127
Percodan Tablets 1130

Pargyline Hydrochloride (Isocarboxazid should not be administered in combination with monoamine oxidase inhibitors. In patients being transferred to isocarboxazid from other MAOI, a medication-free interval of at least 1 week should be allowed, after which isocarboxazid therapy should be started using half the normal starting dosage for at least the first week of therapy. Similarly, at least 1 week should elapse between the discontinuation of isocarboxazid and initiation of another MAOI, or the re-administration of isocarboxazid).
No products indexed under this heading.

Paroxetine Hydrochloride (Isocarboxazid should not be administered in combination with any selective serotonin reuptake inhibitors. At least 2 weeks should be allowed after stopping paroxetine before starting isocarboxazid. In addition, there should be an interval of at least 10 days between discontinuation of isocarboxazid and initiation of SSRIs). Products include:
Paxil 1535
Paxil CR Controlled-Release Tablets 1544

Penbutolol Sulfate (Isocarboxazid should not be used in combination with anti-hypertensive agents, including thiazide diuretics. A marked potentiating effect on these drugs has been reported, resulting in hypotension).
No products indexed under this heading.

Pentobarbital Sodium (Isocarboxazid should not be administered in combination with central nervous system depressants). Products include:
Nembutal Sodium Solution, USP 2494

Perindopril Erbumine (Isocarboxazid should not be used in combination with anti-hypertensive agents, including thiazide diuretics. A marked potentiating effect on these drugs has been reported, resulting in hypotension). Products include:
Aceon Tablets (2 mg, 4 mg, 8 mg)... 3038

Perphenazine (Isocarboxazid should not be administered in combination with central nervous system depressants).
No products indexed under this heading.

Phenelzine Sulfate (Isocarboxazid should not be administered in combination with monoamine oxidase inhibitors. In patients being transferred to isocarboxazid from other MAOI, a medication-free interval of at least 1 week should be allowed, after which isocarboxazid therapy should be started using half the normal starting dosage for at least the first week of therapy. Similarly, at least 1 week should elapse between the discontinuation of isocarboxazid and initiation of another MAOI, or the re-administration of isocarboxazid).
No products indexed under this heading.

Phenobarbital (Isocarboxazid should not be administered in combination with central nervous system depressants). Products include:
Donnatal Extentabs 2507

Phenoxybenzamine Hydrochloride (Isocarboxazid should not be used in combination with anti-hypertensive agents, including thiazide diuretics. A marked potentiating effect on these drugs has been reported, resulting in hypotension). Products include:
Dibenzyline Capsules 3188

Phentolamine Mesylate (Isocarboxazid should not be used in combination with anti-hypertensive agents, including thiazide diuretics. A marked potentiating effect on these drugs has been reported, resulting in hypotension).
No products indexed under this heading.

Phenylephrine Bitartrate (Isocarboxazid should not be administered in combination with sympathomimetics, including amphetamines, or with over-the-counter drugs such as cold, hay fever, or weight-reducing preparations that contain vasoconstrictors).
No products indexed under this heading.

Phenylephrine Hydrochloride (Isocarboxazid should not be administered in combination with sympathomimetics, including amphetamines, or with over-the-counter drugs such as cold, hay fever, or weight-reducing preparations that contain vasoconstrictors). Products include:
Actifed Cold & Allergy Tablets 1895
Benadryl Allergy & Cold Kapgels 1895
Benadryl Allergy & Sinus Headache Kapgels 1895
Benadryl Severe Allergy & Sinus Headache Caplets 1897
Children's Benadryl-D Allergy & Sinus Liquid............................... 1896
Benadryl-D Allergy & Sinus Tablet 1896
PediaCare Children's Allergy & Cold Liquid 1902
PediaCare Children's Decongestant Liquid................... 1902
PediaCare Children's Liquid Multi-Symptom Cold..................... 1902
Sinutab Non-Drying Caplets 1905
Sinutab Sinus Caplets 1905
Children's Sudafed PE Cold & Cough Liquid 1907
Children's Sudafed PE Nasal Decongestant Liquid.................... 1906
Sudafed PE Cold & Cough Caplets... 1907
Sudafed PE Nasal Decongestant Tablets 1907
Sudafed PE Nighttime Cold Caplets... 1907
Sudafed PE Non-Drying Sinus Caplets... 1908
Sudafed PE Severe Cold Caplets 1908
Sudafed PE Sinus & Allergy Tablets 1908
Sudafed PE Sinus Headache Caplets... 1908
Tylenol Allergy Multi-Symptom Caplets with Cool Burst and Rapid Release Gelcaps................ 1916
Tylenol Allergy Multi-Symptom Nighttime Caplets with Cool Burst.. 1916
Children's Tylenol Plus Cold Suspension Liquid 1912
Children's Tylenol Plus Cold & Allergy Suspension Liquid 1914
Children's Tylenol Plus Flu Suspension Liquid 1914
Children's Tylenol Plus Multi-Symptom Cold Suspension Liquid 1912
Tylenol Cold Head Congestion Daytime Caplets with Cool Burst... 1910
Tylenol Cold Head Congestion Nighttime Caplets with Cool Burst... 1910
Tylenol Cold Head Congestion Severe Daytime Caplets with Cool Burst..................................... 1910
Tylenol Cold Multi-Symptom Daytime Caplets with Cool Burst and Rapid Release Gels....... 1913
Tylenol Cold Multi-Symptom Daytime Liquid with Citrus Burst ... 1913
Tylenol Cold Multi-Symptom Nighttime Caplets with Cool Burst... 1913
Tylenol Cold Multi-Symptom Nighttime Liquid with Cool Burst... 1913
Tylenol Cold Multi-Symptom Severe Caplets with Cool Burst..... 1913
Tylenol Cold Multi-Symptom Severe Daytime Liquid with Citrus Burst.. 1913
Tylenol Sinus Congestion & Pain Daytime Caplets with Cool Burst and Gelcaps 1917
Tylenol Sinus Congestion & Pain Nighttime Caplets with Cool Burst... 1917
Tylenol Sinus Congestion & Pain Severe Caplets with Cool Burst..... 1917
Vicks DayQuil Cold & Flu Multi-Symptom Relief 616
Vicks DayQuil LiquiCaps 2567
Vicks DayQuil Liquid 2567
Vicks DayQuil Multi-Symptom Cold/Flu Relief.............................. 2567

Phenylephrine Tannate (Isocarboxazid should not be administered in combination with sympathomimetics, including amphetamines, or with over-the-counter drugs such as cold, hay fever, or weight-reducing preparations that contain vasoconstrictors).
No products indexed under this heading.

Phenylpropanolamine Hydrochloride (Isocarboxazid should not be administered in combination with sympathomimetics, including amphetamines, or with over-the-counter drugs such as cold, hay fever, or weight-reducing preparations that contain vasoconstrictors).
No products indexed under this heading.

Pindolol (Isocarboxazid should not be used in combination with anti-hypertensive agents, including thiazide diuretics. A marked potentiating effect on these drugs has been reported, resulting in hypotension).
No products indexed under this heading.

Pirbuterol Acetate (Isocarboxazid should not be administered in combination with sympathomimetics, including amphetamines, or with over-the-counter drugs such as cold, hay fever, or weight-reducing preparations that contain vasoconstrictors). Products include:

Maxair Autohaler 1705

Polythiazide (Isocarboxazid should not be used in combination with anti-hypertensive agents, including thiazide diuretics. A marked potentiating effect on these drugs has been reported, resulting in hypotension).
No products indexed under this heading.

Prazepam (Isocarboxazid should not be administered in combination with central nervous system depressants).
No products indexed under this heading.

Prazosin Hydrochloride (Isocarboxazid should not be used in combination with anti-hypertensive agents, including thiazide diuretics. A marked potentiating effect on these drugs has been reported, resulting in hypotension).
No products indexed under this heading.

Procarbazine Hydrochloride (Isocarboxazid should not be administered in combination with monoamine oxidase inhibitors. In patients being transferred to isocarboxazid from other MAOI, a medication-free interval of at least 1 week should be allowed, after which isocarboxazid therapy should be started using half the normal starting dosage for at least the first week of therapy. Similarly, at least 1 week should elapse between the discontinuation of isocarboxazid and initiation of another MAOI, or the re-administration of isocarboxazid).
No products indexed under this heading.

Prochlorperazine (Isocarboxazid should not be administered in combination with central nervous system depressants).
No products indexed under this heading.

Promethazine Hydrochloride (Isocarboxazid should not be administered in combination with antihistamines).
No products indexed under this heading.

Propofol (Isocarboxazid should not be administered in combination with anesthetic drugs. Patients taking isocarboxazid should not undergo elective surgery requiring general anesthesia. Also, they should not be given cocaine or local anesthesia containing sympathomimetic vasoconstrictors. The possible combined hypotensive effects of isocarboxazid and spinal anesthesia should be kept in mind. Isocarboxazid should be discontinued at least 10 days before elective surgery).
No products indexed under this heading.

Propoxyphene Hydrochloride (Isocarboxazid should not be administered in combination with some central nervous system depressants including narcotic analgesics).
No products indexed under this heading.

Propoxyphene Napsylate (Isocarboxazid should not be administered in combination with some central nervous system depressants including narcotic analgesics).
No products indexed under this heading.

Propranolol Hydrochloride (Isocarboxazid should not be used in combination with anti-hypertensive agents, including thiazide diuretics. A marked potentiating effect on these drugs has been reported, resulting in hypotension). Products include:
InnoPran XL Extended Release Capsules 1484

Protriptyline Hydrochloride (Isocarboxazid should not be administered in combination with dibenzazepines. In patients being transferred to isocarboxazid from dibenzazepine-related entities, a medication-free interval of at least 1 week should be allowed, after which isocarboxazid therapy should be started using half the normal starting dosage for at least the first week of therapy. Similarly, at least 1 week should elapse between the discontinuation of isocarboxazid and initiation of other dibenzazepine-related entities, or the re-administration of isocarboxazid).
No products indexed under this heading.

Pseudoephedrine Hydrochloride (Isocarboxazid should not be administered in combination with sympathomimetics, including amphetamines, or with over-the-counter drugs such as cold, hay fever, or weight-reducing preparations that contain vasoconstrictors). Products include:
Allegra-D 12 Hour Extended-Release Tablets 2687
Allegra-D 24 Hour Extended-Release Tablets 2690
Children's Motrin Cold Oral Suspension 1899
Sudafed 12 Hour Nasal Decongestant Non-Drowsy Caplets 1909
Sudafed 24 Hour Non-Drowsy Nasal Decongestant Tablets 1906
Children's Sudafed Nasal Decongestant Liquid 1906
Sudafed Nasal Decongestant Tablets 1906
Tylenol Cold Severe Congestion Daytime Caplets with Cool Burst 1912
Tylenol Sinus Severe Congestion Caplets with Cool Burst 1917
Vicks NyQuil LiquiCaps 2567
Vicks NyQuil Liquid 2567
Vicks NyQuil Multi-Symptom Cold/Flu Relief 2567
Zyrtec-D 12 Hour Extended Release Tablets 1923
Zyrtec-D Allergy & Congestion Extended-Release Tablets 1923

Pseudoephedrine Sulfate (Isocarboxazid should not be administered in combination with sympathomimetics, including amphetamines, or with over-the-counter drugs such as cold, hay fever, or weight-reducing preparations that contain vasoconstrictors). Products include:
Clarinex-D 12-Hour Extended-Release Tablets 2831
Clarinex-D 24-Hour Extended-Release Tablets 2834

Pyrilamine Maleate (Isocarboxazid should not be administered in combination with antihistamines).
No products indexed under this heading.

Pyrilamine Tannate (Isocarboxazid should not be administered in combination with antihistamines).
No products indexed under this heading.

Quazepam (Isocarboxazid should not be administered in combination with hypnotics and sedatives).
No products indexed under this heading.

Quetiapine Fumarate (Isocarboxazid should not be administered in combination with central nervous system depressants).
No products indexed under this heading.

Quinapril Hydrochloride (Isocarboxazid should not be used in combination with anti-hypertensive agents, including thiazide diuretics. A marked potentiating effect on these drugs has been reported, resulting in hypotension).
No products indexed under this heading.

Ramelteon (Isocarboxazid should not be administered in combination with hypnotics and sedatives). Products include:
Rozerem Tablets 3091

Ramipril (Isocarboxazid should not be used in combination with anti-hypertensive agents, including thiazide diuretics. A marked potentiating effect on these drugs has been reported, resulting in hypotension).
No products indexed under this heading.

Rasagiline Mesylate (Isocarboxazid should not be administered in combination with monoamine oxidase inhibitors. In patients being transferred to isocarboxazid from other MAOI, a medication-free interval of at least 1 week should be allowed, after which isocarboxazid therapy should be started using half the normal starting dosage for at least the first week of therapy. Similarly, at least 1 week should elapse between the discontinuation of isocarboxazid and initiation of another MAOI, or the re-administration of isocarboxazid). Products include:
Azilect Tablets 3106

Rauwolfia Serpentina (Isocarboxazid should not be used in combination with anti-hypertensive agents, including thiazide diuretics. A marked potentiating effect on these drugs has been reported, resulting in hypotension).
No products indexed under this heading.

Remifentanil Hydrochloride (Isocarboxazid should not be administered in combination with some central nervous system depressants including narcotic analgesics).
No products indexed under this heading.

Rescinnamine (Isocarboxazid should not be used in combination with anti-hypertensive agents, including thiazide diuretics. A marked potentiating effect on these drugs has been reported, resulting in hypotension).
No products indexed under this heading.

Reserpine (Isocarboxazid should not be used in combination with anti-hypertensive agents, including thiazide diuretics. A marked potentiating effect on these drugs has been reported, resulting in hypotension).
No products indexed under this heading.

Risperidone (Isocarboxazid should not be administered in combination with central nervous system depressants). Products include:
Risperdal Consta Long-Acting Injection 1753

Salmeterol Xinafoate (Isocarboxazid should not be administered in combination with sympathomimetics, including amphetamines, or with over-the-counter drugs such as cold, hay fever, or weight-reducing preparations that contain vasoconstrictors). Products include:
Advair Diskus 100/50 1276
Advair Diskus 250/50 1276
Advair Diskus 500/50 1276
Advair HFA 45/21 Inhalation Aerosol 1288
Advair HFA 115/21 Inhalation Aerosol 1288
Advair HFA 230/21 Inhalation Aerosol 1288
Serevent Diskus 1594

Secobarbital Sodium (Isocarboxazid should not be administered in combination with hypnotics and sedatives).
No products indexed under this heading.

Selegiline (Isocarboxazid should not be administered in combination with monoamine oxidase inhibitors. In patients being transferred to isocarboxazid from other MAOI, a medication-free interval of at least 1 week should be allowed, after which isocarboxazid therapy should be started using half the normal starting dosage for at least the first week of therapy. Similarly, at least 1 week should elapse between the discontinuation of isocarboxazid and initiation of another MAOI, or the re-administration of isocarboxazid). Products include:
Emsam Transdermal System 905

Selegiline Hydrochloride (Isocarboxazid should not be administered in combination with monoamine oxidase inhibitors. In patients being transferred to isocarboxazid from other MAOI, a medication-free interval of at least 1 week should be allowed, after which isocarboxazid therapy should be started using half the normal starting dosage for at least the first week of therapy. Similarly, at least 1 week should elapse between the discontinuation of isocarboxazid and initiation of another MAOI, or the re-administration of isocarboxazid). Products include:
Eldepryl Capsules 3052

Sertraline Hydrochloride (Isocarboxazid should not be administered in combination with any selective serotonin reuptake inhibitors. At least 2 weeks should be allowed after stopping sertraline before starting isocarboxazid. In addition, there should be an interval of at least 10 days between discontinuation of isocarboxazid and initiation of SSRIs).
No products indexed under this heading.

Sevoflurane (Isocarboxazid should not be administered in combination with central nervous system depressants). Products include:
Ultane Liquid for Inhalation 524

Sodium Butabarbital (Isocarboxazid should not be administered in combination with hypnotics and sedatives).
No products indexed under this heading.

Sodium Nitroprusside (Isocarboxazid should not be used in combination with anti-hypertensive agents, including thiazide diuretics. A marked potentiating effect on these drugs has been reported, resulting in hypotension).
No products indexed under this heading.

Sodium Oxybate (Isocarboxazid should not be administered in combination with central nervous system depressants). Products include:
Xyrem Oral Solution **1766**

Sotalol Hydrochloride (Isocarboxazid should not be used in combination with anti-hypertensive agents, including thiazide diuretics. A marked potentiating effect on these drugs has been reported, resulting in hypotension).
No products indexed under this heading.

Spirapril Hydrochloride (Isocarboxazid should not be used in combination with anti-hypertensive agents, including thiazide diuretics. A marked potentiating effect on these drugs has been reported, resulting in hypotension).
No products indexed under this heading.

Spironolactone (Isocarboxazid should not be used in combination with anti-hypertensive agents, including thiazide diuretics. A marked potentiating effect on these drugs has been reported, resulting in hypotension).
No products indexed under this heading.

Sufentanil Citrate (Isocarboxazid should not be administered in combination with some central nervous system depressants including narcotic analgesics).
No products indexed under this heading.

Telmisartan (Isocarboxazid should not be used in combination with anti-hypertensive agents, including thiazide diuretics. A marked potentiating effect on these drugs has been reported, resulting in hypotension). Products include:
Micardis Tablets **852**
Micardis HCT Tablets **854**

Temazepam (Isocarboxazid should not be administered in combination with hypnotics and sedatives).
No products indexed under this heading.

Terazosin Hydrochloride (Isocarboxazid should not be used in combination with anti-hypertensive agents, including thiazide diuretics. A marked potentiating effect on these drugs has been reported, resulting in hypotension).
No products indexed under this heading.

Terbutaline Sulfate (Isocarboxazid should not be administered in combination with sympathomimetics, including amphetamines, or with over-the-counter drugs such as cold, hay fever, or weight-reducing preparations that contain vasoconstrictors).
No products indexed under this heading.

Terfenadine (Isocarboxazid should not be administered in combination with antihistamines).
No products indexed under this heading.

Thiamylal Sodium (Isocarboxazid should not be administered in combination with anesthetic drugs. Patients taking isocarboxazid should not undergo elective surgery requiring general anesthesia. Also, they should not be given cocaine or local anesthesia containing sympathomimetic vasoconstrictors. The possible combined hypotensive effects of isocarboxazid and spinal anesthesia should be kept in mind. Isocarboxazid should be discontinued at least 10 days before elective surgery).
No products indexed under this heading.

Thioridazine Hydrochloride (Isocarboxazid should not be administered in combination with central nervous system depressants). Products include:
Thioridazine Hydrochloride Tablets **2195**

Thiothixene (Isocarboxazid should not be administered in combination with central nervous system depressants). Products include:
Thiothixene Capsules **2197**

Timolol Maleate (Isocarboxazid should not be used in combination with anti-hypertensive agents, including thiazide diuretics. A marked potentiating effect on these drugs has been reported, resulting in hypotension). Products include:
Combigan Ophthalmic Solution **553**
Cosopt Sterile Ophthalmic Solution **1969**
Timoptic Sterile Ophthalmic Solution **2121**
Timoptic in Ocudose **2124**
Timoptic-XE Sterile Ophthalmic Gel Forming Solution **2125**

Torsemide (Isocarboxazid should not be used in combination with anti-hypertensive agents, including thiazide diuretics. A marked potentiating effect on these drugs has been reported, resulting in hypotension). Products include:
Demadex Injection **2630**
Demadex Tablets **2630**

Trandolapril (Isocarboxazid should not be used in combination with anti-hypertensive agents, including thiazide diuretics. A marked potentiating effect on these drugs has been reported, resulting in hypotension). Products include:
Mavik Tablets **472**
Tarka Tablets **511**

Tranylcypromine Sulfate (Isocarboxazid should not be administered in combination with monoamine oxidase inhibitors. In patients being transferred to isocarboxazid from other MAOI, a medication-free interval of at least 1 week should be allowed, after which isocarboxazid therapy should be started using half the normal starting dosage for at least the first week of therapy. Similarly, at least 1 week should elapse between the discontinuation of isocarboxazid and initiation of another MAOI, or the re-administration of isocarboxazid). Products include:
Parnate Tablets **1532**

Triamterene (Isocarboxazid should not be used in combination with anti-hypertensive agents, including thiazide diuretics. A marked potentiating effect on these drugs has been reported, resulting in hypotension). Products include:
Dyazide Capsules **1405**
Dyrenium Capsules **3189**

Triazolam (Isocarboxazid should not be administered in combination with hypnotics and sedatives).
No products indexed under this heading.

Trifluoperazine Hydrochloride (Isocarboxazid should not be administered in combination with central nervous system depressants).
No products indexed under this heading.

Trimeprazine Tartrate (Isocarboxazid should not be administered in combination with antihistamines).
No products indexed under this heading.

Trimethaphan Camsylate (Isocarboxazid should not be used in combination with anti-hypertensive agents, including thiazide diuretics. A marked potentiating effect on these drugs has been reported, resulting in hypotension).
No products indexed under this heading.

Trimipramine Maleate (Isocarboxazid should not be administered in combination with dibenzazepines. In patients being transferred to isocarboxazid from dibenzazepine-related entities, a medication-free interval of at least 1 week should be allowed, after which isocarboxazid therapy should be started using half the normal starting dosage for at least the first week of therapy. Similarly, at least 1 week should elapse between the discontinuation of isocarboxazid and initiation of other dibenzazepine-related entities, or the re-administration of isocarboxazid).
No products indexed under this heading.

Tripelennamine Hydrochloride (Isocarboxazid should not be administered in combination with antihistamines).
No products indexed under this heading.

Triprolidine Hydrochloride (Isocarboxazid should not be administered in combination with antihistamines).
No products indexed under this heading.

Valsartan (Isocarboxazid should not be used in combination with anti-hypertensive agents, including thiazide diuretics. A marked potentiating effect on these drugs has been reported, resulting in hypotension). Products include:
Diovan Tablets **2212**
Diovan HCT Tablets **2216**
Exforge Tablets **2238**

Verapamil Hydrochloride (Isocarboxazid should not be used in combination with anti-hypertensive agents, including thiazide diuretics. A marked potentiating effect on these drugs has been reported, resulting in hypotension). Products include:
Tarka Tablets **511**

Zaleplon (Isocarboxazid should not be administered in combination with hypnotics and sedatives).
No products indexed under this heading.

Ziprasidone Hydrochloride (Isocarboxazid should not be administered in combination with central nervous system depressants). Products include:
Geodon Capsules **2520**

Zolpidem Tartrate (Isocarboxazid should not be administered in combination with hypnotics and sedatives). Products include:
Ambien Tablets **2692**
Ambien CR Tablets **2696**

Food Interactions

Alcohol (Isocarboxazid should not be administered in combination with some central nervous systems depressants including alcohol).

Food high in tyramine (Isocarboxazid should not be administered in combination with cheese or other foods with a high tyramine content. Hypertensive crises have sometimes occurred during isocarboxazid therapy after ingestion of foods with a high tyramine content. In general, patients should avoid protein foods in which aging or protein breakdown is used to increase flavor. In particular, patients should be instructed not to take foods such as cheese, sour cream, Chianti wine, sherry, beer (including nonalcoholic beer), liqueurs, pickled herring, anchovies, caviar, liver, canned figs, raisins, bananas or avocados, chocolate, soy sauce, sauerkraut, the pods of broad beans (fava beans), yeast extracts, yogurt, meat extracts, meat prepared with tenderizers, or dry sausage).

MASCULINE CAPSULES

(Amino Acid Preparations, Bee Pollen, Herbals with Minerals, Hydroxypropyl Methylcellulose) **638**
None cited in PDR database.

MASS APPEAL TABLETS

(Amino Acid Preparations, Dicalcium Phosphate, Minerals) **638**
None cited in PDR database.

MAVIK TABLETS

(Trandolapril) **472**
May interact with diuretics, lithium preparations, potassium preparations, potassium sparing diuretics, and certain other agents. Compounds in these categories include:

Amiloride Hydrochloride (Coadministration increases the risk of hyperkalemia; patients on diuretics, especially those on recently instituted diuretic therapy, may experience an excessive reduction in blood pressure after initiation of therapy with trandolapril).
No products indexed under this heading.

Bendroflumethiazide (Patients on diuretics, especially those on recently instituted diuretic therapy, may experience an excessive reduction in blood pressure after initiation of therapy with trandolapril).
No products indexed under this heading.

Bumetanide (Patients on diuretics, especially those on recently instituted diuretic therapy, may experience an excessive reduction in blood pressure after initiation of therapy with trandolapril).
No products indexed under this heading.

Chlorothiazide (Patients on diuretics, especially those on recently instituted diuretic therapy, may experience an excessive reduction in blood pressure after initiation of therapy with trandolapril).
No products indexed under this heading.

Chlorothiazide Sodium (Patients on diuretics, especially those on recently instituted diuretic therapy, may experience an excessive reduction in blood pressure after initiation of therapy with trandolapril). Products include:
Intravenous Sodium Diuril **2490**

Chlorthalidone (Patients on diuretics, especially those on recently instituted diuretic therapy, may experience an excessive reduction in

blood pressure after initiation of therapy with trandolapril). Products include:
Clorpres Tablets 2185

Cimetidine (Co-administration has led to an increase of about 44% in Cmax for trandolapril with no effect on ACE inhibition).
No products indexed under this heading.

Cimetidine Hydrochloride (Co-administration has led to an increase of about 44% in Cmax for trandolapril with no effect on ACE inhibition).
No products indexed under this heading.

Ethacrynic Acid (Patients on diuretics, especially those on recently instituted diuretic therapy, may experience an excessive reduction in blood pressure after initiation of therapy with trandolapril). Products include:
Edecrin Tablets 698

Furosemide (Co-administration has led to an increase of about 25% in the renal clearance of trandolapril with no effect on ACE inhibition; patients on diuretics, especially those on recently instituted diuretic therapy, may experience an excessive reduction in blood pressure after initiation of therapy with trandolapril). Products include:
Furosemide Tablets 2186

Hydrochlorothiazide (Patients on diuretics, especially those on recently instituted diuretic therapy, may experience an excessive reduction in blood pressure after initiation of therapy with trandolapril). Products include:
Atacand HCT 642
Avalide Tablets 892
Avalide Tablets 2713
Benicar HCT Tablets 1010
Diovan HCT Tablets 2216
Dyazide Capsules 1405
Micardis HCT Tablets 854
Prinzide Tablets 2092
Tekturna HCT Tablets 2324
Teveten HCT Tablets 517

Hydroflumethiazide (Patients on diuretics, especially those on recently instituted diuretic therapy, may experience an excessive reduction in blood pressure after initiation of therapy with trandolapril).
No products indexed under this heading.

Indapamide (Patients on diuretics, especially those on recently instituted diuretic therapy, may experience an excessive reduction in blood pressure after initiation of therapy with trandolapril). Products include:
Indapamide Tablets 2188

Lithium (Co-administration of ACE inhibitors and lithium has resulted in increased serum lithium levels and symptoms of lithium toxicity).
No products indexed under this heading.

Lithium Carbonate (Co-administration of ACE inhibitors and lithium has resulted in increased serum lithium levels and symptoms of lithium toxicity).
No products indexed under this heading.

Lithium Citrate (Co-administration of ACE inhibitors and lithium has resulted in increased serum lithium levels and symptoms of lithium toxicity).
No products indexed under this heading.

Methyclothiazide (Patients on diuretics, especially those on recently instituted diuretic therapy, may experience an excessive reduction in blood pressure after initiation of therapy with trandolapril).
No products indexed under this heading.

Metolazone (Patients on diuretics, especially those on recently instituted diuretic therapy, may experience an excessive reduction in blood pressure after initiation of therapy with trandolapril).
No products indexed under this heading.

Polythiazide (Patients on diuretics, especially those on recently instituted diuretic therapy, may experience an excessive reduction in blood pressure after initiation of therapy with trandolapril).
No products indexed under this heading.

Potassium Acid Phosphate (Co-administration increases the risk of hyperkalemia). Products include:
K-Phos Original (Sodium Free) Tablets 814

Potassium Bicarbonate (Co-administration increases the risk of hyperkalemia).
No products indexed under this heading.

Potassium Chloride (Co-administration increases the risk of hyperkalemia). Products include:
MoviPrep Oral Solution 2679

Potassium Citrate (Co-administration increases the risk of hyperkalemia). Products include:
BioLean Free Tablets .... ▣635
Urocit-K Tablets 2176

Potassium Gluconate (Co-administration increases the risk of hyperkalemia).
No products indexed under this heading.

Potassium Phosphate (Co-administration increases the risk of hyperkalemia). Products include:
K-Phos Neutral Tablets 813

Spironolactone (Co-administration increases the risk of hyperkalemia; patients on diuretics, especially those on recently instituted diuretic therapy, may experience an excessive reduction in blood pressure after initiation of therapy with trandolapril).
No products indexed under this heading.

Torsemide (Patients on diuretics, especially those on recently instituted diuretic therapy, may experience an excessive reduction in blood pressure after initiation of therapy with trandolapril). Products include:
Demadex Injection 2630
Demadex Tablets 2630

Triamterene (Co-administration increases the risk of hyperkalemia; patients on diuretics, especially those on recently instituted diuretic therapy, may experience an excessive reduction in blood pressure after initiation of therapy with trandolapril). Products include:
Dyazide Capsules 1405
Dyrenium Capsules 3189

Food Interactions

Food, unspecified (Slows absorption of trandolapril but does not affect AUC or Cmax).

MAXAIR AUTOHALER

(Pirbuterol Acetate) 1705
May interact with beta blockers, monoamine oxidase inhibitors, potassium-depleting diuretics, sympathomimetic aerosol bronchodilators, and tricyclic antidepressants. Compounds in these categories include:

Acebutolol Hydrochloride (Co-administration with beta adrenergic receptor blocking agents blocks the pulmonary effect of pirbuterol and may produce severe bronchospasm in asthmatic patients).
No products indexed under this heading.

Albuterol (Potential for additive effects).
No products indexed under this heading.

Amitriptyline Hydrochloride (Concurrent and/or sequential use with tricyclic antidepressants can result in the potentiation of pirbuterol's action on the vascular system).
No products indexed under this heading.

Amoxapine (Concurrent and/or sequential use with tricyclic antidepressants can result in the potentiation of pirbuterol's action on the vascular system).
No products indexed under this heading.

Atenolol (Co-administration with beta adrenergic receptor blocking agents blocks the pulmonary effect of pirbuterol and may produce severe bronchospasm in asthmatic patients).
No products indexed under this heading.

Bendroflumethiazide (The ECG changes and/or hypokalemia that may result from administration of non-potassium sparing diuretics can be acutely worsened by beta-agonists; clinical significance is not known).
No products indexed under this heading.

Betaxolol Hydrochloride (Co-administration with beta adrenergic receptor blocking agents blocks the pulmonary effect of pirbuterol and may produce severe bronchospasm in asthmatic patients).
No products indexed under this heading.

Bisoprolol Fumarate (Co-administration with beta adrenergic receptor blocking agents blocks the pulmonary effect of pirbuterol and may produce severe bronchospasm in asthmatic patients).
No products indexed under this heading.

Bitolterol Mesylate (Potential for additive effects).
No products indexed under this heading.

Bumetanide (The ECG changes and/or hypokalemia that may result from administration of non-potassium sparing diuretics can be acutely worsened by beta-agonists; clinical significance is not known).
No products indexed under this heading.

Carteolol Hydrochloride (Co-administration with beta adrenergic receptor blocking agents blocks the pulmonary effect of pirbuterol and may produce severe bronchospasm in asthmatic patients).
No products indexed under this heading.

Chlorothiazide (The ECG changes and/or hypokalemia that may result from administration of non-potassium sparing diuretics can be acutely worsened by beta-agonists; clinical significance is not known).
No products indexed under this heading.

Chlorothiazide Sodium (The ECG changes and/or hypokalemia that may result from administration of non-potassium sparing diuretics can be acutely worsened by beta-agonists; clinical significance is not known). Products include:
Intravenous Sodium Diuril 2490

Clomipramine Hydrochloride (Concurrent and/or sequential use with tricyclic antidepressants can result in the potentiation of pirbuterol's action on the vascular system).
No products indexed under this heading.

Desipramine Hydrochloride (Concurrent and/or sequential use with tricyclic antidepressants can result in the potentiation of pirbuterol's action on the vascular system).
No products indexed under this heading.

Doxepin Hydrochloride (Concurrent and/or sequential use with tricyclic antidepressants can result in the potentiation of pirbuterol's action on the vascular system).
No products indexed under this heading.

Esmolol Hydrochloride (Co-administration with beta adrenergic receptor blocking agents blocks the pulmonary effect of pirbuterol and may produce severe bronchospasm in asthmatic patients).
No products indexed under this heading.

Ethacrynic Acid (The ECG changes and/or hypokalemia that may result from administration of non-potassium sparing diuretics can be acutely worsened by beta-agonists; clinical significance is not known). Products include:
Edecrin Tablets 698

Furosemide (The ECG changes and/or hypokalemia that may result from administration of non-potassium sparing diuretics can be acutely worsened by beta-agonists; clinical significance is not known). Products include:
Furosemide Tablets 2186

Hydrochlorothiazide (The ECG changes and/or hypokalemia that may result from administration of non-potassium sparing diuretics can be acutely worsened by beta-agonists; clinical significance is not known). Products include:
Atacand HCT 642
Avalide Tablets 892
Avalide Tablets 2713
Benicar HCT Tablets 1010
Diovan HCT Tablets 2216
Dyazide Capsules 1405
Micardis HCT Tablets 854
Prinzide Tablets 2092
Tekturna HCT Tablets 2324
Teveten HCT Tablets 517

Hydroflumethiazide (The ECG changes and/or hypokalemia that may result from administration of non-potassium sparing diuretics can be acutely worsened by beta-agonists; clinical significance is not known).
No products indexed under this heading.

Imipramine Hydrochloride (Concurrent and/or sequential use with tricyclic antidepressants can result in the potentiation of pirbuterol's action on the vascular system).
No products indexed under this heading.

Imipramine Pamoate (Concurrent and/or sequential use with tricyclic antidepressants can result in the potentiation of pirbuterol's action on the vascular system).
No products indexed under this heading.

Isocarboxazid (Concurrent and/or sequential use with MAO inhibitors can result in the potentiation of pirbuterol's action on the vascular system). Products include:
Marplan Tablets 3177

Isoetharine (Potential for additive effects).
No products indexed under this heading.

Isoproterenol Hydrochloride (Potential for additive effects).
No products indexed under this heading.

Labetalol Hydrochloride (Co-administration with beta adrenergic receptor blocking agents blocks the pulmonary effect of pirbuterol and may produce severe bronchospasm in asthmatic patients).
No products indexed under this heading.

Levalbuterol Hydrochloride (Potential for additive effects). Products include:
Xopenex Inhalation Solution 3001
Xopenex Inhalation Solution Concentrate 3005

Levobunolol Hydrochloride (Co-administration with beta adrenergic receptor blocking agents blocks the pulmonary effect of pirbuterol and may produce severe bronchospasm in asthmatic patients).
No products indexed under this heading.

Maprotiline Hydrochloride (Concurrent and/or sequential use with tricyclic antidepressants can result in the potentiation of pirbuterol's action on the vascular system).
No products indexed under this heading.

Metaproterenol Sulfate (Potential for additive effects).
No products indexed under this heading.

Methyclothiazide (The ECG changes and/or hypokalemia that may result from administration of non-potassium sparing diuretics can be acutely worsened by beta-agonists; clinical significance is not known).
No products indexed under this heading.

Metipranolol Hydrochloride (Co-administration with beta adrenergic receptor blocking agents blocks the pulmonary effect of pirbuterol and may produce severe bronchospasm in asthmatic patients).
No products indexed under this heading.

Metoprolol Succinate (Co-administration with beta adrenergic receptor blocking agents blocks the pulmonary effect of pirbuterol and may produce severe bronchospasm in asthmatic patients). Products include:
Toprol-XL Tablets 666

Metoprolol Tartrate (Co-administration with beta adrenergic receptor blocking agents blocks the pulmonary effect of pirbuterol and may produce severe bronchospasm in asthmatic patients).
No products indexed under this heading.

Moclobemide (Concurrent and/or sequential use with MAO inhibitors can result in the potentiation of pirbuterol's action on the vascular system).
No products indexed under this heading.

Nadolol (Co-administration with beta adrenergic receptor blocking agents blocks the pulmonary effect of pirbuterol and may produce severe bronchospasm in asthmatic patients). Products include:
Nadolol Tablets 2191

Nebivolol (Co-administration with beta adrenergic receptor blocking agents blocks the pulmonary effect of pirbuterol and may produce severe bronchospasm in asthmatic patients). Products include:
Bystolic Tablets 1155

Nortriptyline Hydrochloride (Concurrent and/or sequential use with tricyclic antidepressants can result in the potentiation of pirbuterol's action on the vascular system).
No products indexed under this heading.

Pargyline Hydrochloride (Concurrent and/or sequential use with MAO inhibitors can result in the potentiation of pirbuterol's action on the vascular system).
No products indexed under this heading.

Penbutolol Sulfate (Co-administration with beta adrenergic receptor blocking agents blocks the pulmonary effect of pirbuterol and may produce severe bronchospasm in asthmatic patients).
No products indexed under this heading.

Phenelzine Sulfate (Concurrent and/or sequential use with MAO inhibitors can result in the potentiation of pirbuterol's action on the vascular system).
No products indexed under this heading.

Pindolol (Co-administration with beta adrenergic receptor blocking agents blocks the pulmonary effect of pirbuterol and may produce severe bronchospasm in asthmatic patients).
No products indexed under this heading.

Polythiazide (The ECG changes and/or hypokalemia that may result from administration of non-potassium sparing diuretics can be acutely worsened by beta-agonists; clinical significance is not known).
No products indexed under this heading.

Procarbazine Hydrochloride (Concurrent and/or sequential use with MAO inhibitors can result in the potentiation of pirbuterol's action on the vascular system).
No products indexed under this heading.

Propranolol Hydrochloride (Co-administration with beta adrenergic receptor blocking agents blocks the pulmonary effect of pirbuterol and may produce severe bronchospasm in asthmatic patients). Products include:
InnoPran XL Extended Release Capsules 1484

Protriptyline Hydrochloride (Concurrent and/or sequential use with tricyclic antidepressants can result in the potentiation of pirbuterol's action on the vascular system).
No products indexed under this heading.

Rasagiline Mesylate (Concurrent and/or sequential use with MAO inhibitors can result in the potentiation of pirbuterol's action on the vascular system). Products include:
Azilect Tablets 3106

Salmeterol Xinafoate (Potential for additive effects). Products include:
Advair Diskus 100/50 1276
Advair Diskus 250/50 1276
Advair Diskus 500/50 1276
Advair HFA 45/21 Inhalation Aerosol 1288
Advair HFA 115/21 Inhalation Aerosol 1288
Advair HFA 230/21 Inhalation Aerosol 1288
Serevent Diskus 1594

Selegiline (Concurrent and/or sequential use with MAO inhibitors can result in the potentiation of pirbuterol's action on the vascular system). Products include:
Emsam Transdermal System 905

Selegiline Hydrochloride (Concurrent and/or sequential use with MAO inhibitors can result in the potentiation of pirbuterol's action on the vascular system). Products include:
Eldepryl Capsules 3052

Sotalol Hydrochloride (Co-administration with beta adrenergic receptor blocking agents blocks the pulmonary effect of pirbuterol and may produce severe bronchospasm in asthmatic patients).
No products indexed under this heading.

Terbutaline Sulfate (Potential for additive effects).
No products indexed under this heading.

Timolol Hemihydrate (Co-administration with beta adrenergic receptor blocking agents blocks the pulmonary effect of pirbuterol and may produce severe bronchospasm in asthmatic patients). Products include:
Betimol Ophthalmic Solution 3181

Timolol Maleate (Co-administration with beta adrenergic receptor blocking agents blocks the pulmonary effect of pirbuterol and may produce severe bronchospasm in asthmatic patients). Products include:
Combigan Ophthalmic Solution 553
Cosopt Sterile Ophthalmic Solution 1969
Timoptic Sterile Ophthalmic Solution 2121
Timoptic in Ocudose 2124
Timoptic-XE Sterile Ophthalmic Gel Forming Solution 2125

Torsemide (The ECG changes and/or hypokalemia that may result from administration of non-potassium sparing diuretics can be acutely worsened by beta-agonists; clinical significance is not known). Products include:
Demadex Injection 2630
Demadex Tablets 2630

Tranylcypromine Sulfate (Concurrent and/or sequential use with MAO inhibitors can result in the potentiation of pirbuterol's action on the vascular system). Products include:
Parnate Tablets 1532

Trimipramine Maleate (Concurrent and/or sequential use with tricyclic antidepressants can result in the potentiation of pirbuterol's action on the vascular system).
No products indexed under this heading.

MAXALT TABLETS

(Rizatriptan Benzoate) 2056
May interact with 5HT1-receptor agonists, ergot-containing drugs, monoamine oxidase inhibitors, Serotonin and Norepinephrine Reuptake Inhibitors, selective serotonin reuptake inhibitors, and certain other agents. Compounds in these categories include:

Almotriptan Malate (Co-administration with other 5-HT1 agonists within 24 hours of each other is contraindicated because the vasospastic effects may be additive). Products include:
Axert Tablets 2431

Citalopram Hydrobromide (Co-administration of 5-HT1 agonists with selective serotonin reuptake inhibitors (SSRIs) has resulted, rarely, in hyperreflexia, weakness, and incoordination. The development of a potentially life-threatening serotonin syndrome may occur with triptans, including rizatriptan benzoate treatment, particularly during combined use with SSRIs. If concomitant treatment with rizatriptan benzoate and an SSRI (e.g., fluoxetine, paroxetine, sertraline, fluvoxamine, citalopram escitalopram) is clinically warranted, careful observation of patient is advised, particularly during treatment initiation and dose increases). Products include:
Celexa 1160

Desipramine Hydrochloride (Cases of life-threatening serotonin syndrome have been reported during combined use of serotonin-norepinephrine reuptake inhibitors).
No products indexed under this heading.

Desvenlafaxine Succinate (The development of a potentially life-threatening serotonin syndrome may occur with triptans, including rizatriptan benzoate treatment, particularly during combined use with serotonin norepinephrine reuptake inhibitors (SNRI). If concomitant treatment with rizatriptan benzoate and an SNRI (e.g., venlafaxine, duloxetine) is clinically warranted, careful observation of patient is advised, particularly during treatment initiation and dose increases). Products include:
Pristiq Extended-Release Tablets 3247

IMPORTANT NOTE: Always consult each drug listing in the patient's regimen for possible interactions.

Dihydroergotamine Mesylate (Ergot-containing drugs have been reported to cause prolonged vasospastic reactions; because there is a theoretical basis that these effects may be additive, use of ergot-type agents and rizatriptan within 24 hours is contraindicated).
No products indexed under this heading.

Duloxetine Hydrochloride (The development of a potentially life-threatening serotonin syndrome may occur with triptans, including rizatriptan benzoate treatment, particularly during combined use with serotonin norepinephrine reuptake inhibitors (SNRI). If concomitant treatment with rizatriptan benzoate and an SNRI (e.g., venlafaxine, duloxetine) is clinically warranted, careful observation of patient is advised, particularly during treatment initiation and dose increases). Products include:
Cymbalta Delayed-Release Capsules 1801

Eletriptan Hydrobromide (Co-administration with other 5-HT1 agonists within 24 hours of each other is contraindicated because the vasospastic effects may be additive).
No products indexed under this heading.

Ergonovine Maleate (Ergot-containing drugs have been reported to cause prolonged vasospastic reactions; because there is a theoretical basis that these effects may be additive, use of ergot-type agents and rizatriptan within 24 hours is contraindicated).
No products indexed under this heading.

Ergotamine Tartrate (Ergot-containing drugs have been reported to cause prolonged vasospastic reactions; because there is a theoretical basis that these effects may be additive, use of ergot-type agents and rizatriptan within 24 hours is contraindicated).
No products indexed under this heading.

Escitalopram Oxalate (Co-administration of 5-HT1 agonists with selective serotonin reuptake inhibitors (SSRIs) has resulted, rarely, in hyperreflexia, weakness, and incoordination. The development of a potentially life-threatening serotonin syndrome may occur with triptans, including rizatriptan benzoate treatment, particularly during combined use with SSRIs. If concomitant treatment with rizatriptan benzoate and an SSRI (e.g., fluoxetine, paroxetine, sertraline, fluvoxamine, citalopram escitalopram) is clinically warranted, careful observation of patient is advised, particularly during treatment initiation and dose increases). Products include:
Lexapro Oral Suspension 1174
Lexapro Tablets 1174

Fluoxetine (Co-administration of 5-HT1 agonists with selective serotonin reuptake inhibitors (SSRIs) has resulted, rarely, in hyperreflexia, weakness, and incoordination. The development of a potentially life-threatening serotonin syndrome may occur with triptans, including rizatriptan benzoate treatment, particularly during combined use with SSRIs. If concomitant treatment with rizatriptan benzoate and an SSRI (e.g., fluoxetine, paroxetine, sertraline, fluvoxamine, citalopram escitalopram) is clinically warranted, careful observation of patient is advised, particularly during treatment initiation and dose increases).
No products indexed under this heading.

Fluoxetine Hydrochloride (Co-administration of 5-HT1 agonists with selective serotonin reuptake inhibitors (SSRIs) has resulted, rarely, in hyperreflexia, weakness, and incoordination. The development of a potentially life-threatening serotonin syndrome may occur with triptans, including rizatriptan benzoate treatment, particularly during combined use with SSRIs. If concomitant treatment with rizatriptan benzoate and an SSRI (e.g., fluoxetine, paroxetine, sertraline, fluvoxamine, citalopram escitalopram) is clinically warranted, careful observation of patient is advised, particularly during treatment initiation and dose increases). Products include:
Prozac Weekly Capsules 1852
Prozac Pulvules and Liquid 1852
Symbyax Capsules 1871

Fluvoxamine Maleate (Co-administration of 5-HT1 agonists with selective serotonin reuptake inhibitors (SSRIs) has resulted, rarely, in hyperreflexia, weakness, and incoordination. The development of a potentially life-threatening serotonin syndrome may occur with triptans, including rizatriptan benzoate treatment, particularly during combined use with SSRIs. If concomitant treatment with rizatriptan benzoate and an SSRI (e.g., fluoxetine, paroxetine, sertraline, fluvoxamine, citalopram escitalopram) is clinically warranted, careful observation of patient is advised, particularly during treatment initiation and dose increases). Products include:
Luvox CR Extended-Release Capsules 1759

Frovatriptan Succinate (Co-administration with other 5-HT1 agonists within 24 hours of each other is contraindicated because the vasospastic effects may be additive). Products include:
Frova Tablets 1111

Isocarboxazid (Plasma concentrations of rizatriptan may be increased by MAO inhibitors; concurrent and/or sequential use is contraindicated). Products include:
Marplan Tablets 3177

Methylergonovine Maleate (Ergot-containing drugs have been reported to cause prolonged vasospastic reactions; because there is a theoretical basis that these effects may be additive, use of ergot-type agents and rizatriptan within 24 hours is contraindicated).
No products indexed under this heading.

Methysergide Maleate (Ergot-containing drugs have been reported to cause prolonged vasospastic reactions; because there is a theoretical basis that these effects may be additive, use of ergot-type agents and rizatriptan within 24 hours is contraindicated).
No products indexed under this heading.

Moclobemide (Concomitant therapy with the selective, reversible MAO-A inhibitor, moclobemide, has resulted in increased systemic exposure of rizatriptan and its metabolite; concurrent and/or sequential use is contraindicated).
No products indexed under this heading.

Naratriptan Hydrochloride (Co-administration with other 5-HT1 agonists within 24 hours of each other is contraindicated because the vasospastic effects may be additive). Products include:
Amerge Tablets 1301

Nefazodone Hydrochloride (Cases of life-threatening serotonin syndrome have been reported during combined use of serotonin-norepinephrine reuptake inhibitors).
No products indexed under this heading.

Pargyline Hydrochloride (Plasma concentrations of rizatriptan may be increased by MAO inhibitors; concurrent and/or sequential use is contraindicated).
No products indexed under this heading.

Paroxetine Hydrochloride (Co-administration of 5-HT1 agonists with selective serotonin reuptake inhibitors (SSRIs) has resulted, rarely, in hyperreflexia, weakness, and incoordination; no pharmacokinetic interaction was observed with a single dose study). Products include:
Paxil 1535
Paxil CR Controlled-Release Tablets 1544

Phenelzine Sulfate (Plasma concentrations of rizatriptan may be increased by MAO inhibitors; concurrent and/or sequential use is contraindicated).
No products indexed under this heading.

Procarbazine Hydrochloride (Plasma concentrations of rizatriptan may be increased by MAO inhibitors; concurrent and/or sequential use is contraindicated).
No products indexed under this heading.

Propranolol Hydrochloride (Co-administration has resulted in an increase in mean plasma AUC for rizatriptan by 70%). Products include:
InnoPran XL Extended Release Capsules 1484

Rasagiline Mesylate (Plasma concentrations of rizatriptan may be increased by MAO inhibitors; concurrent and/or sequential use is contraindicated). Products include:
Azilect Tablets 3106

Selegiline (Plasma concentrations of rizatriptan may be increased by MAO inhibitors; concurrent and/or sequential use is contraindicated). Products include:
Emsam Transdermal System 905

Selegiline Hydrochloride (Plasma concentrations of rizatriptan may be increased by MAO inhibitors; concurrent and/or sequential use is contraindicated). Products include:
Eldepryl Capsules 3052

Sertraline Hydrochloride (Co-administration of 5-HT1 agonists with selective serotonin reuptake inhibitors (SSRIs) has resulted, rarely, in hyperreflexia, weakness, and incoordination. The development of a potentially life-threatening serotonin syndrome may occur with triptans, including rizatriptan benzoate treatment, particularly during combined use with SSRIs. If concomitant treatment with rizatriptan benzoate and an SSRI (e.g., fluoxetine, paroxetine, sertraline, fluvoxamine, citalopram escitalopram) is clinically warranted, careful observation of patient is advised, particularly during treatment initiation and dose increases).
No products indexed under this heading.

Sumatriptan (Co-administration with other 5-HT1 agonists within 24 hours of each other is contraindicated because the vasospastic effects may be additive). Products include:
Imitrex Nasal Spray 1470

Sumatriptan Succinate (Co-administration with other 5-HT1 agonists within 24 hours of each other is contraindicated because the vasospastic effects may be additive). Products include:
Imitrex Injection 1465
Imitrex Tablets 1474
Treximet Tablets 1616

Tranylcypromine Sulfate (Plasma concentrations of rizatriptan may be increased by MAO inhibitors; concurrent and/or sequential use is contraindicated). Products include:
Parnate Tablets 1532

Venlafaxine Hydrochloride (The development of a potentially life-threatening serotonin syndrome may occur with triptans, including rizatriptan benzoate treatment, particularly during combined use with serotonin norepinephrine reuptake inhibitors (SNRI). If concomitant treatment with rizatriptan benzoate and an SNRI (e.g., venlafaxine, duloxetine) is clinically warranted, careful observation of patient is advised, particularly during treatment initiation and dose increases). Products include:
Effexor XR Extended-Release Capsules 3195
Venlafaxine Hydrochloride Tablets ... 2199

Zolmitriptan (Co-administration with other 5-HT1 agonists within 24 hours of each other is contraindicated because the vasospastic effects may be additive). Products include:
Zomig Tablets 694
Zomig Nasal Spray 689
Zomig-ZMT Tablets 694

Food Interactions

Food, unspecified (Delays the time to reach peak concentration by an hour; no significant effect on the bioavailability).

MAXALT-MLT ORALLY DISINTEGRATING TABLETS

(Rizatriptan Benzoate) 2056
See Maxalt Tablets

MED OMEGA FISH OIL 2800

(Docosahexaenoic Acid (DHA), Eicosapentaenoic Acid (EPA), Omega-3 Acids)............................... ▣625
None cited in PDR database.

MED OMEGA FISH OIL 2800

(Docosahexaenoic Acid (DHA), Eicosapentaenoic Acid (EPA), Omega-3 Acids)............................... 949
None cited in PDR database.

MEDERMA TOPICAL GEL

(Allantoin, Allium cepa) 2163
None cited in PDR database.

MEDERMA CREAM PLUS SPF 30
(Avobenzone, Octocrylene, Oxybenzone) 2163
None cited in PDR database.

MEDERMA FOR KIDS TOPICAL GEL
(Allantoin, Allium cepa) 2164
None cited in PDR database.

MEDIZYM TABLETS
(Ananas comosus, Bromelains, Carica papaya, Chymotrypsin, Pancreatin, Papain, Trypsin)............... 1894
None cited in PDR database.

MEGA ANTIOXIDANT TABLETS
(Dietary Supplement, Vitamins, Multiple)... 3174
None cited in PDR database.

MEGACE ES ORAL SUSPENSION
(Megestrol Acetate) 2499
May interact with insulin and certain other agents. Compounds in these categories include:

Indinavir Sulfate (A pharmacokinetic study demonstrated that co-administration of megestrol acetate and indinavir results in a significant decrease in the pharmacokinetic parameters (approximately 36% for Cmax and approximately 28% for AUC) of indinavir. Administration of a higher dose of indinavir should be considered when co-administering with megestrol acetate). Products include:
Crixivan Capsules 1979

Insulin (Exacerbation of pre-existing diabetes with increased insulin requirements has been reported in association with concomitant use of megestrol acetate).
No products indexed under this heading.

Insulin, Human, Zinc Suspension (Exacerbation of pre-existing diabetes with increased insulin requirements has been reported in association with concomitant use of megestrol acetate).
No products indexed under this heading.

Insulin, Human (rDNA origin) (Exacerbation of pre-existing diabetes with increased insulin requirements has been reported in association with concomitant use of megestrol acetate). Products include:
Exubera Inhalation Powder 2515

Insulin, Human NPH (Exacerbation of pre-existing diabetes with increased insulin requirements has been reported in association with concomitant use of megestrol acetate). Products include:
Humulin N Vial 1846

Insulin, Human Regular (Exacerbation of pre-existing diabetes with increased insulin requirements has been reported in association with concomitant use of megestrol acetate). Products include:
Humulin R 1849
Humulin R (U-500) 1850

Insulin, Human Regular and Human NPH Mixture (Exacerbation of pre-existing diabetes with increased insulin requirements has been reported in association with concomitant use of megestrol acetate). Products include:
Humulin 50/50, 100 Units 1843
Humulin 70/30 Vial 1844

Insulin, NPH (Exacerbation of pre-existing diabetes with increased insulin requirements has been reported in association with concomitant use of megestrol acetate).
No products indexed under this heading.

Insulin, Regular (Exacerbation of pre-existing diabetes with increased insulin requirements has been reported in association with concomitant use of megestrol acetate).
No products indexed under this heading.

Insulin, Regular and NPH mixture (Exacerbation of pre-existing diabetes with increased insulin requirements has been reported in association with concomitant use of megestrol acetate).
No products indexed under this heading.

Insulin, Zinc Crystals (Exacerbation of pre-existing diabetes with increased insulin requirements has been reported in association with concomitant use of megestrol acetate).
No products indexed under this heading.

Insulin, Zinc Suspension (Exacerbation of pre-existing diabetes with increased insulin requirements has been reported in association with concomitant use of megestrol acetate).
No products indexed under this heading.

Insulin Aspart (Exacerbation of pre-existing diabetes with increased insulin requirements has been reported in association with concomitant use of megestrol acetate).
No products indexed under this heading.

Insulin Aspart, Human (Exacerbation of pre-existing diabetes with increased insulin requirements has been reported in association with concomitant use of megestrol acetate). Products include:
NovoLog Mix 70/30 2364

Insulin Aspart, Human Regular (Exacerbation of pre-existing diabetes with increased insulin requirements has been reported in association with concomitant use of megestrol acetate). Products include:
NovoLog Injection 2359

Insulin Aspart Protamine, Human (Exacerbation of pre-existing diabetes with increased insulin requirements has been reported in association with concomitant use of megestrol acetate). Products include:
NovoLog Mix 70/30 2364

Insulin Detemir (rDNA Origin) (Exacerbation of pre-existing diabetes with increased insulin requirements has been reported in association with concomitant use of megestrol acetate). Products include:
Levemir Injection 2352

Insulin glargine (Exacerbation of pre-existing diabetes with increased insulin requirements has been reported in association with concomitant use of megestrol acetate). Products include:
Lantus Injection 2749

Insulin Glulisine (Exacerbation of pre-existing diabetes with increased insulin requirements has been reported in association with concomitant use of megestrol acetate). Products include:
Apidra Injection 2706

Insulin Lispro, Human (Exacerbation of pre-existing diabetes with increased insulin requirements has been reported in association with concomitant use of megestrol acetate). Products include:
Humalog-Pen and KwikPen 1829
Humalog Mix 50/50-Pen and KwikPen 1833
Humalog Mix 75/25-Pen and KwikPen 1835

Insulin Lispro Protamine, Human (Exacerbation of pre-existing diabetes with increased insulin requirements has been reported in association with concomitant use of megestrol acetate). Products include:
Humalog Mix 50/50-Pen and KwikPen 1833
Humalog Mix 75/25-Pen and KwikPen 1835

MENTAX CREAM
(Butenafine Hydrochloride) 2190
None cited in PDR database.

MEPHYTON TABLETS
(Vitamin K_1) 700
None cited in PDR database.

MEPRON SUSPENSION
(Atovaquone) 1526
May interact with highly protein bound drugs (selected) and certain other agents. Compounds in these categories include:

Amiodarone Hydrochloride (Atovaquone is highly bound to plasma protein (greater than 99.9%); caution is advised when co-administered with other highly protein bound drugs with narrow therapeutic indices).
No products indexed under this heading.

Amitriptyline Hydrochloride (Atovaquone is highly bound to plasma protein (greater than 99.9%); caution is advised when co-administered with other highly protein bound drugs with narrow therapeutic indices).
No products indexed under this heading.

Cefonicid Sodium (Atovaquone is highly bound to plasma protein (greater than 99.9%); caution is advised when co-administered with other highly protein bound drugs with narrow therapeutic indices).
No products indexed under this heading.

Celecoxib (Atovaquone is highly bound to plasma protein (greater than 99.9%); caution is advised when co-administered with other highly protein bound drugs with narrow therapeutic indices). Products include:
Celebrex Capsules 2979

Chlordiazepoxide (Atovaquone is highly bound to plasma protein (greater than 99.9%); caution is advised when co-administered with other highly protein bound drugs with narrow therapeutic indices).
No products indexed under this heading.

Chlordiazepoxide Hydrochloride (Atovaquone is highly bound to plasma protein (greater than 99.9%); caution is advised when co-administered with other highly protein bound drugs with narrow therapeutic indices).
No products indexed under this heading.

Chlorpromazine (Atovaquone is highly bound to plasma protein (greater than 99.9%); caution is advised when co-administered with other highly protein bound drugs with narrow therapeutic indices).
No products indexed under this heading.

Chlorpromazine Hydrochloride (Atovaquone is highly bound to plasma protein (greater than 99.9%); caution is advised when co-administered with other highly protein bound drugs with narrow therapeutic indices).
No products indexed under this heading.

Clomipramine Hydrochloride (Atovaquone is highly bound to plasma protein (greater than 99.9%); caution is advised when co-administered with other highly protein bound drugs with narrow therapeutic indices).
No products indexed under this heading.

Clozapine (Atovaquone is highly bound to plasma protein (greater than 99.9%); caution is advised when co-administered with other highly protein bound drugs with narrow therapeutic indices).
No products indexed under this heading.

Cyclosporine (Atovaquone is highly bound to plasma protein (greater than 99.9%); caution is advised when co-administered with other highly protein bound drugs with narrow therapeutic indices). Products include:
Gengraf Capsules 435
Neoral Oral Solution 2280
Neoral Soft Gelatin Capsules 2280
Restasis Ophthalmic Emulsion 557
Sandimmune 2296

Diazepam (Atovaquone is highly bound to plasma protein (greater than 99.9%); caution is advised when co-administered with other highly protein bound drugs with narrow therapeutic indices). Products include:
Valium Tablets 2658

Diclofenac Potassium (Atovaquone is highly bound to plasma protein (greater than 99.9%); caution is advised when co-administered with other highly protein bound drugs with narrow therapeutic indices).
No products indexed under this heading.

Diclofenac Sodium (Atovaquone is highly bound to plasma protein (greater than 99.9%); caution is advised when co-administered with other highly protein bound drugs with narrow therapeutic indices). Products include:
Diclofenac Sodium Ophthalmic Solution.. ⊙ 240
Voltaren Ophthalmic Solution 2336
Voltaren Tablets 2334
Voltaren-XR Tablets 2337

Dipyridamole (Atovaquone is highly bound to plasma protein (greater than 99.9%); caution is advised when co-administered with other

highly protein bound drugs with narrow therapeutic indices). Products include:

Aggrenox Capsules 819
Persantine Tablets 869

Fenoprofen Calcium (Atovaquone is highly bound to plasma protein (greater than 99.9%); caution is advised when co-administered with other highly protein bound drugs with narrow therapeutic indices). Products include:

Nalfon Capsules 2508

Flurazepam Hydrochloride (Atovaquone is highly bound to plasma protein (greater than 99.9%); caution is advised when co-administered with other highly protein bound drugs with narrow therapeutic indices).

No products indexed under this heading.

Flurbiprofen (Atovaquone is highly bound to plasma protein (greater than 99.9%); caution is advised when co-administered with other highly protein bound drugs with narrow therapeutic indices).

No products indexed under this heading.

Glipizide (Atovaquone is highly bound to plasma protein (greater than 99.9%); caution is advised when co-administered with other highly protein bound drugs with narrow therapeutic indices).

No products indexed under this heading.

Ibuprofen (Atovaquone is highly bound to plasma protein (greater than 99.9%); caution is advised when co-administered with other highly protein bound drugs with narrow therapeutic indices). Products include:

Motrin IB Tablets and Caplets 1900
Children's Motrin Oral Suspension ... 1901
Children's Motrin Non-Staining Dye-Free Oral Suspension............ 1901
Children's Motrin Cold Oral Suspension 1899
Infants' Motrin Concentrated Drops.. 1901
Infants' Motrin Non-Staining Dye-Free Concentrated Drops....... 1901
Junior Strength Motrin Caplets and Chewable Tablets................. 1901
Vicoprofen Tablets 533

Imipramine Hydrochloride (Atovaquone is highly bound to plasma protein (greater than 99.9%); caution is advised when co-administered with other highly protein bound drugs with narrow therapeutic indices).

No products indexed under this heading.

Imipramine Pamoate (Atovaquone is highly bound to plasma protein (greater than 99.9%); caution is advised when co-administered with other highly protein bound drugs with narrow therapeutic indices).

No products indexed under this heading.

Indomethacin (Atovaquone is highly bound to plasma protein (greater than 99.9%); caution is advised when co-administered with other highly protein bound drugs with narrow therapeutic indices). Products include:

Indocin 2024

Indomethacin Sodium Trihydrate (Atovaquone is highly bound to plasma protein (greater than 99.9%); caution is advised when co-administered with other highly protein bound drugs with narrow therapeutic indices). Products include:

Indocin I.V. 2489

Ketoprofen (Atovaquone is highly bound to plasma protein (greater than 99.9%); caution is advised when co-administered with other highly protein bound drugs with narrow therapeutic indices).

No products indexed under this heading.

Ketorolac Tromethamine (Atovaquone is highly bound to plasma protein (greater than 99.9%); caution is advised when co-administered with other highly protein bound drugs with narrow therapeutic indices).

No products indexed under this heading.

Meclofenamate Sodium (Atovaquone is highly bound to plasma protein (greater than 99.9%); caution is advised when co-administered with other highly protein bound drugs with narrow therapeutic indices).

No products indexed under this heading.

Mefenamic Acid (Atovaquone is highly bound to plasma protein (greater than 99.9%); caution is advised when co-administered with other highly protein bound drugs with narrow therapeutic indices).

No products indexed under this heading.

Midazolam Hydrochloride (Atovaquone is highly bound to plasma protein (greater than 99.9%); caution is advised when co-administered with other highly protein bound drugs with narrow therapeutic indices).

No products indexed under this heading.

Naproxen (Atovaquone is highly bound to plasma protein (greater than 99.9%); caution is advised when co-administered with other highly protein bound drugs with narrow therapeutic indices). Products include:

EC-Naprosyn Delayed-Release Tablets 2632
Naprosyn Suspension 2632
Naprosyn Tablets 2632

Naproxen Sodium (Atovaquone is highly bound to plasma protein (greater than 99.9%); caution is advised when co-administered with other highly protein bound drugs with narrow therapeutic indices). Products include:

Anaprox Tablets 2632
Anaprox DS Tablets 2632
Treximet Tablets 1616

Nortriptyline Hydrochloride (Atovaquone is highly bound to plasma protein (greater than 99.9%); caution is advised when co-administered with other highly protein bound drugs with narrow therapeutic indices).

No products indexed under this heading.

Oxaprozin (Atovaquone is highly bound to plasma protein (greater than 99.9%); caution is advised when co-administered with other highly protein bound drugs with narrow therapeutic indices).

No products indexed under this heading.

Oxazepam (Atovaquone is highly bound to plasma protein (greater than 99.9%); caution is advised when co-administered with other highly protein bound drugs with narrow therapeutic indices).

No products indexed under this heading.

Phenylbutazone (Atovaquone is highly bound to plasma protein (greater than 99.9%); caution is advised when co-administered with other highly protein bound drugs with narrow therapeutic indices).

No products indexed under this heading.

Piroxicam (Atovaquone is highly bound to plasma protein (greater than 99.9%); caution is advised when co-administered with other highly protein bound drugs with narrow therapeutic indices).

No products indexed under this heading.

Propranolol Hydrochloride (Atovaquone is highly bound to plasma protein (greater than 99.9%); caution is advised when co-administered with other highly protein bound drugs with narrow therapeutic indices). Products include:

InnoPran XL Extended Release Capsules.................................... 1484

Rifabutin (Due to structural similarity to rifampin, rifabutin may decrease average steady-state plasma atovaquone concentration).

No products indexed under this heading.

Rifampin (Co-administration with oral rifampin in HIV-infected individuals may result in a 52% ± 13% decrease in the average steady-state plasma atovaquone concentration and a 37% +/- 42% increase in the average steady-state plasma rifampin concentration).

No products indexed under this heading.

Sulfamethoxazole (Co-administration with TMP-SMX may result in slight decrease in average steady-state concentrations of TMP-SMX; this effect is minor and would not expect to produce clinically significant events).

No products indexed under this heading.

Sulindac (Atovaquone is highly bound to plasma protein (greater than 99.9%); caution is advised when co-administered with other highly protein bound drugs with narrow therapeutic indices). Products include:

Clinoril Tablets 1962

Temazepam (Atovaquone is highly bound to plasma protein (greater than 99.9%); caution is advised when co-administered with other highly protein bound drugs with narrow therapeutic indices).

No products indexed under this heading.

Tolbutamide (Atovaquone is highly bound to plasma protein (greater than 99.9%); caution is advised when co-administered with other highly protein bound drugs with narrow therapeutic indices).

No products indexed under this heading.

Tolmetin Sodium (Atovaquone is highly bound to plasma protein (greater than 99.9%); caution is advised when co-administered with other highly protein bound drugs with narrow therapeutic indices).

No products indexed under this heading.

Trimethoprim (Co-administration with TMP-SMX may result in slight decrease in average steady-state concentrations of TMP-SMX; this effect is minor and would not expect to produce clinically significant events).

No products indexed under this heading.

Trimipramine Maleate (Atovaquone is highly bound to plasma protein (greater than 99.9%); caution is advised when co-administered with other highly protein bound drugs with narrow therapeutic indices).

No products indexed under this heading.

Warfarin Sodium (Atovaquone is highly bound to plasma protein (greater than 99.9%); caution is advised when co-administered with other highly protein bound drugs with narrow therapeutic indices).

No products indexed under this heading.

Zidovudine (Atovaquone tablets have shown to decrease zidovudine apparent oral clearance leading to an increase in plasma zidovudine AUC; this effect is minor and would not expect to produce clinically significant events). Products include:

Combivir Tablets 1384
Retrovir 1574
Retrovir IV Infusion 1579
Trizivir Tablets 1622

Food Interactions

Food, unspecified (Food enhances absorption by approximately two-fold).

MERIBIN CAPSULES

(Biotin) 2163
None cited in PDR database.

MERIDIA CAPSULES

(Sibutramine Hydrochloride Monohydrate).................................. 475
May interact with anorexiants, erythromycin, lithium preparations, monoamine oxidase inhibitors, serotoninergic agents, and certain other agents. Compounds in these categories include:

Amphetamine Resins (Concurrent use with other centrally acting appetite suppressant drugs is contraindicated).

No products indexed under this heading.

Benzphetamine Hydrochloride (Concurrent use with other centrally acting appetite suppressant drugs is contraindicated).

No products indexed under this heading.

Cimetidine (Co-administration has resulted in small increases in combined (M1 and M2 metabolites) plasma Cmax and AUC).

No products indexed under this heading.

Cimetidine Hydrochloride (Co-administration has resulted in small increases in combined (M1 and M2 metabolites) plasma Cmax and AUC).

No products indexed under this heading.

Citalopram Hydrobromide (Sibutramine inhibits serotonin reuptake and serotonin syndrome, a rare, but serious constellation of symptoms, has been reported with the concomitant use of two SSRIs; concurrent use should be avoided). Products include:

Celexa 1160

Dexfenfluramine Hydrochloride (Concurrent use with other centrally acting appetite suppressant drugs is contraindicated).

No products indexed under this heading.

Dextroamphetamine Sulfate (Concurrent use with other centrally acting appetite suppressant drugs is contraindicated). Products include:

Adderall XR Capsules 3012
Dexedrine 1401

Dextromethorphan Hydrobromide (Sibutramine inhibits serotonin reuptake and combination of SSRIs and dextromethorphan has resulted in serious, sometimes fatal, reactions, serotonin syndrome). Products include:

PediaCare Children's Liquid Multi-Symptom Cold 1902
PediaCare Children's Long-Acting Cough 1902
Children's Sudafed PE Cold & Cough Liquid 1907
Sudafed PE Cold & Cough Caplets 1907
Children's Tylenol Plus Cough & Runny Nose Suspension Liquid 1912
Children's Tylenol Plus Cough & Sore Throat Suspension Liquid 1912
Children's Tylenol Plus Flu Suspension Liquid 1914
Children's Tylenol Plus Multi-Symptom Cold Suspension Liquid 1912
Tylenol Cold Severe Congestion Daytime Caplets with Cool Burst 1912
Tylenol Cold Head Congestion Daytime Caplets with Cool Burst 1910
Tylenol Cold Head Congestion Nighttime Caplets with Cool Burst 1910
Tylenol Cold Head Congestion Severe Daytime Caplets with Cool Burst 1910
Tylenol Cold Multi-Symptom Daytime Caplets with Cool Burst and Rapid Release Gels 1913
Tylenol Cold Multi-Symptom Daytime Liquid with Citrus Burst 1913
Tylenol Cold Multi-Symptom Nighttime Caplets with Cool Burst 1913
Tylenol Cold Multi-Symptom Nighttime Liquid with Cool Burst 1913
Tylenol Cold Multi-Symptom Severe Caplets with Cool Burst 1913
Tylenol Cold Multi-Symptom Severe Daytime Liquid with Citrus Burst 1913
Tylenol Cough & Sore Throat Daytime Liquid with Cool Burst 1918
Tylenol Cough & Sore Throat Nighttime Liquid with Cool Burst 1918
Vicks DayQuil Cold & Flu Multi-Symptom Relief 616
Vicks DayQuil LiquiCaps 2567
Vicks DayQuil Liquid 2567
Vicks DayQuil Multi-Symptom Cold/Flu Relief 2567
Vicks NyQuil Cold & Flu Multi-Symptom Relief 617
Vicks NyQuil LiquiCaps 2567
Vicks NyQuil Liquid 2567
Vicks NyQuil Multi-Symptom Cold/Flu Relief 2567

Dextromethorphan Polistirex (Sibutramine inhibits serotonin reuptake and combination of SSRIs and dextromethorphan has resulted in serious, sometimes fatal, reactions, serotonin syndrome).

No products indexed under this heading.

Diethylpropion Hydrochloride (Concurrent use with other centrally acting appetite suppressant drugs is contraindicated).

No products indexed under this heading.

Dihydroergotamine Mesylate (Sibutramine inhibits serotonin reuptake and combination of SSRIs and agents for migraine, such as dihydroergotamine, has resulted in serious, sometimes fatal, reactions, serotonin syndrome).

No products indexed under this heading.

Erythromycin (Co-administration has resulted in a small increase in the AUC and a small reduction in Cmax of sibutramine metabolites).

No products indexed under this heading.

Erythromycin Estolate (Co-administration has resulted in a small increase in the AUC and a small reduction in Cmax of sibutramine metabolites).

No products indexed under this heading.

Erythromycin Ethylsuccinate (Co-administration has resulted in a small increase in the AUC and a small reduction in Cmax of sibutramine metabolites). Products include:

E.E.S. 433
EryPed 431

Erythromycin Gluceptate (Co-administration has resulted in a small increase in the AUC and a small reduction in Cmax of sibutramine metabolites).

No products indexed under this heading.

Erythromycin Lactobionate (Co-administration has resulted in a small increase in the AUC and a small reduction in Cmax of sibutramine metabolites).

No products indexed under this heading.

Erythromycin Stearate (Co-administration has resulted in a small increase in the AUC and a small reduction in Cmax of sibutramine metabolites).

No products indexed under this heading.

Escitalopram Oxalate (Sibutramine inhibits serotonin reuptake and serotonin syndrome, a rare, but serious constellation of symptoms, has been reported with the concomitant use of two SSRIs; concurrent use should be avoided). Products include:

Lexapro Oral Suspension 1174
Lexapro Tablets 1174

Fenfluramine Hydrochloride (Concurrent use with other centrally acting appetite suppressant drugs is contraindicated).

No products indexed under this heading.

Fentanyl (Sibutramine inhibits serotonin reuptake and combination of SSRIs and certain opioids, such as fentanyl, has resulted in serious, sometimes fatal, reactions, serotonin syndrome). Products include:

Duragesic Transdermal System 2405
Ionsys Transdermal System 2410

Fentanyl Citrate (Sibutramine inhibits serotonin reuptake and combination of SSRIs and certain opioids, such as fentanyl, has resulted in serious, sometimes fatal, reactions, serotonin syndrome). Products include:

Actiq 959
Fentora Tablets 968

Fluoxetine Hydrochloride (Sibutramine inhibits serotonin reuptake and serotonin syndrome, a rare, but serious constellation of symptoms, has been reported with the concomitant use of two SSRIs; concurrent use should be avoided). Products include:

Prozac Weekly Capsules 1852
Prozac Pulvules and Liquid 1852
Symbyax Capsules 1871

Fluvoxamine Maleate (Sibutramine inhibits serotonin reuptake and serotonin syndrome, a rare, but serious constellation of symptoms, has been reported with the concomitant use of two SSRIs; concurrent use should be avoided). Products include:

Luvox CR Extended-Release Capsules 1759

Isocarboxazid (Concurrent and/or sequential use with MAO inhibitors is contraindicated; sibutramine inhibits serotonin reuptake and combination of MAO inhibitor and serotonergic agents has resulted in serious, sometimes fatal, reactions, serotonin syndrome). Products include:

Marplan Tablets 3177

Ketoconazole (Co-administration has resulted in a moderate increase in AUC and Cmax of sibutramine). Products include:

Extina Foam, 2% 3057
Nizoral A-D Shampoo 1901

Lithium (Sibutramine inhibits serotonin reuptake and combination of SSRIs and lithium has resulted in serious, sometimes fatal, reactions, serotonin syndrome).

No products indexed under this heading.

Lithium Carbonate (Sibutramine inhibits serotonin reuptake and combination of SSRIs and lithium has resulted in serious, sometimes fatal, reactions, serotonin syndrome).

No products indexed under this heading.

Lithium Citrate (Sibutramine inhibits serotonin reuptake and combination of SSRIs and lithium has resulted in serious, sometimes fatal, reactions, serotonin syndrome).

No products indexed under this heading.

Mazindol (Concurrent use with other centrally acting appetite suppressant drugs is contraindicated).

No products indexed under this heading.

Meperidine Hydrochloride (Sibutramine inhibits serotonin reuptake and combination of SSRIs and certain opioids, such as meperidine, has resulted in serious, sometimes fatal, reactions, serotonin syndrome).

No products indexed under this heading.

Methamphetamine Hydrochloride (Concurrent use with other centrally acting appetite suppressant drugs is contraindicated).

No products indexed under this heading.

Moclobemide (Concurrent and/or sequential use with MAO inhibitors is contraindicated; sibutramine inhibits serotonin reuptake and combination of MAO inhibitor and serotonergic agents has resulted in serious, sometimes fatal, reactions, serotonin syndrome).

No products indexed under this heading.

Pargyline Hydrochloride (Concurrent and/or sequential use with MAO inhibitors is contraindicated; sibutramine inhibits serotonin reuptake and combination of MAO inhibitor and serotonergic agents has resulted in serious, sometimes fatal, reactions, serotonin syndrome).

No products indexed under this heading.

Paroxetine Hydrochloride (Sibutramine inhibits serotonin reuptake and serotonin syndrome, a rare, but serious constellation of symptoms, has been reported with the concomitant use of two SSRIs; concurrent use should be avoided). Products include:

Paxil 1535
Paxil CR Controlled-Release Tablets 1544

Pentazocine Hydrochloride (Sibutramine inhibits serotonin reuptake and combination of SSRIs and pentazocine has resulted in serious, sometimes fatal, reactions, serotonin syndrome).

No products indexed under this heading.

Phendimetrazine Tartrate (Concurrent use with other centrally acting appetite suppressant drugs is contraindicated).

No products indexed under this heading.

Phenelzine Sulfate (Concurrent and/or sequential use with MAO inhibitors is contraindicated; sibutramine inhibits serotonin reuptake and combination of MAO inhibitor and serotonergic agents has resulted in serious, sometimes fatal, reactions, serotonin syndrome).

No products indexed under this heading.

Phenmetrazine Hydrochloride (Concurrent use with other centrally acting appetite suppressant drugs is contraindicated).

No products indexed under this heading.

Phentermine Hydrochloride (Concurrent use with other centrally acting appetite suppressant drugs is contraindicated). Products include:

Adipex-P 1185

Phentermine Resin (Concurrent use with other centrally acting appetite suppressant drugs is contraindicated).

No products indexed under this heading.

Phenylephrine Hydrochloride (Sibutramine substantially raises blood in some patients and concomitant use of sibutramine and drugs that raise blood pressure and/or heart rate, such as decongestants, requires caution). Products include:

Actifed Cold & Allergy Tablets 1895
Benadryl Allergy & Cold Kapgels 1895
Benadryl Allergy & Sinus Headache Kapgels 1895
Benadryl Severe Allergy & Sinus Headache Caplets 1897
Children's Benadryl-D Allergy & Sinus Liquid 1896

Benadryl-D Allergy & Sinus Tablet 1896
PediaCare Children's Allergy & Cold Liquid 1902
PediaCare Children's Decongestant Liquid 1902
PediaCare Children's Liquid Multi-Symptom Cold 1902
Sinutab Non-Drying Caplets 1905
Sinutab Sinus Caplets 1905
Children's Sudafed PE Cold & Cough Liquid 1907
Children's Sudafed PE Nasal Decongestant Liquid 1906
Sudafed PE Cold & Cough Caplets 1907
Sudafed PE Nasal Decongestant Tablets 1907
Sudafed PE Nighttime Cold Caplets 1907
Sudafed PE Non-Drying Sinus Caplets 1908
Sudafed PE Severe Cold Caplets 1908
Sudafed PE Sinus & Allergy Tablets 1908
Sudafed PE Sinus Headache Caplets 1908
Tylenol Allergy Multi-Symptom Caplets with Cool Burst and Rapid Release Gelcaps 1916
Tylenol Allergy Multi-Symptom Nighttime Caplets with Cool Burst 1916
Children's Tylenol Plus Cold Suspension Liquid 1912
Children's Tylenol Plus Cold & Allergy Suspension Liquid 1914
Children's Tylenol Plus Flu Suspension Liquid 1914
Children's Tylenol Plus Multi-Symptom Cold Suspension Liquid 1912
Tylenol Cold Head Congestion Daytime Caplets with Cool Burst 1910
Tylenol Cold Head Congestion Nighttime Caplets with Cool Burst 1910
Tylenol Cold Head Congestion Severe Daytime Caplets with Cool Burst 1910
Tylenol Cold Multi-Symptom Daytime Caplets with Cool Burst and Rapid Release Gels 1913
Tylenol Cold Multi-Symptom Daytime Liquid with Citrus Burst 1913
Tylenol Cold Multi-Symptom Nighttime Caplets with Cool Burst 1913
Tylenol Cold Multi-Symptom Nighttime Liquid with Cool Burst 1913
Tylenol Cold Multi-Symptom Severe Caplets with Cool Burst 1913
Tylenol Cold Multi-Symptom Severe Daytime Liquid with Citrus Burst 1913
Tylenol Sinus Congestion & Pain Daytime Caplets with Cool Burst and Gelcaps 1917
Tylenol Sinus Congestion & Pain Nighttime Caplets with Cool Burst 1917
Tylenol Sinus Congestion & Pain Severe Caplets with Cool Burst 1917
Vicks DayQuil Cold & Flu Multi-Symptom Relief .... ▣ 616
Vicks DayQuil LiquiCaps 2567
Vicks DayQuil Liquid 2567
Vicks DayQuil Multi-Symptom Cold/Flu Relief 2567

Phenylephrine Tannate (Sibutramine substantially raises blood in some patients and concomitant use of sibutramine and drugs that raise blood pressure and/or heart rate, such as decongestants, requires caution).
No products indexed under this heading.

Phenylpropanolamine Hydrochloride (Sibutramine substantially raises blood in some patients and concomitant use of sibutramine and drugs that raise blood pressure and/or heart rate, such as decongestants, requires caution).
No products indexed under this heading.

Procarbazine Hydrochloride (Concurrent and/or sequential use with MAO inhibitors is contraindicated; sibutramine inhibits serotonin reuptake and combination of MAO inhibitor and serotonergic agents has resulted in serious, sometimes fatal, reactions, serotonin syndrome).
No products indexed under this heading.

Pseudoephedrine Hydrochloride (Sibutramine substantially raises blood in some patients and concomitant use of sibutramine and drugs that raise blood pressure and/or heart rate, such as decongestants, requires caution). Products include:
Allegra-D 12 Hour Extended-Release Tablets 2687
Allegra-D 24 Hour Extended-Release Tablets 2690
Children's Motrin Cold Oral Suspension 1899
Sudafed 12 Hour Nasal Decongestant Non-Drowsy Caplets 1909
Sudafed 24 Hour Non-Drowsy Nasal Decongestant Tablets 1906
Children's Sudafed Nasal Decongestant Liquid 1906
Sudafed Nasal Decongestant Tablets 1906
Tylenol Cold Severe Congestion Daytime Caplets with Cool Burst 1912
Tylenol Sinus Severe Congestion Caplets with Cool Burst 1917
Vicks NyQuil LiquiCaps 2567
Vicks NyQuil Liquid 2567
Vicks NyQuil Multi-Symptom Cold/Flu Relief 2567
Zyrtec-D 12 Hour Extended Release Tablets 1923
Zyrtec-D Allergy & Congestion Extended-Release Tablets 1923

Pseudoephedrine Sulfate (Sibutramine substantially raises blood in some patients and concomitant use of sibutramine and drugs that raise blood pressure and/or heart rate, such as decongestants, requires caution). Products include:
Clarinex-D 12-Hour Extended-Release Tablets 2831
Clarinex-D 24-Hour Extended-Release Tablets 2834

Rasagiline Mesylate (Concurrent and/or sequential use with MAO inhibitors is contraindicated; sibutramine inhibits serotonin reuptake and combination of MAO inhibitor and serotonergic agents has resulted in serious, sometimes fatal, reactions, serotonin syndrome). Products include:
Azilect Tablets 3106

Selegiline (Concurrent and/or sequential use with MAO inhibitors is contraindicated; sibutramine inhibits serotonin reuptake and combination of MAO inhibitor and serotonergic agents has resulted in serious, sometimes fatal, reactions, serotonin syndrome). Products include:
Emsam Transdermal System 905

Selegiline Hydrochloride (Concurrent and/or sequential use with MAO inhibitors is contraindicated; sibutramine inhibits serotonin reuptake and combination of MAO inhibitor and serotonergic agents has resulted in serious, sometimes fatal, reactions, serotonin syndrome). Products include:
Eldepryl Capsules 3052

Sertraline Hydrochloride (Sibutramine inhibits serotonin reuptake and serotonin syndrome, a rare, but serious constellation of symptoms, has been reported with the concomitant use of two SSRIs; concurrent use should be avoided).
No products indexed under this heading.

Sumatriptan (Sibutramine inhibits serotonin reuptake and combination of SSRIs and agents for migraine, such as sumatriptan, has resulted in serious, sometimes fatal, reactions, serotonin syndrome). Products include:
Imitrex Nasal Spray 1470

Sumatriptan Succinate (Sibutramine inhibits serotonin reuptake and combination of SSRIs and agents for migraine, such as sumatriptan, has resulted in serious, sometimes fatal, reactions, serotonin syndrome). Products include:
Imitrex Injection 1465
Imitrex Tablets 1474
Treximet Tablets 1616

Tranylcypromine Sulfate (Concurrent and/or sequential use with MAO inhibitors is contraindicated; sibutramine inhibits serotonin reuptake and combination of MAO inhibitor and serotonergic agents has resulted in serious, sometimes fatal, reactions, serotonin syndrome). Products include:
Parnate Tablets 1532

L-Tryptophan (Sibutramine inhibits serotonin reuptake and combination of SSRIs and tryptophan has resulted in serious, sometimes fatal, reactions, serotonin syndrome).
No products indexed under this heading.

Venlafaxine Hydrochloride (Sibutramine inhibits serotonin reuptake and serotonin syndrome, a rare, but serious constellation of symptoms, has been reported with the concomitant use of two SSRIs; concurrent use should be avoided). Products include:
Effexor XR Extended-Release Capsules 3195
Venlafaxine Hydrochloride Tablets 2199

Food Interactions

Alcohol (Concurrent use has not resulted in psychomotor reactions of clinical significance, however, concomitant use with excessive alcohol is not recommended).

Food, unspecified (Co-administration with a standard breakfast has resulted in reduced peak M1 and M2 amine concentrations and delayed the time to peak by approximately three hours; the AUCs of M1 and M2 were not significantly altered).

MERREM I.V.

(Meropenem) 684
May interact with valproate and certain other agents. Compounds in these categories include:

Divalproex Sodium (A clinically significant reduction in serum valproic acid concentrations has been reported in patients receiving carbapenem antibiotics and may result in loss of seizure control. Although the mechanism of this interaction is not fully understood, data from in vivo and animal studies suggest that carbapenem antibiotics may inhibit valproic acid glucuronide hydrolysis. Serum valproic acid concentrations should be monitored frequently after initiating carbapenem therapy. Alternative antibacterial or anticonvulsant therapy should be considered if serum valproic acid concentrations drop below the therapeutic range or a seizure occurs). Products include:
Depakote ER Tablets 423

Probenecid (Competes with meropenem for active tubular secretion and, thus, inhibits the renal excretion of meropenem. Statistically significant increases in the elimination half-life and the extent of systemic exposure have been reported; co-administration is not recommended).
No products indexed under this heading.

Valproate Sodium (A clinically significant reduction in serum valproic acid concentrations has been reported in patients receiving carbapenem antibiotics and may result in loss of seizure control. Although the mechanism of this interaction is not fully understood, data from in vivo and animal studies suggest that carbapenem antibiotics may inhibit valproic acid glucuronide hydrolysis. Serum valproic acid concentrations should be monitored frequently after initiating carbapenem therapy. Alternative antibacterial or anticonvulsant therapy should be considered if serum valproic acid concentrations drop below the therapeutic range or a seizure occurs).
No products indexed under this heading.

Valproic Acid (A clinically significant reduction in serum valproic acid concentrations has been reported in patients receiving carbapenem antibiotics and may result in loss of seizure control. Although the mechanism of this interaction is not fully understood, data from in vivo and animal studies suggest that carbapenem antibiotics may inhibit valproic acid glucuronide hydrolysis. Serum valproic acid concentrations should be monitored frequently after initiating carbapenem therapy. Alternative antibacterial or anticonvulsant therapy should be considered if serum valproic acid concentrations drop below the therapeutic range or a seizure occurs).
No products indexed under this heading.

MERUVAX II

(Rubella Virus Vaccine Live) 2061
May interact with immunosuppressive agents. Compounds in these categories include:

Azathioprine (Concurrent immunosuppressive therapy is contraindicated).
No products indexed under this heading.

Basiliximab (Concurrent immunosuppressive therapy is contraindicated). Products include:
Simulect for Injection 2306

Cyclosporine (Concurrent immunosuppressive therapy is contraindicated). Products include:
Gengraf Capsules 435
Neoral Oral Solution 2280
Neoral Soft Gelatin Capsules 2280
Restasis Ophthalmic Emulsion 557
Sandimmune 2296

Muromonab-CD3 (Concurrent immunosuppressive therapy is contraindicated). Products include:
Orthoclone OKT3 Sterile Solution 2387

Mycophenolate Mofetil (Concurrent immunosuppressive therapy is contraindicated). Products include:
CellCept Capsules 2622
CellCept Oral Suspension 2622
CellCept Tablets 2622

Sirolimus (Concurrent immunosuppressive therapy is contraindicated). Products include:
Rapamune 3260

Tacrolimus (Concurrent immunosuppressive therapy is contraindicated). Products include:
Prograf Capsules and Injection 622
Protopic Ointment 628

METADATE CD CAPSULES

(Methylphenidate Hydrochloride) 3146

May interact with oral anticoagulants, halogenated hydrocarbon anesthetics, monoamine oxidase inhibitors, phenytoin, selective serotonin reuptake inhibitors, tricyclic antidepressants, urinary alkalinizing agents, vasopressors, and certain other agents. Compounds in these categories include:

Amitriptyline Hydrochloride (Methylphenidate may inhibit the metabolism of tricyclic antidepressants; downward dosage adjustment of tricyclic antidepressants may be required).
No products indexed under this heading.

Ammonium Chloride (Clearance of methylphenidate might be affected by urinary pH, increasing with the use of acidifying agents. This should be considered when methylphenidate is given in combination with agents that alter urinary pH).
No products indexed under this heading.

Amoxapine (Methylphenidate may inhibit the metabolism of tricyclic antidepressants; downward dosage adjustment of tricyclic antidepressants may be required).
No products indexed under this heading.

Anisindione (Methylphenidate may inhibit the metabolism of coumarin anticoagulants; downward dosage adjustment of anticoagulants may be required).
No products indexed under this heading.

Citalopram Hydrobromide (Methylphenidate may inhibit the metabolism of selective serotonin reuptake inhibitors; downward dosage adjustment of SSRI may be required). Products include:
Celexa 1160

Clomipramine Hydrochloride (Methylphenidate may inhibit the metabolism of tricyclic antidepressants; downward dosage adjustment of tricyclic antidepressants may be required).
No products indexed under this heading.

Clonidine (Co-administration has resulted in serious adverse events; the safety of this combination has not been systemically established). Products include:
Catapres-TTS 842

Clonidine Hydrochloride (Co-administration has resulted in serious adverse events; the safety of this combination has not been systemically established). Products include:
Catapres Tablets 841
Clorpres Tablets 2185

Desipramine Hydrochloride (Methylphenidate may inhibit the metabolism of tricyclic antidepressants; downward dosage adjustment of tricyclic antidepressants may be required).
No products indexed under this heading.

Dicumarol (Methylphenidate may inhibit the metabolism of coumarin anticoagulants; downward dosage adjustment of anticoagulants may be required).
No products indexed under this heading.

Dobutamine (Methylphenidate causes rise in blood pressure; co-administration with other pressor agents should be undertaken with caution).
No products indexed under this heading.

Dobutamine Hydrochloride (Methylphenidate causes rise in blood pressure; co-administration with other pressor agents should be undertaken with caution).
No products indexed under this heading.

Dopamine Hydrochloride (Methylphenidate causes rise in blood pressure; co-administration with other pressor agents should be undertaken with caution).
No products indexed under this heading.

Doxepin Hydrochloride (Methylphenidate may inhibit the metabolism of tricyclic antidepressants; downward dosage adjustment of tricyclic antidepressants may be required).
No products indexed under this heading.

Enflurane (There is a risk of sudden blood pressure increase during surgery. If surgery is planned, methylphenidate should not be taken the day of the surgery).
No products indexed under this heading.

Ephedrine Sulfate (Methylphenidate causes rise in blood pressure; co-administration with other pressor agents should be undertaken with caution).
No products indexed under this heading.

Epinephrine Bitartrate (Methylphenidate causes rise in blood pressure; co-administration with other pressor agents should be undertaken with caution).
No products indexed under this heading.

Epinephrine Hydrochloride (Methylphenidate causes rise in blood pressure; co-administration with other pressor agents should be undertaken with caution).
No products indexed under this heading.

Escitalopram Oxalate (Methylphenidate may inhibit the metabolism of selective serotonin reuptake inhibitors; downward dosage adjustment of SSRI may be required). Products include:
Lexapro Oral Suspension 1174
Lexapro Tablets 1174

Fluoxetine (Methylphenidate may inhibit the metabolism of selective serotonin reuptake inhibitors; downward dosage adjustment of SSRI may be required).
No products indexed under this heading.

Fluoxetine Hydrochloride (Methylphenidate may inhibit the metabolism of selective serotonin reuptake inhibitors; downward dosage adjustment of SSRI may be required). Products include:
Prozac Weekly Capsules 1852
Prozac Pulvules and Liquid 1852
Symbyax Capsules 1871

Fluvoxamine Maleate (Methylphenidate may inhibit the metabolism of selective serotonin reuptake inhibitors; downward dosage adjustment of SSRI may be required). Products include:
Luvox CR Extended-Release Capsules 1759

Fosphenytoin Sodium (Methylphenidate may inhibit the metabolism of anticonvulsants, such as phenytoin; additionally methylphenidate may lower the convulsive threshold in patients with prior history of seizures).
No products indexed under this heading.

Guanethidine Monosulfate (Methylphenidate may decrease the hypotensive effect of guanethidine).
No products indexed under this heading.

Halothane (There is a risk of sudden blood pressure increase during surgery. If surgery is planned, methylphenidate should not be taken the day of the surgery).
No products indexed under this heading.

Imipramine Hydrochloride (Methylphenidate may inhibit the metabolism of tricyclic antidepressants; downward dosage adjustment of tricyclic antidepressants may be required).
No products indexed under this heading.

Imipramine Pamoate (Methylphenidate may inhibit the metabolism of tricyclic antidepressants; downward dosage adjustment of tricyclic antidepressants may be required).
No products indexed under this heading.

Isocarboxazid (Co-administration is contraindicated during treatment with monoamine oxidase inhibitors, and also within a minimum of 14 days following discontinuation of a monoamine oxidase inhibitor (hypertensive crises may result)). Products include:
Marplan Tablets 3177

Isoflurane (There is a risk of sudden blood pressure increase during surgery. If surgery is planned, methylphenidate should not be taken the day of the surgery).
No products indexed under this heading.

Isoproterenol Hydrochloride (Methylphenidate causes rise in blood pressure; co-administration with other pressor agents should be undertaken with caution).
No products indexed under this heading.

Isoproterenol Sulfate (Methylphenidate causes rise in blood pressure; co-administration with other pressor agents should be undertaken with caution).
No products indexed under this heading.

Maprotiline Hydrochloride (Methylphenidate may inhibit the metabolism of tricyclic antidepressants; downward dosage adjustment of tricyclic antidepressants may be required).
No products indexed under this heading.

Mephentermine Sulfate (Methylphenidate causes rise in blood pressure; co-administration with other pressor agents should be undertaken with caution).
No products indexed under this heading.

Metaraminol Bitartrate (Methylphenidate causes rise in blood pressure; co-administration with other pressor agents should be undertaken with caution).
No products indexed under this heading.

Methoxamine Hydrochloride (Methylphenidate causes rise in blood pressure; co-administration with other pressor agents should be undertaken with caution).
No products indexed under this heading.

Methoxyflurane (There is a risk of sudden blood pressure increase during surgery. If surgery is planned, methylphenidate should not be taken the day of the surgery).
No products indexed under this heading.

Moclobemide (Co-administration is contraindicated during treatment with monoamine oxidase inhibitors, and also within a minimum of 14 days following discontinuation of a monoamine oxidase inhibitor (hypertensive crises may result)).
No products indexed under this heading.

Norepinephrine Bitartrate (Methylphenidate causes rise in blood pressure; co-administration with other pressor agents should be undertaken with caution).
No products indexed under this heading.

Nortriptyline Hydrochloride (Methylphenidate may inhibit the metabolism of tricyclic antidepressants; downward dosage adjustment of tricyclic antidepressants may be required).
No products indexed under this heading.

Pargyline Hydrochloride (Co-administration is contraindicated during treatment with monoamine oxidase inhibitors, and also within a minimum of 14 days following discontinuation of a monoamine oxidase inhibitor (hypertensive crises may result)).
No products indexed under this heading.

Paroxetine Hydrochloride (Methylphenidate may inhibit the metabolism of selective serotonin reuptake inhibitors; downward dosage adjustment of SSRI may be required). Products include:
Paxil 1535
Paxil CR Controlled-Release Tablets 1544

Phenelzine Sulfate (Co-administration is contraindicated during treatment with monoamine oxidase inhibitors, and also within a minimum of 14 days following discontinuation of a monoamine oxidase inhibitor (hypertensive crises may result)).
No products indexed under this heading.

Phenobarbital (Methylphenidate may inhibit the metabolism of anticonvulsants, such as phenobarbital; additionally methylphenidate may lower the convulsive threshold in patients with prior history of seizures). Products include:
Donnatal Extentabs 2507

Phenylbutazone (Human pharmacologic studies have shown the methylphenidate may inhibit the metabolism of phenylbutazone. Downward dose adjustment of these drugs may be required when given concomitantly with methylphenidate).
No products indexed under this heading.

Phenylephrine Hydrochloride (Methylphenidate causes rise in blood pressure; co-administration with other pressor agents should be undertaken with caution). Products include:
Actifed Cold & Allergy Tablets 1895
Benadryl Allergy & Cold Kapgels 1895
Benadryl Allergy & Sinus Headache Kapgels 1895
Benadryl Severe Allergy & Sinus Headache Caplets 1897
Children's Benadryl-D Allergy & Sinus Liquid 1896
Benadryl-D Allergy & Sinus Tablet 1896
PediaCare Children's Allergy & Cold Liquid 1902
PediaCare Children's Decongestant Liquid.................... 1902
PediaCare Children's Liquid Multi-Symptom Cold.................... 1902
Sinutab Non-Drying Caplets 1905
Sinutab Sinus Caplets 1905
Children's Sudafed PE Cold & Cough Liquid 1907
Children's Sudafed PE Nasal Decongestant Liquid.................... 1906
Sudafed PE Cold & Cough Caplets.. 1907
Sudafed PE Nasal Decongestant Tablets 1907
Sudafed PE Nighttime Cold Caplets.. 1907
Sudafed PE Non-Drying Sinus Caplets.. 1908
Sudafed PE Severe Cold Caplets 1908
Sudafed PE Sinus & Allergy Tablets.. 1908
Sudafed PE Sinus Headache Caplets.. 1908
Tylenol Allergy Multi-Symptom Caplets with Cool Burst and Rapid Release Gelcaps................ 1916
Tylenol Allergy Multi-Symptom Nighttime Caplets with Cool Burst.. 1916
Children's Tylenol Plus Cold Suspension Liquid 1912
Children's Tylenol Plus Cold & Allergy Suspension Liquid............ 1914
Children's Tylenol Plus Flu Suspension Liquid 1914
Children's Tylenol Plus Multi-Symptom Cold Suspension Liquid 1912
Tylenol Cold Head Congestion Daytime Caplets with Cool Burst.. 1910
Tylenol Cold Head Congestion Nighttime Caplets with Cool Burst.. 1910
Tylenol Cold Head Congestion Severe Daytime Caplets with Cool Burst.................................. 1910
Tylenol Cold Multi-Symptom Daytime Caplets with Cool Burst and Rapid Release Gels....... 1913
Tylenol Cold Multi-Symptom Daytime Liquid with Citrus Burst... 1913
Tylenol Cold Multi-Symptom Nighttime Caplets with Cool Burst.. 1913
Tylenol Cold Multi-Symptom Nighttime Liquid with Cool Burst... 1913
Tylenol Cold Multi-Symptom Severe Caplets with Cool Burst..... 1913
Tylenol Cold Multi-Symptom Severe Daytime Liquid with Citrus Burst 1913
Tylenol Sinus Congestion & Pain Daytime Caplets with Cool Burst and Gelcaps..................... 1917
Tylenol Sinus Congestion & Pain Nighttime Caplets with Cool Burst.. 1917
Tylenol Sinus Congestion & Pain Severe Caplets with Cool Burst..... 1917
Vicks DayQuil Cold & Flu Multi-Symptom Relief .... ■616
Vicks DayQuil LiquiCaps 2567
Vicks DayQuil Liquid 2567
Vicks DayQuil Multi-Symptom Cold/Flu Relief............................ 2567

Phenytoin (Methylphenidate may inhibit the metabolism of anticonvulsants, such as phenytoin; additionally methylphenidate may lower the convulsive threshold in patients with prior history of seizures).
No products indexed under this heading.

Phenytoin Sodium (Methylphenidate may inhibit the metabolism of anticonvulsants, such as phenytoin; additionally methylphenidate may lower the convulsive threshold in patients with prior history of seizures). Products include:
Phenytek Capsules 2192

Potassium Citrate (Clearance of methylphenidate might be affected by urinary pH, decreasing with the use of alkalizing agents. This should be considered when methylphenidate is given in combination with agents that alter urinary pH). Products include:
BioLean Free Tablets .... ■635
Urocit-K Tablets 2176

Primidone (Methylphenidate may inhibit the metabolism of anticonvulsants, such as primidone; additionally methylphenidate may lower the convulsive threshold in patients with prior history of seizures).
No products indexed under this heading.

Procarbazine Hydrochloride (Co-administration is contraindicated during treatment with monoamine oxidase inhibitors, and also within a minimum of 14 days following discontinuation of a monoamine oxidase inhibitor (hypertensive crises may result)).
No products indexed under this heading.

Protriptyline Hydrochloride (Methylphenidate may inhibit the metabolism of tricyclic antidepressants; downward dosage adjustment of tricyclic antidepressants may be required).
No products indexed under this heading.

Rasagiline Mesylate (Co-administration is contraindicated during treatment with monoamine oxidase inhibitors, and also within a minimum of 14 days following discontinuation of a monoamine oxidase inhibitor (hypertensive crises may result)). Products include:
Azilect Tablets 3106

Selegiline (Co-administration is contraindicated during treatment with monoamine oxidase inhibitors, and also within a minimum of 14 days following discontinuation of a monoamine oxidase inhibitor (hypertensive crises may result)). Products include:
Emsam Transdermal System 905

Selegiline Hydrochloride (Co-administration is contraindicated during treatment with monoamine oxidase inhibitors, and also within a minimum of 14 days following discontinuation of a monoamine oxidase inhibitor (hypertensive crises may result)). Products include:
Eldepryl Capsules 3052

Sertraline Hydrochloride (Methylphenidate may inhibit the metabolism of selective serotonin reuptake inhibitors; downward dosage adjustment of SSRI may be required).
No products indexed under this heading.

Sodium Acid Phosphate (Clearance of methylphenidate might be affected by urinary pH, increasing with the use of acidifying agents. This should be considered when methylphenidate is given in combination with agents that alter urinary pH). Products include:
Uroqid-Acid No. 2 Tablets 814

Sodium Bicarbonate (Clearance of methylphenidate might be affected by urinary pH, decreasing with the use of alkalizing agents. This should be considered when methylphenidate is given in combination with agents that alter urinary pH). Products include:
Ceo-Two Laxative Suppository 815

Sodium Citrate (Clearance of methylphenidate might be affected by urinary pH, decreasing with the use of alkalizing agents. This should be considered when methylphenidate is given in combination with agents that alter urinary pH).
No products indexed under this heading.

Tranylcypromine Sulfate (Co-administration is contraindicated during treatment with monoamine oxidase inhibitors, and also within a minimum of 14 days following discontinuation of a monoamine oxidase inhibitor (hypertensive crises may result)). Products include:
Parnate Tablets 1532

Trimipramine Maleate (Methylphenidate may inhibit the metabolism of tricyclic antidepressants; downward dosage adjustment of tricyclic antidepressants may be required).
No products indexed under this heading.

Venlafaxine Hydrochloride (Co-administration in a patient on methylphenidate for 18 months has resulted in neuroleptic malignant syndrome within 45 minutes of ingesting his first dose of venlafaxine). Products include:
Effexor XR Extended-Release Capsules.. 3195
Venlafaxine Hydrochloride Tablets ... 2199

Vitamin C (Clearance of methylphenidate might be affected by urinary pH, increasing with the use of acidifying agents. This should be considered when methylphenidate is given in combination with agents that alter urinary pH). Products include:
Bausch & Lomb Ocuvite Adult 50+ Vitamin and Mineral Supplement.................................. ⊙237
Comax Dietary Supplement 995
Ferralet 90 Tablets 2175
Glaucofit Dietary Supplement 995
Glauma Dietary Supplement 995
MoviPrep Oral Solution 2679
Procosa II Tablets 3174
Proflavanol 90 Tablets 3174
Tonox Dietary Supplement 995
Vibe Liquid Multi-Nutrient Supplement.................................. ■626

Warfarin Sodium (Methylphenidate may inhibit the metabolism of coumarin anticoagulants; downward dosage adjustment of anticoagulants may be required).
No products indexed under this heading.

METAMUCIL CAPSULES

(Psyllium Preparations) 2563
None cited in PDR database.

METAMUCIL COARSE MILLED UNFLAVORED POWDER

(Psyllium Preparations) 2563
None cited in PDR database.

METAMUCIL COARSE MILLED ORANGE FLAVOR POWDER

(Psyllium Preparations) 2563
None cited in PDR database.

METAMUCIL DIETARY FIBER SUPPLEMENT

(Psyllium Preparations) 2563
None cited in PDR database.

METAMUCIL SMOOTH TEXTURE ORANGE FLAVOR POWDER

(Psyllium Preparations) 2563
None cited in PDR database.

METAMUCIL SMOOTH TEXTURE SUGAR-FREE UNFLAVORED POWDER

(Psyllium Preparations) 2563
None cited in PDR database.

METAMUCIL SMOOTH TEXTURE SUGAR-FREE ORANGE FLAVOR POWDER

(Psyllium Preparations) 2563
None cited in PDR database.

METAMUCIL WAFERS, APPLE AND CINNAMON FLAVORS

(Psyllium Preparations) 2563
None cited in PDR database.

MEVACOR TABLETS

(Lovastatin) 2063
May interact with azole antifungals, oral anticoagulants, cytochrome p450 3a4 inhibitors (selected), erythromycin, fibrates, protease inhibitors, and certain other agents. Compounds in these categories include:

Acetazolamide (The risk of myopathy/rhabdomyolysis is increased by concomitant use of lovastatin with potent inhibitors of CYP3A4, particularly with higher doses of lovastatin; concomitant use should be avoided unless the benefits of combined therapy outweigh the increased risk).
No products indexed under this heading.

Amiodarone Hydrochloride (The combined use of lovastatin at doses higher than 40 mg daily with amiodarone should be avoided unless the clinical benefit is likely to outweigh the increased risk of myopathy).
No products indexed under this heading.

Amprenavir (The risk of myopathy/ rhabdomyolysis is increased by concomitant use of lovastatin with potent inhibitors of CYP3A4, particularly with higher doses of lovastatin; concomitant use should be avoided unless the benefits of combined therapy outweigh the increased risk).
No products indexed under this heading.

Anastrozole (The risk of myopathy/ rhabdomyolysis is increased by concomitant use of lovastatin with potent inhibitors of CYP3A4, particularly with higher doses of lovastatin; concomitant use should be avoided unless the benefits of combined therapy outweigh the increased risk). Products include:
Arimidex Tablets 672

Anisindione (Co-administration has resulted in bleeding and/or increased prothrombin time in few patients).
No products indexed under this heading.

Aprepitant (The risk of myopathy/ rhabdomyolysis is increased by concomitant use of lovastatin with potent inhibitors of CYP3A4, particularly with higher doses of lovastatin; concomitant use should be avoided unless the benefits of combined therapy outweigh the increased risk). Products include:
Emend Capsules 1992

Atazanavir (The risk of myopathy/ rhabdomyolysis is increased by concomitant use of lovastatin with potent inhibitors of CYP3A4, particularly with higher doses of lovastatin; concomitant use should be avoided unless the benefits of combined therapy outweigh the increased risk).
No products indexed under this heading.

Atazanavir Sulfate (The risk of myopathy/rhabdomyolysis is increased by concomitant use of lovastatin with potent inhibitors of CYP3A4, particularly with higher doses of lovastatin; concomitant use should be avoided unless the benefits of combined therapy outweigh the increased risk). Products include:
Reyataz Capsules 3299

Cimetidine (The risk of myopathy/ rhabdomyolysis is increased by concomitant use of lovastatin with potent inhibitors of CYP3A4, particularly with higher doses of lovastatin; concomitant use should be avoided unless the benefits of combined therapy outweigh the increased risk).
No products indexed under this heading.

Cimetidine Hydrochloride (The risk of myopathy/rhabdomyolysis is increased by concomitant use of lovastatin with potent inhibitors of CYP3A4, particularly with higher doses of lovastatin; concomitant use should be avoided unless the benefits of combined therapy outweigh the increased risk).
No products indexed under this heading.

Ciprofloxacin (The risk of myopathy/rhabdomyolysis is increased by concomitant use of lovastatin with potent inhibitors of CYP3A4, particularly with higher doses of lovastatin; concomitant use should be avoided unless the benefits of combined therapy outweigh the increased risk). Products include:
Cipro I.V. 2817
Cipro Oral Suspension 2810
Cipro XR Tablets 2823
Ciprodex Otic Suspension 541

Clarithromycin (The risk of myopathy appears to be increased by high levels of HMG-CoA reductase inhibitory activity in plasma; lovastatin is metabolized by CYP3A4 isoenzyme, certain agents, such as macrolide antibiotics clarithromycin, share this metabolic pathway and can raise the plasma levels of lovastatin and may increase the risk of myopathy). Products include:
Biaxin/Biaxin XL 411

Clofibrate (The incidence and severity of myopathy are increased by co-administration of HMG-CoA reductase inhibitors with drugs that cause myopathy when given alone, such as fibrates; combined use should be avoided; if used concurrently, the dose of lovastatin should generally not exceed 20 mg).
No products indexed under this heading.

Clotrimazole (The risk of myopathy appears to be increased by high levels of HMG-CoA reductase inhibitory activity in plasma; lovastatin is metabolized by CYP3A4 isoenzyme, certain agents, such as azole antifungals, share this metabolic pathway and can raise the plasma levels of lovastatin and may increase the risk of myopathy). Products include:
Lotrisone 2881

Cyclosporine (The risk of myopathy appears to be increased by high levels of HMG-CoA reductase inhibitory activity in plasma; lovastatin is metabolized by CYP3A4 isoenzyme, certain agents, such as cyclosporine, share this metabolic pathway and can raise the plasma levels of lovastatin and may increase the risk of myopathy; the dose of lovastatin should generally not exceed 20 mg if used concomitantly). Products include:
Gengraf Capsules 435
Neoral Oral Solution 2280
Neoral Soft Gelatin Capsules 2280
Restasis Ophthalmic Emulsion 557
Sandimmune 2296

Dalfopristin (The risk of myopathy/ rhabdomyolysis is increased by concomitant use of lovastatin with potent inhibitors of CYP3A4, particularly with higher doses of lovastatin; concomitant use should be avoided unless the benefits of combined therapy outweigh the increased risk).
No products indexed under this heading.

Danazol (The risk of rhabdomyolysis/myopathy is increased by concomitant administration of danazol, particularly with higher doses of lovastatin. The dose of lovastatin should not exceed 20 mg daily in patients receiving concomitant medication with danazol).
No products indexed under this heading.

Darunavir (The risk of myopathy/ rhabdomyolysis is increased by concomitant use of lovastatin with potent inhibitors of CYP3A4, particularly with higher doses of lovastatin; concomitant use should be avoided unless the benefits of combined therapy outweigh the increased risk).
No products indexed under this heading.

Delavirdine Mesylate (The risk of myopathy/rhabdomyolysis is increased by concomitant use of lovastatin with potent inhibitors of CYP3A4, particularly with higher doses of lovastatin; concomitant use should be avoided unless the benefits of combined therapy outweigh the increased risk).
No products indexed under this heading.

Dicumarol (Co-administration has resulted in bleeding and/or increased prothrombin time in few patients).
No products indexed under this heading.

Diltiazem Hydrochloride (The risk of myopathy/rhabdomyolysis is increased by concomitant use of lovastatin with potent inhibitors of CYP3A4, particularly with higher doses of lovastatin; concomitant use should be avoided unless the benefits of combined therapy outweigh the increased risk). Products include:
Cardizem LA Extended Release Tablets 421

Diltiazem Maleate (The risk of myopathy/rhabdomyolysis is increased by concomitant use of lovastatin with potent inhibitors of CYP3A4, particularly with higher doses of lovastatin; concomitant use should be avoided unless the benefits of combined therapy outweigh the increased risk).
No products indexed under this heading.

Efavirenz (The risk of myopathy/ rhabdomyolysis is increased by concomitant use of lovastatin with potent inhibitors of CYP3A4, particularly with higher doses of lovastatin; concomitant use should be avoided unless the benefits of combined therapy outweigh the increased risk). Products include:
Atripla Tablets 938
Sustiva Capsules 930
Sustiva Tablets 930

Erythromycin (The risk of myopathy/rhabdomyolysis is increased by concomitant use of lovastatin with potent inhibitors of CYP3A4, particularly with higher doses of lovastatin; concomitant use should be avoided unless the benefits of combined therapy outweigh the increased risk).
No products indexed under this heading.

Erythromycin Estolate (The risk of myopathy/rhabdomyolysis is increased by concomitant use of lovastatin with potent inhibitors of CYP3A4, particularly with higher doses of lovastatin; concomitant use should be avoided unless the benefits of combined therapy outweigh the increased risk).
No products indexed under this heading.

Erythromycin Ethylsuccinate (The risk of myopathy/ rhabdomyolysis is increased by concomitant use of lovastatin with potent inhibitors of CYP3A4, particularly with higher doses of lovastatin; concomitant use should be avoided unless the benefits of combined therapy outweigh the increased risk). Products include:
E.E.S. 433
EryPed 431

Erythromycin Gluceptate (The risk of myopathy/rhabdomyolysis is increased by concomitant use of lovastatin with potent inhibitors of CYP3A4, particularly with higher doses of lovastatin; concomitant use should be avoided unless the benefits of combined therapy outweigh the increased risk).
No products indexed under this heading.

Erythromycin Lactobionate (The risk of myopathy/rhabdomyolysis is increased by concomitant use of lovastatin with potent inhibitors of CYP3A4, particularly with higher doses of lovastatin; concomitant use should be avoided unless the benefits of combined therapy outweigh the increased risk).
No products indexed under this heading.

Erythromycin Stearate (The risk of myopathy/rhabdomyolysis is increased by concomitant use of lovastatin with potent inhibitors of CYP3A4, particularly with higher doses of lovastatin; concomitant use should be avoided unless the benefits of combined therapy outweigh the increased risk).
No products indexed under this heading.

Esomeprazole Magnesium (The risk of myopathy/rhabdomyolysis is increased by concomitant use of lovastatin with potent inhibitors of CYP3A4, particularly with higher doses of lovastatin; concomitant use should be avoided unless the benefits of combined therapy outweigh the increased risk). Products include:
Nexium Delayed-Release Capsules 645
Nexium Delayed-Release Oral Suspension 645

Fenofibrate (The incidence and severity of myopathy are increased by co-administration of HMG-CoA reductase inhibitors with drugs that cause myopathy when given alone, such as fibrates; combined use should be avoided; if used concurrently, the dose of lovastatin should generally not exceed 20 mg). Products include:
Fenoglide Tablets 2960
Tricor Tablets 520

Fluconazole (The risk of myopathy appears to be increased by high levels of HMG-CoA reductase inhibitory activity in plasma; lovastatin is metabolized by CYP3A4 isoenzyme, certain agents, such as azole antifungals, share this metabolic pathway and can raise the plasma levels of lovastatin and may increase the risk of myopathy).
No products indexed under this heading.

Fluoxetine (The risk of myopathy/ rhabdomyolysis is increased by concomitant use of lovastatin with potent inhibitors of CYP3A4, particularly with higher doses of lovastatin; concomitant use should be avoided unless the benefits of combined therapy outweigh the increased risk).
No products indexed under this heading.

Fluoxetine Hydrochloride (The risk of myopathy/rhabdomyolysis is increased by concomitant use of lovastatin with potent inhibitors of CYP3A4, particularly with higher doses of lovastatin; concomitant use should be avoided unless the benefits of combined therapy outweigh the increased risk). Products include:

Prozac Weekly Capsules 1852
Prozac Pulvules and Liquid 1852
Symbyax Capsules 1871

Fluvoxamine Maleate (The risk of myopathy/rhabdomyolysis is increased by concomitant use of lovastatin with potent inhibitors of CYP3A4, particularly with higher doses of lovastatin; concomitant use should be avoided unless the benefits of combined therapy outweigh the increased risk). Products include:

Luvox CR Extended-Release Capsules 1759

Fosamprenavir Calcium (The risk of myopathy/rhabdomyolysis is increased by concomitant use of lovastatin with potent inhibitors of CYP3A4, particularly with higher doses of lovastatin; concomitant use should be avoided unless the benefits of combined therapy outweigh the increased risk). Products include:

Lexiva Oral Suspension 1510
Lexiva Tablets 1510

Gemfibrozil (The incidence and severity of myopathy are increased by co-administration of HMG-CoA reductase inhibitors with drugs that cause myopathy when given alone, such as fibrates; combined use should be avoided; if used concurrently, the dose of lovastatin should generally not exceed 20 mg).

No products indexed under this heading.

Indinavir Sulfate (The risk of myopathy/rhabdomyolysis is increased by concomitant use of lovastatin with potent inhibitors of CYP3A4, particularly with higher doses of lovastatin; concomitant use should be avoided unless the benefits of combined therapy outweigh the increased risk). Products include:

Crixivan Capsules 1979

Isoniazid (The risk of myopathy/rhabdomyolysis is increased by concomitant use of lovastatin with potent inhibitors of CYP3A4, particularly with higher doses of lovastatin; concomitant use should be avoided unless the benefits of combined therapy outweigh the increased risk).

No products indexed under this heading.

Itraconazole (The risk of myopathy appears to be increased by high levels of HMG-CoA reductase inhibitory activity in plasma; lovastatin is metabolized by CYP3A4 isoenzyme, certain agents, such as itraconazole, share this metabolic pathway and can raise the plasma levels of lovastatin and may increase the risk of myopathy).

No products indexed under this heading.

Ketoconazole (The risk of myopathy appears to be increased by high levels of HMG-CoA reductase inhibitory activity in plasma; lovastatin is metabolized by CYP3A4 isoenzyme, certain agents, such as ketoconazole, share this metabolic pathway and can raise the plasma levels of lovastatin and may increase the risk of myopathy). Products include:

Extina Foam, 2% 3057
Nizoral A-D Shampoo 1901

Lopinavir (The risk of myopathy/rhabdomyolysis is increased by concomitant use of lovastatin with potent inhibitors of CYP3A4, particularly with higher doses of lovastatin; concomitant use should be avoided unless the benefits of combined therapy outweigh the increased risk). Products include:

Kaletra 452

Loratadine (The risk of myopathy/rhabdomyolysis is increased by concomitant use of lovastatin with potent inhibitors of CYP3A4, particularly with higher doses of lovastatin; concomitant use should be avoided unless the benefits of combined therapy outweigh the increased risk).

No products indexed under this heading.

Metronidazole (The risk of myopathy/rhabdomyolysis is increased by concomitant use of lovastatin with potent inhibitors of CYP3A4, particularly with higher doses of lovastatin; concomitant use should be avoided unless the benefits of combined therapy outweigh the increased risk). Products include:

Pylera Capsules 714

Metronidazole Benzoate (The risk of myopathy/rhabdomyolysis is increased by concomitant use of lovastatin with potent inhibitors of CYP3A4, particularly with higher doses of lovastatin; concomitant use should be avoided unless the benefits of combined therapy outweigh the increased risk).

No products indexed under this heading.

Metronidazole Hydrochloride (The risk of myopathy/rhabdomyolysis is increased by concomitant use of lovastatin with potent inhibitors of CYP3A4, particularly with higher doses of lovastatin; concomitant use should be avoided unless the benefits of combined therapy outweigh the increased risk).

No products indexed under this heading.

Miconazole (The risk of myopathy appears to be increased by high levels of HMG-CoA reductase inhibitory activity in plasma; lovastatin is metabolized by CYP3A4 isoenzyme, certain agents, such as azole antifungals, share this metabolic pathway and can raise the plasma levels of lovastatin and may increase the risk of myopathy).

No products indexed under this heading.

Miconazole Nitrate (The risk of myopathy/rhabdomyolysis is increased by concomitant use of lovastatin with potent inhibitors of CYP3A4, particularly with higher doses of lovastatin; concomitant use should be avoided unless the benefits of combined therapy outweigh the increased risk).

No products indexed under this heading.

Nefazodone Hydrochloride (The risk of myopathy appears to be increased by high levels of HMG-CoA reductase inhibitory activity in plasma; lovastatin is metabolized by CYP3A4 isoenzyme, certain agents, such as antidepressant nefazodone, share this metabolic pathway and can raise the plasma levels of lovastatin and may increase the risk of myopathy).

No products indexed under this heading.

Nelfinavir Mesylate (The risk of myopathy/rhabdomyolysis is increased by concomitant use of lovastatin with potent inhibitors of CYP3A4, particularly with higher doses of lovastatin; concomitant use should be avoided unless the benefits of combined therapy outweigh the increased risk).

No products indexed under this heading.

Nevirapine (The risk of myopathy/rhabdomyolysis is increased by concomitant use of lovastatin with potent inhibitors of CYP3A4, particularly with higher doses of lovastatin; concomitant use should be avoided unless the benefits of combined therapy outweigh the increased risk). Products include:

Viramune Oral Suspension 873
Viramune Tablets 873

Niacin (The incidence and severity of myopathy are increased by co-administration of HMG-CoA reductase inhibitors with drugs that cause myopathy when given alone, such as lipid-lowering doses of niacin; combined use should be avoided; if used concurrently, the dose of lovastatin should generally not exceed 20 mg). Products include:

Advicor Tablets 402
Bausch & Lomb Ocuvite DF Vitamin Supplement .... ⊙ 238
Dismutax Dietary Supplement 995
Niaspan Extended-Release Tablets 480
NT-Kinase Dietary Supplement 995
Simcor Tablets 502

Niacinamide (The risk of myopathy/rhabdomyolysis is increased by concomitant use of lovastatin with potent inhibitors of CYP3A4, particularly with higher doses of lovastatin; concomitant use should be avoided unless the benefits of combined therapy outweigh the increased risk). Products include:

BioLean Free Tablets .... ▣ 635

Nicotinamide (The risk of myopathy/rhabdomyolysis is increased by concomitant use of lovastatin with potent inhibitors of CYP3A4, particularly with higher doses of lovastatin; concomitant use should be avoided unless the benefits of combined therapy outweigh the increased risk).

No products indexed under this heading.

Nifedipine (The risk of myopathy/rhabdomyolysis is increased by concomitant use of lovastatin with potent inhibitors of CYP3A4, particularly with higher doses of lovastatin; concomitant use should be avoided unless the benefits of combined therapy outweigh the increased risk).

No products indexed under this heading.

Norfloxacin (The risk of myopathy/rhabdomyolysis is increased by concomitant use of lovastatin with potent inhibitors of CYP3A4, particularly with higher doses of lovastatin; concomitant use should be avoided unless the benefits of combined therapy outweigh the increased risk). Products include:

Noroxin Tablets 2069

Omeprazole (The risk of myopathy/rhabdomyolysis is increased by concomitant use of lovastatin with potent inhibitors of CYP3A4, particularly with higher doses of lovastatin; concomitant use should be avoided unless the benefits of combined therapy outweigh the increased risk).

No products indexed under this heading.

Oxiconazole Nitrate (The risk of myopathy appears to be increased by high levels of HMG-CoA reductase inhibitory activity in plasma; lovastatin is metabolized by CYP3A4 isoenzyme, certain agents, such as azole antifungals, share this metabolic pathway and can raise the plasma levels of lovastatin and may increase the risk of myopathy).

No products indexed under this heading.

Paroxetine Hydrochloride (The risk of myopathy/rhabdomyolysis is increased by concomitant use of lovastatin with potent inhibitors of CYP3A4, particularly with higher doses of lovastatin; concomitant use should be avoided unless the benefits of combined therapy outweigh the increased risk). Products include:

Paxil 1535
Paxil CR Controlled-Release Tablets 1544

Posaconazole (The risk of myopathy appears to be increased by high levels of HMG-CoA reductase inhibitory activity in plasma; lovastatin is metabolized by CYP3A4 isoenzyme, certain agents, such as azole antifungals, share this metabolic pathway and can raise the plasma levels of lovastatin and may increase the risk of myopathy). Products include:

Noxafil Oral Suspension 2889

Propoxyphene Hydrochloride (The risk of myopathy/rhabdomyolysis is increased by concomitant use of lovastatin with potent inhibitors of CYP3A4, particularly with higher doses of lovastatin; concomitant use should be avoided unless the benefits of combined therapy outweigh the increased risk).

No products indexed under this heading.

Propoxyphene Napsylate (The risk of myopathy/rhabdomyolysis is increased by concomitant use of lovastatin with potent inhibitors of CYP3A4, particularly with higher doses of lovastatin; concomitant use should be avoided unless the benefits of combined therapy outweigh the increased risk).

No products indexed under this heading.

Quinidine (The risk of myopathy/rhabdomyolysis is increased by concomitant use of lovastatin with potent inhibitors of CYP3A4, particularly with higher doses of lovastatin; concomitant use should be avoided unless the benefits of combined therapy outweigh the increased risk).

No products indexed under this heading.

Quinidine Hydrochloride (The risk of myopathy/rhabdomyolysis is increased by concomitant use of lovastatin with potent inhibitors of CYP3A4, particularly with higher doses of lovastatin; concomitant use should be avoided unless the benefits of combined therapy outweigh the increased risk).
No products indexed under this heading.

Quinidine Polygalacturonate (The risk of myopathy/rhabdomyolysis is increased by concomitant use of lovastatin with potent inhibitors of CYP3A4, particularly with higher doses of lovastatin; concomitant use should be avoided unless the benefits of combined therapy outweigh the increased risk).
No products indexed under this heading.

Quinidine Sulfate (The risk of myopathy/rhabdomyolysis is increased by concomitant use of lovastatin with potent inhibitors of CYP3A4, particularly with higher doses of lovastatin; concomitant use should be avoided unless the benefits of combined therapy outweigh the increased risk).
No products indexed under this heading.

Quinine (The risk of myopathy/rhabdomyolysis is increased by concomitant use of lovastatin with potent inhibitors of CYP3A4, particularly with higher doses of lovastatin; concomitant use should be avoided unless the benefits of combined therapy outweigh the increased risk).
No products indexed under this heading.

Quinine Sulfate (The risk of myopathy/rhabdomyolysis is increased by concomitant use of lovastatin with potent inhibitors of CYP3A4, particularly with higher doses of lovastatin; concomitant use should be avoided unless the benefits of combined therapy outweigh the increased risk).
No products indexed under this heading.

Quinupristin (The risk of myopathy/rhabdomyolysis is increased by concomitant use of lovastatin with potent inhibitors of CYP3A4, particularly with higher doses of lovastatin; concomitant use should be avoided unless the benefits of combined therapy outweigh the increased risk).
No products indexed under this heading.

Ranitidine Bismuth Citrate (The risk of myopathy/rhabdomyolysis is increased by concomitant use of lovastatin with potent inhibitors of CYP3A4, particularly with higher doses of lovastatin; concomitant use should be avoided unless the benefits of combined therapy outweigh the increased risk).
No products indexed under this heading.

Ranitidine Hydrochloride (The risk of myopathy/rhabdomyolysis is increased by concomitant use of lovastatin with potent inhibitors of CYP3A4, particularly with higher doses of lovastatin; concomitant use should be avoided unless the benefits of combined therapy outweigh the increased risk). Products include:
Zantac 75 Tablets 603
Zantac **1670**
Zantac Injection **1666**
Zantac Injection Pharmacy Bulk Package **1668**
Maximum Strength Zantac 150 Tablets **603**
Maximum Strength Zantac 150 Cool Mint Tablets **603**

Ritonavir (The risk of myopathy/rhabdomyolysis is increased by concomitant use of lovastatin with potent inhibitors of CYP3A4, particularly with higher doses of lovastatin; concomitant use should be avoided unless the benefits of combined therapy outweigh the increased risk). Products include:
Kaletra **452**
Norvir **489**

Saquinavir (The risk of myopathy/rhabdomyolysis is increased by concomitant use of lovastatin with potent inhibitors of CYP3A4, particularly with higher doses of lovastatin; concomitant use should be avoided unless the benefits of combined therapy outweigh the increased risk).
No products indexed under this heading.

Saquinavir Mesylate (The risk of myopathy/rhabdomyolysis is increased by concomitant use of lovastatin with potent inhibitors of CYP3A4, particularly with higher doses of lovastatin; concomitant use should be avoided unless the benefits of combined therapy outweigh the increased risk).
No products indexed under this heading.

Sertraline Hydrochloride (The risk of myopathy/rhabdomyolysis is increased by concomitant use of lovastatin with potent inhibitors of CYP3A4, particularly with higher doses of lovastatin; concomitant use should be avoided unless the benefits of combined therapy outweigh the increased risk).
No products indexed under this heading.

Sildenafil Citrate (The risk of myopathy/rhabdomyolysis is increased by concomitant use of lovastatin with potent inhibitors of CYP3A4, particularly with higher doses of lovastatin; concomitant use should be avoided unless the benefits of combined therapy outweigh the increased risk).
No products indexed under this heading.

Telithromycin (The risk of myopathy appears to be increased by high levels of HMG-CoA reductase inhibitory activity in plasma; lovastatin is metabolized by CYP3A4 isoenzyme, certain agents, such as macrolide antibiotics telithromycin, share this metabolic pathway and can raise the plasma levels of lovastatin and may increase the risk of myopathy). Products include:
Ketek Tablets **2744**

Terconazole (The risk of myopathy appears to be increased by high levels of HMG-CoA reductase inhibitory activity in plasma; lovastatin is metabolized by CYP3A4 isoenzyme, certain agents, such as azole antifungals, share this metabolic pathway and can raise the plasma levels of lovastatin and may increase the risk of myopathy).
No products indexed under this heading.

Tipranavir (The risk of myopathy/rhabdomyolysis is increased by concomitant use of lovastatin with potent inhibitors of CYP3A4, particularly with higher doses of lovastatin; concomitant use should be avoided unless the benefits of combined therapy outweigh the increased risk). Products include:
Aptivus Capsules **823**
Aptivus Oral Solution **823**

Troglitazone (The risk of myopathy/rhabdomyolysis is increased by concomitant use of lovastatin with potent inhibitors of CYP3A4, particularly with higher doses of lovastatin; concomitant use should be avoided unless the benefits of combined therapy outweigh the increased risk).
No products indexed under this heading.

Troleandomycin (The risk of myopathy/rhabdomyolysis is increased by concomitant use of lovastatin with potent inhibitors of CYP3A4, particularly with higher doses of lovastatin; concomitant use should be avoided unless the benefits of combined therapy outweigh the increased risk).
No products indexed under this heading.

Valproate Sodium (The risk of myopathy/rhabdomyolysis is increased by concomitant use of lovastatin with potent inhibitors of CYP3A4, particularly with higher doses of lovastatin; concomitant use should be avoided unless the benefits of combined therapy outweigh the increased risk).
No products indexed under this heading.

Vardenafil Hydrochloride (The risk of myopathy/rhabdomyolysis is increased by concomitant use of lovastatin with potent inhibitors of CYP3A4, particularly with higher doses of lovastatin; concomitant use should be avoided unless the benefits of combined therapy outweigh the increased risk). Products include:
Levitra Tablets **2876**

Verapamil Hydrochloride (The combined use of lovastatin at doses higher than 40 mg daily with verapamil should be avoided unless the clinical benefit is likely to outweigh the increased risk of myopathy). Products include:
Tarka Tablets **511**

Voriconazole (The risk of myopathy appears to be increased by high levels of HMG-CoA reductase inhibitory activity in plasma; lovastatin is metabolized by CYP3A4 isoenzyme, certain agents, such as azole antifungals, share this metabolic pathway and can raise the plasma levels of lovastatin and may increase the risk of myopathy).
No products indexed under this heading.

Warfarin Sodium (Co-administration has resulted in bleeding and/or increased prothrombin time in few patients).
No products indexed under this heading.

Zafirlukast (The risk of myopathy/rhabdomyolysis is increased by concomitant use of lovastatin with potent inhibitors of CYP3A4, particularly with higher doses of lovastatin; concomitant use should be avoided unless the benefits of combined therapy outweigh the increased risk). Products include:
Accolate Tablets **669**

Zileuton (The risk of myopathy/rhabdomyolysis is increased by concomitant use of lovastatin with potent inhibitors of CYP3A4, particularly with higher doses of lovastatin; concomitant use should be avoided unless the benefits of combined therapy outweigh the increased risk).
No products indexed under this heading.

Food Interactions

Alcohol (Lovastatin should be used with caution in patients who have consumed substantial quantity of alcohol and have a past history of liver disease; active liver disease and unexplained elevation in transaminase are contraindications to the use of lovastatin).

Grapefruit (The risk of myopathy/rhabdomyolysis is increased by concomitant use of lovastatin with potent inhibitors of CYP3A4, particularly with higher doses of lovastatin; concomitant use should be avoided unless the benefits of combined therapy outweigh the increased risk).

Grapefruit Juice (The risk of myopathy/rhabdomyolysis is increased by concomitant use of lovastatin with potent inhibitors of CYP3A4, particularly with higher doses of lovastatin; concomitant use should be avoided unless the benefits of combined therapy outweigh the increased risk).

Meal, unspecified (When lovastatin was given under fasting conditions, plasma concentrations of total inhibitors were on average about two-thirds those found when lovastatin was administered immediately after a standard meal).

MIACALCIN INJECTION

(Calcitonin-Salmon) **2273**
None cited in PDR database.

MIACALCIN NASAL SPRAY

(Calcitonin-Salmon) **2274**
May interact with:

Etidronate Disodium (Diphosphonate) (Prior diphosphonate use may reduce the anti-resorptive response to calcitonin-salmon nasal spray).
No products indexed under this heading.

Pamidronate Disodium (Prior diphosphonate use may reduce the anti-resorptive response to calcitonin-salmon nasal spray).
No products indexed under this heading.

MICARDIS TABLETS

(Telmisartan) **852**
May interact with cytochrome p450 2c19 substrates (selected) and certain other agents. Compounds in these categories include:

Amitriptyline Hydrochloride (Possible inhibition of the metabolism of drugs metabolized by CYP2C19).
No products indexed under this heading.

Amoxapine (Possible inhibition of the metabolism of drugs metabolized by CYP2C19).
No products indexed under this heading.

Carisoprodol (Possible inhibition of the metabolism of drugs metabolized by CYP2C19). Products include:

Soma Tablets 1931

Cilostazol (Possible inhibition of the metabolism of drugs metabolized by CYP2C19). Products include:

Pletal Tablets 2481

Citalopram Hydrobromide (Possible inhibition of the metabolism of drugs metabolized by CYP2C19). Products include:

Celexa 1160

Clomipramine Hydrochloride (Possible inhibition of the metabolism of drugs metabolized by CYP2C19).

No products indexed under this heading.

Cyclophosphamide (Possible inhibition of the metabolism of drugs metabolized by CYP2C19).

No products indexed under this heading.

Desipramine Hydrochloride (Possible inhibition of the metabolism of drugs metabolized by CYP2C19).

No products indexed under this heading.

Dextromethorphan (Possible inhibition of the metabolism of drugs metabolized by CYP2C19).

No products indexed under this heading.

Dextromethorphan Hydrobromide (Possible inhibition of the metabolism of drugs metabolized by CYP2C19). Products include:

PediaCare Children's Liquid Multi-Symptom Cold 1902
PediaCare Children's Long-Acting Cough 1902
Children's Sudafed PE Cold & Cough Liquid 1907
Sudafed PE Cold & Cough Caplets 1907
Children's Tylenol Plus Cough & Runny Nose Suspension Liquid 1912
Children's Tylenol Plus Cough & Sore Throat Suspension Liquid 1912
Children's Tylenol Plus Flu Suspension Liquid 1914
Children's Tylenol Plus Multi-Symptom Cold Suspension Liquid 1912
Tylenol Cold Severe Congestion Daytime Caplets with Cool Burst 1912
Tylenol Cold Head Congestion Daytime Caplets with Cool Burst 1910
Tylenol Cold Head Congestion Nighttime Caplets with Cool Burst 1910
Tylenol Cold Head Congestion Severe Daytime Caplets with Cool Burst 1910
Tylenol Cold Multi-Symptom Daytime Caplets with Cool Burst and Rapid Release Gels 1913
Tylenol Cold Multi-Symptom Daytime Liquid with Citrus Burst ... 1913
Tylenol Cold Multi-Symptom Nighttime Caplets with Cool Burst 1913
Tylenol Cold Multi-Symptom Nighttime Liquid with Cool Burst ... 1913
Tylenol Cold Multi-Symptom Severe Caplets with Cool Burst 1913
Tylenol Cold Multi-Symptom Severe Daytime Liquid with Citrus Burst 1913
Tylenol Cough & Sore Throat Daytime Liquid with Cool Burst...... 1918
Tylenol Cough & Sore Throat Nighttime Liquid with Cool Burst ... 1918
Vicks DayQuil Cold & Flu Multi-Symptom Relief .... ■616
Vicks DayQuil LiquiCaps 2567
Vicks DayQuil Liquid 2567
Vicks DayQuil Multi-Symptom Cold/Flu Relief 2567
Vicks NyQuil Cold & Flu Multi-Symptom Relief .... ■617
Vicks NyQuil LiquiCaps 2567
Vicks NyQuil Liquid 2567
Vicks NyQuil Multi-Symptom Cold/Flu Relief 2567

Diazepam (Possible inhibition of the metabolism of drugs metabolized by CYP2C19). Products include:

Valium Tablets 2658

Digoxin (Co-administration has resulted in median increases in digoxin peak plasma concentration (49%) and in trough concentration (20%); digoxin levels should be monitored when initiating, adjusting, and discontinuing telmisartan to avoid possible over- or under- digitalization). Products include:

Lanoxin Injection 1498
Lanoxin Injection Pediatric 1502
Lanoxin Tablets 1505

Divalproex Sodium (Possible inhibition of the metabolism of drugs metabolized by CYP2C19). Products include:

Depakote ER Tablets 423

Doxepin Hydrochloride (Possible inhibition of the metabolism of drugs metabolized by CYP2C19).

No products indexed under this heading.

Esomeprazole Magnesium (Possible inhibition of the metabolism of drugs metabolized by CYP2C19). Products include:

Nexium Delayed-Release Capsules 645
Nexium Delayed-Release Oral Suspension 645

Ethosuximide (Possible inhibition of the metabolism of drugs metabolized by CYP2C19).

No products indexed under this heading.

Ethotoin (Possible inhibition of the metabolism of drugs metabolized by CYP2C19).

No products indexed under this heading.

Felbamate (Possible inhibition of the metabolism of drugs metabolized by CYP2C19).

No products indexed under this heading.

Formoterol Fumarate (Possible inhibition of the metabolism of drugs metabolized by CYP2C19). Products include:

Foradil Aerolizer 2849
Perforomist Inhalation Solution 1025

Fosphenytoin (Possible inhibition of the metabolism of drugs metabolized by CYP2C19).

No products indexed under this heading.

Fosphenytoin Sodium (Possible inhibition of the metabolism of drugs metabolized by CYP2C19).

No products indexed under this heading.

Gabapentin (Possible inhibition of the metabolism of drugs metabolized by CYP2C19).

No products indexed under this heading.

Imipramine Hydrochloride (Possible inhibition of the metabolism of drugs metabolized by CYP2C19).

No products indexed under this heading.

Imipramine Pamoate (Possible inhibition of the metabolism of drugs metabolized by CYP2C19).

No products indexed under this heading.

Indomethacin (Possible inhibition of the metabolism of drugs metabolized by CYP2C19). Products include:

Indocin 2024

Indomethacin Sodium Trihydrate (Possible inhibition of the metabolism of drugs metabolized by CYP2C19). Products include:

Indocin I.V. 2489

Lamotrigine (Possible inhibition of the metabolism of drugs metabolized by CYP2C19). Products include:

Lamictal 1488

Lansoprazole (Possible inhibition of the metabolism of drugs metabolized by CYP2C19).

No products indexed under this heading.

Levetiracetam (Possible inhibition of the metabolism of drugs metabolized by CYP2C19). Products include:

Keppra Injection 3137
Keppra Oral Solution 3131
Keppra Tablets 3131

Maprotiline Hydrochloride (Possible inhibition of the metabolism of drugs metabolized by CYP2C19).

No products indexed under this heading.

Mephenytoin (Possible inhibition of the metabolism of drugs metabolized by CYP2C19).

No products indexed under this heading.

Mephobarbital (Possible inhibition of the metabolism of drugs metabolized by CYP2C19).

No products indexed under this heading.

Meprobamate (Possible inhibition of the metabolism of drugs metabolized by CYP2C19).

No products indexed under this heading.

Methsuximide (Possible inhibition of the metabolism of drugs metabolized by CYP2C19).

No products indexed under this heading.

Midazolam Hydrochloride (Possible inhibition of the metabolism of drugs metabolized by CYP2C19).

No products indexed under this heading.

Nelfinavir Mesylate (Possible inhibition of the metabolism of drugs metabolized by CYP2C19).

No products indexed under this heading.

Nilutamide (Possible inhibition of the metabolism of drugs metabolized by CYP2C19).

No products indexed under this heading.

Nortriptyline Hydrochloride (Possible inhibition of the metabolism of drugs metabolized by CYP2C19).

No products indexed under this heading.

Omeprazole (Possible inhibition of the metabolism of drugs metabolized by CYP2C19).

No products indexed under this heading.

Oxcarbazepine (Possible inhibition of the metabolism of drugs metabolized by CYP2C19).

No products indexed under this heading.

Pantoprazole Sodium (Possible inhibition of the metabolism of drugs metabolized by CYP2C19). Products include:

Protonix for Delayed-Release Oral Suspension 3254
Protonix Delayed-Release Tablets 3254
Protonix I.V. 3257

Paramethadione (Possible inhibition of the metabolism of drugs metabolized by CYP2C19).

No products indexed under this heading.

Pentamidine Isethionate (Possible inhibition of the metabolism of drugs metabolized by CYP2C19).

No products indexed under this heading.

Phenacemide (Possible inhibition of the metabolism of drugs metabolized by CYP2C19).

No products indexed under this heading.

Phenobarbital (Possible inhibition of the metabolism of drugs metabolized by CYP2C19). Products include:

Donnatal Extentabs 2507

Phenobarbital Sodium (Possible inhibition of the metabolism of drugs metabolized by CYP2C19).

No products indexed under this heading.

Phensuximide (Possible inhibition of the metabolism of drugs metabolized by CYP2C19).

No products indexed under this heading.

Phenytoin (Possible inhibition of the metabolism of drugs metabolized by CYP2C19).

No products indexed under this heading.

Phenytoin Sodium (Possible inhibition of the metabolism of drugs metabolized by CYP2C19). Products include:

Phenytek Capsules 2192

Primidone (Possible inhibition of the metabolism of drugs metabolized by CYP2C19).

No products indexed under this heading.

Progesterone (Possible inhibition of the metabolism of drugs metabolized by CYP2C19). Products include:

Crinone 4% Gel 992
Crinone 8% Gel 992
Prometrium Capsules (100 mg, 200 mg) 3047

Proguanil Hydrochloride (Possible inhibition of the metabolism of drugs metabolized by CYP2C19). Products include:

Malarone Pediatric Tablets 1521
Malarone Tablets 1521

Propranolol Hydrochloride (Possible inhibition of the metabolism of drugs metabolized by CYP2C19). Products include:

InnoPran XL Extended Release Capsules 1484

Protriptyline Hydrochloride (Possible inhibition of the metabolism of drugs metabolized by CYP2C19).

No products indexed under this heading.

Rabeprazole Sodium (Possible inhibition of the metabolism of drugs metabolized by CYP2C19). Products include:

Aciphex Tablets 1053

Sertraline Hydrochloride (Possible inhibition of the metabolism of drugs metabolized by CYP2C19).

No products indexed under this heading.

Teniposide (Possible inhibition of the metabolism of drugs metabolized by CYP2C19).

No products indexed under this heading.

Thioridazine (Possible inhibition of the metabolism of drugs metabolized by CYP2C19).
No products indexed under this heading.

Thioridazine Hydrochloride (Possible inhibition of the metabolism of drugs metabolized by CYP2C19). Products include:
Thioridazine Hydrochloride Tablets 2195

Tiagabine Hydrochloride (Possible inhibition of the metabolism of drugs metabolized by CYP2C19). Products include:
Gabitril Tablets 973

Tolbutamide (Possible inhibition of the metabolism of drugs metabolized by CYP2C19).
No products indexed under this heading.

Tolbutamide Sodium (Possible inhibition of the metabolism of drugs metabolized by CYP2C19).
No products indexed under this heading.

Topiramate (Possible inhibition of the metabolism of drugs metabolized by CYP2C19).
No products indexed under this heading.

Trimethadione (Possible inhibition of the metabolism of drugs metabolized by CYP2C19).
No products indexed under this heading.

Trimipramine Maleate (Possible inhibition of the metabolism of drugs metabolized by CYP2C19).
No products indexed under this heading.

Valproate Sodium (Possible inhibition of the metabolism of drugs metabolized by CYP2C19).
No products indexed under this heading.

Valproic Acid (Possible inhibition of the metabolism of drugs metabolized by CYP2C19).
No products indexed under this heading.

Voriconazole (Possible inhibition of the metabolism of drugs metabolized by CYP2C19).
No products indexed under this heading.

Warfarin Sodium (Co-administration has resulted in slight decrease in the mean warfarin trough plasma concentration; this decrease did not result in a change in INR).
No products indexed under this heading.

Zonisamide (Possible inhibition of the metabolism of drugs metabolized by CYP2C19). Products include:
Zonegran Capsules 1089

Food Interactions

Food, unspecified (Slightly reduces the bioavailability of telmisartan; Micardis tablets may be administered with or without food).

MICARDIS HCT TABLETS

(Hydrochlorothiazide, Telmisartan) 854
May interact with antihypertensives, barbiturates, corticosteroids, cytochrome p450 2c19 substrates (selected), oral hypoglycemic agents, insulin, lithium preparations, narcotic analgesics, nondepolarizing neuromuscular blocking agents, non-steroidal anti-inflammatory agents, potassium preparations, and certain other agents. Compounds in these categories include:

Acarbose (Thiazide diuretics may cause hyperglycemia; dosage adjustment of oral hypoglycemia agents may be required). Products include:
Precose Tablets 792

Acebutolol Hydrochloride (Co-administration with other antihypertensive agents may result in additive effect or potentiation).
No products indexed under this heading.

ACTH (Intensifies electrolyte depletion, particularly hypokalemia).
No products indexed under this heading.

Alfentanil Hydrochloride (Potentiation of orthostatic hypotension).
No products indexed under this heading.

Aliskiren (Co-administration with other antihypertensive agents may result in additive effect or potentiation). Products include:
Tekturna Tablets 2321
Tekturna HCT Tablets 2324

Amitriptyline Hydrochloride (Possible inhibition of the metabolism of drugs metabolized by CYP2C19).
No products indexed under this heading.

Amlodipine Besylate (Co-administration with other antihypertensive agents may result in additive effect or potentiation). Products include:
Azor Tablets 1005
Exforge Tablets 2238

Amoxapine (Possible inhibition of the metabolism of drugs metabolized by CYP2C19).
No products indexed under this heading.

Aprobarbital (Potentiation of orthostatic hypotension).
No products indexed under this heading.

Atenolol (Co-administration with other antihypertensive agents may result in additive effect or potentiation).
No products indexed under this heading.

Atracurium Besylate (Possible increased responsiveness to the muscle relaxants).
No products indexed under this heading.

Benazepril Hydrochloride (Co-administration with other antihypertensive agents may result in additive effect or potentiation).
No products indexed under this heading.

Bendroflumethiazide (Co-administration with other antihypertensive agents may result in additive effect or potentiation).
No products indexed under this heading.

Betamethasone Acetate (Corticosteroids intensify electrolyte depletion, particularly hypokalemia).
No products indexed under this heading.

Betamethasone Sodium Phosphate (Corticosteroids intensify electrolyte depletion, particularly hypokalemia).
No products indexed under this heading.

Betaxolol Hydrochloride (Co-administration with other antihypertensive agents may result in additive effect or potentiation).
No products indexed under this heading.

Bisoprolol Fumarate (Co-administration with other antihypertensive agents may result in additive effect or potentiation).
No products indexed under this heading.

Budesonide (Corticosteroids intensify electrolyte depletion, particularly hypokalemia). Products include:
Pulmicort Flexhaler 654
Symbicort 80/4.5 Inhalation Aerosol 659
Symbicort 160/4.5 Inhalation Aerosol 659

Buprenorphine Hydrochloride (Potentiation of orthostatic hypotension). Products include:
Suboxone Tablets 2601
Subutex Tablets 2601

Butabarbital (Potentiation of orthostatic hypotension).
No products indexed under this heading.

Butalbital (Potentiation of orthostatic hypotension).
No products indexed under this heading.

Candesartan Cilexetil (Co-administration with other antihypertensive agents may result in additive effect or potentiation). Products include:
Atacand Tablets 639
Atacand HCT 642

Captopril (Co-administration with other antihypertensive agents may result in additive effect or potentiation). Products include:
Captopril Tablets 2182

Carisoprodol (Possible inhibition of the metabolism of drugs metabolized by CYP2C19). Products include:
Soma Tablets 1931

Carteolol Hydrochloride (Co-administration with other antihypertensive agents may result in additive effect or potentiation).
No products indexed under this heading.

Celecoxib (Co-administration in some patients can result in reduced diuretic, natriuretic, and antihypertensive effects). Products include:
Celebrex Capsules 2979

Chlorothiazide (Co-administration with other antihypertensive agents may result in additive effect or potentiation).
No products indexed under this heading.

Chlorothiazide Sodium (Co-administration with other antihypertensive agents may result in additive effect or potentiation). Products include:
Intravenous Sodium Diuril 2490

Chlorpropamide (Thiazide diuretics may cause hyperglycemia; dosage adjustment of oral hypoglycemia agents may be required).
No products indexed under this heading.

Chlorthalidone (Co-administration with other antihypertensive agents may result in additive effect or potentiation). Products include:
Clorpres Tablets 2185

Cholestyramine (Absorption of hydrochlorothiazide is impaired in the presence of anionic exchange resins; cholestyramine binds the hydrochlorothiazide from the GI tract by up to 85%).
No products indexed under this heading.

Ciclesonide (Corticosteroids intensify electrolyte depletion, particularly hypokalemia). Products include:
Alvesco Inhalation Aerosol 2985
Omnaris Nasal Spray 2998

Cilostazol (Possible inhibition of the metabolism of drugs metabolized by CYP2C19). Products include:
Pletal Tablets 2481

Cisatracurium Besylate (Possible increased responsiveness to the muscle relaxants). Products include:
Nimbex Injection 484

Citalopram Hydrobromide (Possible inhibition of the metabolism of drugs metabolized by CYP2C19). Products include:
Celexa 1160

Clomipramine Hydrochloride (Possible inhibition of the metabolism of drugs metabolized by CYP2C19).
No products indexed under this heading.

Clonidine (Co-administration with other antihypertensive agents may result in additive effect or potentiation). Products include:
Catapres-TTS 842

Clonidine Hydrochloride (Co-administration with other antihypertensive agents may result in additive effect or potentiation). Products include:
Catapres Tablets 841
Clorpres Tablets 2185

Codeine Phosphate (Potentiation of orthostatic hypotension). Products include:
Tylenol with Codeine Tablets 2427

Colestipol Hydrochloride (Absorption of hydrochlorothiazide is impaired in the presence of anionic exchange resins; colestipol binds the hydroclorothiazide from the GI tract by up to 43%).
No products indexed under this heading.

Cortisone Acetate (Corticosteroids intensify electrolyte depletion, particularly hypokalemia).
No products indexed under this heading.

Cyclophosphamide (Possible inhibition of the metabolism of drugs metabolized by CYP2C19).
No products indexed under this heading.

Deserpidine (Co-administration with other antihypertensive agents may result in additive effect or potentiation).
No products indexed under this heading.

Desipramine Hydrochloride (Possible inhibition of the metabolism of drugs metabolized by CYP2C19).
No products indexed under this heading.

Dexamethasone (Corticosteroids intensify electrolyte depletion, particularly hypokalemia). Products include:

Ciprodex Otic Suspension 541

Dexamethasone Acetate (Corticosteroids intensify electrolyte depletion, particularly hypokalemia).
No products indexed under this heading.

Dexamethasone Sodium Phosphate (Corticosteroids intensify electrolyte depletion, particularly hypokalemia).
No products indexed under this heading.

Dextromethorphan (Possible inhibition of the metabolism of drugs metabolized by CYP2C19).
No products indexed under this heading.

Dextromethorphan Hydrobromide (Possible inhibition of the metabolism of drugs metabolized by CYP2C19). Products include:
PediaCare Children's Liquid Multi-Symptom Cold 1902
PediaCare Children's Long-Acting Cough 1902
Children's Sudafed PE Cold & Cough Liquid 1907
Sudafed PE Cold & Cough Caplets 1907
Children's Tylenol Plus Cough & Runny Nose Suspension Liquid 1912
Children's Tylenol Plus Cough & Sore Throat Suspension Liquid 1912
Children's Tylenol Plus Flu Suspension Liquid 1914
Children's Tylenol Plus Multi-Symptom Cold Suspension Liquid 1912
Tylenol Cold Severe Congestion Daytime Caplets with Cool Burst 1912
Tylenol Cold Head Congestion Daytime Caplets with Cool Burst 1910
Tylenol Cold Head Congestion Nighttime Caplets with Cool Burst 1910
Tylenol Cold Head Congestion Severe Daytime Caplets with Cool Burst 1910
Tylenol Cold Multi-Symptom Daytime Caplets with Cool Burst and Rapid Release Gels 1913
Tylenol Cold Multi-Symptom Daytime Liquid with Citrus Burst ... 1913
Tylenol Cold Multi-Symptom Nighttime Caplets with Cool Burst 1913
Tylenol Cold Multi-Symptom Nighttime Liquid with Cool Burst ... 1913
Tylenol Cold Multi-Symptom Severe Caplets with Cool Burst 1913
Tylenol Cold Multi-Symptom Severe Daytime Liquid with Citrus Burst 1913
Tylenol Cough & Sore Throat Daytime Liquid with Cool Burst 1918
Tylenol Cough & Sore Throat Nighttime Liquid with Cool Burst ... 1918
Vicks DayQuil Cold & Flu Multi-Symptom Relief .... ▣616
Vicks DayQuil LiquiCaps 2567
Vicks DayQuil Liquid 2567
Vicks DayQuil Multi-Symptom Cold/Flu Relief 2567
Vicks NyQuil Cold & Flu Multi-Symptom Relief .... ▣617
Vicks NyQuil LiquiCaps 2567
Vicks NyQuil Liquid 2567
Vicks NyQuil Multi-Symptom Cold/Flu Relief 2567

Dezocine (Potentiation of orthostatic hypotension).
No products indexed under this heading.

Diazepam (Possible inhibition of the metabolism of drugs metabolized by CYP2C19). Products include:
Valium Tablets 2658

Diazoxide (Co-administration with other antihypertensive agents may result in additive effect or potentiation). Products include:
Proglycem Capsules 1185
Proglycem Suspension 1185

Diclofenac Epolamine (Co-administration in some patients can result in reduced diuretic, natriuretic, and antihypertensive effects). Products include:
Flector Patch 561

Diclofenac Potassium (Co-administration in some patients can result in reduced diuretic, natriuretic, and antihypertensive effects).
No products indexed under this heading.

Diclofenac Sodium (Co-administration in some patients can result in reduced diuretic, natriuretic, and antihypertensive effects). Products include:
Diclofenac Sodium Ophthalmic Solution .... ⊙240
Voltaren Ophthalmic Solution 2336
Voltaren Tablets 2334
Voltaren-XR Tablets 2337

Digoxin (Co-administration has resulted in median increases in digoxin peak plasma concentration (49%) and in trough concentration (20%); digoxin levels should be monitored when initiating, adjusting, and discontinuing telmisartan to avoid possible over- or under-digitalization; thiazide-induced hypokalemia exaggerates or sensitizes the response of the heart to the toxic effects of digitalis, i.e., increased ventricular irritability). Products include:
Lanoxin Injection 1498
Lanoxin Injection Pediatric 1502
Lanoxin Tablets 1505

Diltiazem Hydrochloride (Co-administration with other antihypertensive agents may result in additive effect or potentiation). Products include:
Cardizem LA Extended Release Tablets 421

Divalproex Sodium (Possible inhibition of the metabolism of drugs metabolized by CYP2C19). Products include:
Depakote ER Tablets 423

Doxazosin Mesylate (Co-administration with other antihypertensive agents may result in additive effect or potentiation).
No products indexed under this heading.

Doxepin Hydrochloride (Possible inhibition of the metabolism of drugs metabolized by CYP2C19).
No products indexed under this heading.

Enalapril Maleate (Co-administration with other antihypertensive agents may result in additive effect or potentiation).
No products indexed under this heading.

Enalaprilat (Co-administration with other antihypertensive agents may result in additive effect or potentiation).
No products indexed under this heading.

Eprosartan Mesylate (Co-administration with other antihypertensive agents may result in additive effect or potentiation). Products include:
Teveten Tablets 515
Teveten HCT Tablets 517

Esmolol Hydrochloride (Co-administration with other antihypertensive agents may result in additive effect or potentiation).
No products indexed under this heading.

Esomeprazole Magnesium (Possible inhibition of the metabolism of drugs metabolized by CYP2C19). Products include:
Nexium Delayed-Release Capsules 645
Nexium Delayed-Release Oral Suspension 645

Ethosuximide (Possible inhibition of the metabolism of drugs metabolized by CYP2C19).
No products indexed under this heading.

Ethotoin (Possible inhibition of the metabolism of drugs metabolized by CYP2C19).
No products indexed under this heading.

Etodolac (Co-administration in some patients can result in reduced diuretic, natriuretic, and antihypertensive effects).
No products indexed under this heading.

Felbamate (Possible inhibition of the metabolism of drugs metabolized by CYP2C19).
No products indexed under this heading.

Felodipine (Co-administration with other antihypertensive agents may result in additive effect or potentiation).
No products indexed under this heading.

Fenoprofen Calcium (Co-administration in some patients can result in reduced diuretic, natriuretic, and antihypertensive effects). Products include:
Nalfon Capsules 2508

Fentanyl (Potentiation of orthostatic hypotension). Products include:
Duragesic Transdermal System 2405
Ionsys Transdermal System 2410

Fentanyl Citrate (Potentiation of orthostatic hypotension). Products include:
Actiq 959
Fentora Tablets 968

Fludrocortisone Acetate (Corticosteroids intensify electrolyte depletion, particularly hypokalemia).
No products indexed under this heading.

Flunisolide (Corticosteroids intensify electrolyte depletion, particularly hypokalemia). Products include:
Aerobid/Aerobid-M 1153

Flurbiprofen (Co-administration in some patients can result in reduced diuretic, natriuretic, and antihypertensive effects).
No products indexed under this heading.

Fluticasone Propionate (Corticosteroids intensify electrolyte depletion, particularly hypokalemia). Products include:
Advair Diskus 100/50 1276
Advair Diskus 250/50 1276
Advair Diskus 500/50 1276
Advair HFA 45/21 Inhalation Aerosol 1288
Advair HFA 115/21 Inhalation Aerosol 1288
Advair HFA 230/21 Inhalation Aerosol 1288
Flonase Nasal Spray 1431
Flovent Diskus 50 mcg 1435

Fluticasone Propionate HFA (Corticosteroids intensify electrolyte depletion, particularly hypokalemia). Products include:
Flovent HFA 1440

Formoterol Fumarate (Possible inhibition of the metabolism of drugs metabolized by CYP2C19). Products include:
Foradil Aerolizer 2849
Perforomist Inhalation Solution 1025

Fosinopril Sodium (Co-administration with other antihypertensive agents may result in additive effect or potentiation).
No products indexed under this heading.

Fosphenytoin (Possible inhibition of the metabolism of drugs metabolized by CYP2C19).
No products indexed under this heading.

Fosphenytoin Sodium (Possible inhibition of the metabolism of drugs metabolized by CYP2C19).
No products indexed under this heading.

Furosemide (Co-administration with other antihypertensive agents may result in additive effect or potentiation). Products include:
Furosemide Tablets 2186

Gabapentin (Possible inhibition of the metabolism of drugs metabolized by CYP2C19).
No products indexed under this heading.

Glimepiride (Thiazide diuretics may cause hyperglycemia; dosage adjustment of oral hypoglycemia agents may be required). Products include:
Avandaryl Tablets 1344
Duetact Tablets 3085

Glipizide (Thiazide diuretics may cause hyperglycemia; dosage adjustment of oral hypoglycemia agents may be required).
No products indexed under this heading.

Glyburide (Thiazide diuretics may cause hyperglycemia; dosage adjustment of oral hypoglycemia agents may be required).
No products indexed under this heading.

Guanabenz Acetate (Co-administration with other antihypertensive agents may result in additive effect or potentiation).
No products indexed under this heading.

Guanethidine Monosulfate (Co-administration with other antihypertensive agents may result in additive effect or potentiation).
No products indexed under this heading.

Hydralazine Hydrochloride (Co-administration with other antihypertensive agents may result in additive effect or potentiation).
No products indexed under this heading.

Hydrocodone Bitartrate (Potentiation of orthostatic hypotension). Products include:
Lortab 5/500 Tablets 3143
Lortab 7.5/500 Tablets 3144
Lortab 10/500 Tablets 3144
Vicodin Tablets 529
Vicodin ES Tablets 530
Vicodin HP Tablets 531
Vicoprofen Tablets 533
Zydone Tablets 1132

Hydrocodone Polistirex (Potentiation of orthostatic hypotension). Products include:
- Tussionex Pennkinetic Extended-Release Suspension 3154

Hydrocortisone (Corticosteroids intensify electrolyte depletion, particularly hypokalemia).
No products indexed under this heading.

Hydrocortisone Acetate (Corticosteroids intensify electrolyte depletion, particularly hypokalemia). Products include:
- Analpram-HC ... 1140
- Pramosone ... 1141

Hydrocortisone Sodium Phosphate (Corticosteroids intensify electrolyte depletion, particularly hypokalemia).
No products indexed under this heading.

Hydrocortisone Sodium Succinate (Corticosteroids intensify electrolyte depletion, particularly hypokalemia).
No products indexed under this heading.

Hydroflumethiazide (Co-administration with other antihypertensive agents may result in additive effect or potentiation).
No products indexed under this heading.

Hydromorphone Hydrochloride (Potentiation of orthostatic hypotension).
No products indexed under this heading.

Ibuprofen (Co-administration in some patients can result in reduced diuretic, natriuretic, and antihypertensive effects). Products include:
- Motrin IB Tablets and Caplets ... 1900
- Children's Motrin Oral Suspension ... 1901
- Children's Motrin Non-Staining Dye-Free Oral Suspension ... 1901
- Children's Motrin Cold Oral Suspension ... 1899
- Infants' Motrin Concentrated Drops ... 1901
- Infants' Motrin Non-Staining Dye-Free Concentrated Drops ... 1901
- Junior Strength Motrin Caplets and Chewable Tablets ... 1901
- Vicoprofen Tablets ... 533

Imipramine Hydrochloride (Possible inhibition of the metabolism of drugs metabolized by CYP2C19).
No products indexed under this heading.

Imipramine Pamoate (Possible inhibition of the metabolism of drugs metabolized by CYP2C19).
No products indexed under this heading.

Indapamide (Co-administration with other antihypertensive agents may result in additive effect or potentiation). Products include:
- Indapamide Tablets ... 2188

Indomethacin (Possible inhibition of the metabolism of drugs metabolized by CYP2C19). Products include:
- Indocin ... 2024

Indomethacin Sodium Trihydrate (Possible inhibition of the metabolism of drugs metabolized by CYP2C19). Products include:
- Indocin I.V. ... 2489

Insulin (Thiazide diuretics may cause hyperglycemia; dosage adjustment of insulin may be required).
No products indexed under this heading.

Insulin, Human, Zinc Suspension (Thiazide diuretics may cause hyperglycemia; dosage adjustment of insulin may be required).
No products indexed under this heading.

Insulin, Human (rDNA origin) (Thiazide diuretics may cause hyperglycemia; dosage adjustment of insulin may be required). Products include:
- Exubera Inhalation Powder ... 2515

Insulin, Human NPH (Thiazide diuretics may cause hyperglycemia; dosage adjustment of insulin may be required). Products include:
- Humulin N Vial ... 1846

Insulin, Human Regular (Thiazide diuretics may cause hyperglycemia; dosage adjustment of insulin may be required). Products include:
- Humulin R ... 1849
- Humulin R (U-500) ... 1850

Insulin, Human Regular and Human NPH Mixture (Thiazide diuretics may cause hyperglycemia; dosage adjustment of insulin may be required). Products include:
- Humulin 50/50, 100 Units ... 1843
- Humulin 70/30 Vial ... 1844

Insulin, NPH (Thiazide diuretics may cause hyperglycemia; dosage adjustment of insulin may be required).
No products indexed under this heading.

Insulin, Regular (Thiazide diuretics may cause hyperglycemia; dosage adjustment of insulin may be required).
No products indexed under this heading.

Insulin, Regular and NPH mixture (Thiazide diuretics may cause hyperglycemia; dosage adjustment of insulin may be required).
No products indexed under this heading.

Insulin, Zinc Crystals (Thiazide diuretics may cause hyperglycemia; dosage adjustment of insulin may be required).
No products indexed under this heading.

Insulin, Zinc Suspension (Thiazide diuretics may cause hyperglycemia; dosage adjustment of insulin may be required).
No products indexed under this heading.

Insulin Aspart (Thiazide diuretics may cause hyperglycemia; dosage adjustment of insulin may be required).
No products indexed under this heading.

Insulin Aspart, Human (Thiazide diuretics may cause hyperglycemia; dosage adjustment of insulin may be required). Products include:
- NovoLog Mix 70/30 ... 2364

Insulin Aspart, Human Regular (Thiazide diuretics may cause hyperglycemia; dosage adjustment of insulin may be required). Products include:
- NovoLog Injection ... 2359

Insulin Aspart Protamine, Human (Thiazide diuretics may cause hyperglycemia; dosage adjustment of insulin may be required). Products include:
- NovoLog Mix 70/30 ... 2364

Insulin Detemir (rDNA Origin) (Thiazide diuretics may cause hyperglycemia; dosage adjustment of insulin may be required). Products include:
- Levemir Injection ... 2352

Insulin glargine (Thiazide diuretics may cause hyperglycemia; dosage adjustment of insulin may be required). Products include:
- Lantus Injection ... 2749

Insulin Glulisine (Thiazide diuretics may cause hyperglycemia; dosage adjustment of insulin may be required). Products include:
- Apidra Injection ... 2706

Insulin Lispro, Human (Thiazide diuretics may cause hyperglycemia; dosage adjustment of insulin may be required). Products include:
- Humalog-Pen and KwikPen ... 1829
- Humalog Mix 50/50-Pen and KwikPen ... 1833
- Humalog Mix 75/25-Pen and KwikPen ... 1835

Insulin Lispro Protamine, Human (Thiazide diuretics may cause hyperglycemia; dosage adjustment of insulin may be required). Products include:
- Humalog Mix 50/50-Pen and KwikPen ... 1833
- Humalog Mix 75/25-Pen and KwikPen ... 1835

Irbesartan (Co-administration with other antihypertensive agents may result in additive effect or potentiation). Products include:
- Avalide Tablets ... 892
- Avalide Tablets ... 2713
- Avapro Tablets ... 897
- Avapro Tablets ... 2718

Isradipine (Co-administration with other antihypertensive agents may result in additive effect or potentiation). Products include:
- DynaCirc CR Controlled Release Tablets ... 1407

Ketoprofen (Co-administration in some patients can result in reduced diuretic, natriuretic, and antihypertensive effects).
No products indexed under this heading.

Ketorolac Tromethamine (Co-administration in some patients can result in reduced diuretic, natriuretic, and antihypertensive effects).
No products indexed under this heading.

Labetalol Hydrochloride (Co-administration with other antihypertensive agents may result in additive effect or potentiation).
No products indexed under this heading.

Lamotrigine (Possible inhibition of the metabolism of drugs metabolized by CYP2C19). Products include:
- Lamictal ... 1488

Lansoprazole (Possible inhibition of the metabolism of drugs metabolized by CYP2C19).
No products indexed under this heading.

Levetiracetam (Possible inhibition of the metabolism of drugs metabolized by CYP2C19). Products include:
- Keppra Injection ... 3137
- Keppra Oral Solution ... 3131
- Keppra Tablets ... 3131

Levorphanol Tartrate (Potentiation of orthostatic hypotension).
No products indexed under this heading.

Lisinopril (Co-administration with other antihypertensive agents may result in additive effect or potentiation). Products include:
- Prinivil Tablets ... 2087
- Prinzide Tablets ... 2092

Lithium (Diuretics reduce the renal clearance of lithium and add a high risk of lithium toxicity; concurrent use should be avoided).
No products indexed under this heading.

Lithium Carbonate (Diuretics reduce the renal clearance of lithium and add a high risk of lithium toxicity; concurrent use should be avoided).
No products indexed under this heading.

Lithium Citrate (Diuretics reduce the renal clearance of lithium and add a high risk of lithium toxicity; concurrent use should be avoided).
No products indexed under this heading.

Losartan Potassium (Co-administration with other antihypertensive agents may result in additive effect or potentiation). Products include:
- Cozaar Tablets ... 1973

Maprotiline Hydrochloride (Possible inhibition of the metabolism of drugs metabolized by CYP2C19).
No products indexed under this heading.

Mecamylamine Hydrochloride (Co-administration with other antihypertensive agents may result in additive effect or potentiation).
No products indexed under this heading.

Meclofenamate Sodium (Co-administration in some patients can result in reduced diuretic, natriuretic, and antihypertensive effects).
No products indexed under this heading.

Mefenamic Acid (Co-administration in some patients can result in reduced diuretic, natriuretic, and antihypertensive effects).
No products indexed under this heading.

Meloxicam (Co-administration in some patients can result in reduced diuretic, natriuretic, and antihypertensive effects). Products include:
- Mobic Oral Suspension ... 863
- Mobic Tablets ... 863

Meperidine Hydrochloride (Potentiation of orthostatic hypotension).
No products indexed under this heading.

Mephenytoin (Possible inhibition of the metabolism of drugs metabolized by CYP2C19).
No products indexed under this heading.

Mephobarbital (Potentiation of orthostatic hypotension).
No products indexed under this heading.

Meprobamate (Possible inhibition of the metabolism of drugs metabolized by CYP2C19).
No products indexed under this heading.

Metformin Hydrochloride (Thiazide diuretics may cause hyperglycemia; dosage adjustment of oral hypoglycemia agents may be required). Products include:
- ActoPlus Met Tablets ... 3071

IMPORTANT NOTE: Always consult each drug listing in the patient's regimen for possible interactions.

Avandamet Tablets 1336
Janumet Tablets 2041
PrandiMet Tablets 2967

Methadone Hydrochloride (Potentiation of orthostatic hypotension).
No products indexed under this heading.

Methsuximide (Possible inhibition of the metabolism of drugs metabolized by CYP2C19).
No products indexed under this heading.

Methyclothiazide (Co-administration with other antihypertensive agents may result in additive effect or potentiation).
No products indexed under this heading.

Methyldopa (Co-administration with other antihypertensive agents may result in additive effect or potentiation).
No products indexed under this heading.

Methyldopate Hydrochloride (Co-administration with other antihypertensive agents may result in additive effect or potentiation).
No products indexed under this heading.

Methylprednisolone Acetate (Corticosteroids intensify electrolyte depletion, particularly hypokalemia).
No products indexed under this heading.

Methylprednisolone Sodium Succinate (Corticosteroids intensify electrolyte depletion, particularly hypokalemia).
No products indexed under this heading.

Metocurine Iodide (Possible increased responsiveness to the muscle relaxants).
No products indexed under this heading.

Metolazone (Co-administration with other antihypertensive agents may result in additive effect or potentiation).
No products indexed under this heading.

Metoprolol Succinate (Co-administration with other antihypertensive agents may result in additive effect or potentiation). Products include:
Toprol-XL Tablets 666

Metoprolol Tartrate (Co-administration with other antihypertensive agents may result in additive effect or potentiation).
No products indexed under this heading.

Metyrosine (Co-administration with other antihypertensive agents may result in additive effect or potentiation). Products include:
Demser Capsules 1989

Mibefradil Dihydrochloride (Co-administration with other antihypertensive agents may result in additive effect or potentiation).
No products indexed under this heading.

Midazolam Hydrochloride (Possible inhibition of the metabolism of drugs metabolized by CYP2C19).
No products indexed under this heading.

Miglitol (Thiazide diuretics may cause hyperglycemia; dosage adjustment of oral hypoglycemia agents may be required).
No products indexed under this heading.

Minoxidil (Co-administration with other antihypertensive agents may result in additive effect or potentiation).
No products indexed under this heading.

Mivacurium Chloride (Possible increased responsiveness to the muscle relaxants).
No products indexed under this heading.

Moexipril Hydrochloride (Co-administration with other antihypertensive agents may result in additive effect or potentiation).
No products indexed under this heading.

Mometasone Furoate (Corticosteroids intensify electrolyte depletion, particularly hypokalemia). Products include:
Asmanex Twisthaler 2797
Elocon Cream 0.1% 2840
Elocon Lotion 0.1% 2841
Elocon Ointment 0.1% 2842

Mometasone Furoate Monohydrate (Corticosteroids intensify electrolyte depletion, particularly hypokalemia). Products include:
Nasonex Nasal Spray 2883

Morphine Sulfate (Potentiation of orthostatic hypotension). Products include:
Avinza Capsules 1772
DepoDur Injection 1095
MS Contin Tablets 2585

Nabumetone (Co-administration in some patients can result in reduced diuretic, natriuretic, and antihypertensive effects).
No products indexed under this heading.

Nadolol (Co-administration with other antihypertensive agents may result in additive effect or potentiation). Products include:
Nadolol Tablets 2191

Naproxen (Co-administration in some patients can result in reduced diuretic, natriuretic, and antihypertensive effects). Products include:
EC-Naprosyn Delayed-Release Tablets 2632
Naprosyn Suspension 2632
Naprosyn Tablets 2632

Naproxen Sodium (Co-administration in some patients can result in reduced diuretic, natriuretic, and antihypertensive effects). Products include:
Anaprox Tablets 2632
Anaprox DS Tablets 2632
Treximet Tablets 1616

Nateglinide (Thiazide diuretics may cause hyperglycemia; dosage adjustment of oral hypoglycemia agents may be required). Products include:
Starlix Tablets 2314

Nebivolol (Co-administration with other antihypertensive agents may result in additive effect or potentiation). Products include:
Bystolic Tablets 1155

Nelfinavir Mesylate (Possible inhibition of the metabolism of drugs metabolized by CYP2C19).
No products indexed under this heading.

Nicardipine Hydrochloride (Co-administration with other antihypertensive agents may result in additive effect or potentiation). Products include:
Cardene I.V. 1093

Nifedipine (Co-administration with other antihypertensive agents may result in additive effect or potentiation).
No products indexed under this heading.

Nilutamide (Possible inhibition of the metabolism of drugs metabolized by CYP2C19).
No products indexed under this heading.

Nisoldipine (Co-administration with other antihypertensive agents may result in additive effect or potentiation). Products include:
Sular Extended Release Tablets 2975

Nitroglycerin (Co-administration with other antihypertensive agents may result in additive effect or potentiation). Products include:
Nitro-Dur Transdermal Infusion System 2887
Nitrolingual Pumpspray 2965

Norepinephrine Bitartrate (Possible decreased response to pressor amines).
No products indexed under this heading.

Nortriptyline Hydrochloride (Possible inhibition of the metabolism of drugs metabolized by CYP2C19).
No products indexed under this heading.

Omeprazole (Possible inhibition of the metabolism of drugs metabolized by CYP2C19).
No products indexed under this heading.

Oxaprozin (Co-administration in some patients can result in reduced diuretic, natriuretic, and antihypertensive effects).
No products indexed under this heading.

Oxcarbazepine (Possible inhibition of the metabolism of drugs metabolized by CYP2C19).
No products indexed under this heading.

Oxycodone Hydrochloride (Potentiation of orthostatic hypotension). Products include:
OxyContin Tablets 2589
OxyIR Capsules 2593
Percocet Tablets 1127
Percodan Tablets 1130

Pancuronium Bromide (Possible increased responsiveness to the muscle relaxants).
No products indexed under this heading.

Pantoprazole Sodium (Possible inhibition of the metabolism of drugs metabolized by CYP2C19). Products include:
Protonix for Delayed-Release Oral Suspension 3254
Protonix Delayed-Release Tablets 3254
Protonix I.V. 3257

Paramethadione (Possible inhibition of the metabolism of drugs metabolized by CYP2C19).
No products indexed under this heading.

Penbutolol Sulfate (Co-administration with other antihypertensive agents may result in additive effect or potentiation).
No products indexed under this heading.

Pentamidine Isethionate (Possible inhibition of the metabolism of drugs metabolized by CYP2C19).
No products indexed under this heading.

Pentobarbital Sodium (Potentiation of orthostatic hypotension). Products include:
Nembutal Sodium Solution, USP 2494

Perindopril Erbumine (Co-administration with other antihypertensive agents may result in additive effect or potentiation). Products include:
Aceon Tablets (2 mg, 4 mg, 8 mg) 3038

Phenacemide (Possible inhibition of the metabolism of drugs metabolized by CYP2C19).
No products indexed under this heading.

Phenobarbital (Potentiation of orthostatic hypotension). Products include:
Donnatal Extentabs 2507

Phenobarbital Sodium (Possible inhibition of the metabolism of drugs metabolized by CYP2C19).
No products indexed under this heading.

Phenoxybenzamine Hydrochloride (Co-administration with other antihypertensive agents may result in additive effect or potentiation). Products include:
Dibenzyline Capsules 3188

Phensuximide (Possible inhibition of the metabolism of drugs metabolized by CYP2C19).
No products indexed under this heading.

Phentolamine Mesylate (Co-administration with other antihypertensive agents may result in additive effect or potentiation).
No products indexed under this heading.

Phenylbutazone (Co-administration in some patients can result in reduced diuretic, natriuretic, and antihypertensive effects).
No products indexed under this heading.

Phenytoin (Possible inhibition of the metabolism of drugs metabolized by CYP2C19).
No products indexed under this heading.

Phenytoin Sodium (Possible inhibition of the metabolism of drugs metabolized by CYP2C19). Products include:
Phenytek Capsules 2192

Pindolol (Co-administration with other antihypertensive agents may result in additive effect or potentiation).
No products indexed under this heading.

Pioglitazone Hydrochloride (Thiazide diuretics may cause hyperglycemia; dosage adjustment of oral hypoglycemia agents may be required). Products include:
ActoPlus Met Tablets 3071
Actos Tablets 3077
Duetact Tablets 3085

Piroxicam (Co-administration in some patients can result in reduced diuretic, natriuretic, and antihypertensive effects).
No products indexed under this heading.

Polythiazide (Co-administration with other antihypertensive agents may result in additive effect or potentiation).
No products indexed under this heading.

Potassium Acid Phosphate (Concurrent use of potassium supplements or salt substitute is not recommended). Products include:
K-Phos Original (Sodium Free) Tablets 814

Potassium Bicarbonate (Concurrent use of potassium supplements or salt substitute is not recommended).
No products indexed under this heading.

Potassium Chloride (Concurrent use of potassium supplements or salt substitute is not recommended). Products include:
MoviPrep Oral Solution 2679

Potassium Citrate (Concurrent use of potassium supplements or salt substitute is not recommended). Products include:
BioLean Free Tablets 635
Urocit-K Tablets 2176

Potassium Gluconate (Concurrent use of potassium supplements or salt substitute is not recommended).
No products indexed under this heading.

Potassium Phosphate (Concurrent use of potassium supplements or salt substitute is not recommended). Products include:
K-Phos Neutral Tablets 813

Prazosin Hydrochloride (Co-administration with other antihypertensive agents may result in additive effect or potentiation).
No products indexed under this heading.

Prednisolone Acetate (Corticosteroids intensify electrolyte depletion, particularly hypokalemia). Products include:
Pred Forte Ophthalmic Suspension .... ⊙ 227
Pred Mild Ophthalmic Suspension .... ⊙ 230
Pred-G Ophthalmic Ointment .... ⊙ 229
Pred-G Ophthalmic Suspension .... ⊙ 228

Prednisolone Sodium Phosphate (Corticosteroids intensify electrolyte depletion, particularly hypokalemia).
No products indexed under this heading.

Prednisolone Tebutate (Corticosteroids intensify electrolyte depletion, particularly hypokalemia).
No products indexed under this heading.

Prednisone (Corticosteroids intensify electrolyte depletion, particularly hypokalemia).
No products indexed under this heading.

Primidone (Possible inhibition of the metabolism of drugs metabolized by CYP2C19).
No products indexed under this heading.

Progesterone (Possible inhibition of the metabolism of drugs metabolized by CYP2C19). Products include:
Crinone 4% Gel 992
Crinone 8% Gel 992
Prometrium Capsules (100 mg, 200 mg) 3047

Proguanil Hydrochloride (Possible inhibition of the metabolism of drugs metabolized by CYP2C19). Products include:
Malarone Pediatric Tablets 1521
Malarone Tablets 1521

Propoxyphene Hydrochloride (Potentiation of orthostatic hypotension).
No products indexed under this heading.

Propoxyphene Napsylate (Potentiation of orthostatic hypotension).
No products indexed under this heading.

Propranolol Hydrochloride (Possible inhibition of the metabolism of drugs metabolized by CYP2C19). Products include:
InnoPran XL Extended Release Capsules 1484

Protriptyline Hydrochloride (Possible inhibition of the metabolism of drugs metabolized by CYP2C19).
No products indexed under this heading.

Quinapril Hydrochloride (Co-administration with other antihypertensive agents may result in additive effect or potentiation).
No products indexed under this heading.

Rabeprazole Sodium (Possible inhibition of the metabolism of drugs metabolized by CYP2C19). Products include:
Aciphex Tablets 1053

Ramipril (Co-administration with other antihypertensive agents may result in additive effect or potentiation).
No products indexed under this heading.

Rapacuronium Bromide (Possible increased responsiveness to the muscle relaxants).
No products indexed under this heading.

Rauwolfia Serpentina (Co-administration with other antihypertensive agents may result in additive effect or potentiation).
No products indexed under this heading.

Remifentanil Hydrochloride (Potentiation of orthostatic hypotension).
No products indexed under this heading.

Repaglinide (Thiazide diuretics may cause hyperglycemia; dosage adjustment of oral hypoglycemia agents may be required). Products include:
PrandiMet Tablets 2967
Prandin Tablets 2971

Rescinnamine (Co-administration with other antihypertensive agents may result in additive effect or potentiation).
No products indexed under this heading.

Reserpine (Co-administration with other antihypertensive agents may result in additive effect or potentiation).
No products indexed under this heading.

Rocuronium Bromide (Possible increased responsiveness to the muscle relaxants). Products include:
Zemuron Injection 2947

Rofecoxib (Co-administration in some patients can result in reduced diuretic, natriuretic, and antihypertensive effects).
No products indexed under this heading.

Rosiglitazone Maleate (Thiazide diuretics may cause hyperglycemia; dosage adjustment of oral hypoglycemia agents may be required). Products include:
Avandamet Tablets 1336
Avandaryl Tablets 1344
Avandia Tablets 1351

Secobarbital Sodium (Potentiation of orthostatic hypotension).
No products indexed under this heading.

Sertraline Hydrochloride (Possible inhibition of the metabolism of drugs metabolized by CYP2C19).
No products indexed under this heading.

Sitagliptin Phosphate (Thiazide diuretics may cause hyperglycemia; dosage adjustment of oral hypoglycemia agents may be required). Products include:
Janumet Tablets 2041
Januvia Tablets 2048

Sodium Nitroprusside (Co-administration with other antihypertensive agents may result in additive effect or potentiation).
No products indexed under this heading.

Sotalol Hydrochloride (Co-administration with other antihypertensive agents may result in additive effect or potentiation).
No products indexed under this heading.

Spirapril Hydrochloride (Co-administration with other antihypertensive agents may result in additive effect or potentiation).
No products indexed under this heading.

Sufentanil Citrate (Potentiation of orthostatic hypotension).
No products indexed under this heading.

Sulindac (Co-administration in some patients can result in reduced diuretic, natriuretic, and antihypertensive effects). Products include:
Clinoril Tablets 1962

Teniposide (Possible inhibition of the metabolism of drugs metabolized by CYP2C19).
No products indexed under this heading.

Terazosin Hydrochloride (Co-administration with other antihypertensive agents may result in additive effect or potentiation).
No products indexed under this heading.

Thiamylal Sodium (Potentiation of orthostatic hypotension).
No products indexed under this heading.

Thioridazine (Possible inhibition of the metabolism of drugs metabolized by CYP2C19).
No products indexed under this heading.

Thioridazine Hydrochloride (Possible inhibition of the metabolism of drugs metabolized by CYP2C19). Products include:
Thioridazine Hydrochloride Tablets 2195

Tiagabine Hydrochloride (Possible inhibition of the metabolism of drugs metabolized by CYP2C19). Products include:
Gabitril Tablets 973

Timolol Maleate (Co-administration with other antihypertensive agents may result in additive effect or potentiation). Products include:
Combigan Ophthalmic Solution 553
Cosopt Sterile Ophthalmic Solution 1969
Timoptic Sterile Ophthalmic Solution 2121
Timoptic in Ocudose 2124
Timoptic-XE Sterile Ophthalmic Gel Forming Solution 2125

Tolazamide (Thiazide diuretics may cause hyperglycemia; dosage adjustment of oral hypoglycemia agents may be required).
No products indexed under this heading.

Tolbutamide (Possible inhibition of the metabolism of drugs metabolized by CYP2C19).
No products indexed under this heading.

Tolbutamide Sodium (Possible inhibition of the metabolism of drugs metabolized by CYP2C19).
No products indexed under this heading.

Tolmetin Sodium (Co-administration in some patients can result in reduced diuretic, natriuretic, and antihypertensive effects).
No products indexed under this heading.

Topiramate (Possible inhibition of the metabolism of drugs metabolized by CYP2C19).
No products indexed under this heading.

Torsemide (Co-administration with other antihypertensive agents may result in additive effect or potentiation). Products include:
Demadex Injection 2630
Demadex Tablets 2630

Trandolapril (Co-administration with other antihypertensive agents may result in additive effect or potentiation). Products include:
Mavik Tablets 472
Tarka Tablets 511

Triamcinolone (Corticosteroids intensify electrolyte depletion, particularly hypokalemia).
No products indexed under this heading.

Triamcinolone Acetonide (Corticosteroids intensify electrolyte depletion, particularly hypokalemia). Products include:
Azmacort Inhalation Aerosol 407
Nasacort AQ Nasal Spray 2765
Triesence Injectable Suspension .... ⊙ 209

Triamcinolone Diacetate (Corticosteroids intensify electrolyte depletion, particularly hypokalemia).
No products indexed under this heading.

Triamcinolone Hexacetonide (Corticosteroids intensify electrolyte depletion, particularly hypokalemia).
No products indexed under this heading.

Trimethadione (Possible inhibition of the metabolism of drugs metabolized by CYP2C19).
No products indexed under this heading.

Trimethaphan Camsylate (Co-administration with other antihypertensive agents may result in additive effect or potentiation).
No products indexed under this heading.

Trimipramine Maleate (Possible inhibition of the metabolism of drugs metabolized by CYP2C19).
No products indexed under this heading.

Troglitazone (Thiazide diuretics may cause hyperglycemia; dosage adjustment of oral hypoglycemia agents may be required).
No products indexed under this heading.

Valdecoxib (Co-administration in some patients can result in reduced diuretic, natriuretic, and antihypertensive effects).
No products indexed under this heading.

Valproate Sodium (Possible inhibition of the metabolism of drugs metabolized by CYP2C19).
No products indexed under this heading.

Valproic Acid (Possible inhibition of the metabolism of drugs metabolized by CYP2C19).
No products indexed under this heading.

Valsartan (Co-administration with other antihypertensive agents may result in additive effect or potentiation). Products include:
Diovan Tablets **2212**
Diovan HCT Tablets **2216**
Exforge Tablets **2238**

Vecuronium Bromide (Possible increased responsiveness to the muscle relaxants).
No products indexed under this heading.

Verapamil Hydrochloride (Co-administration with other antihypertensive agents may result in additive effect or potentiation). Products include:
Tarka Tablets **511**

Voriconazole (Possible inhibition of the metabolism of drugs metabolized by CYP2C19).
No products indexed under this heading.

Warfarin Sodium (Co-administration has resulted in slight decrease in the mean warfarin trough plasma concentration; this decrease did not result in a change in INR).
No products indexed under this heading.

Zonisamide (Possible inhibition of the metabolism of drugs metabolized by CYP2C19). Products include:
Zonegran Capsules **1089**

Food Interactions

Alcohol (Potentiation of orthostatic hypotension).

Food, unspecified (Slightly reduces the bioavailability of telmisartan with reduction in AUC of about 6%).

MIMYX CREAM

(Glycerin) **3059**
None cited in PDR database.

MIRAPEX TABLETS

(Pramipexole Dihydrochloride) **857**
May interact with dopamine D2 antagonists, quinidine, and certain other agents. Compounds in these categories include:

Amantadine Hydrochloride (Population pharmacokinetic analyses suggest that amantadine may slightly decrease the oral clearance of pramipexole).
No products indexed under this heading.

Chlorpromazine (Co-administration with dopamine antagonists may diminish the effectiveness of pramipexole).
No products indexed under this heading.

Chlorpromazine Hydrochloride (Co-administration with dopamine antagonists may diminish the effectiveness of pramipexole).
No products indexed under this heading.

Chlorprothixene (Co-administration with dopamine antagonists may diminish the effectiveness of pramipexole).
No products indexed under this heading.

Chlorprothixene Hydrochloride (Co-administration with dopamine antagonists may diminish the effectiveness of pramipexole).
No products indexed under this heading.

Cimetidine (Co-administration with cimetidine, a known inhibitor of renal tubular secretion of organic acids via anionic transport, has caused a 50% increase in pramipexole AUC and a 40% increase in half-life).
No products indexed under this heading.

Cimetidine Hydrochloride (Co-administration with cimetidine, a known inhibitor of renal tubular secretion of organic acids via anionic transport, has caused a 50% increase in pramipexole AUC and a 40% increase in half-life).
No products indexed under this heading.

Diltiazem Hydrochloride (Co-administration of drugs that are secreted by the cationic transport system, e.g., diltiazem, decrease the oral clearance of pramipexole by about 20%). Products include:
Cardizem LA Extended Release Tablets **421**

Fluphenazine Decanoate (Co-administration with dopamine antagonists may diminish the effectiveness of pramipexole).
No products indexed under this heading.

Fluphenazine Enanthate (Co-administration with dopamine antagonists may diminish the effectiveness of pramipexole).
No products indexed under this heading.

Fluphenazine Hydrochloride (Co-administration with dopamine antagonists may diminish the effectiveness of pramipexole).
No products indexed under this heading.

Haloperidol (Co-administration with dopamine antagonists may diminish the effectiveness of pramipexole).
No products indexed under this heading.

Haloperidol Decanoate (Co-administration with dopamine antagonists may diminish the effectiveness of pramipexole).
No products indexed under this heading.

Levodopa (Pramipexole may potentiate the dopaminergic side effects of levodopa and may cause or exacerbate pre-existing dyskinesia; pramipexole may cause an increase in levodopa Cmax by about 40% and a decrease in Tmax from 2.5 to 0.6 hours). Products include:
Stalevo Tablets **2309**

Loxapine Hydrochloride (Co-administration with dopamine antagonists may diminish the effectiveness of pramipexole).
No products indexed under this heading.

Loxapine Succinate (Co-administration with dopamine antagonists may diminish the effectiveness of pramipexole).
No products indexed under this heading.

Mesoridazine Besylate (Co-administration with dopamine antagonists may diminish the effectiveness of pramipexole).
No products indexed under this heading.

Methotrimeprazine (Co-administration with dopamine antagonists may diminish the effectiveness of pramipexole).
No products indexed under this heading.

Metoclopramide Hydrochloride (Co-administration with dopamine antagonists may diminish the effectiveness of pramipexole).
No products indexed under this heading.

Molindone Hydrochloride (Co-administration with dopamine antagonists may diminish the effectiveness of pramipexole). Products include:
Moban Tablets **1116**

Perphenazine (Co-administration with dopamine antagonists may diminish the effectiveness of pramipexole).
No products indexed under this heading.

Prochlorperazine (Co-administration with dopamine antagonists may diminish the effectiveness of pramipexole).
No products indexed under this heading.

Promethazine Hydrochloride (Co-administration with dopamine antagonists may diminish the effectiveness of pramipexole).
No products indexed under this heading.

Quetiapine Fumarate (Co-administration with dopamine antagonists may diminish the effectiveness of pramipexole).
No products indexed under this heading.

Quinidine (Co-administration of drugs that are secreted by the cationic transport system, e.g., quinidine, decrease the oral clearance of pramipexole by about 20%).
No products indexed under this heading.

Quinidine Gluconate (Co-administration of drugs that are secreted by the cationic transport system, e.g., quinidine, decrease the oral clearance of pramipexole by about 20%).
No products indexed under this heading.

Quinidine Hydrochloride (Co-administration of drugs that are secreted by the cationic transport system, e.g., quinidine, decrease the oral clearance of pramipexole by about 20%).
No products indexed under this heading.

Quinidine Polygalacturonate (Co-administration of drugs that are secreted by the cationic transport system, e.g., quinidine, decrease the oral clearance of pramipexole by about 20%).
No products indexed under this heading.

Quinidine Sulfate (Co-administration of drugs that are secreted by the cationic transport system, e.g., quinidine, decrease the oral clearance of pramipexole by about 20%).
No products indexed under this heading.

Quinine Sulfate (Co-administration of drugs that are secreted by the cationic transport system, e.g., quinine, decrease the oral clearance of pramipexole by about 20%).
No products indexed under this heading.

Ranitidine Hydrochloride (Co-administration of drugs that are secreted by the cationic transport system, e.g., ranitidine, decrease the oral clearance of pramipexole by about 20%). Products include:
Zantac 75 Tablets .... ■**603**
Zantac **1670**
Zantac Injection **1666**
Zantac Injection Pharmacy Bulk Package **1668**
Maximum Strength Zantac 150 Tablets .... ■**603**
Maximum Strength Zantac 150 Cool Mint Tablets .... ■**603**

Risperidone (Co-administration with dopamine antagonists may diminish the effectiveness of pramipexole). Products include:
Risperdal Consta Long-Acting Injection **1753**

Thioridazine Hydrochloride (Co-administration with dopamine antagonists may diminish the effectiveness of pramipexole). Products include:
Thioridazine Hydrochloride Tablets **2195**

Thiothixene (Co-administration with dopamine antagonists may diminish the effectiveness of pramipexole). Products include:
Thiothixene Capsules **2197**

Triamterene (Co-administration of drugs that are secreted by the cationic transport system, e.g., triamterene, decrease the oral clearance of pramipexole by about 20%). Products include:
Dyazide Capsules **1405**
Dyrenium Capsules **3189**

Trifluoperazine Hydrochloride (Co-administration with dopamine antagonists may diminish the effectiveness of pramipexole).
No products indexed under this heading.

Verapamil Hydrochloride (Co-administration of drugs that are secreted by the cationic transport system, e.g., verapamil, decrease the oral clearance of pramipexole by about 20%). Products include:
Tarka Tablets **511**

Food Interactions

Food, unspecified (Food does not affect the extent of pramipexole absorption, although the time of maximum plasma concentration is increased by about 1 hour when the drug is taken with a meal).

MIRCETTE TABLETS
(Desogestrel, Ethinyl Estradiol) 1034
May interact with barbiturates, tetracyclines, and certain other agents. Compounds in these categories include:

Ampicillin (Potential for reduced efficacy and increased incidence of breakthrough bleeding and menstrual irregularities with concomitant use).
No products indexed under this heading.

Ampicillin Sodium (Potential for reduced efficacy and increased incidence of breakthrough bleeding and menstrual irregularities with concomitant use).
No products indexed under this heading.

Ampicillin Trihydrate (Potential for reduced efficacy and increased incidence of breakthrough bleeding and menstrual irregularities with concomitant use).
No products indexed under this heading.

Aprobarbital (Potential for reduced efficacy and increased incidence of breakthrough bleeding and menstrual irregularities with concomitant use).
No products indexed under this heading.

Butabarbital (Potential for reduced efficacy and increased incidence of breakthrough bleeding and menstrual irregularities with concomitant use).
No products indexed under this heading.

Butalbital (Potential for reduced efficacy and increased incidence of breakthrough bleeding and menstrual irregularities with concomitant use).
No products indexed under this heading.

Carbamazepine (Potential for reduced efficacy and increased incidence of breakthrough bleeding and menstrual irregularities with concomitant use). Products include:
Carbatrol Capsules 3019
Equetro Extended-Release Capsules 3174

Demeclocycline Hydrochloride (Potential for reduced efficacy and increased incidence of breakthrough bleeding and menstrual irregularities with concomitant use).
No products indexed under this heading.

Doxycycline Calcium (Potential for reduced efficacy and increased incidence of breakthrough bleeding and menstrual irregularities with concomitant use).
No products indexed under this heading.

Doxycycline Hyclate (Potential for reduced efficacy and increased incidence of breakthrough bleeding and menstrual irregularities with concomitant use).
No products indexed under this heading.

Doxycycline Monohydrate (Potential for reduced efficacy and increased incidence of breakthrough bleeding and menstrual irregularities with concomitant use).
No products indexed under this heading.

Griseofulvin (Potential for reduced efficacy and increased incidence of breakthrough bleeding and menstrual irregularities with concomitant use). Products include:
Gris-PEG Tablets 2507

Mephobarbital (Potential for reduced efficacy and increased incidence of breakthrough bleeding and menstrual irregularities with concomitant use).
No products indexed under this heading.

Methacycline Hydrochloride (Potential for reduced efficacy and increased incidence of breakthrough bleeding and menstrual irregularities with concomitant use).
No products indexed under this heading.

Minocycline Hydrochloride (Potential for reduced efficacy and increased incidence of breakthrough bleeding and menstrual irregularities with concomitant use). Products include:
Solodyn Extended Release Tablets 1938

Oxytetracycline Hydrochloride (Potential for reduced efficacy and increased incidence of breakthrough bleeding and menstrual irregularities with concomitant use).
No products indexed under this heading.

Pentobarbital Sodium (Potential for reduced efficacy and increased incidence of breakthrough bleeding and menstrual irregularities with concomitant use). Products include:
Nembutal Sodium Solution, USP 2494

Phenobarbital (Potential for reduced efficacy and increased incidence of breakthrough bleeding and menstrual irregularities with concomitant use). Products include:
Donnatal Extentabs 2507

Phenylbutazone (Potential for reduced efficacy and increased incidence of breakthrough bleeding and menstrual irregularities with concomitant use).
No products indexed under this heading.

Phenytoin (Potential for reduced efficacy and increased incidence of breakthrough bleeding and menstrual irregularities with concomitant use).
No products indexed under this heading.

Rifampin (Co-administration with rifampin has been associated with reduced efficacy and increased incidence of breakthrough bleeding and menstrual irregularities).
No products indexed under this heading.

Secobarbital Sodium (Potential for reduced efficacy and increased incidence of breakthrough bleeding and menstrual irregularities with concomitant use).
No products indexed under this heading.

Tetracycline Hydrochloride (Potential for reduced efficacy and increased incidence of breakthrough bleeding and menstrual irregularities with concomitant use). Products include:
Pylera Capsules 714

Thiamylal Sodium (Potential for reduced efficacy and increased incidence of breakthrough bleeding and menstrual irregularities with concomitant use).
No products indexed under this heading.

MIRENA INTRAUTERINE SYSTEM
(Levonorgestrel) 779
May interact with phenytoin and certain other agents. Compounds in these categories include:

Carbamazepine (Co-administration with drugs that induce liver enzymes may impair the effect of hormonal contraceptives). Products include:
Carbatrol Capsules 3019
Equetro Extended-Release Capsules 3174

Fosphenytoin Sodium (Co-administration with drugs that induce liver enzymes may impair the effect of hormonal contraceptives).
No products indexed under this heading.

Phenytoin (Co-administration with drugs that induce liver enzymes may impair the effect of hormonal contraceptives).
No products indexed under this heading.

Phenytoin Sodium (Co-administration with drugs that induce liver enzymes may impair the effect of hormonal contraceptives). Products include:
Phenytek Capsules 2192

Rifampin (Co-administration with drugs that induce liver enzymes may impair the effect of hormonal contraceptives).
No products indexed under this heading.

M-M-R II
(Measles, Mumps & Rubella Virus Vaccine, Live) 2054
May interact with immunosuppressive agents. Compounds in these categories include:

Azathioprine (Concurrent administration with immunosuppressant is contraindicated).
No products indexed under this heading.

Basiliximab (Concurrent administration with immunosuppressant is contraindicated). Products include:
Simulect for Injection 2306

Cyclosporine (Concurrent administration with immunosuppressant is contraindicated). Products include:
Gengraf Capsules 435
Neoral Oral Solution 2280
Neoral Soft Gelatin Capsules 2280
Restasis Ophthalmic Emulsion 557
Sandimmune 2296

Muromonab-CD3 (Concurrent administration with immunosuppressant is contraindicated). Products include:
Orthoclone OKT3 Sterile Solution 2387

Mycophenolate Mofetil (Concurrent administration with immunosuppressant is contraindicated). Products include:
CellCept Capsules 2622
CellCept Oral Suspension 2622
CellCept Tablets 2622

Sirolimus (Concurrent administration with immunosuppressant is contraindicated). Products include:
Rapamune 3260

Tacrolimus (Concurrent administration with immunosuppressant is contraindicated). Products include:
Prograf Capsules and Injection 622
Protopic Ointment 628

MOBAN TABLETS
(Molindone Hydrochloride) 1116
May interact with tetracyclines and certain other agents. Compounds in these categories include:

Demeclocycline Hydrochloride (Calcium sulfate present as an excipient may interfere with the absorption of oral tetracyclines).
No products indexed under this heading.

Doxycycline Calcium (Calcium sulfate present as an excipient may interfere with the absorption of oral tetracyclines).
No products indexed under this heading.

Doxycycline Hyclate (Calcium sulfate present as an excipient may interfere with the absorption of oral tetracyclines).
No products indexed under this heading.

Doxycycline Monohydrate (Calcium sulfate present as an excipient may interfere with the absorption of oral tetracyclines).
No products indexed under this heading.

Methacycline Hydrochloride (Calcium sulfate present as an excipient may interfere with the absorption of oral tetracyclines).
No products indexed under this heading.

Minocycline Hydrochloride (Calcium sulfate present as an excipient may interfere with the absorption of oral tetracyclines). Products include:
Solodyn Extended Release Tablets 1938

Oxytetracycline Hydrochloride (Calcium sulfate present as an excipient may interfere with the absorption of oral tetracyclines).
No products indexed under this heading.

Phenytoin Sodium (Calcium sulfate present as an excipient may interfere with the absorption of oral phenytoin sodium). Products include:
Phenytek Capsules 2192

Tetracycline Hydrochloride (Calcium sulfate present as an excipient may interfere with the absorption of oral tetracyclines). Products include:
Pylera Capsules 714

MOBIC ORAL SUSPENSION
(Meloxicam) 863
See Mobic Tablets

MOBIC TABLETS
(Meloxicam) 863
May interact with ACE inhibitors, lithium preparations, loop diuretics, thiazides, and certain other agents. Compounds in these categories include:

Aspirin (Co-administration of aspirin to healthy volunteers tended to increase the AUC and Cmax of meloxicam; the clinical significance of this interaction is not known; concurrent use may result in an increased rate of GI ulceration or other complications). Products include:
Aggrenox Capsules 819
Bayer Aspirin 750
Percodan Tablets 1130
St. Joseph 81 mg Aspirin Chewable and Enteric Coated Tablets 1903

IMPORTANT NOTE: Always consult each drug listing in the patient's regimen for possible interactions.

Benazepril Hydrochloride (Co-administration of NSAIDs with ACE inhibitors may diminish the antihypertensive effects of ACE inhibitors).

No products indexed under this heading.

Bendroflumethiazide (NSAIDs can reduce the natriuretic effect of thiazide diuretics in some patients. Patients taking thiazides may have impaired response when taking NSAIDs).

No products indexed under this heading.

Bumetanide (Patients taking loop diuretics may have impaired response when taking NSAIDs).

No products indexed under this heading.

Captopril (Co-administration of NSAIDs with ACE inhibitors may diminish the antihypertensive effects of ACE inhibitors). Products include:

Captopril Tablets 2182

Chlorothiazide (NSAIDs can reduce the natriuretic effect of thiazide diuretics in some patients. Patients taking thiazides may have impaired response when taking NSAIDs).

No products indexed under this heading.

Chlorothiazide Sodium (NSAIDs can reduce the natriuretic effect of thiazide diuretics in some patients. Patients taking thiazides may have impaired response when taking NSAIDs). Products include:

Intravenous Sodium Diuril 2490

Cholestyramine (Pretreatment for four days with cholestyramine significantly increased clearance of meloxicam by 50% resulting in a decrease in t1/2 from 19.2 hours to 12.5 hours and a 35% reduction in AUC; the clinical significance of this interaction is not known).

No products indexed under this heading.

Enalapril Maleate (Co-administration of NSAIDs with ACE inhibitors may diminish the antihypertensive effects of ACE inhibitors).

No products indexed under this heading.

Enalaprilat (Co-administration of NSAIDs with ACE inhibitors may diminish the antihypertensive effects of ACE inhibitors).

No products indexed under this heading.

Ethacrynic Acid (Patients taking loop diuretics may have impaired response when taking NSAIDs). Products include:

Edecrin Tablets 698

Fosinopril Sodium (Co-administration of NSAIDs with ACE inhibitors may diminish the antihypertensive effects of ACE inhibitors).

No products indexed under this heading.

Furosemide (NSAIDs can reduce the natriuretic effect of furosemide in some patients; in clinical studies, pharmacokinetics and pharmacodynamics of furosemide were not affected by multiple doses of meloxicam). Products include:

Furosemide Tablets 2186

Hydrochlorothiazide (NSAIDs can reduce the natriuretic effect of thiazide diuretics in some patients. Patients taking thiazides may have impaired response when taking NSAIDs). Products include:

Atacand HCT 642
Avalide Tablets 892
Avalide Tablets 2713
Benicar HCT Tablets 1010
Diovan HCT Tablets 2216
Dyazide Capsules 1405
Micardis HCT Tablets 854
Prinzide Tablets 2092
Tekturna HCT Tablets 2324
Teveten HCT Tablets 517

Hydroflumethiazide (NSAIDs can reduce the natriuretic effect of thiazide diuretics in some patients. Patients taking thiazides may have impaired response when taking NSAIDs).

No products indexed under this heading.

Lisinopril (Co-administration of NSAIDs with ACE inhibitors may diminish the antihypertensive effects of ACE inhibitors). Products include:

Prinivil Tablets 2087
Prinzide Tablets 2092

Lithium (NSAIDs can produce an elevation of plasma lithium levels and a reduction in renal lithium clearance; co-administration in healthy subjects has resulted in increased lithium concentration and AUC).

No products indexed under this heading.

Lithium Carbonate (NSAIDs can produce an elevation of plasma lithium levels and a reduction in renal lithium clearance; co-administration in healthy subjects has resulted in increased lithium concentration and AUC).

No products indexed under this heading.

Lithium Citrate (NSAIDs can produce an elevation of plasma lithium levels and a reduction in renal lithium clearance; co-administration in healthy subjects has resulted in increased lithium concentration and AUC).

No products indexed under this heading.

Methotrexate (Caution should be used when NSAIDs are administered concomitantly with methotrexate).

No products indexed under this heading.

Methotrexate Sodium (Caution should be used when NSAIDs are administered concomitantly with methotrexate).

No products indexed under this heading.

Methyclothiazide (NSAIDs can reduce the natriuretic effect of thiazide diuretics in some patients. Patients taking thiazides may have impaired response when taking NSAIDs).

No products indexed under this heading.

Moexipril Hydrochloride (Co-administration of NSAIDs with ACE inhibitors may diminish the antihypertensive effects of ACE inhibitors).

No products indexed under this heading.

Perindopril Erbumine (Co-administration of NSAIDs with ACE inhibitors may diminish the antihypertensive effects of ACE inhibitors). Products include:

Aceon Tablets (2 mg, 4 mg, 8 mg) 3038

Polythiazide (NSAIDs can reduce the natriuretic effect of thiazide diuretics in some patients. Patients taking thiazides may have impaired response when taking NSAIDs).

No products indexed under this heading.

Quinapril Hydrochloride (Co-administration of NSAIDs with ACE inhibitors may diminish the antihypertensive effects of ACE inhibitors).

No products indexed under this heading.

Ramipril (Co-administration of NSAIDs with ACE inhibitors may diminish the antihypertensive effects of ACE inhibitors).

No products indexed under this heading.

Spirapril Hydrochloride (Co-administration of NSAIDs with ACE inhibitors may diminish the antihypertensive effects of ACE inhibitors).

No products indexed under this heading.

Torsemide (Patients taking loop diuretics may have impaired response when taking NSAIDs). Products include:

Demadex Injection 2630
Demadex Tablets 2630

Trandolapril (Co-administration of NSAIDs with ACE inhibitors may diminish the antihypertensive effects of ACE inhibitors). Products include:

Mavik Tablets 472
Tarka Tablets 511

Warfarin Sodium (Potential for increased risk of bleeding).

No products indexed under this heading.

Food Interactions

Food, unspecified (Co-administration with a high-fat breakfast did not affect extent of absorption of meloxicam capsules but led to 22% higher Cmax values; mean Cmax values were achieved between 5 to 6 hours; Mobic tablets can be administered without regard to timing of meals).

MOTRIN IB TABLETS AND CAPLETS

(Ibuprofen) 1900

May interact with aspirin-acetylsalicylic acid, anticoagulants, corticosteroids, non-steroidal anti-inflammatory agents, and certain other agents. Compounds in these categories include:

Anisindione (Increased risk of stomach bleeding if co-administered with anticoagulants).

No products indexed under this heading.

Ardeparin Sodium (Increased risk of stomach bleeding if co-administered with anticoagulants).

No products indexed under this heading.

Aspirin (Increased risk of stomach bleeding if co-administered with non-steroidal anti-inflammatory drugs; ibuprofen may decrease benefit of aspirin on patients taking it for heart attack or stroke). Products include:

Aggrenox Capsules 819
Bayer Aspirin 750
Percodan Tablets 1130
St. Joseph 81 mg Aspirin Chewable and Enteric Coated Tablets 1903

Aspirin, Enteric Coated (Increased risk of stomach bleeding if co-administered with non-steroidal anti-inflammatory drugs; ibuprofen may decrease benefit of aspirin on patients taking it for heart attack or stroke).

No products indexed under this heading.

Aspirin Buffered (Increased risk of stomach bleeding if co-administered with non-steroidal anti-inflammatory drugs; ibuprofen may decrease benefit of aspirin on patients taking it for heart attack or stroke).

No products indexed under this heading.

Betamethasone Acetate (Increased risk of stomach bleeding if co-administered with steroidal drugs).

No products indexed under this heading.

Betamethasone Sodium Phosphate (Increased risk of stomach bleeding if co-administered with steroidal drugs).

No products indexed under this heading.

Budesonide (Increased risk of stomach bleeding if co-administered with steroidal drugs). Products include:

Pulmicort Flexhaler 654
Symbicort 80/4.5 Inhalation Aerosol 659
Symbicort 160/4.5 Inhalation Aerosol 659

Celecoxib (Increased risk of stomach bleeding if co-administered with non-steroidal anti-inflammatory drugs). Products include:

Celebrex Capsules 2979

Ciclesonide (Increased risk of stomach bleeding if co-administered with steroidal drugs). Products include:

Alvesco Inhalation Aerosol 2985
Omnaris Nasal Spray 2998

Cortisone Acetate (Increased risk of stomach bleeding if co-administered with steroidal drugs).

No products indexed under this heading.

Dalteparin Sodium (Increased risk of stomach bleeding if co-administered with anticoagulants). Products include:

Fragmin Injection 1070

Danaparoid Sodium (Increased risk of stomach bleeding if co-administered with anticoagulants).

No products indexed under this heading.

Dexamethasone (Increased risk of stomach bleeding if co-administered with steroidal drugs). Products include:

Ciprodex Otic Suspension 541

Dexamethasone Acetate (Increased risk of stomach bleeding if co-administered with steroidal drugs).

No products indexed under this heading.

Dexamethasone Sodium Phosphate (Increased risk of stomach bleeding if co-administered with steroidal drugs).

No products indexed under this heading.

Diclofenac Epolamine (Increased risk of stomach bleeding if co-administered with non-steroidal anti-inflammatory drugs). Products include:

Flector Patch 561

Diclofenac Potassium (Increased risk of stomach bleeding if co-administered with non-steroidal anti-inflammatory drugs).
No products indexed under this heading.

Diclofenac Sodium (Increased risk of stomach bleeding if co-administered with non-steroidal anti-inflammatory drugs). Products include:
Diclofenac Sodium Ophthalmic Solution .... ⊙240
Voltaren Ophthalmic Solution 2336
Voltaren Tablets 2334
Voltaren-XR Tablets 2337

Dicumarol (Increased risk of stomach bleeding if co-administered with anticoagulants).
No products indexed under this heading.

Enoxaparin Sodium (Increased risk of stomach bleeding if co-administered with anticoagulants). Products include:
Lovenox Injection 2756

Etodolac (Increased risk of stomach bleeding if co-administered with non-steroidal anti-inflammatory drugs).
No products indexed under this heading.

Fenoprofen Calcium (Increased risk of stomach bleeding if co-administered with non-steroidal anti-inflammatory drugs). Products include:
Nalfon Capsules 2508

Fludrocortisone Acetate (Increased risk of stomach bleeding if co-administered with steroidal drugs).
No products indexed under this heading.

Flunisolide (Increased risk of stomach bleeding if co-administered with steroidal drugs). Products include:
Aerobid/Aerobid-M 1153

Flurbiprofen (Increased risk of stomach bleeding if co-administered with non-steroidal anti-inflammatory drugs).
No products indexed under this heading.

Fluticasone Propionate (Increased risk of stomach bleeding if co-administered with steroidal drugs). Products include:
Advair Diskus 100/50 1276
Advair Diskus 250/50 1276
Advair Diskus 500/50 1276
Advair HFA 45/21 Inhalation Aerosol 1288
Advair HFA 115/21 Inhalation Aerosol 1288
Advair HFA 230/21 Inhalation Aerosol 1288
Flonase Nasal Spray 1431
Flovent Diskus 50 mcg 1435

Fluticasone Propionate HFA (Increased risk of stomach bleeding if co-administered with steroidal drugs). Products include:
Flovent HFA 1440

Fondaparinux Sodium (Increased risk of stomach bleeding if co-administered with anticoagulants). Products include:
Arixtra Injection 1313

Heparin Calcium (Increased risk of stomach bleeding if co-administered with anticoagulants).
No products indexed under this heading.

Heparin Sodium (Increased risk of stomach bleeding if co-administered with anticoagulants).
No products indexed under this heading.

Hydrocortisone (Increased risk of stomach bleeding if co-administered with steroidal drugs).
No products indexed under this heading.

Hydrocortisone Acetate (Increased risk of stomach bleeding if co-administered with steroidal drugs). Products include:
Analpram-HC 1140
Pramosone 1141

Hydrocortisone Sodium Phosphate (Increased risk of stomach bleeding if co-administered with steroidal drugs).
No products indexed under this heading.

Hydrocortisone Sodium Succinate (Increased risk of stomach bleeding if co-administered with steroidal drugs).
No products indexed under this heading.

Indomethacin (Increased risk of stomach bleeding if co-administered with non-steroidal anti-inflammatory drugs). Products include:
Indocin 2024

Indomethacin Sodium Trihydrate (Increased risk of stomach bleeding if co-administered with non-steroidal anti-inflammatory drugs). Products include:
Indocin I.V. 2489

Ketoprofen (Increased risk of stomach bleeding if co-administered with non-steroidal anti-inflammatory drugs).
No products indexed under this heading.

Ketorolac Tromethamine (Increased risk of stomach bleeding if co-administered with non-steroidal anti-inflammatory drugs).
No products indexed under this heading.

Low Molecular Weight Heparins (Increased risk of stomach bleeding if co-administered with anticoagulants).
No products indexed under this heading.

Meclofenamate Sodium (Increased risk of stomach bleeding if co-administered with non-steroidal anti-inflammatory drugs).
No products indexed under this heading.

Mefenamic Acid (Increased risk of stomach bleeding if co-administered with non-steroidal anti-inflammatory drugs).
No products indexed under this heading.

Meloxicam (Increased risk of stomach bleeding if co-administered with non-steroidal anti-inflammatory drugs). Products include:
Mobic Oral Suspension 863
Mobic Tablets 863

Methylprednisolone Acetate (Increased risk of stomach bleeding if co-administered with steroidal drugs).
No products indexed under this heading.

Methylprednisolone Sodium Succinate (Increased risk of stomach bleeding if co-administered with steroidal drugs).
No products indexed under this heading.

Mometasone Furoate (Increased risk of stomach bleeding if co-administered with steroidal drugs). Products include:
Asmanex Twisthaler 2797
Elocon Cream 0.1% 2840
Elocon Lotion 0.1% 2841
Elocon Ointment 0.1% 2842

Mometasone Furoate Monohydrate (Increased risk of stomach bleeding if co-administered with steroidal drugs). Products include:
Nasonex Nasal Spray 2883

Nabumetone (Increased risk of stomach bleeding if co-administered with non-steroidal anti-inflammatory drugs).
No products indexed under this heading.

Naproxen (Increased risk of stomach bleeding if co-administered with non-steroidal anti-inflammatory drugs). Products include:
EC-Naprosyn Delayed-Release Tablets 2632
Naprosyn Suspension 2632
Naprosyn Tablets 2632

Naproxen Sodium (Increased risk of stomach bleeding if co-administered with non-steroidal anti-inflammatory drugs). Products include:
Anaprox Tablets 2632
Anaprox DS Tablets 2632
Treximet Tablets 1616

Oxaprozin (Increased risk of stomach bleeding if co-administered with non-steroidal anti-inflammatory drugs).
No products indexed under this heading.

Phenylbutazone (Increased risk of stomach bleeding if co-administered with non-steroidal anti-inflammatory drugs).
No products indexed under this heading.

Piroxicam (Increased risk of stomach bleeding if co-administered with non-steroidal anti-inflammatory drugs).
No products indexed under this heading.

Prednisolone Acetate (Increased risk of stomach bleeding if co-administered with steroidal drugs). Products include:
Pred Forte Ophthalmic Suspension .... ⊙227
Pred Mild Ophthalmic Suspension .... ⊙230
Pred-G Ophthalmic Ointment .... ⊙229
Pred-G Ophthalmic Suspension .... ⊙228

Prednisolone Sodium Phosphate (Increased risk of stomach bleeding if co-administered with steroidal drugs).
No products indexed under this heading.

Prednisolone Tebutate (Increased risk of stomach bleeding if co-administered with steroidal drugs).
No products indexed under this heading.

Prednisone (Increased risk of stomach bleeding if co-administered with steroidal drugs).
No products indexed under this heading.

Rofecoxib (Increased risk of stomach bleeding if co-administered with non-steroidal anti-inflammatory drugs).
No products indexed under this heading.

Sulindac (Increased risk of stomach bleeding if co-administered with non-steroidal anti-inflammatory drugs). Products include:
Clinoril Tablets 1962

Tinzaparin Sodium (Increased risk of stomach bleeding if co-administered with anticoagulants).
No products indexed under this heading.

Tolmetin Sodium (Increased risk of stomach bleeding if co-administered with non-steroidal anti-inflammatory drugs).
No products indexed under this heading.

Triamcinolone (Increased risk of stomach bleeding if co-administered with steroidal drugs).
No products indexed under this heading.

Triamcinolone Acetonide (Increased risk of stomach bleeding if co-administered with steroidal drugs). Products include:
Azmacort Inhalation Aerosol 407
Nasacort AQ Nasal Spray 2765
Triesence Injectable Suspension .... ⊙209

Triamcinolone Diacetate (Increased risk of stomach bleeding if co-administered with steroidal drugs).
No products indexed under this heading.

Triamcinolone Hexacetonide (Increased risk of stomach bleeding if co-administered with steroidal drugs).
No products indexed under this heading.

Valdecoxib (Increased risk of stomach bleeding if co-administered with non-steroidal anti-inflammatory drugs).
No products indexed under this heading.

Warfarin Sodium (Increased risk of stomach bleeding if co-administered with anticoagulants).
No products indexed under this heading.

CHILDREN'S MOTRIN ORAL SUSPENSION

(Ibuprofen) 1901
None cited in PDR database.

CHILDREN'S MOTRIN NON-STAINING DYE-FREE ORAL SUSPENSION

(Ibuprofen) 1901
See Children's Motrin Oral Suspension

CHILDREN'S MOTRIN COLD ORAL SUSPENSION

(Ibuprofen, Pseudoephedrine Hydrochloride) 1899
May interact with monoamine oxidase inhibitors. Compounds in these categories include:

Isocarboxazid (Concurrent and/or sequential use with MAO inhibitors is not recommended). Products include:
Marplan Tablets 3177

Moclobemide (Concurrent and/or sequential use with MAO inhibitors is not recommended).
No products indexed under this heading.

IMPORTANT NOTE: Always consult each drug listing in the patient's regimen for possible interactions.

Pargyline Hydrochloride (Concurrent and/or sequential use with MAO inhibitors is not recommended).
No products indexed under this heading.

Phenelzine Sulfate (Concurrent and/or sequential use with MAO inhibitors is not recommended).
No products indexed under this heading.

Procarbazine Hydrochloride (Concurrent and/or sequential use with MAO inhibitors is not recommended).
No products indexed under this heading.

Rasagiline Mesylate (Concurrent and/or sequential use with MAO inhibitors is not recommended).
Products include:
Azilect Tablets 3106

Selegiline (Concurrent and/or sequential use with MAO inhibitors is not recommended). Products include:
Emsam Transdermal System 905

Selegiline Hydrochloride (Concurrent and/or sequential use with MAO inhibitors is not recommended).
Products include:
Eldepryl Capsules 3052

Tranylcypromine Sulfate (Concurrent and/or sequential use with MAO inhibitors is not recommended).
Products include:
Parnate Tablets 1532

INFANTS' MOTRIN CONCENTRATED DROPS

(Ibuprofen) 1901
None cited in PDR database.

INFANTS' MOTRIN NON-STAINING DYE-FREE CONCENTRATED DROPS

(Ibuprofen) 1901
None cited in PDR database.

JUNIOR STRENGTH MOTRIN CAPLETS AND CHEWABLE TABLETS

(Ibuprofen) 1901
None cited in PDR database.

MOVIPREP ORAL SOLUTION

(PEG-3350, Potassium Chloride, Sodium Ascorbate, Sodium Chloride, Sodium Sulfate, Vitamin C) 2679
May interact with:

Oral Medications, unspecified (Oral medication administered within 1 hour of the start of administration of MoviPrep may be flushed from the gastrointestinal tract and the medication may not be absorbed).
No products indexed under this heading.

MOXATAG TABLETS

(Amoxicillin) 2165
May interact with chloramphenicol, macrolide antibiotics, oral contraceptives, sulfonamides, tetracyclines, and certain other agents. Compounds in these categories include:

Azithromycin Dihydrate (Macrolides may interfere with the bactericidal effects of penicillin. This has been demonstrated in vitro; however, the clinical significance of this interaction is not well documented).
No products indexed under this heading.

Bendroflumethiazide (Sulfonamides may interfere with the bactericidal effects of penicillin. This has been demonstrated in vitro; however, the clinical significance of this interaction is not well documented).
No products indexed under this heading.

Chloramphenicol (Chloramphenicol may interfere with the bactericidal effects of penicillin. This has been demonstrated in vitro; however, the clinical significance of this interaction is not well documented).
No products indexed under this heading.

Chloramphenicol Palmitate (Chloramphenicol may interfere with the bactericidal effects of penicillin. This has been demonstrated in vitro; however, the clinical significance of this interaction is not well documented).
No products indexed under this heading.

Chloramphenicol Sodium Succinate (Chloramphenicol may interfere with the bactericidal effects of penicillin. This has been demonstrated in vitro; however, the clinical significance of this interaction is not well documented).
No products indexed under this heading.

Chlorothiazide (Sulfonamides may interfere with the bactericidal effects of penicillin. This has been demonstrated in vitro; however, the clinical significance of this interaction is not well documented).
No products indexed under this heading.

Chlorothiazide Sodium (Sulfonamides may interfere with the bactericidal effects of penicillin. This has been demonstrated in vitro; however, the clinical significance of this interaction is not well documented).
Products include:
Intravenous Sodium Diuril 2490

Chlorpropamide (Sulfonamides may interfere with the bactericidal effects of penicillin. This has been demonstrated in vitro; however, the clinical significance of this interaction is not well documented).
No products indexed under this heading.

Clarithromycin (Macrolides may interfere with the bactericidal effects of penicillin. This has been demonstrated in vitro; however, the clinical significance of this interaction is not well documented). Products include:
Biaxin/Biaxin XL 411

Demeclocycline Hydrochloride (Tetracyclines may interfere with the bactericidal effects of penicillin. This has been demonstrated in vitro; however, the clinical significance of this interaction is not well documented).
No products indexed under this heading.

Desogestrel (Amoxicillin may affect the gut flora, leading to lower estrogen reabsorption and potentially resulting in reduced efficacy of combined oral estrogen/progesterone contraceptives). Products include:
Mircette Tablets 1034

Dirithromycin (Macrolides may interfere with the bactericidal effects of penicillin. This has been demonstrated in vitro; however, the clinical significance of this interaction is not well documented).
No products indexed under this heading.

Doxycycline Calcium (Tetracyclines may interfere with the bactericidal effects of penicillin. This has been demonstrated in vitro; however, the clinical significance of this interaction is not well documented).
No products indexed under this heading.

Doxycycline Hyclate (Tetracyclines may interfere with the bactericidal effects of penicillin. This has been demonstrated in vitro; however, the clinical significance of this interaction is not well documented).
No products indexed under this heading.

Doxycycline Monohydrate (Tetracyclines may interfere with the bactericidal effects of penicillin. This has been demonstrated in vitro; however, the clinical significance of this interaction is not well documented).
No products indexed under this heading.

Erythromycin (Macrolides may interfere with the bactericidal effects of penicillin. This has been demonstrated in vitro; however, the clinical significance of this interaction is not well documented).
No products indexed under this heading.

Erythromycin Estolate (Macrolides may interfere with the bactericidal effects of penicillin. This has been demonstrated in vitro; however, the clinical significance of this interaction is not well documented).
No products indexed under this heading.

Erythromycin Ethylsuccinate (Macrolides may interfere with the bactericidal effects of penicillin. This has been demonstrated in vitro; however, the clinical significance of this interaction is not well documented).
Products include:
E.E.S. 433
EryPed 431

Erythromycin Gluceptate (Macrolides may interfere with the bactericidal effects of penicillin. This has been demonstrated in vitro; however, the clinical significance of this interaction is not well documented).
No products indexed under this heading.

Erythromycin Stearate (Macrolides may interfere with the bactericidal effects of penicillin. This has been demonstrated in vitro; however, the clinical significance of this interaction is not well documented).
No products indexed under this heading.

Ethinyl Estradiol (Amoxicillin may affect the gut flora, leading to lower estrogen reabsorption and potentially resulting in reduced efficacy of combined oral estrogen/progesterone contraceptives).
Products include:
Lybrel Tablets 3204
Mircette Tablets 1034
NuvaRing 2897
Ortho-Cyclen/Ortho Tri-Cyclen 2449
Ortho Evra Transdermal System 2437
Ortho Tri-Cyclen Lo Tablets 2458
Seasonique Tablets 1046
Yaz Tablets 805

Ethynodiol Diacetate (Amoxicillin may affect the gut flora, leading to lower estrogen reabsorption and potentially resulting in reduced efficacy of combined oral estrogen/progesterone contraceptives).
No products indexed under this heading.

Glipizide (Sulfonamides may interfere with the bactericidal effects of penicillin. This has been demonstrated in vitro; however, the clinical significance of this interaction is not well documented).
No products indexed under this heading.

Glyburide (Sulfonamides may interfere with the bactericidal effects of penicillin. This has been demonstrated in vitro; however, the clinical significance of this interaction is not well documented).
No products indexed under this heading.

Hydrochlorothiazide (Sulfonamides may interfere with the bactericidal effects of penicillin. This has been demonstrated in vitro; however, the clinical significance of this interaction is not well documented).
Products include:
Atacand HCT 642
Avalide Tablets 892
Avalide Tablets 2713
Benicar HCT Tablets 1010
Diovan HCT Tablets 2216
Dyazide Capsules 1405
Micardis HCT Tablets 854
Prinzide Tablets 2092
Tekturna HCT Tablets 2324
Teveten HCT Tablets 517

Hydroflumethiazide (Sulfonamides may interfere with the bactericidal effects of penicillin. This has been demonstrated in vitro; however, the clinical significance of this interaction is not well documented).
No products indexed under this heading.

Lansoprazole (In a study of healthy adult subjects, amoxicillin AUC was similar whereas Cmax increased approximately 35% following the administration of lansoprazole with amoxicillin extended release tablets given with food).
No products indexed under this heading.

Levonorgestrel (Amoxicillin may affect the gut flora, leading to lower estrogen reabsorption and potentially resulting in reduced efficacy of combined oral estrogen/progesterone contraceptives).
Products include:
Climara Pro Transdermal System 768
Lybrel Tablets 3204
Mirena Intrauterine System 779
Plan B Tablets 1044
Seasonique Tablets 1046

Mestranol (Amoxicillin may affect the gut flora, leading to lower estrogen reabsorption and potentially resulting in reduced efficacy of combined oral estrogen/progesterone contraceptives).
No products indexed under this heading.

Methacycline Hydrochloride (Tetracyclines may interfere with the bactericidal effects of penicillin. This has been demonstrated in vitro; however, the clinical significance of this interaction is not well documented).
No products indexed under this heading.

Methyclothiazide (Sulfonamides may interfere with the bactericidal effects of penicillin. This has been demonstrated in vitro; however, the clinical significance of this interaction is not well documented).
No products indexed under this heading.

Minocycline Hydrochloride (Tetracyclines may interfere with the bactericidal effects of penicillin. This has been demonstrated in vitro; however, the clinical significance of this interaction is not well documented). Products include:
Solodyn Extended Release Tablets 1938

Norethindrone (Amoxicillin may affect the gut flora, leading to lower estrogen reabsorption and potentially resulting in reduced efficacy of combined oral estrogen/progesterone contraceptives). Products include:
Ortho Micronor Tablets 2446

Norethynodrel (Amoxicillin may affect the gut flora, leading to lower estrogen reabsorption and potentially resulting in reduced efficacy of combined oral estrogen/progesterone contraceptives).
No products indexed under this heading.

Norgestimate (Amoxicillin may affect the gut flora, leading to lower estrogen reabsorption and potentially resulting in reduced efficacy of combined oral estrogen/progesterone contraceptives). Products include:
Ortho-Cyclen/Ortho Tri-Cyclen 2449
Ortho Tri-Cyclen Lo Tablets 2458

Norgestrel (Amoxicillin may affect the gut flora, leading to lower estrogen reabsorption and potentially resulting in reduced efficacy of combined oral estrogen/progesterone contraceptives).
No products indexed under this heading.

Oxytetracycline Hydrochloride (Tetracyclines may interfere with the bactericidal effects of penicillin. This has been demonstrated in vitro; however, the clinical significance of this interaction is not well documented).
No products indexed under this heading.

Polythiazide (Sulfonamides may interfere with the bactericidal effects of penicillin. This has been demonstrated in vitro; however, the clinical significance of this interaction is not well documented).
No products indexed under this heading.

Probenecid (Probenecid decreases the renal tubular secretion of amoxicillin. Concurrent use of amoxicillin extended release tablets and probenecid may result in increased and prolonged blood levels of amoxicillin. The clinical relevance of this finding has not been evaluated).
No products indexed under this heading.

Sulfacytine (Sulfonamides may interfere with the bactericidal effects of penicillin. This has been demonstrated in vitro; however, the clinical significance of this interaction is not well documented).
No products indexed under this heading.

Sulfamethizole (Sulfonamides may interfere with the bactericidal effects of penicillin. This has been demonstrated in vitro; however, the clinical significance of this interaction is not well documented).
No products indexed under this heading.

Sulfamethoxazole (Sulfonamides may interfere with the bactericidal effects of penicillin. This has been demonstrated in vitro; however, the clinical significance of this interaction is not well documented).
No products indexed under this heading.

Sulfasalazine (Sulfonamides may interfere with the bactericidal effects of penicillin. This has been demonstrated in vitro; however, the clinical significance of this interaction is not well documented).
No products indexed under this heading.

Sulfinpyrazone (Sulfonamides may interfere with the bactericidal effects of penicillin. This has been demonstrated in vitro; however, the clinical significance of this interaction is not well documented).
No products indexed under this heading.

Sulfisoxazole Acetyl (Sulfonamides may interfere with the bactericidal effects of penicillin. This has been demonstrated in vitro; however, the clinical significance of this interaction is not well documented).
No products indexed under this heading.

Sulfisoxazole Diolamine (Sulfonamides may interfere with the bactericidal effects of penicillin. This has been demonstrated in vitro; however, the clinical significance of this interaction is not well documented).
No products indexed under this heading.

Tetracycline Hydrochloride (Tetracyclines may interfere with the bactericidal effects of penicillin. This has been demonstrated in vitro; however, the clinical significance of this interaction is not well documented). Products include:
Pylera Capsules 714

Tolazamide (Sulfonamides may interfere with the bactericidal effects of penicillin. This has been demonstrated in vitro; however, the clinical significance of this interaction is not well documented).
No products indexed under this heading.

Tolbutamide (Sulfonamides may interfere with the bactericidal effects of penicillin. This has been demonstrated in vitro; however, the clinical significance of this interaction is not well documented).
No products indexed under this heading.

Troleandomycin (Macrolides may interfere with the bactericidal effects of penicillin. This has been demonstrated in vitro; however, the clinical significance of this interaction is not well documented).
No products indexed under this heading.

MS CONTIN TABLETS

(Morphine Sulfate) 2585
May interact with central nervous system depressants, general anesthetics, hypnotics and sedatives, mixed agonist/antagonist opioid analgesics, neuromuscular blocking agents, phenothiazines, tranquilizers, and certain other agents. Compounds in these categories include:

Alfentanil Hydrochloride (Profound sedation, coma, severe hypotension, respiratory depression).
No products indexed under this heading.

Alprazolam (Profound sedation, coma, severe hypotension, respiratory depression).
No products indexed under this heading.

Aprobarbital (Profound sedation, coma, severe hypotension, respiratory depression).
No products indexed under this heading.

Atracurium Besylate (Increased respiratory depression).
No products indexed under this heading.

Buprenorphine Hydrochloride (Mixed agonist/antagonist analgesics may reduce the analgesic effect or may precipitate withdrawal symptoms). Products include:
Suboxone Tablets 2601
Subutex Tablets 2601

Buspirone Hydrochloride (Profound sedation, coma, severe hypotension, respiratory depression).
No products indexed under this heading.

Butabarbital (Profound sedation, coma, severe hypotension, respiratory depression).
No products indexed under this heading.

Butabarbital Sodium (Profound sedation, coma, severe hypotension, respiratory depression).
No products indexed under this heading.

Butalbital (Profound sedation, coma, severe hypotension, respiratory depression).
No products indexed under this heading.

Butorphanol Tartrate (Mixed agonist/antagonist analgesics may reduce the analgesic effect or may precipitate withdrawal symptoms).
No products indexed under this heading.

Chloral Hydrate (Profound sedation, coma, severe hypotension, respiratory depression).
No products indexed under this heading.

Chlordiazepoxide (Profound sedation, coma, severe hypotension, respiratory depression).
No products indexed under this heading.

Chlordiazepoxide Hydrochloride (Profound sedation, coma, severe hypotension, respiratory depression).
No products indexed under this heading.

Chlorpromazine (Profound sedation, coma, severe hypotension, respiratory depression).
No products indexed under this heading.

Chlorpromazine Hydrochloride (Profound sedation, coma, severe hypotension, respiratory depression).
No products indexed under this heading.

Chlorprothixene (Profound sedation, coma, severe hypotension, respiratory depression).
No products indexed under this heading.

Chlorprothixene Hydrochloride (Profound sedation, coma, severe hypotension, respiratory depression).
No products indexed under this heading.

Chlorprothixene Lactate (Profound sedation, coma, severe hypotension, respiratory depression).
No products indexed under this heading.

Cisatracurium Besylate (Increased respiratory depression). Products include:
Nimbex Injection 484

Clorazepate Dipotassium (Profound sedation, coma, severe hypotension, respiratory depression).
No products indexed under this heading.

Clozapine (Profound sedation, coma, severe hypotension, respiratory depression).
No products indexed under this heading.

Codeine Phosphate (Profound sedation, coma, severe hypotension, respiratory depression). Products include:
Tylenol with Codeine Tablets 2427

Desflurane (Profound sedation, coma, severe hypotension, respiratory depression).
No products indexed under this heading.

Dezocine (Profound sedation, coma, severe hypotension, respiratory depression).
No products indexed under this heading.

Diazepam (Profound sedation, coma, severe hypotension, respiratory depression). Products include:
Valium Tablets 2658

Doxacurium Chloride (Increased respiratory depression).
No products indexed under this heading.

Droperidol (Profound sedation, coma, severe hypotension, respiratory depression).
No products indexed under this heading.

Enflurane (Profound sedation, coma, severe hypotension, respiratory depression).
No products indexed under this heading.

Estazolam (Profound sedation, coma, severe hypotension, respiratory depression).
No products indexed under this heading.

Ethanol (Profound sedation, coma, severe hypotension, respiratory depression).
No products indexed under this heading.

Ethchlorvynol (Profound sedation, coma, severe hypotension, respiratory depression).
No products indexed under this heading.

Ethinamate (Profound sedation, coma, severe hypotension, respiratory depression).
No products indexed under this heading.

Ethyl Alcohol (Profound sedation, coma, severe hypotension, respiratory depression).
No products indexed under this heading.

Fentanyl (Profound sedation, coma, severe hypotension, respiratory depression). Products include:
Duragesic Transdermal System 2405
Ionsys Transdermal System 2410

Fentanyl Citrate (Profound sedation, coma, severe hypotension, respiratory depression). Products include:
Actiq 959
Fentora Tablets 968

Fluphenazine Decanoate (Profound sedation, coma, severe hypotension, respiratory depression).
No products indexed under this heading.

Fluphenazine Enanthate (Profound sedation, coma, severe hypotension, respiratory depression).
No products indexed under this heading.

Fluphenazine Hydrochloride (Profound sedation, coma, severe hypotension, respiratory depression).
No products indexed under this heading.

Flurazepam Hydrochloride (Profound sedation, coma, severe hypotension, respiratory depression).
No products indexed under this heading.

Glutethimide (Profound sedation, coma, severe hypotension, respiratory depression).
No products indexed under this heading.

Haloperidol (Profound sedation, coma, severe hypotension, respiratory depression).
No products indexed under this heading.

Haloperidol Decanoate (Profound sedation, coma, severe hypotension, respiratory depression).
No products indexed under this heading.

Hydrocodone Bitartrate (Profound sedation, coma, severe hypotension, respiratory depression). Products include:
Lortab 5/500 Tablets 3143
Lortab 7.5/500 Tablets 3144
Lortab 10/500 Tablets 3144
Vicodin Tablets 529
Vicodin ES Tablets 530
Vicodin HP Tablets 531
Vicoprofen Tablets 533
Zydone Tablets 1132

Hydrocodone Polistirex (Profound sedation, coma, severe hypotension, respiratory depression). Products include:
Tussionex Pennkinetic Extended-Release Suspension 3154

Hydromorphone Hydrochloride (Profound sedation, coma, severe hypotension, respiratory depression).
No products indexed under this heading.

Hydroxyzine Hydrochloride (Profound sedation, coma, severe hypotension, respiratory depression).
No products indexed under this heading.

Isoflurane (Profound sedation, coma, severe hypotension, respiratory depression).
No products indexed under this heading.

Ketamine Hydrochloride (Profound sedation, coma, severe hypotension, respiratory depression).
No products indexed under this heading.

Levomethadyl Acetate Hydrochloride (Profound sedation, coma, severe hypotension, respiratory depression).
No products indexed under this heading.

Levorphanol Tartrate (Profound sedation, coma, severe hypotension, respiratory depression).
No products indexed under this heading.

Lorazepam (Profound sedation, coma, severe hypotension, respiratory depression).
No products indexed under this heading.

Loxapine Hydrochloride (Profound sedation, coma, severe hypotension, respiratory depression).
No products indexed under this heading.

Loxapine Succinate (Profound sedation, coma, severe hypotension, respiratory depression).
No products indexed under this heading.

Meperidine Hydrochloride (Profound sedation, coma, severe hypotension, respiratory depression).
No products indexed under this heading.

Mephobarbital (Profound sedation, coma, severe hypotension, respiratory depression).
No products indexed under this heading.

Meprobamate (Profound sedation, coma, severe hypotension, respiratory depression).
No products indexed under this heading.

Mesoridazine Besylate (Profound sedation, coma, severe hypotension, respiratory depression).
No products indexed under this heading.

Methadone Hydrochloride (Profound sedation, coma, severe hypotension, respiratory depression).
No products indexed under this heading.

Methohexital Sodium (Profound sedation, coma, severe hypotension, respiratory depression).
No products indexed under this heading.

Methotrimeprazine (Profound sedation, coma, severe hypotension, respiratory depression).
No products indexed under this heading.

Methoxyflurane (Profound sedation, coma, severe hypotension, respiratory depression).
No products indexed under this heading.

Metocurine Iodide (Increased respiratory depression).
No products indexed under this heading.

Midazolam Hydrochloride (Profound sedation, coma, severe hypotension, respiratory depression).
No products indexed under this heading.

Mivacurium Chloride (Increased respiratory depression).
No products indexed under this heading.

Molindone Hydrochloride (Profound sedation, coma, severe hypotension, respiratory depression). Products include:
Moban Tablets 1116

Nalbuphine Hydrochloride (Mixed agonist/antagonist analgesics may reduce the analgesic effect or may precipitate withdrawal symptoms).
No products indexed under this heading.

Olanzapine (Profound sedation, coma, severe hypotension, respiratory depression). Products include:
Symbyax Capsules 1871
Zyprexa Tablets 1883
Zyprexa IntraMuscular 1883
Zyprexa ZYDIS Orally Disintegrating Tablets 1883

Oxazepam (Profound sedation, coma, severe hypotension, respiratory depression).
No products indexed under this heading.

Oxycodone Hydrochloride (Profound sedation, coma, severe hypotension, respiratory depression). Products include:
OxyContin Tablets 2589
OxyIR Capsules 2593
Percocet Tablets 1127
Percodan Tablets 1130

Pancuronium Bromide (Increased respiratory depression).
No products indexed under this heading.

Pentazocine Hydrochloride (Mixed agonist/antagonist analgesics may reduce the analgesic effect or may precipitate withdrawal symptoms).
No products indexed under this heading.

Pentazocine Lactate (Mixed agonist/antagonist analgesics may reduce the analgesic effect or may precipitate withdrawal symptoms).
No products indexed under this heading.

Pentobarbital Sodium (Profound sedation, coma, severe hypotension, respiratory depression). Products include:
Nembutal Sodium Solution, USP 2494

Perphenazine (Profound sedation, coma, severe hypotension, respiratory depression).
No products indexed under this heading.

Phenobarbital (Profound sedation, coma, severe hypotension, respiratory depression). Products include:
Donnatal Extentabs 2507

Prazepam (Profound sedation, coma, severe hypotension, respiratory depression).
No products indexed under this heading.

Prochlorperazine (Profound sedation, coma, severe hypotension, respiratory depression).
No products indexed under this heading.

Promethazine Hydrochloride (Profound sedation, coma, severe hypotension, respiratory depression).
No products indexed under this heading.

Propofol (Profound sedation, coma, severe hypotension, respiratory depression).
No products indexed under this heading.

Propoxyphene Hydrochloride (Profound sedation, coma, severe hypotension, respiratory depression).
No products indexed under this heading.

Propoxyphene Napsylate (Profound sedation, coma, severe hypotension, respiratory depression).
No products indexed under this heading.

Quazepam (Profound sedation, coma, severe hypotension, respiratory depression).
No products indexed under this heading.

Quetiapine Fumarate (Profound sedation, coma, severe hypotension, respiratory depression).
No products indexed under this heading.

Ramelteon (Profound sedation, coma, severe hypotension, respiratory depression). Products include:
Rozerem Tablets 3091

Rapacuronium Bromide (Increased respiratory depression).
No products indexed under this heading.

Remifentanil Hydrochloride (Profound sedation, coma, severe hypotension, respiratory depression).
No products indexed under this heading.

Risperidone (Profound sedation, coma, severe hypotension, respiratory depression). Products include:
Risperdal Consta Long-Acting Injection 1753

Rocuronium Bromide (Increased respiratory depression). Products include:
Zemuron Injection 2947

Secobarbital Sodium (Profound sedation, coma, severe hypotension, respiratory depression).
No products indexed under this heading.

Sevoflurane (Profound sedation, coma, severe hypotension, respiratory depression). Products include:
Ultane Liquid for Inhalation 524

Sodium Butabarbital (Profound sedation, coma, severe hypotension, respiratory depression).
No products indexed under this heading.

Sodium Oxybate (Profound sedation, coma, severe hypotension, respiratory depression). Products include:
Xyrem Oral Solution 1766

Succinylcholine Chloride (Increased respiratory depression).
No products indexed under this heading.

Sufentanil Citrate (Profound sedation, coma, severe hypotension, respiratory depression).
No products indexed under this heading.

Temazepam (Profound sedation, coma, severe hypotension, respiratory depression).
No products indexed under this heading.

Thiamylal Sodium (Profound sedation, coma, severe hypotension, respiratory depression).
No products indexed under this heading.

Thioridazine Hydrochloride (Profound sedation, coma, severe hypotension, respiratory depression). Products include:
Thioridazine Hydrochloride Tablets 2195

Thiothixene (Profound sedation, coma, severe hypotension, respiratory depression). Products include:
Thiothixene Capsules 2197

Triazolam (Profound sedation, coma, severe hypotension, respiratory depression).
No products indexed under this heading.

Trifluoperazine Hydrochloride (Profound sedation, coma, severe hypotension, respiratory depression).
No products indexed under this heading.

Vecuronium Bromide (Increased respiratory depression).
No products indexed under this heading.

Zaleplon (Profound sedation, coma, severe hypotension, respiratory depression).
No products indexed under this heading.

Ziprasidone Hydrochloride (Profound sedation, coma, severe hypotension, respiratory depression). Products include:
Geodon Capsules 2520

Zolpidem Tartrate (Profound sedation, coma, severe hypotension, respiratory depression). Products include:
Ambien Tablets 2692
Ambien CR Tablets 2696

Food Interactions

Alcohol (Respiratory depression, hypotension and profound sedation or coma may result).

MUMPSVAX

(Mumps Virus Vaccine, Live) 2068
May interact with immunosuppressive agents. Compounds in these categories include:

Azathioprine (Concurrent immunosuppressive therapy is contraindicated).
No products indexed under this heading.

Basiliximab (Concurrent immunosuppressive therapy is contraindicated). Products include:
Simulect for Injection 2306

Cyclosporine (Concurrent immunosuppressive therapy is contraindicated). Products include:
Gengraf Capsules 435
Neoral Oral Solution 2280
Neoral Soft Gelatin Capsules 2280
Restasis Ophthalmic Emulsion 557
Sandimmune 2296

Muromonab-CD3 (Concurrent immunosuppressive therapy is contraindicated). Products include:
Orthoclone OKT3 Sterile Solution 2387

Mycophenolate Mofetil (Concurrent immunosuppressive therapy is contraindicated). Products include:
CellCept Capsules 2622
CellCept Oral Suspension 2622
CellCept Tablets 2622

Sirolimus (Concurrent immunosuppressive therapy is contraindicated). Products include:
Rapamune 3260

Tacrolimus (Concurrent immunosuppressive therapy is contraindicated). Products include:
Prograf Capsules and Injection 622
Protopic Ointment 628

MURO 128 OPHTHALMIC OINTMENT

(Sodium Chloride) .... ⊙243
None cited in PDR database.

MURO 128 OPHTHALMIC SOLUTION 2% AND 5%

(Sodium Chloride) .... ⊙242
None cited in PDR database.

MUSTARGEN FOR INJECTION

(Mechlorethamine Hydrochloride) 2492
May interact with antineoplastics. Compounds in these categories include:

Altretamine (Hematopoiesis may be further compromised in patients who have been previously treated with chemotherapeutic agents). Products include:
Hexalen Capsules 1078

Anastrozole (Hematopoiesis may be further compromised in patients who have been previously treated with chemotherapeutic agents). Products include:
Arimidex Tablets 672

Asparaginase (Hematopoiesis may be further compromised in patients who have been previously treated with chemotherapeutic agents). Products include:
Elspar for Injection 1990
Elspar for Injection 2488

Bicalutamide (Hematopoiesis may be further compromised in patients who have been previously treated with chemotherapeutic agents). Products include:
No products indexed under this heading.

Bleomycin Sulfate (Hematopoiesis may be further compromised in patients who have been previously treated with chemotherapeutic agents).
No products indexed under this heading.

Busulfan (Hematopoiesis may be further compromised in patients who have been previously treated with chemotherapeutic agents). Products include:
Busulfex Injection 2477
Myleran Tablets 1530

Carboplatin (Hematopoiesis may be further compromised in patients who have been previously treated with chemotherapeutic agents).
No products indexed under this heading.

Carmustine (BCNU) (Hematopoiesis may be further compromised in patients who have been previously treated with chemotherapeutic agents).
No products indexed under this heading.

Chlorambucil (Hematopoiesis may be further compromised in patients who have been previously treated with chemotherapeutic agents). Products include:
Leukeran Tablets 1508

Cisplatin (Hematopoiesis may be further compromised in patients who have been previously treated with chemotherapeutic agents).
No products indexed under this heading.

Cyclophosphamide (Hematopoiesis may be further compromised in patients who have been previously treated with chemotherapeutic agents).
No products indexed under this heading.

Dacarbazine (Hematopoiesis may be further compromised in patients who have been previously treated with chemotherapeutic agents).
No products indexed under this heading.

Daunorubicin Citrate (Hematopoiesis may be further compromised in patients who have been previously treated with chemotherapeutic agents).
No products indexed under this heading.

Daunorubicin Hydrochloride (Hematopoiesis may be further compromised in patients who have been previously treated with chemotherapeutic agents).
No products indexed under this heading.

Denileukin Diftitox (Hematopoiesis may be further compromised in patients who have been previously treated with chemotherapeutic agents). Products include:
Ontak Vials 1079

Docetaxel (Hematopoiesis may be further compromised in patients who have been previously treated with chemotherapeutic agents). Products include:
Taxotere Injection Concentrate 2773

Doxorubicin Hydrochloride (Hematopoiesis may be further compromised in patients who have been previously treated with chemotherapeutic agents).
No products indexed under this heading.

Epirubicin Hydrochloride (Hematopoiesis may be further compromised in patients who have been previously treated with chemotherapeutic agents).
No products indexed under this heading.

Estramustine Phosphate Sodium (Hematopoiesis may be further compromised in patients who have been previously treated with chemotherapeutic agents).
No products indexed under this heading.

Etoposide (Hematopoiesis may be further compromised in patients who have been previously treated with chemotherapeutic agents).
No products indexed under this heading.

Exemestane (Hematopoiesis may be further compromised in patients who have been previously treated with chemotherapeutic agents).
No products indexed under this heading.

Floxuridine (Hematopoiesis may be further compromised in patients who have been previously treated with chemotherapeutic agents).
No products indexed under this heading.

Fluorouracil (Hematopoiesis may be further compromised in patients who have been previously treated with chemotherapeutic agents). Products include:
Carac Cream 0.5% 2722

Flutamide (Hematopoiesis may be further compromised in patients who have been previously treated with chemotherapeutic agents).
No products indexed under this heading.

Gemcitabine Hydrochloride (Hematopoiesis may be further compromised in patients who have been previously treated with chemotherapeutic agents). Products include:
Gemzar for Injection 1820

Hydroxyurea (Hematopoiesis may be further compromised in patients who have been previously treated with chemotherapeutic agents).
No products indexed under this heading.

Idarubicin Hydrochloride (Hematopoiesis may be further compromised in patients who have been previously treated with chemotherapeutic agents).
No products indexed under this heading.

Ifosfamide (Hematopoiesis may be further compromised in patients who have been previously treated with chemotherapeutic agents).
No products indexed under this heading.

Interferon alfa-2a, Recombinant (Hematopoiesis may be further compromised in patients who have been previously treated with chemotherapeutic agents).
No products indexed under this heading.

Interferon alfa-2b, Recombinant (Hematopoiesis may be further compromised in patients who have been previously treated with chemotherapeutic agents). Products include:
Intron A for Injection 2859

Irinotecan Hydrochloride (Hematopoiesis may be further compromised in patients who have been previously treated with chemotherapeutic agents).
No products indexed under this heading.

Levamisole Hydrochloride (Hematopoiesis may be further compromised in patients who have been previously treated with chemotherapeutic agents).
No products indexed under this heading.

Lomustine (CCNU) (Hematopoiesis may be further compromised in patients who have been previously treated with chemotherapeutic agents).
No products indexed under this heading.

Megestrol Acetate (Hematopoiesis may be further compromised in patients who have been previously treated with chemotherapeutic agents). Products include:
Megace ES Oral Suspension 2499

Melphalan (Hematopoiesis may be further compromised in patients who have been previously treated with chemotherapeutic agents).
No products indexed under this heading.

Mercaptopurine (Hematopoiesis may be further compromised in patients who have been previously treated with chemotherapeutic agents).
No products indexed under this heading.

Methotrexate Sodium (Hematopoiesis may be further compromised in patients who have been previously treated with chemotherapeutic agents).
No products indexed under this heading.

Mitomycin (Mitomycin-C) (Hematopoiesis may be further compromised in patients who have been previously treated with chemotherapeutic agents).
No products indexed under this heading.

Mitotane (Hematopoiesis may be further compromised in patients who have been previously treated with chemotherapeutic agents).
No products indexed under this heading.

Mitoxantrone Hydrochloride (Hematopoiesis may be further compromised in patients who have been previously treated with chemotherapeutic agents). Products include:
Novantrone for Injection Concentrate **1100**

Paclitaxel (Hematopoiesis may be further compromised in patients who have been previously treated with chemotherapeutic agents).
No products indexed under this heading.

Procarbazine Hydrochloride (Hematopoiesis may be further compromised in patients who have been previously treated with chemotherapeutic agents).
No products indexed under this heading.

Streptozocin (Hematopoiesis may be further compromised in patients who have been previously treated with chemotherapeutic agents).
No products indexed under this heading.

Tamoxifen Citrate (Hematopoiesis may be further compromised in patients who have been previously treated with chemotherapeutic agents).
No products indexed under this heading.

Teniposide (Hematopoiesis may be further compromised in patients who have been previously treated with chemotherapeutic agents).
No products indexed under this heading.

Thioguanine (Hematopoiesis may be further compromised in patients who have been previously treated with chemotherapeutic agents). Products include:
Tabloid Tablets **1601**

Thiotepa (Hematopoiesis may be further compromised in patients who have been previously treated with chemotherapeutic agents).
No products indexed under this heading.

Topotecan Hydrochloride (Hematopoiesis may be further compromised in patients who have been previously treated with chemotherapeutic agents). Products include:
Hycamtin for Injection **1459**
Hycamtin Capsules **1456**

Toremifene Citrate (Hematopoiesis may be further compromised in patients who have been previously treated with chemotherapeutic agents).
No products indexed under this heading.

Valrubicin (Hematopoiesis may be further compromised in patients who have been previously treated with chemotherapeutic agents). Products include:
Valstar Sterile Solution for Intravesical Instillation **1735**

Vincristine Sulfate (Hematopoiesis may be further compromised in patients who have been previously treated with chemotherapeutic agents).
No products indexed under this heading.

Vinorelbine Tartrate (Hematopoiesis may be further compromised in patients who have been previously treated with chemotherapeutic agents).
No products indexed under this heading.

MYCAMINE FOR INJECTION

(Micafungin Sodium) 616
May interact with:

Itraconazole (When used concomitantly, itraconazole AUC and Cmax were increased by 22% and 11%, respectively. Patients receiving itraconazole in combination with micafungin sodium should be monitored for itraconazole toxicity and itraconazole dosage should be reduced if necessary).
No products indexed under this heading.

Nifedipine (Nifedipine AUC and Cmax were increased by 18% and 42%, respectively, in the presence of steady state micafungin sodium compared with nifedipine alone. Patients receiving nifedipine in combination with micafungin sodium should be monitored for nifedipine toxicity and nifedipine dosage should be reduced if necessary).
No products indexed under this heading.

Sirolimus (Sirolimus AUC was increased by 21% with no effect on Cmax in the presence of steady-state micafungin sodium compared with sirolimus alone. Patients receiving sirolimus in combination with micafungin sodium should be monitored for sirolimus toxicity and sirolimus dosage should be reduced if necessary). Products include:
Rapamune **3260**

MYFORTIC TABLETS

(Mycophenolic Acid) **2276**
May interact with antacids, bacteriostatic antibiotics, bile acid sequestering agents, oral contraceptives, vaccines, live, and certain other agents. Compounds in these categories include:

Acyclovir (May be taken with mycophenolic acid; however, during the period of treatment, physicians should monitor blood cell counts. Both acyclovir and MPAG concentrations are increased in the presence of renal impairment; their coexistence may compete for tubular secretion and further increase in the concentrations of the two). Products include:
Zovirax **1690**
Zovirax Cream **817**
Zovirax Ointment **819**

Acyclovir Sodium (May be taken with mycophenolic acid; however, during the period of treatment, physicians should monitor blood cell counts. Both acyclovir and MPAG concentrations are increased in the presence of renal impairment; their coexistence may compete for tubular secretion and further increase in the concentrations of the two).
No products indexed under this heading.

Aluminum Carbonate (Absorption of a single dose of mycophenolic acid was decreased when administered to stable renal transplant patients also taking magnesium-aluminum containing antacids. Concurrent use with antacids is not recommended).
No products indexed under this heading.

Aluminum Hydroxide (Absorption of a single dose of mycophenolic acid was decreased when administered to stable renal transplant patients also taking magnesium-aluminum containing antacids. Concurrent use with antacids is not recommended).
No products indexed under this heading.

Azathioprine (Given that azathioprine inhibits purine metabolism, it is recommended that mycophenolic acid not be administered concomitantly with azathioprine).
No products indexed under this heading.

Azathioprine Sodium (Given that azathioprine inhibits purine metabolism, it is recommended that mycophenolic acid not be administered concomitantly with azathioprine).
No products indexed under this heading.

BCG Vaccine (During treatment with mycophenolic acid, the use of live attenuated vaccines should be avoided and patients should be advised that vaccinations may be less effective. Influenza vaccination may be of value).
No products indexed under this heading.

Charcoal, Activated (Do not administer mycophenolic acid with agents that may interfere with enterohepatic recirculation, or drugs that may bind bile acids, for example, oral activated charcoal, because of the potential to reduce the efficacy of mycophenolic acid).
No products indexed under this heading.

Chloramphenicol (Drugs that alter the gastrointestinal flora may interact with mycophenolic acid by disrupting enterohepatic recirculation. Interference of MPAG hydrolysis may lead to less mycophenolic acid available for absorption).
No products indexed under this heading.

Chloramphenicol Palmitate (Drugs that alter the gastrointestinal flora may interact with mycophenolic acid by disrupting enterohepatic recirculation. Interference of MPAG hydrolysis may lead to less mycophenolic acid available for absorption).
No products indexed under this heading.

Chloramphenicol Sodium Succinate (Drugs that alter the gastrointestinal flora may interact with mycophenolic acid by disrupting enterohepatic recirculation. Interference of MPAG hydrolysis may lead to less mycophenolic acid available for absorption).
No products indexed under this heading.

Cholestyramine (Do not administer mycophenolic acid with agents that may interfere with enterohepatic recirculation, or drugs that may bind bile acids, for example, bile acid sequestrates, because of the potential to reduce the efficacy of mycophenolic acid).
No products indexed under this heading.

Colesevelam Hydrochloride (Do not administer mycophenolic acid with agents that may interfere with enterohepatic recirculation, or drugs that may bind bile acids, for example, bile acid sequestrates, because of the potential to reduce the efficacy of mycophenolic acid). Products include:
WelChol Tablets **1015**

Colestipol Hydrochloride (Do not administer mycophenolic acid with agents that may interfere with enterohepatic recirculation, or drugs that may bind bile acids, for example, bile acid sequestrates, because of the potential to reduce the efficacy of mycophenolic acid).
No products indexed under this heading.

Demeclocycline Hydrochloride (Drugs that alter the gastrointestinal flora may interact with mycophenolic acid by disrupting enterohepatic recirculation. Interference of MPAG hydrolysis may lead to less mycophenolic acid available for absorption).
No products indexed under this heading.

Desogestrel (In a drug-drug interaction study, mean levonorgesterol AUC was decreased by 15% when co-administered with mycophenolate mofetil; therefore, it is recommended that oral contraceptives are co-administered with mycophenolic acid with caution, and additional birth control methods be considered). Products include:
Mircette Tablets **1034**

Doxycycline Calcium (Drugs that alter the gastrointestinal flora may interact with mycophenolic acid by disrupting enterohepatic recirculation. Interference of MPAG hydrolysis may lead to less mycophenolic acid available for absorption).
No products indexed under this heading.

Doxycycline Hyclate (Drugs that alter the gastrointestinal flora may interact with mycophenolic acid by disrupting enterohepatic recirculation. Interference of MPAG hydrolysis may lead to less mycophenolic acid available for absorption).
No products indexed under this heading.

Doxycycline Monohydrate (Drugs that alter the gastrointestinal flora may interact with mycophenolic acid by disrupting enterohepatic recirculation. Interference of MPAG hydrolysis may lead to less mycophenolic acid available for absorption).
No products indexed under this heading.

Erythromycin (Drugs that alter the gastrointestinal flora may interact with mycophenolic acid by disrupting enterohepatic recirculation. Interference of MPAG hydrolysis may lead to less mycophenolic acid available for absorption).
No products indexed under this heading.

Erythromycin Estolate (Drugs that alter the gastrointestinal flora may interact with mycophenolic acid by disrupting enterohepatic recirculation. Interference of MPAG hydrolysis may lead to less mycophenolic acid available for absorption).
No products indexed under this heading.

Erythromycin Ethylsuccinate (Drugs that alter the gastrointestinal flora may interact with mycophenolic acid by disrupting enterohepatic recirculation. Interference of MPAG hydrolysis may lead to less mycophenolic acid available for absorption). Products include:
E.E.S. 433
EryPed 431

Erythromycin Gluceptate (Drugs that alter the gastrointestinal flora may interact with mycophenolic acid by disrupting enterohepatic recirculation. Interference of MPAG hydrolysis may lead to less mycophenolic acid available for absorption).
No products indexed under this heading.

Erythromycin Stearate (Drugs that alter the gastrointestinal flora may interact with mycophenolic acid by disrupting enterohepatic recirculation. Interference of MPAG hydrolysis may lead to less mycophenolic acid available for absorption).
No products indexed under this heading.

Ethinyl Estradiol (In a drug-drug interaction study, mean levonorgesterol AUC was decreased by 15% when co-administered with mycophenolate mofetil; therefore, it is recommended that oral contraceptives are co-administered with mycophenolic acid with caution, and additional birth control methods be considered). Products include:
Lybrel Tablets 3204
Mircette Tablets 1034
NuvaRing 2897
Ortho-Cyclen/Ortho Tri-Cyclen 2449
Ortho Evra Transdermal System 2437
Ortho Tri-Cyclen Lo Tablets 2458
Seasonique Tablets 1046
Yaz Tablets 805

Ethynodiol Diacetate (In a drug-drug interaction study, mean levonorgesterol AUC was decreased by 15% when co-administered with mycophenolate mofetil; therefore, it is recommended that oral contraceptives are co-administered with mycophenolic acid with caution, and additional birth control methods be considered).
No products indexed under this heading.

Ganciclovir (May be taken with mycophenolic acid; however, during the period of treatment, physicians should monitor blood cell counts. Both ganciclovir and MPAG concentrations are increased in the presence of renal impairment; their coexistence may compete for tubular secretion and further increase in the concentrations of the two).
No products indexed under this heading.

Ganciclovir Sodium (May be taken with mycophenolic acid; however, during the period of treatment, physicians should monitor blood cell counts. Both ganciclovir and MPAG concentrations are increased in the presence of renal impairment; their coexistence may compete for tubular secretion and further increase in the concentrations of the two).
No products indexed under this heading.

Influenza Vaccine, Live Attenuated (During treatment with mycophenolic acid, the use of live attenuated vaccines should be avoided and patients should be advised that vaccinations may be less effective. Influenza vaccination may be of value).
No products indexed under this heading.

Influenza Virus Vaccine Live, Intranasal (During treatment with mycophenolic acid, the use of live attenuated vaccines should be avoided and patients should be advised that vaccinations may be less effective. Influenza vaccination may be of value). Products include:
FluMist Vaccine 1945

Levonorgestrel (In a drug-drug interaction study, mean levonorgesterol AUC was decreased by 15% when co-administered with mycophenolate mofetil; therefore, it is recommended that oral contraceptives are co-administered with mycophenolic acid with caution, and additional birth control methods be considered). Products include:
Climara Pro Transdermal System 768
Lybrel Tablets 3204
Mirena Intrauterine System 779
Plan B Tablets 1044
Seasonique Tablets 1046

Magaldrate (Absorption of a single dose of mycophenolic acid was decreased when administered to stable renal transplant patients also taking magnesium-aluminum containing antacids. Concurrent use with antacids is not recommended).
No products indexed under this heading.

Magnesium Hydroxide (Absorption of a single dose of mycophenolic acid was decreased when administered to stable renal transplant patients also taking magnesium-aluminum containing antacids. Concurrent use with antacids is not recommended). Products include:
Fleet Pedia-Lax Chewable Tablets 1145
Pepcid Complete Chewable Tablets 1771
Extra Strength Rolaids Freshmint Tablets 1903
Rolaids Multi-Symptom Berry Tablets 1903
Rolaids Original Peppermint Tablets 1903

Magnesium Oxide (Absorption of a single dose of mycophenolic acid was decreased when administered to stable renal transplant patients also taking magnesium-aluminum containing antacids. Concurrent use with antacids is not recommended). Products include:
Beelith Tablets 813

Measles, Mumps, Rubella and Varicella Virus Vaccine Live (During treatment with mycophenolic acid, the use of live attenuated vaccines should be avoided and patients should be advised that vaccinations may be less effective. Influenza vaccination may be of value). Products include:
ProQuad 2099

Measles, Mumps & Rubella Virus Vaccine, Live (During treatment with mycophenolic acid, the use of live attenuated vaccines should be avoided and patients should be advised that vaccinations may be less effective. Influenza vaccination may be of value). Products include:
M-M-R II 2054

Measles & Rubella Virus Vaccine Live (During treatment with mycophenolic acid, the use of live attenuated vaccines should be avoided and patients should be advised that vaccinations may be less effective. Influenza vaccination may be of value).
No products indexed under this heading.

Measles Virus Vaccine Live (During treatment with mycophenolic acid, the use of live attenuated vaccines should be avoided and patients should be advised that vaccinations may be less effective. Influenza vaccination may be of value). Products include:
Attenuvax 1951

Mestranol (In a drug-drug interaction study, mean levonorgesterol AUC was decreased by 15% when co-administered with mycophenolate mofetil; therefore, it is recommended that oral contraceptives are co-administered with mycophenolic acid with caution, and additional birth control methods be considered).
No products indexed under this heading.

Methacycline Hydrochloride (Drugs that alter the gastrointestinal flora may interact with mycophenolic acid by disrupting enterohepatic recirculation. Interference of MPAG hydrolysis may lead to less mycophenolic acid available for absorption).
No products indexed under this heading.

Minocycline Hydrochloride (Drugs that alter the gastrointestinal flora may interact with mycophenolic acid by disrupting enterohepatic recirculation. Interference of MPAG hydrolysis may lead to less mycophenolic acid available for absorption). Products include:
Solodyn Extended Release Tablets 1938

Mumps Virus Vaccine, Live (During treatment with mycophenolic acid, the use of live attenuated vaccines should be avoided and patients should be advised that vaccinations may be less effective. Influenza vaccination may be of value). Products include:
Mumpsvax 2068

Mycophenolate Mofetil (Given that mycophenolate mofetil inhibits purine metabolism, it is recommended that mycophenolic acid not be administered concomitantly with mycophenolate mofetil). Products include:
CellCept Capsules 2622
CellCept Oral Suspension 2622
CellCept Tablets 2622

Mycophenolate Mofetil Hydrochloride (Given that mycophenolate mofetil inhibits purine metabolism, it is recommended that mycophenolic acid not be administered concomitantly with mycophenolate mofetil). Products include:
CellCept Intravenous 2622

Norethindrone (In a drug-drug interaction study, mean levonorgesterol AUC was decreased by 15% when co-administered with mycophenolate mofetil; therefore, it is recommended that oral contraceptives are co-administered with mycophenolic acid with caution, and additional birth control methods be considered). Products include:
Ortho Micronor Tablets 2446

Norethynodrel (In a drug-drug interaction study, mean levonorgesterol AUC was decreased by 15% when co-administered with mycophenolate mofetil; therefore, it is recommended that oral contraceptives are co-administered with mycophenolic acid with caution, and additional birth control methods be considered).
No products indexed under this heading.

Norgestimate (In a drug-drug interaction study, mean levonorgesterol AUC was decreased by 15% when co-administered with mycophenolate mofetil; therefore, it is recommended that oral contraceptives are co-administered with mycophenolic acid with caution, and additional birth control methods be considered). Products include:
Ortho-Cyclen/Ortho Tri-Cyclen 2449
Ortho Tri-Cyclen Lo Tablets 2458

Norgestrel (In a drug-drug interaction study, mean levonorgesterol AUC was decreased by 15% when co-administered with mycophenolate mofetil; therefore, it is recommended that oral contraceptives are co-administered with mycophenolic acid with caution, and additional birth control methods be considered).
No products indexed under this heading.

Oxytetracycline Hydrochloride (Drugs that alter the gastrointestinal flora may interact with mycophenolic acid by disrupting enterohepatic recirculation. Interference of MPAG hydrolysis may lead to less mycophenolic acid available for absorption).
No products indexed under this heading.

Poliovirus Vaccine, Live, Oral, Trivalent, Types 1,2,3 (Sabin) (During treatment with mycophenolic acid, the use of live attenuated vaccines should be avoided and patients should be advised that vaccinations may be less effective. Influenza vaccination may be of value).
No products indexed under this heading.

Rotavirus Vaccine, Live, Oral, Tetravalent (During treatment with mycophenolic acid, the use of live attenuated vaccines should be avoided and patients should be advised that vaccinations may be less effective. Influenza vaccination may be of value).
No products indexed under this heading.

Rubella & Mumps Virus Vaccine Live (During treatment with mycophenolic acid, the use of live attenuated vaccines should be avoided and patients should be advised that vaccinations may be less effective. Influenza vaccination may be of value).
No products indexed under this heading.

Rubella Virus Vaccine Live (During treatment with mycophenolic acid, the use of live attenuated vaccines should be avoided and patients should be advised that vaccinations may be less effective. Influenza vaccination may be of value). Products include:
Meruvax II 2061

Smallpox Vaccine (During treatment with mycophenolic acid, the use of live attenuated vaccines should be avoided and patients should be advised that vaccinations may be less effective. Influenza vaccination may be of value).
No products indexed under this heading.

Sodium Bicarbonate (Absorption of a single dose of mycophenolic acid was decreased when administered to stable renal transplant patients also taking magnesium-aluminum containing antacids. Concurrent use with antacids is not recommended). Products include:
Ceo-Two Laxative Suppository 815

Sulfamethizole (Drugs that alter the gastrointestinal flora may interact with mycophenolic acid by disrupting enterohepatic recirculation. Interference of MPAG hydrolysis may lead to less mycophenolic acid available for absorption).
No products indexed under this heading.

Sulfamethoxazole (Drugs that alter the gastrointestinal flora may interact with mycophenolic acid by disrupting enterohepatic recirculation. Interference of MPAG hydrolysis may lead to less mycophenolic acid available for absorption).
No products indexed under this heading.

Sulfisoxazole Acetyl (Drugs that alter the gastrointestinal flora may interact with mycophenolic acid by disrupting enterohepatic recirculation. Interference of MPAG hydrolysis may lead to less mycophenolic acid available for absorption).
No products indexed under this heading.

Tetracycline Hydrochloride (Drugs that alter the gastrointestinal flora may interact with mycophenolic acid by disrupting enterohepatic recirculation. Interference of MPAG hydrolysis may lead to less mycophenolic acid available for absorption). Products include:
Pylera Capsules 714

Typhoid Vaccine (During treatment with mycophenolic acid, the use of live attenuated vaccines should be avoided and patients should be advised that vaccinations may be less effective. Influenza vaccination may be of value).
No products indexed under this heading.

Varicella Virus Vaccine Live (During treatment with mycophenolic acid, the use of live attenuated vaccines should be avoided and patients should be advised that vaccinations may be less effective. Influenza vaccination may be of value). Products include:
Varivax 2133

Yellow Fever Vaccine (During treatment with mycophenolic acid, the use of live attenuated vaccines should be avoided and patients should be advised that vaccinations may be less effective. Influenza vaccination may be of value).
No products indexed under this heading.

Zoster Vaccine Live (During treatment with mycophenolic acid, the use of live attenuated vaccines should be avoided and patients should be advised that vaccinations may be less effective. Influenza vaccination may be of value). Products include:
Zostavax Injection 2145

MYLERAN TABLETS

(Busulfan) 1530

May interact with antineoplastics, cytotoxic drugs, agents associated with myelosuppression, and certain other agents. Compounds in these categories include:

Altretamine (Potential for rare life-threatening hepatic veno-occlusive disease). Products include:
Hexalen Capsules 1078

Anastrozole (Potential for rare life-threatening hepatic veno-occlusive disease). Products include:
Arimidex Tablets 672

Asparaginase (Potential for rare life-threatening hepatic veno-occlusive disease). Products include:
Elspar for Injection 1990
Elspar for Injection 2488

Bicalutamide (Potential for rare life-threatening hepatic veno-occlusive disease). Products include:
No products indexed under this heading.

Bleomycin Sulfate (Busulfan-induced pulmonary toxicity may be additive to the effects produced by other cytotoxic agents).
No products indexed under this heading.

Bone Marrow Depressants, unspecified (Additive myelosuppression).
No products indexed under this heading.

Carboplatin (Potential for rare life-threatening hepatic veno-occlusive disease).
No products indexed under this heading.

Carmustine (BCNU) (Potential for rare life-threatening hepatic veno-occlusive disease).
No products indexed under this heading.

Chlorambucil (Potential for rare life-threatening hepatic veno-occlusive disease). Products include:
Leukeran Tablets 1508

Cisplatin (Potential for rare life-threatening hepatic veno-occlusive disease).
No products indexed under this heading.

Cladribine (Busulfan may cause additive myelosuppression when used with other myelosuppressive drugs). Products include:
Leustatin Injection 2384

Cyclophosphamide (Potential for rare life-threatening hepatic veno-occlusive disease; potential for cardiac temponade; co-administration may result in reduced busulfan clearance).
No products indexed under this heading.

Dacarbazine (Potential for rare life-threatening hepatic veno-occlusive disease).
No products indexed under this heading.

Daunorubicin Citrate (Potential for rare life-threatening hepatic veno-occlusive disease).
No products indexed under this heading.

Daunorubicin Citrate Liposome (Busulfan may cause additive myelosuppression when used with other myelosuppressive drugs).
No products indexed under this heading.

Daunorubicin Hydrochloride (Busulfan-induced pulmonary toxicity may be additive to the effects produced by other cytotoxic agents).
No products indexed under this heading.

Denileukin Diftitox (Potential for rare life-threatening hepatic veno-occlusive disease). Products include:
Ontak Vials 1079

Dexrazoxane (Busulfan may cause additive myelosuppression when used with other myelosuppressive drugs).
No products indexed under this heading.

Docetaxel (Potential for rare life-threatening hepatic veno-occlusive disease). Products include:
Taxotere Injection Concentrate 2773

Doxorubicin Hydrochloride (Busulfan-induced pulmonary toxicity may be additive to the effects produced by other cytotoxic agents).
No products indexed under this heading.

Doxorubicin Hydrochloride Liposome (Busulfan may cause additive myelosuppression when used with other myelosuppressive drugs). Products include:
Doxil Injection 2378

Epirubicin Hydrochloride (Busulfan-induced pulmonary toxicity may be additive to the effects produced by other cytotoxic agents).
No products indexed under this heading.

Estramustine Phosphate Sodium (Potential for rare life-threatening hepatic veno-occlusive disease).
No products indexed under this heading.

Etoposide (Potential for rare life-threatening hepatic veno-occlusive disease).
No products indexed under this heading.

Exemestane (Potential for rare life-threatening hepatic veno-occlusive disease).
No products indexed under this heading.

Floxuridine (Potential for rare life-threatening hepatic veno-occlusive disease).
No products indexed under this heading.

Fludarabine Phosphate (Busulfan may cause additive myelosuppression when used with other myelosuppressive drugs).
No products indexed under this heading.

Fluorouracil (Busulfan-induced pulmonary toxicity may be additive to the effects produced by other cytotoxic agents). Products include:
Carac Cream 0.5% 2722

Flutamide (Potential for rare life-threatening hepatic veno-occlusive disease).
No products indexed under this heading.

Gemcitabine Hydrochloride (Potential for rare life-threatening hepatic veno-occlusive disease). Products include:
Gemzar for Injection 1820

Gemtuzumab Ozogamicin (Busulfan may cause additive myelosuppression when used with other myelosuppressive drugs). Products include:
Mylotarg for Injection 3212

Hydroxyurea (Busulfan-induced pulmonary toxicity may be additive to the effects produced by other cytotoxic agents).
No products indexed under this heading.

Idarubicin Hydrochloride (Potential for rare life-threatening hepatic veno-occlusive disease).
No products indexed under this heading.

Ifosfamide (Potential for rare life-threatening hepatic veno-occlusive disease).
No products indexed under this heading.

Interferon alfa-2a, Recombinant (Potential for rare life-threatening hepatic veno-occlusive disease).
No products indexed under this heading.

Interferon alfa-2b, Recombinant (Potential for rare life-threatening hepatic veno-occlusive disease). Products include:
Intron A for Injection 2859

Irinotecan Hydrochloride (Potential for rare life-threatening hepatic veno-occlusive disease).
No products indexed under this heading.

Itraconazole (The concomitant systemic administration of itraconazole to patients receiving high-dose busulfan may result in reduced busulfan clearance. Patients should be monitored for signs of busulfan toxicity when itraconazole is used concomitantly with busulfan).
No products indexed under this heading.

Levamisole Hydrochloride (Potential for rare life-threatening hepatic veno-occlusive disease).
No products indexed under this heading.

Lomustine (CCNU) (Potential for rare life-threatening hepatic veno-occlusive disease).
No products indexed under this heading.

Mechlorethamine Hydrochloride (Potential for rare life-threatening hepatic veno-occlusive disease). Products include:
Mustargen for Injection 2492

Megestrol Acetate (Potential for rare life-threatening hepatic veno-occlusive disease). Products include:

Megace ES Oral Suspension 2499

Melphalan (Potential for rare life-threatening hepatic veno-occlusive disease).
No products indexed under this heading.

Melphalan Hydrochloride (Busulfan may cause additive myelosuppression when used with other myelosuppressive drugs).
No products indexed under this heading.

Mercaptopurine (Potential for rare life-threatening hepatic veno-occlusive disease).
No products indexed under this heading.

Methotrexate Sodium (Busulfan-induced pulmonary toxicity may be additive to the effects produced by other cytotoxic agents).
No products indexed under this heading.

Metronidazole (The concomitant administration of metronidazole and high-dose busulfan may result in increased trough levels of busulfan and, therefore, it is not recommended). Products include:
Pylera Capsules 714

Metronidazole Benzoate (The concomitant administration of metronidazole and high-dose busulfan may result in increased trough levels of busulfan and, therefore, it is not recommended).
No products indexed under this heading.

Metronidazole Hydrochloride (The concomitant administration of metronidazole and high-dose busulfan may result in increased trough levels of busulfan and, therefore, it is not recommended).
No products indexed under this heading.

Metronidazole Sodium (The concomitant administration of metronidazole and high-dose busulfan may result in increased trough levels of busulfan and, therefore, it is not recommended).
No products indexed under this heading.

Mitomycin (Mitomycin-C) (Potential for rare life-threatening hepatic veno-occlusive disease).
No products indexed under this heading.

Mitotane (Busulfan-induced pulmonary toxicity may be additive to the effects produced by other cytotoxic agents).
No products indexed under this heading.

Mitoxantrone Hydrochloride (Busulfan-induced pulmonary toxicity may be additive to the effects produced by other cytotoxic agents).
Products include:
Novantrone for Injection Concentrate 1100

Oxaliplatin (Potential for rare life-threatening hepatic veno-occlusive disease). Products include:
Eloxatin for Injection 2731

Paclitaxel (Potential for rare life-threatening hepatic veno-occlusive disease).
No products indexed under this heading.

Procarbazine Hydrochloride (Busulfan-induced pulmonary toxicity may be additive to the effects produced by other cytotoxic agents).
No products indexed under this heading.

Streptozocin (Potential for rare life-threatening hepatic veno-occlusive disease).
No products indexed under this heading.

Tamoxifen Citrate (Busulfan-induced pulmonary toxicity may be additive to the effects produced by other cytotoxic agents).
No products indexed under this heading.

Temozolomide (Busulfan may cause additive myelosuppression when used with other myelosuppressive drugs). Products include:
Temodar Capsules 2931

Teniposide (Potential for rare life-threatening hepatic veno-occlusive disease).
No products indexed under this heading.

Thioguanine (Potential for portal hypertension and esophageal varices associated with abnormal liver function tests; potential for rare life-threatening hepatic veno-occlusive disease). Products include:
Tabloid Tablets 1601

Thiotepa (Potential for rare life-threatening hepatic veno-occlusive disease).
No products indexed under this heading.

Topotecan Hydrochloride (Potential for rare life-threatening hepatic veno-occlusive disease). Products include:
Hycamtin for Injection 1459
Hycamtin Capsules 1456

Toremifene Citrate (Potential for rare life-threatening hepatic veno-occlusive disease).
No products indexed under this heading.

Valrubicin (Potential for rare life-threatening hepatic veno-occlusive disease). Products include:
Valstar Sterile Solution for Intravesical Instillation 1735

Vincristine Sulfate (Busulfan-induced pulmonary toxicity may be additive to the effects produced by other cytotoxic agents).
No products indexed under this heading.

Vinorelbine Tartrate (Potential for rare life-threatening hepatic veno-occlusive disease).
No products indexed under this heading.

MYLOTARG FOR INJECTION

(Gemtuzumab Ozogamicin) 3212
May interact with drugs which undergo biotransformation by cytochrome p-450 mixed function oxidase. Compounds in these categories include:

Acarbose (Potential for drug-drug interaction with drugs affected by CYP450 enzymes). Products include:
Precose Tablets 792

Acetaminophen (Potential for drug-drug interaction with drugs affected by CYP450 enzymes). Products include:
Benadryl Allergy & Cold Kapgels 1895
Benadryl Allergy & Sinus Headache Kapgels 1895
Benadryl Severe Allergy & Sinus Headache Caplets 1897
Lortab 5/500 Tablets 3143
Lortab 7.5/500 Tablets 3144
Lortab 10/500 Tablets 3144
Percocet Tablets 1127
Sinutab Sinus Caplets 1905
Sudafed PE Cold & Cough Caplets 1907
Sudafed PE Nighttime Cold Caplets 1907
Sudafed PE Severe Cold Caplets 1908
Sudafed PE Sinus Headache Caplets 1908
Regular Strength Tylenol Tablets 1915
Tylenol 8 Hour Extended Release Caplets 1915
Extra Strength Tylenol Caplets, Cool Caplets, and EZ Tabs 1915
Extra Strength Tylenol Adult Rapid Blast Liquid 1915
Extra Strength Tylenol PM Caplets, Geltabs, Liquid, and Rapid Release Gels 1915
Extra Strength Tylenol Rapid Release Gels 1915
Tylenol with Codeine Tablets 2427
Tylenol Allergy Multi-Symptom Caplets with Cool Burst and Rapid Release Gelcaps 1916
Tylenol Allergy Multi-Symptom Nighttime Caplets with Cool Burst 1916
Tylenol Severe Allergy Caplets 1916
Tylenol Arthritis Pain Extended Release Geltabs/Caplets 1915
Tylenol Chest Congestion Caplets with Cool Burst 1910
Tylenol Chest Congestion Liquid with Cool Burst 1910
Children's Tylenol Plus Cold Suspension Liquid 1912
Children's Tylenol Plus Cold & Allergy Suspension Liquid 1914
Children's Tylenol Plus Cough & Runny Nose Suspension Liquid 1912
Children's Tylenol Plus Cough & Sore Throat Suspension Liquid 1912
Children's Tylenol Plus Flu Suspension Liquid 1914
Children's Tylenol Suspension Liquid 1909
Children's Tylenol Meltaways 1909
Children's Tylenol Plus Multi-Symptom Cold Suspension Liquid 1912
Tylenol Cold Severe Congestion Daytime Caplets with Cool Burst 1912
Tylenol Cold Head Congestion Daytime Caplets with Cool Burst 1910
Tylenol Cold Head Congestion Nighttime Caplets with Cool Burst 1910
Tylenol Cold Head Congestion Severe Daytime Caplets with Cool Burst 1910
Tylenol Cold Multi-Symptom Daytime Caplets with Cool Burst and Rapid Release Gels 1913
Tylenol Cold Multi-Symptom Daytime Liquid with Citrus Burst 1913
Tylenol Cold Multi-Symptom Nighttime Caplets with Cool Burst 1913
Tylenol Cold Multi-Symptom Nighttime Liquid with Cool Burst 1913
Tylenol Cold Multi-Symptom Severe Caplets with Cool Burst 1913
Tylenol Cold Multi-Symptom Severe Daytime Liquid with Citrus Burst 1913
Tylenol Cough & Sore Throat Daytime Liquid with Cool Burst 1918
Tylenol Cough & Sore Throat Nighttime Liquid with Cool Burst 1918
Concentrated Tylenol Infants' Drops 1909
Jr. Tylenol Meltaways 1909
Tylenol Sinus Congestion & Pain Daytime Caplets with Cool Burst and Gelcaps 1917
Tylenol Sinus Congestion & Pain Nighttime Caplets with Cool Burst 1917
Tylenol Sinus Congestion & Pain Severe Caplets with Cool Burst 1917
Tylenol Sinus Severe Congestion Caplets with Cool Burst 1917
Tylenol Sore Throat Daytime Liquid with Cool Burst 1918
Tylenol Sore Throat Nighttime Liquid with Cool Burst 1918
Women's Tylenol Menstrual Relief Caplets 1919
Vicks DayQuil Cold & Flu Multi-Symptom Relief 616
Vicks DayQuil LiquiCaps 2567
Vicks DayQuil Liquid 2567
Vicks DayQuil Multi-Symptom Cold/Flu Relief 2567
Vicks NyQuil Cold & Flu Multi-Symptom Relief 617
Vicks NyQuil LiquiCaps 2567
Vicks NyQuil Liquid 2567
Vicks NyQuil Multi-Symptom Cold/Flu Relief 2567
Vicodin Tablets 529
Vicodin ES Tablets 530
Vicodin HP Tablets 531
Zydone Tablets 1132

Alatrofloxacin Mesylate (Potential for drug-drug interaction with drugs affected by CYP450 enzymes).
No products indexed under this heading.

Alfentanil Hydrochloride (Potential for drug-drug interaction with drugs affected by CYP450 enzymes).
No products indexed under this heading.

Alprazolam (Potential for drug-drug interaction with drugs affected by CYP450 enzymes).
No products indexed under this heading.

Aminophylline (Potential for drug-drug interaction with drugs affected by CYP450 enzymes).
No products indexed under this heading.

Amiodarone Hydrochloride (Potential for drug-drug interaction with drugs affected by CYP450 enzymes).
No products indexed under this heading.

Amitriptyline Hydrochloride (Potential for drug-drug interaction with drugs affected by CYP450 enzymes).
No products indexed under this heading.

Amlodipine Besylate (Potential for drug-drug interaction with drugs affected by CYP450 enzymes). Products include:
Azor Tablets 1005
Exforge Tablets 2238

Amoxapine (Potential for drug-drug interaction with drugs affected by CYP450 enzymes).
No products indexed under this heading.

Amphetamine Aspartate (Potential for drug-drug interaction with drugs affected by CYP450 enzymes). Products include:
Adderall XR Capsules 3012

Amphetamine Aspartate Monohydrate (Potential for drug-drug interaction with drugs affected by CYP450 enzymes).
No products indexed under this heading.

Amphetamine Sulfate (Potential for drug-drug interaction with drugs affected by CYP450 enzymes). Products include:
Adderall XR Capsules 3012

Aprepitant (Potential for drug-drug interaction with drugs affected by CYP450 enzymes). Products include:
Emend Capsules 1992

Astemizole (Potential for drug-drug interaction with drugs affected by CYP450 enzymes).
No products indexed under this heading.

Atomoxetine Hydrochloride (Potential for drug-drug interaction with drugs affected by CYP450 enzymes). Products include:
Strattera Capsules 1864

Atorvastatin Calcium (Potential for drug-drug interaction with drugs affected by CYP450 enzymes). Products include:
Lipitor Tablets 2501

Belladonna Ergotamine (Potential for drug-drug interaction with drugs affected by CYP450 enzymes).
No products indexed under this heading.

Benzphetamine Hydrochloride (Potential for drug-drug interaction with drugs affected by CYP450 enzymes).
No products indexed under this heading.

Bisoprolol Fumarate (Potential for drug-drug interaction with drugs affected by CYP450 enzymes).
No products indexed under this heading.

Buspirone Hydrochloride (Potential for drug-drug interaction with drugs affected by CYP450 enzymes).
No products indexed under this heading.

Busulfan (Potential for drug-drug interaction with drugs affected by CYP450 enzymes). Products include:
Busulfex Injection 2477
Myleran Tablets 1530

Caffeine (Potential for drug-drug interaction with drugs affected by CYP450 enzymes). Products include:
BioLean Free Tablets .... ▣635
BioLean II Tablets .... ▣635
Winrgy Dietary Supplement .... ▣642

Caffeine Anhydrous (Potential for drug-drug interaction with drugs affected by CYP450 enzymes).
No products indexed under this heading.

Caffeine Citrate (Potential for drug-drug interaction with drugs affected by CYP450 enzymes).
No products indexed under this heading.

Candesartan Cilexetil (Potential for drug-drug interaction with drugs affected by CYP450 enzymes). Products include:
Atacand Tablets 639
Atacand HCT 642

Captopril (Potential for drug-drug interaction with drugs affected by CYP450 enzymes). Products include:
Captopril Tablets 2182

Carbamazepine (Potential for drug-drug interaction with drugs affected by CYP450 enzymes). Products include:
Carbatrol Capsules 3019
Equetro Extended-Release Capsules 3174

Carisoprodol (Potential for drug-drug interaction with drugs affected by CYP450 enzymes). Products include:
Soma Tablets 1931

Carvedilol (Potential for drug-drug interaction with drugs affected by CYP450 enzymes). Products include:
Coreg Tablets 1387

Celecoxib (Potential for drug-drug interaction with drugs affected by CYP450 enzymes). Products include:
Celebrex Capsules 2979

Cerivastatin Sodium (Potential for drug-drug interaction with drugs affected by CYP450 enzymes).
No products indexed under this heading.

Cevimeline Hydrochloride (Potential for drug-drug interaction with drugs affected by CYP450 enzymes). Products include:
Evoxac Capsules 1013

Chlordiazepoxide (Potential for drug-drug interaction with drugs affected by CYP450 enzymes).
No products indexed under this heading.

Chlordiazepoxide Hydrochloride (Potential for drug-drug interaction with drugs affected by CYP450 enzymes).
No products indexed under this heading.

Chlorpheniramine (Potential for drug-drug interaction with drugs affected by CYP450 enzymes).
No products indexed under this heading.

Chlorpheniramine Maleate (Potential for drug-drug interaction with drugs affected by CYP450 enzymes). Products include:
Actifed Cold & Allergy Tablets 1895
Sudafed PE Sinus & Allergy Tablets 1908
Tylenol Allergy Multi-Symptom Caplets with Cool Burst and Rapid Release Gelcaps 1916
Children's Tylenol Plus Cold Suspension Liquid 1912
Children's Tylenol Plus Cough & Runny Nose Suspension Liquid 1912
Children's Tylenol Plus Flu Suspension Liquid 1914
Children's Tylenol Plus Multi-Symptom Cold Suspension Liquid 1912
Tylenol Cold Head Congestion Nighttime Caplets with Cool Burst 1910
Tylenol Cold Multi-Symptom Nighttime Caplets with Cool Burst 1913
Tylenol Sinus Congestion & Pain Nighttime Caplets with Cool Burst 1917

Chlorpheniramine Polistirex (Potential for drug-drug interaction with drugs affected by CYP450 enzymes). Products include:
Tussionex Pennkinetic Extended-Release Suspension 3154

Chlorpheniramine Tannate (Potential for drug-drug interaction with drugs affected by CYP450 enzymes).
No products indexed under this heading.

Chlorpromazine (Potential for drug-drug interaction with drugs affected by CYP450 enzymes).
No products indexed under this heading.

Chlorpromazine Hydrochloride (Potential for drug-drug interaction with drugs affected by CYP450 enzymes).
No products indexed under this heading.

Chlorpropamide (Potential for drug-drug interaction with drugs affected by CYP450 enzymes).
No products indexed under this heading.

Cilostazol (Potential for drug-drug interaction with drugs affected by CYP450 enzymes). Products include:
Pletal Tablets 2481

Cimetidine Hydrochloride (Potential for drug-drug interaction with drugs affected by CYP450 enzymes).
No products indexed under this heading.

Ciprofloxacin (Potential for drug-drug interaction with drugs affected by CYP450 enzymes). Products include:
Cipro I.V. 2817
Cipro Oral Suspension 2810
Cipro XR Tablets 2823
Ciprodex Otic Suspension 541

Ciprofloxacin Hydrochloride (Potential for drug-drug interaction with drugs affected by CYP450 enzymes). Products include:
Cipro Tablets 2810

Cisapride (Potential for drug-drug interaction with drugs affected by CYP450 enzymes).
No products indexed under this heading.

Citalopram Hydrobromide (Potential for drug-drug interaction with drugs affected by CYP450 enzymes). Products include:
Celexa 1160

Clarithromycin (Potential for drug-drug interaction with drugs affected by CYP450 enzymes). Products include:
Biaxin/Biaxin XL 411

Clomipramine Hydrochloride (Potential for drug-drug interaction with drugs affected by CYP450 enzymes).
No products indexed under this heading.

Clopidogrel Hydrogen Sulfate (Potential for drug-drug interaction with drugs affected by CYP450 enzymes).
No products indexed under this heading.

Clozapine (Potential for drug-drug interaction with drugs affected by CYP450 enzymes).
No products indexed under this heading.

Codeine Phosphate (Potential for drug-drug interaction with drugs affected by CYP450 enzymes). Products include:
Tylenol with Codeine Tablets 2427

Codeine Sulfate (Potential for drug-drug interaction with drugs affected by CYP450 enzymes).
No products indexed under this heading.

Cyclobenzaprine (Potential for drug-drug interaction with drugs affected by CYP450 enzymes).
No products indexed under this heading.

Cyclobenzaprine Hydrochloride (Potential for drug-drug interaction with drugs affected by CYP450 enzymes). Products include:
Amrix Capsules 966

Cyclophosphamide (Potential for drug-drug interaction with drugs affected by CYP450 enzymes).
No products indexed under this heading.

Cyclosporine (Potential for drug-drug interaction with drugs affected by CYP450 enzymes). Products include:
Gengraf Capsules 435
Neoral Oral Solution 2280
Neoral Soft Gelatin Capsules 2280
Restasis Ophthalmic Emulsion 557
Sandimmune 2296

Desipramine Hydrochloride (Potential for drug-drug interaction with drugs affected by CYP450 enzymes).
No products indexed under this heading.

Desogestrel (Potential for drug-drug interaction with drugs affected by CYP450 enzymes). Products include:
Mircette Tablets 1034

Dexamethasone (Potential for drug-drug interaction with drugs affected by CYP450 enzymes). Products include:
Ciprodex Otic Suspension 541

Dexamethasone Acetate (Potential for drug-drug interaction with drugs affected by CYP450 enzymes).
No products indexed under this heading.

Dexamethasone Phosphate (Potential for drug-drug interaction with drugs affected by CYP450 enzymes).
No products indexed under this heading.

Dexamethasone Sodium (Potential for drug-drug interaction with drugs affected by CYP450 enzymes).
No products indexed under this heading.

Dexamethasone Sodium Phosphate (Potential for drug-drug interaction with drugs affected by CYP450 enzymes).
No products indexed under this heading.

Dexfenfluramine Hydrochloride (Potential for drug-drug interaction with drugs affected by CYP450 enzymes).
No products indexed under this heading.

Dextromethorphan (Potential for drug-drug interaction with drugs affected by CYP450 enzymes).
No products indexed under this heading.

Dextromethorphan Hydrobromide (Potential for drug-drug interaction with drugs affected by CYP450 enzymes). Products include:
PediaCare Children's Liquid Multi-Symptom Cold 1902
PediaCare Children's Long-Acting Cough 1902
Children's Sudafed PE Cold & Cough Liquid 1907
Sudafed PE Cold & Cough Caplets 1907
Children's Tylenol Plus Cough & Runny Nose Suspension Liquid 1912
Children's Tylenol Plus Cough & Sore Throat Suspension Liquid 1912
Children's Tylenol Plus Flu Suspension Liquid 1914
Children's Tylenol Plus Multi-Symptom Cold Suspension Liquid 1912

Tylenol Cold Severe Congestion Daytime Caplets with Cool Burst ... 1912
Tylenol Cold Head Congestion Daytime Caplets with Cool Burst ... 1910
Tylenol Cold Head Congestion Nighttime Caplets with Cool Burst ... 1910
Tylenol Cold Head Congestion Severe Daytime Caplets with Cool Burst ... 1910
Tylenol Cold Multi-Symptom Daytime Caplets with Cool Burst and Rapid Release Gels ... 1913
Tylenol Cold Multi-Symptom Daytime Liquid with Citrus Burst ... 1913
Tylenol Cold Multi-Symptom Nighttime Caplets with Cool Burst ... 1913
Tylenol Cold Multi-Symptom Nighttime Liquid with Cool Burst ... 1913
Tylenol Cold Multi-Symptom Severe Caplets with Cool Burst ... 1913
Tylenol Cold Multi-Symptom Severe Daytime Liquid with Citrus Burst ... 1913
Tylenol Cough & Sore Throat Daytime Liquid with Cool Burst ... 1918
Tylenol Cough & Sore Throat Nighttime Liquid with Cool Burst ... 1918
Vicks DayQuil Cold & Flu Multi-Symptom Relief ... ▣616
Vicks DayQuil LiquiCaps ... 2567
Vicks DayQuil Liquid ... 2567
Vicks DayQuil Multi-Symptom Cold/Flu Relief ... 2567
Vicks NyQuil Cold & Flu Multi-Symptom Relief ... ▣617
Vicks NyQuil LiquiCaps ... 2567
Vicks NyQuil Liquid ... 2567
Vicks NyQuil Multi-Symptom Cold/Flu Relief ... 2567

Dextromethorphan Polistirex (Potential for drug-drug interaction with drugs affected by CYP450 enzymes).
No products indexed under this heading.

Diazepam (Potential for drug-drug interaction with drugs affected by CYP450 enzymes). Products include:
Valium Tablets ... 2658

Diclofenac Potassium (Potential for drug-drug interaction with drugs affected by CYP450 enzymes).
No products indexed under this heading.

Diclofenac Sodium (Potential for drug-drug interaction with drugs affected by CYP450 enzymes). Products include:
Diclofenac Sodium Ophthalmic Solution ... ⊙240
Voltaren Ophthalmic Solution ... 2336
Voltaren Tablets ... 2334
Voltaren-XR Tablets ... 2337

Dihydroergotamine Mesylate (Potential for drug-drug interaction with drugs affected by CYP450 enzymes).
No products indexed under this heading.

Diltiazem Hydrochloride (Potential for drug-drug interaction with drugs affected by CYP450 enzymes). Products include:
Cardizem LA Extended Release Tablets ... 421

Diltiazem Maleate (Potential for drug-drug interaction with drugs affected by CYP450 enzymes).
No products indexed under this heading.

Disopyramide (Potential for drug-drug interaction with drugs affected by CYP450 enzymes).
No products indexed under this heading.

Disopyramide Phosphate (Potential for drug-drug interaction with drugs affected by CYP450 enzymes).
No products indexed under this heading.

Divalproex Sodium (Potential for drug-drug interaction with drugs affected by CYP450 enzymes). Products include:
Depakote ER Tablets ... 423

Docetaxel (Potential for drug-drug interaction with drugs affected by CYP450 enzymes). Products include:
Taxotere Injection Concentrate ... 2773

Dolasetron Mesylate (Potential for drug-drug interaction with drugs affected by CYP450 enzymes). Products include:
Anzemet Injection ... 2701
Anzemet Tablets ... 2704

Donepezil Hydrochloride (Potential for drug-drug interaction with drugs affected by CYP450 enzymes). Products include:
Aricept Tablets ... 1062
Aricept ODT Tablets ... 1062

Doxepin Hydrochloride (Potential for drug-drug interaction with drugs affected by CYP450 enzymes).
No products indexed under this heading.

Doxorubicin Hydrochloride (Potential for drug-drug interaction with drugs affected by CYP450 enzymes).
No products indexed under this heading.

Dronabinol (Potential for drug-drug interaction with drugs affected by CYP450 enzymes). Products include:
Marinol Capsules ... 3163

Drugs that Undergo Biotransformation by Cytochrome P-450 Mixed Function Oxidase (Potential for drug-drug interaction with drugs affected by CYP450 enzymes).
No products indexed under this heading.

Dyphylline (Potential for drug-drug interaction with drugs affected by CYP450 enzymes).
No products indexed under this heading.

Encainide Hydrochloride (Potential for drug-drug interaction with drugs affected by CYP450 enzymes).
No products indexed under this heading.

Enoxacin (Potential for drug-drug interaction with drugs affected by CYP450 enzymes).
No products indexed under this heading.

Eprosartan Mesylate (Potential for drug-drug interaction with drugs affected by CYP450 enzymes). Products include:
Teveten Tablets ... 515
Teveten HCT Tablets ... 517

Ergotamine Tartrate (Potential for drug-drug interaction with drugs affected by CYP450 enzymes).
No products indexed under this heading.

Erythromycin (Potential for drug-drug interaction with drugs affected by CYP450 enzymes).
No products indexed under this heading.

Erythromycin Estolate (Potential for drug-drug interaction with drugs affected by CYP450 enzymes).
No products indexed under this heading.

Erythromycin Ethylsuccinate (Potential for drug-drug interaction with drugs affected by CYP450 enzymes). Products include:
E.E.S. ... 433
EryPed ... 431

Erythromycin Gluceptate (Potential for drug-drug interaction with drugs affected by CYP450 enzymes).
No products indexed under this heading.

Erythromycin Lactobionate (Potential for drug-drug interaction with drugs affected by CYP450 enzymes).
No products indexed under this heading.

Erythromycin Stearate (Potential for drug-drug interaction with drugs affected by CYP450 enzymes).
No products indexed under this heading.

Esomeprazole Magnesium (Potential for drug-drug interaction with drugs affected by CYP450 enzymes). Products include:
Nexium Delayed-Release Capsules ... 645
Nexium Delayed-Release Oral Suspension ... 645

Estradiol (Potential for drug-drug interaction with drugs affected by CYP450 enzymes). Products include:
Activella Tablets ... 2347
Angeliq Tablets ... 751
Climara Transdermal System ... 763
Climara Pro Transdermal System ... 768
Divigel ... 3167
Vagifem Tablets ... 2375

Estradiol Benzoate (Potential for drug-drug interaction with drugs affected by CYP450 enzymes).
No products indexed under this heading.

Estradiol Cypionate (Potential for drug-drug interaction with drugs affected by CYP450 enzymes).
No products indexed under this heading.

Estradiol Valerate (Potential for drug-drug interaction with drugs affected by CYP450 enzymes).
No products indexed under this heading.

Estrogen (Potential for drug-drug interaction with drugs affected by CYP450 enzymes).
No products indexed under this heading.

Estrogens, Conjugated (Potential for drug-drug interaction with drugs affected by CYP450 enzymes). Products include:
Premarin Intravenous ... 3217
Premarin Tablets ... 3221
Premarin Vaginal Cream ... 3228
Premphase Tablets ... 3232
Prempro Tablets ... 3232

Estrogens, Conjugated, Synthetic A (Potential for drug-drug interaction with drugs affected by CYP450 enzymes).
No products indexed under this heading.

Estrogens, Esterified (Potential for drug-drug interaction with drugs affected by CYP450 enzymes). Products include:
Estratest Tablets ... 3043
Estratest H.S. Tablets ... 3043

Ethinyl Estradiol (Potential for drug-drug interaction with drugs affected by CYP450 enzymes). Products include:
Lybrel Tablets ... 3204
Mircette Tablets ... 1034
NuvaRing ... 2897
Ortho-Cyclen/Ortho Tri-Cyclen ... 2449
Ortho Evra Transdermal System ... 2437
Ortho Tri-Cyclen Lo Tablets ... 2458
Seasonique Tablets ... 1046
Yaz Tablets ... 805

Ethosuximide (Potential for drug-drug interaction with drugs affected by CYP450 enzymes).
No products indexed under this heading.

Ethotoin (Potential for drug-drug interaction with drugs affected by CYP450 enzymes).
No products indexed under this heading.

Ethynodiol Diacetate (Potential for drug-drug interaction with drugs affected by CYP450 enzymes).
No products indexed under this heading.

Etodolac (Potential for drug-drug interaction with drugs affected by CYP450 enzymes).
No products indexed under this heading.

Etoposide (Potential for drug-drug interaction with drugs affected by CYP450 enzymes).
No products indexed under this heading.

Etoposide Phosphate (Potential for drug-drug interaction with drugs affected by CYP450 enzymes).
No products indexed under this heading.

Felbamate (Potential for drug-drug interaction with drugs affected by CYP450 enzymes).
No products indexed under this heading.

Felodipine (Potential for drug-drug interaction with drugs affected by CYP450 enzymes).
No products indexed under this heading.

Fenoprofen Calcium (Potential for drug-drug interaction with drugs affected by CYP450 enzymes). Products include:
Nalfon Capsules ... 2508

Fentanyl (Potential for drug-drug interaction with drugs affected by CYP450 enzymes). Products include:
Duragesic Transdermal System ... 2405
Ionsys Transdermal System ... 2410

Fentanyl Citrate (Potential for drug-drug interaction with drugs affected by CYP450 enzymes). Products include:
Actiq ... 959
Fentora Tablets ... 968

Flecainide Acetate (Potential for drug-drug interaction with drugs affected by CYP450 enzymes).
No products indexed under this heading.

Fluoxetine (Potential for drug-drug interaction with drugs affected by CYP450 enzymes).
No products indexed under this heading.

Fluoxetine Hydrochloride (Potential for drug-drug interaction with drugs affected by CYP450 enzymes). Products include:
Prozac Weekly Capsules ... 1852
Prozac Pulvules and Liquid ... 1852
Symbyax Capsules ... 1871

IMPORTANT NOTE: Always consult each drug listing in the patient's regimen for possible interactions.

Fluphenazine Decanoate (Potential for drug-drug interaction with drugs affected by CYP450 enzymes).
No products indexed under this heading.

Fluphenazine Enanthate (Potential for drug-drug interaction with drugs affected by CYP450 enzymes).
No products indexed under this heading.

Fluphenazine Hydrochloride (Potential for drug-drug interaction with drugs affected by CYP450 enzymes).
No products indexed under this heading.

Flurbiprofen (Potential for drug-drug interaction with drugs affected by CYP450 enzymes).
No products indexed under this heading.

Flurbiprofen Sodium (Potential for drug-drug interaction with drugs affected by CYP450 enzymes).
No products indexed under this heading.

Flutamide (Potential for drug-drug interaction with drugs affected by CYP450 enzymes).
No products indexed under this heading.

Fluticasone Propionate (Potential for drug-drug interaction with drugs affected by CYP450 enzymes).
Products include:
Advair Diskus 100/50 .... **1276**
Advair Diskus 250/50 .... **1276**
Advair Diskus 500/50 .... **1276**
Advair HFA 45/21 Inhalation Aerosol.................................. **1288**
Advair HFA 115/21 Inhalation Aerosol.................................. **1288**
Advair HFA 230/21 Inhalation Aerosol.................................. **1288**
Flonase Nasal Spray **1431**
Flovent Diskus 50 mcg **1435**

Fluvastatin Sodium (Potential for drug-drug interaction with drugs affected by CYP450 enzymes).
Products include:
Lescol Capsules **2268**
Lescol XL Tablets **2268**

Fluvoxamine Maleate (Potential for drug-drug interaction with drugs affected by CYP450 enzymes).
Products include:
Luvox CR Extended-Release Capsules.................................. **1759**

Formoterol Fumarate (Potential for drug-drug interaction with drugs affected by CYP450 enzymes).
Products include:
Foradil Aerolizer **2849**
Perforomist Inhalation Solution **1025**

Fosphenytoin (Potential for drug-drug interaction with drugs affected by CYP450 enzymes).
No products indexed under this heading.

Fosphenytoin Sodium (Potential for drug-drug interaction with drugs affected by CYP450 enzymes).
No products indexed under this heading.

Gabapentin (Potential for drug-drug interaction with drugs affected by CYP450 enzymes).
No products indexed under this heading.

Galantamine Hydrobromide (Potential for drug-drug interaction with drugs affected by CYP450 enzymes).
No products indexed under this heading.

Glimepiride (Potential for drug-drug interaction with drugs affected by CYP450 enzymes). Products include:
Avandaryl Tablets **1344**
Duetact Tablets **3085**

Glipizide (Potential for drug-drug interaction with drugs affected by CYP450 enzymes).
No products indexed under this heading.

Glyburide (Potential for drug-drug interaction with drugs affected by CYP450 enzymes).
No products indexed under this heading.

Grepafloxacin Hydrochloride (Potential for drug-drug interaction with drugs affected by CYP450 enzymes).
No products indexed under this heading.

Haloperidol (Potential for drug-drug interaction with drugs affected by CYP450 enzymes).
No products indexed under this heading.

Haloperidol Decanoate (Potential for drug-drug interaction with drugs affected by CYP450 enzymes).
No products indexed under this heading.

Haloperidol Lactate (Potential for drug-drug interaction with drugs affected by CYP450 enzymes).
No products indexed under this heading.

Hydrocodone Bitartrate (Potential for drug-drug interaction with drugs affected by CYP450 enzymes).
Products include:
Lortab 5/500 Tablets **3143**
Lortab 7.5/500 Tablets **3144**
Lortab 10/500 Tablets **3144**
Vicodin Tablets **529**
Vicodin ES Tablets **530**
Vicodin HP Tablets **531**
Vicoprofen Tablets **533**
Zydone Tablets **1132**

Ibuprofen (Potential for drug-drug interaction with drugs affected by CYP450 enzymes). Products include:
Motrin IB Tablets and Caplets **1900**
Children's Motrin Oral Suspension ... **1901**
Children's Motrin Non-Staining Dye-Free Oral Suspension.............. **1901**
Children's Motrin Cold Oral Suspension **1899**
Infants' Motrin Concentrated Drops.. **1901**
Infants' Motrin Non-Staining Dye-Free Concentrated Drops....... **1901**
Junior Strength Motrin Caplets and Chewable Tablets................... **1901**
Vicoprofen Tablets **533**

Imipramine Hydrochloride (Potential for drug-drug interaction with drugs affected by CYP450 enzymes).
No products indexed under this heading.

Imipramine Pamoate (Potential for drug-drug interaction with drugs affected by CYP450 enzymes).
No products indexed under this heading.

Indinavir Sulfate (Potential for drug-drug interaction with drugs affected by CYP450 enzymes).
Products include:
Crixivan Capsules **1979**

Indomethacin (Potential for drug-drug interaction with drugs affected by CYP450 enzymes). Products include:
Indocin **2024**

Indomethacin Sodium Trihydrate (Potential for drug-drug interaction with drugs affected by CYP450 enzymes). Products include:
Indocin I.V. **2489**

Indoramin Hydrochloride (Potential for drug-drug interaction with drugs affected by CYP450 enzymes).
No products indexed under this heading.

Irbesartan (Potential for drug-drug interaction with drugs affected by CYP450 enzymes). Products include:
Avalide Tablets **892**
Avalide Tablets **2713**
Avapro Tablets **897**
Avapro Tablets **2718**

Isotretinoin (Potential for drug-drug interaction with drugs affected by CYP450 enzymes). Products include:
Accutane Capsules **2607**

Isradipine (Potential for drug-drug interaction with drugs affected by CYP450 enzymes). Products include:
DynaCirc CR Controlled Release Tablets **1407**

Itraconazole (Potential for drug-drug interaction with drugs affected by CYP450 enzymes).
No products indexed under this heading.

Ketoconazole (Potential for drug-drug interaction with drugs affected by CYP450 enzymes). Products include:
Extina Foam, 2% **3057**
Nizoral A-D Shampoo **1901**

Ketoprofen (Potential for drug-drug interaction with drugs affected by CYP450 enzymes).
No products indexed under this heading.

Ketorolac Tromethamine (Potential for drug-drug interaction with drugs affected by CYP450 enzymes).
No products indexed under this heading.

Labetalol Hydrochloride (Potential for drug-drug interaction with drugs affected by CYP450 enzymes).
No products indexed under this heading.

Lamotrigine (Potential for drug-drug interaction with drugs affected by CYP450 enzymes). Products include:
Lamictal **1488**

Lansoprazole (Potential for drug-drug interaction with drugs affected by CYP450 enzymes).
No products indexed under this heading.

Levetiracetam (Potential for drug-drug interaction with drugs affected by CYP450 enzymes). Products include:
Keppra Injection **3137**
Keppra Oral Solution **3131**
Keppra Tablets **3131**

Levobupivacaine Hydrochloride (Potential for drug-drug interaction with drugs affected by CYP450 enzymes).
No products indexed under this heading.

Levonorgestrel (Potential for drug-drug interaction with drugs affected by CYP450 enzymes). Products include:
Climara Pro Transdermal System **768**
Lybrel Tablets **3204**
Mirena Intrauterine System **779**
Plan B Tablets **1044**
Seasonique Tablets **1046**

Lidocaine (Potential for drug-drug interaction with drugs affected by CYP450 enzymes). Products include:
Lidoderm Patch **1114**

Lidocaine Base (Potential for drug-drug interaction with drugs affected by CYP450 enzymes).
No products indexed under this heading.

Lidocaine Hydrochloride (Potential for drug-drug interaction with drugs affected by CYP450 enzymes).
No products indexed under this heading.

Lomefloxacin Hydrochloride (Potential for drug-drug interaction with drugs affected by CYP450 enzymes).
No products indexed under this heading.

Losartan Potassium (Potential for drug-drug interaction with drugs affected by CYP450 enzymes).
Products include:
Cozaar Tablets **1973**

Lovastatin (Potential for drug-drug interaction with drugs affected by CYP450 enzymes). Products include:
Advicor Tablets **402**
Mevacor Tablets **2063**

Maprotiline Hydrochloride (Potential for drug-drug interaction with drugs affected by CYP450 enzymes).
No products indexed under this heading.

Meclofenamate Sodium (Potential for drug-drug interaction with drugs affected by CYP450 enzymes).
No products indexed under this heading.

Mefenamic Acid (Potential for drug-drug interaction with drugs affected by CYP450 enzymes).
No products indexed under this heading.

Meloxicam (Potential for drug-drug interaction with drugs affected by CYP450 enzymes). Products include:
Mobic Oral Suspension **863**
Mobic Tablets **863**

Meperidine Hydrochloride (Potential for drug-drug interaction with drugs affected by CYP450 enzymes).
No products indexed under this heading.

Mephenytoin (Potential for drug-drug interaction with drugs affected by CYP450 enzymes).
No products indexed under this heading.

Mephobarbital (Potential for drug-drug interaction with drugs affected by CYP450 enzymes).
No products indexed under this heading.

Meprobamate (Potential for drug-drug interaction with drugs affected by CYP450 enzymes).
No products indexed under this heading.

Mestranol (Potential for drug-drug interaction with drugs affected by CYP450 enzymes).
No products indexed under this heading.

Metformin Hydrochloride (Potential for drug-drug interaction with drugs affected by CYP450 enzymes). Products include:
ActoPlus Met Tablets ... 3071
Avandamet Tablets ... 1336
Janumet Tablets ... 2041
PrandiMet Tablets ... 2967

Methadone Hydrochloride (Potential for drug-drug interaction with drugs affected by CYP450 enzymes).
No products indexed under this heading.

Methamphetamine Hydrochloride (Potential for drug-drug interaction with drugs affected by CYP450 enzymes).
No products indexed under this heading.

Methsuximide (Potential for drug-drug interaction with drugs affected by CYP450 enzymes).
No products indexed under this heading.

Metoprolol Succinate (Potential for drug-drug interaction with drugs affected by CYP450 enzymes). Products include:
Toprol-XL Tablets ... 666

Metoprolol Tartrate (Potential for drug-drug interaction with drugs affected by CYP450 enzymes).
No products indexed under this heading.

Mexiletine Hydrochloride (Potential for drug-drug interaction with drugs affected by CYP450 enzymes).
No products indexed under this heading.

Midazolam Hydrochloride (Potential for drug-drug interaction with drugs affected by CYP450 enzymes).
No products indexed under this heading.

Miglitol (Potential for drug-drug interaction with drugs affected by CYP450 enzymes).
No products indexed under this heading.

Mirtazapine (Potential for drug-drug interaction with drugs affected by CYP450 enzymes). Products include:
Remeron Tablets ... 2924
RemeronSolTab Tablets ... 2927

Montelukast Sodium (Potential for drug-drug interaction with drugs affected by CYP450 enzymes). Products include:
Singulair ... 2114

Morphine Sulfate (Potential for drug-drug interaction with drugs affected by CYP450 enzymes). Products include:
Avinza Capsules ... 1772
DepoDur Injection ... 1095
MS Contin Tablets ... 2585

Moxifloxacin Hydrochloride (Potential for drug-drug interaction with drugs affected by CYP450 enzymes). Products include:
Avelox ... 2803
Vigamox Ophthalmic Solution ... 548

Nabumetone (Potential for drug-drug interaction with drugs affected by CYP450 enzymes).
No products indexed under this heading.

Nafcillin Sodium (Potential for drug-drug interaction with drugs affected by CYP450 enzymes).
No products indexed under this heading.

Naproxen (Potential for drug-drug interaction with drugs affected by CYP450 enzymes). Products include:
EC-Naprosyn Delayed-Release Tablets ... 2632
Naprosyn Suspension ... 2632
Naprosyn Tablets ... 2632

Naproxen Sodium (Potential for drug-drug interaction with drugs affected by CYP450 enzymes). Products include:
Anaprox Tablets ... 2632
Anaprox DS Tablets ... 2632
Treximet Tablets ... 1616

Nateglinide (Potential for drug-drug interaction with drugs affected by CYP450 enzymes). Products include:
Starlix Tablets ... 2314

Nefazodone Hydrochloride (Potential for drug-drug interaction with drugs affected by CYP450 enzymes).
No products indexed under this heading.

Nelfinavir Mesylate (Potential for drug-drug interaction with drugs affected by CYP450 enzymes).
No products indexed under this heading.

Nicardipine (Potential for drug-drug interaction with drugs affected by CYP450 enzymes).
No products indexed under this heading.

Nicardipine Hydrochloride (Potential for drug-drug interaction with drugs affected by CYP450 enzymes). Products include:
Cardene I.V. ... 1093

Nicotine Polacrilex (Potential for drug-drug interaction with drugs affected by CYP450 enzymes).
No products indexed under this heading.

Nicotine Salicylate (Potential for drug-drug interaction with drugs affected by CYP450 enzymes).
No products indexed under this heading.

Nicotine Sulfate (Potential for drug-drug interaction with drugs affected by CYP450 enzymes).
No products indexed under this heading.

Nifedipine (Potential for drug-drug interaction with drugs affected by CYP450 enzymes).
No products indexed under this heading.

Nilutamide (Potential for drug-drug interaction with drugs affected by CYP450 enzymes).
No products indexed under this heading.

Nimodipine (Potential for drug-drug interaction with drugs affected by CYP450 enzymes). Products include:
Nimotop Capsules ... 790

Nisoldipine (Potential for drug-drug interaction with drugs affected by CYP450 enzymes). Products include:
Sular Extended Release Tablets ... 2975

Nitrendipine (Potential for drug-drug interaction with drugs affected by CYP450 enzymes).
No products indexed under this heading.

Norethindrone (Potential for drug-drug interaction with drugs affected by CYP450 enzymes). Products include:
Ortho Micronor Tablets ... 2446

Norethindrone Acetate (Potential for drug-drug interaction with drugs affected by CYP450 enzymes). Products include:
Activella Tablets ... 2347

Norfloxacin (Potential for drug-drug interaction with drugs affected by CYP450 enzymes). Products include:
Noroxin Tablets ... 2069

Norgestrel (Potential for drug-drug interaction with drugs affected by CYP450 enzymes).
No products indexed under this heading.

Nortriptyline Hydrochloride (Potential for drug-drug interaction with drugs affected by CYP450 enzymes).
No products indexed under this heading.

Ofloxacin (Potential for drug-drug interaction with drugs affected by CYP450 enzymes). Products include:
Ofloxacin Ophthalmic Solution 0.3% ... ⊙243

Olanzapine (Potential for drug-drug interaction with drugs affected by CYP450 enzymes). Products include:
Symbyax Capsules ... 1871
Zyprexa Tablets ... 1883
Zyprexa IntraMuscular ... 1883
Zyprexa ZYDIS Orally Disintegrating Tablets ... 1883

Omeprazole (Potential for drug-drug interaction with drugs affected by CYP450 enzymes).
No products indexed under this heading.

Ondansetron (Potential for drug-drug interaction with drugs affected by CYP450 enzymes). Products include:
Zofran ODT Orally Disintegrating Tablets ... 1687

Ondansetron Hydrochloride (Potential for drug-drug interaction with drugs affected by CYP450 enzymes). Products include:
Zofran Injection ... 1682
Zofran ... 1687

Oxaprozin (Potential for drug-drug interaction with drugs affected by CYP450 enzymes).
No products indexed under this heading.

Oxcarbazepine (Potential for drug-drug interaction with drugs affected by CYP450 enzymes).
No products indexed under this heading.

Oxycodone Hydrochloride (Potential for drug-drug interaction with drugs affected by CYP450 enzymes). Products include:
OxyContin Tablets ... 2589
OxyIR Capsules ... 2593
Percocet Tablets ... 1127
Percodan Tablets ... 1130

Paclitaxel (Potential for drug-drug interaction with drugs affected by CYP450 enzymes).
No products indexed under this heading.

Pantoprazole Sodium (Potential for drug-drug interaction with drugs affected by CYP450 enzymes). Products include:
Protonix for Delayed-Release Oral Suspension ... 3254
Protonix Delayed-Release Tablets ... 3254
Protonix I.V. ... 3257

Paramethadione (Potential for drug-drug interaction with drugs affected by CYP450 enzymes).
No products indexed under this heading.

Paroxetine Hydrochloride (Potential for drug-drug interaction with drugs affected by CYP450 enzymes). Products include:
Paxil ... 1535
Paxil CR Controlled-Release Tablets ... 1544

Pentamidine Isethionate (Potential for drug-drug interaction with drugs affected by CYP450 enzymes).
No products indexed under this heading.

Phenacemide (Potential for drug-drug interaction with drugs affected by CYP450 enzymes).
No products indexed under this heading.

Phenobarbital (Potential for drug-drug interaction with drugs affected by CYP450 enzymes). Products include:
Donnatal Extentabs ... 2507

Phenobarbital Sodium (Potential for drug-drug interaction with drugs affected by CYP450 enzymes).
No products indexed under this heading.

Phensuximide (Potential for drug-drug interaction with drugs affected by CYP450 enzymes).
No products indexed under this heading.

Phenylbutazone (Potential for drug-drug interaction with drugs affected by CYP450 enzymes).
No products indexed under this heading.

Phenytoin (Potential for drug-drug interaction with drugs affected by CYP450 enzymes).
No products indexed under this heading.

Phenytoin Sodium (Potential for drug-drug interaction with drugs affected by CYP450 enzymes). Products include:
Phenytek Capsules ... 2192

Pimozide (Potential for drug-drug interaction with drugs affected by CYP450 enzymes).
No products indexed under this heading.

Pindolol (Potential for drug-drug interaction with drugs affected by CYP450 enzymes).
No products indexed under this heading.

Pioglitazone Hydrochloride (Potential for drug-drug interaction with drugs affected by CYP450 enzymes). Products include:
ActoPlus Met Tablets ... 3071
Actos Tablets ... 3077
Duetact Tablets ... 3085

Piroxicam (Potential for drug-drug interaction with drugs affected by CYP450 enzymes).
No products indexed under this heading.

Polyestradiol Phosphate (Potential for drug-drug interaction with drugs affected by CYP450 enzymes).
No products indexed under this heading.

Primidone (Potential for drug-drug interaction with drugs affected by CYP450 enzymes).
No products indexed under this heading.

IMPORTANT NOTE: Always consult each drug listing in the patient's regimen for possible interactions.

Progesterone (Potential for drug-drug interaction with drugs affected by CYP450 enzymes). Products include:
- Crinone 4% Gel 992
- Crinone 8% Gel 992
- Prometrium Capsules (100 mg, 200 mg) 3047

Proguanil Hydrochloride (Potential for drug-drug interaction with drugs affected by CYP450 enzymes). Products include:
- Malarone Pediatric Tablets 1521
- Malarone Tablets 1521

Propafenone Hydrochloride (Potential for drug-drug interaction with drugs affected by CYP450 enzymes). Products include:
- Rythmol Tablets 1586
- Rythmol SR Capsules 1590

Propoxyphene Hydrochloride (Potential for drug-drug interaction with drugs affected by CYP450 enzymes).
No products indexed under this heading.

Propoxyphene Napsylate (Potential for drug-drug interaction with drugs affected by CYP450 enzymes).
No products indexed under this heading.

Propranolol Hydrochloride (Potential for drug-drug interaction with drugs affected by CYP450 enzymes). Products include:
- InnoPran XL Extended Release Capsules 1484

Protriptyline Hydrochloride (Potential for drug-drug interaction with drugs affected by CYP450 enzymes).
No products indexed under this heading.

Quetiapine Fumarate (Potential for drug-drug interaction with drugs affected by CYP450 enzymes).
No products indexed under this heading.

Quinidine Gluconate (Potential for drug-drug interaction with drugs affected by CYP450 enzymes).
No products indexed under this heading.

Quinidine Hydrochloride (Potential for drug-drug interaction with drugs affected by CYP450 enzymes).
No products indexed under this heading.

Quinidine Polygalacturonate (Potential for drug-drug interaction with drugs affected by CYP450 enzymes).
No products indexed under this heading.

Quinidine Sulfate (Potential for drug-drug interaction with drugs affected by CYP450 enzymes).
No products indexed under this heading.

Quinine (Potential for drug-drug interaction with drugs affected by CYP450 enzymes).
No products indexed under this heading.

Quinine Sulfate (Potential for drug-drug interaction with drugs affected by CYP450 enzymes).
No products indexed under this heading.

Rabeprazole Sodium (Potential for drug-drug interaction with drugs affected by CYP450 enzymes). Products include:
- Aciphex Tablets 1053

Repaglinide (Potential for drug-drug interaction with drugs affected by CYP450 enzymes). Products include:
- PrandiMet Tablets 2967
- Prandin Tablets 2971

Rifabutin (Potential for drug-drug interaction with drugs affected by CYP450 enzymes).
No products indexed under this heading.

Riluzole (Potential for drug-drug interaction with drugs affected by CYP450 enzymes). Products include:
- Rilutek Tablets 2771

Risperidone (Potential for drug-drug interaction with drugs affected by CYP450 enzymes). Products include:
- Risperdal Consta Long-Acting Injection 1753

Ritonavir (Potential for drug-drug interaction with drugs affected by CYP450 enzymes). Products include:
- Kaletra 452
- Norvir 489

Rofecoxib (Potential for drug-drug interaction with drugs affected by CYP450 enzymes).
No products indexed under this heading.

Ropinirole Hydrochloride (Potential for drug-drug interaction with drugs affected by CYP450 enzymes). Products include:
- Requip Tablets 1561
- Requip XL Tablets 1568

Ropivacaine Hydrochloride (Potential for drug-drug interaction with drugs affected by CYP450 enzymes).
No products indexed under this heading.

Rosiglitazone Maleate (Potential for drug-drug interaction with drugs affected by CYP450 enzymes). Products include:
- Avandamet Tablets 1336
- Avandaryl Tablets 1344
- Avandia Tablets 1351

Saquinavir (Potential for drug-drug interaction with drugs affected by CYP450 enzymes).
No products indexed under this heading.

Saquinavir Mesylate (Potential for drug-drug interaction with drugs affected by CYP450 enzymes).
No products indexed under this heading.

Sertraline Hydrochloride (Potential for drug-drug interaction with drugs affected by CYP450 enzymes).
No products indexed under this heading.

Sildenafil Citrate (Potential for drug-drug interaction with drugs affected by CYP450 enzymes).
No products indexed under this heading.

Simvastatin (Potential for drug-drug interaction with drugs affected by CYP450 enzymes). Products include:
- Simcor Tablets 502
- Vytorin 10/10 Tablets 2149
- Vytorin 10/10 Tablets 2939
- Vytorin 10/20 Tablets 2149
- Vytorin 10/20 Tablets 2939
- Vytorin 10/40 Tablets 2149
- Vytorin 10/40 Tablets 2939
- Vytorin 10/80 Tablets 2149
- Vytorin 10/80 Tablets 2939
- Zocor Tablets 2136

Sirolimus (Potential for drug-drug interaction with drugs affected by CYP450 enzymes). Products include:
- Rapamune 3260

Sulfamethoxazole (Potential for drug-drug interaction with drugs affected by CYP450 enzymes).
No products indexed under this heading.

Sulindac (Potential for drug-drug interaction with drugs affected by CYP450 enzymes). Products include:
- Clinoril Tablets 1962

Suprofen (Potential for drug-drug interaction with drugs affected by CYP450 enzymes).
No products indexed under this heading.

Tacrine Hydrochloride (Potential for drug-drug interaction with drugs affected by CYP450 enzymes).
No products indexed under this heading.

Tacrolimus (Potential for drug-drug interaction with drugs affected by CYP450 enzymes). Products include:
- Prograf Capsules and Injection 622
- Protopic Ointment 628

Tamoxifen Citrate (Potential for drug-drug interaction with drugs affected by CYP450 enzymes).
No products indexed under this heading.

Telmisartan (Potential for drug-drug interaction with drugs affected by CYP450 enzymes). Products include:
- Micardis Tablets 852
- Micardis HCT Tablets 854

Teniposide (Potential for drug-drug interaction with drugs affected by CYP450 enzymes).
No products indexed under this heading.

Terfenadine (Potential for drug-drug interaction with drugs affected by CYP450 enzymes).
No products indexed under this heading.

Testosterone (Potential for drug-drug interaction with drugs affected by CYP450 enzymes). Products include:
- AndroGel 3159
- Testim 1% Gel 701

Testosterone Cypionate (Potential for drug-drug interaction with drugs affected by CYP450 enzymes).
No products indexed under this heading.

Testosterone Enanthate (Potential for drug-drug interaction with drugs affected by CYP450 enzymes). Products include:
- Delatestryl Injection 1730

Testosterone Propionate (Potential for drug-drug interaction with drugs affected by CYP450 enzymes).
No products indexed under this heading.

Theophylline (Potential for drug-drug interaction with drugs affected by CYP450 enzymes).
No products indexed under this heading.

Theophylline Anhydrous (Potential for drug-drug interaction with drugs affected by CYP450 enzymes). Products include:
- Uniphyl Tablets 2595

Theophylline Sodium Glycinate (Potential for drug-drug interaction with drugs affected by CYP450 enzymes).
No products indexed under this heading.

Thioridazine (Potential for drug-drug interaction with drugs affected by CYP450 enzymes).
No products indexed under this heading.

Thioridazine Hydrochloride (Potential for drug-drug interaction with drugs affected by CYP450 enzymes). Products include:
- Thioridazine Hydrochloride Tablets 2195

Tiagabine Hydrochloride (Potential for drug-drug interaction with drugs affected by CYP450 enzymes). Products include:
- Gabitril Tablets 973

Timolol Maleate (Potential for drug-drug interaction with drugs affected by CYP450 enzymes). Products include:
- Combigan Ophthalmic Solution 553
- Cosopt Sterile Ophthalmic Solution 1969
- Timoptic Sterile Ophthalmic Solution 2121
- Timoptic in Ocudose 2124
- Timoptic-XE Sterile Ophthalmic Gel Forming Solution 2125

Tolazamide (Potential for drug-drug interaction with drugs affected by CYP450 enzymes).
No products indexed under this heading.

Tolbutamide (Potential for drug-drug interaction with drugs affected by CYP450 enzymes).
No products indexed under this heading.

Tolbutamide Sodium (Potential for drug-drug interaction with drugs affected by CYP450 enzymes).
No products indexed under this heading.

Tolmetin Sodium (Potential for drug-drug interaction with drugs affected by CYP450 enzymes).
No products indexed under this heading.

Tolterodine Tartrate (Potential for drug-drug interaction with drugs affected by CYP450 enzymes).
No products indexed under this heading.

Topiramate (Potential for drug-drug interaction with drugs affected by CYP450 enzymes).
No products indexed under this heading.

Torsemide (Potential for drug-drug interaction with drugs affected by CYP450 enzymes). Products include:
- Demadex Injection 2630
- Demadex Tablets 2630

Tramadol Hydrochloride (Potential for drug-drug interaction with drugs affected by CYP450 enzymes). Products include:
- Ultram ER Extended-Release Tablets 2428

Trazodone Hydrochloride (Potential for drug-drug interaction with drugs affected by CYP450 enzymes).
No products indexed under this heading.

Tretinoin (Potential for drug-drug interaction with drugs affected by CYP450 enzymes). Products include:

Vesanoid Capsules 2660
Ziana Gel 1942

Triazolam (Potential for drug-drug interaction with drugs affected by CYP450 enzymes).
No products indexed under this heading.

Trimethadione (Potential for drug-drug interaction with drugs affected by CYP450 enzymes).
No products indexed under this heading.

Trimethaphan Camsylate (Potential for drug-drug interaction with drugs affected by CYP450 enzymes).
No products indexed under this heading.

Trimipramine Maleate (Potential for drug-drug interaction with drugs affected by CYP450 enzymes).
No products indexed under this heading.

Troglitazone (Potential for drug-drug interaction with drugs affected by CYP450 enzymes).
No products indexed under this heading.

Trovafloxacin Mesylate (Potential for drug-drug interaction with drugs affected by CYP450 enzymes).
No products indexed under this heading.

Valdecoxib (Potential for drug-drug interaction with drugs affected by CYP450 enzymes).
No products indexed under this heading.

Valproate Sodium (Potential for drug-drug interaction with drugs affected by CYP450 enzymes).
No products indexed under this heading.

Valproic Acid (Potential for drug-drug interaction with drugs affected by CYP450 enzymes).
No products indexed under this heading.

Valsartan (Potential for drug-drug interaction with drugs affected by CYP450 enzymes). Products include:
Diovan Tablets 2212
Diovan HCT Tablets 2216
Exforge Tablets 2238

Venlafaxine Hydrochloride (Potential for drug-drug interaction with drugs affected by CYP450 enzymes). Products include:
Effexor XR Extended-Release Capsules 3195
Venlafaxine Hydrochloride Tablets ... 2199

Verapamil Hydrochloride (Potential for drug-drug interaction with drugs affected by CYP450 enzymes). Products include:
Tarka Tablets 511

Vinblastine Sulfate (Potential for drug-drug interaction with drugs affected by CYP450 enzymes).
No products indexed under this heading.

Vincristine Sulfate (Potential for drug-drug interaction with drugs affected by CYP450 enzymes).
No products indexed under this heading.

Vitamin A (Potential for drug-drug interaction with drugs affected by CYP450 enzymes). Products include:
Norwegian Cod Liver Oil 949

Vitamin A Acetate (Potential for drug-drug interaction with drugs affected by CYP450 enzymes).
No products indexed under this heading.

Voriconazole (Potential for drug-drug interaction with drugs affected by CYP450 enzymes).
No products indexed under this heading.

Warfarin Sodium (Potential for drug-drug interaction with drugs affected by CYP450 enzymes).
No products indexed under this heading.

Zafirlukast (Potential for drug-drug interaction with drugs affected by CYP450 enzymes). Products include:
Accolate Tablets 669

Zileuton (Potential for drug-drug interaction with drugs affected by CYP450 enzymes).
No products indexed under this heading.

Zolmitriptan (Potential for drug-drug interaction with drugs affected by CYP450 enzymes). Products include:
Zomig Tablets 694
Zomig Nasal Spray 689
Zomig-ZMT Tablets 694

Zonisamide (Potential for drug-drug interaction with drugs affected by CYP450 enzymes). Products include:
Zonegran Capsules 1089

Zopiclone (Potential for drug-drug interaction with drugs affected by CYP450 enzymes).
No products indexed under this heading.

NABI-HB

(Hepatitis B Immune Globulin (Human)).. 815
May interact with:

Mumps Virus Vaccine, Live (H-BIG may interfere with the immune response to vaccination, therefore, vaccination with live virus vaccine should be deferred until approximately 3 months). Products include:
Mumpsvax 2068

Rubella & Mumps Virus Vaccine Live (H-BIG may interfere with the immune response to vaccination, therefore, vaccination with live virus vaccine should be deferred until approximately 3 months).
No products indexed under this heading.

Rubella Virus Vaccine Live (H-BIG may interfere with the immune response to vaccination, therefore, vaccination with live virus vaccine should be deferred until approximately 3 months). Products include:
Meruvax II 2061

NADOLOL TABLETS

(Nadolol) 2191
May interact with general anesthetics, oral hypoglycemic agents, insulin, and certain other agents. Compounds in these categories include:

Acarbose (Beta-adrenergic blockade may prevent the appearance of premonitory signs and symptoms, such as tachycardia and blood pressure changes, of acute hypoglycemia; beta-blockade also reduces the release of insulin in response to hyperglycemia; adjust dosage of oral antidiabetic drugs). Products include:
Precose Tablets 792

Chlorpropamide (Beta-adrenergic blockade may prevent the appearance of premonitory signs and symptoms, such as tachycardia and blood pressure changes, of acute hypoglycemia; beta-blockade also reduces the release of insulin in response to hyperglycemia; adjust dosage of oral antidiabetic drugs).
No products indexed under this heading.

Enflurane (Co-administration may result in exaggeration of the hypotension induced by general anesthetics).
No products indexed under this heading.

Epinephrine (Patients with a history of severe anaphylactic reaction to variety of allergens may be more reactive to repeated challenge; potential for unresponsiveness to the usual dose of epinephrine). Products include:
EpiPen 1024

Epinephrine Hydrochloride (Patients with a history of severe anaphylactic reaction to variety of allergens may be more reactive to repeated challenge; potential for unresponsiveness to the usual dose of epinephrine).
No products indexed under this heading.

Glimepiride (Beta-adrenergic blockade may prevent the appearance of premonitory signs and symptoms, such as tachycardia and blood pressure changes, of acute hypoglycemia; beta-blockade also reduces the release of insulin in response to hyperglycemia; adjust dosage of oral antidiabetic drugs). Products include:
Avandaryl Tablets 1344
Duetact Tablets 3085

Glipizide (Beta-adrenergic blockade may prevent the appearance of premonitory signs and symptoms, such as tachycardia and blood pressure changes, of acute hypoglycemia; beta-blockade also reduces the release of insulin in response to hyperglycemia; adjust dosage of oral antidiabetic drugs).
No products indexed under this heading.

Glyburide (Beta-adrenergic blockade may prevent the appearance of premonitory signs and symptoms, such as tachycardia and blood pressure changes, of acute hypoglycemia; beta-blockade also reduces the release of insulin in response to hyperglycemia; adjust dosage of oral antidiabetic drugs).
No products indexed under this heading.

Insulin (Beta-adrenergic blockade may prevent the appearance of premonitory signs and symptoms, such as tachycardia and blood pressure changes, of acute hypoglycemia; beta-blockade also reduces the release of insulin in response to hyperglycemia; adjust dosage of insulin).
No products indexed under this heading.

Insulin, Human, Zinc Suspension (Beta-adrenergic blockade may prevent the appearance of premonitory signs and symptoms, such as tachycardia and blood pressure changes, of acute hypoglycemia; beta-blockade also reduces the release of insulin in response to hyperglycemia; adjust dosage of insulin).
No products indexed under this heading.

Insulin, Human (rDNA origin) (Beta-adrenergic blockade may prevent the appearance of premonitory signs and symptoms, such as tachycardia and blood pressure changes, of acute hypoglycemia; beta-blockade also reduces the release of insulin in response to hyperglycemia; adjust dosage of insulin). Products include:
Exubera Inhalation Powder 2515

Insulin, Human NPH (Beta-adrenergic blockade may prevent the appearance of premonitory signs and symptoms, such as tachycardia and blood pressure changes, of acute hypoglycemia; beta-blockade also reduces the release of insulin in response to hyperglycemia; adjust dosage of insulin). Products include:
Humulin N Vial 1846

Insulin, Human Regular (Beta-adrenergic blockade may prevent the appearance of premonitory signs and symptoms, such as tachycardia and blood pressure changes, of acute hypoglycemia; beta-blockade also reduces the release of insulin in response to hyperglycemia; adjust dosage of insulin). Products include:
Humulin R 1849
Humulin R (U-500) 1850

Insulin, Human Regular and Human NPH Mixture (Beta-adrenergic blockade may prevent the appearance of premonitory signs and symptoms, such as tachycardia and blood pressure changes, of acute hypoglycemia; beta-blockade also reduces the release of insulin in response to hyperglycemia; adjust dosage of insulin). Products include:
Humulin 50/50, 100 Units 1843
Humulin 70/30 Vial 1844

Insulin, NPH (Beta-adrenergic blockade may prevent the appearance of premonitory signs and symptoms, such as tachycardia and blood pressure changes, of acute hypoglycemia; beta-blockade also reduces the release of insulin in response to hyperglycemia; adjust dosage of insulin).
No products indexed under this heading.

Insulin, Regular (Beta-adrenergic blockade may prevent the appearance of premonitory signs and symptoms, such as tachycardia and blood pressure changes, of acute hypoglycemia; beta-blockade also reduces the release of insulin in response to hyperglycemia; adjust dosage of insulin).
No products indexed under this heading.

Insulin, Regular and NPH mixture (Beta-adrenergic blockade may prevent the appearance of premonitory signs and symptoms, such as tachycardia and blood pressure changes, of acute hypoglycemia; beta-blockade also reduces the release of insulin in response to hyperglycemia; adjust dosage of insulin).
No products indexed under this heading.

Insulin, Zinc Crystals (Beta-adrenergic blockade may prevent the appearance of premonitory signs and symptoms, such as tachycardia and blood pressure changes, of acute hypoglycemia; beta-blockade also reduces the release of insulin in response to hyperglycemia; adjust dosage of insulin).

No products indexed under this heading.

Insulin, Zinc Suspension (Beta-adrenergic blockade may prevent the appearance of premonitory signs and symptoms, such as tachycardia and blood pressure changes, of acute hypoglycemia; beta-blockade also reduces the release of insulin in response to hyperglycemia; adjust dosage of insulin).

No products indexed under this heading.

Insulin Aspart (Beta-adrenergic blockade may prevent the appearance of premonitory signs and symptoms, such as tachycardia and blood pressure changes, of acute hypoglycemia; beta-blockade also reduces the release of insulin in response to hyperglycemia; adjust dosage of insulin).

No products indexed under this heading.

Insulin Aspart, Human (Beta-adrenergic blockade may prevent the appearance of premonitory signs and symptoms, such as tachycardia and blood pressure changes, of acute hypoglycemia; beta-blockade also reduces the release of insulin in response to hyperglycemia; adjust dosage of insulin). Products include:

NovoLog Mix 70/30 2364

Insulin Aspart, Human Regular (Beta-adrenergic blockade may prevent the appearance of premonitory signs and symptoms, such as tachycardia and blood pressure changes, of acute hypoglycemia; beta-blockade also reduces the release of insulin in response to hyperglycemia; adjust dosage of insulin). Products include:

NovoLog Injection 2359

Insulin Aspart Protamine, Human (Beta-adrenergic blockade may prevent the appearance of premonitory signs and symptoms, such as tachycardia and blood pressure changes, of acute hypoglycemia; beta-blockade also reduces the release of insulin in response to hyperglycemia; adjust dosage of insulin). Products include:

NovoLog Mix 70/30 2364

Insulin Detemir (rDNA Origin) (Beta-adrenergic blockade may prevent the appearance of premonitory signs and symptoms, such as tachycardia and blood pressure changes, of acute hypoglycemia; beta-blockade also reduces the release of insulin in response to hyperglycemia; adjust dosage of insulin). Products include:

Levemir Injection 2352

Insulin glargine (Beta-adrenergic blockade may prevent the appearance of premonitory signs and symptoms, such as tachycardia and blood pressure changes, of acute hypoglycemia; beta-blockade also reduces the release of insulin in response to hyperglycemia; adjust dosage of insulin). Products include:

Lantus Injection 2749

Insulin Glulisine (Beta-adrenergic blockade may prevent the appearance of premonitory signs and symptoms, such as tachycardia and blood pressure changes, of acute hypoglycemia; beta-blockade also reduces the release of insulin in response to hyperglycemia; adjust dosage of insulin). Products include:

Apidra Injection 2706

Insulin Lispro, Human (Beta-adrenergic blockade may prevent the appearance of premonitory signs and symptoms, such as tachycardia and blood pressure changes, of acute hypoglycemia; beta-blockade also reduces the release of insulin in response to hyperglycemia; adjust dosage of insulin). Products include:

Humalog-Pen and KwikPen 1829
Humalog Mix 50/50-Pen and KwikPen 1833
Humalog Mix 75/25-Pen and KwikPen 1835

Insulin Lispro Protamine, Human (Beta-adrenergic blockade may prevent the appearance of premonitory signs and symptoms, such as tachycardia and blood pressure changes, of acute hypoglycemia; beta-blockade also reduces the release of insulin in response to hyperglycemia; adjust dosage of insulin). Products include:

Humalog Mix 50/50-Pen and KwikPen 1833
Humalog Mix 75/25-Pen and KwikPen 1835

Isoflurane (Co-administration may result in exaggeration of the hypotension induced by general anesthetics).

No products indexed under this heading.

Ketamine Hydrochloride (Co-administration may result in exaggeration of the hypotension induced by general anesthetics).

No products indexed under this heading.

Metformin Hydrochloride (Beta-adrenergic blockade may prevent the appearance of premonitory signs and symptoms, such as tachycardia and blood pressure changes, of acute hypoglycemia; beta-blockade also reduces the release of insulin in response to hyperglycemia; adjust dosage of oral antidiabetic drugs). Products include:

ActoPlus Met Tablets 3071
Avandamet Tablets 1336
Janumet Tablets 2041
PrandiMet Tablets 2967

Methohexital Sodium (Co-administration may result in exaggeration of the hypotension induced by general anesthetics).

No products indexed under this heading.

Methoxyflurane (Co-administration may result in exaggeration of the hypotension induced by general anesthetics).

No products indexed under this heading.

Miglitol (Beta-adrenergic blockade may prevent the appearance of premonitory signs and symptoms, such as tachycardia and blood pressure changes, of acute hypoglycemia; beta-blockade also reduces the release of insulin in response to hyperglycemia; adjust dosage of oral antidiabetic drugs).

No products indexed under this heading.

Nateglinide (Beta-adrenergic blockade may prevent the appearance of premonitory signs and symptoms, such as tachycardia and blood pressure changes, of acute hypoglycemia; beta-blockade also reduces the release of insulin in response to hyperglycemia; adjust dosage of oral antidiabetic drugs). Products include:

Starlix Tablets 2314

Pioglitazone Hydrochloride (Beta-adrenergic blockade may prevent the appearance of premonitory signs and symptoms, such as tachycardia and blood pressure changes, of acute hypoglycemia; beta-blockade also reduces the release of insulin in response to hyperglycemia; adjust dosage of oral antidiabetic drugs). Products include:

ActoPlus Met Tablets 3071
Actos Tablets 3077
Duetact Tablets 3085

Propofol (Co-administration may result in exaggeration of the hypotension induced by general anesthetics).

No products indexed under this heading.

Repaglinide (Beta-adrenergic blockade may prevent the appearance of premonitory signs and symptoms, such as tachycardia and blood pressure changes, of acute hypoglycemia; beta-blockade also reduces the release of insulin in response to hyperglycemia; adjust dosage of oral antidiabetic drugs). Products include:

PrandiMet Tablets 2967
Prandin Tablets 2971

Reserpine (Potential for additive effects resulting in hypotension and/or excessive bradycardia (vertigo, syncope, postural hypotension)).

No products indexed under this heading.

Rosiglitazone Maleate (Beta-adrenergic blockade may prevent the appearance of premonitory signs and symptoms, such as tachycardia and blood pressure changes, of acute hypoglycemia; beta-blockade also reduces the release of insulin in response to hyperglycemia; adjust dosage of oral antidiabetic drugs). Products include:

Avandamet Tablets 1336
Avandaryl Tablets 1344
Avandia Tablets 1351

Sevoflurane (Co-administration may result in exaggeration of the hypotension induced by general anesthetics). Products include:

Ultane Liquid for Inhalation 524

Sitagliptin Phosphate (Beta-adrenergic blockade may prevent the appearance of premonitory signs and symptoms, such as tachycardia and blood pressure changes, of acute hypoglycemia; beta-blockade also reduces the release of insulin in response to hyperglycemia; adjust dosage of oral antidiabetic drugs). Products include:

Janumet Tablets 2041
Januvia Tablets 2048

Tolazamide (Beta-adrenergic blockade may prevent the appearance of premonitory signs and symptoms, such as tachycardia and blood pressure changes, of acute hypoglycemia; beta-blockade also reduces the release of insulin in response to hyperglycemia; adjust dosage of oral antidiabetic drugs).

No products indexed under this heading.

Tolbutamide (Beta-adrenergic blockade may prevent the appearance of premonitory signs and symptoms, such as tachycardia and blood pressure changes, of acute hypoglycemia; beta-blockade also reduces the release of insulin in response to hyperglycemia; adjust dosage of oral antidiabetic drugs).

No products indexed under this heading.

Troglitazone (Beta-adrenergic blockade may prevent the appearance of premonitory signs and symptoms, such as tachycardia and blood pressure changes, of acute hypoglycemia; beta-blockade also reduces the release of insulin in response to hyperglycemia; adjust dosage of oral antidiabetic drugs).

No products indexed under this heading.

NAFTIN CREAM

(Naftifine Hydrochloride) 2164
None cited in PDR database.

NAFTIN GEL

(Naftifine Hydrochloride) 2164
None cited in PDR database.

NALFON CAPSULES

(Fenoprofen Calcium) 2508
May interact with ACE inhibitors, oral anticoagulants, diuretics, hydantoin anticonvulsants, loop diuretics, salicylates, sulfonamides, sulfonylureas, and certain other agents. Compounds in these categories include:

Amiloride Hydrochloride (Fenoprofen calcium may reduce the natriuretic effect of diuretics. This inhibition has been attributed to inhibition of renal prostaglandin synthesis. During concomitant therapy with NSAIDs, the patient should be observed closely for signs of renal failure, as well as to assure diuretic efficacy).

No products indexed under this heading.

Anisindione (In patients receiving coumarin-type anticoagulants, the addition of fenoprofen calcium to therapy could prolong the prothrombin time. Patients receiving both drugs should be under careful observation).

No products indexed under this heading.

Aspirin (The co-administration of aspirin decreases the biologic half-life of fenoprofen because of an increase in metabolic clearance that results in a greater amount of hydroxylated fenoprofen in the urine. Although the mechanism of interaction between fenoprofen and aspirin is not totally known, enzyme induction and displacement of fenoprofen from plasma albumin binding sites are possibilities. Because fenoprofen calcium has not been shown to produce any additional effect beyond that obtained with aspirin alone and because aspirin increases the rate of excretion of fenoprofen calcium, concomitant use of fenoprofen calcium and salicylates is not recommended). Products include:

Aggrenox Capsules 819
Bayer Aspirin 750
Percodan Tablets 1130
St. Joseph 81 mg Aspirin Chewable and Enteric Coated Tablets 1903

Aspirin, Enteric Coated (The co-administration of aspirin decreases

the biologic half-life of fenoprofen because of an increase in metabolic clearance that results in a greater amount of hydroxylated fenoprofen in the urine. Although the mechanism of interaction between fenoprofen and aspirin is not totally known, enzyme induction and displacement of fenoprofen from plasma albumin binding sites are possibilities. Because fenoprofen calcium has not been shown to produce any additional effect beyond that obtained with aspirin alone and because aspirin increases the rate of excretion of fenoprofen calcium, concomitant use of fenoprofen calcium and salicylates is not recommended).
No products indexed under this heading.

Aspirin Buffered (The co-administration of aspirin decreases the biologic half-life of fenoprofen because of an increase in metabolic clearance that results in a greater amount of hydroxylated fenoprofen in the urine. Although the mechanism of interaction between fenoprofen and aspirin is not totally known, enzyme induction and displacement of fenoprofen from plasma albumin binding sites are possibilities. Because fenoprofen calcium has not been shown to produce any additional effect beyond that obtained with aspirin alone and because aspirin increases the rate of excretion of fenoprofen calcium, concomitant use of fenoprofen calcium and salicylates is not recommended).
No products indexed under this heading.

Benazepril Hydrochloride (Reports suggest that NSAIDs may diminish the antihypertensive effect of ACE-inhibitors. This interaction should be given consideration in patients taking NSAIDs concomitantly with ACE-inhibitors).
No products indexed under this heading.

Bendroflumethiazide (In vitro studies have shown that fenoprofen, because of its affinity for albumin, may displace from their bindings sites other drugs that are also albumin bound, and this may lead to drug interaction. Theoretically, fenoprofen could likewise be displayed. Patients receiving sulfonylureas should be observed for increased activity of these drugs and, therefore, signs of toxicity from these drugs. Fenoprofen calcium may reduce the natriuretic effect of thiazides. This inhibition has been attributed to inhibition of renal prostaglandin synthesis. During concomitant therapy with NSAIDs, the patient should be observed closely for signs of renal failure, as well as to assure diuretic efficacy).
No products indexed under this heading.

Benzthiazide (Fenoprofen calcium may reduce the natriuretic effect of thiazides. This inhibition has been attributed to inhibition of renal prostaglandin synthesis. During concomitant therapy with NSAIDs, the patient should be observed closely for signs of renal failure, as well as to assure diuretic efficacy).
No products indexed under this heading.

Bumetanide (Fenoprofen calcium may reduce the natriuretic effect of diuretics. This inhibition has been attributed to inhibition of renal prostaglandin synthesis. During concomitant therapy with NSAIDs, the patient should be observed closely for signs of renal failure, as well as to assure diuretic efficacy).
No products indexed under this heading.

Captopril (Reports suggest that NSAIDs may diminish the antihypertensive effect of ACE-inhibitors. This interaction should be given consideration in patients taking NSAIDs concomitantly with ACE-inhibitors). Products include:
Captopril Tablets 2182

Chlorothiazide (In vitro studies have shown that fenoprofen, because of its affinity for albumin, may displace from their bindings sites other drugs that are also albumin bound, and this may lead to drug interaction. Theoretically, fenoprofen could likewise be displayed. Patients receiving sulfonylureas should be observed for increased activity of these drugs and, therefore, signs of toxicity from these drugs. Fenoprofen calcium may reduce the natriuretic effect of thiazides. This inhibition has been attributed to inhibition of renal prostaglandin synthesis. During concomitant therapy with NSAIDs, the patient should be observed closely for signs of renal failure, as well as to assure diuretic efficacy).
No products indexed under this heading.

Chlorothiazide Sodium (In vitro studies have shown that fenoprofen, because of its affinity for albumin, may displace from their bindings sites other drugs that are also albumin bound, and this may lead to drug interaction. Theoretically, fenoprofen could likewise be displayed. Patients receiving sulfonylureas should be observed for increased activity of these drugs and, therefore, signs of toxicity from these drugs. Fenoprofen calcium may reduce the natriuretic effect of thiazides. This inhibition has been attributed to inhibition of renal prostaglandin synthesis. During concomitant therapy with NSAIDs, the patient should be observed closely for signs of renal failure, as well as to assure diuretic efficacy). Products include:
Intravenous Sodium Diuril 2490

Chlorpropamide (In vitro studies have shown that fenoprofen, because of its affinity for albumin, may displace from their bindings sites other drugs that are also albumin bound, and this may lead to drug interaction. Theoretically, fenoprofen could likewise be displayed. Patients receiving sulfonamides should be observed for increased activity of these drugs and, therefore, signs of toxicity from these drugs).
No products indexed under this heading.

Chlorthalidone (Fenoprofen calcium may reduce the natriuretic effect of diuretics. This inhibition has been attributed to inhibition of renal prostaglandin synthesis. During concomitant therapy with NSAIDs, the patient should be observed closely for signs of renal failure, as well as to assure diuretic efficacy). Products include:
Clorpres Tablets 2185

Choline Magnesium Trisalicylate (The co-administration of aspirin decreases the biologic half-life of fenoprofen because of an increase in metabolic clearance that results in a greater amount of hydroxylated fenoprofen in the urine. Although the mechanism of interaction between fenoprofen and aspirin is not totally known, enzyme induction and displacement of fenoprofen from plasma albumin binding sites are possibilities. Because fenoprofen calcium has not been shown to produce any additional effect beyond that obtained with aspirin alone and because aspirin increases the rate of excretion of fenoprofen calcium, concomitant use of fenoprofen calcium and salicylates is not recommended).
No products indexed under this heading.

Dicumarol (In patients receiving coumarin-type anticoagulants, the addition of fenoprofen calcium to therapy could prolong the prothrombin time. Patients receiving both drugs should be under careful observation).
No products indexed under this heading.

Diflunisal (The co-administration of aspirin decreases the biologic half-life of fenoprofen because of an increase in metabolic clearance that results in a greater amount of hydroxylated fenoprofen in the urine. Although the mechanism of interaction between fenoprofen and aspirin is not totally known, enzyme induction and displacement of fenoprofen from plasma albumin binding sites are possibilities. Because fenoprofen calcium has not been shown to produce any additional effect beyond that obtained with aspirin alone and because aspirin increases the rate of excretion of fenoprofen calcium, concomitant use of fenoprofen calcium and salicylates is not recommended).
No products indexed under this heading.

Enalapril Maleate (Reports suggest that NSAIDs may diminish the antihypertensive effect of ACE-inhibitors. This interaction should be given consideration in patients taking NSAIDs concomitantly with ACE-inhibitors).
No products indexed under this heading.

Enalaprilat (Reports suggest that NSAIDs may diminish the antihypertensive effect of ACE-inhibitors. This interaction should be given consideration in patients taking NSAIDs concomitantly with ACE-inhibitors).
No products indexed under this heading.

Ethacrynic Acid (Fenoprofen calcium may reduce the natriuretic effect of diuretics. This inhibition has been attributed to inhibition of renal prostaglandin synthesis. During concomitant therapy with NSAIDs, the patient should be observed closely for signs of renal failure, as well as to assure diuretic efficacy). Products include:
Edecrin Tablets 698

Ethotoin (In vitro studies have shown that fenoprofen, because of its affinity for albumin, may displace from their binding sites other drugs that are also albumin bound, and this may lead to drug interaction. Theoretically, fenoprofen could likewise be displayed.Patients receiving hydantins should be observed for increased activity drugs and, therefore, signs of toxicity from these drugs).
No products indexed under this heading.

Fosinopril Sodium (Reports suggest that NSAIDs may diminish the antihypertensive effect of ACE-inhibitors. This interaction should be given consideration in patients taking NSAIDs concomitantly with ACE-inhibitors).
No products indexed under this heading.

Fosphenytoin Sodium (In vitro studies have shown that fenoprofen, because of its affinity for albumin, may displace from their binding sites other drugs that are also albumin bound, and this may lead to drug interaction. Theoretically, fenoprofen could likewise be displayed.Patients receiving hydantins should be observed for increased activity drugs and, therefore, signs of toxicity from these drugs).
No products indexed under this heading.

Furosemide (Fenoprofen calcium may reduce the natriuretic effect of loop diuretics. This inhibition has been attributed to inhibition of renal prostaglandin synthesis. During concomitant therapy with NSAIDs, the patient should be observed closely for signs of renal failure, as well as to assure diuretic efficacy). Products include:
Furosemide Tablets 2186

Glimepiride (In vitro studies have shown that fenoprofen, because of its affinity for albumin, may displace from their bindings sites other drugs that are also albumin bound, and this may lead to drug interaction. Theoretically, fenoprofen could likewise be displayed. Patients receiving sulfonylureas should be observed for increased activity of these drugs and, therefore, signs of toxicity from these drugs). Products include:
Avandaryl Tablets 1344
Duetact Tablets 3085

Glipizide (In vitro studies have shown that fenoprofen, because of its affinity for albumin, may displace from their bindings sites other drugs that are also albumin bound, and this may lead to drug interaction. Theoretically, fenoprofen could likewise be displayed. Patients receiving sulfonamides should be observed for increased activity of these drugs and, therefore, signs of toxicity from these drugs).
No products indexed under this heading.

Glyburide (In vitro studies have shown that fenoprofen, because of its affinity for albumin, may displace from their bindings sites other drugs that are also albumin bound, and this may lead to drug interaction. Theoretically, fenoprofen could likewise be displayed. Patients receiving sulfonamides should be observed for increased activity of these drugs and, therefore, signs of toxicity from these drugs).
No products indexed under this heading.

Hydrochlorothiazide (In vitro studies have shown that fenoprofen, because of its affinity for albumin, may displace from their bindings sites other drugs that are also albumin bound, and this may lead to drug interaction. Theoretically, fenoprofen could likewise be displayed. Patients receiving sulfonylureas should be observed for increased activity of these drugs and, therefore, signs of toxicity from these drugs. Fenoprofen calcium may reduce the natriuretic effect of thiazides. This inhibition has been attributed to inhibition of renal prostaglandin synthesis. During concomitant therapy with NSAIDs, the patient should be observed closely for signs of renal failure, as well as to assure diuretic efficacy). Products include:

Atacand HCT ... 642
Avalide Tablets ... 892
Avalide Tablets ... 2713
Benicar HCT Tablets ... 1010
Diovan HCT Tablets ... 2216
Dyazide Capsules ... 1405
Micardis HCT Tablets ... 854
Prinzide Tablets ... 2092
Tekturna HCT Tablets ... 2324
Teveten HCT Tablets ... 517

Hydroflumethiazide (In vitro studies have shown that fenoprofen, because of its affinity for albumin, may displace from their bindings sites other drugs that are also albumin bound, and this may lead to drug interaction. Theoretically, fenoprofen could likewise be displayed. Patients receiving sulfonylureas should be observed for increased activity of these drugs and, therefore, signs of toxicity from these drugs. Fenoprofen calcium may reduce the natriuretic effect of thiazides. This inhibition has been attributed to inhibition of renal prostaglandin synthesis. During concomitant therapy with NSAIDs, the patient should be observed closely for signs of renal failure, as well as to assure diuretic efficacy).

No products indexed under this heading.

Indapamide (Fenoprofen calcium may reduce the natriuretic effect of diuretics. This inhibition has been attributed to inhibition of renal prostaglandin synthesis. During concomitant therapy with NSAIDs, the patient should be observed closely for signs of renal failure, as well as to assure diuretic efficacy). Products include:

Indapamide Tablets ... 2188

Lisinopril (Reports suggest that NSAIDs may diminish the antihypertensive effect of ACE-inhibitors. This interaction should be given consideration in patients taking NSAIDs concomitantly with ACE-inhibitors). Products include:

Prinivil Tablets ... 2087
Prinzide Tablets ... 2092

Lithium Carbonate (NSAIDs have produced an elevation of plasma lithium levels and a reduction in renal lithium clearance. The mean minimum lithium concentration increased 15% and the renal clearance was decreased by approximately 20%. These effects have been attributed to inhibition of renal prostaglandin synthesis by the NSAID. Thus, when NSAIDs and lithium are administered concurrently, subjects should be observed carefully for signs of lithium toxicity).

No products indexed under this heading.

Lithium Citrate (NSAIDs have produced an elevation of plasma lithium levels and a reduction in renal lithium clearance. The mean minimum lithium concentration increased 15% and the renal clearance was decreased by approximately 20%. These effects have been attributed to inhibition of renal prostaglandin synthesis by the NSAID. Thus, when NSAIDs and lithium are administered concurrently, subjects should be observed carefully for signs of lithium toxicity).

No products indexed under this heading.

Magnesium Salicylate (The co-administration of aspirin decreases the biologic half-life of fenoprofen because of an increase in metabolic clearance that results in a greater amount of hydroxylated fenoprofen in the urine. Although the mechanism of interaction between fenoprofen and aspirin is not totally known, enzyme induction and displacement of fenoprofen from plasma albumin binding sites are possibilities. Because fenoprofen calcium has not been shown to produce any additional effect beyond that obtained with aspirin alone and because aspirin increases the rate of excretion of fenoprofen calcium, concomitant use of fenoprofen calcium and salicylates is not recommended).

No products indexed under this heading.

Mephenytoin (In vitro studies have shown that fenoprofen, because of its affinity for albumin, may displace from their binding sites other drugs that are also albumin bound, and this may lead to drug interaction. Theoretically, fenoprofen could likewise be displayed.Patients receiving hydantins should be observed for increased activity drugs and, therefore, signs of toxicity from these drugs).

No products indexed under this heading.

Methotrexate Sodium (NSAIDs have been reported to competitively inhibit methotrexate accumulation in rabbit kidney slices. This may indicate that they could enhance the toxicity of methotrexate. Caution should be used when NSAIDs are administered concomitantly with methotrexate).

No products indexed under this heading.

Methyclothiazide (In vitro studies have shown that fenoprofen, because of its affinity for albumin, may displace from their bindings sites other drugs that are also albumin bound, and this may lead to drug interaction. Theoretically, fenoprofen could likewise be displayed. Patients receiving sulfonylureas should be observed for increased activity of these drugs and, therefore, signs of toxicity from these drugs. Fenoprofen calcium may reduce the natriuretic effect of thiazides. This inhibition has been attributed to inhibition of renal prostaglandin synthesis. During concomitant therapy with NSAIDs, the patient should be observed closely for signs of renal failure, as well as to assure diuretic efficacy).

No products indexed under this heading.

Metolazone (Fenoprofen calcium may reduce the natriuretic effect of diuretics. This inhibition has been attributed to inhibition of renal prostaglandin synthesis. During concomitant therapy with NSAIDs, the patient should be observed closely for signs of renal failure, as well as to assure diuretic efficacy).

No products indexed under this heading.

Moexipril Hydrochloride (Reports suggest that NSAIDs may diminish the antihypertensive effect of ACE-inhibitors. This interaction should be given consideration in patients taking NSAIDs concomitantly with ACE-inhibitors).

No products indexed under this heading.

Perindopril Erbumine (Reports suggest that NSAIDs may diminish the antihypertensive effect of ACE-inhibitors. This interaction should be given consideration in patients taking NSAIDs concomitantly with ACE-inhibitors). Products include:

Aceon Tablets (2 mg, 4 mg, 8 mg) ... 3038

Phenobarbital (Chronic administration of phenobarbital, a known enzyme inducer, may be associated with a decrease in the plasma half-life of fenoprofen. When phenobarbital is added to or withdrawn from treatment, dosage adjustment of fenoprofen calcium may be required). Products include:

Donnatal Extentabs ... 2507

Phenobarbital Sodium (Chronic administration of phenobarbital, a known enzyme inducer, may be associated with a decrease in the plasma half-life of fenoprofen. When phenobarbital is added to or withdrawn from treatment, dosage adjustment of fenoprofen calcium may be required).

No products indexed under this heading.

Phenytoin (In vitro studies have shown that fenoprofen, because of its affinity for albumin, may displace from their binding sites other drugs that are also albumin bound, and this may lead to drug interaction. Theoretically, fenoprofen could likewise be displayed.Patients receiving hydantins should be observed for increased activity drugs and, therefore, signs of toxicity from these drugs).

No products indexed under this heading.

Phenytoin Sodium (In vitro studies have shown that fenoprofen, because of its affinity for albumin, may displace from their binding sites other drugs that are also albumin bound, and this may lead to drug interaction. Theoretically, fenoprofen could likewise be displayed.Patients receiving hydantins should be observed for increased activity drugs and, therefore, signs of toxicity from these drugs). Products include:

Phenytek Capsules ... 2192

Polythiazide (In vitro studies have shown that fenoprofen, because of its affinity for albumin, may displace from their bindings sites other drugs that are also albumin bound, and this may lead to drug interaction. Theoretically, fenoprofen could likewise be displayed. Patients receiving sulfonylureas should be observed for increased activity of these drugs and, therefore, signs of toxicity from these drugs. Fenoprofen calcium may reduce the natriuretic effect of thiazides. This inhibition has been attributed to inhibition of renal prostaglandin synthesis. During concomitant therapy with NSAIDs, the patient should be observed closely for signs of renal failure, as well as to assure diuretic efficacy).

No products indexed under this heading.

Quinapril Hydrochloride (Reports suggest that NSAIDs may diminish the antihypertensive effect of ACE-inhibitors. This interaction should be given consideration in patients taking NSAIDs concomitantly with ACE-inhibitors).

No products indexed under this heading.

Ramipril (Reports suggest that NSAIDs may diminish the antihypertensive effect of ACE-inhibitors. This interaction should be given consideration in patients taking NSAIDs concomitantly with ACE-inhibitors).

No products indexed under this heading.

Salsalate (The co-administration of aspirin decreases the biologic half-life of fenoprofen because of an increase in metabolic clearance that results in a greater amount of hydroxylated fenoprofen in the urine. Although the mechanism of interaction between fenoprofen and aspirin is not totally known, enzyme induction and displacement of fenoprofen from plasma albumin binding sites are possibilities. Because fenoprofen calcium has not been shown to produce any additional effect beyond that obtained with aspirin alone and because aspirin increases the rate of excretion of fenoprofen calcium, concomitant use of fenoprofen calcium and salicylates is not recommended).

No products indexed under this heading.

Spirapril Hydrochloride (Reports suggest that NSAIDs may diminish the antihypertensive effect of ACE-inhibitors. This interaction should be given consideration in patients taking NSAIDs concomitantly with ACE-inhibitors).

No products indexed under this heading.

Spironolactone (Fenoprofen calcium may reduce the natriuretic effect of diuretics. This inhibition has been attributed to inhibition of renal prostaglandin synthesis. During concomitant therapy with NSAIDs, the patient should be observed closely for signs of renal failure, as well as to assure diuretic efficacy).

No products indexed under this heading.

Sulfacytine (In vitro studies have shown that fenoprofen, because of its affinity for albumin, may displace from their bindings sites other drugs that are also albumin bound, and this may lead to drug interaction. Theoretically, fenoprofen could likewise be displayed. Patients receiving sulfonamides should be observed for increased activity of these drugs and, therefore, signs of toxicity from these drugs).

No products indexed under this heading.

Sulfamethizole (In vitro studies have shown that fenoprofen,

because of its affinity for albumin, may displace from their bindings sites other drugs that are also albumin bound, and this may lead to drug interaction. Theoretically, fenoprofen could likewise be displayed. Patients receiving sulfonamides should be observed for increased activity of these drugs and, therefore, signs of toxicity from these drugs).

No products indexed under this heading.

Sulfamethoxazole (In vitro studies have shown that fenoprofen, because of its affinity for albumin, may displace from their bindings sites other drugs that are also albumin bound, and this may lead to drug interaction. Theoretically, fenoprofen could likewise be displayed. Patients receiving sulfonamides should be observed for increased activity of these drugs and, therefore, signs of toxicity from these drugs).

No products indexed under this heading.

Sulfasalazine (In vitro studies have shown that fenoprofen, because of its affinity for albumin, may displace from their bindings sites other drugs that are also albumin bound, and this may lead to drug interaction. Theoretically, fenoprofen could likewise be displayed. Patients receiving sulfonamides should be observed for increased activity of these drugs and, therefore, signs of toxicity from these drugs).

No products indexed under this heading.

Sulfinpyrazone (In vitro studies have shown that fenoprofen, because of its affinity for albumin, may displace from their bindings sites other drugs that are also albumin bound, and this may lead to drug interaction. Theoretically, fenoprofen could likewise be displayed. Patients receiving sulfonamides should be observed for increased activity of these drugs and, therefore, signs of toxicity from these drugs).

No products indexed under this heading.

Sulfisoxazole Acetyl (In vitro studies have shown that fenoprofen, because of its affinity for albumin, may displace from their bindings sites other drugs that are also albumin bound, and this may lead to drug interaction. Theoretically, fenoprofen could likewise be displayed. Patients receiving sulfonamides should be observed for increased activity of these drugs and, therefore, signs of toxicity from these drugs).

No products indexed under this heading.

Sulfisoxazole Diolamine (In vitro studies have shown that fenoprofen, because of its affinity for albumin, may displace from their bindings sites other drugs that are also albumin bound, and this may lead to drug interaction. Theoretically, fenoprofen could likewise be displayed. Patients receiving sulfonamides should be observed for increased activity of these drugs and, therefore, signs of toxicity from these drugs).

No products indexed under this heading.

Tolazamide (In vitro studies have shown that fenoprofen, because of its affinity for albumin, may displace from their bindings sites other drugs that are also albumin bound, and this may lead to drug interaction. Theoretically, fenoprofen could likewise be displayed. Patients receiving sulfonamides should be observed for increased activity of these drugs and, therefore, signs of toxicity from these drugs).

No products indexed under this heading.

Tolbutamide (In vitro studies have shown that fenoprofen, because of its affinity for albumin, may displace from their bindings sites other drugs that are also albumin bound, and this may lead to drug interaction. Theoretically, fenoprofen could likewise be displayed. Patients receiving sulfonamides should be observed for increased activity of these drugs and, therefore, signs of toxicity from these drugs).

No products indexed under this heading.

Torsemide (Fenoprofen calcium may reduce the natriuretic effect of diuretics. This inhibition has been attributed to inhibition of renal prostaglandin synthesis. During concomitant therapy with NSAIDs, the patient should be observed closely for signs of renal failure, as well as to assure diuretic efficacy). Products include:

Demadex Injection 2630
Demadex Tablets 2630

Trandolapril (Reports suggest that NSAIDs may diminish the antihypertensive effect of ACE-inhibitors. This interaction should be given consideration in patients taking NSAIDs concomitantly with ACE-inhibitors). Products include:

Mavik Tablets 472
Tarka Tablets 511

Triamterene (Fenoprofen calcium may reduce the natriuretic effect of diuretics. This inhibition has been attributed to inhibition of renal prostaglandin synthesis. During concomitant therapy with NSAIDs, the patient should be observed closely for signs of renal failure, as well as to assure diuretic efficacy). Products include:

Dyazide Capsules 1405
Dyrenium Capsules 3189

Trichlormethiazide (In vitro studies have shown that fenoprofen, because of its affinity for albumin, may displace from their bindings sites other drugs that are also albumin bound, and this may lead to drug interaction. Theoretically, fenoprofen could likewise be displayed. Patients receiving sulfonylureas should be observed for increased activity of these drugs and, therefore, signs of toxicity from these drugs. Fenoprofen calcium may reduce the natriuretic effect of thiazides. This inhibition has been attributed to inhibition of renal prostaglandin synthesis. During concomitant therapy with NSAIDs, the patient should be observed closely for signs of renal failure, as well as to assure diuretic efficacy).

No products indexed under this heading.

Warfarin Sodium (In patients receiving coumarin-type anticoagulants, the addition of fenoprofen calcium to therapy could prolong the prothrombin time. Patients receiving both drugs should be under careful observation. The effects of warfarin and NSAIDs on GI bleeding are synergestic, such that users of both drugs together have a risk of serious GI bleeding higher than users of either drug alone).

No products indexed under this heading.

NAMENDA ORAL SOLUTION

(Memantine Hydrochloride) 1180
See Namenda Tablets

NAMENDA TABLETS

(Memantine Hydrochloride) 1180
May interact with carbonic anhydrase inhibitors, quinidine, urinary alkalinizing agents, and certain other agents. Compounds in these categories include:

Acetazolamide (Alterations of urine pH towards the alkaline condition by drugs that make the urine alkaline (e.g., carbonic anhydrase inhibitors) may lead to an accumulation of memantine with a possible increase in adverse effects; use with caution).

No products indexed under this heading.

Amantadine Hydrochloride (The combined use of memantine with other NMDA antagonists, like amantadine, has not been systemically evaluated and such use should be approached with caution).

No products indexed under this heading.

Cimetidine (Co-administration with drugs that use the same renal cationic system, including cimetidine, could potentially result in altered plasma levels of both drugs).

No products indexed under this heading.

Cimetidine Hydrochloride (Co-administration with drugs that use the same renal cationic system, including cimetidine, could potentially result in altered plasma levels of both drugs).

No products indexed under this heading.

Dextromethorphan (The combined use of memantine with other NMDA antagonists, like dextromethorphan, has not been systemically evaluated and such use should be approached with caution).

No products indexed under this heading.

Dextromethorphan Hydrobromide (The combined use of memantine with other NMDA antagonists, like dextromethorphan, has not been systemically evaluated and such use should be approached with caution). Products include:

PediaCare Children's Liquid Multi-Symptom Cold 1902
PediaCare Children's Long-Acting Cough 1902
Children's Sudafed PE Cold & Cough Liquid 1907
Sudafed PE Cold & Cough Caplets 1907
Children's Tylenol Plus Cough & Runny Nose Suspension Liquid 1912
Children's Tylenol Plus Cough & Sore Throat Suspension Liquid 1912
Children's Tylenol Plus Flu Suspension Liquid 1914
Children's Tylenol Plus Multi-Symptom Cold Suspension Liquid 1912
Tylenol Cold Severe Congestion Daytime Caplets with Cool Burst 1912
Tylenol Cold Head Congestion Daytime Caplets with Cool Burst 1910
Tylenol Cold Head Congestion Nighttime Caplets with Cool Burst 1910
Tylenol Cold Head Congestion Severe Daytime Caplets with Cool Burst 1910
Tylenol Cold Multi-Symptom Daytime Caplets with Cool Burst and Rapid Release Gels 1913
Tylenol Cold Multi-Symptom Daytime Liquid with Citrus Burst 1913
Tylenol Cold Multi-Symptom Nighttime Caplets with Cool Burst 1913
Tylenol Cold Multi-Symptom Nighttime Liquid with Cool Burst 1913
Tylenol Cold Multi-Symptom Severe Caplets with Cool Burst 1913
Tylenol Cold Multi-Symptom Severe Daytime Liquid with Citrus Burst 1913
Tylenol Cough & Sore Throat Daytime Liquid with Cool Burst 1918
Tylenol Cough & Sore Throat Nighttime Liquid with Cool Burst 1918
Vicks DayQuil Cold & Flu Multi-Symptom Relief 616
Vicks DayQuil LiquiCaps 2567
Vicks DayQuil Liquid 2567
Vicks DayQuil Multi-Symptom Cold/Flu Relief 2567
Vicks NyQuil Cold & Flu Multi-Symptom Relief 617
Vicks NyQuil LiquiCaps 2567
Vicks NyQuil Liquid 2567
Vicks NyQuil Multi-Symptom Cold/Flu Relief 2567

Dextromethorphan Polistirex (The combined use of memantine with other NMDA antagonists, like dextromethorphan, has not been systemically evaluated and such use should be approached with caution).

No products indexed under this heading.

Dextromethorphan tannate (The combined use of memantine with other NMDA antagonists, like dextromethorphan, has not been systemically evaluated and such use should be approached with caution).

No products indexed under this heading.

Dichlorphenamide (Alterations of urine pH towards the alkaline condition by drugs that make the urine alkaline (e.g., carbonic anhydrase inhibitors) may lead to an accumulation of memantine with a possible increase in adverse effects; use with caution).

No products indexed under this heading.

Dorzolamide Hydrochloride (Alterations of urine pH towards the alkaline condition by drugs that make the urine alkaline (e.g., carbonic anhydrase inhibitors) may lead to an accumulation of memantine with a possible increase in adverse effects; use with caution). Products include:

Cosopt Sterile Ophthalmic Solution 1969
Trusopt Sterile Ophthalmic Solution 2128

Hydrochlorothiazide (Co-administration with drugs that use the same renal cationic system, including hydrochlorothiazide, could potentially result in altered plasma levels of both drugs. The co-administration of memantine and hydrochlorothiazide/triamterene

decreased the bioavailability of hydrochlorothiazide by 20%). Products include:
Atacand HCT ... 642
Avalide Tablets ... 892
Avalide Tablets ... 2713
Benicar HCT Tablets ... 1010
Diovan HCT Tablets ... 2216
Dyazide Capsules ... 1405
Micardis HCT Tablets ... 854
Prinzide Tablets ... 2092
Tekturna HCT Tablets ... 2324
Teveten HCT Tablets ... 517

Hydrochlorothiazide Hydrochloride (Co-administration with drugs that use the same renal cationic system, including hydrochlorothiazide, could potentially result in altered plasma levels of both drugs. The co-administration of memantine and hydrochlorothiazide/triamterene decreased the bioavailability of hydrochlorothiazide by 20%).
No products indexed under this heading.

Ketamine (The combined use of memantine with other NMDA antagonists, like ketamine, has not been systemically evaluated and such use should be approached with caution).
No products indexed under this heading.

Ketamine Hydrochloride (The combined use of memantine with other NMDA antagonists, like ketamine, has not been systemically evaluated and such use should be approached with caution).
No products indexed under this heading.

Methazolamide (Alterations of urine pH towards the alkaline condition by drugs that make the urine alkaline (e.g., carbonic anhydrase inhibitors) may lead to an accumulation of memantine with a possible increase in adverse effects; use with caution).
No products indexed under this heading.

Nicotine (Co-administration with drugs that use the same renal cationic system, including nicotine, could potentially result in altered plasma levels of both drugs).
No products indexed under this heading.

Nicotine Polacrilex (Co-administration with drugs that use the same renal cationic system, including nicotine, could potentially result in altered plasma levels of both drugs).
No products indexed under this heading.

Nicotine Salicylate (Co-administration with drugs that use the same renal cationic system, including nicotine, could potentially result in altered plasma levels of both drugs).
No products indexed under this heading.

Nicotine Sulfate (Co-administration with drugs that use the same renal cationic system, including nicotine, could potentially result in altered plasma levels of both drugs).
No products indexed under this heading.

Potassium Citrate (Alterations of urine pH towards the alkaline condition by drugs that make the urine alkaline may lead to an accumulation of memantine with a possible increase in adverse effects; use with caution). Products include:
BioLean Free Tablets ... ▣635
Urocit-K Tablets ... 2176

Quinidine (Co-administration with drugs that use the same renal cationic system, including quinidine, could potentially result in altered plasma levels of both drugs).
No products indexed under this heading.

Quinidine Gluconate (Co-administration with drugs that use the same renal cationic system, including quinidine, could potentially result in altered plasma levels of both drugs).
No products indexed under this heading.

Quinidine Hydrochloride (Co-administration with drugs that use the same renal cationic system, including quinidine, could potentially result in altered plasma levels of both drugs).
No products indexed under this heading.

Quinidine Polygalacturonate (Co-administration with drugs that use the same renal cationic system, including quinidine, could potentially result in altered plasma levels of both drugs).
No products indexed under this heading.

Quinidine Sulfate (Co-administration with drugs that use the same renal cationic system, including quinidine, could potentially result in altered plasma levels of both drugs).
No products indexed under this heading.

Ranitidine Bismuth Citrate (Co-administration with drugs that use the same renal cationic system, including ranitidine, could potentially result in altered plasma levels of both drugs).
No products indexed under this heading.

Ranitidine Hydrochloride (Co-administration with drugs that use the same renal cationic system, including ranitidine, could potentially result in altered plasma levels of both drugs). Products include:
Zantac 75 Tablets ... ▣603
Zantac ... 1670
Zantac Injection ... 1666
Zantac Injection Pharmacy Bulk Package ... 1668
Maximum Strength Zantac 150 Tablets ... ▣603
Maximum Strength Zantac 150 Cool Mint Tablets ... ▣603

Sodium Bicarbonate (Alterations of urine pH towards the alkaline condition by drugs that make the urine alkaline (e.g., sodium bicarbonate) may lead to an accumulation of memantine with a possible increase in adverse effects; hence, use with caution). Products include:
Ceo-Two Laxative Suppository ... 815

Sodium Citrate (Alterations of urine pH towards the alkaline condition by drugs that make the urine alkaline may lead to an accumulation of memantine with a possible increase in adverse effects; use with caution).
No products indexed under this heading.

Torsemide (Alterations of urine pH towards the alkaline condition by drugs that make the urine alkaline (e.g., carbonic anhydrase inhibitors) may lead to an accumulation of memantine with a possible increase in adverse effects; use with caution). Products include:
Demadex Injection ... 2630
Demadex Tablets ... 2630

Triamterene (Co-administration with drugs that use the same renal cationic system, including triamterene, could potentially result in altered plasma levels of both drugs. However, co-administration of memantine and hydrochlorothiazide/triamterene did not affect the bioavailability of either memantine or triamterene). Products include:
Dyazide Capsules ... 1405
Dyrenium Capsules ... 3189

NAPROSYN SUSPENSION
(Naproxen) ... 2632
See EC-Naprosyn Delayed-Release Tablets

NAPROSYN TABLETS
(Naproxen) ... 2632
See EC-Naprosyn Delayed-Release Tablets

NASACORT AQ NASAL SPRAY
(Triamcinolone Acetonide) ... 2765
None cited in PDR database.

NASONEX NASAL SPRAY
(Mometasone Furoate Monohydrate) ... 2883
None cited in PDR database.

NATACYN ANTIFUNGAL OPHTHALMIC SUSPENSION
(Natamycin) ... ⊙204
None cited in PDR database.

NATRECOR FOR INJECTION
(Nesiritide) ... 2977
None cited in PDR database.

NATURAL JOINT CAPSULES
(Dietary Supplement) ... ▣628
None cited in PDR database.

NATURETHROID TABLETS
(Levothyroxine, Liothyronine, Thyroid) ... 2605
May interact with androgens, corticosteroids, oral anticoagulants, estrogens, oral hypoglycemic agents, insulin, oral contraceptives, salicylates, and certain other agents. Compounds in these categories include:

Acarbose (Initiating thyroid replacement therapy may cause increases in insulin or oral hypoglycemic requirements). Products include:
Precose Tablets ... 792

Anisindione (Thryoid hormones appear to increase catabolism of vitamin K-dependent clotting factors. If oral anticoagulants are also being given, compensatory increases in clotting factor synthesis are impaired).
No products indexed under this heading.

Aspirin (Preparations containing salicylates are known to interfere with laboratory tests performed in patients on thyroid hormone therapy). Products include:
Aggrenox Capsules ... 819
Bayer Aspirin ... 750
Percodan Tablets ... 1130
St. Joseph 81 mg Aspirin Chewable and Enteric Coated Tablets ... 1903

Aspirin, Enteric Coated (Preparations containing salicylates are known to interfere with laboratory tests performed in patients on thyroid hormone therapy).
No products indexed under this heading.

Aspirin Buffered (Preparations containing salicylates are known to interfere with laboratory tests performed in patients on thyroid hormone therapy).
No products indexed under this heading.

Betamethasone Acetate (Corticosteroids are known to interfere with laboratory tests performed in patients on thyroid hormone therapy).
No products indexed under this heading.

Betamethasone Sodium Phosphate (Corticosteroids are known to interfere with laboratory tests performed in patients on thyroid hormone therapy).
No products indexed under this heading.

Budesonide (Corticosteroids are known to interfere with laboratory tests performed in patients on thyroid hormone therapy). Products include:
Pulmicort Flexhaler ... 654
Symbicort 80/4.5 Inhalation Aerosol ... 659
Symbicort 160/4.5 Inhalation Aerosol ... 659

Chlorotrianisene (Patients without a functioning thyroid gland who are on thyroid replacemet therapy may need to increase their thyroid dose if estrogens are given. Estrogens are also known to interfere with laboratory tests performed in patients on thyroid hormone therapy).
No products indexed under this heading.

Chlorpropamide (Initiating thyroid replacement therapy may cause increases in insulin or oral hypoglycemic requirements).
No products indexed under this heading.

Cholestyramine (Cholestyramine binds both levothyroxine and liothyronine in the intestine, thus impairing absorption of these thyroid hormones. Four to five hours should elapse between administration of cholestyramine and thyroid hormones).
No products indexed under this heading.

Choline Magnesium Trisalicylate (Preparations containing salicylates are known to interfere with laboratory tests performed in patients on thyroid hormone therapy).
No products indexed under this heading.

Ciclesonide (Corticosteroids are known to interfere with laboratory tests performed in patients on thyroid hormone therapy). Products include:
Alvesco Inhalation Aerosol ... 2985
Omnaris Nasal Spray ... 2998

Colestipol (Colestipol binds both levothyroxine and liothyronine in the intestine, thus impairing absorption of these thyroid hormones. Four to five hours should elapse between administration of cholestyramine and thyroid hormones).
No products indexed under this heading.

Colestipol Hydrochloride (Colestipol binds both levothyroxine and liothyronine in the intestine, thus impairing absorption of these thyroid hormones. Four to five hours should elapse between administration of cholestyramine and thyroid hormones).
No products indexed under this heading.

Cortisone Acetate (Corticosteroids are known to interfere with laboratory tests performed in patients on thyroid hormone therapy).
No products indexed under this heading.

Desogestrel (Patients without a functioning thyroid gland who are on thyroid replacemet therapy may need to increase their thyroid dose if estrogens containing oral contraceptives are given. Estrogens containing oral contraceptives are also known to interfere with laboratory tests performed in patients on thyroid hormone therapy). Products include:
Mircette Tablets ... 1034

Dexamethasone (Corticosteroids are known to interfere with laboratory tests performed in patients on thyroid hormone therapy). Products include:
Ciprodex Otic Suspension ... 541

Dexamethasone Acetate (Corticosteroids are known to interfere with laboratory tests performed in patients on thryoid hormone therapy).
No products indexed under this heading.

Dexamethasone Sodium Phosphate (Corticosteroids are known to interfere with laboratory tests performed in patients on thryoid hormone therapy).
No products indexed under this heading.

Dicumarol (Thyroid hormones appear to increase catabolism of vitamin K-dependent clotting factors. If oral anticoagulants are also being given, compensatory increases in clotting factor synthesis are impaired).
No products indexed under this heading.

Dienestrol (Patients without a functioning thyroid gland who are on thyroid replacemet therapy may need to increase their thyroid dose if estrogens are given. Estrogens are also known to interfere with laboratory tests performed in patients on thyroid hormone therapy).
No products indexed under this heading.

Diethylstilbestrol (Patients without a functioning thyroid gland who are on thyroid replacemet therapy may need to increase their thyroid dose if estrogens are given. Estrogens are also known to interfere with laboratory tests performed in patients on thyroid hormone therapy).
No products indexed under this heading.

Diflunisal (Preparations containing salicylates are known to interfere with laboratory tests performed in patients on thyroid hormone therapy).
No products indexed under this heading.

Estradiol (Patients without a functioning thyroid gland who are on thyroid replacemet therapy may need to increase their thyroid dose if estrogens are given. Estrogens are also known to interfere with laboratory tests performed in patients on thyroid hormone therapy). Products include:
Activella Tablets ... 2347
Angeliq Tablets ... 751
Climara Transdermal System ... 763
Climara Pro Transdermal System ... 768
Divigel ... 3167
Vagifem Tablets ... 2375

Estrogens, Conjugated (Patients without a functioning thyroid gland who are on thyroid replacemet therapy may need to increase their thyroid dose if estrogens are given. Estrogens are also known to interfere with laboratory tests performed in patients on thyroid hormone therapy). Products include:
Premarin Intravenous ... 3217
Premarin Tablets ... 3221
Premarin Vaginal Cream ... 3228
Premphase Tablets ... 3232
Prempro Tablets ... 3232

Estrogens, Esterified (Patients without a functioning thyroid gland who are on thyroid replacemet therapy may need to increase their thyroid dose if estrogens are given. Estrogens are also known to interfere with laboratory tests performed in patients on thyroid hormone therapy). Products include:
Estratest Tablets ... 3043
Estratest H.S. Tablets ... 3043

Estropipate (Patients without a functioning thyroid gland who are on thyroid replacemet therapy may need to increase their thyroid dose if estrogens are given. Estrogens are also known to interfere with laboratory tests performed in patients on thyroid hormone therapy).
No products indexed under this heading.

Ethinyl Estradiol (Patients without a functioning thyroid gland who are on thyroid replacemet therapy may need to increase their thyroid dose if estrogens are given. Estrogens are also known to interfere with laboratory tests performed in patients on thyroid hormone therapy). Products include:
Lybrel Tablets ... 3204
Mircette Tablets ... 1034
NuvaRing ... 2897
Ortho-Cyclen/Ortho Tri-Cyclen ... 2449
Ortho Evra Transdermal System ... 2437
Ortho Tri-Cyclen Lo Tablets ... 2458
Seasonique Tablets ... 1046
Yaz Tablets ... 805

Ethynodiol Diacetate (Patients without a functioning thyroid gland who are on thyroid replacemet therapy may need to increase their thyroid dose if estrogens containing oral contraceptives are given. Estrogens containing oral contraceptives are also known to interfere with laboratory tests performed in patients on thyroid hormone therapy).
No products indexed under this heading.

Fludrocortisone Acetate (Corticosteroids are known to interfere with laboratory tests performed in patients on thryoid hormone therapy).
No products indexed under this heading.

Flunisolide (Corticosteroids are known to interfere with laboratory tests performed in patients on thryoid hormone therapy). Products include:
Aerobid/Aerobid-M ... 1153

Fluoxymesterone (Androgens are known to interfere with laboratory tests performed in patients on thryoid hormone therapy).
No products indexed under this heading.

Fluticasone Propionate (Corticosteroids are known to interfere with laboratory tests performed in patients on thyroid hormone therapy). Products include:
Advair Diskus 100/50 ... 1276
Advair Diskus 250/50 ... 1276
Advair Diskus 500/50 ... 1276
Advair HFA 45/21 Inhalation Aerosol ... 1288
Advair HFA 115/21 Inhalation Aerosol ... 1288
Advair HFA 230/21 Inhalation Aerosol ... 1288
Flonase Nasal Spray ... 1431
Flovent Diskus 50 mcg ... 1435

Fluticasone Propionate HFA (Corticosteroids are known to interfere with laboratory tests performed in patients on thyroid hormone therapy). Products include:
Flovent HFA ... 1440

Glimepiride (Initiating thyroid replacement therapy may cause increases in insulin or oral hypoglycemic requirements). Products include:
Avandaryl Tablets ... 1344
Duetact Tablets ... 3085

Glipizide (Initiating thyroid replacement therapy may cause increases in insulin or oral hypoglycemic requirements).
No products indexed under this heading.

Glyburide (Initiating thyroid replacement therapy may cause increases in insulin or oral hypoglycemic requirements).
No products indexed under this heading.

Hydrocortisone (Corticosteroids are known to interfere with laboratory tests performed in patients on thryoid hormone therapy).
No products indexed under this heading.

Hydrocortisone Acetate (Corticosteroids are known to interfere with laboratory tests performed in patients on thyroid hormone therapy). Products include:
Analpram-HC ... 1140
Pramosone ... 1141

Hydrocortisone Sodium Phosphate (Corticosteroids are known to interfere with laboratory tests performed in patients on thryoid hormone therapy).
No products indexed under this heading.

Hydrocortisone Sodium Succinate (Corticosteroids are known to interfere with laboratory tests performed in patients on thryoid hormone therapy).
No products indexed under this heading.

Insulin (Initiating thyroid replacement therapy may cause increases in insulin or oral hypoglycemic requirements).
No products indexed under this heading.

Insulin, Human, Zinc Suspension (Initiating thyroid replacement therapy may cause increases in insulin or oral hypoglycemic requirements).
No products indexed under this heading.

Insulin, Human (rDNA origin) (Initiating thyroid replacement therapy may cause increases in insulin or oral hypoglycemic requirements). Products include:
Exubera Inhalation Powder ... 2515

Insulin, Human NPH (Initiating thyroid replacement therapy may cause increases in insulin or oral hypoglycemic requirements). Products include:
Humulin N Vial ... 1846

Insulin, Human Regular (Initiating thyroid replacement therapy may cause increases in insulin or oral hypoglycemic requirements). Products include:
Humulin R ... 1849
Humulin R (U-500) ... 1850

Insulin, Human Regular and Human NPH Mixture (Initiating thyroid replacement therapy may cause increases in insulin or oral hypoglycemic requirements). Products include:
Humulin 50/50, 100 Units ... 1843
Humulin 70/30 Vial ... 1844

Insulin, NPH (Initiating thyroid replacement therapy may cause increases in insulin or oral hypoglycemic requirements).
No products indexed under this heading.

Insulin, Regular (Initiating thyroid replacement therapy may cause increases in insulin or oral hypoglycemic requirements).
No products indexed under this heading.

Insulin, Regular and NPH mixture (Initiating thyroid replacement therapy may cause increases in insulin or oral hypoglycemic requirements).
No products indexed under this heading.

Insulin, Zinc Crystals (Initiating thyroid replacement therapy may cause increases in insulin or oral hypoglycemic requirements).
No products indexed under this heading.

Insulin, Zinc Suspension (Initiating thyroid replacement therapy may cause increases in insulin or oral hypoglycemic requirements).
No products indexed under this heading.

Insulin Aspart (Initiating thyroid replacement therapy may cause increases in insulin or oral hypoglycemic requirements).
No products indexed under this heading.

Insulin Aspart, Human (Initiating thyroid replacement therapy may cause increases in insulin or oral hypoglycemic requirements). Products include:
NovoLog Mix 70/30 ... 2364

Insulin Aspart, Human Regular (Initiating thyroid replacement thera-

py may cause increases in insulin or oral hypoglycemic requirements). Products include:
NovoLog Injection 2359

Insulin Aspart Protamine, Human (Initiating thyroid replacement therapy may cause increases in insulin or oral hypoglycemic requirements). Products include:
NovoLog Mix 70/30 2364

Insulin Detemir (rDNA Origin) (Initiating thyroid replacement therapy may cause increases in insulin or oral hypoglycemic requirements). Products include:
Levemir Injection 2352

Insulin glargine (Initiating thyroid replacement therapy may cause increases in insulin or oral hypoglycemic requirements). Products include:
Lantus Injection 2749

Insulin Glulisine (Initiating thyroid replacement therapy may cause increases in insulin or oral hypoglycemic requirements). Products include:
Apidra Injection 2706

Insulin Lispro, Human (Initiating thyroid replacement therapy may cause increases in insulin or oral hypoglycemic requirements). Products include:
Humalog-Pen and KwikPen 1829
Humalog Mix 50/50-Pen and KwikPen 1833
Humalog Mix 75/25-Pen and KwikPen 1835

Insulin Lispro Protamine, Human (Initiating thyroid replacement therapy may cause increases in insulin or oral hypoglycemic requirements). Products include:
Humalog Mix 50/50-Pen and KwikPen 1833
Humalog Mix 75/25-Pen and KwikPen 1835

Iodine Preparations (Iodine-containing preparations are known to interfere with laboratory tests performed in patients on thyroid hormone therapy).
No products indexed under this heading.

Levonorgestrel (Patients without a functioning thyroid gland who are on thyroid replacemet therapy may need to increase their thyroid dose if estrogens containing oral contraceptives are given. Estrogens containing oral contraceptives are also known to interfere with laboratory tests performed in patients on thyroid hormone therapy). Products include:
Climara Pro Transdermal System 768
Lybrel Tablets 3204
Mirena Intrauterine System 779
Plan B Tablets 1044
Seasonique Tablets 1046

Magnesium Salicylate (Preparations containing salicylates are known to interfere with laboratory tests performed in patients on thyroid hormone therapy).
No products indexed under this heading.

Mestranol (Patients without a functioning thyroid gland who are on thyroid replacemet therapy may need to increase their thyroid dose if estrogens containing oral contraceptives are given. Estrogens containing oral contraceptives are also known to interfere with laboratory tests performed in patients on thyroid hormone therapy).
No products indexed under this heading.

Metformin Hydrochloride (Initiating thyroid replacement therapy may cause increases in insulin or oral hypoglycemic requirements). Products include:
ActoPlus Met Tablets 3071
Avandamet Tablets 1336
Janumet Tablets 2041
PrandiMet Tablets 2967

Methylprednisolone Acetate (Corticosteroids are known to interfere with laboratory tests performed in patients on thyroid hormone therapy).
No products indexed under this heading.

Methylprednisolone Sodium Succinate (Corticosteroids are known to interfere with laboratory tests performed in patients on thyroid hormone therapy).
No products indexed under this heading.

Methyltestosterone (Androgens are known to interfere with laboratory tests performed in patients on thyroid hormone therapy). Products include:
Estratest Tablets 3043
Estratest H.S. Tablets 3043

Miglitol (Initiating thyroid replacement therapy may cause increases in insulin or oral hypoglycemic requirements).
No products indexed under this heading.

Mometasone Furoate (Corticosteroids are known to interfere with laboratory tests performed in patients on thyroid hormone therapy). Products include:
Asmanex Twisthaler 2797
Elocon Cream 0.1% 2840
Elocon Lotion 0.1% 2841
Elocon Ointment 0.1% 2842

Mometasone Furoate Monohydrate (Corticosteroids are known to interfere with laboratory tests performed in patients on thyroid hormone therapy). Products include:
Nasonex Nasal Spray 2883

Nateglinide (Initiating thyroid replacement therapy may cause increases in insulin or oral hypoglycemic requirements). Products include:
Starlix Tablets 2314

Norethindrone (Patients without a functioning thyroid gland who are on thyroid replacemet therapy may need to increase their thyroid dose if estrogens containing oral contraceptives are given. Estrogens containing oral contraceptives are also known to interfere with laboratory tests performed in patients on thyroid hormone therapy). Products include:
Ortho Micronor Tablets 2446

Norethynodrel (Patients without a functioning thyroid gland who are on thyroid replacemet therapy may need to increase their thyroid dose if estrogens containing oral contraceptives are given. Estrogens containing oral contraceptives are also known to interfere with laboratory tests performed in patients on thyroid hormone therapy).
No products indexed under this heading.

Norgestimate (Patients without a functioning thyroid gland who are on thyroid replacemet therapy may need to increase their thyroid dose if estrogens containing oral contraceptives are given. Estrogens containing oral contraceptives are also known to interfere with laboratory tests performed in patients on thyroid hormone therapy). Products include:
Ortho-Cyclen/Ortho Tri-Cyclen 2449
Ortho Tri-Cyclen Lo Tablets 2458

Norgestrel (Patients without a functioning thyroid gland who are on thyroid replacemet therapy may need to increase their thyroid dose if estrogens containing oral contraceptives are given. Estrogens containing oral contraceptives are also known to interfere with laboratory tests performed in patients on thyroid hormone therapy).
No products indexed under this heading.

Oxandrolone (Androgens are known to interfere with laboratory tests performed in patients on thyroid hormone therapy).
No products indexed under this heading.

Oxymetholone (Androgens are known to interfere with laboratory tests performed in patients on thyroid hormone therapy).
No products indexed under this heading.

Pioglitazone Hydrochloride (Initiating thyroid replacement therapy may cause increases in insulin or oral hypoglycemic requirements). Products include:
ActoPlus Met Tablets 3071
Actos Tablets 3077
Duetact Tablets 3085

Polyestradiol Phosphate (Patients without a functioning thyroid gland who are on thyroid replacemet therapy may need to increase their thyroid dose if estrogens are given. Estrogens are also known to interfere with laboratory tests performed in patients on thyroid hormone therapy).
No products indexed under this heading.

Prednisolone Acetate (Corticosteroids are known to interfere with laboratory tests performed in patients on thyroid hormone therapy). Products include:
Pred Forte Ophthalmic Suspension .... ⊙ 227
Pred Mild Ophthalmic Suspension .... ⊙ 230
Pred-G Ophthalmic Ointment .... ⊙ 229
Pred-G Ophthalmic Suspension .... ⊙ 228

Prednisolone Sodium Phosphate (Corticosteroids are known to interfere with laboratory tests performed in patients on thryoid hormone therapy).
No products indexed under this heading.

Prednisolone Tebutate (Corticosteroids are known to interfere with laboratory tests performed in patients on thryoid hormone therapy).
No products indexed under this heading.

Prednisone (Corticosteroids are known to interfere with laboratory tests performed in patients on thyroid hormone therapy).
No products indexed under this heading.

Quinestrol (Patients without a functioning thyroid gland who are on thyroid replacemet therapy may need to increase their thyroid dose if estrogens are given. Estrogens are also known to interfere with laboratory tests performed in patients on thyroid hormone therapy).
No products indexed under this heading.

Repaglinide (Initiating thyroid replacement therapy may cause increases in insulin or oral hypoglycemic requirements). Products include:
PrandiMet Tablets 2967
Prandin Tablets 2971

Rosiglitazone Maleate (Initiating thyroid replacement therapy may cause increases in insulin or oral hypoglycemic requirements). Products include:
Avandamet Tablets 1336
Avandaryl Tablets 1344
Avandia Tablets 1351

Salsalate (Preparations containing salicylates are known to interfere with laboratory tests performed in patients on thyroid hormone therapy).
No products indexed under this heading.

Sitagliptin Phosphate (Initiating thyroid replacement therapy may cause increases in insulin or oral hypoglycemic requirements). Products include:
Janumet Tablets 2041
Januvia Tablets 2048

Stanozolol (Androgens are known to interfere with laboratory tests performed in patients on thyroid hormone therapy).
No products indexed under this heading.

Tolazamide (Initiating thyroid replacement therapy may cause increases in insulin or oral hypoglycemic requirements).
No products indexed under this heading.

Tolbutamide (Initiating thyroid replacement therapy may cause increases in insulin or oral hypoglycemic requirements).
No products indexed under this heading.

Triamcinolone (Corticosteroids are known to interfere with laboratory tests performed in patients on thyroid hormone therapy).
No products indexed under this heading.

Triamcinolone Acetonide (Corticosteroids are known to interfere with laboratory tests performed in patients on thyroid hormone therapy). Products include:
Azmacort Inhalation Aerosol 407
Nasacort AQ Nasal Spray 2765
Triesence Injectable Suspension .... ⊙ 209

Triamcinolone Diacetate (Corticosteroids are known to interfere with laboratory tests performed in patients on thyroid hormone therapy).
No products indexed under this heading.

Triamcinolone Hexacetonide (Corticosteroids are known to interfere with laboratory tests performed in patients on thyroid hormone therapy).
No products indexed under this heading.

Troglitazone (Initiating thyroid replacement therapy may cause increases in insulin or oral hypoglycemic requirements).
No products indexed under this heading.

Warfarin Sodium (Thyroid hormones appear to increase catabolism of vitamin K-dependent clotting factors. If oral anticoagulants are also being given, compensatory increases in clotting factor synthesis are impaired).
No products indexed under this heading.

NEMBUTAL SODIUM SOLUTION, USP

(Pentobarbital Sodium) **2494**

May interact with central nervous system depressants, corticosteroids, oral anticoagulants, doxycycline, estrogens, monoamine oxidase inhibitors, oral contraceptives, phenytoin, and certain other agents. Compounds in these categories include:

Alfentanil Hydrochloride (Concomitant use of other CNS depressants may produce additive depressant effects).
No products indexed under this heading.

Alprazolam (Concomitant use of other CNS depressants may produce additive depressant effects).
No products indexed under this heading.

Anisindione (Barbiturates can induce hepatic microsomal enzymes resulting in increased metabolism and decreased anticoagulant response of oral anticoagulants).
No products indexed under this heading.

Aprobarbital (Concomitant use of other CNS depressants may produce additive depressant effects).
No products indexed under this heading.

Betamethasone Acetate (Barbiturates appear to enhance the metabolism of exogenous corticosteroids probably through the induction of hepatic microsomal enzymes).
No products indexed under this heading.

Betamethasone Sodium Phosphate (Barbiturates appear to enhance the metabolism of exogenous corticosteroids probably through the induction of hepatic microsomal enzymes).
No products indexed under this heading.

Budesonide (Barbiturates appear to enhance the metabolism of exogenous corticosteroids probably through the induction of hepatic microsomal enzymes). Products include:
Pulmicort Flexhaler **654**
Symbicort 80/4.5 Inhalation Aerosol.. **659**
Symbicort 160/4.5 Inhalation Aerosol.. **659**

Buprenorphine Hydrochloride (Concomitant use of other CNS depressants may produce additive depressant effects). Products include:
Suboxone Tablets **2601**
Subutex Tablets **2601**

Buspirone Hydrochloride (Concomitant use of other CNS depressants may produce additive depressant effects).
No products indexed under this heading.

Butabarbital (Concomitant use of other CNS depressants may produce additive depressant effects).
No products indexed under this heading.

Butalbital (Concomitant use of other CNS depressants may produce additive depressant effects).
No products indexed under this heading.

Chlordiazepoxide (Concomitant use of other CNS depressants may produce additive depressant effects).
No products indexed under this heading.

Chlordiazepoxide Hydrochloride (Concomitant use of other CNS depressants may produce additive depressant effects).
No products indexed under this heading.

Chlorotrianisene (Pretreatment with or co-administration of phenobarbital may decrease the effect of estrogen by increasing its metabolism; application of this data to other barbiturates appears valid).
No products indexed under this heading.

Chlorpromazine (Concomitant use of other CNS depressants may produce additive depressant effects).
No products indexed under this heading.

Chlorpromazine Hydrochloride (Concomitant use of other CNS depressants may produce additive depressant effects).
No products indexed under this heading.

Chlorprothixene (Concomitant use of other CNS depressants may produce additive depressant effects).
No products indexed under this heading.

Chlorprothixene Hydrochloride (Concomitant use of other CNS depressants may produce additive depressant effects).
No products indexed under this heading.

Chlorprothixene Lactate (Concomitant use of other CNS depressants may produce additive depressant effects).
No products indexed under this heading.

Ciclesonide (Barbiturates appear to enhance the metabolism of exogenous corticosteroids probably through the induction of hepatic microsomal enzymes). Products include:
Alvesco Inhalation Aerosol **2985**
Omnaris Nasal Spray **2998**

Clorazepate Dipotassium (Concomitant use of other CNS depressants may produce additive depressant effects).
No products indexed under this heading.

Clozapine (Concomitant use of other CNS depressants may produce additive depressant effects).
No products indexed under this heading.

Codeine Phosphate (Concomitant use of other CNS depressants may produce additive depressant effects). Products include:
Tylenol with Codeine Tablets **2427**

Cortisone Acetate (Barbiturates appear to enhance the metabolism of exogenous corticosteroids probably through the induction of hepatic microsomal enzymes).
No products indexed under this heading.

Desflurane (Concomitant use of other CNS depressants may produce additive depressant effects).
No products indexed under this heading.

Desogestrel (Pretreatment with or co-administration of phenobarbital may decrease the effect of estrogen by increasing its metabolism; application of this data to other barbiturates appears valid; higher incidence of pregnancy in patients on co-administration). Products include:
Mircette Tablets **1034**

Dexamethasone (Barbiturates appear to enhance the metabolism of exogenous corticosteroids probably through the induction of hepatic microsomal enzymes). Products include:
Ciprodex Otic Suspension **541**

Dexamethasone Acetate (Barbiturates appear to enhance the metabolism of exogenous corticosteroids probably through the induction of hepatic microsomal enzymes).
No products indexed under this heading.

Dexamethasone Sodium Phosphate (Barbiturates appear to enhance the metabolism of exogenous corticosteroids probably through the induction of hepatic microsomal enzymes).
No products indexed under this heading.

Dezocine (Concomitant use of other CNS depressants may produce additive depressant effects).
No products indexed under this heading.

Diazepam (Concomitant use of other CNS depressants may produce additive depressant effects). Products include:
Valium Tablets **2658**

Dicumarol (Barbiturates can induce hepatic microsomal enzymes resulting in increased metabolism and decreased anticoagulant response of oral anticoagulants).
No products indexed under this heading.

Dienestrol (Pretreatment with or co-administration of phenobarbital may decrease the effect of estrogen by increasing its metabolism; application of this data to other barbiturates appears valid).
No products indexed under this heading.

Diethylstilbestrol (Pretreatment with or co-administration of phenobarbital may decrease the effect of estrogen by increasing its metabolism; application of this data to other barbiturates appears valid).
No products indexed under this heading.

Divalproex Sodium (Valproate appears to decrease barbiturate metabolism). Products include:
Depakote ER Tablets **423**

Doxycycline Calcium (Phenobarbital has been shown to shorten the half-life of doxycycline for as long as 2 weeks after barbiturate therapy is discontinued; application of this data to other barbiturates appears valid).
No products indexed under this heading.

Doxycycline Hyclate (Phenobarbital has been shown to shorten the half-life of doxycycline for as long as 2 weeks after barbiturate therapy is discontinued; application of this data to other barbiturates appears valid).
No products indexed under this heading.

Doxycycline Monohydrate (Phenobarbital has been shown to shorten the half-life of doxycycline for as long as 2 weeks after barbiturate therapy is discontinued; application of this data to other barbiturates appears valid).
No products indexed under this heading.

Droperidol (Concomitant use of other CNS depressants may produce additive depressant effects).
No products indexed under this heading.

Enflurane (Concomitant use of other CNS depressants may produce additive depressant effects).
No products indexed under this heading.

Estazolam (Concomitant use of other CNS depressants may produce additive depressant effects).
No products indexed under this heading.

Estradiol (Pretreatment with or co-administration of phenobarbital may decrease the effect of estrogen by increasing its metabolism; application of this data to other barbiturates appears valid). Products include:
Activella Tablets **2347**
Angeliq Tablets **751**
Climara Transdermal System **763**
Climara Pro Transdermal System **768**
Divigel **3167**
Vagifem Tablets **2375**

Estrogens, Conjugated (Pretreatment with or co-administration of phenobarbital may decrease the effect of estrogen by increasing its metabolism; application of this data to other barbiturates appears valid). Products include:
Premarin Intravenous **3217**
Premarin Tablets **3221**
Premarin Vaginal Cream **3228**
Premphase Tablets **3232**
Prempro Tablets **3232**

Estrogens, Esterified (Pretreatment with or co-administration of phenobarbital may decrease the effect of estrogen by increasing its metabolism; application of this data to other barbiturates appears valid). Products include:
Estratest Tablets **3043**
Estratest H.S. Tablets **3043**

Estropipate (Pretreatment with or co-administration of phenobarbital may decrease the effect of estrogen by increasing its metabolism; application of this data to other barbiturates appears valid).
No products indexed under this heading.

Ethanol (Concomitant use of other CNS depressants may produce additive depressant effects).
No products indexed under this heading.

Ethchlorvynol (Concomitant use of other CNS depressants may produce additive depressant effects).
No products indexed under this heading.

Ethinamate (Concomitant use of other CNS depressants may produce additive depressant effects).
No products indexed under this heading.

Ethinyl Estradiol (Pretreatment with or co-administration of phenobarbital may decrease the effect of estrogen by increasing its metabolism; application of this data to other barbiturates appears valid; higher incidence of pregnancy in patients on co-administration). Products include:
Lybrel Tablets ... 3204
Mircette Tablets ... 1034
NuvaRing ... 2897
Ortho-Cyclen/Ortho Tri-Cyclen ... 2449
Ortho Evra Transdermal System ... 2437
Ortho Tri-Cyclen Lo Tablets ... 2458
Seasonique Tablets ... 1046
Yaz Tablets ... 805

Ethyl Alcohol (Concomitant use of other CNS depressants may produce additive depressant effects).
No products indexed under this heading.

Ethynodiol Diacetate (Pretreatment with or co-administration of phenobarbital may decrease the effect of estrogen by increasing its metabolism; application of this data to other barbiturates appears valid; higher incidence of pregnancy in patients on co-administration).
No products indexed under this heading.

Fentanyl (Concomitant use of other CNS depressants may produce additive depressant effects). Products include:
Duragesic Transdermal System ... 2405
Ionsys Transdermal System ... 2410

Fentanyl Citrate (Concomitant use of other CNS depressants may produce additive depressant effects). Products include:
Actiq ... 959
Fentora Tablets ... 968

Fludrocortisone Acetate (Barbiturates appear to enhance the metabolism of exogenous corticosteroids probably through the induction of hepatic microsomal enzymes).
No products indexed under this heading.

Flunisolide (Barbiturates appear to enhance the metabolism of exogenous corticosteroids probably through the induction of hepatic microsomal enzymes). Products include:
Aerobid/Aerobid-M ... 1153

Fluphenazine Decanoate (Concomitant use of other CNS depressants may produce additive depressant effects).
No products indexed under this heading.

Fluphenazine Enanthate (Concomitant use of other CNS depressants may produce additive depressant effects).
No products indexed under this heading.

Fluphenazine Hydrochloride (Concomitant use of other CNS depressants may produce additive depressant effects).
No products indexed under this heading.

Flurazepam Hydrochloride (Concomitant use of other CNS depressants may produce additive depressant effects).
No products indexed under this heading.

Fluticasone Propionate (Barbiturates appear to enhance the metabolism of exogenous corticosteroids probably through the induction of hepatic microsomal enzymes). Products include:
Advair Diskus 100/50 ... 1276
Advair Diskus 250/50 ... 1276
Advair Diskus 500/50 ... 1276
Advair HFA 45/21 Inhalation Aerosol ... 1288
Advair HFA 115/21 Inhalation Aerosol ... 1288
Advair HFA 230/21 Inhalation Aerosol ... 1288
Flonase Nasal Spray ... 1431
Flovent Diskus 50 mcg ... 1435

Fluticasone Propionate HFA (Barbiturates appear to enhance the metabolism of exogenous corticosteroids probably through the induction of hepatic microsomal enzymes). Products include:
Flovent HFA ... 1440

Fosphenytoin Sodium (The effect of barbiturates on the metabolism of phenytoin appears to be variable).
No products indexed under this heading.

Furazolidone (Co-administration with MAO inhibitors prolongs the effects of barbiturates probably because the metabolism of the barbiturate is inhibited).
No products indexed under this heading.

Glutethimide (Concomitant use of other CNS depressants may produce additive depressant effects).
No products indexed under this heading.

Griseofulvin (Phenobarbital appears to interfere with the absorption of orally administered griseofulvin, thus decreasing its blood level; application of this data to other barbiturates appears valid). Products include:
Gris-PEG Tablets ... 2507

Haloperidol (Concomitant use of other CNS depressants may produce additive depressant effects).
No products indexed under this heading.

Haloperidol Decanoate (Concomitant use of other CNS depressants may produce additive depressant effects).
No products indexed under this heading.

Hydrocodone Bitartrate (Concomitant use of other CNS depressants may produce additive depressant effects). Products include:
Lortab 5/500 Tablets ... 3143
Lortab 7.5/500 Tablets ... 3144
Lortab 10/500 Tablets ... 3144
Vicodin Tablets ... 529
Vicodin ES Tablets ... 530
Vicodin HP Tablets ... 531
Vicoprofen Tablets ... 533
Zydone Tablets ... 1132

Hydrocodone Polistirex (Concomitant use of other CNS depressants may produce additive depressant effects). Products include:
Tussionex Pennkinetic Extended-Release Suspension ... 3154

Hydrocortisone (Barbiturates appear to enhance the metabolism of exogenous corticosteroids probably through the induction of hepatic microsomal enzymes).
No products indexed under this heading.

Hydrocortisone Acetate (Barbiturates appear to enhance the metabolism of exogenous corticosteroids probably through the induction of hepatic microsomal enzymes). Products include:
Analpram-HC ... 1140
Pramosone ... 1141

Hydrocortisone Sodium Phosphate (Barbiturates appear to enhance the metabolism of exogenous corticosteroids probably through the induction of hepatic microsomal enzymes).
No products indexed under this heading.

Hydrocortisone Sodium Succinate (Barbiturates appear to enhance the metabolism of exogenous corticosteroids probably through the induction of hepatic microsomal enzymes).
No products indexed under this heading.

Hydromorphone Hydrochloride (Concomitant use of other CNS depressants may produce additive depressant effects).
No products indexed under this heading.

Hydroxyzine Hydrochloride (Concomitant use of other CNS depressants may produce additive depressant effects).
No products indexed under this heading.

Isocarboxazid (Co-administration with MAO inhibitors prolongs the effects of barbiturates probably because the metabolism of the barbiturate is inhibited). Products include:
Marplan Tablets ... 3177

Isoflurane (Concomitant use of other CNS depressants may produce additive depressant effects).
No products indexed under this heading.

Ketamine Hydrochloride (Concomitant use of other CNS depressants may produce additive depressant effects).
No products indexed under this heading.

Levomethadyl Acetate Hydrochloride (Concomitant use of other CNS depressants may produce additive depressant effects).
No products indexed under this heading.

Levonorgestrel (Pretreatment with or co-administration of phenobarbital may decrease the effect of estrogen by increasing its metabolism; application of this data to other barbiturates appears valid; higher incidence of pregnancy in patients on co-administration). Products include:
Climara Pro Transdermal System ... 768
Lybrel Tablets ... 3204
Mirena Intrauterine System ... 779
Plan B Tablets ... 1044
Seasonique Tablets ... 1046

Levorphanol Tartrate (Concomitant use of other CNS depressants may produce additive depressant effects).
No products indexed under this heading.

Lorazepam (Concomitant use of other CNS depressants may produce additive depressant effects).
No products indexed under this heading.

Loxapine Hydrochloride (Concomitant use of other CNS depressants may produce additive depressant effects).
No products indexed under this heading.

Loxapine Succinate (Concomitant use of other CNS depressants may produce additive depressant effects).
No products indexed under this heading.

Meperidine Hydrochloride (Concomitant use of other CNS depressants may produce additive depressant effects).
No products indexed under this heading.

Mephobarbital (Concomitant use of other CNS depressants may produce additive depressant effects).
No products indexed under this heading.

Meprobamate (Concomitant use of other CNS depressants may produce additive depressant effects).
No products indexed under this heading.

Mesoridazine Besylate (Concomitant use of other CNS depressants may produce additive depressant effects).
No products indexed under this heading.

Mestranol (Pretreatment with or co-administration of phenobarbital may decrease the effect of estrogen by increasing its metabolism; application of this data to other barbiturates appears valid; higher incidence of pregnancy in patients on co-administration).
No products indexed under this heading.

Methadone Hydrochloride (Concomitant use of other CNS depressants may produce additive depressant effects).
No products indexed under this heading.

Methohexital Sodium (Concomitant use of other CNS depressants may produce additive depressant effects).
No products indexed under this heading.

Methotrimeprazine (Concomitant use of other CNS depressants may produce additive depressant effects).
No products indexed under this heading.

Methoxyflurane (Concomitant use of other CNS depressants may produce additive depressant effects).
No products indexed under this heading.

Methylprednisolone Acetate (Barbiturates appear to enhance the metabolism of exogenous corticosteroids probably through the induction of hepatic microsomal enzymes).
No products indexed under this heading.

Methylprednisolone Sodium Succinate (Barbiturates appear to enhance the metabolism of exogenous corticosteroids probably through the induction of hepatic microsomal enzymes).
No products indexed under this heading.

Midazolam Hydrochloride (Concomitant use of other CNS depressants may produce additive depressant effects).
No products indexed under this heading.

Moclobemide (Co-administration with MAO inhibitors prolongs the effects of barbiturates probably because the metabolism of the barbiturate is inhibited).
No products indexed under this heading.

Molindone Hydrochloride (Concomitant use of other CNS depressants may produce additive depressant effects). Products include:
Moban Tablets **1116**

Mometasone Furoate (Barbiturates appear to enhance the metabolism of exogenous corticosteroids probably through the induction of hepatic microsomal enzymes).
Products include:
Asmanex Twisthaler **2797**
Elocon Cream 0.1% **2840**
Elocon Lotion 0.1% **2841**
Elocon Ointment 0.1% **2842**

Mometasone Furoate Monohydrate (Barbiturates appear to enhance the metabolism of exogenous corticosteroids probably through the induction of hepatic microsomal enzymes). Products include:
Nasonex Nasal Spray **2883**

Morphine Sulfate (Concomitant use of other CNS depressants may produce additive depressant effects). Products include:
Avinza Capsules **1772**
DepoDur Injection **1095**
MS Contin Tablets **2585**

Norethindrone (Pretreatment with or co-administration of phenobarbital may decrease the effect of estrogen by increasing its metabolism; application of this data to other barbiturates appears valid; higher incidence of pregnancy in patients on co-administration). Products include:
Ortho Micronor Tablets **2446**

Norethynodrel (Pretreatment with or co-administration of phenobarbital may decrease the effect of estrogen by increasing its metabolism; application of this data to other barbiturates appears valid; higher incidence of pregnancy in patients on co-administration).
No products indexed under this heading.

Norgestimate (Pretreatment with or co-administration of phenobarbital may decrease the effect of estrogen by increasing its metabolism; application of this data to other barbiturates appears valid; higher incidence of pregnancy in patients on co-administration). Products include:
Ortho-Cyclen/Ortho Tri-Cyclen **2449**
Ortho Tri-Cyclen Lo Tablets **2458**

Norgestrel (Pretreatment with or co-administration of phenobarbital may decrease the effect of estrogen by increasing its metabolism; application of this data to other barbiturates appears valid; higher incidence of pregnancy in patients on co-administration).
No products indexed under this heading.

Olanzapine (Concomitant use of other CNS depressants may produce additive depressant effects). Products include:
Symbyax Capsules **1871**
Zyprexa Tablets **1883**
Zyprexa IntraMuscular **1883**
Zyprexa ZYDIS Orally Disintegrating Tablets **1883**

Oxazepam (Concomitant use of other CNS depressants may produce additive depressant effects).
No products indexed under this heading.

Oxycodone Hydrochloride (Concomitant use of other CNS depressants may produce additive depressant effects). Products include:
OxyContin Tablets **2589**
OxyIR Capsules **2593**
Percocet Tablets **1127**
Percodan Tablets **1130**

Pargyline Hydrochloride (Co-administration with MAO inhibitors prolongs the effects of barbiturates probably because the metabolism of the barbiturate is inhibited).
No products indexed under this heading.

Perphenazine (Concomitant use of other CNS depressants may produce additive depressant effects).
No products indexed under this heading.

Phenelzine Sulfate (Co-administration with MAO inhibitors prolongs the effects of barbiturates probably because the metabolism of the barbiturate is inhibited).
No products indexed under this heading.

Phenobarbital (Concomitant use of other CNS depressants may produce additive depressant effects). Products include:
Donnatal Extentabs **2507**

Phenytoin (The effect of barbiturates on the metabolism of phenytoin appears to be variable).
No products indexed under this heading.

Phenytoin Sodium (The effect of barbiturates on the metabolism of phenytoin appears to be variable). Products include:
Phenytek Capsules **2192**

Polyestradiol Phosphate (Pretreatment with or co-administration of phenobarbital may decrease the effect of estrogen by increasing its metabolism; application of this data to other barbiturates appears valid).
No products indexed under this heading.

Prazepam (Concomitant use of other CNS depressants may produce additive depressant effects).
No products indexed under this heading.

Prednisolone Acetate (Barbiturates appear to enhance the metabolism of exogenous corticosteroids probably through the induction of hepatic microsomal enzymes). Products include:
Pred Forte Ophthalmic Suspension .... ⊙ **227**
Pred Mild Ophthalmic Suspension .... ⊙ **230**
Pred-G Ophthalmic Ointment .... ⊙ **229**
Pred-G Ophthalmic Suspension .... ⊙ **228**

Prednisolone Sodium Phosphate (Barbiturates appear to enhance the metabolism of exogenous corticosteroids probably through the induction of hepatic microsomal enzymes).
No products indexed under this heading.

Prednisolone Tebutate (Barbiturates appear to enhance the metabolism of exogenous corticosteroids probably through the induction of hepatic microsomal enzymes).
No products indexed under this heading.

Prednisone (Barbiturates appear to enhance the metabolism of exogenous corticosteroids probably through the induction of hepatic microsomal enzymes).
No products indexed under this heading.

Procarbazine Hydrochloride (Co-administration with MAO inhibitors prolongs the effects of barbiturates probably because the metabolism of the barbiturate is inhibited).
No products indexed under this heading.

Prochlorperazine (Concomitant use of other CNS depressants may produce additive depressant effects).
No products indexed under this heading.

Promethazine Hydrochloride (Concomitant use of other CNS depressants may produce additive depressant effects).
No products indexed under this heading.

Propofol (Concomitant use of other CNS depressants may produce additive depressant effects).
No products indexed under this heading.

Propoxyphene Hydrochloride (Concomitant use of other CNS depressants may produce additive depressant effects).
No products indexed under this heading.

Propoxyphene Napsylate (Concomitant use of other CNS depressants may produce additive depressant effects).
No products indexed under this heading.

Quazepam (Concomitant use of other CNS depressants may produce additive depressant effects).
No products indexed under this heading.

Quetiapine Fumarate (Concomitant use of other CNS depressants may produce additive depressant effects).
No products indexed under this heading.

Quinestrol (Pretreatment with or co-administration of phenobarbital may decrease the effect of estrogen by increasing its metabolism; application of this data to other barbiturates appears valid).
No products indexed under this heading.

Rasagiline Mesylate (Co-administration with MAO inhibitors prolongs the effects of barbiturates probably because the metabolism of the barbiturate is inhibited). Products include:
Azilect Tablets **3106**

Remifentanil Hydrochloride (Concomitant use of other CNS depressants may produce additive depressant effects).
No products indexed under this heading.

Risperidone (Concomitant use of other CNS depressants may produce additive depressant effects). Products include:
Risperdal Consta Long-Acting Injection **1753**

Secobarbital Sodium (Concomitant use of other CNS depressants may produce additive depressant effects).
No products indexed under this heading.

Selegiline (Co-administration with MAO inhibitors prolongs the effects of barbiturates probably because the metabolism of the barbiturate is inhibited). Products include:
Emsam Transdermal System **905**

Selegiline Hydrochloride (Co-administration with MAO inhibitors prolongs the effects of barbiturates probably because the metabolism of the barbiturate is inhibited). Products include:
Eldepryl Capsules **3052**

Sevoflurane (Concomitant use of other CNS depressants may produce additive depressant effects). Products include:
Ultane Liquid for Inhalation **524**

Sufentanil Citrate (Concomitant use of other CNS depressants may produce additive depressant effects).
No products indexed under this heading.

Temazepam (Concomitant use of other CNS depressants may produce additive depressant effects).
No products indexed under this heading.

Thiamylal Sodium (Concomitant use of other CNS depressants may produce additive depressant effects).
No products indexed under this heading.

Thioridazine Hydrochloride (Concomitant use of other CNS depressants may produce additive depressant effects). Products include:
Thioridazine Hydrochloride Tablets **2195**

Thiothixene (Concomitant use of other CNS depressants may produce additive depressant effects). Products include:
Thiothixene Capsules **2197**

Tranylcypromine Sulfate (Co-administration with MAO inhibitors prolongs the effects of barbiturates probably because the metabolism of the barbiturate is inhibited). Products include:
Parnate Tablets **1532**

Triamcinolone (Barbiturates appear to enhance the metabolism of exogenous corticosteroids probably through the induction of hepatic microsomal enzymes).
No products indexed under this heading.

Triamcinolone Acetonide (Barbiturates appear to enhance the metabolism of exogenous corticosteroids probably through the induction of hepatic microsomal enzymes). Products include:

Azmacort Inhalation Aerosol 407
Nasacort AQ Nasal Spray 2765
Triesence Injectable Suspension .... ⊙209

Triamcinolone Diacetate (Barbiturates appear to enhance the metabolism of exogenous corticosteroids probably through the induction of hepatic microsomal enzymes).

No products indexed under this heading.

Triamcinolone Hexacetonide (Barbiturates appear to enhance the metabolism of exogenous corticosteroids probably through the induction of hepatic microsomal enzymes).

No products indexed under this heading.

Triazolam (Concomitant use of other CNS depressants may produce additive depressant effects).

No products indexed under this heading.

Trifluoperazine Hydrochloride (Concomitant use of other CNS depressants may produce additive depressant effects).

No products indexed under this heading.

Valproate Sodium (Valproate appears to decrease barbiturate metabolism).

No products indexed under this heading.

Valproic Acid (Appears to decrease barbiturate metabolism).

No products indexed under this heading.

Warfarin Sodium (Barbiturates can induce hepatic microsomal enzymes resulting in increased metabolism and decreased anticoagulant response of oral anticoagulants).

No products indexed under this heading.

Zaleplon (Concomitant use of other CNS depressants may produce additive depressant effects).

No products indexed under this heading.

Ziprasidone Hydrochloride (Concomitant use of other CNS depressants may produce additive depressant effects). Products include:

Geodon Capsules 2520

Zolpidem Tartrate (Concomitant use of other CNS depressants may produce additive depressant effects). Products include:

Ambien Tablets 2692
Ambien CR Tablets 2696

Food Interactions

Alcohol (Concomitant use of other CNS depressants may produce additive depressant effects. Alcohol should not be consumed while taking barbiturates).

NEOPROFEN INJECTION

(Ibuprofen Lysine) 2496
None cited in PDR database.

NEORAL ORAL SOLUTION

(Cyclosporine) 2280
See Neoral Soft Gelatin Capsules

NEORAL SOFT GELATIN CAPSULES

(Cyclosporine) 2280
May interact with ACE inhibitors, angiotensin-II receptor antagonists, erythromycin, fibrates, HMG-CoA reductase inhibitors, non-steroidal anti-inflammatory agents, oral contraceptives, phenytoin, potassium preparations, protease inhibitors, potassium sparing diuretics, vaccines, live, and certain other agents. Compounds in these categories include:

Allopurinol (Increases cyclosporine concentrations).

No products indexed under this heading.

Amiloride Hydrochloride (Cyclosporine may cause hyperkalemia; concurrent use should be avoided).

No products indexed under this heading.

Amiodarone Hydrochloride (Increases cyclosporine concentrations).

No products indexed under this heading.

Amphotericin B (May potentiate renal dysfunction).

No products indexed under this heading.

Amprenavir (The HIV protease inhibitors are known to inhibit cytochrome P450IIIA and increase the concentration of drugs metabolized by this enzyme system; agents that inhibit this enzyme could decrease metabolism and increase cyclosporine concentrations; this interaction has not been studied; however, care should be exercised).

No products indexed under this heading.

Atorvastatin Calcium (Co-administration may result in myotoxicity; atorvastatin dosage should be reduced according to label recommendations. Atorvastatin needs to be temporarily withheld or discontinued in patients with signs and symptoms of myopathy or those with risk factors predisposing to severe renal injury secondary to rhabdomyolysis). Products include:

Lipitor Tablets 2501

Azapropazon (May potentiate renal dysfunction).

No products indexed under this heading.

Azathioprine (May potentiate renal dysfunction).

No products indexed under this heading.

Azithromycin (Concomitant azithromycin may increase cyclosporine concentrations). Products include:

AzaSite Ophthalmic Drops 1740

BCG Vaccine (The use of live vaccines should be avoided).

No products indexed under this heading.

Benazepril Hydrochloride (Caution is required when cyclosporine is co-administered with potassium-sparing drugs, such as angiotensin-converting enzyme inhibitors).

No products indexed under this heading.

Bromocriptine Mesylate (Increases cyclosporine concentrations).

No products indexed under this heading.

Candesartan Cilexetil (Caution is required when cyclosporine is co-administered with potassium-sparing drugs, such as angiotensin II receptor antagonists). Products include:

Atacand Tablets 639
Atacand HCT 642

Captopril (Caution is required when cyclosporine is co-administered with potassium-sparing drugs, such as angiotensin-converting enzyme inhibitors). Products include:

Captopril Tablets 2182

Carbamazepine (Decreases cyclosporine concentrations). Products include:

Carbatrol Capsules 3019
Equetro Extended-Release Capsules 3174

Celecoxib (Co-administration with NSAID's particularly in the setting of dehydration, may potentiate renal dysfunction). Products include:

Celebrex Capsules 2979

Cimetidine (May potentiate renal dysfunction).

No products indexed under this heading.

Cimetidine Hydrochloride (May potentiate renal dysfunction).

No products indexed under this heading.

Ciprofloxacin (Concomitant ciprofloxacin may potentiate renal dysfunction). Products include:

Cipro I.V. 2817
Cipro Oral Suspension 2810
Cipro XR Tablets 2823
Ciprodex Otic Suspension 541

Ciprofloxacin Hydrochloride (Concomitant ciprofloxacin may potentiate renal dysfunction). Products include:

Cipro Tablets 2810

Clarithromycin (Concomitant clarithromycin may increase cyclosporine concentrations). Products include:

Biaxin/Biaxin XL 411

Clofibrate (Concomitant fibric acid derivatives may potentiate renal dysfunction).

No products indexed under this heading.

Colchicine (Cyclosporine may reduce the clearance of colchicine and enhance the toxic effects of colchicine, such as myopathy and neuropathy, especially in patients with renal dysfunction. Close clinical observation is required during concurrent therapy to enable early detection of colchicine toxicity, followed by reduction of dosage or its withdrawal).

No products indexed under this heading.

Dalfopristin (Co-administration with substrates that inhibit CYP450 3A, such as dalfopristin, could decrease metabolism and increase cyclosporine concentrations).

No products indexed under this heading.

Danazol (Increases cyclosporine concentrations).

No products indexed under this heading.

Darunavir (The HIV protease inhibitors are known to inhibit cytochrome P450IIIA and increase the concentration of drugs metabolized by this enzyme system; agents that inhibit this enzyme could decrease metabolism and increase cyclosporine concentrations; this interaction has not been studied; however, care should be exercised).

No products indexed under this heading.

Desogestrel (Concomitant oral contraceptives may increase cyclosporine concentrations). Products include:

Mircette Tablets 1034

Diclofenac Epolamine (Co-administration with NSAID's particularly in the setting of dehydration, may potentiate renal dysfunction). Products include:

Flector Patch 561

Diclofenac Potassium (Co-administration has been associated with approximate doubling of diclofenac blood levels and occasional reports of reversible decreases in renal function; possible potentiation of renal dysfunction; the dose of diclofenac should be in the lower end of the therapeutic range).

No products indexed under this heading.

Diclofenac Sodium (Co-administration has been associated with approximate doubling of diclofenac blood levels and occasional reports of reversible decreases in renal function; possible potentiation of renal dysfunction; the dose of diclofenac should be in the lower end of the therapeutic range). Products include:

Diclofenac Sodium Ophthalmic Solution .... ⊙240
Voltaren Ophthalmic Solution 2336
Voltaren Tablets 2334
Voltaren-XR Tablets 2337

Digoxin (Cyclosporine may reduce the clearence of digoxin; severe digitalis toxicity may result. Closed clinical observation is required during concurrent therapy to enable early detection of digitalis toxicity, followed by reduction of dosage or its withdrawal). Products include:

Lanoxin Injection 1498
Lanoxin Injection Pediatric 1502
Lanoxin Tablets 1505

Diltiazem Hydrochloride (Increases cyclosporine concentrations). Products include:

Cardizem LA Extended Release Tablets 421

Enalapril Maleate (Caution is required when cyclosporine is co-administered with potassium-sparing drugs, such as angiotensin-converting enzyme inhibitors).

No products indexed under this heading.

Enalaprilat (Caution is required when cyclosporine is co-administered with potassium-sparing drugs, such as angiotensin-converting enzyme inhibitors).

No products indexed under this heading.

Eprosartan Mesylate (Caution is required when cyclosporine is co-administered with potassium-sparing drugs, such as angiotensin II receptor antagonists). Products include:

Teveten Tablets 515
Teveten HCT Tablets 517

Erythromycin (Co-administration with substrates that inhibit CYP450 3A, such as erythromycin, could decrease metabolism and increase cyclosporine concentrations).
No products indexed under this heading.

Erythromycin Estolate (Co-administration with substrates that inhibit CYP450 3A, such as erythromycin, could decrease metabolism and increase cyclosporine concentrations).
No products indexed under this heading.

Erythromycin Ethylsuccinate (Co-administration with substrates that inhibit CYP450 3A, such as erythromycin, could decrease metabolism and increase cyclosporine concentrations). Products include:
E.E.S. 433
EryPed 431

Erythromycin Gluceptate (Co-administration with substrates that inhibit CYP450 3A, such as erythromycin, could decrease metabolism and increase cyclosporine concentrations).
No products indexed under this heading.

Erythromycin Lactobionate (Co-administration with substrates that inhibit CYP450 3A, such as erythromycin, could decrease metabolism and increase cyclosporine concentrations).
No products indexed under this heading.

Erythromycin Stearate (Co-administration with substrates that inhibit CYP450 3A, such as erythromycin, could decrease metabolism and increase cyclosporine concentrations).
No products indexed under this heading.

Ethinyl Estradiol (Concomitant oral contraceptives may increase cyclosporine concentrations). Products include:
Lybrel Tablets 3204
Mircette Tablets 1034
NuvaRing 2897
Ortho-Cyclen/Ortho Tri-Cyclen 2449
Ortho Evra Transdermal System 2437
Ortho Tri-Cyclen Lo Tablets 2458
Seasonique Tablets 1046
Yaz Tablets 805

Ethynodiol Diacetate (Concomitant oral contraceptives may increase cyclosporine concentrations).
No products indexed under this heading.

Etodolac (Co-administration with NSAID's particularly in the setting of dehydration, may potentiate renal dysfunction).
No products indexed under this heading.

Fenofibrate (Concomitant fibric acid derivatives may potentiate renal dysfunction). Products include:
Fenoglide Tablets 2960
Tricor Tablets 520

Fenoprofen Calcium (Co-administration with NSAID's particularly in the setting of dehydration, may potentiate renal dysfunction). Products include:
Nalfon Capsules 2508

Fluconazole (Increases cyclosporine concentrations).
No products indexed under this heading.

Flurbiprofen (Co-administration with NSAID's particularly in the setting of dehydration, may potentiate renal dysfunction).
No products indexed under this heading.

Fluvastatin Sodium (Co-administration may rarely result in myotoxicity; fluvastatin dosage should be reduced according to label recommendations. Fluvastatin needs to be temporarily withheld or discontinued in patients with signs and symptons of myopathy or those with risk factors predisposing to severe renal injury secondary to rhabdomyolysis). Products include:
Lescol Capsules 2268
Lescol XL Tablets 2268

Fosamprenavir Calcium (The HIV protease inhibitors are known to inhibit cytochrome P450IIIA and increase the concentration of drugs metabolized by this enzyme system; agents that inhibit this enzyme could decrease metabolism and increase cyclosporine concentrations; this interaction has not been studied; however, care should be exercised). Products include:
Lexiva Oral Suspension 1510
Lexiva Tablets 1510

Fosinopril Sodium (Caution is required when cyclosporine is co-administered with potassium-sparing drugs, such as angiotensin-converting enzyme inhibitors).
No products indexed under this heading.

Fosphenytoin Sodium (Concomitant use may decrease cyclosporine drug levels).
No products indexed under this heading.

Gemfibrozil (Concomitant fibric acid derivatives may potentiate renal dysfunction).
No products indexed under this heading.

Gentamicin Sulfate (May potentiate renal dysfunction). Products include:
Pred-G Ophthalmic Ointment .... ⊙ 229
Pred-G Ophthalmic Suspension .... ⊙ 228

Hypericum (Co-administration has been reported to produce a marked reduction in blood cyclosporine concentrations, resulting in subtherapeutic levels, rejection of transplanted organs, and graft loss). Products include:
Satiété Tablets 640

Ibuprofen (Co-administration with NSAID's particularly in the setting of dehydration, may potentiate renal dysfunction). Products include:
Motrin IB Tablets and Caplets 1900
Children's Motrin Oral Suspension ... 1901
Children's Motrin Non-Staining Dye-Free Oral Suspension 1901
Children's Motrin Cold Oral Suspension 1899
Infants' Motrin Concentrated Drops 1901
Infants' Motrin Non-Staining Dye-Free Concentrated Drops 1901
Junior Strength Motrin Caplets and Chewable Tablets 1901
Vicoprofen Tablets 533

Imatinib Mesylate (Concomitant imatinib may increase cyclosporine concentrations). Products include:
Gleevec Tablets 2255

Indinavir Sulfate (The HIV protease inhibitors are known to inhibit cytochrome P450IIIA and increase the concentration of drugs metabolized by this enzyme system; agents that inhibit this enzyme could decrease metabolism and increase cyclosporine concentrations; this interaction has not been studied; however, care should be exercised). Products include:
Crixivan Capsules 1979

Indomethacin (Co-administration with NSAID's particularly in the setting of dehydration, may potentiate renal dysfunction). Products include:
Indocin 2024

Indomethacin Sodium Trihydrate (Co-administration with NSAID's particularly in the setting of dehydration, may potentiate renal dysfunction). Products include:
Indocin I.V. 2489

Influenza Vaccine, Live Attenuated (The use of live vaccines should be avoided).
No products indexed under this heading.

Influenza Virus Vaccine Live, Intranasal (The use of live vaccines should be avoided). Products include:
FluMist Vaccine 1945

Irbesartan (Caution is required when cyclosporine is co-administered with potassium-sparing drugs, such as angiotensin II receptor antagonists). Products include:
Avalide Tablets 892
Avalide Tablets 2713
Avapro Tablets 897
Avapro Tablets 2718

Itraconazole (Increases cyclosporine concentrations).
No products indexed under this heading.

Ketoconazole (May potentiate renal dysfunction; co-administration with substrates that inhibit CYP450 3A, such as ketoconazole, could decrease metabolism and increase cyclosporine concentrations). Products include:
Extina Foam, 2% 3057
Nizoral A-D Shampoo 1901

Ketoprofen (Co-administration with NSAID's particularly in the setting of dehydration, may potentiate renal dysfunction).
No products indexed under this heading.

Ketorolac Tromethamine (Co-administration with NSAID's particularly in the setting of dehydration, may potentiate renal dysfunction).
No products indexed under this heading.

Levonorgestrel (Concomitant oral contraceptives may increase cyclosporine concentrations). Products include:
Climara Pro Transdermal System 768
Lybrel Tablets 3204
Mirena Intrauterine System 779
Plan B Tablets 1044
Seasonique Tablets 1046

Lisinopril (Caution is required when cyclosporine is co-administered with potassium-sparing drugs, such as angiotensin-converting enzyme inhibitors). Products include:
Prinivil Tablets 2087
Prinzide Tablets 2092

Lopinavir (The HIV protease inhibitors are known to inhibit cytochrome P450IIIA and increase the concentration of drugs metabolized by this enzyme system; agents that inhibit this enzyme could decrease metabolism and increase cyclosporine concentrations; this interaction has not been studied; however, care should be exercised). Products include:
Kaletra 452

Losartan Potassium (Caution is required when cyclosporine is co-administered with potassium-sparing drugs, such as angiotensin II receptor antagonists). Products include:
Cozaar Tablets 1973

Lovastatin (Co-administration may results in myotoxicity; lovastatin dosage should be reduced according to label recommendations. Lovastatin needs to be temporarily withheld or discontinued in patients with signs and symptoms of myopathy or those with risk factors predisposing to severe renal injury secondary to rhabdomyolysis). Products include:
Advicor Tablets 402
Mevacor Tablets 2063

Measles, Mumps, Rubella and Varicella Virus Vaccine Live (The use of live vaccines should be avoided). Products include:
ProQuad 2099

Measles, Mumps & Rubella Virus Vaccine, Live (The use of live vaccines should be avoided). Products include:
M-M-R II 2054

Measles & Rubella Virus Vaccine Live (The use of live vaccines should be avoided).
No products indexed under this heading.

Measles Virus Vaccine Live (The use of live vaccines should be avoided). Products include:
Attenuvax 1951

Meclofenamate Sodium (Co-administration with NSAID's particularly in the setting of dehydration, may potentiate renal dysfunction).
No products indexed under this heading.

Mefenamic Acid (Co-administration with NSAID's particularly in the setting of dehydration, may potentiate renal dysfunction).
No products indexed under this heading.

Meloxicam (Co-administration with NSAID's particularly in the setting of dehydration, may potentiate renal dysfunction). Products include:
Mobic Oral Suspension 863
Mobic Tablets 863

Melphalan (May potentiate renal dysfunction).
No products indexed under this heading.

Mestranol (Concomitant oral contraceptives may increase cyclosporine concentrations).
No products indexed under this heading.

Methotrexate Sodium (Increased risk of developing skin malignancies in psoriasis patients with concurrent use; in rheumatoid arthritis patients, methotrexate concentrations (AUCs) were increased approximately 30% and concentrations (AUCs) of its metabolites were decreased approximately 80%; the clinical significance is unknown).
No products indexed under this heading.

Methylprednisolone (Convulsions have been reported with high doses of methylprednisolone).
No products indexed under this heading.

Methylprednisolone Acetate (Convulsions have been reported with high doses of methylprednisolone).
No products indexed under this heading.

Methylprednisolone Sodium Succinate (Convulsions have been reported with high doses of methylprednisolone).
No products indexed under this heading.

Metoclopramide Hydrochloride (Increases cyclosporine concentrations).
No products indexed under this heading.

Moexipril Hydrochloride (Caution is required when cyclosporine is co-administered with potassium-sparing drugs, such as angiotensin-converting enzyme inhibitors).
No products indexed under this heading.

Mumps Virus Vaccine, Live (The use of live vaccines should be avoided). Products include:
Mumpsvax **2068**

Muromonab-CD3 (Psoriasis patients receiving other immunosuppressive agents, such as muromonab-CD3, should not receive concurrent cyclosporine because of the possibility of excessive immunosuppression). Products include:
Orthoclone OKT3 Sterile Solution **2387**

Mycophenolate Mofetil (Psoriasis patients receiving other immunosuppressive agents, such as mycophenolate mofetil, should not receive concurrent cyclosporine because of the possibility of excessive immunosuppression). Products include:
CellCept Capsules **2622**
CellCept Oral Suspension **2622**
CellCept Tablets **2622**

Nabumetone (Co-administration with NSAID's particularly in the setting of dehydration, may potentiate renal dysfunction).
No products indexed under this heading.

Nafcillin Sodium (Decreases cyclosporine concentrations).
No products indexed under this heading.

Naproxen (Concomitant use is associated with additive decreases in renal function with possible potentiation of renal dysfunction).
Products include:
EC-Naprosyn Delayed-Release Tablets **2632**
Naprosyn Suspension **2632**
Naprosyn Tablets **2632**

Naproxen Sodium (Concomitant use is associated with additive decreases in renal function with possible potentiation of renal dysfunction). Products include:
Anaprox Tablets **2632**
Anaprox DS Tablets **2632**
Treximet Tablets **1616**

Nelfinavir Mesylate (The HIV protease inhibitors are known to inhibit cytochrome P450IIIA and increase the concentration of drugs metabolized by this enzyme system; agents that inhibit this enzyme could decrease metabolism and increase cyclosporine concentrations; this interaction has not been studied; however, care should be exercised).
No products indexed under this heading.

Nephrotoxic Drugs (Potential for increased nephrotoxicity; careful monitoring of renal function is required).
No products indexed under this heading.

Nicardipine Hydrochloride (Increases cyclosporine concentrations). Products include:
Cardene I.V. **1093**

Nifedipine (Potential for frequent gingival hyperplasia).
No products indexed under this heading.

Norethindrone (Concomitant oral contraceptives may increase cyclosporine concentrations).
Products include:
Ortho Micronor Tablets **2446**

Norethynodrel (Concomitant oral contraceptives may increase cyclosporine concentrations).
No products indexed under this heading.

Norgestimate (Concomitant oral contraceptives may increase cyclosporine concentrations).
Products include:
Ortho-Cyclen/Ortho Tri-Cyclen **2449**
Ortho Tri-Cyclen Lo Tablets **2458**

Norgestrel (Concomitant oral contraceptives may increase cyclosporine concentrations).
No products indexed under this heading.

Octreotide Acetate (Decreases cyclosporine concentrations).
Products include:
Sandostatin Injection **2300**
Sandostatin LAR Depot **2302**

Orlistat (Co-administration can result in decreased absorption of cyclosporine; concomitant use should be avoided). Products include:
Xenical Capsules **2672**

Oxaprozin (Co-administration with NSAID's particularly in the setting of dehydration, may potentiate renal dysfunction).
No products indexed under this heading.

Perindopril Erbumine (Caution is required when cyclosporine is co-administered with potassium-sparing drugs, such as angiotensin-converting enzyme inhibitors).
Products include:
Aceon Tablets (2 mg, 4 mg, 8 mg) **3038**

Phenobarbital (Decreases cyclosporine concentrations).
Products include:
Donnatal Extentabs **2507**

Phenylbutazone (Co-administration with NSAID's particularly in the setting of dehydration, may potentiate renal dysfunction).
No products indexed under this heading.

Phenytoin (Concomitant use may decrease cyclosporine drug levels).
No products indexed under this heading.

Phenytoin Sodium (Concomitant use may decrease cyclosporine drug levels). Products include:
Phenytek Capsules **2192**

Piroxicam (Co-administration with NSAID's particularly in the setting of dehydration, may potentiate renal dysfunction).
No products indexed under this heading.

Poliovirus Vaccine, Live, Oral, Trivalent, Types 1,2,3 (Sabin) (The use of live vaccines should be avoided).
No products indexed under this heading.

Potassium Acid Phosphate (Caution is required when cyclosporine is co-administered with potassium-containing drugs). Products include:
K-Phos Original (Sodium Free) Tablets **814**

Potassium Bicarbonate (Caution is required when cyclosporine is co-administered with potassium-containing drugs).
No products indexed under this heading.

Potassium Chloride (Caution is required when cyclosporine is co-administered with potassium-containing drugs). Products include:
MoviPrep Oral Solution **2679**

Potassium Citrate (Caution is required when cyclosporine is co-administered with potassium-containing drugs). Products include:
BioLean Free Tablets .... ▣**635**
Urocit-K Tablets **2176**

Potassium Gluconate (Caution is required when cyclosporine is co-administered with potassium-containing drugs).
No products indexed under this heading.

Potassium Phosphate (Caution is required when cyclosporine is co-administered with potassium-containing drugs). Products include:
K-Phos Neutral Tablets **813**

Pravastatin Sodium (Co-administration may result in myotoxicity; pravastatin dosage should be reduced according to label recommendations. Pravastatin needs to be temporarily withheld or discontinued in patients with signs and symptoms of myopathy or those with risk factors predisposing to severe renal injury secondary to rhabdomyolysis).
No products indexed under this heading.

Prednisolone (Cyclosporine may reduce the clearance of prednisolone).
No products indexed under this heading.

Prednisolone Acetate (Cyclosporine may reduce the clearance of prednisolone). Products include:
Pred Forte Ophthalmic Suspension .... ⊙**227**
Pred Mild Ophthalmic Suspension .... ⊙**230**
Pred-G Ophthalmic Ointment .... ⊙**229**
Pred-G Ophthalmic Suspension ...... ⊙**228**

Prednisolone Sodium Phosphate (Cyclosporine may reduce the clearance of prednisolone).
No products indexed under this heading.

Quinapril Hydrochloride (Caution is required when cyclosporine is co-administered with potassium-sparing drugs, such as angiotensin-converting enzyme inhibitors).
No products indexed under this heading.

Quinupristin (Co-administration with substrates that inhibit CYP450 3A, such as quinupristin, could decrease metabolism and increase cyclosporine concentrations).
No products indexed under this heading.

Ramipril (Caution is required when cyclosporine is co-administered with potassium-sparing drugs, such as angiotensin-converting enzyme inhibitors).
No products indexed under this heading.

Ranitidine Hydrochloride (May potentiate renal dysfunction).
Products include:
Zantac 75 Tablets .... ▣**603**
Zantac **1670**
Zantac Injection **1666**
Zantac Injection Pharmacy Bulk Package **1668**
Maximum Strength Zantac 150 Tablets .... ▣**603**
Maximum Strength Zantac 150 Cool Mint Tablets .... ▣**603**

Rifabutin (Substances that are inducers of cyctochrome P450 activity could increase metabolism and decrease cyclosporine concentrations; rifabutin is known to increase the metabolism of other drugs metabolized by the cytochrome P450; this interaction has not been studied, however, care should be exercised).
No products indexed under this heading.

Rifampin (Decreases cyclosporine concentrations).
No products indexed under this heading.

Ritonavir (The HIV protease inhibitors are known to inhibit cytochrome P450IIIA and increase the concentration of drugs metabolized by this enzyme system; agents that inhibit this enzyme could decrease metabolism and increase cyclosporine concentrations; this interaction has not been studied; however, care should be exercised). Products include:
Kaletra **452**
Norvir **489**

Rofecoxib (Co-administration with NSAID's particularly in the setting of dehydration, may potentiate renal dysfunction).
No products indexed under this heading.

Rosuvastatin Calcium (Literature and post-marketing cases of myotoxicity, including muscle pain and weakness, myositis, and rhabdomyolysis, have been reported with concomitant administration of cyclosporine with lovastatin, simvastatin, atorvastatin, pravastatin, and rarely, fluvastatin. When concurrently administered with cyclosporine, the dosage of these statins should be reduced according to label recommendations. Statin therapy needs to be temporarily withheld or discontinued in patients with signs and symptoms of myopathy or those with risk factors predisposing to severe renal injury, including renal failure, secondary to rhabomyolysis). Products include:
Crestor Tablets **677**

Rotavirus Vaccine, Live, Oral, Tetravalent (The use of live vaccines should be avoided).
No products indexed under this heading.

Rubella & Mumps Virus Vaccine Live (The use of live vaccines should be avoided).
No products indexed under this heading.

Rubella Virus Vaccine Live (The use of live vaccines should be avoided). Products include:

Meruvax II 2061

Saquinavir (The HIV protease inhibitors are known to inhibit cytochrome P450IIIA and increase the concentration of drugs metabolized by this enzyme system; agents that inhibit this enzyme could decrease metabolism and increase cyclosporine concentrations; this interaction has not been studied; however, care should be exercised).
No products indexed under this heading.

Saquinavir Mesylate (The HIV protease inhibitors are known to inhibit cytochrome P450IIIA and increase the concentration of drugs metabolized by this enzyme system; agents that inhibit this enzyme could decrease metabolism and increase cyclosporine concentrations; this interaction has not been studied; however, care should be exercised).
No products indexed under this heading.

Simvastatin (Co-administration may result in myotoxicity; simvastation dosage should be reduced according to label recommendations. Simvastatin needs to be temporarily withheld or discontinued in patients with signs and symptoms of myopathy or those with risk factors predisposing to severe renal injury secondary to rhabdomyolysis). Products include:
Simcor Tablets 502
Vytorin 10/10 Tablets 2149
Vytorin 10/10 Tablets 2939
Vytorin 10/20 Tablets 2149
Vytorin 10/20 Tablets 2939
Vytorin 10/40 Tablets 2149
Vytorin 10/40 Tablets 2939
Vytorin 10/80 Tablets 2149
Vytorin 10/80 Tablets 2939
Zocor Tablets 2136

Sirolimus (Elevations in serum creatinine were observed in studies using sirolimus in combination with full-dose cyclosporine. The effect is often reversible with cyclosporine dose reduction. Simultaneous coadministration of cyclosproine significantly increases blood levels of sirolimus. To minimize increases in sirolimus blood concentrations, it is recommended that sirolimus be given 4 hours after cyclosporine administration). Products include:
Rapamune 3260

Smallpox Vaccine (The use of live vaccines should be avoided).
No products indexed under this heading.

Spirapril Hydrochloride (Caution is required when cyclosporine is coadministered with potassium-sparing drugs, such as angiotensin-converting enzyme inhibitors).
No products indexed under this heading.

Spironolactone (Cyclosporine may cause hyperkalemia; concurrent use should be avoided).
No products indexed under this heading.

Sulfamethoxazole (Co-administration with trimethoprim/sulfamethoxazole may potentiate renal dysfunction).
No products indexed under this heading.

Sulfinpyrazone (Concomitant sulfinpyrazone may decrease cyclosporine concentrations).
No products indexed under this heading.

Sulindac (Concomitant use is associated with additive decreases in renal function with possible potentiation of renal dysfunction). Products include:
Clinoril Tablets 1962

Tacrolimus (May potentiate renal dysfunction). Products include:
Prograf Capsules and Injection 622
Protopic Ointment 628

Telmisartan (Caution is required when cyclosporine is co-administered with potassium-sparing drugs, such as angiotensin II receptor antagonists). Products include:
Micardis Tablets 852
Micardis HCT Tablets 854

Terbinafine Hydrochloride (Concomitant terbinafine may decrease cyclosporine concentrations). Products include:
Lamisil Oral Granules 2264
Lamisil Tablets 2266

Ticlopidine Hydrochloride (Decreases cyclosporine concentrations).
No products indexed under this heading.

Tipranavir (The HIV protease inhibitors are known to inhibit cytochrome P450IIIA and increase the concentration of drugs metabolized by this enzyme system; agents that inhibit this enzyme could decrease metabolism and increase cyclosporine concentrations; this interaction has not been studied; however, care should be exercised). Products include:
Aptivus Capsules 823
Aptivus Oral Solution 823

Tobramycin (May potentiate renal dysfunction). Products include:
Zylet Ophthalmic Suspension .... ⊙247

Tobramycin Sulfate (May potentiate renal dysfunction).
No products indexed under this heading.

Tolmetin Sodium (Co-administration with NSAID's particularly in the setting of dehydration, may potentiate renal dysfunction).
No products indexed under this heading.

Trandolapril (Caution is required when cyclosporine is co-administered with potassium-sparing drugs, such as angiotensin-converting enzyme inhibitors). Products include:
Mavik Tablets 472
Tarka Tablets 511

Triamterene (Cyclosporine may cause hyperkalemia; concurrent use should be avoided). Products include:
Dyazide Capsules 1405
Dyrenium Capsules 3189

Trimethoprim (Co-administration with trimethoprim/sulfamethoxazole may potentiate renal dysfunction).
No products indexed under this heading.

Typhoid Vaccine (The use of live vaccines should be avoided).
No products indexed under this heading.

Vaccines (Live) (Vaccination may be less effective).
No products indexed under this heading.

Valdecoxib (Co-administration with NSAID's particularly in the setting of dehydration, may potentiate renal dysfunction).
No products indexed under this heading.

Valsartan (Caution is required when cyclosporine is co-administered with potassium-sparing drugs, such as angiotensin II receptor antagonists). Products include:
Diovan Tablets 2212
Diovan HCT Tablets 2216
Exforge Tablets 2238

Vancomycin Hydrochloride (May potentiate renal dysfunction).
No products indexed under this heading.

Varicella Virus Vaccine Live (The use of live vaccines should be avoided). Products include:
Varivax 2133

Verapamil Hydrochloride (Increases cyclosporine concentrations). Products include:
Tarka Tablets 511

Yellow Fever Vaccine (The use of live vaccines should be avoided).
No products indexed under this heading.

Zoster Vaccine Live (The use of live vaccines should be avoided). Products include:
Zostavax Injection 2145

Food Interactions

Diet, high-lipid (A high-fat meal consumed within one-half hour before Neoral administration decreased the AUC by 13% and Cmax by 33%).

Food, unspecified (Administration of food with Neoral decreases the AUC and Cmax).

Grapefruit (Affects the metabolism of cyclosporine and should be avoided).

Grapefruit Juice (Affects the metabolism of cyclosporine and should be avoided).

NEOSPORIN OPHTHALMIC SOLUTION STERILE

(Gramicidin, Neomycin Sulfate, Polymyxin B Sulfate) .... ⊙252
May interact with:

Gentamicin (Allergic cross-reactions may occur which could prevent the use of gentamicin for the treatment of future infections).
No products indexed under this heading.

Kanamycin Sulfate (Allergic cross-reactions may occur which could prevent the use of kanamycin for the treatment of future infections).
No products indexed under this heading.

Paromomycin Sulfate (Allergic cross-reactions may occur which could prevent the use of paromomycin for the treatment of future infections).
No products indexed under this heading.

Streptomycin Sulfate (Allergic cross-reactions may occur which could prevent the use of streptomycin for the treatment of future infections).
No products indexed under this heading.

NEULASTA INJECTION

(Pegfilgrastim) 587
May interact with drugs which potentiate the release of neutrophils. Compounds in these categories include:

Lithium Carbonate (Concurrent use should be undertaken with caution since lithium potentiates the release of neutrophils).
No products indexed under this heading.

Lithium Citrate (Concurrent use should be undertaken with caution since lithium potentiates the release of neutrophils).
No products indexed under this heading.

NEUPOGEN FOR INJECTION

(Filgrastim) 589
May interact with drugs which potentiate the release of neutrophils. Compounds in these categories include:

Lithium Carbonate (Concurrent use should be undertaken with caution since lithium potentiates the release of neutrophils).
No products indexed under this heading.

Lithium Citrate (Concurrent use should be undertaken with caution since lithium potentiates the release of neutrophils).
No products indexed under this heading.

NEUPRO TRANSDERMAL SYSTEM

(Rotigotine) 3149
May interact with cytochrome p450 2c19 substrates (selected), cytochrome p450 2d6 substrates (selected), and dopamine D2 antagonists. Compounds in these categories include:

Amitriptyline Hydrochloride (There is a low risk of inhibition of cyp2c19 catalyzed metabolism of other drugs at therapeutic concentrations).
No products indexed under this heading.

Amoxapine (There is a low risk of inhibition of cyp2c19 catalyzed metabolism of other drugs at therapeutic concentrations).
No products indexed under this heading.

Amphetamine Aspartate (There is a low risk of inhibition of cyp2d6 catalyzed metabolism of other drugs at therapeutic concentrations). Products include:
Adderall XR Capsules 3012

Amphetamine Aspartate Monohydrate (There is a low risk of inhibition of cyp2d6 catalyzed metabolism of other drugs at therapeutic concentrations).
No products indexed under this heading.

Amphetamine Sulfate (There is a low risk of inhibition of cyp2d6 catalyzed metabolism of other drugs at therapeutic concentrations). Products include:
Adderall XR Capsules 3012

Atomoxetine Hydrochloride (There is a low risk of inhibition of cyp2d6 catalyzed metabolism of other drugs at therapeutic concentrations). Products include:
Strattera Capsules 1864

Bisoprolol Fumarate (There is a low risk of inhibition of cyp2d6 catalyzed metabolism of other drugs at therapeutic concentrations).
No products indexed under this heading.

Captopril (There is a low risk of inhibition of cyp2d6 catalyzed metabolism of other drugs at therapeutic concentrations). Products include:

Captopril Tablets 2182

Carisoprodol (There is a low risk of inhibition of cyp2c19 catalyzed metabolism of other drugs at therapeutic concentrations). Products include:
Soma Tablets 1931

Carvedilol (There is a low risk of inhibition of cyp2d6 catalyzed metabolism of other drugs at therapeutic concentrations). Products include:
Coreg Tablets 1387

Cevimeline Hydrochloride (There is a low risk of inhibition of cyp2d6 catalyzed metabolism of other drugs at therapeutic concentrations). Products include:
Evoxac Capsules 1013

Chlorpromazine (It is possible that dopamine antagonists, such as antipsychotics or metoclopramide, could diminish the effectiveness of rotigotine).
No products indexed under this heading.

Chlorpromazine Hydrochloride (It is possible that dopamine antagonists, such as antipsychotics or metoclopramide, could diminish the effectiveness of rotigotine).
No products indexed under this heading.

Chlorpropamide (There is a low risk of inhibition of cyp2d6 catalyzed metabolism of other drugs at therapeutic concentrations).
No products indexed under this heading.

Chlorprothixene (It is possible that dopamine antagonists, such as antipsychotics or metoclopramide, could diminish the effectiveness of rotigotine).
No products indexed under this heading.

Chlorprothixene Hydrochloride (It is possible that dopamine antagonists, such as antipsychotics or metoclopramide, could diminish the effectiveness of rotigotine).
No products indexed under this heading.

Cilostazol (There is a low risk of inhibition of cyp2c19 catalyzed metabolism of other drugs at therapeutic concentrations). Products include:
Pletal Tablets 2481

Citalopram Hydrobromide (There is a low risk of inhibition of cyp2c19 catalyzed metabolism of other drugs at therapeutic concentrations). Products include:
Celexa 1160

Clomipramine Hydrochloride (There is a low risk of inhibition of cyp2c19 catalyzed metabolism of other drugs at therapeutic concentrations).
No products indexed under this heading.

Clozapine (There is a low risk of inhibition of cyp2d6 catalyzed metabolism of other drugs at therapeutic concentrations).
No products indexed under this heading.

Codeine Phosphate (There is a low risk of inhibition of cyp2d6 catalyzed metabolism of other drugs at therapeutic concentrations). Products include:
Tylenol with Codeine Tablets 2427

Codeine Sulfate (There is a low risk of inhibition of cyp2d6 catalyzed metabolism of other drugs at therapeutic concentrations).
No products indexed under this heading.

Cyclobenzaprine Hydrochloride (There is a low risk of inhibition of cyp2d6 catalyzed metabolism of other drugs at therapeutic concentrations). Products include:
Amrix Capsules 966

Cyclophosphamide (There is a low risk of inhibition of cyp2c19 catalyzed metabolism of other drugs at therapeutic concentrations).
No products indexed under this heading.

Desipramine Hydrochloride (There is a low risk of inhibition of cyp2c19 catalyzed metabolism of other drugs at therapeutic concentrations).
No products indexed under this heading.

Dexfenfluramine Hydrochloride (There is a low risk of inhibition of cyp2d6 catalyzed metabolism of other drugs at therapeutic concentrations).
No products indexed under this heading.

Dextromethorphan (There is a low risk of inhibition of cyp2c19 catalyzed metabolism of other drugs at therapeutic concentrations).
No products indexed under this heading.

Dextromethorphan Hydrobromide (There is a low risk of inhibition of cyp2c19 catalyzed metabolism of other drugs at therapeutic concentrations). Products include:
PediaCare Children's Liquid Multi-Symptom Cold 1902
PediaCare Children's Long-Acting Cough 1902
Children's Sudafed PE Cold & Cough Liquid 1907
Sudafed PE Cold & Cough Caplets 1907
Children's Tylenol Plus Cough & Runny Nose Suspension Liquid 1912
Children's Tylenol Plus Cough & Sore Throat Suspension Liquid 1912
Children's Tylenol Plus Flu Suspension Liquid 1914
Children's Tylenol Plus Multi-Symptom Cold Suspension Liquid 1912
Tylenol Cold Severe Congestion Daytime Caplets with Cool Burst 1912
Tylenol Cold Head Congestion Daytime Caplets with Cool Burst 1910
Tylenol Cold Head Congestion Nighttime Caplets with Cool Burst 1910
Tylenol Cold Head Congestion Severe Daytime Caplets with Cool Burst 1910
Tylenol Cold Multi-Symptom Daytime Caplets with Cool Burst and Rapid Release Gels 1913
Tylenol Cold Multi-Symptom Daytime Liquid with Citrus Burst 1913
Tylenol Cold Multi-Symptom Nighttime Caplets with Cool Burst 1913
Tylenol Cold Multi-Symptom Nighttime Liquid with Cool Burst 1913
Tylenol Cold Multi-Symptom Severe Caplets with Cool Burst 1913
Tylenol Cold Multi-Symptom Severe Daytime Liquid with Citrus Burst 1913
Tylenol Cough & Sore Throat Daytime Liquid with Cool Burst 1918
Tylenol Cough & Sore Throat Nighttime Liquid with Cool Burst 1918
Vicks DayQuil Cold & Flu Multi-Symptom Relief .... ▣ 616
Vicks DayQuil LiquiCaps 2567
Vicks DayQuil Liquid 2567
Vicks DayQuil Multi-Symptom Cold/Flu Relief 2567
Vicks NyQuil Cold & Flu Multi-Symptom Relief .... ▣ 617
Vicks NyQuil LiquiCaps 2567
Vicks NyQuil Liquid 2567
Vicks NyQuil Multi-Symptom Cold/Flu Relief 2567

Dextromethorphan Polistirex (There is a low risk of inhibition of cyp2d6 catalyzed metabolism of other drugs at therapeutic concentrations).
No products indexed under this heading.

Diazepam (There is a low risk of inhibition of cyp2c19 catalyzed metabolism of other drugs at therapeutic concentrations). Products include:
Valium Tablets 2658

Divalproex Sodium (There is a low risk of inhibition of cyp2c19 catalyzed metabolism of other drugs at therapeutic concentrations). Products include:
Depakote ER Tablets 423

Dolasetron Mesylate (There is a low risk of inhibition of cyp2d6 catalyzed metabolism of other drugs at therapeutic concentrations). Products include:
Anzemet Injection 2701
Anzemet Tablets 2704

Donepezil Hydrochloride (There is a low risk of inhibition of cyp2d6 catalyzed metabolism of other drugs at therapeutic concentrations). Products include:
Aricept Tablets 1062
Aricept ODT Tablets 1062

Doxepin Hydrochloride (There is a low risk of inhibition of cyp2c19 catalyzed metabolism of other drugs at therapeutic concentrations).
No products indexed under this heading.

Encainide Hydrochloride (There is a low risk of inhibition of cyp2d6 catalyzed metabolism of other drugs at therapeutic concentrations).
No products indexed under this heading.

Esomeprazole Magnesium (There is a low risk of inhibition of cyp2c19 catalyzed metabolism of other drugs at therapeutic concentrations). Products include:
Nexium Delayed-Release Capsules 645
Nexium Delayed-Release Oral Suspension 645

Ethosuximide (There is a low risk of inhibition of cyp2c19 catalyzed metabolism of other drugs at therapeutic concentrations).
No products indexed under this heading.

Ethotoin (There is a low risk of inhibition of cyp2c19 catalyzed metabolism of other drugs at therapeutic concentrations).
No products indexed under this heading.

Felbamate (There is a low risk of inhibition of cyp2c19 catalyzed metabolism of other drugs at therapeutic concentrations).
No products indexed under this heading.

Fentanyl (There is a low risk of inhibition of cyp2d6 catalyzed metabolism of other drugs at therapeutic concentrations). Products include:
Duragesic Transdermal System 2405
Ionsys Transdermal System 2410

Fentanyl Citrate (There is a low risk of inhibition of cyp2d6 catalyzed metabolism of other drugs at therapeutic concentrations). Products include:
Actiq 959
Fentora Tablets 968

Flecainide Acetate (There is a low risk of inhibition of cyp2d6 catalyzed metabolism of other drugs at therapeutic concentrations).
No products indexed under this heading.

Fluoxetine (There is a low risk of inhibition of cyp2d6 catalyzed metabolism of other drugs at therapeutic concentrations).
No products indexed under this heading.

Fluoxetine Hydrochloride (There is a low risk of inhibition of cyp2d6 catalyzed metabolism of other drugs at therapeutic concentrations). Products include:
Prozac Weekly Capsules 1852
Prozac Pulvules and Liquid 1852
Symbyax Capsules 1871

Fluphenazine Decanoate (It is possible that dopamine antagonists, such as antipsychotics or metoclopramide, could diminish the effectiveness of rotigotine).
No products indexed under this heading.

Fluphenazine Enanthate (It is possible that dopamine antagonists, such as antipsychotics or metoclopramide, could diminish the effectiveness of rotigotine).
No products indexed under this heading.

Fluphenazine Hydrochloride (It is possible that dopamine antagonists, such as antipsychotics or metoclopramide, could diminish the effectiveness of rotigotine).
No products indexed under this heading.

Fluvoxamine Maleate (There is a low risk of inhibition of cyp2d6 catalyzed metabolism of other drugs at therapeutic concentrations). Products include:
Luvox CR Extended-Release Capsules 1759

Formoterol Fumarate (There is a low risk of inhibition of cyp2c19 catalyzed metabolism of other drugs at therapeutic concentrations). Products include:
Foradil Aerolizer 2849
Perforomist Inhalation Solution 1025

Fosphenytoin (There is a low risk of inhibition of cyp2c19 catalyzed metabolism of other drugs at therapeutic concentrations).
No products indexed under this heading.

Fosphenytoin Sodium (There is a low risk of inhibition of cyp2c19 catalyzed metabolism of other drugs at therapeutic concentrations).
No products indexed under this heading.

Gabapentin (There is a low risk of inhibition of cyp2c19 catalyzed metabolism of other drugs at therapeutic concentrations).
No products indexed under this heading.

Galantamine Hydrobromide (There is a low risk of inhibition of cyp2d6 catalyzed metabolism of other drugs at therapeutic concentrations).
No products indexed under this heading.

Haloperidol (It is possible that dopamine antagonists, such as antipsychotics or metoclopramide, could diminish the effectiveness of rotigotine).
No products indexed under this heading.

Haloperidol Decanoate (It is possible that dopamine antagonists, such as antipsychotics or metoclopramide, could diminish the effectiveness of rotigotine).
No products indexed under this heading.

Hydrocodone Bitartrate (There is a low risk of inhibition of cyp2d6 catalyzed metabolism of other drugs at therapeutic concentrations).
Products include:
- Lortab 5/500 Tablets **3143**
- Lortab 7.5/500 Tablets **3144**
- Lortab 10/500 Tablets **3144**
- Vicodin Tablets **529**
- Vicodin ES Tablets **530**
- Vicodin HP Tablets **531**
- Vicoprofen Tablets **533**
- Zydone Tablets **1132**

Imipramine Hydrochloride (There is a low risk of inhibition of cyp2c19 catalyzed metabolism of other drugs at therapeutic concentrations).
No products indexed under this heading.

Imipramine Pamoate (There is a low risk of inhibition of cyp2c19 catalyzed metabolism of other drugs at therapeutic concentrations).
No products indexed under this heading.

Indomethacin (There is a low risk of inhibition of cyp2c19 catalyzed metabolism of other drugs at therapeutic concentrations). Products include:
- Indocin **2024**

Indomethacin Sodium Trihydrate (There is a low risk of inhibition of cyp2c19 catalyzed metabolism of other drugs at therapeutic concentrations). Products include:
- Indocin I.V. **2489**

Indoramin Hydrochloride (There is a low risk of inhibition of cyp2d6 catalyzed metabolism of other drugs at therapeutic concentrations).
No products indexed under this heading.

Labetalol Hydrochloride (There is a low risk of inhibition of cyp2d6 catalyzed metabolism of other drugs at therapeutic concentrations).
No products indexed under this heading.

Lamotrigine (There is a low risk of inhibition of cyp2c19 catalyzed metabolism of other drugs at therapeutic concentrations). Products include:
- Lamictal **1488**

Lansoprazole (There is a low risk of inhibition of cyp2c19 catalyzed metabolism of other drugs at therapeutic concentrations).
No products indexed under this heading.

Levetiracetam (There is a low risk of inhibition of cyp2c19 catalyzed metabolism of other drugs at therapeutic concentrations). Products include:
- Keppra Injection **3137**
- Keppra Oral Solution **3131**
- Keppra Tablets **3131**

Lidocaine (There is a low risk of inhibition of cyp2d6 catalyzed metabolism of other drugs at therapeutic concentrations). Products include:
- Lidoderm Patch **1114**

Lidocaine Hydrochloride (There is a low risk of inhibition of cyp2d6 catalyzed metabolism of other drugs at therapeutic concentrations).
No products indexed under this heading.

Loxapine Hydrochloride (It is possible that dopamine antagonists, such as antipsychotics or metoclopramide, could diminish the effectiveness of rotigotine).
No products indexed under this heading.

Loxapine Succinate (It is possible that dopamine antagonists, such as antipsychotics or metoclopramide, could diminish the effectiveness of rotigotine).
No products indexed under this heading.

Maprotiline Hydrochloride (There is a low risk of inhibition of cyp2c19 catalyzed metabolism of other drugs at therapeutic concentrations).
No products indexed under this heading.

Meperidine Hydrochloride (There is a low risk of inhibition of cyp2d6 catalyzed metabolism of other drugs at therapeutic concentrations).
No products indexed under this heading.

Mephenytoin (There is a low risk of inhibition of cyp2c19 catalyzed metabolism of other drugs at therapeutic concentrations).
No products indexed under this heading.

Mephobarbital (There is a low risk of inhibition of cyp2c19 catalyzed metabolism of other drugs at therapeutic concentrations).
No products indexed under this heading.

Meprobamate (There is a low risk of inhibition of cyp2c19 catalyzed metabolism of other drugs at therapeutic concentrations).
No products indexed under this heading.

Mesoridazine Besylate (It is possible that dopamine antagonists, such as antipsychotics or metoclopramide, could diminish the effectiveness of rotigotine).
No products indexed under this heading.

Methadone Hydrochloride (There is a low risk of inhibition of cyp2d6 catalyzed metabolism of other drugs at therapeutic concentrations).
No products indexed under this heading.

Methamphetamine Hydrochloride (There is a low risk of inhibition of cyp2d6 catalyzed metabolism of other drugs at therapeutic concentrations).
No products indexed under this heading.

Methotrimeprazine (It is possible that dopamine antagonists, such as antipsychotics or metoclopramide, could diminish the effectiveness of rotigotine).
No products indexed under this heading.

Methsuximide (There is a low risk of inhibition of cyp2c19 catalyzed metabolism of other drugs at therapeutic concentrations).
No products indexed under this heading.

Metoclopramide Hydrochloride (It is possible that dopamine antagonists, such as antipsychotics or metoclopramide, could diminish the effectiveness of rotigotine).
No products indexed under this heading.

Metoprolol Succinate (There is a low risk of inhibition of cyp2d6 catalyzed metabolism of other drugs at therapeutic concentrations).
Products include:
- Toprol-XL Tablets **666**

Metoprolol Tartrate (There is a low risk of inhibition of cyp2d6 catalyzed metabolism of other drugs at therapeutic concentrations).
No products indexed under this heading.

Mexiletine Hydrochloride (There is a low risk of inhibition of cyp2d6 catalyzed metabolism of other drugs at therapeutic concentrations).
No products indexed under this heading.

Midazolam Hydrochloride (There is a low risk of inhibition of cyp2c19 catalyzed metabolism of other drugs at therapeutic concentrations).
No products indexed under this heading.

Mirtazapine (There is a low risk of inhibition of cyp2d6 catalyzed metabolism of other drugs at therapeutic concentrations). Products include:
- Remeron Tablets **2924**
- RemeronSolTab Tablets **2927**

Molindone Hydrochloride (It is possible that dopamine antagonists, such as antipsychotics or metoclopramide, could diminish the effectiveness of rotigotine). Products include:
- Moban Tablets **1116**

Morphine Sulfate (There is a low risk of inhibition of cyp2d6 catalyzed metabolism of other drugs at therapeutic concentrations). Products include:
- Avinza Capsules **1772**
- DepoDur Injection **1095**
- MS Contin Tablets **2585**

Nelfinavir Mesylate (There is a low risk of inhibition of cyp2c19 catalyzed metabolism of other drugs at therapeutic concentrations).
No products indexed under this heading.

Nilutamide (There is a low risk of inhibition of cyp2c19 catalyzed metabolism of other drugs at therapeutic concentrations).
No products indexed under this heading.

Nortriptyline Hydrochloride (There is a low risk of inhibition of cyp2c19 catalyzed metabolism of other drugs at therapeutic concentrations).
No products indexed under this heading.

Olanzapine (There is a low risk of inhibition of cyp2d6 catalyzed metabolism of other drugs at therapeutic concentrations). Products include:
- Symbyax Capsules **1871**
- Zyprexa Tablets **1883**
- Zyprexa IntraMuscular **1883**
- Zyprexa ZYDIS Orally Disintegrating Tablets **1883**

Omeprazole (There is a low risk of inhibition of cyp2c19 catalyzed metabolism of other drugs at therapeutic concentrations).
No products indexed under this heading.

Ondansetron (There is a low risk of inhibition of cyp2d6 catalyzed metabolism of other drugs at therapeutic concentrations). Products include:
- Zofran ODT Orally Disintegrating Tablets **1687**

Ondansetron Hydrochloride (There is a low risk of inhibition of cyp2d6 catalyzed metabolism of other drugs at therapeutic concentrations). Products include:
- Zofran Injection **1682**
- Zofran **1687**

Oxcarbazepine (There is a low risk of inhibition of cyp2c19 catalyzed metabolism of other drugs at therapeutic concentrations).
No products indexed under this heading.

Oxycodone Hydrochloride (There is a low risk of inhibition of cyp2d6 catalyzed metabolism of other drugs at therapeutic concentrations).
Products include:
- OxyContin Tablets **2589**
- OxyIR Capsules **2593**
- Percocet Tablets **1127**
- Percodan Tablets **1130**

Paclitaxel (There is a low risk of inhibition of cyp2d6 catalyzed metabolism of other drugs at therapeutic concentrations).
No products indexed under this heading.

Pantoprazole Sodium (There is a low risk of inhibition of cyp2c19 catalyzed metabolism of other drugs at therapeutic concentrations).
Products include:
- Protonix for Delayed-Release Oral Suspension **3254**
- Protonix Delayed-Release Tablets **3254**
- Protonix I.V. **3257**

Paramethadione (There is a low risk of inhibition of cyp2c19 catalyzed metabolism of other drugs at therapeutic concentrations).
No products indexed under this heading.

Paroxetine Hydrochloride (There is a low risk of inhibition of cyp2d6 catalyzed metabolism of other drugs at therapeutic concentrations).
Products include:
- Paxil **1535**
- Paxil CR Controlled-Release Tablets **1544**

Pentamidine Isethionate (There is a low risk of inhibition of cyp2c19 catalyzed metabolism of other drugs at therapeutic concentrations).
No products indexed under this heading.

Perphenazine (It is possible that dopamine antagonists, such as antipsychotics or metoclopramide, could diminish the effectiveness of rotigotine).
No products indexed under this heading.

Phenacemide (There is a low risk of inhibition of cyp2c19 catalyzed metabolism of other drugs at therapeutic concentrations).
No products indexed under this heading.

Phenobarbital (There is a low risk of inhibition of cyp2c19 catalyzed

metabolism of other drugs at therapeutic concentrations). Products include:
Donnatal Extentabs 2507

Phenobarbital Sodium (There is a low risk of inhibition of cyp2c19 catalyzed metabolism of other drugs at therapeutic concentrations).
No products indexed under this heading.

Phensuximide (There is a low risk of inhibition of cyp2c19 catalyzed metabolism of other drugs at therapeutic concentrations).
No products indexed under this heading.

Phenytoin (There is a low risk of inhibition of cyp2c19 catalyzed metabolism of other drugs at therapeutic concentrations).
No products indexed under this heading.

Phenytoin Sodium (There is a low risk of inhibition of cyp2c19 catalyzed metabolism of other drugs at therapeutic concentrations).
Products include:
Phenytek Capsules 2192

Pindolol (There is a low risk of inhibition of cyp2d6 catalyzed metabolism of other drugs at therapeutic concentrations).
No products indexed under this heading.

Primidone (There is a low risk of inhibition of cyp2c19 catalyzed metabolism of other drugs at therapeutic concentrations).
No products indexed under this heading.

Prochlorperazine (It is possible that dopamine antagonists, such as antipsychotics or metoclopramide, could diminish the effectiveness of rotigotine).
No products indexed under this heading.

Progesterone (There is a low risk of inhibition of cyp2c19 catalyzed metabolism of other drugs at therapeutic concentrations). Products include:
Crinone 4% Gel 992
Crinone 8% Gel 992
Prometrium Capsules (100 mg, 200 mg) 3047

Proguanil Hydrochloride (There is a low risk of inhibition of cyp2c19 catalyzed metabolism of other drugs at therapeutic concentrations).
Products include:
Malarone Pediatric Tablets 1521
Malarone Tablets 1521

Promethazine Hydrochloride (It is possible that dopamine antagonists, such as antipsychotics or metoclopramide, could diminish the effectiveness of rotigotine).
No products indexed under this heading.

Propafenone Hydrochloride (There is a low risk of inhibition of cyp2d6 catalyzed metabolism of other drugs at therapeutic concentrations). Products include:
Rythmol Tablets 1586
Rythmol SR Capsules 1590

Propoxyphene Hydrochloride (There is a low risk of inhibition of cyp2d6 catalyzed metabolism of other drugs at therapeutic concentrations).
No products indexed under this heading.

Propoxyphene Napsylate (There is a low risk of inhibition of cyp2d6 catalyzed metabolism of other drugs at therapeutic concentrations).
No products indexed under this heading.

Propranolol Hydrochloride (There is a low risk of inhibition of cyp2c19 catalyzed metabolism of other drugs at therapeutic concentrations).
Products include:
InnoPran XL Extended Release Capsules 1484

Protriptyline Hydrochloride (There is a low risk of inhibition of cyp2c19 catalyzed metabolism of other drugs at therapeutic concentrations).
No products indexed under this heading.

Quetiapine Fumarate (It is possible that dopamine antagonists, such as antipsychotics or metoclopramide, could diminish the effectiveness of rotigotine).
No products indexed under this heading.

Quinidine Gluconate (There is a low risk of inhibition of cyp2d6 catalyzed metabolism of other drugs at therapeutic concentrations).
No products indexed under this heading.

Quinidine Hydrochloride (There is a low risk of inhibition of cyp2d6 catalyzed metabolism of other drugs at therapeutic concentrations).
No products indexed under this heading.

Quinidine Polygalacturonate (There is a low risk of inhibition of cyp2d6 catalyzed metabolism of other drugs at therapeutic concentrations).
No products indexed under this heading.

Quinidine Sulfate (There is a low risk of inhibition of cyp2d6 catalyzed metabolism of other drugs at therapeutic concentrations).
No products indexed under this heading.

Rabeprazole Sodium (There is a low risk of inhibition of cyp2c19 catalyzed metabolism of other drugs at therapeutic concentrations).
Products include:
Aciphex Tablets 1053

Risperidone (It is possible that dopamine antagonists, such as antipsychotics or metoclopramide, could diminish the effectiveness of rotigotine). Products include:
Risperdal Consta Long-Acting Injection 1753

Ritonavir (There is a low risk of inhibition of cyp2d6 catalyzed metabolism of other drugs at therapeutic concentrations). Products include:
Kaletra 452
Norvir 489

Sertraline Hydrochloride (There is a low risk of inhibition of cyp2c19 catalyzed metabolism of other drugs at therapeutic concentrations).
No products indexed under this heading.

Tamoxifen Citrate (There is a low risk of inhibition of cyp2d6 catalyzed metabolism of other drugs at therapeutic concentrations).
No products indexed under this heading.

Teniposide (There is a low risk of inhibition of cyp2c19 catalyzed metabolism of other drugs at therapeutic concentrations).
No products indexed under this heading.

Testosterone (There is a low risk of inhibition of cyp2d6 catalyzed metabolism of other drugs at therapeutic concentrations). Products include:
AndroGel 3159
Testim 1% Gel 701

Testosterone Cypionate (There is a low risk of inhibition of cyp2d6 catalyzed metabolism of other drugs at therapeutic concentrations).
No products indexed under this heading.

Testosterone Enanthate (There is a low risk of inhibition of cyp2d6 catalyzed metabolism of other drugs at therapeutic concentrations).
Products include:
Delatestryl Injection 1730

Testosterone Propionate (There is a low risk of inhibition of cyp2d6 catalyzed metabolism of other drugs at therapeutic concentrations).
No products indexed under this heading.

Thioridazine (There is a low risk of inhibition of cyp2c19 catalyzed metabolism of other drugs at therapeutic concentrations).
No products indexed under this heading.

Thioridazine Hydrochloride (It is possible that dopamine antagonists, such as antipsychotics or metoclopramide, could diminish the effectiveness of rotigotine). Products include:
Thioridazine Hydrochloride Tablets 2195

Thiothixene (It is possible that dopamine antagonists, such as antipsychotics or metoclopramide, could diminish the effectiveness of rotigotine). Products include:
Thiothixene Capsules 2197

Tiagabine Hydrochloride (There is a low risk of inhibition of cyp2c19 catalyzed metabolism of other drugs at therapeutic concentrations).
Products include:
Gabitril Tablets 973

Timolol Maleate (There is a low risk of inhibition of cyp2d6 catalyzed metabolism of other drugs at therapeutic concentrations). Products include:
Combigan Ophthalmic Solution 553
Cosopt Sterile Ophthalmic Solution 1969
Timoptic Sterile Ophthalmic Solution 2121
Timoptic in Ocudose 2124
Timoptic-XE Sterile Ophthalmic Gel Forming Solution 2125

Tolbutamide (There is a low risk of inhibition of cyp2c19 catalyzed metabolism of other drugs at therapeutic concentrations).
No products indexed under this heading.

Tolbutamide Sodium (There is a low risk of inhibition of cyp2c19 catalyzed metabolism of other drugs at therapeutic concentrations).
No products indexed under this heading.

Tolterodine Tartrate (There is a low risk of inhibition of cyp2d6 catalyzed metabolism of other drugs at therapeutic concentrations).
No products indexed under this heading.

Topiramate (There is a low risk of inhibition of cyp2c19 catalyzed metabolism of other drugs at therapeutic concentrations).
No products indexed under this heading.

Tramadol Hydrochloride (There is a low risk of inhibition of cyp2d6 catalyzed metabolism of other drugs at therapeutic concentrations).
Products include:
Ultram ER Extended-Release Tablets 2428

Trazodone Hydrochloride (There is a low risk of inhibition of cyp2d6 catalyzed metabolism of other drugs at therapeutic concentrations).
No products indexed under this heading.

Triazolam (There is a low risk of inhibition of cyp2d6 catalyzed metabolism of other drugs at therapeutic concentrations).
No products indexed under this heading.

Trifluoperazine Hydrochloride (It is possible that dopamine antagonists, such as antipsychotics or metoclopramide, could diminish the effectiveness of rotigotine).
No products indexed under this heading.

Trimethadione (There is a low risk of inhibition of cyp2c19 catalyzed metabolism of other drugs at therapeutic concentrations).
No products indexed under this heading.

Trimipramine Maleate (There is a low risk of inhibition of cyp2c19 catalyzed metabolism of other drugs at therapeutic concentrations).
No products indexed under this heading.

Valproate Sodium (There is a low risk of inhibition of cyp2c19 catalyzed metabolism of other drugs at therapeutic concentrations).
No products indexed under this heading.

Valproic Acid (There is a low risk of inhibition of cyp2c19 catalyzed metabolism of other drugs at therapeutic concentrations).
No products indexed under this heading.

Venlafaxine Hydrochloride (There is a low risk of inhibition of cyp2d6 catalyzed metabolism of other drugs at therapeutic concentrations).
Products include:
Effexor XR Extended-Release Capsules 3195
Venlafaxine Hydrochloride Tablets ... 2199

Vinblastine Sulfate (There is a low risk of inhibition of cyp2d6 catalyzed metabolism of other drugs at therapeutic concentrations).
No products indexed under this heading.

Voriconazole (There is a low risk of inhibition of cyp2c19 catalyzed metabolism of other drugs at therapeutic concentrations).
No products indexed under this heading.

Warfarin Sodium (There is a low risk of inhibition of cyp2c19 catalyzed metabolism of other drugs at therapeutic concentrations).
No products indexed under this heading.

Zonisamide (There is a low risk of inhibition of cyp2c19 catalyzed metabolism of other drugs at therapeutic concentrations). Products include:

Zonegran Capsules 1089

NEVANAC OPHTHALMIC SUSPENSION 0.1%
(Nepafenac) .... ⊙205
May interact with anticoagulants and corticosteroids. Compounds in these categories include:

Anisindione (It is recommended that nepafenac ophthalmic suspension be used with caution in patients who are receiving other medications which may prolong bleeding time).
No products indexed under this heading.

Ardeparin Sodium (It is recommended that nepafenac ophthalmic suspension be used with caution in patients who are receiving other medications which may prolong bleeding time).
No products indexed under this heading.

Betamethasone Acetate (Topical nonsteroidal anti-inflammatory drugs (NSAIDs), including nepafenac ophthalmic suspension, may slow or delay healing. Topical corticosteroids are known to slow or delay healing. Concomitant use of topical NSAIDs and topical steroids may increase the potential for healing problems).
No products indexed under this heading.

Betamethasone Sodium Phosphate (Topical nonsteroidal anti-inflammatory drugs (NSAIDs), including nepafenac ophthalmic suspension, may slow or delay healing. Topical corticosteroids are known to slow or delay healing. Concomitant use of topical NSAIDs and topical steroids may increase the potential for healing problems).
No products indexed under this heading.

Budesonide (Topical nonsteroidal anti-inflammatory drugs (NSAIDs), including nepafenac ophthalmic suspension, may slow or delay healing. Topical corticosteroids are known to slow or delay healing. Concomitant use of topical NSAIDs and topical steroids may increase the potential for healing problems). Products include:
Pulmicort Flexhaler 654
Symbicort 80/4.5 Inhalation Aerosol.. 659
Symbicort 160/4.5 Inhalation Aerosol.. 659

Ciclesonide (Topical nonsteroidal anti-inflammatory drugs (NSAIDs), including nepafenac ophthalmic suspension, may slow or delay healing. Topical corticosteroids are known to slow or delay healing. Concomitant use of topical NSAIDs and topical steroids may increase the potential for healing problems). Products include:
Alvesco Inhalation Aerosol 2985
Omnaris Nasal Spray 2998

Cortisone Acetate (Topical nonsteroidal anti-inflammatory drugs (NSAIDs), including nepafenac ophthalmic suspension, may slow or delay healing. Topical corticosteroids are known to slow or delay healing. Concomitant use of topical NSAIDs and topical steroids may increase the potential for healing problems).
No products indexed under this heading.

Dalteparin Sodium (It is recommended that nepafenac ophthalmic suspension be used with caution in patients who are receiving other medications which may prolong bleeding time). Products include:
Fragmin Injection 1070

Danaparoid Sodium (It is recommended that nepafenac ophthalmic suspension be used with caution in patients who are receiving other medications which may prolong bleeding time).
No products indexed under this heading.

Dexamethasone (Topical nonsteroidal anti-inflammatory drugs (NSAIDs), including nepafenac ophthalmic suspension, may slow or delay healing. Topical corticosteroids are known to slow or delay healing. Concomitant use of topical NSAIDs and topical steroids may increase the potential for healing problems). Products include:
Ciprodex Otic Suspension 541

Dexamethasone Acetate (Topical nonsteroidal anti-inflammatory drugs (NSAIDs), including nepafenac ophthalmic suspension, may slow or delay healing. Topical corticosteroids are known to slow or delay healing. Concomitant use of topical NSAIDs and topical steroids may increase the potential for healing problems).
No products indexed under this heading.

Dexamethasone Sodium Phosphate (Topical nonsteroidal anti-inflammatory drugs (NSAIDs), including nepafenac ophthalmic suspension, may slow or delay healing. Topical corticosteroids are known to slow or delay healing. Concomitant use of topical NSAIDs and topical steroids may increase the potential for healing problems).
No products indexed under this heading.

Dicumarol (It is recommended that nepafenac ophthalmic suspension be used with caution in patients who are receiving other medications which may prolong bleeding time).
No products indexed under this heading.

Enoxaparin Sodium (It is recommended that nepafenac ophthalmic suspension be used with caution in patients who are receiving other medications which may prolong bleeding time). Products include:
Lovenox Injection 2756

Fludrocortisone Acetate (Topical nonsteroidal anti-inflammatory drugs (NSAIDs), including nepafenac ophthalmic suspension, may slow or delay healing. Topical corticosteroids are known to slow or delay healing. Concomitant use of topical NSAIDs and topical steroids may increase the potential for healing problems).
No products indexed under this heading.

Flunisolide (Topical nonsteroidal anti-inflammatory drugs (NSAIDs), including nepafenac ophthalmic suspension, may slow or delay healing. Topical corticosteroids are known to slow or delay healing. Concomitant use of topical NSAIDs and topical steroids may increase the potential for healing problems). Products include:
Aerobid/Aerobid-M 1153

Fluticasone Propionate (Topical nonsteroidal anti-inflammatory drugs (NSAIDs), including nepafenac ophthalmic suspension, may slow or delay healing. Topical corticosteroids are known to slow or delay healing. Concomitant use of topical NSAIDs and topical steroids may increase the potential for healing problems). Products include:
Advair Diskus 100/50 1276
Advair Diskus 250/50 1276
Advair Diskus 500/50 1276
Advair HFA 45/21 Inhalation Aerosol.. 1288
Advair HFA 115/21 Inhalation Aerosol.. 1288
Advair HFA 230/21 Inhalation Aerosol.. 1288
Flonase Nasal Spray 1431
Flovent Diskus 50 mcg 1435

Fluticasone Propionate HFA (Topical nonsteroidal anti-inflammatory drugs (NSAIDs), including nepafenac ophthalmic suspension, may slow or delay healing. Topical corticosteroids are known to slow or delay healing. Concomitant use of topical NSAIDs and topical steroids may increase the potential for healing problems). Products include:
Flovent HFA 1440

Fondaparinux Sodium (It is recommended that nepafenac ophthalmic suspension be used with caution in patients who are receiving other medications which may prolong bleeding time). Products include:
Arixtra Injection 1313

Heparin Calcium (It is recommended that nepafenac ophthalmic suspension be used with caution in patients who are receiving other medications which may prolong bleeding time).
No products indexed under this heading.

Heparin Sodium (It is recommended that nepafenac ophthalmic suspension be used with caution in patients who are receiving other medications which may prolong bleeding time).
No products indexed under this heading.

Hydrocortisone (Topical nonsteroidal anti-inflammatory drugs (NSAIDs), including nepafenac ophthalmic suspension, may slow or delay healing. Topical corticosteroids are known to slow or delay healing. Concomitant use of topical NSAIDs and topical steroids may increase the potential for healing problems).
No products indexed under this heading.

Hydrocortisone Acetate (Topical nonsteroidal anti-inflammatory drugs (NSAIDs), including nepafenac ophthalmic suspension, may slow or delay healing. Topical corticosteroids are known to slow or delay healing. Concomitant use of topical NSAIDs and topical steroids may increase the potential for healing problems). Products include:
Analpram-HC 1140
Pramosone 1141

Hydrocortisone Sodium Phosphate (Topical nonsteroidal anti-inflammatory drugs (NSAIDs), including nepafenac ophthalmic suspension, may slow or delay healing. Topical corticosteroids are known to slow or delay healing. Concomitant use of topical NSAIDs and topical steroids may increase the potential for healing problems).
No products indexed under this heading.

Hydrocortisone Sodium Succinate (Topical nonsteroidal anti-inflammatory drugs (NSAIDs), including nepafenac ophthalmic suspension, may slow or delay healing. Topical corticosteroids are known to slow or delay healing. Concomitant use of topical NSAIDs and topical steroids may increase the potential for healing problems).
No products indexed under this heading.

Low Molecular Weight Heparins (It is recommended that nepafenac ophthalmic suspension be used with caution in patients who are receiving other medications which may prolong bleeding time).
No products indexed under this heading.

Methylprednisolone Acetate (Topical nonsteroidal anti-inflammatory drugs (NSAIDs), including nepafenac ophthalmic suspension, may slow or delay healing. Topical corticosteroids are known to slow or delay healing. Concomitant use of topical NSAIDs and topical steroids may increase the potential for healing problems).
No products indexed under this heading.

Methylprednisolone Sodium Succinate (Topical nonsteroidal anti-inflammatory drugs (NSAIDs), including nepafenac ophthalmic suspension, may slow or delay healing. Topical corticosteroids are known to slow or delay healing. Concomitant use of topical NSAIDs and topical steroids may increase the potential for healing problems).
No products indexed under this heading.

Mometasone Furoate (Topical nonsteroidal anti-inflammatory drugs (NSAIDs), including nepafenac ophthalmic suspension, may slow or delay healing. Topical corticosteroids are known to slow or delay healing. Concomitant use of topical NSAIDs and topical steroids may increase the potential for healing problems). Products include:
Asmanex Twisthaler 2797
Elocon Cream 0.1% 2840
Elocon Lotion 0.1% 2841
Elocon Ointment 0.1% 2842

Mometasone Furoate Monohydrate (Topical nonsteroidal anti-inflammatory drugs (NSAIDs), including nepafenac ophthalmic suspension, may slow or delay healing. Topical corticosteroids are known to slow or delay healing. Concomitant use of topical NSAIDs and topical steroids may increase the potential for healing problems). Products include:
Nasonex Nasal Spray 2883

Prednisolone Acetate (Topical nonsteroidal anti-inflammatory drugs (NSAIDs), including nepafenac ophthalmic suspension, may slow or delay healing. Topical corticoster-

oids are known to slow or delay healing. Concomitant use of topical NSAIDs and topical steroids may increase the potential for healing problems). Products include:

Pred Forte Ophthalmic Suspension ⊙ 227
Pred Mild Ophthalmic Suspension ⊙ 230
Pred-G Ophthalmic Ointment ⊙ 229
Pred-G Ophthalmic Suspension ⊙ 228

Prednisolone Sodium Phosphate (Topical nonsteroidal anti-inflammatory drugs (NSAIDs), including nepafenac ophthalmic suspension, may slow or delay healing. Topical corticosteroids are known to slow or delay healing. Concomitant use of topical NSAIDs and topical steroids may increase the potential for healing problems).

No products indexed under this heading.

Prednisolone Tebutate (Topical nonsteroidal anti-inflammatory drugs (NSAIDs), including nepafenac ophthalmic suspension, may slow or delay healing. Topical corticosteroids are known to slow or delay healing. Concomitant use of topical NSAIDs and topical steroids may increase the potential for healing problems).

No products indexed under this heading.

Prednisone (Topical nonsteroidal anti-inflammatory drugs (NSAIDs), including nepafenac ophthalmic suspension, may slow or delay healing. Topical corticosteroids are known to slow or delay healing. Concomitant use of topical NSAIDs and topical steroids may increase the potential for healing problems).

No products indexed under this heading.

Tinzaparin Sodium (It is recommended that nepafenac ophthalmic suspension be used with caution in patients who are receiving other medications which may prolong bleeding time).

No products indexed under this heading.

Triamcinolone (Topical nonsteroidal anti-inflammatory drugs (NSAIDs), including nepafenac ophthalmic suspension, may slow or delay healing. Topical corticosteroids are known to slow or delay healing. Concomitant use of topical NSAIDs and topical steroids may increase the potential for healing problems).

No products indexed under this heading.

Triamcinolone Acetonide (Topical nonsteroidal anti-inflammatory drugs (NSAIDs), including nepafenac ophthalmic suspension, may slow or delay healing. Topical corticosteroids are known to slow or delay healing. Concomitant use of topical NSAIDs and topical steroids may increase the potential for healing problems). Products include:

Azmacort Inhalation Aerosol 407
Nasacort AQ Nasal Spray 2765
Triesence Injectable Suspension ⊙ 209

Triamcinolone Diacetate (Topical nonsteroidal anti-inflammatory drugs (NSAIDs), including nepafenac ophthalmic suspension, may slow or delay healing. Topical corticosteroids are known to slow or delay healing. Concomitant use of topical NSAIDs and topical steroids may increase the potential for healing problems).

No products indexed under this heading.

Triamcinolone Hexacetonide (Topical nonsteroidal anti-inflammatory drugs (NSAIDs), including nepafenac ophthalmic suspension, may slow or delay healing. Topical corticosteroids are known to slow or delay healing. Concomitant use of topical NSAIDs and topical steroids may increase the potential for healing problems).

No products indexed under this heading.

Warfarin Sodium (It is recommended that nepafenac ophthalmic suspension be used with caution in patients who are receiving other medications which may prolong bleeding time).

No products indexed under this heading.

NEXAVAR TABLETS

(Sorafenib) 784

May interact with cytochrome p450 2c8 substrates (selected), cytochrome p450 3a4 inducers (selected), dexamethasone, phenytoin, and certain other agents. Compounds in these categories include:

Allium sativum (Inducers of CYP3A4 activity may increase the metabolism of sorafenib and thus decrease sorafenib concentrations).

No products indexed under this heading.

Amiodarone Hydrochloride (Sorafenib inhibits CYP2B6 and CYP2C8 in vitro with Ki values of 6 and 1-2 μM, respectively. Systemic exposure to substrates of CYP2B6 and CYP2C8 is expected to increase when co-administered with sorafenib. Caution is recommended when administering substrates of CYP2B6 and CYP2C8 with sorafenib).

No products indexed under this heading.

Amitriptyline Hydrochloride (Sorafenib inhibits CYP2B6 and CYP2C8 in vitro with Ki values of 6 and 1-2 μM, respectively. Systemic exposure to substrates of CYP2B6 and CYP2C8 is expected to increase when co-administered with sorafenib. Caution is recommended when administering substrates of CYP2B6 and CYP2C8 with sorafenib).

No products indexed under this heading.

Amoxapine (Sorafenib inhibits CYP2B6 and CYP2C8 in vitro with Ki values of 6 and 1-2 μM, respectively. Systemic exposure to substrates of CYP2B6 and CYP2C8 is expected to increase when co-administered with sorafenib. Caution is recommended when administering substrates of CYP2B6 and CYP2C8 with sorafenib).

No products indexed under this heading.

Aprepitant (Inducers of CYP3A4 activity may increase the metabolism of sorafenib and thus decrease sorafenib concentrations). Products include:

Emend Capsules 1992

Benzphetamine Hydrochloride (Sorafenib inhibits CYP2B6 and CYP2C8 in vitro with Ki values of 6 and 1-2 μM, respectively. Systemic exposure to substrates of CYP2B6 and CYP2C8 is expected to increase when co-administered with sorafenib. Caution is recommended when administering substrates of CYP2B6 and CYP2C8 with sorafenib).

No products indexed under this heading.

Betamethasone Acetate (Inducers of CYP3A4 activity may increase the metabolism of sorafenib and thus decrease sorafenib concentrations).

No products indexed under this heading.

Betamethasone Sodium Phosphate (Inducers of CYP3A4 activity may increase the metabolism of sorafenib and thus decrease sorafenib concentrations).

No products indexed under this heading.

Carbamazepine (Inducers of CYP3A4 activity such as carbamazepine may increase the metabolism of sorafenib and thus decrease sorafenib concentrations). Products include:

Carbatrol Capsules 3019
Equetro Extended-Release Capsules 3174

Ciprofloxacin Hydrochloride (Inducers of CYP3A4 activity may increase the metabolism of sorafenib and thus decrease sorafenib concentrations). Products include:

Cipro Tablets 2810

Cisplatin (Inducers of CYP3A4 activity may increase the metabolism of sorafenib and thus decrease sorafenib concentrations).

No products indexed under this heading.

Clomipramine Hydrochloride (Sorafenib inhibits CYP2B6 and CYP2C8 in vitro with Ki values of 6 and 1-2 μM, respectively. Systemic exposure to substrates of CYP2B6 and CYP2C8 is expected to increase when co-administered with sorafenib. Caution is recommended when administering substrates of CYP2B6 and CYP2C8 with sorafenib).

No products indexed under this heading.

Cortisone Acetate (Inducers of CYP3A4 activity may increase the metabolism of sorafenib and thus decrease sorafenib concentrations).

No products indexed under this heading.

Desipramine Hydrochloride (Sorafenib inhibits CYP2B6 and CYP2C8 in vitro with Ki values of 6 and 1-2 μM, respectively. Systemic exposure to substrates of CYP2B6 and CYP2C8 is expected to increase when co-administered with sorafenib. Caution is recommended when administering substrates of CYP2B6 and CYP2C8 with sorafenib).

No products indexed under this heading.

Dexamethasone (Inducers of CYP3A4 activity such as dexamethasone may increase the metabolism of sorafenib and thus decrease sorafenib concentrations). Products include:

Ciprodex Otic Suspension 541

Dexamethasone Acetate (Inducers of CYP3A4 activity such as dexamethasone may increase the metabolism of sorafenib and thus decrease sorafenib concentrations).

No products indexed under this heading.

Dexamethasone Sodium Phosphate (Inducers of CYP3A4 activity such as dexamethasone may increase the metabolism of sorafenib and thus decrease sorafenib concentrations).

No products indexed under this heading.

Diazepam (Sorafenib inhibits CYP2B6 and CYP2C8 in vitro with Ki values of 6 and 1-2 μM, respectively. Systemic exposure to substrates of CYP2B6 and CYP2C8 is expected to increase when co-administered with sorafenib. Caution is recommended when administering substrates of CYP2B6 and CYP2C8 with sorafenib). Products include:

Valium Tablets 2658

Diclofenac Potassium (Sorafenib inhibits CYP2B6 and CYP2C8 in vitro with Ki values of 6 and 1-2 μM, respectively. Systemic exposure to substrates of CYP2B6 and CYP2C8 is expected to increase when co-administered with sorafenib. Caution is recommended when administering substrates of CYP2B6 and CYP2C8 with sorafenib).

No products indexed under this heading.

Diclofenac Sodium (Sorafenib inhibits CYP2B6 and CYP2C8 in vitro with Ki values of 6 and 1-2 μM, respectively. Systemic exposure to substrates of CYP2B6 and CYP2C8 is expected to increase when co-administered with sorafenib. Caution is recommended when administering substrates of CYP2B6 and CYP2C8 with sorafenib). Products include:

Diclofenac Sodium Ophthalmic Solution ⊙ 240
Voltaren Ophthalmic Solution 2336
Voltaren Tablets 2334
Voltaren-XR Tablets 2337

Docetaxel (Concomitant use of docetaxel (75 or 100 mg/m2 administered every 21 days) with sorafenib (200 or 400 mg b.i.d.), administered with a 3-day break in dosing around administration of docetaxel, resulted in a 36% to 80% increase in docetaxel AUC and a 16% to32% increase in docetaxel Cmax. Caution is recommended when sorafenib is co-administered with docetaxel). Products include:

Taxotere Injection Concentrate 2773

Doxepin Hydrochloride (Sorafenib inhibits CYP2B6 and CYP2C8 in vitro with Ki values of 6 and 1-2 μM, respectively. Systemic exposure to substrates of CYP2B6 and CYP2C8 is expected to increase when co-administered with sorafenib. Caution is recommended when administering substrates of CYP2B6 and CYP2C8 with sorafenib).

No products indexed under this heading.

Doxorubicin Hydrochloride (Concomitant treatment with sorafenib resulted in a 21% increase in the AUC of doxorubicin. Caution is recommended when administering doxorubicin with sorafenib. The clinical significance of these findings is unknown).

No products indexed under this heading.

Doxorubicin Hydrochloride Liposome (Concomitant treatment with sorafenib resulted in a 21% increase in the AUC of doxorubicin. Caution is recommended when administering doxorubicin with sorafenib. The clinical significance of these findings is unknown). Products include:

Doxil Injection **2378**

Efavirenz (Inducers of CYP3A4 activity may increase the metabolism of sorafenib and thus decrease sorafenib concentrations). Products include:

Atripla Tablets **938**
Sustiva Capsules **930**
Sustiva Tablets **930**

Ethosuximide (Inducers of CYP3A4 activity may increase the metabolism of sorafenib and thus decrease sorafenib concentrations).

No products indexed under this heading.

Felbamate (Inducers of CYP3A4 activity may increase the metabolism of sorafenib and thus decrease sorafenib concentrations).

No products indexed under this heading.

Fludrocortisone Acetate (Inducers of CYP3A4 activity may increase the metabolism of sorafenib and thus decrease sorafenib concentrations).

No products indexed under this heading.

Fluorouracil (Both increases (21% to 47%) and decreases (10%) of the AUC of fluorouracil were observed with concomitant treatment with sorafenib. Caution is recommended when sorafenib is co-administered with fluorouracil/leucovorin). Products include:

Carac Cream 0.5% **2722**

Fluvastatin Sodium (Sorafenib inhibits CYP2B6 and CYP2C8 in vitro with Ki values of 6 and 1-2 μM, respectively. Systemic exposure to substrates of CYP2B6 and CYP2C8 is expected to increase when co-administered with sorafenib. Caution is recommended when administering substrates of CYP2B6 and CYP2C8 with sorafenib). Products include:

Lescol Capsules **2268**
Lescol XL Tablets **2268**

Fosphenytoin Sodium (Inducers of CYP3A4 activity such as phenytoin may increase the metabolism of sorafenib and thus decrease sorafenib concentrations).

No products indexed under this heading.

Garlic Extract (Inducers of CYP3A4 activity may increase the metabolism of sorafenib and thus decrease sorafenib concentrations).

No products indexed under this heading.

Garlic Oil (Inducers of CYP3A4 activity may increase the metabolism of sorafenib and thus decrease sorafenib concentrations).

No products indexed under this heading.

Hydrocortisone (Inducers of CYP3A4 activity may increase the metabolism of sorafenib and thus decrease sorafenib concentrations).

No products indexed under this heading.

Hydrocortisone Acetate (Inducers of CYP3A4 activity may increase the metabolism of sorafenib and thus decrease sorafenib concentrations). Products include:

Analpram-HC **1140**
Pramosone **1141**

Hydrocortisone Butyrate (Inducers of CYP3A4 activity may increase the metabolism of sorafenib and thus decrease sorafenib concentrations).

No products indexed under this heading.

Hydrocortisone Cypionate (Inducers of CYP3A4 activity may increase the metabolism of sorafenib and thus decrease sorafenib concentrations).

No products indexed under this heading.

Hydrocortisone Hemisuccinate (Inducers of CYP3A4 activity may increase the metabolism of sorafenib and thus decrease sorafenib concentrations).

No products indexed under this heading.

Hydrocortisone Probutate (Inducers of CYP3A4 activity may increase the metabolism of sorafenib and thus decrease sorafenib concentrations).

No products indexed under this heading.

Hydrocortisone Sodium Phosphate (Inducers of CYP3A4 activity may increase the metabolism of sorafenib and thus decrease sorafenib concentrations).

No products indexed under this heading.

Hydrocortisone Sodium Succinate (Inducers of CYP3A4 activity may increase the metabolism of sorafenib and thus decrease sorafenib concentrations).

No products indexed under this heading.

Hydrocortisone Valerate (Inducers of CYP3A4 activity may increase the metabolism of sorafenib and thus decrease sorafenib concentrations).

No products indexed under this heading.

Hypericum (Inducers of CYP3A4 activity such as hypericum perforatum which is also known as St. John's Wort, may increase the metabolism of sorafenib and thus decrease sorafenib concentrations). Products include:

Satieté Tablets **640**

Hypericum Perforatum (Inducers of CYP3A4 activity such as hypericum perforatum which is also known as St. John's Wort, may increase the metabolism of sorafenib and thus decrease sorafenib concentrations).

No products indexed under this heading.

Imipramine Hydrochloride (Sorafenib inhibits CYP2B6 and CYP2C8 in vitro with Ki values of 6 and 1-2 μM, respectively. Systemic exposure to substrates of CYP2B6 and CYP2C8 is expected to increase when co-administered with sorafenib. Caution is recommended when administering substrates of CYP2B6 and CYP2C8 with sorafenib).

No products indexed under this heading.

Imipramine Pamoate (Sorafenib inhibits CYP2B6 and CYP2C8 in vitro with Ki values of 6 and 1-2 μM, respectively. Systemic exposure to substrates of CYP2B6 and CYP2C8 is expected to increase when co-administered with sorafenib. Caution is recommended when administering substrates of CYP2B6 and CYP2C8 with sorafenib).

No products indexed under this heading.

Irinotecan Hydrochloride (Caution is recommended when administering sorafenib with compounds that are metabolized/eliminated predominantly by the UGT1A1 pathway such as irinotecan. Sorafenib inhibits glucuronidation by the UGT1A1 (Ki value: 1 μM) and UGT1A9 pathways (Ki value: 2μM). Systemic exposure to substrates of UGT1A1 and UGT1A9 may increase when co-administered with sorafenib. In clinical studies, when sorafenib was administered with irinotecan, whose active metabolite SN-38 is further metabolized by the UGT1A1 pathway, there was a 67% to 120% increase in the AUC of SN-38 and a 26% to 42% increase in the AUC of irinotecan. The clinical significance of these findings is unknown).

No products indexed under this heading.

Isotretinoin (Sorafenib inhibits CYP2B6 and CYP2C8 in vitro with Ki values of 6 and 1-2 μM, respectively. Systemic exposure to substrates of CYP2B6 and CYP2C8 is expected to increase when co-administered with sorafenib. Caution is recommended when administering substrates of CYP2B6 and CYP2C8 with sorafenib). Products include:

Accutane Capsules **2607**

Maprotiline Hydrochloride (Sorafenib inhibits CYP2B6 and CYP2C8 in vitro with Ki values of 6 and 1-2 μM, respectively. Systemic exposure to substrates of CYP2B6 and CYP2C8 is expected to increase when co-administered with sorafenib. Caution is recommended when administering substrates of CYP2B6 and CYP2C8 with sorafenib).

No products indexed under this heading.

Mephenytoin (Inducers of CYP3A4 activity may increase the metabolism of sorafenib and thus decrease sorafenib concentrations).

No products indexed under this heading.

Mephobarbital (Sorafenib inhibits CYP2B6 and CYP2C8 in vitro with Ki values of 6 and 1-2 μM, respectively. Systemic exposure to substrates of CYP2B6 and CYP2C8 is expected to increase when co-administered with sorafenib. Caution is recommended when administering substrates of CYP2B6 and CYP2C8 with sorafenib).

No products indexed under this heading.

Methsuximide (Inducers of CYP3A4 activity may increase the metabolism of sorafenib and thus decrease sorafenib concentrations).

No products indexed under this heading.

Methylprednisolone (Inducers of CYP3A4 activity may increase the metabolism of sorafenib and thus decrease sorafenib concentrations).

No products indexed under this heading.

Methylprednisolone Acetate (Inducers of CYP3A4 activity may increase the metabolism of sorafenib and thus decrease sorafenib concentrations).

No products indexed under this heading.

Methylprednisolone Sodium Succinate (Inducers of CYP3A4 activity may increase the metabolism of sorafenib and thus decrease sorafenib concentrations).

No products indexed under this heading.

Modafinil (Inducers of CYP3A4 activity may increase the metabolism of sorafenib and thus decrease sorafenib concentrations). Products include:

Provigil Tablets **977**

Nevirapine (Inducers of CYP3A4 activity may increase the metabolism of sorafenib and thus decrease sorafenib concentrations). Products include:

Viramune Oral Suspension **873**
Viramune Tablets **873**

Nortriptyline Hydrochloride (Sorafenib inhibits CYP2B6 and CYP2C8 in vitro with Ki values of 6 and 1-2 μM, respectively. Systemic exposure to substrates of CYP2B6 and CYP2C8 is expected to increase when co-administered with sorafenib. Caution is recommended when administering substrates of CYP2B6 and CYP2C8 with sorafenib).

No products indexed under this heading.

Omeprazole (Sorafenib inhibits CYP2B6 and CYP2C8 in vitro with Ki values of 6 and 1-2 μM, respectively. Systemic exposure to substrates of CYP2B6 and CYP2C8 is expected to increase when co-administered with sorafenib. Caution is recommended when administering substrates of CYP2B6 and CYP2C8 with sorafenib).

No products indexed under this heading.

Oxcarbazepine (Inducers of CYP3A4 activity may increase the metabolism of sorafenib and thus decrease sorafenib concentrations).

No products indexed under this heading.

Paclitaxel (Sorafenib inhibits CYP2B6 and CYP2C8 in vitro with Ki values of 6 and 1-2 μM, respectively. Systemic exposure to substrates of CYP2B6 and CYP2C8 is expected to increase when co-administered with sorafenib. Caution is recommended when administering substrates of CYP2B6 and CYP2C8 with sorafenib).

No products indexed under this heading.

Phenobarbital (Inducers of CYP3A4 activity such as phenobarbital may increase the metabolism of sorafenib and thus decrease sorafenib concentrations). Products include:

Donnatal Extentabs **2507**

Phenobarbital Sodium (Inducers of CYP3A4 activity such as phenobarbital may increase the metabolism of sorafenib and thus decrease sorafenib concentrations).

No products indexed under this heading.

Phenytoin (Inducers of CYP3A4 activity such as phenytoin may increase the metabolism of sorafenib and thus decrease sorafenib concentrations).
No products indexed under this heading.

Phenytoin Sodium (Inducers of CYP3A4 activity such as phenytoin may increase the metabolism of sorafenib and thus decrease sorafenib concentrations). Products include:
Phenytek Capsules 2192

Pioglitazone Hydrochloride (Sorafenib inhibits CYP2B6 and CYP2C8 in vitro with Ki values of 6 and 1-2 μM, respectively. Systemic exposure to substrates of CYP2B6 and CYP2C8 is expected to increase when co-administered with sorafenib. Caution is recommended when administering substrates of CYP2B6 and CYP2C8 with sorafenib).
Products include:
ActoPlus Met Tablets 3071
Actos Tablets 3077
Duetact Tablets 3085

Prednisolone Acetate (Inducers of CYP3A4 activity may increase the metabolism of sorafenib and thus decrease sorafenib concentrations).
Products include:
Pred Forte Ophthalmic Suspension .... ⊙ 227
Pred Mild Ophthalmic Suspension .... ⊙ 230
Pred-G Ophthalmic Ointment .... ⊙ 229
Pred-G Ophthalmic Suspension ...... ⊙ 228

Prednisolone Sodium Phosphate (Inducers of CYP3A4 activity may increase the metabolism of sorafenib and thus decrease sorafenib concentrations).
No products indexed under this heading.

Prednisolone Tebutate (Inducers of CYP3A4 activity may increase the metabolism of sorafenib and thus decrease sorafenib concentrations).
No products indexed under this heading.

Prednisone (Inducers of CYP3A4 activity may increase the metabolism of sorafenib and thus decrease sorafenib concentrations).
No products indexed under this heading.

Primidone (Inducers of CYP3A4 activity may increase the metabolism of sorafenib and thus decrease sorafenib concentrations).
No products indexed under this heading.

Protriptyline Hydrochloride (Sorafenib inhibits CYP2B6 and CYP2C8 in vitro with Ki values of 6 and 1-2 μM, respectively. Systemic exposure to substrates of CYP2B6 and CYP2C8 is expected to increase when co-administered with sorafenib. Caution is recommended when administering substrates of CYP2B6 and CYP2C8 with sorafenib).
No products indexed under this heading.

Repaglinide (Sorafenib inhibits CYP2B6 and CYP2C8 in vitro with Ki values of 6 and 1-2 μM, respectively. Systemic exposure to substrates of CYP2B6 and CYP2C8 is expected to increase when co-administered with sorafenib. Caution is recommended when administering substrates of CYP2B6 and CYP2C8 with sorafenib). Products include:
PrandiMet Tablets 2967
Prandin Tablets 2971

Rifabutin (Inducers of CYP3A4 activity may increase the metabolism of sorafenib and thus decrease sorafenib concentrations).
No products indexed under this heading.

Rifampicin (Continuous concomitant administration of sorafenib and rifampicin resulted in an average 37% reduction of sorafenib AUC).
No products indexed under this heading.

Rifampin (Inducers of CYP3A4 activity may increase the metabolism of sorafenib and thus decrease sorafenib concentrations).
No products indexed under this heading.

Rifapentine (Inducers of CYP3A4 activity may increase the metabolism of sorafenib and thus decrease sorafenib concentrations).
No products indexed under this heading.

Rosiglitazone Maleate (Sorafenib inhibits CYP2B6 and CYP2C8 in vitro with Ki values of 6 and 1-2 μM, respectively. Systemic exposure to substrates of CYP2B6 and CYP2C8 is expected to increase when co-administered with sorafenib. Caution is recommended when administering substrates of CYP2B6 and CYP2C8 with sorafenib). Products include:
Avandamet Tablets 1336
Avandaryl Tablets 1344
Avandia Tablets 1351

Rosiglitazone/Metformin (Sorafenib inhibits CYP2B6 and CYP2C8 in vitro with Ki values of 6 and 1-2 μM, respectively. Systemic exposure to substrates of CYP2B6 and CYP2C8 is expected to increase when co-administered with sorafenib. Caution is recommended when administering substrates of CYP2B6 and CYP2C8 with sorafenib).
No products indexed under this heading.

Sulfinpyrazone (Inducers of CYP3A4 activity may increase the metabolism of sorafenib and thus decrease sorafenib concentrations).
No products indexed under this heading.

Theophylline (Inducers of CYP3A4 activity may increase the metabolism of sorafenib and thus decrease sorafenib concentrations).
No products indexed under this heading.

Theophylline Anhydrous (Inducers of CYP3A4 activity may increase the metabolism of sorafenib and thus decrease sorafenib concentrations).
Products include:
Uniphyl Tablets 2595

Theophylline Calcium Salicylate (Inducers of CYP3A4 activity may increase the metabolism of sorafenib and thus decrease sorafenib concentrations).
No products indexed under this heading.

Theophylline Dihydroxypropyl (Glyceryl) (Inducers of CYP3A4 activity may increase the metabolism of sorafenib and thus decrease sorafenib concentrations).
No products indexed under this heading.

Theophylline Ethylenediamine (Inducers of CYP3A4 activity may increase the metabolism of sorafenib and thus decrease sorafenib concentrations).
No products indexed under this heading.

Tolbutamide (Sorafenib inhibits CYP2B6 and CYP2C8 in vitro with Ki values of 6 and 1-2 μM, respectively. Systemic exposure to substrates of CYP2B6 and CYP2C8 is expected to increase when co-administered with sorafenib. Caution is recommended when administering substrates of CYP2B6 and CYP2C8 with sorafenib).
No products indexed under this heading.

Tolbutamide Sodium (Sorafenib inhibits CYP2B6 and CYP2C8 in vitro with Ki values of 6 and 1-2 μM, respectively. Systemic exposure to substrates of CYP2B6 and CYP2C8 is expected to increase when co-administered with sorafenib. Caution is recommended when administering substrates of CYP2B6 and CYP2C8 with sorafenib).
No products indexed under this heading.

Tretinoin (Sorafenib inhibits CYP2B6 and CYP2C8 in vitro with Ki values of 6 and 1-2 μM, respectively. Systemic exposure to substrates of CYP2B6 and CYP2C8 is expected to increase when co-administered with sorafenib. Caution is recommended when administering substrates of CYP2B6 and CYP2C8 with sorafenib). Products include:
Vesanoid Capsules 2660
Ziana Gel 1942

Triamcinolone (Inducers of CYP3A4 activity may increase the metabolism of sorafenib and thus decrease sorafenib concentrations).
No products indexed under this heading.

Triamcinolone Acetonide (Inducers of CYP3A4 activity may increase the metabolism of sorafenib and thus decrease sorafenib concentrations). Products include:
Azmacort Inhalation Aerosol 407
Nasacort AQ Nasal Spray 2765
Triesence Injectable Suspension .... ⊙ 209

Triamcinolone Diacetate (Inducers of CYP3A4 activity may increase the metabolism of sorafenib and thus decrease sorafenib concentrations).
No products indexed under this heading.

Triamcinolone Hexacetonide (Inducers of CYP3A4 activity may increase the metabolism of sorafenib and thus decrease sorafenib concentrations).
No products indexed under this heading.

Trimipramine Maleate (Sorafenib inhibits CYP2B6 and CYP2C8 in vitro with Ki values of 6 and 1-2 μM, respectively. Systemic exposure to substrates of CYP2B6 and CYP2C8 is expected to increase when co-administered with sorafenib. Caution is recommended when administering substrates of CYP2B6 and CYP2C8 with sorafenib).
No products indexed under this heading.

Troglitazone (Inducers of CYP3A4 activity may increase the metabolism of sorafenib and thus decrease sorafenib concentrations).
No products indexed under this heading.

Verapamil Hydrochloride (Sorafenib inhibits CYP2B6 and CYP2C8 in vitro with Ki values of 6 and 1-2 μM, respectively. Systemic exposure to substrates of CYP2B6 and CYP2C8 is expected to increase when co-administered with sorafenib. Caution is recommended when administering substrates of CYP2B6 and CYP2C8 with sorafenib).
Products include:
Tarka Tablets 511

Vitamin A (Sorafenib inhibits CYP2B6 and CYP2C8 in vitro with Ki values of 6 and 1-2 μM, respectively. Systemic exposure to substrates of CYP2B6 and CYP2C8 is expected to increase when co-administered with sorafenib. Caution is recommended when administering substrates of CYP2B6 and CYP2C8 with sorafenib). Products include:
Norwegian Cod Liver Oil 949

Vitamin A Acetate (Sorafenib inhibits CYP2B6 and CYP2C8 in vitro with Ki values of 6 and 1-2 μM, respectively. Systemic exposure to substrates of CYP2B6 and CYP2C8 is expected to increase when co-administered with sorafenib. Caution is recommended when administering substrates of CYP2B6 and CYP2C8 with sorafenib).
No products indexed under this heading.

Warfarin Sodium (Infrequent bleeding or elevations in the International Normalized Ratio (INR) have been reported in some patients taking warfarin while on sorafenib therapy. Patients taking concomitant warfarin should be monitored regularly for changes in prothrombin time, INR or clinical bleeding episodes).
No products indexed under this heading.

Zopiclone (Sorafenib inhibits CYP2B6 and CYP2C8 in vitro with Ki values of 6 and 1-2 μM, respectively. Systemic exposure to substrates of CYP2B6 and CYP2C8 is expected to increase when co-administered with sorafenib. Caution is recommended when administering substrates of CYP2B6 and CYP2C8 with sorafenib).
No products indexed under this heading.

NEXIUM DELAYED-RELEASE CAPSULES

(Esomeprazole Magnesium) 645
May interact with iron containing oral preparations and certain other agents. Compounds in these categories include:

Amoxicillin (Co-administration of esomeprazole, clarithromycin, and amoxicillin has resulted in an increase in the plasma levels of esomeprazole and 14-hydroxyclarithromycin; the observed increase in esomeprazole exposure during co-administration with clarithromycin and amoxicillin is not expected to produce safety concerns). Products include:
Amoxil Capsules 1305
Amoxil Chewable Tablets 1305

Amoxil Pediatric Drops for Oral Suspension 1305
Amoxil Powder for Oral Suspension 1305
Amoxil Tablets 1305
Augmentin 1323
Augmentin Tablets 1327
Augmentin XR Extended Release Tablets 1333
Augmentin ES-600 Powder for Oral Suspension 1329
Moxatag Tablets 2165

Amoxicillin Trihydrate (Co-administration of esomeprazole, clarithromycin, and amoxicillin has resulted in an increase in the plasma levels of esomeprazole and 14-hydroxyclarithromycin; the observed increase in esomeprazole exposure during co-administration with clarithromycin and amoxicillin is not expected to produce safety concerns).
No products indexed under this heading.

Atazanavir (Concomitant use of atazanavir and proton pump inhibitors is not recommended. Co-administration of atazanavir with proton pump inhibitors may substantially decrease atazanavir plasma concentrations and may reduce its therapeutic effect).
No products indexed under this heading.

Clarithromycin (Co-administration of esomeprazole, clarithromycin, and amoxicillin has resulted in an increase in the plasma levels of esomeprazole and 14-hydroxyclarithromycin; the observed increase in esomeprazole exposure during co-administration with clarithromycin and amoxicillin is not expected to produce safety concerns). Products include:
Biaxin/Biaxin XL 411

Diazepam (Esomeprazole may interfere with CYP2C19, the major metabolizing enzyme; co-administration of esomeprazole and diazepam, a CYP2C19 substrate, resulted in a 45% decrease in clearance of diazepam; increased plasma levels of diazepam were observed 12 hours after dosing and onwards; however, at that time the plasma levels of diazepam were below the therapeutic interval, and this interaction is unlikely to be of clinical relevance). Products include:
Valium Tablets 2658

Digoxin (Esomeprazole inhibits gastric acid secretion; therefore, esomeprazole may interfere with the absorption of drugs where gastric pH is an important determinant of bioavailability, such as digoxin). Products include:
Lanoxin Injection 1498
Lanoxin Injection Pediatric 1502
Lanoxin Tablets 1505

Ferrous Fumarate (Esomeprazole inhibits gastric acid secretion; therefore, esomeprazole may interfere with the absorption of drugs where gastric pH is an important determinant of bioavailability, such as oral iron salts).
No products indexed under this heading.

Ferrous Gluconate (Esomeprazole inhibits gastric acid secretion; therefore, esomeprazole may interfere with the absorption of drugs where gastric pH is an important determinant of bioavailability, such as oral iron salts). Products include:
CitraNatal DHA Tablets 2175

Ferrous Sulfate (Esomeprazole inhibits gastric acid secretion; therefore, esomeprazole may interfere with the absorption of drugs where gastric pH is an important determinant of bioavailability, such as oral iron salts).
No products indexed under this heading.

Iron (Esomeprazole inhibits gastric acid secretion; therefore, esomeprazole may interfere with the absorption of drugs where gastric pH is an important determinant of bioavailability, such as oral iron salts). Products include:
Phyto-Vite Tablets 639

Ketoconazole (Esomeprazole inhibits gastric acid secretion; therefore, esomeprazole may interfere with the absorption of drugs where gastric pH is an important determinant of bioavailability, such as ketoconazole). Products include:
Extina Foam, 2% 3057
Nizoral A-D Shampoo 1901

Pimozide (Co-administration of clarithromycin-esomeprazole combination with pimozide is contraindicated; concurrent use of clarithromycin and/or erythromycin with pimozide has resulted in cardiac arrhythmias including QT prolongation, ventricular tachycardia, ventricular fibrillations and torsade de pointes).
No products indexed under this heading.

Polysaccharide Iron Complex (Esomeprazole inhibits gastric acid secretion; therefore, esomeprazole may interfere with the absorption of drugs where gastric pH is an important determinant of bioavailability, such as oral iron salts). Products include:
Nu-Iron 150 Capsules 2165

Voriconazole (Concomitant administration of esomeprazole and a combined inhibitor of CYP2C19 and CYP3A4, such as voriconazole, may result in more than doubling of the esomeprazole exposure. dose adjustment of esomeprazole is not normally required. However, in patients with Zollinger-Ellison's syndrome, who may require higher doses up to 240mg/day, dose adjustment may be considered).
No products indexed under this heading.

Warfarin Sodium (Changes in prothrombin measures have been reported among patients on concomitant warfarin and esomeprazole therapy. Increases in INR and prothrombin time may lead to abnormal bleeding and even death. Patients treated with proton pump inhibitors and warfarin concomitantly may need to be monitored for increases in INR and prothrombin time).
No products indexed under this heading.

NEXIUM I.V.

(Esomeprazole Sodium) 652
May interact with iron containing oral preparations and certain other agents. Compounds in these categories include:

Atazanavir (Concomitant administration of esomeprazole may reduce the plasma levels of atazanavir; appropriate clinical monitoring is recommended. Concomitant use of atazanavir and proton pump inhibitors is not recommended).
No products indexed under this heading.

Atazanavir Sulfate (Concomitant administration of esomeprazole may reduce the plasma levels of atazanavir; appropriate clinical monitoring is recommended. Concomitant use of atazanavir and proton pump inhibitors is not recommended). Products include:
Reyataz Capsules 3299

Diazepam (Esomeprazole may interfere with CYP2C19, the major metabolizing enzyme; co-administration of esomeprazole and diazepam, a CYP2C19 substrate, resulted in a 45% decrease in clearance of diazepam; increased plasma levels of diazepam were observed 12 hours after dosing and onwards; however, at that time the plasma levels of diazepam were below the therapeutic interval, and this interaction is unlikely to be of clinical relevance). Products include:
Valium Tablets 2658

Digoxin (Esomeprazole inhibits gastric acid secretion; therefore, esomeprazole may interfere with the absorption of drugs where gastric pH is an important determinant of bioavailability, such as digoxin). Products include:
Lanoxin Injection 1498
Lanoxin Injection Pediatric 1502
Lanoxin Tablets 1505

Ferrous Fumarate (Esomeprazole inhibits gastric acid secretion; therefore, esomeprazole may interfere with the absorption of drugs where gastric pH is an important determinant of bioavailability, such as oral iron salts).
No products indexed under this heading.

Ferrous Gluconate (Esomeprazole inhibits gastric acid secretion; therefore, esomeprazole may interfere with the absorption of drugs where gastric pH is an important determinant of bioavailability, such as oral iron salts). Products include:
CitraNatal DHA Tablets 2175

Ferrous Sulfate (Esomeprazole inhibits gastric acid secretion; therefore, esomeprazole may interfere with the absorption of drugs where gastric pH is an important determinant of bioavailability, such as oral iron salts).
No products indexed under this heading.

Iron (Esomeprazole inhibits gastric acid secretion; therefore, esomeprazole may interfere with the absorption of drugs where gastric pH is an important determinant of bioavailability, such as oral iron salts). Products include:
Phyto-Vite Tablets 639

Ketoconazole (Esomeprazole inhibits gastric acid secretion; therefore, esomeprazole may interfere with the absorption of drugs where gastric pH is an important determinant of bioavailability, such as ketoconazole). Products include:
Extina Foam, 2% 3057
Nizoral A-D Shampoo 1901

Pimozide (Co-administration of clarithromycin-esomeprazole combination with pimozide is contraindicated; concurrent use of clarithromycin and/or erythromycin with pimozide has resulted in cardiac arrhythmias including QT prolongation, ventricular tachycardia, ventricular fibrillations and torsade de pointes).
No products indexed under this heading.

Polysaccharide Iron Complex (Esomeprazole inhibits gastric acid secretion; therefore, esomeprazole may interfere with the absorption of drugs where gastric pH is an important determinant of bioavailability, such as oral iron salts). Products include:
Nu-Iron 150 Capsules 2165

Voriconazole (Concomitant administration of esomeprazole and a combined inhibitor of CYP2C19 and CYP3A4, such as voriconazole, may result in more than doubling of the esomeprazole exposure. Dose adjustment of esomeprazole is not normally required for the recommended doses. However, in patients who may require higher doses, dose adjustment may be considered).
No products indexed under this heading.

Warfarin Sodium (Changes in prothrombin measures have been reported among patients on concomitant warfarin and esomeprazole therapy. Increases in INR and prothrombin time may lead to abnormal bleeding and even death. Patients treated with proton pump inhibitors and warfarin concomitantly may need to be monitored for increases in INR and prothrombin time).
No products indexed under this heading.

NEXIUM DELAYED-RELEASE ORAL SUSPENSION

(Esomeprazole Magnesium) 645
See Nexium Delayed-Release Capsules

NIASPAN EXTENDED-RELEASE TABLETS

(Niacin) 480
May interact with beta blockers, calcium channel blockers, oral anticoagulants, HMG-CoA reductase inhibitors, nitrates and nitrites, and certain other agents. Compounds in these categories include:

Acebutolol Hydrochloride (Co-administration with vasoactive drugs, such as adrenergic blocking agents, may result in postural hypotension, particularly in patients with unstable angina or acute phase of myocardial infarction).
No products indexed under this heading.

Amlodipine Besylate (Co-administration with vasoactive drugs, such as calcium channel blockers, may result in postural hypotension, particularly in patients with unstable angina or acute phase of myocardial infarction). Products include:
Azor Tablets 1005
Exforge Tablets 2238

Amyl Nitrite (Co-administration with vasoactive drugs, such as nitrates, may result in postural hypotension, particularly in patients with unstable angina or acute phase of myocardial infarction).
No products indexed under this heading.

Anisindione (Niacin prolongs prothrombin time; caution should be exercised when used concurrently).
No products indexed under this heading.

Aspirin (Concomitant aspirin may decrease the metabolic clearance of nicotinic acid; the clinical relevance of this finding is unclear). Products include:
Aggrenox Capsules 819
Bayer Aspirin 750
Percodan Tablets 1130
St. Joseph 81 mg Aspirin Chewable and Enteric Coated Tablets 1903

Atenolol (Co-administration with vasoactive drugs, such as adrenergic blocking agents, may result in postural hypotension, particularly in patients with unstable angina or acute phase of myocardial infarction).
No products indexed under this heading.

Atorvastatin Calcium (Co-administration of lipid-altering doses (≥ 1 g/day) of niacin and HMG-CoA reductase inhibitors has resulted in rare cases of rhabdomyolysis). Products include:
Lipitor Tablets 2501

Bepridil Hydrochloride (Co-administration with vasoactive drugs, such as calcium channel blockers, may result in postural hypotension, particularly in patients with unstable angina or acute phase of myocardial infarction).
No products indexed under this heading.

Betaxolol Hydrochloride (Co-administration with vasoactive drugs, such as adrenergic blocking agents, may result in postural hypotension, particularly in patients with unstable angina or acute phase of myocardial infarction).
No products indexed under this heading.

Bisoprolol Fumarate (Co-administration with vasoactive drugs, such as adrenergic blocking agents, may result in postural hypotension, particularly in patients with unstable angina or acute phase of myocardial infarction).
No products indexed under this heading.

Carteolol Hydrochloride (Co-administration with vasoactive drugs, such as adrenergic blocking agents, may result in postural hypotension, particularly in patients with unstable angina or acute phase of myocardial infarction).
No products indexed under this heading.

Cerivastatin Sodium (Co-administration of lipid-altering doses (≥ 1 g/day) of niacin and HMG-CoA reductase inhibitors has resulted in rare cases of rhabdomyolysis).
No products indexed under this heading.

Cholestyramine (*In vitro* study resulted in approximately 10% to 30% of available niacin bound to cholestyramine; 4 to 6 hours or greater should elapse between ingestion of bile acid-binding resins and the administration of Niaspan).
No products indexed under this heading.

Colestipol Hydrochloride (*In vitro* study resulted in approximately 90% of available niacin bound to colestipol; 4 to 6 hours or greater should elapse between ingestion of bile acid-binding resins and the administration of Niaspan).
No products indexed under this heading.

Dicumarol (Niacin prolongs prothrombin time; caution should be exercised when used concurrently).
No products indexed under this heading.

Diltiazem Hydrochloride (Co-administration with vasoactive drugs, such as calcium channel blockers, may result in postural hypotension, particularly in patients with unstable angina or acute phase of myocardial infarction). Products include:
Cardizem LA Extended Release Tablets 421

Erythrityl Tetranitrate (Co-administration with vasoactive drugs, such as nitrates, may result in postural hypotension, particularly in patients with unstable angina or acute phase of myocardial infarction).
No products indexed under this heading.

Esmolol Hydrochloride (Co-administration with vasoactive drugs, such as adrenergic blocking agents, may result in postural hypotension, particularly in patients with unstable angina or acute phase of myocardial infarction).
No products indexed under this heading.

Felodipine (Co-administration with vasoactive drugs, such as calcium channel blockers, may result in postural hypotension, particularly in patients with unstable angina or acute phase of myocardial infarction).
No products indexed under this heading.

Fluvastatin Sodium (Co-administration of lipid-altering doses (≥ 1 g/day) of niacin and HMG-CoA reductase inhibitors has resulted in rare cases of rhabdomyolysis). Products include:
Lescol Capsules 2268
Lescol XL Tablets 2268

Isosorbide Dinitrate (Co-administration with vasoactive drugs, such as nitrates, may result in postural hypotension, particularly in patients with unstable angina or acute phase of myocardial infarction).
No products indexed under this heading.

Isosorbide Mononitrate (Co-administration with vasoactive drugs, such as nitrates, may result in postural hypotension, particularly in patients with unstable angina or acute phase of myocardial infarction).
No products indexed under this heading.

Isradipine (Co-administration with vasoactive drugs, such as calcium channel blockers, may result in postural hypotension, particularly in patients with unstable angina or acute phase of myocardial infarction). Products include:
DynaCirc CR Controlled Release Tablets 1407

Labetalol Hydrochloride (Co-administration with vasoactive drugs, such as adrenergic blocking agents, may result in postural hypotension, particularly in patients with unstable angina or acute phase of myocardial infarction).
No products indexed under this heading.

Levobunolol Hydrochloride (Co-administration with vasoactive drugs, such as adrenergic blocking agents, may result in postural hypotension, particularly in patients with unstable angina or acute phase of myocardial infarction).
No products indexed under this heading.

Lovastatin (Co-administration of lipid-altering doses (≥ 1 g/day) of niacin and HMG-CoA reductase inhibitors has resulted in rare cases of rhabdomyolysis). Products include:
Advicor Tablets 402
Mevacor Tablets 2063

Mecamylamine Hydrochloride (Niacin may potentiate the effects of ganglionic blocking agents, such as mecamylamine, resulting in postural hypotension).
No products indexed under this heading.

Metipranolol Hydrochloride (Co-administration with vasoactive drugs, such as adrenergic blocking agents, may result in postural hypotension, particularly in patients with unstable angina or acute phase of myocardial infarction).
No products indexed under this heading.

Metoprolol Succinate (Co-administration with vasoactive drugs, such as adrenergic blocking agents, may result in postural hypotension, particularly in patients with unstable angina or acute phase of myocardial infarction). Products include:
Toprol-XL Tablets 666

Metoprolol Tartrate (Co-administration with vasoactive drugs, such as adrenergic blocking agents, may result in postural hypotension, particularly in patients with unstable angina or acute phase of myocardial infarction).
No products indexed under this heading.

Mibefradil Dihydrochloride (Co-administration with vasoactive drugs, such as calcium channel blockers, may result in postural hypotension, particularly in patients with unstable angina or acute phase of myocardial infarction).
No products indexed under this heading.

Nadolol (Co-administration with vasoactive drugs, such as adrenergic blocking agents, may result in postural hypotension, particularly in patients with unstable angina or acute phase of myocardial infarction). Products include:
Nadolol Tablets 2191

Nebivolol (Co-administration with vasoactive drugs, such as adrenergic blocking agents, may result in postural hypotension, particularly in patients with unstable angina or acute phase of myocardial infarction). Products include:
Bystolic Tablets 1155

Nicardipine Hydrochloride (Co-administration with vasoactive drugs, such as calcium channel blockers, may result in postural hypotension, particularly in patients with unstable angina or acute phase of myocardial infarction). Products include:
Cardene I.V. 1093

Nicotinamide (May potentiate the adverse effects of Niaspan).
No products indexed under this heading.

Nifedipine (Co-administration with vasoactive drugs, such as calcium channel blockers, may result in postural hypotension, particularly in patients with unstable angina or acute phase of myocardial infarction).
No products indexed under this heading.

Nimodipine (Co-administration with vasoactive drugs, such as calcium channel blockers, may result in postural hypotension, particularly in patients with unstable angina or acute phase of myocardial infarction). Products include:
Nimotop Capsules 790

Nisoldipine (Co-administration with vasoactive drugs, such as calcium channel blockers, may result in postural hypotension, particularly in patients with unstable angina or acute phase of myocardial infarction). Products include:
Sular Extended Release Tablets 2975

Nitroglycerin (Co-administration with vasoactive drugs, such as nitrates, may result in postural hypotension, particularly in patients with unstable angina or acute phase of myocardial infarction). Products include:
Nitro-Dur Transdermal Infusion System 2887
Nitrolingual Pumpspray 2965

Penbutolol Sulfate (Co-administration with vasoactive drugs, such as adrenergic blocking agents, may result in postural hypotension, particularly in patients with unstable angina or acute phase of myocardial infarction).
No products indexed under this heading.

Pentaerythritol Tetranitrate (Co-administration with vasoactive drugs, such as nitrates, may result in postural hypotension, particularly in patients with unstable angina or acute phase of myocardial infarction).
No products indexed under this heading.

Pindolol (Co-administration with vasoactive drugs, such as adrenergic blocking agents, may result in postural hypotension, particularly in patients with unstable angina or acute phase of myocardial infarction).
No products indexed under this heading.

Pravastatin Sodium (Co-administration of lipid-altering doses (≥ 1 g/day) of niacin and HMG-CoA reductase inhibitors has resulted in rare cases of rhabdomyolysis).
No products indexed under this heading.

Propranolol Hydrochloride (Co-administration with vasoactive drugs, such as adrenergic blocking agents, may result in postural hypotension, particularly in patients with unstable angina or acute phase of myocardial infarction). Products include:

InnoPran XL Extended Release Capsules 1484

Rosuvastatin Calcium (Co-administration of lipid-altering doses ($\geq$ 1 g/day) of niacin and HMG-CoA reductase inhibitors has resulted in rare cases of rhabdomyolysis). Products include:

Crestor Tablets 677

Simvastatin (Co-administration of lipid-altering doses ($\geq$ 1 g/day) of niacin and HMG-CoA reductase inhibitors has resulted in rare cases of rhabdomyolysis). Products include:

Simcor Tablets 502
Vytorin 10/10 Tablets 2149
Vytorin 10/10 Tablets 2939
Vytorin 10/20 Tablets 2149
Vytorin 10/20 Tablets 2939
Vytorin 10/40 Tablets 2149
Vytorin 10/40 Tablets 2939
Vytorin 10/80 Tablets 2149
Vytorin 10/80 Tablets 2939
Zocor Tablets 2136

Sotalol Hydrochloride (Co-administration with vasoactive drugs, such as adrenergic blocking agents, may result in postural hypotension, particularly in patients with unstable angina or acute phase of myocardial infarction).

No products indexed under this heading.

Timolol Hemihydrate (Co-administration with vasoactive drugs, such as adrenergic blocking agents, may result in postural hypotension, particularly in patients with unstable angina or acute phase of myocardial infarction). Products include:

Betimol Ophthalmic Solution 3181

Timolol Maleate (Co-administration with vasoactive drugs, such as adrenergic blocking agents, may result in postural hypotension, particularly in patients with unstable angina or acute phase of myocardial infarction). Products include:

Combigan Ophthalmic Solution 553
Cosopt Sterile Ophthalmic Solution 1969
Timoptic Sterile Ophthalmic Solution 2121
Timoptic in Ocudose 2124
Timoptic-XE Sterile Ophthalmic Gel Forming Solution 2125

Verapamil Hydrochloride (Co-administration with vasoactive drugs, such as calcium channel blockers, may result in postural hypotension, particularly in patients with unstable angina or acute phase of myocardial infarction). Products include:

Tarka Tablets 511

Warfarin Sodium (Niacin prolongs prothrombin time; caution should be exercised when used concurrently).

No products indexed under this heading.

Food Interactions

Alcohol (Concomitant alcohol may increase the side effects of flushing and pruritus and should be avoided around the time of Niaspan ingestion).

Drinks, hot, unspecified (Concomitant hot drinks may increase the side effects of flushing and pruritus and should be avoided around the time of Niaspan ingestion).

NIMBEX INJECTION

(Cisatracurium Besylate) 484

May interact with aminoglycosides, lithium preparations, local anesthetics, phenytoin, tetracyclines, and certain other agents. Compounds in these categories include:

Amikacin Sulfate (Enhances neuromuscular blocking action).

No products indexed under this heading.

Bacitracin (Enhances neuromuscular blocking action).

No products indexed under this heading.

Bupivacaine Hydrochloride (Enhances neuromuscular blocking action).

No products indexed under this heading.

Carbamazepine (Chronic administration of carbamazepine may produce resistance to the neuromuscular blocking action; slightly shorter durations of neuromuscular block may be anticipated). Products include:

Carbatrol Capsules 3019
Equetro Extended-Release Capsules 3174

Chloroprocaine Hydrochloride (Enhances neuromuscular blocking action).

No products indexed under this heading.

Clindamycin Hydrochloride (Enhances neuromuscular blocking action).

No products indexed under this heading.

Clindamycin Palmitate Hydrochloride (Enhances neuromuscular blocking action).

No products indexed under this heading.

Clindamycin Phosphate (Enhances neuromuscular blocking action). Products include:

Benzaclin Topical Gel 2721
Evoclin Foam, 1% 3056
Ziana Gel 1942

Colistimethate Sodium (Enhances neuromuscular blocking action).

No products indexed under this heading.

Colistin Sulfate (Enhances neuromuscular blocking action).

No products indexed under this heading.

Demeclocycline Hydrochloride (Enhances neuromuscular blocking action).

No products indexed under this heading.

Doxycycline Calcium (Enhances neuromuscular blocking action).

No products indexed under this heading.

Doxycycline Hyclate (Enhances neuromuscular blocking action).

No products indexed under this heading.

Doxycycline Monohydrate (Enhances neuromuscular blocking action).

No products indexed under this heading.

Enflurane (Enflurane administered with nitrous oxide/oxygen may prolong the clinically effective duration of action of initial and maintenance doses of cisatracurium and decrease the required infusion rate of cisatracurium).

No products indexed under this heading.

Etidocaine Hydrochloride (Enhances neuromuscular blocking action).

No products indexed under this heading.

Fosphenytoin Sodium (Chronic administration of phenytoin may produce resistance to the neuromuscular blocking action; slightly shorter durations of neuromuscular block may be anticipated).

No products indexed under this heading.

Gentamicin Sulfate (Enhances neuromuscular blocking action). Products include:

Pred-G Ophthalmic Ointment .... ⊙ 229
Pred-G Ophthalmic Suspension .... ⊙ 228

Isoflurane (Isoflurane administered with nitrous oxide/oxygen may prolong the clinically effective duration of action of initial and maintenance doses of cisatracurium and decrease the required infusion rate of cisatracurium).

No products indexed under this heading.

Kanamycin Sulfate (Enhances neuromuscular blocking action).

No products indexed under this heading.

Levobupivacaine Hydrochloride (Enhances neuromuscular blocking action).

No products indexed under this heading.

Lidocaine Hydrochloride (Enhances neuromuscular blocking action).

No products indexed under this heading.

Lincomycin Hydrochloride (Enhances neuromuscular blocking action).

No products indexed under this heading.

Lithium (Enhances neuromuscular blocking action).

No products indexed under this heading.

Lithium Carbonate (Enhances neuromuscular blocking action).

No products indexed under this heading.

Lithium Citrate (Enhances neuromuscular blocking action).

No products indexed under this heading.

Magnesium Salts (Enhances neuromuscular blocking action).

No products indexed under this heading.

Mepivacaine Hydrochloride (Enhances neuromuscular blocking action).

No products indexed under this heading.

Methacycline Hydrochloride (Enhances neuromuscular blocking action).

No products indexed under this heading.

Minocycline Hydrochloride (Enhances neuromuscular blocking action). Products include:

Solodyn Extended Release Tablets 1938

Oxytetracycline Hydrochloride (Enhances neuromuscular blocking action).

No products indexed under this heading.

Phenytoin (Chronic administration of phenytoin may produce resistance to the neuromuscular blocking action; slightly shorter durations of neuromuscular block may be anticipated).

No products indexed under this heading.

Phenytoin Sodium (Chronic administration of phenytoin may produce resistance to the neuromuscular blocking action; slightly shorter durations of neuromuscular block may be anticipated). Products include:

Phenytek Capsules 2192

Polymyxin Preparations (Enhances neuromuscular blocking action).

No products indexed under this heading.

Procainamide Hydrochloride (Enhances neuromuscular blocking action).

No products indexed under this heading.

Procaine Hydrochloride (Enhances neuromuscular blocking action).

No products indexed under this heading.

Quinidine Gluconate (Enhances neuromuscular blocking action).

No products indexed under this heading.

Quinidine Polygalacturonate (Enhances neuromuscular blocking action).

No products indexed under this heading.

Quinidine Sulfate (Enhances neuromuscular blocking action).

No products indexed under this heading.

Streptomycin Sulfate (Enhances neuromuscular blocking action).

No products indexed under this heading.

Tetracaine Hydrochloride (Enhances neuromuscular blocking action).

No products indexed under this heading.

Tetracycline Hydrochloride (Enhances neuromuscular blocking action). Products include:

Pylera Capsules 714

Tobramycin (Enhances neuromuscular blocking action). Products include:

Zylet Ophthalmic Suspension .... ⊙ 247

Tobramycin Sulfate (Enhances neuromuscular blocking action).

No products indexed under this heading.

NIMOTOP CAPSULES

(Nimodipine) 790

May interact with ACE inhibitors, alpha adrenergic blockers, antihypertensives, azole antifungals, beta blockers, calcium channel blockers, cytochrome p450 3a4 inducers (selected), cytochrome p450 3a4 inhibitors (selected), diuretics, macrolide antibiotics, PDE5 inhibitors, phenytoin, protease inhibitors, and certain other agents. Compounds in these categories include:

Acebutolol Hydrochloride (Nimodipine may increase the blood pressure lowering effect of concomitantly administered anti-hypertensives such as beta blockers. However, if a combination of this type proves unavoidable, particularly careful monitoring of the patient is necessary).

No products indexed under this heading.

Acetazolamide (Nimodipine is metabolized via cytochrome P450 3A4 system located both in the intestinal mucosa and in the liver. Plasma concentrations of drugs which are known inhibitors of the cytochrome P450 3A4 system may be increased. Upon co-administration of drugs which are known inhibitors of cytochrome P450 3A4, the blood pressure should be monitored and, if necessary, a reduction of the nimodipine dose should be considered).
No products indexed under this heading.

Aliskiren (Nimodipine may increase the blood presure lowering effect of concomitantly administered anti-hypertensives. However, if a combination of this type proves undavoidable particularly careful monitoring of the patient is necessary). Products include:
Tekturna Tablets ... 2321
Tekturna HCT Tablets ... 2324

Allium sativum (Nimodipine is metabolized via the cytochrome P450 3A4 system located both in the intestinal mucosa and in the liver. Drugs that are known to induce cytochrome P450 3A4 may therefore alter the first pass or the clearance of nimodipine).
No products indexed under this heading.

Amiloride Hydrochloride (Nimodipine may increase the blood pressure lowering effect of concomitantly administered anti-hypertensives such as diuretics. However, if a combination of this type proves unavoidable, particularly careful monitoring of the patient is necessary).
No products indexed under this heading.

Amiodarone Hydrochloride (Nimodipine is metabolized via cytochrome P450 3A4 system located both in the intestinal mucosa and in the liver. Plasma concentrations of drugs which are known inhibitors of the cytochrome P450 3A4 system may be increased. Upon co-administration of drugs which are known inhibitors of cytochrome P450 3A4, the blood pressure should be monitored and, if necessary, a reduction of the nimodipine dose should be considered).
No products indexed under this heading.

Amlodipine Besylate (Nimodipine may increase the blood pressure lowering effect of concomitantly administered anti-hypertensives such as other calcium antagonists. However, if a combination of this type proves unavoidable particularly careful monitoring of the patient is necessary). Products include:
Azor Tablets ... 1005
Exforge Tablets ... 2238

Amprenavir (No formal studies have been performed to investigate the potential interaction between nimodipine and anti-HIV protease inhibitors. Drugs of this class have been reported to be potent inhibitors of the cytochrome P450 3A4 system. Therefore, the potential for a marked and clinically relevant increase in nimodipine plasma concentrations upon co-administration with these protease inhibitors cannot be excluded. Upon co-administration with protease inhibitors, which are inhibitors of the cytochrome P450 3A4 system, blood pressure should be monitored and, if necessary, an adjustment in the nimodipine dose should be considered).
No products indexed under this heading.

Anastrozole (Nimodipine is metabolized via cytochrome P450 3A4 system located both in the intestinal mucosa and in the liver. Plasma concentrations of drugs which are known inhibitors of the cytochrome P450 3A4 system may be increased. Upon co-administration of drugs which are known inhibitors of cytochrome P450 3A4, the blood pressure should be monitored and, if necessary, a reduction of the nimodipine dose should be considered). Products include:
Arimidex Tablets ... 672

Aprepitant (Nimodipine is metabolized via cytochrome P450 3A4 system located both in the intestinal mucosa and in the liver. Plasma concentrations of drugs which are known inhibitors of the cytochrome P450 3A4 system may be increased. Upon co-administration of drugs which are known inhibitors of cytochrome P450 3A4, the blood pressure should be monitored and, if necessary, a reduction of the nimodipine dose should be considered). Products include:
Emend Capsules ... 1992

Atazanavir (Nimodipine is metabolized via cytochrome P450 3A4 system located both in the intestinal mucosa and in the liver. Plasma concentrations of drugs which are known inhibitors of the cytochrome P450 3A4 system may be increased. Upon co-administration of drugs which are known inhibitors of cytochrome P450 3A4, the blood pressure should be monitored and, if necessary, a reduction of the nimodipine dose should be considered).
No products indexed under this heading.

Atazanavir Sulfate (Nimodipine is metabolized via cytochrome P450 3A4 system located both in the intestinal mucosa and in the liver. Plasma concentrations of drugs which are known inhibitors of the cytochrome P450 3A4 system may be increased. Upon co-administration of drugs which are known inhibitors of cytochrome P450 3A4, the blood pressure should be monitored and, if necessary, a reduction of the nimodipine dose should be considered). Products include:
Reyataz Capsules ... 3299

Atenolol (Nimodipine may increase the blood pressure lowering effect of concomitantly administered anti-hypertensives such as beta blockers. However, if a combination of this type proves unavoidable, particularly careful monitoring of the patient is necessary).
No products indexed under this heading.

Azithromycin Dihydrate (No interaction studies have been carried out between nimodipine and macrolide antibiotics. Certain macrolide antibiotics are known to inhibit cytochrome P450 3A4 system and the potential for drug interaction cannot be ruled out at this stage. Therefore, macrolide antibiotics should not be used in combination with nimodipine. However, if macrolide antibiotics which are inhibitors of the cytochrome P450 3A4 system are co-administered with nimodipine, blood pressure should be monitored and, if necessary, an adjustment in the nimodipine dose should be considered. Azithromycin, although structurally related to the class of macrolide, is void of CYP3A4 inhibition).
No products indexed under this heading.

Benazepril Hydrochloride (Nimodipine may increase the blood pressure lowering effect of concomitantly administered anti-hypertensives such as ACE inhibitors. However, if a combination of this type proves unavoidable, particularly careful monitoring of the patient is necessary).
No products indexed under this heading.

Bendroflumethiazide (Nimodipine may increase the blood pressure lowering effect of concomitantly administered anti-hypertensives such as diuretics. However, if a combination of this type proves unavoidable, particularly careful monitoring of the patient is necessary).
No products indexed under this heading.

Bepridil Hydrochloride (Nimodipine may increase the blood pressure lowering effect of concomitantly administered anti-hypertensives such as other calcium antagonists. However, if a combination of this type proves unavoidable particularly careful monitoring of the patient is necessary).
No products indexed under this heading.

Betamethasone Acetate (Nimodipine is metabolized via the cytochrome P450 3A4 system located both in the intestinal mucosa and in the liver. Drugs that are known to induce cytochrome P450 3A4 may therefore alter the first pass or the clearance of nimodipine).
No products indexed under this heading.

Betamethasone Sodium Phosphate (Nimodipine is metabolized via the cytochrome P450 3A4 system located both in the intestinal mucosa and in the liver. Drugs that are known to induce cytochrome P450 3A4 may therefore alter the first pass or the clearance of nimodipine).
No products indexed under this heading.

Betaxolol Hydrochloride (Nimodipine may increase the blood pressure lowering effect of concomitantly administered anti-hypertensives such as beta blockers. However, if a combination of this type proves unavoidable, particularly careful monitoring of the patient is necessary).
No products indexed under this heading.

Bisoprolol Fumarate (Nimodipine may increase the blood pressure lowering effect of concomitantly administered anti-hypertensives such as beta blockers. However, if a combination of this type proves unavoidable, particularly careful monitoring of the patient is necessary).
No products indexed under this heading.

Bumetanide (Nimodipine may increase the blood pressure lowering effect of concomitantly administered anti-hypertensives such as diuretics. However, if a combination of this type proves unavoidable, particularly careful monitoring of the patient is necessary).
No products indexed under this heading.

Candesartan Cilexetil (Nimodipine may increase the blood presure lowering effect of concomitantly administered anti-hypertensives. However, if a combination of this type proves undavoidable particularly careful monitoring of the patient is necessary). Products include:
Atacand Tablets ... 639
Atacand HCT ... 642

Captopril (Nimodipine may increase the blood pressure lowering effect of concomitantly administered anti-hypertensives such as ACE inhibitors. However, if a combination of this type proves unavoidable, particularly careful monitoring of the patient is necessary). Products include:
Captopril Tablets ... 2182

Carbamazepine (Previous chronic administration of the antiepileptic drug carbamazepine markedly reduces the bioavailability of orally administered nimodipine. Therefore, the concomitant use of oral nimodipine and carbamazepine is contraindicated). Products include:
Carbatrol Capsules ... 3019
Equetro Extended-Release Capsules ... 3174

Carteolol Hydrochloride (Nimodipine may increase the blood pressure lowering effect of concomitantly administered anti-hypertensives such as beta blockers. However, if a combination of this type proves unavoidable, particularly careful monitoring of the patient is necessary).
No products indexed under this heading.

Chlorothiazide (Nimodipine may increase the blood pressure lowering effect of concomitantly administered anti-hypertensives such as diuretics. However, if a combination of this type proves unavoidable, particularly careful monitoring of the patient is necessary).
No products indexed under this heading.

Chlorothiazide Sodium (Nimodipine may increase the blood pressure lowering effect of concomitantly administered anti-hypertensives such as diuretics. However, if a combination of this type proves unavoidable, particularly careful monitoring of the patient is necessary). Products include:
Intravenous Sodium Diuril ... 2490

Chlorthalidone (Nimodipine may increase the blood pressure lowering effect of concomitantly administered anti-hypertensives such as diuretics. However, if a combination of this type proves unavoidable, particularly careful monitoring of the patient is necessary). Products include:
Clorpres Tablets ... 2185

Cimetidine (The simultaneous administration of the H2-antagonist cimetidine can lead to an increase in the plasma nimodipine concentration. A study in eight healthy volunteers has shown a 50% increase in mean peak nimodipine plasma concentrations and a 90% increase in mean area under the curve, after a one week course of cimetidine at 1,000 mg/day and nimodipine at 90 mg/day. This effect may be mediated by the known inhibition of hepatic cytochrome P-450 by cimetidine, which could decrease first-pass metabolism of nimodipine. Upon co-administration with cimetidine, blood pressure should be monitored and, if necessary, an adjustment in the nimodipine dose should be considered).

No products indexed under this heading.

Cimetidine Hydrochloride (The simultaneous administration of the H2-antagonist cimetidine can lead to an increase in the plasma nimodipine concentration. A study in eight healthy volunteers has shown a 50% increase in mean peak nimodipine plasma concentrations and a 90% increase in mean area under the curve, after a one week course of cimetidine at 1,000 mg/day and nimodipine at 90 mg/day. This effect may be mediated by the known inhibition of hepatic cytochrome P-450 by cimetidine, which could decrease first-pass metabolism of nimodipine. Upon co-administration with cimetidine, blood pressure should be monitored and, if necessary, an adjustment in the nimodipine dose should be considered).

No products indexed under this heading.

Ciprofloxacin (Nimodipine is metabolized via cytochrome P450 3A4 system located both in the intestinal mucosa and in the liver. Plasma concentrations of drugs which are known inhibitors of the cytochrome P450 3A4 system may be increased. Upon co-administration of drugs which are known inhibitors of cytochrome P450 3A4, the blood pressure should be monitored and, if necessary, a reduction of the nimodipine dose should be considered). Products include:

Cipro I.V. ... **2817**
Cipro Oral Suspension ... **2810**
Cipro XR Tablets ... **2823**
Ciprodex Otic Suspension ... **541**

Ciprofloxacin Hydrochloride (Nimodipine is metabolized via the cytochrome P450 3A4 system located both in the intestinal mucosa and in the liver. Drugs that are known to induce cytochrome P450 3A4 may therefore alter the first pass or the clearance of nimodipine). Products include:

Cipro Tablets ... **2810**

Cisplatin (Nimodipine is metabolized via the cytochrome P450 3A4 system located both in the intestinal mucosa and in the liver. Drugs that are known to induce cytochrome P450 3A4 may therefore alter the first pass or the clearance of nimodipine).

No products indexed under this heading.

Clarithromycin (No interaction studies have been carried out between nimodipine and macrolide antibiotics. Certain macrolide antibiotics are known to inhibit cytochrome P450 3A4 system and the potential for drug interaction cannot be ruled out at this stage. Therefore, macrolide antibiotics should not be used in combination with nimodipine. However, if macrolide antibiotics which are inhibitors of the cytochrome P450 3A4 system are co-administered with nimodipine, blood pressure should be monitored and, if necessary, an adjustment in the nimodipine dose should be considered. Azithromycin, although structurally related to the class of macrolide, is void of CYP3A4 inhibition). Products include:

Biaxin/Biaxin XL ... **411**

Clonidine (Nimodipine may increase the blood presure lowering effect of concomitantly administered anti-hypertensives. However, if a combination of this type proves undavoidable particularly careful monitoring of the patient is necessary). Products include:

Catapres-TTS ... **842**

Clonidine Hydrochloride (Nimodipine may increase the blood presure lowering effect of concomitantly administered anti-hypertensives. However, if a combination of this type proves undavoidable particularly careful monitoring of the patient is necessary). Products include:

Catapres Tablets ... **841**
Clorpres Tablets ... **2185**

Clotrimazole (A formal interaction study investigating the potential of drug interaction between nimodipine and ketoconazole has not been performed. Azole anti-mycotics are known to inhibit the cytochrome P450 3A4 system, and various interactions have been reported for other dihydropyridine calcium antagonists. Therefore, when administered together with oral nimodipine, a substantial increase in systemic bioavailability of nimodipine due to a decreased first-pass metabolism cannot be excluded. Upon co-administration with azole anti-mycotics which are inhibitors of the cytochrome P450 3A4 system, blood pressure should be monitored and, if necessary, an adjustment in the nimodipine dose should be considered). Products include:

Lotrisone ... **2881**

Cortisone Acetate (Nimodipine is metabolized via the cytochrome P450 3A4 system located both in the intestinal mucosa and in the liver. Drugs that are known to induce cytochrome P450 3A4 may therefore alter the first pass or the clearance of nimodipine).

No products indexed under this heading.

Cyclosporine (Nimodipine is metabolized via cytochrome P450 3A4 system located both in the intestinal mucosa and in the liver. Plasma concentrations of drugs which are known inhibitors of the cytochrome P450 3A4 system may be increased. Upon co-administration of drugs which are known inhibitors of cytochrome P450 3A4, the blood pressure should be monitored and, if necessary, a reduction of the nimodipine dose should be considered). Products include:

Gengraf Capsules ... **435**
Neoral Oral Solution ... **2280**
Neoral Soft Gelatin Capsules ... **2280**
Restasis Ophthalmic Emulsion ... **557**
Sandimmune ... **2296**

Dalfopristin (Based on experience with the calcium-antagonist nifedipine, co-administration of dalfopristin may lead to increased plasma concentrations of nimodipine. Upon co-administration with dalfopristin, blood pressure should be monitored and, if necessary, an adjustment in the nimodipine dose should be considered).

No products indexed under this heading.

Danazol (Nimodipine is metabolized via cytochrome P450 3A4 system located both in the intestinal mucosa and in the liver. Plasma concentrations of drugs which are known inhibitors of the cytochrome P450 3A4 system may be increased. Upon co-administration of drugs which are known inhibitors of cytochrome P450 3A4, the blood pressure should be monitored and, if necessary, a reduction of the nimodipine dose should be considered).

No products indexed under this heading.

Darunavir (No formal studies have been performed to investigate the potential interaction between nimodipine and anti-HIV protease inhibitors. Drugs of this class have been reported to be potent inhibitors of the cytochrome P450 3A4 system. Therefore, the potential for a marked and clinically relevant increase in nimodipine plasma concentrations upon co-administration with these protease inhibitors cannot be excluded. Upon co-administration with protease inhibitors, which are inhibitors of the cytochrome P450 3A4 system, blood pressure should be monitored and, if necessary, an adjustment in the nimodipine dose should be considered).

No products indexed under this heading.

Delavirdine Mesylate (Nimodipine is metabolized via cytochrome P450 3A4 system located both in the intestinal mucosa and in the liver. Plasma concentrations of drugs which are known inhibitors of the cytochrome P450 3A4 system may be increased. Upon co-administration of drugs which are known inhibitors of cytochrome P450 3A4, the blood pressure should be monitored and, if necessary, a reduction of the nimodipine dose should be considered).

No products indexed under this heading.

Deserpidine (Nimodipine may increase the blood presure lowering effect of concomitantly administered anti-hypertensives. However, if a combination of this type proves undavoidable particularly careful monitoring of the patient is necessary).

No products indexed under this heading.

Dexamethasone (Nimodipine is metabolized via the cytochrome P450 3A4 system located both in the intestinal mucosa and in the liver. Drugs that are known to induce cytochrome P450 3A4 may therefore alter the first pass or the clearance of nimodipine). Products include:

Ciprodex Otic Suspension ... **541**

Dexamethasone Acetate (Nimodipine is metabolized via the cytochrome P450 3A4 system located both in the intestinal mucosa and in the liver. Drugs that are known to induce cytochrome P450 3A4 may therefore alter the first pass or the clearance of nimodipine).

No products indexed under this heading.

Dexamethasone Sodium Phosphate (Nimodipine is metabolized via the cytochrome P450 3A4 system located both in the intestinal mucosa and in the liver. Drugs that are known to induce cytochrome P450 3A4 may therefore alter the first pass or the clearance of nimodipine).

No products indexed under this heading.

Diazoxide (Nimodipine may increase the blood presure lowering effect of concomitantly administered anti-hypertensives. However, if a combination of this type proves undavoidable particularly careful monitoring of the patient is necessary). Products include:

Proglycem Capsules ... **1185**
Proglycem Suspension ... **1185**

Diltiazem Hydrochloride (Nimodipine may increase the blood pressure lowering effect of concomitantly administered anti-hypertensives such as other calcium antagonists. However, if a combination of this type proves unavoidable particularly careful monitoring of the patient is necessary). Products include:

Cardizem LA Extended Release Tablets ... **421**

Diltiazem Maleate (Nimodipine is metabolized via cytochrome P450 3A4 system located both in the intestinal mucosa and in the liver. Plasma concentrations of drugs which are known inhibitors of the cytochrome P450 3A4 system may be increased. Upon co-administration of drugs which are known inhibitors of cytochrome P450 3A4, the blood pressure should be monitored and, if necessary, a reduction of the nimodipine dose should be considered).

No products indexed under this heading.

Dirithromycin (No interaction studies have been carried out between nimodipine and macrolide antibiotics. Certain macrolide antibiotics are known to inhibit cytochrome P450 3A4 system and the potential for drug interaction cannot be ruled out at this stage. Therefore, macrolide antibiotics should not be used in combination with nimodipine. However, if macrolide antibiotics which are inhibitors of the cytochrome P450 3A4 system are co-administered with nimodipine, blood pressure should be monitored and, if necessary, an adjustment in the nimodipine dose should be considered. Azithromycin, although structurally related to the class of macrolide, is void of CYP3A4 inhibition).

No products indexed under this heading.

Doxazosin Mesylate (Nimodipine may increase the blood pressure lowering effect of concomitantly administered anti-hypertensives such as alpha adrenergic blocking agents. However, if a combination of this type proves unavoidable, particularly careful monitoring of the patient is necessary).
No products indexed under this heading.

Doxorubicin Hydrochloride (Nimodipine is metabolized via the cytochrome P450 3A4 system located both in the intestinal mucosa and in the liver. Drugs that are known to induce cytochrome P450 3A4 may therefore alter the first pass or the clearance of nimodipine).
No products indexed under this heading.

Efavirenz (Nimodipine is metabolized via cytochrome P450 3A4 system located both in the intestinal mucosa and in the liver. Plasma concentrations of drugs which are known inhibitors of the cytochrome P450 3A4 system may be increased. Upon co-administration of drugs which are known inhibitors of cytochrome P450 3A4, the blood pressure should be monitored and, if necessary, a reduction of the nimodipine dose should be considered). Products include:
Atripla Tablets **938**
Sustiva Capsules **930**
Sustiva Tablets **930**

Enalapril Maleate (Nimodipine may increase the blood pressure lowering effect of concomitantly administered anti-hypertensives such as ACE inhibitors. However, if a combination of this type proves unavoidable, particularly careful monitoring of the patient is necessary).
No products indexed under this heading.

Enalaprilat (Nimodipine may increase the blood pressure lowering effect of concomitantly administered anti-hypertensives such as ACE inhibitors. However, if a combination of this type proves unavoidable, particularly careful monitoring of the patient is necessary).
No products indexed under this heading.

Eprosartan Mesylate (Nimodipine may increase the blood presure lowering effect of concomitantly administered anti-hypertensives. However, if a combination of this type proves undavoidable particularly careful monitoring of the patient is necessary). Products include:
Teveten Tablets **515**
Teveten HCT Tablets **517**

Erythromycin (No interaction studies have been carried out between nimodipine and macrolide antibiotics. Certain macrolide antibiotics are known to inhibit cytochrome P450 3A4 system and the potential for drug interaction cannot be ruled out at this stage. Therefore, macrolide antibiotics should not be used in combination with nimodipine. However, if macrolide antibiotics which are inhibitors of the cytochrome P450 3A4 system are co-administered with nimodipine, blood pressure should be monitored and, if necessary, an adjustment in the nimodipine dose should be considered. Azithromycin, although structurally related to the class of macrolide, is void of CYP3A4 inhibition).
No products indexed under this heading.

Erythromycin Estolate (No interaction studies have been carried out between nimodipine and macrolide antibiotics. Certain macrolide antibiotics are known to inhibit cytochrome P450 3A4 system and the potential for drug interaction cannot be ruled out at this stage. Therefore, macrolide antibiotics should not be used in combination with nimodipine. However, if macrolide antibiotics which are inhibitors of the cytochrome P450 3A4 system are co-administered with nimodipine, blood pressure should be monitored and, if necessary, an adjustment in the nimodipine dose should be considered. Azithromycin, although structurally related to the class of macrolide, is void of CYP3A4 inhibition).
No products indexed under this heading.

Erythromycin Ethylsuccinate (No interaction studies have been carried out between nimodipine and macrolide antibiotics. Certain macrolide antibiotics are known to inhibit cytochrome P450 3A4 system and the potential for drug interaction cannot be ruled out at this stage. Therefore, macrolide antibiotics should not be used in combination with nimodipine. However, if macrolide antibiotics which are inhibitors of the cytochrome P450 3A4 system are co-administered with nimodipine, blood pressure should be monitored and, if necessary, an adjustment in the nimodipine dose should be considered. Azithromycin, although structurally related to the class of macrolide, is void of CYP3A4 inhibition). Products include:
E.E.S. **433**
EryPed **431**

Erythromycin Gluceptate (No interaction studies have been carried out between nimodipine and macrolide antibiotics. Certain macrolide antibiotics are known to inhibit cytochrome P450 3A4 system and the potential for drug interaction cannot be ruled out at this stage. Therefore, macrolide antibiotics should not be used in combination with nimodipine. However, if macrolide antibiotics which are inhibitors of the cytochrome P450 3A4 system are co-administered with nimodipine, blood pressure should be monitored and, if necessary, an adjustment in the nimodipine dose should be considered. Azithromycin, although structurally related to the class of macrolide, is void of CYP3A4 inhibition).
No products indexed under this heading.

Erythromycin Lactobionate (Nimodipine is metabolized via cytochrome P450 3A4 system located both in the intestinal mucosa and in the liver. Plasma concentrations of drugs which are known inhibitors of the cytochrome P450 3A4 system may be increased. Upon co-administration of drugs which are known inhibitors of cytochrome P450 3A4, the blood pressure should be monitored and, if necessary, a reduction of the nimodipine dose should be considered).
No products indexed under this heading.

Erythromycin Stearate (No interaction studies have been carried out between nimodipine and macrolide antibiotics. Certain macrolide antibiotics are known to inhibit cytochrome P450 3A4 system and the potential for drug interaction cannot be ruled out at this stage. Therefore, macrolide antibiotics should not be used in combination with nimodipine. However, if macrolide antibiotics which are inhibitors of the cytochrome P450 3A4 system are co-administered with nimodipine, blood pressure should be monitored and, if necessary, an adjustment in the nimodipine dose should be considered. Azithromycin, although structurally related to the class of macrolide, is void of CYP3A4 inhibition).
No products indexed under this heading.

Esmolol Hydrochloride (Nimodipine may increase the blood pressure lowering effect of concomitantly administered anti-hypertensives such as beta blockers. However, if a combination of this type proves unavoidable, particularly careful monitoring of the patient is necessary).
No products indexed under this heading.

Esomeprazole Magnesium (Nimodipine is metabolized via cytochrome P450 3A4 system located both in the intestinal mucosa and in the liver. Plasma concentrations of drugs which are known inhibitors of the cytochrome P450 3A4 system may be increased. Upon co-administration of drugs which are known inhibitors of cytochrome P450 3A4, the blood pressure should be monitored and, if necessary, a reduction of the nimodipine dose should be considered). Products include:
Nexium Delayed-Release Capsules **645**
Nexium Delayed-Release Oral Suspension **645**

Ethacrynic Acid (Nimodipine may increase the blood pressure lowering effect of concomitantly administered anti-hypertensives such as diuretics. However, if a combination of this type proves unavoidable, particularly careful monitoring of the patient is necessary). Products include:
Edecrin Tablets **698**

Ethosuximide (Nimodipine is metabolized via the cytochrome P450 3A4 system located both in the intestinal mucosa and in the liver. Drugs that are known to induce cytochrome P450 3A4 may therefore alter the first pass or the clearance of nimodipine).
No products indexed under this heading.

Felbamate (Nimodipine is metabolized via the cytochrome P450 3A4 system located both in the intestinal mucosa and in the liver. Drugs that are known to induce cytochrome P450 3A4 may therefore alter the first pass or the clearance of nimodipine).
No products indexed under this heading.

Felodipine (Nimodipine may increase the blood pressure lowering effect of concomitantly administered anti-hypertensives such as other calcium antagonists. However, if a combination of this type proves unavoidable particularly careful monitoring of the patient is necessary).
No products indexed under this heading.

Fluconazole (A formal interaction study investigating the potential of drug interaction between nimodipine and ketoconazole has not been performed. Azole anti-mycotics are known to inhibit the cytochrome P450 3A4 system, and various interactions have been reported for other dihydropyridine calcium antagonists. Therefore, when administered together with oral nimodipine, a substantial increase in systemic bioavailability of nimodipine due to a decreased first-pass metabolism cannot be excluded. Upon co-administration with azole anti-mycotics which are inhibitors of the cytochrome P450 3A4 system, blood pressure should be monitored and, if necessary, an adjustment in the nimodipine dose should be considered).
No products indexed under this heading.

Fludrocortisone Acetate (Nimodipine is metabolized via the cytochrome P450 3A4 system located both in the intestinal mucosa and in the liver. Drugs that are known to induce cytochrome P450 3A4 may therefore alter the first pass or the clearance of nimodipine).
No products indexed under this heading.

Fluoxetine (Nimodipine is metabolized via cytochrome P450 3A4 system located both in the intestinal mucosa and in the liver. Fluoxetine is a known inhibitor of cytochrome P450 3A4. The steady-state concomitant administration of nimodipine with fluoxetine led to about 50% higher nimodipine plasma concentrations. Fluoxetine exposure was markedly decreased, while its active metabolite norfloxetine was not affected. Upon co-administration with fluoxetine, blood pressure should be monitored and, if necessary, an adjustment in the nimodipine dose should be considered).
No products indexed under this heading.

Fluoxetine Hydrochloride (Nimodipine is metabolized via cytochrome P450 3A4 system located both in the intestinal mucosa and in the liver. Fluoxetine is a known inhibitor of cytochrome P450 3A4. The steady-state concomitant administration of nimodipine with fluoxetine led to about 50% higher nimodipine plasma concentrations. Fluoxetine exposure was markedly decreased, while its active metabolite norfloxetine was not affected. Upon co-administration with fluoxetine, blood pressure should be monitored and, if necessary, an adjustment in the nimodipine dose should be considered). Products include:
Prozac Weekly Capsules **1852**
Prozac Pulvules and Liquid **1852**
Symbyax Capsules **1871**

Fluvoxamine Maleate (Nimodipine is metabolized via cytochrome P450 3A4 system located both in the intestinal mucosa and in the liver. Plasma concentrations of drugs which are known inhibitors of the cytochrome P450 3A4 system may be increased. Upon co-administration of drugs which are known inhibitors of cytochrome P450 3A4, the blood pressure should be monitored and, if neces-

sary, a reduction of the nimodipine dose should be considered). Products include:

Luvox CR Extended-Release Capsules **1759**

Fosamprenavir Calcium (No formal studies have been performed to investigate the potential interaction between nimodipine and anti-HIV protease inhibitors. Drugs of this class have been reported to be potent inhibitors of the cytochrome P450 3A4 system. Therefore, the potential for a marked and clinically relevant increase in nimodipine plasma concentrations upon co-administration with these protease inhibitors cannot be excluded. Upon co-administration with protease inhibitors, which are inhibitors of the cytochrome P450 3A4 system, blood pressure should be monitored and, if necessary, an adjustment in the nimodipine dose should be considered). Products include:

Lexiva Oral Suspension **1510**
Lexiva Tablets **1510**

Fosinopril Sodium (Nimodipine may increase the blood pressure lowering effect of concomitantly administered anti-hypertensives such as ACE inhibitors. However, if a combination of this type proves unavoidable, particularly careful monitoring of the patient is necessary).

No products indexed under this heading.

Fosphenytoin Sodium (Previous chronic administration of the antiepileptic drug phenytoin markedly reduces the bioavailability of orally administered nimodipine. Therefore, the concomitant use of oral nimodipine and phenytoin is contraindicated).

No products indexed under this heading.

Furosemide (Nimodipine may increase the blood pressure lowering effect of concomitantly administered anti-hypertensives such as diuretics. However, if a combination of this type proves unavoidable, particularly careful monitoring of the patient is necessary). Products include:

Furosemide Tablets **2186**

Garlic Extract (Nimodipine is metabolized via the cytochrome P450 3A4 system located both in the intestinal mucosa and in the liver. Drugs that are known to induce cytochrome P450 3A4 may therefore alter the first pass or the clearance of nimodipine).

No products indexed under this heading.

Garlic Oil (Nimodipine is metabolized via the cytochrome P450 3A4 system located both in the intestinal mucosa and in the liver. Drugs that are known to induce cytochrome P450 3A4 may therefore alter the first pass or the clearance of nimodipine).

No products indexed under this heading.

Guanabenz Acetate (Nimodipine may increase the blood presure lowering effect of concomitantly administered anti-hypertensives. However, if a combination of this type proves undavoidable particularly careful monitoring of the patient is necessary).

No products indexed under this heading.

Guanethidine Monosulfate (Nimodipine may increase the blood presure lowering effect of concomitantly administered anti-hypertensives. However, if a combination of this type proves undavoidable particularly careful monitoring of the patient is necessary).

No products indexed under this heading.

Hydralazine Hydrochloride (Nimodipine may increase the blood presure lowering effect of concomitantly administered anti-hypertensives. However, if a combination of this type proves undavoidable particularly careful monitoring of the patient is necessary).

No products indexed under this heading.

Hydrochlorothiazide (Nimodipine may increase the blood pressure lowering effect of concomitantly administered anti-hypertensives such as diuretics. However, if a combination of this type proves unavoidable, particularly careful monitoring of the patient is necessary). Products include:

Atacand HCT **642**
Avalide Tablets **892**
Avalide Tablets **2713**
Benicar HCT Tablets **1010**
Diovan HCT Tablets **2216**
Dyazide Capsules **1405**
Micardis HCT Tablets **854**
Prinzide Tablets **2092**
Tekturna HCT Tablets **2324**
Teveten HCT Tablets **517**

Hydrocortisone (Nimodipine is metabolized via the cytochrome P450 3A4 system located both in the intestinal mucosa and in the liver. Drugs that are known to induce cytochrome P450 3A4 may therefore alter the first pass or the clearance of nimodipine).

No products indexed under this heading.

Hydrocortisone Acetate (Nimodipine is metabolized via the cytochrome P450 3A4 system located both in the intestinal mucosa and in the liver. Drugs that are known to induce cytochrome P450 3A4 may therefore alter the first pass or the clearance of nimodipine). Products include:

Analpram-HC **1140**
Pramosone **1141**

Hydrocortisone Butyrate (Nimodipine is metabolized via the cytochrome P450 3A4 system located both in the intestinal mucosa and in the liver. Drugs that are known to induce cytochrome P450 3A4 may therefore alter the first pass or the clearance of nimodipine).

No products indexed under this heading.

Hydrocortisone Cypionate (Nimodipine is metabolized via the cytochrome P450 3A4 system located both in the intestinal mucosa and in the liver. Drugs that are known to induce cytochrome P450 3A4 may therefore alter the first pass or the clearance of nimodipine).

No products indexed under this heading.

Hydrocortisone Hemisuccinate (Nimodipine is metabolized via the cytochrome P450 3A4 system located both in the intestinal mucosa and in the liver. Drugs that are known to induce cytochrome P450 3A4 may therefore alter the first pass or the clearance of nimodipine).

No products indexed under this heading.

Hydrocortisone Probutate (Nimodipine is metabolized via the cytochrome P450 3A4 system located both in the intestinal mucosa and in the liver. Drugs that are known to induce cytochrome P450 3A4 may therefore alter the first pass or the clearance of nimodipine).

No products indexed under this heading.

Hydrocortisone Sodium Phosphate (Nimodipine is metabolized via the cytochrome P450 3A4 system located both in the intestinal mucosa and in the liver. Drugs that are known to induce cytochrome P450 3A4 may therefore alter the first pass or the clearance of nimodipine).

No products indexed under this heading.

Hydrocortisone Sodium Succinate (Nimodipine is metabolized via the cytochrome P450 3A4 system located both in the intestinal mucosa and in the liver. Drugs that are known to induce cytochrome P450 3A4 may therefore alter the first pass or the clearance of nimodipine).

No products indexed under this heading.

Hydrocortisone Valerate (Nimodipine is metabolized via the cytochrome P450 3A4 system located both in the intestinal mucosa and in the liver. Drugs that are known to induce cytochrome P450 3A4 may therefore alter the first pass or the clearance of nimodipine).

No products indexed under this heading.

Hydroflumethiazide (Nimodipine may increase the blood pressure lowering effect of concomitantly administered anti-hypertensives such as diuretics. However, if a combination of this type proves unavoidable, particularly careful monitoring of the patient is necessary).

No products indexed under this heading.

Hypericum (Nimodipine is metabolized via the cytochrome P450 3A4 system located both in the intestinal mucosa and in the liver. Drugs that are known to induce cytochrome P450 3A4 may therefore alter the first pass or the clearance of nimodipine). Products include:

Satieté Tablets **640**

Hypericum Perforatum (Nimodipine is metabolized via the cytochrome P450 3A4 system located both in the intestinal mucosa and in the liver. Drugs that are known to induce cytochrome P450 3A4 may therefore alter the first pass or the clearance of nimodipine).

No products indexed under this heading.

Indapamide (Nimodipine may increase the blood pressure lowering effect of concomitantly administered anti-hypertensives such as diuretics. However, if a combination of this type proves unavoidable, particularly careful monitoring of the patient is necessary). Products include:

Indapamide Tablets **2188**

Indinavir Sulfate (No formal studies have been performed to investigate the potential interaction between nimodipine and anti-HIV protease inhibitors. Drugs of this class have been reported to be potent inhibitors of the cytochrome P450 3A4 system. Therefore, the potential for a marked and clinically relevant increase in nimodipine plasma concentrations upon co-administration with these protease inhibitors cannot be excluded. Upon co-administration with protease inhibitors, which are inhibitors of the cytochrome P450 3A4 system, blood pressure should be monitored and, if necessary, an adjustment in the nimodipine dose should be considered). Products include:

Crixivan Capsules **1979**

Irbesartan (Nimodipine may increase the blood presure lowering effect of concomitantly administered anti-hypertensives. However, if a combination of this type proves undavoidable particularly careful monitoring of the patient is necessary). Products include:

Avalide Tablets **892**
Avalide Tablets **2713**
Avapro Tablets **897**
Avapro Tablets **2718**

Isoniazid (Nimodipine is metabolized via cytochrome P450 3A4 system located both in the intestinal mucosa and in the liver. Plasma concentrations of drugs which are known inhibitors of the cytochrome P450 3A4 system may be increased. Upon co-administration of drugs which are known inhibitors of cytochrome P450 3A4, the blood pressure should be monitored and, if necessary, a reduction of the nimodipine dose should be considered).

No products indexed under this heading.

Isradipine (Nimodipine may increase the blood pressure lowering effect of concomitantly administered anti-hypertensives such as other calcium antagonists. However, if a combination of this type proves unavoidable particularly careful monitoring of the patient is necessary). Products include:

DynaCirc CR Controlled Release Tablets **1407**

Itraconazole (A formal interaction study investigating the potential of drug interaction between nimodipine and ketoconazole has not been performed. Azole anti-mycotics are known to inhibit the cytochrome P450 3A4 system, and various interactions have been reported for other dihydropyridine calcium antagonists. Therefore, when administered together with oral nimodipine, a substantial increase in systemic bioavailability of nimodipine due to a decreased first-pass metabolism cannot be excluded. Upon co-administration with azole anti-mycotics which are inhibitors of the cytochrome P450 3A4 system, blood pressure should be monitored and, if necessary, an adjustment in the nimodipine dose should be considered).

No products indexed under this heading.

Ketoconazole (A formal interaction study investigating the potential of drug interaction between nimodipine and ketoconazole has not been performed. Azole anti-mycotics are known to inhibit the cytochrome P450 3A4 system, and various interactions have been reported for other dihydropyridine calcium antagonists. Therefore, when administered together with oral nimodipine, a substantial increase in systemic bioavailability of nimodipine due to a decreased first-pass metabolism cannot be excluded. Upon co-administration with azole anti-mycotics which are inhibitors of the cytochrome P450 3A4 system, blood pressure should be monitored and, if necessary, an adjustment in the nimodipine dose should be considered). Products include:
Extina Foam, 2% 3057
Nizoral A-D Shampoo 1901

Labetalol Hydrochloride (Nimodipine may increase the blood pressure lowering effect of concomitantly administered anti-hypertensives such as beta blockers. However, if a combination of this type proves unavoidable, particularly careful monitoring of the patient is necessary).
No products indexed under this heading.

Levobunolol Hydrochloride (Nimodipine may increase the blood pressure lowering effect of concomitantly administered anti-hypertensives such as beta blockers. However, if a combination of this type proves unavoidable, particularly careful monitoring of the patient is necessary).
No products indexed under this heading.

Lisinopril (Nimodipine may increase the blood pressure lowering effect of concomitantly administered anti-hypertensives such as ACE inhibitors. However, if a combination of this type proves unavoidable, particularly careful monitoring of the patient is necessary). Products include:
Prinivil Tablets 2087
Prinzide Tablets 2092

Lopinavir (No formal studies have been performed to investigate the potential interaction between nimodipine and anti-HIV protease inhibitors. Drugs of this class have been reported to be potent inhibitors of the cytochrome P450 3A4 system. Therefore, the potential for a marked and clinically relevant increase in nimodipine plasma concentrations upon co-administration with these protease inhibitors cannot be excluded. Upon co-administration with protease inhibitors, which are inhibitors of the cytochrome P450 3A4 system, blood pressure should be monitored and, if necessary, an adjustment in the nimodipine dose should be considered). Products include:
Kaletra 452

Loratadine (Nimodipine is metabolized via cytochrome P450 3A4 system located both in the intestinal mucosa and in the liver. Plasma concentrations of drugs which are known inhibitors of the cytochrome P450 3A4 system may be increased. Upon co-administration of drugs which are known inhibitors of cytochrome P450 3A4, the blood pressure should be monitored and, if necessary, a reduction of the nimodipine dose should be considered).
No products indexed under this heading.

Losartan Potassium (Nimodipine may increase the blood presure lowering effect of concomitantly administered anti-hypertensives. However, if a combination of this type proves undavoidable particularly careful monitoring of the patient is necessary). Products include:
Cozaar Tablets 1973

Mecamylamine Hydrochloride (Nimodipine may increase the blood presure lowering effect of concomitantly administered anti-hypertensives. However, if a combination of this type proves undavoidable particularly careful monitoring of the patient is necessary).
No products indexed under this heading.

Mephenytoin (Nimodipine is metabolized via the cytochrome P450 3A4 system located both in the intestinal mucosa and in the liver. Drugs that are known to induce cytochrome P450 3A4 may therefore alter the first pass or the clearance of nimodipine).
No products indexed under this heading.

Methsuximide (Nimodipine is metabolized via the cytochrome P450 3A4 system located both in the intestinal mucosa and in the liver. Drugs that are known to induce cytochrome P450 3A4 may therefore alter the first pass or the clearance of nimodipine).
No products indexed under this heading.

Methyclothiazide (Nimodipine may increase the blood pressure lowering effect of concomitantly administered anti-hypertensives such as diuretics. However, if a combination of this type proves unavoidable, particularly careful monitoring of the patient is necessary).
No products indexed under this heading.

Methyldopa (Nimodipine may increase the blood pressure lowering effect of concomitantly administered anti-hypertensives such as methyldopa. However, if a combination of this type proves unavoidable particularly careful monitoring of the patient is necessary).
No products indexed under this heading.

Methyldopate Hydrochloride (Nimodipine may increase the blood presure lowering effect of concomitantly administered anti-hypertensives. However, if a combination of this type proves undavoidable particularly careful monitoring of the patient is necessary).
No products indexed under this heading.

Methylprednisolone (Nimodipine is metabolized via the cytochrome P450 3A4 system located both in the intestinal mucosa and in the liver. Drugs that are known to induce cytochrome P450 3A4 may therefore alter the first pass or the clearance of nimodipine).
No products indexed under this heading.

Methylprednisolone Acetate (Nimodipine is metabolized via the cytochrome P450 3A4 system located both in the intestinal mucosa and in the liver. Drugs that are known to induce cytochrome P450 3A4 may therefore alter the first pass or the clearance of nimodipine).
No products indexed under this heading.

Methylprednisolone Sodium Succinate (Nimodipine is metabolized via the cytochrome P450 3A4 system located both in the intestinal mucosa and in the liver. Drugs that are known to induce cytochrome P450 3A4 may therefore alter the first pass or the clearance of nimodipine).
No products indexed under this heading.

Metipranolol Hydrochloride (Nimodipine may increase the blood pressure lowering effect of concomitantly administered anti-hypertensives such as beta blockers. However, if a combination of this type proves unavoidable, particularly careful monitoring of the patient is necessary).
No products indexed under this heading.

Metolazone (Nimodipine may increase the blood pressure lowering effect of concomitantly administered anti-hypertensives such as diuretics. However, if a combination of this type proves unavoidable, particularly careful monitoring of the patient is necessary).
No products indexed under this heading.

Metoprolol Succinate (Nimodipine may increase the blood pressure lowering effect of concomitantly administered anti-hypertensives such as beta blockers. However, if a combination of this type proves unavoidable, particularly careful monitoring of the patient is necessary). Products include:
Toprol-XL Tablets 666

Metoprolol Tartrate (Nimodipine may increase the blood pressure lowering effect of concomitantly administered anti-hypertensives such as beta blockers. However, if a combination of this type proves unavoidable, particularly careful monitoring of the patient is necessary).
No products indexed under this heading.

Metronidazole (Nimodipine is metabolized via cytochrome P450 3A4 system located both in the intestinal mucosa and in the liver. Plasma concentrations of drugs which are known inhibitors of the cytochrome P450 3A4 system may be increased. Upon co-administration of drugs which are known inhibitors of cytochrome P450 3A4, the blood pressure should be monitored and, if necessary, a reduction of the nimodipine dose should be considered). Products include:
Pylera Capsules 714

Metronidazole Benzoate (Nimodipine is metabolized via cytochrome P450 3A4 system located both in the intestinal mucosa and in the liver. Plasma concentrations of drugs which are known inhibitors of the cytochrome P450 3A4 system may be increased. Upon co-administration of drugs which are known inhibitors of cytochrome P450 3A4, the blood pressure should be monitored and, if necessary, a reduction of the nimodipine dose should be considered).
No products indexed under this heading.

Metronidazole Hydrochloride (Nimodipine is metabolized via cytochrome P450 3A4 system located both in the intestinal mucosa and in the liver. Plasma concentrations of drugs which are known inhibitors of the cytochrome P450 3A4 system may be increased. Upon co-administration of drugs which are known inhibitors of cytochrome P450 3A4, the blood pressure should be monitored and, if necessary, a reduction of the nimodipine dose should be considered).
No products indexed under this heading.

Metronidazole Sodium (Nimodipine is metabolized via cytochrome P450 3A4 system located both in the intestinal mucosa and in the liver. Plasma concentrations of drugs which are known inhibitors of the cytochrome P450 3A4 system may be increased. Upon co-administration of drugs which are known inhibitors of cytochrome P450 3A4, the blood pressure should be monitored and, if necessary, a reduction of the nimodipine dose should be considered).
No products indexed under this heading.

Metyrosine (Nimodipine may increase the blood presure lowering effect of concomitantly administered anti-hypertensives. However, if a combination of this type proves undavoidable particularly careful monitoring of the patient is necessary). Products include:
Demser Capsules 1989

Mibefradil Dihydrochloride (Nimodipine may increase the blood pressure lowering effect of concomitantly administered anti-hypertensives such as other calcium antagonists. However, if a combination of this type proves unavoidable particularly careful monitoring of the patient is necessary).
No products indexed under this heading.

Miconazole (A formal interaction study investigating the potential of drug interaction between nimodipine and ketoconazole has not been performed. Azole anti-mycotics are known to inhibit the cytochrome P450 3A4 system, and various interactions have been reported for other dihydropyridine calcium antagonists. Therefore, when administered together with oral nimodipine, a substantial increase in systemic bioavailability of nimodipine due to a decreased first-pass metabolism cannot be excluded. Upon co-administration with azole anti-mycotics which are inhibitors of the cytochrome P450 3A4 system, blood pressure should be monitored and, if necessary, an adjustment in the nimodipine dose should be considered).
No products indexed under this heading.

Miconazole Nitrate (Nimodipine is metabolized via cytochrome P450 3A4 system located both in the intestinal mucosa and in the liver. Plasma concentrations of drugs

which are known inhibitors of the cytochrome P450 3A4 system may be increased. Upon co-administration of drugs which are known inhibitors of cytochrome P450 3A4, the blood pressure should be monitored and, if necessary, a reduction of the nimodipine dose should be considered).
No products indexed under this heading.

Minoxidil (Nimodipine may increase the blood presure lowering effect of concomitantly administered anti-hypertensives. However, if a combination of this type proves undavoidable particularly careful monitoring of the patient is necessary).
No products indexed under this heading.

Modafinil (Nimodipine is metabolized via the cytochrome P450 3A4 system located both in the intestinal mucosa and in the liver. Drugs that are known to induce cytochrome P450 3A4 may therefore alter the first pass or the clearance of nimodipine). Products include:
Provigil Tablets 977

Moexipril Hydrochloride (Nimodipine may increase the blood pressure lowering effect of concomitantly administered anti-hypertensives such as ACE inhibitors. However, if a combination of this type proves unavoidable, particularly careful monitoring of the patient is necessary).
No products indexed under this heading.

Nadolol (Nimodipine may increase the blood pressure lowering effect of concomitantly administered anti-hypertensives such as beta blockers. However, if a combination of this type proves unavoidable, particularly careful monitoring of the patient is necessary). Products include:
Nadolol Tablets 2191

Nebivolol (Nimodipine may increase the blood pressure lowering effect of concomitantly administered anti-hypertensives such as beta blockers. However, if a combination of this type proves unavoidable, particularly careful monitoring of the patient is necessary). Products include:
Bystolic Tablets 1155

Nefazodone Hydrochloride (No formal studies have been performed to investigate the potential interaction between nimodipine and nefazodone. This antidepressant drug has been reported to be a potent inhibitor of the cytochrome P450 3A4. Therefore, the potential for an increase in nimodipine plasma concentrations upon co-administration with nefazodone cannot be excluded. Upon co-administration with nefazodone, blood pressure should be monitored and, if necessary, an adjustment in nimodipine dose should be considered).
No products indexed under this heading.

Nelfinavir Mesylate (No formal studies have been performed to investigate the potential interaction between nimodipine and anti-HIV protease inhibitors. Drugs of this class have been reported to be potent inhibitors of the cytochrome P450 3A4 system. Therefore, the potential for a marked and clinically relevant increase in nimodipine plasma concentrations upon co-administration with these protease inhibitors cannot be excluded. Upon co-administration with protease inhibitors, which are inhibitors of the cytochrome P450 3A4 system, blood pressure should be monitored and, if necessary, an adjustment in the nimodipine dose should be considered).
No products indexed under this heading.

Nevirapine (Nimodipine is metabolized via cytochrome P450 3A4 system located both in the intestinal mucosa and in the liver. Plasma concentrations of drugs which are known inhibitors of the cytochrome P450 3A4 system may be increased. Upon co-administration of drugs which are known inhibitors of cytochrome P450 3A4, the blood pressure should be monitored and, if necessary, a reduction of the nimodipine dose should be considered). Products include:
Viramune Oral Suspension 873
Viramune Tablets 873

Niacinamide (Nimodipine is metabolized via cytochrome P450 3A4 system located both in the intestinal mucosa and in the liver. Plasma concentrations of drugs which are known inhibitors of the cytochrome P450 3A4 system may be increased. Upon co-administration of drugs which are known inhibitors of cytochrome P450 3A4, the blood pressure should be monitored and, if necessary, a reduction of the nimodipine dose should be considered). Products include:
BioLean Free Tablets 635

Nicardipine Hydrochloride (Nimodipine may increase the blood pressure lowering effect of concomitantly administered anti-hypertensives such as other calcium antagonists. However, if a combination of this type proves unavoidable particularly careful monitoring of the patient is necessary). Products include:
Cardene I.V. 1093

Nicotinamide (Nimodipine is metabolized via cytochrome P450 3A4 system located both in the intestinal mucosa and in the liver. Plasma concentrations of drugs which are known inhibitors of the cytochrome P450 3A4 system may be increased. Upon co-administration of drugs which are known inhibitors of cytochrome P450 3A4, the blood pressure should be monitored and, if necessary, a reduction of the nimodipine dose should be considered).
No products indexed under this heading.

Nifedipine (Nimodipine may increase the blood pressure lowering effect of concomitantly administered anti-hypertensives such as other calcium antagonists. However, if a combination of this type proves unavoidable particularly careful monitoring of the patient is necessary).
No products indexed under this heading.

Nisoldipine (Nimodipine may increase the blood pressure lowering effect of concomitantly administered anti-hypertensives such as other calcium antagonists. However, if a combination of this type proves unavoidable particularly careful monitoring of the patient is necessary). Products include:
Sular Extended Release Tablets 2975

Nitroglycerin (Nimodipine may increase the blood presure lowering effect of concomitantly administered anti-hypertensives. However, if a combination of this type proves undavoidable particularly careful monitoring of the patient is necessary). Products include:
Nitro-Dur Transdermal Infusion System 2887
Nitrolingual Pumpspray 2965

Norfloxacin (Nimodipine is metabolized via cytochrome P450 3A4 system located both in the intestinal mucosa and in the liver. Plasma concentrations of drugs which are known inhibitors of the cytochrome P450 3A4 system may be increased. Upon co-administration of drugs which are known inhibitors of cytochrome P450 3A4, the blood pressure should be monitored and, if necessary, a reduction of the nimodipine dose should be considered). Products include:
Noroxin Tablets 2069

Nortriptyline Hydrochloride (The steady-state concomitant administration of nimodpine and nortriptyline led to a slight decrease in nimodipine exposure with unaffected nortriptyline plasma concentrations).
No products indexed under this heading.

Omeprazole (Nimodipine is metabolized via cytochrome P450 3A4 system located both in the intestinal mucosa and in the liver. Plasma concentrations of drugs which are known inhibitors of the cytochrome P450 3A4 system may be increased. Upon co-administration of drugs which are known inhibitors of cytochrome P450 3A4, the blood pressure should be monitored and, if necessary, a reduction of the nimodipine dose should be considered).
No products indexed under this heading.

Oxcarbazepine (Nimodipine is metabolized via the cytochrome P450 3A4 system located both in the intestinal mucosa and in the liver. Drugs that are known to induce cytochrome P450 3A4 may therefore alter the first pass or the clearance of nimodipine).
No products indexed under this heading.

Oxiconazole Nitrate (A formal interaction study investigating the potential of drug interaction between nimodipine and ketoconazole has not been performed. Azole antimycotics are known to inhibit the cytochrome P450 3A4 system, and various interactions have been reported for other dihydropyridine calcium antagonists. Therefore, when administered together with oral nimodipine, a substantial increase in systemic bioavailability of nimodipine due to a decreased first-pass metabolism cannot be excluded. Upon co-administration with azole antimycotics which are inhibitors of the cytochrome P450 3A4 system, blood pressure should be monitored and, if necessary, an adjustment in the nimodipine dose should be considered).
No products indexed under this heading.

Paroxetine Hydrochloride (Nimodipine is metabolized via cytochrome P450 3A4 system located both in the intestinal mucosa and in the liver. Plasma concentrations of drugs which are known inhibitors of the cytochrome P450 3A4 system may be increased. Upon co-administration of drugs which are known inhibitors of cytochrome P450 3A4, the blood pressure should be monitored and, if necessary, a reduction of the nimodipine dose should be considered). Products include:
Paxil 1535
Paxil CR Controlled-Release Tablets 1544

Penbutolol Sulfate (Nimodipine may increase the blood pressure lowering effect of concomitantly administered anti-hypertensives such as beta blockers. However, if a combination of this type proves unavoidable, particularly careful monitoring of the patient is necessary).
No products indexed under this heading.

Perindopril Erbumine (Nimodipine may increase the blood pressure lowering effect of concomitantly administered anti-hypertensives such as ACE inhibitors. However, if a combination of this type proves unavoidable, particularly careful monitoring of the patient is necessary). Products include:
Aceon Tablets (2 mg, 4 mg, 8 mg) 3038

Phenobarbital (Previous chronic administration of the antiepileptic drug phenobarbital markedly reduces the bioavailability of orally administered nimodipine. Therefore, the concomitant use of oral nimodipine and phenytoin is contraindicated). Products include:
Donnatal Extentabs 2507

Phenobarbital Sodium (Previous chronic administration of the antiepileptic drug phenobarbital markedly reduces the bioavailability of orally administered nimodipine. Therefore, the concomitant use of oral nimodipine and phenytoin is contraindicated).
No products indexed under this heading.

Phenoxybenzamine Hydrochloride (Nimodipine may increase the blood presure lowering effect of concomitantly administered anti-hypertensives. However, if a combination of this type proves undavoidable particularly careful monitoring of the patient is necessary). Products include:
Dibenzyline Capsules 3188

Phentolamine Mesylate (Nimodipine may increase the blood presure lowering effect of concomitantly administered anti-hypertensives. However, if a combination of this type proves undavoidable particularly careful monitoring of the patient is necessary).
No products indexed under this heading.

Phenytoin (Previous chronic administration of the antiepileptic drug phenytoin markedly reduces the bioavailability of orally administered nimodipine. Therefore, the concomitant use of oral nimodipine and phenytoin is contraindicated).
No products indexed under this heading.

Phenytoin Sodium (Previous chronic administration of the antiepileptic drug phenytoin markedly reduces the bioavailability of orally administered nimodipine. Therefore, the concomitant use of oral nimodipine and phenytoin is contraindicated). Products include:

Phenytek Capsules 2192

Pindolol (Nimodipine may increase the blood pressure lowering effect of concomitantly administered anti-hypertensives such as beta blockers. However, if a combination of this type proves unavoidable, particularly careful monitoring of the patient is necessary).

No products indexed under this heading.

Polythiazide (Nimodipine may increase the blood pressure lowering effect of concomitantly administered anti-hypertensives such as diuretics. However, if a combination of this type proves unavoidable, particularly careful monitoring of the patient is necessary).

No products indexed under this heading.

Posaconazole (A formal interaction study investigating the potential of drug interaction between nimodipine and ketoconazole has not been performed. Azole anti-mycotics are known to inhibit the cytochrome P450 3A4 system, and various interactions have been reported for other dihydropyridine calcium antagonists. Therefore, when administered together with oral nimodipine, a substantial increase in systemic bioavailability of nimodipine due to a decreased first-pass metabolism cannot be excluded. Upon co-administration with azole anti-mycotics which are inhibitors of the cytochrome P450 3A4 system, blood pressure should be monitored and, if necessary, an adjustment in the nimodipine dose should be considered). Products include:

Noxafil Oral Suspension 2889

Prazosin Hydrochloride (Nimodipine may increase the blood pressure lowering effect of concomitantly administered anti-hypertensives such as alpha adrenergic blocking agents. However, if a combination of this type proves unavoidable, particularly careful monitoring of the patient is necessary).

No products indexed under this heading.

Prednisolone Acetate (Nimodipine is metabolized via the cytochrome P450 3A4 system located both in the intestinal mucosa and in the liver. Drugs that are known to induce cytochrome P450 3A4 may therefore alter the first pass or the clearance of nimodipine). Products include:

Pred Forte Ophthalmic Suspension .... ⊙227
Pred Mild Ophthalmic Suspension .... ⊙230
Pred-G Ophthalmic Ointment .... ⊙229
Pred-G Ophthalmic Suspension ...... ⊙228

Prednisolone Sodium Phosphate (Nimodipine is metabolized via the cytochrome P450 3A4 system located both in the intestinal mucosa and in the liver. Drugs that are known to induce cytochrome P450 3A4 may therefore alter the first pass or the clearance of nimodipine).

No products indexed under this heading.

Prednisolone Tebutate (Nimodipine is metabolized via the cytochrome P450 3A4 system located both in the intestinal mucosa and in the liver. Drugs that are known to induce cytochrome P450 3A4 may therefore alter the first pass or the clearance of nimodipine).

No products indexed under this heading.

Prednisone (Nimodipine is metabolized via the cytochrome P450 3A4 system located both in the intestinal mucosa and in the liver. Drugs that are known to induce cytochrome P450 3A4 may therefore alter the first pass or the clearance of nimodipine).

No products indexed under this heading.

Primidone (Nimodipine is metabolized via the cytochrome P450 3A4 system located both in the intestinal mucosa and in the liver. Drugs that are known to induce cytochrome P450 3A4 may therefore alter the first pass or the clearance of nimodipine).

No products indexed under this heading.

Propoxyphene Hydrochloride (Nimodipine is metabolized via cytochrome P450 3A4 system located both in the intestinal mucosa and in the liver. Plasma concentrations of drugs which are known inhibitors of the cytochrome P450 3A4 system may be increased. Upon co-administration of drugs which are known inhibitors of cytochrome P450 3A4, the blood pressure should be monitored and, if necessary, a reduction of the nimodipine dose should be considered).

No products indexed under this heading.

Propoxyphene Napsylate (Nimodipine is metabolized via cytochrome P450 3A4 system located both in the intestinal mucosa and in the liver. Plasma concentrations of drugs which are known inhibitors of the cytochrome P450 3A4 system may be increased. Upon co-administration of drugs which are known inhibitors of cytochrome P450 3A4, the blood pressure should be monitored and, if necessary, a reduction of the nimodipine dose should be considered).

No products indexed under this heading.

Propranolol Hydrochloride (Nimodipine may increase the blood pressure lowering effect of concomitantly administered anti-hypertensives such as beta blockers. However, if a combination of this type proves unavoidable, particularly careful monitoring of the patient is necessary). Products include:

InnoPran XL Extended Release Capsules 1484

Quinapril Hydrochloride (Nimodipine may increase the blood pressure lowering effect of concomitantly administered anti-hypertensives such as ACE inhibitors. However, if a combination of this type proves unavoidable, particularly careful monitoring of the patient is necessary).

No products indexed under this heading.

Quinidine (Nimodipine is metabolized via cytochrome P450 3A4 system located both in the intestinal mucosa and in the liver. Plasma concentrations of drugs which are known inhibitors of the cytochrome P450 3A4 system may be increased. Upon co-administration of drugs which are known inhibitors of cytochrome P450 3A4, the blood pressure should be monitored and, if necessary, a reduction of the nimodipine dose should be considered).

No products indexed under this heading.

Quinidine Hydrochloride (Nimodipine is metabolized via cytochrome P450 3A4 system located both in the intestinal mucosa and in the liver. Plasma concentrations of drugs which are known inhibitors of the cytochrome P450 3A4 system may be increased. Upon co-administration of drugs which are known inhibitors of cytochrome P450 3A4, the blood pressure should be monitored and, if necessary, a reduction of the nimodipine dose should be considered).

No products indexed under this heading.

Quinidine Polygalacturonate (Nimodipine is metabolized via cytochrome P450 3A4 system located both in the intestinal mucosa and in the liver. Plasma concentrations of drugs which are known inhibitors of the cytochrome P450 3A4 system may be increased. Upon co-administration of drugs which are known inhibitors of cytochrome P450 3A4, the blood pressure should be monitored and, if necessary, a reduction of the nimodipine dose should be considered).

No products indexed under this heading.

Quinidine Sulfate (Nimodipine is metabolized via cytochrome P450 3A4 system located both in the intestinal mucosa and in the liver. Plasma concentrations of drugs which are known inhibitors of the cytochrome P450 3A4 system may be increased. Upon co-administration of drugs which are known inhibitors of cytochrome P450 3A4, the blood pressure should be monitored and, if necessary, a reduction of the nimodipine dose should be considered).

No products indexed under this heading.

Quinine (Nimodipine is metabolized via cytochrome P450 3A4 system located both in the intestinal mucosa and in the liver. Plasma concentrations of drugs which are known inhibitors of the cytochrome P450 3A4 system may be increased. Upon co-administration of drugs which are known inhibitors of cytochrome P450 3A4, the blood pressure should be monitored and, if necessary, a reduction of the nimodipine dose should be considered).

No products indexed under this heading.

Quinine Sulfate (Nimodipine is metabolized via cytochrome P450 3A4 system located both in the intestinal mucosa and in the liver. Plasma concentrations of drugs which are known inhibitors of the cytochrome P450 3A4 system may be increased. Upon co-administration of drugs which are known inhibitors of cytochrome P450 3A4, the blood pressure should be monitored and, if necessary, a reduction of the nimodipine dose should be considered).

No products indexed under this heading.

Quinupristin (Based on experience with the calcium-antagonist nifedipine, co-administration of quinupristin may lead to increased plasma concentrations of nimodipine. Upon co-administration with quinupristin, blood pressure should be monitored and, if necessary, an adjustment in the nimodipine dose should be considered).

No products indexed under this heading.

Ramipril (Nimodipine may increase the blood pressure lowering effect of concomitantly administered anti-hypertensives such as ACE inhibitors. However, if a combination of this type proves unavoidable, particularly careful monitoring of the patient is necessary).

No products indexed under this heading.

Ranitidine Bismuth Citrate (Nimodipine is metabolized via cytochrome P450 3A4 system located both in the intestinal mucosa and in the liver. Plasma concentrations of drugs which are known inhibitors of the cytochrome P450 3A4 system may be increased. Upon co-administration of drugs which are known inhibitors of cytochrome P450 3A4, the blood pressure should be monitored and, if necessary, a reduction of the nimodipine dose should be considered).

No products indexed under this heading.

Ranitidine Hydrochloride (Nimodipine is metabolized via cytochrome P450 3A4 system located both in the intestinal mucosa and in the liver. Plasma concentrations of drugs which are known inhibitors of the cytochrome P450 3A4 system may be increased. Upon co-administration of drugs which are known inhibitors of cytochrome P450 3A4, the blood pressure should be monitored and, if necessary, a reduction of the nimodipine dose should be considered). Products include:

Zantac 75 Tablets .... ▣603
Zantac 1670
Zantac Injection 1666
Zantac Injection Pharmacy Bulk Package 1668
Maximum Strength Zantac 150 Tablets .... ▣603
Maximum Strength Zantac 150 Cool Mint Tablets .... ▣603

Rauwolfia Serpentina (Nimodipine may increase the blood presure lowering effect of concomitantly administered anti-hypertensives. However, if a combination of this type proves undavoidable particularly careful monitoring of the patient is necessary).

No products indexed under this heading.

Rescinnamine (Nimodipine may increase the blood presure lowering effect of concomitantly administered anti-hypertensives. However, if a combination of this type proves undavoidable particularly careful monitoring of the patient is necessary).

No products indexed under this heading.

Reserpine (Nimodipine may increase the blood presure lowering effect of concomitantly administered anti-hypertensives. However, if a combination of this type proves undavoidable particularly careful monitoring of the patient is necessary).
No products indexed under this heading.

Rifabutin (Nimodipine is metabolized via the cytochrome P450 3A4 system located both in the intestinal mucosa and in the liver. Drugs that are known to induce cytochrome P450 3A4 may therefore alter the first pass or the clearance of nimodipine).
No products indexed under this heading.

Rifampicin (Nimodipine is metabolized via the cytochrome P450 3A4 system located both in the intestinal mucosa and in the liver. Drugs that are known to induce cytochrome P450 3A4 may therefore alter the first pass or the clearance of nimodipine).
No products indexed under this heading.

Rifampin (From the experience with other calcium antagonists it has to be expected that rifampin accelerates the metabolism of nimodipine due to enzyme induction. Thus, efficacy of nimodipine could be significantly reduced when concomitantly administered with rifampin. The use of nimodipine in combination with rifampin is therefore contraindicated).
No products indexed under this heading.

Rifapentine (Nimodipine is metabolized via the cytochrome P450 3A4 system located both in the intestinal mucosa and in the liver. Drugs that are known to induce cytochrome P450 3A4 may therefore alter the first pass or the clearance of nimodipine).
No products indexed under this heading.

Ritonavir (No formal studies have been performed to investigate the potential interaction between nimodipine and anti-HIV protease inhibitors. Drugs of this class have been reported to be potent inhibitors of the cytochrome P450 3A4 system. Therefore, the potential for a marked and clinically relevant increase in nimodipine plasma concentrations upon co-administration with these protease inhibitors cannot be excluded. Upon co-administration with protease inhibitors, which are inhibitors of the cytochrome P450 3A4 system, blood pressure should be monitored and, if necessary, an adjustment in the nimodipine dose should be considered). Products include:
Kaletra 452
Norvir 489

Saquinavir (No formal studies have been performed to investigate the potential interaction between nimodipine and anti-HIV protease inhibitors. Drugs of this class have been reported to be potent inhibitors of the cytochrome P450 3A4 system. Therefore, the potential for a marked and clinically relevant increase in nimodipine plasma concentrations upon co-administration with these protease inhibitors cannot be excluded. Upon co-administration with protease inhibitors, which are inhibitors of the cytochrome P450 3A4 system, blood pressure should be monitored and, if necessary, an adjustment in the nimodipine dose should be considered).
No products indexed under this heading.

Saquinavir Mesylate (No formal studies have been performed to investigate the potential interaction between nimodipine and anti-HIV protease inhibitors. Drugs of this class have been reported to be potent inhibitors of the cytochrome P450 3A4 system. Therefore, the potential for a marked and clinically relevant increase in nimodipine plasma concentrations upon co-administration with these protease inhibitors cannot be excluded. Upon co-administration with protease inhibitors, which are inhibitors of the cytochrome P450 3A4 system, blood pressure should be monitored and, if necessary, an adjustment in the nimodipine dose should be considered).
No products indexed under this heading.

Sertraline Hydrochloride (Nimodipine is metabolized via cytochrome P450 3A4 system located both in the intestinal mucosa and in the liver. Plasma concentrations of drugs which are known inhibitors of the cytochrome P450 3A4 system may be increased. Upon co-administration of drugs which are known inhibitors of cytochrome P450 3A4, the blood pressure should be monitored and, if necessary, a reduction of the nimodipine dose should be considered).
No products indexed under this heading.

Sildenafil Citrate (Nimodipine may increase the blood pressure lowering effect of concomitantly administered anti-hypertensives such as phosphodiesterase type 5 inhibitors. However, if a combination of this type proves unavoidable, particularly careful monitoring of the patient is necessary).
No products indexed under this heading.

Sodium Nitroprusside (Nimodipine may increase the blood presure lowering effect of concomitantly administered anti-hypertensives. However, if a combination of this type proves undavoidable particularly careful monitoring of the patient is necessary).
No products indexed under this heading.

Sotalol Hydrochloride (Nimodipine may increase the blood pressure lowering effect of concomitantly administered anti-hypertensives such as beta blockers. However, if a combination of this type proves unavoidable, particularly careful monitoring of the patient is necessary).
No products indexed under this heading.

Spirapril Hydrochloride (Nimodipine may increase the blood pressure lowering effect of concomitantly administered anti-hypertensives such as ACE inhibitors. However, if a combination of this type proves unavoidable, particularly careful monitoring of the patient is necessary).
No products indexed under this heading.

Spironolactone (Nimodipine may increase the blood pressure lowering effect of concomitantly administered anti-hypertensives such as diuretics. However, if a combination of this type proves unavoidable, particularly careful monitoring of the patient is necessary).
No products indexed under this heading.

Sulfinpyrazone (Nimodipine is metabolized via the cytochrome P450 3A4 system located both in the intestinal mucosa and in the liver. Drugs that are known to induce cytochrome P450 3A4 may therefore alter the first pass or the clearance of nimodipine).
No products indexed under this heading.

Tadalafil (Nimodipine may increase the blood pressure lowering effect of concomitantly administered anti-hypertensives such as phosphodiesterase type 5 inhibitors. However, if a combination of this type proves unavoidable, particularly careful monitoring of the patient is necessary). Products include:
Cialis Tablets 1792

Tamsulosin Hydrochloride (Nimodipine may increase the blood pressure lowering effect of concomitantly administered anti-hypertensives such as alpha adrenergic blocking agents. However, if a combination of this type proves unavoidable, particularly careful monitoring of the patient is necessary). Products include:
Flomax Capsules 848

Telithromycin (Nimodipine is metabolized via cytochrome P450 3A4 system located both in the intestinal mucosa and in the liver. Plasma concentrations of drugs which are known inhibitors of the cytochrome P450 3A4 system may be increased. Upon co-administration of drugs which are known inhibitors of cytochrome P450 3A4, the blood pressure should be monitored and, if necessary, a reduction of the nimodipine dose should be considered). Products include:
Ketek Tablets 2744

Telmisartan (Nimodipine may increase the blood presure lowering effect of concomitantly administered anti-hypertensives. However, if a combination of this type proves undavoidable particularly careful monitoring of the patient is necessary). Products include:
Micardis Tablets 852
Micardis HCT Tablets 854

Terazosin Hydrochloride (Nimodipine may increase the blood pressure lowering effect of concomitantly administered anti-hypertensives such as alpha adrenergic blocking agents. However, if a combination of this type proves unavoidable, particularly careful monitoring of the patient is necessary).
No products indexed under this heading.

Terconazole (A formal interaction study investigating the potential of drug interaction between nimodipine and ketoconazole has not been performed. Azole anti-mycotics are known to inhibit the cytochrome P450 3A4 system, and various interactions have been reported for other dihydropyridine calcium antagonists. Therefore, when administered together with oral nimodipine, a substantial increase in systemic bioavailability of nimodipine due to a decreased first-pass metabolism cannot be excluded. Upon co-administration with azole anti-mycotics which are inhibitors of the cytochrome P450 3A4 system, blood pressure should be monitored and, if necessary, an adjustment in the nimodipine dose should be considered).
No products indexed under this heading.

Theophylline (Nimodipine is metabolized via the cytochrome P450 3A4 system located both in the intestinal mucosa and in the liver. Drugs that are known to induce cytochrome P450 3A4 may therefore alter the first pass or the clearance of nimodipine).
No products indexed under this heading.

Theophylline Anhydrous (Nimodipine is metabolized via the cytochrome P450 3A4 system located both in the intestinal mucosa and in the liver. Drugs that are known to induce cytochrome P450 3A4 may therefore alter the first pass or the clearance of nimodipine). Products include:
Uniphyl Tablets 2595

Theophylline Calcium Salicylate (Nimodipine is metabolized via the cytochrome P450 3A4 system located both in the intestinal mucosa and in the liver. Drugs that are known to induce cytochrome P450 3A4 may therefore alter the first pass or the clearance of nimodipine).
No products indexed under this heading.

Theophylline Dihydroxypropyl (Glyceryl) (Nimodipine is metabolized via the cytochrome P450 3A4 system located both in the intestinal mucosa and in the liver. Drugs that are known to induce cytochrome P450 3A4 may therefore alter the first pass or the clearance of nimodipine).
No products indexed under this heading.

Theophylline Ethylenediamine (Nimodipine is metabolized via the cytochrome P450 3A4 system located both in the intestinal mucosa and in the liver. Drugs that are known to induce cytochrome P450 3A4 may therefore alter the first pass or the clearance of nimodipine).
No products indexed under this heading.

Timolol Hemihydrate (Nimodipine may increase the blood pressure lowering effect of concomitantly administered anti-hypertensives such as beta blockers. However, if a combination of this type proves unavoidable, particularly careful monitoring of the patient is necessary). Products include:
Betimol Ophthalmic Solution 3181

Timolol Maleate (Nimodipine may increase the blood pressure lowering effect of concomitantly administered anti-hypertensives such as beta blockers. However, if a combination of this type proves unavoidable, particularly careful monitoring of the patient is necessary). Products include:
Combigan Ophthalmic Solution 553
Cosopt Sterile Ophthalmic Solution 1969

Timoptic Sterile Ophthalmic Solution **2121**
Timoptic in Ocudose **2124**
Timoptic-XE Sterile Ophthalmic Gel Forming Solution **2125**

Tipranavir (No formal studies have been performed to investigate the potential interaction between nimodipine and anti-HIV protease inhibitors. Drugs of this class have been reported to be potent inhibitors of the cytochrome P450 3A4 system. Therefore, the potential for a marked and clinically relevant increase in nimodipine plasma concentrations upon co-administration with these protease inhibitors cannot be excluded. Upon co-administration with protease inhibitors, which are inhibitors of the cytochrome P450 3A4 system, blood pressure should be monitored and, if necessary, an adjustment in the nimodipine dose should be considered). Products include:
Aptivus Capsules **823**
Aptivus Oral Solution **823**

Torsemide (Nimodipine may increase the blood pressure lowering effect of concomitantly administered anti-hypertensives such as diuretics. However, if a combination of this type proves unavoidable, particularly careful monitoring of the patient is necessary). Products include:
Demadex Injection **2630**
Demadex Tablets **2630**

Trandolapril (Nimodipine may increase the blood pressure lowering effect of concomitantly administered anti-hypertensives such as ACE inhibitors. However, if a combination of this type proves unavoidable, particularly careful monitoring of the patient is necessary). Products include:
Mavik Tablets **472**
Tarka Tablets **511**

Triamcinolone (Nimodipine is metabolized via the cytochrome P450 3A4 system located both in the intestinal mucosa and in the liver. Drugs that are known to induce cytochrome P450 3A4 may therefore alter the first pass or the clearance of nimodipine).
No products indexed under this heading.

Triamcinolone Acetonide (Nimodipine is metabolized via the cytochrome P450 3A4 system located both in the intestinal mucosa and in the liver. Drugs that are known to induce cytochrome P450 3A4 may therefore alter the first pass or the clearance of nimodipine). Products include:
Azmacort Inhalation Aerosol **407**
Nasacort AQ Nasal Spray **2765**
Triesence Injectable Suspension .... ⊙ **209**

Triamcinolone Diacetate (Nimodipine is metabolized via the cytochrome P450 3A4 system located both in the intestinal mucosa and in the liver. Drugs that are known to induce cytochrome P450 3A4 may therefore alter the first pass or the clearance of nimodipine).
No products indexed under this heading.

Triamcinolone Hexacetonide (Nimodipine is metabolized via the cytochrome P450 3A4 system located both in the intestinal mucosa and in the liver. Drugs that are known to induce cytochrome P450 3A4 may therefore alter the first pass or the clearance of nimodipine).
No products indexed under this heading.

Triamterene (Nimodipine may increase the blood pressure lowering effect of concomitantly administered anti-hypertensives such as diuretics. However, if a combination of this type proves unavoidable, particularly careful monitoring of the patient is necessary). Products include:
Dyazide Capsules **1405**
Dyrenium Capsules **3189**

Trimethaphan Camsylate (Nimodipine may increase the blood presure lowering effect of concomitantly administered anti-hypertensives. However, if a combination of this type proves undavoidable particularly careful monitoring of the patient is necessary).
No products indexed under this heading.

Troglitazone (Nimodipine is metabolized via cytochrome P450 3A4 system located both in the intestinal mucosa and in the liver. Plasma concentrations of drugs which are known inhibitors of the cytochrome P450 3A4 system may be increased. Upon co-administration of drugs which are known inhibitors of cytochrome P450 3A4, the blood pressure should be monitored and, if necessary, a reduction of the nimodipine dose should be considered).
No products indexed under this heading.

Troleandomycin (No interaction studies have been carried out between nimodipine and macrolide antibiotics. Certain macrolide antibiotics are known to inhibit cytochrome P450 3A4 system and the potential for drug interaction cannot be ruled out at this stage. Therefore, macrolide antibiotics should not be used in combination with nimodipine. However, if macrolide antibiotics which are inhibitors of the cytochrome P450 3A4 system are co-administered with nimodipine, blood pressure should be monitored and, if necessary, an adjustment in the nimodipine dose should be considered. Azithromycin, although structurally related to the class of macrolide, is void of CYP3A4 inhibition).
No products indexed under this heading.

Valproate Sodium (Nimodipine is metabolized via cytochrome P450 3A4 system located both in the intestinal mucosa and in the liver. Plasma concentrations of drugs which are known inhibitors of the cytochrome P450 3A4 system may be increased. Upon co-administration of drugs which are known inhibitors of cytochrome P450 3A4, the blood pressure should be monitored and, if necessary, a reduction of the nimodipine dose should be considered).
No products indexed under this heading.

Valproic Acid (The simulatenous administration of the anti-convulsant valproic acid can lead to increase in the plamsa nimodipine concentration. Upon co-administration with valproic acid, the blood pressure should be monitored and, if necessary, an adjustment in the nimodipine dose should be considered).
No products indexed under this heading.

Valsartan (Nimodipine may increase the blood presure lowering effect of concomitantly administered anti-hypertensives. However, if a combination of this type proves undavoidable particularly careful monitoring of the patient is necessary). Products include:
Diovan Tablets **2212**
Diovan HCT Tablets **2216**
Exforge Tablets **2238**

Vardenafil Hydrochloride (Nimodipine may increase the blood pressure lowering effect of concomitantly administered anti-hypertensives such as phosphodiesterase type 5 inhibitors. However, if a combination of this type proves unavoidable, particularly careful monitoring of the patient is necessary). Products include:
Levitra Tablets **2876**

Verapamil Hydrochloride (Nimodipine may increase the blood pressure lowering effect of concomitantly administered anti-hypertensives such as other calcium antagonists. However, if a combination of this type proves unavoidable particularly careful monitoring of the patient is necessary). Products include:
Tarka Tablets **511**

Voriconazole (A formal interaction study investigating the potential of drug interaction between nimodipine and ketoconazole has not been performed. Azole anti-mycotics are known to inhibit the cytochrome P450 3A4 system, and various interactions have been reported for other dihydropyridine calcium antagonists. Therefore, when administered together with oral nimodipine, a substantial increase in systemic bioavailability of nimodipine due to a decreased first-pass metabolism cannot be excluded. Upon co-administration with azole anti-mycotics which are inhibitors of the cytochrome P450 3A4 system, blood pressure should be monitored and, if necessary, an adjustment in the nimodipine dose should be considered).
No products indexed under this heading.

Zafirlukast (Nimodipine is metabolized via cytochrome P450 3A4 system located both in the intestinal mucosa and in the liver. Plasma concentrations of drugs which are known inhibitors of the cytochrome P450 3A4 system may be increased. Upon co-administration of drugs which are known inhibitors of cytochrome P450 3A4, the blood pressure should be monitored and, if necessary, a reduction of the nimodipine dose should be considered). Products include:
Accolate Tablets **669**

Zidovudine (In an animal study, simulateneous administration of the anti-HIV drug zidovudine i.v. and nimodipine bolus i.v. resulted in significantly higher AUC of zidovudine, whereas the distribution volume and clearance were significantly reduced). Products include:
Combivir Tablets **1384**
Retrovir **1574**
Retrovir IV Infusion **1579**
Trizivir Tablets **1622**

Zileuton (Nimodipine is metabolized via cytochrome P450 3A4 system located both in the intestinal mucosa and in the liver. Plasma concentrations of drugs which are known inhibitors of the cytochrome P450 3A4 system may be increased. Upon co-administration of drugs which are known inhibitors of cytochrome P450 3A4, the blood pressure should be monitored and, if necessary, a reduction of the nimodipine dose should be considered).
No products indexed under this heading.

Food Interactions

Grapefruit (Grapefruit juice inhibits the cytochrome P450 3A4 system. Administration of dihydropyridine calcium antagonists together with grapefruit juice thus results in elevated concentrations and prolonged action of nimodipine due to a decreased first pass metabolism or reduced clearance. As a consequence, the blood pressure lowering effect may be increased. After intake of grapefruit juice this effect may last for at least 4 days after the last ingestion of grapefruit juice. Ingestion of grapefruit/grapefruit juice is therefore to be avoided while taking nimodipine).

Grapefruit Juice (Grapefruit juice inhibits the cytochrome P450 3A4 system. Administration of dihydropyridine calcium antagonists together with grapefruit juice thus results in elevated concentrations and prolonged action of nimodipine due to a decreased first pass metabolism or reduced clearance. As a consequence, the blood pressure lowering effect may be increased. After intake of grapefruit juice this effect may last for at least 4 days after the last ingestion of grapefruit juice. Ingestion of grapefruit/grapefruit juice is therefore to be avoided while taking nimodipine).

Meal, unspecified (In a study of 24 healthy volunteers, administration of nimodipine capsules following a standard breakfast resulted in a 68% lower peak plasma concentrations and 38% lower bioavailability relative to dosing under fasted conditions. In general, nimodipine capsules should be swallowed whole with little liquid, preferably not less than one hour before or two hours after meals).

NITRO-DUR TRANSDERMAL INFUSION SYSTEM

(Nitroglycerin) **2887**
May interact with calcium channel blockers, vasodilators, and certain other agents. Compounds in these categories include:

Amlodipine Besylate (Vasodilating effects of nitroglycerin may be additive with those of other vasodilators). Products include:
Azor Tablets **1005**
Exforge Tablets **2238**

Amyl Nitrite (Vasodilating effects of nitroglycerin may be additive with those of other vasodilators).
No products indexed under this heading.

Bepridil Hydrochloride (Vasodilating effects of nitroglycerin may be additive with those of other vasodilators).
No products indexed under this heading.

Diazoxide (Vasodilating effects of nitroglycerin may be additive with those of other vasodilators). Products include:
Proglycem Capsules **1185**
Proglycem Suspension **1185**

Diltiazem Hydrochloride (Vasodilating effects of nitroglycerin may be additive with those of other vasodilators). Products include:

Cardizem LA Extended Release Tablets 421

Epoprostenol Sodium (Vasodilating effects of nitroglycerin may be additive with those of other vasodilators). Products include:

Flolan for Injection 1426

Ethaverine Hydrochloride (Vasodilating effects of nitroglycerin may be additive with those of other vasodilators).

No products indexed under this heading.

Felodipine (Vasodilating effects of nitroglycerin may be additive with those of other vasodilators).

No products indexed under this heading.

Hydralazine Hydrochloride (Vasodilating effects of nitroglycerin may be additive with those of other vasodilators).

No products indexed under this heading.

Isosorbide Dinitrate (Vasodilating effects of nitroglycerin may be additive with those of other vasodilators).

No products indexed under this heading.

Isosorbide Mononitrate (Vasodilating effects of nitroglycerin may be additive with those of other vasodilators).

No products indexed under this heading.

Isoxsuprine Hydrochloride (Vasodilating effects of nitroglycerin may be additive with those of other vasodilators).

No products indexed under this heading.

Isradipine (Vasodilating effects of nitroglycerin may be additive with those of other vasodilators). Products include:

DynaCirc CR Controlled Release Tablets 1407

Mibefradil Dihydrochloride (Vasodilating effects of nitroglycerin may be additive with those of other vasodilators).

No products indexed under this heading.

Minoxidil (Vasodilating effects of nitroglycerin may be additive with those of other vasodilators).

No products indexed under this heading.

Nicardipine Hydrochloride (Vasodilating effects of nitroglycerin may be additive with those of other vasodilators). Products include:

Cardene I.V. 1093

Nifedipine (Vasodilating effects of nitroglycerin may be additive with those of other vasodilators).

No products indexed under this heading.

Nimodipine (Vasodilating effects of nitroglycerin may be additive with those of other vasodilators). Products include:

Nimotop Capsules 790

Nisoldipine (Vasodilating effects of nitroglycerin may be additive with those of other vasodilators). Products include:

Sular Extended Release Tablets 2975

Nitroglycerin, long-acting formulations (Vasodilating effects of nitroglycerin may be additive with those of other vasodilators).

No products indexed under this heading.

Nitroglycerin Intravenous (Vasodilating effects of nitroglycerin may be additive with those of other vasodilators).

No products indexed under this heading.

Papaverine (Vasodilating effects of nitroglycerin may be additive with those of other vasodilators).

No products indexed under this heading.

Papaverine Hydrochloride (Vasodilating effects of nitroglycerin may be additive with those of other vasodilators).

No products indexed under this heading.

Sildenafil Citrate (Amplification of the vasodilatory effects of the nitroglycerin patch by sildenafil can result in severe hypotension).

No products indexed under this heading.

Tolazoline Hydrochloride (Vasodilating effects of nitroglycerin may be additive with those of other vasodilators).

No products indexed under this heading.

Verapamil Hydrochloride (Vasodilating effects of nitroglycerin may be additive with those of other vasodilators). Products include:

Tarka Tablets 511

Food Interactions

Alcohol (Enhances sensitivity to the hypotensive effects).

NITROLINGUAL PUMPSPRAY

(Nitroglycerin) 2965

May interact with calcium channel blockers and certain other agents. Compounds in these categories include:

Amlodipine Besylate (Marked symptomatic orthostatic hypotension). Products include:

Azor Tablets 1005
Exforge Tablets 2238

Bepridil Hydrochloride (Marked symptomatic orthostatic hypotension).

No products indexed under this heading.

Diltiazem Hydrochloride (Marked symptomatic orthostatic hypotension). Products include:

Cardizem LA Extended Release Tablets 421

Drugs Depending On Vascular Smooth Muscle (Decreased or increased effect).

No products indexed under this heading.

Felodipine (Marked symptomatic orthostatic hypotension).

No products indexed under this heading.

Isradipine (Marked symptomatic orthostatic hypotension). Products include:

DynaCirc CR Controlled Release Tablets 1407

Mibefradil Dihydrochloride (Marked symptomatic orthostatic hypotension).

No products indexed under this heading.

Nicardipine Hydrochloride (Marked symptomatic orthostatic hypotension). Products include:

Cardene I.V. 1093

Nifedipine (Marked symptomatic orthostatic hypotension).

No products indexed under this heading.

Nimodipine (Marked symptomatic orthostatic hypotension). Products include:

Nimotop Capsules 790

Nisoldipine (Marked symptomatic orthostatic hypotension). Products include:

Sular Extended Release Tablets 2975

Sildenafil Citrate (Concomitant administration with phosphodiesterase inhibitors can cause severe hypotension. The time, course and dose dependency of this interaction are not known. Concurrent use is contraindicated).

No products indexed under this heading.

Tadalafil (Concomitant administration with phosphodiesterase inhibitors can cause severe hypotension. The time, course and dose dependency of this interaction are not known. Concurrent use is contraindicated). Products include:

Cialis Tablets 1792

Vardenafil Hydrochloride (Concomitant administration with phosphodiesterase inhibitors can cause severe hypotension. The time, course and dose dependency of this interaction are not known. Concurrent use is contraindicated). Products include:

Levitra Tablets 2876

Verapamil Hydrochloride (Marked symptomatic orthostatic hypotension). Products include:

Tarka Tablets 511

Food Interactions

Alcohol (Enhanced sensitivity to hypotensive effects).

NIZORAL A-D SHAMPOO

(Ketoconazole) 1901

None cited in PDR database.

NORDITROPIN CARTRIDGES

(Somatropin (rDNA Origin)) 2354

May interact with corticosteroids, cytochrome p450 3a4 substrates (selected), anticonvulsants, estrogens, oral hypoglycemic agents, insulin, and sex steroids. Compounds in these categories include:

Acarbose (In patients with diabetes mellitus requiring drug therapy, the dose of insulin and/or oral agents may require adjustment when somatropin therapy is initiated). Products include:

Precose Tablets 792

Alfentanil Hydrochloride (Limited published data indicate that somatropin treatment increases cytochrome P450 (CYP450)-mediated antipyrine clearance in man. This data suggests that somatropin administration may alter the clearance of compounds known to be metabolized by CYP450 liver enzymes (eg, corticosteroids, sex steroids, anticonvulsants, cyclosporine). Careful monitoring is advisable when somatropin is administered in combination with other drugs known to be metabolized by CYP450 liver enzymes).

No products indexed under this heading.

Alprazolam (Limited published data indicate that somatropin treatment increases cytochrome P450 (CYP450)-mediated antipyrine clearance in man. This data suggests that somatropin administration may alter the clearance of compounds known to be metabolized by CYP450 liver enzymes (eg, corticosteroids, sex steroids, anticonvulsants, cyclosporine). Careful monitoring is advisable when somatropin is administered in combination with other drugs known to be metabolized by CYP450 liver enzymes).

No products indexed under this heading.

Amiodarone Hydrochloride (Limited published data indicate that somatropin treatment increases cytochrome P450 (CYP450)-mediated antipyrine clearance in man. This data suggests that somatropin administration may alter the clearance of compounds known to be metabolized by CYP450 liver enzymes (eg, corticosteroids, sex steroids, anticonvulsants, cyclosporine). Careful monitoring is advisable when somatropin is administered in combination with other drugs known to be metabolized by CYP450 liver enzymes).

No products indexed under this heading.

Amitriptyline Hydrochloride (Limited published data indicate that somatropin treatment increases cytochrome P450 (CYP450)-mediated antipyrine clearance in man. This data suggests that somatropin administration may alter the clearance of compounds known to be metabolized by CYP450 liver enzymes (eg, corticosteroids, sex steroids, anticonvulsants, cyclosporine). Careful monitoring is advisable when somatropin is administered in combination with other drugs known to be metabolized by CYP450 liver enzymes).

No products indexed under this heading.

Amlodipine Besylate (Limited published data indicate that somatropin treatment increases cytochrome P450 (CYP450)-mediated antipyrine clearance in man. This data suggests that somatropin administration may alter the clearance of compounds known to be metabolized by CYP450 liver enzymes (eg, corticosteroids, sex steroids, anticonvulsants, cyclosporine). Careful monitoring is advisable when somatropin is administered in combination with other drugs known to be metabolized by CYP450 liver enzymes). Products include:

Azor Tablets 1005
Exforge Tablets 2238

Aprepitant (Limited published data indicate that somatropin treatment increases cytochrome P450 (CYP450)-mediated antipyrine clearance in man. This data suggests that somatropin administration may alter the clearance of compounds known to be metabolized by CYP450 liver enzymes (eg, corticosteroids, sex steroids, anticonvulsants, cyclosporine). Careful monitoring is advisable when somatropin is administered in combination with other drugs known to be metabolized by CYP450 liver enzymes). Products include:

Emend Capsules 1992

Astemizole (Limited published data indicate that somatropin treatment increases cytochrome P450 (CYP450)-mediated antipyrine clearance in man. This data suggests that somatropin administration may alter the clearance of compounds known to be metabolized by CYP450 liver enzymes (eg, corticosteroids, sex steroids, anticonvulsants, cyclosporine). Careful monitoring is advisable when somatropin is administered in combination with other drugs known to be metabolized by CYP450 liver enzymes).

No products indexed under this heading.

Atorvastatin Calcium (Limited published data indicate that somatropin treatment increases cytochrome P450 (CYP450)-mediated antipyrine clearance in man. This data suggests that somatropin administration may alter the clearance of compounds known to be metabolized by CYP450 liver enzymes (eg, corticosteroids, sex steroids, anticonvulsants, cyclosporine). Careful monitoring is advisable when somatropin is administered in combination with other drugs known to be metabolized by CYP450 liver enzymes). Products include:

Lipitor Tablets **2501**

Belladonna Ergotamine (Limited published data indicate that somatropin treatment increases cytochrome P450 (CYP450)-mediated antipyrine clearance in man. This data suggests that somatropin administration may alter the clearance of compounds known to be metabolized by CYP450 liver enzymes (eg, corticosteroids, sex steroids, anticonvulsants, cyclosporine). Careful monitoring is advisable when somatropin is administered in combination with other drugs known to be metabolized by CYP450 liver enzymes).

No products indexed under this heading.

Betamethasone Acetate (Limited published data indicate that somatropin treatment increases cytochrome P450 (CYP450)-mediated antipyrine clearance in man. This data suggests that somatropin administration may alter the clearance of compounds known to be metabolized by CYP450 liver enzymes (eg, corticosteroids). Careful monitoring is advisable when somatropin is administered in combination with other drugs known to be metabolized by CYP450 liver enzymes. Excessive glucocorticoid therapy may attenuate the growth promoting effects of somatropin in children).

No products indexed under this heading.

Betamethasone Sodium Phosphate (Limited published data indicate that somatropin treatment increases cytochrome P450 (CYP450)-mediated antipyrine clearance in man. This data suggests that somatropin administration may alter the clearance of compounds known to be metabolized by CYP450 liver enzymes (eg, corticosteroids). Careful monitoring is advisable when somatropin is administered in combination with other drugs known to be metabolized by CYP450 liver enzymes. Excessive glucocorticoid therapy may attenuate the growth promoting effects of somatropin in children).

No products indexed under this heading.

Budesonide (Limited published data indicate that somatropin treatment increases cytochrome P450 (CYP450)-mediated antipyrine clearance in man. This data suggests that somatropin administration may alter the clearance of compounds known to be metabolized by CYP450 liver enzymes (eg, corticosteroids). Careful monitoring is advisable when somatropin is administered in combination with other drugs known to be metabolized by CYP450 liver enzymes. Excessive glucocorticoid therapy may attenuate the growth promoting effects of somatropin in children). Products include:

Pulmicort Flexhaler **654**
Symbicort 80/4.5 Inhalation Aerosol.. **659**
Symbicort 160/4.5 Inhalation Aerosol.. **659**

Buspirone Hydrochloride (Limited published data indicate that somatropin treatment increases cytochrome P450 (CYP450)-mediated antipyrine clearance in man. This data suggests that somatropin administration may alter the clearance of compounds known to be metabolized by CYP450 liver enzymes (eg, corticosteroids, sex steroids, anticonvulsants, cyclosporine). Careful monitoring is advisable when somatropin is administered in combination with other drugs known to be metabolized by CYP450 liver enzymes).

No products indexed under this heading.

Busulfan (Limited published data indicate that somatropin treatment increases cytochrome P450 (CYP450)-mediated antipyrine clearance in man. This data suggests that somatropin administration may alter the clearance of compounds known to be metabolized by CYP450 liver enzymes (eg, corticosteroids, sex steroids, anticonvulsants, cyclosporine). Careful monitoring is advisable when somatropin is administered in combination with other drugs known to be metabolized by CYP450 liver enzymes). Products include:

Busulfex Injection **2477**
Myleran Tablets **1530**

Carbamazepine (Limited published data indicate that somatropin treatment increases cytochrome P450 (CYP450)-mediated antipyrine clearance in man. This data suggests that somatropin administration may alter the clearance of compounds known to be metabolized by CYP450 liver enzymes (eg, anticonvulsants). Careful monitoring is advisable when somatropin is administered in combination with other drugs known to be metabolized by CYP450 liver enzymes). Products include:

Carbatrol Capsules **3019**
Equetro Extended-Release Capsules.................................... **3174**

Cerivastatin Sodium (Limited published data indicate that somatropin treatment increases cytochrome P450 (CYP450)-mediated antipyrine clearance in man. This data suggests that somatropin administration may alter the clearance of compounds known to be metabolized by CYP450 liver enzymes (eg, corticosteroids, sex steroids, anticonvulsants, cyclosporine). Careful monitoring is advisable when somatropin is administered in combination with other drugs known to be metabolized by CYP450 liver enzymes).

No products indexed under this heading.

Chlorotrianisene (In adult women on oral estrogen replacement, a larger dose of somatropin may be required to achieve the defined treatment goal).

No products indexed under this heading.

Chlorpheniramine (Limited published data indicate that somatropin treatment increases cytochrome P450 (CYP450)-mediated antipyrine clearance in man. This data suggests that somatropin administration may alter the clearance of compounds known to be metabolized by CYP450 liver enzymes (eg, corticosteroids, sex steroids, anticonvulsants, cyclosporine). Careful monitoring is advisable when somatropin is administered in combination with other drugs known to be metabolized by CYP450 liver enzymes).

No products indexed under this heading.

Chlorpheniramine Maleate (Limited published data indicate that somatropin treatment increases cytochrome P450 (CYP450)-mediated antipyrine clearance in man. This data suggests that somatropin administration may alter the clearance of compounds known to be metabolized by CYP450 liver enzymes (eg, corticosteroids, sex steroids, anticonvulsants, cyclosporine). Careful monitoring is advisable when somatropin is administered in combination with other drugs known to be metabolized by CYP450 liver enzymes). Products include:

Actifed Cold & Allergy Tablets **1895**
Sudafed PE Sinus & Allergy Tablets.. **1908**
Tylenol Allergy Multi-Symptom Caplets with Cool Burst and Rapid Release Gelcaps................ **1916**
Children's Tylenol Plus Cold Suspension Liquid **1912**
Children's Tylenol Plus Cough & Runny Nose Suspension Liquid..... **1912**
Children's Tylenol Plus Flu Suspension Liquid **1914**
Children's Tylenol Plus Multi-Symptom Cold Suspension Liquid **1912**
Tylenol Cold Head Congestion Nighttime Caplets with Cool Burst.. **1910**
Tylenol Cold Multi-Symptom Nighttime Caplets with Cool Burst.. **1913**
Tylenol Sinus Congestion & Pain Nighttime Caplets with Cool Burst.. **1917**

Chlorpheniramine Polistirex (Limited published data indicate that somatropin treatment increases cytochrome P450 (CYP450)-mediated antipyrine clearance in man. This data suggests that somatropin administration may alter the clearance of compounds known to be metabolized by CYP450 liver enzymes (eg, corticosteroids, sex steroids, anticonvulsants, cyclosporine). Careful monitoring is advisable when somatropin is administered in combination with other drugs known to be metabolized by CYP450 liver enzymes). Products include:

Tussionex Pennkinetic Extended-Release Suspension...... **3154**

Chlorpheniramine Tannate (Limited published data indicate that somatropin treatment increases cytochrome P450 (CYP450)-mediated antipyrine clearance in man. This data suggests that somatropin administration may alter the clearance of compounds known to be metabolized by CYP450 liver enzymes (eg, corticosteroids, sex steroids, anticonvulsants, cyclosporine). Careful monitoring is advisable when somatropin is administered in combination with other drugs known to be metabolized by CYP450 liver enzymes).

No products indexed under this heading.

Chlorpropamide (In patients with diabetes mellitus requiring drug therapy, the dose of insulin and/or oral agents may require adjustment when somatropin therapy is initiated).

No products indexed under this heading.

Ciclesonide (Limited published data indicate that somatropin treatment increases cytochrome P450 (CYP450)-mediated antipyrine clearance in man. This data suggests that somatropin administration may alter the clearance of compounds known to be metabolized by CYP450 liver enzymes (eg, corticosteroids). Careful monitoring is advisable when somatropin is administered in combination with other drugs known to be metabolized by CYP450 liver enzymes. Excessive glucocorticoid therapy may attenuate the growth promoting effects of somatropin in children). Products include:

Alvesco Inhalation Aerosol **2985**
Omnaris Nasal Spray **2998**

Cisapride (Limited published data indicate that somatropin treatment increases cytochrome P450 (CYP450)-mediated antipyrine clearance in man. This data suggests that somatropin administration may alter the clearance of compounds known to be metabolized by CYP450 liver enzymes (eg, corticosteroids, sex steroids, anticonvulsants, cyclosporine). Careful monitoring is advisable when somatropin is administered in combination with other drugs known to be metabolized by CYP450 liver enzymes).

No products indexed under this heading.

Clarithromycin (Limited published data indicate that somatropin treatment increases cytochrome P450 (CYP450)-mediated antipyrine clearance in man. This data suggests that somatropin administration may alter the clearance of compounds known to be metabolized by CYP450 liver enzymes (eg, corticosteroids, sex steroids, anticonvulsants, cyclosporine). Careful monitoring is advisable when somatropin is administered in combination with other drugs known to be metabolized by CYP450 liver enzymes). Products include:

Biaxin/Biaxin XL **411**

Cortisone Acetate (Limited published data indicate that somatropin treatment increases cytochrome P450 (CYP450)-mediated antipyrine clearance in man. This data suggests that somatropin administration may alter the clearance of compounds known to be metabolized by CYP450 liver enzymes (eg, corticosteroids). Careful monitoring is advisable when somatropin is administered in combination with other drugs known to be metabolized by CYP450 liver enzymes. Excessive glucocorticoid therapy may attenuate the growth promoting effects of somatropin in children).

No products indexed under this heading.

Cyclosporine (Limited published data indicate that somatropin treatment increases cytochrome P450 (CYP450)-mediated antipyrine clearance in man. This data suggests that somatropin administration may alter the clearance of compounds known to be metabolized by CYP450 liver enzymes (eg, corticosteroids, sex steroids, anticonvulsants, cyclosporine). Careful monitoring is advisable when somatropin is administered in combination with other drugs known to be metabolized by CYP450 liver enzymes). Products include:

Gengraf Capsules 435
Neoral Oral Solution 2280
Neoral Soft Gelatin Capsules 2280
Restasis Ophthalmic Emulsion 557
Sandimmune 2296

Desogestrel (Limited published data indicate that somatropin treatment increases cytochrome P450 (CYP450)-mediated antipyrine clearance in man. This data suggests that somatropin administration may alter the clearance of compounds known to be metabolized by CYP450 liver enzymes (eg, sex steroids). Careful monitoring is advisable when somatropin is administered in combination with other drugs known to be metabolized by CYP450 liver enzymes). Products include:

Mircette Tablets 1034

Dexamethasone (Limited published data indicate that somatropin treatment increases cytochrome P450 (CYP450)-mediated antipyrine clearance in man. This data suggests that somatropin administration may alter the clearance of compounds known to be metabolized by CYP450 liver enzymes (eg, corticosteroids). Careful monitoring is advisable when somatropin is administered in combination with other drugs known to be metabolized by CYP450 liver enzymes. Excessive glucocorticoid therapy may attenuate the growth promoting effects of somatropin in children). Products include:

Ciprodex Otic Suspension 541

Dexamethasone Acetate (Limited published data indicate that somatropin treatment increases cytochrome P450 (CYP450)-mediated antipyrine clearance in man. This data suggests that somatropin administration may alter the clearance of compounds known to be metabolized by CYP450 liver enzymes (eg, corticosteroids). Careful monitoring is advisable when somatropin is administered in combination with other drugs known to be metabolized by CYP450 liver enzymes. Excessive glucocorticoid therapy may attenuate the growth promoting effects of somatropin in children).

No products indexed under this heading.

Dexamethasone Sodium Phosphate (Limited published data indicate that somatropin treatment increases cytochrome P450 (CYP450)-mediated antipyrine clearance in man. This data suggests that somatropin administration may alter the clearance of compounds known to be metabolized by CYP450 liver enzymes (eg, corticosteroids). Careful monitoring is advisable when somatropin is administered in combination with other drugs known to be metabolized by CYP450 liver enzymes. Excessive glucocorticoid therapy may attenuate the growth promoting effects of somatropin in children).

No products indexed under this heading.

Diazepam (Limited published data indicate that somatropin treatment increases cytochrome P450 (CYP450)-mediated antipyrine clearance in man. This data suggests that somatropin administration may alter the clearance of compounds known to be metabolized by CYP450 liver enzymes (eg, corticosteroids, sex steroids, anticonvulsants, cyclosporine). Careful monitoring is advisable when somatropin is administered in combination with other drugs known to be metabolized by CYP450 liver enzymes). Products include:

Valium Tablets 2658

Dienestrol (In adult women on oral estrogen replacement, a larger dose of somatropin may be required to achieve the defined treatment goal).

No products indexed under this heading.

Diethylstilbestrol (In adult women on oral estrogen replacement, a larger dose of somatropin may be required to achieve the defined treatment goal).

No products indexed under this heading.

Dihydroergotamine Mesylate (Limited published data indicate that somatropin treatment increases cytochrome P450 (CYP450)-mediated antipyrine clearance in man. This data suggests that somatropin administration may alter the clearance of compounds known to be metabolized by CYP450 liver enzymes (eg, corticosteroids, sex steroids, anticonvulsants, cyclosporine). Careful monitoring is advisable when somatropin is administered in combination with other drugs known to be metabolized by CYP450 liver enzymes).

No products indexed under this heading.

Diltiazem Hydrochloride (Limited published data indicate that somatropin treatment increases cytochrome P450 (CYP450)-mediated antipyrine clearance in man. This data suggests that somatropin administration may alter the clearance of compounds known to be metabolized by CYP450 liver enzymes (eg, corticosteroids, sex steroids, anticonvulsants, cyclosporine). Careful monitoring is advisable when somatropin is administered in combination with other drugs known to be metabolized by CYP450 liver enzymes). Products include:

Cardizem LA Extended Release Tablets 421

Diltiazem Maleate (Limited published data indicate that somatropin treatment increases cytochrome P450 (CYP450)-mediated antipyrine clearance in man. This data suggests that somatropin administration may alter the clearance of compounds known to be metabolized by CYP450 liver enzymes (eg, corticosteroids, sex steroids, anticonvulsants, cyclosporine). Careful monitoring is advisable when somatropin is administered in combination with other drugs known to be metabolized by CYP450 liver enzymes).

No products indexed under this heading.

Disopyramide (Limited published data indicate that somatropin treatment increases cytochrome P450 (CYP450)-mediated antipyrine clearance in man. This data suggests that somatropin administration may alter the clearance of compounds known to be metabolized by CYP450 liver enzymes (eg, corticosteroids, sex steroids, anticonvulsants, cyclosporine). Careful monitoring is advisable when somatropin is administered in combination with other drugs known to be metabolized by CYP450 liver enzymes).

No products indexed under this heading.

Disopyramide Phosphate (Limited published data indicate that somatropin treatment increases cytochrome P450 (CYP450)-mediated antipyrine clearance in man. This data suggests that somatropin administration may alter the clearance of compounds known to be metabolized by CYP450 liver enzymes (eg, corticosteroids, sex steroids, anticonvulsants, cyclosporine). Careful monitoring is advisable when somatropin is administered in combination with other drugs known to be metabolized by CYP450 liver enzymes).

No products indexed under this heading.

Disulfiram (Limited published data indicate that somatropin treatment increases cytochrome P450 (CYP450)-mediated antipyrine clearance in man. This data suggests that somatropin administration may alter the clearance of compounds known to be metabolized by CYP450 liver enzymes (eg, corticosteroids, sex steroids, anticonvulsants, cyclosporine). Careful monitoring is advisable when somatropin is administered in combination with other drugs known to be metabolized by CYP450 liver enzymes).

No products indexed under this heading.

Divalproex Sodium (Limited published data indicate that somatropin treatment increases cytochrome P450 (CYP450)-mediated antipyrine clearance in man. This data suggests that somatropin administration may alter the clearance of compounds known to be metabolized by CYP450 liver enzymes (eg, anticonvulsants). Careful monitoring is advisable when somatropin is administered in combination with other drugs known to be metabolized by CYP450 liver enzymes). Products include:

Depakote ER Tablets 423

Doxorubicin Hydrochloride (Limited published data indicate that somatropin treatment increases cytochrome P450 (CYP450)-mediated antipyrine clearance in man. This data suggests that somatropin administration may alter the clearance of compounds known to be metabolized by CYP450 liver enzymes (eg, corticosteroids, sex steroids, anticonvulsants, cyclosporine). Careful monitoring is advisable when somatropin is administered in combination with other drugs known to be metabolized by CYP450 liver enzymes).

No products indexed under this heading.

Dronabinol (Limited published data indicate that somatropin treatment increases cytochrome P450 (CYP450)-mediated antipyrine clearance in man. This data suggests that somatropin administration may alter the clearance of compounds known to be metabolized by CYP450 liver enzymes (eg, corticosteroids, sex steroids, anticonvulsants, cyclosporine). Careful monitoring is advisable when somatropin is administered in combination with other drugs known to be metabolized by CYP450 liver enzymes). Products include:

Marinol Capsules 3163

Ergotamine Tartrate (Limited published data indicate that somatropin treatment increases cytochrome P450 (CYP450)-mediated antipyrine clearance in man. This data suggests that somatropin administration may alter the clearance of compounds known to be metabolized by CYP450 liver enzymes (eg, corticosteroids, sex steroids, anticonvulsants, cyclosporine). Careful monitoring is advisable when somatropin is administered in combination with other drugs known to be metabolized by CYP450 liver enzymes).

No products indexed under this heading.

Erythromycin (Limited published data indicate that somatropin treatment increases cytochrome P450 (CYP450)-mediated antipyrine clearance in man. This data suggests that somatropin administration may alter the clearance of compounds known to be metabolized by CYP450 liver enzymes (eg, corticosteroids, sex steroids, anticonvulsants, cyclosporine). Careful monitoring is advisable when somatropin is administered in combination with other drugs known to be metabolized by CYP450 liver enzymes).

No products indexed under this heading.

Erythromycin Estolate (Limited published data indicate that somatropin treatment increases cytochrome P450 (CYP450)-mediated antipyrine clearance in man. This data suggests that somatropin administration may alter the clearance of compounds known to be metabolized by CYP450 liver enzymes (eg, corticosteroids, sex steroids, anticonvulsants, cyclosporine). Careful monitoring is advisable when somatropin is administered in combination with other drugs known to be metabolized by CYP450 liver enzymes).

No products indexed under this heading.

Erythromycin Ethylsuccinate (Limited published data indicate that somatropin treatment increases cytochrome P450 (CYP450)-mediated antipyrine clearance in man. This data suggests that somatropin administration may alter the clearance of compounds known to be metabolized by CYP450 liver enzymes (eg, corticosteroids, sex steroids, anticonvulsants, cyclosporine). Careful monitoring is advisable when somatropin is administered in combination with other drugs known to be metabolized by CYP450 liver enzymes). Products include:

E.E.S. 433
EryPed 431

Erythromycin Gluceptate (Limited published data indicate that somatropin treatment increases cytochrome P450 (CYP450)-mediated antipyrine clearance in man. This data sug-

gests that somatropin administration may alter the clearance of compounds known to be metabolized by CYP450 liver enzymes (eg, corticosteroids, sex steroids, anticonvulsants, cyclosporine). Careful monitoring is advisable when somatropin is administered in combination with other drugs known to be metabolized by CYP450 liver enzymes).

No products indexed under this heading.

Erythromycin Lactobionate (Limited published data indicate that somatropin treatment increases cytochrome P450 (CYP450)-mediated antipyrine clearance in man. This data suggests that somatropin administration may alter the clearance of compounds known to be metabolized by CYP450 liver enzymes (eg, corticosteroids, sex steroids, anticonvulsants, cyclosporine). Careful monitoring is advisable when somatropin is administered in combination with other drugs known to be metabolized by CYP450 liver enzymes).

No products indexed under this heading.

Erythromycin Stearate (Limited published data indicate that somatropin treatment increases cytochrome P450 (CYP450)-mediated antipyrine clearance in man. This data suggests that somatropin administration may alter the clearance of compounds known to be metabolized by CYP450 liver enzymes (eg, corticosteroids, sex steroids, anticonvulsants, cyclosporine). Careful monitoring is advisable when somatropin is administered in combination with other drugs known to be metabolized by CYP450 liver enzymes).

No products indexed under this heading.

Estradiol (In adult women on oral estrogen replacement, a larger dose of somatropin may be required to achieve the defined treatment goal). Products include:

Activella Tablets **2347**
Angeliq Tablets **751**
Climara Transdermal System **763**
Climara Pro Transdermal System **768**
Divigel **3167**
Vagifem Tablets **2375**

Estradiol Benzoate (Limited published data indicate that somatropin treatment increases cytochrome P450 (CYP450)-mediated antipyrine clearance in man. This data suggests that somatropin administration may alter the clearance of compounds known to be metabolized by CYP450 liver enzymes (eg, corticosteroids, sex steroids, anticonvulsants, cyclosporine). Careful monitoring is advisable when somatropin is administered in combination with other drugs known to be metabolized by CYP450 liver enzymes).

No products indexed under this heading.

Estradiol Cypionate (Limited published data indicate that somatropin treatment increases cytochrome P450 (CYP450)-mediated antipyrine clearance in man. This data suggests that somatropin administration may alter the clearance of compounds known to be metabolized by CYP450 liver enzymes (eg, corticosteroids, sex steroids, anticonvulsants, cyclosporine). Careful monitoring is advisable when somatropin is administered in combination with other drugs known to be metabolized by CYP450 liver enzymes).

No products indexed under this heading.

Estradiol Valerate (Limited published data indicate that somatropin treatment increases cytochrome P450 (CYP450)-mediated antipyrine clearance in man. This data suggests that somatropin administration may alter the clearance of compounds known to be metabolized by CYP450 liver enzymes (eg, corticosteroids, sex steroids, anticonvulsants, cyclosporine). Careful monitoring is advisable when somatropin is administered in combination with other drugs known to be metabolized by CYP450 liver enzymes).

No products indexed under this heading.

Estrogens, Conjugated (In adult women on oral estrogen replacement, a larger dose of somatropin may be required to achieve the defined treatment goal). Products include:

Premarin Intravenous **3217**
Premarin Tablets **3221**
Premarin Vaginal Cream **3228**
Premphase Tablets **3232**
Prempro Tablets **3232**

Estrogens, Esterified (In adult women on oral estrogen replacement, a larger dose of somatropin may be required to achieve the defined treatment goal). Products include:

Estratest Tablets **3043**
Estratest H.S. Tablets **3043**

Estropipate (In adult women on oral estrogen replacement, a larger dose of somatropin may be required to achieve the defined treatment goal).

No products indexed under this heading.

Ethinyl Estradiol (In adult women on oral estrogen replacement, a larger dose of somatropin may be required to achieve the defined treatment goal). Products include:

Lybrel Tablets **3204**
Mircette Tablets **1034**
NuvaRing **2897**
Ortho-Cyclen/Ortho Tri-Cyclen **2449**
Ortho Evra Transdermal System **2437**
Ortho Tri-Cyclen Lo Tablets **2458**
Seasonique Tablets **1046**
Yaz Tablets **805**

Ethosuximide (Limited published data indicate that somatropin treatment increases cytochrome P450 (CYP450)-mediated antipyrine clearance in man. This data suggests that somatropin administration may alter the clearance of compounds known to be metabolized by CYP450 liver enzymes (eg, anticonvulsants). Careful monitoring is advisable when somatropin is administered in combination with other drugs known to be metabolized by CYP450 liver enzymes).

No products indexed under this heading.

Ethotoin (Limited published data indicate that somatropin treatment increases cytochrome P450 (CYP450)-mediated antipyrine clearance in man. This data suggests that somatropin administration may alter the clearance of compounds known to be metabolized by CYP450 liver enzymes (eg, anticonvulsants). Careful monitoring is advisable when somatropin is administered in combination with other drugs known to be metabolized by CYP450 liver enzymes).

No products indexed under this heading.

Ethynodiol Diacetate (Limited published data indicate that somatropin treatment increases cytochrome P450 (CYP450)-mediated antipyrine clearance in man. This data suggests that somatropin administration may alter the clearance of compounds known to be metabolized by CYP450 liver enzymes (eg, sex steroids). Careful monitoring is advisable when somatropin is administered in combination with other drugs known to be metabolized by CYP450 liver enzymes).

No products indexed under this heading.

Etoposide (Limited published data indicate that somatropin treatment increases cytochrome P450 (CYP450)-mediated antipyrine clearance in man. This data suggests that somatropin administration may alter the clearance of compounds known to be metabolized by CYP450 liver enzymes (eg, corticosteroids, sex steroids, anticonvulsants, cyclosporine). Careful monitoring is advisable when somatropin is administered in combination with other drugs known to be metabolized by CYP450 liver enzymes).

No products indexed under this heading.

Etoposide Phosphate (Limited published data indicate that somatropin treatment increases cytochrome P450 (CYP450)-mediated antipyrine clearance in man. This data suggests that somatropin administration may alter the clearance of compounds known to be metabolized by CYP450 liver enzymes (eg, corticosteroids, sex steroids, anticonvulsants, cyclosporine). Careful monitoring is advisable when somatropin is administered in combination with other drugs known to be metabolized by CYP450 liver enzymes).

No products indexed under this heading.

Felbamate (Limited published data indicate that somatropin treatment increases cytochrome P450 (CYP450)-mediated antipyrine clearance in man. This data suggests that somatropin administration may alter the clearance of compounds known to be metabolized by CYP450 liver enzymes (eg, anticonvulsants). Careful monitoring is advisable when somatropin is administered in combination with other drugs known to be metabolized by CYP450 liver enzymes).

No products indexed under this heading.

Felodipine (Limited published data indicate that somatropin treatment increases cytochrome P450 (CYP450)-mediated antipyrine clearance in man. This data suggests that somatropin administration may alter the clearance of compounds known to be metabolized by CYP450 liver enzymes (eg, corticosteroids, sex steroids, anticonvulsants, cyclosporine). Careful monitoring is advisable when somatropin is administered in combination with other drugs known to be metabolized by CYP450 liver enzymes).

No products indexed under this heading.

Fentanyl (Limited published data indicate that somatropin treatment increases cytochrome P450 (CYP450)-mediated antipyrine clearance in man. This data suggests that somatropin administration may alter the clearance of compounds known to be metabolized by CYP450 liver enzymes (eg, corticosteroids, sex steroids, anticonvulsants, cyclosporine). Careful monitoring is advisable when somatropin is administered in combination with other drugs known to be metabolized by CYP450 liver enzymes). Products include:

Duragesic Transdermal System **2405**
Ionsys Transdermal System **2410**

Fentanyl Citrate (Limited published data indicate that somatropin treatment increases cytochrome P450 (CYP450)-mediated antipyrine clearance in man. This data suggests that somatropin administration may alter the clearance of compounds known to be metabolized by CYP450 liver enzymes (eg, corticosteroids, sex steroids, anticonvulsants, cyclosporine). Careful monitoring is advisable when somatropin is administered in combination with other drugs known to be metabolized by CYP450 liver enzymes). Products include:

Actiq **959**
Fentora Tablets **968**

Fludrocortisone Acetate (Limited published data indicate that somatropin treatment increases cytochrome P450 (CYP450)-mediated antipyrine clearance in man. This data suggests that somatropin administration may alter the clearance of compounds known to be metabolized by CYP450 liver enzymes (eg, corticosteroids). Careful monitoring is advisable when somatropin is administered in combination with other drugs known to be metabolized by CYP450 liver enzymes. Excessive glucocorticoid therapy may attenuate the growth promoting effects of somatropin in children).

No products indexed under this heading.

Flunisolide (Limited published data indicate that somatropin treatment increases cytochrome P450 (CYP450)-mediated antipyrine clearance in man. This data suggests that somatropin administration may alter the clearance of compounds known to be metabolized by CYP450 liver enzymes (eg, corticosteroids). Careful monitoring is advisable when somatropin is administered in combination with other drugs known to be metabolized by CYP450 liver enzymes. Excessive glucocorticoid therapy may attenuate the growth promoting effects of somatropin in children). Products include:

Aerobid/Aerobid-M **1153**

Fluoxymesterone (Limited published data indicate that somatropin treatment increases cytochrome P450 (CYP450)-mediated antipyrine clearance in man. This data suggests that somatropin administration may alter the clearance of compounds known to be metabolized by CYP450 liver enzymes (eg, sex steroids). Careful monitoring is advisable when somatropin is administered in combination with other drugs known to be metabolized by CYP450 liver enzymes).

No products indexed under this heading.

Fluticasone Propionate (Limited published data indicate that somatropin treatment increases cytochrome

P450 (CYP450)-mediated antipyrine clearance in man. This data suggests that somatropin administration may alter the clearance of compounds known to be metabolized by CYP450 liver enzymes (eg, corticosteroids). Careful monitoring is advisable when somatropin is administered in combination with other drugs known to be metabolized by CYP450 liver enzymes. Excessive glucocorticoid therapy may attenuate the growth promoting effects of somatropin in children). Products include:

Advair Diskus 100/50 .... **1276**
Advair Diskus 250/50 .... **1276**
Advair Diskus 500/50 .... **1276**
Advair HFA 45/21 Inhalation Aerosol.................................. **1288**
Advair HFA 115/21 Inhalation Aerosol.................................. **1288**
Advair HFA 230/21 Inhalation Aerosol.................................. **1288**
Flonase Nasal Spray **1431**
Flovent Diskus 50 mcg **1435**

Fluticasone Propionate HFA (Limited published data indicate that somatropin treatment increases cytochrome P450 (CYP450)-mediated antipyrine clearance in man. This data suggests that somatropin administration may alter the clearance of compounds known to be metabolized by CYP450 liver enzymes (eg, corticosteroids). Careful monitoring is advisable when somatropin is administered in combination with other drugs known to be metabolized by CYP450 liver enzymes. Excessive glucocorticoid therapy may attenuate the growth promoting effects of somatropin in children). Products include:

Flovent HFA **1440**

Fosphenytoin (Limited published data indicate that somatropin treatment increases cytochrome P450 (CYP450)-mediated antipyrine clearance in man. This data suggests that somatropin administration may alter the clearance of compounds known to be metabolized by CYP450 liver enzymes (eg, anticonvulsants). Careful monitoring is advisable when somatropin is administered in combination with other drugs known to be metabolized by CYP450 liver enzymes).

No products indexed under this heading.

Fosphenytoin Sodium (Limited published data indicate that somatropin treatment increases cytochrome P450 (CYP450)-mediated antipyrine clearance in man. This data suggests that somatropin administration may alter the clearance of compounds known to be metabolized by CYP450 liver enzymes (eg, anticonvulsants). Careful monitoring is advisable when somatropin is administered in combination with other drugs known to be metabolized by CYP450 liver enzymes).

No products indexed under this heading.

Gabapentin (Limited published data indicate that somatropin treatment increases cytochrome P450 (CYP450)-mediated antipyrine clearance in man. This data suggests that somatropin administration may alter the clearance of compounds known to be metabolized by CYP450 liver enzymes (eg, anticonvulsants). Careful monitoring is advisable when somatropin is administered in combination with other drugs known to be metabolized by CYP450 liver enzymes).

No products indexed under this heading.

Glimepiride (In patients with diabetes mellitus requiring drug therapy, the dose of insulin and/or oral agents may require adjustment when somatropin therapy is initiated). Products include:

Avandaryl Tablets **1344**
Duetact Tablets **3085**

Glipizide (In patients with diabetes mellitus requiring drug therapy, the dose of insulin and/or oral agents may require adjustment when somatropin therapy is initiated).

No products indexed under this heading.

Glyburide (In patients with diabetes mellitus requiring drug therapy, the dose of insulin and/or oral agents may require adjustment when somatropin therapy is initiated).

No products indexed under this heading.

Haloperidol (Limited published data indicate that somatropin treatment increases cytochrome P450 (CYP450)-mediated antipyrine clearance in man. This data suggests that somatropin administration may alter the clearance of compounds known to be metabolized by CYP450 liver enzymes (eg, corticosteroids, sex steroids, anticonvulsants, cyclosporine). Careful monitoring is advisable when somatropin is administered in combination with other drugs known to be metabolized by CYP450 liver enzymes).

No products indexed under this heading.

Haloperidol Decanoate (Limited published data indicate that somatropin treatment increases cytochrome P450 (CYP450)-mediated antipyrine clearance in man. This data suggests that somatropin administration may alter the clearance of compounds known to be metabolized by CYP450 liver enzymes (eg, corticosteroids, sex steroids, anticonvulsants, cyclosporine). Careful monitoring is advisable when somatropin is administered in combination with other drugs known to be metabolized by CYP450 liver enzymes).

No products indexed under this heading.

Haloperidol Lactate (Limited published data indicate that somatropin treatment increases cytochrome P450 (CYP450)-mediated antipyrine clearance in man. This data suggests that somatropin administration may alter the clearance of compounds known to be metabolized by CYP450 liver enzymes (eg, corticosteroids, sex steroids, anticonvulsants, cyclosporine). Careful monitoring is advisable when somatropin is administered in combination with other drugs known to be metabolized by CYP450 liver enzymes).

No products indexed under this heading.

Hydrocortisone (Limited published data indicate that somatropin treatment increases cytochrome P450 (CYP450)-mediated antipyrine clearance in man. This data suggests that somatropin administration may alter the clearance of compounds known to be metabolized by CYP450 liver enzymes (eg, corticosteroids). Careful monitoring is advisable when somatropin is administered in combination with other drugs known to be metabolized by CYP450 liver enzymes. Excessive glucocorticoid therapy may attenuate the growth promoting effects of somatropin in children).

No products indexed under this heading.

Hydrocortisone Acetate (Limited published data indicate that somatropin treatment increases cytochrome P450 (CYP450)-mediated antipyrine clearance in man. This data suggests that somatropin administration may alter the clearance of compounds known to be metabolized by CYP450 liver enzymes (eg, corticosteroids). Careful monitoring is advisable when somatropin is administered in combination with other drugs known to be metabolized by CYP450 liver enzymes. Excessive glucocorticoid therapy may attenuate the growth promoting effects of somatropin in children). Products include:

Analpram-HC **1140**
Pramosone **1141**

Hydrocortisone Sodium Phosphate (Limited published data indicate that somatropin treatment increases cytochrome P450 (CYP450)-mediated antipyrine clearance in man. This data suggests that somatropin administration may alter the clearance of compounds known to be metabolized by CYP450 liver enzymes (eg, corticosteroids). Careful monitoring is advisable when somatropin is administered in combination with other drugs known to be metabolized by CYP450 liver enzymes. Excessive glucocorticoid therapy may attenuate the growth promoting effects of somatropin in children).

No products indexed under this heading.

Hydrocortisone Sodium Succinate (Limited published data indicate that somatropin treatment increases cytochrome P450 (CYP450)-mediated antipyrine clearance in man. This data suggests that somatropin administration may alter the clearance of compounds known to be metabolized by CYP450 liver enzymes (eg, corticosteroids). Careful monitoring is advisable when somatropin is administered in combination with other drugs known to be metabolized by CYP450 liver enzymes. Excessive glucocorticoid therapy may attenuate the growth promoting effects of somatropin in children).

No products indexed under this heading.

Indinavir Sulfate (Limited published data indicate that somatropin treatment increases cytochrome P450 (CYP450)-mediated antipyrine clearance in man. This data suggests that somatropin administration may alter the clearance of compounds known to be metabolized by CYP450 liver enzymes (eg, corticosteroids, sex steroids, anticonvulsants, cyclosporine). Careful monitoring is advisable when somatropin is administered in combination with other drugs known to be metabolized by CYP450 liver enzymes). Products include:

Crixivan Capsules **1979**

Insulin (In patients with diabetes mellitus requiring drug therapy, the dose of insulin and/or oral agents may require adjustment when somatropin therapy is initiated).

No products indexed under this heading.

Insulin, Human, Zinc Suspension (In patients with diabetes mellitus requiring drug therapy, the dose of insulin and/or oral agents may require adjustment when somatropin therapy is initiated).

No products indexed under this heading.

Insulin, Human (rDNA origin) (In patients with diabetes mellitus requiring drug therapy, the dose of insulin and/or oral agents may require adjustment when somatropin therapy is initiated). Products include:

Exubera Inhalation Powder **2515**

Insulin, Human NPH (In patients with diabetes mellitus requiring drug therapy, the dose of insulin and/or oral agents may require adjustment when somatropin therapy is initiated). Products include:

Humulin N Vial **1846**

Insulin, Human Regular (In patients with diabetes mellitus requiring drug therapy, the dose of insulin and/or oral agents may require adjustment when somatropin therapy is initiated). Products include:

Humulin R **1849**
Humulin R (U-500) **1850**

Insulin, Human Regular and Human NPH Mixture (In patients with diabetes mellitus requiring drug therapy, the dose of insulin and/or oral agents may require adjustment when somatropin therapy is initiated). Products include:

Humulin 50/50, 100 Units **1843**
Humulin 70/30 Vial **1844**

Insulin, NPH (In patients with diabetes mellitus requiring drug therapy, the dose of insulin and/or oral agents may require adjustment when somatropin therapy is initiated).

No products indexed under this heading.

Insulin, Regular (In patients with diabetes mellitus requiring drug therapy, the dose of insulin and/or oral agents may require adjustment when somatropin therapy is initiated).

No products indexed under this heading.

Insulin, Regular and NPH mixture (In patients with diabetes mellitus requiring drug therapy, the dose of insulin and/or oral agents may require adjustment when somatropin therapy is initiated).

No products indexed under this heading.

Insulin, Zinc Crystals (In patients with diabetes mellitus requiring drug therapy, the dose of insulin and/or oral agents may require adjustment when somatropin therapy is initiated).

No products indexed under this heading.

Insulin, Zinc Suspension (In patients with diabetes mellitus requiring drug therapy, the dose of insulin and/or oral agents may require adjustment when somatropin therapy is initiated).

No products indexed under this heading.

Insulin Aspart (In patients with diabetes mellitus requiring drug therapy, the dose of insulin and/or oral agents may require adjustment when somatropin therapy is initiated).

No products indexed under this heading.

Insulin Aspart, Human (In patients with diabetes mellitus requiring drug therapy, the dose of insulin and/or oral agents may require adjustment when somatropin therapy is initiated). Products include:

NovoLog Mix 70/30 2364

Insulin Aspart, Human Regular (In patients with diabetes mellitus requiring drug therapy, the dose of insulin and/or oral agents may require adjustment when somatropin therapy is initiated). Products include:

NovoLog Injection 2359

Insulin Aspart Protamine, Human (In patients with diabetes mellitus requiring drug therapy, the dose of insulin and/or oral agents may require adjustment when somatropin therapy is initiated). Products include:

NovoLog Mix 70/30 2364

Insulin Detemir (rDNA Origin) (In patients with diabetes mellitus requiring drug therapy, the dose of insulin and/or oral agents may require adjustment when somatropin therapy is initiated). Products include:

Levemir Injection 2352

Insulin glargine (In patients with diabetes mellitus requiring drug therapy, the dose of insulin and/or oral agents may require adjustment when somatropin therapy is initiated). Products include:

Lantus Injection 2749

Insulin Glulisine (In patients with diabetes mellitus requiring drug therapy, the dose of insulin and/or oral agents may require adjustment when somatropin therapy is initiated). Products include:

Apidra Injection 2706

Insulin Lispro, Human (In patients with diabetes mellitus requiring drug therapy, the dose of insulin and/or oral agents may require adjustment when somatropin therapy is initiated). Products include:

Humalog-Pen and KwikPen 1829
Humalog Mix 50/50-Pen and KwikPen 1833
Humalog Mix 75/25-Pen and KwikPen 1835

Insulin Lispro Protamine, Human (In patients with diabetes mellitus requiring drug therapy, the dose of insulin and/or oral agents may require adjustment when somatropin therapy is initiated). Products include:

Humalog Mix 50/50-Pen and KwikPen 1833
Humalog Mix 75/25-Pen and KwikPen 1835

Isradipine (Limited published data indicate that somatropin treatment increases cytochrome P450 (CYP450)-mediated antipyrine clearance in man. This data suggests that somatropin administration may alter the clearance of compounds known to be metabolized by CYP450 liver enzymes (eg, corticosteroids, sex steroids, anticonvulsants, cyclosporine). Careful monitoring is advisable when somatropin is administered in combination with other drugs known to be metabolized by CYP450 liver enzymes). Products include:

DynaCirc CR Controlled Release Tablets 1407

Itraconazole (Limited published data indicate that somatropin treatment increases cytochrome P450 (CYP450)-mediated antipyrine clearance in man. This data suggests that somatropin administration may alter the clearance of compounds known to be metabolized by CYP450 liver enzymes (eg, corticosteroids, sex steroids, anticonvulsants, cyclosporine). Careful monitoring is advisable when somatropin is administered in combination with other drugs known to be metabolized by CYP450 liver enzymes).

No products indexed under this heading.

Ixabepilone (Limited published data indicate that somatropin treatment increases cytochrome P450 (CYP450)-mediated antipyrine clearance in man. This data suggests that somatropin administration may alter the clearance of compounds known to be metabolized by CYP450 liver enzymes (eg, corticosteroids, sex steroids, anticonvulsants, cyclosporine). Careful monitoring is advisable when somatropin is administered in combination with other drugs known to be metabolized by CYP450 liver enzymes). Products include:

Ixempra Kit for Injection 915

Ketoconazole (Limited published data indicate that somatropin treatment increases cytochrome P450 (CYP450)-mediated antipyrine clearance in man. This data suggests that somatropin administration may alter the clearance of compounds known to be metabolized by CYP450 liver enzymes (eg, corticosteroids, sex steroids, anticonvulsants, cyclosporine). Careful monitoring is advisable when somatropin is administered in combination with other drugs known to be metabolized by CYP450 liver enzymes). Products include:

Extina Foam, 2% 3057
Nizoral A-D Shampoo 1901

Lamotrigine (Limited published data indicate that somatropin treatment increases cytochrome P450 (CYP450)-mediated antipyrine clearance in man. This data suggests that somatropin administration may alter the clearance of compounds known to be metabolized by CYP450 liver enzymes (eg, anticonvulsants). Careful monitoring is advisable when somatropin is administered in combination with other drugs known to be metabolized by CYP450 liver enzymes). Products include:

Lamictal 1488

Levetiracetam (Limited published data indicate that somatropin treatment increases cytochrome P450 (CYP450)-mediated antipyrine clearance in man. This data suggests that somatropin administration may alter the clearance of compounds known to be metabolized by CYP450 liver enzymes (eg, anticonvulsants). Careful monitoring is advisable when somatropin is administered in combination with other drugs known to be metabolized by CYP450 liver enzymes). Products include:

Keppra Injection 3137
Keppra Oral Solution 3131
Keppra Tablets 3131

Levonorgestrel (Limited published data indicate that somatropin treatment increases cytochrome P450 (CYP450)-mediated antipyrine clearance in man. This data suggests that somatropin administration may alter the clearance of compounds known to be metabolized by CYP450 liver enzymes (eg, sex steroids). Careful monitoring is advisable when somatropin is administered in combination with other drugs known to be metabolized by CYP450 liver enzymes). Products include:

Climara Pro Transdermal System 768
Lybrel Tablets 3204
Mirena Intrauterine System 779
Plan B Tablets 1044
Seasonique Tablets 1046

Lidocaine (Limited published data indicate that somatropin treatment increases cytochrome P450 (CYP450)-mediated antipyrine clearance in man. This data suggests that somatropin administration may alter the clearance of compounds known to be metabolized by CYP450 liver enzymes (eg, corticosteroids, sex steroids, anticonvulsants, cyclosporine). Careful monitoring is advisable when somatropin is administered in combination with other drugs known to be metabolized by CYP450 liver enzymes). Products include:

Lidoderm Patch 1114

Lidocaine Hydrochloride (Limited published data indicate that somatropin treatment increases cytochrome P450 (CYP450)-mediated antipyrine clearance in man. This data suggests that somatropin administration may alter the clearance of compounds known to be metabolized by CYP450 liver enzymes (eg, corticosteroids, sex steroids, anticonvulsants, cyclosporine). Careful monitoring is advisable when somatropin is administered in combination with other drugs known to be metabolized by CYP450 liver enzymes).

No products indexed under this heading.

Lovastatin (Limited published data indicate that somatropin treatment increases cytochrome P450 (CYP450)-mediated antipyrine clearance in man. This data suggests that somatropin administration may alter the clearance of compounds known to be metabolized by CYP450 liver enzymes (eg, corticosteroids, sex steroids, anticonvulsants, cyclosporine). Careful monitoring is advisable when somatropin is administered in combination with other drugs known to be metabolized by CYP450 liver enzymes). Products include:

Advicor Tablets 402
Mevacor Tablets 2063

Mephenytoin (Limited published data indicate that somatropin treatment increases cytochrome P450 (CYP450)-mediated antipyrine clearance in man. This data suggests that somatropin administration may alter the clearance of compounds known to be metabolized by CYP450 liver enzymes (eg, anticonvulsants). Careful monitoring is advisable when somatropin is administered in combination with other drugs known to be metabolized by CYP450 liver enzymes).

No products indexed under this heading.

Mestranol (Limited published data indicate that somatropin treatment increases cytochrome P450 (CYP450)-mediated antipyrine clearance in man. This data suggests that somatropin administration may alter the clearance of compounds known to be metabolized by CYP450 liver enzymes (eg, sex steroids). Careful monitoring is advisable when somatropin is administered in combination with other drugs known to be metabolized by CYP450 liver enzymes).

No products indexed under this heading.

Metformin Hydrochloride (In patients with diabetes mellitus requiring drug therapy, the dose of insulin and/or oral agents may require adjustment when somatropin therapy is initiated). Products include:

ActoPlus Met Tablets 3071
Avandamet Tablets 1336
Janumet Tablets 2041
PrandiMet Tablets 2967

Methadone Hydrochloride (Limited published data indicate that somatropin treatment increases cytochrome P450 (CYP450)-mediated antipyrine clearance in man. This data suggests that somatropin administration may alter the clearance of compounds known to be metabolized by CYP450 liver enzymes (eg, corticosteroids, sex steroids, anticonvulsants, cyclosporine). Careful monitoring is advisable when somatropin is administered in combination with other drugs known to be metabolized by CYP450 liver enzymes).

No products indexed under this heading.

Methsuximide (Limited published data indicate that somatropin treatment increases cytochrome P450 (CYP450)-mediated antipyrine clearance in man. This data suggests that somatropin administration may alter the clearance of compounds known to be metabolized by CYP450 liver enzymes (eg, anticonvulsants). Careful monitoring is advisable when somatropin is administered in combination with other drugs known to be metabolized by CYP450 liver enzymes).

No products indexed under this heading.

Methylprednisolone Acetate (Limited published data indicate that somatropin treatment increases cytochrome P450 (CYP450)-mediated antipyrine clearance in man. This data suggests that somatropin administration may alter the clearance of compounds known to be metabolized by CYP450 liver enzymes (eg, corticosteroids). Careful monitoring is advisable when somatropin is administered in combination with other drugs known to be metabolized by CYP450 liver enzymes. Excessive glucocorticoid therapy may attenuate the growth promoting effects of somatropin in children).

No products indexed under this heading.

Methylprednisolone Sodium Succinate (Limited published data indicate that somatropin treatment increases cytochrome P450 (CYP450)-mediated antipyrine clearance in man. This data suggests that somatropin administration may alter the clearance of compounds known to be metabolized by CYP450 liver enzymes (eg, corticosteroids). Careful monitoring is advisable when somatropin is administered in combination with other drugs known to be metabolized by CYP450 liver enzymes. Excessive glucocorticoid therapy may attenuate the growth

promoting effects of somatropin in children).

No products indexed under this heading.

Methyltestosterone (Limited published data indicate that somatropin treatment increases cytochrome P450 (CYP450)-mediated antipyrine clearance in man. This data suggests that somatropin administration may alter the clearance of compounds known to be metabolized by CYP450 liver enzymes (eg, sex steroids). Careful monitoring is advisable when somatropin is administered in combination with other drugs known to be metabolized by CYP450 liver enzymes). Products include:

Estratest Tablets **3043**
Estratest H.S. Tablets **3043**

Midazolam Hydrochloride (Limited published data indicate that somatropin treatment increases cytochrome P450 (CYP450)-mediated antipyrine clearance in man. This data suggests that somatropin administration may alter the clearance of compounds known to be metabolized by CYP450 liver enzymes (eg, corticosteroids, sex steroids, anticonvulsants, cyclosporine). Careful monitoring is advisable when somatropin is administered in combination with other drugs known to be metabolized by CYP450 liver enzymes).

No products indexed under this heading.

Miglitol (In patients with diabetes mellitus requiring drug therapy, the dose of insulin and/or oral agents may require adjustment when somatropin therapy is initiated).

No products indexed under this heading.

Mometasone Furoate (Limited published data indicate that somatropin treatment increases cytochrome P450 (CYP450)-mediated antipyrine clearance in man. This data suggests that somatropin administration may alter the clearance of compounds known to be metabolized by CYP450 liver enzymes (eg, corticosteroids). Careful monitoring is advisable when somatropin is administered in combination with other drugs known to be metabolized by CYP450 liver enzymes. Excessive glucocorticoid therapy may attenuate the growth promoting effects of somatropin in children). Products include:

Asmanex Twisthaler **2797**
Elocon Cream 0.1% **2840**
Elocon Lotion 0.1% **2841**
Elocon Ointment 0.1% **2842**

Mometasone Furoate Monohydrate (Limited published data indicate that somatropin treatment increases cytochrome P450 (CYP450)-mediated antipyrine clearance in man. This data suggests that somatropin administration may alter the clearance of compounds known to be metabolized by CYP450 liver enzymes (eg, corticosteroids). Careful monitoring is advisable when somatropin is administered in combination with other drugs known to be metabolized by CYP450 liver enzymes. Excessive glucocorticoid therapy may attenuate the growth promoting effects of somatropin in children). Products include:

Nasonex Nasal Spray **2883**

Nateglinide (In patients with diabetes mellitus requiring drug therapy, the dose of insulin and/or oral agents may require adjustment when somatropin therapy is initiated). Products include:

Starlix Tablets **2314**

Nefazodone Hydrochloride (Limited published data indicate that somatropin treatment increases cytochrome P450 (CYP450)-mediated antipyrine clearance in man. This data suggests that somatropin administration may alter the clearance of compounds known to be metabolized by CYP450 liver enzymes (eg, corticosteroids, sex steroids, anticonvulsants, cyclosporine). Careful monitoring is advisable when somatropin is administered in combination with other drugs known to be metabolized by CYP450 liver enzymes).

No products indexed under this heading.

Nelfinavir Mesylate (Limited published data indicate that somatropin treatment increases cytochrome P450 (CYP450)-mediated antipyrine clearance in man. This data suggests that somatropin administration may alter the clearance of compounds known to be metabolized by CYP450 liver enzymes (eg, corticosteroids, sex steroids, anticonvulsants, cyclosporine). Careful monitoring is advisable when somatropin is administered in combination with other drugs known to be metabolized by CYP450 liver enzymes).

No products indexed under this heading.

Nicardipine Hydrochloride (Limited published data indicate that somatropin treatment increases cytochrome P450 (CYP450)-mediated antipyrine clearance in man. This data suggests that somatropin administration may alter the clearance of compounds known to be metabolized by CYP450 liver enzymes (eg, corticosteroids, sex steroids, anticonvulsants, cyclosporine). Careful monitoring is advisable when somatropin is administered in combination with other drugs known to be metabolized by CYP450 liver enzymes). Products include:

Cardene I.V. **1093**

Nifedipine (Limited published data indicate that somatropin treatment increases cytochrome P450 (CYP450)-mediated antipyrine clearance in man. This data suggests that somatropin administration may alter the clearance of compounds known to be metabolized by CYP450 liver enzymes (eg, corticosteroids, sex steroids, anticonvulsants, cyclosporine). Careful monitoring is advisable when somatropin is administered in combination with other drugs known to be metabolized by CYP450 liver enzymes).

No products indexed under this heading.

Nimodipine (Limited published data indicate that somatropin treatment increases cytochrome P450 (CYP450)-mediated antipyrine clearance in man. This data suggests that somatropin administration may alter the clearance of compounds known to be metabolized by CYP450 liver enzymes (eg, corticosteroids, sex steroids, anticonvulsants, cyclosporine). Careful monitoring is advisable when somatropin is administered in combination with other drugs known to be metabolized by CYP450 liver enzymes). Products include:

Nimotop Capsules **790**

Nisoldipine (Limited published data indicate that somatropin treatment increases cytochrome P450 (CYP450)-mediated antipyrine clearance in man. This data suggests that somatropin administration may alter the clearance of compounds known to be metabolized by CYP450 liver enzymes (eg, corticosteroids, sex steroids, anticonvulsants, cyclosporine). Careful monitoring is advisable when somatropin is administered in combination with other drugs known to be metabolized by CYP450 liver enzymes). Products include:

Sular Extended Release Tablets **2975**

Nitrendipine (Limited published data indicate that somatropin treatment increases cytochrome P450 (CYP450)-mediated antipyrine clearance in man. This data suggests that somatropin administration may alter the clearance of compounds known to be metabolized by CYP450 liver enzymes (eg, corticosteroids, sex steroids, anticonvulsants, cyclosporine). Careful monitoring is advisable when somatropin is administered in combination with other drugs known to be metabolized by CYP450 liver enzymes).

No products indexed under this heading.

Norethindrone (Limited published data indicate that somatropin treatment increases cytochrome P450 (CYP450)-mediated antipyrine clearance in man. This data suggests that somatropin administration may alter the clearance of compounds known to be metabolized by CYP450 liver enzymes (eg, sex steroids). Careful monitoring is advisable when somatropin is administered in combination with other drugs known to be metabolized by CYP450 liver enzymes). Products include:

Ortho Micronor Tablets **2446**

Norethindrone Acetate (Limited published data indicate that somatropin treatment increases cytochrome P450 (CYP450)-mediated antipyrine clearance in man. This data suggests that somatropin administration may alter the clearance of compounds known to be metabolized by CYP450 liver enzymes (eg, sex steroids). Careful monitoring is advisable when somatropin is administered in combination with other drugs known to be metabolized by CYP450 liver enzymes). Products include:

Activella Tablets **2347**

Norgestimate (Limited published data indicate that somatropin treatment increases cytochrome P450 (CYP450)-mediated antipyrine clearance in man. This data suggests that somatropin administration may alter the clearance of compounds known to be metabolized by CYP450 liver enzymes (eg, sex steroids). Careful monitoring is advisable when somatropin is administered in combination with other drugs known to be metabolized by CYP450 liver enzymes). Products include:

Ortho-Cyclen/Ortho Tri-Cyclen **2449**
Ortho Tri-Cyclen Lo Tablets **2458**

Norgestrel (Limited published data indicate that somatropin treatment increases cytochrome P450 (CYP450)-mediated antipyrine clearance in man. This data suggests that somatropin administration may alter the clearance of compounds known to be metabolized by CYP450 liver enzymes (eg, corticosteroids, sex steroids, anticonvulsants, cyclosporine). Careful monitoring is advisable when somatropin is administered in combination with other drugs known to be metabolized by CYP450 liver enzymes).

No products indexed under this heading.

Ondansetron (Limited published data indicate that somatropin treatment increases cytochrome P450 (CYP450)-mediated antipyrine clearance in man. This data suggests that somatropin administration may alter the clearance of compounds known to be metabolized by CYP450 liver enzymes (eg, corticosteroids, sex steroids, anticonvulsants, cyclosporine). Careful monitoring is advisable when somatropin is administered in combination with other drugs known to be metabolized by CYP450 liver enzymes). Products include:

Zofran ODT Orally Disintegrating Tablets **1687**

Ondansetron Hydrochloride (Limited published data indicate that somatropin treatment increases cytochrome P450 (CYP450)-mediated antipyrine clearance in man. This data suggests that somatropin administration may alter the clearance of compounds known to be metabolized by CYP450 liver enzymes (eg, corticosteroids, sex steroids, anticonvulsants, cyclosporine). Careful monitoring is advisable when somatropin is administered in combination with other drugs known to be metabolized by CYP450 liver enzymes). Products include:

Zofran Injection **1682**
Zofran **1687**

Oxcarbazepine (Limited published data indicate that somatropin treatment increases cytochrome P450 (CYP450)-mediated antipyrine clearance in man. This data suggests that somatropin administration may alter the clearance of compounds known to be metabolized by CYP450 liver enzymes (eg, anticonvulsants). Careful monitoring is advisable when somatropin is administered in combination with other drugs known to be metabolized by CYP450 liver enzymes).

No products indexed under this heading.

Paclitaxel (Limited published data indicate that somatropin treatment increases cytochrome P450 (CYP450)-mediated antipyrine clearance in man. This data suggests that somatropin administration may alter the clearance of compounds known to be metabolized by CYP450 liver enzymes (eg, corticosteroids, sex steroids, anticonvulsants, cyclosporine). Careful monitoring is advisable when somatropin is administered in combination with other drugs known to be metabolized by CYP450 liver enzymes).

No products indexed under this heading.

Paramethadione (Limited published data indicate that somatropin treatment increases cytochrome P450 (CYP450)-mediated antipyrine clearance in man. This data suggests that somatropin administration may alter the clearance of compounds known to be metabolized by CYP450 liver enzymes (eg, anticonvulsants). Careful monitoring is advisable when somatropin is administered in combination with other drugs known to be metabolized by CYP450 liver enzymes).

No products indexed under this heading.

Phenacemide (Limited published data indicate that somatropin treatment increases cytochrome P450 (CYP450)-mediated antipyrine clearance in man. This data suggests that somatropin administration may alter the clearance of compounds known to be metabolized by CYP450 liver enzymes (eg, anticonvulsants). Careful monitoring is advisable when somatropin is administered in combination with other drugs known to be metabolized by CYP450 liver enzymes).

No products indexed under this heading.

Phenobarbital (Limited published data indicate that somatropin treatment increases cytochrome P450 (CYP450)-mediated antipyrine clearance in man. This data suggests that somatropin administration may alter the clearance of compounds known to be metabolized by CYP450 liver enzymes (eg, anticonvulsants). Careful monitoring is advisable when somatropin is administered in combination with other drugs known to be metabolized by CYP450 liver enzymes). Products include:

Donnatal Extentabs **2507**

Phensuximide (Limited published data indicate that somatropin treatment increases cytochrome P450 (CYP450)-mediated antipyrine clearance in man. This data suggests that somatropin administration may alter the clearance of compounds known to be metabolized by CYP450 liver enzymes (eg, anticonvulsants). Careful monitoring is advisable when somatropin is administered in combination with other drugs known to be metabolized by CYP450 liver enzymes).

No products indexed under this heading.

Phenytoin (Limited published data indicate that somatropin treatment increases cytochrome P450 (CYP450)-mediated antipyrine clearance in man. This data suggests that somatropin administration may alter the clearance of compounds known to be metabolized by CYP450 liver enzymes (eg, anticonvulsants). Careful monitoring is advisable when somatropin is administered in combination with other drugs known to be metabolized by CYP450 liver enzymes).

No products indexed under this heading.

Phenytoin Sodium (Limited published data indicate that somatropin treatment increases cytochrome P450 (CYP450)-mediated antipyrine clearance in man. This data suggests that somatropin administration may alter the clearance of compounds known to be metabolized by CYP450 liver enzymes (eg, anticonvulsants). Careful monitoring is advisable when somatropin is administered in combination with other drugs known to be metabolized by CYP450 liver enzymes). Products include:

Phenytek Capsules **2192**

Pimozide (Limited published data indicate that somatropin treatment increases cytochrome P450 (CYP450)-mediated antipyrine clearance in man. This data suggests that somatropin administration may alter the clearance of compounds known to be metabolized by CYP450 liver enzymes (eg, corticosteroids, sex steroids, anticonvulsants, cyclosporine). Careful monitoring is advisable when somatropin is administered in combination with other drugs known to be metabolized by CYP450 liver enzymes).

No products indexed under this heading.

Pioglitazone Hydrochloride (In patients with diabetes mellitus requiring drug therapy, the dose of insulin and/or oral agents may require adjustment when somatropin therapy is initiated). Products include:

ActoPlus Met Tablets **3071**
Actos Tablets **3077**
Duetact Tablets **3085**

Polyestradiol Phosphate (In adult women on oral estrogen replacement, a larger dose of somatropin may be required to achieve the defined treatment goal).

No products indexed under this heading.

Prednisolone Acetate (Limited published data indicate that somatropin treatment increases cytochrome P450 (CYP450)-mediated antipyrine clearance in man. This data suggests that somatropin administration may alter the clearance of compounds known to be metabolized by CYP450 liver enzymes (eg, corticosteroids). Careful monitoring is advisable when somatropin is administered in combination with other drugs known to be metabolized by CYP450 liver enzymes. Excessive glucocorticoid therapy may attenuate the growth promoting effects of somatropin in children). Products include:

Pred Forte Ophthalmic Suspension .... ⊙ **227**
Pred Mild Ophthalmic Suspension .... ⊙ **230**
Pred-G Ophthalmic Ointment .... ⊙ **229**
Pred-G Ophthalmic Suspension .... ⊙ **228**

Prednisolone Sodium Phosphate (Limited published data indicate that somatropin treatment increases cytochrome P450 (CYP450)-mediated antipyrine clearance in man. This data suggests that somatropin administration may alter the clearance of compounds known to be metabolized by CYP450 liver enzymes (eg, corticosteroids). Careful monitoring is advisable when somatropin is administered in combination with other drugs known to be metabolized by CYP450 liver enzymes. Excessive glucocorticoid therapy may attenuate the growth promoting effects of somatropin in children).

No products indexed under this heading.

Prednisolone Tebutate (Limited published data indicate that somatropin treatment increases cytochrome P450 (CYP450)-mediated antipyrine clearance in man. This data suggests that somatropin administration may alter the clearance of compounds known to be metabolized by CYP450 liver enzymes (eg, corticosteroids). Careful monitoring is advisable when somatropin is administered in combination with other drugs known to be metabolized by CYP450 liver enzymes. Excessive glucocorticoid therapy may attenuate the growth promoting effects of somatropin in children).

No products indexed under this heading.

Prednisone (Limited published data indicate that somatropin treatment increases cytochrome P450 (CYP450)-mediated antipyrine clearance in man. This data suggests that somatropin administration may alter the clearance of compounds known to be metabolized by CYP450 liver enzymes (eg, corticosteroids). Careful monitoring is advisable when somatropin is administered in combination with other drugs known to be metabolized by CYP450 liver enzymes. Excessive glucocorticoid therapy may attenuate the growth promoting effects of somatropin in children).

No products indexed under this heading.

Primidone (Limited published data indicate that somatropin treatment increases cytochrome P450 (CYP450)-mediated antipyrine clearance in man. This data suggests that somatropin administration may alter the clearance of compounds known to be metabolized by CYP450 liver enzymes (eg, anticonvulsants). Careful monitoring is advisable when somatropin is administered in combination with other drugs known to be metabolized by CYP450 liver enzymes).

No products indexed under this heading.

Quinestrol (In adult women on oral estrogen replacement, a larger dose of somatropin may be required to achieve the defined treatment goal).

No products indexed under this heading.

Quinidine Gluconate (Limited published data indicate that somatropin treatment increases cytochrome P450 (CYP450)-mediated antipyrine clearance in man. This data suggests that somatropin administration may alter the clearance of compounds known to be metabolized by CYP450 liver enzymes (eg, corticosteroids, sex steroids, anticonvulsants, cyclosporine). Careful monitoring is advisable when somatropin is administered in combination with other drugs known to be metabolized by CYP450 liver enzymes).

No products indexed under this heading.

Quinidine Polygalacturonate (Limited published data indicate that somatropin treatment increases cytochrome P450 (CYP450)-mediated antipyrine clearance in man. This data suggests that somatropin administration may alter the clearance of compounds known to be metabolized by CYP450 liver enzymes (eg, corticosteroids, sex steroids, anticonvulsants, cyclosporine). Careful monitoring is advisable when somatropin is administered in combination with other drugs known to be metabolized by CYP450 liver enzymes).

No products indexed under this heading.

Quinidine Sulfate (Limited published data indicate that somatropin treatment increases cytochrome P450 (CYP450)-mediated antipyrine clearance in man. This data suggests that somatropin administration may alter the clearance of compounds known to be metabolized by CYP450 liver enzymes (eg, corticosteroids, sex steroids, anticonvulsants, cyclosporine). Careful monitoring is advisable when somatropin is administered in combination with other drugs known to be metabolized by CYP450 liver enzymes).

No products indexed under this heading.

Repaglinide (In patients with diabetes mellitus requiring drug therapy, the dose of insulin and/or oral agents may require adjustment when somatropin therapy is initiated). Products include:

PrandiMet Tablets **2967**
Prandin Tablets **2971**

Rifabutin (Limited published data indicate that somatropin treatment increases cytochrome P450 (CYP450)-mediated antipyrine clearance in man. This data suggests that somatropin administration may alter the clearance of compounds known to be metabolized by CYP450 liver enzymes (eg, corticosteroids, sex steroids, anticonvulsants, cyclosporine). Careful monitoring is advisable when somatropin is administered in combination with other drugs known to be metabolized by CYP450 liver enzymes).

No products indexed under this heading.

Ritonavir (Limited published data indicate that somatropin treatment increases cytochrome P450 (CYP450)-mediated antipyrine clearance in man. This data suggests that somatropin administration may alter the clearance of compounds known to be metabolized by CYP450 liver enzymes (eg, corticosteroids, sex steroids, anticonvulsants, cyclosporine). Careful monitoring is advisable when somatropin is administered in combination with other drugs known to be metabolized by CYP450 liver enzymes). Products include:

Kaletra **452**
Norvir **489**

Rosiglitazone Maleate (In patients with diabetes mellitus requiring drug therapy, the dose of insulin and/or oral agents may require adjustment when somatropin therapy is initiated). Products include:

Avandamet Tablets **1336**
Avandaryl Tablets **1344**
Avandia Tablets **1351**

Saquinavir (Limited published data indicate that somatropin treatment increases cytochrome P450 (CYP450)-mediated antipyrine clearance in man. This data suggests that somatropin administration may alter the clearance of compounds known to be metabolized by CYP450 liver enzymes (eg, corticosteroids, sex steroids, anticonvulsants, cyclosporine). Careful monitoring is advisable when somatropin is administered in combination with other drugs known to be metabolized by CYP450 liver enzymes).

No products indexed under this heading.

Saquinavir Mesylate (Limited published data indicate that somatropin treatment increases cytochrome P450 (CYP450)-mediated antipyrine clearance in man. This data suggests that somatropin administration

may alter the clearance of compounds known to be metabolized by CYP450 liver enzymes (eg, corticosteroids, sex steroids, anticonvulsants, cyclosporine). Careful monitoring is advisable when somatropin is administered in combination with other drugs known to be metabolized by CYP450 liver enzymes).
No products indexed under this heading.

Sertraline Hydrochloride (Limited published data indicate that somatropin treatment increases cytochrome P450 (CYP450)-mediated antipyrine clearance in man. This data suggests that somatropin administration may alter the clearance of compounds known to be metabolized by CYP450 liver enzymes (eg, corticosteroids, sex steroids, anticonvulsants, cyclosporine). Careful monitoring is advisable when somatropin is administered in combination with other drugs known to be metabolized by CYP450 liver enzymes).
No products indexed under this heading.

Sildenafil Citrate (Limited published data indicate that somatropin treatment increases cytochrome P450 (CYP450)-mediated antipyrine clearance in man. This data suggests that somatropin administration may alter the clearance of compounds known to be metabolized by CYP450 liver enzymes (eg, corticosteroids, sex steroids, anticonvulsants, cyclosporine). Careful monitoring is advisable when somatropin is administered in combination with other drugs known to be metabolized by CYP450 liver enzymes).
No products indexed under this heading.

Simvastatin (Limited published data indicate that somatropin treatment increases cytochrome P450 (CYP450)-mediated antipyrine clearance in man. This data suggests that somatropin administration may alter the clearance of compounds known to be metabolized by CYP450 liver enzymes (eg, corticosteroids, sex steroids, anticonvulsants, cyclosporine). Careful monitoring is advisable when somatropin is administered in combination with other drugs known to be metabolized by CYP450 liver enzymes). Products include:
Simcor Tablets 502
Vytorin 10/10 Tablets 2149
Vytorin 10/10 Tablets 2939
Vytorin 10/20 Tablets 2149
Vytorin 10/20 Tablets 2939
Vytorin 10/40 Tablets 2149
Vytorin 10/40 Tablets 2939
Vytorin 10/80 Tablets 2149
Vytorin 10/80 Tablets 2939
Zocor Tablets 2136

Sirolimus (Limited published data indicate that somatropin treatment increases cytochrome P450 (CYP450)-mediated antipyrine clearance in man. This data suggests that somatropin administration may alter the clearance of compounds known to be metabolized by CYP450 liver enzymes (eg, corticosteroids, sex steroids, anticonvulsants, cyclosporine). Careful monitoring is advisable when somatropin is administered in combination with other drugs known to be metabolized by CYP450 liver enzymes). Products include:
Rapamune 3260

Sitagliptin Phosphate (In patients with diabetes mellitus requiring drug therapy, the dose of insulin and/or oral agents may require adjustment when somatropin therapy is initiated). Products include:
Janumet Tablets 2041
Januvia Tablets 2048

Tacrolimus (Limited published data indicate that somatropin treatment increases cytochrome P450 (CYP450)-mediated antipyrine clearance in man. This data suggests that somatropin administration may alter the clearance of compounds known to be metabolized by CYP450 liver enzymes (eg, corticosteroids, sex steroids, anticonvulsants, cyclosporine). Careful monitoring is advisable when somatropin is administered in combination with other drugs known to be metabolized by CYP450 liver enzymes). Products include:
Prograf Capsules and Injection 622
Protopic Ointment 628

Tadalafil (Limited published data indicate that somatropin treatment increases cytochrome P450 (CYP450)-mediated antipyrine clearance in man. This data suggests that somatropin administration may alter the clearance of compounds known to be metabolized by CYP450 liver enzymes (eg, corticosteroids, sex steroids, anticonvulsants, cyclosporine). Careful monitoring is advisable when somatropin is administered in combination with other drugs known to be metabolized by CYP450 liver enzymes). Products include:
Cialis Tablets 1792

Tamoxifen Citrate (Limited published data indicate that somatropin treatment increases cytochrome P450 (CYP450)-mediated antipyrine clearance in man. This data suggests that somatropin administration may alter the clearance of compounds known to be metabolized by CYP450 liver enzymes (eg, corticosteroids, sex steroids, anticonvulsants, cyclosporine). Careful monitoring is advisable when somatropin is administered in combination with other drugs known to be metabolized by CYP450 liver enzymes).
No products indexed under this heading.

Testosterone (Limited published data indicate that somatropin treatment increases cytochrome P450 (CYP450)-mediated antipyrine clearance in man. This data suggests that somatropin administration may alter the clearance of compounds known to be metabolized by CYP450 liver enzymes (eg, sex steroids). Careful monitoring is advisable when somatropin is administered in combination with other drugs known to be metabolized by CYP450 liver enzymes). Products include:
AndroGel 3159
Testim 1% Gel 701

Tiagabine Hydrochloride (Limited published data indicate that somatropin treatment increases cytochrome P450 (CYP450)-mediated antipyrine clearance in man. This data suggests that somatropin administration may alter the clearance of compounds known to be metabolized by CYP450 liver enzymes (eg, anticonvulsants). Careful monitoring is advisable when somatropin is administered in combination with other drugs known to be metabolized by CYP450 liver enzymes). Products include:
Gabitril Tablets 973

Tolazamide (In patients with diabetes mellitus requiring drug therapy, the dose of insulin and/or oral agents may require adjustment when somatropin therapy is initiated).
No products indexed under this heading.

Tolbutamide (In patients with diabetes mellitus requiring drug therapy, the dose of insulin and/or oral agents may require adjustment when somatropin therapy is initiated).
No products indexed under this heading.

Tolterodine Tartrate (Limited published data indicate that somatropin treatment increases cytochrome P450 (CYP450)-mediated antipyrine clearance in man. This data suggests that somatropin administration may alter the clearance of compounds known to be metabolized by CYP450 liver enzymes (eg, corticosteroids, sex steroids, anticonvulsants, cyclosporine). Careful monitoring is advisable when somatropin is administered in combination with other drugs known to be metabolized by CYP450 liver enzymes).
No products indexed under this heading.

Topiramate (Limited published data indicate that somatropin treatment increases cytochrome P450 (CYP450)-mediated antipyrine clearance in man. This data suggests that somatropin administration may alter the clearance of compounds known to be metabolized by CYP450 liver enzymes (eg, anticonvulsants). Careful monitoring is advisable when somatropin is administered in combination with other drugs known to be metabolized by CYP450 liver enzymes).
No products indexed under this heading.

Trazodone Hydrochloride (Limited published data indicate that somatropin treatment increases cytochrome P450 (CYP450)-mediated antipyrine clearance in man. This data suggests that somatropin administration may alter the clearance of compounds known to be metabolized by CYP450 liver enzymes (eg, corticosteroids, sex steroids, anticonvulsants, cyclosporine). Careful monitoring is advisable when somatropin is administered in combination with other drugs known to be metabolized by CYP450 liver enzymes).
No products indexed under this heading.

Triamcinolone (Limited published data indicate that somatropin treatment increases cytochrome P450 (CYP450)-mediated antipyrine clearance in man. This data suggests that somatropin administration may alter the clearance of compounds known to be metabolized by CYP450 liver enzymes (eg, corticosteroids). Careful monitoring is advisable when somatropin is administered in combination with other drugs known to be metabolized by CYP450 liver enzymes. Excessive glucocorticoid therapy may attenuate the growth promoting effects of somatropin in children).
No products indexed under this heading.

Triamcinolone Acetonide (Limited published data indicate that somatropin treatment increases cytochrome P450 (CYP450)-mediated antipyrine clearance in man. This data suggests that somatropin administration may alter the clearance of compounds known to be metabolized by CYP450 liver enzymes (eg, corticosteroids). Careful monitoring is advisable when somatropin is administered in combination with other drugs known to be metabolized by CYP450 liver enzymes. Excessive glucocorticoid therapy may attenuate the growth promoting effects of somatropin in children). Products include:
Azmacort Inhalation Aerosol 407
Nasacort AQ Nasal Spray 2765
Triesence Injectable Suspension .... ⊙ 209

Triamcinolone Diacetate (Limited published data indicate that somatropin treatment increases cytochrome P450 (CYP450)-mediated antipyrine clearance in man. This data suggests that somatropin administration may alter the clearance of compounds known to be metabolized by CYP450 liver enzymes (eg, corticosteroids). Careful monitoring is advisable when somatropin is administered in combination with other drugs known to be metabolized by CYP450 liver enzymes. Excessive glucocorticoid therapy may attenuate the growth promoting effects of somatropin in children).
No products indexed under this heading.

Triamcinolone Hexacetonide (Limited published data indicate that somatropin treatment increases cytochrome P450 (CYP450)-mediated antipyrine clearance in man. This data suggests that somatropin administration may alter the clearance of compounds known to be metabolized by CYP450 liver enzymes (eg, corticosteroids). Careful monitoring is advisable when somatropin is administered in combination with other drugs known to be metabolized by CYP450 liver enzymes. Excessive glucocorticoid therapy may attenuate the growth promoting effects of somatropin in children).
No products indexed under this heading.

Triazolam (Limited published data indicate that somatropin treatment increases cytochrome P450 (CYP450)-mediated antipyrine clearance in man. This data suggests that somatropin administration may alter the clearance of compounds known to be metabolized by CYP450 liver enzymes (eg, corticosteroids, sex steroids, anticonvulsants, cyclosporine). Careful monitoring is advisable when somatropin is administered in combination with other drugs known to be metabolized by CYP450 liver enzymes).
No products indexed under this heading.

Trimethadione (Limited published data indicate that somatropin treatment increases cytochrome P450 (CYP450)-mediated antipyrine clearance in man. This data suggests that somatropin administration may alter the clearance of compounds known to be metabolized by CYP450 liver enzymes (eg, anticonvulsants). Careful monitoring is advisable when somatropin is administered in combination with other drugs known to be metabolized by CYP450 liver

enzymes).
No products indexed under this heading.

Troglitazone (In patients with diabetes mellitus requiring drug therapy, the dose of insulin and/or oral agents may require adjustment when somatropin therapy is initiated).
No products indexed under this heading.

Valproate Sodium (Limited published data indicate that somatropin treatment increases cytochrome P450 (CYP450)-mediated antipyrine clearance in man. This data suggests that somatropin administration may alter the clearance of compounds known to be metabolized by CYP450 liver enzymes (eg, anticonvulsants). Careful monitoring is advisable when somatropin is administered in combination with other drugs known to be metabolized by CYP450 liver enzymes).
No products indexed under this heading.

Valproic Acid (Limited published data indicate that somatropin treatment increases cytochrome P450 (CYP450)-mediated antipyrine clearance in man. This data suggests that somatropin administration may alter the clearance of compounds known to be metabolized by CYP450 liver enzymes (eg, anticonvulsants). Careful monitoring is advisable when somatropin is administered in combination with other drugs known to be metabolized by CYP450 liver enzymes).
No products indexed under this heading.

Vardenafil Hydrochloride (Limited published data indicate that somatropin treatment increases cytochrome P450 (CYP450)-mediated antipyrine clearance in man. This data suggests that somatropin administration may alter the clearance of compounds known to be metabolized by CYP450 liver enzymes (eg, corticosteroids, sex steroids, anticonvulsants, cyclosporine). Careful monitoring is advisable when somatropin is administered in combination with other drugs known to be metabolized by CYP450 liver enzymes). Products include:
Levitra Tablets 2876

Verapamil Hydrochloride (Limited published data indicate that somatropin treatment increases cytochrome P450 (CYP450)-mediated antipyrine clearance in man. This data suggests that somatropin administration may alter the clearance of compounds known to be metabolized by CYP450 liver enzymes (eg, corticosteroids, sex steroids, anticonvulsants, cyclosporine). Careful monitoring is advisable when somatropin is administered in combination with other drugs known to be metabolized by CYP450 liver enzymes). Products include:
Tarka Tablets 511

Vinblastine Sulfate (Limited published data indicate that somatropin treatment increases cytochrome P450 (CYP450)-mediated antipyrine clearance in man. This data suggests that somatropin administration may alter the clearance of compounds known to be metabolized by CYP450 liver enzymes (eg, corticosteroids, sex steroids, anticonvulsants, cyclosporine). Careful monitoring is advisable when somatropin is administered in combination with other drugs known to be metabolized by CYP450 liver enzymes).
No products indexed under this heading.

Vincristine Sulfate (Limited published data indicate that somatropin treatment increases cytochrome P450 (CYP450)-mediated antipyrine clearance in man. This data suggests that somatropin administration may alter the clearance of compounds known to be metabolized by CYP450 liver enzymes (eg, corticosteroids, sex steroids, anticonvulsants, cyclosporine). Careful monitoring is advisable when somatropin is administered in combination with other drugs known to be metabolized by CYP450 liver enzymes).
No products indexed under this heading.

Warfarin Sodium (Limited published data indicate that somatropin treatment increases cytochrome P450 (CYP450)-mediated antipyrine clearance in man. This data suggests that somatropin administration may alter the clearance of compounds known to be metabolized by CYP450 liver enzymes (eg, corticosteroids, sex steroids, anticonvulsants, cyclosporine). Careful monitoring is advisable when somatropin is administered in combination with other drugs known to be metabolized by CYP450 liver enzymes).
No products indexed under this heading.

Zonisamide (Limited published data indicate that somatropin treatment increases cytochrome P450 (CYP450)-mediated antipyrine clearance in man. This data suggests that somatropin administration may alter the clearance of compounds known to be metabolized by CYP450 liver enzymes (eg, anticonvulsants). Careful monitoring is advisable when somatropin is administered in combination with other drugs known to be metabolized by CYP450 liver enzymes). Products include:
Zonegran Capsules 1089

NOROXIN TABLETS

(Norfloxacin) 2069

May interact with antacids containing aluminum, calcium and magnesium, class 1A antiarrhythmics, class III antiarrhythmics, corticosteroids, oral anticoagulants, erythromycin, iron containing oral preparations, antipsychotic agents, non-steroidal anti-inflammatory agents, drugs that prolong the QT interval, tricyclic antidepressants, xanthines, and certain other agents. Compounds in these categories include:

Alprazolam (Precaution should be taken in elderly patients when using norfloxacin concomitantly with drugs that can result in prolongation of the QTc interval (e.g., Class IA or Class III antiarrhythmics) or in patients with risk factors for torsades de pointes (e.g., known QTc prolongation, uncorrected hypokalemia).
No products indexed under this heading.

Aluminum Carbonate (May interfere with absorption resulting in lower serum and urine levels of norfloxacin; antacids should not be administered concomitantly with, or within 2 hours of, the administration of norfloxacin).
No products indexed under this heading.

Aluminum Hydroxide (May interfere with absorption resulting in lower serum and urine levels of norfloxacin; antacids should not be administered concomitantly with, or within 2 hours of, the administration of norfloxacin).
No products indexed under this heading.

Aminophylline (Co-administration of quinolone with theophylline has resulted in elevated plasma levels of theophylline resulting in theophylline-related side effects).
No products indexed under this heading.

Amiodarone Hydrochloride (Risk of developing arrhythmias with norfloxacin may be reduced by avoiding concurrent treatment with class III antiarrhythmic agents).
No products indexed under this heading.

Amitriptyline Hydrochloride (Norfloxacin should be used with caution in subjects receiving drugs that affect the QTc interval, such as tricyclic antidepressants).
No products indexed under this heading.

Amoxapine (Norfloxacin should be used with caution in subjects receiving drugs that affect the QTc interval, such as tricyclic antidepressants).
No products indexed under this heading.

Anisindione (Co-administration may enhance the effects of oral anticoagulants).
No products indexed under this heading.

Aripiprazole (Norfloxacin should be used with caution in subjects receiving drugs that affect the QTc interval, such as antipsychotics).
Products include:
Abilify Injection 881
Abilify Injection 2466
Abilify Oral Solution 881
Abilify Oral Solution 2466
Abilify Discmelt Orally Disintegrating Tablets 881
Abilify Discmelt Orally Disintegrating Tablets 2466
Abilify Tablets 881
Abilify Tablets 2466

Astemizole (Precaution should be taken in elderly patients when using norfloxacin concomitantly with drugs that can result in prolongation of the QTc interval (e.g., Class IA or Class III antiarrhythmics) or in patients with risk factors for torsades de pointes (e.g., known QTc prolongation, uncorrected hypokalemia).
No products indexed under this heading.

Betamethasone Acetate (The risk of ruptures of the shoulder, hand or Achilles tendons may be increased in patients receiving concomitant corticosteroids, especially in the elderly).
No products indexed under this heading.

Betamethasone Sodium Phosphate (The risk of ruptures of the shoulder, hand or Achilles tendons may be increased in patients receiving concomitant corticosteroids, especially in the elderly).
No products indexed under this heading.

Bretylium Tosylate (Risk of developing arrhythmias with norfloxacin may be reduced by avoiding concurrent treatment with class III antiarrhythmic agents).
No products indexed under this heading.

Budesonide (The risk of ruptures of the shoulder, hand or Achilles tendons may be increased in patients receiving concomitant corticosteroids, especially in the elderly).
Products include:
Pulmicort Flexhaler 654
Symbicort 80/4.5 Inhalation Aerosol 659
Symbicort 160/4.5 Inhalation Aerosol 659

Buspirone Hydrochloride (Precaution should be taken in elderly patients when using norfloxacin concomitantly with drugs that can result in prolongation of the QTc interval (e.g., Class IA or Class III antiarrhythmics) or in patients with risk factors for torsades de pointes (e.g., known QTc prolongation, uncorrected hypokalemia).
No products indexed under this heading.

Caffeine (Some quinolones have been shown to interfere with the metabolism of caffeine leading to reduced clearance of caffeine and a prolongation of its plasma half-life, which may lead to accumulation of caffeine in plasma when products containing caffeine are consumed while taking norfloxacin). Products include:
BioLean Free Tablets .... ▣ 635
BioLean II Tablets .... ▣ 635
Winrgy Dietary Supplement .... ▣ 642

Celecoxib (The concomitant administration of a non-steroidal anti-inflammatory drug (NSAID) with a quinolone, including norfloxacin, may increase the risk of CNS stimulation and convulsive seizures. Therefore, norfloxacin should be used with caution in individuals receiving NSAIDs concomitantly). Products include:
Celebrex Capsules 2979

Chlordiazepoxide (Precaution should be taken in elderly patients when using norfloxacin concomitantly with drugs that can result in prolongation of the QTc interval (e.g., Class IA or Class III antiarrhythmics) or in patients with risk factors for torsades de pointes (e.g., known QTc prolongation, uncorrected hypokalemia).
No products indexed under this heading.

Chlordiazepoxide Hydrochloride (Precaution should be taken in elderly patients when using norfloxacin concomitantly with drugs that can result in prolongation of the QTc interval (e.g., Class IA or Class III antiarrhythmics) or in patients with risk factors for torsades de pointes (e.g., known QTc prolongation, uncorrected hypokalemia).
No products indexed under this heading.

Chlorpromazine (Precaution should be taken in elderly patients when using norfloxacin concomitantly with drugs that can result in prolongation of the QTc interval (e.g., Class IA or Class III antiarrhythmics) or in patients with risk factors for torsades de pointes (e.g., known QTc prolongation, uncorrected hypokalemia).
No products indexed under this heading.

Chlorpromazine Hydrochloride (Precaution should be taken in elderly patients when using norfloxacin concomitantly with drugs that can result in prolongation of the QTc interval (e.g., Class IA or Class III antiarrhythmics) or in patients with risk factors for torsades de pointes (e.g., known QTc prolongation, uncorrected hypokalemia).
No products indexed under this heading.

Chlorprothixene (Precaution should be taken in elderly patients when using norfloxacin concomitantly with drugs that can result in prolongation of the QTc interval (e.g., Class IA or Class III antiarrhythmics) or in patients with risk factors for torsades de pointes (e.g., known QTc prolongation, uncorrected hypokalemia).
No products indexed under this heading.

Chlorprothixene Hydrochloride (Precaution should be taken in elderly patients when using norfloxacin concomitantly with drugs that can result in prolongation of the QTc interval (e.g., Class IA or Class III antiarrhythmics) or in patients with risk factors for torsades de pointes (e.g., known QTc prolongation, uncorrected hypokalemia).
No products indexed under this heading.

Ciclesonide (The risk of ruptures of the shoulder, hand or Achilles tendons may be increased in patients receiving concomitant corticosteroids, especially in the elderly). Products include:
Alvesco Inhalation Aerosol 2985
Omnaris Nasal Spray 2998

Cisapride (Norfloxacin should be used with caution in subjects receiving drugs that affect the QTc interval, such as cisapride).
No products indexed under this heading.

Clomipramine Hydrochloride (Norfloxacin should be used with caution in subjects receiving drugs that affect the QTc interval, such as tricyclic antidepressants).
No products indexed under this heading.

Clorazepate Dipotassium (Precaution should be taken in elderly patients when using norfloxacin concomitantly with drugs that can result in prolongation of the QTc interval (e.g., Class IA or Class III antiarrhythmics) or in patients with risk factors for torsades de pointes (e.g., known QTc prolongation, uncorrected hypokalemia).
No products indexed under this heading.

Clozapine (Precaution should be taken in elderly patients when using norfloxacin concomitantly with drugs that can result in prolongation of the QTc interval (e.g., Class IA or Class III antiarrhythmics) or in patients with risk factors for torsades de pointes (e.g., known QTc prolongation, uncorrected hypokalemia).
No products indexed under this heading.

Cortisone Acetate (The risk of ruptures of the shoulder, hand or Achilles tendons may be increased in patients receiving concomitant corticosteroids, especially in the elderly).
No products indexed under this heading.

Cyclosporine (Co-administration has resulted in elevated serum levels of cyclosporine). Products include:
Gengraf Capsules 435
Neoral Oral Solution 2280
Neoral Soft Gelatin Capsules 2280
Restasis Ophthalmic Emulsion 557
Sandimmune 2296

Desipramine Hydrochloride (Norfloxacin should be used with caution in subjects receiving drugs that affect the QTc interval, such as tricyclic antidepressants).
No products indexed under this heading.

Dexamethasone (The risk of ruptures of the shoulder, hand or Achilles tendons may be increased in patients receiving concomitant corticosteroids, especially in the elderly). Products include:
Ciprodex Otic Suspension 541

Dexamethasone Acetate (The risk of ruptures of the shoulder, hand or Achilles tendons may be increased in patients receiving concomitant corticosteroids, especially in the elderly).
No products indexed under this heading.

Dexamethasone Sodium Phosphate (The risk of ruptures of the shoulder, hand or Achilles tendons may be increased in patients receiving concomitant corticosteroids, especially in the elderly).
No products indexed under this heading.

Diazepam (Precaution should be taken in elderly patients when using norfloxacin concomitantly with drugs that can result in prolongation of the QTc interval (e.g., Class IA or Class III antiarrhythmics) or in patients with risk factors for torsades de pointes (e.g., known QTc prolongation, uncorrected hypokalemia). Products include:
Valium Tablets 2658

Diclofenac Epolamine (The concomitant administration of a non-steroidal anti-inflammatory drug (NSAID) with a quinolone, including norfloxacin, may increase the risk of CNS stimulation and convulsive seizures. Therefore, norfloxacin should be used with caution in individuals receiving NSAIDs concomitantly). Products include:
Flector Patch 561

Diclofenac Potassium (The concomitant administration of a non-steroidal anti-inflammatory drug (NSAID) with a quinolone, including norfloxacin, may increase the risk of CNS stimulation and convulsive seizures. Therefore, norfloxacin should be used with caution in individuals receiving NSAIDs concomitantly).
No products indexed under this heading.

Diclofenac Sodium (The concomitant administration of a non-steroidal anti-inflammatory drug (NSAID) with a quinolone, including norfloxacin, may increase the risk of CNS stimulation and convulsive seizures. Therefore, norfloxacin should be used with caution in individuals receiving NSAIDs concomitantly). Products include:
Diclofenac Sodium Ophthalmic Solution..................................... ⊙ 240
Voltaren Ophthalmic Solution 2336
Voltaren Tablets 2334
Voltaren-XR Tablets 2337

Dicumarol (Co-administration may enhance the effects of oral anticoagulants).
No products indexed under this heading.

Didanosine (Co-administration with Videx, didanosine chewable/buffered tablets or the pediatric powder for oral solution may interfere with absorption resulting in lower serum and urine levels of norfloxacin; this combination should not be administered concomitantly or within 2 hours of administration of norfloxacin).
No products indexed under this heading.

Disopyramide (Risk of developing arrhythmias with norfloxacin may be reduced by avoiding concurrent treatment with class IA antiarrhythmic agents).
No products indexed under this heading.

Disopyramide Phosphate (Precaution should be taken in elderly patients when using norfloxacin concomitantly with drugs that can result in prolongation of the QTc interval (e.g., Class IA or Class III antiarrhythmics) or in patients with risk factors for torsades de pointes (e.g., known QTc prolongation, uncorrected hypokalemia).
No products indexed under this heading.

Dofetilide (Precaution should be taken in elderly patients when using norfloxacin concomitantly with drugs that can result in prolongation of the QTc interval (e.g., Class IA or Class III antiarrhythmics) or in patients with risk factors for torsades de pointes (e.g., known QTc prolongation, uncorrected hypokalemia).
No products indexed under this heading.

Doxepin Hydrochloride (Norfloxacin should be used with caution in subjects receiving drugs that affect the QTc interval, such as tricyclic antidepressants).
No products indexed under this heading.

Droperidol (Precaution should be taken in elderly patients when using norfloxacin concomitantly with drugs that can result in prolongation of the QTc interval (e.g., Class IA or Class III antiarrhythmics) or in patients with risk factors for torsades de pointes (e.g., known QTc prolongation, uncorrected hypokalemia).
No products indexed under this heading.

Dyphylline (Co-administration of quinolone with theophylline has resulted in elevated plasma levels of theophylline resulting in theophylline-related side effects).
No products indexed under this heading.

Erythromycin (Norfloxacin should be used with caution in subjects receiving drugs that affect the QTc interval, such as erythromycin).
No products indexed under this heading.

Erythromycin Estolate (Norfloxacin should be used with caution in subjects receiving drugs that affect the QTc interval, such as erythromycin).
No products indexed under this heading.

Erythromycin Ethylsuccinate (Norfloxacin should be used with caution in subjects receiving drugs that affect the QTc interval, such as erythromycin). Products include:
E.E.S. 433
EryPed 431

Erythromycin Gluceptate (Norfloxacin should be used with caution in subjects receiving drugs that affect the QTc interval, such as erythromycin).
No products indexed under this heading.

Erythromycin Lactobionate (Norfloxacin should be used with caution in subjects receiving drugs that affect the QTc interval, such as erythromycin).
No products indexed under this heading.

Erythromycin Stearate (Norfloxacin should be used with caution in subjects receiving drugs that affect the QTc interval, such as erythromycin).
No products indexed under this heading.

Etodolac (The concomitant administration of a non-steroidal anti-inflammatory drug (NSAID) with a quinolone, including norfloxacin, may increase the risk of CNS stimulation and convulsive seizures. Therefore, norfloxacin should be used with caution in individuals receiving NSAIDs concomitantly).
No products indexed under this heading.

Fenoprofen Calcium (The concomitant administration of a non-steroidal anti-inflammatory drug (NSAID) with a quinolone, including norfloxacin, may increase the risk of CNS stimulation and convulsive seizures. Therefore, norfloxacin should be used with caution in individuals receiving NSAIDs concomitantly). Products include:
Nalfon Capsules 2508

Ferrous Fumarate (May interfere with absorption resulting in lower serum and urine levels of norfloxacin; iron-containing products should not be administered concomitantly with, or within 2 hours of, the administration of norfloxacin).
No products indexed under this heading.

Ferrous Gluconate (May interfere with absorption resulting in lower serum and urine levels of norfloxacin; iron-containing products should not be administered concomitantly with, or within 2 hours of, the administration of norfloxacin). Products include:
CitraNatal DHA Tablets 2175

Ferrous Sulfate (May interfere with absorption resulting in lower serum and urine levels of norfloxacin; iron-containing products should not be administered concomitantly with, or within 2 hours of, the administration of norfloxacin).
No products indexed under this heading.

Flecainide Acetate (Precaution should be taken in elderly patients when using norfloxacin concomitantly with drugs that can result in prolongation of the QTc interval (e.g., Class IA or Class III antiarrhythmics) or in patients with risk factors for torsades de pointes (e.g., known QTc prolongation, uncorrected hypokalemia).
No products indexed under this heading.

Fludrocortisone Acetate (The risk of ruptures of the shoulder, hand or Achilles tendons may be increased in patients receiving concomitant corticosteroids, especially in the elderly).
No products indexed under this heading.

Flunisolide (The risk of ruptures of the shoulder, hand or Achilles tendons may be increased in patients receiving concomitant corticosteroids, especially in the elderly).
Products include:
Aerobid/Aerobid-M 1153

Fluphenazine Decanoate (Precaution should be taken in elderly patients when using norfloxacin concomitantly with drugs that can result in prolongation of the QTc interval (e.g., Class IA or Class III antiarrhythmics) or in patients with risk factors for torsades de pointes (e.g., known QTc prolongation, uncorrected hypokalemia).
No products indexed under this heading.

Fluphenazine Enanthate (Precaution should be taken in elderly patients when using norfloxacin concomitantly with drugs that can result in prolongation of the QTc interval (e.g., Class IA or Class III antiarrhythmics) or in patients with risk factors for torsades de pointes (e.g., known QTc prolongation, uncorrected hypokalemia).
No products indexed under this heading.

Fluphenazine Hydrochloride (Precaution should be taken in elderly patients when using norfloxacin concomitantly with drugs that can result in prolongation of the QTc interval (e.g., Class IA or Class III antiarrhythmics) or in patients with risk factors for torsades de pointes (e.g., known QTc prolongation, uncorrected hypokalemia).
No products indexed under this heading.

Flurbiprofen (The concomitant administration of a non-steroidal anti-inflammatory drug (NSAID) with a quinolone, including norfloxacin, may increase the risk of CNS stimulation and convulsive seizures. Therefore, norfloxacin should be used with caution in individuals receiving NSAIDs concomitantly).
No products indexed under this heading.

Fluticasone Propionate (The risk of ruptures of the shoulder, hand or Achilles tendons may be increased in patients receiving concomitant corticosteroids, especially in the elderly).
Products include:
Advair Diskus 100/50 1276
Advair Diskus 250/50 1276
Advair Diskus 500/50 1276
Advair HFA 45/21 Inhalation Aerosol 1288
Advair HFA 115/21 Inhalation Aerosol 1288
Advair HFA 230/21 Inhalation Aerosol 1288
Flonase Nasal Spray 1431
Flovent Diskus 50 mcg 1435

Fluticasone Propionate HFA (The risk of ruptures of the shoulder, hand or Achilles tendons may be increased in patients receiving concomitant corticosteroids, especially in the elderly). Products include:
Flovent HFA 1440

Glyburide (Concomitant administration of norfloxacin with glyburide has rarely resulted in severe hypoglycemia; monitoring of blood glucose is recommended when these agents are co-administered).
No products indexed under this heading.

Haloperidol (Precaution should be taken in elderly patients when using norfloxacin concomitantly with drugs that can result in prolongation of the QTc interval (e.g., Class IA or Class III antiarrhythmics) or in patients with risk factors for torsades de pointes (e.g., known QTc prolongation, uncorrected hypokalemia).
No products indexed under this heading.

Haloperidol Decanoate (Precaution should be taken in elderly patients when using norfloxacin concomitantly with drugs that can result in prolongation of the QTc interval (e.g., Class IA or Class III antiarrhythmics) or in patients with risk factors for torsades de pointes (e.g., known QTc prolongation, uncorrected hypokalemia).
No products indexed under this heading.

Hydrocortisone (The risk of ruptures of the shoulder, hand or Achilles tendons may be increased in patients receiving concomitant corticosteroids, especially in the elderly).
No products indexed under this heading.

Hydrocortisone Acetate (The risk of ruptures of the shoulder, hand or Achilles tendons may be increased in patients receiving concomitant corticosteroids, especially in the elderly).
Products include:
Analpram-HC 1140
Pramosone 1141

Hydrocortisone Sodium Phosphate (The risk of ruptures of the shoulder, hand or Achilles tendons may be increased in patients receiving concomitant corticosteroids, especially in the elderly).
No products indexed under this heading.

Hydrocortisone Sodium Succinate (The risk of ruptures of the shoulder, hand or Achilles tendons may be increased in patients receiving concomitant corticosteroids, especially in the elderly).
No products indexed under this heading.

Hydroxyzine Hydrochloride (Precaution should be taken in elderly patients when using norfloxacin concomitantly with drugs that can result in prolongation of the QTc interval (e.g., Class IA or Class III antiarrhythmics) or in patients with risk factors for torsades de pointes (e.g., known QTc prolongation, uncorrected hypokalemia).
No products indexed under this heading.

Ibuprofen (The concomitant administration of a non-steroidal anti-inflammatory drug (NSAID) with a quinolone, including norfloxacin, may increase the risk of CNS stimulation and convulsive seizures. Therefore, norfloxacin should be used with caution in individuals receiving NSAIDs concomitantly). Products include:
Motrin IB Tablets and Caplets 1900
Children's Motrin Oral Suspension ... 1901
Children's Motrin Non-Staining Dye-Free Oral Suspension 1901
Children's Motrin Cold Oral Suspension 1899
Infants' Motrin Concentrated Drops 1901
Infants' Motrin Non-Staining Dye-Free Concentrated Drops....... 1901
Junior Strength Motrin Caplets and Chewable Tablets 1901
Vicoprofen Tablets 533

Imipramine Hydrochloride (Norfloxacin should be used with caution in subjects receiving drugs that affect the QTc interval, such as tricyclic antidepressants).
No products indexed under this heading.

Imipramine Pamoate (Norfloxacin should be used with caution in subjects receiving drugs that affect the QTc interval, such as tricyclic antidepressants).
No products indexed under this heading.

Indomethacin (The concomitant administration of a non-steroidal anti-inflammatory drug (NSAID) with a quinolone, including norfloxacin, may increase the risk of CNS stimulation and convulsive seizures. Therefore, norfloxacin should be used with caution in individuals receiving NSAIDs concomitantly). Products include:
Indocin 2024

Indomethacin Sodium Trihydrate (The concomitant administration of a non-steroidal anti-inflammatory drug (NSAID) with a quinolone, including norfloxacin, may increase the risk of CNS stimulation and convulsive seizures. Therefore, norfloxacin should be used with caution in individuals receiving NSAIDs concomitantly). Products include:
Indocin I.V. 2489

Iron (May interfere with absorption resulting in lower serum and urine levels of norfloxacin; iron-containing products should not be administered concomitantly with, or within 2 hours of, the administration of norfloxacin).
Products include:
Phyto-Vite Tablets .... ■639

Isocarboxazid (Precaution should be taken in elderly patients when using norfloxacin concomitantly with drugs that can result in prolongation of the QTc interval (e.g., Class IA or Class III antiarrhythmics) or in patients with risk factors for torsades de pointes (e.g., known QTc prolongation, uncorrected hypokalemia). Products include:
Marplan Tablets 3177

Ketoprofen (The concomitant administration of a non-steroidal anti-inflammatory drug (NSAID) with a quinolone, including norfloxacin, may increase the risk of CNS stimulation and convulsive seizures. Therefore, norfloxacin should be used with caution in individuals receiving NSAIDs concomitantly).
No products indexed under this heading.

Ketorolac Tromethamine (The concomitant administration of a non-steroidal anti-inflammatory drug (NSAID) with a quinolone, including norfloxacin, may increase the risk of CNS stimulation and convulsive seizures. Therefore, norfloxacin should be used with caution in individuals receiving NSAIDs concomitantly).
No products indexed under this heading.

Lidocaine Hydrochloride (Precaution should be taken in elderly patients when using norfloxacin concomitantly with drugs that can result in prolongation of the QTc interval (e.g., Class IA or Class III antiarrhythmics) or in patients with risk factors for torsades de pointes (e.g., known QTc prolongation, uncorrected hypokalemia).
No products indexed under this heading.

Lithium Carbonate (Precaution should be taken in elderly patients when using norfloxacin concomitantly with drugs that can result in prolongation of the QTc interval (e.g., Class IA or Class III antiarrhythmics) or in patients with risk factors for torsades de pointes (e.g., known QTc prolongation, uncorrected hypokalemia).
No products indexed under this heading.

Lithium Citrate (Precaution should be taken in elderly patients when using norfloxacin concomitantly with drugs that can result in prolongation of the QTc interval (e.g., Class IA or Class III antiarrhythmics) or in patients with risk factors for torsades de pointes (e.g., known QTc prolongation, uncorrected hypokalemia).
No products indexed under this heading.

Lorazepam (Precaution should be taken in elderly patients when using norfloxacin concomitantly with drugs that can result in prolongation of the QTc interval (e.g., Class IA or Class III antiarrhythmics) or in patients with risk factors for torsades de pointes (e.g., known QTc prolongation, uncorrected hypokalemia).
No products indexed under this heading.

Loxapine Hydrochloride (Precaution should be taken in elderly patients when using norfloxacin concomitantly with drugs that can result in prolongation of the QTc interval (e.g., Class IA or Class III antiarrhythmics) or in patients with risk factors for torsades de pointes (e.g., known QTc prolongation, uncorrected hypokalemia).
No products indexed under this heading.

Loxapine Succinate (Precaution should be taken in elderly patients when using norfloxacin concomitantly with drugs that can result in prolongation of the QTc interval (e.g., Class IA or Class III antiarrhythmics) or in patients with risk factors for torsades de pointes (e.g., known QTc prolongation, uncorrected hypokalemia).
No products indexed under this heading.

Magaldrate (May interfere with absorption resulting in lower serum and urine levels of norfloxacin; antacids should not be administered concomitantly with, or within 2 hours of, the administration of norfloxacin).
No products indexed under this heading.

Magnesium Hydroxide (May interfere with absorption resulting in lower serum and urine levels of norfloxacin; antacids should not be administered concomitantly with, or within 2 hours of, the administration of norfloxacin). Products include:
Fleet Pedia-Lax Chewable Tablets 1145

Pepcid Complete Chewable Tablets 1771
Extra Strength Rolaids Freshmint Tablets 1903
Rolaids Multi-Symptom Berry Tablets 1903
Rolaids Original Peppermint Tablets 1903

Magnesium Oxide (May interfere with absorption resulting in lower serum and urine levels of norfloxacin; antacids should not be administered concomitantly with, or within 2 hours of, the administration of norfloxacin). Products include:
Beelith Tablets 813

Maprotiline Hydrochloride (Norfloxacin should be used with caution in subjects receiving drugs that affect the QTc interval, such as tricyclic antidepressants).
No products indexed under this heading.

Meclofenamate Sodium (The concomitant administration of a non-steroidal anti-inflammatory drug (NSAID) with a quinolone, including norfloxacin, may increase the risk of CNS stimulation and convulsive seizures. Therefore, norfloxacin should be used with caution in individuals receiving NSAIDs concomitantly).
No products indexed under this heading.

Mefenamic Acid (The concomitant administration of a non-steroidal anti-inflammatory drug (NSAID) with a quinolone, including norfloxacin, may increase the risk of CNS stimulation and convulsive seizures. Therefore, norfloxacin should be used with caution in individuals receiving NSAIDs concomitantly).
No products indexed under this heading.

Meloxicam (The concomitant administration of a non-steroidal anti-inflammatory drug (NSAID) with a quinolone, including norfloxacin, may increase the risk of CNS stimulation and convulsive seizures. Therefore, norfloxacin should be used with caution in individuals receiving NSAIDs concomitantly). Products include:
Mobic Oral Suspension 863
Mobic Tablets 863

Meprobamate (Precaution should be taken in elderly patients when using norfloxacin concomitantly with drugs that can result in prolongation of the QTc interval (e.g., Class IA or Class III antiarrhythmics) or in patients with risk factors for torsades de pointes (e.g., known QTc prolongation, uncorrected hypokalemia).
No products indexed under this heading.

Mesoridazine Besylate (Precaution should be taken in elderly patients when using norfloxacin concomitantly with drugs that can result in prolongation of the QTc interval (e.g., Class IA or Class III antiarrhythmics) or in patients with risk factors for torsades de pointes (e.g., known QTc prolongation, uncorrected hypokalemia).
No products indexed under this heading.

Methotrimeprazine (Norfloxacin should be used with caution in subjects receiving drugs that affect the QTc interval, such as antipsychotics).
No products indexed under this heading.

Methylprednisolone Acetate (The risk of ruptures of the shoulder, hand or Achilles tendons may be increased in patients receiving concomitant corticosteroids, especially in the elderly).
No products indexed under this heading.

Methylprednisolone Sodium Succinate (The risk of ruptures of the shoulder, hand or Achilles tendons may be increased in patients receiving concomitant corticosteroids, especially in the elderly).
No products indexed under this heading.

Mexiletine Hydrochloride (Precaution should be taken in elderly patients when using norfloxacin concomitantly with drugs that can result in prolongation of the QTc interval (e.g., Class IA or Class III antiarrhythmics) or in patients with risk factors for torsades de pointes (e.g., known QTc prolongation, uncorrected hypokalemia).
No products indexed under this heading.

Midazolam Hydrochloride (Precaution should be taken in elderly patients when using norfloxacin concomitantly with drugs that can result in prolongation of the QTc interval (e.g., Class IA or Class III antiarrhythmics) or in patients with risk factors for torsades de pointes (e.g., known QTc prolongation, uncorrected hypokalemia).
No products indexed under this heading.

Molindone Hydrochloride (Precaution should be taken in elderly patients when using norfloxacin concomitantly with drugs that can result in prolongation of the QTc interval (e.g., Class IA or Class III antiarrhythmics) or in patients with risk factors for torsades de pointes (e.g., known QTc prolongation, uncorrected hypokalemia). Products include:
Moban Tablets 1116

Mometasone Furoate (The risk of ruptures of the shoulder, hand or Achilles tendons may be increased in patients receiving concomitant corticosteroids, especially in the elderly). Products include:
Asmanex Twisthaler 2797
Elocon Cream 0.1% 2840
Elocon Lotion 0.1% 2841
Elocon Ointment 0.1% 2842

Mometasone Furoate Monohydrate (The risk of ruptures of the shoulder, hand or Achilles tendons may be increased in patients receiving concomitant corticosteroids, especially in the elderly). Products include:
Nasonex Nasal Spray 2883

Moricizine Hydrochloride (Risk of developing arrhythmias with norfloxacin may be reduced by avoiding concurrent treatment with class IA antiarrhythmic agents).
No products indexed under this heading.

Nabumetone (The concomitant administration of a non-steroidal anti-inflammatory drug (NSAID) with a quinolone, including norfloxacin, may increase the risk of CNS stimulation and convulsive seizures. Therefore, norfloxacin should be used with caution in individuals receiving NSAIDs concomitantly).
No products indexed under this heading.

Naproxen (The concomitant administration of a non-steroidal anti-inflammatory drug (NSAID) with a quinolone, including norfloxacin, may increase the risk of CNS stimulation and convulsive seizures. Therefore, norfloxacin should be used with caution in individuals receiving NSAIDs concomitantly). Products include:
EC-Naprosyn Delayed-Release Tablets 2632
Naprosyn Suspension 2632
Naprosyn Tablets 2632

Naproxen Sodium (The concomitant administration of a non-steroidal anti-inflammatory drug (NSAID) with a quinolone, including norfloxacin, may increase the risk of CNS stimulation and convulsive seizures. Therefore, norfloxacin should be used with caution in individuals receiving NSAIDs concomitantly). Products include:
Anaprox Tablets 2632
Anaprox DS Tablets 2632
Treximet Tablets 1616

Nitrofurantoin (Nitrofurantoin may antagonize the antibacterial effect of norfloxacin in the urinary tract; concurrent use is not recommended).
No products indexed under this heading.

Nortriptyline Hydrochloride (Norfloxacin should be used with caution in subjects receiving drugs that affect the QTc interval, such as tricyclic antidepressants).
No products indexed under this heading.

Olanzapine (Precaution should be taken in elderly patients when using norfloxacin concomitantly with drugs that can result in prolongation of the QTc interval (e.g., Class IA or Class III antiarrhythmics) or in patients with risk factors for torsades de pointes (e.g., known QTc prolongation, uncorrected hypokalemia). Products include:
Symbyax Capsules 1871
Zyprexa Tablets 1883
Zyprexa IntraMuscular 1883
Zyprexa ZYDIS Orally Disintegrating Tablets 1883

Oxaprozin (The concomitant administration of a non-steroidal anti-inflammatory drug (NSAID) with a quinolone, including norfloxacin, may increase the risk of CNS stimulation and convulsive seizures. Therefore, norfloxacin should be used with caution in individuals receiving NSAIDs concomitantly).
No products indexed under this heading.

Oxazepam (Precaution should be taken in elderly patients when using norfloxacin concomitantly with drugs that can result in prolongation of the QTc interval (e.g., Class IA or Class III antiarrhythmics) or in patients with risk factors for torsades de pointes (e.g., known QTc prolongation, uncorrected hypokalemia).
No products indexed under this heading.

Paliperidone (Norfloxacin should be used with caution in subjects receiving drugs that affect the QTc interval, such as antipsychotics). Products include:
Invega Extended-Release Tablets 1748

Perphenazine (Precaution should be taken in elderly patients when using norfloxacin concomitantly with drugs that can result in prolongation of the QTc interval (e.g., Class IA or Class III antiarrhythmics) or in patients with risk factors for torsades de pointes (e.g., known QTc prolongation, uncorrected hypokalemia).
No products indexed under this heading.

Phenelzine Sulfate (Precaution should be taken in elderly patients when using norfloxacin concomitantly with drugs that can result in prolongation of the QTc interval (e.g., Class IA or Class III antiarrhythmics) or in patients with risk factors for torsades de pointes (e.g., known QTc prolongation, uncorrected hypokalemia).
No products indexed under this heading.

Phenylbutazone (The concomitant administration of a non-steroidal anti-inflammatory drug (NSAID) with a quinolone, including norfloxacin, may increase the risk of CNS stimulation and convulsive seizures. Therefore, norfloxacin should be used with caution in individuals receiving NSAIDs concomitantly).
No products indexed under this heading.

Pimozide (Norfloxacin should be used with caution in subjects receiving drugs that affect the QTc interval, such as antipsychotics).
No products indexed under this heading.

Piroxicam (The concomitant administration of a non-steroidal anti-inflammatory drug (NSAID) with a quinolone, including norfloxacin, may increase the risk of CNS stimulation and convulsive seizures. Therefore, norfloxacin should be used with caution in individuals receiving NSAIDs concomitantly).
No products indexed under this heading.

Polysaccharide Iron Complex (May interfere with absorption resulting in lower serum and urine levels of norfloxacin; iron-containing products should not be administered concomitantly with, or within 2 hours of, the administration of norfloxacin). Products include:
Nu-Iron 150 Capsules 2165

Prazepam (Precaution should be taken in elderly patients when using norfloxacin concomitantly with drugs that can result in prolongation of the QTc interval (e.g., Class IA or Class III antiarrhythmics) or in patients with risk factors for torsades de pointes (e.g., known QTc prolongation, uncorrected hypokalemia).
No products indexed under this heading.

Prednisolone Acetate (The risk of ruptures of the shoulder, hand or Achilles tendons may be increased in patients receiving concomitant corticosteroids, especially in the elderly). Products include:
Pred Forte Ophthalmic Suspension .... ⊙ 227
Pred Mild Ophthalmic Suspension .... ⊙ 230
Pred-G Ophthalmic Ointment .... ⊙ 229
Pred-G Ophthalmic Suspension .... ⊙ 228

Prednisolone Sodium Phosphate (The risk of ruptures of the shoulder, hand or Achilles tendons may be increased in patients receiving concomitant corticosteroids, especially in the elderly).
No products indexed under this heading.

Prednisolone Tebutate (The risk of ruptures of the shoulder, hand or Achilles tendons may be increased in patients receiving concomitant corticosteroids, especially in the elderly).
No products indexed under this heading.

Prednisone (The risk of ruptures of the shoulder, hand or Achilles tendons may be increased in patients receiving concomitant corticosteroids, especially in the elderly).
No products indexed under this heading.

Probenecid (Co-administration with probenecid has resulted in diminished urinary excretion).
No products indexed under this heading.

Procainamide (Risk of developing arrhythmias with norfloxacin may be reduced by avoiding concurrent treatment with class IA antiarrhythmic agents).
No products indexed under this heading.

Procainamide Hydrochloride (Precaution should be taken in elderly patients when using norfloxacin concomitantly with drugs that can result in prolongation of the QTc interval (e.g., Class IA or Class III antiarrhythmics) or in patients with risk factors for torsades de pointes (e.g., known QTc prolongation, uncorrected hypokalemia).
No products indexed under this heading.

Prochlorperazine (Precaution should be taken in elderly patients when using norfloxacin concomitantly with drugs that can result in prolongation of the QTc interval (e.g., Class IA or Class III antiarrhythmics) or in patients with risk factors for torsades de pointes (e.g., known QTc prolongation, uncorrected hypokalemia).
No products indexed under this heading.

Promethazine Hydrochloride (Precaution should be taken in elderly patients when using norfloxacin concomitantly with drugs that can result in prolongation of the QTc interval (e.g., Class IA or Class III antiarrhythmics) or in patients with risk factors for torsades de pointes (e.g., known QTc prolongation, uncorrected hypokalemia).
No products indexed under this heading.

Propafenone Hydrochloride (Precaution should be taken in elderly patients when using norfloxacin concomitantly with drugs that can result in prolongation of the QTc interval (e.g., Class IA or Class III antiarrhythmics) or in patients with risk factors for torsades de pointes (e.g., known QTc prolongation, uncorrected hypokalemia). Products include:
Rythmol Tablets 1586
Rythmol SR Capsules 1590

Protriptyline Hydrochloride (Norfloxacin should be used with caution in subjects receiving drugs that affect the QTc interval, such as tricyclic antidepressants).
No products indexed under this heading.

Quetiapine Fumarate (Precaution should be taken in elderly patients when using norfloxacin concomitantly with drugs that can result in prolongation of the QTc interval (e.g., Class IA or Class III antiarrhythmics) or in patients with risk factors for torsades de pointes (e.g., known QTc prolongation, uncorrected hypokalemia).
No products indexed under this heading.

Quinidine (Risk of developing arrhythmias with norfloxacin may be reduced by avoiding concurrent treatment with class IA antiarrhythmic agents).
No products indexed under this heading.

Quinidine Gluconate (Risk of developing arrhythmias with norfloxacin may be reduced by avoiding concurrent treatment with class IA antiarrhythmic agents).
No products indexed under this heading.

Quinidine Hydrochloride (Risk of developing arrhythmias with norfloxacin may be reduced by avoiding concurrent treatment with class IA antiarrhythmic agents).
No products indexed under this heading.

Quinidine Polygalacturonate (Risk of developing arrhythmias with norfloxacin may be reduced by avoiding concurrent treatment with class IA antiarrhythmic agents).
No products indexed under this heading.

Quinidine Sulfate (Risk of developing arrhythmias with norfloxacin may be reduced by avoiding concurrent treatment with class IA antiarrhythmic agents).
No products indexed under this heading.

Risperidone (Precaution should be taken in elderly patients when using norfloxacin concomitantly with drugs that can result in prolongation of the QTc interval (e.g., Class IA or Class III antiarrhythmics) or in patients with risk factors for torsades de pointes (e.g., known QTc prolongation, uncorrected hypokalemia). Products include:
Risperdal Consta Long-Acting Injection 1753

Rofecoxib (The concomitant administration of a non-steroidal anti-inflammatory drug (NSAID) with a quinolone, including norfloxacin, may increase the risk of CNS stimulation and convulsive seizures. Therefore, norfloxacin should be used with caution in individuals receiving NSAIDs concomitantly).
No products indexed under this heading.

Sotalol Hydrochloride (Risk of developing arrhythmias with norfloxacin may be reduced by avoiding concurrent treatment with class III antiarrhythmic agents).
No products indexed under this heading.

Sucralfate (May interfere with absorption resulting in lower serum and urine levels of norfloxacin; sucralfate should not be administered concomitantly with, or within 2 hours of, the administration of norfloxacin). Products include:
Carafate Suspension 706
Carafate Tablets 707

Sulindac (The concomitant administration of a non-steroidal anti-inflammatory drug (NSAID) with a quinolone, including norfloxacin, may increase the risk of CNS stimulation and convulsive seizures. Therefore, norfloxacin should be used with caution in individuals receiving NSAIDs concomitantly). Products include:
Clinoril Tablets 1962

Theophylline (Co-administration of quinolone with theophylline has resulted in elevated plasma levels of theophylline resulting in theophylline-related side effects).
No products indexed under this heading.

Theophylline Anhydrous (Co-administration of quinolone with theophylline has resulted in elevated plasma levels of theophylline resulting in theophylline-related side effects). Products include:
Uniphyl Tablets 2595

Theophylline Calcium Salicylate (Co-administration of quinolone with theophylline has resulted in elevated plasma levels of theophylline resulting in theophylline-related side effects).
No products indexed under this heading.

Theophylline Dihydroxypropyl (Glyceryl) (Co-administration of quinolone with theophylline has resulted in elevated plasma levels of theophylline resulting in theophylline-related side effects).
No products indexed under this heading.

Theophylline Ethylenediamine (Co-administration of quinolone with theophylline has resulted in elevated plasma levels of theophylline resulting in theophylline-related side effects).
No products indexed under this heading.

Theophylline Sodium Glycinate (Co-administration of quinolone with theophylline has resulted in elevated plasma levels of theophylline resulting in theophylline-related side effects).
No products indexed under this heading.

Thioridazine Hydrochloride (Precaution should be taken in elderly patients when using norfloxacin concomitantly with drugs that can result in prolongation of the QTc interval (e.g., Class IA or Class III antiarrhythmics) or in patients with risk factors for torsades de pointes (e.g., known QTc prolongation, uncorrected hypokalemia). Products include:
Thioridazine Hydrochloride Tablets 2195

Thiothixene (Precaution should be taken in elderly patients when using norfloxacin concomitantly with drugs that can result in prolongation of the QTc interval (e.g., Class IA or Class III antiarrhythmics) or in patients with risk factors for torsades de pointes (e.g., known QTc prolongation, uncorrected hypokalemia). Products include:
Thiothixene Capsules 2197

Tocainide Hydrochloride (Precaution should be taken in elderly patients when using norfloxacin concomitantly with drugs that can result in prolongation of the QTc interval (e.g., Class IA or Class III antiarrhythmics) or in patients with risk factors for torsades de pointes (e.g., known QTc prolongation, uncorrected hypokalemia).
No products indexed under this heading.

Tolmetin Sodium (The concomitant administration of a non-steroidal anti-inflammatory drug (NSAID) with a quinolone, including norfloxacin, may increase the risk of CNS stimulation and convulsive seizures. Therefore, norfloxacin should be used with caution in individuals receiving NSAIDs concomitantly).
No products indexed under this heading.

Tranylcypromine Sulfate (Precaution should be taken in elderly patients when using norfloxacin concomitantly with drugs that can result in prolongation of the QTc interval (e.g., Class IA or Class III antiarrhythmics) or in patients with risk factors for torsades de pointes (e.g., known QTc prolongation, uncorrected hypokalemia). Products include:
Parnate Tablets 1532

Triamcinolone (The risk of ruptures of the shoulder, hand or Achilles tendons may be increased in patients receiving concomitant corticosteroids, especially in the elderly).
No products indexed under this heading.

Triamcinolone Acetonide (The risk of ruptures of the shoulder, hand or Achilles tendons may be increased in patients receiving concomitant corticosteroids, especially in the elderly). Products include:
Azmacort Inhalation Aerosol 407
Nasacort AQ Nasal Spray 2765
Triesence Injectable Suspension ..... ⊙209

Triamcinolone Diacetate (The risk of ruptures of the shoulder, hand or Achilles tendons may be increased in patients receiving concomitant corticosteroids, especially in the elderly).
No products indexed under this heading.

Triamcinolone Hexacetonide (The risk of ruptures of the shoulder, hand or Achilles tendons may be increased in patients receiving concomitant corticosteroids, especially in the elderly).
No products indexed under this heading.

Trifluoperazine Hydrochloride (Precaution should be taken in elderly patients when using norfloxacin concomitantly with drugs that can result in prolongation of the QTc interval (e.g., Class IA or Class III antiarrhythmics) or in patients with risk factors for torsades de pointes (e.g., known QTc prolongation, uncorrected hypokalemia).
No products indexed under this heading.

Trimipramine Maleate (Norfloxacin should be used with caution in subjects receiving drugs that affect the QTc interval, such as tricyclic antidepressants).
No products indexed under this heading.

Valdecoxib (The concomitant administration of a non-steroidal anti-inflammatory drug (NSAID) with a quinolone, including norfloxacin, may increase the risk of CNS stimulation and convulsive seizures. Therefore, norfloxacin should be used with caution in individuals receiving NSAIDs concomitantly).
No products indexed under this heading.

Warfarin Sodium (Co-administration may enhance the effects of oral anticoagulants).
No products indexed under this heading.

Zinc Sulfate (May interfere with absorption resulting in lower serum and urine levels of norfloxacin; zinc-containing oral products should not be administered concomitantly with, or within 2 hours of, the administration of norfloxacin). Products include:
Clear Eyes Itchy Eye Relief .... ⊙255
Zinc-220 Capsules 564

Ziprasidone Hydrochloride (Precaution should be taken in elderly patients when using norfloxacin concomitantly with drugs that can result in prolongation of the QTc interval (e.g., Class IA or Class III antiarrhythmics) or in patients with risk factors for torsades de pointes (e.g., known QTc prolongation, uncorrected hypokalemia). Products include:
Geodon Capsules 2520

Food Interactions

Dairy products (Avoid simultaneous ingestion; administer norfloxacin at least one hour before or two hours after ingestion of milk and/or other dairy products).

Food, unspecified (Co-administration may decrease the absorption of norfloxacin; administer at least one hour before or two hours after a meal).

NORVIR ORAL SOLUTION

(Ritonavir) 489
See Norvir Soft Gelatin Capsules

NORVIR SOFT GELATIN CAPSULES

(Ritonavir) 489
May interact with beta blockers, cytochrome p450 2d6 substrates (selected), cytochrome p450 3a inducers (selected), cytochrome p450 3a substrates (selected), dexamethasone, ergot-containing drugs, erythromycin, HMG-CoA reductase inhibitors, oral hypoglycemic agents, highly metabolized sedatives and hypnotics, insulin, phenytoin, quinidine, selective serotonin reuptake inhibitors, tricyclic antidepressants, valproate, xanthines, and certain other agents. Compounds in these categories include:

Acarbose (New onset diabetes mellitus, exacerbation of pre-existing diabetes, and hyperglycemia have been reported with protease inhibitors; dosage adjustment of oral hypoglycemic agents may be required). Products include:
Precose Tablets 792

Acebutolol Hydrochloride (Co-administration with beta-blockers has resulted in cardiac and neurologic events).
No products indexed under this heading.

Albendazole (Co-administration results in a possible increase in AUC of albendazole; dosage adjustments may be required). Products include:
Albenza Tablets 1297

Alfentanil Hydrochloride (Co-administration results in a large increase (> 3x) in AUC of alfentanil; dosage adjustments may be required).
No products indexed under this heading.

Alfuzosin Hydrochloride (Co-administration is contraindicated due to the potential for serious reactions such as hypotension). Products include:
Uroxatral Tablets 2786

Allium sativum (Potential for increase in the clearance of ritonavir resulting in decreased ritonavir plasma concentrations).
No products indexed under this heading.

Alprazolam (Co-administration is likely to produce large increases in highly metabolized sedatives and hypnotics resulting in extreme sedation and respiratory depression; concurrent use is contraindicated).
No products indexed under this heading.

Aminophylline (Co-administration results in the reduction of the average AUC of theophylline; increased dosage of theophylline may be required and therapeutic monitoring should be considered).
No products indexed under this heading.

Amiodarone Hydrochloride (Co-administration is contraindicated due to potential for serious and/or life-threatening reactions, such as cardiac arrhythmias).
No products indexed under this heading.

Amitriptyline Hydrochloride (Co-administration may result in increased tricyclic antidepressants' plasma concentrations; dose decrease of tricyclics may be needed. Use with caution).
No products indexed under this heading.

Amlodipine Besylate (Co-administration of ritonavir and a drug primarily metabolized by CYP3A may result in a large increase in the AUC (>3x) of the other drug that could increase or prolong its therapeutic and adverse effects. Dose adjustment may be required). Products include:
Azor Tablets 1005
Exforge Tablets 2238

Amoxapine (Co-administration may result in increased tricyclic antidepressants' plasma concentrations; dose decrease of tricyclics may be needed. Use with caution).
No products indexed under this heading.

Amphetamine Aspartate (Co-administration of substrates of CYP2D6 with ritonavir could result in increases (up to 2x) in the AUC of the other agent that could increase or prolong its therapeutic and adverse effects. Dose adjustment may be required). Products include:
Adderall XR Capsules 3012

Amphetamine Aspartate Monohydrate (Co-administration of substrates of CYP2D6 with ritonavir could result in increases (up to 2x) in the AUC of the other agent that could increase or prolong its therapeutic and adverse effects. Dose adjustment may be required).
No products indexed under this heading.

Amphetamine Sulfate (Co-administration of substrates of CYP2D6 with ritonavir could result in increases (up to 2x) in the AUC of the other agent that could increase or prolong its therapeutic and adverse effects. Dose adjustment may be required). Products include:
Adderall XR Capsules 3012

Aprepitant (Potential for increase in the clearance of ritonavir resulting in decreased ritonavir plasma concentrations). Products include:
Emend Capsules 1992

Astemizole (Co-administration is contraindicated due to potential for serious and/or life-threatening reactions, such as cardiac arrhythmias).
No products indexed under this heading.

Atenolol (Co-administration with beta-blockers has resulted in cardiac and neurologic events).
No products indexed under this heading.

Atomoxetine Hydrochloride (Co-administration of substrates of CYP2D6 with ritonavir could result in increases (up to 2x) in the AUC of the other agent that could increase or prolong its therapeutic and adverse effects. Dose adjustment may be required). Products include:
Strattera Capsules 1864

Atorvastatin Calcium (Co-administration may result in increased plasma concentrations of atorvastatin calcium; the risk of myopathy, including rhabdomyolysis, may be increased. Dosage adjustment may be needed. Use with caution). Products include:
Lipitor Tablets 2501

Atovaquone (Co-administration may result in decreased atovaquone plasma concentrations; dose increase of atovaquone may be needed. Use with caution). Products include:
Malarone Pediatric Tablets 1521
Malarone Tablets 1521
Mepron Suspension 1526

Bepridil Hydrochloride (Co-administration is contraindicated due to potential for serious and/or life-threatening reactions, such as cardiac arrhythmias).
No products indexed under this heading.

Betaxolol Hydrochloride (Co-administration results in a possible increase in AUC of betaxolol; dosage adjustments may be required).
No products indexed under this heading.

Bisoprolol Fumarate (Co-administration with beta-blockers has resulted in cardiac and neurologic events).
No products indexed under this heading.

Bromocriptine Mesylate (Co-administration results in a large increase (> 3x) in AUC of bromocriptine; dosage adjustments may be required).
No products indexed under this heading.

Bupropion Hydrochloride (Co-administration may result in increased bupropion plasma concentrations; dose decrease of bupropion may be needed. Use with caution). Products include:
Wellbutrin Tablets 1648
Wellbutrin SR Sustained-Release Tablets 1653
Wellbutrin XL Extended-Release Tablets 1659
Zyban Sustained-Release Tablets 1692

Buspirone Hydrochloride (Co-administration may result in increased buspirone plasma concentrations; dose decrease of buspirone may be needed. Use with caution).
No products indexed under this heading.

Busulfan (Co-administration of ritonavir and a drug primarily metabolized by CYP3A may result in a large increase in the AUC (>3x) of the other drug that could increase or prolong its therapeutic and adverse effects. Dose adjustment may be required). Products include:
Busulfex Injection 2477
Myleran Tablets 1530

Captopril (Co-administration of substrates of CYP2D6 with ritonavir could result in increases (up to 2x) in the AUC of the other agent that could increase or prolong its therapeutic and adverse effects. Dose adjustment may be required). Products include:
Captopril Tablets 2182

Carbamazepine (Co-administration may result in increased carbamazepine plasma concentrations; dose decrease of carbamazepine may be needed. Use with caution). Products include:
Carbatrol Capsules 3019
Equetro Extended-Release Capsules 3174

Carteolol Hydrochloride (Co-administration with beta-blockers has resulted in cardiac and neurologic events).
No products indexed under this heading.

Carvedilol (Co-administration of substrates of CYP2D6 with ritonavir could result in increases (up to 2x) in the AUC of the other agent that could increase or prolong its therapeutic and adverse effects. Dose adjustment may be required). Products include:
Coreg Tablets 1387

Cerivastatin Sodium (Co-administration may result in increased plasma concentrations of cerivastatin; the risk of myopathy, including rhabdomyolysis, may be increased. Dosage adjustment may be needed. Use with caution).
No products indexed under this heading.

Cevimeline Hydrochloride (Co-administration of substrates of CYP2D6 with ritonavir could result in increases (up to 2x) in the AUC of the other agent that could increase or prolong its therapeutic and adverse effects. Dose adjustment may be required). Products include:
Evoxac Capsules 1013

Chloroquine Hydrochloride (Co-administration results in a possible increase in AUC of chloroquine; dosage adjustments may be required).
No products indexed under this heading.

Chloroquine Phosphate (Co-administration results in a possible increase in AUC of chloroquine; dosage adjustments may be required).
No products indexed under this heading.

Chlorpheniramine (Co-administration of ritonavir and a drug primarily metabolized by CYP3A may result in a large increase in the AUC (>3x) of the other drug that could increase or prolong its therapeutic and adverse effects. Dose adjustment may be required).
No products indexed under this heading.

Chlorpheniramine Maleate (Co-administration of ritonavir and a drug primarily metabolized by CYP3A may result in a large increase in the AUC (>3x) of the other drug that could increase or prolong its therapeutic and adverse effects. Dose adjustment may be required). Products include:
- Actifed Cold & Allergy Tablets 1895
- Sudafed PE Sinus & Allergy Tablets 1908
- Tylenol Allergy Multi-Symptom Caplets with Cool Burst and Rapid Release Gelcaps 1916
- Children's Tylenol Plus Cold Suspension Liquid 1912
- Children's Tylenol Plus Cough & Runny Nose Suspension Liquid 1912
- Children's Tylenol Plus Flu Suspension Liquid 1914
- Children's Tylenol Plus Multi-Symptom Cold Suspension Liquid 1912
- Tylenol Cold Head Congestion Nighttime Caplets with Cool Burst 1910
- Tylenol Cold Multi-Symptom Nighttime Caplets with Cool Burst 1913
- Tylenol Sinus Congestion & Pain Nighttime Caplets with Cool Burst 1917

Chlorpheniramine Polistirex (Co-administration of ritonavir and a drug primarily metabolized by CYP3A may result in a large increase in the AUC (>3x) of the other drug that could increase or prolong its therapeutic and adverse effects. Dose adjustment may be required). Products include:
- Tussionex Pennkinetic Extended-Release Suspension 3154

Chlorpheniramine Tannate (Co-administration of ritonavir and a drug primarily metabolized by CYP3A may result in a large increase in the AUC (>3x) of the other drug that could increase or prolong its therapeutic and adverse effects. Dose adjustment may be required).
No products indexed under this heading.

Chlorpromazine (Co-administration results in a moderate increase (1.5 to 3x) in AUC of chlorpromazine; dosage adjustments may be required).
No products indexed under this heading.

Chlorpromazine Hydrochloride (Co-administration results in a moderate increase (1.5 to 3x) in AUC of chlorpromazine; dosage adjustments may be required).
No products indexed under this heading.

Chlorpropamide (New onset diabetes mellitus, exacerbation of pre-existing diabetes, and hyperglycemia have been reported with protease inhibitors; dosage adjustment of oral hypoglycemic agents may be required).
No products indexed under this heading.

Cisapride (Co-administration is contraindicated due to potential for serious and/or life-threatening reactions, such as cardiac arrhythmias).
No products indexed under this heading.

Citalopram Hydrobromide (Co-administration may result in increased selective serotonin reuptake inhibitors' plasma concentrations; dose decrease of SSRIs may be needed. Use with caution). Products include:
- Celexa 1160

Clarithromycin (Co-administration may result in increased clarithromycin concentration; for patients with renal impairment, dosage adjustments should be considered). Products include:
- Biaxin/Biaxin XL 411

Clofibrate (Ritonavir may increase the activity of glucuronosyltransferase; co-administration results in a decrease in AUC of clofibrate; dosage adjustments may be required).
No products indexed under this heading.

Clomipramine Hydrochloride (Co-administration may result in increased tricyclic antidepressants' plasma concentrations; dose decrease of tricyclics may be needed. Use with caution).
No products indexed under this heading.

Clonazepam (Co-administration may result in increased clonazepam plasma concentrations; dose decrease of clonazepam may be needed. Use with caution). Products include:
- Klonopin 2639

Clorazepate Dipotassium (Co-administration may result in increased clorazepate plasma concentrations; dose decrease of clorazepate may be needed. Use with caution).
No products indexed under this heading.

Clozapine (Ritonavir is expected to produce a large increase in the plasma clozapine concentrations; clozapine has recognized risk to induce hematologic abnormalities; co-administration is contraindicated).
No products indexed under this heading.

Codeine Phosphate (Ritonavir may increase the activity of glucuronosyltransferase; co-administration results in possible decrease in AUC of codeine; possible need for dosage alterations of codeine). Products include:
- Tylenol with Codeine Tablets 2427

Codeine Sulfate (Co-administration of substrates of CYP2D6 with ritonavir could result in increases (up to 2x) in the AUC of the other agent that could increase or prolong its therapeutic and adverse effects. Dose adjustment may be required).
No products indexed under this heading.

Cyclobenzaprine Hydrochloride (Co-administration of substrates of CYP2D6 with ritonavir could result in increases (up to 2x) in the AUC of the other agent that could increase or prolong its therapeutic and adverse effects. Dose adjustment may be required). Products include:
- Amrix Capsules 966

Cyclophosphamide (An increase in the AUC of cyclophosphamide, activated by CYP, may correspond to a decrease in the AUC of the active metabolite(s) and a possible decrease in efficacy of cyclophosphamide).
No products indexed under this heading.

Cyclosporine (Co-administration may result in increased cyclosporine plasma concentrations; dose decrease of cyclosporine may be needed. Use with caution). Products include:
- Gengraf Capsules 435
- Neoral Oral Solution 2280
- Neoral Soft Gelatin Capsules 2280
- Restasis Ophthalmic Emulsion 557
- Sandimmune 2296

Daunorubicin Hydrochloride (Co-administration results in a possible increase in AUC of daunorubicin; dosage adjustments may be required).
No products indexed under this heading.

Desipramine Hydrochloride (Co-administration may lead to increased desipramine levels. Dosage reduction and concentration monitoring of desipramine is recommended).
No products indexed under this heading.

Desogestrel (Co-administration of ritonavir and a drug primarily metabolized by CYP3A may result in a large increase in the AUC (>3x) of the other drug that could increase or prolong its therapeutic and adverse effects. Dose adjustment may be required). Products include:
- Mircette Tablets 1034

Dexamethasone (Co-administration may result in increased dexamethasone plasma concentrations; dose decrease of dexamethasone may be needed. Use with caution). Products include:
- Ciprodex Otic Suspension 541

Dexamethasone Acetate (Co-administration may result in increased dexamethasone plasma concentrations; dose decrease of dexamethasone may be needed. Use with caution).
No products indexed under this heading.

Dexamethasone Phosphate (Co-administration of ritonavir and a drug primarily metabolized by CYP3A may result in a large increase in the AUC (>3x) of the other drug that could increase or prolong its therapeutic and adverse effects. Dose adjustment may be required).
No products indexed under this heading.

Dexamethasone Sodium (Co-administration of ritonavir and a drug primarily metabolized by CYP3A may result in a large increase in the AUC (>3x) of the other drug that could increase or prolong its therapeutic and adverse effects. Dose adjustment may be required).
No products indexed under this heading.

Dexamethasone Sodium Phosphate (Co-administration may result in increased dexamethasone plasma concentrations; dose decrease of dexamethasone may be needed. Use with caution).
No products indexed under this heading.

Dexfenfluramine Hydrochloride (Co-administration may lead to increased desipramine levels. Dosage reduction and concentration monitoring of desipramine is recommended).
No products indexed under this heading.

Dextromethorphan Hydrobromide (Co-administration of substrates of CYP2D6 with ritonavir could result in increases (up to 2x) in the AUC of the other agent that could increase or prolong its therapeutic and adverse effects. Dose adjustment may be required). Products include:
- PediaCare Children's Liquid Multi-Symptom Cold 1902
- PediaCare Children's Long-Acting Cough 1902
- Children's Sudafed PE Cold & Cough Liquid 1907
- Sudafed PE Cold & Cough Caplets 1907
- Children's Tylenol Plus Cough & Runny Nose Suspension Liquid 1912
- Children's Tylenol Plus Cough & Sore Throat Suspension Liquid 1912
- Children's Tylenol Plus Flu Suspension Liquid 1914
- Children's Tylenol Plus Multi-Symptom Cold Suspension Liquid 1912
- Tylenol Cold Severe Congestion Daytime Caplets with Cool Burst 1912
- Tylenol Cold Head Congestion Daytime Caplets with Cool Burst 1910
- Tylenol Cold Head Congestion Nighttime Caplets with Cool Burst 1910
- Tylenol Cold Head Congestion Severe Daytime Caplets with Cool Burst 1910
- Tylenol Cold Multi-Symptom Daytime Caplets with Cool Burst and Rapid Release Gels 1913
- Tylenol Cold Multi-Symptom Daytime Liquid with Citrus Burst 1913
- Tylenol Cold Multi-Symptom Nighttime Caplets with Cool Burst 1913
- Tylenol Cold Multi-Symptom Nighttime Liquid with Cool Burst 1913
- Tylenol Cold Multi-Symptom Severe Caplets with Cool Burst 1913
- Tylenol Cold Multi-Symptom Severe Daytime Liquid with Citrus Burst 1913
- Tylenol Cough & Sore Throat Daytime Liquid with Cool Burst 1918
- Tylenol Cough & Sore Throat Nighttime Liquid with Cool Burst 1918
- Vicks DayQuil Cold & Flu Multi-Symptom Relief .... ▣616
- Vicks DayQuil LiquiCaps 2567
- Vicks DayQuil Liquid 2567
- Vicks DayQuil Multi-Symptom Cold/Flu Relief 2567
- Vicks NyQuil Cold & Flu Multi-Symptom Relief .... ▣617
- Vicks NyQuil LiquiCaps 2567
- Vicks NyQuil Liquid 2567
- Vicks NyQuil Multi-Symptom Cold/Flu Relief 2567

Dextromethorphan Polistirex (Co-administration of substrates of CYP2D6 with ritonavir could result in increases (up to 2x) in the AUC of the other agent that could increase or prolong its therapeutic and adverse effects. Dose adjustment may be required).
No products indexed under this heading.

Diazepam (Co-administration may result in increased diazepam plasma concentrations; dose decrease of diazepam may be needed. Use with caution). Products include:
Valium Tablets ... 2658

Diclofenac Potassium (Co-administration results in a moderate (1.5 to 3x) increase or decrease in AUC of diclofenac).
No products indexed under this heading.

Diclofenac Sodium (Co-administration results in a moderate (1.5 to 3x) increase or decrease in AUC of diclofenac). Products include:
Diclofenac Sodium Ophthalmic Solution ... ⊙240
Voltaren Ophthalmic Solution ... 2336
Voltaren Tablets ... 2334
Voltaren-XR Tablets ... 2337

Didanosine (Dosing of these two drugs should be separated by 2.5 hours to avoid formulation incompatability).
No products indexed under this heading.

Digoxin (Co-administration may result in increased digoxin levels. Caution should be exercised when co-administering ritonavir with digoxin, with appropriate monitoring of serum digoxin levels). Products include:
Lanoxin Injection ... 1498
Lanoxin Injection Pediatric ... 1502
Lanoxin Tablets ... 1505

Dihydroergotamine Mesylate (Co-administration is contraindicated due to potential for serious and/or life-threatening reactions, such as acute ergot toxicity characterized by vasospasm and ischemia of the extremities and other tissues including the CNS).
No products indexed under this heading.

Diltiazem Hydrochloride (Co-administration may result in increased diltiazem plasma concentrations; dose decrease of diltiazem may be needed. Use with caution). Products include:
Cardizem LA Extended Release Tablets ... 421

Diltiazem Maleate (Co-administration of ritonavir and a drug primarily metabolized by CYP3A may result in a large increase in the AUC (>3x) of the other drug that could increase or prolong its therapeutic and adverse effects. Dose adjustment may be required).
No products indexed under this heading.

Diphenoxylate Hydrochloride (Ritonavir may increase the activity of glucuronosyltransferase; co-administration results in a decrease in AUC of diphenoxylate; dosage adjustments may be required).
No products indexed under this heading.

Disopyramide Phosphate (Co-administration may result in increased disopyramide plasma concentrations; cardiac and neurologic events have been reported with co-administration. Dosage adjustment may be needed. Use with caution).
No products indexed under this heading.

Disulfiram (Potential for disulfiram-like reactions due to the presence of ethanol in the ritonavir formulations).
No products indexed under this heading.

Divalproex Sodium (Co-administration may result in decreased valproate plasma concentrations; dose increase of valproate may be needed. Use with caution). Products include:
Depakote ER Tablets ... 423

Dolasetron Mesylate (Co-administration of substrates of CYP2D6 with ritonavir could result in increases (up to 2x) in the AUC of the other agent that could increase or prolong its therapeutic and adverse effects. Dose adjustment may be required). Products include:
Anzemet Injection ... 2701
Anzemet Tablets ... 2704

Donepezil Hydrochloride (Co-administration of substrates of CYP2D6 with ritonavir could result in increases (up to 2x) in the AUC of the other agent that could increase or prolong its therapeutic and adverse effects. Dose adjustment may be required). Products include:
Aricept Tablets ... 1062
Aricept ODT Tablets ... 1062

Doxazosin Mesylate (Co-administration results in a possible increase in AUC of doxazosin; dosage adjustments may be required).
No products indexed under this heading.

Doxepin Hydrochloride (Co-administration results in a possible increase in the AUC of doxepin; dosage adjustment of doxepin may be required).
No products indexed under this heading.

Doxorubicin Hydrochloride (Co-administration results in a possible increase in AUC of doxorubicin; dosage adjustments may be required).
No products indexed under this heading.

Dronabinol (Co-administration may result in increased dronabinol plasma concentrations; dose decrease of dronabinol may be needed. Use with caution). Products include:
Marinol Capsules ... 3163

Dyphylline (Co-administration results in the reduction of the average AUC of theophylline; increased dosage of theophylline may be required and therapeutic monitoring should be considered).
No products indexed under this heading.

Efavirenz (Potential for increase in the clearance of ritonavir resulting in decreased ritonavir plasma concentrations). Products include:
Atripla Tablets ... 938
Sustiva Capsules ... 930
Sustiva Tablets ... 930

Encainide Hydrochloride (Ritonavir is expected to produce a large increase in the plasma concentrations of encainide; concurrent use is contraindicated).
No products indexed under this heading.

Ergonovine Maleate (Co-administration may result in a possible increase in concentrations of ergonovine; in general, concurrent use with ergot alkaloid preparations is contraindicated).
No products indexed under this heading.

Ergotamine Tartrate (Co-administration is contraindicated due to potential for serious and/or life-threatening reactions, such as acute ergot toxicity characterized by vasospasm and ischemia of the extremities and other tissues including the CNS).
No products indexed under this heading.

Erythromycin (Co-administration results in a large increase (> 3x) in AUC of erythromycin; dosage adjustments may be required).
No products indexed under this heading.

Erythromycin Estolate (Co-administration results in a large increase (> 3x) in AUC of erythromycin; dosage adjustments may be required).
No products indexed under this heading.

Erythromycin Ethylsuccinate (Co-administration results in a large increase (> 3x) in AUC of erythromycin; dosage adjustments may be required). Products include:
E.E.S. ... 433
EryPed ... 431

Erythromycin Gluceptate (Co-administration results in a large increase (> 3x) in AUC of erythromycin; dosage adjustments may be required).
No products indexed under this heading.

Erythromycin Lactobionate (Co-administration results in a large increase (> 3x) in AUC of erythromycin; dosage adjustments may be required).
No products indexed under this heading.

Erythromycin Stearate (Co-administration results in a large increase (> 3x) in AUC of erythromycin; dosage adjustments may be required).
No products indexed under this heading.

Escitalopram Oxalate (Co-administration may result in increased selective serotonin reuptake inhibitors' plasma concentrations; dose decrease of SSRIs may be needed. Use with caution). Products include:
Lexapro Oral Suspension ... 1174
Lexapro Tablets ... 1174

Esmolol Hydrochloride (Co-administration with beta-blockers has resulted in cardiac and neurologic events).
No products indexed under this heading.

Estazolam (Co-administration may result in increased estazolam plasma concentrations; dose decrease of estazolam may be needed. Use with caution).
No products indexed under this heading.

Estrogen (Co-administration of ritonavir and a drug primarily metabolized by CYP3A may result in a large increase in the AUC (>3x) of the other drug that could increase or prolong its therapeutic and adverse effects. Dose adjustment may be required).
No products indexed under this heading.

Estrogens, Conjugated (Co-administration of ritonavir and a drug primarily metabolized by CYP3A may result in a large increase in the AUC (>3x) of the other drug that could increase or prolong its therapeutic and adverse effects. Dose adjustment may be required). Products include:
Premarin Intravenous ... 3217
Premarin Tablets ... 3221
Premarin Vaginal Cream ... 3228
Premphase Tablets ... 3232
Prempro Tablets ... 3232

Estrogens, Conjugated, Synthetic A (Co-administration of ritonavir and a drug primarily metabolized by CYP3A may result in a large increase in the AUC (>3x) of the other drug that could increase or prolong its therapeutic and adverse effects. Dose adjustment may be required).
No products indexed under this heading.

Estrogens, Esterified (Co-administration of ritonavir and a drug primarily metabolized by CYP3A may result in a large increase in the AUC (>3x) of the other drug that could increase or prolong its therapeutic and adverse effects. Dose adjustment may be required). Products include:
Estratest Tablets ... 3043
Estratest H.S. Tablets ... 3043

Ethinyl Estradiol (Co-administration may result in the reduction of ethinyl estradiol levels; dosage increase or alternate contraceptive measures should be considered). Products include:
Lybrel Tablets ... 3204
Mircette Tablets ... 1034
NuvaRing ... 2897
Ortho-Cyclen/Ortho Tri-Cyclen ... 2449
Ortho Evra Transdermal System ... 2437
Ortho Tri-Cyclen Lo Tablets ... 2458
Seasonique Tablets ... 1046
Yaz Tablets ... 805

Ethosuximide (Co-administration may result in increased ethosuximide plasma concentrations; dose decrease of ethosuximide may be needed. Use with caution).
No products indexed under this heading.

Ethynodiol Diacetate (Co-administration of ritonavir and a drug primarily metabolized by CYP3A may result in a large increase in the AUC (>3x) of the other drug that could increase or prolong its therapeutic and adverse effects. Dose adjustment may be required).
No products indexed under this heading.

Etoposide (Co-administration results in a large increase (> 3x) in AUC of etoposide; dosage adjustments may be required).
No products indexed under this heading.

Etoposide Phosphate (Co-administration of ritonavir and a drug primarily metabolized by CYP3A may result in a large increase in the AUC (>3x) of the other drug that could increase or prolong its therapeutic and adverse effects. Dose adjustment may be required).
No products indexed under this heading.

Felodipine (Co-administration of ritonavir and a drug primarily metabolized by CYP3A may result in a large increase in the AUC (>3x) of the other drug that could increase or prolong its therapeutic and adverse effects. Dose adjustment may be required).
No products indexed under this heading.

Fentanyl (Co-administration results in a large increase (> 3x) in AUC of fentanyl; dosage adjustments may be required). Products include:
Duragesic Transdermal System 2405
Ionsys Transdermal System 2410

Fentanyl Citrate (Co-administration results in a large increase (> 3x) in AUC of fentanyl; dosage adjustments may be required). Products include:
Actiq 959
Fentora Tablets 968

Flecainide Acetate (Co-administration is contraindicated due to potential for serious and/or life-threatening reactions, such as cardiac arrhythmias).
No products indexed under this heading.

Fluconazole (Co-administration has resulted in an increase in AUC and Cmax of ritonavir by 12% and 15%, respectively).
No products indexed under this heading.

Fluoxetine (Co-administration may result in increased selective serotonin reuptake inhibitors' plasma concentrations; dose decrease of SSRIs may be needed. Use with caution).
No products indexed under this heading.

Fluoxetine Hydrochloride (Cardiac and neurologic events have been reported when ritonavir has been co-administered with fluoxetine, Co-administration may result in increased selective serotonin reuptake inhibitors' plasma concentrations; dose decrease of SSRIs may be needed. Use with caution). Products include:
Prozac Weekly Capsules 1852
Prozac Pulvules and Liquid 1852
Symbyax Capsules 1871

Fluphenazine Decanoate (Co-administration of substrates of CYP2D6 with ritonavir could result in increases (up to 2x) in the AUC of the other agent that could increase or prolong its therapeutic and adverse effects. Dose adjustment may be required).
No products indexed under this heading.

Fluphenazine Enanthate (Co-administration of substrates of CYP2D6 with ritonavir could result in increases (up to 2x) in the AUC of the other agent that could increase or prolong its therapeutic and adverse effects. Dose adjustment may be required).
No products indexed under this heading.

Fluphenazine Hydrochloride (Co-administration of substrates of CYP2D6 with ritonavir could result in increases (up to 2x) in the AUC of the other agent that could increase or prolong its therapeutic and adverse effects. Dose adjustment may be required).
No products indexed under this heading.

Flurazepam Hydrochloride (Co-administration may result in increased flurazepam plasma concentrations; dose decrease of flurazepam may be needed. Use with caution).
No products indexed under this heading.

Flurbiprofen (Co-administration results in a moderate (1.5 to 3x) increase or decrease in AUC of flurbiprofen).
No products indexed under this heading.

Fluticasone Propionate (Co-administration increases plasma fluticasone proprionate exposures, resulting in significantly decreased serum cortisol concentrations and leading to systemic corticosteroid effects, including Cushing's syndrome and adrenal suppression). Products include:
Advair Diskus 100/50 1276
Advair Diskus 250/50 1276
Advair Diskus 500/50 1276
Advair HFA 45/21 Inhalation Aerosol.. 1288
Advair HFA 115/21 Inhalation Aerosol.. 1288
Advair HFA 230/21 Inhalation Aerosol.. 1288
Flonase Nasal Spray 1431
Flovent Diskus 50 mcg 1435

Fluvastatin Sodium (Co-administration results in a possible increase in AUC of fluvastatin; dosage adjustments may be required). Products include:
Lescol Capsules 2268
Lescol XL Tablets 2268

Fluvoxamine Maleate (Co-administration may result in increased selective serotonin reuptake inhibitors' plasma concentrations; dose decrease of SSRIs may be needed. Use with caution). Products include:
Luvox CR Extended-Release Capsules.................................... 1759

Formoterol Fumarate (Co-administration of substrates of CYP2D6 with ritonavir could result in increases (up to 2x) in the AUC of the other agent that could increase or prolong its therapeutic and adverse effects. Dose adjustment may be required). Products include:
Foradil Aerolizer 2849
Perforomist Inhalation Solution 1025

Fosphenytoin Sodium (Co-administration results in a moderate increase or decrease in AUC of phenytoin; dosage adjustments may be required; potential for increase in the clearance of ritonavir resulting in decreased ritonavir plasma concentrations).
No products indexed under this heading.

Galantamine Hydrobromide (Co-administration of substrates of CYP2D6 with ritonavir could result in increases (up to 2x) in the AUC of the other agent that could increase or prolong its therapeutic and adverse effects. Dose adjustment may be required).
No products indexed under this heading.

Gemfibrozil (Co-administration results in a possible increase in AUC of gemfibrozil; dosage adjustments may be required).
No products indexed under this heading.

Glimepiride (Co-administration results in a moderate increase or decrease in AUC of glimepiride; dosage adjustments may be required). Products include:
Avandaryl Tablets 1344
Duetact Tablets 3085

Glipizide (Co-administration results in a moderate increase or decrease in AUC of glipizide; dosage adjustments may be required).
No products indexed under this heading.

Glyburide (Co-administration results in a moderate increase or decrease in AUC of glyburide; dosage adjustments may be required).
No products indexed under this heading.

Haloperidol (Co-administration results in a moderate increase (1.5 to 3x) in AUC of haloperidol; dosage adjustments may be required).
No products indexed under this heading.

Haloperidol Decanoate (Co-administration results in a moderate increase (1.5 to 3x) in AUC of haloperidol; dosage adjustments may be required).
No products indexed under this heading.

Hydrocodone Bitartrate (Co-administration results in a moderate increase (1.5 to 3x) in AUC of hydrocodone; dosage adjustments may be required). Products include:
Lortab 5/500 Tablets 3143
Lortab 7.5/500 Tablets 3144
Lortab 10/500 Tablets 3144
Vicodin Tablets 529
Vicodin ES Tablets 530
Vicodin HP Tablets 531
Vicoprofen Tablets 533
Zydone Tablets 1132

Hydromorphone Hydrochloride (Ritonavir may increase the activity of glucuronosyltransferase; co-administration results in possible decrease in AUC of hydromorphone; possible need for dosage alterations of hydromorphone).
No products indexed under this heading.

Hypericum (May lead to loss of virologic response and possible resistance to ritonavir or to the class of protease inhibitors). Products include:
Satieté Tablets 640

Ibuprofen (Co-administration results in a moderate (1.5 to 3x) increase or decrease in AUC of ibuprofen). Products include:
Motrin IB Tablets and Caplets 1900
Children's Motrin Oral Suspension ... 1901
Children's Motrin Non-Staining Dye-Free Oral Suspension............. 1901
Children's Motrin Cold Oral Suspension 1899
Infants' Motrin Concentrated Drops.. 1901
Infants' Motrin Non-Staining Dye-Free Concentrated Drops....... 1901
Junior Strength Motrin Caplets and Chewable Tablets.................. 1901
Vicoprofen Tablets 533

Ifosfamide (An increase in the AUC of ifosfamide, activated by CYP, may correspond to a decrease in the AUC of the active metabolite(s) and a possible decrease in efficacy of ifosfamide).
No products indexed under this heading.

Imipramine Hydrochloride (Co-administration may result in increased tricyclic antidepressants' plasma concentrations; dose decrease of tricyclics may be needed. Use with caution).
No products indexed under this heading.

Imipramine Pamoate (Co-administration may result in increased tricyclic antidepressants' plasma concentrations; dose decrease of tricyclics may be needed. Use with caution).
No products indexed under this heading.

Indinavir Sulfate (When co-administered with reduced doses of indinavir, ritonavir increased indinavir concentration, decreased Cmax, and increased Cmin; appropriate doses for this combination with respect to efficacy and safety have not been established). Products include:
Crixivan Capsules 1979

Indomethacin (Co-administration results in a moderate (1.5 to 3x) increase or decrease in AUC of indomethacin). Products include:
Indocin 2024

Indoramin Hydrochloride (Co-administration of substrates of CYP2D6 with ritonavir could result in increases (up to 2x) in the AUC of the other agent that could increase or prolong its therapeutic and adverse effects. Dose adjustment may be required).
No products indexed under this heading.

Insulin (New onset diabetes mellitus, exacerbation of pre-existing diabetes, and hyperglycemia have been reported with protease inhibitors; dosage adjustment of insulin may be required).
No products indexed under this heading.

Insulin, Human, Zinc Suspension (New onset diabetes mellitus, exacerbation of pre-existing diabetes, and hyperglycemia have been reported with protease inhibitors; dosage adjustment of insulin may be required).
No products indexed under this heading.

Insulin, Human (rDNA origin) (New onset diabetes mellitus, exacerbation of pre-existing diabetes, and hyperglycemia have been reported with protease inhibitors; dosage adjustment of insulin may be required). Products include:
Exubera Inhalation Powder 2515

Insulin, Human NPH (New onset diabetes mellitus, exacerbation of pre-existing diabetes, and hyperglycemia have been reported with protease inhibitors; dosage adjustment of insulin may be required). Products include:
Humulin N Vial 1846

Insulin, Human Regular (New onset diabetes mellitus, exacerbation of pre-existing diabetes, and hyperglycemia have been reported with protease inhibitors; dosage adjustment of insulin may be required). Products include:
Humulin R 1849
Humulin R (U-500) 1850

Insulin, Human Regular and Human NPH Mixture (New onset diabetes mellitus, exacerbation of pre-existing diabetes, and hyperglycemia have been reported with protease inhibitors; dosage adjustment of insulin may be required). Products include:
Humulin 50/50, 100 Units 1843
Humulin 70/30 Vial 1844

Insulin, NPH (New onset diabetes mellitus, exacerbation of pre-existing diabetes, and hyperglycemia have been reported with protease inhibitors; dosage adjustment of insulin may be required).
No products indexed under this heading.

Insulin, Regular (New onset diabetes mellitus, exacerbation of pre-existing diabetes, and hyperglycemia have been reported with protease inhibitors; dosage adjustment of insulin may be required).
No products indexed under this heading.

Insulin, Regular and NPH mixture (New onset diabetes mellitus, exacerbation of pre-existing diabetes, and hyperglycemia have been reported with protease inhibitors; dosage adjustment of insulin may be required).
No products indexed under this heading.

Insulin, Zinc Crystals (New onset diabetes mellitus, exacerbation of pre-existing diabetes, and hyperglycemia have been reported with protease inhibitors; dosage adjustment of insulin may be required).
No products indexed under this heading.

Insulin, Zinc Suspension (New onset diabetes mellitus, exacerbation of pre-existing diabetes, and hyperglycemia have been reported with protease inhibitors; dosage adjustment of insulin may be required).
No products indexed under this heading.

Insulin Aspart (New onset diabetes mellitus, exacerbation of pre-existing diabetes, and hyperglycemia have been reported with protease inhibitors; dosage adjustment of insulin may be required).
No products indexed under this heading.

Insulin Aspart, Human (New onset diabetes mellitus, exacerbation of pre-existing diabetes, and hyperglycemia have been reported with protease inhibitors; dosage adjustment of insulin may be required). Products include:
NovoLog Mix 70/30 .... **2364**

Insulin Aspart, Human Regular (New onset diabetes mellitus, exacerbation of pre-existing diabetes, and hyperglycemia have been reported with protease inhibitors; dosage adjustment of insulin may be required). Products include:
NovoLog Injection **2359**

Insulin Aspart Protamine, Human (New onset diabetes mellitus, exacerbation of pre-existing diabetes, and hyperglycemia have been reported with protease inhibitors; dosage adjustment of insulin may be required). Products include:
NovoLog Mix 70/30 .... **2364**

Insulin Detemir (rDNA Origin) (New onset diabetes mellitus, exacerbation of pre-existing diabetes, and hyperglycemia have been reported with protease inhibitors; dosage adjustment of insulin may be required). Products include:
Levemir Injection **2352**

Insulin glargine (New onset diabetes mellitus, exacerbation of pre-existing diabetes, and hyperglycemia have been reported with protease inhibitors; dosage adjustment of insulin may be required). Products include:
Lantus Injection **2749**

Insulin Glulisine (New onset diabetes mellitus, exacerbation of pre-existing diabetes, and hyperglycemia have been reported with protease inhibitors; dosage adjustment of insulin may be required). Products include:
Apidra Injection **2706**

Insulin Lispro, Human (New onset diabetes mellitus, exacerbation of pre-existing diabetes, and hyperglycemia have been reported with protease inhibitors; dosage adjustment of insulin may be required). Products include:
Humalog-Pen and KwikPen **1829**
Humalog Mix 50/50-Pen and KwikPen **1833**
Humalog Mix 75/25-Pen and KwikPen **1835**

Insulin Lispro Protamine, Human (New onset diabetes mellitus, exacerbation of pre-existing diabetes, and hyperglycemia have been reported with protease inhibitors; dosage adjustment of insulin may be required). Products include:
Humalog Mix 50/50-Pen and KwikPen **1833**
Humalog Mix 75/25-Pen and KwikPen **1835**

Isradipine (Co-administration of ritonavir and a drug primarily metabolized by CYP3A may result in a large increase in the AUC (>3x) of the other drug that could increase or prolong its therapeutic and adverse effects. Dose adjustment may be required). Products include:
DynaCirc CR Controlled Release Tablets **1407**

Itraconazole (Co-administration may result in a possible increase in plasma concentrations of itraconazole; dosage adjustment may be required. Use with caution).
No products indexed under this heading.

Ketoconazole (Co-administration may result in increased ketoconazole concentration; high doses of ketoconazole (>200 mg/day) are not recommended). Products include:
Extina Foam, 2% **3057**
Nizoral A-D Shampoo **1901**

Ketoprofen (Ritonavir may increase the activity of glucuronosyltransferase; co-administration results in possible decrease in AUC of ketoprofen; possible need for dosage alterations of ketoprofen).
No products indexed under this heading.

Ketorolac Tromethamine (Ritonavir may increase the activity of glucuronosyltransferase; co-administration results in possible decrease in AUC of ketorolac; possible need for dosage alterations of ketorolac).
No products indexed under this heading.

Labetalol Hydrochloride (Co-administration with beta-blockers has resulted in cardiac and neurologic events).
No products indexed under this heading.

Lamotrigine (Co-administration may result in decreased lamotrigine plasma concentrations; dose increase of lamotrigine may be needed. Use with caution). Products include:
Lamictal **1488**

Lansoprazole (Co-administration results in a moderate increase or decrease in AUC of lansoprazole; dosage adjustments may be required).
No products indexed under this heading.

Levobunolol Hydrochloride (Co-administration with beta-blockers has resulted in cardiac and neurologic events).
No products indexed under this heading.

Levonorgestrel (Co-administration of ritonavir and a drug primarily metabolized by CYP3A may result in a large increase in the AUC (>3x) of the other drug that could increase or prolong its therapeutic and adverse effects. Dose adjustment may be required). Products include:
Climara Pro Transdermal System **768**
Lybrel Tablets **3204**
Mirena Intrauterine System **779**
Plan B Tablets **1044**
Seasonique Tablets **1046**

Lidocaine (Co-administration of ritonavir and a drug primarily metabolized by CYP3A may result in a large increase in the AUC (>3x) of the other drug that could increase or prolong its therapeutic and adverse effects. Dose adjustment may be required). Products include:
Lidoderm Patch **1114**

Lidocaine Hydrochloride (Co-administration may result in an increase in plasma concentrations of lidocaine; dosage adjustments may be required. Use with caution).
No products indexed under this heading.

Loperamide Hydrochloride (Co-administration results in a decrease in AUC of loperamide). Products include:
Imodium A-D Liquid, Caplets, and EZ Chews **1898**
Imodium Multi-Symptom Relief Caplets and Chewable Tablets...... **1899**

Loratadine (Ritonavir is expected to produce a large increase (> 3x) in the plasma concentrations of loratadine; dosage adjustments may be required).
No products indexed under this heading.

Lorazepam (Ritonavir may increase the activity of glucuronosyltransferase; co-administration results in a decrease in AUC of lorazepam; dosage adjustments may be required).
No products indexed under this heading.

Losartan Potassium (Co-administration results in a moderate increase or decrease in AUC of losartan; dosage adjustments may be required). Products include:
Cozaar Tablets **1973**

Lovastatin (Co-administration results in increased plasma concentrations of lovastatin; the risk of myopathy, including rhabdomyolysis, may be increased). Products include:
Advicor Tablets **402**
Mevacor Tablets **2063**

Maprotiline Hydrochloride (Co-administration may result in increased tricyclic antidepressants' plasma concentrations; dose decrease of tricyclics may be needed. Use with caution).
No products indexed under this heading.

Meperidine Hydrochloride (Co-administration results in decreased meperidine concentration and increased normeperidine concentration; dosage increase and long-term use of meperidine with ritonavir are not recommended due to the increased concentrations of the metabolite normeperidine which has both analgesic activity and CNS stimulant activity, such as seizures).
No products indexed under this heading.

Mestranol (Co-administration of ritonavir and a drug primarily metabolized by CYP3A may result in a large increase in the AUC (>3x) of the other drug that could increase or prolong its therapeutic and adverse effects. Dose adjustment may be required).
No products indexed under this heading.

Metformin Hydrochloride (New onset diabetes mellitus, exacerbation of pre-existing diabetes, and hyperglycemia have been reported with protease inhibitors; dosage adjustment of oral hypoglycemic agents may be required). Products include:
ActoPlus Met Tablets **3071**
Avandamet Tablets **1336**
Janumet Tablets **2041**
PrandiMet Tablets **2967**

Methadone Hydrochloride (Co-administration may result may result in decreased methadone concentration; dosage increase of methadone may be considered).
No products indexed under this heading.

Methamphetamine Hydrochloride (Co-administration may result in increased methamphetamine plasma concentrations; dose decrease of methamphetamine may be needed. Use with caution).
No products indexed under this heading.

Methylergonovine Maleate (Co-administration is contraindicated due to potential for serious and/or life-threatening reactions, such as acute ergot toxicity characterized by vasospasm and ischemia of the extremities and other tissues including the CNS).
No products indexed under this heading.

Methylphenidate Hydrochloride (Co-administration results in a possible increase in AUC of methylphenidate; dosage adjustments may be required). Products include:
Concerta Extended-Release Tablets **1925**
Metadate CD Capsules **3146**

Methysergide Maleate (Co-administration is contraindicated due to potential for serious and/or life-threatening reactions, such as acute ergot toxicity characterized by vasospasm and ischemia of the extremities and other tissues including the CNS).
No products indexed under this heading.

Metipranolol Hydrochloride (Co-administration with beta-blockers has resulted in cardiac and neurologic events).
No products indexed under this heading.

Metoclopramide Hydrochloride (Ritonavir may increase the activity of glucuronosyltransferase; co-administration results in a decrease in AUC of metoclopramide; dosage adjustments may be required).
No products indexed under this heading.

Metoprolol Succinate (Co-administration may result in increased metoprolol plasma concentrations; cardiac and neurologic events have been reported with co-administration. Dosage adjustment may be needed. Use with caution). Products include:
Toprol-XL Tablets 666

Metoprolol Tartrate (Co-administration may result in increased metoprolol plasma concentrations; cardiac and neurologic events have been reported with co-administration. Dosage adjustment may be needed. Use with caution).
No products indexed under this heading.

Metronidazole (Potential for disulfiram-like reactions due to the presence of ethanol in the ritonavir formulations). Products include:
Pylera Capsules 714

Metronidazole Hydrochloride (Potential for disulfiram-like reactions due to the presence of ethanol in the ritonavir formulations).
No products indexed under this heading.

Mexiletine Hydrochloride (Co-administration may result in increased mexiletine plasma concentrations; cardiac and neurologic events have been reported with co-administration. Dosage adjustment may be needed. Use with caution).
No products indexed under this heading.

Miconazole (Co-administration results in a possible increase in AUC of miconazole; dosage adjustments may be required).
No products indexed under this heading.

Miconazole Nitrate (Co-administration results in a possible increase in AUC of miconazole; dosage adjustments may be required).
No products indexed under this heading.

Midazolam Hydrochloride (Co-administration is contraindicated due to potential for prolonged or increased sedation and/or respiratory depression).
No products indexed under this heading.

Miglitol (New onset diabetes mellitus, exacerbation of pre-existing diabetes, and hyperglycemia have been reported with protease inhibitors; dosage adjustment of oral hypoglycemic agents may be required).
No products indexed under this heading.

Mirtazapine (Co-administration of substrates of CYP2D6 with ritonavir could result in increases (up to 2x) in the AUC of the other agent that could increase or prolong its therapeutic and adverse effects. Dose adjustment may be required). Products include:
Remeron Tablets 2924
RemeronSolTab Tablets 2927

Modafinil (Potential for increase in the clearance of ritonavir resulting in decreased ritonavir plasma concentrations). Products include:
Provigil Tablets 977

Morphine Sulfate (Ritonavir may increase the activity of glucuronosyltransferase; co-administration results in possible decrease in AUC of morphine; possible need for dosage alterations of morphine). Products include:
Avinza Capsules 1772
DepoDur Injection 1095
MS Contin Tablets 2585

Nadolol (Co-administration with beta-blockers has resulted in cardiac and neurologic events). Products include:
Nadolol Tablets 2191

Naproxen (Ritonavir may increase the activity of glucuronosyltransferase; co-administration results in possible decrease in AUC of naproxen; possible need for dosage alterations of naproxen). Products include:
EC-Naprosyn Delayed-Release Tablets 2632
Naprosyn Suspension 2632
Naprosyn Tablets 2632

Naproxen Sodium (Ritonavir may increase the activity of glucuronosyltransferase; co-administration results in possible decrease in AUC of naproxen; possible need for dosage alterations of naproxen). Products include:
Anaprox Tablets 2632
Anaprox DS Tablets 2632
Treximet Tablets 1616

Nateglinide (New onset diabetes mellitus, exacerbation of pre-existing diabetes, and hyperglycemia have been reported with protease inhibitors; dosage adjustment of oral hypoglycemic agents may be required). Products include:
Starlix Tablets 2314

Nebivolol (Co-administration with beta-blockers has resulted in cardiac and neurologic events). Products include:
Bystolic Tablets 1155

Nefazodone Hydrochloride (Co-administration may result in increased nefazodone plasma concentrations; cardiac and neurologic events have been reported with co-administration. Dosage adjustment may be needed. Use with caution).
No products indexed under this heading.

Nelfinavir Mesylate (Co-administration of ritonavir and a drug primarily metabolized by CYP3A may result in a large increase in the AUC (>3x) of the other drug that could increase or prolong its therapeutic and adverse effects. Dose adjustment may be required).
No products indexed under this heading.

Nevirapine (Co-administration may result in a possible increase in concentrations of nevirapine). Products include:
Viramune Oral Suspension 873
Viramune Tablets 873

Nicardipine (Co-administration of ritonavir and a drug primarily metabolized by CYP3A may result in a large increase in the AUC (>3x) of the other drug that could increase or prolong its therapeutic and adverse effects. Dose adjustment may be required).
No products indexed under this heading.

Nicardipine Hydrochloride (Co-administration of ritonavir and a drug primarily metabolized by CYP3A may result in a large increase in the AUC (>3x) of the other drug that could increase or prolong its therapeutic and adverse effects. Dose adjustment may be required). Products include:
Cardene I.V. 1093

Nifedipine (Co-administration may result in increased nifedipine plasma concentrations; dose decrease of nifedipine may be needed. Use with caution).
No products indexed under this heading.

Nimodipine (Co-administration of ritonavir and a drug primarily metabolized by CYP3A may result in a large increase in the AUC (>3x) of the other drug that could increase or prolong its therapeutic and adverse effects. Dose adjustment may be required). Products include:
Nimotop Capsules 790

Nisoldipine (Co-administration of ritonavir and a drug primarily metabolized by CYP3A may result in a large increase in the AUC (>3x) of the other drug that could increase or prolong its therapeutic and adverse effects. Dose adjustment may be required). Products include:
Sular Extended Release Tablets 2975

Nitrendipine (Co-administration results in a large increase (> 3x) in AUC of nitrendipine; dosage adjustments may be required).
No products indexed under this heading.

Norethindrone (Co-administration of ritonavir and a drug primarily metabolized by CYP3A may result in a large increase in the AUC (>3x) of the other drug that could increase or prolong its therapeutic and adverse effects. Dose adjustment may be required). Products include:
Ortho Micronor Tablets 2446

Norgestrel (Co-administration of ritonavir and a drug primarily metabolized by CYP3A may result in a large increase in the AUC (>3x) of the other drug that could increase or prolong its therapeutic and adverse effects. Dose adjustment may be required).
No products indexed under this heading.

Nortriptyline Hydrochloride (Co-administration may result in increased tricyclic antidepressants' plasma concentrations; dose decrease of tricyclics may be needed. Use with caution).
No products indexed under this heading.

Olanzapine (Co-administration of substrates of CYP2D6 with ritonavir could result in increases (up to 2x) in the AUC of the other agent that could increase or prolong its therapeutic and adverse effects. Dose adjustment may be required). Products include:
Symbyax Capsules 1871
Zyprexa Tablets 1883
Zyprexa IntraMuscular 1883
Zyprexa ZYDIS Orally Disintegrating Tablets 1883

Omeprazole (Co-administration results in a moderate increase or decrease in AUC of omeprazole; dosage adjustments may be required).
No products indexed under this heading.

Ondansetron (Co-administration of substrates of CYP2D6 with ritonavir could result in increases (up to 2x) in the AUC of the other agent that could increase or prolong its therapeutic and adverse effects. Dose adjustment may be required). Products include:
Zofran ODT Orally Disintegrating Tablets 1687

Ondansetron Hydrochloride (Co-administration results in a large increase (> 3x) in AUC of ondansetron; dosage adjustments may be required). Products include:
Zofran Injection 1682
Zofran 1687

Oxazepam (Ritonavir may increase the activity of glucuronosyltransferase; co-administration results in a decrease in AUC of oxazepam; dosage adjustments may be required).
No products indexed under this heading.

Oxycodone Hydrochloride (Co-administration results in a moderate increase (1.5 to 3x) in AUC of oxycodone; dosage adjustments may be required). Products include:
OxyContin Tablets 2589
OxyIR Capsules 2593
Percocet Tablets 1127
Percodan Tablets 1130

Paclitaxel (Co-administration results in a large increase (> 3x) in AUC of paclitaxel; dosage adjustments may be required).
No products indexed under this heading.

Paroxetine Hydrochloride (Co-administration results in a moderate increase (1.5 to 3x) in AUC of paroxetine; dosage adjustments may be required). Products include:
Paxil 1535
Paxil CR Controlled-Release Tablets 1544

Penbutolol Sulfate (Co-administration results in a possible increase in AUC of penbutolol; dosage adjustments may be required).
No products indexed under this heading.

Pentoxifylline (Co-administration results in a possible increase in AUC of pentoxifylline; dosage adjustments may be required).
No products indexed under this heading.

Perphenazine (Co-administration may result in increased perphenazine plasma concentrations; dose decrease of perphenazine may be needed).
No products indexed under this heading.

Phenobarbital (Co-administration results in a possible increase in AUC of phenobarbital; dosage adjustments may be required; potential for increase in the clearance of ritonavir resulting in decreased ritonavir plasma concentrations). Products include:
Donnatal Extentabs 2507

Phenytoin (Co-administration may result in decreased phenytoin plasma concentrations; dose increase of phenytoin may be needed. Use with caution).
No products indexed under this heading.

Phenytoin Sodium (Co-administration may result in decreased phenytoin plasma concentrations; dose increase of phenytoin may be needed. Use with caution). Products include:
Phenytek Capsules 2192

Pimozide (Co-administration is contraindicated due to potential for serious and/or life-threatening reactions, such as cardiac arrhythmias).
No products indexed under this heading.

Pindolol (Co-administration results in a possible increase in AUC of pindolol; dosage adjustments may be required).
No products indexed under this heading.

Pioglitazone Hydrochloride (New onset diabetes mellitus, exacerbation of pre-existing diabetes, and hyperglycemia have been reported with protease inhibitors; dosage adjustment of oral hypoglycemic agents may be required). Products include:
ActoPlus Met Tablets 3071
Actos Tablets 3077
Duetact Tablets 3085

Piroxicam (Ritonavir is expected to produce a large increase in the plasma concentrations of piroxicam; concurrent use is contraindicated).
No products indexed under this heading.

Pravastatin Sodium (Co-administration results in a large increase (> 3x) in AUC of pravastatin; dosage adjustments may be required).
No products indexed under this heading.

Prazosin Hydrochloride (Co-administration results in a possible increase in AUC of prazosin; dosage adjustments may be required).
No products indexed under this heading.

Prednisone (Co-administration may result in increased prednisone plasma concentrations; dose decrease of prednisone may be needed. Use with caution).
No products indexed under this heading.

Primaquine Phosphate (Co-administration results in a possible increase in AUC of primaquine; dosage adjustments may be required).
No products indexed under this heading.

Prochlorperazine (Co-administration results in a possible increase in AUC of prochlorperazine; dosage adjustments may be required).
No products indexed under this heading.

Proguanil (Co-administration results in a moderate increase or decrease in AUC of proguanil; dosage adjustments may be required).
No products indexed under this heading.

Promethazine Hydrochloride (Co-administration results in a possible increase in AUC of promethazine; dosage adjustments may be required).
No products indexed under this heading.

Propafenone Hydrochloride (Co-administration is contraindicated due to potential for serious and/or life-threatening reactions, such as cardiac arrhythmias). Products include:
Rythmol Tablets 1586
Rythmol SR Capsules 1590

Propofol (Ritonavir may increase the activity of glucuronosyltransferase; co-administration results in a decrease in AUC of propofol; dosage adjustments may be required).
No products indexed under this heading.

Propoxyphene Hydrochloride (Ritonavir may produce an increase in the plasma concentrations of propoxyphene. Dosage adjustment may be needed. Use with caution).
No products indexed under this heading.

Propoxyphene Napsylate (Ritonavir may produce an increase in the plasma concentrations of propoxyphene. Dosage adjustment may be needed. Use with caution).
No products indexed under this heading.

Propranolol Hydrochloride (Co-administration results in a moderate increase (1.5 to 3x) in AUC of propranolol; dosage adjustments may be required). Products include:
InnoPran XL Extended Release Capsules 1484

Protriptyline Hydrochloride (Co-administration may result in increased tricyclic antidepressants' plasma concentrations; dose decrease of tricyclics may be needed. Use with caution).
No products indexed under this heading.

Pyrimethamine (Co-administration results in a possible increase in AUC of pyrimethamine; dosage adjustments may be required). Products include:
Daraprim Tablets 1400
Fansidar Tablets 2636

Quetiapine Fumarate (Co-administration of substrates of CYP2D6 with ritonavir could result in increases (up to 2x) in the AUC of the other agent that could increase or prolong its therapeutic and adverse effects. Dose adjustment may be required).
No products indexed under this heading.

Quinidine (Co-administration is contraindicated due to potential for serious and/or life-threatening reactions, such as cardiac arrhythmias).
No products indexed under this heading.

Quinidine Gluconate (Co-administration is contraindicated due to potential for serious and/or life-threatening reactions, such as cardiac arrhythmias).
No products indexed under this heading.

Quinidine Hydrochloride (Co-administration is contraindicated due to potential for serious and/or life-threatening reactions, such as cardiac arrhythmias).
No products indexed under this heading.

Quinidine Polygalacturonate (Co-administration is contraindicated due to potential for serious and/or life-threatening reactions, such as cardiac arrhythmias).
No products indexed under this heading.

Quinidine Sulfate (Co-administration is contraindicated due to potential for serious and/or life-threatening reactions, such as cardiac arrhythmias).
No products indexed under this heading.

Quinine (Co-administration of ritonavir and a drug primarily metabolized by CYP3A may result in a large increase in the AUC (>3x) of the other drug that could increase or prolong its therapeutic and adverse effects. Dose adjustment may be required).
No products indexed under this heading.

Quinine Sulfate (Co-administration may result in increased quinine plasma concentrations; dose decrease of quinine may be needed. Use with caution).
No products indexed under this heading.

Rapamycin (Co-administration may result in increased rapamycin plasma concentrations; dose decrease of rapamycin may be needed. Use with caution).
No products indexed under this heading.

Repaglinide (New onset diabetes mellitus, exacerbation of pre-existing diabetes, and hyperglycemia have been reported with protease inhibitors; dosage adjustment of oral hypoglycemic agents may be required). Products include:
PrandiMet Tablets 2967
Prandin Tablets 2971

Rifabutin (Co-administration results in increased rifabutin and rifabutin metabolite concentration; dosage reduction of rifabutin by at least three-quarters of the usual dose of 300 mg/day is recommended).
No products indexed under this heading.

Rifampicin (Potential for increase in the clearance of ritonavir resulting in decreased ritonavir plasma concentrations).
No products indexed under this heading.

Rifampin (Co-administration has resulted in decreased ritonavir concentration leading to loss of virologic response. Consider alternate antimyobacterial agents).
No products indexed under this heading.

Rifapentine (Potential for increase in the clearance of ritonavir resulting in decreased ritonavir plasma concentrations).
No products indexed under this heading.

Risperidone (Co-administration may result in increased risperidone plasma concentrations; dose decrease of risperidone may be needed. Use with caution). Products include:
Risperdal Consta Long-Acting Injection 1753

Rosiglitazone Maleate (New onset diabetes mellitus, exacerbation of pre-existing diabetes, and hyperglycemia have been reported with protease inhibitors; dosage adjustment of oral hypoglycemic agents may be required). Products include:
Avandamet Tablets 1336
Avandaryl Tablets 1344
Avandia Tablets 1351

Rosuvastatin Calcium (Use the lowest possible dose of atrovastatin or rosuvastatin with careful monitoring or consider other HMG-CoA reductase inhibitors such as provastatin or fluvastatin in combination with Ritonavir. Potential for serious reactions such as risk of myopathyin rhabdomyolysis). Products include:
Crestor Tablets 677

Saquinavir (When co-administered with reduced doses of saquinavir and ritonavir increased saquinavir concentration, increased AUC, Cmax, and Cmin have resulted).
No products indexed under this heading.

Saquinavir Mesylate (When co-administered with reduced doses of saquinavir and ritonavir, increased saquinavir concentration, increased AUC, Cmax, and Cmin have resulted).
No products indexed under this heading.

Sertraline Hydrochloride (Co-administration results in a large increase (> 3x) in AUC of sertraline; dosage adjustments may be required).
No products indexed under this heading.

Sildenafil Citrate (Co-administration is expected to substantially increase PDE 5 inhibitor concentrations and may result in an increase in adverse events, including hypotension, syncope, visual changes, and prolonged erection).
No products indexed under this heading.

Simvastatin (Co-administration results in increased plasma concentrations of simvastatin; the risk of myopathy, including rhabdomyolysis, may be increased). Products include:
Simcor Tablets 502
Vytorin 10/10 Tablets 2149
Vytorin 10/10 Tablets 2939
Vytorin 10/20 Tablets 2149
Vytorin 10/20 Tablets 2939
Vytorin 10/40 Tablets 2149
Vytorin 10/40 Tablets 2939
Vytorin 10/80 Tablets 2149
Vytorin 10/80 Tablets 2939
Zocor Tablets 2136

Sirolimus (Co-administration may result in increased sirolimus plasma concentrations; dose decrease of sirolimus may be needed. Use with caution). Products include:
Rapamune 3260

Sitagliptin Phosphate (New onset diabetes mellitus, exacerbation of pre-existing diabetes, and hyperglycemia have been reported with protease inhibitors; dosage adjustment of oral hypoglycemic agents may be required). Products include:
Janumet Tablets 2041
Januvia Tablets 2048

Sotalol Hydrochloride (Co-administration with beta-blockers has resulted in cardiac and neurologic events).
No products indexed under this heading.

Sulfamethoxazole (Co-administration with a combination tablet containing sulfamethoxazole and trimethoprim has resulted in decreased AUC of sulfamethoxazole by 20% and no change in AUC).
No products indexed under this heading.

Tacrolimus (Co-administration may result in increased tacrolimus plasma concentrations; dose decrease of tacrolimus may be needed. Use with caution). Products include:
Prograf Capsules and Injection 622
Protopic Ointment 628

Tadalafil (Co-administration is expected to substantially increase PDE 5 inhibitor concentrations and may result in an increase in adverse events, including hypotension, syncope, visual changes, and prolonged erection). Products include:
Cialis Tablets 1792

Tamoxifen Citrate (Co-administration results in a large increase (> 3x) in AUC of tamoxifen; dosage adjustments may be required).
No products indexed under this heading.

Temazepam (Ritonavir may increase the activity of glucuronosyltransferase; co-administration results in a decrease in AUC of temazepam; dosage adjustments may be required).
No products indexed under this heading.

Teniposide (Co-administration of substrates of CYP2D6 with ritonavir could result in increases (up to 2x) in the AUC of the other agent that could increase or prolong its therapeutic and adverse effects. Dose adjustment may be required).
No products indexed under this heading.

Terazosin Hydrochloride (Co-administration results in a possible increase in AUC of terazosin; dosage adjustments may be required).
No products indexed under this heading.

Terfenadine (Co-administration is contraindicated due to potential for serious and/or life-threatening reactions, such as cardiac arrhythmias).
No products indexed under this heading.

Testosterone (Co-administration of ritonavir and a drug primarily metabolized by CYP3A may result in a large increase in the AUC (>3x) of the other drug that could increase or prolong its therapeutic and adverse effects. Dose adjustment may be required). Products include:
AndroGel 3159
Testim 1% Gel 701

Testosterone Cypionate (Co-administration of ritonavir and a drug primarily metabolized by CYP3A may result in a large increase in the AUC (>3x) of the other drug that could increase or prolong its therapeutic and adverse effects. Dose adjustment may be required).
No products indexed under this heading.

Testosterone Enanthate (Co-administration of ritonavir and a drug primarily metabolized by CYP3A may result in a large increase in the AUC (>3x) of the other drug that could increase or prolong its therapeutic and adverse effects. Dose adjustment may be required). Products include:
Delatestryl Injection 1730

Testosterone Propionate (Co-administration of ritonavir and a drug primarily metabolized by CYP3A may result in a large increase in the AUC (>3x) of the other drug that could increase or prolong its therapeutic and adverse effects. Dose adjustment may be required).
No products indexed under this heading.

Theophylline (Co-administration results in the reduction of the average AUC of theophylline; increased dosage of theophylline may be required and therapeutic monitoring should be considered).
No products indexed under this heading.

Theophylline Anhydrous (Co-administration results in the reduction of the average AUC of theophylline; increased dosage of theophylline may be required and therapeutic monitoring should be considered). Products include:
Uniphyl Tablets 2595

Theophylline Calcium Salicylate (Co-administration results in the reduction of the average AUC of theophylline; increased dosage of theophylline may be required and therapeutic monitoring should be considered).
No products indexed under this heading.

Theophylline Dihydroxypropyl (Glyceryl) (Co-administration results in the reduction of the average AUC of theophylline; increased dosage of theophylline may be required and therapeutic monitoring should be considered).
No products indexed under this heading.

Theophylline Ethylenediamine (Co-administration results in the reduction of the average AUC of theophylline; increased dosage of theophylline may be required and therapeutic monitoring should be considered).
No products indexed under this heading.

Theophylline Sodium Glycinate (Co-administration results in the reduction of the average AUC of theophylline; increased dosage of theophylline may be required and therapeutic monitoring should be considered).
No products indexed under this heading.

Thioridazine (Co-administration of substrates of CYP2D6 with ritonavir could result in increases (up to 2x) in the AUC of the other agent that could increase or prolong its therapeutic and adverse effects. Dose adjustment may be required).
No products indexed under this heading.

Thioridazine Hydrochloride (Co-administration may result in increased thioridazine plasma concentrations; dose decrease of thioridazine may be needed. Use with caution). Products include:
Thioridazine Hydrochloride Tablets 2195

Tiagabine Hydrochloride (Co-administration of ritonavir and a drug primarily metabolized by CYP3A may result in a large increase in the AUC (>3x) of the other drug that could increase or prolong its therapeutic and adverse effects. Dose adjustment may be required). Products include:
Gabitril Tablets 973

Timolol Hemihydrate (Co-administration may result in increased timolol plasma concentrations; cardiac and neurologic events have been reported with co-administration. Dosage adjustment may be needed. Use with caution). Products include:
Betimol Ophthalmic Solution 3181

Timolol Maleate (Co-administration may result in increased timolol plasma concentrations; dosage adjustment may be needed). Products include:
Combigan Ophthalmic Solution 553
Cosopt Sterile Ophthalmic Solution 1969
Timoptic Sterile Ophthalmic Solution 2121
Timoptic in Ocudose 2124
Timoptic-XE Sterile Ophthalmic Gel Forming Solution 2125

Tipranavir (Tipranavir co-administered with 200mg of ritonavir has been associated with reports of clinical hepatitis and hepatic decompensation including some fatalities. Extra vigilance is warranted in patients with chronic hepatitis B or hepatitis C co-infection). Products include:
Aptivus Capsules 823
Aptivus Oral Solution 823

Tocainide Hydrochloride (Co-administration results in a possible increase in AUC of tocainide; dosage adjustments may be required).
No products indexed under this heading.

Tolazamide (New onset diabetes mellitus, exacerbation of pre-existing diabetes, and hyperglycemia have been reported with protease inhibitors; dosage adjustment of oral hypoglycemic agents may be required).
No products indexed under this heading.

Tolbutamide (Co-administration results in a moderate increase or decrease in AUC of tolbutamide; dosage adjustments may be required).
No products indexed under this heading.

Tolterodine Tartrate (Co-administration of ritonavir and a drug primarily metabolized by CYP3A may result in a large increase in the AUC (>3x) of the other drug that could increase or prolong its therapeutic and adverse effects. Dose adjustment may be required).
No products indexed under this heading.

Tramadol Hydrochloride (Co-administration may result in an increase in AUC of tramadol; dosage adjustments may be required. Use with caution). Products include:
Ultram ER Extended-Release Tablets 2428

Trazodone Hydrochloride (Co-administration results in a large increase (> 3x) in AUC of trazodone; dosage adjustments may be required).
No products indexed under this heading.

Triazolam (Co-administration is contraindicated due to potential for prolonged or increased sedation and/or respiratory depression).
No products indexed under this heading.

Trimethoprim (Co-administration with a combination tablet containing sulfamethoxazole and trimethoprim has resulted in increased AUC of trimethoprim by 20% and no change in AUC of ritonavir).
No products indexed under this heading.

Trimipramine Maleate (Co-administration may result in increased tricyclic antidepressants' plasma concentrations; dose decrease of tricyclics may be needed. Use with caution).
No products indexed under this heading.

Troglitazone (New onset diabetes mellitus, exacerbation of pre-existing diabetes, and hyperglycemia have been reported with protease inhibitors; dosage adjustment of oral hypoglycemic agents may be required).
No products indexed under this heading.

Valproate Sodium (Co-administration may result in decreased valproate plasma concentrations; dose increase of valproate may be needed. Use with caution).
No products indexed under this heading.

Valproic Acid (Co-administration may result in decreased valproate plasma concentrations; dose increase of valproate may be needed. Use with caution).
No products indexed under this heading.

Vardenafil Hydrochloride (Co-administration is expected to substantially increase PDE 5 inhibitor concentrations and may result in an increase in adverse events, including hypotension, syncope, visual changes, and prolonged erection). Products include:
Levitra Tablets 2876

Venlafaxine Hydrochloride (Co-administration results in a moderate increase (1.5 to 3x) in AUC of venlafaxine; dosage adjustments may be required). Products include:
Effexor XR Extended-Release Capsules 3195
Venlafaxine Hydrochloride Tablets ... 2199

Verapamil Hydrochloride (Co-administration may result in increased verapamil plasma concentrations; dose decrease of verapamil may be needed. Use with caution). Products include:
Tarka Tablets 511

Vinblastine Sulfate (Co-administration results in a large increase (> 3x) in AUC of vinblastine; dosage adjustments may be required).
No products indexed under this heading.

Vincristine Sulfate (Co-administration results in a large increase (> 3x) in AUC of vincristine; dosage adjustments may be required).
No products indexed under this heading.

Voriconazole (Co-administration is contraindicated due to significant decreases in voriconazole plasma concentrations and may lead to loss of antifungal response).
No products indexed under this heading.

Warfarin Sodium (Co-administration may result in decreased warfarin plasma concentrations; initial frequent monitoring of the INR during ritonavir and nartarin co-administration is indicated).
No products indexed under this heading.

Zidovudine (Co-administration has resulted in decreased AUC and Cmax of zidovudine by 25% and 27%, respectively, and no change in ritonavir AUC and/or Cmax). Products include:
Combivir Tablets 1384
Retrovir 1574
Retrovir IV Infusion 1579
Trizivir Tablets 1622

Zolpidem Tartrate (Co-administration may result in increased zolpidem plasma concentrations; dose decrease of zolpidem may be needed. Use with caution). Products include:
Ambien Tablets 2692
Ambien CR Tablets 2696

Zonisamide (Co-administration of substrates of CYP2D6 with ritonavir could result in increases (up to 2x) in the AUC of the other agent that could increase or prolong its therapeutic and adverse effects. Dose adjustment may be required). Products include:
Zonegran Capsules 1089

Food Interactions

Meal, unspecified (Relative to fasting conditions, the extent of absorption of ritonavir from capsule formulation was 15% higher when administered with a meal; decreased peak ritonavir concentrations when oral solution was given under non-fasting condition).

NORWEGIAN COD LIVER OIL

(ALA (Alpha-Linolenic Acid), Cod Liver Oil, Docosahexaenoic Acid (DHA), Eicosapentaenoic Acid (EPA), Omega-3 Acids, Vitamin A, Vitamin D, Vitamin E) 949
None cited in PDR database.

NOSMO[KING] STOP SMOKING AID

(Herbals, Multiple) 630
None cited in PDR database.

NOVANTRONE FOR INJECTION CONCENTRATE

(Mitoxantrone Hydrochloride) 1100
None cited in PDR database.

NOVOLOG MIX 70/30

(Insulin Aspart, Human, Insulin Aspart Protamine, Human) 2364
May interact with ACE inhibitors, beta blockers, corticosteroids, diuretics, estrogens, fibrates, monoamine oxidase inhibitors, oral contraceptives, phenothiazines, progestins, sulfonamides, sympathomimetics, thyroid preparations, and certain other agents. Compounds in these categories include:

Acebutolol Hydrochloride (May potentiate or weaken the blood-glucose-lowering effect of insulin. The signs of hypoglycemia may be reduced or absent).
No products indexed under this heading.

Albuterol (Substances that may reduce the blood-glucose-lowering effect).
No products indexed under this heading.

Albuterol Sulfate (Substances that may reduce the blood-glucose-lowering effect). Products include:
Combivent Inhalation Aerosol 845
ProAir HFA Inhalation Aerosol 3113
Proventil HFA Inhalation Aerosol 2914
Ventolin HFA Inhalation Aerosol 1638

Amiloride Hydrochloride (Substances that may reduce the blood-glucose-lowering effect).
No products indexed under this heading.

Atenolol (May potentiate or weaken the blood-glucose-lowering effect of insulin. The signs of hypoglycemia may be reduced or absent).
No products indexed under this heading.

Benazepril Hydrochloride (Substances that may increase the blood-glucose-lowering effect and susceptibility to hypoglycemia).
No products indexed under this heading.

Bendroflumethiazide (Substances that may increase the blood-glucose-lowering effect and susceptibility to hypoglycemia).
No products indexed under this heading.

Betamethasone Acetate (Substances that may reduce the blood-glucose-lowering effect).
No products indexed under this heading.

Betamethasone Sodium Phosphate (Substances that may reduce the blood-glucose-lowering effect).
No products indexed under this heading.

Betaxolol Hydrochloride (May potentiate or weaken the blood-glucose-lowering effect of insulin. The signs of hypoglycemia may be reduced or absent).
No products indexed under this heading.

Bisoprolol Fumarate (May potentiate or weaken the blood-glucose-lowering effect of insulin. The signs of hypoglycemia may be reduced or absent).
No products indexed under this heading.

Budesonide (Substances that may reduce the blood-glucose-lowering effect). Products include:
Pulmicort Flexhaler 654
Symbicort 80/4.5 Inhalation Aerosol 659
Symbicort 160/4.5 Inhalation Aerosol 659

Bumetanide (Substances that may reduce the blood-glucose-lowering effect).
No products indexed under this heading.

Captopril (Substances that may increase the blood-glucose-lowering effect and susceptibility to hypoglycemia). Products include:
Captopril Tablets 2182

Carteolol Hydrochloride (May potentiate or weaken the blood-glucose-lowering effect of insulin. The signs of hypoglycemia may be reduced or absent).
No products indexed under this heading.

Chlorothiazide (Substances that may increase the blood-glucose-lowering effect and susceptibility to hypoglycemia).
No products indexed under this heading.

Chlorothiazide Sodium (Substances that may increase the blood-glucose-lowering effect and susceptibility to hypoglycemia). Products include:
Intravenous Sodium Diuril 2490

Chlorotrianisene (Substances that may reduce the blood-glucose-lowering effect).
No products indexed under this heading.

Chlorpromazine (Substances that may reduce the blood-glucose-lowering effect).
No products indexed under this heading.

Chlorpromazine Hydrochloride (Substances that may reduce the blood-glucose-lowering effect).
No products indexed under this heading.

Chlorpropamide (Substances that may increase the blood-glucose-lowering effect and susceptibility to hypoglycemia).
No products indexed under this heading.

Chlorthalidone (Substances that may reduce the blood-glucose-lowering effect). Products include:
Clorpres Tablets 2185

Ciclesonide (Substances that may reduce the blood-glucose-lowering effect). Products include:
Alvesco Inhalation Aerosol 2985
Omnaris Nasal Spray 2998

Clofibrate (Substances that may increase the blood-glucose-lowering effect and susceptibility to hypoglycemia).
No products indexed under this heading.

Clonidine Hydrochloride (May potentiate or weaken the blood-glucose-lowering effect of insulin. The signs of hypoglycemia may be reduced or absent). Products include:
Catapres Tablets 841
Clorpres Tablets 2185

Cortisone Acetate (Substances that may reduce the blood-glucose-lowering effect).
No products indexed under this heading.

Danazol (Substances that may reduce the blood-glucose-lowering effect).
No products indexed under this heading.

Desogestrel (Substances that may reduce the blood-glucose-lowering effect). Products include:
Mircette Tablets 1034

Dexamethasone (Substances that may reduce the blood-glucose-lowering effect). Products include:
Ciprodex Otic Suspension 541

Dexamethasone Acetate (Substances that may reduce the blood-glucose-lowering effect).
No products indexed under this heading.

Dexamethasone Sodium Phosphate (Substances that may reduce the blood-glucose-lowering effect).
No products indexed under this heading.

Dienestrol (Substances that may reduce the blood-glucose-lowering effect).
No products indexed under this heading.

Diethylstilbestrol (Substances that may reduce the blood-glucose-lowering effect).
No products indexed under this heading.

Disopyramide Phosphate (Substances that may increase the blood-glucose-lowering effect and susceptibility to hypoglycemia).
No products indexed under this heading.

Dobutamine Hydrochloride (Substances that may reduce the blood-glucose-lowering effect).
No products indexed under this heading.

Dopamine Hydrochloride (Substances that may reduce the blood-glucose-lowering effect).
No products indexed under this heading.

Enalapril Maleate (Substances that may increase the blood-glucose-lowering effect and susceptibility to hypoglycemia).
No products indexed under this heading.

Enalaprilat (Substances that may increase the blood-glucose-lowering effect and susceptibility to hypoglycemia).
No products indexed under this heading.

Ephedrine Hydrochloride (Substances that may reduce the blood-glucose-lowering effect).
No products indexed under this heading.

Ephedrine Sulfate (Substances that may reduce the blood-glucose-lowering effect).
No products indexed under this heading.

Ephedrine Tannate (Substances that may reduce the blood-glucose-lowering effect).
No products indexed under this heading.

Epinephrine (Substances that may reduce the blood-glucose-lowering effect). Products include:
EpiPen 1024

Epinephrine Bitartrate (Substances that may reduce the blood-glucose-lowering effect).
No products indexed under this heading.

Epinephrine Hydrochloride (Substances that may reduce the blood-glucose-lowering effect).
No products indexed under this heading.

Esmolol Hydrochloride (May potentiate or weaken the blood-glucose-lowering effect of insulin. The signs of hypoglycemia may be reduced or absent).
No products indexed under this heading.

IMPORTANT NOTE: Always consult each drug listing in the patient's regimen for possible interactions.

Estradiol (Substances that may reduce the blood-glucose-lowering effect). Products include:
Activella Tablets 2347
Angeliq Tablets 751
Climara Transdermal System 763
Climara Pro Transdermal System 768
Divigel 3167
Vagifem Tablets 2375

Estrogens, Conjugated (Substances that may reduce the blood-glucose-lowering effect). Products include:
Premarin Intravenous 3217
Premarin Tablets 3221
Premarin Vaginal Cream 3228
Premphase Tablets 3232
Prempro Tablets 3232

Estrogens, Esterified (Substances that may reduce the blood-glucose-lowering effect). Products include:
Estratest Tablets 3043
Estratest H.S. Tablets 3043

Estropipate (Substances that may reduce the blood-glucose-lowering effect).
No products indexed under this heading.

Ethacrynic Acid (Substances that may reduce the blood-glucose-lowering effect). Products include:
Edecrin Tablets 698

Ethinyl Estradiol (Substances that may reduce the blood-glucose-lowering effect). Products include:
Lybrel Tablets 3204
Mircette Tablets 1034
NuvaRing 2897
Ortho-Cyclen/Ortho Tri-Cyclen 2449
Ortho Evra Transdermal System 2437
Ortho Tri-Cyclen Lo Tablets 2458
Seasonique Tablets 1046
Yaz Tablets 805

Ethynodiol Diacetate (Substances that may reduce the blood-glucose-lowering effect).
No products indexed under this heading.

Fenofibrate (Substances that may increase the blood-glucose-lowering effect and susceptibility to hypoglycemia). Products include:
Fenoglide Tablets 2960
Tricor Tablets 520

Fludrocortisone Acetate (Substances that may reduce the blood-glucose-lowering effect).
No products indexed under this heading.

Flunisolide (Substances that may reduce the blood-glucose-lowering effect). Products include:
Aerobid/Aerobid-M 1153

Fluoxetine Hydrochloride (Substances that may increase the blood-glucose-lowering effect and susceptibility to hypoglycemia). Products include:
Prozac Weekly Capsules 1852
Prozac Pulvules and Liquid 1852
Symbyax Capsules 1871

Fluphenazine Decanoate (Substances that may reduce the blood-glucose-lowering effect).
No products indexed under this heading.

Fluphenazine Enanthate (Substances that may reduce the blood-glucose-lowering effect).
No products indexed under this heading.

Fluphenazine Hydrochloride (Substances that may reduce the blood-glucose-lowering effect).
No products indexed under this heading.

Fluticasone Propionate (Substances that may reduce the blood-glucose-lowering effect). Products include:
Advair Diskus 100/50 1276
Advair Diskus 250/50 1276
Advair Diskus 500/50 1276
Advair HFA 45/21 Inhalation Aerosol 1288
Advair HFA 115/21 Inhalation Aerosol 1288
Advair HFA 230/21 Inhalation Aerosol 1288
Flonase Nasal Spray 1431
Flovent Diskus 50 mcg 1435

Fluticasone Propionate HFA (Substances that may reduce the blood-glucose-lowering effect). Products include:
Flovent HFA 1440

Fosinopril Sodium (Substances that may increase the blood-glucose-lowering effect and susceptibility to hypoglycemia).
No products indexed under this heading.

Furosemide (Substances that may reduce the blood-glucose-lowering effect). Products include:
Furosemide Tablets 2186

Gemfibrozil (Substances that may increase the blood-glucose-lowering effect and susceptibility to hypoglycemia).
No products indexed under this heading.

Glipizide (Substances that may increase the blood-glucose-lowering effect and susceptibility to hypoglycemia).
No products indexed under this heading.

Glyburide (Substances that may increase the blood-glucose-lowering effect and susceptibility to hypoglycemia).
No products indexed under this heading.

Guanethidine Monosulfate (The signs of hypoglycemia may be reduced or absent when under the influence of guanethidine).
No products indexed under this heading.

Hydrochlorothiazide (Substances that may increase the blood-glucose-lowering effect and susceptibility to hypoglycemia). Products include:
Atacand HCT 642
Avalide Tablets 892
Avalide Tablets 2713
Benicar HCT Tablets 1010
Diovan HCT Tablets 2216
Dyazide Capsules 1405
Micardis HCT Tablets 854
Prinzide Tablets 2092
Tekturna HCT Tablets 2324
Teveten HCT Tablets 517

Hydrocortisone (Substances that may reduce the blood-glucose-lowering effect).
No products indexed under this heading.

Hydrocortisone Acetate (Substances that may reduce the blood-glucose-lowering effect). Products include:
Analpram-HC 1140
Pramosone 1141

Hydrocortisone Sodium Phosphate (Substances that may reduce the blood-glucose-lowering effect).
No products indexed under this heading.

Hydrocortisone Sodium Succinate (Substances that may reduce the blood-glucose-lowering effect).
No products indexed under this heading.

Hydroflumethiazide (Substances that may increase the blood-glucose-lowering effect and susceptibility to hypoglycemia).
No products indexed under this heading.

Indapamide (Substances that may reduce the blood-glucose-lowering effect). Products include:
Indapamide Tablets 2188

Isocarboxazid (Substances that may increase the blood-glucose-lowering effect and susceptibility to hypoglycemia). Products include:
Marplan Tablets 3177

Isoniazid (Substances that may reduce the blood-glucose-lowering effect).
No products indexed under this heading.

Isoproterenol Hydrochloride (Substances that may reduce the blood-glucose-lowering effect).
No products indexed under this heading.

Isoproterenol Sulfate (Substances that may reduce the blood-glucose-lowering effect).
No products indexed under this heading.

Labetalol Hydrochloride (May potentiate or weaken the blood-glucose-lowering effect of insulin. The signs of hypoglycemia may be reduced or absent).
No products indexed under this heading.

Levalbuterol Hydrochloride (Substances that may reduce the blood-glucose-lowering effect). Products include:
Xopenex Inhalation Solution 3001
Xopenex Inhalation Solution Concentrate 3005

Levobunolol Hydrochloride (May potentiate or weaken the blood-glucose-lowering effect of insulin. The signs of hypoglycemia may be reduced or absent).
No products indexed under this heading.

Levonorgestrel (Substances that may reduce the blood-glucose-lowering effect). Products include:
Climara Pro Transdermal System 768
Lybrel Tablets 3204
Mirena Intrauterine System 779
Plan B Tablets 1044
Seasonique Tablets 1046

Levothyroxine Sodium (Substances that may reduce the blood-glucose-lowering effect). Products include:
Levothroid Tablets 1170
Levoxyl Tablets 1780
Synthroid Tablets 507

Liothyronine Sodium (Substances that may reduce the blood-glucose-lowering effect). Products include:
Cytomel Tablets 1778

Liotrix (Substances that may reduce the blood-glucose-lowering effect).
No products indexed under this heading.

Lisinopril (Substances that may increase the blood-glucose-lowering effect and susceptibility to hypoglycemia). Products include:
Prinivil Tablets 2087
Prinzide Tablets 2092

Lithium Carbonate (May potentiate or weaken the blood-glucose-lowering effect of insulin).
No products indexed under this heading.

Lithium Citrate (May potentiate or weaken the blood-glucose-lowering effect of insulin).
No products indexed under this heading.

Medroxyprogesterone Acetate (Substances that may reduce the blood-glucose-lowering effect). Products include:
Premphase Tablets 3232
Prempro Tablets 3232

Megestrol Acetate (Substances that may reduce the blood-glucose-lowering effect). Products include:
Megace ES Oral Suspension 2499

Mesoridazine Besylate (Substances that may reduce the blood-glucose-lowering effect).
No products indexed under this heading.

Mestranol (Substances that may reduce the blood-glucose-lowering effect).
No products indexed under this heading.

Metaproterenol Sulfate (Substances that may reduce the blood-glucose-lowering effect).
No products indexed under this heading.

Metaraminol Bitartrate (Substances that may reduce the blood-glucose-lowering effect).
No products indexed under this heading.

Methotrimeprazine (Substances that may reduce the blood-glucose-lowering effect).
No products indexed under this heading.

Methoxamine Hydrochloride (Substances that may reduce the blood-glucose-lowering effect).
No products indexed under this heading.

Methyclothiazide (Substances that may increase the blood-glucose-lowering effect and susceptibility to hypoglycemia).
No products indexed under this heading.

Methylprednisolone Acetate (Substances that may reduce the blood-glucose-lowering effect).
No products indexed under this heading.

Methylprednisolone Sodium Succinate (Substances that may reduce the blood-glucose-lowering effect).
No products indexed under this heading.

Metipranolol Hydrochloride (May potentiate or weaken the blood-glucose-lowering effect of insulin. The signs of hypoglycemia may be reduced or absent).
No products indexed under this heading.

Metolazone (Substances that may reduce the blood-glucose-lowering effect).
No products indexed under this heading.

Metoprolol Succinate (May potentiate or weaken the blood-glucose-lowering effect of insulin. The signs of hypoglycemia may be reduced or absent). Products include:
Toprol-XL Tablets 666

Metoprolol Tartrate (May potentiate or weaken the blood-glucose-lowering effect of insulin. The signs of hypoglycemia may be reduced or absent).
No products indexed under this heading.

Moclobemide (Substances that may increase the blood-glucose-lowering effect and susceptibility to hypoglycemia).
No products indexed under this heading.

Moexipril Hydrochloride (Substances that may increase the blood-glucose-lowering effect and susceptibility to hypoglycemia).
No products indexed under this heading.

Mometasone Furoate (Substances that may reduce the blood-glucose-lowering effect). Products include:
Asmanex Twisthaler **2797**
Elocon Cream 0.1% **2840**
Elocon Lotion 0.1% **2841**
Elocon Ointment 0.1% **2842**

Mometasone Furoate Monohydrate (Substances that may reduce the blood-glucose-lowering effect). Products include:
Nasonex Nasal Spray **2883**

Nadolol (May potentiate or weaken the blood-glucose-lowering effect of insulin. The signs of hypoglycemia may be reduced or absent). Products include:
Nadolol Tablets **2191**

Nebivolol (May potentiate or weaken the blood-glucose-lowering effect of insulin. The signs of hypoglycemia may be reduced or absent). Products include:
Bystolic Tablets **1155**

Niacin (Substances that may reduce the blood-glucose-lowering effect). Products include:
Advicor Tablets **402**
Bausch & Lomb Ocuvite DF Vitamin Supplement .... ⊙**238**
Dismutax Dietary Supplement **995**
Niaspan Extended-Release Tablets **480**
NT-Kinase Dietary Supplement **995**
Simcor Tablets **502**

Norepinephrine Bitartrate (Substances that may reduce the blood-glucose-lowering effect).
No products indexed under this heading.

Norethindrone (Substances that may reduce the blood-glucose-lowering effect). Products include:
Ortho Micronor Tablets **2446**

Norethynodrel (Substances that may reduce the blood-glucose-lowering effect).
No products indexed under this heading.

Norgestimate (Substances that may reduce the blood-glucose-lowering effect). Products include:
Ortho-Cyclen/Ortho Tri-Cyclen **2449**
Ortho Tri-Cyclen Lo Tablets **2458**

Norgestrel (Substances that may reduce the blood-glucose-lowering effect).
No products indexed under this heading.

Octreotide Acetate (Substances that may increase the blood-glucose-lowering effect and susceptibility to hypoglycemia). Products include:
Sandostatin Injection **2300**
Sandostatin LAR Depot **2302**

Pargyline Hydrochloride (Substances that may increase the blood-glucose-lowering effect and susceptibility to hypoglycemia).
No products indexed under this heading.

Penbutolol Sulfate (May potentiate or weaken the blood-glucose-lowering effect of insulin. The signs of hypoglycemia may be reduced or absent).
No products indexed under this heading.

Pentamidine Isethionate (May cause hypoglycemia, which may sometimes be followed by hyperglycemia).
No products indexed under this heading.

Perindopril Erbumine (Substances that may increase the blood-glucose-lowering effect and susceptibility to hypoglycemia). Products include:
Aceon Tablets (2 mg, 4 mg, 8 mg) **3038**

Perphenazine (Substances that may reduce the blood-glucose-lowering effect).
No products indexed under this heading.

Phenelzine Sulfate (Substances that may increase the blood-glucose-lowering effect and susceptibility to hypoglycemia).
No products indexed under this heading.

Phenylephrine Bitartrate (Substances that may reduce the blood-glucose-lowering effect).
No products indexed under this heading.

Phenylephrine Hydrochloride (Substances that may reduce the blood-glucose-lowering effect). Products include:
Actifed Cold & Allergy Tablets **1895**
Benadryl Allergy & Cold Kapgels **1895**
Benadryl Allergy & Sinus Headache Kapgels **1895**
Benadryl Severe Allergy & Sinus Headache Caplets **1897**
Children's Benadryl-D Allergy & Sinus Liquid **1896**
Benadryl-D Allergy & Sinus Tablet **1896**
PediaCare Children's Allergy & Cold Liquid **1902**
PediaCare Children's Decongestant Liquid **1902**
PediaCare Children's Liquid Multi-Symptom Cold **1902**
Sinutab Non-Drying Caplets **1905**
Sinutab Sinus Caplets **1905**
Children's Sudafed PE Cold & Cough Liquid **1907**
Children's Sudafed PE Nasal Decongestant Liquid **1906**
Sudafed PE Cold & Cough Caplets **1907**
Sudafed PE Nasal Decongestant Tablets **1907**
Sudafed PE Nighttime Cold Caplets **1907**
Sudafed PE Non-Drying Sinus Caplets **1908**
Sudafed PE Severe Cold Caplets **1908**
Sudafed PE Sinus & Allergy Tablets **1908**
Sudafed PE Sinus Headache Caplets **1908**
Tylenol Allergy Multi-Symptom Caplets with Cool Burst and Rapid Release Gelcaps **1916**
Tylenol Allergy Multi-Symptom Nighttime Caplets with Cool Burst **1916**
Children's Tylenol Plus Cold Suspension Liquid **1912**
Children's Tylenol Plus Cold & Allergy Suspension Liquid **1914**
Children's Tylenol Plus Flu Suspension Liquid **1914**
Children's Tylenol Plus Multi-Symptom Cold Suspension Liquid **1912**
Tylenol Cold Head Congestion Daytime Caplets with Cool Burst **1910**
Tylenol Cold Head Congestion Nighttime Caplets with Cool Burst **1910**
Tylenol Cold Head Congestion Severe Daytime Caplets with Cool Burst **1910**
Tylenol Cold Multi-Symptom Daytime Caplets with Cool Burst and Rapid Release Gels **1913**
Tylenol Cold Multi-Symptom Daytime Liquid with Citrus Burst **1913**
Tylenol Cold Multi-Symptom Nighttime Caplets with Cool Burst **1913**
Tylenol Cold Multi-Symptom Nighttime Liquid with Cool Burst **1913**
Tylenol Cold Multi-Symptom Severe Caplets with Cool Burst **1913**
Tylenol Cold Multi-Symptom Severe Daytime Liquid with Citrus Burst **1913**
Tylenol Sinus Congestion & Pain Daytime Caplets with Cool Burst and Gelcaps **1917**
Tylenol Sinus Congestion & Pain Nighttime Caplets with Cool Burst **1917**
Tylenol Sinus Congestion & Pain Severe Caplets with Cool Burst **1917**
Vicks DayQuil Cold & Flu Multi-Symptom Relief .... ▣**616**
Vicks DayQuil LiquiCaps **2567**
Vicks DayQuil Liquid **2567**
Vicks DayQuil Multi-Symptom Cold/Flu Relief **2567**

Phenylephrine Tannate (Substances that may reduce the blood-glucose-lowering effect).
No products indexed under this heading.

Phenylpropanolamine Hydrochloride (Substances that may reduce the blood-glucose-lowering effect).
No products indexed under this heading.

Pindolol (May potentiate or weaken the blood-glucose-lowering effect of insulin. The signs of hypoglycemia may be reduced or absent).
No products indexed under this heading.

Pirbuterol Acetate (Substances that may reduce the blood-glucose-lowering effect). Products include:
Maxair Autohaler **1705**

Polyestradiol Phosphate (Substances that may reduce the blood-glucose-lowering effect).
No products indexed under this heading.

Polythiazide (Substances that may increase the blood-glucose-lowering effect and susceptibility to hypoglycemia).
No products indexed under this heading.

Prednisolone Acetate (Substances that may reduce the blood-glucose-lowering effect). Products include:
Pred Forte Ophthalmic Suspension .... ⊙**227**
Pred Mild Ophthalmic Suspension .... ⊙**230**
Pred-G Ophthalmic Ointment .... ⊙**229**
Pred-G Ophthalmic Suspension .... ⊙**228**

Prednisolone Sodium Phosphate (Substances that may reduce the blood-glucose-lowering effect).
No products indexed under this heading.

Prednisolone Tebutate (Substances that may reduce the blood-glucose-lowering effect).
No products indexed under this heading.

Prednisone (Substances that may reduce the blood-glucose-lowering effect).
No products indexed under this heading.

Procarbazine Hydrochloride (Substances that may increase the blood-glucose-lowering effect and susceptibility to hypoglycemia).
No products indexed under this heading.

Prochlorperazine (Substances that may reduce the blood-glucose-lowering effect).
No products indexed under this heading.

Promethazine Hydrochloride (Substances that may reduce the blood-glucose-lowering effect).
No products indexed under this heading.

Propoxyphene Hydrochloride (Substances that may increase the blood-glucose-lowering effect and susceptibility to hypoglycemia).
No products indexed under this heading.

Propoxyphene Napsylate (Substances that may increase the blood-glucose-lowering effect and susceptibility to hypoglycemia).
No products indexed under this heading.

Propranolol Hydrochloride (May potentiate or weaken the blood-glucose-lowering effect of insulin. The signs of hypoglycemia may be reduced or absent). Products include:
InnoPran XL Extended Release Capsules **1484**

Pseudoephedrine Hydrochloride (Substances that may reduce the blood-glucose-lowering effect). Products include:
Allegra-D 12 Hour Extended-Release Tablets **2687**
Allegra-D 24 Hour Extended-Release Tablets **2690**
Children's Motrin Cold Oral Suspension **1899**
Sudafed 12 Hour Nasal Decongestant Non-Drowsy Caplets **1909**
Sudafed 24 Hour Non-Drowsy Nasal Decongestant Tablets **1906**
Children's Sudafed Nasal Decongestant Liquid **1906**
Sudafed Nasal Decongestant Tablets **1906**
Tylenol Cold Severe Congestion Daytime Caplets with Cool Burst **1912**
Tylenol Sinus Severe Congestion Caplets with Cool Burst **1917**
Vicks NyQuil LiquiCaps **2567**
Vicks NyQuil Liquid **2567**
Vicks NyQuil Multi-Symptom Cold/Flu Relief **2567**
Zyrtec-D 12 Hour Extended Release Tablets **1923**
Zyrtec-D Allergy & Congestion Extended-Release Tablets **1923**

Pseudoephedrine Sulfate (Substances that may reduce the blood-glucose-lowering effect). Products include:
Clarinex-D 12-Hour Extended-Release Tablets **2831**
Clarinex-D 24-Hour Extended-Release Tablets **2834**

Quinapril Hydrochloride (Substances that may increase the blood-glucose-lowering effect and susceptibility to hypoglycemia).
No products indexed under this heading.

Quinestrol (Substances that may reduce the blood-glucose-lowering effect).
No products indexed under this heading.

Ramipril (Substances that may increase the blood-glucose-lowering effect and susceptibility to hypoglycemia).
No products indexed under this heading.

Rasagiline Mesylate (Substances that may increase the blood-glucose-lowering effect and susceptibility to hypoglycemia). Products include:
Azilect Tablets ... 3106

Reserpine (The signs of hypoglycemia may be reduced or absent when under the influence of reserpine).
No products indexed under this heading.

Salmeterol Xinafoate (Substances that may reduce the blood-glucose-lowering effect). Products include:
Advair Diskus 100/50 ... 1276
Advair Diskus 250/50 ... 1276
Advair Diskus 500/50 ... 1276
Advair HFA 45/21 Inhalation Aerosol ... 1288
Advair HFA 115/21 Inhalation Aerosol ... 1288
Advair HFA 230/21 Inhalation Aerosol ... 1288
Serevent Diskus ... 1594

Selegiline (Substances that may increase the blood-glucose-lowering effect and susceptibility to hypoglycemia). Products include:
Emsam Transdermal System ... 905

Selegiline Hydrochloride (Substances that may increase the blood-glucose-lowering effect and susceptibility to hypoglycemia). Products include:
Eldepryl Capsules ... 3052

Somatropin (Substances that may reduce the blood-glucose-lowering effect). Products include:
Genotropin Lyophilized Powder ... 2547
Humatrope Vials and Cartridges ... 1838
Nutropin for Injection ... 1208
Nutropin AQ Injection ... 1212
Nutropin AQ NuSpin Injection ... 1212
Nutropin AQ Pen ... 1212
Nutropin AQ Pen Cartridge ... 1212

Sotalol Hydrochloride (May potentiate or weaken the blood-glucose-lowering effect of insulin. The signs of hypoglycemia may be reduced or absent).
No products indexed under this heading.

Spirapril Hydrochloride (Substances that may increase the blood-glucose-lowering effect and susceptibility to hypoglycemia).
No products indexed under this heading.

Spironolactone (Substances that may reduce the blood-glucose-lowering effect).
No products indexed under this heading.

Sulfacytine (Substances that may increase the blood-glucose-lowering effect and susceptibility to hypoglycemia).
No products indexed under this heading.

Sulfamethizole (Substances that may increase the blood-glucose-lowering effect and susceptibility to hypoglycemia).
No products indexed under this heading.

Sulfamethoxazole (Substances that may increase the blood-glucose-lowering effect and susceptibility to hypoglycemia).
No products indexed under this heading.

Sulfasalazine (Substances that may increase the blood-glucose-lowering effect and susceptibility to hypoglycemia).
No products indexed under this heading.

Sulfinpyrazone (Substances that may increase the blood-glucose-lowering effect and susceptibility to hypoglycemia).
No products indexed under this heading.

Sulfisoxazole Acetyl (Substances that may increase the blood-glucose-lowering effect and susceptibility to hypoglycemia).
No products indexed under this heading.

Sulfisoxazole Diolamine (Substances that may increase the blood-glucose-lowering effect and susceptibility to hypoglycemia).
No products indexed under this heading.

Terbutaline Sulfate (Substances that may reduce the blood-glucose-lowering effect).
No products indexed under this heading.

Thioridazine Hydrochloride (Substances that may reduce the blood-glucose-lowering effect). Products include:
Thioridazine Hydrochloride Tablets ... 2195

Thyroglobulin (Substances that may reduce the blood-glucose-lowering effect).
No products indexed under this heading.

Thyroid (Substances that may reduce the blood-glucose-lowering effect). Products include:
Naturethroid Tablets ... 2605

Thyroxine (Substances that may reduce the blood-glucose-lowering effect).
No products indexed under this heading.

Thyroxine Sodium (Substances that may reduce the blood-glucose-lowering effect).
No products indexed under this heading.

Timolol Hemihydrate (May potentiate or weaken the blood-glucose-lowering effect of insulin. The signs of hypoglycemia may be reduced or absent). Products include:
Betimol Ophthalmic Solution ... 3181

Timolol Maleate (May potentiate or weaken the blood-glucose-lowering effect of insulin. The signs of hypoglycemia may be reduced or absent). Products include:
Combigan Ophthalmic Solution ... 553
Cosopt Sterile Ophthalmic Solution ... 1969
Timoptic Sterile Ophthalmic Solution ... 2121
Timoptic in Ocudose ... 2124
Timoptic-XE Sterile Ophthalmic Gel Forming Solution ... 2125

Tolazamide (Substances that may increase the blood-glucose-lowering effect and susceptibility to hypoglycemia).
No products indexed under this heading.

Tolbutamide (Substances that may increase the blood-glucose-lowering effect and susceptibility to hypoglycemia).
No products indexed under this heading.

Torsemide (Substances that may reduce the blood-glucose-lowering effect). Products include:
Demadex Injection ... 2630
Demadex Tablets ... 2630

Trandolapril (Substances that may increase the blood-glucose-lowering effect and susceptibility to hypoglycemia). Products include:
Mavik Tablets ... 472
Tarka Tablets ... 511

Tranylcypromine Sulfate (Substances that may increase the blood-glucose-lowering effect and susceptibility to hypoglycemia). Products include:
Parnate Tablets ... 1532

Triamcinolone (Substances that may reduce the blood-glucose-lowering effect).
No products indexed under this heading.

Triamcinolone Acetonide (Substances that may reduce the blood-glucose-lowering effect). Products include:
Azmacort Inhalation Aerosol ... 407
Nasacort AQ Nasal Spray ... 2765
Triesence Injectable Suspension ... ⊙209

Triamcinolone Diacetate (Substances that may reduce the blood-glucose-lowering effect).
No products indexed under this heading.

Triamcinolone Hexacetonide (Substances that may reduce the blood-glucose-lowering effect).
No products indexed under this heading.

Triamterene (Substances that may reduce the blood-glucose-lowering effect). Products include:
Dyazide Capsules ... 1405
Dyrenium Capsules ... 3189

Trifluoperazine Hydrochloride (Substances that may reduce the blood-glucose-lowering effect).
No products indexed under this heading.

NOVOLOG INJECTION

(Insulin Aspart, Human Regular) ... 2359
May interact with ACE inhibitors, beta blockers, corticosteroids, diuretics, fibrates, oral hypoglycemic agents, lithium preparations, monoamine oxidase inhibitors, oral contraceptives, phenothiazines, salicylates, sympathomimetics, thyroid preparations, and certain other agents. Compounds in these categories include:

Acarbose (May increase the blood-glucose-lowering effect and susceptibility to hypoglycemia). Products include:
Precose Tablets ... 792

Acebutolol Hydrochloride (Beta-blockers may either potentiate or weaken the blood-glucose-lowering effect of insulin; signs of hypoglycemia may be reduced or absent with co-administration).
No products indexed under this heading.

Albuterol (Sympathomimetic agents may reduce the blood-glucose-lowering effect of insulin).
No products indexed under this heading.

Albuterol Sulfate (Sympathomimetic agents may reduce the blood-glucose-lowering effect of insulin). Products include:
Combivent Inhalation Aerosol ... 845
ProAir HFA Inhalation Aerosol ... 3113
Proventil HFA Inhalation Aerosol ... 2914
Ventolin HFA Inhalation Aerosol ... 1638

Amiloride Hydrochloride (Diuretics may reduce the blood-glucose-lowering effect of insulin).
No products indexed under this heading.

Aspirin (May increase the blood-glucose-lowering effect and susceptibility to hypoglycemia). Products include:
Aggrenox Capsules ... 819
Bayer Aspirin ... 750
Percodan Tablets ... 1130
St. Joseph 81 mg Aspirin Chewable and Enteric Coated Tablets ... 1903

Aspirin, Enteric Coated (May increase the blood-glucose-lowering effect and susceptibility to hypoglycemia).
No products indexed under this heading.

Aspirin Buffered (May increase the blood-glucose-lowering effect and susceptibility to hypoglycemia).
No products indexed under this heading.

Atenolol (Beta-blockers may either potentiate or weaken the blood-glucose-lowering effect of insulin; signs of hypoglycemia may be reduced or absent with co-administration).
No products indexed under this heading.

Benazepril Hydrochloride (May increase the blood-glucose-lowering effect and susceptibility to hypoglycemia).
No products indexed under this heading.

Bendroflumethiazide (Diuretics may reduce the blood-glucose-lowering effect of insulin).
No products indexed under this heading.

Betamethasone Acetate (Co-administration with corticosteroids may reduce the blood-glucose-lowering effect of insulin).
No products indexed under this heading.

Betamethasone Sodium Phosphate (Co-administration with corticosteroids may reduce the blood-glucose-lowering effect of insulin).
No products indexed under this heading.

Betaxolol Hydrochloride (Beta-blockers may either potentiate or weaken the blood-glucose-lowering effect of insulin; signs of hypoglycemia may be reduced or absent with co-administration).
No products indexed under this heading.

Bisoprolol Fumarate (Beta-blockers may either potentiate or weaken the blood-glucose-lowering effect of insulin; signs of hypoglycemia may be reduced or absent with co-administration).
No products indexed under this heading.

Budesonide (Co-administration with corticosteroids may reduce the blood-glucose-lowering effect of insulin). Products include:
Pulmicort Flexhaler 654
Symbicort 80/4.5 Inhalation Aerosol.... 659
Symbicort 160/4.5 Inhalation Aerosol.... 659

Bumetanide (Diuretics may reduce the blood-glucose-lowering effect of insulin).
No products indexed under this heading.

Captopril (May increase the blood-glucose-lowering effect and susceptibility to hypoglycemia). Products include:
Captopril Tablets 2182

Carteolol Hydrochloride (Beta-blockers may either potentiate or weaken the blood-glucose-lowering effect of insulin; signs of hypoglycemia may be reduced or absent with co-administration).
No products indexed under this heading.

Chlorothiazide (Diuretics may reduce the blood-glucose-lowering effect of insulin).
No products indexed under this heading.

Chlorothiazide Sodium (Diuretics may reduce the blood-glucose-lowering effect of insulin). Products include:
Intravenous Sodium Diuril 2490

Chlorpromazine (Phenothiazine derivatives may reduce the blood-glucose-lowering effect of insulin).
No products indexed under this heading.

Chlorpromazine Hydrochloride (Phenothiazine derivatives may reduce the blood-glucose-lowering effect of insulin).
No products indexed under this heading.

Chlorpropamide (May increase the blood-glucose-lowering effect and susceptibility to hypoglycemia).
No products indexed under this heading.

Chlorthalidone (Diuretics may reduce the blood-glucose-lowering effect of insulin). Products include:
Clorpres Tablets 2185

Choline Magnesium Trisalicylate (May increase the blood-glucose-lowering effect and susceptibility to hypoglycemia).
No products indexed under this heading.

Ciclesonide (Co-administration with corticosteroids may reduce the blood-glucose-lowering effect of insulin). Products include:
Alvesco Inhalation Aerosol 2985
Omnaris Nasal Spray 2998

Clofibrate (May increase the blood-glucose-lowering effect and susceptibility to hypoglycemia).
No products indexed under this heading.

Clonidine (May either potentiate or weaken the blood glucose lowering effect of insulin). Products include:
Catapres-TTS 842

Clonidine Hydrochloride (May either potentiate or weaken the blood glucose lowering effect of insulin). Products include:
Catapres Tablets 841
Clorpres Tablets 2185

Cortisone Acetate (Co-administration with corticosteroids may reduce the blood-glucose-lowering effect of insulin).
No products indexed under this heading.

Danazol (May reduce the blood-glucose-lowering effect of insulin).
No products indexed under this heading.

Desogestrel (Oral contraceptives may reduce the blood-glucose-lowering effect of insulin). Products include:
Mircette Tablets 1034

Dexamethasone (Co-administration with corticosteroids may reduce the blood-glucose-lowering effect of insulin). Products include:
Ciprodex Otic Suspension 541

Dexamethasone Acetate (Co-administration with corticosteroids may reduce the blood-glucose-lowering effect of insulin).
No products indexed under this heading.

Dexamethasone Sodium Phosphate (Co-administration with corticosteroids may reduce the blood-glucose-lowering effect of insulin).
No products indexed under this heading.

Diflunisal (May increase the blood-glucose-lowering effect and susceptibility to hypoglycemia).
No products indexed under this heading.

Disopyramide Phosphate (May increase the blood-glucose-lowering effect and susceptibility to hypoglycemia).
No products indexed under this heading.

Dobutamine Hydrochloride (Sympathomimetic agents may reduce the blood-glucose-lowering effect of insulin).
No products indexed under this heading.

Dopamine Hydrochloride (Sympathomimetic agents may reduce the blood-glucose-lowering effect of insulin).
No products indexed under this heading.

Enalapril Maleate (May increase the blood-glucose-lowering effect and susceptibility to hypoglycemia).
No products indexed under this heading.

Enalaprilat (May increase the blood-glucose-lowering effect and susceptibility to hypoglycemia).
No products indexed under this heading.

Ephedrine Hydrochloride (Sympathomimetic agents may reduce the blood-glucose-lowering effect of insulin).
No products indexed under this heading.

Ephedrine Sulfate (Sympathomimetic agents may reduce the blood-glucose-lowering effect of insulin).
No products indexed under this heading.

Ephedrine Tannate (Sympathomimetic agents may reduce the blood-glucose-lowering effect of insulin).
No products indexed under this heading.

Epinephrine (Sympathomimetic agents may reduce the blood-glucose-lowering effect of insulin). Products include:
EpiPen 1024

Epinephrine Bitartrate (Sympathomimetic agents may reduce the blood-glucose-lowering effect of insulin).
No products indexed under this heading.

Epinephrine Hydrochloride (Sympathomimetic agents may reduce the blood-glucose-lowering effect of insulin).
No products indexed under this heading.

Esmolol Hydrochloride (Beta-blockers may either potentiate or weaken the blood-glucose-lowering effect of insulin; signs of hypoglycemia may be reduced or absent with co-administration).
No products indexed under this heading.

Estradiol (May reduce the blood glucose lowering effect). Products include:
Activella Tablets 2347
Angeliq Tablets 751
Climara Transdermal System 763
Climara Pro Transdermal System 768
Divigel 3167
Vagifem Tablets 2375

Estradiol Acetate (May reduce the blood glucose lowering effect).
No products indexed under this heading.

Estradiol Benzoate (May reduce the blood glucose lowering effect).
No products indexed under this heading.

Estradiol Cypionate (May reduce the blood glucose lowering effect).
No products indexed under this heading.

Estradiol Valerate (May reduce the blood glucose lowering effect).
No products indexed under this heading.

Estrogen (May reduce the blood glucose lowering effect).
No products indexed under this heading.

Estrogens, Conjugated (May reduce the blood glucose lowering effect). Products include:
Premarin Intravenous 3217
Premarin Tablets 3221
Premarin Vaginal Cream 3228
Premphase Tablets 3232
Prempro Tablets 3232

Estrogens, Conjugated, Synthetic A (May reduce the blood glucose lowering effect).
No products indexed under this heading.

Estrogens, Conjugated, Synthetic B (May reduce the blood glucose lowering effect). Products include:
Enjuvia Tablets 1029

Estrogens, Esterified (May reduce the blood glucose lowering effect). Products include:
Estratest Tablets 3043
Estratest H.S. Tablets 3043

Estrone (May reduce the blood glucose lowering effect).
No products indexed under this heading.

Ethacrynic Acid (Diuretics may reduce the blood-glucose-lowering effect of insulin). Products include:
Edecrin Tablets 698

Ethinyl Estradiol (Oral contraceptives may reduce the blood-glucose-lowering effect of insulin). Products include:
Lybrel Tablets 3204
Mircette Tablets 1034
NuvaRing 2897
Ortho-Cyclen/Ortho Tri-Cyclen 2449
Ortho Evra Transdermal System 2437
Ortho Tri-Cyclen Lo Tablets 2458
Seasonique Tablets 1046
Yaz Tablets 805

Ethynodiol Diacetate (Oral contraceptives may reduce the blood-glucose-lowering effect of insulin).
No products indexed under this heading.

Fenofibrate (May increase the blood-glucose-lowering effect and susceptibility to hypoglycemia). Products include:
Fenoglide Tablets 2960
Tricor Tablets 520

Fludrocortisone Acetate (Co-administration with corticosteroids may reduce the blood-glucose-lowering effect of insulin).
No products indexed under this heading.

Flunisolide (Co-administration with corticosteroids may reduce the blood-glucose-lowering effect of insulin). Products include:
Aerobid/Aerobid-M 1153

Fluoxetine Hydrochloride (May increase the blood-glucose-lowering effect and susceptibility to hypoglycemia). Products include:
Prozac Weekly Capsules 1852
Prozac Pulvules and Liquid 1852
Symbyax Capsules 1871

Fluphenazine Decanoate (Phenothiazine derivatives may reduce the blood-glucose-lowering effect of insulin).
No products indexed under this heading.

Fluphenazine Enanthate (Phenothiazine derivatives may reduce the blood-glucose-lowering effect of insulin).
No products indexed under this heading.

Fluphenazine Hydrochloride (Phenothiazine derivatives may reduce the blood-glucose-lowering effect of insulin).
No products indexed under this heading.

Fluticasone Propionate (Co-administration with corticosteroids may reduce the blood-glucose-lowering effect of insulin). Products include:
Advair Diskus 100/50 1276
Advair Diskus 250/50 1276
Advair Diskus 500/50 1276
Advair HFA 45/21 Inhalation Aerosol.... 1288
Advair HFA 115/21 Inhalation Aerosol.... 1288
Advair HFA 230/21 Inhalation Aerosol.... 1288
Flonase Nasal Spray 1431
Flovent Diskus 50 mcg 1435

Fluticasone Propionate HFA (Co-administration with corticosteroids may reduce the blood-glucose-lowering effect of insulin). Products include:
Flovent HFA 1440

Fosinopril Sodium (May increase the blood-glucose-lowering effect and susceptibility to hypoglycemia).
No products indexed under this heading.

Furosemide (Diuretics may reduce the blood-glucose-lowering effect of insulin). Products include:
Furosemide Tablets 2186

IMPORTANT NOTE: Always consult each drug listing in the patient's regimen for possible interactions.

Gemfibrozil (May increase the blood-glucose-lowering effect and susceptibility to hypoglycemia).
No products indexed under this heading.

Glimepiride (May increase the blood-glucose-lowering effect and susceptibility to hypoglycemia). Products include:
Avandaryl Tablets ... 1344
Duetact Tablets ... 3085

Glipizide (May increase the blood-glucose-lowering effect and susceptibility to hypoglycemia).
No products indexed under this heading.

Glyburide (May increase the blood-glucose-lowering effect and susceptibility to hypoglycemia).
No products indexed under this heading.

Guanethidine Monosulfate (Signs of hypoglycemia may be reduced or absent with co-administration).
No products indexed under this heading.

Hydrochlorothiazide (Diuretics may reduce the blood-glucose-lowering effect of insulin). Products include:
Atacand HCT ... 642
Avalide Tablets ... 892
Avalide Tablets ... 2713
Benicar HCT Tablets ... 1010
Diovan HCT Tablets ... 2216
Dyazide Capsules ... 1405
Micardis HCT Tablets ... 854
Prinzide Tablets ... 2092
Tekturna HCT Tablets ... 2324
Teveten HCT Tablets ... 517

Hydrocortisone (Co-administration with corticosteroids may reduce the blood-glucose-lowering effect of insulin).
No products indexed under this heading.

Hydrocortisone Acetate (Co-administration with corticosteroids may reduce the blood-glucose-lowering effect of insulin). Products include:
Analpram-HC ... 1140
Pramosone ... 1141

Hydrocortisone Sodium Phosphate (Co-administration with corticosteroids may reduce the blood-glucose-lowering effect of insulin).
No products indexed under this heading.

Hydrocortisone Sodium Succinate (Co-administration with corticosteroids may reduce the blood-glucose-lowering effect of insulin).
No products indexed under this heading.

Hydroflumethiazide (Diuretics may reduce the blood-glucose-lowering effect of insulin).
No products indexed under this heading.

Indapamide (Diuretics may reduce the blood-glucose-lowering effect of insulin). Products include:
Indapamide Tablets ... 2188

Isocarboxazid (May increase the blood-glucose-lowering effect and susceptibility to hypoglycemia). Products include:
Marplan Tablets ... 3177

Isoniazid (May reduce the blood-glucose-lowering effect of insulin).
No products indexed under this heading.

Isoproterenol Hydrochloride (Sympathomimetic agents may reduce the blood-glucose-lowering effect of insulin).
No products indexed under this heading.

Isoproterenol Sulfate (Sympathomimetic agents may reduce the blood-glucose-lowering effect of insulin).
No products indexed under this heading.

Labetalol Hydrochloride (Beta-blockers may either potentiate or weaken the blood-glucose-lowering effect of insulin; signs of hypoglycemia may be reduced or absent with co-administration).
No products indexed under this heading.

Levalbuterol Hydrochloride (Sympathomimetic agents may reduce the blood-glucose-lowering effect of insulin). Products include:
Xopenex Inhalation Solution ... 3001
Xopenex Inhalation Solution Concentrate ... 3005

Levobunolol Hydrochloride (Beta-blockers may either potentiate or weaken the blood-glucose-lowering effect of insulin; signs of hypoglycemia may be reduced or absent with co-administration).
No products indexed under this heading.

Levonorgestrel (Oral contraceptives may reduce the blood-glucose-lowering effect of insulin). Products include:
Climara Pro Transdermal System ... 768
Lybrel Tablets ... 3204
Mirena Intrauterine System ... 779
Plan B Tablets ... 1044
Seasonique Tablets ... 1046

Levothyroxine Sodium (May reduce the blood-glucose-lowering effect of insulin). Products include:
Levothroid Tablets ... 1170
Levoxyl Tablets ... 1780
Synthroid Tablets ... 507

Liothyronine Sodium (May reduce the blood-glucose-lowering effect of insulin). Products include:
Cytomel Tablets ... 1778

Liotrix (May reduce the blood-glucose-lowering effect of insulin).
No products indexed under this heading.

Lisinopril (May increase the blood-glucose-lowering effect and susceptibility to hypoglycemia). Products include:
Prinivil Tablets ... 2087
Prinzide Tablets ... 2092

Lithium (May either potentiate or weaken the blood-glucose-lowering effect of insulin).
No products indexed under this heading.

Lithium Carbonate (May either potentiate or weaken the blood-glucose-lowering effect of insulin).
No products indexed under this heading.

Lithium Citrate (May either potentiate or weaken the blood-glucose-lowering effect of insulin).
No products indexed under this heading.

Magnesium Salicylate (May increase the blood-glucose-lowering effect and susceptibility to hypoglycemia).
No products indexed under this heading.

Mesoridazine Besylate (Phenothiazine derivatives may reduce the blood-glucose-lowering effect of insulin).
No products indexed under this heading.

Mestranol (Oral contraceptives may reduce the blood-glucose-lowering effect of insulin).
No products indexed under this heading.

Metaproterenol Sulfate (Sympathomimetic agents may reduce the blood-glucose-lowering effect of insulin).
No products indexed under this heading.

Metaraminol Bitartrate (Sympathomimetic agents may reduce the blood-glucose-lowering effect of insulin).
No products indexed under this heading.

Metformin Hydrochloride (May increase the blood-glucose-lowering effect and susceptibility to hypoglycemia). Products include:
ActoPlus Met Tablets ... 3071
Avandamet Tablets ... 1336
Janumet Tablets ... 2041
PrandiMet Tablets ... 2967

Methotrimeprazine (Phenothiazine derivatives may reduce the blood-glucose-lowering effect of insulin).
No products indexed under this heading.

Methoxamine Hydrochloride (Sympathomimetic agents may reduce the blood-glucose-lowering effect of insulin).
No products indexed under this heading.

Methyclothiazide (Diuretics may reduce the blood-glucose-lowering effect of insulin).
No products indexed under this heading.

Methylprednisolone Acetate (Co-administration with corticosteroids may reduce the blood-glucose-lowering effect of insulin).
No products indexed under this heading.

Methylprednisolone Sodium Succinate (Co-administration with corticosteroids may reduce the blood-glucose-lowering effect of insulin).
No products indexed under this heading.

Metipranolol Hydrochloride (Beta-blockers may either potentiate or weaken the blood-glucose-lowering effect of insulin; signs of hypoglycemia may be reduced or absent with co-administration).
No products indexed under this heading.

Metolazone (Diuretics may reduce the blood-glucose-lowering effect of insulin).
No products indexed under this heading.

Metoprolol Succinate (Beta-blockers may either potentiate or weaken the blood-glucose-lowering effect of insulin; signs of hypoglycemia may be reduced or absent with co-administration). Products include:
Toprol-XL Tablets ... 666

Metoprolol Tartrate (Beta-blockers may either potentiate or weaken the blood-glucose-lowering effect of insulin; signs of hypoglycemia may be reduced or absent with co-administration).
No products indexed under this heading.

Miglitol (May increase the blood-glucose-lowering effect and susceptibility to hypoglycemia).
No products indexed under this heading.

Moclobemide (May increase the blood-glucose-lowering effect and susceptibility to hypoglycemia).
No products indexed under this heading.

Moexipril Hydrochloride (May increase the blood-glucose-lowering effect and susceptibility to hypoglycemia).
No products indexed under this heading.

Mometasone Furoate (Co-administration with corticosteroids may reduce the blood-glucose-lowering effect of insulin). Products include:
Asmanex Twisthaler ... 2797
Elocon Cream 0.1% ... 2840
Elocon Lotion 0.1% ... 2841
Elocon Ointment 0.1% ... 2842

Mometasone Furoate Monohydrate (Co-administration with corticosteroids may reduce the blood-glucose-lowering effect of insulin). Products include:
Nasonex Nasal Spray ... 2883

Nadolol (Beta-blockers may either potentiate or weaken the blood-glucose-lowering effect of insulin; signs of hypoglycemia may be reduced or absent with co-administration). Products include:
Nadolol Tablets ... 2191

Nateglinide (May increase the blood-glucose-lowering effect and susceptibility to hypoglycemia). Products include:
Starlix Tablets ... 2314

Nebivolol (Beta-blockers may either potentiate or weaken the blood-glucose-lowering effect of insulin; signs of hypoglycemia may be reduced or absent with co-administration). Products include:
Bystolic Tablets ... 1155

Niacin (May reduce the blood-glucose-lowering effect of insulin). Products include:
Advicor Tablets ... 402
Bausch & Lomb Ocuvite DF Vitamin Supplement ... ⊙ 238
Dismutax Dietary Supplement ... 995
Niaspan Extended-Release Tablets ... 480
NT-Kinase Dietary Supplement ... 995
Simcor Tablets ... 502

Norepinephrine Bitartrate (Sympathomimetic agents may reduce the blood-glucose-lowering effect of insulin).
No products indexed under this heading.

Norethindrone (Oral contraceptives may reduce the blood-glucose-lowering effect of insulin). Products include:
Ortho Micronor Tablets ... 2446

Norethynodrel (Oral contraceptives may reduce the blood-glucose-lowering effect of insulin).
No products indexed under this heading.

Norgestimate (Oral contraceptives may reduce the blood-glucose-lowering effect of insulin). Products include:
- Ortho-Cyclen/Ortho Tri-Cyclen 2449
- Ortho Tri-Cyclen Lo Tablets 2458

Norgestrel (Oral contraceptives may reduce the blood-glucose-lowering effect of insulin).
- No products indexed under this heading.

Octreotide Acetate (May increase the blood-glucose-lowering effect and susceptibility to hypoglycemia). Products include:
- Sandostatin Injection 2300
- Sandostatin LAR Depot 2302

Pargyline Hydrochloride (May increase the blood-glucose-lowering effect and susceptibility to hypoglycemia).
- No products indexed under this heading.

Penbutolol Sulfate (Beta-blockers may either potentiate or weaken the blood-glucose-lowering effect of insulin; signs of hypoglycemia may be reduced or absent with co-administration).
- No products indexed under this heading.

Pentamidine Isethionate (May cause hypoglycemia, which may sometimes be followed by hyperglycemia).
- No products indexed under this heading.

Perindopril Erbumine (May increase the blood-glucose-lowering effect and susceptibility to hypoglycemia). Products include:
- Aceon Tablets (2 mg, 4 mg, 8 mg) 3038

Perphenazine (Phenothiazine derivatives may reduce the blood-glucose-lowering effect of insulin).
- No products indexed under this heading.

Phenelzine Sulfate (May increase the blood-glucose-lowering effect and susceptibility to hypoglycemia).
- No products indexed under this heading.

Phenylephrine Bitartrate (Sympathomimetic agents may reduce the blood-glucose-lowering effect of insulin).
- No products indexed under this heading.

Phenylephrine Hydrochloride (Sympathomimetic agents may reduce the blood-glucose-lowering effect of insulin). Products include:
- Actifed Cold & Allergy Tablets 1895
- Benadryl Allergy & Cold Kapgels 1895
- Benadryl Allergy & Sinus Headache Kapgels 1895
- Benadryl Severe Allergy & Sinus Headache Caplets 1897
- Children's Benadryl-D Allergy & Sinus Liquid 1896
- Benadryl-D Allergy & Sinus Tablet 1896
- PediaCare Children's Allergy & Cold Liquid 1902
- PediaCare Children's Decongestant Liquid.................... 1902
- PediaCare Children's Liquid Multi-Symptom Cold..................... 1902
- Sinutab Non-Drying Caplets 1905
- Sinutab Sinus Caplets 1905
- Children's Sudafed PE Cold & Cough Liquid 1907
- Children's Sudafed PE Nasal Decongestant Liquid.................... 1906
- Sudafed PE Cold & Cough Caplets.. 1907
- Sudafed PE Nasal Decongestant Tablets... 1907
- Sudafed PE Nighttime Cold Caplets.. 1907
- Sudafed PE Non-Drying Sinus Caplets.. 1908
- Sudafed PE Severe Cold Caplets 1908
- Sudafed PE Sinus & Allergy Tablets 1908
- Sudafed PE Sinus Headache Caplets.. 1908
- Tylenol Allergy Multi-Symptom Caplets with Cool Burst and Rapid Release Gelcaps 1916
- Tylenol Allergy Multi-Symptom Nighttime Caplets with Cool Burst 1916
- Children's Tylenol Plus Cold Suspension Liquid 1912
- Children's Tylenol Plus Cold & Allergy Suspension Liquid 1914
- Children's Tylenol Plus Flu Suspension Liquid 1914
- Children's Tylenol Plus Multi-Symptom Cold Suspension Liquid........................ 1912
- Tylenol Cold Head Congestion Daytime Caplets with Cool Burst... 1910
- Tylenol Cold Head Congestion Nighttime Caplets with Cool Burst... 1910
- Tylenol Cold Head Congestion Severe Daytime Caplets with Cool Burst.................................. 1910
- Tylenol Cold Multi-Symptom Daytime Caplets with Cool Burst and Rapid Release Gels 1913
- Tylenol Cold Multi-Symptom Daytime Liquid with Citrus Burst ... 1913
- Tylenol Cold Multi-Symptom Nighttime Caplets with Cool Burst... 1913
- Tylenol Cold Multi-Symptom Nighttime Liquid with Cool Burst ... 1913
- Tylenol Cold Multi-Symptom Severe Caplets with Cool Burst..... 1913
- Tylenol Cold Multi-Symptom Severe Daytime Liquid with Citrus Burst 1913
- Tylenol Sinus Congestion & Pain Daytime Caplets with Cool Burst and Gelcaps 1917
- Tylenol Sinus Congestion & Pain Nighttime Caplets with Cool Burst... 1917
- Tylenol Sinus Congestion & Pain Severe Caplets with Cool Burst..... 1917
- Vicks DayQuil Cold & Flu Multi-Symptom Relief 616
- Vicks DayQuil LiquiCaps 2567
- Vicks DayQuil Liquid 2567
- Vicks DayQuil Multi-Symptom Cold/Flu Relief............................. 2567

Phenylephrine Tannate (Sympathomimetic agents may reduce the blood-glucose-lowering effect of insulin).
- No products indexed under this heading.

Phenylpropanolamine Hydrochloride (Sympathomimetic agents may reduce the blood-glucose-lowering effect of insulin).
- No products indexed under this heading.

Pindolol (Beta-blockers may either potentiate or weaken the blood-glucose-lowering effect of insulin; signs of hypoglycemia may be reduced or absent with co-administration).
- No products indexed under this heading.

Pioglitazone Hydrochloride (May increase the blood-glucose-lowering effect and susceptibility to hypoglycemia). Products include:
- ActoPlus Met Tablets 3071
- Actos Tablets 3077
- Duetact Tablets............................... 3085

Pirbuterol Acetate (Sympathomimetic agents may reduce the blood-glucose-lowering effect of insulin). Products include:
- Maxair Autohaler 1705

Polythiazide (Diuretics may reduce the blood-glucose-lowering effect of insulin).
- No products indexed under this heading.

Pramlintide Acetate (May reduce the blood glucose lowering effect and susceptibility to hypoglycemia).
- No products indexed under this heading.

Prednisolone Acetate (Co-administration with corticosteroids may reduce the blood-glucose-lowering effect of insulin). Products include:
- Pred Forte Ophthalmic Suspension .... ⊙227
- Pred Mild Ophthalmic Suspension .... ⊙230
- Pred-G Ophthalmic Ointment .... ⊙229
- Pred-G Ophthalmic Suspension ...... ⊙228

Prednisolone Sodium Phosphate (Co-administration with corticosteroids may reduce the blood-glucose-lowering effect of insulin).
- No products indexed under this heading.

Prednisolone Tebutate (Co-administration with corticosteroids may reduce the blood-glucose-lowering effect of insulin).
- No products indexed under this heading.

Prednisone (Co-administration with corticosteroids may reduce the blood-glucose-lowering effect of insulin).
- No products indexed under this heading.

Procarbazine Hydrochloride (May increase the blood-glucose-lowering effect and susceptibility to hypoglycemia).
- No products indexed under this heading.

Prochlorperazine (Phenothiazine derivatives may reduce the blood-glucose-lowering effect of insulin).
- No products indexed under this heading.

Progesterone (May reduce the blood glucose lowering effect). Products include:
- Crinone 4% Gel 992
- Crinone 8% Gel 992
- Prometrium Capsules (100 mg, 200 mg)... 3047

Progestins (May reduce the blood glucose lowering effect).
- No products indexed under this heading.

Promethazine Hydrochloride (Phenothiazine derivatives may reduce the blood-glucose-lowering effect of insulin).
- No products indexed under this heading.

Propoxyphene Hydrochloride (May increase the blood-glucose-lowering effect and susceptibility to hypoglycemia).
- No products indexed under this heading.

Propoxyphene Napsylate (May increase the blood-glucose-lowering effect and susceptibility to hypoglycemia).
- No products indexed under this heading.

Propranolol Hydrochloride (Beta-blockers may either potentiate or weaken the blood-glucose-lowering effect of insulin; signs of hypoglycemia may be reduced or absent with co-administration). Products include:
- InnoPran XL Extended Release Capsules 1484

Pseudoephedrine Hydrochloride (Sympathomimetic agents may reduce the blood-glucose-lowering effect of insulin). Products include:
- Allegra-D 12 Hour Extended-Release Tablets............ 2687
- Allegra-D 24 Hour Extended-Release Tablets............ 2690
- Children's Motrin Cold Oral Suspension 1899
- Sudafed 12 Hour Nasal Decongestant Non-Drowsy Caplets.. 1909
- Sudafed 24 Hour Non-Drowsy Nasal Decongestant Tablets......... 1906
- Children's Sudafed Nasal Decongestant Liquid.................... 1906
- Sudafed Nasal Decongestant Tablets... 1906
- Tylenol Cold Severe Congestion Daytime Caplets with Cool Burst... 1912
- Tylenol Sinus Severe Congestion Caplets with Cool Burst.............. 1917
- Vicks NyQuil LiquiCaps 2567
- Vicks NyQuil Liquid 2567
- Vicks NyQuil Multi-Symptom Cold/Flu Relief............................. 2567
- Zyrtec-D 12 Hour Extended Release Tablets.......................... 1923
- Zyrtec-D Allergy & Congestion Extended-Release Tablets............ 1923

Pseudoephedrine Sulfate (Sympathomimetic agents may reduce the blood-glucose-lowering effect of insulin). Products include:
- Clarinex-D 12-Hour Extended-Release Tablets............ 2831
- Clarinex-D 24-Hour Extended-Release Tablets............ 2834

Quinapril Hydrochloride (May increase the blood-glucose-lowering effect and susceptibility to hypoglycemia).
- No products indexed under this heading.

Ramipril (May increase the blood-glucose-lowering effect and susceptibility to hypoglycemia).
- No products indexed under this heading.

Rasagiline Mesylate (May increase the blood-glucose-lowering effect and susceptibility to hypoglycemia). Products include:
- Azilect Tablets 3106

Repaglinide (May increase the blood-glucose-lowering effect and susceptibility to hypoglycemia). Products include:
- PrandiMet Tablets 2967
- Prandin Tablets 2971

Reserpine (Signs of hypoglycemia may be reduced or absent with co-administration).
- No products indexed under this heading.

Rosiglitazone Maleate (May increase the blood-glucose-lowering effect and susceptibility to hypoglycemia). Products include:
- Avandamet Tablets 1336
- Avandaryl Tablets 1344
- Avandia Tablets 1351

Salmeterol Xinafoate (Sympathomimetic agents may reduce the blood-glucose-lowering effect of insulin). Products include:
- Advair Diskus 100/50 1276
- Advair Diskus 250/50 1276
- Advair Diskus 500/50 1276
- Advair HFA 45/21 Inhalation Aerosol.. 1288
- Advair HFA 115/21 Inhalation Aerosol.. 1288
- Advair HFA 230/21 Inhalation Aerosol.. 1288
- Serevent Diskus 1594

IMPORTANT NOTE: Always consult each drug listing in the patient's regimen for possible interactions.

Salsalate (May increase the blood-glucose-lowering effect and susceptibility to hypoglycemia).
No products indexed under this heading.

Selegiline (May increase the blood-glucose-lowering effect and susceptibility to hypoglycemia). Products include:
Emsam Transdermal System 905

Selegiline Hydrochloride (May increase the blood-glucose-lowering effect and susceptibility to hypoglycemia). Products include:
Eldepryl Capsules 3052

Sitagliptin Phosphate (May increase the blood-glucose-lowering effect and susceptibility to hypoglycemia). Products include:
Janumet Tablets 2041
Januvia Tablets 2048

Somatropin (May reduce the blood-glucose-lowering effect of insulin). Products include:
Genotropin Lyophilized Powder 2547
Humatrope Vials and Cartridges 1838
Nutropin for Injection 1208
Nutropin AQ Injection 1212
Nutropin AQ NuSpin Injection 1212
Nutropin AQ Pen 1212
Nutropin AQ Pen Cartridge 1212

Sotalol Hydrochloride (Beta-blockers may either potentiate or weaken the blood-glucose-lowering effect of insulin; signs of hypoglycemia may be reduced or absent with co-administration).
No products indexed under this heading.

Spirapril Hydrochloride (May increase the blood-glucose-lowering effect and susceptibility to hypoglycemia).
No products indexed under this heading.

Spironolactone (Diuretics may reduce the blood-glucose-lowering effect of insulin).
No products indexed under this heading.

Sulfamethoxazole (Co-administration with sulfonamide antibiotics may increase the blood-glucose-lowering effect and susceptibility to hypoglycemia).
No products indexed under this heading.

Sulfisoxazole Acetyl (Co-administration with sulfonamide antibiotics may increase the blood-glucose-lowering effect and susceptibility to hypoglycemia).
No products indexed under this heading.

Terbutaline Sulfate (Sympathomimetic agents may reduce the blood-glucose-lowering effect of insulin).
No products indexed under this heading.

Thioridazine Hydrochloride (Phenothiazine derivatives may reduce the blood-glucose-lowering effect of insulin). Products include:
Thioridazine Hydrochloride Tablets 2195

Thyroglobulin (May reduce the blood-glucose-lowering effect of insulin).
No products indexed under this heading.

Thyroid (May reduce the blood-glucose-lowering effect of insulin). Products include:
Naturethroid Tablets 2605

Thyroxine (May reduce the blood-glucose-lowering effect of insulin).
No products indexed under this heading.

Thyroxine Sodium (May reduce the blood-glucose-lowering effect of insulin).
No products indexed under this heading.

Timolol Hemihydrate (Beta-blockers may either potentiate or weaken the blood-glucose-lowering effect of insulin; signs of hypoglycemia may be reduced or absent with co-administration). Products include:
Betimol Ophthalmic Solution 3181

Timolol Maleate (Beta-blockers may either potentiate or weaken the blood-glucose-lowering effect of insulin; signs of hypoglycemia may be reduced or absent with co-administration). Products include:
Combigan Ophthalmic Solution 553
Cosopt Sterile Ophthalmic Solution 1969
Timoptic Sterile Ophthalmic Solution 2121
Timoptic in Ocudose 2124
Timoptic-XE Sterile Ophthalmic Gel Forming Solution 2125

Tolazamide (May increase the blood-glucose-lowering effect and susceptibility to hypoglycemia).
No products indexed under this heading.

Tolbutamide (May increase the blood-glucose-lowering effect and susceptibility to hypoglycemia).
No products indexed under this heading.

Torsemide (Diuretics may reduce the blood-glucose-lowering effect of insulin). Products include:
Demadex Injection 2630
Demadex Tablets 2630

Trandolapril (May increase the blood-glucose-lowering effect and susceptibility to hypoglycemia). Products include:
Mavik Tablets 472
Tarka Tablets 511

Tranylcypromine Sulfate (May increase the blood-glucose-lowering effect and susceptibility to hypoglycemia). Products include:
Parnate Tablets 1532

Triamcinolone (Co-administration with corticosteroids may reduce the blood-glucose-lowering effect of insulin).
No products indexed under this heading.

Triamcinolone Acetonide (Co-administration with corticosteroids may reduce the blood-glucose-lowering effect of insulin). Products include:
Azmacort Inhalation Aerosol 407
Nasacort AQ Nasal Spray 2765
Triesence Injectable Suspension .... ⊙ 209

Triamcinolone Diacetate (Co-administration with corticosteroids may reduce the blood-glucose-lowering effect of insulin).
No products indexed under this heading.

Triamcinolone Hexacetonide (Co-administration with corticosteroids may reduce the blood-glucose-lowering effect of insulin).
No products indexed under this heading.

Triamterene (Diuretics may reduce the blood-glucose-lowering effect of insulin). Products include:
Dyazide Capsules 1405
Dyrenium Capsules 3189

Trifluoperazine Hydrochloride (Phenothiazine derivatives may reduce the blood-glucose-lowering effect of insulin).
No products indexed under this heading.

Troglitazone (May increase the blood-glucose-lowering effect and susceptibility to hypoglycemia).
No products indexed under this heading.

Food Interactions

Alcohol (May either potentiate or weaken the blood-glucose-lowering effect of insulin).

NOVOSEVEN

(Antihemophilic Factor (Recombinant)) 2367
None cited in PDR database.

NOVOSEVEN RT

(Coagulation Factor VIIa, Recombinant) 2370
May interact with:

Prothrombin complex concentrates (The risk of a potential interaction between rFVIIa and coagulation factor concentrates has not been adequately evaluated in preclinical or clinical studies. Simultaneous use of prothrombin complex concentrates or activated prothrombin complex concentrates should be avoided).
No products indexed under this heading.

NOXAFIL ORAL SUSPENSION

(Posaconazole) 2889
May interact with benzodiazepine that are metabolized by CYP3A4, calcium channel blockers, cytochrome p450 3a4 substrates (selected), ergot-containing drugs, HMG-CoA reductase inhibitors, P-glycoprotein inducers, P-glycoprotein inhibitors, phenytoin, drugs that prolong the QT interval, quinidine, vinca alkaloids, and certain other agents. Compounds in these categories include:

Alfentanil Hydrochloride (A clinical study in healthy volunteers indicates that posaconazole is a strong CYP3A4 inhibitor. Therefore, plasma concentrations of drugs predominantly metabolized by CYP3A4 may be increased by posaconazole).
No products indexed under this heading.

Alprazolam (Frequent monitoring of adverse effects of benzodiazepines metabolized by CYP3A4 should be performed and dose reduction of these benzodiazepines should be considered during co-administration with posaconazole).
No products indexed under this heading.

Amiodarone Hydrochloride (Some azoles, including posaconazole, have been associated with prolongation of the QT interval on the electrocardiogram. Posaconazole should not be administered with drugs that are known to prolong the QTc interval and are metabolized through CYP3A4).
No products indexed under this heading.

Amitriptyline Hydrochloride (Some azoles, including posaconazole, have been associated with prolongation of the QT interval on the electrocardiogram. Posaconazole should not be administered with drugs that are known to prolong the QTc interval and are metabolized through CYP3A4).
No products indexed under this heading.

Amlodipine Besylate (Frequent monitoring for adverse events and toxicity related to calcium channel blockers which are metabolized through CYP3A4 is recommended during co-administration. Dose reduction of calcium channel blockers which are metabolized through CYP3A4 may be needed). Products include:
Azor Tablets 1005
Exforge Tablets 2238

Amoxapine (Some azoles, including posaconazole, have been associated with prolongation of the QT interval on the electrocardiogram. Posaconazole should not be administered with drugs that are known to prolong the QTc interval and are metabolized through CYP3A4).
No products indexed under this heading.

Aprepitant (A clinical study in healthy volunteers indicates that posaconazole is a strong CYP3A4 inhibitor. Therefore, plasma concentrations of drugs predominantly metabolized by CYP3A4 may be increased by posaconazole). Products include:
Emend Capsules 1992

Astemizole (Co-administration of the CYP3A4 substrate astemizole with posaconazole is contraindicated since it may result in increased plasma concentrations of astemizole, leading to QTc prolongation and rare occurrences of torsades de pointes).
No products indexed under this heading.

Atazanavir (Frequent monitoring of adverse effects and toxicity of atazanavir should be performed during co-administration with posaconazole).
No products indexed under this heading.

Atazanavir Sulfate (Frequent monitoring of adverse effects and toxicity of atazanavir should be performed during co-administration with posaconazole). Products include:
Reyataz Capsules 3299

Atenolol (Posaconazole is a substrate for p-glycoprotein (P-gp) efflux. Therefore, inhibitors of p-glycoprotein may affect posaconazole plasma concentrations).
No products indexed under this heading.

Atorvastatin Calcium (It is recommended that dose reduction of statins metabolized through CYP3A4 be considered during co-administration. Increased statin concentrations in plasma can be associated with rhabdomyolysis). Products include:
Lipitor Tablets 2501

Azithromycin Dihydrate (Posaconazole is a substrate for p-glycoprotein (P-gp) efflux. Therefore, inhibitors of p-glycoprotein may affect posaconazole plasma concentrations).
No products indexed under this heading.

Belladonna Ergotamine (A clinical study in healthy volunteers indicates that posaconazole is a strong CYP3A4 inhibitor. Therefore, plasma concentrations of drugs predominantly metabolized by CYP3A4 may be increased by posaconazole).
No products indexed under this heading.

Bepridil Hydrochloride (Frequent monitoring for adverse events and toxicity related to calcium channel blockers which are metabolized through CYP3A4 is recommended during co-administration. Dose reduction of calcium channel blockers which are metabolized through CYP3A4 may be needed).
No products indexed under this heading.

Bretylium Tosylate (Some azoles, including posaconazole, have been associated with prolongation of the QT interval on the electrocardiogram. Posaconazole should not be administered with drugs that are known to prolong the QTc interval and are metabolized through CYP3A4).
No products indexed under this heading.

Buspirone Hydrochloride (Some azoles, including posaconazole, have been associated with prolongation of the QT interval on the electrocardiogram. Posaconazole should not be administered with drugs that are known to prolong the QTc interval and are metabolized through CYP3A4).
No products indexed under this heading.

Busulfan (A clinical study in healthy volunteers indicates that posaconazole is a strong CYP3A4 inhibitor. Therefore, plasma concentrations of drugs predominantly metabolized by CYP3A4 may be increased by posaconazole). Products include:
Busulfex Injection 2477
Myleran Tablets 1530

Carbamazepine (A clinical study in healthy volunteers indicates that posaconazole is a strong CYP3A4 inhibitor. Therefore, plasma concentrations of drugs predominantly metabolized by CYP3A4 may be increased by posaconazole).
Products include:
Carbatrol Capsules 3019
Equetro Extended-Release Capsules 3174

Cerivastatin Sodium (It is recommended that dose reduction of statins metabolized through CYP3A4 be considered during co-administration. Increased statin concentrations in plasma can be associated with rhabdomyolysis).
No products indexed under this heading.

Chlordiazepoxide (Some azoles, including posaconazole, have been associated with prolongation of the QT interval on the electrocardiogram. Posaconazole should not be administered with drugs that are known to prolong the QTc interval and are metabolized through CYP3A4).
No products indexed under this heading.

Chlordiazepoxide Hydrochloride (Some azoles, including posaconazole, have been associated with prolongation of the QT interval on the electrocardiogram. Posaconazole should not be administered with drugs that are known to prolong the QTc interval and are metabolized through CYP3A4).
No products indexed under this heading.

Chlorpheniramine (A clinical study in healthy volunteers indicates that posaconazole is a strong CYP3A4 inhibitor. Therefore, plasma concentrations of drugs predominantly metabolized by CYP3A4 may be increased by posaconazole).
No products indexed under this heading.

Chlorpheniramine Maleate (A clinical study in healthy volunteers indicates that posaconazole is a strong CYP3A4 inhibitor. Therefore, plasma concentrations of drugs predominantly metabolized by CYP3A4 may be increased by posaconazole).
Products include:
Actifed Cold & Allergy Tablets 1895
Sudafed PE Sinus & Allergy Tablets 1908
Tylenol Allergy Multi-Symptom Caplets with Cool Burst and Rapid Release Gelcaps 1916
Children's Tylenol Plus Cold Suspension Liquid 1912
Children's Tylenol Plus Cough & Runny Nose Suspension Liquid 1912
Children's Tylenol Plus Flu Suspension Liquid 1914
Children's Tylenol Plus Multi-Symptom Cold Suspension Liquid 1912
Tylenol Cold Head Congestion Nighttime Caplets with Cool Burst 1910
Tylenol Cold Multi-Symptom Nighttime Caplets with Cool Burst 1913
Tylenol Sinus Congestion & Pain Nighttime Caplets with Cool Burst 1917

Chlorpheniramine Polistirex (A clinical study in healthy volunteers indicates that posaconazole is a strong CYP3A4 inhibitor. Therefore, plasma concentrations of drugs predominantly metabolized by CYP3A4 may be increased by posaconazole).
Products include:
Tussionex Pennkinetic Extended-Release Suspension 3154

Chlorpheniramine Tannate (A clinical study in healthy volunteers indicates that posaconazole is a strong CYP3A4 inhibitor. Therefore, plasma concentrations of drugs predominantly metabolized by CYP3A4 may be increased by posaconazole).
No products indexed under this heading.

Chlorpromazine (Some azoles, including posaconazole, have been associated with prolongation of the QT interval on the electrocardiogram. Posaconazole should not be administered with drugs that are known to prolong the QTc interval and are metabolized through CYP3A4).
No products indexed under this heading.

Chlorpromazine Hydrochloride (Some azoles, including posaconazole, have been associated with prolongation of the QT interval on the electrocardiogram. Posaconazole should not be administered with drugs that are known to prolong the QTc interval and are metabolized through CYP3A4).
No products indexed under this heading.

Chlorprothixene (Some azoles, including posaconazole, have been associated with prolongation of the QT interval on the electrocardiogram. Posaconazole should not be administered with drugs that are known to prolong the QTc interval and are metabolized through CYP3A4).
No products indexed under this heading.

Chlorprothixene Hydrochloride (Some azoles, including posaconazole, have been associated with prolongation of the QT interval on the electrocardiogram. Posaconazole should not be administered with drugs that are known to prolong the QTc interval and are metabolized through CYP3A4).
No products indexed under this heading.

Cimetidine (Co-administration of cimetidine with posaconazole may result in lower plasma concentrations of posaconazole; avoid concomitant use unless the benefits outweigh the risks).
No products indexed under this heading.

Cimetidine Hydrochloride (Co-administration of cimetidine with posaconazole may result in lower plasma concentrations of posaconazole; avoid concomitant use unless the benefits outweigh the risks).
No products indexed under this heading.

Cisapride (Co-administration of the CYP3A4 substrate cisapride with posaconazole is contraindicated since it may result in increased plasma concentrations of cisapride, leading to QTc prolongation and rare occurrences of torsades de pointes).
No products indexed under this heading.

Clarithromycin (A clinical study in healthy volunteers indicates that posaconazole is a strong CYP3A4 inhibitor. Therefore, plasma concentrations of drugs predominantly metabolized by CYP3A4 may be increased by posaconazole).
Products include:
Biaxin/Biaxin XL 411

Clomipramine Hydrochloride (Some azoles, including posaconazole, have been associated with prolongation of the QT interval on the electrocardiogram. Posaconazole should not be administered with drugs that are known to prolong the QTc interval and are metabolized through CYP3A4).
No products indexed under this heading.

Clorazepate Dipotassium (Some azoles, including posaconazole, have been associated with prolongation of the QT interval on the electrocardiogram. Posaconazole should not be administered with drugs that are known to prolong the QTc interval and are metabolized through CYP3A4).
No products indexed under this heading.

Clozapine (Some azoles, including posaconazole, have been associated with prolongation of the QT interval on the electrocardiogram. Posaconazole should not be administered with drugs that are known to prolong the QTc interval and are metabolized through CYP3A4).
No products indexed under this heading.

Cyclosporine (Increased cyclosporine concentrations resulted in cyclosporine dose reductions in heart transplant patients co-administered posaconazole. At initiation of posaconazole treatment, reduce the cyclosporine dose to approximately 3/4 of the original dose. Frequent monitoring of cyclosporine whole blood trough concentrations should be performed during and at discontinuation of posaconazole treatment and the cyclosporine dose adjusted accordingly). Products include:
Gengraf Capsules 435
Neoral Oral Solution 2280
Neoral Soft Gelatin Capsules 2280
Restasis Ophthalmic Emulsion 557
Sandimmune 2296

Desipramine Hydrochloride (Some azoles, including posaconazole, have been associated with prolongation of the QT interval on the electrocardiogram. Posaconazole should not be administered with drugs that are known to prolong the QTc interval and are metabolized through CYP3A4).
No products indexed under this heading.

Desogestrel (A clinical study in healthy volunteers indicates that posaconazole is a strong CYP3A4 inhibitor. Therefore, plasma concentrations of drugs predominantly metabolized by CYP3A4 may be increased by posaconazole).
Products include:
Mircette Tablets 1034

Diazepam (Frequent monitoring of adverse effects of benzodiazepines metabolized by CYP3A4 should be performed and dose reduction of these benzodiazepines should be considered during co-administration with posaconazole). Products include:
Valium Tablets 2658

Digoxin (Increased plasma concentrations of digoxin have been reported in patients receiving digoxin and posaconazole. Therefore, monitoring of digoxin plasma concentrations is recommended during co-administration). Products include:
Lanoxin Injection 1498
Lanoxin Injection Pediatric 1502
Lanoxin Tablets 1505

Dihydroergotamine Mesylate (Co-administration of posaconazole with ergot alkaloids is contraindicated. Posaconazole may increase the plasma concentrations of ergot alkaloids which may lead to ergotism).
No products indexed under this heading.

Diltiazem Hydrochloride (Frequent monitoring for adverse events and toxicity related to calcium channel blockers which are metabolized through CYP3A4 is recommended during co-administration. Dose reduction of calcium channel blockers which are metabolized through CYP3A4 may be needed). Products include:
Cardizem LA Extended Release Tablets 421

Diltiazem Maleate (A clinical study in healthy volunteers indicates that posaconazole is a strong CYP3A4 inhibitor. Therefore, plasma concentrations of drugs predominantly metabolized by CYP3A4 may be increased by posaconazole).
No products indexed under this heading.

Dirithromycin (Posaconazole is a substrate for p-glycoprotein (P-gp) efflux. Therefore, inhibitors of p-glycoprotein may affect posaconazole plasma concentrations).
No products indexed under this heading.

Disopyramide (A clinical study in healthy volunteers indicates that posaconazole is a strong CYP3A4 inhibitor. Therefore, plasma concentrations of drugs predominantly metabolized by CYP3A4 may be increased by posaconazole).
No products indexed under this heading.

Disopyramide Phosphate (Some azoles, including posaconazole, have been associated with prolongation of the QT interval on the electrocardiogram. Posaconazole should not be administered with drugs that are known to prolong the QTc interval and are metabolized through CYP3A4).
No products indexed under this heading.

Disulfiram (A clinical study in healthy volunteers indicates that posaconazole is a strong CYP3A4 inhibitor. Therefore, plasma concentrations of drugs predominantly metabolized by CYP3A4 may be increased by posaconazole).
No products indexed under this heading.

Dofetilide (Some azoles, including posaconazole, have been associated with prolongation of the QT interval on the electrocardiogram. Posaconazole should not be administered with drugs that are known to prolong the QTc interval and are metabolized through CYP3A4).
No products indexed under this heading.

Doxepin Hydrochloride (Some azoles, including posaconazole, have been associated with prolongation of the QT interval on the electrocardiogram. Posaconazole should not be administered with drugs that are known to prolong the QTc interval and are metabolized through CYP3A4).
No products indexed under this heading.

Doxorubicin Hydrochloride (A clinical study in healthy volunteers indicates that posaconazole is a strong CYP3A4 inhibitor. Therefore, plasma concentrations of drugs predominantly metabolized by CYP3A4 may be increased by posaconazole).
No products indexed under this heading.

Dronabinol (A clinical study in healthy volunteers indicates that posaconazole is a strong CYP3A4 inhibitor. Therefore, plasma concentrations of drugs predominantly metabolized by CYP3A4 may be increased by posaconazole). Products include:
Marinol Capsules 3163

Droperidol (Some azoles, including posaconazole, have been associated with prolongation of the QT interval on the electrocardiogram. Posaconazole should not be administered with drugs that are known to prolong the QTc interval and are metabolized through CYP3A4).
No products indexed under this heading.

Efavirenz (Co-administration of efavirenz with posaconazole may result in lower plasma concentrations of posaconazole; avoid concomitant use unless the benefits outweigh the risks). Products include:
Atripla Tablets 938
Sustiva Capsules 930
Sustiva Tablets 930

Elacridar (Posaconazole is a substrate for p-glycoprotein (P-gp) efflux. Therefore, inhibitors of p-glycoprotein may affect posaconazole plasma concentrations).
No products indexed under this heading.

Ergonovine Maleate (Co-administration of posaconazole with ergot alkaloids is contraindicated. Posaconazole may increase the plasma concentrations of ergot alkaloids which may lead to ergotism).
No products indexed under this heading.

Ergotamine Tartrate (Co-administration of posaconazole with ergot alkaloids is contraindicated. Posaconazole may increase the plasma concentrations of ergot alkaloids which may lead to ergotism).
No products indexed under this heading.

Erythromycin (Some azoles, including posaconazole, have been associated with prolongation of the QT interval on the electrocardiogram. Posaconazole should not be administered with drugs that are known to prolong the QTc interval and are metabolized through CYP3A4).
No products indexed under this heading.

Erythromycin Estolate (Some azoles, including posaconazole, have been associated with prolongation of the QT interval on the electrocardiogram. Posaconazole should not be administered with drugs that are known to prolong the QTc interval and are metabolized through CYP3A4).
No products indexed under this heading.

Erythromycin Ethylsuccinate (Some azoles, including posaconazole, have been associated with prolongation of the QT interval on the electrocardiogram. Posaconazole should not be administered with drugs that are known to prolong the QTc interval and are metabolized through CYP3A4). Products include:
E.E.S. 433
EryPed 431

Erythromycin Gluceptate (Some azoles, including posaconazole, have been associated with prolongation of the QT interval on the electrocardiogram. Posaconazole should not be administered with drugs that are known to prolong the QTc interval and are metabolized through CYP3A4).
No products indexed under this heading.

Erythromycin Lactobionate (Some azoles, including posaconazole, have been associated with prolongation of the QT interval on the electrocardiogram. Posaconazole should not be administered with drugs that are known to prolong the QTc interval and are metabolized through CYP3A4).
No products indexed under this heading.

Erythromycin Stearate (Some azoles, including posaconazole, have been associated with prolongation of the QT interval on the electrocardiogram. Posaconazole should not be administered with drugs that are known to prolong the QTc interval and are metabolized through CYP3A4).
No products indexed under this heading.

Estradiol (A clinical study in healthy volunteers indicates that posaconazole is a strong CYP3A4 inhibitor. Therefore, plasma concentrations of drugs predominantly metabolized by CYP3A4 may be increased by posaconazole). Products include:
Activella Tablets 2347
Angeliq Tablets 751
Climara Transdermal System 763
Climara Pro Transdermal System 768
Divigel 3167
Vagifem Tablets 2375

Estradiol Benzoate (A clinical study in healthy volunteers indicates that posaconazole is a strong CYP3A4 inhibitor. Therefore, plasma concentrations of drugs predominantly metabolized by CYP3A4 may be increased by posaconazole).
No products indexed under this heading.

Estradiol Cypionate (A clinical study in healthy volunteers indicates that posaconazole is a strong CYP3A4 inhibitor. Therefore, plasma concentrations of drugs predominantly metabolized by CYP3A4 may be increased by posaconazole).
No products indexed under this heading.

Estradiol Valerate (A clinical study in healthy volunteers indicates that posaconazole is a strong CYP3A4 inhibitor. Therefore, plasma concentrations of drugs predominantly metabolized by CYP3A4 may be increased by posaconazole).
No products indexed under this heading.

Ethinyl Estradiol (A clinical study in healthy volunteers indicates that posaconazole is a strong CYP3A4 inhibitor. Therefore, plasma concentrations of drugs predominantly metabolized by CYP3A4 may be increased by posaconazole). Products include:
Lybrel Tablets 3204
Mircette Tablets 1034
NuvaRing 2897
Ortho-Cyclen/Ortho Tri-Cyclen 2449
Ortho Evra Transdermal System 2437
Ortho Tri-Cyclen Lo Tablets 2458
Seasonique Tablets 1046
Yaz Tablets 805

Ethosuximide (A clinical study in healthy volunteers indicates that posaconazole is a strong CYP3A4 inhibitor. Therefore, plasma concentrations of drugs predominantly metabolized by CYP3A4 may be increased by posaconazole).
No products indexed under this heading.

Ethynodiol Diacetate (A clinical study in healthy volunteers indicates that posaconazole is a strong CYP3A4 inhibitor. Therefore, plasma concentrations of drugs predominantly metabolized by CYP3A4 may be increased by posaconazole).
No products indexed under this heading.

Etoposide (A clinical study in healthy volunteers indicates that posaconazole is a strong CYP3A4 inhibitor. Therefore, plasma concentrations of drugs predominantly metabolized by CYP3A4 may be increased by posaconazole).
No products indexed under this heading.

Etoposide Phosphate (A clinical study in healthy volunteers indicates that posaconazole is a strong CYP3A4 inhibitor. Therefore, plasma concentrations of drugs predominantly metabolized by CYP3A4 may be increased by posaconazole).
No products indexed under this heading.

Felodipine (Frequent monitoring for adverse events and toxicity related to calcium channel blockers which are metabolized through CYP3A4 is recommended during co-administration. Dose reduction of calcium channel blockers which are metabolized through CYP3A4 may be needed).
No products indexed under this heading.

Fentanyl (A clinical study in healthy volunteers indicates that posaconazole is a strong CYP3A4 inhibitor. Therefore, plasma concentrations of drugs predominantly metabolized by CYP3A4 may be increased by posaconazole). Products include:
Duragesic Transdermal System 2405
Ionsys Transdermal System 2410

Fentanyl Citrate (A clinical study in healthy volunteers indicates that posaconazole is a strong CYP3A4 inhibitor. Therefore, plasma concentrations of drugs predominantly

metabolized by CYP3A4 may be increased by posaconazole). Products include:

Actiq 959
Fentora Tablets 968

Flecainide Acetate (Some azoles, including posaconazole, have been associated with prolongation of the QT interval on the electrocardiogram. Posaconazole should not be administered with drugs that are known to prolong the QTc interval and are metabolized through CYP3A4).

No products indexed under this heading.

Fluphenazine Decanoate (Some azoles, including posaconazole, have been associated with prolongation of the QT interval on the electrocardiogram. Posaconazole should not be administered with drugs that are known to prolong the QTc interval and are metabolized through CYP3A4).

No products indexed under this heading.

Fluphenazine Enanthate (Some azoles, including posaconazole, have been associated with prolongation of the QT interval on the electrocardiogram. Posaconazole should not be administered with drugs that are known to prolong the QTc interval and are metabolized through CYP3A4).

No products indexed under this heading.

Fluphenazine Hydrochloride (Some azoles, including posaconazole, have been associated with prolongation of the QT interval on the electrocardiogram. Posaconazole should not be administered with drugs that are known to prolong the QTc interval and are metabolized through CYP3A4).

No products indexed under this heading.

Fluvastatin Sodium (It is recommended that dose reduction of statins metabolized through CYP3A4 be considered during co-administration. Increased statin concentrations in plasma can be associated with rhabdomyolysis). Products include:

Lescol Capsules 2268
Lescol XL Tablets 2268

Fosphenytoin Sodium (Co-administration of posaconazole with phenytoin may result in lower plasma concentrations of posaconazole. Avoid concomitant use unless the benefits outweigh the risks. Frequent monitoring of phenytoin concentrations should be performed while co-administered with posaconazole and dose reduction of phenytoin should be considered).

No products indexed under this heading.

Glipizide (Posaconazole administration with glipizide does not require a dose adjustment in either drug, however glucose concentrations decreased in some healthy volunteers administered the combination. Therefore, glucose concentrations should be monitored in accordance with the current standard of care for patients with diabetes when posaconazole is co-administered with glipizide).

No products indexed under this heading.

Halofantrine (Co-administration of the CYP3A4 substrate halofantrine with posaconazole is contraindicated since it may result in increased plasma concentrations of halofantrine, leading to QTc prolongation and rare occurrences of torsades de pointes).

No products indexed under this heading.

Halofantrine Hydrochloride (Co-administration of the CYP3A4 substrate halofantrine with posaconazole is contraindicated since it may result in increased plasma concentrations of halofantrine, leading to QTc prolongation and rare occurrences of torsades de pointes).

No products indexed under this heading.

Haloperidol (Some azoles, including posaconazole, have been associated with prolongation of the QT interval on the electrocardiogram. Posaconazole should not be administered with drugs that are known to prolong the QTc interval and are metabolized through CYP3A4).

No products indexed under this heading.

Haloperidol Decanoate (Some azoles, including posaconazole, have been associated with prolongation of the QT interval on the electrocardiogram. Posaconazole should not be administered with drugs that are known to prolong the QTc interval and are metabolized through CYP3A4).

No products indexed under this heading.

Haloperidol Lactate (A clinical study in healthy volunteers indicates that posaconazole is a strong CYP3A4 inhibitor. Therefore, plasma concentrations of drugs predominantly metabolized by CYP3A4 may be increased by posaconazole).

No products indexed under this heading.

Hydroxyzine Hydrochloride (Some azoles, including posaconazole, have been associated with prolongation of the QT interval on the electrocardiogram. Posaconazole should not be administered with drugs that are known to prolong the QTc interval and are metabolized through CYP3A4).

No products indexed under this heading.

Hypericum (Posaconazole is a substrate for p-glycoprotein (P-gp) efflux. Therefore, inducers of p-glycoprotein may affect posaconazole plasma concentrations). Products include:

Satieté Tablets 640

Hypericum Perforatum (Posaconazole is a substrate for p-glycoprotein (P-gp) efflux. Therefore, inducers of p-glycoprotein may affect posaconazole plasma concentrations).

No products indexed under this heading.

Imipramine Hydrochloride (Some azoles, including posaconazole, have been associated with prolongation of the QT interval on the electrocardiogram. Posaconazole should not be administered with drugs that are known to prolong the QTc interval and are metabolized through CYP3A4).

No products indexed under this heading.

Imipramine Pamoate (Some azoles, including posaconazole, have been associated with prolongation of the QT interval on the electrocardiogram. Posaconazole should not be administered with drugs that are known to prolong the QTc interval and are metabolized through CYP3A4).

No products indexed under this heading.

Indinavir Sulfate (A clinical study in healthy volunteers indicates that posaconazole is a strong CYP3A4 inhibitor. Therefore, plasma concentrations of drugs predominantly metabolized by CYP3A4 may be increased by posaconazole). Products include:

Crixivan Capsules 1979

Isocarboxazid (Some azoles, including posaconazole, have been associated with prolongation of the QT interval on the electrocardiogram. Posaconazole should not be administered with drugs that are known to prolong the QTc interval and are metabolized through CYP3A4). Products include:

Marplan Tablets 3177

Isradipine (Frequent monitoring for adverse events and toxicity related to calcium channel blockers which are metabolized through CYP3A4 is recommended during co-administration. Dose reduction of calcium channel blockers which are metabolized through CYP3A4 may be needed). Products include:

DynaCirc CR Controlled Release Tablets 1407

Itraconazole (A clinical study in healthy volunteers indicates that posaconazole is a strong CYP3A4 inhibitor. Therefore, plasma concentrations of drugs predominantly metabolized by CYP3A4 may be increased by posaconazole).

No products indexed under this heading.

Ixabepilone (A clinical study in healthy volunteers indicates that posaconazole is a strong CYP3A4 inhibitor. Therefore, plasma concentrations of drugs predominantly metabolized by CYP3A4 may be increased by posaconazole). Products include:

Ixempra Kit for Injection 915

Ketoconazole (A clinical study in healthy volunteers indicates that posaconazole is a strong CYP3A4 inhibitor. Therefore, plasma concentrations of drugs predominantly metabolized by CYP3A4 may be increased by posaconazole). Products include:

Extina Foam, 2% 3057
Nizoral A-D Shampoo 1901

Levonorgestrel (A clinical study in healthy volunteers indicates that posaconazole is a strong CYP3A4 inhibitor. Therefore, plasma concentrations of drugs predominantly metabolized by CYP3A4 may be increased by posaconazole). Products include:

Climara Pro Transdermal System 768
Lybrel Tablets 3204
Mirena Intrauterine System 779
Plan B Tablets 1044
Seasonique Tablets 1046

Lidocaine (A clinical study in healthy volunteers indicates that posaconazole is a strong CYP3A4 inhibitor. Therefore, plasma concentrations of drugs predominantly metabolized by CYP3A4 may be increased by posaconazole). Products include:

Lidoderm Patch 1114

Lidocaine Hydrochloride (Some azoles, including posaconazole, have been associated with prolongation of the QT interval on the electrocardiogram. Posaconazole should not be administered with drugs that are known to prolong the QTc interval and are metabolized through CYP3A4).

No products indexed under this heading.

Lithium Carbonate (Some azoles, including posaconazole, have been associated with prolongation of the QT interval on the electrocardiogram. Posaconazole should not be administered with drugs that are known to prolong the QTc interval and are metabolized through CYP3A4).

No products indexed under this heading.

Lithium Citrate (Some azoles, including posaconazole, have been associated with prolongation of the QT interval on the electrocardiogram. Posaconazole should not be administered with drugs that are known to prolong the QTc interval and are metabolized through CYP3A4).

No products indexed under this heading.

Lorazepam (Some azoles, including posaconazole, have been associated with prolongation of the QT interval on the electrocardiogram. Posaconazole should not be administered with drugs that are known to prolong the QTc interval and are metabolized through CYP3A4).

No products indexed under this heading.

Lovastatin (It is recommended that dose reduction of statins metabolized through CYP3A4 be considered during co-administration. Increased statin concentrations in plasma can be associated with rhabdomyolysis). Products include:

Advicor Tablets 402
Mevacor Tablets 2063

Loxapine Hydrochloride (Some azoles, including posaconazole, have been associated with prolongation of the QT interval on the electrocardiogram. Posaconazole should not be administered with drugs that are known to prolong the QTc interval and are metabolized through CYP3A4).

No products indexed under this heading.

Loxapine Succinate (Some azoles, including posaconazole, have been associated with prolongation of the QT interval on the electrocardiogram. Posaconazole should not be administered with drugs that are known to prolong the QTc interval and are metabolized through CYP3A4).

No products indexed under this heading.

Maprotiline Hydrochloride (Some azoles, including posaconazole, have been associated with prolongation of the QT interval on the electrocardiogram. Posaconazole should not be administered with drugs that are known to prolong the QTc interval and are metabolized through CYP3A4).

No products indexed under this heading.

Meprobamate (Some azoles, including posaconazole, have been associated with prolongation of the QT interval on the electrocardiogram. Posaconazole should not be administered with drugs that are known to prolong the QTc interval and are metabolized through CYP3A4).
No products indexed under this heading.

Mesoridazine Besylate (Some azoles, including posaconazole, have been associated with prolongation of the QT interval on the electrocardiogram. Posaconazole should not be administered with drugs that are known to prolong the QTc interval and are metabolized through CYP3A4).
No products indexed under this heading.

Mestranol (A clinical study in healthy volunteers indicates that posaconazole is a strong CYP3A4 inhibitor. Therefore, plasma concentrations of drugs predominantly metabolized by CYP3A4 may be increased by posaconazole).
No products indexed under this heading.

Methadone Hydrochloride (A clinical study in healthy volunteers indicates that posaconazole is a strong CYP3A4 inhibitor. Therefore, plasma concentrations of drugs predominantly metabolized by CYP3A4 may be increased by posaconazole).
No products indexed under this heading.

Methylergonovine Maleate (Co-administration of posaconazole with ergot alkaloids is contraindicated. Posaconazole may increase the plasma concentrations of ergot alkaloids which may lead to ergotism).
No products indexed under this heading.

Methysergide Maleate (Co-administration of posaconazole with ergot alkaloids is contraindicated. Posaconazole may increase the plasma concentrations of ergot alkaloids which may lead to ergotism).
No products indexed under this heading.

Mexiletine Hydrochloride (Some azoles, including posaconazole, have been associated with prolongation of the QT interval on the electrocardiogram. Posaconazole should not be administered with drugs that are known to prolong the QTc interval and are metabolized through CYP3A4).
No products indexed under this heading.

Mibefradil Dihydrochloride (Frequent monitoring for adverse events and toxicity related to calcium channel blockers which are metabolized through CYP3A4 is recommended during co-administration. Dose reduction of calcium channel blockers which are metabolized through CYP3A4 may be needed).
No products indexed under this heading.

Midazolam Hydrochloride (Frequent monitoring of adverse effects of benzodiazepines metabolized by CYP3A4 should be performed and dose reduction of these benzodiazepines should be considered during co-administration with posaconazole).
No products indexed under this heading.

Molindone Hydrochloride (Some azoles, including posaconazole, have been associated with prolongation of the QT interval on the electrocardiogram. Posaconazole should not be administered with drugs that are known to prolong the QTc interval and are metabolized through CYP3A4). Products include:
Moban Tablets **1116**

Nefazodone Hydrochloride (A clinical study in healthy volunteers indicates that posaconazole is a strong CYP3A4 inhibitor. Therefore, plasma concentrations of drugs predominantly metabolized by CYP3A4 may be increased by posaconazole).
No products indexed under this heading.

Nelfinavir Mesylate (A clinical study in healthy volunteers indicates that posaconazole is a strong CYP3A4 inhibitor. Therefore, plasma concentrations of drugs predominantly metabolized by CYP3A4 may be increased by posaconazole).
No products indexed under this heading.

Nicardipine Hydrochloride (Frequent monitoring for adverse events and toxicity related to calcium channel blockers which are metabolized through CYP3A4 is recommended during co-administration. Dose reduction of calcium channel blockers which are metabolized through CYP3A4 may be needed). Products include:
Cardene I.V. **1093**

Nifedipine (Frequent monitoring for adverse events and toxicity related to calcium channel blockers which are metabolized through CYP3A4 is recommended during co-administration. Dose reduction of calcium channel blockers which are metabolized through CYP3A4 may be needed).
No products indexed under this heading.

Nimodipine (Frequent monitoring for adverse events and toxicity related to calcium channel blockers which are metabolized through CYP3A4 is recommended during co-administration. Dose reduction of calcium channel blockers which are metabolized through CYP3A4 may be needed). Products include:
Nimotop Capsules **790**

Nisoldipine (Frequent monitoring for adverse events and toxicity related to calcium channel blockers which are metabolized through CYP3A4 is recommended during co-administration. Dose reduction of calcium channel blockers which are metabolized through CYP3A4 may be needed). Products include:
Sular Extended Release Tablets **2975**

Nitrendipine (A clinical study in healthy volunteers indicates that posaconazole is a strong CYP3A4 inhibitor. Therefore, plasma concentrations of drugs predominantly metabolized by CYP3A4 may be increased by posaconazole).
No products indexed under this heading.

Norethindrone (A clinical study in healthy volunteers indicates that posaconazole is a strong CYP3A4 inhibitor. Therefore, plasma concentrations of drugs predominantly metabolized by CYP3A4 may be increased by posaconazole). Products include:
Ortho Micronor Tablets **2446**

Norethindrone Acetate (A clinical study in healthy volunteers indicates that posaconazole is a strong CYP3A4 inhibitor. Therefore, plasma concentrations of drugs predominantly metabolized by CYP3A4 may be increased by posaconazole). Products include:
Activella Tablets **2347**

Norgestrel (A clinical study in healthy volunteers indicates that posaconazole is a strong CYP3A4 inhibitor. Therefore, plasma concentrations of drugs predominantly metabolized by CYP3A4 may be increased by posaconazole).
No products indexed under this heading.

Nortriptyline Hydrochloride (Some azoles, including posaconazole, have been associated with prolongation of the QT interval on the electrocardiogram. Posaconazole should not be administered with drugs that are known to prolong the QTc interval and are metabolized through CYP3A4).
No products indexed under this heading.

Olanzapine (Some azoles, including posaconazole, have been associated with prolongation of the QT interval on the electrocardiogram. Posaconazole should not be administered with drugs that are known to prolong the QTc interval and are metabolized through CYP3A4). Products include:
Symbyax Capsules **1871**
Zyprexa Tablets **1883**
Zyprexa IntraMuscular **1883**
Zyprexa ZYDIS Orally Disintegrating Tablets **1883**

Ondansetron (A clinical study in healthy volunteers indicates that posaconazole is a strong CYP3A4 inhibitor. Therefore, plasma concentrations of drugs predominantly metabolized by CYP3A4 may be increased by posaconazole). Products include:
Zofran ODT Orally Disintegrating Tablets **1687**

Ondansetron Hydrochloride (A clinical study in healthy volunteers indicates that posaconazole is a strong CYP3A4 inhibitor. Therefore, plasma concentrations of drugs predominantly metabolized by CYP3A4 may be increased by posaconazole). Products include:
Zofran Injection **1682**
Zofran **1687**

Oxazepam (Some azoles, including posaconazole, have been associated with prolongation of the QT interval on the electrocardiogram. Posaconazole should not be administered with drugs that are known to prolong the QTc interval and are metabolized through CYP3A4).
No products indexed under this heading.

Paclitaxel (A clinical study in healthy volunteers indicates that posaconazole is a strong CYP3A4 inhibitor. Therefore, plasma concentrations of drugs predominantly metabolized by CYP3A4 may be increased by posaconazole).
No products indexed under this heading.

Perphenazine (Some azoles, including posaconazole, have been associated with prolongation of the QT interval on the electrocardiogram. Posaconazole should not be administered with drugs that are known to prolong the QTc interval and are metabolized through CYP3A4).
No products indexed under this heading.

Phenelzine Sulfate (Some azoles, including posaconazole, have been associated with prolongation of the QT interval on the electrocardiogram. Posaconazole should not be administered with drugs that are known to prolong the QTc interval and are metabolized through CYP3A4).
No products indexed under this heading.

Phenytoin (Co-administration of posaconazole with phenytoin may result in lower plasma concentrations of posaconazole. Avoid concomitant use unless the benefits outweigh the risks. Frequent monitoring of phenytoin concentrations should be performed while co-administered with posaconazole and dose reduction of phenytoin should be considered).
No products indexed under this heading.

Phenytoin Sodium (Co-administration of posaconazole with phenytoin may result in lower plasma concentrations of posaconazole. Avoid concomitant use unless the benefits outweigh the risks. Frequent monitoring of phenytoin concentrations should be performed while co-administered with posaconazole and dose reduction of phenytoin should be considered). Products include:
Phenytek Capsules **2192**

Pimozide (Co-administration of the CYP3A4 substrate pimozide with posaconazole is contraindicated since it may result in increased plasma concentrations of pimozide, leading to QTc prolongation and rare occurrences of torsades de pointes).
No products indexed under this heading.

Polyestradiol Phosphate (A clinical study in healthy volunteers indicates that posaconazole is a strong CYP3A4 inhibitor. Therefore, plasma concentrations of drugs predominantly metabolized by CYP3A4 may be increased by posaconazole).
No products indexed under this heading.

Pravastatin Sodium (It is recommended that dose reduction of statins metabolized through CYP3A4 be considered during co-administration. Increased statin concentrations in plasma can be associated with rhabdomyolysis).
No products indexed under this heading.

Prazepam (Some azoles, including posaconazole, have been associated with prolongation of the QT interval on the electrocardiogram. Posaconazole should not be administered with drugs that are known to prolong the QTc interval and are metabolized through CYP3A4).
No products indexed under this heading.

Procainamide Hydrochloride (Some azoles, including posaconazole, have been associated with prolongation of the QT interval on the electrocardiogram. Posaconazole should not be administered with drugs that are known to prolong the QTc interval and are metabolized through CYP3A4).
No products indexed under this heading.

Prochlorperazine (Some azoles, including posaconazole, have been associated with prolongation of the QT interval on the electrocardiogram. Posaconazole should not be administered with drugs that are known to prolong the QTc interval and are metabolized through CYP3A4).
No products indexed under this heading.

Promethazine Hydrochloride (Some azoles, including posaconazole, have been associated with prolongation of the QT interval on the electrocardiogram. Posaconazole should not be administered with drugs that are known to prolong the QTc interval and are metabolized through CYP3A4).
No products indexed under this heading.

Propafenone Hydrochloride (Some azoles, including posaconazole, have been associated with prolongation of the QT interval on the electrocardiogram. Posaconazole should not be administered with drugs that are known to prolong the QTc interval and are metabolized through CYP3A4). Products include:
Rythmol Tablets **1586**
Rythmol SR Capsules **1590**

Protriptyline Hydrochloride (Some azoles, including posaconazole, have been associated with prolongation of the QT interval on the electrocardiogram. Posaconazole should not be administered with drugs that are known to prolong the QTc interval and are metabolized through CYP3A4).
No products indexed under this heading.

Quetiapine Fumarate (Some azoles, including posaconazole, have been associated with prolongation of the QT interval on the electrocardiogram. Posaconazole should not be administered with drugs that are known to prolong the QTc interval and are metabolized through CYP3A4).
No products indexed under this heading.

Quinidine (Co-administration of the CYP3A4 substrate quinidine with posaconazole is contraindicated since it may result in increased plasma concentrations of quinidine, leading to QTc prolongation and rare occurrences of torsades de pointes).
No products indexed under this heading.

Quinidine Gluconate (Some azoles, including posaconazole, have been associated with prolongation of the QT interval on the electrocardiogram. Posaconazole should not be administered with drugs that are known to prolong the QTc interval and are metabolized through CYP3A4).
No products indexed under this heading.

Quinidine Hydrochloride (Co-administration of the CYP3A4 substrate quinidine with posaconazole is contraindicated since it may result in increased plasma concentrations of quinidine, leading to QTc prolongation and rare occurrences of torsades de pointes).
No products indexed under this heading.

Quinidine Polygalacturonate (Some azoles, including posaconazole, have been associated with prolongation of the QT interval on the electrocardiogram. Posaconazole should not be administered with drugs that are known to prolong the QTc interval and are metabolized through CYP3A4).
No products indexed under this heading.

Quinidine Sulfate (Some azoles, including posaconazole, have been associated with prolongation of the QT interval on the electrocardiogram. Posaconazole should not be administered with drugs that are known to prolong the QTc interval and are metabolized through CYP3A4).
No products indexed under this heading.

Rifabutin (Concomitant use of posaconazole and rifabutin should be avoided unless the benefit to the patient outweighs the risk. However, if concomitant administration is required, frequent monitoring of full blood counts and adverse events due to increased rifabutin levels (eg, uveitis, leukopenia) is recommended. Co-administration may also result in lower plasma concentrations of posaconazole).
No products indexed under this heading.

Rifampicin (Posaconazole is a substrate for p-glycoprotein (P-gp) efflux. Therefore, inducers of p-glycoprotein may affect posaconazole plasma concentrations).
No products indexed under this heading.

Risperidone (Some azoles, including posaconazole, have been associated with prolongation of the QT interval on the electrocardiogram. Posaconazole should not be administered with drugs that are known to prolong the QTc interval and are metabolized through CYP3A4). Products include:
Risperdal Consta Long-Acting Injection **1753**

Ritonavir (Frequent monitoring of adverse effects and toxicity of ritonavir should be performed during co-administration with posaconazole). Products include:
Kaletra **452**
Norvir **489**

Rosuvastatin Calcium (It is recommended that dose reduction of statins metabolized through CYP3A4 be considered during co-administration. Increased statin concentrations in plasma can be associated with rhabdomyolysis). Products include:
Crestor Tablets **677**

Saquinavir (A clinical study in healthy volunteers indicates that posaconazole is a strong CYP3A4 inhibitor. Therefore, plasma concentrations of drugs predominantly metabolized by CYP3A4 may be increased by posaconazole).
No products indexed under this heading.

Saquinavir Mesylate (A clinical study in healthy volunteers indicates that posaconazole is a strong CYP3A4 inhibitor. Therefore, plasma concentrations of drugs predominantly metabolized by CYP3A4 may be increased by posaconazole).
No products indexed under this heading.

Sertraline Hydrochloride (A clinical study in healthy volunteers indicates that posaconazole is a strong CYP3A4 inhibitor. Therefore, plasma concentrations of drugs predominantly metabolized by CYP3A4 may be increased by posaconazole).
No products indexed under this heading.

Sildenafil Citrate (A clinical study in healthy volunteers indicates that posaconazole is a strong CYP3A4 inhibitor. Therefore, plasma concentrations of drugs predominantly metabolized by CYP3A4 may be increased by posaconazole).
No products indexed under this heading.

Simvastatin (It is recommended that dose reduction of statins metabolized through CYP3A4 be considered during co-administration. Increased statin concentrations in plasma can be associated with rhabdomyolysis). Products include:
Simcor Tablets **502**
Vytorin 10/10 Tablets **2149**
Vytorin 10/10 Tablets **2939**
Vytorin 10/20 Tablets **2149**
Vytorin 10/20 Tablets **2939**
Vytorin 10/40 Tablets **2149**
Vytorin 10/40 Tablets **2939**
Vytorin 10/80 Tablets **2149**
Vytorin 10/80 Tablets **2939**
Zocor Tablets **2136**

Sirolimus (Co-administration of posaconazole with sirolimus is contraindicated. Concomitant use of posaconazole with sirolimus may increase mean Cmax and mean AUC of sirolimus). Products include:
Rapamune **3260**

Tacrolimus (Posaconazole has been shown to increase Cmax and AUC of tacrolimus significantly. At initiation of posaconazole treatment, reduce the tacrolimus dose to approximately 1/3 of the original dose. Frequent monitoring of tacrolimus whole blood trough concentrations should be performed during and at discontinuation of posaconazole treatment and the tacrolimus dose adjusted accordingly). Products include:
Prograf Capsules and Injection **622**
Protopic Ointment **628**

Tadalafil (A clinical study in healthy volunteers indicates that posaconazole is a strong CYP3A4 inhibitor. Therefore, plasma concentrations of drugs predominantly metabolized by CYP3A4 may be increased by posaconazole). Products include:
Cialis Tablets **1792**

Tamoxifen Citrate (A clinical study in healthy volunteers indicates that posaconazole is a strong CYP3A4 inhibitor. Therefore, plasma concentrations of drugs predominantly metabolized by CYP3A4 may be increased by posaconazole).
No products indexed under this heading.

Terfenadine (Co-administration of the CYP3A4 substrate terfenadine with posaconazole is contraindicated since it may result in increased plasma concentrations of terfenadine, leading to QTc prolongation and rare occurrences of torsades de pointes).
No products indexed under this heading.

Thioridazine Hydrochloride (Some azoles, including posaconazole, have been associated with prolongation of the QT interval on the electrocardiogram. Posaconazole should not be administered with drugs that are known to prolong the QTc interval and are metabolized through CYP3A4). Products include:
Thioridazine Hydrochloride Tablets **2195**

Thiothixene (Some azoles, including posaconazole, have been associated with prolongation of the QT interval on the electrocardiogram. Posaconazole should not be administered with drugs that are known to prolong the QTc interval and are metabolized through CYP3A4). Products include:
Thiothixene Capsules **2197**

Tiagabine Hydrochloride (A clinical study in healthy volunteers indicates that posaconazole is a strong CYP3A4 inhibitor. Therefore, plasma concentrations of drugs predominantly metabolized by CYP3A4 may be increased by posaconazole). Products include:
Gabitril Tablets **973**

Tocainide Hydrochloride (Some azoles, including posaconazole, have been associated with prolongation of the QT interval on the electrocardiogram. Posaconazole should not be administered with drugs that are known to prolong the QTc interval and are metabolized through CYP3A4).
No products indexed under this heading.

Tolterodine Tartrate (A clinical study in healthy volunteers indicates that posaconazole is a strong CYP3A4 inhibitor. Therefore, plasma concentrations of drugs predominantly metabolized by CYP3A4 may be increased by posaconazole).
No products indexed under this heading.

Tranylcypromine Sulfate (Some azoles, including posaconazole, have been associated with prolongation of the QT interval on the electrocardiogram. Posaconazole should not be administered with drugs that are known to prolong the QTc interval and are metabolized through CYP3A4). Products include:
Parnate Tablets **1532**

Trazodone Hydrochloride (A clinical study in healthy volunteers indicates that posaconazole is a strong CYP3A4 inhibitor. Therefore, plasma concentrations of drugs predominantly metabolized by CYP3A4 may be increased by posaconazole).
No products indexed under this heading.

Triazolam (Frequent monitoring of adverse effects of benzodiazepines metabolized by CYP3A4 should be performed and dose reduction of these benzodiazepines should be considered during co-administration with posaconazole).
No products indexed under this heading.

Trifluoperazine Hydrochloride (Some azoles, including posaconazole, have been associated with prolongation of the QT interval on the electrocardiogram. Posaconazole should not be administered with drugs that are known to prolong the QTc interval and are metabolized through CYP3A4).
No products indexed under this heading.

Trimipramine Maleate (Some azoles, including posaconazole, have been associated with prolongation of the QT interval on the electrocardiogram. Posaconazole should not be administered with drugs that are known to prolong the QTc interval and are metabolized through CYP3A4).
No products indexed under this heading.

Troleandomycin (Posaconazole is a substrate for p-glycoprotein (P-gp) efflux. Therefore, inhibitors of p-glycoprotein may affect posaconazole plasma concentrations).
No products indexed under this heading.

Vardenafil Hydrochloride (A clinical study in healthy volunteers indicates that posaconazole is a strong CYP3A4 inhibitor. Therefore, plasma concentrations of drugs predominantly metabolized by CYP3A4 may be increased by posaconazole). Products include:
Levitra Tablets 2876

Verapamil Hydrochloride (Frequent monitoring for adverse events and toxicity related to calcium channel blockers which are metabolized through CYP3A4 is recommended during co-administration. Dose reduction of calcium channel blockers which are metabolized through CYP3A4 may be needed). Products include:
Tarka Tablets 511

Vinblastine Sulfate (Posaconazole may increase the plasma concentrations of vinca alkaloids which may lead to neurotoxicity. Therefore, it is recommended that the dose adjustment of the vinca alkaloid be considered).
No products indexed under this heading.

Vincristine Sulfate (Posaconazole may increase the plasma concentrations of vinca alkaloids which may lead to neurotoxicity. Therefore, it is recommended that the dose adjustment of the vinca alkaloid be considered).
No products indexed under this heading.

Vinorelbine Tartrate (Posaconazole may increase the plasma concentrations of vinca alkaloids which may lead to neurotoxicity. Therefore, it is recommended that the dose adjustment of the vinca alkaloid be considered).
No products indexed under this heading.

Warfarin Sodium (A clinical study in healthy volunteers indicates that posaconazole is a strong CYP3A4 inhibitor. Therefore, plasma concentrations of drugs predominantly metabolized by CYP3A4 may be increased by posaconazole).
No products indexed under this heading.

Ziprasidone Hydrochloride (Some azoles, including posaconazole, have been associated with prolongation of the QT interval on the electrocardiogram. Posaconazole should not be administered with drugs that are known to prolong the QTc interval and are metabolized through CYP3A4). Products include:
Geodon Capsules 2520

NT-KINASE DIETARY SUPPLEMENT
(Coenzyme Q-10, L-Arginine, Minerals, Niacin, Superoxide Dismutase)........ 995
None cited in PDR database.

NU-IRON 150 CAPSULES
(Polysaccharide Iron Complex) 2165
None cited in PDR database.

NUTROPIN FOR INJECTION
(Somatropin) 1208
May interact with corticosteroids, phenytoin, and certain other agents. Compounds in these categories include:

Betamethasone Acetate (Excessive glucocorticoid therapy will inhibit the growth-promoting effect of human growth hormone).
No products indexed under this heading.

Betamethasone Sodium Phosphate (Excessive glucocorticoid therapy will inhibit the growth-promoting effect of human growth hormone).
No products indexed under this heading.

Budesonide (Excessive glucocorticoid therapy will inhibit the growth-promoting effect of human growth hormone). Products include:
Pulmicort Flexhaler 654
Symbicort 80/4.5 Inhalation Aerosol 659
Symbicort 160/4.5 Inhalation Aerosol 659

Carbamazepine (Limited published data suggests that growth hormone treatment increased CYP450 mediated antipyrine clearance in man; therefore, growth hormone administration may alter the clearance of compounds known to be metabolized by CYP450 liver enzymes, such as anticonvulsanta including carbamazepine). Products include:
Carbatrol Capsules 3019
Equetro Extended-Release Capsules 3174

Ciclesonide (Excessive glucocorticoid therapy will inhibit the growth-promoting effect of human growth hormone). Products include:
Alvesco Inhalation Aerosol 2985
Omnaris Nasal Spray 2998

Cortisone Acetate (Excessive glucocorticoid therapy will inhibit the growth-promoting effect of human growth hormone).
No products indexed under this heading.

Cyclosporine (Limited published data suggests that growth hormone treatment increases CYP450 mediated antipyrine clearance in man, therefore, growth hormone administration may alter the clearance of compounds known to be metabolized by CYP450 liver enzymes, such as cyclosporine). Products include:
Gengraf Capsules 435
Neoral Oral Solution 2280
Neoral Soft Gelatin Capsules 2280
Restasis Ophthalmic Emulsion 557
Sandimmune 2296

Dexamethasone (Excessive glucocorticoid therapy will inhibit the growth-promoting effect of human growth hormone). Products include:
Ciprodex Otic Suspension 541

Dexamethasone Acetate (Excessive glucocorticoid therapy will inhibit the growth-promoting effect of human growth hormone).
No products indexed under this heading.

Dexamethasone Sodium Phosphate (Excessive glucocorticoid therapy will inhibit the growth-promoting effect of human growth hormone).
No products indexed under this heading.

Fludrocortisone Acetate (Excessive glucocorticoid therapy will inhibit the growth-promoting effect of human growth hormone).
No products indexed under this heading.

Flunisolide (Excessive glucocorticoid therapy will inhibit the growth-promoting effect of human growth hormone). Products include:
Aerobid/Aerobid-M 1153

Fluticasone Propionate (Excessive glucocorticoid therapy will inhibit the growth-promoting effect of human growth hormone). Products include:
Advair Diskus 100/50 1276
Advair Diskus 250/50 1276
Advair Diskus 500/50 1276
Advair HFA 45/21 Inhalation Aerosol 1288
Advair HFA 115/21 Inhalation Aerosol 1288
Advair HFA 230/21 Inhalation Aerosol 1288
Flonase Nasal Spray 1431
Flovent Diskus 50 mcg 1435

Fluticasone Propionate HFA (Excessive glucocorticoid therapy will inhibit the growth-promoting effect of human growth hormone). Products include:
Flovent HFA 1440

Fosphenytoin Sodium (Limited published data suggests that growth hormone treatment increases CYP450 mediated antipyrine clearance in man; therefore, growth hormone administration may alter the clearance of compounds known to be metabolized by CYP450 liver enzymes, such as anticonvulsants, including phenytoin).
No products indexed under this heading.

Hydrocortisone (Excessive glucocorticoid therapy will inhibit the growth-promoting effect of human growth hormone).
No products indexed under this heading.

Hydrocortisone Acetate (Excessive glucocorticoid therapy will inhibit the growth-promoting effect of human growth hormone). Products include:
Analpram-HC 1140
Pramosone 1141

Hydrocortisone Sodium Phosphate (Excessive glucocorticoid therapy will inhibit the growth-promoting effect of human growth hormone).
No products indexed under this heading.

Hydrocortisone Sodium Succinate (Excessive glucocorticoid therapy will inhibit the growth-promoting effect of human growth hormone).
No products indexed under this heading.

Methylprednisolone Acetate (Excessive glucocorticoid therapy will inhibit the growth-promoting effect of human growth hormone).
No products indexed under this heading.

Methylprednisolone Sodium Succinate (Excessive glucocorticoid therapy will inhibit the growth-promoting effect of human growth hormone).
No products indexed under this heading.

Mometasone Furoate (Excessive glucocorticoid therapy will inhibit the growth-promoting effect of human growth hormone). Products include:
Asmanex Twisthaler 2797
Elocon Cream 0.1% 2840
Elocon Lotion 0.1% 2841
Elocon Ointment 0.1% 2842

Mometasone Furoate Monohydrate (Excessive glucocorticoid therapy will inhibit the growth-promoting effect of human growth hormone). Products include:
Nasonex Nasal Spray 2883

Phenytoin (Limited published data suggests that growth hormone treatment increases CYP450 mediated antipyrine clearance in man; therefore, growth hormone administration may alter the clearance of compounds known to be metabolized by CYP450 liver enzymes, such as anticonvulsants, including phenytoin).
No products indexed under this heading.

Phenytoin Sodium (Limited published data suggests that growth hormone treatment increases CYP450 mediated antipyrine clearance in man; therefore, growth hormone administration may alter the clearance of compounds known to be metabolized by CYP450 liver enzymes, such as anticonvulsants, including phenytoin). Products include:
Phenytek Capsules 2192

Prednisolone Acetate (Excessive glucocorticoid therapy will inhibit the growth-promoting effect of human growth hormone). Products include:
Pred Forte Ophthalmic Suspension .... ⊙227
Pred Mild Ophthalmic Suspension .... ⊙230
Pred-G Ophthalmic Ointment .... ⊙229
Pred-G Ophthalmic Suspension .... ⊙228

Prednisolone Sodium Phosphate (Excessive glucocorticoid therapy will inhibit the growth-promoting effect of human growth hormone).
No products indexed under this heading.

Prednisolone Tebutate (Excessive glucocorticoid therapy will inhibit the growth-promoting effect of human growth hormone).
No products indexed under this heading.

Prednisone (Excessive glucocorticoid therapy will inhibit the growth-promoting effect of human growth hormone).
No products indexed under this heading.

Triamcinolone (Excessive glucocorticoid therapy will inhibit the growth-promoting effect of human growth hormone).
No products indexed under this heading.

Triamcinolone Acetonide (Excessive glucocorticoid therapy will inhibit the growth-promoting effect of human growth hormone). Products include:
Azmacort Inhalation Aerosol 407
Nasacort AQ Nasal Spray 2765
Triesence Injectable Suspension .... ⊙209

Triamcinolone Diacetate (Excessive glucocorticoid therapy will inhibit the growth-promoting effect of human growth hormone).
No products indexed under this heading.

Triamcinolone Hexacetonide (Excessive glucocorticoid therapy will inhibit the growth-promoting effect of human growth hormone).
No products indexed under this heading.

NUTROPIN AQ INJECTION
(Somatropin) 1212
See Nutropin for Injection

NUTROPIN AQ NUSPIN INJECTION
(Somatropin) 1212
See Nutropin for Injection

NUTROPIN AQ PEN
(Somatropin) 1212
See Nutropin for Injection

NUTROPIN AQ PEN CARTRIDGE
(Somatropin) 1212
See Nutropin for Injection

NUVARING
(Ethinyl Estradiol, Etonogestrel) 2897
May interact with azole antifungals, barbiturates, cytochrome p450 3a4 inhibitors (selected), anticonvulsants, protease inhibitors, theophyllines, and certain other agents. Compounds in these categories include:

Acetaminophen (Acetaminophen may increase plasma ethinyl estradiol levels. Decreased plasma concentrations of acetaminophen have been noted when administered with oral contraceptives). Products include:
Benadryl Allergy & Cold Kapgels 1895
Benadryl Allergy & Sinus Headache Kapgels 1895
Benadryl Severe Allergy & Sinus Headache Caplets 1897
Lortab 5/500 Tablets 3143
Lortab 7.5/500 Tablets 3144
Lortab 10/500 Tablets 3144
Percocet Tablets 1127
Sinutab Sinus Caplets 1905
Sudafed PE Cold & Cough Caplets 1907
Sudafed PE Nighttime Cold Caplets 1907
Sudafed PE Severe Cold Caplets 1908
Sudafed PE Sinus Headache Caplets 1908
Regular Strength Tylenol Tablets 1915
Tylenol 8 Hour Extended Release Caplets 1915
Extra Strength Tylenol Caplets, Cool Caplets, and EZ Tabs 1915
Extra Strength Tylenol Adult Rapid Blast Liquid 1915
Extra Strength Tylenol PM Caplets, Geltabs, Liquid, and Rapid Release Gels 1915
Extra Strength Tylenol Rapid Release Gels 1915
Tylenol with Codeine Tablets 2427
Tylenol Allergy Multi-Symptom Caplets with Cool Burst and Rapid Release Gelcaps 1916
Tylenol Allergy Multi-Symptom Nighttime Caplets with Cool Burst 1916
Tylenol Severe Allergy Caplets 1916
Tylenol Arthritis Pain Extended Release Geltabs/Caplets 1915
Tylenol Chest Congestion Caplets with Cool Burst 1910
Tylenol Chest Congestion Liquid with Cool Burst 1910
Children's Tylenol Plus Cold Suspension Liquid 1912
Children's Tylenol Plus Cold & Allergy Suspension Liquid 1914
Children's Tylenol Plus Cough & Runny Nose Suspension Liquid 1912
Children's Tylenol Plus Cough & Sore Throat Suspension Liquid 1912
Children's Tylenol Plus Flu Suspension Liquid 1914
Children's Tylenol Suspension Liquid 1909
Children's Tylenol Meltaways 1909
Children's Tylenol Plus Multi-Symptom Cold Suspension Liquid 1912
Tylenol Cold Severe Congestion Daytime Caplets with Cool Burst 1912
Tylenol Cold Head Congestion Daytime Caplets with Cool Burst 1910
Tylenol Cold Head Congestion Nighttime Caplets with Cool Burst 1910
Tylenol Cold Head Congestion Severe Daytime Caplets with Cool Burst 1910
Tylenol Cold Multi-Symptom Daytime Caplets with Cool Burst and Rapid Release Gels 1913
Tylenol Cold Multi-Symptom Daytime Liquid with Citrus Burst ... 1913
Tylenol Cold Multi-Symptom Nighttime Caplets with Cool Burst 1913
Tylenol Cold Multi-Symptom Nighttime Liquid with Cool Burst ... 1913
Tylenol Cold Multi-Symptom Severe Caplets with Cool Burst..... 1913
Tylenol Cold Multi-Symptom Severe Daytime Liquid with Citrus Burst 1913
Tylenol Cough & Sore Throat Daytime Liquid with Cool Burst...... 1918
Tylenol Cough & Sore Throat Nighttime Liquid with Cool Burst ... 1918
Concentrated Tylenol Infants' Drops 1909
Jr. Tylenol Meltaways 1909
Tylenol Sinus Congestion & Pain Daytime Caplets with Cool Burst and Gelcaps 1917
Tylenol Sinus Congestion & Pain Nighttime Caplets with Cool Burst 1917
Tylenol Sinus Congestion & Pain Severe Caplets with Cool Burst..... 1917
Tylenol Sinus Severe Congestion Caplets with Cool Burst 1917
Tylenol Sore Throat Daytime Liquid with Cool Burst 1918
Tylenol Sore Throat Nighttime Liquid with Cool Burst 1918
Women's Tylenol Menstrual Relief Caplets 1919
Vicks DayQuil Cold & Flu Multi-Symptom Relief 616
Vicks DayQuil LiquiCaps 2567
Vicks DayQuil Liquid 2567
Vicks DayQuil Multi-Symptom Cold/Flu Relief 2567
Vicks NyQuil Cold & Flu Multi-Symptom Relief 617
Vicks NyQuil LiquiCaps 2567
Vicks NyQuil Liquid 2567
Vicks NyQuil Multi-Symptom Cold/Flu Relief 2567
Vicodin Tablets 529
Vicodin ES Tablets 530
Vicodin HP Tablets 531
Zydone Tablets 1132

Acetazolamide (CYP3A4 inhibitors may increase plasma hormone levels).
No products indexed under this heading.

Amiodarone Hydrochloride (CYP3A4 inhibitors may increase plasma hormone levels).
No products indexed under this heading.

Amprenavir (Several of the anti-HIV protease inhibitors have been studied with co-administration of oral combination hormonal contraceptives; significant changes (increases and decreases) in the mean AUC of the estrogen and progestin have been noted in some cases. The efficacy and safety of oral contraceptive products may be affected; it is not known whether this applies to NuvaRing).
No products indexed under this heading.

Anastrozole (CYP3A4 inhibitors may increase plasma hormone levels). Products include:
Arimidex Tablets 672

Aprepitant (CYP3A4 inhibitors may increase plasma hormone levels). Products include:
Emend Capsules 1992

Aprobarbital (Contraceptive effectiveness may be reduced when hormonal contraceptives are co-administered with drugs that increase the metabolism of contraceptive steroids. This could result in unintended pregnancy or breakthrough bleeding. Women may need to use anadditional contraceptive method).
No products indexed under this heading.

Ascorbic Acid (Ascorbic acid may increase plasma ethinyl estradiol levels).
No products indexed under this heading.

Atazanavir (CYP3A4 inhibitors may increase plasma hormone levels).
No products indexed under this heading.

Atazanavir Sulfate (CYP3A4 inhibitors may increase plasma hormone levels). Products include:
Reyataz Capsules 3299

Atorvastatin Calcium (Co-administration of atorvastatin and certain oral contraceptives containing ethinyl estradiol increase AUC values for ethinyl estradiol by approximately 20%). Products include:
Lipitor Tablets 2501

Butabarbital (Contraceptive effectiveness may be reduced when hormonal contraceptives are co-administered with drugs that increase the metabolism of contraceptive steroids. This could result in unintended pregnancy or breakthrough bleeding. Women may need to use anadditional contraceptive method).
No products indexed under this heading.

Butalbital (Contraceptive effectiveness may be reduced when hormonal contraceptives are co-administered with drugs that increase the metabolism of contraceptive steroids. This could result in unintended pregnancy or breakthrough bleeding. Women may need to use anadditional contraceptive method).
No products indexed under this heading.

Carbamazepine (Contraceptive effectiveness may be reduced when hormonal contraceptives are co-administered with some anticonvulsants and other drugs that increase the metabolism of contraceptive steroids. This could result in unintended pregnancy or breakthrough bleeding. Women may need to use an additional contraceptive method). Products include:
Carbatrol Capsules 3019
Equetro Extended-Release Capsules 3174

Cimetidine (CYP3A4 inhibitors may increase plasma hormone levels).
No products indexed under this heading.

Cimetidine Hydrochloride (CYP3A4 inhibitors may increase plasma hormone levels).
No products indexed under this heading.

Ciprofloxacin (CYP3A4 inhibitors may increase plasma hormone levels). Products include:
Cipro I.V. 2817
Cipro Oral Suspension 2810
Cipro XR Tablets 2823
Ciprodex Otic Suspension 541

Clarithromycin (CYP3A4 inhibitors may increase plasma hormone levels). Products include:
Biaxin/Biaxin XL 411

Clofibric Acid (Increased clearance of clofibric acid have been noted when administered with oral contraceptives).
No products indexed under this heading.

Clotrimazole (Contraceptive effectiveness may be reduced when hormonal contraceptives are co-administered with some antifungals and other drugs that increase the metabolism of contraceptive steroids. This could result in unintended pregnancy or breakthrough bleeding. Women may need to use an additional contraceptive method). Products include:
Lotrisone 2881

Cyclosporine (Combination hormonal contraceptives containing some synthetic estrogens may inhibit the metabolism of other compounds. Increased plasma concentrations of cyclosporine have been reported with concomitant administration of oral contraceptives). Products include:
Gengraf Capsules 435
Neoral Oral Solution 2280
Neoral Soft Gelatin Capsules 2280
Restasis Ophthalmic Emulsion 557
Sandimmune 2296

Dalfopristin (CYP3A4 inhibitors may increase plasma hormone levels).
No products indexed under this heading.

Danazol (CYP3A4 inhibitors may increase plasma hormone levels).
No products indexed under this heading.

Darunavir (Several of the anti-HIV protease inhibitors have been studied with co-administration of oral combination hormonal contraceptives; significant changes (increases and decreases) in the mean AUC of the estrogen and progestin have been noted in some cases. The efficacy and safety of oral contraceptive products may be affected; it is not known whether this applies to NuvaRing).
No products indexed under this heading.

Delavirdine Mesylate (CYP3A4 inhibitors may increase plasma hormone levels).
No products indexed under this heading.

Diltiazem Hydrochloride (CYP3A4 inhibitors may increase plasma hormone levels). Products include:
Cardizem LA Extended Release Tablets 421

Diltiazem Maleate (CYP3A4 inhibitors may increase plasma hormone levels).
No products indexed under this heading.

Divalproex Sodium (Contraceptive effectiveness may be reduced when hormonal contraceptives are co-administered with some anticonvulsants and other drugs that increase the metabolism of contraceptive steroids. This could result in unintended pregnancy or breakthrough bleeding. Women may need to use an additional contraceptive method). Products include:
Depakote ER Tablets 423

Efavirenz (CYP3A4 inhibitors may increase plasma hormone levels). Products include:
Atripla Tablets 938
Sustiva Capsules 930
Sustiva Tablets 930

Erythromycin (CYP3A4 inhibitors may increase plasma hormone levels).
No products indexed under this heading.

Erythromycin Estolate (CYP3A4 inhibitors may increase plasma hormone levels).
No products indexed under this heading.

Erythromycin Ethylsuccinate (CYP3A4 inhibitors may increase plasma hormone levels). Products include:
E.E.S. 433
EryPed 431

Erythromycin Gluceptate (CYP3A4 inhibitors may increase plasma hormone levels).
No products indexed under this heading.

Erythromycin Lactobionate (CYP3A4 inhibitors may increase plasma hormone levels).
No products indexed under this heading.

Erythromycin Stearate (CYP3A4 inhibitors may increase plasma hormone levels).
No products indexed under this heading.

Esomeprazole Magnesium (CYP3A4 inhibitors may increase plasma hormone levels). Products include:
Nexium Delayed-Release Capsules 645
Nexium Delayed-Release Oral Suspension 645

Ethosuximide (Contraceptive effectiveness may be reduced when hormonal contraceptives are co-administered with some anticonvulsants and other drugs that increase the metabolism of contraceptive steroids. This could result in unintended pregnancy or breakthrough bleeding. Women may need to use an additional contraceptive method).
No products indexed under this heading.

Ethotoin (Contraceptive effectiveness may be reduced when hormonal contraceptives are co-administered with some anticonvulsants and other drugs that increase the metabolism of contraceptive steroids. This could result in unintended pregnancy or breakthrough bleeding. Women may need to use an additional contraceptive method).
No products indexed under this heading.

Felbamate (Contraceptive effectiveness may be reduced when hormonal contraceptives are co-administered with some anticonvulsants and other drugs that increase the metabolism of contraceptive steroids. This could result in unintended pregnancy or breakthrough bleeding. Women may need to use an additional contraceptive method).
No products indexed under this heading.

Fluconazole (Contraceptive effectiveness may be reduced when hormonal contraceptives are co-administered with some antifungals and other drugs that increase the metabolism of contraceptive steroids. This could result in unintended pregnancy or breakthrough bleeding. Women may need to use an additional contraceptive method).
No products indexed under this heading.

Fluoxetine (CYP3A4 inhibitors may increase plasma hormone levels).
No products indexed under this heading.

Fluoxetine Hydrochloride (CYP3A4 inhibitors may increase plasma hormone levels). Products include:
Prozac Weekly Capsules 1852
Prozac Pulvules and Liquid 1852
Symbyax Capsules 1871

Fluvoxamine Maleate (CYP3A4 inhibitors may increase plasma hormone levels). Products include:
Luvox CR Extended-Release Capsules 1759

Fosamprenavir Calcium (Several of the anti-HIV protease inhibitors have been studied with co-administration of oral combination hormonal contraceptives; significant changes (increases and decreases) in the mean AUC of the estrogen and progestin have been noted in some cases. The efficacy and safety of oral contraceptive products may be affected; it is not known whether this applies to NuvaRing). Products include:
Lexiva Oral Suspension 1510
Lexiva Tablets 1510

Fosphenytoin (Contraceptive effectiveness may be reduced when hormonal contraceptives are co-administered with some anticonvulsants and other drugs that increase the metabolism of contraceptive steroids. This could result in unintended pregnancy or breakthrough bleeding. Women may need to use an additional contraceptive method).
No products indexed under this heading.

Fosphenytoin Sodium (Contraceptive effectiveness may be reduced when hormonal contraceptives are co-administered with some anticonvulsants and other drugs that increase the metabolism of contraceptive steroids. This could result in unintended pregnancy or breakthrough bleeding. Women may need to use an additional contraceptive method).
No products indexed under this heading.

Gabapentin (Contraceptive effectiveness may be reduced when hormonal contraceptives are co-administered with some anticonvulsants and other drugs that increase the metabolism of contraceptive steroids. This could result in unintended pregnancy or breakthrough bleeding. Women may need to use an additional contraceptive method).
No products indexed under this heading.

Griseofulvin (Contraceptive effectiveness may be reduced when hormonal contraceptives are co-administered with drugs that increase the metabolism of contraceptive steroids. This could result in unintended pregnancy or breakthrough bleeding. Women may need to use an additional contraceptive method). Products include:
Gris-PEG Tablets 2507

Hypericum (Herbal products containing St. John's Wort may induce hepatic enzymes (cytochrome P450) and p-glycoprotein transporter and may reduce the effectiveness of contraceptive steroids. This may also result in breakthrough bleeding). Products include:
Satieté Tablets .... ▣ 640

Hypericum Perforatum (Herbal products containing St. John's Wort may induce hepatic enzymes (cytochrome P450) and p-glycoprotein transporter and may reduce the effectiveness of contraceptive steroids. This may also result in breakthrough bleeding).
No products indexed under this heading.

Indinavir Sulfate (Several of the anti-HIV protease inhibitors have been studied with co-administration of oral combination hormonal contraceptives; significant changes (increases and decreases) in the mean AUC of the estrogen and progestin have been noted in some cases. The efficacy and safety of oral contraceptive products may be affected; it is not known whether this applies to NuvaRing). Products include:
Crixivan Capsules 1979

Isoniazid (CYP3A4 inhibitors may increase plasma hormone levels).
No products indexed under this heading.

Itraconazole (Contraceptive effectiveness may be reduced when hormonal contraceptives are co-administered with some antifungals and other drugs that increase the metabolism of contraceptive steroids. This could result in unintended pregnancy or breakthrough bleeding. Women may need to use an additional contraceptive method).
No products indexed under this heading.

Ketoconazole (Contraceptive effectiveness may be reduced when hormonal contraceptives are co-administered with some antifungals and other drugs that increase the metabolism of contraceptive steroids. This could result in unintended pregnancy or breakthrough bleeding. Women may need to use an additional contraceptive method). Products include:
Extina Foam, 2% 3057
Nizoral A-D Shampoo 1901

Lamotrigine (Contraceptive effectiveness may be reduced when hormonal contraceptives are co-administered with some anticonvulsants and other drugs that increase the metabolism of contraceptive steroids. This could result in unintended pregnancy or breakthrough bleeding. Women may need to use an additional contraceptive method). Products include:
Lamictal 1488

Levetiracetam (Contraceptive effectiveness may be reduced when hormonal contraceptives are co-administered with some anticonvulsants and other drugs that increase the metabolism of contraceptive steroids. This could result in unintended pregnancy or breakthrough bleeding. Women may need to use an additional contraceptive method). Products include:
Keppra Injection 3137
Keppra Oral Solution 3131
Keppra Tablets 3131

Lopinavir (Several of the anti-HIV protease inhibitors have been studied with co-administration of oral combination hormonal contraceptives; significant changes (increases and decreases) in the mean AUC of the estrogen and progestin have been noted in some cases. The efficacy and safety of oral contraceptive products may be affected; it is not known whether this applies to NuvaRing). Products include:
Kaletra 452

Loratadine (CYP3A4 inhibitors may increase plasma hormone levels).
No products indexed under this heading.

Mephenytoin (Contraceptive effectiveness may be reduced when hormonal contraceptives are co-administered with some anticonvulsants and other drugs that increase the metabolism of contraceptive steroids. This could result in unintended pregnancy or breakthrough bleeding. Women may need to use an additional contraceptive method).
No products indexed under this heading.

Mephobarbital (Contraceptive effectiveness may be reduced when hormonal contraceptives are co-administered with drugs that increase the metabolism of contraceptive steroids. This could result in unintended pregnancy or breakthrough bleeding. Women may need to use anadditional contraceptive method).
No products indexed under this heading.

Methsuximide (Contraceptive effectiveness may be reduced when hormonal contraceptives are co-administered with some anticonvulsants and other drugs that increase the metabolism of contraceptive steroids. This could result in unintended pregnancy or breakthrough bleeding. Women may need to use an additional contraceptive method).
No products indexed under this heading.

Metronidazole (CYP3A4 inhibitors may increase plasma hormone levels). Products include:
Pylera Capsules 714

Metronidazole Benzoate (CYP3A4 inhibitors may increase plasma hormone levels).
No products indexed under this heading.

Metronidazole Hydrochloride (CYP3A4 inhibitors may increase plasma hormone levels).
No products indexed under this heading.

Metronidazole Sodium (CYP3A4 inhibitors may increase plasma hormone levels).
No products indexed under this heading.

Miconazole (Contraceptive effectiveness may be reduced when hormonal contraceptives are co-administered with some antifungals and other drugs that increase the metabolism of contraceptive steroids. This could result in unintended pregnancy or breakthrough bleeding. Women may need to use an additional contraceptive method).
No products indexed under this heading.

Miconazole Nitrate (Co-administration of vaginal miconazole nitrate increases the serum concentrations of etonogestrel and ethinyl estradiol by up to 40%).
No products indexed under this heading.

Modafinil (Contraceptive effectiveness may be reduced when hormonal contraceptives are co-administered with drugs that increase the metabolism of contraceptive steroids. This could result in unintended pregnancy or breakthrough bleeding. Women may need to use an additional contraceptive method). Products include:
Provigil Tablets 977

Morphine Sulfate (Increased clearance of morphine has been noted when administered with oral contraceptives). Products include:
Avinza Capsules 1772
DepoDur Injection 1095
MS Contin Tablets 2585

Nefazodone Hydrochloride (CYP3A4 inhibitors may increase plasma hormone levels).
No products indexed under this heading.

Nelfinavir Mesylate (Several of the anti-HIV protease inhibitors have been studied with co-administration of oral combination hormonal contraceptives; significant changes (increases and decreases) in the mean AUC of the estrogen and progestin have been noted in some cases. The efficacy and safety of oral contraceptive products may be affected; it is not known whether this applies to NuvaRing).
No products indexed under this heading.

Nevirapine (CYP3A4 inhibitors may increase plasma hormone levels). Products include:
Viramune Oral Suspension 873
Viramune Tablets 873

Niacinamide (CYP3A4 inhibitors may increase plasma hormone levels). Products include:
BioLean Free Tablets 635

Nicotinamide (CYP3A4 inhibitors may increase plasma hormone levels).
No products indexed under this heading.

Nifedipine (CYP3A4 inhibitors may increase plasma hormone levels).
No products indexed under this heading.

Norfloxacin (CYP3A4 inhibitors may increase plasma hormone levels). Products include:
Noroxin Tablets 2069

Omeprazole (CYP3A4 inhibitors may increase plasma hormone levels).
No products indexed under this heading.

Oxcarbazepine (Contraceptive effectiveness may be reduced when hormonal contraceptives are co-administered with some anticonvulsants and other drugs that increase the metabolism of contraceptive steroids. This could result in unintended pregnancy or breakthrough bleeding. Women may need to use an additional contraceptive method).
No products indexed under this heading.

Oxiconazole Nitrate (Contraceptive effectiveness may be reduced when hormonal contraceptives are co-administered with some antifungals and other drugs that increase the metabolism of contraceptive steroids. This could result in unintended pregnancy or breakthrough bleeding. Women may need to use an additional contraceptive method).
No products indexed under this heading.

Paramethadione (Contraceptive effectiveness may be reduced when hormonal contraceptives are co-administered with some anticonvulsants and other drugs that increase the metabolism of contraceptive steroids. This could result in unintended pregnancy or breakthrough bleeding. Women may need to use an additional contraceptive method).
No products indexed under this heading.

Paroxetine Hydrochloride (CYP3A4 inhibitors may increase plasma hormone levels). Products include:
Paxil 1535
Paxil CR Controlled-Release Tablets 1544

Pentobarbital Sodium (Contraceptive effectiveness may be reduced when hormonal contraceptives are co-administered with drugs that increase the metabolism of contraceptive steroids. This could result in unintended pregnancy or breakthrough bleeding. Women may need to use anadditional contraceptive method). Products include:
Nembutal Sodium Solution, USP 2494

Phenacemide (Contraceptive effectiveness may be reduced when hormonal contraceptives are co-administered with some anticonvulsants and other drugs that increase the metabolism of contraceptive steroids. This could result in unintended pregnancy or breakthrough bleeding. Women may need to use an additional contraceptive method).
No products indexed under this heading.

Phenobarbital (Contraceptive effectiveness may be reduced when hormonal contraceptives are co-administered with some anticonvulsants and other drugs that increase the metabolism of contraceptive steroids. This could result in unintended pregnancy or breakthrough bleeding. Women may need to use an additional contraceptive method). Products include:
Donnatal Extentabs 2507

Phensuximide (Contraceptive effectiveness may be reduced when hormonal contraceptives are co-administered with some anticonvulsants and other drugs that increase the metabolism of contraceptive steroids. This could result in unintended pregnancy or breakthrough bleeding. Women may need to use an additional contraceptive method).
No products indexed under this heading.

Phenylbutazone (Contraceptive effectiveness may be reduced when hormonal contraceptives are co-administered with drugs that increase the metabolism of contraceptive steroids. This could result in unintended pregnancy or breakthrough bleeding. Women may need to use an additional contraceptive method).
No products indexed under this heading.

Phenytoin (Contraceptive effectiveness may be reduced when hormonal contraceptives are co-administered with some anticonvulsants and other drugs that increase the metabolism of contraceptive steroids. This could result in unintended pregnancy or breakthrough bleeding. Women may need to use an additional contraceptive method).
No products indexed under this heading.

Phenytoin Sodium (Contraceptive effectiveness may be reduced when hormonal contraceptives are co-administered with some anticonvulsants and other drugs that increase the metabolism of contraceptive steroids. This could result in unintended pregnancy or breakthrough bleeding. Women may need to use an additional contraceptive method). Products include:
Phenytek Capsules 2192

Posaconazole (Contraceptive effectiveness may be reduced when hormonal contraceptives are co-administered with some antifungals and other drugs that increase the metabolism of contraceptive steroids. This could result in unintended pregnancy or breakthrough bleeding. Women may need to use an additional contraceptive method). Products include:
Noxafil Oral Suspension 2889

Prednisolone (Combination hormonal contraceptives containing some synthetic estrogens may inhibit the metabolism of other compounds. Increased plasma concentrations of prednisolone have been reported with concomitant administration of oral contraceptives).
No products indexed under this heading.

Prednisolone Acetate (Combination hormonal contraceptives containing some synthetic estrogens may inhibit the metabolism of other compounds. Increased plasma concentrations of prednisolone have been reported with concomitant administration of oral contraceptives). Products include:
Pred Forte Ophthalmic Suspension .... ⊙ 227
Pred Mild Ophthalmic Suspension .... ⊙ 230
Pred-G Ophthalmic Ointment .... ⊙ 229
Pred-G Ophthalmic Suspension .... ⊙ 228

Prednisolone Sodium Phosphate (Combination hormonal contraceptives containing some synthetic estrogens may inhibit the metabolism of other compounds. Increased plasma concentrations of prednisolone have been reported with concomitant administration of oral contraceptives).
No products indexed under this heading.

Prednisolone Tebutate (Combination hormonal contraceptives containing some synthetic estrogens may inhibit the metabolism of other compounds. Increased plasma concentrations of prednisolone have been reported with concomitant administration of oral contraceptives).
No products indexed under this heading.

Primidone (Contraceptive effectiveness may be reduced when hormonal contraceptives are co-administered with some anticonvulsants and other drugs that increase the metabolism of contraceptive steroids. This could result in unintended pregnancy or breakthrough bleeding. Women may need to use an additional contraceptive method).
No products indexed under this heading.

Propoxyphene Hydrochloride (CYP3A4 inhibitors may increase plasma hormone levels).
No products indexed under this heading.

Propoxyphene Napsylate (CYP3A4 inhibitors may increase plasma hormone levels).
No products indexed under this heading.

Quinidine (CYP3A4 inhibitors may increase plasma hormone levels).
No products indexed under this heading.

Quinidine Hydrochloride (CYP3A4 inhibitors may increase plasma hormone levels).
No products indexed under this heading.

Quinidine Polygalacturonate (CYP3A4 inhibitors may increase plasma hormone levels).
No products indexed under this heading.

Quinidine Sulfate (CYP3A4 inhibitors may increase plasma hormone levels).
No products indexed under this heading.

Quinine (CYP3A4 inhibitors may increase plasma hormone levels).
No products indexed under this heading.

Quinine Sulfate (CYP3A4 inhibitors may increase plasma hormone levels).
No products indexed under this heading.

Quinupristin (CYP3A4 inhibitors may increase plasma hormone levels).
No products indexed under this heading.

Ranitidine Bismuth Citrate (CYP3A4 inhibitors may increase plasma hormone levels).
No products indexed under this heading.

Ranitidine Hydrochloride (CYP3A4 inhibitors may increase plasma hormone levels). Products include:
Zantac 75 Tablets .... ▣603
Zantac 1670
Zantac Injection 1666
Zantac Injection Pharmacy Bulk Package 1668
Maximum Strength Zantac 150 Tablets .... ▣603
Maximum Strength Zantac 150 Cool Mint Tablets .... ▣603

Rifampin (Contraceptive effectiveness may be reduced when hormonal contraceptives are co-administered with drugs that increase the metabolism of contraceptive steroids. This could result in unintended pregnancy or breakthrough bleeding. Women may need to use an additional contraceptive method).
No products indexed under this heading.

Ritonavir (Several of the anti-HIV protease inhibitors have been studied with co-administration of oral combination hormonal contraceptives; significant changes (increases and decreases) in the mean AUC of the estrogen and progestin have been noted in some cases. The efficacy and safety of oral contraceptive products may be affected; it is not known whether this applies to NuvaRing). Products include:
Kaletra 452
Norvir 489

Salicylic Acid (Increased clearance of salicylic acid has been noted when administered with oral contraceptives).
No products indexed under this heading.

Saquinavir (Several of the anti-HIV protease inhibitors have been studied with co-administration of oral combination hormonal contraceptives; significant changes (increases and decreases) in the mean AUC of the estrogen and progestin have been noted in some cases. The efficacy and safety of oral contraceptive products may be affected; it is not known whether this applies to NuvaRing).
No products indexed under this heading.

Saquinavir Mesylate (Several of the anti-HIV protease inhibitors have been studied with co-administration of oral combination hormonal contraceptives; significant changes (increases and decreases) in the mean AUC of the estrogen and progestin have been noted in some cases. The efficacy and safety of oral contraceptive products may be affected; it is not known whether this applies to NuvaRing).
No products indexed under this heading.

Secobarbital Sodium (Contraceptive effectiveness may be reduced when hormonal contraceptives are co-administered with drugs that increase the metabolism of contraceptive steroids. This could result in unintended pregnancy or breakthrough bleeding. Women may need to use anadditional contraceptive method).
No products indexed under this heading.

Sertraline Hydrochloride (CYP3A4 inhibitors may increase plasma hormone levels).
No products indexed under this heading.

Sildenafil Citrate (CYP3A4 inhibitors may increase plasma hormone levels).
No products indexed under this heading.

Telithromycin (CYP3A4 inhibitors may increase plasma hormone levels). Products include:
Ketek Tablets 2744

Temazepam (Increased clearance of temazepam has been noted when administered with oral contraceptives).
No products indexed under this heading.

Terconazole (Contraceptive effectiveness may be reduced when hormonal contraceptives are co-administered with some antifungals and other drugs that increase the metabolism of contraceptive steroids. This could result in unintended pregnancy or breakthrough bleeding. Women may need to use an additional contraceptive method).
No products indexed under this heading.

Theophylline (Combination hormonal contraceptives containing some synthetic estrogens may inhibit the metabolism of other compounds. Increased plasma concentrations of theophylline have been reported with concomitant administration of oral contraceptives).
No products indexed under this heading.

Theophylline Anhydrous (Combination hormonal contraceptives containing some synthetic estrogens may inhibit the metabolism of other compounds. Increased plasma concentrations of theophylline have been reported with concomitant administration of oral contraceptives). Products include:
Uniphyl Tablets 2595

Theophylline Calcium Salicylate (Combination hormonal contraceptives containing some synthetic estrogens may inhibit the metabolism of other compounds. Increased plasma concentrations of theophylline have been reported with concomitant administration of oral contraceptives).
No products indexed under this heading.

Theophylline Dihydroxypropyl (Glyceryl) (Combination hormonal contraceptives containing some synthetic estrogens may inhibit the metabolism of other compounds. Increased plasma concentrations of theophylline have been reported with concomitant administration of oral contraceptives).
No products indexed under this heading.

Theophylline Ethylenediamine (Combination hormonal contraceptives containing some synthetic estrogens may inhibit the metabolism of other compounds. Increased plasma concentrations of theophylline have been reported with concomitant administration of oral contraceptives).
No products indexed under this heading.

Theophylline Sodium Glycinate (Combination hormonal contraceptives containing some synthetic estrogens may inhibit the metabolism of other compounds. Increased plasma concentrations of theophylline have been reported with concomitant administration of oral contraceptives).
No products indexed under this heading.

Thiamylal Sodium (Contraceptive effectiveness may be reduced when hormonal contraceptives are co-administered with drugs that increase the metabolism of contraceptive steroids. This could result in unintended pregnancy or breakthrough bleeding. Women may need to use anadditional contraceptive method).
No products indexed under this heading.

Tiagabine Hydrochloride (Contraceptive effectiveness may be reduced when hormonal contraceptives are co-administered with some anticonvulsants and other drugs that increase the metabolism of contraceptive steroids. This could result in unintended pregnancy or breakthrough bleeding. Women may need to use an additional contraceptive method). Products include:
Gabitril Tablets 973

Tipranavir (Several of the anti-HIV protease inhibitors have been studied with co-administration of oral combination hormonal contraceptives; significant changes (increases and decreases) in the mean AUC of the estrogen and progestin have been noted in some cases. The efficacy and safety of oral contraceptive products may be affected; it is not known whether this applies to NuvaRing). Products include:
Aptivus Capsules 823
Aptivus Oral Solution 823

Topiramate (Contraceptive effectiveness may be reduced when hormonal contraceptives are co-administered with some anticonvulsants and other drugs that increase the metabolism of contraceptive steroids. This could result in unintended pregnancy or breakthrough bleeding. Women may need to use an additional contraceptive method).
No products indexed under this heading.

Trimethadione (Contraceptive effectiveness may be reduced when hormonal contraceptives are co-administered with some anticonvulsants and other drugs that increase the metabolism of contraceptive steroids. This could result in unintended pregnancy or breakthrough bleeding. Women may need to use an additional contraceptive method).
No products indexed under this heading.

Troglitazone (CYP3A4 inhibitors may increase plasma hormone levels).
No products indexed under this heading.

Troleandomycin (CYP3A4 inhibitors may increase plasma hormone levels).
No products indexed under this heading.

Valproate Sodium (Contraceptive effectiveness may be reduced when hormonal contraceptives are co-administered with some anticonvulsants and other drugs that increase the metabolism of contraceptive steroids. This could result in unintended pregnancy or breakthrough bleeding. Women may need to use an additional contraceptive method).
No products indexed under this heading.

Valproic Acid (Contraceptive effectiveness may be reduced when hormonal contraceptives are co-administered with some anticonvulsants and other drugs that increase the metabolism of contraceptive steroids. This could result in unintended pregnancy or breakthrough bleeding. Women may need to use an additional contraceptive method).
No products indexed under this heading.

Vardenafil Hydrochloride (CYP3A4 inhibitors may increase plasma hormone levels). Products include:
Levitra Tablets 2876

Verapamil Hydrochloride (CYP3A4 inhibitors may increase plasma hormone levels). Products include:
Tarka Tablets 511

Vitamin C (Ascorbic acid may increase plasma ethinyl estradiol levels). Products include:
Bausch & Lomb Ocuvite Adult 50+ Vitamin and Mineral Supplement .... ⊙237
Comax Dietary Supplement 995
Ferralet 90 Tablets 2175
Glaucofit Dietary Supplement 995
Glauma Dietary Supplement 995
MoviPrep Oral Solution 2679
Procosa II Tablets 3174
Proflavanol 90 Tablets 3174
Tonox Dietary Supplement 995
Vibe Liquid Multi-Nutrient Supplement .... ▣626

Voriconazole (Contraceptive effectiveness may be reduced when hormonal contraceptives are co-administered with some antifungals and other drugs that increase the metabolism of contraceptive steroids. This could result in unintended pregnancy or breakthrough bleeding. Women may need to use an additional contraceptive method).
No products indexed under this heading.

Zafirlukast (CYP3A4 inhibitors may increase plasma hormone levels). Products include:

Accolate Tablets 669

Zileuton (CYP3A4 inhibitors may increase plasma hormone levels).
No products indexed under this heading.

Zonisamide (Contraceptive effectiveness may be reduced when hormonal contraceptives are co-administered with some anticonvulsants and other drugs that increase the metabolism of contraceptive steroids. This could result in unintended pregnancy or breakthrough bleeding. Women may need to use an additional contraceptive method). Products include:
Zonegran Capsules 1089

Food Interactions

Grapefruit (CYP3A4 inhibitors may increase plasma hormone levels).

Grapefruit Juice (CYP3A4 inhibitors may increase plasma hormone levels).

NYSTOP TOPICAL POWDER USP

(Nystatin) 2498
None cited in PDR database.

OFLOXACIN OPHTHALMIC SOLUTION 0.3%

(Ofloxacin) 243
May interact with xanthines and certain other agents. Compounds in these categories include:

Aminophylline (Systemic administration of some quinolones has been shown to elevate plasma concentrations of theophylline).
No products indexed under this heading.

Caffeine (Systemic administration of some quinolones has been shown to interfere with the metabolism of caffeine). Products include:
BioLean Free Tablets 635
BioLean II Tablets 635
Winrgy Dietary Supplement 642

Caffeine Citrate (Systemic administration of some quinolones has been shown to interfere with the metabolism of caffeine).
No products indexed under this heading.

Cyclosporine (Systemic administration of some quinolones has been associated with transient elevations of serum creatinine in patients receiving systemic cyclosporine concomitantly). Products include:
Gengraf Capsules 435
Neoral Oral Solution 2280
Neoral Soft Gelatin Capsules 2280
Restasis Ophthalmic Emulsion 557
Sandimmune 2296

Dyphylline (Systemic administration of some quinolones has been shown to elevate plasma concentrations of theophylline).
No products indexed under this heading.

Theophylline (Systemic administration of some quinolones has been shown to elevate plasma concentrations of theophylline).
No products indexed under this heading.

Theophylline Anhydrous (Systemic administration of some quinolones has been shown to elevate plasma concentrations of theophylline). Products include:
Uniphyl Tablets 2595

Theophylline Calcium Salicylate (Systemic administration of some quinolones has been shown to elevate plasma concentrations of theophylline).
No products indexed under this heading.

Theophylline Dihydroxypropyl (Glyceryl) (Systemic administration of some quinolones has been shown to elevate plasma concentrations of theophylline).
No products indexed under this heading.

Theophylline Ethylenediamine (Systemic administration of some quinolones has been shown to elevate plasma concentrations of theophylline).
No products indexed under this heading.

Theophylline Sodium Glycinate (Systemic administration of some quinolones has been shown to elevate plasma concentrations of theophylline).
No products indexed under this heading.

Warfarin Sodium (Systemic administration of some quinolones has been shown to enhance the effects of the oral anticoagulant warfarin).
No products indexed under this heading.

OLUX FOAM

(Clobetasol Propionate) 3061
None cited in PDR database.

OLUX-E FOAM

(Clobetasol Propionate) 3059
None cited in PDR database.

OMEGA 3-10 SOFTGELS

(Coenzyme Q-10, Omega-3 Acids) 632
None cited in PDR database.

OMNARIS NASAL SPRAY

(Ciclesonide) 2998
May interact with:

Ketoconazole (In one study, co-administration of orally inhaled ciclesonide and oral ketoconazole, a potent inhibitor of cytochrome P450 3A4, increase the exposure (AUC) of desciclesonide by approximately 3.6-fold at steady state, while levels of ciclesonide remained unchanged. Therefore, ketoconazole should be administered with caution with intranasal ciclesonide). Products include:
Extina Foam, 2% 3057
Nizoral A-D Shampoo 1901

OMNICEF CAPSULES

(Cefdinir) 497
May interact with antacids containing aluminum, calcium and magnesium, iron containing oral preparations, and certain other agents. Compounds in these categories include:

Aluminum Carbonate (Antacids (aluminum- or magnesium-containing) interfere with the absorption of cefdinir; Omnicef should be taken at least 2 hours before or after the antacids).
No products indexed under this heading.

Aluminum Hydroxide (Antacids (aluminum- or magnesium-containing) interfere with the absorption of cefdinir; Omnicef should be taken at least 2 hours before or after the antacids).
No products indexed under this heading.

Ferrous Fumarate (Iron supplements, including multivitamins that contain iron, interfere with the absorption of cefdinir; Omnicef should be taken at least 2 hours before or after the administration of iron-containing products).
No products indexed under this heading.

Ferrous Gluconate (Iron supplements, including multivitamins that contain iron, interfere with the absorption of cefdinir; Omnicef should be taken at least 2 hours before or after the administration of iron-containing products). Products include:
CitraNatal DHA Tablets 2175

Ferrous Sulfate (Iron supplements, including multivitamins that contain iron, interfere with the absorption of cefdinir; Omnicef should be taken at least 2 hours before or after the administration of iron-containing products).
No products indexed under this heading.

Iron (Iron supplements, including multivitamins that contain iron, interfere with the absorption of cefdinir; Omnicef should be taken at least 2 hours before or after the administration of iron-containing products). Products include:
Phyto-Vite Tablets 639

Magaldrate (Antacids (aluminum- or magnesium-containing) interfere with the absorption of cefdinir; Omnicef should be taken at least 2 hours before or after the antacids).
No products indexed under this heading.

Magnesium Hydroxide (Antacids (aluminum- or magnesium-containing) interfere with the absorption of cefdinir; Omnicef should be taken at least 2 hours before or after the antacids). Products include:
Fleet Pedia-Lax Chewable Tablets 1145
Pepcid Complete Chewable Tablets 1771
Extra Strength Rolaids Freshmint Tablets 1903
Rolaids Multi-Symptom Berry Tablets 1903
Rolaids Original Peppermint Tablets 1903

Magnesium Oxide (Antacids (aluminum- or magnesium-containing) interfere with the absorption of cefdinir; Omnicef should be taken at least 2 hours before or after the antacids). Products include:
Beelith Tablets 813

Polysaccharide Iron Complex (Iron supplements, including multivitamins that contain iron, interfere with the absorption of cefdinir; Omnicef should be taken at least 2 hours before or after the administration of iron-containing products). Products include:
Nu-Iron 150 Capsules 2165

Probenecid (Inhibits renal excretion of cefdinir, resulting in an approximate doubling in AUC, a 54% increase in peak cefdinir plasma levels, and a 50% prolongation in the apparent elimination).
No products indexed under this heading.

Food Interactions

Food, unspecified (Although Cmax and AUC of cefdinir absorption from capsules are reduced by 44% and 33%, respectively, when given with a high-fat meal, the magnitude of these reductions is not likely to be clinically significant; therefore, cefdinir may be taken without regard to food).

OMNICEF FOR ORAL SUSPENSION

(Cefdinir) 497
See Omnicef Capsules

ONCASPAR INJECTION

(Pegaspargase) 1138
May interact with antineoplastics, anticoagulants, non-steroidal anti-inflammatory agents, highly protein bound drugs (selected), and certain other agents. Compounds in these categories include:

Altretamine (Potential for unspecified unfavorable interactions). Products include:
Hexalen Capsules 1078

Amiodarone Hydrochloride (Depletion of serum proteins by pegaspargase may increase the toxicity of other drugs which are protein bound).
No products indexed under this heading.

Amitriptyline Hydrochloride (Depletion of serum proteins by pegaspargase may increase the toxicity of other drugs which are protein bound).
No products indexed under this heading.

Anastrozole (Potential for unspecified unfavorable interactions). Products include:
Arimidex Tablets 672

Anisindione (Increased risk of bleeding and/or thrombosis).
No products indexed under this heading.

Ardeparin Sodium (Increased risk of bleeding and/or thrombosis).
No products indexed under this heading.

Asparaginase (Potential for unspecified unfavorable interactions). Products include:
Elspar for Injection 1990
Elspar for Injection 2488

Aspirin (Increased risk of bleeding and/or thrombosis). Products include:
Aggrenox Capsules 819
Bayer Aspirin 750
Percodan Tablets 1130
St. Joseph 81 mg Aspirin Chewable and Enteric Coated Tablets 1903

Atovaquone (Depletion of serum proteins by pegaspargase may increase the toxicity of other drugs which are protein bound). Products include:
Malarone Pediatric Tablets 1521
Malarone Tablets 1521
Mepron Suspension 1526

Bicalutamide (Potential for unspecified unfavorable interac-

tions). Products include:
No products indexed under this heading.

Bleomycin Sulfate (Potential for unspecified unfavorable interactions).
No products indexed under this heading.

Busulfan (Potential for unspecified unfavorable interactions). Products include:
Busulfex Injection 2477
Myleran Tablets 1530

Carboplatin (Potential for unspecified unfavorable interactions).
No products indexed under this heading.

Carmustine (BCNU) (Potential for unspecified unfavorable interactions).
No products indexed under this heading.

Cefonicid Sodium (Depletion of serum proteins by pegaspargase may increase the toxicity of other drugs which are protein bound).
No products indexed under this heading.

Celecoxib (Increased risk of bleeding and/or thrombosis). Products include:
Celebrex Capsules 2979

Chlorambucil (Potential for unspecified unfavorable interactions). Products include:
Leukeran Tablets 1508

Chlordiazepoxide (Depletion of serum proteins by pegaspargase may increase the toxicity of other drugs which are protein bound).
No products indexed under this heading.

Chlordiazepoxide Hydrochloride (Depletion of serum proteins by pegaspargase may increase the toxicity of other drugs which are protein bound).
No products indexed under this heading.

Chlorpromazine (Depletion of serum proteins by pegaspargase may increase the toxicity of other drugs which are protein bound).
No products indexed under this heading.

Chlorpromazine Hydrochloride (Depletion of serum proteins by pegaspargase may increase the toxicity of other drugs which are protein bound).
No products indexed under this heading.

Cisplatin (Potential for unspecified unfavorable interactions).
No products indexed under this heading.

Clomipramine Hydrochloride (Depletion of serum proteins by pegaspargase may increase the toxicity of other drugs which are protein bound).
No products indexed under this heading.

Clozapine (Depletion of serum proteins by pegaspargase may increase the toxicity of other drugs which are protein bound).
No products indexed under this heading.

Cyclophosphamide (Potential for unspecified unfavorable interactions).
No products indexed under this heading.

Cyclosporine (Depletion of serum proteins by pegaspargase may increase the toxicity of other drugs which are protein bound). Products include:
Gengraf Capsules 435
Neoral Oral Solution 2280
Neoral Soft Gelatin Capsules 2280
Restasis Ophthalmic Emulsion 557
Sandimmune 2296

Dacarbazine (Potential for unspecified unfavorable interactions).
No products indexed under this heading.

Dalteparin Sodium (Increased risk of bleeding and/or thrombosis). Products include:
Fragmin Injection 1070

Danaparoid Sodium (Increased risk of bleeding and/or thrombosis).
No products indexed under this heading.

Daunorubicin Citrate (Potential for unspecified unfavorable interactions).
No products indexed under this heading.

Daunorubicin Hydrochloride (Potential for unspecified unfavorable interactions).
No products indexed under this heading.

Denileukin Diftitox (Potential for unspecified unfavorable interactions). Products include:
Ontak Vials 1079

Diazepam (Depletion of serum proteins by pegaspargase may increase the toxicity of other drugs which are protein bound). Products include:
Valium Tablets 2658

Diclofenac Epolamine (Increased risk of bleeding and/or thrombosis). Products include:
Flector Patch 561

Diclofenac Potassium (Depletion of serum proteins by pegaspargase may increase the toxicity of other drugs which are protein bound; increased risk of bleeding and/or thrombosis).
No products indexed under this heading.

Diclofenac Sodium (Depletion of serum proteins by pegaspargase may increase the toxicity of other drugs which are protein bound; increased risk of bleeding and/or thrombosis). Products include:
Diclofenac Sodium Ophthalmic Solution .... ⊙ 240
Voltaren Ophthalmic Solution 2336
Voltaren Tablets 2334
Voltaren-XR Tablets 2337

Dicumarol (Increased risk of bleeding and/or thrombosis).
No products indexed under this heading.

Dipyridamole (Depletion of serum proteins by pegaspargase may increase the toxicity of other drugs which are protein bound). Products include:
Aggrenox Capsules 819
Persantine Tablets 869

Docetaxel (Potential for unspecified unfavorable interactions). Products include:
Taxotere Injection Concentrate 2773

Doxorubicin Hydrochloride (Potential for unspecified unfavorable interactions).
No products indexed under this heading.

Enoxaparin Sodium (Increased risk of bleeding and/or thrombosis). Products include:
Lovenox Injection 2756

Epirubicin Hydrochloride (Potential for unspecified unfavorable interactions).
No products indexed under this heading.

Estramustine Phosphate Sodium (Potential for unspecified unfavorable interactions).
No products indexed under this heading.

Etodolac (Increased risk of bleeding and/or thrombosis).
No products indexed under this heading.

Etoposide (Potential for unspecified unfavorable interactions).
No products indexed under this heading.

Exemestane (Potential for unspecified unfavorable interactions).
No products indexed under this heading.

Fenoprofen Calcium (Depletion of serum proteins by pegaspargase may increase the toxicity of other drugs which are protein bound; increased risk of bleeding and/or thrombosis). Products include:
Nalfon Capsules 2508

Floxuridine (Potential for unspecified unfavorable interactions).
No products indexed under this heading.

Fluorouracil (Potential for unspecified unfavorable interactions). Products include:
Carac Cream 0.5% 2722

Flurazepam Hydrochloride (Depletion of serum proteins by pegaspargase may increase the toxicity of other drugs which are protein bound).
No products indexed under this heading.

Flurbiprofen (Depletion of serum proteins by pegaspargase may increase the toxicity of other drugs which are protein bound; increased risk of bleeding and/or thrombosis).
No products indexed under this heading.

Flutamide (Potential for unspecified unfavorable interactions).
No products indexed under this heading.

Fondaparinux Sodium (Increased risk of bleeding and/or thrombosis). Products include:
Arixtra Injection 1313

Gemcitabine Hydrochloride (Potential for unspecified unfavorable interactions). Products include:
Gemzar for Injection 1820

Glipizide (Depletion of serum proteins by pegaspargase may increase the toxicity of other drugs which are protein bound).
No products indexed under this heading.

Heparin Calcium (Increased risk of bleeding and/or thrombosis).
No products indexed under this heading.

Heparin Sodium (Increased risk of bleeding and/or thrombosis).
No products indexed under this heading.

Hydroxyurea (Potential for unspecified unfavorable interactions).
No products indexed under this heading.

Ibuprofen (Depletion of serum proteins by pegaspargase may increase the toxicity of other drugs which are protein bound; increased risk of bleeding and/or thrombosis). Products include:
Motrin IB Tablets and Caplets 1900
Children's Motrin Oral Suspension 1901
Children's Motrin Non-Staining Dye-Free Oral Suspension 1901
Children's Motrin Cold Oral Suspension 1899
Infants' Motrin Concentrated Drops 1901
Infants' Motrin Non-Staining Dye-Free Concentrated Drops 1901
Junior Strength Motrin Caplets and Chewable Tablets 1901
Vicoprofen Tablets 533

Idarubicin Hydrochloride (Potential for unspecified unfavorable interactions).
No products indexed under this heading.

Ifosfamide (Potential for unspecified unfavorable interactions).
No products indexed under this heading.

Imipramine Hydrochloride (Depletion of serum proteins by pegaspargase may increase the toxicity of other drugs which are protein bound).
No products indexed under this heading.

Imipramine Pamoate (Depletion of serum proteins by pegaspargase may increase the toxicity of other drugs which are protein bound).
No products indexed under this heading.

Indomethacin (Depletion of serum proteins by pegaspargase may increase the toxicity of other drugs which are protein bound; increased risk of bleeding and/or thrombosis). Products include:
Indocin 2024

Indomethacin Sodium Trihydrate (Depletion of serum proteins by pegaspargase may increase the toxicity of other drugs which are protein bound; increased risk of bleeding and/or thrombosis). Products include:
Indocin I.V. 2489

Interferon alfa-2a, Recombinant (Potential for unspecified unfavorable interactions).
No products indexed under this heading.

Interferon alfa-2b, Recombinant (Potential for unspecified unfavorable interactions). Products include:
Intron A for Injection 2859

Irinotecan Hydrochloride (Potential for unspecified unfavorable interactions).
No products indexed under this heading.

Ketoprofen (Depletion of serum proteins by pegaspargase may increase the toxicity of other drugs which are protein bound; increased risk of bleeding and/or thrombosis).
No products indexed under this heading.

Ketorolac Tromethamine (Depletion of serum proteins by pegaspargase may increase the toxicity of other drugs which are protein bound; increased risk of bleeding and/or thrombosis).
No products indexed under this heading.

Levamisole Hydrochloride (Potential for unspecified unfavorable interactions).
No products indexed under this heading.

Lomustine (CCNU) (Potential for unspecified unfavorable interactions).
No products indexed under this heading.

Low Molecular Weight Heparins (Increased risk of bleeding and/or thrombosis).
No products indexed under this heading.

Mechlorethamine Hydrochloride (Potential for unspecified unfavorable interactions). Products include:
Mustargen for Injection 2492

Meclofenamate Sodium (Depletion of serum proteins by pegaspargase may increase the toxicity of other drugs which are protein bound; increased risk of bleeding and/or thrombosis).
No products indexed under this heading.

Mefenamic Acid (Depletion of serum proteins by pegaspargase may increase the toxicity of other drugs which are protein bound; increased risk of bleeding and/or thrombosis).
No products indexed under this heading.

Megestrol Acetate (Potential for unspecified unfavorable interactions). Products include:
Megace ES Oral Suspension 2499

Meloxicam (Increased risk of bleeding and/or thrombosis). Products include:
Mobic Oral Suspension 863
Mobic Tablets 863

Melphalan (Potential for unspecified unfavorable interactions).
No products indexed under this heading.

Mercaptopurine (Potential for unspecified unfavorable interactions).
No products indexed under this heading.

Methotrexate Sodium (Pegaspargase inhibits protein synthesis and cell replication and thus interferes with the action of methotrexate which requires cell replication for its lethal effect; potential for unspecified unfavorable interactions).
No products indexed under this heading.

Midazolam Hydrochloride (Depletion of serum proteins by pegaspargase may increase the toxicity of other drugs which are protein bound).
No products indexed under this heading.

Mitomycin (Mitomycin-C) (Potential for unspecified unfavorable interactions).
No products indexed under this heading.

Mitotane (Potential for unspecified unfavorable interactions).
No products indexed under this heading.

Mitoxantrone Hydrochloride (Potential for unspecified unfavorable interactions). Products include:
Novantrone for Injection Concentrate 1100

Nabumetone (Increased risk of bleeding and/or thrombosis).
No products indexed under this heading.

Naproxen (Depletion of serum proteins by pegaspargase may increase the toxicity of other drugs which are protein bound; increased risk of bleeding and/or thrombosis). Products include:
EC-Naprosyn Delayed-Release Tablets 2632
Naprosyn Suspension 2632
Naprosyn Tablets 2632

Naproxen Sodium (Depletion of serum proteins by pegaspargase may increase the toxicity of other drugs which are protein bound; increased risk of bleeding and/or thrombosis). Products include:
Anaprox Tablets 2632
Anaprox DS Tablets 2632
Treximet Tablets 1616

Nortriptyline Hydrochloride (Depletion of serum proteins by pegaspargase may increase the toxicity of other drugs which are protein bound).
No products indexed under this heading.

Oxaliplatin (Potential for unspecified unfavorable interactions). Products include:
Eloxatin for Injection 2731

Oxaprozin (Depletion of serum proteins by pegaspargase may increase the toxicity of other drugs which are protein bound; increased risk of bleeding and/or thrombosis).
No products indexed under this heading.

Oxazepam (Depletion of serum proteins by pegaspargase may increase the toxicity of other drugs which are protein bound).
No products indexed under this heading.

Paclitaxel (Potential for unspecified unfavorable interactions).
No products indexed under this heading.

Phenylbutazone (Depletion of serum proteins by pegaspargase may increase the toxicity of other drugs which are protein bound; increased risk of bleeding and/or thrombosis).
No products indexed under this heading.

Piroxicam (Depletion of serum proteins by pegaspargase may increase the toxicity of other drugs which are protein bound; increased risk of bleeding and/or thrombosis).
No products indexed under this heading.

Procarbazine Hydrochloride (Potential for unspecified unfavorable interactions).
No products indexed under this heading.

Propranolol Hydrochloride (Depletion of serum proteins by pegaspargase may increase the toxicity of other drugs which are protein bound). Products include:
InnoPran XL Extended Release Capsules 1484

Rofecoxib (Increased risk of bleeding and/or thrombosis).
No products indexed under this heading.

Streptozocin (Potential for unspecified unfavorable interactions).
No products indexed under this heading.

Sulindac (Depletion of serum proteins by pegaspargase may increase the toxicity of other drugs which are protein bound; increased risk of bleeding and/or thrombosis). Products include:
Clinoril Tablets 1962

Tamoxifen Citrate (Potential for unspecified unfavorable interactions).
No products indexed under this heading.

Temazepam (Depletion of serum proteins by pegaspargase may increase the toxicity of other drugs which are protein bound).
No products indexed under this heading.

Teniposide (Potential for unspecified unfavorable interactions).
No products indexed under this heading.

Thioguanine (Potential for unspecified unfavorable interactions). Products include:
Tabloid Tablets 1601

Thiotepa (Potential for unspecified unfavorable interactions).
No products indexed under this heading.

Tinzaparin Sodium (Increased risk of bleeding and/or thrombosis).
No products indexed under this heading.

Tolbutamide (Depletion of serum proteins by pegaspargase may increase the toxicity of other drugs which are protein bound).
No products indexed under this heading.

Tolmetin Sodium (Depletion of serum proteins by pegaspargase may increase the toxicity of other drugs which are protein bound; increased risk of bleeding and/or thrombosis).
No products indexed under this heading.

Topotecan Hydrochloride (Potential for unspecified unfavorable interactions). Products include:
Hycamtin for Injection 1459
Hycamtin Capsules 1456

Toremifene Citrate (Potential for unspecified unfavorable interactions).
No products indexed under this heading.

Trimipramine Maleate (Depletion of serum proteins by pegaspargase may increase the toxicity of other drugs which are protein bound).
No products indexed under this heading.

Valdecoxib (Increased risk of bleeding and/or thrombosis).
No products indexed under this heading.

Valrubicin (Potential for unspecified unfavorable interactions). Products include:
Valstar Sterile Solution for Intravesical Instillation.................. 1735

Vincristine Sulfate (Potential for unspecified unfavorable interactions).
No products indexed under this heading.

Vinorelbine Tartrate (Potential for unspecified unfavorable interactions).
No products indexed under this heading.

Warfarin Sodium (Depletion of serum proteins by pegaspargase may increase the toxicity of other drugs which are protein bound; increased risk of bleeding and/or thrombosis).
No products indexed under this heading.

ONTAK VIALS

(Denileukin Diftitox) 1079
None cited in PDR database.

OPANA TABLETS

(Oxymorphone Hydrochloride) 1117
May interact with anesthetics, anticholinergics, central nervous system depressants, hypnotics and sedatives, monoamine oxidase inhibitors, mixed agonist/antagonist opioid analgesics, narcotic analgesics, phenothiazines, tranquilizers, and certain other agents. Compounds in these categories include:

Alfentanil Hydrochloride (The concomitant use of other CNS depressants including sedatives, hypnotics, tranquilizers, general anesthetics, phenothiazines, other opioids, and alcohol may produce additive CNS depressant effects. Additive effects resulting in respiratory depression, hypotension, profound sedation or coma may result if these drugs are taken in combination with the usual doses of oxymorphone hydrochloride).
No products indexed under this heading.

Alprazolam (The concomitant use of other CNS depressants including sedatives, hypnotics, tranquilizers, general anesthetics, phenothiazines, other opioids, and alcohol may produce additive CNS depressant effects. Additive effects resulting in respiratory depression, hypotension, profound sedation or coma may result if these drugs are taken in combination with the usual doses of oxymorphone hydrochloride).
No products indexed under this heading.

Aprobarbital (The concomitant use of other CNS depressants including sedatives, hypnotics, tranquilizers, general anesthetics, phenothiazines, other opioids, and alcohol may produce additive CNS depressant effects. Additive effects resulting in respiratory depression, hypotension, profound sedation or coma may result if these drugs are taken in combination with the usual dose of oxymorphone hydrochloride).
No products indexed under this heading.

Atropine Sulfate (Anticholinergics or other medications with anticholinergic activity when used concurrently with opioid analgesics may result in increased risk of urinary retention and/or severe constipation, which may lead to paralytic ileus). Products include:
Donnatal Extentabs 2507

Belladonna Alkaloids (Anticholinergics or other medications with anticholinergic activity when used concurrently with opioid analgesics may result in increased risk of urinary retention and/or severe constipation, which may lead to paralytic ileus). Products include:
Hyland's Teething Tablets 621

Benztropine Mesylate (Anticholinergics or other medications with anticholinergic activity when used concurrently with opioid analgesics may result in increased risk of urinary retention and/or severe constipation, which may lead to paralytic ileus).
No products indexed under this heading.

Biperiden Hydrochloride (Anticholinergics or other medications with anticholinergic activity when used concurrently with opioid analgesics may result in increased risk of urinary retention and/or severe constipation, which may lead to paralytic ileus).

No products indexed under this heading.

Buprenorphine Hydrochloride (The concomitant use of other CNS depressants including sedatives, hypnotics, tranquilizers, general anesthetics, phenothiazines, other opioids, and alcohol may produce additive CNS depressant effects. Additive effects resulting in respiratory depression, hypotension, profound sedation or coma may result if these drugs are taken in combination with the usual doses of oxymorphone hydrochloride). Products include:

Suboxone Tablets **2601**
Subutex Tablets **2601**

Buspirone Hydrochloride (The concomitant use of other CNS depressants including sedatives, hypnotics, tranquilizers, general anesthetics, phenothiazines, other opioids, and alcohol may produce additive CNS depressant effects. Additive effects resulting in respiratory depression, hypotension, profound sedation or coma may result if these drugs are taken in combination with the usual doses of oxymorphone hydrochloride).

No products indexed under this heading.

Butabarbital (The concomitant use of other CNS depressants including sedatives, hypnotics, tranquilizers, general anesthetics, phenothiazines, other opioids, and alcohol may produce additive CNS depressant effects. Additive effects resulting in respiratory depression, hypotension, profound sedation or coma may result if these drugs are taken in combination with the usual doses of oxymorphone hydrochloride).

No products indexed under this heading.

Butabarbital Sodium (The concomitant use of other CNS depressants including sedatives, hypnotics, tranquilizers, general anesthetics, phenothiazines, other opioids, and alcohol may produce additive CNS depressant effects. Additive effects resulting in respiratory depression, hypotension, profound sedation or coma may result if these drugs are taken in combination with the usual doses of oxymorphone hydrochloride).

No products indexed under this heading.

Butalbital (The concomitant use of other CNS depressants including sedatives, hypnotics, tranquilizers, general anesthetics, phenothiazines, other opioids, and alcohol may produce additive CNS depressant effects. Additive effects resulting in respiratory depression, hypotension, profound sedation or coma may result if these drugs are taken in combination with the usual dose of oxymorphone hydrochloride).

No products indexed under this heading.

Butorphanol Tartrate (Agonist/antagonist analgesics should not be administered to patients who have received or are receiving a course of therapy with pure opioid agonist analgesic, such as oxymorphone hydrochloride. In this situation, mixed agonist/antagonist analgesics may reduce the analgesic effect of oxymorphone hydrochloride and/or may precipitate withdrawal symptoms).

No products indexed under this heading.

Chloral Hydrate (The concomitant use of other CNS depressants including sedatives, hypnotics, tranquilizers, general anesthetics, phenothiazines, other opioids, and alcohol may produce additive CNS depressant effects. Additive effects resulting in respiratory depression, hypotension, profound sedation or coma may result if these drugs are taken in combination with the usual doses of oxymorphone hydrochloride).

No products indexed under this heading.

Chlordiazepoxide (The concomitant use of other CNS depressants including sedatives, hypnotics, tranquilizers, general anesthetics, phenothiazines, other opioids, and alcohol may produce additive CNS depressant effects. Additive effects resulting in respiratory depression, hypotension, profound sedation or coma may result if these drugs are taken in combination with the usual doses of oxymorphone hydrochloride).

No products indexed under this heading.

Chlordiazepoxide Hydrochloride (The concomitant use of other CNS depressants including sedatives, hypnotics, tranquilizers, general anesthetics, phenothiazines, other opioids, and alcohol may produce additive CNS depressant effects. Additive effects resulting in respiratory depression, hypotension, profound sedation or coma may result if these drugs are taken in combination with the usual doses of oxymorphone hydrochloride).

No products indexed under this heading.

Chlorpromazine (The concomitant use of other CNS depressants including sedatives, hypnotics, tranquilizers, general anesthetics, phenothiazines, other opioids, and alcohol may produce additive CNS depressant effects. Additive effects resulting in respiratory depression, hypotension, profound sedation or coma may result if these drugs are taken in combination with the usual doses of oxymorphone hydrochloride).

No products indexed under this heading.

Chlorpromazine Hydrochloride (The concomitant use of other CNS depressants including sedatives, hypnotics, tranquilizers, general anesthetics, phenothiazines, other opioids, and alcohol may produce additive CNS depressant effects. Additive effects resulting in respiratory depression, hypotension, profound sedation or coma may result if these drugs are taken in combination with the usual doses of oxymorphone hydrochloride).

No products indexed under this heading.

Chlorprothixene (The concomitant use of other CNS depressants including sedatives, hypnotics, tranquilizers, general anesthetics, phenothiazines, other opioids, and alcohol may produce additive CNS depressant effects. Additive effects resulting in respiratory depression, hypotension, profound sedation or coma may result if these drugs are taken in combination with the usual doses of oxymorphone hydrochloride).

No products indexed under this heading.

Chlorprothixene Hydrochloride (The concomitant use of other CNS depressants including sedatives, hypnotics, tranquilizers, general anesthetics, phenothiazines, other opioids, and alcohol may produce additive CNS depressant effects. Additive effects resulting in respiratory depression, hypotension, profound sedation or coma may result if these drugs are taken in combination with the usual doses of oxymorphone hydrochloride).

No products indexed under this heading.

Chlorprothixene Lactate (The concomitant use of other CNS depressants including sedatives, hypnotics, tranquilizers, general anesthetics, phenothiazines, other opioids, and alcohol may produce additive CNS depressant effects. Additive effects resulting in respiratory depression, hypotension, profound sedation or coma may result if these drugs are taken in combination with the usual dose of oxymorphone hydrochloride).

No products indexed under this heading.

Clidinium Bromide (Anticholinergics or other medications with anticholinergic activity when used concurrently with opioid analgesics may result in increased risk of urinary retention and/or severe constipation, which may lead to paralytic ileus).

No products indexed under this heading.

Clorazepate Dipotassium (The concomitant use of other CNS depressants including sedatives, hypnotics, tranquilizers, general anesthetics, phenothiazines, other opioids, and alcohol may produce additive CNS depressant effects. Additive effects resulting in respiratory depression, hypotension, profound sedation or coma may result if these drugs are taken in combination with the usual doses of oxymorphone hydrochloride).

No products indexed under this heading.

Clozapine (The concomitant use of other CNS depressants including sedatives, hypnotics, tranquilizers, general anesthetics, phenothiazines, other opioids, and alcohol may produce additive CNS depressant effects. Additive effects resulting in respiratory depression, hypotension, profound sedation or coma may result if these drugs are taken in combination with the usual dose of oxymorphone hydrochloride).

No products indexed under this heading.

Codeine Phosphate (The concomitant use of other CNS depressants including sedatives, hypnotics, tranquilizers, general anesthetics, phenothiazines, other opioids, and alcohol may produce additive CNS depressant effects. Additive effects resulting in respiratory depression, hypotension, profound sedation or coma may result if these drugs are taken in combination with the usual doses of oxymorphone hydrochloride). Products include:

Tylenol with Codeine Tablets **2427**

Desflurane (The concomitant use of other CNS depressants including sedatives, hypnotics, tranquilizers, general anesthetics, phenothiazines, other opioids, and alcohol may produce additive CNS depressant effects. Additive effects resulting in respiratory depression, hypotension, profound sedation or coma may result if these drugs are taken in combination with the usual dose of oxymorphone hydrochloride).

No products indexed under this heading.

Dezocine (The concomitant use of other CNS depressants including sedatives, hypnotics, tranquilizers, general anesthetics, phenothiazines, other opioids, and alcohol may produce additive CNS depressant effects. Additive effects resulting in respiratory depression, hypotension, profound sedation or coma may result if these drugs are taken in combination with the usual doses of oxymorphone hydrochloride).

No products indexed under this heading.

Diazepam (The concomitant use of other CNS depressants including sedatives, hypnotics, tranquilizers, general anesthetics, phenothiazines, other opioids, and alcohol may produce additive CNS depressant effects. Additive effects resulting in respiratory depression, hypotension, profound sedation or coma may result if these drugs are taken in combination with the usual doses of oxymorphone hydrochloride). Products include:

Valium Tablets **2658**

Dicyclomine Hydrochloride (Anticholinergics or other medications with anticholinergic activity when used concurrently with opioid analgesics may result in increased risk of urinary retention and/or severe constipation, which may lead to paralytic ileus). Products include:

Bentyl Capsules **703**
Bentyl Injection **703**
Bentyl Syrup **703**
Bentyl Tablets **703**

Droperidol (The concomitant use of other CNS depressants including sedatives, hypnotics, tranquilizers, general anesthetics, phenothiazines, other opioids, and alcohol may produce additive CNS depressant effects. Additive effects resulting in respiratory depression, hypotension, profound sedation or coma may result if these drugs are taken in combination with the usual doses of oxymorphone hydrochloride).

No products indexed under this heading.

Enflurane (The concomitant use of other CNS depressants including sedatives, hypnotics, tranquilizers, general anesthetics, phenothiazines, other opioids, and alcohol may produce additive CNS depressant

effects. Additive effects resulting in respiratory depression, hypotension, profound sedation or coma may result if these drugs are taken in combination with the usual doses of oxymorphone hydrochloride).

No products indexed under this heading.

Estazolam (The concomitant use of other CNS depressants including sedatives, hypnotics, tranquilizers, general anesthetics, phenothiazines, other opioids, and alcohol may produce additive CNS depressant effects. Additive effects resulting in respiratory depression, hypotension, profound sedation or coma may result if these drugs are taken in combination with the usual doses of oxymorphone hydrochloride).

No products indexed under this heading.

Ethanol (The concomitant use of other CNS depressants including sedatives, hypnotics, tranquilizers, general anesthetics, phenothiazines, other opioids, and alcohol may produce additive CNS depressant effects. Additive effects resulting in respiratory depression, hypotension, profound sedation or coma may result if these drugs are taken in combination with the usual dose of oxymorphone hydrochloride).

No products indexed under this heading.

Ethchlorvynol (The concomitant use of other CNS depressants including sedatives, hypnotics, tranquilizers, general anesthetics, phenothiazines, other opioids, and alcohol may produce additive CNS depressant effects. Additive effects resulting in respiratory depression, hypotension, profound sedation or coma may result if these drugs are taken in combination with the usual doses of oxymorphone hydrochloride).

No products indexed under this heading.

Ethinamate (The concomitant use of other CNS depressants including sedatives, hypnotics, tranquilizers, general anesthetics, phenothiazines, other opioids, and alcohol may produce additive CNS depressant effects. Additive effects resulting in respiratory depression, hypotension, profound sedation or coma may result if these drugs are taken in combination with the usual doses of oxymorphone hydrochloride).

No products indexed under this heading.

Ethyl Alcohol (The concomitant use of other CNS depressants including sedatives, hypnotics, tranquilizers, general anesthetics, phenothiazines, other opioids, and alcohol may produce additive CNS depressant effects. Additive effects resulting in respiratory depression, hypotension, profound sedation or coma may result if these drugs are taken in combination with the usual dose of oxymorphone hydrochloride).

No products indexed under this heading.

Fentanyl (The concomitant use of other CNS depressants including sedatives, hypnotics, tranquilizers, general anesthetics, phenothiazines, other opioids, and alcohol may produce additive CNS depressant effects. Additive effects resulting in respiratory depression, hypotension, profound sedation or coma may result if these drugs are taken in combination with the usual doses of oxymorphone hydrochloride). Products include:

Duragesic Transdermal System **2405**
Ionsys Transdermal System **2410**

Fentanyl Citrate (The concomitant use of other CNS depressants including sedatives, hypnotics, tranquilizers, general anesthetics, phenothiazines, other opioids, and alcohol may produce additive CNS depressant effects. Additive effects resulting in respiratory depression, hypotension, profound sedation or coma may result if these drugs are taken in combination with the usual doses of oxymorphone hydrochloride). Products include:

Actiq **959**
Fentora Tablets **968**

Fluphenazine Decanoate (The concomitant use of other CNS depressants including sedatives, hypnotics, tranquilizers, general anesthetics, phenothiazines, other opioids, and alcohol may produce additive CNS depressant effects. Additive effects resulting in respiratory depression, hypotension, profound sedation or coma may result if these drugs are taken in combination with the usual doses of oxymorphone hydrochloride).

No products indexed under this heading.

Fluphenazine Enanthate (The concomitant use of other CNS depressants including sedatives, hypnotics, tranquilizers, general anesthetics, phenothiazines, other opioids, and alcohol may produce additive CNS depressant effects. Additive effects resulting in respiratory depression, hypotension, profound sedation or coma may result if these drugs are taken in combination with the usual doses of oxymorphone hydrochloride).

No products indexed under this heading.

Fluphenazine Hydrochloride (The concomitant use of other CNS depressants including sedatives, hypnotics, tranquilizers, general anesthetics, phenothiazines, other opioids, and alcohol may produce additive CNS depressant effects. Additive effects resulting in respiratory depression, hypotension, profound sedation or coma may result if these drugs are taken in combination with the usual doses of oxymorphone hydrochloride).

No products indexed under this heading.

Flurazepam Hydrochloride (The concomitant use of other CNS depressants including sedatives, hypnotics, tranquilizers, general anesthetics, phenothiazines, other opioids, and alcohol may produce additive CNS depressant effects. Additive effects resulting in respiratory depression, hypotension, profound sedation or coma may result if these drugs are taken in combination with the usual doses of oxymorphone hydrochloride).

No products indexed under this heading.

Glutethimide (The concomitant use of other CNS depressants including sedatives, hypnotics, tranquilizers, general anesthetics, phenothiazines, other opioids, and alcohol may produce additive CNS depressant effects. Additive effects resulting in respiratory depression, hypotension, profound sedation or coma may result if these drugs are taken in combination with the usual doses of oxymorphone hydrochloride).

No products indexed under this heading.

Glycopyrrolate (Anticholinergics or other medications with anticholinergic activity when used concurrently with opioid analgesics may result in increased risk of urinary retention and/or severe constipation, which may lead to paralytic ileus).

No products indexed under this heading.

Haloperidol (The concomitant use of other CNS depressants including sedatives, hypnotics, tranquilizers, general anesthetics, phenothiazines, other opioids, and alcohol may produce additive CNS depressant effects. Additive effects resulting in respiratory depression, hypotension, profound sedation or coma may result if these drugs are taken in combination with the usual doses of oxymorphone hydrochloride).

No products indexed under this heading.

Haloperidol Decanoate (The concomitant use of other CNS depressants including sedatives, hypnotics, tranquilizers, general anesthetics, phenothiazines, other opioids, and alcohol may produce additive CNS depressant effects. Additive effects resulting in respiratory depression, hypotension, profound sedation or coma may result if these drugs are taken in combination with the usual doses of oxymorphone hydrochloride).

No products indexed under this heading.

Halothane (The concomitant use of other CNS depressants including sedatives, hypnotics, tranquilizers, general anesthetics, phenothiazines, other opioids, and alcohol may produce additive CNS depressant effects. Additive effects resulting in respiratory depression, hypotension, profound sedation or coma may result if these drugs are taken in combination with the usual doses of oxymorphone hydrochloride).

No products indexed under this heading.

Hydrocodone Bitartrate (The concomitant use of other CNS depressants including sedatives, hypnotics, tranquilizers, general anesthetics, phenothiazines, other opioids, and alcohol may produce additive CNS depressant effects. Additive effects resulting in respiratory depression, hypotension, profound sedation or coma may result if these drugs are taken in combination with the usual doses of oxymorphone hydrochloride). Products include:

Lortab 5/500 Tablets **3143**
Lortab 7.5/500 Tablets **3144**
Lortab 10/500 Tablets **3144**
Vicodin Tablets **529**
Vicodin ES Tablets **530**
Vicodin HP Tablets **531**
Vicoprofen Tablets **533**
Zydone Tablets **1132**

Hydrocodone Polistirex (The concomitant use of other CNS depressants including sedatives, hypnotics, tranquilizers, general anesthetics, phenothiazines, other opioids, and alcohol may produce additive CNS depressant effects. Additive effects resulting in respiratory depression, hypotension, profound sedation or coma may result if these drugs are taken in combination with the usual doses of oxymorphone hydrochloride). Products include:

Tussionex Pennkinetic Extended-Release Suspension **3154**

Hydromorphone Hydrochloride (The concomitant use of other CNS depressants including sedatives, hypnotics, tranquilizers, general anesthetics, phenothiazines, other opioids, and alcohol may produce additive CNS depressant effects. Additive effects resulting in respiratory depression, hypotension, profound sedation or coma may result if these drugs are taken in combination with the usual doses of oxymorphone hydrochloride).

No products indexed under this heading.

Hydroxyzine Hydrochloride (The concomitant use of other CNS depressants including sedatives, hypnotics, tranquilizers, general anesthetics, phenothiazines, other opioids, and alcohol may produce additive CNS depressant effects. Additive effects resulting in respiratory depression, hypotension, profound sedation or coma may result if these drugs are taken in combination with the usual doses of oxymorphone hydrochloride).

No products indexed under this heading.

Hyoscyamine (Anticholinergics or other medications with anticholinergic activity when used concurrently with opioid analgesics may result in increased risk of urinary retention and/or severe constipation, which may lead to paralytic ileus).

No products indexed under this heading.

Hyoscyamine Sulfate (Anticholinergics or other medications with anticholinergic activity when used concurrently with opioid analgesics may result in increased risk of urinary retention and/or severe constipation, which may lead to paralytic ileus). Products include:

Donnatal Extentabs **2507**

Ipratropium Bromide (Anticholinergics or other medications with anticholinergic activity when used concurrently with opioid analgesics may result in increased risk of urinary retention and/or severe constipation, which may lead to paralytic ileus). Products include:

Atrovent HFA Inhalation Aerosol **839**
Atrovent Nasal Spray 0.03% **834**
Atrovent Nasal Spray 0.06% **836**
Combivent Inhalation Aerosol **845**

Isocarboxazid (No specific interaction between oxymorphone and monoamine oxidase inhibitors has been observed, but caution in the use of any opioid in patients taking this class of drugs is appropriate). Products include:

Marplan Tablets **3177**

Isoflurane (The concomitant use of other CNS depressants including sedatives, hypnotics, tranquilizers, general anesthetics, phenothiazines, other opioids, and alcohol may produce additive CNS depressant effects. Additive effects resulting in respiratory depression, hypotension, profound sedation or coma may result if these drugs are taken in combination with the usual doses of

oxymorphone hydrochloride).
No products indexed under this heading.

Ketamine Hydrochloride (The concomitant use of other CNS depressants including sedatives, hypnotics, tranquilizers, general anesthetics, phenothiazines, other opioids, and alcohol may produce additive CNS depressant effects. Additive effects resulting in respiratory depression, hypotension, profound sedation or coma may result if these drugs are taken in combination with the usual doses of oxymorphone hydrochloride).
No products indexed under this heading.

Levomethadyl Acetate Hydrochloride (The concomitant use of other CNS depressants including sedatives, hypnotics, tranquilizers, general anesthetics, phenothiazines, other opioids, and alcohol may produce additive CNS depressant effects. Additive effects resulting in respiratory depression, hypotension, profound sedation or coma may result if these drugs are taken in combination with the usual dose of oxymorphone hydrochloride).
No products indexed under this heading.

Levorphanol Tartrate (The concomitant use of other CNS depressants including sedatives, hypnotics, tranquilizers, general anesthetics, phenothiazines, other opioids, and alcohol may produce additive CNS depressant effects. Additive effects resulting in respiratory depression, hypotension, profound sedation or coma may result if these drugs are taken in combination with the usual doses of oxymorphone hydrochloride).
No products indexed under this heading.

Lorazepam (The concomitant use of other CNS depressants including sedatives, hypnotics, tranquilizers, general anesthetics, phenothiazines, other opioids, and alcohol may produce additive CNS depressant effects. Additive effects resulting in respiratory depression, hypotension, profound sedation or coma may result if these drugs are taken in combination with the usual doses of oxymorphone hydrochloride).
No products indexed under this heading.

Loxapine Hydrochloride (The concomitant use of other CNS depressants including sedatives, hypnotics, tranquilizers, general anesthetics, phenothiazines, other opioids, and alcohol may produce additive CNS depressant effects. Additive effects resulting in respiratory depression, hypotension, profound sedation or coma may result if these drugs are taken in combination with the usual doses of oxymorphone hydrochloride).
No products indexed under this heading.

Loxapine Succinate (The concomitant use of other CNS depressants including sedatives, hypnotics, tranquilizers, general anesthetics, phenothiazines, other opioids, and alcohol may produce additive CNS depressant effects. Additive effects resulting in respiratory depression, hypotension, profound sedation or coma may result if these drugs are taken in combination with the usual doses of oxymorphone hydrochloride).
No products indexed under this heading.

Mepenzolate Bromide (Anticholinergics or other medications with anticholinergic activity when used concurrently with opioid analgesics may result in increased risk of urinary retention and/or severe constipation, which may lead to paralytic ileus).
No products indexed under this heading.

Meperidine Hydrochloride (The concomitant use of other CNS depressants including sedatives, hypnotics, tranquilizers, general anesthetics, phenothiazines, other opioids, and alcohol may produce additive CNS depressant effects. Additive effects resulting in respiratory depression, hypotension, profound sedation or coma may result if these drugs are taken in combination with the usual doses of oxymorphone hydrochloride).
No products indexed under this heading.

Mephobarbital (The concomitant use of other CNS depressants including sedatives, hypnotics, tranquilizers, general anesthetics, phenothiazines, other opioids, and alcohol may produce additive CNS depressant effects. Additive effects resulting in respiratory depression, hypotension, profound sedation or coma may result if these drugs are taken in combination with the usual dose of oxymorphone hydrochloride).
No products indexed under this heading.

Meprobamate (The concomitant use of other CNS depressants including sedatives, hypnotics, tranquilizers, general anesthetics, phenothiazines, other opioids, and alcohol may produce additive CNS depressant effects. Additive effects resulting in respiratory depression, hypotension, profound sedation or coma may result if these drugs are taken in combination with the usual doses of oxymorphone hydrochloride).
No products indexed under this heading.

Mesoridazine Besylate (The concomitant use of other CNS depressants including sedatives, hypnotics, tranquilizers, general anesthetics, phenothiazines, other opioids, and alcohol may produce additive CNS depressant effects. Additive effects resulting in respiratory depression, hypotension, profound sedation or coma may result if these drugs are taken in combination with the usual doses of oxymorphone hydrochloride).
No products indexed under this heading.

Methadone Hydrochloride (The concomitant use of other CNS depressants including sedatives, hypnotics, tranquilizers, general anesthetics, phenothiazines, other opioids, and alcohol may produce additive CNS depressant effects. Additive effects resulting in respiratory depression, hypotension, profound sedation or coma may result if these drugs are taken in combination with the usual doses of oxymorphone hydrochloride).
No products indexed under this heading.

Methohexital Sodium (The concomitant use of other CNS depressants including sedatives, hypnotics, tranquilizers, general anesthetics, phenothiazines, other opioids, and alcohol may produce additive CNS depressant effects. Additive effects resulting in respiratory depression, hypotension, profound sedation or coma may result if these drugs are taken in combination with the usual doses of oxymorphone hydrochloride).
No products indexed under this heading.

Methotrimeprazine (The concomitant use of other CNS depressants including sedatives, hypnotics, tranquilizers, general anesthetics, phenothiazines, other opioids, and alcohol may produce additive CNS depressant effects. Additive effects resulting in respiratory depression, hypotension, profound sedation or coma may result if these drugs are taken in combination with the usual doses of oxymorphone hydrochloride).
No products indexed under this heading.

Methoxyflurane (The concomitant use of other CNS depressants including sedatives, hypnotics, tranquilizers, general anesthetics, phenothiazines, other opioids, and alcohol may produce additive CNS depressant effects. Additive effects resulting in respiratory depression, hypotension, profound sedation or coma may result if these drugs are taken in combination with the usual dose of oxymorphone hydrochloride).
No products indexed under this heading.

Midazolam Hydrochloride (The concomitant use of other CNS depressants including sedatives, hypnotics, tranquilizers, general anesthetics, phenothiazines, other opioids, and alcohol may produce additive CNS depressant effects. Additive effects resulting in respiratory depression, hypotension, profound sedation or coma may result if these drugs are taken in combination with the usual doses of oxymorphone hydrochloride).
No products indexed under this heading.

Moclobemide (No specific interaction between oxymorphone and monoamine oxidase inhibitors has been observed, but caution in the use of any opioid in patients taking this class of drugs is appropriate).
No products indexed under this heading.

Molindone Hydrochloride (The concomitant use of other CNS depressants including sedatives, hypnotics, tranquilizers, general anesthetics, phenothiazines, other opioids, and alcohol may produce additive CNS depressant effects. Additive effects resulting in respiratory depression, hypotension, profound sedation or coma may result if these drugs are taken in combination with the usual doses of oxymorphone hydrochloride). Products include:
Moban Tablets ... 1116

Morphine Sulfate (The concomitant use of other CNS depressants including sedatives, hypnotics, tranquilizers, general anesthetics, phenothiazines, other opioids, and alcohol may produce additive CNS depressant effects. Additive effects resulting in respiratory depression, hypotension, profound sedation or coma may result if these drugs are taken in combination with the usual doses of oxymorphone hydrochloride). Products include:
Avinza Capsules ... 1772
DepoDur Injection ... 1095
MS Contin Tablets ... 2585

Nalbuphine Hydrochloride (Agonist/antagonist analgesics should not be administered to patients who have received or are receiving a course of therapy with pure opioid agonist analgesic, such as oxymorphone hydrochloride. In this situation, mixed agonist/antagonist analgesics may reduce the analgesic effect of oxymorphone hydrochloride and/or may precipitate withdrawal symptoms).
No products indexed under this heading.

Olanzapine (The concomitant use of other CNS depressants including sedatives, hypnotics, tranquilizers, general anesthetics, phenothiazines, other opioids, and alcohol may produce additive CNS depressant effects. Additive effects resulting in respiratory depression, hypotension, profound sedation or coma may result if these drugs are taken in combination with the usual dose of oxymorphone hydrochloride). Products include:
Symbyax Capsules ... 1871
Zyprexa Tablets ... 1883
Zyprexa IntraMuscular ... 1883
Zyprexa ZYDIS Orally Disintegrating Tablets ... 1883

Oxazepam (The concomitant use of other CNS depressants including sedatives, hypnotics, tranquilizers, general anesthetics, phenothiazines, other opioids, and alcohol may produce additive CNS depressant effects. Additive effects resulting in respiratory depression, hypotension, profound sedation or coma may result if these drugs are taken in combination with the usual doses of oxymorphone hydrochloride).
No products indexed under this heading.

Oxybutynin Chloride (Anticholinergics or other medications with anticholinergic activity when used concurrently with opioid analgesics may result in increased risk of urinary retention and/or severe constipation, which may lead to paralytic ileus).
No products indexed under this heading.

Oxycodone Hydrochloride (The concomitant use of other CNS depressants including sedatives, hypnotics, tranquilizers, general anesthetics, phenothiazines, other opioids, and alcohol may produce additive CNS depressant effects. Additive effects resulting in respiratory depression, hypotension, profound sedation or coma may result if these drugs are taken in combination with the usual doses of oxymorphone hydrochloride). Products include:
OxyContin Tablets ... 2589
OxyIR Capsules ... 2593

Percocet Tablets 1127
Percodan Tablets 1130

Pargyline Hydrochloride (No specific interaction between oxymorphone and monoamine oxidase inhibitors has been observed, but caution in the use of any opioid in patients taking this class of drugs is appropriate).
No products indexed under this heading.

Pentazocine Hydrochloride (Agonist/antagonist analgesics should not be administered to patients who have received or are receiving a course of therapy with pure opioid agonist analgesic, such as oxymorphone hydrochloride. In this situation, mixed agonist/antagonist analgesics may reduce the analgesic effect of oxymorphone hydrochloride and/or may precipitate withdrawal symptoms).
No products indexed under this heading.

Pentazocine Lactate (Agonist/antagonist analgesics should not be administered to patients who have received or are receiving a course of therapy with pure opioid agonist analgesic, such as oxymorphone hydrochloride. In this situation, mixed agonist/antagonist analgesics may reduce the analgesic effect of oxymorphone hydrochloride and/or may precipitate withdrawal symptoms).
No products indexed under this heading.

Pentobarbital Sodium (The concomitant use of other CNS depressants including sedatives, hypnotics, tranquilizers, general anesthetics, phenothiazines, other opioids, and alcohol may produce additive CNS depressant effects. Additive effects resulting in respiratory depression, hypotension, profound sedation or coma may result if these drugs are taken in combination with the usual dose of oxymorphone hydrochloride). Products include:
Nembutal Sodium Solution, USP 2494

Perphenazine (The concomitant use of other CNS depressants including sedatives, hypnotics, tranquilizers, general anesthetics, phenothiazines, other opioids, and alcohol may produce additive CNS depressant effects. Additive effects resulting in respiratory depression, hypotension, profound sedation or coma may result if these drugs are taken in combination with the usual doses of oxymorphone hydrochloride).
No products indexed under this heading.

Phenelzine Sulfate (No specific interaction between oxymorphone and monoamine oxidase inhibitors has been observed, but caution in the use of any opioid in patients taking this class of drugs is appropriate).
No products indexed under this heading.

Phenobarbital (The concomitant use of other CNS depressants including sedatives, hypnotics, tranquilizers, general anesthetics, phenothiazines, other opioids, and alcohol may produce additive CNS depressant effects. Additive effects resulting in respiratory depression, hypotension, profound sedation or coma may result if these drugs are taken in combination with the usual dose of oxymorphone hydrochloride). Products include:
Donnatal Extentabs 2507

Prazepam (The concomitant use of other CNS depressants including sedatives, hypnotics, tranquilizers, general anesthetics, phenothiazines, other opioids, and alcohol may produce additive CNS depressant effects. Additive effects resulting in respiratory depression, hypotension, profound sedation or coma may result if these drugs are taken in combination with the usual doses of oxymorphone hydrochloride).
No products indexed under this heading.

Procarbazine Hydrochloride (No specific interaction between oxymorphone and monoamine oxidase inhibitors has been observed, but caution in the use of any opioid in patients taking this class of drugs is appropriate).
No products indexed under this heading.

Prochlorperazine (The concomitant use of other CNS depressants including sedatives, hypnotics, tranquilizers, general anesthetics, phenothiazines, other opioids, and alcohol may produce additive CNS depressant effects. Additive effects resulting in respiratory depression, hypotension, profound sedation or coma may result if these drugs are taken in combination with the usual doses of oxymorphone hydrochloride).
No products indexed under this heading.

Procyclidine Hydrochloride (Anticholinergics or other medications with anticholinergic activity when used concurrently with opioid analgesics may result in increased risk of urinary retention and/or severe constipation, which may lead to paralytic ileus).
No products indexed under this heading.

Promethazine Hydrochloride (The concomitant use of other CNS depressants including sedatives, hypnotics, tranquilizers, general anesthetics, phenothiazines, other opioids, and alcohol may produce additive CNS depressant effects. Additive effects resulting in respiratory depression, hypotension, profound sedation or coma may result if these drugs are taken in combination with the usual doses of oxymorphone hydrochloride).
No products indexed under this heading.

Propantheline Bromide (Anticholinergics or other medications with anticholinergic activity when used concurrently with opioid analgesics may result in increased risk of urinary retention and/or severe constipation, which may lead to paralytic ileus).
No products indexed under this heading.

Propofol (The concomitant use of other CNS depressants including sedatives, hypnotics, tranquilizers, general anesthetics, phenothiazines, other opioids, and alcohol may produce additive CNS depressant effects. Additive effects resulting in respiratory depression, hypotension, profound sedation or coma may result if these drugs are taken in combination with the usual doses of oxymorphone hydrochloride).
No products indexed under this heading.

Propoxyphene Hydrochloride (The concomitant use of other CNS depressants including sedatives, hypnotics, tranquilizers, general anesthetics, phenothiazines, other opioids, and alcohol may produce additive CNS depressant effects. Additive effects resulting in respiratory depression, hypotension, profound sedation or coma may result if these drugs are taken in combination with the usual doses of oxymorphone hydrochloride).
No products indexed under this heading.

Propoxyphene Napsylate (The concomitant use of other CNS depressants including sedatives, hypnotics, tranquilizers, general anesthetics, phenothiazines, other opioids, and alcohol may produce additive CNS depressant effects. Additive effects resulting in respiratory depression, hypotension, profound sedation or coma may result if these drugs are taken in combination with the usual doses of oxymorphone hydrochloride).
No products indexed under this heading.

Quazepam (The concomitant use of other CNS depressants including sedatives, hypnotics, tranquilizers, general anesthetics, phenothiazines, other opioids, and alcohol may produce additive CNS depressant effects. Additive effects resulting in respiratory depression, hypotension, profound sedation or coma may result if these drugs are taken in combination with the usual doses of oxymorphone hydrochloride).
No products indexed under this heading.

Quetiapine Fumarate (The concomitant use of other CNS depressants including sedatives, hypnotics, tranquilizers, general anesthetics, phenothiazines, other opioids, and alcohol may produce additive CNS depressant effects. Additive effects resulting in respiratory depression, hypotension, profound sedation or coma may result if these drugs are taken in combination with the usual dose of oxymorphone hydrochloride).
No products indexed under this heading.

Ramelteon (The concomitant use of other CNS depressants including sedatives, hypnotics, tranquilizers, general anesthetics, phenothiazines, other opioids, and alcohol may produce additive CNS depressant effects. Additive effects resulting in respiratory depression, hypotension, profound sedation or coma may result if these drugs are taken in combination with the usual doses of oxymorphone hydrochloride). Products include:
Rozerem Tablets 3091

Rasagiline Mesylate (No specific interaction between oxymorphone and monoamine oxidase inhibitors has been observed, but caution in the use of any opioid in patients taking this class of drugs is appropriate). Products include:
Azilect Tablets 3106

Remifentanil Hydrochloride (The concomitant use of other CNS depressants including sedatives, hypnotics, tranquilizers, general anesthetics, phenothiazines, other opioids, and alcohol may produce additive CNS depressant effects. Additive effects resulting in respiratory depression, hypotension, profound sedation or coma may result if these drugs are taken in combination with the usual doses of oxymorphone hydrochloride).
No products indexed under this heading.

Risperidone (The concomitant use of other CNS depressants including sedatives, hypnotics, tranquilizers, general anesthetics, phenothiazines, other opioids, and alcohol may produce additive CNS depressant effects. Additive effects resulting in respiratory depression, hypotension, profound sedation or coma may result if these drugs are taken in combination with the usual dose of oxymorphone hydrochloride). Products include:
Risperdal Consta Long-Acting Injection 1753

Scopolamine (Anticholinergics or other medications with anticholinergic activity when used concurrently with opioid analgesics may result in increased risk of urinary retention and/or severe constipation, which may lead to paralytic ileus). Products include:
Transderm Scōp Transdermal Therapeutic System 2206

Scopolamine Hydrobromide (Anticholinergics or other medications with anticholinergic activity when used concurrently with opioid analgesics may result in increased risk of urinary retention and/or severe constipation, which may lead to paralytic ileus). Products include:
Donnatal Extentabs 2507

Secobarbital Sodium (The concomitant use of other CNS depressants including sedatives, hypnotics, tranquilizers, general anesthetics, phenothiazines, other opioids, and alcohol may produce additive CNS depressant effects. Additive effects resulting in respiratory depression, hypotension, profound sedation or coma may result if these drugs are taken in combination with the usual doses of oxymorphone hydrochloride).
No products indexed under this heading.

Selegiline (No specific interaction between oxymorphone and monoamine oxidase inhibitors has been observed, but caution in the use of any opioid in patients taking this class of drugs is appropriate). Products include:
Emsam Transdermal System 905

Selegiline Hydrochloride (No specific interaction between oxymorphone and monoamine oxidase inhibitors has been observed, but caution in the use of any opioid in patients taking this class of drugs is appropriate). Products include:
Eldepryl Capsules 3052

Sevoflurane (The concomitant use of other CNS depressants including sedatives, hypnotics, tranquilizers, general anesthetics, phenothiazines, other opioids, and alcohol may produce additive CNS depressant effects. Additive effects resulting in respiratory depression, hypotension, profound sedation or coma may result if these drugs are taken in

combination with the usual dose of oxymorphone hydrochloride). Products include:

Ultane Liquid for Inhalation 524

Sodium Butabarbital (The concomitant use of other CNS depressants including sedatives, hypnotics, tranquilizers, general anesthetics, phenothiazines, other opioids, and alcohol may produce additive CNS depressant effects. Additive effects resulting in respiratory depression, hypotension, profound sedation or coma may result if these drugs are taken in combination with the usual doses of oxymorphone hydrochloride).

No products indexed under this heading.

Sodium Oxybate (The concomitant use of other CNS depressants including sedatives, hypnotics, tranquilizers, general anesthetics, phenothiazines, other opioids, and alcohol may produce additive CNS depressant effects. Additive effects resulting in respiratory depression, hypotension, profound sedation or coma may result if these drugs are taken in combination with the usual dose of oxymorphone hydrochloride). Products include:

Xyrem Oral Solution 1766

Sufentanil Citrate (The concomitant use of other CNS depressants including sedatives, hypnotics, tranquilizers, general anesthetics, phenothiazines, other opioids, and alcohol may produce additive CNS depressant effects. Additive effects resulting in respiratory depression, hypotension, profound sedation or coma may result if these drugs are taken in combination with the usual doses of oxymorphone hydrochloride).

No products indexed under this heading.

Temazepam (The concomitant use of other CNS depressants including sedatives, hypnotics, tranquilizers, general anesthetics, phenothiazines, other opioids, and alcohol may produce additive CNS depressant effects. Additive effects resulting in respiratory depression, hypotension, profound sedation or coma may result if these drugs are taken in combination with the usual doses of oxymorphone hydrochloride).

No products indexed under this heading.

Thiamylal Sodium (The concomitant use of other CNS depressants including sedatives, hypnotics, tranquilizers, general anesthetics, phenothiazines, other opioids, and alcohol may produce additive CNS depressant effects. Additive effects resulting in respiratory depression, hypotension, profound sedation or coma may result if these drugs are taken in combination with the usual doses of oxymorphone hydrochloride).

No products indexed under this heading.

Thioridazine Hydrochloride (The concomitant use of other CNS depressants including sedatives, hypnotics, tranquilizers, general anesthetics, phenothiazines, other opioids, and alcohol may produce additive CNS depressant effects. Additive effects resulting in respiratory depression, hypotension, profound sedation or coma may result if these drugs are taken in combination with the usual doses of oxymorphone hydrochloride). Products include:

Thioridazine Hydrochloride Tablets 2195

Thiothixene (The concomitant use of other CNS depressants including sedatives, hypnotics, tranquilizers, general anesthetics, phenothiazines, other opioids, and alcohol may produce additive CNS depressant effects. Additive effects resulting in respiratory depression, hypotension, profound sedation or coma may result if these drugs are taken in combination with the usual doses of oxymorphone hydrochloride). Products include:

Thiothixene Capsules 2197

Tolterodine Tartrate (Anticholinergics or other medications with anticholinergic activity when used concurrently with opioid analgesics may result in increased risk of urinary retention and/or severe constipation, which may lead to paralytic ileus).

No products indexed under this heading.

Tranylcypromine Sulfate (No specific interaction between oxymorphone and monoamine oxidase inhibitors has been observed, but caution in the use of any opioid in patients taking this class of drugs is appropriate). Products include:

Parnate Tablets 1532

Triazolam (The concomitant use of other CNS depressants including sedatives, hypnotics, tranquilizers, general anesthetics, phenothiazines, other opioids, and alcohol may produce additive CNS depressant effects. Additive effects resulting in respiratory depression, hypotension, profound sedation or coma may result if these drugs are taken in combination with the usual doses of oxymorphone hydrochloride).

No products indexed under this heading.

Tridihexethyl Chloride (Anticholinergics or other medications with anticholinergic activity when used concurrently with opioid analgesics may result in increased risk of urinary retention and/or severe constipation, which may lead to paralytic ileus).

No products indexed under this heading.

Trifluoperazine Hydrochloride (The concomitant use of other CNS depressants including sedatives, hypnotics, tranquilizers, general anesthetics, phenothiazines, other opioids, and alcohol may produce additive CNS depressant effects. Additive effects resulting in respiratory depression, hypotension, profound sedation or coma may result if these drugs are taken in combination with the usual doses of oxymorphone hydrochloride).

No products indexed under this heading.

Trihexyphenidyl Hydrochloride (Anticholinergics or other medications with anticholinergic activity when used concurrently with opioid analgesics may result in increased risk of urinary retention and/or severe constipation, which may lead to paralytic ileus).

No products indexed under this heading.

Zaleplon (The concomitant use of other CNS depressants including sedatives, hypnotics, tranquilizers, general anesthetics, phenothiazines, other opioids, and alcohol may produce additive CNS depressant effects. Additive effects resulting in respiratory depression, hypotension, profound sedation or coma may result if these drugs are taken in combination with the usual doses of oxymorphone hydrochloride).

No products indexed under this heading.

Ziprasidone Hydrochloride (The concomitant use of other CNS depressants including sedatives, hypnotics, tranquilizers, general anesthetics, phenothiazines, other opioids, and alcohol may produce additive CNS depressant effects. Additive effects resulting in respiratory depression, hypotension, profound sedation or coma may result if these drugs are taken in combination with the usual dose of oxymorphone hydrochloride). Products include:

Geodon Capsules 2520

Zolpidem Tartrate (The concomitant use of other CNS depressants including sedatives, hypnotics, tranquilizers, general anesthetics, phenothiazines, other opioids, and alcohol may produce additive CNS depressant effects. Additive effects resulting in respiratory depression, hypotension, profound sedation or coma may result if these drugs are taken in combination with the usual doses of oxymorphone hydrochloride). Products include:

Ambien Tablets 2692
Ambien CR Tablets 2696

Food Interactions

Alcohol (The concomitant use of other CNS depressants including sedatives, hypnotics, tranquilizers, general anesthetics, phenothiazines, other opioids, and alcohol may produce additive CNS depressant effects. Additive effects resulting in respiratory depression, hypotension, profound sedation or coma may result if these drugs are taken in combination with the usual doses of oxymorphone hydrochloride).

OPANA ER TABLETS

(Oxymorphone Hydrochloride) 1121
See Opana Tablets

OPTIGOLD MEGA-30 MG PLUS MCT DIETARY SUPPLEMENT

(Lutein, Medium-Chain Triglycerides, Vitamins with Minerals, Zeaxanthin)........................ 995
None cited in PDR database.

OPTIPRANOLOL METIPRANOLOL OPHTHALMIC SOLUTION 0.3%

(Metipranolol) .... ⊙245
May interact with adrenergic augmenting psychotropics, beta blockers, calcium channel blockers, cardiac glycosides, and certain other agents. Compounds in these categories include:

Acebutolol Hydrochloride (Co-administration with oral beta blockers may result in additive effects or systemic beta blockade).

No products indexed under this heading.

Amlodipine Besylate (Co-administration with oral or intravenous calcium channel antagonists may result in possible precipitation of left ventricular failure and hypotension). Products include:

Azor Tablets 1005
Exforge Tablets 2238

Atenolol (Co-administration with oral beta blockers may result in additive effects or systemic beta blockade).

No products indexed under this heading.

Bepridil Hydrochloride (Co-administration with oral or intravenous calcium channel antagonists may result in possible precipitation of left ventricular failure and hypotension).

No products indexed under this heading.

Betaxolol Hydrochloride (Co-administration with oral beta blockers may result in additive effects or systemic beta blockade).

No products indexed under this heading.

Bisoprolol Fumarate (Co-administration with oral beta blockers may result in additive effects or systemic beta blockade).

No products indexed under this heading.

Carteolol Hydrochloride (Co-administration with oral beta blockers may result in additive effects or systemic beta blockade).

No products indexed under this heading.

Deserpidine (Possible additive effects and production of hypotension and/or bradycardia when beta blocker is concurrently used with catecholamine-depleting drugs).

No products indexed under this heading.

Deslanoside (Concomitant use of beta blockers with digitalis and calcium channel blockers may result in additive effects in prolonging atrioventricular conduction time).

No products indexed under this heading.

Digitalis Glycoside Preparations (Concomitant use of beta blockers with digitalis and calcium channel blockers may result in additive effects in prolonging atrioventricular conduction time).

No products indexed under this heading.

Digitoxin (Concomitant use of beta blockers with digitalis and calcium channel blockers may result in additive effects in prolonging atrioventricular conduction time).

No products indexed under this heading.

Digoxin (Concomitant use of beta blockers with digitalis and calcium channel blockers may result in additive effects in prolonging atrioventricular conduction time). Products include:

Lanoxin Injection 1498
Lanoxin Injection Pediatric 1502
Lanoxin Tablets 1505

Diltiazem Hydrochloride (Co-administration with oral or intravenous calcium channel antagonists may result in possible precipitation of left ventricular failure and hypotension). Products include:

Cardizem LA Extended Release Tablets 421

Epinephrine (Concurrent use in patients with history of atopy or severe anaphylactic reaction to allergens may be unresponsive to the

usual doses of epinephrine used to treat anaphylactic reaction). Products include:

EpiPen 1024

Epinephrine Hydrochloride (Concurrent use in patients with history of atopy or severe anaphylactic reaction to allergens may be unresponsive to the usual doses of epinephrine used to treat anaphylactic reaction).

No products indexed under this heading.

Esmolol Hydrochloride (Co-administration with oral beta blockers may result in additive effects or systemic beta blockade).

No products indexed under this heading.

Felodipine (Co-administration with oral or intravenous calcium channel antagonists may result in possible precipitation of left ventricular failure and hypotension).

No products indexed under this heading.

Isocarboxazid (Exercise caution when used concurrently with adrenergic psychotropic drugs). Products include:

Marplan Tablets 3177

Isradipine (Co-administration with oral or intravenous calcium channel antagonists may result in possible precipitation of left ventricular failure and hypotension). Products include:

DynaCirc CR Controlled Release Tablets 1407

Labetalol Hydrochloride (Co-administration with oral beta blockers may result in additive effects or systemic beta blockade).

No products indexed under this heading.

Levobunolol Hydrochloride (Co-administration with oral beta blockers may result in additive effects or systemic beta blockade).

No products indexed under this heading.

Metoprolol Succinate (Co-administration with oral beta blockers may result in additive effects or systemic beta blockade). Products include:

Toprol-XL Tablets 666

Metoprolol Tartrate (Co-administration with oral beta blockers may result in additive effects or systemic beta blockade).

No products indexed under this heading.

Mibefradil Dihydrochloride (Co-administration with oral or intravenous calcium channel antagonists may result in possible precipitation of left ventricular failure and hypotension).

No products indexed under this heading.

Nadolol (Co-administration with oral beta blockers may result in additive effects or systemic beta blockade). Products include:

Nadolol Tablets 2191

Nebivolol (Co-administration with oral beta blockers may result in additive effects or systemic beta blockade). Products include:

Bystolic Tablets 1155

Nicardipine Hydrochloride (Co-administration with oral or intravenous calcium channel antagonists may result in possible precipitation of left ventricular failure and hypotension). Products include:

Cardene I.V. 1093

Nifedipine (Co-administration with oral or intravenous calcium channel antagonists may result in possible precipitation of left ventricular failure and hypotension).

No products indexed under this heading.

Nimodipine (Co-administration with oral or intravenous calcium channel antagonists may result in possible precipitation of left ventricular failure and hypotension). Products include:

Nimotop Capsules 790

Nisoldipine (Co-administration with oral or intravenous calcium channel antagonists may result in possible precipitation of left ventricular failure and hypotension). Products include:

Sular Extended Release Tablets 2975

Pargyline Hydrochloride (Exercise caution when used concurrently with adrenergic psychotropic drugs).

No products indexed under this heading.

Penbutolol Sulfate (Co-administration with oral beta blockers may result in additive effects or systemic beta blockade).

No products indexed under this heading.

Phenelzine Sulfate (Exercise caution when used concurrently with adrenergic psychotropic drugs).

No products indexed under this heading.

Pindolol (Co-administration with oral beta blockers may result in additive effects or systemic beta blockade).

No products indexed under this heading.

Propranolol Hydrochloride (Co-administration with oral beta blockers may result in additive effects or systemic beta blockade). Products include:

InnoPran XL Extended Release Capsules 1484

Rauwolfia Serpentina (Possible additive effects and production of hypotension and/or bradycardia when beta blocker is concurrently used with catecholamine-depleting drugs).

No products indexed under this heading.

Rescinnamine (Possible additive effects and production of hypotension and/or bradycardia when beta blocker is concurrently used with catecholamine-depleting drugs).

No products indexed under this heading.

Reserpine (Possible additive effects and production of hypotension and/or bradycardia when beta blocker is concurrently used with catecholamine-depleting drugs).

No products indexed under this heading.

Sotalol Hydrochloride (Co-administration with oral beta blockers may result in additive effects or systemic beta blockade).

No products indexed under this heading.

Timolol Hemihydrate (Co-administration with oral beta blockers may result in additive effects or systemic beta blockade). Products include:

Betimol Ophthalmic Solution 3181

Timolol Maleate (Co-administration with oral beta blockers may result in additive effects or systemic beta blockade). Products include:

Combigan Ophthalmic Solution 553

Cosopt Sterile Ophthalmic Solution 1969

Timoptic Sterile Ophthalmic Solution 2121

Timoptic in Ocudose 2124

Timoptic-XE Sterile Ophthalmic Gel Forming Solution 2125

Tranylcypromine Sulfate (Exercise caution when used concurrently with adrenergic psychotropic drugs). Products include:

Parnate Tablets 1532

Verapamil Hydrochloride (Co-administration with oral or intravenous calcium channel antagonists may result in possible precipitation of left ventricular failure and hypotension). Products include:

Tarka Tablets 511

OPTIVAR OPHTHALMIC SOLUTION

(Azelastine Hydrochloride) .... ⊙254

None cited in PDR database.

OPTIVE LUBRICANT EYE DROPS

(Carboxymethylcellulose Sodium, Glycerin)... ⊙227

None cited in PDR database.

OPTIVE SENSITIVE LUBRICANT EYE DROPS

(Carboxymethylcellulose Sodium, Glycerin)... ⊙227

None cited in PDR database.

ORENCIA POWDER FOR INTRAVENOUS INFUSION

(Abatacept) 921

May interact with TNF antagonists, vaccines, live, and certain other agents. Compounds in these categories include:

Adalimumab (Concurrent administration of TNF antagonists with abatacept has been associated with an increased risk of serious infections and no significant additional efficacy over use of the TNF antagonists alone. Concurrent therapy with abatacept and TNF antagonists is not recommended). Products include:

Humira Injection 442

Anakinra (There is insufficient experience to assess the safety and efficacy of abatacept concurrently administered with anakinra. Concurrent use is not recommended). Products include:

Kineret Injection 585

BCG Vaccine (Live vaccines should not be given concurrently or within 3 months of discontinuation of abatacept).

No products indexed under this heading.

Etanercept (Concurrent administration of TNF antagonists with abatacept has been associated with an increased risk of serious infections and no significant additional efficacy over use of the TNF antagonists alone. Concurrent therapy with abatacept and TNF antagonists is not recommended). Products include:

Enbrel for Injection 569

Infliximab (Concurrent administration of TNF antagonists with abatacept has been associated with an increased risk of serious infections and no significant additional efficacy over use of the TNF antagonists alone. Concurrent therapy with abatacept and TNF antagonists is not recommended). Products include:

Remicade for IV Injection 950

Influenza Vaccine, Live Attenuated (Live vaccines should not be given concurrently or within 3 months of discontinuation of abatacept).

No products indexed under this heading.

Influenza Virus Vaccine Live, Intranasal (Live vaccines should not be given concurrently or within 3 months of discontinuation of abatacept). Products include:

FluMist Vaccine 1945

Measles, Mumps, Rubella and Varicella Virus Vaccine Live (Avoid administration of live vaccines). Products include:

ProQuad 2099

Measles, Mumps & Rubella Virus Vaccine, Live (Live vaccines should not be given concurrently or within 3 months of discontinuation of abatacept). Products include:

M-M-R II 2054

Measles & Rubella Virus Vaccine Live (Live vaccines should not be given concurrently or within 3 months of discontinuation of abatacept).

No products indexed under this heading.

Measles Virus Vaccine Live (Live vaccines should not be given concurrently or within 3 months of discontinuation of abatacept). Products include:

Attenuvax 1951

Mumps Virus Vaccine, Live (Live vaccines should not be given concurrently or within 3 months of discontinuation of abatacept). Products include:

Mumpsvax 2068

Poliovirus Vaccine, Live, Oral, Trivalent, Types 1,2,3 (Sabin) (Live vaccines should not be given concurrently or within 3 months of discontinuation of abatacept).

No products indexed under this heading.

Rotavirus Vaccine, Live, Oral, Tetravalent (Live vaccines should not be given concurrently or within 3 months of discontinuation of abatacept).

No products indexed under this heading.

Rubella & Mumps Virus Vaccine Live (Live vaccines should not be given concurrently or within 3 months of discontinuation of abatacept).

No products indexed under this heading.

Rubella Virus Vaccine Live (Live vaccines should not be given concurrently or within 3 months of discontinuation of abatacept). Products include:

Meruvax II 2061

Smallpox Vaccine (Live vaccines should not be given concurrently or within 3 months of discontinuation of abatacept).

No products indexed under this heading.

Typhoid Vaccine (Live vaccines should not be given concurrently or within 3 months of discontinuation of abatacept).

No products indexed under this heading.

Varicella Virus Vaccine Live (Live vaccines should not be given concurrently or within 3 months of discontinuation of abatacept). Products include:

Varivax 2133

Yellow Fever Vaccine (Live vaccines should not be given concurrently or within 3 months of discontinuation of abatacept).

No products indexed under this heading.

Zoster Vaccine Live (Live vaccines should not be given concurrently or within 3 months of discontinuation of abatacept). Products include:

Zostavax Injection 2145

ORTHO-CYCLEN TABLETS

(Ethinyl Estradiol, Norgestimate) 2449

May interact with bacteriostatic antibiotics, barbiturates, beta-lactams antibiotics, cephalosporins, cytochrome p450 3a4 inhibitors (selected), anticonvulsants, fluoroquinolone antibiotics, macrolide antibiotics, penicillins, protease inhibitors, tetracyclines, and theophyllines. Compounds in these categories include:

Acetaminophen (Acetaminophen may increase plasma ethinyl estraiol levels. Decreased plasma concentrations of acetaminophen have been reported when co-administered with oral contraceptives). Products include:

Benadryl Allergy & Cold Kapgels 1895
Benadryl Allergy & Sinus Headache Kapgels 1895
Benadryl Severe Allergy & Sinus Headache Caplets 1897
Lortab 5/500 Tablets 3143
Lortab 7.5/500 Tablets 3144
Lortab 10/500 Tablets 3144
Percocet Tablets 1127
Sinutab Sinus Caplets 1905
Sudafed PE Cold & Cough Caplets 1907
Sudafed PE Nighttime Cold Caplets 1907
Sudafed PE Severe Cold Caplets 1908
Sudafed PE Sinus Headache Caplets 1908
Regular Strength Tylenol Tablets 1915
Tylenol 8 Hour Extended Release Caplets 1915
Extra Strength Tylenol Caplets, Cool Caplets, and EZ Tabs 1915
Extra Strength Tylenol Adult Rapid Blast Liquid 1915
Extra Strength Tylenol PM Caplets, Geltabs, Liquid, and Rapid Release Gels 1915
Extra Strength Tylenol Rapid Release Gels 1915
Tylenol with Codeine Tablets 2427
Tylenol Allergy Multi-Symptom Caplets with Cool Burst and Rapid Release Gelcaps 1916
Tylenol Allergy Multi-Symptom Nighttime Caplets with Cool Burst 1916
Tylenol Severe Allergy Caplets 1916
Tylenol Arthritis Pain Extended Release Geltabs/Caplets 1915
Tylenol Chest Congestion Caplets with Cool Burst 1910
Tylenol Chest Congestion Liquid with Cool Burst 1910
Children's Tylenol Plus Cold Suspension Liquid 1912
Children's Tylenol Plus Cold & Allergy Suspension Liquid 1914
Children's Tylenol Plus Cough & Runny Nose Suspension Liquid 1912
Children's Tylenol Plus Cough & Sore Throat Suspension Liquid 1912
Children's Tylenol Plus Flu Suspension Liquid 1914
Children's Tylenol Suspension Liquid 1909
Children's Tylenol Meltaways 1909
Children's Tylenol Plus Multi-Symptom Cold Suspension Liquid 1912
Tylenol Cold Severe Congestion Daytime Caplets with Cool Burst 1912
Tylenol Cold Head Congestion Daytime Caplets with Cool Burst 1910
Tylenol Cold Head Congestion Nighttime Caplets with Cool Burst 1910
Tylenol Cold Head Congestion Severe Daytime Caplets with Cool Burst 1910
Tylenol Cold Multi-Symptom Daytime Caplets with Cool Burst and Rapid Release Gels 1913
Tylenol Cold Multi-Symptom Daytime Liquid with Citrus Burst ... 1913
Tylenol Cold Multi-Symptom Nighttime Caplets with Cool Burst 1913
Tylenol Cold Multi-Symptom Nighttime Liquid with Cool Burst ... 1913
Tylenol Cold Multi-Symptom Severe Caplets with Cool Burst 1913
Tylenol Cold Multi-Symptom Severe Daytime Liquid with Citrus Burst 1913
Tylenol Cough & Sore Throat Daytime Liquid with Cool Burst 1918
Tylenol Cough & Sore Throat Nighttime Liquid with Cool Burst ... 1918
Concentrated Tylenol Infants' Drops 1909
Jr. Tylenol Meltaways 1909
Tylenol Sinus Congestion & Pain Daytime Caplets with Cool Burst and Gelcaps 1917
Tylenol Sinus Congestion & Pain Nighttime Caplets with Cool Burst 1917
Tylenol Sinus Congestion & Pain Severe Caplets with Cool Burst 1917
Tylenol Sinus Severe Congestion Caplets with Cool Burst 1917
Tylenol Sore Throat Daytime Liquid with Cool Burst 1918
Tylenol Sore Throat Nighttime Liquid with Cool Burst 1918
Women's Tylenol Menstrual Relief Caplets 1919
Vicks DayQuil Cold & Flu Multi-Symptom Relief .... ■ 616
Vicks DayQuil LiquiCaps 2567
Vicks DayQuil Liquid 2567
Vicks DayQuil Multi-Symptom Cold/Flu Relief 2567
Vicks NyQuil Cold & Flu Multi-Symptom Relief .... ■ 617
Vicks NyQuil LiquiCaps 2567
Vicks NyQuil Liquid 2567
Vicks NyQuil Multi-Symptom Cold/Flu Relief 2567
Vicodin Tablets 529
Vicodin ES Tablets 530
Vicodin HP Tablets 531
Zydone Tablets 1132

Acetaminophen-containing products (Acetaminophen may increase plasma ethinyl estraiol levels. Decreased plasma concentrations of acetaminophen have been reported when co-administered with oral contraceptives).

No products indexed under this heading.

Acetazolamide (CYP3A4 inhibitors such as itraconazole or ketoconazole may increase plasma hormone levels).

No products indexed under this heading.

Alatrofloxacin Mesylate (Contraceptive effectiveness may be reduced when hormonal contraceptives are co-administered with antibiotics, anti-convulsants, and other drugs that increase the metabolism of contraceptive steroids. This could result in unintended pregnancy or breakthrough bleeding).

No products indexed under this heading.

5-Amino-Salicylic Acid (Contraceptive effectiveness may be reduced when hormonal contraceptives are co-administered with antibiotics, anti-convulsants, and other drugs that increase the metabolism of contraceptive steroids. This could result in unintended pregnancy or breakthrough bleeding).

No products indexed under this heading.

Amiodarone Hydrochloride (CYP3A4 inhibitors such as itraconazole or ketoconazole may increase plasma hormone levels).

No products indexed under this heading.

Amoxicillin (Contraceptive effectiveness may be reduced when hormonal contraceptives are co-administered with antibiotics, anti-convulsants, and other drugs that increase the metabolism of contraceptive steroids. This could result in unintended pregnancy or breakthrough bleeding). Products include:

Amoxil Capsules 1305
Amoxil Chewable Tablets 1305
Amoxil Pediatric Drops for Oral Suspension 1305
Amoxil Powder for Oral Suspension 1305
Amoxil Tablets 1305
Augmentin 1323
Augmentin Tablets 1327
Augmentin XR Extended Release Tablets 1333
Augmentin ES-600 Powder for Oral Suspension 1329
Moxatag Tablets 2165

Amoxicillin Trihydrate (Contraceptive effectiveness may be reduced when hormonal contraceptives are co-administered with antibiotics, anti-convulsants, and other drugs that increase the metabolism of contraceptive steroids. This could result in unintended pregnancy or breakthrough bleeding).

No products indexed under this heading.

Ampicillin (Contraceptive effectiveness may be reduced when hormonal contraceptives are co-administered with antibiotics, anti-convulsants, and other drugs that increase the metabolism of contraceptive steroids. This could result in unintended pregnancy or breakthrough bleeding).

No products indexed under this heading.

Ampicillin Sodium (Contraceptive effectiveness may be reduced when hormonal contraceptives are co-administered with antibiotics, anti-convulsants, and other drugs that increase the metabolism of contraceptive steroids. This could result in unintended pregnancy or breakthrough bleeding).

No products indexed under this heading.

Ampicillin Trihydrate (Contraceptive effectiveness may be reduced when hormonal contraceptives are co-administered with antibiotics, anti-convulsants, and other drugs that increase the metabolism of contraceptive steroids. This could result in unintended pregnancy or breakthrough bleeding).

No products indexed under this heading.

Amprenavir (Several of the anti-HIV protease inhibitors have been studied with co-administration of oral combination hormonal contraceptives; significant changes (increase and decrease) in the plasma levels of the estrogen and progestin have been noted in some cases. The safety and efficacy of oral contraceptive products may be affected with co-administration of anti-HIV protease inhibitors).

No products indexed under this heading.

Anastrozole (CYP3A4 inhibitors such as itraconazole or ketoconazole may increase plasma hormone levels). Products include:

Arimidex Tablets 672

Aprepitant (CYP3A4 inhibitors such as itraconazole or ketoconazole may increase plasma hormone levels). Products include:

Emend Capsules 1992

Aprobarbital (Contraceptive effectiveness may be reduced when hormonal contraceptives are co-administered with antibiotics, anti-convulsants, and other drugs that increase the metabolism of contraceptive steroids. This could result in unintended pregnancy or breakthrough bleeding).

No products indexed under this heading.

Ascorbate (Ascorbic acid may increase plasma ethinyl estradiol levels).

No products indexed under this heading.

Ascorbic Acid (Ascorbic acid may increase plasma ethinyl estradiol levels).

No products indexed under this heading.

Atazanavir (CYP3A4 inhibitors such as itraconazole or ketoconazole may increase plasma hormone levels).

No products indexed under this heading.

Atazanavir Sulfate (CYP3A4 inhibitors such as itraconazole or ketoconazole may increase plasma hormone levels). Products include:

Reyataz Capsules 3299

Atorvastatin Calcium (Co-administration of atorvastatin and certain oral contraceptives containing ethinyl estradiol increase AUC values for ethinyl estradiol by approximately 20%). Products include:

Lipitor Tablets 2501

Azithromycin Dihydrate (Contraceptive effectiveness may be reduced when hormonal contraceptives are co-administered with antibiotics, anti-convulsants, and other drugs that increase the metabolism of contraceptive steroids. This could result in unintended pregnancy or breakthrough bleeding).

No products indexed under this heading.

Azlocillin Sodium (Contraceptive effectiveness may be reduced when hormonal contraceptives are co-administered with antibiotics, anti-convulsants, and other drugs that increase the metabolism of contraceptive steroids. This could result in unintended pregnancy or breakthrough bleeding).

No products indexed under this heading.

Aztreonam (Contraceptive effectiveness may be reduced when hormonal contraceptives are co-administered with antibiotics, anti-convulsants, and other drugs that increase the metabolism of contraceptive steroids. This could result in unintended pregnancy or breakthrough bleeding).
No products indexed under this heading.

Bacampicillin Hydrochloride (Contraceptive effectiveness may be reduced when hormonal contraceptives are co-administered with antibiotics, anti-convulsants, and other drugs that increase the metabolism of contraceptive steroids. This could result in unintended pregnancy or breakthrough bleeding).
No products indexed under this heading.

Bosentan (Contraceptive effectiveness may be reduced when hormonal contraceptives are co-administered with drugs that increase the metabolism of contraceptive steroids such as bosentan. Concurrent use of bosentan and ethinyl estradiol containing products may result in decreased concentration of these contraceptive hormones thereby increasing the risk of unintended pregnancy and unscheduled bleeding). Products include:
Tracleer Tablets 3289

Butabarbital (Contraceptive effectiveness may be reduced when hormonal contraceptives are co-administered with antibiotics, anti-convulsants, and other drugs that increase the metabolism of contraceptive steroids. This could result in unintended pregnancy or breakthrough bleeding).
No products indexed under this heading.

Butalbital (Contraceptive effectiveness may be reduced when hormonal contraceptives are co-administered with antibiotics, anti-convulsants, and other drugs that increase the metabolism of contraceptive steroids. This could result in unintended pregnancy or breakthrough bleeding).
No products indexed under this heading.

Carbamazepine (Contraceptive effectiveness may be reduced when hormonal contraceptives are co-administered with antibiotics, anti-convulsants, and other drugs that increase the metabolism of contraceptive steroids. This could result in unintended pregnancy or breakthrough bleeding). Products include:
Carbatrol Capsules 3019
Equetro Extended-Release Capsules 3174

Carbenicillin Disodium (Contraceptive effectiveness may be reduced when hormonal contraceptives are co-administered with antibiotics, anti-convulsants, and other drugs that increase the metabolism of contraceptive steroids. This could result in unintended pregnancy or breakthrough bleeding).
No products indexed under this heading.

Carbenicillin Indanyl Sodium (Contraceptive effectiveness may be reduced when hormonal contraceptives are co-administered with antibiotics, anti-convulsants, and other drugs that increase the metabolism of contraceptive steroids. This could result in unintended pregnancy or breakthrough bleeding).
No products indexed under this heading.

Cefaclor (Contraceptive effectiveness may be reduced when hormonal contraceptives are co-administered with antibiotics, anti-convulsants, and other drugs that increase the metabolism of contraceptive steroids. This could result in unintended pregnancy or breakthrough bleeding).
No products indexed under this heading.

Cefadroxil (Contraceptive effectiveness may be reduced when hormonal contraceptives are co-administered with antibiotics, anti-convulsants, and other drugs that increase the metabolism of contraceptive steroids. This could result in unintended pregnancy or breakthrough bleeding).
No products indexed under this heading.

Cefamandole Nafate (Contraceptive effectiveness may be reduced when hormonal contraceptives are co-administered with antibiotics, anti-convulsants, and other drugs that increase the metabolism of contraceptive steroids. This could result in unintended pregnancy or breakthrough bleeding).
No products indexed under this heading.

Cefazolin Sodium (Contraceptive effectiveness may be reduced when hormonal contraceptives are co-administered with antibiotics, anti-convulsants, and other drugs that increase the metabolism of contraceptive steroids. This could result in unintended pregnancy or breakthrough bleeding).
No products indexed under this heading.

Cefdinir (Contraceptive effectiveness may be reduced when hormonal contraceptives are co-administered with antibiotics, anti-convulsants, and other drugs that increase the metabolism of contraceptive steroids. This could result in unintended pregnancy or breakthrough bleeding). Products include:
Omnicef Capsules 497
Omnicef for Oral Suspension 497

Cefepime Hydrochloride (Contraceptive effectiveness may be reduced when hormonal contraceptives are co-administered with antibiotics, anti-convulsants, and other drugs that increase the metabolism of contraceptive steroids. This could result in unintended pregnancy or breakthrough bleeding).
No products indexed under this heading.

Cefixime (Contraceptive effectiveness may be reduced when hormonal contraceptives are co-administered with antibiotics, anti-convulsants, and other drugs that increase the metabolism of contraceptive steroids. This could result in unintended pregnancy or breakthrough bleeding). Products include:
Suprax for Oral Suspension 1891
Suprax Tablets 1891

Cefmetazole Sodium (Contraceptive effectiveness may be reduced when hormonal contraceptives are co-administered with antibiotics, anti-convulsants, and other drugs that increase the metabolism of contraceptive steroids. This could result in unintended pregnancy or breakthrough bleeding).
No products indexed under this heading.

Cefonicid Sodium (Contraceptive effectiveness may be reduced when hormonal contraceptives are co-administered with antibiotics, anti-convulsants, and other drugs that increase the metabolism of contraceptive steroids. This could result in unintended pregnancy or breakthrough bleeding).
No products indexed under this heading.

Cefoperazone Sodium (Contraceptive effectiveness may be reduced when hormonal contraceptives are co-administered with antibiotics, anti-convulsants, and other drugs that increase the metabolism of contraceptive steroids. This could result in unintended pregnancy or breakthrough bleeding).
No products indexed under this heading.

Ceforanide (Contraceptive effectiveness may be reduced when hormonal contraceptives are co-administered with antibiotics, anti-convulsants, and other drugs that increase the metabolism of contraceptive steroids. This could result in unintended pregnancy or breakthrough bleeding).
No products indexed under this heading.

Cefotaxime Sodium (Contraceptive effectiveness may be reduced when hormonal contraceptives are co-administered with antibiotics, anti-convulsants, and other drugs that increase the metabolism of contraceptive steroids. This could result in unintended pregnancy or breakthrough bleeding).
No products indexed under this heading.

Cefotetan (Contraceptive effectiveness may be reduced when hormonal contraceptives are co-administered with antibiotics, anti-convulsants, and other drugs that increase the metabolism of contraceptive steroids. This could result in unintended pregnancy or breakthrough bleeding).
No products indexed under this heading.

Cefoxitin Sodium (Contraceptive effectiveness may be reduced when hormonal contraceptives are co-administered with antibiotics, anti-convulsants, and other drugs that increase the metabolism of contraceptive steroids. This could result in unintended pregnancy or breakthrough bleeding).
No products indexed under this heading.

Cefpodoxime Proxetil (Contraceptive effectiveness may be reduced when hormonal contraceptives are co-administered with antibiotics, anti-convulsants, and other drugs that increase the metabolism of contraceptive steroids. This could result in unintended pregnancy or breakthrough bleeding).
No products indexed under this heading.

Cefprozil (Contraceptive effectiveness may be reduced when hormonal contraceptives are co-administered with antibiotics, anti-convulsants, and other drugs that increase the metabolism of contraceptive steroids. This could result in unintended pregnancy or breakthrough bleeding).
No products indexed under this heading.

Ceftazidime (Contraceptive effectiveness may be reduced when hormonal contraceptives are co-administered with antibiotics, anti-convulsants, and other drugs that increase the metabolism of contraceptive steroids. This could result in unintended pregnancy or breakthrough bleeding). Products include:
Fortaz 1450

Ceftizoxime Sodium (Contraceptive effectiveness may be reduced when hormonal contraceptives are co-administered with antibiotics, anti-convulsants, and other drugs that increase the metabolism of contraceptive steroids. This could result in unintended pregnancy or breakthrough bleeding).
No products indexed under this heading.

Ceftriaxone Sodium (Contraceptive effectiveness may be reduced when hormonal contraceptives are co-administered with antibiotics, anti-convulsants, and other drugs that increase the metabolism of contraceptive steroids. This could result in unintended pregnancy or breakthrough bleeding). Products include:
Rocephin Injectable Vials, ADD-Vantage, Galaxy, Bulk 2642

Cefuroxime Axetil (Contraceptive effectiveness may be reduced when hormonal contraceptives are co-administered with antibiotics, anti-convulsants, and other drugs that increase the metabolism of contraceptive steroids. This could result in unintended pregnancy or breakthrough bleeding). Products include:
Ceftin 1380

Cefuroxime Sodium (Contraceptive effectiveness may be reduced when hormonal contraceptives are co-administered with antibiotics, anti-convulsants, and other drugs that increase the metabolism of contraceptive steroids. This could result in unintended pregnancy or breakthrough bleeding).
No products indexed under this heading.

Cephalexin (Contraceptive effectiveness may be reduced when hormonal contraceptives are co-administered with antibiotics, anti-convulsants, and other drugs that increase the metabolism of contraceptive steroids. This could result in unintended pregnancy or breakthrough bleeding).
No products indexed under this heading.

Cephalothin Sodium (Contraceptive effectiveness may be reduced when hormonal contraceptives are co-administered with antibiotics, anti-convulsants, and other drugs that increase the metabolism of contraceptive steroids. This could result in unintended pregnancy or breakthrough bleeding).
No products indexed under this heading.

Cephapirin Sodium (Contraceptive effectiveness may be reduced when hormonal contraceptives are co-administered with antibiotics, anti-convulsants, and other drugs that increase the metabolism of contraceptive steroids. This could result in unintended pregnancy or breakthrough bleeding).
No products indexed under this heading.

Cephradine (Contraceptive effectiveness may be reduced when hormonal contraceptives are co-administered with antibiotics, anti-convulsants, and other drugs that increase the metabolism of contraceptive steroids. This could result in unintended pregnancy or breakthrough bleeding).
No products indexed under this heading.

Chloramphenicol (Contraceptive effectiveness may be reduced when hormonal contraceptives are co-administered with antibiotics, anti-convulsants, and other drugs that increase the metabolism of contraceptive steroids. This could result in unintended pregnancy or breakthrough bleeding).
No products indexed under this heading.

Chloramphenicol Palmitate (Contraceptive effectiveness may be reduced when hormonal contraceptives are co-administered with antibiotics, anti-convulsants, and other drugs that increase the metabolism of contraceptive steroids. This could result in unintended pregnancy or breakthrough bleeding).
No products indexed under this heading.

Chloramphenicol Sodium Succinate (Contraceptive effectiveness may be reduced when hormonal contraceptives are co-administered with antibiotics, anti-convulsants, and other drugs that increase the metabolism of contraceptive steroids. This could result in unintended pregnancy or breakthrough bleeding).
No products indexed under this heading.

Cilastatin Sodium (Contraceptive effectiveness may be reduced when hormonal contraceptives are co-administered with antibiotics, anti-convulsants, and other drugs that increase the metabolism of contraceptive steroids. This could result in unintended pregnancy or breakthrough bleeding). Products include:
Primaxin I.M. 2080
Primaxin I.V. 2083

Cimetidine (CYP3A4 inhibitors such as itraconazole or ketoconazole may increase plasma hormone levels).
No products indexed under this heading.

Cimetidine Hydrochloride (CYP3A4 inhibitors such as itraconazole or ketoconazole may increase plasma hormone levels).
No products indexed under this heading.

Ciprofloxacin (Contraceptive effectiveness may be reduced when hormonal contraceptives are co-administered with antibiotics, anti-convulsants, and other drugs that increase the metabolism of contraceptive steroids. This could result in unintended pregnancy or breakthrough bleeding). Products include:
Cipro I.V. 2817
Cipro Oral Suspension 2810
Cipro XR Tablets 2823
Ciprodex Otic Suspension 541

Ciprofloxacin Hydrochloride (Contraceptive effectiveness may be reduced when hormonal contraceptives are co-administered with antibiotics, anti-convulsants, and other drugs that increase the metabolism of contraceptive steroids. This could result in unintended pregnancy or breakthrough bleeding). Products include:
Cipro Tablets 2810

Clarithromycin (Contraceptive effectiveness may be reduced when hormonal contraceptives are co-administered with antibiotics, anti-convulsants, and other drugs that increase the metabolism of contraceptive steroids. This could result in unintended pregnancy or breakthrough bleeding). Products include:
Biaxin/Biaxin XL 411

Clofibrate (Increased clearance of clofibric acid has been reported when co-administered with oral contraceptives).
No products indexed under this heading.

Clofibric Acid (Increased clearance of clofibric acid has been reported when co-administered with oral contraceptives).
No products indexed under this heading.

Clotrimazole (CYP3A4 inhibitors such as itraconazole or ketoconazole may increase plasma hormone levels). Products include:
Lotrisone 2881

Cyclosporine (Combination hormonal contraceptives containing some synthetic estrogens (e.g., ethinyl estradiol) may inhibit the metabolism of some compounds. Increased plasma concentrations of cyclosporine have been reported with concomitant administration of oral contraceptives). Products include:
Gengraf Capsules 435
Neoral Oral Solution 2280
Neoral Soft Gelatin Capsules 2280
Restasis Ophthalmic Emulsion 557
Sandimmune 2296

Dalfopristin (CYP3A4 inhibitors such as itraconazole or ketoconazole may increase plasma hormone levels).
No products indexed under this heading.

Danazol (CYP3A4 inhibitors such as itraconazole or ketoconazole may increase plasma hormone levels).
No products indexed under this heading.

Darunavir (Several of the anti-HIV protease inhibitors have been studied with co-administration of oral combination hormonal contraceptives; significant changes (increase and decrease) in the plasma levels of the estrogen and progestin have been noted in some cases. The safety and efficacy of oral contraceptive products may be affected with co-administration of anti-HIV protease inhibitors).
No products indexed under this heading.

Delavirdine Mesylate (CYP3A4 inhibitors such as itraconazole or ketoconazole may increase plasma hormone levels).
No products indexed under this heading.

Demeclocycline Hydrochloride (Contraceptive effectiveness may be reduced when hormonal contraceptives are co-administered with antibiotics, anti-convulsants, and other drugs that increase the metabolism of contraceptive steroids. This could result in unintended pregnancy or breakthrough bleeding).
No products indexed under this heading.

Dicloxacillin Sodium (Contraceptive effectiveness may be reduced when hormonal contraceptives are co-administered with antibiotics, anti-convulsants, and other drugs that increase the metabolism of contraceptive steroids. This could result in unintended pregnancy or breakthrough bleeding).
No products indexed under this heading.

Diltiazem Hydrochloride (CYP3A4 inhibitors such as itraconazole or ketoconazole may increase plasma hormone levels). Products include:
Cardizem LA Extended Release Tablets 421

Diltiazem Maleate (CYP3A4 inhibitors such as itraconazole or ketoconazole may increase plasma hormone levels).
No products indexed under this heading.

Dirithromycin (Contraceptive effectiveness may be reduced when hormonal contraceptives are co-administered with antibiotics, anti-convulsants, and other drugs that increase the metabolism of contraceptive steroids. This could result in unintended pregnancy or breakthrough bleeding).
No products indexed under this heading.

Divalproex Sodium (Contraceptive effectiveness may be reduced when hormonal contraceptives are co-administered with antibiotics, anti-convulsants, and other drugs that increase the metabolism of contraceptive steroids. This could result in unintended pregnancy or breakthrough bleeding). Products include:
Depakote ER Tablets 423

Doxycycline Calcium (Contraceptive effectiveness may be reduced when hormonal contraceptives are co-administered with antibiotics, anti-convulsants, and other drugs that increase the metabolism of contraceptive steroids. This could result in unintended pregnancy or breakthrough bleeding).
No products indexed under this heading.

Doxycycline Hyclate (Contraceptive effectiveness may be reduced when hormonal contraceptives are co-administered with antibiotics, anti-convulsants, and other drugs that increase the metabolism of contraceptive steroids. This could result in unintended pregnancy or breakthrough bleeding).
No products indexed under this heading.

Doxycycline Monohydrate (Contraceptive effectiveness may be reduced when hormonal contraceptives are co-administered with antibiotics, anti-convulsants, and other drugs that increase the metabolism of contraceptive steroids. This could result in unintended pregnancy or breakthrough bleeding).
No products indexed under this heading.

Efavirenz (CYP3A4 inhibitors such as itraconazole or ketoconazole may increase plasma hormone levels). Products include:
Atripla Tablets 938
Sustiva Capsules 930
Sustiva Tablets 930

Enoxacin (Contraceptive effectiveness may be reduced when hormonal contraceptives are co-administered with antibiotics, anti-convulsants, and other drugs that increase the metabolism of contraceptive steroids. This could result in unintended pregnancy or breakthrough bleeding).
No products indexed under this heading.

Erythromycin (Contraceptive effectiveness may be reduced when hormonal contraceptives are co-administered with antibiotics, anti-convulsants, and other drugs that increase the metabolism of contraceptive steroids. This could result in unintended pregnancy or breakthrough bleeding).
No products indexed under this heading.

Erythromycin Estolate (Contraceptive effectiveness may be reduced when hormonal contraceptives are co-administered with antibiotics, anti-convulsants, and other drugs that increase the metabolism of contraceptive steroids. This could result in unintended pregnancy or breakthrough bleeding).
No products indexed under this heading.

Erythromycin Ethylsuccinate (Contraceptive effectiveness may be reduced when hormonal contraceptives are co-administered with antibiotics, anti-convulsants, and other drugs that increase the metabolism of contraceptive steroids. This could result in unintended pregnancy or breakthrough bleeding). Products include:
E.E.S. 433
EryPed 431

Erythromycin Gluceptate (Contraceptive effectiveness may be reduced when hormonal contraceptives are co-administered with antibiotics, anti-convulsants, and other drugs that increase the metabolism of contraceptive steroids. This could result in unintended pregnancy or breakthrough bleeding).
No products indexed under this heading.

Erythromycin Lactobionate (CYP3A4 inhibitors such as itraconazole or ketoconazole may increase plasma hormone levels).
No products indexed under this heading.

Erythromycin Stearate (Contraceptive effectiveness may be reduced when hormonal contraceptives are co-administered with antibiotics, anti-convulsants, and other drugs that increase the metabolism of contraceptive steroids. This could result in unintended pregnancy or breakthrough bleeding).
No products indexed under this heading.

Esomeprazole Magnesium (CYP3A4 inhibitors such as itraconazole or ketoconazole may increase plasma hormone levels). Products include:
Nexium Delayed-Release Capsules 645

Nexium Delayed-Release Oral Suspension 645

Ethosuximide (Contraceptive effectiveness may be reduced when hormonal contraceptives are co-administered with antibiotics, anti-convulsants, and other drugs that increase the metabolism of contraceptive steroids. This could result in unintended pregnancy or breakthrough bleeding).
No products indexed under this heading.

Ethotoin (Contraceptive effectiveness may be reduced when hormonal contraceptives are co-administered with antibiotics, anti-convulsants, and other drugs that increase the metabolism of contraceptive steroids. This could result in unintended pregnancy or breakthrough bleeding).
No products indexed under this heading.

Felbamate (Contraceptive effectiveness may be reduced when hormonal contraceptives are co-administered with antibiotics, anti-convulsants, and other drugs that increase the metabolism of contraceptive steroids. This could result in unintended pregnancy or breakthrough bleeding).
No products indexed under this heading.

Fluconazole (CYP3A4 inhibitors such as itraconazole or ketoconazole may increase plasma hormone levels).
No products indexed under this heading.

Fluoxetine (CYP3A4 inhibitors such as itraconazole or ketoconazole may increase plasma hormone levels).
No products indexed under this heading.

Fluoxetine Hydrochloride (CYP3A4 inhibitors such as itraconazole or ketoconazole may increase plasma hormone levels). Products include:
Prozac Weekly Capsules 1852
Prozac Pulvules and Liquid 1852
Symbyax Capsules 1871

Fluvoxamine Maleate (CYP3A4 inhibitors such as itraconazole or ketoconazole may increase plasma hormone levels). Products include:
Luvox CR Extended-Release Capsules 1759

Fosamprenavir Calcium (Several of the anti-HIV protease inhibitors have been studied with co-administration of oral combination hormonal contraceptives; significant changes (increase and decrease) in the plasma levels of the estrogen and progestin have been noted in some cases. The safety and efficacy of oral contraceptive products may be affected with co-administration of anti-HIV protease inhibitors). Products include:
Lexiva Oral Suspension 1510
Lexiva Tablets 1510

Fosphenytoin (Contraceptive effectiveness may be reduced when hormonal contraceptives are co-administered with antibiotics, anti-convulsants, and other drugs that increase the metabolism of contraceptive steroids. This could result in unintended pregnancy or breakthrough bleeding).
No products indexed under this heading.

Fosphenytoin Sodium (Contraceptive effectiveness may be reduced when hormonal contraceptives are co-administered with antibiotics, anti-convulsants, and other drugs that increase the metabolism of contraceptive steroids. This could result in unintended pregnancy or breakthrough bleeding).
No products indexed under this heading.

Gabapentin (Contraceptive effectiveness may be reduced when hormonal contraceptives are co-administered with antibiotics, anti-convulsants, and other drugs that increase the metabolism of contraceptive steroids. This could result in unintended pregnancy or breakthrough bleeding).
No products indexed under this heading.

Gatifloxacin (Contraceptive effectiveness may be reduced when hormonal contraceptives are co-administered with antibiotics, anti-convulsants, and other drugs that increase the metabolism of contraceptive steroids. This could result in unintended pregnancy or breakthrough bleeding).
No products indexed under this heading.

Grepafloxacin Hydrochloride (Contraceptive effectiveness may be reduced when hormonal contraceptives are co-administered with antibiotics, anti-convulsants, and other drugs that increase the metabolism of contraceptive steroids. This could result in unintended pregnancy or breakthrough bleeding).
No products indexed under this heading.

Griseofulvin (Contraceptive effectiveness may be reduced when hormonal contraceptives are co-administered with antibiotics, anti-convulsants, and other drugs that increase the metabolism of contraceptive steroids. This could result in unintended pregnancy or breakthrough bleeding). Products include:
Gris-PEG Tablets 2507

Hypericum (Herbal products containing St. John's Wort (hypericum perforatum) may induce hepatic enzymes (cytochrome P450) and p-glycoprotein transporter and may reduce the effectiveness of contraceptive steroids. This may also result in breakthrough bleeding). Products include:
Satieté Tablets 640

Hypericum Perforatum (Herbal products containing St. John's Wort (hypericum perforatum) may induce hepatic enzymes (cytochrome P450) and p-glycoprotein transporter and may reduce the effectiveness of contraceptive steroids. This may also result in breakthrough bleeding).
No products indexed under this heading.

Imipenem (Contraceptive effectiveness may be reduced when hormonal contraceptives are co-administered with antibiotics, anti-convulsants, and other drugs that increase the metabolism of contraceptive steroids. This could result in unintended pregnancy or breakthrough bleeding). Products include:
Primaxin I.M. 2080
Primaxin I.V. 2083

Indinavir Sulfate (Several of the anti-HIV protease inhibitors have been studied with co-administration of oral combination hormonal contraceptives; significant changes (increase and decrease) in the plasma levels of the estrogen and progestin have been noted in some cases. The safety and efficacy of oral contraceptive products may be affected with co-administration of anti-HIV protease inhibitors). Products include:
Crixivan Capsules 1979

Isoniazid (CYP3A4 inhibitors such as itraconazole or ketoconazole may increase plasma hormone levels).
No products indexed under this heading.

Itraconazole (CYP3A4 inhibitors such as itraconazole or ketoconazole may increase plasma hormone levels).
No products indexed under this heading.

Ketoconazole (CYP3A4 inhibitors such as itraconazole or ketoconazole may increase plasma hormone levels). Products include:
Extina Foam, 2% 3057
Nizoral A-D Shampoo 1901

Lamotrigine (Contraceptive effectiveness may be reduced when hormonal contraceptives are co-administered with antibiotics, anti-convulsants, and other drugs that increase the metabolism of contraceptive steroids. This could result in unintended pregnancy or breakthrough bleeding). Products include:
Lamictal 1488

Levetiracetam (Contraceptive effectiveness may be reduced when hormonal contraceptives are co-administered with antibiotics, anti-convulsants, and other drugs that increase the metabolism of contraceptive steroids. This could result in unintended pregnancy or breakthrough bleeding). Products include:
Keppra Injection 3137
Keppra Oral Solution 3131
Keppra Tablets 3131

Levofloxacin (Contraceptive effectiveness may be reduced when hormonal contraceptives are co-administered with antibiotics, anti-convulsants, and other drugs that increase the metabolism of contraceptive steroids. This could result in unintended pregnancy or breakthrough bleeding). Products include:
Iquix Ophthalmic Solution 3183
Levaquin 2416
Levaquin in 5% Dextrose Injection 2416
Quixin Ophthalmic Solution 3184

Lomefloxacin Hydrochloride (Contraceptive effectiveness may be reduced when hormonal contraceptives are co-administered with antibiotics, anti-convulsants, and other drugs that increase the metabolism of contraceptive steroids. This could result in unintended pregnancy or breakthrough bleeding).
No products indexed under this heading.

Lopinavir (Several of the anti-HIV protease inhibitors have been studied with co-administration of oral combination hormonal contraceptives; significant changes (increase and decrease) in the plasma levels of the estrogen and progestin have been noted in some cases. The safety and efficacy of oral contraceptive products may be affected with co-administration of anti-HIV protease inhibitors). Products include:
Kaletra 452

Loracarbef (Contraceptive effectiveness may be reduced when hormonal contraceptives are co-administered with antibiotics, anti-convulsants, and other drugs that increase the metabolism of contraceptive steroids. This could result in unintended pregnancy or breakthrough bleeding).
No products indexed under this heading.

Loratadine (CYP3A4 inhibitors such as itraconazole or ketoconazole may increase plasma hormone levels).
No products indexed under this heading.

Mephenytoin (Contraceptive effectiveness may be reduced when hormonal contraceptives are co-administered with antibiotics, anti-convulsants, and other drugs that increase the metabolism of contraceptive steroids. This could result in unintended pregnancy or breakthrough bleeding).
No products indexed under this heading.

Mephobarbital (Contraceptive effectiveness may be reduced when hormonal contraceptives are co-administered with antibiotics, anti-convulsants, and other drugs that increase the metabolism of contraceptive steroids. This could result in unintended pregnancy or breakthrough bleeding).
No products indexed under this heading.

Methacycline Hydrochloride (Contraceptive effectiveness may be reduced when hormonal contraceptives are co-administered with antibiotics, anti-convulsants, and other drugs that increase the metabolism of contraceptive steroids. This could result in unintended pregnancy or breakthrough bleeding).
No products indexed under this heading.

Methsuximide (Contraceptive effectiveness may be reduced when hormonal contraceptives are co-administered with antibiotics, anti-convulsants, and other drugs that increase the metabolism of contraceptive steroids. This could result in unintended pregnancy or breakthrough bleeding).
No products indexed under this heading.

Metronidazole (CYP3A4 inhibitors such as itraconazole or ketoconazole may increase plasma hormone levels). Products include:
Pylera Capsules 714

Metronidazole Benzoate (CYP3A4 inhibitors such as itraconazole or ketoconazole may increase plasma hormone levels).
No products indexed under this heading.

Metronidazole Hydrochloride (CYP3A4 inhibitors such as itraconazole or ketoconazole may increase plasma hormone levels).
No products indexed under this heading.

Metronidazole Sodium (CYP3A4 inhibitors such as itraconazole or ketoconazole may increase plasma hormone levels).
No products indexed under this heading.

Mezlocillin Sodium (Contraceptive effectiveness may be reduced when hormonal contraceptives are co-administered with antibiotics, anti-convulsants, and other drugs that increase the metabolism of contraceptive steroids. This could result in unintended pregnancy or break-through bleeding).
No products indexed under this heading.

Miconazole (CYP3A4 inhibitors such as itraconazole or ketoconazole may increase plasma hormone levels).
No products indexed under this heading.

Miconazole Nitrate (CYP3A4 inhibitors such as itraconazole or ketoconazole may increase plasma hormone levels).
No products indexed under this heading.

Minocycline Hydrochloride (Contraceptive effectiveness may be reduced when hormonal contraceptives are co-administered with antibiotics, anti-convulsants, and other drugs that increase the metabolism of contraceptive steroids. This could result in unintended pregnancy or breakthrough bleeding). Products include:
Solodyn Extended Release Tablets 1938

Morphine Sulfate (Increased clearance of morphine has been reported when co-administered with oral contraceptives). Products include:
Avinza Capsules 1772
DepoDur Injection 1095
MS Contin Tablets 2585

Moxifloxacin Hydrochloride (Contraceptive effectiveness may be reduced when hormonal contraceptives are co-administered with antibiotics, anti-convulsants, and other drugs that increase the metabolism of contraceptive steroids. This could result in unintended pregnancy or breakthrough bleeding). Products include:
Avelox 2803
Vigamox Ophthalmic Solution 548

Nafcillin Sodium (Contraceptive effectiveness may be reduced when hormonal contraceptives are co-administered with antibiotics, anti-convulsants, and other drugs that increase the metabolism of contraceptive steroids. This could result in unintended pregnancy or break-through bleeding).
No products indexed under this heading.

Nefazodone Hydrochloride (CYP3A4 inhibitors such as itraconazole or ketoconazole may increase plasma hormone levels).
No products indexed under this heading.

Nelfinavir Mesylate (Several of the anti-HIV protease inhibitors have been studied with co-administration of oral combination hormonal contraceptives; significant changes (increase and decrease) in the plasma levels of the estrogen and progestin have been noted in some cases. The safety and efficacy of oral contraceptive products may be affected with co-administration of anti-HIV protease inhibitors).
No products indexed under this heading.

Nevirapine (CYP3A4 inhibitors such as itraconazole or ketoconazole may increase plasma hormone levels). Products include:
Viramune Oral Suspension 873
Viramune Tablets 873

Niacinamide (CYP3A4 inhibitors such as itraconazole or ketoconazole may increase plasma hormone levels). Products include:
BioLean Free Tablets .... ▣635

Nicotinamide (CYP3A4 inhibitors such as itraconazole or ketoconazole may increase plasma hormone levels).
No products indexed under this heading.

Nifedipine (CYP3A4 inhibitors such as itraconazole or ketoconazole may increase plasma hormone levels).
No products indexed under this heading.

Norfloxacin (Contraceptive effectiveness may be reduced when hormonal contraceptives are co-administered with antibiotics, anti-convulsants, and other drugs that increase the metabolism of contraceptive steroids. This could result in unintended pregnancy or break-through bleeding). Products include:
Noroxin Tablets 2069

Ofloxacin (Contraceptive effectiveness may be reduced when hormonal contraceptives are co-administered with antibiotics, anti-convulsants, and other drugs that increase the metabolism of contraceptive steroids. This could result in unintended pregnancy or break-through bleeding). Products include:
Ofloxacin Ophthalmic Solution 0.3% .... ⊙243

Omeprazole (CYP3A4 inhibitors such as itraconazole or ketoconazole may increase plasma hormone levels).
No products indexed under this heading.

Oxcarbazepine (Contraceptive effectiveness may be reduced when hormonal contraceptives are co-administered with antibiotics, anti-convulsants, and other drugs that increase the metabolism of contraceptive steroids. This could result in unintended pregnancy or break-through bleeding).
No products indexed under this heading.

Oxytetracycline Hydrochloride (Contraceptive effectiveness may be reduced when hormonal contraceptives are co-administered with antibiotics, anti-convulsants, and other drugs that increase the metabolism of contraceptive steroids. This could result in unintended pregnancy or breakthrough bleeding).
No products indexed under this heading.

Paramethadione (Contraceptive effectiveness may be reduced when hormonal contraceptives are co-administered with antibiotics, anti-convulsants, and other drugs that increase the metabolism of contraceptive steroids. This could result in unintended pregnancy or break-through bleeding).
No products indexed under this heading.

Paroxetine Hydrochloride (CYP3A4 inhibitors such as itraconazole or ketoconazole may increase plasma hormone levels). Products include:
Paxil 1535
Paxil CR Controlled-Release Tablets 1544

Penicillin G Benzathine (Contraceptive effectiveness may be reduced when hormonal contraceptives are co-administered with antibiotics, anti-convulsants, and other drugs that increase the metabolism of contraceptive steroids. This could result in unintended pregnancy or breakthrough bleeding). Products include:
Bicillin C-R Injectable Suspension 1775
Bicillin L-A Injection 1777

Penicillin G Potassium (Contraceptive effectiveness may be reduced when hormonal contraceptives are co-administered with antibiotics, anti-convulsants, and other drugs that increase the metabolism of contraceptive steroids. This could result in unintended pregnancy or breakthrough bleeding).
No products indexed under this heading.

Penicillin G Procaine (Contraceptive effectiveness may be reduced when hormonal contraceptives are co-administered with antibiotics, anti-convulsants, and other drugs that increase the metabolism of contraceptive steroids. This could result in unintended pregnancy or break-through bleeding). Products include:
Bicillin C-R Injectable Suspension 1775
Bicillin L-A Injection 1777

Penicillin G Sodium (Contraceptive effectiveness may be reduced when hormonal contraceptives are co-administered with antibiotics, anti-convulsants, and other drugs that increase the metabolism of contraceptive steroids. This could result in unintended pregnancy or break-through bleeding).
No products indexed under this heading.

Penicillin V Potassium (Contraceptive effectiveness may be reduced when hormonal contraceptives are co-administered with antibiotics, anti-convulsants, and other drugs that increase the metabolism of contraceptive steroids. This could result in unintended pregnancy or breakthrough bleeding).
No products indexed under this heading.

Pentobarbital Sodium (Contraceptive effectiveness may be reduced when hormonal contraceptives are co-administered with antibiotics, anti-convulsants, and other drugs that increase the metabolism of contraceptive steroids. This could result in unintended pregnancy or break-through bleeding). Products include:
Nembutal Sodium Solution, USP 2494

Phenacemide (Contraceptive effectiveness may be reduced when hormonal contraceptives are co-administered with antibiotics, anti-convulsants, and other drugs that increase the metabolism of contraceptive steroids. This could result in unintended pregnancy or break-through bleeding).
No products indexed under this heading.

Phenobarbital (Contraceptive effectiveness may be reduced when hormonal contraceptives are co-administered with antibiotics, anti-convulsants, and other drugs that increase the metabolism of contraceptive steroids. This could result in unintended pregnancy or break-through bleeding). Products include:
Donnatal Extentabs 2507

Phensuximide (Contraceptive effectiveness may be reduced when hormonal contraceptives are co-administered with antibiotics, anti-convulsants, and other drugs that increase the metabolism of contraceptive steroids. This could result in unintended pregnancy or break-through bleeding).
No products indexed under this heading.

Phenylbutazone (Contraceptive effectiveness may be reduced when hormonal contraceptives are co-administered with antibiotics, anti-convulsants, and other drugs that increase the metabolism of contraceptive steroids. This could result in unintended pregnancy or break-through bleeding).
No products indexed under this heading.

Phenytoin (Contraceptive effectiveness may be reduced when hormonal contraceptives are co-administered with antibiotics, anti-convulsants, and other drugs that increase the metabolism of contraceptive steroids. This could result in unintended pregnancy or break-through bleeding).
No products indexed under this heading.

Phenytoin Sodium (Contraceptive effectiveness may be reduced when hormonal contraceptives are co-administered with antibiotics, anti-convulsants, and other drugs that increase the metabolism of contraceptive steroids. This could result in unintended pregnancy or break-through bleeding). Products include:
Phenytek Capsules 2192

Prednisolone (Combination hormonal contraceptives containing some synthetic estrogens (e.g., ethinyl estradiol) may inhibit the metabolism of some compounds. Increased plasma concentrations of cyclosporine have been reported with concomitant administration of oral contraceptives).
No products indexed under this heading.

Primidone (Contraceptive effectiveness may be reduced when hormonal contraceptives are co-administered with antibiotics, anti-convulsants, and other drugs that increase the metabolism of contraceptive steroids. This could result in unintended pregnancy or break-through bleeding).
No products indexed under this heading.

Propoxyphene Hydrochloride (CYP3A4 inhibitors such as itraconazole or ketoconazole may increase plasma hormone levels).
No products indexed under this heading.

Propoxyphene Napsylate (CYP3A4 inhibitors such as itraconazole or ketoconazole may increase plasma hormone levels).
No products indexed under this heading.

Quinidine (CYP3A4 inhibitors such as itraconazole or ketoconazole may increase plasma hormone levels).
No products indexed under this heading.

Quinidine Hydrochloride (CYP3A4 inhibitors such as itraconazole or ketoconazole may increase plasma hormone levels).
No products indexed under this heading.

Quinidine Polygalacturonate (CYP3A4 inhibitors such as itraconazole or ketoconazole may increase plasma hormone levels).
No products indexed under this heading.

Quinidine Sulfate (CYP3A4 inhibitors such as itraconazole or ketoconazole may increase plasma hormone levels).
No products indexed under this heading.

Quinine (CYP3A4 inhibitors such as itraconazole or ketoconazole may increase plasma hormone levels).
No products indexed under this heading.

Quinine Sulfate (CYP3A4 inhibitors such as itraconazole or ketoconazole may increase plasma hormone levels).
No products indexed under this heading.

Quinupristin (CYP3A4 inhibitors such as itraconazole or ketoconazole may increase plasma hormone levels).
No products indexed under this heading.

Ranitidine Bismuth Citrate (CYP3A4 inhibitors such as itraconazole or ketoconazole may increase plasma hormone levels).
No products indexed under this heading.

Ranitidine Hydrochloride (CYP3A4 inhibitors such as itraconazole or ketoconazole may increase plasma hormone levels). Products include:
Zantac 75 Tablets 603
Zantac **1670**
Zantac Injection **1666**
Zantac Injection Pharmacy Bulk Package **1668**
Maximum Strength Zantac 150 Tablets 603
Maximum Strength Zantac 150 Cool Mint Tablets 603

Rifampin (Contraceptive effectiveness may be reduced when hormonal contraceptives are co-administered with antibiotics, anti-convulsants, and other drugs that increase the metabolism of contraceptive steroids. This could result in unintended pregnancy or breakthrough bleeding).
No products indexed under this heading.

Ritonavir (Several of the anti-HIV protease inhibitors have been studied with co-administration of oral combination hormonal contraceptives; significant changes (increase and decrease) in the plasma levels of the estrogen and progestin have been noted in some cases. The safety and efficacy of oral contraceptive products may be affected with co-administration of anti-HIV protease inhibitors). Products include:
Kaletra **452**
Norvir **489**

Salicylic Acid (Increased clearance of salicylic acid has been reported when co-administered with oral contraceptives).
No products indexed under this heading.

Saquinavir (Several of the anti-HIV protease inhibitors have been studied with co-administration of oral combination hormonal contraceptives; significant changes (increase and decrease) in the plasma levels of the estrogen and progestin have been noted in some cases. The safety and efficacy of oral contraceptive products may be affected with co-administration of anti-HIV protease inhibitors).
No products indexed under this heading.

Saquinavir Mesylate (Several of the anti-HIV protease inhibitors have been studied with co-administration of oral combination hormonal contraceptives; significant changes (increase and decrease) in the plasma levels of the estrogen and progestin have been noted in some cases. The safety and efficacy of oral contraceptive products may be affected with co-administration of anti-HIV protease inhibitors).
No products indexed under this heading.

Secobarbital Sodium (Contraceptive effectiveness may be reduced when hormonal contraceptives are co-administered with antibiotics, anti-convulsants, and other drugs that increase the metabolism of contraceptive steroids. This could result in unintended pregnancy or breakthrough bleeding).
No products indexed under this heading.

Sertraline Hydrochloride (CYP3A4 inhibitors such as itraconazole or ketoconazole may increase plasma hormone levels).
No products indexed under this heading.

Sildenafil Citrate (CYP3A4 inhibitors such as itraconazole or ketoconazole may increase plasma hormone levels).
No products indexed under this heading.

Sulfamethizole (Contraceptive effectiveness may be reduced when hormonal contraceptives are co-administered with antibiotics, anti-convulsants, and other drugs that increase the metabolism of contraceptive steroids. This could result in unintended pregnancy or breakthrough bleeding).
No products indexed under this heading.

Sulfamethoxazole (Contraceptive effectiveness may be reduced when hormonal contraceptives are co-administered with antibiotics, anti-convulsants, and other drugs that increase the metabolism of contraceptive steroids. This could result in unintended pregnancy or breakthrough bleeding).
No products indexed under this heading.

Sulfisoxazole Acetyl (Contraceptive effectiveness may be reduced when hormonal contraceptives are co-administered with antibiotics, anti-convulsants, and other drugs that increase the metabolism of contraceptive steroids. This could result in unintended pregnancy or breakthrough bleeding).
No products indexed under this heading.

Telithromycin (CYP3A4 inhibitors such as itraconazole or ketoconazole may increase plasma hormone levels). Products include:
Ketek Tablets **2744**

Temazepam (Increased clearance of temazepam has been reported when co-administered with oral contraceptives).
No products indexed under this heading.

Tetracycline Hydrochloride (Contraceptive effectiveness may be reduced when hormonal contraceptives are co-administered with antibiotics, anti-convulsants, and other drugs that increase the metabolism of contraceptive steroids. This could result in unintended pregnancy or breakthrough bleeding). Products include:
Pylera Capsules **714**

Theophylline (Combination hormonal contraceptives containing some synthetic estrogens (e.g., ethinyl estradiol) may inhibit the metabolism of some compounds. Increased plasma concentrations of theophylline have been reported with concomitant administration of oral contraceptives).
No products indexed under this heading.

Theophylline Anhydrous (Combination hormonal contraceptives containing some synthetic estrogens (e.g., ethinyl estradiol) may inhibit the metabolism of some compounds. Increased plasma concentrations of theophylline have been reported with concomitant administration of oral contraceptives). Products include:
Uniphyl Tablets **2595**

Theophylline Calcium Salicylate (Combination hormonal contraceptives containing some synthetic estrogens (e.g., ethinyl estradiol) may inhibit the metabolism of some compounds. Increased plasma concentrations of theophylline have been reported with concomitant administration of oral contraceptives).
No products indexed under this heading.

Theophylline Dihydroxypropyl (Glyceryl) (Combination hormonal contraceptives containing some synthetic estrogens (e.g., ethinyl estradiol) may inhibit the metabolism of some compounds. Increased plasma concentrations of theophylline have been reported with concomitant administration of oral contraceptives).
No products indexed under this heading.

Theophylline Ethylenediamine (Combination hormonal contraceptives containing some synthetic estrogens (e.g., ethinyl estradiol) may inhibit the metabolism of some compounds. Increased plasma concentrations of theophylline have been reported with concomitant administration of oral contraceptives).
No products indexed under this heading.

Theophylline Sodium Glycinate (Combination hormonal contraceptives containing some synthetic estrogens (e.g., ethinyl estradiol) may inhibit the metabolism of some compounds. Increased plasma concentrations of theophylline have been reported with concomitant administration of oral contraceptives).
No products indexed under this heading.

Thiamylal Sodium (Contraceptive effectiveness may be reduced when hormonal contraceptives are co-administered with antibiotics, anti-convulsants, and other drugs that increase the metabolism of contraceptive steroids. This could result in unintended pregnancy or breakthrough bleeding).
No products indexed under this heading.

Tiagabine Hydrochloride (Contraceptive effectiveness may be reduced when hormonal contraceptives are co-administered with antibiotics, anti-convulsants, and other drugs that increase the metabolism of contraceptive steroids. This could result in unintended pregnancy or breakthrough bleeding). Products include:
Gabitril Tablets **973**

Ticarcillin Disodium (Contraceptive effectiveness may be reduced when hormonal contraceptives are co-administered with antibiotics, anti-convulsants, and other drugs that increase the metabolism of contraceptive steroids. This could result in unintended pregnancy or breakthrough bleeding). Products include:
Timentin ADD-Vantage **1606**
Timentin Injection Galaxy Container **1609**
Timentin IV Infusion **1603**
Timentin Pharmacy Bulk Package **1613**

Tipranavir (Several of the anti-HIV protease inhibitors have been studied with co-administration of oral combination hormonal contraceptives; significant changes (increase and decrease) in the plasma levels of the estrogen and progestin have been noted in some cases. The safety and efficacy of oral contraceptive products may be affected with co-administration of anti-HIV protease inhibitors). Products include:
Aptivus Capsules **823**
Aptivus Oral Solution **823**

Topiramate (Contraceptive effectiveness may be reduced when hormonal contraceptives are co-administered with antibiotics, anti-convulsants, and other drugs that increase the metabolism of contraceptive steroids. This could result in unintended pregnancy or breakthrough bleeding).
No products indexed under this heading.

Trimethadione (Contraceptive effectiveness may be reduced when hormonal contraceptives are co-administered with antibiotics, anti-convulsants, and other drugs that increase the metabolism of contraceptive steroids. This could result in unintended pregnancy or breakthrough bleeding).
No products indexed under this heading.

Troglitazone (CYP3A4 inhibitors such as itraconazole or ketoconazole may increase plasma hormone levels).
No products indexed under this heading.

Troleandomycin (Contraceptive effectiveness may be reduced when hormonal contraceptives are co-administered with antibiotics, anti-convulsants, and other drugs that increase the metabolism of contraceptive steroids. This could result in unintended pregnancy or breakthrough bleeding).
No products indexed under this heading.

Trovafloxacin Mesylate (Contraceptive effectiveness may be reduced when hormonal contraceptives are co-administered with antibiotics, anti-convulsants, and other drugs that increase the metabolism of contraceptive steroids. This could result in unintended pregnancy or breakthrough bleeding).
No products indexed under this heading.

Valproate Sodium (Contraceptive effectiveness may be reduced when hormonal contraceptives are co-administered with antibiotics, anti-convulsants, and other drugs that increase the metabolism of contraceptive steroids. This could result in unintended pregnancy or breakthrough bleeding).
No products indexed under this heading.

Valproic Acid (Contraceptive effectiveness may be reduced when hormonal contraceptives are co-administered with antibiotics, anti-convulsants, and other drugs that increase the metabolism of contraceptive steroids. This could result in unintended pregnancy or breakthrough bleeding).
No products indexed under this heading.

Vardenafil Hydrochloride (CYP3A4 inhibitors such as itraconazole or ketoconazole may increase plasma hormone levels). Products include:
Levitra Tablets 2876

Verapamil Hydrochloride (CYP3A4 inhibitors such as itraconazole or ketoconazole may increase plasma hormone levels). Products include:
Tarka Tablets 511

Vitamin C (Ascorbic acid may increase plasma ethinyl estradiol levels). Products include:
Bausch & Lomb Ocuvite Adult 50+ Vitamin and Mineral Supplement .... ⊙237
Comax Dietary Supplement 995
Ferralet 90 Tablets 2175
Glaucofit Dietary Supplement 995
Glauma Dietary Supplement 995
MoviPrep Oral Solution 2679
Procosa II Tablets 3174
Proflavanol 90 Tablets 3174
Tonox Dietary Supplement 995
Vibe Liquid Multi-Nutrient Supplement .... ▣626

Voriconazole (CYP3A4 inhibitors such as itraconazole or ketoconazole may increase plasma hormone levels).
No products indexed under this heading.

Zafirlukast (CYP3A4 inhibitors such as itraconazole or ketoconazole may increase plasma hormone levels). Products include:
Accolate Tablets 669

Zileuton (CYP3A4 inhibitors such as itraconazole or ketoconazole may increase plasma hormone levels).
No products indexed under this heading.

Zonisamide (Contraceptive effectiveness may be reduced when hormonal contraceptives are co-administered with antibiotics, anti-convulsants, and other drugs that increase the metabolism of contraceptive steroids. This could result in unintended pregnancy or breakthrough bleeding). Products include:
Zonegran Capsules 1089

Food Interactions

Grapefruit (CYP3A4 inhibitors such as itraconazole or ketoconazole may increase plasma hormone levels).

Grapefruit Juice (CYP3A4 inhibitors such as itraconazole or ketoconazole may increase plasma hormone levels).

ORTHO EVRA TRANSDERMAL SYSTEM

(Ethinyl Estradiol, Norelgestromin) 2437
May interact with barbiturates, phenytoin, prednisolone, protease inhibitors, xanthines, and certain other agents. Compounds in these categories include:

Acetaminophen (Co-administration with certain oral contraceptives containing ethinyl estradiol increases plasma ethinyl estradiol levels possibly by inhibition of conjugation; decreased plasma levels of acetaminophen). Products include:
Benadryl Allergy & Cold Kapgels 1895
Benadryl Allergy & Sinus Headache Kapgels 1895
Benadryl Severe Allergy & Sinus Headache Caplets 1897
Lortab 5/500 Tablets 3143
Lortab 7.5/500 Tablets 3144
Lortab 10/500 Tablets 3144
Percocet Tablets 1127
Sinutab Sinus Caplets 1905
Sudafed PE Cold & Cough Caplets 1907
Sudafed PE Nighttime Cold Caplets 1907
Sudafed PE Severe Cold Caplets 1908
Sudafed PE Sinus Headache Caplets 1908
Regular Strength Tylenol Tablets 1915
Tylenol 8 Hour Extended Release Caplets 1915
Extra Strength Tylenol Caplets, Cool Caplets, and EZ Tabs 1915
Extra Strength Tylenol Adult Rapid Blast Liquid 1915
Extra Strength Tylenol PM Caplets, Geltabs, Liquid, and Rapid Release Gels 1915
Extra Strength Tylenol Rapid Release Gels 1915
Tylenol with Codeine Tablets 2427
Tylenol Allergy Multi-Symptom Caplets with Cool Burst and Rapid Release Gelcaps 1916
Tylenol Allergy Multi-Symptom Nighttime Caplets with Cool Burst 1916
Tylenol Severe Allergy Caplets 1916
Tylenol Arthritis Pain Extended Release Geltabs/Caplets 1915
Tylenol Chest Congestion Caplets with Cool Burst 1910
Tylenol Chest Congestion Liquid with Cool Burst 1910
Children's Tylenol Plus Cold Suspension Liquid 1912
Children's Tylenol Plus Cold & Allergy Suspension Liquid 1914
Children's Tylenol Plus Cough & Runny Nose Suspension Liquid 1912
Children's Tylenol Plus Cough & Sore Throat Suspension Liquid 1912
Children's Tylenol Plus Flu Suspension Liquid 1914
Children's Tylenol Suspension Liquid 1909
Children's Tylenol Meltaways 1909
Children's Tylenol Plus Multi-Symptom Cold Suspension Liquid 1912
Tylenol Cold Severe Congestion Daytime Caplets with Cool Burst 1912
Tylenol Cold Head Congestion Daytime Caplets with Cool Burst 1910
Tylenol Cold Head Congestion Nighttime Caplets with Cool Burst 1910
Tylenol Cold Head Congestion Severe Daytime Caplets with Cool Burst 1910
Tylenol Cold Multi-Symptom Daytime Caplets with Cool Burst and Rapid Release Gels 1913
Tylenol Cold Multi-Symptom Daytime Liquid with Citrus Burst 1913
Tylenol Cold Multi-Symptom Nighttime Caplets with Cool Burst 1913
Tylenol Cold Multi-Symptom Nighttime Liquid with Cool Burst 1913
Tylenol Cold Multi-Symptom Severe Caplets with Cool Burst 1913
Tylenol Cold Multi-Symptom Severe Daytime Liquid with Citrus Burst 1913
Tylenol Cough & Sore Throat Daytime Liquid with Cool Burst 1918
Tylenol Cough & Sore Throat Nighttime Liquid with Cool Burst 1918
Concentrated Tylenol Infants' Drops 1909
Jr. Tylenol Meltaways 1909
Tylenol Sinus Congestion & Pain Daytime Caplets with Cool Burst and Gelcaps 1917
Tylenol Sinus Congestion & Pain Nighttime Caplets with Cool Burst 1917
Tylenol Sinus Congestion & Pain Severe Caplets with Cool Burst 1917
Tylenol Sinus Severe Congestion Caplets with Cool Burst 1917
Tylenol Sore Throat Daytime Liquid with Cool Burst 1918
Tylenol Sore Throat Nighttime Liquid with Cool Burst 1918
Women's Tylenol Menstrual Relief Caplets 1919
Vicks DayQuil Cold & Flu Multi-Symptom Relief .... ▣616
Vicks DayQuil LiquiCaps 2567
Vicks DayQuil Liquid 2567
Vicks DayQuil Multi-Symptom Cold/Flu Relief 2567
Vicks NyQuil Cold & Flu Multi-Symptom Relief .... ▣617
Vicks NyQuil LiquiCaps 2567
Vicks NyQuil Liquid 2567
Vicks NyQuil Multi-Symptom Cold/Flu Relief 2567
Vicodin Tablets 529
Vicodin ES Tablets 530
Vicodin HP Tablets 531
Zydone Tablets 1132

Aminophylline (Co-administration increases the plasma concentrations of theophylline).
No products indexed under this heading.

Ampicillin (Increases the metabolism of contraceptive steroids resulting in reduced contraceptive effectiveness which could precipitate unintended pregnancy).
No products indexed under this heading.

Ampicillin Sodium (Increases the metabolism of contraceptive steroids resulting in reduced contraceptive effectiveness which could precipitate unintended pregnancy).
No products indexed under this heading.

Amprenavir (Several of the protease inhibitors have induced significant changes in the AUC of the estrogen and progestins in some cases; it is not known if this applies to Ortho Evra).
No products indexed under this heading.

Aprobarbital (Barbiturates increase the metabolism of contraceptive steroids resulting in reduced contraceptive effectiveness which could precipitate unintended pregnancy).
No products indexed under this heading.

Atorvastatin Calcium (Co-administration with certain oral contraceptives containing ethinyl estradiol increases AUC values for ethinyl estradiol by approximately 20%). Products include:
Lipitor Tablets 2501

Bosentan (Bosentan, used to treat pulmonary hypertension, may interact with hormonal contraceptives to make them less effective in preventing pregnancy or cause an increase in breakthrough bleeding). Products include:
Tracleer Tablets 3289

Butabarbital (Barbiturates increase the metabolism of contraceptive steroids resulting in reduced contraceptive effectiveness which could precipitate unintended pregnancy).
No products indexed under this heading.

Butalbital (Barbiturates increase the metabolism of contraceptive steroids resulting in reduced contraceptive effectiveness which could precipitate unintended pregnancy).
No products indexed under this heading.

Carbamazepine (Increases the metabolism of contraceptive steroids resulting in reduced contraceptive effectiveness which could precipitate unintended pregnancy). Products include:
Carbatrol Capsules 3019
Equetro Extended-Release Capsules 3174

Clofibrate (Increased clearance of clofibric acid).
No products indexed under this heading.

Cyclosporine (Co-administration increases the plasma concentrations of cyclosporine). Products include:
Gengraf Capsules 435
Neoral Oral Solution 2280
Neoral Soft Gelatin Capsules 2280
Restasis Ophthalmic Emulsion 557
Sandimmune 2296

Darunavir (Several of the protease inhibitors have induced significant changes in the AUC of the estrogen and progestins in some cases; it is not known if this applies to Ortho Evra).
No products indexed under this heading.

Dyphylline (Co-administration increases the plasma concentrations of theophylline).
No products indexed under this heading.

Fosamprenavir Calcium (Several of the protease inhibitors have induced significant changes in the AUC of the estrogen and progestins in some cases; it is not known if this applies to Ortho Evra). Products include:
Lexiva Oral Suspension 1510
Lexiva Tablets 1510

Fosphenytoin Sodium (Increases the metabolism of contraceptive steroids resulting in reduced contraceptive effectiveness which could precipitate unintended pregnancy).
No products indexed under this heading.

Griseofulvin (Increases the metabolism of contraceptive steroids resulting in reduced contraceptive effectiveness which could precipitate unintended pregnancy). Products include:
Gris-PEG Tablets 2507

Hypericum (May induce hepatic enzymes and p-glycoprotein transporter and may reduce the effective-

ness of contraceptive steroids which may result in breakthrough bleeding). Products include:
Satieté Tablets 640

Indinavir Sulfate (Several of the protease inhibitors have induced significant changes in the AUC of the estrogen and progestins in some cases; it is not known if this applies to Ortho Evra). Products include:
Crixivan Capsules 1979

Itraconazole (Co-administration with CYP 3A4 inhibitors may increase plasma hormone levels).
No products indexed under this heading.

Ketoconazole (Co-administration with CYP 3A4 inhibitors may increase plasma hormone levels). Products include:
Extina Foam, 2% 3057
Nizoral A-D Shampoo 1901

Lamotrigine (Combined hormonal contraceptives have been shown to significantly decrease plasma concentrations of lamotrigine when co-administered due to induction of lamotrigine glucouronidation. This may reduce seizure control; therefore, dosage adjustments of lamotrigine may be necessary). Products include:
Lamictal 1488

Lopinavir (Several of the protease inhibitors have induced significant changes in the AUC of the estrogen and progestins in some cases; it is not known if this applies to Ortho Evra). Products include:
Kaletra 452

Mephobarbital (Barbiturates increase the metabolism of contraceptive steroids resulting in reduced contraceptive effectiveness which could precipitate unintended pregnancy).
No products indexed under this heading.

Morphine Sulfate (Increased clearance of morphine). Products include:
Avinza Capsules 1772
DepoDur Injection 1095
MS Contin Tablets 2585

Nelfinavir Mesylate (Several of the protease inhibitors have induced significant changes in the AUC of the estrogen and progestins in some cases; it is not known if this applies to Ortho Evra).
No products indexed under this heading.

Pentobarbital Sodium (Barbiturates increase the metabolism of contraceptive steroids resulting in reduced contraceptive effectiveness which could precipitate unintended pregnancy). Products include:
Nembutal Sodium Solution, USP 2494

Phenobarbital (Barbiturates increase the metabolism of contraceptive steroids resulting in reduced contraceptive effectiveness which could precipitate unintended pregnancy). Products include:
Donnatal Extentabs 2507

Phenylbutazone (Increases the metabolism of contraceptive steroids resulting in reduced contraceptive effectiveness which could precipitate unintended pregnancy).
No products indexed under this heading.

Phenytoin (Increases the metabolism of contraceptive steroids resulting in reduced contraceptive effectiveness which could precipitate unintended pregnancy).
No products indexed under this heading.

Phenytoin Sodium (Increases the metabolism of contraceptive steroids resulting in reduced contraceptive effectiveness which could precipitate unintended pregnancy). Products include:
Phenytek Capsules 2192

Prednisolone (Co-administration increases the plasma concentrations of prednisolone).
No products indexed under this heading.

Prednisolone Acetate (Co-administration increases the plasma concentrations of prednisolone). Products include:
Pred Forte Ophthalmic Suspension .... ⊙227
Pred Mild Ophthalmic Suspension .... ⊙230
Pred-G Ophthalmic Ointment .... ⊙229
Pred-G Ophthalmic Suspension .... ⊙228

Prednisolone Sodium Phosphate (Co-administration increases the plasma concentrations of prednisolone).
No products indexed under this heading.

Prednisolone Tebutate (Co-administration increases the plasma concentrations of prednisolone).
No products indexed under this heading.

Rifampin (Increases the metabolism of contraceptive steroids resulting in reduced contraceptive effectiveness which could precipitate unintended pregnancy).
No products indexed under this heading.

Ritonavir (Several of the protease inhibitors have induced significant changes in the AUC of the estrogen and progestins in some cases; it is not known if this applies to Ortho Evra). Products include:
Kaletra 452
Norvir 489

Salicylic Acid (Increased clearance of salicylic acid).
No products indexed under this heading.

Saquinavir (Several of the protease inhibitors have induced significant changes in the AUC of the estrogen and progestins in some cases; it is not known if this applies to Ortho Evra).
No products indexed under this heading.

Saquinavir Mesylate (Several of the protease inhibitors have induced significant changes in the AUC of the estrogen and progestins in some cases; it is not known if this applies to Ortho Evra).
No products indexed under this heading.

Secobarbital Sodium (Barbiturates increase the metabolism of contraceptive steroids resulting in reduced contraceptive effectiveness which could precipitate unintended pregnancy).
No products indexed under this heading.

Temazepam (Increased clearance of temazepam).
No products indexed under this heading.

Theophylline (Co-administration increases the plasma concentrations of theophylline).
No products indexed under this heading.

Theophylline Anhydrous (Co-administration increases the plasma concentrations of theophylline). Products include:
Uniphyl Tablets 2595

Theophylline Calcium Salicylate (Co-administration increases the plasma concentrations of theophylline).
No products indexed under this heading.

Theophylline Dihydroxypropyl (Glyceryl) (Co-administration increases the plasma concentrations of theophylline).
No products indexed under this heading.

Theophylline Ethylenediamine (Co-administration increases the plasma concentrations of theophylline).
No products indexed under this heading.

Theophylline Sodium Glycinate (Co-administration increases the plasma concentrations of theophylline).
No products indexed under this heading.

Thiamylal Sodium (Barbiturates increase the metabolism of contraceptive steroids resulting in reduced contraceptive effectiveness which could precipitate unintended pregnancy).
No products indexed under this heading.

Tipranavir (Several of the protease inhibitors have induced significant changes in the AUC of the estrogen and progestins in some cases; it is not known if this applies to Ortho Evra). Products include:
Aptivus Capsules 823
Aptivus Oral Solution 823

Topiramate (Increases the metabolism of contraceptive steroids resulting in reduced contraceptive effectiveness which could precipitate unintended pregnancy).
No products indexed under this heading.

Vitamin C (Co-administration with certain oral contraceptives containing ethinyl estradiol increases plasma ethinyl estradiol levels possibly by inhibition of conjugation). Products include:
Bausch & Lomb Ocuvite Adult 50+ Vitamin and Mineral Supplement .... ⊙237
Comax Dietary Supplement 995
Ferralet 90 Tablets 2175
Glaucofit Dietary Supplement 995
Glauma Dietary Supplement 995
MoviPrep Oral Solution 2679
Procosa II Tablets 3174
Proflavanol 90 Tablets 3174
Tonox Dietary Supplement 995
Vibe Liquid Multi-Nutrient Supplement 626

ORTHO MICRONOR TABLETS

(Norethindrone) 2446

May interact with barbiturates, phenytoin, and certain other agents. Compounds in these categories include:

Aprobarbital (The effectiveness of progestin-only oral contraceptives is reduced by hepatic enzyme-inducing agents such as barbiturates).
No products indexed under this heading.

Bosentan (Concurrent use of bosentan and norethindrone-containing products may result in decreased concentrations of these contraceptive hormones thereby increasing the risk of unintended pregnancy and unscheduled bleeding). Products include:
Tracleer Tablets 3289

Butabarbital (The effectiveness of progestin-only oral contraceptives is reduced by hepatic enzyme-inducing agents such as barbiturates).
No products indexed under this heading.

Butalbital (The effectiveness of progestin-only oral contraceptives is reduced by hepatic enzyme-inducing agents such as barbiturates).
No products indexed under this heading.

Carbamazepine (The effectiveness of progestin-only oral contraceptives is reduced by hepatic enzyme-inducing agents such as carbamazepine). Products include:
Carbatrol Capsules 3019
Equetro Extended-Release Capsules 3174

Fosphenytoin Sodium (The effectiveness of progestin-only oral contraceptives is reduced by hepatic enzyme-inducing agents such as phenytoin).
No products indexed under this heading.

Hypericum (Herbal products containing St. John's Wort (hypericum perforatum) may induce hepatic enzymes (cytochrome P450) and p-glycoprotein transporter and may reduce the effectiveness of contraceptive steroids. This may also result in breakthrough bleeding). Products include:
Satieté Tablets 640

Hypericum Perforatum (Herbal products containing St. John's Wort (hypericum perforatum) may induce hepatic enzymes (cytochrome P450) and p-glycoprotein transporter and may reduce the effectiveness of contraceptive steroids. This may also result in breakthrough bleeding).
No products indexed under this heading.

Mephobarbital (The effectiveness of progestin-only oral contraceptives is reduced by hepatic enzyme-inducing agents such as barbiturates).
No products indexed under this heading.

Pentobarbital Sodium (The effectiveness of progestin-only oral contraceptives is reduced by hepatic enzyme-inducing agents such as barbiturates). Products include:
Nembutal Sodium Solution, USP 2494

Phenobarbital (The effectiveness of progestin-only oral contraceptives

is reduced by hepatic enzyme-inducing agents such as barbiturates). Products include:
Donnatal Extentabs **2507**

Phenytoin (The effectiveness of progestin-only oral contraceptives is reduced by hepatic enzyme-inducing agents such as phenytoin).
No products indexed under this heading.

Phenytoin Sodium (The effectiveness of progestin-only oral contraceptives is reduced by hepatic enzyme-inducing agents such as phenytoin). Products include:
Phenytek Capsules **2192**

Rifampin (The effectiveness of progestin-only oral contraceptives is reduced by hepatic enzyme-inducing agents such as rifampin).
No products indexed under this heading.

Secobarbital Sodium (The effectiveness of progestin-only oral contraceptives is reduced by hepatic enzyme-inducing agents such as barbiturates).
No products indexed under this heading.

Thiamylal Sodium (The effectiveness of progestin-only oral contraceptives is reduced by hepatic enzyme-inducing agents such as barbiturates).
No products indexed under this heading.

ORTHO TRI-CYCLEN TABLETS

(Ethinyl Estradiol, Norgestimate) **2449**
May interact with barbiturates, phenytoin, prednisolone, protease inhibitors, tetracyclines, xanthines, and certain other agents. Compounds in these categories include:

Acetaminophen (Co-administration with certain oral contraceptives containing ethinyl estradiol increases plasma ethinyl estradiol levels possibly by inhibition of conjugation; decreased plasma levels of acetaminophen). Products include:
Benadryl Allergy & Cold Kapgels **1895**
Benadryl Allergy & Sinus Headache Kapgels **1895**
Benadryl Severe Allergy & Sinus Headache Caplets **1897**
Lortab 5/500 Tablets **3143**
Lortab 7.5/500 Tablets **3144**
Lortab 10/500 Tablets **3144**
Percocet Tablets **1127**
Sinutab Sinus Caplets **1905**
Sudafed PE Cold & Cough Caplets.. **1907**
Sudafed PE Nighttime Cold Caplets.. **1907**
Sudafed PE Severe Cold Caplets **1908**
Sudafed PE Sinus Headache Caplets.. **1908**
Regular Strength Tylenol Tablets **1915**
Tylenol 8 Hour Extended Release Caplets.. **1915**
Extra Strength Tylenol Caplets, Cool Caplets, and EZ Tabs........... **1915**
Extra Strength Tylenol Adult Rapid Blast Liquid.................................. **1915**
Extra Strength Tylenol PM Caplets, Geltabs, Liquid, and Rapid Release Gels...................... **1915**
Extra Strength Tylenol Rapid Release Gels **1915**
Tylenol with Codeine Tablets **2427**
Tylenol Allergy Multi-Symptom Caplets with Cool Burst and Rapid Release Gelcaps............... **1916**
Tylenol Allergy Multi-Symptom Nighttime Caplets with Cool Burst.. **1916**
Tylenol Severe Allergy Caplets **1916**
Tylenol Arthritis Pain Extended Release Geltabs/Caplets **1915**
Tylenol Chest Congestion Caplets with Cool Burst........................... **1910**
Tylenol Chest Congestion Liquid with Cool Burst........................... **1910**
Children's Tylenol Plus Cold Suspension Liquid **1912**
Children's Tylenol Plus Cold & Allergy Suspension Liquid **1914**
Children's Tylenol Plus Cough & Runny Nose Suspension Liquid..... **1912**
Children's Tylenol Plus Cough & Sore Throat Suspension Liquid..... **1912**
Children's Tylenol Plus Flu Suspension Liquid **1914**
Children's Tylenol Suspension Liquid **1909**
Children's Tylenol Meltaways **1909**
Children's Tylenol Plus Multi-Symptom Cold Suspension Liquid **1912**
Tylenol Cold Severe Congestion Daytime Caplets with Cool Burst... **1912**
Tylenol Cold Head Congestion Daytime Caplets with Cool Burst... **1910**
Tylenol Cold Head Congestion Nighttime Caplets with Cool Burst... **1910**
Tylenol Cold Head Congestion Severe Daytime Caplets with Cool Burst................................... **1910**
Tylenol Cold Multi-Symptom Daytime Caplets with Cool Burst and Rapid Release Gels....... **1913**
Tylenol Cold Multi-Symptom Daytime Liquid with Citrus Burst... **1913**
Tylenol Cold Multi-Symptom Nighttime Caplets with Cool Burst... **1913**
Tylenol Cold Multi-Symptom Nighttime Liquid with Cool Burst... **1913**
Tylenol Cold Multi-Symptom Severe Caplets with Cool Burst..... **1913**
Tylenol Cold Multi-Symptom Severe Daytime Liquid with Citrus Burst................................ **1913**
Tylenol Cough & Sore Throat Daytime Liquid with Cool Burst...... **1918**
Tylenol Cough & Sore Throat Nighttime Liquid with Cool Burst... **1918**
Concentrated Tylenol Infants' Drops.. **1909**
Jr. Tylenol Meltaways **1909**
Tylenol Sinus Congestion & Pain Daytime Caplets with Cool Burst and Gelcaps....................... **1917**
Tylenol Sinus Congestion & Pain Nighttime Caplets with Cool Burst... **1917**
Tylenol Sinus Congestion & Pain Severe Caplets with Cool Burst..... **1917**
Tylenol Sinus Severe Congestion Caplets with Cool Burst **1917**
Tylenol Sore Throat Daytime Liquid with Cool Burst.................. **1918**
Tylenol Sore Throat Nighttime Liquid with Cool Burst.................. **1918**
Women's Tylenol Menstrual Relief Caplets.. **1919**
Vicks DayQuil Cold & Flu Multi-Symptom Relief .... ▣ **616**
Vicks DayQuil LiquiCaps **2567**
Vicks DayQuil Liquid **2567**
Vicks DayQuil Multi-Symptom Cold/Flu Relief............................ **2567**
Vicks NyQuil Cold & Flu Multi-Symptom Relief .... ▣ **617**
Vicks NyQuil LiquiCaps **2567**
Vicks NyQuil Liquid **2567**
Vicks NyQuil Multi-Symptom Cold/Flu Relief............................ **2567**
Vicodin Tablets **529**
Vicodin ES Tablets **530**
Vicodin HP Tablets **531**
Zydone Tablets **1132**

Aminophylline (Co-administration increases the plasma concentrations of theophylline).
No products indexed under this heading.

Ampicillin (Several cases of contraceptive failure and breakthrough bleeding have been reported in the literature with concomitant administration of antibiotics, such as tetracyclines. However, clinical pharmacology studies investigating drug interaction between combined oral contraceptives and tetracyclines have reported inconsistent results).
No products indexed under this heading.

Ampicillin Sodium (Several cases of contraceptive failure and breakthrough bleeding have been reported in the literature with concomitant administration of antibiotics, such as tetracyclines. However, clinical pharmacology studies investigating drug interaction between combined oral contraceptives and tetracyclines have reported inconsistent results).
No products indexed under this heading.

Amprenavir (Several of the protease inhibitors have induced significant changes in the AUC of the estrogen and progestins in some cases; co-administration may affect safety and efficacy of oral contraceptives).
No products indexed under this heading.

Aprobarbital (Barbiturates increase the metabolism of contraceptive steroids resulting in reduced contraceptive effectiveness and this could precipitate unintended pregnancy or breakthrough bleeding).
No products indexed under this heading.

Atorvastatin Calcium (Co-administration with certain oral contraceptives containing ethinyl estradiol increases AUC values for ethinyl estradiol by approximately 20%). Products include:
Lipitor Tablets **2501**

Bosentan (Contraceptive effectiveness may be reduced when hormonal contraceptives are co-administered with drugs that increase the metabolism of contraceptive steroids such as bosentan. Concurrent use of bosentan and ethinyl estradiol containing products may result in decrease concentration of these contraceptive hormones thereby increasing the risk of unintended pregnancy and unscheduled bleeding). Products include:
Tracleer Tablets **3289**

Butabarbital (Barbiturates increase the metabolism of contraceptive steroids resulting in reduced contraceptive effectiveness and this could precipitate unintended pregnancy or breakthrough bleeding).
No products indexed under this heading.

Butalbital (Barbiturates increase the metabolism of contraceptive steroids resulting in reduced contraceptive effectiveness and this could precipitate unintended pregnancy or breakthrough bleeding).
No products indexed under this heading.

Carbamazepine (Increases the metabolism of contraceptive steroids resulting in reduced contraceptive effectiveness and this could precipitate unintended pregnancy or breakthrough bleeding). Products include:
Carbatrol Capsules **3019**
Equetro Extended-Release Capsules **3174**

Clofibrate (Increased clearance of clofibric acid).
No products indexed under this heading.

Cyclosporine (Co-administration increases the plasma concentrations of cyclosporine). Products include:
Gengraf Capsules **435**
Neoral Oral Solution **2280**
Neoral Soft Gelatin Capsules **2280**
Restasis Ophthalmic Emulsion **557**
Sandimmune **2296**

Darunavir (Several of the protease inhibitors have induced significant changes in the AUC of the estrogen and progestins in some cases; co-administration may affect safety and efficacy of oral contraceptives).
No products indexed under this heading.

Demeclocycline Hydrochloride (Several cases of contraceptive failure and breakthrough bleeding have been reported in the literature with concomitant administration of antibiotics, such as tetracyclines. However, clinical pharmacology studies investigating drug interaction between combined oral contraceptives and tetracyclines have reported inconsistent results).
No products indexed under this heading.

Doxycycline Calcium (Several cases of contraceptive failure and breakthrough bleeding have been reported in the literature with concomitant administration of antibiotics, such as tetracyclines. However, clinical pharmacology studies investigating drug interaction between combined oral contraceptives and tetracyclines have reported inconsistent results).
No products indexed under this heading.

Doxycycline Hyclate (Several cases of contraceptive failure and breakthrough bleeding have been reported in the literature with concomitant administration of antibiotics, such as tetracyclines. However, clinical pharmacology studies investigating drug interaction between combined oral contraceptives and tetracyclines have reported inconsistent results).
No products indexed under this heading.

Doxycycline Monohydrate (Several cases of contraceptive failure and breakthrough bleeding have been reported in the literature with concomitant administration of antibiotics, such as tetracyclines. However, clinical pharmacology studies investigating drug interaction between combined oral contraceptives and tetracyclines have reported inconsistent results).
No products indexed under this heading.

Dyphylline (Co-administration increases the plasma concentrations of theophylline).
No products indexed under this heading.

Felbamate (Increases the metabolism of contraceptive steroids resulting in reduced contraceptive effectiveness and this could precipitate unintended pregnancy or breakthrough bleeding).
No products indexed under this heading.

Fosamprenavir Calcium (Several of the protease inhibitors have induced significant changes in the AUC of the estrogen and progestins in some cases; co-administration may affect safety and efficacy of oral contraceptives). Products include:
- Lexiva Oral Suspension 1510
- Lexiva Tablets 1510

Fosphenytoin Sodium (Increases the metabolism of contraceptive steroids resulting in reduced contraceptive effectiveness and this could precipitate unintended pregnancy or breakthrough bleeding).
No products indexed under this heading.

Griseofulvin (Increases the metabolism of contraceptive steroids resulting in reduced contraceptive effectiveness and this could precipitate unintended pregnancy or breakthrough bleeding). Products include:
- Gris-PEG Tablets 2507

Hypericum (May induce hepatic enzymes and p-glycoprotein transporter and may reduce the effectiveness of contraceptive steroids and this may result in breakthrough bleeding). Products include:
- Satieté Tablets 640

Indinavir Sulfate (Several of the protease inhibitors have induced significant changes in the AUC of the estrogen and progestins in some cases; co-administration may affect safety and efficacy of oral contraceptives). Products include:
- Crixivan Capsules 1979

Itraconazole (Co-administration with CYP 3A4 inhibitors may increase plasma hormone levels).
No products indexed under this heading.

Ketoconazole (Co-administration with CYP 3A4 inhibitors may increase plasma hormone levels). Products include:
- Extina Foam, 2% 3057
- Nizoral A-D Shampoo 1901

Lopinavir (Several of the protease inhibitors have induced significant changes in the AUC of the estrogen and progestins in some cases; co-administration may affect safety and efficacy of oral contraceptives). Products include:
- Kaletra 452

Mephobarbital (Barbiturates increase the metabolism of contraceptive steroids resulting in reduced contraceptive effectiveness and this could precipitate unintended pregnancy or breakthrough bleeding).
No products indexed under this heading.

Methacycline Hydrochloride (Several cases of contraceptive failure and breakthrough bleeding have been reported in the literature with concomitant administration of antibiotics, such as tetracyclines. However, clinical pharmacology studies investigating drug interaction between combined oral contraceptives and tetracyclines have reported inconsistent results).
No products indexed under this heading.

Minocycline Hydrochloride (Several cases of contraceptive failure and breakthrough bleeding have been reported in the literature with concomitant administration of antibiotics, such as tetracyclines. However, clinical pharmacology studies investigating drug interaction between combined oral contraceptives and tetracyclines have reported inconsistent results). Products include:
- Solodyn Extended Release Tablets 1938

Morphine Sulfate (Increased clearance of morphine). Products include:
- Avinza Capsules 1772
- DepoDur Injection 1095
- MS Contin Tablets 2585

Nelfinavir Mesylate (Several of the protease inhibitors have induced significant changes in the AUC of the estrogen and progestins in some cases; co-administration may affect safety and efficacy of oral contraceptives).
No products indexed under this heading.

Oxcarbazepine (Increases the metabolism of contraceptive steroids resulting in reduced contraceptive effectiveness and this could precipitate unintended pregnancy or breakthrough bleeding).
No products indexed under this heading.

Oxytetracycline Hydrochloride (Several cases of contraceptive failure and breakthrough bleeding have been reported in the literature with concomitant administration of antibiotics, such as tetracyclines. However, clinical pharmacology studies investigating drug interaction between combined oral contraceptives and tetracyclines have reported inconsistent results).
No products indexed under this heading.

Pentobarbital Sodium (Barbiturates increase the metabolism of contraceptive steroids resulting in reduced contraceptive effectiveness and this could precipitate unintended pregnancy or breakthrough bleeding). Products include:
- Nembutal Sodium Solution, USP 2494

Phenobarbital (Barbiturates increase the metabolism of contraceptive steroids resulting in reduced contraceptive effectiveness and this could precipitate unintended pregnancy or breakthrough bleeding). Products include:
- Donnatal Extentabs 2507

Phenylbutazone (Increases the metabolism of contraceptive steroids resulting in reduced contraceptive effectiveness and this could precipitate unintended pregnancy or breakthrough bleeding).
No products indexed under this heading.

Phenytoin (Increases the metabolism of contraceptive steroids resulting in reduced contraceptive effectiveness and this could precipitate unintended pregnancy or breakthrough bleeding).
No products indexed under this heading.

Phenytoin Sodium (Increases the metabolism of contraceptive steroids resulting in reduced contraceptive effectiveness and this could precipitate unintended pregnancy or breakthrough bleeding). Products include:
- Phenytek Capsules 2192

Prednisolone (Co-administration increases the plasma concentrations of prednisolone).
No products indexed under this heading.

Prednisolone Acetate (Co-administration increases the plasma concentrations of prednisolone). Products include:
- Pred Forte Ophthalmic Suspension .... ⊙ 227
- Pred Mild Ophthalmic Suspension .... ⊙ 230
- Pred-G Ophthalmic Ointment .... ⊙ 229
- Pred-G Ophthalmic Suspension ...... ⊙ 228

Prednisolone Sodium Phosphate (Co-administration increases the plasma concentrations of prednisolone).
No products indexed under this heading.

Prednisolone Tebutate (Co-administration increases the plasma concentrations of prednisolone).
No products indexed under this heading.

Rifampin (Increases the metabolism of contraceptive steroids resulting in reduced contraceptive effectiveness and this could precipitate unintended pregnancy or breakthrough bleeding).
No products indexed under this heading.

Ritonavir (Several of the protease inhibitors have induced significant changes in the AUC of the estrogen and progestins in some cases; co-administration may affect safety and efficacy of oral contraceptives). Products include:
- Kaletra 452
- Norvir 489

Salicylic Acid (Increased clearance of salicylic acid).
No products indexed under this heading.

Saquinavir (Several of the protease inhibitors have induced significant changes in the AUC of the estrogen and progestins in some cases; co-administration may affect safety and efficacy of oral contraceptives).
No products indexed under this heading.

Saquinavir Mesylate (Several of the protease inhibitors have induced significant changes in the AUC of the estrogen and progestins in some cases; co-administration may affect safety and efficacy of oral contraceptives).
No products indexed under this heading.

Secobarbital Sodium (Barbiturates increase the metabolism of contraceptive steroids resulting in reduced contraceptive effectiveness and this could precipitate unintended pregnancy or breakthrough bleeding).
No products indexed under this heading.

Temazepam (Increased clearance of temazepam).
No products indexed under this heading.

Tetracycline Hydrochloride (Several cases of contraceptive failure and breakthrough bleeding have been reported in the literature with concomitant administration of antibiotics, such as tetracyclines. However, clinical pharmacology studies investigating drug interaction between combined oral contraceptives and tetracyclines have reported inconsistent results). Products include:
- Pylera Capsules 714

Theophylline (Co-administration increases the plasma concentrations of theophylline).
No products indexed under this heading.

Theophylline Anhydrous (Co-administration increases the plasma concentrations of theophylline). Products include:
- Uniphyl Tablets 2595

Theophylline Calcium Salicylate (Co-administration increases the plasma concentrations of theophylline).
No products indexed under this heading.

Theophylline Dihydroxypropyl (Glyceryl) (Co-administration increases the plasma concentrations of theophylline).
No products indexed under this heading.

Theophylline Ethylenediamine (Co-administration increases the plasma concentrations of theophylline).
No products indexed under this heading.

Theophylline Sodium Glycinate (Co-administration increases the plasma concentrations of theophylline).
No products indexed under this heading.

Thiamylal Sodium (Barbiturates increase the metabolism of contraceptive steroids resulting in reduced contraceptive effectiveness and this could precipitate unintended pregnancy or breakthrough bleeding).
No products indexed under this heading.

Tipranavir (Several of the protease inhibitors have induced significant changes in the AUC of the estrogen and progestins in some cases; co-administration may affect safety and efficacy of oral contraceptives). Products include:
- Aptivus Capsules 823
- Aptivus Oral Solution 823

Topiramate (Increases the metabolism of contraceptive steroids resulting in reduced contraceptive effectiveness and this could precipitate unintended pregnancy or breakthrough bleeding).
No products indexed under this heading.

Vitamin C (Co-administration with certain oral contraceptives containing ethinyl estradiol increases plasma ethinyl estradiol levels possibly by inhibition of conjugation). Products include:
- Bausch & Lomb Ocuvite Adult 50+ Vitamin and Mineral Supplement................................ ⊙ 237
- Comax Dietary Supplement 995
- Ferralet 90 Tablets 2175
- Glaucofit Dietary Supplement 995
- Glauma Dietary Supplement 995
- MoviPrep Oral Solution 2679
- Procosa II Tablets 3174
- Proflavanol 90 Tablets 3174
- Tonox Dietary Supplement 995
- Vibe Liquid Multi-Nutrient Supplement 626

ORTHO TRI-CYCLEN LO TABLETS
(Ethinyl Estradiol, Norgestimate) 2458
May interact with barbiturates, phenytoin, prednisolone, protease inhibitors, tetracyclines, xanthines, and certain other agents. Compounds in these categories include:

Acetaminophen (Co-administration with certain oral contraceptives containing ethinyl estradiol increases plasma ethinyl estradiol levels possibly by inhibition of conjugation; decreased plasma levels of acetaminophen). Products include:
Benadryl Allergy & Cold Kapgels 1895
Benadryl Allergy & Sinus Headache Kapgels 1895
Benadryl Severe Allergy & Sinus Headache Caplets 1897
Lortab 5/500 Tablets 3143
Lortab 7.5/500 Tablets 3144
Lortab 10/500 Tablets 3144
Percocet Tablets 1127
Sinutab Sinus Caplets 1905
Sudafed PE Cold & Cough Caplets 1907
Sudafed PE Nighttime Cold Caplets 1907
Sudafed PE Severe Cold Caplets 1908
Sudafed PE Sinus Headache Caplets 1908
Regular Strength Tylenol Tablets 1915
Tylenol 8 Hour Extended Release Caplets 1915
Extra Strength Tylenol Caplets, Cool Caplets, and EZ Tabs 1915
Extra Strength Tylenol Adult Rapid Blast Liquid 1915
Extra Strength Tylenol PM Caplets, Geltabs, Liquid, and Rapid Release Gels 1915
Extra Strength Tylenol Rapid Release Gels 1915
Tylenol with Codeine Tablets 2427
Tylenol Allergy Multi-Symptom Caplets with Cool Burst and Rapid Release Gelcaps 1916
Tylenol Allergy Multi-Symptom Nighttime Caplets with Cool Burst 1916
Tylenol Severe Allergy Caplets 1916
Tylenol Arthritis Pain Extended Release Geltabs/Caplets 1915
Tylenol Chest Congestion Caplets with Cool Burst 1910
Tylenol Chest Congestion Liquid with Cool Burst 1910
Children's Tylenol Plus Cold Suspension Liquid 1912
Children's Tylenol Plus Cold & Allergy Suspension Liquid 1914
Children's Tylenol Plus Cough & Runny Nose Suspension Liquid 1912
Children's Tylenol Plus Cough & Sore Throat Suspension Liquid 1912
Children's Tylenol Plus Flu Suspension Liquid 1914
Children's Tylenol Suspension Liquid 1909
Children's Tylenol Meltaways 1909
Children's Tylenol Plus Multi-Symptom Cold Suspension Liquid 1912
Tylenol Cold Severe Congestion Daytime Caplets with Cool Burst 1912
Tylenol Cold Head Congestion Daytime Caplets with Cool Burst 1910
Tylenol Cold Head Congestion Nighttime Caplets with Cool Burst 1910
Tylenol Cold Head Congestion Severe Daytime Caplets with Cool Burst 1910
Tylenol Cold Multi-Symptom Daytime Caplets with Cool Burst and Rapid Release Gels 1913
Tylenol Cold Multi-Symptom Daytime Liquid with Citrus Burst ... 1913
Tylenol Cold Multi-Symptom Nighttime Caplets with Cool Burst 1913
Tylenol Cold Multi-Symptom Nighttime Liquid with Cool Burst ... 1913
Tylenol Cold Multi-Symptom Severe Caplets with Cool Burst 1913
Tylenol Cold Multi-Symptom Severe Daytime Liquid with Citrus Burst 1913
Tylenol Cough & Sore Throat Daytime Liquid with Cool Burst 1918
Tylenol Cough & Sore Throat Nighttime Liquid with Cool Burst ... 1918
Concentrated Tylenol Infants' Drops 1909
Jr. Tylenol Meltaways 1909
Tylenol Sinus Congestion & Pain Daytime Caplets with Cool Burst and Gelcaps 1917
Tylenol Sinus Congestion & Pain Nighttime Caplets with Cool Burst 1917
Tylenol Sinus Congestion & Pain Severe Caplets with Cool Burst 1917
Tylenol Sinus Severe Congestion Caplets with Cool Burst 1917
Tylenol Sore Throat Daytime Liquid with Cool Burst 1918
Tylenol Sore Throat Nighttime Liquid with Cool Burst 1918
Women's Tylenol Menstrual Relief Caplets 1919
Vicks DayQuil Cold & Flu Multi-Symptom Relief .... ▣616
Vicks DayQuil LiquiCaps 2567
Vicks DayQuil Liquid 2567
Vicks DayQuil Multi-Symptom Cold/Flu Relief 2567
Vicks NyQuil Cold & Flu Multi-Symptom Relief .... ▣617
Vicks NyQuil LiquiCaps 2567
Vicks NyQuil Liquid 2567
Vicks NyQuil Multi-Symptom Cold/Flu Relief 2567
Vicodin Tablets 529
Vicodin ES Tablets 530
Vicodin HP Tablets 531
Zydone Tablets 1132

Aminophylline (Co-administration increases the plasma concentrations of theophylline).
No products indexed under this heading.

Ampicillin (Several cases of contraceptive failure and breakthrough bleeding have been reported in the literature with concomitant administration of antibiotics, such as tetracyclines. However, clinical pharmacology studies investigating drug interaction between combined oral contraceptives and tetracyclines have reported inconsistent results).
No products indexed under this heading.

Ampicillin Sodium (Several cases of contraceptive failure and breakthrough bleeding have been reported in the literature with concomitant administration of antibiotics, such as tetracyclines. However, clinical pharmacology studies investigating drug interaction between combined oral contraceptives and tetracyclines have reported inconsistent results).
No products indexed under this heading.

Amprenavir (Several of the protease inhibitors have induced significant changes in the AUC of the estrogen and progestins in some cases; co-administration may affect safety and efficacy of oral contraceptives).
No products indexed under this heading.

Aprobarbital (Barbiturates increase the metabolism of contraceptive steroids resulting in reduced contraceptive effectiveness and this could precipitate unintended pregnancy or breakthrough bleeding).
No products indexed under this heading.

Atorvastatin Calcium (Co-administration with certain oral contraceptives containing ethinyl estradiol increases AUC values for ethinyl estradiol by approximately 20%). Products include:
Lipitor Tablets 2501

Bosentan (Concurrent use of bosentan and ethinyl estradiol containing products may result in decreased concentrations of these contraceptive hormones thereby increasing the risk of unintended pregnancy and unscheduled bleeding). Products include:
Tracleer Tablets 3289

Butabarbital (Barbiturates increase the metabolism of contraceptive steroids resulting in reduced contraceptive effectiveness and this could precipitate unintended pregnancy or breakthrough bleeding).
No products indexed under this heading.

Butalbital (Barbiturates increase the metabolism of contraceptive steroids resulting in reduced contraceptive effectiveness and this could precipitate unintended pregnancy or breakthrough bleeding).
No products indexed under this heading.

Carbamazepine (Increases the metabolism of contraceptive steroids resulting in reduced contraceptive effectiveness and this could precipitate unintended pregnancy or breakthrough bleeding). Products include:
Carbatrol Capsules 3019
Equetro Extended-Release Capsules 3174

Clofibrate (Increased clearance of clofibric acid).
No products indexed under this heading.

Cyclosporine (Co-administration increases the plasma concentrations of cyclosporine). Products include:
Gengraf Capsules 435
Neoral Oral Solution 2280
Neoral Soft Gelatin Capsules 2280
Restasis Ophthalmic Emulsion 557
Sandimmune 2296

Darunavir (Several of the protease inhibitors have induced significant changes in the AUC of the estrogen and progestins in some cases; co-administration may affect safety and efficacy of oral contraceptives).
No products indexed under this heading.

Demeclocycline Hydrochloride (Several cases of contraceptive failure and breakthrough bleeding have been reported in the literature with concomitant administration of antibiotics, such as tetracyclines. However, clinical pharmacology studies investigating drug interaction between combined oral contraceptives and tetracyclines have reported inconsistent results).
No products indexed under this heading.

Doxycycline Calcium (Several cases of contraceptive failure and breakthrough bleeding have been reported in the literature with concomitant administration of antibiotics, such as tetracyclines. However, clinical pharmacology studies investigating drug interaction between combined oral contraceptives and tetracyclines have reported inconsistent results).
No products indexed under this heading.

Doxycycline Hyclate (Several cases of contraceptive failure and breakthrough bleeding have been reported in the literature with concomitant administration of antibiotics, such as tetracyclines. However, clinical pharmacology studies investigating drug interaction between combined oral contraceptives and tetracyclines have reported inconsistent results).
No products indexed under this heading.

Doxycycline Monohydrate (Several cases of contraceptive failure and breakthrough bleeding have been reported in the literature with concomitant administration of antibiotics, such as tetracyclines. However, clinical pharmacology studies investigating drug interaction between combined oral contraceptives and tetracyclines have reported inconsistent results).
No products indexed under this heading.

Dyphylline (Co-administration increases the plasma concentrations of theophylline).
No products indexed under this heading.

Felbamate (Increases the metabolism of contraceptive steroids resulting in reduced contraceptive effectiveness and this could precipitate unintended pregnancy or breakthrough bleeding).
No products indexed under this heading.

Fosamprenavir Calcium (Several of the protease inhibitors have induced significant changes in the AUC of the estrogen and progestins in some cases; co-administration may affect safety and efficacy of oral contraceptives). Products include:
Lexiva Oral Suspension 1510
Lexiva Tablets 1510

Fosphenytoin Sodium (Increases the metabolism of contraceptive steroids resulting in reduced contraceptive effectiveness and this could precipitate unintended pregnancy or breakthrough bleeding).
No products indexed under this heading.

Griseofulvin (Increases the metabolism of contraceptive steroids resulting in reduced contraceptive effectiveness and this could precipitate unintended pregnancy or breakthrough bleeding). Products include:
Gris-PEG Tablets 2507

Hypericum (Herbal products containing St. John's Wort (hypericum perforatum) may induce hepatic enzymes (cytochrome P450) and p-glycoprotein transporter and may reduce the effectiveness of contraceptive steroids. This may also result in breakthrough bleeding). Products include:
Satieté Tablets .... ▣640

Hypericum Perforatum (Herbal products containing St. John's Wort (hypericum perforatum) may induce hepatic enzymes (cytochrome P450) and p-glycoprotein transporter and may reduce the effectiveness of contraceptive steroids. This may also result in breakthrough bleeding).
No products indexed under this heading.

Indinavir Sulfate (Several of the protease inhibitors have induced significant changes in the AUC of the estrogen and progestins in some cases; co-administration may affect safety and efficacy of oral contraceptives). Products include:

Crixivan Capsules 1979

Itraconazole (Co-administration with CYP 3A4 inhibitors may increase plasma hormone levels).

No products indexed under this heading.

Ketoconazole (Co-administration with CYP 3A4 inhibitors may increase plasma hormone levels). Products include:

Extina Foam, 2% 3057
Nizoral A-D Shampoo 1901

Lopinavir (Several of the protease inhibitors have induced significant changes in the AUC of the estrogen and progestins in some cases; co-administration may affect safety and efficacy of oral contraceptives). Products include:

Kaletra 452

Mephobarbital (Barbiturates increase the metabolism of contraceptive steroids resulting in reduced contraceptive effectiveness and this could precipitate unintended pregnancy or breakthrough bleeding).

No products indexed under this heading.

Methacycline Hydrochloride (Several cases of contraceptive failure and breakthrough bleeding have been reported in the literature with concomitant administration of antibiotics, such as tetracyclines. However, clinical pharmacology studies investigating drug interaction between combined oral contraceptives and tetracyclines have reported inconsistent results).

No products indexed under this heading.

Minocycline Hydrochloride (Several cases of contraceptive failure and breakthrough bleeding have been reported in the literature with concomitant administration of antibiotics, such as tetracyclines. However, clinical pharmacology studies investigating drug interaction between combined oral contraceptives and tetracyclines have reported inconsistent results). Products include:

Solodyn Extended Release Tablets 1938

Morphine Sulfate (Increased clearance of morphine). Products include:

Avinza Capsules 1772
DepoDur Injection 1095
MS Contin Tablets 2585

Nelfinavir Mesylate (Several of the protease inhibitors have induced significant changes in the AUC of the estrogen and progestins in some cases; co-administration may affect safety and efficacy of oral contraceptives).

No products indexed under this heading.

Oxcarbazepine (Increases the metabolism of contraceptive steroids resulting in reduced contraceptive effectiveness and this could precipitate unintended pregnancy or breakthrough bleeding).

No products indexed under this heading.

Oxytetracycline Hydrochloride (Several cases of contraceptive failure and breakthrough bleeding have been reported in the literature with concomitant administration of antibiotics, such as tetracyclines. However, clinical pharmacology studies investigating drug interaction between combined oral contraceptives and tetracyclines have reported inconsistent results).

No products indexed under this heading.

Pentobarbital Sodium (Barbiturates increase the metabolism of contraceptive steroids resulting in reduced contraceptive effectiveness and this could precipitate unintended pregnancy or breakthrough bleeding). Products include:

Nembutal Sodium Solution, USP 2494

Phenobarbital (Barbiturates increase the metabolism of contraceptive steroids resulting in reduced contraceptive effectiveness and this could precipitate unintended pregnancy or breakthrough bleeding). Products include:

Donnatal Extentabs 2507

Phenylbutazone (Increases the metabolism of contraceptive steroids resulting in reduced contraceptive effectiveness and this could precipitate unintended pregnancy or breakthrough bleeding).

No products indexed under this heading.

Phenytoin (Increases the metabolism of contraceptive steroids resulting in reduced contraceptive effectiveness and this could precipitate unintended pregnancy or breakthrough bleeding).

No products indexed under this heading.

Phenytoin Sodium (Increases the metabolism of contraceptive steroids resulting in reduced contraceptive effectiveness and this could precipitate unintended pregnancy or breakthrough bleeding). Products include:

Phenytek Capsules 2192

Prednisolone (Co-administration increases the plasma concentrations of prednisolone).

No products indexed under this heading.

Prednisolone Acetate (Co-administration increases the plasma concentrations of prednisolone). Products include:

Pred Forte Ophthalmic Suspension .... ⊙227
Pred Mild Ophthalmic Suspension .... ⊙230
Pred-G Ophthalmic Ointment .... ⊙229
Pred-G Ophthalmic Suspension .... ⊙228

Prednisolone Sodium Phosphate (Co-administration increases the plasma concentrations of prednisolone).

No products indexed under this heading.

Prednisolone Tebutate (Co-administration increases the plasma concentrations of prednisolone).

No products indexed under this heading.

Rifampin (Increases the metabolism of contraceptive steroids resulting in reduced contraceptive effectiveness and this could precipitate unintended pregnancy or breakthrough bleeding).

No products indexed under this heading.

Ritonavir (Several of the protease inhibitors have induced significant changes in the AUC of the estrogen and progestins in some cases; co-administration may affect safety and efficacy of oral contraceptives). Products include:

Kaletra 452
Norvir 489

Salicylic Acid (Increased clearance of salicylic acid).

No products indexed under this heading.

Saquinavir (Several of the protease inhibitors have induced significant changes in the AUC of the estrogen and progestins in some cases; co-administration may affect safety and efficacy of oral contraceptives).

No products indexed under this heading.

Saquinavir Mesylate (Several of the protease inhibitors have induced significant changes in the AUC of the estrogen and progestins in some cases; co-administration may affect safety and efficacy of oral contraceptives).

No products indexed under this heading.

Secobarbital Sodium (Barbiturates increase the metabolism of contraceptive steroids resulting in reduced contraceptive effectiveness and this could precipitate unintended pregnancy or breakthrough bleeding).

No products indexed under this heading.

Temazepam (Increased clearance of temazepam).

No products indexed under this heading.

Tetracycline Hydrochloride (Several cases of contraceptive failure and breakthrough bleeding have been reported in the literature with concomitant administration of antibiotics, such as tetracyclines. However, clinical pharmacology studies investigating drug interaction between combined oral contraceptives and tetracyclines have reported inconsistent results). Products include:

Pylera Capsules 714

Theophylline (Co-administration increases the plasma concentrations of theophylline).

No products indexed under this heading.

Theophylline Anhydrous (Co-administration increases the plasma concentrations of theophylline). Products include:

Uniphyl Tablets 2595

Theophylline Calcium Salicylate (Co-administration increases the plasma concentrations of theophylline).

No products indexed under this heading.

Theophylline Dihydroxypropyl (Glyceryl) (Co-administration increases the plasma concentrations of theophylline).

No products indexed under this heading.

Theophylline Ethylenediamine (Co-administration increases the plasma concentrations of theophylline).

No products indexed under this heading.

Theophylline Sodium Glycinate (Co-administration increases the plasma concentrations of theophylline).

No products indexed under this heading.

Thiamylal Sodium (Barbiturates increase the metabolism of contraceptive steroids resulting in reduced contraceptive effectiveness and this could precipitate unintended pregnancy or breakthrough bleeding).

No products indexed under this heading.

Tipranavir (Several of the protease inhibitors have induced significant changes in the AUC of the estrogen and progestins in some cases; co-administration may affect safety and efficacy of oral contraceptives). Products include:

Aptivus Capsules 823
Aptivus Oral Solution 823

Topiramate (Increases the metabolism of contraceptive steroids resulting in reduced contraceptive effectiveness and this could precipitate unintended pregnancy or breakthrough bleeding).

No products indexed under this heading.

Vitamin C (Co-administration with certain oral contraceptives containing ethinyl estradiol increases plasma ethinyl estradiol levels possibly by inhibition of conjugation). Products include:

Bausch & Lomb Ocuvite Adult 50+ Vitamin and Mineral Supplement .... ⊙237
Comax Dietary Supplement 995
Ferralet 90 Tablets 2175
Glaucofit Dietary Supplement 995
Glauma Dietary Supplement 995
MoviPrep Oral Solution 2679
Procosa II Tablets 3174
Proflavanol 90 Tablets 3174
Tonox Dietary Supplement 995
Vibe Liquid Multi-Nutrient Supplement 626

ORTHOCLONE OKT3 STERILE SOLUTION

(Muromonab-CD3) 2387

May interact with corticosteroids and certain other agents. Compounds in these categories include:

Azathioprine (Infection or malignancies have been reported with azathioprine alone and in conjunction with muromonab-CD3).

No products indexed under this heading.

Betamethasone Acetate (Psychosis and infection have been reported in patients treated with corticosteroids alone and in conjunction with muromonab-CD3).

No products indexed under this heading.

Betamethasone Sodium Phosphate (Psychosis and infection have been reported in patients treated with corticosteroids alone and in conjunction with muromonab-CD3).

No products indexed under this heading.

Budesonide (Psychosis and infection have been reported in patients treated with corticosteroids alone and in conjunction with muromonab-CD3). Products include:

Pulmicort Flexhaler 654
Symbicort 80/4.5 Inhalation Aerosol 659
Symbicort 160/4.5 Inhalation Aerosol 659

Ciclesonide (Psychosis and infection have been reported in patients treated with corticosteroids alone and in conjunction with muromonab-CD3). Products include:
Alvesco Inhalation Aerosol 2985
Omnaris Nasal Spray 2998

Cortisone Acetate (Psychosis and infection have been reported in patients treated with corticosteroids alone and in conjunction with muromonab-CD3).
No products indexed under this heading.

Cyclosporine (Seizures, encephalopathy, infections, malignancies, and thrombotic events have been reported in patients receiving cyclosporine alone and in conjunction with muromonab-CD3). Products include:
Gengraf Capsules 435
Neoral Oral Solution 2280
Neoral Soft Gelatin Capsules 2280
Restasis Ophthalmic Emulsion 557
Sandimmune 2296

Dexamethasone (Psychosis and infection have been reported in patients treated with corticosteroids alone and in conjunction with muromonab-CD3). Products include:
Ciprodex Otic Suspension 541

Dexamethasone Acetate (Psychosis and infection have been reported in patients treated with corticosteroids alone and in conjunction with muromonab-CD3).
No products indexed under this heading.

Dexamethasone Sodium Phosphate (Psychosis and infection have been reported in patients treated with corticosteroids alone and in conjunction with muromonab-CD3).
No products indexed under this heading.

Fludrocortisone Acetate (Psychosis and infection have been reported in patients treated with corticosteroids alone and in conjunction with muromonab-CD3).
No products indexed under this heading.

Flunisolide (Psychosis and infection have been reported in patients treated with corticosteroids alone and in conjunction with muromonab-CD3). Products include:
Aerobid/Aerobid-M 1153

Fluticasone Propionate (Psychosis and infection have been reported in patients treated with corticosteroids alone and in conjunction with muromonab-CD3). Products include:
Advair Diskus 100/50 1276
Advair Diskus 250/50 1276
Advair Diskus 500/50 1276
Advair HFA 45/21 Inhalation Aerosol 1288
Advair HFA 115/21 Inhalation Aerosol 1288
Advair HFA 230/21 Inhalation Aerosol 1288
Flonase Nasal Spray 1431
Flovent Diskus 50 mcg 1435

Fluticasone Propionate HFA (Psychosis and infection have been reported in patients treated with corticosteroids alone and in conjunction with muromonab-CD3). Products include:
Flovent HFA 1440

Hydrocortisone (Psychosis and infection have been reported in patients treated with corticosteroids alone and in conjunction with muromonab-CD3).
No products indexed under this heading.

Hydrocortisone Acetate (Psychosis and infection have been reported in patients treated with corticosteroids alone and in conjunction with muromonab-CD3). Products include:
Analpram-HC 1140
Pramosone 1141

Hydrocortisone Sodium Phosphate (Psychosis and infection have been reported in patients treated with corticosteroids alone and in conjunction with muromonab-CD3).
No products indexed under this heading.

Hydrocortisone Sodium Succinate (Psychosis and infection have been reported in patients treated with corticosteroids alone and in conjunction with muromonab-CD3).
No products indexed under this heading.

Indomethacin (Encephalopathy and other CNS effects have been reported in patients treated with indomethacin alone and in conjunction with muromonab-CD3). Products include:
Indocin 2024

Indomethacin Sodium Trihydrate (Encephalopathy and other CNS effects have been reported in patients treated with indomethacin alone and in conjunction with muromonab-CD3). Products include:
Indocin I.V. 2489

Methylprednisolone Acetate (Psychosis and infection have been reported in patients treated with corticosteroids alone and in conjunction with muromonab-CD3).
No products indexed under this heading.

Methylprednisolone Sodium Succinate (Psychosis and infection have been reported in patients treated with corticosteroids alone and in conjunction with muromonab-CD3).
No products indexed under this heading.

Mometasone Furoate (Psychosis and infection have been reported in patients treated with corticosteroids alone and in conjunction with muromonab-CD3). Products include:
Asmanex Twisthaler 2797
Elocon Cream 0.1% 2840
Elocon Lotion 0.1% 2841
Elocon Ointment 0.1% 2842

Mometasone Furoate Monohydrate (Psychosis and infection have been reported in patients treated with corticosteroids alone and in conjunction with muromonab-CD3). Products include:
Nasonex Nasal Spray 2883

Prednisolone Acetate (Psychosis and infection have been reported in patients treated with corticosteroids alone and in conjunction with muromonab-CD3). Products include:
Pred Forte Ophthalmic Suspension .... ⊙227
Pred Mild Ophthalmic Suspension .... ⊙230
Pred-G Ophthalmic Ointment .... ⊙229
Pred-G Ophthalmic Suspension ...... ⊙228

Prednisolone Sodium Phosphate (Psychosis and infection have been reported in patients treated with corticosteroids alone and in conjunction with muromonab-CD3).
No products indexed under this heading.

Prednisolone Tebutate (Psychosis and infection have been reported in patients treated with corticosteroids alone and in conjunction with muromonab-CD3).
No products indexed under this heading.

Prednisone (Psychosis and infection have been reported in patients treated with corticosteroids alone and in conjunction with muromonab-CD3).
No products indexed under this heading.

Triamcinolone (Psychosis and infection have been reported in patients treated with corticosteroids alone and in conjunction with muromonab-CD3).
No products indexed under this heading.

Triamcinolone Acetonide (Psychosis and infection have been reported in patients treated with corticosteroids alone and in conjunction with muromonab-CD3). Products include:
Azmacort Inhalation Aerosol 407
Nasacort AQ Nasal Spray 2765
Triesence Injectable Suspension .... ⊙209

Triamcinolone Diacetate (Psychosis and infection have been reported in patients treated with corticosteroids alone and in conjunction with muromonab-CD3).
No products indexed under this heading.

Triamcinolone Hexacetonide (Psychosis and infection have been reported in patients treated with corticosteroids alone and in conjunction with muromonab-CD3).
No products indexed under this heading.

OSCILLOCOCCINUM
(Anas Barbariae Hepatis et Cordis Extractum) .... ▣604
None cited in PDR database.

OSMOPREP TABLETS
(Sodium Phosphate) 2680
May interact with drugs that prolong the QT interval, drugs which lower seizure threshold, and certain other agents. Compounds in these categories include:

Alprazolam (Sodium phosphate should be used with caution in patients using concomitant medications that lower seizure threshold).
No products indexed under this heading.

Amiodarone Hydrochloride (Sodium phosphate should be used with caution in patients who are taking medications known to prolong the QT interval, since serious complications may occur).
No products indexed under this heading.

Amitriptyline Hydrochloride (Sodium phosphate should be used with caution in patients using concomitant medications that lower seizure threshold).
No products indexed under this heading.

Amoxapine (Sodium phosphate should be used with caution in patients using concomitant medications that lower seizure threshold).
No products indexed under this heading.

Buspirone Hydrochloride (Sodium phosphate should be used with caution in patients who are taking medications known to prolong the QT interval, since serious complications may occur).
No products indexed under this heading.

Chlordiazepoxide (Sodium phosphate should be used with caution in patients using concomitant medications that lower seizure threshold).
No products indexed under this heading.

Chlordiazepoxide Hydrochloride (Sodium phosphate should be used with caution in patients using concomitant medications that lower seizure threshold).
No products indexed under this heading.

Chlorpromazine (Sodium phosphate should be used with caution in patients using concomitant medications that lower seizure threshold).
No products indexed under this heading.

Chlorpromazine Hydrochloride (Sodium phosphate should be used with caution in patients using concomitant medications that lower seizure threshold).
No products indexed under this heading.

Chlorprothixene (Sodium phosphate should be used with caution in patients who are taking medications known to prolong the QT interval, since serious complications may occur).
No products indexed under this heading.

Chlorprothixene Hydrochloride (Sodium phosphate should be used with caution in patients who are taking medications known to prolong the QT interval, since serious complications may occur).
No products indexed under this heading.

Clorazepate Dipotassium (Sodium phosphate should be used with caution in patients who are taking medications known to prolong the QT interval, since serious complications may occur).
No products indexed under this heading.

Clozapine (Sodium phosphate should be used with caution in patients who are taking medications known to prolong the QT interval, since serious complications may occur).
No products indexed under this heading.

Desipramine Hydrochloride (Sodium phosphate should be used with caution in patients using concomitant medications that lower seizure threshold).
No products indexed under this heading.

Diazepam (Sodium phosphate should be used with caution in patients using concomitant medications that lower seizure threshold). Products include:
Valium Tablets 2658

Doxepin Hydrochloride (Sodium phosphate should be used with caution in patients using concomitant medications that lower seizure threshold).

No products indexed under this heading.

Droperidol (Sodium phosphate should be used with caution in patients who are taking medications known to prolong the QT interval, since serious complications may occur).

No products indexed under this heading.

Erythromycin (Sodium phosphate should be used with caution in patients who are taking medications known to prolong the QT interval, since serious complications may occur).

No products indexed under this heading.

Erythromycin Estolate (Sodium phosphate should be used with caution in patients who are taking medications known to prolong the QT interval, since serious complications may occur).

No products indexed under this heading.

Erythromycin Ethylsuccinate (Sodium phosphate should be used with caution in patients who are taking medications known to prolong the QT interval, since serious complications may occur). Products include:

E.E.S. 433
EryPed 431

Erythromycin Gluceptate (Sodium phosphate should be used with caution in patients who are taking medications known to prolong the QT interval, since serious complications may occur).

No products indexed under this heading.

Erythromycin Lactobionate (Sodium phosphate should be used with caution in patients who are taking medications known to prolong the QT interval, since serious complications may occur).

No products indexed under this heading.

Erythromycin Stearate (Sodium phosphate should be used with caution in patients who are taking medications known to prolong the QT interval, since serious complications may occur).

No products indexed under this heading.

Fluoxetine Hydrochloride (Sodium phosphate should be used with caution in patients using concomitant medications that lower seizure threshold). Products include:

Prozac Weekly Capsules 1852
Prozac Pulvules and Liquid 1852
Symbyax Capsules 1871

Fluphenazine Decanoate (Sodium phosphate should be used with caution in patients using concomitant medications that lower seizure threshold).

No products indexed under this heading.

Fluphenazine Enanthate (Sodium phosphate should be used with caution in patients using concomitant medications that lower seizure threshold).

No products indexed under this heading.

Fluphenazine Hydrochloride (Sodium phosphate should be used with caution in patients using concomitant medications that lower seizure threshold).

No products indexed under this heading.

Haloperidol (Sodium phosphate should be used with caution in patients using concomitant medications that lower seizure threshold).

No products indexed under this heading.

Haloperidol Decanoate (Sodium phosphate should be used with caution in patients using concomitant medications that lower seizure threshold).

No products indexed under this heading.

Hydroxyzine Hydrochloride (Sodium phosphate should be used with caution in patients who are taking medications known to prolong the QT interval, since serious complications may occur).

No products indexed under this heading.

Imipramine Hydrochloride (Sodium phosphate should be used with caution in patients using concomitant medications that lower seizure threshold).

No products indexed under this heading.

Imipramine Pamoate (Sodium phosphate should be used with caution in patients using concomitant medications that lower seizure threshold).

No products indexed under this heading.

Isocarboxazid (Sodium phosphate should be used with caution in patients who are taking medications known to prolong the QT interval, since serious complications may occur). Products include:

Marplan Tablets 3177

Lithium Carbonate (Sodium phosphate should be used with caution in patients who are taking medications known to prolong the QT interval, since serious complications may occur).

No products indexed under this heading.

Lithium Citrate (Sodium phosphate should be used with caution in patients who are taking medications known to prolong the QT interval, since serious complications may occur).

No products indexed under this heading.

Lorazepam (Sodium phosphate should be used with caution in patients using concomitant medications that lower seizure threshold).

No products indexed under this heading.

Loxapine Hydrochloride (Sodium phosphate should be used with caution in patients who are taking medications known to prolong the QT interval, since serious complications may occur).

No products indexed under this heading.

Loxapine Succinate (Sodium phosphate should be used with caution in patients who are taking medications known to prolong the QT interval, since serious complications may occur).

No products indexed under this heading.

Maprotiline Hydrochloride (Sodium phosphate should be used with caution in patients using concomitant medications that lower seizure threshold).

No products indexed under this heading.

Meprobamate (Sodium phosphate should be used with caution in patients who are taking medications known to prolong the QT interval, since serious complications may occur).

No products indexed under this heading.

Mesoridazine Besylate (Sodium phosphate should be used with caution in patients using concomitant medications that lower seizure threshold).

No products indexed under this heading.

Midazolam Hydrochloride (Sodium phosphate should be used with caution in patients who are taking medications known to prolong the QT interval, since serious complications may occur).

No products indexed under this heading.

Molindone Hydrochloride (Sodium phosphate should be used with caution in patients who are taking medications known to prolong the QT interval, since serious complications may occur). Products include:

Moban Tablets 1116

Nortriptyline Hydrochloride (Sodium phosphate should be used with caution in patients using concomitant medications that lower seizure threshold).

No products indexed under this heading.

Olanzapine (Sodium phosphate should be used with caution in patients who are taking medications known to prolong the QT interval, since serious complications may occur). Products include:

Symbyax Capsules 1871
Zyprexa Tablets 1883
Zyprexa IntraMuscular 1883
Zyprexa ZYDIS Orally Disintegrating Tablets 1883

Oral Medications, unspecified (Medications administered in close proximity to OsmoPrep tablets may not be absorbed from the gastrointestinal tract due to the rapid intestinal peristalsis and watery diarrhea induced by the purgative agent).

No products indexed under this heading.

Oxazepam (Sodium phosphate should be used with caution in patients using concomitant medications that lower seizure threshold).

No products indexed under this heading.

Perphenazine (Sodium phosphate should be used with caution in patients using concomitant medications that lower seizure threshold).

No products indexed under this heading.

Phenelzine Sulfate (Sodium phosphate should be used with caution in patients who are taking medications known to prolong the QT interval, since serious complications may occur).

No products indexed under this heading.

Prazepam (Sodium phosphate should be used with caution in patients using concomitant medications that lower seizure threshold).

No products indexed under this heading.

Prochlorperazine (Sodium phosphate should be used with caution in patients using concomitant medications that lower seizure threshold).

No products indexed under this heading.

Promethazine Hydrochloride (Sodium phosphate should be used with caution in patients using concomitant medications that lower seizure threshold).

No products indexed under this heading.

Protriptyline Hydrochloride (Sodium phosphate should be used with caution in patients using concomitant medications that lower seizure threshold).

No products indexed under this heading.

Quetiapine Fumarate (Sodium phosphate should be used with caution in patients who are taking medications known to prolong the QT interval, since serious complications may occur).

No products indexed under this heading.

Risperidone (Sodium phosphate should be used with caution in patients who are taking medications known to prolong the QT interval, since serious complications may occur). Products include:

Risperdal Consta Long-Acting Injection 1753

Thioridazine Hydrochloride (Sodium phosphate should be used with caution in patients using concomitant medications that lower seizure threshold). Products include:

Thioridazine Hydrochloride Tablets 2195

Thiothixene (Sodium phosphate should be used with caution in patients who are taking medications known to prolong the QT interval, since serious complications may occur). Products include:

Thiothixene Capsules 2197

Tranylcypromine Sulfate (Sodium phosphate should be used with caution in patients who are taking medications known to prolong the QT interval, since serious complications may occur). Products include:

Parnate Tablets 1532

Trazodone Hydrochloride (Sodium phosphate should be used with caution in patients using concomitant medications that lower seizure threshold).

No products indexed under this heading.

Trifluoperazine Hydrochloride (Sodium phosphate should be used with caution in patients using concomitant medications that lower seizure threshold).

No products indexed under this heading.

Trimipramine Maleate (Sodium phosphate should be used with caution in patients using concomitant medications that lower seizure threshold).

No products indexed under this heading.

IMPORTANT NOTE: Always consult each drug listing in the patient's regimen for possible interactions.

OXYCONTIN TABLETS
(Oxycodone Hydrochloride) 2589
May interact with central nervous system depressants, cytochrome p450 2d6 inhibitors (selected), general anesthetics, hypnotics and sedatives, mixed agonist/antagonist opioid analgesics, phenothiazines, tranquilizers, and certain other agents. Compounds in these categories include:

Alfentanil Hydrochloride (Concurrent use with the usual dose of OxyContin may result in respiratory depression, profound sedation or coma; reduced dosage (1/3 to 1/2 of the usual dosage) may be necessary).
No products indexed under this heading.

Alprazolam (Concurrent use with the usual dose of OxyContin may result in respiratory depression, profound sedation or coma; reduced dosage (1/3 to 1/2 of the usual dosage) may be necessary).
No products indexed under this heading.

Amiodarone Hydrochloride (Concurrent use with CYP2D6 inhibitors may block metabolism of oxycodone).
No products indexed under this heading.

Amitriptyline Hydrochloride (Concurrent use with CYP2D6 inhibitors may block metabolism of oxycodone).
No products indexed under this heading.

Amoxapine (Concurrent use with CYP2D6 inhibitors may block metabolism of oxycodone).
No products indexed under this heading.

Aprobarbital (Concurrent use with the usual dose of OxyContin may result in respiratory depression, profound sedation or coma; reduced dosage (1/3 to 1/2 of the usual dosage) may be necessary).
No products indexed under this heading.

Buprenorphine Hydrochloride (Mixed agonist/antagonist analgesics may reduce the analgesic effect of oxycodone and/or may precipitate withdrawal symptoms).
Products include:
Suboxone Tablets 2601
Subutex Tablets 2601

Bupropion Hydrochloride (Concurrent use with CYP2D6 inhibitors may block metabolism of oxycodone). Products include:
Wellbutrin Tablets 1648
Wellbutrin SR Sustained-Release Tablets 1653
Wellbutrin XL Extended-Release Tablets 1659
Zyban Sustained-Release Tablets 1692

Buspirone Hydrochloride (Concurrent use with the usual dose of OxyContin may result in respiratory depression, profound sedation or coma; reduced dosage (1/3 to 1/2 of the usual dosage) may be necessary).
No products indexed under this heading.

Butabarbital (Concurrent use with the usual dose of OxyContin may result in respiratory depression, profound sedation or coma; reduced dosage (1/3 to 1/2 of the usual dosage) may be necessary).
No products indexed under this heading.

Butabarbital Sodium (Concurrent use with the usual dose of OxyContin may result in respiratory depression, profound sedation or coma; reduced dosage (1/3 to 1/2 of the usual dosage) may be necessary).
No products indexed under this heading.

Butalbital (Concurrent use with the usual dose of OxyContin may result in respiratory depression, profound sedation or coma; reduced dosage (1/3 to 1/2 of the usual dosage) may be necessary).
No products indexed under this heading.

Butorphanol Tartrate (Mixed agonist/antagonist analgesics may reduce the analgesic effect of oxycodone and/or may precipitate withdrawal symptoms).
No products indexed under this heading.

Celecoxib (Concurrent use with CYP2D6 inhibitors may block metabolism of oxycodone). Products include:
Celebrex Capsules 2979

Chloral Hydrate (Concurrent use with the usual dose of OxyContin may result in respiratory depression, profound sedation or coma; reduced dosage (1/3 to 1/2 of the usual dosage) may be necessary).
No products indexed under this heading.

Chlordiazepoxide (Concurrent use with the usual dose of OxyContin may result in respiratory depression, profound sedation or coma; reduced dosage (1/3 to 1/2 of the usual dosage) may be necessary).
No products indexed under this heading.

Chlordiazepoxide Hydrochloride (Concurrent use with the usual dose of OxyContin may result in respiratory depression, profound sedation or coma; reduced dosage (1/3 to 1/2 of the usual dosage) may be necessary).
No products indexed under this heading.

Chloroquine Hydrochloride (Concurrent use with CYP2D6 inhibitors may block metabolism of oxycodone).
No products indexed under this heading.

Chloroquine Phosphate (Concurrent use with CYP2D6 inhibitors may block metabolism of oxycodone).
No products indexed under this heading.

Chlorpheniramine (Concurrent use with CYP2D6 inhibitors may block metabolism of oxycodone).
No products indexed under this heading.

Chlorpheniramine Maleate (Concurrent use with CYP2D6 inhibitors may block metabolism of oxycodone). Products include:
Actifed Cold & Allergy Tablets 1895
Sudafed PE Sinus & Allergy Tablets 1908
Tylenol Allergy Multi-Symptom Caplets with Cool Burst and Rapid Release Gelcaps 1916
Children's Tylenol Plus Cold Suspension Liquid 1912
Children's Tylenol Plus Cough & Runny Nose Suspension Liquid 1912
Children's Tylenol Plus Flu Suspension Liquid 1914
Children's Tylenol Plus Multi-Symptom Cold Suspension Liquid 1912
Tylenol Cold Head Congestion Nighttime Caplets with Cool Burst 1910
Tylenol Cold Multi-Symptom Nighttime Caplets with Cool Burst 1913
Tylenol Sinus Congestion & Pain Nighttime Caplets with Cool Burst 1917

Chlorpheniramine Polistirex (Concurrent use with CYP2D6 inhibitors may block metabolism of oxycodone). Products include:
Tussionex Pennkinetic Extended-Release Suspension 3154

Chlorpheniramine Tannate (Concurrent use with CYP2D6 inhibitors may block metabolism of oxycodone).
No products indexed under this heading.

Chlorpromazine (Concurrent use with the usual dose of OxyContin may result in respiratory depression, profound sedation or coma; reduced dosage (1/3 to 1/2 of the usual dosage) may be necessary).
No products indexed under this heading.

Chlorpromazine Hydrochloride (Concurrent use with the usual dose of OxyContin may result in respiratory depression, profound sedation or coma; reduced dosage (1/3 to 1/2 of the usual dosage) may be necessary).
No products indexed under this heading.

Chlorprothixene (Concurrent use with the usual dose of OxyContin may result in respiratory depression, profound sedation or coma; reduced dosage (1/3 to 1/2 of the usual dosage) may be necessary).
No products indexed under this heading.

Chlorprothixene Hydrochloride (Concurrent use with the usual dose of OxyContin may result in respiratory depression, profound sedation or coma; reduced dosage (1/3 to 1/2 of the usual dosage) may be necessary).
No products indexed under this heading.

Chlorprothixene Lactate (Concurrent use with the usual dose of OxyContin may result in respiratory depression, profound sedation or coma; reduced dosage (1/3 to 1/2 of the usual dosage) may be necessary).
No products indexed under this heading.

Cimetidine (Concurrent use with CYP2D6 inhibitors may block metabolism of oxycodone).
No products indexed under this heading.

Cimetidine Hydrochloride (Concurrent use with CYP2D6 inhibitors may block metabolism of oxycodone).
No products indexed under this heading.

Citalopram Hydrobromide (Concurrent use with CYP2D6 inhibitors may block metabolism of oxycodone). Products include:
Celexa 1160

Clomipramine Hydrochloride (Concurrent use with CYP2D6 inhibitors may block metabolism of oxycodone).
No products indexed under this heading.

Clorazepate Dipotassium (Concurrent use with the usual dose of OxyContin may result in respiratory depression, profound sedation or coma; reduced dosage (1/3 to 1/2 of the usual dosage) may be necessary).
No products indexed under this heading.

Clozapine (Concurrent use with the usual dose of OxyContin may result in respiratory depression, profound sedation or coma; reduced dosage (1/3 to 1/2 of the usual dosage) may be necessary).
No products indexed under this heading.

Cocaine Hydrochloride (Concurrent use with CYP2D6 inhibitors may block metabolism of oxycodone).
No products indexed under this heading.

Codeine Phosphate (Concurrent use with the usual dose of OxyContin may result in respiratory depression, profound sedation or coma; reduced dosage (1/3 to 1/2 of the usual dosage) may be necessary). Products include:
Tylenol with Codeine Tablets 2427

Desflurane (Concurrent use with the usual dose of OxyContin may result in respiratory depression, profound sedation or coma; reduced dosage (1/3 to 1/2 of the usual dosage) may be necessary).
No products indexed under this heading.

Desipramine Hydrochloride (Concurrent use with CYP2D6 inhibitors may block metabolism of oxycodone).
No products indexed under this heading.

Dezocine (Concurrent use with the usual dose of OxyContin may result in respiratory depression, profound sedation or coma; reduced dosage (1/3 to 1/2 of the usual dosage) may be necessary).
No products indexed under this heading.

Diazepam (Concurrent use with the usual dose of OxyContin may result in respiratory depression, profound sedation or coma; reduced dosage (1/3 to 1/2 of the usual dosage) may be necessary). Products include:
Valium Tablets 2658

Diphenhydramine (Concurrent use with CYP2D6 inhibitors may block metabolism of oxycodone).
No products indexed under this heading.

Diphenhydramine Hydrochloride (Concurrent use with CYP2D6 inhibitors may block metabolism of oxycodone). Products include:
Benadryl Allergy & Cold Kapgels 1895
Benadryl Allergy & Sinus Headache Kapgels 1895
Benadryl Severe Allergy & Sinus Headache Caplets 1897
Benadryl Dye-Free Allergy Liqui-gels Softgels 1897
Benadryl Allergy Kapgels 1895
Benadryl Allergy Quick Dissolve Strips 1896
Benadryl Allergy Ultratab Tablets 1896
Children's Benadryl Dye-Free Allergy Liquid 1897
Children's Benadryl Allergy Fastmelts 1897
Children's Benadryl Allergy Liquid 1898
Children's Benadryl Allergy Perfect Measure 1896

Children's Benadryl-D Allergy & Sinus Liquid 1896
Benadryl-D Allergy & Sinus Tablet 1896
PediaCare Children's Allergy & Cold Liquid 1902
PediaCare Children's Allergy Liquid 1902
Simply Sleep Caplets 1905
Sudafed PE Nighttime Cold Caplets 1907
Sudafed PE Severe Cold Caplets 1908
Extra Strength Tylenol PM Caplets, Geltabs, Liquid, and Rapid Release Gels 1915
Tylenol Allergy Multi-Symptom Nighttime Caplets with Cool Burst 1916
Tylenol Severe Allergy Caplets 1916
Children's Tylenol Plus Cold & Allergy Suspension Liquid 1914
Tylenol Sore Throat Nighttime Liquid with Cool Burst 1918

Doxepin Hydrochloride (Concurrent use with CYP2D6 inhibitors may block metabolism of oxycodone).
No products indexed under this heading.

Droperidol (Concurrent use with the usual dose of OxyContin may result in respiratory depression, profound sedation or coma; reduced dosage (1/3 to 1/2 of the usual dosage) may be necessary).
No products indexed under this heading.

Enflurane (Concurrent use with the usual dose of OxyContin may result in respiratory depression, profound sedation or coma; reduced dosage (1/3 to 1/2 of the usual dosage) may be necessary).
No products indexed under this heading.

Escitalopram Oxalate (Concurrent use with CYP2D6 inhibitors may block metabolism of oxycodone). Products include:
Lexapro Oral Suspension 1174
Lexapro Tablets 1174

Estazolam (Concurrent use with the usual dose of OxyContin may result in respiratory depression, profound sedation or coma; reduced dosage (1/3 to 1/2 of the usual dosage) may be necessary).
No products indexed under this heading.

Ethanol (Concurrent use with the usual dose of OxyContin may result in respiratory depression, profound sedation or coma; reduced dosage (1/3 to 1/2 of the usual dosage) may be necessary).
No products indexed under this heading.

Ethchlorvynol (Concurrent use with the usual dose of OxyContin may result in respiratory depression, profound sedation or coma; reduced dosage (1/3 to 1/2 of the usual dosage) may be necessary).
No products indexed under this heading.

Ethinamate (Concurrent use with the usual dose of OxyContin may result in respiratory depression, profound sedation or coma; reduced dosage (1/3 to 1/2 of the usual dosage) may be necessary).
No products indexed under this heading.

Ethyl Alcohol (Concurrent use with the usual dose of OxyContin may result in respiratory depression, profound sedation or coma; reduced dosage (1/3 to 1/2 of the usual dosage) may be necessary).
No products indexed under this heading.

Fentanyl (Concurrent use with the usual dose of OxyContin may result in respiratory depression, profound sedation or coma; reduced dosage (1/3 to 1/2 of the usual dosage) may be necessary). Products include:
Duragesic Transdermal System 2405
Ionsys Transdermal System 2410

Fentanyl Citrate (Concurrent use with the usual dose of OxyContin may result in respiratory depression, profound sedation or coma; reduced dosage (1/3 to 1/2 of the usual dosage) may be necessary). Products include:
Actiq 959
Fentora Tablets 968

Fluoxetine (Concurrent use with CYP2D6 inhibitors may block metabolism of oxycodone).
No products indexed under this heading.

Fluoxetine Hydrochloride (Concurrent use with CYP2D6 inhibitors may block metabolism of oxycodone). Products include:
Prozac Weekly Capsules 1852
Prozac Pulvules and Liquid 1852
Symbyax Capsules 1871

Fluphenazine Decanoate (Concurrent use with the usual dose of OxyContin may result in respiratory depression, profound sedation or coma; reduced dosage (1/3 to 1/2 of the usual dosage) may be necessary).
No products indexed under this heading.

Fluphenazine Enanthate (Concurrent use with the usual dose of OxyContin may result in respiratory depression, profound sedation or coma; reduced dosage (1/3 to 1/2 of the usual dosage) may be necessary).
No products indexed under this heading.

Fluphenazine Hydrochloride (Concurrent use with the usual dose of OxyContin may result in respiratory depression, profound sedation or coma; reduced dosage (1/3 to 1/2 of the usual dosage) may be necessary).
No products indexed under this heading.

Flurazepam Hydrochloride (Concurrent use with the usual dose of OxyContin may result in respiratory depression, profound sedation or coma; reduced dosage (1/3 to 1/2 of the usual dosage) may be necessary).
No products indexed under this heading.

Fluvoxamine Maleate (Concurrent use with CYP2D6 inhibitors may block metabolism of oxycodone). Products include:
Luvox CR Extended-Release Capsules 1759

Glutethimide (Concurrent use with the usual dose of OxyContin may result in respiratory depression, profound sedation or coma; reduced dosage (1/3 to 1/2 of the usual dosage) may be necessary).
No products indexed under this heading.

Halofantrine Hydrochloride (Concurrent use with CYP2D6 inhibitors may block metabolism of oxycodone).
No products indexed under this heading.

Haloperidol (Concurrent use with the usual dose of OxyContin may result in respiratory depression, profound sedation or coma; reduced dosage (1/3 to 1/2 of the usual dosage) may be necessary).
No products indexed under this heading.

Haloperidol Decanoate (Concurrent use with the usual dose of OxyContin may result in respiratory depression, profound sedation or coma; reduced dosage (1/3 to 1/2 of the usual dosage) may be necessary).
No products indexed under this heading.

Hydrocodone Bitartrate (Concurrent use with the usual dose of OxyContin may result in respiratory depression, profound sedation or coma; reduced dosage (1/3 to 1/2 of the usual dosage) may be necessary). Products include:
Lortab 5/500 Tablets 3143
Lortab 7.5/500 Tablets 3144
Lortab 10/500 Tablets 3144
Vicodin Tablets 529
Vicodin ES Tablets 530
Vicodin HP Tablets 531
Vicoprofen Tablets 533
Zydone Tablets 1132

Hydrocodone Polistirex (Concurrent use with the usual dose of OxyContin may result in respiratory depression, profound sedation or coma; reduced dosage (1/3 to 1/2 of the usual dosage) may be necessary). Products include:
Tussionex Pennkinetic Extended-Release Suspension 3154

Hydromorphone Hydrochloride (Concurrent use with the usual dose of OxyContin may result in respiratory depression, profound sedation or coma; reduced dosage (1/3 to 1/2 of the usual dosage) may be necessary).
No products indexed under this heading.

Hydroxychloroquine Sulfate (Concurrent use with CYP2D6 inhibitors may block metabolism of oxycodone).
No products indexed under this heading.

Hydroxyzine Hydrochloride (Concurrent use with the usual dose of OxyContin may result in respiratory depression, profound sedation or coma; reduced dosage (1/3 to 1/2 of the usual dosage) may be necessary).
No products indexed under this heading.

Imatinib Mesylate (Concurrent use with CYP2D6 inhibitors may block metabolism of oxycodone). Products include:
Gleevec Tablets 2255

Imipramine Hydrochloride (Concurrent use with CYP2D6 inhibitors may block metabolism of oxycodone).
No products indexed under this heading.

Imipramine Pamoate (Concurrent use with CYP2D6 inhibitors may block metabolism of oxycodone).
No products indexed under this heading.

Isoflurane (Concurrent use with the usual dose of OxyContin may result in respiratory depression, profound sedation or coma; reduced dosage (1/3 to 1/2 of the usual dosage) may be necessary).
No products indexed under this heading.

Ketamine Hydrochloride (Concurrent use with the usual dose of OxyContin may result in respiratory depression, profound sedation or coma; reduced dosage (1/3 to 1/2 of the usual dosage) may be necessary).
No products indexed under this heading.

Levomethadyl Acetate Hydrochloride (Concurrent use with the usual dose of OxyContin may result in respiratory depression, profound sedation or coma; reduced dosage (1/3 to 1/2 of the usual dosage) may be necessary).
No products indexed under this heading.

Levorphanol Tartrate (Concurrent use with the usual dose of OxyContin may result in respiratory depression, profound sedation or coma; reduced dosage (1/3 to 1/2 of the usual dosage) may be necessary).
No products indexed under this heading.

Lorazepam (Concurrent use with the usual dose of OxyContin may result in respiratory depression, profound sedation or coma; reduced dosage (1/3 to 1/2 of the usual dosage) may be necessary).
No products indexed under this heading.

Loxapine Hydrochloride (Concurrent use with the usual dose of OxyContin may result in respiratory depression, profound sedation or coma; reduced dosage (1/3 to 1/2 of the usual dosage) may be necessary).
No products indexed under this heading.

Loxapine Succinate (Concurrent use with the usual dose of OxyContin may result in respiratory depression, profound sedation or coma; reduced dosage (1/3 to 1/2 of the usual dosage) may be necessary).
No products indexed under this heading.

Maprotiline Hydrochloride (Concurrent use with CYP2D6 inhibitors may block metabolism of oxycodone).
No products indexed under this heading.

Meperidine Hydrochloride (Concurrent use with the usual dose of OxyContin may result in respiratory depression, profound sedation or coma; reduced dosage (1/3 to 1/2 of the usual dosage) may be necessary).
No products indexed under this heading.

Mephobarbital (Concurrent use with the usual dose of OxyContin may result in respiratory depression, profound sedation or coma; reduced dosage (1/3 to 1/2 of the usual dosage) may be necessary).
No products indexed under this heading.

Meprobamate (Concurrent use with the usual dose of OxyContin may result in respiratory depression, profound sedation or coma; reduced dosage (1/3 to 1/2 of the usual dosage) may be necessary).
No products indexed under this heading.

Mesoridazine Besylate (Concurrent use with the usual dose of OxyContin may result in respiratory depression, profound sedation or coma; reduced dosage (1/3 to 1/2 of the usual dosage) may be necessary).
No products indexed under this heading.

Methadone Hydrochloride (Concurrent use with the usual dose of OxyContin may result in respiratory depression, profound sedation or coma; reduced dosage (1/3 to 1/2 of the usual dosage) may be necessary).
No products indexed under this heading.

Methohexital Sodium (Concurrent use with the usual dose of OxyContin may result in respiratory depression, profound sedation or coma; reduced dosage (1/3 to 1/2 of the usual dosage) may be necessary).
No products indexed under this heading.

Methotrimeprazine (Concurrent use with the usual dose of OxyContin may result in respiratory depression, profound sedation or coma; reduced dosage (1/3 to 1/2 of the usual dosage) may be necessary).
No products indexed under this heading.

Methoxyflurane (Concurrent use with the usual dose of OxyContin may result in respiratory depression, profound sedation or coma; reduced dosage (1/3 to 1/2 of the usual dosage) may be necessary).
No products indexed under this heading.

Mibefradil Dihydrochloride (Concurrent use with CYP2D6 inhibitors may block metabolism of oxycodone).
No products indexed under this heading.

Midazolam Hydrochloride (Concurrent use with the usual dose of OxyContin may result in respiratory depression, profound sedation or coma; reduced dosage (1/3 to 1/2 of the usual dosage) may be necessary).
No products indexed under this heading.

Moclobemide (Concurrent use with CYP2D6 inhibitors may block metabolism of oxycodone).
No products indexed under this heading.

Molindone Hydrochloride (Concurrent use with the usual dose of OxyContin may result in respiratory depression, profound sedation or coma; reduced dosage (1/3 to 1/2 of the usual dosage) may be necessary). Products include:
Moban Tablets 1116

Morphine Sulfate (Concurrent use with the usual dose of OxyContin may result in respiratory depression, profound sedation or coma; reduced dosage (1/3 to 1/2 of the usual dosage) may be necessary). Products include:
Avinza Capsules 1772
DepoDur Injection 1095
MS Contin Tablets 2585

Nalbuphine Hydrochloride (Mixed agonist/antagonist analgesics may reduce the analgesic effect of oxycodone and/or may precipitate withdrawal symptoms).
No products indexed under this heading.

Nortriptyline Hydrochloride (Concurrent use with CYP2D6 inhibitors may block metabolism of oxycodone).
No products indexed under this heading.

Olanzapine (Concurrent use with the usual dose of OxyContin may result in respiratory depression, profound sedation or coma; reduced dosage (1/3 to 1/2 of the usual dosage) may be necessary). Products include:
Symbyax Capsules 1871
Zyprexa Tablets 1883
Zyprexa IntraMuscular 1883
Zyprexa ZYDIS Orally Disintegrating Tablets 1883

Oxazepam (Concurrent use with the usual dose of OxyContin may result in respiratory depression, profound sedation or coma; reduced dosage (1/3 to 1/2 of the usual dosage) may be necessary).
No products indexed under this heading.

Paroxetine Hydrochloride (Concurrent use with CYP2D6 inhibitors may block metabolism of oxycodone). Products include:
Paxil 1535
Paxil CR Controlled-Release Tablets 1544

Pentazocine Hydrochloride (Mixed agonist/antagonist analgesics may reduce the analgesic effect of oxycodone and/or may precipitate withdrawal symptoms).
No products indexed under this heading.

Pentazocine Lactate (Mixed agonist/antagonist analgesics may reduce the analgesic effect of oxycodone and/or may precipitate withdrawal symptoms).
No products indexed under this heading.

Pentobarbital Sodium (Concurrent use with the usual dose of OxyContin may result in respiratory depression, profound sedation or coma; reduced dosage (1/3 to 1/2 of the usual dosage) may be necessary). Products include:
Nembutal Sodium Solution, USP 2494

Perphenazine (Concurrent use with the usual dose of OxyContin may result in respiratory depression, profound sedation or coma; reduced dosage (1/3 to 1/2 of the usual dosage) may be necessary).
No products indexed under this heading.

Phenobarbital (Concurrent use with the usual dose of OxyContin may result in respiratory depression, profound sedation or coma; reduced dosage (1/3 to 1/2 of the usual dosage) may be necessary). Products include:
Donnatal Extentabs 2507

Prazepam (Concurrent use with the usual dose of OxyContin may result in respiratory depression, profound sedation or coma; reduced dosage (1/3 to 1/2 of the usual dosage) may be necessary).
No products indexed under this heading.

Prochlorperazine (Concurrent use with the usual dose of OxyContin may result in respiratory depression, profound sedation or coma; reduced dosage (1/3 to 1/2 of the usual dosage) may be necessary).
No products indexed under this heading.

Promethazine Hydrochloride (Concurrent use with the usual dose of OxyContin may result in respiratory depression, profound sedation or coma; reduced dosage (1/3 to 1/2 of the usual dosage) may be necessary).
No products indexed under this heading.

Propafenone Hydrochloride (Concurrent use with CYP2D6 inhibitors may block metabolism of oxycodone). Products include:
Rythmol Tablets 1586
Rythmol SR Capsules 1590

Propofol (Concurrent use with the usual dose of OxyContin may result in respiratory depression, profound sedation or coma; reduced dosage (1/3 to 1/2 of the usual dosage) may be necessary).
No products indexed under this heading.

Propoxyphene Hydrochloride (Concurrent use with the usual dose of OxyContin may result in respiratory depression, profound sedation or coma; reduced dosage (1/3 to 1/2 of the usual dosage) may be necessary).
No products indexed under this heading.

Propoxyphene Napsylate (Concurrent use with the usual dose of OxyContin may result in respiratory depression, profound sedation or coma; reduced dosage (1/3 to 1/2 of the usual dosage) may be necessary).
No products indexed under this heading.

Protriptyline Hydrochloride (Concurrent use with CYP2D6 inhibitors may block metabolism of oxycodone).
No products indexed under this heading.

Quazepam (Concurrent use with the usual dose of OxyContin may result in respiratory depression, profound sedation or coma; reduced dosage (1/3 to 1/2 of the usual dosage) may be necessary).
No products indexed under this heading.

Quetiapine Fumarate (Concurrent use with the usual dose of OxyContin may result in respiratory depression, profound sedation or coma; reduced dosage (1/3 to 1/2 of the usual dosage) may be necessary).
No products indexed under this heading.

Quinacrine Hydrochloride (Concurrent use with CYP2D6 inhibitors may block metabolism of oxycodone).
No products indexed under this heading.

Quinidine Gluconate (Concurrent use with CYP2D6 inhibitors may block metabolism of oxycodone).
No products indexed under this heading.

Quinidine Hydrochloride (Concurrent use with CYP2D6 inhibitors may block metabolism of oxycodone).
No products indexed under this heading.

Quinidine Polygalacturonate (Concurrent use with CYP2D6 inhibitors may block metabolism of oxycodone).
No products indexed under this heading.

Quinidine Sulfate (Concurrent use with CYP2D6 inhibitors may block metabolism of oxycodone).
No products indexed under this heading.

Ramelteon (Concurrent use with the usual dose of OxyContin may result in respiratory depression, profound sedation or coma; reduced dosage (1/3 to 1/2 of the usual dosage) may be necessary). Products include:
Rozerem Tablets 3091

Ranitidine Bismuth Citrate (Concurrent use with CYP2D6 inhibitors may block metabolism of oxycodone).
No products indexed under this heading.

Ranitidine Hydrochloride (Concurrent use with CYP2D6 inhibitors may block metabolism of oxycodone). Products include:
Zantac 75 Tablets .... ▣603
Zantac 1670
Zantac Injection 1666
Zantac Injection Pharmacy Bulk Package 1668
Maximum Strength Zantac 150 Tablets .... ▣603
Maximum Strength Zantac 150 Cool Mint Tablets .... ▣603

Remifentanil Hydrochloride (Concurrent use with the usual dose of OxyContin may result in respiratory depression, profound sedation or coma; reduced dosage (1/3 to 1/2 of the usual dosage) may be necessary).
No products indexed under this heading.

Risperidone (Concurrent use with the usual dose of OxyContin may result in respiratory depression, profound sedation or coma; reduced dosage (1/3 to 1/2 of the usual dosage) may be necessary). Products include:
Risperdal Consta Long-Acting Injection 1753

Ritonavir (Concurrent use with CYP2D6 inhibitors may block metabolism of oxycodone). Products include:
Kaletra 452
Norvir 489

Secobarbital Sodium (Concurrent use with the usual dose of OxyContin may result in respiratory depression, profound sedation or coma; reduced dosage (1/3 to 1/2 of the usual dosage) may be necessary).
No products indexed under this heading.

Sertraline Hydrochloride (Concurrent use with CYP2D6 inhibitors may block metabolism of oxycodone).
No products indexed under this heading.

Sevoflurane (Concurrent use with the usual dose of OxyContin may

result in respiratory depression, profound sedation or coma; reduced dosage (1/3 to 1/2 of the usual dosage) may be necessary). Products include:
Ultane Liquid for Inhalation 524

Sildenafil Citrate (Concurrent use with CYP2D6 inhibitors may block metabolism of oxycodone).
No products indexed under this heading.

Sodium Butabarbital (Concurrent use with the usual dose of OxyContin may result in respiratory depression, profound sedation or coma; reduced dosage (1/3 to 1/2 of the usual dosage) may be necessary).
No products indexed under this heading.

Sodium Oxybate (Concurrent use with the usual dose of OxyContin may result in respiratory depression, profound sedation or coma; reduced dosage (1/3 to 1/2 of the usual dosage) may be necessary). Products include:
Xyrem Oral Solution 1766

Sufentanil Citrate (Concurrent use with the usual dose of OxyContin may result in respiratory depression, profound sedation or coma; reduced dosage (1/3 to 1/2 of the usual dosage) may be necessary).
No products indexed under this heading.

Temazepam (Concurrent use with the usual dose of OxyContin may result in respiratory depression, profound sedation or coma; reduced dosage (1/3 to 1/2 of the usual dosage) may be necessary).
No products indexed under this heading.

Terbinafine Hydrochloride (Concurrent use with CYP2D6 inhibitors may block metabolism of oxycodone). Products include:
Lamisil Oral Granules 2264
Lamisil Tablets 2266

Thiamylal Sodium (Concurrent use with the usual dose of OxyContin may result in respiratory depression, profound sedation or coma; reduced dosage (1/3 to 1/2 of the usual dosage) may be necessary).
No products indexed under this heading.

Thioridazine Hydrochloride (Concurrent use with the usual dose of OxyContin may result in respiratory depression, profound sedation or coma; reduced dosage (1/3 to 1/2 of the usual dosage) may be necessary). Products include:
Thioridazine Hydrochloride Tablets 2195

Thiothixene (Concurrent use with the usual dose of OxyContin may result in respiratory depression, profound sedation or coma; reduced dosage (1/3 to 1/2 of the usual dosage) may be necessary). Products include:
Thiothixene Capsules 2197

Triazolam (Concurrent use with the usual dose of OxyContin may result in respiratory depression, profound sedation or coma; reduced dosage (1/3 to 1/2 of the usual dosage) may be necessary).
No products indexed under this heading.

Trifluoperazine Hydrochloride (Concurrent use with the usual dose of OxyContin may result in respiratory depression, profound sedation or coma; reduced dosage (1/3 to 1/2 of the usual dosage) may be necessary).
No products indexed under this heading.

Trimipramine Maleate (Concurrent use with CYP2D6 inhibitors may block metabolism of oxycodone).
No products indexed under this heading.

Vardenafil Hydrochloride (Concurrent use with CYP2D6 inhibitors may block metabolism of oxycodone). Products include:
Levitra Tablets 2876

Zaleplon (Concurrent use with the usual dose of OxyContin may result in respiratory depression, profound sedation or coma; reduced dosage (1/3 to 1/2 of the usual dosage) may be necessary).
No products indexed under this heading.

Ziprasidone Hydrochloride (Concurrent use with the usual dose of OxyContin may result in respiratory depression, profound sedation or coma; reduced dosage (1/3 to 1/2 of the usual dosage) may be necessary). Products include:
Geodon Capsules 2520

Zolpidem Tartrate (Concurrent use with the usual dose of OxyContin may result in respiratory depression, profound sedation or coma; reduced dosage (1/3 to 1/2 of the usual dosage) may be necessary). Products include:
Ambien Tablets 2692
Ambien CR Tablets 2696

Food Interactions

Alcohol (Concurrent use with the usual dose of OxyContin may result in respiratory depression, profound sedation or coma).

OXYIR CAPSULES

(Oxycodone Hydrochloride) 2593
May interact with central nervous system depressants, general anesthetics, hypnotics and sedatives, mixed agonist/antagonist opioid analgesics, narcotic analgesics, phenothiazines, tranquilizers, and certain other agents. Compounds in these categories include:

Alfentanil Hydrochloride (Concomitant use may exhibit an additive CNS depression).
No products indexed under this heading.

Alprazolam (Concomitant use may exhibit an additive CNS depression).
No products indexed under this heading.

Aprobarbital (Concomitant use may exhibit an additive CNS depression).
No products indexed under this heading.

Buprenorphine Hydrochloride (Co-administration with mixed agonist/antagonist analgesics may reduce the analgesic effect of oxycodone and/or may precipitate withdrawal symptoms). Products include:
Suboxone Tablets 2601
Subutex Tablets 2601

Buspirone Hydrochloride (Concomitant use may exhibit an additive CNS depression).
No products indexed under this heading.

Butabarbital (Concomitant use may exhibit an additive CNS depression).
No products indexed under this heading.

Butabarbital Sodium (Concomitant use may exhibit an additive CNS depression).
No products indexed under this heading.

Butalbital (Concomitant use may exhibit an additive CNS depression).
No products indexed under this heading.

Butorphanol Tartrate (Co-administration with mixed agonist/antagonist analgesics may reduce the analgesic effect of oxycodone and/or may precipitate withdrawal symptoms).
No products indexed under this heading.

Chloral Hydrate (Concomitant use may exhibit an additive CNS depression).
No products indexed under this heading.

Chlordiazepoxide (Concomitant use may exhibit an additive CNS depression).
No products indexed under this heading.

Chlordiazepoxide Hydrochloride (Concomitant use may exhibit an additive CNS depression).
No products indexed under this heading.

Chlorpromazine (Concomitant use may exhibit an additive CNS depression).
No products indexed under this heading.

Chlorpromazine Hydrochloride (Concomitant use may exhibit an additive CNS depression).
No products indexed under this heading.

Chlorprothixene (Concomitant use may exhibit an additive CNS depression).
No products indexed under this heading.

Chlorprothixene Hydrochloride (Concomitant use may exhibit an additive CNS depression).
No products indexed under this heading.

Chlorprothixene Lactate (Concomitant use may exhibit an additive CNS depression).
No products indexed under this heading.

Clorazepate Dipotassium (Concomitant use may exhibit an additive CNS depression).
No products indexed under this heading.

Clozapine (Concomitant use may exhibit an additive CNS depression).
No products indexed under this heading.

Codeine Phosphate (Concomitant use may exhibit an additive CNS depression). Products include:
Tylenol with Codeine Tablets 2427

Desflurane (Concomitant use may exhibit an additive CNS depression).
No products indexed under this heading.

Dezocine (Concomitant use may exhibit an additive CNS depression).
No products indexed under this heading.

Diazepam (Concomitant use may exhibit an additive CNS depression). Products include:
Valium Tablets 2658

Droperidol (Concomitant use may exhibit an additive CNS depression).
No products indexed under this heading.

Enflurane (Concomitant use may exhibit an additive CNS depression).
No products indexed under this heading.

Estazolam (Concomitant use may exhibit an additive CNS depression).
No products indexed under this heading.

Ethanol (Concomitant use may exhibit an additive CNS depression).
No products indexed under this heading.

Ethchlorvynol (Concomitant use may exhibit an additive CNS depression).
No products indexed under this heading.

Ethinamate (Concomitant use may exhibit an additive CNS depression).
No products indexed under this heading.

Ethyl Alcohol (Concomitant use may exhibit an additive CNS depression).
No products indexed under this heading.

Fentanyl (Concomitant use may exhibit an additive CNS depression). Products include:
Duragesic Transdermal System 2405
Ionsys Transdermal System 2410

Fentanyl Citrate (Concomitant use may exhibit an additive CNS depression). Products include:
Actiq 959
Fentora Tablets 968

Fluphenazine Decanoate (Concomitant use may exhibit an additive CNS depression).
No products indexed under this heading.

Fluphenazine Enanthate (Concomitant use may exhibit an additive CNS depression).
No products indexed under this heading.

Fluphenazine Hydrochloride (Concomitant use may exhibit an additive CNS depression).
No products indexed under this heading.

Flurazepam Hydrochloride (Concomitant use may exhibit an additive CNS depression).
No products indexed under this heading.

Glutethimide (Concomitant use may exhibit an additive CNS depression).
No products indexed under this heading.

Haloperidol (Concomitant use may exhibit an additive CNS depression).
No products indexed under this heading.

Haloperidol Decanoate (Concomitant use may exhibit an additive CNS depression).
No products indexed under this heading.

Hydrocodone Bitartrate (Concomitant use may exhibit an additive CNS depression). Products include:
Lortab 5/500 Tablets 3143
Lortab 7.5/500 Tablets 3144
Lortab 10/500 Tablets 3144
Vicodin Tablets 529
Vicodin ES Tablets 530
Vicodin HP Tablets 531
Vicoprofen Tablets 533

Zydone Tablets 1132

Hydrocodone Polistirex (Concomitant use may exhibit an additive CNS depression). Products include:

Tussionex Pennkinetic Extended-Release Suspension 3154

Hydromorphone Hydrochloride (Concomitant use may exhibit an additive CNS depression).

No products indexed under this heading.

Hydroxyzine Hydrochloride (Concomitant use may exhibit an additive CNS depression).

No products indexed under this heading.

Isoflurane (Concomitant use may exhibit an additive CNS depression).

No products indexed under this heading.

Ketamine Hydrochloride (Concomitant use may exhibit an additive CNS depression).

No products indexed under this heading.

Levomethadyl Acetate Hydrochloride (Concomitant use may exhibit an additive CNS depression).

No products indexed under this heading.

Levorphanol Tartrate (Concomitant use may exhibit an additive CNS depression).

No products indexed under this heading.

Lorazepam (Concomitant use may exhibit an additive CNS depression).

No products indexed under this heading.

Loxapine Hydrochloride (Concomitant use may exhibit an additive CNS depression).

No products indexed under this heading.

Loxapine Succinate (Concomitant use may exhibit an additive CNS depression).

No products indexed under this heading.

Meperidine Hydrochloride (Concomitant use may exhibit an additive CNS depression).

No products indexed under this heading.

Mephobarbital (Concomitant use may exhibit an additive CNS depression).

No products indexed under this heading.

Meprobamate (Concomitant use may exhibit an additive CNS depression).

No products indexed under this heading.

Mesoridazine Besylate (Concomitant use may exhibit an additive CNS depression).

No products indexed under this heading.

Methadone Hydrochloride (Concomitant use may exhibit an additive CNS depression).

No products indexed under this heading.

Methohexital Sodium (Concomitant use may exhibit an additive CNS depression).

No products indexed under this heading.

Methotrimeprazine (Concomitant use may exhibit an additive CNS depression).

No products indexed under this heading.

Methoxyflurane (Concomitant use may exhibit an additive CNS depression).

No products indexed under this heading.

Midazolam Hydrochloride (Concomitant use may exhibit an additive CNS depression).

No products indexed under this heading.

Molindone Hydrochloride (Concomitant use may exhibit an additive CNS depression). Products include:

Moban Tablets 1116

Morphine Sulfate (Concomitant use may exhibit an additive CNS depression). Products include:

Avinza Capsules 1772
DepoDur Injection 1095
MS Contin Tablets 2585

Nalbuphine Hydrochloride (Coadministration with mixed agonist/antagonist analgesics may reduce the analgesic effect of oxycodone and/or may precipitate withdrawal symptoms).

No products indexed under this heading.

Olanzapine (Concomitant use may exhibit an additive CNS depression). Products include:

Symbyax Capsules 1871
Zyprexa Tablets 1883
Zyprexa IntraMuscular 1883
Zyprexa ZYDIS Orally Disintegrating Tablets 1883

Oxazepam (Concomitant use may exhibit an additive CNS depression).

No products indexed under this heading.

Pentazocine Hydrochloride (Coadministration with mixed agonist/antagonist analgesics may reduce the analgesic effect of oxycodone and/or may precipitate withdrawal symptoms).

No products indexed under this heading.

Pentazocine Lactate (Coadministration with mixed agonist/antagonist analgesics may reduce the analgesic effect of oxycodone and/or may precipitate withdrawal symptoms).

No products indexed under this heading.

Pentobarbital Sodium (Concomitant use may exhibit an additive CNS depression). Products include:

Nembutal Sodium Solution, USP 2494

Perphenazine (Concomitant use may exhibit an additive CNS depression).

No products indexed under this heading.

Phenobarbital (Concomitant use may exhibit an additive CNS depression). Products include:

Donnatal Extentabs 2507

Prazepam (Concomitant use may exhibit an additive CNS depression).

No products indexed under this heading.

Prochlorperazine (Concomitant use may exhibit an additive CNS depression).

No products indexed under this heading.

Promethazine Hydrochloride (Concomitant use may exhibit an additive CNS depression).

No products indexed under this heading.

Propofol (Concomitant use may exhibit an additive CNS depression).

No products indexed under this heading.

Propoxyphene Hydrochloride (Concomitant use may exhibit an additive CNS depression).

No products indexed under this heading.

Propoxyphene Napsylate (Concomitant use may exhibit an additive CNS depression).

No products indexed under this heading.

Quazepam (Concomitant use may exhibit an additive CNS depression).

No products indexed under this heading.

Quetiapine Fumarate (Concomitant use may exhibit an additive CNS depression).

No products indexed under this heading.

Ramelteon (Concomitant use may exhibit an additive CNS depression). Products include:

Rozerem Tablets 3091

Remifentanil Hydrochloride (Concomitant use may exhibit an additive CNS depression).

No products indexed under this heading.

Risperidone (Concomitant use may exhibit an additive CNS depression). Products include:

Risperdal Consta Long-Acting Injection 1753

Secobarbital Sodium (Concomitant use may exhibit an additive CNS depression).

No products indexed under this heading.

Sevoflurane (Concomitant use may exhibit an additive CNS depression). Products include:

Ultane Liquid for Inhalation 524

Sodium Butabarbital (Concomitant use may exhibit an additive CNS depression).

No products indexed under this heading.

Sufentanil Citrate (Concomitant use may exhibit an additive CNS depression).

No products indexed under this heading.

Temazepam (Concomitant use may exhibit an additive CNS depression).

No products indexed under this heading.

Thiamylal Sodium (Concomitant use may exhibit an additive CNS depression).

No products indexed under this heading.

Thioridazine Hydrochloride (Concomitant use may exhibit an additive CNS depression). Products include:

Thioridazine Hydrochloride Tablets 2195

Thiothixene (Concomitant use may exhibit an additive CNS depression). Products include:

Thiothixene Capsules 2197

Triazolam (Concomitant use may exhibit an additive CNS depression).

No products indexed under this heading.

Trifluoperazine Hydrochloride (Concomitant use may exhibit an additive CNS depression).

No products indexed under this heading.

Zaleplon (Concomitant use may exhibit an additive CNS depression).

No products indexed under this heading.

Ziprasidone Hydrochloride (Concomitant use may exhibit an additive CNS depression). Products include:

Geodon Capsules 2520

Zolpidem Tartrate (Concomitant use may exhibit an additive CNS depression). Products include:

Ambien Tablets 2692
Ambien CR Tablets 2696

Food Interactions

Alcohol (Concomitant use may exhibit an additive CNS depression).

PANAFIL OINTMENT

(Chlorophyllin Copper Complex Sodium, Papain, Urea)........................ 1723

May interact with:

Heavy metal salts, unspecified (Papain may be inactivated by the salts of heavy metals).

No products indexed under this heading.

Hydrogen Peroxide (May inactivate papain).

No products indexed under this heading.

PANAFIL SE SPRAY EMULSION

(Chlorophyllin Copper Complex Sodium, Papain, Urea)........................ 1724

See Panafil Ointment

PANHEMATIN FOR INJECTION

(Hemin) 2497

May interact with barbiturates, oral anticoagulants, and estrogens. Compounds in these categories include:

Anisindione (Hemin exhibits transient, mild anticoagulant effects, therefore, concurrent anticoagulant therapy should be avoided).

No products indexed under this heading.

Aprobarbital (Hemin inhibits the enzyme delta-aminolevulinic acid synthetase; concurrent use with drugs that increase the activity of delta-aminolevulinic acid synthetase, such as barbiturates, should be avoided).

No products indexed under this heading.

Butabarbital (Hemin inhibits the enzyme delta-aminolevulinic acid synthetase; concurrent use with drugs that increase the activity of delta-aminolevulinic acid synthetase, such as barbiturates, should be avoided).

No products indexed under this heading.

Butalbital (Hemin inhibits the enzyme delta-aminolevulinic acid synthetase; concurrent use with drugs that increase the activity of delta-aminolevulinic acid synthetase, such as barbiturates, should be avoided).

No products indexed under this heading.

Chlorotrianisene (Hemin inhibits the enzyme delta-aminolevulinic acid synthetase; concurrent use with drugs that increase the activity of delta-aminolevulinic acid synthetase, such as estrogens, should be avoided).

No products indexed under this heading.

Dicumarol (Hemin exhibits transient, mild anticoagulant effects, therefore, concurrent anticoagulant therapy should be avoided).

No products indexed under this heading.

Dienestrol (Hemin inhibits the enzyme delta-aminolevulinic acid synthetase; concurrent use with drugs that increase the activity of delta-aminolevulinic acid synthetase, such as estrogens, should be avoided).
No products indexed under this heading.

Diethylstilbestrol (Hemin inhibits the enzyme delta-aminolevulinic acid synthetase; concurrent use with drugs that increase the activity of delta-aminolevulinic acid synthetase, such as estrogens, should be avoided).
No products indexed under this heading.

Estradiol (Hemin inhibits the enzyme delta-aminolevulinic acid synthetase; concurrent use with drugs that increase the activity of delta-aminolevulinic acid synthetase, such as estrogens, should be avoided). Products include:
Activella Tablets ... 2347
Angeliq Tablets ... 751
Climara Transdermal System ... 763
Climara Pro Transdermal System ... 768
Divigel ... 3167
Vagifem Tablets ... 2375

Estrogens, Conjugated (Hemin inhibits the enzyme delta-aminolevulinic acid synthetase; concurrent use with drugs that increase the activity of delta-aminolevulinic acid synthetase, such as estrogens, should be avoided). Products include:
Premarin Intravenous ... 3217
Premarin Tablets ... 3221
Premarin Vaginal Cream ... 3228
Premphase Tablets ... 3232
Prempro Tablets ... 3232

Estrogens, Esterified (Hemin inhibits the enzyme delta-aminolevulinic acid synthetase; concurrent use with drugs that increase the activity of delta-aminolevulinic acid synthetase, such as estrogens, should be avoided). Products include:
Estratest Tablets ... 3043
Estratest H.S. Tablets ... 3043

Estropipate (Hemin inhibits the enzyme delta-aminolevulinic acid synthetase; concurrent use with drugs that increase the activity of delta-aminolevulinic acid synthetase, such as estrogens, should be avoided).
No products indexed under this heading.

Ethinyl Estradiol (Hemin inhibits the enzyme delta-aminolevulinic acid synthetase; concurrent use with drugs that increase the activity of delta-aminolevulinic acid synthetase, such as estrogens, should be avoided). Products include:
Lybrel Tablets ... 3204
Mircette Tablets ... 1034
NuvaRing ... 2897
Ortho-Cyclen/Ortho Tri-Cyclen ... 2449
Ortho Evra Transdermal System ... 2437
Ortho Tri-Cyclen Lo Tablets ... 2458
Seasonique Tablets ... 1046
Yaz Tablets ... 805

Mephobarbital (Hemin inhibits the enzyme delta-aminolevulinic acid synthetase; concurrent use with drugs that increase the activity of delta-aminolevulinic acid synthetase, such as barbiturates, should be avoided).
No products indexed under this heading.

Pentobarbital Sodium (Hemin inhibits the enzyme delta-aminolevulinic acid synthetase; concurrent use with drugs that increase the activity of delta-aminolevulinic acid synthetase, such as barbiturates, should be avoided). Products include:
Nembutal Sodium Solution, USP ... 2494

Phenobarbital (Hemin inhibits the enzyme delta-aminolevulinic acid synthetase; concurrent use with drugs that increase the activity of delta-aminolevulinic acid synthetase, such as barbiturates, should be avoided). Products include:
Donnatal Extentabs ... 2507

Polyestradiol Phosphate (Hemin inhibits the enzyme delta-aminolevulinic acid synthetase; concurrent use with drugs that increase the activity of delta-aminolevulinic acid synthetase, such as estrogens, should be avoided).
No products indexed under this heading.

Quinestrol (Hemin inhibits the enzyme delta-aminolevulinic acid synthetase; concurrent use with drugs that increase the activity of delta-aminolevulinic acid synthetase, such as estrogens, should be avoided).
No products indexed under this heading.

Secobarbital Sodium (Hemin inhibits the enzyme delta-aminolevulinic acid synthetase; concurrent use with drugs that increase the activity of delta-aminolevulinic acid synthetase, such as barbiturates, should be avoided).
No products indexed under this heading.

Thiamylal Sodium (Hemin inhibits the enzyme delta-aminolevulinic acid synthetase; concurrent use with drugs that increase the activity of delta-aminolevulinic acid synthetase, such as barbiturates, should be avoided).
No products indexed under this heading.

Warfarin Sodium (Hemin exhibits transient, mild anticoagulant effects, therefore, concurrent anticoagulant therapy should be avoided).
No products indexed under this heading.

PANRETIN GEL 0.1%
(Alitretinoin) ... 1081
May interact with:

DEET (N,N-diethyl-m-toluamide) (Avoid DEET (N,N-diethyl-m-toluamide) containing products (e.g., insect repellent). Alitretinoin may increase DEET toxicity).
No products indexed under this heading.

PARAGARD T 380A INTRAUTERINE COPPER CONTRACEPTIVE
(Copper, Intrauterine) ... 1041
None cited in PDR database.

PARNATE TABLETS
(Tranylcypromine Sulfate) ... 1532
May interact with alpha adrenergic stimulants, amphetamines, anesthetics, anorexiants, antihistamines, antihypertensives, anticholinergic-type antiparkinsonism drugs, dibenzazepines, diuretics, oral hypoglycemic agents, hypnotics and sedatives, insulin, monoamine oxidase inhibitors, narcotic analgesics, phenothiazines, selective serotonin reuptake inhibitors, sympathomimetics, tricyclic antidepressants, and certain other agents. Compounds in these categories include:

Acarbose (Some MAO inhibitors have contributed to hypoglycemic episodes in diabetic patients receiving oral hypoglycemic agents). Products include:
Precose Tablets ... 792

Acebutolol Hydrochloride (Concurrent use with hypotensive agents is contraindicated; a marked potentiating effect on these classes of drugs has been reported).
No products indexed under this heading.

Acrivastine (Concurrent use is contraindicated).
No products indexed under this heading.

Albuterol (Concurrent and/or sequential use is contraindicated; combination therapy may precipitate hypertension, headache and related symptoms).
No products indexed under this heading.

Albuterol Sulfate (Concurrent and/or sequential use is contraindicated; combination therapy may precipitate hypertension, headache and related symptoms). Products include:
Combivent Inhalation Aerosol ... 845
ProAir HFA Inhalation Aerosol ... 3113
Proventil HFA Inhalation Aerosol ... 2914
Ventolin HFA Inhalation Aerosol ... 1638

Alfentanil Hydrochloride (Concurrent use is contraindicated; a marked potentiating effect on these classes of drugs has been reported).
No products indexed under this heading.

Aliskiren (Concurrent use with hypotensive agents is contraindicated; a marked potentiating effect on these classes of drugs has been reported). Products include:
Tekturna Tablets ... 2321
Tekturna HCT Tablets ... 2324

Amiloride Hydrochloride (Concurrent use with hypotensive agents is contraindicated; a marked potentiating effect on these classes of drugs has been reported).
No products indexed under this heading.

Amitriptyline Hydrochloride (Concurrent use with dibenzazepine-related entities may result in hypertensive crises or severe convulsive seizures; concurrent and/or sequential use is contraindicated).
No products indexed under this heading.

Amlodipine Besylate (Concurrent use with hypotensive agents is contraindicated; a marked potentiating effect on these classes of drugs has been reported). Products include:
Azor Tablets ... 1005
Exforge Tablets ... 2238

Amoxapine (Concurrent use with dibenzazepine-related entities may result in hypertensive crises or severe convulsive seizures; concurrent and/or sequential use is contraindicated).
No products indexed under this heading.

Amphetamine Resins (Concurrent and/or sequential use is contraindicated).
No products indexed under this heading.

Amphetamine Sulfate (Concurrent and/or sequential use is contraindicated). Products include:
Adderall XR Capsules ... 3012

Astemizole (Concurrent use is contraindicated).
No products indexed under this heading.

Atenolol (Concurrent use with hypotensive agents is contraindicated; a marked potentiating effect on these classes of drugs has been reported).
No products indexed under this heading.

Azatadine Maleate (Concurrent use is contraindicated).
No products indexed under this heading.

Benazepril Hydrochloride (Concurrent use with hypotensive agents is contraindicated; a marked potentiating effect on these classes of drugs has been reported).
No products indexed under this heading.

Bendroflumethiazide (Concurrent use with hypotensive agents is contraindicated; a marked potentiating effect on these classes of drugs has been reported).
No products indexed under this heading.

Benzphetamine Hydrochloride (Concurrent and/or sequential use is contraindicated).
No products indexed under this heading.

Benztropine Mesylate (Anti-Parkinsonism drugs should be used with caution in patients receiving Parnate since severe reactions have been reported).
No products indexed under this heading.

Betaxolol Hydrochloride (Concurrent use with hypotensive agents is contraindicated; a marked potentiating effect on these classes of drugs has been reported).
No products indexed under this heading.

Biperiden Hydrochloride (Anti-Parkinsonism drugs should be used with caution in patients receiving Parnate since severe reactions have been reported).
No products indexed under this heading.

Bisoprolol Fumarate (Concurrent use with hypotensive agents is contraindicated; a marked potentiating effect on these classes of drugs has been reported).
No products indexed under this heading.

Bromodiphenhydramine Hydrochloride (Concurrent use is contraindicated).
No products indexed under this heading.

Brompheniramine Maleate (Concurrent use is contraindicated).
No products indexed under this heading.

Bumetanide (Concurrent use with hypotensive agents is contraindicated; a marked potentiating effect on these classes of drugs has been reported).
No products indexed under this heading.

Buprenorphine Hydrochloride (Concurrent use is contraindicated; a marked potentiating effect on these classes of drugs has been reported). Products include:
Suboxone Tablets ... 2601
Subutex Tablets ... 2601

Bupropion Hydrochloride (Concurrent use is contraindicated; at least 14 days should elapse between discontinuation of an MAO inhibitor and initiation of treatment with bupropion). Products include:

Wellbutrin Tablets 1648
Wellbutrin SR Sustained-Release Tablets 1653
Wellbutrin XL Extended-Release Tablets 1659
Zyban Sustained-Release Tablets 1692

Buspirone Hydrochloride (Concurrent use of buspirone and an MAO inhibitor has resulted in several cases of hypertension; concurrent use is contraindicated; at least 10 days should elapse between the discontinuation of Parnate and the initiation of buspirone).
No products indexed under this heading.

Butabarbital (Concurrent use is contraindicated).
No products indexed under this heading.

Butabarbital Sodium (Concurrent use is contraindicated).
No products indexed under this heading.

Caffeine (Excessive use of caffeine in any form is contraindicated). Products include:
BioLean Free Tablets .... ▣635
BioLean II Tablets .... ▣635
Winrgy Dietary Supplement .... ▣642

Candesartan Cilexetil (Concurrent use with hypotensive agents is contraindicated; a marked potentiating effect on these classes of drugs has been reported). Products include:
Atacand Tablets 639
Atacand HCT 642

Captopril (Concurrent use with hypotensive agents is contraindicated; a marked potentiating effect on these classes of drugs has been reported). Products include:
Captopril Tablets 2182

Carbamazepine (Concurrent use with dibenzazepine-related entities may result in hypertensive crises or severe convulsive seizures; concurrent and/or sequential use is contraindicated). Products include:
Carbatrol Capsules 3019
Equetro Extended-Release Capsules 3174

Carteolol Hydrochloride (Concurrent use with hypotensive agents is contraindicated; a marked potentiating effect on these classes of drugs has been reported).
No products indexed under this heading.

Cetirizine Hydrochloride (Concurrent use is contraindicated). Products include:
Zyrtec Allergy Tablets 1919
Zyrtec Chewable Tablets 1920
Children's Zyrtec Allergy Chewable Tablets 1922
Children's Zyrtec Allergy Syrup 1920
Children's Zyrtec Hives Relief Syrup 1920
Zyrtec Syrup 1920
Zyrtec Tablets 1920
Zyrtec-D 12 Hour Extended Release Tablets 1923
Zyrtec-D Allergy & Congestion Extended-Release Tablets 1923

Chloral Hydrate (Concurrent use is contraindicated).
No products indexed under this heading.

Chlorothiazide (Concurrent use with hypotensive agents is contraindicated; a marked potentiating effect on these classes of drugs has been reported).
No products indexed under this heading.

Chlorothiazide Sodium (Concurrent use with hypotensive agents is contraindicated; a marked potentiating effect on these classes of drugs has been reported). Products include:
Intravenous Sodium Diuril 2490

Chlorpheniramine Maleate (Concurrent use is contraindicated). Products include:
Actifed Cold & Allergy Tablets 1895
Sudafed PE Sinus & Allergy Tablets 1908
Tylenol Allergy Multi-Symptom Caplets with Cool Burst and Rapid Release Gelcaps 1916
Children's Tylenol Plus Cold Suspension Liquid 1912
Children's Tylenol Plus Cough & Runny Nose Suspension Liquid 1912
Children's Tylenol Plus Flu Suspension Liquid 1914
Children's Tylenol Plus Multi-Symptom Cold Suspension Liquid 1912
Tylenol Cold Head Congestion Nighttime Caplets with Cool Burst 1910
Tylenol Cold Multi-Symptom Nighttime Caplets with Cool Burst 1913
Tylenol Sinus Congestion & Pain Nighttime Caplets with Cool Burst 1917

Chlorpheniramine Polistirex (Concurrent use is contraindicated). Products include:
Tussionex Pennkinetic Extended-Release Suspension 3154

Chlorpheniramine Tannate (Concurrent use is contraindicated).
No products indexed under this heading.

Chlorpromazine (Possibility of additive hypotensive effects).
No products indexed under this heading.

Chlorpromazine Hydrochloride (Possibility of additive hypotensive effects).
No products indexed under this heading.

Chlorpropamide (Some MAO inhibitors have contributed to hypoglycemic episodes in diabetic patients receiving oral hypoglycemic agents).
No products indexed under this heading.

Chlorthalidone (Concurrent use with hypotensive agents is contraindicated; a marked potentiating effect on these classes of drugs has been reported). Products include:
Clorpres Tablets 2185

Citalopram Hydrobromide (Concurrent and/or sequential use is contraindicated; potential for serious, sometimes fatal, reactions including hyperthermia, rigidity, myoclonus, and other toxicities). Products include:
Celexa 1160

Clemastine Fumarate (Concurrent use is contraindicated).
No products indexed under this heading.

Clomipramine Hydrochloride (Concurrent use with dibenzazepine-related entities may result in hypertensive crises or severe convulsive seizures; concurrent and/or sequential use is contraindicated).
No products indexed under this heading.

Clonidine (Concurrent use with hypotensive agents is contraindicated; a marked potentiating effect on these classes of drugs has been reported). Products include:
Catapres-TTS 842

Clonidine Hydrochloride (Concurrent use with hypotensive agents is contraindicated; a marked potentiating effect on these classes of drugs has been reported). Products include:
Catapres Tablets 841
Clorpres Tablets 2185

Clozapine (Concurrent use with dibenzazepine-related entities may result in hypertensive crises or severe convulsive seizures; concurrent and/or sequential use is contraindicated).
No products indexed under this heading.

Cocaine Hydrochloride (Concurrent use is contraindicated).
No products indexed under this heading.

Codeine Phosphate (Concurrent use is contraindicated; a marked potentiating effect on these classes of drugs has been reported). Products include:
Tylenol with Codeine Tablets 2427

Cyclobenzaprine Hydrochloride (Concurrent use with dibenzazepine-related entities may result in hypertensive crises or severe convulsive seizures; concurrent and/or sequential use is contraindicated). Products include:
Amrix Capsules 966

Cyproheptadine Hydrochloride (Concurrent use is contraindicated).
No products indexed under this heading.

Deserpidine (Concurrent use with hypotensive agents is contraindicated; a marked potentiating effect on these classes of drugs has been reported).
No products indexed under this heading.

Desipramine Hydrochloride (Concurrent use with dibenzazepine-related entities may result in hypertensive crises or severe convulsive seizures; concurrent and/or sequential use is contraindicated).
No products indexed under this heading.

Dexchlorpheniramine Maleate (Concurrent use is contraindicated).
No products indexed under this heading.

Dexfenfluramine Hydrochloride (Co-administration with dexfenfluramine, a serotonin releaser and reuptake inhibitor, is contraindicated).
No products indexed under this heading.

Dextroamphetamine Sulfate (Concurrent and/or sequential use is contraindicated). Products include:
Adderall XR Capsules 3012
Dexedrine 1401

Dextromethorphan Hydrobromide (The combination of dextromethorphan and MAO inhibitors has been reported to cause brief episodes of psychosis or bizzare behavior; concurrent use is contraindicated). Products include:
PediaCare Children's Liquid Multi-Symptom Cold 1902
PediaCare Children's Long-Acting Cough 1902
Children's Sudafed PE Cold & Cough Liquid 1907
Sudafed PE Cold & Cough Caplets 1907
Children's Tylenol Plus Cough & Runny Nose Suspension Liquid 1912
Children's Tylenol Plus Cough & Sore Throat Suspension Liquid 1912
Children's Tylenol Plus Flu Suspension Liquid 1914
Children's Tylenol Plus Multi-Symptom Cold Suspension Liquid 1912
Tylenol Cold Severe Congestion Daytime Caplets with Cool Burst 1912
Tylenol Cold Head Congestion Daytime Caplets with Cool Burst 1910
Tylenol Cold Head Congestion Nighttime Caplets with Cool Burst 1910
Tylenol Cold Head Congestion Severe Daytime Caplets with Cool Burst 1910
Tylenol Cold Multi-Symptom Daytime Caplets with Cool Burst and Rapid Release Gels 1913
Tylenol Cold Multi-Symptom Daytime Liquid with Citrus Burst ... 1913
Tylenol Cold Multi-Symptom Nighttime Caplets with Cool Burst 1913
Tylenol Cold Multi-Symptom Nighttime Liquid with Cool Burst ... 1913
Tylenol Cold Multi-Symptom Severe Caplets with Cool Burst 1913
Tylenol Cold Multi-Symptom Severe Daytime Liquid with Citrus Burst 1913
Tylenol Cough & Sore Throat Daytime Liquid with Cool Burst 1918
Tylenol Cough & Sore Throat Nighttime Liquid with Cool Burst ... 1918
Vicks DayQuil Cold & Flu Multi-Symptom Relief .... ▣616
Vicks DayQuil LiquiCaps 2567
Vicks DayQuil Liquid 2567
Vicks DayQuil Multi-Symptom Cold/Flu Relief 2567
Vicks NyQuil Cold & Flu Multi-Symptom Relief .... ▣617
Vicks NyQuil LiquiCaps 2567
Vicks NyQuil Liquid 2567
Vicks NyQuil Multi-Symptom Cold/Flu Relief 2567

Dextromethorphan Polistirex (The combination of dextromethorphan and MAO inhibitors has been reported to cause brief episodes of psychosis or bizzare behavior; concurrent use is contraindicated).
No products indexed under this heading.

Dezocine (Concurrent use is contraindicated; a marked potentiating effect on these classes of drugs has been reported).
No products indexed under this heading.

Diazoxide (Concurrent use with hypotensive agents is contraindicated; a marked potentiating effect on these classes of drugs has been reported). Products include:
Proglycem Capsules 1185
Proglycem Suspension 1185

Diethylpropion Hydrochloride (Concurrent and/or sequential use is contraindicated).
No products indexed under this heading.

Diltiazem Hydrochloride (Concurrent use with hypotensive agents is contraindicated; a marked potentiating effect on these classes of drugs has been reported). Products include:
Cardizem LA Extended Release Tablets 421

Diphenhydramine Citrate (Concurrent use is contraindicated).
No products indexed under this heading.

Diphenhydramine Hydrochloride (Anti-Parkinsonism drugs should be used with caution in patients receiv-

ing Parnate since severe reactions have been reported). Products include:
- Benadryl Allergy & Cold Kapgels **1895**
- Benadryl Allergy & Sinus Headache Kapgels **1895**
- Benadryl Severe Allergy & Sinus Headache Caplets **1897**
- Benadryl Dye-Free Allergy Liqui-gels Softgels **1897**
- Benadryl Allergy Kapgels **1895**
- Benadryl Allergy Quick Dissolve Strips **1896**
- Benadryl Allergy Ultratab Tablets **1896**
- Children's Benadryl Dye-Free Allergy Liquid **1897**
- Children's Benadryl Allergy Fastmelts **1897**
- Children's Benadryl Allergy Liquid **1898**
- Children's Benadryl Allergy Perfect Measure **1896**
- Children's Benadryl-D Allergy & Sinus Liquid **1896**
- Benadryl-D Allergy & Sinus Tablet **1896**
- PediaCare Children's Allergy & Cold Liquid **1902**
- PediaCare Children's Allergy Liquid **1902**
- Simply Sleep Caplets **1905**
- Sudafed PE Nighttime Cold Caplets **1907**
- Sudafed PE Severe Cold Caplets **1908**
- Extra Strength Tylenol PM Caplets, Geltabs, Liquid, and Rapid Release Gels **1915**
- Tylenol Allergy Multi-Symptom Nighttime Caplets with Cool Burst **1916**
- Tylenol Severe Allergy Caplets **1916**
- Children's Tylenol Plus Cold & Allergy Suspension Liquid **1914**
- Tylenol Sore Throat Nighttime Liquid with Cool Burst **1918**

Diphenylpyraline Hydrochloride (Concurrent use is contraindicated).
No products indexed under this heading.

Disulfiram (Concurrent use requires caution; co-administration in animal models has resulted in severe toxicity, including convulsions and death).
No products indexed under this heading.

Dobutamine Hydrochloride (Concurrent and/or sequential use is contraindicated; combination therapy may precipitate hypertension, headache and related symptoms).
No products indexed under this heading.

Dopamine Hydrochloride (Concurrent and/or sequential use is contraindicated; combination therapy may precipitate hypertension, headache and related symptoms).
No products indexed under this heading.

Doxazosin Mesylate (Concurrent use with hypotensive agents is contraindicated; a marked potentiating effect on these classes of drugs has been reported).
No products indexed under this heading.

Doxepin Hydrochloride (Concurrent use with dibenzazepine-related entities may result in hypertensive crises or severe convulsive seizures; concurrent and/or sequential use is contraindicated).
No products indexed under this heading.

Enalapril Maleate (Concurrent use with hypotensive agents is contraindicated; a marked potentiating effect on these classes of drugs has been reported).
No products indexed under this heading.

Enalaprilat (Concurrent use with hypotensive agents is contraindicated; a marked potentiating effect on these classes of drugs has been reported).
No products indexed under this heading.

Enflurane (Patients taking tranylcypromine should not undergo elective surgery requiring general anesthesia; the possible combined hypotensive effects of tranylcypromine should be kept in mind; Parnate should be discontinued at least 10 days prior to elective surgery).
No products indexed under this heading.

Ephedrine Hydrochloride (Concurrent and/or sequential use is contraindicated; combination therapy may precipitate hypertension, headache and related symptoms).
No products indexed under this heading.

Ephedrine Sulfate (Concurrent and/or sequential use is contraindicated; combination therapy may precipitate hypertension, headache and related symptoms).
No products indexed under this heading.

Ephedrine Tannate (Concurrent and/or sequential use is contraindicated; combination therapy may precipitate hypertension, headache and related symptoms).
No products indexed under this heading.

Epinephrine (Concurrent and/or sequential use is contraindicated; combination therapy may precipitate hypertension, headache and related symptoms). Products include:
- EpiPen **1024**

Epinephrine Bitartrate (Concurrent and/or sequential use is contraindicated; combination therapy may precipitate hypertension, headache and related symptoms).
No products indexed under this heading.

Epinephrine Hydrochloride (Concurrent and/or sequential use is contraindicated; combination therapy may precipitate hypertension, headache and related symptoms).
No products indexed under this heading.

Eprosartan Mesylate (Concurrent use with hypotensive agents is contraindicated; a marked potentiating effect on these classes of drugs has been reported). Products include:
- Teveten Tablets **515**
- Teveten HCT Tablets **517**

Escitalopram Oxalate (Concurrent and/or sequential use is contraindicated; potential for serious, sometimes fatal, reactions including hyperthermia, rigidity, myoclonus, and other toxicities). Products include:
- Lexapro Oral Suspension **1174**
- Lexapro Tablets **1174**

Esmolol Hydrochloride (Concurrent use with hypotensive agents is contraindicated; a marked potentiating effect on these classes of drugs has been reported).
No products indexed under this heading.

Estazolam (Concurrent use is contraindicated).
No products indexed under this heading.

Ethacrynic Acid (Concurrent use with hypotensive agents is contraindicated; a marked potentiating effect on these classes of drugs has been reported). Products include:
- Edecrin Tablets **698**

Ethchlorvynol (Concurrent use is contraindicated).
No products indexed under this heading.

Ethinamate (Concurrent use is contraindicated).
No products indexed under this heading.

Felodipine (Concurrent use with hypotensive agents is contraindicated; a marked potentiating effect on these classes of drugs has been reported).
No products indexed under this heading.

Fenfluramine Hydrochloride (Concurrent and/or sequential use is contraindicated).
No products indexed under this heading.

Fentanyl (Concurrent use is contraindicated; a marked potentiating effect on these classes of drugs has been reported). Products include:
- Duragesic Transdermal System **2405**
- Ionsys Transdermal System **2410**

Fentanyl Citrate (Concurrent use is contraindicated; a marked potentiating effect on these classes of drugs has been reported). Products include:
- Actiq **959**
- Fentora Tablets **968**

Fexofenadine Hydrochloride (Concurrent use is contraindicated). Products include:
- Allegra Oral Solution **2684**
- Allegra Tablets **2684**
- Allegra-D 12 Hour Extended-Release Tablets **2687**
- Allegra-D 24 Hour Extended-Release Tablets **2690**

Fluoxetine (Concurrent and/or sequential use is contraindicated; potential for serious, sometimes fatal, reactions including hyperthermia, rigidity, myoclonus, and other toxicities).
No products indexed under this heading.

Fluoxetine Hydrochloride (Concurrent use has resulted in serious, sometimes fatal, reactions, including hyperthermia, rigidity, myoclonus, autonomic instability with possible rapid fluctuations of vital signs and mental status; concurrent use is contraindicated; at least 5 weeks should be allowed after stopping fluoxetine before starting an MAO inhibitor). Products include:
- Prozac Weekly Capsules **1852**
- Prozac Pulvules and Liquid **1852**
- Symbyax Capsules **1871**

Fluphenazine Decanoate (Possibility of additive hypotensive effects).
No products indexed under this heading.

Fluphenazine Enanthate (Possibility of additive hypotensive effects).
No products indexed under this heading.

Fluphenazine Hydrochloride (Possibility of additive hypotensive effects).
No products indexed under this heading.

Flurazepam Hydrochloride (Concurrent use is contraindicated).
No products indexed under this heading.

Fluvoxamine Maleate (Concurrent and/or sequential use is contraindicated; potential for serious, sometimes fatal, reactions including hyperthermia, rigidity, myoclonus, and other toxicities). Products include:
- Luvox CR Extended-Release Capsules **1759**

Fosinopril Sodium (Concurrent use with hypotensive agents is contraindicated; a marked potentiating effect on these classes of drugs has been reported).
No products indexed under this heading.

Furazolidone (Concurrent use with another MAO inhibitor may result in hypertensive crises or severe convulsive seizures; concurrent and/or sequential use is contraindicated).
No products indexed under this heading.

Furosemide (Concurrent use with hypotensive agents is contraindicated; a marked potentiating effect on these classes of drugs has been reported). Products include:
- Furosemide Tablets **2186**

Glimepiride (Some MAO inhibitors have contributed to hypoglycemic episodes in diabetic patients receiving oral hypoglycemic agents). Products include:
- Avandaryl Tablets **1344**
- Duetact Tablets **3085**

Glipizide (Some MAO inhibitors have contributed to hypoglycemic episodes in diabetic patients receiving oral hypoglycemic agents).
No products indexed under this heading.

Glutethimide (Concurrent use is contraindicated).
No products indexed under this heading.

Glyburide (Some MAO inhibitors have contributed to hypoglycemic episodes in diabetic patients receiving oral hypoglycemic agents).
No products indexed under this heading.

Guanabenz Acetate (Concurrent use with hypotensive agents is contraindicated; a marked potentiating effect on these classes of drugs has been reported).
No products indexed under this heading.

Guanethidine Monosulfate (Concurrent and/or sequential use is contraindicated; combination therapy may precipitate hypertension, headache and related symptoms).
No products indexed under this heading.

Halothane (Patients taking tranylcypromine should not undergo elective surgery requiring general anesthesia; the possible combined hypotensive effects of tranylcypromine should be kept in mind; Parnate should be discontinued at least 10 days prior to elective surgery).
No products indexed under this heading.

Hydralazine Hydrochloride (Concurrent use with hypotensive agents is contraindicated; a marked potentiating effect on these classes of drugs has been reported).
No products indexed under this heading.

Hydrochlorothiazide (Concurrent use with hypotensive agents is contraindicated; a marked potentiating effect on these classes of drugs has been reported). Products include:

Atacand HCT 642
Avalide Tablets 892
Avalide Tablets 2713
Benicar HCT Tablets 1010
Diovan HCT Tablets 2216
Dyazide Capsules 1405
Micardis HCT Tablets 854
Prinzide Tablets 2092
Tekturna HCT Tablets 2324
Teveten HCT Tablets 517

Hydrocodone Bitartrate (Concurrent use is contraindicated; a marked potentiating effect on these classes of drugs has been reported). Products include:
Lortab 5/500 Tablets 3143
Lortab 7.5/500 Tablets 3144
Lortab 10/500 Tablets 3144
Vicodin Tablets 529
Vicodin ES Tablets 530
Vicodin HP Tablets 531
Vicoprofen Tablets 533
Zydone Tablets 1132

Hydrocodone Polistirex (Concurrent use is contraindicated; a marked potentiating effect on these classes of drugs has been reported). Products include:
Tussionex Pennkinetic Extended-Release Suspension 3154

Hydroflumethiazide (Concurrent use with hypotensive agents is contraindicated; a marked potentiating effect on these classes of drugs has been reported).
No products indexed under this heading.

Hydromorphone Hydrochloride (Concurrent use is contraindicated; a marked potentiating effect on these classes of drugs has been reported).
No products indexed under this heading.

Imipramine Hydrochloride (Concurrent use with dibenzazepine-related entities may result in hypertensive crises or severe convulsive seizures; concurrent and/or sequential use is contraindicated).
No products indexed under this heading.

Imipramine Pamoate (Concurrent use with dibenzazepine-related entities may result in hypertensive crises or severe convulsive seizures; concurrent and/or sequential use is contraindicated).
No products indexed under this heading.

Indapamide (Concurrent use with hypotensive agents is contraindicated; a marked potentiating effect on these classes of drugs has been reported). Products include:
Indapamide Tablets 2188

Insulin (Some MAO inhibitors have contributed to hypoglycemic episodes in diabetic patients receiving insulin).
No products indexed under this heading.

Insulin, Human, Zinc Suspension (Some MAO inhibitors have contributed to hypoglycemic episodes in diabetic patients receiving insulin).
No products indexed under this heading.

Insulin, Human (rDNA origin) (Some MAO inhibitors have contributed to hypoglycemic episodes in diabetic patients receiving insulin). Products include:
Exubera Inhalation Powder 2515

Insulin, Human NPH (Some MAO inhibitors have contributed to hypoglycemic episodes in diabetic patients receiving insulin). Products include:
Humulin N Vial 1846

Insulin, Human Regular (Some MAO inhibitors have contributed to hypoglycemic episodes in diabetic patients receiving insulin). Products include:
Humulin R 1849
Humulin R (U-500) 1850

Insulin, Human Regular and Human NPH Mixture (Some MAO inhibitors have contributed to hypoglycemic episodes in diabetic patients receiving insulin). Products include:
Humulin 50/50, 100 Units 1843
Humulin 70/30 Vial 1844

Insulin, NPH (Some MAO inhibitors have contributed to hypoglycemic episodes in diabetic patients receiving insulin).
No products indexed under this heading.

Insulin, Regular (Some MAO inhibitors have contributed to hypoglycemic episodes in diabetic patients receiving insulin).
No products indexed under this heading.

Insulin, Regular and NPH mixture (Some MAO inhibitors have contributed to hypoglycemic episodes in diabetic patients receiving insulin).
No products indexed under this heading.

Insulin, Zinc Crystals (Some MAO inhibitors have contributed to hypoglycemic episodes in diabetic patients receiving insulin).
No products indexed under this heading.

Insulin, Zinc Suspension (Some MAO inhibitors have contributed to hypoglycemic episodes in diabetic patients receiving insulin).
No products indexed under this heading.

Insulin Aspart (Some MAO inhibitors have contributed to hypoglycemic episodes in diabetic patients receiving insulin).
No products indexed under this heading.

Insulin Aspart, Human (Some MAO inhibitors have contributed to hypoglycemic episodes in diabetic patients receiving insulin). Products include:
NovoLog Mix 70/30 2364

Insulin Aspart, Human Regular (Some MAO inhibitors have contributed to hypoglycemic episodes in diabetic patients receiving insulin). Products include:
NovoLog Injection 2359

Insulin Aspart Protamine, Human (Some MAO inhibitors have contributed to hypoglycemic episodes in diabetic patients receiving insulin). Products include:
NovoLog Mix 70/30 2364

Insulin Detemir (rDNA Origin) (Some MAO inhibitors have contributed to hypoglycemic episodes in diabetic patients receiving insulin). Products include:
Levemir Injection 2352

Insulin glargine (Some MAO inhibitors have contributed to hypoglycemic episodes in diabetic patients receiving insulin). Products include:
Lantus Injection 2749

Insulin Glulisine (Some MAO inhibitors have contributed to hypoglycemic episodes in diabetic patients receiving insulin). Products include:
Apidra Injection 2706

Insulin Lispro, Human (Some MAO inhibitors have contributed to hypoglycemic episodes in diabetic patients receiving insulin). Products include:
Humalog-Pen and KwikPen 1829
Humalog Mix 50/50-Pen and KwikPen 1833
Humalog Mix 75/25-Pen and KwikPen 1835

Insulin Lispro Protamine, Human (Some MAO inhibitors have contributed to hypoglycemic episodes in diabetic patients receiving insulin). Products include:
Humalog Mix 50/50-Pen and KwikPen 1833
Humalog Mix 75/25-Pen and KwikPen 1835

Irbesartan (Concurrent use with hypotensive agents is contraindicated; a marked potentiating effect on these classes of drugs has been reported). Products include:
Avalide Tablets 892
Avalide Tablets 2713
Avapro Tablets 897
Avapro Tablets 2718

Isocarboxazid (Concurrent use with another MAO inhibitor may result in hypertensive crises or severe convulsive seizures; concurrent and/or sequential use is contraindicated). Products include:
Marplan Tablets 3177

Isoflurane (Patients taking tranylcypromine should not undergo elective surgery requiring general anesthesia; the possible combined hypotensive effects of tranylcypromine should be kept in mind; Parnate should be discontinued at least 10 days prior to elective surgery).
No products indexed under this heading.

Isoproterenol Hydrochloride (Concurrent and/or sequential use is contraindicated; combination therapy may precipitate hypertension, headache and related symptoms).
No products indexed under this heading.

Isoproterenol Sulfate (Concurrent and/or sequential use is contraindicated; combination therapy may precipitate hypertension, headache and related symptoms).
No products indexed under this heading.

Isradipine (Concurrent use with hypotensive agents is contraindicated; a marked potentiating effect on these classes of drugs has been reported). Products include:
DynaCirc CR Controlled Release Tablets 1407

Ketamine Hydrochloride (Patients taking tranylcypromine should not undergo elective surgery requiring general anesthesia; the possible combined hypotensive effects of tranylcypromine should be kept in mind; Parnate should be discontinued at least 10 days prior to elective surgery).
No products indexed under this heading.

Labetalol Hydrochloride (Concurrent use with hypotensive agents is contraindicated; a marked potentiating effect on these classes of drugs has been reported).
No products indexed under this heading.

Levalbuterol Hydrochloride (Concurrent and/or sequential use is contraindicated; combination therapy may precipitate hypertension, headache and related symptoms). Products include:
Xopenex Inhalation Solution 3001
Xopenex Inhalation Solution Concentrate 3005

Levodopa (Concurrent and/or sequential use is contraindicated; combination therapy may precipitate hypertension, headache and related symptoms). Products include:
Stalevo Tablets 2309

Levorphanol Tartrate (Concurrent use is contraindicated; a marked potentiating effect on these classes of drugs has been reported).
No products indexed under this heading.

Lisinopril (Concurrent use with hypotensive agents is contraindicated; a marked potentiating effect on these classes of drugs has been reported). Products include:
Prinivil Tablets 2087
Prinzide Tablets 2092

Loratadine (Concurrent use is contraindicated).
No products indexed under this heading.

Lorazepam (Concurrent use is contraindicated).
No products indexed under this heading.

Losartan Potassium (Concurrent use with hypotensive agents is contraindicated; a marked potentiating effect on these classes of drugs has been reported). Products include:
Cozaar Tablets 1973

Maprotiline Hydrochloride (Concurrent use with dibenzazepine-related entities may result in hypertensive crises or severe convulsive seizures; concurrent and/or sequential use is contraindicated).
No products indexed under this heading.

Mazindol (Concurrent and/or sequential use is contraindicated).
No products indexed under this heading.

Mecamylamine Hydrochloride (Concurrent use with hypotensive agents is contraindicated; a marked potentiating effect on these classes of drugs has been reported).
No products indexed under this heading.

Meperidine Hydrochloride (Concomitant use or within 2 or 3 weeks following MAOI therapy is contraindicated; serious reactions including coma, severe hypertension or hypotension, convulsion, severe respiratory depression, malignant hyperplexia, excitation, peripheral vascular collapse, and death have been reported with combined use).
No products indexed under this heading.

Mesoridazine Besylate (Possibility of additive hypotensive effects).
No products indexed under this heading.

Metaproterenol Sulfate (Concurrent and/or sequential use is contraindicated; combination therapy may precipitate hypertension, headache and related symptoms).
No products indexed under this heading.

Metaraminol Bitartrate (Concurrent and/or sequential use is contraindicated; combination therapy may precipitate hypertension, headache and related symptoms).
No products indexed under this heading.

Metformin Hydrochloride (Some MAO inhibitors have contributed to hypoglycemic episodes in diabetic patients receiving oral hypoglycemic agents). Products include:
ActoPlus Met Tablets 3071
Avandamet Tablets 1336
Janumet Tablets 2041
PrandiMet Tablets 2967

Methadone Hydrochloride (Concurrent use is contraindicated; a marked potentiating effect on these classes of drugs has been reported).
No products indexed under this heading.

Methamphetamine Hydrochloride (Concurrent and/or sequential use is contraindicated).
No products indexed under this heading.

Methdilazine Hydrochloride (Concurrent use is contraindicated).
No products indexed under this heading.

Methohexital Sodium (Patients taking tranylcypromine should not undergo elective surgery requiring general anesthesia; the possible combined hypotensive effects of tranylcypromine should be kept in mind; Parnate should be discontinued at least 10 days prior to elective surgery).
No products indexed under this heading.

Methotrimeprazine (Possibility of additive hypotensive effects).
No products indexed under this heading.

Methoxamine Hydrochloride (Concurrent and/or sequential use is contraindicated; combination therapy may precipitate hypertension, headache and related symptoms).
No products indexed under this heading.

Methyclothiazide (Concurrent use with hypotensive agents is contraindicated; a marked potentiating effect on these classes of drugs has been reported).
No products indexed under this heading.

Methyldopa (Concurrent and/or sequential use is contraindicated; combination therapy may precipitate hypertension, headache and related symptoms).
No products indexed under this heading.

Methyldopate Hydrochloride (Concurrent and/or sequential use is contraindicated; combination therapy may precipitate hypertension, headache and related symptoms).
No products indexed under this heading.

Metolazone (Concurrent use with hypotensive agents is contraindicated; a marked potentiating effect on these classes of drugs has been reported).
No products indexed under this heading.

Metoprolol Succinate (Concurrent use with hypotensive agents is contraindicated; a marked potentiating effect on these classes of drugs has been reported). Products include:
Toprol-XL Tablets 666

Metoprolol Tartrate (Concurrent use with hypotensive agents is contraindicated; a marked potentiating effect on these classes of drugs has been reported).
No products indexed under this heading.

Metrizamide (Concurrent use with drugs which lower seizure threshold, including MAO inhibitors, should not be used with metrizamide).
No products indexed under this heading.

Metyrosine (Concurrent use with hypotensive agents is contraindicated; a marked potentiating effect on these classes of drugs has been reported). Products include:
Demser Capsules 1989

Mibefradil Dihydrochloride (Concurrent use with hypotensive agents is contraindicated; a marked potentiating effect on these classes of drugs has been reported).
No products indexed under this heading.

Midazolam Hydrochloride (Patients taking tranylcypromine should not undergo elective surgery requiring general anesthesia; the possible combined hypotensive effects of tranylcypromine should be kept in mind; Parnate should be discontinued at least 10 days prior to elective surgery).
No products indexed under this heading.

Miglitol (Some MAO inhibitors have contributed to hypoglycemic episodes in diabetic patients receiving oral hypoglycemic agents).
No products indexed under this heading.

Minoxidil (Concurrent use with hypotensive agents is contraindicated; a marked potentiating effect on these classes of drugs has been reported).
No products indexed under this heading.

Moclobemide (Concurrent use with another MAO inhibitor may result in hypertensive crises or severe convulsive seizures; concurrent and/or sequential use is contraindicated).
No products indexed under this heading.

Moexipril Hydrochloride (Concurrent use with hypotensive agents is contraindicated; a marked potentiating effect on these classes of drugs has been reported).
No products indexed under this heading.

Morphine Sulfate (Concurrent use is contraindicated; a marked potentiating effect on these classes of drugs has been reported). Products include:
Avinza Capsules 1772
DepoDur Injection 1095
MS Contin Tablets 2585

Nadolol (Concurrent use with hypotensive agents is contraindicated; a marked potentiating effect on these classes of drugs has been reported). Products include:
Nadolol Tablets 2191

Naphazoline Hydrochloride (Concurrent and/or sequential use is contraindicated; combination therapy may precipitate hypertension, headache and related symptoms). Products include:
Clear Eyes Itchy Eye Relief .... ⊙255

Nateglinide (Some MAO inhibitors have contributed to hypoglycemic episodes in diabetic patients receiving oral hypoglycemic agents). Products include:
Starlix Tablets 2314

Nebivolol (Concurrent use with hypotensive agents is contraindicated; a marked potentiating effect on these classes of drugs has been reported). Products include:
Bystolic Tablets 1155

Nicardipine Hydrochloride (Concurrent use with hypotensive agents is contraindicated; a marked potentiating effect on these classes of drugs has been reported). Products include:
Cardene I.V. 1093

Nifedipine (Concurrent use with hypotensive agents is contraindicated; a marked potentiating effect on these classes of drugs has been reported).
No products indexed under this heading.

Nisoldipine (Concurrent use with hypotensive agents is contraindicated; a marked potentiating effect on these classes of drugs has been reported). Products include:
Sular Extended Release Tablets 2975

Nitroglycerin (Concurrent use with hypotensive agents is contraindicated; a marked potentiating effect on these classes of drugs has been reported). Products include:
Nitro-Dur Transdermal Infusion System 2887
Nitrolingual Pumpspray 2965

Norepinephrine Bitartrate (Concurrent and/or sequential use is contraindicated; combination therapy may precipitate hypertension, headache and related symptoms).
No products indexed under this heading.

Nortriptyline Hydrochloride (Concurrent use with dibenzazepine-related entities may result in hypertensive crises or severe convulsive seizures; concurrent and/or sequential use is contraindicated).
No products indexed under this heading.

Oxycodone Hydrochloride (Concurrent use is contraindicated; a marked potentiating effect on these classes of drugs has been reported). Products include:
OxyContin Tablets 2589
OxyIR Capsules 2593
Percocet Tablets 1127
Percodan Tablets 1130

Oxymetazoline Hydrochloride (Concurrent and/or sequential use is contraindicated; combination therapy may precipitate hypertension, headache and related symptoms). Products include:
Sudafed OM Sinus Cold Moisturizing Nasal Spray 1906
Sudafed OM Sinus Congestion Moisturizing Nasal Spray 1906

Pargyline Hydrochloride (Concurrent use with another MAO inhibitor may result in hypertensive crises or severe convulsive seizures; concurrent and/or sequential use is contraindicated).
No products indexed under this heading.

Paroxetine Hydrochloride (Concurrent and/or sequential use is contraindicated; potential for serious, sometimes fatal, reactions including hyperthermia, rigidity, myoclonus, and other toxicities; at least 2 weeks should be allowed after stopping paroxetine before starting an MAO inhibitor). Products include:
Paxil 1535
Paxil CR Controlled-Release Tablets 1544

Penbutolol Sulfate (Concurrent use with hypotensive agents is contraindicated; a marked potentiating effect on these classes of drugs has been reported).
No products indexed under this heading.

Perindopril Erbumine (Concurrent use with hypotensive agents is contraindicated; a marked potentiating effect on these classes of drugs has been reported). Products include:
Aceon Tablets (2 mg, 4 mg, 8 mg) 3038

Perphenazine (Possibility of additive hypotensive effects).
No products indexed under this heading.

Phendimetrazine Tartrate (Concurrent and/or sequential use is contraindicated).
No products indexed under this heading.

Phenelzine Sulfate (Concurrent use with another MAO inhibitor may result in hypertensive crises or severe convulsive seizures; concurrent and/or sequential use is contraindicated).
No products indexed under this heading.

Phenmetrazine Hydrochloride (Concurrent and/or sequential use is contraindicated).
No products indexed under this heading.

Phenoxybenzamine Hydrochloride (Concurrent use with hypotensive agents is contraindicated; a marked potentiating effect on these classes of drugs has been reported). Products include:
Dibenzyline Capsules 3188

Phentolamine Mesylate (Concurrent use with hypotensive agents is contraindicated; a marked potentiating effect on these classes of drugs has been reported).
No products indexed under this heading.

Phenylephrine Bitartrate (Concurrent and/or sequential use is contraindicated; combination therapy may precipitate hypertension, headache and related symptoms).
No products indexed under this heading.

Phenylephrine Hydrochloride (Concurrent and/or sequential use is contraindicated; combination therapy may precipitate hypertension, headache and related symptoms). Products include:
Actifed Cold & Allergy Tablets 1895
Benadryl Allergy & Cold Kapgels 1895
Benadryl Allergy & Sinus Headache Kapgels 1895
Benadryl Severe Allergy & Sinus Headache Caplets 1897
Children's Benadryl-D Allergy & Sinus Liquid 1896
Benadryl-D Allergy & Sinus Tablet 1896
PediaCare Children's Allergy & Cold Liquid 1902
PediaCare Children's Decongestant Liquid 1902
PediaCare Children's Liquid Multi-Symptom Cold 1902
Sinutab Non-Drying Caplets 1905
Sinutab Sinus Caplets 1905

Children's Sudafed PE Cold & Cough Liquid 1907
Children's Sudafed PE Nasal Decongestant Liquid 1906
Sudafed PE Cold & Cough Caplets 1907
Sudafed PE Nasal Decongestant Tablets 1907
Sudafed PE Nighttime Cold Caplets 1907
Sudafed PE Non-Drying Sinus Caplets 1908
Sudafed PE Severe Cold Caplets 1908
Sudafed PE Sinus & Allergy Tablets 1908
Sudafed PE Sinus Headache Caplets 1908
Tylenol Allergy Multi-Symptom Caplets with Cool Burst and Rapid Release Gelcaps 1916
Tylenol Allergy Multi-Symptom Nighttime Caplets with Cool Burst 1916
Children's Tylenol Plus Cold Suspension Liquid 1912
Children's Tylenol Plus Cold & Allergy Suspension Liquid 1914
Children's Tylenol Plus Flu Suspension Liquid 1914
Children's Tylenol Plus Multi-Symptom Cold Suspension Liquid 1912
Tylenol Cold Head Congestion Daytime Caplets with Cool Burst 1910
Tylenol Cold Head Congestion Nighttime Caplets with Cool Burst 1910
Tylenol Cold Head Congestion Severe Daytime Caplets with Cool Burst 1910
Tylenol Cold Multi-Symptom Daytime Caplets with Cool Burst and Rapid Release Gels 1913
Tylenol Cold Multi-Symptom Daytime Liquid with Citrus Burst 1913
Tylenol Cold Multi-Symptom Nighttime Caplets with Cool Burst 1913
Tylenol Cold Multi-Symptom Nighttime Liquid with Cool Burst 1913
Tylenol Cold Multi-Symptom Severe Caplets with Cool Burst 1913
Tylenol Cold Multi-Symptom Severe Daytime Liquid with Citrus Burst 1913
Tylenol Sinus Congestion & Pain Daytime Caplets with Cool Burst and Gelcaps 1917
Tylenol Sinus Congestion & Pain Nighttime Caplets with Cool Burst 1917
Tylenol Sinus Congestion & Pain Severe Caplets with Cool Burst 1917
Vicks DayQuil Cold & Flu Multi-Symptom Relief .... ▣616
Vicks DayQuil LiquiCaps 2567
Vicks DayQuil Liquid 2567
Vicks DayQuil Multi-Symptom Cold/Flu Relief 2567

Phenylephrine Tannate (Concurrent and/or sequential use is contraindicated; combination therapy may precipitate hypertension, headache and related symptoms).
No products indexed under this heading.

Phenylpropanolamine Hydrochloride (Concurrent and/or sequential use is contraindicated; combination therapy may precipitate hypertension, headache and related symptoms).
No products indexed under this heading.

Pindolol (Concurrent use with hypotensive agents is contraindicated; a marked potentiating effect on these classes of drugs has been reported).
No products indexed under this heading.

Pioglitazone Hydrochloride (Some MAO inhibitors have contributed to hypoglycemic episodes in diabetic patients receiving oral hypoglycemic agents). Products include:
ActoPlus Met Tablets 3071
Actos Tablets 3077
Duetact Tablets 3085

Pirbuterol Acetate (Concurrent and/or sequential use is contraindicated; combination therapy may precipitate hypertension, headache and related symptoms). Products include:
Maxair Autohaler 1705

Polythiazide (Concurrent use with hypotensive agents is contraindicated; a marked potentiating effect on these classes of drugs has been reported).
No products indexed under this heading.

Prazosin Hydrochloride (Concurrent use with hypotensive agents is contraindicated; a marked potentiating effect on these classes of drugs has been reported).
No products indexed under this heading.

Procarbazine Hydrochloride (Concurrent use with another MAO inhibitor may result in hypertensive crises or severe convulsive seizures; concurrent and/or sequential use is contraindicated).
No products indexed under this heading.

Prochlorperazine (Possibility of additive hypotensive effects).
No products indexed under this heading.

Procyclidine Hydrochloride (Anti-Parkinsonism drugs should be used with caution in patients receiving Parnate since severe reactions have been reported).
No products indexed under this heading.

Promethazine Hydrochloride (Concurrent use is contraindicated).
No products indexed under this heading.

Propofol (Patients taking tranylcypromine should not undergo elective surgery requiring general anesthesia; the possible combined hypotensive effects of tranylcypromine should be kept in mind; Parnate should be discontinued at least 10 days prior to elective surgery).
No products indexed under this heading.

Propoxyphene Hydrochloride (Concurrent use is contraindicated; a marked potentiating effect on these classes of drugs has been reported).
No products indexed under this heading.

Propoxyphene Napsylate (Concurrent use is contraindicated; a marked potentiating effect on these classes of drugs has been reported).
No products indexed under this heading.

Propranolol Hydrochloride (Concurrent use with hypotensive agents is contraindicated; a marked potentiating effect on these classes of drugs has been reported). Products include:
InnoPran XL Extended Release Capsules 1484

Protriptyline Hydrochloride (Concurrent use with dibenzazepine-related entities may result in hypertensive crises or severe convulsive seizures; concurrent and/or sequential use is contraindicated).
No products indexed under this heading.

Pseudoephedrine Hydrochloride (Concurrent and/or sequential use is contraindicated; combination therapy may precipitate hypertension, headache and related symptoms). Products include:
Allegra-D 12 Hour Extended-Release Tablets 2687
Allegra-D 24 Hour Extended-Release Tablets 2690
Children's Motrin Cold Oral Suspension 1899
Sudafed 12 Hour Nasal Decongestant Non-Drowsy Caplets 1909
Sudafed 24 Hour Non-Drowsy Nasal Decongestant Tablets 1906
Children's Sudafed Nasal Decongestant Liquid 1906
Sudafed Nasal Decongestant Tablets 1906
Tylenol Cold Severe Congestion Daytime Caplets with Cool Burst 1912
Tylenol Sinus Severe Congestion Caplets with Cool Burst 1917
Vicks NyQuil LiquiCaps 2567
Vicks NyQuil Liquid 2567
Vicks NyQuil Multi-Symptom Cold/Flu Relief 2567
Zyrtec-D 12 Hour Extended Release Tablets 1923
Zyrtec-D Allergy & Congestion Extended-Release Tablets 1923

Pseudoephedrine Sulfate (Concurrent and/or sequential use is contraindicated; combination therapy may precipitate hypertension, headache and related symptoms). Products include:
Clarinex-D 12-Hour Extended-Release Tablets 2831
Clarinex-D 24-Hour Extended-Release Tablets 2834

Pyrilamine Maleate (Concurrent use is contraindicated).
No products indexed under this heading.

Pyrilamine Tannate (Concurrent use is contraindicated).
No products indexed under this heading.

Quazepam (Concurrent use is contraindicated).
No products indexed under this heading.

Quinapril Hydrochloride (Concurrent use with hypotensive agents is contraindicated; a marked potentiating effect on these classes of drugs has been reported).
No products indexed under this heading.

Ramelteon (Concurrent use is contraindicated). Products include:
Rozerem Tablets 3091

Ramipril (Concurrent use with hypotensive agents is contraindicated; a marked potentiating effect on these classes of drugs has been reported).
No products indexed under this heading.

Rasagiline Mesylate (Concurrent use with another MAO inhibitor may result in hypertensive crises or severe convulsive seizures; concurrent and/or sequential use is contraindicated). Products include:
Azilect Tablets 3106

Rauwolfia Serpentina (Concurrent use with hypotensive agents is contraindicated; a marked potentiating effect on these classes of drugs has been reported).
No products indexed under this heading.

Remifentanil Hydrochloride (Concurrent use is contraindicated; a marked potentiating effect on these classes of drugs has been reported).
No products indexed under this heading.

Repaglinide (Some MAO inhibitors have contributed to hypoglycemic episodes in diabetic patients receiving oral hypoglycemic agents). Products include:
PrandiMet Tablets 2967
Prandin Tablets 2971

Rescinnamine (Concurrent use with hypotensive agents is contraindicated; a marked potentiating effect on these classes of drugs has been reported).
No products indexed under this heading.

Reserpine (Concurrent and/or sequential use is contraindicated; combination therapy may precipitate hypertension, headache and related symptoms).
No products indexed under this heading.

Rosiglitazone Maleate (Some MAO inhibitors have contributed to hypoglycemic episodes in diabetic patients receiving oral hypoglycemic agents). Products include:
Avandamet Tablets 1336
Avandaryl Tablets 1344
Avandia Tablets 1351

Salmeterol Xinafoate (Concurrent and/or sequential use is contraindicated; combination therapy may precipitate hypertension, headache and related symptoms). Products include:
Advair Diskus 100/50 1276
Advair Diskus 250/50 1276
Advair Diskus 500/50 1276
Advair HFA 45/21 Inhalation Aerosol 1288
Advair HFA 115/21 Inhalation Aerosol 1288
Advair HFA 230/21 Inhalation Aerosol 1288
Serevent Diskus 1594

Secobarbital Sodium (Concurrent use is contraindicated).
No products indexed under this heading.

Selegiline (Concurrent use with another MAO inhibitor may result in hypertensive crises or severe convulsive seizures; concurrent and/or sequential use is contraindicated). Products include:
Emsam Transdermal System 905

Selegiline Hydrochloride (Concurrent use with another MAO inhibitor may result in hypertensive crises or severe convulsive seizures; concurrent and/or sequential use is contraindicated). Products include:
Eldepryl Capsules 3052

Sertraline Hydrochloride (Concurrent and/or sequential use is contraindicated; potential for serious, sometimes fatal, reactions, including hyperthermia, rigidity, myoclonus, and other toxicities; at least 2 weeks should be allowed after stopping sertraline before starting an MAO inhibitor).
No products indexed under this heading.

Sibutramine Hydrochloride Monohydrate (Concurrent and/or sequential use is contraindicated). Products include:
Meridia Capsules 475

Sitagliptin Phosphate (Some MAO inhibitors have contributed to hypoglycemic episodes in diabetic patients receiving oral hypoglycemic agents). Products include:
Janumet Tablets 2041
Januvia Tablets 2048

Sodium Butabarbital (Concurrent use is contraindicated).
No products indexed under this heading.

Sodium Nitroprusside (Concurrent use with hypotensive agents is contraindicated; a marked potentiating effect on these classes of drugs has been reported).
No products indexed under this heading.

Sotalol Hydrochloride (Concurrent use with hypotensive agents is contraindicated; a marked potentiating effect on these classes of drugs has been reported).
No products indexed under this heading.

Spirapril Hydrochloride (Concurrent use with hypotensive agents is contraindicated; a marked potentiating effect on these classes of drugs has been reported).
No products indexed under this heading.

Spironolactone (Concurrent use with hypotensive agents is contraindicated; a marked potentiating effect on these classes of drugs has been reported).
No products indexed under this heading.

Sufentanil Citrate (Concurrent use is contraindicated; a marked potentiating effect on these classes of drugs has been reported).
No products indexed under this heading.

Telmisartan (Concurrent use with hypotensive agents is contraindicated; a marked potentiating effect on these classes of drugs has been reported). Products include:
Micardis Tablets 852
Micardis HCT Tablets 854

Temazepam (Concurrent use is contraindicated).
No products indexed under this heading.

Terazosin Hydrochloride (Concurrent use with hypotensive agents is contraindicated; a marked potentiating effect on these classes of drugs has been reported).
No products indexed under this heading.

Terbutaline Sulfate (Concurrent and/or sequential use is contraindicated; combination therapy may precipitate hypertension, headache and related symptoms).
No products indexed under this heading.

Terfenadine (Concurrent use is contraindicated).
No products indexed under this heading.

Tetrahydrozoline Hydrochloride (Concurrent and/or sequential use is contraindicated; combination therapy may precipitate hypertension, headache and related symptoms). Products include:
Clear Eyes Triple Action Relief .... ⊙255

Thiamylal Sodium (Patients taking tranylcypromine should not undergo elective surgery requiring general anesthesia; the possible combined hypotensive effects of tranylcypromine should be kept in mind; Parnate should be discontinued at least 10 days prior to elective surgery).
No products indexed under this heading.

Thioridazine Hydrochloride (Possibility of additive hypotensive effects). Products include:
Thioridazine Hydrochloride Tablets 2195

Timolol Maleate (Concurrent use with hypotensive agents is contraindicated; a marked potentiating effect on these classes of drugs has been reported). Products include:
Combigan Ophthalmic Solution 553
Cosopt Sterile Ophthalmic Solution 1969
Timoptic Sterile Ophthalmic Solution 2121
Timoptic in Ocudose 2124
Timoptic-XE Sterile Ophthalmic Gel Forming Solution 2125

Tolazamide (Some MAO inhibitors have contributed to hypoglycemic episodes in diabetic patients receiving oral hypoglycemic agents).
No products indexed under this heading.

Tolbutamide (Some MAO inhibitors have contributed to hypoglycemic episodes in diabetic patients receiving oral hypoglycemic agents).
No products indexed under this heading.

Torsemide (Concurrent use with hypotensive agents is contraindicated; a marked potentiating effect on these classes of drugs has been reported). Products include:
Demadex Injection 2630
Demadex Tablets 2630

Trandolapril (Concurrent use with hypotensive agents is contraindicated; a marked potentiating effect on these classes of drugs has been reported). Products include:
Mavik Tablets 472
Tarka Tablets 511

Triamterene (Concurrent use with hypotensive agents is contraindicated; a marked potentiating effect on these classes of drugs has been reported). Products include:
Dyazide Capsules 1405
Dyrenium Capsules 3189

Triazolam (Concurrent use is contraindicated).
No products indexed under this heading.

Tridihexethyl Chloride (Anti-Parkinsonism drugs should be used with caution in patients receiving Parnate since severe reactions have been reported).
No products indexed under this heading.

Trifluoperazine Hydrochloride (Possibility of additive hypotensive effects).
No products indexed under this heading.

Trihexyphenidyl Hydrochloride (Anti-Parkinsonism drugs should be used with caution in patients receiving Parnate since severe reactions have been reported).
No products indexed under this heading.

Trimeprazine Tartrate (Concurrent use is contraindicated).
No products indexed under this heading.

Trimethaphan Camsylate (Concurrent use with hypotensive agents is contraindicated; a marked potentiating effect on these classes of drugs has been reported).
No products indexed under this heading.

Trimipramine Maleate (Concurrent use with dibenzazepine-related entities may result in hypertensive crises or severe convulsive seizures; concurrent and/or sequential use is contraindicated).
No products indexed under this heading.

Tripelennamine Hydrochloride (Concurrent use is contraindicated).
No products indexed under this heading.

Triprolidine Hydrochloride (Concurrent use is contraindicated).
No products indexed under this heading.

Troglitazone (Some MAO inhibitors have contributed to hypoglycemic episodes in diabetic patients receiving oral hypoglycemic agents).
No products indexed under this heading.

L-Tryptophan (Concurrent and/or sequential use is contraindicated; combination therapy may precipitate hypertension, disorientation, memory impairment, other neurologic and behavioral changes, headache and related symptoms).
No products indexed under this heading.

Tyramine (Concurrent use is contraindicated).
No products indexed under this heading.

Valsartan (Concurrent use with hypotensive agents is contraindicated; a marked potentiating effect on these classes of drugs has been reported). Products include:
Diovan Tablets 2212
Diovan HCT Tablets 2216
Exforge Tablets 2238

Verapamil Hydrochloride (Concurrent use with hypotensive agents is contraindicated; a marked potentiating effect on these classes of drugs has been reported). Products include:
Tarka Tablets 511

Zaleplon (Concurrent use is contraindicated).
No products indexed under this heading.

Zolpidem Tartrate (Concurrent use is contraindicated). Products include:
Ambien Tablets 2692
Ambien CR Tablets 2696

Food Interactions

Alcohol (Concurrent use is contraindicated; a marked potentiating effect on alcohol has been reported).

Anchovies (Potential for hypertensive crisis; concurrent use is contraindicated).

Avocados (Potential for hypertensive crisis; concurrent use is contraindicated).

Bananas (Potential for hypertensive crisis; concurrent use is contraindicated).

Beans, broad (Potential for hypertensive crisis; concurrent use is contraindicated).

Beans, Fava (Potential for hypertensive crisis; concurrent use is contraindicated).

Beer, alcohol-free (Potential for hypertensive crisis; concurrent use is contraindicated).

Beer, unspecified (Potential for hypertensive crisis; concurrent use is contraindicated).

Beverages, caffeine-containing (Potential for hypertensive crisis; concurrent use is contraindicated).

Caviar (Potential for hypertensive crisis; concurrent use is contraindicated).

Cheese, aged (Potential for hypertensive crisis; concurrent use is contraindicated).

Cheese, strong, unpasteurized (Potential for hypertensive crisis; concurrent use is contraindicated).

Cheese, unspecified (Potential for hypertensive crisis; concurrent use is contraindicated).

Chocolate (Potential for hypertensive crisis; concurrent use is contraindicated).

Cream, sour (Potential for hypertensive crisis; concurrent use is contraindicated).

Figs, canned (Potential for hypertensive crisis; concurrent use is contraindicated).

Food with high concentration of tyramine (Potential for hypertensive crisis; concurrent use is contraindicated).

Fruits, dried (Potential for hypertensive crisis; concurrent use is contraindicated).

Fruits, overripe (Potential for hypertensive crisis; concurrent use is contraindicated).

Herring, pickled (Potential for hypertensive crisis; concurrent use is contraindicated).

Liqueurs (Potential for hypertensive crisis; concurrent use is contraindicated).

Liver (Potential for hypertensive crisis; concurrent use is contraindicated).

Meat extracts (Potential for hypertensive crisis; concurrent use is contraindicated).

Meat prepared with tenderizers (Potential for hypertensive crisis; concurrent use is contraindicated).

Prunes (Potential for hypertensive crisis; concurrent use is contraindicated).

Raisins (Potential for hypertensive crisis; concurrent use is contraindicated).

Raspberries (Potential for hypertensive crisis; concurrent use is contraindicated).

Sauerkraut (Potential for hypertensive crisis; concurrent use is contraindicated).

Sherry (Potential for hypertensive crisis; concurrent use is contraindicated).

Soy Sauce (Potential for hypertensive crisis; concurrent use is contraindicated).

Wine, Chianti (Potential for hypertensive crisis; concurrent use is contraindicated).

Yeast Extract (Potential for hypertensive crisis; concurrent use is contraindicated).

Yogurt (Potential for hypertensive crisis; concurrent use is contraindicated).

PASER GRANULES

(Aminosalicylic Acid) 1747
May interact with:

Digoxin (Potential for reduced digoxin levels). Products include:

Lanoxin Injection 1498
Lanoxin Injection Pediatric 1502
Lanoxin Tablets 1505

Isoniazid (Concurrent use with a rapidly available form of aminosalicylic acid has been reported to produce a 20% reduction in the acetylation of INH; the lower serum levels produced by delayed release preparation will result in a reduced effect on the acetylation of INH).
No products indexed under this heading.

Rifampin (May block the absorption of rifampin; PASER granules do not contain excipient that blocks the absorption).
No products indexed under this heading.

Vitamin B_{12} (Reduced absorption of vitamin B_{12} with clinically significant erythrocyte abnormalities developing after depletion). Products include:
Animi-3 Capsules 2506
Authia Cream 3190
Bevitamel Tablets 3190
Comax Dietary Supplement 995
Ferralet 90 Tablets 2175
Glaucofit Dietary Supplement 995
Glauma Dietary Supplement 995
Tonox Dietary Supplement 995

PATADAY OPHTHALMIC SOLUTION

(Olopatadine Hydrochloride) 543
None cited in PDR database.

PATANASE NASAL SPRAY

(Olopatadine Hydrochloride) 544
May interact with central nervous system depressants and certain other agents. Compounds in these categories include:

Alfentanil Hydrochloride (Concurrent use of olopatadine nasal spray with other central nervous system depressants should be avoided because additional reductions in alertness and additional impairment of central nervous system performance may occur).
No products indexed under this heading.

Alprazolam (Concurrent use of olopatadine nasal spray with other central nervous system depressants should be avoided because additional reductions in alertness and additional impairment of central nervous system performance may occur).
No products indexed under this heading.

Aprobarbital (Concurrent use of olopatadine nasal spray with other central nervous system depressants should be avoided because additional reductions in alertness and additional impairment of central nervous system performance may occur).
No products indexed under this heading.

Buprenorphine Hydrochloride (Concurrent use of olopatadine nasal spray with other central nervous system depressants should be avoided because additional reductions in alertness and additional impairment of central nervous system performance may occur). Products include:
Suboxone Tablets 2601
Subutex Tablets 2601

Buspirone Hydrochloride (Concurrent use of olopatadine nasal spray with other central nervous system depressants should be avoided because additional reductions in alertness and additional impairment of central nervous system performance may occur).
No products indexed under this heading.

Butabarbital (Concurrent use of olopatadine nasal spray with other central nervous system depressants should be avoided because additional reductions in alertness and additional impairment of central nervous system performance may occur).
No products indexed under this heading.

Butalbital (Concurrent use of olopatadine nasal spray with other central nervous system depressants should be avoided because additional reductions in alertness and additional impairment of central nervous system performance may occur).
No products indexed under this heading.

Chlordiazepoxide (Concurrent use of olopatadine nasal spray with other central nervous system depressants should be avoided because additional reductions in alertness and additional impairment of central nervous system performance may occur).
No products indexed under this heading.

Chlordiazepoxide Hydrochloride (Concurrent use of olopatadine nasal spray with other central nervous system depressants should be avoided because additional reductions in alertness and additional impairment of central nervous system performance may occur).
No products indexed under this heading.

Chlorpromazine (Concurrent use of olopatadine nasal spray with other central nervous system depressants should be avoided because additional reductions in alertness and additional impairment of central nervous system performance may occur).
No products indexed under this heading.

Chlorpromazine Hydrochloride (Concurrent use of olopatadine nasal spray with other central nervous system depressants should be avoided because additional reductions in alertness and additional impairment of central nervous system performance may occur).
No products indexed under this heading.

Chlorprothixene (Concurrent use of olopatadine nasal spray with other central nervous system depressants should be avoided because additional reductions in alertness and additional impairment of central nervous system performance may occur).
No products indexed under this heading.

Chlorprothixene Hydrochloride (Concurrent use of olopatadine nasal spray with other central nervous system depressants should be avoided because additional reductions in alertness and additional impairment of central nervous system performance may occur).
No products indexed under this heading.

Chlorprothixene Lactate (Concurrent use of olopatadine nasal spray with other central nervous system depressants should be avoided because additional reductions in alertness and additional impairment of central nervous system performance may occur).
No products indexed under this heading.

Clorazepate Dipotassium (Concurrent use of olopatadine nasal spray with other central nervous system depressants should be avoided because additional reductions in alertness and additional impairment of central nervous system performance may occur).
No products indexed under this heading.

Clozapine (Concurrent use of olopatadine nasal spray with other central nervous system depressants should be avoided because additional reductions in alertness and additional impairment of central nervous system performance may occur).
No products indexed under this heading.

Codeine Phosphate (Concurrent use of olopatadine nasal spray with other central nervous system depressants should be avoided because additional reductions in alertness and additional impairment of central nervous system performance may occur). Products include:
Tylenol with Codeine Tablets 2427

Desflurane (Concurrent use of olopatadine nasal spray with other central nervous system depressants should be avoided because additional reductions in alertness and additional impairment of central nervous system performance may occur).
No products indexed under this heading.

Dezocine (Concurrent use of olopatadine nasal spray with other central nervous system depressants should be avoided because additional reductions in alertness and additional impairment of central nervous system performance may occur).
No products indexed under this heading.

Diazepam (Concurrent use of olopatadine nasal spray with other central nervous system depressants should be avoided because additional reductions in alertness and additional impairment of central nervous system performance may occur). Products include:
Valium Tablets 2658

Droperidol (Concurrent use of olopatadine nasal spray with other central nervous system depressants should be avoided because additional reductions in alertness and additional impairment of central nervous system performance may occur).
No products indexed under this heading.

Enflurane (Concurrent use of olopatadine nasal spray with other central nervous system depressants should be avoided because additional reductions in alertness and additional impairment of central nervous system performance may occur).
No products indexed under this heading.

Estazolam (Concurrent use of olopatadine nasal spray with other central nervous system depressants should be avoided because additional reductions in alertness and additional impairment of central nervous system performance may occur).
No products indexed under this heading.

Ethanol (Concurrent use of olopatadine nasal spray with alcohol should be avoided because additional reductions in alertness and additional impairment of central nervous system performance may occur).
No products indexed under this heading.

Ethchlorvynol (Concurrent use of olopatadine nasal spray with other central nervous system depressants should be avoided because additional reductions in alertness and additional impairment of central nervous system performance may occur).
No products indexed under this heading.

Ethinamate (Concurrent use of olopatadine nasal spray with other central nervous system depressants should be avoided because additional reductions in alertness and additional impairment of central nervous system performance may occur).
No products indexed under this heading.

Ethyl Alcohol (Concurrent use of olopatadine nasal spray with alcohol should be avoided because additional reductions in alertness and additional impairment of central nervous system performance may occur).
No products indexed under this heading.

Fentanyl (Concurrent use of olopatadine nasal spray with other central nervous system depressants should be avoided because additional reductions in alertness and additional impairment of central nervous system performance may occur). Products include:
Duragesic Transdermal System 2405
Ionsys Transdermal System 2410

Fentanyl Citrate (Concurrent use of olopatadine nasal spray with other central nervous system depressants should be avoided because additional reductions in alertness and additional impairment of central nervous system performance may occur). Products include:
Actiq 959
Fentora Tablets 968

Fluphenazine Decanoate (Concurrent use of olopatadine nasal spray with other central nervous system depressants should be avoided because additional reductions in alertness and additional impairment of central nervous system performance may occur).
No products indexed under this heading.

Fluphenazine Enanthate (Concurrent use of olopatadine nasal spray with other central nervous system depressants should be avoided because additional reductions in alertness and additional impairment of central nervous system performance may occur).
No products indexed under this heading.

Fluphenazine Hydrochloride (Concurrent use of olopatadine nasal spray with other central nervous system depressants should be avoided because additional reductions in alertness and additional impairment of central nervous system performance may occur).
No products indexed under this heading.

Flurazepam Hydrochloride (Concurrent use of olopatadine nasal spray with other central nervous system depressants should be avoided because additional reductions in alertness and additional impairment of central nervous system performance may occur).
No products indexed under this heading.

Glutethimide (Concurrent use of olopatadine nasal spray with other central nervous system depressants should be avoided because additional reductions in alertness and additional impairment of central nervous system performance may occur).
No products indexed under this heading.

Haloperidol (Concurrent use of olopatadine nasal spray with other central nervous system depressants should be avoided because additional reductions in alertness and additional impairment of central nervous system performance may occur).
No products indexed under this heading.

Haloperidol Decanoate (Concurrent use of olopatadine nasal spray with other central nervous system depressants should be avoided because additional reductions in alertness and additional impairment of central nervous system performance may occur).
No products indexed under this heading.

Hydrocodone Bitartrate (Concurrent use of olopatadine nasal spray with other central nervous system depressants should be avoided because additional reductions in alertness and additional impairment of central nervous system performance may occur). Products include:

Lortab 5/500 Tablets **3143**
Lortab 7.5/500 Tablets **3144**
Lortab 10/500 Tablets **3144**
Vicodin Tablets **529**
Vicodin ES Tablets **530**
Vicodin HP Tablets **531**
Vicoprofen Tablets **533**
Zydone Tablets **1132**

Hydrocodone Polistirex (Concurrent use of olopatadine nasal spray with other central nervous system depressants should be avoided because additional reductions in alertness and additional impairment of central nervous system performance may occur). Products include:

Tussionex Pennkinetic Extended-Release Suspension **3154**

Hydromorphone Hydrochloride (Concurrent use of olopatadine nasal spray with other central nervous system depressants should be avoided because additional reductions in alertness and additional impairment of central nervous system performance may occur).
No products indexed under this heading.

Hydroxyzine Hydrochloride (Concurrent use of olopatadine nasal spray with other central nervous system depressants should be avoided because additional reductions in alertness and additional impairment of central nervous system performance may occur).
No products indexed under this heading.

Isoflurane (Concurrent use of olopatadine nasal spray with other central nervous system depressants should be avoided because additional reductions in alertness and additional impairment of central nervous system performance may occur).
No products indexed under this heading.

Ketamine Hydrochloride (Concurrent use of olopatadine nasal spray with other central nervous system depressants should be avoided because additional reductions in alertness and additional impairment of central nervous system performance may occur).
No products indexed under this heading.

Levomethadyl Acetate Hydrochloride (Concurrent use of olopatadine nasal spray with other central nervous system depressants should be avoided because additional reductions in alertness and additional impairment of central nervous system performance may occur).
No products indexed under this heading.

Levorphanol Tartrate (Concurrent use of olopatadine nasal spray with other central nervous system depressants should be avoided because additional reductions in alertness and additional impairment of central nervous system performance may occur).
No products indexed under this heading.

Lorazepam (Concurrent use of olopatadine nasal spray with other central nervous system depressants should be avoided because additional reductions in alertness and additional impairment of central nervous system performance may occur).
No products indexed under this heading.

Loxapine Hydrochloride (Concurrent use of olopatadine nasal spray with other central nervous system depressants should be avoided because additional reductions in alertness and additional impairment of central nervous system performance may occur).
No products indexed under this heading.

Loxapine Succinate (Concurrent use of olopatadine nasal spray with other central nervous system depressants should be avoided because additional reductions in alertness and additional impairment of central nervous system performance may occur).
No products indexed under this heading.

Meperidine Hydrochloride (Concurrent use of olopatadine nasal spray with other central nervous system depressants should be avoided because additional reductions in alertness and additional impairment of central nervous system performance may occur).
No products indexed under this heading.

Mephobarbital (Concurrent use of olopatadine nasal spray with other central nervous system depressants should be avoided because additional reductions in alertness and additional impairment of central nervous system performance may occur).
No products indexed under this heading.

Meprobamate (Concurrent use of olopatadine nasal spray with other central nervous system depressants should be avoided because additional reductions in alertness and additional impairment of central nervous system performance may occur).
No products indexed under this heading.

Mesoridazine Besylate (Concurrent use of olopatadine nasal spray with other central nervous system depressants should be avoided because additional reductions in alertness and additional impairment of central nervous system performance may occur).
No products indexed under this heading.

Methadone Hydrochloride (Concurrent use of olopatadine nasal spray with other central nervous system depressants should be avoided because additional reductions in alertness and additional impairment of central nervous system performance may occur).
No products indexed under this heading.

Methohexital Sodium (Concurrent use of olopatadine nasal spray with other central nervous system depressants should be avoided because additional reductions in alertness and additional impairment of central nervous system performance may occur).
No products indexed under this heading.

Methotrimeprazine (Concurrent use of olopatadine nasal spray with other central nervous system depressants should be avoided because additional reductions in alertness and additional impairment of central nervous system performance may occur).
No products indexed under this heading.

Methoxyflurane (Concurrent use of olopatadine nasal spray with other central nervous system depressants should be avoided because additional reductions in alertness and additional impairment of central nervous system performance may occur).
No products indexed under this heading.

Midazolam Hydrochloride (Concurrent use of olopatadine nasal spray with other central nervous system depressants should be avoided because additional reductions in alertness and additional impairment of central nervous system performance may occur).
No products indexed under this heading.

Molindone Hydrochloride (Concurrent use of olopatadine nasal spray with other central nervous system depressants should be avoided because additional reductions in alertness and additional impairment of central nervous system performance may occur). Products include:

Moban Tablets **1116**

Morphine Sulfate (Concurrent use of olopatadine nasal spray with other central nervous system depressants should be avoided because additional reductions in alertness and additional impairment of central nervous system performance may occur). Products include:

Avinza Capsules **1772**
DepoDur Injection **1095**
MS Contin Tablets **2585**

Olanzapine (Concurrent use of olopatadine nasal spray with other central nervous system depressants should be avoided because additional reductions in alertness and additional impairment of central nervous system performance may occur). Products include:

Symbyax Capsules **1871**
Zyprexa Tablets **1883**
Zyprexa IntraMuscular **1883**
Zyprexa ZYDIS Orally Disintegrating Tablets **1883**

Oxazepam (Concurrent use of olopatadine nasal spray with other central nervous system depressants should be avoided because additional reductions in alertness and additional impairment of central nervous system performance may occur).
No products indexed under this heading.

Oxycodone Hydrochloride (Concurrent use of olopatadine nasal spray with other central nervous system depressants should be avoided because additional reductions in alertness and additional impairment of central nervous system performance may occur). Products include:

OxyContin Tablets **2589**
OxyIR Capsules **2593**
Percocet Tablets **1127**
Percodan Tablets **1130**

Pentobarbital Sodium (Concurrent use of olopatadine nasal spray with other central nervous system depressants should be avoided because additional reductions in alertness and additional impairment of central nervous system performance may occur). Products include:

Nembutal Sodium Solution, USP **2494**

Perphenazine (Concurrent use of olopatadine nasal spray with other central nervous system depressants should be avoided because additional reductions in alertness and additional impairment of central nervous system performance may occur).
No products indexed under this heading.

Phenobarbital (Concurrent use of olopatadine nasal spray with other central nervous system depressants should be avoided because additional reductions in alertness and additional impairment of central nervous system performance may occur). Products include:

Donnatal Extentabs **2507**

Prazepam (Concurrent use of olopatadine nasal spray with other central nervous system depressants should be avoided because additional reductions in alertness and additional impairment of central nervous system performance may occur).
No products indexed under this heading.

Prochlorperazine (Concurrent use of olopatadine nasal spray with other central nervous system depressants should be avoided because additional reductions in alertness and additional impairment of central nervous system performance may occur).
No products indexed under this heading.

Promethazine Hydrochloride (Concurrent use of olopatadine nasal spray with other central nervous system depressants should be avoided because additional reductions in alertness and additional impairment of central nervous system performance may occur).
No products indexed under this heading.

Propofol (Concurrent use of olopatadine nasal spray with other central nervous system depressants should be avoided because additional reductions in alertness and additional impairment of central nervous system performance may occur).
No products indexed under this heading.

Propoxyphene Hydrochloride (Concurrent use of olopatadine nasal spray with other central nervous system depressants should be avoided because additional reductions in alertness and additional impairment of central nervous system performance may occur).
No products indexed under this heading.

Propoxyphene Napsylate (Concurrent use of olopatadine nasal spray with other central nervous system depressants should be avoided because additional reductions in alertness and additional impairment of central nervous system performance may occur).
No products indexed under this heading.

Quazepam (Concurrent use of olopatadine nasal spray with other central nervous system depressants should be avoided because additional reductions in alertness and additional impairment of central nervous system performance may occur).
No products indexed under this heading.

Quetiapine Fumarate (Concurrent use of olopatadine nasal spray with other central nervous system depressants should be avoided because additional reductions in alertness and additional impairment of central nervous system performance may occur).
No products indexed under this heading.

Remifentanil Hydrochloride (Concurrent use of olopatadine nasal spray with other central nervous system depressants should be avoided because additional reductions in alertness and additional impairment of central nervous system performance may occur).
No products indexed under this heading.

Risperidone (Concurrent use of olopatadine nasal spray with other central nervous system depressants should be avoided because additional reductions in alertness and additional impairment of central nervous system performance may occur).
Products include:
Risperdal Consta Long-Acting Injection 1753

Secobarbital Sodium (Concurrent use of olopatadine nasal spray with other central nervous system depressants should be avoided because additional reductions in alertness and additional impairment of central nervous system performance may occur).
No products indexed under this heading.

Sevoflurane (Concurrent use of olopatadine nasal spray with other central nervous system depressants should be avoided because additional reductions in alertness and additional impairment of central nervous system performance may occur).
Products include:
Ultane Liquid for Inhalation 524

Sodium Oxybate (Concurrent use of olopatadine nasal spray with other central nervous system depressants should be avoided because additional reductions in alertness and additional impairment of central nervous system performance may occur).
Products include:
Xyrem Oral Solution 1766

Sufentanil Citrate (Concurrent use of olopatadine nasal spray with other central nervous system depressants should be avoided because additional reductions in alertness and additional impairment of central nervous system performance may occur).
No products indexed under this heading.

Temazepam (Concurrent use of olopatadine nasal spray with other central nervous system depressants should be avoided because additional reductions in alertness and additional impairment of central nervous system performance may occur).
No products indexed under this heading.

Thiamylal Sodium (Concurrent use of olopatadine nasal spray with other central nervous system depressants should be avoided because additional reductions in alertness and additional impairment of central nervous system performance may occur).
No products indexed under this heading.

Thioridazine Hydrochloride (Concurrent use of olopatadine nasal spray with other central nervous system depressants should be avoided because additional reductions in alertness and additional impairment of central nervous system performance may occur). Products include:
Thioridazine Hydrochloride Tablets 2195

Thiothixene (Concurrent use of olopatadine nasal spray with other central nervous system depressants should be avoided because additional reductions in alertness and additional impairment of central nervous system performance may occur).
Products include:
Thiothixene Capsules 2197

Triazolam (Concurrent use of olopatadine nasal spray with other central nervous system depressants should be avoided because additional reductions in alertness and additional impairment of central nervous system performance may occur).
No products indexed under this heading.

Trifluoperazine Hydrochloride (Concurrent use of olopatadine nasal spray with other central nervous system depressants should be avoided because additional reductions in alertness and additional impairment of central nervous system performance may occur).
No products indexed under this heading.

Zaleplon (Concurrent use of olopatadine nasal spray with other central nervous system depressants should be avoided because additional reductions in alertness and additional impairment of central nervous system performance may occur).
No products indexed under this heading.

Ziprasidone Hydrochloride (Concurrent use of olopatadine nasal spray with other central nervous system depressants should be avoided because additional reductions in alertness and additional impairment of central nervous system performance may occur). Products include:
Geodon Capsules 2520

Zolpidem Tartrate (Concurrent use of olopatadine nasal spray with other central nervous system depressants should be avoided because additional reductions in alertness and additional impairment of central nervous system performance may occur).
Products include:
Ambien Tablets 2692
Ambien CR Tablets 2696

Food Interactions

Alcohol (Concurrent use of olopatadine nasal spray with alcohol should be avoided because additional reductions in alertness and additional impairment of central nervous system performance may occur).

PATANOL OPHTHALMIC SOLUTION

(Olopatadine Hydrochloride) 546
None cited in PDR database.

PAXIL ORAL SUSPENSION

(Paroxetine Hydrochloride) 1535
See Paxil Tablets

PAXIL TABLETS

(Paroxetine Hydrochloride) 1535
May interact with monoamine oxidase inhibitors, non-steroidal anti-inflammatory agents, phenothiazines, phenytoin, highly protein bound drugs (selected), serotoninergic agents, selective serotonin reuptake inhibitors, tricyclic antidepressants, triptans, xanthines, and certain other agents. Compounds in these categories include:

Almotriptan Malate (There have been rare postmarketing reports of serotonin syndrome with the use of an SSRI and a triptan. If concomitant use of paroxetine hydrochloride with a triptan is clinically warranted, careful observation of the patient is advised, particularly during treatment initiation and dose increases).
Products include:
Axert Tablets 2431

Aminophylline (There have been reports of elevated theophylline levels associated with co-administration; monitor theophylline levels when these drugs are concurrently administered).
No products indexed under this heading.

Amiodarone Hydrochloride (Paroxetine is metabolized by the cytochrome P450 isoenzyme CYP2D6. Therefore, co-administration of paroxetine with other drugs that inhibit this enzyme should be approached with caution).
No products indexed under this heading.

Amitriptyline Hydrochloride (Caution is indicated in the co-administration of tricyclic antidepressants with paroxetine because paroxetine may inhibit TCA metabolism. Plasma TCA concentrations may need to be monitored and the dose of TCA may need to be reduced if a TCA is co-administered with paroxetine).
No products indexed under this heading.

Amoxapine (Caution is indicated in the co-administration of tricyclic antidepressants with paroxetine because paroxetine may inhibit TCA metabolism. Plasma TCA concentrations may need to be monitored and the dose of TCA may need to be reduced if a TCA is co-administered with paroxetine).
No products indexed under this heading.

Amphetamine Aspartate (Paroxetine may significantly inhibit the activity of the cytochrome P450 2D6 isoenzyme. Concomitant use of paroxetine with other drugs metabolized by cytochrome CYP2D6 has not been formally studied but may require lower doses than usually prescribed for either paroxetine or the other drug. Therefore, co-administration of paroxetine with other drugs that are metabolized by this isozyme should be approached with caution). Products include:
Adderall XR Capsules 3012

Amphetamine Aspartate Monohydrate (Paroxetine may significantly inhibit the activity of the cytochrome P450 2D6 isoenzyme. Concomitant use of paroxetine with other drugs metabolized by cytochrome CYP2D6 has not been formally studied but may require lower doses than usually prescribed for either paroxetine or the other drug. Therefore, co-administration of paroxetine with other drugs that are metabolized by this isozyme should be approached with caution).
No products indexed under this heading.

Amphetamine Sulfate (Paroxetine may significantly inhibit the activity of the cytochrome P450 2D6 isoenzyme. Concomitant use of paroxetine with other drugs metabolized by cytochrome CYP2D6 has not been formally studied but may require lower doses than usually prescribed for either paroxetine or the other drug. Therefore, co-administration of paroxetine with other drugs that are metabolized by this isozyme should be approached with caution).
Products include:
Adderall XR Capsules 3012

Anisindione (The combined use of psychotropic drugs that interfere with serotonin reuptake and drugs that affect coagulation has been associated with an increased risk of bleeding; concomitant administration should be undertaken with caution).
No products indexed under this heading.

Ardeparin Sodium (The combined use of psychotropic drugs that interfere with serotonin reuptake and drugs that affect coagulation has been associated with an increased risk of bleeding; concomitant administration should be undertaken with caution).
No products indexed under this heading.

Aspirin (The combined use of psychotropic drugs that interfere with serotonin reuptake and drugs that affect coagulation has been associated with an increased risk of bleeding). Products include:
Aggrenox Capsules 819
Bayer Aspirin 750
Percodan Tablets 1130
St. Joseph 81 mg Aspirin Chewable and Enteric Coated Tablets 1903

Aspirin, Enteric Coated (The combined use of psychotropic drugs that interfere with serotonin reuptake and drugs that affect coagulation has been associated with an increased risk of bleeding).
No products indexed under this heading.

Aspirin Buffered (The combined use of psychotropic drugs that interfere with serotonin reuptake and drugs that affect coagulation has been associated with an increased risk of bleeding).
No products indexed under this heading.

Atomoxetine Hydrochloride (Paroxetine may significantly inhibit the activity of the cytochrome P450 2D6 isoenzyme. Concomitant use of paroxetine with other drugs metabolized by cytochrome CYP2D6 has not been formally studied but may require lower doses than usually prescribed for either paroxetine or the other drug. Therefore, co-administration of paroxetine with other drugs that are metabolized by this isozyme should be approached with caution). Products include:
Strattera Capsules 1864

Atovaquone (Co-administration with another drug that is highly protein bound may increase free concentrations of the other drug or paroxetine potentially resulting in adverse events). Products include:
Malarone Pediatric Tablets 1521
Malarone Tablets 1521
Mepron Suspension 1526

Bisoprolol Fumarate (Paroxetine may significantly inhibit the activity of the cytochrome P450 2D6 isoenzyme. Concomitant use of paroxetine with other drugs metabolized by cytochrome CYP2D6 has not been formally studied but may require lower doses than usually prescribed for either paroxetine or the other drug. Therefore, co-administration of paroxetine with other drugs that are metabolized by this isozyme should be approached with caution).
No products indexed under this heading.

Bupropion Hydrochloride (Paroxetine is metabolized by the cytochrome P450 isoenzyme CYP2D6. Therefore, co-administration of paroxetine with other drugs that inhibit this enzyme should be approached with caution). Products include:
Wellbutrin Tablets 1648
Wellbutrin SR Sustained-Release Tablets 1653
Wellbutrin XL Extended-Release Tablets 1659
Zyban Sustained-Release Tablets 1692

Captopril (Paroxetine may significantly inhibit the activity of the cytochrome P450 2D6 isoenzyme. Concomitant use of paroxetine with other drugs metabolized by cytochrome CYP2D6 has not been formally studied but may require lower doses than usually prescribed for either paroxetine or the other drug. Therefore, co-administration of paroxetine with other drugs that are metabolized by this isozyme should be approached with caution). Products include:
Captopril Tablets 2182

Carvedilol (Paroxetine may significantly inhibit the activity of the cytochrome P450 2D6 isoenzyme. Concomitant use of paroxetine with other drugs metabolized by cytochrome CYP2D6 has not been formally studied but may require lower doses than usually prescribed for either paroxetine or the other drug. Therefore, co-administration of paroxetine with other drugs that are metabolized by this isozyme should be approached with caution). Products include:
Coreg Tablets 1387

Cefonicid Sodium (Co-administration with another drug that is highly protein bound may increase free concentrations of the other drug or paroxetine potentially resulting in adverse events).
No products indexed under this heading.

Celecoxib (Paroxetine is metabolized by the cytochrome P450 isoenzyme CYP2D6. Therefore, co-administration of paroxetine with other drugs that inhibit this enzyme should be approached with caution). Products include:
Celebrex Capsules 2979

Cevimeline Hydrochloride (Paroxetine may significantly inhibit the activity of the cytochrome P450 2D6 isoenzyme. Concomitant use of paroxetine with other drugs metabolized by cytochrome CYP2D6 has not been formally studied but may require lower doses than usually prescribed for either paroxetine or the other drug. Therefore, co-administration of paroxetine with other drugs that are metabolized by this isozyme should be approached with caution). Products include:
Evoxac Capsules 1013

Chlordiazepoxide (Co-administration with another drug that is highly protein bound may increase free concentrations of the other drug or paroxetine potentially resulting in adverse events).
No products indexed under this heading.

Chlordiazepoxide Hydrochloride (Co-administration with another drug that is highly protein bound may increase free concentrations of the other drug or paroxetine potentially resulting in adverse events).
No products indexed under this heading.

Chloroquine Hydrochloride (Paroxetine is metabolized by the cytochrome P450 isoenzyme CYP2D6. Therefore, co-administration of paroxetine with other drugs that inhibit this enzyme should be approached with caution).
No products indexed under this heading.

Chloroquine Phosphate (Paroxetine is metabolized by the cytochrome P450 isoenzyme CYP2D6. Therefore, co-administration of paroxetine with other drugs that inhibit this enzyme should be approached with caution).
No products indexed under this heading.

Chlorpheniramine (Paroxetine is metabolized by the cytochrome P450 isoenzyme CYP2D6. Therefore, co-administration of paroxetine with other drugs that inhibit this enzyme should be approached with caution).
No products indexed under this heading.

Chlorpheniramine Maleate (Paroxetine is metabolized by the cytochrome P450 isoenzyme CYP2D6. Therefore, co-administration of paroxetine with other drugs that inhibit this enzyme should be approached with caution). Products include:
Actifed Cold & Allergy Tablets 1895
Sudafed PE Sinus & Allergy Tablets 1908
Tylenol Allergy Multi-Symptom Caplets with Cool Burst and Rapid Release Gelcaps 1916
Children's Tylenol Plus Cold Suspension Liquid 1912
Children's Tylenol Plus Cough & Runny Nose Suspension Liquid 1912
Children's Tylenol Plus Flu Suspension Liquid 1914
Children's Tylenol Plus Multi-Symptom Cold Suspension Liquid 1912
Tylenol Cold Head Congestion Nighttime Caplets with Cool Burst 1910
Tylenol Cold Multi-Symptom Nighttime Caplets with Cool Burst 1913
Tylenol Sinus Congestion & Pain Nighttime Caplets with Cool Burst 1917

Chlorpheniramine Polistirex (Paroxetine is metabolized by the cytochrome P450 isoenzyme CYP2D6. Therefore, co-administration of paroxetine with other drugs that inhibit this enzyme should be approached with caution). Products include:
Tussionex Pennkinetic Extended-Release Suspension 3154

Chlorpheniramine Tannate (Paroxetine is metabolized by the cytochrome P450 isoenzyme CYP2D6. Therefore, co-administration of paroxetine with other drugs that inhibit this enzyme should be approached with caution).
No products indexed under this heading.

Chlorpromazine (Paroxetine may significantly inhibit the activity of cytochrome P450 2D6 isoenzyme. Concomitant use of paroxetine with other drugs metabolized by cytochrome CYP2D6 has not been formally studied but may require lower doses than usually prescribed for either paroxetine or the other drug. Therefore, co-administration of paroxetine with other drugs that are metabolized by this isozyme should be approached with caution).
No products indexed under this heading.

Chlorpromazine Hydrochloride (Paroxetine may significantly inhibit the activity of cytochrome P450 2D6 isoenzyme. Concomitant use of paroxetine with other drugs metabolized by cytochrome CYP2D6 has not been formally studied but may require lower doses than usually prescribed for either paroxetine or the other drug. Therefore, co-administration of paroxetine with other drugs that are metabolized by this isozyme should be approached with caution).
No products indexed under this heading.

Chlorpropamide (Paroxetine may significantly inhibit the activity of the cytochrome P450 2D6 isoenzyme. Concomitant use of paroxetine with other drugs metabolized by cytochrome CYP2D6 has not been formally studied but may require lower doses than usually prescribed for either paroxetine or the other drug. Therefore, co-administration of paroxetine with other drugs that are metabolized by this isozyme should be approached with caution).
No products indexed under this heading.

Cimetidine (Co-administration with oral cimetidine has resulted in an increase in steady-state plasma concentrations of paroxetine).
No products indexed under this heading.

Cimetidine Hydrochloride (Co-administration with oral cimetidine has resulted in an increase in steady-state plasma concentrations of paroxetine).
No products indexed under this heading.

Citalopram Hydrobromide (Paroxetine is metabolized by the cytochrome P450 isoenzyme CYP2D6. Therefore, co-administration of paroxetine with other drugs that inhibit this enzyme should be approached with caution). Products include:
Celexa 1160

Clomipramine Hydrochloride (Caution is indicated in the co-administration of tricyclic antidepressants with paroxetine because paroxetine may inhibit TCA metabolism. Plasma TCA concentrations may need to be monitored and the dose of TCA may need to be reduced if a TCA is co-administered with paroxetine).
No products indexed under this heading.

Clozapine (Paroxetine may significantly inhibit the activity of the cytochrome P450 2D6 isoenzyme. Concomitant use of paroxetine with other drugs metabolized by cytochrome CYP2D6 has not been formally studied but may require lower doses than usually prescribed for either paroxetine or the other drug. Therefore, co-administration of paroxetine with other drugs that are metabolized by this isozyme should be approached with caution).
No products indexed under this heading.

Cocaine Hydrochloride (Paroxetine is metabolized by the cytochrome P450 isoenzyme CYP2D6. Therefore, co-administration of paroxetine with other drugs that inhibit this enzyme should be approached with caution).
No products indexed under this heading.

Codeine Phosphate (Paroxetine may significantly inhibit the activity of the cytochrome P450 2D6 isoenzyme. Concomitant use of paroxetine with other drugs metabolized by cytochrome CYP2D6 has not been formally studied but may require low-

er doses than usually prescribed for either paroxetine or the other drug. Therefore, co-administration of paroxetine with other drugs that are metabolized by this isozyme should be approached with caution). Products include:

Tylenol with Codeine Tablets **2427**

Codeine Sulfate (Paroxetine may significantly inhibit the activity of the cytochrome P450 2D6 isoenzyme. Concomitant use of paroxetine with other drugs metabolized by cytochrome CYP2D6 has not been formally studied but may require lower doses than usually prescribed for either paroxetine or the other drug. Therefore, co-administration of paroxetine with other drugs that are metabolized by this isozyme should be approached with caution).

No products indexed under this heading.

Cyclobenzaprine Hydrochloride (Paroxetine may significantly inhibit the activity of the cytochrome P450 2D6 isoenzyme. Concomitant use of paroxetine with other drugs metabolized by cytochrome CYP2D6 has not been formally studied but may require lower doses than usually prescribed for either paroxetine or the other drug. Therefore, co-administration of paroxetine with other drugs that are metabolized by this isozyme should be approached with caution). Products include:

Amrix Capsules **966**

Cyclosporine (Co-administration with another drug that is highly protein bound may increase free concentrations of the other drug or paroxetine potentially resulting in adverse events). Products include:

Gengraf Capsules **435**
Neoral Oral Solution **2280**
Neoral Soft Gelatin Capsules **2280**
Restasis Ophthalmic Emulsion **557**
Sandimmune **2296**

Dalteparin Sodium (The combined use of psychotropic drugs that interfere with serotonin reuptake and drugs that affect coagulation has been associated with an increased risk of bleeding; concomitant administration should be undertaken with caution). Products include:

Fragmin Injection **1070**

Danaparoid Sodium (The combined use of psychotropic drugs that interfere with serotonin reuptake and drugs that affect coagulation has been associated with an increased risk of bleeding; concomitant administration should be undertaken with caution).

No products indexed under this heading.

Desipramine Hydrochloride (Co-administration with desipramine has resulted in an increase in Cmax, AUC and T1/2 by an average of approximately two-, five- and three-fold, respectively).

No products indexed under this heading.

Dexfenfluramine Hydrochloride (Paroxetine may significantly inhibit the activity of the cytochrome P450 2D6 isoenzyme. Concomitant use of paroxetine with other drugs metabolized by cytochrome CYP2D6 has not been formally studied but may require lower doses than usually prescribed for either paroxetine or the other drug. Therefore, co-administration of paroxetine with other drugs that are metabolized by this isozyme should be approached with caution).

No products indexed under this heading.

Dextromethorphan Hydrobromide (Paroxetine may significantly inhibit the activity of the cytochrome P450 2D6 isoenzyme. Concomitant use of paroxetine with other drugs metabolized by cytochrome CYP2D6 has not been formally studied but may require lower doses than usually prescribed for either paroxetine or the other drug. Therefore, co-administration of paroxetine with other drugs that are metabolized by this isozyme should be approached with caution). Products include:

PediaCare Children's Liquid Multi-Symptom Cold..................... **1902**
PediaCare Children's Long-Acting Cough.. **1902**
Children's Sudafed PE Cold & Cough Liquid.............................. **1907**
Sudafed PE Cold & Cough Caplets.. **1907**
Children's Tylenol Plus Cough & Runny Nose Suspension Liquid..... **1912**
Children's Tylenol Plus Cough & Sore Throat Suspension Liquid..... **1912**
Children's Tylenol Plus Flu Suspension Liquid....................... **1914**
Children's Tylenol Plus Multi-Symptom Cold Suspension Liquid....................... **1912**
Tylenol Cold Severe Congestion Daytime Caplets with Cool Burst... **1912**
Tylenol Cold Head Congestion Daytime Caplets with Cool Burst... **1910**
Tylenol Cold Head Congestion Nighttime Caplets with Cool Burst... **1910**
Tylenol Cold Head Congestion Severe Daytime Caplets with Cool Burst................................... **1910**
Tylenol Cold Multi-Symptom Daytime Caplets with Cool Burst and Rapid Release Gels...... **1913**
Tylenol Cold Multi-Symptom Daytime Liquid with Citrus Burst... **1913**
Tylenol Cold Multi-Symptom Nighttime Caplets with Cool Burst... **1913**
Tylenol Cold Multi-Symptom Nighttime Liquid with Cool Burst... **1913**
Tylenol Cold Multi-Symptom Severe Caplets with Cool Burst..... **1913**
Tylenol Cold Multi-Symptom Severe Daytime Liquid with Citrus Burst.................................... **1913**
Tylenol Cough & Sore Throat Daytime Liquid with Cool Burst...... **1918**
Tylenol Cough & Sore Throat Nighttime Liquid with Cool Burst... **1918**
Vicks DayQuil Cold & Flu Multi-Symptom Relief................. ▣ **616**
Vicks DayQuil LiquiCaps **2567**
Vicks DayQuil Liquid **2567**
Vicks DayQuil Multi-Symptom Cold/Flu Relief............................ **2567**
Vicks NyQuil Cold & Flu Multi-Symptom Relief................. ▣ **617**
Vicks NyQuil LiquiCaps **2567**
Vicks NyQuil Liquid **2567**
Vicks NyQuil Multi-Symptom Cold/Flu Relief............................ **2567**

Dextromethorphan Polistirex (Paroxetine may significantly inhibit the activity of the cytochrome P450 2D6 isoenzyme. Concomitant use of paroxetine with other drugs metabolized by cytochrome CYP2D6 has not been formally studied but may require lower doses than usually prescribed for either paroxetine or the other drug. Therefore, co-administration of paroxetine with other drugs that are metabolized by this isozyme should be approached with caution).

No products indexed under this heading.

Diazepam (Co-administration with another drug that is highly protein bound may increase free concentrations of the other drug or paroxetine potentially resulting in adverse events). Products include:

Valium Tablets **2658**

Diclofenac Epolamine (The combined use of psychotropic drugs that interfere with serotonin reuptake and drugs that affect coagulation has been associated with an increased risk of bleeding). Products include:

Flector Patch **561**

Diclofenac Potassium (The combined use of psychotropic drugs that interfere with serotonin reuptake and drugs that affect coagulation has been associated with an increased risk of bleeding).

No products indexed under this heading.

Diclofenac Sodium (The combined use of psychotropic drugs that interfere with serotonin reuptake and drugs that affect coagulation has been associated with an increased risk of bleeding). Products include:

Diclofenac Sodium Ophthalmic Solution.. ⊙ **240**
Voltaren Ophthalmic Solution **2336**
Voltaren Tablets **2334**
Voltaren-XR Tablets **2337**

Dicumarol (The combined use of psychotropic drugs that interfere with serotonin reuptake and drugs that affect coagulation has been associated with an increased risk of bleeding; concomitant administration should be undertaken with caution).

No products indexed under this heading.

Digoxin (The steady-state pharmacokinetics of paroxetine was not altered when administered with digoxin at steady state. Mean digoxin AUC at steady state decreased by 15% in the presence of paroxetine. Since there is little clinical experience, the concurrent administration of paroxetine and digoxin should be undertaken with caution). Products include:

Lanoxin Injection **1498**
Lanoxin Injection Pediatric **1502**
Lanoxin Tablets **1505**

Diphenhydramine (Paroxetine is metabolized by the cytochrome P450 isoenzyme CYP2D6. Therefore, co-administration of paroxetine with other drugs that inhibit this enzyme should be approached with caution).

No products indexed under this heading.

Diphenhydramine Hydrochloride (Paroxetine is metabolized by the cytochrome P450 isoenzyme CYP2D6. Therefore, co-administration of paroxetine with other drugs that inhibit this enzyme should be approached with caution). Products include:

Benadryl Allergy & Cold Kapgels...... **1895**
Benadryl Allergy & Sinus Headache Kapgels........................ **1895**
Benadryl Severe Allergy & Sinus Headache Caplets........................ **1897**
Benadryl Dye-Free Allergy Liqui-gels Softgels........................ **1897**
Benadryl Allergy Kapgels **1895**
Benadryl Allergy Quick Dissolve Strips... **1896**
Benadryl Allergy Ultratab Tablets **1896**
Children's Benadryl Dye-Free Allergy Liquid.................................. **1897**
Children's Benadryl Allergy Fastmelts.................................... **1897**
Children's Benadryl Allergy Liquid **1898**
Children's Benadryl Allergy Perfect Measure............................. **1896**
Children's Benadryl-D Allergy & Sinus Liquid................................. **1896**
Benadryl-D Allergy & Sinus Tablet **1896**
PediaCare Children's Allergy & Cold Liquid.................................... **1902**
PediaCare Children's Allergy Liquid.. **1902**
Simply Sleep Caplets **1905**
Sudafed PE Nighttime Cold Caplets.. **1907**
Sudafed PE Severe Cold Caplets **1908**
Extra Strength Tylenol PM Caplets, Geltabs, Liquid, and Rapid Release Gels....................... **1915**
Tylenol Allergy Multi-Symptom Nighttime Caplets with Cool Burst... **1916**
Tylenol Severe Allergy Caplets **1916**
Children's Tylenol Plus Cold & Allergy Suspension Liquid............ **1914**
Tylenol Sore Throat Nighttime Liquid with Cool Burst................... **1918**

Dipyridamole (Co-administration with another drug that is highly protein bound may increase free concentrations of the other drug or paroxetine potentially resulting in adverse events). Products include:

Aggrenox Capsules **819**
Persantine Tablets **869**

Dolasetron Mesylate (Paroxetine may significantly inhibit the activity of the cytochrome P450 2D6 isoenzyme. Concomitant use of paroxetine with other drugs metabolized by cytochrome CYP2D6 has not been formally studied but may require lower doses than usually prescribed for either paroxetine or the other drug. Therefore, co-administration of paroxetine with other drugs that are metabolized by this isozyme should be approached with caution). Products include:

Anzemet Injection **2701**
Anzemet Tablets **2704**

Donepezil Hydrochloride (Paroxetine may significantly inhibit the activity of the cytochrome P450 2D6 isoenzyme. Concomitant use of paroxetine with other drugs metabolized by cytochrome CYP2D6 has not been formally studied but may require lower doses than usually prescribed for either paroxetine or the other drug. Therefore, co-administration of paroxetine with other drugs that are metabolized by this isozyme should be approached with caution). Products include:

Aricept Tablets **1062**
Aricept ODT Tablets **1062**

Doxepin Hydrochloride (Caution is indicated in the co-administration of tricyclic antidepressants with paroxetine because paroxetine may inhibit TCA metabolism. Plasma TCA concentrations may need to be monitored and the dose of TCA may need to be reduced if a TCA is co-administered with paroxetine).

No products indexed under this heading.

Dyphylline (There have been reports of elevated theophylline levels associated with co-administration; monitor theophylline levels when these drugs are concurrently administered).

No products indexed under this heading.

Eletriptan Hydrobromide (There have been rare postmarketing reports of serotonin syndrome with the use of an SSRI and a triptan. If concomitant use of paroxetine hydrochloride with a triptan is clinically warranted, careful observation of the patient is advised, particularly during treatment initiation and dose increases).
No products indexed under this heading.

Encainide Hydrochloride (Paroxetine may significantly inhibit the activity of the cytochrome P450 2D6 isoenzyme. Concomitant use of paroxetine with other drugs metabolized by cytochrome CYP2D6 has not been formally studied but may require lower doses than usually prescribed for either paroxetine or the other drug. Therefore, co-administration of paroxetine with other drugs that are metabolized by this isozyme should be approached with caution).
No products indexed under this heading.

Enoxaparin Sodium (The combined use of psychotropic drugs that interfere with serotonin reuptake and drugs that affect coagulation has been associated with an increased risk of bleeding; concomitant administration should be undertaken with caution). Products include:
Lovenox Injection ... **2756**

Escitalopram Oxalate (Paroxetine is metabolized by the cytochrome P450 isoenzyme CYP2D6. Therefore, co-administration of paroxetine with other drugs that inhibit this enzyme should be approached with caution). Products include:
Lexapro Oral Suspension ... **1174**
Lexapro Tablets ... **1174**

Etodolac (The combined use of psychotropic drugs that interfere with serotonin reuptake and drugs that affect coagulation has been associated with an increased risk of bleeding).
No products indexed under this heading.

Fenoprofen Calcium (The combined use of psychotropic drugs that interfere with serotonin reuptake and drugs that affect coagulation has been associated with an increased risk of bleeding). Products include:
Nalfon Capsules ... **2508**

Fentanyl (Paroxetine may significantly inhibit the activity of the cytochrome P450 2D6 isoenzyme. Concomitant use of paroxetine with other drugs metabolized by cytochrome CYP2D6 has not been formally studied but may require lower doses than usually prescribed for either paroxetine or the other drug. Therefore, co-administration of paroxetine with other drugs that are metabolized by this isozyme should be approached with caution). Products include:
Duragesic Transdermal System ... **2405**
Ionsys Transdermal System ... **2410**

Fentanyl Citrate (Paroxetine may significantly inhibit the activity of the cytochrome P450 2D6 isoenzyme. Concomitant use of paroxetine with other drugs metabolized by cytochrome CYP2D6 has not been formally studied but may require lower doses than usually prescribed for either paroxetine or the other drug. Therefore, co-administration of paroxetine with other drugs that are metabolized by this isozyme should be approached with caution). Products include:
Actiq ... **959**
Fentora Tablets ... **968**

Flecainide Acetate (Paroxetine may significantly inhibit the activity of the cytochrome P450 2D6 isoenzyme. Concomitant use of paroxetine with other drugs metabolized by cytochrome CYP2D6 has not been formally studied but may require lower doses than usually prescribed for either paroxetine or the other drug. Therefore, co-administration of paroxetine with other drugs that are metabolized by this isozyme should be approached with caution).
No products indexed under this heading.

Fluoxetine (Paroxetine is metabolized by the cytochrome P450 isoenzyme CYP2D6. Therefore, co-administration of paroxetine with other drugs that inhibit this enzyme should be approached with caution).
No products indexed under this heading.

Fluoxetine Hydrochloride (Paroxetine is metabolized by the cytochrome P450 isoenzyme CYP2D6. Therefore, co-administration of paroxetine with other drugs that inhibit this enzyme should be approached with caution). Products include:
Prozac Weekly Capsules ... **1852**
Prozac Pulvules and Liquid ... **1852**
Symbyax Capsules ... **1871**

Fluphenazine Decanoate (Paroxetine is metabolized by the cytochrome P450 isoenzyme CYP2D6. Therefore, co-administration of paroxetine with other drugs that inhibit this enzyme should be approached with caution).
No products indexed under this heading.

Fluphenazine Enanthate (Paroxetine is metabolized by the cytochrome P450 isoenzyme CYP2D6. Therefore, co-administration of paroxetine with other drugs that inhibit this enzyme should be approached with caution).
No products indexed under this heading.

Fluphenazine Hydrochloride (Paroxetine is metabolized by the cytochrome P450 isoenzyme CYP2D6. Therefore, co-administration of paroxetine with other drugs that inhibit this enzyme should be approached with caution).
No products indexed under this heading.

Flurazepam Hydrochloride (Co-administration with another drug that is highly protein bound may increase free concentrations of the other drug or paroxetine potentially resulting in adverse events).
No products indexed under this heading.

Flurbiprofen (The combined use of psychotropic drugs that interfere with serotonin reuptake and drugs that affect coagulation has been associated with an increased risk of bleeding).
No products indexed under this heading.

Fluvoxamine Maleate (Paroxetine is metabolized by the cytochrome P450 isoenzyme CYP2D6. Therefore, co-administration of paroxetine with other drugs that inhibit this enzyme should be approached with caution). Products include:
Luvox CR Extended-Release Capsules ... **1759**

Fondaparinux Sodium (The combined use of psychotropic drugs that interfere with serotonin reuptake and drugs that affect coagulation has been associated with an increased risk of bleeding; concomitant administration should be undertaken with caution). Products include:
Arixtra Injection ... **1313**

Formoterol Fumarate (Paroxetine may significantly inhibit the activity of the cytochrome P450 2D6 isoenzyme. Concomitant use of paroxetine with other drugs metabolized by cytochrome CYP2D6 has not been formally studied but may require lower doses than usually prescribed for either paroxetine or the other drug. Therefore, co-administration of paroxetine with other drugs that are metabolized by this isozyme should be approached with caution). Products include:
Foradil Aerolizer ... **2849**
Perforomist Inhalation Solution ... **1025**

Fosamprenavir Calcium (Co-administration of fosamprenavir with paroxetine significantly decreased plasma levels of paroxetine. Any dose adjustment should be guided by clinical effect (tolerability and efficacy)). Products include:
Lexiva Oral Suspension ... **1510**
Lexiva Tablets ... **1510**

Fosphenytoin Sodium (Co-administration has resulted in reduction of paroxetine AUC and T1/2; potential for elevated phenytoin levels or slight reduction in phenytoin AUC).
No products indexed under this heading.

Frovatriptan Succinate (There have been rare postmarketing reports of serotonin syndrome with the use of an SSRI and a triptan. If concomitant use of paroxetine hydrochloride with a triptan is clinically warranted, careful observation of the patient is advised, particularly during treatment initiation and dose increases). Products include:
Frova Tablets ... **1111**

Galantamine Hydrobromide (Paroxetine may significantly inhibit the activity of the cytochrome P450 2D6 isoenzyme. Concomitant use of paroxetine with other drugs metabolized by cytochrome CYP2D6 has not been formally studied but may require lower doses than usually prescribed for either paroxetine or the other drug. Therefore, co-administration of paroxetine with other drugs that are metabolized by this isozyme should be approached with caution).
No products indexed under this heading.

Glipizide (Co-administration with another drug that is highly protein bound may increase free concentrations of the other drug or paroxetine potentially resulting in adverse events).
No products indexed under this heading.

Halofantrine Hydrochloride (Paroxetine is metabolized by the cytochrome P450 isoenzyme CYP2D6. Therefore, co-administration of paroxetine with other drugs that inhibit this enzyme should be approached with caution).
No products indexed under this heading.

Haloperidol (Paroxetine is metabolized by the cytochrome P450 isoenzyme CYP2D6. Therefore, co-administration of paroxetine with other drugs that inhibit this enzyme should be approached with caution).
No products indexed under this heading.

Haloperidol Decanoate (Paroxetine is metabolized by the cytochrome P450 isoenzyme CYP2D6. Therefore, co-administration of paroxetine with other drugs that inhibit this enzyme should be approached with caution).
No products indexed under this heading.

Heparin Calcium (The combined use of psychotropic drugs that interfere with serotonin reuptake and drugs that affect coagulation has been associated with an increased risk of bleeding; concomitant administration should be undertaken with caution).
No products indexed under this heading.

Heparin Sodium (The combined use of psychotropic drugs that interfere with serotonin reuptake and drugs that affect coagulation has been associated with an increased risk of bleeding; concomitant administration should be undertaken with caution).
No products indexed under this heading.

Hydrocodone Bitartrate (Paroxetine may significantly inhibit the activity of the cytochrome P450 2D6 isoenzyme. Concomitant use of paroxetine with other drugs metabolized by cytochrome CYP2D6 has not been formally studied but may require lower doses than usually prescribed for either paroxetine or the other drug. Therefore, co-administration of paroxetine with other drugs that are metabolized by this isozyme should be approached with caution). Products include:
Lortab 5/500 Tablets ... **3143**
Lortab 7.5/500 Tablets ... **3144**
Lortab 10/500 Tablets ... **3144**
Vicodin Tablets ... **529**
Vicodin ES Tablets ... **530**
Vicodin HP Tablets ... **531**
Vicoprofen Tablets ... **533**
Zydone Tablets ... **1132**

Hydroxychloroquine Sulfate (Paroxetine is metabolized by the cytochrome P450 isoenzyme CYP2D6. Therefore, co-administration of paroxetine with other drugs that inhibit this enzyme should be approached with caution).
No products indexed under this heading.

Hypericum (Based on the mechanism of action of paroxetine and the potential for serotonin syndrome, caution is advised when paroxetine hydrochloride is co-administered with other drugs or agents that may affect the serotonergic neurotransmitter systems, such as St. John's Wort). Products include:
Satieté Tablets ... **640**

Ibuprofen (The combined use of psychotropic drugs that interfere with serotonin reuptake and drugs that affect coagulation has been associated with an increased risk of bleeding). Products include:

Motrin IB Tablets and Caplets 1900
Children's Motrin Oral Suspension ... 1901
Children's Motrin Non-Staining Dye-Free Oral Suspension............ 1901
Children's Motrin Cold Oral Suspension 1899
Infants' Motrin Concentrated Drops.. 1901
Infants' Motrin Non-Staining Dye-Free Concentrated Drops....... 1901
Junior Strength Motrin Caplets and Chewable Tablets.................. 1901
Vicoprofen Tablets 533

Imatinib Mesylate (Paroxetine is metabolized by the cytochrome P450 isoenzyme CYP2D6. Therefore, co-administration of paroxetine with other drugs that inhibit this enzyme should be approached with caution). Products include:

Gleevec Tablets 2255

Imipramine Hydrochloride (Caution is indicated in the co-administration of tricyclic antidepressants with paroxetine because paroxetine may inhibit TCA metabolism. Plasma TCA concentrations may need to be monitored and the dose of TCA may need to be reduced if a TCA is co-administered with paroxetine).

No products indexed under this heading.

Imipramine Pamoate (Caution is indicated in the co-administration of tricyclic antidepressants with paroxetine because paroxetine may inhibit TCA metabolism. Plasma TCA concentrations may need to be monitored and the dose of TCA may need to be reduced if a TCA is co-administered with paroxetine).

No products indexed under this heading.

Indomethacin (The combined use of psychotropic drugs that interfere with serotonin reuptake and drugs that affect coagulation has been associated with an increased risk of bleeding). Products include:

Indocin 2024

Indomethacin Sodium Trihydrate (The combined use of psychotropic drugs that interfere with serotonin reuptake and drugs that affect coagulation has been associated with an increased risk of bleeding). Products include:

Indocin I.V. 2489

Indoramin Hydrochloride (Paroxetine may significantly inhibit the activity of the cytochrome P450 2D6 isoenzyme. Concomitant use of paroxetine with other drugs metabolized by cytochrome CYP2D6 has not been formally studied but may require lower doses than usually prescribed for either paroxetine or the other drug. Therefore, co-administration of paroxetine with other drugs that are metabolized by this isozyme should be approached with caution).

No products indexed under this heading.

Isocarboxazid (Concomitant use of paroxetine hydrochloride and MAOIs intended to treat depression is contraindicated. Potential for serious and/or fatal reactions, including hyperthermia, rigidity, myoclonus, and other serious reactions; therefore, it is recommended that paroxetine hydrochloride not be used in combination with a MAOI, or within 14 days of discontinuing treatment with a MAOI. At least 2 weeks should be allowed after stopping paroxetine hydrochloride before starting a MAOI). Products include:

Marplan Tablets 3177

Ketoprofen (The combined use of psychotropic drugs that interfere with serotonin reuptake and drugs that affect coagulation has been associated with an increased risk of bleeding).

No products indexed under this heading.

Ketorolac Tromethamine (The combined use of psychotropic drugs that interfere with serotonin reuptake and drugs that affect coagulation has been associated with an increased risk of bleeding).

No products indexed under this heading.

Labetalol Hydrochloride (Paroxetine may significantly inhibit the activity of the cytochrome P450 2D6 isoenzyme. Concomitant use of paroxetine with other drugs metabolized by cytochrome CYP2D6 has not been formally studied but may require lower doses than usually prescribed for either paroxetine or the other drug. Therefore, co-administration of paroxetine with other drugs that are metabolized by this isozyme should be approached with caution).

No products indexed under this heading.

Lidocaine (Paroxetine may significantly inhibit the activity of the cytochrome P450 2D6 isoenzyme. Concomitant use of paroxetine with other drugs metabolized by cytochrome CYP2D6 has not been formally studied but may require lower doses than usually prescribed for either paroxetine or the other drug. Therefore, co-administration of paroxetine with other drugs that are metabolized by this isozyme should be approached with caution). Products include:

Lidoderm Patch 1114

Lidocaine Hydrochloride (Paroxetine may significantly inhibit the activity of the cytochrome P450 2D6 isoenzyme. Concomitant use of paroxetine with other drugs metabolized by cytochrome CYP2D6 has not been formally studied but may require lower doses than usually prescribed for either paroxetine or the other drug. Therefore, co-administration of paroxetine with other drugs that are metabolized by this isozyme should be approached with caution).

No products indexed under this heading.

Linezolid (Concomitant use of paroxetine in patients taking linezolid is contraindicated). Products include:

Zyvox 2552

Lithium (A multiple-dose study has shown that there is no pharmacokinetic interaction between paroxetine and lithium carbonate. However, due to the potential for serotonin syndrome, caution is advised when paroxetine is co-administered with lithium).

No products indexed under this heading.

Lithium Carbonate (A multiple-dose study has shown that there is no pharmacokinetic interaction between paroxetine and lithium carbonate. However, due to the potential for serotonin syndrome, caution is advised when paroxetine is co-administered with lithium).

No products indexed under this heading.

Lithium Citrate (A multiple-dose study has shown that there is no pharmacokinetic interaction between paroxetine and lithium carbonate. However, due to the potential for serotonin syndrome, caution is advised when paroxetine is co-administered with lithium).

No products indexed under this heading.

Low Molecular Weight Heparins (The combined use of psychotropic drugs that interfere with serotonin reuptake and drugs that affect coagulation has been associated with an increased risk of bleeding; concomitant administration should be undertaken with caution).

No products indexed under this heading.

Maprotiline Hydrochloride (Caution is indicated in the co-administration of tricyclic antidepressants with paroxetine because paroxetine may inhibit TCA metabolism. Plasma TCA concentrations may need to be monitored and the dose of TCA may need to be reduced if a TCA is co-administered with paroxetine).

No products indexed under this heading.

Meclofenamate Sodium (The combined use of psychotropic drugs that interfere with serotonin reuptake and drugs that affect coagulation has been associated with an increased risk of bleeding).

No products indexed under this heading.

Mefenamic Acid (The combined use of psychotropic drugs that interfere with serotonin reuptake and drugs that affect coagulation has been associated with an increased risk of bleeding).

No products indexed under this heading.

Meloxicam (The combined use of psychotropic drugs that interfere with serotonin reuptake and drugs that affect coagulation has been associated with an increased risk of bleeding). Products include:

Mobic Oral Suspension 863
Mobic Tablets 863

Meperidine Hydrochloride (Paroxetine may significantly inhibit the activity of the cytochrome P450 2D6 isoenzyme. Concomitant use of paroxetine with other drugs metabolized by cytochrome CYP2D6 has not been formally studied but may require lower doses than usually prescribed for either paroxetine or the other drug. Therefore, co-administration of paroxetine with other drugs that are metabolized by this isozyme should be approached with caution).

No products indexed under this heading.

Mesoridazine Besylate (Paroxetine may significantly inhibit the activity of cytochrome P450 2D6 isoenzyme. Concomitant use of paroxetine with other drugs metabolized by cytochrome CYP2D6 has not been formally studied but may require lower doses than usually prescribed for either paroxetine or the other drug. Therefore, co-administration of paroxetine with other drugs that are metabolized by this isozyme should be approached with caution).

No products indexed under this heading.

Methadone Hydrochloride (Paroxetine is metabolized by the cytochrome P450 isoenzyme CYP2D6. Therefore, co-administration of paroxetine with other drugs that inhibit this enzyme should be approached with caution).

No products indexed under this heading.

Methamphetamine Hydrochloride (Paroxetine may significantly inhibit the activity of the cytochrome P450 2D6 isoenzyme. Concomitant use of paroxetine with other drugs metabolized by cytochrome CYP2D6 has not been formally studied but may require lower doses than usually prescribed for either paroxetine or the other drug. Therefore, co-administration of paroxetine with other drugs that are metabolized by this isozyme should be approached with caution).

No products indexed under this heading.

Methotrimeprazine (Paroxetine may significantly inhibit the activity of cytochrome P450 2D6 isoenzyme. Concomitant use of paroxetine with other drugs metabolized by cytochrome CYP2D6 has not been formally studied but may require lower doses than usually prescribed for either paroxetine or the other drug. Therefore, co-administration of paroxetine with other drugs that are metabolized by this isozyme should be approached with caution).

No products indexed under this heading.

Metoprolol Succinate (There has been a case report of severe hypotension when immediate-release paroxetine was added to chronic metoprolol treatment). Products include:

Toprol-XL Tablets 666

Metoprolol Tartrate (There has been a case report of severe hypotension when immediate-release paroxetine was added to chronic metoprolol treatment).

No products indexed under this heading.

Mexiletine Hydrochloride (Paroxetine may significantly inhibit the activity of the cytochrome P450 2D6 isoenzyme. Concomitant use of paroxetine with other drugs metabolized by cytochrome CYP2D6 has not been formally studied but may require lower doses than usually prescribed for either paroxetine or the other drug. Therefore, co-administration of paroxetine with other drugs that are metabolized by this isozyme should be approached with caution).

No products indexed under this heading.

Mibefradil Dihydrochloride (Paroxetine is metabolized by the cytochrome P450 isoenzyme CYP2D6. Therefore, co-administration of paroxetine with other drugs that inhibit this enzyme should be approached with caution).

No products indexed under this heading.

Midazolam Hydrochloride (Co-administration with another drug that is highly protein bound may increase free concentrations of the other drug or paroxetine potentially resulting in adverse events).
No products indexed under this heading.

Mirtazapine (Paroxetine may significantly inhibit the activity of the cytochrome P450 2D6 isoenzyme. Concomitant use of paroxetine with other drugs metabolized by cytochrome CYP2D6 has not been formally studied but may require lower doses than usually prescribed for either paroxetine or the other drug. Therefore, co-administration of paroxetine with other drugs that are metabolized by this isozyme should be approached with caution).
Products include:
Remeron Tablets **2924**
RemeronSolTab Tablets **2927**

Moclobemide (Concomitant use of paroxetine hydrochloride and MAOIs intended to treat depression is contraindicated. Potential for serious and/or fatal reactions, including hyperthermia, rigidity, myoclonus, and other serious reactions; therefore, it is recommended that paroxetine hydrochloride not be used in combination with a MAOI, or within 14 days of discontinuing treatment with a MAOI. At least 2 weeks should be allowed after stopping paroxetine hydrochloride before starting a MAOI).
No products indexed under this heading.

Morphine Sulfate (Paroxetine may significantly inhibit the activity of the cytochrome P450 2D6 isoenzyme. Concomitant use of paroxetine with other drugs metabolized by cytochrome CYP2D6 has not been formally studied but may require lower doses than usually prescribed for either paroxetine or the other drug. Therefore, co-administration of paroxetine with other drugs that are metabolized by this isozyme should be approached with caution).
Products include:
Avinza Capsules **1772**
DepoDur Injection **1095**
MS Contin Tablets **2585**

Nabumetone (The combined use of psychotropic drugs that interfere with serotonin reuptake and drugs that affect coagulation has been associated with an increased risk of bleeding).
No products indexed under this heading.

Naproxen (The combined use of psychotropic drugs that interfere with serotonin reuptake and drugs that affect coagulation has been associated with an increased risk of bleeding). Products include:
EC-Naprosyn Delayed-Release Tablets **2632**
Naprosyn Suspension **2632**
Naprosyn Tablets **2632**

Naproxen Sodium (The combined use of psychotropic drugs that interfere with serotonin reuptake and drugs that affect coagulation has been associated with an increased risk of bleeding). Products include:
Anaprox Tablets **2632**
Anaprox DS Tablets **2632**
Treximet Tablets **1616**

Naratriptan Hydrochloride (There have been rare postmarketing reports of serotonin syndrome with the use of an SSRI and a triptan. If concomitant use of paroxetine hydrochloride with a triptan is clinically warranted, careful observation of the patient is advised, particularly during treatment initiation and dose increases). Products include:
Amerge Tablets **1301**

Nelfinavir Mesylate (Paroxetine may significantly inhibit the activity of the cytochrome P450 2D6 isoenzyme. Concomitant use of paroxetine with other drugs metabolized by cytochrome CYP2D6 has not been formally studied but may require lower doses than usually prescribed for either paroxetine or the other drug. Therefore, co-administration of paroxetine with other drugs that are metabolized by this isozyme should be approached with caution).
No products indexed under this heading.

Nortriptyline Hydrochloride (Caution is indicated in the co-administration of tricyclic antidepressants with paroxetine because paroxetine may inhibit TCA metabolism. Plasma TCA concentrations may need to be monitored and the dose of TCA may need to be reduced if a TCA is co-administered with paroxetine).
No products indexed under this heading.

Olanzapine (Paroxetine may significantly inhibit the activity of the cytochrome P450 2D6 isoenzyme. Concomitant use of paroxetine with other drugs metabolized by cytochrome CYP2D6 has not been formally studied but may require lower doses than usually prescribed for either paroxetine or the other drug. Therefore, co-administration of paroxetine with other drugs that are metabolized by this isozyme should be approached with caution).
Products include:
Symbyax Capsules **1871**
Zyprexa Tablets **1883**
Zyprexa IntraMuscular **1883**
Zyprexa ZYDIS Orally Disintegrating Tablets **1883**

Omeprazole (Paroxetine may significantly inhibit the activity of the cytochrome P450 2D6 isoenzyme. Concomitant use of paroxetine with other drugs metabolized by cytochrome CYP2D6 has not been formally studied but may require lower doses than usually prescribed for either paroxetine or the other drug. Therefore, co-administration of paroxetine with other drugs that are metabolized by this isozyme should be approached with caution).
No products indexed under this heading.

Ondansetron (Paroxetine may significantly inhibit the activity of the cytochrome P450 2D6 isoenzyme. Concomitant use of paroxetine with other drugs metabolized by cytochrome CYP2D6 has not been formally studied but may require lower doses than usually prescribed for either paroxetine or the other drug. Therefore, co-administration of paroxetine with other drugs that are metabolized by this isozyme should be approached with caution).
Products include:
Zofran ODT Orally Disintegrating Tablets **1687**

Ondansetron Hydrochloride (Paroxetine may significantly inhibit the activity of the cytochrome P450 2D6 isoenzyme. Concomitant use of paroxetine with other drugs metabolized by cytochrome CYP2D6 has not been formally studied but may require lower doses than usually prescribed for either paroxetine or the other drug. Therefore, co-administration of paroxetine with other drugs that are metabolized by this isozyme should be approached with caution). Products include:
Zofran Injection **1682**
Zofran **1687**

Oxaprozin (The combined use of psychotropic drugs that interfere with serotonin reuptake and drugs that affect coagulation has been associated with an increased risk of bleeding).
No products indexed under this heading.

Oxazepam (Co-administration with another drug that is highly protein bound may increase free concentrations of the other drug or paroxetine potentially resulting in adverse events).
No products indexed under this heading.

Oxycodone Hydrochloride (Paroxetine may significantly inhibit the activity of the cytochrome P450 2D6 isoenzyme. Concomitant use of paroxetine with other drugs metabolized by cytochrome CYP2D6 has not been formally studied but may require lower doses than usually prescribed for either paroxetine or the other drug. Therefore, co-administration of paroxetine with other drugs that are metabolized by this isozyme should be approached with caution). Products include:
OxyContin Tablets **2589**
OxyIR Capsules **2593**
Percocet Tablets **1127**
Percodan Tablets **1130**

Paclitaxel (Paroxetine may significantly inhibit the activity of the cytochrome P450 2D6 isoenzyme. Concomitant use of paroxetine with other drugs metabolized by cytochrome CYP2D6 has not been formally studied but may require lower doses than usually prescribed for either paroxetine or the other drug. Therefore, co-administration of paroxetine with other drugs that are metabolized by this isozyme should be approached with caution).
No products indexed under this heading.

Pargyline Hydrochloride (Concomitant use of paroxetine hydrochloride and MAOIs intended to treat depression is contraindicated. Potential for serious and/or fatal reactions, including hyperthermia, rigidity, myoclonus, and other serious reactions; therefore, it is recommended that paroxetine hydrochloride not be used in combination with a MAOI, or within 14 days of discontinuing treatment with a MAOI. At least 2 weeks should be allowed after stopping paroxetine hydrochloride before starting a MAOI).
No products indexed under this heading.

Perphenazine (Paroxetine is metabolized by the cytochrome P450 isoenzyme CYP2D6. Therefore, co-administration of paroxetine with other drugs that inhibit this enzyme should be approached with caution).
No products indexed under this heading.

Phenelzine Sulfate (Concomitant use of paroxetine hydrochloride and MAOIs intended to treat depression is contraindicated. Potential for serious and/or fatal reactions, including hyperthermia, rigidity, myoclonus, and other serious reactions; therefore, it is recommended that paroxetine hydrochloride not be used in combination with a MAOI, or within 14 days of discontinuing treatment with a MAOI. At least 2 weeks should be allowed after stopping paroxetine hydrochloride before starting a MAOI).
No products indexed under this heading.

Phenobarbital (Co-administration has resulted in reduction of paroxetine AUC and T1/2). Products include:
Donnatal Extentabs **2507**

Phenylbutazone (The combined use of psychotropic drugs that interfere with serotonin reuptake and drugs that affect coagulation has been associated with an increased risk of bleeding).
No products indexed under this heading.

Phenytoin (Co-administration has resulted in reduction of paroxetine AUC and T1/2; potential for elevated phenytoin levels or slight reduction in phenytoin AUC).
No products indexed under this heading.

Phenytoin Sodium (Co-administration has resulted in reduction of paroxetine AUC and T1/2; potential for elevated phenytoin levels or slight reduction in phenytoin AUC). Products include:
Phenytek Capsules **2192**

Pimozide (Due to the narrow therapeutic index of pimozide and its known ability to prolong the QT interval, concomitant use of pimozide and paroxetine hydrocholoride is contraindicated).
No products indexed under this heading.

Pindolol (Paroxetine may significantly inhibit the activity of the cytochrome P450 2D6 isoenzyme. Concomitant use of paroxetine with other drugs metabolized by cytochrome CYP2D6 has not been formally studied but may require lower doses than usually prescribed for either paroxetine or the other drug. Therefore, co-administration of paroxetine with other drugs that are metabolized by this isozyme should be approached with caution).
No products indexed under this heading.

Piroxicam (The combined use of psychotropic drugs that interfere with serotonin reuptake and drugs that affect coagulation has been associated with an increased risk of bleeding).
No products indexed under this heading.

Procarbazine Hydrochloride (Concomitant use of paroxetine hydrochloride and MAOIs intended to treat depression is contraindicated. Potential for serious and/or fatal reactions, including hyperthermia, rigidity, myoclonus, and other serious reactions; therefore, it is recommended that paroxetine hydrochloride not be used in combination with a MAOI, or within 14 days of discontinuing treatment with a MAOI. At

least 2 weeks should be allowed after stopping paroxetine hydrochloride before starting a MAOI).
No products indexed under this heading.

Prochlorperazine (Paroxetine may significantly inhibit the activity of cytochrome P450 2D6 isoenzyme. Concomitant use of paroxetine with other drugs metabolized by cytochrome CYP2D6 has not been formally studied but may require lower doses than usually prescribed for either paroxetine or the other drug. Therefore, co-administration of paroxetine with other drugs that are metabolized by this isozyme should be approached with caution).
No products indexed under this heading.

Procyclidine Hydrochloride (Increased steady-state AUC, Cmax and Cmin values of procyclidine with concurrent use).
No products indexed under this heading.

Promethazine Hydrochloride (Paroxetine may significantly inhibit the activity of cytochrome P450 2D6 isoenzyme. Concomitant use of paroxetine with other drugs metabolized by cytochrome CYP2D6 has not been formally studied but may require lower doses than usually prescribed for either paroxetine or the other drug. Therefore, co-administration of paroxetine with other drugs that are metabolized by this isozyme should be approached with caution).
No products indexed under this heading.

Propafenone Hydrochloride (Paroxetine is metabolized by the cytochrome P450 isoenzyme CYP2D6. Therefore, co-administration of paroxetine with other drugs that inhibit this enzyme should be approached with caution). Products include:
Rythmol Tablets 1586
Rythmol SR Capsules 1590

Propoxyphene Hydrochloride (Paroxetine is metabolized by the cytochrome P450 isoenzyme CYP2D6. Therefore, co-administration of paroxetine with other drugs that inhibit this enzyme should be approached with caution).
No products indexed under this heading.

Propoxyphene Napsylate (Paroxetine is metabolized by the cytochrome P450 isoenzyme CYP2D6. Therefore, co-administration of paroxetine with other drugs that inhibit this enzyme should be approached with caution).
No products indexed under this heading.

Propranolol Hydrochloride (Paroxetine may significantly inhibit the activity of the cytochrome P450 2D6 isoenzyme. Concomitant use of paroxetine with other drugs metabolized by cytochrome CYP2D6 has not been formally studied but may require lower doses than usually prescribed for either paroxetine or the other drug. Therefore, co-administration of paroxetine with other drugs that are metabolized by this isozyme should be approached with caution). Products include:
InnoPran XL Extended Release Capsules 1484

Protriptyline Hydrochloride (Caution is indicated in the co-administration of tricyclic antidepressants with paroxetine because paroxetine may inhibit TCA metabolism. Plasma TCA concentrations may need to be monitored and the dose of TCA may need to be reduced if a TCA is co-administered with paroxetine).
No products indexed under this heading.

Quetiapine Fumarate (Paroxetine may significantly inhibit the activity of the cytochrome P450 2D6 isoenzyme. Concomitant use of paroxetine with other drugs metabolized by cytochrome CYP2D6 has not been formally studied but may require lower doses than usually prescribed for either paroxetine or the other drug. Therefore, co-administration of paroxetine with other drugs that are metabolized by this isozyme should be approached with caution).
No products indexed under this heading.

Quinacrine Hydrochloride (Paroxetine is metabolized by the cytochrome P450 isoenzyme CYP2D6. Therefore, co-administration of paroxetine with other drugs that inhibit this enzyme should be approached with caution).
No products indexed under this heading.

Quinidine Gluconate (Paroxetine is metabolized by the cytochrome P450 isoenzyme CYP2D6. Therefore, co-administration of paroxetine with other drugs that inhibit this enzyme should be approached with caution).
No products indexed under this heading.

Quinidine Hydrochloride (Paroxetine is metabolized by the cytochrome P450 isoenzyme CYP2D6. Therefore, co-administration of paroxetine with other drugs that inhibit this enzyme should be approached with caution).
No products indexed under this heading.

Quinidine Polygalacturonate (Paroxetine is metabolized by the cytochrome P450 isoenzyme CYP2D6. Therefore, co-administration of paroxetine with other drugs that inhibit this enzyme should be approached with caution).
No products indexed under this heading.

Quinidine Sulfate (Paroxetine is metabolized by the cytochrome P450 isoenzyme CYP2D6. Therefore, co-administration of paroxetine with other drugs that inhibit this enzyme should be approached with caution).
No products indexed under this heading.

Ranitidine Bismuth Citrate (Paroxetine is metabolized by the cytochrome P450 isoenzyme CYP2D6. Therefore, co-administration of paroxetine with other drugs that inhibit this enzyme should be approached with caution).
No products indexed under this heading.

Ranitidine Hydrochloride (Paroxetine is metabolized by the cytochrome P450 isoenzyme CYP2D6. Therefore, co-administration of paroxetine with other drugs that inhibit this enzyme should be approached with caution). Products include:
Zantac 75 Tablets .... ▣ 603
Zantac 1670
Zantac Injection 1666
Zantac Injection Pharmacy Bulk Package 1668
Maximum Strength Zantac 150 Tablets .... ▣ 603
Maximum Strength Zantac 150 Cool Mint Tablets .... ▣ 603

Rasagiline Mesylate (Concomitant use of paroxetine hydrochloride and MAOIs intended to treat depression is contraindicated. Potential for serious and/or fatal reactions, including hyperthermia, rigidity, myoclonus, and other serious reactions; therefore, it is recommended that paroxetine hydrochloride not be used in combination with a MAOI, or within 14 days of discontinuing treatment with a MAOI. At least 2 weeks should be allowed after stopping paroxetine hydrochloride before starting a MAOI). Products include:
Azilect Tablets 3106

Risperidone (Paroxetine may significantly inhibit the activity of the cytochrome P450 2D6 isoenzyme. Concomitant use of paroxetine with other drugs metabolized by cytochrome CYP2D6 has not been formally studied but may require lower doses than usually prescribed for either paroxetine or the other drug. Therefore, co-administration of paroxetine with other drugs that are metabolized by this isozyme should be approached with caution). Products include:
Risperdal Consta Long-Acting Injection 1753

Ritonavir (Co-administration of ritonavir with paroxetine significantly decreased plasma levels of paroxetine. Any dose adjustment should be guided by clinical effect (tolerability and efficacy)). Products include:
Kaletra 452
Norvir 489

Rizatriptan Benzoate (There have been rare postmarketing reports of serotonin syndrome with the use of an SSRI and a triptan. If concomitant use of paroxetine hydrochloride with a triptan is clinically warranted, careful observation of the patient is advised, particularly during treatment initiation and dose increases). Products include:
Maxalt Tablets 2056
Maxalt-MLT Orally Disintegrating Tablets 2056

Rofecoxib (The combined use of psychotropic drugs that interfere with serotonin reuptake and drugs that affect coagulation has been associated with an increased risk of bleeding).
No products indexed under this heading.

Selegiline (Concomitant use of paroxetine hydrochloride and MAOIs intended to treat depression is contraindicated. Potential for serious and/or fatal reactions, including hyperthermia, rigidity, myoclonus, and other serious reactions; therefore, it is recommended that paroxetine hydrochloride not be used in combination with a MAOI, or within 14 days of discontinuing treatment with a MAOI. At least 2 weeks should be allowed after stopping paroxetine hydrochloride before starting a MAOI). Products include:
Emsam Transdermal System 905

Selegiline Hydrochloride (Concomitant use of paroxetine hydrochloride and MAOIs intended to treat depression is contraindicated. Potential for serious and/or fatal reactions, including hyperthermia, rigidity, myoclonus, and other serious reactions; therefore, it is recommended that paroxetine hydrochloride not be used in combination with a MAOI, or within 14 days of discontinuing treatment with a MAOI. At least 2 weeks should be allowed after stopping paroxetine hydrochloride before starting a MAOI). Products include:
Eldepryl Capsules 3052

Sertraline Hydrochloride (Paroxetine is metabolized by the cytochrome P450 isoenzyme CYP2D6. Therefore, co-administration of paroxetine with other drugs that inhibit this enzyme should be approached with caution).
No products indexed under this heading.

Sildenafil Citrate (Paroxetine is metabolized by the cytochrome P450 isoenzyme CYP2D6. Therefore, co-administration of paroxetine with other drugs that inhibit this enzyme should be approached with caution).
No products indexed under this heading.

Sulindac (The combined use of psychotropic drugs that interfere with serotonin reuptake and drugs that affect coagulation has been associated with an increased risk of bleeding). Products include:
Clinoril Tablets 1962

Sumatriptan (Co-administration of a selective serotonin reuptake inhibitor (SSRI) and sumatriptan has resulted in weakness, hyperreflexia, and incoordination). Products include:
Imitrex Nasal Spray 1470

Sumatriptan Succinate (Co-administration of a selective serotonin reuptake inhibitor (SSRI) and sumatriptan has resulted in weakness, hyperreflexia, and incoordination). Products include:
Imitrex Injection 1465
Imitrex Tablets 1474
Treximet Tablets 1616

Tamoxifen Citrate (Paroxetine may significantly inhibit the activity of the cytochrome P450 2D6 isoenzyme. Concomitant use of paroxetine with other drugs metabolized by cytochrome CYP2D6 has not been formally studied but may require lower doses than usually prescribed for either paroxetine or the other drug. Therefore, co-administration of paroxetine with other drugs that are metabolized by this isozyme should be approached with caution).
No products indexed under this heading.

Temazepam (Co-administration with another drug that is highly protein bound may increase free concentrations of the other drug or paroxetine potentially resulting in adverse events).
No products indexed under this heading.

Teniposide (Paroxetine may significantly inhibit the activity of the cytochrome P450 2D6 isoenzyme. Concomitant use of paroxetine with other drugs metabolized by cytochrome CYP2D6 has not been formally studied but may require lower doses than usually prescribed for either paroxetine or the other drug. Therefore, co-administration of par-

oxetine with other drugs that are metabolized by this isozyme should be approached with caution).
No products indexed under this heading.

Terbinafine Hydrochloride (Paroxetine is metabolized by the cytochrome P450 isoenzyme CYP2D6. Therefore, co-administration of paroxetine with other drugs that inhibit this enzyme should be approached with caution). Products include:
Lamisil Oral Granules **2264**
Lamisil Tablets **2266**

Testosterone (Paroxetine may significantly inhibit the activity of the cytochrome P450 2D6 isoenzyme. Concomitant use of paroxetine with other drugs metabolized by cytochrome CYP2D6 has not been formally studied but may require lower doses than usually prescribed for either paroxetine or the other drug. Therefore, co-administration of paroxetine with other drugs that are metabolized by this isozyme should be approached with caution). Products include:
AndroGel **3159**
Testim 1% Gel **701**

Testosterone Cypionate (Paroxetine may significantly inhibit the activity of the cytochrome P450 2D6 isoenzyme. Concomitant use of paroxetine with other drugs metabolized by cytochrome CYP2D6 has not been formally studied but may require lower doses than usually prescribed for either paroxetine or the other drug. Therefore, co-administration of paroxetine with other drugs that are metabolized by this isozyme should be approached with caution).
No products indexed under this heading.

Testosterone Enanthate (Paroxetine may significantly inhibit the activity of the cytochrome P450 2D6 isoenzyme. Concomitant use of paroxetine with other drugs metabolized by cytochrome CYP2D6 has not been formally studied but may require lower doses than usually prescribed for either paroxetine or the other drug. Therefore, co-administration of paroxetine with other drugs that are metabolized by this isozyme should be approached with caution). Products include:
Delatestryl Injection **1730**

Testosterone Propionate (Paroxetine may significantly inhibit the activity of the cytochrome P450 2D6 isoenzyme. Concomitant use of paroxetine with other drugs metabolized by cytochrome CYP2D6 has not been formally studied but may require lower doses than usually prescribed for either paroxetine or the other drug. Therefore, co-administration of paroxetine with other drugs that are metabolized by this isozyme should be approached with caution).
No products indexed under this heading.

Theophylline (There have been reports of elevated theophylline levels associated with co-administration; monitor theophylline levels when these drugs are concurrently administered).
No products indexed under this heading.

Theophylline Anhydrous (There have been reports of elevated theophylline levels associated with co-administration; monitor theophylline levels when these drugs are concurrently administered). Products include:
Uniphyl Tablets **2595**

Theophylline Calcium Salicylate (There have been reports of elevated theophylline levels associated with co-administration; monitor theophylline levels when these drugs are concurrently administered).
No products indexed under this heading.

Theophylline Dihydroxypropyl (Glyceryl) (There have been reports of elevated theophylline levels associated with co-administration; monitor theophylline levels when these drugs are concurrently administered).
No products indexed under this heading.

Theophylline Ethylenediamine (There have been reports of elevated theophylline levels associated with co-administration; monitor theophylline levels when these drugs are concurrently administered).
No products indexed under this heading.

Theophylline Sodium Glycinate (There have been reports of elevated theophylline levels associated with co-administration; monitor theophylline levels when these drugs are concurrently administered).
No products indexed under this heading.

Thioridazine (Co-administration of drugs which inhibit CYP450IID6, such as paroxetine, will elevate plasma levels of thioridazine because thioridazine administration produces a dose-related prolongation of the QTc interval which is associated with serious ventricular arrhythmias, such as torsade de pointes-type arrhythmias, and sudden death; concurrent use is contraindicated).
No products indexed under this heading.

Thioridazine Hydrochloride (Co-administration of drugs which inhibit CYP450IID6, such as paroxetine, will elevate plasma levels of thioridazine because thioridazine administration produces a dose-related prolongation of the QTc interval which is associated with serious ventricular arrhythmias, such as torsade de pointes-type arrhythmias, and sudden death; concurrent use is contraindicated). Products include:
Thioridazine Hydrochloride Tablets **2195**

Timolol Maleate (Paroxetine may significantly inhibit the activity of the cytochrome P450 2D6 isoenzyme. Concomitant use of paroxetine with other drugs metabolized by cytochrome CYP2D6 has not been formally studied but may require lower doses than usually prescribed for either paroxetine or the other drug. Therefore, co-administration of paroxetine with other drugs that are metabolized by this isozyme should be approached with caution). Products include:
Combigan Ophthalmic Solution **553**
Cosopt Sterile Ophthalmic Solution **1969**
Timoptic Sterile Ophthalmic Solution **2121**
Timoptic in Ocudose **2124**
Timoptic-XE Sterile Ophthalmic Gel Forming Solution **2125**

Tinzaparin Sodium (The combined use of psychotropic drugs that interfere with serotonin reuptake and drugs that affect coagulation has been associated with an increased risk of bleeding; concomitant administration should be undertaken with caution).
No products indexed under this heading.

Tolbutamide (Co-administration with another drug that is highly protein bound may increase free concentrations of the other drug or paroxetine potentially resulting in adverse events).
No products indexed under this heading.

Tolmetin Sodium (The combined use of psychotropic drugs that interfere with serotonin reuptake and drugs that affect coagulation has been associated with an increased risk of bleeding).
No products indexed under this heading.

Tolterodine Tartrate (Paroxetine may significantly inhibit the activity of the cytochrome P450 2D6 isoenzyme. Concomitant use of paroxetine with other drugs metabolized by cytochrome CYP2D6 has not been formally studied but may require lower doses than usually prescribed for either paroxetine or the other drug. Therefore, co-administration of paroxetine with other drugs that are metabolized by this isozyme should be approached with caution).
No products indexed under this heading.

Tramadol Hydrochloride (Based on the mechanism of action of paroxetine and the potential for serotonin syndrome, caution is advised when paroxetine hydrochloride is co-administered with other drugs or agents that may affect the serotonergic neurotransmitter systems, such as tramadol). Products include:
Ultram ER Extended-Release Tablets **2428**

Tranylcypromine Sulfate (Concomitant use of paroxetine hydrochloride and MAOIs intended to treat depression is contraindicated. Potential for serious and/or fatal reactions, including hyperthermia, rigidity, myoclonus, and other serious reactions; therefore, it is recommended that paroxetine hydrochloride not be used in combination with a MAOI, or within 14 days of discontinuing treatment with a MAOI. At least 2 weeks should be allowed after stopping paroxetine hydrochloride before starting a MAOI). Products include:
Parnate Tablets **1532**

Trazodone Hydrochloride (Paroxetine may significantly inhibit the activity of the cytochrome P450 2D6 isoenzyme. Concomitant use of paroxetine with other drugs metabolized by cytochrome CYP2D6 has not been formally studied but may require lower doses than usually prescribed for either paroxetine or the other drug. Therefore, co-administration of paroxetine with other drugs that are metabolized by this isozyme should be approached with caution).
No products indexed under this heading.

Triazolam (Paroxetine may significantly inhibit the activity of the cytochrome P450 2D6 isoenzyme. Concomitant use of paroxetine with other drugs metabolized by cytochrome CYP2D6 has not been formally studied but may require lower doses than usually prescribed for either paroxetine or the other drug. Therefore, co-administration of paroxetine with other drugs that are metabolized by this isozyme should be approached with caution).
No products indexed under this heading.

Trifluoperazine Hydrochloride (Paroxetine may significantly inhibit the activity of cytochrome P450 2D6 isoenzyme. Concomitant use of paroxetine with other drugs metabolized by cytochrome CYP2D6 has not been formally studied but may require lower doses than usually prescribed for either paroxetine or the other drug. Therefore, co-administration of paroxetine with other drugs that are metabolized by this isozyme should be approached with caution).
No products indexed under this heading.

Trimipramine Maleate (Caution is indicated in the co-administration of tricyclic antidepressants with paroxetine because paroxetine may inhibit TCA metabolism. Plasma TCA concentrations may need to be monitored and the dose of TCA may need to be reduced if a TCA is co-administered with paroxetine).
No products indexed under this heading.

L-Tryptophan (Potential for headache, nausea, sweating and dizziness; concomitant use is not recommended).
No products indexed under this heading.

Valdecoxib (The combined use of psychotropic drugs that interfere with serotonin reuptake and drugs that affect coagulation has been associated with an increased risk of bleeding).
No products indexed under this heading.

Vardenafil Hydrochloride (Paroxetine is metabolized by the cytochrome P450 isoenzyme CYP2D6. Therefore, co-administration of paroxetine with other drugs that inhibit this enzyme should be approached with caution). Products include:
Levitra Tablets **2876**

Venlafaxine Hydrochloride (Paroxetine may significantly inhibit the activity of the cytochrome P450 2D6 isoenzyme. Concomitant use of paroxetine with other drugs metabolized by cytochrome CYP2D6 has not been formally studied but may require lower doses than usually prescribed for either paroxetine or the other drug. Therefore, co-administration of paroxetine with other drugs that are metabolized by this isozyme should be approached with caution). Products include:
Effexor XR Extended-Release Capsules **3195**
Venlafaxine Hydrochloride Tablets ... **2199**

Vinblastine Sulfate (Paroxetine may significantly inhibit the activity of the cytochrome P450 2D6 isoenzyme. Concomitant use of paroxetine with other drugs metabolized by cytochrome CYP2D6 has not been formally studied but may require lower doses than usually prescribed for either paroxetine or the other drug. Therefore, co-administration of par-

oxetine with other drugs that are metabolized by this isozyme should be approached with caution).
No products indexed under this heading.

Warfarin Sodium (Preliminary data suggest that there may be a pharmacodynamic interaction (that causes an increased bleeding diathesis in the face of unaltered prothrombin time) between paroxetine and warfarin. Since there is little clinical experience, the concomitant administration of paroxetine and warfarin should be undertaken with caution).
No products indexed under this heading.

Zolmitriptan (There have been rare postmarketing reports of serotonin syndrome with the use of an SSRI and a triptan. If concomitant use of paroxetine hydrochloride with a triptan is clinically warranted, careful observation of the patient is advised, particularly during treatment initiation and dose increases). Products include:
Zomig Tablets 694
Zomig Nasal Spray 689
Zomig-ZMT Tablets 694

Zonisamide (Paroxetine may significantly inhibit the activity of the cytochrome P450 2D6 isoenzyme. Concomitant use of paroxetine with other drugs metabolized by cytochrome CYP2D6 has not been formally studied but may require lower doses than usually prescribed for either paroxetine or the other drug. Therefore, co-administration of paroxetine with other drugs that are metabolized by this isozyme should be approached with caution). Products include:
Zonegran Capsules 1089

Food Interactions

Alcohol (Concurrent use should be avoided).

Food, unspecified (Co-administration with food resulted in a slight increase (6%) in AUC, but Cmax was 29% greater; time to reach peak plasma concentration decreased from 6.4 hours post-dosing to 4.9 hours).

PAXIL CR CONTROLLED-RELEASE TABLETS

(Paroxetine Hydrochloride) 1544
See Paxil Tablets

PEDIACARE CHILDREN'S ALLERGY & COLD LIQUID

(Diphenhydramine Hydrochloride, Phenylephrine Hydrochloride) 1902
May interact with hypnotics and sedatives, monoamine oxidase inhibitors, and tranquilizers. Compounds in these categories include:

Alprazolam (May increase drowsiness effect).
No products indexed under this heading.

Buspirone Hydrochloride (May increase drowsiness effect).
No products indexed under this heading.

Butabarbital (May increase the drowsiness effect).
No products indexed under this heading.

Butabarbital Sodium (May increase the drowsiness effect).
No products indexed under this heading.

Chloral Hydrate (May increase the drowsiness effect).
No products indexed under this heading.

Chlordiazepoxide (May increase drowsiness effect).
No products indexed under this heading.

Chlordiazepoxide Hydrochloride (May increase drowsiness effect).
No products indexed under this heading.

Chlorpromazine (May increase drowsiness effect).
No products indexed under this heading.

Chlorpromazine Hydrochloride (May increase drowsiness effect).
No products indexed under this heading.

Chlorprothixene (May increase drowsiness effect).
No products indexed under this heading.

Chlorprothixene Hydrochloride (May increase drowsiness effect).
No products indexed under this heading.

Clorazepate Dipotassium (May increase drowsiness effect).
No products indexed under this heading.

Diazepam (May increase drowsiness effect). Products include:
Valium Tablets 2658

Droperidol (May increase drowsiness effect).
No products indexed under this heading.

Estazolam (May increase the drowsiness effect).
No products indexed under this heading.

Ethchlorvynol (May increase the drowsiness effect).
No products indexed under this heading.

Ethinamate (May increase the drowsiness effect).
No products indexed under this heading.

Fluphenazine Decanoate (May increase drowsiness effect).
No products indexed under this heading.

Fluphenazine Enanthate (May increase drowsiness effect).
No products indexed under this heading.

Fluphenazine Hydrochloride (May increase drowsiness effect).
No products indexed under this heading.

Flurazepam Hydrochloride (May increase the drowsiness effect).
No products indexed under this heading.

Glutethimide (May increase the drowsiness effect).
No products indexed under this heading.

Haloperidol (May increase drowsiness effect).
No products indexed under this heading.

Haloperidol Decanoate (May increase drowsiness effect).
No products indexed under this heading.

Hydroxyzine Hydrochloride (May increase drowsiness effect).
No products indexed under this heading.

Isocarboxazid (Avoid use with monoamine oxidase inhibitor (MAOI) or for two weeks after stopping the MAOI drug). Products include:
Marplan Tablets 3177

Lorazepam (May increase the drowsiness effect).
No products indexed under this heading.

Loxapine Hydrochloride (May increase drowsiness effect).
No products indexed under this heading.

Loxapine Succinate (May increase drowsiness effect).
No products indexed under this heading.

Meprobamate (May increase drowsiness effect).
No products indexed under this heading.

Mesoridazine Besylate (May increase drowsiness effect).
No products indexed under this heading.

Midazolam Hydrochloride (May increase the drowsiness effect).
No products indexed under this heading.

Moclobemide (Avoid use with monoamine oxidase inhibitor (MAOI) or for two weeks after stopping the MAOI drug).
No products indexed under this heading.

Molindone Hydrochloride (May increase drowsiness effect). Products include:
Moban Tablets 1116

Oxazepam (May increase drowsiness effect).
No products indexed under this heading.

Pargyline Hydrochloride (Avoid use with monoamine oxidase inhibitor (MAOI) or for two weeks after stopping the MAOI drug).
No products indexed under this heading.

Perphenazine (May increase drowsiness effect).
No products indexed under this heading.

Phenelzine Sulfate (Avoid use with monoamine oxidase inhibitor (MAOI) or for two weeks after stopping the MAOI drug).
No products indexed under this heading.

Prazepam (May increase drowsiness effect).
No products indexed under this heading.

Procarbazine Hydrochloride (Avoid use with monoamine oxidase inhibitor (MAOI) or for two weeks after stopping the MAOI drug).
No products indexed under this heading.

Prochlorperazine (May increase drowsiness effect).
No products indexed under this heading.

Promethazine Hydrochloride (May increase drowsiness effect).
No products indexed under this heading.

Propofol (May increase the drowsiness effect).
No products indexed under this heading.

Quazepam (May increase the drowsiness effect).
No products indexed under this heading.

Ramelteon (May increase the drowsiness effect). Products include:
Rozerem Tablets 3091

Rasagiline Mesylate (Avoid use with monoamine oxidase inhibitor (MAOI) or for two weeks after stopping the MAOI drug). Products include:
Azilect Tablets 3106

Secobarbital Sodium (May increase the drowsiness effect).
No products indexed under this heading.

Selegiline (Avoid use with monoamine oxidase inhibitor (MAOI) or for two weeks after stopping the MAOI drug). Products include:
Emsam Transdermal System 905

Selegiline Hydrochloride (Avoid use with monoamine oxidase inhibitor (MAOI) or for two weeks after stopping the MAOI drug). Products include:
Eldepryl Capsules 3052

Sodium Butabarbital (May increase the drowsiness effect).
No products indexed under this heading.

Temazepam (May increase the drowsiness effect).
No products indexed under this heading.

Thioridazine Hydrochloride (May increase drowsiness effect). Products include:
Thioridazine Hydrochloride Tablets 2195

Thiothixene (May increase drowsiness effect). Products include:
Thiothixene Capsules 2197

Tranylcypromine Sulfate (Avoid use with monoamine oxidase inhibitor (MAOI) or for two weeks after stopping the MAOI drug). Products include:
Parnate Tablets 1532

Triazolam (May increase the drowsiness effect).
No products indexed under this heading.

Trifluoperazine Hydrochloride (May increase drowsiness effect).
No products indexed under this heading.

Zaleplon (May increase the drowsiness effect).
No products indexed under this heading.

Zolpidem Tartrate (May increase the drowsiness effect). Products include:
Ambien Tablets 2692
Ambien CR Tablets 2696

PEDIACARE CHILDREN'S ALLERGY LIQUID

(Diphenhydramine Hydrochloride) 1902
May interact with hypnotics and sedatives and tranquilizers. Compounds in these categories include:

Alprazolam (May increase the drowsiness effect).
No products indexed under this heading.

Buspirone Hydrochloride (May increase the drowsiness effect).
No products indexed under this heading.

Butabarbital (May increase the drowsiness effect).
No products indexed under this heading.

Butabarbital Sodium (May increase the drowsiness effect).
No products indexed under this heading.

Chloral Hydrate (May increase the drowsiness effect).
No products indexed under this heading.

Chlordiazepoxide (May increase the drowsiness effect).
No products indexed under this heading.

Chlordiazepoxide Hydrochloride (May increase the drowsiness effect).
No products indexed under this heading.

Chlorpromazine (May increase the drowsiness effect).
No products indexed under this heading.

Chlorpromazine Hydrochloride (May increase the drowsiness effect).
No products indexed under this heading.

Chlorprothixene (May increase the drowsiness effect).
No products indexed under this heading.

Chlorprothixene Hydrochloride (May increase the drowsiness effect).
No products indexed under this heading.

Clorazepate Dipotassium (May increase the drowsiness effect).
No products indexed under this heading.

Diazepam (May increase the drowsiness effect). Products include:
Valium Tablets 2658

Droperidol (May increase the drowsiness effect).
No products indexed under this heading.

Estazolam (May increase the drowsiness effect).
No products indexed under this heading.

Ethchlorvynol (May increase the drowsiness effect).
No products indexed under this heading.

Ethinamate (May increase the drowsiness effect).
No products indexed under this heading.

Fluphenazine Decanoate (May increase the drowsiness effect).
No products indexed under this heading.

Fluphenazine Enanthate (May increase the drowsiness effect).
No products indexed under this heading.

Fluphenazine Hydrochloride (May increase the drowsiness effect).
No products indexed under this heading.

Flurazepam Hydrochloride (May increase the drowsiness effect).
No products indexed under this heading.

Glutethimide (May increase the drowsiness effect).
No products indexed under this heading.

Haloperidol (May increase the drowsiness effect).
No products indexed under this heading.

Haloperidol Decanoate (May increase the drowsiness effect).
No products indexed under this heading.

Hydroxyzine Hydrochloride (May increase the drowsiness effect).
No products indexed under this heading.

Lorazepam (May increase the drowsiness effect).
No products indexed under this heading.

Loxapine Hydrochloride (May increase the drowsiness effect).
No products indexed under this heading.

Loxapine Succinate (May increase the drowsiness effect).
No products indexed under this heading.

Meprobamate (May increase the drowsiness effect).
No products indexed under this heading.

Mesoridazine Besylate (May increase the drowsiness effect).
No products indexed under this heading.

Midazolam Hydrochloride (May increase the drowsiness effect).
No products indexed under this heading.

Molindone Hydrochloride (May increase the drowsiness effect). Products include:
Moban Tablets 1116

Oxazepam (May increase the drowsiness effect).
No products indexed under this heading.

Perphenazine (May increase the drowsiness effect).
No products indexed under this heading.

Prazepam (May increase the drowsiness effect).
No products indexed under this heading.

Prochlorperazine (May increase the drowsiness effect).
No products indexed under this heading.

Promethazine Hydrochloride (May increase the drowsiness effect).
No products indexed under this heading.

Propofol (May increase the drowsiness effect).
No products indexed under this heading.

Quazepam (May increase the drowsiness effect).
No products indexed under this heading.

Ramelteon (May increase the drowsiness effect). Products include:
Rozerem Tablets 3091

Secobarbital Sodium (May increase the drowsiness effect).
No products indexed under this heading.

Sodium Butabarbital (May increase the drowsiness effect).
No products indexed under this heading.

Temazepam (May increase the drowsiness effect).
No products indexed under this heading.

Thioridazine Hydrochloride (May increase the drowsiness effect). Products include:
Thioridazine Hydrochloride Tablets 2195

Thiothixene (May increase the drowsiness effect). Products include:
Thiothixene Capsules 2197

Triazolam (May increase the drowsiness effect).
No products indexed under this heading.

Trifluoperazine Hydrochloride (May increase the drowsiness effect).
No products indexed under this heading.

Zaleplon (May increase the drowsiness effect).
No products indexed under this heading.

Zolpidem Tartrate (May increase the drowsiness effect). Products include:
Ambien Tablets 2692
Ambien CR Tablets 2696

PEDIACARE CHILDREN'S DECONGESTANT LIQUID

(Phenylephrine Hydrochloride) 1902
May interact with monoamine oxidase inhibitors. Compounds in these categories include:

Isocarboxazid (Concurrent and/or sequential use with MAO inhibitors is not recommended). Products include:
Marplan Tablets 3177

Moclobemide (Concurrent and/or sequential use with MAO inhibitors is not recommended).
No products indexed under this heading.

Pargyline Hydrochloride (Concurrent and/or sequential use with MAO inhibitors is not recommended).
No products indexed under this heading.

Phenelzine Sulfate (Concurrent and/or sequential use with MAO inhibitors is not recommended).
No products indexed under this heading.

Procarbazine Hydrochloride (Concurrent and/or sequential use with MAO inhibitors is not recommended).
No products indexed under this heading.

Rasagiline Mesylate (Concurrent and/or sequential use with MAO inhibitors is not recommended). Products include:
Azilect Tablets 3106

Selegiline (Concurrent and/or sequential use with MAO inhibitors is not recommended). Products include:
Emsam Transdermal System 905

Selegiline Hydrochloride (Concurrent and/or sequential use with MAO inhibitors is not recommended). Products include:
Eldepryl Capsules 3052

Tranylcypromine Sulfate (Concurrent and/or sequential use with MAO inhibitors is not recommended). Products include:
Parnate Tablets 1532

PEDIACARE CHILDREN'S LIQUID MULTI-SYMPTOM COLD

(Dextromethorphan Hydrobromide, Phenylephrine Hydrochloride) 1902
May interact with monoamine oxidase inhibitors. Compounds in these categories include:

Isocarboxazid (Avoid concurrent use with MAO inhibitor or for 2 weeks after MAO inhibitor). Products include:
Marplan Tablets 3177

Moclobemide (Avoid concurrent use with MAO inhibitor or for 2 weeks after MAO inhibitor).
No products indexed under this heading.

Pargyline Hydrochloride (Avoid concurrent use with MAO inhibitor or for 2 weeks after MAO inhibitor).
No products indexed under this heading.

Phenelzine Sulfate (Avoid concurrent use with MAO inhibitor or for 2 weeks after MAO inhibitor).
No products indexed under this heading.

Procarbazine Hydrochloride (Avoid concurrent use with MAO inhibitor or for 2 weeks after MAO inhibitor).
No products indexed under this heading.

Rasagiline Mesylate (Avoid concurrent use with MAO inhibitor or for 2 weeks after MAO inhibitor). Products include:
Azilect Tablets 3106

Selegiline (Avoid concurrent use with MAO inhibitor or for 2 weeks after MAO inhibitor). Products include:
Emsam Transdermal System 905

Selegiline Hydrochloride (Avoid concurrent use with MAO inhibitor or for 2 weeks after MAO inhibitor). Products include:
Eldepryl Capsules 3052

Tranylcypromine Sulfate (Avoid concurrent use with MAO inhibitor or for 2 weeks after MAO inhibitor). Products include:
Parnate Tablets 1532

PEDIACARE CHILDREN'S LONG-ACTING COUGH

(Dextromethorphan Hydrobromide) ... 1902
May interact with monoamine oxidase inhibitors. Compounds in these categories include:

Isocarboxazid (Avoid use with monoamine oxidase inhibitor (MAOI) or for two weeks after stopping the MAOI drug). Products include:
Marplan Tablets 3177

Moclobemide (Avoid use with monoamine oxidase inhibitor (MAOI) or for two weeks after stopping the MAOI drug).
No products indexed under this heading.

Pargyline Hydrochloride (Avoid use with monoamine oxidase inhibitor (MAOI) or for two weeks after stopping the MAOI drug).
No products indexed under this heading.

Phenelzine Sulfate (Avoid use with monoamine oxidase inhibitor (MAOI) or for two weeks after stopping the MAOI drug).
No products indexed under this heading.

Procarbazine Hydrochloride (Avoid use with monoamine oxidase inhibitor (MAOI) or for two weeks after stopping the MAOI drug).
No products indexed under this heading.

Rasagiline Mesylate (Avoid use with monoamine oxidase inhibitor (MAOI) or for two weeks after stopping the MAOI drug). Products include:
Azilect Tablets 3106

Selegiline (Avoid use with monoamine oxidase inhibitor (MAOI) or for two weeks after stopping the MAOI drug). Products include:
Emsam Transdermal System 905

Selegiline Hydrochloride (Avoid use with monoamine oxidase inhibitor (MAOI) or for two weeks after stopping the MAOI drug). Products include:
Eldepryl Capsules 3052

Tranylcypromine Sulfate (Avoid use with monoamine oxidase inhibitor (MAOI) or for two weeks after stopping the MAOI drug). Products include:
Parnate Tablets 1532

PEDIARIX VACCINE
(Diphtheria & Tetanus Toxoids and Acellular Pertussis Vaccine Adsorbed, Hepatitis B Vaccine, Recombinant, Poliovirus Vaccine Inactivated).. 1552

May interact with alkylating agents, antimetabolites, corticosteroids, cytotoxic drugs, immunosuppressive agents, and certain other agents. Compounds in these categories include:

Azathioprine (May reduce immune response to vaccines. When administered to patients who are receiving immunosuppressive therapy, who have an immunodeficiency disorder, or who have received a recent injection of immune globulin, an adequate immunologic response may not be obtained).
No products indexed under this heading.

Basiliximab (May reduce immune response to vaccines. When administered to patients who are receiving immunosuppressive therapy, who have an immunodeficiency disorder, or who have received a recent injection of immune globulin, an adequate immunologic response may not be obtained). Products include:
Simulect for Injection 2306

Betamethasone Acetate (May reduce immune response to vaccines. When administered to patients who are receiving immunosuppressive therapy, who have an immunodeficiency disorder, or who have received a recent injection of immune globulin, an adequate immunologic response may not be obtained).
No products indexed under this heading.

Betamethasone Sodium Phosphate (May reduce immune response to vaccines. When administered to patients who are receiving immunosuppressive therapy, who have an immunodeficiency disorder, or who have received a recent injection of immune globulin, an adequate immunologic response may not be obtained).
No products indexed under this heading.

Bleomycin Sulfate (May reduce immune response to vaccines. When administered to patients who are receiving immunosuppressive therapy, who have an immunodeficiency disorder, or who have received a recent injection of immune globulin, an adequate immunologic response may not be obtained).
No products indexed under this heading.

Budesonide (May reduce immune response to vaccines. When administered to patients who are receiving immunosuppressive therapy, who have an immunodeficiency disorder, or who have received a recent injection of immune globulin, an adequate immunologic response may not be obtained). Products include:
Pulmicort Flexhaler 654
Symbicort 80/4.5 Inhalation Aerosol... 659
Symbicort 160/4.5 Inhalation Aerosol... 659

Busulfan (May reduce immune response to vaccines. When administered to patients who are receiving immunosuppressive therapy, who have an immunodeficiency disorder, or who have received a recent injection of immune globulin, an adequate immunologic response may not be obtained). Products include:
Busulfex Injection 2477
Myleran Tablets 1530

Capecitabine (May reduce immune response to vaccines. When administered to patients who are receiving immunosuppressive therapy, who have an immunodeficiency disorder, or who have received a recent injection of immune globulin, an adequate immunologic response may not be obtained). Products include:
Xeloda Tablets 2662

Carmustine (BCNU) (May reduce immune response to vaccines. When administered to patients who are receiving immunosuppressive therapy, who have an immunodeficiency disorder, or who have received a recent injection of immune globulin, an adequate immunologic response may not be obtained).
No products indexed under this heading.

Chlorambucil (May reduce immune response to vaccines. When administered to patients who are receiving immunosuppressive therapy, who have an immunodeficiency disorder, or who have received a recent injection of immune globulin, an adequate immunologic response may not be obtained). Products include:
Leukeran Tablets 1508

Ciclesonide (May reduce immune response to vaccines. When administered to patients who are receiving immunosuppressive therapy, who have an immunodeficiency disorder, or who have received a recent injection of immune globulin, an adequate immunologic response may not be obtained). Products include:
Alvesco Inhalation Aerosol 2985
Omnaris Nasal Spray 2998

Cladribine (May reduce immune response to vaccines. When administered to patients who are receiving immunosuppressive therapy, who have an immunodeficiency disorder, or who have received a recent injection of immune globulin, an adequate immunologic response may not be obtained). Products include:
Leustatin Injection 2384

Cortisone Acetate (May reduce immune response to vaccines. When administered to patients who are receiving immunosuppressive therapy, who have an immunodeficiency disorder, or who have received a recent injection of immune globulin, an adequate immunologic response may not be obtained).
No products indexed under this heading.

Cyclophosphamide (May reduce immune response to vaccines. When administered to patients who are receiving immunosuppressive therapy, who have an immunodeficiency disorder, or who have received a recent injection of immune globulin, an adequate immunologic response may not be obtained).
No products indexed under this heading.

Cyclosporine (May reduce immune response to vaccines. When administered to patients who are receiving immunosuppressive therapy, who have an immunodeficiency disorder, or who have received a recent injection of immune globulin, an adequate immunologic response may not be obtained). Products include:
Gengraf Capsules 435
Neoral Oral Solution 2280
Neoral Soft Gelatin Capsules 2280
Restasis Ophthalmic Emulsion 557
Sandimmune 2296

Cytarabine (May reduce immune response to vaccines. When administered to patients who are receiving immunosuppressive therapy, who have an immunodeficiency disorder, or who have received a recent injection of immune globulin, an adequate immunologic response may not be obtained).
No products indexed under this heading.

Dacarbazine (May reduce immune response to vaccines. When administered to patients who are receiving immunosuppressive therapy, who have an immunodeficiency disorder, or who have received a recent injection of immune globulin, an adequate immunologic response may not be obtained).
No products indexed under this heading.

Daunorubicin Hydrochloride (May reduce immune response to vaccines. When administered to patients who are receiving immunosuppressive therapy, who have an immunodeficiency disorder, or who have received a recent injection of immune globulin, an adequate immunologic response may not be obtained).
No products indexed under this heading.

Dexamethasone (May reduce immune response to vaccines. When administered to patients who are receiving immunosuppressive therapy, who have an immunodeficiency disorder, or who have received a recent injection of immune globulin, an adequate immunologic response may not be obtained). Products include:
Ciprodex Otic Suspension 541

Dexamethasone Acetate (May reduce immune response to vaccines. When administered to patients who are receiving immunosuppressive therapy, who have an immunodeficiency disorder, or who have received a recent injection of immune globulin, an adequate immunologic response may not be obtained).
No products indexed under this heading.

Dexamethasone Sodium Phosphate (May reduce immune response to vaccines. When administered to patients who are receiving immunosuppressive therapy, who have an immunodeficiency disorder, or who have received a recent injection of immune globulin, an adequate immunologic response may not be obtained).
No products indexed under this heading.

Doxorubicin Hydrochloride (May reduce immune response to vaccines. When administered to patients who are receiving immunosuppressive therapy, who have an immunodeficiency disorder, or who have received a recent injection of immune globulin, an adequate immunologic response may not be obtained).
No products indexed under this heading.

Epirubicin Hydrochloride (May reduce immune response to vaccines. When administered to patients who are receiving immunosuppressive therapy, who have an immunodeficiency disorder, or who have received a recent injection of immune globulin, an adequate immunologic response may not be obtained).
No products indexed under this heading.

Floxuridine (May reduce immune response to vaccines. When administered to patients who are receiving immunosuppressive therapy, who have an immunodeficiency disorder, or who have received a recent injection of immune globulin, an adequate immunologic response may not be obtained).
No products indexed under this heading.

Fludarabine Phosphate (May reduce immune response to vaccines. When administered to patients who are receiving immunosuppressive therapy, who have an immunodeficiency disorder, or who have received a recent injection of immune globulin, an adequate immunologic response may not be obtained).
No products indexed under this heading.

Fludrocortisone Acetate (May reduce immune response to vaccines. When administered to patients who are receiving immunosuppressive therapy, who have an immunodeficiency disorder, or who have received a recent injection of immune globulin, an adequate immunologic response may not be obtained).
No products indexed under this heading.

Flunisolide (May reduce immune response to vaccines. When administered to patients who are receiving immunosuppressive therapy, who have an immunodeficiency disorder, or who have received a recent injection of immune globulin, an adequate immunologic response may not be obtained). Products include:
Aerobid/Aerobid-M 1153

Fluorouracil (May reduce immune response to vaccines. When administered to patients who are receiving immunosuppressive therapy, who have an immunodeficiency disorder, or who have received a recent injec-

tion of immune globulin, an adequate immunologic response may not be obtained). Products include:

Carac Cream 0.5% 2722

Fluticasone Propionate (May reduce immune response to vaccines. When administered to patients who are receiving immunosuppressive therapy, who have an immunodeficiency disorder, or who have received a recent injection of immune globulin, an adequate immunologic response may not be obtained). Products include:

Advair Diskus 100/50 1276
Advair Diskus 250/50 1276
Advair Diskus 500/50 1276
Advair HFA 45/21 Inhalation Aerosol 1288
Advair HFA 115/21 Inhalation Aerosol 1288
Advair HFA 230/21 Inhalation Aerosol 1288
Flonase Nasal Spray 1431
Flovent Diskus 50 mcg 1435

Fluticasone Propionate HFA (May reduce immune response to vaccines. When administered to patients who are receiving immunosuppressive therapy, who have an immunodeficiency disorder, or who have received a recent injection of immune globulin, an adequate immunologic response may not be obtained). Products include:

Flovent HFA 1440

Gemcitabine Hydrochloride (May reduce immune response to vaccines. When administered to patients who are receiving immunosuppressive therapy, who have an immunodeficiency disorder, or who have received a recent injection of immune globulin, an adequate immunologic response may not be obtained). Products include:

Gemzar for Injection 1820

Hydrocortisone (May reduce immune response to vaccines. When administered to patients who are receiving immunosuppressive therapy, who have an immunodeficiency disorder, or who have received a recent injection of immune globulin, an adequate immunologic response may not be obtained).

No products indexed under this heading.

Hydrocortisone Acetate (May reduce immune response to vaccines. When administered to patients who are receiving immunosuppressive therapy, who have an immunodeficiency disorder, or who have received a recent injection of immune globulin, an adequate immunologic response may not be obtained). Products include:

Analpram-HC 1140
Pramosone 1141

Hydrocortisone Sodium Phosphate (May reduce immune response to vaccines. When administered to patients who are receiving immunosuppressive therapy, who have an immunodeficiency disorder, or who have received a recent injection of immune globulin, an adequate immunologic response may not be obtained).

No products indexed under this heading.

Hydrocortisone Sodium Succinate (May reduce immune response to vaccines. When administered to patients who are receiving immunosuppressive therapy, who have an immunodeficiency disorder, or who have received a recent injection of immune globulin, an adequate immunologic response may not be obtained).

No products indexed under this heading.

Hydroxyurea (May reduce immune response to vaccines. When administered to patients who are receiving immunosuppressive therapy, who have an immunodeficiency disorder, or who have received a recent injection of immune globulin, an adequate immunologic response may not be obtained).

No products indexed under this heading.

Immune Globulin Intravenous (Human) (May reduce immune response to vaccines. When administered to patients who are receiving immunosuppressive therapy, who have an immunodeficiency disorder, or who have received a recent injection of immune globulin, an adequate immunologic response may not be obtained). Products include:

Flebogamma 5% DIF 1718
Gammagard Liquid 730
Gammagard S/D 734
Gamunex 3094

Lomustine (CCNU) (May reduce immune response to vaccines. When administered to patients who are receiving immunosuppressive therapy, who have an immunodeficiency disorder, or who have received a recent injection of immune globulin, an adequate immunologic response may not be obtained).

No products indexed under this heading.

Mechlorethamine Hydrochloride (May reduce immune response to vaccines. When administered to patients who are receiving immunosuppressive therapy, who have an immunodeficiency disorder, or who have received a recent injection of immune globulin, an adequate immunologic response may not be obtained). Products include:

Mustargen for Injection 2492

Melphalan (May reduce immune response to vaccines. When administered to patients who are receiving immunosuppressive therapy, who have an immunodeficiency disorder, or who have received a recent injection of immune globulin, an adequate immunologic response may not be obtained).

No products indexed under this heading.

Mercaptopurine (May reduce immune response to vaccines. When administered to patients who are receiving immunosuppressive therapy, who have an immunodeficiency disorder, or who have received a recent injection of immune globulin, an adequate immunologic response may not be obtained).

No products indexed under this heading.

Methotrexate (May reduce immune response to vaccines. When administered to patients who are receiving immunosuppressive therapy, who have an immunodeficiency disorder, or who have received a recent injection of immune globulin, an adequate immunologic response may not be obtained).

No products indexed under this heading.

Methotrexate Sodium (May reduce immune response to vaccines. When administered to patients who are receiving immunosuppressive therapy, who have an immunodeficiency disorder, or who have received a recent injection of immune globulin, an adequate immunologic response may not be obtained).

No products indexed under this heading.

Methylprednisolone Acetate (May reduce immune response to vaccines. When administered to patients who are receiving immunosuppressive therapy, who have an immunodeficiency disorder, or who have received a recent injection of immune globulin, an adequate immunologic response may not be obtained).

No products indexed under this heading.

Methylprednisolone Sodium Succinate (May reduce immune response to vaccines. When administered to patients who are receiving immunosuppressive therapy, who have an immunodeficiency disorder, or who have received a recent injection of immune globulin, an adequate immunologic response may not be obtained).

No products indexed under this heading.

Mitotane (May reduce immune response to vaccines. When administered to patients who are receiving immunosuppressive therapy, who have an immunodeficiency disorder, or who have received a recent injection of immune globulin, an adequate immunologic response may not be obtained).

No products indexed under this heading.

Mitoxantrone Hydrochloride (May reduce immune response to vaccines. When administered to patients who are receiving immunosuppressive therapy, who have an immunodeficiency disorder, or who have received a recent injection of immune globulin, an adequate immunologic response may not be obtained). Products include:

Novantrone for Injection Concentrate 1100

Mometasone Furoate (May reduce immune response to vaccines. When administered to patients who are receiving immunosuppressive therapy, who have an immunodeficiency disorder, or who have received a recent injection of immune globulin, an adequate immunologic response may not be obtained). Products include:

Asmanex Twisthaler 2797
Elocon Cream 0.1% 2840
Elocon Lotion 0.1% 2841
Elocon Ointment 0.1% 2842

Mometasone Furoate Monohydrate (May reduce immune response to vaccines. When administered to patients who are receiving immunosuppressive therapy, who have an immunodeficiency disorder, or who have received a recent injection of immune globulin, an adequate immunologic response may not be obtained). Products include:

Nasonex Nasal Spray 2883

Muromonab-CD3 (May reduce immune response to vaccines. When administered to patients who are receiving immunosuppressive therapy, who have an immunodeficiency disorder, or who have received a recent injection of immune globulin, an adequate immunologic response may not be obtained). Products include:

Orthoclone OKT3 Sterile Solution 2387

Mycophenolate Mofetil (May reduce immune response to vaccines. When administered to patients who are receiving immunosuppressive therapy, who have an immunodeficiency disorder, or who have received a recent injection of immune globulin, an adequate immunologic response may not be obtained). Products include:

CellCept Capsules 2622
CellCept Oral Suspension 2622
CellCept Tablets 2622

Pentostatin (May reduce immune response to vaccines. When administered to patients who are receiving immunosuppressive therapy, who have an immunodeficiency disorder, or who have received a recent injection of immune globulin, an adequate immunologic response may not be obtained).

No products indexed under this heading.

Prednisolone Acetate (May reduce immune response to vaccines. When administered to patients who are receiving immunosuppressive therapy, who have an immunodeficiency disorder, or who have received a recent injection of immune globulin, an adequate immunologic response may not be obtained). Products include:

Pred Forte Ophthalmic Suspension .... ⊙ 227
Pred Mild Ophthalmic Suspension .... ⊙ 230
Pred-G Ophthalmic Ointment .... ⊙ 229
Pred-G Ophthalmic Suspension .... ⊙ 228

Prednisolone Sodium Phosphate (May reduce immune response to vaccines. When administered to patients who are receiving immunosuppressive therapy, who have an immunodeficiency disorder, or who have received a recent injection of immune globulin, an adequate immunologic response may not be obtained).

No products indexed under this heading.

Prednisolone Tebutate (May reduce immune response to vaccines. When administered to patients who are receiving immunosuppressive therapy, who have an immunodeficiency disorder, or who have received a recent injection of immune globulin, an adequate immunologic response may not be obtained).

No products indexed under this heading.

Prednisone (May reduce immune response to vaccines. When administered to patients who are receiving immunosuppressive therapy, who have an immunodeficiency disorder, or who have received a recent injection of immune globulin, an adequate immunologic response may not be obtained).
No products indexed under this heading.

Procarbazine Hydrochloride (May reduce immune response to vaccines. When administered to patients who are receiving immunosuppressive therapy, who have an immunodeficiency disorder, or who have received a recent injection of immune globulin, an adequate immunologic response may not be obtained).
No products indexed under this heading.

Sirolimus (May reduce immune response to vaccines. When administered to patients who are receiving immunosuppressive therapy, who have an immunodeficiency disorder, or who have received a recent injection of immune globulin, an adequate immunologic response may not be obtained). Products include:
Rapamune 3260

Tacrolimus (May reduce immune response to vaccines. When administered to patients who are receiving immunosuppressive therapy, who have an immunodeficiency disorder, or who have received a recent injection of immune globulin, an adequate immunologic response may not be obtained). Products include:
Prograf Capsules and Injection 622
Protopic Ointment 628

Tamoxifen Citrate (May reduce immune response to vaccines. When administered to patients who are receiving immunosuppressive therapy, who have an immunodeficiency disorder, or who have received a recent injection of immune globulin, an adequate immunologic response may not be obtained).
No products indexed under this heading.

Thioguanine (May reduce immune response to vaccines. When administered to patients who are receiving immunosuppressive therapy, who have an immunodeficiency disorder, or who have received a recent injection of immune globulin, an adequate immunologic response may not be obtained). Products include:
Tabloid Tablets 1601

Thiotepa (May reduce immune response to vaccines. When administered to patients who are receiving immunosuppressive therapy, who have an immunodeficiency disorder, or who have received a recent injection of immune globulin, an adequate immunologic response may not be obtained).
No products indexed under this heading.

Triamcinolone (May reduce immune response to vaccines. When administered to patients who are receiving immunosuppressive therapy, who have an immunodeficiency disorder, or who have received a recent injection of immune globulin, an adequate immunologic response may not be obtained).
No products indexed under this heading.

Triamcinolone Acetonide (May reduce immune response to vaccines. When administered to patients who are receiving immunosuppressive therapy, who have an immunodeficiency disorder, or who have received a recent injection of immune globulin, an adequate immunologic response may not be obtained). Products include:
Azmacort Inhalation Aerosol 407
Nasacort AQ Nasal Spray 2765
Triesence Injectable Suspension .... ⊙209

Triamcinolone Diacetate (May reduce immune response to vaccines. When administered to patients who are receiving immunosuppressive therapy, who have an immunodeficiency disorder, or who have received a recent injection of immune globulin, an adequate immunologic response may not be obtained).
No products indexed under this heading.

Triamcinolone Hexacetonide (May reduce immune response to vaccines. When administered to patients who are receiving immunosuppressive therapy, who have an immunodeficiency disorder, or who have received a recent injection of immune globulin, an adequate immunologic response may not be obtained).
No products indexed under this heading.

Vincristine Sulfate (May reduce immune response to vaccines. When administered to patients who are receiving immunosuppressive therapy, who have an immunodeficiency disorder, or who have received a recent injection of immune globulin, an adequate immunologic response may not be obtained).
No products indexed under this heading.

LIQUID PEDVAXHIB

(Haemophilus B Conjugate Vaccine).. 2073
None cited in PDR database.

PEGINTRON POWDER FOR INJECTION

(Peginterferon Alfa-2b) 2903
May interact with cytochrome p450 2c8 substrates (selected), cytochrome p450 2c9 substrates (selected), cytochrome p450 2d6 substrates (selected), nucleoside analogue reverse transcriptase inhibitors, and certain other agents. Compounds in these categories include:

Acarbose (Peginterferon alpha-2b treatment has been reported to result in a 28% (mean) increase in a measure of CYP2C9 activity. Caution should be used when administering peginterferon alpha-2b with medications metabolized by CYP2C9). Products include:
Precose Tablets 792

Amiodarone Hydrochloride (Peginterferon alpha-2b treatment has been reported to result in a 28% (mean) increase in a measure of CYP2C8 activity. Caution should be used when administering peginterferon alpha-2b with medications metabolized by CYP2C8).
No products indexed under this heading.

Amitriptyline Hydrochloride (Peginterferon alpha-2b treatment has been reported to result in a 28% (mean) increase in a measure of CYP2C8 activity. Caution should be used when administering peginterferon alpha-2b with medications metabolized by CYP2C8).
No products indexed under this heading.

Amoxapine (Peginterferon alpha-2b treatment has been reported to result in a 28% (mean) increase in a measure of CYP2C8 activity. Caution should be used when administering peginterferon alpha-2b with medications metabolized by CYP2C8).
No products indexed under this heading.

Amphetamine Aspartate (Peginterferon alpha-2b treatment has been reported to result in a 66% (mean) increase in the measure of CYP2D6 activity. Caution should be used when administering peginterferon alpha 2b with medications metabolized by CYP2D6). Products include:
Adderall XR Capsules 3012

Amphetamine Aspartate Monohydrate (Peginterferon alpha-2b treatment has been reported to result in a 66% (mean) increase in the measure of CYP2D6 activity. Caution should be used when administering peginterferon alpha 2b with medications metabolized by CYP2D6).
No products indexed under this heading.

Amphetamine Sulfate (Peginterferon alpha-2b treatment has been reported to result in a 66% (mean) increase in the measure of CYP2D6 activity. Caution should be used when administering peginterferon alpha 2b with medications metabolized by CYP2D6). Products include:
Adderall XR Capsules 3012

Atomoxetine Hydrochloride (Peginterferon alpha-2b treatment has been reported to result in a 66% (mean) increase in the measure of CYP2D6 activity. Caution should be used when administering peginterferon alpha 2b with medications metabolized by CYP2D6). Products include:
Strattera Capsules 1864

Benzphetamine Hydrochloride (Peginterferon alpha-2b treatment has been reported to result in a 28% (mean) increase in a measure of CYP2C8 activity. Caution should be used when administering peginterferon alpha-2b with medications metabolized by CYP2C8).
No products indexed under this heading.

Bisoprolol Fumarate (Peginterferon alpha-2b treatment has been reported to result in a 66% (mean) increase in the measure of CYP2D6 activity. Caution should be used when administering peginterferon alpha 2b with medications metabolized by CYP2D6).
No products indexed under this heading.

Candesartan Cilexetil (Peginterferon alpha-2b treatment has been reported to result in a 28% (mean) increase in a measure of CYP2C9 activity. Caution should be used when administering peginterferon alpha-2b with medications metabolized by CYP2C9). Products include:
Atacand Tablets 639
Atacand HCT 642

Captopril (Peginterferon alpha-2b treatment has been reported to result in a 66% (mean) increase in the measure of CYP2D6 activity. Caution should be used when administering peginterferon alpha 2b with medications metabolized by CYP2D6). Products include:
Captopril Tablets 2182

Carbamazepine (Peginterferon alpha-2b treatment has been reported to result in a 28% (mean) increase in a measure of CYP2C8 activity. Caution should be used when administering peginterferon alpha-2b with medications metabolized by CYP2C8). Products include:
Carbatrol Capsules 3019
Equetro Extended-Release Capsules................................... 3174

Carvedilol (Peginterferon alpha-2b treatment has been reported to result in a 28% (mean) increase in a measure of CYP2C9 activity. Caution should be used when administering peginterferon alpha-2b with medications metabolized by CYP2C9). Products include:
Coreg Tablets 1387

Celecoxib (Peginterferon alpha-2b treatment has been reported to result in a 28% (mean) increase in a measure of CYP2C9 activity. Caution should be used when administering peginterferon alpha-2b with medications metabolized by CYP2C9). Products include:
Celebrex Capsules 2979

Cevimeline Hydrochloride (Peginterferon alpha-2b treatment has been reported to result in a 66% (mean) increase in the measure of CYP2D6 activity. Caution should be used when administering peginterferon alpha 2b with medications metabolized by CYP2D6). Products include:
Evoxac Capsules 1013

Chlorpromazine (Peginterferon alpha-2b treatment has been reported to result in a 66% (mean) increase in the measure of CYP2D6 activity. Caution should be used when administering peginterferon alpha 2b with medications metabolized by CYP2D6).
No products indexed under this heading.

Chlorpromazine Hydrochloride (Peginterferon alpha-2b treatment has been reported to result in a 66% (mean) increase in the measure of CYP2D6 activity. Caution should be used when administering peginterferon alpha 2b with medications metabolized by CYP2D6).
No products indexed under this heading.

Chlorpropamide (Peginterferon alpha-2b treatment has been reported to result in a 28% (mean) increase in a measure of CYP2C9 activity. Caution should be used when administering peginterferon alpha-2b with medications metabolized by CYP2C9).
No products indexed under this heading.

Clomipramine Hydrochloride (Peginterferon alpha-2b treatment has been reported to result in a 28% (mean) increase in a measure of CYP2C8 activity. Caution should be used when administering peginterferon alpha-2b with medications metabolized by CYP2C8).
No products indexed under this heading.

Clozapine (Peginterferon alpha-2b treatment has been reported to result in a 66% (mean) increase in the measure of CYP2D6 activity. Caution should be used when administering peginterferon alpha 2b with medications metabolized by CYP2D6).
No products indexed under this heading.

Codeine Phosphate (Peginterferon alpha-2b treatment has been reported to result in a 66% (mean) increase in the measure of CYP2D6 activity. Caution should be used when administering peginterferon alpha 2b with medications metabolized by CYP2D6). Products include:
Tylenol with Codeine Tablets 2427

Codeine Sulfate (Peginterferon alpha-2b treatment has been reported to result in a 66% (mean) increase in the measure of CYP2D6 activity. Caution should be used when administering peginterferon alpha 2b with medications metabolized by CYP2D6).
No products indexed under this heading.

Cyclobenzaprine Hydrochloride (Peginterferon alpha-2b treatment has been reported to result in a 66% (mean) increase in the measure of CYP2D6 activity. Caution should be used when administering peginterferon alpha 2b with medications metabolized by CYP2D6). Products include:
Amrix Capsules 966

Dapsone (The pharmacokinetics of representative drugs metabolized by N-acetyltransferase (e.g., dapsone) was studied in 22 patients with chronic hepatitis C who received peginterferon alpha-2b (1.5 mcg/kg) once weekly for four weeks. Peginterferon alpha-2b treatment resulted in a 28% (mean) increase in a measure of N-acetyltransferase activity). Products include:
Aczone Gel 5% 3296
Dapsone Tablets USP 1746

Desipramine Hydrochloride (Peginterferon alpha-2b treatment has been reported to result in a 28% (mean) increase in a measure of CYP2C8 activity. Caution should be used when administering peginterferon alpha-2b with medications metabolized by CYP2C8).
No products indexed under this heading.

Desogestrel (Peginterferon alpha-2b treatment has been reported to result in a 28% (mean) increase in a measure of CYP2C9 activity. Caution should be used when administering peginterferon alpha-2b with medications metabolized by CYP2C9). Products include:
Mircette Tablets 1034

Dexfenfluramine Hydrochloride (Peginterferon alpha-2b treatment has been reported to result in a 66% (mean) increase in the measure of CYP2D6 activity. Caution should be used when administering peginterferon alpha 2b with medications metabolized by CYP2D6).
No products indexed under this heading.

Dextromethorphan (Peginterferon alpha-2b treatment has been reported to result in a 28% (mean) increase in a measure of CYP2C9 activity. Caution should be used when administering peginterferon alpha-2b with medications metabolized by CYP2C9).
No products indexed under this heading.

Dextromethorphan Hydrobromide (Peginterferon alpha-2b treatment has been reported to result in a 66% (mean) increase in the measure of CYP2D6 activity. Caution should be used when administering peginterferon alpha 2b with medications metabolized by CYP2D6). Products include:
PediaCare Children's Liquid Multi-Symptom Cold..................... 1902
PediaCare Children's Long-Acting Cough 1902
Children's Sudafed PE Cold & Cough Liquid 1907
Sudafed PE Cold & Cough Caplets.. 1907
Children's Tylenol Plus Cough & Runny Nose Suspension Liquid..... 1912
Children's Tylenol Plus Cough & Sore Throat Suspension Liquid..... 1912
Children's Tylenol Plus Flu Suspension Liquid 1914
Children's Tylenol Plus Multi-Symptom Cold Suspension Liquid 1912
Tylenol Cold Severe Congestion Daytime Caplets with Cool Burst.. 1912
Tylenol Cold Head Congestion Daytime Caplets with Cool Burst.. 1910
Tylenol Cold Head Congestion Nighttime Caplets with Cool Burst.. 1910
Tylenol Cold Head Congestion Severe Daytime Caplets with Cool Burst................................. 1910
Tylenol Cold Multi-Symptom Daytime Caplets with Cool Burst and Rapid Release Gels....... 1913
Tylenol Cold Multi-Symptom Daytime Liquid with Citrus Burst... 1913
Tylenol Cold Multi-Symptom Nighttime Caplets with Cool Burst.. 1913
Tylenol Cold Multi-Symptom Nighttime Liquid with Cool Burst... 1913
Tylenol Cold Multi-Symptom Severe Caplets with Cool Burst..... 1913
Tylenol Cold Multi-Symptom Severe Daytime Liquid with Citrus Burst................................ 1913
Tylenol Cough & Sore Throat Daytime Liquid with Cool Burst...... 1918
Tylenol Cough & Sore Throat Nighttime Liquid with Cool Burst... 1918
Vicks DayQuil Cold & Flu Multi-Symptom Relief .... ▣616
Vicks DayQuil LiquiCaps 2567
Vicks DayQuil Liquid 2567
Vicks DayQuil Multi-Symptom Cold/Flu Relief.................................. 2567
Vicks NyQuil Cold & Flu Multi-Symptom Relief .... ▣617
Vicks NyQuil LiquiCaps 2567
Vicks NyQuil Liquid 2567
Vicks NyQuil Multi-Symptom Cold/Flu Relief.......................... 2567

Dextromethorphan Polistirex (Peginterferon alpha-2b treatment has been reported to result in a 66% (mean) increase in the measure of CYP2D6 activity. Caution should be used when administering peginterferon alpha 2b with medications metabolized by CYP2D6).
No products indexed under this heading.

Diazepam (Peginterferon alpha-2b treatment has been reported to result in a 28% (mean) increase in a measure of CYP2C8 activity. Caution should be used when administering peginterferon alpha-2b with medications metabolized by CYP2C8). Products include:
Valium Tablets 2658

Diclofenac Potassium (Peginterferon alpha-2b treatment has been reported to result in a 28% (mean) increase in a measure of CYP2C8 activity. Caution should be used when administering peginterferon alpha-2b with medications metabolized by CYP2C8).
No products indexed under this heading.

Diclofenac Sodium (Peginterferon alpha-2b treatment has been reported to result in a 28% (mean) increase in a measure of CYP2C8 activity. Caution should be used when administering peginterferon alpha-2b with medications metabolized by CYP2C8). Products include:
Diclofenac Sodium Ophthalmic Solution..................................... ⊙ 240
Voltaren Ophthalmic Solution 2336
Voltaren Tablets 2334
Voltaren-XR Tablets 2337

Didanosine (Patients receiving interferon with ribavirin and nucleoside reverse transcriptase inhibitors (NRTIs) should be closely monitored for treamtent-associated toxicities, especially hepatic decompensation and anemia. Discontinuation of NRTIs should be considered as medically appropriate (see individual NRTI product information). Dose reduction or discontinuation of interferon, ribavirin, or both should also be considered if worsening clinical toxicities are observed, including hepatic decompensation (e.g., Child-Pugh>6)).
No products indexed under this heading.

Docetaxel (Peginterferon alpha-2b treatment has been reported to result in a 28% (mean) increase in a measure of CYP2C8 activity. Caution should be used when administering peginterferon alpha-2b with medications metabolized by CYP2C8). Products include:
Taxotere Injection Concentrate 2773

Dolasetron Mesylate (Peginterferon alpha-2b treatment has been reported to result in a 66% (mean) increase in the measure of CYP2D6 activity. Caution should be used when administering peginterferon alpha 2b with medications metabolized by CYP2D6). Products include:
Anzemet Injection 2701
Anzemet Tablets 2704

Donepezil Hydrochloride (Peginterferon alpha-2b treatment has been reported to result in a 66% (mean) increase in the measure of CYP2D6 activity. Caution should be used when administering peginterferon alpha 2b with medications metabolized by CYP2D6). Products include:
Aricept Tablets 1062
Aricept ODT Tablets 1062

Doxepin Hydrochloride (Peginterferon alpha-2b treatment has been reported to result in a 28% (mean) increase in a measure of CYP2C8 activity. Caution should be used when administering peginterferon alpha-2b with medications metabolized by CYP2C8).
No products indexed under this heading.

Dronabinol (Peginterferon alpha-2b treatment has been reported to result in a 28% (mean) increase in a measure of CYP2C9 activity. Caution should be used when administering peginterferon alpha-2b with medications metabolized by CYP2C9). Products include:
Marinol Capsules 3163

Encainide Hydrochloride (Peginterferon alpha-2b treatment has been reported to result in a 66% (mean) increase in the measure of CYP2D6 activity. Caution should be used when administering peginterferon alpha 2b with medications metabolized by CYP2D6).
No products indexed under this heading.

Eprosartan Mesylate (Peginterferon alpha-2b treatment has been reported to result in a 28% (mean) increase in a measure of CYP2C9 activity. Caution should be used when administering peginterferon alpha-2b with medications metabolized by CYP2C9). Products include:
Teveten Tablets 515
Teveten HCT Tablets 517

Etodolac (Peginterferon alpha-2b treatment has been reported to result in a 28% (mean) increase in a measure of CYP2C9 activity. Caution should be used when administering peginterferon alpha-2b with medications metabolized by CYP2C9).
No products indexed under this heading.

Fenoprofen Calcium (Peginterferon alpha-2b treatment has been reported to result in a 28% (mean) increase in a measure of CYP2C9 activity. Caution should be used when administering peginterferon alpha-2b with medications metabolized by CYP2C9). Products include:
Nalfon Capsules 2508

Fentanyl (Peginterferon alpha-2b treatment has been reported to result in a 66% (mean) increase in the measure of CYP2D6 activity. Caution should be used when administering peginterferon alpha 2b with medications metabolized by CYP2D6). Products include:
Duragesic Transdermal System 2405
Ionsys Transdermal System 2410

Fentanyl Citrate (Peginterferon alpha-2b treatment has been reported to result in a 66% (mean) increase in the measure of CYP2D6 activity. Caution should be used when administering peginterferon alpha 2b with medications metabolized by CYP2D6). Products include:
Actiq 959
Fentora Tablets 968

Flecainide Acetate (Peginterferon alpha-2b treatment has been reported to result in a 66% (mean) increase in the measure of CYP2D6 activity. Caution should be used when administering peginterferon alpha 2b with medications metabolized by CYP2D6).
No products indexed under this heading.

Fluoxetine (Peginterferon alpha-2b treatment has been reported to result in a 66% (mean) increase in the measure of CYP2D6 activity. Caution should be used when administering peginterferon alpha 2b with medications metabolized by CYP2D6).
No products indexed under this heading.

Fluoxetine Hydrochloride (Peginterferon alpha-2b treatment has been reported to result in a 28% (mean) increase in a measure of CYP2C9 activity. Caution should be used when administering peginterferon alpha-2b with medications metabolized by CYP2C9). Products include:
Prozac Weekly Capsules 1852
Prozac Pulvules and Liquid 1852
Symbyax Capsules 1871

Fluphenazine Decanoate (Peginterferon alpha-2b treatment has been reported to result in a 66% (mean) increase in the measure of CYP2D6 activity. Caution should be used when administering peginterferon alpha 2b with medications metabolized by CYP2D6).
No products indexed under this heading.

Fluphenazine Enanthate (Peginterferon alpha-2b treatment has been reported to result in a 66% (mean) increase in the measure of CYP2D6 activity. Caution should be used when administering peginterferon alpha 2b with medications metabolized by CYP2D6).
No products indexed under this heading.

Fluphenazine Hydrochloride (Peginterferon alpha-2b treatment has been reported to result in a 66% (mean) increase in the measure of CYP2D6 activity. Caution should be used when administering peginterferon alpha 2b with medications metabolized by CYP2D6).
No products indexed under this heading.

Flurbiprofen (Peginterferon alpha-2b treatment has been reported to result in a 28% (mean) increase in a measure of CYP2C9 activity. Caution should be used when administering peginterferon alpha-2b with medications metabolized by CYP2C9).
No products indexed under this heading.

Flurbiprofen Sodium (Peginterferon alpha-2b treatment has been reported to result in a 28% (mean) increase in a measure of CYP2C9 activity. Caution should be used when administering peginterferon alpha-2b with medications metabolized by CYP2C9).
No products indexed under this heading.

Fluvastatin Sodium (Peginterferon alpha-2b treatment has been reported to result in a 28% (mean) increase in a measure of CYP2C8 activity. Caution should be used when administering peginterferon alpha-2b with medications metabolized by CYP2C8). Products include:
Lescol Capsules 2268
Lescol XL Tablets 2268

Fluvoxamine Maleate (Peginterferon alpha-2b treatment has been reported to result in a 66% (mean) increase in the measure of CYP2D6 activity. Caution should be used when administering peginterferon alpha 2b with medications metabolized by CYP2D6). Products include:
Luvox CR Extended-Release Capsules 1759

Formoterol Fumarate (Peginterferon alpha-2b treatment has been reported to result in a 66% (mean) increase in the measure of CYP2D6 activity. Caution should be used when administering peginterferon alpha 2b with medications metabolized by CYP2D6). Products include:
Foradil Aerolizer 2849
Perforomist Inhalation Solution 1025

Galantamine Hydrobromide (Peginterferon alpha-2b treatment has been reported to result in a 66% (mean) increase in the measure of CYP2D6 activity. Caution should be used when administering peginterferon alpha 2b with medications metabolized by CYP2D6).
No products indexed under this heading.

Glimepiride (Peginterferon alpha-2b treatment has been reported to result in a 28% (mean) increase in a measure of CYP2C9 activity. Caution should be used when administering peginterferon alpha-2b with medications metabolized by CYP2C9). Products include:
Avandaryl Tablets 1344
Duetact Tablets 3085

Glipizide (Peginterferon alpha-2b treatment has been reported to result in a 28% (mean) increase in a measure of CYP2C9 activity. Caution should be used when administering peginterferon alpha-2b with medications metabolized by CYP2C9).
No products indexed under this heading.

Haloperidol (Peginterferon alpha-2b treatment has been reported to result in a 66% (mean) increase in the measure of CYP2D6 activity. Caution should be used when administering peginterferon alpha 2b with medications metabolized by CYP2D6).
No products indexed under this heading.

Haloperidol Decanoate (Peginterferon alpha-2b treatment has been reported to result in a 66% (mean) increase in the measure of CYP2D6 activity. Caution should be used when administering peginterferon alpha 2b with medications metabolized by CYP2D6).
No products indexed under this heading.

Hydrocodone Bitartrate (Peginterferon alpha-2b treatment has been reported to result in a 66% (mean) increase in the measure of CYP2D6 activity. Caution should be used when administering peginterferon alpha 2b with medications metabolized by CYP2D6). Products include:
Lortab 5/500 Tablets 3143
Lortab 7.5/500 Tablets 3144
Lortab 10/500 Tablets 3144
Vicodin Tablets 529
Vicodin ES Tablets 530
Vicodin HP Tablets 531
Vicoprofen Tablets 533
Zydone Tablets 1132

Ibuprofen (Peginterferon alpha-2b treatment has been reported to result in a 28% (mean) increase in a measure of CYP2C9 activity. Caution should be used when administering peginterferon alpha-2b with medications metabolized by CYP2C9). Products include:
Motrin IB Tablets and Caplets 1900
Children's Motrin Oral Suspension ... 1901
Children's Motrin Non-Staining Dye-Free Oral Suspension 1901
Children's Motrin Cold Oral Suspension 1899
Infants' Motrin Concentrated Drops 1901
Infants' Motrin Non-Staining Dye-Free Concentrated Drops 1901
Junior Strength Motrin Caplets and Chewable Tablets 1901
Vicoprofen Tablets 533

Imipramine Hydrochloride (Peginterferon alpha-2b treatment has been reported to result in a 28% (mean) increase in a measure of CYP2C8 activity. Caution should be used when administering peginterferon alpha-2b with medications metabolized by CYP2C8).
No products indexed under this heading.

Imipramine Pamoate (Peginterferon alpha-2b treatment has been reported to result in a 28% (mean) increase in a measure of CYP2C8 activity. Caution should be used when administering peginterferon alpha-2b with medications metabolized by CYP2C8).
No products indexed under this heading.

Indomethacin (Peginterferon alpha-2b treatment has been reported to result in a 28% (mean) increase in a measure of CYP2C9 activity. Caution should be used when administering peginterferon alpha-2b with medications metabolized by CYP2C9). Products include:
Indocin 2024

Indomethacin Sodium Trihydrate (Peginterferon alpha-2b treatment has been reported to result in a 28% (mean) increase in a measure of CYP2C9 activity. Caution should be used when administering peginterferon alpha-2b with medications metabolized by CYP2C9). Products include:
Indocin I.V. 2489

Indoramin Hydrochloride (Peginterferon alpha-2b treatment has been reported to result in a 66% (mean) increase in the measure of CYP2D6 activity. Caution should be used when administering peginterferon alpha 2b with medications metabolized by CYP2D6).
No products indexed under this heading.

Irbesartan (Peginterferon alpha-2b treatment has been reported to result in a 28% (mean) increase in a measure of CYP2C9 activity. Caution should be used when administering peginterferon alpha-2b with medications metabolized by CYP2C9). Products include:
Avalide Tablets 892
Avalide Tablets 2713
Avapro Tablets 897
Avapro Tablets 2718

Isotretinoin (Peginterferon alpha-2b treatment has been reported to result in a 28% (mean) increase in a measure of CYP2C8 activity. Caution should be used when administering peginterferon alpha-2b with medications metabolized by CYP2C8). Products include:
Accutane Capsules 2607

Ketoprofen (Peginterferon alpha-2b treatment has been reported to result in a 28% (mean) increase in a measure of CYP2C9 activity. Caution should be used when administering peginterferon alpha-2b with medications metabolized by CYP2C9).
No products indexed under this heading.

Ketorolac Tromethamine (Peginterferon alpha-2b treatment has been reported to result in a 28% (mean) increase in a measure of CYP2C9 activity. Caution should be used when administering peginterferon alpha-2b with medications metabolized by CYP2C9).
No products indexed under this heading.

Labetalol Hydrochloride (Peginterferon alpha-2b treatment has been reported to result in a 66% (mean) increase in the measure of CYP2D6 activity. Caution should be used when administering peginterferon alpha 2b with medications metabolized by CYP2D6).
No products indexed under this heading.

Lamivudine (Patients receiving interferon with ribavirin and nucleoside reverse transcriptase inhibitors (NRTIs) should be closely monitored for treamtent-associated toxicities, especially hepatic decompensation and anemia. Discontinuation of NRTIs should be considered as medically appropriate (see individual NRTI product information). Dose reduction or discontinuation of interferon, ribavirin, or both should also be considered if worsening clinical toxicities are observed, including hepatic decompensation (e.g., Child-Pugh>6)). Products include:
Combivir Tablets 1384
Epivir 1412
Epivir-HBV 1417
Epzicom Tablets 1422
Trizivir Tablets 1622

Lansoprazole (Peginterferon alpha-2b treatment has been reported to result in a 28% (mean) increase in a measure of CYP2C9 activity. Caution should be used when administering peginterferon alpha-2b with medications metabolized by CYP2C9).
No products indexed under this heading.

Lidocaine (Peginterferon alpha-2b treatment has been reported to result in a 66% (mean) increase in the measure of CYP2D6 activity. Caution should be used when administering peginterferon alpha 2b with medications metabolized by CYP2D6). Products include:
Lidoderm Patch 1114

Lidocaine Hydrochloride (Peginterferon alpha-2b treatment has been reported to result in a 66% (mean) increase in the measure of CYP2D6 activity. Caution should be used when administering peginterferon alpha 2b with medications metabolized by CYP2D6).
No products indexed under this heading.

Losartan Potassium (Peginterferon alpha-2b treatment has been reported to result in a 28% (mean)

increase in a measure of CYP2C9 activity. Caution should be used when administering peginterferon alpha-2b with medications metabolized by CYP2C9). Products include:

Cozaar Tablets 1973

Maprotiline Hydrochloride (Peginterferon alpha-2b treatment has been reported to result in a 28% (mean) increase in a measure of CYP2C8 activity. Caution should be used when administering peginterferon alpha-2b with medications metabolized by CYP2C8).

No products indexed under this heading.

Meclofenamate Sodium (Peginterferon alpha-2b treatment has been reported to result in a 28% (mean) increase in a measure of CYP2C9 activity. Caution should be used when administering peginterferon alpha-2b with medications metabolized by CYP2C9).

No products indexed under this heading.

Mefenamic Acid (Peginterferon alpha-2b treatment has been reported to result in a 28% (mean) increase in a measure of CYP2C9 activity. Caution should be used when administering peginterferon alpha-2b with medications metabolized by CYP2C9).

No products indexed under this heading.

Meloxicam (Peginterferon alpha-2b treatment has been reported to result in a 28% (mean) increase in a measure of CYP2C9 activity. Caution should be used when administering peginterferon alpha-2b with medications metabolized by CYP2C9). Products include:

Mobic Oral Suspension 863
Mobic Tablets 863

Meperidine Hydrochloride (Peginterferon alpha-2b treatment has been reported to result in a 66% (mean) increase in the measure of CYP2D6 activity. Caution should be used when administering peginterferon alpha 2b with medications metabolized by CYP2D6).

No products indexed under this heading.

Mephobarbital (Peginterferon alpha-2b treatment has been reported to result in a 28% (mean) increase in a measure of CYP2C8 activity. Caution should be used when administering peginterferon alpha-2b with medications metabolized by CYP2C8).

No products indexed under this heading.

Metformin Hydrochloride (Peginterferon alpha-2b treatment has been reported to result in a 28% (mean) increase in a measure of CYP2C9 activity. Caution should be used when administering peginterferon alpha-2b with medications metabolized by CYP2C9). Products include:

ActoPlus Met Tablets 3071
Avandamet Tablets 1336
Janumet Tablets 2041
PrandiMet Tablets 2967

Methadone Hydrochloride (In a pharmacokinetic study of 18 chronic hepatitis C patients concomitantly receiving methadone, treatment with PEG-Intron once weekly for four weeks was associated with a mean increase of 16% in methadone AUC. In two out of 18 patients, methadone AUC doubled. The clinical significance of this finding is unknown; however, patients should be monitored for the signs and symptoms of increased narcotic effect).

No products indexed under this heading.

Methamphetamine Hydrochloride (Peginterferon alpha-2b treatment has been reported to result in a 66% (mean) increase in the measure of CYP2D6 activity. Caution should be used when administering peginterferon alpha 2b with medications metabolized by CYP2D6).

No products indexed under this heading.

Metoprolol Succinate (Peginterferon alpha-2b treatment has been reported to result in a 66% (mean) increase in the measure of CYP2D6 activity. Caution should be used when administering peginterferon alpha 2b with medications metabolized by CYP2D6). Products include:

Toprol-XL Tablets 666

Metoprolol Tartrate (Peginterferon alpha-2b treatment has been reported to result in a 66% (mean) increase in the measure of CYP2D6 activity. Caution should be used when administering peginterferon alpha 2b with medications metabolized by CYP2D6).

No products indexed under this heading.

Mexiletine Hydrochloride (Peginterferon alpha-2b treatment has been reported to result in a 66% (mean) increase in the measure of CYP2D6 activity. Caution should be used when administering peginterferon alpha 2b with medications metabolized by CYP2D6).

No products indexed under this heading.

Miglitol (Peginterferon alpha-2b treatment has been reported to result in a 28% (mean) increase in a measure of CYP2C9 activity. Caution should be used when administering peginterferon alpha-2b with medications metabolized by CYP2C9).

No products indexed under this heading.

Mirtazapine (Peginterferon alpha-2b treatment has been reported to result in a 28% (mean) increase in a measure of CYP2C9 activity. Caution should be used when administering peginterferon alpha-2b with medications metabolized by CYP2C9). Products include:

Remeron Tablets 2924
RemeronSolTab Tablets 2927

Montelukast Sodium (Peginterferon alpha-2b treatment has been reported to result in a 28% (mean) increase in a measure of CYP2C9 activity. Caution should be used when administering peginterferon alpha-2b with medications metabolized by CYP2C9). Products include:

Singulair 2114

Morphine Sulfate (Peginterferon alpha-2b treatment has been reported to result in a 66% (mean) increase in the measure of CYP2D6 activity. Caution should be used when administering peginterferon alpha 2b with medications metabolized by CYP2D6). Products include:

Avinza Capsules 1772
DepoDur Injection 1095
MS Contin Tablets 2585

Nabumetone (Peginterferon alpha-2b treatment has been reported to result in a 28% (mean) increase in a measure of CYP2C9 activity. Caution should be used when administering peginterferon alpha-2b with medications metabolized by CYP2C9).

No products indexed under this heading.

Naproxen (Peginterferon alpha-2b treatment has been reported to result in a 28% (mean) increase in a measure of CYP2C9 activity. Caution should be used when administering peginterferon alpha-2b with medications metabolized by CYP2C9). Products include:

EC-Naprosyn Delayed-Release Tablets 2632
Naprosyn Suspension 2632
Naprosyn Tablets 2632

Naproxen Sodium (Peginterferon alpha-2b treatment has been reported to result in a 28% (mean) increase in a measure of CYP2C9 activity. Caution should be used when administering peginterferon alpha-2b with medications metabolized by CYP2C9). Products include:

Anaprox Tablets 2632
Anaprox DS Tablets 2632
Treximet Tablets 1616

Nateglinide (Peginterferon alpha-2b treatment has been reported to result in a 28% (mean) increase in a measure of CYP2C9 activity. Caution should be used when administering peginterferon alpha-2b with medications metabolized by CYP2C9). Products include:

Starlix Tablets 2314

Nelfinavir Mesylate (Peginterferon alpha-2b treatment has been reported to result in a 66% (mean) increase in the measure of CYP2D6 activity. Caution should be used when administering peginterferon alpha 2b with medications metabolized by CYP2D6).

No products indexed under this heading.

Nifedipine (Peginterferon alpha-2b treatment has been reported to result in a 28% (mean) increase in a measure of CYP2C9 activity. Caution should be used when administering peginterferon alpha-2b with medications metabolized by CYP2C9).

No products indexed under this heading.

Nortriptyline Hydrochloride (Peginterferon alpha-2b treatment has been reported to result in a 28% (mean) increase in a measure of CYP2C8 activity. Caution should be used when administering peginterferon alpha-2b with medications metabolized by CYP2C8).

No products indexed under this heading.

Olanzapine (Peginterferon alpha-2b treatment has been reported to result in a 66% (mean) increase in the measure of CYP2D6 activity. Caution should be used when administering peginterferon alpha 2b with medications metabolized by CYP2D6). Products include:

Symbyax Capsules 1871
Zyprexa Tablets 1883
Zyprexa IntraMuscular 1883
Zyprexa ZYDIS Orally Disintegrating Tablets 1883

Omeprazole (Peginterferon alpha-2b treatment has been reported to result in a 28% (mean) increase in a measure of CYP2C8 activity. Caution should be used when administering peginterferon alpha-2b with medications metabolized by CYP2C8).

No products indexed under this heading.

Ondansetron (Peginterferon alpha-2b treatment has been reported to result in a 66% (mean) increase in the measure of CYP2D6 activity. Caution should be used when administering peginterferon alpha 2b with medications metabolized by CYP2D6). Products include:

Zofran ODT Orally Disintegrating Tablets 1687

Ondansetron Hydrochloride (Peginterferon alpha-2b treatment has been reported to result in a 66% (mean) increase in the measure of CYP2D6 activity. Caution should be used when administering peginterferon alpha 2b with medications metabolized by CYP2D6). Products include:

Zofran Injection 1682
Zofran 1687

Oxaprozin (Peginterferon alpha-2b treatment has been reported to result in a 28% (mean) increase in a measure of CYP2C9 activity. Caution should be used when administering peginterferon alpha-2b with medications metabolized by CYP2C9).

No products indexed under this heading.

Oxycodone Hydrochloride (Peginterferon alpha-2b treatment has been reported to result in a 66% (mean) increase in the measure of CYP2D6 activity. Caution should be used when administering peginterferon alpha 2b with medications metabolized by CYP2D6). Products include:

OxyContin Tablets 2589
OxyIR Capsules 2593
Percocet Tablets 1127
Percodan Tablets 1130

Paclitaxel (Peginterferon alpha-2b treatment has been reported to result in a 28% (mean) increase in a measure of CYP2C8 activity. Caution should be used when administering peginterferon alpha-2b with medications metabolized by CYP2C8).

No products indexed under this heading.

Paroxetine Hydrochloride (Peginterferon alpha-2b treatment has been reported to result in a 66% (mean) increase in the measure of CYP2D6 activity. Caution should be used when administering peginterferon alpha 2b with medications metabolized by CYP2D6). Products include:

Paxil 1535
Paxil CR Controlled-Release Tablets 1544

Phenylbutazone (Peginterferon alpha-2b treatment has been reported to result in a 28% (mean) increase in a measure of CYP2C9 activity. Caution should be used when administering peginterferon alpha-2b with medications metabolized by CYP2C9).

No products indexed under this heading.

Phenytoin (Peginterferon alpha-2b treatment has been reported to result in a 28% (mean) increase in a measure of CYP2C8 activity. Caution should be used when administering peginterferon alpha-2b with medications metabolized by CYP2C8).

No products indexed under this heading.

Phenytoin Sodium (Peginterferon alpha-2b treatment has been reported to result in a 28% (mean) increase in a measure of CYP2C8 activity. Caution should be used when administering peginterferon alpha-2b with medications metabolized by CYP2C8). Products include:

Phenytek Capsules **2192**

Pindolol (Peginterferon alpha-2b treatment has been reported to result in a 66% (mean) increase in the measure of CYP2D6 activity. Caution should be used when administering peginterferon alpha 2b with medications metabolized by CYP2D6).

No products indexed under this heading.

Pioglitazone Hydrochloride (Peginterferon alpha-2b treatment has been reported to result in a 28% (mean) increase in a measure of CYP2C8 activity. Caution should be used when administering peginterferon alpha-2b with medications metabolized by CYP2C8). Products include:

ActoPlus Met Tablets **3071**
Actos Tablets **3077**
Duetact Tablets **3085**

Piroxicam (Peginterferon alpha-2b treatment has been reported to result in a 28% (mean) increase in a measure of CYP2C9 activity. Caution should be used when administering peginterferon alpha-2b with medications metabolized by CYP2C9).

No products indexed under this heading.

Propafenone Hydrochloride (Peginterferon alpha-2b treatment has been reported to result in a 66% (mean) increase in the measure of CYP2D6 activity. Caution should be used when administering peginterferon alpha 2b with medications metabolized by CYP2D6). Products include:

Rythmol Tablets **1586**
Rythmol SR Capsules **1590**

Propoxyphene Hydrochloride (Peginterferon alpha-2b treatment has been reported to result in a 66% (mean) increase in the measure of CYP2D6 activity. Caution should be used when administering peginterferon alpha 2b with medications metabolized by CYP2D6).

No products indexed under this heading.

Propoxyphene Napsylate (Peginterferon alpha-2b treatment has been reported to result in a 66% (mean) increase in the measure of CYP2D6 activity. Caution should be used when administering peginterferon alpha 2b with medications metabolized by CYP2D6).

No products indexed under this heading.

Propranolol Hydrochloride (Peginterferon alpha-2b treatment has been reported to result in a 66% (mean) increase in the measure of CYP2D6 activity. Caution should be used when administering peginterferon alpha 2b with medications metabolized by CYP2D6). Products include:

InnoPran XL Extended Release Capsules **1484**

Protriptyline Hydrochloride (Peginterferon alpha-2b treatment has been reported to result in a 28% (mean) increase in a measure of CYP2C8 activity. Caution should be used when administering peginterferon alpha-2b with medications metabolized by CYP2C8).

No products indexed under this heading.

Quetiapine Fumarate (Peginterferon alpha-2b treatment has been reported to result in a 66% (mean) increase in the measure of CYP2D6 activity. Caution should be used when administering peginterferon alpha 2b with medications metabolized by CYP2D6).

No products indexed under this heading.

Quinidine Gluconate (Peginterferon alpha-2b treatment has been reported to result in a 66% (mean) increase in the measure of CYP2D6 activity. Caution should be used when administering peginterferon alpha 2b with medications metabolized by CYP2D6).

No products indexed under this heading.

Quinidine Hydrochloride (Peginterferon alpha-2b treatment has been reported to result in a 66% (mean) increase in the measure of CYP2D6 activity. Caution should be used when administering peginterferon alpha 2b with medications metabolized by CYP2D6).

No products indexed under this heading.

Quinidine Polygalacturonate (Peginterferon alpha-2b treatment has been reported to result in a 66% (mean) increase in the measure of CYP2D6 activity. Caution should be used when administering peginterferon alpha 2b with medications metabolized by CYP2D6).

No products indexed under this heading.

Quinidine Sulfate (Peginterferon alpha-2b treatment has been reported to result in a 66% (mean) increase in the measure of CYP2D6 activity. Caution should be used when administering peginterferon alpha 2b with medications metabolized by CYP2D6).

No products indexed under this heading.

Repaglinide (Peginterferon alpha-2b treatment has been reported to result in a 28% (mean) increase in a measure of CYP2C8 activity. Caution should be used when administering peginterferon alpha-2b with medications metabolized by CYP2C8). Products include:

PrandiMet Tablets **2967**
Prandin Tablets **2971**

Ribavirin (Hepatic decompensation (some fatal) has occurred in cirrhotic HIV/HCV co-infected patients receiving combination antiretoviral therapy for HIV and interferon alpha and ribavirin. Adding treatment with alpha interferons alone or in combination with ribavirin may increase the risk in this patient subset). Products include:

Rebetol **2917**

Risperidone (Peginterferon alpha-2b treatment has been reported to result in a 66% (mean) increase in the measure of CYP2D6 activity. Caution should be used when administering peginterferon alpha 2b with medications metabolized by CYP2D6). Products include:

Risperdal Consta Long-Acting Injection **1753**

Ritonavir (Peginterferon alpha-2b treatment has been reported to result in a 66% (mean) increase in the measure of CYP2D6 activity. Caution should be used when administering peginterferon alpha 2b with medications metabolized by CYP2D6). Products include:

Kaletra **452**
Norvir **489**

Rofecoxib (Peginterferon alpha-2b treatment has been reported to result in a 28% (mean) increase in a measure of CYP2C9 activity. Caution should be used when administering peginterferon alpha-2b with medications metabolized by CYP2C9).

No products indexed under this heading.

Rosiglitazone Maleate (Peginterferon alpha-2b treatment has been reported to result in a 28% (mean) increase in a measure of CYP2C8 activity. Caution should be used when administering peginterferon alpha-2b with medications metabolized by CYP2C8). Products include:

Avandamet Tablets **1336**
Avandaryl Tablets **1344**
Avandia Tablets **1351**

Rosiglitazone/Metformin (Peginterferon alpha-2b treatment has been reported to result in a 28% (mean) increase in a measure of CYP2C8 activity. Caution should be used when administering peginterferon alpha-2b with medications metabolized by CYP2C8).

No products indexed under this heading.

Sildenafil Citrate (Peginterferon alpha-2b treatment has been reported to result in a 28% (mean) increase in a measure of CYP2C9 activity. Caution should be used when administering peginterferon alpha-2b with medications metabolized by CYP2C9).

No products indexed under this heading.

Stavudine (Patients receiving interferon with ribavirin and nucleoside reverse transcriptase inhibitors (NRTIs) should be closely monitored for treamtent-associated toxicities, especially hepatic decompensation and anemia. Discontinuation of NRTIs should be considered as medically appropriate (see individual NRTI product information). Dose reduction or discontinuation of interferon, ribavirin, or both should also be considered if worsening clinical toxicities are observed, including hepatic decompensation (e.g., Child-Pugh>6)).

No products indexed under this heading.

Sulfamethoxazole (Peginterferon alpha-2b treatment has been reported to result in a 28% (mean) increase in a measure of CYP2C9 activity. Caution should be used when administering peginterferon alpha-2b with medications metabolized by CYP2C9).

No products indexed under this heading.

Sulindac (Peginterferon alpha-2b treatment has been reported to result in a 28% (mean) increase in a measure of CYP2C9 activity. Caution should be used when administering peginterferon alpha-2b with medications metabolized by CYP2C9). Products include:

Clinoril Tablets **1962**

Suprofen (Peginterferon alpha-2b treatment has been reported to result in a 28% (mean) increase in a measure of CYP2C9 activity. Caution should be used when administering peginterferon alpha-2b with medications metabolized by CYP2C9).

No products indexed under this heading.

Tamoxifen Citrate (Peginterferon alpha-2b treatment has been reported to result in a 28% (mean) increase in a measure of CYP2C9 activity. Caution should be used when administering peginterferon alpha-2b with medications metabolized by CYP2C9).

No products indexed under this heading.

Telmisartan (Peginterferon alpha-2b treatment has been reported to result in a 28% (mean) increase in a measure of CYP2C9 activity. Caution should be used when administering peginterferon alpha-2b with medications metabolized by CYP2C9). Products include:

Micardis Tablets **852**
Micardis HCT Tablets **854**

Teniposide (Peginterferon alpha-2b treatment has been reported to result in a 66% (mean) increase in the measure of CYP2D6 activity. Caution should be used when administering peginterferon alpha 2b with medications metabolized by CYP2D6).

No products indexed under this heading.

Testosterone (Peginterferon alpha-2b treatment has been reported to result in a 66% (mean) increase in the measure of CYP2D6 activity. Caution should be used when administering peginterferon alpha 2b with medications metabolized by CYP2D6). Products include:

AndroGel **3159**
Testim 1% Gel **701**

Testosterone Cypionate (Peginterferon alpha-2b treatment has been reported to result in a 66% (mean) increase in the measure of CYP2D6 activity. Caution should be used when administering peginterferon alpha 2b with medications metabolized by CYP2D6).

No products indexed under this heading.

Testosterone Enanthate (Peginterferon alpha-2b treatment has been reported to result in a 66% (mean) increase in the measure of CYP2D6 activity. Caution should be used when administering peginterferon alpha 2b with medications metabolized by CYP2D6). Products include:

Delatestryl Injection **1730**

Testosterone Propionate (Peginterferon alpha-2b treatment has been reported to result in a 66% (mean) increase in the measure of CYP2D6 activity. Caution should be used when administering peginterferon alpha 2b with medications metabolized by CYP2D6).

No products indexed under this heading.

Thioridazine (Peginterferon alpha-2b treatment has been reported to result in a 66% (mean) increase in the measure of CYP2D6 activity. Caution should be used when administering peginterferon alpha 2b with medications metabolized by CYP2D6).
No products indexed under this heading.

Thioridazine Hydrochloride (Peginterferon alpha-2b treatment has been reported to result in a 66% (mean) increase in the measure of CYP2D6 activity. Caution should be used when administering peginterferon alpha 2b with medications metabolized by CYP2D6). Products include:
Thioridazine Hydrochloride Tablets ... 2195

Timolol Maleate (Peginterferon alpha-2b treatment has been reported to result in a 66% (mean) increase in the measure of CYP2D6 activity. Caution should be used when administering peginterferon alpha 2b with medications metabolized by CYP2D6). Products include:
Combigan Ophthalmic Solution ... 553
Cosopt Sterile Ophthalmic Solution ... 1969
Timoptic Sterile Ophthalmic Solution ... 2121
Timoptic in Ocudose ... 2124
Timoptic-XE Sterile Ophthalmic Gel Forming Solution ... 2125

Tolazamide (Peginterferon alpha-2b treatment has been reported to result in a 28% (mean) increase in a measure of CYP2C9 activity. Caution should be used when administering peginterferon alpha-2b with medications metabolized by CYP2C9).
No products indexed under this heading.

Tolbutamide (Peginterferon alpha-2b treatment has been reported to result in a 28% (mean) increase in a measure of CYP2C8 activity. Caution should be used when administering peginterferon alpha-2b with medications metabolized by CYP2C8).
No products indexed under this heading.

Tolbutamide Sodium (Peginterferon alpha-2b treatment has been reported to result in a 28% (mean) increase in a measure of CYP2C8 activity. Caution should be used when administering peginterferon alpha-2b with medications metabolized by CYP2C8).
No products indexed under this heading.

Tolmetin Sodium (Peginterferon alpha-2b treatment has been reported to result in a 28% (mean) increase in a measure of CYP2C9 activity. Caution should be used when administering peginterferon alpha-2b with medications metabolized by CYP2C9).
No products indexed under this heading.

Tolterodine Tartrate (Peginterferon alpha-2b treatment has been reported to result in a 66% (mean) increase in the measure of CYP2D6 activity. Caution should be used when administering peginterferon alpha 2b with medications metabolized by CYP2D6).
No products indexed under this heading.

Torsemide (Peginterferon alpha-2b treatment has been reported to result in a 28% (mean) increase in a measure of CYP2C9 activity. Caution should be used when administering peginterferon alpha-2b with medications metabolized by CYP2C9). Products include:
Demadex Injection ... 2630
Demadex Tablets ... 2630

Tramadol Hydrochloride (Peginterferon alpha-2b treatment has been reported to result in a 66% (mean) increase in the measure of CYP2D6 activity. Caution should be used when administering peginterferon alpha 2b with medications metabolized by CYP2D6). Products include:
Ultram ER Extended-Release Tablets ... 2428

Trazodone Hydrochloride (Peginterferon alpha-2b treatment has been reported to result in a 66% (mean) increase in the measure of CYP2D6 activity. Caution should be used when administering peginterferon alpha 2b with medications metabolized by CYP2D6).
No products indexed under this heading.

Tretinoin (Peginterferon alpha-2b treatment has been reported to result in a 28% (mean) increase in a measure of CYP2C8 activity. Caution should be used when administering peginterferon alpha-2b with medications metabolized by CYP2C8). Products include:
Vesanoid Capsules ... 2660
Ziana Gel ... 1942

Triazolam (Peginterferon alpha-2b treatment has been reported to result in a 66% (mean) increase in the measure of CYP2D6 activity. Caution should be used when administering peginterferon alpha 2b with medications metabolized by CYP2D6).
No products indexed under this heading.

Trimipramine Maleate (Peginterferon alpha-2b treatment has been reported to result in a 28% (mean) increase in a measure of CYP2C8 activity. Caution should be used when administering peginterferon alpha-2b with medications metabolized by CYP2C8).
No products indexed under this heading.

Troglitazone (Peginterferon alpha-2b treatment has been reported to result in a 28% (mean) increase in a measure of CYP2C9 activity. Caution should be used when administering peginterferon alpha-2b with medications metabolized by CYP2C9).
No products indexed under this heading.

Valdecoxib (Peginterferon alpha-2b treatment has been reported to result in a 28% (mean) increase in a measure of CYP2C9 activity. Caution should be used when administering peginterferon alpha-2b with medications metabolized by CYP2C9).
No products indexed under this heading.

Valsartan (Peginterferon alpha-2b treatment has been reported to result in a 28% (mean) increase in a measure of CYP2C9 activity. Caution should be used when administering peginterferon alpha-2b with medications metabolized by CYP2C9). Products include:
Diovan Tablets ... 2212
Diovan HCT Tablets ... 2216
Exforge Tablets ... 2238

Vardenafil Hydrochloride (Peginterferon alpha-2b treatment has been reported to result in a 28% (mean) increase in a measure of CYP2C9 activity. Caution should be used when administering peginterferon alpha-2b with medications metabolized by CYP2C9). Products include:
Levitra Tablets ... 2876

Venlafaxine Hydrochloride (Peginterferon alpha-2b treatment has been reported to result in a 66% (mean) increase in the measure of CYP2D6 activity. Caution should be used when administering peginterferon alpha 2b with medications metabolized by CYP2D6). Products include:
Effexor XR Extended-Release Capsules ... 3195
Venlafaxine Hydrochloride Tablets ... 2199

Verapamil Hydrochloride (Peginterferon alpha-2b treatment has been reported to result in a 28% (mean) increase in a measure of CYP2C8 activity. Caution should be used when administering peginterferon alpha-2b with medications metabolized by CYP2C8). Products include:
Tarka Tablets ... 511

Vinblastine Sulfate (Peginterferon alpha-2b treatment has been reported to result in a 66% (mean) increase in the measure of CYP2D6 activity. Caution should be used when administering peginterferon alpha 2b with medications metabolized by CYP2D6).
No products indexed under this heading.

Vitamin A (Peginterferon alpha-2b treatment has been reported to result in a 28% (mean) increase in a measure of CYP2C8 activity. Caution should be used when administering peginterferon alpha-2b with medications metabolized by CYP2C8). Products include:
Norwegian Cod Liver Oil ... 949

Vitamin A Acetate (Peginterferon alpha-2b treatment has been reported to result in a 28% (mean) increase in a measure of CYP2C8 activity. Caution should be used when administering peginterferon alpha-2b with medications metabolized by CYP2C8).
No products indexed under this heading.

Voriconazole (Peginterferon alpha-2b treatment has been reported to result in a 28% (mean) increase in a measure of CYP2C9 activity. Caution should be used when administering peginterferon alpha-2b with medications metabolized by CYP2C9).
No products indexed under this heading.

Warfarin Sodium (Peginterferon alpha-2b treatment has been reported to result in a 28% (mean) increase in a measure of CYP2C8 activity. Caution should be used when administering peginterferon alpha-2b with medications metabolized by CYP2C8).
No products indexed under this heading.

Zafirlukast (Peginterferon alpha-2b treatment has been reported to result in a 28% (mean) increase in a measure of CYP2C9 activity. Caution should be used when administering peginterferon alpha-2b with medications metabolized by CYP2C9). Products include:
Accolate Tablets ... 669

Zalcitabine (Patients receiving interferon with ribavirin and nucleoside reverse transcriptase inhibitors (NRTIs) should be closely monitored for treamtent-associated toxicities, especially hepatic decompensation and anemia. Discontinuation of NRTIs should be considered as medically appropriate (see individual NRTI product information). Dose reduction or discontinuation of interferon, ribavirin, or both should also be considered if worsening clinical toxicities are observed, including hepatic decompensation (e.g., Child-Pugh>6)).
No products indexed under this heading.

Zidovudine (Although there was no evidence of loss of HIV/HCV virologic suppression when ribavirin was co-administered with zidovudine, HIV/HCV co-infected patients who are administered zidovudine in combination with pegylated interferon alpha and ribavirin developed severe neutropenia (ANC less than 500) and severe anemia (Hgb less than 8 g/dL) more frequently than similar patients not receiving zidovudine). Products include:
Combivir Tablets ... 1384
Retrovir ... 1574
Retrovir IV Infusion ... 1579
Trizivir Tablets ... 1622

Zileuton (Peginterferon alpha-2b treatment has been reported to result in a 28% (mean) increase in a measure of CYP2C9 activity. Caution should be used when administering peginterferon alpha-2b with medications metabolized by CYP2C9).
No products indexed under this heading.

Zonisamide (Peginterferon alpha-2b treatment has been reported to result in a 66% (mean) increase in the measure of CYP2D6 activity. Caution should be used when administering peginterferon alpha 2b with medications metabolized by CYP2D6). Products include:
Zonegran Capsules ... 1089

Zopiclone (Peginterferon alpha-2b treatment has been reported to result in a 28% (mean) increase in a measure of CYP2C8 activity. Caution should be used when administering peginterferon alpha-2b with medications metabolized by CYP2C8).
No products indexed under this heading.

PENTACEL

(Diphtheria and Tetanus Toxoids and Acellular Pertussis Adsorbed, Inactivated Poliovirus and Haemophilus b Conjugate (Tetanus Toxoid Conjugate) Vaccine) ... 2792
May interact with alkylating agents, antimetabolites, corticosteroids, cytotoxic drugs, immunosuppressive agents, and certain other agents. Compounds in these categories include:

Azathioprine (Immunosuppressive therapies may reduce the immune response to Pentacel vaccine).
No products indexed under this heading.

Basiliximab (Immunosuppressive therapies may reduce the immune response to Pentacel vaccine). Products include:

Simulect for Injection 2306

Betamethasone Acetate (Corticosteroids (used in greater than physiologic doses) may reduce the immune response to Pentacel vaccine).
No products indexed under this heading.

Betamethasone Sodium Phosphate (Corticosteroids (used in greater than physiologic doses) may reduce the immune response to Pentacel vaccine).
No products indexed under this heading.

Bleomycin Sulfate (Cytotoxic drugs may reduce the immune response to Pentacel vaccine).
No products indexed under this heading.

Budesonide (Corticosteroids (used in greater than physiologic doses) may reduce the immune response to Pentacel vaccine). Products include:
Pulmicort Flexhaler 654
Symbicort 80/4.5 Inhalation Aerosol.. 659
Symbicort 160/4.5 Inhalation Aerosol.. 659

Busulfan (Alkylating agents may reduce the immune response to Pentacel vaccine). Products include:
Busulfex Injection 2477
Myleran Tablets 1530

Capecitabine (Antimetabolites may reduce the immune response to Pentacel vaccine). Products include:
Xeloda Tablets 2662

Carmustine (BCNU) (Alkylating agents may reduce the immune response to Pentacel vaccine).
No products indexed under this heading.

Chlorambucil (Alkylating agents may reduce the immune response to Pentacel vaccine). Products include:
Leukeran Tablets 1508

Ciclesonide (Corticosteroids (used in greater than physiologic doses) may reduce the immune response to Pentacel vaccine). Products include:
Alvesco Inhalation Aerosol 2985
Omnaris Nasal Spray 2998

Cladribine (Antimetabolites may reduce the immune response to Pentacel vaccine). Products include:
Leustatin Injection 2384

Cortisone Acetate (Corticosteroids (used in greater than physiologic doses) may reduce the immune response to Pentacel vaccine).
No products indexed under this heading.

Cyclophosphamide (Alkylating agents may reduce the immune response to Pentacel vaccine).
No products indexed under this heading.

Cyclosporine (Immunosuppressive therapies may reduce the immune response to Pentacel vaccine). Products include:
Gengraf Capsules 435
Neoral Oral Solution 2280
Neoral Soft Gelatin Capsules 2280
Restasis Ophthalmic Emulsion 557
Sandimmune 2296

Cytarabine (Antimetabolites may reduce the immune response to Pentacel vaccine).
No products indexed under this heading.

Dacarbazine (Alkylating agents may reduce the immune response to Pentacel vaccine).
No products indexed under this heading.

Daunorubicin Hydrochloride (Cytotoxic drugs may reduce the immune response to Pentacel vaccine).
No products indexed under this heading.

Dexamethasone (Corticosteroids (used in greater than physiologic doses) may reduce the immune response to Pentacel vaccine). Products include:
Ciprodex Otic Suspension 541

Dexamethasone Acetate (Corticosteroids (used in greater than physiologic doses) may reduce the immune response to Pentacel vaccine).
No products indexed under this heading.

Dexamethasone Sodium Phosphate (Corticosteroids (used in greater than physiologic doses) may reduce the immune response to Pentacel vaccine).
No products indexed under this heading.

Doxorubicin Hydrochloride (Cytotoxic drugs may reduce the immune response to Pentacel vaccine).
No products indexed under this heading.

Epirubicin Hydrochloride (Cytotoxic drugs may reduce the immune response to Pentacel vaccine).
No products indexed under this heading.

Floxuridine (Antimetabolites may reduce the immune response to Pentacel vaccine).
No products indexed under this heading.

Fludarabine Phosphate (Antimetabolites may reduce the immune response to Pentacel vaccine).
No products indexed under this heading.

Fludrocortisone Acetate (Corticosteroids (used in greater than physiologic doses) may reduce the immune response to Pentacel vaccine).
No products indexed under this heading.

Flunisolide (Corticosteroids (used in greater than physiologic doses) may reduce the immune response to Pentacel vaccine). Products include:
Aerobid/Aerobid-M 1153

Fluorouracil (Antimetabolites may reduce the immune response to Pentacel vaccine). Products include:
Carac Cream 0.5% 2722

Fluticasone Propionate (Corticosteroids (used in greater than physiologic doses) may reduce the immune response to Pentacel vaccine). Products include:
Advair Diskus 100/50 1276
Advair Diskus 250/50 1276
Advair Diskus 500/50 1276
Advair HFA 45/21 Inhalation Aerosol.. 1288
Advair HFA 115/21 Inhalation Aerosol.. 1288
Advair HFA 230/21 Inhalation Aerosol.. 1288
Flonase Nasal Spray 1431
Flovent Diskus 50 mcg 1435

Fluticasone Propionate HFA (Corticosteroids (used in greater than physiologic doses) may reduce the immune response to Pentacel vaccine). Products include:
Flovent HFA 1440

Gemcitabine Hydrochloride (Antimetabolites may reduce the immune response to Pentacel vaccine). Products include:
Gemzar for Injection 1820

Hydrocortisone (Corticosteroids (used in greater than physiologic doses) may reduce the immune response to Pentacel vaccine).
No products indexed under this heading.

Hydrocortisone Acetate (Corticosteroids (used in greater than physiologic doses) may reduce the immune response to Pentacel vaccine). Products include:
Analpram-HC 1140
Pramosone 1141

Hydrocortisone Sodium Phosphate (Corticosteroids (used in greater than physiologic doses) may reduce the immune response to Pentacel vaccine).
No products indexed under this heading.

Hydrocortisone Sodium Succinate (Corticosteroids (used in greater than physiologic doses) may reduce the immune response to Pentacel vaccine).
No products indexed under this heading.

Hydroxyurea (Cytotoxic drugs may reduce the immune response to Pentacel vaccine).
No products indexed under this heading.

Lomustine (CCNU) (Alkylating agents may reduce the immune response to Pentacel vaccine).
No products indexed under this heading.

Mechlorethamine Hydrochloride (Alkylating agents may reduce the immune response to Pentacel vaccine). Products include:
Mustargen for Injection 2492

Melphalan (Alkylating agents may reduce the immune response to Pentacel vaccine).
No products indexed under this heading.

Mercaptopurine (Antimetabolites may reduce the immune response to Pentacel vaccine).
No products indexed under this heading.

Methotrexate (Antimetabolites may reduce the immune response to Pentacel vaccine).
No products indexed under this heading.

Methotrexate Sodium (Cytotoxic drugs may reduce the immune response to Pentacel vaccine).
No products indexed under this heading.

Methylprednisolone Acetate (Corticosteroids (used in greater than physiologic doses) may reduce the immune response to Pentacel vaccine).
No products indexed under this heading.

Methylprednisolone Sodium Succinate (Corticosteroids (used in greater than physiologic doses) may reduce the immune response to Pentacel vaccine).
No products indexed under this heading.

Mitotane (Cytotoxic drugs may reduce the immune response to Pentacel vaccine).
No products indexed under this heading.

Mitoxantrone Hydrochloride (Cytotoxic drugs may reduce the immune response to Pentacel vaccine). Products include:
Novantrone for Injection Concentrate 1100

Mometasone Furoate (Corticosteroids (used in greater than physiologic doses) may reduce the immune response to Pentacel vaccine). Products include:
Asmanex Twisthaler 2797
Elocon Cream 0.1% 2840
Elocon Lotion 0.1% 2841
Elocon Ointment 0.1% 2842

Mometasone Furoate Monohydrate (Corticosteroids (used in greater than physiologic doses) may reduce the immune response to Pentacel vaccine). Products include:
Nasonex Nasal Spray 2883

Muromonab-CD3 (Immunosuppressive therapies may reduce the immune response to Pentacel vaccine). Products include:
Orthoclone OKT3 Sterile Solution 2387

Mycophenolate Mofetil (Immunosuppressive therapies may reduce the immune response to Pentacel vaccine). Products include:
CellCept Capsules 2622
CellCept Oral Suspension 2622
CellCept Tablets 2622

Pentostatin (Antimetabolites may reduce the immune response to Pentacel vaccine).
No products indexed under this heading.

Prednisolone Acetate (Corticosteroids (used in greater than physiologic doses) may reduce the immune response to Pentacel vaccine). Products include:
Pred Forte Ophthalmic Suspension................................ ⊙227
Pred Mild Ophthalmic Suspension................................ ⊙230
Pred-G Ophthalmic Ointment .... ⊙229
Pred-G Ophthalmic Suspension ...... ⊙228

Prednisolone Sodium Phosphate (Corticosteroids (used in greater than physiologic doses) may reduce the immune response to Pentacel vaccine).
No products indexed under this heading.

Prednisolone Tebutate (Corticosteroids (used in greater than physiologic doses) may reduce the immune response to Pentacel vaccine).
No products indexed under this heading.

Prednisone (Corticosteroids (used in greater than physiologic doses) may reduce the immune response to Pentacel vaccine).
No products indexed under this heading.

Procarbazine Hydrochloride (Cytotoxic drugs may reduce the immune response to Pentacel vaccine).
No products indexed under this heading.

Radiation (Irradiation may reduce the immune response to pentacel vaccine).
No products indexed under this heading.

Sirolimus (Immunosuppressive therapies may reduce the immune response to Pentacel vaccine). Products include:
Rapamune 3260

Tacrolimus (Immunosuppressive therapies may reduce the immune response to Pentacel vaccine). Products include:
- Prograf Capsules and Injection 622
- Protopic Ointment 628

Tamoxifen Citrate (Cytotoxic drugs may reduce the immune response to Pentacel vaccine).
No products indexed under this heading.

Thioguanine (Antimetabolites may reduce the immune response to Pentacel vaccine). Products include:
- Tabloid Tablets 1601

Thiotepa (Alkylating agents may reduce the immune response to Pentacel vaccine).
No products indexed under this heading.

Triamcinolone (Corticosteroids (used in greater than physiologic doses) may reduce the immune response to Pentacel vaccine).
No products indexed under this heading.

Triamcinolone Acetonide (Corticosteroids (used in greater than physiologic doses) may reduce the immune response to Pentacel vaccine). Products include:
- Azmacort Inhalation Aerosol 407
- Nasacort AQ Nasal Spray 2765
- Triesence Injectable Suspension .... ⊙ 209

Triamcinolone Diacetate (Corticosteroids (used in greater than physiologic doses) may reduce the immune response to Pentacel vaccine).
No products indexed under this heading.

Triamcinolone Hexacetonide (Corticosteroids (used in greater than physiologic doses) may reduce the immune response to Pentacel vaccine).
No products indexed under this heading.

Vincristine Sulfate (Cytotoxic drugs may reduce the immune response to Pentacel vaccine).
No products indexed under this heading.

PENTASA CAPSULES

(Mesalamine) 3030
None cited in PDR database.

PEPCID TABLETS

(Famotidine) 2075
May interact with antacids and certain other agents. Compounds in these categories include:

Aluminum Carbonate (Bioavailability may be slightly decreased by antacids).
No products indexed under this heading.

Aluminum Hydroxide (Bioavailability may be slightly decreased by antacids).
No products indexed under this heading.

Magaldrate (Bioavailability may be slightly decreased by antacids).
No products indexed under this heading.

Magnesium Hydroxide (Bioavailability may be slightly decreased by antacids). Products include:
- Fleet Pedia-Lax Chewable Tablets 1145
- Pepcid Complete Chewable Tablets 1771
- Extra Strength Rolaids Freshmint Tablets 1903
- Rolaids Multi-Symptom Berry Tablets 1903
- Rolaids Original Peppermint Tablets 1903

Magnesium Oxide (Bioavailability may be slightly decreased by antacids). Products include:
- Beelith Tablets 813

Sodium Bicarbonate (Bioavailability may be slightly decreased by antacids). Products include:
- Ceo-Two Laxative Suppository 815

Food Interactions

Food, unspecified (Bioavailability may be slightly increased by antacids).

ORIGINAL STRENGTH PEPCID AC GELCAPS

(Famotidine) 1771
None cited in PDR database.

ORIGINAL STRENGTH PEPCID AC TABLETS

(Famotidine) 1771
None cited in PDR database.

MAXIMUM STRENGTH PEPCID AC TABLETS

(Famotidine) 1771
None cited in PDR database.

PEPCID COMPLETE CHEWABLE TABLETS

(Calcium Carbonate, Famotidine, Magnesium Hydroxide) 1771
May interact with:

Prescription Drugs, unspecified (Antacids contained in Pepcid Complete may interact with certain prescription drugs).
No products indexed under this heading.

PEPTO-BISMOL ORIGINAL LIQUID, MAXIMUM STRENGTH LIQUID, ORIGINAL AND CHERRY TABLETS, CHEWABLE TABLETS AND EASY-TO-SWALLOW CAPLETS

(Bismuth Subsalicylate) 2564
May interact with oral anticoagulants, antigout agents, and oral hypoglycemic agents. Compounds in these categories include:

Acarbose (Concurrent use should be undertaken with physician's supervision). Products include:
- Precose Tablets 792

Allopurinol (Concurrent use should be undertaken with physician's supervision).
No products indexed under this heading.

Anisindione (Concurrent use should be undertaken with physician's supervision).
No products indexed under this heading.

Chlorpropamide (Concurrent use should be undertaken with physician's supervision).
No products indexed under this heading.

Dicumarol (Concurrent use should be undertaken with physician's supervision).
No products indexed under this heading.

Glimepiride (Concurrent use should be undertaken with physician's supervision). Products include:
- Avandaryl Tablets 1344
- Duetact Tablets 3085

Glipizide (Concurrent use should be undertaken with physician's supervision).
No products indexed under this heading.

Glyburide (Concurrent use should be undertaken with physician's supervision).
No products indexed under this heading.

Metformin Hydrochloride (Concurrent use should be undertaken with physician's supervision). Products include:
- ActoPlus Met Tablets 3071
- Avandamet Tablets 1336
- Janumet Tablets 2041
- PrandiMet Tablets 2967

Miglitol (Concurrent use should be undertaken with physician's supervision).
No products indexed under this heading.

Nateglinide (Concurrent use should be undertaken with physician's supervision). Products include:
- Starlix Tablets 2314

Pioglitazone Hydrochloride (Concurrent use should be undertaken with physician's supervision). Products include:
- ActoPlus Met Tablets 3071
- Actos Tablets 3077
- Duetact Tablets 3085

Probenecid (Concurrent use should be undertaken with physician's supervision).
No products indexed under this heading.

Repaglinide (Concurrent use should be undertaken with physician's supervision). Products include:
- PrandiMet Tablets 2967
- Prandin Tablets 2971

Rosiglitazone Maleate (Concurrent use should be undertaken with physician's supervision). Products include:
- Avandamet Tablets 1336
- Avandaryl Tablets 1344
- Avandia Tablets 1351

Sitagliptin Phosphate (Concurrent use should be undertaken with physician's supervision). Products include:
- Janumet Tablets 2041
- Januvia Tablets 2048

Sulfinpyrazone (Concurrent use should be undertaken with physician's supervision).
No products indexed under this heading.

Tolazamide (Concurrent use should be undertaken with physician's supervision).
No products indexed under this heading.

Tolbutamide (Concurrent use should be undertaken with physician's supervision).
No products indexed under this heading.

Troglitazone (Concurrent use should be undertaken with physician's supervision).
No products indexed under this heading.

Warfarin Sodium (Concurrent use should be undertaken with physician's supervision).
No products indexed under this heading.

PEPTO-BISMOL ORIGINAL LIQUID, ORIGINAL AND CHERRY CHEWABLE TABLETS & CAPLETS

(Bismuth Subsalicylate) .... ▣613
None cited in PDR database.

PEPTO-BISMOL MAXIMUM STRENGTH LIQUID

(Bismuth Subsalicylate) .... ▣613
None cited in PDR database.

PERCOCET TABLETS

(Acetaminophen, Oxycodone Hydrochloride) 1127
May interact with narcotic analgesics, oral contraceptives, phenothiazines, tranquilizers, tricyclic antidepressants, vasodilators, and certain other agents. Compounds in these categories include:

Alfentanil Hydrochloride (Additive CNS depression; dose of one or both agents should be reduced).
No products indexed under this heading.

Alprazolam (Additive CNS depression; dose of one or both agents should be reduced).
No products indexed under this heading.

Amitriptyline Hydrochloride (Increased effect of antidepressant or oxycodone).
No products indexed under this heading.

Amoxapine (Increased effect of antidepressant or oxycodone).
No products indexed under this heading.

Amyl Nitrite (Oxycodone may cause severe hypotension after concurrent administration with drugs which compromise vasomotor tone).
No products indexed under this heading.

Aprobarbital (Additive CNS depression; dose of one or both agents should be reduced).
No products indexed under this heading.

Atropine Sulfate (May produce paralytic ileus). Products include:
- Donnatal Extentabs 2507

Belladonna Alkaloids (May produce paralytic ileus). Products include:
- Hyland's Teething Tablets .... ▣621

Benztropine Mesylate (May produce paralytic ileus).
No products indexed under this heading.

Biperiden Hydrochloride (May produce paralytic ileus).
No products indexed under this heading.

Bumetanide (The effects of loop diuretics may be decreased).
No products indexed under this heading.

Buprenorphine Hydrochloride (Additive CNS depression; dose of one or both agents should be reduced). Products include:
- Suboxone Tablets 2601
- Subutex Tablets 2601

Buspirone Hydrochloride (Additive CNS depression; dose of one or both agents should be reduced).
No products indexed under this heading.

Butabarbital (Additive CNS depression; dose of one or both agents should be reduced).
No products indexed under this heading.

Butabarbital Sodium (Additive CNS depression; dose of one or both agents should be reduced).
No products indexed under this heading.

Butalbital (Additive CNS depression; dose of one or both agents should be reduced).
No products indexed under this heading.

Butorphanol Tartrate (Mixed agonist/antagonist analgesics may reduce the analgesic effect of oxycodone and/or may precipitate withdrawal symptoms in these patients).
No products indexed under this heading.

Chloral Hydrate (Additive CNS depression; dose of one or both agents should be reduced).
No products indexed under this heading.

Chlordiazepoxide (Additive CNS depression; dose of one or both agents should be reduced).
No products indexed under this heading.

Chlordiazepoxide Hydrochloride (Additive CNS depression; dose of one or both agents should be reduced).
No products indexed under this heading.

Chlorpromazine (Additive CNS depression; dose of one or both agents should be reduced).
No products indexed under this heading.

Chlorpromazine Hydrochloride (Additive CNS depression; dose of one or both agents should be reduced).
No products indexed under this heading.

Chlorprothixene (Additive CNS depression; dose of one or both agents should be reduced).
No products indexed under this heading.

Chlorprothixene Hydrochloride (Additive CNS depression; dose of one or both agents should be reduced).
No products indexed under this heading.

Chlorprothixene Lactate (Additive CNS depression; dose of one or both agents should be reduced).
No products indexed under this heading.

Clidinium Bromide (May produce paralytic ileus).
No products indexed under this heading.

Clomipramine Hydrochloride (Increased effect of antidepressant or oxycodone).
No products indexed under this heading.

Clorazepate Dipotassium (Additive CNS depression; dose of one or both agents should be reduced).
No products indexed under this heading.

Clozapine (Additive CNS depression; dose of one or both agents should be reduced).
No products indexed under this heading.

Codeine Phosphate (Additive CNS depression; dose of one or both agents should be reduced). Products include:
Tylenol with Codeine Tablets 2427

Desflurane (Additive CNS depression; dose of one or both agents should be reduced).
No products indexed under this heading.

Desipramine Hydrochloride (Increased effect of antidepressant or oxycodone).
No products indexed under this heading.

Desogestrel (Increase in glucoronidation resulting in increased plasma clearance and a decreased half-life of acetaminophen). Products include:
Mircette Tablets 1034

Dezocine (Additive CNS depression; dose of one or both agents should be reduced).
No products indexed under this heading.

Diazepam (Additive CNS depression; dose of one or both agents should be reduced). Products include:
Valium Tablets 2658

Diazoxide (Oxycodone may cause severe hypotension after concurrent administration with drugs which compromise vasomotor tone). Products include:
Proglycem Capsules 1185
Proglycem Suspension 1185

Dicyclomine Hydrochloride (May produce paralytic ileus). Products include:
Bentyl Capsules 703
Bentyl Injection 703
Bentyl Syrup 703
Bentyl Tablets 703

Doxepin Hydrochloride (Increased effect of antidepressant or oxycodone).
No products indexed under this heading.

Droperidol (Additive CNS depression; dose of one or both agents should be reduced).
No products indexed under this heading.

Enflurane (Additive CNS depression; dose of one or both agents should be reduced).
No products indexed under this heading.

Epoprostenol Sodium (Oxycodone may cause severe hypotension after concurrent administration with drugs which compromise vasomotor tone). Products include:
Flolan for Injection 1426

Estazolam (Additive CNS depression; dose of one or both agents should be reduced).
No products indexed under this heading.

Ethacrynic Acid (The effects of loop diuretics may be decreased). Products include:
Edecrin Tablets 698

Ethanol (Additive CNS depression; dose of one or both agents should be reduced).
No products indexed under this heading.

Ethaverine Hydrochloride (Oxycodone may cause severe hypotension after concurrent administration with drugs which compromise vasomotor tone).
No products indexed under this heading.

Ethchlorvynol (Additive CNS depression; dose of one or both agents should be reduced).
No products indexed under this heading.

Ethinamate (Additive CNS depression; dose of one or both agents should be reduced).
No products indexed under this heading.

Ethinyl Estradiol (Increase in glucoronidation resulting in increased plasma clearance and a decreased half-life of acetaminophen). Products include:
Lybrel Tablets 3204
Mircette Tablets 1034
NuvaRing 2897
Ortho-Cyclen/Ortho Tri-Cyclen 2449
Ortho Evra Transdermal System 2437
Ortho Tri-Cyclen Lo Tablets 2458
Seasonique Tablets 1046
Yaz Tablets 805

Ethopropazine Hydrochloride (May produce paralytic ileus).
No products indexed under this heading.

Ethyl Alcohol (Additive CNS depression; dose of one or both agents should be reduced).
No products indexed under this heading.

Ethynodiol Diacetate (Increase in glucoronidation resulting in increased plasma clearance and a decreased half-life of acetaminophen).
No products indexed under this heading.

Fentanyl (Additive CNS depression; dose of one or both agents should be reduced). Products include:
Duragesic Transdermal System 2405
Ionsys Transdermal System 2410

Fentanyl Citrate (Additive CNS depression; dose of one or both agents should be reduced). Products include:
Actiq 959
Fentora Tablets 968

Fluphenazine Decanoate (Additive CNS depression; dose of one or both agents should be reduced).
No products indexed under this heading.

Fluphenazine Enanthate (Additive CNS depression; dose of one or both agents should be reduced).
No products indexed under this heading.

Fluphenazine Hydrochloride (Additive CNS depression; dose of one or both agents should be reduced).
No products indexed under this heading.

Flurazepam Hydrochloride (Additive CNS depression; dose of one or both agents should be reduced).
No products indexed under this heading.

Furosemide (The effects of loop diuretics may be decreased). Products include:
Furosemide Tablets 2186

Glutethimide (Additive CNS depression; dose of one or both agents should be reduced).
No products indexed under this heading.

Glycopyrrolate (May produce paralytic ileus).
No products indexed under this heading.

Haloperidol (Additive CNS depression; dose of one or both agents should be reduced).
No products indexed under this heading.

Haloperidol Decanoate (Additive CNS depression; dose of one or both agents should be reduced).
No products indexed under this heading.

Hydralazine Hydrochloride (Oxycodone may cause severe hypotension after concurrent administration with drugs which compromise vasomotor tone).
No products indexed under this heading.

Hydrocodone Bitartrate (Additive CNS depression; dose of one or both agents should be reduced). Products include:
Lortab 5/500 Tablets 3143
Lortab 7.5/500 Tablets 3144
Lortab 10/500 Tablets 3144
Vicodin Tablets 529
Vicodin ES Tablets 530
Vicodin HP Tablets 531
Vicoprofen Tablets 533
Zydone Tablets 1132

Hydrocodone Polistirex (Additive CNS depression; dose of one or both agents should be reduced). Products include:
Tussionex Pennkinetic Extended-Release Suspension 3154

Hydromorphone Hydrochloride (Additive CNS depression; dose of one or both agents should be reduced).
No products indexed under this heading.

Hydroxyzine Hydrochloride (Additive CNS depression; dose of one or both agents should be reduced).
No products indexed under this heading.

Hyoscyamine (May produce paralytic ileus).
No products indexed under this heading.

Hyoscyamine Sulfate (May produce paralytic ileus). Products include:
Donnatal Extentabs 2507

Imipramine Hydrochloride (Increased effect of antidepressant or oxycodone).
No products indexed under this heading.

Imipramine Pamoate (Increased effect of antidepressant or oxycodone).
No products indexed under this heading.

Ipratropium Bromide (May produce paralytic ileus). Products include:
Atrovent HFA Inhalation Aerosol 839
Atrovent Nasal Spray 0.03% 834
Atrovent Nasal Spray 0.06% 836
Combivent Inhalation Aerosol 845

Isocarboxazid (Increased effect of either oxycodone or MAO inhibitor). Products include:
Marplan Tablets 3177

Isoflurane (Additive CNS depression; dose of one or both agents should be reduced).
No products indexed under this heading.

Isosorbide Dinitrate (Oxycodone may cause severe hypotension after concurrent administration with drugs which compromise vasomotor tone).
No products indexed under this heading.

Isosorbide Mononitrate (Oxycodone may cause severe hypotension after concurrent administration with drugs which compromise vasomotor tone).
No products indexed under this heading.

Isoxsuprine Hydrochloride (Oxycodone may cause severe hypotension after concurrent administration with drugs which compromise vasomotor tone).
No products indexed under this heading.

Ketamine Hydrochloride (Additive CNS depression; dose of one or both agents should be reduced).
No products indexed under this heading.

Lamotrigine (Serum lamotrigine concentrations may be reduced, producing a decrease in therapeutic effects). Products include:
Lamictal **1488**

Levomethadyl Acetate Hydrochloride (Additive CNS depression; dose of one or both agents should be reduced).
No products indexed under this heading.

Levonorgestrel (Increase in glucoronidation resulting in increased plasma clearance and a decreased half-life of acetaminophen). Products include:
Climara Pro Transdermal System **768**
Lybrel Tablets **3204**
Mirena Intrauterine System **779**
Plan B Tablets **1044**
Seasonique Tablets **1046**

Levorphanol Tartrate (Additive CNS depression; dose of one or both agents should be reduced).
No products indexed under this heading.

Lorazepam (Additive CNS depression; dose of one or both agents should be reduced).
No products indexed under this heading.

Loxapine Hydrochloride (Additive CNS depression; dose of one or both agents should be reduced).
No products indexed under this heading.

Loxapine Succinate (Additive CNS depression; dose of one or both agents should be reduced).
No products indexed under this heading.

Maprotiline Hydrochloride (Increased effect of antidepressant or oxycodone).
No products indexed under this heading.

Mepenzolate Bromide (May produce paralytic ileus).
No products indexed under this heading.

Meperidine Hydrochloride (Additive CNS depression; dose of one or both agents should be reduced).
No products indexed under this heading.

Mephobarbital (Additive CNS depression; dose of one or both agents should be reduced).
No products indexed under this heading.

Meprobamate (Additive CNS depression; dose of one or both agents should be reduced).
No products indexed under this heading.

Mesoridazine Besylate (Additive CNS depression; dose of one or both agents should be reduced).
No products indexed under this heading.

Mestranol (Increase in glucoronidation resulting in increased plasma clearance and a decreased half-life of acetaminophen).
No products indexed under this heading.

Methadone Hydrochloride (Additive CNS depression; dose of one or both agents should be reduced).
No products indexed under this heading.

Methohexital Sodium (Additive CNS depression; dose of one or both agents should be reduced).
No products indexed under this heading.

Methotrimeprazine (Additive CNS depression; dose of one or both agents should be reduced).
No products indexed under this heading.

Methoxyflurane (Additive CNS depression; dose of one or both agents should be reduced).
No products indexed under this heading.

Midazolam Hydrochloride (Additive CNS depression; dose of one or both agents should be reduced).
No products indexed under this heading.

Minoxidil (Oxycodone may cause severe hypotension after concurrent administration with drugs which compromise vasomotor tone).
No products indexed under this heading.

Moclobemide (Increased effect of either oxycodone or MAO inhibitor).
No products indexed under this heading.

Molindone Hydrochloride (Additive CNS depression; dose of one or both agents should be reduced). Products include:
Moban Tablets **1116**

Morphine Sulfate (Additive CNS depression; dose of one or both agents should be reduced). Products include:
Avinza Capsules **1772**
DepoDur Injection **1095**
MS Contin Tablets **2585**

Nalbuphine Hydrochloride (Mixed agonist/antagonist analgesics may reduce the analgesic effect of oxycodone and/or may precipitate withdrawal symptoms in these patients).
No products indexed under this heading.

Nitroglycerin (Oxycodone may cause severe hypotension after concurrent administration with drugs which compromise vasomotor tone). Products include:
Nitro-Dur Transdermal Infusion System **2887**
Nitrolingual Pumpspray **2965**

Nitroglycerin, long-acting formulations (Oxycodone may cause severe hypotension after concurrent administration with drugs which compromise vasomotor tone).
No products indexed under this heading.

Nitroglycerin Intravenous (Oxycodone may cause severe hypotension after concurrent administration with drugs which compromise vasomotor tone).
No products indexed under this heading.

Norethindrone (Increase in glucoronidation resulting in increased plasma clearance and a decreased half-life of acetaminophen). Products include:
Ortho Micronor Tablets **2446**

Norethynodrel (Increase in glucoronidation resulting in increased plasma clearance and a decreased half-life of acetaminophen).
No products indexed under this heading.

Norgestimate (Increase in glucoronidation resulting in increased plasma clearance and a decreased half-life of acetaminophen). Products include:
Ortho-Cyclen/Ortho Tri-Cyclen **2449**
Ortho Tri-Cyclen Lo Tablets **2458**

Norgestrel (Increase in glucoronidation resulting in increased plasma clearance and a decreased half-life of acetaminophen).
No products indexed under this heading.

Nortriptyline Hydrochloride (Increased effect of antidepressant or oxycodone).
No products indexed under this heading.

Olanzapine (Additive CNS depression; dose of one or both agents should be reduced). Products include:
Symbyax Capsules **1871**
Zyprexa Tablets **1883**
Zyprexa IntraMuscular **1883**
Zyprexa ZYDIS Orally Disintegrating Tablets **1883**

Oxazepam (Additive CNS depression; dose of one or both agents should be reduced; increased effect of antidepressant).
No products indexed under this heading.

Oxybutynin Chloride (May produce paralytic ileus).
No products indexed under this heading.

Oxyphenonium Bromide (May produce paralytic ileus).
No products indexed under this heading.

Papaverine (Oxycodone may cause severe hypotension after concurrent administration with drugs which compromise vasomotor tone).
No products indexed under this heading.

Papaverine Hydrochloride (Oxycodone may cause severe hypotension after concurrent administration with drugs which compromise vasomotor tone).
No products indexed under this heading.

Pargyline Hydrochloride (Increased effect of either oxycodone or MAO inhibitor).
No products indexed under this heading.

Pentazocine Hydrochloride (Mixed agonist/antagonist analgesics may reduce the analgesic effect of oxycodone and/or may precipitate withdrawal symptoms in these patients).
No products indexed under this heading.

Pentazocine Lactate (Mixed agonist/antagonist analgesics may reduce the analgesic effect of oxycodone and/or may precipitate withdrawal symptoms in these patients).
No products indexed under this heading.

Pentobarbital Sodium (Additive CNS depression; dose of one or both agents should be reduced). Products include:
Nembutal Sodium Solution, USP **2494**

Perphenazine (Additive CNS depression; dose of one or both agents should be reduced).
No products indexed under this heading.

Phenelzine Sulfate (Increased effect of either oxycodone or MAO inhibitor).
No products indexed under this heading.

Phenobarbital (Additive CNS depression; dose of one or both agents should be reduced). Products include:
Donnatal Extentabs **2507**

Prazepam (Additive CNS depression; dose of one or both agents should be reduced).
No products indexed under this heading.

Probenecid (Probenicid may increase the therapeutic effectiveness of acetaminophen slightly).
No products indexed under this heading.

Procarbazine Hydrochloride (Increased effect of either oxycodone or MAO inhibitor).
No products indexed under this heading.

Prochlorperazine (Additive CNS depression; dose of one or both agents should be reduced).
No products indexed under this heading.

Procyclidine Hydrochloride (May produce paralytic ileus).
No products indexed under this heading.

Promethazine Hydrochloride (Additive CNS depression; dose of one or both agents should be reduced).
No products indexed under this heading.

Propantheline Bromide (May produce paralytic ileus).
No products indexed under this heading.

Propofol (Additive CNS depression; dose of one or both agents should be reduced).
No products indexed under this heading.

Propoxyphene Hydrochloride (Additive CNS depression; dose of one or both agents should be reduced).
No products indexed under this heading.

Propoxyphene Napsylate (Additive CNS depression; dose of one or both agents should be reduced).
No products indexed under this heading.

Propranolol (Propanolol appears to inhibit the enzyme system responsible for the metabolism of acetaminophen. Therefore, the pharmacologic effects of acetaminophen may be increased).
No products indexed under this heading.

Protriptyline Hydrochloride (Increased effect of antidepressant or oxycodone).
No products indexed under this heading.

Quazepam (Additive CNS depression; dose of one or both agents should be reduced).
No products indexed under this heading.

Quetiapine Fumarate (Additive CNS depression; dose of one or both agents should be reduced).
No products indexed under this heading.

Ramelteon (Additive CNS depression; dose of one or both agents should be reduced). Products include:
Rozerem Tablets 3091

Rasagiline Mesylate (Increased effect of either oxycodone or MAO inhibitor). Products include:
Azilect Tablets 3106

Remifentanil Hydrochloride (Additive CNS depression; dose of one or both agents should be reduced).
No products indexed under this heading.

Risperidone (Additive CNS depression; dose of one or both agents should be reduced). Products include:
Risperdal Consta Long-Acting Injection 1753

Scopolamine (May produce paralytic ileus). Products include:
Transderm Scōp Transdermal Therapeutic System 2206

Scopolamine Hydrobromide (May produce paralytic ileus). Products include:
Donnatal Extentabs 2507

Secobarbital Sodium (Additive CNS depression; dose of one or both agents should be reduced).
No products indexed under this heading.

Selegiline (Increased effect of either oxycodone or MAO inhibitor). Products include:
Emsam Transdermal System 905

Selegiline Hydrochloride (Increased effect of either oxycodone or MAO inhibitor). Products include:
Eldepryl Capsules 3052

Sevoflurane (Additive CNS depression; dose of one or both agents should be reduced). Products include:
Ultane Liquid for Inhalation 524

Sodium Butabarbital (Additive CNS depression; dose of one or both agents should be reduced).
No products indexed under this heading.

Sodium Oxybate (Additive CNS depression; dose of one or both agents should be reduced). Products include:
Xyrem Oral Solution 1766

Sufentanil Citrate (Additive CNS depression; dose of one or both agents should be reduced).
No products indexed under this heading.

Temazepam (Additive CNS depression; dose of one or both agents should be reduced).
No products indexed under this heading.

Thiamylal Sodium (Additive CNS depression; dose of one or both agents should be reduced).
No products indexed under this heading.

Thioridazine Hydrochloride (Additive CNS depression; dose of one or both agents should be reduced). Products include:
Thioridazine Hydrochloride Tablets 2195

Thiothixene (Additive CNS depression; dose of one or both agents should be reduced). Products include:
Thiothixene Capsules 2197

Tolazoline Hydrochloride (Oxycodone may cause severe hypotension after concurrent administration with drugs which compromise vasomotor tone).
No products indexed under this heading.

Tolterodine Tartrate (May produce paralytic ileus).
No products indexed under this heading.

Torsemide (The effects of loop diuretics may be decreased). Products include:
Demadex Injection 2630
Demadex Tablets 2630

Tranylcypromine Sulfate (Increased effect of either oxycodone or MAO inhibitor). Products include:
Parnate Tablets 1532

Triazolam (Additive CNS depression; dose of one or both agents should be reduced).
No products indexed under this heading.

Tridihexethyl Chloride (May produce paralytic ileus).
No products indexed under this heading.

Trifluoperazine Hydrochloride (Additive CNS depression; dose of one or both agents should be reduced).
No products indexed under this heading.

Trihexyphenidyl Hydrochloride (May produce paralytic ileus).
No products indexed under this heading.

Trimipramine Maleate (Increased effect of antidepressant or oxycodone).
No products indexed under this heading.

Zaleplon (Additive CNS depression; dose of one or both agents should be reduced).
No products indexed under this heading.

Zidovudine (The pharmacologic effects of zidovudine may be decreased because of enhanced non-hepatic or renal clearance of zidovudine). Products include:
Combivir Tablets 1384
Retrovir 1574
Retrovir IV Infusion 1579
Trizivir Tablets 1622

Ziprasidone Hydrochloride (Additive CNS depression; dose of one or both agents should be reduced). Products include:
Geodon Capsules 2520

Zolpidem Tartrate (Additive CNS depression; dose of one or both agents should be reduced). Products include:
Ambien Tablets 2692
Ambien CR Tablets 2696

Food Interactions

Alcohol (Additive CNS depression).

PERCODAN TABLETS

(Aspirin, Oxycodone Hydrochloride) ... 1130
May interact with ACE inhibitors, beta blockers, central nervous system depressants, anticoagulants, diuretics, anticonvulsants, general anesthetics, antigout agents, oral hypoglycemic agents, hypnotics and sedatives, mixed agonist/antagonist opioid analgesics, narcotic analgesics, non-steroidal anti-inflammatory agents, phenothiazines, tranquilizers, and certain other agents. Compounds in these categories include:

Acarbose (Aspirin may increase the serum glucose-lowering action of insulin and sulfonylureas leading to hypoglycemia). Products include:
Precose Tablets 792

Acebutolol Hydrochloride (The hypotensive effects of beta blockers may be diminished by concomitant administration of aspirin).
No products indexed under this heading.

Acetazolamide (Concurrent use of acetazolamide can lead to high serum levels of acetazolamide and toxicity).
No products indexed under this heading.

Acetazolamide Sodium (Concurrent use of acetazolamide can lead to high serum levels of acetazolamide and toxicity).
No products indexed under this heading.

Alfentanil Hydrochloride (Additive CNS depression).
No products indexed under this heading.

Allopurinol (Salicylates antagonize the uricosuric action of uricosuric agents).
No products indexed under this heading.

Alprazolam (Additive CNS depression).
No products indexed under this heading.

Amiloride Hydrochloride (The effectiveness of diuretics in patients with underlying renal or cardiovascular disease may by diminished by the concomitant administration of aspirin).
No products indexed under this heading.

Anisindione (Enhanced effect of anticoagulant).
No products indexed under this heading.

Aprobarbital (Additive CNS depression).
No products indexed under this heading.

Ardeparin Sodium (Enhanced effect of anticoagulant).
No products indexed under this heading.

Atenolol (The hypotensive effects of beta blockers may be diminished by concomitant administration of aspirin).
No products indexed under this heading.

Benazepril Hydrochloride (Reports suggested that NSAIDs may diminish the hyponatremic and hypotensive effect of ACE inhibitors).
No products indexed under this heading.

Bendroflumethiazide (The effectiveness of diuretics in patients with underlying renal or cardiovascular disease may by diminished by the concomitant administration of aspirin).
No products indexed under this heading.

Betaxolol Hydrochloride (The hypotensive effects of beta blockers may be diminished by concomitant administration of aspirin).
No products indexed under this heading.

Bisoprolol Fumarate (The hypotensive effects of beta blockers may be diminished by concomitant administration of aspirin).
No products indexed under this heading.

Bumetanide (The effectiveness of diuretics in patients with underlying renal or cardiovascular disease may by diminished by the concomitant administration of aspirin).
No products indexed under this heading.

Buprenorphine Hydrochloride (Additive CNS depression). Products include:
Suboxone Tablets 2601
Subutex Tablets 2601

Buspirone Hydrochloride (Additive CNS depression).
No products indexed under this heading.

Butabarbital (Additive CNS depression).
No products indexed under this heading.

Butabarbital Sodium (Additive CNS depression).
No products indexed under this heading.

Butalbital (Additive CNS depression).
No products indexed under this heading.

Butorphanol Tartrate (Agonist/antagonist analgesics may reduce the analgesic effect of oxycodone or may precipitate withdrawal symptoms).
No products indexed under this heading.

Captopril (Reports suggested that NSAIDs may diminish the hyponatremic and hypotensive effect of ACE inhibitors). Products include:
Captopril Tablets 2182

Carbamazepine (Salicylate can displace protein-bound phenytoin and valproic acid, leading to a decrease in the total concentration of phenytoin and an increase in serum valproic acid levels). Products include:
Carbatrol Capsules 3019
Equetro Extended-Release Capsules 3174

Carteolol Hydrochloride (The hypotensive effects of beta blockers may be diminished by concomitant administration of aspirin).
No products indexed under this heading.

Celecoxib (The concurrent use of aspirin with other NSAIDs should be avoided because this may increase bleeding or lead to decreased renal function). Products include:
Celebrex Capsules 2979

Chloral Hydrate (Additive CNS depression).
No products indexed under this heading.

Chlordiazepoxide (Additive CNS depression).
No products indexed under this heading.

Chlordiazepoxide Hydrochloride (Additive CNS depression).
No products indexed under this heading.

Chlorothiazide (The effectiveness of diuretics in patients with underlying renal or cardiovascular disease may by diminished by the concomitant administration of aspirin).
No products indexed under this heading.

Chlorothiazide Sodium (The effectiveness of diuretics in patients with underlying renal or cardiovascular disease may by diminished by the concomitant administration of aspirin). Products include:
Intravenous Sodium Diuril **2490**

Chlorpromazine (Additive CNS depression).
No products indexed under this heading.

Chlorpromazine Hydrochloride (Additive CNS depression).
No products indexed under this heading.

Chlorpropamide (Aspirin may increase the serum glucose-lowering action of insulin and sulfonylureas leading to hypoglycemia).
No products indexed under this heading.

Chlorprothixene (Additive CNS depression).
No products indexed under this heading.

Chlorprothixene Hydrochloride (Additive CNS depression).
No products indexed under this heading.

Chlorprothixene Lactate (Additive CNS depression).
No products indexed under this heading.

Chlorthalidone (The effectiveness of diuretics in patients with underlying renal or cardiovascular disease may by diminished by the concomitant administration of aspirin). Products include:
Clorpres Tablets **2185**

Clorazepate Dipotassium (Additive CNS depression).
No products indexed under this heading.

Clozapine (Additive CNS depression).
No products indexed under this heading.

Codeine Phosphate (Additive CNS depression). Products include:
Tylenol with Codeine Tablets **2427**

Dalteparin Sodium (Enhanced effect of anticoagulant). Products include:
Fragmin Injection **1070**

Danaparoid Sodium (Enhanced effect of anticoagulant).
No products indexed under this heading.

Desflurane (Additive CNS depression).
No products indexed under this heading.

Dezocine (Additive CNS depression).
No products indexed under this heading.

Diazepam (Additive CNS depression). Products include:
Valium Tablets **2658**

Diclofenac Epolamine (The concurrent use of aspirin with other NSAIDs should be avoided because this may increase bleeding or lead to decreased renal function). Products include:
Flector Patch **561**

Diclofenac Potassium (The concurrent use of aspirin with other NSAIDs should be avoided because this may increase bleeding or lead to decreased renal function).
No products indexed under this heading.

Diclofenac Sodium (The concurrent use of aspirin with other NSAIDs should be avoided because this may increase bleeding or lead to decreased renal function). Products include:
Diclofenac Sodium Ophthalmic Solution.................................... ⊙**240**
Voltaren Ophthalmic Solution **2336**
Voltaren Tablets **2334**
Voltaren-XR Tablets **2337**

Dicumarol (Enhanced effect of anticoagulant).
No products indexed under this heading.

Divalproex Sodium (Salicylate can displace protein-bound phenytoin and valproic acid, leading to a decrease in the total concentration of phenytoin and an increase in serum valproic acid levels). Products include:
Depakote ER Tablets **423**

Droperidol (Additive CNS depression).
No products indexed under this heading.

Enalapril Maleate (Reports suggested that NSAIDs may diminish the hyponatremic and hypotensive effect of ACE inhibitors).
No products indexed under this heading.

Enalaprilat (Reports suggested that NSAIDs may diminish the hyponatremic and hypotensive effect of ACE inhibitors).
No products indexed under this heading.

Enflurane (Additive CNS depression).
No products indexed under this heading.

Enoxaparin Sodium (Enhanced effect of anticoagulant). Products include:
Lovenox Injection **2756**

Esmolol Hydrochloride (The hypotensive effects of beta blockers may be diminished by concomitant administration of aspirin).
No products indexed under this heading.

Estazolam (Additive CNS depression).
No products indexed under this heading.

Ethacrynic Acid (The effectiveness of diuretics in patients with underlying renal or cardiovascular disease may by diminished by the concomitant administration of aspirin). Products include:
Edecrin Tablets **698**

Ethanol (Additive CNS depression).
No products indexed under this heading.

Ethchlorvynol (Additive CNS depression).
No products indexed under this heading.

Ethinamate (Additive CNS depression).
No products indexed under this heading.

Ethosuximide (Salicylate can displace protein-bound phenytoin and valproic acid, leading to a decrease in the total concentration of phenytoin and an increase in serum valproic acid levels).
No products indexed under this heading.

Ethotoin (Salicylate can displace protein-bound phenytoin and valproic acid, leading to a decrease in the total concentration of phenytoin and an increase in serum valproic acid levels).
No products indexed under this heading.

Ethyl Alcohol (Additive CNS depression).
No products indexed under this heading.

Etodolac (The concurrent use of aspirin with other NSAIDs should be avoided because this may increase bleeding or lead to decreased renal function).
No products indexed under this heading.

Felbamate (Salicylate can displace protein-bound phenytoin and valproic acid, leading to a decrease in the total concentration of phenytoin and an increase in serum valproic acid levels).
No products indexed under this heading.

Fenoprofen Calcium (The concurrent use of aspirin with other NSAIDs should be avoided because this may increase bleeding or lead to decreased renal function). Products include:
Nalfon Capsules **2508**

Fentanyl (Additive CNS depression). Products include:
Duragesic Transdermal System....... **2405**
Ionsys Transdermal System **2410**

Fentanyl Citrate (Additive CNS depression). Products include:
Actiq **959**
Fentora Tablets **968**

Fluphenazine Decanoate (Additive CNS depression).
No products indexed under this heading.

Fluphenazine Enanthate (Additive CNS depression).
No products indexed under this heading.

Fluphenazine Hydrochloride (Additive CNS depression).
No products indexed under this heading.

Flurazepam Hydrochloride (Additive CNS depression).
No products indexed under this heading.

Flurbiprofen (The concurrent use of aspirin with other NSAIDs should be avoided because this may increase bleeding or lead to decreased renal function).
No products indexed under this heading.

Fondaparinux Sodium (Enhanced effect of anticoagulant). Products include:
Arixtra Injection **1313**

Fosinopril Sodium (Reports suggested that NSAIDs may diminish the hyponatremic and hypotensive effect of ACE inhibitors).
No products indexed under this heading.

Fosphenytoin (Salicylate can displace protein-bound phenytoin and valproic acid, leading to a decrease in the total concentration of phenytoin and an increase in serum valproic acid levels).
No products indexed under this heading.

Fosphenytoin Sodium (Salicylate can displace protein-bound phenytoin and valproic acid, leading to a decrease in the total concentration of phenytoin and an increase in serum valproic acid levels).
No products indexed under this heading.

Furosemide (The effectiveness of diuretics in patients with underlying renal or cardiovascular disease may by diminished by the concomitant administration of aspirin). Products include:
Furosemide Tablets **2186**

Gabapentin (Salicylate can displace protein-bound phenytoin and valproic acid, leading to a decrease in the total concentration of phenytoin and an increase in serum valproic acid levels).
No products indexed under this heading.

Glimepiride (Aspirin may increase the serum glucose-lowering action of insulin and sulfonylureas leading to hypoglycemia). Products include:
Avandaryl Tablets **1344**
Duetact Tablets **3085**

Glipizide (Aspirin may increase the serum glucose-lowering action of insulin and sulfonylureas leading to hypoglycemia).
No products indexed under this heading.

Glutethimide (Additive CNS depression).
No products indexed under this heading.

Glyburide (Aspirin may increase the serum glucose-lowering action of insulin and sulfonylureas leading to hypoglycemia).
No products indexed under this heading.

Haloperidol (Additive CNS depression).
No products indexed under this heading.

Haloperidol Decanoate (Additive CNS depression).
No products indexed under this heading.

Heparin Calcium (Enhanced effect of anticoagulant).
No products indexed under this heading.

Heparin Sodium (Enhanced effect of anticoagulant).
No products indexed under this heading.

Hydrochlorothiazide (The effectiveness of diuretics in patients with underlying renal or cardiovascular disease may by diminished by the concomitant administration of aspirin). Products include:
Atacand HCT **642**
Avalide Tablets **892**
Avalide Tablets **2713**
Benicar HCT Tablets **1010**
Diovan HCT Tablets **2216**

Dyazide Capsules 1405
Micardis HCT Tablets 854
Prinzide Tablets 2092
Tekturna HCT Tablets 2324
Teveten HCT Tablets 517

Hydrocodone Bitartrate (Additive CNS depression). Products include:
Lortab 5/500 Tablets 3143
Lortab 7.5/500 Tablets 3144
Lortab 10/500 Tablets 3144
Vicodin Tablets 529
Vicodin ES Tablets 530
Vicodin HP Tablets 531
Vicoprofen Tablets 533
Zydone Tablets 1132

Hydrocodone Polistirex (Additive CNS depression). Products include:
Tussionex Pennkinetic Extended-Release Suspension 3154

Hydroflumethiazide (The effectiveness of diuretics in patients with underlying renal or cardiovascular disease may by diminished by the concomitant administration of aspirin).
No products indexed under this heading.

Hydromorphone Hydrochloride (Additive CNS depression).
No products indexed under this heading.

Hydroxyzine Hydrochloride (Additive CNS depression).
No products indexed under this heading.

Ibuprofen (The concurrent use of aspirin with other NSAIDs should be avoided because this may increase bleeding or lead to decreased renal function). Products include:
Motrin IB Tablets and Caplets 1900
Children's Motrin Oral Suspension ... 1901
Children's Motrin Non-Staining Dye-Free Oral Suspension 1901
Children's Motrin Cold Oral Suspension 1899
Infants' Motrin Concentrated Drops 1901
Infants' Motrin Non-Staining Dye-Free Concentrated Drops 1901
Junior Strength Motrin Caplets and Chewable Tablets 1901
Vicoprofen Tablets 533

Indapamide (The effectiveness of diuretics in patients with underlying renal or cardiovascular disease may by diminished by the concomitant administration of aspirin). Products include:
Indapamide Tablets 2188

Indomethacin (The concurrent use of aspirin with other NSAIDs should be avoided because this may increase bleeding or lead to decreased renal function). Products include:
Indocin 2024

Indomethacin Sodium Trihydrate (The concurrent use of aspirin with other NSAIDs should be avoided because this may increase bleeding or lead to decreased renal function). Products include:
Indocin I.V. 2489

Isoflurane (Additive CNS depression).
No products indexed under this heading.

Ketamine Hydrochloride (Additive CNS depression).
No products indexed under this heading.

Ketoprofen (The concurrent use of aspirin with other NSAIDs should be avoided because this may increase bleeding or lead to decreased renal function).
No products indexed under this heading.

Ketorolac Tromethamine (The concurrent use of aspirin with other NSAIDs should be avoided because this may increase bleeding or lead to decreased renal function).
No products indexed under this heading.

Labetalol Hydrochloride (The hypotensive effects of beta blockers may be diminished by concomitant administration of aspirin).
No products indexed under this heading.

Lamotrigine (Salicylate can displace protein-bound phenytoin and valproic acid, leading to a decrease in the total concentration of phenytoin and an increase in serum valproic acid levels). Products include:
Lamictal 1488

Levetiracetam (Salicylate can displace protein-bound phenytoin and valproic acid, leading to a decrease in the total concentration of phenytoin and an increase in serum valproic acid levels). Products include:
Keppra Injection 3137
Keppra Oral Solution 3131
Keppra Tablets 3131

Levobunolol Hydrochloride (The hypotensive effects of beta blockers may be diminished by concomitant administration of aspirin).
No products indexed under this heading.

Levomethadyl Acetate Hydrochloride (Additive CNS depression).
No products indexed under this heading.

Levorphanol Tartrate (Additive CNS depression).
No products indexed under this heading.

Lisinopril (Reports suggested that NSAIDs may diminish the hyponatremic and hypotensive effect of ACE inhibitors). Products include:
Prinivil Tablets 2087
Prinzide Tablets 2092

Lorazepam (Additive CNS depression).
No products indexed under this heading.

Low Molecular Weight Heparins (Enhanced effect of anticoagulant).
No products indexed under this heading.

Loxapine Hydrochloride (Additive CNS depression).
No products indexed under this heading.

Loxapine Succinate (Additive CNS depression).
No products indexed under this heading.

Meclofenamate Sodium (The concurrent use of aspirin with other NSAIDs should be avoided because this may increase bleeding or lead to decreased renal function).
No products indexed under this heading.

Mefenamic Acid (The concurrent use of aspirin with other NSAIDs should be avoided because this may increase bleeding or lead to decreased renal function).
No products indexed under this heading.

Meloxicam (The concurrent use of aspirin with other NSAIDs should be avoided because this may increase bleeding or lead to decreased renal function). Products include:
Mobic Oral Suspension 863
Mobic Tablets 863

Meperidine Hydrochloride (Additive CNS depression).
No products indexed under this heading.

Mephenytoin (Salicylate can displace protein-bound phenytoin and valproic acid, leading to a decrease in the total concentration of phenytoin and an increase in serum valproic acid levels).
No products indexed under this heading.

Mephobarbital (Additive CNS depression).
No products indexed under this heading.

Meprobamate (Additive CNS depression).
No products indexed under this heading.

Mesoridazine Besylate (Additive CNS depression).
No products indexed under this heading.

Metformin Hydrochloride (Aspirin may increase the serum glucose-lowering action of insulin and sulfonylureas leading to hypoglycemia). Products include:
ActoPlus Met Tablets 3071
Avandamet Tablets 1336
Janumet Tablets 2041
PrandiMet Tablets 2967

Methadone Hydrochloride (Additive CNS depression).
No products indexed under this heading.

Methohexital Sodium (Additive CNS depression).
No products indexed under this heading.

Methotrexate (Salicylate can inhibit renal clearance of methotrexate, leading to bone marrow toxicity, especially in the elderly or renal impaired).
No products indexed under this heading.

Methotrexate Sodium (Salicylate can inhibit renal clearance of methotrexate, leading to bone marrow toxicity, especially in the elderly or renal impaired).
No products indexed under this heading.

Methotrimeprazine (Additive CNS depression).
No products indexed under this heading.

Methoxyflurane (Additive CNS depression).
No products indexed under this heading.

Methsuximide (Salicylate can displace protein-bound phenytoin and valproic acid, leading to a decrease in the total concentration of phenytoin and an increase in serum valproic acid levels).
No products indexed under this heading.

Methyclothiazide (The effectiveness of diuretics in patients with underlying renal or cardiovascular disease may by diminished by the concomitant administration of aspirin).
No products indexed under this heading.

Metipranolol Hydrochloride (The hypotensive effects of beta blockers may be diminished by concomitant administration of aspirin).
No products indexed under this heading.

Metolazone (The effectiveness of diuretics in patients with underlying renal or cardiovascular disease may by diminished by the concomitant administration of aspirin).
No products indexed under this heading.

Metoprolol Succinate (The hypotensive effects of beta blockers may be diminished by concomitant administration of aspirin). Products include:
Toprol-XL Tablets 666

Metoprolol Tartrate (The hypotensive effects of beta blockers may be diminished by concomitant administration of aspirin).
No products indexed under this heading.

Midazolam Hydrochloride (Additive CNS depression).
No products indexed under this heading.

Miglitol (Aspirin may increase the serum glucose-lowering action of insulin and sulfonylureas leading to hypoglycemia).
No products indexed under this heading.

Moexipril Hydrochloride (Reports suggested that NSAIDs may diminish the hyponatremic and hypotensive effect of ACE inhibitors).
No products indexed under this heading.

Molindone Hydrochloride (Additive CNS depression). Products include:
Moban Tablets 1116

Morphine Sulfate (Additive CNS depression). Products include:
Avinza Capsules 1772
DepoDur Injection 1095
MS Contin Tablets 2585

Nabumetone (The concurrent use of aspirin with other NSAIDs should be avoided because this may increase bleeding or lead to decreased renal function).
No products indexed under this heading.

Nadolol (The hypotensive effects of beta blockers may be diminished by concomitant administration of aspirin). Products include:
Nadolol Tablets 2191

Nalbuphine Hydrochloride (Agonist/antagonist analgesics may reduce the analgesic effect of oxycodone or may precipitate withdrawal symptoms).
No products indexed under this heading.

Naproxen (The concurrent use of aspirin with other NSAIDs should be avoided because this may increase bleeding or lead to decreased renal function). Products include:
EC-Naprosyn Delayed-Release Tablets 2632
Naprosyn Suspension 2632
Naprosyn Tablets 2632

Naproxen Sodium (The concurrent use of aspirin with other NSAIDs should be avoided because this may increase bleeding or lead to decreased renal function). Products include:
Anaprox Tablets 2632
Anaprox DS Tablets 2632
Treximet Tablets 1616

Nateglinide (Aspirin may increase the serum glucose-lowering action of insulin and sulfonylureas leading to hypoglycemia). Products include:
Starlix Tablets 2314

Nebivolol (The hypotensive effects of beta blockers may be diminished by concomitant administration of aspirin). Products include:
Bystolic Tablets ... 1155

Olanzapine (Additive CNS depression). Products include:
Symbyax Capsules ... 1871
Zyprexa Tablets ... 1883
Zyprexa IntraMuscular ... 1883
Zyprexa ZYDIS Orally Disintegrating Tablets ... 1883

Oxaprozin (The concurrent use of aspirin with other NSAIDs should be avoided because this may increase bleeding or lead to decreased renal function).
No products indexed under this heading.

Oxazepam (Additive CNS depression).
No products indexed under this heading.

Oxcarbazepine (Salicylate can displace protein-bound phenytoin and valproic acid, leading to a decrease in the total concentration of phenytoin and an increase in serum valproic acid levels).
No products indexed under this heading.

Paramethadione (Salicylate can displace protein-bound phenytoin and valproic acid, leading to a decrease in the total concentration of phenytoin and an increase in serum valproic acid levels).
No products indexed under this heading.

Penbutolol Sulfate (The hypotensive effects of beta blockers may be diminished by concomitant administration of aspirin).
No products indexed under this heading.

Pentazocine Hydrochloride (Agonist/antagonist analgesics may reduce the analgesic effect of oxycodone or may precipitate withdrawal symptoms).
No products indexed under this heading.

Pentazocine Lactate (Agonist/antagonist analgesics may reduce the analgesic effect of oxycodone or may precipitate withdrawal symptoms).
No products indexed under this heading.

Pentobarbital Sodium (Additive CNS depression). Products include:
Nembutal Sodium Solution, USP ... 2494

Perindopril Erbumine (Reports suggested that NSAIDs may diminish the hyponatremic and hypotensive effect of ACE inhibitors). Products include:
Aceon Tablets (2 mg, 4 mg, 8 mg) ... 3038

Perphenazine (Additive CNS depression).
No products indexed under this heading.

Phenacemide (Salicylate can displace protein-bound phenytoin and valproic acid, leading to a decrease in the total concentration of phenytoin and an increase in serum valproic acid levels).
No products indexed under this heading.

Phenobarbital (Additive CNS depression). Products include:
Donnatal Extentabs ... 2507

Phensuximide (Salicylate can displace protein-bound phenytoin and valproic acid, leading to a decrease in the total concentration of phenytoin and an increase in serum valproic acid levels).
No products indexed under this heading.

Phenylbutazone (The concurrent use of aspirin with other NSAIDs should be avoided because this may increase bleeding or lead to decreased renal function).
No products indexed under this heading.

Phenytoin (Salicylate can displace protein-bound phenytoin and valproic acid, leading to a decrease in the total concentration of phenytoin and an increase in serum valproic acid levels).
No products indexed under this heading.

Phenytoin Sodium (Salicylate can displace protein-bound phenytoin and valproic acid, leading to a decrease in the total concentration of phenytoin and an increase in serum valproic acid levels). Products include:
Phenytek Capsules ... 2192

Pindolol (The hypotensive effects of beta blockers may be diminished by concomitant administration of aspirin).
No products indexed under this heading.

Pioglitazone Hydrochloride (Aspirin may increase the serum glucose-lowering action of insulin and sulfonylureas leading to hypoglycemia). Products include:
ActoPlus Met Tablets ... 3071
Actos Tablets ... 3077
Duetact Tablets ... 3085

Piroxicam (The concurrent use of aspirin with other NSAIDs should be avoided because this may increase bleeding or lead to decreased renal function).
No products indexed under this heading.

Polythiazide (The effectiveness of diuretics in patients with underlying renal or cardiovascular disease may by diminished by the concomitant administration of aspirin).
No products indexed under this heading.

Prazepam (Additive CNS depression).
No products indexed under this heading.

Primidone (Salicylate can displace protein-bound phenytoin and valproic acid, leading to a decrease in the total concentration of phenytoin and an increase in serum valproic acid levels).
No products indexed under this heading.

Probenecid (Aspirin may inhibit the uricosuric effects).
No products indexed under this heading.

Prochlorperazine (Additive CNS depression).
No products indexed under this heading.

Promethazine Hydrochloride (Additive CNS depression).
No products indexed under this heading.

Propofol (Additive CNS depression).
No products indexed under this heading.

Propoxyphene Hydrochloride (Additive CNS depression).
No products indexed under this heading.

Propoxyphene Napsylate (Additive CNS depression).
No products indexed under this heading.

Propranolol Hydrochloride (The hypotensive effects of beta blockers may be diminished by concomitant administration of aspirin). Products include:
InnoPran XL Extended Release Capsules ... 1484

Quazepam (Additive CNS depression).
No products indexed under this heading.

Quetiapine Fumarate (Additive CNS depression).
No products indexed under this heading.

Quinapril Hydrochloride (Reports suggested that NSAIDs may diminish the hyponatremic and hypotensive effect of ACE inhibitors).
No products indexed under this heading.

Ramelteon (Additive CNS depression). Products include:
Rozerem Tablets ... 3091

Ramipril (Reports suggested that NSAIDs may diminish the hyponatremic and hypotensive effect of ACE inhibitors).
No products indexed under this heading.

Remifentanil Hydrochloride (Additive CNS depression).
No products indexed under this heading.

Repaglinide (Aspirin may increase the serum glucose-lowering action of insulin and sulfonylureas leading to hypoglycemia). Products include:
PrandiMet Tablets ... 2967
Prandin Tablets ... 2971

Risperidone (Additive CNS depression). Products include:
Risperdal Consta Long-Acting Injection ... 1753

Rofecoxib (The concurrent use of aspirin with other NSAIDs should be avoided because this may increase bleeding or lead to decreased renal function).
No products indexed under this heading.

Rosiglitazone Maleate (Aspirin may increase the serum glucose-lowering action of insulin and sulfonylureas leading to hypoglycemia). Products include:
Avandamet Tablets ... 1336
Avandaryl Tablets ... 1344
Avandia Tablets ... 1351

Secobarbital Sodium (Additive CNS depression).
No products indexed under this heading.

Sevoflurane (Additive CNS depression). Products include:
Ultane Liquid for Inhalation ... 524

Sitagliptin Phosphate (Aspirin may increase the serum glucose-lowering action of insulin and sulfonylureas leading to hypoglycemia). Products include:
Janumet Tablets ... 2041
Januvia Tablets ... 2048

Sodium Butabarbital (Additive CNS depression).
No products indexed under this heading.

Sodium Oxybate (Additive CNS depression). Products include:
Xyrem Oral Solution ... 1766

Sotalol Hydrochloride (The hypotensive effects of beta blockers may be diminished by concomitant administration of aspirin).
No products indexed under this heading.

Spirapril Hydrochloride (Reports suggested that NSAIDs may diminish the hyponatremic and hypotensive effect of ACE inhibitors).
No products indexed under this heading.

Spironolactone (The effectiveness of diuretics in patients with underlying renal or cardiovascular disease may by diminished by the concomitant administration of aspirin).
No products indexed under this heading.

Sufentanil Citrate (Additive CNS depression).
No products indexed under this heading.

Sulfinpyrazone (Aspirin may inhibit the uricosuric effects).
No products indexed under this heading.

Sulindac (The concurrent use of aspirin with other NSAIDs should be avoided because this may increase bleeding or lead to decreased renal function). Products include:
Clinoril Tablets ... 1962

Temazepam (Additive CNS depression).
No products indexed under this heading.

Thiamylal Sodium (Additive CNS depression).
No products indexed under this heading.

Thioridazine Hydrochloride (Additive CNS depression). Products include:
Thioridazine Hydrochloride Tablets ... 2195

Thiothixene (Additive CNS depression). Products include:
Thiothixene Capsules ... 2197

Tiagabine Hydrochloride (Salicylate can displace protein-bound phenytoin and valproic acid, leading to a decrease in the total concentration of phenytoin and an increase in serum valproic acid levels). Products include:
Gabitril Tablets ... 973

Timolol Hemihydrate (The hypotensive effects of beta blockers may be diminished by concomitant administration of aspirin). Products include:
Betimol Ophthalmic Solution ... 3181

Timolol Maleate (The hypotensive effects of beta blockers may be diminished by concomitant administration of aspirin). Products include:
Combigan Ophthalmic Solution ... 553
Cosopt Sterile Ophthalmic Solution ... 1969
Timoptic Sterile Ophthalmic Solution ... 2121
Timoptic in Ocudose ... 2124
Timoptic-XE Sterile Ophthalmic Gel Forming Solution ... 2125

Tinzaparin Sodium (Enhanced effect of anticoagulant).
No products indexed under this heading.

Tolazamide (Aspirin may increase the serum glucose-lowering action of insulin and sulfonylureas leading to hypoglycemia).
No products indexed under this heading.

Tolbutamide (Aspirin may increase the serum glucose-lowering action of insulin and sulfonylureas leading to hypoglycemia).
No products indexed under this heading.

Tolmetin Sodium (The concurrent use of aspirin with other NSAIDs should be avoided because this may increase bleeding or lead to decreased renal function).
No products indexed under this heading.

Topiramate (Salicylate can displace protein-bound phenytoin and valproic acid, leading to a decrease in the total concentration of phenytoin and an increase in serum valproic acid levels).
No products indexed under this heading.

Torsemide (The effectiveness of diuretics in patients with underlying renal or cardiovascular disease may by diminished by the concomitant administration of aspirin). Products include:
Demadex Injection ... 2630
Demadex Tablets ... 2630

Trandolapril (Reports suggested that NSAIDs may diminish the hyponatremic and hypotensive effect of ACE inhibitors). Products include:
Mavik Tablets ... 472
Tarka Tablets ... 511

Triamterene (The effectiveness of diuretics in patients with underlying renal or cardiovascular disease may by diminished by the concomitant administration of aspirin). Products include:
Dyazide Capsules ... 1405
Dyrenium Capsules ... 3189

Triazolam (Additive CNS depression).
No products indexed under this heading.

Trifluoperazine Hydrochloride (Additive CNS depression).
No products indexed under this heading.

Trimethadione (Salicylate can displace protein-bound phenytoin and valproic acid, leading to a decrease in the total concentration of phenytoin and an increase in serum valproic acid levels).
No products indexed under this heading.

Troglitazone (Aspirin may increase the serum glucose-lowering action of insulin and sulfonylureas leading to hypoglycemia).
No products indexed under this heading.

Valdecoxib (The concurrent use of aspirin with other NSAIDs should be avoided because this may increase bleeding or lead to decreased renal function).
No products indexed under this heading.

Valproate Sodium (Salicylate can displace protein-bound phenytoin and valproic acid, leading to a decrease in the total concentration of phenytoin and an increase in serum valproic acid levels).
No products indexed under this heading.

Valproic Acid (Salicylate can displace protein-bound phenytoin and valproic acid, leading to a decrease in the total concentration of phenytoin and an increase in serum valproic acid levels).
No products indexed under this heading.

Warfarin Sodium (Enhanced effect of anticoagulant).
No products indexed under this heading.

Zaleplon (Additive CNS depression).
No products indexed under this heading.

Ziprasidone Hydrochloride (Additive CNS depression). Products include:
Geodon Capsules ... 2520

Zolpidem Tartrate (Additive CNS depression). Products include:
Ambien Tablets ... 2692
Ambien CR Tablets ... 2696

Zonisamide (Salicylate can displace protein-bound phenytoin and valproic acid, leading to a decrease in the total concentration of phenytoin and an increase in serum valproic acid levels). Products include:
Zonegran Capsules ... 1089

Food Interactions

Alcohol (Additive CNS depression).

PERFOROMIST INHALATION SOLUTION

(Formoterol Fumarate) ... 1025
May interact with beta blockers, diuretics, glucocorticoids, monoamine oxidase inhibitors, nonpotassium-sparing diuretics, drugs that prolong the QT interval, sympathomimetics, tricyclic antidepressants, and xanthines. Compounds in these categories include:

Acebutolol Hydrochloride (Co-administration with beta-blockers may inhibit the effect of each other. Beta-blockers not only block the therapeutic effect of beta-agonists, such as formoterol, but may produce severe bronchospasm in patients with asthma).
No products indexed under this heading.

Albuterol (Co-administration with additional adrenergic drugs may potentiate the sympathetic effects of formoterol).
No products indexed under this heading.

Albuterol Sulfate (Co-administration with additional adrenergic drugs may potentiate the sympathetic effects of formoterol). Products include:
Combivent Inhalation Aerosol ... 845
ProAir HFA Inhalation Aerosol ... 3113
Proventil HFA Inhalation Aerosol ... 2914
Ventolin HFA Inhalation Aerosol ... 1638

Alprazolam (Co-administration with drugs known to prolong the QTc interval may lead to an increased risk of ventricular arrhythmias; co-administer with extreme caution).
No products indexed under this heading.

Amiloride Hydrochloride (Concomitant treatment with diuretics may potentiate any hypokalemic effect of adrenergic agonists).
No products indexed under this heading.

Aminophylline (Co-administration with xanthine derivatives may potentiate hypokalemic effect of adrenergic agonists).
No products indexed under this heading.

Amiodarone Hydrochloride (Co-administration with drugs known to prolong the QTc interval may lead to an increased risk of ventricular arrhythmias; co-administer with extreme caution).
No products indexed under this heading.

Amitriptyline Hydrochloride (Concurrent and/or sequential administration with tricyclic antidepressants may potentiate the action of adrenergic agonists on the cardiovascular system; co-administer with extreme caution).
No products indexed under this heading.

Amoxapine (Concurrent and/or sequential administration with tricyclic antidepressants may potentiate the action of adrenergic agonists on the cardiovascular system; co-administer with extreme caution).
No products indexed under this heading.

Astemizole (Co-administration with drugs known to prolong the QTc interval may lead to an increased risk of ventricular arrhythmias; co-administer with extreme caution).
No products indexed under this heading.

Atenolol (Co-administration with beta-blockers may inhibit the effect of each other. Beta-blockers not only block the therapeutic effect of beta-agonists, such as formoterol, but may produce severe bronchospasm in patients with asthma).
No products indexed under this heading.

Bendroflumethiazide (The ECG changes and/or hypokalemia that may result from the administration of non-potassium sparing diuretics can be acutely worsened by beta-agonists, especially when the recommended dose of beta-agonist is exceeded).
No products indexed under this heading.

Betamethasone Acetate (Co-administration with glucocorticosteroids may potentiate hypokalemic effect of adrenergic agonists).
No products indexed under this heading.

Betamethasone Sodium Phosphate (Co-administration with glucocorticosteroids may potentiate hypokalemic effect of adrenergic agonists).
No products indexed under this heading.

Betaxolol Hydrochloride (Co-administration with beta-blockers may inhibit the effect of each other. Beta-blockers not only block the therapeutic effect of beta-agonists, such as formoterol, but may produce severe bronchospasm in patients with asthma).
No products indexed under this heading.

Bisoprolol Fumarate (Co-administration with beta-blockers may inhibit the effect of each other. Beta-blockers not only block the therapeutic effect of beta-agonists, such as formoterol, but may produce severe bronchospasm in patients with asthma).
No products indexed under this heading.

Bretylium Tosylate (Co-administration with drugs known to prolong the QTc interval may lead to an increased risk of ventricular arrhythmias; co-administer with extreme caution).
No products indexed under this heading.

Bumetanide (The ECG changes and/or hypokalemia that may result from the administration of non-potassium sparing diuretics can be acutely worsened by beta-agonists, especially when the recommended dose of beta-agonist is exceeded).
No products indexed under this heading.

Buspirone Hydrochloride (Co-administration with drugs known to prolong the QTc interval may lead to an increased risk of ventricular arrhythmias; co-administer with extreme caution).
No products indexed under this heading.

Carteolol Hydrochloride (Co-administration with beta-blockers may inhibit the effect of each other. Beta-blockers not only block the therapeutic effect of beta-agonists, such as formoterol, but may produce severe bronchospasm in patients with asthma).
No products indexed under this heading.

Chlordiazepoxide (Co-administration with drugs known to prolong the QTc interval may lead to an increased risk of ventricular arrhythmias; co-administer with extreme caution).
No products indexed under this heading.

Chlordiazepoxide Hydrochloride (Co-administration with drugs known to prolong the QTc interval may lead to an increased risk of ventricular arrhythmias; co-administer with extreme caution).
No products indexed under this heading.

Chlorothiazide (The ECG changes and/or hypokalemia that may result from the administration of non-potassium sparing diuretics can be acutely worsened by beta-agonists, especially when the recommended dose of beta-agonist is exceeded).
No products indexed under this heading.

Chlorothiazide Sodium (The ECG changes and/or hypokalemia that may result from the administration of non-potassium sparing diuretics can be acutely worsened by beta-agonists, especially when the recommended dose of beta-agonist is exceeded). Products include:
Intravenous Sodium Diuril ... 2490

Chlorpromazine (Co-administration with drugs known to prolong the QTc interval may lead to an increased risk of ventricular arrhythmias; co-administer with extreme caution).
No products indexed under this heading.

Chlorpromazine Hydrochloride (Co-administration with drugs known to prolong the QTc interval may lead to an increased risk of ventricular arrhythmias; co-administer with extreme caution).
No products indexed under this heading.

Chlorprothixene (Co-administration with drugs known to prolong the QTc interval may lead to an increased risk of ventricular arrhythmias; co-administer with extreme caution).
No products indexed under this heading.

Chlorprothixene Hydrochloride (Co-administration with drugs known to prolong the QTc interval may lead to an increased risk of ventricular arrhythmias; co-administer with extreme caution).
No products indexed under this heading.

Chlorthalidone (Concomitant treatment with diuretics may potentiate any hypokalemic effect of adrenergic agonists). Products include:
Clorpres Tablets **2185**

Clomipramine Hydrochloride (Concurrent and/or sequential administration with tricyclic antidepressants may potentiate the action of adrenergic agonists on the cardiovascular system; co-administer with extreme caution).
No products indexed under this heading.

Clorazepate Dipotassium (Co-administration with drugs known to prolong the QTc interval may lead to an increased risk of ventricular arrhythmias; co-administer with extreme caution).
No products indexed under this heading.

Clozapine (Co-administration with drugs known to prolong the QTc interval may lead to an increased risk of ventricular arrhythmias; co-administer with extreme caution).
No products indexed under this heading.

Cortisone Acetate (Co-administration with glucocorticosteroids may potentiate hypokalemic effect of adrenergic agonists).
No products indexed under this heading.

Desipramine Hydrochloride (Concurrent and/or sequential administration with tricyclic antidepressants may potentiate the action of adrenergic agonists on the cardiovascular system; co-administer with extreme caution).
No products indexed under this heading.

Dexamethasone (Co-administration with glucocorticosteroids may potentiate hypokalemic effect of adrenergic agonists). Products include:
Ciprodex Otic Suspension **541**

Dexamethasone Acetate (Co-administration with glucocorticosteroids may potentiate hypokalemic effect of adrenergic agonists).
No products indexed under this heading.

Dexamethasone Sodium Phosphate (Co-administration with glucocorticosteroids may potentiate hypokalemic effect of adrenergic agonists).
No products indexed under this heading.

Diazepam (Co-administration with drugs known to prolong the QTc interval may lead to an increased risk of ventricular arrhythmias; co-administer with extreme caution). Products include:
Valium Tablets **2658**

Disopyramide Phosphate (Co-administration with drugs known to prolong the QTc interval may lead to an increased risk of ventricular arrhythmias; co-administer with extreme caution).
No products indexed under this heading.

Dobutamine Hydrochloride (Co-administration with additional adrenergic drugs may potentiate the sympathetic effects of formoterol).
No products indexed under this heading.

Dofetilide (Co-administration with drugs known to prolong the QTc interval may lead to an increased risk of ventricular arrhythmias; co-administer with extreme caution).
No products indexed under this heading.

Dopamine Hydrochloride (Co-administration with additional adrenergic drugs may potentiate the sympathetic effects of formoterol).
No products indexed under this heading.

Doxepin Hydrochloride (Concurrent and/or sequential administration with tricyclic antidepressants may potentiate the action of adrenergic agonists on the cardiovascular system; co-administer with extreme caution).
No products indexed under this heading.

Droperidol (Co-administration with drugs known to prolong the QTc interval may lead to an increased risk of ventricular arrhythmias; co-administer with extreme caution).
No products indexed under this heading.

Dyphylline (Co-administration with xanthine derivatives may potentiate hypokalemic effect of adrenergic agonists).
No products indexed under this heading.

Ephedrine Hydrochloride (Co-administration with additional adrenergic drugs may potentiate the sympathetic effects of formoterol).
No products indexed under this heading.

Ephedrine Sulfate (Co-administration with additional adrenergic drugs may potentiate the sympathetic effects of formoterol).
No products indexed under this heading.

Ephedrine Tannate (Co-administration with additional adrenergic drugs may potentiate the sympathetic effects of formoterol).
No products indexed under this heading.

Epinephrine (Co-administration with additional adrenergic drugs may potentiate the sympathetic effects of formoterol). Products include:
EpiPen **1024**

Epinephrine Bitartrate (Co-administration with additional adrenergic drugs may potentiate the sympathetic effects of formoterol).
No products indexed under this heading.

Epinephrine Hydrochloride (Co-administration with additional adrenergic drugs may potentiate the sympathetic effects of formoterol).
No products indexed under this heading.

Erythromycin (Co-administration with drugs known to prolong the QTc interval may lead to an increased risk of ventricular arrhythmias; co-administer with extreme caution).
No products indexed under this heading.

Erythromycin Estolate (Co-administration with drugs known to prolong the QTc interval may lead to an increased risk of ventricular arrhythmias; co-administer with extreme caution).
No products indexed under this heading.

Erythromycin Ethylsuccinate (Co-administration with drugs known to prolong the QTc interval may lead to an increased risk of ventricular arrhythmias; co-administer with extreme caution). Products include:
E.E.S. **433**
EryPed **431**

Erythromycin Gluceptate (Co-administration with drugs known to prolong the QTc interval may lead to an increased risk of ventricular arrhythmias; co-administer with extreme caution).
No products indexed under this heading.

Erythromycin Lactobionate (Co-administration with drugs known to prolong the QTc interval may lead to an increased risk of ventricular arrhythmias; co-administer with extreme caution).
No products indexed under this heading.

Erythromycin Stearate (Co-administration with drugs known to prolong the QTc interval may lead to an increased risk of ventricular arrhythmias; co-administer with extreme caution).
No products indexed under this heading.

Esmolol Hydrochloride (Co-administration with beta-blockers may inhibit the effect of each other. Beta-blockers not only block the therapeutic effect of beta-agonists, such as formoterol, but may produce severe bronchospasm in patients with asthma).
No products indexed under this heading.

Ethacrynic Acid (The ECG changes and/or hypokalemia that may result from the administration of non-potassium sparing diuretics can be acutely worsened by beta-agonists, especially when the recommended dose of beta-agonist is exceeded). Products include:
Edecrin Tablets **698**

Flecainide Acetate (Co-administration with drugs known to prolong the QTc interval may lead to an increased risk of ventricular arrhythmias; co-administer with extreme caution).
No products indexed under this heading.

Fludrocortisone Acetate (Co-administration with glucocorticosteroids may potentiate hypokalemic effect of adrenergic agonists).
No products indexed under this heading.

Fluphenazine Decanoate (Co-administration with drugs known to prolong the QTc interval may lead to an increased risk of ventricular arrhythmias; co-administer with extreme caution).
No products indexed under this heading.

Fluphenazine Enanthate (Co-administration with drugs known to prolong the QTc interval may lead to an increased risk of ventricular arrhythmias; co-administer with extreme caution).
No products indexed under this heading.

Fluphenazine Hydrochloride (Co-administration with drugs known to prolong the QTc interval may lead to an increased risk of ventricular arrhythmias; co-administer with extreme caution).
No products indexed under this heading.

Furosemide (The ECG changes and/or hypokalemia that may result from the administration of non-potassium sparing diuretics can be acutely worsened by beta-agonists, especially when the recommended dose of beta-agonist is exceeded). Products include:
Furosemide Tablets **2186**

Haloperidol (Co-administration with drugs known to prolong the QTc interval may lead to an increased risk of ventricular arrhythmias; co-administer with extreme caution).
No products indexed under this heading.

Haloperidol Decanoate (Co-administration with drugs known to prolong the QTc interval may lead to an increased risk of ventricular arrhythmias; co-administer with extreme caution).
No products indexed under this heading.

Hydrochlorothiazide (The ECG changes and/or hypokalemia that may result from the administration of non-potassium sparing diuretics can be acutely worsened by beta-agonists, especially when the recommended dose of beta-agonist is exceeded). Products include:
Atacand HCT **642**
Avalide Tablets **892**
Avalide Tablets **2713**
Benicar HCT Tablets **1010**
Diovan HCT Tablets **2216**
Dyazide Capsules **1405**
Micardis HCT Tablets **854**
Prinzide Tablets **2092**
Tekturna HCT Tablets **2324**
Teveten HCT Tablets **517**

Hydrocortisone (Co-administration with glucocorticosteroids may potentiate hypokalemic effect of adrenergic agonists).
No products indexed under this heading.

Hydrocortisone Acetate (Co-administration with glucocorticosteroids may potentiate hypokalemic effect of adrenergic agonists). Products include:
Analpram-HC **1140**
Pramosone **1141**

Hydrocortisone Sodium Phosphate (Co-administration with glucocorticosteroids may potentiate hypokalemic effect of adrenergic agonists).
No products indexed under this heading.

Perphenazine (Co-administration with drugs known to prolong the QTc interval may lead to an increased risk of ventricular arrhythmias; co-administer with extreme caution).
No products indexed under this heading.

Phenelzine Sulfate (Concurent and/or sequential administration with MAO inhibitors may potentiate the action of adrenergic agonists on the cardiovascular system; co-administer with extreme caution).
No products indexed under this heading.

Phenylephrine Bitartrate (Co-administration with additional adrenergic drugs may potentiate the sympathetic effects of formoterol).
No products indexed under this heading.

Phenylephrine Hydrochloride (Co-administration with additional adrenergic drugs may potentiate the sympathetic effects of formoterol).
Products include:
Actifed Cold & Allergy Tablets 1895
Benadryl Allergy & Cold Kapgels 1895
Benadryl Allergy & Sinus Headache Kapgels 1895
Benadryl Severe Allergy & Sinus Headache Caplets 1897
Children's Benadryl-D Allergy & Sinus Liquid 1896
Benadryl-D Allergy & Sinus Tablet 1896
PediaCare Children's Allergy & Cold Liquid 1902
PediaCare Children's Decongestant Liquid.................... 1902
PediaCare Children's Liquid Multi-Symptom Cold.................... 1902
Sinutab Non-Drying Caplets 1905
Sinutab Sinus Caplets 1905
Children's Sudafed PE Cold & Cough Liquid 1907
Children's Sudafed PE Nasal Decongestant Liquid.................... 1906
Sudafed PE Cold & Cough Caplets.. 1907
Sudafed PE Nasal Decongestant Tablets.. 1907
Sudafed PE Nighttime Cold Caplets.. 1907
Sudafed PE Non-Drying Sinus Caplets.. 1908
Sudafed PE Severe Cold Caplets 1908
Sudafed PE Sinus & Allergy Tablets.. 1908
Sudafed PE Sinus Headache Caplets.. 1908
Tylenol Allergy Multi-Symptom Caplets with Cool Burst and Rapid Release Gelcaps.................... 1916
Tylenol Allergy Multi-Symptom Nighttime Caplets with Cool Burst.. 1916
Children's Tylenol Plus Cold Suspension Liquid 1912
Children's Tylenol Plus Cold & Allergy Suspension Liquid 1914
Children's Tylenol Plus Flu Suspension Liquid 1914
Children's Tylenol Plus Multi-Symptom Cold Suspension Liquid 1912
Tylenol Cold Head Congestion Daytime Caplets with Cool Burst.. 1910
Tylenol Cold Head Congestion Nighttime Caplets with Cool Burst.. 1910
Tylenol Cold Head Congestion Severe Daytime Caplets with Cool Burst.. 1910
Tylenol Cold Multi-Symptom Daytime Caplets with Cool Burst and Rapid Release Gels....... 1913
Tylenol Cold Multi-Symptom Daytime Liquid with Citrus Burst ... 1913
Tylenol Cold Multi-Symptom Nighttime Caplets with Cool Burst.. 1913
Tylenol Cold Multi-Symptom Nighttime Liquid with Cool Burst ... 1913
Tylenol Cold Multi-Symptom Severe Caplets with Cool Burst..... 1913
Tylenol Cold Multi-Symptom Severe Daytime Liquid with Citrus Burst................................ 1913
Tylenol Sinus Congestion & Pain Daytime Caplets with Cool Burst and Gelcaps...................... 1917
Tylenol Sinus Congestion & Pain Nighttime Caplets with Cool Burst.. 1917
Tylenol Sinus Congestion & Pain Severe Caplets with Cool Burst..... 1917
Vicks DayQuil Cold & Flu Multi-Symptom Relief .... ■616
Vicks DayQuil LiquiCaps 2567
Vicks DayQuil Liquid 2567
Vicks DayQuil Multi-Symptom Cold/Flu Relief................................ 2567

Phenylephrine Tannate (Co-administration with additional adrenergic drugs may potentiate the sympathetic effects of formoterol).
No products indexed under this heading.

Phenylpropanolamine Hydrochloride (Co-administration with additional adrenergic drugs may potentiate the sympathetic effects of formoterol).
No products indexed under this heading.

Pindolol (Co-administration with beta-blockers may inhibit the effect of each other. Beta-blockers not only block the therapeutic effect of beta-agonists, such as formoterol, but may produce severe bronchospasm in patients with asthma).
No products indexed under this heading.

Pirbuterol Acetate (Co-administration with additional adrenergic drugs may potentiate the sympathetic effects of formoterol).
Products include:
Maxair Autohaler 1705

Polythiazide (The ECG changes and/or hypokalemia that may result from the administration of non-potassium sparing diuretics can be acutely worsened by beta-agonists, especially when the recommended dose of beta-agonist is exceeded).
No products indexed under this heading.

Prazepam (Co-administration with drugs known to prolong the QTc interval may lead to an increased risk of ventricular arrhythmias; co-administer with extreme caution).
No products indexed under this heading.

Prednisolone Acetate (Co-administration with glucocorticosteroids may potentiate hypokalemic effect of adrenergic agonists).
Products include:
Pred Forte Ophthalmic Suspension .... ⊙227
Pred Mild Ophthalmic Suspension .... ⊙230
Pred-G Ophthalmic Ointment .... ⊙229
Pred-G Ophthalmic Suspension ...... ⊙228

Prednisolone Sodium Phosphate (Co-administration with glucocorticosteroids may potentiate hypokalemic effect of adrenergic agonists).
No products indexed under this heading.

Prednisolone Tebutate (Co-administration with glucocorticosteroids may potentiate hypokalemic effect of adrenergic agonists).
No products indexed under this heading.

Prednisone (Co-administration with glucocorticosteroids may potentiate hypokalemic effect of adrenergic agonists).
No products indexed under this heading.

Procainamide Hydrochloride (Co-administration with drugs known to prolong the QTc interval may lead to an increased risk of ventricular arrhythmias; co-administer with extreme caution).
No products indexed under this heading.

Procarbazine Hydrochloride (Concurent and/or sequential administration with MAO inhibitors may potentiate the action of adrenergic agonists on the cardiovascular system; co-administer with extreme caution).
No products indexed under this heading.

Prochlorperazine (Co-administration with drugs known to prolong the QTc interval may lead to an increased risk of ventricular arrhythmias; co-administer with extreme caution).
No products indexed under this heading.

Promethazine Hydrochloride (Co-administration with drugs known to prolong the QTc interval may lead to an increased risk of ventricular arrhythmias; co-administer with extreme caution).
No products indexed under this heading.

Propafenone Hydrochloride (Co-administration with drugs known to prolong the QTc interval may lead to an increased risk of ventricular arrhythmias; co-administer with extreme caution). Products include:
Rythmol Tablets 1586
Rythmol SR Capsules 1590

Propranolol Hydrochloride (Co-administration with beta-blockers may inhibit the effect of each other. Beta-blockers not only block the therapeutic effect of beta-agonists, such as formoterol, but may produce severe bronchospasm in patients with asthma). Products include:
InnoPran XL Extended Release Capsules.................................... 1484

Protriptyline Hydrochloride (Concurrent and/or sequential administration with tricyclic antidepressants may potentiate the action of adrenergic agonists on the cardiovascular system; co-administer with extreme caution).
No products indexed under this heading.

Pseudoephedrine Hydrochloride (Co-administration with additional adrenergic drugs may potentiate the sympathetic effects of formoterol).
Products include:
Allegra-D 12 Hour Extended-Release Tablets............ 2687
Allegra-D 24 Hour Extended-Release Tablets............ 2690
Children's Motrin Cold Oral Suspension 1899
Sudafed 12 Hour Nasal Decongestant Non-Drowsy Caplets.. 1909
Sudafed 24 Hour Non-Drowsy Nasal Decongestant Tablets......... 1906
Children's Sudafed Nasal Decongestant Liquid.................... 1906
Sudafed Nasal Decongestant Tablets.. 1906
Tylenol Cold Severe Congestion Daytime Caplets with Cool Burst.. 1912
Tylenol Sinus Severe Congestion Caplets with Cool Burst............... 1917
Vicks NyQuil LiquiCaps 2567
Vicks NyQuil Liquid 2567
Vicks NyQuil Multi-Symptom Cold/Flu Relief................................ 2567
Zyrtec-D 12 Hour Extended Release Tablets 1923
Zyrtec-D Allergy & Congestion Extended-Release Tablets............... 1923

Pseudoephedrine Sulfate (Co-administration with additional adrenergic drugs may potentiate the sympathetic effects of formoterol).
Products include:
Clarinex-D 12-Hour Extended-Release Tablets............ 2831
Clarinex-D 24-Hour Extended-Release Tablets............ 2834

Quetiapine Fumarate (Co-administration with drugs known to prolong the QTc interval may lead to an increased risk of ventricular arrhythmias; co-administer with extreme caution).
No products indexed under this heading.

Quinidine Gluconate (Co-administration with drugs known to prolong the QTc interval may lead to an increased risk of ventricular arrhythmias; co-administer with extreme caution).
No products indexed under this heading.

Quinidine Polygalacturonate (Co-administration with drugs known to prolong the QTc interval may lead to an increased risk of ventricular arrhythmias; co-administer with extreme caution).
No products indexed under this heading.

Quinidine Sulfate (Co-administration with drugs known to prolong the QTc interval may lead to an increased risk of ventricular arrhythmias; co-administer with extreme caution).
No products indexed under this heading.

Rasagiline Mesylate (Concurent and/or sequential administration with MAO inhibitors may potentiate the action of adrenergic agonists on the cardiovascular system; co-administer with extreme caution).
Products include:
Azilect Tablets 3106

Risperidone (Co-administration with drugs known to prolong the QTc interval may lead to an increased risk of ventricular arrhythmias; co-administer with extreme caution).
Products include:
Risperdal Consta Long-Acting Injection 1753

Salmeterol Xinafoate (Co-administration with additional adrenergic drugs may potentiate the sympathetic effects of formoterol).
Products include:
Advair Diskus 100/50 1276
Advair Diskus 250/50 1276
Advair Diskus 500/50 1276
Advair HFA 45/21 Inhalation Aerosol.. 1288
Advair HFA 115/21 Inhalation Aerosol.. 1288
Advair HFA 230/21 Inhalation Aerosol.. 1288
Serevent Diskus 1594

Selegiline (Concurent and/or sequential administration with MAO inhibitors may potentiate the action of adrenergic agonists on the cardio-

vascular system; co-administer with extreme caution). Products include:
Emsam Transdermal System 905

Selegiline Hydrochloride (Concurent and/or sequential administration with MAO inhibitors may potentiate the action of adrenergic agonists on the cardiovascular system; co-administer with extreme caution). Products include:
Eldepryl Capsules 3052

Sotalol Hydrochloride (Co-administration with beta-blockers may inhibit the effect of each other. Beta-blockers not only block the therapeutic effect of beta-agonists, such as formoterol, but may produce severe bronchospasm in patients with asthma).
No products indexed under this heading.

Spironolactone (Concomitant treatment with diuretics may potentiate any hypokalemic effect of adrenergic agonists).
No products indexed under this heading.

Terbutaline Sulfate (Co-administration with additional adrenergic drugs may potentiate the sympathetic effects of formoterol).
No products indexed under this heading.

Theophylline (Co-administration with xanthine derivatives may potentiate hypokalemic effect of adrenergic agonists).
No products indexed under this heading.

Theophylline Anhydrous (Co-administration with xanthine derivatives may potentiate hypokalemic effect of adrenergic agonists). Products include:
Uniphyl Tablets 2595

Theophylline Calcium Salicylate (Co-administration with xanthine derivatives may potentiate hypokalemic effect of adrenergic agonists).
No products indexed under this heading.

Theophylline Dihydroxypropyl (Glyceryl) (Co-administration with xanthine derivatives may potentiate hypokalemic effect of adrenergic agonists).
No products indexed under this heading.

Theophylline Ethylenediamine (Co-administration with xanthine derivatives may potentiate hypokalemic effect of adrenergic agonists).
No products indexed under this heading.

Theophylline Sodium Glycinate (Co-administration with xanthine derivatives may potentiate hypokalemic effect of adrenergic agonists).
No products indexed under this heading.

Thioridazine Hydrochloride (Co-administration with drugs known to prolong the QTc interval may lead to an increased risk of ventricular arrhythmias; co-administer with extreme caution). Products include:
Thioridazine Hydrochloride Tablets 2195

Thiothixene (Co-administration with drugs known to prolong the QTc interval may lead to an increased risk of ventricular arrhythmias; co-administer with extreme caution). Products include:
Thiothixene Capsules 2197

Timolol Hemihydrate (Co-administration with beta-blockers may inhibit the effect of each other. Beta-blockers not only block the therapeutic effect of beta-agonists, such as formoterol, but may produce severe bronchospasm in patients with asthma). Products include:
Betimol Ophthalmic Solution 3181

Timolol Maleate (Co-administration with beta-blockers may inhibit the effect of each other. Beta-blockers not only block the therapeutic effect of beta-agonists, such as formoterol, but may produce severe bronchospasm in patients with asthma). Products include:
Combigan Ophthalmic Solution 553
Cosopt Sterile Ophthalmic Solution....................................... 1969
Timoptic Sterile Ophthalmic Solution....................................... 2121
Timoptic in Ocudose 2124
Timoptic-XE Sterile Ophthalmic Gel Forming Solution 2125

Tocainide Hydrochloride (Co-administration with drugs known to prolong the QTc interval may lead to an increased risk of ventricular arrhythmias; co-administer with extreme caution).
No products indexed under this heading.

Torsemide (The ECG changes and/or hypokalemia that may result from the administration of non-potassium sparing diuretics can be acutely worsened by beta-agonists, especially when the recommended dose of beta-agonist is exceeded). Products include:
Demadex Injection 2630
Demadex Tablets 2630

Tranylcypromine Sulfate (Concurent and/or sequential administration with MAO inhibitors may potentiate the action of adrenergic agonists on the cardiovascular system; co-administer with extreme caution). Products include:
Parnate Tablets 1532

Triamcinolone (Co-administration with glucocorticosteroids may potentiate hypokalemic effect of adrenergic agonists).
No products indexed under this heading.

Triamcinolone Acetonide (Co-administration with glucocorticosteroids may potentiate hypokalemic effect of adrenergic agonists). Products include:
Azmacort Inhalation Aerosol 407
Nasacort AQ Nasal Spray 2765
Triesence Injectable Suspension .... ⊙209

Triamcinolone Diacetate (Co-administration with glucocorticosteroids may potentiate hypokalemic effect of adrenergic agonists).
No products indexed under this heading.

Triamcinolone Hexacetonide (Co-administration with glucocorticosteroids may potentiate hypokalemic effect of adrenergic agonists).
No products indexed under this heading.

Triamterene (Concomitant treatment with diuretics may potentiate any hypokalemic effect of adrenergic agonists). Products include:
Dyazide Capsules 1405
Dyrenium Capsules 3189

Trifluoperazine Hydrochloride (Co-administration with drugs known to prolong the QTc interval may lead to an increased risk of ventricular arrhythmias; co-administer with extreme caution).
No products indexed under this heading.

Trimipramine Maleate (Concurrent and/or sequential administration with tricyclic antidepressants may potentiate the action of adrenergic agonists on the cardiovascular system; co-administer with extreme caution).
No products indexed under this heading.

Ziprasidone Hydrochloride (Co-administration with drugs known to prolong the QTc interval may lead to an increased risk of ventricular arrhythmias; co-administer with extreme caution). Products include:
Geodon Capsules 2520

PERSANTINE TABLETS

(Dipyridamole) 869
May interact with anticholinesterase drugs and certain other agents. Compounds in these categories include:

Adenosine (Dipyridamole has been reported to increase the plasma levels and cardiovascular effects of adenosine. Adjustment of adenosine dosage may be necessary). Products include:
Adenocard IV Injection 603
Adenoscan 605

Donepezil Hydrochloride (Dipyridamole may counteract the anticholinesterase effect of cholinesterase inhibitors, thereby potentially aggravating myasthenia gravis). Products include:
Aricept Tablets 1062
Aricept ODT Tablets 1062

Galantamine Hydrobromide (Dipyridamole may counteract the anticholinesterase effect of cholinesterase inhibitors, thereby potentially aggravating myasthenia gravis).
No products indexed under this heading.

Neostigmine Bromide (Dipyridamole may counteract the anticholinesterase effect of cholinesterase inhibitors, thereby potentially aggravating myasthenia gravis).
No products indexed under this heading.

Neostigmine Methylsulfate (Dipyridamole may counteract the anticholinesterase effect of cholinesterase inhibitors, thereby potentially aggravating myasthenia gravis).
No products indexed under this heading.

Pyridostigmine Bromide (Dipyridamole may counteract the anticholinesterase effect of cholinesterase inhibitors, thereby potentially aggravating myasthenia gravis).
No products indexed under this heading.

Rivastigmine Tartrate (Dipyridamole may counteract the anticholinesterase effect of cholinesterase inhibitors, thereby potentially aggravating myasthenia gravis). Products include:
Exelon Capsules 2229
Exelon Oral Solution 2229
Exelon Patch 2233

Tacrine Hydrochloride (Dipyridamole may counteract the anticholinesterase effect of cholinesterase inhibitors, thereby potentially aggravating myasthenia gravis).
No products indexed under this heading.

PHENYTEK CAPSULES

(Phenytoin Sodium) 2192
May interact with chloramphenicol, corticosteroids, oral anticoagulants, doxycycline, estrogens, histamine H_2-receptor antagonists, oral contraceptives, phenothiazines, quinidine, salicylates, succinimides, tricyclic antidepressants, valproate, xanthines, and certain other agents. Compounds in these categories include:

Aminophylline (Phenytoin impairs efficacy of theophylline).
No products indexed under this heading.

Amiodarone Hydrochloride (May increase phenytoin serum levels).
No products indexed under this heading.

Amitriptyline Hydrochloride (Tricyclic antidepressants may precipitate seizures in susceptible patients and phenytoin dosage may need to be adjusted).
No products indexed under this heading.

Amoxapine (Tricyclic antidepressants may precipitate seizures in susceptible patients and phenytoin dosage may need to be adjusted).
No products indexed under this heading.

Anisindione (Phenytoin impairs efficacy of oral anticoagulants).
No products indexed under this heading.

Aspirin (May increase phenytoin serum levels). Products include:
Aggrenox Capsules 819
Bayer Aspirin 750
Percodan Tablets 1130
St. Joseph 81 mg Aspirin Chewable and Enteric Coated Tablets 1903

Aspirin, Enteric Coated (May increase phenytoin serum levels).
No products indexed under this heading.

Aspirin Buffered (May increase phenytoin serum levels).
No products indexed under this heading.

Betamethasone Acetate (Phenytoin impairs efficacy of corticosteroids).
No products indexed under this heading.

Betamethasone Sodium Phosphate (Phenytoin impairs efficacy of corticosteroids).
No products indexed under this heading.

Budesonide (Phenytoin impairs efficacy of corticosteroids). Products include:
Pulmicort Flexhaler 654
Symbicort 80/4.5 Inhalation Aerosol.. 659
Symbicort 160/4.5 Inhalation Aerosol.. 659

Calcium Carbonate (Ingestion times of phenytoin and antacid preparations containing calcium should be staggered in patients with low phenytoin levels to prevent absorption problems). Products include:
Accelerator Tablets .... ■634

Actonel with Calcium Tablets 2574
BioLean II Tablets 635
Calcet Triple Calcium + Vitamin D Tablets 629
D-Cal Chewable Caplets 624
Elixir Capsules 636
Pepcid Complete Chewable Tablets 1771
Extra Strength Rolaids Plus Gas Relief Tropical Fruit Softchews 1903
Extra Strength Rolaids Softchews Vanilla Creme 1903
Extra Strength Rolaids Freshmint Tablets 1903
Rolaids Multi-Symptom Berry Tablets 1903
Rolaids Original Peppermint Tablets 1903

Carbamazepine (May increase phenytoin serum levels). Products include:
Carbatrol Capsules 3019
Equetro Extended-Release Capsules 3174

Chloramphenicol (May increase phenytoin serum levels).
No products indexed under this heading.

Chloramphenicol Palmitate (May increase phenytoin serum levels).
No products indexed under this heading.

Chloramphenicol Sodium Succinate (May increase phenytoin serum levels).
No products indexed under this heading.

Chlordiazepoxide (May increase phenytoin serum levels).
No products indexed under this heading.

Chlordiazepoxide Hydrochloride (May increase phenytoin serum levels).
No products indexed under this heading.

Chlorotrianisene (May increase phenytoin serum levels; phenytoin impairs efficacy of estrogens).
No products indexed under this heading.

Chlorpromazine (Phenothiazines may increase phenytoin serum levels).
No products indexed under this heading.

Chlorpromazine Hydrochloride (Phenothiazines may increase phenytoin serum levels).
No products indexed under this heading.

Choline Magnesium Trisalicylate (May increase phenytoin serum levels).
No products indexed under this heading.

Ciclesonide (Phenytoin impairs efficacy of corticosteroids). Products include:
Alvesco Inhalation Aerosol 2985
Omnaris Nasal Spray 2998

Cimetidine (May increase phenytoin serum levels).
No products indexed under this heading.

Cimetidine Hydrochloride (May increase phenytoin serum levels).
No products indexed under this heading.

Clomipramine Hydrochloride (Tricyclic antidepressants may precipitate seizures in susceptible patients and phenytoin dosage may need to be adjusted).
No products indexed under this heading.

Cortisone Acetate (Phenytoin impairs efficacy of corticosteroids).
No products indexed under this heading.

Desipramine Hydrochloride (Tricyclic antidepressants may precipitate seizures in susceptible patients and phenytoin dosage may need to be adjusted).
No products indexed under this heading.

Desogestrel (Phenytoin impairs efficacy of oral contraceptives). Products include:
Mircette Tablets 1034

Dexamethasone (Phenytoin impairs efficacy of corticosteroids). Products include:
Ciprodex Otic Suspension 541

Dexamethasone Acetate (Phenytoin impairs efficacy of corticosteroids).
No products indexed under this heading.

Dexamethasone Sodium Phosphate (Phenytoin impairs efficacy of corticosteroids).
No products indexed under this heading.

Diazepam (May increase phenytoin serum levels). Products include:
Valium Tablets 2658

Dicumarol (May increase phenytoin serum levels; phenytoin impairs efficacy of oral anticoagulants).
No products indexed under this heading.

Dienestrol (May increase phenytoin serum levels; phenytoin impairs efficacy of estrogens).
No products indexed under this heading.

Diethylstilbestrol (May increase phenytoin serum levels; phenytoin impairs efficacy of estrogens).
No products indexed under this heading.

Diflunisal (May increase phenytoin serum levels).
No products indexed under this heading.

Digitoxin (Phenytoin impairs efficacy of digitoxin).
No products indexed under this heading.

Disulfiram (May increase phenytoin serum levels).
No products indexed under this heading.

Divalproex Sodium (May decrease or increase phenytoin serum levels; the effect of phenytoin on valproate serum levels is unpredictable). Products include:
Depakote ER Tablets 423

Doxepin Hydrochloride (Tricyclic antidepressants may precipitate seizures in susceptible patients and phenytoin dosage may need to be adjusted).
No products indexed under this heading.

Doxycycline Calcium (Phenytoin impairs efficacy of doxycycline).
No products indexed under this heading.

Doxycycline Hyclate (Phenytoin impairs efficacy of doxycycline).
No products indexed under this heading.

Doxycycline Monohydrate (Phenytoin impairs efficacy of doxycycline).
No products indexed under this heading.

Dyphylline (Phenytoin impairs efficacy of theophylline).
No products indexed under this heading.

Estradiol (May increase phenytoin serum levels; phenytoin impairs efficacy of estrogens). Products include:
Activella Tablets 2347
Angeliq Tablets 751
Climara Transdermal System 763
Climara Pro Transdermal System 768
Divigel 3167
Vagifem Tablets 2375

Estrogens, Conjugated (May increase phenytoin serum levels; phenytoin impairs efficacy of estrogens). Products include:
Premarin Intravenous 3217
Premarin Tablets 3221
Premarin Vaginal Cream 3228
Premphase Tablets 3232
Prempro Tablets 3232

Estrogens, Esterified (May increase phenytoin serum levels; phenytoin impairs efficacy of estrogens). Products include:
Estratest Tablets 3043
Estratest H.S. Tablets 3043

Estropipate (May increase phenytoin serum levels; phenytoin impairs efficacy of estrogens).
No products indexed under this heading.

Ethinyl Estradiol (May increase phenytoin serum levels; phenytoin impairs efficacy of estrogens). Products include:
Lybrel Tablets 3204
Mircette Tablets 1034
NuvaRing 2897
Ortho-Cyclen/Ortho Tri-Cyclen 2449
Ortho Evra Transdermal System 2437
Ortho Tri-Cyclen Lo Tablets 2458
Seasonique Tablets 1046
Yaz Tablets 805

Ethosuximide (May increase phenytoin serum levels).
No products indexed under this heading.

Ethynodiol Diacetate (Phenytoin impairs efficacy of oral contraceptives).
No products indexed under this heading.

Famotidine (May increase phenytoin serum levels). Products include:
Pepcid Tablets 2075
Original Strength Pepcid AC Gelcaps 1771
Original Strength Pepcid AC Tablets 1771
Maximum Strength Pepcid AC Tablets 1771
Pepcid Complete Chewable Tablets 1771

Fludrocortisone Acetate (Phenytoin impairs efficacy of corticosteroids).
No products indexed under this heading.

Flunisolide (Phenytoin impairs efficacy of corticosteroids). Products include:
Aerobid/Aerobid-M 1153

Fluphenazine Decanoate (Phenothiazines may increase phenytoin serum levels).
No products indexed under this heading.

Fluphenazine Enanthate (Phenothiazines may increase phenytoin serum levels).
No products indexed under this heading.

Fluphenazine Hydrochloride (Phenothiazines may increase phenytoin serum levels).
No products indexed under this heading.

Fluticasone Propionate (Phenytoin impairs efficacy of corticosteroids). Products include:
Advair Diskus 100/50 1276
Advair Diskus 250/50 1276
Advair Diskus 500/50 1276
Advair HFA 45/21 Inhalation Aerosol 1288
Advair HFA 115/21 Inhalation Aerosol 1288
Advair HFA 230/21 Inhalation Aerosol 1288
Flonase Nasal Spray 1431
Flovent Diskus 50 mcg 1435

Fluticasone Propionate HFA (Phenytoin impairs efficacy of corticosteroids). Products include:
Flovent HFA 1440

Furosemide (Phenytoin impairs efficacy of furosemide). Products include:
Furosemide Tablets 2186

Halothane (May increase phenytoin serum levels).
No products indexed under this heading.

Hydrocortisone (Phenytoin impairs efficacy of corticosteroids).
No products indexed under this heading.

Hydrocortisone Acetate (Phenytoin impairs efficacy of corticosteroids). Products include:
Analpram-HC 1140
Pramosone 1141

Hydrocortisone Sodium Phosphate (Phenytoin impairs efficacy of corticosteroids).
No products indexed under this heading.

Hydrocortisone Sodium Succinate (Phenytoin impairs efficacy of corticosteroids).
No products indexed under this heading.

Imipramine Hydrochloride (Tricyclic antidepressants may precipitate seizures in susceptible patients and phenytoin dosage may need to be adjusted).
No products indexed under this heading.

Imipramine Pamoate (Tricyclic antidepressants may precipitate seizures in susceptible patients and phenytoin dosage may need to be adjusted).
No products indexed under this heading.

Isoniazid (May increase phenytoin serum levels).
No products indexed under this heading.

Levonorgestrel (Phenytoin impairs efficacy of oral contraceptives). Products include:
Climara Pro Transdermal System 768
Lybrel Tablets 3204
Mirena Intrauterine System 779
Plan B Tablets 1044
Seasonique Tablets 1046

Magnesium Salicylate (May increase phenytoin serum levels).
No products indexed under this heading.

Maprotiline Hydrochloride (Tricyclic antidepressants may precipitate seizures in susceptible patients and phenytoin dosage may need to be adjusted).
No products indexed under this heading.

IMPORTANT NOTE: Always consult each drug listing in the patient's regimen for possible interactions.

Mesoridazine Besylate (Phenothiazines may increase phenytoin serum levels).
No products indexed under this heading.

Mestranol (Phenytoin impairs efficacy of oral contraceptives).
No products indexed under this heading.

Methotrimeprazine (Phenothiazines may increase phenytoin serum levels).
No products indexed under this heading.

Methsuximide (May increase phenytoin serum levels).
No products indexed under this heading.

Methylphenidate Hydrochloride (May increase phenytoin serum levels). Products include:
Concerta Extended-Release Tablets 1925
Metadate CD Capsules 3146

Methylprednisolone Acetate (Phenytoin impairs efficacy of corticosteroids).
No products indexed under this heading.

Methylprednisolone Sodium Succinate (Phenytoin impairs efficacy of corticosteroids).
No products indexed under this heading.

Molindone Hydrochloride (Contains calcium ions which may decrease phenytoin serum levels). Products include:
Moban Tablets 1116

Mometasone Furoate (Phenytoin impairs efficacy of corticosteroids). Products include:
Asmanex Twisthaler 2797
Elocon Cream 0.1% 2840
Elocon Lotion 0.1% 2841
Elocon Ointment 0.1% 2842

Mometasone Furoate Monohydrate (Phenytoin impairs efficacy of corticosteroids). Products include:
Nasonex Nasal Spray 2883

Nizatidine (May increase phenytoin serum levels). Products include:
Axid Capsules 1364

Norethindrone (Phenytoin impairs efficacy of oral contraceptives). Products include:
Ortho Micronor Tablets 2446

Norethynodrel (Phenytoin impairs efficacy of oral contraceptives).
No products indexed under this heading.

Norgestimate (Phenytoin impairs efficacy of oral contraceptives). Products include:
Ortho-Cyclen/Ortho Tri-Cyclen 2449
Ortho Tri-Cyclen Lo Tablets 2458

Norgestrel (Phenytoin impairs efficacy of oral contraceptives).
No products indexed under this heading.

Nortriptyline Hydrochloride (Tricyclic antidepressants may precipitate seizures in susceptible patients and phenytoin dosage may need to be adjusted).
No products indexed under this heading.

Perphenazine (Phenothiazines may increase phenytoin serum levels).
No products indexed under this heading.

Phenobarbital (May decrease or increase phenytoin serum levels; the effect of phenytoin on phenobarbital serum levels is unpredictable). Products include:
Donnatal Extentabs 2507

Phensuximide (May increase phenytoin serum levels).
No products indexed under this heading.

Phenylbutazone (May increase phenytoin serum levels).
No products indexed under this heading.

Polyestradiol Phosphate (May increase phenytoin serum levels; phenytoin impairs efficacy of estrogens).
No products indexed under this heading.

Prednisolone Acetate (Phenytoin impairs efficacy of corticosteroids). Products include:
Pred Forte Ophthalmic Suspension .... ⊙227
Pred Mild Ophthalmic Suspension .... ⊙230
Pred-G Ophthalmic Ointment .... ⊙229
Pred-G Ophthalmic Suspension .... ⊙228

Prednisolone Sodium Phosphate (Phenytoin impairs efficacy of corticosteroids).
No products indexed under this heading.

Prednisolone Tebutate (Phenytoin impairs efficacy of corticosteroids).
No products indexed under this heading.

Prednisone (Phenytoin impairs efficacy of corticosteroids).
No products indexed under this heading.

Prochlorperazine (Phenothiazines may increase phenytoin serum levels).
No products indexed under this heading.

Promethazine Hydrochloride (Phenothiazines may increase phenytoin serum levels).
No products indexed under this heading.

Protriptyline Hydrochloride (Tricyclic antidepressants may precipitate seizures in susceptible patients and phenytoin dosage may need to be adjusted).
No products indexed under this heading.

Quinestrol (May increase phenytoin serum levels; phenytoin impairs efficacy of estrogens).
No products indexed under this heading.

Quinidine (Phenytoin impairs efficacy of quinidine).
No products indexed under this heading.

Quinidine Gluconate (Phenytoin impairs efficacy of quinidine).
No products indexed under this heading.

Quinidine Hydrochloride (Phenytoin impairs efficacy of quinidine).
No products indexed under this heading.

Quinidine Polygalacturonate (Phenytoin impairs efficacy of quinidine).
No products indexed under this heading.

Quinidine Sulfate (Phenytoin impairs efficacy of quinidine).
No products indexed under this heading.

Ranitidine Bismuth Citrate (May increase phenytoin serum levels).
No products indexed under this heading.

Ranitidine Hydrochloride (May increase phenytoin serum levels). Products include:
Zantac 75 Tablets .... ▣603
Zantac 1670
Zantac Injection 1666
Zantac Injection Pharmacy Bulk Package 1668
Maximum Strength Zantac 150 Tablets .... ▣603
Maximum Strength Zantac 150 Cool Mint Tablets .... ▣603

Reserpine (May increase phenytoin serum levels).
No products indexed under this heading.

Rifampin (Phenytoin impairs efficacy of rifampin).
No products indexed under this heading.

Salsalate (May increase phenytoin serum levels).
No products indexed under this heading.

Sucralfate (May increase phenytoin serum levels). Products include:
Carafate Suspension 706
Carafate Tablets 707

Sulfamethizole (May increase phenytoin serum levels).
No products indexed under this heading.

Sulfamethoxazole (May increase phenytoin serum levels).
No products indexed under this heading.

Sulfisoxazole Acetyl (May increase phenytoin serum levels).
No products indexed under this heading.

Theophylline (Phenytoin impairs efficacy of theophylline).
No products indexed under this heading.

Theophylline Anhydrous (Phenytoin impairs efficacy of theophylline). Products include:
Uniphyl Tablets 2595

Theophylline Calcium Salicylate (Phenytoin impairs efficacy of theophylline).
No products indexed under this heading.

Theophylline Dihydroxypropyl (Glyceryl) (Phenytoin impairs efficacy of theophylline).
No products indexed under this heading.

Theophylline Ethylenediamine (Phenytoin impairs efficacy of theophylline).
No products indexed under this heading.

Theophylline Sodium Glycinate (Phenytoin impairs efficacy of theophylline).
No products indexed under this heading.

Thioridazine Hydrochloride (Phenothiazines may increase phenytoin serum levels). Products include:
Thioridazine Hydrochloride Tablets 2195

Tolbutamide (May increase phenytoin serum levels).
No products indexed under this heading.

Trazodone Hydrochloride (May increase phenytoin serum levels).
No products indexed under this heading.

Triamcinolone (Phenytoin impairs efficacy of corticosteroids).
No products indexed under this heading.

Triamcinolone Acetonide (Phenytoin impairs efficacy of corticosteroids). Products include:
Azmacort Inhalation Aerosol 407
Nasacort AQ Nasal Spray 2765
Triesence Injectable Suspension .... ⊙209

Triamcinolone Diacetate (Phenytoin impairs efficacy of corticosteroids).
No products indexed under this heading.

Triamcinolone Hexacetonide (Phenytoin impairs efficacy of corticosteroids).
No products indexed under this heading.

Trifluoperazine Hydrochloride (Phenothiazines may increase phenytoin serum levels).
No products indexed under this heading.

Trimipramine Maleate (Tricyclic antidepressants may precipitate seizures in susceptible patients and phenytoin dosage may need to be adjusted).
No products indexed under this heading.

Valproate Sodium (May decrease or increase phenytoin serum levels; the effect of phenytoin on valproate serum levels is unpredictable).
No products indexed under this heading.

Valproic Acid (May decrease or increase phenytoin serum levels; the effect of phenytoin on valproate serum levels is unpredictable).
No products indexed under this heading.

Vitamin D (Phenytoin impairs efficacy of vitamin D). Products include:
Active Calcium Tablets 3173
D-Cal Chewable Caplets .... ▣624
Norwegian Cod Liver Oil 949

Warfarin Sodium (Phenytoin impairs efficacy of oral anticoagulants).
No products indexed under this heading.

Food Interactions

Alcohol (Acute alcohol intake may increase phenytoin serum levels; chronic alcohol abuse may decrease phenytoin serum levels).

PHOSLO GELCAPS

(Calcium Acetate) 1184
May interact with calcium preparations, cardiac glycosides, tetracyclines, and certain other agents. Compounds in these categories include:

Antacids, unspecified (Concurrent use should be avoided).
No products indexed under this heading.

Calcium Carbonate (Potential for increased risk of hypercalcemia; concurrent use with other calcium supplements is not recommended). Products include:
Accelerator Tablets .... ▣634
Actonel with Calcium Tablets 2574
BioLean II Tablets .... ▣635
Calcet Triple Calcium + Vitamin D Tablets .... ▣629
D-Cal Chewable Caplets .... ▣624
Elixir Capsules .... ▣636
Pepcid Complete Chewable Tablets 1771
Extra Strength Rolaids Plus Gas Relief Tropical Fruit Softchews 1903
Extra Strength Rolaids Softchews Vanilla Creme 1903
Extra Strength Rolaids Freshmint Tablets 1903
Rolaids Multi-Symptom Berry Tablets 1903

Rolaids Original Peppermint Tablets 1903

Calcium Chloride (Potential for increased risk of hypercalcemia; concurrent use with other calcium supplements is not recommended).
No products indexed under this heading.

Calcium Citrate (Potential for increased risk of hypercalcemia; concurrent use with other calcium supplements is not recommended). Products include:
Active Calcium Tablets 3173
CitraNatal DHA Tablets 2175
CitraNatal 90 DHA Tablets 2175

Calcium Glubionate (Potential for increased risk of hypercalcemia; concurrent use with other calcium supplements is not recommended).
No products indexed under this heading.

Demeclocycline Hydrochloride (Bioavailability of oral tetracyclines may be decreased).
No products indexed under this heading.

Deslanoside (Hypercalcemia may precipitate cardiac arrhythmia).
No products indexed under this heading.

Digitalis Glycoside Preparations (Hypercalcemia may precipitate cardiac arrhythmia).
No products indexed under this heading.

Digitoxin (Hypercalcemia may precipitate cardiac arrhythmia).
No products indexed under this heading.

Digoxin (Hypercalcemia may precipitate cardiac arrhythmia). Products include:
Lanoxin Injection 1498
Lanoxin Injection Pediatric 1502
Lanoxin Tablets 1505

Doxycycline Calcium (Bioavailability of oral tetracyclines may be decreased).
No products indexed under this heading.

Doxycycline Hyclate (Bioavailability of oral tetracyclines may be decreased).
No products indexed under this heading.

Doxycycline Monohydrate (Bioavailability of oral tetracyclines may be decreased).
No products indexed under this heading.

Methacycline Hydrochloride (Bioavailability of oral tetracyclines may be decreased).
No products indexed under this heading.

Minocycline Hydrochloride (Bioavailability of oral tetracyclines may be decreased). Products include:
Solodyn Extended Release Tablets 1938

Oxytetracycline Hydrochloride (Bioavailability of oral tetracyclines may be decreased).
No products indexed under this heading.

Tetracycline Hydrochloride (Bioavailability of oral tetracyclines may be decreased). Products include:
Pylera Capsules 714

PHOTOFRIN FOR INJECTION

(Porfimer Sodium) 708
May interact with calcium channel blockers, glucocorticoids, drugs known to be photosensitizers, inhibitors of endogenous prostaglandin synthesis, and certain other agents. Compounds in these categories include:

Acetazolamide (Co-administration with other photosensitizing agents could increase the photosensitivity reactions).
No products indexed under this heading.

Acitretin (Co-administration with other photosensitizing agents could increase the photosensitivity reactions). Products include:
Soriatane Capsules 3062

Alatrofloxacin Mesylate (Co-administration with other photosensitizing agents could increase the photosensitivity reactions).
No products indexed under this heading.

Allopurinol (Could interfere with porfimer photodynamic therapy).
No products indexed under this heading.

Amlodipine Besylate (Could interfere with porfimer photodynamic therapy). Products include:
Azor Tablets 1005
Exforge Tablets 2238

Anthralin (Co-administration with other photosensitizing agents could increase the photosensitivity reactions).
No products indexed under this heading.

Aspirin (Some prostaglandin synthesis inhibitors could interfere with porfimer photodynamic therapy). Products include:
Aggrenox Capsules 819
Bayer Aspirin 750
Percodan Tablets 1130
St. Joseph 81 mg Aspirin Chewable and Enteric Coated Tablets 1903

Bendroflumethiazide (Co-administration with other photosensitizing agents could increase the photosensitivity reactions).
No products indexed under this heading.

Bepridil Hydrochloride (Could interfere with porfimer photodynamic therapy).
No products indexed under this heading.

Beta-Carotene (Compounds that quench active oxygen species or scavenge radicals, such as b-carotene, would be expected to decrease photodynamic therapy; no human data available to support or rebut this possibility).
No products indexed under this heading.

Betamethasone Acetate (Glucocorticoid hormone given before or concomitantly with photodynamic therapy may decrease the efficacy of the treatment).
No products indexed under this heading.

Betamethasone Sodium Phosphate (Glucocorticoid hormone given before or concomitantly with photodynamic therapy may decrease the efficacy of the treatment).
No products indexed under this heading.

Celecoxib (Some prostaglandin synthesis inhibitors could interfere with porfimer photodynamic therapy). Products include:
Celebrex Capsules 2979

Chlorothiazide (Co-administration with other photosensitizing agents could increase the photosensitivity reactions).
No products indexed under this heading.

Chlorothiazide Sodium (Co-administration with other photosensitizing agents could increase the photosensitivity reactions). Products include:
Intravenous Sodium Diuril 2490

Chlorpromazine (Co-administration with other photosensitizing agents could increase the photosensitivity reactions).
No products indexed under this heading.

Chlorpromazine Hydrochloride (Co-administration with other photosensitizing agents could increase the photosensitivity reactions).
No products indexed under this heading.

Chlorpropamide (Co-administration with other photosensitizing agents could increase the photosensitivity reactions).
No products indexed under this heading.

Ciprofloxacin (Co-administration with other photosensitizing agents could increase the photosensitivity reactions). Products include:
Cipro I.V. 2817
Cipro Oral Suspension 2810
Cipro XR Tablets 2823
Ciprodex Otic Suspension 541

Ciprofloxacin Hydrochloride (Co-administration with other photosensitizing agents could increase the photosensitivity reactions). Products include:
Cipro Tablets 2810

Coal Tar (Co-administration with other photosensitizing agents could increase the photosensitivity reactions).
No products indexed under this heading.

Cortisone Acetate (Glucocorticoid hormone given before or concomitantly with photodynamic therapy may decrease the efficacy of the treatment).
No products indexed under this heading.

Demeclocycline Hydrochloride (Co-administration with other photosensitizing agents could increase the photosensitivity reactions).
No products indexed under this heading.

Dexamethasone (Glucocorticoid hormone given before or concomitantly with photodynamic therapy may decrease the efficacy of the treatment). Products include:
Ciprodex Otic Suspension 541

Dexamethasone Acetate (Glucocorticoid hormone given before or concomitantly with photodynamic therapy may decrease the efficacy of the treatment).
No products indexed under this heading.

Dexamethasone Sodium Phosphate (Glucocorticoid hormone given before or concomitantly with photodynamic therapy may decrease the efficacy of the treatment).
No products indexed under this heading.

Diclofenac Potassium (Some prostaglandin synthesis inhibitors could interfere with porfimer photodynamic therapy).
No products indexed under this heading.

Diclofenac Sodium (Some prostaglandin synthesis inhibitors could interfere with porfimer photodynamic therapy). Products include:
Diclofenac Sodium Ophthalmic Solution .... ⊙240
Voltaren Ophthalmic Solution 2336
Voltaren Tablets 2334
Voltaren-XR Tablets 2337

Diltiazem Hydrochloride (Could interfere with porfimer photodynamic therapy). Products include:
Cardizem LA Extended Release Tablets 421

Dimethyl Sulfoxide (Compounds that quench active oxygen species or scavenge radicals, such as DMSO, would be expected to decrease photodynamic therapy; no human data available to support or rebut this possibility).
No products indexed under this heading.

Doxycycline Calcium (Co-administration with other photosensitizing agents could increase the photosensitivity reactions).
No products indexed under this heading.

Doxycycline Hyclate (Co-administration with other photosensitizing agents could increase the photosensitivity reactions).
No products indexed under this heading.

Doxycycline Monohydrate (Co-administration with other photosensitizing agents could increase the photosensitivity reactions).
No products indexed under this heading.

Enoxacin (Co-administration with other photosensitizing agents could increase the photosensitivity reactions).
No products indexed under this heading.

Felodipine (Could interfere with porfimer photodynamic therapy).
No products indexed under this heading.

Fenoprofen Calcium (Some prostaglandin synthesis inhibitors could interfere with porfimer photodynamic therapy). Products include:
Nalfon Capsules 2508

Fludrocortisone Acetate (Glucocorticoid hormone given before or concomitantly with photodynamic therapy may decrease the efficacy of the treatment).
No products indexed under this heading.

Fluphenazine Decanoate (Co-administration with other photosensitizing agents could increase the photosensitivity reactions).
No products indexed under this heading.

Fluphenazine Enanthate (Co-administration with other photosensitizing agents could increase the photosensitivity reactions).
No products indexed under this heading.

Fluphenazine Hydrochloride (Co-administration with other photosensitizing agents could increase the photosensitivity reactions).
No products indexed under this heading.

Flurbiprofen (Some prostaglandin synthesis inhibitors could interfere with porfimer photodynamic therapy).
No products indexed under this heading.

Furosemide (Co-administration with other photosensitizing agents could increase the photosensitivity reactions). Products include:
Furosemide Tablets 2186

Glipizide (Co-administration with other photosensitizing agents could increase the photosensitivity reactions).
No products indexed under this heading.

Glyburide (Co-administration with other photosensitizing agents could increase the photosensitivity reactions).
No products indexed under this heading.

Grepafloxacin Hydrochloride (Co-administration with other photosensitizing agents could increase the photosensitivity reactions).
No products indexed under this heading.

Griseofulvin (Co-administration with other photosensitizing agents could increase the photosensitivity reactions). Products include:
Gris-PEG Tablets 2507

Hydrochlorothiazide (Co-administration with other photosensitizing agents could increase the photosensitivity reactions). Products include:
Atacand HCT 642
Avalide Tablets 892
Avalide Tablets 2713
Benicar HCT Tablets 1010
Diovan HCT Tablets 2216
Dyazide Capsules 1405
Micardis HCT Tablets 854
Prinzide Tablets 2092
Tekturna HCT Tablets 2324
Teveten HCT Tablets 517

Hydrocortisone (Glucocorticoid hormone given before or concomitantly with photodynamic therapy may decrease the efficacy of the treatment).
No products indexed under this heading.

Hydrocortisone Acetate (Glucocorticoid hormone given before or concomitantly with photodynamic therapy may decrease the efficacy of the treatment). Products include:
Analpram-HC 1140
Pramosone 1141

Hydrocortisone Sodium Phosphate (Glucocorticoid hormone given before or concomitantly with photodynamic therapy may decrease the efficacy of the treatment).
No products indexed under this heading.

Hydrocortisone Sodium Succinate (Glucocorticoid hormone given before or concomitantly with photodynamic therapy may decrease the efficacy of the treatment).
No products indexed under this heading.

Hydroflumethiazide (Co-administration with other photosensitizing agents could increase the photosensitivity reactions).
No products indexed under this heading.

Ibuprofen (Some prostaglandin synthesis inhibitors could interfere with porfimer photodynamic therapy). Products include:
Motrin IB Tablets and Caplets 1900
Children's Motrin Oral Suspension ... 1901
Children's Motrin Non-Staining Dye-Free Oral Suspension 1901
Children's Motrin Cold Oral Suspension 1899
Infants' Motrin Concentrated Drops 1901
Infants' Motrin Non-Staining Dye-Free Concentrated Drops 1901
Junior Strength Motrin Caplets and Chewable Tablets 1901
Vicoprofen Tablets 533

Indomethacin (Some prostaglandin synthesis inhibitors could interfere with porfimer photodynamic therapy). Products include:
Indocin 2024

Indomethacin Sodium Trihydrate (Some prostaglandin synthesis inhibitors could interfere with porfimer photodynamic therapy). Products include:
Indocin I.V. 2489

Isradipine (Could interfere with porfimer photodynamic therapy). Products include:
DynaCirc CR Controlled Release Tablets 1407

Ketoprofen (Some prostaglandin synthesis inhibitors could interfere with porfimer photodynamic therapy).
No products indexed under this heading.

Lomefloxacin Hydrochloride (Co-administration with other photosensitizing agents could increase the photosensitivity reactions).
No products indexed under this heading.

Mannitol (Compounds that quench active oxygen species or scavenge radicals, such as mannitol, would be expected to decrease photodynamic therapy; no human data available to support or rebut this possibility).
No products indexed under this heading.

Meclofenamate Sodium (Some prostaglandin synthesis inhibitors could interfere with porfimer photodynamic therapy).
No products indexed under this heading.

Mefenamic Acid (Some prostaglandin synthesis inhibitors could interfere with porfimer photodynamic therapy).
No products indexed under this heading.

Mesoridazine Besylate (Co-administration with other photosensitizing agents could increase the photosensitivity reactions).
No products indexed under this heading.

Metabromsalan (Co-administration with other photosensitizing agents could increase the photosensitivity reactions).
No products indexed under this heading.

Methacycline Hydrochloride (Co-administration with other photosensitizing agents could increase the photosensitivity reactions).
No products indexed under this heading.

Methotrimeprazine (Co-administration with other photosensitizing agents could increase the photosensitivity reactions).
No products indexed under this heading.

Methyclothiazide (Co-administration with other photosensitizing agents could increase the photosensitivity reactions).
No products indexed under this heading.

Methylprednisolone Acetate (Glucocorticoid hormone given before or concomitantly with photodynamic therapy may decrease the efficacy of the treatment).
No products indexed under this heading.

Methylprednisolone Sodium Succinate (Glucocorticoid hormone given before or concomitantly with photodynamic therapy may decrease the efficacy of the treatment).
No products indexed under this heading.

Mibefradil Dihydrochloride (Could interfere with porfimer photodynamic therapy).
No products indexed under this heading.

Minocycline Hydrochloride (Co-administration with other photosensitizing agents could increase the photosensitivity reactions). Products include:
Solodyn Extended Release Tablets 1938

Nalidixic Acid (Co-administration with other photosensitizing agents could increase the photosensitivity reactions).
No products indexed under this heading.

Naproxen (Some prostaglandin synthesis inhibitors could interfere with porfimer photodynamic therapy). Products include:
EC-Naprosyn Delayed-Release Tablets 2632
Naprosyn Suspension 2632
Naprosyn Tablets 2632

Naproxen Sodium (Some prostaglandin synthesis inhibitors could interfere with porfimer photodynamic therapy). Products include:
Anaprox Tablets 2632
Anaprox DS Tablets 2632
Treximet Tablets 1616

Nicardipine Hydrochloride (Could interfere with porfimer photodynamic therapy). Products include:
Cardene I.V. 1093

Nifedipine (Could interfere with porfimer photodynamic therapy).
No products indexed under this heading.

Nimodipine (Could interfere with porfimer photodynamic therapy). Products include:
Nimotop Capsules 790

Nisoldipine (Could interfere with porfimer photodynamic therapy). Products include:
Sular Extended Release Tablets 2975

Norfloxacin (Co-administration with other photosensitizing agents could increase the photosensitivity reactions). Products include:
Noroxin Tablets 2069

Ofloxacin (Co-administration with other photosensitizing agents could increase the photosensitivity reactions). Products include:
Ofloxacin Ophthalmic Solution 0.3% .... ⊙ 243

Oxytetracycline Hydrochloride (Co-administration with other photosensitizing agents could increase the photosensitivity reactions).
No products indexed under this heading.

Perphenazine (Co-administration with other photosensitizing agents could increase the photosensitivity reactions).
No products indexed under this heading.

Phenylbutazone (Some prostaglandin synthesis inhibitors could interfere with porfimer photodynamic therapy).
No products indexed under this heading.

Piroxicam (Some prostaglandin synthesis inhibitors could interfere with porfimer photodynamic therapy).
No products indexed under this heading.

Polythiazide (Co-administration with other photosensitizing agents could increase the photosensitivity reactions).
No products indexed under this heading.

Prednisolone Acetate (Glucocorticoid hormone given before or concomitantly with photodynamic therapy may decrease the efficacy of the treatment). Products include:
Pred Forte Ophthalmic Suspension .... ⊙ 227
Pred Mild Ophthalmic Suspension .... ⊙ 230
Pred-G Ophthalmic Ointment .... ⊙ 229
Pred-G Ophthalmic Suspension .... ⊙ 228

Prednisolone Sodium Phosphate (Glucocorticoid hormone given before or concomitantly with photodynamic therapy may decrease the efficacy of the treatment).
No products indexed under this heading.

Prednisolone Tebutate (Glucocorticoid hormone given before or concomitantly with photodynamic therapy may decrease the efficacy of the treatment).
No products indexed under this heading.

Prednisone (Glucocorticoid hormone given before or concomitantly with photodynamic therapy may decrease the efficacy of the treatment).
No products indexed under this heading.

Prochlorperazine (Co-administration with other photosensitizing agents could increase the photosensitivity reactions).
No products indexed under this heading.

Promethazine Hydrochloride (Co-administration with other photosensitizing agents could increase the photosensitivity reactions).
No products indexed under this heading.

Sulfamethizole (Co-administration with other photosensitizing agents could increase the photosensitivity reactions).
No products indexed under this heading.

Sulfamethoxazole (Co-administration with other photosensitizing agents could increase the photosensitivity reactions).
No products indexed under this heading.

Sulfasalazine (Co-administration with other photosensitizing agents could increase the photosensitivity reactions).
No products indexed under this heading.

Sulfinpyrazone (Co-administration with other photosensitizing agents could increase the photosensitivity reactions).
No products indexed under this heading.

Sulfisoxazole Acetyl (Co-administration with other photosensitizing agents could increase the photosensitivity reactions).
No products indexed under this heading.

Sulfisoxazole Diolamine (Co-administration with other photosensitizing agents could increase the photosensitivity reactions).
No products indexed under this heading.

Sulindac (Some prostaglandin synthesis inhibitors could interfere with porfimer photodynamic therapy). Products include:
Clinoril Tablets **1962**

Tetrachlorosalicylanilide (Co-administration with other photosensitizing agents could increase the photosensitivity reactions).
No products indexed under this heading.

Tetracycline Hydrochloride (Co-administration with other photosensitizing agents could increase the photosensitivity reactions). Products include:
Pylera Capsules **714**

Thioridazine Hydrochloride (Co-administration with other photosensitizing agents could increase the photosensitivity reactions). Products include:
Thioridazine Hydrochloride Tablets **2195**

Tolazamide (Co-administration with other photosensitizing agents could increase the photosensitivity reactions).
No products indexed under this heading.

Tolbutamide (Co-administration with other photosensitizing agents could increase the photosensitivity reactions).
No products indexed under this heading.

Tolmetin Sodium (Some prostaglandin synthesis inhibitors could interfere with porfimer photodynamic therapy).
No products indexed under this heading.

Triamcinolone (Glucocorticoid hormone given before or concomitantly with photodynamic therapy may decrease the efficacy of the treatment).
No products indexed under this heading.

Triamcinolone Acetonide (Glucocorticoid hormone given before or concomitantly with photodynamic therapy may decrease the efficacy of the treatment). Products include:
Azmacort Inhalation Aerosol **407**
Nasacort AQ Nasal Spray **2765**
Triesence Injectable Suspension .... ⊙**209**

Triamcinolone Diacetate (Glucocorticoid hormone given before or concomitantly with photodynamic therapy may decrease the efficacy of the treatment).
No products indexed under this heading.

Triamcinolone Hexacetonide (Glucocorticoid hormone given before or concomitantly with photodynamic therapy may decrease the efficacy of the treatment).
No products indexed under this heading.

Trifluoperazine Hydrochloride (Co-administration with other photosensitizing agents could increase the photosensitivity reactions).
No products indexed under this heading.

Trovafloxacin Mesylate (Co-administration with other photosensitizing agents could increase the photosensitivity reactions).
No products indexed under this heading.

Verapamil Hydrochloride (Could interfere with porfimer photodynamic therapy). Products include:
Tarka Tablets **511**

Food Interactions

Alcohol (Compounds that quench active oxygen species or scavenge radicals, such as ethanol, would be expected to decrease photodynamic therapy; no human data available to support or rebut this possibility).

PHYTO-VITE TABLETS

(Antioxidants, Bioflavonoids, Calcium, Folate, Ginkgo biloba, Herbals with Vitamins & Minerals, Iron, Phytonutrients, Potassium, Soy Extract)................................... ▣**639**
None cited in PDR database.

PLAN B TABLETS

(Levonorgestrel) **1044**
May interact with barbiturates and hepatic microsomal enzyme inducers. Compounds in these categories include:

Aprobarbital (Hepatic enzyme-inducing drugs (e.g., barbiturates) may reduce the effectiveness of low-dose progestin-only pills).
No products indexed under this heading.

Butabarbital (Hepatic enzyme-inducing drugs (e.g., barbiturates) may reduce the effectiveness of low-dose progestin-only pills).
No products indexed under this heading.

Butalbital (Hepatic enzyme-inducing drugs (e.g., barbiturates) may reduce the effectiveness of low-dose progestin-only pills).
No products indexed under this heading.

Carbamazepine (Hepatic enzyme-inducing drugs may reduce the effectiveness of low-dose progestin-only pills). Products include:
Carbatrol Capsules **3019**
Equetro Extended-Release Capsules.................................. **3174**

Chlorpropamide (Hepatic enzyme-inducing drugs may reduce the effectiveness of low-dose progestin-only pills).
No products indexed under this heading.

Ethanol (Hepatic enzyme-inducing drugs may reduce the effectiveness of low-dose progestin-only pills).
No products indexed under this heading.

Fosphenytoin Sodium (Hepatic enzyme-inducing drugs may reduce the effectiveness of low-dose progestin-only pills).
No products indexed under this heading.

Glipizide (Hepatic enzyme-inducing drugs may reduce the effectiveness of low-dose progestin-only pills).
No products indexed under this heading.

Glyburide (Hepatic enzyme-inducing drugs may reduce the effectiveness of low-dose progestin-only pills).
No products indexed under this heading.

Mephobarbital (Hepatic enzyme-inducing drugs (e.g., barbiturates) may reduce the effectiveness of low-dose progestin-only pills).
No products indexed under this heading.

Pentobarbital Sodium (Hepatic enzyme-inducing drugs (e.g., barbiturates) may reduce the effectiveness of low-dose progestin-only pills). Products include:
Nembutal Sodium Solution, USP **2494**

Phenobarbital (Hepatic enzyme-inducing drugs may reduce the effectiveness of low-dose progestin-only pills). Products include:
Donnatal Extentabs **2507**

Phenylbutazone (Hepatic enzyme-inducing drugs may reduce the effectiveness of low-dose progestin-only pills).
No products indexed under this heading.

Phenytoin (Hepatic enzyme-inducing drugs may reduce the effectiveness of low-dose progestin-only pills).
No products indexed under this heading.

Phenytoin Sodium (Hepatic enzyme-inducing drugs may reduce the effectiveness of low-dose progestin-only pills). Products include:
Phenytek Capsules **2192**

Rifampin (Hepatic enzyme-inducing drugs may reduce the effectiveness of low-dose progestin-only pills).
No products indexed under this heading.

Rifapentine (Hepatic enzyme-inducing drugs may reduce the effectiveness of low-dose progestin-only pills).
No products indexed under this heading.

Secobarbital Sodium (Hepatic enzyme-inducing drugs (e.g., barbiturates) may reduce the effectiveness of low-dose progestin-only pills).
No products indexed under this heading.

Thiamylal Sodium (Hepatic enzyme-inducing drugs (e.g., barbiturates) may reduce the effectiveness of low-dose progestin-only pills).
No products indexed under this heading.

Tolazamide (Hepatic enzyme-inducing drugs may reduce the effectiveness of low-dose progestin-only pills).
No products indexed under this heading.

Tolbutamide (Hepatic enzyme-inducing drugs may reduce the effectiveness of low-dose progestin-only pills).
No products indexed under this heading.

PLAVIX TABLETS

(Clopidogrel Bisulfate) **926**
May interact with aspirin-acetylsalicylic acid, non-steroidal anti-inflammatory agents, phenytoin, and certain other agents. Compounds in these categories include:

Aspirin (Aspirin did not modify the clopidogrel-mediated inhibition of ADP-induced platelet aggregation. Concomitant administration of 500 mg of aspirin twice a day for one day did not significantly increase the prolongation of bleeding time induced by clopidogrel bisulfate. Clopidogrel bisulfate potentiated the effect of aspirin on a collagen-induced platelet aggregation. Clopidogrel bisulfate and aspirin have been administered together for up to one year). Products include:
Aggrenox Capsules **819**
Bayer Aspirin **750**
Percodan Tablets **1130**
St. Joseph 81 mg Aspirin Chewable and Enteric Coated Tablets **1903**

Aspirin, Enteric Coated (Aspirin did not modify the clopidogrel-mediated inhibition of ADP-induced platelet aggregation. Concomitant administration of 500 mg of aspirin twice a day for one day did not significantly increase the prolongation of bleeding time induced by clopidogrel bisulfate. Clopidogrel bisulfate potentiated the effect of aspirin on a collagen-induced platelet aggregation. Clopidogrel bisulfate and aspirin have been administered together for up to one year).
No products indexed under this heading.

Aspirin Buffered (Aspirin did not modify the clopidogrel-mediated inhibition of ADP-induced platelet aggregation. Concomitant administration of 500 mg of aspirin twice a day for one day did not significantly increase the prolongation of bleeding time induced by clopidogrel bisulfate. Clopidogrel bisulfate potentiated the effect of aspirin on a collagen-induced platelet aggregation. Clopidogrel bisulfate and aspirin have been administered together for up to one year).
No products indexed under this heading.

Celecoxib (Co-administration can be associated with increased occult gastrointestinal blood loss. At high concentrations in vitro, clopidogrel inhibits P450IIC9; accordingly, it may interfere with the metabolism of many non-steroidal anti-inflammatory agents. Use caution when co-administering with clopidogrel). Products include:

Celebrex Capsules 2979

Diclofenac Epolamine (Co-administration can be associated with increased occult gastrointestinal blood loss. At high concentrations in vitro, clopidogrel inhibits P450IIC9; accordingly, it may interfere with the metabolism of many non-steroidal anti-inflammatory agents. Use caution when co-administering with clopidogrel). Products include:

Flector Patch 561

Diclofenac Potassium (Co-administration can be associated with increased occult gastrointestinal blood loss. At high concentrations in vitro, clopidogrel inhibits P450IIC9; accordingly, it may interfere with the metabolism of many non-steroidal anti-inflammatory agents. Use caution when co-administering with clopidogrel).

No products indexed under this heading.

Diclofenac Sodium (Co-administration can be associated with increased occult gastrointestinal blood loss. At high concentrations in vitro, clopidogrel inhibits P450IIC9; accordingly, it may interfere with the metabolism of many non-steroidal anti-inflammatory agents. Use caution when co-administering with clopidogrel). Products include:

Diclofenac Sodium Ophthalmic Solution .... ⊙240
Voltaren Ophthalmic Solution 2336
Voltaren Tablets 2334
Voltaren-XR Tablets 2337

Etodolac (Co-administration can be associated with increased occult gastrointestinal blood loss. At high concentrations in vitro, clopidogrel inhibits P450IIC9; accordingly, it may interfere with the metabolism of many non-steroidal anti-inflammatory agents. Use caution when co-administering with clopidogrel).

No products indexed under this heading.

Fenoprofen Calcium (Co-administration can be associated with increased occult gastrointestinal blood loss. At high concentrations in vitro, clopidogrel inhibits P450IIC9; accordingly, it may interfere with the metabolism of many non-steroidal anti-inflammatory agents. Use caution when co-administering with clopidogrel). Products include:

Nalfon Capsules 2508

Flurbiprofen (Co-administration can be associated with increased occult gastrointestinal blood loss. At high concentrations in vitro, clopidogrel inhibits P450IIC9; accordingly, it may interfere with the metabolism of many non-steroidal anti-inflammatory agents. Use caution when co-administering with clopidogrel).

No products indexed under this heading.

Fluvastatin Sodium (At high concentrations in vitro, clopidogrel inhibits P450IIC9; accordingly, it may interfere with the metabolism of fluvastatin). Products include:

Lescol Capsules 2268
Lescol XL Tablets 2268

Fosphenytoin Sodium (At high concentrations in vitro, clopidogrel inhibits P450IIC9; accordingly, it may interfere with the metabolism of phenytoin. Use caution when co-administering with clopidogrel).

No products indexed under this heading.

Heparin Sodium (Co-administration should be undertaken with caution; concomitant heparin has no effect on inhibition of platelet aggregation induced by clopidogrel).

No products indexed under this heading.

Ibuprofen (Co-administration can be associated with increased occult gastrointestinal blood loss. At high concentrations in vitro, clopidogrel inhibits P450IIC9; accordingly, it may interfere with the metabolism of many non-steroidal anti-inflammatory agents. Use caution when co-administering with clopidogrel). Products include:

Motrin IB Tablets and Caplets 1900
Children's Motrin Oral Suspension ... 1901
Children's Motrin Non-Staining Dye-Free Oral Suspension............ 1901
Children's Motrin Cold Oral Suspension 1899
Infants' Motrin Concentrated Drops 1901
Infants' Motrin Non-Staining Dye-Free Concentrated Drops....... 1901
Junior Strength Motrin Caplets and Chewable Tablets................. 1901
Vicoprofen Tablets 533

Indomethacin (Co-administration can be associated with increased occult gastrointestinal blood loss. At high concentrations in vitro, clopidogrel inhibits P450IIC9; accordingly, it may interfere with the metabolism of many non-steroidal anti-inflammatory agents. Use caution when co-administering with clopidogrel). Products include:

Indocin 2024

Indomethacin Sodium Trihydrate (Co-administration can be associated with increased occult gastrointestinal blood loss. At high concentrations in vitro, clopidogrel inhibits P450IIC9; accordingly, it may interfere with the metabolism of many non-steroidal anti-inflammatory agents. Use caution when co-administering with clopidogrel). Products include:

Indocin I.V. 2489

Ketoprofen (Co-administration can be associated with increased occult gastrointestinal blood loss. At high concentrations in vitro, clopidogrel inhibits P450IIC9; accordingly, it may interfere with the metabolism of many non-steroidal anti-inflammatory agents. Use caution when co-administering with clopidogrel).

No products indexed under this heading.

Ketorolac Tromethamine (Co-administration can be associated with increased occult gastrointestinal blood loss. At high concentrations in vitro, clopidogrel inhibits P450IIC9; accordingly, it may interfere with the metabolism of many non-steroidal anti-inflammatory agents. Use caution when co-administering with clopidogrel).

No products indexed under this heading.

Meclofenamate Sodium (Co-administration can be associated with increased occult gastrointestinal blood loss. At high concentrations in vitro, clopidogrel inhibits P450IIC9; accordingly, it may interfere with the metabolism of many non-steroidal anti-inflammatory agents. Use caution when co-administering with clopidogrel).

No products indexed under this heading.

Mefenamic Acid (Co-administration can be associated with increased occult gastrointestinal blood loss. At high concentrations in vitro, clopidogrel inhibits P450IIC9; accordingly, it may interfere with the metabolism of many non-steroidal anti-inflammatory agents. Use caution when co-administering with clopidogrel).

No products indexed under this heading.

Meloxicam (Co-administration can be associated with increased occult gastrointestinal blood loss. At high concentrations in vitro, clopidogrel inhibits P450IIC9; accordingly, it may interfere with the metabolism of many non-steroidal anti-inflammatory agents. Use caution when co-administering with clopidogrel). Products include:

Mobic Oral Suspension 863
Mobic Tablets 863

Nabumetone (Co-administration can be associated with increased occult gastrointestinal blood loss. At high concentrations in vitro, clopidogrel inhibits P450IIC9; accordingly, it may interfere with the metabolism of many non-steroidal anti-inflammatory agents. Use caution when co-administering with clopidogrel).

No products indexed under this heading.

Naproxen (Co-administration can be associated with increased occult gastrointestinal blood loss. At high concentrations in vitro, clopidogrel inhibits P450IIC9; accordingly, it may interfere with the metabolism of many non-steroidal anti-inflammatory agents. Use caution when co-administering with clopidogrel). Products include:

EC-Naprosyn Delayed-Release Tablets.. 2632
Naprosyn Suspension 2632
Naprosyn Tablets 2632

Naproxen Sodium (Co-administration can be associated with increased occult gastrointestinal blood loss. At high concentrations in vitro, clopidogrel inhibits P450IIC9; accordingly, it may interfere with the metabolism of many non-steroidal anti-inflammatory agents. Use caution when co-administering with clopidogrel). Products include:

Anaprox Tablets 2632
Anaprox DS Tablets 2632
Treximet Tablets 1616

Oxaprozin (Co-administration can be associated with increased occult gastrointestinal blood loss. At high concentrations in vitro, clopidogrel inhibits P450IIC9; accordingly, it may interfere with the metabolism of many non-steroidal anti-inflammatory agents. Use caution when co-administering with clopidogrel).

No products indexed under this heading.

Phenylbutazone (Co-administration can be associated with increased occult gastrointestinal blood loss. At high concentrations in vitro, clopidogrel inhibits P450IIC9; accordingly, it may interfere with the metabolism of many non-steroidal anti-inflammatory agents. Use caution when co-administering with clopidogrel).

No products indexed under this heading.

Phenytoin (At high concentrations in vitro, clopidogrel inhibits P450IIC9; accordingly, it may interfere with the metabolism of phenytoin. Use caution when co-administering with clopidogrel).

No products indexed under this heading.

Phenytoin Sodium (At high concentrations in vitro, clopidogrel inhibits P450IIC9; accordingly, it may interfere with the metabolism of phenytoin. Use caution when co-administering with clopidogrel). Products include:

Phenytek Capsules 2192

Piroxicam (Co-administration can be associated with increased occult gastrointestinal blood loss. At high concentrations in vitro, clopidogrel inhibits P450IIC9; accordingly, it may interfere with the metabolism of many non-steroidal anti-inflammatory agents. Use caution when co-administering with clopidogrel).

No products indexed under this heading.

Rofecoxib (Co-administration can be associated with increased occult gastrointestinal blood loss. At high concentrations in vitro, clopidogrel inhibits P450IIC9; accordingly, it may interfere with the metabolism of many non-steroidal anti-inflammatory agents. Use caution when co-administering with clopidogrel).

No products indexed under this heading.

Sulindac (Co-administration can be associated with increased occult gastrointestinal blood loss. At high concentrations in vitro, clopidogrel inhibits P450IIC9; accordingly, it may interfere with the metabolism of many non-steroidal anti-inflammatory agents. Use caution when co-administering with clopidogrel). Products include:

Clinoril Tablets 1962

Tamoxifen Citrate (At high concentrations in vitro, clopidogrel inhibits P450IIC9; accordingly, it may interfere with the metabolism of tamoxifen).

No products indexed under this heading.

Tolbutamide (At high concentrations in vitro, clopidogrel inhibits P450IIC9; accordingly, it may interfere with the metabolism of tolbutamide).

No products indexed under this heading.

Tolmetin Sodium (Co-administration can be associated with increased occult gastrointestinal blood loss. At high concentrations in vitro, clopidogrel inhibits P450IIC9; accordingly, it may interfere with the metabolism of many non-steroidal anti-inflammatory agents. Use caution when co-administering with clopidogrel).

No products indexed under this heading.

Torsemide (At high concentrations in vitro, clopidogrel inhibits P450IIC9; accordingly, it may interfere with the metabolism of torsemide). Products include:

Demadex Injection 2630
Demadex Tablets 2630

Valdecoxib (Co-administration can be associated with increased occult gastrointestinal blood loss. At high concentrations in vitro, clopidogrel inhibits P450IIC9; accordingly, it may interfere with the metabolism of many non-steroidal anti-inflammatory agents. Use caution when co-administering with clopidrogel).

No products indexed under this heading.

Warfarin Sodium (Co-administration should be undertaken with caution due to the increased risk of bleeding; at high concentrations in vitro, clopidogrel inhibits P450IIC9; accordingly, it may interfere with the metabolism of warfarin).

No products indexed under this heading.

PLAVIX TABLETS

(Clopidogrel Bisulfate) 2767

May interact with aspirin-acetylsalicylic acid, non-steroidal anti-inflammatory agents, phenytoin, and certain other agents. Compounds in these categories include:

Aspirin (Aspirin did not modify the clopidogrel-mediated inhibition of ADP-induced platelet aggregation. Concomitant administration of 500 mg of aspirin twice a day for one day did not significantly increase the prolongation of bleeding time induced by clopidogrel bisulfate. Clopidogrel bisulfate potentiated the effect of aspirin on a collagen-induced platelet aggregation. Clopidogrel bisulfate and aspirin have been administered together for up to one year). Products include:

Aggrenox Capsules 819
Bayer Aspirin 750
Percodan Tablets 1130
St. Joseph 81 mg Aspirin Chewable and Enteric Coated Tablets 1903

Aspirin, Enteric Coated (Aspirin did not modify the clopidogrel-mediated inhibition of ADP-induced platelet aggregation. Concomitant administration of 500 mg of aspirin twice a day for one day did not significantly increase the prolongation of bleeding time induced by clopidogrel bisulfate. Clopidogrel bisulfate potentiated the effect of aspirin on a collagen-induced platelet aggregation. Clopidogrel bisulfate and aspirin have been administered together for up to one year).

No products indexed under this heading.

Aspirin Buffered (Aspirin did not modify the clopidogrel-mediated inhibition of ADP-induced platelet aggregation. Concomitant administration of 500 mg of aspirin twice a day for one day did not significantly increase the prolongation of bleeding time induced by clopidogrel bisulfate. Clopidogrel bisulfate potentiated the effect of aspirin on a collagen-induced platelet aggregation. Clopidogrel bisulfate and aspirin have been administered together for up to one year).

No products indexed under this heading.

Celecoxib (Co-administration can be associated with increased occult gastrointestinal blood loss; at high concentrations in vitro, clopidogrel inhibits P450IIC9; accordingly, it may interfere with the metabolism of many non-steroidal anti-inflammatory agents. Use caution when co-adminstering with clopidrogel). Products include:

Celebrex Capsules 2979

Diclofenac Epolamine (Co-administration can be associated with increased occult gastrointestinal blood loss; at high concentrations in vitro, clopidogrel inhibits P450IIC9; accordingly, it may interfere with the metabolism of many non-steroidal anti-inflammatory agents. Use caution when co-adminstering with clopidrogel). Products include:

Flector Patch 561

Diclofenac Potassium (Co-administration can be associated with increased occult gastrointestinal blood loss; at high concentrations in vitro, clopidogrel inhibits P450IIC9; accordingly, it may interfere with the metabolism of many non-steroidal anti-inflammatory agents. Use caution when co-adminstering with clopidrogel).

No products indexed under this heading.

Diclofenac Sodium (Co-administration can be associated with increased occult gastrointestinal blood loss; at high concentrations in vitro, clopidogrel inhibits P450IIC9; accordingly, it may interfere with the metabolism of many non-steroidal anti-inflammatory agents. Use caution when co-adminstering with clopidrogel). Products include:

Diclofenac Sodium Ophthalmic Solution .... ⊙ 240
Voltaren Ophthalmic Solution 2336
Voltaren Tablets 2334
Voltaren-XR Tablets 2337

Etodolac (Co-administration can be associated with increased occult gastrointestinal blood loss; at high concentrations in vitro, clopidogrel inhibits P450IIC9; accordingly, it may interfere with the metabolism of many non-steroidal anti-inflammatory agents. Use caution when co-adminstering with clopidrogel).

No products indexed under this heading.

Fenoprofen Calcium (Co-administration can be associated with increased occult gastrointestinal blood loss; at high concentrations in vitro, clopidogrel inhibits P450IIC9; accordingly, it may interfere with the metabolism of many non-steroidal anti-inflammatory agents. Use caution when co-adminstering with clopidrogel). Products include:

Nalfon Capsules 2508

Flurbiprofen (Co-administration can be associated with increased occult gastrointestinal blood loss; at high concentrations in vitro, clopidogrel inhibits P450IIC9; accordingly, it may interfere with the metabolism of many non-steroidal anti-inflammatory agents. Use caution when co-adminstering with clopidrogel).

No products indexed under this heading.

Fluvastatin Sodium (At high concentrations in vitro, clopidogrel inhibits P450IIC9; accordingly, it may interfere with the metabolism of fluvastatin. Use caution when co-administering with clopidrogel). Products include:

Lescol Capsules 2268
Lescol XL Tablets 2268

Fosphenytoin Sodium (At high concentrations in vitro, clopidogrel inhibits P450IIC9; accordingly, it may interfere with the metabolism of phenytoin. Use caution when co-administering with clopidrogel).

No products indexed under this heading.

Ibuprofen (Co-administration can be associated with increased occult gastrointestinal blood loss; at high concentrations in vitro, clopidogrel inhibits P450IIC9; accordingly, it may interfere with the metabolism of many non-steroidal anti-inflammatory agents. Use caution when co-adminstering with clopidrogel). Products include:

Motrin IB Tablets and Caplets 1900
Children's Motrin Oral Suspension 1901
Children's Motrin Non-Staining Dye-Free Oral Suspension 1901
Children's Motrin Cold Oral Suspension 1899
Infants' Motrin Concentrated Drops 1901
Infants' Motrin Non-Staining Dye-Free Concentrated Drops 1901
Junior Strength Motrin Caplets and Chewable Tablets 1901
Vicoprofen Tablets 533

Indomethacin (Co-administration can be associated with increased occult gastrointestinal blood loss; at high concentrations in vitro, clopidogrel inhibits P450IIC9; accordingly, it may interfere with the metabolism of many non-steroidal anti-inflammatory agents. Use caution when co-adminstering with clopidrogel). Products include:

Indocin 2024

Indomethacin Sodium Trihydrate (Co-administration can be associated with increased occult gastrointestinal blood loss; at high concentrations in vitro, clopidogrel inhibits P450IIC9; accordingly, it may interfere with the metabolism of many non-steroidal anti-inflammatory agents. Use caution when co-adminstering with clopidrogel). Products include:

Indocin I.V. 2489

Ketoprofen (Co-administration can be associated with increased occult gastrointestinal blood loss; at high concentrations in vitro, clopidogrel inhibits P450IIC9; accordingly, it may interfere with the metabolism of many non-steroidal anti-inflammatory agents. Use caution when co-adminstering with clopidrogel).

No products indexed under this heading.

Ketorolac Tromethamine (Co-administration can be associated with increased occult gastrointestinal blood loss; at high concentrations in vitro, clopidogrel inhibits P450IIC9; accordingly, it may interfere with the metabolism of many non-steroidal anti-inflammatory agents. Use caution when co-adminstering with clopidrogel).

No products indexed under this heading.

Meclofenamate Sodium (Co-administration can be associated with increased occult gastrointestinal blood loss; at high concentrations in vitro, clopidogrel inhibits P450IIC9; accordingly, it may interfere with the metabolism of many non-steroidal anti-inflammatory agents. Use caution when co-adminstering with clopidrogel).

No products indexed under this heading.

Mefenamic Acid (Co-administration can be associated with increased occult gastrointestinal blood loss; at high concentrations in vitro, clopidogrel inhibits P450IIC9; accordingly, it may interfere with the metabolism of many non-steroidal anti-inflammatory agents. Use caution when co-adminstering with clopidrogel).

No products indexed under this heading.

Meloxicam (Co-administration can be associated with increased occult gastrointestinal blood loss; at high concentrations in vitro, clopidogrel inhibits P450IIC9; accordingly, it may interfere with the metabolism of many non-steroidal anti-inflammatory agents. Use caution when co-adminstering with clopidrogel). Products include:

Mobic Oral Suspension 863
Mobic Tablets 863

Nabumetone (Co-administration can be associated with increased occult gastrointestinal blood loss; at high concentrations in vitro, clopidogrel inhibits P450IIC9; accordingly, it may interfere with the metabolism of many non-steroidal anti-inflammatory agents. Use caution when co-adminstering with clopidrogel).

No products indexed under this heading.

Naproxen (Co-administration can be associated with increased occult gastrointestinal blood loss; at high concentrations in vitro, clopidogrel inhibits P450IIC9; accordingly, it may interfere with the metabolism of many non-steroidal anti-inflammatory agents. Use caution when co-adminstering with clopidrogel). Products include:

EC-Naprosyn Delayed-Release Tablets 2632
Naprosyn Suspension 2632
Naprosyn Tablets 2632

Naproxen Sodium (Co-administration can be associated with increased occult gastrointestinal blood loss; at high concentrations in vitro, clopidogrel inhibits P450IIC9; accordingly, it may interfere with the metabolism of many non-steroidal anti-inflammatory agents. Use caution when co-adminstering with clopidrogel). Products include:

Anaprox Tablets 2632
Anaprox DS Tablets 2632
Treximet Tablets 1616

Oxaprozin (Co-administration can be associated with increased occult gastrointestinal blood loss; at high concentrations in vitro, clopidogrel inhibits P450IIC9; accordingly, it may interfere with the metabolism of many non-steroidal anti-inflammatory agents. Use caution when co-adminstering with clopidrogel).

No products indexed under this heading.

Phenylbutazone (Co-administration can be associated with increased occult gastrointestinal blood loss; at high concentrations in vitro, clopidogrel inhibits P450IIC9; accordingly, it may interfere with the metabolism of many non-steroidal anti-inflammatory agents. Use caution when co-adminstering with clopidrogel).
No products indexed under this heading.

Phenytoin (At high concentrations in vitro, clopidogrel inhibits P450IIC9; accordingly, it may interfere with the metabolism of phenytoin. Use caution when co-administering with clopidrogel).
No products indexed under this heading.

Phenytoin Sodium (At high concentrations in vitro, clopidogrel inhibits P450IIC9; accordingly, it may interfere with the metabolism of phenytoin. Use caution when co-administering with clopidrogel). Products include:
Phenytek Capsules 2192

Piroxicam (Co-administration can be associated with increased occult gastrointestinal blood loss; at high concentrations in vitro, clopidogrel inhibits P450IIC9; accordingly, it may interfere with the metabolism of many non-steroidal anti-inflammatory agents. Use caution when co-adminstering with clopidrogel).
No products indexed under this heading.

Rofecoxib (Co-administration can be associated with increased occult gastrointestinal blood loss; at high concentrations in vitro, clopidogrel inhibits P450IIC9; accordingly, it may interfere with the metabolism of many non-steroidal anti-inflammatory agents. Use caution when co-adminstering with clopidrogel).
No products indexed under this heading.

Sulindac (Co-administration can be associated with increased occult gastrointestinal blood loss; at high concentrations in vitro, clopidogrel inhibits P450IIC9; accordingly, it may interfere with the metabolism of many non-steroidal anti-inflammatory agents. Use caution when co-adminstering with clopidrogel). Products include:
Clinoril Tablets 1962

Tamoxifen Citrate (At high concentrations in vitro, clopidogrel inhibits P450IIC9; accordingly, it may interfere with the metabolism of tamoxifen. Use caution when co-administering with clopidrogel).
No products indexed under this heading.

Tolbutamide (At high concentrations in vitro, clopidogrel inhibits P450IIC9; accordingly, it may interfere with the metabolism of tolbutamide. Use caution when co-administering with clopidrogel).
No products indexed under this heading.

Tolmetin Sodium (Co-administration can be associated with increased occult gastrointestinal blood loss; at high concentrations in vitro, clopidogrel inhibits P450IIC9; accordingly, it may interfere with the metabolism of many non-steroidal anti-inflammatory agents. Use caution when co-adminstering with clopidrogel).
No products indexed under this heading.

Torsemide (At high concentrations in vitro, clopidogrel inhibits P450IIC9; accordingly, it may interfere with the metabolism of torsemide. Use caution when co-administering with clopidrogel). Products include:
Demadex Injection 2630
Demadex Tablets 2630

Valdecoxib (Co-administration can be associated with increased occult gastrointestinal blood loss; at high concentrations in vitro, clopidogrel inhibits P450IIC9; accordingly, it may interfere with the metabolism of many non-steroidal anti-inflammatory agents. Use caution when co-adminstering with clopidrogel).
No products indexed under this heading.

Warfarin Sodium (Because of the increased risk of bleeding, the concomitant administration of warfarin with clopidrogel should be undertaken with caution).
No products indexed under this heading.

PLETAL TABLETS

(Cilostazol) 2481
May interact with cytochrome p450 2c9 inhibitors (selected), cytochrome p450 3a4 inhibitors (selected), erythromycin, platelet inhibitors, and certain other agents. Compounds in these categories include:

Acetazolamide (A reduced dose of cilostazol should be considered when taken concomitantly with CYP3A4 inhibitors).
No products indexed under this heading.

Amiodarone Hydrochloride (A reduced dose of cilostazol should be considered when taken concomitantly with CYP3A4 inhibitors).
No products indexed under this heading.

Amprenavir (A reduced dose of cilostazol should be considered when taken concomitantly with CYP3A4 inhibitors).
No products indexed under this heading.

Anastrozole (A reduced dose of cilostazol should be considered when taken concomitantly with CYP3A4 inhibitors). Products include:
Arimidex Tablets 672

Aprepitant (A reduced dose of cilostazol should be considered when taken concomitantly with CYP3A4 inhibitors). Products include:
Emend Capsules 1992

Aspirin (Short-term (less than or equal to 4 days) co-administration has shown a 22% to 37% increase in inhibition of ADP-induced ex vivo platelet aggregation compared to aspirin alone; no clinically significant impact on bleeding time, PT, or aPTT was noted; there was no apparent greater incidence of hemorrhagic adverse effects in patients on cilostazol and aspirin compared to patients taking placebo and aspirin). Products include:
Aggrenox Capsules 819
Bayer Aspirin 750
Percodan Tablets 1130
St. Joseph 81 mg Aspirin Chewable and Enteric Coated Tablets 1903

Aspirin, Enteric Coated (Caution is advised in patients receiving both cilostazol and any other antiplatelet agent).
No products indexed under this heading.

Aspirin Buffered (Caution is advised in patients receiving both cilostazol and any other antiplatelet agent).
No products indexed under this heading.

Atazanavir (A reduced dose of cilostazol should be considered when taken concomitantly with CYP3A4 inhibitors).
No products indexed under this heading.

Atazanavir Sulfate (A reduced dose of cilostazol should be considered when taken concomitantly with CYP3A4 inhibitors). Products include:
Reyataz Capsules 3299

Azlocillin Sodium (Caution is advised in patients receiving both cilostazol and any other antiplatelet agent).
No products indexed under this heading.

Bendroflumethiazide (A reduced dose of cilostazol should be considered when taken concomitantly with CYP2C19 inhibitors).
No products indexed under this heading.

Carbenicillin Indanyl Sodium (Caution is advised in patients receiving both cilostazol and any other antiplatelet agent).
No products indexed under this heading.

Chloramphenicol (A reduced dose of cilostazol should be considered when taken concomitantly with CYP2C19 inhibitors).
No products indexed under this heading.

Chlorothiazide (A reduced dose of cilostazol should be considered when taken concomitantly with CYP2C19 inhibitors).
No products indexed under this heading.

Chlorothiazide Sodium (A reduced dose of cilostazol should be considered when taken concomitantly with CYP2C19 inhibitors). Products include:
Intravenous Sodium Diuril 2490

Chlorpropamide (A reduced dose of cilostazol should be considered when taken concomitantly with CYP2C19 inhibitors).
No products indexed under this heading.

Choline Magnesium Trisalicylate (Caution is advised in patients receiving both cilostazol and any other antiplatelet agent).
No products indexed under this heading.

Cimetidine (A reduced dose of cilostazol should be considered when taken concomitantly with CYP3A4 inhibitors).
No products indexed under this heading.

Cimetidine Hydrochloride (A reduced dose of cilostazol should be considered when taken concomitantly with CYP3A4 inhibitors).
No products indexed under this heading.

Ciprofloxacin (A reduced dose of cilostazol should be considered when taken concomitantly with CYP3A4 inhibitors). Products include:
Cipro I.V. 2817
Cipro Oral Suspension 2810
Cipro XR Tablets 2823
Ciprodex Otic Suspension 541

Clarithromycin (Co-administration of cilostazol with moderate inhibitors of CYP3A4, such as clarithromycin, a macrolide antibiotic, may result in significant increases in the systemic exposure of cilostazol and/or its major metabolites; caution should be exercised if concurrently used). Products include:
Biaxin/Biaxin XL 411

Clopidogrel Bisulfate (Althought it cannot be determined whether there was an additive effect on bleeding times during concomitant administration, caution should be advised for checking bleeding times). Products include:
Plavix Tablets 926
Plavix Tablets 2767

Clopidogrel Hydrogen Sulfate (Althought it cannot be determined whether there was an additive effect on bleeding times during concomitant administration, caution should be advised for checking bleeding times).
No products indexed under this heading.

Clotrimazole (A reduced dose of cilostazol should be considered when taken concomitantly with CYP3A4 inhibitors). Products include:
Lotrisone 2881

Cyclosporine (A reduced dose of cilostazol should be considered when taken concomitantly with CYP3A4 inhibitors). Products include:
Gengraf Capsules 435
Neoral Oral Solution 2280
Neoral Soft Gelatin Capsules 2280
Restasis Ophthalmic Emulsion 557
Sandimmune 2296

Dalfopristin (A reduced dose of cilostazol should be considered when taken concomitantly with CYP3A4 inhibitors).
No products indexed under this heading.

Danazol (A reduced dose of cilostazol should be considered when taken concomitantly with CYP3A4 inhibitors).
No products indexed under this heading.

Delavirdine Mesylate (A reduced dose of cilostazol should be considered when taken concomitantly with CYP3A4 inhibitors).
No products indexed under this heading.

Diclofenac Potassium (Caution is advised in patients receiving both cilostazol and any other antiplatelet agent).
No products indexed under this heading.

Diclofenac Sodium (Caution is advised in patients receiving both cilostazol and any other antiplatelet agent). Products include:
Diclofenac Sodium Ophthalmic Solution.. ⊙240
Voltaren Ophthalmic Solution 2336
Voltaren Tablets 2334
Voltaren-XR Tablets 2337

Diflunisal (Caution is advised in patients receiving both cilostazol and any other antiplatelet agent).
No products indexed under this heading.

Diltiazem Hydrochloride (Co-administration of cilostazol with moderate inhibitors of CYP3A4, such as diltiazem, has been shown to increase cilostazol plasma concentrations by approximately 30%). Products include:
Cardizem LA Extended Release Tablets ... 421

Diltiazem Maleate (Co-administration of cilostazol with moderate inhibitors of CYP3A4, such as diltiazem, has been shown to increase cilostazol plasma concentrations by approximately 30%).
No products indexed under this heading.

Dipyridamole (Caution is advised in patients receiving both cilostazol and any other antiplatelet agent). Products include:
Aggrenox Capsules ... 819
Persantine Tablets ... 869

Disulfiram (A reduced dose of cilostazol should be considered when taken concomitantly with CYP2C19 inhibitors).
No products indexed under this heading.

Efavirenz (A reduced dose of cilostazol should be considered when taken concomitantly with CYP3A4 inhibitors). Products include:
Atripla Tablets ... 938
Sustiva Capsules ... 930
Sustiva Tablets ... 930

Erythromycin (Co-administration of cilostazol with moderately strong inhibitors of CYP3A4, such as erythromycin, significantly increases the systemic exposure of cilostazol and/or its major metabolites; caution should be exercised if concurrently used).
No products indexed under this heading.

Erythromycin Estolate (Co-administration of cilostazol with moderately strong inhibitors of CYP3A4, such as erythromycin, significantly increases the systemic exposure of cilostazol and/or its major metabolites; caution should be exercised if concurrently used).
No products indexed under this heading.

Erythromycin Ethylsuccinate (Co-administration of cilostazol with moderately strong inhibitors of CYP3A4, such as erythromycin, significantly increases the systemic exposure of cilostazol and/or its major metabolites; caution should be exercised if concurrently used). Products include:
E.E.S. ... 433
EryPed ... 431

Erythromycin Gluceptate (Co-administration of cilostazol with moderately strong inhibitors of CYP3A4, such as erythromycin, significantly increases the systemic exposure of cilostazol and/or its major metabolites; caution should be exercised if concurrently used).
No products indexed under this heading.

Erythromycin Lactobionate (Co-administration of cilostazol with moderately strong inhibitors of CYP3A4, such as erythromycin, significantly increases the systemic exposure of cilostazol and/or its major metabolites; caution should be exercised if concurrently used).
No products indexed under this heading.

Erythromycin Stearate (Co-administration of cilostazol with moderately strong inhibitors of CYP3A4, such as erythromycin, significantly increases the systemic exposure of cilostazol and/or its major metabolites; caution should be exercised if concurrently used).
No products indexed under this heading.

Esomeprazole Magnesium (A reduced dose of cilostazol should be considered when taken concomitantly with CYP3A4 inhibitors). Products include:
Nexium Delayed-Release Capsules ... 645
Nexium Delayed-Release Oral Suspension ... 645

Fenofibrate (A reduced dose of cilostazol should be considered when taken concomitantly with CYP2C19 inhibitors). Products include:
Fenoglide Tablets ... 2960
Tricor Tablets ... 520

Fenoprofen Calcium (Caution is advised in patients receiving both cilostazol and any other antiplatelet agent). Products include:
Nalfon Capsules ... 2508

Fluconazole (Co-administration of cilostazol with strong inhibitors of CYP3A4, such as fluconazole, would be expected to cause an increase in cilostazol Cmax and AUC).
No products indexed under this heading.

Fluorouracil (A reduced dose of cilostazol should be considered when taken concomitantly with CYP2C19 inhibitors). Products include:
Carac Cream 0.5% ... 2722

Fluoxetine (A reduced dose of cilostazol should be considered when taken concomitantly with CYP3A4 inhibitors).
No products indexed under this heading.

Fluoxetine Hydrochloride (Co-administration of cilostazol with strong inhibitors of CYP3A4, such as fluoxetine, would be expected to cause an increase in cilostazol Cmax and AUC). Products include:
Prozac Weekly Capsules ... 1852
Prozac Pulvules and Liquid ... 1852
Symbyax Capsules ... 1871

Flurbiprofen (Caution is advised in patients receiving both cilostazol and any other antiplatelet agent).
No products indexed under this heading.

Flurbiprofen Sodium (A reduced dose of cilostazol should be considered when taken concomitantly with CYP2C19 inhibitors).
No products indexed under this heading.

Fluvastatin Sodium (A reduced dose of cilostazol should be considered when taken concomitantly with CYP2C19 inhibitors). Products include:
Lescol Capsules ... 2268
Lescol XL Tablets ... 2268

Fluvoxamine Maleate (Co-administration of cilostazol with strong inhibitors of CYP3A4, such as fluvoxamine, would be expected to cause an increase in cilostazol Cmax and AUC). Products include:
Luvox CR Extended-Release Capsules ... 1759

Fosamprenavir Calcium (A reduced dose of cilostazol should be considered when taken concomitantly with CYP3A4 inhibitors). Products include:
Lexiva Oral Suspension ... 1510
Lexiva Tablets ... 1510

Gemfibrozil (A reduced dose of cilostazol should be considered when taken concomitantly with CYP2C19 inhibitors).
No products indexed under this heading.

Glipizide (A reduced dose of cilostazol should be considered when taken concomitantly with CYP2C19 inhibitors).
No products indexed under this heading.

Glyburide (A reduced dose of cilostazol should be considered when taken concomitantly with CYP2C19 inhibitors).
No products indexed under this heading.

Hydrochlorothiazide (A reduced dose of cilostazol should be considered when taken concomitantly with CYP2C19 inhibitors). Products include:
Atacand HCT ... 642
Avalide Tablets ... 892
Avalide Tablets ... 2713
Benicar HCT Tablets ... 1010
Diovan HCT Tablets ... 2216
Dyazide Capsules ... 1405
Micardis HCT Tablets ... 854
Prinzide Tablets ... 2092
Tekturna HCT Tablets ... 2324
Teveten HCT Tablets ... 517

Hydroflumethiazide (A reduced dose of cilostazol should be considered when taken concomitantly with CYP2C19 inhibitors).
No products indexed under this heading.

Ibuprofen (Caution is advised in patients receiving both cilostazol and any other antiplatelet agent). Products include:
Motrin IB Tablets and Caplets ... 1900
Children's Motrin Oral Suspension ... 1901
Children's Motrin Non-Staining Dye-Free Oral Suspension ... 1901
Children's Motrin Cold Oral Suspension ... 1899
Infants' Motrin Concentrated Drops ... 1901
Infants' Motrin Non-Staining Dye-Free Concentrated Drops ... 1901
Junior Strength Motrin Caplets and Chewable Tablets ... 1901
Vicoprofen Tablets ... 533

Imatinib Mesylate (A reduced dose of cilostazol should be considered when taken concomitantly with CYP2C19 inhibitors). Products include:
Gleevec Tablets ... 2255

Indinavir Sulfate (A reduced dose of cilostazol should be considered when taken concomitantly with CYP3A4 inhibitors). Products include:
Crixivan Capsules ... 1979

Indomethacin (Caution is advised in patients receiving both cilostazol and any other antiplatelet agent). Products include:
Indocin ... 2024

Indomethacin Sodium Trihydrate (Caution is advised in patients receiving both cilostazol and any other antiplatelet agent). Products include:
Indocin I.V. ... 2489

Isoniazid (A reduced dose of cilostazol should be considered when taken concomitantly with CYP3A4 inhibitors).
No products indexed under this heading.

Itraconazole (Co-administration of cilostazol with strong inhibitors of CYP3A4, such as itraconazole, would be expected to cause an increase in cilostazol Cmax and AUC).
No products indexed under this heading.

Ketoconazole (Co-administration of cilostazol with strong inhibitors of CYP3A4, such as ketoconazole increased cilostazol Cmax and AUC). Products include:
Extina Foam, 2% ... 3057
Nizoral A-D Shampoo ... 1901

Ketoprofen (Caution is advised in patients receiving both cilostazol and any other antiplatelet agent).
No products indexed under this heading.

Leflunomide (A reduced dose of cilostazol should be considered when taken concomitantly with CYP2C19 inhibitors).
No products indexed under this heading.

Lopinavir (A reduced dose of cilostazol should be considered when taken concomitantly with CYP3A4 inhibitors). Products include:
Kaletra ... 452

Loratadine (A reduced dose of cilostazol should be considered when taken concomitantly with CYP3A4 inhibitors).
No products indexed under this heading.

Lovastatin (A reduced dose of cilostazol should be considered when taken concomitantly with CYP2C19 inhibitors). Products include:
Advicor Tablets ... 402
Mevacor Tablets ... 2063

Magnesium Salicylate (Caution is advised in patients receiving both cilostazol and any other antiplatelet agent).
No products indexed under this heading.

Meclofenamate Sodium (Caution is advised in patients receiving both cilostazol and any other antiplatelet agent).
No products indexed under this heading.

Mefenamic Acid (Caution is advised in patients receiving both cilostazol and any other antiplatelet agent).
No products indexed under this heading.

Methyclothiazide (A reduced dose of cilostazol should be considered when taken concomitantly with CYP2C19 inhibitors).
No products indexed under this heading.

Metronidazole (A reduced dose of cilostazol should be considered when taken concomitantly with CYP3A4 inhibitors). Products include:
Pylera Capsules ... 714

Metronidazole Benzoate (A reduced dose of cilostazol should be considered when taken concomitantly with CYP3A4 inhibitors).
No products indexed under this heading.

Metronidazole Hydrochloride (A reduced dose of cilostazol should be considered when taken concomitantly with CYP3A4 inhibitors).
No products indexed under this heading.

Mezlocillin Sodium (Caution is advised in patients receiving both cilostazol and any other antiplatelet agent).
No products indexed under this heading.

Miconazole (Co-administration of cilostazol with strong inhibitors of CYP3A4, such as miconazole, would be expected to cause an increase in Cmax and AUC).
No products indexed under this heading.

Miconazole Nitrate (A reduced dose of cilostazol should be considered when taken concomitantly with CYP3A4 inhibitors).
No products indexed under this heading.

Modafinil (A reduced dose of cilostazol should be considered when taken concomitantly with CYP2C19 inhibitors). Products include:
Provigil Tablets 977

Nafcillin Sodium (Caution is advised in patients receiving both cilostazol and any other antiplatelet agent).
No products indexed under this heading.

Naproxen (Caution is advised in patients receiving both cilostazol and any other antiplatelet agent). Products include:
EC-Naprosyn Delayed-Release Tablets 2632
Naprosyn Suspension 2632
Naprosyn Tablets 2632

Naproxen Sodium (Caution is advised in patients receiving both cilostazol and any other antiplatelet agent). Products include:
Anaprox Tablets 2632
Anaprox DS Tablets 2632
Treximet Tablets 1616

Nefazodone Hydrochloride (Co-administration of cilostazol with strong inhibitors of CYP3A4, such as nefazodone, would be expected to cause an increase cilostazol Cmax and AUC).
No products indexed under this heading.

Nelfinavir Mesylate (A reduced dose of cilostazol should be considered when taken concomitantly with CYP3A4 inhibitors).
No products indexed under this heading.

Nevirapine (A reduced dose of cilostazol should be considered when taken concomitantly with CYP3A4 inhibitors). Products include:
Viramune Oral Suspension 873
Viramune Tablets 873

Niacinamide (A reduced dose of cilostazol should be considered when taken concomitantly with CYP3A4 inhibitors). Products include:
BioLean Free Tablets .... ▣635

Nicotinamide (A reduced dose of cilostazol should be considered when taken concomitantly with CYP3A4 inhibitors).
No products indexed under this heading.

Nifedipine (A reduced dose of cilostazol should be considered when taken concomitantly with CYP3A4 inhibitors).
No products indexed under this heading.

Norfloxacin (A reduced dose of cilostazol should be considered when taken concomitantly with CYP3A4 inhibitors). Products include:
Noroxin Tablets 2069

Omeprazole (Co-administration with potent inhibitors of CYP2C19, such as omeprazole, has increased the systemic exposure to 3,4 dehydro-cilostazol by 69%).
No products indexed under this heading.

Oxiconazole Nitrate (A reduced dose of cilostazol should be considered when taken concomitantly with CYP2C19 inhibitors).
No products indexed under this heading.

Paroxetine Hydrochloride (A reduced dose of cilostazol should be considered when taken concomitantly with CYP3A4 inhibitors). Products include:
Paxil 1535
Paxil CR Controlled-Release Tablets 1544

Penicillin G Benzathine (Caution is advised in patients receiving both cilostazol and any other antiplatelet agent). Products include:
Bicillin C-R Injectable Suspension 1775
Bicillin L-A Injection 1777

Penicillin G Procaine (Caution is advised in patients receiving both cilostazol and any other antiplatelet agent). Products include:
Bicillin C-R Injectable Suspension 1775
Bicillin L-A Injection 1777

Phenylbutazone (Caution is advised in patients receiving both cilostazol and any other antiplatelet agent).
No products indexed under this heading.

Piroxicam (Caution is advised in patients receiving both cilostazol and any other antiplatelet agent).
No products indexed under this heading.

Polythiazide (A reduced dose of cilostazol should be considered when taken concomitantly with CYP2C19 inhibitors).
No products indexed under this heading.

Propoxyphene Hydrochloride (A reduced dose of cilostazol should be considered when taken concomitantly with CYP3A4 inhibitors).
No products indexed under this heading.

Propoxyphene Napsylate (A reduced dose of cilostazol should be considered when taken concomitantly with CYP3A4 inhibitors).
No products indexed under this heading.

Quinidine (A reduced dose of cilostazol should be considered when taken concomitantly with CYP3A4 inhibitors).
No products indexed under this heading.

Quinidine Hydrochloride (A reduced dose of cilostazol should be considered when taken concomitantly with CYP3A4 inhibitors).
No products indexed under this heading.

Quinidine Polygalacturonate (A reduced dose of cilostazol should be considered when taken concomitantly with CYP3A4 inhibitors).
No products indexed under this heading.

Quinidine Sulfate (A reduced dose of cilostazol should be considered when taken concomitantly with CYP3A4 inhibitors).
No products indexed under this heading.

Quinine (A reduced dose of cilostazol should be considered when taken concomitantly with CYP3A4 inhibitors).
No products indexed under this heading.

Quinine Sulfate (A reduced dose of cilostazol should be considered when taken concomitantly with CYP3A4 inhibitors).
No products indexed under this heading.

Quinupristin (A reduced dose of cilostazol should be considered when taken concomitantly with CYP3A4 inhibitors).
No products indexed under this heading.

Ranitidine Bismuth Citrate (A reduced dose of cilostazol should be considered when taken concomitantly with CYP3A4 inhibitors).
No products indexed under this heading.

Ranitidine Hydrochloride (A reduced dose of cilostazol should be considered when taken concomitantly with CYP3A4 inhibitors). Products include:
Zantac 75 Tablets .... ▣603
Zantac 1670
Zantac Injection 1666
Zantac Injection Pharmacy Bulk Package 1668
Maximum Strength Zantac 150 Tablets .... ▣603
Maximum Strength Zantac 150 Cool Mint Tablets .... ▣603

Ritonavir (A reduced dose of cilostazol should be considered when taken concomitantly with CYP3A4 inhibitors). Products include:
Kaletra 452
Norvir 489

Salsalate (Caution is advised in patients receiving both cilostazol and any other antiplatelet agent).
No products indexed under this heading.

Saquinavir (A reduced dose of cilostazol should be considered when taken concomitantly with CYP3A4 inhibitors).
No products indexed under this heading.

Saquinavir Mesylate (A reduced dose of cilostazol should be considered when taken concomitantly with CYP3A4 inhibitors).
No products indexed under this heading.

Sertraline Hydrochloride (Co-administration of cilostazol with strong inhibitors of CYP3A4, such as sertraline, would be expected to cause an increase in cilostazol Cmax and AUC).
No products indexed under this heading.

Sildenafil Citrate (A reduced dose of cilostazol should be considered when taken concomitantly with CYP3A4 inhibitors).
No products indexed under this heading.

Sulfacytine (A reduced dose of cilostazol should be considered when taken concomitantly with CYP2C19 inhibitors).
No products indexed under this heading.

Sulfamethizole (A reduced dose of cilostazol should be considered when taken concomitantly with CYP2C19 inhibitors).
No products indexed under this heading.

Sulfamethoxazole (A reduced dose of cilostazol should be considered when taken concomitantly with CYP2C19 inhibitors).
No products indexed under this heading.

Sulfasalazine (A reduced dose of cilostazol should be considered when taken concomitantly with CYP2C19 inhibitors).
No products indexed under this heading.

Sulfinpyrazone (A reduced dose of cilostazol should be considered when taken concomitantly with CYP2C19 inhibitors).
No products indexed under this heading.

Sulfisoxazole Acetyl (A reduced dose of cilostazol should be considered when taken concomitantly with CYP2C19 inhibitors).
No products indexed under this heading.

Sulfisoxazole Diolamine (A reduced dose of cilostazol should be considered when taken concomitantly with CYP2C19 inhibitors).
No products indexed under this heading.

Sulindac (Caution is advised in patients receiving both cilostazol and any other antiplatelet agent). Products include:
Clinoril Tablets 1962

Telithromycin (A reduced dose of cilostazol should be considered when taken concomitantly with CYP3A4 inhibitors). Products include:
Ketek Tablets 2744

Terconazole (A reduced dose of cilostazol should be considered when taken concomitantly with CYP2C19 inhibitors).
No products indexed under this heading.

Ticarcillin Disodium (Caution is advised in patients receiving both cilostazol and any other antiplatelet agent). Products include:
Timentin ADD-Vantage 1606
Timentin Injection Galaxy Container 1609
Timentin IV Infusion 1603
Timentin Pharmacy Bulk Package 1613

Ticlopidine Hydrochloride (Caution is advised in patients receiving both cilostazol and any other antiplatelet agent).
No products indexed under this heading.

Tolazamide (A reduced dose of cilostazol should be considered when taken concomitantly with CYP2C19 inhibitors).
No products indexed under this heading.

Tolbutamide (A reduced dose of cilostazol should be considered when taken concomitantly with CYP2C19 inhibitors).
No products indexed under this heading.

Tolbutamide Sodium (A reduced dose of cilostazol should be considered when taken concomitantly with CYP2C19 inhibitors).
No products indexed under this heading.

Tolmetin Sodium (Caution is advised in patients receiving both cilostazol and any other antiplatelet agent).
No products indexed under this heading.

Troglitazone (A reduced dose of cilostazol should be considered when taken concomitantly with CYP3A4 inhibitors).
No products indexed under this heading.

Troleandomycin (A reduced dose of cilostazol should be considered when taken concomitantly with CYP3A4 inhibitors).
No products indexed under this heading.

Valproate Sodium (A reduced dose of cilostazol should be considered when taken concomitantly with CYP3A4 inhibitors).
No products indexed under this heading.

Vardenafil Hydrochloride (A reduced dose of cilostazol should be considered when taken concomitantly with CYP3A4 inhibitors). Products include:
Levitra Tablets 2876

Verapamil Hydrochloride (A reduced dose of cilostazol should be considered when taken concomitantly with CYP3A4 inhibitors). Products include:
Tarka Tablets 511

Voriconazole (A reduced dose of cilostazol should be considered when taken concomitantly with CYP3A4 inhibitors).
No products indexed under this heading.

Zafirlukast (A reduced dose of cilostazol should be considered when taken concomitantly with CYP3A4 inhibitors). Products include:
Accolate Tablets 669

Zileuton (A reduced dose of cilostazol should be considered when taken concomitantly with CYP3A4 inhibitors).
No products indexed under this heading.

Food Interactions

Food, unspecified (Co-administration with a high-fat meal increases absorption, with an approximately 90% increase in Cmax and a 25% increase in AUC; patients should be advised to take Pletal at least one hour before or two hours after breakfast and dinner).

Grapefruit (A reduced dose of cilostazol should be considered when taken concomitantly with CYP3A4 inhibitors).

Grapefruit Juice (Co-administration of cilostazol with inhibitors of CYP3A4, such as grapefruit juice, increase cilostazol plasma concentration by 50%; concurrent consumption of grapefruit juice should be avoided).

PNEUMOVAX 23
(Pneumococcal Vaccine, Polyvalent).......... 2078
May interact with:

Azathioprine (Co-administration of vaccine in patients receiving immunosuppressive therapy may not result in expected serum antibody response; potential impairment of future immune responses to pneumococcal antigens may occur).
No products indexed under this heading.

Cyclosporine (Co-administration of vaccine in patients receiving immunosuppressive therapy may not result in expected serum antibody response; potential impairment of future immune responses to pneumococcal antigens may occur). Products include:
Gengraf Capsules 435
Neoral Oral Solution 2280
Neoral Soft Gelatin Capsules 2280
Restasis Ophthalmic Emulsion 557
Sandimmune 2296

Muromonab-CD3 (Co-administration of vaccine in patients receiving immunosuppressive therapy may not result in expected serum antibody response; potential impairment of future immune responses to pneumococcal antigens may occur). Products include:
Orthoclone OKT3 Sterile Solution 2387

Mycophenolate Mofetil (Co-administration of vaccine in patients receiving immunosuppressive therapy may not result in expected serum antibody response; potential impairment of future immune responses to pneumococcal antigens may occur). Products include:
CellCept Capsules 2622
CellCept Oral Suspension 2622
CellCept Tablets 2622

Tacrolimus (Co-administration of vaccine in patients receiving immunosuppressive therapy may not result in expected serum antibody response; potential impairment of future immune responses to pneumococcal antigens may occur). Products include:
Prograf Capsules and Injection 622
Protopic Ointment 628

POTABA CAPSULES
(Aminobenzoate Potassium) 1698
May interact with sulfonamides. Compounds in these categories include:

Bendroflumethiazide (Co-administration with sulfonamides is contraindicated).
No products indexed under this heading.

Chlorothiazide (Co-administration with sulfonamides is contraindicated).
No products indexed under this heading.

Chlorothiazide Sodium (Co-administration with sulfonamides is contraindicated). Products include:
Intravenous Sodium Diuril 2490

Chlorpropamide (Co-administration with sulfonamides is contraindicated).
No products indexed under this heading.

Glipizide (Co-administration with sulfonamides is contraindicated).
No products indexed under this heading.

Glyburide (Co-administration with sulfonamides is contraindicated).
No products indexed under this heading.

Hydrochlorothiazide (Co-administration with sulfonamides is contraindicated). Products include:
Atacand HCT 642
Avalide Tablets 892
Avalide Tablets 2713
Benicar HCT Tablets 1010
Diovan HCT Tablets 2216
Dyazide Capsules 1405
Micardis HCT Tablets 854
Prinzide Tablets 2092
Tekturna HCT Tablets 2324
Teveten HCT Tablets 517

Hydroflumethiazide (Co-administration with sulfonamides is contraindicated).
No products indexed under this heading.

Methyclothiazide (Co-administration with sulfonamides is contraindicated).
No products indexed under this heading.

Polythiazide (Co-administration with sulfonamides is contraindicated).
No products indexed under this heading.

Sulfacytine (Co-administration with sulfonamides is contraindicated).
No products indexed under this heading.

Sulfamethizole (Co-administration with sulfonamides is contraindicated).
No products indexed under this heading.

Sulfamethoxazole (Co-administration with sulfonamides is contraindicated).
No products indexed under this heading.

Sulfasalazine (Co-administration with sulfonamides is contraindicated).
No products indexed under this heading.

Sulfinpyrazone (Co-administration with sulfonamides is contraindicated).
No products indexed under this heading.

Sulfisoxazole Acetyl (Co-administration with sulfonamides is contraindicated).
No products indexed under this heading.

Sulfisoxazole Diolamine (Co-administration with sulfonamides is contraindicated).
No products indexed under this heading.

Tolazamide (Co-administration with sulfonamides is contraindicated).
No products indexed under this heading.

Tolbutamide (Co-administration with sulfonamides is contraindicated).
No products indexed under this heading.

POTABA ENVULES
(Aminobenzoate Potassium) 1698
See Potaba Capsules

POTABA TABLETS
(Aminobenzoate Potassium) 1698
See Potaba Capsules

PRAMOSONE CREAM 1% AND 2.5%
(Hydrocortisone Acetate, Pramoxine Hydrochloride).......... 1141
None cited in PDR database.

PRAMOSONE LOTION 1% AND 2.5%
(Hydrocortisone Acetate, Pramoxine Hydrochloride).......... 1141
See Pramosone Cream 1% and 2.5%

PRAMOSONE OINTMENT 1% AND 2.5%
(Hydrocortisone Acetate, Pramoxine Hydrochloride).......... 1141
See Pramosone Cream 1% and 2.5%

PRANDIMET TABLETS
(Metformin Hydrochloride, Repaglinide).......... 2967
May interact with cationic drugs that are eliminated by renal tubular, cytochrome p450 2c8 inducers (selected), cytochrome p450 2c8 inhibitors (selected), cytochrome p450 3a4 inducers (selected), cytochrome p450 3a4 inhibitors (selected), and certain other agents. Compounds in these categories include:

Acetazolamide (Repaglinide is metabolized by CYP2C8 and to a lesser extent by CYP3A4. Drugs that inhibit 3A4 may alter the pharmacokinetics and pharmacodynamics of repaglinide).
No products indexed under this heading.

Allium sativum (Repaglinide is metabolized by CYP2C8 and to a lesser extent by CYP3A4. Drugs that induce CYP3A4 may alter the pharmacokinetics and pharmacodynamics of repaglinide).
No products indexed under this heading.

Amiloride Hydrochloride (Cationic drugs that are eliminated by renal tubular secretion theoretically have the potential for interaction with metformin by competing for common renal tubular transport systems. Careful patient monitoring and dose adjustment of PrandiMet and/or the interfering drug is recommended in patients who are taking cationic medications that are excreted via the proximal renal tubular secretory system).
No products indexed under this heading.

Amiodarone Hydrochloride (Repaglinide is metabolized by CYP2C8 and to a lesser extent by CYP3A4. Drugs that inhibit 3A4 may alter the pharmacokinetics and pharmacodynamics of repaglinide).
No products indexed under this heading.

Amprenavir (Repaglinide is metabolized by CYP2C8 and to a lesser extent by CYP3A4. Drugs that inhibit 3A4 may alter the pharmacokinetics and pharmacodynamics of repaglinide).
No products indexed under this heading.

Anastrozole (Repaglinide is metabolized by CYP2C8 and to a lesser extent by CYP3A4. Drugs that inhibit 2C8 may alter the pharmacokinetics and pharmacodynamics of repaglinide). Products include:
Arimidex Tablets 672

Aprepitant (Repaglinide is metabolized by CYP2C8 and to a lesser

extent by CYP3A4. Drugs that inhibit 3A4 may alter the pharmacokinetics and pharmacodynamics of repaglinide). Products include:

Emend Capsules 1992

Atazanavir (Repaglinide is metabolized by CYP2C8 and to a lesser extent by CYP3A4. Drugs that inhibit 3A4 may alter the pharmacokinetics and pharmacodynamics of repaglinide).

No products indexed under this heading.

Atazanavir Sulfate (Repaglinide is metabolized by CYP2C8 and to a lesser extent by CYP3A4. Drugs that inhibit 3A4 may alter the pharmacokinetics and pharmacodynamics of repaglinide). Products include:

Reyataz Capsules 3299

Betamethasone Acetate (Repaglinide is metabolized by CYP2C8 and to a lesser extent by CYP3A4. Drugs that induce CYP3A4 may alter the pharmacokinetics and pharmacodynamics of repaglinide).

No products indexed under this heading.

Betamethasone Sodium Phosphate (Repaglinide is metabolized by CYP2C8 and to a lesser extent by CYP3A4. Drugs that induce CYP3A4 may alter the pharmacokinetics and pharmacodynamics of repaglinide).

No products indexed under this heading.

Carbamazepine (Repaglinide is metabolized by CYP2C8 and to a lesser extent by CYP3A4. Drugs that induce CYP2C8 may alter the pharmacokinetics and pharmacodynamics of repaglinide). Products include:

Carbatrol Capsules 3019
Equetro Extended-Release Capsules 3174

Cimetidine (Repaglinide is metabolized by CYP2C8 and to a lesser extent by CYP3A4. Drugs that inhibit 2C8 may alter the pharmacokinetics and pharmacodynamics of repaglinide).

No products indexed under this heading.

Cimetidine Hydrochloride (Repaglinide is metabolized by CYP2C8 and to a lesser extent by CYP3A4. Drugs that inhibit 2C8 may alter the pharmacokinetics and pharmacodynamics of repaglinide).

No products indexed under this heading.

Ciprofloxacin (Repaglinide is metabolized by CYP2C8 and to a lesser extent by CYP3A4. Drugs that inhibit 3A4 may alter the pharmacokinetics and pharmacodynamics of repaglinide). Products include:

Cipro I.V. 2817
Cipro Oral Suspension 2810
Cipro XR Tablets 2823
Ciprodex Otic Suspension 541

Ciprofloxacin Hydrochloride (Repaglinide is metabolized by CYP2C8 and to a lesser extent by CYP3A4. Drugs that induce CYP3A4 may alter the pharmacokinetics and pharmacodynamics of repaglinide). Products include:

Cipro Tablets 2810

Cisplatin (Repaglinide is metabolized by CYP2C8 and to a lesser extent by CYP3A4. Drugs that induce CYP3A4 may alter the pharmacokinetics and pharmacodynamics of repaglinide).

No products indexed under this heading.

Clarithromycin (Repaglinide is metabolized by CYP2C8 and to a lesser extent by CYP3A4. Drugs that inhibit 3A4 may alter the pharmacokinetics and pharmacodynamics of repaglinide). Products include:

Biaxin/Biaxin XL 411

Clotrimazole (Repaglinide is metabolized by CYP2C8 and to a lesser extent by CYP3A4. Drugs that inhibit 3A4 may alter the pharmacokinetics and pharmacodynamics of repaglinide). Products include:

Lotrisone 2881

Cortisone Acetate (Repaglinide is metabolized by CYP2C8 and to a lesser extent by CYP3A4. Drugs that induce CYP3A4 may alter the pharmacokinetics and pharmacodynamics of repaglinide).

No products indexed under this heading.

Cyclosporine (Repaglinide is metabolized by CYP2C8 and to a lesser extent by CYP3A4. Drugs that inhibit 3A4 may alter the pharmacokinetics and pharmacodynamics of repaglinide). Products include:

Gengraf Capsules 435
Neoral Oral Solution 2280
Neoral Soft Gelatin Capsules 2280
Restasis Ophthalmic Emulsion 557
Sandimmune 2296

Dalfopristin (Repaglinide is metabolized by CYP2C8 and to a lesser extent by CYP3A4. Drugs that inhibit 3A4 may alter the pharmacokinetics and pharmacodynamics of repaglinide).

No products indexed under this heading.

Danazol (Repaglinide is metabolized by CYP2C8 and to a lesser extent by CYP3A4. Drugs that inhibit 3A4 may alter the pharmacokinetics and pharmacodynamics of repaglinide).

No products indexed under this heading.

Delavirdine Mesylate (Repaglinide is metabolized by CYP2C8 and to a lesser extent by CYP3A4. Drugs that inhibit 3A4 may alter the pharmacokinetics and pharmacodynamics of repaglinide).

No products indexed under this heading.

Dexamethasone (Repaglinide is metabolized by CYP2C8 and to a lesser extent by CYP3A4. Drugs that induce CYP3A4 may alter the pharmacokinetics and pharmacodynamics of repaglinide). Products include:

Ciprodex Otic Suspension 541

Dexamethasone Acetate (Repaglinide is metabolized by CYP2C8 and to a lesser extent by CYP3A4. Drugs that induce CYP3A4 may alter the pharmacokinetics and pharmacodynamics of repaglinide).

No products indexed under this heading.

Dexamethasone Sodium Phosphate (Repaglinide is metabolized by CYP2C8 and to a lesser extent by CYP3A4. Drugs that induce CYP3A4 may alter the pharmacokinetics and pharmacodynamics of repaglinide).

No products indexed under this heading.

Digoxin (Cationic drugs that are eliminated by renal tubular secretion theoretically have the potential for interaction with metformin by competing for common renal tubular transport systems. Careful patient monitoring and dose adjustment of PrandiMet and/or the interfering drug is recommended in patients who are taking cationic medications that are excreted via the proximal renal tubular secretory system). Products include:

Lanoxin Injection 1498
Lanoxin Injection Pediatric 1502
Lanoxin Tablets 1505

Diltiazem Hydrochloride (Repaglinide is metabolized by CYP2C8 and to a lesser extent by CYP3A4. Drugs that inhibit 3A4 may alter the pharmacokinetics and pharmacodynamics of repaglinide). Products include:

Cardizem LA Extended Release Tablets 421

Diltiazem Maleate (Repaglinide is metabolized by CYP2C8 and to a lesser extent by CYP3A4. Drugs that inhibit 3A4 may alter the pharmacokinetics and pharmacodynamics of repaglinide).

No products indexed under this heading.

Doxorubicin Hydrochloride (Repaglinide is metabolized by CYP2C8 and to a lesser extent by CYP3A4. Drugs that induce CYP3A4 may alter the pharmacokinetics and pharmacodynamics of repaglinide).

No products indexed under this heading.

Efavirenz (Repaglinide is metabolized by CYP2C8 and to a lesser extent by CYP3A4. Drugs that inhibit 3A4 may alter the pharmacokinetics and pharmacodynamics of repaglinide). Products include:

Atripla Tablets 938
Sustiva Capsules 930
Sustiva Tablets 930

Erythromycin (Repaglinide is metabolized by CYP2C8 and to a lesser extent by CYP3A4. Drugs that inhibit 3A4 may alter the pharmacokinetics and pharmacodynamics of repaglinide).

No products indexed under this heading.

Erythromycin Estolate (Repaglinide is metabolized by CYP2C8 and to a lesser extent by CYP3A4. Drugs that inhibit 3A4 may alter the pharmacokinetics and pharmacodynamics of repaglinide).

No products indexed under this heading.

Erythromycin Ethylsuccinate (Repaglinide is metabolized by CYP2C8 and to a lesser extent by CYP3A4. Drugs that inhibit 3A4 may alter the pharmacokinetics and pharmacodynamics of repaglinide). Products include:

E.E.S. 433
EryPed 431

Erythromycin Gluceptate (Repaglinide is metabolized by CYP2C8 and to a lesser extent by CYP3A4. Drugs that inhibit 3A4 may alter the pharmacokinetics and pharmacodynamics of repaglinide).

No products indexed under this heading.

Erythromycin Lactobionate (Repaglinide is metabolized by CYP2C8 and to a lesser extent by CYP3A4. Drugs that inhibit 3A4 may alter the pharmacokinetics and pharmacodynamics of repaglinide).

No products indexed under this heading.

Erythromycin Stearate (Repaglinide is metabolized by CYP2C8 and to a lesser extent by CYP3A4. Drugs that inhibit 3A4 may alter the pharmacokinetics and pharmacodynamics of repaglinide).

No products indexed under this heading.

Esomeprazole Magnesium (Repaglinide is metabolized by CYP2C8 and to a lesser extent by CYP3A4. Drugs that inhibit 3A4 may alter the pharmacokinetics and pharmacodynamics of repaglinide). Products include:

Nexium Delayed-Release Capsules 645
Nexium Delayed-Release Oral Suspension 645

Ethanol (Alcohol potentiates the effect of metformin on lactate metabolism. Patients should be warned against excessive alcohol intake while receiving PrandiMet).

No products indexed under this heading.

Ethosuximide (Repaglinide is metabolized by CYP2C8 and to a lesser extent by CYP3A4. Drugs that induce CYP3A4 may alter the pharmacokinetics and pharmacodynamics of repaglinide).

No products indexed under this heading.

Ethyl Alcohol (Alcohol potentiates the effect of metformin on lactate metabolism. Patients should be warned against excessive alcohol intake while receiving PrandiMet).

No products indexed under this heading.

Felbamate (Repaglinide is metabolized by CYP2C8 and to a lesser extent by CYP3A4. Drugs that induce CYP3A4 may alter the pharmacokinetics and pharmacodynamics of repaglinide).

No products indexed under this heading.

Fluconazole (Repaglinide is metabolized by CYP2C8 and to a lesser extent by CYP3A4. Drugs that inhibit 3A4 may alter the pharmacokinetics and pharmacodynamics of repaglinide).

No products indexed under this heading.

Fludrocortisone Acetate (Repaglinide is metabolized by CYP2C8 and to a lesser extent by CYP3A4. Drugs that induce CYP3A4 may alter the pharmacokinetics and pharmacodynamics of repaglinide).

No products indexed under this heading.

Fluoxetine (Repaglinide is metabolized by CYP2C8 and to a lesser extent by CYP3A4. Drugs that inhibit 3A4 may alter the pharmacokinetics and pharmacodynamics of repaglinide).

No products indexed under this heading.

Fluoxetine Hydrochloride (Repaglinide is metabolized by CYP2C8 and to a lesser extent by CYP3A4. Drugs that inhibit 3A4 may alter the pharmacokinetics and pharmacodynamics of repaglinide). Products include:

Prozac Weekly Capsules 1852
Prozac Pulvules and Liquid 1852
Symbyax Capsules 1871

Fluvoxamine Maleate (Repaglinide is metabolized by CYP2C8 and to a lesser extent by CYP3A4. Drugs that inhibit 3A4 may alter the phar-

macokinetics and pharmacodynamics of repaglinide). Products include:
Luvox CR Extended-Release Capsules 1759

Fosamprenavir Calcium (Repaglinide is metabolized by CYP2C8 and to a lesser extent by CYP3A4. Drugs that inhibit 3A4 may alter the pharmacokinetics and pharmacodynamics of repaglinide). Products include:
Lexiva Oral Suspension 1510
Lexiva Tablets 1510

Fosphenytoin Sodium (Repaglinide is metabolized by CYP2C8 and to a lesser extent by CYP3A4. Drugs that induce CYP3A4 may alter the pharmacokinetics and pharmacodynamics of repaglinide).
No products indexed under this heading.

Garlic Extract (Repaglinide is metabolized by CYP2C8 and to a lesser extent by CYP3A4. Drugs that induce CYP3A4 may alter the pharmacokinetics and pharmacodynamics of repaglinide).
No products indexed under this heading.

Garlic Oil (Repaglinide is metabolized by CYP2C8 and to a lesser extent by CYP3A4. Drugs that induce CYP3A4 may alter the pharmacokinetics and pharmacodynamics of repaglinide).
No products indexed under this heading.

Gemfibrozil (Gemfibrozil increases exposures to repaglinide, one of the components of PrandiMet, which may enhance and prolong the blood glucose lowering effects of repaglinide. Post-marketing events of serious hypoglycemia have been reported in patients taking both repaglinide and gemfibrozil. Administration of PrandiMet and gemfibrozil to the same patient is not recommended. Repaglinide exposures are increased more than 20-fold in patients taking both gemfibrozil and itraconazole. Therefore, do not use PrandiMet in patients taking both gemfibrozil and intraconazole).
No products indexed under this heading.

Hydrocortisone (Repaglinide is metabolized by CYP2C8 and to a lesser extent by CYP3A4. Drugs that induce CYP3A4 may alter the pharmacokinetics and pharmacodynamics of repaglinide).
No products indexed under this heading.

Hydrocortisone Acetate (Repaglinide is metabolized by CYP2C8 and to a lesser extent by CYP3A4. Drugs that induce CYP3A4 may alter the pharmacokinetics and pharmacodynamics of repaglinide). Products include:
Analpram-HC 1140
Pramosone 1141

Hydrocortisone Butyrate (Repaglinide is metabolized by CYP2C8 and to a lesser extent by CYP3A4. Drugs that induce CYP3A4 may alter the pharmacokinetics and pharmacodynamics of repaglinide).
No products indexed under this heading.

Hydrocortisone Cypionate (Repaglinide is metabolized by CYP2C8 and to a lesser extent by CYP3A4. Drugs that induce CYP3A4 may alter the pharmacokinetics and pharmacodynamics of repaglinide).
No products indexed under this heading.

Hydrocortisone Hemisuccinate (Repaglinide is metabolized by CYP2C8 and to a lesser extent by CYP3A4. Drugs that induce CYP3A4 may alter the pharmacokinetics and pharmacodynamics of repaglinide).
No products indexed under this heading.

Hydrocortisone Probutate (Repaglinide is metabolized by CYP2C8 and to a lesser extent by CYP3A4. Drugs that induce CYP3A4 may alter the pharmacokinetics and pharmacodynamics of repaglinide).
No products indexed under this heading.

Hydrocortisone Sodium Phosphate (Repaglinide is metabolized by CYP2C8 and to a lesser extent by CYP3A4. Drugs that induce CYP3A4 may alter the pharmacokinetics and pharmacodynamics of repaglinide).
No products indexed under this heading.

Hydrocortisone Sodium Succinate (Repaglinide is metabolized by CYP2C8 and to a lesser extent by CYP3A4. Drugs that induce CYP3A4 may alter the pharmacokinetics and pharmacodynamics of repaglinide).
No products indexed under this heading.

Hydrocortisone Valerate (Repaglinide is metabolized by CYP2C8 and to a lesser extent by CYP3A4. Drugs that induce CYP3A4 may alter the pharmacokinetics and pharmacodynamics of repaglinide).
No products indexed under this heading.

Hypericum (Repaglinide is metabolized by CYP2C8 and to a lesser extent by CYP3A4. Drugs that induce CYP3A4 may alter the pharmacokinetics and pharmacodynamics of repaglinide). Products include:
Satieté Tablets 640

Hypericum Perforatum (Repaglinide is metabolized by CYP2C8 and to a lesser extent by CYP3A4. Drugs that induce CYP3A4 may alter the pharmacokinetics and pharmacodynamics of repaglinide).
No products indexed under this heading.

Indinavir Sulfate (Repaglinide is metabolized by CYP2C8 and to a lesser extent by CYP3A4. Drugs that inhibit 3A4 may alter the pharmacokinetics and pharmacodynamics of repaglinide). Products include:
Crixivan Capsules 1979

Insulin, Human NPH (Repaglinide is not indicated for use in combination with NPH-insulin. Across seven controlled clinical trials, there were six serious adverse events (1.4%) of myocardial ischemia with repaglinide in combination with NPH-insulin to one event (0.3%) in patients using insulin alone). Products include:
Humulin N Vial 1846

Iodine, radiolabeled (Intravascular contrast studies with iodinated materials can lead to acute alteration of renal function and have been associated with lactic acidosis in patients receiving metformin hydrochloride. Therefore, in patients whom any such study is planned, PrandiMet should be temporarily discontinued at the time of or prior to the procedure, and withheld for 48 hours subsequent to the procedure and reinstituted only after renal function has been re-evaluated and found to be normal).
No products indexed under this heading.

Isoniazid (Repaglinide is metabolized by CYP2C8 and to a lesser extent by CYP3A4. Drugs that inhibit 3A4 may alter the pharmacokinetics and pharmacodynamics of repaglinide).
No products indexed under this heading.

Itraconazole (Repaglinide exposures are increased more than 20-fold in patients taking both gemfibrozil and intraconazole. Therefore, do not use PrandiMet in patients taking both gemfibrozil and itraconzole).
No products indexed under this heading.

Ketoconazole (Repaglinide is metabolized by CYP2C8 and to a lesser extent by CYP3A4. Drugs that inhibit 3A4 may alter the pharmacokinetics and pharmacodynamics of repaglinide). Products include:
Extina Foam, 2% 3057
Nizoral A-D Shampoo 1901

Lopinavir (Repaglinide is metabolized by CYP2C8 and to a lesser extent by CYP3A4. Drugs that inhibit 3A4 may alter the pharmacokinetics and pharmacodynamics of repaglinide). Products include:
Kaletra 452

Loratadine (Repaglinide is metabolized by CYP2C8 and to a lesser extent by CYP3A4. Drugs that inhibit 3A4 may alter the pharmacokinetics and pharmacodynamics of repaglinide).
No products indexed under this heading.

Mephenytoin (Repaglinide is metabolized by CYP2C8 and to a lesser extent by CYP3A4. Drugs that induce CYP3A4 may alter the pharmacokinetics and pharmacodynamics of repaglinide).
No products indexed under this heading.

Methsuximide (Repaglinide is metabolized by CYP2C8 and to a lesser extent by CYP3A4. Drugs that induce CYP3A4 may alter the pharmacokinetics and pharmacodynamics of repaglinide).
No products indexed under this heading.

Methylprednisolone (Repaglinide is metabolized by CYP2C8 and to a lesser extent by CYP3A4. Drugs that induce CYP3A4 may alter the pharmacokinetics and pharmacodynamics of repaglinide).
No products indexed under this heading.

Methylprednisolone Acetate (Repaglinide is metabolized by CYP2C8 and to a lesser extent by CYP3A4. Drugs that induce CYP3A4 may alter the pharmacokinetics and pharmacodynamics of repaglinide).
No products indexed under this heading.

Methylprednisolone Sodium Succinate (Repaglinide is metabolized by CYP2C8 and to a lesser extent by CYP3A4. Drugs that induce CYP3A4 may alter the pharmacokinetics and pharmacodynamics of repaglinide).
No products indexed under this heading.

Metronidazole (Repaglinide is metabolized by CYP2C8 and to a lesser extent by CYP3A4. Drugs that inhibit 3A4 may alter the pharmacokinetics and pharmacodynamics of repaglinide). Products include:
Pylera Capsules 714

Metronidazole Benzoate (Repaglinide is metabolized by CYP2C8 and to a lesser extent by CYP3A4. Drugs that inhibit 3A4 may alter the pharmacokinetics and pharmacodynamics of repaglinide).
No products indexed under this heading.

Metronidazole Hydrochloride (Repaglinide is metabolized by CYP2C8 and to a lesser extent by CYP3A4. Drugs that inhibit 3A4 may alter the pharmacokinetics and pharmacodynamics of repaglinide).
No products indexed under this heading.

Metronidazole Sodium (Repaglinide is metabolized by CYP2C8 and to a lesser extent by CYP3A4. Drugs that inhibit 3A4 may alter the pharmacokinetics and pharmacodynamics of repaglinide).
No products indexed under this heading.

Miconazole (Repaglinide is metabolized by CYP2C8 and to a lesser extent by CYP3A4. Drugs that inhibit 3A4 may alter the pharmacokinetics and pharmacodynamics of repaglinide).
No products indexed under this heading.

Miconazole Nitrate (Repaglinide is metabolized by CYP2C8 and to a lesser extent by CYP3A4. Drugs that inhibit 3A4 may alter the pharmacokinetics and pharmacodynamics of repaglinide).
No products indexed under this heading.

Modafinil (Repaglinide is metabolized by CYP2C8 and to a lesser extent by CYP3A4. Drugs that induce CYP3A4 may alter the pharmacokinetics and pharmacodynamics of repaglinide). Products include:
Provigil Tablets 977

Morphine Sulfate (Cationic drugs that are eliminated by renal tubular secretion theoretically have the potential for interaction with metformin by competing for common renal tubular transport systems. Careful patient monitoring and dose adjustment of PrandiMet and/or the interfering drug is recommended in patients who are taking cationic medications that are excreted via the proximal renal tubular secretory system). Products include:
Avinza Capsules 1772
DepoDur Injection 1095
MS Contin Tablets 2585

Nefazodone Hydrochloride (Repaglinide is metabolized by CYP2C8 and to a lesser extent by CYP3A4. Drugs that inhibit 3A4 may alter the pharmacokinetics and pharmacodynamics of repaglinide).
No products indexed under this heading.

Nelfinavir Mesylate (Repaglinide is metabolized by CYP2C8 and to a lesser extent by CYP3A4. Drugs that inhibit 3A4 may alter the pharmacokinetics and pharmacodynamics of repaglinide).
No products indexed under this heading.

Nevirapine (Repaglinide is metabolized by CYP2C8 and to a lesser extent by CYP3A4. Drugs that inhibit 3A4 may alter the pharmacokinetics and pharmacodynamics of repaglinide). Products include:
Viramune Oral Suspension 873
Viramune Tablets 873

Niacinamide (Repaglinide is metabolized by CYP2C8 and to a lesser extent by CYP3A4. Drugs that inhibit 3A4 may alter the pharmacokinetics and pharmacodynamics of repaglinide). Products include:
BioLean Free Tablets .... ▣635

Nicardipine Hydrochloride (Repaglinide is metabolized by CYP2C8 and to a lesser extent by CYP3A4. Drugs that inhibit 2C8 may alter the pharmacokinetics and pharmacodynamics of repaglinide). Products include:
Cardene I.V. 1093

Nicotinamide (Repaglinide is metabolized by CYP2C8 and to a lesser extent by CYP3A4. Drugs that inhibit 3A4 may alter the pharmacokinetics and pharmacodynamics of repaglinide).
No products indexed under this heading.

Nifedipine (Repaglinide is metabolized by CYP2C8 and to a lesser extent by CYP3A4. Drugs that inhibit 3A4 may alter the pharmacokinetics and pharmacodynamics of repaglinide).
No products indexed under this heading.

Norfloxacin (Repaglinide is metabolized by CYP2C8 and to a lesser extent by CYP3A4. Drugs that inhibit 3A4 may alter the pharmacokinetics and pharmacodynamics of repaglinide). Products include:
Noroxin Tablets 2069

Omeprazole (Repaglinide is metabolized by CYP2C8 and to a lesser extent by CYP3A4. Drugs that inhibit 2C8 may alter the pharmacokinetics and pharmacodynamics of repaglinide).
No products indexed under this heading.

Oxcarbazepine (Repaglinide is metabolized by CYP2C8 and to a lesser extent by CYP3A4. Drugs that induce CYP3A4 may alter the pharmacokinetics and pharmacodynamics of repaglinide).
No products indexed under this heading.

Paroxetine Hydrochloride (Repaglinide is metabolized by CYP2C8 and to a lesser extent by CYP3A4. Drugs that inhibit 3A4 may alter the pharmacokinetics and pharmacodynamics of repaglinide). Products include:
Paxil 1535
Paxil CR Controlled-Release Tablets 1544

Phenobarbital (Repaglinide is metabolized by CYP2C8 and to a lesser extent by CYP3A4. Drugs that induce CYP2C8 may alter the pharmacokinetics and pharmacodynamics of repaglinide). Products include:
Donnatal Extentabs 2507

Phenobarbital Sodium (Repaglinide is metabolized by CYP2C8 and to a lesser extent by CYP3A4. Drugs that induce CYP3A4 may alter the pharmacokinetics and pharmacodynamics of repaglinide).
No products indexed under this heading.

Phenytoin (Repaglinide is metabolized by CYP2C8 and to a lesser extent by CYP3A4. Drugs that induce CYP3A4 may alter the pharmacokinetics and pharmacodynamics of repaglinide).
No products indexed under this heading.

Phenytoin Sodium (Repaglinide is metabolized by CYP2C8 and to a lesser extent by CYP3A4. Drugs that induce CYP3A4 may alter the pharmacokinetics and pharmacodynamics of repaglinide). Products include:
Phenytek Capsules 2192

Prednisolone Acetate (Repaglinide is metabolized by CYP2C8 and to a lesser extent by CYP3A4. Drugs that induce CYP3A4 may alter the pharmacokinetics and pharmacodynamics of repaglinide). Products include:
Pred Forte Ophthalmic Suspension .... ⊙227
Pred Mild Ophthalmic Suspension .... ⊙230
Pred-G Ophthalmic Ointment .... ⊙229
Pred-G Ophthalmic Suspension ...... ⊙228

Prednisolone Sodium Phosphate (Repaglinide is metabolized by CYP2C8 and to a lesser extent by CYP3A4. Drugs that induce CYP3A4 may alter the pharmacokinetics and pharmacodynamics of repaglinide).
No products indexed under this heading.

Prednisolone Tebutate (Repaglinide is metabolized by CYP2C8 and to a lesser extent by CYP3A4. Drugs that induce CYP3A4 may alter the pharmacokinetics and pharmacodynamics of repaglinide).
No products indexed under this heading.

Prednisone (Repaglinide is metabolized by CYP2C8 and to a lesser extent by CYP3A4. Drugs that induce CYP3A4 may alter the pharmacokinetics and pharmacodynamics of repaglinide).
No products indexed under this heading.

Primidone (Repaglinide is metabolized by CYP2C8 and to a lesser extent by CYP3A4. Drugs that induce CYP2C8 may alter the pharmacokinetics and pharmacodynamics of repaglinide).
No products indexed under this heading.

Procainamide Hydrochloride (Cationic drugs that are eliminated by renal tubular secretion theoretically have the potential for interaction with metformin by competing for common renal tubular transport systems. Careful patient monitoring and dose adjustment of PrandiMet and/or the interfering drug is recommended in patients who are taking cationic medications that are excreted via the proximal renal tubular secretory system).
No products indexed under this heading.

Propoxyphene Hydrochloride (Repaglinide is metabolized by CYP2C8 and to a lesser extent by CYP3A4. Drugs that inhibit 3A4 may alter the pharmacokinetics and pharmacodynamics of repaglinide).
No products indexed under this heading.

Propoxyphene Napsylate (Repaglinide is metabolized by CYP2C8 and to a lesser extent by CYP3A4. Drugs that inhibit 3A4 may alter the pharmacokinetics and pharmacodynamics of repaglinide).
No products indexed under this heading.

Quercetin (Repaglinide is metabolized by CYP2C8 and to a lesser extent by CYP3A4. Drugs that inhibit 2C8 may alter the pharmacokinetics and pharmacodynamics of repaglinide).
No products indexed under this heading.

Quinidine (Repaglinide is metabolized by CYP2C8 and to a lesser extent by CYP3A4. Drugs that inhibit 3A4 may alter the pharmacokinetics and pharmacodynamics of repaglinide).
No products indexed under this heading.

Quinidine Gluconate (Cationic drugs that are eliminated by renal tubular secretion theoretically have the potential for interaction with metformin by competing for common renal tubular transport systems. Careful patient monitoring and dose adjustment of PrandiMet and/or the interfering drug is recommended in patients who are taking cationic medications that are excreted via the proximal renal tubular secretory system).
No products indexed under this heading.

Quinidine Hydrochloride (Repaglinide is metabolized by CYP2C8 and to a lesser extent by CYP3A4. Drugs that inhibit 3A4 may alter the pharmacokinetics and pharmacodynamics of repaglinide).
No products indexed under this heading.

Quinidine Polygalacturonate (Cationic drugs that are eliminated by renal tubular secretion theoretically have the potential for interaction with metformin by competing for common renal tubular transport systems. Careful patient monitoring and dose adjustment of PrandiMet and/or the interfering drug is recommended in patients who are taking cationic medications that are excreted via the proximal renal tubular secretory system).
No products indexed under this heading.

Quinidine Sulfate (Cationic drugs that are eliminated by renal tubular secretion theoretically have the potential for interaction with metformin by competing for common renal tubular transport systems. Careful patient monitoring and dose adjustment of PrandiMet and/or the interfering drug is recommended in patients who are taking cationic medications that are excreted via the proximal renal tubular secretory system).
No products indexed under this heading.

Quinine (Repaglinide is metabolized by CYP2C8 and to a lesser extent by CYP3A4. Drugs that inhibit 3A4 may alter the pharmacokinetics and pharmacodynamics of repaglinide).
No products indexed under this heading.

Quinine Sulfate (Cationic drugs that are eliminated by renal tubular secretion theoretically have the potential for interaction with metformin by competing for common renal tubular transport systems. Careful patient monitoring and dose adjustment of PrandiMet and/or the interfering drug is recommended in patients who are taking cationic medications that are excreted via the proximal renal tubular secretory system).
No products indexed under this heading.

Quinupristin (Repaglinide is metabolized by CYP2C8 and to a lesser extent by CYP3A4. Drugs that inhibit 3A4 may alter the pharmacokinetics and pharmacodynamics of repaglinide).
No products indexed under this heading.

Ranitidine Bismuth Citrate (Repaglinide is metabolized by CYP2C8 and to a lesser extent by CYP3A4. Drugs that inhibit 3A4 may alter the pharmacokinetics and pharmacodynamics of repaglinide).
No products indexed under this heading.

Ranitidine Hydrochloride (Cationic drugs that are eliminated by renal tubular secretion theoretically have the potential for interaction with metformin by competing for common renal tubular transport systems. Careful patient monitoring and dose adjustment of PrandiMet and/or the interfering drug is recommended in patients who are taking cationic medications that are excreted via the proximal renal tubular secretory system). Products include:
Zantac 75 Tablets .... ▣603
Zantac 1670
Zantac Injection 1666
Zantac Injection Pharmacy Bulk Package 1668
Maximum Strength Zantac 150 Tablets .... ▣603
Maximum Strength Zantac 150 Cool Mint Tablets .... ▣603

Rifabutin (Repaglinide is metabolized by CYP2C8 and to a lesser extent by CYP3A4. Drugs that induce CYP2C8 may alter the pharmacokinetics and pharmacodynamics of repaglinide).
No products indexed under this heading.

Rifampicin (Repaglinide is metabolized by CYP2C8 and to a lesser extent by CYP3A4. Drugs that induce CYP3A4 may alter the pharmacokinetics and pharmacodynamics of repaglinide).
No products indexed under this heading.

Rifampin (Repaglinide is metabolized by CYP2C8 and to a lesser extent by CYP3A4. Drugs that induce CYP2C8 may alter the pharmacokinetics and pharmacodynamics of repaglinide).
No products indexed under this heading.

Rifapentine (Repaglinide is metabolized by CYP2C8 and to a lesser extent by CYP3A4. Drugs that induce CYP3A4 may alter the pharmacokinetics and pharmacodynamics of repaglinide).
No products indexed under this heading.

Ritonavir (Repaglinide is metabolized by CYP2C8 and to a lesser extent by CYP3A4. Drugs that inhibit 3A4 may alter the pharmacokinetics and pharmacodynamics of repaglinide). Products include:
Kaletra 452
Norvir 489

Saquinavir (Repaglinide is metabolized by CYP2C8 and to a lesser extent by CYP3A4. Drugs that inhibit 3A4 may alter the pharmacokinetics and pharmacodynamics of repaglinide).
No products indexed under this heading.

Saquinavir Mesylate (Repaglinide is metabolized by CYP2C8 and to a lesser extent by CYP3A4. Drugs that inhibit 3A4 may alter the pharmacokinetics and pharmacodynamics of repaglinide).
No products indexed under this heading.

Sertraline Hydrochloride (Repaglinide is metabolized by CYP2C8 and to a lesser extent by CYP3A4. Drugs that inhibit 3A4 may alter the pharmacokinetics and pharmacodynamics of repaglinide).
No products indexed under this heading.

Sildenafil Citrate (Repaglinide is metabolized by CYP2C8 and to a lesser extent by CYP3A4. Drugs that inhibit 3A4 may alter the pharmacokinetics and pharmacodynamics of repaglinide).
No products indexed under this heading.

Sulfaphenazole (Repaglinide is metabolized by CYP2C8 and to a lesser extent by CYP3A4. Drugs that inhibit 2C8 may alter the pharmacokinetics and pharmacodynamics of repaglinide).
No products indexed under this heading.

Sulfinpyrazone (Repaglinide is metabolized by CYP2C8 and to a lesser extent by CYP3A4. Drugs that inhibit 2C8 may alter the pharmacokinetics and pharmacodynamics of repaglinide).
No products indexed under this heading.

Telithromycin (Repaglinide is metabolized by CYP2C8 and to a lesser extent by CYP3A4. Drugs that inhibit 3A4 may alter the pharmacokinetics and pharmacodynamics of repaglinide). Products include:
Ketek Tablets 2744

Theophylline (Repaglinide is metabolized by CYP2C8 and to a lesser extent by CYP3A4. Drugs that induce CYP3A4 may alter the pharmacokinetics and pharmacodynamics of repaglinide).
No products indexed under this heading.

Theophylline Anhydrous (Repaglinide is metabolized by CYP2C8 and to a lesser extent by CYP3A4. Drugs that induce CYP3A4 may alter the pharmacokinetics and pharmacodynamics of repaglinide). Products include:
Uniphyl Tablets 2595

Theophylline Calcium Salicylate (Repaglinide is metabolized by CYP2C8 and to a lesser extent by CYP3A4. Drugs that induce CYP3A4 may alter the pharmacokinetics and pharmacodynamics of repaglinide).
No products indexed under this heading.

Theophylline Dihydroxypropyl (Glyceryl) (Repaglinide is metabolized by CYP2C8 and to a lesser extent by CYP3A4. Drugs that induce CYP3A4 may alter the pharmacokinetics and pharmacodynamics of repaglinide).
No products indexed under this heading.

Theophylline Ethylenediamine (Repaglinide is metabolized by CYP2C8 and to a lesser extent by CYP3A4. Drugs that induce CYP3A4 may alter the pharmacokinetics and pharmacodynamics of repaglinide).
No products indexed under this heading.

Triamcinolone (Repaglinide is metabolized by CYP2C8 and to a lesser extent by CYP3A4. Drugs that induce CYP3A4 may alter the pharmacokinetics and pharmacodynamics of repaglinide).
No products indexed under this heading.

Triamcinolone Acetonide (Repaglinide is metabolized by CYP2C8 and to a lesser extent by CYP3A4. Drugs that induce CYP3A4 may alter the pharmacokinetics and pharmacodynamics of repaglinide). Products include:
Azmacort Inhalation Aerosol 407
Nasacort AQ Nasal Spray 2765
Triesence Injectable Suspension .... ⊙209

Triamcinolone Diacetate (Repaglinide is metabolized by CYP2C8 and to a lesser extent by CYP3A4. Drugs that induce CYP3A4 may alter the pharmacokinetics and pharmacodynamics of repaglinide).
No products indexed under this heading.

Triamcinolone Hexacetonide (Repaglinide is metabolized by CYP2C8 and to a lesser extent by CYP3A4. Drugs that induce CYP3A4 may alter the pharmacokinetics and pharmacodynamics of repaglinide).
No products indexed under this heading.

Triamterene (Cationic drugs that are eliminated by renal tubular secretion theoretically have the potential for interaction with metformin by competing for common renal tubular transport systems. Careful patient monitoring and dose adjustment of PrandiMet and/or the interfering drug is recommended in patients who are taking cationic medications that are excreted via the proximal renal tubular secretory system). Products include:
Dyazide Capsules 1405
Dyrenium Capsules 3189

Trimethoprim (Cationic drugs that are eliminated by renal tubular secretion theoretically have the potential for interaction with metformin by competing for common renal tubular transport systems. Careful patient monitoring and dose adjustment of PrandiMet and/or the interfering drug is recommended in patients who are taking cationic medications that are excreted via the proximal renal tubular secretory system).
No products indexed under this heading.

Trimethoprim Hydrochloride (Repaglinide is metabolized by CYP2C8 and to a lesser extent by CYP3A4. Drugs that inhibit 2C8 may alter the pharmacokinetics and pharmacodynamics of repaglinide).
No products indexed under this heading.

Trimethoprim Sulfate (Cationic drugs that are eliminated by renal tubular secretion theoretically have the potential for interaction with metformin by competing for common renal tubular transport systems. Careful patient monitoring and dose adjustment of PrandiMet and/or the interfering drug is recommended in patients who are taking cationic medications that are excreted via the proximal renal tubular secretory system).
No products indexed under this heading.

Troglitazone (Repaglinide is metabolized by CYP2C8 and to a lesser extent by CYP3A4. Drugs that inhibit 3A4 may alter the pharmacokinetics and pharmacodynamics of repaglinide).
No products indexed under this heading.

Troleandomycin (Repaglinide is metabolized by CYP2C8 and to a lesser extent by CYP3A4. Drugs that inhibit 3A4 may alter the pharmacokinetics and pharmacodynamics of repaglinide).
No products indexed under this heading.

Valproate Sodium (Repaglinide is metabolized by CYP2C8 and to a lesser extent by CYP3A4. Drugs that inhibit 3A4 may alter the pharmacokinetics and pharmacodynamics of repaglinide).
No products indexed under this heading.

Vancomycin Hydrochloride (Cationic drugs that are eliminated by renal tubular secretion theoretically have the potential for interaction with metformin by competing for common renal tubular transport systems. Careful patient monitoring and dose adjustment of PrandiMet and/or the interfering drug is recommended in patients who are taking cationic medications that are excreted via the proximal renal tubular secretory system).
No products indexed under this heading.

Vardenafil Hydrochloride (Repaglinide is metabolized by CYP2C8 and to a lesser extent by CYP3A4. Drugs that inhibit 3A4 may alter the pharmacokinetics and pharmacodynamics of repaglinide). Products include:
Levitra Tablets 2876

Verapamil Hydrochloride (Repaglinide is metabolized by CYP2C8 and to a lesser extent by CYP3A4. Drugs that inhibit 3A4 may alter the pharmacokinetics and pharmacodynamics of repaglinide). Products include:
Tarka Tablets 511

Voriconazole (Repaglinide is metabolized by CYP2C8 and to a lesser extent by CYP3A4. Drugs that inhibit 3A4 may alter the pharmacokinetics and pharmacodynamics of repaglinide).
No products indexed under this heading.

Zafirlukast (Repaglinide is metabolized by CYP2C8 and to a lesser extent by CYP3A4. Drugs that inhibit 3A4 may alter the pharmacokinetics and pharmacodynamics of repaglinide). Products include:
Accolate Tablets 669

Zileuton (Repaglinide is metabolized by CYP2C8 and to a lesser extent by CYP3A4. Drugs that inhibit 3A4 may alter the pharmacokinetics and pharmacodynamics of repaglinide).
No products indexed under this heading.

Food Interactions

Alcohol (Alcohol potentiates the effect of metformin on lactate metabolism. Patients should be warned against excessive alcohol intake while receiving PrandiMet).

Grapefruit (Repaglinide is metabolized by CYP2C8 and to a lesser extent by CYP3A4. Drugs that inhibit 3A4 may alter the pharmacokinetics and pharmacodynamics of repaglinide).

Grapefruit Juice (Repaglinide is metabolized by CYP2C8 and to a lesser extent by CYP3A4. Drugs that inhibit 3A4 may alter the pharmacokinetics and pharmacodynamics of repaglinide).

PRANDIN TABLETS

(Repaglinide) 2971
May interact with barbiturates, beta blockers, calcium channel blockers, corticosteroids, cytochrome p450 2c8 inducers (selected), cytochrome p450 2c8 inhibitors (selected), cytochrome p450 3a4 inducers (selected), cytochrome p450 3a4 inhibitors (selected), diuretics, erythromycin, estrogens, monoamine oxidase inhibitors, non-steroidal anti-inflammatory agents, oral contraceptives, phenothiazines, phenytoin, highly protein bound drugs (selected), salicylates, sulfonamides, sympathomimetics, thyroid preparations, and certain other agents. Compounds in these categories include:

Acebutolol Hydrochloride (The hypoglycemic action of oral blood glucose-lowering agents may be potentiated by beta adrenergic blocking agents. When administered to a patient receiving an oral blood glucose-lowering agent, the patient should be observed closely for hypoglycemia. When a beta adrenergic blocking agent is withdrawn from a patient receiving an oral blood glucose-lowering agent, the patient should be observed closely for loss of glycemic control).
No products indexed under this heading.

Acetazolamide (Repaglinide is metabolized by the cytochrome P4502C8 and 3A4 enzymes. Consequently, repaglinide metabolism may be altered by drugs that are CYP3A4 inhibitors. Caution should be used in patients concomitantly using repaglinide and a CYP3A4 inhibitor. The effect may be very significant if both CYP3A4 and CYP2C8 are inhibited at the same time).
No products indexed under this heading.

Albuterol (Sympathomimetics tend to produce hyperglycemia and may lead to loss of glycemic control. When administered to a patient receiving an oral blood glucose-lowering agent, the patient should be observed for loss of glycemic control. When a sympathomimeticsis withdrawn from a patient receiving an oral blood glucose-lowering agent, the patient should be observed closely for hypoglycemia).
No products indexed under this heading.

Albuterol Sulfate (Sympathomimetics tend to produce hyperglycemia and may lead to loss of glycemic control. When administered to a patient receiving an oral blood glucose-lowering agent, the patient should be observed for loss of glycemic control. When a sympathomimeticsis withdrawn from a patient receiving an oral blood glucose-lowering agent, the patient should be observed closely for hypoglycemia). Products include:
Combivent Inhalation Aerosol 845
ProAir HFA Inhalation Aerosol 3113
Proventil HFA Inhalation Aerosol 2914
Ventolin HFA Inhalation Aerosol 1638

Allium sativum (Repaglinide is metabolized by the cytochrome P4502C8 and 3A4 enzymes. Consequently, repaglinide metabolism may be altered by drugs that are CYP3A4 inducers. Caution should be used in patients concomitantly using repaglinide and a CYP3A4 inducer).
No products indexed under this heading.

Amiloride Hydrochloride (Diuretics tend to produce hyperglycemia and may lead to loss of glycemic control. When administered to a patient receiving an oral blood glucose-lowering agent, the patient should be observed for loss of glycemic control. When a diuretic drug is withdrawn from a patient receiving an oral blood glucose-lowering agent, the patient should be observed closely for hypoglycemia).
No products indexed under this heading.

Amiodarone Hydrochloride (Repaglinide is metabolized by the cytochrome P4502C8 and 3A4 enzymes. Consequently, repaglinide metabolism may be altered by drugs that are CYP3A4 inhibitors. Caution should be used in patients concomitantly using repaglinide and a CYP3A4 inhibitor. The effect may be very significant if both CYP3A4 and CYP2C8 are inhibited at the same time).
No products indexed under this heading.

Amitriptyline Hydrochloride (The hypoglycemic action of oral blood glucose-lowering agents may be potentiated by highly protein bounded drugs. When administered to a patient receiving an oral blood glucose-lowering agent, the patient should be observed closely for hypoglycemia. When a highly protein bound drug is withdrawn from a patient receiving an oral blood glucose-lowering agent, the patient should be observed closely for loss of glycemic control).
No products indexed under this heading.

Amlodipine Besylate (Calcium channel blockers tend to produce hyperglycemia and may lead to loss of glycemic control. When administered to a patient receiving an oral blood glucose-lowering agent, the patient should be observed for loss of glycemic control. When a calcium channel blocker is withdrawn from a patient receiving an oral blood glucose-lowering agent, the patient should be observed closely for hypoglycemia). Products include:
Azor Tablets 1005
Exforge Tablets 2238

Amprenavir (Repaglinide is metabolized by the cytochrome P4502C8 and 3A4 enzymes. Consequently, repaglinide metabolism may be altered by drugs that are CYP3A4 inhibitors. Caution should be used in patients concomitantly using repaglinide and a CYP3A4 inhibitor. The effect may be very significant if both CYP3A4 and CYP2C8 are inhibited at the same time).
No products indexed under this heading.

Anastrozole (Repaglinide is metabolized by the cytochrome P4502C8 and 3A4 enzymes. Consequently, repaglinide metabolism may be altered by drugs that are CYP3A4 inhibitors. Caution should be used in patients concomitantly using repaglinide and a CYP3A4 inhibitor. The effect may be very significant if both CYP3A4 and CYP2C8 are inhibited at the same time). Products include:
Arimidex Tablets 672

Aprepitant (Repaglinide is metabolized by the cytochrome P4502C8 and 3A4 enzymes. Consequently, repaglinide metabolism may be altered by drugs that are CYP3A4 inducers. Caution should be used in patients concomitantly using repaglinide and a CYP3A4 inducer). Products include:
Emend Capsules 1992

Aprobarbital (Concomitant use with barbiturates which are inducers of CYP3A4 and/or CYP2C8 may alter the metabolism of repaglinide; caution with use).
No products indexed under this heading.

Aspirin (The hypoglycemic action of oral blood glucose-lowering agents may be potentiated by salicylates. When administered to a patient receiving an oral blood glucose-lowering agent, the patient should be observed closely for hypoglycemia. When a salicylate is withdrawn from a patient receiving an oral blood glucose-lowering agent, the patient should be observed closely for loss of glycemic control). Products include:
Aggrenox Capsules 819
Bayer Aspirin 750
Percodan Tablets 1130
St. Joseph 81 mg Aspirin Chewable and Enteric Coated Tablets 1903

Aspirin, Enteric Coated (The hypoglycemic action of oral blood glucose-lowering agents may be potentiated by salicylates. When administered to a patient receiving an oral blood glucose-lowering agent, the patient should be observed closely for hypoglycemia. When a salicylate is withdrawn from a patient receiving an oral blood glucose-lowering agent, the patient should be observed closely for loss of glycemic control).
No products indexed under this heading.

Aspirin Buffered (The hypoglycemic action of oral blood glucose-lowering agents may be potentiated by salicylates. When administered to a patient receiving an oral blood glucose-lowering agent, the patient should be observed closely for hypoglycemia. When a salicylate is withdrawn from a patient receiving an oral blood glucose-lowering agent, the patient should be observed closely for loss of glycemic control).
No products indexed under this heading.

Atazanavir (Repaglinide is metabolized by the cytochrome P4502C8 and 3A4 enzymes. Consequently, repaglinide metabolism may be altered by drugs that are CYP3A4 inhibitors. Caution should be used in patients concomitantly using repaglinide and a CYP3A4 inhibitor. The effect may be very significant if both CYP3A4 and CYP2C8 are inhibited at the same time).
No products indexed under this heading.

Atazanavir Sulfate (Repaglinide is metabolized by the cytochrome P4502C8 and 3A4 enzymes. Consequently, repaglinide metabolism may be altered by drugs that are CYP3A4 inhibitors. Caution should be used in patients concomitantly using repaglinide and a CYP3A4 inhibitor. The effect may be very significant if both CYP3A4 and CYP2C8 are inhibited at the same time). Products include:
Reyataz Capsules 3299

Atenolol (The hypoglycemic action of oral blood glucose-lowering agents may be potentiated by beta adrenergic blocking agents. When administered to a patient receiving an oral blood glucose-lowering agent, the patient should be observed closely for hypoglycemia. When a beta adrenergic blocking agent is withdrawn from a patient receiving an oral blood glucose-lowering agent, the patient should be observed closely for loss of glycemic control).
No products indexed under this heading.

Atovaquone (The hypoglycemic action of oral blood glucose-lowering agents may be potentiated by highly protein bounded drugs. When administered to a patient receiving an oral blood glucose-lowering agent, the patient should be observed closely for hypoglycemia. When a highly protein bound drug is withdrawn from a patient receiving an oral blood glucose-lowering agent, the patient should be observed closely for loss of glycemic control). Products include:
Malarone Pediatric Tablets 1521
Malarone Tablets 1521
Mepron Suspension 1526

Bendroflumethiazide (The hypoglycemic action of oral blood glucose-lowering agents may be potentiated by sulfonamides. When administered to a patient receiving an oral blood glucose-lowering agent, the patient should be observed closely for hypoglycemia. When a sulfonamideis withdrawn from a patient receiving an oral blood glucose-lowering agent, the patient should be observed closely for loss of glycemic control).
No products indexed under this heading.

Bepridil Hydrochloride (Calcium channel blockers tend to produce hyperglycemia and may lead to loss of glycemic control. When administered to a patient receiving an oral blood glucose-lowering agent, the patient should be observed for loss of glycemic control. When a calcium channel blocker is withdrawn from a patient receiving an oral blood glucose-lowering agent, the patient should be observed closely for hypoglycemia).
No products indexed under this heading.

Betamethasone Acetate (Repaglinide is metabolized by the cytochrome P4502C8 and 3A4 enzymes. Consequently, repaglinide metabolism may be altered by drugs that are CYP3A4 inducers. Caution should be used in patients concomitantly using repaglinide and a CYP3A4 inducer).
No products indexed under this heading.

Betamethasone Sodium Phosphate (Repaglinide is metabolized by the cytochrome P4502C8 and 3A4 enzymes. Consequently, repaglinide metabolism may be altered by drugs that are CYP3A4 inducers. Caution should be used in patients concomitantly using repaglinide and a CYP3A4 inducer).
No products indexed under this heading.

Betaxolol Hydrochloride (The hypoglycemic action of oral blood glucose-lowering agents may be potentiated by beta adrenergic blocking agents. When administered to a patient receiving an oral blood glucose-lowering agent, the patient should be observed closely for hypoglycemia. When a beta adrenergic blocking agent is withdrawn from a patient receiving an oral blood glucose-lowering agent, the patient should be observed closely for loss of glycemic control).
No products indexed under this heading.

Bisoprolol Fumarate (The hypoglycemic action of oral blood glucose-lowering agents may be potentiated by beta adrenergic blocking agents. When administered to a patient receiving an oral blood glucose-lowering agent, the patient should be observed closely for hypoglycemia. When a beta adrenergic blocking agent is withdrawn from a patient receiving an oral blood glucose-lowering agent, the patient should be observed closely for loss of glycemic control).
No products indexed under this heading.

Budesonide (Corticosteroids tend to produce hyperglycemia and may lead to loss of glycemic control. When administered to a patient receiving an oral blood glucose-lowering agent, the patient should be observed for loss of glycemic control. When a corticosteroid iswithdrawn from a patient receiving an oral blood glucose-lowering agent, the patient should be observed closely for hypoglycemia). Products include:
Pulmicort Flexhaler 654
Symbicort 80/4.5 Inhalation Aerosol 659
Symbicort 160/4.5 Inhalation Aerosol 659

Bumetanide (Diuretics tend to produce hyperglycemia and may lead to loss of glycemic control. When administered to a patient receiving an oral blood glucose-lowering agent, the patient should be observed for loss of glycemic control. When a diuretic drug is withdrawn from a patient receiving an oral blood glucose-lowering agent, the patient should be observed closely for hypoglycemia).
No products indexed under this heading.

Butabarbital (Concomitant use with barbiturates which are inducers of CYP3A4 and/or CYP2C8 may alter the metabolism of repaglinide; caution with use).
No products indexed under this heading.

Butalbital (Concomitant use with barbiturates which are inducers of CYP3A4 and/or CYP2C8 may alter the metabolism of repaglinide; caution with use).
No products indexed under this heading.

Carbamazepine (Concomitant use with carbamazepine, a CYP3A4 and CYP2C8 inducer, may alter the metabolism of repaglinide; caution with use). Products include:
Carbatrol Capsules **3019**
Equetro Extended-Release Capsules **3174**

Carteolol Hydrochloride (The hypoglycemic action of oral blood glucose-lowering agents may be potentiated by beta adrenergic blocking agents. When administered to a patient receiving an oral blood glucose-lowering agent, the patient should be observed closely for hypoglycemia. When a beta adrenergic blocking agent is withdrawn from a patient receiving an oral blood glucose-lowering agent, the patient should be observed closely for loss of glycemic control).
No products indexed under this heading.

Cefonicid Sodium (The hypoglycemic action of oral blood glucose-lowering agents may be potentiated by highly protein bounded drugs. When administered to a patient receiving an oral blood glucose-lowering agent, the patient should be observed closely for hypoglycemia. When a highly protein bound drug is withdrawn from a patient receiving an oral blood glucose-lowering agent, the patient should be observed closely for loss of glycemic control).
No products indexed under this heading.

Celecoxib (The hypoglycemic action of oral blood glucose-lowering agents may be potentiated by nonsteroidal anti-inflammatory agents. When administered to a patient receiving an oral blood glucose-lowering agent, the patient should be observed closely for hypoglycemia. When a nonsteroidal anti-inflammatory agent is withdrawn from a patient receiving an oral blood glucose-lowering agent, the patient should be observed closely for loss of glycemic control). Products include:
Celebrex Capsules **2979**

Chloramphenicol (The hypoglycemic action of oral blood glucose-lowering agents may be potentiated by chloramphenicol. When administered to a patient receiving an oral blood glucose-lowering agent, the patient should be observed closely for hypoglycemia. When chloramphenicol is withdrawn from a patient receiving an oral blood glucose-lowering agent, the patient should be observed closely for loss of glycemic control).
No products indexed under this heading.

Chloramphenicol Palmitate (The hypoglycemic action of oral blood glucose-lowering agents may be potentiated by chloramphenicol. When administered to a patient receiving an oral blood glucose-lowering agent, the patient should be observed closely for hypoglycemia. When chloramphenicol is withdrawn from a patient receiving an oral blood glucose-lowering agent, the patient should be observed closely for loss of glycemic control).
No products indexed under this heading.

Chloramphenicol Sodium Succinate (The hypoglycemic action of oral blood glucose-lowering agents may be potentiated by chloramphenicol. When administered to a patient receiving an oral blood glucose-lowering agent, the patient should be observed closely for hypoglycemia. When chloramphenicol is withdrawn from a patient receiving an oral blood glucose-lowering agent, the patient should be observed closely for loss of glycemic control).
No products indexed under this heading.

Chlordiazepoxide (The hypoglycemic action of oral blood glucose-lowering agents may be potentiated by highly protein bounded drugs. When administered to a patient receiving an oral blood glucose-lowering agent, the patient should be observed closely for hypoglycemia. When a highly protein bound drug is withdrawn from a patient receiving an oral blood glucose-lowering agent, the patient should be observed closely for loss of glycemic control).
No products indexed under this heading.

Chlordiazepoxide Hydrochloride (The hypoglycemic action of oral blood glucose-lowering agents may be potentiated by highly protein bounded drugs. When administered to a patient receiving an oral blood glucose-lowering agent, the patient should be observed closely for hypoglycemia. When a highly protein bound drug is withdrawn from a patient receiving an oral blood glucose-lowering agent, the patient should be observed closely for loss of glycemic control).
No products indexed under this heading.

Chlorothiazide (The hypoglycemic action of oral blood glucose-lowering agents may be potentiated by sulfonamides. When administered to a patient receiving an oral blood glucose-lowering agent, the patient should be observed closely for hypoglycemia. When a sulfonamideis withdrawn from a patient receiving an oral blood glucose-lowering agent, the patient should be observed closely for loss of glycemic control).
No products indexed under this heading.

Chlorothiazide Sodium (The hypoglycemic action of oral blood glucose-lowering agents may be potentiated by sulfonamides. When administered to a patient receiving an oral blood glucose-lowering agent, the patient should be observed closely for hypoglycemia. When a sulfonamideis withdrawn from a patient receiving an oral blood glucose-lowering agent, the patient should be observed closely for loss of glycemic control). Products include:
Intravenous Sodium Diuril **2490**

Chlorotrianisene (Estrogens and oral contraceptives tend to produce hyperglycemia and may lead to loss of glycemic control. When administered to a patient receiving an oral blood glucose-lowering agent, the patient should be observed for loss of glycemic control. When an estrogen is withdrawn from a patient receiving an oral blood glucose-lowering agent, the patient should be observed closely for hypoglycemia).
No products indexed under this heading.

Chlorpromazine (The hypoglycemic action of oral blood glucose-lowering agents may be potentiated by highly protein bounded drugs. When administered to a patient receiving an oral blood glucose-lowering agent, the patient should be observed closely for hypoglycemia. When a highly protein bound drug is withdrawn from a patient receiving an oral blood glucose-lowering agent, the patient should be observed closely for loss of glycemic control).
No products indexed under this heading.

Chlorpromazine Hydrochloride (The hypoglycemic action of oral blood glucose-lowering agents may be potentiated by highly protein bounded drugs. When administered to a patient receiving an oral blood glucose-lowering agent, the patient should be observed closely for hypoglycemia. When a highly protein bound drug is withdrawn from a patient receiving an oral blood glucose-lowering agent, the patient should be observed closely for loss of glycemic control).
No products indexed under this heading.

Chlorpropamide (The hypoglycemic action of oral blood glucose-lowering agents may be potentiated by sulfonamides. When administered to a patient receiving an oral blood glucose-lowering agent, the patient should be observed closely for hypoglycemia. When a sulfonamideis withdrawn from a patient receiving an oral blood glucose-lowering agent, the patient should be observed closely for loss of glycemic control).
No products indexed under this heading.

Chlorthalidone (Diuretics tend to produce hyperglycemia and may lead to loss of glycemic control. When administered to a patient receiving an oral blood glucose-lowering agent, the patient should be observed for loss of glycemic control. When a diuretic drug is withdrawn from a patient receiving an oral blood glucose-lowering agent, the patient should be observed closely for hypoglycemia). Products include:
Clorpres Tablets **2185**

Choline Magnesium Trisalicylate (The hypoglycemic action of oral blood glucose-lowering agents may be potentiated by salicylates. When administered to a patient receiving an oral blood glucose-lowering agent, the patient should be observed closely for hypoglycemia. When a salicylate is withdrawn from a patient receiving an oral blood glucose-lowering agent, the patient should be observed closely for loss of glycemic control).
No products indexed under this heading.

Ciclesonide (Corticosteroids tend to produce hyperglycemia and may lead to loss of glycemic control. When administered to a patient receiving an oral blood glucose-lowering agent, the patient should be observed for loss of glycemic control. When a corticosteroid iswithdrawn from a patient receiving an oral blood glucose-lowering agent, the patient should be observed closely for hypoglycemia). Products include:
Alvesco Inhalation Aerosol **2985**
Omnaris Nasal Spray **2998**

Cimetidine (Repaglinide is metabolized by the cytochrome P4502C8 and 3A4 enzymes. Consequently, repaglinide metabolism may be altered by drugs that are CYP3A4 inhibitors. Caution should be used in patients concomitantly using repaglinide and a CYP3A4 inhibitor. The effect may be very significant if both CYP3A4 and CYP2C8 are inhibited at the same time).
No products indexed under this heading.

Cimetidine Hydrochloride (Repaglinide is metabolized by the cytochrome P4502C8 and 3A4 enzymes. Consequently, repaglinide metabolism may be altered by drugs that are CYP3A4 inhibitors. Caution should be used in patients concomitantly using repaglinide and a CYP3A4 inhibitor. The effect may be very significant if both CYP3A4 and CYP2C8 are inhibited at the same time).
No products indexed under this heading.

Ciprofloxacin (Repaglinide is metabolized by the cytochrome P4502C8 and 3A4 enzymes. Consequently, repaglinide metabolism may be altered by drugs that are CYP3A4 inhibitors. Caution should be used in patients concomitantly using repaglinide and a CYP3A4 inhibitor. The effect may be very significant if both CYP3A4 and CYP2C8 are inhibited at the same time). Products include:
Cipro I.V. **2817**
Cipro Oral Suspension **2810**
Cipro XR Tablets **2823**
Ciprodex Otic Suspension **541**

Ciprofloxacin Hydrochloride (Repaglinide is metabolized by the cytochrome P4502C8 and 3A4 enzymes. Consequently, repaglinide metabolism may be altered by drugs that are CYP3A4 inducers. Caution should be used in patients concomitantly using repaglinide and a CYP3A4 inducer). Products include:
Cipro Tablets **2810**

Cisplatin (Repaglinide is metabolized by the cytochrome P4502C8 and 3A4 enzymes. Consequently, repaglinide metabolism may be altered by drugs that are CYP3A4 inducers. Caution should be used in patients concomitantly using repaglinide and a CYP3A4 inducer).
No products indexed under this heading.

Clarithromycin (Co-administration of 250 mg clarithromycin and a single dose of 0.25 mg repaglinide (after 4 days of twice-daily clarithromycin 250 mg) resulted in a 40% and 67% increase in repaglinide AUC and Cmax, respectively. The increase in AUC was from 5.3 ng/mL*hr to 7.5 ng/mL*hr for AUC and the increase in Cmax was from 4.4 ng/mL to 7.3 ng/mL. These increases in repaglinide plasma levels may necessitate a dose adjustment of repaglinide). Products include:
Biaxin/Biaxin XL 411

Clomipramine Hydrochloride (The hypoglycemic action of oral blood glucose-lowering agents may be potentiated by highly protein bounded drugs. When administered to a patient receiving an oral blood glucose-lowering agent, the patient should be observed closely for hypoglycemia. When a highly protein bound drug is withdrawn from a patient receiving an oral blood glucose-lowering agent, the patient should be observed closely for loss of glycemic control).
No products indexed under this heading.

Clotrimazole (Repaglinide is metabolized by the cytochrome P4502C8 and 3A4 enzymes. Consequently, repaglinide metabolism may be altered by drugs that are CYP3A4 inhibitors. Caution should be used in patients concomitantly using repaglinide and a CYP3A4 inhibitor. The effect may be very significant if both CYP3A4 and CYP2C8 are inhibited at the same time). Products include:
Lotrisone 2881

Clozapine (The hypoglycemic action of oral blood glucose-lowering agents may be potentiated by highly protein bounded drugs. When administered to a patient receiving an oral blood glucose-lowering agent, the patient should be observed closely for hypoglycemia. When a highly protein bound drug is withdrawn from a patient receiving an oral blood glucose-lowering agent, the patient should be observed closely for loss of glycemic control).
No products indexed under this heading.

Cortisone Acetate (Repaglinide is metabolized by the cytochrome P4502C8 and 3A4 enzymes. Consequently, repaglinide metabolism may be altered by drugs that are CYP3A4 inducers. Caution should be used in patients concomitantly using repaglinide and a CYP3A4 inducer).
No products indexed under this heading.

Coumarin Derivatives (The hypoglycemic action of oral blood glucose-lowering agents may be potentiated by coumarins. When administered to a patient receiving an oral blood glucose-lowering agent, the patient should be observed closely for hypoglycemia. When coumarins are withdrawn from a patient receiving an oral blood glucose-lowering agent, the patient should be observed closely for loss of glycemic control).
No products indexed under this heading.

Cyclosporine (Repaglinide is metabolized by the cytochrome P4502C8 and 3A4 enzymes. Consequently, repaglinide metabolism may be altered by drugs that are CYP3A4 inhibitors. Caution should be used in patients concomitantly using repaglinide and a CYP3A4 inhibitor. The effect may be very significant if both CYP3A4 and CYP2C8 are inhibited at the same time). Products include:
Gengraf Capsules 435
Neoral Oral Solution 2280
Neoral Soft Gelatin Capsules 2280
Restasis Ophthalmic Emulsion 557
Sandimmune 2296

Dalfopristin (Repaglinide is metabolized by the cytochrome P4502C8 and 3A4 enzymes. Consequently, repaglinide metabolism may be altered by drugs that are CYP3A4 inhibitors. Caution should be used in patients concomitantly using repaglinide and a CYP3A4 inhibitor. The effect may be very significant if both CYP3A4 and CYP2C8 are inhibited at the same time).
No products indexed under this heading.

Danazol (Repaglinide is metabolized by the cytochrome P4502C8 and 3A4 enzymes. Consequently, repaglinide metabolism may be altered by drugs that are CYP3A4 inhibitors. Caution should be used in patients concomitantly using repaglinide and a CYP3A4 inhibitor. The effect may be very significant if both CYP3A4 and CYP2C8 are inhibited at the same time).
No products indexed under this heading.

Delavirdine Mesylate (Repaglinide is metabolized by the cytochrome P4502C8 and 3A4 enzymes. Consequently, repaglinide metabolism may be altered by drugs that are CYP3A4 inhibitors. Caution should be used in patients concomitantly using repaglinide and a CYP3A4 inhibitor. The effect may be very significant if both CYP3A4 and CYP2C8 are inhibited at the same time).
No products indexed under this heading.

Desogestrel (Estrogens and oral contraceptives tend to produce hyperglycemia and may lead to loss of glycemic control. When administered to a patient receiving an oral blood glucose-lowering agent, the patient should be observed for loss of gylcemic control. When an oral contraceptive is withdrawn from a patient receiving an oral blood glucose-lowering agent, the patient should be observed closely for hypoglycemia). Products include:
Mircette Tablets 1034

Dexamethasone (Repaglinide is metabolized by the cytochrome P4502C8 and 3A4 enzymes. Consequently, repaglinide metabolism may be altered by drugs that are CYP3A4 inducers. Caution should be used in patients concomitantly using repaglinide and a CYP3A4 inducer). Products include:
Ciprodex Otic Suspension 541

Dexamethasone Acetate (Repaglinide is metabolized by the cytochrome P4502C8 and 3A4 enzymes. Consequently, repaglinide metabolism may be altered by drugs that are CYP3A4 inducers. Caution should be used in patients concomitantly using repaglinide and a CYP3A4 inducer).
No products indexed under this heading.

Dexamethasone Sodium Phosphate (Repaglinide is metabolized by the cytochrome P4502C8 and 3A4 enzymes. Consequently, repaglinide metabolism may be altered by drugs that are CYP3A4 inducers. Caution should be used in patients concomitantly using repaglinide and a CYP3A4 inducer).
No products indexed under this heading.

Diazepam (The hypoglycemic action of oral blood glucose-lowering agents may be potentiated by highly protein bounded drugs. When administered to a patient receiving an oral blood glucose-lowering agent, the patient should be observed closely for hypoglycemia. When a highly protein bound drug is withdrawn from a patient receiving an oral blood glucose-lowering agent, the patient should be observed closely for loss of glycemic control). Products include:
Valium Tablets 2658

Diclofenac Epolamine (The hypoglycemic action of oral blood glucose-lowering agents may be potentiated by nonsteroidal anti-inflammatory agents. When administered to a patient receiving an oral blood glucose-lowering agent, the patient should be observed closely for hypoglycemia. When a nonsteroidal anti-inflammatory agent is withdrawn from a patient receiving an oral blood glucose-lowering agent, the patient should be observed closely for loss of glycemic control). Products include:
Flector Patch 561

Diclofenac Potassium (The hypoglycemic action of oral blood glucose-lowering agents may be potentiated by nonsteroidal anti-inflammatory agents. When administered to a patient receiving an oral blood glucose-lowering agent, the patient should be observed closely for hypoglycemia. When a nonsteroidal anti-inflammatory agent is withdrawn from a patient receiving an oral blood glucose-lowering agent, the patient should be observed closely for loss of glycemic control).
No products indexed under this heading.

Diclofenac Sodium (The hypoglycemic action of oral blood glucose-lowering agents may be potentiated by nonsteroidal anti-inflammatory agents. When administered to a patient receiving an oral blood glucose-lowering agent, the patient should be observed closely for hypoglycemia. When a nonsteroidal anti-inflammatory agent is withdrawn from a patient receiving an oral blood glucose-lowering agent, the patient should be observed closely for loss of glycemic control). Products include:
Diclofenac Sodium Ophthalmic Solution .... ⊙240
Voltaren Ophthalmic Solution 2336
Voltaren Tablets 2334
Voltaren-XR Tablets 2337

Dienestrol (Estrogens and oral contraceptives tend to produce hyperglycemia and may lead to loss of glycemic control. When administered to a patient receiving an oral blood glucose-lowering agent, the patient should be observed for loss of glycemic control. When an estrogen is withdrawn from a patient receiving an oral blood glucose-lowering agent, the patient should be observed closely for hypoglycemia).
No products indexed under this heading.

Diethylstilbestrol (Estrogens and oral contraceptives tend to produce hyperglycemia and may lead to loss of glycemic control. When administered to a patient receiving an oral blood glucose-lowering agent, the patient should be observed for loss of glycemic control. When an estrogen is withdrawn from a patient receiving an oral blood glucose-lowering agent, the patient should be observed closely for hypoglycemia).
No products indexed under this heading.

Diflunisal (The hypoglycemic action of oral blood glucose-lowering agents may be potentiated by salicylates. When administered to a patient receiving an oral blood glucose-lowering agent, the patient should be observed closely for hypoglycemia. When a salicylate is withdrawn from a patient receiving an oral blood glucose-lowering agent, the patient should be observed closely for loss of glycemic control).
No products indexed under this heading.

Diltiazem Hydrochloride (Repaglinide is metabolized by the cytochrome P4502C8 and 3A4 enzymes. Consequently, repaglinide metabolism may be altered by drugs that are CYP3A4 inhibitors. Caution should be used in patients concomitantly using repaglinide and a CYP3A4 inhibitor. The effect may be very significant if both CYP3A4 and CYP2C8 are inhibited at the same time). Products include:
Cardizem LA Extended Release Tablets 421

Diltiazem Maleate (Repaglinide is metabolized by the cytochrome P4502C8 and 3A4 enzymes. Consequently, repaglinide metabolism may be altered by drugs that are CYP3A4 inhibitors. Caution should be used in patients concomitantly using repaglinide and a CYP3A4 inhibitor. The effect may be very significant if both CYP3A4 and CYP2C8 are inhibited at the same time).
No products indexed under this heading.

Dipyridamole (The hypoglycemic action of oral blood glucose-lowering agents may be potentiated by highly protein bounded drugs. When administered to a patient receiving an oral blood glucose-lowering agent, the patient should be observed closely for hypoglycemia. When a highly protein bound drug is withdrawn from a patient receiving an oral blood glucose-lowering agent, the patient should be observed closely for loss of glycemic control). Products include:
Aggrenox Capsules 819
Persantine Tablets 869

Dobutamine Hydrochloride (Sympathomimetics tend to produce

hyperglycemia and may lead to loss of glycemic control. When administered to a patient receiving an oral blood glucose-lowering agent, the patient should be observed for loss of glycemic control. When a sympathomimeticsis withdrawn from a patient receiving an oral blood glucose-lowering agent, the patient should be observed closely for hypoglycemia).
No products indexed under this heading.

Dopamine Hydrochloride (Sympathomimetics tend to produce hyperglycemia and may lead to loss of glycemic control. When administered to a patient receiving an oral blood glucose-lowering agent, the patient should be observed for loss of glycemic control. When a sympathomimeticsis withdrawn from a patient receiving an oral blood glucose-lowering agent, the patient should be observed closely for hypoglycemia).
No products indexed under this heading.

Doxorubicin Hydrochloride (Repaglinide is metabolized by the cytochrome P4502C8 and 3A4 enzymes. Consequently, repaglinide metabolism may be altered by drugs that are CYP3A4 inducers. Caution should be used in patients concomitantly using repaglinide and a CYP3A4 inducer).
No products indexed under this heading.

Efavirenz (Repaglinide is metabolized by the cytochrome P4502C8 and 3A4 enzymes. Consequently, repaglinide metabolism may be altered by drugs that are CYP3A4 inducers. Caution should be used in patients concomitantly using repaglinide and a CYP3A4 inducer). Products include:
Atripla Tablets ... **938**
Sustiva Capsules ... **930**
Sustiva Tablets ... **930**

Ephedrine Hydrochloride (Sympathomimetics tend to produce hyperglycemia and may lead to loss of glycemic control. When administered to a patient receiving an oral blood glucose-lowering agent, the patient should be observed for loss of glycemic control. When a sympathomimeticsis withdrawn from a patient receiving an oral blood glucose-lowering agent, the patient should be observed closely for hypoglycemia).
No products indexed under this heading.

Ephedrine Sulfate (Sympathomimetics tend to produce hyperglycemia and may lead to loss of glycemic control. When administered to a patient receiving an oral blood glucose-lowering agent, the patient should be observed for loss of glycemic control. When a sympathomimeticsis withdrawn from a patient receiving an oral blood glucose-lowering agent, the patient should be observed closely for hypoglycemia).
No products indexed under this heading.

Ephedrine Tannate (Sympathomimetics tend to produce hyperglycemia and may lead to loss of glycemic control. When administered to a patient receiving an oral blood glucose-lowering agent, the patient should be observed for loss of glycemic control. When a sympathomimeticsis withdrawn from a patient receiving an oral blood glucose-lowering agent, the patient should be observed closely for hypoglycemia).
No products indexed under this heading.

Epinephrine (Sympathomimetics tend to produce hyperglycemia and may lead to loss of glycemic control. When administered to a patient receiving an oral blood glucose-lowering agent, the patient should be observed for loss of glycemic control. When a sympathomimeticsis withdrawn from a patient receiving an oral blood glucose-lowering agent, the patient should be observed closely for hypoglycemia). Products include:
EpiPen ... **1024**

Epinephrine Bitartrate (Sympathomimetics tend to produce hyperglycemia and may lead to loss of glycemic control. When administered to a patient receiving an oral blood glucose-lowering agent, the patient should be observed for loss of glycemic control. When a sympathomimeticsis withdrawn from a patient receiving an oral blood glucose-lowering agent, the patient should be observed closely for hypoglycemia).
No products indexed under this heading.

Epinephrine Hydrochloride (Sympathomimetics tend to produce hyperglycemia and may lead to loss of glycemic control. When administered to a patient receiving an oral blood glucose-lowering agent, the patient should be observed for loss of glycemic control. When a sympathomimeticsis withdrawn from a patient receiving an oral blood glucose-lowering agent, the patient should be observed closely for hypoglycemia).
No products indexed under this heading.

Erythromycin (Repaglinide is metabolized by the cytochrome P4502C8 and 3A4 enzymes. Consequently, repaglinide metabolism may be altered by drugs that are CYP3A4 inhibitors. Caution should be used in patients concomitantly using repaglinide and a CYP3A4 inhibitor. The effect may be very significant if both CYP3A4 and CYP2C8 are inhibited at the same time).
No products indexed under this heading.

Erythromycin Estolate (Repaglinide is metabolized by the cytochrome P4502C8 and 3A4 enzymes. Consequently, repaglinide metabolism may be altered by drugs that are CYP3A4 inhibitors. Caution should be used in patients concomitantly using repaglinide and a CYP3A4 inhibitor. The effect may be very significant if both CYP3A4 and CYP2C8 are inhibited at the same time).
No products indexed under this heading.

Erythromycin Ethylsuccinate (Repaglinide is metabolized by the cytochrome P4502C8 and 3A4 enzymes. Consequently, repaglinide metabolism may be altered by drugs that are CYP3A4 inhibitors. Caution should be used in patients concomitantly using repaglinide and a CYP3A4 inhibitor. The effect may be very significant if both CYP3A4 and CYP2C8 are inhibited at the same time). Products include:
E.E.S. ... **433**
EryPed ... **431**

Erythromycin Gluceptate (Repaglinide is metabolized by the cytochrome P4502C8 and 3A4 enzymes. Consequently, repaglinide metabolism may be altered by drugs that are CYP3A4 inhibitors. Caution should be used in patients concomitantly using repaglinide and a CYP3A4 inhibitor. The effect may be very significant if both CYP3A4 and CYP2C8 are inhibited at the same time).
No products indexed under this heading.

Erythromycin Lactobionate (Repaglinide is metabolized by the cytochrome P4502C8 and 3A4 enzymes. Consequently, repaglinide metabolism may be altered by drugs that are CYP3A4 inhibitors. Caution should be used in patients concomitantly using repaglinide and a CYP3A4 inhibitor. The effect may be very significant if both CYP3A4 and CYP2C8 are inhibited at the same time).
No products indexed under this heading.

Erythromycin Stearate (Repaglinide is metabolized by the cytochrome P4502C8 and 3A4 enzymes. Consequently, repaglinide metabolism may be altered by drugs that are CYP3A4 inhibitors. Caution should be used in patients concomitantly using repaglinide and a CYP3A4 inhibitor. The effect may be very significant if both CYP3A4 and CYP2C8 are inhibited at the same time).
No products indexed under this heading.

Esmolol Hydrochloride (The hypoglycemic action of oral blood glucose-lowering agents may be potentiated by beta adrenergic blocking agents. When administered to a patient receiving an oral blood glucose-lowering agent, the patient should be observed closely for hypoglycemia. When a beta adrenergic blocking agent is withdrawn from a patient receiving an oral blood glucose-lowering agent, the patient should be observed closely for loss of glycemic control).
No products indexed under this heading.

Esomeprazole Magnesium (Repaglinide is metabolized by the cytochrome P4502C8 and 3A4 enzymes. Consequently, repaglinide metabolism may be altered by drugs that are CYP3A4 inhibitors. Caution should be used in patients concomitantly using repaglinide and a CYP3A4 inhibitor. The effect may be very significant if both CYP3A4 and CYP2C8 are inhibited at the same time). Products include:
Nexium Delayed-Release Capsules ... **645**
Nexium Delayed-Release Oral Suspension ... **645**

Estradiol (Estrogens and oral contraceptives tend to produce hyperglycemia and may lead to loss of glycemic control. When administered to a patient receiving an oral blood glucose-lowering agent, the patient should be observed for loss of glycemic control. When an estrogen is withdrawn from a patient receiving an oral blood glucose-lowering agent, the patient should be observed closely for hypoglycemia). Products include:
Activella Tablets ... **2347**
Angeliq Tablets ... **751**
Climara Transdermal System ... **763**
Climara Pro Transdermal System ... **768**
Divigel ... **3167**
Vagifem Tablets ... **2375**

Estrogens, Conjugated (Estrogens and oral contraceptives tend to produce hyperglycemia and may lead to loss of glycemic control. When administered to a patient receiving an oral blood glucose-lowering agent, the patient should be observed for loss of glycemic control. When an estrogen is withdrawn from a patient receiving an oral blood glucose-lowering agent, the patient should be observed closely for hypoglycemia). Products include:
Premarin Intravenous ... **3217**
Premarin Tablets ... **3221**
Premarin Vaginal Cream ... **3228**
Premphase Tablets ... **3232**
Prempro Tablets ... **3232**

Estrogens, Esterified (Estrogens and oral contraceptives tend to produce hyperglycemia and may lead to loss of glycemic control. When administered to a patient receiving an oral blood glucose-lowering agent, the patient should be observed for loss of glycemic control. When an estrogen is withdrawn from a patient receiving an oral blood glucose-lowering agent, the patient should be observed closely for hypoglycemia). Products include:
Estratest Tablets ... **3043**
Estratest H.S. Tablets ... **3043**

Estropipate (Estrogens and oral contraceptives tend to produce hyperglycemia and may lead to loss of glycemic control. When administered to a patient receiving an oral blood glucose-lowering agent, the patient should be observed for loss of glycemic control. When an estrogen is withdrawn from a patient receiving an oral blood glucose-lowering agent, the patient should be observed closely for hypoglycemia).
No products indexed under this heading.

Ethacrynic Acid (Diuretics tend to produce hyperglycemia and may lead to loss of glycemic control. When administered to a patient receiving an oral blood glucose-lowering agent, the patient should be observed for loss of glycemic control. When a diuretic drug is withdrawn from a patient receiving an oral blood glucose-lowering agent, the patient should be observed closely for hypoglycemia). Products include:
Edecrin Tablets ... **698**

Ethinyl Estradiol (Coadministration of a combination tablet of levonorgestrel and ethinyl estradiol administered q.d. for 21 days with repaglinide administered t.i.d (days 1-4) and a single dose on day 5 resulted in 20% increases in repaglinide, levonorgestrel, and ethinyl estradiol Cmax. Ethinyl estradiol AUC parameters were increased by 20%, while repaglinide and levonorgestrel AUC values remained unchanged. Estrogens tend to produce hyperglycemia and may lead to loss of glycemic control when an oral blood glucose-lowering agent is administered. Patient should be

observed for loss of glycemic control. When an estrogen is withdrawn from a patient receiving an oral blood glucose lowering agent, the patient should be observed closely for hypoglycemia). Products include:

Lybrel Tablets **3204**
Mircette Tablets **1034**
NuvaRing **2897**
Ortho-Cyclen/Ortho Tri-Cyclen **2449**
Ortho Evra Transdermal System **2437**
Ortho Tri-Cyclen Lo Tablets **2458**
Seasonique Tablets **1046**
Yaz Tablets **805**

Ethosuximide (Repaglinide is metabolized by the cytochrome P4502C8 and 3A4 enzymes. Consequently, repaglinide metabolism may be altered by drugs that are CYP3A4 inducers. Caution should be used in patients concomitantly using repaglinide and a CYP3A4 inducer).

No products indexed under this heading.

Ethynodiol Diacetate (Estrogens and oral contraceptives tend to produce hyperglycemia and may lead to loss of glycemic control. When administered to a patient receiving an oral blood glucose-lowering agent, the patient should be observed for loss of gylcemic control. When an oral contraceptive is withdrawn from a patient receiving an oral blood glucose-lowering agent, the patient should be observed closely for hypoglycemia).

No products indexed under this heading.

Etodolac (The hypoglycemic action of oral blood glucose-lowering agents may be potentiated by nonsteroidal anti-inflammatory agents. When administered to a patient receiving an oral blood glucose-lowering agent, the patient should be observed closely for hypoglycemia. When a nonsteroidal anti-inflammatory agent is withdrawn from a patient receiving an oral blood glucose-lowering agent, the patient should be observed closely for loss of glycemic control).

No products indexed under this heading.

Felbamate (Repaglinide is metabolized by the cytochrome P4502C8 and 3A4 enzymes. Consequently, repaglinide metabolism may be altered by drugs that are CYP3A4 inducers. Caution should be used in patients concomitantly using repaglinide and a CYP3A4 inducer).

No products indexed under this heading.

Felodipine (Calcium channel blockers tend to produce hyperglycemia and may lead to loss of glycemic control. When administered to a patient receiving an oral blood glucose-lowering agent, the patient should be observed for loss of glycemic control. When a calcium channel blocker is withdrawn from a patient receiving an oral blood glucose-lowering agent, the patient should be observed closely for hypoglycemia).

No products indexed under this heading.

Fenoprofen Calcium (The hypoglycemic action of oral blood glucose-lowering agents may be potentiated by nonsteroidal anti-inflammatory agents. When administered to a patient receiving an oral blood glucose-lowering agent, the patient should be observed closely for hypoglycemia. When a nonsteroidal anti-inflammatory agent is withdrawn from a patient receiving an oral blood glucose-lowering agent, the patient should be observed closely for loss of glycemic control). Products include:

Nalfon Capsules **2508**

Fluconazole (Repaglinide is metabolized by the cytochrome P4502C8 and 3A4 enzymes. Consequently, repaglinide metabolism may be altered by drugs that are CYP3A4 inhibitors. Caution should be used in patients concomitantly using repaglinide and a CYP3A4 inhibitor. The effect may be very significant if both CYP3A4 and CYP2C8 are inhibited at the same time).

No products indexed under this heading.

Fludrocortisone Acetate (Repaglinide is metabolized by the cytochrome P4502C8 and 3A4 enzymes. Consequently, repaglinide metabolism may be altered by drugs that are CYP3A4 inducers. Caution should be used in patients concomitantly using repaglinide and a CYP3A4 inducer).

No products indexed under this heading.

Flunisolide (Corticosteroids tend to produce hyperglycemia and may lead to loss of glycemic control. When administered to a patient receiving an oral blood glucose-lowering agent, the patient should be observed for loss of glycemic control. When a corticosteroid iswithdrawn from a patient receiving an oral blood glucose-lowering agent, the patient should be observed closely for hypoglycemia). Products include:

Aerobid/Aerobid-M **1153**

Fluoxetine (Repaglinide is metabolized by the cytochrome P4502C8 and 3A4 enzymes. Consequently, repaglinide metabolism may be altered by drugs that are CYP3A4 inhibitors. Caution should be used in patients concomitantly using repaglinide and a CYP3A4 inhibitor. The effect may be very significant if both CYP3A4 and CYP2C8 are inhibited at the same time).

No products indexed under this heading.

Fluoxetine Hydrochloride (Repaglinide is metabolized by the cytochrome P4502C8 and 3A4 enzymes. Consequently, repaglinide metabolism may be altered by drugs that are CYP3A4 inhibitors. Caution should be used in patients concomitantly using repaglinide and a CYP3A4 inhibitor. The effect may be very significant if both CYP3A4 and CYP2C8 are inhibited at the same time). Products include:

Prozac Weekly Capsules **1852**
Prozac Pulvules and Liquid **1852**
Symbyax Capsules **1871**

Fluphenazine Decanoate (Phenothiazines tend to produce hyperglycemia and may lead to loss of glycemic control. When administered to a patient receiving an oral blood glucose-lowering agent, the patient should be observed for loss of glycemic control. When a phenothiazine is withdrawn from a patient receiving an oral blood glucose-lowering agent, the patient should be observed closely for loss of hypoglycemia).

No products indexed under this heading.

Fluphenazine Enanthate (Phenothiazines tend to produce hyperglycemia and may lead to loss of glycemic control. When administered to a patient receiving an oral blood glucose-lowering agent, the patient should be observed for loss of glycemic control. When a phenothiazine is withdrawn from a patient receiving an oral blood glucose-lowering agent, the patient should be observed closely for loss of hypoglycemia).

No products indexed under this heading.

Fluphenazine Hydrochloride (Phenothiazines tend to produce hyperglycemia and may lead to loss of glycemic control. When administered to a patient receiving an oral blood glucose-lowering agent, the patient should be observed for loss of glycemic control. When a phenothiazine is withdrawn from a patient receiving an oral blood glucose-lowering agent, the patient should be observed closely for loss of hypoglycemia).

No products indexed under this heading.

Flurazepam Hydrochloride (The hypoglycemic action of oral blood glucose-lowering agents may be potentiated by highly protein bounded drugs. When administered to a patient receiving an oral blood glucose-lowering agent, the patient should be observed closely for hypoglycemia. When a highly protein bound drug is withdrawn from a patient receiving an oral blood glucose-lowering agent, the patient should be observed closely for loss of glycemic control).

No products indexed under this heading.

Flurbiprofen (The hypoglycemic action of oral blood glucose-lowering agents may be potentiated by nonsteroidal anti-inflammatory agents. When administered to a patient receiving an oral blood glucose-lowering agent, the patient should be observed closely for hypoglycemia. When a nonsteroidal anti-inflammatory agent is withdrawn from a patient receiving an oral blood glucose-lowering agent, the patient should be observed closely for loss of glycemic control).

No products indexed under this heading.

Fluticasone Propionate (Corticosteroids tend to produce hyperglycemia and may lead to loss of glycemic control. When administered to a patient receiving an oral blood glucose-lowering agent, the patient should be observed for loss of glycemic control. When a corticosteroid iswithdrawn from a patient receiving an oral blood glucose-lowering agent, the patient should be observed closely for hypoglycemia). Products include:

Advair Diskus 100/50 .... **1276**
Advair Diskus 250/50 .... **1276**
Advair Diskus 500/50 .... **1276**
Advair HFA 45/21 Inhalation Aerosol... **1288**
Advair HFA 115/21 Inhalation Aerosol... **1288**
Advair HFA 230/21 Inhalation Aerosol... **1288**
Flonase Nasal Spray **1431**
Flovent Diskus 50 mcg **1435**

Fluticasone Propionate HFA (Corticosteroids tend to produce hyperglycemia and may lead to loss of glycemic control. When administered to a patient receiving an oral blood glucose-lowering agent, the patient should be observed for loss of glycemic control. When a corticosteroid iswithdrawn from a patient receiving an oral blood glucose-lowering agent, the patient should be observed closely for hypoglycemia). Products include:

Flovent HFA **1440**

Fluvoxamine Maleate (Repaglinide is metabolized by the cytochrome P4502C8 and 3A4 enzymes. Consequently, repaglinide metabolism may be altered by drugs that are CYP3A4 inhibitors. Caution should be used in patients concomitantly using repaglinide and a CYP3A4 inhibitor. The effect may be very significant if both CYP3A4 and CYP2C8 are inhibited at the same time). Products include:

Luvox CR Extended-Release Capsules **1759**

Fosamprenavir Calcium (Repaglinide is metabolized by the cytochrome P4502C8 and 3A4 enzymes. Consequently, repaglinide metabolism may be altered by drugs that are CYP3A4 inhibitors. Caution should be used in patients concomitantly using repaglinide and a CYP3A4 inhibitor. The effect may be very significant if both CYP3A4 and CYP2C8 are inhibited at the same time). Products include:

Lexiva Oral Suspension **1510**
Lexiva Tablets **1510**

Fosphenytoin Sodium (Repaglinide is metabolized by the cytochrome P4502C8 and 3A4 enzymes. Consequently, repaglinide metabolism may be altered by drugs that are CYP3A4 inducers. Caution should be used in patients concomitantly using repaglinide and a CYP3A4 inducer).

No products indexed under this heading.

Furosemide (Diuretics tend to produce hyperglycemia and may lead to loss of glycemic control. When administered to a patient receiving an oral blood glucose-lowering agent, the patient should be observed for loss of glycemic control. When a diuretic drug is withdrawn from a patient receiving an oral blood glucose-lowering agent, the patient should be observed closely for hypoglycemia). Products include:

Furosemide Tablets **2186**

Garlic Extract (Repaglinide is metabolized by the cytochrome P4502C8 and 3A4 enzymes. Consequently, repaglinide metabolism may be altered by drugs that are CYP3A4 inducers. Caution should be used in patients concomitantly using repaglinide and a CYP3A4 inducer).

No products indexed under this heading.

Garlic Oil (Repaglinide is metabolized by the cytochrome P4502C8 and 3A4 enzymes. Consequently, repaglinide metabolism may be altered by drugs that are CYP3A4 inducers. Caution should be used in patients concomitantly using repaglinide and a CYP3A4 inducer).

No products indexed under this heading.

Gemfibrozil (Co-administration of gemfibrozil (600 mg) and a single dose of 0.25 mg repaglinide (after 3

days of twice-daily 600 mg gemfibrozil) resulted in an 8.1-fold higher repaglinide AUC and prolonged repaglinide half-life from 1.3 to 3.7 hours. Patients taking repaglinide should not start taking gemfibrozil; patients taking gemfibrozil should not start taking repaglinide. Concomitant use may result in enhanced and prolonged blood glucose-lowering effects of repaglinide. Caution should be used in patients already on repaglinide and gemfibrozil; blood glucose levels should be monitored and repaglinide dose adjustment may be needed).

No products indexed under this heading.

Glipizide (The hypoglycemic action of oral blood glucose-lowering agents may be potentiated by highly protein bounded drugs. When administered to a patient receiving an oral blood glucose-lowering agent, the patient should be observed closely for hypoglycemia. When a highly protein bound drug is withdrawn from a patient receiving an oral blood glucose-lowering agent, the patient should be observed closely for loss of glycemic control).

No products indexed under this heading.

Glyburide (The hypoglycemic action of oral blood glucose-lowering agents may be potentiated by sulfonamides. When administered to a patient receiving an oral blood glucose-lowering agent, the patient should be observed closely for hypoglycemia. When a sulfonamideis withdrawn from a patient receiving an oral blood glucose-lowering agent, the patient should be observed closely for loss of glycemic control).

No products indexed under this heading.

Hydrochlorothiazide (The hypoglycemic action of oral blood glucose-lowering agents may be potentiated by sulfonamides. When administered to a patient receiving an oral blood glucose-lowering agent, the patient should be observed closely for hypoglycemia. When a sulfonamideis withdrawn from a patient receiving an oral blood glucose-lowering agent, the patient should be observed closely for loss of glycemic control). Products include:

Atacand HCT 642
Avalide Tablets 892
Avalide Tablets 2713
Benicar HCT Tablets 1010
Diovan HCT Tablets 2216
Dyazide Capsules 1405
Micardis HCT Tablets 854
Prinzide Tablets 2092
Tekturna HCT Tablets 2324
Teveten HCT Tablets 517

Hydrocortisone (Repaglinide is metabolized by the cytochrome P4502C8 and 3A4 enzymes. Consequently, repaglinide metabolism may be altered by drugs that are CYP3A4 inducers. Caution should be used in patients concomitantly using repaglinide and a CYP3A4 inducer).

No products indexed under this heading.

Hydrocortisone Acetate (Repaglinide is metabolized by the cytochrome P4502C8 and 3A4 enzymes. Consequently, repaglinide metabolism may be altered by drugs that are CYP3A4 inducers. Caution should be used in patients concomitantly using repaglinide and a CYP3A4 inducer). Products include:

Analpram-HC 1140
Pramosone 1141

Hydrocortisone Butyrate (Repaglinide is metabolized by the cytochrome P4502C8 and 3A4 enzymes. Consequently, repaglinide metabolism may be altered by drugs that are CYP3A4 inducers. Caution should be used in patients concomitantly using repaglinide and a CYP3A4 inducer).

No products indexed under this heading.

Hydrocortisone Cypionate (Repaglinide is metabolized by the cytochrome P4502C8 and 3A4 enzymes. Consequently, repaglinide metabolism may be altered by drugs that are CYP3A4 inducers. Caution should be used in patients concomitantly using repaglinide and a CYP3A4 inducer).

No products indexed under this heading.

Hydrocortisone Hemisuccinate (Repaglinide is metabolized by the cytochrome P4502C8 and 3A4 enzymes. Consequently, repaglinide metabolism may be altered by drugs that are CYP3A4 inducers. Caution should be used in patients concomitantly using repaglinide and a CYP3A4 inducer).

No products indexed under this heading.

Hydrocortisone Probutate (Repaglinide is metabolized by the cytochrome P4502C8 and 3A4 enzymes. Consequently, repaglinide metabolism may be altered by drugs that are CYP3A4 inducers. Caution should be used in patients concomitantly using repaglinide and a CYP3A4 inducer).

No products indexed under this heading.

Hydrocortisone Sodium Phosphate (Repaglinide is metabolized by the cytochrome P4502C8 and 3A4 enzymes. Consequently, repaglinide metabolism may be altered by drugs that are CYP3A4 inducers. Caution should be used in patients concomitantly using repaglinide and a CYP3A4 inducer).

No products indexed under this heading.

Hydrocortisone Sodium Succinate (Repaglinide is metabolized by the cytochrome P4502C8 and 3A4 enzymes. Consequently, repaglinide metabolism may be altered by drugs that are CYP3A4 inducers. Caution should be used in patients concomitantly using repaglinide and a CYP3A4 inducer).

No products indexed under this heading.

Hydrocortisone Valerate (Repaglinide is metabolized by the cytochrome P4502C8 and 3A4 enzymes. Consequently, repaglinide metabolism may be altered by drugs that are CYP3A4 inducers. Caution should be used in patients concomitantly using repaglinide and a CYP3A4 inducer).

No products indexed under this heading.

Hydroflumethiazide (The hypoglycemic action of oral blood glucose-lowering agents may be potentiated by sulfonamides. When administered to a patient receiving an oral blood glucose-lowering agent, the patient should be observed closely for hypoglycemia. When a sulfonamideis withdrawn from a patient receiving an oral blood glucose-lowering agent, the patient should be observed closely for loss of glycemic control).

No products indexed under this heading.

Hypericum (Repaglinide is metabolized by the cytochrome P4502C8 and 3A4 enzymes. Consequently, repaglinide metabolism may be altered by drugs that are CYP3A4 inducers. Caution should be used in patients concomitantly using repaglinide and a CYP3A4 inducer). Products include:

Satieté Tablets 640

Hypericum Perforatum (Repaglinide is metabolized by the cytochrome P4502C8 and 3A4 enzymes. Consequently, repaglinide metabolism may be altered by drugs that are CYP3A4 inducers. Caution should be used in patients concomitantly using repaglinide and a CYP3A4 inducer).

No products indexed under this heading.

Ibuprofen (The hypoglycemic action of oral blood glucose-lowering agents may be potentiated by nonsteroidal anti-inflammatory agents. When administered to a patient receiving an oral blood glucose-lowering agent, the patient should be observed closely for hypoglycemia. When a nonsteroidal anti-inflammatory agent is withdrawn from a patient receiving an oral blood glucose-lowering agent, the patient should be observed closely for loss of glycemic control). Products include:

Motrin IB Tablets and Caplets 1900
Children's Motrin Oral Suspension ... 1901
Children's Motrin Non-Staining Dye-Free Oral Suspension 1901
Children's Motrin Cold Oral Suspension 1899
Infants' Motrin Concentrated Drops 1901
Infants' Motrin Non-Staining Dye-Free Concentrated Drops 1901
Junior Strength Motrin Caplets and Chewable Tablets 1901
Vicoprofen Tablets 533

Imipramine Hydrochloride (The hypoglycemic action of oral blood glucose-lowering agents may be potentiated by highly protein bounded drugs. When administered to a patient receiving an oral blood glucose-lowering agent, the patient should be observed closely for hypoglycemia. When a highly protein bound drug is withdrawn from a patient receiving an oral blood glucose-lowering agent, the patient should be observed closely for loss of glycemic control).

No products indexed under this heading.

Imipramine Pamoate (The hypoglycemic action of oral blood glucose-lowering agents may be potentiated by highly protein bounded drugs. When administered to a patient receiving an oral blood glucose-lowering agent, the patient should be observed closely for hypoglycemia. When a highly protein bound drug is withdrawn from a patient receiving an oral blood glucose-lowering agent, the patient should be observed closely for loss of glycemic control).

No products indexed under this heading.

Indapamide (Diuretics tend to produce hyperglycemia and may lead to loss of glycemic control. When administered to a patient receiving an oral blood glucose-lowering agent, the patient should be observed for loss of glycemic control. When a diuretic drug is withdrawn from a patient receiving an oral blood glucose-lowering agent, the patient should be observed closely for hypoglycemia). Products include:

Indapamide Tablets 2188

Indinavir Sulfate (Repaglinide is metabolized by the cytochrome P4502C8 and 3A4 enzymes. Consequently, repaglinide metabolism may be altered by drugs that are CYP3A4 inhibitors. Caution should be used in patients concomitantly using repaglinide and a CYP3A4 inhibitor. The effect may be very significant if both CYP3A4 and CYP2C8 are inhibited at the same time). Products include:

Crixivan Capsules 1979

Indomethacin (The hypoglycemic action of oral blood glucose-lowering agents may be potentiated by nonsteroidal anti-inflammatory agents. When administered to a patient receiving an oral blood glucose-lowering agent, the patient should be observed closely for hypoglycemia. When a nonsteroidal anti-inflammatory agent is withdrawn from a patient receiving an oral blood glucose-lowering agent, the patient should be observed closely for loss of glycemic control). Products include:

Indocin 2024

Indomethacin Sodium Trihydrate (The hypoglycemic action of oral blood glucose-lowering agents may be potentiated by nonsteroidal anti-inflammatory agents. When administered to a patient receiving an oral blood glucose-lowering agent, the patient should be observed closely for hypoglycemia. When a nonsteroidal anti-inflammatory agent is withdrawn from a patient receiving an oral blood glucose-lowering agent, the patient should be observed closely for loss of glycemic control). Products include:

Indocin I.V. 2489

Isocarboxazid (The hypoglycemic action of oral blood glucose-lowering agents may be potentiated by MAO inhibitors. When administered to a patient receiving an oral blood glucose-lowering agent, the patient should be observed closely for hypoglycemia. When an MAO inhibitor is withdrawn from a patient receiving an oral blood glucose-lowering agent, the patient should be observed closely for loss of glycemic control). Products include:

Marplan Tablets 3177

Isoniazid (Isoniazid tends to produce hyperglycemia and may lead to loss of glycemic control. When administered to a patient receiving an oral blood glucose-lowering agent, the patient should be observed for loss of glycemic control. When isoniazid is withdrawn from a patient receiving an oral blood glucose-lowering agent, the patient should be observed closely for hypoglycemia).

No products indexed under this heading.

Isoproterenol Hydrochloride (Sympathomimetics tend to produce hyperglycemia and may lead to loss

of glycemic control. When administered to a patient receiving an oral blood glucose-lowering agent, the patient should be observed for loss of glycemic control. When a sympathomimeticsis withdrawn from a patient receiving an oral blood glucose-lowering agent, the patient should be observed closely for hypoglycemia).
No products indexed under this heading.

Isoproterenol Sulfate (Sympathomimetics tend to produce hyperglycemia and may lead to loss of glycemic control. When administered to a patient receiving an oral blood glucose-lowering agent, the patient should be observed for loss of glycemic control. When a sympathomimeticsis withdrawn from a patient receiving an oral blood glucose-lowering agent, the patient should be observed closely for hypoglycemia).
No products indexed under this heading.

Isradipine (Calcium channel blockers tend to produce hyperglycemia and may lead to loss of glycemic control. When administered to a patient receiving an oral blood glucose-lowering agent, the patient should be observed for loss of glycemic control. When a calcium channel blocker is withdrawn from a patient receiving an oral blood glucose-lowering agent, the patient should be observed closely for hypoglycemia). Products include:
DynaCirc CR Controlled Release Tablets 1407

Itraconazole (Gemfibrozil and itraconazole had a synergistic metabolic inhibitory effect on repaglinide. Therefore, patients taking repaglinide and gemfibrozil should not take itraconazole).
No products indexed under this heading.

Ketoconazole (Co-administration of 200 mg ketoconazole and a single dose of 2 mg repaglinide (after 4 days of once-daily ketoconazole 200 mg) resulted in a 15% and 16% increase in repaglinide AUC and Cmax, respectively. The increases were from 20.2 ng/mL to 23.5 ng/mL for Cmax and from 38.9 ng/mL*hr to 44.9 ng/mL*hr for AUC). Products include:
Extina Foam, 2% 3057
Nizoral A-D Shampoo 1901

Ketoprofen (The hypoglycemic action of oral blood glucose-lowering agents may be potentiated by nonsteroidal anti-inflammatory agents. When administered to a patient receiving an oral blood glucose-lowering agent, the patient should be observed closely for hypoglycemia. When a nonsteroidal anti-inflammatory agent is withdrawn from a patient receiving an oral blood glucose-lowering agent, the patient should be observed closely for loss of glycemic control).
No products indexed under this heading.

Ketorolac Tromethamine (The hypoglycemic action of oral blood glucose-lowering agents may be potentiated by nonsteroidal anti-inflammatory agents. When administered to a patient receiving an oral blood glucose-lowering agent, the patient should be observed closely for hypoglycemia. When a nonsteroidal anti-inflammatory agent is withdrawn from a patient receiving an oral blood glucose-lowering agent, the patient should be observed closely for loss of glycemic control).
No products indexed under this heading.

Labetalol Hydrochloride (The hypoglycemic action of oral blood glucose-lowering agents may be potentiated by beta adrenergic blocking agents. When administered to a patient receiving an oral blood glucose-lowering agent, the patient should be observed closely for hypoglycemia. When a beta adrenergic blocking agent is withdrawn from a patient receiving an oral blood glucose-lowering agent, the patient should be observed closely for loss of glycemic control).
No products indexed under this heading.

Levalbuterol Hydrochloride (Sympathomimetics tend to produce hyperglycemia and may lead to loss of glycemic control. When administered to a patient receiving an oral blood glucose-lowering agent, the patient should be observed for loss of glycemic control. When a sympathomimeticsis withdrawn from a patient receiving an oral blood glucose-lowering agent, the patient should be observed closely for hypoglycemia). Products include:
Xopenex Inhalation Solution 3001
Xopenex Inhalation Solution Concentrate 3005

Levobunolol Hydrochloride (The hypoglycemic action of oral blood glucose-lowering agents may be potentiated by beta adrenergic blocking agents. When administered to a patient receiving an oral blood glucose-lowering agent, the patient should be observed closely for hypoglycemia. When a beta adrenergic blocking agent is withdrawn from a patient receiving an oral blood glucose-lowering agent, the patient should be observed closely for loss of glycemic control).
No products indexed under this heading.

Levonorgestrel (Co-administration of a combination tablet of levonorgestrel and ethinyl estradiol administered q.d. for 21 days with repaglinide administered t.i.d (days 1-4) and a single dose on day 5 resulted in 20% increases in repaglinide, levonorgestrel, and ethinyl estradiol Cmax. Ethinyl estradiol AUC parameters were increased by 20%, while repaglinide and levonorgestrel AUC values remained unchanged. Estrogens tend to produce hyperglycemia and may lead to loss of glycemic control when an oral blood glucose-lowering agent is administered. Patient should be observed for loss of glycemic control. When an estrogen is withdrawn from a patient receiving an oral blood glucose lowering agent, the patient should be observed closely for hypoglycemia). Products include:
Climara Pro Transdermal System 768
Lybrel Tablets 3204
Mirena Intrauterine System 779
Plan B Tablets 1044
Seasonique Tablets 1046

Levothyroxine Sodium (Thyroid products tend to produce hyperglycemia and may lead to loss of glycemic control. When administered to a patient receiving an oral blood glucose-lowering agent, the patient should be observed for loss of glycemic control. When a thyroid product is withdrawn from a patient receiving an oral blood glucose-lowering agent, the patient should be observed closely for hypoglycemia). Products include:
Levothroid Tablets 1170
Levoxyl Tablets 1780
Synthroid Tablets 507

Liothyronine Sodium (Thyroid products tend to produce hyperglycemia and may lead to loss of glycemic control. When administered to a patient receiving an oral blood glucose-lowering agent, the patient should be observed for loss of glycemic control. When a thyroid product is withdrawn from a patient receiving an oral blood glucose-lowering agent, the patient should be observed closely for hypoglycemia). Products include:
Cytomel Tablets 1778

Liotrix (Thyroid products tend to produce hyperglycemia and may lead to loss of glycemic control. When administered to a patient receiving an oral blood glucose-lowering agent, the patient should be observed for loss of glycemic control. When a thyroid product is withdrawn from a patient receiving an oral blood glucose-lowering agent, the patient should be observed closely for hypoglycemia).
No products indexed under this heading.

Lopinavir (Repaglinide is metabolized by the cytochrome P4502C8 and 3A4 enzymes. Consequently, repaglinide metabolism may be altered by drugs that are CYP3A4 inhibitors. Caution should be used in patients concomitantly using repaglinide and a CYP3A4 inhibitor. The effect may be very significant if both CYP3A4 and CYP2C8 are inhibited at the same time). Products include:
Kaletra 452

Loratadine (Repaglinide is metabolized by the cytochrome P4502C8 and 3A4 enzymes. Consequently, repaglinide metabolism may be altered by drugs that are CYP3A4 inhibitors. Caution should be used in patients concomitantly using repaglinide and a CYP3A4 inhibitor. The effect may be very significant if both CYP3A4 and CYP2C8 are inhibited at the same time).
No products indexed under this heading.

Magnesium Salicylate (The hypoglycemic action of oral blood glucose-lowering agents may be potentiated by salicylates. When administered to a patient receiving an oral blood glucose-lowering agent, the patient should be observed closely for hypoglycemia. When a salicylate is withdrawn from a patient receiving an oral blood glucose-lowering agent, the patient should be observed closely for loss of glycemic control).
No products indexed under this heading.

Meclofenamate Sodium (The hypoglycemic action of oral blood glucose-lowering agents may be potentiated by nonsteroidal anti-inflammatory agents. When administered to a patient receiving an oral blood glucose-lowering agent, the patient should be observed closely for hypoglycemia. When a nonsteroidal anti-inflammatory agent is withdrawn from a patient receiving an oral blood glucose-lowering agent, the patient should be observed closely for loss of glycemic control).
No products indexed under this heading.

Mefenamic Acid (The hypoglycemic action of oral blood glucose-lowering agents may be potentiated by nonsteroidal anti-inflammatory agents. When administered to a patient receiving an oral blood glucose-lowering agent, the patient should be observed closely for hypoglycemia. When a nonsteroidal anti-inflammatory agent is withdrawn from a patient receiving an oral blood glucose-lowering agent, the patient should be observed closely for loss of glycemic control).
No products indexed under this heading.

Meloxicam (The hypoglycemic action of oral blood glucose-lowering agents may be potentiated by nonsteroidal anti-inflammatory agents. When administered to a patient receiving an oral blood glucose-lowering agent, the patient should be observed closely for hypoglycemia. When a nonsteroidal anti-inflammatory agent is withdrawn from a patient receiving an oral blood glucose-lowering agent, the patient should be observed closely for loss of glycemic control). Products include:
Mobic Oral Suspension 863
Mobic Tablets 863

Mephenytoin (Repaglinide is metabolized by the cytochrome P4502C8 and 3A4 enzymes. Consequently, repaglinide metabolism may be altered by drugs that are CYP3A4 inducers. Caution should be used in patients concomitantly using repaglinide and a CYP3A4 inducer).
No products indexed under this heading.

Mephobarbital (Concomitant use with barbiturates which are inducers of CYP3A4 and/or CYP2C8 may alter the metabolism of repaglinide; caution with use).
No products indexed under this heading.

Mesoridazine Besylate (Phenothiazines tend to produce hyperglycemia and may lead to loss of glycemic control. When administered to a patient receiving an oral blood glucose-lowering agent, the patient should be observed for loss of glycemic control. When a phenothiazine is withdrawn from a patient receiving an oral blood glucose-lowering agent, the patient should be observed closely for loss of hypoglycemia).
No products indexed under this heading.

Mestranol (Estrogens and oral contraceptives tend to produce hyperglycemia and may lead to loss of glycemic control. When administered to a patient receiving an oral blood glucose-lowering agent, the patient should be observed for loss of gylcemic control. When an oral contraceptive is withdrawn from a patient receiving an oral blood glucose-lowering agent, the patient should be observed closely for hypoglycemia).
No products indexed under this heading.

Metaproterenol Sulfate (Sympathomimetics tend to produce hyperglycemia and may lead to loss of glycemic control. When adminis-

tered to a patient receiving an oral blood glucose-lowering agent, the patient should be observed for loss of glycemic control. When a sympathomimeticsis withdrawn from a patient receiving an oral blood glucose-lowering agent, the patient should be observed closely for hypoglycemia).
No products indexed under this heading.

Metaraminol Bitartrate (Sympathomimetics tend to produce hyperglycemia and may lead to loss of glycemic control. When administered to a patient receiving an oral blood glucose-lowering agent, the patient should be observed for loss of glycemic control. When a sympathomimeticsis withdrawn from a patient receiving an oral blood glucose-lowering agent, the patient should be observed closely for hypoglycemia).
No products indexed under this heading.

Methotrimeprazine (Phenothiazines tend to produce hyperglycemia and may lead to loss of glycemic control. When administered to a patient receiving an oral blood glucose-lowering agent, the patient should be observed for loss of glycemic control. When a phenothiazine is withdrawn from a patient receiving an oral blood glucose-lowering agent, the patient should be observed closely for loss of hypoglycemia).
No products indexed under this heading.

Methoxamine Hydrochloride (Sympathomimetics tend to produce hyperglycemia and may lead to loss of glycemic control. When administered to a patient receiving an oral blood glucose-lowering agent, the patient should be observed for loss of glycemic control. When a sympathomimeticsis withdrawn from a patient receiving an oral blood glucose-lowering agent, the patient should be observed closely for hypoglycemia).
No products indexed under this heading.

Methsuximide (Repaglinide is metabolized by the cytochrome P4502C8 and 3A4 enzymes. Consequently, repaglinide metabolism may be altered by drugs that are CYP3A4 inducers. Caution should be used in patients concomitantly using repaglinide and a CYP3A4 inducer).
No products indexed under this heading.

Methyclothiazide (The hypoglycemic action of oral blood glucose-lowering agents may be potentiated by sulfonamides. When administered to a patient receiving an oral blood glucose-lowering agent, the patient should be observed closely for hypoglycemia. When a sulfonamideis withdrawn from a patient receiving an oral blood glucose-lowering agent, the patient should be observed closely for loss of glycemic control).
No products indexed under this heading.

Methylprednisolone (Repaglinide is metabolized by the cytochrome P4502C8 and 3A4 enzymes. Consequently, repaglinide metabolism may be altered by drugs that are CYP3A4 inducers. Caution should be used in patients concomitantly using repaglinide and a CYP3A4 inducer).
No products indexed under this heading.

Methylprednisolone Acetate (Repaglinide is metabolized by the cytochrome P4502C8 and 3A4 enzymes. Consequently, repaglinide metabolism may be altered by drugs that are CYP3A4 inducers. Caution should be used in patients concomitantly using repaglinide and a CYP3A4 inducer).
No products indexed under this heading.

Methylprednisolone Sodium Succinate (Repaglinide is metabolized by the cytochrome P4502C8 and 3A4 enzymes. Consequently, repaglinide metabolism may be altered by drugs that are CYP3A4 inducers. Caution should be used in patients concomitantly using repaglinide and a CYP3A4 inducer).
No products indexed under this heading.

Metipranolol Hydrochloride (The hypoglycemic action of oral blood glucose-lowering agents may be potentiated by beta adrenergic blocking agents. When administered to a patient receiving an oral blood glucose-lowering agent, the patient should be observed closely for hypoglycemia. When a beta adrenergic blocking agent is withdrawn from a patient receiving an oral blood glucose-lowering agent, the patient should be observed closely for loss of glycemic control).
No products indexed under this heading.

Metolazone (Diuretics tend to produce hyperglycemia and may lead to loss of glycemic control. When administered to a patient receiving an oral blood glucose-lowering agent, the patient should be observed for loss of glycemic control. When a diuretic drug is withdrawn from a patient receiving an oral blood glucose-lowering agent, the patient should be observed closely for hypoglycemia).
No products indexed under this heading.

Metoprolol Succinate (The hypoglycemic action of oral blood glucose-lowering agents may be potentiated by beta adrenergic blocking agents. When administered to a patient receiving an oral blood glucose-lowering agent, the patient should be observed closely for hypoglycemia. When a beta adrenergic blocking agent is withdrawn from a patient receiving an oral blood glucose-lowering agent, the patient should be observed closely for loss of glycemic control). Products include:
Toprol-XL Tablets **666**

Metoprolol Tartrate (The hypoglycemic action of oral blood glucose-lowering agents may be potentiated by beta adrenergic blocking agents. When administered to a patient receiving an oral blood glucose-lowering agent, the patient should be observed closely for hypoglycemia. When a beta adrenergic blocking agent is withdrawn from a patient receiving an oral blood glucose-lowering agent, the patient should be observed closely for loss of glycemic control).
No products indexed under this heading.

Metronidazole (Repaglinide is metabolized by the cytochrome P4502C8 and 3A4 enzymes. Consequently, repaglinide metabolism may be altered by drugs that are CYP3A4 inhibitors. Caution should be used in patients concomitantly using repaglinide and a CYP3A4 inhibitor. The effect may be very significant if both CYP3A4 and CYP2C8 are inhibited at the same time). Products include:
Pylera Capsules **714**

Metronidazole Benzoate (Repaglinide is metabolized by the cytochrome P4502C8 and 3A4 enzymes. Consequently, repaglinide metabolism may be altered by drugs that are CYP3A4 inhibitors. Caution should be used in patients concomitantly using repaglinide and a CYP3A4 inhibitor. The effect may be very significant if both CYP3A4 and CYP2C8 are inhibited at the same time).
No products indexed under this heading.

Metronidazole Hydrochloride (Repaglinide is metabolized by the cytochrome P4502C8 and 3A4 enzymes. Consequently, repaglinide metabolism may be altered by drugs that are CYP3A4 inhibitors. Caution should be used in patients concomitantly using repaglinide and a CYP3A4 inhibitor. The effect may be very significant if both CYP3A4 and CYP2C8 are inhibited at the same time).
No products indexed under this heading.

Metronidazole Sodium (Repaglinide is metabolized by the cytochrome P4502C8 and 3A4 enzymes. Consequently, repaglinide metabolism may be altered by drugs that are CYP3A4 inhibitors. Caution should be used in patients concomitantly using repaglinide and a CYP3A4 inhibitor. The effect may be very significant if both CYP3A4 and CYP2C8 are inhibited at the same time).
No products indexed under this heading.

Mibefradil Dihydrochloride (Calcium channel blockers tend to produce hyperglycemia and may lead to loss of glycemic control. When administered to a patient receiving an oral blood glucose-lowering agent, the patient should be observed for loss of glycemic control. When a calcium channel blocker is withdrawn from a patient receiving an oral blood glucose-lowering agent, the patient should be observed closely for hypoglycemia).
No products indexed under this heading.

Miconazole (Repaglinide is metabolized by the cytochrome P4502C8 and 3A4 enzymes. Consequently, repaglinide metabolism may be altered by drugs that are CYP3A4 inhibitors. Caution should be used in patients concomitantly using repaglinide and a CYP3A4 inhibitor. The effect may be very significant if both CYP3A4 and CYP2C8 are inhibited at the same time).
No products indexed under this heading.

Miconazole Nitrate (Repaglinide is metabolized by the cytochrome P4502C8 and 3A4 enzymes. Consequently, repaglinide metabolism may be altered by drugs that are CYP3A4 inhibitors. Caution should be used in patients concomitantly using repaglinide and a CYP3A4 inhibitor. The effect may be very significant if both CYP3A4 and CYP2C8 are inhibited at the same time).
No products indexed under this heading.

Midazolam Hydrochloride (The hypoglycemic action of oral blood glucose-lowering agents may be potentiated by highly protein bounded drugs. When administered to a patient receiving an oral blood glucose-lowering agent, the patient should be observed closely for hypoglycemia. When a highly protein bound drug is withdrawn from a patient receiving an oral blood glucose-lowering agent, the patient should be observed closely for loss of glycemic control).
No products indexed under this heading.

Moclobemide (The hypoglycemic action of oral blood glucose-lowering agents may be potentiated by MAO inhibitors. When administered to a patient receiving an oral blood glucose-lowering agent, the patient should be observed closely for hypoglycemia. When an MAO inhibitor is withdrawn from a patient receiving an oral blood glucose-lowering agent, the patient should be observed closely for loss of glycemic control).
No products indexed under this heading.

Modafinil (Repaglinide is metabolized by the cytochrome P4502C8 and 3A4 enzymes. Consequently, repaglinide metabolism may be altered by drugs that are CYP3A4 inducers. Caution should be used in patients concomitantly using repaglinide and a CYP3A4 inducer). Products include:
Provigil Tablets **977**

Mometasone Furoate (Corticosteroids tend to produce hyperglycemia and may lead to loss of glycemic control. When administered to a patient receiving an oral blood glucose-lowering agent, the patient should be observed for loss of glycemic control. When a corticosteroid iswithdrawn from a patient receiving an oral blood glucose-lowering agent, the patient should be observed closely for hypoglycemia). Products include:
Asmanex Twisthaler **2797**
Elocon Cream 0.1% **2840**
Elocon Lotion 0.1% **2841**
Elocon Ointment 0.1% **2842**

Mometasone Furoate Monohydrate (Corticosteroids tend to produce hyperglycemia and may lead to loss of glycemic control. When administered to a patient receiving an oral blood glucose-lowering agent, the patient should be observed for loss of glycemic control. When a corticosteroid iswithdrawn from a patient receiving an oral blood glucose-lowering agent, the patient should be observed closely for hypoglycemia). Products include:
Nasonex Nasal Spray **2883**

Montelukast Sodium (Concomitant use with montelukast, a

CYP2C8 inhibitor, may alter the metabolism of repaglinide; caution with use). Products include:

Singulair 2114

Nabumetone (The hypoglycemic action of oral blood glucose-lowering agents may be potentiated by nonsteroidal anti-inflammatory agents. When administered to a patient receiving an oral blood glucose-lowering agent, the patient should be observed closely for hypoglycemia. When a nonsteroidal anti-inflammatory agent is withdrawn from a patient receiving an oral blood glucose-lowering agent, the patient should be observed closely for loss of glycemic control).

No products indexed under this heading.

Nadolol (The hypoglycemic action of oral blood glucose-lowering agents may be potentiated by beta adrenergic blocking agents. When administered to a patient receiving an oral blood glucose-lowering agent, the patient should be observed closely for hypoglycemia. When a beta adrenergic blocking agent is withdrawn from a patient receiving an oral blood glucose-lowering agent, the patient should be observed closely for loss of glycemic control). Products include:

Nadolol Tablets 2191

Naproxen (The hypoglycemic action of oral blood glucose-lowering agents may be potentiated by nonsteroidal anti-inflammatory agents. When administered to a patient receiving an oral blood glucose-lowering agent, the patient should be observed closely for hypoglycemia. When a nonsteroidal anti-inflammatory agent is withdrawn from a patient receiving an oral blood glucose-lowering agent, the patient should be observed closely for loss of glycemic control). Products include:

EC-Naprosyn Delayed-Release Tablets 2632
Naprosyn Suspension 2632
Naprosyn Tablets 2632

Naproxen Sodium (The hypoglycemic action of oral blood glucose-lowering agents may be potentiated by nonsteroidal anti-inflammatory agents. When administered to a patient receiving an oral blood glucose-lowering agent, the patient should be observed closely for hypoglycemia. When a nonsteroidal anti-inflammatory agent is withdrawn from a patient receiving an oral blood glucose-lowering agent, the patient should be observed closely for loss of glycemic control). Products include:

Anaprox Tablets 2632
Anaprox DS Tablets 2632
Treximet Tablets 1616

Nebivolol (The hypoglycemic action of oral blood glucose-lowering agents may be potentiated by beta adrenergic blocking agents. When administered to a patient receiving an oral blood glucose-lowering agent, the patient should be observed closely for hypoglycemia. When a beta adrenergic blocking agent is withdrawn from a patient receiving an oral blood glucose-lowering agent, the patient should be observed closely for loss of glycemic control). Products include:

Bystolic Tablets 1155

Nefazodone Hydrochloride (Repaglinide is metabolized by the cytochrome P4502C8 and 3A4 enzymes. Consequently, repaglinide metabolism may be altered by drugs that are CYP3A4 inhibitors. Caution should be used in patients concomitantly using repaglinide and a CYP3A4 inhibitor. The effect may be very significant if both CYP3A4 and CYP2C8 are inhibited at the same time).

No products indexed under this heading.

Nelfinavir Mesylate (Repaglinide is metabolized by the cytochrome P4502C8 and 3A4 enzymes. Consequently, repaglinide metabolism may be altered by drugs that are CYP3A4 inhibitors. Caution should be used in patients concomitantly using repaglinide and a CYP3A4 inhibitor. The effect may be very significant if both CYP3A4 and CYP2C8 are inhibited at the same time).

No products indexed under this heading.

Nevirapine (Repaglinide is metabolized by the cytochrome P4502C8 and 3A4 enzymes. Consequently, repaglinide metabolism may be altered by drugs that are CYP3A4 inducers. Caution should be used in patients concomitantly using repaglinide and a CYP3A4 inducer). Products include:

Viramune Oral Suspension 873
Viramune Tablets 873

Niacinamide (Repaglinide is metabolized by the cytochrome P4502C8 and 3A4 enzymes. Consequently, repaglinide metabolism may be altered by drugs that are CYP3A4 inhibitors. Caution should be used in patients concomitantly using repaglinide and a CYP3A4 inhibitor. The effect may be very significant if both CYP3A4 and CYP2C8 are inhibited at the same time). Products include:

BioLean Free Tablets .... ▣ 635

Nicardipine Hydrochloride (Repaglinide is metabolized by the cytochrome P4502C8 and 3A4 enzymes. Consequently, repaglinide metabolism may be altered by drugs that are CYP2C8 inhibitors. Caution should be used in patients concomitantly using repaglinide and a CYP2C8 inhibitor. The effect may be very significant if both CYP3A4 and CYP2C8 are inhibited at the same time). Products include:

Cardene I.V. 1093

Nicotinamide (Repaglinide is metabolized by the cytochrome P4502C8 and 3A4 enzymes. Consequently, repaglinide metabolism may be altered by drugs that are CYP3A4 inhibitors. Caution should be used in patients concomitantly using repaglinide and a CYP3A4 inhibitor. The effect may be very significant if both CYP3A4 and CYP2C8 are inhibited at the same time).

No products indexed under this heading.

Nicotinic Acid (Nicotinic acid tends to produce hyperglycemia and may lead to loss of glycemic control. When administered to a patient receiving an oral blood glucose-lowering agent, the patient should be observed for loss of glycemic control. When nicotinic acid is withdrawn from a patient receiving an oral blood glucose-lowering agent, the patient should be observed closely for hypoglycemia).

No products indexed under this heading.

Nifedipine (Co-administration of 10 mg nifedipine with a single dose of 2 mg repaglinide (after 4 days of t.i.d nifedipine 10 mg and t.i.d. repaglinide 2 mg) resulted in unchanged AUC and Cmax values for both drugs).

No products indexed under this heading.

Nimodipine (Calcium channel blockers tend to produce hyperglycemia and may lead to loss of glycemic control. When administered to a patient receiving an oral blood glucose-lowering agent, the patient should be observed for loss of glycemic control. When a calcium channel blocker is withdrawn from a patient receiving an oral blood glucose-lowering agent, the patient should be observed closely for hypoglycemia). Products include:

Nimotop Capsules 790

Nisoldipine (Calcium channel blockers tend to produce hyperglycemia and may lead to loss of glycemic control. When administered to a patient receiving an oral blood glucose-lowering agent, the patient should be observed for loss of glycemic control. When a calcium channel blocker is withdrawn from a patient receiving an oral blood glucose-lowering agent, the patient should be observed closely for hypoglycemia). Products include:

Sular Extended Release Tablets 2975

Norepinephrine Bitartrate (Sympathomimetics tend to produce hyperglycemia and may lead to loss of glycemic control. When administered to a patient receiving an oral blood glucose-lowering agent, the patient should be observed for loss of glycemic control. When a sympathomimeticsis withdrawn from a patient receiving an oral blood glucose-lowering agent, the patient should be observed closely for hypoglycemia).

No products indexed under this heading.

Norethindrone (Estrogens and oral contraceptives tend to produce hyperglycemia and may lead to loss of glycemic control. When administered to a patient receiving an oral blood glucose-lowering agent, the patient should be observed for loss of gylcemic control. When an oral contraceptive is withdrawn from a patient receiving an oral blood glucose-lowering agent, the patient should be observed closely for hypoglycemia). Products include:

Ortho Micronor Tablets 2446

Norethynodrel (Estrogens and oral contraceptives tend to produce hyperglycemia and may lead to loss of glycemic control. When administered to a patient receiving an oral blood glucose-lowering agent, the patient should be observed for loss of gylcemic control. When an oral contraceptive is withdrawn from a patient receiving an oral blood glucose-lowering agent, the patient should be observed closely for hypoglycemia).

No products indexed under this heading.

Norfloxacin (Repaglinide is metabolized by the cytochrome P4502C8 and 3A4 enzymes. Consequently, repaglinide metabolism may be altered by drugs that are CYP3A4 inhibitors. Caution should be used in patients concomitantly using repaglinide and a CYP3A4 inhibitor. The effect may be very significant if both CYP3A4 and CYP2C8 are inhibited at the same time). Products include:

Noroxin Tablets 2069

Norgestimate (Estrogens and oral contraceptives tend to produce hyperglycemia and may lead to loss of glycemic control. When administered to a patient receiving an oral blood glucose-lowering agent, the patient should be observed for loss of gylcemic control. When an oral contraceptive is withdrawn from a patient receiving an oral blood glucose-lowering agent, the patient should be observed closely for hypoglycemia). Products include:

Ortho-Cyclen/Ortho Tri-Cyclen 2449
Ortho Tri-Cyclen Lo Tablets 2458

Norgestrel (Estrogens and oral contraceptives tend to produce hyperglycemia and may lead to loss of glycemic control. When administered to a patient receiving an oral blood glucose-lowering agent, the patient should be observed for loss of gylcemic control. When an oral contraceptive is withdrawn from a patient receiving an oral blood glucose-lowering agent, the patient should be observed closely for hypoglycemia).

No products indexed under this heading.

Nortriptyline Hydrochloride (The hypoglycemic action of oral blood glucose-lowering agents may be potentiated by highly protein bounded drugs. When administered to a patient receiving an oral blood glucose-lowering agent, the patient should be observed closely for hypoglycemia. When a highly protein bound drug is withdrawn from a patient receiving an oral blood glucose-lowering agent, the patient should be observed closely for loss of glycemic control).

No products indexed under this heading.

Omeprazole (Repaglinide is metabolized by the cytochrome P4502C8 and 3A4 enzymes. Consequently, repaglinide metabolism may be altered by drugs that are CYP3A4 inhibitors. Caution should be used in patients concomitantly using repaglinide and a CYP3A4 inhibitor. The effect may be very significant if both CYP3A4 and CYP2C8 are inhibited at the same time).

No products indexed under this heading.

Oxaprozin (The hypoglycemic action of oral blood glucose-lowering agents may be potentiated by nonsteroidal anti-inflammatory agents. When administered to a patient receiving an oral blood glucose-lowering agent, the patient should be observed closely for hypoglycemia. When a nonsteroidal anti-inflammatory agent is withdrawn from a patient receiving an oral blood glucose-lowering agent, the patient should be observed closely for loss of glycemic control).

No products indexed under this heading.

Oxazepam (The hypoglycemic action of oral blood glucose-lowering agents may be potentiated by highly protein bounded drugs. When administered to a patient receiving an oral blood glucose-lowering agent, the patient should be observed closely for hypoglycemia. When a highly protein bound drug is withdrawn from a patient receiving an oral blood glucose-lowering agent, the patient should be observed closely for loss of glycemic control).

No products indexed under this heading.

Oxcarbazepine (Repaglinide is metabolized by the cytochrome P4502C8 and 3A4 enzymes. Consequently, repaglinide metabolism may be altered by drugs that are CYP3A4 inducers. Caution should be used in patients concomitantly using repaglinide and a CYP3A4 inducer).

No products indexed under this heading.

Pargyline Hydrochloride (The hypoglycemic action of oral blood glucose-lowering agents may be potentiated by MAO inhibitors. When administered to a patient receiving an oral blood glucose-lowering agent, the patient should be observed closely for hypoglycemia. When an MAO inhibitor is withdrawn from a patient receiving an oral blood glucose-lowering agent, the patient should be observed closely for loss of glycemic control).

No products indexed under this heading.

Paroxetine Hydrochloride (Repaglinide is metabolized by the cytochrome P4502C8 and 3A4 enzymes. Consequently, repaglinide metabolism may be altered by drugs that are CYP3A4 inhibitors. Caution should be used in patients concomitantly using repaglinide and a CYP3A4 inhibitor. The effect may be very significant if both CYP3A4 and CYP2C8 are inhibited at the same time). Products include:

Paxil **1535**
Paxil CR Controlled-Release Tablets **1544**

Penbutolol Sulfate (The hypoglycemic action of oral blood glucose-lowering agents may be potentiated by beta adrenergic blocking agents. When administered to a patient receiving an oral blood glucose-lowering agent, the patient should be observed closely for hypoglycemia. When a beta adrenergic blocking agent is withdrawn from a patient receiving an oral blood glucose-lowering agent, the patient should be observed closely for loss of glycemic control).

No products indexed under this heading.

Pentobarbital Sodium (Concomitant use with barbiturates which are inducers of CYP3A4 and/or CYP2C8 may alter the metabolism of repaglinide; caution with use). Products include:

Nembutal Sodium Solution, USP **2494**

Perphenazine (Phenothiazines tend to produce hyperglycemia and may lead to loss of glycemic control. When administered to a patient receiving an oral blood glucose-lowering agent, the patient should be observed for loss of glycemic control. When a phenothiazine is withdrawn from a patient receiving an oral blood glucose-lowering agent, the patient should be observed closely for loss of hypoglycemia).

No products indexed under this heading.

Phenelzine Sulfate (The hypoglycemic action of oral blood glucose-lowering agents may be potentiated by MAO inhibitors. When administered to a patient receiving an oral blood glucose-lowering agent, the patient should be observed closely for hypoglycemia. When an MAO inhibitor is withdrawn from a patient receiving an oral blood glucose-lowering agent, the patient should be observed closely for loss of glycemic control).

No products indexed under this heading.

Phenobarbital (Repaglinide is metabolized by the cytochrome P4502C8 and 3A4 enzymes. Consequently, repaglinide metabolism may be altered by drugs that are CYP3A4 inducers. Caution should be used in patients concomitantly using repaglinide and a CYP3A4 inducer). Products include:

Donnatal Extentabs **2507**

Phenobarbital Sodium (Repaglinide is metabolized by the cytochrome P4502C8 and 3A4 enzymes. Consequently, repaglinide metabolism may be altered by drugs that are CYP3A4 inducers. Caution should be used in patients concomitantly using repaglinide and a CYP3A4 inducer).

No products indexed under this heading.

Phenylbutazone (The hypoglycemic action of oral blood glucose-lowering agents may be potentiated by nonsteroidal anti-inflammatory agents. When administered to a patient receiving an oral blood glucose-lowering agent, the patient should be observed closely for hypoglycemia. When a nonsteroidal anti-inflammatory agent is withdrawn from a patient receiving an oral blood glucose-lowering agent, the patient should be observed closely for loss of glycemic control).

No products indexed under this heading.

Phenylephrine Bitartrate (Sympathomimetics tend to produce hyperglycemia and may lead to loss of glycemic control. When administered to a patient receiving an oral blood glucose-lowering agent, the patient should be observed for loss of glycemic control. When a sympathomimeticsis withdrawn from a patient receiving an oral blood glucose-lowering agent, the patient should be observed closely for hypoglycemia).

No products indexed under this heading.

Phenylephrine Hydrochloride (Sympathomimetics tend to produce hyperglycemia and may lead to loss of glycemic control. When administered to a patient receiving an oral blood glucose-lowering agent, the patient should be observed for loss of glycemic control. When a sympathomimeticsis withdrawn from a patient receiving an oral blood glucose-lowering agent, the patient should be observed closely for hypoglycemia). Products include:

Actifed Cold & Allergy Tablets **1895**
Benadryl Allergy & Cold Kapgels **1895**
Benadryl Allergy & Sinus Headache Kapgels **1895**
Benadryl Severe Allergy & Sinus Headache Caplets **1897**
Children's Benadryl-D Allergy & Sinus Liquid **1896**
Benadryl-D Allergy & Sinus Tablet **1896**
PediaCare Children's Allergy & Cold Liquid **1902**
PediaCare Children's Decongestant Liquid **1902**
PediaCare Children's Liquid Multi-Symptom Cold **1902**
Sinutab Non-Drying Caplets **1905**
Sinutab Sinus Caplets **1905**
Children's Sudafed PE Cold & Cough Liquid **1907**
Children's Sudafed PE Nasal Decongestant Liquid **1906**
Sudafed PE Cold & Cough Caplets **1907**
Sudafed PE Nasal Decongestant Tablets **1907**
Sudafed PE Nighttime Cold Caplets **1907**
Sudafed PE Non-Drying Sinus Caplets **1908**
Sudafed PE Severe Cold Caplets **1908**
Sudafed PE Sinus & Allergy Tablets **1908**
Sudafed PE Sinus Headache Caplets **1908**
Tylenol Allergy Multi-Symptom Caplets with Cool Burst and Rapid Release Gelcaps **1916**
Tylenol Allergy Multi-Symptom Nighttime Caplets with Cool Burst **1916**
Children's Tylenol Plus Cold Suspension Liquid **1912**
Children's Tylenol Plus Cold & Allergy Suspension Liquid **1914**
Children's Tylenol Plus Flu Suspension Liquid **1914**
Children's Tylenol Plus Multi-Symptom Cold Suspension Liquid **1912**
Tylenol Cold Head Congestion Daytime Caplets with Cool Burst **1910**
Tylenol Cold Head Congestion Nighttime Caplets with Cool Burst **1910**
Tylenol Cold Head Congestion Severe Daytime Caplets with Cool Burst **1910**
Tylenol Cold Multi-Symptom Daytime Caplets with Cool Burst and Rapid Release Gels **1913**
Tylenol Cold Multi-Symptom Daytime Liquid with Citrus Burst ... **1913**
Tylenol Cold Multi-Symptom Nighttime Caplets with Cool Burst **1913**
Tylenol Cold Multi-Symptom Nighttime Liquid with Cool Burst ... **1913**
Tylenol Cold Multi-Symptom Severe Caplets with Cool Burst..... **1913**
Tylenol Cold Multi-Symptom Severe Daytime Liquid with Citrus Burst **1913**
Tylenol Sinus Congestion & Pain Daytime Caplets with Cool Burst and Gelcaps **1917**
Tylenol Sinus Congestion & Pain Nighttime Caplets with Cool Burst **1917**
Tylenol Sinus Congestion & Pain Severe Caplets with Cool Burst..... **1917**
Vicks DayQuil Cold & Flu Multi-Symptom Relief **616**
Vicks DayQuil LiquiCaps **2567**
Vicks DayQuil Liquid **2567**
Vicks DayQuil Multi-Symptom Cold/Flu Relief **2567**

Phenylephrine Tannate (Sympathomimetics tend to produce hyperglycemia and may lead to loss of glycemic control. When administered to a patient receiving an oral blood glucose-lowering agent, the patient should be observed for loss of glycemic control. When a sympathomimeticsis withdrawn from a patient receiving an oral blood glucose-lowering agent, the patient should be observed closely for hypoglycemia).

No products indexed under this heading.

Phenylpropanolamine Hydrochloride (Sympathomimetics tend to produce hyperglycemia and may lead to loss of glycemic control. When administered to a patient receiving an oral blood glucose-lowering agent, the patient should be observed for loss of glycemic control. When a sympathomimeticsis withdrawn from a patient receiving an oral blood glucose-lowering agent, the patient should be observed closely for hypoglycemia).

No products indexed under this heading.

Phenytoin (Repaglinide is metabolized by the cytochrome P4502C8 and 3A4 enzymes. Consequently, repaglinide metabolism may be altered by drugs that are CYP3A4 inducers. Caution should be used in patients concomitantly using repaglinide and a CYP3A4 inducer).

No products indexed under this heading.

Phenytoin Sodium (Repaglinide is metabolized by the cytochrome P4502C8 and 3A4 enzymes. Consequently, repaglinide metabolism may be altered by drugs that are CYP3A4 inducers. Caution should be used in patients concomitantly using repaglinide and a CYP3A4 inducer). Products include:

Phenytek Capsules **2192**

Pindolol (The hypoglycemic action of oral blood glucose-lowering agents may be potentiated by beta adrenergic blocking agents. When administered to a patient receiving an oral blood glucose-lowering agent, the patient should be observed closely for hypoglycemia. When a beta adrenergic blocking agent is withdrawn from a patient receiving an oral blood glucose-lowering agent, the patient should be observed closely for loss of glycemic control).

No products indexed under this heading.

Pirbuterol Acetate (Sympathomimetics tend to produce hyperglycemia and may lead to loss of glycemic control. When administered to a patient receiving an oral blood glucose-lowering agent, the patient should be observed for loss of glycemic control. When a sympathomimeticsis withdrawn from a patient receiving an oral blood glucose-lowering agent, the patient should be observed closely for hypoglycemia). Products include:

Maxair Autohaler **1705**

Piroxicam (The hypoglycemic action of oral blood glucose-lowering agents may be potentiated by nonsteroidal anti-inflammatory agents. When administered to a patient receiving an oral blood glucose-lowering agent, the patient should be observed closely for hypoglycemia. When a nonsteroidal anti-inflammatory agent is withdrawn from a patient receiving an oral blood glucose-lowering agent, the patient should be observed closely for loss of glycemic control).

No products indexed under this heading.

Polyestradiol Phosphate (Estrogens and oral contraceptives tend to produce hyperglycemia and may lead to loss of glycemic control. When administered to a patient receiving an oral blood glucose-lowering agent, the patient should be observed for loss of glycemic control. When an estrogen is withdrawn

from a patient receiving an oral blood glucose-lowering agent, the patient should be observed closely for hypoglycemia).
No products indexed under this heading.

Polythiazide (The hypoglycemic action of oral blood glucose-lowering agents may be potentiated by sulfonamides. When administered to a patient receiving an oral blood glucose-lowering agent, the patient should be observed closely for hypoglycemia. When a sulfonamideis withdrawn from a patient receiving an oral blood glucose-lowering agent, the patient should be observed closely for loss of glycemic control).
No products indexed under this heading.

Prednisolone Acetate (Repaglinide is metabolized by the cytochrome P4502C8 and 3A4 enzymes. Consequently, repaglinide metabolism may be altered by drugs that are CYP3A4 inducers. Caution should be used in patients concomitantly using repaglinide and a CYP3A4 inducer). Products include:
Pred Forte Ophthalmic Suspension .... ⊙227
Pred Mild Ophthalmic Suspension .... ⊙230
Pred-G Ophthalmic Ointment .... ⊙229
Pred-G Ophthalmic Suspension .... ⊙228

Prednisolone Sodium Phosphate (Repaglinide is metabolized by the cytochrome P4502C8 and 3A4 enzymes. Consequently, repaglinide metabolism may be altered by drugs that are CYP3A4 inducers. Caution should be used in patients concomitantly using repaglinide and a CYP3A4 inducer).
No products indexed under this heading.

Prednisolone Tebutate (Repaglinide is metabolized by the cytochrome P4502C8 and 3A4 enzymes. Consequently, repaglinide metabolism may be altered by drugs that are CYP3A4 inducers. Caution should be used in patients concomitantly using repaglinide and a CYP3A4 inducer).
No products indexed under this heading.

Prednisone (Repaglinide is metabolized by the cytochrome P4502C8 and 3A4 enzymes. Consequently, repaglinide metabolism may be altered by drugs that are CYP3A4 inducers. Caution should be used in patients concomitantly using repaglinide and a CYP3A4 inducer).
No products indexed under this heading.

Primidone (Repaglinide is metabolized by the cytochrome P4502C8 and 3A4 enzymes. Consequently, repaglinide metabolism may be altered by drugs that are CYP3A4 inducers. Caution should be used in patients concomitantly using repaglinide and a CYP3A4 inducer).
No products indexed under this heading.

Probenecid (The hypoglycemic action of oral blood glucose-lowering agents may be potentiated by probenecid. When administered to a patient receiving an oral blood glucose-lowering agent, the patient should be observed closely for hypoglycemia. When probenecid is withdrawn from a patient receiving an oral blood glucose-lowering agent, the patient should be observed closely for loss of glycemic control).
No products indexed under this heading.

Procarbazine Hydrochloride (The hypoglycemic action of oral blood glucose-lowering agents may be potentiated by MAO inhibitors. When administered to a patient receiving an oral blood glucose-lowering agent, the patient should be observed closely for hypoglycemia. When an MAO inhibitor is withdrawn from a patient receiving an oral blood glucose-lowering agent, the patient should be observed closely for loss of glycemic control).
No products indexed under this heading.

Prochlorperazine (Phenothiazines tend to produce hyperglycemia and may lead to loss of glycemic control. When administered to a patient receiving an oral blood glucose-lowering agent, the patient should be observed for loss of glycemic control. When a phenothiazine is withdrawn from a patient receiving an oral blood glucose-lowering agent, the patient should be observed closely for loss of hypoglycemia).
No products indexed under this heading.

Promethazine Hydrochloride (Phenothiazines tend to produce hyperglycemia and may lead to loss of glycemic control. When administered to a patient receiving an oral blood glucose-lowering agent, the patient should be observed for loss of glycemic control. When a phenothiazine is withdrawn from a patient receiving an oral blood glucose-lowering agent, the patient should be observed closely for loss of hypoglycemia).
No products indexed under this heading.

Propoxyphene Hydrochloride (Repaglinide is metabolized by the cytochrome P4502C8 and 3A4 enzymes. Consequently, repaglinide metabolism may be altered by drugs that are CYP3A4 inhibitors. Caution should be used in patients concomitantly using repaglinide and a CYP3A4 inhibitor. The effect may be very significant if both CYP3A4 and CYP2C8 are inhibited at the same time).
No products indexed under this heading.

Propoxyphene Napsylate (Repaglinide is metabolized by the cytochrome P4502C8 and 3A4 enzymes. Consequently, repaglinide metabolism may be altered by drugs that are CYP3A4 inhibitors. Caution should be used in patients concomitantly using repaglinide and a CYP3A4 inhibitor. The effect may be very significant if both CYP3A4 and CYP2C8 are inhibited at the same time).
No products indexed under this heading.

Propranolol Hydrochloride (The hypoglycemic action of oral blood glucose-lowering agents may be potentiated by highly protein bounded drugs. When administered to a patient receiving an oral blood glucose-lowering agent, the patient should be observed closely for hypoglycemia. When a highly protein bound drug is withdrawn from a patient receiving an oral blood glucose-lowering agent, the patient should be observed closely for loss of glycemic control). Products include:
InnoPran XL Extended Release Capsules 1484

Pseudoephedrine Hydrochloride (Sympathomimetics tend to produce hyperglycemia and may lead to loss of glycemic control. When administered to a patient receiving an oral blood glucose-lowering agent, the patient should be observed for loss of glycemic control. When a sympathomimeticsis withdrawn from a patient receiving an oral blood glucose-lowering agent, the patient should be observed closely for hypoglycemia). Products include:
Allegra-D 12 Hour Extended-Release Tablets 2687
Allegra-D 24 Hour Extended-Release Tablets 2690
Children's Motrin Cold Oral Suspension 1899
Sudafed 12 Hour Nasal Decongestant Non-Drowsy Caplets 1909
Sudafed 24 Hour Non-Drowsy Nasal Decongestant Tablets 1906
Children's Sudafed Nasal Decongestant Liquid 1906
Sudafed Nasal Decongestant Tablets 1906
Tylenol Cold Severe Congestion Daytime Caplets with Cool Burst 1912
Tylenol Sinus Severe Congestion Caplets with Cool Burst 1917
Vicks NyQuil LiquiCaps 2567
Vicks NyQuil Liquid 2567
Vicks NyQuil Multi-Symptom Cold/Flu Relief 2567
Zyrtec-D 12 Hour Extended Release Tablets 1923
Zyrtec-D Allergy & Congestion Extended-Release Tablets 1923

Pseudoephedrine Sulfate (Sympathomimetics tend to produce hyperglycemia and may lead to loss of glycemic control. When administered to a patient receiving an oral blood glucose-lowering agent, the patient should be observed for loss of glycemic control. When a sympathomimeticsis withdrawn from a patient receiving an oral blood glucose-lowering agent, the patient should be observed closely for hypoglycemia). Products include:
Clarinex-D 12-Hour Extended-Release Tablets 2831
Clarinex-D 24-Hour Extended-Release Tablets 2834

Quercetin (Repaglinide is metabolized by the cytochrome P4502C8 and 3A4 enzymes. Consequently, repaglinide metabolism may be altered by drugs that are CYP2C8 inhibitors. Caution should be used in patients concomitantly using repaglinide and a CYP2C8 inhibitor. The effect may be very significant if both CYP3A4 and CYP2C8 are inhibited at the same time).
No products indexed under this heading.

Quinestrol (Estrogens and oral contraceptives tend to produce hyperglycemia and may lead to loss of glycemic control. When administered to a patient receiving an oral blood glucose-lowering agent, the patient should be observed for loss of glycemic control. When an estrogen is withdrawn from a patient receiving an oral blood glucose-lowering agent, the patient should be observed closely for hypoglycemia).
No products indexed under this heading.

Quinidine (Repaglinide is metabolized by the cytochrome P4502C8 and 3A4 enzymes. Consequently, repaglinide metabolism may be altered by drugs that are CYP3A4 inhibitors. Caution should be used in patients concomitantly using repaglinide and a CYP3A4 inhibitor. The effect may be very significant if both CYP3A4 and CYP2C8 are inhibited at the same time).
No products indexed under this heading.

Quinidine Hydrochloride (Repaglinide is metabolized by the cytochrome P4502C8 and 3A4 enzymes. Consequently, repaglinide metabolism may be altered by drugs that are CYP3A4 inhibitors. Caution should be used in patients concomitantly using repaglinide and a CYP3A4 inhibitor. The effect may be very significant if both CYP3A4 and CYP2C8 are inhibited at the same time).
No products indexed under this heading.

Quinidine Polygalacturonate (Repaglinide is metabolized by the cytochrome P4502C8 and 3A4 enzymes. Consequently, repaglinide metabolism may be altered by drugs that are CYP3A4 inhibitors. Caution should be used in patients concomitantly using repaglinide and a CYP3A4 inhibitor. The effect may be very significant if both CYP3A4 and CYP2C8 are inhibited at the same time).
No products indexed under this heading.

Quinidine Sulfate (Repaglinide is metabolized by the cytochrome P4502C8 and 3A4 enzymes. Consequently, repaglinide metabolism may be altered by drugs that are CYP3A4 inhibitors. Caution should be used in patients concomitantly using repaglinide and a CYP3A4 inhibitor. The effect may be very significant if both CYP3A4 and CYP2C8 are inhibited at the same time).
No products indexed under this heading.

Quinine (Repaglinide is metabolized by the cytochrome P4502C8 and 3A4 enzymes. Consequently, repaglinide metabolism may be altered by drugs that are CYP3A4 inhibitors. Caution should be used in patients concomitantly using repaglinide and a CYP3A4 inhibitor. The effect may be very significant if both CYP3A4 and CYP2C8 are inhibited at the same time).
No products indexed under this heading.

Quinine Sulfate (Repaglinide is metabolized by the cytochrome P4502C8 and 3A4 enzymes. Consequently, repaglinide metabolism may be altered by drugs that are CYP3A4 inhibitors. Caution should be used in patients concomitantly using repaglinide and a CYP3A4 inhibitor. The effect may be very significant if both CYP3A4 and CYP2C8 are inhibited at the same time).
No products indexed under this heading.

Quinupristin (Repaglinide is metabolized by the cytochrome P4502C8 and 3A4 enzymes. Consequently, repaglinide metabolism may be altered by drugs that are CYP3A4 inhibitors. Caution should be used in patients concomitantly using repaglinide and a CYP3A4 inhibitor. The effect may be very significant if both CYP3A4 and CYP2C8 are inhibited at the same time).
No products indexed under this heading.

Ranitidine Bismuth Citrate (Repaglinide is metabolized by the cytochrome P4502C8 and 3A4 enzymes. Consequently, repaglinide metabolism may be altered by drugs that are CYP3A4 inhibitors. Caution should be used in patients concomitantly using repaglinide and a CYP3A4 inhibitor. The effect may be very significant if both CYP3A4 and CYP2C8 are inhibited at the same time).
No products indexed under this heading.

Ranitidine Hydrochloride (Repaglinide is metabolized by the cytochrome P4502C8 and 3A4 enzymes. Consequently, repaglinide metabolism may be altered by drugs that are CYP3A4 inhibitors. Caution should be used in patients concomitantly using repaglinide and a CYP3A4 inhibitor. The effect may be very significant if both CYP3A4 and CYP2C8 are inhibited at the same time). Products include:
Zantac 75 Tablets 603
Zantac 1670
Zantac Injection 1666
Zantac Injection Pharmacy Bulk Package 1668
Maximum Strength Zantac 150 Tablets 603
Maximum Strength Zantac 150 Cool Mint Tablets 603

Rasagiline Mesylate (The hypoglycemic action of oral blood glucose-lowering agents may be potentiated by MAO inhibitors. When administered to a patient receiving an oral blood glucose-lowering agent, the patient should be observed closely for hypoglycemia. When an MAO inhibitor is withdrawn from a patient receiving an oral blood glucose-lowering agent, the patient should be observed closely for loss of glycemic control). Products include:
Azilect Tablets 3106

Rifabutin (Repaglinide is metabolized by the cytochrome P4502C8 and 3A4 enzymes. Consequently, repaglinide metabolism may be altered by drugs that are CYP3A4 inducers. Caution should be used in patients concomitantly using repaglinide and a CYP3A4 inducer).
No products indexed under this heading.

Rifampicin (Repaglinide is metabolized by the cytochrome P4502C8 and 3A4 enzymes. Consequently, repaglinide metabolism may be altered by drugs that are CYP3A4 inducers. Caution should be used in patients concomitantly using repaglinide and a CYP3A4 inducer).
No products indexed under this heading.

Rifampin (Co-administration of 600 mg rifampin and a single dose of 4 mg repaglinide (after 6 days of once-daily rifampin 600 mg) resulted in a 32% and 26% decrease in repaglinide AUC and Cmax, respectively. The decreases were from 40.4 ng/mL to 29.7 ng/mL for Cmax and 56.8 ng/mL*hr to 38.7 ng/mL*hr for AUC. Concomitant use with rifampin, a CYP3A4 and CYP2C8 inducer, may alter the metabolism of repaglinide; use with caution).
No products indexed under this heading.

Rifapentine (Repaglinide is metabolized by the cytochrome P4502C8 and 3A4 enzymes. Consequently, repaglinide metabolism may be altered by drugs that are CYP3A4 inducers. Caution should be used in patients concomitantly using repaglinide and a CYP3A4 inducer).
No products indexed under this heading.

Ritonavir (Repaglinide is metabolized by the cytochrome P4502C8 and 3A4 enzymes. Consequently, repaglinide metabolism may be altered by drugs that are CYP3A4 inhibitors. Caution should be used in patients concomitantly using repaglinide and a CYP3A4 inhibitor. The effect may be very significant if both CYP3A4 and CYP2C8 are inhibited at the same time). Products include:
Kaletra 452
Norvir 489

Rofecoxib (The hypoglycemic action of oral blood glucose-lowering agents may be potentiated by nonsteroidal anti-inflammatory agents. When administered to a patient receiving an oral blood glucose-lowering agent, the patient should be observed closely for hypoglycemia. When a nonsteroidal anti-inflammatory agent is withdrawn from a patient receiving an oral blood glucose-lowering agent, the patient should be observed closely for loss of glycemic control).
No products indexed under this heading.

Salmeterol Xinafoate (Sympathomimetics tend to produce hyperglycemia and may lead to loss of glycemic control. When administered to a patient receiving an oral blood glucose-lowering agent, the patient should be observed for loss of glycemic control. When a sympathomimeticsis withdrawn from a patient receiving an oral blood glucose-lowering agent, the patient should be observed closely for hypoglycemia). Products include:
Advair Diskus 100/50 1276
Advair Diskus 250/50 1276
Advair Diskus 500/50 1276
Advair HFA 45/21 Inhalation Aerosol 1288
Advair HFA 115/21 Inhalation Aerosol 1288
Advair HFA 230/21 Inhalation Aerosol 1288
Serevent Diskus 1594

Salsalate (The hypoglycemic action of oral blood glucose-lowering agents may be potentiated by salicylates. When administered to a patient receiving an oral blood glucose-lowering agent, the patient should be observed closely for hypoglycemia. When a salicylate is withdrawn from a patient receiving an oral blood glucose-lowering agent, the patient should be observed closely for loss of glycemic control).
No products indexed under this heading.

Saquinavir (Repaglinide is metabolized by the cytochrome P4502C8 and 3A4 enzymes. Consequently, repaglinide metabolism may be altered by drugs that are CYP3A4 inhibitors. Caution should be used in patients concomitantly using repaglinide and a CYP3A4 inhibitor. The effect may be very significant if both CYP3A4 and CYP2C8 are inhibited at the same time).
No products indexed under this heading.

Saquinavir Mesylate (Repaglinide is metabolized by the cytochrome P4502C8 and 3A4 enzymes. Consequently, repaglinide metabolism may be altered by drugs that are CYP3A4 inhibitors. Caution should be used in patients concomitantly using repaglinide and a CYP3A4 inhibitor. The effect may be very significant if both CYP3A4 and CYP2C8 are inhibited at the same time).
No products indexed under this heading.

Secobarbital Sodium (Concomitant use with barbiturates which are inducers of CYP3A4 and/or CYP2C8 may alter the metabolism of repaglinide; caution with use).
No products indexed under this heading.

Selegiline (The hypoglycemic action of oral blood glucose-lowering agents may be potentiated by MAO inhibitors. When administered to a patient receiving an oral blood glucose-lowering agent, the patient should be observed closely for hypoglycemia. When an MAO inhibitor is withdrawn from a patient receiving an oral blood glucose-lowering agent, the patient should be observed closely for loss of glycemic control). Products include:
Emsam Transdermal System 905

Selegiline Hydrochloride (The hypoglycemic action of oral blood glucose-lowering agents may be potentiated by MAO inhibitors. When administered to a patient receiving an oral blood glucose-lowering agent, the patient should be observed closely for hypoglycemia. When an MAO inhibitor is withdrawn from a patient receiving an oral blood glucose-lowering agent, the patient should be observed closely for loss of glycemic control). Products include:
Eldepryl Capsules 3052

Sertraline Hydrochloride (Repaglinide is metabolized by the cytochrome P4502C8 and 3A4 enzymes. Consequently, repaglinide metabolism may be altered by drugs that are CYP3A4 inhibitors. Caution should be used in patients concomitantly using repaglinide and a CYP3A4 inhibitor. The effect may be very significant if both CYP3A4 and CYP2C8 are inhibited at the same time).
No products indexed under this heading.

Sildenafil Citrate (Repaglinide is metabolized by the cytochrome P4502C8 and 3A4 enzymes. Consequently, repaglinide metabolism may be altered by drugs that are CYP3A4 inhibitors. Caution should be used in patients concomitantly using repaglinide and a CYP3A4 inhibitor. The effect may be very significant if both CYP3A4 and CYP2C8 are inhibited at the same time).
No products indexed under this heading.

Simvastatin (Co-administration of 20 mg simvastatin and single dose of 2 mg repaglinide (after 4 days of once-daily simvastatin 20 mg and t.i.d. repaglinide 2 mg) resulted in a 26% increase in repaglinide Cmax from 23.6 ng/mL to 29.7 ng/mL. AUC was unchanged). Products include:
Simcor Tablets 502
Vytorin 10/10 Tablets 2149
Vytorin 10/10 Tablets 2939
Vytorin 10/20 Tablets 2149
Vytorin 10/20 Tablets 2939
Vytorin 10/40 Tablets 2149
Vytorin 10/40 Tablets 2939
Vytorin 10/80 Tablets 2149
Vytorin 10/80 Tablets 2939
Zocor Tablets 2136

Sotalol Hydrochloride (The hypoglycemic action of oral blood glucose-lowering agents may be potentiated by beta adrenergic blocking agents. When administered to a patient receiving an oral blood glucose-lowering agent, the patient should be observed closely for hypoglycemia. When a beta adrenergic blocking agent is withdrawn from a patient receiving an oral blood glucose-lowering agent, the patient should be observed closely for loss of glycemic control).
No products indexed under this heading.

Spironolactone (Diuretics tend to produce hyperglycemia and may lead to loss of glycemic control. When administered to a patient receiving an oral blood glucose-lowering agent, the patient should be observed for loss of glycemic control. When a diuretic drug is withdrawn from a patient receiving an oral blood glucose-lowering agent, the patient should be observed closely for hypoglycemia).
No products indexed under this heading.

Sulfacytine (The hypoglycemic action of oral blood glucose-lowering agents may be potentiated by sulfonamides. When administered to a patient receiving an oral blood glucose-lowering agent, the patient should be observed closely for hypoglycemia. When a sulfonamideis withdrawn from a patient receiving an oral blood glucose-lowering agent, the patient should be observed closely for loss of glycemic control).
No products indexed under this heading.

Sulfamethizole (The hypoglycemic action of oral blood glucose-lowering agents may be potentiated by sulfonamides. When administered to a patient receiving an oral blood glucose-lowering agent, the patient should be observed closely for hypoglycemia. When a sulfonamideis withdrawn from a patient receiving an oral blood glucose-lowering agent, the patient should be observed closely for loss of glycemic control).
No products indexed under this heading.

Sulfamethoxazole (The hypoglycemic action of oral blood glucose-lowering agents may be potentiated by sulfonamides. When administered to a patient receiving an oral blood glucose-lowering agent, the patient should be observed closely for hypoglycemia. When a sulfonamideis withdrawn from a patient receiving an oral blood glucose-lowering agent, the patient should be observed

closely for loss of glycemic control).
No products indexed under this heading.

Sulfaphenazole (Repaglinide is metabolized by the cytochrome P4502C8 and 3A4 enzymes. Consequently, repaglinide metabolism may be altered by drugs that are CYP2C8 inhibitors. Caution should be used in patients concomitantly using repaglinide and a CYP2C8 inhibitor. The effect may be very significant if both CYP3A4 and CYP2C8 are inhibited at the same time).
No products indexed under this heading.

Sulfasalazine (The hypoglycemic action of oral blood glucose-lowering agents may be potentiated by sulfonamides. When administered to a patient receiving an oral blood glucose-lowering agent, the patient should be observed closely for hypoglycemia. When a sulfonamideis withdrawn from a patient receiving an oral blood glucose-lowering agent, the patient should be observed closely for loss of glycemic control).
No products indexed under this heading.

Sulfinpyrazone (Repaglinide is metabolized by the cytochrome P4502C8 and 3A4 enzymes. Consequently, repaglinide metabolism may be altered by drugs that are CYP3A4 inducers. Caution should be used in patients concomitantly using repaglinide and a CYP3A4 inducer).
No products indexed under this heading.

Sulfisoxazole Acetyl (The hypoglycemic action of oral blood glucose-lowering agents may be potentiated by sulfonamides. When administered to a patient receiving an oral blood glucose-lowering agent, the patient should be observed closely for hypoglycemia. When a sulfonamideis withdrawn from a patient receiving an oral blood glucose-lowering agent, the patient should be observed closely for loss of glycemic control).
No products indexed under this heading.

Sulfisoxazole Diolamine (The hypoglycemic action of oral blood glucose-lowering agents may be potentiated by sulfonamides. When administered to a patient receiving an oral blood glucose-lowering agent, the patient should be observed closely for hypoglycemia. When a sulfonamideis withdrawn from a patient receiving an oral blood glucose-lowering agent, the patient should be observed closely for loss of glycemic control).
No products indexed under this heading.

Sulindac (The hypoglycemic action of oral blood glucose-lowering agents may be potentiated by nonsteroidal anti-inflammatory agents. When administered to a patient receiving an oral blood glucose-lowering agent, the patient should be observed closely for hypoglycemia. When a nonsteroidal anti-inflammatory agent is withdrawn from a patient receiving an oral blood glucose-lowering agent, the patient should be observed closely for loss of glycemic control). Products include:
Clinoril Tablets 1962

Telithromycin (Repaglinide is metabolized by the cytochrome P4502C8 and 3A4 enzymes. Consequently, repaglinide metabolism may be altered by drugs that are CYP3A4 inhibitors. Caution should be used in patients concomitantly using repaglinide and a CYP3A4 inhibitor. The effect may be very significant if both CYP3A4 and CYP2C8 are inhibited at the same time). Products include:
Ketek Tablets 2744

Temazepam (The hypoglycemic action of oral blood glucose-lowering agents may be potentiated by highly protein bounded drugs. When administered to a patient receiving an oral blood glucose-lowering agent, the patient should be observed closely for hypoglycemia. When a highly protein bound drug is withdrawn from a patient receiving an oral blood glucose-lowering agent, the patient should be observed closely for loss of glycemic control).
No products indexed under this heading.

Terbutaline Sulfate (Sympathomimetics tend to produce hyperglycemia and may lead to loss of glycemic control. When administered to a patient receiving an oral blood glucose-lowering agent, the patient should be observed for loss of glycemic control. When a sympathomimeticsis withdrawn from a patient receiving an oral blood glucose-lowering agent, the patient should be observed closely for hypoglycemia).
No products indexed under this heading.

Theophylline (Repaglinide is metabolized by the cytochrome P4502C8 and 3A4 enzymes. Consequently, repaglinide metabolism may be altered by drugs that are CYP3A4 inducers. Caution should be used in patients concomitantly using repaglinide and a CYP3A4 inducer).
No products indexed under this heading.

Theophylline Anhydrous (Repaglinide is metabolized by the cytochrome P4502C8 and 3A4 enzymes. Consequently, repaglinide metabolism may be altered by drugs that are CYP3A4 inducers. Caution should be used in patients concomitantly using repaglinide and a CYP3A4 inducer). Products include:
Uniphyl Tablets 2595

Theophylline Calcium Salicylate (Repaglinide is metabolized by the cytochrome P4502C8 and 3A4 enzymes. Consequently, repaglinide metabolism may be altered by drugs that are CYP3A4 inducers. Caution should be used in patients concomitantly using repaglinide and a CYP3A4 inducer).
No products indexed under this heading.

Theophylline Dihydroxypropyl (Glyceryl) (Repaglinide is metabolized by the cytochrome P4502C8 and 3A4 enzymes. Consequently, repaglinide metabolism may be altered by drugs that are CYP3A4 inducers. Caution should be used in patients concomitantly using repaglinide and a CYP3A4 inducer).
No products indexed under this heading.

Theophylline Ethylenediamine (Repaglinide is metabolized by the cytochrome P4502C8 and 3A4 enzymes. Consequently, repaglinide metabolism may be altered by drugs that are CYP3A4 inducers. Caution should be used in patients concomitantly using repaglinide and a CYP3A4 inducer).
No products indexed under this heading.

Thiamylal Sodium (Concomitant use with barbiturates which are inducers of CYP3A4 and/or CYP2C8 may alter the metabolism of repaglinide; caution with use).
No products indexed under this heading.

Thioridazine Hydrochloride (Phenothiazines tend to produce hyperglycemia and may lead to loss of glycemic control. When administered to a patient receiving an oral blood glucose-lowering agent, the patient should be observed for loss of glycemic control. When a phenothiazine is withdrawn from a patient receiving an oral blood glucose-lowering agent, the patient should be observed closely for loss of hypoglycemia). Products include:
Thioridazine Hydrochloride Tablets 2195

Thyroglobulin (Thyroid products tend to produce hyperglycemia and may lead to loss of glycemic control. When administered to a patient receiving an oral blood glucose-lowering agent, the patient should be observed for loss of glycemic control. When a thyroid product is withdrawn from a patient receiving an oral blood glucose-lowering agent, the patient should be observed closely for hypoglycemia).
No products indexed under this heading.

Thyroid (Thyroid products tend to produce hyperglycemia and may lead to loss of glycemic control. When administered to a patient receiving an oral blood glucose-lowering agent, the patient should be observed for loss of glycemic control. When a thyroid product is withdrawn from a patient receiving an oral blood glucose-lowering agent, the patient should be observed closely for hypoglycemia). Products include:
Naturethroid Tablets 2605

Thyroxine (Thyroid products tend to produce hyperglycemia and may lead to loss of glycemic control. When administered to a patient receiving an oral blood glucose-lowering agent, the patient should be observed for loss of glycemic control. When a thyroid product is withdrawn from a patient receiving an oral blood glucose-lowering agent, the patient should be observed closely for hypoglycemia).
No products indexed under this heading.

Thyroxine Sodium (Thyroid products tend to produce hyperglycemia and may lead to loss of glycemic control. When administered to a patient receiving an oral blood glucose-lowering agent, the patient should be observed for loss of glycemic control. When a thyroid product is withdrawn from a patient receiving an oral blood glucose-lowering agent, the patient should be observed closely for hypoglycemia).
No products indexed under this heading.

Timolol Hemihydrate (The hypoglycemic action of oral blood glucose-lowering agents may be potentiated by beta adrenergic blocking agents. When administered to a patient receiving an oral blood glucose-lowering agent, the patient should be observed closely for hypoglycemia. When a beta adrenergic blocking agent is withdrawn from a patient receiving an oral blood glucose-lowering agent, the patient should be observed closely for loss of glycemic control). Products include:
Betimol Ophthalmic Solution 3181

Timolol Maleate (The hypoglycemic action of oral blood glucose-lowering agents may be potentiated by beta adrenergic blocking agents. When administered to a patient receiving an oral blood glucose-lowering agent, the patient should be observed closely for hypoglycemia. When a beta adrenergic blocking agent is withdrawn from a patient receiving an oral blood glucose-lowering agent, the patient should be observed closely for loss of glycemic control). Products include:
Combigan Ophthalmic Solution 553
Cosopt Sterile Ophthalmic Solution 1969
Timoptic Sterile Ophthalmic Solution 2121
Timoptic in Ocudose 2124
Timoptic-XE Sterile Ophthalmic Gel Forming Solution 2125

Tolazamide (The hypoglycemic action of oral blood glucose-lowering agents may be potentiated by sulfonamides. When administered to a patient receiving an oral blood glucose-lowering agent, the patient should be observed closely for hypoglycemia. When a sulfonamideis withdrawn from a patient receiving an oral blood glucose-lowering agent, the patient should be observed closely for loss of glycemic control).
No products indexed under this heading.

Tolbutamide (The hypoglycemic action of oral blood glucose-lowering agents may be potentiated by highly protein bounded drugs. When administered to a patient receiving an oral blood glucose-lowering agent, the patient should be observed closely for hypoglycemia. When a highly protein bound drug is withdrawn from a patient receiving an oral blood glucose-lowering agent, the patient should be observed closely for loss of glycemic control).
No products indexed under this heading.

Tolmetin Sodium (The hypoglycemic action of oral blood glucose-lowering agents may be potentiated by nonsteroidal anti-inflammatory agents. When administered to a patient receiving an oral blood glucose-lowering agent, the patient should be observed closely for hypoglycemia. When a nonsteroidal anti-inflammatory agent is withdrawn from a patient receiving an oral blood glucose-lowering agent, the patient should be observed closely for loss of glycemic control).
No products indexed under this heading.

Torsemide (Diuretics tend to produce hyperglycemia and may lead to loss of glycemic control. When administered to a patient receiving an oral blood glucose-lowering agent, the patient should be observed for loss of glycemic control. When a diuretic drug is withdrawn from a patient receiving an oral blood glucose-lowering agent, the patient should be observed closely for hypoglycemia). Products include:

Demadex Injection 2630
Demadex Tablets 2630

Tranylcypromine Sulfate (The hypoglycemic action of oral blood glucose-lowering agents may be potentiated by MAO inhibitors. When administered to a patient receiving an oral blood glucose-lowering agent, the patient should be observed closely for hypoglycemia. When an MAO inhibitor is withdrawn from a patient receiving an oral blood glucose-lowering agent, the patient should be observed closely for loss of glycemic control). Products include:

Parnate Tablets 1532

Triamcinolone (Repaglinide is metabolized by the cytochrome P4502C8 and 3A4 enzymes. Consequently, repaglinide metabolism may be altered by drugs that are CYP3A4 inducers. Caution should be used in patients concomitantly using repaglinide and a CYP3A4 inducer).

No products indexed under this heading.

Triamcinolone Acetonide (Repaglinide is metabolized by the cytochrome P4502C8 and 3A4 enzymes. Consequently, repaglinide metabolism may be altered by drugs that are CYP3A4 inducers. Caution should be used in patients concomitantly using repaglinide and a CYP3A4 inducer). Products include:

Azmacort Inhalation Aerosol 407
Nasacort AQ Nasal Spray 2765
Triesence Injectable Suspension .... ⊙ 209

Triamcinolone Diacetate (Repaglinide is metabolized by the cytochrome P4502C8 and 3A4 enzymes. Consequently, repaglinide metabolism may be altered by drugs that are CYP3A4 inducers. Caution should be used in patients concomitantly using repaglinide and a CYP3A4 inducer).

No products indexed under this heading.

Triamcinolone Hexacetonide (Repaglinide is metabolized by the cytochrome P4502C8 and 3A4 enzymes. Consequently, repaglinide metabolism may be altered by drugs that are CYP3A4 inducers. Caution should be used in patients concomitantly using repaglinide and a CYP3A4 inducer).

No products indexed under this heading.

Triamterene (Diuretics tend to produce hyperglycemia and may lead to loss of glycemic control. When administered to a patient receiving an oral blood glucose-lowering agent, the patient should be observed for loss of glycemic control. When a diuretic drug is withdrawn from a patient receiving an oral blood glucose-lowering agent, the patient should be observed closely for hypoglycemia). Products include:

Dyazide Capsules 1405
Dyrenium Capsules 3189

Trifluoperazine Hydrochloride (Phenothiazines tend to produce hyperglycemia and may lead to loss of glycemic control. When administered to a patient receiving an oral blood glucose-lowering agent, the patient should be observed for loss of glycemic control. When a phenothiazine is withdrawn from a patient receiving an oral blood glucose-lowering agent, the patient should be observed closely for loss of hypoglycemia).

No products indexed under this heading.

Trimethoprim (Co-administration of 160 mg trimethroprim and a single dose of 0.25 mg repaglinide (after 2 days of twice-daily and one dose on the third day of trimethoprim 160 mg) resulted in a 61% and 41% increase in repaglinide AUC and Cmax, respectively. The increase in AUC was from 5.9 ng/mL*hr to 9.6 ng/mL*hr for AUC and the increase in Cmax was from 4.7 ng/mL to 6.6 ng/mL. These increases in repaglinide plasma levels may necessitate a repaglinide dose adjustment).

No products indexed under this heading.

Trimethoprim Hydrochloride (Co-administration of 160 mg trimethroprim and a single dose of 0.25 mg repaglinide (after 2 days of twice-daily and one dose on the third day of trimethoprim 160 mg) resulted in a 61% and 41% increase in repaglinide AUC and Cmax, respectively. The increase in AUC was from 5.9 ng/mL*hr to 9.6 ng/mL*hr for AUC and the increase in Cmax was from 4.7 ng/mL to 6.6 ng/mL. These increases in repaglinide plasma levels may necessitate a repaglinide dose adjustment).

No products indexed under this heading.

Trimethoprim Sulfate (Co-administration of 160 mg trimethroprim and a single dose of 0.25 mg repaglinide (after 2 days of twice-daily and one dose on the third day of trimethoprim 160 mg) resulted in a 61% and 41% increase in repaglinide AUC and Cmax, respectively. The increase in AUC was from 5.9 ng/mL*hr to 9.6 ng/mL*hr for AUC and the increase in Cmax was from 4.7 ng/mL to 6.6 ng/mL. These increases in repaglinide plasma levels may necessitate a repaglinide dose adjustment).

No products indexed under this heading.

Trimipramine Maleate (The hypoglycemic action of oral blood glucose-lowering agents may be potentiated by highly protein bounded drugs. When administered to a patient receiving an oral blood glucose-lowering agent, the patient should be observed closely for hypoglycemia. When a highly protein bound drug is withdrawn from a patient receiving an oral blood glucose-lowering agent, the patient should be observed closely for loss of glycemic control).

No products indexed under this heading.

Troglitazone (Repaglinide is metabolized by the cytochrome P4502C8 and 3A4 enzymes. Consequently, repaglinide metabolism may be altered by drugs that are CYP3A4 inducers. Caution should be used in patients concomitantly using repaglinide and a CYP3A4 inducer).

No products indexed under this heading.

Troleandomycin (Repaglinide is metabolized by the cytochrome P4502C8 and 3A4 enzymes. Consequently, repaglinide metabolism may be altered by drugs that are CYP3A4 inhibitors. Caution should be used in patients concomitantly using repaglinide and a CYP3A4 inhibitor. The effect may be very significant if both CYP3A4 and CYP2C8 are inhibited at the same time).

No products indexed under this heading.

Valdecoxib (The hypoglycemic action of oral blood glucose-lowering agents may be potentiated by nonsteroidal anti-inflammatory agents. When administered to a patient receiving an oral blood glucose-lowering agent, the patient should be observed closely for hypoglycemia. When a nonsteroidal anti-inflammatory agent is withdrawn from a patient receiving an oral blood glucose-lowering agent, the patient should be observed closely for loss of glycemic control).

No products indexed under this heading.

Valproate Sodium (Repaglinide is metabolized by the cytochrome P4502C8 and 3A4 enzymes. Consequently, repaglinide metabolism may be altered by drugs that are CYP3A4 inhibitors. Caution should be used in patients concomitantly using repaglinide and a CYP3A4 inhibitor. The effect may be very significant if both CYP3A4 and CYP2C8 are inhibited at the same time).

No products indexed under this heading.

Vardenafil Hydrochloride (Repaglinide is metabolized by the cytochrome P4502C8 and 3A4 enzymes. Consequently, repaglinide metabolism may be altered by drugs that are CYP3A4 inhibitors. Caution should be used in patients concomitantly using repaglinide and a CYP3A4 inhibitor. The effect may be very significant if both CYP3A4 and CYP2C8 are inhibited at the same time). Products include:

Levitra Tablets 2876

Verapamil Hydrochloride (Repaglinide is metabolized by the cytochrome P4502C8 and 3A4 enzymes. Consequently, repaglinide metabolism may be altered by drugs that are CYP3A4 inhibitors. Caution should be used in patients concomitantly using repaglinide and a CYP3A4 inhibitor. The effect may be very significant if both CYP3A4 and CYP2C8 are inhibited at the same time). Products include:

Tarka Tablets 511

Voriconazole (Repaglinide is metabolized by the cytochrome P4502C8 and 3A4 enzymes. Consequently, repaglinide metabolism may be altered by drugs that are CYP3A4 inhibitors. Caution should be used in patients concomitantly using repaglinide and a CYP3A4 inhibitor. The effect may be very significant if both CYP3A4 and CYP2C8 are inhibited at the same time).

No products indexed under this heading.

Warfarin Sodium (The hypoglycemic action of oral blood glucose-lowering agents may be potentiated by highly protein bounded drugs. When administered to a patient receiving an oral blood glucose-lowering agent, the patient should be observed closely for hypoglycemia. When a highly protein bound drug is withdrawn from a patient receiving an oral blood glucose-lowering agent, the patient should be observed closely for loss of glycemic control).

No products indexed under this heading.

Zafirlukast (Repaglinide is metabolized by the cytochrome P4502C8 and 3A4 enzymes. Consequently, repaglinide metabolism may be altered by drugs that are CYP3A4 inhibitors. Caution should be used in patients concomitantly using repaglinide and a CYP3A4 inhibitor. The effect may be very significant if both CYP3A4 and CYP2C8 are inhibited at the same time). Products include:

Accolate Tablets 669

Zileuton (Repaglinide is metabolized by the cytochrome P4502C8 and 3A4 enzymes. Consequently, repaglinide metabolism may be altered by drugs that are CYP3A4 inhibitors. Caution should be used in patients concomitantly using repaglinide and a CYP3A4 inhibitor. The effect may be very significant if both CYP3A4 and CYP2C8 are inhibited at the same time).

No products indexed under this heading.

Food Interactions

Grapefruit (Repaglinide is metabolized by the cytochrome P4502C8 and 3A4 enzymes. Consequently, repaglinide metabolism may be altered by drugs that are CYP3A4 inhibitors. Caution should be used in patients concomitantly using repaglinide and a CYP3A4 inhibitor. The effect may be very significant if both CYP3A4 and CYP2C8 are inhibited at the same time).

Grapefruit Juice (Repaglinide is metabolized by the cytochrome P4502C8 and 3A4 enzymes. Consequently, repaglinide metabolism may be altered by drugs that are CYP3A4 inhibitors. Caution should be used in patients concomitantly using repaglinide and a CYP3A4 inhibitor. The effect may be very significant if both CYP3A4 and CYP2C8 are inhibited at the same time).

PRECOSE TABLETS

(Acarbose) 792

May interact with calcium channel blockers, corticosteroids, estrogens, oral contraceptives, phenothiazines, phenytoin, sympathomimetics, thiazides, thyroid preparations, and certain other agents. Compounds in these categories include:

Albuterol (Sympathomimetics tend to produce hyperglycemia leading to loss of control; patients on concurrent therapy should be closely observed for loss of control).

No products indexed under this heading.

Albuterol Sulfate (Sympathomimetics tend to produce hyperglycemia leading to loss of control; patients on concurrent therapy should be closely observed for loss of control). Products include:
- Combivent Inhalation Aerosol 845
- ProAir HFA Inhalation Aerosol 3113
- Proventil HFA Inhalation Aerosol 2914
- Ventolin HFA Inhalation Aerosol 1638

Amlodipine Besylate (Calcium channel blockers tend to produce hyperglycemia leading to loss of control; patients on concurrent therapy should be closely observed for loss of control). Products include:
- Azor Tablets 1005
- Exforge Tablets 2238

Amylase (Amylase, a carbohydrate splitting enzyme, may reduce the effect of acarbose and should not be taken concurrently).
No products indexed under this heading.

Bendroflumethiazide (Thiazide diuretics tend to produce hyperglycemia leading to loss of control; patients on concurrent therapy should be closely observed for loss of control).
No products indexed under this heading.

Bepridil Hydrochloride (Calcium channel blockers tend to produce hyperglycemia leading to loss of control; patients on concurrent therapy should be closely observed for loss of control).
No products indexed under this heading.

Betamethasone Acetate (Corticosteroids tend to produce hyperglycemia leading to loss of control; patients on concurrent therapy should be closely observed for loss of control).
No products indexed under this heading.

Betamethasone Sodium Phosphate (Corticosteroids tend to produce hyperglycemia leading to loss of control; patients on concurrent therapy should be closely observed for loss of control).
No products indexed under this heading.

Budesonide (Corticosteroids tend to produce hyperglycemia leading to loss of control; patients on concurrent therapy should be closely observed for loss of control). Products include:
- Pulmicort Flexhaler 654
- Symbicort 80/4.5 Inhalation Aerosol.. 659
- Symbicort 160/4.5 Inhalation Aerosol.. 659

Charcoal, Activated (Charcoal, an intestinal adsorbent, may reduce the effect of acarbose and should not be taken concurrently).
No products indexed under this heading.

Chlorothiazide (Thiazide diuretics tend to produce hyperglycemia leading to loss of control; patients on concurrent therapy should be closely observed for loss of control).
No products indexed under this heading.

Chlorothiazide Sodium (Thiazide diuretics tend to produce hyperglycemia leading to loss of control; patients on concurrent therapy should be closely observed for loss of control). Products include:
- Intravenous Sodium Diuril 2490

Chlorotrianisene (Estrogens tend to produce hyperglycemia leading to loss of control; patients on concurrent therapy should be closely observed for loss of control).
No products indexed under this heading.

Chlorpromazine (Phenothiazines tend to produce hyperglycemia leading to loss of control; patients on concurrent therapy should be closely observed for loss of control).
No products indexed under this heading.

Chlorpromazine Hydrochloride (Phenothiazines tend to produce hyperglycemia leading to loss of control; patients on concurrent therapy should be closely observed for loss of control).
No products indexed under this heading.

Ciclesonide (Corticosteroids tend to produce hyperglycemia leading to loss of control; patients on concurrent therapy should be closely observed for loss of control). Products include:
- Alvesco Inhalation Aerosol 2985
- Omnaris Nasal Spray 2998

Cortisone Acetate (Corticosteroids tend to produce hyperglycemia leading to loss of control; patients on concurrent therapy should be closely observed for loss of control).
No products indexed under this heading.

Desogestrel (Oral contraceptives tend to produce hyperglycemia leading to loss of control; patients on concurrent therapy should be closely observed for loss of control). Products include:
- Mircette Tablets 1034

Dexamethasone (Corticosteroids tend to produce hyperglycemia leading to loss of control; patients on concurrent therapy should be closely observed for loss of control). Products include:
- Ciprodex Otic Suspension 541

Dexamethasone Acetate (Corticosteroids tend to produce hyperglycemia leading to loss of control; patients on concurrent therapy should be closely observed for loss of control).
No products indexed under this heading.

Dexamethasone Sodium Phosphate (Corticosteroids tend to produce hyperglycemia leading to loss of control; patients on concurrent therapy should be closely observed for loss of control).
No products indexed under this heading.

Dienestrol (Estrogens tend to produce hyperglycemia leading to loss of control; patients on concurrent therapy should be closely observed for loss of control).
No products indexed under this heading.

Diethylstilbestrol (Estrogens tend to produce hyperglycemia leading to loss of control; patients on concurrent therapy should be closely observed for loss of control).
No products indexed under this heading.

Digoxin (Precose has been shown to change the bioavailability of digoxin when they are co-administered, which may require digoxin dose adjustment). Products include:
- Lanoxin Injection 1498
- Lanoxin Injection Pediatric 1502
- Lanoxin Tablets 1505

Diltiazem Hydrochloride (Calcium channel blockers tend to produce hyperglycemia leading to loss of control; patients on concurrent therapy should be closely observed for loss of control). Products include:
- Cardizem LA Extended Release Tablets.. 421

Dobutamine Hydrochloride (Sympathomimetics tend to produce hyperglycemia leading to loss of control; patients on concurrent therapy should be closely observed for loss of control).
No products indexed under this heading.

Dopamine Hydrochloride (Sympathomimetics tend to produce hyperglycemia leading to loss of control; patients on concurrent therapy should be closely observed for loss of control).
No products indexed under this heading.

Ephedrine Hydrochloride (Sympathomimetics tend to produce hyperglycemia leading to loss of control; patients on concurrent therapy should be closely observed for loss of control).
No products indexed under this heading.

Ephedrine Sulfate (Sympathomimetics tend to produce hyperglycemia leading to loss of control; patients on concurrent therapy should be closely observed for loss of control).
No products indexed under this heading.

Ephedrine Tannate (Sympathomimetics tend to produce hyperglycemia leading to loss of control; patients on concurrent therapy should be closely observed for loss of control).
No products indexed under this heading.

Epinephrine (Sympathomimetics tend to produce hyperglycemia leading to loss of control; patients on concurrent therapy should be closely observed for loss of control). Products include:
- EpiPen 1024

Epinephrine Bitartrate (Sympathomimetics tend to produce hyperglycemia leading to loss of control; patients on concurrent therapy should be closely observed for loss of control).
No products indexed under this heading.

Epinephrine Hydrochloride (Sympathomimetics tend to produce hyperglycemia leading to loss of control; patients on concurrent therapy should be closely observed for loss of control).
No products indexed under this heading.

Estradiol (Estrogens tend to produce hyperglycemia leading to loss of control; patients on concurrent therapy should be closely observed for loss of control). Products include:
- Activella Tablets 2347
- Angeliq Tablets 751
- Climara Transdermal System 763
- Climara Pro Transdermal System 768
- Divigel 3167
- Vagifem Tablets 2375

Estrogens, Conjugated (Estrogens tend to produce hyperglycemia leading to loss of control; patients on concurrent therapy should be closely observed for loss of control). Products include:
- Premarin Intravenous 3217
- Premarin Tablets 3221
- Premarin Vaginal Cream 3228
- Premphase Tablets 3232
- Prempro Tablets 3232

Estrogens, Esterified (Estrogens tend to produce hyperglycemia leading to loss of control; patients on concurrent therapy should be closely observed for loss of control). Products include:
- Estratest Tablets 3043
- Estratest H.S. Tablets 3043

Estropipate (Estrogens tend to produce hyperglycemia leading to loss of control; patients on concurrent therapy should be closely observed for loss of control).
No products indexed under this heading.

Ethinyl Estradiol (Estrogens tend to produce hyperglycemia leading to loss of control; patients on concurrent therapy should be closely observed for loss of control). Products include:
- Lybrel Tablets 3204
- Mircette Tablets 1034
- NuvaRing 2897
- Ortho-Cyclen/Ortho Tri-Cyclen 2449
- Ortho Evra Transdermal System 2437
- Ortho Tri-Cyclen Lo Tablets 2458
- Seasonique Tablets 1046
- Yaz Tablets 805

Ethynodiol Diacetate (Oral contraceptives tend to produce hyperglycemia leading to loss of control; patients on concurrent therapy should be closely observed for loss of control).
No products indexed under this heading.

Felodipine (Calcium channel blockers tend to produce hyperglycemia leading to loss of control; patients on concurrent therapy should be closely observed for loss of control).
No products indexed under this heading.

Fludrocortisone Acetate (Corticosteroids tend to produce hyperglycemia leading to loss of control; patients on concurrent therapy should be closely observed for loss of control).
No products indexed under this heading.

Flunisolide (Corticosteroids tend to produce hyperglycemia leading to loss of control; patients on concurrent therapy should be closely observed for loss of control). Products include:
- Aerobid/Aerobid-M 1153

Fluphenazine Decanoate (Phenothiazines tend to produce hyperglycemia leading to loss of control; patients on concurrent therapy should be closely observed for loss of control).
No products indexed under this heading.

Fluphenazine Enanthate (Phenothiazines tend to produce hyperglycemia leading to loss of control; patients on concurrent therapy should be closely observed for loss of control).
No products indexed under this heading.

Fluphenazine Hydrochloride (Phenothiazines tend to produce hyperglycemia leading to loss of control; patients on concurrent therapy should be closely observed for loss of control).
No products indexed under this heading.

Fluticasone Propionate (Corticosteroids tend to produce hyperglycemia leading to loss of control; patients on concurrent therapy should be closely observed for loss of control). Products include:
Advair Diskus 100/50 1276
Advair Diskus 250/50 1276
Advair Diskus 500/50 1276
Advair HFA 45/21 Inhalation Aerosol.. 1288
Advair HFA 115/21 Inhalation Aerosol.. 1288
Advair HFA 230/21 Inhalation Aerosol.. 1288
Flonase Nasal Spray 1431
Flovent Diskus 50 mcg 1435

Fluticasone Propionate HFA (Corticosteroids tend to produce hyperglycemia leading to loss of control; patients on concurrent therapy should be closely observed for loss of control). Products include:
Flovent HFA 1440

Fosphenytoin Sodium (Phenytoin tends to produce hyperglycemia leading to loss of control; patients on concurrent therapy should be closely observed for loss of control).
No products indexed under this heading.

Hydrochlorothiazide (Thiazide diuretics tend to produce hyperglycemia leading to loss of control; patients on concurrent therapy should be closely observed for loss of control). Products include:
Atacand HCT 642
Avalide Tablets 892
Avalide Tablets 2713
Benicar HCT Tablets 1010
Diovan HCT Tablets 2216
Dyazide Capsules 1405
Micardis HCT Tablets 854
Prinzide Tablets 2092
Tekturna HCT Tablets 2324
Teveten HCT Tablets 517

Hydrocortisone (Corticosteroids tend to produce hyperglycemia leading to loss of control; patients on concurrent therapy should be closely observed for loss of control).
No products indexed under this heading.

Hydrocortisone Acetate (Corticosteroids tend to produce hyperglycemia leading to loss of control; patients on concurrent therapy should be closely observed for loss of control). Products include:
Analpram-HC 1140
Pramosone 1141

Hydrocortisone Sodium Phosphate (Corticosteroids tend to produce hyperglycemia leading to loss of control; patients on concurrent therapy should be closely observed for loss of control).
No products indexed under this heading.

Hydrocortisone Sodium Succinate (Corticosteroids tend to produce hyperglycemia leading to loss of control; patients on concurrent therapy should be closely observed for loss of control).
No products indexed under this heading.

Hydroflumethiazide (Thiazide diuretics tend to produce hyperglycemia leading to loss of control; patients on concurrent therapy should be closely observed for loss of control).
No products indexed under this heading.

Isoniazid (Isoniazid tends to produce hyperglycemia leading to loss of control; patients on concurrent therapy should be closely observed for loss of control).
No products indexed under this heading.

Isoproterenol Hydrochloride (Sympathomimetics tend to produce hyperglycemia leading to loss of control; patients on concurrent therapy should be closely observed for loss of control).
No products indexed under this heading.

Isoproterenol Sulfate (Sympathomimetics tend to produce hyperglycemia leading to loss of control; patients on concurrent therapy should be closely observed for loss of control).
No products indexed under this heading.

Isradipine (Calcium channel blockers tend to produce hyperglycemia leading to loss of control; patients on concurrent therapy should be closely observed for loss of control). Products include:
DynaCirc CR Controlled Release Tablets.. 1407

Levalbuterol Hydrochloride (Sympathomimetics tend to produce hyperglycemia leading to loss of control; patients on concurrent therapy should be closely observed for loss of control). Products include:
Xopenex Inhalation Solution 3001
Xopenex Inhalation Solution Concentrate 3005

Levonorgestrel (Oral contraceptives tend to produce hyperglycemia leading to loss of control; patients on concurrent therapy should be closely observed for loss of control). Products include:
Climara Pro Transdermal System 768
Lybrel Tablets 3204
Mirena Intrauterine System 779
Plan B Tablets 1044
Seasonique Tablets 1046

Levothyroxine Sodium (Thyroid products tend to produce hyperglycemia leading to loss of control; patients on concurrent therapy should be closely observed for loss of control). Products include:
Levothroid Tablets 1170
Levoxyl Tablets 1780
Synthroid Tablets 507

Liothyronine Sodium (Thyroid products tend to produce hyperglycemia leading to loss of control; patients on concurrent therapy should be closely observed for loss of control). Products include:
Cytomel Tablets 1778

Liotrix (Thyroid products tend to produce hyperglycemia leading to loss of control; patients on concurrent therapy should be closely observed for loss of control).
No products indexed under this heading.

Mesoridazine Besylate (Phenothiazines tend to produce hyperglycemia leading to loss of control; patients on concurrent therapy should be closely observed for loss of control).
No products indexed under this heading.

Mestranol (Oral contraceptives tend to produce hyperglycemia leading to loss of control; patients on concurrent therapy should be closely observed for loss of control).
No products indexed under this heading.

Metaproterenol Sulfate (Sympathomimetics tend to produce hyperglycemia leading to loss of control; patients on concurrent therapy should be closely observed for loss of control).
No products indexed under this heading.

Metaraminol Bitartrate (Sympathomimetics tend to produce hyperglycemia leading to loss of control; patients on concurrent therapy should be closely observed for loss of control).
No products indexed under this heading.

Methotrimeprazine (Phenothiazines tend to produce hyperglycemia leading to loss of control; patients on concurrent therapy should be closely observed for loss of control).
No products indexed under this heading.

Methoxamine Hydrochloride (Sympathomimetics tend to produce hyperglycemia leading to loss of control; patients on concurrent therapy should be closely observed for loss of control).
No products indexed under this heading.

Methyclothiazide (Thiazide diuretics tend to produce hyperglycemia leading to loss of control; patients on concurrent therapy should be closely observed for loss of control).
No products indexed under this heading.

Methylprednisolone Acetate (Corticosteroids tend to produce hyperglycemia leading to loss of control; patients on concurrent therapy should be closely observed for loss of control).
No products indexed under this heading.

Methylprednisolone Sodium Succinate (Corticosteroids tend to produce hyperglycemia leading to loss of control; patients on concurrent therapy should be closely observed for loss of control).
No products indexed under this heading.

Mibefradil Dihydrochloride (Calcium channel blockers tend to produce hyperglycemia leading to loss of control; patients on concurrent therapy should be closely observed for loss of control).
No products indexed under this heading.

Mometasone Furoate (Corticosteroids tend to produce hyperglycemia leading to loss of control; patients on concurrent therapy should be closely observed for loss of control). Products include:
Asmanex Twisthaler 2797
Elocon Cream 0.1% 2840
Elocon Lotion 0.1% 2841
Elocon Ointment 0.1% 2842

Mometasone Furoate Monohydrate (Corticosteroids tend to produce hyperglycemia leading to loss of control; patients on concurrent therapy should be closely observed for loss of control). Products include:
Nasonex Nasal Spray 2883

Nicardipine Hydrochloride (Calcium channel blockers tend to produce hyperglycemia leading to loss of control; patients on concurrent therapy should be closely observed for loss of control). Products include:
Cardene I.V. 1093

Nicotinic Acid (Nicotinic acid tends to produce hyperglycemia leading to loss of control; patients on concurrent therapy should be closely observed for loss of control).
No products indexed under this heading.

Nifedipine (Calcium channel blockers tend to produce hyperglycemia leading to loss of control; patients on concurrent therapy should be closely observed for loss of control).
No products indexed under this heading.

Nimodipine (Calcium channel blockers tend to produce hyperglycemia leading to loss of control; patients on concurrent therapy should be closely observed for loss of control). Products include:
Nimotop Capsules 790

Nisoldipine (Calcium channel blockers tend to produce hyperglycemia leading to loss of control; patients on concurrent therapy should be closely observed for loss of control). Products include:
Sular Extended Release Tablets 2975

Norepinephrine Bitartrate (Sympathomimetics tend to produce hyperglycemia leading to loss of control; patients on concurrent therapy should be closely observed for loss of control).
No products indexed under this heading.

Norethindrone (Oral contraceptives tend to produce hyperglycemia leading to loss of control; patients on concurrent therapy should be closely observed for loss of control). Products include:
Ortho Micronor Tablets 2446

Norethynodrel (Oral contraceptives tend to produce hyperglycemia leading to loss of control; patients on concurrent therapy should be closely observed for loss of control).
No products indexed under this heading.

Norgestimate (Oral contraceptives tend to produce hyperglycemia leading to loss of control; patients on concurrent therapy should be closely observed for loss of control). Products include:
Ortho-Cyclen/Ortho Tri-Cyclen 2449
Ortho Tri-Cyclen Lo Tablets 2458

Norgestrel (Oral contraceptives tend to produce hyperglycemia leading to loss of control; patients on concurrent therapy should be closely observed for loss of control).
No products indexed under this heading.

Pancreatin (Pancreatin, a carbohydrate splitting enzyme, may reduce the effect of acarbose and should not be taken concurrently). Products include:
Medizym Tablets 1894

Perphenazine (Phenothiazines tend to produce hyperglycemia leading to loss of control; patients on concurrent therapy should be closely observed for loss of control).
No products indexed under this heading.

Phenylephrine Bitartrate (Sympathomimetics tend to produce hyperglycemia leading to loss of control; patients on concurrent therapy should be closely observed for loss of control).
No products indexed under this heading.

Phenylephrine Hydrochloride (Sympathomimetics tend to produce hyperglycemia leading to loss of control; patients on concurrent therapy should be closely observed for loss of control). Products include:
- Actifed Cold & Allergy Tablets 1895
- Benadryl Allergy & Cold Kapgels 1895
- Benadryl Allergy & Sinus Headache Kapgels 1895
- Benadryl Severe Allergy & Sinus Headache Caplets 1897
- Children's Benadryl-D Allergy & Sinus Liquid 1896
- Benadryl-D Allergy & Sinus Tablet 1896
- PediaCare Children's Allergy & Cold Liquid 1902
- PediaCare Children's Decongestant Liquid 1902
- PediaCare Children's Liquid Multi-Symptom Cold 1902
- Sinutab Non-Drying Caplets 1905
- Sinutab Sinus Caplets 1905
- Children's Sudafed PE Cold & Cough Liquid 1907
- Children's Sudafed PE Nasal Decongestant Liquid 1906
- Sudafed PE Cold & Cough Caplets.. 1907
- Sudafed PE Nasal Decongestant Tablets 1907
- Sudafed PE Nighttime Cold Caplets.. 1907
- Sudafed PE Non-Drying Sinus Caplets.. 1908
- Sudafed PE Severe Cold Caplets 1908
- Sudafed PE Sinus & Allergy Tablets 1908
- Sudafed PE Sinus Headache Caplets.. 1908
- Tylenol Allergy Multi-Symptom Caplets with Cool Burst and Rapid Release Gelcaps................ 1916
- Tylenol Allergy Multi-Symptom Nighttime Caplets with Cool Burst.. 1916
- Children's Tylenol Plus Cold Suspension Liquid 1912
- Children's Tylenol Plus Cold & Allergy Suspension Liquid............ 1914
- Children's Tylenol Plus Flu Suspension Liquid 1914
- Children's Tylenol Plus Multi-Symptom Cold Suspension Liquid 1912
- Tylenol Cold Head Congestion Daytime Caplets with Cool Burst.. 1910
- Tylenol Cold Head Congestion Nighttime Caplets with Cool Burst.. 1910
- Tylenol Cold Head Congestion Severe Daytime Caplets with Cool Burst.................................. 1910
- Tylenol Cold Multi-Symptom Daytime Caplets with Cool Burst and Rapid Release Gels....... 1913
- Tylenol Cold Multi-Symptom Daytime Liquid with Citrus Burst... 1913
- Tylenol Cold Multi-Symptom Nighttime Caplets with Cool Burst.. 1913
- Tylenol Cold Multi-Symptom Nighttime Liquid with Cool Burst... 1913
- Tylenol Cold Multi-Symptom Severe Caplets with Cool Burst..... 1913
- Tylenol Cold Multi-Symptom Severe Daytime Liquid with Citrus Burst.................................. 1913
- Tylenol Sinus Congestion & Pain Daytime Caplets with Cool Burst and Gelcaps....................... 1917
- Tylenol Sinus Congestion & Pain Nighttime Caplets with Cool Burst.. 1917
- Tylenol Sinus Congestion & Pain Severe Caplets with Cool Burst..... 1917
- Vicks DayQuil Cold & Flu Multi-Symptom Relief.................. ■616
- Vicks DayQuil LiquiCaps 2567
- Vicks DayQuil Liquid 2567
- Vicks DayQuil Multi-Symptom Cold/Flu Relief............................ 2567

Phenylephrine Tannate (Sympathomimetics tend to produce hyperglycemia leading to loss of control; patients on concurrent therapy should be closely observed for loss of control).
No products indexed under this heading.

Phenylpropanolamine Hydrochloride (Sympathomimetics tend to produce hyperglycemia leading to loss of control; patients on concurrent therapy should be closely observed for loss of control).
No products indexed under this heading.

Phenytoin (Phenytoin tends to produce hyperglycemia leading to loss of control; patients on concurrent therapy should be closely observed for loss of control).
No products indexed under this heading.

Phenytoin Sodium (Phenytoin tends to produce hyperglycemia leading to loss of control; patients on concurrent therapy should be closely observed for loss of control). Products include:
- Phenytek Capsules 2192

Pirbuterol Acetate (Sympathomimetics tend to produce hyperglycemia leading to loss of control; patients on concurrent therapy should be closely observed for loss of control). Products include:
- Maxair Autohaler 1705

Polyestradiol Phosphate (Estrogens tend to produce hyperglycemia leading to loss of control; patients on concurrent therapy should be closely observed for loss of control).
No products indexed under this heading.

Polythiazide (Thiazide diuretics tend to produce hyperglycemia leading to loss of control; patients on concurrent therapy should be closely observed for loss of control).
No products indexed under this heading.

Prednisolone Acetate (Corticosteroids tend to produce hyperglycemia leading to loss of control; patients on concurrent therapy should be closely observed for loss of control). Products include:
- Pred Forte Ophthalmic Suspension .... ⊙227
- Pred Mild Ophthalmic Suspension .... ⊙230
- Pred-G Ophthalmic Ointment .... ⊙229
- Pred-G Ophthalmic Suspension ...... ⊙228

Prednisolone Sodium Phosphate (Corticosteroids tend to produce hyperglycemia leading to loss of control; patients on concurrent therapy should be closely observed for loss of control).
No products indexed under this heading.

Prednisolone Tebutate (Corticosteroids tend to produce hyperglycemia leading to loss of control; patients on concurrent therapy should be closely observed for loss of control).
No products indexed under this heading.

Prednisone (Corticosteroids tend to produce hyperglycemia leading to loss of control; patients on concurrent therapy should be closely observed for loss of control).
No products indexed under this heading.

Prochlorperazine (Phenothiazines tend to produce hyperglycemia leading to loss of control; patients on concurrent therapy should be closely observed for loss of control).
No products indexed under this heading.

Promethazine Hydrochloride (Phenothiazines tend to produce hyperglycemia leading to loss of control; patients on concurrent therapy should be closely observed for loss of control).
No products indexed under this heading.

Pseudoephedrine Hydrochloride (Sympathomimetics tend to produce hyperglycemia leading to loss of control; patients on concurrent therapy should be closely observed for loss of control). Products include:
- Allegra-D 12 Hour Extended-Release Tablets............ 2687
- Allegra-D 24 Hour Extended-Release Tablets............ 2690
- Children's Motrin Cold Oral Suspension 1899
- Sudafed 12 Hour Nasal Decongestant Non-Drowsy Caplets.. 1909
- Sudafed 24 Hour Non-Drowsy Nasal Decongestant Tablets......... 1906
- Children's Sudafed Nasal Decongestant Liquid..................... 1906
- Sudafed Nasal Decongestant Tablets 1906
- Tylenol Cold Severe Congestion Daytime Caplets with Cool Burst.. 1912
- Tylenol Sinus Severe Congestion Caplets with Cool Burst.............. 1917
- Vicks NyQuil LiquiCaps 2567
- Vicks NyQuil Liquid 2567
- Vicks NyQuil Multi-Symptom Cold/Flu Relief............................ 2567
- Zyrtec-D 12 Hour Extended Release Tablets............................ 1923
- Zyrtec-D Allergy & Congestion Extended-Release Tablets............ 1923

Pseudoephedrine Sulfate (Sympathomimetics tend to produce hyperglycemia leading to loss of control; patients on concurrent therapy should be closely observed for loss of control). Products include:
- Clarinex-D 12-Hour Extended-Release Tablets............ 2831
- Clarinex-D 24-Hour Extended-Release Tablets............ 2834

Quinestrol (Estrogens tend to produce hyperglycemia leading to loss of control; patients on concurrent therapy should be closely observed for loss of control).
No products indexed under this heading.

Salmeterol Xinafoate (Sympathomimetics tend to produce hyperglycemia leading to loss of control; patients on concurrent therapy should be closely observed for loss of control). Products include:
- Advair Diskus 100/50 1276
- Advair Diskus 250/50 1276
- Advair Diskus 500/50 1276
- Advair HFA 45/21 Inhalation Aerosol.. 1288
- Advair HFA 115/21 Inhalation Aerosol.. 1288
- Advair HFA 230/21 Inhalation Aerosol.. 1288
- Serevent Diskus 1594

Terbutaline Sulfate (Sympathomimetics tend to produce hyperglycemia leading to loss of control; patients on concurrent therapy should be closely observed for loss of control).
No products indexed under this heading.

Thioridazine Hydrochloride (Phenothiazines tend to produce hyperglycemia leading to loss of control; patients on concurrent therapy should be closely observed for loss of control). Products include:
- Thioridazine Hydrochloride Tablets 2195

Thyroglobulin (Thyroid products tend to produce hyperglycemia leading to loss of control; patients on concurrent therapy should be closely observed for loss of control).
No products indexed under this heading.

Thyroid (Thyroid products tend to produce hyperglycemia leading to loss of control; patients on concurrent therapy should be closely observed for loss of control). Products include:
- Naturethroid Tablets 2605

Thyroxine (Thyroid products tend to produce hyperglycemia leading to loss of control; patients on concurrent therapy should be closely observed for loss of control).
No products indexed under this heading.

Thyroxine Sodium (Thyroid products tend to produce hyperglycemia leading to loss of control; patients on concurrent therapy should be closely observed for loss of control).
No products indexed under this heading.

Triamcinolone (Corticosteroids tend to produce hyperglycemia leading to loss of control; patients on concurrent therapy should be closely observed for loss of control).
No products indexed under this heading.

Triamcinolone Acetonide (Corticosteroids tend to produce hyperglycemia leading to loss of control; patients on concurrent therapy should be closely observed for loss of control). Products include:
- Azmacort Inhalation Aerosol 407
- Nasacort AQ Nasal Spray 2765
- Triesence Injectable Suspension .... ⊙209

Triamcinolone Diacetate (Corticosteroids tend to produce hyperglycemia leading to loss of control; patients on concurrent therapy should be closely observed for loss of control).
No products indexed under this heading.

Triamcinolone Hexacetonide (Corticosteroids tend to produce hyperglycemia leading to loss of control; patients on concurrent therapy should be closely observed for loss of control).
No products indexed under this heading.

Trifluoperazine Hydrochloride (Phenothiazines tend to produce hyperglycemia leading to loss of control; patients on concurrent therapy should be closely observed for loss of control).
No products indexed under this heading.

Verapamil Hydrochloride (Calcium channel blockers tend to produce hyperglycemia leading to loss of control; patients on concurrent therapy should be closely observed for loss of control). Products include:
Tarka Tablets 511

PRED FORTE OPHTHALMIC SUSPENSION

(Prednisolone Acetate) .... ⊙227
None cited in PDR database.

PRED MILD OPHTHALMIC SUSPENSION

(Prednisolone Acetate) .... ⊙230
None cited in PDR database.

PRED-G OPHTHALMIC OINTMENT

(Gentamicin Sulfate, Prednisolone Acetate).. ⊙229
None cited in PDR database.

PRED-G OPHTHALMIC SUSPENSION

(Gentamicin Sulfate, Prednisolone Acetate).. ⊙228
None cited in PDR database.

PREMARIN INTRAVENOUS

(Estrogens, Conjugated) 3217
See Premarin Tablets

PREMARIN TABLETS

(Estrogens, Conjugated) 3221
May interact with cytochrome p450 3a4 inducers (selected), cytochrome p450 3a4 inhibitors (selected), and certain other agents. Compounds in these categories include:

Acetazolamide (Co-administration of inhibitors of CYP3A4 with estrogens may affect estrogen drug metabolism. Inhibitors of CYP3A4 may increase plasma concentrations of estrogens and may result in side effects).
No products indexed under this heading.

Allium sativum (Co-administration of inducers of CYP3A4 with estrogens may affect estrogen drug metabolism. Inducers of CYP3A4 may reduce plasma concentrations of estrogens, possibly resulting in a decrease in therapeutic effects and/or changes in the uterine bleeding profile).
No products indexed under this heading.

Amiodarone Hydrochloride (Co-administration of inhibitors of CYP3A4 with estrogens may affect estrogen drug metabolism. Inhibitors of CYP3A4 may increase plasma concentrations of estrogens and may result in side effects).
No products indexed under this heading.

Amprenavir (Co-administration of inhibitors of CYP3A4 with estrogens may affect estrogen drug metabolism. Inhibitors of CYP3A4 may increase plasma concentrations of estrogens and may result in side effects).
No products indexed under this heading.

Anastrozole (Co-administration of inhibitors of CYP3A4 with estrogens may affect estrogen drug metabolism. Inhibitors of CYP3A4 may increase plasma concentrations of estrogens and may result in side effects). Products include:
Arimidex Tablets 672

Aprepitant (Co-administration of inducers of CYP3A4 with estrogens may affect estrogen drug metabolism. Inducers of CYP3A4 may reduce plasma concentrations of estrogens, possibly resulting in a decrease in therapeutic effects and/or changes in the uterine bleeding profile). Products include:
Emend Capsules 1992

Atazanavir (Co-administration of inhibitors of CYP3A4 with estrogens may affect estrogen drug metabolism. Inhibitors of CYP3A4 may increase plasma concentrations of estrogens and may result in side effects).
No products indexed under this heading.

Atazanavir Sulfate (Co-administration of inhibitors of CYP3A4 with estrogens may affect estrogen drug metabolism. Inhibitors of CYP3A4 may increase plasma concentrations of estrogens and may result in side effects). Products include:
Reyataz Capsules 3299

Betamethasone Acetate (Co-administration of inducers of CYP3A4 with estrogens may affect estrogen drug metabolism. Inducers of CYP3A4 may reduce plasma concentrations of estrogens, possibly resulting in a decrease in therapeutic effects and/or changes in the uterine bleeding profile).
No products indexed under this heading.

Betamethasone Sodium Phosphate (Co-administration of inducers of CYP3A4 with estrogens may affect estrogen drug metabolism. Inducers of CYP3A4 may reduce plasma concentrations of estrogens, possibly resulting in a decrease in therapeutic effects and/or changes in the uterine bleeding profile).
No products indexed under this heading.

Carbamazepine (Co-administration of inducers of CYP3A4 with estrogens may affect estrogen drug metabolism. Inducers of CYP3A4 may reduce plasma concentrations of estrogens, possibly resulting in a decrease in therapeutic effects and/or changes in the uterine bleeding profile). Products include:
Carbatrol Capsules 3019
Equetro Extended-Release Capsules................................... 3174

Cimetidine (Co-administration of inhibitors of CYP3A4 with estrogens may affect estrogen drug metabolism. Inhibitors of CYP3A4 may increase plasma concentrations of estrogens and may result in side effects).
No products indexed under this heading.

Cimetidine Hydrochloride (Co-administration of inhibitors of CYP3A4 with estrogens may affect estrogen drug metabolism. Inhibitors of CYP3A4 may increase plasma concentrations of estrogens and may result in side effects).
No products indexed under this heading.

Ciprofloxacin (Co-administration of inhibitors of CYP3A4 with estrogens may affect estrogen drug metabolism. Inhibitors of CYP3A4 may increase plasma concentrations of estrogens and may result in side effects). Products include:
Cipro I.V. 2817
Cipro Oral Suspension 2810
Cipro XR Tablets 2823
Ciprodex Otic Suspension 541

Ciprofloxacin Hydrochloride (Co-administration of inducers of CYP3A4 with estrogens may affect estrogen drug metabolism. Inducers of CYP3A4 may reduce plasma concentrations of estrogens, possibly resulting in a decrease in therapeutic effects and/or changes in the uterine bleeding profile). Products include:
Cipro Tablets 2810

Cisplatin (Co-administration of inducers of CYP3A4 with estrogens may affect estrogen drug metabolism. Inducers of CYP3A4 may reduce plasma concentrations of estrogens, possibly resulting in a decrease in therapeutic effects and/or changes in the uterine bleeding profile).
No products indexed under this heading.

Clarithromycin (Co-administration of inhibitors of CYP3A4 with estrogens may affect estrogen drug metabolism. Inhibitors of CYP3A4 may increase plasma concentrations of estrogens and may result in side effects). Products include:
Biaxin/Biaxin XL 411

Clotrimazole (Co-administration of inhibitors of CYP3A4 with estrogens may affect estrogen drug metabolism. Inhibitors of CYP3A4 may increase plasma concentrations of estrogens and may result in side effects). Products include:
Lotrisone 2881

Cortisone Acetate (Co-administration of inducers of CYP3A4 with estrogens may affect estrogen drug metabolism. Inducers of CYP3A4 may reduce plasma concentrations of estrogens, possibly resulting in a decrease in therapeutic effects and/or changes in the uterine bleeding profile).
No products indexed under this heading.

Cyclosporine (Co-administration of inhibitors of CYP3A4 with estrogens may affect estrogen drug metabolism. Inhibitors of CYP3A4 may increase plasma concentrations of estrogens and may result in side effects). Products include:
Gengraf Capsules 435
Neoral Oral Solution 2280
Neoral Soft Gelatin Capsules 2280
Restasis Ophthalmic Emulsion 557
Sandimmune 2296

Dalfopristin (Co-administration of inhibitors of CYP3A4 with estrogens may affect estrogen drug metabolism. Inhibitors of CYP3A4 may increase plasma concentrations of estrogens and may result in side effects).
No products indexed under this heading.

Danazol (Co-administration of inhibitors of CYP3A4 with estrogens may affect estrogen drug metabolism. Inhibitors of CYP3A4 may increase plasma concentrations of estrogens and may result in side effects).
No products indexed under this heading.

Delavirdine Mesylate (Co-administration of inhibitors of CYP3A4 with estrogens may affect estrogen drug metabolism. Inhibitors of CYP3A4 may increase plasma concentrations of estrogens and may result in side effects).
No products indexed under this heading.

Dexamethasone (Co-administration of inducers of CYP3A4 with estrogens may affect estrogen drug metabolism. Inducers of CYP3A4 may reduce plasma concentrations of estrogens, possibly resulting in a decrease in therapeutic effects and/or changes in the uterine bleeding profile). Products include:
Ciprodex Otic Suspension 541

Dexamethasone Acetate (Co-administration of inducers of CYP3A4 with estrogens may affect estrogen drug metabolism. Inducers of CYP3A4 may reduce plasma concentrations of estrogens, possibly resulting in a decrease in therapeutic effects and/or changes in the uterine bleeding profile).
No products indexed under this heading.

Dexamethasone Sodium Phosphate (Co-administration of inducers of CYP3A4 with estrogens may affect estrogen drug metabolism. Inducers of CYP3A4 may reduce plasma concentrations of estrogens, possibly resulting in a decrease in therapeutic effects and/or changes in the uterine bleeding profile).
No products indexed under this heading.

Diltiazem Hydrochloride (Co-administration of inhibitors of CYP3A4 with estrogens may affect estrogen drug metabolism. Inhibitors of CYP3A4 may increase plasma concentrations of estrogens and may result in side effects). Products include:
Cardizem LA Extended Release Tablets.. 421

Diltiazem Maleate (Co-administration of inhibitors of CYP3A4 with estrogens may affect estrogen drug metabolism. Inhibitors of CYP3A4 may increase plasma concentrations of estrogens and may result in side effects).
No products indexed under this heading.

Doxorubicin Hydrochloride (Co-administration of inducers of CYP3A4 with estrogens may affect estrogen drug metabolism. Inducers of CYP3A4 may reduce plasma concentrations of estrogens, possibly resulting in a decrease in therapeutic effects and/or changes in the uterine bleeding profile).
No products indexed under this heading.

Efavirenz (Co-administration of inducers of CYP3A4 with estrogens may affect estrogen drug metabolism. Inducers of CYP3A4 may reduce plasma concentrations of estrogens, possibly resulting in a decrease in therapeutic effects and/ or changes in the uterine bleeding profile). Products include:

Atripla Tablets 938
Sustiva Capsules 930
Sustiva Tablets 930

Erythromycin (Co-administration of inhibitors of CYP3A4 with estrogens may affect estrogen drug metabolism. Inhibitors of CYP3A4 may increase plasma concentrations of estrogens and may result in side effects).
No products indexed under this heading.

Erythromycin Estolate (Co-administration of inhibitors of CYP3A4 with estrogens may affect estrogen drug metabolism. Inhibitors of CYP3A4 may increase plasma concentrations of estrogens and may result in side effects).
No products indexed under this heading.

Erythromycin Ethylsuccinate (Co-administration of inhibitors of CYP3A4 with estrogens may affect estrogen drug metabolism. Inhibitors of CYP3A4 may increase plasma concentrations of estrogens and may result in side effects). Products include:

E.E.S. 433
EryPed 431

Erythromycin Gluceptate (Co-administration of inhibitors of CYP3A4 with estrogens may affect estrogen drug metabolism. Inhibitors of CYP3A4 may increase plasma concentrations of estrogens and may result in side effects).
No products indexed under this heading.

Erythromycin Lactobionate (Co-administration of inhibitors of CYP3A4 with estrogens may affect estrogen drug metabolism. Inhibitors of CYP3A4 may increase plasma concentrations of estrogens and may result in side effects).
No products indexed under this heading.

Erythromycin Stearate (Co-administration of inhibitors of CYP3A4 with estrogens may affect estrogen drug metabolism. Inhibitors of CYP3A4 may increase plasma concentrations of estrogens and may result in side effects).
No products indexed under this heading.

Esomeprazole Magnesium (Co-administration of inhibitors of CYP3A4 with estrogens may affect estrogen drug metabolism. Inhibitors of CYP3A4 may increase plasma concentrations of estrogens and may result in side effects). Products include:

Nexium Delayed-Release Capsules 645
Nexium Delayed-Release Oral Suspension 645

Ethosuximide (Co-administration of inducers of CYP3A4 with estrogens may affect estrogen drug metabolism. Inducers of CYP3A4 may reduce plasma concentrations of estrogens, possibly resulting in a decrease in therapeutic effects and/ or changes in the uterine bleeding profile).
No products indexed under this heading.

Felbamate (Co-administration of inducers of CYP3A4 with estrogens may affect estrogen drug metabolism. Inducers of CYP3A4 may reduce plasma concentrations of estrogens, possibly resulting in a decrease in therapeutic effects and/ or changes in the uterine bleeding profile).
No products indexed under this heading.

Fluconazole (Co-administration of inhibitors of CYP3A4 with estrogens may affect estrogen drug metabolism. Inhibitors of CYP3A4 may increase plasma concentrations of estrogens and may result in side effects).
No products indexed under this heading.

Fludrocortisone Acetate (Co-administration of inducers of CYP3A4 with estrogens may affect estrogen drug metabolism. Inducers of CYP3A4 may reduce plasma concentrations of estrogens, possibly resulting in a decrease in therapeutic effects and/or changes in the uterine bleeding profile).
No products indexed under this heading.

Fluoxetine (Co-administration of inhibitors of CYP3A4 with estrogens may affect estrogen drug metabolism. Inhibitors of CYP3A4 may increase plasma concentrations of estrogens and may result in side effects).
No products indexed under this heading.

Fluoxetine Hydrochloride (Co-administration of inhibitors of CYP3A4 with estrogens may affect estrogen drug metabolism. Inhibitors of CYP3A4 may increase plasma concentrations of estrogens and may result in side effects). Products include:

Prozac Weekly Capsules 1852
Prozac Pulvules and Liquid 1852
Symbyax Capsules 1871

Fluvoxamine Maleate (Co-administration of inhibitors of CYP3A4 with estrogens may affect estrogen drug metabolism. Inhibitors of CYP3A4 may increase plasma concentrations of estrogens and may result in side effects). Products include:

Luvox CR Extended-Release Capsules 1759

Fosamprenavir Calcium (Co-administration of inhibitors of CYP3A4 with estrogens may affect estrogen drug metabolism. Inhibitors of CYP3A4 may increase plasma concentrations of estrogens and may result in side effects). Products include:

Lexiva Oral Suspension 1510
Lexiva Tablets 1510

Fosphenytoin Sodium (Co-administration of inducers of CYP3A4 with estrogens may affect estrogen drug metabolism. Inducers of CYP3A4 may reduce plasma concentrations of estrogens, possibly resulting in a decrease in therapeutic effects and/or changes in the uterine bleeding profile).
No products indexed under this heading.

Garlic Extract (Co-administration of inducers of CYP3A4 with estrogens may affect estrogen drug metabolism. Inducers of CYP3A4 may reduce plasma concentrations of estrogens, possibly resulting in a decrease in therapeutic effects and/ or changes in the uterine bleeding profile).
No products indexed under this heading.

Garlic Oil (Co-administration of inducers of CYP3A4 with estrogens may affect estrogen drug metabolism. Inducers of CYP3A4 may reduce plasma concentrations of estrogens, possibly resulting in a decrease in therapeutic effects and/ or changes in the uterine bleeding profile).
No products indexed under this heading.

Hydrocortisone (Co-administration of inducers of CYP3A4 with estrogens may affect estrogen drug metabolism. Inducers of CYP3A4 may reduce plasma concentrations of estrogens, possibly resulting in a decrease in therapeutic effects and/ or changes in the uterine bleeding profile).
No products indexed under this heading.

Hydrocortisone Acetate (Co-administration of inducers of CYP3A4 with estrogens may affect estrogen drug metabolism. Inducers of CYP3A4 may reduce plasma concentrations of estrogens, possibly resulting in a decrease in therapeutic effects and/or changes in the uterine bleeding profile). Products include:

Analpram-HC 1140
Pramosone 1141

Hydrocortisone Butyrate (Co-administration of inducers of CYP3A4 with estrogens may affect estrogen drug metabolism. Inducers of CYP3A4 may reduce plasma concentrations of estrogens, possibly resulting in a decrease in therapeutic effects and/or changes in the uterine bleeding profile).
No products indexed under this heading.

Hydrocortisone Cypionate (Co-administration of inducers of CYP3A4 with estrogens may affect estrogen drug metabolism. Inducers of CYP3A4 may reduce plasma concentrations of estrogens, possibly resulting in a decrease in therapeutic effects and/or changes in the uterine bleeding profile).
No products indexed under this heading.

Hydrocortisone Hemisuccinate (Co-administration of inducers of CYP3A4 with estrogens may affect estrogen drug metabolism. Inducers of CYP3A4 may reduce plasma concentrations of estrogens, possibly resulting in a decrease in therapeutic effects and/or changes in the uterine bleeding profile).
No products indexed under this heading.

Hydrocortisone Probutate (Co-administration of inducers of CYP3A4 with estrogens may affect estrogen drug metabolism. Inducers of CYP3A4 may reduce plasma concentrations of estrogens, possibly resulting in a decrease in therapeutic effects and/or changes in the uterine bleeding profile).
No products indexed under this heading.

Hydrocortisone Sodium Phosphate (Co-administration of inducers of CYP3A4 with estrogens may affect estrogen drug metabolism. Inducers of CYP3A4 may reduce plasma concentrations of estrogens, possibly resulting in a decrease in therapeutic effects and/or changes in the uterine bleeding profile).
No products indexed under this heading.

Hydrocortisone Sodium Succinate (Co-administration of inducers of CYP3A4 with estrogens may affect estrogen drug metabolism. Inducers of CYP3A4 may reduce plasma concentrations of estrogens, possibly resulting in a decrease in therapeutic effects and/or changes in the uterine bleeding profile).
No products indexed under this heading.

Hydrocortisone Valerate (Co-administration of inducers of CYP3A4 with estrogens may affect estrogen drug metabolism. Inducers of CYP3A4 may reduce plasma concentrations of estrogens, possibly resulting in a decrease in therapeutic effects and/or changes in the uterine bleeding profile).
No products indexed under this heading.

Hypericum (Co-administration of inducers of CYP3A4 with estrogens may affect estrogen drug metabolism. Inducers of CYP3A4 may reduce plasma concentrations of estrogens, possibly resulting in a decrease in therapeutic effects and/ or changes in the uterine bleeding profile). Products include:

Satieté Tablets .... ▣ 640

Hypericum Perforatum (Co-administration of inducers of CYP3A4 with estrogens may affect estrogen drug metabolism. Inducers of CYP3A4 may reduce plasma concentrations of estrogens, possibly resulting in a decrease in therapeutic effects and/or changes in the uterine bleeding profile).
No products indexed under this heading.

Indinavir Sulfate (Co-administration of inhibitors of CYP3A4 with estrogens may affect estrogen drug metabolism. Inhibitors of CYP3A4 may increase plasma concentrations of estrogens and may result in side effects). Products include:

Crixivan Capsules 1979

Isoniazid (Co-administration of inhibitors of CYP3A4 with estrogens may affect estrogen drug metabolism. Inhibitors of CYP3A4 may increase plasma concentrations of estrogens and may result in side effects).
No products indexed under this heading.

Itraconazole (Co-administration of inhibitors of CYP3A4 with estrogens may affect estrogen drug metabolism. Inhibitors of CYP3A4 may increase plasma concentrations of estrogens and may result in side effects).

No products indexed under this heading.

Ketoconazole (Co-administration of inhibitors of CYP3A4 with estrogens may affect estrogen drug metabolism. Inhibitors of CYP3A4 may increase plasma concentrations of estrogens and may result in side effects). Products include:

Extina Foam, 2% **3057**
Nizoral A-D Shampoo **1901**

Lopinavir (Co-administration of inhibitors of CYP3A4 with estrogens may affect estrogen drug metabolism. Inhibitors of CYP3A4 may increase plasma concentrations of estrogens and may result in side effects). Products include:

Kaletra **452**

Loratadine (Co-administration of inhibitors of CYP3A4 with estrogens may affect estrogen drug metabolism. Inhibitors of CYP3A4 may increase plasma concentrations of estrogens and may result in side effects).

No products indexed under this heading.

Mephenytoin (Co-administration of inducers of CYP3A4 with estrogens may affect estrogen drug metabolism. Inducers of CYP3A4 may reduce plasma concentrations of estrogens, possibly resulting in a decrease in therapeutic effects and/or changes in the uterine bleeding profile).

No products indexed under this heading.

Methsuximide (Co-administration of inducers of CYP3A4 with estrogens may affect estrogen drug metabolism. Inducers of CYP3A4 may reduce plasma concentrations of estrogens, possibly resulting in a decrease in therapeutic effects and/or changes in the uterine bleeding profile).

No products indexed under this heading.

Methylprednisolone (Co-administration of inducers of CYP3A4 with estrogens may affect estrogen drug metabolism. Inducers of CYP3A4 may reduce plasma concentrations of estrogens, possibly resulting in a decrease in therapeutic effects and/or changes in the uterine bleeding profile).

No products indexed under this heading.

Methylprednisolone Acetate (Co-administration of inducers of CYP3A4 with estrogens may affect estrogen drug metabolism. Inducers of CYP3A4 may reduce plasma concentrations of estrogens, possibly resulting in a decrease in therapeutic effects and/or changes in the uterine bleeding profile).

No products indexed under this heading.

Methylprednisolone Sodium Succinate (Co-administration of inducers of CYP3A4 with estrogens may affect estrogen drug metabolism. Inducers of CYP3A4 may reduce plasma concentrations of estrogens, possibly resulting in a decrease in therapeutic effects and/or changes in the uterine bleeding profile).

No products indexed under this heading.

Metronidazole (Co-administration of inhibitors of CYP3A4 with estrogens may affect estrogen drug metabolism. Inhibitors of CYP3A4 may increase plasma concentrations of estrogens and may result in side effects). Products include:

Pylera Capsules **714**

Metronidazole Benzoate (Co-administration of inhibitors of CYP3A4 with estrogens may affect estrogen drug metabolism. Inhibitors of CYP3A4 may increase plasma concentrations of estrogens and may result in side effects).

No products indexed under this heading.

Metronidazole Hydrochloride (Co-administration of inhibitors of CYP3A4 with estrogens may affect estrogen drug metabolism. Inhibitors of CYP3A4 may increase plasma concentrations of estrogens and may result in side effects).

No products indexed under this heading.

Miconazole (Co-administration of inhibitors of CYP3A4 with estrogens may affect estrogen drug metabolism. Inhibitors of CYP3A4 may increase plasma concentrations of estrogens and may result in side effects).

No products indexed under this heading.

Miconazole Nitrate (Co-administration of inhibitors of CYP3A4 with estrogens may affect estrogen drug metabolism. Inhibitors of CYP3A4 may increase plasma concentrations of estrogens and may result in side effects).

No products indexed under this heading.

Modafinil (Co-administration of inducers of CYP3A4 with estrogens may affect estrogen drug metabolism. Inducers of CYP3A4 may reduce plasma concentrations of estrogens, possibly resulting in a decrease in therapeutic effects and/or changes in the uterine bleeding profile). Products include:

Provigil Tablets **977**

Nefazodone Hydrochloride (Co-administration of inhibitors of CYP3A4 with estrogens may affect estrogen drug metabolism. Inhibitors of CYP3A4 may increase plasma concentrations of estrogens and may result in side effects).

No products indexed under this heading.

Nelfinavir Mesylate (Co-administration of inhibitors of CYP3A4 with estrogens may affect estrogen drug metabolism. Inhibitors of CYP3A4 may increase plasma concentrations of estrogens and may result in side effects).

No products indexed under this heading.

Nevirapine (Co-administration of inducers of CYP3A4 with estrogens may affect estrogen drug metabolism. Inducers of CYP3A4 may reduce plasma concentrations of estrogens, possibly resulting in a decrease in therapeutic effects and/or changes in the uterine bleeding profile). Products include:

Viramune Oral Suspension **873**
Viramune Tablets **873**

Niacinamide (Co-administration of inhibitors of CYP3A4 with estrogens may affect estrogen drug metabolism. Inhibitors of CYP3A4 may increase plasma concentrations of estrogens and may result in side effects). Products include:

BioLean Free Tablets **635**

Nicotinamide (Co-administration of inhibitors of CYP3A4 with estrogens may affect estrogen drug metabolism. Inhibitors of CYP3A4 may increase plasma concentrations of estrogens and may result in side effects).

No products indexed under this heading.

Nifedipine (Co-administration of inhibitors of CYP3A4 with estrogens may affect estrogen drug metabolism. Inhibitors of CYP3A4 may increase plasma concentrations of estrogens and may result in side effects).

No products indexed under this heading.

Norfloxacin (Co-administration of inhibitors of CYP3A4 with estrogens may affect estrogen drug metabolism. Inhibitors of CYP3A4 may increase plasma concentrations of estrogens and may result in side effects). Products include:

Noroxin Tablets **2069**

Omeprazole (Co-administration of inhibitors of CYP3A4 with estrogens may affect estrogen drug metabolism. Inhibitors of CYP3A4 may increase plasma concentrations of estrogens and may result in side effects).

No products indexed under this heading.

Oxcarbazepine (Co-administration of inducers of CYP3A4 with estrogens may affect estrogen drug metabolism. Inducers of CYP3A4 may reduce plasma concentrations of estrogens, possibly resulting in a decrease in therapeutic effects and/or changes in the uterine bleeding profile).

No products indexed under this heading.

Paroxetine Hydrochloride (Co-administration of inhibitors of CYP3A4 with estrogens may affect estrogen drug metabolism. Inhibitors of CYP3A4 may increase plasma concentrations of estrogens and may result in side effects). Products include:

Paxil **1535**
Paxil CR Controlled-Release Tablets **1544**

Phenobarbital (Co-administration of inducers of CYP3A4 with estrogens may affect estrogen drug metabolism. Inducers of CYP3A4 may reduce plasma concentrations of estrogens, possibly resulting in a decrease in therapeutic effects and/or changes in the uterine bleeding profile). Products include:

Donnatal Extentabs **2507**

Phenobarbital Sodium (Co-administration of inducers of CYP3A4 with estrogens may affect estrogen drug metabolism. Inducers of CYP3A4 may reduce plasma concentrations of estrogens, possibly resulting in a decrease in therapeutic effects and/or changes in the uterine bleeding profile).

No products indexed under this heading.

Phenytoin (Co-administration of inducers of CYP3A4 with estrogens may affect estrogen drug metabolism. Inducers of CYP3A4 may reduce plasma concentrations of estrogens, possibly resulting in a decrease in therapeutic effects and/or changes in the uterine bleeding profile).

No products indexed under this heading.

Phenytoin Sodium (Co-administration of inducers of CYP3A4 with estrogens may affect estrogen drug metabolism. Inducers of CYP3A4 may reduce plasma concentrations of estrogens, possibly resulting in a decrease in therapeutic effects and/or changes in the uterine bleeding profile). Products include:

Phenytek Capsules **2192**

Prednisolone Acetate (Co-administration of inducers of CYP3A4 with estrogens may affect estrogen drug metabolism. Inducers of CYP3A4 may reduce plasma concentrations of estrogens, possibly resulting in a decrease in therapeutic effects and/or changes in the uterine bleeding profile). Products include:

Pred Forte Ophthalmic Suspension .... ⊙**227**
Pred Mild Ophthalmic Suspension .... ⊙**230**
Pred-G Ophthalmic Ointment .... ⊙**229**
Pred-G Ophthalmic Suspension ...... ⊙**228**

Prednisolone Sodium Phosphate (Co-administration of inducers of CYP3A4 with estrogens may affect estrogen drug metabolism. Inducers of CYP3A4 may reduce plasma concentrations of estrogens, possibly resulting in a decrease in therapeutic effects and/or changes in the uterine bleeding profile).

No products indexed under this heading.

Prednisolone Tebutate (Co-administration of inducers of CYP3A4 with estrogens may affect estrogen drug metabolism. Inducers of CYP3A4 may reduce plasma concentrations of estrogens, possibly resulting in a decrease in therapeutic effects and/or changes in the uterine bleeding profile).

No products indexed under this heading.

Prednisone (Co-administration of inducers of CYP3A4 with estrogens may affect estrogen drug metabolism. Inducers of CYP3A4 may reduce plasma concentrations of estrogens, possibly resulting in a decrease in therapeutic effects and/or changes in the uterine bleeding profile).

No products indexed under this heading.

Primidone (Co-administration of inducers of CYP3A4 with estrogens may affect estrogen drug metabolism. Inducers of CYP3A4 may reduce plasma concentrations of estrogens, possibly resulting in a decrease in therapeutic effects and/ or changes in the uterine bleeding profile).
No products indexed under this heading.

Propoxyphene Hydrochloride (Co-administration of inhibitors of CYP3A4 with estrogens may affect estrogen drug metabolism. Inhibitors of CYP3A4 may increase plasma concentrations of estrogens and may result in side effects).
No products indexed under this heading.

Propoxyphene Napsylate (Co-administration of inhibitors of CYP3A4 with estrogens may affect estrogen drug metabolism. Inhibitors of CYP3A4 may increase plasma concentrations of estrogens and may result in side effects).
No products indexed under this heading.

Quinidine (Co-administration of inhibitors of CYP3A4 with estrogens may affect estrogen drug metabolism. Inhibitors of CYP3A4 may increase plasma concentrations of estrogens and may result in side effects).
No products indexed under this heading.

Quinidine Hydrochloride (Co-administration of inhibitors of CYP3A4 with estrogens may affect estrogen drug metabolism. Inhibitors of CYP3A4 may increase plasma concentrations of estrogens and may result in side effects).
No products indexed under this heading.

Quinidine Polygalacturonate (Co-administration of inhibitors of CYP3A4 with estrogens may affect estrogen drug metabolism. Inhibitors of CYP3A4 may increase plasma concentrations of estrogens and may result in side effects).
No products indexed under this heading.

Quinidine Sulfate (Co-administration of inhibitors of CYP3A4 with estrogens may affect estrogen drug metabolism. Inhibitors of CYP3A4 may increase plasma concentrations of estrogens and may result in side effects).
No products indexed under this heading.

Quinine (Co-administration of inhibitors of CYP3A4 with estrogens may affect estrogen drug metabolism. Inhibitors of CYP3A4 may increase plasma concentrations of estrogens and may result in side effects).
No products indexed under this heading.

Quinine Sulfate (Co-administration of inhibitors of CYP3A4 with estrogens may affect estrogen drug metabolism. Inhibitors of CYP3A4 may increase plasma concentrations of estrogens and may result in side effects).
No products indexed under this heading.

Quinupristin (Co-administration of inhibitors of CYP3A4 with estrogens may affect estrogen drug metabolism. Inhibitors of CYP3A4 may increase plasma concentrations of estrogens and may result in side effects).
No products indexed under this heading.

Ranitidine Bismuth Citrate (Co-administration of inhibitors of CYP3A4 with estrogens may affect estrogen drug metabolism. Inhibitors of CYP3A4 may increase plasma concentrations of estrogens and may result in side effects).
No products indexed under this heading.

Ranitidine Hydrochloride (Co-administration of inhibitors of CYP3A4 with estrogens may affect estrogen drug metabolism. Inhibitors of CYP3A4 may increase plasma concentrations of estrogens and may result in side effects). Products include:

Zantac 75 Tablets .... ◘**603**
Zantac **1670**
Zantac Injection **1666**
Zantac Injection Pharmacy Bulk Package **1668**
Maximum Strength Zantac 150 Tablets .... ◘**603**
Maximum Strength Zantac 150 Cool Mint Tablets .... ◘**603**

Rifabutin (Co-administration of inducers of CYP3A4 with estrogens may affect estrogen drug metabolism. Inducers of CYP3A4 may reduce plasma concentrations of estrogens, possibly resulting in a decrease in therapeutic effects and/ or changes in the uterine bleeding profile).
No products indexed under this heading.

Rifampicin (Co-administration of inducers of CYP3A4 with estrogens may affect estrogen drug metabolism. Inducers of CYP3A4 may reduce plasma concentrations of estrogens, possibly resulting in a decrease in therapeutic effects and/ or changes in the uterine bleeding profile).
No products indexed under this heading.

Rifampin (Co-administration of inducers of CYP3A4 with estrogens may affect estrogen drug metabolism. Inducers of CYP3A4 may reduce plasma concentrations of estrogens, possibly resulting in a decrease in therapeutic effects and/ or changes in the uterine bleeding profile).
No products indexed under this heading.

Rifapentine (Co-administration of inducers of CYP3A4 with estrogens may affect estrogen drug metabolism. Inducers of CYP3A4 may reduce plasma concentrations of estrogens, possibly resulting in a decrease in therapeutic effects and/ or changes in the uterine bleeding profile).
No products indexed under this heading.

Ritonavir (Co-administration of inhibitors of CYP3A4 with estrogens may affect estrogen drug metabolism. Inhibitors of CYP3A4 may increase plasma concentrations of estrogens and may result in side effects). Products include:

Kaletra **452**
Norvir **489**

Saquinavir (Co-administration of inhibitors of CYP3A4 with estrogens may affect estrogen drug metabolism. Inhibitors of CYP3A4 may increase plasma concentrations of estrogens and may result in side effects).
No products indexed under this heading.

Saquinavir Mesylate (Co-administration of inhibitors of CYP3A4 with estrogens may affect estrogen drug metabolism. Inhibitors of CYP3A4 may increase plasma concentrations of estrogens and may result in side effects).
No products indexed under this heading.

Sertraline Hydrochloride (Co-administration of inhibitors of CYP3A4 with estrogens may affect estrogen drug metabolism. Inhibitors of CYP3A4 may increase plasma concentrations of estrogens and may result in side effects).
No products indexed under this heading.

Sildenafil Citrate (Co-administration of inhibitors of CYP3A4 with estrogens may affect estrogen drug metabolism. Inhibitors of CYP3A4 may increase plasma concentrations of estrogens and may result in side effects).
No products indexed under this heading.

Sulfinpyrazone (Co-administration of inducers of CYP3A4 with estrogens may affect estrogen drug metabolism. Inducers of CYP3A4 may reduce plasma concentrations of estrogens, possibly resulting in a decrease in therapeutic effects and/ or changes in the uterine bleeding profile).
No products indexed under this heading.

Telithromycin (Co-administration of inhibitors of CYP3A4 with estrogens may affect estrogen drug metabolism. Inhibitors of CYP3A4 may increase plasma concentrations of estrogens and may result in side effects). Products include:

Ketek Tablets **2744**

Theophylline (Co-administration of inducers of CYP3A4 with estrogens may affect estrogen drug metabolism. Inducers of CYP3A4 may reduce plasma concentrations of estrogens, possibly resulting in a decrease in therapeutic effects and/ or changes in the uterine bleeding profile).
No products indexed under this heading.

Theophylline Anhydrous (Co-administration of inducers of CYP3A4 with estrogens may affect estrogen drug metabolism. Inducers of CYP3A4 may reduce plasma concentrations of estrogens, possibly resulting in a decrease in therapeutic effects and/or changes in the uterine bleeding profile). Products include:

Uniphyl Tablets **2595**

Theophylline Calcium Salicylate (Co-administration of inducers of CYP3A4 with estrogens may affect estrogen drug metabolism. Inducers of CYP3A4 may reduce plasma concentrations of estrogens, possibly resulting in a decrease in therapeutic effects and/or changes in the uterine bleeding profile).
No products indexed under this heading.

Theophylline Dihydroxypropyl (Glyceryl) (Co-administration of inducers of CYP3A4 with estrogens may affect estrogen drug metabolism. Inducers of CYP3A4 may reduce plasma concentrations of estrogens, possibly resulting in a decrease in therapeutic effects and/ or changes in the uterine bleeding profile).
No products indexed under this heading.

Theophylline Ethylenediamine (Co-administration of inducers of CYP3A4 with estrogens may affect estrogen drug metabolism. Inducers of CYP3A4 may reduce plasma concentrations of estrogens, possibly resulting in a decrease in therapeutic effects and/or changes in the uterine bleeding profile).
No products indexed under this heading.

Triamcinolone (Co-administration of inducers of CYP3A4 with estrogens may affect estrogen drug metabolism. Inducers of CYP3A4 may reduce plasma concentrations of estrogens, possibly resulting in a decrease in therapeutic effects and/ or changes in the uterine bleeding profile).
No products indexed under this heading.

Triamcinolone Acetonide (Co-administration of inducers of CYP3A4 with estrogens may affect estrogen drug metabolism. Inducers of CYP3A4 may reduce plasma concentrations of estrogens, possibly resulting in a decrease in therapeutic effects and/or changes in the uterine bleeding profile). Products include:

Azmacort Inhalation Aerosol **407**
Nasacort AQ Nasal Spray **2765**
Triesence Injectable Suspension .... ⊙**209**

Triamcinolone Diacetate (Co-administration of inducers of CYP3A4 with estrogens may affect estrogen drug metabolism. Inducers of CYP3A4 may reduce plasma concentrations of estrogens, possibly resulting in a decrease in therapeutic effects and/or changes in the uterine bleeding profile).
No products indexed under this heading.

Triamcinolone Hexacetonide (Co-administration of inducers of CYP3A4 with estrogens may affect estrogen drug metabolism. Inducers of CYP3A4 may reduce plasma concentrations of estrogens, possibly resulting in a decrease in therapeutic effects and/or changes in the uterine bleeding profile).
No products indexed under this heading.

Troglitazone (Co-administration of inducers of CYP3A4 with estrogens may affect estrogen drug metabolism. Inducers of CYP3A4 may reduce plasma concentrations of estrogens, possibly resulting in a decrease in therapeutic effects and/ or changes in the uterine bleeding profile).
No products indexed under this heading.

Troleandomycin (Co-administration of inhibitors of CYP3A4 with estrogens may affect estrogen drug metabolism. Inhibitors of CYP3A4 may increase plasma concentrations of estrogens and may result in side effects).
No products indexed under this heading.

Valproate Sodium (Co-administration of inhibitors of CYP3A4 with estrogens may affect estrogen drug metabolism. Inhibitors of CYP3A4 may increase plasma concentrations of estrogens and may result in side effects).
No products indexed under this heading.

Vardenafil Hydrochloride (Co-administration of inhibitors of CYP3A4 with estrogens may affect estrogen drug metabolism. Inhibitors of CYP3A4 may increase plasma concentrations of estrogens and may result in side effects). Products include:
Levitra Tablets **2876**

Verapamil Hydrochloride (Co-administration of inhibitors of CYP3A4 with estrogens may affect estrogen drug metabolism. Inhibitors of CYP3A4 may increase plasma concentrations of estrogens and may result in side effects). Products include:
Tarka Tablets **511**

Voriconazole (Co-administration of inhibitors of CYP3A4 with estrogens may affect estrogen drug metabolism. Inhibitors of CYP3A4 may increase plasma concentrations of estrogens and may result in side effects).
No products indexed under this heading.

Zafirlukast (Co-administration of inhibitors of CYP3A4 with estrogens may affect estrogen drug metabolism. Inhibitors of CYP3A4 may increase plasma concentrations of estrogens and may result in side effects). Products include:
Accolate Tablets **669**

Zileuton (Co-administration of inhibitors of CYP3A4 with estrogens may affect estrogen drug metabolism. Inhibitors of CYP3A4 may increase plasma concentrations of estrogens and may result in side effects).
No products indexed under this heading.

Food Interactions

Grapefruit (Co-administration of inhibitors of CYP3A4 with estrogens may affect estrogen drug metabolism. Inhibitors of CYP3A4 may increase plasma concentrations of estrogens and may result in side effects).

Grapefruit Juice (Co-administration of grapefruit juice with estrogens may increase plasma concentrations of estrogens and may result in side effects).

PREMARIN VAGINAL CREAM

(Estrogens, Conjugated) **3228**
See Premarin Tablets

PREMPHASE TABLETS

(Estrogens, Conjugated, Medroxyprogesterone Acetate).......... **3232**
May interact with cytochrome p450 3a4 inducers (selected), cytochrome p450 3a4 inhibitors (selected), and certain other agents. Compounds in these categories include:

Acetazolamide (Co-administration of estrogens with inhibitors of CYP3A4 may increase plasma concentrations of estrogens and may result in side effects).
No products indexed under this heading.

Allium sativum (Co-administration of estrogens with inducers of CYP3A4 may reduce plasma concentrations of estrogens, possibly resulting in a decrease in therapeutic effects and/or changes in the uterine bleeding profile).
No products indexed under this heading.

Aminoglutethimide (Aminoglutethimide administered concomitantly with medroxyprogesterone acetate (MPA) may significantly depress the bioavailability of MPA).
No products indexed under this heading.

Amiodarone Hydrochloride (Co-administration of estrogens with inhibitors of CYP3A4 may increase plasma concentrations of estrogens and may result in side effects).
No products indexed under this heading.

Amprenavir (Co-administration of estrogens with inhibitors of CYP3A4 may increase plasma concentrations of estrogens and may result in side effects).
No products indexed under this heading.

Anastrozole (Co-administration of estrogens with inhibitors of CYP3A4 may increase plasma concentrations of estrogens and may result in side effects). Products include:
Arimidex Tablets **672**

Aprepitant (Co-administration of estrogens with inducers of CYP3A4 may reduce plasma concentrations of estrogens, possibly resulting in a decrease in therapeutic effects and/or changes in the uterine bleeding profile). Products include:
Emend Capsules **1992**

Atazanavir (Co-administration of estrogens with inhibitors of CYP3A4 may increase plasma concentrations of estrogens and may result in side effects).
No products indexed under this heading.

Atazanavir Sulfate (Co-administration of estrogens with inhibitors of CYP3A4 may increase plasma concentrations of estrogens and may result in side effects). Products include:
Reyataz Capsules **3299**

Betamethasone Acetate (Co-administration of estrogens with inducers of CYP3A4 may reduce plasma concentrations of estrogens, possibly resulting in a decrease in therapeutic effects and/or changes in the uterine bleeding profile).
No products indexed under this heading.

Betamethasone Sodium Phosphate (Co-administration of estrogens with inducers of CYP3A4 may reduce plasma concentrations of estrogens, possibly resulting in a decrease in therapeutic effects and/or changes in the uterine bleeding profile).
No products indexed under this heading.

Carbamazepine (Co-administration of estrogens with inducers of CYP3A4 may reduce plasma concentrations of estrogens, possibly resulting in a decrease in therapeutic effects and/or changes in the uterine bleeding profile). Products include:
Carbatrol Capsules **3019**
Equetro Extended-Release Capsules **3174**

Cimetidine (Co-administration of estrogens with inhibitors of CYP3A4 may increase plasma concentrations of estrogens and may result in side effects).
No products indexed under this heading.

Cimetidine Hydrochloride (Co-administration of estrogens with inhibitors of CYP3A4 may increase plasma concentrations of estrogens and may result in side effects).
No products indexed under this heading.

Ciprofloxacin (Co-administration of estrogens with inhibitors of CYP3A4 may increase plasma concentrations of estrogens and may result in side effects). Products include:
Cipro I.V. **2817**
Cipro Oral Suspension **2810**
Cipro XR Tablets **2823**
Ciprodex Otic Suspension **541**

Ciprofloxacin Hydrochloride (Co-administration of estrogens with inducers of CYP3A4 may reduce plasma concentrations of estrogens, possibly resulting in a decrease in therapeutic effects and/or changes in the uterine bleeding profile). Products include:
Cipro Tablets **2810**

Cisplatin (Co-administration of estrogens with inducers of CYP3A4 may reduce plasma concentrations of estrogens, possibly resulting in a decrease in therapeutic effects and/or changes in the uterine bleeding profile).
No products indexed under this heading.

Clarithromycin (Co-administration of estrogens with inhibitors of CYP3A4 may increase plasma concentrations of estrogens and may result in side effects). Products include:
Biaxin/Biaxin XL **411**

Clotrimazole (Co-administration of estrogens with inhibitors of CYP3A4 may increase plasma concentrations of estrogens and may result in side effects). Products include:
Lotrisone **2881**

Cortisone Acetate (Co-administration of estrogens with inducers of CYP3A4 may reduce plasma concentrations of estrogens, possibly resulting in a decrease in therapeutic effects and/or changes in the uterine bleeding profile).
No products indexed under this heading.

Cyclosporine (Co-administration of estrogens with inhibitors of CYP3A4 may increase plasma concentrations of estrogens and may result in side effects). Products include:
Gengraf Capsules **435**
Neoral Oral Solution **2280**
Neoral Soft Gelatin Capsules **2280**
Restasis Ophthalmic Emulsion **557**
Sandimmune **2296**

Dalfopristin (Co-administration of estrogens with inhibitors of CYP3A4 may increase plasma concentrations of estrogens and may result in side effects).
No products indexed under this heading.

Danazol (Co-administration of estrogens with inhibitors of CYP3A4 may increase plasma concentrations of estrogens and may result in side effects).
No products indexed under this heading.

Delavirdine Mesylate (Co-administration of estrogens with inhibitors of CYP3A4 may increase plasma concentrations of estrogens and may result in side effects).
No products indexed under this heading.

Dexamethasone (Co-administration of estrogens with inducers of CYP3A4 may reduce plasma concentrations of estrogens, possibly resulting in a decrease in therapeutic effects and/or changes in the uterine bleeding profile). Products include:
Ciprodex Otic Suspension **541**

Dexamethasone Acetate (Co-administration of estrogens with inducers of CYP3A4 may reduce plasma concentrations of estrogens, possibly resulting in a decrease in therapeutic effects and/or changes in the uterine bleeding profile).
No products indexed under this heading.

Dexamethasone Sodium Phosphate (Co-administration of estrogens with inducers of CYP3A4 may reduce plasma concentrations of estrogens, possibly resulting in a decrease in therapeutic effects and/or changes in the uterine bleeding profile).
No products indexed under this heading.

Diltiazem Hydrochloride (Co-administration of estrogens with inhibitors of CYP3A4 may increase plasma concentrations of estrogens and may result in side effects). Products include:
Cardizem LA Extended Release Tablets **421**

Diltiazem Maleate (Co-administration of estrogens with inhibitors of CYP3A4 may increase plasma concentrations of estrogens and may result in side effects).
No products indexed under this heading.

Doxorubicin Hydrochloride (Co-administration of estrogens with inducers of CYP3A4 may reduce plasma concentrations of estrogens, possibly resulting in a decrease in therapeutic effects and/or changes in the uterine bleeding profile).
No products indexed under this heading.

Efavirenz (Co-administration of estrogens with inducers of CYP3A4 may reduce plasma concentrations of estrogens, possibly resulting in a decrease in therapeutic effects and/or changes in the uterine bleeding profile). Products include:
Atripla Tablets **938**
Sustiva Capsules **930**
Sustiva Tablets **930**

Erythromycin (Co-administration of estrogens with inhibitors of CYP3A4 may increase plasma concentrations of estrogens and may result in side effects).
No products indexed under this heading.

Erythromycin Estolate (Co-administration of estrogens with inhibitors of CYP3A4 may increase plasma concentrations of estrogens and may result in side effects).
No products indexed under this heading.

Erythromycin Ethylsuccinate (Co-administration of estrogens with inhibitors of CYP3A4 may increase plasma concentrations of estrogens and may result in side effects).
Products include:
E.E.S. 433
EryPed 431

Erythromycin Gluceptate (Co-administration of estrogens with inhibitors of CYP3A4 may increase plasma concentrations of estrogens and may result in side effects).
No products indexed under this heading.

Erythromycin Lactobionate (Co-administration of estrogens with inhibitors of CYP3A4 may increase plasma concentrations of estrogens and may result in side effects).
No products indexed under this heading.

Erythromycin Stearate (Co-administration of estrogens with inhibitors of CYP3A4 may increase plasma concentrations of estrogens and may result in side effects).
No products indexed under this heading.

Esomeprazole Magnesium (Co-administration of estrogens with inhibitors of CYP3A4 may increase plasma concentrations of estrogens and may result in side effects).
Products include:
Nexium Delayed-Release Capsules 645
Nexium Delayed-Release Oral Suspension 645

Ethosuximide (Co-administration of estrogens with inducers of CYP3A4 may reduce plasma concentrations of estrogens, possibly resulting in a decrease in therapeutic effects and/or changes in the uterine bleeding profile).
No products indexed under this heading.

Felbamate (Co-administration of estrogens with inducers of CYP3A4 may reduce plasma concentrations of estrogens, possibly resulting in a decrease in therapeutic effects and/or changes in the uterine bleeding profile).
No products indexed under this heading.

Fluconazole (Co-administration of estrogens with inhibitors of CYP3A4 may increase plasma concentrations of estrogens and may result in side effects).
No products indexed under this heading.

Fludrocortisone Acetate (Co-administration of estrogens with inducers of CYP3A4 may reduce plasma concentrations of estrogens, possibly resulting in a decrease in therapeutic effects and/or changes in the uterine bleeding profile).
No products indexed under this heading.

Fluoxetine (Co-administration of estrogens with inhibitors of CYP3A4 may increase plasma concentrations of estrogens and may result in side effects).
No products indexed under this heading.

Fluoxetine Hydrochloride (Co-administration of estrogens with inhibitors of CYP3A4 may increase plasma concentrations of estrogens and may result in side effects).
Products include:
Prozac Weekly Capsules 1852
Prozac Pulvules and Liquid 1852
Symbyax Capsules 1871

Fluvoxamine Maleate (Co-administration of estrogens with inhibitors of CYP3A4 may increase plasma concentrations of estrogens and may result in side effects).
Products include:
Luvox CR Extended-Release Capsules 1759

Fosamprenavir Calcium (Co-administration of estrogens with inhibitors of CYP3A4 may increase plasma concentrations of estrogens and may result in side effects).
Products include:
Lexiva Oral Suspension 1510
Lexiva Tablets 1510

Fosphenytoin Sodium (Co-administration of estrogens with inducers of CYP3A4 may reduce plasma concentrations of estrogens, possibly resulting in a decrease in therapeutic effects and/or changes in the uterine bleeding profile).
No products indexed under this heading.

Garlic Extract (Co-administration of estrogens with inducers of CYP3A4 may reduce plasma concentrations of estrogens, possibly resulting in a decrease in therapeutic effects and/or changes in the uterine bleeding profile).
No products indexed under this heading.

Garlic Oil (Co-administration of estrogens with inducers of CYP3A4 may reduce plasma concentrations of estrogens, possibly resulting in a decrease in therapeutic effects and/or changes in the uterine bleeding profile).
No products indexed under this heading.

Hydrocortisone (Co-administration of estrogens with inducers of CYP3A4 may reduce plasma concentrations of estrogens, possibly resulting in a decrease in therapeutic effects and/or changes in the uterine bleeding profile).
No products indexed under this heading.

Hydrocortisone Acetate (Co-administration of estrogens with inducers of CYP3A4 may reduce plasma concentrations of estrogens, possibly resulting in a decrease in therapeutic effects and/or changes in the uterine bleeding profile).
Products include:
Analpram-HC 1140
Pramosone 1141

Hydrocortisone Butyrate (Co-administration of estrogens with inducers of CYP3A4 may reduce plasma concentrations of estrogens, possibly resulting in a decrease in therapeutic effects and/or changes in the uterine bleeding profile).
No products indexed under this heading.

Hydrocortisone Cypionate (Co-administration of estrogens with inducers of CYP3A4 may reduce plasma concentrations of estrogens, possibly resulting in a decrease in therapeutic effects and/or changes in the uterine bleeding profile).
No products indexed under this heading.

Hydrocortisone Hemisuccinate (Co-administration of estrogens with inducers of CYP3A4 may reduce plasma concentrations of estrogens, possibly resulting in a decrease in therapeutic effects and/or changes in the uterine bleeding profile).
No products indexed under this heading.

Hydrocortisone Probutate (Co-administration of estrogens with inducers of CYP3A4 may reduce plasma concentrations of estrogens, possibly resulting in a decrease in therapeutic effects and/or changes in the uterine bleeding profile).
No products indexed under this heading.

Hydrocortisone Sodium Phosphate (Co-administration of estrogens with inducers of CYP3A4 may reduce plasma concentrations of estrogens, possibly resulting in a decrease in therapeutic effects and/or changes in the uterine bleeding profile).
No products indexed under this heading.

Hydrocortisone Sodium Succinate (Co-administration of estrogens with inducers of CYP3A4 may reduce plasma concentrations of estrogens, possibly resulting in a decrease in therapeutic effects and/or changes in the uterine bleeding profile).
No products indexed under this heading.

Hydrocortisone Valerate (Co-administration of estrogens with inducers of CYP3A4 may reduce plasma concentrations of estrogens, possibly resulting in a decrease in therapeutic effects and/or changes in the uterine bleeding profile).
No products indexed under this heading.

Hypericum (Co-administration of estrogens with inducers of CYP3A4 may reduce plasma concentrations of estrogens, possibly resulting in a decrease in therapeutic effects and/or changes in the uterine bleeding profile). Products include:
Satieté Tablets .... ▣640

Hypericum Perforatum (Co-administration of estrogens with inducers of CYP3A4 may reduce plasma concentrations of estrogens, possibly resulting in a decrease in therapeutic effects and/or changes in the uterine bleeding profile).
No products indexed under this heading.

Indinavir Sulfate (Co-administration of estrogens with inhibitors of CYP3A4 may increase plasma concentrations of estrogens and may result in side effects).
Products include:
Crixivan Capsules 1979

Isoniazid (Co-administration of estrogens with inhibitors of CYP3A4 may increase plasma concentrations of estrogens and may result in side effects).
No products indexed under this heading.

Itraconazole (Co-administration of estrogens with inhibitors of CYP3A4 may increase plasma concentrations of estrogens and may result in side effects).
No products indexed under this heading.

Ketoconazole (Co-administration of estrogens with inhibitors of CYP3A4 may increase plasma concentrations of estrogens and may result in side effects). Products include:
Extina Foam, 2% 3057
Nizoral A-D Shampoo 1901

Lopinavir (Co-administration of estrogens with inhibitors of CYP3A4 may increase plasma concentrations of estrogens and may result in side effects). Products include:
Kaletra 452

Loratadine (Co-administration of estrogens with inhibitors of CYP3A4 may increase plasma concentrations of estrogens and may result in side effects).
No products indexed under this heading.

Mephenytoin (Co-administration of estrogens with inducers of CYP3A4 may reduce plasma concentrations of estrogens, possibly resulting in a decrease in therapeutic effects and/or changes in the uterine bleeding profile).
No products indexed under this heading.

Methsuximide (Co-administration of estrogens with inducers of CYP3A4 may reduce plasma concentrations of estrogens, possibly resulting in a decrease in therapeutic effects and/or changes in the uterine bleeding profile).
No products indexed under this heading.

Methylprednisolone (Co-administration of estrogens with inducers of CYP3A4 may reduce plasma concentrations of estrogens, possibly resulting in a decrease in therapeutic effects and/or changes in the uterine bleeding profile).
No products indexed under this heading.

Methylprednisolone Acetate (Co-administration of estrogens with inducers of CYP3A4 may reduce plasma concentrations of estrogens, possibly resulting in a decrease in therapeutic effects and/or changes in the uterine bleeding profile).
No products indexed under this heading.

Methylprednisolone Sodium Succinate (Co-administration of estrogens with inducers of CYP3A4 may reduce plasma concentrations of estrogens, possibly resulting in a decrease in therapeutic effects and/or changes in the uterine bleeding profile).
No products indexed under this heading.

Metronidazole (Co-administration of estrogens with inhibitors of CYP3A4 may increase plasma concentrations of estrogens and may result in side effects). Products include:
Pylera Capsules 714

Metronidazole Benzoate (Co-administration of estrogens with inhibitors of CYP3A4 may increase plasma concentrations of estrogens and may result in side effects).
No products indexed under this heading.

Metronidazole Hydrochloride (Co-administration of estrogens with inhibitors of CYP3A4 may increase plasma concentrations of estrogens and may result in side effects).
No products indexed under this heading.

Miconazole (Co-administration of estrogens with inhibitors of CYP3A4 may increase plasma concentrations of estrogens and may result in side effects).
No products indexed under this heading.

Miconazole Nitrate (Co-administration of estrogens with inhibitors of CYP3A4 may increase plasma concentrations of estrogens and may result in side effects).
No products indexed under this heading.

Modafinil (Co-administration of estrogens with inducers of CYP3A4 may reduce plasma concentrations of estrogens, possibly resulting in a decrease in therapeutic effects and/or changes in the uterine bleeding profile). Products include:
Provigil Tablets 977

Nefazodone Hydrochloride (Co-administration of estrogens with inhibitors of CYP3A4 may increase plasma concentrations of estrogens and may result in side effects).
No products indexed under this heading.

Nelfinavir Mesylate (Co-administration of estrogens with inhibitors of CYP3A4 may increase plasma concentrations of estrogens and may result in side effects).
No products indexed under this heading.

Nevirapine (Co-administration of estrogens with inducers of CYP3A4 may reduce plasma concentrations of estrogens, possibly resulting in a decrease in therapeutic effects and/or changes in the uterine bleeding profile). Products include:
Viramune Oral Suspension 873
Viramune Tablets 873

Niacinamide (Co-administration of estrogens with inhibitors of CYP3A4 may increase plasma concentrations of estrogens and may result in side effects). Products include:
BioLean Free Tablets 635

Nicotinamide (Co-administration of estrogens with inhibitors of CYP3A4 may increase plasma concentrations of estrogens and may result in side effects).
No products indexed under this heading.

Nifedipine (Co-administration of estrogens with inhibitors of CYP3A4 may increase plasma concentrations of estrogens and may result in side effects).
No products indexed under this heading.

Norfloxacin (Co-administration of estrogens with inhibitors of CYP3A4 may increase plasma concentrations of estrogens and may result in side effects). Products include:
Noroxin Tablets 2069

Omeprazole (Co-administration of estrogens with inhibitors of CYP3A4 may increase plasma concentrations of estrogens and may result in side effects).
No products indexed under this heading.

Oxcarbazepine (Co-administration of estrogens with inducers of CYP3A4 may reduce plasma concentrations of estrogens, possibly resulting in a decrease in therapeutic effects and/or changes in the uterine bleeding profile).
No products indexed under this heading.

Paroxetine Hydrochloride (Co-administration of estrogens with inhibitors of CYP3A4 may increase plasma concentrations of estrogens and may result in side effects). Products include:
Paxil 1535
Paxil CR Controlled-Release Tablets 1544

Phenobarbital (Co-administration of estrogens with inducers of CYP3A4 may reduce plasma concentrations of estrogens, possibly resulting in a decrease in therapeutic effects and/or changes in the uterine bleeding profile). Products include:
Donnatal Extentabs 2507

Phenobarbital Sodium (Co-administration of estrogens with inducers of CYP3A4 may reduce plasma concentrations of estrogens, possibly resulting in a decrease in therapeutic effects and/or changes in the uterine bleeding profile).
No products indexed under this heading.

Phenytoin (Co-administration of estrogens with inducers of CYP3A4 may reduce plasma concentrations of estrogens, possibly resulting in a decrease in therapeutic effects and/or changes in the uterine bleeding profile).
No products indexed under this heading.

Phenytoin Sodium (Co-administration of estrogens with inducers of CYP3A4 may reduce plasma concentrations of estrogens, possibly resulting in a decrease in therapeutic effects and/or changes in the uterine bleeding profile). Products include:
Phenytek Capsules 2192

Prednisolone Acetate (Co-administration of estrogens with inducers of CYP3A4 may reduce plasma concentrations of estrogens, possibly resulting in a decrease in therapeutic effects and/or changes in the uterine bleeding profile). Products include:
Pred Forte Ophthalmic Suspension .... ⊙227
Pred Mild Ophthalmic Suspension .... ⊙230
Pred-G Ophthalmic Ointment .... ⊙229
Pred-G Ophthalmic Suspension .... ⊙228

Prednisolone Sodium Phosphate (Co-administration of estrogens with inducers of CYP3A4 may reduce plasma concentrations of estrogens, possibly resulting in a decrease in therapeutic effects and/or changes in the uterine bleeding profile).
No products indexed under this heading.

Prednisolone Tebutate (Co-administration of estrogens with inducers of CYP3A4 may reduce plasma concentrations of estrogens, possibly resulting in a decrease in therapeutic effects and/or changes in the uterine bleeding profile).
No products indexed under this heading.

Prednisone (Co-administration of estrogens with inducers of CYP3A4 may reduce plasma concentrations of estrogens, possibly resulting in a decrease in therapeutic effects and/or changes in the uterine bleeding profile).
No products indexed under this heading.

Primidone (Co-administration of estrogens with inducers of CYP3A4 may reduce plasma concentrations of estrogens, possibly resulting in a decrease in therapeutic effects and/or changes in the uterine bleeding profile).
No products indexed under this heading.

Propoxyphene Hydrochloride (Co-administration of estrogens with inhibitors of CYP3A4 may increase plasma concentrations of estrogens and may result in side effects).
No products indexed under this heading.

Propoxyphene Napsylate (Co-administration of estrogens with inhibitors of CYP3A4 may increase plasma concentrations of estrogens and may result in side effects).
No products indexed under this heading.

Quinidine (Co-administration of estrogens with inhibitors of CYP3A4 may increase plasma concentrations of estrogens and may result in side effects).
No products indexed under this heading.

Quinidine Hydrochloride (Co-administration of estrogens with inhibitors of CYP3A4 may increase plasma concentrations of estrogens and may result in side effects).
No products indexed under this heading.

Quinidine Polygalacturonate (Co-administration of estrogens with inhibitors of CYP3A4 may increase plasma concentrations of estrogens and may result in side effects).
No products indexed under this heading.

Quinidine Sulfate (Co-administration of estrogens with inhibitors of CYP3A4 may increase plasma concentrations of estrogens and may result in side effects).
No products indexed under this heading.

Quinine (Co-administration of estrogens with inhibitors of CYP3A4 may increase plasma concentrations of estrogens and may result in side effects).
No products indexed under this heading.

Quinine Sulfate (Co-administration of estrogens with inhibitors of CYP3A4 may increase plasma concentrations of estrogens and may result in side effects).
No products indexed under this heading.

Quinupristin (Co-administration of estrogens with inhibitors of CYP3A4 may increase plasma concentrations of estrogens and may result in side effects).
No products indexed under this heading.

Ranitidine Bismuth Citrate (Co-administration of estrogens with inhibitors of CYP3A4 may increase plasma concentrations of estrogens and may result in side effects).
No products indexed under this heading.

Ranitidine Hydrochloride (Co-administration of estrogens with inhibitors of CYP3A4 may increase plasma concentrations of estrogens and may result in side effects). Products include:
Zantac 75 Tablets 603
Zantac 1670
Zantac Injection 1666
Zantac Injection Pharmacy Bulk Package 1668
Maximum Strength Zantac 150 Tablets 603
Maximum Strength Zantac 150 Cool Mint Tablets 603

Rifabutin (Co-administration of estrogens with inducers of CYP3A4 may reduce plasma concentrations of estrogens, possibly resulting in a decrease in therapeutic effects and/or changes in the uterine bleeding profile).
No products indexed under this heading.

Rifampicin (Co-administration of estrogens with inducers of CYP3A4 may reduce plasma concentrations of estrogens, possibly resulting in a decrease in therapeutic effects and/or changes in the uterine bleeding profile).
No products indexed under this heading.

Rifampin (Co-administration of estrogens with inducers of CYP3A4 may reduce plasma concentrations of estrogens, possibly resulting in a decrease in therapeutic effects and/or changes in the uterine bleeding profile).
No products indexed under this heading.

Rifapentine (Co-administration of estrogens with inducers of CYP3A4 may reduce plasma concentrations of estrogens, possibly resulting in a decrease in therapeutic effects and/or changes in the uterine bleeding profile).
No products indexed under this heading.

Ritonavir (Co-administration of estrogens with inhibitors of CYP3A4 may increase plasma concentrations of estrogens and may result in side effects). Products include:
Kaletra 452
Norvir 489

Saquinavir (Co-administration of estrogens with inhibitors of CYP3A4 may increase plasma concentrations of estrogens and may result in side effects).
No products indexed under this heading.

Saquinavir Mesylate (Co-administration of estrogens with inhibitors of CYP3A4 may increase plasma concentrations of estrogens and may result in side effects).
No products indexed under this heading.

Sertraline Hydrochloride (Co-administration of estrogens with inhibitors of CYP3A4 may increase plasma concentrations of estrogens and may result in side effects).
No products indexed under this heading.

Sildenafil Citrate (Co-administration of estrogens with inhibitors of CYP3A4 may increase plasma concentrations of estrogens and may result in side effects).
No products indexed under this heading.

Sulfinpyrazone (Co-administration of estrogens with inducers of CYP3A4 may reduce plasma concentrations of estrogens, possibly resulting in a decrease in therapeutic effects and/or changes in the uterine bleeding profile).
No products indexed under this heading.

Telithromycin (Co-administration of estrogens with inhibitors of CYP3A4 may increase plasma concentrations of estrogens and may result in side effects). Products include:
Ketek Tablets 2744

Theophylline (Co-administration of estrogens with inducers of CYP3A4 may reduce plasma concentrations of estrogens, possibly resulting in a decrease in therapeutic effects and/or changes in the uterine bleeding profile).
No products indexed under this heading.

Theophylline Anhydrous (Co-administration of estrogens with inducers of CYP3A4 may reduce plasma concentrations of estrogens, possibly resulting in a decrease in therapeutic effects and/or changes in the uterine bleeding profile). Products include:
Uniphyl Tablets 2595

Theophylline Calcium Salicylate (Co-administration of estrogens with inducers of CYP3A4 may reduce plasma concentrations of estrogens, possibly resulting in a decrease in therapeutic effects and/or changes in the uterine bleeding profile).
No products indexed under this heading.

Theophylline Dihydroxypropyl (Glyceryl) (Co-administration of estrogens with inducers of CYP3A4 may reduce plasma concentrations of estrogens, possibly resulting in a decrease in therapeutic effects and/or changes in the uterine bleeding profile).
No products indexed under this heading.

Theophylline Ethylenediamine (Co-administration of estrogens with inducers of CYP3A4 may reduce plasma concentrations of estrogens, possibly resulting in a decrease in therapeutic effects and/or changes in the uterine bleeding profile).
No products indexed under this heading.

Triamcinolone (Co-administration of estrogens with inducers of CYP3A4 may reduce plasma concentrations of estrogens, possibly resulting in a decrease in therapeutic effects and/or changes in the uterine bleeding profile).
No products indexed under this heading.

Triamcinolone Acetonide (Co-administration of estrogens with inducers of CYP3A4 may reduce plasma concentrations of estrogens, possibly resulting in a decrease in therapeutic effects and/or changes in the uterine bleeding profile). Products include:
Azmacort Inhalation Aerosol 407
Nasacort AQ Nasal Spray 2765
Triesence Injectable Suspension .... ⊙ 209

Triamcinolone Diacetate (Co-administration of estrogens with inducers of CYP3A4 may reduce plasma concentrations of estrogens, possibly resulting in a decrease in therapeutic effects and/or changes in the uterine bleeding profile).
No products indexed under this heading.

Triamcinolone Hexacetonide (Co-administration of estrogens with inducers of CYP3A4 may reduce plasma concentrations of estrogens, possibly resulting in a decrease in therapeutic effects and/or changes in the uterine bleeding profile).
No products indexed under this heading.

Troglitazone (Co-administration of estrogens with inducers of CYP3A4 may reduce plasma concentrations of estrogens, possibly resulting in a decrease in therapeutic effects and/or changes in the uterine bleeding profile).
No products indexed under this heading.

Troleandomycin (Co-administration of estrogens with inhibitors of CYP3A4 may increase plasma concentrations of estrogens and may result in side effects).
No products indexed under this heading.

Valproate Sodium (Co-administration of estrogens with inhibitors of CYP3A4 may increase plasma concentrations of estrogens and may result in side effects).
No products indexed under this heading.

Vardenafil Hydrochloride (Co-administration of estrogens with inhibitors of CYP3A4 may increase plasma concentrations of estrogens and may result in side effects). Products include:
Levitra Tablets 2876

Verapamil Hydrochloride (Co-administration of estrogens with inhibitors of CYP3A4 may increase plasma concentrations of estrogens and may result in side effects). Products include:
Tarka Tablets 511

Voriconazole (Co-administration of estrogens with inhibitors of CYP3A4 may increase plasma concentrations of estrogens and may result in side effects).
No products indexed under this heading.

Zafirlukast (Co-administration of estrogens with inhibitors of CYP3A4 may increase plasma concentrations of estrogens and may result in side effects). Products include:
Accolate Tablets 669

Zileuton (Co-administration of estrogens with inhibitors of CYP3A4 may increase plasma concentrations of estrogens and may result in side effects).
No products indexed under this heading.

Food Interactions

Food, unspecified (Administration with a high fat breakfast decreased total estrone Cmax and increased total equilin Cmax compared to fasting state, no other effect on rate or extent of absorption; administration with food doubles MPA Cmax and increases MPA AUC).

Grapefruit (Co-administration of estrogens with inhibitors of CYP3A4 may increase plasma concentrations of estrogens and may result in side effects).

Grapefruit Juice (Co-administration of estrogens with inhibitors of CYP3A4, such as grapefruit juice, may increase plasma concentrations of estrogens and may result in side effects).

PREMPRO TABLETS
(Estrogens, Conjugated, Medroxyprogesterone Acetate).......... 3232
May interact with cytochrome p450 3a4 inducers (selected), cytochrome p450 3a4 inhibitors (selected), and certain other agents. Compounds in these categories include:

Acetazolamide (Co-administration of estrogens with inhibitors of CYP3A4 may increase plasma concentrations of estrogens and may result in side effects).
No products indexed under this heading.

Allium sativum (Co-administration of estrogens with inducers of CYP3A4 may reduce plasma concentrations of estrogens, possibly resulting in a decrease in therapeutic effects and/or changes in the uterine bleeding profile).
No products indexed under this heading.

Aminoglutethimide (Aminoglutethimide administered concomitantly with medroxyprogesterone acetate (MPA) may significantly depress the bioavailability of MPA).
No products indexed under this heading.

Amiodarone Hydrochloride (Co-administration of estrogens with inhibitors of CYP3A4 may increase plasma concentrations of estrogens and may result in side effects).
No products indexed under this heading.

Amprenavir (Co-administration of estrogens with inhibitors of CYP3A4 may increase plasma concentrations of estrogens and may result in side effects).
No products indexed under this heading.

Anastrozole (Co-administration of estrogens with inhibitors of CYP3A4 may increase plasma concentrations of estrogens and may result in side effects). Products include:
Arimidex Tablets 672

Aprepitant (Co-administration of estrogens with inducers of CYP3A4 may reduce plasma concentrations of estrogens, possibly resulting in a decrease in therapeutic effects and/or changes in the uterine bleeding profile). Products include:
Emend Capsules 1992

Atazanavir (Co-administration of estrogens with inhibitors of CYP3A4 may increase plasma concentrations of estrogens and may result in side effects).
No products indexed under this heading.

Atazanavir Sulfate (Co-administration of estrogens with inhibitors of CYP3A4 may increase plasma concentrations of estrogens and may result in side effects). Products include:
Reyataz Capsules 3299

Betamethasone Acetate (Co-administration of estrogens with inducers of CYP3A4 may reduce plasma concentrations of estrogens, possibly resulting in a decrease in therapeutic effects and/or changes in the uterine bleeding profile).
No products indexed under this heading.

Betamethasone Sodium Phosphate (Co-administration of estrogens with inducers of CYP3A4 may reduce plasma concentrations of estrogens, possibly resulting in a decrease in therapeutic effects and/or changes in the uterine bleeding profile).
No products indexed under this heading.

Carbamazepine (Co-administration of estrogens with inducers of CYP3A4 may reduce plasma concentrations of estrogens, possibly resulting in a decrease in therapeutic effects and/or changes in the uterine bleeding profile). Products include:
Carbatrol Capsules 3019
Equetro Extended-Release Capsules 3174

Cimetidine (Co-administration of estrogens with inhibitors of CYP3A4 may increase plasma concentrations of estrogens and may result in side effects).
No products indexed under this heading.

Cimetidine Hydrochloride (Co-administration of estrogens with inhibitors of CYP3A4 may increase plasma concentrations of estrogens and may result in side effects).
No products indexed under this heading.

Ciprofloxacin (Co-administration of estrogens with inhibitors of CYP3A4 may increase plasma concentrations of estrogens and may result in side effects). Products include:
Cipro I.V. 2817
Cipro Oral Suspension 2810
Cipro XR Tablets 2823
Ciprodex Otic Suspension 541

Ciprofloxacin Hydrochloride (Co-administration of estrogens with inducers of CYP3A4 may reduce plasma concentrations of estrogens, possibly resulting in a decrease in therapeutic effects and/or changes in the uterine bleeding profile). Products include:
Cipro Tablets 2810

Cisplatin (Co-administration of estrogens with inducers of CYP3A4 may reduce plasma concentrations of estrogens, possibly resulting in a decrease in therapeutic effects and/or changes in the uterine bleeding profile).
No products indexed under this heading.

Clarithromycin (Co-administration of estrogens with inhibitors of CYP3A4 may increase plasma concentrations of estrogens and may result in side effects). Products include:
Biaxin/Biaxin XL 411

Clotrimazole (Co-administration of estrogens with inhibitors of CYP3A4 may increase plasma concentrations of estrogens and may result in side effects). Products include:
Lotrisone 2881

Cortisone Acetate (Co-administration of estrogens with inducers of CYP3A4 may reduce plasma concentrations of estrogens, possibly resulting in a decrease in therapeutic effects and/or changes in the uterine bleeding profile).
No products indexed under this heading.

Cyclosporine (Co-administration of estrogens with inhibitors of CYP3A4 may increase plasma concentrations of estrogens and may result in side effects). Products include:
Gengraf Capsules 435
Neoral Oral Solution 2280
Neoral Soft Gelatin Capsules 2280
Restasis Ophthalmic Emulsion 557
Sandimmune 2296

Dalfopristin (Co-administration of estrogens with inhibitors of CYP3A4 may increase plasma concentrations of estrogens and may result in side effects).
No products indexed under this heading.

Danazol (Co-administration of estrogens with inhibitors of CYP3A4 may increase plasma concentrations of estrogens and may result in side effects).
No products indexed under this heading.

Delavirdine Mesylate (Co-administration of estrogens with inhibitors of CYP3A4 may increase plasma concentrations of estrogens and may result in side effects).
No products indexed under this heading.

Dexamethasone (Co-administration of estrogens with inducers of CYP3A4 may reduce plasma concentrations of estrogens, possibly resulting in a decrease in therapeutic effects and/or changes in the uterine bleeding profile). Products include:
Ciprodex Otic Suspension 541

Dexamethasone Acetate (Co-administration of estrogens with inducers of CYP3A4 may reduce plasma concentrations of estrogens, possibly resulting in a decrease in therapeutic effects and/or changes in the uterine bleeding profile).
No products indexed under this heading.

Dexamethasone Sodium Phosphate (Co-administration of estrogens with inducers of CYP3A4 may reduce plasma concentrations of estrogens, possibly resulting in a decrease in therapeutic effects and/or changes in the uterine bleeding profile).
No products indexed under this heading.

Diltiazem Hydrochloride (Co-administration of estrogens with inhibitors of CYP3A4 may increase plasma concentrations of estrogens and may result in side effects). Products include:
Cardizem LA Extended Release Tablets 421

Diltiazem Maleate (Co-administration of estrogens with inhibitors of CYP3A4 may increase plasma concentrations of estrogens and may result in side effects).
No products indexed under this heading.

Doxorubicin Hydrochloride (Co-administration of estrogens with inducers of CYP3A4 may reduce plasma concentrations of estrogens, possibly resulting in a decrease in therapeutic effects and/or changes in the uterine bleeding profile).
No products indexed under this heading.

Efavirenz (Co-administration of estrogens with inducers of CYP3A4 may reduce plasma concentrations of estrogens, possibly resulting in a decrease in therapeutic effects and/or changes in the uterine bleeding profile). Products include:
Atripla Tablets 938
Sustiva Capsules 930
Sustiva Tablets 930

Erythromycin (Co-administration of estrogens with inhibitors of CYP3A4 may increase plasma concentrations of estrogens and may result in side effects).
No products indexed under this heading.

Erythromycin Estolate (Co-administration of estrogens with inhibitors of CYP3A4 may increase plasma concentrations of estrogens and may result in side effects).
No products indexed under this heading.

Erythromycin Ethylsuccinate (Co-administration of estrogens with inhibitors of CYP3A4 may increase plasma concentrations of estrogens and may result in side effects). Products include:
E.E.S. 433
EryPed 431

Erythromycin Gluceptate (Co-administration of estrogens with inhibitors of CYP3A4 may increase plasma concentrations of estrogens and may result in side effects).
No products indexed under this heading.

Erythromycin Lactobionate (Co-administration of estrogens with inhibitors of CYP3A4 may increase plasma concentrations of estrogens and may result in side effects).
No products indexed under this heading.

Erythromycin Stearate (Co-administration of estrogens with inhibitors of CYP3A4 may increase plasma concentrations of estrogens and may result in side effects).
No products indexed under this heading.

Esomeprazole Magnesium (Co-administration of estrogens with inhibitors of CYP3A4 may increase plasma concentrations of estrogens and may result in side effects). Products include:
Nexium Delayed-Release Capsules 645
Nexium Delayed-Release Oral Suspension 645

Ethosuximide (Co-administration of estrogens with inducers of CYP3A4 may reduce plasma concentrations of estrogens, possibly resulting in a decrease in therapeutic effects and/or changes in the uterine bleeding profile).
No products indexed under this heading.

Felbamate (Co-administration of estrogens with inducers of CYP3A4 may reduce plasma concentrations of estrogens, possibly resulting in a decrease in therapeutic effects and/or changes in the uterine bleeding profile).
No products indexed under this heading.

Fluconazole (Co-administration of estrogens with inhibitors of CYP3A4 may increase plasma concentrations of estrogens and may result in side effects).
No products indexed under this heading.

Fludrocortisone Acetate (Co-administration of estrogens with inducers of CYP3A4 may reduce plasma concentrations of estrogens, possibly resulting in a decrease in therapeutic effects and/or changes in the uterine bleeding profile).
No products indexed under this heading.

Fluoxetine (Co-administration of estrogens with inhibitors of CYP3A4 may increase plasma concentrations of estrogens and may result in side effects).
No products indexed under this heading.

Fluoxetine Hydrochloride (Co-administration of estrogens with inhibitors of CYP3A4 may increase plasma concentrations of estrogens and may result in side effects). Products include:
Prozac Weekly Capsules 1852
Prozac Pulvules and Liquid 1852
Symbyax Capsules 1871

Fluvoxamine Maleate (Co-administration of estrogens with inhibitors of CYP3A4 may increase plasma concentrations of estrogens and may result in side effects). Products include:
Luvox CR Extended-Release Capsules 1759

Fosamprenavir Calcium (Co-administration of estrogens with inhibitors of CYP3A4 may increase plasma concentrations of estrogens and may result in side effects). Products include:
Lexiva Oral Suspension 1510
Lexiva Tablets 1510

Fosphenytoin Sodium (Co-administration of estrogens with inducers of CYP3A4 may reduce plasma concentrations of estrogens, possibly resulting in a decrease in therapeutic effects and/or changes in the uterine bleeding profile).
No products indexed under this heading.

Garlic Extract (Co-administration of estrogens with inducers of CYP3A4 may reduce plasma concentrations of estrogens, possibly resulting in a decrease in therapeutic effects and/or changes in the uterine bleeding profile).
No products indexed under this heading.

Garlic Oil (Co-administration of estrogens with inducers of CYP3A4 may reduce plasma concentrations of estrogens, possibly resulting in a decrease in therapeutic effects and/or changes in the uterine bleeding profile).
No products indexed under this heading.

Hydrocortisone (Co-administration of estrogens with inducers of CYP3A4 may reduce plasma concentrations of estrogens, possibly resulting in a decrease in therapeutic effects and/or changes in the uterine bleeding profile).
No products indexed under this heading.

Hydrocortisone Acetate (Co-administration of estrogens with inducers of CYP3A4 may reduce plasma concentrations of estrogens, possibly resulting in a decrease in therapeutic effects and/or changes in the uterine bleeding profile). Products include:
Analpram-HC 1140
Pramosone 1141

Hydrocortisone Butyrate (Co-administration of estrogens with inducers of CYP3A4 may reduce plasma concentrations of estrogens, possibly resulting in a decrease in therapeutic effects and/or changes in the uterine bleeding profile).
No products indexed under this heading.

Hydrocortisone Cypionate (Co-administration of estrogens with inducers of CYP3A4 may reduce plasma concentrations of estrogens, possibly resulting in a decrease in therapeutic effects and/or changes in the uterine bleeding profile).
No products indexed under this heading.

Hydrocortisone Hemisuccinate (Co-administration of estrogens with inducers of CYP3A4 may reduce plasma concentrations of estrogens, possibly resulting in a decrease in therapeutic effects and/or changes in the uterine bleeding profile).
No products indexed under this heading.

Hydrocortisone Probutate (Co-administration of estrogens with inducers of CYP3A4 may reduce plasma concentrations of estrogens, possibly resulting in a decrease in therapeutic effects and/or changes in the uterine bleeding profile).
No products indexed under this heading.

Hydrocortisone Sodium Phosphate (Co-administration of estrogens with inducers of CYP3A4 may reduce plasma concentrations of estrogens, possibly resulting in a decrease in therapeutic effects and/or changes in the uterine bleeding profile).
No products indexed under this heading.

Hydrocortisone Sodium Succinate (Co-administration of estrogens with inducers of CYP3A4 may reduce plasma concentrations of estrogens, possibly resulting in a decrease in therapeutic effects and/or changes in the uterine bleeding profile).
No products indexed under this heading.

Hydrocortisone Valerate (Co-administration of estrogens with inducers of CYP3A4 may reduce plasma concentrations of estrogens, possibly resulting in a decrease in therapeutic effects and/or changes in the uterine bleeding profile).
No products indexed under this heading.

Hypericum (Co-administration of estrogens with inducers of CYP3A4 may reduce plasma concentrations

of estrogens, possibly resulting in a decrease in therapeutic effects and/or changes in the uterine bleeding profile). Products include:

Satieté Tablets .... ◙640

Hypericum Perforatum (Co-administration of estrogens with inducers of CYP3A4 may reduce plasma concentrations of estrogens, possibly resulting in a decrease in therapeutic effects and/or changes in the uterine bleeding profile).

No products indexed under this heading.

Indinavir Sulfate (Co-administration of estrogens with inhibitors of CYP3A4 may increase plasma concentrations of estrogens and may result in side effects). Products include:

Crixivan Capsules 1979

Isoniazid (Co-administration of estrogens with inhibitors of CYP3A4 may increase plasma concentrations of estrogens and may result in side effects).

No products indexed under this heading.

Itraconazole (Co-administration of estrogens with inhibitors of CYP3A4 may increase plasma concentrations of estrogens and may result in side effects).

No products indexed under this heading.

Ketoconazole (Co-administration of estrogens with inhibitors of CYP3A4 may increase plasma concentrations of estrogens and may result in side effects). Products include:

Extina Foam, 2% 3057
Nizoral A-D Shampoo 1901

Lopinavir (Co-administration of estrogens with inhibitors of CYP3A4 may increase plasma concentrations of estrogens and may result in side effects). Products include:

Kaletra 452

Loratadine (Co-administration of estrogens with inhibitors of CYP3A4 may increase plasma concentrations of estrogens and may result in side effects).

No products indexed under this heading.

Mephenytoin (Co-administration of estrogens with inducers of CYP3A4 may reduce plasma concentrations of estrogens, possibly resulting in a decrease in therapeutic effects and/or changes in the uterine bleeding profile).

No products indexed under this heading.

Methsuximide (Co-administration of estrogens with inducers of CYP3A4 may reduce plasma concentrations of estrogens, possibly resulting in a decrease in therapeutic effects and/or changes in the uterine bleeding profile).

No products indexed under this heading.

Methylprednisolone (Co-administration of estrogens with inducers of CYP3A4 may reduce plasma concentrations of estrogens, possibly resulting in a decrease in therapeutic effects and/or changes in the uterine bleeding profile).

No products indexed under this heading.

Methylprednisolone Acetate (Co-administration of estrogens with inducers of CYP3A4 may reduce plasma concentrations of estrogens, possibly resulting in a decrease in therapeutic effects and/or changes in the uterine bleeding profile).

No products indexed under this heading.

Methylprednisolone Sodium Succinate (Co-administration of estrogens with inducers of CYP3A4 may reduce plasma concentrations of estrogens, possibly resulting in a decrease in therapeutic effects and/or changes in the uterine bleeding profile).

No products indexed under this heading.

Metronidazole (Co-administration of estrogens with inhibitors of CYP3A4 may increase plasma concentrations of estrogens and may result in side effects). Products include:

Pylera Capsules 714

Metronidazole Benzoate (Co-administration of estrogens with inhibitors of CYP3A4 may increase plasma concentrations of estrogens and may result in side effects).

No products indexed under this heading.

Metronidazole Hydrochloride (Co-administration of estrogens with inhibitors of CYP3A4 may increase plasma concentrations of estrogens and may result in side effects).

No products indexed under this heading.

Miconazole (Co-administration of estrogens with inhibitors of CYP3A4 may increase plasma concentrations of estrogens and may result in side effects).

No products indexed under this heading.

Miconazole Nitrate (Co-administration of estrogens with inhibitors of CYP3A4 may increase plasma concentrations of estrogens and may result in side effects).

No products indexed under this heading.

Modafinil (Co-administration of estrogens with inducers of CYP3A4 may reduce plasma concentrations of estrogens, possibly resulting in a decrease in therapeutic effects and/or changes in the uterine bleeding profile). Products include:

Provigil Tablets 977

Nefazodone Hydrochloride (Co-administration of estrogens with inhibitors of CYP3A4 may increase plasma concentrations of estrogens and may result in side effects).

No products indexed under this heading.

Nelfinavir Mesylate (Co-administration of estrogens with inhibitors of CYP3A4 may increase plasma concentrations of estrogens and may result in side effects).

No products indexed under this heading.

Nevirapine (Co-administration of estrogens with inducers of CYP3A4 may reduce plasma concentrations of estrogens, possibly resulting in a decrease in therapeutic effects and/or changes in the uterine bleeding profile). Products include:

Viramune Oral Suspension 873
Viramune Tablets 873

Niacinamide (Co-administration of estrogens with inhibitors of CYP3A4 may increase plasma concentrations of estrogens and may result in side effects). Products include:

BioLean Free Tablets .... ◙635

Nicotinamide (Co-administration of estrogens with inhibitors of CYP3A4 may increase plasma concentrations of estrogens and may result in side effects).

No products indexed under this heading.

Nifedipine (Co-administration of estrogens with inhibitors of CYP3A4 may increase plasma concentrations of estrogens and may result in side effects).

No products indexed under this heading.

Norfloxacin (Co-administration of estrogens with inhibitors of CYP3A4 may increase plasma concentrations of estrogens and may result in side effects). Products include:

Noroxin Tablets 2069

Omeprazole (Co-administration of estrogens with inhibitors of CYP3A4 may increase plasma concentrations of estrogens and may result in side effects).

No products indexed under this heading.

Oxcarbazepine (Co-administration of estrogens with inducers of CYP3A4 may reduce plasma concentrations of estrogens, possibly resulting in a decrease in therapeutic effects and/or changes in the uterine bleeding profile).

No products indexed under this heading.

Paroxetine Hydrochloride (Co-administration of estrogens with inhibitors of CYP3A4 may increase plasma concentrations of estrogens and may result in side effects). Products include:

Paxil 1535
Paxil CR Controlled-Release Tablets 1544

Phenobarbital (Co-administration of estrogens with inducers of CYP3A4 may reduce plasma concentrations of estrogens, possibly resulting in a decrease in therapeutic effects and/or changes in the uterine bleeding profile). Products include:

Donnatal Extentabs 2507

Phenobarbital Sodium (Co-administration of estrogens with inducers of CYP3A4 may reduce plasma concentrations of estrogens, possibly resulting in a decrease in therapeutic effects and/or changes in the uterine bleeding profile).

No products indexed under this heading.

Phenytoin (Co-administration of estrogens with inducers of CYP3A4 may reduce plasma concentrations of estrogens, possibly resulting in a decrease in therapeutic effects and/or changes in the uterine bleeding profile).

No products indexed under this heading.

Phenytoin Sodium (Co-administration of estrogens with inducers of CYP3A4 may reduce plasma concentrations of estrogens, possibly resulting in a decrease in therapeutic effects and/or changes in the uterine bleeding profile). Products include:

Phenytek Capsules 2192

Prednisolone Acetate (Co-administration of estrogens with inducers of CYP3A4 may reduce plasma concentrations of estrogens, possibly resulting in a decrease in therapeutic effects and/or changes in the uterine bleeding profile). Products include:

Pred Forte Ophthalmic Suspension .... ⊙227
Pred Mild Ophthalmic Suspension .... ⊙230
Pred-G Ophthalmic Ointment .... ⊙229
Pred-G Ophthalmic Suspension ...... ⊙228

Prednisolone Sodium Phosphate (Co-administration of estrogens with inducers of CYP3A4 may reduce plasma concentrations of estrogens, possibly resulting in a decrease in therapeutic effects and/or changes in the uterine bleeding profile).

No products indexed under this heading.

Prednisolone Tebutate (Co-administration of estrogens with inducers of CYP3A4 may reduce plasma concentrations of estrogens, possibly resulting in a decrease in therapeutic effects and/or changes in the uterine bleeding profile).

No products indexed under this heading.

Prednisone (Co-administration of estrogens with inducers of CYP3A4 may reduce plasma concentrations of estrogens, possibly resulting in a decrease in therapeutic effects and/or changes in the uterine bleeding profile).

No products indexed under this heading.

Primidone (Co-administration of estrogens with inducers of CYP3A4 may reduce plasma concentrations of estrogens, possibly resulting in a decrease in therapeutic effects and/or changes in the uterine bleeding profile).

No products indexed under this heading.

Propoxyphene Hydrochloride (Co-administration of estrogens with inhibitors of CYP3A4 may increase plasma concentrations of estrogens and may result in side effects).

No products indexed under this heading.

Propoxyphene Napsylate (Co-administration of estrogens with inhibitors of CYP3A4 may increase plasma concentrations of estrogens and may result in side effects).

No products indexed under this heading.

Quinidine (Co-administration of estrogens with inhibitors of CYP3A4 may increase plasma concentrations of estrogens and may result in side effects).

No products indexed under this heading.

Quinidine Hydrochloride (Co-administration of estrogens with inhibitors of CYP3A4 may increase plasma concentrations of estrogens and may result in side effects).

No products indexed under this heading.

Quinidine Polygalacturonate (Co-administration of estrogens with inhibitors of CYP3A4 may increase plasma concentrations of estrogens and may result in side effects).

No products indexed under this heading.

Quinidine Sulfate (Co-administration of estrogens with inhibitors of CYP3A4 may increase plasma concentrations of estrogens and may result in side effects).
No products indexed under this heading.

Quinine (Co-administration of estrogens with inhibitors of CYP3A4 may increase plasma concentrations of estrogens and may result in side effects).
No products indexed under this heading.

Quinine Sulfate (Co-administration of estrogens with inhibitors of CYP3A4 may increase plasma concentrations of estrogens and may result in side effects).
No products indexed under this heading.

Quinupristin (Co-administration of estrogens with inhibitors of CYP3A4 may increase plasma concentrations of estrogens and may result in side effects).
No products indexed under this heading.

Ranitidine Bismuth Citrate (Co-administration of estrogens with inhibitors of CYP3A4 may increase plasma concentrations of estrogens and may result in side effects).
No products indexed under this heading.

Ranitidine Hydrochloride (Co-administration of estrogens with inhibitors of CYP3A4 may increase plasma concentrations of estrogens and may result in side effects). Products include:
Zantac 75 Tablets 603
Zantac 1670
Zantac Injection 1666
Zantac Injection Pharmacy Bulk Package 1668
Maximum Strength Zantac 150 Tablets 603
Maximum Strength Zantac 150 Cool Mint Tablets 603

Rifabutin (Co-administration of estrogens with inducers of CYP3A4 may reduce plasma concentrations of estrogens, possibly resulting in a decrease in therapeutic effects and/or changes in the uterine bleeding profile).
No products indexed under this heading.

Rifampicin (Co-administration of estrogens with inducers of CYP3A4 may reduce plasma concentrations of estrogens, possibly resulting in a decrease in therapeutic effects and/or changes in the uterine bleeding profile).
No products indexed under this heading.

Rifampin (Co-administration of estrogens with inducers of CYP3A4 may reduce plasma concentrations of estrogens, possibly resulting in a decrease in therapeutic effects and/or changes in the uterine bleeding profile).
No products indexed under this heading.

Rifapentine (Co-administration of estrogens with inducers of CYP3A4 may reduce plasma concentrations of estrogens, possibly resulting in a decrease in therapeutic effects and/or changes in the uterine bleeding profile).
No products indexed under this heading.

Ritonavir (Co-administration of estrogens with inhibitors of CYP3A4 may increase plasma concentrations of estrogens and may result in side effects). Products include:
Kaletra 452
Norvir 489

Saquinavir (Co-administration of estrogens with inhibitors of CYP3A4 may increase plasma concentrations of estrogens and may result in side effects).
No products indexed under this heading.

Saquinavir Mesylate (Co-administration of estrogens with inhibitors of CYP3A4 may increase plasma concentrations of estrogens and may result in side effects).
No products indexed under this heading.

Sertraline Hydrochloride (Co-administration of estrogens with inhibitors of CYP3A4 may increase plasma concentrations of estrogens and may result in side effects).
No products indexed under this heading.

Sildenafil Citrate (Co-administration of estrogens with inhibitors of CYP3A4 may increase plasma concentrations of estrogens and may result in side effects).
No products indexed under this heading.

Sulfinpyrazone (Co-administration of estrogens with inducers of CYP3A4 may reduce plasma concentrations of estrogens, possibly resulting in a decrease in therapeutic effects and/or changes in the uterine bleeding profile).
No products indexed under this heading.

Telithromycin (Co-administration of estrogens with inhibitors of CYP3A4 may increase plasma concentrations of estrogens and may result in side effects). Products include:
Ketek Tablets 2744

Theophylline (Co-administration of estrogens with inducers of CYP3A4 may reduce plasma concentrations of estrogens, possibly resulting in a decrease in therapeutic effects and/or changes in the uterine bleeding profile).
No products indexed under this heading.

Theophylline Anhydrous (Co-administration of estrogens with inducers of CYP3A4 may reduce plasma concentrations of estrogens, possibly resulting in a decrease in therapeutic effects and/or changes in the uterine bleeding profile). Products include:
Uniphyl Tablets 2595

Theophylline Calcium Salicylate (Co-administration of estrogens with inducers of CYP3A4 may reduce plasma concentrations of estrogens, possibly resulting in a decrease in therapeutic effects and/or changes in the uterine bleeding profile).
No products indexed under this heading.

Theophylline Dihydroxypropyl (Glyceryl) (Co-administration of estrogens with inducers of CYP3A4 may reduce plasma concentrations of estrogens, possibly resulting in a decrease in therapeutic effects and/or changes in the uterine bleeding profile).
No products indexed under this heading.

Theophylline Ethylenediamine (Co-administration of estrogens with inducers of CYP3A4 may reduce plasma concentrations of estrogens, possibly resulting in a decrease in therapeutic effects and/or changes in the uterine bleeding profile).
No products indexed under this heading.

Triamcinolone (Co-administration of estrogens with inducers of CYP3A4 may reduce plasma concentrations of estrogens, possibly resulting in a decrease in therapeutic effects and/or changes in the uterine bleeding profile).
No products indexed under this heading.

Triamcinolone Acetonide (Co-administration of estrogens with inducers of CYP3A4 may reduce plasma concentrations of estrogens, possibly resulting in a decrease in therapeutic effects and/or changes in the uterine bleeding profile). Products include:
Azmacort Inhalation Aerosol 407
Nasacort AQ Nasal Spray 2765
Triesence Injectable Suspension .... ⊙ 209

Triamcinolone Diacetate (Co-administration of estrogens with inducers of CYP3A4 may reduce plasma concentrations of estrogens, possibly resulting in a decrease in therapeutic effects and/or changes in the uterine bleeding profile).
No products indexed under this heading.

Triamcinolone Hexacetonide (Co-administration of estrogens with inducers of CYP3A4 may reduce plasma concentrations of estrogens, possibly resulting in a decrease in therapeutic effects and/or changes in the uterine bleeding profile).
No products indexed under this heading.

Troglitazone (Co-administration of estrogens with inducers of CYP3A4 may reduce plasma concentrations of estrogens, possibly resulting in a decrease in therapeutic effects and/or changes in the uterine bleeding profile).
No products indexed under this heading.

Troleandomycin (Co-administration of estrogens with inhibitors of CYP3A4 may increase plasma concentrations of estrogens and may result in side effects).
No products indexed under this heading.

Valproate Sodium (Co-administration of estrogens with inhibitors of CYP3A4 may increase plasma concentrations of estrogens and may result in side effects).
No products indexed under this heading.

Vardenafil Hydrochloride (Co-administration of estrogens with inhibitors of CYP3A4 may increase plasma concentrations of estrogens and may result in side effects). Products include:
Levitra Tablets 2876

Verapamil Hydrochloride (Co-administration of estrogens with inhibitors of CYP3A4 may increase plasma concentrations of estrogens and may result in side effects). Products include:
Tarka Tablets 511

Voriconazole (Co-administration of estrogens with inhibitors of CYP3A4 may increase plasma concentrations of estrogens and may result in side effects).
No products indexed under this heading.

Zafirlukast (Co-administration of estrogens with inhibitors of CYP3A4 may increase plasma concentrations of estrogens and may result in side effects). Products include:
Accolate Tablets 669

Zileuton (Co-administration of estrogens with inhibitors of CYP3A4 may increase plasma concentrations of estrogens and may result in side effects).
No products indexed under this heading.

Food Interactions

Food, unspecified (Administration with food decreased Cmax of total estrone compared to fasting state, no other effect on rate or extent of absorption; administration with food doubles MPA Cmax and increases MPA AUC).

Grapefruit (Co-administration of estrogens with inhibitors of CYP3A4 may increase plasma concentrations of estrogens and may result in side effects).

Grapefruit Juice (Co-administration of estrogens with inhibitors of CYP3A4, such as grapefruit juice, may increase plasma concentrations of estrogens and may result in side effects).

PREVNAR

(Pneumococcal vaccine, diphtheria conjugate) 3241
May interact with alkylating agents, antimetabolites, anticoagulants, corticosteroids, cytotoxic drugs, and immunosuppressive agents. Compounds in these categories include:

Anisindione (Prevnar should be given with caution to children on anticoagulant therapy).
No products indexed under this heading.

Ardeparin Sodium (Prevnar should be given with caution to children on anticoagulant therapy).
No products indexed under this heading.

Azathioprine (Children receiving immunosuppressive therapy may not respond optimally to active immunization).
No products indexed under this heading.

Basiliximab (Children receiving immunosuppressive therapy may not respond optimally to active immunization). Products include:
Simulect for Injection 2306

Betamethasone Acetate (Children receiving large doses of corticosteroids for immunosuppressive therapy may not respond optimally to active immunization).
No products indexed under this heading.

Betamethasone Sodium Phosphate (Children receiving large doses of corticosteroids for immunosuppressive therapy may not respond optimally to active immunization).
No products indexed under this heading.

Bleomycin Sulfate (Children receiving cytotoxic agents may not respond optimally to active immunization).
No products indexed under this heading.

Budesonide (Children receiving large doses of corticosteroids for immunosuppressive therapy may not respond optimally to active immunization). Products include:
Pulmicort Flexhaler 654
Symbicort 80/4.5 Inhalation Aerosol 659
Symbicort 160/4.5 Inhalation Aerosol 659

Busulfan (Children receiving alkylating agents may not respond optimally to active immunization). Products include:
Busulfex Injection 2477
Myleran Tablets 1530

Capecitabine (Children receiving antimetabolite agents may not respond optimally to active immunization). Products include:
Xeloda Tablets 2662

Carmustine (BCNU) (Children receiving alkylating agents may not respond optimally to active immunization).
No products indexed under this heading.

Chlorambucil (Children receiving alkylating agents may not respond optimally to active immunization). Products include:
Leukeran Tablets 1508

Ciclesonide (Children receiving large doses of corticosteroids for immunosuppressive therapy may not respond optimally to active immunization). Products include:
Alvesco Inhalation Aerosol 2985
Omnaris Nasal Spray 2998

Cladribine (Children receiving antimetabolite agents may not respond optimally to active immunization). Products include:
Leustatin Injection 2384

Cortisone Acetate (Children receiving large doses of corticosteroids for immunosuppressive therapy may not respond optimally to active immunization).
No products indexed under this heading.

Cyclophosphamide (Children receiving cytotoxic agents may not respond optimally to active immunization).
No products indexed under this heading.

Cyclosporine (Children receiving immunosuppressive therapy may not respond optimally to active immunization). Products include:
Gengraf Capsules 435
Neoral Oral Solution 2280
Neoral Soft Gelatin Capsules 2280
Restasis Ophthalmic Emulsion 557
Sandimmune 2296

Cytarabine (Children receiving antimetabolite agents may not respond optimally to active immunization).
No products indexed under this heading.

Dacarbazine (Children receiving alkylating agents may not respond optimally to active immunization).
No products indexed under this heading.

Dalteparin Sodium (Prevnar should be given with caution to children on anticoagulant therapy). Products include:
Fragmin Injection 1070

Danaparoid Sodium (Prevnar should be given with caution to children on anticoagulant therapy).
No products indexed under this heading.

Daunorubicin Hydrochloride (Children receiving cytotoxic agents may not respond optimally to active immunization).
No products indexed under this heading.

Dexamethasone (Children receiving large doses of corticosteroids for immunosuppressive therapy may not respond optimally to active immunization). Products include:
Ciprodex Otic Suspension 541

Dexamethasone Acetate (Children receiving large doses of corticosteroids for immunosuppressive therapy may not respond optimally to active immunization).
No products indexed under this heading.

Dexamethasone Sodium Phosphate (Children receiving large doses of corticosteroids for immunosuppressive therapy may not respond optimally to active immunization).
No products indexed under this heading.

Dicumarol (Prevnar should be given with caution to children on anticoagulant therapy).
No products indexed under this heading.

Doxorubicin Hydrochloride (Children receiving cytotoxic agents may not respond optimally to active immunization).
No products indexed under this heading.

Enoxaparin Sodium (Prevnar should be given with caution to children on anticoagulant therapy). Products include:
Lovenox Injection 2756

Epirubicin Hydrochloride (Children receiving cytotoxic agents may not respond optimally to active immunization).
No products indexed under this heading.

Floxuridine (Children receiving antimetabolite agents may not respond optimally to active immunization).
No products indexed under this heading.

Fludarabine Phosphate (Children receiving antimetabolite agents may not respond optimally to active immunization).
No products indexed under this heading.

Fludrocortisone Acetate (Children receiving large doses of corticosteroids for immunosuppressive therapy may not respond optimally to active immunization).
No products indexed under this heading.

Flunisolide (Children receiving large doses of corticosteroids for immunosuppressive therapy may not respond optimally to active immunization). Products include:
Aerobid/Aerobid-M 1153

Fluorouracil (Children receiving cytotoxic agents may not respond optimally to active immunization). Products include:
Carac Cream 0.5% 2722

Fluticasone Propionate (Children receiving large doses of corticosteroids for immunosuppressive therapy may not respond optimally to active immunization). Products include:
Advair Diskus 100/50 1276
Advair Diskus 250/50 1276
Advair Diskus 500/50 1276
Advair HFA 45/21 Inhalation Aerosol 1288
Advair HFA 115/21 Inhalation Aerosol 1288
Advair HFA 230/21 Inhalation Aerosol 1288
Flonase Nasal Spray 1431
Flovent Diskus 50 mcg 1435

Fluticasone Propionate HFA (Children receiving large doses of corticosteroids for immunosuppressive therapy may not respond optimally to active immunization). Products include:
Flovent HFA 1440

Fondaparinux Sodium (Prevnar should be given with caution to children on anticoagulant therapy). Products include:
Arixtra Injection 1313

Gemcitabine Hydrochloride (Children receiving antimetabolite agents may not respond optimally to active immunization). Products include:
Gemzar for Injection 1820

Heparin Calcium (Prevnar should be given with caution to children on anticoagulant therapy).
No products indexed under this heading.

Heparin Sodium (Prevnar should be given with caution to children on anticoagulant therapy).
No products indexed under this heading.

Hydrocortisone (Children receiving large doses of corticosteroids for immunosuppressive therapy may not respond optimally to active immunization).
No products indexed under this heading.

Hydrocortisone Acetate (Children receiving large doses of corticosteroids for immunosuppressive therapy may not respond optimally to active immunization). Products include:
Analpram-HC 1140
Pramosone 1141

Hydrocortisone Sodium Phosphate (Children receiving large doses of corticosteroids for immunosuppressive therapy may not respond optimally to active immunization).
No products indexed under this heading.

Hydrocortisone Sodium Succinate (Children receiving large doses of corticosteroids for immunosuppressive therapy may not respond optimally to active immunization).
No products indexed under this heading.

Hydroxyurea (Children receiving cytotoxic agents may not respond optimally to active immunization).
No products indexed under this heading.

Lomustine (CCNU) (Children receiving alkylating agents may not respond optimally to active immunization).
No products indexed under this heading.

Low Molecular Weight Heparins (Prevnar should be given with caution to children on anticoagulant therapy).
No products indexed under this heading.

Mechlorethamine Hydrochloride (Children receiving alkylating agents may not respond optimally to active immunization). Products include:
Mustargen for Injection 2492

Melphalan (Children receiving alkylating agents may not respond optimally to active immunization).
No products indexed under this heading.

Mercaptopurine (Children receiving antimetabolite agents may not respond optimally to active immunization).
No products indexed under this heading.

Methotrexate (Children receiving antimetabolite agents may not respond optimally to active immunization).
No products indexed under this heading.

Methotrexate Sodium (Children receiving cytotoxic agents may not respond optimally to active immunization).
No products indexed under this heading.

Methylprednisolone Acetate (Children receiving large doses of corticosteroids for immunosuppressive therapy may not respond optimally to active immunization).
No products indexed under this heading.

Methylprednisolone Sodium Succinate (Children receiving large doses of corticosteroids for immunosuppressive therapy may not respond optimally to active immunization).
No products indexed under this heading.

Mitotane (Children receiving cytotoxic agents may not respond optimally to active immunization).
No products indexed under this heading.

Mitoxantrone Hydrochloride (Children receiving cytotoxic agents may not respond optimally to active immunization). Products include:
Novantrone for Injection Concentrate 1100

Mometasone Furoate (Children receiving large doses of corticosteroids for immunosuppressive therapy may not respond optimally to active immunization). Products include:
Asmanex Twisthaler 2797
Elocon Cream 0.1% 2840
Elocon Lotion 0.1% 2841
Elocon Ointment 0.1% 2842

Mometasone Furoate Monohydrate (Children receiving large doses of corticosteroids for immunosuppressive therapy may not respond optimally to active immunization). Products include:
Nasonex Nasal Spray 2883

Muromonab-CD3 (Children receiving immunosuppressive therapy may not respond optimally to active immunization). Products include:
Orthoclone OKT3 Sterile Solution 2387

Mycophenolate Mofetil (Children receiving immunosuppressive therapy may not respond optimally to active immunization). Products include:
CellCept Capsules 2622
CellCept Oral Suspension 2622
CellCept Tablets 2622

Pentostatin (Children receiving antimetabolite agents may not respond optimally to active immunization).
No products indexed under this heading.

Prednisolone Acetate (Children receiving large doses of corticosteroids for immunosuppressive therapy may not respond optimally to active immunization). Products include:
Pred Forte Ophthalmic Suspension .... ⊙ 227
Pred Mild Ophthalmic Suspension .... ⊙ 230
Pred-G Ophthalmic Ointment .... ⊙ 229
Pred-G Ophthalmic Suspension ...... ⊙ 228

Prednisolone Sodium Phosphate (Children receiving large doses of corticosteroids for immunosuppressive therapy may not respond optimally to active immunization).
No products indexed under this heading.

Prednisolone Tebutate (Children receiving large doses of corticosteroids for immunosuppressive therapy may not respond optimally to active immunization).
No products indexed under this heading.

Prednisone (Children receiving large doses of corticosteroids for immunosuppressive therapy may not respond optimally to active immunization).
No products indexed under this heading.

Procarbazine Hydrochloride (Children receiving cytotoxic agents may not respond optimally to active immunization).
No products indexed under this heading.

Sirolimus (Children receiving immunosuppressive therapy may not respond optimally to active immunization). Products include:
Rapamune 3260

Tacrolimus (Children receiving immunosuppressive therapy may not respond optimally to active immunization). Products include:
Prograf Capsules and Injection 622
Protopic Ointment 628

Tamoxifen Citrate (Children receiving cytotoxic agents may not respond optimally to active immunization).
No products indexed under this heading.

Thioguanine (Children receiving antimetabolite agents may not respond optimally to active immunization). Products include:
Tabloid Tablets 1601

Thiotepa (Children receiving alkylating agents may not respond optimally to active immunization).
No products indexed under this heading.

Tinzaparin Sodium (Prevnar should be given with caution to children on anticoagulant therapy).
No products indexed under this heading.

Triamcinolone (Children receiving large doses of corticosteroids for immunosuppressive therapy may not respond optimally to active immunization).
No products indexed under this heading.

Triamcinolone Acetonide (Children receiving large doses of corticosteroids for immunosuppressive therapy may not respond optimally to active immunization). Products include:
Azmacort Inhalation Aerosol 407
Nasacort AQ Nasal Spray 2765
Triesence Injectable Suspension .... ⊙ 209

Triamcinolone Diacetate (Children receiving large doses of corticosteroids for immunosuppressive therapy may not respond optimally to active immunization).
No products indexed under this heading.

Triamcinolone Hexacetonide (Children receiving large doses of corticosteroids for immunosuppressive therapy may not respond optimally to active immunization).
No products indexed under this heading.

Vincristine Sulfate (Children receiving cytotoxic agents may not respond optimally to active immunization).
No products indexed under this heading.

Warfarin Sodium (Prevnar should be given with caution to children on anticoagulant therapy).
No products indexed under this heading.

PRILOSEC OTC TABLETS

(Omeprazole Magnesium) 2565
None cited in PDR database.

PRIMAXIN I.M.

(Cilastatin Sodium, Imipenem) 2080
See Primaxin I.V.

PRIMAXIN I.V.

(Cilastatin Sodium, Imipenem) 2083
May interact with:

Ganciclovir Sodium (Concomitant administration may result in generalized seizures).
No products indexed under this heading.

Probenecid (Concomitant administration results in only minimal increase in plasma levels of imipenem; concomitant administration not recommended).
No products indexed under this heading.

Valproic Acid (Decreased serum levels of valproic acid have been reported when co-administered with carbapenem antibiotics. Seizure may result due to co-administration. Careful monitoring of serum levels of valproic acid should be considered if imipenem is to be co-administered with valproic acid).
No products indexed under this heading.

PRINIVIL TABLETS

(Lisinopril) 2087
May interact with diuretics, oral hypoglycemic agents, insulin, lithium preparations, non-steroidal anti-inflammatory agents, potassium preparations, potassium sparing diuretics, thiazides, and certain other agents. Compounds in these categories include:

Acarbose (Epidemiological studies have suggested that concomitant administration of ACE inhibitors and antidiabetic medicines (insulins, oral hypoglycemic agents) may cause an increased blood-glucose-lowering effect with risk of hypoglycemia. This phenomenon appeared to be more likely to occur during the first weeks of combined treatment and in patients with renal impairment. In diabetic patients treated with oral antidiabetic agents or insulin, glycemic control should be closely monitored for hypoglycemia, especially during the first month of treatment with an ACE inhibitor). Products include:
Precose Tablets 792

Amiloride Hydrochloride (Use of lisinopril with potassium-sparing diuretics (such as spironolactone, triamterene or amiloride), potassium supplements or potassium-containing salt substitutes may lead to significant increases in serum potassium. Therefore, if concomitant use of these agents is indicated because of demonstrated hypokalemia, they should be used with caution and with frequent monitoring of serum potassium. Potassium-sparing agents should generally not be used in patients with heart failure who are receiving lisinopril).
No products indexed under this heading.

Bendroflumethiazide (Thiazide-induced potassium loss attenuated; possibility of excessive reduction in blood pressure).
No products indexed under this heading.

Bumetanide (Possibility of excessive reduction in blood pressure).
No products indexed under this heading.

Celecoxib (Reports suggest that NSAIDs, including selective COX-2 inhibitors, may diminish the antihypertensive effect of ACE inhibitors, including lisinopril. This interaction should be given consideration in patients taking NSAIDs or selective COX-2 inhibitors concomitantly with ACE inhibitors. In some patients with compromised renal function who are being treated with NSAIDs, including selective COX-2 inhibitors, the co-administration of angiotensin II receptor antagonists or ACE inhibitors, may result in further deterioration of renal function, including possible acute renal failure. These effects are usually reversible. Therefore, the combination should be administered with caution, especially in the elderly). Products include:
Celebrex Capsules 2979

Chlorothiazide (Thiazide-induced potassium loss attenuated; possibility of excessive reduction in blood pressure).
No products indexed under this heading.

Chlorothiazide Sodium (Thiazide-induced potassium loss attenuated; possibility of excessive reduction in blood pressure). Products include:
Intravenous Sodium Diuril 2490

Chlorpropamide (Epidemiological studies have suggested that concomitant administration of ACE inhibitors and antidiabetic medicines (insulins, oral hypoglycemic agents) may cause an increased blood-glucose-lowering effect with risk of hypoglycemia. This phenomenon appeared to be more likely to occur during the first weeks of combined treatment and in patients with renal impairment. In diabetic patients treated with oral antidiabetic agents or insulin, glycemic control should be closely monitored for hypoglycemia, especially during the first month of treatment with an ACE inhibitor).
No products indexed under this heading.

Chlorthalidone (Possibility of excessive reduction in blood pressure). Products include:
Clorpres Tablets 2185

Diclofenac Epolamine (Reports suggest that NSAIDs, including selective COX-2 inhibitors, may diminish the antihypertensive effect of ACE inhibitors, including lisinopril. This interaction should be given consideration in patients taking NSAIDs or selective COX-2 inhibitors concomitantly with ACE inhibitors. In some patients with compromised renal function who are being treated with NSAIDs, including selective COX-2 inhibitors, the co-administration of angiotensin II receptor antagonists or ACE inhibitors, may result in further deterioration of renal function, including possible acute renal failure. These effects are usually reversible. Therefore, the combination should be administered with caution, especially in the elderly). Products include:
Flector Patch 561

Diclofenac Potassium (Reports suggest that NSAIDs, including selective COX-2 inhibitors, may diminish the antihypertensive effect of ACE inhibitors, including lisinopril. This interaction should be given consideration in patients taking NSAIDs or selective COX-2 inhibitors concomitantly with ACE inhibitors. In some patients with compromised renal function who are being treated with NSAIDs, including selective COX-2 inhibitors, the co-administration of angiotensin II receptor antagonists or ACE inhibitors, may result in further deterioration of renal function, including possible acute renal failure. These effects are usually reversible. Therefore, the combination should be administered with caution, especially in the elderly).
No products indexed under this heading.

Diclofenac Sodium (Reports suggest that NSAIDs, including selective COX-2 inhibitors, may diminish the antihypertensive effect of ACE inhibitors, including lisinopril. This interaction should be given consideration in patients taking NSAIDs or selective COX-2 inhibitors concomitantly with ACE inhibitors. In some patients with compromised renal function who are being treated with NSAIDs, including selective COX-2 inhibitors, the co-administration of angiotensin II receptor antagonists or ACE inhibitors, may result in further deterioration of renal function, including possible acute renal failure. These effects are usually reversible. Therefore, the combination should be administered with caution, especially in the elderly). Products include:
Diclofenac Sodium Ophthalmic Solution .... ⊙ 240
Voltaren Ophthalmic Solution 2336
Voltaren Tablets 2334
Voltaren-XR Tablets 2337

Eplerenone (Use of lisinopril with potassium-sparing diuretics (such as spironolactone, triamterene or amiloride), potassium supplements or potassium-containing salt substitutes may lead to significant increases in serum potassium. Therefore, if concomitant use of

these agents is indicated because of demonstrated hypokalemia, they should be used with caution and with frequent monitoring of serum potassium. Potassium-sparing agents should generally not be used in patients with heart failure who are receiving lisinopril).
No products indexed under this heading.

Ethacrynic Acid (Possibility of excessive reduction in blood pressure). Products include:
Edecrin Tablets 698

Etodolac (Reports suggest that NSAIDs, including selective COX-2 inhibitors, may diminish the antihypertensive effect of ACE inhibitors, including lisinopril. This interaction should be given consideration in patients taking NSAIDs or selective COX-2 inhibitors concomitantly with ACE inhibitors. In some patients with compromised renal function who are being treated with NSAIDs, including selective COX-2 inhibitors, the co-administration of angiotensin II receptor antagonists or ACE inhibitors, may result in further deterioration of renal function, including possible acute renal failure. These effects are usually reversible. Therefore, the combination should be administered with caution, especially in the elderly).
No products indexed under this heading.

Fenoprofen Calcium (Reports suggest that NSAIDs, including selective COX-2 inhibitors, may diminish the antihypertensive effect of ACE inhibitors, including lisinopril. This interaction should be given consideration in patients taking NSAIDs or selective COX-2 inhibitors concomitantly with ACE inhibitors. In some patients with compromised renal function who are being treated with NSAIDs, including selective COX-2 inhibitors, the co-administration of angiotensin II receptor antagonists or ACE inhibitors, may result in further deterioration of renal function, including possible acute renal failure. These effects are usually reversible. Therefore, the combination should be administered with caution, especially in the elderly). Products include:
Nalfon Capsules 2508

Flurbiprofen (Reports suggest that NSAIDs, including selective COX-2 inhibitors, may diminish the antihypertensive effect of ACE inhibitors, including lisinopril. This interaction should be given consideration in patients taking NSAIDs or selective COX-2 inhibitors concomitantly with ACE inhibitors. In some patients with compromised renal function who are being treated with NSAIDs, including selective COX-2 inhibitors, the co-administration of angiotensin II receptor antagonists or ACE inhibitors, may result in further deterioration of renal function, including possible acute renal failure. These effects are usually reversible. Therefore, the combination should be administered with caution, especially in the elderly).
No products indexed under this heading.

Furosemide (Possibility of excessive reduction in blood pressure). Products include:
Furosemide Tablets 2186

Glimepiride (Epidemiological studies have suggested that concomitant administration of ACE inhibitors and antidiabetic medicines (insulins, oral hypoglycemic agents) may cause an increased blood-glucose-lowering effect with risk of hypoglycemia. This phenomenon appeared to be more likely to occur during the first weeks of combined treatment and in patients with renal impairment. In diabetic patients treated with oral antidiabetic agents or insulin, glycemic control should be closely monitored for hypoglycemia, especially during the first month of treatment with an ACE inhibitor). Products include:
Avandaryl Tablets 1344
Duetact Tablets 3085

Glipizide (Epidemiological studies have suggested that concomitant administration of ACE inhibitors and antidiabetic medicines (insulins, oral hypoglycemic agents) may cause an increased blood-glucose-lowering effect with risk of hypoglycemia. This phenomenon appeared to be more likely to occur during the first weeks of combined treatment and in patients with renal impairment. In diabetic patients treated with oral antidiabetic agents or insulin, glycemic control should be closely monitored for hypoglycemia, especially during the first month of treatment with an ACE inhibitor).
No products indexed under this heading.

Glyburide (Epidemiological studies have suggested that concomitant administration of ACE inhibitors and antidiabetic medicines (insulins, oral hypoglycemic agents) may cause an increased blood-glucose-lowering effect with risk of hypoglycemia. This phenomenon appeared to be more likely to occur during the first weeks of combined treatment and in patients with renal impairment. In diabetic patients treated with oral antidiabetic agents or insulin, glycemic control should be closely monitored for hypoglycemia, especially during the first month of treatment with an ACE inhibitor).
No products indexed under this heading.

Gold Sodium Thiomalate (Nitroid reactions (symptoms include facial flushing, nausea, vomiting and hypotension) have been reported rarely in patients on therapy with injectable gold and concomitant ACE inhibitor therapy including lisinopril).
No products indexed under this heading.

Gold Therapy (Nitroid reactions (symptoms include facial flushing, nausea, vomiting and hypotension) have been reported rarely in patients on therapy with injectable gold and concomitant ACE inhibitor therapy including lisinopril).
No products indexed under this heading.

Hydrochlorothiazide (Thiazide-induced potassium loss attenuated; possibility of excessive reduction in blood pressure). Products include:
Atacand HCT 642
Avalide Tablets 892
Avalide Tablets 2713
Benicar HCT Tablets 1010
Diovan HCT Tablets 2216
Dyazide Capsules 1405
Micardis HCT Tablets 854
Prinzide Tablets 2092
Tekturna HCT Tablets 2324
Teveten HCT Tablets 517

Hydroflumethiazide (Thiazide-induced potassium loss attenuated; possibility of excessive reduction in blood pressure).
No products indexed under this heading.

Ibuprofen (Reports suggest that NSAIDs, including selective COX-2 inhibitors, may diminish the antihypertensive effect of ACE inhibitors, including lisinopril. This interaction should be given consideration in patients taking NSAIDs or selective COX-2 inhibitors concomitantly with ACE inhibitors. In some patients with compromised renal function who are being treated with NSAIDs, including selective COX-2 inhibitors, the co-administration of angiotensin II receptor antagonists or ACE inhibitors, may result in further deterioration of renal function, including possible acute renal failure. These effects are usually reversible. Therefore, the combination should be administered with caution, especially in the elderly). Products include:
Motrin IB Tablets and Caplets 1900
Children's Motrin Oral Suspension 1901
Children's Motrin Non-Staining Dye-Free Oral Suspension 1901
Children's Motrin Cold Oral Suspension 1899
Infants' Motrin Concentrated Drops 1901
Infants' Motrin Non-Staining Dye-Free Concentrated Drops 1901
Junior Strength Motrin Caplets and Chewable Tablets 1901
Vicoprofen Tablets 533

Indapamide (Possibility of excessive reduction in blood pressure). Products include:
Indapamide Tablets 2188

Indomethacin (Co-administration in some patients with compromised renal function who are being treated with NSAIDs may result in a further deterioration of renal function. In a study, the use of indomethacin was associated with a reduced antihypertensive effect, although the difference between lisinopril alone to lisinopril given concomitantly with indomethacin was not significant). Products include:
Indocin 2024

Indomethacin Sodium Trihydrate (Reports suggest that NSAIDs, including selective COX-2 inhibitors, may diminish the antihypertensive effect of ACE inhibitors, including lisinopril. This interaction should be given consideration in patients taking NSAIDs or selective COX-2 inhibitors concomitantly with ACE inhibitors. In some patients with compromised renal function who are being treated with NSAIDs, including selective COX-2 inhibitors, the co-administration of angiotensin II receptor antagonists or ACE inhibitors, may result in further deterioration of renal function, including possible acute renal failure. These effects are usually reversible. Therefore, the combination should be administered with caution, especially in the elderly). Products include:
Indocin I.V. 2489

Insulin (Epidemiological studies have suggested that concomitant administration of ACE inhibitors and antidiabetic medicines (insulins, oral hypoglycemic agents) may cause an increased blood-glucose-lowering effect with risk of hypoglycemia. This phenomenon appeared to be more likely to occur during the first weeks of combined treatment and in patients with renal impairment. In diabetic patients treated with oral antidiabetic agents or insulin, glycemic control should be closely monitored for hypoglycemia, especially during the first month of treatment with an ACE inhibitor).
No products indexed under this heading.

Insulin, Human, Zinc Suspension (Epidemiological studies have suggested that concomitant administration of ACE inhibitors and antidiabetic medicines (insulins, oral hypoglycemic agents) may cause an increased blood-glucose-lowering effect with risk of hypoglycemia. This phenomenon appeared to be more likely to occur during the first weeks of combined treatment and in patients with renal impairment. In diabetic patients treated with oral antidiabetic agents or insulin, glycemic control should be closely monitored for hypoglycemia, especially during the first month of treatment with an ACE inhibitor).
No products indexed under this heading.

Insulin, Human (rDNA origin) (Epidemiological studies have suggested that concomitant administration of ACE inhibitors and antidiabetic medicines (insulins, oral hypoglycemic agents) may cause an increased blood-glucose-lowering effect with risk of hypoglycemia. This phenomenon appeared to be more likely to occur during the first weeks of combined treatment and in patients with renal impairment. In diabetic patients treated with oral antidiabetic agents or insulin, glycemic control should be closely monitored for hypoglycemia, especially during the first month of treatment with an ACE inhibitor). Products include:
Exubera Inhalation Powder 2515

Insulin, Human NPH (Epidemiological studies have suggested that concomitant administration of ACE inhibitors and antidiabetic medicines (insulins, oral hypoglycemic agents) may cause an increased blood-glucose-lowering effect with risk of hypoglycemia. This phenomenon appeared to be more likely to occur during the first weeks of combined treatment and in patients with renal impairment. In diabetic patients treated with oral antidiabetic agents or insulin, glycemic control should be closely monitored for hypoglycemia, especially during the first month of treatment with an ACE inhibitor). Products include:
Humulin N Vial 1846

Insulin, Human Regular (Epidemiological studies have suggested that concomitant administration of ACE inhibitors and antidiabetic medicines (insulins, oral hypoglycemic agents) may cause an increased blood-glucose-lowering effect with risk of hypoglycemia. This phenomenon appeared to be more likely to occur during the first weeks of combined treatment and in patients with renal impairment. In diabetic patients treated with oral antidiabetic agents or insulin, glycemic control should be closely monitored for hypoglyce-

mia, especially during the first month of treatment with an ACE inhibitor). Products include:

Humulin R 1849
Humulin R (U-500) 1850

Insulin, Human Regular and Human NPH Mixture (Epidemiological studies have suggested that concomitant administration of ACE inhibitors and antidiabetic medicines (insulins, oral hypoglycemic agents) may cause an increased blood-glucose-lowering effect with risk of hypoglycemia. This phenomenon appeared to be more likely to occur during the first weeks of combined treatment and in patients with renal impairment. In diabetic patients treated with oral antidiabetic agents or insulin, glycemic control should be closely monitored for hypoglycemia, especially during the first month of treatment with an ACE inhibitor). Products include:

Humulin 50/50, 100 Units 1843
Humulin 70/30 Vial 1844

Insulin, NPH (Epidemiological studies have suggested that concomitant administration of ACE inhibitors and antidiabetic medicines (insulins, oral hypoglycemic agents) may cause an increased blood-glucose-lowering effect with risk of hypoglycemia. This phenomenon appeared to be more likely to occur during the first weeks of combined treatment and in patients with renal impairment. In diabetic patients treated with oral antidiabetic agents or insulin, glycemic control should be closely monitored for hypoglycemia, especially during the first month of treatment with an ACE inhibitor).

No products indexed under this heading.

Insulin, Regular (Epidemiological studies have suggested that concomitant administration of ACE inhibitors and antidiabetic medicines (insulins, oral hypoglycemic agents) may cause an increased blood-glucose-lowering effect with risk of hypoglycemia. This phenomenon appeared to be more likely to occur during the first weeks of combined treatment and in patients with renal impairment. In diabetic patients treated with oral antidiabetic agents or insulin, glycemic control should be closely monitored for hypoglycemia, especially during the first month of treatment with an ACE inhibitor).

No products indexed under this heading.

Insulin, Regular and NPH mixture (Epidemiological studies have suggested that concomitant administration of ACE inhibitors and antidiabetic medicines (insulins, oral hypoglycemic agents) may cause an increased blood-glucose-lowering effect with risk of hypoglycemia. This phenomenon appeared to be more likely to occur during the first weeks of combined treatment and in patients with renal impairment. In diabetic patients treated with oral antidiabetic agents or insulin, glycemic control should be closely monitored for hypoglycemia, especially during the first month of treatment with an ACE inhibitor).

No products indexed under this heading.

Insulin, Zinc Crystals (Epidemiological studies have suggested that concomitant administration of ACE inhibitors and antidiabetic medicines (insulins, oral hypoglycemic agents) may cause an increased blood-glucose-lowering effect with risk of hypoglycemia. This phenomenon appeared to be more likely to occur during the first weeks of combined treatment and in patients with renal impairment. In diabetic patients treated with oral antidiabetic agents or insulin, glycemic control should be closely monitored for hypoglycemia, especially during the first month of treatment with an ACE inhibitor).

No products indexed under this heading.

Insulin, Zinc Suspension (Epidemiological studies have suggested that concomitant administration of ACE inhibitors and antidiabetic medicines (insulins, oral hypoglycemic agents) may cause an increased blood-glucose-lowering effect with risk of hypoglycemia. This phenomenon appeared to be more likely to occur during the first weeks of combined treatment and in patients with renal impairment. In diabetic patients treated with oral antidiabetic agents or insulin, glycemic control should be closely monitored for hypoglycemia, especially during the first month of treatment with an ACE inhibitor).

No products indexed under this heading.

Insulin Aspart (Epidemiological studies have suggested that concomitant administration of ACE inhibitors and antidiabetic medicines (insulins, oral hypoglycemic agents) may cause an increased blood-glucose-lowering effect with risk of hypoglycemia. This phenomenon appeared to be more likely to occur during the first weeks of combined treatment and in patients with renal impairment. In diabetic patients treated with oral antidiabetic agents or insulin, glycemic control should be closely monitored for hypoglycemia, especially during the first month of treatment with an ACE inhibitor).

No products indexed under this heading.

Insulin Aspart, Human (Epidemiological studies have suggested that concomitant administration of ACE inhibitors and antidiabetic medicines (insulins, oral hypoglycemic agents) may cause an increased blood-glucose-lowering effect with risk of hypoglycemia. This phenomenon appeared to be more likely to occur during the first weeks of combined treatment and in patients with renal impairment. In diabetic patients treated with oral antidiabetic agents or insulin, glycemic control should be closely monitored for hypoglycemia, especially during the first month of treatment with an ACE inhibitor). Products include:

NovoLog Mix 70/30 2364

Insulin Aspart, Human Regular (Epidemiological studies have suggested that concomitant administration of ACE inhibitors and antidiabetic medicines (insulins, oral hypoglycemic agents) may cause an increased blood-glucose-lowering effect with risk of hypoglycemia. This phenomenon appeared to be more likely to occur during the first weeks of combined treatment and in patients with renal impairment. In diabetic patients treated with oral antidiabetic agents or insulin, glycemic control should be closely monitored for hypoglycemia, especially during the first month of treatment with an ACE inhibitor). Products include:

NovoLog Injection 2359

Insulin Aspart Protamine, Human (Epidemiological studies have suggested that concomitant administration of ACE inhibitors and antidiabetic medicines (insulins, oral hypoglycemic agents) may cause an increased blood-glucose-lowering effect with risk of hypoglycemia. This phenomenon appeared to be more likely to occur during the first weeks of combined treatment and in patients with renal impairment. In diabetic patients treated with oral antidiabetic agents or insulin, glycemic control should be closely monitored for hypoglycemia, especially during the first month of treatment with an ACE inhibitor). Products include:

NovoLog Mix 70/30 2364

Insulin Detemir (rDNA Origin) (Epidemiological studies have suggested that concomitant administration of ACE inhibitors and antidiabetic medicines (insulins, oral hypoglycemic agents) may cause an increased blood-glucose-lowering effect with risk of hypoglycemia. This phenomenon appeared to be more likely to occur during the first weeks of combined treatment and in patients with renal impairment. In diabetic patients treated with oral antidiabetic agents or insulin, glycemic control should be closely monitored for hypoglycemia, especially during the first month of treatment with an ACE inhibitor). Products include:

Levemir Injection 2352

Insulin glargine (Epidemiological studies have suggested that concomitant administration of ACE inhibitors and antidiabetic medicines (insulins, oral hypoglycemic agents) may cause an increased blood-glucose-lowering effect with risk of hypoglycemia. This phenomenon appeared to be more likely to occur during the first weeks of combined treatment and in patients with renal impairment. In diabetic patients treated with oral antidiabetic agents or insulin, glycemic control should be closely monitored for hypoglycemia, especially during the first month of treatment with an ACE inhibitor). Products include:

Lantus Injection 2749

Insulin Glulisine (Epidemiological studies have suggested that concomitant administration of ACE inhibitors and antidiabetic medicines (insulins, oral hypoglycemic agents) may cause an increased blood-glucose-lowering effect with risk of hypoglycemia. This phenomenon appeared to be more likely to occur during the first weeks of combined treatment and in patients with renal impairment. In diabetic patients treated with oral antidiabetic agents or insulin, glycemic control should be closely monitored for hypoglycemia, especially during the first month of treatment with an ACE inhibitor). Products include:

Apidra Injection 2706

Insulin Lispro, Human (Epidemiological studies have suggested that concomitant administration of ACE inhibitors and antidiabetic medicines (insulins, oral hypoglycemic agents) may cause an increased blood-glucose-lowering effect with risk of hypoglycemia. This phenomenon appeared to be more likely to occur during the first weeks of combined treatment and in patients with renal impairment. In diabetic patients treated with oral antidiabetic agents or insulin, glycemic control should be closely monitored for hypoglycemia, especially during the first month of treatment with an ACE inhibitor). Products include:

Humalog-Pen and KwikPen 1829
Humalog Mix 50/50-Pen and KwikPen 1833
Humalog Mix 75/25-Pen and KwikPen 1835

Insulin Lispro Protamine, Human (Epidemiological studies have suggested that concomitant administration of ACE inhibitors and antidiabetic medicines (insulins, oral hypoglycemic agents) may cause an increased blood-glucose-lowering effect with risk of hypoglycemia. This phenomenon appeared to be more likely to occur during the first weeks of combined treatment and in patients with renal impairment. In diabetic patients treated with oral antidiabetic agents or insulin, glycemic control should be closely monitored for hypoglycemia, especially during the first month of treatment with an ACE inhibitor). Products include:

Humalog Mix 50/50-Pen and KwikPen 1833
Humalog Mix 75/25-Pen and KwikPen 1835

Ketoprofen (Reports suggest that NSAIDs, including selective COX-2 inhibitors, may diminish the antihypertensive effect of ACE inhibitors, including lisinopril. This interaction should be given consideration in patients taking NSAIDs or selective COX-2 inhibitors concomitantly with ACE inhibitors. In some patients with compromised renal function who are being treated with NSAIDs, including selective COX-2 inhibitors, the co-administration of angiotensin II receptor antagonists or ACE inhibitors, may result in further deterioration of renal function, including possible acute renal failure. These effects are usually reversible. Therefore, the combination should be administered with caution, especially in the elderly).

No products indexed under this heading.

Ketorolac Tromethamine (Reports suggest that NSAIDs, including selective COX-2 inhibitors, may diminish the antihypertensive effect of ACE inhibitors, including lisinopril. This interaction should be given consideration in patients taking NSAIDs or selective COX-2 inhibitors concomitantly with ACE inhibitors. In some patients with compromised renal function who are being treated with NSAIDs, including selective COX-2 inhibitors, the co-administration of angiotensin II receptor antagonists or ACE inhibitors, may result in further deterioration of renal function, including possible acute renal failure. These effects are usually reversible. Therefore, the combination should be administered with caution, especially in the elderly).

No products indexed under this heading.

Lithium (Potential for reversible lithium toxicity; frequent monitoring of lithium levels is recommended).
No products indexed under this heading.

Lithium Carbonate (Potential for reversible lithium toxicity; frequent monitoring of lithium levels is recommended).
No products indexed under this heading.

Lithium Citrate (Potential for reversible lithium toxicity; frequent monitoring of lithium levels is recommended).
No products indexed under this heading.

Meclofenamate Sodium (Reports suggest that NSAIDs, including selective COX-2 inhibitors, may diminish the antihypertensive effect of ACE inhibitors, including lisinopril. This interaction should be given consideration in patients taking NSAIDs or selective COX-2 inhibitors concomitantly with ACE inhibitors. In some patients with compromised renal function who are being treated with NSAIDs, including selective COX-2 inhibitors, the co-administration of angiotensin II receptor antagonists or ACE inhibitors, may result in further deterioration of renal function, including possible acute renal failure. These effects are usually reversible. Therefore, the combination should be administered with caution, especially in the elderly).
No products indexed under this heading.

Mefenamic Acid (Reports suggest that NSAIDs, including selective COX-2 inhibitors, may diminish the antihypertensive effect of ACE inhibitors, including lisinopril. This interaction should be given consideration in patients taking NSAIDs or selective COX-2 inhibitors concomitantly with ACE inhibitors. In some patients with compromised renal function who are being treated with NSAIDs, including selective COX-2 inhibitors, the co-administration of angiotensin II receptor antagonists or ACE inhibitors, may result in further deterioration of renal function, including possible acute renal failure. These effects are usually reversible. Therefore, the combination should be administered with caution, especially in the elderly).
No products indexed under this heading.

Meloxicam (Reports suggest that NSAIDs, including selective COX-2 inhibitors, may diminish the antihypertensive effect of ACE inhibitors, including lisinopril. This interaction should be given consideration in patients taking NSAIDs or selective COX-2 inhibitors concomitantly with ACE inhibitors. In some patients with compromised renal function who are being treated with NSAIDs, including selective COX-2 inhibitors, the co-administration of angiotensin II receptor antagonists or ACE inhibitors, may result in further deterioration of renal function, including possible acute renal failure. These effects are usually reversible. Therefore, the combination should be administered with caution, especially in the elderly). Products include:
Mobic Oral Suspension **863**
Mobic Tablets **863**

Metformin Hydrochloride (Epidemiological studies have suggested that concomitant administration of ACE inhibitors and antidiabetic medicines (insulins, oral hypoglycemic agents) may cause an increased blood-glucose-lowering effect with risk of hypoglycemia. This phenomenon appeared to be more likely to occur during the first weeks of combined treatment and in patients with renal impairment. In diabetic patients treated with oral antidiabetic agents or insulin, glycemic control should be closely monitored for hypoglycemia, especially during the first month of treatment with an ACE inhibitor). Products include:
ActoPlus Met Tablets **3071**
Avandamet Tablets **1336**
Janumet Tablets **2041**
PrandiMet Tablets **2967**

Methyclothiazide (Thiazide-induced potassium loss attenuated; possibility of excessive reduction in blood pressure).
No products indexed under this heading.

Metolazone (Possibility of excessive reduction in blood pressure).
No products indexed under this heading.

Miglitol (Epidemiological studies have suggested that concomitant administration of ACE inhibitors and antidiabetic medicines (insulins, oral hypoglycemic agents) may cause an increased blood-glucose-lowering effect with risk of hypoglycemia. This phenomenon appeared to be more likely to occur during the first weeks of combined treatment and in patients with renal impairment. In diabetic patients treated with oral antidiabetic agents or insulin, glycemic control should be closely monitored for hypoglycemia, especially during the first month of treatment with an ACE inhibitor).
No products indexed under this heading.

Nabumetone (Reports suggest that NSAIDs, including selective COX-2 inhibitors, may diminish the antihypertensive effect of ACE inhibitors, including lisinopril. This interaction should be given consideration in patients taking NSAIDs or selective COX-2 inhibitors concomitantly with ACE inhibitors. In some patients with compromised renal function who are being treated with NSAIDs, including selective COX-2 inhibitors, the co-administration of angiotensin II receptor antagonists or ACE inhibitors, may result in further deterioration of renal function, including possible acute renal failure. These effects are usually reversible. Therefore, the combination should be administered with caution, especially in the elderly).
No products indexed under this heading.

Naproxen (Reports suggest that NSAIDs, including selective COX-2 inhibitors, may diminish the antihypertensive effect of ACE inhibitors, including lisinopril. This interaction should be given consideration in patients taking NSAIDs or selective COX-2 inhibitors concomitantly with ACE inhibitors. In some patients with compromised renal function who are being treated with NSAIDs, including selective COX-2 inhibitors, the co-administration of angiotensin II receptor antagonists or ACE inhibitors, may result in further deterioration of renal function, including possible acute renal failure. These effects are usually reversible. Therefore, the combination should be administered with caution, especially in the elderly). Products include:
EC-Naprosyn Delayed-Release Tablets **2632**
Naprosyn Suspension **2632**
Naprosyn Tablets **2632**

Naproxen Sodium (Reports suggest that NSAIDs, including selective COX-2 inhibitors, may diminish the antihypertensive effect of ACE inhibitors, including lisinopril. This interaction should be given consideration in patients taking NSAIDs or selective COX-2 inhibitors concomitantly with ACE inhibitors. In some patients with compromised renal function who are being treated with NSAIDs, including selective COX-2 inhibitors, the co-administration of angiotensin II receptor antagonists or ACE inhibitors, may result in further deterioration of renal function, including possible acute renal failure. These effects are usually reversible. Therefore, the combination should be administered with caution, especially in the elderly). Products include:
Anaprox Tablets **2632**
Anaprox DS Tablets **2632**
Treximet Tablets **1616**

Nateglinide (Epidemiological studies have suggested that concomitant administration of ACE inhibitors and antidiabetic medicines (insulins, oral hypoglycemic agents) may cause an increased blood-glucose-lowering effect with risk of hypoglycemia. This phenomenon appeared to be more likely to occur during the first weeks of combined treatment and in patients with renal impairment. In diabetic patients treated with oral antidiabetic agents or insulin, glycemic control should be closely monitored for hypoglycemia, especially during the first month of treatment with an ACE inhibitor). Products include:
Starlix Tablets **2314**

Oxaprozin (Reports suggest that NSAIDs, including selective COX-2 inhibitors, may diminish the antihypertensive effect of ACE inhibitors, including lisinopril. This interaction should be given consideration in patients taking NSAIDs or selective COX-2 inhibitors concomitantly with ACE inhibitors. In some patients with compromised renal function who are being treated with NSAIDs, including selective COX-2 inhibitors, the co-administration of angiotensin II receptor antagonists or ACE inhibitors, may result in further deterioration of renal function, including possible acute renal failure. These effects are usually reversible. Therefore, the combination should be administered with caution, especially in the elderly).
No products indexed under this heading.

Phenylbutazone (Reports suggest that NSAIDs, including selective COX-2 inhibitors, may diminish the antihypertensive effect of ACE inhibitors, including lisinopril. This interaction should be given consideration in patients taking NSAIDs or selective COX-2 inhibitors concomitantly with ACE inhibitors. In some patients with compromised renal function who are being treated with NSAIDs, including selective COX-2 inhibitors, the co-administration of angiotensin II receptor antagonists or ACE inhibitors, may result in further deterioration of renal function, including possible acute renal failure. These effects are usually reversible. Therefore, the combination should be administered with caution, especially in the elderly).
No products indexed under this heading.

Pioglitazone Hydrochloride (Epidemiological studies have suggested that concomitant administration of ACE inhibitors and antidiabetic medicines (insulins, oral hypoglycemic agents) may cause an increased blood-glucose-lowering effect with risk of hypoglycemia. This phenomenon appeared to be more likely to occur during the first weeks of combined treatment and in patients with renal impairment. In diabetic patients treated with oral antidiabetic agents or insulin, glycemic control should be closely monitored for hypoglycemia, especially during the first month of treatment with an ACE inhibitor). Products include:
ActoPlus Met Tablets **3071**
Actos Tablets **3077**
Duetact Tablets **3085**

Piroxicam (Reports suggest that NSAIDs, including selective COX-2 inhibitors, may diminish the antihypertensive effect of ACE inhibitors, including lisinopril. This interaction should be given consideration in patients taking NSAIDs or selective COX-2 inhibitors concomitantly with ACE inhibitors. In some patients with compromised renal function who are being treated with NSAIDs, including selective COX-2 inhibitors, the co-administration of angiotensin II receptor antagonists or ACE inhibitors, may result in further deterioration of renal function, including possible acute renal failure. These effects are usually reversible. Therefore, the combination should be administered with caution, especially in the elderly).
No products indexed under this heading.

Polythiazide (Thiazide-induced potassium loss attenuated; possibility of excessive reduction in blood pressure).
No products indexed under this heading.

Potassium Acid Phosphate (Use of lisinopril with potassium-sparing diuretics (such as spironolactone, triamterene or amiloride), potassium supplements or potassium-containing salt substitutes may lead to significant increases in serum potassium. Therefore, if concomitant use of these agents is indicated because of demonstrated hypokalemia, they should be used with caution and with frequent monitoring of serum potassium. Potassium-sparing agents should generally not be used in patients with heart failure who are receiving lisinopril). Products include:
K-Phos Original (Sodium Free) Tablets **814**

Potassium Bicarbonate (Use of lisinopril with potassium-sparing diuretics (such as spironolactone, triamterene or amiloride), potassium supplements or potassium-containing salt substitutes may lead

to significant increases in serum potassium. Therefore, if concomitant use of these agents is indicated because of demonstrated hypokalemia, they should be used with caution and with frequent monitoring of serum potassium. Potassium-sparing agents should generally not be used in patients with heart failure who are receiving lisinopril).

No products indexed under this heading.

Potassium Chloride (Use of lisinopril with potassium-sparing diuretics (such as spironolactone, triamterene or amiloride), potassium supplements or potassium-containing salt substitutes may lead to significant increases in serum potassium. Therefore, if concomitant use of these agents is indicated because of demonstrated hypokalemia, they should be used with caution and with frequent monitoring of serum potassium. Potassium-sparing agents should generally not be used in patients with heart failure who are receiving lisinopril). Products include:

MoviPrep Oral Solution 2679

Potassium Citrate (Use of lisinopril with potassium-sparing diuretics (such as spironolactone, triamterene or amiloride), potassium supplements or potassium-containing salt substitutes may lead to significant increases in serum potassium. Therefore, if concomitant use of these agents is indicated because of demonstrated hypokalemia, they should be used with caution and with frequent monitoring of serum potassium. Potassium-sparing agents should generally not be used in patients with heart failure who are receiving lisinopril). Products include:

BioLean Free Tablets 635
Urocit-K Tablets 2176

Potassium Gluconate (Use of lisinopril with potassium-sparing diuretics (such as spironolactone, triamterene or amiloride), potassium supplements or potassium-containing salt substitutes may lead to significant increases in serum potassium. Therefore, if concomitant use of these agents is indicated because of demonstrated hypokalemia, they should be used with caution and with frequent monitoring of serum potassium. Potassium-sparing agents should generally not be used in patients with heart failure who are receiving lisinopril).

No products indexed under this heading.

Potassium Phosphate (Use of lisinopril with potassium-sparing diuretics (such as spironolactone, triamterene or amiloride), potassium supplements or potassium-containing salt substitutes may lead to significant increases in serum potassium. Therefore, if concomitant use of these agents is indicated because of demonstrated hypokalemia, they should be used with caution and with frequent monitoring of serum potassium. Potassium-sparing agents should generally not be used in patients with heart failure who are receiving lisinopril). Products include:

K-Phos Neutral Tablets 813

Repaglinide (Epidemiological studies have suggested that concomitant administration of ACE inhibitors and antidiabetic medicines (insulins, oral hypoglycemic agents) may cause an increased blood-glucose-lowering effect with risk of hypoglycemia. This phenomenon appeared to be more likely to occur during the first weeks of combined treatment and in patients with renal impairment. In diabetic patients treated with oral antidiabetic agents or insulin, glycemic control should be closely monitored for hypoglycemia, especially during the first month of treatment with an ACE inhibitor). Products include:

PrandiMet Tablets 2967
Prandin Tablets 2971

Rofecoxib (Reports suggest that NSAIDs, including selective COX-2 inhibitors, may diminish the antihypertensive effect of ACE inhibitors, including lisinopril. This interaction should be given consideration in patients taking NSAIDs or selective COX-2 inhibitors concomitantly with ACE inhibitors. In some patients with compromised renal function who are being treated with NSAIDs, including selective COX-2 inhibitors, the co-administration of angiotensin II receptor antagonists or ACE inhibitors, may result in further deterioration of renal function, including possible acute renal failure. These effects are usually reversible. Therefore, the combination should be administered with caution, especially in the elderly).

No products indexed under this heading.

Rosiglitazone Maleate (Epidemiological studies have suggested that concomitant administration of ACE inhibitors and antidiabetic medicines (insulins, oral hypoglycemic agents) may cause an increased blood-glucose-lowering effect with risk of hypoglycemia. This phenomenon appeared to be more likely to occur during the first weeks of combined treatment and in patients with renal impairment. In diabetic patients treated with oral antidiabetic agents or insulin, glycemic control should be closely monitored for hypoglycemia, especially during the first month of treatment with an ACE inhibitor). Products include:

Avandamet Tablets 1336
Avandaryl Tablets 1344
Avandia Tablets 1351

Sitagliptin Phosphate (Epidemiological studies have suggested that concomitant administration of ACE inhibitors and antidiabetic medicines (insulins, oral hypoglycemic agents) may cause an increased blood-glucose-lowering effect with risk of hypoglycemia. This phenomenon appeared to be more likely to occur during the first weeks of combined treatment and in patients with renal impairment. In diabetic patients treated with oral antidiabetic agents or insulin, glycemic control should be closely monitored for hypoglycemia, especially during the first month of treatment with an ACE inhibitor). Products include:

Janumet Tablets 2041
Januvia Tablets 2048

Spironolactone (Use of lisinopril with potassium-sparing diuretics (such as spironolactone, triamterene or amiloride), potassium supplements or potassium-containing salt substitutes may lead to significant increases in serum potassium. Therefore, if concomitant use of these agents is indicated because of demonstrated hypokalemia, they should be used with caution and with frequent monitoring of serum potassium. Potassium-sparing agents should generally not be used in patients with heart failure who are receiving lisinopril).

No products indexed under this heading.

Sulindac (Reports suggest that NSAIDs, including selective COX-2 inhibitors, may diminish the antihypertensive effect of ACE inhibitors, including lisinopril. This interaction should be given consideration in patients taking NSAIDs or selective COX-2 inhibitors concomitantly with ACE inhibitors. In some patients with compromised renal function who are being treated with NSAIDs, including selective COX-2 inhibitors, the co-administration of angiotensin II receptor antagonists or ACE inhibitors, may result in further deterioration of renal function, including possible acute renal failure. These effects are usually reversible. Therefore, the combination should be administered with caution, especially in the elderly). Products include:

Clinoril Tablets 1962

Tolazamide (Epidemiological studies have suggested that concomitant administration of ACE inhibitors and antidiabetic medicines (insulins, oral hypoglycemic agents) may cause an increased blood-glucose-lowering effect with risk of hypoglycemia. This phenomenon appeared to be more likely to occur during the first weeks of combined treatment and in patients with renal impairment. In diabetic patients treated with oral antidiabetic agents or insulin, glycemic control should be closely monitored for hypoglycemia, especially during the first month of treatment with an ACE inhibitor).

No products indexed under this heading.

Tolbutamide (Epidemiological studies have suggested that concomitant administration of ACE inhibitors and antidiabetic medicines (insulins, oral hypoglycemic agents) may cause an increased blood-glucose-lowering effect with risk of hypoglycemia. This phenomenon appeared to be more likely to occur during the first weeks of combined treatment and in patients with renal impairment. In diabetic patients treated with oral antidiabetic agents or insulin, glycemic control should be closely monitored for hypoglycemia, especially during the first month of treatment with an ACE inhibitor).

No products indexed under this heading.

Tolmetin Sodium (Reports suggest that NSAIDs, including selective COX-2 inhibitors, may diminish the antihypertensive effect of ACE inhibitors, including lisinopril. This interaction should be given consideration in patients taking NSAIDs or selective COX-2 inhibitors concomitantly with ACE inhibitors. In some patients with compromised renal function who are being treated with NSAIDs, including selective COX-2 inhibitors, the co-administration of angiotensin II receptor antagonists or ACE inhibitors, may result in further deterioration of renal function, including possible acute renal failure. These effects are usually reversible. Therefore, the combination should be administered with caution, especially in the elderly).

No products indexed under this heading.

Torsemide (Possibility of excessive reduction in blood pressure). Products include:

Demadex Injection 2630
Demadex Tablets 2630

Triamterene (Use of lisinopril with potassium-sparing diuretics (such as spironolactone, triamterene or amiloride), potassium supplements or potassium-containing salt substitutes may lead to significant increases in serum potassium. Therefore, if concomitant use of these agents is indicated because of demonstrated hypokalemia, they should be used with caution and with frequent monitoring of serum potassium. Potassium-sparing agents should generally not be used in patients with heart failure who are receiving lisinopril). Products include:

Dyazide Capsules 1405
Dyrenium Capsules 3189

Troglitazone (Epidemiological studies have suggested that concomitant administration of ACE inhibitors and antidiabetic medicines (insulins, oral hypoglycemic agents) may cause an increased blood-glucose-lowering effect with risk of hypoglycemia. This phenomenon appeared to be more likely to occur during the first weeks of combined treatment and in patients with renal impairment. In diabetic patients treated with oral antidiabetic agents or insulin, glycemic control should be closely monitored for hypoglycemia, especially during the first month of treatment with an ACE inhibitor).

No products indexed under this heading.

Valdecoxib (Reports suggest that NSAIDs, including selective COX-2 inhibitors, may diminish the antihypertensive effect of ACE inhibitors, including lisinopril. This interaction should be given consideration in patients taking NSAIDs or selective COX-2 inhibitors concomitantly with ACE inhibitors. In some patients with compromised renal function who are being treated with NSAIDs, including selective COX-2 inhibitors, the co-administration of angiotensin II receptor antagonists or ACE inhibitors, may result in further deterioration of renal function, including possible acute renal failure. These effects are usually reversible. Therefore, the combination should be administered with caution, especially in the elderly).

No products indexed under this heading.

Food Interactions

Salt Substitutes, Potassium-Containing (Use of lisinopril with potassium-sparing diuretics (such as spironolactone, triamterene or amiloride), potassium supplements or potassium-containing salt substitutes may lead to significant increases in serum potassium. Therefore, if concomitant use of these agents is indicated because of demonstrated hypokalemia, they should be used with caution and with frequent monitoring of serum potassium. Potassium-sparing agents should generally not be used in patients with heart failure who are receiving lisinopril).

PRINZIDE TABLETS
(Hydrochlorothiazide, Lisinopril) 2092
May interact with antihypertensives, barbiturates, corticosteroids, diuretics, cardiac glycosides, oral hypoglycemic agents, insulin, lithium preparations, narcotic analgesics, nondepolarizing neuromuscular blocking agents, non-steroidal anti-inflammatory agents, potassium preparations, potassium sparing diuretics, and certain other agents. Compounds in these categories include:

Acarbose (Hyperglycemia may occur with thiazide diuretics; dosage adjustment of oral hypoglycemic agents may be required). Products include:
Precose Tablets 792

Acebutolol Hydrochloride (Co-administration of thiazide and other antihypertensive agents can lead to additive effect or potentiation).
No products indexed under this heading.

ACTH (Co-administration of thiazide diuretics with ACTH intensifies electrolyte depletion, particularly potassium).
No products indexed under this heading.

Alfentanil Hydrochloride (Co-administration of thiazide and narcotics may potentiate orthostatic hypotension).
No products indexed under this heading.

Aliskiren (Co-administration of thiazide and other antihypertensive agents can lead to additive effect or potentiation). Products include:
Tekturna Tablets 2321
Tekturna HCT Tablets 2324

Amiloride Hydrochloride (Risk factors for the development of hyperkalemia include the concomitant use of potassium-sparing diuretics, potassium supplements and/or potassium-containing salt substitutes. Hyperkalemia can cause serious, sometimes, fatal, arrhythmias. Prinzide should be used cautiously, if at all, with these agents and with frequent monitoring of serum potassium).
No products indexed under this heading.

Amlodipine Besylate (Co-administration of thiazide and other antihypertensive agents can lead to additive effect or potentiation). Products include:
Azor Tablets 1005
Exforge Tablets 2238

Aprobarbital (Co-administration of thiazide and barbiturates may potentiate orthostatic hypotension).
No products indexed under this heading.

Atenolol (Co-administration of thiazide and other antihypertensive agents can lead to additive effect or potentiation).
No products indexed under this heading.

Atracurium Besylate (Co-administration with nondepolarizing skeletal muscle relaxants may result in possible increased responsiveness to the muscle relaxant).
No products indexed under this heading.

Benazepril Hydrochloride (Co-administration of thiazide and other antihypertensive agents can lead to additive effect or potentiation).
No products indexed under this heading.

Bendroflumethiazide (Co-administration of lisinopril in patients on diuretics, especially those in whom diuretic therapy was recently instituted, may occasionally experience excessive hypotension; antihypertensive effects of lisinopril are augmented by antihypertensive agents that cause renin release).
No products indexed under this heading.

Betamethasone Acetate (Co-administration of thiazide diuretics with corticosteroids intensifies electrolyte depletion, particularly potassium).
No products indexed under this heading.

Betamethasone Sodium Phosphate (Co-administration of thiazide diuretics with corticosteroids intensifies electrolyte depletion, particularly potassium).
No products indexed under this heading.

Betaxolol Hydrochloride (Co-administration of thiazide and other antihypertensive agents can lead to additive effect or potentiation).
No products indexed under this heading.

Bisoprolol Fumarate (Co-administration of thiazide and other antihypertensive agents can lead to additive effect or potentiation).
No products indexed under this heading.

Budesonide (Co-administration of thiazide diuretics with corticosteroids intensifies electrolyte depletion, particularly potassium). Products include:
Pulmicort Flexhaler 654
Symbicort 80/4.5 Inhalation Aerosol.. 659
Symbicort 160/4.5 Inhalation Aerosol.. 659

Bumetanide (Co-administration of lisinopril in patients on diuretics, especially those in whom diuretic therapy was recently instituted, may occasionally experience excessive hypotension; antihypertensive effects of lisinopril are augmented by antihypertensive agents that cause renin release).
No products indexed under this heading.

Buprenorphine Hydrochloride (Co-administration of thiazide and narcotics may potentiate orthostatic hypotension). Products include:
Suboxone Tablets 2601
Subutex Tablets 2601

Butabarbital (Co-administration of thiazide and barbiturates may potentiate orthostatic hypotension).
No products indexed under this heading.

Butalbital (Co-administration of thiazide and barbiturates may potentiate orthostatic hypotension).
No products indexed under this heading.

Candesartan Cilexetil (Co-administration of thiazide and other antihypertensive agents can lead to additive effect or potentiation). Products include:
Atacand Tablets 639
Atacand HCT 642

Captopril (Co-administration of thiazide and other antihypertensive agents can lead to additive effect or potentiation). Products include:
Captopril Tablets 2182

Carteolol Hydrochloride (Co-administration of thiazide and other antihypertensive agents can lead to additive effect or potentiation).
No products indexed under this heading.

Celecoxib (Reports suggest that NSAIDs, including selective COX-2 inhibitors, may diminish the antihypertensive effect of ACE inhibitors, including lisinopril. This interaction should be given consideration in patients taking NSAIDs or selective COX-2 inhibitors concomitantly with ACE inhibitors. In some patients with compromised renal function who are being treated with NSAIDs, including selective COX-2 inhibitors, the co-administration of angiotensin II receptor antagonists or ACE inhibitors, may result in further deterioration of renal function, including possible acute renal failure. These effects are usually reversible. Therefore, the combination should be administered with caution, especially in the elderly). Products include:
Celebrex Capsules 2979

Chlorothiazide (Co-administration of lisinopril in patients on diuretics, especially those in whom diuretic therapy was recently instituted, may occasionally experience excessive hypotension; antihypertensive effects of lisinopril are augmented by antihypertensive agents that cause renin release).
No products indexed under this heading.

Chlorothiazide Sodium (Co-administration of lisinopril in patients on diuretics, especially those in whom diuretic therapy was recently instituted, may occasionally experience excessive hypotension; antihypertensive effects of lisinopril are augmented by antihypertensive agents that cause renin release). Products include:
Intravenous Sodium Diuril 2490

Chlorpropamide (Hyperglycemia may occur with thiazide diuretics; dosage adjustment of oral hypoglycemic agents may be required).
No products indexed under this heading.

Chlorthalidone (Co-administration of lisinopril in patients on diuretics, especially those in whom diuretic therapy was recently instituted, may occasionally experience excessive hypotension; antihypertensive effects of lisinopril are augmented by antihypertensive agents that cause renin release). Products include:
Clorpres Tablets 2185

Cholestyramine (Absorption of hydrochlorothiazide is impaired in the presence of anionic exchange resins; these resins bind the hydrochlorothiazide and reduce its absorption from GI tract).
No products indexed under this heading.

Ciclesonide (Co-administration of thiazide diuretics with corticosteroids intensifies electrolyte depletion, particularly potassium). Products include:
Alvesco Inhalation Aerosol 2985
Omnaris Nasal Spray 2998

Cisatracurium Besylate (Co-administration with nondepolarizing skeletal muscle relaxants may result in possible increased responsiveness to the muscle relaxant). Products include:
Nimbex Injection 484

Clonidine (Co-administration of thiazide and other antihypertensive agents can lead to additive effect or potentiation). Products include:
Catapres-TTS 842

Clonidine Hydrochloride (Co-administration of thiazide and other antihypertensive agents can lead to additive effect or potentiation). Products include:
Catapres Tablets 841
Clorpres Tablets 2185

Codeine Phosphate (Co-administration of thiazide and narcotics may potentiate orthostatic hypotension). Products include:
Tylenol with Codeine Tablets 2427

Colestipol Hydrochloride (Absorption of hydrochlorothiazide is impaired in the presence of anionic exchange resins; these resins bind the hydrochlorothiazide and reduce its absorption from GI tract).
No products indexed under this heading.

Cortisone Acetate (Co-administration of thiazide diuretics with corticosteroids intensifies electrolyte depletion, particularly potassium).
No products indexed under this heading.

Deserpidine (Co-administration of thiazide and other antihypertensive agents can lead to additive effect or potentiation).
No products indexed under this heading.

Deslanoside (Hypokalemia induced by thiazide diuretics may cause cardiac arrhythmia and may also sensitize or exaggerate the response to the heart to the toxic effects of digitalis, such as ventricular irritability).
No products indexed under this heading.

Dexamethasone (Co-administration of thiazide diuretics with corticosteroids intensifies electrolyte depletion, particularly potassium). Products include:
Ciprodex Otic Suspension 541

Dexamethasone Acetate (Co-administration of thiazide diuretics with corticosteroids intensifies electrolyte depletion, particularly potassium).
No products indexed under this heading.

Dexamethasone Sodium Phosphate (Co-administration of thiazide diuretics with corticosteroids intensifies electrolyte depletion, particularly potassium).
No products indexed under this heading.

Dezocine (Co-administration of thiazide and narcotics may potentiate orthostatic hypotension).
No products indexed under this heading.

Diazoxide (Co-administration of thiazide and other antihypertensive agents can lead to additive effect or potentiation). Products include:
Proglycem Capsules 1185
Proglycem Suspension 1185

Diclofenac Epolamine (Reports suggest that NSAIDs, including selective COX-2 inhibitors, may diminish the antihypertensive effect of ACE inhibitors, including lisinopril. This interaction should be given consideration in patients taking NSAIDs or selective COX-2 inhibitors concomitantly with ACE inhibitors. In some patients with compromised renal function who are being treated with NSAIDs, including selective COX-2 inhibitors, the co-administration of angiotensin II receptor antagonists or ACE inhibitors, may result in further deterioration of renal function, including possible acute renal failure. These effects are usually reversible. Therefore, the combination should be administered with caution, especially in the elderly). Products include:
- Flector Patch 561

Diclofenac Potassium (Reports suggest that NSAIDs, including selective COX-2 inhibitors, may diminish the antihypertensive effect of ACE inhibitors, including lisinopril. This interaction should be given consideration in patients taking NSAIDs or selective COX-2 inhibitors concomitantly with ACE inhibitors. In some patients with compromised renal function who are being treated with NSAIDs, including selective COX-2 inhibitors, the co-administration of angiotensin II receptor antagonists or ACE inhibitors, may result in further deterioration of renal function, including possible acute renal failure. These effects are usually reversible. Therefore, the combination should be administered with caution, especially in the elderly).
- No products indexed under this heading.

Diclofenac Sodium (Reports suggest that NSAIDs, including selective COX-2 inhibitors, may diminish the antihypertensive effect of ACE inhibitors, including lisinopril. This interaction should be given consideration in patients taking NSAIDs or selective COX-2 inhibitors concomitantly with ACE inhibitors. In some patients with compromised renal function who are being treated with NSAIDs, including selective COX-2 inhibitors, the co-administration of angiotensin II receptor antagonists or ACE inhibitors, may result in further deterioration of renal function, including possible acute renal failure. These effects are usually reversible. Therefore, the combination should be administered with caution, especially in the elderly). Products include:
- Diclofenac Sodium Ophthalmic Solution .... ⊙ 240
- Voltaren Ophthalmic Solution 2336
- Voltaren Tablets 2334
- Voltaren-XR Tablets 2337

Digitalis Glycoside Preparations (Hypokalemia induced by thiazide diuretics may cause cardiac arrhythmia and may also sensitize or exaggerate the response to the heart to the toxic effects of digitalis, such as ventricular irritability).
- No products indexed under this heading.

Digitoxin (Hypokalemia induced by thiazide diuretics may cause cardiac arrhythmia and may also sensitize or exaggerate the response to the heart to the toxic effects of digitalis, such as ventricular irritability).
- No products indexed under this heading.

Digoxin (Hypokalemia induced by thiazide diuretics may cause cardiac arrhythmia and may also sensitize or exaggerate the response to the heart to the toxic effects of digitalis, such as ventricular irritability). Products include:
- Lanoxin Injection 1498
- Lanoxin Injection Pediatric 1502
- Lanoxin Tablets 1505

Diltiazem Hydrochloride (Co-administration of thiazide and other antihypertensive agents can lead to additive effect or potentiation). Products include:
- Cardizem LA Extended Release Tablets 421

Doxazosin Mesylate (Co-administration of thiazide and other antihypertensive agents can lead to additive effect or potentiation).
- No products indexed under this heading.

Enalapril Maleate (Co-administration of thiazide and other antihypertensive agents can lead to additive effect or potentiation).
- No products indexed under this heading.

Enalaprilat (Co-administration of thiazide and other antihypertensive agents can lead to additive effect or potentiation).
- No products indexed under this heading.

Eplerenone (Use of lisinopril with potassium-sparing diuretics (such as spironolactone, triamterene or amiloride), potassium supplements or potassium-containing salt substitutes may lead to significant increases in serum potassium. Therefore, if concomitant use of these agents is indicated because of demonstrated hypokalemia, they should be used with caution and with frequent monitoring of serum potassium. Potassium-sparing agents should generally not be used in patients with heart failure who are receiving lisinopril).
- No products indexed under this heading.

Eprosartan Mesylate (Co-administration of thiazide and other antihypertensive agents can lead to additive effect or potentiation). Products include:
- Teveten Tablets 515
- Teveten HCT Tablets 517

Esmolol Hydrochloride (Co-administration of thiazide and other antihypertensive agents can lead to additive effect or potentiation).
- No products indexed under this heading.

Ethacrynic Acid (Co-administration of lisinopril in patients on diuretics, especially those in whom diuretic therapy was recently instituted, may occasionally experience excessive hypotension; antihypertensive effects of lisinopril are augmented by antihypertensive agents that cause renin release). Products include:
- Edecrin Tablets 698

Etodolac (Reports suggest that NSAIDs, including selective COX-2 inhibitors, may diminish the antihypertensive effect of ACE inhibitors, including lisinopril. This interaction should be given consideration in patients taking NSAIDs or selective COX-2 inhibitors concomitantly with ACE inhibitors. In some patients with compromised renal function who are being treated with NSAIDs, including selective COX-2 inhibitors, the co-administration of angiotensin II receptor antagonists or ACE inhibitors, may result in further deterioration of renal function, including possible acute renal failure. These effects are usually reversible. Therefore, the combination should be administered with caution, especially in the elderly).
- No products indexed under this heading.

Felodipine (Co-administration of thiazide and other antihypertensive agents can lead to additive effect or potentiation).
- No products indexed under this heading.

Fenoprofen Calcium (Reports suggest that NSAIDs, including selective COX-2 inhibitors, may diminish the antihypertensive effect of ACE inhibitors, including lisinopril. This interaction should be given consideration in patients taking NSAIDs or selective COX-2 inhibitors concomitantly with ACE inhibitors. In some patients with compromised renal function who are being treated with NSAIDs, including selective COX-2 inhibitors, the co-administration of angiotensin II receptor antagonists or ACE inhibitors, may result in further deterioration of renal function, including possible acute renal failure. These effects are usually reversible. Therefore, the combination should be administered with caution, especially in the elderly). Products include:
- Nalfon Capsules 2508

Fentanyl (Co-administration of thiazide and narcotics may potentiate orthostatic hypotension). Products include:
- Duragesic Transdermal System 2405
- Ionsys Transdermal System 2410

Fentanyl Citrate (Co-administration of thiazide and narcotics may potentiate orthostatic hypotension). Products include:
- Actiq 959
- Fentora Tablets 968

Fludrocortisone Acetate (Co-administration of thiazide diuretics with corticosteroids intensifies electrolyte depletion, particularly potassium).
- No products indexed under this heading.

Flunisolide (Co-administration of thiazide diuretics with corticosteroids intensifies electrolyte depletion, particularly potassium). Products include:
- Aerobid/Aerobid-M 1153

Flurbiprofen (Reports suggest that NSAIDs, including selective COX-2 inhibitors, may diminish the antihypertensive effect of ACE inhibitors, including lisinopril. This interaction should be given consideration in patients taking NSAIDs or selective COX-2 inhibitors concomitantly with ACE inhibitors. In some patients with compromised renal function who are being treated with NSAIDs, including selective COX-2 inhibitors, the co-administration of angiotensin II receptor antagonists or ACE inhibitors, may result in further deterioration of renal function, including possible acute renal failure. These effects are usually reversible. Therefore, the combination should be administered with caution, especially in the elderly).
- No products indexed under this heading.

Fluticasone Propionate (Co-administration of thiazide diuretics with corticosteroids intensifies electrolyte depletion, particularly potassium). Products include:
- Advair Diskus 100/50 1276
- Advair Diskus 250/50 1276
- Advair Diskus 500/50 1276
- Advair HFA 45/21 Inhalation Aerosol 1288
- Advair HFA 115/21 Inhalation Aerosol 1288
- Advair HFA 230/21 Inhalation Aerosol 1288
- Flonase Nasal Spray 1431
- Flovent Diskus 50 mcg 1435

Fluticasone Propionate HFA (Co-administration of thiazide diuretics with corticosteroids intensifies electrolyte depletion, particularly potassium). Products include:
- Flovent HFA 1440

Fosinopril Sodium (Co-administration of thiazide and other antihypertensive agents can lead to additive effect or potentiation).
- No products indexed under this heading.

Furosemide (Co-administration of lisinopril in patients on diuretics, especially those in whom diuretic therapy was recently instituted, may occasionally experience excessive hypotension; antihypertensive effects of lisinopril are augmented by antihypertensive agents that cause renin release). Products include:
- Furosemide Tablets 2186

Glimepiride (Hyperglycemia may occur with thiazide diuretics; dosage adjustment of oral hypoglycemic agents may be required). Products include:
- Avandaryl Tablets 1344
- Duetact Tablets 3085

Glipizide (Hyperglycemia may occur with thiazide diuretics; dosage adjustment of oral hypoglycemic agents may be required).
- No products indexed under this heading.

Glyburide (Hyperglycemia may occur with thiazide diuretics; dosage adjustment of oral hypoglycemic agents may be required).
- No products indexed under this heading.

Guanabenz Acetate (Co-administration of thiazide and other antihypertensive agents can lead to additive effect or potentiation).
- No products indexed under this heading.

Guanethidine Monosulfate (Co-administration of thiazide and other antihypertensive agents can lead to additive effect or potentiation).
- No products indexed under this heading.

Hydralazine Hydrochloride (Co-administration of thiazide and other antihypertensive agents can lead to additive effect or potentiation).
- No products indexed under this heading.

Hydrocodone Bitartrate (Co-administration of thiazide and narcotics may potentiate orthostatic hypotension). Products include:
- Lortab 5/500 Tablets 3143
- Lortab 7.5/500 Tablets 3144
- Lortab 10/500 Tablets 3144
- Vicodin Tablets 529

Vicodin ES Tablets 530
Vicodin HP Tablets 531
Vicoprofen Tablets 533
Zydone Tablets 1132

Hydrocodone Polistirex (Co-administration of thiazide and narcotics may potentiate orthostatic hypotension). Products include:
Tussionex Pennkinetic Extended-Release Suspension 3154

Hydrocortisone (Co-administration of thiazide diuretics with corticosteroids intensifies electrolyte depletion, particularly potassium).
No products indexed under this heading.

Hydrocortisone Acetate (Co-administration of thiazide diuretics with corticosteroids intensifies electrolyte depletion, particularly potassium). Products include:
Analpram-HC 1140
Pramosone 1141

Hydrocortisone Sodium Phosphate (Co-administration of thiazide diuretics with corticosteroids intensifies electrolyte depletion, particularly potassium).
No products indexed under this heading.

Hydrocortisone Sodium Succinate (Co-administration of thiazide diuretics with corticosteroids intensifies electrolyte depletion, particularly potassium).
No products indexed under this heading.

Hydroflumethiazide (Co-administration of lisinopril in patients on diuretics, especially those in whom diuretic therapy was recently instituted, may occasionally experience excessive hypotension; antihypertensive effects of lisinopril are augmented by antihypertensive agents that cause renin release).
No products indexed under this heading.

Hydromorphone Hydrochloride (Co-administration of thiazide and narcotics may potentiate orthostatic hypotension).
No products indexed under this heading.

Ibuprofen (Reports suggest that NSAIDs, including selective COX-2 inhibitors, may diminish the antihypertensive effect of ACE inhibitors, including lisinopril. This interaction should be given consideration in patients taking NSAIDs or selective COX-2 inhibitors concomitantly with ACE inhibitors. In some patients with compromised renal function who are being treated with NSAIDs, including selective COX-2 inhibitors, the co-administration of angiotensin II receptor antagonists or ACE inhibitors, may result in further deterioration of renal function, including possible acute renal failure. These effects are usually reversible. Therefore, the combination should be administered with caution, especially in the elderly). Products include:
Motrin IB Tablets and Caplets 1900
Children's Motrin Oral Suspension ... 1901
Children's Motrin Non-Staining Dye-Free Oral Suspension 1901
Children's Motrin Cold Oral Suspension 1899
Infants' Motrin Concentrated Drops 1901
Infants' Motrin Non-Staining Dye-Free Concentrated Drops....... 1901
Junior Strength Motrin Caplets and Chewable Tablets.................. 1901
Vicoprofen Tablets 533

Indapamide (Co-administration of lisinopril in patients on diuretics, especially those in whom diuretic therapy was recently instituted, may occasionally experience excessive hypotension; antihypertensive effects of lisinopril are augmented by antihypertensive agents that cause renin release). Products include:
Indapamide Tablets 2188

Indomethacin (Reports suggest that NSAIDs, including selective COX-2 inhibitors, may diminish the antihypertensive effect of ACE inhibitors, including lisinopril. This interaction should be given consideration in patients taking NSAIDs or selective COX-2 inhibitors concomitantly with ACE inhibitors. In some patients with compromised renal function who are being treated with NSAIDs, including selective COX-2 inhibitors, the co-administration of angiotensin II receptor antagonists or ACE inhibitors, may result in further deterioration of renal function, including possible acute renal failure. These effects are usually reversible. Therefore, the combination should be administered with caution, especially in the elderly). Products include:
Indocin 2024

Indomethacin Sodium Trihydrate (Reports suggest that NSAIDs, including selective COX-2 inhibitors, may diminish the antihypertensive effect of ACE inhibitors, including lisinopril. This interaction should be given consideration in patients taking NSAIDs or selective COX-2 inhibitors concomitantly with ACE inhibitors. In some patients with compromised renal function who are being treated with NSAIDs, including selective COX-2 inhibitors, the co-administration of angiotensin II receptor antagonists or ACE inhibitors, may result in further deterioration of renal function, including possible acute renal failure. These effects are usually reversible. Therefore, the combination should be administered with caution, especially in the elderly). Products include:
Indocin I.V. 2489

Insulin (Hyperglycemia may occur with thiazide diuretics; dosage adjustment of insulin may be required).
No products indexed under this heading.

Insulin, Human, Zinc Suspension (Hyperglycemia may occur with thiazide diuretics; dosage adjustment of insulin may be required).
No products indexed under this heading.

Insulin, Human (rDNA origin) (Hyperglycemia may occur with thiazide diuretics; dosage adjustment of insulin may be required). Products include:
Exubera Inhalation Powder 2515

Insulin, Human NPH (Hyperglycemia may occur with thiazide diuretics; dosage adjustment of insulin may be required). Products include:
Humulin N Vial 1846

Insulin, Human Regular (Hyperglycemia may occur with thiazide diuretics; dosage adjustment of insulin may be required). Products include:
Humulin R 1849
Humulin R (U-500) 1850

Insulin, Human Regular and Human NPH Mixture (Hyperglycemia may occur with thiazide diuretics; dosage adjustment of insulin may be required). Products include:
Humulin 50/50, 100 Units 1843
Humulin 70/30 Vial 1844

Insulin, NPH (Hyperglycemia may occur with thiazide diuretics; dosage adjustment of insulin may be required).
No products indexed under this heading.

Insulin, Regular (Hyperglycemia may occur with thiazide diuretics; dosage adjustment of insulin may be required).
No products indexed under this heading.

Insulin, Regular and NPH mixture (Hyperglycemia may occur with thiazide diuretics; dosage adjustment of insulin may be required).
No products indexed under this heading.

Insulin, Zinc Crystals (Hyperglycemia may occur with thiazide diuretics; dosage adjustment of insulin may be required).
No products indexed under this heading.

Insulin, Zinc Suspension (Hyperglycemia may occur with thiazide diuretics; dosage adjustment of insulin may be required).
No products indexed under this heading.

Insulin Aspart (Hyperglycemia may occur with thiazide diuretics; dosage adjustment of insulin may be required).
No products indexed under this heading.

Insulin Aspart, Human (Hyperglycemia may occur with thiazide diuretics; dosage adjustment of insulin may be required). Products include:
NovoLog Mix 70/30 2364

Insulin Aspart, Human Regular (Hyperglycemia may occur with thiazide diuretics; dosage adjustment of insulin may be required). Products include:
NovoLog Injection 2359

Insulin Aspart Protamine, Human (Hyperglycemia may occur with thiazide diuretics; dosage adjustment of insulin may be required). Products include:
NovoLog Mix 70/30 2364

Insulin Detemir (rDNA Origin) (Hyperglycemia may occur with thiazide diuretics; dosage adjustment of insulin may be required). Products include:
Levemir Injection 2352

Insulin glargine (Hyperglycemia may occur with thiazide diuretics; dosage adjustment of insulin may be required). Products include:
Lantus Injection 2749

Insulin Glulisine (Hyperglycemia may occur with thiazide diuretics; dosage adjustment of insulin may be required). Products include:
Apidra Injection 2706

Insulin Lispro, Human (Hyperglycemia may occur with thiazide diuretics; dosage adjustment of insulin may be required). Products include:
Humalog-Pen and KwikPen 1829
Humalog Mix 50/50-Pen and KwikPen 1833
Humalog Mix 75/25-Pen and KwikPen 1835

Insulin Lispro Protamine, Human (Hyperglycemia may occur with thiazide diuretics; dosage adjustment of insulin may be required). Products include:
Humalog Mix 50/50-Pen and KwikPen 1833
Humalog Mix 75/25-Pen and KwikPen 1835

Irbesartan (Co-administration of thiazide and other antihypertensive agents can lead to additive effect or potentiation). Products include:
Avalide Tablets 892
Avalide Tablets 2713
Avapro Tablets 897
Avapro Tablets 2718

Isradipine (Co-administration of thiazide and other antihypertensive agents can lead to additive effect or potentiation). Products include:
DynaCirc CR Controlled Release Tablets 1407

Ketoprofen (Reports suggest that NSAIDs, including selective COX-2 inhibitors, may diminish the antihypertensive effect of ACE inhibitors, including lisinopril. This interaction should be given consideration in patients taking NSAIDs or selective COX-2 inhibitors concomitantly with ACE inhibitors. In some patients with compromised renal function who are being treated with NSAIDs, including selective COX-2 inhibitors, the co-administration of angiotensin II receptor antagonists or ACE inhibitors, may result in further deterioration of renal function, including possible acute renal failure. These effects are usually reversible. Therefore, the combination should be administered with caution, especially in the elderly).
No products indexed under this heading.

Ketorolac Tromethamine (Reports suggest that NSAIDs, including selective COX-2 inhibitors, may diminish the antihypertensive effect of ACE inhibitors, including lisinopril. This interaction should be given consideration in patients taking NSAIDs or selective COX-2 inhibitors concomitantly with ACE inhibitors. In some patients with compromised renal function who are being treated with NSAIDs, including selective COX-2 inhibitors, the co-administration of angiotensin II receptor antagonists or ACE inhibitors, may result in further deterioration of renal function, including possible acute renal failure. These effects are usually reversible. Therefore, the combination should be administered with caution, especially in the elderly).
No products indexed under this heading.

Labetalol Hydrochloride (Co-administration of thiazide and other antihypertensive agents can lead to additive effect or potentiation).
No products indexed under this heading.

Levorphanol Tartrate (Co-administration of thiazide and narcotics may potentiate orthostatic hypotension).
No products indexed under this heading.

Lithium (Co-administration of lithium with drugs that cause elimination of sodium, including ACE inhibitors, can lead to lithium toxicity; diuretics can reduce renal clearance of lithium and add a high risk of lithium toxicity).
No products indexed under this heading.

Lithium Carbonate (Co-administration of lithium with drugs that cause elimination of sodium, including ACE inhibitors, can lead to lithium toxicity; diuretics can reduce renal clearance of lithium and add a high risk of lithium toxicity).
No products indexed under this heading.

Lithium Citrate (Co-administration of lithium with drugs that cause elimination of sodium, including ACE inhibitors, can lead to lithium toxicity; diuretics can reduce renal clearance of lithium and add a high risk of lithium toxicity).
No products indexed under this heading.

Losartan Potassium (Co-administration of thiazide and other antihypertensive agents can lead to additive effect or potentiation). Products include:
Cozaar Tablets 1973

Mecamylamine Hydrochloride (Co-administration of thiazide and other antihypertensive agents can lead to additive effect or potentiation).
No products indexed under this heading.

Meclofenamate Sodium (Reports suggest that NSAIDs, including selective COX-2 inhibitors, may diminish the antihypertensive effect of ACE inhibitors, including lisinopril. This interaction should be given consideration in patients taking NSAIDs or selective COX-2 inhibitors concomitantly with ACE inhibitors. In some patients with compromised renal function who are being treated with NSAIDs, including selective COX-2 inhibitors, the co-administration of angiotensin II receptor antagonists or ACE inhibitors, may result in further deterioration of renal function, including possible acute renal failure. These effects are usually reversible. Therefore, the combination should be administered with caution, especially in the elderly).
No products indexed under this heading.

Mefenamic Acid (Reports suggest that NSAIDs, including selective COX-2 inhibitors, may diminish the antihypertensive effect of ACE inhibitors, including lisinopril. This interaction should be given consideration in patients taking NSAIDs or selective COX-2 inhibitors concomitantly with ACE inhibitors. In some patients with compromised renal function who are being treated with NSAIDs, including selective COX-2 inhibitors, the co-administration of angiotensin II receptor antagonists or ACE inhibitors, may result in further deterioration of renal function, including possible acute renal failure. These effects are usually reversible. Therefore, the combination should be administered with caution, especially in the elderly).
No products indexed under this heading.

Meloxicam (Reports suggest that NSAIDs, including selective COX-2 inhibitors, may diminish the antihypertensive effect of ACE inhibitors, including lisinopril. This interaction should be given consideration in patients taking NSAIDs or selective COX-2 inhibitors concomitantly with ACE inhibitors. In some patients with compromised renal function who are being treated with NSAIDs, including selective COX-2 inhibitors, the co-administration of angiotensin II receptor antagonists or ACE inhibitors, may result in further deterioration of renal function, including possible acute renal failure. These effects are usually reversible. Therefore, the combination should be administered with caution, especially in the elderly). Products include:
Mobic Oral Suspension 863
Mobic Tablets 863

Meperidine Hydrochloride (Co-administration of thiazide and narcotics may potentiate orthostatic hypotension).
No products indexed under this heading.

Mephobarbital (Co-administration of thiazide and barbiturates may potentiate orthostatic hypotension).
No products indexed under this heading.

Metformin Hydrochloride (Hyperglycemia may occur with thiazide diuretics; dosage adjustment of oral hypoglycemic agents may be required). Products include:
ActoPlus Met Tablets 3071
Avandamet Tablets 1336
Janumet Tablets 2041
PrandiMet Tablets 2967

Methadone Hydrochloride (Co-administration of thiazide and narcotics may potentiate orthostatic hypotension).
No products indexed under this heading.

Methyclothiazide (Co-administration of lisinopril in patients on diuretics, especially those in whom diuretic therapy was recently instituted, may occasionally experience excessive hypotension; antihypertensive effects of lisinopril are augmented by antihypertensive agents that cause renin release).
No products indexed under this heading.

Methyldopa (Co-administration of thiazide and other antihypertensive agents can lead to additive effect or potentiation).
No products indexed under this heading.

Methyldopate Hydrochloride (Co-administration of thiazide and other antihypertensive agents can lead to additive effect or potentiation).
No products indexed under this heading.

Methylprednisolone Acetate (Co-administration of thiazide diuretics with corticosteroids intensifies electrolyte depletion, particularly potassium).
No products indexed under this heading.

Methylprednisolone Sodium Succinate (Co-administration of thiazide diuretics with corticosteroids intensifies electrolyte depletion, particularly potassium).
No products indexed under this heading.

Metocurine Iodide (Co-administration with nondepolarizing skeletal muscle relaxants may result in possible increased responsiveness to the muscle relaxant).
No products indexed under this heading.

Metolazone (Co-administration of lisinopril in patients on diuretics, especially those in whom diuretic therapy was recently instituted, may occasionally experience excessive hypotension; antihypertensive effects of lisinopril are augmented by antihypertensive agents that cause renin release).
No products indexed under this heading.

Metoprolol Succinate (Co-administration of thiazide and other antihypertensive agents can lead to additive effect or potentiation). Products include:
Toprol-XL Tablets 666

Metoprolol Tartrate (Co-administration of thiazide and other antihypertensive agents can lead to additive effect or potentiation).
No products indexed under this heading.

Metyrosine (Co-administration of thiazide and other antihypertensive agents can lead to additive effect or potentiation). Products include:
Demser Capsules 1989

Mibefradil Dihydrochloride (Co-administration of thiazide and other antihypertensive agents can lead to additive effect or potentiation).
No products indexed under this heading.

Miglitol (Hyperglycemia may occur with thiazide diuretics; dosage adjustment of oral hypoglycemic agents may be required).
No products indexed under this heading.

Minoxidil (Co-administration of thiazide and other antihypertensive agents can lead to additive effect or potentiation).
No products indexed under this heading.

Mivacurium Chloride (Co-administration with nondepolarizing skeletal muscle relaxants may result in possible increased responsiveness to the muscle relaxant).
No products indexed under this heading.

Moexipril Hydrochloride (Co-administration of thiazide and other antihypertensive agents can lead to additive effect or potentiation).
No products indexed under this heading.

Mometasone Furoate (Co-administration of thiazide diuretics with corticosteroids intensifies electrolyte depletion, particularly potassium). Products include:
Asmanex Twisthaler 2797
Elocon Cream 0.1% 2840
Elocon Lotion 0.1% 2841
Elocon Ointment 0.1% 2842

Mometasone Furoate Monohydrate (Co-administration of thiazide diuretics with corticosteroids intensifies electrolyte depletion, particularly potassium). Products include:
Nasonex Nasal Spray 2883

Morphine Sulfate (Co-administration of thiazide and narcotics may potentiate orthostatic hypotension). Products include:
Avinza Capsules 1772
DepoDur Injection 1095
MS Contin Tablets 2585

Nabumetone (Reports suggest that NSAIDs, including selective COX-2 inhibitors, may diminish the antihypertensive effect of ACE inhibitors, including lisinopril. This interaction should be given consideration in patients taking NSAIDs or selective COX-2 inhibitors concomitantly with ACE inhibitors. In some patients with compromised renal function who are being treated with NSAIDs, including selective COX-2 inhibitors, the co-administration of angiotensin II receptor antagonists or ACE inhibitors, may result in further deterioration of renal function, including possible acute renal failure. These effects are usually reversible. Therefore, the combination should be administered with caution, especially in the elderly).
No products indexed under this heading.

Nadolol (Co-administration of thiazide and other antihypertensive agents can lead to additive effect or potentiation). Products include:
Nadolol Tablets 2191

Naproxen (Reports suggest that NSAIDs, including selective COX-2 inhibitors, may diminish the antihypertensive effect of ACE inhibitors, including lisinopril. This interaction should be given consideration in patients taking NSAIDs or selective COX-2 inhibitors concomitantly with ACE inhibitors. In some patients with compromised renal function who are being treated with NSAIDs, including selective COX-2 inhibitors, the co-administration of angiotensin II receptor antagonists or ACE inhibitors, may result in further deterioration of renal function, including possible acute renal failure. These effects are usually reversible. Therefore, the combination should be administered with caution, especially in the elderly). Products include:
EC-Naprosyn Delayed-Release Tablets 2632
Naprosyn Suspension 2632
Naprosyn Tablets 2632

Naproxen Sodium (Reports suggest that NSAIDs, including selective COX-2 inhibitors, may diminish the antihypertensive effect of ACE inhibitors, including lisinopril. This interaction should be given consideration in patients taking NSAIDs or selective COX-2 inhibitors concomitantly with ACE inhibitors. In some patients with compromised renal function who are being treated with NSAIDs, including selective COX-2 inhibitors, the co-administration of angiotensin II receptor antagonists or ACE inhibitors, may result in further deterioration of renal function, including possible acute renal failure. These effects are usually reversible. Therefore, the combination should be administered with caution, especially in the elderly). Products include:
Anaprox Tablets 2632
Anaprox DS Tablets 2632
Treximet Tablets 1616

Nateglinide (Hyperglycemia may occur with thiazide diuretics; dosage adjustment of oral hypoglycemic agents may be required). Products include:
Starlix Tablets 2314

Nebivolol (Co-administration of thiazide and other antihypertensive agents can lead to additive effect or potentiation). Products include:
Bystolic Tablets 1155

Nicardipine Hydrochloride (Co-administration of thiazide and other antihypertensive agents can lead to additive effect or potentiation). Products include:

Cardene I.V. 1093

Nifedipine (Co-administration of thiazide and other antihypertensive agents can lead to additive effect or potentiation).
No products indexed under this heading.

Nisoldipine (Co-administration of thiazide and other antihypertensive agents can lead to additive effect or potentiation). Products include:
Sular Extended Release Tablets 2975

Nitroglycerin (Co-administration of thiazide and other antihypertensive agents can lead to additive effect or potentiation). Products include:
Nitro-Dur Transdermal Infusion System.. 2887
Nitrolingual Pumpspray 2965

Norepinephrine Bitartrate (Possible decreased response to pressor amines but not sufficient to preclude pressor amine use).
No products indexed under this heading.

Oxaprozin (Reports suggest that NSAIDs, including selective COX-2 inhibitors, may diminish the antihypertensive effect of ACE inhibitors, including lisinopril. This interaction should be given consideration in patients taking NSAIDs or selective COX-2 inhibitors concomitantly with ACE inhibitors. In some patients with compromised renal function who are being treated with NSAIDs, including selective COX-2 inhibitors, the co-administration of angiotensin II receptor antagonists or ACE inhibitors, may result in further deterioration of renal function, including possible acute renal failure. These effects are usually reversible. Therefore, the combination should be administered with caution, especially in the elderly).
No products indexed under this heading.

Oxycodone Hydrochloride (Co-administration of thiazide and narcotics may potentiate orthostatic hypotension). Products include:
OxyContin Tablets 2589
OxyIR Capsules 2593
Percocet Tablets 1127
Percodan Tablets 1130

Pancuronium Bromide (Co-administration with nondepolarizing skeletal muscle relaxants may result in possible increased responsiveness to the muscle relaxant).
No products indexed under this heading.

Penbutolol Sulfate (Co-administration of thiazide and other antihypertensive agents can lead to additive effect or potentiation).
No products indexed under this heading.

Pentobarbital Sodium (Co-administration of thiazide and barbiturates may potentiate orthostatic hypotension). Products include:
Nembutal Sodium Solution, USP 2494

Perindopril Erbumine (Co-administration of thiazide and other antihypertensive agents can lead to additive effect or potentiation). Products include:
Aceon Tablets (2 mg, 4 mg, 8 mg)... 3038

Phenobarbital (Co-administration of thiazide and barbiturates may potentiate orthostatic hypotension). Products include:
Donnatal Extentabs 2507

Phenoxybenzamine Hydrochloride (Co-administration of thiazide and other antihypertensive agents can lead to additive effect or potentiation). Products include:
Dibenzyline Capsules 3188

Phentolamine Mesylate (Co-administration of thiazide and other antihypertensive agents can lead to additive effect or potentiation).
No products indexed under this heading.

Phenylbutazone (Reports suggest that NSAIDs, including selective COX-2 inhibitors, may diminish the antihypertensive effect of ACE inhibitors, including lisinopril. This interaction should be given consideration in patients taking NSAIDs or selective COX-2 inhibitors concomitantly with ACE inhibitors. In some patients with compromised renal function who are being treated with NSAIDs, including selective COX-2 inhibitors, the co-administration of angiotensin II receptor antagonists or ACE inhibitors, may result in further deterioration of renal function, including possible acute renal failure. These effects are usually reversible. Therefore, the combination should be administered with caution, especially in the elderly).
No products indexed under this heading.

Pindolol (Co-administration of thiazide and other antihypertensive agents can lead to additive effect or potentiation).
No products indexed under this heading.

Pioglitazone Hydrochloride (Hyperglycemia may occur with thiazide diuretics; dosage adjustment of oral hypoglycemic agents may be required). Products include:
ActoPlus Met Tablets 3071
Actos Tablets 3077
Duetact Tablets 3085

Piroxicam (Reports suggest that NSAIDs, including selective COX-2 inhibitors, may diminish the antihypertensive effect of ACE inhibitors, including lisinopril. This interaction should be given consideration in patients taking NSAIDs or selective COX-2 inhibitors concomitantly with ACE inhibitors. In some patients with compromised renal function who are being treated with NSAIDs, including selective COX-2 inhibitors, the co-administration of angiotensin II receptor antagonists or ACE inhibitors, may result in further deterioration of renal function, including possible acute renal failure. These effects are usually reversible. Therefore, the combination should be administered with caution, especially in the elderly).
No products indexed under this heading.

Polythiazide (Co-administration of lisinopril in patients on diuretics, especially those in whom diuretic therapy was recently instituted, may occasionally experience excessive hypotension; antihypertensive effects of lisinopril are augmented by antihypertensive agents that cause renin release).
No products indexed under this heading.

Potassium Acid Phosphate (Risk factors for the development of hyperkalemia include the concomitant use of potassium-sparing diuretics, potassium supplements and/or potassium-containing salt substitutes. Hyperkalemia can cause serious, sometimes, fatal, arrhythmias. Prinzide should be used cautiously, if at all, with these agents and with frequent monitoring of serum potassium). Products include:
K-Phos Original (Sodium Free) Tablets 814

Potassium Bicarbonate (Risk factors for the development of hyperkalemia include the concomitant use of potassium-sparing diuretics, potassium supplements and/or potassium-containing salt substitutes. Hyperkalemia can cause serious, sometimes, fatal, arrhythmias. Prinzide should be used cautiously, if at all, with these agents and with frequent monitoring of serum potassium).
No products indexed under this heading.

Potassium Chloride (Risk factors for the development of hyperkalemia include the concomitant use of potassium-sparing diuretics, potassium supplements and/or potassium-containing salt substitutes. Hyperkalemia can cause serious, sometimes, fatal, arrhythmias. Prinzide should be used cautiously, if at all, with these agents and with frequent monitoring of serum potassium). Products include:
MoviPrep Oral Solution 2679

Potassium Citrate (Risk factors for the development of hyperkalemia include the concomitant use of potassium-sparing diuretics, potassium supplements and/or potassium-containing salt substitutes. Hyperkalemia can cause serious, sometimes, fatal, arrhythmias. Prinzide should be used cautiously, if at all, with these agents and with frequent monitoring of serum potassium). Products include:
BioLean Free Tablets .... ▣635
Urocit-K Tablets 2176

Potassium Gluconate (Risk factors for the development of hyperkalemia include the concomitant use of potassium-sparing diuretics, potassium supplements and/or potassium-containing salt substitutes. Hyperkalemia can cause serious, sometimes, fatal, arrhythmias. Prinzide should be used cautiously, if at all, with these agents and with frequent monitoring of serum potassium).
No products indexed under this heading.

Potassium Phosphate (Risk factors for the development of hyperkalemia include the concomitant use of potassium-sparing diuretics, potassium supplements and/or potassium-containing salt substitutes. Hyperkalemia can cause serious, sometimes, fatal, arrhythmias. Prinzide should be used cautiously, if at all, with these agents and with frequent monitoring of serum potassium). Products include:
K-Phos Neutral Tablets 813

Prazosin Hydrochloride (Co-administration of thiazide and other antihypertensive agents can lead to additive effect or potentiation).
No products indexed under this heading.

Prednisolone Acetate (Co-administration of thiazide diuretics with corticosteroids intensifies electrolyte depletion, particularly potassium). Products include:
Pred Forte Ophthalmic Suspension .... ⊙227
Pred Mild Ophthalmic Suspension .... ⊙230
Pred-G Ophthalmic Ointment .... ⊙229
Pred-G Ophthalmic Suspension ...... ⊙228

Prednisolone Sodium Phosphate (Co-administration of thiazide diuretics with corticosteroids intensifies electrolyte depletion, particularly potassium).
No products indexed under this heading.

Prednisolone Tebutate (Co-administration of thiazide diuretics with corticosteroids intensifies electrolyte depletion, particularly potassium).
No products indexed under this heading.

Prednisone (Co-administration of thiazide diuretics with corticosteroids intensifies electrolyte depletion, particularly potassium).
No products indexed under this heading.

Propoxyphene Hydrochloride (Co-administration of thiazide and narcotics may potentiate orthostatic hypotension).
No products indexed under this heading.

Propoxyphene Napsylate (Co-administration of thiazide and narcotics may potentiate orthostatic hypotension).
No products indexed under this heading.

Propranolol Hydrochloride (Co-administration of thiazide and other antihypertensive agents can lead to additive effect or potentiation). Products include:
InnoPran XL Extended Release Capsules.................................... 1484

Quinapril Hydrochloride (Co-administration of thiazide and other antihypertensive agents can lead to additive effect or potentiation).
No products indexed under this heading.

Ramipril (Co-administration of thiazide and other antihypertensive agents can lead to additive effect or potentiation).
No products indexed under this heading.

Rapacuronium Bromide (Co-administration with nondepolarizing skeletal muscle relaxants may result in possible increased responsiveness to the muscle relaxant).
No products indexed under this heading.

Rauwolfia Serpentina (Co-administration of thiazide and other antihypertensive agents can lead to additive effect or potentiation).
No products indexed under this heading.

Remifentanil Hydrochloride (Co-administration of thiazide and narcotics may potentiate orthostatic hypotension).
No products indexed under this heading.

Repaglinide (Hyperglycemia may occur with thiazide diuretics; dosage

adjustment of oral hypoglycemic agents may be required). Products include:
PrandiMet Tablets 2967
Prandin Tablets 2971

Rescinnamine (Co-administration of thiazide and other antihypertensive agents can lead to additive effect or potentiation).
No products indexed under this heading.

Reserpine (Co-administration of thiazide and other antihypertensive agents can lead to additive effect or potentiation).
No products indexed under this heading.

Rocuronium Bromide (Co-administration with nondepolarizing skeletal muscle relaxants may result in possible increased responsiveness to the muscle relaxant). Products include:
Zemuron Injection 2947

Rofecoxib (Reports suggest that NSAIDs, including selective COX-2 inhibitors, may diminish the antihypertensive effect of ACE inhibitors, including lisinopril. This interaction should be given consideration in patients taking NSAIDs or selective COX-2 inhibitors concomitantly with ACE inhibitors. In some patients with compromised renal function who are being treated with NSAIDs, including selective COX-2 inhibitors, the co-administration of angiotensin II receptor antagonists or ACE inhibitors, may result in further deterioration of renal function, including possible acute renal failure. These effects are usually reversible. Therefore, the combination should be administered with caution, especially in the elderly).
No products indexed under this heading.

Rosiglitazone Maleate (Hyperglycemia may occur with thiazide diuretics; dosage adjustment of oral hypoglycemic agents may be required). Products include:
Avandamet Tablets 1336
Avandaryl Tablets 1344
Avandia Tablets 1351

Secobarbital Sodium (Co-administration of thiazide and barbiturates may potentiate orthostatic hypotension).
No products indexed under this heading.

Sitagliptin Phosphate (Hyperglycemia may occur with thiazide diuretics; dosage adjustment of oral hypoglycemic agents may be required). Products include:
Janumet Tablets 2041
Januvia Tablets 2048

Sodium Nitroprusside (Co-administration of thiazide and other antihypertensive agents can lead to additive effect or potentiation).
No products indexed under this heading.

Sotalol Hydrochloride (Co-administration of thiazide and other antihypertensive agents can lead to additive effect or potentiation).
No products indexed under this heading.

Spirapril Hydrochloride (Co-administration of thiazide and other antihypertensive agents can lead to additive effect or potentiation).
No products indexed under this heading.

Spironolactone (Risk factors for the development of hyperkalemia include the concomitant use of potassium-sparing diuretics, potassium supplements and/or potassium-containing salt substitutes. Hyperkalemia can cause serious, sometimes, fatal, arrhythmias. Prinzide should be used cautiously, if at all, with these agents and with frequent monitoring of serum potassium).
No products indexed under this heading.

Sufentanil Citrate (Co-administration of thiazide and narcotics may potentiate orthostatic hypotension).
No products indexed under this heading.

Sulindac (Reports suggest that NSAIDs, including selective COX-2 inhibitors, may diminish the antihypertensive effect of ACE inhibitors, including lisinopril. This interaction should be given consideration in patients taking NSAIDs or selective COX-2 inhibitors concomitantly with ACE inhibitors. In some patients with compromised renal function who are being treated with NSAIDs, including selective COX-2 inhibitors, the co-administration of angiotensin II receptor antagonists or ACE inhibitors, may result in further deterioration of renal function, including possible acute renal failure. These effects are usually reversible. Therefore, the combination should be administered with caution, especially in the elderly). Products include:
Clinoril Tablets 1962

Telmisartan (Co-administration of thiazide and other antihypertensive agents can lead to additive effect or potentiation). Products include:
Micardis Tablets 852
Micardis HCT Tablets 854

Terazosin Hydrochloride (Co-administration of thiazide and other antihypertensive agents can lead to additive effect or potentiation).
No products indexed under this heading.

Thiamylal Sodium (Co-administration of thiazide and barbiturates may potentiate orthostatic hypotension).
No products indexed under this heading.

Timolol Maleate (Co-administration of thiazide and other antihypertensive agents can lead to additive effect or potentiation). Products include:
Combigan Ophthalmic Solution 553
Cosopt Sterile Ophthalmic Solution 1969
Timoptic Sterile Ophthalmic Solution 2121
Timoptic in Ocudose 2124
Timoptic-XE Sterile Ophthalmic Gel Forming Solution 2125

Tolazamide (Hyperglycemia may occur with thiazide diuretics; dosage adjustment of oral hypoglycemic agents may be required).
No products indexed under this heading.

Tolbutamide (Hyperglycemia may occur with thiazide diuretics; dosage adjustment of oral hypoglycemic agents may be required).
No products indexed under this heading.

Tolmetin Sodium (Reports suggest that NSAIDs, including selective COX-2 inhibitors, may diminish the antihypertensive effect of ACE inhibitors, including lisinopril. This interaction should be given consideration in patients taking NSAIDs or selective COX-2 inhibitors concomitantly with ACE inhibitors. In some patients with compromised renal function who are being treated with NSAIDs, including selective COX-2 inhibitors, the co-administration of angiotensin II receptor antagonists or ACE inhibitors, may result in further deterioration of renal function, including possible acute renal failure. These effects are usually reversible. Therefore, the combination should be administered with caution, especially in the elderly).
No products indexed under this heading.

Torsemide (Co-administration of lisinopril in patients on diuretics, especially those in whom diuretic therapy was recently instituted, may occasionally experience excessive hypotension; antihypertensive effects of lisinopril are augmented by antihypertensive agents that cause renin release). Products include:
Demadex Injection 2630
Demadex Tablets 2630

Trandolapril (Co-administration of thiazide and other antihypertensive agents can lead to additive effect or potentiation). Products include:
Mavik Tablets 472
Tarka Tablets 511

Triamcinolone (Co-administration of thiazide diuretics with corticosteroids intensifies electrolyte depletion, particularly potassium).
No products indexed under this heading.

Triamcinolone Acetonide (Co-administration of thiazide diuretics with corticosteroids intensifies electrolyte depletion, particularly potassium). Products include:
Azmacort Inhalation Aerosol 407
Nasacort AQ Nasal Spray 2765
Triesence Injectable Suspension .... ⊙209

Triamcinolone Diacetate (Co-administration of thiazide diuretics with corticosteroids intensifies electrolyte depletion, particularly potassium).
No products indexed under this heading.

Triamcinolone Hexacetonide (Co-administration of thiazide diuretics with corticosteroids intensifies electrolyte depletion, particularly potassium).
No products indexed under this heading.

Triamterene (Risk factors for the development of hyperkalemia include the concomitant use of potassium-sparing diuretics, potassium supplements and/or potassium-containing salt substitutes. Hyperkalemia can cause serious, sometimes, fatal, arrhythmias. Prinzide should be used cautiously, if at all, with these agents and with frequent monitoring of serum potassium). Products include:
Dyazide Capsules 1405
Dyrenium Capsules 3189

Trimethaphan Camsylate (Co-administration of thiazide and other antihypertensive agents can lead to additive effect or potentiation).
No products indexed under this heading.

Troglitazone (Hyperglycemia may occur with thiazide diuretics; dosage adjustment of oral hypoglycemic agents may be required).
No products indexed under this heading.

Valdecoxib (Reports suggest that NSAIDs, including selective COX-2 inhibitors, may diminish the antihypertensive effect of ACE inhibitors, including lisinopril. This interaction should be given consideration in patients taking NSAIDs or selective COX-2 inhibitors concomitantly with ACE inhibitors. In some patients with compromised renal function who are being treated with NSAIDs, including selective COX-2 inhibitors, the co-administration of angiotensin II receptor antagonists or ACE inhibitors, may result in further deterioration of renal function, including possible acute renal failure. These effects are usually reversible. Therefore, the combination should be administered with caution, especially in the elderly).
No products indexed under this heading.

Valsartan (Co-administration of thiazide and other antihypertensive agents can lead to additive effect or potentiation). Products include:
Diovan Tablets 2212
Diovan HCT Tablets 2216
Exforge Tablets 2238

Vecuronium Bromide (Co-administration with nondepolarizing skeletal muscle relaxants may result in possible increased responsiveness to the muscle relaxant).
No products indexed under this heading.

Verapamil Hydrochloride (Co-administration of thiazide and other antihypertensive agents can lead to additive effect or potentiation). Products include:
Tarka Tablets 511

Food Interactions

Alcohol (Co-administration of thiazide and alcohol may potentiate orthostatic hypotension).

Salt Substitutes, Potassium-Containing (Risk factors for the development of hyperkalemia include the concomitant use of potassium-sparing diuretics, potassium supplements and/or potassium-containing salt substitutes. Hyperkalemia can cause serious, sometimes, fatal, arrhythmias. Prinzide should be used cautiously, if at all, with these agents and with frequent monitoring of serum potassium).

PRISTIQ EXTENDED-RELEASE TABLETS
(Desvenlafaxine Succinate) 3247
May interact with aspirin-acetylsalicylic acid, central nervous system depressants, central nervous system stimulants, cytochrome p450 2d6 substrates (selected), cytochrome p450 3a4 inhibitors (selected), cytochrome p450 3a4 substrates (selected), monoamine oxidase inhibitors, non-steroidal anti-inflammatory agents, Serotonin and Norepinephrine Reuptake Inhibitors, selective serotonin reuptake inhibitors, triptans, and certain other agents. Compounds in these categories include:

5-hydroxytryptophan (Concomitant use of desvenlafaxine with serotonin precursors (such as tryptophan supplements) is not recommended).
No products indexed under this heading.

Acetazolamide (CYP3A4 is a minor pathway for the metabolism of desvenlafaxine. In a clinical study, ketoconazole (200 mg b.i.d.) increased the area under the concentration vs. time curve AUC of desvenlafaxine (400 mg single dose) by about 43% and Cmax by about 8%. Concomitant use of desvenlafaxine with potent inhibitors of CYP3A4 may result in higher concentrations of desvenlafaxine).
No products indexed under this heading.

Alfentanil Hydrochloride (Caution is advised when desvenlafaxine is taken in combination with other CNS-active drugs).
No products indexed under this heading.

Almotriptan Malate (The development of potentially life-threatening serotonin syndrome may occur when desvenlafaxine is used concomitantly with triptans. Serotonin syndrome symptoms may include mental status changes, autonomic instability, neuromuscular aberrations, and/or gastrointestinal symptoms. If concomitant treatment with desvenlafaxine and a triptan is clinically warranted, careful observation of the patient is advised, particularly during treatment initiation and dose increases). Products include:
Axert Tablets 2431

Alprazolam (Caution is advised when desvenlafaxine is taken in combination with other CNS-active drugs).
No products indexed under this heading.

Amiodarone Hydrochloride (CYP3A4 is a minor pathway for the metabolism of desvenlafaxine. In a clinical study, ketoconazole (200 mg b.i.d.) increased the area under the concentration vs. time curve AUC of desvenlafaxine (400 mg single dose) by about 43% and Cmax by about 8%. Concomitant use of desvenlafaxine with potent inhibitors of CYP3A4 may result in higher concentrations of desvenlafaxine).
No products indexed under this heading.

Amitriptyline Hydrochloride (Concomitant use of desvenlafaxine with a drug metabolized by CYP2D6 can result in higher concentrations of that drug).
No products indexed under this heading.

Amlodipine Besylate (Concomitant use of desvenlafaxine with a drug metabolized by CYP3A4 can result in lower exposures to that drug). Products include:
Azor Tablets 1005
Exforge Tablets 2238

Amphetamine Aspartate (Concomitant use of desvenlafaxine with a drug metabolized by CYP2D6 can result in higher concentrations of that drug). Products include:
Adderall XR Capsules 3012

Amphetamine Aspartate Monohydrate (Concomitant use of desvenlafaxine with a drug metabolized by CYP2D6 can result in higher concentrations of that drug).
No products indexed under this heading.

Amphetamine Resins (Caution is advised when desvenlafaxine is taken in combination with other CNS-active drugs).
No products indexed under this heading.

Amphetamine Sulfate (Concomitant use of desvenlafaxine with a drug metabolized by CYP2D6 can result in higher concentrations of that drug). Products include:
Adderall XR Capsules 3012

Amprenavir (CYP3A4 is a minor pathway for the metabolism of desvenlafaxine. In a clinical study, ketoconazole (200 mg b.i.d.) increased the area under the concentration vs. time curve AUC of desvenlafaxine (400 mg single dose) by about 43% and Cmax by about 8%. Concomitant use of desvenlafaxine with potent inhibitors of CYP3A4 may result in higher concentrations of desvenlafaxine).
No products indexed under this heading.

Anastrozole (CYP3A4 is a minor pathway for the metabolism of desvenlafaxine. In a clinical study, ketoconazole (200 mg b.i.d.) increased the area under the concentration vs. time curve AUC of desvenlafaxine (400 mg single dose) by about 43% and Cmax by about 8%. Concomitant use of desvenlafaxine with potent inhibitors of CYP3A4 may result in higher concentrations of desvenlafaxine). Products include:
Arimidex Tablets 672

Aprepitant (CYP3A4 is a minor pathway for the metabolism of desvenlafaxine. In a clinical study, ketoconazole (200 mg b.i.d.) increased the area under the concentration vs. time curve AUC of desvenlafaxine (400 mg single dose) by about 43% and Cmax by about 8%. Concomitant use of desvenlafaxine with potent inhibitors of CYP3A4 may result in higher concentrations of desvenlafaxine). Products include:
Emend Capsules 1992

Aprobarbital (Caution is advised when desvenlafaxine is taken in combination with other CNS-active drugs).
No products indexed under this heading.

Aspirin (Studies have shown that concurrent use of aspirin may potentiate the risk of upper GI bleeding. Patients should be cautioned about the concomitant use of desvenlafaxine with aspirin). Products include:
Aggrenox Capsules 819
Bayer Aspirin 750
Percodan Tablets 1130
St. Joseph 81 mg Aspirin Chewable and Enteric Coated Tablets 1903

Aspirin, Enteric Coated (Studies have shown that concurrent use of aspirin may potentiate the risk of upper GI bleeding. Patients should be cautioned about the concomitant use of desvenlafaxine with aspirin).
No products indexed under this heading.

Aspirin Buffered (Studies have shown that concurrent use of aspirin may potentiate the risk of upper GI bleeding. Patients should be cautioned about the concomitant use of desvenlafaxine with aspirin).
No products indexed under this heading.

Astemizole (Concomitant use of desvenlafaxine with a drug metabolized by CYP3A4 can result in lower exposures to that drug).
No products indexed under this heading.

Atazanavir (CYP3A4 is a minor pathway for the metabolism of desvenlafaxine. In a clinical study, ketoconazole (200 mg b.i.d.) increased the area under the concentration vs. time curve AUC of desvenlafaxine (400 mg single dose) by about 43% and Cmax by about 8%. Concomitant use of desvenlafaxine with potent inhibitors of CYP3A4 may result in higher concentrations of desvenlafaxine).
No products indexed under this heading.

Atazanavir Sulfate (CYP3A4 is a minor pathway for the metabolism of desvenlafaxine. In a clinical study, ketoconazole (200 mg b.i.d.) increased the area under the concentration vs. time curve AUC of desvenlafaxine (400 mg single dose) by about 43% and Cmax by about 8%. Concomitant use of desvenlafaxine with potent inhibitors of CYP3A4 may result in higher concentrations of desvenlafaxine). Products include:
Reyataz Capsules 3299

Atomoxetine Hydrochloride (Concomitant use of desvenlafaxine with a drug metabolized by CYP2D6 can result in higher concentrations of that drug). Products include:
Strattera Capsules 1864

Atorvastatin Calcium (Concomitant use of desvenlafaxine with a drug metabolized by CYP3A4 can result in lower exposures to that drug). Products include:
Lipitor Tablets 2501

Belladonna Ergotamine (Concomitant use of desvenlafaxine with a drug metabolized by CYP3A4 can result in lower exposures to that drug).
No products indexed under this heading.

Bisoprolol Fumarate (Concomitant use of desvenlafaxine with a drug metabolized by CYP2D6 can result in higher concentrations of that drug).
No products indexed under this heading.

Buprenorphine Hydrochloride (Caution is advised when desvenlafaxine is taken in combination with other CNS-active drugs). Products include:
Suboxone Tablets 2601
Subutex Tablets 2601

Buspirone Hydrochloride (Caution is advised when desvenlafaxine is taken in combination with other CNS-active drugs).
No products indexed under this heading.

Busulfan (Concomitant use of desvenlafaxine with a drug metabolized by CYP3A4 can result in lower exposures to that drug). Products include:
Busulfex Injection 2477
Myleran Tablets 1530

Butabarbital (Caution is advised when desvenlafaxine is taken in combination with other CNS-active drugs).
No products indexed under this heading.

Butalbital (Caution is advised when desvenlafaxine is taken in combination with other CNS-active drugs).
No products indexed under this heading.

Captopril (Concomitant use of desvenlafaxine with a drug metabolized by CYP2D6 can result in higher concentrations of that drug). Products include:
Captopril Tablets 2182

Carbamazepine (Concomitant use of desvenlafaxine with a drug metabolized by CYP3A4 can result in lower exposures to that drug). Products include:
Carbatrol Capsules 3019
Equetro Extended-Release Capsules 3174

Carvedilol (Concomitant use of desvenlafaxine with a drug metabolized by CYP2D6 can result in higher concentrations of that drug). Products include:
Coreg Tablets 1387

Celecoxib (Studies have shown that concurrent use of an NSAID may potentiate the risk of upper GI bleeding. Patients should be cautioned about the concomitant use of desvenlafaxine with NSAIDs). Products include:
Celebrex Capsules 2979

Cerivastatin Sodium (Concomitant use of desvenlafaxine with a drug metabolized by CYP3A4 can result in lower exposures to that drug).
No products indexed under this heading.

Cevimeline Hydrochloride (Concomitant use of desvenlafaxine with a drug metabolized by CYP2D6 can result in higher concentrations of that drug). Products include:
Evoxac Capsules 1013

Chlordiazepoxide (Caution is advised when desvenlafaxine is taken in combination with other CNS-active drugs).
No products indexed under this heading.

Chlordiazepoxide Hydrochloride (Caution is advised when desvenlafaxine is taken in combination with other CNS-active drugs).
No products indexed under this heading.

Chlorpheniramine (Concomitant use of desvenlafaxine with a drug metabolized by CYP3A4 can result in lower exposures to that drug).
No products indexed under this heading.

Chlorpheniramine Maleate (Concomitant use of desvenlafaxine with a drug metabolized by CYP3A4 can result in lower exposures to that drug). Products include:
Actifed Cold & Allergy Tablets 1895
Sudafed PE Sinus & Allergy Tablets 1908
Tylenol Allergy Multi-Symptom Caplets with Cool Burst and Rapid Release Gelcaps 1916
Children's Tylenol Plus Cold Suspension Liquid 1912
Children's Tylenol Plus Cough & Runny Nose Suspension Liquid 1912
Children's Tylenol Plus Flu Suspension Liquid 1914
Children's Tylenol Plus Multi-Symptom Cold Suspension Liquid 1912
Tylenol Cold Head Congestion Nighttime Caplets with Cool Burst 1910
Tylenol Cold Multi-Symptom Nighttime Caplets with Cool Burst 1913
Tylenol Sinus Congestion & Pain Nighttime Caplets with Cool Burst 1917

Chlorpheniramine Polistirex (Concomitant use of desvenlafaxine with a drug metabolized by CYP3A4 can result in lower exposures to that drug). Products include:
Tussionex Pennkinetic Extended-Release Suspension 3154

Chlorpheniramine Tannate (Concomitant use of desvenlafaxine with a drug metabolized by CYP3A4 can result in lower exposures to that drug).
No products indexed under this heading.

Chlorpromazine (Caution is advised when desvenlafaxine is taken in combination with other CNS-active drugs).
No products indexed under this heading.

Chlorpromazine Hydrochloride (Caution is advised when desvenlafaxine is taken in combination with other CNS-active drugs).
No products indexed under this heading.

Chlorpropamide (Concomitant use of desvenlafaxine with a drug metabolized by CYP2D6 can result in higher concentrations of that drug).
No products indexed under this heading.

Chlorprothixene (Caution is advised when desvenlafaxine is taken in combination with other CNS-active drugs).
No products indexed under this heading.

Chlorprothixene Hydrochloride (Caution is advised when desvenlafaxine is taken in combination with other CNS-active drugs).
No products indexed under this heading.

Chlorprothixene Lactate (Caution is advised when desvenlafaxine is taken in combination with other CNS-active drugs).
No products indexed under this heading.

Cimetidine (CYP3A4 is a minor pathway for the metabolism of desvenlafaxine. In a clinical study, ketoconazole (200 mg b.i.d.) increased the area under the concentration vs. time curve AUC of desvenlafaxine (400 mg single dose) by about 43% and Cmax by about 8%. Concomitant use of desvenlafaxine with potent inhibitors of CYP3A4 may result in higher concentrations of desvenlafaxine).
No products indexed under this heading.

Cimetidine Hydrochloride (CYP3A4 is a minor pathway for the metabolism of desvenlafaxine. In a clinical study, ketoconazole (200 mg b.i.d.) increased the area under the concentration vs. time curve AUC of desvenlafaxine (400 mg single dose) by about 43% and Cmax by about 8%. Concomitant use of desvenlafaxine with potent inhibitors of CYP3A4 may result in higher concentrations of desvenlafaxine).
No products indexed under this heading.

Ciprofloxacin (CYP3A4 is a minor pathway for the metabolism of desvenlafaxine. In a clinical study, ketoconazole (200 mg b.i.d.) increased the area under the concentration vs. time curve AUC of desvenlafaxine (400 mg single dose) by about 43% and Cmax by about 8%. Concomitant use of desvenlafaxine with potent inhibitors of CYP3A4 may result in higher concentrations of desvenlafaxine). Products include:
Cipro I.V. 2817
Cipro Oral Suspension 2810
Cipro XR Tablets 2823
Ciprodex Otic Suspension 541

Cisapride (Concomitant use of desvenlafaxine with a drug metabolized by CYP3A4 can result in lower exposures to that drug).
No products indexed under this heading.

Citalopram Hydrobromide (The development of potentially life-threatening serotonin syndrome may occur when desvenlafaxine is used concomitantly with SSRIs. Serotonin syndrome symptoms may include mental status changes, autonomic instability, neuromuscular aberrations, and/or gastrointestinal symptoms. If concomitant treatment with desvenlafaxine and an SSRI is clinically warranted, careful observation of the patient is advised, particularly during treatment initiation and dose increases). Products include:
Celexa 1160

Clarithromycin (CYP3A4 is a minor pathway for the metabolism of desvenlafaxine. In a clinical study, ketoconazole (200 mg b.i.d.) increased the area under the concentration vs. time curve AUC of desvenlafaxine (400 mg single dose) by about 43% and Cmax by about 8%. Concomitant use of desvenlafaxine with potent inhibitors of CYP3A4 may result in higher concentrations of desvenlafaxine). Products include:
Biaxin/Biaxin XL 411

Clomipramine Hydrochloride (Concomitant use of desvenlafaxine with a drug metabolized by CYP2D6 can result in higher concentrations of that drug).
No products indexed under this heading.

Clorazepate Dipotassium (Caution is advised when desvenlafaxine is taken in combination with other CNS-active drugs).
No products indexed under this heading.

Clotrimazole (CYP3A4 is a minor pathway for the metabolism of desvenlafaxine. In a clinical study, ketoconazole (200 mg b.i.d.) increased the area under the concentration vs. time curve AUC of desvenlafaxine (400 mg single dose) by about 43% and Cmax by about 8%. Concomitant use of desvenlafaxine with potent inhibitors of CYP3A4 may result in higher concentrations of desvenlafaxine). Products include:
Lotrisone 2881

Clozapine (Caution is advised when desvenlafaxine is taken in combination with other CNS-active drugs).
No products indexed under this heading.

Codeine Phosphate (Caution is advised when desvenlafaxine is taken in combination with other CNS-active drugs). Products include:
Tylenol with Codeine Tablets 2427

Codeine Sulfate (Concomitant use of desvenlafaxine with a drug metabolized by CYP2D6 can result in higher concentrations of that drug).
No products indexed under this heading.

Cyclobenzaprine Hydrochloride (Concomitant use of desvenlafaxine with a drug metabolized by CYP2D6 can result in higher concentrations of that drug). Products include:
Amrix Capsules 966

Cyclosporine (CYP3A4 is a minor pathway for the metabolism of desvenlafaxine. In a clinical study, ketoconazole (200 mg b.i.d.) increased the area under the concentration vs. time curve AUC of desvenlafaxine (400 mg single dose) by about 43% and Cmax by about 8%. Concomitant use of desvenlafaxine with potent inhibitors of CYP3A4 may result in higher concentrations of desvenlafaxine). Products include:
Gengraf Capsules 435
Neoral Oral Solution 2280
Neoral Soft Gelatin Capsules 2280
Restasis Ophthalmic Emulsion 557
Sandimmune 2296

Dalfopristin (CYP3A4 is a minor pathway for the metabolism of desvenlafaxine. In a clinical study, ketoconazole (200 mg b.i.d.) increased the area under the concentration vs. time curve AUC of desvenlafaxine (400 mg single dose) by about 43% and Cmax by about 8%. Concomitant use of desvenlafaxine with potent inhibitors of CYP3A4 may result in higher concentrations of desvenlafaxine).
No products indexed under this heading.

Danazol (CYP3A4 is a minor pathway for the metabolism of desvenlafaxine. In a clinical study, ketoconazole (200 mg b.i.d.) increased the area under the concentration vs. time curve AUC of desvenlafaxine (400 mg single dose) by about 43% and Cmax by about 8%. Concomitant use of desvenlafaxine with potent inhibitors of CYP3A4 may result in higher concentrations of desvenlafaxine).
No products indexed under this heading.

Delavirdine Mesylate (CYP3A4 is a minor pathway for the metabolism of desvenlafaxine. In a clinical study, ketoconazole (200 mg b.i.d.) increased the area under the concentration vs. time curve AUC of desvenlafaxine (400 mg single dose) by about 43% and Cmax by about 8%. Concomitant use of desvenlafaxine with potent inhibitors of CYP3A4 may result in higher concentrations of desvenlafaxine).
No products indexed under this heading.

Desflurane (Caution is advised when desvenlafaxine is taken in combination with other CNS-active drugs).
No products indexed under this heading.

Desipramine Hydrochloride (When desvenlafaxine succinate was administered at a dose of 100 mg daily in conjunction with a single 50 mg dose of desipramine, the Cmax and AUC of desipramine increased approximately 25% and 17%, respectively. When 400 mg (8 times the recommended 50 mg dose) was administered, the Cmax and AUC of desipramine increased approximately 50% and 90%, respectively).
No products indexed under this heading.

Desogestrel (Concomitant use of desvenlafaxine with a drug metabolized by CYP3A4 can result in lower exposures to that drug). Products include:
Mircette Tablets 1034

Dexfenfluramine Hydrochloride (Concomitant use of desvenlafaxine with a drug metabolized by CYP2D6 can result in higher concentrations of that drug).
No products indexed under this heading.

Dextroamphetamine Sulfate (Caution is advised when desvenlafaxine is taken in combination with other CNS-active drugs). Products include:
Adderall XR Capsules 3012
Dexedrine 1401

Dextromethorphan Hydrobromide (Concomitant use of desvenlafaxine with a drug metabolized by CYP2D6 can result in higher concentrations of that drug). Products include:
PediaCare Children's Liquid Multi-Symptom Cold 1902
PediaCare Children's Long-Acting Cough 1902
Children's Sudafed PE Cold & Cough Liquid 1907
Sudafed PE Cold & Cough Caplets 1907
Children's Tylenol Plus Cough & Runny Nose Suspension Liquid 1912
Children's Tylenol Plus Cough & Sore Throat Suspension Liquid 1912
Children's Tylenol Plus Flu Suspension Liquid 1914
Children's Tylenol Plus Multi-Symptom Cold Suspension Liquid 1912

IMPORTANT NOTE: Always consult each drug listing in the patient's regimen for possible interactions.

Tylenol Cold Severe Congestion Daytime Caplets with Cool Burst.......... 1912
Tylenol Cold Head Congestion Daytime Caplets with Cool Burst.......... 1910
Tylenol Cold Head Congestion Nighttime Caplets with Cool Burst.......... 1910
Tylenol Cold Head Congestion Severe Daytime Caplets with Cool Burst.......... 1910
Tylenol Cold Multi-Symptom Daytime Caplets with Cool Burst and Rapid Release Gels....... 1913
Tylenol Cold Multi-Symptom Daytime Liquid with Citrus Burst... 1913
Tylenol Cold Multi-Symptom Nighttime Caplets with Cool Burst.......... 1913
Tylenol Cold Multi-Symptom Nighttime Liquid with Cool Burst... 1913
Tylenol Cold Multi-Symptom Severe Caplets with Cool Burst..... 1913
Tylenol Cold Multi-Symptom Severe Daytime Liquid with Citrus Burst.......... 1913
Tylenol Cough & Sore Throat Daytime Liquid with Cool Burst...... 1918
Tylenol Cough & Sore Throat Nighttime Liquid with Cool Burst... 1918
Vicks DayQuil Cold & Flu Multi-Symptom Relief.......... ▣616
Vicks DayQuil LiquiCaps.......... 2567
Vicks DayQuil Liquid.......... 2567
Vicks DayQuil Multi-Symptom Cold/Flu Relief.......... 2567
Vicks NyQuil Cold & Flu Multi-Symptom Relief.......... ▣617
Vicks NyQuil LiquiCaps.......... 2567
Vicks NyQuil Liquid.......... 2567
Vicks NyQuil Multi-Symptom Cold/Flu Relief.......... 2567

Dextromethorphan Polistirex (Concomitant use of desvenlafaxine with a drug metabolized by CYP2D6 can result in higher concentrations of that drug).
No products indexed under this heading.

Dezocine (Caution is advised when desvenlafaxine is taken in combination with other CNS-active drugs).
No products indexed under this heading.

Diazepam (Caution is advised when desvenlafaxine is taken in combination with other CNS-active drugs). Products include:
Valium Tablets.......... 2658

Diclofenac Epolamine (Studies have shown that concurrent use of an NSAID may potentiate the risk of upper GI bleeding. Patients should be cautioned about the concomitant use of desvenlafaxine with NSAIDs). Products include:
Flector Patch.......... 561

Diclofenac Potassium (Studies have shown that concurrent use of an NSAID may potentiate the risk of upper GI bleeding. Patients should be cautioned about the concomitant use of desvenlafaxine with NSAIDs).
No products indexed under this heading.

Diclofenac Sodium (Studies have shown that concurrent use of an NSAID may potentiate the risk of upper GI bleeding. Patients should be cautioned about the concomitant use of desvenlafaxine with NSAIDs). Products include:
Diclofenac Sodium Ophthalmic Solution.......... ⊙240
Voltaren Ophthalmic Solution.......... 2336
Voltaren Tablets.......... 2334
Voltaren-XR Tablets.......... 2337

Dihydroergotamine Mesylate (Concomitant use of desvenlafaxine with a drug metabolized by CYP3A4 can result in lower exposures to that drug).
No products indexed under this heading.

Diltiazem Hydrochloride (CYP3A4 is a minor pathway for the metabolism of desvenlafaxine. In a clinical study, ketoconazole (200 mg b.i.d.) increased the area under the concentration vs. time curve AUC of desvenlafaxine (400 mg single dose) by about 43% and Cmax by about 8%. Concomitant use of desvenlafaxine with potent inhibitors of CYP3A4 may result in higher concentrations of desvenlafaxine). Products include:
Cardizem LA Extended Release Tablets.......... 421

Diltiazem Maleate (CYP3A4 is a minor pathway for the metabolism of desvenlafaxine. In a clinical study, ketoconazole (200 mg b.i.d.) increased the area under the concentration vs. time curve AUC of desvenlafaxine (400 mg single dose) by about 43% and Cmax by about 8%. Concomitant use of desvenlafaxine with potent inhibitors of CYP3A4 may result in higher concentrations of desvenlafaxine).
No products indexed under this heading.

Disopyramide (Concomitant use of desvenlafaxine with a drug metabolized by CYP3A4 can result in lower exposures to that drug).
No products indexed under this heading.

Disopyramide Phosphate (Concomitant use of desvenlafaxine with a drug metabolized by CYP3A4 can result in lower exposures to that drug).
No products indexed under this heading.

Disulfiram (Concomitant use of desvenlafaxine with a drug metabolized by CYP3A4 can result in lower exposures to that drug).
No products indexed under this heading.

Dolasetron Mesylate (Concomitant use of desvenlafaxine with a drug metabolized by CYP2D6 can result in higher concentrations of that drug). Products include:
Anzemet Injection.......... 2701
Anzemet Tablets.......... 2704

Donepezil Hydrochloride (Concomitant use of desvenlafaxine with a drug metabolized by CYP2D6 can result in higher concentrations of that drug). Products include:
Aricept Tablets.......... 1062
Aricept ODT Tablets.......... 1062

Doxepin Hydrochloride (Concomitant use of desvenlafaxine with a drug metabolized by CYP2D6 can result in higher concentrations of that drug).
No products indexed under this heading.

Doxorubicin Hydrochloride (Concomitant use of desvenlafaxine with a drug metabolized by CYP3A4 can result in lower exposures to that drug).
No products indexed under this heading.

Dronabinol (Concomitant use of desvenlafaxine with a drug metabolized by CYP3A4 can result in lower exposures to that drug). Products include:
Marinol Capsules.......... 3163

Droperidol (Caution is advised when desvenlafaxine is taken in combination with other CNS-active drugs).
No products indexed under this heading.

Duloxetine Hydrochloride (The development of potentially life-threatening serotonin syndrome may occur when desvenlafaxine is used concomitantly with other SNRIs. Serotonin syndrome symptoms may include mental status changes, autonomic instability, neuromuscular aberrations, and/or gastrointestinal symptoms. If concomitant treatment with desvenlafaxine and another SNRI is clinically warranted, careful observation of the patient is advised, particularly during treatment initiation and dose increases). Products include:
Cymbalta Delayed-Release Capsules.......... 1801

Efavirenz (CYP3A4 is a minor pathway for the metabolism of desvenlafaxine. In a clinical study, ketoconazole (200 mg b.i.d.) increased the area under the concentration vs. time curve AUC of desvenlafaxine (400 mg single dose) by about 43% and Cmax by about 8%. Concomitant use of desvenlafaxine with potent inhibitors of CYP3A4 may result in higher concentrations of desvenlafaxine). Products include:
Atripla Tablets.......... 938
Sustiva Capsules.......... 930
Sustiva Tablets.......... 930

Eletriptan Hydrobromide (The development of potentially life-threatening serotonin syndrome may occur when desvenlafaxine is used concomitantly with triptans. Serotonin syndrome symptoms may include mental status changes, autonomic instability, neuromuscular aberrations, and/or gastrointestinal symptoms. If concomitant treatment with desvenlafaxine and a triptan is clinically warranted, careful observation of the patient is advised, particularly during treatment initiation and dose increases).
No products indexed under this heading.

Encainide Hydrochloride (Concomitant use of desvenlafaxine with a drug metabolized by CYP2D6 can result in higher concentrations of that drug).
No products indexed under this heading.

Enflurane (Caution is advised when desvenlafaxine is taken in combination with other CNS-active drugs).
No products indexed under this heading.

Ergotamine Tartrate (Concomitant use of desvenlafaxine with a drug metabolized by CYP3A4 can result in lower exposures to that drug).
No products indexed under this heading.

Erythromycin (CYP3A4 is a minor pathway for the metabolism of desvenlafaxine. In a clinical study, ketoconazole (200 mg b.i.d.) increased the area under the concentration vs. time curve AUC of desvenlafaxine (400 mg single dose) by about 43% and Cmax by about 8%. Concomitant use of desvenlafaxine with potent inhibitors of CYP3A4 may result in higher concentrations of desvenlafaxine).
No products indexed under this heading.

Erythromycin Estolate (CYP3A4 is a minor pathway for the metabolism of desvenlafaxine. In a clinical study, ketoconazole (200 mg b.i.d.) increased the area under the concentration vs. time curve AUC of desvenlafaxine (400 mg single dose) by about 43% and Cmax by about 8%. Concomitant use of desvenlafaxine with potent inhibitors of CYP3A4 may result in higher concentrations of desvenlafaxine).
No products indexed under this heading.

Erythromycin Ethylsuccinate (CYP3A4 is a minor pathway for the metabolism of desvenlafaxine. In a clinical study, ketoconazole (200 mg b.i.d.) increased the area under the concentration vs. time curve AUC of desvenlafaxine (400 mg single dose) by about 43% and Cmax by about 8%. Concomitant use of desvenlafaxine with potent inhibitors of CYP3A4 may result in higher concentrations of desvenlafaxine). Products include:
E.E.S... 433
EryPed.......... 431

Erythromycin Gluceptate (CYP3A4 is a minor pathway for the metabolism of desvenlafaxine. In a clinical study, ketoconazole (200 mg b.i.d.) increased the area under the concentration vs. time curve AUC of desvenlafaxine (400 mg single dose) by about 43% and Cmax by about 8%. Concomitant use of desvenlafaxine with potent inhibitors of CYP3A4 may result in higher concentrations of desvenlafaxine).
No products indexed under this heading.

Erythromycin Lactobionate (CYP3A4 is a minor pathway for the metabolism of desvenlafaxine. In a clinical study, ketoconazole (200 mg b.i.d.) increased the area under the concentration vs. time curve AUC of desvenlafaxine (400 mg single dose) by about 43% and Cmax by about 8%. Concomitant use of desvenlafaxine with potent inhibitors of CYP3A4 may result in higher concentrations of desvenlafaxine).
No products indexed under this heading.

Erythromycin Stearate (CYP3A4 is a minor pathway for the metabolism of desvenlafaxine. In a clinical study, ketoconazole (200 mg b.i.d.) increased the area under the concentration vs. time curve AUC of desvenlafaxine (400 mg single dose) by about 43% and Cmax by about 8%. Concomitant use of desvenlafaxine with potent inhibitors of CYP3A4 may result in higher concentrations of desvenlafaxine).
No products indexed under this heading.

Escitalopram Oxalate (The development of potentially life-threatening serotonin syndrome may occur when desvenlafaxine is used concomitantly with SSRIs. Serotonin syndrome symptoms may include mental status changes, autonomic instability, neuromuscular aberrations, and/or gastrointestinal symptoms. If concomitant treatment with desvenlafaxine and an SSRI is clinically warranted, careful observation of the patient is advised, particularly during treatment initiation and dose increases). Products include:

Lexapro Oral Suspension 1174
Lexapro Tablets 1174

Esomeprazole Magnesium (CYP3A4 is a minor pathway for the metabolism of desvenlafaxine. In a clinical study, ketoconazole (200 mg b.i.d.) increased the area under the concentration vs. time curve AUC of desvenlafaxine (400 mg single dose) by about 43% and Cmax by about 8%. Concomitant use of desvenlafaxine with potent inhibitors of CYP3A4 may result in higher concentrations of desvenlafaxine). Products include:
Nexium Delayed-Release Capsules 645
Nexium Delayed-Release Oral Suspension................................. 645

Estazolam (Caution is advised when desvenlafaxine is taken in combination with other CNS-active drugs).
No products indexed under this heading.

Estradiol (Concomitant use of desvenlafaxine with a drug metabolized by CYP3A4 can result in lower exposures to that drug). Products include:
Activella Tablets 2347
Angeliq Tablets 751
Climara Transdermal System 763
Climara Pro Transdermal System 768
Divigel 3167
Vagifem Tablets 2375

Estradiol Benzoate (Concomitant use of desvenlafaxine with a drug metabolized by CYP3A4 can result in lower exposures to that drug).
No products indexed under this heading.

Estradiol Cypionate (Concomitant use of desvenlafaxine with a drug metabolized by CYP3A4 can result in lower exposures to that drug).
No products indexed under this heading.

Estradiol Valerate (Concomitant use of desvenlafaxine with a drug metabolized by CYP3A4 can result in lower exposures to that drug).
No products indexed under this heading.

Ethanol (A clinical study has shown that desvenlafaxine does not increase the impairment of mental and motor skills caused by ethanol. However, patients should be advised to avoid alcohol consumption while taking desvenlafaxine).
No products indexed under this heading.

Ethchlorvynol (Caution is advised when desvenlafaxine is taken in combination with other CNS-active drugs).
No products indexed under this heading.

Ethinamate (Caution is advised when desvenlafaxine is taken in combination with other CNS-active drugs).
No products indexed under this heading.

Ethinyl Estradiol (Concomitant use of desvenlafaxine with a drug metabolized by CYP3A4 can result in lower exposures to that drug). Products include:
Lybrel Tablets 3204
Mircette Tablets 1034
NuvaRing 2897
Ortho-Cyclen/Ortho Tri-Cyclen 2449
Ortho Evra Transdermal System 2437
Ortho Tri-Cyclen Lo Tablets 2458
Seasonique Tablets 1046
Yaz Tablets 805

Ethosuximide (Concomitant use of desvenlafaxine with a drug metabolized by CYP3A4 can result in lower exposures to that drug).
No products indexed under this heading.

Ethyl Alcohol (Caution is advised when desvenlafaxine is taken in combination with other CNS-active drugs).
No products indexed under this heading.

Ethynodiol Diacetate (Concomitant use of desvenlafaxine with a drug metabolized by CYP3A4 can result in lower exposures to that drug).
No products indexed under this heading.

Etodolac (Studies have shown that concurrent use of an NSAID may potentiate the risk of upper GI bleeding. Patients should be cautioned about the concomitant use of desvenlafaxine with NSAIDs).
No products indexed under this heading.

Etoposide (Concomitant use of desvenlafaxine with a drug metabolized by CYP3A4 can result in lower exposures to that drug).
No products indexed under this heading.

Etoposide Phosphate (Concomitant use of desvenlafaxine with a drug metabolized by CYP3A4 can result in lower exposures to that drug).
No products indexed under this heading.

Felodipine (Concomitant use of desvenlafaxine with a drug metabolized by CYP3A4 can result in lower exposures to that drug).
No products indexed under this heading.

Fenoprofen Calcium (Studies have shown that concurrent use of an NSAID may potentiate the risk of upper GI bleeding. Patients should be cautioned about the concomitant use of desvenlafaxine with NSAIDs). Products include:
Nalfon Capsules 2508

Fentanyl (Caution is advised when desvenlafaxine is taken in combination with other CNS-active drugs). Products include:
Duragesic Transdermal System 2405
Ionsys Transdermal System 2410

Fentanyl Citrate (Caution is advised when desvenlafaxine is taken in combination with other CNS-active drugs). Products include:
Actiq 959
Fentora Tablets 968

Flecainide Acetate (Concomitant use of desvenlafaxine with a drug metabolized by CYP2D6 can result in higher concentrations of that drug).
No products indexed under this heading.

Fluconazole (CYP3A4 is a minor pathway for the metabolism of desvenlafaxine. In a clinical study, ketoconazole (200 mg b.i.d.) increased the area under the concentration vs. time curve AUC of desvenlafaxine (400 mg single dose) by about 43% and Cmax by about 8%. Concomitant use of desvenlafaxine with potent inhibitors of CYP3A4 may result in higher concentrations of desvenlafaxine).
No products indexed under this heading.

Fluoxetine (The development of potentially life-threatening serotonin syndrome may occur when desvenlafaxine is used concomitantly with SSRIs. Serotonin syndrome symptoms may include mental status changes, autonomic instability, neuromuscular aberrations, and/or gastrointestinal symptoms. If concomitant treatment with desvenlafaxine and an SSRI is clinically warranted, careful observation of the patient is advised, particularly during treatment initiation and dose increases).
No products indexed under this heading.

Fluoxetine Hydrochloride (The development of potentially life-threatening serotonin syndrome may occur when desvenlafaxine is used concomitantly with SSRIs. Serotonin syndrome symptoms may include mental status changes, autonomic instability, neuromuscular aberrations, and/or gastrointestinal symptoms. If concomitant treatment with desvenlafaxine and an SSRI is clinically warranted, careful observation of the patient is advised, particularly during treatment initiation and dose increases). Products include:
Prozac Weekly Capsules 1852
Prozac Pulvules and Liquid 1852
Symbyax Capsules 1871

Fluphenazine Decanoate (Caution is advised when desvenlafaxine is taken in combination with other CNS-active drugs).
No products indexed under this heading.

Fluphenazine Enanthate (Caution is advised when desvenlafaxine is taken in combination with other CNS-active drugs).
No products indexed under this heading.

Fluphenazine Hydrochloride (Caution is advised when desvenlafaxine is taken in combination with other CNS-active drugs).
No products indexed under this heading.

Flurazepam Hydrochloride (Caution is advised when desvenlafaxine is taken in combination with other CNS-active drugs).
No products indexed under this heading.

Flurbiprofen (Studies have shown that concurrent use of an NSAID may potentiate the risk of upper GI bleeding. Patients should be cautioned about the concomitant use of desvenlafaxine with NSAIDs).
No products indexed under this heading.

Fluvoxamine Maleate (The development of potentially life-threatening serotonin syndrome may occur when desvenlafaxine is used concomitantly with SSRIs. Serotonin syndrome symptoms may include mental status changes, autonomic instability, neuromuscular aberrations, and/or gastrointestinal symptoms. If concomitant treatment with desvenlafaxine and an SSRI is clinically warranted, careful observation of the patient is advised, particularly during treatment initiation and dose increases). Products include:
Luvox CR Extended-Release Capsules 1759

Formoterol Fumarate (Concomitant use of desvenlafaxine with a drug metabolized by CYP2D6 can result in higher concentrations of that drug). Products include:
Foradil Aerolizer 2849
Perforomist Inhalation Solution 1025

Fosamprenavir Calcium (CYP3A4 is a minor pathway for the metabolism of desvenlafaxine. In a clinical study, ketoconazole (200 mg b.i.d.) increased the area under the concentration vs. time curve AUC of desvenlafaxine (400 mg single dose) by about 43% and Cmax by about 8%. Concomitant use of desvenlafaxine with potent inhibitors of CYP3A4 may result in higher concentrations of desvenlafaxine). Products include:
Lexiva Oral Suspension 1510
Lexiva Tablets 1510

Frovatriptan Succinate (The development of potentially life-threatening serotonin syndrome may occur when desvenlafaxine is used concomitantly with triptans. Serotonin syndrome symptoms may include mental status changes, autonomic instability, neuromuscular aberrations, and/or gastrointestinal symptoms. If concomitant treatment with desvenlafaxine and a triptan is clinically warranted, careful observation of the patient is advised, particularly during treatment initiation and dose increases). Products include:
Frova Tablets 1111

Galantamine Hydrobromide (Concomitant use of desvenlafaxine with a drug metabolized by CYP2D6 can result in higher concentrations of that drug).
No products indexed under this heading.

Glutethimide (Caution is advised when desvenlafaxine is taken in combination with other CNS-active drugs).
No products indexed under this heading.

Haloperidol (Caution is advised when desvenlafaxine is taken in combination with other CNS-active drugs).
No products indexed under this heading.

Haloperidol Decanoate (Caution is advised when desvenlafaxine is taken in combination with other CNS-active drugs).
No products indexed under this heading.

Haloperidol Lactate (Concomitant use of desvenlafaxine with a drug metabolized by CYP3A4 can result in lower exposures to that drug).
No products indexed under this heading.

Hydrocodone Bitartrate (Caution is advised when desvenlafaxine is taken in combination with other CNS-active drugs). Products include:
Lortab 5/500 Tablets 3143
Lortab 7.5/500 Tablets 3144
Lortab 10/500 Tablets 3144
Vicodin Tablets 529
Vicodin ES Tablets 530
Vicodin HP Tablets 531
Vicoprofen Tablets 533
Zydone Tablets 1132

Hydrocodone Polistirex (Caution is advised when desvenlafaxine is taken in combination with other CNS-active drugs). Products include:
Tussionex Pennkinetic Extended-Release Suspension...... 3154

Hydromorphone Hydrochloride (Caution is advised when desvenlafaxine is taken in combination with other CNS-active drugs).
No products indexed under this heading.

Hydroxyzine Hydrochloride (Caution is advised when desvenlafaxine is taken in combination with other CNS-active drugs).
No products indexed under this heading.

Ibuprofen (Studies have shown that concurrent use of an NSAID may potentiate the risk of upper GI bleeding. Patients should be cautioned about the concomitant use of desvenlafaxine with NSAIDs). Products include:
Motrin IB Tablets and Caplets 1900
Children's Motrin Oral Suspension ... 1901
Children's Motrin Non-Staining Dye-Free Oral Suspension 1901
Children's Motrin Cold Oral Suspension 1899
Infants' Motrin Concentrated Drops 1901
Infants' Motrin Non-Staining Dye-Free Concentrated Drops 1901
Junior Strength Motrin Caplets and Chewable Tablets 1901
Vicoprofen Tablets 533

Imipramine Hydrochloride (Concomitant use of desvenlafaxine with a drug metabolized by CYP2D6 can result in higher concentrations of that drug).
No products indexed under this heading.

Imipramine Pamoate (Concomitant use of desvenlafaxine with a drug metabolized by CYP2D6 can result in higher concentrations of that drug).
No products indexed under this heading.

Indinavir Sulfate (CYP3A4 is a minor pathway for the metabolism of desvenlafaxine. In a clinical study, ketoconazole (200 mg b.i.d.) increased the area under the concentration vs. time curve AUC of desvenlafaxine (400 mg single dose) by about 43% and Cmax by about 8%. Concomitant use of desvenlafaxine with potent inhibitors of CYP3A4 may result in higher concentrations of desvenlafaxine). Products include:
Crixivan Capsules 1979

Indomethacin (Studies have shown that concurrent use of an NSAID may potentiate the risk of upper GI bleeding. Patients should be cautioned about the concomitant use of desvenlafaxine with NSAIDs). Products include:
Indocin 2024

Indomethacin Sodium Trihydrate (Studies have shown that concurrent use of an NSAID may potentiate the risk of upper GI bleeding. Patients should be cautioned about the concomitant use of desvenlafaxine with NSAIDs). Products include:
Indocin I.V. 2489

Indoramin Hydrochloride (Concomitant use of desvenlafaxine with a drug metabolized by CYP2D6 can result in higher concentrations of that drug).
No products indexed under this heading.

Isocarboxazid (Desvenlafaxine must not be used concomitantly in patients taking monoamine oxidase inhibitors (MAOIs) or in patients who have taken MAOIs in the preceding 14 days due to the risk of serious, sometimes fatal, drug interactions with an SNRI. These interactions have been associated with symptoms that include tremor, myoclonus, diaphoresis, nausea, vomiting, flushing, dizziness, hyperthermia with features resembling neuroleptic malignant syndrome, seizures, rigidity, autonomic instability with possible rapid fluctuations of vital signs, and mental status changes. Based on the half-life of desvenlafaxine, at least 7 days should be allowed after stopping desvenlafaxine before starting an MAOI). Products include:
Marplan Tablets 3177

Isoflurane (Caution is advised when desvenlafaxine is taken in combination with other CNS-active drugs).
No products indexed under this heading.

Isoniazid (CYP3A4 is a minor pathway for the metabolism of desvenlafaxine. In a clinical study, ketoconazole (200 mg b.i.d.) increased the area under the concentration vs. time curve AUC of desvenlafaxine (400 mg single dose) by about 43% and Cmax by about 8%. Concomitant use of desvenlafaxine with potent inhibitors of CYP3A4 may result in higher concentrations of desvenlafaxine).
No products indexed under this heading.

Isradipine (Concomitant use of desvenlafaxine with a drug metabolized by CYP3A4 can result in lower exposures to that drug). Products include:
DynaCirc CR Controlled Release Tablets 1407

Itraconazole (CYP3A4 is a minor pathway for the metabolism of desvenlafaxine. In a clinical study, ketoconazole (200 mg b.i.d.) increased the area under the concentration vs. time curve AUC of desvenlafaxine (400 mg single dose) by about 43% and Cmax by about 8%. Concomitant use of desvenlafaxine with potent inhibitors of CYP3A4 may result in higher concentrations of desvenlafaxine).
No products indexed under this heading.

Ixabepilone (Concomitant use of desvenlafaxine with a drug metabolized by CYP3A4 can result in lower exposures to that drug). Products include:
Ixempra Kit for Injection 915

Ketamine Hydrochloride (Caution is advised when desvenlafaxine is taken in combination with other CNS-active drugs).
No products indexed under this heading.

Ketoconazole (CYP3A4 is a minor pathway for the metabolism of desvenlafaxine. In a clinical study, ketoconazole (200 mg b.i.d.) increased the area under the concentration vs. time curve AUC of desvenlafaxine (400 mg single dose) by about 43% and Cmax by about 8%. Concomitant use of desvenlafaxine with potent inhibitors of CYP3A4 may result in higher concentrations of desvenlafaxine). Products include:
Extina Foam, 2% 3057
Nizoral A-D Shampoo 1901

Ketoprofen (Studies have shown that concurrent use of an NSAID may potentiate the risk of upper GI bleeding. Patients should be cautioned about the concomitant use of desvenlafaxine with NSAIDs).
No products indexed under this heading.

Ketorolac Tromethamine (Studies have shown that concurrent use of an NSAID may potentiate the risk of upper GI bleeding. Patients should be cautioned about the concomitant use of desvenlafaxine with NSAIDs).
No products indexed under this heading.

Labetalol Hydrochloride (Concomitant use of desvenlafaxine with a drug metabolized by CYP2D6 can result in higher concentrations of that drug).
No products indexed under this heading.

Levomethadyl Acetate Hydrochloride (Caution is advised when desvenlafaxine is taken in combination with other CNS-active drugs).
No products indexed under this heading.

Levonorgestrel (Concomitant use of desvenlafaxine with a drug metabolized by CYP3A4 can result in lower exposures to that drug). Products include:
Climara Pro Transdermal System 768
Lybrel Tablets 3204
Mirena Intrauterine System 779
Plan B Tablets 1044
Seasonique Tablets 1046

Levorphanol Tartrate (Caution is advised when desvenlafaxine is taken in combination with other CNS-active drugs).
No products indexed under this heading.

Lidocaine (Concomitant use of desvenlafaxine with a drug metabolized by CYP2D6 can result in higher concentrations of that drug). Products include:
Lidoderm Patch 1114

Lidocaine Hydrochloride (Concomitant use of desvenlafaxine with a drug metabolized by CYP2D6 can result in higher concentrations of that drug).
No products indexed under this heading.

Lopinavir (CYP3A4 is a minor pathway for the metabolism of desvenlafaxine. In a clinical study, ketoconazole (200 mg b.i.d.) increased the area under the concentration vs. time curve AUC of desvenlafaxine (400 mg single dose) by about 43% and Cmax by about 8%. Concomitant use of desvenlafaxine with potent inhibitors of CYP3A4 may result in higher concentrations of desvenlafaxine). Products include:
Kaletra 452

Loratadine (CYP3A4 is a minor pathway for the metabolism of desvenlafaxine. In a clinical study, ketoconazole (200 mg b.i.d.) increased the area under the concentration vs. time curve AUC of desvenlafaxine (400 mg single dose) by about 43% and Cmax by about 8%. Concomitant use of desvenlafaxine with potent inhibitors of CYP3A4 may result in higher concentrations of desvenlafaxine).
No products indexed under this heading.

Lorazepam (Caution is advised when desvenlafaxine is taken in combination with other CNS-active drugs).
No products indexed under this heading.

Lovastatin (Concomitant use of desvenlafaxine with a drug metabolized by CYP3A4 can result in lower exposures to that drug). Products include:
Advicor Tablets 402
Mevacor Tablets 2063

Loxapine Hydrochloride (Caution is advised when desvenlafaxine is taken in combination with other CNS-active drugs).
No products indexed under this heading.

Loxapine Succinate (Caution is advised when desvenlafaxine is taken in combination with other CNS-active drugs).
No products indexed under this heading.

Maprotiline Hydrochloride (Concomitant use of desvenlafaxine with a drug metabolized by CYP2D6 can result in higher concentrations of that drug).
No products indexed under this heading.

Meclofenamate Sodium (Studies have shown that concurrent use of an NSAID may potentiate the risk of upper GI bleeding. Patients should be cautioned about the concomitant use of desvenlafaxine with NSAIDs).
No products indexed under this heading.

Mefenamic Acid (Studies have shown that concurrent use of an NSAID may potentiate the risk of upper GI bleeding. Patients should be cautioned about the concomitant use of desvenlafaxine with NSAIDs).
No products indexed under this heading.

Meloxicam (Studies have shown that concurrent use of an NSAID may potentiate the risk of upper GI bleeding. Patients should be cautioned about the concomitant use of desvenlafaxine with NSAIDs). Products include:
Mobic Oral Suspension 863
Mobic Tablets 863

Meperidine Hydrochloride (Caution is advised when desvenlafaxine is taken in combination with other CNS-active drugs).
No products indexed under this heading.

Mephobarbital (Caution is advised when desvenlafaxine is taken in combination with other CNS-active drugs).
No products indexed under this heading.

Meprobamate (Caution is advised when desvenlafaxine is taken in combination with other CNS-active drugs).
No products indexed under this heading.

Mesoridazine Besylate (Caution is advised when desvenlafaxine is taken in combination with other CNS-active drugs).
No products indexed under this heading.

Mestranol (Concomitant use of desvenlafaxine with a drug metabolized by CYP3A4 can result in lower exposures to that drug).
No products indexed under this heading.

Methadone Hydrochloride (Caution is advised when desvenlafaxine is taken in combination with other CNS-active drugs).
No products indexed under this heading.

Methamphetamine Hydrochloride (Caution is advised when desvenlafaxine is taken in combination with other CNS-active drugs).
No products indexed under this heading.

Methohexital Sodium (Caution is advised when desvenlafaxine is taken in combination with other CNS-active drugs).
No products indexed under this heading.

Methotrimeprazine (Caution is advised when desvenlafaxine is taken in combination with other CNS-active drugs).
No products indexed under this heading.

Methoxyflurane (Caution is advised when desvenlafaxine is taken in combination with other CNS-active drugs).
No products indexed under this heading.

Methylphenidate (Caution is advised when desvenlafaxine is taken in combination with other CNS-active drugs). Products include:
Daytrana Transdermal Patch **3022**

Methylphenidate Hydrochloride (Caution is advised when desvenlafaxine is taken in combination with other CNS-active drugs). Products include:
Concerta Extended-Release Tablets **1925**
Metadate CD Capsules **3146**

Metoprolol Succinate (Concomitant use of desvenlafaxine with a drug metabolized by CYP2D6 can result in higher concentrations of that drug). Products include:
Toprol-XL Tablets **666**

Metoprolol Tartrate (Concomitant use of desvenlafaxine with a drug metabolized by CYP2D6 can result in higher concentrations of that drug).
No products indexed under this heading.

Metronidazole (CYP3A4 is a minor pathway for the metabolism of desvenlafaxine. In a clinical study, ketoconazole (200 mg b.i.d.) increased the area under the concentration vs. time curve AUC of desvenlafaxine (400 mg single dose) by about 43% and Cmax by about 8%. Concomitant use of desvenlafaxine with potent inhibitors of CYP3A4 may result in higher concentrations of desvenlafaxine). Products include:
Pylera Capsules **714**

Metronidazole Benzoate (CYP3A4 is a minor pathway for the metabolism of desvenlafaxine. In a clinical study, ketoconazole (200 mg b.i.d.) increased the area under the concentration vs. time curve AUC of desvenlafaxine (400 mg single dose) by about 43% and Cmax by about 8%. Concomitant use of desvenlafaxine with potent inhibitors of CYP3A4 may result in higher concentrations of desvenlafaxine).
No products indexed under this heading.

Metronidazole Hydrochloride (CYP3A4 is a minor pathway for the metabolism of desvenlafaxine. In a clinical study, ketoconazole (200 mg b.i.d.) increased the area under the concentration vs. time curve AUC of desvenlafaxine (400 mg single dose) by about 43% and Cmax by about 8%. Concomitant use of desvenlafaxine with potent inhibitors of CYP3A4 may result in higher concentrations of desvenlafaxine).
No products indexed under this heading.

Metronidazole Sodium (CYP3A4 is a minor pathway for the metabolism of desvenlafaxine. In a clinical study, ketoconazole (200 mg b.i.d.) increased the area under the concentration vs. time curve AUC of desvenlafaxine (400 mg single dose) by about 43% and Cmax by about 8%. Concomitant use of desvenlafaxine with potent inhibitors of CYP3A4 may result in higher concentrations of desvenlafaxine).
No products indexed under this heading.

Mexiletine Hydrochloride (Concomitant use of desvenlafaxine with a drug metabolized by CYP2D6 can result in higher concentrations of that drug).
No products indexed under this heading.

Miconazole (CYP3A4 is a minor pathway for the metabolism of desvenlafaxine. In a clinical study, ketoconazole (200 mg b.i.d.) increased the area under the concentration vs. time curve AUC of desvenlafaxine (400 mg single dose) by about 43% and Cmax by about 8%. Concomitant use of desvenlafaxine with potent inhibitors of CYP3A4 may result in higher concentrations of desvenlafaxine).
No products indexed under this heading.

Miconazole Nitrate (CYP3A4 is a minor pathway for the metabolism of desvenlafaxine. In a clinical study, ketoconazole (200 mg b.i.d.) increased the area under the concentration vs. time curve AUC of desvenlafaxine (400 mg single dose) by about 43% and Cmax by about 8%. Concomitant use of desvenlafaxine with potent inhibitors of CYP3A4 may result in higher concentrations of desvenlafaxine).
No products indexed under this heading.

Midazolam Hydrochloride (In a clinical study, desvenlafaxine 400 mg daily (8 times the recommended 50 mg dose) was co-administered with a single 4 mg dose of midazolam. The AUC and Cmax of midazolam decreased by approximately 31% and 16%, respectively).
No products indexed under this heading.

Mirtazapine (Concomitant use of desvenlafaxine with a drug metabolized by CYP2D6 can result in higher concentrations of that drug). Products include:
Remeron Tablets **2924**
RemeronSolTab Tablets **2927**

Moclobemide (Desvenlafaxine must not be used concomitantly in patients taking monoamine oxidase inhibitors (MAOIs) or in patients who have taken MAOIs in the preceding 14 days due to the risk of serious, sometimes fatal, drug interactions with an SNRI. These interactions have been associated with symptoms that include tremor, myoclonus, diaphoresis, nausea, vomiting, flushing, dizziness, hyperthermia with features resembling neuroleptic malignant syndrome, seizures, rigidity, autonomic instability with possible rapid fluctuations of vital signs, and mental status changes. Based on the half-life of desvenlafaxine, at least 7 days should be allowed after stopping desvenlafaxine before starting an MAOI).
No products indexed under this heading.

Molindone Hydrochloride (Caution is advised when desvenlafaxine is taken in combination with other CNS-active drugs). Products include:
Moban Tablets **1116**

Morphine Sulfate (Caution is advised when desvenlafaxine is taken in combination with other CNS-active drugs). Products include:
Avinza Capsules **1772**
DepoDur Injection **1095**
MS Contin Tablets **2585**

Nabumetone (Studies have shown that concurrent use of an NSAID may potentiate the risk of upper GI bleeding. Patients should be cautioned about the concomitant use of desvenlafaxine with NSAIDs).
No products indexed under this heading.

Naproxen (Studies have shown that concurrent use of an NSAID may potentiate the risk of upper GI bleeding. Patients should be cautioned about the concomitant use of desvenlafaxine with NSAIDs). Products include:
EC-Naprosyn Delayed-Release Tablets **2632**
Naprosyn Suspension **2632**
Naprosyn Tablets **2632**

Naproxen Sodium (Studies have shown that concurrent use of an NSAID may potentiate the risk of upper GI bleeding. Patients should be cautioned about the concomitant use of desvenlafaxine with NSAIDs). Products include:
Anaprox Tablets **2632**
Anaprox DS Tablets **2632**
Treximet Tablets **1616**

Naratriptan Hydrochloride (The development of potentially life-threatening serotonin syndrome may occur when desvenlafaxine is used concomitantly with triptans. Serotonin syndrome symptoms may include mental status changes, autonomic instability, neuromuscular aberrations, and/or gastrointestinal symptoms. If concomitant treatment with desvenlafaxine and a triptan is clinically warranted, careful observation of the patient is advised, particularly during treatment initiation and dose increases). Products include:
Amerge Tablets **1301**

Nefazodone Hydrochloride (The development of potentially life-threatening serotonin syndrome may occur when desvenlafaxine is used concomitantly with other SNRIs. Serotonin syndrome symptoms may include mental status changes, autonomic instability, neuromuscular aberrations, and/or gastrointestinal symptoms. If concomitant treatment with desvenlafaxine and another SNRI is clinically warranted, careful observation of the patient is advised, particularly during treatment initiation and dose increases).
No products indexed under this heading.

Nelfinavir Mesylate (CYP3A4 is a minor pathway for the metabolism of desvenlafaxine. In a clinical study, ketoconazole (200 mg b.i.d.) increased the area under the concentration vs. time curve AUC of desvenlafaxine (400 mg single dose) by about 43% and Cmax by about 8%. Concomitant use of desvenlafaxine with potent inhibitors of CYP3A4 may result in higher concentrations of desvenlafaxine).
No products indexed under this heading.

Nevirapine (CYP3A4 is a minor pathway for the metabolism of desvenlafaxine. In a clinical study, ketoconazole (200 mg b.i.d.) increased the area under the concentration vs. time curve AUC of desvenlafaxine (400 mg single dose) by about 43% and Cmax by about 8%. Concomitant use of desvenlafaxine with potent inhibitors of CYP3A4 may result in higher concentrations of desvenlafaxine). Products include:
Viramune Oral Suspension **873**
Viramune Tablets **873**

Niacinamide (CYP3A4 is a minor pathway for the metabolism of desvenlafaxine. In a clinical study, ketoconazole (200 mg b.i.d.) increased the area under the concentration vs. time curve AUC of desvenlafaxine (400 mg single dose) by about 43% and Cmax by about 8%. Concomitant use of desvenlafaxine with potent inhibitors of CYP3A4 may result in higher concentrations of desvenlafaxine). Products include:
BioLean Free Tablets **635**

Nicardipine Hydrochloride (Concomitant use of desvenlafaxine with a drug metabolized by CYP3A4 can result in lower exposures to that drug). Products include:
Cardene I.V. **1093**

Nicotinamide (CYP3A4 is a minor pathway for the metabolism of desvenlafaxine. In a clinical study, ketoconazole (200 mg b.i.d.) increased the area under the concentration vs. time curve AUC of desvenlafaxine (400 mg single dose) by about 43% and Cmax by about 8%. Concomitant use of desvenlafaxine with potent inhibitors of CYP3A4 may result in higher concentrations of desvenlafaxine).
No products indexed under this heading.

Nifedipine (CYP3A4 is a minor pathway for the metabolism of desvenlafaxine. In a clinical study, ketoconazole (200 mg b.i.d.) increased the area under the concentration vs. time curve AUC of desvenlafaxine (400 mg single dose) by about 43% and Cmax by about 8%. Concomitant use of desvenlafaxine with potent inhibitors of CYP3A4 may result in higher concentrations of desvenlafaxine).
No products indexed under this heading.

Nimodipine (Concomitant use of desvenlafaxine with a drug metabolized by CYP3A4 can result in lower exposures to that drug). Products include:
Nimotop Capsules **790**

Nisoldipine (Concomitant use of desvenlafaxine with a drug metabolized by CYP3A4 can result in lower exposures to that drug). Products include:
Sular Extended Release Tablets **2975**

Nitrendipine (Concomitant use of desvenlafaxine with a drug metabolized by CYP3A4 can result in lower exposures to that drug).
No products indexed under this heading.

Norethindrone (Concomitant use of desvenlafaxine with a drug metabolized by CYP3A4 can result in lower exposures to that drug). Products include:
Ortho Micronor Tablets 2446

Norethindrone Acetate (Concomitant use of desvenlafaxine with a drug metabolized by CYP3A4 can result in lower exposures to that drug). Products include:
Activella Tablets 2347

Norfloxacin (CYP3A4 is a minor pathway for the metabolism of desvenlafaxine. In a clinical study, ketoconazole (200 mg b.i.d.) increased the area under the concentration vs. time curve AUC of desvenlafaxine (400 mg single dose) by about 43% and Cmax by about 8%. Concomitant use of desvenlafaxine with potent inhibitors of CYP3A4 may result in higher concentrations of desvenlafaxine). Products include:
Noroxin Tablets 2069

Norgestrel (Concomitant use of desvenlafaxine with a drug metabolized by CYP3A4 can result in lower exposures to that drug).
No products indexed under this heading.

Nortriptyline Hydrochloride (Concomitant use of desvenlafaxine with a drug metabolized by CYP2D6 can result in higher concentrations of that drug).
No products indexed under this heading.

Olanzapine (Caution is advised when desvenlafaxine is taken in combination with other CNS-active drugs). Products include:
Symbyax Capsules 1871
Zyprexa Tablets 1883
Zyprexa IntraMuscular 1883
Zyprexa ZYDIS Orally Disintegrating Tablets 1883

Omeprazole (CYP3A4 is a minor pathway for the metabolism of desvenlafaxine. In a clinical study, ketoconazole (200 mg b.i.d.) increased the area under the concentration vs. time curve AUC of desvenlafaxine (400 mg single dose) by about 43% and Cmax by about 8%. Concomitant use of desvenlafaxine with potent inhibitors of CYP3A4 may result in higher concentrations of desvenlafaxine).
No products indexed under this heading.

Ondansetron (Concomitant use of desvenlafaxine with a drug metabolized by CYP2D6 can result in higher concentrations of that drug). Products include:
Zofran ODT Orally Disintegrating Tablets 1687

Ondansetron Hydrochloride (Concomitant use of desvenlafaxine with a drug metabolized by CYP2D6 can result in higher concentrations of that drug). Products include:
Zofran Injection 1682
Zofran 1687

Oxaprozin (Studies have shown that concurrent use of an NSAID may potentiate the risk of upper GI bleeding. Patients should be cautioned about the concomitant use of desvenlafaxine with NSAIDs).
No products indexed under this heading.

Oxazepam (Caution is advised when desvenlafaxine is taken in combination with other CNS-active drugs).
No products indexed under this heading.

Oxycodone Hydrochloride (Caution is advised when desvenlafaxine is taken in combination with other CNS-active drugs). Products include:
OxyContin Tablets 2589
OxyIR Capsules 2593
Percocet Tablets 1127
Percodan Tablets 1130

Paclitaxel (Concomitant use of desvenlafaxine with a drug metabolized by CYP2D6 can result in higher concentrations of that drug).
No products indexed under this heading.

Pargyline Hydrochloride (Desvenlafaxine must not be used concomitantly in patients taking monoamine oxidase inhibitors (MAOIs) or in patients who have taken MAOIs in the preceding 14 days due to the risk of serious, sometimes fatal, drug interactions with an SNRI. These interactions have been associated with symptoms that include tremor, myoclonus, diaphoresis, nausea, vomiting, flushing, dizziness, hyperthermia with features resembling neuroleptic malignant syndrome, seizures, rigidity, autonomic instability with possible rapid fluctuations of vital signs, and mental status changes. Based on the half-life of desvenlafaxine, at least 7 days should be allowed after stopping desvenlafaxine before starting an MAOI).
No products indexed under this heading.

Paroxetine Hydrochloride (The development of potentially life-threatening serotonin syndrome may occur when desvenlafaxine is used concomitantly with SSRIs. Serotonin syndrome symptoms may include mental status changes, autonomic instability, neuromuscular aberrations, and/or gastrointestinal symptoms. If concomitant treatment with desvenlafaxine and an SSRI is clinically warranted, careful observation of the patient is advised, particularly during treatment initiation and dose increases). Products include:
Paxil 1535
Paxil CR Controlled-Release Tablets 1544

Pemoline (Caution is advised when desvenlafaxine is taken in combination with other CNS-active drugs).
No products indexed under this heading.

Pentobarbital Sodium (Caution is advised when desvenlafaxine is taken in combination with other CNS-active drugs). Products include:
Nembutal Sodium Solution, USP 2494

Perphenazine (Caution is advised when desvenlafaxine is taken in combination with other CNS-active drugs).
No products indexed under this heading.

Phenelzine Sulfate (Desvenlafaxine must not be used concomitantly in patients taking monoamine oxidase inhibitors (MAOIs) or in patients who have taken MAOIs in the preceding 14 days due to the risk of serious, sometimes fatal, drug interactions with an SNRI. These interactions have been associated with symptoms that include tremor, myoclonus, diaphoresis, nausea, vomiting, flushing, dizziness, hyperthermia with features resembling neuroleptic malignant syndrome, seizures, rigidity, autonomic instability with possible rapid fluctuations of vital signs, and mental status changes. Based on the half-life of desvenlafaxine, at least 7 days should be allowed after stopping desvenlafaxine before starting an MAOI).
No products indexed under this heading.

Phenobarbital (Caution is advised when desvenlafaxine is taken in combination with other CNS-active drugs). Products include:
Donnatal Extentabs 2507

Phenylbutazone (Studies have shown that concurrent use of an NSAID may potentiate the risk of upper GI bleeding. Patients should be cautioned about the concomitant use of desvenlafaxine with NSAIDs).
No products indexed under this heading.

Pimozide (Concomitant use of desvenlafaxine with a drug metabolized by CYP3A4 can result in lower exposures to that drug).
No products indexed under this heading.

Pindolol (Concomitant use of desvenlafaxine with a drug metabolized by CYP2D6 can result in higher concentrations of that drug).
No products indexed under this heading.

Piroxicam (Studies have shown that concurrent use of an NSAID may potentiate the risk of upper GI bleeding. Patients should be cautioned about the concomitant use of desvenlafaxine with NSAIDs).
No products indexed under this heading.

Polyestradiol Phosphate (Concomitant use of desvenlafaxine with a drug metabolized by CYP3A4 can result in lower exposures to that drug).
No products indexed under this heading.

Prazepam (Caution is advised when desvenlafaxine is taken in combination with other CNS-active drugs).
No products indexed under this heading.

Procarbazine Hydrochloride (Desvenlafaxine must not be used concomitantly in patients taking monoamine oxidase inhibitors (MAOIs) or in patients who have taken MAOIs in the preceding 14 days due to the risk of serious, sometimes fatal, drug interactions with an SNRI. These interactions have been associated with symptoms that include tremor, myoclonus, diaphoresis, nausea, vomiting, flushing, dizziness, hyperthermia with features resembling neuroleptic malignant syndrome, seizures, rigidity, autonomic instability with possible rapid fluctuations of vital signs, and mental status changes. Based on the half-life of desvenlafaxine, at least 7 days should be allowed after stopping desvenlafaxine before starting an MAOI).
No products indexed under this heading.

Prochlorperazine (Caution is advised when desvenlafaxine is taken in combination with other CNS-active drugs).
No products indexed under this heading.

Promethazine Hydrochloride (Caution is advised when desvenlafaxine is taken in combination with other CNS-active drugs).
No products indexed under this heading.

Propafenone Hydrochloride (Concomitant use of desvenlafaxine with a drug metabolized by CYP2D6 can result in higher concentrations of that drug). Products include:
Rythmol Tablets 1586
Rythmol SR Capsules 1590

Propofol (Caution is advised when desvenlafaxine is taken in combination with other CNS-active drugs).
No products indexed under this heading.

Propoxyphene Hydrochloride (Caution is advised when desvenlafaxine is taken in combination with other CNS-active drugs).
No products indexed under this heading.

Propoxyphene Napsylate (Caution is advised when desvenlafaxine is taken in combination with other CNS-active drugs).
No products indexed under this heading.

Propranolol Hydrochloride (Concomitant use of desvenlafaxine with a drug metabolized by CYP2D6 can result in higher concentrations of that drug). Products include:
InnoPran XL Extended Release Capsules 1484

Quazepam (Caution is advised when desvenlafaxine is taken in combination with other CNS-active drugs).
No products indexed under this heading.

Quetiapine Fumarate (Caution is advised when desvenlafaxine is taken in combination with other CNS-active drugs).
No products indexed under this heading.

Quinidine (CYP3A4 is a minor pathway for the metabolism of desvenlafaxine. In a clinical study, ketoconazole (200 mg b.i.d.) increased the area under the concentration vs. time curve AUC of desvenlafaxine (400 mg single dose) by about 43% and Cmax by about 8%. Concomitant use of desvenlafaxine with potent inhibitors of CYP3A4 may result in higher concentrations of desvenlafaxine).
No products indexed under this heading.

Quinidine Gluconate (Concomitant use of desvenlafaxine with a drug metabolized by CYP2D6 can result in higher concentrations of that drug).
No products indexed under this heading.

Quinidine Hydrochloride (CYP3A4 is a minor pathway for the metabolism of desvenlafaxine. In a clinical study, ketoconazole (200 mg b.i.d.) increased the area under the concentration vs. time curve AUC of desvenlafaxine (400 mg single dose) by about 43% and Cmax by about

8%. Concomitant use of desvenlafaxine with potent inhibitors of CYP3A4 may result in higher concentrations of desvenlafaxine).

No products indexed under this heading.

Quinidine Polygalacturonate (CYP3A4 is a minor pathway for the metabolism of desvenlafaxine. In a clinical study, ketoconazole (200 mg b.i.d.) increased the area under the concentration vs. time curve AUC of desvenlafaxine (400 mg single dose) by about 43% and Cmax by about 8%. Concomitant use of desvenlafaxine with potent inhibitors of CYP3A4 may result in higher concentrations of desvenlafaxine).

No products indexed under this heading.

Quinidine Sulfate (CYP3A4 is a minor pathway for the metabolism of desvenlafaxine. In a clinical study, ketoconazole (200 mg b.i.d.) increased the area under the concentration vs. time curve AUC of desvenlafaxine (400 mg single dose) by about 43% and Cmax by about 8%. Concomitant use of desvenlafaxine with potent inhibitors of CYP3A4 may result in higher concentrations of desvenlafaxine).

No products indexed under this heading.

Quinine (CYP3A4 is a minor pathway for the metabolism of desvenlafaxine. In a clinical study, ketoconazole (200 mg b.i.d.) increased the area under the concentration vs. time curve AUC of desvenlafaxine (400 mg single dose) by about 43% and Cmax by about 8%. Concomitant use of desvenlafaxine with potent inhibitors of CYP3A4 may result in higher concentrations of desvenlafaxine).

No products indexed under this heading.

Quinine Sulfate (CYP3A4 is a minor pathway for the metabolism of desvenlafaxine. In a clinical study, ketoconazole (200 mg b.i.d.) increased the area under the concentration vs. time curve AUC of desvenlafaxine (400 mg single dose) by about 43% and Cmax by about 8%. Concomitant use of desvenlafaxine with potent inhibitors of CYP3A4 may result in higher concentrations of desvenlafaxine).

No products indexed under this heading.

Quinupristin (CYP3A4 is a minor pathway for the metabolism of desvenlafaxine. In a clinical study, ketoconazole (200 mg b.i.d.) increased the area under the concentration vs. time curve AUC of desvenlafaxine (400 mg single dose) by about 43% and Cmax by about 8%. Concomitant use of desvenlafaxine with potent inhibitors of CYP3A4 may result in higher concentrations of desvenlafaxine).

No products indexed under this heading.

Ranitidine Bismuth Citrate (CYP3A4 is a minor pathway for the metabolism of desvenlafaxine. In a clinical study, ketoconazole (200 mg b.i.d.) increased the area under the concentration vs. time curve AUC of desvenlafaxine (400 mg single dose) by about 43% and Cmax by about 8%. Concomitant use of desvenlafaxine with potent inhibitors of CYP3A4 may result in higher concentrations of desvenlafaxine).

No products indexed under this heading.

Ranitidine Hydrochloride (CYP3A4 is a minor pathway for the metabolism of desvenlafaxine. In a clinical study, ketoconazole (200 mg b.i.d.) increased the area under the concentration vs. time curve AUC of desvenlafaxine (400 mg single dose) by about 43% and Cmax by about 8%. Concomitant use of desvenlafaxine with potent inhibitors of CYP3A4 may result in higher concentrations of desvenlafaxine). Products include:

Zantac 75 Tablets 603
Zantac 1670
Zantac Injection 1666
Zantac Injection Pharmacy Bulk Package 1668
Maximum Strength Zantac 150 Tablets 603
Maximum Strength Zantac 150 Cool Mint Tablets 603

Rasagiline Mesylate (Desvenlafaxine must not be used concomitantly in patients taking monoamine oxidase inhibitors (MAOIs) or in patients who have taken MAOIs in the preceding 14 days due to the risk of serious, sometimes fatal, drug interactions with an SNRI. These interactions have been associated with symptoms that include tremor, myoclonus, diaphoresis, nausea, vomiting, flushing, dizziness, hyperthermia with features resembling neuroleptic malignant syndrome, seizures, rigidity, autonomic instability with possible rapid fluctuations of vital signs, and mental status changes. Based on the half-life of desvenlafaxine, at least 7 days should be allowed after stopping desvenlafaxine before starting an MAOI). Products include:

Azilect Tablets 3106

Remifentanil Hydrochloride (Caution is advised when desvenlafaxine is taken in combination with other CNS-active drugs).

No products indexed under this heading.

Rifabutin (Concomitant use of desvenlafaxine with a drug metabolized by CYP3A4 can result in lower exposures to that drug).

No products indexed under this heading.

Risperidone (Caution is advised when desvenlafaxine is taken in combination with other CNS-active drugs). Products include:

Risperdal Consta Long-Acting Injection 1753

Ritonavir (CYP3A4 is a minor pathway for the metabolism of desvenlafaxine. In a clinical study, ketoconazole (200 mg b.i.d.) increased the area under the concentration vs. time curve AUC of desvenlafaxine (400 mg single dose) by about 43% and Cmax by about 8%. Concomitant use of desvenlafaxine with potent inhibitors of CYP3A4 may result in higher concentrations of desvenlafaxine). Products include:

Kaletra 452
Norvir 489

Rizatriptan Benzoate (The development of potentially life-threatening serotonin syndrome may occur when desvenlafaxine is used concomitantly with triptans. Serotonin syndrome symptoms may include mental status changes, autonomic instability, neuromuscular aberrations, and/or gastrointestinal symptoms. If concomitant treatment with desvenlafaxine and a triptan is clinically warranted, careful observation of the patient is advised, particularly during treatment initiation and dose increases). Products include:

Maxalt Tablets 2056
Maxalt-MLT Orally Disintegrating Tablets 2056

Rofecoxib (Studies have shown that concurrent use of an NSAID may potentiate the risk of upper GI bleeding. Patients should be cautioned about the concomitant use of desvenlafaxine with NSAIDs).

No products indexed under this heading.

Saquinavir (CYP3A4 is a minor pathway for the metabolism of desvenlafaxine. In a clinical study, ketoconazole (200 mg b.i.d.) increased the area under the concentration vs. time curve AUC of desvenlafaxine (400 mg single dose) by about 43% and Cmax by about 8%. Concomitant use of desvenlafaxine with potent inhibitors of CYP3A4 may result in higher concentrations of desvenlafaxine).

No products indexed under this heading.

Saquinavir Mesylate (CYP3A4 is a minor pathway for the metabolism of desvenlafaxine. In a clinical study, ketoconazole (200 mg b.i.d.) increased the area under the concentration vs. time curve AUC of desvenlafaxine (400 mg single dose) by about 43% and Cmax by about 8%. Concomitant use of desvenlafaxine with potent inhibitors of CYP3A4 may result in higher concentrations of desvenlafaxine).

No products indexed under this heading.

Secobarbital Sodium (Caution is advised when desvenlafaxine is taken in combination with other CNS-active drugs).

No products indexed under this heading.

Selegiline (Desvenlafaxine must not be used concomitantly in patients taking monoamine oxidase inhibitors (MAOIs) or in patients who have taken MAOIs in the preceding 14 days due to the risk of serious, sometimes fatal, drug interactions with an SNRI. These interactions have been associated with symptoms that include tremor, myoclonus, diaphoresis, nausea, vomiting, flushing, dizziness, hyperthermia with features resembling neuroleptic malignant syndrome, seizures, rigidity, autonomic instability with possible rapid fluctuations of vital signs, and mental status changes. Based on the half-life of desvenlafaxine, at least 7 days should be allowed after stopping desvenlafaxine before starting an MAOI). Products include:

Emsam Transdermal System 905

Selegiline Hydrochloride (Desvenlafaxine must not be used concomitantly in patients taking monoamine oxidase inhibitors (MAOIs) or in patients who have taken MAOIs in the preceding 14 days due to the risk of serious, sometimes fatal, drug interactions with an SNRI. These interactions have been associated with symptoms that include tremor, myoclonus, diaphoresis, nausea, vomiting, flushing, dizziness, hyperthermia with features resembling neuroleptic malignant syndrome, seizures, rigidity, autonomic instability with possible rapid fluctuations of vital signs, and mental status changes. Based on the half-life of desvenlafaxine, at least 7 days should be allowed after stopping desvenlafaxine before starting an MAOI). Products include:

Eldepryl Capsules 3052

Sertraline Hydrochloride (The development of potentially life-threatening serotonin syndrome may occur when desvenlafaxine is used concomitantly with SSRIs. Serotonin syndrome symptoms may include mental status changes, autonomic instability, neuromuscular aberrations, and/or gastrointestinal symptoms. If concomitant treatment with desvenlafaxine and an SSRI is clinically warranted, careful observation of the patient is advised, particularly during treatment initiation and dose increases).

No products indexed under this heading.

Sevoflurane (Caution is advised when desvenlafaxine is taken in combination with other CNS-active drugs). Products include:

Ultane Liquid for Inhalation 524

Sildenafil Citrate (CYP3A4 is a minor pathway for the metabolism of desvenlafaxine. In a clinical study, ketoconazole (200 mg b.i.d.) increased the area under the concentration vs. time curve AUC of desvenlafaxine (400 mg single dose) by about 43% and Cmax by about 8%. Concomitant use of desvenlafaxine with potent inhibitors of CYP3A4 may result in higher concentrations of desvenlafaxine).

No products indexed under this heading.

Simvastatin (Concomitant use of desvenlafaxine with a drug metabolized by CYP3A4 can result in lower exposures to that drug). Products include:

Simcor Tablets 502
Vytorin 10/10 Tablets 2149
Vytorin 10/10 Tablets 2939
Vytorin 10/20 Tablets 2149
Vytorin 10/20 Tablets 2939
Vytorin 10/40 Tablets 2149
Vytorin 10/40 Tablets 2939
Vytorin 10/80 Tablets 2149
Vytorin 10/80 Tablets 2939
Zocor Tablets 2136

Sirolimus (Concomitant use of desvenlafaxine with a drug metabolized by CYP3A4 can result in lower exposures to that drug). Products include:

Rapamune 3260

Sodium Oxybate (Caution is advised when desvenlafaxine is taken in combination with other CNS-active drugs). Products include:

Xyrem Oral Solution 1766

Sufentanil Citrate (Caution is advised when desvenlafaxine is taken in combination with other CNS-active drugs).

No products indexed under this heading.

Sulindac (Studies have shown that concurrent use of an NSAID may potentiate the risk of upper GI bleeding. Patients should be cautioned about the concomitant use of desvenlafaxine with NSAIDs). Products include:

Clinoril Tablets 1962

Sumatriptan (The development of potentially life-threatening serotonin syndrome may occur when desvenlafaxine is used concomitantly with triptans. Serotonin syndrome symptoms may include mental status changes, autonomic instability, neuromuscular aberrations, and/or gastrointestinal symptoms. If concomitant treatment with desvenlafaxine and a triptan is clinically warranted, careful observation of the patient is advised, particularly during treatment initiation and dose increases). Products include:

Imitrex Nasal Spray 1470

Sumatriptan Succinate (The development of potentially life-threatening serotonin syndrome may occur when desvenlafaxine is used concomitantly with triptans. Serotonin syndrome symptoms may include mental status changes, autonomic instability, neuromuscular aberrations, and/or gastrointestinal symptoms. If concomitant treatment with desvenlafaxine and a triptan is clinically warranted, careful observation of the patient is advised, particularly during treatment initiation and dose increases). Products include:

Imitrex Injection 1465
Imitrex Tablets 1474
Treximet Tablets 1616

Tacrolimus (Concomitant use of desvenlafaxine with a drug metabolized by CYP3A4 can result in lower exposures to that drug). Products include:

Prograf Capsules and Injection 622
Protopic Ointment 628

Tadalafil (Concomitant use of desvenlafaxine with a drug metabolized by CYP3A4 can result in lower exposures to that drug). Products include:

Cialis Tablets 1792

Tamoxifen Citrate (Concomitant use of desvenlafaxine with a drug metabolized by CYP2D6 can result in higher concentrations of that drug).

No products indexed under this heading.

Telithromycin (CYP3A4 is a minor pathway for the metabolism of desvenlafaxine. In a clinical study, ketoconazole (200 mg b.i.d.) increased the area under the concentration vs. time curve AUC of desvenlafaxine (400 mg single dose) by about 43% and Cmax by about 8%. Concomitant use of desvenlafaxine with potent inhibitors of CYP3A4 may result in higher concentrations of desvenlafaxine). Products include:

Ketek Tablets 2744

Temazepam (Caution is advised when desvenlafaxine is taken in combination with other CNS-active drugs).

No products indexed under this heading.

Teniposide (Concomitant use of desvenlafaxine with a drug metabolized by CYP2D6 can result in higher concentrations of that drug).

No products indexed under this heading.

Testosterone (Concomitant use of desvenlafaxine with a drug metabolized by CYP2D6 can result in higher concentrations of that drug). Products include:

AndroGel 3159
Testim 1% Gel 701

Testosterone Cypionate (Concomitant use of desvenlafaxine with a drug metabolized by CYP2D6 can result in higher concentrations of that drug).

No products indexed under this heading.

Testosterone Enanthate (Concomitant use of desvenlafaxine with a drug metabolized by CYP2D6 can result in higher concentrations of that drug). Products include:

Delatestryl Injection 1730

Testosterone Propionate (Concomitant use of desvenlafaxine with a drug metabolized by CYP2D6 can result in higher concentrations of that drug).

No products indexed under this heading.

Thiamylal Sodium (Caution is advised when desvenlafaxine is taken in combination with other CNS-active drugs).

No products indexed under this heading.

Thioridazine (Concomitant use of desvenlafaxine with a drug metabolized by CYP2D6 can result in higher concentrations of that drug).

No products indexed under this heading.

Thioridazine Hydrochloride (Caution is advised when desvenlafaxine is taken in combination with other CNS-active drugs). Products include:

Thioridazine Hydrochloride Tablets 2195

Thiothixene (Caution is advised when desvenlafaxine is taken in combination with other CNS-active drugs). Products include:

Thiothixene Capsules 2197

Tiagabine Hydrochloride (Concomitant use of desvenlafaxine with a drug metabolized by CYP3A4 can result in lower exposures to that drug). Products include:

Gabitril Tablets 973

Timolol Maleate (Concomitant use of desvenlafaxine with a drug metabolized by CYP2D6 can result in higher concentrations of that drug). Products include:

Combigan Ophthalmic Solution 553
Cosopt Sterile Ophthalmic Solution 1969
Timoptic Sterile Ophthalmic Solution 2121
Timoptic in Ocudose 2124
Timoptic-XE Sterile Ophthalmic Gel Forming Solution 2125

Tolmetin Sodium (Studies have shown that concurrent use of an NSAID may potentiate the risk of upper GI bleeding. Patients should be cautioned about the concomitant use of desvenlafaxine with NSAIDs).

No products indexed under this heading.

Tolterodine Tartrate (Concomitant use of desvenlafaxine with a drug metabolized by CYP2D6 can result in higher concentrations of that drug).

No products indexed under this heading.

Tramadol Hydrochloride (Concomitant use of desvenlafaxine with a drug metabolized by CYP2D6 can result in higher concentrations of that drug). Products include:

Ultram ER Extended-Release Tablets 2428

Tranylcypromine Sulfate (Desvenlafaxine must not be used concomitantly in patients taking monoamine oxidase inhibitors (MAOIs) or in patients who have taken MAOIs in the preceding 14 days due to the risk of serious, sometimes fatal, drug interactions with an SNRI. These interactions have been associated with symptoms that include tremor, myoclonus, diaphoresis, nausea, vomiting, flushing, dizziness, hyperthermia with features resembling neuroleptic malignant syndrome, seizures, rigidity, autonomic instability with possible rapid fluctuations of vital signs, and mental status changes. Based on the half-life of desvenlafaxine, at least 7 days should be allowed after stopping desvenlafaxine before starting an MAOI). Products include:

Parnate Tablets 1532

Trazodone Hydrochloride (Concomitant use of desvenlafaxine with a drug metabolized by CYP2D6 can result in higher concentrations of that drug).

No products indexed under this heading.

Triazolam (Caution is advised when desvenlafaxine is taken in combination with other CNS-active drugs).

No products indexed under this heading.

Trifluoperazine Hydrochloride (Caution is advised when desvenlafaxine is taken in combination with other CNS-active drugs).

No products indexed under this heading.

Trimipramine Maleate (Concomitant use of desvenlafaxine with a drug metabolized by CYP2D6 can result in higher concentrations of that drug).

No products indexed under this heading.

Troglitazone (CYP3A4 is a minor pathway for the metabolism of desvenlafaxine. In a clinical study, ketoconazole (200 mg b.i.d.) increased the area under the concentration vs. time curve AUC of desvenlafaxine (400 mg single dose) by about 43% and Cmax by about 8%. Concomitant use of desvenlafaxine with potent inhibitors of CYP3A4 may result in higher concentrations of desvenlafaxine).

No products indexed under this heading.

Troleandomycin (CYP3A4 is a minor pathway for the metabolism of desvenlafaxine. In a clinical study, ketoconazole (200 mg b.i.d.) increased the area under the concentration vs. time curve AUC of desvenlafaxine (400 mg single dose) by about 43% and Cmax by about 8%. Concomitant use of desvenlafaxine with potent inhibitors of CYP3A4 may result in higher concentrations of desvenlafaxine).

No products indexed under this heading.

Tryptophan (Concomitant use of desvenlafaxine with serotonin precursors (such as tryptophan supplements) is not recommended).

No products indexed under this heading.

Valdecoxib (Studies have shown that concurrent use of an NSAID may potentiate the risk of upper GI bleeding. Patients should be cautioned about the concomitant use of desvenlafaxine with NSAIDs).

No products indexed under this heading.

Valproate Sodium (CYP3A4 is a minor pathway for the metabolism of desvenlafaxine. In a clinical study, ketoconazole (200 mg b.i.d.) increased the area under the concentration vs. time curve AUC of desvenlafaxine (400 mg single dose) by about 43% and Cmax by about 8%. Concomitant use of desvenlafaxine with potent inhibitors of CYP3A4 may result in higher concentrations of desvenlafaxine).

No products indexed under this heading.

Vardenafil Hydrochloride (CYP3A4 is a minor pathway for the metabolism of desvenlafaxine. In a clinical study, ketoconazole (200 mg b.i.d.) increased the area under the concentration vs. time curve AUC of desvenlafaxine (400 mg single dose) by about 43% and Cmax by about 8%. Concomitant use of desvenlafaxine with potent inhibitors of CYP3A4 may result in higher concentrations of desvenlafaxine). Products include:

Levitra Tablets 2876

Venlafaxine Hydrochloride (The development of potentially life-threatening serotonin syndrome may occur when desvenlafaxine is used concomitantly with other SNRIs. Serotonin syndrome symptoms may include mental status changes, autonomic instability, neuromuscular aberrations, and/or gastrointestinal symptoms. If concomitant treatment with desvenlafaxine and another SNRI is clinically warranted, careful observation of the patient is advised, particularly during treatment initiation and dose increases). Products include:

Effexor XR Extended-Release Capsules 3195
Venlafaxine Hydrochloride Tablets ... 2199

Verapamil Hydrochloride (CYP3A4 is a minor pathway for the metabolism of desvenlafaxine. In a clinical study, ketoconazole (200 mg b.i.d.) increased the area under the concentration vs. time curve AUC of desvenlafaxine (400 mg single dose) by about 43% and Cmax by about 8%. Concomitant use of desvenlafaxine with potent inhibitors of CYP3A4 may result in higher concentrations of desvenlafaxine). Products include:

Tarka Tablets 511

Vinblastine Sulfate (Concomitant use of desvenlafaxine with a drug metabolized by CYP2D6 can result in higher concentrations of that drug).

No products indexed under this heading.

Vincristine Sulfate (Concomitant use of desvenlafaxine with a drug metabolized by CYP3A4 can result in lower exposures to that drug).

No products indexed under this heading.

Voriconazole (CYP3A4 is a minor pathway for the metabolism of desvenlafaxine. In a clinical study, ketoconazole (200 mg b.i.d.) increased the area under the concentration vs. time curve AUC of desvenlafaxine (400 mg single dose) by about 43% and Cmax by about 8%. Concomitant use of desvenlafaxine with potent inhibitors of CYP3A4 may result in higher concentrations of desvenlafaxine).

No products indexed under this heading.

Warfarin Sodium (Altered anticoagulant effects, including increased bleeding, have been reported when SNRIs are co-administered with warfarin. Patients receiving warfarin therapy should be carefully monitored when desvenlafaxine is initiated or discontinued).
No products indexed under this heading.

Zafirlukast (CYP3A4 is a minor pathway for the metabolism of desvenlafaxine. In a clinical study, ketoconazole (200 mg b.i.d.) increased the area under the concentration vs. time curve AUC of desvenlafaxine (400 mg single dose) by about 43% and Cmax by about 8%. Concomitant use of desvenlafaxine with potent inhibitors of CYP3A4 may result in higher concentrations of desvenlafaxine). Products include:
Accolate Tablets 669

Zaleplon (Caution is advised when desvenlafaxine is taken in combination with other CNS-active drugs).
No products indexed under this heading.

Zileuton (CYP3A4 is a minor pathway for the metabolism of desvenlafaxine. In a clinical study, ketoconazole (200 mg b.i.d.) increased the area under the concentration vs. time curve AUC of desvenlafaxine (400 mg single dose) by about 43% and Cmax by about 8%. Concomitant use of desvenlafaxine with potent inhibitors of CYP3A4 may result in higher concentrations of desvenlafaxine).
No products indexed under this heading.

Ziprasidone Hydrochloride (Caution is advised when desvenlafaxine is taken in combination with other CNS-active drugs). Products include:
Geodon Capsules 2520

Zolmitriptan (The development of potentially life-threatening serotonin syndrome may occur when desvenlafaxine is used concomitantly with triptans. Serotonin syndrome symptoms may include mental status changes, autonomic instability, neuromuscular aberrations, and/or gastrointestinal symptoms. If concomitant treatment with desvenlafaxine and a triptan is clinically warranted, careful observation of the patient is advised, particularly during treatment initiation and dose increases). Products include:
Zomig Tablets 694
Zomig Nasal Spray 689
Zomig-ZMT Tablets 694

Zolpidem Tartrate (Caution is advised when desvenlafaxine is taken in combination with other CNS-active drugs). Products include:
Ambien Tablets 2692
Ambien CR Tablets 2696

Zonisamide (Concomitant use of desvenlafaxine with a drug metabolized by CYP2D6 can result in higher concentrations of that drug). Products include:
Zonegran Capsules 1089

Food Interactions

Alcohol (Caution is advised when desvenlafaxine is taken in combination with other CNS-active drugs).

Grapefruit (CYP3A4 is a minor pathway for the metabolism of desvenlafaxine. In a clinical study, ketoconazole (200 mg b.i.d.) increased the area under the concentration vs. time curve AUC of desvenlafaxine (400 mg single dose) by about 43% and Cmax by about 8%. Concomitant use of desvenlafaxine with potent inhibitors of CYP3A4 may result in higher concentrations of desvenlafaxine).

Grapefruit Juice (CYP3A4 is a minor pathway for the metabolism of desvenlafaxine. In a clinical study, ketoconazole (200 mg b.i.d.) increased the area under the concentration vs. time curve AUC of desvenlafaxine (400 mg single dose) by about 43% and Cmax by about 8%. Concomitant use of desvenlafaxine with potent inhibitors of CYP3A4 may result in higher concentrations of desvenlafaxine).

PROAIR HFA INHALATION AEROSOL

(Albuterol Sulfate) 3113
May interact with beta blockers, monoamine oxidase inhibitors, non-potassium-sparing diuretics, sympathomimetic aerosol bronchodilators, tricyclic antidepressants, and certain other agents. Compounds in these categories include:

Acebutolol Hydrochloride (Beta-adrenergic-receptor blocking agents not only block the pulmonary effect of beta-agonists, such as albuterol sulfate, but may produce severe bronchospasm in asthmatic patients. Therefore, patients with asthma should not normally be treated with beta-blockers. However, under certain circumstances, e.g., as prophylaxis after myocardial infarction, there may be no acceptable alternatives to the use of beta-adrenergic-blocking agents in patients with asthma. In this setting, cardioselective beta-blockers should be considered, although they should be administered with caution).
No products indexed under this heading.

Albuterol (Other short-acting sympathomimetic aerosol bronchodilators should not be used concomitantly with albuterol sulfate. If additional adrenergic drugs are to be administered by any route, they should be used with caution to avoid deleterious cardiovascular effects).
No products indexed under this heading.

Amitriptyline Hydrochloride (Albuterol sulfate should be administered with extreme caution to patients being treated with monoamine oxidase inhibitors or tricyclic antidepressants, or within 2 weeks of discontinuation of such agents, because the action of albuterol on the cardiovascular system may be potentiated).
No products indexed under this heading.

Amoxapine (Albuterol sulfate should be administered with extreme caution to patients being treated with monoamine oxidase inhibitors or tricyclic antidepressants, or within 2 weeks of discontinuation of such agents, because the action of albuterol on the cardiovascular system may be potentiated).
No products indexed under this heading.

Atenolol (Beta-adrenergic-receptor blocking agents not only block the pulmonary effect of beta-agonists, such as albuterol sulfate, but may produce severe bronchospasm in asthmatic patients. Therefore, patients with asthma should not normally be treated with beta-blockers. However, under certain circumstances, e.g., as prophylaxis after myocardial infarction, there may be no acceptable alternatives to the use of beta-adrenergic-blocking agents in patients with asthma. In this setting, cardioselective beta-blockers should be considered, although they should be administered with caution).
No products indexed under this heading.

Bendroflumethiazide (The ECG changes and/or hypokalemia which may result from the administration of non-potassium sparing diuretics (such as loop or thiazide diuretics) can be acutely worsened by beta-agonists, especially when the recommended dose of beta-agonist is exceeded. Although the clinical significance of these effects is not known, caution is advised in the co-administration of beta-agonists with non-potassium sparing diuretics).
No products indexed under this heading.

Betaxolol Hydrochloride (Beta-adrenergic-receptor blocking agents not only block the pulmonary effect of beta-agonists, such as albuterol sulfate, but may produce severe bronchospasm in asthmatic patients. Therefore, patients with asthma should not normally be treated with beta-blockers. However, under certain circumstances, e.g., as prophylaxis after myocardial infarction, there may be no acceptable alternatives to the use of beta-adrenergic-blocking agents in patients with asthma. In this setting, cardioselective beta-blockers should be considered, although they should be administered with caution).
No products indexed under this heading.

Bisoprolol Fumarate (Beta-adrenergic-receptor blocking agents not only block the pulmonary effect of beta-agonists, such as albuterol sulfate, but may produce severe bronchospasm in asthmatic patients. Therefore, patients with asthma should not normally be treated with beta-blockers. However, under certain circumstances, e.g., as prophylaxis after myocardial infarction, there may be no acceptable alternatives to the use of beta-adrenergic-blocking agents in patients with asthma. In this setting, cardioselective beta-blockers should be considered, although they should be administered with caution).
No products indexed under this heading.

Bitolterol Mesylate (Other short-acting sympathomimetic aerosol bronchodilators should not be used concomitantly with albuterol sulfate. If additional adrenergic drugs are to be administered by any route, they should be used with caution to avoid deleterious cardiovascular effects).
No products indexed under this heading.

Bumetanide (The ECG changes and/or hypokalemia which may result from the administration of non-potassium sparing diuretics (such as loop or thiazide diuretics) can be acutely worsened by beta-agonists, especially when the recommended dose of beta-agonist is exceeded. Although the clinical significance of these effects is not known, caution is advised in the co-administration of beta-agonists with non-potassium sparing diuretics).
No products indexed under this heading.

Carteolol Hydrochloride (Beta-adrenergic-receptor blocking agents not only block the pulmonary effect of beta-agonists, such as albuterol sulfate, but may produce severe bronchospasm in asthmatic patients. Therefore, patients with asthma should not normally be treated with beta-blockers. However, under certain circumstances, e.g., as prophylaxis after myocardial infarction, there may be no acceptable alternatives to the use of beta-adrenergic-blocking agents in patients with asthma. In this setting, cardioselective beta-blockers should be considered, although they should be administered with caution).
No products indexed under this heading.

Chlorothiazide (The ECG changes and/or hypokalemia which may result from the administration of non-potassium sparing diuretics (such as loop or thiazide diuretics) can be acutely worsened by beta-agonists, especially when the recommended dose of beta-agonist is exceeded. Although the clinical significance of these effects is not known, caution is advised in the co-administration of beta-agonists with non-potassium sparing diuretics).
No products indexed under this heading.

Chlorothiazide Sodium (The ECG changes and/or hypokalemia which may result from the administration of non-potassium sparing diuretics (such as loop or thiazide diuretics) can be acutely worsened by beta-agonists, especially when the recommended dose of beta-agonist is exceeded. Although the clinical significance of these effects is not known, caution is advised in the co-administration of beta-agonists with non-potassium sparing diuretics). Products include:
Intravenous Sodium Diuril 2490

Clomipramine Hydrochloride (Albuterol sulfate should be administered with extreme caution to patients being treated with monoamine oxidase inhibitors or tricyclic antidepressants, or within 2 weeks of discontinuation of such agents, because the action of albuterol on the cardiovascular system may be potentiated).
No products indexed under this heading.

Desipramine Hydrochloride (Albuterol sulfate should be administered with extreme caution to patients being treated with monoamine oxidase inhibitors or tricyclic antidepressants, or within 2 weeks of discontinuation of such agents, because the action of albuterol on the cardiovascular system may be potentiated).
No products indexed under this heading.

Digoxin (Mean decreases of 16% and 22% in serum digoxin levels were demonstrated after single dose intravenous and oral administration of albuterol, respectively, to normal volunteers who had received digoxin for 10 days. The clinical significance of these findings for patients with obstructive airway disease who are receiving albuterol and digoxin on a chronic basis is unclear. Neverthe-

less, it would be prudent to carefully evaluate the serum digoxin levels in patients who are currently receiving digoxin and albuterol sulfate). Products include:
Lanoxin Injection ... 1498
Lanoxin Injection Pediatric ... 1502
Lanoxin Tablets ... 1505

Doxepin Hydrochloride (Albuterol sulfate should be administered with extreme caution to patients being treated with monoamine oxidase inhibitors or tricyclic antidepressants, or within 2 weeks of discontinuation of such agents, because the action of albuterol on the cardiovascular system may be potentiated).
No products indexed under this heading.

Esmolol Hydrochloride (Beta-adrenergic-receptor blocking agents not only block the pulmonary effect of beta-agonists, such as albuterol sulfate, but may produce severe bronchospasm in asthmatic patients. Therefore, patients with asthma should not normally be treated with beta-blockers. However, under certain circumstances, e.g., as prophylaxis after myocardial infarction, there may be no acceptable alternatives to the use of beta-adrenergic-blocking agents in patients with asthma. In this setting, cardioselective beta-blockers should be considered, although they should be administered with caution).
No products indexed under this heading.

Ethacrynic Acid (The ECG changes and/or hypokalemia which may result from the administration of non-potassium sparing diuretics (such as loop or thiazide diuretics) can be acutely worsened by beta-agonists, especially when the recommended dose of beta-agonist is exceeded. Although the clinical significance of these effects is not known, caution is advised in the co-administration of beta-agonists with non-potassium sparing diuretics). Products include:
Edecrin Tablets ... 698

Furosemide (The ECG changes and/or hypokalemia which may result from the administration of non-potassium sparing diuretics (such as loop or thiazide diuretics) can be acutely worsened by beta-agonists, especially when the recommended dose of beta-agonist is exceeded. Although the clinical significance of these effects is not known, caution is advised in the co-administration of beta-agonists with non-potassium sparing diuretics). Products include:
Furosemide Tablets ... 2186

Hydrochlorothiazide (The ECG changes and/or hypokalemia which may result from the administration of non-potassium sparing diuretics (such as loop or thiazide diuretics) can be acutely worsened by beta-agonists, especially when the recommended dose of beta-agonist is exceeded. Although the clinical significance of these effects is not known, caution is advised in the co-administration of beta-agonists with non-potassium sparing diuretics). Products include:
Atacand HCT ... 642
Avalide Tablets ... 892
Avalide Tablets ... 2713
Benicar HCT Tablets ... 1010
Diovan HCT Tablets ... 2216
Dyazide Capsules ... 1405
Micardis HCT Tablets ... 854
Prinzide Tablets ... 2092
Tekturna HCT Tablets ... 2324
Teveten HCT Tablets ... 517

Hydroflumethiazide (The ECG changes and/or hypokalemia which may result from the administration of non-potassium sparing diuretics (such as loop or thiazide diuretics) can be acutely worsened by beta-agonists, especially when the recommended dose of beta-agonist is exceeded. Although the clinical significance of these effects is not known, caution is advised in the co-administration of beta-agonists with non-potassium sparing diuretics).
No products indexed under this heading.

Imipramine Hydrochloride (Albuterol sulfate should be administered with extreme caution to patients being treated with monoamine oxidase inhibitors or tricyclic antidepressants, or within 2 weeks of discontinuation of such agents, because the action of albuterol on the cardiovascular system may be potentiated).
No products indexed under this heading.

Imipramine Pamoate (Albuterol sulfate should be administered with extreme caution to patients being treated with monoamine oxidase inhibitors or tricyclic antidepressants, or within 2 weeks of discontinuation of such agents, because the action of albuterol on the cardiovascular system may be potentiated).
No products indexed under this heading.

Isocarboxazid (Albuterol sulfate should be administered with extreme caution to patients being treated with monoamine oxidase inhibitors or tricyclic antidepressants, or within 2 weeks of discontinuation of such agents, because the action of albuterol on the cardiovascular system may be potentiated). Products include:
Marplan Tablets ... 3177

Isoetharine (Other short-acting sympathomimetic aerosol bronchodilators should not be used concomitantly with albuterol sulfate. If additional adrenergic drugs are to be administered by any route, they should be used with caution to avoid deleterious cardiovascular effects).
No products indexed under this heading.

Isoproterenol Hydrochloride (Other short-acting sympathomimetic aerosol bronchodilators should not be used concomitantly with albuterol sulfate. If additional adrenergic drugs are to be administered by any route, they should be used with caution to avoid deleterious cardiovascular effects).
No products indexed under this heading.

Labetalol Hydrochloride (Beta-adrenergic-receptor blocking agents not only block the pulmonary effect of beta-agonists, such as albuterol sulfate, but may produce severe bronchospasm in asthmatic patients. Therefore, patients with asthma should not normally be treated with beta-blockers. However, under certain circumstances, e.g., as prophylaxis after myocardial infarction, there may be no acceptable alternatives to the use of beta-adrenergic-blocking agents in patients with asthma. In this setting, cardioselective beta-blockers should be considered, although they should be administered with caution).
No products indexed under this heading.

Levalbuterol Hydrochloride (Other short-acting sympathomimetic aerosol bronchodilators should not be used concomitantly with albuterol sulfate. If additional adrenergic drugs are to be administered by any route, they should be used with caution to avoid deleterious cardiovascular effects). Products include:
Xopenex Inhalation Solution ... 3001
Xopenex Inhalation Solution Concentrate ... 3005

Levobunolol Hydrochloride (Beta-adrenergic-receptor blocking agents not only block the pulmonary effect of beta-agonists, such as albuterol sulfate, but may produce severe bronchospasm in asthmatic patients. Therefore, patients with asthma should not normally be treated with beta-blockers. However, under certain circumstances, e.g., as prophylaxis after myocardial infarction, there may be no acceptable alternatives to the use of beta-adrenergic-blocking agents in patients with asthma. In this setting, cardioselective beta-blockers should be considered, although they should be administered with caution).
No products indexed under this heading.

Maprotiline Hydrochloride (Albuterol sulfate should be administered with extreme caution to patients being treated with monoamine oxidase inhibitors or tricyclic antidepressants, or within 2 weeks of discontinuation of such agents, because the action of albuterol on the cardiovascular system may be potentiated).
No products indexed under this heading.

Metaproterenol Sulfate (Other short-acting sympathomimetic aerosol bronchodilators should not be used concomitantly with albuterol sulfate. If additional adrenergic drugs are to be administered by any route, they should be used with caution to avoid deleterious cardiovascular effects).
No products indexed under this heading.

Methyclothiazide (The ECG changes and/or hypokalemia which may result from the administration of non-potassium sparing diuretics (such as loop or thiazide diuretics) can be acutely worsened by beta-agonists, especially when the recommended dose of beta-agonist is exceeded. Although the clinical significance of these effects is not known, caution is advised in the co-administration of beta-agonists with non-potassium sparing diuretics).
No products indexed under this heading.

Metipranolol Hydrochloride (Beta-adrenergic-receptor blocking agents not only block the pulmonary effect of beta-agonists, such as albuterol sulfate, but may produce severe bronchospasm in asthmatic patients. Therefore, patients with asthma should not normally be treated with beta-blockers. However, under certain circumstances, e.g., as prophylaxis after myocardial infarction, there may be no acceptable alternatives to the use of beta-adrenergic-blocking agents in patients with asthma. In this setting, cardioselective beta-blockers should be considered, although they should be administered with caution).
No products indexed under this heading.

Metoprolol Succinate (Beta-adrenergic-receptor blocking agents not only block the pulmonary effect of beta-agonists, such as albuterol sulfate, but may produce severe bronchospasm in asthmatic patients. Therefore, patients with asthma should not normally be treated with beta-blockers. However, under certain circumstances, e.g., as prophylaxis after myocardial infarction, there may be no acceptable alternatives to the use of beta-adrenergic-blocking agents in patients with asthma. In this setting, cardioselective beta-blockers should be considered, although they should be administered with caution). Products include:
Toprol-XL Tablets ... 666

Metoprolol Tartrate (Beta-adrenergic-receptor blocking agents not only block the pulmonary effect of beta-agonists, such as albuterol sulfate, but may produce severe bronchospasm in asthmatic patients. Therefore, patients with asthma should not normally be treated with beta-blockers. However, under certain circumstances, e.g., as prophylaxis after myocardial infarction, there may be no acceptable alternatives to the use of beta-adrenergic-blocking agents in patients with asthma. In this setting, cardioselective beta-blockers should be considered, although they should be administered with caution).
No products indexed under this heading.

Moclobemide (Albuterol sulfate should be administered with extreme caution to patients being treated with monoamine oxidase inhibitors or tricyclic antidepressants, or within 2 weeks of discontinuation of such agents, because the action of albuterol on the cardiovascular system may be potentiated).
No products indexed under this heading.

Nadolol (Beta-adrenergic-receptor blocking agents not only block the pulmonary effect of beta-agonists, such as albuterol sulfate, but may produce severe bronchospasm in asthmatic patients. Therefore, patients with asthma should not normally be treated with beta-blockers. However, under certain circumstances, e.g., as prophylaxis after myocardial infarction, there may be no acceptable alternatives to the use of beta-adrenergic-blocking agents in patients with asthma. In this setting, cardioselective beta-blockers should be considered, although they should be administered with caution). Products include:
Nadolol Tablets ... 2191

Nebivolol (Beta-adrenergic-receptor blocking agents not only block the pulmonary effect of beta-agonists, such as albuterol sulfate, but may produce severe bronchospasm in asthmatic patients. Therefore, patients with asthma should not normally be treated with beta-blockers. However, under certain circumstanc-

es, e.g., as prophylaxis after myocardial infarction, there may be no acceptable alternatives to the use of beta-adrenergic-blocking agents in patients with asthma. In this setting, cardioselective beta-blockers should be considered, although they should be administered with caution). Products include:
Bystolic Tablets 1155

Nortriptyline Hydrochloride (Albuterol sulfate should be administered with extreme caution to patients being treated with monoamine oxidase inhibitors or tricyclic antidepressants, or within 2 weeks of discontinuation of such agents, because the action of albuterol on the cardiovascular system may be potentiated).
No products indexed under this heading.

Pargyline Hydrochloride (Albuterol sulfate should be administered with extreme caution to patients being treated with monoamine oxidase inhibitors or tricyclic antidepressants, or within 2 weeks of discontinuation of such agents, because the action of albuterol on the cardiovascular system may be potentiated).
No products indexed under this heading.

Penbutolol Sulfate (Beta-adrenergic-receptor blocking agents not only block the pulmonary effect of beta-agonists, such as albuterol sulfate, but may produce severe bronchospasm in asthmatic patients. Therefore, patients with asthma should not normally be treated with beta-blockers. However, under certain circumstances, e.g., as prophylaxis after myocardial infarction, there may be no acceptable alternatives to the use of beta-adrenergic-blocking agents in patients with asthma. In this setting, cardioselective beta-blockers should be considered, although they should be administered with caution).
No products indexed under this heading.

Phenelzine Sulfate (Albuterol sulfate should be administered with extreme caution to patients being treated with monoamine oxidase inhibitors or tricyclic antidepressants, or within 2 weeks of discontinuation of such agents, because the action of albuterol on the cardiovascular system may be potentiated).
No products indexed under this heading.

Pindolol (Beta-adrenergic-receptor blocking agents not only block the pulmonary effect of beta-agonists, such as albuterol sulfate, but may produce severe bronchospasm in asthmatic patients. Therefore, patients with asthma should not normally be treated with beta-blockers. However, under certain circumstances, e.g., as prophylaxis after myocardial infarction, there may be no acceptable alternatives to the use of beta-adrenergic-blocking agents in patients with asthma. In this setting, cardioselective beta-blockers should be considered, although they should be administered with caution).
No products indexed under this heading.

Pirbuterol Acetate (Other short-acting sympathomimetic aerosol bronchodilators should not be used concomitantly with albuterol sulfate. If additional adrenergic drugs are to be administered by any route, they should be used with caution to avoid deleterious cardiovascular effects). Products include:
Maxair Autohaler 1705

Polythiazide (The ECG changes and/or hypokalemia which may result from the administration of non-potassium sparing diuretics (such as loop or thiazide diuretics) can be acutely worsened by beta-agonists, especially when the recommended dose of beta-agonist is exceeded. Although the clinical significance of these effects is not known, caution is advised in the co-administration of beta-agonists with non-potassium sparing diuretics).
No products indexed under this heading.

Procarbazine Hydrochloride (Albuterol sulfate should be administered with extreme caution to patients being treated with monoamine oxidase inhibitors or tricyclic antidepressants, or within 2 weeks of discontinuation of such agents, because the action of albuterol on the cardiovascular system may be potentiated).
No products indexed under this heading.

Propranolol Hydrochloride (Beta-adrenergic-receptor blocking agents not only block the pulmonary effect of beta-agonists, such as albuterol sulfate, but may produce severe bronchospasm in asthmatic patients. Therefore, patients with asthma should not normally be treated with beta-blockers. However, under certain circumstances, e.g., as prophylaxis after myocardial infarction, there may be no acceptable alternatives to the use of beta-adrenergic-blocking agents in patients with asthma. In this setting, cardioselective beta-blockers should be considered, although they should be administered with caution). Products include:
InnoPran XL Extended Release Capsules 1484

Protriptyline Hydrochloride (Albuterol sulfate should be administered with extreme caution to patients being treated with monoamine oxidase inhibitors or tricyclic antidepressants, or within 2 weeks of discontinuation of such agents, because the action of albuterol on the cardiovascular system may be potentiated).
No products indexed under this heading.

Rasagiline Mesylate (Albuterol sulfate should be administered with extreme caution to patients being treated with monoamine oxidase inhibitors or tricyclic antidepressants, or within 2 weeks of discontinuation of such agents, because the action of albuterol on the cardiovascular system may be potentiated). Products include:
Azilect Tablets 3106

Salmeterol Xinafoate (Other short-acting sympathomimetic aerosol bronchodilators should not be used concomitantly with albuterol sulfate. If additional adrenergic drugs are to be administered by any route, they should be used with caution to avoid deleterious cardiovascular effects). Products include:
Advair Diskus 100/50 1276
Advair Diskus 250/50 1276
Advair Diskus 500/50 1276
Advair HFA 45/21 Inhalation Aerosol 1288
Advair HFA 115/21 Inhalation Aerosol 1288
Advair HFA 230/21 Inhalation Aerosol 1288
Serevent Diskus 1594

Selegiline (Albuterol sulfate should be administered with extreme caution to patients being treated with monoamine oxidase inhibitors or tricyclic antidepressants, or within 2 weeks of discontinuation of such agents, because the action of albuterol on the cardiovascular system may be potentiated). Products include:
Emsam Transdermal System 905

Selegiline Hydrochloride (Albuterol sulfate should be administered with extreme caution to patients being treated with monoamine oxidase inhibitors or tricyclic antidepressants, or within 2 weeks of discontinuation of such agents, because the action of albuterol on the cardiovascular system may be potentiated). Products include:
Eldepryl Capsules 3052

Sotalol Hydrochloride (Beta-adrenergic-receptor blocking agents not only block the pulmonary effect of beta-agonists, such as albuterol sulfate, but may produce severe bronchospasm in asthmatic patients. Therefore, patients with asthma should not normally be treated with beta-blockers. However, under certain circumstances, e.g., as prophylaxis after myocardial infarction, there may be no acceptable alternatives to the use of beta-adrenergic-blocking agents in patients with asthma. In this setting, cardioselective beta-blockers should be considered, although they should be administered with caution).
No products indexed under this heading.

Terbutaline Sulfate (Other short-acting sympathomimetic aerosol bronchodilators should not be used concomitantly with albuterol sulfate. If additional adrenergic drugs are to be administered by any route, they should be used with caution to avoid deleterious cardiovascular effects).
No products indexed under this heading.

Timolol Hemihydrate (Beta-adrenergic-receptor blocking agents not only block the pulmonary effect of beta-agonists, such as albuterol sulfate, but may produce severe bronchospasm in asthmatic patients. Therefore, patients with asthma should not normally be treated with beta-blockers. However, under certain circumstances, e.g., as prophylaxis after myocardial infarction, there may be no acceptable alternatives to the use of beta-adrenergic-blocking agents in patients with asthma. In this setting, cardioselective beta-blockers should be considered, although they should be administered with caution). Products include:
Betimol Ophthalmic Solution 3181

Timolol Maleate (Beta-adrenergic-receptor blocking agents not only block the pulmonary effect of beta-agonists, such as albuterol sulfate, but may produce severe bronchospasm in asthmatic patients. Therefore, patients with asthma should not normally be treated with beta-blockers. However, under certain circumstances, e.g., as prophylaxis after myocardial infarction, there may be no acceptable alternatives to the use of beta-adrenergic-blocking agents in patients with asthma. In this setting, cardioselective beta-blockers should be considered, although they should be administered with caution). Products include:
Combigan Ophthalmic Solution 553
Cosopt Sterile Ophthalmic Solution 1969
Timoptic Sterile Ophthalmic Solution 2121
Timoptic in Ocudose 2124
Timoptic-XE Sterile Ophthalmic Gel Forming Solution 2125

Torsemide (The ECG changes and/or hypokalemia which may result from the administration of non-potassium sparing diuretics (such as loop or thiazide diuretics) can be acutely worsened by beta-agonists, especially when the recommended dose of beta-agonist is exceeded. Although the clinical significance of these effects is not known, caution is advised in the co-administration of beta-agonists with non-potassium sparing diuretics). Products include:
Demadex Injection 2630
Demadex Tablets 2630

Tranylcypromine Sulfate (Albuterol sulfate should be administered with extreme caution to patients being treated with monoamine oxidase inhibitors or tricyclic antidepressants, or within 2 weeks of discontinuation of such agents, because the action of albuterol on the cardiovascular system may be potentiated). Products include:
Parnate Tablets 1532

Trimipramine Maleate (Albuterol sulfate should be administered with extreme caution to patients being treated with monoamine oxidase inhibitors or tricyclic antidepressants, or within 2 weeks of discontinuation of such agents, because the action of albuterol on the cardiovascular system may be potentiated).
No products indexed under this heading.

PROAMATINE TABLETS
(Midodrine Hydrochloride) 3032
May interact with alpha adrenergic blockers, cardiac glycosides, quinidine, and certain other agents. Compounds in these categories include:

Cimetidine (The high renal clearance of desglymidodrine is due to active tubular secretion by the base-secreting system also responsible for the secretion of cimetidine; possibility of drug interaction exists with co-administration).
No products indexed under this heading.

Deslanoside (Co-administration with cardiac glycosides may enhance or precipitate bradycardia, AV block or arrhythmia).
No products indexed under this heading.

Digitalis Glycoside Preparations (Co-administration with cardiac glycosides may enhance or precipitate bradycardia, AV block or arrhythmia).
No products indexed under this heading.

Digitoxin (Co-administration with cardiac glycosides may enhance or precipitate bradycardia, AV block or arrhythmia).
No products indexed under this heading.

Digoxin (Co-administration with cardiac glycosides may enhance or precipitate bradycardia, AV block or arrhythmia). Products include:
- Lanoxin Injection **1498**
- Lanoxin Injection Pediatric **1502**
- Lanoxin Tablets **1505**

Dihydroergotamine Mesylate (Co-administration with alpha-adrenergic receptor stimulants may enhance or potentiate pressor effects of midodrine).
No products indexed under this heading.

Doxazosin Mesylate (Alpha adrenergic blocking agents can antagonize the effects of midodrine).
No products indexed under this heading.

Ephedrine Hydrochloride (Co-administration with alpha-adrenergic receptor stimulants may enhance or potentiate pressor effects of midodrine).
No products indexed under this heading.

Ephedrine Sulfate (Co-administration with alpha-adrenergic receptor stimulants may enhance or potentiate pressor effects of midodrine).
No products indexed under this heading.

Ephedrine Tannate (Co-administration with alpha-adrenergic receptor stimulants may enhance or potentiate pressor effects of midodrine).
No products indexed under this heading.

Flecainide Acetate (The high renal clearance of desglymidodrine is due to active tubular secretion by the base-secreting system also responsible for the secretion of flecainide; possibility of drug interaction exists with co-administration).
No products indexed under this heading.

Fludrocortisone Acetate (Co-administration with salt-retaining steroid therapy increases the potential for supine hypertension; this can be minimized by reducing the dose of fludrocortisone or decreasing salt intake).
No products indexed under this heading.

Metformin (The high renal clearance of desglymidodrine is due to active tubular secretion by the base-secreting system also responsible for the secretion of metformin; possibility of drug interaction exists with co-administration).
No products indexed under this heading.

Phenylephrine Hydrochloride (Co-administration with alpha-adrenergic receptor stimulants may enhance or potentiate pressor effects of midodrine). Products include:
- Actifed Cold & Allergy Tablets **1895**
- Benadryl Allergy & Cold Kapgels **1895**
- Benadryl Allergy & Sinus Headache Kapgels **1895**
- Benadryl Severe Allergy & Sinus Headache Caplets **1897**
- Children's Benadryl-D Allergy & Sinus Liquid **1896**
- Benadryl-D Allergy & Sinus Tablet **1896**
- PediaCare Children's Allergy & Cold Liquid **1902**
- PediaCare Children's Decongestant Liquid **1902**
- PediaCare Children's Liquid Multi-Symptom Cold **1902**
- Sinutab Non-Drying Caplets **1905**
- Sinutab Sinus Caplets **1905**
- Children's Sudafed PE Cold & Cough Liquid **1907**
- Children's Sudafed PE Nasal Decongestant Liquid **1906**
- Sudafed PE Cold & Cough Caplets **1907**
- Sudafed PE Nasal Decongestant Tablets **1907**
- Sudafed PE Nighttime Cold Caplets **1907**
- Sudafed PE Non-Drying Sinus Caplets **1908**
- Sudafed PE Severe Cold Caplets **1908**
- Sudafed PE Sinus & Allergy Tablets **1908**
- Sudafed PE Sinus Headache Caplets **1908**
- Tylenol Allergy Multi-Symptom Caplets with Cool Burst and Rapid Release Gelcaps **1916**
- Tylenol Allergy Multi-Symptom Nighttime Caplets with Cool Burst **1916**
- Children's Tylenol Plus Cold Suspension Liquid **1912**
- Children's Tylenol Plus Cold & Allergy Suspension Liquid **1914**
- Children's Tylenol Plus Flu Suspension Liquid **1914**
- Children's Tylenol Plus Multi-Symptom Cold Suspension Liquid **1912**
- Tylenol Cold Head Congestion Daytime Caplets with Cool Burst **1910**
- Tylenol Cold Head Congestion Nighttime Caplets with Cool Burst **1910**
- Tylenol Cold Head Congestion Severe Daytime Caplets with Cool Burst **1910**
- Tylenol Cold Multi-Symptom Daytime Caplets with Cool Burst and Rapid Release Gels **1913**
- Tylenol Cold Multi-Symptom Daytime Liquid with Citrus Burst **1913**
- Tylenol Cold Multi-Symptom Nighttime Caplets with Cool Burst **1913**
- Tylenol Cold Multi-Symptom Nighttime Liquid with Cool Burst **1913**
- Tylenol Cold Multi-Symptom Severe Caplets with Cool Burst **1913**
- Tylenol Cold Multi-Symptom Severe Daytime Liquid with Citrus Burst **1913**
- Tylenol Sinus Congestion & Pain Daytime Caplets with Cool Burst and Gelcaps **1917**
- Tylenol Sinus Congestion & Pain Nighttime Caplets with Cool Burst **1917**
- Tylenol Sinus Congestion & Pain Severe Caplets with Cool Burst **1917**
- Vicks DayQuil Cold & Flu Multi-Symptom Relief .... ■□ **616**
- Vicks DayQuil LiquiCaps **2567**
- Vicks DayQuil Liquid **2567**
- Vicks DayQuil Multi-Symptom Cold/Flu Relief **2567**

Phenylephrine Tannate (Co-administration with alpha-adrenergic receptor stimulants may enhance or potentiate pressor effects of midodrine).
No products indexed under this heading.

Prazosin Hydrochloride (Alpha adrenergic blocking agents can antagonize the effects of midodrine).
No products indexed under this heading.

Procainamide Hydrochloride (The high renal clearance of desglymidodrine is due to active tubular secretion by the base-secreting system also responsible for the secretion of procainamide; possibility of drug interaction exists with co-administration).
No products indexed under this heading.

Pseudoephedrine Hydrochloride (Co-administration with alpha-adrenergic receptor stimulants may enhance or potentiate pressor effects of midodrine). Products include:
- Allegra-D 12 Hour Extended-Release Tablets **2687**
- Allegra-D 24 Hour Extended-Release Tablets **2690**
- Children's Motrin Cold Oral Suspension **1899**
- Sudafed 12 Hour Nasal Decongestant Non-Drowsy Caplets **1909**
- Sudafed 24 Hour Non-Drowsy Nasal Decongestant Tablets **1906**
- Children's Sudafed Nasal Decongestant Liquid **1906**
- Sudafed Nasal Decongestant Tablets **1906**
- Tylenol Cold Severe Congestion Daytime Caplets with Cool Burst **1912**
- Tylenol Sinus Severe Congestion Caplets with Cool Burst **1917**
- Vicks NyQuil LiquiCaps **2567**
- Vicks NyQuil Liquid **2567**
- Vicks NyQuil Multi-Symptom Cold/Flu Relief **2567**
- Zyrtec-D 12 Hour Extended Release Tablets **1923**
- Zyrtec-D Allergy & Congestion Extended-Release Tablets **1923**

Pseudoephedrine Sulfate (Co-administration with alpha-adrenergic receptor stimulants may enhance or potentiate pressor effects of midodrine). Products include:
- Clarinex-D 12-Hour Extended-Release Tablets **2831**
- Clarinex-D 24-Hour Extended-Release Tablets **2834**

Quinidine (The high renal clearance of desglymidodrine is due to active tubular secretion by the base-secreting system also responsible for the secretion of quinidine; possibility of drug interaction exists with co-administration).
No products indexed under this heading.

Quinidine Gluconate (The high renal clearance of desglymidodrine is due to active tubular secretion by the base-secreting system also responsible for the secretion of quinidine; possibility of drug interaction exists with co-administration).
No products indexed under this heading.

Quinidine Hydrochloride (The high renal clearance of desglymidodrine is due to active tubular secretion by the base-secreting system also responsible for the secretion of quinidine; possibility of drug interaction exists with co-administration).
No products indexed under this heading.

Quinidine Polygalacturonate (The high renal clearance of desglymidodrine is due to active tubular secretion by the base-secreting system also responsible for the secretion of quinidine; possibility of drug interaction exists with co-administration).
No products indexed under this heading.

Quinidine Sulfate (The high renal clearance of desglymidodrine is due to active tubular secretion by the base-secreting system also responsible for the secretion of quinidine; possibility of drug interaction exists with co-administration).
No products indexed under this heading.

Ranitidine Hydrochloride (The high renal clearance of desglymidodrine is due to active tubular secretion by the base-secreting system also responsible for the secretion of ranitidine; possibility of drug interaction exists with co-administration). Products include:
- Zantac 75 Tablets .... ■□ **603**
- Zantac **1670**
- Zantac Injection **1666**
- Zantac Injection Pharmacy Bulk Package **1668**
- Maximum Strength Zantac 150 Tablets .... ■□ **603**
- Maximum Strength Zantac 150 Cool Mint Tablets .... ■□ **603**

Tamsulosin Hydrochloride (Alpha adrenergic blocking agents can antagonize the effects of midodrine). Products include:
- Flomax Capsules **848**

Terazosin Hydrochloride (Alpha adrenergic blocking agents can antagonize the effects of midodrine).
No products indexed under this heading.

Triamterene (The high renal clearance of desglymidodrine is due to active tubular secretion by the base-secreting system also responsible for the secretion of triamterene; possibility of drug interaction exists with co-administration). Products include:
- Dyazide Capsules **1405**
- Dyrenium Capsules **3189**

PROCOSA II TABLETS

(Glucosamine Sulfate, Manganese, Vitamin C) **3174**
None cited in PDR database.

PROCRIT FOR INJECTION

(Epoetin Alfa) **2391**
None cited in PDR database.

PROFILNINE SD SOLVENT DETERGENT

(Factor IX Complex) **1721**
None cited in PDR database.

PROFLAVANOL 90 TABLETS

(Dietary Supplement, Herbals with Vitamins & Minerals, Vitamin C) **3174**
None cited in PDR database.

PROGLYCEM CAPSULES

(Diazoxide) **1185**
May interact with diuretics, highly protein bound drugs (selected), thiazides, and certain other agents. Compounds in these categories include:

Amiloride Hydrochloride (The concomitant administration of commonly used diuretics may potentiate the hyperglycemic effects of diazoxide).
No products indexed under this heading.

Amiodarone Hydrochloride (Since diazoxide is highly bound to serum proteins, it may displace other substances which are also bound to protein, resulting in higher blood levels of these substances).
No products indexed under this heading.

Amitriptyline Hydrochloride (Since diazoxide is highly bound to serum proteins, it may displace other substances which are also bound to protein, resulting in higher blood levels of these substances).
No products indexed under this heading.

Atovaquone (Since diazoxide is highly bound to serum proteins, it may displace other substances which are also bound to protein, resulting in higher blood levels of these substances). Products include:
Malarone Pediatric Tablets **1521**
Malarone Tablets **1521**
Mepron Suspension **1526**

Bendroflumethiazide (The concomitant administration of thiazides may potentiate the hyperglycemic and hyperuricemic effects of diazoxide).
No products indexed under this heading.

Bumetanide (The concomitant administration of commonly used diuretics may potentiate the hyperglycemic effects of diazoxide).
No products indexed under this heading.

Cefonicid Sodium (Since diazoxide is highly bound to serum proteins, it may displace other substances which are also bound to protein, resulting in higher blood levels of these substances).
No products indexed under this heading.

Celecoxib (Since diazoxide is highly bound to serum proteins, it may displace other substances which are also bound to protein, resulting in higher blood levels of these substances). Products include:
Celebrex Capsules **2979**

Chlordiazepoxide (Since diazoxide is highly bound to serum proteins, it may displace other substances which are also bound to protein, resulting in higher blood levels of these substances).
No products indexed under this heading.

Chlordiazepoxide Hydrochloride (Since diazoxide is highly bound to serum proteins, it may displace other substances which are also bound to protein, resulting in higher blood levels of these substances).
No products indexed under this heading.

Chlorothiazide (The concomitant administration of thiazides may potentiate the hyperglycemic and hyperuricemic effects of diazoxide).
No products indexed under this heading.

Chlorothiazide Sodium (The concomitant administration of thiazides may potentiate the hyperglycemic and hyperuricemic effects of diazoxide). Products include:
Intravenous Sodium Diuril **2490**

Chlorpromazine (Since diazoxide is highly bound to serum proteins, it may displace other substances which are also bound to protein, resulting in higher blood levels of these substances).
No products indexed under this heading.

Chlorpromazine Hydrochloride (Since diazoxide is highly bound to serum proteins, it may displace other substances which are also bound to protein, resulting in higher blood levels of these substances).
No products indexed under this heading.

Chlorthalidone (The concomitant administration of commonly used diuretics may potentiate the hyperglycemic effects of diazoxide). Products include:
Clorpres Tablets **2185**

Clomipramine Hydrochloride (Since diazoxide is highly bound to serum proteins, it may displace other substances which are also bound to protein, resulting in higher blood levels of these substances).
No products indexed under this heading.

Clozapine (Since diazoxide is highly bound to serum proteins, it may displace other substances which are also bound to protein, resulting in higher blood levels of these substances).
No products indexed under this heading.

Cyclosporine (Since diazoxide is highly bound to serum proteins, it may displace other substances which are also bound to protein, resulting in higher blood levels of these substances). Products include:
Gengraf Capsules **435**
Neoral Oral Solution **2280**
Neoral Soft Gelatin Capsules **2280**
Restasis Ophthalmic Emulsion **557**
Sandimmune **2296**

Diazepam (Since diazoxide is highly bound to serum proteins, it may displace other substances which are also bound to protein, resulting in higher blood levels of these substances). Products include:
Valium Tablets **2658**

Diclofenac Potassium (Since diazoxide is highly bound to serum proteins, it may displace other substances which are also bound to protein, resulting in higher blood levels of these substances).
No products indexed under this heading.

Diclofenac Sodium (Since diazoxide is highly bound to serum proteins, it may displace other substances which are also bound to protein, resulting in higher blood levels of these substances). Products include:
Diclofenac Sodium Ophthalmic Solution .... ⊙ **240**
Voltaren Ophthalmic Solution **2336**
Voltaren Tablets **2334**
Voltaren-XR Tablets **2337**

Diphenylhydantoin (Concomitant administration of oral diazoxide and diphenylhydantoin may result in a loss of seizure control).
No products indexed under this heading.

Diphenylhydantoin Sodium (Concomitant administration of oral diazoxide and diphenylhydantoin may result in a loss of seizure control).
No products indexed under this heading.

Dipyridamole (Since diazoxide is highly bound to serum proteins, it may displace other substances which are also bound to protein, resulting in higher blood levels of these substances). Products include:
Aggrenox Capsules **819**
Persantine Tablets **869**

Ethacrynic Acid (The concomitant administration of commonly used diuretics may potentiate the hyperglycemic effects of diazoxide). Products include:
Edecrin Tablets **698**

Fenoprofen Calcium (Since diazoxide is highly bound to serum proteins, it may displace other substances which are also bound to protein, resulting in higher blood levels of these substances). Products include:
Nalfon Capsules **2508**

Flurazepam Hydrochloride (Since diazoxide is highly bound to serum proteins, it may displace other substances which are also bound to protein, resulting in higher blood levels of these substances).
No products indexed under this heading.

Flurbiprofen (Since diazoxide is highly bound to serum proteins, it may displace other substances which are also bound to protein, resulting in higher blood levels of these substances).
No products indexed under this heading.

Furosemide (The concomitant administration of commonly used diuretics may potentiate the hyperglycemic effects of diazoxide). Products include:
Furosemide Tablets **2186**

Glipizide (Since diazoxide is highly bound to serum proteins, it may displace other substances which are also bound to protein, resulting in higher blood levels of these substances).
No products indexed under this heading.

Hydrochlorothiazide (The concomitant administration of thiazides may potentiate the hyperglycemic and hyperuricemic effects of diazoxide). Products include:
Atacand HCT **642**
Avalide Tablets **892**
Avalide Tablets **2713**
Benicar HCT Tablets **1010**
Diovan HCT Tablets **2216**
Dyazide Capsules **1405**
Micardis HCT Tablets **854**
Prinzide Tablets **2092**
Tekturna HCT Tablets **2324**
Teveten HCT Tablets **517**

Hydroflumethiazide (The concomitant administration of thiazides may potentiate the hyperglycemic and hyperuricemic effects of diazoxide).
No products indexed under this heading.

Ibuprofen (Since diazoxide is highly bound to serum proteins, it may displace other substances which are also bound to protein, resulting in higher blood levels of these substances). Products include:
Motrin IB Tablets and Caplets **1900**
Children's Motrin Oral Suspension **1901**
Children's Motrin Non-Staining Dye-Free Oral Suspension **1901**
Children's Motrin Cold Oral Suspension **1899**
Infants' Motrin Concentrated Drops **1901**
Infants' Motrin Non-Staining Dye-Free Concentrated Drops **1901**
Junior Strength Motrin Caplets and Chewable Tablets **1901**
Vicoprofen Tablets **533**

Imipramine Hydrochloride (Since diazoxide is highly bound to serum proteins, it may displace other substances which are also bound to protein, resulting in higher blood levels of these substances).
No products indexed under this heading.

Imipramine Pamoate (Since diazoxide is highly bound to serum proteins, it may displace other substances which are also bound to protein, resulting in higher blood levels of these substances).
No products indexed under this heading.

Indapamide (The concomitant administration of commonly used diuretics may potentiate the hyperglycemic effects of diazoxide). Products include:
Indapamide Tablets **2188**

Indomethacin (Since diazoxide is highly bound to serum proteins, it may displace other substances which are also bound to protein, resulting in higher blood levels of these substances). Products include:
Indocin **2024**

Indomethacin Sodium Trihydrate (Since diazoxide is highly bound to serum proteins, it may displace other substances which are also bound to protein, resulting in higher blood levels of these substances). Products include:
Indocin I.V. **2489**

Ketoprofen (Since diazoxide is highly bound to serum proteins, it may displace other substances which are also bound to protein, resulting in higher blood levels of these substances).
No products indexed under this heading.

Ketorolac Tromethamine (Since diazoxide is highly bound to serum proteins, it may displace other substances which are also bound to protein, resulting in higher blood levels of these substances).
No products indexed under this heading.

Meclofenamate Sodium (Since diazoxide is highly bound to serum proteins, it may displace other substances which are also bound to protein, resulting in higher blood levels of these substances).
No products indexed under this heading.

Mefenamic Acid (Since diazoxide is highly bound to serum proteins, it may displace other substances which are also bound to protein, resulting in higher blood levels of these substances).
No products indexed under this heading.

Methyclothiazide (The concomitant administration of thiazides may potentiate the hyperglycemic and hyperuricemic effects of diazoxide).
No products indexed under this heading.

Metolazone (The concomitant administration of commonly used diuretics may potentiate the hyperglycemic effects of diazoxide).
No products indexed under this heading.

Midazolam Hydrochloride (Since diazoxide is highly bound to serum proteins, it may displace other substances which are also bound to protein, resulting in higher blood levels of these substances).
No products indexed under this heading.

Naproxen (Since diazoxide is highly bound to serum proteins, it may displace other substances which are also bound to protein, resulting in higher blood levels of these substances). Products include:
EC-Naprosyn Delayed-Release Tablets 2632
Naprosyn Suspension 2632
Naprosyn Tablets 2632

Naproxen Sodium (Since diazoxide is highly bound to serum proteins, it may displace other substances which are also bound to protein, resulting in higher blood levels of these substances).
Products include:
Anaprox Tablets 2632
Anaprox DS Tablets 2632
Treximet Tablets 1616

Nortriptyline Hydrochloride (Since diazoxide is highly bound to serum proteins, it may displace other substances which are also bound to protein, resulting in higher blood levels of these substances).
No products indexed under this heading.

Oxaprozin (Since diazoxide is highly bound to serum proteins, it may displace other substances which are also bound to protein, resulting in higher blood levels of these substances).
No products indexed under this heading.

Oxazepam (Since diazoxide is highly bound to serum proteins, it may displace other substances which are also bound to protein, resulting in higher blood levels of these substances).
No products indexed under this heading.

Phenylbutazone (Since diazoxide is highly bound to serum proteins, it may displace other substances which are also bound to protein, resulting in higher blood levels of these substances).
No products indexed under this heading.

Piroxicam (Since diazoxide is highly bound to serum proteins, it may displace other substances which are also bound to protein, resulting in higher blood levels of these substances).
No products indexed under this heading.

Polythiazide (The concomitant administration of thiazides may potentiate the hyperglycemic and hyperuricemic effects of diazoxide).
No products indexed under this heading.

Propranolol Hydrochloride (Since diazoxide is highly bound to serum proteins, it may displace other substances which are also bound to protein, resulting in higher blood levels of these substances).
Products include:
InnoPran XL Extended Release Capsules 1484

Spironolactone (The concomitant administration of commonly used diuretics may potentiate the hyperglycemic effects of diazoxide).
No products indexed under this heading.

Sulindac (Since diazoxide is highly bound to serum proteins, it may displace other substances which are also bound to protein, resulting in higher blood levels of these substances). Products include:
Clinoril Tablets 1962

Temazepam (Since diazoxide is highly bound to serum proteins, it may displace other substances which are also bound to protein, resulting in higher blood levels of these substances).
No products indexed under this heading.

Tolbutamide (Since diazoxide is highly bound to serum proteins, it may displace other substances which are also bound to protein, resulting in higher blood levels of these substances).
No products indexed under this heading.

Tolmetin Sodium (Since diazoxide is highly bound to serum proteins, it may displace other substances which are also bound to protein, resulting in higher blood levels of these substances).
No products indexed under this heading.

Torsemide (The concomitant administration of commonly used diuretics may potentiate the hyperglycemic effects of diazoxide).
Products include:
Demadex Injection 2630
Demadex Tablets 2630

Triamterene (The concomitant administration of commonly used diuretics may potentiate the hyperglycemic effects of diazoxide).
Products include:
Dyazide Capsules 1405
Dyrenium Capsules 3189

Trimipramine Maleate (Since diazoxide is highly bound to serum proteins, it may displace other substances which are also bound to protein, resulting in higher blood levels of these substances).
No products indexed under this heading.

Warfarin Sodium (Since diazoxide is highly bound to serum proteins, it may displace other substances which are also bound to protein, resulting in higher blood levels of these substances).
No products indexed under this heading.

PROGLYCEM SUSPENSION

(Diazoxide) 1185
See Proglycem Capsules

PROGRAF CAPSULES AND INJECTION

(Tacrolimus) 622
May interact with aminoglycosides, calcium channel blockers, cytochrome p450 3a inducers (selected), cytochrome p450 3a inhibitors (selected), erythromycin, methylprednisolone, phenytoin, protease inhibitors, potassium sparing diuretics, vaccines, live, and certain other agents. Compounds in these categories include:

Allium sativum (Since tacrolimus is metabolized mainly by the CYP3A enzyme systems, drugs known to induce these enzymes may result in an increased metabolism of tacrolimus or decreased bioavailability as indicated by decreased whole blood or plasma concentrations. Monitoring of blood concentrations and appropriate dosage adjustments are essential when such drugs are used concomitantly).
No products indexed under this heading.

Aluminum Hydroxide (Co-administration has resulted in a 21% increase in the mean tacrolimus AUC and a 10% decrease in the Cmax).
No products indexed under this heading.

Amikacin Sulfate (Potential for additive or synergistic impairment of renal function).
No products indexed under this heading.

Amiloride Hydrochloride (Mild to severe hyperkalemia has been reported with tacrolimus; concurrent use with potassium-sparing diuretics should be avoided).
No products indexed under this heading.

Amiodarone Hydrochloride (Since tacrolimus is metabolized mainly by the CYP3A enzyme systems, substances known to inhibit these enzymes may decrease the metabolism or increase bioavailability of tacrolimus as indicated by increased whole blood or plasma concentrations. Monitoringof blood concentrations and appropriate dosage adjustments are essential when such drugs are used concomitantly).
No products indexed under this heading.

Amlodipine Besylate (While calcium-channel blocking agents can be effective in treating tacrolimus-associated hypertension, care should be taken since interference with tacrolimus metabolism may require dosage reduction). Products include:
Azor Tablets 1005
Exforge Tablets 2238

Amphotericin B (Potential for additive or synergistic impairment of renal function).
No products indexed under this heading.

Amprenavir (Co-administration with drugs known to inhibit CYP3A enzyme systems, such as protease inhibitors, may increase tacrolimus blood concentrations).
No products indexed under this heading.

Aprepitant (Since tacrolimus is metabolized mainly by the CYP3A enzyme systems, substances known to inhibit these enzymes may decrease the metabolism or increase bioavailability of tacrolimus as indicated by increased whole blood or plasma concentrations. Monitoringof blood concentrations and appropriate dosage adjustments are essential when such drugs are used concomitantly). Products include:
Emend Capsules 1992

BCG Vaccine (Immunosupressants may affect vaccination. Therefore, during treatment with tacrolimus, vaccination may be less effective. The use of live vaccines should be avoided).
No products indexed under this heading.

Bepridil Hydrochloride (While calcium-channel blocking agents can be effective in treating tacrolimus-associated hypertension, care should be taken since interference with tacrolimus metabolism may require dosage reduction).
No products indexed under this heading.

Bromocriptine Mesylate (Co-administration with drugs known to inhibit CYP3A enzyme systems, such as bromocriptine, may increase tacrolimus blood concentrations).
No products indexed under this heading.

Carbamazepine (Co-administration with drugs known to induce CYP3A enzyme systems, such as carbamazepine, may result in increased metabolism of tacrolimus and decreased blood or plasma concentrations). Products include:
Carbatrol Capsules 3019
Equetro Extended-Release Capsules 3174

Caspofungin acetate (Co-administration has resulted in a significant decrease in oral tacrolimus blood concentrations). Products include:
Cancidas for Injection 1953

Chloramphenicol (Co-administration with drugs known to inhibit CYP3A enzyme systems, such as chloramphenicol, may increase tacrolimus blood concentrations).
No products indexed under this heading.

Chloramphenicol Palmitate (Co-administration with drugs known to inhibit CYP3A enzyme systems, such as chloramphenicol, may increase tacrolimus blood concentrations).
No products indexed under this heading.

Chloramphenicol Sodium Succinate (Co-administration with drugs known to inhibit CYP3A enzyme systems, such as chloramphenicol, may increase tacrolimus blood concentrations).
No products indexed under this heading.

Cimetidine (Co-administration with drugs known to inhibit CYP3A enzyme systems, such as cimetidine, may increase tacrolimus blood concentrations).
No products indexed under this heading.

Cimetidine Hydrochloride (Co-administration with drugs known to inhibit CYP3A enzyme systems, such as cimetidine, may increase tacrolimus blood concentrations).
No products indexed under this heading.

Ciprofloxacin (Since tacrolimus is metabolized mainly by the CYP3A enzyme systems, substances known to inhibit these enzymes may decrease the metabolism or increase bioavailability of tacrolimus as indicated by increased whole blood or plasma concentrations. Monitoringof blood concentrations and appropriate dosage adjustments are essential when such drugs are used concomitantly). Products include:
Cipro I.V. 2817
Cipro Oral Suspension 2810
Cipro XR Tablets 2823
Ciprodex Otic Suspension 541

Ciprofloxacin Hydrochloride (Since tacrolimus is metabolized mainly by the CYP3A enzyme systems, substances known to inhibit these enzymes may decrease the metabolism or increase bioavailability of tacrolimus as indicated by increased whole blood or plasma concentrations. Monitoringof blood concentrations and appropriate dosage adjustments are essential when such drugs are used concomitantly). Products include:

Cipro Tablets **2810**

Cisapride (Co-administration with drugs known to inhibit CYP3A enzyme systems, such as cisapride, may increase tacrolimus blood concentrations).

No products indexed under this heading.

Cisplatin (Potential for additive or synergistic impairment of renal function).

No products indexed under this heading.

Clarithromycin (Co-administration with drugs known to inhibit CYP3A enzyme systems, such as clarithromycin, may increase tacrolimus blood concentrations). Products include:

Biaxin/Biaxin XL **411**

Clotrimazole (Co-administration with drugs known to inhibit CYP3A enzyme systems, such as clotrimazole, may increase tacrolimus blood concentrations). Products include:

Lotrisone **2881**

Cyclosporine (Increases tacrolimus blood levels resulting in additive/synergistic nephrotoxicity; Prograf should not be used simultaneously with cyclosporine; Prograf or cyclosporine should be discontinued at least 24 hours or more prior to initiating the other). Products include:

Gengraf Capsules **435**
Neoral Oral Solution **2280**
Neoral Soft Gelatin Capsules **2280**
Restasis Ophthalmic Emulsion **557**
Sandimmune **2296**

Danazol (Co-administration with drugs known to inhibit CYP3A enzyme systems, such as danazol, may increase tacrolimus blood concentrations).

No products indexed under this heading.

Darunavir (Co-administration with drugs known to inhibit CYP3A enzyme systems, such as protease inhibitors, may increase tacrolimus blood concentrations).

No products indexed under this heading.

Delavirdine Mesylate (Since tacrolimus is metabolized mainly by the CYP3A enzyme systems, substances known to inhibit these enzymes may decrease the metabolism or increase bioavailability of tacrolimus as indicated by increased whole blood or plasma concentrations. Monitoringof blood concentrations and appropriate dosage adjustments are essential when such drugs are used concomitantly).

No products indexed under this heading.

Dexamethasone (Since tacrolimus is metabolized mainly by the CYP3A enzyme systems, drugs known to induce these enzymes may result in an increased metabolism of tacrolimus or decreased bioavailability as indicated by decreased whole blood or plasma concentrations. Monitoring of blood concentrations and appropriate dosage adjustments are essential when such drugs are used concomitantly). Products include:

Ciprodex Otic Suspension **541**

Diltiazem Hydrochloride (Co-administration with drugs known to inhibit CYP3A enzyme systems, such as diltiazem, may increase tacrolimus blood concentrations). Products include:

Cardizem LA Extended Release Tablets **421**

Diltiazem Maleate (Since tacrolimus is metabolized mainly by the CYP3A enzyme systems, substances known to inhibit these enzymes may decrease the metabolism or increase bioavailability of tacrolimus as indicated by increased whole blood or plasma concentrations. Monitoringof blood concentrations and appropriate dosage adjustments are essential when such drugs are used concomitantly).

No products indexed under this heading.

Efavirenz (Since tacrolimus is metabolized mainly by the CYP3A enzyme systems, substances known to inhibit these enzymes may decrease the metabolism or increase bioavailability of tacrolimus as indicated by increased whole blood or plasma concentrations. Monitoringof blood concentrations and appropriate dosage adjustments are essential when such drugs are used concomitantly). Products include:

Atripla Tablets **938**
Sustiva Capsules **930**
Sustiva Tablets **930**

Erythromycin (Co-administration with drugs known to inhibit CYP3A enzyme systems, such as erythromycin, may increase tacrolimus blood concentrations).

No products indexed under this heading.

Erythromycin Estolate (Co-administration with drugs known to inhibit CYP3A enzyme systems, such as erythromycin, may increase tacrolimus blood concentrations).

No products indexed under this heading.

Erythromycin Ethylsuccinate (Co-administration with drugs known to inhibit CYP3A enzyme systems, such as erythromycin, may increase tacrolimus blood concentrations). Products include:

E.E.S. **433**
EryPed **431**

Erythromycin Gluceptate (Co-administration with drugs known to inhibit CYP3A enzyme systems, such as erythromycin, may increase tacrolimus blood concentrations).

No products indexed under this heading.

Erythromycin Lactobionate (Co-administration with drugs known to inhibit CYP3A enzyme systems, such as erythromycin, may increase tacrolimus blood concentrations).

No products indexed under this heading.

Erythromycin Stearate (Co-administration with drugs known to inhibit CYP3A enzyme systems, such as erythromycin, may increase tacrolimus blood concentrations).

No products indexed under this heading.

Ethinyl Estradiol (May increase tacrolimus blood concentrations). Products include:

Lybrel Tablets **3204**
Mircette Tablets **1034**
NuvaRing **2897**
Ortho-Cyclen/Ortho Tri-Cyclen **2449**
Ortho Evra Transdermal System **2437**
Ortho Tri-Cyclen Lo Tablets **2458**
Seasonique Tablets **1046**
Yaz Tablets **805**

Ethosuximide (Since tacrolimus is metabolized mainly by the CYP3A enzyme systems, drugs known to induce these enzymes may result in an increased metabolism of tacrolimus or decreased bioavailability as indicated by decreased whole blood or plasma concentrations. Monitoring of blood concentrations and appropriate dosage adjustments are essential when such drugs are used concomitantly).

No products indexed under this heading.

Felodipine (While calcium-channel blocking agents can be effective in treating tacrolimus-associated hypertension, care should be taken since interference with tacrolimus metabolism may require dosage reduction).

No products indexed under this heading.

Fluconazole (Co-administration with drugs known to inhibit CYP3A enzyme systems, such as fluconazole, may increase tacrolimus blood concentrations).

No products indexed under this heading.

Fluoxetine (Since tacrolimus is metabolized mainly by the CYP3A enzyme systems, substances known to inhibit these enzymes may decrease the metabolism or increase bioavailability of tacrolimus as indicated by increased whole blood or plasma concentrations. Monitoringof blood concentrations and appropriate dosage adjustments are essential when such drugs are used concomitantly).

No products indexed under this heading.

Fluoxetine Hydrochloride (Since tacrolimus is metabolized mainly by the CYP3A enzyme systems, substances known to inhibit these enzymes may decrease the metabolism or increase bioavailability of tacrolimus as indicated by increased whole blood or plasma concentrations. Monitoringof blood concentrations and appropriate dosage adjustments are essential when such drugs are used concomitantly). Products include:

Prozac Weekly Capsules **1852**
Prozac Pulvules and Liquid **1852**
Symbyax Capsules **1871**

Fluvoxamine Maleate (Since tacrolimus is metabolized mainly by the CYP3A enzyme systems, substances known to inhibit these enzymes may decrease the metabolism or increase bioavailability of tacrolimus as indicated by increased whole blood or plasma concentrations. Monitoringof blood concentrations and appropriate dosage adjustments are essential when such drugs are used concomitantly). Products include:

Luvox CR Extended-Release Capsules **1759**

Fosamprenavir Calcium (Co-administration with drugs known to inhibit CYP3A enzyme systems, such as protease inhibitors, may increase tacrolimus blood concentrations). Products include:

Lexiva Oral Suspension **1510**
Lexiva Tablets **1510**

Fosphenytoin Sodium (Co-administration may result in increased metabolism of tacrolimus and decreased plasma levels; tacrolimus may increase the plasma phenytoin levels).

No products indexed under this heading.

Ganciclovir (May increase nephrotoxicity).

No products indexed under this heading.

Ganciclovir Sodium (May increase nephrotoxicity).

No products indexed under this heading.

Gentamicin Sulfate (Potential for additive or synergistic impairment of renal function). Products include:

Pred-G Ophthalmic Ointment .... ⊙ **229**
Pred-G Ophthalmic Suspension .... ⊙ **228**

Hypericum (Co-administration with St. John's Wort may result in decreased tacrolimus blood concentrations). Products include:

Satieté Tablets **640**

Indinavir Sulfate (Co-administration with drugs known to inhibit CYP3A enzyme systems, such as protease inhibitors, may increase tacrolimus blood concentrations). Products include:

Crixivan Capsules **1979**

Influenza Vaccine, Live Attenuated (Immunosupressants may affect vaccination. Therefore, during treatment with tacrolimus, vaccination may be less effective. The use of live vaccines should be avoided).

No products indexed under this heading.

Influenza Virus Vaccine Live, Intranasal (Immunosupressants may affect vaccination. Therefore, during treatment with tacrolimus, vaccination may be less effective. The use of live vaccines should be avoided). Products include:

FluMist Vaccine **1945**

Isoniazid (Since tacrolimus is metabolized mainly by the CYP3A enzyme systems, substances known to inhibit these enzymes may decrease the metabolism or increase bioavailability of tacrolimus as indicated by increased whole blood or plasma concentrations. Monitoringof blood concentrations and appropriate dosage adjustments are essential when such drugs are used concomitantly).

No products indexed under this heading.

Isradipine (While calcium-channel blocking agents can be effective in treating tacrolimus-associated hypertension, care should be taken since interference with tacrolimus metabolism may require dosage reduction). Products include:

DynaCirc CR Controlled Release Tablets **1407**

Itraconazole (Co-administration with drugs known to inhibit CYP3A enzyme systems, such as itraconazole, may increase tacrolimus blood concentrations).

No products indexed under this heading.

Kanamycin Sulfate (Potential for additive or synergistic impairment of renal function).

No products indexed under this heading.

Ketoconazole (Co-administration has resulted in a significant increase in tacrolimus bioavailability and significant decrease in clearance; overall IV clearance of tacrolimus was not significantly changed by ketoconazole, although it was highly variable between patients). Products include:

Extina Foam, 2% 3057
Nizoral A-D Shampoo 1901

Lopinavir (Co-administration with drugs known to inhibit CYP3A enzyme systems, such as protease inhibitors, may increase tacrolimus blood concentrations). Products include:

Kaletra 452

Magnesium Hydroxide (Co-administration has resulted in a 21% increase in the mean tacrolimus AUC and a 10% decrease in the Cmax). Products include:

Fleet Pedia-Lax Chewable Tablets 1145
Pepcid Complete Chewable Tablets 1771
Extra Strength Rolaids Freshmint Tablets 1903
Rolaids Multi-Symptom Berry Tablets 1903
Rolaids Original Peppermint Tablets 1903

Measles, Mumps, Rubella and Varicella Virus Vaccine Live (Immunosupressants may affect vaccination. Therefore, during treatment with tacrolimus, vaccination may be less effective. The use of live vaccines should be avoided). Products include:

ProQuad 2099

Measles, Mumps & Rubella Virus Vaccine, Live (During treatment with tacrolimus, vaccination may be less effective). Products include:

M-M-R II 2054

Measles & Rubella Virus Vaccine Live (During treatment with tacrolimus, vaccination may be less effective).

No products indexed under this heading.

Measles Virus Vaccine Live (During treatment with tacrolimus, vaccination may be less effective). Products include:

Attenuvax 1951

Methylprednisolone (May increase tacrolimus blood concentrations).

No products indexed under this heading.

Methylprednisolone Acetate (May increase tacrolimus blood concentrations).

No products indexed under this heading.

Methylprednisolone Sodium Succinate (May increase tacrolimus blood concentrations).

No products indexed under this heading.

Metoclopramide Hydrochloride (Co-administration with drugs known to inhibit CYP3A enzyme systems, such as metoclopramide, may increase tacrolimus blood concentrations).

No products indexed under this heading.

Metronidazole (Since tacrolimus is metabolized mainly by the CYP3A enzyme systems, substances known to inhibit these enzymes may decrease the metabolism or increase bioavailability of tacrolimus as indicated by increased whole blood or plasma concentrations. Monitoringof blood concentrations and appropriate dosage adjustments are essential when such drugs are used concomitantly). Products include:

Pylera Capsules 714

Metronidazole Benzoate (Since tacrolimus is metabolized mainly by the CYP3A enzyme systems, substances known to inhibit these enzymes may decrease the metabolism or increase bioavailability of tacrolimus as indicated by increased whole blood or plasma concentrations. Monitoringof blood concentrations and appropriate dosage adjustments are essential when such drugs are used concomitantly).

No products indexed under this heading.

Metronidazole Hydrochloride (Since tacrolimus is metabolized mainly by the CYP3A enzyme systems, substances known to inhibit these enzymes may decrease the metabolism or increase bioavailability of tacrolimus as indicated by increased whole blood or plasma concentrations. Monitoringof blood concentrations and appropriate dosage adjustments are essential when such drugs are used concomitantly).

No products indexed under this heading.

Mibefradil Dihydrochloride (While calcium-channel blocking agents can be effective in treating tacrolimus-associated hypertension, care should be taken since interference with tacrolimus metabolism may require dosage reduction).

No products indexed under this heading.

Miconazole (Since tacrolimus is metabolized mainly by the CYP3A enzyme systems, substances known to inhibit these enzymes may decrease the metabolism or increase bioavailability of tacrolimus as indicated by increased whole blood or plasma concentrations. Monitoringof blood concentrations and appropriate dosage adjustments are essential when such drugs are used concomitantly).

No products indexed under this heading.

Modafinil (Since tacrolimus is metabolized mainly by the CYP3A enzyme systems, drugs known to induce these enzymes may result in an increased metabolism of tacrolimus or decreased bioavailability as indicated by decreased whole blood or plasma concentrations. Monitoring of blood concentrations and appropriate dosage adjustments are essential when such drugs are used concomitantly). Products include:

Provigil Tablets 977

Mumps Virus Vaccine, Live (Immunosupressants may affect vaccination. Therefore, during treatment with tacrolimus, vaccination may be less effective. The use of live vaccines should be avoided). Products include:

Mumpsvax 2068

Nefazodone Hydrochloride (May increase tacrolimus blood concentrations).

No products indexed under this heading.

Nelfinavir Mesylate (Co-administration has resulted in a significant increase in oral tacrolimus blood concentrations).

No products indexed under this heading.

Nevirapine (Since tacrolimus is metabolized mainly by the CYP3A enzyme systems, drugs known to induce these enzymes may result in an increased metabolism of tacrolimus or decreased bioavailability as indicated by decreased whole blood or plasma concentrations. Monitoring of blood concentrations and appropriate dosage adjustments are essential when such drugs are used concomitantly). Products include:

Viramune Oral Suspension 873
Viramune Tablets 873

Nicardipine Hydrochloride (Co-administration with drugs known to inhibit CYP3A enzyme systems, such as nicardipine, may increase tacrolimus blood concentrations). Products include:

Cardene I.V. 1093

Nifedipine (Co-administration with drugs known to inhibit CYP3A enzyme systems, such as nifedipine, may increase tacrolimus blood concentrations).

No products indexed under this heading.

Nimodipine (While calcium-channel blocking agents can be effective in treating tacrolimus-associated hypertension, care should be taken since interference with tacrolimus metabolism may require dosage reduction). Products include:

Nimotop Capsules 790

Nisoldipine (While calcium-channel blocking agents can be effective in treating tacrolimus-associated hypertension, care should be taken since interference with tacrolimus metabolism may require dosage reduction). Products include:

Sular Extended Release Tablets 2975

Norfloxacin (Since tacrolimus is metabolized mainly by the CYP3A enzyme systems, substances known to inhibit these enzymes may decrease the metabolism or increase bioavailability of tacrolimus as indicated by increased whole blood or plasma concentrations. Monitoringof blood concentrations and appropriate dosage adjustments are essential when such drugs are used concomitantly). Products include:

Noroxin Tablets 2069

Omeprazole (May increase tacrolimus blood concentrations).

No products indexed under this heading.

Paroxetine Hydrochloride (Since tacrolimus is metabolized mainly by the CYP3A enzyme systems, substances known to inhibit these enzymes may decrease the metabolism or increase bioavailability of tacrolimus as indicated by increased whole blood or plasma concentrations. Monitoringof blood concentrations and appropriate dosage adjustments are essential when such drugs are used concomitantly). Products include:

Paxil 1535
Paxil CR Controlled-Release Tablets 1544

Phenobarbital (Co-administration with drugs known to induce CYP3A enzyme systems, such as phenobarbital, may result in increased metabolism of tacrolimus and decreased blood or plasma concentrations). Products include:

Donnatal Extentabs 2507

Phenytoin (Co-administration may result in increased metabolism of tacrolimus and decreased plasma levels; tacrolimus may increase the plasma phenytoin levels).

No products indexed under this heading.

Phenytoin Sodium (Co-administration may result in increased metabolism of tacrolimus and decreased plasma levels; tacrolimus may increase the plasma phenytoin levels). Products include:

Phenytek Capsules 2192

Poliovirus Vaccine, Live, Oral, Trivalent, Types 1,2,3 (Sabin) (During treatment with tacrolimus, vaccination may be less effective).

No products indexed under this heading.

Poliovirus Vaccine Inactivated (During treatment with tacrolimus, vaccination may be less effective). Products include:

Pediarix Vaccine 1552

Quinine (Since tacrolimus is metabolized mainly by the CYP3A enzyme systems, substances known to inhibit these enzymes may decrease the metabolism or increase bioavailability of tacrolimus as indicated by increased whole blood or plasma concentrations. Monitoringof blood concentrations and appropriate dosage adjustments are essential when such drugs are used concomitantly).

No products indexed under this heading.

Quinine Sulfate (Since tacrolimus is metabolized mainly by the CYP3A enzyme systems, substances known to inhibit these enzymes may decrease the metabolism or increase bioavailability of tacrolimus as indicated by increased whole blood or plasma concentrations. Monitoringof blood concentrations and appropriate dosage adjustments are essential when such drugs are used concomitantly).

No products indexed under this heading.

Rifabutin (Co-administration with drugs known to induce CYP3A enzyme systems, such as rifabutin, may result in increased metabolism of tacrolimus and decreased blood or plasma concentrations).

No products indexed under this heading.

Rifampicin (Since tacrolimus is metabolized mainly by the CYP3A enzyme systems, drugs known to induce these enzymes may result in an increased metabolism of tacrolimus or decreased bioavailability as indicated by decreased whole blood or plasma concentrations. Monitoring of blood concentrations and appropriate dosage adjustments are essential when such drugs are used concomitantly).

No products indexed under this heading.

Rifampin (Co-administration has resulted in a significant decrease in oral tacrolimus bioavailability and significant increase in clearance).
No products indexed under this heading.

Rifapentine (Since tacrolimus is metabolized mainly by the CYP3A enzyme systems, drugs known to induce these enzymes may result in an increased metabolism of tacrolimus or decreased bioavailability as indicated by decreased whole blood or plasma concentrations. Monitoring of blood concentrations and appropriate dosage adjustments are essential when such drugs are used concomitantly).
No products indexed under this heading.

Ritonavir (Co-administration with drugs known to inhibit CYP3A enzyme systems, such as protease inhibitors, may increase tacrolimus blood concentrations). Products include:
Kaletra 452
Norvir 489

Rotavirus Vaccine, Live, Oral, Tetravalent (Immunosupressants may affect vaccination. Therefore, during treatment with tacrolimus, vaccination may be less effective. The use of live vaccines should be avoided).
No products indexed under this heading.

Rubella & Mumps Virus Vaccine Live (Immunosupressants may affect vaccination. Therefore, during treatment with tacrolimus, vaccination may be less effective. The use of live vaccines should be avoided).
No products indexed under this heading.

Rubella Virus Vaccine Live (Immunosupressants may affect vaccination. Therefore, during treatment with tacrolimus, vaccination may be less effective. The use of live vaccines should be avoided). Products include:
Meruvax II 2061

Saquinavir (Co-administration with drugs known to inhibit CYP3A enzyme systems, such as protease inhibitors, may increase tacrolimus blood concentrations).
No products indexed under this heading.

Saquinavir Mesylate (Co-administration with drugs known to inhibit CYP3A enzyme systems, such as protease inhibitors, may increase tacrolimus blood concentrations).
No products indexed under this heading.

Sertraline Hydrochloride (Since tacrolimus is metabolized mainly by the CYP3A enzyme systems, substances known to inhibit these enzymes may decrease the metabolism or increase bioavailability of tacrolimus as indicated by increased whole blood or plasma concentrations. Monitoringof blood concentrations and appropriate dosage adjustments are essential when such drugs are used concomitantly).
No products indexed under this heading.

Sirolimus (Co-administration has resulted in a 30% decrease in oral tacrolimus AUC(0-12) and Cmin). Products include:
Rapamune 3260

Smallpox Vaccine (Immunosupressants may affect vaccination. Therefore, during treatment with tacrolimus, vaccination may be less effective. The use of live vaccines should be avoided).
No products indexed under this heading.

Spironolactone (Mild to severe hyperkalemia has been reported with tacrolimus; concurrent use with potassium-sparing diuretics should be avoided).
No products indexed under this heading.

Streptomycin Sulfate (Potential for additive or synergistic impairment of renal function).
No products indexed under this heading.

Tipranavir (Co-administration with drugs known to inhibit CYP3A enzyme systems, such as protease inhibitors, may increase tacrolimus blood concentrations). Products include:
Aptivus Capsules 823
Aptivus Oral Solution 823

Tobramycin (Potential for additive or synergistic impairment of renal function). Products include:
Zylet Ophthalmic Suspension .... ⊙247

Tobramycin Sulfate (Potential for additive or synergistic impairment of renal function).
No products indexed under this heading.

Triamterene (Mild to severe hyperkalemia has been reported with tacrolimus; concurrent use with potassium-sparing diuretics should be avoided). Products include:
Dyazide Capsules 1405
Dyrenium Capsules 3189

Troleandomycin (Co-administration with drugs known to inhibit CYP3A enzyme systems, such as troleandomycin, may increase tacrolimus blood concentrations).
No products indexed under this heading.

Typhoid Vaccine (Immunosupressants may affect vaccination. Therefore, during treatment with tacrolimus, vaccination may be less effective. The use of live vaccines should be avoided).
No products indexed under this heading.

Typhoid Vaccine Live Oral TY21a (During treatment with tacrolimus, vaccination may be less effective).
No products indexed under this heading.

Vaccines (Live) (During treatment with tacrolimus, vaccination may be less effective).
No products indexed under this heading.

Varicella Virus Vaccine Live (Immunosupressants may affect vaccination. Therefore, during treatment with tacrolimus, vaccination may be less effective. The use of live vaccines should be avoided). Products include:
Varivax 2133

Venlafaxine Hydrochloride (Since tacrolimus is metabolized mainly by the CYP3A enzyme systems, substances known to inhibit these enzymes may decrease the metabolism or increase bioavailability of tacrolimus as indicated by increased whole blood or plasma concentrations. Monitoringof blood concentrations and appropriate dosage adjustments are essential when such drugs are used concomitantly). Products include:
Effexor XR Extended-Release Capsules 3195
Venlafaxine Hydrochloride Tablets ... 2199

Verapamil Hydrochloride (Co-administration with drugs known to inhibit CYP3A enzyme systems, such as verapamil, may increase tacrolimus blood concentrations). Products include:
Tarka Tablets 511

Voriconazole (Co-administration with drugs known to inhibit CYP3A enzyme systems, such as voriconazole, may increase tacrolimus blood concentrations).
No products indexed under this heading.

Yellow Fever Vaccine (During treatment with tacrolimus, vaccination may be less effective).
No products indexed under this heading.

Zafirlukast (Since tacrolimus is metabolized mainly by the CYP3A enzyme systems, substances known to inhibit these enzymes may decrease the metabolism or increase bioavailability of tacrolimus as indicated by increased whole blood or plasma concentrations. Monitoringof blood concentrations and appropriate dosage adjustments are essential when such drugs are used concomitantly). Products include:
Accolate Tablets 669

Zileuton (Since tacrolimus is metabolized mainly by the CYP3A enzyme systems, substances known to inhibit these enzymes may decrease the metabolism or increase bioavailability of tacrolimus as indicated by increased whole blood or plasma concentrations. Monitoringof blood concentrations and appropriate dosage adjustments are essential when such drugs are used concomitantly).
No products indexed under this heading.

Zoster Vaccine Live (Immunosupressants may affect vaccination. Therefore, during treatment with tacrolimus, vaccination may be less effective. The use of live vaccines should be avoided). Products include:
Zostavax Injection 2145

Food Interactions

Food, unspecified (The presence and composition of food has decreased both the rate and extent of tacrolimus absorption; this effect was most pronounced with a high-fat meal; the rate and extent of tacrolimus absorption were greatest under fasted conditions).

Grapefruit (Since tacrolimus is metabolized mainly by the CYP3A enzyme systems, substances known to inhibit these enzymes may decrease the metabolism or increase bioavailability of tacrolimus as indicated by increased whole blood or plasma concentrations. Monitoringof blood concentrations and appropriate dosage adjustments are essential when such drugs are used concomitantly).

Grapefruit Juice (Co-administered grapefruit juice has been reported to increase tacrolimus blood trough concentrations in liver transplant patients; grapefruit juice should be avoided).

PROLASTIN

(Alpha$_1$-Proteinase Inhibitor (Human)) 3099
None cited in PDR database.

PROLEUKIN FOR INJECTION

(Aldesleukin) 2287

May interact with aminoglycosides, antihypertensives, beta blockers, antineoplastics, cytotoxic drugs, glucocorticoids, hypnotics and sedatives, agents associated with myelosuppression, narcotic analgesics, nephrotoxic agents, parenteral analgesics, psychotropics, radiographic iodinated contrast media, tranquilizers, and certain other agents. Compounds in these categories include:

Abacavir Sulfate (Concurrent administration of drugs possessing nephrotoxic effects with aldesleukin may increase the potential for nephrotoxicity). Products include:
Epzicom Tablets 1422
Trizivir Tablets 1622
Ziagen 1673

Acebutolol Hydrochloride (Beta-blockers may potentiate the hypotension seen with aldesleukin).
No products indexed under this heading.

Acyclovir (Concurrent administration of drugs possessing nephrotoxic effects with aldesleukin may increase the potential for nephrotoxicity). Products include:
Zovirax 1690
Zovirax Cream 817
Zovirax Ointment 819

Acyclovir Sodium (Concurrent administration of drugs possessing nephrotoxic effects with aldesleukin may increase the potential for nephrotoxicity).
No products indexed under this heading.

Alatrofloxacin Mesylate (Concurrent administration of drugs possessing nephrotoxic effects with aldesleukin may increase the potential for nephrotoxicity).
No products indexed under this heading.

Alfentanil Hydrochloride (Aldesleukin may affect central nervous function. Therefore, interactions could occur following concomitant administration of narcotics).
No products indexed under this heading.

Aliskiren (Concurrent use with antihypertensive drugs may potentiate the hypotension seen with aldesleukin). Products include:
Tekturna Tablets 2321
Tekturna HCT Tablets 2324

Alprazolam (Aldesleukin may affect central nervous function. Therefore, interactions could occur following concomitant administration of psychotropic drugs).
No products indexed under this heading.

Altretamine (Concurrent administration of drugs possessing myelotoxic effects with aldesleukin may increase the potential for myelotoxicity). Products include:
Hexalen Capsules 1078

Amikacin Sulfate (Concurrent administration of drugs possessing nephrotoxic effects with aldesleukin may increase the potential for nephrotoxicity).
No products indexed under this heading.

Amitriptyline Hydrochloride (Aldesleukin may affect central nervous function. Therefore, interactions could occur following concomitant administration of psychotropic drugs).
No products indexed under this heading.

Amlodipine Besylate (Concurrent use with antihypertensive drugs may potentiate the hypotension seen with aldesleukin). Products include:
Azor Tablets 1005
Exforge Tablets 2238

Amoxapine (Aldesleukin may affect central nervous function. Therefore, interactions could occur following concomitant administration of psychotropic drugs).
No products indexed under this heading.

Amoxicillin (Concurrent administration of drugs possessing nephrotoxic effects with aldesleukin may increase the potential for nephrotoxicity). Products include:
Amoxil Capsules 1305
Amoxil Chewable Tablets 1305
Amoxil Pediatric Drops for Oral Suspension 1305
Amoxil Powder for Oral Suspension 1305
Amoxil Tablets 1305
Augmentin 1323
Augmentin Tablets 1327
Augmentin XR Extended Release Tablets 1333
Augmentin ES-600 Powder for Oral Suspension 1329
Moxatag Tablets 2165

Amoxicillin Trihydrate (Concurrent administration of drugs possessing nephrotoxic effects with aldesleukin may increase the potential for nephrotoxicity).
No products indexed under this heading.

Amphotericin B (Concurrent administration of drugs possessing nephrotoxic effects with aldesleukin may increase the potential for nephrotoxicity).
No products indexed under this heading.

Amphotericin B, liposomal (Concurrent administration of drugs possessing nephrotoxic effects with aldesleukin may increase the potential for nephrotoxicity). Products include:
AmBisome for Injection 606

Amphotericin B Cholesteryl Sulfate (Concurrent administration of drugs possessing nephrotoxic effects with aldesleukin may increase the potential for nephrotoxicity).
No products indexed under this heading.

Amphotericin B Lipid Complex (Concurrent administration of drugs possessing nephrotoxic effects with aldesleukin may increase the potential for nephrotoxicity). Products include:
Abelcet Injection 1134

Ampicillin (Concurrent administration of drugs possessing nephrotoxic effects with aldesleukin may increase the potential for nephrotoxicity).
No products indexed under this heading.

Ampicillin Sodium (Concurrent administration of drugs possessing nephrotoxic effects with aldesleukin may increase the potential for nephrotoxicity).
No products indexed under this heading.

Ampicillin Trihydrate (Concurrent administration of drugs possessing nephrotoxic effects with aldesleukin may increase the potential for nephrotoxicity).
No products indexed under this heading.

Amprenavir (Concurrent administration of drugs possessing nephrotoxic effects with aldesleukin may increase the potential for nephrotoxicity).
No products indexed under this heading.

Anastrozole (Hypersensitivity reactions have been reported in patients receiving combination regimens containing sequential high dose aldesleukin and antineoplastic agents. These reactions consisted of erythema, pruritus, and hypotension and occurred within hours of administration of chemotherapy. These events required medical intervention in some patients). Products include:
Arimidex Tablets 672

Asparaginase (Concurrent administration of drugs possessing hepatotoxic effects with aldesleukin may increase the potential for hepatotoxicity). Products include:
Elspar for Injection 1990
Elspar for Injection 2488

Aspirin (Concurrent administration of drugs possessing nephrotoxic effects with aldesleukin may increase the potential for nephrotoxicity). Products include:
Aggrenox Capsules 819
Bayer Aspirin 750
Percodan Tablets 1130
St. Joseph 81 mg Aspirin Chewable and Enteric Coated Tablets 1903

Atazanavir (Concurrent administration of drugs possessing nephrotoxic effects with aldesleukin may increase the potential for nephrotoxicity).
No products indexed under this heading.

Atenolol (Beta-blockers may potentiate the hypotension seen with aldesleukin).
No products indexed under this heading.

Atorvastatin Calcium (Concurrent administration of drugs possessing nephrotoxic effects with aldesleukin may increase the potential for nephrotoxicity). Products include:
Lipitor Tablets 2501

Azithromycin Dihydrate (Concurrent administration of drugs possessing nephrotoxic effects with aldesleukin may increase the potential for nephrotoxicity).
No products indexed under this heading.

Azlocillin Sodium (Concurrent administration of drugs possessing nephrotoxic effects with aldesleukin may increase the potential for nephrotoxicity).
No products indexed under this heading.

Aztreonam (Concurrent administration of drugs possessing nephrotoxic effects with aldesleukin may increase the potential for nephrotoxicity).
No products indexed under this heading.

Bacampicillin Hydrochloride (Concurrent administration of drugs possessing nephrotoxic effects with aldesleukin may increase the potential for nephrotoxicity).
No products indexed under this heading.

Balsalazide Disodium (Concurrent administration of drugs possessing nephrotoxic effects with aldesleukin may increase the potential for nephrotoxicity).
No products indexed under this heading.

Benazepril Hydrochloride (Concurrent administration of drugs possessing nephrotoxic effects with aldesleukin may increase the potential for nephrotoxicity).
No products indexed under this heading.

Bendroflumethiazide (Concurrent administration of drugs possessing nephrotoxic effects with aldesleukin may increase the potential for nephrotoxicity).
No products indexed under this heading.

Betamethasone Acetate (Although glucocorticoids have been shown to reduce aldesleukin-induced side effects including fever, renal insufficiency, hyperbilirubinemia, confusion, and dyspnea, concomitant administration of these agents with aldesleukin may reduce the antitumor effectiveness of aldesleukin and thus should be avoided).
No products indexed under this heading.

Betamethasone Sodium Phosphate (Although glucocorticoids have been shown to reduce aldesleukin-induced side effects including fever, renal insufficiency, hyperbilirubinemia, confusion, and dyspnea, concomitant administration of these agents with aldesleukin may reduce the antitumor effectiveness of aldesleukin and thus should be avoided).
No products indexed under this heading.

Betaxolol Hydrochloride (Beta-blockers may potentiate the hypotension seen with aldesleukin).
No products indexed under this heading.

Bicalutamide (Hypersensitivity reactions have been reported in patients receiving combination regimens containing sequential high dose aldesleukin and antineoplastic agents. These reactions consisted of erythema, pruritus, and hypotension and occurred within hours of administration of chemotherapy. These events required medical intervention in some patients). Products include:
No products indexed under this heading.

Bisoprolol Fumarate (Beta-blockers may potentiate the hypotension seen with aldesleukin).
No products indexed under this heading.

Bleomycin Sulfate (Concurrent administration of drugs possessing myelotoxic effects with aldesleukin may increase the potential for myelotoxicity).
No products indexed under this heading.

Buprenorphine Hydrochloride (Aldesleukin may affect central nervous function. Therefore, interactions could occur following concomitant administration of narcotics). Products include:
Suboxone Tablets 2601
Subutex Tablets 2601

Buspirone Hydrochloride (Aldesleukin may affect central nervous function. Therefore, interactions could occur following concomitant administration of psychotropic drugs).
No products indexed under this heading.

Busulfan (Concurrent administration of drugs possessing myelotoxic effects with aldesleukin may increase the potential for myelotoxicity). Products include:
Busulfex Injection 2477
Myleran Tablets 1530

Butabarbital (Aldesleukin may affect central nervous function. Therefore, interactions could occur following concomitant administration of psychotropic drugs).
No products indexed under this heading.

Butabarbital Sodium (Aldesleukin may affect central nervous function. Therefore, interactions could occur following concomitant administration of psychotropic drugs).
No products indexed under this heading.

Butorphanol Tartrate (Aldesleukin may affect central nervous function. Therefore, interactions could occur following concomitant administration of analgesics).
No products indexed under this heading.

Caffeine (Concurrent administration of drugs possessing nephrotoxic effects with aldesleukin may increase the potential for nephrotoxicity). Products include:
BioLean Free Tablets .... ▣635
BioLean II Tablets .... ▣635
Winrgy Dietary Supplement .... ▣642

Candesartan Cilexetil (Concurrent use with antihypertensive drugs may potentiate the hypotension seen with aldesleukin). Products include:
Atacand Tablets 639
Atacand HCT 642

Captopril (Concurrent administration of drugs possessing nephrotoxic effects with aldesleukin may increase the potential for nephrotoxicity). Products include:
Captopril Tablets 2182

Carbenicillin Disodium (Concurrent administration of drugs possessing nephrotoxic effects with aldesleukin may increase the potential for nephrotoxicity).
No products indexed under this heading.

Carbenicillin Indanyl Sodium (Concurrent administration of drugs possessing nephrotoxic effects with aldesleukin may increase the potential for nephrotoxicity).
No products indexed under this heading.

Carboplatin (Concurrent administration of drugs possessing nephrotoxic effects with aldesleukin may increase the potential for nephrotoxicity).
No products indexed under this heading.

Carmustine (BCNU) (Concurrent administration of drugs possessing nephrotoxic effects with aldesleukin may increase the potential for nephrotoxicity).
No products indexed under this heading.

Carteolol Hydrochloride (Beta-blockers may potentiate the hypotension seen with aldesleukin).
No products indexed under this heading.

Cefaclor (Concurrent administration of drugs possessing nephrotoxic effects with aldesleukin may increase the potential for nephrotoxicity).
No products indexed under this heading.

Cefadroxil (Concurrent administration of drugs possessing nephrotoxic effects with aldesleukin may increase the potential for nephrotoxicity).
No products indexed under this heading.

Cefamandole Nafate (Concurrent administration of drugs possessing nephrotoxic effects with aldesleukin may increase the potential for nephrotoxicity).
No products indexed under this heading.

Cefazolin Sodium (Concurrent administration of drugs possessing nephrotoxic effects with aldesleukin may increase the potential for nephrotoxicity).
No products indexed under this heading.

Cefdinir (Concurrent administration of drugs possessing nephrotoxic effects with aldesleukin may increase the potential for nephrotoxicity). Products include:
Omnicef Capsules 497
Omnicef for Oral Suspension 497

Cefepime Hydrochloride (Concurrent administration of drugs possessing nephrotoxic effects with aldesleukin may increase the potential for nephrotoxicity).
No products indexed under this heading.

Cefixime (Concurrent administration of drugs possessing nephrotoxic effects with aldesleukin may increase the potential for nephrotoxicity). Products include:
Suprax for Oral Suspension 1891
Suprax Tablets 1891

Cefmetazole Sodium (Concurrent administration of drugs possessing nephrotoxic effects with aldesleukin may increase the potential for nephrotoxicity).
No products indexed under this heading.

Cefonicid Sodium (Concurrent administration of drugs possessing nephrotoxic effects with aldesleukin may increase the potential for nephrotoxicity).
No products indexed under this heading.

Cefoperazone Sodium (Concurrent administration of drugs possessing nephrotoxic effects with aldesleukin may increase the potential for nephrotoxicity).
No products indexed under this heading.

Ceforanide (Concurrent administration of drugs possessing nephrotoxic effects with aldesleukin may increase the potential for nephrotoxicity).
No products indexed under this heading.

Cefotaxime Sodium (Concurrent administration of drugs possessing nephrotoxic effects with aldesleukin may increase the potential for nephrotoxicity).
No products indexed under this heading.

Cefotetan (Concurrent administration of drugs possessing nephrotoxic effects with aldesleukin may increase the potential for nephrotoxicity).
No products indexed under this heading.

Cefoxitin Sodium (Concurrent administration of drugs possessing nephrotoxic effects with aldesleukin may increase the potential for nephrotoxicity).
No products indexed under this heading.

Cefpodoxime Proxetil (Concurrent administration of drugs possessing nephrotoxic effects with aldesleukin may increase the potential for nephrotoxicity).
No products indexed under this heading.

Cefprozil (Concurrent administration of drugs possessing nephrotoxic effects with aldesleukin may increase the potential for nephrotoxicity).
No products indexed under this heading.

Ceftazidime (Concurrent administration of drugs possessing nephrotoxic effects with aldesleukin may increase the potential for nephrotoxicity). Products include:
Fortaz 1450

Ceftizoxime Sodium (Concurrent administration of drugs possessing nephrotoxic effects with aldesleukin may increase the potential for nephrotoxicity).
No products indexed under this heading.

Ceftriaxone Sodium (Concurrent administration of drugs possessing nephrotoxic effects with aldesleukin may increase the potential for nephrotoxicity). Products include:
Rocephin Injectable Vials, ADD-Vantage, Galaxy, Bulk 2642

Cefuroxime Axetil (Concurrent administration of drugs possessing nephrotoxic effects with aldesleukin may increase the potential for nephrotoxicity). Products include:
Ceftin 1380

Cefuroxime Sodium (Concurrent administration of drugs possessing nephrotoxic effects with aldesleukin may increase the potential for nephrotoxicity).
No products indexed under this heading.

Celecoxib (Concurrent administration of drugs possessing nephrotoxic effects with aldesleukin may increase the potential for nephrotoxicity). Products include:
Celebrex Capsules 2979

Cephalexin (Concurrent administration of drugs possessing nephrotoxic effects with aldesleukin may increase the potential for nephrotoxicity).
No products indexed under this heading.

Cephalothin Sodium (Concurrent administration of drugs possessing nephrotoxic effects with aldesleukin may increase the potential for nephrotoxicity).
No products indexed under this heading.

Cephapirin Sodium (Concurrent administration of drugs possessing nephrotoxic effects with aldesleukin may increase the potential for nephrotoxicity).
No products indexed under this heading.

Cephradine (Concurrent administration of drugs possessing nephrotoxic effects with aldesleukin may increase the potential for nephrotoxicity).
No products indexed under this heading.

Cerivastatin Sodium (Concurrent administration of drugs possessing nephrotoxic effects with aldesleukin may increase the potential for nephrotoxicity).
No products indexed under this heading.

Chloral Hydrate (Aldesleukin may affect central nervous function. Therefore, interactions could occur following concomitant administration of psychotropic drugs).
No products indexed under this heading.

Chlorambucil (Concurrent administration of drugs possessing myelotoxic effects with aldesleukin may increase the potential for myelotoxicity). Products include:
Leukeran Tablets 1508

Chlordiazepoxide (Aldesleukin may affect central nervous function. Therefore, interactions could occur following concomitant administration of psychotropic drugs).
No products indexed under this heading.

Chlordiazepoxide Hydrochloride (Aldesleukin may affect central nervous function. Therefore, interactions could occur following concomitant administration of psychotropic drugs).
No products indexed under this heading.

Chlorothiazide (Concurrent administration of drugs possessing nephrotoxic effects with aldesleukin may increase the potential for nephrotoxicity).
No products indexed under this heading.

Chlorothiazide Sodium (Concurrent administration of drugs possessing nephrotoxic effects with aldesleukin may increase the potential for nephrotoxicity). Products include:
Intravenous Sodium Diuril 2490

Chlorpromazine (Aldesleukin may affect central nervous function. Therefore, interactions could occur following concomitant administration of psychotropic drugs).
No products indexed under this heading.

Chlorpromazine Hydrochloride (Aldesleukin may affect central nervous function. Therefore, interactions could occur following concomitant administration of psychotropic drugs).
No products indexed under this heading.

Chlorpropamide (Concurrent administration of drugs possessing nephrotoxic effects with aldesleukin may increase the potential for nephrotoxicity).
No products indexed under this heading.

Chlorprothixene (Aldesleukin may affect central nervous function. Therefore, interactions could occur following concomitant administration of psychotropic drugs).
No products indexed under this heading.

Chlorprothixene Hydrochloride (Aldesleukin may affect central nervous function. Therefore, interactions could occur following concomitant administration of psychotropic drugs).
No products indexed under this heading.

Chlorthalidone (Concurrent use with antihypertensive drugs may potentiate the hypotension seen with aldesleukin). Products include:
Clorpres Tablets 2185

Cidofovir (Concurrent administration of drugs possessing nephrotoxic effects with aldesleukin may increase the potential for nephrotoxicity).
No products indexed under this heading.

Cilastatin Sodium (Concurrent administration of drugs possessing nephrotoxic effects with aldesleukin may increase the potential for nephrotoxicity). Products include:
Primaxin I.M. 2080
Primaxin I.V. 2083

Cimetidine (Concurrent administration of drugs possessing nephrotoxic effects with aldesleukin may increase the potential for nephrotoxicity).
No products indexed under this heading.

Cimetidine Hydrochloride (Concurrent administration of drugs possessing nephrotoxic effects with aldesleukin may increase the potential for nephrotoxicity).
No products indexed under this heading.

Cisplatin (Hypersensitivity reactions have been reported in patients receiving combination regimens containing sequential high dose aldesleukin and antineoplastic agents, specifically cisplatin. These reactions consisted of erythema, pruritis, and hypotension and occurred within hours of administration of chemotherapy. These events required medical intervention in some patients).
No products indexed under this heading.

Cladribine (Concurrent administration of drugs possessing nephrotoxic effects with aldesleukin may increase the potential for nephrotoxicity). Products include:
Leustatin Injection 2384

Clonidine (Concurrent use with antihypertensive drugs may potentiate the hypotension seen with aldesleukin). Products include:

Catapres-TTS 842

Clonidine Hydrochloride (Aldesleukin may affect central nervous function. Therefore, interactions could occur following concomitant administration of analgesics). Products include:
Catapres Tablets 841
Clorpres Tablets 2185

Clorazepate Dipotassium (Aldesleukin may affect central nervous function. Therefore, interactions could occur following concomitant administration of psychotropic drugs).
No products indexed under this heading.

Clozapine (Aldesleukin may affect central nervous function. Therefore, interactions could occur following concomitant administration of psychotropic drugs).
No products indexed under this heading.

Codeine Phosphate (Aldesleukin may affect central nervous function. Therefore, interactions could occur following concomitant administration of narcotics). Products include:
Tylenol with Codeine Tablets 2427

Colistimethate Sodium (Concurrent administration of drugs possessing nephrotoxic effects with aldesleukin may increase the potential for nephrotoxicity).
No products indexed under this heading.

Colistin Sulfate (Concurrent administration of drugs possessing nephrotoxic effects with aldesleukin may increase the potential for nephrotoxicity).
No products indexed under this heading.

Cortisone Acetate (Although glucocorticoids have been shown to reduce aldesleukin-induced side effects including fever, renal insufficiency, hyperbilirubinemia, confusion, and dyspnea, concomitant administration of these agents with aldesleukin may reduce the antitumor effectiveness of aldesleukin and thus should be avoided).
No products indexed under this heading.

Cyclophosphamide (Concurrent administration of drugs possessing nephrotoxic effects with aldesleukin may increase the potential for nephrotoxicity).
No products indexed under this heading.

Cyclosporine (Concurrent administration of drugs possessing nephrotoxic effects with aldesleukin may increase the potential for nephrotoxicity). Products include:
Gengraf Capsules 435
Neoral Oral Solution 2280
Neoral Soft Gelatin Capsules 2280
Restasis Ophthalmic Emulsion 557
Sandimmune 2296

Cytarabine (Concurrent administration of drugs possessing nephrotoxic effects with aldesleukin may increase the potential for nephrotoxicity).
No products indexed under this heading.

Cytarabine Liposome (Concurrent administration of drugs possessing nephrotoxic effects with aldesleukin may increase the potential for nephrotoxicity). Products include:
DepoCyt Injection 1136

Dacarbazine (Hypersensitivity reactions have been reported in patients receiving combination regimens containing sequential high dose aldesleukin and antineoplastic agents, specifically dacarbazine. These reactions consisted of erythema, pruritis, and hypotension and occurred within hours of administration of chemotherapy. These events required medical intervention in some patients).
No products indexed under this heading.

Daunorubicin Citrate (Hypersensitivity reactions have been reported in patients receiving combination regimens containing sequential high dose aldesleukin and antineoplastic agents. These reactions consisted of erythema, pruritus, and hypotension and occurred within hours of administration of chemotherapy. These events required medical intervention in some patients).
No products indexed under this heading.

Daunorubicin Citrate Liposome (Concurrent administration of drugs possessing myelotoxic effects with aldesleukin may increase the potential for myelotoxicity).
No products indexed under this heading.

Daunorubicin Hydrochloride (Concurrent administration of drugs possessing myelotoxic effects with aldesleukin may increase the potential for myelotoxicity).
No products indexed under this heading.

Delavirdine Mesylate (Concurrent administration of drugs possessing nephrotoxic effects with aldesleukin may increase the potential for nephrotoxicity).
No products indexed under this heading.

Denileukin Diftitox (Hypersensitivity reactions have been reported in patients receiving combination regimens containing sequential high dose aldesleukin and antineoplastic agents. These reactions consisted of erythema, pruritus, and hypotension and occurred within hours of administration of chemotherapy. These events required medical intervention in some patients). Products include:
Ontak Vials 1079

Deserpidine (Concurrent use with antihypertensive drugs may potentiate the hypotension seen with aldesleukin).
No products indexed under this heading.

Desipramine Hydrochloride (Aldesleukin may affect central nervous function. Therefore, interactions could occur following concomitant administration of psychotropic drugs).
No products indexed under this heading.

Dexamethasone (Although glucocorticoids have been shown to reduce aldesleukin-induced side effects including fever, renal insufficiency, hyperbilirubinemia, confusion, and dyspnea, concomitant administration of these agents with aldesleukin may reduce the antitumor effectiveness of aldesleukin and thus should be avoided). Products include:
Ciprodex Otic Suspension 541

Dexamethasone Acetate (Although glucocorticoids have been shown to reduce aldesleukin-induced side effects including fever, renal insufficiency, hyperbilirubinemia, confusion, and dyspnea, concomitant administration of these agents with aldesleukin may reduce the antitumor effectiveness of aldesleukin and thus should be avoided).
No products indexed under this heading.

Dexamethasone Sodium Phosphate (Although glucocorticoids have been shown to reduce aldesleukin-induced side effects including fever, renal insufficiency, hyperbilirubinemia, confusion, and dyspnea, concomitant administration of these agents with aldesleukin may reduce the antitumor effectiveness of aldesleukin and thus should be avoided).
No products indexed under this heading.

Dexrazoxane (Concurrent administration of drugs possessing myelotoxic effects with aldesleukin may increase the potential for myelotoxicity).
No products indexed under this heading.

Dezocine (Aldesleukin may affect central nervous function. Therefore, interactions could occur following concomitant administration of narcotics).
No products indexed under this heading.

Diatrizoate Meglumine (Concurrent administration of drugs possessing nephrotoxic effects with aldesleukin may increase the potential for nephrotoxicity).
No products indexed under this heading.

Diatrizoate Sodium (Concurrent administration of drugs possessing nephrotoxic effects with aldesleukin may increase the potential for nephrotoxicity).
No products indexed under this heading.

Diazepam (Aldesleukin may affect central nervous function. Therefore, interactions could occur following concomitant administration of psychotropic drugs). Products include:
Valium Tablets 2658

Diazoxide (Concurrent use with antihypertensive drugs may potentiate the hypotension seen with aldesleukin). Products include:
Proglycem Capsules 1185
Proglycem Suspension 1185

Diclofenac Potassium (Concurrent administration of drugs possessing nephrotoxic effects with aldesleukin may increase the potential for nephrotoxicity).
No products indexed under this heading.

Diclofenac Sodium (Concurrent administration of drugs possessing nephrotoxic effects with aldesleukin may increase the potential for nephrotoxicity). Products include:
Diclofenac Sodium Ophthalmic Solution................................ ⊙ 240
Voltaren Ophthalmic Solution 2336
Voltaren Tablets 2334
Voltaren-XR Tablets 2337

Dicloxacillin Sodium (Concurrent administration of drugs possessing nephrotoxic effects with aldesleukin may increase the potential for nephrotoxicity).
No products indexed under this heading.

Didanosine (Concurrent administration of drugs possessing nephrotoxic effects with aldesleukin may increase the potential for nephrotoxicity).
No products indexed under this heading.

Diltiazem Hydrochloride (Concurrent use with antihypertensive drugs may potentiate the hypotension seen with aldesleukin). Products include:
Cardizem LA Extended Release Tablets 421

Docetaxel (Hypersensitivity reactions have been reported in patients receiving combination regimens containing sequential high dose aldesleukin and antineoplastic agents. These reactions consisted of erythema, pruritus, and hypotension and occurred within hours of administration of chemotherapy. These events required medical intervention in some patients). Products include:
Taxotere Injection Concentrate 2773

Doxazosin Mesylate (Concurrent use with antihypertensive drugs may potentiate the hypotension seen with aldesleukin).
No products indexed under this heading.

Doxepin Hydrochloride (Aldesleukin may affect central nervous function. Therefore, interactions could occur following concomitant administration of psychotropic drugs).
No products indexed under this heading.

Doxorubicin Hydrochloride (Concurrent administration of drugs possessing cardiotoxic effects with aldesleukin may increase the potential for cardiotoxicity).
No products indexed under this heading.

Doxorubicin Hydrochloride Liposome (Concurrent administration of drugs possessing cardiotoxic effects with aldesleukin may increase the potential for cardiotoxicity). Products include:
Doxil Injection 2378

Droperidol (Aldesleukin may affect central nervous function. Therefore, interactions could occur following concomitant administration of psychotropic drugs).
No products indexed under this heading.

Efavirenz (Concurrent administration of drugs possessing nephrotoxic effects with aldesleukin may increase the potential for nephrotoxicity). Products include:
Atripla Tablets 938
Sustiva Capsules 930
Sustiva Tablets 930

Emtricitabine (Concurrent administration of drugs possessing nephrotoxic effects with aldesleukin may increase the potential for nephrotoxicity). Products include:
Atripla Tablets 938
Emtriva Capsules 1246
Emtriva Oral Solution 1246
Truvada Tablets 1262

Enalapril Maleate (Concurrent administration of drugs possessing nephrotoxic effects with aldesleukin may increase the potential for nephrotoxicity).
No products indexed under this heading.

Enalaprilat (Concurrent administration of drugs possessing nephrotoxic effects with aldesleukin may increase the potential for nephrotoxicity).
No products indexed under this heading.

Enfuvirtide (Concurrent administration of drugs possessing nephrotoxic effects with aldesleukin may increase the potential for nephrotoxicity).
No products indexed under this heading.

Epirubicin Hydrochloride (Concurrent administration of drugs possessing myelotoxic effects with aldesleukin may increase the potential for myelotoxicity).
No products indexed under this heading.

Eprosartan Mesylate (Concurrent use with antihypertensive drugs may potentiate the hypotension seen with aldesleukin). Products include:
Teveten Tablets 515
Teveten HCT Tablets 517

Esmolol Hydrochloride (Beta-blockers may potentiate the hypotension seen with aldesleukin).
No products indexed under this heading.

Estazolam (Aldesleukin may affect central nervous function. Therefore, interactions could occur following concomitant administration of psychotropic drugs).
No products indexed under this heading.

Estramustine Phosphate Sodium (Hypersensitivity reactions have been reported in patients receiving combination regimens containing sequential high dose aldesleukin and antineoplastic agents. These reactions consisted of erythema, pruritus, and hypotension and occurred within hours of administration of chemotherapy. These events required medical intervention in some patients).
No products indexed under this heading.

Ethchlorvynol (Aldesleukin may affect central nervous function. Therefore, interactions could occur following concomitant administration of psychotropic drugs).
No products indexed under this heading.

Ethinamate (Aldesleukin may affect central nervous function. Therefore, interactions could occur following concomitant administration of psychotropic drugs).
No products indexed under this heading.

Ethiodized Oil (Concurrent administration of drugs possessing nephrotoxic effects with aldesleukin may increase the potential for nephrotoxicity).
No products indexed under this heading.

Etodolac (Concurrent administration of drugs possessing nephrotoxic effects with aldesleukin may increase the potential for nephrotoxicity).
No products indexed under this heading.

Etoposide (Hypersensitivity reactions have been reported in patients receiving combination regimens containing sequential high dose aldesleukin and antineoplastic agents. These reactions consisted of erythema, pruritus, and hypotension and occurred within hours of administration of chemotherapy. These events required medical intervention in some patients).
No products indexed under this heading.

Exemestane (Hypersensitivity reactions have been reported in patients receiving combination regimens containing sequential high dose aldesleukin and antineoplastic agents. These reactions consisted of erythema, pruritus, and hypotension and occurred within hours of administration of chemotherapy. These events required medical intervention in some patients).
No products indexed under this heading.

Felodipine (Concurrent use with antihypertensive drugs may potentiate the hypotension seen with aldesleukin).
No products indexed under this heading.

Fenoprofen Calcium (Concurrent administration of drugs possessing nephrotoxic effects with aldesleukin may increase the potential for nephrotoxicity). Products include:
Nalfon Capsules 2508

Fentanyl (Aldesleukin may affect central nervous function. Therefore, interactions could occur following concomitant administration of narcotics). Products include:
Duragesic Transdermal System 2405
Ionsys Transdermal System 2410

Fentanyl Citrate (Aldesleukin may affect central nervous function. Therefore, interactions could occur following concomitant administration of narcotics). Products include:
Actiq 959
Fentora Tablets 968

Filgrastim (Concurrent administration of drugs possessing nephrotoxic effects with aldesleukin may increase the potential for nephrotoxicity). Products include:
Neupogen for Injection 589

Floxuridine (Hypersensitivity reactions have been reported in patients receiving combination regimens containing sequential high dose aldesleukin and antineoplastic agents. These reactions consisted of erythema, pruritus, and hypotension and occurred within hours of administration of chemotherapy. These events required medical intervention in some patients).
No products indexed under this heading.

Fludarabine Phosphate (Concurrent administration of drugs possessing myelotoxic effects with aldesleukin may increase the potential for myelotoxicity).
No products indexed under this heading.

Fludrocortisone Acetate (Although glucocorticoids have been shown to reduce aldesleukin-induced side effects including fever, renal insufficiency, hyperbilirubinemia, confusion, and dyspnea, concomitant administration of these agents with aldesleukin may reduce the antitumor effectiveness of aldesleukin and thus should be avoided).
No products indexed under this heading.

Fluorouracil (Concurrent administration of drugs possessing nephrotoxic effects with aldesleukin may increase the potential for nephrotoxicity). Products include:
Carac Cream 0.5% 2722

Fluphenazine Decanoate (Aldesleukin may affect central nervous function. Therefore, interactions could occur following concomitant administration of psychotropic drugs).
No products indexed under this heading.

Fluphenazine Enanthate (Aldesleukin may affect central nervous function. Therefore, interactions could occur following concomitant administration of psychotropic drugs).
No products indexed under this heading.

Fluphenazine Hydrochloride (Aldesleukin may affect central nervous function. Therefore, interactions could occur following concomitant administration of psychotropic drugs).
No products indexed under this heading.

Flurazepam Hydrochloride (Aldesleukin may affect central nervous function. Therefore, interactions could occur following concomitant administration of psychotropic drugs).
No products indexed under this heading.

Flurbiprofen (Concurrent administration of drugs possessing nephrotoxic effects with aldesleukin may increase the potential for nephrotoxicity).
No products indexed under this heading.

Flutamide (Hypersensitivity reactions have been reported in patients receiving combination regimens containing sequential high dose aldesleukin and antineoplastic agents. These reactions consisted of erythema, pruritus, and hypotension and occurred within hours of administration of chemotherapy. These events required medical intervention in some patients).
No products indexed under this heading.

Fluvastatin Sodium (Concurrent administration of drugs possessing nephrotoxic effects with aldesleukin may increase the potential for nephrotoxicity). Products include:
Lescol Capsules 2268
Lescol XL Tablets 2268

Foscarnet Sodium (Concurrent administration of drugs possessing nephrotoxic effects with aldesleukin may increase the potential for nephrotoxicity).
No products indexed under this heading.

Fosinopril Sodium (Concurrent administration of drugs possessing nephrotoxic effects with aldesleukin may increase the potential for nephrotoxicity).
No products indexed under this heading.

Furosemide (Concurrent administration of drugs possessing nephrotoxic effects with aldesleukin may increase the potential for nephrotoxicity). Products include:
Furosemide Tablets 2186

Gadopentetate Dimeglumine (Concurrent administration of drugs possessing nephrotoxic effects with aldesleukin may increase the potential for nephrotoxicity).
No products indexed under this heading.

Gemcitabine Hydrochloride (Concurrent administration of drugs possessing myelotoxic effects with aldesleukin may increase the potential for myelotoxicity). Products include:
Gemzar for Injection 1820

Gemtuzumab Ozogamicin (Concurrent administration of drugs possessing myelotoxic effects with aldesleukin may increase the potential for myelotoxicity). Products include:
Mylotarg for Injection 3212

Gentamicin (Concurrent administration of drugs possessing nephrotoxic effects with aldesleukin may increase the potential for nephrotoxicity).
No products indexed under this heading.

Gentamicin Sulfate (Concurrent administration of drugs possessing nephrotoxic effects with aldesleukin may increase the potential for nephrotoxicity). Products include:
Pred-G Ophthalmic Ointment .... ⊙ 229
Pred-G Ophthalmic Suspension ...... ⊙ 228

Glipizide (Concurrent administration of drugs possessing nephrotoxic effects with aldesleukin may increase the potential for nephrotoxicity).
No products indexed under this heading.

Globulin, Immune (Human) (Concurrent administration of drugs possessing nephrotoxic effects with aldesleukin may increase the potential for nephrotoxicity). Products include:
Flebogamma 5% 1715

Glutethimide (Aldesleukin may affect central nervous function. Therefore, interactions could occur following concomitant administration of psychotropic drugs).
No products indexed under this heading.

Glyburide (Concurrent administration of drugs possessing nephrotoxic effects with aldesleukin may increase the potential for nephrotoxicity).
No products indexed under this heading.

Gold Therapy (Concurrent administration of drugs possessing nephrotoxic effects with aldesleukin may increase the potential for nephrotoxicity).
No products indexed under this heading.

Guanabenz Acetate (Concurrent use with antihypertensive drugs may potentiate the hypotension seen with aldesleukin).
No products indexed under this heading.

Guanethidine Monosulfate (Concurrent use with antihypertensive drugs may potentiate the hypotension seen with aldesleukin).
No products indexed under this heading.

Haloperidol (Aldesleukin may affect central nervous function. Therefore, interactions could occur following concomitant administration of psychotropic drugs).
No products indexed under this heading.

Haloperidol Decanoate (Aldesleukin may affect central nervous function. Therefore, interactions could occur following concomitant administration of psychotropic drugs).
No products indexed under this heading.

HMG-CoA Reductase Inhibitors (Concurrent administration of drugs possessing nephrotoxic effects with aldesleukin may increase the potential for nephrotoxicity).
No products indexed under this heading.

Hydralazine Hydrochloride (Concurrent use with antihypertensive drugs may potentiate the hypotension seen with aldesleukin).
No products indexed under this heading.

Hydrochlorothiazide (Concurrent administration of drugs possessing nephrotoxic effects with aldesleukin may increase the potential for nephrotoxicity). Products include:
Atacand HCT 642
Avalide Tablets 892
Avalide Tablets 2713
Benicar HCT Tablets 1010
Diovan HCT Tablets 2216
Dyazide Capsules 1405
Micardis HCT Tablets 854
Prinzide Tablets 2092
Tekturna HCT Tablets 2324
Teveten HCT Tablets 517

Hydrocodone Bitartrate (Aldesleukin may affect central nervous function. Therefore, interactions could occur following concomitant administration of narcotics). Products include:
Lortab 5/500 Tablets 3143
Lortab 7.5/500 Tablets 3144
Lortab 10/500 Tablets 3144
Vicodin Tablets 529
Vicodin ES Tablets 530
Vicodin HP Tablets 531
Vicoprofen Tablets 533
Zydone Tablets 1132

Hydrocodone Polistirex (Aldesleukin may affect central nervous function. Therefore, interactions could occur following concomitant administration of narcotics). Products include:
Tussionex Pennkinetic Extended-Release Suspension 3154

Hydrocortisone (Although glucocorticoids have been shown to reduce aldesleukin-induced side effects including fever, renal insufficiency, hyperbilirubinemia, confusion, and dyspnea, concomitant administration of these agents with aldesleukin may reduce the antitumor effectiveness of aldesleukin and thus should be avoided).
No products indexed under this heading.

Hydrocortisone Acetate (Although glucocorticoids have been shown to reduce aldesleukin-induced side effects including fever, renal insufficiency, hyperbilirubinemia, confusion, and dyspnea, concomitant administration of these agents with aldesleukin may reduce the antitumor effectiveness of aldesleukin and thus should be avoided). Products include:
Analpram-HC 1140
Pramosone 1141

Hydrocortisone Sodium Phosphate (Although glucocorticoids have been shown to reduce aldesleukin-induced side effects including fever, renal insufficiency, hyperbilirubinemia, confusion, and dyspnea, concomitant administration of these agents with aldesleukin may reduce the antitumor effectiveness of aldesleukin and thus should be avoided).
No products indexed under this heading.

Hydrocortisone Sodium Succinate (Although glucocorticoids have been shown to reduce aldesleukin-induced side effects including fever, renal insufficiency, hyperbilirubinemia, confusion, and dyspnea, concomitant administration of these agents with aldesleukin may reduce the antitumor effectiveness of aldesleukin and thus should be avoided).
No products indexed under this heading.

Hydroflumethiazide (Concurrent administration of drugs possessing nephrotoxic effects with aldesleukin may increase the potential for nephrotoxicity).
No products indexed under this heading.

Hydromorphone Hydrochloride (Aldesleukin may affect central nervous function. Therefore, interactions could occur following concomitant administration of narcotics).
No products indexed under this heading.

Hydroxyurea (Concurrent administration of drugs possessing myelotoxic effects with aldesleukin may increase the potential for myelotoxicity).
No products indexed under this heading.

Hydroxyzine Hydrochloride (Aldesleukin may affect central nervous function. Therefore, interactions could occur following concomitant administration of psychotropic drugs).
No products indexed under this heading.

Ibuprofen (Concurrent administration of drugs possessing nephrotoxic effects with aldesleukin may increase the potential for nephrotoxicity). Products include:
Motrin IB Tablets and Caplets 1900
Children's Motrin Oral Suspension 1901
Children's Motrin Non-Staining Dye-Free Oral Suspension 1901
Children's Motrin Cold Oral Suspension 1899
Infants' Motrin Concentrated Drops 1901
Infants' Motrin Non-Staining Dye-Free Concentrated Drops 1901
Junior Strength Motrin Caplets and Chewable Tablets 1901
Vicoprofen Tablets 533

Idarubicin Hydrochloride (Concurrent administration of drugs possessing nephrotoxic effects with aldesleukin may increase the potential for nephrotoxicity).
No products indexed under this heading.

Ifosfamide (Concurrent administration of drugs possessing nephrotoxic effects with aldesleukin may increase the potential for nephrotoxicity).
No products indexed under this heading.

Imipenem (Concurrent administration of drugs possessing nephrotoxic effects with aldesleukin may increase the potential for nephrotoxicity). Products include:
Primaxin I.M. 2080
Primaxin I.V. 2083

Imipramine Hydrochloride (Aldesleukin may affect central nervous function. Therefore, interactions could occur following concomitant administration of psychotropic drugs).
No products indexed under this heading.

Imipramine Pamoate (Aldesleukin may affect central nervous function. Therefore, interactions could occur following concomitant administration of psychotropic drugs).
No products indexed under this heading.

Immune Globulin Intravenous (Human) (Concurrent administration of drugs possessing nephrotoxic effects with aldesleukin may increase the potential for nephrotoxicity). Products include:
Flebogamma 5% DIF 1718
Gammagard Liquid 730
Gammagard S/D 734
Gamunex 3094

Indapamide (Concurrent use with antihypertensive drugs may potentiate the hypotension seen with aldesleukin). Products include:
Indapamide Tablets 2188

Indinavir Sulfate (Concurrent administration of drugs possessing nephrotoxic effects with aldesleukin may increase the potential for nephrotoxicity). Products include:
Crixivan Capsules 1979

Indomethacin (Concurrent administration of drugs possessing nephrotoxic effects with aldesleukin may increase the potential for nephrotoxicity). Products include:
Indocin 2024

Indomethacin Sodium Trihydrate (Concurrent administration of drugs possessing nephrotoxic effects with aldesleukin may increase the potential for nephrotoxicity). Products include:
Indocin I.V. 2489

Interferon alfa-2a, Recombinant (Myocardial injury and severe rhabdomyolysis appear to be increased with concurrent use of aldesleukin and interferon-alfa. Also, hypersensitivity reactions have been reported in patients receiving combination regimens containing sequential high dose aldesleukin and interferon-alfa. These reactions consisted of erythema, pruritus, and hypotension and occurred within hours of administration of chemotherapy. In addition, exacerbation of the initial presentation of a number of autoimmune and inflammatory disorders has been observed following concurrent use of interferon-alfa and aldesleukin, including crescentic IgA glomerulonephritis, oculo-bulbar myasthenia gravis, inflammatory arthritis, thyroiditis, bullous pemphigoid, and Stevens-Johnson syndrome).
No products indexed under this heading.

Interferon alfa-2b, Recombinant (Myocardial injury and severe rhabdomyolysis appear to be increased with concurrent use of aldesleukin and interferon-alfa. Also, hypersensitivity reactions have been reported in patients receiving combination regimens containing sequential high dose aldesleukin and interferon-alfa. These reactions consisted of erythema, pruritus, and hypotension and occurred within hours of administration of chemotherapy. In addition, exacerbation of the initial presentation of a number of autoimmune and inflammatory disorders has been observed following concurrent use of interferon-alfa and aldesleukin, including crescentic IgA glomerulonephritis, oculo-bulbar myasthenia gravis, inflammatory arthritis, thyroiditis, bullous pemphigoid, and Stevens-Johnson syndrome). Products include:
Intron A for Injection 2859

Interferon Beta-1b (Concurrent administration of drugs possessing nephrotoxic effects with aldesleukin may increase the potential for nephrotoxicity). Products include:
Betaseron for SC Injection 756

Interleuken-2 (Concurrent administration of drugs possessing nephrotoxic effects with aldesleukin may increase the potential for nephrotoxicity).
No products indexed under this heading.

Iodamide Meglumine (Concurrent administration of drugs possessing nephrotoxic effects with aldesleukin may increase the potential for nephrotoxicity).
No products indexed under this heading.

Iohexol (Concurrent administration of drugs possessing nephrotoxic effects with aldesleukin may increase the potential for nephrotoxicity).
No products indexed under this heading.

Iopamidol (Concurrent administration of drugs possessing nephrotoxic effects with aldesleukin may increase the potential for nephrotoxicity).
No products indexed under this heading.

Iopanoic Acid (Concurrent administration of drugs possessing nephrotoxic effects with aldesleukin may increase the potential for nephrotoxicity).
No products indexed under this heading.

Iothalamate Meglumine (Concurrent administration of drugs possessing nephrotoxic effects with aldesleukin may increase the potential for nephrotoxicity).
No products indexed under this heading.

Ioxaglate Meglumine (Concurrent administration of drugs possessing nephrotoxic effects with aldesleukin may increase the potential for nephrotoxicity).
No products indexed under this heading.

Ioxaglate Sodium (Concurrent administration of drugs possessing nephrotoxic effects with aldesleukin may increase the potential for nephrotoxicity).
No products indexed under this heading.

Irbesartan (Concurrent use with antihypertensive drugs may potentiate the hypotension seen with aldesleukin). Products include:
Avalide Tablets 892
Avalide Tablets 2713
Avapro Tablets 897
Avapro Tablets 2718

Irinotecan Hydrochloride (Concurrent administration of drugs possessing myelotoxic effects with aldesleukin may increase the potential for myelotoxicity).
No products indexed under this heading.

Isocarboxazid (Aldesleukin may affect central nervous function. Therefore, interactions could occur following concomitant administration of psychotropic drugs). Products include:
Marplan Tablets 3177

Isradipine (Concurrent use with antihypertensive drugs may potentiate the hypotension seen with aldesleukin). Products include:
DynaCirc CR Controlled Release Tablets 1407

Kanamycin Sulfate (Concurrent administration of drugs possessing nephrotoxic effects with aldesleukin may increase the potential for nephrotoxicity).
No products indexed under this heading.

Ketoprofen (Concurrent administration of drugs possessing nephrotoxic effects with aldesleukin may increase the potential for nephrotoxicity).
No products indexed under this heading.

Ketorolac Tromethamine (Concurrent administration of drugs possessing nephrotoxic effects with aldesleukin may increase the potential for nephrotoxicity).
No products indexed under this heading.

Labetalol Hydrochloride (Beta-blockers may potentiate the hypotension seen with aldesleukin).
No products indexed under this heading.

Lamium album (Concurrent administration of drugs possessing nephrotoxic effects with aldesleukin may increase the potential for nephrotoxicity).
No products indexed under this heading.

Levamisole Hydrochloride (Hypersensitivity reactions have been reported in patients receiving combination regimens containing sequential high dose aldesleukin and antineoplastic agents. These reactions consisted of erythema, pruritus, and hypotension and occurred within hours of administration of chemotherapy. These events required medical intervention in some patients).
No products indexed under this heading.

Levobunolol Hydrochloride (Beta-blockers may potentiate the hypotension seen with aldesleukin).
No products indexed under this heading.

Levorphanol Tartrate (Aldesleukin may affect central nervous function. Therefore, interactions could occur following concomitant administration of narcotics).
No products indexed under this heading.

Lisinopril (Concurrent administration of drugs possessing nephrotoxic effects with aldesleukin may increase the potential for nephrotoxicity). Products include:
Prinivil Tablets 2087
Prinzide Tablets 2092

Lithium (Concurrent administration of drugs possessing nephrotoxic effects with aldesleukin may increase the potential for nephrotoxicity).
No products indexed under this heading.

Lithium Carbonate (Aldesleukin may affect central nervous function. Therefore, interactions could occur following concomitant administration of psychotropic drugs).
No products indexed under this heading.

Lithium Citrate (Aldesleukin may affect central nervous function. Therefore, interactions could occur following concomitant administration of psychotropic drugs).
No products indexed under this heading.

Lomustine (CCNU) (Hypersensitivity reactions have been reported in patients receiving combination regimens containing sequential high dose aldesleukin and antineoplastic agents. These reactions consisted of erythema, pruritus, and hypotension and occurred within hours of administration of chemotherapy. These events required medical intervention in some patients).
No products indexed under this heading.

Lopinavir (Concurrent administration of drugs possessing nephrotoxic effects with aldesleukin may increase the potential for nephrotoxicity). Products include:
Kaletra 452

Loracarbef (Concurrent administration of drugs possessing nephrotoxic effects with aldesleukin may increase the potential for nephrotoxicity).
No products indexed under this heading.

Lorazepam (Aldesleukin may affect central nervous function. Therefore, interactions could occur following concomitant administration of psychotropic drugs).
No products indexed under this heading.

Losartan Potassium (Concurrent use with antihypertensive drugs may potentiate the hypotension seen with aldesleukin). Products include:
Cozaar Tablets 1973

Lovastatin (Concurrent administration of drugs possessing nephrotoxic effects with aldesleukin may increase the potential for nephrotoxicity). Products include:
Advicor Tablets 402
Mevacor Tablets 2063

Loxapine Hydrochloride (Aldesleukin may affect central nervous function. Therefore, interactions could occur following concomitant administration of psychotropic drugs).
No products indexed under this heading.

Loxapine Succinate (Aldesleukin may affect central nervous function. Therefore, interactions could occur following concomitant administration of psychotropic drugs).
No products indexed under this heading.

Maprotiline Hydrochloride (Aldesleukin may affect central nervous function. Therefore, interactions could occur following concomitant administration of psychotropic drugs).
No products indexed under this heading.

Mecamylamine Hydrochloride (Concurrent use with antihypertensive drugs may potentiate the hypotension seen with aldesleukin).
No products indexed under this heading.

Mechlorethamine Hydrochloride (Hypersensitivity reactions have been reported in patients receiving combination regimens containing sequential high dose aldesleukin and antineoplastic agents. These reactions consisted of erythema, pruritus, and hypotension and occurred within hours of administration of chemotherapy. These events required medical intervention in some patients). Products include:
Mustargen for Injection 2492

Meclofenamate Sodium (Concurrent administration of drugs possessing nephrotoxic effects with aldesleukin may increase the potential for nephrotoxicity).
No products indexed under this heading.

Mefenamic Acid (Concurrent administration of drugs possessing nephrotoxic effects with aldesleukin may increase the potential for nephrotoxicity).
No products indexed under this heading.

Megestrol Acetate (Hypersensitivity reactions have been reported in patients receiving combination regimens containing sequential high dose aldesleukin and antineoplastic agents. These reactions consisted of erythema, pruritus, and hypotension and occurred within hours of administration of chemotherapy. These events required medical intervention in some patients). Products include:
Megace ES Oral Suspension 2499

Meloxicam (Concurrent administration of drugs possessing nephrotoxic effects with aldesleukin may increase the potential for nephrotoxicity). Products include:
Mobic Oral Suspension 863
Mobic Tablets 863

Melphalan (Hypersensitivity reactions have been reported in patients receiving combination regimens containing sequential high dose aldesleukin and antineoplastic agents. These reactions consisted of erythema, pruritus, and hypotension and occurred within hours of administration of chemotherapy. These events required medical intervention in some patients).
No products indexed under this heading.

Melphalan Hydrochloride (Concurrent administration of drugs possessing nephrotoxic effects with aldesleukin may increase the potential for nephrotoxicity).
No products indexed under this heading.

Meperidine Hydrochloride (Aldesleukin may affect central nervous function. Therefore, interactions could occur following concomitant administration of narcotics).
No products indexed under this heading.

Meprobamate (Aldesleukin may affect central nervous function. Therefore, interactions could occur following concomitant administration of psychotropic drugs).
No products indexed under this heading.

Mercaptopurine (Concurrent administration of drugs possessing myelotoxic effects with aldesleukin may increase the potential for myelotoxicity).
No products indexed under this heading.

Mesalamine (Concurrent administration of drugs possessing nephrotoxic effects with aldesleukin may increase the potential for nephrotoxicity). Products include:
Asacol Delayed-Release Tablets 2579
Canasa Rectal Suppositories 705
Lialda Tablets 3029
Pentasa Capsules 3030

Mesoridazine Besylate (Aldesleukin may affect central nervous function. Therefore, interactions could occur following concomitant administration of psychotropic drugs).
No products indexed under this heading.

Methadone Hydrochloride (Aldesleukin may affect central nervous function. Therefore, interactions could occur following concomitant administration of narcotics).
No products indexed under this heading.

Methimazole (Concurrent administration of drugs possessing nephrotoxic effects with aldesleukin may increase the potential for nephrotoxicity).
No products indexed under this heading.

Methotrexate (Concurrent administration of drugs possessing hepatotoxic effects with aldesleukin may increase the potential for hepatotoxicity).
No products indexed under this heading.

Methotrexate Sodium (Concurrent administration of drugs possessing nephrotoxic effects with aldesleukin may increase the potential for nephrotoxicity).
No products indexed under this heading.

Methyclothiazide (Concurrent administration of drugs possessing nephrotoxic effects with aldesleukin may increase the potential for nephrotoxicity).
No products indexed under this heading.

Methyldopa (Concurrent use with antihypertensive drugs may potentiate the hypotension seen with aldesleukin).
No products indexed under this heading.

Methyldopate Hydrochloride (Concurrent use with antihypertensive drugs may potentiate the hypotension seen with aldesleukin).
No products indexed under this heading.

Methylprednisolone Acetate (Although glucocorticoids have been shown to reduce aldesleukin-induced side effects including fever, renal insufficiency, hyperbilirubinemia, confusion, and dyspnea, concomitant administration of these agents with aldesleukin may reduce the antitumor effectiveness of aldesleukin and thus should be avoided).
No products indexed under this heading.

Methylprednisolone Sodium Succinate (Although glucocorticoids have been shown to reduce aldesleukin-induced side effects including fever, renal insufficiency, hyperbilirubinemia, confusion, and dyspnea, concomitant administration of these agents with aldesleukin may reduce the antitumor effectiveness of aldesleukin and thus should be avoided).
No products indexed under this heading.

Metipranolol Hydrochloride (Beta-blockers may potentiate the hypotension seen with aldesleukin).
No products indexed under this heading.

Metolazone (Concurrent use with antihypertensive drugs may potentiate the hypotension seen with aldesleukin).
No products indexed under this heading.

Metoprolol Succinate (Beta-blockers may potentiate the hypotension seen with aldesleukin). Products include:
Toprol-XL Tablets **666**

Metoprolol Tartrate (Beta-blockers may potentiate the hypotension seen with aldesleukin).
No products indexed under this heading.

Metyrosine (Concurrent use with antihypertensive drugs may potentiate the hypotension seen with aldesleukin). Products include:
Demser Capsules **1989**

Mezlocillin Sodium (Concurrent administration of drugs possessing nephrotoxic effects with aldesleukin may increase the potential for nephrotoxicity).
No products indexed under this heading.

Mibefradil Dihydrochloride (Concurrent use with antihypertensive drugs may potentiate the hypotension seen with aldesleukin).
No products indexed under this heading.

Midazolam Hydrochloride (Aldesleukin may affect central nervous function. Therefore, interactions could occur following concomitant administration of psychotropic drugs).
No products indexed under this heading.

Minocycline Hydrochloride (Concurrent administration of drugs possessing nephrotoxic effects with aldesleukin may increase the potential for nephrotoxicity). Products include:
Solodyn Extended Release Tablets **1938**

Minoxidil (Concurrent use with antihypertensive drugs may potentiate the hypotension seen with aldesleukin).
No products indexed under this heading.

Mitomycin (Mitomycin-C) (Concurrent administration of drugs possessing nephrotoxic effects with aldesleukin may increase the potential for nephrotoxicity).
No products indexed under this heading.

Mitotane (Concurrent administration of drugs possessing myelotoxic effects with aldesleukin may increase the potential for myelotoxicity).
No products indexed under this heading.

Mitoxantrone Hydrochloride (Concurrent administration of drugs possessing myelotoxic effects with aldesleukin may increase the potential for myelotoxicity). Products include:
Novantrone for Injection Concentrate **1100**

Moexipril Hydrochloride (Concurrent administration of drugs possessing nephrotoxic effects with aldesleukin may increase the potential for nephrotoxicity).
No products indexed under this heading.

Molindone Hydrochloride (Aldesleukin may affect central nervous function. Therefore, interactions could occur following concomitant administration of psychotropic drugs). Products include:
Moban Tablets **1116**

Morphine Sulfate (Aldesleukin may affect central nervous function. Therefore, interactions could occur following concomitant administration of narcotics). Products include:
Avinza Capsules **1772**
DepoDur Injection **1095**
MS Contin Tablets **2585**

Muromonab-CD3 (Concurrent administration of drugs possessing nephrotoxic effects with aldesleukin may increase the potential for nephrotoxicity). Products include:
Orthoclone OKT3 Sterile Solution **2387**

Nabumetone (Concurrent administration of drugs possessing nephrotoxic effects with aldesleukin may increase the potential for nephrotoxicity).
No products indexed under this heading.

Nadolol (Beta-blockers may potentiate the hypotension seen with aldesleukin). Products include:
Nadolol Tablets **2191**

Nafcillin Sodium (Concurrent administration of drugs possessing nephrotoxic effects with aldesleukin may increase the potential for nephrotoxicity).
No products indexed under this heading.

Nalbuphine Hydrochloride (Aldesleukin may affect central nervous function. Therefore, interactions could occur following concomitant administration of analgesics).
No products indexed under this heading.

Naproxen (Concurrent administration of drugs possessing nephrotoxic effects with aldesleukin may increase the potential for nephrotoxicity). Products include:
EC-Naprosyn Delayed-Release Tablets **2632**
Naprosyn Suspension **2632**
Naprosyn Tablets **2632**

Naproxen Sodium (Concurrent administration of drugs possessing nephrotoxic effects with aldesleukin may increase the potential for nephrotoxicity). Products include:
Anaprox Tablets **2632**
Anaprox DS Tablets **2632**
Treximet Tablets **1616**

Nebivolol (Beta-blockers may potentiate the hypotension seen with aldesleukin). Products include:
Bystolic Tablets **1155**

Nelfinavir Mesylate (Concurrent administration of drugs possessing nephrotoxic effects with aldesleukin may increase the potential for nephrotoxicity).
No products indexed under this heading.

Neomycin (Concurrent administration of drugs possessing nephrotoxic effects with aldesleukin may increase the potential for nephrotoxicity).
No products indexed under this heading.

Neomycin, oral (Concurrent administration of drugs possessing nephrotoxic effects with aldesleukin may increase the potential for nephrotoxicity).
No products indexed under this heading.

Neomycin Sulfate (Concurrent administration of drugs possessing nephrotoxic effects with aldesleukin may increase the potential for nephrotoxicity). Products include:
Neosporin Ophthalmic Solution Sterile .... ⊙ **252**

Nevirapine (Concurrent administration of drugs possessing nephrotoxic effects with aldesleukin may increase the potential for nephrotoxicity). Products include:
Viramune Oral Suspension **873**
Viramune Tablets **873**

Nicardipine Hydrochloride (Concurrent use with antihypertensive drugs may potentiate the hypotension seen with aldesleukin). Products include:
Cardene I.V. **1093**

Nifedipine (Concurrent use with antihypertensive drugs may potentiate the hypotension seen with aldesleukin).
No products indexed under this heading.

Nisoldipine (Concurrent use with antihypertensive drugs may potentiate the hypotension seen with aldesleukin). Products include:
Sular Extended Release Tablets **2975**

Nitroglycerin (Concurrent use with antihypertensive drugs may potentiate the hypotension seen with aldesleukin). Products include:
Nitro-Dur Transdermal Infusion System **2887**
Nitrolingual Pumpspray **2965**

Norfloxacin (Concurrent administration of drugs possessing nephrotoxic effects with aldesleukin may increase the potential for nephrotoxicity). Products include:
Noroxin Tablets **2069**

Nortriptyline Hydrochloride (Aldesleukin may affect central nervous function. Therefore, interactions could occur following concomitant administration of psychotropic drugs).
No products indexed under this heading.

Olanzapine (Aldesleukin may affect central nervous function. Therefore, interactions could occur following concomitant administration of psychotropic drugs). Products include:
Symbyax Capsules **1871**
Zyprexa Tablets **1883**
Zyprexa IntraMuscular **1883**
Zyprexa ZYDIS Orally Disintegrating Tablets **1883**

Olsalazine Sodium (Concurrent administration of drugs possessing nephrotoxic effects with aldesleukin may increase the potential for nephrotoxicity).
No products indexed under this heading.

Omeprazole (Concurrent administration of drugs possessing nephrotoxic effects with aldesleukin may increase the potential for nephrotoxicity).
No products indexed under this heading.

Oxaliplatin (Hypersensitivity reactions have been reported in patients receiving combination regimens containing sequential high dose aldesleukin and antineoplastic agents. These reactions consisted of erythema, pruritus, and hypotension and occurred within hours of administration of chemotherapy. These events required medical intervention in some patients). Products include:
Eloxatin for Injection **2731**

Oxaprozin (Concurrent administration of drugs possessing nephrotoxic effects with aldesleukin may increase the potential for nephrotoxicity).
No products indexed under this heading.

Oxazepam (Aldesleukin may affect central nervous function. Therefore, interactions could occur following concomitant administration of psychotropic drugs).
No products indexed under this heading.

Oxycodone Hydrochloride (Aldesleukin may affect central nervous function. Therefore, interactions could occur following concomitant administration of narcotics). Products include:
OxyContin Tablets **2589**
OxyIR Capsules **2593**
Percocet Tablets **1127**
Percodan Tablets **1130**

Oxymorphone Hydrochloride (Aldesleukin may affect central nervous function. Therefore, interac-

tions could occur following concomitant administration of analgesics). Products include:
Opana Tablets 1117
Opana ER Tablets 1121

Paclitaxel (Hypersensitivity reactions have been reported in patients receiving combination regimens containing sequential high dose aldesleukin and antineoplastic agents. These reactions consisted of erythema, pruritus, and hypotension and occurred within hours of administration of chemotherapy. These events required medical intervention in some patients).
No products indexed under this heading.

Paliperidone (Aldesleukin may affect central nervous function. Therefore, interactions could occur following concomitant administration of psychotropic drugs). Products include:
Invega Extended-Release Tablets 1748

Pamidronate Disodium (Concurrent administration of drugs possessing nephrotoxic effects with aldesleukin may increase the potential for nephrotoxicity).
No products indexed under this heading.

Paroxetine Hydrochloride (Concurrent administration of drugs possessing nephrotoxic effects with aldesleukin may increase the potential for nephrotoxicity). Products include:
Paxil 1535
Paxil CR Controlled-Release Tablets 1544

Penbutolol Sulfate (Beta-blockers may potentiate the hypotension seen with aldesleukin).
No products indexed under this heading.

Penicillamine (Concurrent administration of drugs possessing nephrotoxic effects with aldesleukin may increase the potential for nephrotoxicity). Products include:
Cuprimine Capsules 1986

Penicillin G Benzathine (Concurrent administration of drugs possessing nephrotoxic effects with aldesleukin may increase the potential for nephrotoxicity). Products include:
Bicillin C-R Injectable Suspension 1775
Bicillin L-A Injection 1777

Penicillin G Potassium (Concurrent administration of drugs possessing nephrotoxic effects with aldesleukin may increase the potential for nephrotoxicity).
No products indexed under this heading.

Penicillin G Procaine (Concurrent administration of drugs possessing nephrotoxic effects with aldesleukin may increase the potential for nephrotoxicity). Products include:
Bicillin C-R Injectable Suspension 1775
Bicillin L-A Injection 1777

Penicillin G Sodium (Concurrent administration of drugs possessing nephrotoxic effects with aldesleukin may increase the potential for nephrotoxicity).
No products indexed under this heading.

Penicillin V Potassium (Concurrent administration of drugs possessing nephrotoxic effects with aldesleukin may increase the potential for nephrotoxicity).
No products indexed under this heading.

Pentamidine Isethionate (Concurrent administration of drugs possessing nephrotoxic effects with aldesleukin may increase the potential for nephrotoxicity).
No products indexed under this heading.

Pentazocine Hydrochloride (Aldesleukin may affect central nervous function. Therefore, interactions could occur following concomitant administration of analgesics).
No products indexed under this heading.

Perindopril Erbumine (Concurrent administration of drugs possessing nephrotoxic effects with aldesleukin may increase the potential for nephrotoxicity). Products include:
Aceon Tablets (2 mg, 4 mg, 8 mg) 3038

Perphenazine (Aldesleukin may affect central nervous function. Therefore, interactions could occur following concomitant administration of psychotropic drugs).
No products indexed under this heading.

Phenelzine Sulfate (Aldesleukin may affect central nervous function. Therefore, interactions could occur following concomitant administration of psychotropic drugs).
No products indexed under this heading.

Phenoxybenzamine Hydrochloride (Concurrent use with antihypertensive drugs may potentiate the hypotension seen with aldesleukin). Products include:
Dibenzyline Capsules 3188

Phentolamine Mesylate (Concurrent use with antihypertensive drugs may potentiate the hypotension seen with aldesleukin).
No products indexed under this heading.

Phenylbutazone (Concurrent administration of drugs possessing nephrotoxic effects with aldesleukin may increase the potential for nephrotoxicity).
No products indexed under this heading.

Pindolol (Beta-blockers may potentiate the hypotension seen with aldesleukin).
No products indexed under this heading.

Piroxicam (Concurrent administration of drugs possessing nephrotoxic effects with aldesleukin may increase the potential for nephrotoxicity).
No products indexed under this heading.

Plicamycin (Concurrent administration of drugs possessing nephrotoxic effects with aldesleukin may increase the potential for nephrotoxicity).
No products indexed under this heading.

Polymyxin (Concurrent administration of drugs possessing nephrotoxic effects with aldesleukin may increase the potential for nephrotoxicity).
No products indexed under this heading.

Polymyxin B Sulfate (Concurrent administration of drugs possessing nephrotoxic effects with aldesleukin may increase the potential for nephrotoxicity). Products include:
Neosporin Ophthalmic Solution Sterile .... ⊙252

Polythiazide (Concurrent administration of drugs possessing nephrotoxic effects with aldesleukin may increase the potential for nephrotoxicity).
No products indexed under this heading.

Pravastatin Sodium (Concurrent administration of drugs possessing nephrotoxic effects with aldesleukin may increase the potential for nephrotoxicity).
No products indexed under this heading.

Prazepam (Aldesleukin may affect central nervous function. Therefore, interactions could occur following concomitant administration of psychotropic drugs).
No products indexed under this heading.

Prazosin Hydrochloride (Concurrent use with antihypertensive drugs may potentiate the hypotension seen with aldesleukin).
No products indexed under this heading.

Prednisolone Acetate (Although glucocorticoids have been shown to reduce aldesleukin-induced side effects including fever, renal insufficiency, hyperbilirubinemia, confusion, and dyspnea, concomitant administration of these agents with aldesleukin may reduce the antitumor effectiveness of aldesleukin and thus should be avoided). Products include:
Pred Forte Ophthalmic Suspension .... ⊙227
Pred Mild Ophthalmic Suspension .... ⊙230
Pred-G Ophthalmic Ointment .... ⊙229
Pred-G Ophthalmic Suspension ...... ⊙228

Prednisolone Sodium Phosphate (Although glucocorticoids have been shown to reduce aldesleukin-induced side effects including fever, renal insufficiency, hyperbilirubinemia, confusion, and dyspnea, concomitant administration of these agents with aldesleukin may reduce the antitumor effectiveness of aldesleukin and thus should be avoided).
No products indexed under this heading.

Prednisolone Tebutate (Although glucocorticoids have been shown to reduce aldesleukin-induced side effects including fever, renal insufficiency, hyperbilirubinemia, confusion, and dyspnea, concomitant administration of these agents with aldesleukin may reduce the antitumor effectiveness of aldesleukin and thus should be avoided).
No products indexed under this heading.

Prednisone (Although glucocorticoids have been shown to reduce aldesleukin-induced side effects including fever, renal insufficiency, hyperbilirubinemia, confusion, and dyspnea, concomitant administration of these agents with aldesleukin may reduce the antitumor effectiveness of aldesleukin and thus should be avoided).
No products indexed under this heading.

Probenecid (Concurrent administration of drugs possessing nephrotoxic effects with aldesleukin may increase the potential for nephrotoxicity).
No products indexed under this heading.

Procarbazine Hydrochloride (Concurrent administration of drugs possessing myelotoxic effects with aldesleukin may increase the potential for myelotoxicity).
No products indexed under this heading.

Prochlorperazine (Aldesleukin may affect central nervous function. Therefore, interactions could occur following concomitant administration of psychotropic drugs).
No products indexed under this heading.

Promethazine Hydrochloride (Aldesleukin may affect central nervous function. Therefore, interactions could occur following concomitant administration of psychotropic drugs).
No products indexed under this heading.

Propofol (Aldesleukin may affect central nervous function. Therefore, interactions could occur following concomitant administration of psychotropic drugs).
No products indexed under this heading.

Propoxyphene Hydrochloride (Aldesleukin may affect central nervous function. Therefore, interactions could occur following concomitant administration of narcotics).
No products indexed under this heading.

Propoxyphene Napsylate (Aldesleukin may affect central nervous function. Therefore, interactions could occur following concomitant administration of narcotics).
No products indexed under this heading.

Propranolol Hydrochloride (Beta-blockers may potentiate the hypotension seen with aldesleukin). Products include:
InnoPran XL Extended Release Capsules 1484

Protriptyline Hydrochloride (Aldesleukin may affect central nervous function. Therefore, interactions could occur following concomitant administration of psychotropic drugs).
No products indexed under this heading.

Quazepam (Aldesleukin may affect central nervous function. Therefore, interactions could occur following concomitant administration of psychotropic drugs).
No products indexed under this heading.

Quetiapine Fumarate (Aldesleukin may affect central nervous function. Therefore, interactions could occur following concomitant administration of psychotropic drugs).
No products indexed under this heading.

Quinapril Hydrochloride (Concurrent administration of drugs possessing nephrotoxic effects with aldesleukin may increase the potential for nephrotoxicity).
No products indexed under this heading.

Rabeprazole Sodium (Concurrent administration of drugs possessing

nephrotoxic effects with aldesleukin may increase the potential for nephrotoxicity). Products include:
Aciphex Tablets 1053

Ramelteon (Aldesleukin may affect central nervous function. Therefore, interactions could occur following concomitant administration of psychotropic drugs). Products include:
Rozerem Tablets 3091

Ramipril (Concurrent administration of drugs possessing nephrotoxic effects with aldesleukin may increase the potential for nephrotoxicity).
No products indexed under this heading.

Rauwolfia Serpentina (Concurrent use with antihypertensive drugs may potentiate the hypotension seen with aldesleukin).
No products indexed under this heading.

Remifentanil Hydrochloride (Aldesleukin may affect central nervous function. Therefore, interactions could occur following concomitant administration of narcotics).
No products indexed under this heading.

Rescinnamine (Concurrent use with antihypertensive drugs may potentiate the hypotension seen with aldesleukin).
No products indexed under this heading.

Reserpine (Concurrent use with antihypertensive drugs may potentiate the hypotension seen with aldesleukin).
No products indexed under this heading.

Rifampin (Concurrent administration of drugs possessing nephrotoxic effects with aldesleukin may increase the potential for nephrotoxicity).
No products indexed under this heading.

Riluzole (Concurrent administration of drugs possessing nephrotoxic effects with aldesleukin may increase the potential for nephrotoxicity). Products include:
Rilutek Tablets 2771

Risperidone (Aldesleukin may affect central nervous function. Therefore, interactions could occur following concomitant administration of psychotropic drugs). Products include:
Risperdal Consta Long-Acting Injection 1753

Ritonavir (Concurrent administration of drugs possessing nephrotoxic effects with aldesleukin may increase the potential for nephrotoxicity). Products include:
Kaletra 452
Norvir 489

Rofecoxib (Concurrent administration of drugs possessing nephrotoxic effects with aldesleukin may increase the potential for nephrotoxicity).
No products indexed under this heading.

Saquinavir (Concurrent administration of drugs possessing nephrotoxic effects with aldesleukin may increase the potential for nephrotoxicity).
No products indexed under this heading.

Secobarbital Sodium (Aldesleukin may affect central nervous function. Therefore, interactions could occur following concomitant administration of psychotropic drugs).
No products indexed under this heading.

Sibutramine Hydrochloride Monohydrate (Concurrent administration of drugs possessing nephrotoxic effects with aldesleukin may increase the potential for nephrotoxicity). Products include:
Meridia Capsules 475

Simvastatin (Concurrent administration of drugs possessing nephrotoxic effects with aldesleukin may increase the potential for nephrotoxicity). Products include:
Simcor Tablets 502
Vytorin 10/10 Tablets 2149
Vytorin 10/10 Tablets 2939
Vytorin 10/20 Tablets 2149
Vytorin 10/20 Tablets 2939
Vytorin 10/40 Tablets 2149
Vytorin 10/40 Tablets 2939
Vytorin 10/80 Tablets 2149
Vytorin 10/80 Tablets 2939
Zocor Tablets 2136

Sodium Butabarbital (Aldesleukin may affect central nervous function. Therefore, interactions could occur following concomitant administration of psychotropic drugs).
No products indexed under this heading.

Sodium Nitroprusside (Concurrent use with antihypertensive drugs may potentiate the hypotension seen with aldesleukin).
No products indexed under this heading.

Sotalol Hydrochloride (Beta-blockers may potentiate the hypotension seen with aldesleukin).
No products indexed under this heading.

Spirapril Hydrochloride (Concurrent administration of drugs possessing nephrotoxic effects with aldesleukin may increase the potential for nephrotoxicity).
No products indexed under this heading.

Stavudine (Concurrent administration of drugs possessing nephrotoxic effects with aldesleukin may increase the potential for nephrotoxicity).
No products indexed under this heading.

Streptomycin Sulfate (Concurrent administration of drugs possessing nephrotoxic effects with aldesleukin may increase the potential for nephrotoxicity).
No products indexed under this heading.

Streptozocin (Concurrent administration of drugs possessing nephrotoxic effects with aldesleukin may increase the potential for nephrotoxicity).
No products indexed under this heading.

Sufentanil Citrate (Aldesleukin may affect central nervous function. Therefore, interactions could occur following concomitant administration of narcotics).
No products indexed under this heading.

Sulfacytine (Concurrent administration of drugs possessing nephrotoxic effects with aldesleukin may increase the potential for nephrotoxicity).
No products indexed under this heading.

Sulfamethizole (Concurrent administration of drugs possessing nephrotoxic effects with aldesleukin may increase the potential for nephrotoxicity).
No products indexed under this heading.

Sulfamethoxazole (Concurrent administration of drugs possessing nephrotoxic effects with aldesleukin may increase the potential for nephrotoxicity).
No products indexed under this heading.

Sulfasalazine (Concurrent administration of drugs possessing nephrotoxic effects with aldesleukin may increase the potential for nephrotoxicity).
No products indexed under this heading.

Sulfinpyrazone (Concurrent administration of drugs possessing nephrotoxic effects with aldesleukin may increase the potential for nephrotoxicity).
No products indexed under this heading.

Sulfisoxazole Acetyl (Concurrent administration of drugs possessing nephrotoxic effects with aldesleukin may increase the potential for nephrotoxicity).
No products indexed under this heading.

Sulfisoxazole Diolamine (Concurrent administration of drugs possessing nephrotoxic effects with aldesleukin may increase the potential for nephrotoxicity).
No products indexed under this heading.

Sulindac (Concurrent administration of drugs possessing nephrotoxic effects with aldesleukin may increase the potential for nephrotoxicity). Products include:
Clinoril Tablets 1962

Tacrolimus (Concurrent administration of drugs possessing nephrotoxic effects with aldesleukin may increase the potential for nephrotoxicity). Products include:
Prograf Capsules and Injection 622
Protopic Ointment 628

Tamoxifen Citrate (Hypersensitivity reactions have been reported in patients receiving combination regimens containing sequential high dose aldesleukin and antineoplastic agents, specifically tamoxifen. These reactions consisted of erythema, pruritus, and hypotension and occurred within hours of administration of chemotherapy. These events required medical intervention in some patients).
No products indexed under this heading.

Telmisartan (Concurrent use with antihypertensive drugs may potentiate the hypotension seen with aldesleukin). Products include:
Micardis Tablets 852
Micardis HCT Tablets 854

Temazepam (Aldesleukin may affect central nervous function. Therefore, interactions could occur following concomitant administration of psychotropic drugs).
No products indexed under this heading.

Temozolomide (Concurrent administration of drugs possessing myelotoxic effects with aldesleukin may increase the potential for myelotoxicity). Products include:
Temodar Capsules 2931

Teniposide (Hypersensitivity reactions have been reported in patients receiving combination regimens containing sequential high dose aldesleukin and antineoplastic agents. These reactions consisted of erythema, pruritus, and hypotension and occurred within hours of administration of chemotherapy. These events required medical intervention in some patients).
No products indexed under this heading.

Tenofovir Disoproxil Fumarate (Concurrent administration of drugs possessing nephrotoxic effects with aldesleukin may increase the potential for nephrotoxicity). Products include:
Atripla Tablets 938
Truvada Tablets 1262
Viread Tablets 1268

Terazosin Hydrochloride (Concurrent use with antihypertensive drugs may potentiate the hypotension seen with aldesleukin).
No products indexed under this heading.

Thioguanine (Concurrent administration of drugs possessing nephrotoxic effects with aldesleukin may increase the potential for nephrotoxicity). Products include:
Tabloid Tablets 1601

Thioridazine Hydrochloride (Aldesleukin may affect central nervous function. Therefore, interactions could occur following concomitant administration of psychotropic drugs). Products include:
Thioridazine Hydrochloride Tablets 2195

Thiotepa (Hypersensitivity reactions have been reported in patients receiving combination regimens containing sequential high dose aldesleukin and antineoplastic agents. These reactions consisted of erythema, pruritus, and hypotension and occurred within hours of administration of chemotherapy. These events required medical intervention in some patients).
No products indexed under this heading.

Thiothixene (Aldesleukin may affect central nervous function. Therefore, interactions could occur following concomitant administration of psychotropic drugs). Products include:
Thiothixene Capsules 2197

Ticarcillin Disodium (Concurrent administration of drugs possessing nephrotoxic effects with aldesleukin may increase the potential for nephrotoxicity). Products include:
Timentin ADD-Vantage 1606
Timentin Injection Galaxy Container 1609
Timentin IV Infusion 1603
Timentin Pharmacy Bulk Package 1613

Timolol Hemihydrate (Beta-blockers may potentiate the hypotension seen with aldesleukin). Products include:
- Betimol Ophthalmic Solution 3181

Timolol Maleate (Beta-blockers may potentiate the hypotension seen with aldesleukin). Products include:
- Combigan Ophthalmic Solution 553
- Cosopt Sterile Ophthalmic Solution 1969
- Timoptic Sterile Ophthalmic Solution 2121
- Timoptic in Ocudose 2124
- Timoptic-XE Sterile Ophthalmic Gel Forming Solution 2125

Tobramycin (Concurrent administration of drugs possessing nephrotoxic effects with aldesleukin may increase the potential for nephrotoxicity). Products include:
- Zylet Ophthalmic Suspension .... ⊙247

Tobramycin Sulfate (Concurrent administration of drugs possessing nephrotoxic effects with aldesleukin may increase the potential for nephrotoxicity).
No products indexed under this heading.

Tolazamide (Concurrent administration of drugs possessing nephrotoxic effects with aldesleukin may increase the potential for nephrotoxicity).
No products indexed under this heading.

Tolbutamide (Concurrent administration of drugs possessing nephrotoxic effects with aldesleukin may increase the potential for nephrotoxicity).
No products indexed under this heading.

Tolmetin Sodium (Concurrent administration of drugs possessing nephrotoxic effects with aldesleukin may increase the potential for nephrotoxicity).
No products indexed under this heading.

Topotecan Hydrochloride (Hypersensitivity reactions have been reported in patients receiving combination regimens containing sequential high dose aldesleukin and antineoplastic agents. These reactions consisted of erythema, pruritus, and hypotension and occurred within hours of administration of chemotherapy. These events required medical intervention in some patients). Products include:
- Hycamtin for Injection 1459
- Hycamtin Capsules 1456

Toremifene Citrate (Hypersensitivity reactions have been reported in patients receiving combination regimens containing sequential high dose aldesleukin and antineoplastic agents. These reactions consisted of erythema, pruritus, and hypotension and occurred within hours of administration of chemotherapy. These events required medical intervention in some patients).
No products indexed under this heading.

Torsemide (Concurrent use with antihypertensive drugs may potentiate the hypotension seen with aldesleukin). Products include:
- Demadex Injection 2630
- Demadex Tablets 2630

Trandolapril (Concurrent administration of drugs possessing nephrotoxic effects with aldesleukin may increase the potential for nephrotoxicity). Products include:
- Mavik Tablets 472
- Tarka Tablets 511

Tranylcypromine Sulfate (Aldesleukin may affect central nervous function. Therefore, interactions could occur following concomitant administration of psychotropic drugs). Products include:
- Parnate Tablets 1532

Triamcinolone (Although glucocorticoids have been shown to reduce aldesleukin-induced side effects including fever, renal insufficiency, hyperbilirubinemia, confusion, and dyspnea, concomitant administration of these agents with aldesleukin may reduce the antitumor effectiveness of aldesleukin and thus should be avoided).
No products indexed under this heading.

Triamcinolone Acetonide (Although glucocorticoids have been shown to reduce aldesleukin-induced side effects including fever, renal insufficiency, hyperbilirubinemia, confusion, and dyspnea, concomitant administration of these agents with aldesleukin may reduce the antitumor effectiveness of aldesleukin and thus should be avoided). Products include:
- Azmacort Inhalation Aerosol 407
- Nasacort AQ Nasal Spray 2765
- Triesence Injectable Suspension .... ⊙209

Triamcinolone Diacetate (Although glucocorticoids have been shown to reduce aldesleukin-induced side effects including fever, renal insufficiency, hyperbilirubinemia, confusion, and dyspnea, concomitant administration of these agents with aldesleukin may reduce the antitumor effectiveness of aldesleukin and thus should be avoided).
No products indexed under this heading.

Triamcinolone Hexacetonide (Although glucocorticoids have been shown to reduce aldesleukin-induced side effects including fever, renal insufficiency, hyperbilirubinemia, confusion, and dyspnea, concomitant administration of these agents with aldesleukin may reduce the antitumor effectiveness of aldesleukin and thus should be avoided).
No products indexed under this heading.

Triamterene (Concurrent administration of drugs possessing nephrotoxic effects with aldesleukin may increase the potential for nephrotoxicity). Products include:
- Dyazide Capsules 1405
- Dyrenium Capsules 3189

Triazolam (Aldesleukin may affect central nervous function. Therefore, interactions could occur following concomitant administration of psychotropic drugs).
No products indexed under this heading.

Trifluoperazine Hydrochloride (Aldesleukin may affect central nervous function. Therefore, interactions could occur following concomitant administration of psychotropic drugs).
No products indexed under this heading.

Trimethadione (Concurrent administration of drugs possessing nephrotoxic effects with aldesleukin may increase the potential for nephrotoxicity).
No products indexed under this heading.

Trimethaphan Camsylate (Concurrent use with antihypertensive drugs may potentiate the hypotension seen with aldesleukin).
No products indexed under this heading.

Trimipramine Maleate (Aldesleukin may affect central nervous function. Therefore, interactions could occur following concomitant administration of psychotropic drugs).
No products indexed under this heading.

Trovafloxacin Mesylate (Concurrent administration of drugs possessing nephrotoxic effects with aldesleukin may increase the potential for nephrotoxicity).
No products indexed under this heading.

Tyropanoate Sodium (Concurrent administration of drugs possessing nephrotoxic effects with aldesleukin may increase the potential for nephrotoxicity).
No products indexed under this heading.

Valacyclovir Hydrochloride (Concurrent administration of drugs possessing nephrotoxic effects with aldesleukin may increase the potential for nephrotoxicity). Products include:
- Valtrex Caplets 1635

Valdecoxib (Concurrent administration of drugs possessing nephrotoxic effects with aldesleukin may increase the potential for nephrotoxicity).
No products indexed under this heading.

Valrubicin (Hypersensitivity reactions have been reported in patients receiving combination regimens containing sequential high dose aldesleukin and antineoplastic agents. These reactions consisted of erythema, pruritus, and hypotension and occurred within hours of administration of chemotherapy. These events required medical intervention in some patients). Products include:
- Valstar Sterile Solution for Intravesical Instillation 1735

Valsartan (Concurrent use with antihypertensive drugs may potentiate the hypotension seen with aldesleukin). Products include:
- Diovan Tablets 2212
- Diovan HCT Tablets 2216
- Exforge Tablets 2238

Vancomycin Hydrochloride (Concurrent administration of drugs possessing nephrotoxic effects with aldesleukin may increase the potential for nephrotoxicity).
No products indexed under this heading.

Verapamil Hydrochloride (Concurrent use with antihypertensive drugs may potentiate the hypotension seen with aldesleukin). Products include:
- Tarka Tablets 511

Vincristine Sulfate (Concurrent administration of drugs possessing myelotoxic effects with aldesleukin may increase the potential for myelotoxicity).
No products indexed under this heading.

Vinorelbine Tartrate (Concurrent administration of drugs possessing myelotoxic effects with aldesleukin may increase the potential for myelotoxicity).
No products indexed under this heading.

Voriconazole (Concurrent administration of drugs possessing nephrotoxic effects with aldesleukin may increase the potential for nephrotoxicity).
No products indexed under this heading.

Zalcitabine (Concurrent administration of drugs possessing nephrotoxic effects with aldesleukin may increase the potential for nephrotoxicity).
No products indexed under this heading.

Zaleplon (Aldesleukin may affect central nervous function. Therefore, interactions could occur following concomitant administration of psychotropic drugs).
No products indexed under this heading.

Zidovudine (Concurrent administration of drugs possessing nephrotoxic effects with aldesleukin may increase the potential for nephrotoxicity). Products include:
- Combivir Tablets 1384
- Retrovir 1574
- Retrovir IV Infusion 1579
- Trizivir Tablets 1622

Ziprasidone Hydrochloride (Aldesleukin may affect central nervous function. Therefore, interactions could occur following concomitant administration of psychotropic drugs). Products include:
- Geodon Capsules 2520

Zoledronic acid (Concurrent administration of drugs possessing nephrotoxic effects with aldesleukin may increase the potential for nephrotoxicity). Products include:
- Reclast Injection 2291
- Zometa for Intravenous Infusion 2341

Zolpidem Tartrate (Aldesleukin may affect central nervous function. Therefore, interactions could occur following concomitant administration of psychotropic drugs). Products include:
- Ambien Tablets 2692
- Ambien CR Tablets 2696

PROMETRIUM CAPSULES (100 MG, 200 MG)

(Progesterone) 3047
May interact with:

Estrogens, Conjugated (Coadministration has resulted in an increase in total estrone and equilin concentrations and decrease in circulating 17β estradiol concentrations). Products include:
- Premarin Intravenous 3217
- Premarin Tablets 3221
- Premarin Vaginal Cream 3228
- Premphase Tablets 3232
- Prempro Tablets 3232

Ketoconazole (The metabolism of progesterone by human liver microsomes is inhibited by ketoconazole, a known inhibitor of CYP4503A4; the clinical relevance of the in vitro findings is unknown). Products include:
- Extina Foam, 2% 3057
- Nizoral A-D Shampoo 1901

Food Interactions

Food, unspecified (Concomitant food ingestion increases the bioavailability of Prometrium Capsules relative to the fasting state).

PRONUTRA PROTEIN SUPPLEMENT

(Vitamins with Minerals, Whey Protein Isolate) 1730
None cited in PDR database.

PROPECIA TABLETS

(Finasteride) 2095
None cited in PDR database.

PROQUAD

(Measles, Mumps, Rubella and Varicella Virus Vaccine Live) 2099
May interact with corticosteroids, immunosuppressive agents, salicylates, and certain other agents. Compounds in these categories include:

Aspirin (Reye's syndrome has been reported following the use of salicylates during wild-type varicella infection. Vaccine recipients should avoid use of salicylates for 6 weeks after vaccination with Measles, Mumps, Rubella, and Varicella Virus Vaccine, Live). Products include:
Aggrenox Capsules 819
Bayer Aspirin 750
Percodan Tablets 1130
St. Joseph 81 mg Aspirin Chewable and Enteric Coated Tablets 1903

Aspirin, Enteric Coated (Reye's syndrome has been reported following the use of salicylates during wild-type varicella infection. Vaccine recipients should avoid use of salicylates for 6 weeks after vaccination with Measles, Mumps, Rubella, and Varicella Virus Vaccine, Live).
No products indexed under this heading.

Aspirin Buffered (Reye's syndrome has been reported following the use of salicylates during wild-type varicella infection. Vaccine recipients should avoid use of salicylates for 6 weeks after vaccination with Measles, Mumps, Rubella, and Varicella Virus Vaccine, Live).
No products indexed under this heading.

Azathioprine (Measles, Mumps, Rubella, and Varicella Virus Vaccine, Live may be used in individuals who are receiving topical corticosteroids or low-dose corticosteroids for asthma prophylaxis or replacement therapy, (e.g., for Addison's disease). Measles, Mumps, Rubella, and Varicella Virus Vaccine, Live should not be given to individuals receiving immunosuppressive doses of corticosteroids or other immunosuppressive drugs).
No products indexed under this heading.

Basiliximab (Measles, Mumps, Rubella, and Varicella Virus Vaccine, Live may be used in individuals who are receiving topical corticosteroids or low-dose corticosteroids for asthma prophylaxis or replacement therapy, (e.g., for Addison's disease). Measles, Mumps, Rubella, and Varicella Virus Vaccine, Live should not be given to individuals receiving immunosuppressive doses of corticosteroids or other immunosuppressive drugs). Products include:
Simulect for Injection 2306

Betamethasone Acetate (Measles, Mumps, Rubella, and Varicella Virus Vaccine, Live may be used in individuals who are receiving topical corticosteroids or low-dose corticosteroids for asthma prophylaxis or replacement therapy, (e.g., for Addison's disease). Measles, Mumps, Rubella, and Varicella Virus Vaccine, Live should not be given to individuals receiving immunosuppressive doses of corticosteroids or other immunosuppressive drugs).
No products indexed under this heading.

Betamethasone Sodium Phosphate (Measles, Mumps, Rubella, and Varicella Virus Vaccine, Live may be used in individuals who are receiving topical corticosteroids or low-dose corticosteroids for asthma prophylaxis or replacement therapy, (e.g., for Addison's disease). Measles, Mumps, Rubella, and Varicella Virus Vaccine, Live should not be given to individuals receiving immunosuppressive doses of corticosteroids or other immunosuppressive drugs).
No products indexed under this heading.

Budesonide (Measles, Mumps, Rubella, and Varicella Virus Vaccine, Live may be used in individuals who are receiving topical corticosteroids or low-dose corticosteroids for asthma prophylaxis or replacement therapy, (e.g., for Addison's disease). Measles, Mumps, Rubella, and Varicella Virus Vaccine, Live should not be given to individuals receiving immunosuppressive doses of corticosteroids or other immunosuppressive drugs). Products include:
Pulmicort Flexhaler 654
Symbicort 80/4.5 Inhalation Aerosol 659
Symbicort 160/4.5 Inhalation Aerosol 659

Choline Magnesium Trisalicylate (Reye's syndrome has been reported following the use of salicylates during wild-type varicella infection. Vaccine recipients should avoid use of salicylates for 6 weeks after vaccination with Measles, Mumps, Rubella, and Varicella Virus Vaccine, Live).
No products indexed under this heading.

Ciclesonide (Measles, Mumps, Rubella, and Varicella Virus Vaccine, Live may be used in individuals who are receiving topical corticosteroids or low-dose corticosteroids for asthma prophylaxis or replacement therapy, (e.g., for Addison's disease). Measles, Mumps, Rubella, and Varicella Virus Vaccine, Live should not be given to individuals receiving immunosuppressive doses of corticosteroids or other immunosuppressive drugs). Products include:
Alvesco Inhalation Aerosol 2985
Omnaris Nasal Spray 2998

Cortisone Acetate (Measles, Mumps, Rubella, and Varicella Virus Vaccine, Live may be used in individuals who are receiving topical corticosteroids or low-dose corticosteroids for asthma prophylaxis or replacement therapy, (e.g., for Addison's disease). Measles, Mumps, Rubella, and Varicella Virus Vaccine, Live should not be given to individuals receiving immunosuppressive doses of corticosteroids or other immunosuppressive drugs).
No products indexed under this heading.

Cyclosporine (Measles, Mumps, Rubella, and Varicella Virus Vaccine, Live may be used in individuals who are receiving topical corticosteroids or low-dose corticosteroids for asthma prophylaxis or replacement therapy, (e.g., for Addison's disease). Measles, Mumps, Rubella, and Varicella Virus Vaccine, Live should not be given to individuals receiving immunosuppressive doses of corticosteroids or other immunosuppressive drugs). Products include:
Gengraf Capsules 435
Neoral Oral Solution 2280
Neoral Soft Gelatin Capsules 2280
Restasis Ophthalmic Emulsion 557
Sandimmune 2296

Dexamethasone (Measles, Mumps, Rubella, and Varicella Virus Vaccine, Live may be used in individuals who are receiving topical corticosteroids or low-dose corticosteroids for asthma prophylaxis or replacement therapy, (e.g., for Addison's disease). Measles, Mumps, Rubella, and Varicella Virus Vaccine, Live should not be given to individuals receiving immunosuppressive doses of corticosteroids or other immunosuppressive drugs).
Products include:
Ciprodex Otic Suspension 541

Dexamethasone Acetate (Measles, Mumps, Rubella, and Varicella Virus Vaccine, Live may be used in individuals who are receiving topical corticosteroids or low-dose corticosteroids for asthma prophylaxis or replacement therapy, (e.g., for Addison's disease). Measles, Mumps, Rubella, and Varicella Virus Vaccine, Live should not be given to individuals receiving immunosuppressive doses of corticosteroids or other immunosuppressive drugs).
No products indexed under this heading.

Dexamethasone Sodium Phosphate (Measles, Mumps, Rubella, and Varicella Virus Vaccine, Live may be used in individuals who are receiving topical corticosteroids or low-dose corticosteroids for asthma prophylaxis or replacement therapy, (e.g., for Addison's disease). Measles, Mumps, Rubella, and Varicella Virus Vaccine, Live should not be given to individuals receiving immunosuppressive doses of corticosteroids or other immunosuppressive drugs).
No products indexed under this heading.

Diflunisal (Reye's syndrome has been reported following the use of salicylates during wild-type varicella infection. Vaccine recipients should avoid use of salicylates for 6 weeks after vaccination with Measles, Mumps, Rubella, and Varicella Virus Vaccine, Live).
No products indexed under this heading.

Fludrocortisone Acetate (Measles, Mumps, Rubella, and Varicella Virus Vaccine, Live may be used in individuals who are receiving topical corticosteroids or low-dose corticosteroids for asthma prophylaxis or replacement therapy, (e.g., for Addison's disease). Measles, Mumps, Rubella, and Varicella Virus Vaccine, Live should not be given to individuals receiving immunosuppressive doses of corticosteroids or other immunosuppressive drugs).
No products indexed under this heading.

Flunisolide (Measles, Mumps, Rubella, and Varicella Virus Vaccine, Live may be used in individuals who are receiving topical corticosteroids or low-dose corticosteroids for asthma prophylaxis or replacement therapy, (e.g., for Addison's disease). Measles, Mumps, Rubella, and Varicella Virus Vaccine, Live should not be given to individuals receiving immunosuppressive doses of corticosteroids or other immunosuppressive drugs). Products include:
Aerobid/Aerobid-M 1153

Fluticasone Propionate (Measles, Mumps, Rubella, and Varicella Virus Vaccine, Live may be used in individuals who are receiving topical corticosteroids or low-dose corticosteroids for asthma prophylaxis or replacement therapy, (e.g., for Addison's disease). Measles, Mumps, Rubella, and Varicella Virus Vaccine, Live should not be given to individuals receiving immunosuppressive doses of corticosteroids or other immunosuppressive drugs).
Products include:
Advair Diskus 100/50 1276
Advair Diskus 250/50 1276
Advair Diskus 500/50 1276
Advair HFA 45/21 Inhalation Aerosol 1288
Advair HFA 115/21 Inhalation Aerosol 1288
Advair HFA 230/21 Inhalation Aerosol 1288
Flonase Nasal Spray 1431
Flovent Diskus 50 mcg 1435

Fluticasone Propionate HFA (Measles, Mumps, Rubella, and Varicella Virus Vaccine, Live may be used in individuals who are receiving topical corticosteroids or low-dose corticosteroids for asthma prophylaxis or replacement therapy, (e.g., for Addison's disease). Measles, Mumps, Rubella, and Varicella Virus Vaccine, Live should not be given to individuals receiving immunosuppressive doses of corticosteroids or other immunosuppressive drugs).
Products include:
Flovent HFA 1440

Globulin, Immune (Human) (Immune globulins administered concomitantly with Measles, Mumps, Rubella, and Varicella Virus Vaccine, Live may interfere with the expected immune response. Vaccination should be deferred for at least 3 months following blood plasma transfusions, or administration of immune globulins (IG)). Products include:
Flebogamma 5% 1715

Hydrocortisone (Measles, Mumps, Rubella, and Varicella Virus Vaccine, Live may be used in individuals who are receiving topical corticosteroids or low-dose corticosteroids for asthma prophylaxis or replacement therapy, (e.g., for Addison's disease). Measles, Mumps, Rubella, and Varicella Virus Vaccine, Live should not be given to individuals receiving immunosuppressive doses of corticosteroids or other immunosuppressive drugs).
No products indexed under this heading.

Hydrocortisone Acetate (Measles, Mumps, Rubella, and Varicella Virus Vaccine, Live may be used in

individuals who are receiving topical corticosteroids or low-dose corticosteroids for asthma prophylaxis or replacement therapy, (e.g., for Addison's disease). Measles, Mumps, Rubella, and Varicella Virus Vaccine, Live should not be given to individuals receiving immunosuppressive doses of corticosteroids or other immunosuppressive drugs).
Products include:
Analpram-HC 1140
Pramosone 1141

Hydrocortisone Sodium Phosphate (Measles, Mumps, Rubella, and Varicella Virus Vaccine, Live may be used in individuals who are receiving topical corticosteroids or low-dose corticosteroids for asthma prophylaxis or replacement therapy, (e.g., for Addison's disease). Measles, Mumps, Rubella, and Varicella Virus Vaccine, Live should not be given to individuals receiving immunosuppressive doses of corticosteroids or other immunosuppressive drugs).
No products indexed under this heading.

Hydrocortisone Sodium Succinate (Measles, Mumps, Rubella, and Varicella Virus Vaccine, Live may be used in individuals who are receiving topical corticosteroids or low-dose corticosteroids for asthma prophylaxis or replacement therapy, (e.g., for Addison's disease). Measles, Mumps, Rubella, and Varicella Virus Vaccine, Live should not be given to individuals receiving immunosuppressive doses of corticosteroids or other immunosuppressive drugs).
No products indexed under this heading.

Magnesium Salicylate (Reye's syndrome has been reported following the use of salicylates during wild-type varicella infection. Vaccine recipients should avoid use of salicylates for 6 weeks after vaccination with Measles, Mumps, Rubella, and Varicella Virus Vaccine, Live).
No products indexed under this heading.

Methylprednisolone Acetate (Measles, Mumps, Rubella, and Varicella Virus Vaccine, Live may be used in individuals who are receiving topical corticosteroids or low-dose corticosteroids for asthma prophylaxis or replacement therapy, (e.g., for Addison's disease). Measles, Mumps, Rubella, and Varicella Virus Vaccine, Live should not be given to individuals receiving immunosuppressive doses of corticosteroids or other immunosuppressive drugs).
No products indexed under this heading.

Methylprednisolone Sodium Succinate (Measles, Mumps, Rubella, and Varicella Virus Vaccine, Live may be used in individuals who are receiving topical corticosteroids or low-dose corticosteroids for asthma prophylaxis or replacement therapy, (e.g., for Addison's disease). Measles, Mumps, Rubella, and Varicella Virus Vaccine, Live should not be given to individuals receiving immunosuppressive doses of corticosteroids or other immunosuppressive drugs).
No products indexed under this heading.

Mometasone Furoate (Measles, Mumps, Rubella, and Varicella Virus Vaccine, Live may be used in individuals who are receiving topical corticosteroids or low-dose corticosteroids for asthma prophylaxis or replacement therapy, (e.g., for Addison's disease). Measles, Mumps, Rubella, and Varicella Virus Vaccine, Live should not be given to individuals receiving immunosuppressive doses of corticosteroids or other immunosuppressive drugs).
Products include:
Asmanex Twisthaler 2797
Elocon Cream 0.1% 2840
Elocon Lotion 0.1% 2841
Elocon Ointment 0.1% 2842

Mometasone Furoate Monohydrate (Measles, Mumps, Rubella, and Varicella Virus Vaccine, Live may be used in individuals who are receiving topical corticosteroids or low-dose corticosteroids for asthma prophylaxis or replacement therapy, (e.g., for Addison's disease). Measles, Mumps, Rubella, and Varicella Virus Vaccine, Live should not be given to individuals receiving immunosuppressive doses of corticosteroids or other immunosuppressive drugs). Products include:
Nasonex Nasal Spray 2883

Muromonab-CD3 (Measles, Mumps, Rubella, and Varicella Virus Vaccine, Live may be used in individuals who are receiving topical corticosteroids or low-dose corticosteroids for asthma prophylaxis or replacement therapy, (e.g., for Addison's disease). Measles, Mumps, Rubella, and Varicella Virus Vaccine, Live should not be given to individuals receiving immunosuppressive doses of corticosteroids or other immunosuppressive drugs).
Products include:
Orthoclone OKT3 Sterile Solution 2387

Mycophenolate Mofetil (Measles, Mumps, Rubella, and Varicella Virus Vaccine, Live may be used in individuals who are receiving topical corticosteroids or low-dose corticosteroids for asthma prophylaxis or replacement therapy, (e.g., for Addison's disease). Measles, Mumps, Rubella, and Varicella Virus Vaccine, Live should not be given to individuals receiving immunosuppressive doses of corticosteroids or other immunosuppressive drugs).
Products include:
CellCept Capsules 2622
CellCept Oral Suspension 2622
CellCept Tablets 2622

Prednisolone Acetate (Measles, Mumps, Rubella, and Varicella Virus Vaccine, Live may be used in individuals who are receiving topical corticosteroids or low-dose corticosteroids for asthma prophylaxis or replacement therapy, (e.g., for Addison's disease). Measles, Mumps, Rubella, and Varicella Virus Vaccine, Live should not be given to individuals receiving immunosuppressive doses of corticosteroids or other immunosuppressive drugs).
Products include:
Pred Forte Ophthalmic Suspension .... ⊙227
Pred Mild Ophthalmic Suspension .... ⊙230
Pred-G Ophthalmic Ointment .... ⊙229
Pred-G Ophthalmic Suspension .... ⊙228

Prednisolone Sodium Phosphate (Measles, Mumps, Rubella, and Varicella Virus Vaccine, Live may be used in individuals who are receiving topical corticosteroids or low-dose corticosteroids for asthma prophylaxis or replacement therapy, (e.g., for Addison's disease). Measles, Mumps, Rubella, and Varicella Virus Vaccine, Live should not be given to individuals receiving immunosuppressive doses of corticosteroids or other immunosuppressive drugs).
No products indexed under this heading.

Prednisolone Tebutate (Measles, Mumps, Rubella, and Varicella Virus Vaccine, Live may be used in individuals who are receiving topical corticosteroids or low-dose corticosteroids for asthma prophylaxis or replacement therapy, (e.g., for Addison's disease). Measles, Mumps, Rubella, and Varicella Virus Vaccine, Live should not be given to individuals receiving immunosuppressive doses of corticosteroids or other immunosuppressive drugs).
No products indexed under this heading.

Prednisone (Measles, Mumps, Rubella, and Varicella Virus Vaccine, Live may be used in individuals who are receiving topical corticosteroids or low-dose corticosteroids for asthma prophylaxis or replacement therapy, (e.g., for Addison's disease). Measles, Mumps, Rubella, and Varicella Virus Vaccine, Live should not be given to individuals receiving immunosuppressive doses of corticosteroids or other immunosuppressive drugs).
No products indexed under this heading.

Salsalate (Reye's syndrome has been reported following the use of salicylates during wild-type varicella infection. Vaccine recipients should avoid use of salicylates for 6 weeks after vaccination with Measles, Mumps, Rubella, and Varicella Virus Vaccine, Live).
No products indexed under this heading.

Sirolimus (Measles, Mumps, Rubella, and Varicella Virus Vaccine, Live may be used in individuals who are receiving topical corticosteroids or low-dose corticosteroids for asthma prophylaxis or replacement therapy, (e.g., for Addison's disease). Measles, Mumps, Rubella, and Varicella Virus Vaccine, Live should not be given to individuals receiving immunosuppressive doses of corticosteroids or other immunosuppressive drugs). Products include:
Rapamune 3260

Tacrolimus (Measles, Mumps, Rubella, and Varicella Virus Vaccine, Live may be used in individuals who are receiving topical corticosteroids or low-dose corticosteroids for asthma prophylaxis or replacement therapy, (e.g., for Addison's disease). Measles, Mumps, Rubella, and Varicella Virus Vaccine, Live should not be given to individuals receiving immunosuppressive doses of corticosteroids or other immunosuppressive drugs). Products include:
Prograf Capsules and Injection 622
Protopic Ointment 628

Triamcinolone (Measles, Mumps, Rubella, and Varicella Virus Vaccine, Live may be used in individuals who are receiving topical corticosteroids or low-dose corticosteroids for asthma prophylaxis or replacement therapy, (e.g., for Addison's disease). Measles, Mumps, Rubella, and Varicella Virus Vaccine, Live should not be given to individuals receiving immunosuppressive doses of corticosteroids or other immunosuppressive drugs).
No products indexed under this heading.

Triamcinolone Acetonide (Measles, Mumps, Rubella, and Varicella Virus Vaccine, Live may be used in individuals who are receiving topical corticosteroids or low-dose corticosteroids for asthma prophylaxis or replacement therapy, (e.g., for Addison's disease). Measles, Mumps, Rubella, and Varicella Virus Vaccine, Live should not be given to individuals receiving immunosuppressive doses of corticosteroids or other immunosuppressive drugs).
Products include:
Azmacort Inhalation Aerosol 407
Nasacort AQ Nasal Spray 2765
Triesence Injectable Suspension .... ⊙209

Triamcinolone Diacetate (Measles, Mumps, Rubella, and Varicella Virus Vaccine, Live may be used in individuals who are receiving topical corticosteroids or low-dose corticosteroids for asthma prophylaxis or replacement therapy, (e.g., for Addison's disease). Measles, Mumps, Rubella, and Varicella Virus Vaccine, Live should not be given to individuals receiving immunosuppressive doses of corticosteroids or other immunosuppressive drugs).
No products indexed under this heading.

Triamcinolone Hexacetonide (Measles, Mumps, Rubella, and Varicella Virus Vaccine, Live may be used in individuals who are receiving topical corticosteroids or low-dose corticosteroids for asthma prophylaxis or replacement therapy, (e.g., for Addison's disease). Measles, Mumps, Rubella, and Varicella Virus Vaccine, Live should not be given to individuals receiving immunosuppressive doses of corticosteroids or other immunosuppressive drugs).
No products indexed under this heading.

PROSCAR TABLETS

(Finasteride) 2102
None cited in PDR database.

PROSTATE OLYMPUS DIETARY SUPPLEMENT

(Herbals, Multiple) 628
None cited in PDR database.

PROTECTOR CAPSULES

(Amino Acid Preparations, Astragalus, Bee Pollen, Cellulose, Herbals, Multiple, Hydroxypropyl Methylcellulose, Magnesium, Silicon Dioxide, Soy-containing dietary supplements, Stearic Acid).... 639
None cited in PDR database.

PROTONIX FOR DELAYED-RELEASE ORAL SUSPENSION

(Pantoprazole Sodium) 3254
See Protonix Delayed-Release Tablets

PROTONIX DELAYED-RELEASE TABLETS
(Pantoprazole Sodium) **3254**
May interact with iron containing oral preparations and certain other agents. Compounds in these categories include:

Atazanavir (Concomitant administration of pantoprazole may reduce the plasma levels of atazanavir. Concomitant use of atazanavir and proton pump inhibitors is not recommended. Concomitant use may substantially decrease atazanavir concentration and thereby reduce its therapeutic effect).
No products indexed under this heading.

Atazanavir Sulfate (Concomitant administration of pantoprazole may reduce the plasma levels of atazanavir. Appropriate clinical monitoring is recommended). Products include:
Reyataz Capsules **3299**

Bacampicillin Hydrochloride (Pantoprazole produces sustained inhibition of gastric acid secretion; pantoprazole may interfere with the absorption of certain drugs, such as ampicillin esters, where gastric pH is an important determinant of the bioavailability).
No products indexed under this heading.

Ferrous Fumarate (Pantoprazole produces sustained inhibition of gastric acid secretion; pantoprazole may interfere with the absorption of certain drugs, such as iron salts, where gastric pH is an important determinant of the bioavailability).
No products indexed under this heading.

Ferrous Gluconate (Pantoprazole produces sustained inhibition of gastric acid secretion; pantoprazole may interfere with the absorption of certain drugs, such as iron salts, where gastric pH is an important determinant of the bioavailability). Products include:
CitraNatal DHA Tablets **2175**

Ferrous Sulfate (Pantoprazole produces sustained inhibition of gastric acid secretion; pantoprazole may interfere with the absorption of certain drugs, such as iron salts, where gastric pH is an important determinant of the bioavailability).
No products indexed under this heading.

Iron (Pantoprazole produces sustained inhibition of gastric acid secretion; pantoprazole may interfere with the absorption of certain drugs, such as iron salts, where gastric pH is an important determinant of the bioavailability). Products include:
Phyto-Vite Tablets .... ▣ **639**

Ketoconazole (Pantoprazole produces sustained inhibition of gastric acid secretion; pantoprazole may interfere with the absorption of certain drugs, such as ketoconazole, where gastric pH is an important determinant of the bioavailability). Products include:
Extina Foam, 2% **3057**
Nizoral A-D Shampoo **1901**

Polysaccharide Iron Complex (Pantoprazole produces sustained inhibition of gastric acid secretion; pantoprazole may interfere with the absorption of certain drugs, such as iron salts, where gastric pH is an important determinant of the bioavailability). Products include:
Nu-Iron 150 Capsules **2165**

Warfarin Sodium (There have been reports of increased INR and prothrombin time in patients receiving proton pump inhibitors, including pantoprazole and warfarin concomitantly. Patients treated with proton pump inhibitors and warfarin concomitantly should be monitored for increases in INR and prothrombin time).
No products indexed under this heading.

PROTONIX I.V.
(Pantoprazole Sodium) **3257**
See Protonix Delayed-Release Tablets

PROTOPIC OINTMENT
(Tacrolimus) **628**
May interact with calcium channel blockers, erythromycin, and certain other agents. Compounds in these categories include:

Amlodipine Besylate (Co-administration of known CYP3A4 inhibitors, such as calcium channel blockers, in patients with widespread and/or erythrodermic disease should be done with caution; based on its minimal extent of absorption, interactions of Protopic Ointment with systemically administered drugs are unlikely to occur but cannot be ruled out). Products include:
Azor Tablets **1005**
Exforge Tablets **2238**

Bepridil Hydrochloride (Co-administration of known CYP3A4 inhibitors, such as calcium channel blockers, in patients with widespread and/or erythrodermic disease should be done with caution; based on its minimal extent of absorption, interactions of Protopic Ointment with systemically administered drugs are unlikely to occur but cannot be ruled out).
No products indexed under this heading.

Cimetidine (Co-administration of known CYP3A4 inhibitors, such as cimetidine, in patients with widespread and/or erythrodermic disease should be done with caution; based on its minimal extent of absorption, interactions of Protopic Ointment with systemically administered drugs are unlikely to occur but cannot be ruled out).
No products indexed under this heading.

Cimetidine Hydrochloride (Co-administration of known CYP3A4 inhibitors, such as cimetidine, in patients with widespread and/or erythrodermic disease should be done with caution; based on its minimal extent of absorption, interactions of Protopic Ointment with systemically administered drugs are unlikely to occur but cannot be ruled out).
No products indexed under this heading.

Diltiazem Hydrochloride (Co-administration of known CYP3A4 inhibitors, such as calcium channel blockers, in patients with widespread and/or erythrodermic disease should be done with caution; based on its minimal extent of absorption, interactions of Protopic Ointment with systemically administered drugs are unlikely to occur but cannot be ruled out). Products include:
Cardizem LA Extended Release Tablets **421**

Erythromycin (Co-administration of known CYP3A4 inhibitors, such as erythromycin, in patients with widespread and/or erythrodermic disease should be done with caution; based on its minimal extent of absorption, interactions of Protopic Ointment with systemically administered drugs are unlikely to occur but cannot be ruled out).
No products indexed under this heading.

Erythromycin Estolate (Co-administration of known CYP3A4 inhibitors, such as erythromycin, in patients with widespread and/or erythrodermic disease should be done with caution; based on its minimal extent of absorption, interactions of Protopic Ointment with systemically administered drugs are unlikely to occur but cannot be ruled out).
No products indexed under this heading.

Erythromycin Ethylsuccinate (Co-administration of known CYP3A4 inhibitors, such as erythromycin, in patients with widespread and/or erythrodermic disease should be done with caution; based on its minimal extent of absorption, interactions of Protopic Ointment with systemically administered drugs are unlikely to occur but cannot be ruled out). Products include:
E.E.S. **433**
EryPed **431**

Erythromycin Gluceptate (Co-administration of known CYP3A4 inhibitors, such as erythromycin, in patients with widespread and/or erythrodermic disease should be done with caution; based on its minimal extent of absorption, interactions of Protopic Ointment with systemically administered drugs are unlikely to occur but cannot be ruled out).
No products indexed under this heading.

Erythromycin Lactobionate (Co-administration of known CYP3A4 inhibitors, such as erythromycin, in patients with widespread and/or erythrodermic disease should be done with caution; based on its minimal extent of absorption, interactions of Protopic Ointment with systemically administered drugs are unlikely to occur but cannot be ruled out).
No products indexed under this heading.

Erythromycin Stearate (Co-administration of known CYP3A4 inhibitors, such as erythromycin, in patients with widespread and/or erythrodermic disease should be done with caution; based on its minimal extent of absorption, interactions of Protopic Ointment with systemically administered drugs are unlikely to occur but cannot be ruled out).
No products indexed under this heading.

Felodipine (Co-administration of known CYP3A4 inhibitors, such as calcium channel blockers, in patients with widespread and/or erythrodermic disease should be done with caution; based on its minimal extent of absorption, interactions of Protopic Ointment with systemically administered drugs are unlikely to occur but cannot be ruled out).
No products indexed under this heading.

Fluconazole (Co-administration of known CYP3A4 inhibitors, such as fluconazole, in patients with widespread and/or erythrodermic disease should be done with caution; based on its minimal extent of absorption, interactions of Protopic Ointment with systemically administered drugs are unlikely to occur but cannot be ruled out).
No products indexed under this heading.

Isradipine (Co-administration of known CYP3A4 inhibitors, such as calcium channel blockers, in patients with widespread and/or erythrodermic disease should be done with caution; based on its minimal extent of absorption, interactions of Protopic Ointment with systemically administered drugs are unlikely to occur but cannot be ruled out). Products include:
DynaCirc CR Controlled Release Tablets **1407**

Itraconazole (Co-administration of known CYP3A4 inhibitors, such as itraconazole, in patients with widespread and/or erythrodermic disease should be done with caution; based on its minimal extent of absorption, interactions of Protopic Ointment with systemically administered drugs are unlikely to occur but cannot be ruled out).
No products indexed under this heading.

Ketoconazole (Co-administration of known CYP3A4 inhibitors, such as ketoconazole, in patients with widespread and/or erythrodermic disease should be done with caution; based on its minimal extent of absorption, interactions of Protopic Ointment with systemically administered drugs are unlikely to occur but cannot be ruled out). Products include:
Extina Foam, 2% **3057**
Nizoral A-D Shampoo **1901**

Mibefradil Dihydrochloride (Co-administration of known CYP3A4 inhibitors, such as calcium channel blockers, in patients with widespread and/or erythrodermic disease should be done with caution; based on its minimal extent of absorption, interactions of Protopic Ointment with systemically administered drugs are unlikely to occur but cannot be ruled out).
No products indexed under this heading.

Nicardipine Hydrochloride (Co-administration of known CYP3A4 inhibitors, such as calcium channel blockers, in patients with widespread and/or erythrodermic disease should be done with caution; based on its minimal extent of absorption, interactions of Protopic Ointment with systemically administered drugs are unlikely to occur but cannot be ruled out). Products include:
Cardene I.V. **1093**

Nifedipine (Co-administration of known CYP3A4 inhibitors, such as calcium channel blockers, in patients with widespread and/or erythrodermic disease should be done with caution; based on its minimal extent of absorption, interactions of Protopic Ointment with systemically administered drugs are unlikely to occur but cannot be ruled out).
No products indexed under this heading.

Nimodipine (Co-administration of known CYP3A4 inhibitors, such as calcium channel blockers, in patients with widespread and/or erythrodermic disease should be done with caution; based on its minimal extent of absorption, interactions of Protopic Ointment with systemically administered drugs are unlikely to occur but cannot be ruled out). Products include:
Nimotop Capsules 790

Nisoldipine (Co-administration of known CYP3A4 inhibitors, such as calcium channel blockers, in patients with widespread and/or erythrodermic disease should be done with caution; based on its minimal extent of absorption, interactions of Protopic Ointment with systemically administered drugs are unlikely to occur but cannot be ruled out). Products include:
Sular Extended Release Tablets 2975

Verapamil Hydrochloride (Co-administration of known CYP3A4 inhibitors, such as calcium channel blockers, in patients with widespread and/or erythrodermic disease should be done with caution; based on its minimal extent of absorption, interactions of Protopic Ointment with systemically administered drugs are unlikely to occur but cannot be ruled out). Products include:
Tarka Tablets 511

PROVENTIL HFA INHALATION AEROSOL

(Albuterol Sulfate) 2914
May interact with beta blockers, loop diuretics, monoamine oxidase inhibitors, nonpotassium-sparing diuretics, thiazides, tricyclic antidepressants, and certain other agents. Compounds in these categories include:

Acebutolol Hydrochloride (Co-administration with beta adrenergic blocking agent blocks the pulmonary effect of beta agonists and may produce severe bronchospasm in asthmatic patients; co-administer with caution).
No products indexed under this heading.

Amitriptyline Hydrochloride (Action of albuterol on the cardiovascular system may be potentiated by tricyclic antidepressants; co-administer with caution).
No products indexed under this heading.

Amoxapine (Action of albuterol on the cardiovascular system may be potentiated by tricyclic antidepressants; co-administer with caution).
No products indexed under this heading.

Atenolol (Co-administration with beta adrenergic blocking agent blocks the pulmonary effect of beta agonists and may produce severe bronchospasm in asthmatic patients; co-administer with caution).
No products indexed under this heading.

Bendroflumethiazide (The ECG changes and hypokalemia which may result from administration of nonpotassium-sparing diuretics can be acutely worsened by beta agonists. Caution is advised in the co-administration of beta agonists with nonpotassium-sparing diuretics).
No products indexed under this heading.

Betaxolol Hydrochloride (Co-administration with beta adrenergic blocking agent blocks the pulmonary effect of beta agonists and may produce severe bronchospasm in asthmatic patients; co-administer with caution).
No products indexed under this heading.

Bisoprolol Fumarate (Co-administration with beta adrenergic blocking agent blocks the pulmonary effect of beta agonists and may produce severe bronchospasm in asthmatic patients; co-administer with caution).
No products indexed under this heading.

Bumetanide (The ECG changes and hypokalemia which may result from administration of nonpotassium-sparing diuretics can be acutely worsened by beta agonists. Caution is advised in the co-administration of beta agonists with nonpotassium-sparing diuretics).
No products indexed under this heading.

Carteolol Hydrochloride (Co-administration with beta adrenergic blocking agent blocks the pulmonary effect of beta agonists and may produce severe bronchospasm in asthmatic patients; co-administer with caution).
No products indexed under this heading.

Chlorothiazide (The ECG changes and hypokalemia which may result from administration of nonpotassium-sparing diuretics can be acutely worsened by beta agonists. Caution is advised in the co-administration of beta agonists with nonpotassium-sparing diuretics).
No products indexed under this heading.

Chlorothiazide Sodium (The ECG changes and hypokalemia which may result from administration of nonpotassium-sparing diuretics can be acutely worsened by beta agonists. Caution is advised in the co-administration of beta agonists with nonpotassium-sparing diuretics).
Products include:
Intravenous Sodium Diuril 2490

Clomipramine Hydrochloride (Action of albuterol on the cardiovascular system may be potentiated by tricyclic antidepressants; co-administer with caution).
No products indexed under this heading.

Desipramine Hydrochloride (Action of albuterol on the cardiovascular system may be potentiated by tricyclic antidepressants; co-administer with caution).
No products indexed under this heading.

Digoxin (Mean decreases in serum digoxin levels have been demonstrated with intravenous and oral albuterol). Products include:
Lanoxin Injection 1498
Lanoxin Injection Pediatric 1502
Lanoxin Tablets 1505

Doxepin Hydrochloride (Action of albuterol on the cardiovascular system may be potentiated by tricyclic antidepressants; co-administer with caution).
No products indexed under this heading.

Esmolol Hydrochloride (Co-administration with beta adrenergic blocking agent blocks the pulmonary effect of beta agonists and may produce severe bronchospasm in asthmatic patients; co-administer with caution).
No products indexed under this heading.

Ethacrynic Acid (The ECG changes and hypokalemia which may result from administration of nonpotassium-sparing diuretics can be acutely worsened by beta agonists. Caution is advised in the co-administration of beta agonists with nonpotassium-sparing diuretics).
Products include:
Edecrin Tablets 698

Furosemide (The ECG changes and hypokalemia which may result from administration of nonpotassium-sparing diuretics can be acutely worsened by beta agonists. Caution is advised in the co-administration of beta agonists with nonpotassium-sparing diuretics). Products include:
Furosemide Tablets 2186

Hydrochlorothiazide (The ECG changes and hypokalemia which may result from administration of nonpotassium-sparing diuretics can be acutely worsened by beta agonists. Caution is advised in the co-administration of beta agonists with nonpotassium-sparing diuretics).
Products include:
Atacand HCT 642
Avalide Tablets 892
Avalide Tablets 2713
Benicar HCT Tablets 1010
Diovan HCT Tablets 2216
Dyazide Capsules 1405
Micardis HCT Tablets 854
Prinzide Tablets 2092
Tekturna HCT Tablets 2324
Teveten HCT Tablets 517

Hydroflumethiazide (The ECG changes and hypokalemia which may result from administration of nonpotassium-sparing diuretics can be acutely worsened by beta agonists. Caution is advised in the co-administration of beta agonists with nonpotassium-sparing diuretics).
No products indexed under this heading.

Imipramine Hydrochloride (Action of albuterol on the cardiovascular system may be potentiated by tricyclic antidepressants; co-administer with caution).
No products indexed under this heading.

Imipramine Pamoate (Action of albuterol on the cardiovascular system may be potentiated by tricyclic antidepressants; co-administer with caution).
No products indexed under this heading.

Isocarboxazid (Action of albuterol on the cardiovascular system may be potentiated by MAO inhibitors; co-administer with caution). Products include:
Marplan Tablets 3177

Labetalol Hydrochloride (Co-administration with beta adrenergic blocking agent blocks the pulmonary effect of beta agonists and may produce severe bronchospasm in asthmatic patients; co-administer with caution).
No products indexed under this heading.

Levobunolol Hydrochloride (Co-administration with beta adrenergic blocking agent blocks the pulmonary effect of beta agonists and may produce severe bronchospasm in asthmatic patients; co-administer with caution).
No products indexed under this heading.

Maprotiline Hydrochloride (Action of albuterol on the cardiovascular system may be potentiated by tricyclic antidepressants; co-administer with caution).
No products indexed under this heading.

Methyclothiazide (The ECG changes and hypokalemia which may result from administration of nonpotassium-sparing diuretics can be acutely worsened by beta agonists. Caution is advised in the co-administration of beta agonists with nonpotassium-sparing diuretics).
No products indexed under this heading.

Metipranolol Hydrochloride (Co-administration with beta adrenergic blocking agent blocks the pulmonary effect of beta agonists and may produce severe bronchospasm in asthmatic patients; co-administer with caution).
No products indexed under this heading.

Metoprolol Succinate (Co-administration with beta adrenergic blocking agent blocks the pulmonary effect of beta agonists and may produce severe bronchospasm in asthmatic patients; co-administer with caution). Products include:
Toprol-XL Tablets 666

Metoprolol Tartrate (Co-administration with beta adrenergic blocking agent blocks the pulmonary effect of beta agonists and may produce severe bronchospasm in asthmatic patients; co-administer with caution).
No products indexed under this heading.

Moclobemide (Action of albuterol on the cardiovascular system may be potentiated by MAO inhibitors; co-administer with caution).
No products indexed under this heading.

Nadolol (Co-administration with beta adrenergic blocking agent blocks the pulmonary effect of beta agonists and may produce severe bronchospasm in asthmatic patients; co-administer with caution). Products include:

Nadolol Tablets 2191

Nebivolol (Co-administration with beta adrenergic blocking agent blocks the pulmonary effect of beta agonists and may produce severe bronchospasm in asthmatic patients; co-administer with caution). Products include:

Bystolic Tablets 1155

Nortriptyline Hydrochloride (Action of albuterol on the cardiovascular system may be potentiated by tricyclic antidepressants; co-administer with caution).

No products indexed under this heading.

Pargyline Hydrochloride (Action of albuterol on the cardiovascular system may be potentiated by MAO inhibitors; co-administer with caution).

No products indexed under this heading.

Penbutolol Sulfate (Co-administration with beta adrenergic blocking agent blocks the pulmonary effect of beta agonists and may produce severe bronchospasm in asthmatic patients; co-administer with caution).

No products indexed under this heading.

Phenelzine Sulfate (Action of albuterol on the cardiovascular system may be potentiated by MAO inhibitors; co-administer with caution).

No products indexed under this heading.

Pindolol (Co-administration with beta adrenergic blocking agent blocks the pulmonary effect of beta agonists and may produce severe bronchospasm in asthmatic patients; co-administer with caution).

No products indexed under this heading.

Polythiazide (The ECG changes and hypokalemia which may result from administration of nonpotassium-sparing diuretics can be acutely worsened by beta agonists. Caution is advised in the co-administration of beta agonists with nonpotassium-sparing diuretics).

No products indexed under this heading.

Procarbazine Hydrochloride (Action of albuterol on the cardiovascular system may be potentiated by MAO inhibitors; co-administer with caution).

No products indexed under this heading.

Propranolol Hydrochloride (Co-administration with beta adrenergic blocking agent blocks the pulmonary effect of beta agonists and may produce severe bronchospasm in asthmatic patients; co-administer with caution). Products include:

InnoPran XL Extended Release Capsules 1484

Protriptyline Hydrochloride (Action of albuterol on the cardiovascular system may be potentiated by tricyclic antidepressants; co-administer with caution).

No products indexed under this heading.

Rasagiline Mesylate (Action of albuterol on the cardiovascular system may be potentiated by MAO inhibitors; co-administer with caution). Products include:

Azilect Tablets 3106

Selegiline (Action of albuterol on the cardiovascular system may be potentiated by MAO inhibitors; co-administer with caution). Products include:

Emsam Transdermal System 905

Selegiline Hydrochloride (Action of albuterol on the cardiovascular system may be potentiated by MAO inhibitors; co-administer with caution). Products include:

Eldepryl Capsules 3052

Sotalol Hydrochloride (Co-administration with beta adrenergic blocking agent blocks the pulmonary effect of beta agonists and may produce severe bronchospasm in asthmatic patients; co-administer with caution).

No products indexed under this heading.

Timolol Hemihydrate (Co-administration with beta adrenergic blocking agent blocks the pulmonary effect of beta agonists and may produce severe bronchospasm in asthmatic patients; co-administer with caution). Products include:

Betimol Ophthalmic Solution 3181

Timolol Maleate (Co-administration with beta adrenergic blocking agent blocks the pulmonary effect of beta agonists and may produce severe bronchospasm in asthmatic patients; co-administer with caution). Products include:

Combigan Ophthalmic Solution 553

Cosopt Sterile Ophthalmic Solution 1969

Timoptic Sterile Ophthalmic Solution 2121

Timoptic in Ocudose 2124

Timoptic-XE Sterile Ophthalmic Gel Forming Solution 2125

Torsemide (The ECG changes and hypokalemia which may result from administration of nonpotassium-sparing diuretics can be acutely worsened by beta agonists. Caution is advised in the co-administration of beta agonists with nonpotassium-sparing diuretics). Products include:

Demadex Injection 2630

Demadex Tablets 2630

Tranylcypromine Sulfate (Action of albuterol on the cardiovascular system may be potentiated by MAO inhibitors; co-administer with caution). Products include:

Parnate Tablets 1532

Trimipramine Maleate (Action of albuterol on the cardiovascular system may be potentiated by tricyclic antidepressants; co-administer with caution).

No products indexed under this heading.

PROVIGIL TABLETS

(Modafinil) 977

May interact with cytochrome p450 2c9 substrates (selected), cytochrome p450 3a4 inducers (selected), cytochrome p450 3a4 inhibitors (selected), cytochrome p450 3a4 substrates (selected), monoamine oxidase inhibitors, oral contraceptives, phenytoin, selective serotonin reuptake inhibitors, tricyclic antidepressants, xanthines, and certain other agents. Compounds in these categories include:

Acarbose (An apparent concentration-related suppression of CYP2C9 activity was observed in human hepatocytes after exposure to modafinil in vitro suggesting that there is a potential for a metabolic interaction between modafinil and substrates of CYP2C9). Products include:

Precose Tablets 792

Acetazolamide (Co-administration of potent inhibitors of CYP3A4 could alter the plasma levels of modafinil).

No products indexed under this heading.

Alfentanil Hydrochloride (Chronic administration of modafinil can increase the elimination of substrates of CYP3A4. Dose adjustments may be necessary for patients being treated with these and similar medications).

No products indexed under this heading.

Allium sativum (Co-administration of potent inducers of CYP3A4 could alter the plasma levels of modafinil).

No products indexed under this heading.

Alprazolam (Chronic administration of modafinil can increase the elimination of substrates of CYP3A4. Dose adjustments may be necessary for patients being treated with these and similar medications).

No products indexed under this heading.

Aminophylline (Chronic administration of modafinil may cause modest induction of CYP3A4, thus reducing the levels, to a lesser degree, of co-administered substrate for that enzyme system, such as theophylline).

No products indexed under this heading.

Amiodarone Hydrochloride (Chronic administration of modafinil can increase the elimination of substrates of CYP3A4. Dose adjustments may be necessary for patients being treated with these and similar medications).

No products indexed under this heading.

Amitriptyline Hydrochloride (CYP2C19 provides an ancillary pathway for the metabolism of certain tricyclic antidepressants that are primarily metabolized by CYP2D6. In tricyclic-treated patients deficient in CYP2D6, the amount of metabolism by CYP2C19 may be substantially increased. Modafinil may cause elevation of the levels of these tricyclics in this subset of patients. A reduction in the dose of tricyclic agents might be needed in these patients).

No products indexed under this heading.

Amlodipine Besylate (Chronic administration of modafinil can increase the elimination of substrates of CYP3A4. Dose adjustments may be necessary for patients being treated with these and similar medications). Products include:

Azor Tablets 1005

Exforge Tablets 2238

Amoxapine (CYP2C19 provides an ancillary pathway for the metabolism of certain tricyclic antidepressants that are primarily metabolized by CYP2D6. In tricyclic-treated patients deficient in CYP2D6, the amount of metabolism by CYP2C19 may be substantially increased. Modafinil may cause elevation of the levels of these tricyclics in this subset of patients. A reduction in the dose of tricyclic agents might be needed in these patients).

No products indexed under this heading.

Amprenavir (Co-administration of potent inhibitors of CYP3A4 could alter the plasma levels of modafinil).

No products indexed under this heading.

Anastrozole (Co-administration of potent inhibitors of CYP3A4 could alter the plasma levels of modafinil). Products include:

Arimidex Tablets 672

Aprepitant (Chronic administration of modafinil can increase the elimination of substrates of CYP3A4. Dose adjustments may be necessary for patients being treated with these and similar medications). Products include:

Emend Capsules 1992

Astemizole (Chronic administration of modafinil can increase the elimination of substrates of CYP3A4. Dose adjustments may be necessary for patients being treated with these and similar medications).

No products indexed under this heading.

Atazanavir (Co-administration of potent inhibitors of CYP3A4 could alter the plasma levels of modafinil).

No products indexed under this heading.

Atazanavir Sulfate (Co-administration of potent inhibitors of CYP3A4 could alter the plasma levels of modafinil). Products include:

Reyataz Capsules 3299

Atorvastatin Calcium (Chronic administration of modafinil can increase the elimination of substrates of CYP3A4. Dose adjustments may be necessary for patients being treated with these and similar medications). Products include:

Lipitor Tablets 2501

Belladonna Ergotamine (Chronic administration of modafinil can increase the elimination of substrates of CYP3A4. Dose adjustments may be necessary for patients being treated with these and similar medications).

No products indexed under this heading.

Betamethasone Acetate (Co-administration of potent inducers of CYP3A4 could alter the plasma levels of modafinil).

No products indexed under this heading.

Betamethasone Sodium Phosphate (Co-administration of potent inducers of CYP3A4 could alter the plasma levels of modafinil).

No products indexed under this heading.

Buspirone Hydrochloride (Chronic administration of modafinil can increase the elimination of substrates of CYP3A4. Dose adjustments may be necessary for patients being treated with these and similar medications).

No products indexed under this heading.

Busulfan (Chronic administration of modafinil can increase the elimination of substrates of CYP3A4. Dose adjustments may be necessary for patients being treated with these and similar medications). Products include:

Busulfex Injection 2477

Myleran Tablets **1530**

Candesartan Cilexetil (An apparent concentration-related suppression of CYP2C9 activity was observed in human hepatocytes after exposure to modafinil in vitro suggesting that there is a potential for a metabolic interaction between modafinil and substrates of CYP2C9). Products include:

Atacand Tablets **639**
Atacand HCT **642**

Carbamazepine (Chronic administration of modafinil may cause induction of its metabolism; co-administration of potent inducers of CYP3A4, such as carbamazepine, could alter the levels of modafinil due to the partial involvement of that enzyme in the metabolic elimination of the compound). Products include:

Carbatrol Capsules **3019**
Equetro Extended-Release Capsules **3174**

Carvedilol (An apparent concentration-related suppression of CYP2C9 activity was observed in human hepatocytes after exposure to modafinil in vitro suggesting that there is a potential for a metabolic interaction between modafinil and substrates of CYP2C9). Products include:

Coreg Tablets **1387**

Celecoxib (An apparent concentration-related suppression of CYP2C9 activity was observed in human hepatocytes after exposure to modafinil in vitro suggesting that there is a potential for a metabolic interaction between modafinil and substrates of CYP2C9). Products include:

Celebrex Capsules **2979**

Cerivastatin Sodium (Chronic administration of modafinil can increase the elimination of substrates of CYP3A4. Dose adjustments may be necessary for patients being treated with these and similar medications).

No products indexed under this heading.

Chlorpheniramine (Chronic administration of modafinil can increase the elimination of substrates of CYP3A4. Dose adjustments may be necessary for patients being treated with these and similar medications).

No products indexed under this heading.

Chlorpheniramine Maleate (Chronic administration of modafinil can increase the elimination of substrates of CYP3A4. Dose adjustments may be necessary for patients being treated with these and similar medications). Products include:

Actifed Cold & Allergy Tablets **1895**
Sudafed PE Sinus & Allergy Tablets **1908**
Tylenol Allergy Multi-Symptom Caplets with Cool Burst and Rapid Release Gelcaps **1916**
Children's Tylenol Plus Cold Suspension Liquid **1912**
Children's Tylenol Plus Cough & Runny Nose Suspension Liquid **1912**
Children's Tylenol Plus Flu Suspension Liquid **1914**
Children's Tylenol Plus Multi-Symptom Cold Suspension Liquid **1912**
Tylenol Cold Head Congestion Nighttime Caplets with Cool Burst **1910**
Tylenol Cold Multi-Symptom Nighttime Caplets with Cool Burst **1913**
Tylenol Sinus Congestion & Pain Nighttime Caplets with Cool Burst **1917**

Chlorpheniramine Polistirex (Chronic administration of modafinil can increase the elimination of substrates of CYP3A4. Dose adjustments may be necessary for patients being treated with these and similar medications). Products include:

Tussionex Pennkinetic Extended-Release Suspension **3154**

Chlorpheniramine Tannate (Chronic administration of modafinil can increase the elimination of substrates of CYP3A4. Dose adjustments may be necessary for patients being treated with these and similar medications).

No products indexed under this heading.

Chlorpropamide (An apparent concentration-related suppression of CYP2C9 activity was observed in human hepatocytes after exposure to modafinil in vitro suggesting that there is a potential for a metabolic interaction between modafinil and substrates of CYP2C9).

No products indexed under this heading.

Cimetidine (Co-administration of potent inhibitors of CYP3A4 could alter the plasma levels of modafinil).

No products indexed under this heading.

Cimetidine Hydrochloride (Co-administration of potent inhibitors of CYP3A4 could alter the plasma levels of modafinil).

No products indexed under this heading.

Ciprofloxacin (Co-administration of potent inhibitors of CYP3A4 could alter the plasma levels of modafinil). Products include:

Cipro I.V. **2817**
Cipro Oral Suspension **2810**
Cipro XR Tablets **2823**
Ciprodex Otic Suspension **541**

Ciprofloxacin Hydrochloride (Co-administration of potent inducers of CYP3A4 could alter the plasma levels of modafinil). Products include:

Cipro Tablets **2810**

Cisapride (Chronic administration of modafinil can increase the elimination of substrates of CYP3A4. Dose adjustments may be necessary for patients being treated with these and similar medications).

No products indexed under this heading.

Cisplatin (Co-administration of potent inducers of CYP3A4 could alter the plasma levels of modafinil).

No products indexed under this heading.

Citalopram Hydrobromide (Modafinil is a reversible inhibitor of the CYP2C19; the levels of CYP2D6 substrates, such as selective serotonin reuptake inhibitors, which have ancillary routes of elimination through CYP2D6, may be increased by co-administration of modafinil). Products include:

Celexa **1160**

Clarithromycin (Chronic administration of modafinil can increase the elimination of substrates of CYP3A4. Dose adjustments may be necessary for patients being treated with these and similar medications). Products include:

Biaxin/Biaxin XL **411**

Clomipramine Hydrochloride (Co-administration has resulted in one incident of increased levels of clomipramine and its active metabolite desmethylclomipramine).

No products indexed under this heading.

Clotrimazole (Co-administration of potent inhibitors of CYP3A4 could alter the plasma levels of modafinil). Products include:

Lotrisone **2881**

Cortisone Acetate (Co-administration of potent inducers of CYP3A4 could alter the plasma levels of modafinil).

No products indexed under this heading.

Cyclosporine (The blood levels of cyclosporine may be reduced when used with modafinil. Monitoring of circulating cyclosporine concentrations and appropriate dosage adjustment for cyclosporine should be considered when these drugs are used concomitantly). Products include:

Gengraf Capsules **435**
Neoral Oral Solution **2280**
Neoral Soft Gelatin Capsules **2280**
Restasis Ophthalmic Emulsion **557**
Sandimmune **2296**

Dalfopristin (Co-administration of potent inhibitors of CYP3A4 could alter the plasma levels of modafinil).

No products indexed under this heading.

Danazol (Co-administration of potent inhibitors of CYP3A4 could alter the plasma levels of modafinil).

No products indexed under this heading.

Delavirdine Mesylate (Co-administration of potent inhibitors of CYP3A4 could alter the plasma levels of modafinil).

No products indexed under this heading.

Desipramine Hydrochloride (CYP2C19 provides an ancillary pathway for the metabolism of certain tricyclic antidepressants that are primarily metabolized by CYP2D6. In tricyclic-treated patients deficient in CYP2D6, the amount of metabolism by CYP2C19 may be substantially increased. Modafinil may cause elevation of the levels of these tricyclics in this subset of patients. A reduction in the dose of tricyclic agents might be needed in these patients).

No products indexed under this heading.

Desogestrel (The effectiveness of steroidal contraceptives may be reduced when used with modafinil tablets and for one month after discontinuation of therapy. Alternative or concomitant methods of contraception are recommended for patients treated with modafinil tablets and for one month after discontinuation of modafinil). Products include:

Mircette Tablets **1034**

Dexamethasone (Co-administration of potent inducers of CYP3A4 could alter the plasma levels of modafinil). Products include:

Ciprodex Otic Suspension **541**

Dexamethasone Acetate (Co-administration of potent inducers of CYP3A4 could alter the plasma levels of modafinil).

No products indexed under this heading.

Dexamethasone Sodium Phosphate (Co-administration of potent inducers of CYP3A4 could alter the plasma levels of modafinil).

No products indexed under this heading.

Dextroamphetamine (Absorption of modafinil may be delayed by approximately one hour when co-administered with dextroamphetamine).

No products indexed under this heading.

Dextroamphetamine Saccharate (Absorption of modafinil may be delayed by approximately one hour when co-administered with dextroamphetamine). Products include:

Adderall XR Capsules **3012**

Dextroamphetamine Sulfate (Absorption of modafinil may be delayed by approximately one hour when co-administered with dextroamphetamine). Products include:

Adderall XR Capsules **3012**
Dexedrine **1401**

Dextromethorphan (An apparent concentration-related suppression of CYP2C9 activity was observed in human hepatocytes after exposure to modafinil in vitro suggesting that there is a potential for a metabolic interaction between modafinil and substrates of CYP2C9).

No products indexed under this heading.

Diazepam (Modafinil is a reversible inhibitor of the CYP2C19; co-administration with drugs that are largely eliminated via this pathway, such as diazepam, may increase the circulating levels of diazepam). Products include:

Valium Tablets **2658**

Diclofenac Potassium (An apparent concentration-related suppression of CYP2C9 activity was observed in human hepatocytes after exposure to modafinil in vitro suggesting that there is a potential for a metabolic interaction between modafinil and substrates of CYP2C9).

No products indexed under this heading.

Diclofenac Sodium (An apparent concentration-related suppression of CYP2C9 activity was observed in human hepatocytes after exposure to modafinil in vitro suggesting that there is a potential for a metabolic interaction between modafinil and substrates of CYP2C9). Products include:

Diclofenac Sodium Ophthalmic Solution..................................... ⊙ **240**
Voltaren Ophthalmic Solution **2336**
Voltaren Tablets **2334**
Voltaren-XR Tablets **2337**

Dihydroergotamine Mesylate (Chronic administration of modafinil can increase the elimination of substrates of CYP3A4. Dose adjustments may be necessary for patients being treated with these and similar medications).

No products indexed under this heading.

Diltiazem Hydrochloride (Chronic administration of modafinil can increase the elimination of sub-

IMPORTANT NOTE: Always consult each drug listing in the patient's regimen for possible interactions.

strates of CYP3A4. Dose adjustments may be necessary for patients being treated with these and similar medications). Products include:

Cardizem LA Extended Release Tablets ... 421

Diltiazem Maleate (Chronic administration of modafinil can increase the elimination of substrates of CYP3A4. Dose adjustments may be necessary for patients being treated with these and similar medications).

No products indexed under this heading.

Disopyramide (Chronic administration of modafinil can increase the elimination of substrates of CYP3A4. Dose adjustments may be necessary for patients being treated with these and similar medications).

No products indexed under this heading.

Disopyramide Phosphate (Chronic administration of modafinil can increase the elimination of substrates of CYP3A4. Dose adjustments may be necessary for patients being treated with these and similar medications).

No products indexed under this heading.

Disulfiram (Chronic administration of modafinil can increase the elimination of substrates of CYP3A4. Dose adjustments may be necessary for patients being treated with these and similar medications).

No products indexed under this heading.

Doxepin Hydrochloride (CYP2C19 provides an ancillary pathway for the metabolism of certain tricyclic antidepressants that are primarily metabolized by CYP2D6. In tricyclic-treated patients deficient in CYP2D6, the amount of metabolism by CYP2C19 may be substantially increased. Modafinil may cause elevation of the levels of these tricyclics in this subset of patients. A reduction in the dose of tricyclic agents might be needed in these patients).

No products indexed under this heading.

Doxorubicin Hydrochloride (Chronic administration of modafinil can increase the elimination of substrates of CYP3A4. Dose adjustments may be necessary for patients being treated with these and similar medications).

No products indexed under this heading.

Dronabinol (Chronic administration of modafinil can increase the elimination of substrates of CYP3A4. Dose adjustments may be necessary for patients being treated with these and similar medications). Products include:

Marinol Capsules ... 3163

Dyphylline (Chronic administration of modafinil may cause modest induction of CYP3A4, thus reducing the levels, to a lesser degree, of co-administered substrate for that enzyme system, such as theophylline).

No products indexed under this heading.

Efavirenz (Co-administration of potent inducers of CYP3A4 could alter the plasma levels of modafinil). Products include:

Atripla Tablets ... 938
Sustiva Capsules ... 930
Sustiva Tablets ... 930

Eprosartan Mesylate (An apparent concentration-related suppression of CYP2C9 activity was observed in human hepatocytes after exposure to modafinil in vitro suggesting that there is a potential for a metabolic interaction between modafinil and substrates of CYP2C9). Products include:

Teveten Tablets ... 515
Teveten HCT Tablets ... 517

Ergotamine Tartrate (Chronic administration of modafinil can increase the elimination of substrates of CYP3A4. Dose adjustments may be necessary for patients being treated with these and similar medications).

No products indexed under this heading.

Erythromycin (Chronic administration of modafinil can increase the elimination of substrates of CYP3A4. Dose adjustments may be necessary for patients being treated with these and similar medications).

No products indexed under this heading.

Erythromycin Estolate (Chronic administration of modafinil can increase the elimination of substrates of CYP3A4. Dose adjustments may be necessary for patients being treated with these and similar medications).

No products indexed under this heading.

Erythromycin Ethylsuccinate (Chronic administration of modafinil can increase the elimination of substrates of CYP3A4. Dose adjustments may be necessary for patients being treated with these and similar medications). Products include:

E.E.S. ... 433
EryPed ... 431

Erythromycin Gluceptate (Chronic administration of modafinil can increase the elimination of substrates of CYP3A4. Dose adjustments may be necessary for patients being treated with these and similar medications).

No products indexed under this heading.

Erythromycin Lactobionate (Chronic administration of modafinil can increase the elimination of substrates of CYP3A4. Dose adjustments may be necessary for patients being treated with these and similar medications).

No products indexed under this heading.

Erythromycin Stearate (Chronic administration of modafinil can increase the elimination of substrates of CYP3A4. Dose adjustments may be necessary for patients being treated with these and similar medications).

No products indexed under this heading.

Escitalopram Oxalate (Modafinil is a reversible inhibitor of the CYP2C19; the levels of CYP2D6 substrates, such as selective serotonin reuptake inhibitors, which have ancillary routes of elimination through CYP2D6, may be increased by co-administration of modafinil). Products include:

Lexapro Oral Suspension ... 1174
Lexapro Tablets ... 1174

Esomeprazole Magnesium (Co-administration of potent inhibitors of CYP3A4 could alter the plasma levels of modafinil). Products include:

Nexium Delayed-Release Capsules ... 645
Nexium Delayed-Release Oral Suspension ... 645

Estradiol (Chronic administration of modafinil can increase the elimination of substrates of CYP3A4. Dose adjustments may be necessary for patients being treated with these and similar medications). Products include:

Activella Tablets ... 2347
Angeliq Tablets ... 751
Climara Transdermal System ... 763
Climara Pro Transdermal System ... 768
Divigel ... 3167
Vagifem Tablets ... 2375

Estradiol Benzoate (Chronic administration of modafinil can increase the elimination of substrates of CYP3A4. Dose adjustments may be necessary for patients being treated with these and similar medications).

No products indexed under this heading.

Estradiol Cypionate (Chronic administration of modafinil can increase the elimination of substrates of CYP3A4. Dose adjustments may be necessary for patients being treated with these and similar medications).

No products indexed under this heading.

Estradiol Valerate (Chronic administration of modafinil can increase the elimination of substrates of CYP3A4. Dose adjustments may be necessary for patients being treated with these and similar medications).

No products indexed under this heading.

Ethinyl Estradiol (Administration of modafinil to female volunteers resulted in a mean 11% decrease in Cmax and an 18% decrease in AUC of ethinyl estradiol. There was no apparent change in the elimination rate of ethinyl estradiol). Products include:

Lybrel Tablets ... 3204
Mircette Tablets ... 1034
NuvaRing ... 2897
Ortho-Cyclen/Ortho Tri-Cyclen ... 2449
Ortho Evra Transdermal System ... 2437
Ortho Tri-Cyclen Lo Tablets ... 2458
Seasonique Tablets ... 1046
Yaz Tablets ... 805

Ethosuximide (Chronic administration of modafinil can increase the elimination of substrates of CYP3A4. Dose adjustments may be necessary for patients being treated with these and similar medications).

No products indexed under this heading.

Ethynodiol Diacetate (The effectiveness of steroidal contraceptives may be reduced when used with modafinil tablets and for one month after discontinuation of therapy. Alternative or concomitant methods of contraception are recommended for patients treated with modafinil tablets and for one month after discontinuation of modafinil).

No products indexed under this heading.

Etodolac (An apparent concentration-related suppression of CYP2C9 activity was observed in human hepatocytes after exposure to modafinil in vitro suggesting that there is a potential for a metabolic interaction between modafinil and substrates of CYP2C9).

No products indexed under this heading.

Etoposide (Chronic administration of modafinil can increase the elimination of substrates of CYP3A4. Dose adjustments may be necessary for patients being treated with these and similar medications).

No products indexed under this heading.

Etoposide Phosphate (Chronic administration of modafinil can increase the elimination of substrates of CYP3A4. Dose adjustments may be necessary for patients being treated with these and similar medications).

No products indexed under this heading.

Felbamate (Co-administration of potent inducers of CYP3A4 could alter the plasma levels of modafinil).

No products indexed under this heading.

Felodipine (Chronic administration of modafinil can increase the elimination of substrates of CYP3A4. Dose adjustments may be necessary for patients being treated with these and similar medications).

No products indexed under this heading.

Fenoprofen Calcium (An apparent concentration-related suppression of CYP2C9 activity was observed in human hepatocytes after exposure to modafinil in vitro suggesting that there is a potential for a metabolic interaction between modafinil and substrates of CYP2C9). Products include:

Nalfon Capsules ... 2508

Fentanyl (Chronic administration of modafinil can increase the elimination of substrates of CYP3A4. Dose adjustments may be necessary for patients being treated with these and similar medications). Products include:

Duragesic Transdermal System ... 2405
Ionsys Transdermal System ... 2410

Fentanyl Citrate (Chronic administration of modafinil can increase the elimination of substrates of CYP3A4. Dose adjustments may be necessary for patients being treated with these and similar medications). Products include:

Actiq ... 959
Fentora Tablets ... 968

Fluconazole (Co-administration of potent inhibitors of CYP3A4 could alter the plasma levels of modafinil).

No products indexed under this heading.

Fludrocortisone Acetate (Co-administration of potent inducers of CYP3A4 could alter the plasma levels of modafinil).

No products indexed under this heading.

Fluoxetine (Modafinil is a reversible inhibitor of the CYP2C19; the levels of CYP2D6 substrates, such as selective serotonin reuptake inhibitors, which have ancillary routes of elimination through CYP2D6, may be increased by co-administration of modafinil).
No products indexed under this heading.

Fluoxetine Hydrochloride (Modafinil is a reversible inhibitor of the CYP2C19; the levels of CYP2D6 substrates, such as selective serotonin reuptake inhibitors, which have ancillary routes of elimination through CYP2D6, may be increased by co-administration of modafinil). Products include:
Prozac Weekly Capsules ... 1852
Prozac Pulvules and Liquid ... 1852
Symbyax Capsules ... 1871

Flurbiprofen (An apparent concentration-related suppression of CYP2C9 activity was observed in human hepatocytes after exposure to modafinil in vitro suggesting that there is a potential for a metabolic interaction between modafinil and substrates of CYP2C9).
No products indexed under this heading.

Flurbiprofen Sodium (An apparent concentration-related suppression of CYP2C9 activity was observed in human hepatocytes after exposure to modafinil in vitro suggesting that there is a potential for a metabolic interaction between modafinil and substrates of CYP2C9).
No products indexed under this heading.

Fluvastatin Sodium (An apparent concentration-related suppression of CYP2C9 activity was observed in human hepatocytes after exposure to modafinil in vitro suggesting that there is a potential for a metabolic interaction between modafinil and substrates of CYP2C9). Products include:
Lescol Capsules ... 2268
Lescol XL Tablets ... 2268

Fluvoxamine Maleate (Modafinil is a reversible inhibitor of the CYP2C19; the levels of CYP2D6 substrates, such as selective serotonin reuptake inhibitors, which have ancillary routes of elimination through CYP2D6, may be increased by co-administration of modafinil). Products include:
Luvox CR Extended-Release Capsules ... 1759

Fosamprenavir Calcium (Co-administration of potent inhibitors of CYP3A4 could alter the plasma levels of modafinil). Products include:
Lexiva Oral Suspension ... 1510
Lexiva Tablets ... 1510

Fosphenytoin Sodium (Modafinil is a reversible inhibitor of the CYP2C19; co-administration with drugs that are largely eliminated via this pathway, such as phenytoin, may increase the circulating levels of phenytoin).
No products indexed under this heading.

Garlic Extract (Co-administration of potent inducers of CYP3A4 could alter the plasma levels of modafinil).
No products indexed under this heading.

Garlic Oil (Co-administration of potent inducers of CYP3A4 could alter the plasma levels of modafinil).
No products indexed under this heading.

Glimepiride (An apparent concentration-related suppression of CYP2C9 activity was observed in human hepatocytes after exposure to modafinil in vitro suggesting that there is a potential for a metabolic interaction between modafinil and substrates of CYP2C9). Products include:
Avandaryl Tablets ... 1344
Duetact Tablets ... 3085

Glipizide (An apparent concentration-related suppression of CYP2C9 activity was observed in human hepatocytes after exposure to modafinil in vitro suggesting that there is a potential for a metabolic interaction between modafinil and substrates of CYP2C9).
No products indexed under this heading.

Haloperidol (Chronic administration of modafinil can increase the elimination of substrates of CYP3A4. Dose adjustments may be necessary for patients being treated with these and similar medications).
No products indexed under this heading.

Haloperidol Decanoate (Chronic administration of modafinil can increase the elimination of substrates of CYP3A4. Dose adjustments may be necessary for patients being treated with these and similar medications).
No products indexed under this heading.

Haloperidol Lactate (Chronic administration of modafinil can increase the elimination of substrates of CYP3A4. Dose adjustments may be necessary for patients being treated with these and similar medications).
No products indexed under this heading.

Hydrocortisone (Co-administration of potent inducers of CYP3A4 could alter the plasma levels of modafinil).
No products indexed under this heading.

Hydrocortisone Acetate (Co-administration of potent inducers of CYP3A4 could alter the plasma levels of modafinil). Products include:
Analpram-HC ... 1140
Pramosone ... 1141

Hydrocortisone Butyrate (Co-administration of potent inducers of CYP3A4 could alter the plasma levels of modafinil).
No products indexed under this heading.

Hydrocortisone Cypionate (Co-administration of potent inducers of CYP3A4 could alter the plasma levels of modafinil).
No products indexed under this heading.

Hydrocortisone Hemisuccinate (Co-administration of potent inducers of CYP3A4 could alter the plasma levels of modafinil).
No products indexed under this heading.

Hydrocortisone Probutate (Co-administration of potent inducers of CYP3A4 could alter the plasma levels of modafinil).
No products indexed under this heading.

Hydrocortisone Sodium Phosphate (Co-administration of potent inducers of CYP3A4 could alter the plasma levels of modafinil).
No products indexed under this heading.

Hydrocortisone Sodium Succinate (Co-administration of potent inducers of CYP3A4 could alter the plasma levels of modafinil).
No products indexed under this heading.

Hydrocortisone Valerate (Co-administration of potent inducers of CYP3A4 could alter the plasma levels of modafinil).
No products indexed under this heading.

Hypericum (Co-administration of potent inducers of CYP3A4 could alter the plasma levels of modafinil). Products include:
Satieté Tablets ... 640

Hypericum Perforatum (Co-administration of potent inducers of CYP3A4 could alter the plasma levels of modafinil).
No products indexed under this heading.

Ibuprofen (An apparent concentration-related suppression of CYP2C9 activity was observed in human hepatocytes after exposure to modafinil in vitro suggesting that there is a potential for a metabolic interaction between modafinil and substrates of CYP2C9). Products include:
Motrin IB Tablets and Caplets ... 1900
Children's Motrin Oral Suspension ... 1901
Children's Motrin Non-Staining Dye-Free Oral Suspension ... 1901
Children's Motrin Cold Oral Suspension ... 1899
Infants' Motrin Concentrated Drops ... 1901
Infants' Motrin Non-Staining Dye-Free Concentrated Drops ... 1901
Junior Strength Motrin Caplets and Chewable Tablets ... 1901
Vicoprofen Tablets ... 533

Imipramine Hydrochloride (CYP2C19 provides an ancillary pathway for the metabolism of certain tricyclic antidepressants that are primarily metabolized by CYP2D6. In tricyclic-treated patients deficient in CYP2D6, the amount of metabolism by CYP2C19 may be substantially increased. Modafinil may cause elevation of the levels of these tricyclics in this subset of patients. A reduction in the dose of tricyclic agents might be needed in these patients).
No products indexed under this heading.

Imipramine Pamoate (CYP2C19 provides an ancillary pathway for the metabolism of certain tricyclic antidepressants that are primarily metabolized by CYP2D6. In tricyclic-treated patients deficient in CYP2D6, the amount of metabolism by CYP2C19 may be substantially increased. Modafinil may cause elevation of the levels of these tricyclics in this subset of patients. A reduction in the dose of tricyclic agents might be needed in these patients).
No products indexed under this heading.

Indinavir Sulfate (Chronic administration of modafinil can increase the elimination of substrates of CYP3A4. Dose adjustments may be necessary for patients being treated with these and similar medications). Products include:
Crixivan Capsules ... 1979

Indomethacin (An apparent concentration-related suppression of CYP2C9 activity was observed in human hepatocytes after exposure to modafinil in vitro suggesting that there is a potential for a metabolic interaction between modafinil and substrates of CYP2C9). Products include:
Indocin ... 2024

Indomethacin Sodium Trihydrate (An apparent concentration-related suppression of CYP2C9 activity was observed in human hepatocytes after exposure to modafinil in vitro suggesting that there is a potential for a metabolic interaction between modafinil and substrates of CYP2C9). Products include:
Indocin I.V. ... 2489

Irbesartan (An apparent concentration-related suppression of CYP2C9 activity was observed in human hepatocytes after exposure to modafinil in vitro suggesting that there is a potential for a metabolic interaction between modafinil and substrates of CYP2C9). Products include:
Avalide Tablets ... 892
Avalide Tablets ... 2713
Avapro Tablets ... 897
Avapro Tablets ... 2718

Isocarboxazid (Co-administration requires caution; no interaction studies have been performed). Products include:
Marplan Tablets ... 3177

Isoniazid (Co-administration of potent inhibitors of CYP3A4 could alter the plasma levels of modafinil).
No products indexed under this heading.

Isradipine (Chronic administration of modafinil can increase the elimination of substrates of CYP3A4. Dose adjustments may be necessary for patients being treated with these and similar medications). Products include:
DynaCirc CR Controlled Release Tablets ... 1407

Itraconazole (Chronic administration of modafinil may cause induction of its metabolism; co-administration of potent inhibitors of CYP3A4, such as itraconazole, could alter the levels of modafinil due to the partial involvement of that enzyme in the metabolic elimination of the compound).
No products indexed under this heading.

Ixabepilone (Chronic administration of modafinil can increase the elimination of substrates of CYP3A4. Dose adjustments may be necessary for patients being treated with these and similar medications). Products include:
Ixempra Kit for Injection ... 915

Ketoconazole (Chronic administration of modafinil may cause induction of its metabolism; co-administration of potent inhibitors of CYP3A4, such as ketoconazole, could alter the levels of modafinil due to the partial involvement of that enzyme in the metabolic elimination of the compound). Products include:
Extina Foam, 2% ... 3057
Nizoral A-D Shampoo ... 1901

Ketoprofen (An apparent concentration-related suppression of CYP2C9 activity was observed in human hepatocytes after exposure to modafinil in vitro suggesting that there is a potential for a metabolic interaction between modafinil and substrates of CYP2C9).
No products indexed under this heading.

Ketorolac Tromethamine (An apparent concentration-related suppression of CYP2C9 activity was observed in human hepatocytes after exposure to modafinil in vitro suggesting that there is a potential for a metabolic interaction between modafinil and substrates of CYP2C9).
No products indexed under this heading.

Lansoprazole (An apparent concentration-related suppression of CYP2C9 activity was observed in human hepatocytes after exposure to modafinil in vitro suggesting that there is a potential for a metabolic interaction between modafinil and substrates of CYP2C9).
No products indexed under this heading.

Levonorgestrel (The effectiveness of steroidal contraceptives may be reduced when used with modafinil tablets and for one month after discontinuation of therapy. Alternative or concomitant methods of contraception are recommended for patients treated with modafinil tablets and for one month after discontinuation of modafinil). Products include:
Climara Pro Transdermal System 768
Lybrel Tablets 3204
Mirena Intrauterine System 779
Plan B Tablets 1044
Seasonique Tablets 1046

Lidocaine (Chronic administration of modafinil can increase the elimination of substrates of CYP3A4. Dose adjustments may be necessary for patients being treated with these and similar medications). Products include:
Lidoderm Patch 1114

Lidocaine Hydrochloride (Chronic administration of modafinil can increase the elimination of substrates of CYP3A4. Dose adjustments may be necessary for patients being treated with these and similar medications).
No products indexed under this heading.

Lopinavir (Co-administration of potent inhibitors of CYP3A4 could alter the plasma levels of modafinil). Products include:
Kaletra 452

Loratadine (Co-administration of potent inhibitors of CYP3A4 could alter the plasma levels of modafinil).
No products indexed under this heading.

Losartan Potassium (An apparent concentration-related suppression of CYP2C9 activity was observed in human hepatocytes after exposure to modafinil in vitro suggesting that there is a potential for a metabolic interaction between modafinil and substrates of CYP2C9). Products include:
Cozaar Tablets 1973

Lovastatin (Chronic administration of modafinil can increase the elimination of substrates of CYP3A4. Dose adjustments may be necessary for patients being treated with these and similar medications). Products include:
Advicor Tablets 402
Mevacor Tablets 2063

Maprotiline Hydrochloride (CYP2C19 provides an ancillary pathway for the metabolism of certain tricyclic antidepressants that are primarily metabolized by CYP2D6. In tricyclic-treated patients deficient in CYP2D6, the amount of metabolism by CYP2C19 may be substantially increased. Modafinil may cause elevation of the levels of these tricyclics in this subset of patients. A reduction in the dose of tricyclic agents might be needed in these patients).
No products indexed under this heading.

Meclofenamate Sodium (An apparent concentration-related suppression of CYP2C9 activity was observed in human hepatocytes after exposure to modafinil in vitro suggesting that there is a potential for a metabolic interaction between modafinil and substrates of CYP2C9).
No products indexed under this heading.

Mefenamic Acid (An apparent concentration-related suppression of CYP2C9 activity was observed in human hepatocytes after exposure to modafinil in vitro suggesting that there is a potential for a metabolic interaction between modafinil and substrates of CYP2C9).
No products indexed under this heading.

Meloxicam (An apparent concentration-related suppression of CYP2C9 activity was observed in human hepatocytes after exposure to modafinil in vitro suggesting that there is a potential for a metabolic interaction between modafinil and substrates of CYP2C9). Products include:
Mobic Oral Suspension 863
Mobic Tablets 863

Mephenytoin (Co-administration of potent inducers of CYP3A4 could alter the plasma levels of modafinil).
No products indexed under this heading.

Mestranol (The effectiveness of steroidal contraceptives may be reduced when used with modafinil tablets and for one month after discontinuation of therapy. Alternative or concomitant methods of contraception are recommended for patients treated with modafinil tablets and for one month after discontinuation of modafinil).
No products indexed under this heading.

Metformin Hydrochloride (An apparent concentration-related suppression of CYP2C9 activity was observed in human hepatocytes after exposure to modafinil in vitro suggesting that there is a potential for a metabolic interaction between modafinil and substrates of CYP2C9). Products include:
ActoPlus Met Tablets 3071
Avandamet Tablets 1336
Janumet Tablets 2041
PrandiMet Tablets 2967

Methadone Hydrochloride (Chronic administration of modafinil can increase the elimination of substrates of CYP3A4. Dose adjustments may be necessary for patients being treated with these and similar medications).
No products indexed under this heading.

Methsuximide (Co-administration of potent inducers of CYP3A4 could alter the plasma levels of modafinil).
No products indexed under this heading.

Methylphenidate Hydrochloride (May delay absorption of modafinil by approximately one hour; no significant alterations in pharmacokinetics of either drug). Products include:
Concerta Extended-Release Tablets 1925
Metadate CD Capsules 3146

Methylprednisolone (Co-administration of potent inducers of CYP3A4 could alter the plasma levels of modafinil).
No products indexed under this heading.

Methylprednisolone Acetate (Co-administration of potent inducers of CYP3A4 could alter the plasma levels of modafinil).
No products indexed under this heading.

Methylprednisolone Sodium Succinate (Co-administration of potent inducers of CYP3A4 could alter the plasma levels of modafinil).
No products indexed under this heading.

Metronidazole (Co-administration of potent inhibitors of CYP3A4 could alter the plasma levels of modafinil). Products include:
Pylera Capsules 714

Metronidazole Benzoate (Co-administration of potent inhibitors of CYP3A4 could alter the plasma levels of modafinil).
No products indexed under this heading.

Metronidazole Hydrochloride (Co-administration of potent inhibitors of CYP3A4 could alter the plasma levels of modafinil).
No products indexed under this heading.

Miconazole (Co-administration of potent inhibitors of CYP3A4 could alter the plasma levels of modafinil).
No products indexed under this heading.

Miconazole Nitrate (Co-administration of potent inhibitors of CYP3A4 could alter the plasma levels of modafinil).
No products indexed under this heading.

Midazolam Hydrochloride (Chronic administration of modafinil can increase the elimination of substrates of CYP3A4. Dose adjustments may be necessary for patients being treated with these and similar medications).
No products indexed under this heading.

Miglitol (An apparent concentration-related suppression of CYP2C9 activity was observed in human hepatocytes after exposure to modafinil in vitro suggesting that there is a potential for a metabolic interaction between modafinil and substrates of CYP2C9).
No products indexed under this heading.

Mirtazapine (An apparent concentration-related suppression of CYP2C9 activity was observed in human hepatocytes after exposure to modafinil in vitro suggesting that there is a potential for a metabolic interaction between modafinil and substrates of CYP2C9). Products include:
Remeron Tablets 2924
RemeronSolTab Tablets 2927

Moclobemide (Co-administration requires caution; no interaction studies have been performed).
No products indexed under this heading.

Montelukast Sodium (An apparent concentration-related suppression of CYP2C9 activity was observed in human hepatocytes after exposure to modafinil in vitro suggesting that there is a potential for a metabolic interaction between modafinil and substrates of CYP2C9). Products include:
Singulair 2114

Nabumetone (An apparent concentration-related suppression of CYP2C9 activity was observed in human hepatocytes after exposure to modafinil in vitro suggesting that there is a potential for a metabolic interaction between modafinil and substrates of CYP2C9).
No products indexed under this heading.

Naproxen (An apparent concentration-related suppression of CYP2C9 activity was observed in human hepatocytes after exposure to modafinil in vitro suggesting that there is a potential for a metabolic interaction between modafinil and substrates of CYP2C9). Products include:
EC-Naprosyn Delayed-Release Tablets 2632
Naprosyn Suspension 2632
Naprosyn Tablets 2632

Naproxen Sodium (An apparent concentration-related suppression of CYP2C9 activity was observed in human hepatocytes after exposure to modafinil in vitro suggesting that there is a potential for a metabolic interaction between modafinil and substrates of CYP2C9). Products include:
Anaprox Tablets 2632
Anaprox DS Tablets 2632
Treximet Tablets 1616

Nateglinide (An apparent concentration-related suppression of CYP2C9 activity was observed in human hepatocytes after exposure to modafinil in vitro suggesting that there is a potential for a metabolic interaction between modafinil and substrates of CYP2C9). Products include:
Starlix Tablets 2314

Nefazodone Hydrochloride (Chronic administration of modafinil can increase the elimination of substrates of CYP3A4. Dose adjustments may be necessary for patients being treated with these and similar medications).
No products indexed under this heading.

Nelfinavir Mesylate (Chronic administration of modafinil can increase the elimination of substrates of CYP3A4. Dose adjustments may be necessary for patients being treated with these and similar medications).
No products indexed under this heading.

Nevirapine (Co-administration of potent inducers of CYP3A4 could alter the plasma levels of modafinil). Products include:
Viramune Oral Suspension 873
Viramune Tablets 873

Niacinamide (Co-administration of potent inhibitors of CYP3A4 could alter the plasma levels of modafinil). Products include:
BioLean Free Tablets .... ■635

Nicardipine Hydrochloride (Chronic administration of modafinil can increase the elimination of substrates of CYP3A4. Dose adjustments may be necessary for patients being treated with these and similar medications). Products include:
Cardene I.V. 1093

Nicotinamide (Co-administration of potent inhibitors of CYP3A4 could alter the plasma levels of modafinil).
No products indexed under this heading.

Nifedipine (Chronic administration of modafinil can increase the elimination of substrates of CYP3A4. Dose adjustments may be necessary for patients being treated with these and similar medications).
No products indexed under this heading.

Nimodipine (Chronic administration of modafinil can increase the elimination of substrates of CYP3A4. Dose adjustments may be necessary for patients being treated with these and similar medications). Products include:
Nimotop Capsules 790

Nisoldipine (Chronic administration of modafinil can increase the elimination of substrates of CYP3A4. Dose adjustments may be necessary for patients being treated with these and similar medications). Products include:
Sular Extended Release Tablets 2975

Nitrendipine (Chronic administration of modafinil can increase the elimination of substrates of CYP3A4. Dose adjustments may be necessary for patients being treated with these and similar medications).
No products indexed under this heading.

Norethindrone (The effectiveness of steroidal contraceptives may be reduced when used with modafinil tablets and for one month after discontinuation of therapy. Alternative or concomitant methods of contraception are recommended for patients treated with modafinil tablets and for one month after discontinuation of modafinil). Products include:
Ortho Micronor Tablets 2446

Norethindrone Acetate (Chronic administration of modafinil can increase the elimination of substrates of CYP3A4. Dose adjustments may be necessary for patients being treated with these and similar medications). Products include:
Activella Tablets 2347

Norethynodrel (The effectiveness of steroidal contraceptives may be reduced when used with modafinil tablets and for one month after discontinuation of therapy. Alternative or concomitant methods of contraception are recommended for patients treated with modafinil tablets and for one month after discontinuation of modafinil).
No products indexed under this heading.

Norfloxacin (Co-administration of potent inhibitors of CYP3A4 could alter the plasma levels of modafinil). Products include:
Noroxin Tablets 2069

Norgestimate (The effectiveness of steroidal contraceptives may be reduced when used with modafinil tablets and for one month after discontinuation of therapy. Alternative or concomitant methods of contraception are recommended for patients treated with modafinil tablets and for one month after discontinuation of modafinil). Products include:
Ortho-Cyclen/Ortho Tri-Cyclen 2449
Ortho Tri-Cyclen Lo Tablets 2458

Norgestrel (The effectiveness of steroidal contraceptives may be reduced when used with modafinil tablets and for one month after discontinuation of therapy. Alternative or concomitant methods of contraception are recommended for patients treated with modafinil tablets and for one month after discontinuation of modafinil).
No products indexed under this heading.

Nortriptyline Hydrochloride (CYP2C19 provides an ancillary pathway for the metabolism of certain tricyclic antidepressants that are primarily metabolized by CYP2D6. In tricyclic-treated patients deficient in CYP2D6, the amount of metabolism by CYP2C19 may be substantially increased. Modafinil may cause elevation of the levels of these tricyclics in this subset of patients. A reduction in the dose of tricyclic agents might be needed in these patients).
No products indexed under this heading.

Omeprazole (An apparent concentration-related suppression of CYP2C9 activity was observed in human hepatocytes after exposure to modafinil in vitro suggesting that there is a potential for a metabolic interaction between modafinil and substrates of CYP2C9).
No products indexed under this heading.

Ondansetron (Chronic administration of modafinil can increase the elimination of substrates of CYP3A4. Dose adjustments may be necessary for patients being treated with these and similar medications). Products include:
Zofran ODT Orally Disintegrating Tablets 1687

Ondansetron Hydrochloride (Chronic administration of modafinil can increase the elimination of substrates of CYP3A4. Dose adjustments may be necessary for patients being treated with these and similar medications). Products include:
Zofran Injection 1682
Zofran 1687

Oxaprozin (An apparent concentration-related suppression of CYP2C9 activity was observed in human hepatocytes after exposure to modafinil in vitro suggesting that there is a potential for a metabolic interaction between modafinil and substrates of CYP2C9).
No products indexed under this heading.

Oxcarbazepine (Co-administration of potent inducers of CYP3A4 could alter the plasma levels of modafinil).
No products indexed under this heading.

Paclitaxel (Chronic administration of modafinil can increase the elimination of substrates of CYP3A4. Dose adjustments may be necessary for patients being treated with these and similar medications).
No products indexed under this heading.

Pargyline Hydrochloride (Co-administration requires caution; no interaction studies have been performed).
No products indexed under this heading.

Paroxetine Hydrochloride (Modafinil is a reversible inhibitor of the CYP2C19; the levels of CYP2D6 substrates, such as selective serotonin reuptake inhibitors, which have ancillary routes of elimination through CYP2D6, may be increased by co-administration of modafinil). Products include:
Paxil 1535
Paxil CR Controlled-Release Tablets 1544

Phenelzine Sulfate (Co-administration requires caution; no interaction studies have been performed).
No products indexed under this heading.

Phenobarbital (Chronic administration of modafinil may cause induction of its metabolism; co-administration of potent inducers of CYP3A4, such as phenobarbital, could alter the levels of modafinil due to the partial involvement of that enzyme in the metabolic elimination of the compound). Products include:
Donnatal Extentabs 2507

Phenobarbital Sodium (Co-administration of potent inducers of CYP3A4 could alter the plasma levels of modafinil).
No products indexed under this heading.

Phenylbutazone (An apparent concentration-related suppression of CYP2C9 activity was observed in human hepatocytes after exposure to modafinil in vitro suggesting that there is a potential for a metabolic interaction between modafinil and substrates of CYP2C9).
No products indexed under this heading.

Phenytoin (Modafinil is a reversible inhibitor of the CYP2C19; co-administration with drugs that are largely eliminated via this pathway, such as phenytoin, may increase the circulating levels of phenytoin).
No products indexed under this heading.

Phenytoin Sodium (Modafinil is a reversible inhibitor of the CYP2C19; co-administration with drugs that are largely eliminated via this pathway, such as phenytoin, may increase the circulating levels of phenytoin). Products include:
Phenytek Capsules 2192

Pimozide (Chronic administration of modafinil can increase the elimination of substrates of CYP3A4. Dose adjustments may be necessary for patients being treated with these and similar medications).
No products indexed under this heading.

Pioglitazone Hydrochloride (An apparent concentration-related suppression of CYP2C9 activity was observed in human hepatocytes after exposure to modafinil in vitro suggesting that there is a potential for a metabolic interaction between modafinil and substrates of CYP2C9). Products include:
ActoPlus Met Tablets 3071
Actos Tablets 3077
Duetact Tablets 3085

Piroxicam (An apparent concentration-related suppression of CYP2C9 activity was observed in human hepatocytes after exposure to modafinil in vitro suggesting that there is a potential for a metabolic interaction between modafinil and substrates of CYP2C9).
No products indexed under this heading.

Polyestradiol Phosphate (Chronic administration of modafinil can increase the elimination of substrates of CYP3A4. Dose adjustments may be necessary for patients being treated with these and similar medications).
No products indexed under this heading.

Prednisolone Acetate (Co-administration of potent inducers of CYP3A4 could alter the plasma levels of modafinil). Products include:
Pred Forte Ophthalmic Suspension .... ⊙227
Pred Mild Ophthalmic Suspension .... ⊙230
Pred-G Ophthalmic Ointment .... ⊙229
Pred-G Ophthalmic Suspension ...... ⊙228

Prednisolone Sodium Phosphate (Co-administration of potent inducers of CYP3A4 could alter the plasma levels of modafinil).
No products indexed under this heading.

Prednisolone Tebutate (Co-administration of potent inducers of CYP3A4 could alter the plasma levels of modafinil).
No products indexed under this heading.

Prednisone (Co-administration of potent inducers of CYP3A4 could alter the plasma levels of modafinil).
No products indexed under this heading.

Primidone (Co-administration of potent inducers of CYP3A4 could alter the plasma levels of modafinil).
No products indexed under this heading.

Procarbazine Hydrochloride (Co-administration requires caution; no interaction studies have been performed).
No products indexed under this heading.

Propoxyphene Hydrochloride (Co-administration of potent inhibitors of CYP3A4 could alter the plasma levels of modafinil).
No products indexed under this heading.

Propoxyphene Napsylate (Co-administration of potent inhibitors of CYP3A4 could alter the plasma levels of modafinil).
No products indexed under this heading.

Propranolol Hydrochloride (Modafinil is a reversible inhibitor of the CYP2C19; co-administration with drugs that are largely eliminated via this pathway, such as propranolol, may increase the circulating levels of propranolol). Products include:
InnoPran XL Extended Release Capsules 1484

Protriptyline Hydrochloride (CYP2C19 provides an ancillary pathway for the metabolism of certain tricyclic antidepressants that are primarily metabolized by CYP2D6. In tricyclic-treated patients deficient in CYP2D6, the amount of metabolism by CYP2C19 may be substantially increased. Modafinil may cause elevation of the levels of these tricyclics in this subset of patients. A reduction in the dose of tricyclic agents might be needed in these patients).
No products indexed under this heading.

Quinidine (Co-administration of potent inhibitors of CYP3A4 could alter the plasma levels of modafinil).
No products indexed under this heading.

Quinidine Gluconate (Chronic administration of modafinil can increase the elimination of substrates of CYP3A4. Dose adjustments may be necessary for patients being treated with these and similar medications).
No products indexed under this heading.

Quinidine Hydrochloride (Co-administration of potent inhibitors of CYP3A4 could alter the plasma levels of modafinil).
No products indexed under this heading.

Quinidine Polygalacturonate (Chronic administration of modafinil can increase the elimination of substrates of CYP3A4. Dose adjustments may be necessary for patients being treated with these and similar medications).
No products indexed under this heading.

Quinidine Sulfate (Chronic administration of modafinil can increase the elimination of substrates of CYP3A4. Dose adjustments may be necessary for patients being treated with these and similar medications).
No products indexed under this heading.

Quinine (Co-administration of potent inhibitors of CYP3A4 could alter the plasma levels of modafinil).
No products indexed under this heading.

Quinine Sulfate (Co-administration of potent inhibitors of CYP3A4 could alter the plasma levels of modafinil).
No products indexed under this heading.

Quinupristin (Co-administration of potent inhibitors of CYP3A4 could alter the plasma levels of modafinil).
No products indexed under this heading.

Ranitidine Bismuth Citrate (Co-administration of potent inhibitors of CYP3A4 could alter the plasma levels of modafinil).
No products indexed under this heading.

Ranitidine Hydrochloride (Co-administration of potent inhibitors of CYP3A4 could alter the plasma levels of modafinil). Products include:
Zantac 75 Tablets .... ▣ 603
Zantac 1670
Zantac Injection 1666
Zantac Injection Pharmacy Bulk Package 1668
Maximum Strength Zantac 150 Tablets .... ▣ 603
Maximum Strength Zantac 150 Cool Mint Tablets .... ▣ 603

Rasagiline Mesylate (Co-administration requires caution; no interaction studies have been performed). Products include:
Azilect Tablets 3106

Repaglinide (An apparent concentration-related suppression of CYP2C9 activity was observed in human hepatocytes after exposure to modafinil in vitro suggesting that there is a potential for a metabolic interaction between modafinil and substrates of CYP2C9). Products include:
PrandiMet Tablets 2967
Prandin Tablets 2971

Rifabutin (Chronic administration of modafinil can increase the elimination of substrates of CYP3A4. Dose adjustments may be necessary for patients being treated with these and similar medications).
No products indexed under this heading.

Rifampicin (Co-administration of potent inducers of CYP3A4 could alter the plasma levels of modafinil).
No products indexed under this heading.

Rifampin (Chronic administration of modafinil may cause induction of its metabolism; co-administration of potent inducers of CYP3A4, such as rifampin, could alter the levels of modafinil due to the partial involvement of that enzyme in the metabolic elimination of the compound).
No products indexed under this heading.

Rifapentine (Co-administration of potent inducers of CYP3A4 could alter the plasma levels of modafinil).
No products indexed under this heading.

Ritonavir (Chronic administration of modafinil can increase the elimination of substrates of CYP3A4. Dose adjustments may be necessary for patients being treated with these and similar medications). Products include:
Kaletra 452
Norvir 489

Rofecoxib (An apparent concentration-related suppression of CYP2C9 activity was observed in human hepatocytes after exposure to modafinil in vitro suggesting that there is a potential for a metabolic interaction between modafinil and substrates of CYP2C9).
No products indexed under this heading.

Rosiglitazone Maleate (An apparent concentration-related suppression of CYP2C9 activity was observed in human hepatocytes after exposure to modafinil in vitro suggesting that there is a potential for a metabolic interaction between modafinil and substrates of CYP2C9). Products include:
Avandamet Tablets 1336
Avandaryl Tablets 1344
Avandia Tablets 1351

Saquinavir (Chronic administration of modafinil can increase the elimination of substrates of CYP3A4. Dose adjustments may be necessary for patients being treated with these and similar medications).
No products indexed under this heading.

Saquinavir Mesylate (Chronic administration of modafinil can increase the elimination of substrates of CYP3A4. Dose adjustments may be necessary for patients being treated with these and similar medications).
No products indexed under this heading.

Selegiline (Co-administration requires caution; no interaction studies have been performed). Products include:
Emsam Transdermal System 905

Selegiline Hydrochloride (Co-administration requires caution; no interaction studies have been performed). Products include:
Eldepryl Capsules 3052

Sertraline Hydrochloride (Modafinil is a reversible inhibitor of the CYP2C19; the levels of CYP2D6 substrates, such as selective serotonin reuptake inhibitors, which have ancillary routes of elimination through CYP2D6, may be increased by co-administration of modafinil).
No products indexed under this heading.

Sildenafil Citrate (Chronic administration of modafinil can increase the elimination of substrates of CYP3A4. Dose adjustments may be necessary for patients being treated with these and similar medications).
No products indexed under this heading.

Simvastatin (Chronic administration of modafinil can increase the elimination of substrates of CYP3A4. Dose adjustments may be necessary for patients being treated with these and similar medications). Products include:
Simcor Tablets 502
Vytorin 10/10 Tablets 2149
Vytorin 10/10 Tablets 2939
Vytorin 10/20 Tablets 2149
Vytorin 10/20 Tablets 2939
Vytorin 10/40 Tablets 2149
Vytorin 10/40 Tablets 2939
Vytorin 10/80 Tablets 2149
Vytorin 10/80 Tablets 2939
Zocor Tablets 2136

Sirolimus (Chronic administration of modafinil can increase the elimination of substrates of CYP3A4. Dose adjustments may be necessary for patients being treated with these and similar medications). Products include:
Rapamune 3260

Sulfamethoxazole (An apparent concentration-related suppression of CYP2C9 activity was observed in human hepatocytes after exposure to modafinil in vitro suggesting that there is a potential for a metabolic interaction between modafinil and substrates of CYP2C9).
No products indexed under this heading.

Sulfinpyrazone (Co-administration of potent inducers of CYP3A4 could alter the plasma levels of modafinil).
No products indexed under this heading.

Sulindac (An apparent concentration-related suppression of CYP2C9 activity was observed in human hepatocytes after exposure to modafinil in vitro suggesting that there is a potential for a metabolic interaction between modafinil and substrates of CYP2C9). Products include:
Clinoril Tablets 1962

Suprofen (An apparent concentration-related suppression of CYP2C9 activity was observed in human hepatocytes after exposure to modafinil in vitro suggesting that there is a potential for a metabolic interaction between modafinil and substrates of CYP2C9).
No products indexed under this heading.

Tacrolimus (Chronic administration of modafinil can increase the elimination of substrates of CYP3A4. Dose adjustments may be necessary for patients being treated with these and similar medications). Products include:
Prograf Capsules and Injection 622
Protopic Ointment 628

Tadalafil (Chronic administration of modafinil can increase the elimination of substrates of CYP3A4. Dose adjustments may be necessary for patients being treated with these and similar medications). Products include:
Cialis Tablets 1792

Tamoxifen Citrate (Chronic administration of modafinil can increase the elimination of substrates of CYP3A4. Dose adjustments may be necessary for patients being treated with these and similar medications).
No products indexed under this heading.

Telithromycin (Co-administration of potent inhibitors of CYP3A4 could alter the plasma levels of modafinil). Products include:
Ketek Tablets 2744

Telmisartan (An apparent concentration-related suppression of CYP2C9 activity was observed in human hepatocytes after exposure to modafinil in vitro suggesting that there is a potential for a metabolic interaction between modafinil and substrates of CYP2C9). Products include:
Micardis Tablets 852
Micardis HCT Tablets 854

Theophylline (Chronic administration of modafinil may cause modest induction of CYP3A4, thus reducing the levels, to a lesser degree, of co-administered substrate for that enzyme system, such as theophylline).
No products indexed under this heading.

Theophylline Anhydrous (Chronic administration of modafinil may cause modest induction of CYP3A4, thus reducing the levels, to a lesser degree, of co-administered substrate for that enzyme system, such as theophylline). Products include:
Uniphyl Tablets 2595

Theophylline Calcium Salicylate (Chronic administration of modafinil may cause modest induction of CYP3A4, thus reducing the levels, to a lesser degree, of co-administered substrate for that enzyme system, such as theophylline).
No products indexed under this heading.

Theophylline Dihydroxypropyl (Glyceryl) (Chronic administration of modafinil may cause modest induction of CYP3A4, thus reducing the levels, to a lesser degree, of co-administered substrate for that enzyme system, such as theophylline).
No products indexed under this heading.

Theophylline Ethylenediamine (Chronic administration of modafinil may cause modest induction of CYP3A4, thus reducing the levels, to a lesser degree, of co-administered substrate for that enzyme system, such as theophylline).
No products indexed under this heading.

Theophylline Sodium Glycinate (Chronic administration of modafinil may cause modest induction of CYP3A4, thus reducing the levels, to a lesser degree, of co-administered substrate for that enzyme system, such as theophylline).
No products indexed under this heading.

Tiagabine Hydrochloride (Chronic administration of modafinil can increase the elimination of substrates of CYP3A4. Dose adjustments may be necessary for patients being treated with these and similar medications). Products include:
Gabitril Tablets 973

Tolazamide (An apparent concentration-related suppression of CYP2C9 activity was observed in human hepatocytes after exposure to modafinil in vitro suggesting that there is a potential for a metabolic interaction between modafinil and substrates of CYP2C9).
No products indexed under this heading.

Tolbutamide (An apparent concentration-related suppression of CYP2C9 activity was observed in human hepatocytes after exposure to modafinil in vitro suggesting that there is a potential for a metabolic interaction between modafinil and substrates of CYP2C9).
No products indexed under this heading.

Tolbutamide Sodium (An apparent concentration-related suppression of CYP2C9 activity was observed in human hepatocytes after exposure to modafinil in vitro suggesting that there is a potential for a metabolic interaction between modafinil and substrates of CYP2C9).
No products indexed under this heading.

Tolmetin Sodium (An apparent concentration-related suppression of CYP2C9 activity was observed in human hepatocytes after exposure to modafinil in vitro suggesting that there is a potential for a metabolic interaction between modafinil and substrates of CYP2C9).
No products indexed under this heading.

Tolterodine Tartrate (Chronic administration of modafinil can increase the elimination of substrates of CYP3A4. Dose adjustments may be necessary for patients being treated with these and similar medications).
No products indexed under this heading.

Torsemide (An apparent concentration-related suppression of CYP2C9 activity was observed in human hepatocytes after exposure to modafinil in vitro suggesting that there is a potential for a metabolic interaction between modafinil and substrates of CYP2C9). Products include:
Demadex Injection 2630
Demadex Tablets 2630

Tranylcypromine Sulfate (Co-administration requires caution; no interaction studies have been performed). Products include:
Parnate Tablets 1532

Trazodone Hydrochloride (Chronic administration of modafinil can increase the elimination of substrates of CYP3A4. Dose adjustments may be necessary for patients being treated with these and similar medications).
No products indexed under this heading.

Triamcinolone (Co-administration of potent inducers of CYP3A4 could alter the plasma levels of modafinil).
No products indexed under this heading.

Triamcinolone Acetonide (Co-administration of potent inducers of CYP3A4 could alter the plasma levels of modafinil). Products include:
Azmacort Inhalation Aerosol 407
Nasacort AQ Nasal Spray 2765
Triesence Injectable Suspension .... ⊙209

Triamcinolone Diacetate (Co-administration of potent inducers of CYP3A4 could alter the plasma levels of modafinil).
No products indexed under this heading.

Triamcinolone Hexacetonide (Co-administration of potent inducers of CYP3A4 could alter the plasma levels of modafinil).
No products indexed under this heading.

Triazolam (When modafinil was administered concurrently with triazolam, mean Cmax and AUC of triazolam were decreased by 42% and 59%, respectively, and its elimination half-life was decreased by approximately an hour after the modafinil treatment).
No products indexed under this heading.

Trimipramine Maleate (CYP2C19 provides an ancillary pathway for the metabolism of certain tricyclic antidepressants that are primarily metabolized by CYP2D6. In tricyclic-treated patients deficient in CYP2D6, the amount of metabolism by CYP2C19 may be substantially increased. Modafinil may cause elevation of the levels of these tricyclics in this subset of patients. A reduction in the dose of tricyclic agents might be needed in these patients).
No products indexed under this heading.

Troglitazone (An apparent concentration-related suppression of CYP2C9 activity was observed in human hepatocytes after exposure to modafinil in vitro suggesting that there is a potential for a metabolic interaction between modafinil and substrates of CYP2C9).
No products indexed under this heading.

Troleandomycin (Co-administration of potent inhibitors of CYP3A4 could alter the plasma levels of modafinil).
No products indexed under this heading.

Valdecoxib (An apparent concentration-related suppression of CYP2C9 activity was observed in human hepatocytes after exposure to modafinil in vitro suggesting that there is a potential for a metabolic interaction between modafinil and substrates of CYP2C9).
No products indexed under this heading.

Valproate Sodium (Co-administration of potent inhibitors of CYP3A4 could alter the plasma levels of modafinil).
No products indexed under this heading.

Valsartan (An apparent concentration-related suppression of CYP2C9 activity was observed in human hepatocytes after exposure to modafinil in vitro suggesting that there is a potential for a metabolic interaction between modafinil and substrates of CYP2C9). Products include:
Diovan Tablets 2212
Diovan HCT Tablets 2216
Exforge Tablets 2238

Vardenafil Hydrochloride (Chronic administration of modafinil can increase the elimination of substrates of CYP3A4. Dose adjustments may be necessary for patients being treated with these and similar medications). Products include:
Levitra Tablets 2876

Verapamil Hydrochloride (Chronic administration of modafinil can increase the elimination of substrates of CYP3A4. Dose adjustments may be necessary for patients being treated with these and similar medications). Products include:
Tarka Tablets 511

Vinblastine Sulfate (Chronic administration of modafinil can increase the elimination of substrates of CYP3A4. Dose adjustments may be necessary for patients being treated with these and similar medications).
No products indexed under this heading.

Vincristine Sulfate (Chronic administration of modafinil can increase the elimination of substrates of CYP3A4. Dose adjustments may be necessary for patients being treated with these and similar medications).
No products indexed under this heading.

Voriconazole (An apparent concentration-related suppression of CYP2C9 activity was observed in human hepatocytes after exposure to modafinil in vitro suggesting that there is a potential for a metabolic interaction between modafinil and substrates of CYP2C9).
No products indexed under this heading.

Warfarin Sodium (There were no significant changes in the pharmacokinetic profile of warfarin in healthy subjects given a single dose of warfarin following chronic administration of modafinil relative to the profiles in subjects given placebo. However, more frequent monitoring of prothrombin times/INR is advisable whenever modafinil is co-administered with warfarin).
No products indexed under this heading.

Zafirlukast (An apparent concentration-related suppression of CYP2C9 activity was observed in human hepatocytes after exposure to modafinil in vitro suggesting that there is a potential for a metabolic interaction between modafinil and substrates of CYP2C9). Products include:
Accolate Tablets 669

Zileuton (An apparent concentration-related suppression of CYP2C9 activity was observed in human hepatocytes after exposure to modafinil in vitro suggesting that there is a potential for a metabolic interaction between modafinil and substrates of CYP2C9).
No products indexed under this heading.

Food Interactions

Alcohol (The use of modafinil in combination with alcohol has not been studied. It is advisable to avoid alcohol while taking modafinil).

Food, unspecified (Delays the absorption (tmax) by approximately one hour; no effect on overall bioavailability).

Grapefruit (Co-administration of potent inhibitors of CYP3A4 could alter the plasma levels of modafinil).

Grapefruit Juice (Co-administration of potent inhibitors of CYP3A4 could alter the plasma levels of modafinil).

PROXTREME PROTEIN SUPPLEMENT

(Amino Acid Preparations, Folic Acid, Protein Preparations, Vitamins with Minerals)...................... ▣639
None cited in PDR database.

PROZAC WEEKLY CAPSULES

(Fluoxetine Hydrochloride) 1852
May interact with aspirin-acetylsalicylic acid, central nervous system depressants, central nervous system stimulants, anticoagulants, cytochrome p450 2d6 substrates (selected), diuretics, oral hypoglycemic agents, insulin, lithium preparations, monoamine oxidase inhibitors, nonsteroidal anti-inflammatory agents, phenothiazines, phenytoin, highly protein bound drugs (selected), serotoninergic agents, Serotonin and Norepinephrine Reuptake Inhibitors, selective serotonin reuptake inhibitors, tricyclic antidepressants, triptans, and certain other agents. Compounds in these categories include:

Acarbose (In patients with diabetes, fluoxetine may alter glycemic control. Hypoglycemia has occurred during therapy with fluoxetine, and hyperglycemia has developed following discontinuation of the drug. As is true with many other types of medication when taken concurrently by patients with diabetes, oral hypoglycemic dosage may need to be adjusted when therapy with fluoxetine is instituted or discontinued). Products include:

Precose Tablets **792**

Alfentanil Hydrochloride (The risk of using fluoxetine in combination with other CNS active drugs has not been systematically evaluated. Nonetheless, caution is advised if the concomitant administration of fluoxetine and such drugs is required. In evaluating individual cases, consideration should be given to using lower initial doses of the concomitantly administered drugs, using conservative titration schedules, and monitoring of clinical status).
No products indexed under this heading.

Almotriptan Malate (There have been rare postmarketing reports of serotonin syndrome with use of an SSRI and a triptan. If concomitant treatment of fluoxetine with a triptan is clinically warranted, careful observation of the patient is advised, particularly during treatment initiation and dose increases). Products include:
Axert Tablets **2431**

Alprazolam (Co-administration of alprazolam and fluoxetine has resulted in increased alprazolam plasma concentrations and in further psychomotor performance decrement due to increase alprazolam levels).
No products indexed under this heading.

Amiloride Hydrochloride (Hyponatremia may occur as a result of treatment with SSRIs, including fluoxetine. In many cases this hyponatremia appears to be the result of the syndrome of inappropriate antidiuretic hormone secretion (SIADH). Cases with serum sodium lower than 110 mmol/L have been reported and appeared to be reversible when fluoxetine was discontinued. Patients taking diuretics may be at greater risk. Discontinuation of fluoxetine should be considered in patients with symptomatic hyponatremia and appropriate medical intervention should be instituted).
No products indexed under this heading.

Amiodarone Hydrochloride (Because fluoxetine is tightly bound to plasma protein, the administration of fluoxetine to a patient taking another drugs that is tightly bound to protein may cause a shift in plasma concentrations potentially resulting in an adverse effect. Conversely,adverse effects may result from displacement of protein-bound fluoxetine by other tightly-bound drugs).
No products indexed under this heading.

Amitriptyline Hydrochloride (Fluoxetine inhibits the activity of CYP2D6, and may make individuals with normal CYP2D6 metabolic activity resemble a poor metabolizer. Co-administration of fluoxetine with other drugs that are metabolized by CYP2D6, including TCAs, should be approached with caution. Therapy with medications that are predominantly metabolized by the CYP2D6 system and that have a relatively narrow therapeutic index (eg, TCAs) should be initiated at the low end of the dose range if a patient is receiving fluoxetine concurrently or has taken it in the previous 5 weeks. If fluoxetine is added to the treatment regimen of a patient already receiving a drug metabolized by CYP2D6, the need for decreased dose of the original medication should be considered).
No products indexed under this heading.

Amoxapine (Fluoxetine inhibits the activity of CYP2D6, and may make individuals with normal CYP2D6 metabolic activity resemble a poor metabolizer. Co-administration of fluoxetine with other drugs that are metabolized by CYP2D6, including TCAs, should be approached with caution. Therapy with medications that are predominantly metabolized by the CYP2D6 system and that have a relatively narrow therapeutic index (eg, TCAs) should be initiated at the low end of the dose range if a patient is receiving fluoxetine concurrently or has taken it in the previous 5 weeks. If fluoxetine is added to the treatment regimen of a patient already receiving a drug metabolized by CYP2D6, the need for decreased dose of the original medication should be considered).
No products indexed under this heading.

Amphetamine Aspartate (Fluoxetine inhibits the activity of CYP2D6, and may make individuals with normal CYP2D6 metabolic activity resemble a poor metabolizer. Co-administration of fluoxetine with other drugs that are metabolized by CYP2D6 should be approached with caution. Therapy with medications that are predominantly metabolized by the CYP2D6 system and that have a relatively narrow therapeutic index should be initiated at the low end of the dose range if a patient is receiving fluoxetine concurrently or has taken it in the previous 5 weeks. If fluoxetine is added to the treatment regimen of a patient already receiving a drug metabolized by CYP2D6, the need for decreased dose of the original medication should be considered). Products include:
Adderall XR Capsules **3012**

Amphetamine Aspartate Monohydrate (Fluoxetine inhibits the activity of CYP2D6, and may make individuals with normal CYP2D6 metabolic activity resemble a poor metabolizer. Co-administration of fluoxetine with other drugs that are metabolized by CYP2D6 should be approached with caution. Therapy with medications that are predominantly metabolized by the CYP2D6 system and that have a relatively narrow therapeutic index should be initiated at the low end of the dose range if a patient is receiving fluoxetine concurrently or has taken it in the previous 5 weeks. If fluoxetine is added to the treatment regimen of a patient already receiving a drug metabolized by CYP2D6, the need for decreased dose of the original medication should be considered).
No products indexed under this heading.

Amphetamine Resins (The risk of using fluoxetine in combination with other CNS active drugs has not been systematically evaluated. Nonetheless, caution is advised if the concomitant administration of fluoxetine and such drugs is required. In evaluating individual cases, consideration should be given to using lower initial doses of the concomitantly administered drugs, using conservative titration schedules, and monitoring of clinical status).
No products indexed under this heading.

Amphetamine Sulfate (Fluoxetine inhibits the activity of CYP2D6, and may make individuals with normal CYP2D6 metabolic activity resemble a poor metabolizer. Co-administration of fluoxetine with other drugs that are metabolized by CYP2D6 should be approached with caution. Therapy with medications that are predominantly metabolized by the CYP2D6 system and that have a relatively narrow therapeutic index should be initiated at the low end of the dose range if a patient is receiving fluoxetine concurrently or has taken it in the previous 5 weeks. If fluoxetine is added to the treatment regimen of a patient already receiving a drug metabolized by CYP2D6, the need for decreased dose of the original medication should be considered). Products include:
Adderall XR Capsules **3012**

Anisindione (Case reports and epidemiological studies (case-control and cohort design) have demonstrated an association between use of drugs that interfere with serotonin reuptake and the occurrence of gastrointestinal bleeding. Bleeding events related to SSRI use have ranged from ecchymoses, hematomas, epistaxis, and petechiae to live-threatening hemorrhages. Patients should be cautioned about the risk of bleeding associated with the concomitant use of fluoxetine and other drugs that affect coagulation).
No products indexed under this heading.

Aprobarbital (The risk of using fluoxetine in combination with other CNS active drugs has not been systematically evaluated. Nonetheless, caution is advised if the concomitant administration of fluoxetine and such drugs is required. In evaluating individual cases, consideration should be given to using lower initial doses of the concomitantly administered drugs, using conservative titration schedules, and monitoring of clinical status).
No products indexed under this heading.

Ardeparin Sodium (Case reports and epidemiological studies (case-control and cohort design) have demonstrated an association between use of drugs that interfere with serotonin reuptake and the occurrence of gastrointestinal bleeding. Bleeding events related to SSRI use have ranged from ecchymoses, hematomas, epistaxis, and petechiae to live-threatening hemorrhages. Patients should be cautioned about the risk of bleeding associated with the concomitant use of fluoxetine and other drugs that affect coagulation).
No products indexed under this heading.

Aspirin (SSRIs, including fluoxetine, may increase the risk of bleeding events. Concomitant use of aspirin may add to this risk. Case reports and epidemiological studies (case-control and cohort design) have demonstrated an association between use of drugs thatinterfere with serotonin reuptake and the occurrence of gastrointestinal bleeding. Bleeding events related to SSRI use have ranged from ecchymoses, hematomas, epistaxis, and petechiae to live-threatening hemorrhages. Patients should be cautioned about the risk of bleeding associated with the concomitant use of fluoxetine and aspirin). Products include:
Aggrenox Capsules **819**
Bayer Aspirin **750**
Percodan Tablets **1130**
St. Joseph 81 mg Aspirin Chewable and Enteric Coated Tablets **1903**

Aspirin, Enteric Coated (SSRIs, including fluoxetine, may increase the risk of bleeding events. Concomitant use of aspirin may add to this risk. Case reports and epidemiological studies (case-control and cohort design) have demonstrated an association between use of drugs thatinterfere with serotonin reuptake and the occurrence of gastrointestinal bleeding. Bleeding events related to SSRI use have ranged from ecchymoses, hematomas, epistaxis, and petechiae to live-threatening hemorrhages. Patients should be cautioned about the risk of bleeding associated with the concomitant use of fluoxetine and aspirin).
No products indexed under this heading.

Aspirin Buffered (SSRIs, including fluoxetine, may increase the risk of bleeding events. Concomitant use of aspirin may add to this risk. Case reports and epidemiological studies (case-control and cohort design) have demonstrated an association between use of drugs thatinterfere with serotonin reuptake and the occurrence of gastrointestinal bleeding. Bleeding events related to SSRI use have ranged from ecchymoses, hematomas, epistaxis, and petechiae to live-threatening hemorrhages. Patients should be cautioned about the risk of bleeding associated with the concomitant use of fluoxetine and aspirin).
No products indexed under this heading.

Atomoxetine Hydrochloride (Fluoxetine inhibits the activity of CYP2D6, and may make individuals with normal CYP2D6 metabolic activity resemble a poor metabolizer. Co-administration of fluoxetine with other drugs that are metabolized by CYP2D6 should be approached with caution. Therapy with medications that are predominantly metabolized by the CYP2D6 system and that have a relatively narrow therapeutic index should be initiated at the low end of the dose range if a patient is receiving fluoxetine concurrently or has taken it in the previous 5 weeks. If fluoxetine is added to the treatment regimen of a patient already receiving a drug metabolized by CYP2D6, the need for decreased dose of the original medication should be considered). Products include:
Strattera Capsules **1864**

Atovaquone (Because fluoxetine is tightly bound to plasma protein, the administration of fluoxetine to a patient taking another drugs that is tightly bound to protein may cause a shift in plasma concentrations potentially resulting in an adverse effect. Conversely,adverse effects may

result from displacement of protein-bound fluoxetine by other tightly-bound drugs). Products include:
Malarone Pediatric Tablets 1521
Malarone Tablets 1521
Mepron Suspension 1526

Bendroflumethiazide (Hyponatremia may occur as a result of treatment with SSRIs, including fluoxetine. In many cases this hyponatremia appears to be the result of the syndrome of inappropriate antidiuretic hormone secretion (SIADH). Cases with serum sodium lower than 110 mmol/L have been reported and appeared to be reversible when fluoxetine was discontinued. Patients taking diuretics may be at greater risk. Discontinuation of fluoxetine should be considered in patients with symptomatic hyponatremia and appropriate medical intervention should be instituted).
No products indexed under this heading.

Bisoprolol Fumarate (Fluoxetine inhibits the activity of CYP2D6, and may make individuals with normal CYP2D6 metabolic activity resemble a poor metabolizer. Co-administration of fluoxetine with other drugs that are metabolized by CYP2D6 should be approached with caution. Therapy with medications that are predominantly metabolized by the CYP2D6 system and that have a relatively narrow therapeutic index should be initiated at the low end of the dose range if a patient is receiving fluoxetine concurrently or has taken it in the previous 5 weeks. If fluoxetine is added to the treatment regimen of a patient already receiving a drug metabolized by CYP2D6, the need for decreased dose of the original medication should be considered).
No products indexed under this heading.

Bumetanide (Hyponatremia may occur as a result of treatment with SSRIs, including fluoxetine. In many cases this hyponatremia appears to be the result of the syndrome of inappropriate antidiuretic hormone secretion (SIADH). Cases with serum sodium lower than 110 mmol/L have been reported and appeared to be reversible when fluoxetine was discontinued. Patients taking diuretics may be at greater risk. Discontinuation of fluoxetine should be considered in patients with symptomatic hyponatremia and appropriate medical intervention should be instituted).
No products indexed under this heading.

Buprenorphine Hydrochloride (The risk of using fluoxetine in combination with other CNS active drugs has not been systematically evaluated. Nonetheless, caution is advised if the concomitant administration of fluoxetine and such drugs is required. In evaluating individual cases, consideration should be given to using lower initial doses of the concomitantly administered drugs, using conservative titration schedules, and monitoring of clinical status). Products include:
Suboxone Tablets 2601
Subutex Tablets 2601

Buspirone Hydrochloride (The risk of using fluoxetine in combination with other CNS active drugs has not been systematically evaluated. Nonetheless, caution is advised if the concomitant administration of fluoxetine and such drugs is required. In evaluating individual cases, consideration should be given to using lower initial doses of the concomitantly administered drugs, using conservative titration schedules, and monitoring of clinical status).
No products indexed under this heading.

Butabarbital (The risk of using fluoxetine in combination with other CNS active drugs has not been systematically evaluated. Nonetheless, caution is advised if the concomitant administration of fluoxetine and such drugs is required. In evaluating individual cases, consideration should be given to using lower initial doses of the concomitantly administered drugs, using conservative titration schedules, and monitoring of clinical status).
No products indexed under this heading.

Butalbital (The risk of using fluoxetine in combination with other CNS active drugs has not been systematically evaluated. Nonetheless, caution is advised if the concomitant administration of fluoxetine and such drugs is required. In evaluating individual cases, consideration should be given to using lower initial doses of the concomitantly administered drugs, using conservative titration schedules, and monitoring of clinical status).
No products indexed under this heading.

Captopril (Fluoxetine inhibits the activity of CYP2D6, and may make individuals with normal CYP2D6 metabolic activity resemble a poor metabolizer. Co-administration of fluoxetine with other drugs that are metabolized by CYP2D6 should be approached with caution. Therapy with medications that are predominantly metabolized by the CYP2D6 system and that have a relatively narrow therapeutic index should be initiated at the low end of the dose range if a patient is receiving fluoxetine concurrently or has taken it in the previous 5 weeks. If fluoxetine is added to the treatment regimen of a patient already receiving a drug metabolized by CYP2D6, the need for decreased dose of the original medication should be considered). Products include:
Captopril Tablets 2182

Carbamazepine (Patients on stable doses of carbamazepine have developed elevated plasma anticonvulsant concentrations and clinical anticonvulsant toxicity following initiation of concomitant fluoxetine treatment). Products include:
Carbatrol Capsules 3019
Equetro Extended-Release Capsules 3174

Carvedilol (Fluoxetine inhibits the activity of CYP2D6, and may make individuals with normal CYP2D6 metabolic activity resemble a poor metabolizer. Co-administration of fluoxetine with other drugs that are metabolized by CYP2D6 should be approached with caution. Therapy with medications that are predominantly metabolized by the CYP2D6 system and that have a relatively narrow therapeutic index should be initiated at the low end of the dose range if a patient is receiving fluoxetine concurrently or has taken it in the previous 5 weeks. If fluoxetine is added to the treatment regimen of a patient already receiving a drug metabolized by CYP2D6, the need for decreased dose of the original medication should be considered). Products include:
Coreg Tablets 1387

Cefonicid Sodium (Because fluoxetine is tightly bound to plasma protein, the administration of fluoxetine to a patient taking another drugs that is tightly bound to protein may cause a shift in plasma concentrations potentially resulting in an adverse effect. Conversely,adverse effects may result from displacement of protein-bound fluoxetine by other tightly-bound drugs).
No products indexed under this heading.

Celecoxib (SSRIs, including fluoxetine, may increase the risk of bleeding events. Concomitant use of non-steroidal anti-inflammatory drugs may add to this risk. Case reports and epidemiological studies (case-control and cohort design) have demonstrated an association between use of drugs that interfere with serotonin reuptake and the occurrence of gastrointestinal bleeding. Bleeding events related to SSRI use have ranged from ecchymoses, hematomas, epistaxis, and petechiae to live-threatening hemorrhages. Patients should be cautioned about the risk of bleeding associated with the concomitant use of fluoxetine and NSAIDs). Products include:
Celebrex Capsules 2979

Cevimeline Hydrochloride (Fluoxetine inhibits the activity of CYP2D6, and may make individuals with normal CYP2D6 metabolic activity resemble a poor metabolizer. Co-administration of fluoxetine with other drugs that are metabolized by CYP2D6 should be approached with caution. Therapy with medications that are predominantly metabolized by the CYP2D6 system and that have a relatively narrow therapeutic index should be initiated at the low end of the dose range if a patient is receiving fluoxetine concurrently or has taken it in the previous 5 weeks. If fluoxetine is added to the treatment regimen of a patient already receiving a drug metabolized by CYP2D6, the need for decreased dose of the original medication should be considered). Products include:
Evoxac Capsules 1013

Chlordiazepoxide (The risk of using fluoxetine in combination with other CNS active drugs has not been systematically evaluated. Nonetheless, caution is advised if the concomitant administration of fluoxetine and such drugs is required. In evaluating individual cases, consideration should be given to using lower initial doses of the concomitantly administered drugs, using conservative titration schedules, and monitoring of clinical status).
No products indexed under this heading.

Chlordiazepoxide Hydrochloride (The risk of using fluoxetine in combination with other CNS active drugs has not been systematically evaluated. Nonetheless, caution is advised if the concomitant administration of fluoxetine and such drugs is required. In evaluating individual cases, consideration should be given to using lower initial doses of the concomitantly administered drugs, using conservative titration schedules, and monitoring of clinical status).
No products indexed under this heading.

Chlorothiazide (Hyponatremia may occur as a result of treatment with SSRIs, including fluoxetine. In many cases this hyponatremia appears to be the result of the syndrome of inappropriate antidiuretic hormone secretion (SIADH). Cases with serum sodium lower than 110 mmol/L have been reported and appeared to be reversible when fluoxetine was discontinued. Patients taking diuretics may be at greater risk. Discontinuation of fluoxetine should be considered in patients with symptomatic hyponatremia and appropriate medical intervention should be instituted).
No products indexed under this heading.

Chlorothiazide Sodium (Hyponatremia may occur as a result of treatment with SSRIs, including fluoxetine. In many cases this hyponatremia appears to be the result of the syndrome of inappropriate antidiuretic hormone secretion (SIADH). Cases with serum sodium lower than 110 mmol/L have been reported and appeared to be reversible when fluoxetine was discontinued. Patients taking diuretics may be at greater risk. Discontinuation of fluoxetine should be considered in patients with symptomatic hyponatremia and appropriate medical intervention should be instituted). Products include:
Intravenous Sodium Diuril 2490

Chlorpromazine (Fluoxetine inhibits the activity of CYP2D6, and may make individuals with normal CYP2D6 metabolic activity resemble a poor metabolizer. Co-administration of fluoxetine with other drugs that are metabolized by CYP2D6, including phenothiazines, should be approached with caution. If fluoxetine is added to the treatment regimen of a patient already receiving a drug metabolized by CYP2D6, the need for decreased dose of the original medication should be considered).
No products indexed under this heading.

Chlorpromazine Hydrochloride (Fluoxetine inhibits the activity of CYP2D6, and may make individuals with normal CYP2D6 metabolic activity resemble a poor metabolizer. Co-administration of fluoxetine with other drugs that are metabolized by CYP2D6, including phenothiazines, should be approached with caution. If fluoxetine is added to the treatment regimen of a patient already receiving a drug metabolized by CYP2D6, the need for decreased dose of the original medication should be considered).
No products indexed under this heading.

Chlorpropamide (Fluoxetine inhibits the activity of CYP2D6, and may make individuals with normal CYP2D6 metabolic activity resemble a poor metabolizer. Co-administration of fluoxetine with other drugs that are metabolized by

CYP2D6 should be approached with caution. Therapy with medications that are predominantly metabolized by the CYP2D6 system and that have a relatively narrow therapeutic index should be initiated at the low end of the dose range if a patient is receiving fluoxetine concurrently or has taken it in the previous 5 weeks. If fluoxetine is added to the treatment regimen of a patient already receiving a drug metabolized by CYP2D6, the need for decreased dose of the original medication should be considered).

No products indexed under this heading.

Chlorprothixene (The risk of using fluoxetine in combination with other CNS active drugs has not been systematically evaluated. Nonetheless, caution is advised if the concomitant administration of fluoxetine and such drugs is required. In evaluating individual cases, consideration should be given to using lower initial doses of the concomitantly administered drugs, using conservative titration schedules, and monitoring of clinical status).

No products indexed under this heading.

Chlorprothixene Hydrochloride (The risk of using fluoxetine in combination with other CNS active drugs has not been systematically evaluated. Nonetheless, caution is advised if the concomitant administration of fluoxetine and such drugs is required. In evaluating individual cases, consideration should be given to using lower initial doses of the concomitantly administered drugs, using conservative titration schedules, and monitoring of clinical status).

No products indexed under this heading.

Chlorprothixene Lactate (The risk of using fluoxetine in combination with other CNS active drugs has not been systematically evaluated. Nonetheless, caution is advised if the concomitant administration of fluoxetine and such drugs is required. In evaluating individual cases, consideration should be given to using lower initial doses of the concomitantly administered drugs, using conservative titration schedules, and monitoring of clinical status).

No products indexed under this heading.

Chlorthalidone (Hyponatremia may occur as a result of treatment with SSRIs, including fluoxetine. In many cases this hyponatremia appears to be the result of the syndrome of inappropriate antidiuretic hormone secretion (SIADH). Cases with serum sodium lower than 110 mmol/L have been reported and appeared to be reversible when fluoxetine was discontinued. Patients taking diuretics may be at greater risk. Discontinuation of fluoxetine should be considered in patients with symptomatic hyponatremia and appropriate medical intervention should be instituted). Products include:

Clorpres Tablets 2185

Citalopram Hydrobromide (Based on the mechanism of action of SSRIs, including fluoxetine, and the potential for serotonin syndrome, caution is advised when fluoxetine is co-administered with other drugs that may affect serotonergic neurotransmitter systems. The Concomitant use of fluoxetine with other SSRIs is not recommended). Products include:

Celexa 1160

Clomipramine Hydrochloride (Fluoxetine inhibits the activity of CYP2D6, and may make individuals with normal CYP2D6 metabolic activity resemble a poor metabolizer. Co-administration of fluoxetine with other drugs that are metabolized by CYP2D6, including TCAs, should be approached with caution. Therapy with medications that are predominantly metabolized by the CYP2D6 system and that have a relatively narrow therapeutic index (eg, TCAs) should be initiated at the low end of the dose range if a patient is receiving fluoxetine concurrently or has taken it in the previous 5 weeks. If fluoxetine is added to the treatment regimen of a patient already receiving a drug metabolized by CYP2D6, the need for decreased dose of the original medication should be considered).

No products indexed under this heading.

Clorazepate Dipotassium (The risk of using fluoxetine in combination with other CNS active drugs has not been systematically evaluated. Nonetheless, caution is advised if the concomitant administration of fluoxetine and such drugs is required. In evaluating individual cases, consideration should be given to using lower initial doses of the concomitantly administered drugs, using conservative titration schedules, and monitoring of clinical status).

No products indexed under this heading.

Clozapine (Some clinical data suggests a possible pharmacodynamic and/or pharmacokinetic interaction between SSRIs and antipsychotics. Elevation of blood levels of clozapine has been observed in patients receiving concomitant fluoxetine).

No products indexed under this heading.

Codeine Phosphate (The risk of using fluoxetine in combination with other CNS active drugs has not been systematically evaluated. Nonetheless, caution is advised if the concomitant administration of fluoxetine and such drugs is required. In evaluating individual cases, consideration should be given to using lower initial doses of the concomitantly administered drugs, using conservative titration schedules, and monitoring of clinical status). Products include:

Tylenol with Codeine Tablets 2427

Codeine Sulfate (Fluoxetine inhibits the activity of CYP2D6, and may make individuals with normal CYP2D6 metabolic activity resemble a poor metabolizer. Co-administration of fluoxetine with other drugs that are metabolized by CYP2D6 should be approached with caution. Therapy with medications that are predominantly metabolized by the CYP2D6 system and that have a relatively narrow therapeutic index should be initiated at the low end of the dose range if a patient is receiving fluoxetine concurrently or has taken it in the previous 5 weeks. If fluoxetine is added to the treatment regimen of a patient already receiving a drug metabolized by CYP2D6, the need for decreased dose of the original medication should be considered).

No products indexed under this heading.

Cyclobenzaprine Hydrochloride (Fluoxetine inhibits the activity of CYP2D6, and may make individuals with normal CYP2D6 metabolic activity resemble a poor metabolizer. Co-administration of fluoxetine with other drugs that are metabolized by CYP2D6 should be approached with caution. Therapy with medications that are predominantly metabolized by the CYP2D6 system and that have a relatively narrow therapeutic index should be initiated at the low end of the dose range if a patient is receiving fluoxetine concurrently or has taken it in the previous 5 weeks. If fluoxetine is added to the treatment regimen of a patient already receiving a drug metabolized by CYP2D6, the need for decreased dose of the original medication should be considered). Products include:

Amrix Capsules 966

Cyclosporine (Because fluoxetine is tightly bound to plasma protein, the administration of fluoxetine to a patient taking another drugs that is tightly bound to protein may cause a shift in plasma concentrations potentially resulting in an adverse effect. Conversely,adverse effects may result from displacement of protein-bound fluoxetine by other tightly-bound drugs). Products include:

Gengraf Capsules 435
Neoral Oral Solution 2280
Neoral Soft Gelatin Capsules 2280
Restasis Ophthalmic Emulsion 557
Sandimmune 2296

Dalteparin Sodium (Case reports and epidemiological studies (case-control and cohort design) have demonstrated an association between use of drugs that interfere with serotonin reuptake and the occurrence of gastrointestinal bleeding. Bleeding events related to SSRI use have ranged from ecchymoses, hematomas, epistaxis, and petechiae to live-threatening hemorrhages. Patients should be cautioned about the risk of bleeding associated with the concomitant use of fluoxetine and other drugs that affect coagulation). Products include:

Fragmin Injection 1070

Danaparoid Sodium (Case reports and epidemiological studies (case-control and cohort design) have demonstrated an association between use of drugs that interfere with serotonin reuptake and the occurrence of gastrointestinal bleeding. Bleeding events related to SSRI use have ranged from ecchymoses, hematomas, epistaxis, and petechiae to live-threatening hemorrhages. Patients should be cautioned about the risk of bleeding associated with the concomitant use of fluoxetine and other drugs that affect coagulation).

No products indexed under this heading.

Desflurane (The risk of using fluoxetine in combination with other CNS active drugs has not been systematically evaluated. Nonetheless, caution is advised if the concomitant administration of fluoxetine and such drugs is required. In evaluating individual cases, consideration should be given to using lower initial doses of the concomitantly administered drugs, using conservative titration schedules, and monitoring of clinical status).

No products indexed under this heading.

Desipramine Hydrochloride (Fluoxetine inhibits the activity of CYP2D6, and may make individuals with normal CYP2D6 metabolic activity resemble a poor metabolizer. Co-administration of fluoxetine with other drugs that are metabolized by CYP2D6, including TCAs, should be approached with caution. Therapy with medications that are predominantly metabolized by the CYP2D6 system and that have a relatively narrow therapeutic index (eg, TCAs) should be initiated at the low end of the dose range if a patient is receiving fluoxetine concurrently or has taken it in the previous 5 weeks. If fluoxetine is added to the treatment regimen of a patient already receiving a drug metabolized by CYP2D6, the need for decreased dose of the original medication should be considered).

No products indexed under this heading.

Desvenlafaxine Succinate (Based on the mechanism of action of SSRIs, including Prozac, and the potential for serotonin syndrome, caution is advised when fluoxetine is co-administered with other drugs that may affect serotonergic neurotransmitter systems. The Concimitant use of fluoxetine with SNRIs is not recommended). Products include:

Pristiq Extended-Release Tablets 3247

Dexfenfluramine Hydrochloride (Fluoxetine inhibits the activity of CYP2D6, and may make individuals with normal CYP2D6 metabolic activity resemble a poor metabolizer. Co-administration of fluoxetine with other drugs that are metabolized by CYP2D6 should be approached with caution. Therapy with medications that are predominantly metabolized by the CYP2D6 system and that have a relatively narrow therapeutic index should be initiated at the low end of the dose range if a patient is receiving fluoxetine concurrently or has taken it in the previous 5 weeks. If fluoxetine is added to the treatment regimen of a patient already receiving a drug metabolized by CYP2D6, the need for decreased dose of the original medication should be considered).

No products indexed under this heading.

Dextroamphetamine Sulfate (The risk of using fluoxetine in combination with other CNS active drugs has not been systematically evaluated. Nonetheless, caution is advised if the concomitant administration of fluoxetine and such drugs is required. In evaluating individual cases, consideration should be given to using lower initial doses of the concomitantly administered drugs, using conservative titration schedules, and monitoring of clinical status). Products include:

Adderall XR Capsules 3012
Dexedrine 1401

Dextromethorphan Hydrobromide (Fluoxetine inhibits the activity of CYP2D6, and may make individuals with normal CYP2D6 metabolic activity resemble a poor metabolizer. Co-administration of fluoxetine with other drugs that are metabolized by CYP2D6 should be approached with caution. Therapy with medications that are predominantly metabolized by the CYP2D6 system and that have a relatively narrow therapeutic index should be initiated at the low end of the dose range if a patient is receiving fluoxetine concurrently or has taken it in the previous 5 weeks. If fluoxetine is added to the treatment regimen of a patient already receiving a drug metabolized by CYP2D6, the need for decreased dose of the original medication should be considered). Products include:

- PediaCare Children's Liquid Multi-Symptom Cold 1902
- PediaCare Children's Long-Acting Cough 1902
- Children's Sudafed PE Cold & Cough Liquid 1907
- Sudafed PE Cold & Cough Caplets 1907
- Children's Tylenol Plus Cough & Runny Nose Suspension Liquid 1912
- Children's Tylenol Plus Cough & Sore Throat Suspension Liquid 1912
- Children's Tylenol Plus Flu Suspension Liquid 1914
- Children's Tylenol Plus Multi-Symptom Cold Suspension Liquid 1912
- Tylenol Cold Severe Congestion Daytime Caplets with Cool Burst 1912
- Tylenol Cold Head Congestion Daytime Caplets with Cool Burst 1910
- Tylenol Cold Head Congestion Nighttime Caplets with Cool Burst 1910
- Tylenol Cold Head Congestion Severe Daytime Caplets with Cool Burst 1910
- Tylenol Cold Multi-Symptom Daytime Caplets with Cool Burst and Rapid Release Gels 1913
- Tylenol Cold Multi-Symptom Daytime Liquid with Citrus Burst ... 1913
- Tylenol Cold Multi-Symptom Nighttime Caplets with Cool Burst 1913
- Tylenol Cold Multi-Symptom Nighttime Liquid with Cool Burst ... 1913
- Tylenol Cold Multi-Symptom Severe Caplets with Cool Burst 1913
- Tylenol Cold Multi-Symptom Severe Daytime Liquid with Citrus Burst 1913
- Tylenol Cough & Sore Throat Daytime Liquid with Cool Burst 1918
- Tylenol Cough & Sore Throat Nighttime Liquid with Cool Burst ... 1918
- Vicks DayQuil Cold & Flu Multi-Symptom Relief ...... ▣616
- Vicks DayQuil LiquiCaps 2567
- Vicks DayQuil Liquid 2567
- Vicks DayQuil Multi-Symptom Cold/Flu Relief 2567
- Vicks NyQuil Cold & Flu Multi-Symptom Relief ...... ▣617
- Vicks NyQuil LiquiCaps 2567
- Vicks NyQuil Liquid 2567
- Vicks NyQuil Multi-Symptom Cold/Flu Relief 2567

Dextromethorphan Polistirex (Fluoxetine inhibits the activity of CYP2D6, and may make individuals with normal CYP2D6 metabolic activity resemble a poor metabolizer. Co-administration of fluoxetine with other drugs that are metabolized by CYP2D6 should be approached with caution. Therapy with medications that are predominantly metabolized by the CYP2D6 system and that have a relatively narrow therapeutic index should be initiated at the low end of the dose range if a patient is receiving fluoxetine concurrently or has taken it in the previous 5 weeks. If fluoxetine is added to the treatment regimen of a patient already receiving a drug metabolized by CYP2D6, the need for decreased dose of the original medication should be considered).

No products indexed under this heading.

Dezocine (The risk of using fluoxetine in combination with other CNS active drugs has not been systematically evaluated. Nonetheless, caution is advised if the concomitant administration of fluoxetine and such drugs is required. In evaluating individual cases, consideration should be given to using lower initial doses of the concomitantly administered drugs, using conservative titration schedules, and monitoring of clinical status).

No products indexed under this heading.

Diazepam (The half-life of concurrently administered diazepam may be prolonged in some patients). Products include:

- Valium Tablets 2658

Diclofenac Epolamine (SSRIs, including fluoxetine, may increase the risk of bleeding events. Concomitant use of nonsteroidal anti-inflammatory drugs may add to this risk. Case reports and epidemiological studies (case-control and cohort design) have demonstrated an association between use of drugs that interfere with serotonin reuptake and the occurrence of gastrointestinal bleeding. Bleeding events related to SSRI use have ranged from ecchymoses, hematomas, epistaxis, and petechiae to live-threatening hemorrhages. Patients should be cautioned about the risk of bleeding associated with the concomitant use of fluoxetine and NSAIDs). Products include:

- Flector Patch 561

Diclofenac Potassium (SSRIs, including fluoxetine, may increase the risk of bleeding events. Concomitant use of nonsteroidal anti-inflammatory drugs may add to this risk. Case reports and epidemiological studies (case-control and cohort design) have demonstrated an association between use of drugs that interfere with serotonin reuptake and the occurrence of gastrointestinal bleeding. Bleeding events related to SSRI use have ranged from ecchymoses, hematomas, epistaxis, and petechiae to live-threatening hemorrhages. Patients should be cautioned about the risk of bleeding associated with the concomitant use of fluoxetine and NSAIDs).

No products indexed under this heading.

Diclofenac Sodium (SSRIs, including fluoxetine, may increase the risk of bleeding events. Concomitant use of nonsteroidal anti-inflammatory drugs may add to this risk. Case reports and epidemiological studies (case-control and cohort design) have demonstrated an association between use of drugs that interfere with serotonin reuptake and the occurrence of gastrointestinal bleeding. Bleeding events related to SSRI use have ranged from ecchymoses, hematomas, epistaxis, and petechiae to live-threatening hemorrhages. Patients should be cautioned about the risk of bleeding associated with the concomitant use of fluoxetine and NSAIDs). Products include:

- Diclofenac Sodium Ophthalmic Solution ...... ⊙240
- Voltaren Ophthalmic Solution 2336
- Voltaren Tablets 2334
- Voltaren-XR Tablets 2337

Dicumarol (Case reports and epidemiological studies (case-control and cohort design) have demonstrated an association between use of drugs that interfere with serotonin reuptake and the occurrence of gastrointestinal bleeding. Bleeding events related to SSRI use have ranged from ecchymoses, hematomas, epistaxis, and petechiae to live-threatening hemorrhages. Patients should be cautioned about the risk of bleeding associated with the concomitant use of fluoxetine and other drugs that affect coagulation).

No products indexed under this heading.

Digitoxin (Because fluoxetine is tightly bound to plasma protein, the administration of fluoxetine to a patient taking another drug that is tightly bound to protein (eg, digitoxin) may cause a shift in plasma concentrations potentially resulting in an adverse effect. Conversely, adverse effects may result from displacement of protein-bound fluoxetine by other tightly-bound drugs).

No products indexed under this heading.

Dipyridamole (Because fluoxetine is tightly bound to plasma protein, the administration of fluoxetine to a patient taking another drugs that is tightly bound to protein may cause a shift in plasma concentrations potentially resulting in an adverse effect. Conversely,adverse effects may result from displacement of protein-bound fluoxetine by other tightly-bound drugs). Products include:

- Aggrenox Capsules 819
- Persantine Tablets 869

Dolasetron Mesylate (Fluoxetine inhibits the activity of CYP2D6, and may make individuals with normal CYP2D6 metabolic activity resemble a poor metabolizer. Co-administration of fluoxetine with other drugs that are metabolized by CYP2D6 should be approached with caution. Therapy with medications that are predominantly metabolized by the CYP2D6 system and that have a relatively narrow therapeutic index should be initiated at the low end of the dose range if a patient is receiving fluoxetine concurrently or has taken it in the previous 5 weeks. If fluoxetine is added to the treatment regimen of a patient already receiving a drug metabolized by CYP2D6, the need for decreased dose of the original medication should be considered). Products include:

- Anzemet Injection 2701
- Anzemet Tablets 2704

Donepezil Hydrochloride (Fluoxetine inhibits the activity of CYP2D6, and may make individuals with normal CYP2D6 metabolic activity resemble a poor metabolizer. Co-administration of fluoxetine with other drugs that are metabolized by CYP2D6 should be approached with caution. Therapy with medications that are predominantly metabolized by the CYP2D6 system and that have a relatively narrow therapeutic index should be initiated at the low end of the dose range if a patient is receiving fluoxetine concurrently or has taken it in the previous 5 weeks. If fluoxetine is added to the treatment regimen of a patient already receiving a drug metabolized by CYP2D6, the need for decreased dose of the original medication should be considered). Products include:

- Aricept Tablets 1062
- Aricept ODT Tablets 1062

Doxepin Hydrochloride (Fluoxetine inhibits the activity of CYP2D6, and may make individuals with normal CYP2D6 metabolic activity resemble a poor metabolizer. Co-administration of fluoxetine with other drugs that are metabolized by CYP2D6, including TCAs, should be approached with caution. Therapy with medications that are predominantly metabolized by the CYP2D6 system and that have a relatively narrow therapeutic index (eg, TCAs) should be initiated at the low end of the dose range if a patient is receiving fluoxetine concurrently or has taken it in the previous 5 weeks. If fluoxetine is added to the treatment regimen of a patient already receiving a drug metabolized by CYP2D6, the need for decreased dose of the original medication should be considered).

No products indexed under this heading.

Droperidol (The risk of using fluoxetine in combination with other CNS active drugs has not been systematically evaluated. Nonetheless, caution is advised if the concomitant administration of fluoxetine and such drugs is required. In evaluating individual cases, consideration should be given to using lower initial doses of the concomitantly administered drugs, using conservative titration schedules, and monitoring of clinical status).

No products indexed under this heading.

Duloxetine Hydrochloride (Based on the mechanism of action of SSRIs, including Prozac, and the potential for serotonin syndrome, caution is advised when fluoxetine is co-administered with other drugs that may affect serotonergic neurotransmitter systems. The Concimitant use of fluoxetine with SNRIs is not recommended). Products include:

- Cymbalta Delayed-Release Capsules 1801

Eletriptan Hydrobromide (There have been rare postmarketing reports of serotonin syndrome with use of an SSRI and a triptan. If concomitant treatment of fluoxetine with a triptan is clinically warranted, careful observation of the patient is advised, particularly during treatment initiation and dose increases).

No products indexed under this heading.

Encainide Hydrochloride (Fluoxetine inhibits the activity of CYP2D6, and may make individuals with normal CYP2D6 metabolic activity resemble a poor metabolizer. Co-administration of fluoxetine with other drugs that are metabolized by CYP2D6 should be approached with caution. Therapy with medications that are predominantly metabolized by the CYP2D6 system and that have a relatively narrow therapeutic index should be initiated at the low end of the dose range if a patient is receiving fluoxetine concurrently or has taken it in the previous 5 weeks. If fluoxetine is added to the treatment regimen of a patient already receiving a drug metabolized by CYP2D6, the need for decreased dose of the original medication should be considered).

No products indexed under this heading.

Enflurane (The risk of using fluoxetine in combination with other CNS active drugs has not been systematically evaluated. Nonetheless, caution is advised if the concomitant administration of fluoxetine and such drugs is required. In evaluating individual cases, consideration should be given to using lower initial doses of the concomitantly administered drugs, using conservative titration schedules, and monitoring of clinical status).

No products indexed under this heading.

Enoxaparin Sodium (Case reports and epidemiological studies (case-control and cohort design) have demonstrated an association between use of drugs that interfere with serotonin reuptake and the occurrence of gastrointestinal bleeding. Bleeding events related to SSRI use have ranged from ecchymoses, hematomas, epistaxis, and petechiae to live-threatening hemorrhages. Patients should be cautioned about the risk of bleeding associated with the concomitant use of fluoxetine and other drugs that affect coagulation). Products include:

Lovenox Injection 2756

Escitalopram Oxalate (Based on the mechanism of action of SSRIs, including fluoxetine, and the potential for serotonin syndrome, caution is advised when fluoxetine is co-administered with other drugs that may affect serotonergic neurotransmitter systems. The Concomitant use of fluoxetine with other SSRIs is not recommended). Products include:

Lexapro Oral Suspension 1174
Lexapro Tablets 1174

Estazolam (The risk of using fluoxetine in combination with other CNS active drugs has not been systematically evaluated. Nonetheless, caution is advised if the concomitant administration of fluoxetine and such drugs is required. In evaluating individual cases, consideration should be given to using lower initial doses of the concomitantly administered drugs, using conservative titration schedules, and monitoring of clinical status).

No products indexed under this heading.

Ethacrynic Acid (Hyponatremia may occur as a result of treatment with SSRIs, including fluoxetine. In many cases this hyponatremia appears to be the result of the syndrome of inappropriate antidiuretic hormone secretion (SIADH). Cases with serum sodium lower than 110 mmol/L have been reported and appeared to be reversible when fluoxetine was discontinued. Patients taking diuretics may be at greater risk. Discontinuation of fluoxetine should be considered in patients with symptomatic hyponatremia and appropriate medical intervention should be instituted). Products include:

Edecrin Tablets 698

Ethanol (The risk of using fluoxetine in combination with other CNS active drugs has not been systematically evaluated. Nonetheless, caution is advised if the concomitant administration of fluoxetine and such drugs is required. In evaluating individual cases, consideration should be given to using lower initial doses of the concomitantly administered drugs, using conservative titration schedules, and monitoring of clinical status).

No products indexed under this heading.

Ethchlorvynol (The risk of using fluoxetine in combination with other CNS active drugs has not been systematically evaluated. Nonetheless, caution is advised if the concomitant administration of fluoxetine and such drugs is required. In evaluating individual cases, consideration should be given to using lower initial doses of the concomitantly administered drugs, using conservative titration schedules, and monitoring of clinical status).

No products indexed under this heading.

Ethinamate (The risk of using fluoxetine in combination with other CNS active drugs has not been systematically evaluated. Nonetheless, caution is advised if the concomitant administration of fluoxetine and such drugs is required. In evaluating individual cases, consideration should be given to using lower initial doses of the concomitantly administered drugs, using conservative titration schedules, and monitoring of clinical status).

No products indexed under this heading.

Ethyl Alcohol (The risk of using fluoxetine in combination with other CNS active drugs has not been systematically evaluated. Nonetheless, caution is advised if the concomitant administration of fluoxetine and such drugs is required. In evaluating individual cases, consideration should be given to using lower initial doses of the concomitantly administered drugs, using conservative titration schedules, and monitoring of clinical status).

No products indexed under this heading.

Etodolac (SSRIs, including fluoxetine, may increase the risk of bleeding events. Concomitant use of nonsteroidal anti-inflammatory drugs may add to this risk. Case reports and epidemiological studies (case-control and cohort design) have demonstrated an association between use of drugs that interfere with serotonin reuptake and the occurrence of gastrointestinal bleeding. Bleeding events related to SSRI use have ranged from ecchymoses, hematomas, epistaxis, and petechiae to live-threatening hemorrhages. Patients should be cautioned about the risk of bleeding associated with the concomitant use of fluoxetine and NSAIDs).

No products indexed under this heading.

Fenoprofen Calcium (SSRIs, including fluoxetine, may increase the risk of bleeding events. Concomitant use of nonsteroidal anti-inflammatory drugs may add to this risk. Case reports and epidemiological studies (case-control and cohort design) have demonstrated an association between use of drugs that interfere with serotonin reuptake and the occurrence of gastrointestinal bleeding. Bleeding events related to SSRI use have ranged from ecchymoses, hematomas, epistaxis, and petechiae to live-threatening hemorrhages. Patients should be cautioned about the risk of bleeding associated with the concomitant use of fluoxetine and NSAIDs). Products include:

Nalfon Capsules 2508

Fentanyl (The risk of using fluoxetine in combination with other CNS active drugs has not been systematically evaluated. Nonetheless, caution is advised if the concomitant administration of fluoxetine and such drugs is required. In evaluating individual cases, consideration should be given to using lower initial doses of the concomitantly administered drugs, using conservative titration schedules, and monitoring of clinical status). Products include:

Duragesic Transdermal System 2405
Ionsys Transdermal System 2410

Fentanyl Citrate (The risk of using fluoxetine in combination with other CNS active drugs has not been systematically evaluated. Nonetheless, caution is advised if the concomitant administration of fluoxetine and such drugs is required. In evaluating individual cases, consideration should be given to using lower initial doses of the concomitantly administered drugs, using conservative titration schedules, and monitoring of clinical status). Products include:

Actiq 959
Fentora Tablets 968

Flecainide Acetate (Fluoxetine inhibits the activity of CYP2D6 and may make individuals with normal CYP2D6 metabolic activity resemble a poor metabolizer. Co-administration of fluoxetine with other drugs that are metabolized by CYP2D6, including flecainide, should be approached with caution. Therapy with medications that are predominantly metabolized by the CYP2D6 system and that have a relatively narrow therapeutic index (eg, flecainide) should be initiated at the low end of the dose range if a patient is receiving fluoxetine concurrently or has taken it in the previous 5 weeks. If fluoxetine is added to the treatment regimen of a patient already receiving a drug metabolized CYP2D6, the need for decreased dose of the original medication should be considered).

No products indexed under this heading.

Fluoxetine (Based on the mechanism of action of SSRIs, including fluoxetine, and the potential for serotonin syndrome, caution is advised when fluoxetine is co-administered with other drugs that may affect serotonergic neurotransmitter systems. The Concomitant use of fluoxetine with other SSRIs is not recommended).

No products indexed under this heading.

Fluphenazine Decanoate (Fluoxetine inhibits the activity of CYP2D6, and may make individuals with normal CYP2D6 metabolic activity resemble a poor metabolizer. Co-administration of fluoxetine with other drugs that are metabolized by CYP2D6, including phenothiazines, should be approached with caution. If fluoxetine is added to the treatment regimen of a patient already receiving a drug metabolized by CYP2D6, the need for decreased dose of the original medication should be considered).

No products indexed under this heading.

Fluphenazine Enanthate (Fluoxetine inhibits the activity of CYP2D6, and may make individuals with normal CYP2D6 metabolic activity resemble a poor metabolizer. Co-administration of fluoxetine with other drugs that are metabolized by CYP2D6, including phenothiazines, should be approached with caution. If fluoxetine is added to the treatment regimen of a patient already receiving a drug metabolized by CYP2D6, the need for decreased dose of the original medication should be considered).

No products indexed under this heading.

Fluphenazine Hydrochloride (Fluoxetine inhibits the activity of CYP2D6, and may make individuals with normal CYP2D6 metabolic activity resemble a poor metabolizer. Co-administration of fluoxetine with other drugs that are metabolized by CYP2D6, including phenothiazines, should be approached with caution. If fluoxetine is added to the treatment regimen of a patient already receiving a drug metabolized by CYP2D6, the need for decreased dose of the original medication should be considered).

No products indexed under this heading.

Flurazepam Hydrochloride (The risk of using fluoxetine in combination with other CNS active drugs has not been systematically evaluated. Nonetheless, caution is advised if the concomitant administration of fluoxetine and such drugs is required. In evaluating individual cases, consideration should be given to using lower initial doses of the concomitantly administered drugs, using conservative titration schedules, and monitoring of clinical status).

No products indexed under this heading.

Flurbiprofen (SSRIs, including fluoxetine, may increase the risk of bleeding events. Concomitant use of nonsteroidal anti-inflammatory drugs may add to this risk. Case reports and epidemiological studies (case-control and cohort design) have demonstrated an association between use of drugs that interfere with serotonin reuptake and the occurrence of gastrointestinal bleeding. Bleeding events related to SSRI use have ranged from ecchymoses, hematomas, epistaxis, and petechiae to live-threatening hemorrhages. Patients should be cautioned about the risk of bleeding associated with the concomitant use of fluoxetine and NSAIDs).

No products indexed under this heading.

Fluvoxamine Maleate (Based on the mechanism of action of SSRIs, including fluoxetine, and the potential for serotonin syndrome, caution is advised when fluoxetine is co-administered with other drugs that may affect serotonergic neurotransmitter systems. The Concomitant use of fluoxetine with other SSRIs is not recommended). Products include:

Luvox CR Extended-Release Capsules 1759

Fondaparinux Sodium (Case reports and epidemiological studies (case-control and cohort design) have demonstrated an association between use of drugs that interfere with serotonin reuptake and the occurrence of gastrointestinal bleeding. Bleeding events related to SSRI use have ranged from ecchymoses, hematomas, epistaxis, and petechiae to live-threatening hemorrhages. Patients should be cautioned about the risk of bleeding associated with the concomitant use of fluoxetine and other drugs that affect coagulation). Products include:

Arixtra Injection 1313

Formoterol Fumarate (Fluoxetine inhibits the activity of CYP2D6, and may make individuals with normal CYP2D6 metabolic activity resemble a poor metabolizer. Co-administration of fluoxetine with other drugs that are metabolized by CYP2D6 should be approached with caution. Therapy with medications that are predominantly metabolized by the CYP2D6 system and that have a relatively narrow therapeutic index should be initiated at the low end of the dose range if a patient is receiving fluoxetine concurrently or has taken it in the previous 5 weeks. If fluoxetine is added to the treatment regimen of a patient already receiving a drug metabolized by CYP2D6, the need for decreased dose of the original medication should be considered). Products include:

Foradil Aerolizer 2849
Perforomist Inhalation Solution 1025

Fosphenytoin Sodium (Patients on stable doses of phenytoin have developed elevated plasma anticonvulsant concentrations and clinical anticonvulsant toxicity following initiation of concomitant fluoxetine treatment).

No products indexed under this heading.

Frovatriptan Succinate (There have been rare postmarketing reports of serotonin syndrome with use of an SSRI and a triptan. If concomitant treatment of fluoxetine with a triptan is clinically warranted, careful observation of the patient is advised, particularly during treatment initiation and dose increases). Products include:

Frova Tablets 1111

Furosemide (Hyponatremia may occur as a result of treatment with SSRIs, including fluoxetine. In many cases this hyponatremia appears to be the result of the syndrome of inappropriate antidiuretic hormone secretion (SIADH). Cases with serum sodium lower than 110 mmol/L have been reported and appeared to be reversible when fluoxetine was discontinued. Patients taking diuretics may be at greater risk. Discontinuation of fluoxetine should be considered in patients with symptomatic hyponatremia and appropriate medical intervention should be instituted). Products include:

Furosemide Tablets 2186

Galantamine Hydrobromide (Fluoxetine inhibits the activity of CYP2D6, and may make individuals with normal CYP2D6 metabolic activity resemble a poor metabolizer. Co-administration of fluoxetine with other drugs that are metabolized by CYP2D6 should be approached with caution. Therapy with medications that are predominantly metabolized by the CYP2D6 system and that have a relatively narrow therapeutic index should be initiated at the low end of the dose range if a patient is receiving fluoxetine concurrently or has taken it in the previous 5 weeks. If fluoxetine is added to the treatment regimen of a patient already receiving a drug metabolized by CYP2D6, the need for decreased dose of the original medication should be considered).

No products indexed under this heading.

Glimepiride (In patients with diabetes, fluoxetine may alter glycemic control. Hypoglycemia has occurred during therapy with fluoxetine, and hyperglycemia has developed following discontinuation of the drug. As is true with many other types of medication when taken concurrently by patients with diabetes, oral hypoglycemic dosage may need to be adjusted when therapy with fluoxetine is instituted or discontinued). Products include:

Avandaryl Tablets 1344
Duetact Tablets 3085

Glipizide (Because fluoxetine is tightly bound to plasma protein, the administration of fluoxetine to a patient taking another drugs that is tightly bound to protein may cause a shift in plasma concentrations potentially resulting in an adverse effect. Conversely,adverse effects may result from displacement of protein-bound fluoxetine by other tightly-bound drugs).

No products indexed under this heading.

Glutethimide (The risk of using fluoxetine in combination with other CNS active drugs has not been systematically evaluated. Nonetheless, caution is advised if the concomitant administration of fluoxetine and such drugs is required. In evaluating individual cases, consideration should be given to using lower initial doses of the concomitantly administered drugs, using conservative titration schedules, and monitoring of clinical status).

No products indexed under this heading.

Glyburide (In patients with diabetes, fluoxetine may alter glycemic control. Hypoglycemia has occurred during therapy with fluoxetine, and hyperglycemia has developed following discontinuation of the drug. As is true with many other types of medication when taken concurrently by patients with diabetes, oral hypoglycemic dosage may need to be adjusted when therapy with fluoxetine is instituted or discontinued).

No products indexed under this heading.

Haloperidol (Some clinical data suggests a possible pharmacodynamic and/or pharmacokinetic interaction between SSRIs and antipsychotics. Elevation of blood levels of haloperidol has been observed in patients receiving concomitant fluoxetine).

No products indexed under this heading.

Haloperidol Decanoate (Some clinical data suggests a possible pharmacodynamic and/or pharmacokinetic interaction between SSRIs and antipsychotics. Elevation of blood levels of haloperidol has been observed in patients receiving concomitant fluoxetine).

No products indexed under this heading.

Haloperidol Lactate (Some clinical data suggests a possible pharmacodynamic and/or pharmacokinetic interaction between SSRIs and antipsychotics. Elevation of blood levels of haloperidol has been observed in patients receiving concomitant fluoxetine).

No products indexed under this heading.

Heparin Calcium (Case reports and epidemiological studies (case-control and cohort design) have demonstrated an association between use of drugs that interfere with serotonin reuptake and the occurrence of gastrointestinal bleeding. Bleeding events related to SSRI use have ranged from ecchymoses, hematomas, epistaxis, and petechiae to live-threatening hemorrhages. Patients should be cautioned about the risk of bleeding associated with the concomitant use of fluoxetine and other drugs that affect coagulation).

No products indexed under this heading.

Heparin Sodium (Case reports and epidemiological studies (case-control and cohort design) have demonstrated an association between use of drugs that interfere with serotonin reuptake and the occurrence of gastrointestinal bleeding. Bleeding events related to SSRI use have ranged from ecchymoses, hematomas, epistaxis, and petechiae to live-threatening hemorrhages. Patients should be cautioned about the risk of bleeding associated with the concomitant use of fluoxetine and other drugs that affect coagulation).

No products indexed under this heading.

Hydrochlorothiazide (Hyponatremia may occur as a result of treatment with SSRIs, including fluoxetine. In many cases this hyponatremia appears to be the result of the syndrome of inappropriate antidiuretic hormone secretion (SIADH). Cases with serum sodium lower than 110 mmol/L have been reported and appeared to be reversible when fluoxetine was discontinued. Patients taking diuretics may be at greater risk. Discontinuation of fluoxetine should be considered in patients with symptomatic hyponatremia and appropriate medical intervention should be instituted). Products include:

Atacand HCT 642
Avalide Tablets 892
Avalide Tablets 2713
Benicar HCT Tablets 1010
Diovan HCT Tablets 2216
Dyazide Capsules 1405
Micardis HCT Tablets 854
Prinzide Tablets 2092
Tekturna HCT Tablets 2324
Teveten HCT Tablets 517

Hydrocodone Bitartrate (The risk of using fluoxetine in combination with other CNS active drugs has not been systematically evaluated. Nonetheless, caution is advised if the concomitant administration of fluoxetine and such drugs is required. In evaluating individual cases, consideration should be given to using lower initial doses of the concomitantly administered drugs, using conservative titration schedules, and monitoring of clinical status). Products include:

Lortab 5/500 Tablets 3143
Lortab 7.5/500 Tablets 3144
Lortab 10/500 Tablets 3144
Vicodin Tablets 529
Vicodin ES Tablets 530
Vicodin HP Tablets 531
Vicoprofen Tablets 533
Zydone Tablets 1132

Hydrocodone Polistirex (The risk of using fluoxetine in combination with other CNS active drugs has not been systematically evaluated. Nonetheless, caution is advised if the concomitant administration of fluoxetine and such drugs is required. In evaluating individual cases, consideration should be given to using lower initial doses of the concomitantly administered drugs, using conservative titration schedules, and monitoring of clinical status). Products include:

Tussionex Pennkinetic Extended-Release Suspension 3154

Hydroflumethiazide (Hyponatremia may occur as a result of treatment with SSRIs, including fluoxetine. In many cases this hyponatremia appears to be the result of the syndrome of inappropriate antidiuretic hormone secretion (SIADH). Cases with serum sodium lower than 110 mmol/L have been reported and appeared to be reversible when fluoxetine was discontinued. Patients taking diuretics may be at greater risk. Discontinuation of fluoxetine should be considered in patients with symptomatic hyponatremia and appropriate medical intervention should be instituted).

No products indexed under this heading.

Hydromorphone Hydrochloride (The risk of using fluoxetine in combination with other CNS active drugs has not been systematically evaluated. Nonetheless, caution is advised if the concomitant administration of fluoxetine and such drugs is required. In evaluating individual cases, consideration should be given to using lower initial doses of the concomitantly administered drugs, using conservative titration schedules, and monitoring of clinical status).

No products indexed under this heading.

Hydroxyzine Hydrochloride (The risk of using fluoxetine in combination with other CNS active drugs has not been systematically evaluated. Nonetheless, caution is advised if the concomitant administration of fluoxetine and such drugs is required. In evaluating individual cases, consideration should be given to using lower initial doses of the concomitantly administered drugs, using conservative titration sched-

ules, and monitoring of clinical status).
No products indexed under this heading.

Hypericum (Based on the mechanism of action of SSRIs, including fluoxetine, and the potential for serotonin syndrome, caution is advised when fluoxetine is co-administered with other drugs that may affect serotonergic neurotransmitter systems, such as St. John's Wort). Products include:
Satieté Tablets .... ▣ 640

Ibuprofen (SSRIs, including fluoxetine, may increase the risk of bleeding events. Concomitant use of nonsteroidal anti-inflammatory drugs may add to this risk. Case reports and epidemiological studies (case-control and cohort design) have demonstrated an association between use of drugs that interfere with serotonin reuptake and the occurrence of gastrointestinal bleeding. Bleeding events related to SSRI use have ranged from ecchymoses, hematomas, epistaxis, and petechiae to life-threatening hemorrhages. Patients should be cautioned about the risk of bleeding associated with the concomitant use of fluoxetine and NSAIDs). Products include:
Motrin IB Tablets and Caplets **1900**
Children's Motrin Oral Suspension ... **1901**
Children's Motrin Non-Staining Dye-Free Oral Suspension............ **1901**
Children's Motrin Cold Oral Suspension **1899**
Infants' Motrin Concentrated Drops........................ **1901**
Infants' Motrin Non-Staining Dye-Free Concentrated Drops....... **1901**
Junior Strength Motrin Caplets and Chewable Tablets.................. **1901**
Vicoprofen Tablets **533**

Imipramine Hydrochloride (Fluoxetine inhibits the activity of CYP2D6, and may make individuals with normal CYP2D6 metabolic activity resemble a poor metabolizer. Co-administration of fluoxetine with other drugs that are metabolized by CYP2D6, including TCAs, should be approached with caution. Therapy with medications that are predominantly metabolized by the CYP2D6 system and that have a relatively narrow therapeutic index (eg, TCAs) should be initiated at the low end of the dose range if a patient is receiving fluoxetine concurrently or has taken it in the previous 5 weeks. If fluoxetine is added to the treatment regimen of a patient already receiving a drug metabolized by CYP2D6, the need for decreased dose of the original medication should be considered).
No products indexed under this heading.

Imipramine Pamoate (Fluoxetine inhibits the activity of CYP2D6, and may make individuals with normal CYP2D6 metabolic activity resemble a poor metabolizer. Co-administration of fluoxetine with other drugs that are metabolized by CYP2D6, including TCAs, should be approached with caution. Therapy with medications that are predominantly metabolized by the CYP2D6 system and that have a relatively narrow therapeutic index (eg, TCAs) should be initiated at the low end of the dose range if a patient is receiving fluoxetine concurrently or has taken it in the previous 5 weeks. If fluoxetine is added to the treatment regimen of a patient already receiving a drug metabolized by CYP2D6, the need for decreased dose of the original medication should be considered).
No products indexed under this heading.

Indapamide (Hyponatremia may occur as a result of treatment with SSRIs, including fluoxetine. In many cases this hyponatremia appears to be the result of the syndrome of inappropriate antidiuretic hormone secretion (SIADH). Cases with serum sodium lower than 110 mmol/L have been reported and appeared to be reversible when fluoxetine was discontinued. Patients taking diuretics may be at greater risk. Discontinuation of fluoxetine should be considered in patients with symptomatic hyponatremia and appropriate medical intervention should be instituted). Products include:
Indapamide Tablets **2188**

Indomethacin (SSRIs, including fluoxetine, may increase the risk of bleeding events. Concomitant use of nonsteroidal anti-inflammatory drugs may add to this risk. Case reports and epidemiological studies (case-control and cohort design) have demonstrated an association between use of drugs that interfere with serotonin reuptake and the occurrence of gastrointestinal bleeding. Bleeding events related to SSRI use have ranged from ecchymoses, hematomas, epistaxis, and petechiae to live-threatening hemorrhages. Patients should be cautioned about the risk of bleeding associated with the concomitant use of fluoxetine and NSAIDs). Products include:
Indocin **2024**

Indomethacin Sodium Trihydrate (SSRIs, including fluoxetine, may increase the risk of bleeding events. Concomitant use of nonsteroidal anti-inflammatory drugs may add to this risk. Case reports and epidemiological studies (case-control and cohort design) have demonstrated an association between use of drugs that interfere with serotonin reuptake and the occurrence of gastrointestinal bleeding. Bleeding events related to SSRI use have ranged from ecchymoses, hematomas, epistaxis, and petechiae to live-threatening hemorrhages. Patients should be cautioned about the risk of bleeding associated with the concomitant use of fluoxetine and NSAIDs). Products include:
Indocin I.V. **2489**

Indoramin Hydrochloride (Fluoxetine inhibits the activity of CYP2D6, and may make individuals with normal CYP2D6 metabolic activity resemble a poor metabolizer. Co-administration of fluoxetine with other drugs that are metabolized by CYP2D6 should be approached with caution. Therapy with medications that are predominantly metabolized by the CYP2D6 system and that have a relatively narrow therapeutic index should be initiated at the low end of the dose range if a patient is receiving fluoxetine concurrently or has taken it in the previous 5 weeks. If fluoxetine is added to the treatment regimen of a patient already receiving a drug metabolized by CYP2D6, the need for decreased dose of the original medication should be considered).
No products indexed under this heading.

Insulin (In patients with diabetes, fluoxetine may alter glycemic control. Hypoglycemia has occurred during therapy with fluoxetine, and hyperglycemia has developed following discontinuation of the drug. Insulin dosage may need to be adjusted when therapy with fluoxetine is instituted or discontinued).
No products indexed under this heading.

Insulin, Human, Zinc Suspension (In patients with diabetes, fluoxetine may alter glycemic control. Hypoglycemia has occurred during therapy with fluoxetine, and hyperglycemia has developed following discontinuation of the drug. Insulin dosage may need to be adjusted when therapy with fluoxetine is instituted or discontinued).
No products indexed under this heading.

Insulin, Human (rDNA origin) (In patients with diabetes, fluoxetine may alter glycemic control. Hypoglycemia has occurred during therapy with fluoxetine, and hyperglycemia has developed following discontinuation of the drug. Insulin dosage may need to be adjusted when therapy with fluoxetine is instituted or discontinued). Products include:
Exubera Inhalation Powder **2515**

Insulin, Human NPH (In patients with diabetes, fluoxetine may alter glycemic control. Hypoglycemia has occurred during therapy with fluoxetine, and hyperglycemia has developed following discontinuation of the drug. Insulin dosage may need to be adjusted when therapy with fluoxetine is instituted or discontinued). Products include:
Humulin N Vial **1846**

Insulin, Human Regular (In patients with diabetes, fluoxetine may alter glycemic control. Hypoglycemia has occurred during therapy with fluoxetine, and hyperglycemia has developed following discontinuation of the drug. Insulin dosage may need to be adjusted when therapy with fluoxetine is instituted or discontinued). Products include:
Humulin R **1849**
Humulin R (U-500) **1850**

Insulin, Human Regular and Human NPH Mixture (In patients with diabetes, fluoxetine may alter glycemic control. Hypoglycemia has occurred during therapy with fluoxetine, and hyperglycemia has developed following discontinuation of the drug. Insulin dosage may need to be adjusted when therapy with fluoxetine is instituted or discontinued). Products include:
Humulin 50/50, 100 Units **1843**
Humulin 70/30 Vial **1844**

Insulin, NPH (In patients with diabetes, fluoxetine may alter glycemic control. Hypoglycemia has occurred during therapy with fluoxetine, and hyperglycemia has developed following discontinuation of the drug. Insulin dosage may need to be adjusted when therapy with fluoxetine is instituted or discontinued).
No products indexed under this heading.

Insulin, Regular (In patients with diabetes, fluoxetine may alter glycemic control. Hypoglycemia has occurred during therapy with fluoxetine, and hyperglycemia has developed following discontinuation of the drug. Insulin dosage may need to be adjusted when therapy with fluoxetine is instituted or discontinued).
No products indexed under this heading.

Insulin, Regular and NPH mixture (In patients with diabetes, fluoxetine may alter glycemic control. Hypoglycemia has occurred during therapy with fluoxetine, and hyperglycemia has developed following discontinuation of the drug. Insulin dosage may need to be adjusted when therapy with fluoxetine is instituted or discontinued).
No products indexed under this heading.

Insulin, Zinc Crystals (In patients with diabetes, fluoxetine may alter glycemic control. Hypoglycemia has occurred during therapy with fluoxetine, and hyperglycemia has developed following discontinuation of the drug. Insulin dosage may need to be adjusted when therapy with fluoxetine is instituted or discontinued).
No products indexed under this heading.

Insulin, Zinc Suspension (In patients with diabetes, fluoxetine may alter glycemic control. Hypoglycemia has occurred during therapy with fluoxetine, and hyperglycemia has developed following discontinuation of the drug. Insulin dosage may need to be adjusted when therapy with fluoxetine is instituted or discontinued).
No products indexed under this heading.

Insulin Aspart (In patients with diabetes, fluoxetine may alter glycemic control. Hypoglycemia has occurred during therapy with fluoxetine, and hyperglycemia has developed following discontinuation of the drug. Insulin dosage may need to be adjusted when therapy with fluoxetine is instituted or discontinued).
No products indexed under this heading.

Insulin Aspart, Human (In patients with diabetes, fluoxetine may alter glycemic control. Hypoglycemia has occurred during therapy with fluoxetine, and hyperglycemia has developed following discontinuation of the drug. Insulin dosage may need to be adjusted when therapy with fluoxetine is instituted or discontinued). Products include:
NovoLog Mix 70/30 .... **2364**

Insulin Aspart, Human Regular (In patients with diabetes, fluoxetine may alter glycemic control. Hypoglycemia has occurred during therapy with fluoxetine, and hyperglycemia has developed following discontinuation of the drug. Insulin dosage may need to be adjusted when therapy with fluoxetine is instituted or discontinued). Products include:
NovoLog Injection **2359**

Insulin Aspart Protamine, Human (In patients with diabetes, fluoxetine may alter glycemic control. Hypoglycemia has occurred during therapy with fluoxetine, and hyperglycemia has developed following discontinuation of the drug. Insulin dosage may need to be adjusted when therapy with fluoxetine is instituted or discontinued). Products include:

NovoLog Mix 70/30 2364

Insulin Detemir (rDNA Origin) (In patients with diabetes, fluoxetine may alter glycemic control. Hypoglycemia has occurred during therapy with fluoxetine, and hyperglycemia has developed following discontinuation of the drug. Insulin dosage may need to be adjusted when therapy with fluoxetine is instituted or discontinued). Products include:

Levemir Injection 2352

Insulin glargine (In patients with diabetes, fluoxetine may alter glycemic control. Hypoglycemia has occurred during therapy with fluoxetine, and hyperglycemia has developed following discontinuation of the drug. Insulin dosage may need to be adjusted when therapy with fluoxetine is instituted or discontinued). Products include:

Lantus Injection 2749

Insulin Glulisine (In patients with diabetes, fluoxetine may alter glycemic control. Hypoglycemia has occurred during therapy with fluoxetine, and hyperglycemia has developed following discontinuation of the drug. Insulin dosage may need to be adjusted when therapy with fluoxetine is instituted or discontinued). Products include:

Apidra Injection 2706

Insulin Lispro, Human (In patients with diabetes, fluoxetine may alter glycemic control. Hypoglycemia has occurred during therapy with fluoxetine, and hyperglycemia has developed following discontinuation of the drug. Insulin dosage may need to be adjusted when therapy with fluoxetine is instituted or discontinued). Products include:

Humalog-Pen and KwikPen 1829

Humalog Mix 50/50-Pen and KwikPen 1833

Humalog Mix 75/25-Pen and KwikPen 1835

Insulin Lispro Protamine, Human (In patients with diabetes, fluoxetine may alter glycemic control. Hypoglycemia has occurred during therapy with fluoxetine, and hyperglycemia has developed following discontinuation of the drug. Insulin dosage may need to be adjusted when therapy with fluoxetine is instituted or discontinued). Products include:

Humalog Mix 50/50-Pen and KwikPen 1833

Humalog Mix 75/25-Pen and KwikPen 1835

Isocarboxazid (Use with MAOIs is contraindicated. There have been reports of serious, sometimes fatal, reactions in patients receiving fluoxetine in combination with a monoamine oxidase inhibitor (MAOI), and in patients who have recently discontinued fluoxetine and are then started on an MAOI. Some cases presented with features resembling neuroleptic malignant syndrome. Therefore fluoxetine should not be used in combination with an MAOI, or within a minimum of 14 days of discontinuing therapy with an MAOI. Since fluoxetine and its major metabolite have very long elimination half-lives, at least 5 weeks or longer, (especially if fluoxetine has been prescribed chronically and/or at higher doses) should be allowed after stopping fluoxetine before starting an MAOI). Products include:

Marplan Tablets 3177

Isoflurane (The risk of using fluoxetine in combination with other CNS active drugs has not been systematically evaluated. Nonetheless, caution is advised if the concomitant administration of fluoxetine and such drugs is required. In evaluating individual cases, consideration should be given to using lower initial doses of the concomitantly administered drugs, using conservative titration schedules, and monitoring of clinical status).

No products indexed under this heading.

Ketamine Hydrochloride (The risk of using fluoxetine in combination with other CNS active drugs has not been systematically evaluated. Nonetheless, caution is advised if the concomitant administration of fluoxetine and such drugs is required. In evaluating individual cases, consideration should be given to using lower initial doses of the concomitantly administered drugs, using conservative titration schedules, and monitoring of clinical status).

No products indexed under this heading.

Ketoprofen (SSRIs, including fluoxetine, may increase the risk of bleeding events. Concomitant use of nonsteroidal anti-inflammatory drugs may add to this risk. Case reports and epidemiological studies (case-control and cohort design) have demonstrated an association between use of drugs that interfere with serotonin reuptake and the occurrence of gastrointestinal bleeding. Bleeding events related to SSRI use have ranged from ecchymoses, hematomas, epistaxis, and petechiae to live-threatening hemorrhages. Patients should be cautioned about the risk of bleeding associated with the concomitant use of fluoxetine and NSAIDs).

No products indexed under this heading.

Ketorolac Tromethamine (SSRIs, including fluoxetine, may increase the risk of bleeding events. Concomitant use of nonsteroidal anti-inflammatory drugs may add to this risk. Case reports and epidemiological studies (case-control and cohort design) have demonstrated an association between use of drugs that interfere with serotonin reuptake and the occurrence of gastrointestinal bleeding. Bleeding events related to SSRI use have ranged from ecchymoses, hematomas, epistaxis, and petechiae to live-threatening hemorrhages. Patients should be cautioned about the risk of bleeding associated with the concomitant use of fluoxetine and NSAIDs).

No products indexed under this heading.

Labetalol Hydrochloride (Fluoxetine inhibits the activity of CYP2D6, and may make individuals with normal CYP2D6 metabolic activity resemble a poor metabolizer. Co-administration of fluoxetine with other drugs that are metabolized by CYP2D6 should be approached with caution. Therapy with medications that are predominantly metabolized by the CYP2D6 system and that have a relatively narrow therapeutic index should be initiated at the low end of the dose range if a patient is receiving fluoxetine concurrently or has taken it in the previous 5 weeks. If fluoxetine is added to the treatment regimen of a patient already receiving a drug metabolized by CYP2D6, the need for decreased dose of the original medication should be considered).

No products indexed under this heading.

Levomethadyl Acetate Hydrochloride (The risk of using fluoxetine in combination with other CNS active drugs has not been systematically evaluated. Nonetheless, caution is advised if the concomitant administration of fluoxetine and such drugs is required. In evaluating individual cases, consideration should be given to using lower initial doses of the concomitantly administered drugs, using conservative titration schedules, and monitoring of clinical status).

No products indexed under this heading.

Levorphanol Tartrate (The risk of using fluoxetine in combination with other CNS active drugs has not been systematically evaluated. Nonetheless, caution is advised if the concomitant administration of fluoxetine and such drugs is required. In evaluating individual cases, consideration should be given to using lower initial doses of the concomitantly administered drugs, using conservative titration schedules, and monitoring of clinical status).

No products indexed under this heading.

Lidocaine (Fluoxetine inhibits the activity of CYP2D6, and may make individuals with normal CYP2D6 metabolic activity resemble a poor metabolizer. Co-administration of fluoxetine with other drugs that are metabolized by CYP2D6 should be approached with caution. Therapy with medications that are predominantly metabolized by the CYP2D6 system and that have a relatively narrow therapeutic index should be initiated at the low end of the dose range if a patient is receiving fluoxetine concurrently or has taken it in the previous 5 weeks. If fluoxetine is added to the treatment regimen of a patient already receiving a drug metabolized by CYP2D6, the need for decreased dose of the original medication should be considered). Products include:

Lidoderm Patch 1114

Lidocaine Hydrochloride (Fluoxetine inhibits the activity of CYP2D6, and may make individuals with normal CYP2D6 metabolic activity resemble a poor metabolizer. Co-administration of fluoxetine with other drugs that are metabolized by CYP2D6 should be approached with caution. Therapy with medications that are predominantly metabolized by the CYP2D6 system and that have a relatively narrow therapeutic index should be initiated at the low end of the dose range if a patient is receiving fluoxetine concurrently or has taken it in the previous 5 weeks. If fluoxetine is added to the treatment regimen of a patient already receiving a drug metabolized by CYP2D6, the need for decreased dose of the original medication should be considered).

No products indexed under this heading.

Linezolid (Based on the mechanism of action of SSRIs, including fluoxetine, and the potential for serotonin syndrome, caution is advised when fluoxetine is co-administered with other drugs that may affect serotonergic neurotransmitter systems, such as linezolid (an antibiotic which is a reversible non-selective MAOI)). Products include:

Zyvox 2552

Lithium (Based on the mechanism of action of SSRIs, including fluoxetine, and the potential for serotonin syndrome, caution is advised when fluoxetine is co-administered with other drugs that may affect serotonergic neurotransmitter systems, such as lithium. There have been reports of both increased and decreased lithium levels when lithium was used concomitantly with fluoxetine. Cases of lithium toxicity and increased serotonergic effects have been reported. Lithium levels should be monitored when these drugs are administered concomitantly).

No products indexed under this heading.

Lithium Carbonate (Based on the mechanism of action of SSRIs, including fluoxetine, and the potential for serotonin syndrome, caution is advised when fluoxetine is co-administered with other drugs that may affect serotonergic neurotransmitter systems, such as lithium. There have been reports of both increased and decreased lithium levels when lithium was used concomitantly with fluoxetine. Cases of lithium toxicity and increased serotonergic effects have been reported. Lithium levels should be monitored when these drugs are administered concomitantly).

No products indexed under this heading.

Lithium Citrate (Based on the mechanism of action of SSRIs, including fluoxetine, and the potential for serotonin syndrome, caution is advised when fluoxetine is co-administered with other drugs that may affect serotonergic neurotransmitter systems, such as lithium. There have been reports of both increased and decreased lithium levels when lithium was used concomitantly with fluoxetine. Cases of lithium toxicity and increased serotonergic effects have been reported. Lithium levels should be monitored when these drugs are administered concomitantly).

No products indexed under this heading.

Lorazepam (The risk of using fluoxetine in combination with other CNS active drugs has not been systematically evaluated. Nonetheless, caution is advised if the concomitant administration of fluoxetine and such drugs is required. In evaluating individual cases, consideration should be given to using lower initial doses of the concomitantly administered drugs, using conservative titration schedules, and monitoring of clinical status).

No products indexed under this heading.

Low Molecular Weight Heparins (Case reports and epidemiological studies (case-control and cohort

design) have demonstrated an association between use of drugs that interfere with serotonin reuptake and the occurrence of gastrointestinal bleeding. Bleeding events related to SSRI use have ranged from ecchymoses, hematomas, epistaxis, and petechiae to life-threatening hemorrhages. Patients should be cautioned about the risk of bleeding associated with the concomitant use of fluoxetine and other drugs that affect coagulation).
No products indexed under this heading.

Loxapine Hydrochloride (The risk of using fluoxetine in combination with other CNS active drugs has not been systematically evaluated. Nonetheless, caution is advised if the concomitant administration of fluoxetine and such drugs is required. In evaluating individual cases, consideration should be given to using lower initial doses of the concomitantly administered drugs, using conservative titration schedules, and monitoring of clinical status).
No products indexed under this heading.

Loxapine Succinate (The risk of using fluoxetine in combination with other CNS active drugs has not been systematically evaluated. Nonetheless, caution is advised if the concomitant administration of fluoxetine and such drugs is required. In evaluating individual cases, consideration should be given to using lower initial doses of the concomitantly administered drugs, using conservative titration schedules, and monitoring of clinical status).
No products indexed under this heading.

Maprotiline Hydrochloride (Fluoxetine inhibits the activity of CYP2D6, and may make individuals with normal CYP2D6 metabolic activity resemble a poor metabolizer. Coadministration of fluoxetine with other drugs that are metabolized by CYP2D6, including TCAs, should be approached with caution. Therapy with medications that are predominantly metabolized by the CYP2D6 system and that have a relatively narrow therapeutic index (eg, TCAs) should be initiated at the low end of the dose range if a patient is receiving fluoxetine concurrently or has taken it in the previous 5 weeks. If fluoxetine is added to the treatment regimen of a patient already receiving a drug metabolized by CYP2D6, the need for decreased dose of the original medication should be considered).
No products indexed under this heading.

Meclofenamate Sodium (SSRIs, including fluoxetine, may increase the risk of bleeding events. Concomitant use of nonsteroidal anti-inflammatory drugs may add to this risk. Case reports and epidemiological studies (case-control and cohort design) have demonstrated an association between use of drugs that interfere with serotonin reuptake and the occurrence of gastrointestinal bleeding. Bleeding events related to SSRI use have ranged from ecchymoses, hematomas, epistaxis, and petechiae to life-threatening hemorrhages. Patients should be cautioned about the risk of bleeding associated with the concomitant use of fluoxetine and NSAIDs).
No products indexed under this heading.

Mefenamic Acid (SSRIs, including fluoxetine, may increase the risk of bleeding events. Concomitant use of nonsteroidal anti-inflammatory drugs may add to this risk. Case reports and epidemiological studies (case-control and cohort design) have demonstrated an association between use of drugs that interfere with serotonin reuptake and the occurrence of gastrointestinal bleeding. Bleeding events related to SSRI use have ranged from ecchymoses, hematomas, epistaxis, and petechiae to life-threatening hemorrhages. Patients should be cautioned about the risk of bleeding associated with the concomitant use of fluoxetine and NSAIDs).
No products indexed under this heading.

Meloxicam (SSRIs, including fluoxetine, may increase the risk of bleeding events. Concomitant use of nonsteroidal anti-inflammatory drugs may add to this risk. Case reports and epidemiological studies (case-control and cohort design) have demonstrated an association between use of drugs that interfere with serotonin reuptake and the occurrence of gastrointestinal bleeding. Bleeding events related to SSRI use have ranged from ecchymoses, hematomas, epistaxis, and petechiae to life-threatening hemorrhages. Patients should be cautioned about the risk of bleeding associated with the concomitant use of fluoxetine and NSAIDs). Products include:
Mobic Oral Suspension 863
Mobic Tablets 863

Meperidine Hydrochloride (The risk of using fluoxetine in combination with other CNS active drugs has not been systematically evaluated. Nonetheless, caution is advised if the concomitant administration of fluoxetine and such drugs is required. In evaluating individual cases, consideration should be given to using lower initial doses of the concomitantly administered drugs, using conservative titration schedules, and monitoring of clinical status).
No products indexed under this heading.

Mephobarbital (The risk of using fluoxetine in combination with other CNS active drugs has not been systematically evaluated. Nonetheless, caution is advised if the concomitant administration of fluoxetine and such drugs is required. In evaluating individual cases, consideration should be given to using lower initial doses of the concomitantly administered drugs, using conservative titration schedules, and monitoring of clinical status).
No products indexed under this heading.

Meprobamate (The risk of using fluoxetine in combination with other CNS active drugs has not been systematically evaluated. Nonetheless, caution is advised if the concomitant administration of fluoxetine and such drugs is required. In evaluating individual cases, consideration should be given to using lower initial doses of the concomitantly administered drugs, using conservative titration schedules, and monitoring of clinical status).
No products indexed under this heading.

Mesoridazine Besylate (Fluoxetine inhibits the activity of CYP2D6, and may make individuals with normal CYP2D6 metabolic activity resemble a poor metabolizer. Coadministration of fluoxetine with other drugs that are metabolized by CYP2D6, including phenothiazines, should be approached with caution. If fluoxetine is added to the treatment regimen of a patient already receiving a drug metabolized by CYP2D6, the need for decreased dose of the original medication should be considered).
No products indexed under this heading.

Metformin Hydrochloride (In patients with diabetes, fluoxetine may alter glycemic control. Hypoglycemia has occurred during therapy with fluoxetine, and hyperglycemia has developed following discontinuation of the drug. As is true with many other types of medication when taken concurrently by patients with diabetes, oral hypoglycemic dosage may need to be adjusted when therapy with fluoxetine is instituted or discontinued). Products include:
ActoPlus Met Tablets 3071
Avandamet Tablets 1336
Janumet Tablets 2041
PrandiMet Tablets 2967

Methadone Hydrochloride (The risk of using fluoxetine in combination with other CNS active drugs has not been systematically evaluated. Nonetheless, caution is advised if the concomitant administration of fluoxetine and such drugs is required. In evaluating individual cases, consideration should be given to using lower initial doses of the concomitantly administered drugs, using conservative titration schedules, and monitoring of clinical status).
No products indexed under this heading.

Methamphetamine Hydrochloride (The risk of using fluoxetine in combination with other CNS active drugs has not been systematically evaluated. Nonetheless, caution is advised if the concomitant administration of fluoxetine and such drugs is required. In evaluating individual cases, consideration should be given to using lower initial doses of the concomitantly administered drugs, using conservative titration schedules, and monitoring of clinical status).
No products indexed under this heading.

Methohexital Sodium (The risk of using fluoxetine in combination with other CNS active drugs has not been systematically evaluated. Nonetheless, caution is advised if the concomitant administration of fluoxetine and such drugs is required. In evaluating individual cases, consideration should be given to using lower initial doses of the concomitantly administered drugs, using conservative titration schedules, and monitoring of clinical status).
No products indexed under this heading.

Methotrimeprazine (Fluoxetine inhibits the activity of CYP2D6, and may make individuals with normal CYP2D6 metabolic activity resemble a poor metabolizer. Coadministration of fluoxetine with other drugs that are metabolized by CYP2D6, including phenothiazines, should be approached with caution. If fluoxetine is added to the treatment regimen of a patient already receiving a drug metabolized by CYP2D6, the need for decreased dose of the original medication should be considered).
No products indexed under this heading.

Methoxyflurane (The risk of using fluoxetine in combination with other CNS active drugs has not been systematically evaluated. Nonetheless, caution is advised if the concomitant administration of fluoxetine and such drugs is required. In evaluating individual cases, consideration should be given to using lower initial doses of the concomitantly administered drugs, using conservative titration schedules, and monitoring of clinical status).
No products indexed under this heading.

Methyclothiazide (Hyponatremia may occur as a result of treatment with SSRIs, including fluoxetine. In many cases this hyponatremia appears to be the result of the syndrome of inappropriate antidiuretic hormone secretion (SIADH). Cases with serum sodium lower than 110 mmol/L have been reported and appeared to be reversible when fluoxetine was discontinued. Patients taking diuretics may be at greater risk. Discontinuation of fluoxetine should be considered in patients with symptomatic hyponatremia and appropriate medical intervention should be instituted).
No products indexed under this heading.

Methylphenidate (The risk of using fluoxetine in combination with other CNS active drugs has not been systematically evaluated. Nonetheless, caution is advised if the concomitant administration of fluoxetine and such drugs is required. In evaluating individual cases, consideration should be given to using lower initial doses of the concomitantly administered drugs, using conservative titration schedules, and monitoring of clinical status). Products include:
Daytrana Transdermal Patch 3022

Methylphenidate Hydrochloride (The risk of using fluoxetine in combination with other CNS active drugs has not been systematically evaluated. Nonetheless, caution is advised if the concomitant administration of fluoxetine and such drugs is required. In evaluating individual cases, consideration should be given to using lower initial doses of the concomitantly administered drugs, using conservative titration schedules, and monitoring of clinical status). Products include:
Concerta Extended-Release Tablets 1925
Metadate CD Capsules 3146

Metolazone (Hyponatremia may occur as a result of treatment with SSRIs, including fluoxetine. In many cases this hyponatremia appears to be the result of the syndrome of inappropriate antidiuretic hormone secretion (SIADH). Cases with serum sodium lower than 110 mmol/L have been reported and appeared to be

reversible when fluoxetine was discontinued. Patients taking diuretics may be at greater risk. Discontinuation of fluoxetine should be considered in patients with symptomatic hyponatremia and appropriate medical intervention should be instituted).

No products indexed under this heading.

Metoprolol Succinate (Fluoxetine inhibits the activity of CYP2D6, and may make individuals with normal CYP2D6 metabolic activity resemble a poor metabolizer. Co-administration of fluoxetine with other drugs that are metabolized by CYP2D6 should be approached with caution. Therapy with medications that are predominantly metabolized by the CYP2D6 system and that have a relatively narrow therapeutic index should be initiated at the low end of the dose range if a patient is receiving fluoxetine concurrently or has taken it in the previous 5 weeks. If fluoxetine is added to the treatment regimen of a patient already receiving a drug metabolized by CYP2D6, the need for decreased dose of the original medication should be considered). Products include:

Toprol-XL Tablets 666

Metoprolol Tartrate (Fluoxetine inhibits the activity of CYP2D6, and may make individuals with normal CYP2D6 metabolic activity resemble a poor metabolizer. Co-administration of fluoxetine with other drugs that are metabolized by CYP2D6 should be approached with caution. Therapy with medications that are predominantly metabolized by the CYP2D6 system and that have a relatively narrow therapeutic index should be initiated at the low end of the dose range if a patient is receiving fluoxetine concurrently or has taken it in the previous 5 weeks. If fluoxetine is added to the treatment regimen of a patient already receiving a drug metabolized by CYP2D6, the need for decreased dose of the original medication should be considered).

No products indexed under this heading.

Mexiletine Hydrochloride (Fluoxetine inhibits the activity of CYP2D6, and may make individuals with normal CYP2D6 metabolic activity resemble a poor metabolizer. Co-administration of fluoxetine with other drugs that are metabolized by CYP2D6 should be approached with caution. Therapy with medications that are predominantly metabolized by the CYP2D6 system and that have a relatively narrow therapeutic index should be initiated at the low end of the dose range if a patient is receiving fluoxetine concurrently or has taken it in the previous 5 weeks. If fluoxetine is added to the treatment regimen of a patient already receiving a drug metabolized by CYP2D6, the need for decreased dose of the original medication should be considered).

No products indexed under this heading.

Midazolam Hydrochloride (The risk of using fluoxetine in combination with other CNS active drugs has not been systematically evaluated. Nonetheless, caution is advised if the concomitant administration of fluoxetine and such drugs is required. In evaluating individual cases, consideration should be given to using lower initial doses of the concomitantly administered drugs, using conservative titration schedules, and monitoring of clinical status).

No products indexed under this heading.

Miglitol (In patients with diabetes, fluoxetine may alter glycemic control. Hypoglycemia has occurred during therapy with fluoxetine, and hyperglycemia has developed following discontinuation of the drug. As is true with many other types of medication when taken concurrently by patients with diabetes, oral hypoglycemic dosage may need to be adjusted when therapy with fluoxetine is instituted or discontinued).

No products indexed under this heading.

Mirtazapine (Fluoxetine inhibits the activity of CYP2D6, and may make individuals with normal CYP2D6 metabolic activity resemble a poor metabolizer. Co-administration of fluoxetine with other drugs that are metabolized by CYP2D6 should be approached with caution. Therapy with medications that are predominantly metabolized by the CYP2D6 system and that have a relatively narrow therapeutic index should be initiated at the low end of the dose range if a patient is receiving fluoxetine concurrently or has taken it in the previous 5 weeks. If fluoxetine is added to the treatment regimen of a patient already receiving a drug metabolized by CYP2D6, the need for decreased dose of the original medication should be considered). Products include:

Remeron Tablets 2924
RemeronSolTab Tablets 2927

Moclobemide (Use with MAOIs is contraindicated. There have been reports of serious, sometimes fatal, reactions in patients receiving fluoxetine in combination with a monoamine oxidase inhibitor (MAOI), and in patients who have recently discontinued fluoxetine and are then started on an MAOI. Some cases presented with features resembling neuroleptic malignant syndrome. Therefore fluoxetine should not be used in combination with an MAOI, or within a minimum of 14 days of discontinuing therapy with an MAOI. Since fluoxetine and its major metabolite have very long elimination half-lives, at least 5 weeks or longer, (especially if fluoxetine has been prescribed chronically and/or at higher doses) should be allowed after stopping fluoxetine before starting an MAOI).

No products indexed under this heading.

Molindone Hydrochloride (The risk of using fluoxetine in combination with other CNS active drugs has not been systematically evaluated. Nonetheless, caution is advised if the concomitant administration of fluoxetine and such drugs is required. In evaluating individual cases, consideration should be given to using lower initial doses of the concomitantly administered drugs, using conservative titration schedules, and monitoring of clinical status). Products include:

Moban Tablets 1116

Morphine Sulfate (The risk of using fluoxetine in combination with other CNS active drugs has not been systematically evaluated. Nonetheless, caution is advised if the concomitant administration of fluoxetine and such drugs is required. In evaluating individual cases, consideration should be given to using lower initial doses of the concomitantly administered drugs, using conservative titration schedules, and monitoring of clinical status). Products include:

Avinza Capsules 1772
DepoDur Injection 1095
MS Contin Tablets 2585

Nabumetone (SSRIs, including fluoxetine, may increase the risk of bleeding events. Concomitant use of nonsteroidal anti-inflammatory drugs may add to this risk. Case reports and epidemiological studies (case-control and cohort design) have demonstrated an association between use of drugs that interfere with serotonin reuptake and the occurrence of gastrointestinal bleeding. Bleeding events related to SSRI use have ranged from ecchymoses, hematomas, epistaxis, and petechiae to life-threatening hemorrhages. Patients should be cautioned about the risk of bleeding associated with the concomitant use of fluoxetine and NSAIDs).

No products indexed under this heading.

Naproxen (SSRIs, including fluoxetine, may increase the risk of bleeding events. Concomitant use of nonsteroidal anti-inflammatory drugs may add to this risk. Case reports and epidemiological studies (case-control and cohort design) have demonstrated an association between use of drugs that interfere with serotonin reuptake and the occurrence of gastrointestinal bleeding. Bleeding events related to SSRI use have ranged from ecchymoses, hematomas, epistaxis, and petechiae to life-threatening hemorrhages. Patients should be cautioned about the risk of bleeding associated with the concomitant use of fluoxetine and NSAIDs). Products include:

EC-Naprosyn Delayed-Release Tablets 2632
Naprosyn Suspension 2632
Naprosyn Tablets 2632

Naproxen Sodium (SSRIs, including fluoxetine, may increase the risk of bleeding events. Concomitant use of nonsteroidal anti-inflammatory drugs may add to this risk. Case reports and epidemiological studies (case-control and cohort design) have demonstrated an association between use of drugs that interfere with serotonin reuptake and the occurrence of gastrointestinal bleeding. Bleeding events related to SSRI use have ranged from ecchymoses, hematomas, epistaxis, and petechiae to life-threatening hemorrhages. Patients should be cautioned about the risk of bleeding associated with the concomitant use of fluoxetine and NSAIDs). Products include:

Anaprox Tablets 2632
Anaprox DS Tablets 2632
Treximet Tablets 1616

Naratriptan Hydrochloride (There have been rare postmarketing reports of serotonin syndrome with use of an SSRI and a triptan. If concomitant treatment of fluoxetine with a triptan is clinically warranted, careful observation of the patient is advised, particularly during treatment initiation and dose increases). Products include:

Amerge Tablets 1301

Nateglinide (In patients with diabetes, fluoxetine may alter glycemic control. Hypoglycemia has occurred during therapy with fluoxetine, and hyperglycemia has developed following discontinuation of the drug. As is true with many other types of medication when taken concurrently by patients with diabetes, oral hypoglycemic dosage may need to be adjusted when therapy with fluoxetine is instituted or discontinued). Products include:

Starlix Tablets 2314

Nefazodone Hydrochloride (Based on the mechanism of action of SSRIs, including Prozac, and the potential for serotonin syndrome, caution is advised when fluoxetine is co-administered with other drugs that may affect serotonergic neurotransmitter systems. The Concimitant use of fluoxetine with SNRIs is not recommended).

No products indexed under this heading.

Nelfinavir Mesylate (Fluoxetine inhibits the activity of CYP2D6, and may make individuals with normal CYP2D6 metabolic activity resemble a poor metabolizer. Co-administration of fluoxetine with other drugs that are metabolized by CYP2D6 should be approached with caution. Therapy with medications that are predominantly metabolized by the CYP2D6 system and that have a relatively narrow therapeutic index should be initiated at the low end of the dose range if a patient is receiving fluoxetine concurrently or has taken it in the previous 5 weeks. If fluoxetine is added to the treatment regimen of a patient already receiving a drug metabolized by CYP2D6, the need for decreased dose of the original medication should be considered).

No products indexed under this heading.

Nortriptyline Hydrochloride (Fluoxetine inhibits the activity of CYP2D6, and may make individuals with normal CYP2D6 metabolic activity resemble a poor metabolizer. Co-administration of fluoxetine with other drugs that are metabolized by CYP2D6, including TCAs, should be approached with caution. Therapy with medications that are predominantly metabolized by the CYP2D6 system and that have a relatively narrow therapeutic index (eg, TCAs) should be initiated at the low end of the dose range if a patient is receiving fluoxetine concurrently or has taken it in the previous 5 weeks. If fluoxetine is added to the treatment regimen of a patient already receiving a drug metabolized by CYP2D6, the need for decreased dose of the original medication should be considered).

No products indexed under this heading.

Olanzapine (The risk of using fluoxetine in combination with other CNS active drugs has not been systematically evaluated. Nonetheless, caution is advised if the concomitant administration of fluoxetine and such drugs is required. In evaluating individual cases, consideration should be given to using lower initial doses of the concomitantly administered drugs, using conservative titration schedules, and monitoring of clinical status). Products include:

Symbyax Capsules 1871
Zyprexa Tablets 1883
Zyprexa IntraMuscular 1883
Zyprexa ZYDIS Orally Disintegrating Tablets 1883

Omeprazole (Fluoxetine inhibits the activity of CYP2D6, and may make individuals with normal CYP2D6 metabolic activity resemble a poor metabolizer. Co-administration of fluoxetine with other drugs that are metabolized by CYP2D6 should be approached with caution. Therapy with medications that are predominantly metabolized by the CYP2D6 system and that have a relatively narrow therapeutic index should be initiated at the low end of the dose range if a patient is receiving fluoxetine concurrently or has taken it in the previous 5 weeks. If fluoxetine is added to the treatment regimen of a patient already receiving a drug metabolized by CYP2D6, the need for decreased dose of the original medication should be considered).

No products indexed under this heading.

Ondansetron (Fluoxetine inhibits the activity of CYP2D6, and may make individuals with normal CYP2D6 metabolic activity resemble a poor metabolizer. Co-administration of fluoxetine with other drugs that are metabolized by CYP2D6 should be approached with caution. Therapy with medications that are predominantly metabolized by the CYP2D6 system and that have a relatively narrow therapeutic index should be initiated at the low end of the dose range if a patient is receiving fluoxetine concurrently or has taken it in the previous 5 weeks. If fluoxetine is added to the treatment regimen of a patient already receiving a drug metabolized by CYP2D6, the need for decreased dose of the original medication should be considered). Products include:

Zofran ODT Orally Disintegrating Tablets 1687

Ondansetron Hydrochloride (Fluoxetine inhibits the activity of CYP2D6, and may make individuals with normal CYP2D6 metabolic activity resemble a poor metabolizer. Co-administration of fluoxetine with other drugs that are metabolized by CYP2D6 should be approached with caution. Therapy with medications that are predominantly metabolized by the CYP2D6 system and that have a relatively narrow therapeutic index should be initiated at the low end of the dose range if a patient is receiving fluoxetine concurrently or has taken it in the previous 5 weeks. If fluoxetine is added to the treatment regimen of a patient already receiving a drug metabolized by CYP2D6, the need for decreased dose of the original medication should be considered). Products include:

Zofran Injection 1682
Zofran 1687

Oxaprozin (SSRIs, including fluoxetine, may increase the risk of bleeding events. Concomitant use of nonsteroidal anti-inflammatory drugs may add to this risk. Case reports and epidemiological studies (case-control and cohort design) have demonstrated an association between use of drugs that interfere with serotonin reuptake and the occurrence of gastrointestinal bleeding. Bleeding events related to SSRI use have ranged from ecchymoses, hematomas, epistaxis, and petechiae to life-threatening hemorrhages. Patients should be cautioned about the risk of bleeding associated with the concomitant use of fluoxetine and NSAIDs).

No products indexed under this heading.

Oxazepam (The risk of using fluoxetine in combination with other CNS active drugs has not been systematically evaluated. Nonetheless, caution is advised if the concomitant administration of fluoxetine and such drugs is required. In evaluating individual cases, consideration should be given to using lower initial doses of the concomitantly administered drugs, using conservative titration schedules, and monitoring of clinical status).

No products indexed under this heading.

Oxycodone Hydrochloride (The risk of using fluoxetine in combination with other CNS active drugs has not been systematically evaluated. Nonetheless, caution is advised if the concomitant administration of fluoxetine and such drugs is required. In evaluating individual cases, consideration should be given to using lower initial doses of the concomitantly administered drugs, using conservative titration schedules, and monitoring of clinical status). Products include:

OxyContin Tablets 2589
OxyIR Capsules 2593
Percocet Tablets 1127
Percodan Tablets 1130

Paclitaxel (Fluoxetine inhibits the activity of CYP2D6, and may make individuals with normal CYP2D6 metabolic activity resemble a poor metabolizer. Co-administration of fluoxetine with other drugs that are metabolized by CYP2D6 should be approached with caution. Therapy with medications that are predominantly metabolized by the CYP2D6 system and that have a relatively narrow therapeutic index should be initiated at the low end of the dose range if a patient is receiving fluoxetine concurrently or has taken it in the previous 5 weeks. If fluoxetine is added to the treatment regimen of a patient already receiving a drug metabolized by CYP2D6, the need for decreased dose of the original medication should be considered).

No products indexed under this heading.

Pargyline Hydrochloride (Use with MAOIs is contraindicated. There have been reports of serious, sometimes fatal, reactions in patients receiving fluoxetine in combination with a monoamine oxidase inhibitor (MAOI), and in patients who have recently discontinued fluoxetine and are then started on an MAOI. Some cases presented with features resembling neuroleptic malignant syndrome. Therefore fluoxetine should not be used in combination with an MAOI, or within a minimum of 14 days of discontinuing therapy with an MAOI. Since fluoxetine and its major metabolite have very long elimination half-lives, at least 5 weeks or longer, (especially if fluoxetine has been prescribed chronically and/or at higher doses) should be allowed after stopping fluoxetine before starting an MAOI).

No products indexed under this heading.

Paroxetine Hydrochloride (Based on the mechanism of action of SSRIs, including fluoxetine, and the potential for serotonin syndrome, caution is advised when fluoxetine is co-administered with other drugs that may affect serotonergic neurotransmitter systems. The Concomitant use of fluoxetine with other SSRIs is not recommended). Products include:

Paxil 1535
Paxil CR Controlled-Release Tablets 1544

Pemoline (The risk of using fluoxetine in combination with other CNS active drugs has not been systematically evaluated. Nonetheless, caution is advised if the concomitant administration of fluoxetine and such drugs is required. In evaluating individual cases, consideration should be given to using lower initial doses of the concomitantly administered drugs, using conservative titration schedules, and monitoring of clinical status).

No products indexed under this heading.

Pentobarbital Sodium (The risk of using fluoxetine in combination with other CNS active drugs has not been systematically evaluated. Nonetheless, caution is advised if the concomitant administration of fluoxetine and such drugs is required. In evaluating individual cases, consideration should be given to using lower initial doses of the concomitantly administered drugs, using conservative titration schedules, and monitoring of clinical status). Products include:

Nembutal Sodium Solution, USP 2494

Perphenazine (Fluoxetine inhibits the activity of CYP2D6, and may make individuals with normal CYP2D6 metabolic activity resemble a poor metabolizer. Co-administration of fluoxetine with other drugs that are metabolized by CYP2D6, including phenothiazines, should be approached with caution. If fluoxetine is added to the treatment regimen of a patient already receiving a drug metabolized by CYP2D6, the need for decreased dose of the original medication should be considered).

No products indexed under this heading.

Phenelzine Sulfate (Use with MAOIs is contraindicated. There have been reports of serious, sometimes fatal, reactions in patients receiving fluoxetine in combination with a monoamine oxidase inhibitor (MAOI), and in patients who have recently discontinued fluoxetine and are then started on an MAOI. Some cases presented with features resembling neuroleptic malignant syndrome. Therefore fluoxetine should not be used in combination with an MAOI, or within a minimum of 14 days of discontinuing therapy with an MAOI. Since fluoxetine and its major metabolite have very long elimination half-lives, at least 5 weeks or longer, (especially if fluoxetine has been prescribed chronically and/or at higher doses) should be allowed after stopping fluoxetine before starting an MAOI).

No products indexed under this heading.

Phenobarbital (The risk of using fluoxetine in combination with other CNS active drugs has not been systematically evaluated. Nonetheless, caution is advised if the concomitant administration of fluoxetine and such drugs is required. In evaluating individual cases, consideration should be given to using lower initial doses of the concomitantly administered drugs, using conservative titration schedules, and monitoring of clinical status). Products include:

Donnatal Extentabs 2507

Phenylbutazone (SSRIs, including fluoxetine, may increase the risk of bleeding events. Concomitant use of nonsteroidal anti-inflammatory drugs may add to this risk. Case reports and epidemiological studies (case-control and cohort design) have demonstrated an association between use of drugs that interfere with serotonin reuptake and the occurrence of gastrointestinal bleeding. Bleeding events related to SSRI use have ranged from ecchymoses, hematomas, epistaxis, and petechiae to life-threatening hemorrhages. Patients should be cautioned about the risk of bleeding associated with the concomitant use of fluoxetine and NSAIDs).

No products indexed under this heading.

Phenytoin (Patients on stable doses of phenytoin have developed elevated plasma anticonvulsant concentrations and clinical anticonvulsant toxicity following initiation of concomitant fluoxetine treatment).

No products indexed under this heading.

Phenytoin Sodium (Patients on stable doses of phenytoin have developed elevated plasma anticonvulsant concentrations and clinical anticonvulsant toxicity following initiation of concomitant fluoxetine treatment). Products include:

Phenytek Capsules 2192

Pimozide (Concomitant use of fluoxetine and pimozide is contraindicated. Clinical studies of pimozide with other antidepressants demonstrate an increase in drug interaction or QTc prolongation. While a specific study with pimozide and fluoxetine has not been conducted, the potential for drug interactions or QTc prolongation warrants restricting the concurrent use of pimozide and fluoxetine).

No products indexed under this heading.

Pindolol (Fluoxetine inhibits the activity of CYP2D6, and may make individuals with normal CYP2D6 metabolic activity resemble a poor metabolizer. Co-administration of fluoxetine with other drugs that are metabolized by CYP2D6 should be approached with caution. Therapy with medications that are predominantly metabolized by the CYP2D6 system and that have a relatively narrow therapeutic index should be initiated at the low end of the dose range if a patient is receiving fluoxetine concurrently or has taken it in the previous 5 weeks. If fluoxetine is added to the treatment regimen of a patient already receiving a drug metabolized by CYP2D6, the need for decreased dose of the original medication should be considered).

No products indexed under this heading.

Pioglitazone Hydrochloride (In patients with diabetes, fluoxetine may alter glycemic control. Hypoglycemia has occurred during therapy with fluoxetine, and hyperglycemia has developed following discontinuation of the drug. As is true with many other types of medication when taken concurrently by patients with diabetes, oral hypoglycemic dosage may need to be adjusted when therapy with fluoxetine is instituted or discontinued). Products include:

ActoPlus Met Tablets **3071**
Actos Tablets **3077**
Duetact Tablets **3085**

Piroxicam (SSRIs, including fluoxetine, may increase the risk of bleeding events. Concomitant use of nonsteroidal anti-inflammatory drugs may add to this risk. Case reports and epidemiological studies (case-control and cohort design) have demonstrated an association between use of drugs that interfere with serotonin reuptake and the occurrence of gastrointestinal bleeding. Bleeding events related to SSRI use have ranged from ecchymoses, hematomas, epistaxis, and petechiae to live-threatening hemorrhages. Patients should be cautioned about the risk of bleeding associated with the concomitant use of fluoxetine and NSAIDs).

No products indexed under this heading.

Polythiazide (Hyponatremia may occur as a result of treatment with SSRIs, including fluoxetine. In many cases this hyponatremia appears to be the result of the syndrome of inappropriate antidiuretic hormone secretion (SIADH). Cases with serum sodium lower than 110 mmol/L have been reported and appeared to be reversible when fluoxetine was discontinued. Patients taking diuretics may be at greater risk. Discontinuation of fluoxetine should be considered in patients with symptomatic hyponatremia and appropriate medical intervention should be instituted).

No products indexed under this heading.

Prazepam (The risk of using fluoxetine in combination with other CNS active drugs has not been systematically evaluated. Nonetheless, caution is advised if the concomitant administration of fluoxetine and such drugs is required. In evaluating individual cases, consideration should be given to using lower initial doses of the concomitantly administered drugs, using conservative titration schedules, and monitoring of clinical status).

No products indexed under this heading.

Procarbazine Hydrochloride (Use with MAOIs is contraindicated. There have been reports of serious, sometimes fatal, reactions in patients receiving fluoxetine in combination with a monoamine oxidase inhibitor (MAOI), and in patients who have recently discontinued fluoxetine and are then started on an MAOI. Some cases presented with features resembling neuroleptic malignant syndrome. Therefore fluoxetine should not be used in combination with an MAOI, or within a minimum of 14 days of discontinuing therapy with an MAOI. Since fluoxetine and its major metabolite have very long elimination half-lives, at least 5 weeks or longer, (especially if fluoxetine has been prescribed chronically and/or at higher doses) should be allowed after stopping fluoxetine before starting an MAOI).

No products indexed under this heading.

Prochlorperazine (Fluoxetine inhibits the activity of CYP2D6, and may make individuals with normal CYP2D6 metabolic activity resemble a poor metabolizer. Co-administration of fluoxetine with other drugs that are metabolized by CYP2D6, including phenothiazines, should be approached with caution. If fluoxetine is added to the treatment regimen of a patient already receiving a drug metabolized by CYP2D6, the need for decreased dose of the original medication should be considered).

No products indexed under this heading.

Promethazine Hydrochloride (Fluoxetine inhibits the activity of CYP2D6, and may make individuals with normal CYP2D6 metabolic activity resemble a poor metabolizer. Co-administration of fluoxetine with other drugs that are metabolized by CYP2D6, including phenothiazines, should be approached with caution. If fluoxetine is added to the treatment regimen of a patient already receiving a drug metabolized by CYP2D6, the need for decreased dose of the original medication should be considered).

No products indexed under this heading.

Propafenone Hydrochloride (Fluoxetine inhibits the activity of CYP2D6 and may make individuals with normal CYP2D6 metabolic activity resemble a poor metabolizer. Co-administration of fluoxetine with other drugs that are metabolized by CYP2D6, including propafenone, should be approached with caution. Therapy with medications that are predominantly metabolized by the CYP2D6 system and that have a relatively narrow therapeutic index (eg, propafenone) should be initiated at the low end of the dose range if a patient is receiving fluoxetine concurrently or has taken it in the previous 5 weeks. If fluoxetine is added to the treatment regimen of a patient already receiving a drug metabolized CYP2D6, the need for decreased dose of the original medication should be considered). Products include:

Rythmol Tablets **1586**
Rythmol SR Capsules **1590**

Propofol (The risk of using fluoxetine in combination with other CNS active drugs has not been systematically evaluated. Nonetheless, caution is advised if the concomitant administration of fluoxetine and such drugs is required. In evaluating individual cases, consideration should be given to using lower initial doses of the concomitantly administered drugs, using conservative titration schedules, and monitoring of clinical status).

No products indexed under this heading.

Propoxyphene Hydrochloride (The risk of using fluoxetine in combination with other CNS active drugs has not been systematically evaluated. Nonetheless, caution is advised if the concomitant administration of fluoxetine and such drugs is required. In evaluating individual cases, consideration should be given to using lower initial doses of the concomitantly administered drugs, using conservative titration schedules, and monitoring of clinical status).

No products indexed under this heading.

Propoxyphene Napsylate (The risk of using fluoxetine in combination with other CNS active drugs has not been systematically evaluated. Nonetheless, caution is advised if the concomitant administration of fluoxetine and such drugs is required. In evaluating individual cases, consideration should be given to using lower initial doses of the concomitantly administered drugs, using conservative titration schedules, and monitoring of clinical status).

No products indexed under this heading.

Propranolol Hydrochloride (Fluoxetine inhibits the activity of CYP2D6, and may make individuals with normal CYP2D6 metabolic activity resemble a poor metabolizer. Co-administration of fluoxetine with other drugs that are metabolized by CYP2D6 should be approached with caution. Therapy with medications that are predominantly metabolized by the CYP2D6 system and that have a relatively narrow therapeutic index should be initiated at the low end of the dose range if a patient is receiving fluoxetine concurrently or has taken it in the previous 5 weeks. If fluoxetine is added to the treatment regimen of a patient already receiving a drug metabolized by CYP2D6, the need for decreased dose of the original medication should be considered). Products include:

InnoPran XL Extended Release Capsules **1484**

Protriptyline Hydrochloride (Fluoxetine inhibits the activity of CYP2D6, and may make individuals with normal CYP2D6 metabolic activity resemble a poor metabolizer. Co-administration of fluoxetine with other drugs that are metabolized by CYP2D6, including TCAs, should be approached with caution. Therapy with medications that are predominantly metabolized by the CYP2D6 system and that have a relatively narrow therapeutic index (eg, TCAs) should be initiated at the low end of the dose range if a patient is receiving fluoxetine concurrently or has taken it in the previous 5 weeks. If fluoxetine is added to the treatment regimen of a patient already receiving a drug metabolized by CYP2D6, the need for decreased dose of the original medication should be considered).

No products indexed under this heading.

Quazepam (The risk of using fluoxetine in combination with other CNS active drugs has not been systematically evaluated. Nonetheless, caution is advised if the concomitant administration of fluoxetine and such drugs is required. In evaluating individual cases, consideration should be given to using lower initial doses of the concomitantly administered drugs, using conservative titration schedules, and monitoring of clinical status).

No products indexed under this heading.

Quetiapine Fumarate (The risk of using fluoxetine in combination with other CNS active drugs has not been systematically evaluated. Nonetheless, caution is advised if the concomitant administration of fluoxetine and such drugs is required. In evaluating individual cases, consideration should be given to using lower initial doses of the concomitantly administered drugs, using conservative titration schedules, and monitoring of clinical status).

No products indexed under this heading.

Quinidine Gluconate (Fluoxetine inhibits the activity of CYP2D6, and may make individuals with normal CYP2D6 metabolic activity resemble a poor metabolizer. Co-administration of fluoxetine with other drugs that are metabolized by CYP2D6 should be approached with caution. Therapy with medications that are predominantly metabolized by the CYP2D6 system and that have a relatively narrow therapeutic index should be initiated at the low end of the dose range if a patient is receiving fluoxetine concurrently or has taken it in the previous 5 weeks. If fluoxetine is added to the treatment regimen of a patient already receiving a drug metabolized by CYP2D6, the need for decreased dose of the original medication should be considered).

No products indexed under this heading.

Quinidine Hydrochloride (Fluoxetine inhibits the activity of CYP2D6, and may make individuals with normal CYP2D6 metabolic activity resemble a poor metabolizer. Co-administration of fluoxetine with other drugs that are metabolized by CYP2D6 should be approached with caution. Therapy with medications that are predominantly metabolized by the CYP2D6 system and that have a relatively narrow therapeutic index should be initiated at the low end of the dose range if a patient is receiving fluoxetine concurrently or has taken it in the previous 5 weeks. If fluoxetine is added to the treatment regimen of a patient already receiving a drug metabolized by CYP2D6, the need for decreased dose of the original medication should be considered).

No products indexed under this heading.

Quinidine Polygalacturonate (Fluoxetine inhibits the activity of CYP2D6, and may make individuals with normal CYP2D6 metabolic activity resemble a poor metabolizer. Co-administration of fluoxetine with other drugs that are metabolized by CYP2D6 should be approached with caution. Therapy with medications that are predominantly metabolized by the CYP2D6 system and that have a relatively narrow therapeutic index should be initiated at the low

end of the dose range if a patient is receiving fluoxetine concurrently or has taken it in the previous 5 weeks. If fluoxetine is added to the treatment regimen of a patient already receiving a drug metabolized by CYP2D6, the need for decreased dose of the original medication should be considered).
No products indexed under this heading.

Quinidine Sulfate (Fluoxetine inhibits the activity of CYP2D6, and may make individuals with normal CYP2D6 metabolic activity resemble a poor metabolizer. Co-administration of fluoxetine with other drugs that are metabolized by CYP2D6 should be approached with caution. Therapy with medications that are predominantly metabolized by the CYP2D6 system and that have a relatively narrow therapeutic index should be initiated at the low end of the dose range if a patient is receiving fluoxetine concurrently or has taken it in the previous 5 weeks. If fluoxetine is added to the treatment regimen of a patient already receiving a drug metabolized by CYP2D6, the need for decreased dose of the original medication should be considered).
No products indexed under this heading.

Rasagiline Mesylate (Use with MAOIs is contraindicated. There have been reports of serious, sometimes fatal, reactions in patients receiving fluoxetine in combination with a monoamine oxidase inhibitor (MAOI), and in patients who have recently discontinued fluoxetine and are then started on an MAOI. Some cases presented with features resembling neuroleptic malignant syndrome. Therefore fluoxetine should not be used in combination with an MAOI, or within a minimum of 14 days of discontinuing therapy with an MAOI. Since fluoxetine and its major metabolite have very long elimination half-lives, at least 5 weeks or longer, (especially if fluoxetine has been prescribed chronically and/or at higher doses) should be allowed after stopping fluoxetine before starting an MAOI). Products include:
Azilect Tablets 3106

Remifentanil Hydrochloride (The risk of using fluoxetine in combination with other CNS active drugs has not been systematically evaluated. Nonetheless, caution is advised if the concomitant administration of fluoxetine and such drugs is required. In evaluating individual cases, consideration should be given to using lower initial doses of the concomitantly administered drugs, using conservative titration schedules, and monitoring of clinical status).
No products indexed under this heading.

Repaglinide (In patients with diabetes, fluoxetine may alter glycemic control. Hypoglycemia has occurred during therapy with fluoxetine, and hyperglycemia has developed following discontinuation of the drug. As is true with many other types of medication when taken concurrently by patients with diabetes, oral hypoglycemic dosage may need to be adjusted when therapy with fluoxetine is instituted or discontinued). Products include:
PrandiMet Tablets 2967
Prandin Tablets 2971

Risperidone (The risk of using fluoxetine in combination with other CNS active drugs has not been systematically evaluated. Nonetheless, caution is advised if the concomitant administration of fluoxetine and such drugs is required. In evaluating individual cases, consideration should be given to using lower initial doses of the concomitantly administered drugs, using conservative titration schedules, and monitoring of clinical status). Products include:
Risperdal Consta Long-Acting Injection 1753

Ritonavir (Fluoxetine inhibits the activity of CYP2D6, and may make individuals with normal CYP2D6 metabolic activity resemble a poor metabolizer. Co-administration of fluoxetine with other drugs that are metabolized by CYP2D6 should be approached with caution. Therapy with medications that are predominantly metabolized by the CYP2D6 system and that have a relatively narrow therapeutic index should be initiated at the low end of the dose range if a patient is receiving fluoxetine concurrently or has taken it in the previous 5 weeks. If fluoxetine is added to the treatment regimen of a patient already receiving a drug metabolized by CYP2D6, the need for decreased dose of the original medication should be considered). Products include:
Kaletra 452
Norvir 489

Rizatriptan Benzoate (There have been rare postmarketing reports of serotonin syndrome with use of an SSRI and a triptan. If concomitant treatment of fluoxetine with a triptan is clinically warranted, careful observation of the patient is advised, particularly during treatment initiation and dose increases). Products include:
Maxalt Tablets 2056
Maxalt-MLT Orally Disintegrating Tablets 2056

Rofecoxib (SSRIs, including fluoxetine, may increase the risk of bleeding events. Concomitant use of nonsteroidal anti-inflammatory drugs may add to this risk. Case reports and epidemiological studies (case-control and cohort design) have demonstrated an association between use of drugs that interfere with serotonin reuptake and the occurrence of gastrointestinal bleeding. Bleeding events related to SSRI use have ranged from ecchymoses, hematomas, epistaxis, and petechiae to live-threatening hemorrhages. Patients should be cautioned about the risk of bleeding associated with the concomitant use of fluoxetine and NSAIDs).
No products indexed under this heading.

Rosiglitazone Maleate (In patients with diabetes, fluoxetine may alter glycemic control. Hypoglycemia has occurred during therapy with fluoxetine, and hyperglycemia has developed following discontinuation of the drug. As is true with many other types of medication when taken concurrently by patients with diabetes, oral hypoglycemic dosage may need to be adjusted when therapy with fluoxetine is instituted or discontinued). Products include:
Avandamet Tablets 1336
Avandaryl Tablets 1344
Avandia Tablets 1351

Secobarbital Sodium (The risk of using fluoxetine in combination with other CNS active drugs has not been systematically evaluated. Nonetheless, caution is advised if the concomitant administration of fluoxetine and such drugs is required. In evaluating individual cases, consideration should be given to using lower initial doses of the concomitantly administered drugs, using conservative titration schedules, and monitoring of clinical status).
No products indexed under this heading.

Selegiline (Use with MAOIs is contraindicated. There have been reports of serious, sometimes fatal, reactions in patients receiving fluoxetine in combination with a monoamine oxidase inhibitor (MAOI), and in patients who have recently discontinued fluoxetine and are then started on an MAOI. Some cases presented with features resembling neuroleptic malignant syndrome. Therefore fluoxetine should not be used in combination with an MAOI, or within a minimum of 14 days of discontinuing therapy with an MAOI. Since fluoxetine and its major metabolite have very long elimination half-lives, at least 5 weeks or longer, (especially if fluoxetine has been prescribed chronically and/or at higher doses) should be allowed after stopping fluoxetine before starting an MAOI). Products include:
Emsam Transdermal System 905

Selegiline Hydrochloride (Use with MAOIs is contraindicated. There have been reports of serious, sometimes fatal, reactions in patients receiving fluoxetine in combination with a monoamine oxidase inhibitor (MAOI), and in patients who have recently discontinued fluoxetine and are then started on an MAOI. Some cases presented with features resembling neuroleptic malignant syndrome. Therefore fluoxetine should not be used in combination with an MAOI, or within a minimum of 14 days of discontinuing therapy with an MAOI. Since fluoxetine and its major metabolite have very long elimination half-lives, at least 5 weeks or longer, (especially if fluoxetine has been prescribed chronically and/or at higher doses) should be allowed after stopping fluoxetine before starting an MAOI). Products include:
Eldepryl Capsules 3052

Sertraline Hydrochloride (Based on the mechanism of action of SSRIs, including fluoxetine, and the potential for serotonin syndrome, caution is advised when fluoxetine is co-administered with other drugs that may affect serotonergic neurotransmitter systems. The Concomitant use of fluoxetine with other SSRIs is not recommended).
No products indexed under this heading.

Sevoflurane (The risk of using fluoxetine in combination with other CNS active drugs has not been systematically evaluated. Nonetheless, caution is advised if the concomitant administration of fluoxetine and such drugs is required. In evaluating individual cases, consideration should be given to using lower initial doses of the concomitantly administered drugs, using conservative titration schedules, and monitoring of clinical status). Products include:
Ultane Liquid for Inhalation 524

Sitagliptin Phosphate (In patients with diabetes, fluoxetine may alter glycemic control. Hypoglycemia has occurred during therapy with fluoxetine, and hyperglycemia has developed following discontinuation of the drug. As is true with many other types of medication when taken concurrently by patients with diabetes, oral hypoglycemic dosage may need to be adjusted when therapy with fluoxetine is instituted or discontinued). Products include:
Janumet Tablets 2041
Januvia Tablets 2048

Sodium Oxybate (The risk of using fluoxetine in combination with other CNS active drugs has not been systematically evaluated. Nonetheless, caution is advised if the concomitant administration of fluoxetine and such drugs is required. In evaluating individual cases, consideration should be given to using lower initial doses of the concomitantly administered drugs, using conservative titration schedules, and monitoring of clinical status). Products include:
Xyrem Oral Solution 1766

Spironolactone (Hyponatremia may occur as a result of treatment with SSRIs, including fluoxetine. In many cases this hyponatremia appears to be the result of the syndrome of inappropriate antidiuretic hormone secretion (SIADH). Cases with serum sodium lower than 110 mmol/L have been reported and appeared to be reversible when fluoxetine was discontinued. Patients taking diuretics may be at greater risk. Discontinuation of fluoxetine should be considered in patients with symptomatic hyponatremia and appropriate medical intervention should be instituted).
No products indexed under this heading.

Sufentanil Citrate (The risk of using fluoxetine in combination with other CNS active drugs has not been systematically evaluated. Nonetheless, caution is advised if the concomitant administration of fluoxetine and such drugs is required. In evaluating individual cases, consideration should be given to using lower initial doses of the concomitantly administered drugs, using conservative titration schedules, and monitoring of clinical status).
No products indexed under this heading.

Sulindac (SSRIs, including fluoxetine, may increase the risk of bleeding events. Concomitant use of nonsteroidal anti-inflammatory drugs may add to this risk. Case reports and epidemiological studies (case-control and cohort design) have demonstrated an association between use of drugs that interfere with serotonin reuptake and the occurrence of gastrointestinal bleeding. Bleeding events related to SSRI use have ranged from ecchymoses, hematomas, epistaxis, and petechiae to live-threatening hemorrhages. Patients should be cautioned about the risk of bleeding

associated with the concomitant use of fluoxetine and NSAIDs). Products include:
Clinoril Tablets 1962

Sumatriptan (There have been rare postmarketing reports of serotonin syndrome with use of an SSRI and a triptan. If concomitant treatment of fluoxetine with a triptan is clinically warranted, careful observation of the patient is advised, particularly during treatment initiation and dose increases). Products include:
Imitrex Nasal Spray 1470

Sumatriptan Succinate (There have been rare postmarketing reports of serotonin syndrome with use of an SSRI and a triptan. If concomitant treatment of fluoxetine with a triptan is clinically warranted, careful observation of the patient is advised, particularly during treatment initiation and dose increases). Products include:
Imitrex Injection 1465
Imitrex Tablets 1474
Treximet Tablets 1616

Tamoxifen Citrate (Fluoxetine inhibits the activity of CYP2D6, and may make individuals with normal CYP2D6 metabolic activity resemble a poor metabolizer. Co-administration of fluoxetine with other drugs that are metabolized by CYP2D6 should be approached with caution. Therapy with medications that are predominantly metabolized by the CYP2D6 system and that have a relatively narrow therapeutic index should be initiated at the low end of the dose range if a patient is receiving fluoxetine concurrently or has taken it in the previous 5 weeks. If fluoxetine is added to the treatment regimen of a patient already receiving a drug metabolized by CYP2D6, the need for decreased dose of the original medication should be considered).
No products indexed under this heading.

Temazepam (The risk of using fluoxetine in combination with other CNS active drugs has not been systematically evaluated. Nonetheless, caution is advised if the concomitant administration of fluoxetine and such drugs is required. In evaluating individual cases, consideration should be given to using lower initial doses of the concomitantly administered drugs, using conservative titration schedules, and monitoring of clinical status).
No products indexed under this heading.

Teniposide (Fluoxetine inhibits the activity of CYP2D6, and may make individuals with normal CYP2D6 metabolic activity resemble a poor metabolizer. Co-administration of fluoxetine with other drugs that are metabolized by CYP2D6 should be approached with caution. Therapy with medications that are predominantly metabolized by the CYP2D6 system and that have a relatively narrow therapeutic index should be initiated at the low end of the dose range if a patient is receiving fluoxetine concurrently or has taken it in the previous 5 weeks. If fluoxetine is added to the treatment regimen of a patient already receiving a drug metabolized by CYP2D6, the need for decreased dose of the original medication should be considered).
No products indexed under this heading.

Testosterone (Fluoxetine inhibits the activity of CYP2D6, and may make individuals with normal CYP2D6 metabolic activity resemble a poor metabolizer. Co-administration of fluoxetine with other drugs that are metabolized by CYP2D6 should be approached with caution. Therapy with medications that are predominantly metabolized by the CYP2D6 system and that have a relatively narrow therapeutic index should be initiated at the low end of the dose range if a patient is receiving fluoxetine concurrently or has taken it in the previous 5 weeks. If fluoxetine is added to the treatment regimen of a patient already receiving a drug metabolized by CYP2D6, the need for decreased dose of the original medication should be considered). Products include:
AndroGel 3159
Testim 1% Gel 701

Testosterone Cypionate (Fluoxetine inhibits the activity of CYP2D6, and may make individuals with normal CYP2D6 metabolic activity resemble a poor metabolizer. Co-administration of fluoxetine with other drugs that are metabolized by CYP2D6 should be approached with caution. Therapy with medications that are predominantly metabolized by the CYP2D6 system and that have a relatively narrow therapeutic index should be initiated at the low end of the dose range if a patient is receiving fluoxetine concurrently or has taken it in the previous 5 weeks. If fluoxetine is added to the treatment regimen of a patient already receiving a drug metabolized by CYP2D6, the need for decreased dose of the original medication should be considered).
No products indexed under this heading.

Testosterone Enanthate (Fluoxetine inhibits the activity of CYP2D6, and may make individuals with normal CYP2D6 metabolic activity resemble a poor metabolizer. Co-administration of fluoxetine with other drugs that are metabolized by CYP2D6 should be approached with caution. Therapy with medications that are predominantly metabolized by the CYP2D6 system and that have a relatively narrow therapeutic index should be initiated at the low end of the dose range if a patient is receiving fluoxetine concurrently or has taken it in the previous 5 weeks. If fluoxetine is added to the treatment regimen of a patient already receiving a drug metabolized by CYP2D6, the need for decreased dose of the original medication should be considered). Products include:
Delatestryl Injection 1730

Testosterone Propionate (Fluoxetine inhibits the activity of CYP2D6, and may make individuals with normal CYP2D6 metabolic activity resemble a poor metabolizer. Co-administration of fluoxetine with other drugs that are metabolized by CYP2D6 should be approached with caution. Therapy with medications that are predominantly metabolized by the CYP2D6 system and that have a relatively narrow therapeutic index should be initiated at the low end of the dose range if a patient is receiving fluoxetine concurrently or has taken it in the previous 5 weeks. If fluoxetine is added to the treatment regimen of a patient already receiving a drug metabolized by CYP2D6, the need for decreased dose of the original medication should be considered).
No products indexed under this heading.

Thiamylal Sodium (The risk of using fluoxetine in combination with other CNS active drugs has not been systematically evaluated. Nonetheless, caution is advised if the concomitant administration of fluoxetine and such drugs is required. In evaluating individual cases, consideration should be given to using lower initial doses of the concomitantly administered drugs, using conservative titration schedules, and monitoring of clinical status).
No products indexed under this heading.

Thioridazine (In a study of 19 healthy male subjects, which included 6 slow and 13 rapid hydroxylators of debrisoquin, a single 25-mg oral dose of thioridazine produced a 2.4-fold higher Cmax and a 4.5-fold higher AUC for thioridazine in the slow hydroxylators compared with rapid hydroxylators. The rate of debrisoquin hydroxylation is felt to depend on the level of CYP2D6 isozyme activity. Thus, this study suggests that drugs which inhibit CYP2D6, such as SSRIs, including fluoxetine, will produce elevated plasma levels of thioridazine. Thioridazine should not be administered with fluoxetine or within a minimum of 5 weeks after fluoxetine has been discontinued).
No products indexed under this heading.

Thioridazine Hydrochloride (In a study of 19 healthy male subjects, which included 6 slow and 13 rapid hydroxylators of debrisoquin, a single 25-mg oral dose of thioridazine produced a 2.4-fold higher Cmax and a 4.5-fold higher AUC for thioridazine in the slow hydroxylators compared with rapid hydroxylators. The rate of debrisoquin hydroxylation is felt to depend on the level of CYP2D6 isozyme activity. Thus, this study suggests that drugs which inhibit CYP2D6, such as SSRIs, including fluoxetine, will produce elevated plasma levels of thioridazine. Thioridazine should not be administered with fluoxetine or within a minimum of 5 weeks after fluoxetine has been discontinued). Products include:
Thioridazine Hydrochloride Tablets 2195

Thiothixene (The risk of using fluoxetine in combination with other CNS active drugs has not been systematically evaluated. Nonetheless, caution is advised if the concomitant administration of fluoxetine and such drugs is required. In evaluating individual cases, consideration should be given to using lower initial doses of the concomitantly administered drugs, using conservative titration schedules, and monitoring of clinical status). Products include:
Thiothixene Capsules 2197

Timolol Maleate (Fluoxetine inhibits the activity of CYP2D6, and may make individuals with normal CYP2D6 metabolic activity resemble a poor metabolizer. Co-administration of fluoxetine with other drugs that are metabolized by CYP2D6 should be approached with caution. Therapy with medications that are predominantly metabolized by the CYP2D6 system and that have a relatively narrow therapeutic index should be initiated at the low end of the dose range if a patient is receiving fluoxetine concurrently or has taken it in the previous 5 weeks. If fluoxetine is added to the treatment regimen of a patient already receiving a drug metabolized by CYP2D6, the need for decreased dose of the original medication should be considered). Products include:
Combigan Ophthalmic Solution 553
Cosopt Sterile Ophthalmic Solution 1969
Timoptic Sterile Ophthalmic Solution 2121
Timoptic in Ocudose 2124
Timoptic-XE Sterile Ophthalmic Gel Forming Solution 2125

Tinzaparin Sodium (Case reports and epidemiological studies (case-control and cohort design) have demonstrated an association between use of drugs that interfere with serotonin reuptake and the occurrence of gastrointestinal bleeding. Bleeding events related to SSRI use have ranged from ecchymoses, hematomas, epistaxis, and petechiae to live-threatening hemorrhages. Patients should be cautioned about the risk of bleeding associated with the concomitant use of fluoxetine and other drugs that affect coagulation).
No products indexed under this heading.

Tolazamide (In patients with diabetes, fluoxetine may alter glycemic control. Hypoglycemia has occurred during therapy with fluoxetine, and hyperglycemia has developed following discontinuation of the drug. As is true with many other types of medication when taken concurrently by patients with diabetes, oral hypoglycemic dosage may need to be adjusted when therapy with fluoxetine is instituted or discontinued).
No products indexed under this heading.

Tolbutamide (Because fluoxetine is tightly bound to plasma protein, the administration of fluoxetine to a patient taking another drugs that is tightly bound to protein may cause a shift in plasma concentrations potentially resulting in an adverse effect. Conversely,adverse effects may result from displacement of protein-bound fluoxetine by other tightly-bound drugs).
No products indexed under this heading.

Tolmetin Sodium (SSRIs, including fluoxetine, may increase the risk of bleeding events. Concomitant use of nonsteroidal anti-inflammatory drugs may add to this risk. Case reports and epidemiological studies (case-control and cohort design) have demonstrated an association between use of drugs that interfere with serotonin reuptake and the occurrence of gastrointestinal bleeding. Bleeding events related to SSRI use have ranged from ecchymoses, hematomas, epistaxis, and petechiae to live-threatening hemor-

rhages. Patients should be cautioned about the risk of bleeding associated with the concomitant use of fluoxetine and NSAIDs).
No products indexed under this heading.

Tolterodine Tartrate (Fluoxetine inhibits the activity of CYP2D6, and may make individuals with normal CYP2D6 metabolic activity resemble a poor metabolizer. Co-administration of fluoxetine with other drugs that are metabolized by CYP2D6 should be approached with caution. Therapy with medications that are predominantly metabolized by the CYP2D6 system and that have a relatively narrow therapeutic index should be initiated at the low end of the dose range if a patient is receiving fluoxetine concurrently or has taken it in the previous 5 weeks. If fluoxetine is added to the treatment regimen of a patient already receiving a drug metabolized by CYP2D6, the need for decreased dose of the original medication should be considered).
No products indexed under this heading.

Torsemide (Hyponatremia may occur as a result of treatment with SSRIs, including fluoxetine. In many cases this hyponatremia appears to be the result of the syndrome of inappropriate antidiuretic hormone secretion (SIADH). Cases with serum sodium lower than 110 mmol/L have been reported and appeared to be reversible when fluoxetine was discontinued. Patients taking diuretics may be at greater risk. Discontinuation of fluoxetine should be considered in patients with symptomatic hyponatremia and appropriate medical intervention should be instituted). Products include:
Demadex Injection 2630
Demadex Tablets 2630

Tramadol Hydrochloride (Based on the mechanism of action of SSRIs, including fluoxetine, and the potential for serotonin syndrome, caution is advised when fluoxetine is co-administered with other drugs that may affect serotonergic neurotransmitter systems, such as tramadol). Products include:
Ultram ER Extended-Release Tablets 2428

Tranylcypromine Sulfate (Use with MAOIs is contraindicated. There have been reports of serious, sometimes fatal, reactions in patients receiving fluoxetine in combination with a monoamine oxidase inhibitor (MAOI), and in patients who have recently discontinued fluoxetine and are then started on an MAOI. Some cases presented with features resembling neuroleptic malignant syndrome. Therefore fluoxetine should not be used in combination with an MAOI, or within a minimum of 14 days of discontinuing therapy with an MAOI. Since fluoxetine and its major metabolite have very long elimination half-lives, at least 5 weeks or longer, (especially if fluoxetine has been prescribed chronically and/or at higher doses) should be allowed after stopping fluoxetine before starting an MAOI). Products include:
Parnate Tablets 1532

Trazodone Hydrochloride (Fluoxetine inhibits the activity of CYP2D6, and may make individuals with normal CYP2D6 metabolic activity resemble a poor metabolizer. Co-administration of fluoxetine with other drugs that are metabolized by CYP2D6 should be approached with caution. Therapy with medications that are predominantly metabolized by the CYP2D6 system and that have a relatively narrow therapeutic index should be initiated at the low end of the dose range if a patient is receiving fluoxetine concurrently or has taken it in the previous 5 weeks. If fluoxetine is added to the treatment regimen of a patient already receiving a drug metabolized by CYP2D6, the need for decreased dose of the original medication should be considered).
No products indexed under this heading.

Triamterene (Hyponatremia may occur as a result of treatment with SSRIs, including fluoxetine. In many cases this hyponatremia appears to be the result of the syndrome of inappropriate antidiuretic hormone secretion (SIADH). Cases with serum sodium lower than 110 mmol/L have been reported and appeared to be reversible when fluoxetine was discontinued. Patients taking diuretics may be at greater risk. Discontinuation of fluoxetine should be considered in patients with symptomatic hyponatremia and appropriate medical intervention should be instituted). Products include:
Dyazide Capsules 1405
Dyrenium Capsules 3189

Triazolam (The risk of using fluoxetine in combination with other CNS active drugs has not been systematically evaluated. Nonetheless, caution is advised if the concomitant administration of fluoxetine and such drugs is required. In evaluating individual cases, consideration should be given to using lower initial doses of the concomitantly administered drugs, using conservative titration schedules, and monitoring of clinical status).
No products indexed under this heading.

Trifluoperazine Hydrochloride (Fluoxetine inhibits the activity of CYP2D6, and may make individuals with normal CYP2D6 metabolic activity resemble a poor metabolizer. Co-administration of fluoxetine with other drugs that are metabolized by CYP2D6, including phenothiazines, should be approached with caution. If fluoxetine is added to the treatment regimen of a patient already receiving a drug metabolized by CYP2D6, the need for decreased dose of the original medication should be considered).
No products indexed under this heading.

Trimipramine Maleate (Fluoxetine inhibits the activity of CYP2D6, and may make individuals with normal CYP2D6 metabolic activity resemble a poor metabolizer. Co-administration of fluoxetine with other drugs that are metabolized by CYP2D6, including TCAs, should be approached with caution. Therapy with medications that are predominantly metabolized by the CYP2D6 system and that have a relatively narrow therapeutic index (eg, TCAs) should be initiated at the low end of the dose range if a patient is receiving fluoxetine concurrently or has taken it in the previous 5 weeks. If fluoxetine is added to the treatment regimen of a patient already receiving a drug metabolized by CYP2D6, the need for decreased dose of the original medication should be considered).
No products indexed under this heading.

Troglitazone (In patients with diabetes, fluoxetine may alter glycemic control. Hypoglycemia has occurred during therapy with fluoxetine, and hyperglycemia has developed following discontinuation of the drug. As is true with many other types of medication when taken concurrently by patients with diabetes, oral hypoglycemic dosage may need to be adjusted when therapy with fluoxetine is instituted or discontinued).
No products indexed under this heading.

Tryptophan (Five patients receiving fluoxetine in combination with tryptophan experienced adverse reactions, including agitation, restlessness, and gastrointestinal distress. The concomitant use of fluoxetine with serotonin precursors (such as tryptophan) is not recommended).
No products indexed under this heading.

L-Tryptophan (Five patients receiving fluoxetine in combination with tryptophan experienced adverse reactions, including agitation, restlessness, and gastrointestinal distress. The concomitant use of fluoxetine with serotonin precursors (such as tryptophan) is not recommended).
No products indexed under this heading.

Valdecoxib (SSRIs, including fluoxetine, may increase the risk of bleeding events. Concomitant use of nonsteroidal anti-inflammatory drugs may add to this risk. Case reports and epidemiological studies (case-control and cohort design) have demonstrated an association between use of drugs that interfere with serotonin reuptake and the occurrence of gastrointestinal bleeding. Bleeding events related to SSRI use have ranged from ecchymoses, hematomas, epistaxis, and petechiae to life-threatening hemorrhages. Patients should be cautioned about the risk of bleeding associated with the concomitant use of fluoxetine and NSAIDs).
No products indexed under this heading.

Venlafaxine Hydrochloride (Based on the mechanism of action of SSRIs, including fluoxetine, and the potential for serotonin syndrome, caution is advised when fluoxetine is co-administered with other drugs that may affect serotonergic neurotransmitter systems. The concomitant use of fluoxetine with other SSRIs, SNRIs or tryptophan is not recommended). Products include:
Effexor XR Extended-Release Capsules 3195
Venlafaxine Hydrochloride Tablets ... 2199

Vinblastine Sulfate (Fluoxetine inhibits the activity of CYP2D6 and may make individuals with normal CYP2D6 metabolic activity resemble a poor metabolizer. Co-administration of fluoxetine with other drugs that are metabolized by CYP2D6, including vinblastine, should be approached with caution. Therapy with medications that are predominantly metabolized by the CYP2D6 system and that have a relatively narrow therapeutic index (eg, vinblastine) should be initiated at the low end of the dose range if a patient is receiving fluoxetine concurrently or has taken it in the previous 5 weeks. If fluoxetine is added to the treatment regimen of a patient already receiving a drug metabolized CYP2D6, the need for decreased dose of the original medication should be considered).
No products indexed under this heading.

Warfarin Sodium (Altered anticoagulant effects, including increased bleeding, have been reported when SSRIs are co-administered with warfarin. Patients receiving warfarin therapy should be carefully monitored when fluoxetine is initiated or discontinued).
No products indexed under this heading.

Zaleplon (The risk of using fluoxetine in combination with other CNS active drugs has not been systematically evaluated. Nonetheless, caution is advised if the concomitant administration of fluoxetine and such drugs is required. In evaluating individual cases, consideration should be given to using lower initial doses of the concomitantly administered drugs, using conservative titration schedules, and monitoring of clinical status).
No products indexed under this heading.

Ziprasidone Hydrochloride (The risk of using fluoxetine in combination with other CNS active drugs has not been systematically evaluated. Nonetheless, caution is advised if the concomitant administration of fluoxetine and such drugs is required. In evaluating individual cases, consideration should be given to using lower initial doses of the concomitantly administered drugs, using conservative titration schedules, and monitoring of clinical status). Products include:
Geodon Capsules 2520

Zolmitriptan (There have been rare postmarketing reports of serotonin syndrome with use of an SSRI and a triptan. If concomitant treatment of fluoxetine with a triptan is clinically warranted, careful observation of the patient is advised, particularly during treatment initiation and dose increases). Products include:
Zomig Tablets 694
Zomig Nasal Spray 689
Zomig-ZMT Tablets 694

Zolpidem Tartrate (The risk of using fluoxetine in combination with other CNS active drugs has not been systematically evaluated. Nonetheless, caution is advised if the concomitant administration of fluoxetine and such drugs is required. In evaluating individual cases, consideration should be given to using lower initial doses of the concomitantly administered drugs, using conservative titration schedules, and monitoring of clinical status). Products include:
Ambien Tablets 2692
Ambien CR Tablets 2696

Zonisamide (Fluoxetine inhibits the activity of CYP2D6, and may make individuals with normal CYP2D6 metabolic activity resemble a poor metabolizer. Co-administration of fluoxetine with other drugs that are

metabolized by CYP2D6 should be approached with caution. Therapy with medications that are predominantly metabolized by the CYP2D6 system and that have a relatively narrow therapeutic index should be initiated at the low end of the dose range if a patient is receiving fluoxetine concurrently or has taken it in the previous 5 weeks. If fluoxetine is added to the treatment regimen of a patient already receiving a drug metabolized by CYP2D6, the need for decreased dose of the original medication should be considered). Products include:

Zonegran Capsules 1089

Food Interactions

Alcohol (The risk of using fluoxetine in combination with other CNS active drugs has not been systematically evaluated. Nonetheless, caution is advised if the concomitant administration of fluoxetine and such drugs is required. In evaluating individual cases, consideration should be given to using lower initial doses of the concomitantly administered drugs, using conservative titration schedules, and monitoring of clinical status).

PROZAC PULVULES AND LIQUID

(Fluoxetine Hydrochloride) 1852

May interact with anticoagulants, cytochrome p450 2d6 substrates (selected), oral hypoglycemic agents, insulin, lithium preparations, monoamine oxidase inhibitors, non-steroidal anti-inflammatory agents, phenytoin, highly protein bound drugs (selected), serotoninergic agents, Serotonin and Norepinephrine Reuptake Inhibitors, selective serotonin reuptake inhibitors, tricyclic antidepressants, triptans, and certain other agents. Compounds in these categories include:

Acarbose (Fluoxetine may alter glycemic control in diabetics; hypoglycemia has occurred during therapy with fluoxetine and hyperglycemia has developed following discontinuation of the drug; hypoglycemia dosage may need to be adjusted). Products include:

Precose Tablets 792

Almotriptan Malate (If concomitant treatment of fluoxetine with a triptan is clinically warranted, careful observation of the patient is advised, particularly during treatment initiation and dose increases). Products include:

Axert Tablets 2431

Alprazolam (Co-administration has resulted in increased alprazolam plasma concentrations and further psychomotor performance decrement due to increased alprazolam levels).

No products indexed under this heading.

Amiodarone Hydrochloride (The administration of fluoxetine to a patient taking another drug that is tightly bound to protein may cause a shift in plasma concentrations potentially resulting in an adverse effect. Conversely, adverse effects may result from displacement of protein-bound fluoxetine by other tightly-bound drugs).

No products indexed under this heading.

Amitriptyline Hydrochloride (Fluoxetine inhibits the activity of P450 IID6 isoenzyme making normal metabolizers resemble "poor metabolizers"; therapy with drugs that are predominantly metabolized by the P450 IID6 isoenzyme, such as tricyclic antidepressants, and have a relatively narrow therapeutic index should be initiated at low end of the dose range if a patient is receiving fluoxetine concurrently or has taken it in the previous 5 weeks).

No products indexed under this heading.

Amoxapine (Fluoxetine inhibits the activity of P450 IID6 isoenzyme making normal metabolizers resemble "poor metabolizers"; therapy with drugs that are predominantly metabolized by the P450 IID6 isoenzyme, such as tricyclic antidepressants, and have a relatively narrow therapeutic index should be initiated at low end of the dose range if a patient is receiving fluoxetine concurrently or has taken it in the previous 5 weeks).

No products indexed under this heading.

Amphetamine Aspartate (If fluoxetine is added to the treatment regimen of a patient already receiving a drug metabolized by CYP2D6, the need for decreased dose of the original medication should be considered. Fluoxetine is metabolized by this isoenzyme; thus, both the pharmacokinetic properties and relative proportion of metabolites are altered in poor metabolizers of CYP2D6). Products include:

Adderall XR Capsules 3012

Amphetamine Aspartate Monohydrate (If fluoxetine is added to the treatment regimen of a patient already receiving a drug metabolized by CYP2D6, the need for decreased dose of the original medication should be considered. Fluoxetine is metabolized by this isoenzyme; thus, both the pharmacokinetic properties and relative proportion of metabolites are altered in poor metabolizers of CYP2D6).

No products indexed under this heading.

Amphetamine Sulfate (If fluoxetine is added to the treatment regimen of a patient already receiving a drug metabolized by CYP2D6, the need for decreased dose of the original medication should be considered. Fluoxetine is metabolized by this isoenzyme; thus, both the pharmacokinetic properties and relative proportion of metabolites are altered in poor metabolizers of CYP2D6). Products include:

Adderall XR Capsules 3012

Anisindione (SSRIs and SNRIs, including fluoxetine, may increase the risk of bleeding events. Concomitant use of anti-coagulants may add to this risk. Case reports and epidemiological studies (case-control and cohort design) have demonstrated an association betweenuse of drugs that interfere with serotonin reuptake and the occurrence of gastrointestinal bleeding. Bleeding events related to SSRIs and SNRIs use have ranged from ecchymoses, hematomas, epistaxis, and petechiae to life-threatening hemorrhages. Patients should be cautioned about the risk of bleeding associated with the concomitant use of fluoxetine and drugs that affect coagulation).

No products indexed under this heading.

Ardeparin Sodium (SSRIs and SNRIs, including fluoxetine, may increase the risk of bleeding events. Concomitant use of anti-coagulants may add to this risk. Case reports and epidemiological studies (case-control and cohort design) have demonstrated an association betweenuse of drugs that interfere with serotonin reuptake and the occurrence of gastrointestinal bleeding. Bleeding events related to SSRIs and SNRIs use have ranged from ecchymoses, hematomas, epistaxis, and petechiae to life-threatening hemorrhages. Patients should be cautioned about the risk of bleeding associated with the concomitant use of fluoxetine and drugs that affect coagulation).

No products indexed under this heading.

Aspirin (SSRIs and SNRIs, including fluoxetine, may increase the risk of bleeding events. Concomitant use of aspirin, nonsteroidal anti-inflammatory drugs, warfarin, and other anti-coagulants may add to this risk. Case reports and epidemiological studies (case-control and cohort design) have demonstrated an association between use of drugs that interfere with serotonin reuptake and the occurrence of gastrointestinal bleeding. Bleeding events related to SSRIs and SNRIs use have ranged from ecchymoses, hematomas, epistaxis, and petechiae to life-threatening hemorrhages. Patients should be cautioned about the risk of bleeding associated with the concomitant use of fluoxetine and NSAIDs, aspirin, and other drugs that affect coagulation). Products include:

Aggrenox Capsules 819
Bayer Aspirin 750
Percodan Tablets 1130
St. Joseph 81 mg Aspirin Chewable and Enteric Coated Tablets 1903

Aspirin, Enteric Coated (SSRIs and SNRIs, including fluoxetine, may increase the risk of bleeding events. Concomitant use of aspirin, nonsteroidal anti-inflammatory drugs, warfarin, and other anti-coagulants may add to this risk. Case reports and epidemiological studies (case-control and cohort design) have demonstrated an association between use of drugs that interfere with serotonin reuptake and the occurrence of gastrointestinal bleeding. Bleeding events related to SSRIs and SNRIs use have ranged from ecchymoses, hematomas, epistaxis, and petechiae to life-threatening hemorrhages. Patients should be cautioned about the risk of bleeding associated with the concomitant use of fluoxetine and NSAIDs, aspirin, and other drugs that affect coagulation).

No products indexed under this heading.

Aspirin Buffered (SSRIs and SNRIs, including fluoxetine, may increase the risk of bleeding events. Concomitant use of aspirin may add to this risk. Case reports and epidemiological studies (case-control and cohort design) have demonstrated an association between use of drugs that interfere with serotonin reuptake and the occurrence of gastrointestinal bleeding. Bleeding events related to SSRIs and SNRIs use have ranged from ecchymoses, hematomas, epistaxis, and petechiae to life-threatening hemorrhages. Patients shouldbe cautioned about the risk of bleeding associated with the concomitant use of fluoxetine and aspirin).

No products indexed under this heading.

Atomoxetine Hydrochloride (If fluoxetine is added to the treatment regimen of a patient already receiving a drug metabolized by CYP2D6, the need for decreased dose of the original medication should be considered. Fluoxetine is metabolized by this isoenzyme; thus, both the pharmacokinetic properties and relative proportion of metabolites are altered in poor metabolizers of CYP2D6). Products include:

Strattera Capsules 1864

Atovaquone (The administration of fluoxetine to a patient taking another drug that is tightly bound to protein may cause a shift in plasma concentrations potentially resulting in an adverse effect. Conversely, adverse effects may result from displacement of protein-bound fluoxetine by other tightly-bound drugs). Products include:

Malarone Pediatric Tablets 1521
Malarone Tablets 1521
Mepron Suspension 1526

Bisoprolol Fumarate (If fluoxetine is added to the treatment regimen of a patient already receiving a drug metabolized by CYP2D6, the need for decreased dose of the original medication should be considered. Fluoxetine is metabolized by this isoenzyme; thus, both the pharmacokinetic properties and relative proportion of metabolites are altered in poor metabolizers of CYP2D6).

No products indexed under this heading.

Captopril (If fluoxetine is added to the treatment regimen of a patient already receiving a drug metabolized by CYP2D6, the need for decreased dose of the original medication should be considered. Fluoxetine is metabolized by this isoenzyme; thus, both the pharmacokinetic properties and relative proportion of metabolites are altered in poor metabolizers of CYP2D6). Products include:

Captopril Tablets 2182

Carbamazepine (Patients stable on doses of carbamazepine have developed elevated plasma carbamazepine concentrations and clinical anticonvulsant toxicity following initiation of concomitant fluoxetine therapy). Products include:

Carbatrol Capsules 3019
Equetro Extended-Release Capsules 3174

Carvedilol (If fluoxetine is added to the treatment regimen of a patient already receiving a drug metabolized by CYP2D6, the need for decreased dose of the original medication should be considered. Fluoxetine is metabolized by this isoenzyme; thus, both the pharmacokinetic properties and relative proportion of metabolites are altered in poor metabolizers of CYP2D6). Products include:

Coreg Tablets 1387

Cefonicid Sodium (The administration of fluoxetine to a patient taking another drug that is tightly bound to protein may cause a shift in plasma concentrations potentially resulting in an adverse effect. Conversely, adverse effects may result from displacement of protein-bound fluoxetine by other tightly-bound drugs).

No products indexed under this heading.

Celecoxib (SSRIs and SNRIs, including fluoxetine, may increase the risk of bleeding events. Concomitant use of nonsteroidal anti-inflammatory drugs may add to this risk. Case reports and epidemiological studies (case-control and cohort design) have demonstrated an association between use of drugs that interfere with serotonin reuptake and the occurrence of gastrointestinal bleeding. Bleeding events related to SSRIs and SNRIs use have ranged from ecchymoses, hematomas, epistaxis, and petechiae to life-threateninghemorrhages. Patients should be cautioned about the risk of bleeding associated with the concomitant use of fluoxetine and NSAIDs). Products include:

Celebrex Capsules **2979**

Cevimeline Hydrochloride (If fluoxetine is added to the treatment regimen of a patient already receiving a drug metabolized by CYP2D6, the need for decreased dose of the original medication should be considered. Fluoxetine is metabolized by this isoenzyme; thus, both the pharmacokinetic properties and relative proportion of metabolites are altered in poor metabolizers of CYP2D6). Products include:

Evoxac Capsules **1013**

Chlordiazepoxide (The administration of fluoxetine to a patient taking another drug that is tightly bound to protein may cause a shift in plasma concentrations potentially resulting in an adverse effect. Conversely, adverse effects may result from displacement of protein-bound fluoxetine by other tightly-bound drugs).

No products indexed under this heading.

Chlordiazepoxide Hydrochloride (The administration of fluoxetine to a patient taking another drug that is tightly bound to protein may cause a shift in plasma concentrations potentially resulting in an adverse effect. Conversely, adverse effects may result from displacement of protein-bound fluoxetine by other tightly-bound drugs).

No products indexed under this heading.

Chlorpromazine (The administration of fluoxetine to a patient taking another drug that is tightly bound to protein may cause a shift in plasma concentrations potentially resulting in an adverse effect. Conversely, adverse effects may result from displacement of protein-bound fluoxetine by other tightly-bound drugs).

No products indexed under this heading.

Chlorpromazine Hydrochloride (The administration of fluoxetine to a patient taking another drug that is tightly bound to protein may cause a shift in plasma concentrations potentially resulting in an adverse effect. Conversely, adverse effects may result from displacement of protein-bound fluoxetine by other tightly-bound drugs).

No products indexed under this heading.

Chlorpropamide (Fluoxetine may alter glycemic control in diabetics; hypoglycemia has occurred during therapy with fluoxetine and hyperglycemia has developed following discontinuation of the drug; hypoglycemia dosage may need to be adjusted).

No products indexed under this heading.

Citalopram Hydrobromide (Based on the mechanism of action of SNRIs and SSRIs and the potential for serotonin syndrome, caution is advised when fluoxetine is co-administered with other drugs that may effect the serotonergic neurotransmitter systems). Products include:

Celexa **1160**

Clomipramine Hydrochloride (Fluoxetine inhibits the activity of P450 IID6 isoenzyme making normal metabolizers resemble "poor metabolizers"; therapy with drugs that are predominantly metabolized by the P450 IID6 isoenzyme, such as tricyclic antidepressants, and have a relatively narrow therapeutic index should be initiated at low end of the dose range if a patient is receiving fluoxetine concurrently or has taken it in the previous 5 weeks).

No products indexed under this heading.

Clozapine (Co-administration of SSRIs, fluoxetine, and antipsychotics, such as clozapine, has resulted in elevation of blood levels of clozapine).

No products indexed under this heading.

Codeine Phosphate (If fluoxetine is added to the treatment regimen of a patient already receiving a drug metabolized by CYP2D6, the need for decreased dose of the original medication should be considered. Fluoxetine is metabolized by this isoenzyme; thus, both the pharmacokinetic properties and relative proportion of metabolites are altered in poor metabolizers of CYP2D6). Products include:

Tylenol with Codeine Tablets **2427**

Codeine Sulfate (If fluoxetine is added to the treatment regimen of a patient already receiving a drug metabolized by CYP2D6, the need for decreased dose of the original medication should be considered. Fluoxetine is metabolized by this isoenzyme; thus, both the pharmacokinetic properties and relative proportion of metabolites are altered in poor metabolizers of CYP2D6).

No products indexed under this heading.

Cyclobenzaprine Hydrochloride (If fluoxetine is added to the treatment regimen of a patient already receiving a drug metabolized by CYP2D6, the need for decreased dose of the original medication should be considered. Fluoxetine is metabolized by this isoenzyme; thus, both the pharmacokinetic properties and relative proportion of metabolites are altered in poor metabolizers of CYP2D6). Products include:

Amrix Capsules **966**

Cyclosporine (The administration of fluoxetine to a patient taking another drug that is tightly bound to protein may cause a shift in plasma concentrations potentially resulting in an adverse effect. Conversely, adverse effects may result from displacement of protein-bound fluoxetine by other tightly-bound drugs). Products include:

Gengraf Capsules **435**
Neoral Oral Solution **2280**
Neoral Soft Gelatin Capsules **2280**
Restasis Ophthalmic Emulsion **557**
Sandimmune **2296**

Dalteparin Sodium (SSRIs and SNRIs, including fluoxetine, may increase the risk of bleeding events. Concomitant use of anti-coagulants may add to this risk. Case reports and epidemiological studies (case-control and cohort design) have demonstrated an association betweenuse of drugs that interfere with serotonin reuptake and the occurrence of gastrointestinal bleeding. Bleeding events related to SSRIs and SNRIs use have ranged from ecchymoses, hematomas, epistaxis, and petechiae to life-threatening hemorrhages. Patients should be cautioned about the risk of bleeding associated with the concomitant use of fluoxetine and drugs that affect coagulation). Products include:

Fragmin Injection **1070**

Danaparoid Sodium (SSRIs and SNRIs, including fluoxetine, may increase the risk of bleeding events. Concomitant use of anti-coagulants may add to this risk. Case reports and epidemiological studies (case-control and cohort design) have demonstrated an association betweenuse of drugs that interfere with serotonin reuptake and the occurrence of gastrointestinal bleeding. Bleeding events related to SSRIs and SNRIs use have ranged from ecchymoses, hematomas, epistaxis, and petechiae to life-threatening hemorrhages. Patients should be cautioned about the risk of bleeding associated with the concomitant use of fluoxetine and drugs that affect coagulation).

No products indexed under this heading.

Desipramine Hydrochloride (Fluoxetine inhibits the activity of P450 IID6 isoenzyme making normal metabolizers resemble "poor metabolizers"; therapy with drugs that are predominantly metabolized by the P450 IID6 isoenzyme, such as tricyclic antidepressants, and have a relatively narrow therapeutic index should be initiated at low end of the dose range if a patient is receiving fluoxetine concurrently or has taken it in the previous 5 weeks).

No products indexed under this heading.

Desvenlafaxine Succinate (Based on the mechanism of action of SNRIs and SSRIs and the potential for serotonin syndrome, caution is advised when fluoxetine is co-administered with other frugs that may effect the serotonergic neurotransmitter systems). Products include:

Pristiq Extended-Release Tablets **3247**

Dexfenfluramine Hydrochloride (If fluoxetine is added to the treatment regimen of a patient already receiving a drug metabolized by CYP2D6, the need for decreased dose of the original medication should be considered. Fluoxetine is metabolized by this isoenzyme; thus, both the pharmacokinetic properties and relative proportion of metabolites are altered in poor metabolizers of CYP2D6).

No products indexed under this heading.

Dextromethorphan Hydrobromide (If fluoxetine is added to the treatment regimen of a patient already receiving a drug metabolized by CYP2D6, the need for decreased dose of the original medication should be considered. Fluoxetine is metabolized by this isoenzyme; thus, both the pharmacokinetic properties and relative proportion of metabolites are altered in poor metabolizers of CYP2D6). Products include:

PediaCare Children's Liquid Multi-Symptom Cold **1902**
PediaCare Children's Long-Acting Cough **1902**
Children's Sudafed PE Cold & Cough Liquid **1907**
Sudafed PE Cold & Cough Caplets **1907**
Children's Tylenol Plus Cough & Runny Nose Suspension Liquid **1912**
Children's Tylenol Plus Cough & Sore Throat Suspension Liquid **1912**
Children's Tylenol Plus Flu Suspension Liquid **1914**
Children's Tylenol Plus Multi-Symptom Cold Suspension Liquid **1912**
Tylenol Cold Severe Congestion Daytime Caplets with Cool Burst **1912**
Tylenol Cold Head Congestion Daytime Caplets with Cool Burst **1910**
Tylenol Cold Head Congestion Nighttime Caplets with Cool Burst **1910**
Tylenol Cold Head Congestion Severe Daytime Caplets with Cool Burst **1910**
Tylenol Cold Multi-Symptom Daytime Caplets with Cool Burst and Rapid Release Gels **1913**
Tylenol Cold Multi-Symptom Daytime Liquid with Citrus Burst **1913**
Tylenol Cold Multi-Symptom Nighttime Caplets with Cool Burst **1913**
Tylenol Cold Multi-Symptom Nighttime Liquid with Cool Burst **1913**
Tylenol Cold Multi-Symptom Severe Caplets with Cool Burst **1913**
Tylenol Cold Multi-Symptom Severe Daytime Liquid with Citrus Burst **1913**
Tylenol Cough & Sore Throat Daytime Liquid with Cool Burst **1918**
Tylenol Cough & Sore Throat Nighttime Liquid with Cool Burst **1918**
Vicks DayQuil Cold & Flu Multi-Symptom Relief .... ▣**616**
Vicks DayQuil LiquiCaps **2567**
Vicks DayQuil Liquid **2567**
Vicks DayQuil Multi-Symptom Cold/Flu Relief **2567**
Vicks NyQuil Cold & Flu Multi-Symptom Relief .... ▣**617**
Vicks NyQuil LiquiCaps **2567**
Vicks NyQuil Liquid **2567**
Vicks NyQuil Multi-Symptom Cold/Flu Relief **2567**

Dextromethorphan Polistirex (If fluoxetine is added to the treatment regimen of a patient already receiving a drug metabolized by CYP2D6, the need for decreased dose of the original medication should be considered. Fluoxetine is metabolized by this isoenzyme; thus, both the pharmacokinetic properties and relative proportion of metabolites are altered in poor metabolizers of CYP2D6).
No products indexed under this heading.

Diazepam (Co-administration results in prolonged half-life of diazepam). Products include:
Valium Tablets 2658

Diclofenac Epolamine (SSRIs and SNRIs, including fluoxetine, may increase the risk of bleeding events. Concomitant use of nonsteroidal anti-inflammatory drugs may add to this risk. Case reports and epidemiological studies (case-control and cohort design) have demonstrated an association between use of drugs that interfere with serotonin reuptake and the occurrence of gastrointestinal bleeding. Bleeding events related to SSRIs and SNRIs use have ranged from ecchymoses, hematomas, epistaxis, and petechiae to life-threateninghemorrhages. Patients should be cautioned about the risk of bleeding associated with the concomitant use of fluoxetine and NSAIDs). Products include:
Flector Patch 561

Diclofenac Potassium (SSRIs and SNRIs, including fluoxetine, may increase the risk of bleeding events. Concomitant use of nonsteroidal anti-inflammatory drugs may add to this risk. Case reports and epidemiological studies (case-control and cohort design) have demonstrated an association between use of drugs that interfere with serotonin reuptake and the occurrence of gastrointestinal bleeding. Bleeding events related to SSRIs and SNRIs use have ranged from ecchymoses, hematomas, epistaxis, and petechiae to life-threateninghemorrhages. Patients should be cautioned about the risk of bleeding associated with the concomitant use of fluoxetine and NSAIDs).
No products indexed under this heading.

Diclofenac Sodium (SSRIs and SNRIs, including fluoxetine, may increase the risk of bleeding events. Concomitant use of nonsteroidal anti-inflammatory drugs may add to this risk. Case reports and epidemiological studies (case-control and cohort design) have demonstrated an association between use of drugs that interfere with serotonin reuptake and the occurrence of gastrointestinal bleeding. Bleeding events related to SSRIs and SNRIs use have ranged from ecchymoses, hematomas, epistaxis, and petechiae to life-threateninghemorrhages. Patients should be cautioned about the risk of bleeding associated with the concomitant use of fluoxetine and NSAIDs). Products include:
Diclofenac Sodium Ophthalmic Solution .... ⊙ 240
Voltaren Ophthalmic Solution 2336
Voltaren Tablets 2334
Voltaren-XR Tablets 2337

Dicumarol (SSRIs and SNRIs, including fluoxetine, may increase the risk of bleeding events. Concomitant use of anti-coagulants may add to this risk. Case reports and epidemiological studies (case-control and cohort design) have demonstrated an association betweenuse of drugs that interfere with serotonin reuptake and the occurrence of gastrointestinal bleeding. Bleeding events related to SSRIs and SNRIs use have ranged from ecchymoses, hematomas, epistaxis, and petechiae to life-threatening hemorrhages. Patients should be cautioned about the risk of bleeding associated with the concomitant use of fluoxetine and drugs that affect coagulation).
No products indexed under this heading.

Digitoxin (Fluoxetine is tightly bound to protein; co-administration may cause shift in plasma concentrations resulting in potential adverse effects).
No products indexed under this heading.

Dipyridamole (The administration of fluoxetine to a patient taking another drug that is tightly bound to protein may cause a shift in plasma concentrations potentially resulting in an adverse effect. Conversely, adverse effects may result from displacement of protein-bound fluoxetine by other tightly-bound drugs). Products include:
Aggrenox Capsules 819
Persantine Tablets 869

Dolasetron Mesylate (If fluoxetine is added to the treatment regimen of a patient already receiving a drug metabolized by CYP2D6, the need for decreased dose of the original medication should be considered. Fluoxetine is metabolized by this isoenzyme; thus, both the pharmacokinetic properties and relative proportion of metabolites are altered in poor metabolizers of CYP2D6). Products include:
Anzemet Injection 2701
Anzemet Tablets 2704

Donepezil Hydrochloride (If fluoxetine is added to the treatment regimen of a patient already receiving a drug metabolized by CYP2D6, the need for decreased dose of the original medication should be considered. Fluoxetine is metabolized by this isoenzyme; thus, both the pharmacokinetic properties and relative proportion of metabolites are altered in poor metabolizers of CYP2D6). Products include:
Aricept Tablets 1062
Aricept ODT Tablets 1062

Doxepin Hydrochloride (Fluoxetine inhibits the activity of P450 IID6 isoenzyme making normal metabolizers resemble "poor metabolizers"; therapy with drugs that are predominantly metabolized by the P450 IID6 isoenzyme, such as tricyclic antidepressants, and have a relatively narrow therapeutic index should be initiated at low end of the dose range if a patient is receiving fluoxetine concurrently or has taken it in the previous 5 weeks).
No products indexed under this heading.

Duloxetine Hydrochloride (Based on the mechanism of action of SNRIs and SSRIs and the potential for serotonin syndrome, caution is advised when fluoxetine is co-administered with other frugs that may effect the serotonergic neurotransmitter systems). Products include:
Cymbalta Delayed-Release Capsules 1801

Eletriptan Hydrobromide (If concomitant treatment of fluoxetine with a triptan is clinically warranted, careful observation of the patient is advised, particularly during treatment initiation and dose increases).
No products indexed under this heading.

Encainide Hydrochloride (If fluoxetine is added to the treatment regimen of a patient already receiving a drug metabolized by CYP2D6, the need for decreased dose of the original medication should be considered. Fluoxetine is metabolized by this isoenzyme; thus, both the pharmacokinetic properties and relative proportion of metabolites are altered in poor metabolizers of CYP2D6).
No products indexed under this heading.

Enoxaparin Sodium (SSRIs and SNRIs, including fluoxetine, may increase the risk of bleeding events. Concomitant use of anti-coagulants may add to this risk. Case reports and epidemiological studies (case-control and cohort design) have demonstrated an association betweenuse of drugs that interfere with serotonin reuptake and the occurrence of gastrointestinal bleeding. Bleeding events related to SSRIs and SNRIs use have ranged from ecchymoses, hematomas, epistaxis, and petechiae to life-threatening hemorrhages. Patients should be cautioned about the risk of bleeding associated with the concomitant use of fluoxetine and drugs that affect coagulation). Products include:
Lovenox Injection 2756

Escitalopram Oxalate (Based on the mechanism of action of SNRIs and SSRIs and the potential for serotonin syndrome, caution is advised when fluoxetine is co-administered with other drugs that may effect the serotonergic neurotransmitter systems). Products include:
Lexapro Oral Suspension 1174
Lexapro Tablets 1174

Etodolac (SSRIs and SNRIs, including fluoxetine, may increase the risk of bleeding events. Concomitant use of nonsteroidal anti-inflammatory drugs may add to this risk. Case reports and epidemiological studies (case-control and cohort design) have demonstrated an association between use of drugs that interfere with serotonin reuptake and the occurrence of gastrointestinal bleeding. Bleeding events related to SSRIs and SNRIs use have ranged from ecchymoses, hematomas, epistaxis, and petechiae to life-threateninghemorrhages. Patients should be cautioned about the risk of bleeding associated with the concomitant use of fluoxetine and NSAIDs).
No products indexed under this heading.

Fenoprofen Calcium (SSRIs and SNRIs, including fluoxetine, may increase the risk of bleeding events. Concomitant use of nonsteroidal anti-inflammatory drugs may add to this risk. Case reports and epidemiological studies (case-control and cohort design) have demonstrated an association between use of drugs that interfere with serotonin reuptake and the occurrence of gastrointestinal bleeding. Bleeding events related to SSRIs and SNRIs use have ranged from ecchymoses, hematomas, epistaxis, and petechiae to life-threateninghemorrhages. Patients should be cautioned about the risk of bleeding associated with the concomitant use of fluoxetine and NSAIDs). Products include:
Nalfon Capsules 2508

Fentanyl (If fluoxetine is added to the treatment regimen of a patient already receiving a drug metabolized by CYP2D6, the need for decreased dose of the original medication should be considered. Fluoxetine is metabolized by this isoenzyme; thus, both the pharmacokinetic properties and relative proportion of metabolites are altered in poor metabolizers of CYP2D6). Products include:
Duragesic Transdermal System 2405
Ionsys Transdermal System 2410

Fentanyl Citrate (If fluoxetine is added to the treatment regimen of a patient already receiving a drug metabolized by CYP2D6, the need for decreased dose of the original medication should be considered. Fluoxetine is metabolized by this isoenzyme; thus, both the pharmacokinetic properties and relative proportion of metabolites are altered in poor metabolizers of CYP2D6). Products include:
Actiq 959
Fentora Tablets 968

Flecainide Acetate (Fluoxetine inhibits the activity of P450 IID6 isoenzyme making normal metabolizers resemble "poor metabolizers"; therapy with drugs that are predominantly metabolized by the P450 IID6 isoenzyme, such as flecainide, and have a relatively narrow therapeutic index should be initiated at low end of the dose range if a patient is receiving fluoxetine concurrently or has taken it in the previous 5 weeks).
No products indexed under this heading.

Fluoxetine (Based on the mechanism of action of SNRIs and SSRIs and the potential for serotonin syndrome, caution is advised when fluoxetine is co-administered with other drugs that may effect the serotonergic neurotransmitter systems).
No products indexed under this heading.

Fluphenazine Decanoate (If fluoxetine is added to the treatment regimen of a patient already receiving a drug metabolized by CYP2D6, the need for decreased dose of the original medication should be considered. Fluoxetine is metabolized by this isoenzyme; thus, both the pharmacokinetic properties and relative proportion of metabolites are altered in poor metabolizers of CYP2D6).
No products indexed under this heading.

Fluphenazine Enanthate (If fluoxetine is added to the treatment regimen of a patient already receiving a drug metabolized by CYP2D6, the need for decreased dose of the original medication should be considered. Fluoxetine is metabolized by this isoenzyme; thus, both the pharmacokinetic properties and relative proportion of metabolites are altered in poor metabolizers of CYP2D6).
No products indexed under this heading.

Fluphenazine Hydrochloride (If fluoxetine is added to the treatment regimen of a patient already receiving a drug metabolized by CYP2D6, the need for decreased dose of the original medication should be considered. Fluoxetine is metabolized by this isoenzyme; thus, both the pharmacokinetic properties and relative proportion of metabolites are altered in poor metabolizers of CYP2D6).
No products indexed under this heading.

Flurazepam Hydrochloride (The administration of fluoxetine to a patient taking another drug that is tightly bound to protein may cause a shift in plasma concentrations potentially resulting in an adverse effect. Conversely, adverse effects may result from displacement of protein-bound fluoxetine by other tightly-bound drugs).
No products indexed under this heading.

Flurbiprofen (SSRIs and SNRIs, including fluoxetine, may increase the risk of bleeding events. Concomitant use of nonsteroidal anti-inflammatory drugs may add to this risk. Case reports and epidemiological studies (case-control and cohort design) have demonstrated an association between use of drugs that interfere with serotonin reuptake and the occurrence of gastrointestinal bleeding. Bleeding events related to SSRIs and SNRIs use have ranged from ecchymoses, hematomas, epistaxis, and petechiae to life-threateninghemorrhages. Patients should be cautioned about the risk of bleeding associated with the concomitant use of fluoxetine and NSAIDs).
No products indexed under this heading.

Fluvoxamine Maleate (Based on the mechanism of action of SNRIs and SSRIs and the potential for serotonin syndrome, caution is advised when fluoxetine is co-administered with other drugs that may effect the serotonergic neurotransmitter systems). Products include:
Luvox CR Extended-Release Capsules 1759

Fondaparinux Sodium (SSRIs and SNRIs, including fluoxetine, may increase the risk of bleeding events. Concomitant use of anti-coagulants may add to this risk. Case reports and epidemiological studies (case-control and cohort design) have demonstrated an association betweenuse of drugs that interfere with serotonin reuptake and the occurrence of gastrointestinal bleeding. Bleeding events related to SSRIs and SNRIs use have ranged from ecchymoses, hematomas, epistaxis, and petechiae to life-threatening hemorrhages. Patients should be cautioned about the risk of bleeding associated with the concomitant use of fluoxetine and drugs that affect coagulation). Products include:
Arixtra Injection 1313

Formoterol Fumarate (If fluoxetine is added to the treatment regimen of a patient already receiving a drug metabolized by CYP2D6, the need for decreased dose of the original medication should be considered. Fluoxetine is metabolized by this isoenzyme; thus, both the pharmacokinetic properties and relative proportion of metabolites are altered in poor metabolizers of CYP2D6). Products include:
Foradil Aerolizer 2849
Perforomist Inhalation Solution 1025

Fosphenytoin Sodium (Patients stable on doses of phenytoin have developed elevated plasma phenytoin concentrations and clinical anticonvulsant toxicity following initiation of concomitant fluoxetine therapy).
No products indexed under this heading.

Frovatriptan Succinate (If concomitant treatment of fluoxetine with a triptan is clinically warranted, careful observation of the patient is advised, particularly during treatment initiation and dose increases). Products include:
Frova Tablets 1111

Galantamine Hydrobromide (If fluoxetine is added to the treatment regimen of a patient already receiving a drug metabolized by CYP2D6, the need for decreased dose of the original medication should be considered. Fluoxetine is metabolized by this isoenzyme; thus, both the pharmacokinetic properties and relative proportion of metabolites are altered in poor metabolizers of CYP2D6).
No products indexed under this heading.

Glimepiride (Fluoxetine may alter glycemic control in diabetics; hypoglycemia has occurred during therapy with fluoxetine and hyperglycemia has developed following discontinuation of the drug; hypoglycemia dosage may need to be adjusted). Products include:
Avandaryl Tablets 1344
Duetact Tablets 3085

Glipizide (Fluoxetine may alter glycemic control in diabetics; hypoglycemia has occurred during therapy with fluoxetine and hyperglycemia has developed following discontinuation of the drug; hypoglycemia dosage may need to be adjusted).
No products indexed under this heading.

Glyburide (Fluoxetine may alter glycemic control in diabetics; hypoglycemia has occurred during therapy with fluoxetine and hyperglycemia has developed following discontinuation of the drug; hypoglycemia dosage may need to be adjusted).
No products indexed under this heading.

Haloperidol (Co-administration of SSRIs, fluoxetine, and antipsychotics, such as haloperidol, has resulted in elevation of blood levels of haloperidol).
No products indexed under this heading.

Haloperidol Decanoate (Co-administration of SSRIs, fluoxetine, and antipsychotics, such as haloperidol, has resulted in elevation of blood levels of haloperidol).
No products indexed under this heading.

Heparin Calcium (SSRIs and SNRIs, including fluoxetine, may increase the risk of bleeding events. Concomitant use of anti-coagulants may add to this risk. Case reports and epidemiological studies (case-control and cohort design) have demonstrated an association betweenuse of drugs that interfere with serotonin reuptake and the occurrence of gastrointestinal bleeding. Bleeding events related to SSRIs and SNRIs use have ranged from ecchymoses, hematomas, epistaxis, and petechiae to life-threatening hemorrhages. Patients should be cautioned about the risk of bleeding associated with the concomitant use of fluoxetine and drugs that affect coagulation).
No products indexed under this heading.

Heparin Sodium (SSRIs and SNRIs, including fluoxetine, may increase the risk of bleeding events. Concomitant use of anti-coagulants may add to this risk. Case reports and epidemiological studies (case-control and cohort design) have demonstrated an association betweenuse of drugs that interfere with serotonin reuptake and the occurrence of gastrointestinal bleeding. Bleeding events related to SSRIs and SNRIs use have ranged from ecchymoses, hematomas, epistaxis, and petechiae to life-threatening hemorrhages. Patients should be cautioned about the risk of bleeding associated with the concomitant use of fluoxetine and drugs that affect coagulation).
No products indexed under this heading.

Hydrocodone Bitartrate (If fluoxetine is added to the treatment regimen of a patient already receiving a drug metabolized by CYP2D6, the need for decreased dose of the original medication should be considered. Fluoxetine is metabolized by this isoenzyme; thus, both the pharmacokinetic properties and relative proportion of metabolites are altered in poor metabolizers of CYP2D6). Products include:
Lortab 5/500 Tablets 3143
Lortab 7.5/500 Tablets 3144
Lortab 10/500 Tablets 3144
Vicodin Tablets 529
Vicodin ES Tablets 530
Vicodin HP Tablets 531
Vicoprofen Tablets 533
Zydone Tablets 1132

Hypericum (Based on the mechanism of action of SNRIs and SSRIs and the potential for serotonin syndrome, caution is advised when fluoxetine is co-administered with other drugs that may effect the serotonergic neurotransmitter systems, such as St. John's Wort). Products include:
Satieté Tablets .... ▣640

Hypericum Perforatum (Based on the mechanism of action of SNRIs and SSRIs and the potential for serotonin syndrome, caution is advised when fluoxetine is co-administered with other drugs that may effect the serotonergic neurotransmitter systems, such as St. John's Wort).
No products indexed under this heading.

Ibuprofen (SSRIs and SNRIs, including fluoxetine, may increase the risk of bleeding events. Concomitant use of nonsteroidal anti-inflammatory drugs may add to this risk. Case reports and epidemiological studies (case-control and cohort design) have demonstrated an association between use of drugs that interfere with serotonin reuptake and the occurrence of gastrointestinal bleeding. Bleeding events related to SSRIs and SNRIs use have ranged from ecchymoses, hematomas, epistaxis, and petechiae to life-threateninghemorrhages. Patients should be cautioned about the risk of bleeding associated with the concomitant use of fluoxetine and NSAIDs). Products include:
Motrin IB Tablets and Caplets 1900
Children's Motrin Oral Suspension ... 1901
Children's Motrin Non-Staining Dye-Free Oral Suspension 1901
Children's Motrin Cold Oral Suspension 1899
Infants' Motrin Concentrated Drops 1901
Infants' Motrin Non-Staining Dye-Free Concentrated Drops 1901
Junior Strength Motrin Caplets and Chewable Tablets 1901
Vicoprofen Tablets 533

Imipramine Hydrochloride (Fluoxetine inhibits the activity of P450 IID6 isoenzyme making normal metabolizers resemble "poor metabolizers"; therapy with drugs that are predominantly metabolized by the P450 IID6 isoenzyme, such as tricyclic antidepressants, and have a relatively narrow therapeutic index should be initiated at low end of the dose range if a patient is receiving fluoxetine concurrently or has taken it in the previous 5 weeks).
No products indexed under this heading.

Imipramine Pamoate (Fluoxetine inhibits the activity of P450 IID6 isoenzyme making normal metabolizers resemble "poor metabolizers"; therapy with drugs that are predominantly metabolized by the P450 IID6 isoenzyme, such as tricyclic antidepressants, and have a relatively narrow therapeutic index should be initiated at low end of the dose range if a patient is receiving fluoxetine concurrently or has taken it in the previous 5 weeks).
No products indexed under this heading.

Indomethacin (SSRIs and SNRIs, including fluoxetine, may increase the risk of bleeding events. Concomitant use of nonsteroidal anti-inflammatory drugs may add to this risk. Case reports and epidemiological studies (case-control and cohort design) have demonstrated an association between use of drugs that interfere with serotonin reuptake and the occurrence of gastrointestinal bleeding. Bleeding events related to SSRIs and SNRIs use have ranged from ecchymoses, hematomas, epistaxis, and petechiae to life-threateninghemorrhages. Patients should be cautioned about the risk of bleeding associated with the concomitant use of fluoxetine and NSAIDs). Products include:
Indocin 2024

Indomethacin Sodium Trihydrate (SSRIs and SNRIs, including fluoxetine, may increase the risk of bleeding events. Concomitant use of nonsteroidal anti-inflammatory drugs may add to this risk. Case reports and epidemiological studies (case-control and cohort design) have demonstrated an association between use of drugs that interfere with serotonin reuptake and the occurrence of gastrointestinal bleeding. Bleeding events related to SSRIs and SNRIs use have ranged from ecchymoses, hematomas, epistaxis, and petechiae to life-threateninghemorrhages. Patients should be cautioned about the risk of bleeding associated with the concomitant use of fluoxetine and NSAIDs). Products include:

Indocin I.V. 2489

Indoramin Hydrochloride (If fluoxetine is added to the treatment regimen of a patient already receiving a drug metabolized by CYP2D6, the need for decreased dose of the original medication should be considered. Fluoxetine is metabolized by this isoenzyme; thus, both the pharmacokinetic properties and relative proportion of metabolites are altered in poor metabolizers of CYP2D6).
No products indexed under this heading.

Insulin (Fluoxetine may alter glycemic control in diabetics; hypoglycemia has occurred during therapy with fluoxetine and hyperglycemia has developed following discontinuation of the drug; insulin dosage may need to be adjusted).
No products indexed under this heading.

Insulin, Human, Zinc Suspension (Fluoxetine may alter glycemic control in diabetics; hypoglycemia has occurred during therapy with fluoxetine and hyperglycemia has developed following discontinuation of the drug; insulin dosage may need to be adjusted).
No products indexed under this heading.

Insulin, Human (rDNA origin) (Fluoxetine may alter glycemic control in diabetics; hypoglycemia has occurred during therapy with fluoxetine and hyperglycemia has developed following discontinuation of the drug; insulin dosage may need to be adjusted). Products include:
Exubera Inhalation Powder 2515

Insulin, Human NPH (Fluoxetine may alter glycemic control in diabetics; hypoglycemia has occurred during therapy with fluoxetine and hyperglycemia has developed following discontinuation of the drug; insulin dosage may need to be adjusted). Products include:
Humulin N Vial 1846

Insulin, Human Regular (Fluoxetine may alter glycemic control in diabetics; hypoglycemia has occurred during therapy with fluoxetine and hyperglycemia has developed following discontinuation of the drug; insulin dosage may need to be adjusted). Products include:
Humulin R 1849
Humulin R (U-500) 1850

Insulin, Human Regular and Human NPH Mixture (Fluoxetine may alter glycemic control in diabetics; hypoglycemia has occurred during therapy with fluoxetine and hyperglycemia has developed following discontinuation of the drug; insulin dosage may need to be adjusted). Products include:
Humulin 50/50, 100 Units 1843
Humulin 70/30 Vial 1844

Insulin, NPH (Fluoxetine may alter glycemic control in diabetics; hypoglycemia has occurred during therapy with fluoxetine and hyperglycemia has developed following discontinuation of the drug; insulin dosage may need to be adjusted).
No products indexed under this heading.

Insulin, Regular (Fluoxetine may alter glycemic control in diabetics; hypoglycemia has occurred during therapy with fluoxetine and hyperglycemia has developed following discontinuation of the drug; insulin dosage may need to be adjusted).
No products indexed under this heading.

Insulin, Regular and NPH mixture (Fluoxetine may alter glycemic control in diabetics; hypoglycemia has occurred during therapy with fluoxetine and hyperglycemia has developed following discontinuation of the drug; insulin dosage may need to be adjusted).
No products indexed under this heading.

Insulin, Zinc Crystals (Fluoxetine may alter glycemic control in diabetics; hypoglycemia has occurred during therapy with fluoxetine and hyperglycemia has developed following discontinuation of the drug; insulin dosage may need to be adjusted).
No products indexed under this heading.

Insulin, Zinc Suspension (Fluoxetine may alter glycemic control in diabetics; hypoglycemia has occurred during therapy with fluoxetine and hyperglycemia has developed following discontinuation of the drug; insulin dosage may need to be adjusted).
No products indexed under this heading.

Insulin Aspart (Fluoxetine may alter glycemic control in diabetics; hypoglycemia has occurred during therapy with fluoxetine and hyperglycemia has developed following discontinuation of the drug; insulin dosage may need to be adjusted).
No products indexed under this heading.

Insulin Aspart, Human (Fluoxetine may alter glycemic control in diabetics; hypoglycemia has occurred during therapy with fluoxetine and hyperglycemia has developed following discontinuation of the drug; insulin dosage may need to be adjusted). Products include:
NovoLog Mix 70/30 2364

Insulin Aspart, Human Regular (Fluoxetine may alter glycemic control in diabetics; hypoglycemia has occurred during therapy with fluoxetine and hyperglycemia has developed following discontinuation of the drug; insulin dosage may need to be adjusted). Products include:
NovoLog Injection 2359

Insulin Aspart Protamine, Human (Fluoxetine may alter glycemic control in diabetics; hypoglycemia has occurred during therapy with fluoxetine and hyperglycemia has developed following discontinuation of the drug; insulin dosage may need to be adjusted). Products include:
NovoLog Mix 70/30 2364

Insulin Detemir (rDNA Origin) (Fluoxetine may alter glycemic control in diabetics; hypoglycemia has occurred during therapy with fluoxetine and hyperglycemia has developed following discontinuation of the drug; insulin dosage may need to be adjusted). Products include:
Levemir Injection 2352

Insulin glargine (Fluoxetine may alter glycemic control in diabetics; hypoglycemia has occurred during therapy with fluoxetine and hyperglycemia has developed following discontinuation of the drug; insulin dosage may need to be adjusted). Products include:
Lantus Injection 2749

Insulin Glulisine (Fluoxetine may alter glycemic control in diabetics; hypoglycemia has occurred during therapy with fluoxetine and hyperglycemia has developed following discontinuation of the drug; insulin dosage may need to be adjusted). Products include:
Apidra Injection 2706

Insulin Lispro, Human (Fluoxetine may alter glycemic control in diabetics; hypoglycemia has occurred during therapy with fluoxetine and hyperglycemia has developed following discontinuation of the drug; insulin dosage may need to be adjusted). Products include:
Humalog-Pen and KwikPen 1829
Humalog Mix 50/50-Pen and KwikPen 1833
Humalog Mix 75/25-Pen and KwikPen 1835

Insulin Lispro Protamine, Human (Fluoxetine may alter glycemic control in diabetics; hypoglycemia has occurred during therapy with fluoxetine and hyperglycemia has developed following discontinuation of the drug; insulin dosage may need to be adjusted). Products include:
Humalog Mix 50/50-Pen and KwikPen 1833
Humalog Mix 75/25-Pen and KwikPen 1835

Isocarboxazid (Co-administration with MAO inhibitors has resulted in serious, sometimes fatal, reactions, including hyperthermia, rigidity, extreme agitation, delirium, coma, and features resembling neuroleptic malignant syndrome; concurrent and/or sequential use is contraindicated). Products include:
Marplan Tablets 3177

Ketoprofen (SSRIs and SNRIs, including fluoxetine, may increase the risk of bleeding events. Concomitant use of nonsteroidal anti-inflammatory drugs may add to this risk. Case reports and epidemiological studies (case-control and cohort design) have demonstrated an association between use of drugs that interfere with serotonin reuptake and the occurrence of gastrointestinal bleeding. Bleeding events related to SSRIs and SNRIs use have ranged from ecchymoses, hematomas, epistaxis, and petechiae to life-threateninghemorrhages. Patients should be cautioned about the risk of bleeding associated with the concomitant use of fluoxetine and NSAIDs).
No products indexed under this heading.

Ketorolac Tromethamine (SSRIs and SNRIs, including fluoxetine, may increase the risk of bleeding events. Concomitant use of nonsteroidal anti-inflammatory drugs may add to this risk. Case reports and epidemiological studies (case-control and cohort design) have demonstrated an association between use of drugs that interfere with serotonin reuptake and the occurrence of gastrointestinal bleeding. Bleeding events related to SSRIs and SNRIs use have ranged from ecchymoses, hematomas, epistaxis, and petechiae to life-threateninghemorrhages. Patients should be cautioned about the risk of bleeding associated with the concomitant use of fluoxetine and NSAIDs).
No products indexed under this heading.

Labetalol Hydrochloride (If fluoxetine is added to the treatment regimen of a patient already receiving a drug metabolized by CYP2D6, the need for decreased dose of the original medication should be considered. Fluoxetine is metabolized by this isoenzyme; thus, both the pharmacokinetic properties and relative proportion of metabolites are altered in poor metabolizers of CYP2D6).
No products indexed under this heading.

Lidocaine (If fluoxetine is added to the treatment regimen of a patient already receiving a drug metabolized by CYP2D6, the need for decreased dose of the original medication should be considered. Fluoxetine is metabolized by this isoenzyme; thus, both the pharmacokinetic properties and relative proportion of metabolites are altered in poor metabolizers of CYP2D6). Products include:
Lidoderm Patch 1114

Lidocaine Hydrochloride (If fluoxetine is added to the treatment regimen of a patient already receiving a drug metabolized by CYP2D6, the need for decreased dose of the original medication should be considered. Fluoxetine is metabolized by this isoenzyme; thus, both the pharmacokinetic properties and relative proportion of metabolites are altered in poor metabolizers of CYP2D6).
No products indexed under this heading.

Linezolid (Based on the mechanism of action of SNRIs and SSRIs and the potential for serotonin syndrome, caution is advised when fluoxetine is co-administered with other drugs that may effect the serotonergic neurotransmitter systems, such as linezolid). Products include:
Zyvox 2552

Lithium (Co-administration has resulted in reports of both increased and decreased lithium levels; cases of lithium toxicity have been reported).
No products indexed under this heading.

Lithium Carbonate (Co-administration has resulted in reports of both increased and decreased lithium levels; cases of lithium toxicity have been reported).
No products indexed under this heading.

Lithium Citrate (Co-administration has resulted in reports of both increased and decreased lithium levels; cases of lithium toxicity have been reported).
No products indexed under this heading.

Low Molecular Weight Heparins (SSRIs and SNRIs, including fluoxetine, may increase the risk of bleeding events. Concomitant use of anticoagulants may add to this risk. Case reports and epidemiological studies (case-control and cohort design) have demonstrated an association betweenuse of drugs that interfere with serotonin reuptake and the occurrence of gastrointestinal bleeding. Bleeding events related to SSRIs and SNRIs use have ranged from ecchymoses, hematomas, epi-

staxis, and petechiae to life-threatening hemorrhages. Patients should be cautioned about the risk of bleeding associated with the concomitant use of fluoxetine and drugs that affect coagulation).

No products indexed under this heading.

Maprotiline Hydrochloride (Fluoxetine inhibits the activity of P450 IID6 isoenzyme making normal metabolizers resemble "poor metabolizers"; therapy with drugs that are predominantly metabolized by the P450 IID6 isoenzyme, such as tricyclic antidepressants, and have a relatively narrow therapeutic index should be initiated at low end of the dose range if a patient is receiving fluoxetine concurrently or has taken it in the previous 5 weeks).

No products indexed under this heading.

Meclofenamate Sodium (SSRIs and SNRIs, including fluoxetine, may increase the risk of bleeding events. Concomitant use of nonsteroidal anti-inflammatory drugs may add to this risk. Case reports and epidemiological studies (case-control and cohort design) have demonstrated an association between use of drugs that interfere with serotonin reuptake and the occurrence of gastrointestinal bleeding. Bleeding events related to SSRIs and SNRIs use have ranged from ecchymoses, hematomas, epistaxis, and petechiae to life-threateninghemorrhages. Patients should be cautioned about the risk of bleeding associated with the concomitant use of fluoxetine and NSAIDs).

No products indexed under this heading.

Mefenamic Acid (SSRIs and SNRIs, including fluoxetine, may increase the risk of bleeding events. Concomitant use of nonsteroidal anti-inflammatory drugs may add to this risk. Case reports and epidemiological studies (case-control and cohort design) have demonstrated an association between use of drugs that interfere with serotonin reuptake and the occurrence of gastrointestinal bleeding. Bleeding events related to SSRIs and SNRIs use have ranged from ecchymoses, hematomas, epistaxis, and petechiae to life-threateninghemorrhages. Patients should be cautioned about the risk of bleeding associated with the concomitant use of fluoxetine and NSAIDs).

No products indexed under this heading.

Meloxicam (SSRIs and SNRIs, including fluoxetine, may increase the risk of bleeding events. Concomitant use of nonsteroidal anti-inflammatory drugs may add to this risk. Case reports and epidemiological studies (case-control and cohort design) have demonstrated an association between use of drugs that interfere with serotonin reuptake and the occurrence of gastrointestinal bleeding. Bleeding events related to SSRIs and SNRIs use have ranged from ecchymoses, hematomas, epistaxis, and petechiae to life-threateninghemorrhages. Patients should be cautioned about the risk of bleeding associated with the concomitant use of fluoxetine and NSAIDs). Products include:

Mobic Oral Suspension 863
Mobic Tablets 863

Meperidine Hydrochloride (If fluoxetine is added to the treatment regimen of a patient already receiving a drug metabolized by CYP2D6, the need for decreased dose of the original medication should be considered. Fluoxetine is metabolized by this isoenzyme; thus, both the pharmacokinetic properties and relative proportion of metabolites are altered in poor metabolizers of CYP2D6).

No products indexed under this heading.

Metformin Hydrochloride (Fluoxetine may alter glycemic control in diabetics; hypoglycemia has occurred during therapy with fluoxetine and hyperglycemia has developed following discontinuation of the drug; hypoglycemia dosage may need to be adjusted). Products include:

ActoPlus Met Tablets 3071
Avandamet Tablets 1336
Janumet Tablets 2041
PrandiMet Tablets 2967

Methadone Hydrochloride (If fluoxetine is added to the treatment regimen of a patient already receiving a drug metabolized by CYP2D6, the need for decreased dose of the original medication should be considered. Fluoxetine is metabolized by this isoenzyme; thus, both the pharmacokinetic properties and relative proportion of metabolites are altered in poor metabolizers of CYP2D6).

No products indexed under this heading.

Methamphetamine Hydrochloride (If fluoxetine is added to the treatment regimen of a patient already receiving a drug metabolized by CYP2D6, the need for decreased dose of the original medication should be considered. Fluoxetine is metabolized by this isoenzyme; thus, both the pharmacokinetic properties and relative proportion of metabolites are altered in poor metabolizers of CYP2D6).

No products indexed under this heading.

Metoprolol Succinate (If fluoxetine is added to the treatment regimen of a patient already receiving a drug metabolized by CYP2D6, the need for decreased dose of the original medication should be considered. Fluoxetine is metabolized by this isoenzyme; thus, both the pharmacokinetic properties and relative proportion of metabolites are altered in poor metabolizers of CYP2D6). Products include:

Toprol-XL Tablets 666

Metoprolol Tartrate (If fluoxetine is added to the treatment regimen of a patient already receiving a drug metabolized by CYP2D6, the need for decreased dose of the original medication should be considered. Fluoxetine is metabolized by this isoenzyme; thus, both the pharmacokinetic properties and relative proportion of metabolites are altered in poor metabolizers of CYP2D6).

No products indexed under this heading.

Mexiletine Hydrochloride (If fluoxetine is added to the treatment regimen of a patient already receiving a drug metabolized by CYP2D6, the need for decreased dose of the original medication should be considered. Fluoxetine is metabolized by this isoenzyme; thus, both the pharmacokinetic properties and relative proportion of metabolites are altered in poor metabolizers of CYP2D6).

No products indexed under this heading.

Midazolam Hydrochloride (The administration of fluoxetine to a patient taking another drug that is tightly bound to protein may cause a shift in plasma concentrations potentially resulting in an adverse effect. Conversely, adverse effects may result from displacement of protein-bound fluoxetine by other tightly-bound drugs).

No products indexed under this heading.

Miglitol (Fluoxetine may alter glycemic control in diabetics; hypoglycemia has occurred during therapy with fluoxetine and hyperglycemia has developed following discontinuation of the drug; hypoglycemia dosage may need to be adjusted).

No products indexed under this heading.

Mirtazapine (If fluoxetine is added to the treatment regimen of a patient already receiving a drug metabolized by CYP2D6, the need for decreased dose of the original medication should be considered. Fluoxetine is metabolized by this isoenzyme; thus, both the pharmacokinetic properties and relative proportion of metabolites are altered in poor metabolizers of CYP2D6). Products include:

Remeron Tablets 2924
RemeronSolTab Tablets 2927

Moclobemide (Co-administration with MAO inhibitors has resulted in serious, sometimes fatal, reactions, including hyperthermia, rigidity, extreme agitation, delirium, coma, and features resembling neuroleptic malignant syndrome; concurrent and/or sequential use is contraindicated).

No products indexed under this heading.

Morphine Sulfate (If fluoxetine is added to the treatment regimen of a patient already receiving a drug metabolized by CYP2D6, the need for decreased dose of the original medication should be considered. Fluoxetine is metabolized by this isoenzyme; thus, both the pharmacokinetic properties and relative proportion of metabolites are altered in poor metabolizers of CYP2D6). Products include:

Avinza Capsules 1772
DepoDur Injection 1095
MS Contin Tablets 2585

Nabumetone (SSRIs and SNRIs, including fluoxetine, may increase the risk of bleeding events. Concomitant use of nonsteroidal anti-inflammatory drugs may add to this risk. Case reports and epidemiological studies (case-control and cohort design) have demonstrated an association between use of drugs that interfere with serotonin reuptake and the occurrence of gastrointestinal bleeding. Bleeding events related to SSRIs and SNRIs use have ranged from ecchymoses, hematomas, epistaxis, and petechiae to life-threateninghemorrhages. Patients should be cautioned about the risk of bleeding associated with the concomitant use of fluoxetine and NSAIDs).

No products indexed under this heading.

Naproxen (SSRIs and SNRIs, including fluoxetine, may increase the risk of bleeding events. Concomitant use of nonsteroidal anti-inflammatory drugs may add to this risk. Case reports and epidemiological studies (case-control and cohort design) have demonstrated an association between use of drugs that interfere with serotonin reuptake and the occurrence of gastrointestinal bleeding. Bleeding events related to SSRIs and SNRIs use have ranged from ecchymoses, hematomas, epistaxis, and petechiae to life-threateninghemorrhages. Patients should be cautioned about the risk of bleeding associated with the concomitant use of fluoxetine and NSAIDs). Products include:

EC-Naprosyn Delayed-Release Tablets 2632
Naprosyn Suspension 2632
Naprosyn Tablets 2632

Naproxen Sodium (SSRIs and SNRIs, including fluoxetine, may increase the risk of bleeding events. Concomitant use of nonsteroidal anti-inflammatory drugs may add to this risk. Case reports and epidemiological studies (case-control and cohort design) have demonstrated an association between use of drugs that interfere with serotonin reuptake and the occurrence of gastrointestinal bleeding. Bleeding events related to SSRIs and SNRIs use have ranged from ecchymoses, hematomas, epistaxis, and petechiae to life-threateninghemorrhages. Patients should be cautioned about the risk of bleeding associated with the concomitant use of fluoxetine and NSAIDs). Products include:

Anaprox Tablets 2632
Anaprox DS Tablets 2632
Treximet Tablets 1616

Naratriptan Hydrochloride (If concomitant treatment of fluoxetine with a triptan is clinically warranted, careful observation of the patient is advised, particularly during treatment initiation and dose increases). Products include:

Amerge Tablets 1301

Nateglinide (Fluoxetine may alter glycemic control in diabetics; hypoglycemia has occurred during therapy with fluoxetine and hyperglycemia has developed following discontinuation of the drug; hypoglycemia dosage may need to be adjusted). Products include:

Starlix Tablets 2314

Nefazodone Hydrochloride (Based on the mechanism of action of SNRIs and SSRIs and the potential for serotonin syndrome, caution is advised when fluoxetine is co-administered with other frugs that may effect the serotonergic neurotransmitter systems).

No products indexed under this heading.

Nelfinavir Mesylate (If fluoxetine is added to the treatment regimen of a patient already receiving a drug metabolized by CYP2D6, the need for decreased dose of the original medication should be considered. Fluoxetine is metabolized by this isoenzyme; thus, both the pharmacokinetic properties and relative proportion of metabolites are altered in poor metabolizers of CYP2D6).
No products indexed under this heading.

Nortriptyline Hydrochloride (Fluoxetine inhibits the activity of P450 IID6 isoenzyme making normal metabolizers resemble "poor metabolizers"; therapy with drugs that are predominantly metabolized by the P450 IID6 isoenzyme, such as tricyclic antidepressants, and have a relatively narrow therapeutic index should be initiated at low end of the dose range if a patient is receiving fluoxetine concurrently or has taken it in the previous 5 weeks).
No products indexed under this heading.

Olanzapine (If fluoxetine is added to the treatment regimen of a patient already receiving a drug metabolized by CYP2D6, the need for decreased dose of the original medication should be considered. Fluoxetine is metabolized by this isoenzyme; thus, both the pharmacokinetic properties and relative proportion of metabolites are altered in poor metabolizers of CYP2D6). Products include:
Symbyax Capsules 1871
Zyprexa Tablets 1883
Zyprexa IntraMuscular 1883
Zyprexa ZYDIS Orally Disintegrating Tablets 1883

Omeprazole (If fluoxetine is added to the treatment regimen of a patient already receiving a drug metabolized by CYP2D6, the need for decreased dose of the original medication should be considered. Fluoxetine is metabolized by this isoenzyme; thus, both the pharmacokinetic properties and relative proportion of metabolites are altered in poor metabolizers of CYP2D6).
No products indexed under this heading.

Ondansetron (If fluoxetine is added to the treatment regimen of a patient already receiving a drug metabolized by CYP2D6, the need for decreased dose of the original medication should be considered. Fluoxetine is metabolized by this isoenzyme; thus, both the pharmacokinetic properties and relative proportion of metabolites are altered in poor metabolizers of CYP2D6). Products include:
Zofran ODT Orally Disintegrating Tablets 1687

Ondansetron Hydrochloride (If fluoxetine is added to the treatment regimen of a patient already receiving a drug metabolized by CYP2D6, the need for decreased dose of the original medication should be considered. Fluoxetine is metabolized by this isoenzyme; thus, both the pharmacokinetic properties and relative proportion of metabolites are altered in poor metabolizers of CYP2D6). Products include:
Zofran Injection 1682
Zofran 1687

Oxaprozin (SSRIs and SNRIs, including fluoxetine, may increase the risk of bleeding events. Concomitant use of nonsteroidal anti-inflammatory drugs may add to this risk. Case reports and epidemiological studies (case-control and cohort design) have demonstrated an association between use of drugs that interfere with serotonin reuptake and the occurrence of gastrointestinal bleeding. Bleeding events related to SSRIs and SNRIs use have ranged from ecchymoses, hematomas, epistaxis, and petechiae to life-threateninghemorrhages. Patients should be cautioned about the risk of bleeding associated with the concomitant use of fluoxetine and NSAIDs).
No products indexed under this heading.

Oxazepam (The administration of fluoxetine to a patient taking another drug that is tightly bound to protein may cause a shift in plasma concentrations potentially resulting in an adverse effect. Conversely, adverse effects may result from displacement of protein-bound fluoxetine by other tightly-bound drugs).
No products indexed under this heading.

Oxycodone Hydrochloride (If fluoxetine is added to the treatment regimen of a patient already receiving a drug metabolized by CYP2D6, the need for decreased dose of the original medication should be considered. Fluoxetine is metabolized by this isoenzyme; thus, both the pharmacokinetic properties and relative proportion of metabolites are altered in poor metabolizers of CYP2D6). Products include:
OxyContin Tablets 2589
OxyIR Capsules 2593
Percocet Tablets 1127
Percodan Tablets 1130

Paclitaxel (If fluoxetine is added to the treatment regimen of a patient already receiving a drug metabolized by CYP2D6, the need for decreased dose of the original medication should be considered. Fluoxetine is metabolized by this isoenzyme; thus, both the pharmacokinetic properties and relative proportion of metabolites are altered in poor metabolizers of CYP2D6).
No products indexed under this heading.

Pargyline Hydrochloride (Co-administration with MAO inhibitors has resulted in serious, sometimes fatal, reactions, including hyperthermia, rigidity, extreme agitation, delirium, coma, and features resembling neuroleptic malignant syndrome; concurrent and/or sequential use is contraindicated).
No products indexed under this heading.

Paroxetine Hydrochloride (Based on the mechanism of action of SNRIs and SSRIs and the potential for serotonin syndrome, caution is advised when fluoxetine is co-administered with other drugs that may effect the serotonergic neurotransmitter systems). Products include:
Paxil 1535
Paxil CR Controlled-Release Tablets 1544

Phenelzine Sulfate (Co-administration with MAO inhibitors has resulted in serious, sometimes fatal, reactions, including hyperthermia, rigidity, extreme agitation, delirium, coma, and features resembling neuroleptic malignant syndrome; concurrent and/or sequential use is contraindicated).
No products indexed under this heading.

Phenylbutazone (SSRIs and SNRIs, including fluoxetine, may increase the risk of bleeding events. Concomitant use of nonsteroidal anti-inflammatory drugs may add to this risk. Case reports and epidemiological studies (case-control and cohort design) have demonstrated an association between use of drugs that interfere with serotonin reuptake and the occurrence of gastrointestinal bleeding. Bleeding events related to SSRIs and SNRIs use have ranged from ecchymoses, hematomas, epistaxis, and petechiae to life-threateninghemorrhages. Patients should be cautioned about the risk of bleeding associated with the concomitant use of fluoxetine and NSAIDs).
No products indexed under this heading.

Phenytoin (Patients stable on doses of phenytoin have developed elevated plasma phenytoin concentrations and clinical anticonvulsant toxicity following initiation of concomitant fluoxetine therapy).
No products indexed under this heading.

Phenytoin Sodium (Patients stable on doses of phenytoin have developed elevated plasma phenytoin concentrations and clinical anticonvulsant toxicity following initiation of concomitant fluoxetine therapy). Products include:
Phenytek Capsules 2192

Pimozide (Co-administration has resulted in a single case report of possible additive effects of pimozide leading to bradycardia; concomitant use in patients taking Pimozide is contraindicated).
No products indexed under this heading.

Pindolol (If fluoxetine is added to the treatment regimen of a patient already receiving a drug metabolized by CYP2D6, the need for decreased dose of the original medication should be considered. Fluoxetine is metabolized by this isoenzyme; thus, both the pharmacokinetic properties and relative proportion of metabolites are altered in poor metabolizers of CYP2D6).
No products indexed under this heading.

Pioglitazone Hydrochloride (Fluoxetine may alter glycemic control in diabetics; hypoglycemia has occurred during therapy with fluoxetine and hyperglycemia has developed following discontinuation of the drug; hypoglycemia dosage may need to be adjusted). Products include:
ActoPlus Met Tablets 3071
Actos Tablets 3077
Duetact Tablets 3085

Piroxicam (SSRIs and SNRIs, including fluoxetine, may increase the risk of bleeding events. Concomitant use of nonsteroidal anti-inflammatory drugs may add to this risk. Case reports and epidemiological studies (case-control and cohort design) have demonstrated an association between use of drugs that interfere with serotonin reuptake and the occurrence of gastrointestinal bleeding. Bleeding events related to SSRIs and SNRIs use have ranged from ecchymoses, hematomas, epistaxis, and petechiae to life-threateninghemorrhages. Patients should be cautioned about the risk of bleeding associated with the concomitant use of fluoxetine and NSAIDs).
No products indexed under this heading.

Procarbazine Hydrochloride (Co-administration with MAO inhibitors has resulted in serious, sometimes fatal, reactions, including hyperthermia, rigidity, extreme agitation, delirium, coma, and features resembling neuroleptic malignant syndrome; concurrent and/or sequential use is contraindicated).
No products indexed under this heading.

Propafenone Hydrochloride (If fluoxetine is added to the treatment regimen of a patient already receiving a drug metabolized by CYP2D6, the need for decreased dose of the original medication should be considered. Fluoxetine is metabolized by this isoenzyme; thus, both the pharmacokinetic properties and relative proportion of metabolites are altered in poor metabolizers of CYP2D6). Products include:
Rythmol Tablets 1586
Rythmol SR Capsules 1590

Propoxyphene Hydrochloride (If fluoxetine is added to the treatment regimen of a patient already receiving a drug metabolized by CYP2D6, the need for decreased dose of the original medication should be considered. Fluoxetine is metabolized by this isoenzyme; thus, both the pharmacokinetic properties and relative proportion of metabolites are altered in poor metabolizers of CYP2D6).
No products indexed under this heading.

Propoxyphene Napsylate (If fluoxetine is added to the treatment regimen of a patient already receiving a drug metabolized by CYP2D6, the need for decreased dose of the original medication should be considered. Fluoxetine is metabolized by this isoenzyme; thus, both the pharmacokinetic properties and relative proportion of metabolites are altered in poor metabolizers of CYP2D6).
No products indexed under this heading.

Propranolol Hydrochloride (The administration of fluoxetine to a patient taking another drug that is tightly bound to protein may cause a shift in plasma concentrations potentially resulting in an adverse effect. Conversely, adverse effects may result from displacement of protein-bound fluoxetine by other tightly-bound drugs). Products include:
InnoPran XL Extended Release Capsules 1484

Protriptyline Hydrochloride (Fluoxetine inhibits the activity of P450 IID6 isoenzyme making normal metabolizers resemble "poor metabolizers"; therapy with drugs that are predominantly metabolized by the P450 IID6 isoenzyme, such as tricyclic antidepressants, and

have a relatively narrow therapeutic index should be initiated at low end of the dose range if a patient is receiving fluoxetine concurrently or has taken it in the previous 5 weeks).

No products indexed under this heading.

Quetiapine Fumarate (If fluoxetine is added to the treatment regimen of a patient already receiving a drug metabolized by CYP2D6, the need for decreased dose of the original medication should be considered. Fluoxetine is metabolized by this isoenzyme; thus, both the pharmacokinetic properties and relative proportion of metabolites are altered in poor metabolizers of CYP2D6).

No products indexed under this heading.

Quinidine Gluconate (If fluoxetine is added to the treatment regimen of a patient already receiving a drug metabolized by CYP2D6, the need for decreased dose of the original medication should be considered. Fluoxetine is metabolized by this isoenzyme; thus, both the pharmacokinetic properties and relative proportion of metabolites are altered in poor metabolizers of CYP2D6).

No products indexed under this heading.

Quinidine Hydrochloride (If fluoxetine is added to the treatment regimen of a patient already receiving a drug metabolized by CYP2D6, the need for decreased dose of the original medication should be considered. Fluoxetine is metabolized by this isoenzyme; thus, both the pharmacokinetic properties and relative proportion of metabolites are altered in poor metabolizers of CYP2D6).

No products indexed under this heading.

Quinidine Polygalacturonate (If fluoxetine is added to the treatment regimen of a patient already receiving a drug metabolized by CYP2D6, the need for decreased dose of the original medication should be considered. Fluoxetine is metabolized by this isoenzyme; thus, both the pharmacokinetic properties and relative proportion of metabolites are altered in poor metabolizers of CYP2D6).

No products indexed under this heading.

Quinidine Sulfate (If fluoxetine is added to the treatment regimen of a patient already receiving a drug metabolized by CYP2D6, the need for decreased dose of the original medication should be considered. Fluoxetine is metabolized by this isoenzyme; thus, both the pharmacokinetic properties and relative proportion of metabolites are altered in poor metabolizers of CYP2D6).

No products indexed under this heading.

Rasagiline Mesylate (Co-administration with MAO inhibitors has resulted in serious, sometimes fatal, reactions, including hyperthermia, rigidity, extreme agitation, delirium, coma, and features resembling neuroleptic malignant syndrome; concurrent and/or sequential use is contraindicated). Products include:

Azilect Tablets **3106**

Repaglinide (Fluoxetine may alter glycemic control in diabetics; hypoglycemia has occurred during therapy with fluoxetine and hyperglycemia has developed following discontinuation of the drug; hypoglycemia dosage may need to be adjusted). Products include:

PrandiMet Tablets **2967**
Prandin Tablets **2971**

Risperidone (If fluoxetine is added to the treatment regimen of a patient already receiving a drug metabolized by CYP2D6, the need for decreased dose of the original medication should be considered. Fluoxetine is metabolized by this isoenzyme; thus, both the pharmacokinetic properties and relative proportion of metabolites are altered in poor metabolizers of CYP2D6). Products include:

Risperdal Consta Long-Acting Injection **1753**

Ritonavir (If fluoxetine is added to the treatment regimen of a patient already receiving a drug metabolized by CYP2D6, the need for decreased dose of the original medication should be considered. Fluoxetine is metabolized by this isoenzyme; thus, both the pharmacokinetic properties and relative proportion of metabolites are altered in poor metabolizers of CYP2D6). Products include:

Kaletra **452**
Norvir **489**

Rizatriptan Benzoate (If concomitant treatment of fluoxetine with a triptan is clinically warranted, careful observation of the patient is advised, particularly during treatment initiation and dose increases). Products include:

Maxalt Tablets **2056**
Maxalt-MLT Orally Disintegrating Tablets **2056**

Rofecoxib (SSRIs and SNRIs, including fluoxetine, may increase the risk of bleeding events. Concomitant use of nonsteroidal anti-inflammatory drugs may add to this risk. Case reports and epidemiological studies (case-control and cohort design) have demonstrated an association between use of drugs that interfere with serotonin reuptake and the occurrence of gastrointestinal bleeding. Bleeding events related to SSRIs and SNRIs use have ranged from ecchymoses, hematomas, epistaxis, and petechiae to life-threateninghemorrhages. Patients should be cautioned about the risk of bleeding associated with the concomitant use of fluoxetine and NSAIDs).

No products indexed under this heading.

Rosiglitazone Maleate (Fluoxetine may alter glycemic control in diabetics; hypoglycemia has occurred during therapy with fluoxetine and hyperglycemia has developed following discontinuation of the drug; hypoglycemia dosage may need to be adjusted). Products include:

Avandamet Tablets **1336**
Avandaryl Tablets **1344**
Avandia Tablets **1351**

Selegiline (Co-administration with MAO inhibitors has resulted in serious, sometimes fatal, reactions, including hyperthermia, rigidity, extreme agitation, delirium, coma, and features resembling neuroleptic malignant syndrome; concurrent and/or sequential use is contraindicated). Products include:

Emsam Transdermal System **905**

Selegiline Hydrochloride (Co-administration with MAO inhibitors has resulted in serious, sometimes fatal, reactions, including hyperthermia, rigidity, extreme agitation, delirium, coma, and features resembling neuroleptic malignant syndrome; concurrent and/or sequential use is contraindicated). Products include:

Eldepryl Capsules **3052**

Sertraline Hydrochloride (Based on the mechanism of action of SNRIs and SSRIs and the potential for serotonin syndrome, caution is advised when fluoxetine is co-administered with other drugs that may effect the serotonergic neurotransmitter systems).

No products indexed under this heading.

Sitagliptin Phosphate (Fluoxetine may alter glycemic control in diabetics; hypoglycemia has occurred during therapy with fluoxetine and hyperglycemia has developed following discontinuation of the drug; hypoglycemia dosage may need to be adjusted). Products include:

Janumet Tablets **2041**
Januvia Tablets **2048**

Sulindac (SSRIs and SNRIs, including fluoxetine, may increase the risk of bleeding events. Concomitant use of nonsteroidal anti-inflammatory drugs may add to this risk. Case reports and epidemiological studies (case-control and cohort design) have demonstrated an association between use of drugs that interfere with serotonin reuptake and the occurrence of gastrointestinal bleeding. Bleeding events related to SSRIs and SNRIs use have ranged from ecchymoses, hematomas, epistaxis, and petechiae to life-threateninghemorrhages. Patients should be cautioned about the risk of bleeding associated with the concomitant use of fluoxetine and NSAIDs). Products include:

Clinoril Tablets **1962**

Sumatriptan (Co-administration of SSRIs and sumatriptan has resulted in weakness, hyperreflexia, and incoordination). Products include:

Imitrex Nasal Spray **1470**

Sumatriptan Succinate (Co-administration of SSRIs and sumatriptan has resulted in weakness, hyperreflexia, and incoordination). Products include:

Imitrex Injection **1465**
Imitrex Tablets **1474**
Treximet Tablets **1616**

Tamoxifen Citrate (If fluoxetine is added to the treatment regimen of a patient already receiving a drug metabolized by CYP2D6, the need for decreased dose of the original medication should be considered. Fluoxetine is metabolized by this isoenzyme; thus, both the pharmacokinetic properties and relative proportion of metabolites are altered in poor metabolizers of CYP2D6).

No products indexed under this heading.

Temazepam (The administration of fluoxetine to a patient taking another drug that is tightly bound to protein may cause a shift in plasma concentrations potentially resulting in an adverse effect. Conversely, adverse effects may result from displacement of protein-bound fluoxetine by other tightly-bound drugs).

No products indexed under this heading.

Teniposide (If fluoxetine is added to the treatment regimen of a patient already receiving a drug metabolized by CYP2D6, the need for decreased dose of the original medication should be considered. Fluoxetine is metabolized by this isoenzyme; thus, both the pharmacokinetic properties and relative proportion of metabolites are altered in poor metabolizers of CYP2D6).

No products indexed under this heading.

Testosterone (If fluoxetine is added to the treatment regimen of a patient already receiving a drug metabolized by CYP2D6, the need for decreased dose of the original medication should be considered. Fluoxetine is metabolized by this isoenzyme; thus, both the pharmacokinetic properties and relative proportion of metabolites are altered in poor metabolizers of CYP2D6). Products include:

AndroGel **3159**
Testim 1% Gel **701**

Testosterone Cypionate (If fluoxetine is added to the treatment regimen of a patient already receiving a drug metabolized by CYP2D6, the need for decreased dose of the original medication should be considered. Fluoxetine is metabolized by this isoenzyme; thus, both the pharmacokinetic properties and relative proportion of metabolites are altered in poor metabolizers of CYP2D6).

No products indexed under this heading.

Testosterone Enanthate (If fluoxetine is added to the treatment regimen of a patient already receiving a drug metabolized by CYP2D6, the need for decreased dose of the original medication should be considered. Fluoxetine is metabolized by this isoenzyme; thus, both the pharmacokinetic properties and relative proportion of metabolites are altered in poor metabolizers of CYP2D6). Products include:

Delatestryl Injection **1730**

Testosterone Propionate (If fluoxetine is added to the treatment regimen of a patient already receiving a drug metabolized by CYP2D6, the need for decreased dose of the original medication should be considered. Fluoxetine is metabolized by this isoenzyme; thus, both the pharmacokinetic properties and relative proportion of metabolites are altered in poor metabolizers of CYP2D6).

No products indexed under this heading.

Thioridazine (If fluoxetine is added to the treatment regimen of a patient already receiving a drug metabolized by CYP2D6, the need for decreased dose of the original medication should be considered. Fluoxetine is metabolized by this isoenzyme; thus, both the pharmacokinetic properties and relative proportion of metabolites are altered in poor metabolizers of CYP2D6).

No products indexed under this heading.

Thioridazine Hydrochloride (Co-administration of fluoxetine with thioridazine has produced a 2.4-fold higher Cmax and a 4.5-fold higher AUC for thioridazine; because thioridazine administration produces a dose-related prolongation of the QTc interval, which is associated with serious ventricular arrhythmias such as torsade de pointes-type arrhyth-

mias and sudden death; concurrent and/or sequential use within a minimum of 5 weeks of Prozac is contraindicated). Products include:
Thioridazine Hydrochloride Tablets 2195

Timolol Maleate (If fluoxetine is added to the treatment regimen of a patient already receiving a drug metabolized by CYP2D6, the need for decreased dose of the original medication should be considered. Fluoxetine is metabolized by this isoenzyme; thus, both the pharmacokinetic properties and relative proportion of metabolites are altered in poor metabolizers of CYP2D6). Products include:
Combigan Ophthalmic Solution 553
Cosopt Sterile Ophthalmic Solution 1969
Timoptic Sterile Ophthalmic Solution 2121
Timoptic in Ocudose 2124
Timoptic-XE Sterile Ophthalmic Gel Forming Solution 2125

Tinzaparin Sodium (SSRIs and SNRIs, including fluoxetine, may increase the risk of bleeding events. Concomitant use of anti-coagulants may add to this risk. Case reports and epidemiological studies (case-control and cohort design) have demonstrated an association betweenuse of drugs that interfere with serotonin reuptake and the occurrence of gastrointestinal bleeding. Bleeding events related to SSRIs and SNRIs use have ranged from ecchymoses, hematomas, epistaxis, and petechiae to life-threatening hemorrhages. Patients should be cautioned about the risk of bleeding associated with the concomitant use of fluoxetine and drugs that affect coagulation).
No products indexed under this heading.

Tolazamide (Fluoxetine may alter glycemic control in diabetics; hypoglycemia has occurred during therapy with fluoxetine and hyperglycemia has developed following discontinuation of the drug; hypoglycemia dosage may need to be adjusted).
No products indexed under this heading.

Tolbutamide (Fluoxetine may alter glycemic control in diabetics; hypoglycemia has occurred during therapy with fluoxetine and hyperglycemia has developed following discontinuation of the drug; hypoglycemia dosage may need to be adjusted).
No products indexed under this heading.

Tolmetin Sodium (SSRIs and SNRIs, including fluoxetine, may increase the risk of bleeding events. Concomitant use of nonsteroidal anti-inflammatory drugs may add to this risk. Case reports and epidemiological studies (case-control and cohort design) have demonstrated an association between use of drugs that interfere with serotonin reuptake and the occurrence of gastrointestinal bleeding. Bleeding events related to SSRIs and SNRIs use have ranged from ecchymoses, hematomas, epistaxis, and petechiae to life-threateninghemorrhages. Patients should be cautioned about the risk of bleeding associated with the concomitant use of fluoxetine and NSAIDs).
No products indexed under this heading.

Tolterodine Tartrate (If fluoxetine is added to the treatment regimen of a patient already receiving a drug metabolized by CYP2D6, the need for decreased dose of the original medication should be considered. Fluoxetine is metabolized by this isoenzyme; thus, both the pharmacokinetic properties and relative proportion of metabolites are altered in poor metabolizers of CYP2D6).
No products indexed under this heading.

Tramadol Hydrochloride (Based on the mechanism of action of SNRIs and SSRIs and the potential for serotonin syndrome, caution is advised when fluoxetine is co-administered with other drugs that may effect the serotonergic neurotransmitter systems, such as tramadol). Products include:
Ultram ER Extended-Release Tablets 2428

Tranylcypromine Sulfate (Co-administration with MAO inhibitors has resulted in serious, sometimes fatal, reactions, including hyperthermia, rigidity, extreme agitation, delirium, coma, and features resembling neuroleptic malignant syndrome; concurrent and/or sequential use is contraindicated). Products include:
Parnate Tablets 1532

Trazodone Hydrochloride (If fluoxetine is added to the treatment regimen of a patient already receiving a drug metabolized by CYP2D6, the need for decreased dose of the original medication should be considered. Fluoxetine is metabolized by this isoenzyme; thus, both the pharmacokinetic properties and relative proportion of metabolites are altered in poor metabolizers of CYP2D6).
No products indexed under this heading.

Triazolam (If fluoxetine is added to the treatment regimen of a patient already receiving a drug metabolized by CYP2D6, the need for decreased dose of the original medication should be considered. Fluoxetine is metabolized by this isoenzyme; thus, both the pharmacokinetic properties and relative proportion of metabolites are altered in poor metabolizers of CYP2D6).
No products indexed under this heading.

Trimipramine Maleate (Fluoxetine inhibits the activity of P450 IID6 isoenzyme making normal metabolizers resemble "poor metabolizers"; therapy with drugs that are predominantly metabolized by the P450 IID6 isoenzyme, such as tricyclic antidepressants, and have a relatively narrow therapeutic index should be initiated at low end of the dose range if a patient is receiving fluoxetine concurrently or has taken it in the previous 5 weeks).
No products indexed under this heading.

Troglitazone (Fluoxetine may alter glycemic control in diabetics; hypoglycemia has occurred during therapy with fluoxetine and hyperglycemia has developed following discontinuation of the drug; hypoglycemia dosage may need to be adjusted).
No products indexed under this heading.

L-Tryptophan (Co-administration has resulted in adverse reactions, including agitation, restlessness, and gastrointestinal distress).
No products indexed under this heading.

Valdecoxib (SSRIs and SNRIs, including fluoxetine, may increase the risk of bleeding events. Concomitant use of nonsteroidal anti-inflammatory drugs may add to this risk. Case reports and epidemiological studies (case-control and cohort design) have demonstrated an association between use of drugs that interfere with serotonin reuptake and the occurrence of gastrointestinal bleeding. Bleeding events related to SSRIs and SNRIs use have ranged from ecchymoses, hematomas, epistaxis, and petechiae to life-threateninghemorrhages. Patients should be cautioned about the risk of bleeding associated with the concomitant use of fluoxetine and NSAIDs).
No products indexed under this heading.

Venlafaxine Hydrochloride (Based on the mechanism of action of SNRIs and SSRIs and the potential for serotonin syndrome, caution is advised when fluoxetine is co-administered with other frugs that may effect the serotonergic neurotransmitter systems). Products include:
Effexor XR Extended-Release Capsules 3195
Venlafaxine Hydrochloride Tablets ... 2199

Vinblastine Sulfate (Fluoxetine inhibits the activity of P450 IID6 isoenzyme making normal metabolizers resemble "poor metabolizers"; therapy with drugs that are predominantly metabolized by the P450 IID6 isoenzyme such as vinblastine, and have a relatively narrow therapeutic index, should be initiated at low end of the dose range if a patient is receiving fluoxetine concurrently or has taken it in the previous 5 weeks).
No products indexed under this heading.

Warfarin Sodium (SSRIs and SNRIs, including fluoxetine, may increase the risk of bleeding events. Concomitant use of aspirin, nonsteroidal anti-inflammatory drugs, warfarin, and other anti-coagulants may add to this risk. Case reports and epidemiological studies (case-control and cohort design) have demonstrated an association between use of drugs that interfere with serotonin reuptake and the occurrence of gastrointestinal bleeding. Bleeding events related to SSRIs and SNRIs use have ranged from ecchymoses, hematomas, epistaxis, and petechiae to life-threatening hemorrhages. Patients should be cautioned about the risk of bleeding associated wit the concomitant use of fluoxetine and NSAIDs, aspirin, and other drugs that affect coagulation).
No products indexed under this heading.

Zolmitriptan (If concomitant treatment of fluoxetine with a triptan is clinically warranted, careful observation of the patient is advised, particularly during treatment initiation and dose increases). Products include:
Zomig Tablets 694
Zomig Nasal Spray 689
Zomig-ZMT Tablets 694

Zonisamide (If fluoxetine is added to the treatment regimen of a patient already receiving a drug metabolized by CYP2D6, the need for decreased dose of the original medication should be considered. Fluoxetine is metabolized by this isoenzyme; thus, both the pharmacokinetic properties and relative proportion of metabolites are altered in poor metabolizers of CYP2D6). Products include:
Zonegran Capsules 1089

Food Interactions

Alcohol (Concurrent use with CNS active agents, such as alcohol, requires caution).

Food, unspecified (May delay absorption of fluoxetine inconsequentially; Prozac may be administered with or without food).

PULMICORT FLEXHALER

(Budesonide) 654
May interact with cytochrome p450 3a4 inhibitors (selected) and certain other agents. Compounds in these categories include:

Acetazolamide (Concomitant administration of budesonide with known inhibitors of CYP3A4 may inhibit the metabolism of, and increase the systemic exposure to, budesonide; care should be exercised).
No products indexed under this heading.

Amiodarone Hydrochloride (Concomitant administration of budesonide with known inhibitors of CYP3A4 may inhibit the metabolism of, and increase the systemic exposure to, budesonide; care should be exercised).
No products indexed under this heading.

Amprenavir (Concomitant administration of budesonide with known inhibitors of CYP3A4 may inhibit the metabolism of, and increase the systemic exposure to, budesonide; care should be exercised).
No products indexed under this heading.

Anastrozole (Concomitant administration of budesonide with known inhibitors of CYP3A4 may inhibit the metabolism of, and increase the systemic exposure to, budesonide; care should be exercised). Products include:
Arimidex Tablets 672

Aprepitant (Concomitant administration of budesonide with known inhibitors of CYP3A4 may inhibit the metabolism of, and increase the systemic exposure to, budesonide; care should be exercised). Products include:
Emend Capsules 1992

Atazanavir (Concomitant administration of budesonide with known inhibitors of CYP3A4 may inhibit the metabolism of, and increase the systemic exposure to, budesonide; care should be exercised).
No products indexed under this heading.

Atazanavir Sulfate (Concomitant administration of budesonide with known inhibitors of CYP3A4 may inhibit the metabolism of, and increase the systemic exposure to, budesonide; care should be exercised). Products include:
Reyataz Capsules 3299

Cimetidine (Co-administration of budesonide with cimetidine caused a slight decrease in budesonide clearance and a corresponding increase in its oral bioavailability).
No products indexed under this heading.

Cimetidine Hydrochloride (Concomitant administration of budesonide with known inhibitors of CYP3A4 may inhibit the metabolism of, and increase the systemic exposure to, budesonide; care should be exercised).
No products indexed under this heading.

Ciprofloxacin (Concomitant administration of budesonide with known inhibitors of CYP3A4 may inhibit the metabolism of, and increase the systemic exposure to, budesonide; care should be exercised). Products include:
Cipro I.V. 2817
Cipro Oral Suspension 2810
Cipro XR Tablets 2823
Ciprodex Otic Suspension 541

Clarithromycin (Concomitant administration of budesonide with known inhibitors of CYP3A4 may inhibit the metabolism of, and increase the systemic exposure to, budesonide; care should be exercised). Products include:
Biaxin/Biaxin XL 411

Clotrimazole (Concomitant administration of budesonide with known inhibitors of CYP3A4 may inhibit the metabolism of, and increase the systemic exposure to, budesonide; care should be exercised). Products include:
Lotrisone 2881

Cyclosporine (Concomitant administration of budesonide with known inhibitors of CYP3A4 may inhibit the metabolism of, and increase the systemic exposure to, budesonide; care should be exercised). Products include:
Gengraf Capsules 435
Neoral Oral Solution 2280
Neoral Soft Gelatin Capsules 2280
Restasis Ophthalmic Emulsion 557
Sandimmune 2296

Dalfopristin (Concomitant administration of budesonide with known inhibitors of CYP3A4 may inhibit the metabolism of, and increase the systemic exposure to, budesonide; care should be exercised).
No products indexed under this heading.

Danazol (Concomitant administration of budesonide with known inhibitors of CYP3A4 may inhibit the metabolism of, and increase the systemic exposure to, budesonide; care should be exercised).
No products indexed under this heading.

Delavirdine Mesylate (Concomitant administration of budesonide with known inhibitors of CYP3A4 may inhibit the metabolism of, and increase the systemic exposure to, budesonide; care should be exercised).
No products indexed under this heading.

Diltiazem Hydrochloride (Concomitant administration of budesonide with known inhibitors of CYP3A4 may inhibit the metabolism of, and increase the systemic exposure to, budesonide; care should be exercised). Products include:
Cardizem LA Extended Release Tablets 421

Diltiazem Maleate (Concomitant administration of budesonide with known inhibitors of CYP3A4 may inhibit the metabolism of, and increase the systemic exposure to, budesonide; care should be exercised).
No products indexed under this heading.

Efavirenz (Concomitant administration of budesonide with known inhibitors of CYP3A4 may inhibit the metabolism of, and increase the systemic exposure to, budesonide; care should be exercised). Products include:
Atripla 938
Sustiva Capsules 930
Sustiva Tablets 930

Erythromycin (Concomitant administration of budesonide with known inhibitors of CYP3A4 may inhibit the metabolism of, and increase the systemic exposure to, budesonide; care should be exercised).
No products indexed under this heading.

Erythromycin Estolate (Concomitant administration of budesonide with known inhibitors of CYP3A4 may inhibit the metabolism of, and increase the systemic exposure to, budesonide; care should be exercised).
No products indexed under this heading.

Erythromycin Ethylsuccinate (Concomitant administration of budesonide with known inhibitors of CYP3A4 may inhibit the metabolism of, and increase the systemic exposure to, budesonide; care should be exercised). Products include:
E.E.S. 433
EryPed 431

Erythromycin Gluceptate (Concomitant administration of budesonide with known inhibitors of CYP3A4 may inhibit the metabolism of, and increase the systemic exposure to, budesonide; care should be exercised).
No products indexed under this heading.

Erythromycin Lactobionate (Concomitant administration of budesonide with known inhibitors of CYP3A4 may inhibit the metabolism of, and increase the systemic exposure to, budesonide; care should be exercised).
No products indexed under this heading.

Erythromycin Stearate (Concomitant administration of budesonide with known inhibitors of CYP3A4 may inhibit the metabolism of, and increase the systemic exposure to, budesonide; care should be exercised).
No products indexed under this heading.

Esomeprazole Magnesium (Concomitant administration of budesonide with known inhibitors of CYP3A4 may inhibit the metabolism of, and increase the systemic exposure to, budesonide; care should be exercised). Products include:
Nexium Delayed-Release Capsules 645
Nexium Delayed-Release Oral Suspension 645

Fluconazole (Concomitant administration of budesonide with known inhibitors of CYP3A4 may inhibit the metabolism of, and increase the systemic exposure to, budesonide; care should be exercised).
No products indexed under this heading.

Fluoxetine Hydrochloride (Concomitant administration of budesonide with known inhibitors of CYP3A4 may inhibit the metabolism of, and increase the systemic exposure to, budesonide; care should be exercised). Products include:
Prozac Pulvules and Liquid 1852
Prozac Weekly Capsules 1852
Symbyax Capsules 1871

Fluvoxamine Maleate (Concomitant administration of budesonide with known inhibitors of CYP3A4 may inhibit the metabolism of, and increase the systemic exposure to, budesonide; care should be exercised). Products include:
Luvox CR Extended-Release Capsules 1759

Fosamprenavir Calcium (Concomitant administration of budesonide with known inhibitors of CYP3A4 may inhibit the metabolism of, and increase the systemic exposure to, budesonide; care should be exercised). Products include:
Lexiva Oral Suspension 1510
Lexiva Tablets 1510

Indinavir Sulfate (Concomitant administration of budesonide with known inhibitors of CYP3A4 may inhibit the metabolism of, and increase the systemic exposure to, budesonide; care should be exercised). Products include:
Crixivan Capsules 1979

Isoniazid (Concomitant administration of budesonide with known inhibitors of CYP3A4 may inhibit the metabolism of, and increase the systemic exposure to, budesonide; care should be exercised).
No products indexed under this heading.

Itraconazole (Concomitant administration of budesonide with known inhibitors of CYP3A4 may inhibit the metabolism of, and increase the systemic exposure to, budesonide; care should be exercised).
No products indexed under this heading.

Ketoconazole (Concomitant administration of budesonide with known inhibitors of CYP3A4 may inhibit the metabolism of, and increase the systemic exposure to, budesonide; care should be exercised). Products include:
Extina Foam, 2% 3057
Nizoral A-D Shampoo 1901

Lopinavir (Concomitant administration of budesonide with known inhibitors of CYP3A4 may inhibit the metabolism of, and increase the systemic exposure to, budesonide; care should be exercised). Products include:
Kaletra 452

Loratadine (Concomitant administration of budesonide with known inhibitors of CYP3A4 may inhibit the metabolism of, and increase the systemic exposure to, budesonide; care should be exercised).
No products indexed under this heading.

Metronidazole (Concomitant administration of budesonide with known inhibitors of CYP3A4 may inhibit the metabolism of, and increase the systemic exposure to, budesonide; care should be exercised). Products include:
Pylera Capsules 714

Metronidazole Benzoate (Concomitant administration of budesonide with known inhibitors of CYP3A4 may inhibit the metabolism of, and increase the systemic exposure to, budesonide; care should be exercised).
No products indexed under this heading.

Metronidazole Hydrochloride (Concomitant administration of budesonide with known inhibitors of CYP3A4 may inhibit the metabolism of, and increase the systemic exposure to, budesonide; care should be exercised).
No products indexed under this heading.

Miconazole (Concomitant administration of budesonide with known inhibitors of CYP3A4 may inhibit the metabolism of, and increase the systemic exposure to, budesonide; care should be exercised).
No products indexed under this heading.

Miconazole Nitrate (Concomitant administration of budesonide with known inhibitors of CYP3A4 may inhibit the metabolism of, and increase the systemic exposure to, budesonide; care should be exercised).
No products indexed under this heading.

Nefazodone Hydrochloride (Concomitant administration of budesonide with known inhibitors of CYP3A4 may inhibit the metabolism of, and increase the systemic exposure to, budesonide; care should be exercised).
No products indexed under this heading.

Nelfinavir Mesylate (Concomitant administration of budesonide with known inhibitors of CYP3A4 may inhibit the metabolism of, and increase the systemic exposure to, budesonide; care should be exercised).
No products indexed under this heading.

Nevirapine (Concomitant administration of budesonide with known inhibitors of CYP3A4 may inhibit the metabolism of, and increase the systemic exposure to, budesonide; care should be exercised). Products include:
Viramune Oral Suspension 873
Viramune Tablets 873

Niacinamide (Concomitant administration of budesonide with known inhibitors of CYP3A4 may inhibit the metabolism of, and increase the systemic exposure to, budesonide; care should be exercised). Products include:
BioLean Free Tablets .... ▣635

Nicotinamide (Concomitant administration of budesonide with known inhibitors of CYP3A4 may inhibit the metabolism of, and increase the systemic exposure to, budesonide; care should be exercised).
No products indexed under this heading.

Nifedipine (Concomitant administration of budesonide with known inhibitors of CYP3A4 may inhibit the metabolism of, and increase the systemic exposure to, budesonide; care should be exercised).
No products indexed under this heading.

Norfloxacin (Concomitant administration of budesonide with known inhibitors of CYP3A4 may inhibit the metabolism of, and increase the systemic exposure to, budesonide; care should be exercised). Products include:
Noroxin Tablets **2069**

Omeprazole (Concomitant administration of budesonide with known inhibitors of CYP3A4 may inhibit the metabolism of, and increase the systemic exposure to, budesonide; care should be exercised).
No products indexed under this heading.

Paroxetine Hydrochloride (Concomitant administration of budesonide with known inhibitors of CYP3A4 may inhibit the metabolism of, and increase the systemic exposure to, budesonide; care should be exercised). Products include:
Paxil CR Controlled-Release Tablets **1544**
Paxil **1535**

Propoxyphene Hydrochloride (Concomitant administration of budesonide with known inhibitors of CYP3A4 may inhibit the metabolism of, and increase the systemic exposure to, budesonide; care should be exercised).
No products indexed under this heading.

Propoxyphene Napsylate (Concomitant administration of budesonide with known inhibitors of CYP3A4 may inhibit the metabolism of, and increase the systemic exposure to, budesonide; care should be exercised).
No products indexed under this heading.

Quinidine (Concomitant administration of budesonide with known inhibitors of CYP3A4 may inhibit the metabolism of, and increase the systemic exposure to, budesonide; care should be exercised).
No products indexed under this heading.

Quinidine Hydrochloride (Concomitant administration of budesonide with known inhibitors of CYP3A4 may inhibit the metabolism of, and increase the systemic exposure to, budesonide; care should be exercised).
No products indexed under this heading.

Quinidine Polygalacturonate (Concomitant administration of budesonide with known inhibitors of CYP3A4 may inhibit the metabolism of, and increase the systemic exposure to, budesonide; care should be exercised).
No products indexed under this heading.

Quinidine Sulfate (Concomitant administration of budesonide with known inhibitors of CYP3A4 may inhibit the metabolism of, and increase the systemic exposure to, budesonide; care should be exercised).
No products indexed under this heading.

Quinine (Concomitant administration of budesonide with known inhibitors of CYP3A4 may inhibit the metabolism of, and increase the systemic exposure to, budesonide; care should be exercised).
No products indexed under this heading.

Quinine Sulfate (Concomitant administration of budesonide with known inhibitors of CYP3A4 may inhibit the metabolism of, and increase the systemic exposure to, budesonide; care should be exercised).
No products indexed under this heading.

Quinupristin (Concomitant administration of budesonide with known inhibitors of CYP3A4 may inhibit the metabolism of, and increase the systemic exposure to, budesonide; care should be exercised).
No products indexed under this heading.

Ranitidine Bismuth Citrate (Concomitant administration of budesonide with known inhibitors of CYP3A4 may inhibit the metabolism of, and increase the systemic exposure to, budesonide; care should be exercised).
No products indexed under this heading.

Ranitidine Hydrochloride (Concomitant administration of budesonide with known inhibitors of CYP3A4 may inhibit the metabolism of, and increase the systemic exposure to, budesonide; care should be exercised). Products include:
Zantac 75 Tablets **603**
Zantac **1670**
Zantac Injection **1666**
Zantac Injection Pharmacy Bulk Package **1668**
Maximum Strength Zantac 150 Tablets **603**
Maximum Strength Zantac 150 Cool Mint Tablets **603**

Ritonavir (Concomitant administration of budesonide with known inhibitors of CYP3A4 may inhibit the metabolism of, and increase the systemic exposure to, budesonide; care should be exercised). Products include:
Kaletra **452**
Norvir **489**

Saquinavir (Concomitant administration of budesonide with known inhibitors of CYP3A4 may inhibit the metabolism of, and increase the systemic exposure to, budesonide; care should be exercised).
No products indexed under this heading.

Saquinavir Mesylate (Concomitant administration of budesonide with known inhibitors of CYP3A4 may inhibit the metabolism of, and increase the systemic exposure to, budesonide; care should be exercised).
No products indexed under this heading.

Sertraline Hydrochloride (Concomitant administration of budesonide with known inhibitors of CYP3A4 may inhibit the metabolism of, and increase the systemic exposure to, budesonide; care should be exercised).
No products indexed under this heading.

Telithromycin (Concomitant administration of budesonide with known inhibitors of CYP3A4 may inhibit the metabolism of, and increase the systemic exposure to, budesonide; care should be exercised). Products include:
Ketek Tablets **2744**

Troglitazone (Concomitant administration of budesonide with known inhibitors of CYP3A4 may inhibit the metabolism of, and increase the systemic exposure to, budesonide; care should be exercised).
No products indexed under this heading.

Troleandomycin (Concomitant administration of budesonide with known inhibitors of CYP3A4 may inhibit the metabolism of, and increase the systemic exposure to, budesonide; care should be exercised).
No products indexed under this heading.

Valproate Sodium (Concomitant administration of budesonide with known inhibitors of CYP3A4 may inhibit the metabolism of, and increase the systemic exposure to, budesonide; care should be exercised).
No products indexed under this heading.

Verapamil Hydrochloride (Concomitant administration of budesonide with known inhibitors of CYP3A4 may inhibit the metabolism of, and increase the systemic exposure to, budesonide; care should be exercised). Products include:
Tarka Tablets **511**

Voriconazole (Concomitant administration of budesonide with known inhibitors of CYP3A4 may inhibit the metabolism of, and increase the systemic exposure to, budesonide; care should be exercised).
No products indexed under this heading.

Zafirlukast (Concomitant administration of budesonide with known inhibitors of CYP3A4 may inhibit the metabolism of, and increase the systemic exposure to, budesonide; care should be exercised). Products include:
Accolate Tablets **669**

Zileuton (Concomitant administration of budesonide with known inhibitors of CYP3A4 may inhibit the metabolism of, and increase the systemic exposure to, budesonide; care should be exercised).
No products indexed under this heading.

Food Interactions

Grapefruit (Concomitant administration of budesonide with known inhibitors of CYP3A4 may inhibit the metabolism of, and increase the systemic exposure to, budesonide; care should be exercised).

Grapefruit Juice (Concomitant administration of budesonide with known inhibitors of CYP3A4 may inhibit the metabolism of, and increase the systemic exposure to, budesonide; care should be exercised).

PULMOZYME INHALATION SOLUTION

(Dornase Alfa) **1217**
None cited in PDR database.

PURE GARDENS CREAM

(Herbals with Vitamins) **624**
None cited in PDR database.

PURETRIM MEDITERRANEAN WELLNESS SHAKE

(Antioxidants, Fatty Acids, Rice Protein) **624**
None cited in PDR database.

PYLERA CAPSULES

(Bismuth Subcitrate Potassium, Metronidazole, Tetracycline Hydrochloride) **714**
May interact with antacids, anticoagulants, lithium preparations, oral contraceptives, penicillins, phenytoin, and certain other agents. Compounds in these categories include:

Aluminum Carbonate (Absorption of Pylera is impaired by antacids containing aluminum, calcium, or magnesium).
No products indexed under this heading.

Aluminum Hydroxide (Absorption of Pylera is impaired by antacids containing aluminum, calcium, or magnesium).
No products indexed under this heading.

5-Amino-Salicylic Acid (Since bacteriostatic drugs, such as Pylera class of antibiotics, may interfere with the bactericidal action of penicillin, it is not advisable to administer these drugs concomitantly).
No products indexed under this heading.

Amoxicillin (Since bacteriostatic drugs, such as Pylera class of antibiotics, may interfere with the bactericidal action of penicillin, it is not advisable to administer these drugs concomitantly). Products include:
Amoxil Capsules **1305**
Amoxil Chewable Tablets **1305**
Amoxil Pediatric Drops for Oral Suspension **1305**
Amoxil Powder for Oral Suspension **1305**
Amoxil Tablets **1305**
Augmentin **1323**
Augmentin Tablets **1327**
Augmentin XR Extended Release Tablets **1333**
Augmentin ES-600 Powder for Oral Suspension **1329**
Moxatag Tablets **2165**

Amoxicillin Trihydrate (Since bacteriostatic drugs, such as Pylera class of antibiotics, may interfere with the bactericidal action of penicillin, it is not advisable to administer these drugs concomitantly).
No products indexed under this heading.

Ampicillin (Since bacteriostatic drugs, such as Pylera class of antibiotics, may interfere with the bactericidal action of penicillin, it is not advisable to administer these drugs concomitantly).
No products indexed under this heading.

Ampicillin Sodium (Since bacteriostatic drugs, such as Pylera class of antibiotics, may interfere with the bactericidal action of penicillin, it is not advisable to administer these drugs concomitantly).
No products indexed under this heading.

Ampicillin Trihydrate (Since bacteriostatic drugs, such as Pylera class of antibiotics, may interfere with the bactericidal action of penicillin, it is not advisable to administer these drugs concomitantly).
No products indexed under this heading.

Anisindione (Pylera has been reported to potentiate the anticoagulant effect of warfarin and other oral coumarin anticoagulant, resulting in a prolongation of prothrombin time. Therefore, frequent monitoring therapy with appropriate adjustment of the anticoagulant dosage is warranted with initiation of Pylera).
No products indexed under this heading.

Ardeparin Sodium (Pylera has been reported to potentiate the anticoagulant effect of warfarin and other oral coumarin anticoagulant, resulting in a prolongation of prothrombin time. Therefore, frequent monitoring therapy with appropriate adjustment of the anticoagulant dosage is warranted with initiation of Pylera).
No products indexed under this heading.

Azlocillin Sodium (Since bacteriostatic drugs, such as Pylera class of antibiotics, may interfere with the bactericidal action of penicillin, it is not advisable to administer these drugs concomitantly).
No products indexed under this heading.

Bacampicillin Hydrochloride (Since bacteriostatic drugs, such as Pylera class of antibiotics, may interfere with the bactericidal action of penicillin, it is not advisable to administer these drugs concomitantly).
No products indexed under this heading.

Carbenicillin Disodium (Since bacteriostatic drugs, such as Pylera class of antibiotics, may interfere with the bactericidal action of penicillin, it is not advisable to administer these drugs concomitantly).
No products indexed under this heading.

Carbenicillin Indanyl Sodium (Since bacteriostatic drugs, such as Pylera class of antibiotics, may interfere with the bactericidal action of penicillin, it is not advisable to administer these drugs concomitantly).
No products indexed under this heading.

Cimetidine (The simultaneous administration of drugs that decrease microsomal liver enzyme activity, such as cimetidine, may prolong the half-life and decrease plasma clearance of pylera).
No products indexed under this heading.

Dalteparin Sodium (Pylera has been reported to potentiate the anticoagulant effect of warfarin and other oral coumarin anticoagulant, resulting in a prolongation of prothrombin time. Therefore, frequent monitoring therapy with appropriate adjustment of the anticoagulant dosage is warranted with initiation of Pylera). Products include:
Fragmin Injection 1070

Danaparoid Sodium (Pylera has been reported to potentiate the anticoagulant effect of warfarin and other oral coumarin anticoagulant, resulting in a prolongation of prothrombin time. Therefore, frequent monitoring therapy with appropriate adjustment of the anticoagulant dosage is warranted with initiation of Pylera).
No products indexed under this heading.

Desogestrel (Concurrent use of Pylera may render oral contraceptives less effective. Patients should be advised to use a different or additional form of contraceptives). Products include:
Mircette Tablets 1034

Dicloxacillin Sodium (Since bacteriostatic drugs, such as Pylera class of antibiotics, may interfere with the bactericidal action of penicillin, it is not advisable to administer these drugs concomitantly).
No products indexed under this heading.

Dicumarol (Pylera has been reported to potentiate the anticoagulant effect of warfarin and other oral coumarin anticoagulant, resulting in a prolongation of prothrombin time. Therefore, frequent monitoring therapy with appropriate adjustment of the anticoagulant dosage is warranted with initiation of Pylera).
No products indexed under this heading.

Enoxaparin Sodium (Pylera has been reported to potentiate the anticoagulant effect of warfarin and other oral coumarin anticoagulant, resulting in a prolongation of prothrombin time. Therefore, frequent monitoring therapy with appropriate adjustment of the anticoagulant dosage is warranted with initiation of Pylera). Products include:
Lovenox Injection 2756

Ethinyl Estradiol (Concurrent use of Pylera may render oral contraceptives less effective. Patients should be advised to use a different or additional form of contraceptives). Products include:
Lybrel Tablets 3204
Mircette Tablets 1034
NuvaRing 2897
Ortho-Cyclen/Ortho Tri-Cyclen 2449
Ortho Evra Transdermal System 2437
Ortho Tri-Cyclen Lo Tablets 2458
Seasonique Tablets 1046
Yaz Tablets 805

Ethynodiol Diacetate (Concurrent use of Pylera may render oral contraceptives less effective. Patients should be advised to use a different or additional form of contraceptives).
No products indexed under this heading.

Fondaparinux Sodium (Pylera has been reported to potentiate the anticoagulant effect of warfarin and other oral coumarin anticoagulant, resulting in a prolongation of prothrombin time. Therefore, frequent monitoring therapy with appropriate adjustment of the anticoagulant dosage is warranted with initiation of Pylera). Products include:
Arixtra Injection 1313

Fosphenytoin Sodium (The simultaneous administration of drugs that induce microsomal liver enzymes, such as phenytoin, may accelerate the elimination of Pylera, resulting in reduced plasma levels. Impaired clearance of phenytoin has also been reported in this situation).
No products indexed under this heading.

Heparin Calcium (Pylera has been reported to potentiate the anticoagulant effect of warfarin and other oral coumarin anticoagulant, resulting in a prolongation of prothrombin time. Therefore, frequent monitoring therapy with appropriate adjustment of the anticoagulant dosage is warranted with initiation of Pylera).
No products indexed under this heading.

Heparin Sodium (Pylera has been reported to potentiate the anticoagulant effect of warfarin and other oral coumarin anticoagulant, resulting in a prolongation of prothrombin time. Therefore, frequent monitoring therapy with appropriate adjustment of the anticoagulant dosage is warranted with initiation of Pylera).
No products indexed under this heading.

Levonorgestrel (Concurrent use of Pylera may render oral contraceptives less effective. Patients should be advised to use a different or additional form of contraceptives). Products include:
Climara Pro Transdermal System 768
Lybrel Tablets 3204
Mirena Intrauterine System 779
Plan B Tablets 1044
Seasonique Tablets 1046

Lithium (In patients stabilized on relatively high doses of lithium, short-term Pylera therapy has been associated with elevation of serum lithium and, in a few cases, signs of lithium toxicity).
No products indexed under this heading.

Lithium Carbonate (In patients stabilized on relatively high doses of lithium, short-term Pylera therapy has been associated with elevation of serum lithium and, in a few cases, signs of lithium toxicity).
No products indexed under this heading.

Lithium Citrate (In patients stabilized on relatively high doses of lithium, short-term Pylera therapy has been associated with elevation of serum lithium and, in a few cases, signs of lithium toxicity).
No products indexed under this heading.

Low Molecular Weight Heparins (Pylera has been reported to potentiate the anticoagulant effect of warfarin and other oral coumarin anticoagulant, resulting in a prolongation of prothrombin time. Therefore, frequent monitoring therapy with appropriate adjustment of the anticoagulant dosage is warranted with initiation of Pylera).
No products indexed under this heading.

Magaldrate (Absorption of Pylera is impaired by antacids containing aluminum, calcium, or magnesium).
No products indexed under this heading.

Magnesium Hydroxide (Absorption of Pylera is impaired by antacids containing aluminum, calcium, or magnesium). Products include:
Fleet Pedia-Lax Chewable Tablets 1145
Pepcid Complete Chewable Tablets 1771
Extra Strength Rolaids Freshmint Tablets 1903
Rolaids Multi-Symptom Berry Tablets 1903
Rolaids Original Peppermint Tablets 1903

Magnesium Oxide (Absorption of Pylera is impaired by antacids containing aluminum, calcium, or magnesium). Products include:
Beelith Tablets 813

Mestranol (Concurrent use of Pylera may render oral contraceptives less effective. Patients should be advised to use a different or additional form of contraceptives).
No products indexed under this heading.

Methoxyflurane (The concurrent use of tetracycline and methoxyflurane has been reported to result in fatal renal toxicity).
No products indexed under this heading.

Mezlocillin Sodium (Since bacteriostatic drugs, such as Pylera class of antibiotics, may interfere with the bactericidal action of penicillin, it is not advisable to administer these drugs concomitantly).
No products indexed under this heading.

Nafcillin Sodium (Since bacteriostatic drugs, such as Pylera class of antibiotics, may interfere with the bactericidal action of penicillin, it is not advisable to administer these drugs concomitantly).
No products indexed under this heading.

Norethindrone (Concurrent use of Pylera may render oral contraceptives less effective. Patients should be advised to use a different or additional form of contraceptives). Products include:
Ortho Micronor Tablets 2446

Norethynodrel (Concurrent use of Pylera may render oral contraceptives less effective. Patients should be advised to use a different or additional form of contraceptives).
No products indexed under this heading.

Norgestimate (Concurrent use of Pylera may render oral contraceptives less effective. Patients should be advised to use a different or additional form of contraceptives). Products include:
Ortho-Cyclen/Ortho Tri-Cyclen 2449
Ortho Tri-Cyclen Lo Tablets 2458

Norgestrel (Concurrent use of Pylera may render oral contraceptives less effective. Patients should be advised to use a different or additional form of contraceptives).
No products indexed under this heading.

Penicillin G Benzathine (Since bacteriostatic drugs, such as Pylera class of antibiotics, may interfere with the bactericidal action of penicillin, it is not advisable to administer these drugs concomitantly). Products include:
Bicillin C-R Injectable Suspension 1775
Bicillin L-A Injection 1777

Penicillin G Potassium (Since bacteriostatic drugs, such as Pylera class of antibiotics, may interfere with the bactericidal action of penicillin, it is not advisable to administer these drugs concomitantly).
No products indexed under this heading.

Penicillin G Procaine (Since bacteriostatic drugs, such as Pylera class of antibiotics, may interfere with the bactericidal action of penicillin, it is not advisable to administer these drugs concomitantly). Products include:

Bicillin C-R Injectable Suspension 1775
Bicillin L-A Injection 1777

Penicillin G Sodium (Since bacteriostatic drugs, such as Pylera class of antibiotics, may interfere with the bactericidal action of penicillin, it is not advisable to administer these drugs concomitantly).
No products indexed under this heading.

Penicillin V Potassium (Since bacteriostatic drugs, such as Pylera class of antibiotics, may interfere with the bactericidal action of penicillin, it is not advisable to administer these drugs concomitantly).
No products indexed under this heading.

Phenobarbital (The simultaneous administration of drugs that induce microsomal liver enzymes, such as phenobarbital, may accelerate the elimination of pylera, resulting in reduced plasma levels. Impaired clearance of phenobarbital has also been reported in this situation). Products include:
Donnatal Extentabs 2507

Phenytoin (The simultaneous administration of drugs that induce microsomal liver enzymes, such as phenytoin, may accelerate the elimination of Pylera, resulting in reduced plasma levels. Impaired clearance of phenytoin has also been reported in this situation).
No products indexed under this heading.

Phenytoin Sodium (The simultaneous administration of drugs that induce microsomal liver enzymes, such as phenytoin, may accelerate the elimination of Pylera, resulting in reduced plasma levels. Impaired clearance of phenytoin has also been reported in this situation). Products include:
Phenytek Capsules 2192

Sodium Bicarbonate (Absorption of Pylera is impaired by antacids containing aluminum, calcium, or magnesium). Products include:
Ceo-Two Laxative Suppository 815

Ticarcillin Disodium (Since bacteriostatic drugs, such as Pylera class of antibiotics, may interfere with the bactericidal action of penicillin, it is not advisable to administer these drugs concomitantly). Products include:
Timentin ADD-Vantage 1606
Timentin Injection Galaxy Container 1609
Timentin IV Infusion 1603
Timentin Pharmacy Bulk Package 1613

Tinzaparin Sodium (Pylera has been reported to potentiate the anticoagulant effect of warfarin and other oral coumarin anticoagulant, resulting in a prolongation of prothrombin time. Therefore, frequent monitoring therapy with appropriate adjustment of the anticoagulant dosage is warranted with initiation of Pylera).
No products indexed under this heading.

Vitamins, Multiple (Absorption of Pylera is impaired by preparations containing iron, zinc, or sodium bicarbonate). Products include:
Bausch & Lomb Ocuvite DF Vitamin Supplement..................... ⊙238
Mega Antioxidant Tablets 3174
Vibe Liquid Multi-Nutrient Supplement .... ▣626

Warfarin Sodium (Pylera has been reported to potentiate the anticoagulant effect of warfarin and other oral coumarin anticoagulant, resulting in a prolongation of prothrombin time. Therefore, frequent monitoring therapy with appropriate adjustment of the anticoagulant dosage is warranted with initiation of Pylera).
No products indexed under this heading.

Food Interactions

Alcohol (Alcoholic beverages should not be consumed during Pylera therapy and for at least 1 day afterward. Psychotic reactions have been reported in alcoholic patients who are using Pylera and disulfiram concurrently. Pylera should not be given to patients who have taken disulfiram within the last 2 weeks).

Dairy products (Absorption of Pylera is impaired by milk or dairy products).

QUIXIN OPHTHALMIC SOLUTION

(Levofloxacin) 3184
May interact with xanthines and certain other agents. Compounds in these categories include:

Aminophylline (Systemic administration of some quinolones has been shown to elevate plasma concentrations of theophylline).
No products indexed under this heading.

Caffeine (Systemic administration of some quinolones has been shown to interfere with the metabolism of caffeine). Products include:
BioLean Free Tablets .... ▣635
BioLean II Tablets .... ▣635
Winrgy Dietary Supplement .... ▣642

Caffeine Citrate (Systemic administration of some quinolones has been shown to interfere with the metabolism of caffeine).
No products indexed under this heading.

Cyclosporine (Systemic administration of some quinolones has been associated with transient elevations of serum creatinine in patients receiving systemic cyclosporine concomitantly). Products include:
Gengraf Capsules 435
Neoral Oral Solution 2280
Neoral Soft Gelatin Capsules 2280
Restasis Ophthalmic Emulsion 557
Sandimmune 2296

Dyphylline (Systemic administration of some quinolones has been shown to elevate plasma concentrations of theophylline).
No products indexed under this heading.

Theophylline (Systemic administration of some quinolones has been shown to elevate plasma concentrations of theophylline).
No products indexed under this heading.

Theophylline Anhydrous (Systemic administration of some quinolones has been shown to elevate plasma concentrations of theophylline). Products include:
Uniphyl Tablets 2595

Theophylline Calcium Salicylate (Systemic administration of some quinolones has been shown to elevate plasma concentrations of theophylline).
No products indexed under this heading.

Theophylline Dihydroxypropyl (Glyceryl) (Systemic administration of some quinolones has been shown to elevate plasma concentrations of theophylline).
No products indexed under this heading.

Theophylline Ethylenediamine (Systemic administration of some quinolones has been shown to elevate plasma concentrations of theophylline).
No products indexed under this heading.

Theophylline Sodium Glycinate (Systemic administration of some quinolones has been shown to elevate plasma concentrations of theophylline).
No products indexed under this heading.

Warfarin Sodium (Systemic administration of some quinolones has been shown to enhance the effects of the oral anticoagulant warfarin).
No products indexed under this heading.

QVAR INHALATION AEROSOL

(Beclomethasone Dipropionate) 3116
None cited in PDR database.

RAPAMUNE ORAL SOLUTION

(Sirolimus) 3260
See Rapamune Tablets

RAPAMUNE TABLETS

(Sirolimus) 3260
May interact with ACE inhibitors, cytochrome p450 3a4 inducers (selected), cytochrome p450 3a4 inhibitors, potent, cytochrome p450 3a4 substrates (selected), erythromycin, fibrates, HMG-CoA reductase inhibitors, P-glycoprotein inhibitors, phenytoin, protease inhibitors, vaccines, live, and certain other agents. Compounds in these categories include:

Alfentanil Hydrochloride (Care should be exercised when drugs or other substances that are substrates of CYP3A4 are administered concomitantly with sirolimus).
No products indexed under this heading.

Allium sativum (Sirolimus is known to be a substrate for cytochrome P-450 3A4 (CYP3A4). Inducers of CYP3A4 may decrease sirolimus concentrations. Co-administration of sirolimus with strong inducers of CYP3A4 is not recommended).
No products indexed under this heading.

Alprazolam (Care should be exercised when drugs or other substances that are substrates of CYP3A4 are administered concomitantly with sirolimus).
No products indexed under this heading.

Amiodarone Hydrochloride (Care should be exercised when drugs or other substances that are substrates of CYP3A4 are administered concomitantly with sirolimus).
No products indexed under this heading.

Amitriptyline Hydrochloride (Care should be exercised when drugs or other substances that are substrates of CYP3A4 are administered concomitantly with sirolimus).
No products indexed under this heading.

Amlodipine Besylate (Sirolimus is known to be a substrate for p-glycoprotein (P-gp). Inhibitors of P-gp may increase sirolimus concentrations. Co-administration of sirolimus with strong inhibitors of P-gp is not recommended). Products include:
Azor Tablets 1005
Exforge Tablets 2238

Amprenavir (Exercise caution when using sirolimus with drugs or agents that are modulators of CYP3A4. Co-administration of sirolimus with HIV protease inhibitors may increase sirolimus blood concentrations. The dosage of sirolimus and/or the HIV protease inhibitor may need to be adjusted).
No products indexed under this heading.

Aprepitant (Care should be exercised when drugs or other substances that are substrates of CYP3A4 are administered concomitantly with sirolimus). Products include:
Emend Capsules 1992

Astemizole (Care should be exercised when drugs or other substances that are substrates of CYP3A4 are administered concomitantly with sirolimus).
No products indexed under this heading.

Atazanavir (Sirolimus is known to be a substrate for cytochrome P-450 3A4 (CYP3A4). Inhibitors of CYP3A4 may increase sirolimus concentrations. Co-administration of sirolimus with strong inhibitors of CYP3A4 is not recommended).
No products indexed under this heading.

Atazanavir Sulfate (Sirolimus is known to be a substrate for cytochrome P-450 3A4 (CYP3A4). Inhibitors of CYP3A4 may increase sirolimus concentrations. Co-administration of sirolimus with strong inhibitors of CYP3A4 is not recommended). Products include:
Reyataz Capsules 3299

Atenolol (Sirolimus is known to be a substrate for p-glycoprotein (P-gp). Inhibitors of P-gp may increase sirolimus concentrations. Co-administration of sirolimus with strong inhibitors of P-gp is not recommended).
No products indexed under this heading.

Atorvastatin Calcium (Sirolimus is known to be a substrate for p-glycoprotein (P-gp). Inhibitors of P-gp may increase sirolimus concentrations. Co-administration of sirolimus with strong inhibitors of P-gp is not recommended). Products include:
Lipitor Tablets 2501

Azithromycin Dihydrate (Sirolimus is known to be a substrate for p-glycoprotein (P-gp). Inhibitors of P-gp may increase sirolimus concentrations. Co-administration of sirolimus with strong inhibitors of P-gp is not recommended).
No products indexed under this heading.

BCG Vaccine (Immunosuppressants may affect response to vaccination. Therefore, during treatment with sirolimus, vaccination may be less effective. The use of live vaccines should be avoided).
No products indexed under this heading.

Belladonna Ergotamine (Care should be exercised when drugs or other substances that are substrates of CYP3A4 are administered concomitantly with sirolimus).
No products indexed under this heading.

Benazepril Hydrochloride (Sirolimus has been associated with the development of angioedema. The concomitant use of sirolimus with other drugs known to cause angioedema, such as ACE-inhibitors, may increase the risk of developing angioedema).
No products indexed under this heading.

Betamethasone Acetate (Sirolimus is known to be a substrate for cytochrome P-450 3A4 (CYP3A4). Inducers of CYP3A4 may decrease sirolimus concentrations. Co-administration of sirolimus with strong inducers of CYP3A4 is not recommended).
No products indexed under this heading.

Betamethasone Sodium Phosphate (Sirolimus is known to be a substrate for cytochrome P-450 3A4 (CYP3A4). Inducers of CYP3A4 may decrease sirolimus concentrations. Co-administration of sirolimus with strong inducers of CYP3A4 is not recommended).
No products indexed under this heading.

Bromocriptine Mesylate (Exercise caution when using sirolimus with drugs or agents that are modulators of CYP3A4. Co-administration of sirolimus with bromocriptine may increase sirolimus blood concentrations. The dosage of sirolimus and/or bromocriptine may need to be adjusted).
No products indexed under this heading.

Buspirone Hydrochloride (Care should be exercised when drugs or other substances that are substrates of CYP3A4 are administered concomitantly with sirolimus).
No products indexed under this heading.

Busulfan (Care should be exercised when drugs or other substances that are substrates of CYP3A4 are administered concomitantly with sirolimus). Products include:
Busulfex Injection 2477
Myleran Tablets 1530

Captopril (Sirolimus has been associated with the development of angioedema. The concomitant use of sirolimus with other drugs known to cause angioedema, such as ACE-inhibitors, may increase the risk of developing angioedema). Products include:
Captopril Tablets 2182

Carbamazepine (Exercise caution when using sirolimus with drugs or agents that are modulators of CYP3A4. Co-administration of sirolimus with carbamazepine may decrease sirolimus blood concentrations. The dosage of sirolimus and/or carbamazepine may need to be adjusted). Products include:
Carbatrol Capsules 3019
Equetro Extended-Release Capsules 3174

Cerivastatin Sodium (During sirolimus therapy with cyclosporine, patients administered an HMG-CoA reductase inhibitor and/or fibrate should be monitored for the possible development of rhabdomyolysis and other adverse effects. In clinical trials, the concomitant administration of sirolimus and HMG-CoA reductase inhibitors appeared to be well-tolerated).
No products indexed under this heading.

Chlorpheniramine (Care should be exercised when drugs or other substances that are substrates of CYP3A4 are administered concomitantly with sirolimus).
No products indexed under this heading.

Chlorpheniramine Maleate (Care should be exercised when drugs or other substances that are substrates of CYP3A4 are administered concomitantly with sirolimus). Products include:
Actifed Cold & Allergy Tablets 1895
Sudafed PE Sinus & Allergy Tablets 1908
Tylenol Allergy Multi-Symptom Caplets with Cool Burst and Rapid Release Gelcaps 1916
Children's Tylenol Plus Cold Suspension Liquid 1912
Children's Tylenol Plus Cough & Runny Nose Suspension Liquid 1912
Children's Tylenol Plus Flu Suspension Liquid 1914
Children's Tylenol Plus Multi-Symptom Cold Suspension Liquid 1912
Tylenol Cold Head Congestion Nighttime Caplets with Cool Burst 1910
Tylenol Cold Multi-Symptom Nighttime Caplets with Cool Burst 1913
Tylenol Sinus Congestion & Pain Nighttime Caplets with Cool Burst 1917

Chlorpheniramine Polistirex (Care should be exercised when drugs or other substances that are substrates of CYP3A4 are administered concomitantly with sirolimus). Products include:
Tussionex Pennkinetic Extended-Release Suspension 3154

Chlorpheniramine Tannate (Care should be exercised when drugs or other substances that are substrates of CYP3A4 are administered concomitantly with sirolimus).
No products indexed under this heading.

Cimetidine (Exercise caution when using sirolimus with drugs or agents that are modulators of CYP3A4. Co-administration of sirolimus with cimetidine may increase sirolimus blood concentrations. The dosage of sirolimus and/or cimetidine may need to be adjusted).
No products indexed under this heading.

Cimetidine Hydrochloride (Exercise caution when using sirolimus with drugs or agents that are modulators of CYP3A4. Co-administration of sirolimus with cimetidine may increase sirolimus blood concentrations. The dosage of sirolimus and/or cimetidine may need to be adjusted).
No products indexed under this heading.

Ciprofloxacin Hydrochloride (Sirolimus is known to be a substrate for cytochrome P-450 3A4 (CYP3A4). Inducers of CYP3A4 may decrease sirolimus concentrations. Co-administration of sirolimus with strong inducers of CYP3A4 is not recommended). Products include:
Cipro Tablets 2810

Cisapride (Exercise caution when using sirolimus with drugs or agents that are modulators of CYP3A4. Co-administration of sirolimus with cisapride may increase sirolimus blood concentrations. The dosage of sirolimus and/or cisapride may need to be adjusted).
No products indexed under this heading.

Cisplatin (Sirolimus is known to be a substrate for cytochrome P-450 3A4 (CYP3A4). Inducers of CYP3A4 may decrease sirolimus concentrations. Co-administration of sirolimus with strong inducers of CYP3A4 is not recommended).
No products indexed under this heading.

Clarithromycin (Sirolimus is known to be a substrate for cytochrome P-450 3A4 (CYP3A4). Co-administration of sirolimus with strong inhibitors of CYP3A4 such as clarithromycin is not recommended). Products include:
Biaxin/Biaxin XL 411

Clofibrate (During sirolimus therapy with cyclosporine, patients administered a fibrate should be monitored for the possible development of rhabdomyolysis and other adverse effects. In clinical trials, the concomitant administration of sirolimus and fibrates appeared to be well-tolerated).
No products indexed under this heading.

Clotrimazole (Exercise caution when using sirolimus with drugs or agents that are modulators of CYP3A4. Co-administration of sirolimus with clotrimazole may increase sirolimus blood concentrations. The dosage of sirolimus and/or clotrimazole may need to be adjusted). Products include:
Lotrisone 2881

Cortisone Acetate (Sirolimus is known to be a substrate for cytochrome P-450 3A4 (CYP3A4). Inducers of CYP3A4 may decrease sirolimus concentrations. Co-administration of sirolimus with strong inducers of CYP3A4 is not recommended).
No products indexed under this heading.

Cyclosporine (Cyclosporine, a substrate and inhibitor of CYP3A4 and P-gp, was shown to increase sirolimus concentrations when co-administered with sirolimus. To reduce this, it is recommended that sirolimus be taken 4 hours after administration of cyclosporine oral solution, modified and/or cyclosporine capsules, modified. If cyclosporine is withdrawn from combination therapy with sirolimus, higher doses of sirolimus are needed to maintain recommended sirolimus trough concentration ranges. In studies of de novo livertransplant patients, the use of sirolimus in combination with cyclosporine, was associated with an increase in HAT (Hepatic Artery Thrombosis), (7% in combination vs. 2% in the control arm). Use of sirolimus in liver transplant patients is not recommended). Products include:
Gengraf Capsules 435
Neoral Oral Solution 2280
Neoral Soft Gelatin Capsules 2280
Restasis Ophthalmic Emulsion 557
Sandimmune 2296

Danazol (Exercise caution when using sirolimus with drugs or agents that are modulators of CYP3A4. Co-administration of sirolimus with danazol may increase sirolimus blood concentrations. The dosage of sirolimus and/or danazol may need to be adjusted).
No products indexed under this heading.

Darunavir (Exercise caution when using sirolimus with drugs or agents that are modulators of CYP3A4. Co-administration of sirolimus with HIV protease inhibitors may increase sirolimus blood concentrations. The dosage of sirolimus and/or the HIV protease inhibitor may need to be adjusted).
No products indexed under this heading.

Delavirdine Mesylate (Sirolimus is known to be a substrate for cytochrome P-450 3A4 (CYP3A4). Inhibitors of CYP3A4 may increase sirolimus concentrations. Co-administration of sirolimus with strong inhibitors of CYP3A4 is not recommended).
No products indexed under this heading.

Delavirine (Sirolimus is known to be a substrate for cytochrome P-450 3A4 (CYP3A4). Inhibitors of CYP3A4 may increase sirolimus concentrations. Co-administration of sirolimus with strong inhibitors of CYP3A4 is not recommended).
No products indexed under this heading.

Desogestrel (Care should be exercised when drugs or other substances that are substrates of CYP3A4 are administered concomitantly with sirolimus). Products include:
Mircette Tablets 1034

Dexamethasone (Sirolimus is known to be a substrate for cytochrome P-450 3A4 (CYP3A4). Inducers of CYP3A4 may decrease sirolimus concentrations. Co-administration of sirolimus with strong inducers of CYP3A4 is not recommended). Products include:
Ciprodex Otic Suspension 541

Dexamethasone Acetate (Sirolimus is known to be a substrate for cytochrome P-450 3A4 (CYP3A4). Inducers of CYP3A4 may decrease sirolimus concentrations. Co-administration of sirolimus with strong inducers of CYP3A4 is not recommended).
No products indexed under this heading.

Dexamethasone Sodium Phosphate (Sirolimus is known to be a substrate for cytochrome P-450 3A4 (CYP3A4). Inducers of CYP3A4 may decrease sirolimus concentrations. Co-administration of sirolimus with strong inducers of CYP3A4 is not recommended).
No products indexed under this heading.

Diazepam (Care should be exercised when drugs or other substances that are substrates of

CYP3A4 are administered concomitantly with sirolimus). Products include:
Valium Tablets ... 2658

Digoxin (Sirolimus is known to be a substrate for p-glycoprotein (P-gp). Inhibitors of P-gp may increase sirolimus concentrations. Co-administration of sirolimus with strong inhibitors of P-gp is not recommended). Products include:
Lanoxin Injection ... 1498
Lanoxin Injection Pediatric ... 1502
Lanoxin Tablets ... 1505

Dihydroergotamine Mesylate (Care should be exercised when drugs or other substances that are substrates of CYP3A4 are administered concomitantly with sirolimus).
No products indexed under this heading.

Diltiazem Hydrochloride (Diltiazem is a substrate and inhibitor of CYP3A4 and P-gp; sirolimus concentrations should be monitored and a dose adjustment may be necessary. The simultaneous oral administration of 10 mg of sirolimus oral solution and 120 mg of diltiazem to 18 healthy volunteers significantly affected the bioavailability of sirolimus. Sirolimus Cmax, tmax, and AUC were increased 1.4-, 1.3-, and 1.6-fold, respectively. Sirolimus did not affect the pharmacokinetics of either diltiazem or its metabolites desacetyldiltiazem and desmethyldiltiazem). Products include:
Cardizem LA Extended Release Tablets ... 421

Diltiazem Maleate (Diltiazem is a substrate and inhibitor of CYP3A4 and P-gp; sirolimus concentrations should be monitored and a dose adjustment may be necessary. The simultaneous oral administration of 10 mg of sirolimus oral solution and 120 mg of diltiazem to 18 healthy volunteers significantly affected the bioavailability of sirolimus. Sirolimus Cmax, tmax, and AUC were increased 1.4-, 1.3-, and 1.6-fold, respectively. Sirolimus did not affect the pharmacokinetics of either diltiazem or its metabolites desacetyldiltiazem and desmethyldiltiazem).
No products indexed under this heading.

Dirithromycin (Sirolimus is known to be a substrate for p-glycoprotein (P-gp). Inhibitors of P-gp may increase sirolimus concentrations. Co-administration of sirolimus with strong inhibitors of P-gp is not recommended).
No products indexed under this heading.

Disopyramide (Care should be exercised when drugs or other substances that are substrates of CYP3A4 are administered concomitantly with sirolimus).
No products indexed under this heading.

Disopyramide Phosphate (Care should be exercised when drugs or other substances that are substrates of CYP3A4 are administered concomitantly with sirolimus).
No products indexed under this heading.

Disulfiram (Care should be exercised when drugs or other substances that are substrates of CYP3A4 are administered concomitantly with sirolimus).
No products indexed under this heading.

Doxorubicin Hydrochloride (Care should be exercised when drugs or other substances that are substrates of CYP3A4 are administered concomitantly with sirolimus).
No products indexed under this heading.

Dronabinol (Care should be exercised when drugs or other substances that are substrates of CYP3A4 are administered concomitantly with sirolimus). Products include:
Marinol Capsules ... 3163

Efavirenz (Sirolimus is known to be a substrate for cytochrome P-450 3A4 (CYP3A4). Inducers of CYP3A4 may decrease sirolimus concentrations. Co-administration of sirolimus with strong inducers of CYP3A4 is not recommended). Products include:
Atripla Tablets ... 938
Sustiva Capsules ... 930
Sustiva Tablets ... 930

Elacridar (Sirolimus is known to be a substrate for p-glycoprotein (P-gp). Inhibitors of P-gp may increase sirolimus concentrations. Co-administration of sirolimus with strong inhibitors of P-gp is not recommended).
No products indexed under this heading.

Enalapril Maleate (Sirolimus has been associated with the development of angioedema. The concomitant use of sirolimus with other drugs known to cause angioedema, such as ACE-inhibitors, may increase the risk of developing angioedema).
No products indexed under this heading.

Enalaprilat (Sirolimus has been associated with the development of angioedema. The concomitant use of sirolimus with other drugs known to cause angioedema, such as ACE-inhibitors, may increase the risk of developing angioedema).
No products indexed under this heading.

Ergotamine Tartrate (Care should be exercised when drugs or other substances that are substrates of CYP3A4 are administered concomitantly with sirolimus).
No products indexed under this heading.

Erythromycin (Erythromycin is a substrate and inhibitor of CYP3A4 and P-gp; co-administration of sirolimus oral solution or tablets and erythromycin is not recommended. The simultaneous oral administration of 2 mg daily of sirolimus oral solution and 800 mg q 8h of erythromycin as erythromycin ethylsuccinate tablets at steady state to 24 healthy volunteers significantly affected the bioavailability of sirolimus and erythromycin. Sirolimus Cmax and AUC were increased 4.4- and 4.2-fold, respectively, and tmax was increased by 0.4 hr. Erythromycin Cmax and AUC were increased 1.6- and 1.7-fold, respectively, and tmax was increased by 0.3 hr).
No products indexed under this heading.

Erythromycin Estolate (Erythromycin is a substrate and inhibitor of CYP3A4 and P-gp; co-administration of sirolimus oral solution or tablets and erythromycin is not recommended. The simultaneous oral administration of 2 mg daily of sirolimus oral solution and 800 mg q 8h of erythromycin as erythromycin ethylsuccinate tablets at steady state to 24 healthy volunteers significantly affected the bioavailability of sirolimus and erythromycin. Sirolimus Cmax and AUC were increased 4.4- and 4.2-fold, respectively, and tmax was increased by 0.4 hr. Erythromycin Cmax and AUC were increased 1.6- and 1.7-fold, respectively, and tmax was increased by 0.3 hr).
No products indexed under this heading.

Erythromycin Ethylsuccinate (Erythromycin is a substrate and inhibitor of CYP3A4 and P-gp; co-administration of sirolimus oral solution or tablets and erythromycin is not recommended. The simultaneous oral administration of 2 mg daily of sirolimus oral solution and 800 mg q 8h of erythromycin as erythromycin ethylsuccinate tablets at steady state to 24 healthy volunteers significantly affected the bioavailability of sirolimus and erythromycin. Sirolimus Cmax and AUC were increased 4.4- and 4.2-fold, respectively, and tmax was increased by 0.4 hr. Erythromycin Cmax and AUC were increased 1.6- and 1.7-fold, respectively, and tmax was increased by 0.3 hr). Products include:
E.E.S. ... 433
EryPed ... 431

Erythromycin Gluceptate (Erythromycin is a substrate and inhibitor of CYP3A4 and P-gp; co-administration of sirolimus oral solution or tablets and erythromycin is not recommended. The simultaneous oral administration of 2 mg daily of sirolimus oral solution and 800 mg q 8h of erythromycin as erythromycin ethylsuccinate tablets at steady state to 24 healthy volunteers significantly affected the bioavailability of sirolimus and erythromycin. Sirolimus Cmax and AUC were increased 4.4- and 4.2-fold, respectively, and tmax was increased by 0.4 hr. Erythromycin Cmax and AUC were increased 1.6- and 1.7-fold, respectively, and tmax was increased by 0.3 hr).
No products indexed under this heading.

Erythromycin Lactobionate (Erythromycin is a substrate and inhibitor of CYP3A4 and P-gp; co-administration of sirolimus oral solution or tablets and erythromycin is not recommended. The simultaneous oral administration of 2 mg daily of sirolimus oral solution and 800 mg q 8h of erythromycin as erythromycin ethylsuccinate tablets at steady state to 24 healthy volunteers significantly affected the bioavailability of sirolimus and erythromycin. Sirolimus Cmax and AUC were increased 4.4- and 4.2-fold, respectively, and tmax was increased by 0.4 hr. Erythromycin Cmax and AUC were increased 1.6- and 1.7-fold, respectively, and tmax was increased by 0.3 hr).
No products indexed under this heading.

Erythromycin Stearate (Erythromycin is a substrate and inhibitor of CYP3A4 and P-gp; co-administration of sirolimus oral solution or tablets and erythromycin is not recommended. The simultaneous oral administration of 2 mg daily of sirolimus oral solution and 800 mg q 8h of erythromycin as erythromycin ethylsuccinate tablets at steady state to 24 healthy volunteers significantly affected the bioavailability of sirolimus and erythromycin. Sirolimus Cmax and AUC were increased 4.4- and 4.2-fold, respectively, and tmax was increased by 0.4 hr. Erythromycin Cmax and AUC were increased 1.6- and 1.7-fold, respectively, and tmax was increased by 0.3 hr).
No products indexed under this heading.

Estradiol (Care should be exercised when drugs or other substances that are substrates of CYP3A4 are administered concomitantly with sirolimus). Products include:
Activella Tablets ... 2347
Angeliq Tablets ... 751
Climara Transdermal System ... 763
Climara Pro Transdermal System ... 768
Divigel ... 3167
Vagifem Tablets ... 2375

Estradiol Benzoate (Care should be exercised when drugs or other substances that are substrates of CYP3A4 are administered concomitantly with sirolimus).
No products indexed under this heading.

Estradiol Cypionate (Care should be exercised when drugs or other substances that are substrates of CYP3A4 are administered concomitantly with sirolimus).
No products indexed under this heading.

Estradiol Valerate (Care should be exercised when drugs or other substances that are substrates of CYP3A4 are administered concomitantly with sirolimus).
No products indexed under this heading.

Ethinyl Estradiol (Care should be exercised when drugs or other substances that are substrates of CYP3A4 are administered concomitantly with sirolimus). Products include:
Lybrel Tablets ... 3204
Mircette Tablets ... 1034
NuvaRing ... 2897
Ortho-Cyclen/Ortho Tri-Cyclen ... 2449
Ortho Evra Transdermal System ... 2437
Ortho Tri-Cyclen Lo Tablets ... 2458
Seasonique Tablets ... 1046
Yaz Tablets ... 805

Ethosuximide (Care should be exercised when drugs or other substances that are substrates of CYP3A4 are administered concomitantly with sirolimus).
No products indexed under this heading.

Ethynodiol Diacetate (Care should be exercised when drugs or other substances that are substrates of CYP3A4 are administered concomitantly with sirolimus).
No products indexed under this heading.

Etoposide (Care should be exercised when drugs or other substances that are substrates of CYP3A4 are administered concomitantly with sirolimus).
No products indexed under this heading.

Etoposide Phosphate (Care should be exercised when drugs or other substances that are substrates of CYP3A4 are administered concomitantly with sirolimus).
No products indexed under this heading.

Felbamate (Sirolimus is known to be a substrate for cytochrome P-450 3A4 (CYP3A4). Inducers of CYP3A4 may decrease sirolimus concentrations. Co-administration of sirolimus with strong inducers of CYP3A4 is not recommended).
No products indexed under this heading.

Felodipine (Care should be exercised when drugs or other substances that are substrates of CYP3A4 are administered concomitantly with sirolimus).
No products indexed under this heading.

Fenofibrate (During sirolimus therapy with cyclosporine, patients administered a fibrate should be monitored for the possible development of rhabdomyolysis and other adverse effects. In clinical trials, the concomitant administration of sirolimus and fibrates appeared to be well-tolerated). Products include:
Fenoglide Tablets 2960
Tricor Tablets 520

Fentanyl (Care should be exercised when drugs or other substances that are substrates of CYP3A4 are administered concomitantly with sirolimus). Products include:
Duragesic Transdermal System 2405
Ionsys Transdermal System 2410

Fentanyl Citrate (Care should be exercised when drugs or other substances that are substrates of CYP3A4 are administered concomitantly with sirolimus). Products include:
Actiq 959
Fentora Tablets 968

Fluconazole (Exercise caution when using sirolimus with drugs or agents that are modulators of CYP3A4. Co-administration of sirolimus with fluconazole may increase sirolimus blood concentrations. The dosage of sirolimus and/or fluconazole may need to be adjusted).
No products indexed under this heading.

Fludrocortisone Acetate (Sirolimus is known to be a substrate for cytochrome P-450 3A4 (CYP3A4). Inducers of CYP3A4 may decrease sirolimus concentrations. Co-administration of sirolimus with strong inducers of CYP3A4 is not recommended).
No products indexed under this heading.

Fluvastatin Sodium (During sirolimus therapy with cyclosporine, patients administered an HMG-CoA reductase inhibitor and/or fibrate should be monitored for the possible development of rhabdomyolysis and other adverse effects. In clinical trials, the concomitant administration of sirolimus and HMG-CoA reductase inhibitors appeared to be well-tolerated). Products include:
Lescol Capsules 2268
Lescol XL Tablets 2268

Fosamprenavir Calcium (Exercise caution when using sirolimus with drugs or agents that are modulators of CYP3A4. Co-administration of sirolimus with HIV protease inhibitors may increase sirolimus blood concentrations. The dosage of sirolimus and/or the HIV protease inhibitor may need to be adjusted). Products include:
Lexiva Oral Suspension 1510
Lexiva Tablets 1510

Fosinopril Sodium (Sirolimus has been associated with the development of angioedema. The concomitant use of sirolimus with other drugs known to cause angioedema, such as ACE-inhibitors, may increase the risk of developing angioedema).
No products indexed under this heading.

Fosphenytoin Sodium (Exercise caution when using sirolimus with drugs or agents that are modulators of CYP3A4. Co-administration of sirolimus with phenytoin may decrease sirolimus blood concentrations. The dosage of sirolimus and/or phenytoin may need to be adjusted).
No products indexed under this heading.

Garlic Extract (Sirolimus is known to be a substrate for cytochrome P-450 3A4 (CYP3A4). Inducers of CYP3A4 may decrease sirolimus concentrations. Co-administration of sirolimus with strong inducers of CYP3A4 is not recommended).
No products indexed under this heading.

Garlic Oil (Sirolimus is known to be a substrate for cytochrome P-450 3A4 (CYP3A4). Inducers of CYP3A4 may decrease sirolimus concentrations. Co-administration of sirolimus with strong inducers of CYP3A4 is not recommended).
No products indexed under this heading.

Gemfibrozil (During sirolimus therapy with cyclosporine, patients administered a fibrate should be monitored for the possible development of rhabdomyolysis and other adverse effects. In clinical trials, the concomitant administration of sirolimus and fibrates appeared to be well-tolerated).
No products indexed under this heading.

Haloperidol (Care should be exercised when drugs or other substances that are substrates of CYP3A4 are administered concomitantly with sirolimus).
No products indexed under this heading.

Haloperidol Decanoate (Care should be exercised when drugs or other substances that are substrates of CYP3A4 are administered concomitantly with sirolimus).
No products indexed under this heading.

Haloperidol Lactate (Care should be exercised when drugs or other substances that are substrates of CYP3A4 are administered concomitantly with sirolimus).
No products indexed under this heading.

Hydrocortisone (Sirolimus is known to be a substrate for cytochrome P-450 3A4 (CYP3A4). Inducers of CYP3A4 may decrease sirolimus concentrations. Co-administration of sirolimus with strong inducers of CYP3A4 is not recommended).
No products indexed under this heading.

Hydrocortisone Acetate (Sirolimus is known to be a substrate for cytochrome P-450 3A4 (CYP3A4). Inducers of CYP3A4 may decrease sirolimus concentrations. Co-administration of sirolimus with strong inducers of CYP3A4 is not recommended). Products include:
Analpram-HC 1140
Pramosone 1141

Hydrocortisone Butyrate (Sirolimus is known to be a substrate for cytochrome P-450 3A4 (CYP3A4). Inducers of CYP3A4 may decrease sirolimus concentrations. Co-administration of sirolimus with strong inducers of CYP3A4 is not recommended).
No products indexed under this heading.

Hydrocortisone Cypionate (Sirolimus is known to be a substrate for cytochrome P-450 3A4 (CYP3A4). Inducers of CYP3A4 may decrease sirolimus concentrations. Co-administration of sirolimus with strong inducers of CYP3A4 is not recommended).
No products indexed under this heading.

Hydrocortisone Hemisuccinate (Sirolimus is known to be a substrate for cytochrome P-450 3A4 (CYP3A4). Inducers of CYP3A4 may decrease sirolimus concentrations. Co-administration of sirolimus with strong inducers of CYP3A4 is not recommended).
No products indexed under this heading.

Hydrocortisone Probutate (Sirolimus is known to be a substrate for cytochrome P-450 3A4 (CYP3A4). Inducers of CYP3A4 may decrease sirolimus concentrations. Co-administration of sirolimus with strong inducers of CYP3A4 is not recommended).
No products indexed under this heading.

Hydrocortisone Sodium Phosphate (Sirolimus is known to be a substrate for cytochrome P-450 3A4 (CYP3A4). Inducers of CYP3A4 may decrease sirolimus concentrations. Co-administration of sirolimus with strong inducers of CYP3A4 is not recommended).
No products indexed under this heading.

Hydrocortisone Sodium Succinate (Sirolimus is known to be a substrate for cytochrome P-450 3A4 (CYP3A4). Inducers of CYP3A4 may decrease sirolimus concentrations. Co-administration of sirolimus with strong inducers of CYP3A4 is not recommended).
No products indexed under this heading.

Hydrocortisone Valerate (Sirolimus is known to be a substrate for cytochrome P-450 3A4 (CYP3A4). Inducers of CYP3A4 may decrease sirolimus concentrations. Co-administration of sirolimus with strong inducers of CYP3A4 is not recommended).
No products indexed under this heading.

Hypericum (St. John's Wort (hypericum perforatum) induces CYP3A4 and P-gp. Since sirolimus is a substrate for both cytochrome CYP3A4 and P-gp, there is the potential that the use of St. John's Wort in patients receiving sirolimus could result in reduced sirolimus concentrations). Products include:
Satieté Tablets .... ■□640

Hypericum Perforatum (Sirolimus is known to be a substrate for cytochrome P-450 3A4 (CYP3A4). Inducers of CYP3A4 may decrease sirolimus concentrations. Co-administration of sirolimus with strong inducers of CYP3A4 is not recommended).
No products indexed under this heading.

Indinavir Sulfate (Exercise caution when using sirolimus with drugs or agents that are modulators of CYP3A4. Co-administration of sirolimus with HIV protease inhibitors may increase sirolimus blood concentrations. The dosage of sirolimus and/or the HIV protease inhibitor may need to be adjusted). Products include:
Crixivan Capsules 1979

Influenza Vaccine, Live Attenuated (Immunosuppressants may affect response to vaccination. Therefore, during treatment with sirolimus, vaccination may be less effective. The use of live vaccines should be avoided).
No products indexed under this heading.

Influenza Virus Vaccine Live, Intranasal (Immunosuppressants may affect response to vaccination. Therefore, during treatment with sirolimus, vaccination may be less effective. The use of live vaccines should be avoided). Products include:
FluMist Vaccine 1945

Isradipine (Care should be exercised when drugs or other substances that are substrates of CYP3A4 are administered concomitantly with sirolimus). Products include:
DynaCirc CR Controlled Release Tablets 1407

Itraconazole (Sirolimus is known to be a substrate for cytochrome P-450 3A4 (CYP3A4). Co-administration of sirolimus with strong inhibitors of CYP3A4 such as itraconazole is not recommended).
No products indexed under this heading.

Ixabepilone (Care should be exercised when drugs or other substances that are substrates of CYP3A4 are administered concomitantly with sirolimus). Products include:
Ixempra Kit for Injection 915

Ketoconazole (Ketoconazole is a strong inhibitor of CYP3A4 and P-gp; co-administration of sirolimus oral solution or tablets and ketoconazole is not recommended. Multiple-dose ketoconazole administration significantly affected the rate and extent of absorption and sirolimus exposure after administration of sirolimus oral solution, as reflected by increases in sirolimus Cmax, tmax, and AUC of 4.3-fold, 38%, and 10.9-fold, respectively. However, the terminal t1/2 of sirolimus was not changed. Single-dose sirolimus did not affect steady-state 12-hour plasma ketoconazole concentrations). Products include:
Extina Foam, 2% 3057
Nizoral A-D Shampoo 1901

Levonorgestrel (Care should be exercised when drugs or other sub-

stances that are substrates of CYP3A4 are administered concomitantly with sirolimus). Products include:
Climara Pro Transdermal System 768
Lybrel Tablets 3204
Mirena Intrauterine System 779
Plan B Tablets 1044
Seasonique Tablets 1046

Lidocaine (Care should be exercised when drugs or other substances that are substrates of CYP3A4 are administered concomitantly with sirolimus). Products include:
Lidoderm Patch 1114

Lidocaine Hydrochloride (Care should be exercised when drugs or other substances that are substrates of CYP3A4 are administered concomitantly with sirolimus).
No products indexed under this heading.

Lisinopril (Sirolimus has been associated with the development of angioedema. The concomitant use of sirolimus with other drugs known to cause angioedema, such as ACE-inhibitors, may increase the risk of developing angioedema). Products include:
Prinivil Tablets 2087
Prinzide Tablets 2092

Lopinavir (Exercise caution when using sirolimus with drugs or agents that are modulators of CYP3A4. Co-administration of sirolimus with HIV protease inhibitors may increase sirolimus blood concentrations. The dosage of sirolimus and/or the HIV protease inhibitor may need to be adjusted). Products include:
Kaletra 452

Lovastatin (During sirolimus therapy with cyclosporine, patients administered an HMG-CoA reductase inhibitor and/or fibrate should be monitored for the possible development of rhabdomyolysis and other adverse effects. In clinical trials, the concomitant administration of sirolimus and HMG-CoA reductase inhibitors appeared to be well-tolerated). Products include:
Advicor Tablets 402
Mevacor Tablets 2063

Measles, Mumps, Rubella and Varicella Virus Vaccine Live (Immunosuppressants may affect response to vaccination. Therefore, during treatment with sirolimus, vaccination may be less effective. The use of live vaccines should be avoided). Products include:
ProQuad 2099

Measles, Mumps & Rubella Virus Vaccine, Live (Immunosuppressants may affect response to vaccination. Therefore, during treatment with sirolimus, vaccination may be less effective. The use of live vaccines should be avoided). Products include:
M-M-R II 2054

Measles & Rubella Virus Vaccine Live (Immunosuppressants may affect response to vaccination. Therefore, during treatment with sirolimus, vaccination may be less effective. The use of live vaccines should be avoided).
No products indexed under this heading.

Measles Virus Vaccine Live (Immunosuppressants may affect response to vaccination. Therefore, during treatment with sirolimus, vaccination may be less effective. The use of live vaccines should be avoided). Products include:
Attenuvax 1951

Mephenytoin (Sirolimus is known to be a substrate for cytochrome P-450 3A4 (CYP3A4). Inducers of CYP3A4 may decrease sirolimus concentrations. Co-administration of sirolimus with strong inducers of CYP3A4 is not recommended).
No products indexed under this heading.

Mestranol (Care should be exercised when drugs or other substances that are substrates of CYP3A4 are administered concomitantly with sirolimus).
No products indexed under this heading.

Methadone Hydrochloride (Care should be exercised when drugs or other substances that are substrates of CYP3A4 are administered concomitantly with sirolimus).
No products indexed under this heading.

Methsuximide (Sirolimus is known to be a substrate for cytochrome P-450 3A4 (CYP3A4). Inducers of CYP3A4 may decrease sirolimus concentrations. Co-administration of sirolimus with strong inducers of CYP3A4 is not recommended).
No products indexed under this heading.

Methylprednisolone (Sirolimus is known to be a substrate for cytochrome P-450 3A4 (CYP3A4). Inducers of CYP3A4 may decrease sirolimus concentrations.
Co-administration of sirolimus with strong inducers of CYP3A4 is not recommended).
No products indexed under this heading.

Methylprednisolone Acetate (Sirolimus is known to be a substrate for cytochrome P-450 3A4 (CYP3A4). Inducers of CYP3A4 may decrease sirolimus concentrations. Co-administration of sirolimus with strong inducers of CYP3A4 is not recommended).
No products indexed under this heading.

Methylprednisolone Sodium Succinate (Sirolimus is known to be a substrate for cytochrome P-450 3A4 (CYP3A4). Inducers of CYP3A4 may decrease sirolimus concentrations. Co-administration of sirolimus with strong inducers of CYP3A4 is not recommended).
No products indexed under this heading.

Metoclopramide Hydrochloride (Exercise caution when using sirolimus with drugs or agents that are modulators of CYP3A4. Co-administration of sirolimus with metoclopramide may increase sirolimus blood concentrations. The dosage of sirolimus and/or metoclopramide may need to be adjusted).
No products indexed under this heading.

Mibefradil Dihydrochloride (Sirolimus is known to be a substrate for p-glycoprotein (P-gp). Inhibitors of P-gp may increase sirolimus concentrations. Co-administration of sirolimus with strong inhibitors of P-gp is not recommended).
No products indexed under this heading.

Midazolam Hydrochloride (Care should be exercised when drugs or other substances that are substrates of CYP3A4 are administered concomitantly with sirolimus).
No products indexed under this heading.

Modafinil (Sirolimus is known to be a substrate for cytochrome P-450 3A4 (CYP3A4). Inducers of CYP3A4 may decrease sirolimus concentrations. Co-administration of sirolimus with strong inducers of CYP3A4 is not recommended). Products include:
Provigil Tablets 977

Moexipril Hydrochloride (Sirolimus has been associated with the development of angioedema. The concomitant use of sirolimus with other drugs known to cause angioedema, such as ACE-inhibitors, may increase the risk of developing angioedema).
No products indexed under this heading.

Mumps Virus Vaccine, Live (Immunosuppressants may affect response to vaccination. Therefore, during treatment with sirolimus, vaccination may be less effective. The use of live vaccines should be avoided). Products include:
Mumpsvax 2068

Nefazodone Hydrochloride (Care should be exercised when drugs or other substances that are substrates of CYP3A4 are administered concomitantly with sirolimus).
No products indexed under this heading.

Nelfinavir Mesylate (Exercise caution when using sirolimus with drugs or agents that are modulators of CYP3A4. Co-administration of sirolimus with HIV protease inhibitors may increase sirolimus blood concentrations. The dosage of sirolimus and/or the HIV protease inhibitor may need to be adjusted).
No products indexed under this heading.

Nevirapine (Sirolimus is known to be a substrate for cytochrome P-450 3A4 (CYP3A4). Inducers of CYP3A4 may decrease sirolimus concentrations. Co-administration of sirolimus with strong inducers of CYP3A4 is not recommended). Products include:
Viramune Oral Suspension 873
Viramune Tablets 873

Nicardipine (Exercise caution when using sirolimus with drugs or agents that are modulators of CYP3A4. Co-administration of sirolimus with nicardipine may increase sirolimus blood concentrations. The dosage of sirolimus and/or nicardipine may need to be adjusted).
No products indexed under this heading.

Nicardipine Hydrochloride (Exercise caution when using sirolimus with drugs or agents that are modulators of CYP3A4. Co-administration of sirolimus with nicardipine may increase sirolimus blood concentrations. The dosage of sirolimus and/or nicardipine may need to be adjusted). Products include:
Cardene I.V. 1093

Nifedipine (Care should be exercised when drugs or other substances that are substrates of CYP3A4 are administered concomitantly with sirolimus).
No products indexed under this heading.

Nimodipine (Care should be exercised when drugs or other substances that are substrates of CYP3A4 are administered concomitantly with sirolimus). Products include:
Nimotop Capsules 790

Nisoldipine (Care should be exercised when drugs or other substances that are substrates of CYP3A4 are administered concomitantly with sirolimus). Products include:
Sular Extended Release Tablets 2975

Nitrendipine (Care should be exercised when drugs or other substances that are substrates of CYP3A4 are administered concomitantly with sirolimus).
No products indexed under this heading.

Norethindrone (Care should be exercised when drugs or other substances that are substrates of CYP3A4 are administered concomitantly with sirolimus). Products include:
Ortho Micronor Tablets 2446

Norethindrone Acetate (Care should be exercised when drugs or other substances that are substrates of CYP3A4 are administered concomitantly with sirolimus). Products include:
Activella Tablets 2347

Norgestrel (Care should be exercised when drugs or other substances that are substrates of CYP3A4 are administered concomitantly with sirolimus).
No products indexed under this heading.

Ondansetron (Care should be exercised when drugs or other substances that are substrates of CYP3A4 are administered concomitantly with sirolimus). Products include:
Zofran ODT Orally Disintegrating Tablets 1687

Ondansetron Hydrochloride (Care should be exercised when drugs or other substances that are substrates of CYP3A4 are administered concomitantly with sirolimus). Products include:
Zofran Injection 1682
Zofran 1687

Oxcarbazepine (Sirolimus is known to be a substrate for cytochrome P-450 3A4 (CYP3A4). Inducers of CYP3A4 may decrease sirolimus concentrations.
Co-administration of sirolimus with strong inducers of CYP3A4 is not recommended).
No products indexed under this heading.

Paclitaxel (Care should be exercised when drugs or other substances that are substrates of CYP3A4 are administered concomitantly with sirolimus).
No products indexed under this heading.

Perindopril Erbumine (Sirolimus has been associated with the development of angioedema. The concomitant use of sirolimus with other drugs known to cause angioedema,

Food Interactions

RAPTIVA FOR INJECTION
(Efalizumab) 1218
May interact with immunosuppressive agents and vaccines, live. Compounds in these categories include:

Azathioprine (Patients receiving other immunosuppressive agents should not receive concurrent therapy with efalizumab because of the possibility of increased risk of infections and malignancies).
No products indexed under this heading.

Basiliximab (Patients receiving other immunosuppressive agents should not receive concurrent therapy with efalizumab because of the possibility of increased risk of infections and malignancies). Products include:
Simulect for Injection 2306

BCG Vaccine (Acellular, live and live-attenuated vaccines should not be administered during efalizumab treatment).
No products indexed under this heading.

Cyclosporine (Patients receiving other immunosuppressive agents should not receive concurrent therapy with efalizumab because of the possibility of increased risk of infections and malignancies). Products include:
Gengraf Capsules 435
Neoral Oral Solution 2280
Neoral Soft Gelatin Capsules 2280
Restasis Ophthalmic Emulsion 557
Sandimmune 2296

Influenza Vaccine, Live Attenuated (Acellular, live and live-attenuated vaccines should not be administered during efalizumab treatment).
No products indexed under this heading.

Influenza Virus Vaccine Live, Intranasal (Acellular, live and live-attenuated vaccines should not be administered during efalizumab treatment). Products include:
FluMist Vaccine 1945

Measles, Mumps, Rubella and Varicella Virus Vaccine Live (Acellular, live and live-attenuated vaccines should not be administered during efalizumab treatment). Products include:
ProQuad 2099

Measles, Mumps & Rubella Virus Vaccine, Live (Acellular, live and live-attenuated vaccines should not be administered during efalizumab treatment). Products include:
M-M-R II 2054

Measles & Rubella Virus Vaccine Live (Acellular, live and live-attenuated vaccines should not be administered during efalizumab treatment).
No products indexed under this heading.

Measles Virus Vaccine Live (Acellular, live and live-attenuated vaccines should not be administered during efalizumab treatment). Products include:
Attenuvax 1951

Mumps Virus Vaccine, Live (Acellular, live and live-attenuated vaccines should not be administered during efalizumab treatment). Products include:
Mumpsvax 2068

Muromonab-CD3 (Patients receiving other immunosuppressive agents should not receive concurrent therapy with efalizumab because of the possibility of increased risk of infections and malignancies). Products include:
Orthoclone OKT3 Sterile Solution 2387

Mycophenolate Mofetil (Patients receiving other immunosuppressive agents should not receive concurrent therapy with efalizumab because of the possibility of increased risk of infections and malignancies). Products include:
CellCept Capsules 2622
CellCept Oral Suspension 2622
CellCept Tablets 2622

Poliovirus Vaccine, Live, Oral, Trivalent, Types 1,2,3 (Sabin) (Acellular, live and live-attenuated vaccines should not be administered during efalizumab treatment).
No products indexed under this heading.

Rotavirus Vaccine, Live, Oral, Tetravalent (Acellular, live and live-attenuated vaccines should not be administered during efalizumab treatment).
No products indexed under this heading.

Rubella & Mumps Virus Vaccine Live (Acellular, live and live-attenuated vaccines should not be administered during efalizumab treatment).
No products indexed under this heading.

Rubella Virus Vaccine Live (Acellular, live and live-attenuated vaccines should not be administered during efalizumab treatment). Products include:
Meruvax II 2061

Sirolimus (Patients receiving other immunosuppressive agents should not receive concurrent therapy with efalizumab because of the possibility of increased risk of infections and malignancies). Products include:
Rapamune 3260

Smallpox Vaccine (Acellular, live and live-attenuated vaccines should not be administered during efalizumab treatment).
No products indexed under this heading.

Tacrolimus (Patients receiving other immunosuppressive agents should not receive concurrent therapy with efalizumab because of the possibility of increased risk of infections and malignancies). Products include:
Prograf Capsules and Injection 622
Protopic Ointment 628

Typhoid Vaccine (Acellular, live and live-attenuated vaccines should not be administered during efalizumab treatment).
No products indexed under this heading.

Varicella Virus Vaccine Live (Acellular, live and live-attenuated vaccines should not be administered during efalizumab treatment). Products include:
Varivax 2133

Yellow Fever Vaccine (Acellular, live and live-attenuated vaccines should not be administered during efalizumab treatment).
No products indexed under this heading.

Zoster Vaccine Live (Acellular, live and live-attenuated vaccines should not be administered during efalizumab treatment). Products include:
Zostavax Injection 2145

REBETOL CAPSULES
(Ribavirin) 2917
May interact with antacids. Compounds in these categories include:

Aluminum Carbonate (Co-administration of ribavirin capsules with an antacid containing magnesium, aluminum and simethicone resulted in a 14% decrease in mean ribavirin AUC. The clinical relevance of results from this study is unknown).
No products indexed under this heading.

Aluminum Hydroxide (Co-administration of ribavirin capsules with an antacid containing magnesium, aluminum and simethicone resulted in a 14% decrease in mean ribavirin AUC. The clinical relevance of results from this study is unknown).
No products indexed under this heading.

Didanosine (Co-administration of ribavirin and didanosine is not recommended due to reports of fatal hepatic failure, peripheral neuropathy, pancreatitis, and symptomatic hyperlactactemia/lactic acidosis in clinical trials).
No products indexed under this heading.

Magaldrate (Co-administration of ribavirin capsules with an antacid containing magnesium, aluminum and simethicone resulted in a 14% decrease in mean ribavirin AUC. The clinical relevance of results from this study is unknown).
No products indexed under this heading.

Magnesium Hydroxide (Co-administration of ribavirin capsules with an antacid containing magnesium, aluminum and simethicone resulted in a 14% decrease in mean ribavirin AUC. The clinical relevance of results from this study is unknown). Products include:
Fleet Pedia-Lax Chewable Tablets 1145
Pepcid Complete Chewable Tablets 1771
Extra Strength Rolaids Freshmint Tablets 1903
Rolaids Multi-Symptom Berry Tablets 1903
Rolaids Original Peppermint Tablets 1903

Magnesium Oxide (Co-administration of ribavirin capsules with an antacid containing magnesium, aluminum and simethicone resulted in a 14% decrease in mean ribavirin AUC. The clinical relevance of results from this study is unknown). Products include:
Beelith Tablets 813

Sodium Bicarbonate (Co-administration of ribavirin capsules with an antacid containing magnesium, aluminum and simethicone resulted in a 14% decrease in mean ribavirin AUC. The clinical relevance of results from this study is unknown). Products include:
Ceo-Two Laxative Suppository 815

Stavudine (Ribavirin may antagonize the in vitro anti-viral activity of stavudine against HIV; concomitant use of ribavirin with stavudine should be used with caution).
No products indexed under this heading.

Zidovudine (Ribavirin may antagonize the in vitro anti-viral activity of zidovudine against HIV; concomitant use of ribavirin with zidovudine should be used with caution). Products include:
Combivir Tablets 1384
Retrovir 1574
Retrovir IV Infusion 1579
Trizivir Tablets 1622

REBETOL ORAL SOLUTION
(Ribavirin) 2917
See Rebetol Capsules

REBIF PREFILLED SYRINGE FOR INJECTION
(Interferon Beta-1a) 1107
May interact with agents associated with myelosuppression. Compounds in these categories include:

Altretamine (Due to its potential to cause neutropenia and lymphopenia, proper monitoring of patients is required if interferon beta-1 is given in combination with myelosuppressive agents). Products include:
Hexalen Capsules 1078

Busulfan (Due to its potential to cause neutropenia and lymphopenia, proper monitoring of patients is required if interferon beta-1 is given in combination with myelosuppressive agents). Products include:
Busulfex Injection 2477
Myleran Tablets 1530

Chlorambucil (Due to its potential to cause neutropenia and lymphopenia, proper monitoring of patients is required if interferon beta-1 is given in combination with myelosuppressive agents). Products include:
Leukeran Tablets 1508

Cladribine (Due to its potential to cause neutropenia and lymphopenia, proper monitoring of patients is required if interferon beta-1 is given in combination with myelosuppressive agents). Products include:
Leustatin Injection 2384

Daunorubicin Citrate Liposome (Due to its potential to cause neutropenia and lymphopenia, proper monitoring of patients is required if interferon beta-1 is given in combination with myelosuppressive agents).
No products indexed under this heading.

Daunorubicin Hydrochloride (Due to its potential to cause neutropenia and lymphopenia, proper monitoring of patients is required if interferon beta-1 is given in combination with myelosuppressive agents).
No products indexed under this heading.

Dexrazoxane (Due to its potential to cause neutropenia and lymphopenia, proper monitoring of patients is required if interferon beta-1 is given in combination with myelosuppressive agents).
No products indexed under this heading.

Doxorubicin Hydrochloride (Due to its potential to cause neutropenia and lymphopenia, proper monitoring of patients is required if interferon beta-1 is given in combination with myelosuppressive agents).
No products indexed under this heading.

Doxorubicin Hydrochloride Liposome (Due to its potential to cause neutropenia and lymphopenia, proper monitoring of patients is required if interferon beta-1 is given in combination with myelosuppressive agents). Products include:

Doxil Injection ... 2378

Fludarabine Phosphate (Due to its potential to cause neutropenia and lymphopenia, proper monitoring of patients is required if interferon beta-1 is given in combination with myelosuppressive agents).

No products indexed under this heading.

Gemcitabine Hydrochloride (Due to its potential to cause neutropenia and lymphopenia, proper monitoring of patients is required if interferon beta-1 is given in combination with myelosuppressive agents). Products include:

Gemzar for Injection ... 1820

Gemtuzumab Ozogamicin (Due to its potential to cause neutropenia and lymphopenia, proper monitoring of patients is required if interferon beta-1 is given in combination with myelosuppressive agents). Products include:

Mylotarg for Injection ... 3212

Idarubicin Hydrochloride (Due to its potential to cause neutropenia and lymphopenia, proper monitoring of patients is required if interferon beta-1 is given in combination with myelosuppressive agents).

No products indexed under this heading.

Interferon alfa-2a, Recombinant (Due to its potential to cause neutropenia and lymphopenia, proper monitoring of patients is required if interferon beta-1 is given in combination with myelosuppressive agents).

No products indexed under this heading.

Irinotecan Hydrochloride (Due to its potential to cause neutropenia and lymphopenia, proper monitoring of patients is required if interferon beta-1 is given in combination with myelosuppressive agents).

No products indexed under this heading.

Melphalan Hydrochloride (Due to its potential to cause neutropenia and lymphopenia, proper monitoring of patients is required if interferon beta-1 is given in combination with myelosuppressive agents).

No products indexed under this heading.

Mercaptopurine (Due to its potential to cause neutropenia and lymphopenia, proper monitoring of patients is required if interferon beta-1 is given in combination with myelosuppressive agents).

No products indexed under this heading.

Mitoxantrone Hydrochloride (Due to its potential to cause neutropenia and lymphopenia, proper monitoring of patients is required if interferon beta-1 is given in combination with myelosuppressive agents). Products include:

Novantrone for Injection Concentrate ... 1100

Temozolomide (Due to its potential to cause neutropenia and lymphopenia, proper monitoring of patients is required if interferon beta-1 is given in combination with myelosuppressive agents). Products include:

Temodar Capsules ... 2931

Thioguanine (Due to its potential to cause neutropenia and lymphopenia, proper monitoring of patients is required if interferon beta-1 is given in combination with myelosuppressive agents). Products include:

Tabloid Tablets ... 1601

Vinorelbine Tartrate (Due to its potential to cause neutropenia and lymphopenia, proper monitoring of patients is required if interferon beta-1 is given in combination with myelosuppressive agents).

No products indexed under this heading.

RECLAST INJECTION

(Zoledronic acid) ... 2291

May interact with aminoglycosides, loop diuretics, and nephrotoxic agents. Compounds in these categories include:

Abacavir Sulfate (Caution is indicated when zoledronic acid is used with other potentially nephrotoxic drugs). Products include:

Epzicom Tablets ... 1422
Trizivir Tablets ... 1622
Ziagen ... 1673

Acyclovir (Caution is indicated when zoledronic acid is used with other potentially nephrotoxic drugs). Products include:

Zovirax ... 1690
Zovirax Cream ... 817
Zovirax Ointment ... 819

Acyclovir Sodium (Caution is indicated when zoledronic acid is used with other potentially nephrotoxic drugs).

No products indexed under this heading.

Alatrofloxacin Mesylate (Caution is indicated when zoledronic acid is used with other potentially nephrotoxic drugs).

No products indexed under this heading.

Aldesleukin (Caution is indicated when zoledronic acid is used with other potentially nephrotoxic drugs). Products include:

Proleukin for Injection ... 2287

Amikacin Sulfate (Caution is advised when bisphosphonates are administered with aminoglycosides, since these agents may have an additive effect to lower serum calcium level for prolonged periods).

No products indexed under this heading.

Amoxicillin (Caution is indicated when zoledronic acid is used with other potentially nephrotoxic drugs). Products include:

Amoxil Capsules ... 1305
Amoxil Chewable Tablets ... 1305
Amoxil Pediatric Drops for Oral Suspension ... 1305
Amoxil Powder for Oral Suspension ... 1305
Amoxil Tablets ... 1305
Augmentin ... 1323
Augmentin Tablets ... 1327
Augmentin XR Extended Release Tablets ... 1333
Augmentin ES-600 Powder for Oral Suspension ... 1329
Moxatag Tablets ... 2165

Amoxicillin Trihydrate (Caution is indicated when zoledronic acid is used with other potentially nephrotoxic drugs).

No products indexed under this heading.

Amphotericin B (Caution is indicated when zoledronic acid is used with other potentially nephrotoxic drugs).

No products indexed under this heading.

Amphotericin B, liposomal (Caution is indicated when zoledronic acid is used with other potentially nephrotoxic drugs). Products include:

AmBisome for Injection ... 606

Amphotericin B Cholesteryl Sulfate (Caution is indicated when zoledronic acid is used with other potentially nephrotoxic drugs).

No products indexed under this heading.

Amphotericin B Lipid Complex (Caution is indicated when zoledronic acid is used with other potentially nephrotoxic drugs). Products include:

Abelcet Injection ... 1134

Ampicillin (Caution is indicated when zoledronic acid is used with other potentially nephrotoxic drugs).

No products indexed under this heading.

Ampicillin Sodium (Caution is indicated when zoledronic acid is used with other potentially nephrotoxic drugs).

No products indexed under this heading.

Ampicillin Trihydrate (Caution is indicated when zoledronic acid is used with other potentially nephrotoxic drugs).

No products indexed under this heading.

Amprenavir (Caution is indicated when zoledronic acid is used with other potentially nephrotoxic drugs).

No products indexed under this heading.

Aspirin (Caution is indicated when zoledronic acid is used with other potentially nephrotoxic drugs). Products include:

Aggrenox Capsules ... 819
Bayer Aspirin ... 750
Percodan Tablets ... 1130
St. Joseph 81 mg Aspirin Chewable and Enteric Coated Tablets ... 1903

Atazanavir (Caution is indicated when zoledronic acid is used with other potentially nephrotoxic drugs).

No products indexed under this heading.

Atorvastatin Calcium (Caution is indicated when zoledronic acid is used with other potentially nephrotoxic drugs). Products include:

Lipitor Tablets ... 2501

Azithromycin Dihydrate (Caution is indicated when zoledronic acid is used with other potentially nephrotoxic drugs).

No products indexed under this heading.

Azlocillin Sodium (Caution is indicated when zoledronic acid is used with other potentially nephrotoxic drugs).

No products indexed under this heading.

Aztreonam (Caution is indicated when zoledronic acid is used with other potentially nephrotoxic drugs).

No products indexed under this heading.

Bacampicillin Hydrochloride (Caution is indicated when zoledronic acid is used with other potentially nephrotoxic drugs).

No products indexed under this heading.

Balsalazide Disodium (Caution is indicated when zoledronic acid is used with other potentially nephrotoxic drugs).

No products indexed under this heading.

Benazepril Hydrochloride (Caution is indicated when zoledronic acid is used with other potentially nephrotoxic drugs).

No products indexed under this heading.

Bendroflumethiazide (Caution is indicated when zoledronic acid is used with other potentially nephrotoxic drugs).

No products indexed under this heading.

Bumetanide (Caution should be exercised when zoledronic acid is used in combination with loop diuretics due to an increased risk of hypocalcemia).

No products indexed under this heading.

Caffeine (Caution is indicated when zoledronic acid is used with other potentially nephrotoxic drugs). Products include:

BioLean Free Tablets ... 635
BioLean II Tablets ... 635
Winrgy Dietary Supplement ... 642

Captopril (Caution is indicated when zoledronic acid is used with other potentially nephrotoxic drugs). Products include:

Captopril Tablets ... 2182

Carbenicillin Disodium (Caution is indicated when zoledronic acid is used with other potentially nephrotoxic drugs).

No products indexed under this heading.

Carbenicillin Indanyl Sodium (Caution is indicated when zoledronic acid is used with other potentially nephrotoxic drugs).

No products indexed under this heading.

Carboplatin (Caution is indicated when zoledronic acid is used with other potentially nephrotoxic drugs).

No products indexed under this heading.

Carmustine (BCNU) (Caution is indicated when zoledronic acid is used with other potentially nephrotoxic drugs).

No products indexed under this heading.

Cefaclor (Caution is indicated when zoledronic acid is used with other potentially nephrotoxic drugs).

No products indexed under this heading.

Cefadroxil (Caution is indicated when zoledronic acid is used with other potentially nephrotoxic drugs).

No products indexed under this heading.

Cefamandole Nafate (Caution is indicated when zoledronic acid is used with other potentially nephrotoxic drugs).

No products indexed under this heading.

Cefazolin Sodium (Caution is indicated when zoledronic acid is used with other potentially nephrotoxic drugs).

No products indexed under this heading.

Cefdinir (Caution is indicated when zoledronic acid is used with other potentially nephrotoxic drugs). Products include:

Omnicef Capsules ... 497
Omnicef for Oral Suspension ... 497

Cefepime Hydrochloride (Caution is indicated when zoledronic acid is used with other potentially nephrotoxic drugs).
No products indexed under this heading.

Cefixime (Caution is indicated when zoledronic acid is used with other potentially nephrotoxic drugs).
Products include:
Suprax for Oral Suspension 1891
Suprax Tablets 1891

Cefmetazole Sodium (Caution is indicated when zoledronic acid is used with other potentially nephrotoxic drugs).
No products indexed under this heading.

Cefonicid Sodium (Caution is indicated when zoledronic acid is used with other potentially nephrotoxic drugs).
No products indexed under this heading.

Cefoperazone Sodium (Caution is indicated when zoledronic acid is used with other potentially nephrotoxic drugs).
No products indexed under this heading.

Ceforanide (Caution is indicated when zoledronic acid is used with other potentially nephrotoxic drugs).
No products indexed under this heading.

Cefotaxime Sodium (Caution is indicated when zoledronic acid is used with other potentially nephrotoxic drugs).
No products indexed under this heading.

Cefotetan (Caution is indicated when zoledronic acid is used with other potentially nephrotoxic drugs).
No products indexed under this heading.

Cefoxitin Sodium (Caution is indicated when zoledronic acid is used with other potentially nephrotoxic drugs).
No products indexed under this heading.

Cefpodoxime Proxetil (Caution is indicated when zoledronic acid is used with other potentially nephrotoxic drugs).
No products indexed under this heading.

Cefprozil (Caution is indicated when zoledronic acid is used with other potentially nephrotoxic drugs).
No products indexed under this heading.

Ceftazidime (Caution is indicated when zoledronic acid is used with other potentially nephrotoxic drugs).
Products include:
Fortaz 1450

Ceftizoxime Sodium (Caution is indicated when zoledronic acid is used with other potentially nephrotoxic drugs).
No products indexed under this heading.

Ceftriaxone Sodium (Caution is indicated when zoledronic acid is used with other potentially nephrotoxic drugs). Products include:
Rocephin Injectable Vials, ADD-Vantage, Galaxy, Bulk............ 2642

Cefuroxime Axetil (Caution is indicated when zoledronic acid is used with other potentially nephrotoxic drugs). Products include:
Ceftin 1380

Cefuroxime Sodium (Caution is indicated when zoledronic acid is used with other potentially nephrotoxic drugs).
No products indexed under this heading.

Celecoxib (Caution is indicated when zoledronic acid is used with other potentially nephrotoxic drugs).
Products include:
Celebrex Capsules 2979

Cephalexin (Caution is indicated when zoledronic acid is used with other potentially nephrotoxic drugs).
No products indexed under this heading.

Cephalothin Sodium (Caution is indicated when zoledronic acid is used with other potentially nephrotoxic drugs).
No products indexed under this heading.

Cephapirin Sodium (Caution is indicated when zoledronic acid is used with other potentially nephrotoxic drugs).
No products indexed under this heading.

Cephradine (Caution is indicated when zoledronic acid is used with other potentially nephrotoxic drugs).
No products indexed under this heading.

Cerivastatin Sodium (Caution is indicated when zoledronic acid is used with other potentially nephrotoxic drugs).
No products indexed under this heading.

Chlorothiazide (Caution is indicated when zoledronic acid is used with other potentially nephrotoxic drugs).
No products indexed under this heading.

Chlorothiazide Sodium (Caution is indicated when zoledronic acid is used with other potentially nephrotoxic drugs). Products include:
Intravenous Sodium Diuril 2490

Chlorpropamide (Caution is indicated when zoledronic acid is used with other potentially nephrotoxic drugs).
No products indexed under this heading.

Cidofovir (Caution is indicated when zoledronic acid is used with other potentially nephrotoxic drugs).
No products indexed under this heading.

Cilastatin Sodium (Caution is indicated when zoledronic acid is used with other potentially nephrotoxic drugs). Products include:
Primaxin I.M. 2080
Primaxin I.V. 2083

Cimetidine (Caution is indicated when zoledronic acid is used with other potentially nephrotoxic drugs).
No products indexed under this heading.

Cimetidine Hydrochloride (Caution is indicated when zoledronic acid is used with other potentially nephrotoxic drugs).
No products indexed under this heading.

Cisplatin (Caution is indicated when zoledronic acid is used with other potentially nephrotoxic drugs).
No products indexed under this heading.

Cladribine (Caution is indicated when zoledronic acid is used with other potentially nephrotoxic drugs).
Products include:
Leustatin Injection 2384

Clozapine (Caution is indicated when zoledronic acid is used with other potentially nephrotoxic drugs).
No products indexed under this heading.

Colistimethate Sodium (Caution is indicated when zoledronic acid is used with other potentially nephrotoxic drugs).
No products indexed under this heading.

Colistin Sulfate (Caution is indicated when zoledronic acid is used with other potentially nephrotoxic drugs).
No products indexed under this heading.

Cyclophosphamide (Caution is indicated when zoledronic acid is used with other potentially nephrotoxic drugs).
No products indexed under this heading.

Cyclosporine (Caution is indicated when zoledronic acid is used with other potentially nephrotoxic drugs).
Products include:
Gengraf Capsules 435
Neoral Oral Solution 2280
Neoral Soft Gelatin Capsules 2280
Restasis Ophthalmic Emulsion 557
Sandimmune 2296

Cytarabine (Caution is indicated when zoledronic acid is used with other potentially nephrotoxic drugs).
No products indexed under this heading.

Cytarabine Liposome (Caution is indicated when zoledronic acid is used with other potentially nephrotoxic drugs). Products include:
DepoCyt Injection 1136

Delavirdine Mesylate (Caution is indicated when zoledronic acid is used with other potentially nephrotoxic drugs).
No products indexed under this heading.

Diatrizoate Meglumine (Caution is indicated when zoledronic acid is used with other potentially nephrotoxic drugs).
No products indexed under this heading.

Diatrizoate Sodium (Caution is indicated when zoledronic acid is used with other potentially nephrotoxic drugs).
No products indexed under this heading.

Diclofenac Potassium (Caution is indicated when zoledronic acid is used with other potentially nephrotoxic drugs).
No products indexed under this heading.

Diclofenac Sodium (Caution is indicated when zoledronic acid is used with other potentially nephrotoxic drugs). Products include:
Diclofenac Sodium Ophthalmic Solution............ ⊙ 240
Voltaren Ophthalmic Solution 2336
Voltaren Tablets 2334
Voltaren-XR Tablets 2337

Dicloxacillin Sodium (Caution is indicated when zoledronic acid is used with other potentially nephrotoxic drugs).
No products indexed under this heading.

Didanosine (Caution is indicated when zoledronic acid is used with other potentially nephrotoxic drugs).
No products indexed under this heading.

Efavirenz (Caution is indicated when zoledronic acid is used with other potentially nephrotoxic drugs).
Products include:
Atripla Tablets 938
Sustiva Capsules 930
Sustiva Tablets 930

Emtricitabine (Caution is indicated when zoledronic acid is used with other potentially nephrotoxic drugs).
Products include:
Atripla Tablets 938
Emtriva Capsules 1246
Emtriva Oral Solution 1246
Truvada Tablets 1262

Enalapril Maleate (Caution is indicated when zoledronic acid is used with other potentially nephrotoxic drugs).
No products indexed under this heading.

Enalaprilat (Caution is indicated when zoledronic acid is used with other potentially nephrotoxic drugs).
No products indexed under this heading.

Enfuvirtide (Caution is indicated when zoledronic acid is used with other potentially nephrotoxic drugs).
No products indexed under this heading.

Ethacrynic Acid (Caution should be exercised when zoledronic acid is used in combination with loop diuretics due to an increased risk of hypocalcemia). Products include:
Edecrin Tablets 698

Ethiodized Oil (Caution is indicated when zoledronic acid is used with other potentially nephrotoxic drugs).
No products indexed under this heading.

Etodolac (Caution is indicated when zoledronic acid is used with other potentially nephrotoxic drugs).
No products indexed under this heading.

Fenoprofen Calcium (Caution is indicated when zoledronic acid is used with other potentially nephrotoxic drugs). Products include:
Nalfon Capsules 2508

Filgrastim (Caution is indicated when zoledronic acid is used with other potentially nephrotoxic drugs).
Products include:
Neupogen for Injection 589

Fluorouracil (Caution is indicated when zoledronic acid is used with other potentially nephrotoxic drugs).
Products include:
Carac Cream 0.5% 2722

Flurbiprofen (Caution is indicated when zoledronic acid is used with other potentially nephrotoxic drugs).
No products indexed under this heading.

Fluvastatin Sodium (Caution is indicated when zoledronic acid is used with other potentially nephrotoxic drugs). Products include:
Lescol Capsules 2268
Lescol XL Tablets 2268

Foscarnet Sodium (Caution is indicated when zoledronic acid is used with other potentially nephrotoxic drugs).
No products indexed under this heading.

Fosinopril Sodium (Caution is indicated when zoledronic acid is used with other potentially nephrotoxic drugs).
No products indexed under this heading.

Furosemide (Caution should be exercised when zoledronic acid is used in combination with loop diuretics due to an increased risk of hypocalcemia). Products include:
Furosemide Tablets 2186

Gadopentetate Dimeglumine (Caution is indicated when zoledronic acid is used with other potentially nephrotoxic drugs).
No products indexed under this heading.

Gentamicin (Caution is indicated when zoledronic acid is used with other potentially nephrotoxic drugs).
No products indexed under this heading.

Gentamicin Sulfate (Caution is advised when bisphosphonates are administered with aminoglycosides, since these agents may have an additive effect to lower serum calcium level for prolonged periods). Products include:
Pred-G Ophthalmic Ointment .... ⊙229
Pred-G Ophthalmic Suspension .... ⊙228

Glipizide (Caution is indicated when zoledronic acid is used with other potentially nephrotoxic drugs).
No products indexed under this heading.

Globulin, Immune (Human) (Caution is indicated when zoledronic acid is used with other potentially nephrotoxic drugs). Products include:
Flebogamma 5% 1715

Glyburide (Caution is indicated when zoledronic acid is used with other potentially nephrotoxic drugs).
No products indexed under this heading.

Gold Therapy (Caution is indicated when zoledronic acid is used with other potentially nephrotoxic drugs).
No products indexed under this heading.

HMG-CoA Reductase Inhibitors (Caution is indicated when zoledronic acid is used with other potentially nephrotoxic drugs).
No products indexed under this heading.

Hydrochlorothiazide (Caution is indicated when zoledronic acid is used with other potentially nephrotoxic drugs). Products include:
Atacand HCT 642
Avalide Tablets 892
Avalide Tablets 2713
Benicar HCT Tablets 1010
Diovan HCT Tablets 2216
Dyazide Capsules 1405
Micardis HCT Tablets 854
Prinzide Tablets 2092
Tekturna HCT Tablets 2324
Teveten HCT Tablets 517

Hydroflumethiazide (Caution is indicated when zoledronic acid is used with other potentially nephrotoxic drugs).
No products indexed under this heading.

Ibuprofen (Caution is indicated when zoledronic acid is used with other potentially nephrotoxic drugs). Products include:
Motrin IB Tablets and Caplets 1900
Children's Motrin Oral Suspension ... 1901
Children's Motrin Non-Staining Dye-Free Oral Suspension 1901
Children's Motrin Cold Oral Suspension 1899
Infants' Motrin Concentrated Drops 1901
Infants' Motrin Non-Staining Dye-Free Concentrated Drops 1901
Junior Strength Motrin Caplets and Chewable Tablets 1901
Vicoprofen Tablets 533

Idarubicin Hydrochloride (Caution is indicated when zoledronic acid is used with other potentially nephrotoxic drugs).
No products indexed under this heading.

Ifosfamide (Caution is indicated when zoledronic acid is used with other potentially nephrotoxic drugs).
No products indexed under this heading.

Imipenem (Caution is indicated when zoledronic acid is used with other potentially nephrotoxic drugs). Products include:
Primaxin I.M. 2080
Primaxin I.V. 2083

Immune Globulin Intravenous (Human) (Caution is indicated when zoledronic acid is used with other potentially nephrotoxic drugs). Products include:
Flebogamma 5% DIF 1718
Gammagard Liquid 730
Gammagard S/D 734
Gamunex 3094

Indinavir Sulfate (Caution is indicated when zoledronic acid is used with other potentially nephrotoxic drugs). Products include:
Crixivan Capsules 1979

Indomethacin (Caution is indicated when zoledronic acid is used with other potentially nephrotoxic drugs). Products include:
Indocin 2024

Indomethacin Sodium Trihydrate (Caution is indicated when zoledronic acid is used with other potentially nephrotoxic drugs). Products include:
Indocin I.V. 2489

Interferon Beta-1b (Caution is indicated when zoledronic acid is used with other potentially nephrotoxic drugs). Products include:
Betaseron for SC Injection 756

Interleuken-2 (Caution is indicated when zoledronic acid is used with other potentially nephrotoxic drugs).
No products indexed under this heading.

Iodamide Meglumine (Caution is indicated when zoledronic acid is used with other potentially nephrotoxic drugs).
No products indexed under this heading.

Iohexol (Caution is indicated when zoledronic acid is used with other potentially nephrotoxic drugs).
No products indexed under this heading.

Iopamidol (Caution is indicated when zoledronic acid is used with other potentially nephrotoxic drugs).
No products indexed under this heading.

Iopanoic Acid (Caution is indicated when zoledronic acid is used with other potentially nephrotoxic drugs).
No products indexed under this heading.

Iothalamate Meglumine (Caution is indicated when zoledronic acid is used with other potentially nephrotoxic drugs).
No products indexed under this heading.

Ioxaglate Meglumine (Caution is indicated when zoledronic acid is used with other potentially nephrotoxic drugs).
No products indexed under this heading.

Ioxaglate Sodium (Caution is indicated when zoledronic acid is used with other potentially nephrotoxic drugs).
No products indexed under this heading.

Kanamycin Sulfate (Caution is advised when bisphosphonates are administered with aminoglycosides, since these agents may have an additive effect to lower serum calcium level for prolonged periods).
No products indexed under this heading.

Ketoprofen (Caution is indicated when zoledronic acid is used with other potentially nephrotoxic drugs).
No products indexed under this heading.

Ketorolac Tromethamine (Caution is indicated when zoledronic acid is used with other potentially nephrotoxic drugs).
No products indexed under this heading.

Lamium album (Caution is indicated when zoledronic acid is used with other potentially nephrotoxic drugs).
No products indexed under this heading.

Lisinopril (Caution is indicated when zoledronic acid is used with other potentially nephrotoxic drugs). Products include:
Prinivil Tablets 2087
Prinzide Tablets 2092

Lithium (Caution is indicated when zoledronic acid is used with other potentially nephrotoxic drugs).
No products indexed under this heading.

Lithium Carbonate (Caution is indicated when zoledronic acid is used with other potentially nephrotoxic drugs).
No products indexed under this heading.

Lithium Citrate (Caution is indicated when zoledronic acid is used with other potentially nephrotoxic drugs).
No products indexed under this heading.

Lopinavir (Caution is indicated when zoledronic acid is used with other potentially nephrotoxic drugs). Products include:
Kaletra 452

Loracarbef (Caution is indicated when zoledronic acid is used with other potentially nephrotoxic drugs).
No products indexed under this heading.

Lovastatin (Caution is indicated when zoledronic acid is used with other potentially nephrotoxic drugs). Products include:
Advicor Tablets 402
Mevacor Tablets 2063

Meclofenamate Sodium (Caution is indicated when zoledronic acid is used with other potentially nephrotoxic drugs).
No products indexed under this heading.

Mefenamic Acid (Caution is indicated when zoledronic acid is used with other potentially nephrotoxic drugs).
No products indexed under this heading.

Meloxicam (Caution is indicated when zoledronic acid is used with other potentially nephrotoxic drugs). Products include:
Mobic Oral Suspension 863
Mobic Tablets 863

Melphalan Hydrochloride (Caution is indicated when zoledronic acid is used with other potentially nephrotoxic drugs).
No products indexed under this heading.

Mesalamine (Caution is indicated when zoledronic acid is used with other potentially nephrotoxic drugs). Products include:
Asacol Delayed-Release Tablets 2579
Canasa Rectal Suppositories 705
Lialda Tablets 3029
Pentasa Capsules 3030

Methimazole (Caution is indicated when zoledronic acid is used with other potentially nephrotoxic drugs).
No products indexed under this heading.

Methotrexate (Caution is indicated when zoledronic acid is used with other potentially nephrotoxic drugs).
No products indexed under this heading.

Methotrexate Sodium (Caution is indicated when zoledronic acid is used with other potentially nephrotoxic drugs).
No products indexed under this heading.

Methyclothiazide (Caution is indicated when zoledronic acid is used with other potentially nephrotoxic drugs).
No products indexed under this heading.

Mezlocillin Sodium (Caution is indicated when zoledronic acid is used with other potentially nephrotoxic drugs).
No products indexed under this heading.

Minocycline Hydrochloride (Caution is indicated when zoledronic acid is used with other potentially nephrotoxic drugs). Products include:
Solodyn Extended Release Tablets 1938

Mitomycin (Mitomycin-C) (Caution is indicated when zoledronic acid is used with other potentially nephrotoxic drugs).
No products indexed under this heading.

Moexipril Hydrochloride (Caution is indicated when zoledronic acid is used with other potentially nephrotoxic drugs).
No products indexed under this heading.

Muromonab-CD3 (Caution is indicated when zoledronic acid is used with other potentially nephrotoxic drugs). Products include:
Orthoclone OKT3 Sterile Solution 2387

Nabumetone (Caution is indicated when zoledronic acid is used with other potentially nephrotoxic drugs).
No products indexed under this heading.

Nafcillin Sodium (Caution is indicated when zoledronic acid is used with other potentially nephrotoxic drugs).
No products indexed under this heading.

Naproxen (Caution is indicated when zoledronic acid is used with other potentially nephrotoxic drugs). Products include:
EC-Naprosyn Delayed-Release Tablets **2632**
Naprosyn Suspension **2632**
Naprosyn Tablets **2632**

Naproxen Sodium (Caution is indicated when zoledronic acid is used with other potentially nephrotoxic drugs). Products include:
Anaprox Tablets **2632**
Anaprox DS Tablets **2632**
Treximet Tablets **1616**

Nelfinavir Mesylate (Caution is indicated when zoledronic acid is used with other potentially nephrotoxic drugs).
No products indexed under this heading.

Neomycin (Caution is indicated when zoledronic acid is used with other potentially nephrotoxic drugs).
No products indexed under this heading.

Neomycin, oral (Caution is indicated when zoledronic acid is used with other potentially nephrotoxic drugs).
No products indexed under this heading.

Neomycin Sulfate (Caution is indicated when zoledronic acid is used with other potentially nephrotoxic drugs). Products include:
Neosporin Ophthalmic Solution Sterile .... ⊙**252**

Nevirapine (Caution is indicated when zoledronic acid is used with other potentially nephrotoxic drugs).
Products include:
Viramune Oral Suspension **873**
Viramune Tablets **873**

Norfloxacin (Caution is indicated when zoledronic acid is used with other potentially nephrotoxic drugs).
Products include:
Noroxin Tablets **2069**

Olsalazine Sodium (Caution is indicated when zoledronic acid is used with other potentially nephrotoxic drugs).
No products indexed under this heading.

Omeprazole (Caution is indicated when zoledronic acid is used with other potentially nephrotoxic drugs).
No products indexed under this heading.

Oxaprozin (Caution is indicated when zoledronic acid is used with other potentially nephrotoxic drugs).
No products indexed under this heading.

Pamidronate Disodium (Caution is indicated when zoledronic acid is used with other potentially nephrotoxic drugs).
No products indexed under this heading.

Paroxetine Hydrochloride (Caution is indicated when zoledronic acid is used with other potentially nephrotoxic drugs). Products include:
Paxil **1535**
Paxil CR Controlled-Release Tablets **1544**

Penicillamine (Caution is indicated when zoledronic acid is used with other potentially nephrotoxic drugs).
Products include:
Cuprimine Capsules **1986**

Penicillin G Benzathine (Caution is indicated when zoledronic acid is used with other potentially nephrotoxic drugs). Products include:
Bicillin C-R Injectable Suspension **1775**
Bicillin L-A Injection **1777**

Penicillin G Potassium (Caution is indicated when zoledronic acid is used with other potentially nephrotoxic drugs).
No products indexed under this heading.

Penicillin G Procaine (Caution is indicated when zoledronic acid is used with other potentially nephrotoxic drugs). Products include:
Bicillin C-R Injectable Suspension **1775**
Bicillin L-A Injection **1777**

Penicillin G Sodium (Caution is indicated when zoledronic acid is used with other potentially nephrotoxic drugs).
No products indexed under this heading.

Penicillin V Potassium (Caution is indicated when zoledronic acid is used with other potentially nephrotoxic drugs).
No products indexed under this heading.

Pentamidine Isethionate (Caution is indicated when zoledronic acid is used with other potentially nephrotoxic drugs).
No products indexed under this heading.

Perindopril Erbumine (Caution is indicated when zoledronic acid is used with other potentially nephrotoxic drugs). Products include:
Aceon Tablets (2 mg, 4 mg, 8 mg) **3038**

Phenylbutazone (Caution is indicated when zoledronic acid is used with other potentially nephrotoxic drugs).
No products indexed under this heading.

Piroxicam (Caution is indicated when zoledronic acid is used with other potentially nephrotoxic drugs).
No products indexed under this heading.

Plicamycin (Caution is indicated when zoledronic acid is used with other potentially nephrotoxic drugs).
No products indexed under this heading.

Polymyxin (Caution is indicated when zoledronic acid is used with other potentially nephrotoxic drugs).
No products indexed under this heading.

Polymyxin B Sulfate (Caution is indicated when zoledronic acid is used with other potentially nephrotoxic drugs). Products include:
Neosporin Ophthalmic Solution Sterile .... ⊙**252**

Polythiazide (Caution is indicated when zoledronic acid is used with other potentially nephrotoxic drugs).
No products indexed under this heading.

Pravastatin Sodium (Caution is indicated when zoledronic acid is used with other potentially nephrotoxic drugs).
No products indexed under this heading.

Probenecid (Caution is indicated when zoledronic acid is used with other potentially nephrotoxic drugs).
No products indexed under this heading.

Quinapril Hydrochloride (Caution is indicated when zoledronic acid is used with other potentially nephrotoxic drugs).
No products indexed under this heading.

Rabeprazole Sodium (Caution is indicated when zoledronic acid is used with other potentially nephrotoxic drugs). Products include:
Aciphex Tablets **1053**

Ramipril (Caution is indicated when zoledronic acid is used with other potentially nephrotoxic drugs).
No products indexed under this heading.

Rifampin (Caution is indicated when zoledronic acid is used with other potentially nephrotoxic drugs).
No products indexed under this heading.

Riluzole (Caution is indicated when zoledronic acid is used with other potentially nephrotoxic drugs).
Products include:
Rilutek Tablets **2771**

Ritonavir (Caution is indicated when zoledronic acid is used with other potentially nephrotoxic drugs).
Products include:
Kaletra **452**
Norvir **489**

Rofecoxib (Caution is indicated when zoledronic acid is used with other potentially nephrotoxic drugs).
No products indexed under this heading.

Saquinavir (Caution is indicated when zoledronic acid is used with other potentially nephrotoxic drugs).
No products indexed under this heading.

Sibutramine Hydrochloride Monohydrate (Caution is indicated when zoledronic acid is used with other potentially nephrotoxic drugs).
Products include:
Meridia Capsules **475**

Simvastatin (Caution is indicated when zoledronic acid is used with other potentially nephrotoxic drugs).
Products include:
Simcor Tablets **502**
Vytorin 10/10 Tablets **2149**
Vytorin 10/10 Tablets **2939**
Vytorin 10/20 Tablets **2149**
Vytorin 10/20 Tablets **2939**
Vytorin 10/40 Tablets **2149**
Vytorin 10/40 Tablets **2939**
Vytorin 10/80 Tablets **2149**
Vytorin 10/80 Tablets **2939**
Zocor Tablets **2136**

Spirapril Hydrochloride (Caution is indicated when zoledronic acid is used with other potentially nephrotoxic drugs).
No products indexed under this heading.

Stavudine (Caution is indicated when zoledronic acid is used with other potentially nephrotoxic drugs).
No products indexed under this heading.

Streptomycin Sulfate (Caution is advised when bisphosphonates are administered with aminoglycosides, since these agents may have an additive effect to lower serum calcium level for prolonged periods).
No products indexed under this heading.

Streptozocin (Caution is indicated when zoledronic acid is used with other potentially nephrotoxic drugs).
No products indexed under this heading.

Sulfacytine (Caution is indicated when zoledronic acid is used with other potentially nephrotoxic drugs).
No products indexed under this heading.

Sulfamethizole (Caution is indicated when zoledronic acid is used with other potentially nephrotoxic drugs).
No products indexed under this heading.

Sulfamethoxazole (Caution is indicated when zoledronic acid is used with other potentially nephrotoxic drugs).
No products indexed under this heading.

Sulfasalazine (Caution is indicated when zoledronic acid is used with other potentially nephrotoxic drugs).
No products indexed under this heading.

Sulfinpyrazone (Caution is indicated when zoledronic acid is used with other potentially nephrotoxic drugs).
No products indexed under this heading.

Sulfisoxazole Acetyl (Caution is indicated when zoledronic acid is used with other potentially nephrotoxic drugs).
No products indexed under this heading.

Sulfisoxazole Diolamine (Caution is indicated when zoledronic acid is used with other potentially nephrotoxic drugs).
No products indexed under this heading.

Sulindac (Caution is indicated when zoledronic acid is used with other potentially nephrotoxic drugs).
Products include:
Clinoril Tablets **1962**

Tacrolimus (Caution is indicated when zoledronic acid is used with other potentially nephrotoxic drugs).
Products include:
Prograf Capsules and Injection **622**
Protopic Ointment **628**

Tenofovir Disoproxil Fumarate (Caution is indicated when zoledronic acid is used with other potentially nephrotoxic drugs). Products include:
Atripla Tablets **938**
Truvada Tablets **1262**
Viread Tablets **1268**

Thioguanine (Caution is indicated when zoledronic acid is used with other potentially nephrotoxic drugs).
Products include:
Tabloid Tablets **1601**

Ticarcillin Disodium (Caution is indicated when zoledronic acid is used with other potentially nephrotoxic drugs). Products include:
Timentin ADD-Vantage **1606**
Timentin Injection Galaxy Container **1609**
Timentin IV Infusion **1603**
Timentin Pharmacy Bulk Package **1613**

Tobramycin (Caution is advised when bisphosphonates are administered with aminoglycosides, since these agents may have an additive effect to lower serum calcium level for prolonged periods). Products include:
Zylet Ophthalmic Suspension .... ⊙**247**

Tobramycin Sulfate (Caution is advised when bisphosphonates are administered with aminoglycosides, since these agents may have an additive effect to lower serum calcium level for prolonged periods).
No products indexed under this heading.

Tolazamide (Caution is indicated when zoledronic acid is used with other potentially nephrotoxic drugs).
No products indexed under this heading.

Tolbutamide (Caution is indicated when zoledronic acid is used with other potentially nephrotoxic drugs).
No products indexed under this heading.

Tolmetin Sodium (Caution is indicated when zoledronic acid is used with other potentially nephrotoxic drugs).
No products indexed under this heading.

Torsemide (Caution should be exercised when zoledronic acid is used in combination with loop diuretics due to an increased risk of hypocalcemia). Products include:
- Demadex Injection 2630
- Demadex Tablets 2630

Trandolapril (Caution is indicated when zoledronic acid is used with other potentially nephrotoxic drugs). Products include:
- Mavik Tablets 472
- Tarka Tablets 511

Triamterene (Caution is indicated when zoledronic acid is used with other potentially nephrotoxic drugs). Products include:
- Dyazide Capsules 1405
- Dyrenium Capsules 3189

Trimethadione (Caution is indicated when zoledronic acid is used with other potentially nephrotoxic drugs).
No products indexed under this heading.

Trovafloxacin Mesylate (Caution is indicated when zoledronic acid is used with other potentially nephrotoxic drugs).
No products indexed under this heading.

Tyropanoate Sodium (Caution is indicated when zoledronic acid is used with other potentially nephrotoxic drugs).
No products indexed under this heading.

Valacyclovir Hydrochloride (Caution is indicated when zoledronic acid is used with other potentially nephrotoxic drugs). Products include:
- Valtrex Caplets 1635

Valdecoxib (Caution is indicated when zoledronic acid is used with other potentially nephrotoxic drugs).
No products indexed under this heading.

Vancomycin Hydrochloride (Caution is indicated when zoledronic acid is used with other potentially nephrotoxic drugs).
No products indexed under this heading.

Voriconazole (Caution is indicated when zoledronic acid is used with other potentially nephrotoxic drugs).
No products indexed under this heading.

Zalcitabine (Caution is indicated when zoledronic acid is used with other potentially nephrotoxic drugs).
No products indexed under this heading.

Zidovudine (Caution is indicated when zoledronic acid is used with other potentially nephrotoxic drugs). Products include:
- Combivir Tablets 1384
- Retrovir 1574
- Retrovir IV Infusion 1579
- Trizivir Tablets 1622

RECOMBINATE

(Antihemophilic Factor (Recombinant)) 738
None cited in PDR database.

RECOMBIVAX HB

(Hepatitis B Vaccine, Recombinant) ... 2107
None cited in PDR database.

REESE'S PINWORM TREATMENTS

(Pyrantel Pamoate) .... ⊡618
None cited in PDR database.

REFACTO VIALS

(Antihemophilic Factor (Recombinant)) 3269
None cited in PDR database.

REFLUDAN FOR INJECTION

(Lepirudin) 795
May interact with oral anticoagulants, non-steroidal anti-inflammatory agents, thrombolytics, and certain other agents. Compounds in these categories include:

Alteplase (Concomitant therapy with thrombolytics may increase the risk of bleeding complications and considerably enhance the effect of Refludan on aPTT prolongation). Products include:
- Activase I.V. 1188
- Cathflo Activase 1198

Anisindione (Concomitant therapy with oral anticoagulants may increase the risk of bleeding).
No products indexed under this heading.

Anistreplase (Concomitant therapy with thrombolytics may increase the risk of bleeding complications and considerably enhance the effect of Refludan on aPTT prolongation).
No products indexed under this heading.

Aspirin (Concomitant therapy with drugs that affect platelet function, such as aspirin, may increase the risk of bleeding). Products include:
- Aggrenox Capsules 819
- Bayer Aspirin 750
- Percodan Tablets 1130
- St. Joseph 81 mg Aspirin Chewable and Enteric Coated Tablets 1903

Bivalirudin (Concomitant therapy with thrombolytics may increase the risk of bleeding complications and considerably enhance the effect of Refludan on aPTT prolongation). Products include:
- Angiomax for Injection 1933

Celecoxib (Concomitant therapy with drugs that affect platelet function, such as non-steroid anti-inflammatory agents, may increase the risk of bleeding). Products include:
- Celebrex Capsules 2979

Clopidogrel Bisulfate (Concomitant therapy with drugs that affect platelet function, such as clopidogrel, may increase the risk of bleeding). Products include:
- Plavix Tablets 926
- Plavix Tablets 2767

Diclofenac Epolamine (Concomitant therapy with drugs that affect platelet function, such as non-steroid anti-inflammatory agents, may increase the risk of bleeding). Products include:
- Flector Patch 561

Diclofenac Potassium (Concomitant therapy with drugs that affect platelet function, such as non-steroid anti-inflammatory agents, may increase the risk of bleeding).
No products indexed under this heading.

Diclofenac Sodium (Concomitant therapy with drugs that affect platelet function, such as non-steroid anti-inflammatory agents, may increase the risk of bleeding). Products include:
- Diclofenac Sodium Ophthalmic Solution .... ⊙240
- Voltaren Ophthalmic Solution 2336
- Voltaren Tablets 2334
- Voltaren-XR Tablets 2337

Dicumarol (Concomitant therapy with oral anticoagulants may increase the risk of bleeding).
No products indexed under this heading.

Dipyridamole (Concomitant therapy with drugs that affect platelet function, such as dipyridamole, may increase the risk of bleeding). Products include:
- Aggrenox Capsules 819
- Persantine Tablets 869

Etodolac (Concomitant therapy with drugs that affect platelet function, such as non-steroid anti-inflammatory agents, may increase the risk of bleeding).
No products indexed under this heading.

Fenoprofen Calcium (Concomitant therapy with drugs that affect platelet function, such as non-steroid anti-inflammatory agents, may increase the risk of bleeding). Products include:
- Nalfon Capsules 2508

Flurbiprofen (Concomitant therapy with drugs that affect platelet function, such as non-steroid anti-inflammatory agents, may increase the risk of bleeding).
No products indexed under this heading.

Ibuprofen (Concomitant therapy with drugs that affect platelet function, such as non-steroid anti-inflammatory agents, may increase the risk of bleeding). Products include:
- Motrin IB Tablets and Caplets 1900
- Children's Motrin Oral Suspension ... 1901
- Children's Motrin Non-Staining Dye-Free Oral Suspension 1901
- Children's Motrin Cold Oral Suspension 1899
- Infants' Motrin Concentrated Drops 1901
- Infants' Motrin Non-Staining Dye-Free Concentrated Drops 1901
- Junior Strength Motrin Caplets and Chewable Tablets 1901
- Vicoprofen Tablets 533

Indomethacin (Concomitant therapy with drugs that affect platelet function, such as non-steroid anti-inflammatory agents, may increase the risk of bleeding). Products include:
- Indocin 2024

Indomethacin Sodium Trihydrate (Concomitant therapy with drugs that affect platelet function, such as non-steroid anti-inflammatory agents, may increase the risk of bleeding). Products include:
- Indocin I.V. 2489

Ketoprofen (Concomitant therapy with drugs that affect platelet function, such as non-steroid anti-inflammatory agents, may increase the risk of bleeding).
No products indexed under this heading.

Ketorolac Tromethamine (Concomitant therapy with drugs that affect platelet function, such as non-steroid anti-inflammatory agents, may increase the risk of bleeding).
No products indexed under this heading.

Meclofenamate Sodium (Concomitant therapy with drugs that affect platelet function, such as non-steroid anti-inflammatory agents, may increase the risk of bleeding).
No products indexed under this heading.

Mefenamic Acid (Concomitant therapy with drugs that affect platelet function, such as non-steroid anti-inflammatory agents, may increase the risk of bleeding).
No products indexed under this heading.

Meloxicam (Concomitant therapy with drugs that affect platelet function, such as non-steroid anti-inflammatory agents, may increase the risk of bleeding). Products include:
- Mobic Oral Suspension 863
- Mobic Tablets 863

Nabumetone (Concomitant therapy with drugs that affect platelet function, such as non-steroid anti-inflammatory agents, may increase the risk of bleeding).
No products indexed under this heading.

Naproxen (Concomitant therapy with drugs that affect platelet function, such as non-steroid anti-inflammatory agents, may increase the risk of bleeding). Products include:
- EC-Naprosyn Delayed-Release Tablets 2632
- Naprosyn Suspension 2632
- Naprosyn Tablets 2632

Naproxen Sodium (Concomitant therapy with drugs that affect platelet function, such as non-steroid anti-inflammatory agents, may increase the risk of bleeding). Products include:
- Anaprox Tablets 2632
- Anaprox DS Tablets 2632
- Treximet Tablets 1616

Oxaprozin (Concomitant therapy with drugs that affect platelet function, such as non-steroid anti-inflammatory agents, may increase the risk of bleeding).
No products indexed under this heading.

Phenylbutazone (Concomitant therapy with drugs that affect platelet function, such as non-steroid anti-inflammatory agents, may increase the risk of bleeding).
No products indexed under this heading.

Piroxicam (Concomitant therapy with drugs that affect platelet function, such as non-steroid anti-inflammatory agents, may increase the risk of bleeding).
No products indexed under this heading.

Reteplase (Concomitant therapy with thrombolytics may increase the risk of bleeding complications and considerably enhance the effect of Refludan on aPTT prolongation).
No products indexed under this heading.

Rofecoxib (Concomitant therapy with drugs that affect platelet function, such as non-steroid anti-inflammatory agents, may increase the risk of bleeding).
No products indexed under this heading.

Streptokinase (Concomitant therapy with thrombolytics may increase the risk of bleeding complications and considerably enhance the effect of Refludan on aPTT prolongation).
No products indexed under this heading.

Sulindac (Concomitant therapy with drugs that affect platelet function, such as non-steroid anti-inflammatory agents, may increase the risk of bleeding). Products include:
Clinoril Tablets 1962

Tolmetin Sodium (Concomitant therapy with drugs that affect platelet function, such as non-steroid anti-inflammatory agents, may increase the risk of bleeding).
No products indexed under this heading.

Urokinase (Concomitant therapy with thrombolytics may increase the risk of bleeding complications and considerably enhance the effect of Refludan on aPTT prolongation).
No products indexed under this heading.

Valdecoxib (Concomitant therapy with drugs that affect platelet function, such as non-steroid anti-inflammatory agents, may increase the risk of bleeding).
No products indexed under this heading.

Warfarin Sodium (Concomitant therapy with oral anticoagulants may increase the risk of bleeding).
No products indexed under this heading.

REFRESH CELLUVISC LUBRICANT EYE DROPS
(Carboxymethylcellulose Sodium) ..... ⊙231
None cited in PDR database.

REFRESH EYE ITCH RELIEF
(Ketotifen Fumarate) .... ⊙231
None cited in PDR database.

REFRESH PLUS LUBRICANT EYE DROPS
(Carboxymethylcellulose Sodium) ..... ⊙232
None cited in PDR database.

REFRESH TEARS LUBRICANT EYE DROPS
(Carboxymethylcellulose Sodium) ..... ⊙232
None cited in PDR database.

REISHIMAX CAPSULES
(Ganoderma lucinum mushroom extract) 2561
May interact with immunosuppressive agents. Compounds in these categories include:

Azathioprine (Concurrent use with immunosuppressive agents requires consultation with a physician).
No products indexed under this heading.

Basiliximab (Concurrent use with immunosuppressive agents requires consultation with a physician). Products include:
Simulect for Injection 2306

Cyclosporine (Concurrent use with immunosuppressive agents requires consultation with a physician). Products include:
Gengraf Capsules 435
Neoral Oral Solution 2280
Neoral Soft Gelatin Capsules 2280
Restasis Ophthalmic Emulsion 557
Sandimmune 2296

Muromonab-CD3 (Concurrent use with immunosuppressive agents requires consultation with a physician). Products include:
Orthoclone OKT3 Sterile Solution 2387

Mycophenolate Mofetil (Concurrent use with immunosuppressive agents requires consultation with a physician). Products include:
CellCept Capsules 2622
CellCept Oral Suspension 2622
CellCept Tablets 2622

Sirolimus (Concurrent use with immunosuppressive agents requires consultation with a physician). Products include:
Rapamune 3260

Tacrolimus (Concurrent use with immunosuppressive agents requires consultation with a physician). Products include:
Prograf Capsules and Injection 622
Protopic Ointment 628

RELENZA INHALATION POWDER
(Zanamivir) 1556
May interact with:

Influenza Virus Vaccine Live, Intranasal (Because of potential interference between zanamivir and the influenza virus vaccine live, the live attenuated influenza virus (LAIV) should not be administered within 2 weeks before or 48 hour after administration of zanamivir, unless medically indicated). Products include:
FluMist Vaccine 1945

RELIEF CAPSULES
(Amino Acid Preparations, Herbals with Vitamins, Psyllium Preparations) .... ▣641
None cited in PDR database.

RELISTOR INJECTION
(Methylnaltrexone Bromide) 3310
May interact with cytochrome p450 2d6 substrates (selected). Compounds in these categories include:

Amitriptyline Hydrochloride (Methylnaltrexone bromide is a weak inhibitor of CYP2D6).
No products indexed under this heading.

Amphetamine Aspartate (Methylnaltrexone bromide is a weak inhibitor of CYP2D6). Products include:
Adderall XR Capsules 3012

Amphetamine Aspartate Monohydrate (Methylnaltrexone bromide is a weak inhibitor of CYP2D6).
No products indexed under this heading.

Amphetamine Sulfate (Methylnaltrexone bromide is a weak inhibitor of CYP2D6). Products include:
Adderall XR Capsules 3012

Atomoxetine Hydrochloride (Methylnaltrexone bromide is a weak inhibitor of CYP2D6). Products include:
Strattera Capsules 1864

Bisoprolol Fumarate (Methylnaltrexone bromide is a weak inhibitor of CYP2D6).
No products indexed under this heading.

Captopril (Methylnaltrexone bromide is a weak inhibitor of CYP2D6). Products include:
Captopril Tablets 2182

Carvedilol (Methylnaltrexone bromide is a weak inhibitor of CYP2D6). Products include:
Coreg Tablets 1387

Cevimeline Hydrochloride (Methylnaltrexone bromide is a weak inhibitor of CYP2D6). Products include:
Evoxac Capsules 1013

Chlorpromazine (Methylnaltrexone bromide is a weak inhibitor of CYP2D6).
No products indexed under this heading.

Chlorpromazine Hydrochloride (Methylnaltrexone bromide is a weak inhibitor of CYP2D6).
No products indexed under this heading.

Chlorpropamide (Methylnaltrexone bromide is a weak inhibitor of CYP2D6).
No products indexed under this heading.

Clomipramine Hydrochloride (Methylnaltrexone bromide is a weak inhibitor of CYP2D6).
No products indexed under this heading.

Clozapine (Methylnaltrexone bromide is a weak inhibitor of CYP2D6).
No products indexed under this heading.

Codeine Phosphate (Methylnaltrexone bromide is a weak inhibitor of CYP2D6). Products include:
Tylenol with Codeine Tablets 2427

Codeine Sulfate (Methylnaltrexone bromide is a weak inhibitor of CYP2D6).
No products indexed under this heading.

Cyclobenzaprine Hydrochloride (Methylnaltrexone bromide is a weak inhibitor of CYP2D6). Products include:
Amrix Capsules 966

Desipramine Hydrochloride (Methylnaltrexone bromide is a weak inhibitor of CYP2D6).
No products indexed under this heading.

Dexfenfluramine Hydrochloride (Methylnaltrexone bromide is a weak inhibitor of CYP2D6).
No products indexed under this heading.

Dextromethorphan Hydrobromide (Methylnaltrexone bromide is a weak inhibitor of CYP2D6). Products include:
PediaCare Children's Liquid Multi-Symptom Cold 1902
PediaCare Children's Long-Acting Cough 1902
Children's Sudafed PE Cold & Cough Liquid 1907
Sudafed PE Cold & Cough Caplets 1907
Children's Tylenol Plus Cough & Runny Nose Suspension Liquid 1912
Children's Tylenol Plus Cough & Sore Throat Suspension Liquid 1912
Children's Tylenol Plus Flu Suspension Liquid 1914
Children's Tylenol Plus Multi-Symptom Cold Suspension Liquid 1912
Tylenol Cold Severe Congestion Daytime Caplets with Cool Burst 1912
Tylenol Cold Head Congestion Daytime Caplets with Cool Burst 1910
Tylenol Cold Head Congestion Nighttime Caplets with Cool Burst 1910
Tylenol Cold Head Congestion Severe Daytime Caplets with Cool Burst 1910
Tylenol Cold Multi-Symptom Daytime Caplets with Cool Burst and Rapid Release Gels 1913
Tylenol Cold Multi-Symptom Daytime Liquid with Citrus Burst ... 1913
Tylenol Cold Multi-Symptom Nighttime Caplets with Cool Burst 1913
Tylenol Cold Multi-Symptom Nighttime Liquid with Cool Burst ... 1913
Tylenol Cold Multi-Symptom Severe Caplets with Cool Burst 1913
Tylenol Cold Multi-Symptom Severe Daytime Liquid with Citrus Burst 1913
Tylenol Cough & Sore Throat Daytime Liquid with Cool Burst 1918
Tylenol Cough & Sore Throat Nighttime Liquid with Cool Burst ... 1918
Vicks DayQuil Cold & Flu Multi-Symptom Relief .... ▣616
Vicks DayQuil LiquiCaps 2567
Vicks DayQuil Liquid 2567
Vicks DayQuil Multi-Symptom Cold/Flu Relief 2567
Vicks NyQuil Cold & Flu Multi-Symptom Relief .... ▣617
Vicks NyQuil LiquiCaps 2567
Vicks NyQuil Liquid 2567
Vicks NyQuil Multi-Symptom Cold/Flu Relief 2567

Dextromethorphan Polistirex (Methylnaltrexone bromide is a weak inhibitor of CYP2D6).
No products indexed under this heading.

Dolasetron Mesylate (Methylnaltrexone bromide is a weak inhibitor of CYP2D6). Products include:
Anzemet Injection 2701
Anzemet Tablets 2704

Donepezil Hydrochloride (Methylnaltrexone bromide is a weak inhibitor of CYP2D6). Products include:
Aricept Tablets 1062
Aricept ODT Tablets 1062

Doxepin Hydrochloride (Methylnaltrexone bromide is a weak inhibitor of CYP2D6).
No products indexed under this heading.

Encainide Hydrochloride (Methylnaltrexone bromide is a weak inhibitor of CYP2D6).
No products indexed under this heading.

Fentanyl (Methylnaltrexone bromide is a weak inhibitor of CYP2D6). Products include:
Duragesic Transdermal System 2405
Ionsys Transdermal System 2410

Fentanyl Citrate (Methylnaltrexone bromide is a weak inhibitor of CYP2D6). Products include:

Actiq ... 959
Fentora Tablets ... 968

Flecainide Acetate (Methylnaltrexone bromide is a weak inhibitor of CYP2D6).
No products indexed under this heading.

Fluoxetine (Methylnaltrexone bromide is a weak inhibitor of CYP2D6).
No products indexed under this heading.

Fluoxetine Hydrochloride (Methylnaltrexone bromide is a weak inhibitor of CYP2D6). Products include:
Prozac Weekly Capsules ... 1852
Prozac Pulvules and Liquid ... 1852
Symbyax Capsules ... 1871

Fluphenazine Decanoate (Methylnaltrexone bromide is a weak inhibitor of CYP2D6).
No products indexed under this heading.

Fluphenazine Enanthate (Methylnaltrexone bromide is a weak inhibitor of CYP2D6).
No products indexed under this heading.

Fluphenazine Hydrochloride (Methylnaltrexone bromide is a weak inhibitor of CYP2D6).
No products indexed under this heading.

Fluvoxamine Maleate (Methylnaltrexone bromide is a weak inhibitor of CYP2D6). Products include:
Luvox CR Extended-Release Capsules ... 1759

Formoterol Fumarate (Methylnaltrexone bromide is a weak inhibitor of CYP2D6). Products include:
Foradil Aerolizer ... 2849
Perforomist Inhalation Solution ... 1025

Galantamine Hydrobromide (Methylnaltrexone bromide is a weak inhibitor of CYP2D6).
No products indexed under this heading.

Haloperidol (Methylnaltrexone bromide is a weak inhibitor of CYP2D6).
No products indexed under this heading.

Haloperidol Decanoate (Methylnaltrexone bromide is a weak inhibitor of CYP2D6).
No products indexed under this heading.

Hydrocodone Bitartrate (Methylnaltrexone bromide is a weak inhibitor of CYP2D6). Products include:
Lortab 5/500 Tablets ... 3143
Lortab 7.5/500 Tablets ... 3144
Lortab 10/500 Tablets ... 3144
Vicodin Tablets ... 529
Vicodin ES Tablets ... 530
Vicodin HP Tablets ... 531
Vicoprofen Tablets ... 533
Zydone Tablets ... 1132

Imipramine Hydrochloride (Methylnaltrexone bromide is a weak inhibitor of CYP2D6).
No products indexed under this heading.

Imipramine Pamoate (Methylnaltrexone bromide is a weak inhibitor of CYP2D6).
No products indexed under this heading.

Indoramin Hydrochloride (Methylnaltrexone bromide is a weak inhibitor of CYP2D6).
No products indexed under this heading.

Labetalol Hydrochloride (Methylnaltrexone bromide is a weak inhibitor of CYP2D6).
No products indexed under this heading.

Lidocaine (Methylnaltrexone bromide is a weak inhibitor of CYP2D6). Products include:
Lidoderm Patch ... 1114

Lidocaine Hydrochloride (Methylnaltrexone bromide is a weak inhibitor of CYP2D6).
No products indexed under this heading.

Maprotiline Hydrochloride (Methylnaltrexone bromide is a weak inhibitor of CYP2D6).
No products indexed under this heading.

Meperidine Hydrochloride (Methylnaltrexone bromide is a weak inhibitor of CYP2D6).
No products indexed under this heading.

Methadone Hydrochloride (Methylnaltrexone bromide is a weak inhibitor of CYP2D6).
No products indexed under this heading.

Methamphetamine Hydrochloride (Methylnaltrexone bromide is a weak inhibitor of CYP2D6).
No products indexed under this heading.

Metoprolol Succinate (Methylnaltrexone bromide is a weak inhibitor of CYP2D6). Products include:
Toprol-XL Tablets ... 666

Metoprolol Tartrate (Methylnaltrexone bromide is a weak inhibitor of CYP2D6).
No products indexed under this heading.

Mexiletine Hydrochloride (Methylnaltrexone bromide is a weak inhibitor of CYP2D6).
No products indexed under this heading.

Mirtazapine (Methylnaltrexone bromide is a weak inhibitor of CYP2D6). Products include:
Remeron Tablets ... 2924
RemeronSolTab Tablets ... 2927

Morphine Sulfate (Methylnaltrexone bromide is a weak inhibitor of CYP2D6). Products include:
Avinza Capsules ... 1772
DepoDur Injection ... 1095
MS Contin Tablets ... 2585

Nelfinavir Mesylate (Methylnaltrexone bromide is a weak inhibitor of CYP2D6).
No products indexed under this heading.

Nortriptyline Hydrochloride (Methylnaltrexone bromide is a weak inhibitor of CYP2D6).
No products indexed under this heading.

Olanzapine (Methylnaltrexone bromide is a weak inhibitor of CYP2D6). Products include:
Symbyax Capsules ... 1871
Zyprexa Tablets ... 1883
Zyprexa IntraMuscular ... 1883
Zyprexa ZYDIS Orally Disintegrating Tablets ... 1883

Omeprazole (Methylnaltrexone bromide is a weak inhibitor of CYP2D6).
No products indexed under this heading.

Ondansetron (Methylnaltrexone bromide is a weak inhibitor of CYP2D6). Products include:
Zofran ODT Orally Disintegrating Tablets ... 1687

Ondansetron Hydrochloride (Methylnaltrexone bromide is a weak inhibitor of CYP2D6). Products include:
Zofran Injection ... 1682
Zofran ... 1687

Oxycodone Hydrochloride (Methylnaltrexone bromide is a weak inhibitor of CYP2D6). Products include:
OxyContin Tablets ... 2589
OxyIR Capsules ... 2593
Percocet Tablets ... 1127
Percodan Tablets ... 1130

Paclitaxel (Methylnaltrexone bromide is a weak inhibitor of CYP2D6).
No products indexed under this heading.

Paroxetine Hydrochloride (Methylnaltrexone bromide is a weak inhibitor of CYP2D6). Products include:
Paxil ... 1535
Paxil CR Controlled-Release Tablets ... 1544

Pindolol (Methylnaltrexone bromide is a weak inhibitor of CYP2D6).
No products indexed under this heading.

Propafenone Hydrochloride (Methylnaltrexone bromide is a weak inhibitor of CYP2D6). Products include:
Rythmol Tablets ... 1586
Rythmol SR Capsules ... 1590

Propoxyphene Hydrochloride (Methylnaltrexone bromide is a weak inhibitor of CYP2D6).
No products indexed under this heading.

Propoxyphene Napsylate (Methylnaltrexone bromide is a weak inhibitor of CYP2D6).
No products indexed under this heading.

Propranolol Hydrochloride (Methylnaltrexone bromide is a weak inhibitor of CYP2D6). Products include:
InnoPran XL Extended Release Capsules ... 1484

Quetiapine Fumarate (Methylnaltrexone bromide is a weak inhibitor of CYP2D6).
No products indexed under this heading.

Quinidine Gluconate (Methylnaltrexone bromide is a weak inhibitor of CYP2D6).
No products indexed under this heading.

Quinidine Hydrochloride (Methylnaltrexone bromide is a weak inhibitor of CYP2D6).
No products indexed under this heading.

Quinidine Polygalacturonate (Methylnaltrexone bromide is a weak inhibitor of CYP2D6).
No products indexed under this heading.

Quinidine Sulfate (Methylnaltrexone bromide is a weak inhibitor of CYP2D6).
No products indexed under this heading.

Risperidone (Methylnaltrexone bromide is a weak inhibitor of CYP2D6). Products include:
Risperdal Consta Long-Acting Injection ... 1753

Ritonavir (Methylnaltrexone bromide is a weak inhibitor of CYP2D6). Products include:
Kaletra ... 452
Norvir ... 489

Tamoxifen Citrate (Methylnaltrexone bromide is a weak inhibitor of CYP2D6).
No products indexed under this heading.

Teniposide (Methylnaltrexone bromide is a weak inhibitor of CYP2D6).
No products indexed under this heading.

Testosterone (Methylnaltrexone bromide is a weak inhibitor of CYP2D6). Products include:
AndroGel ... 3159
Testim 1% Gel ... 701

Testosterone Cypionate (Methylnaltrexone bromide is a weak inhibitor of CYP2D6).
No products indexed under this heading.

Testosterone Enanthate (Methylnaltrexone bromide is a weak inhibitor of CYP2D6). Products include:
Delatestryl Injection ... 1730

Testosterone Propionate (Methylnaltrexone bromide is a weak inhibitor of CYP2D6).
No products indexed under this heading.

Thioridazine (Methylnaltrexone bromide is a weak inhibitor of CYP2D6).
No products indexed under this heading.

Thioridazine Hydrochloride (Methylnaltrexone bromide is a weak inhibitor of CYP2D6). Products include:
Thioridazine Hydrochloride Tablets ... 2195

Timolol Maleate (Methylnaltrexone bromide is a weak inhibitor of CYP2D6). Products include:
Combigan Ophthalmic Solution ... 553
Cosopt Sterile Ophthalmic Solution ... 1969
Timoptic Sterile Ophthalmic Solution ... 2121
Timoptic in Ocudose ... 2124
Timoptic-XE Sterile Ophthalmic Gel Forming Solution ... 2125

Tolterodine Tartrate (Methylnaltrexone bromide is a weak inhibitor of CYP2D6).
No products indexed under this heading.

Tramadol Hydrochloride (Methylnaltrexone bromide is a weak inhibitor of CYP2D6). Products include:
Ultram ER Extended-Release Tablets ... 2428

Trazodone Hydrochloride (Methylnaltrexone bromide is a weak inhibitor of CYP2D6).
No products indexed under this heading.

Triazolam (Methylnaltrexone bromide is a weak inhibitor of CYP2D6).
No products indexed under this heading.

Trimipramine Maleate (Methylnaltrexone bromide is a weak inhibitor of CYP2D6).
No products indexed under this heading.

Venlafaxine Hydrochloride (Methylnaltrexone bromide is a weak inhibitor of CYP2D6). Products include:
Effexor XR Extended-Release Capsules ... 3195
Venlafaxine Hydrochloride Tablets ... 2199

Vinblastine Sulfate (Methylnaltrexone bromide is a weak inhibitor of CYP2D6).
No products indexed under this heading.

Zonisamide (Methylnaltrexone bromide is a weak inhibitor of CYP2D6). Products include:
Zonegran Capsules ... 1089

REMERON TABLETS
(Mirtazapine) 2924
May interact with central nervous system depressants, monoamine oxidase inhibitors, and certain other agents. Compounds in these categories include:

Alfentanil Hydrochloride (Co-administration may result in an additive impairment of motor skills).
No products indexed under this heading.

Alprazolam (Co-administration may result in an additive impairment of motor skills).
No products indexed under this heading.

Aprobarbital (Co-administration may result in an additive impairment of motor skills).
No products indexed under this heading.

Buprenorphine Hydrochloride (Co-administration may result in an additive impairment of motor skills). Products include:
Suboxone Tablets 2601
Subutex Tablets 2601

Buspirone Hydrochloride (Co-administration may result in an additive impairment of motor skills).
No products indexed under this heading.

Butabarbital (Co-administration may result in an additive impairment of motor skills).
No products indexed under this heading.

Butalbital (Co-administration may result in an additive impairment of motor skills).
No products indexed under this heading.

Chlordiazepoxide (Co-administration may result in an additive impairment of motor skills).
No products indexed under this heading.

Chlordiazepoxide Hydrochloride (Co-administration may result in an additive impairment of motor skills).
No products indexed under this heading.

Chlorpromazine (Co-administration may result in an additive impairment of motor skills).
No products indexed under this heading.

Chlorpromazine Hydrochloride (Co-administration may result in an additive impairment of motor skills).
No products indexed under this heading.

Chlorprothixene (Co-administration may result in an additive impairment of motor skills).
No products indexed under this heading.

Chlorprothixene Hydrochloride (Co-administration may result in an additive impairment of motor skills).
No products indexed under this heading.

Chlorprothixene Lactate (Co-administration may result in an additive impairment of motor skills).
No products indexed under this heading.

Clorazepate Dipotassium (Co-administration may result in an additive impairment of motor skills).
No products indexed under this heading.

Clozapine (Co-administration may result in an additive impairment of motor skills).
No products indexed under this heading.

Codeine Phosphate (Co-administration may result in an additive impairment of motor skills). Products include:
Tylenol with Codeine Tablets 2427

Desflurane (Co-administration may result in an additive impairment of motor skills).
No products indexed under this heading.

Dezocine (Co-administration may result in an additive impairment of motor skills).
No products indexed under this heading.

Diazepam (Co-administration has shown to result in an additive impairment of motor skills). Products include:
Valium Tablets 2658

Droperidol (Co-administration may result in an additive impairment of motor skills).
No products indexed under this heading.

Enflurane (Co-administration may result in an additive impairment of motor skills).
No products indexed under this heading.

Estazolam (Co-administration may result in an additive impairment of motor skills).
No products indexed under this heading.

Ethanol (Co-administration may result in an additive impairment of motor skills).
No products indexed under this heading.

Ethchlorvynol (Co-administration may result in an additive impairment of motor skills).
No products indexed under this heading.

Ethinamate (Co-administration may result in an additive impairment of motor skills).
No products indexed under this heading.

Ethyl Alcohol (Co-administration may result in an additive impairment of motor skills).
No products indexed under this heading.

Fentanyl (Co-administration may result in an additive impairment of motor skills). Products include:
Duragesic Transdermal System 2405
Ionsys Transdermal System 2410

Fentanyl Citrate (Co-administration may result in an additive impairment of motor skills). Products include:
Actiq 959
Fentora Tablets 968

Fluphenazine Decanoate (Co-administration may result in an additive impairment of motor skills).
No products indexed under this heading.

Fluphenazine Enanthate (Co-administration may result in an additive impairment of motor skills).
No products indexed under this heading.

Fluphenazine Hydrochloride (Co-administration may result in an additive impairment of motor skills).
No products indexed under this heading.

Flurazepam Hydrochloride (Co-administration may result in an additive impairment of motor skills).
No products indexed under this heading.

Glutethimide (Co-administration may result in an additive impairment of motor skills).
No products indexed under this heading.

Haloperidol (Co-administration may result in an additive impairment of motor skills).
No products indexed under this heading.

Haloperidol Decanoate (Co-administration may result in an additive impairment of motor skills).
No products indexed under this heading.

Hydrocodone Bitartrate (Co-administration may result in an additive impairment of motor skills). Products include:
Lortab 5/500 Tablets 3143
Lortab 7.5/500 Tablets 3144
Lortab 10/500 Tablets 3144
Vicodin Tablets 529
Vicodin ES Tablets 530
Vicodin HP Tablets 531
Vicoprofen Tablets 533
Zydone Tablets 1132

Hydrocodone Polistirex (Co-administration may result in an additive impairment of motor skills). Products include:
Tussionex Pennkinetic Extended-Release Suspension 3154

Hydromorphone Hydrochloride (Co-administration may result in an additive impairment of motor skills).
No products indexed under this heading.

Hydroxyzine Hydrochloride (Co-administration may result in an additive impairment of motor skills).
No products indexed under this heading.

Isocarboxazid (Co-administration of antidepressants and MAO inhibitors has resulted in serious, and sometimes fatal, reactions including hyperthermia, autonomic instability, seizures, agitation, and coma; concurrent and/or sequential use is contraindicated). Products include:
Marplan Tablets 3177

Isoflurane (Co-administration may result in an additive impairment of motor skills).
No products indexed under this heading.

Ketamine Hydrochloride (Co-administration may result in an additive impairment of motor skills).
No products indexed under this heading.

Levomethadyl Acetate Hydrochloride (Co-administration may result in an additive impairment of motor skills).
No products indexed under this heading.

Levorphanol Tartrate (Co-administration may result in an additive impairment of motor skills).
No products indexed under this heading.

Lorazepam (Co-administration may result in an additive impairment of motor skills).
No products indexed under this heading.

Loxapine Hydrochloride (Co-administration may result in an additive impairment of motor skills).
No products indexed under this heading.

Loxapine Succinate (Co-administration may result in an additive impairment of motor skills).
No products indexed under this heading.

Meperidine Hydrochloride (Co-administration may result in an additive impairment of motor skills).
No products indexed under this heading.

Mephobarbital (Co-administration may result in an additive impairment of motor skills).
No products indexed under this heading.

Meprobamate (Co-administration may result in an additive impairment of motor skills).
No products indexed under this heading.

Mesoridazine Besylate (Co-administration may result in an additive impairment of motor skills).
No products indexed under this heading.

Methadone Hydrochloride (Co-administration may result in an additive impairment of motor skills).
No products indexed under this heading.

Methohexital Sodium (Co-administration may result in an additive impairment of motor skills).
No products indexed under this heading.

Methotrimeprazine (Co-administration may result in an additive impairment of motor skills).
No products indexed under this heading.

Methoxyflurane (Co-administration may result in an additive impairment of motor skills).
No products indexed under this heading.

Midazolam Hydrochloride (Co-administration may result in an additive impairment of motor skills).
No products indexed under this heading.

Moclobemide (Co-administration of antidepressants and MAO inhibitors has resulted in serious, and sometimes fatal, reactions including hyperthermia, autonomic instability, seizures, agitation, and coma; concurrent and/or sequential use is contraindicated).
No products indexed under this heading.

Molindone Hydrochloride (Co-administration may result in an additive impairment of motor skills). Products include:
Moban Tablets 1116

Morphine Sulfate (Co-administration may result in an additive impairment of motor skills). Products include:
Avinza Capsules 1772
DepoDur Injection 1095
MS Contin Tablets 2585

Olanzapine (Co-administration may result in an additive impairment of motor skills). Products include:
Symbyax Capsules 1871
Zyprexa Tablets 1883
Zyprexa IntraMuscular 1883
Zyprexa ZYDIS Orally Disintegrating Tablets 1883

Oxazepam (Co-administration may result in an additive impairment of motor skills).
No products indexed under this heading.

Oxycodone Hydrochloride (Co-administration may result in an additive impairment of motor skills).
Products include:
OxyContin Tablets 2589
OxyIR Capsules 2593
Percocet Tablets 1127
Percodan Tablets 1130

Pargyline Hydrochloride (Co-administration of antidepressants and MAO inhibitors has resulted in serious, and sometimes fatal, reactions including hyperthermia, autonomic instability, seizures, agitation, and coma; concurrent and/or sequential use is contraindicated).
No products indexed under this heading.

Pentobarbital Sodium (Co-administration may result in an additive impairment of motor skills).
Products include:
Nembutal Sodium Solution, USP 2494

Perphenazine (Co-administration may result in an additive impairment of motor skills).
No products indexed under this heading.

Phenelzine Sulfate (Co-administration of antidepressants and MAO inhibitors has resulted in serious, and sometimes fatal, reactions including hyperthermia, autonomic instability, seizures, agitation, and coma; concurrent and/or sequential use is contraindicated).
No products indexed under this heading.

Phenobarbital (Co-administration may result in an additive impairment of motor skills). Products include:
Donnatal Extentabs 2507

Prazepam (Co-administration may result in an additive impairment of motor skills).
No products indexed under this heading.

Procarbazine Hydrochloride (Co-administration of antidepressants and MAO inhibitors has resulted in serious, and sometimes fatal, reactions including hyperthermia, autonomic instability, seizures, agitation, and coma; concurrent and/or sequential use is contraindicated).
No products indexed under this heading.

Prochlorperazine (Co-administration may result in an additive impairment of motor skills).
No products indexed under this heading.

Promethazine Hydrochloride (Co-administration may result in an additive impairment of motor skills).
No products indexed under this heading.

Propofol (Co-administration may result in an additive impairment of motor skills).
No products indexed under this heading.

Propoxyphene Hydrochloride (Co-administration may result in an additive impairment of motor skills).
No products indexed under this heading.

Propoxyphene Napsylate (Co-administration may result in an additive impairment of motor skills).
No products indexed under this heading.

Quazepam (Co-administration may result in an additive impairment of motor skills).
No products indexed under this heading.

Quetiapine Fumarate (Co-administration may result in an additive impairment of motor skills).
No products indexed under this heading.

Remifentanil Hydrochloride (Co-administration may result in an additive impairment of motor skills).
No products indexed under this heading.

Risperidone (Co-administration may result in an additive impairment of motor skills). Products include:
Risperdal Consta Long-Acting Injection 1753

Secobarbital Sodium (Co-administration may result in an additive impairment of motor skills).
No products indexed under this heading.

Selegiline Hydrochloride (Co-administration of antidepressants and MAO inhibitors has resulted in serious, and sometimes fatal, reactions including hyperthermia, autonomic instability, seizures, agitation, and coma; concurrent and/or sequential use is contraindicated).
Products include:
Eldepryl Capsules 3052

Sevoflurane (Co-administration may result in an additive impairment of motor skills). Products include:
Ultane Liquid for Inhalation 524

Sufentanil Citrate (Co-administration may result in an additive impairment of motor skills).
No products indexed under this heading.

Temazepam (Co-administration may result in an additive impairment of motor skills).
No products indexed under this heading.

Thiamylal Sodium (Co-administration may result in an additive impairment of motor skills).
No products indexed under this heading.

Thioridazine Hydrochloride (Co-administration may result in an additive impairment of motor skills).
Products include:
Thioridazine Hydrochloride Tablets 2195

Thiothixene (Co-administration may result in an additive impairment of motor skills). Products include:
Thiothixene Capsules 2197

Tranylcypromine Sulfate (Co-administration of antidepressants and MAO inhibitors has resulted in serious, and sometimes fatal, reactions including hyperthermia, autonomic instability, seizures, agitation, and coma; concurrent and/or sequential use is contraindicated).
Products include:
Parnate Tablets 1532

Triazolam (Co-administration may result in an additive impairment of motor skills).
No products indexed under this heading.

Trifluoperazine Hydrochloride (Co-administration may result in an additive impairment of motor skills).
No products indexed under this heading.

Zaleplon (Co-administration may result in an additive impairment of motor skills).
No products indexed under this heading.

Ziprasidone Hydrochloride (Co-administration may result in an additive impairment of motor skills).
Products include:
Geodon Capsules 2520

Zolpidem Tartrate (Co-administration may result in an additive impairment of motor skills).
Products include:
Ambien Tablets 2692
Ambien CR Tablets 2696

Food Interactions

Alcohol (Co-administration has shown to result in an additive impairment of motor skills).

Food, unspecified (The presence of food in the stomach has a minimal effect on both the rate and extent of absorption and does not require a dosage adjustment).

REMERONSOLTAB TABLETS

(Mirtazapine) 2927
See Remeron Tablets

REMICADE FOR IV INJECTION

(Infliximab) 950
May interact with:

2-Amino-6-Mercaptopurine (Rare postmarketing cases of hepatosplenic T-cell lymphoma have been reported in adolescent and young adult patients with Crohns's disease treated with Remicade; all of these hepatosplenic T-cell lymphomas with Remicade have occurred in patients on concomitant treatment with azathioprine or 6-mercaptopurine).
No products indexed under this heading.

Anakinra (Serious infections were seen with concurrent use of anakinra and another TNF2-blocking agent, etanercept. Similar toxicities may also result from the combination of anakinra and other TNF2-blocking agents; therefore, concurrent use of anakinra and infliximab is not recommended). Products include:
Kineret Injection 585

Azathioprine (Rare postmarketing cases of hepatosplenic T-cell lymphoma have been reported in adolescent and young adult patients with Crohns's disease treated with Remicade; all of these hepatosplenic T-cell lymphomas with Remicade have occurred in patients on concomitant treatment with azathioprine or 6-mercaptopurine).
No products indexed under this heading.

Azathioprine Sodium (Rare postmarketing cases of hepatosplenic T-cell lymphoma have been reported in adolescent and young adult patients with Crohns's disease treated with Remicade; all of these hepatosplenic T-cell lymphomas with Remicade have occurred in patients on concomitant treatment with azathioprine or 6-mercaptopurine).
No products indexed under this heading.

Mercaptopurine (Rare postmarketing cases of hepatosplenic T-cell lymphoma have been reported in adolescent and young adult patients with Crohns's disease treated with Remicade; all of these hepatosplenic T-cell lymphomas with Remicade have occurred in patients on concomitant treatment with azathioprine or 6-mercaptopurine).
No products indexed under this heading.

REOPRO VIALS

(Abciximab) 1860
May interact with anticoagulants, oral anticoagulants, non-steroidal anti-inflammatory agents, thrombolytics, and certain other agents. Compounds in these categories include:

Alteplase (Co-administration with thrombolytics may be associated with an increase in bleeding).
Products include:
Activase I.V. 1188
Cathflo Activase 1198

Anisindione (Co-administration of oral anticoagulants within seven days is contraindicated unless prothrombin time is less than or equal to 1.2 times control; concurrent use with other anticoagulant agents may be associated with an increase in bleeding).
No products indexed under this heading.

Anistreplase (Co-administration with thrombolytics may be associated with an increase in bleeding).
No products indexed under this heading.

Ardeparin Sodium (Co-administration with other anticoagulant agents may be associated with an increase in bleeding).
No products indexed under this heading.

Aspirin (Co-administration with antiplatelet agents, such as aspirin, may be associated with an increase in bleeding). Products include:
Aggrenox Capsules 819
Bayer Aspirin 750
Percodan Tablets 1130
St. Joseph 81 mg Aspirin Chewable and Enteric Coated Tablets 1903

Bivalirudin (Co-administration with thrombolytics may be associated with an increase in bleeding).
Products include:
Angiomax for Injection 1933

Celecoxib (Co-administration with antiplatelet agents, such as non-steroidal anti-inflammatory agents, may be associated with an increase in bleeding). Products include:
Celebrex Capsules 2979

Clopidogrel Bisulfate (Co-administration with antiplatelet agents, such as clopidogrel, may be associated with an increase in bleeding). Products include:
Plavix Tablets 926
Plavix Tablets 2767

Dalteparin Sodium (Co-administration with other anticoagulant agents may be associated with an increase in bleeding). Products include:
Fragmin Injection 1070

Danaparoid Sodium (Co-administration with other anticoagulant agents may be associated with an increase in bleeding).
No products indexed under this heading.

Dextran (Co-administration with intravenous dextran before percutaneous coronary intervention, or intent to use it during an intervention is contraindicated).
No products indexed under this heading.

Diclofenac Epolamine (Co-administration with antiplatelet agents, such as non-steroidal anti-inflammatory agents, may be associated with an increase in bleeding). Products include:
Flector Patch 561

Diclofenac Potassium (Co-administration with antiplatelet agents, such as non-steroidal anti-inflammatory agents, may be associated with an increase in bleeding).
No products indexed under this heading.

Diclofenac Sodium (Co-administration with antiplatelet agents, such as non-steroidal anti-inflammatory agents, may be associated with an increase in bleeding). Products include:
Diclofenac Sodium Ophthalmic Solution .... ⊙240
Voltaren Ophthalmic Solution 2336
Voltaren Tablets 2334
Voltaren-XR Tablets 2337

Dicumarol (Co-administration of oral anticoagulants within seven days is contraindicated unless prothrombin time is less than or equal to 1.2 times control; concurrent use with other anticoagulant agents may be associated with an increase in bleeding).
No products indexed under this heading.

Dipyridamole (Co-administration with antiplatelet agents, such as dipyridamole, may be associated with an increase in bleeding). Products include:
Aggrenox Capsules 819
Persantine Tablets 869

Enoxaparin Sodium (Co-administration with other anticoagulant agents may be associated with an increase in bleeding). Products include:
Lovenox Injection 2756

Etodolac (Co-administration with antiplatelet agents, such as non-steroidal anti-inflammatory agents, may be associated with an increase in bleeding).
No products indexed under this heading.

Fenoprofen Calcium (Co-administration with antiplatelet agents, such as non-steroidal anti-inflammatory agents, may be associated with an increase in bleeding). Products include:
Nalfon Capsules 2508

Flurbiprofen (Co-administration with antiplatelet agents, such as non-steroidal anti-inflammatory agents, may be associated with an increase in bleeding).
No products indexed under this heading.

Fondaparinux Sodium (Co-administration with other anticoagulant agents may be associated with an increase in bleeding). Products include:
Arixtra Injection 1313

Heparin Calcium (Co-administration with other anticoagulant agents may be associated with an increase in bleeding).
No products indexed under this heading.

Heparin Sodium (Co-administration with other anticoagulant agents may be associated with an increase in bleeding).
No products indexed under this heading.

Ibuprofen (Co-administration with antiplatelet agents, such as non-steroidal anti-inflammatory agents, may be associated with an increase in bleeding). Products include:
Motrin IB Tablets and Caplets 1900
Children's Motrin Oral Suspension ... 1901
Children's Motrin Non-Staining Dye-Free Oral Suspension 1901
Children's Motrin Cold Oral Suspension 1899
Infants' Motrin Concentrated Drops 1901
Infants' Motrin Non-Staining Dye-Free Concentrated Drops 1901
Junior Strength Motrin Caplets and Chewable Tablets 1901
Vicoprofen Tablets 533

Indomethacin (Co-administration with antiplatelet agents, such as non-steroidal anti-inflammatory agents, may be associated with an increase in bleeding). Products include:
Indocin 2024

Indomethacin Sodium Trihydrate (Co-administration with antiplatelet agents, such as non-steroidal anti-inflammatory agents, may be associated with an increase in bleeding). Products include:
Indocin I.V. 2489

Ketoprofen (Co-administration with antiplatelet agents, such as non-steroidal anti-inflammatory agents, may be associated with an increase in bleeding).
No products indexed under this heading.

Ketorolac Tromethamine (Co-administration with antiplatelet agents, such as non-steroidal anti-inflammatory agents, may be associated with an increase in bleeding).
No products indexed under this heading.

Low Molecular Weight Heparins (Co-administration with other anticoagulant agents may be associated with an increase in bleeding).
No products indexed under this heading.

Meclofenamate Sodium (Co-administration with antiplatelet agents, such as non-steroidal anti-inflammatory agents, may be associated with an increase in bleeding).
No products indexed under this heading.

Mefenamic Acid (Co-administration with antiplatelet agents, such as non-steroidal anti-inflammatory agents, may be associated with an increase in bleeding).
No products indexed under this heading.

Meloxicam (Co-administration with antiplatelet agents, such as non-steroidal anti-inflammatory agents, may be associated with an increase in bleeding). Products include:
Mobic Oral Suspension 863
Mobic Tablets 863

Nabumetone (Co-administration with antiplatelet agents, such as non-steroidal anti-inflammatory agents, may be associated with an increase in bleeding).
No products indexed under this heading.

Naproxen (Co-administration with antiplatelet agents, such as non-steroidal anti-inflammatory agents, may be associated with an increase in bleeding). Products include:
EC-Naprosyn Delayed-Release Tablets 2632
Naprosyn Suspension 2632
Naprosyn Tablets 2632

Naproxen Sodium (Co-administration with antiplatelet agents, such as non-steroidal anti-inflammatory agents, may be associated with an increase in bleeding). Products include:
Anaprox Tablets 2632
Anaprox DS Tablets 2632
Treximet Tablets 1616

Oxaprozin (Co-administration with antiplatelet agents, such as non-steroidal anti-inflammatory agents, may be associated with an increase in bleeding).
No products indexed under this heading.

Phenylbutazone (Co-administration with antiplatelet agents, such as non-steroidal anti-inflammatory agents, may be associated with an increase in bleeding).
No products indexed under this heading.

Piroxicam (Co-administration with antiplatelet agents, such as non-steroidal anti-inflammatory agents, may be associated with an increase in bleeding).
No products indexed under this heading.

Reteplase (Co-administration with thrombolytics may be associated with an increase in bleeding).
No products indexed under this heading.

Rofecoxib (Co-administration with antiplatelet agents, such as non-steroidal anti-inflammatory agents, may be associated with an increase in bleeding).
No products indexed under this heading.

Streptokinase (Co-administration with thrombolytics may be associated with an increase in bleeding).
No products indexed under this heading.

Sulindac (Co-administration with antiplatelet agents, such as non-steroidal anti-inflammatory agents, may be associated with an increase in bleeding). Products include:
Clinoril Tablets 1962

Ticlopidine Hydrochloride (Co-administration with antiplatelet agents, such as ticlopidine, may be associated with an increase in bleeding).
No products indexed under this heading.

Tinzaparin Sodium (Co-administration with other anticoagulant agents may be associated with an increase in bleeding).
No products indexed under this heading.

Tolmetin Sodium (Co-administration with antiplatelet agents, such as non-steroidal anti-inflammatory agents, may be associated with an increase in bleeding).
No products indexed under this heading.

Urokinase (Co-administration with thrombolytics may be associated with an increase in bleeding).
No products indexed under this heading.

Valdecoxib (Co-administration with antiplatelet agents, such as non-steroidal anti-inflammatory agents, may be associated with an increase in bleeding).
No products indexed under this heading.

Warfarin Sodium (Co-administration of oral anticoagulants within seven days is contraindicated unless prothrombin time is less than or equal to 1.2 times control; concurrent use with other anticoagulant agents may be associated with an increase in bleeding).
No products indexed under this heading.

REQUIP TABLETS

(Ropinirole Hydrochloride) 1561
May interact with benzodiazepines, butyrophenones, central nervous system depressants, cytochrome p450 1a2 inducers (selected), cytochrome p450 1a2 inhibitors (selected), antidepressant drugs, dopamine D2 antagonists, estrogens, phenothiazines, psychotropics, and certain other agents. Compounds in these categories include:

Alatrofloxacin Mesylate (In vitro metabolism studies showed that CYP1A2 is the major enzyme responsible for the metabolism of ropinirole. There is thus the potential for inducers or inhibitors of this enzyme to alter the clearance of ropinirole. Therefore, if therapy with a drug known to be a potent inducer or inhibitor of CYP1A2 is stopped or started during treatment with ropinirole, adjustment of the dose of ropinirole may be required).
No products indexed under this heading.

Alfentanil Hydrochloride (Sedating medications (such as alcohol or CNS depressants), the presence of sleeping disorders, or other medications that increase plasma levels of ropinirole, may increase the risk of somnlence or falling asleep while engaged in activities of daily living. Because of possible additive effects, caution should be advised when patients are taking other sedating medications, alcohol, or other CNS depressants (e.g., benzodiazepines, antipsychotics, antidepressants) in combination with ropinirole).
No products indexed under this heading.

Alprazolam (Sedating medications (such as alcohol or CNS depressants), the presence of sleeping disorders, or other medications that increase plasma levels of ropinirole, may increase the risk of somnlence or falling asleep while engaged in activities of daily living. Because of possible additive effects, caution should be advised when patients are taking other sedating medications, alcohol, or other CNS depressants (e.g., benzodiazepines, antipsychotics, antidepressants) in combination

with ropinirole).
No products indexed under this heading.

Amiodarone Hydrochloride (In vitro metabolism studies showed that CYP1A2 is the major enzyme responsible for the metabolism of ropinirole. There is thus the potential for inducers or inhibitors of this enzyme to alter the clearance of ropinirole. Therefore, if therapy with a drug known to be a potent inducer or inhibitor of CYP1A2 is stopped or started during treatment with ropinirole, adjustment of the dose of ropinirole may be required).
No products indexed under this heading.

Amitriptyline Hydrochloride (Because of possible additive effects, caution should be advised when patients are taking other sedating medications, alcohol, or other CNS depressants (e.g., benzodiazepines, antipsychotics, antidepressants) in combination with ropinirole).
No products indexed under this heading.

Amoxapine (Because of possible additive effects, caution should be advised when patients are taking other sedating medications, alcohol, or other CNS depressants (e.g., benzodiazepines, antipsychotics, antidepressants) in combination with ropinirole).
No products indexed under this heading.

Anastrozole (In vitro metabolism studies showed that CYP1A2 is the major enzyme responsible for the metabolism of ropinirole. There is thus the potential for inducers or inhibitors of this enzyme to alter the clearance of ropinirole. Therefore, if therapy with a drug known to be a potent inducer or inhibitor of CYP1A2 is stopped or started during treatment with ropinirole, adjustment of the dose of ropinirole may be required). Products include:
Arimidex Tablets 672

Aprobarbital (Sedating medications (such as alcohol or CNS depressants), the presence of sleeping disorders, or other medications that increase plasma levels of ropinirole, may increase the risk of somnlence or falling asleep while engaged in activities of daily living. Because of possible additive effects, caution should be advised when patients are taking other sedating medications, alcohol, or other CNS depressants (e.g., benzodiazepines, antipsychotics, antidepressants) in combination with ropinirole).
No products indexed under this heading.

Buprenorphine Hydrochloride (Sedating medications (such as alcohol or CNS depressants), the presence of sleeping disorders, or other medications that increase plasma levels of ropinirole, may increase the risk of somnlence or falling asleep while engaged in activities of daily living. Because of possible additive effects, caution should be advised when patients are taking other sedating medications, alcohol, or other CNS depressants (e.g., benzodiazepines, antipsychotics, antidepressants) in combination with ropinirole). Products include:
Suboxone Tablets 2601
Subutex Tablets 2601

Bupropion Hydrochloride (Because of possible additive effects, caution should be advised when patients are taking other sedating medications, alcohol, or other CNS depressants (e.g., benzodiazepines, antipsychotics, antidepressants) in combination with ropinirole). Products include:
Wellbutrin Tablets 1648
Wellbutrin SR Sustained-Release Tablets 1653
Wellbutrin XL Extended-Release Tablets 1659
Zyban Sustained-Release Tablets 1692

Buspirone Hydrochloride (Sedating medications (such as alcohol or CNS depressants), the presence of sleeping disorders, or other medications that increase plasma levels of ropinirole, may increase the risk of somnlence or falling asleep while engaged in activities of daily living. Because of possible additive effects, caution should be advised when patients are taking other sedating medications, alcohol, or other CNS depressants (e.g., benzodiazepines, antipsychotics, antidepressants) in combination with ropinirole).
No products indexed under this heading.

Butabarbital (Sedating medications (such as alcohol or CNS depressants), the presence of sleeping disorders, or other medications that increase plasma levels of ropinirole, may increase the risk of somnlence or falling asleep while engaged in activities of daily living. Because of possible additive effects, caution should be advised when patients are taking other sedating medications, alcohol, or other CNS depressants (e.g., benzodiazepines, antipsychotics, antidepressants) in combination with ropinirole).
No products indexed under this heading.

Butalbital (Sedating medications (such as alcohol or CNS depressants), the presence of sleeping disorders, or other medications that increase plasma levels of ropinirole, may increase the risk of somnlence or falling asleep while engaged in activities of daily living. Because of possible additive effects, caution should be advised when patients are taking other sedating medications, alcohol, or other CNS depressants (e.g., benzodiazepines, antipsychotics, antidepressants) in combination with ropinirole).
No products indexed under this heading.

Carbamazepine (In vitro metabolism studies showed that CYP1A2 is the major enzyme responsible for the metabolism of ropinirole. There is thus the potential for inducers or inhibitors of this enzyme to alter the clearance of ropinirole. Therefore, if therapy with a drug known to be a potent inducer or inhibitor of CYP1A2 is stopped or started during treatment with ropinirole, adjustment of the dose of ropinirole may be required). Products include:
Carbatrol Capsules 3019
Equetro Extended-Release Capsules 3174

Chlordiazepoxide (Sedating medications (such as alcohol or CNS depressants), the presence of sleeping disorders, or other medications that increase plasma levels of ropinirole, may increase the risk of somnlence or falling asleep while engaged in activities of daily living. Because of possible additive effects, caution should be advised when patients are taking other sedating medications, alcohol, or other CNS depressants (e.g., benzodiazepines, antipsychotics, antidepressants) in combination with ropinirole).
No products indexed under this heading.

Chlordiazepoxide Hydrochloride (Sedating medications (such as alcohol or CNS depressants), the presence of sleeping disorders, or other medications that increase plasma levels of ropinirole, may increase the risk of somnlence or falling asleep while engaged in activities of daily living. Because of possible additive effects, caution should be advised when patients are taking other sedating medications, alcohol, or other CNS depressants (e.g., benzodiazepines, antipsychotics, antidepressants) in combination with ropinirole).
No products indexed under this heading.

Chlorotrianisene (Population pharmacokinetic analysis revealed that higher doses of estrogens (usually associated with hormone replacement therapy) reduced the oral clearance of ropinirole by approximately 35%. Dosage adjustment is not needed for initiating ropinirole in patients on estrogen therapy because patients are individually titrated with ropinirole to tolerance or adequate effect. If estrogen therapy is stopped or started during treatment with ropinirole, then adjustment of the dose of ropinirole may be required).
No products indexed under this heading.

Chlorpromazine (Sedating medications (such as alcohol or CNS depressants), the presence of sleeping disorders, or other medications that increase plasma levels of ropinirole, may increase the risk of somnlence or falling asleep while engaged in activities of daily living. Because of possible additive effects, caution should be advised when patients are taking other sedating medications, alcohol, or other CNS depressants (e.g., benzodiazepines, antipsychotics, antidepressants) in combination with ropinirole).
No products indexed under this heading.

Chlorpromazine Hydrochloride (Sedating medications (such as alcohol or CNS depressants), the presence of sleeping disorders, or other medications that increase plasma levels of ropinirole, may increase the risk of somnlence or falling asleep while engaged in activities of daily living. Because of possible additive effects, caution should be advised when patients are taking other sedating medications, alcohol, or other CNS depressants (e.g., benzodiazepines, antipsychotics, antidepressants) in combination with ropinirole).
No products indexed under this heading.

Chlorprothixene (Sedating medications (such as alcohol or CNS depressants), the presence of sleeping disorders, or other medications that increase plasma levels of ropinirole, may increase the risk of somnlence or falling asleep while engaged in activities of daily living. Because of possible additive effects, caution should be advised when patients are taking other sedating medications, alcohol, or other CNS depressants (e.g., benzodiazepines, antipsychotics, antidepressants) in combination with ropinirole).
No products indexed under this heading.

Chlorprothixene Hydrochloride (Sedating medications (such as alcohol or CNS depressants), the presence of sleeping disorders, or other medications that increase plasma levels of ropinirole, may increase the risk of somnlence or falling asleep while engaged in activities of daily living. Because of possible additive effects, caution should be advised when patients are taking other sedating medications, alcohol, or other CNS depressants (e.g., benzodiazepines, antipsychotics, antidepressants) in combination with ropinirole).
No products indexed under this heading.

Chlorprothixene Lactate (Sedating medications (such as alcohol or CNS depressants), the presence of sleeping disorders, or other medications that increase plasma levels of ropinirole, may increase the risk of somnlence or falling asleep while engaged in activities of daily living. Because of possible additive effects, caution should be advised when patients are taking other sedating medications, alcohol, or other CNS depressants (e.g., benzodiazepines, antipsychotics, antidepressants) in combination with ropinirole).
No products indexed under this heading.

Cimetidine (In vitro metabolism studies showed that CYP1A2 is the major enzyme responsible for the metabolism of ropinirole. There is thus the potential for inducers or inhibitors of this enzyme to alter the clearance of ropinirole. Therefore, if therapy with a drug known to be a potent inducer or inhibitor of CYP1A2 is stopped or started during treatment with ropinirole, adjustment of the dose of ropinirole may be required).
No products indexed under this heading.

Cimetidine Hydrochloride (In vitro metabolism studies showed that CYP1A2 is the major enzyme responsible for the metabolism of ropinirole. There is thus the potential for inducers or inhibitors of this enzyme to alter the clearance of ropinirole. Therefore, if therapy with a drug known to be a potent inducer or inhibitor of CYP1A2 is stopped or started during treatment with ropinirole, adjustment of the dose of ropinirole may be required).
No products indexed under this heading.

Ciprofloxacin (In vitro metabolism studies showed that CYP1A2 is the major enzyme responsible for the metabolism of ropinirole. There is thus the potential for inducers or inhibitors of this enzyme to alter the clearance of ropinirole. Therefore, if therapy with a drug known to be a potent inducer or inhibitor of CYP1A2 is stopped or started during treatment with ropinirole, adjustment

CYP1A2 is the major enzyme responsible for the metabolism of ropinirole. There is thus the potential for inducers or inhibitors of this enzyme to alter the clearance of ropinirole. Therefore, if therapy with a drug known to be a potent inducer or inhibitor of CYP1A2 is stopped or started during treatment with ropinirole, adjustment of the dose of ropinirole may be required).

No products indexed under this heading.

Erythromycin Lactobionate (In vitro metabolism studies showed that CYP1A2 is the major enzyme responsible for the metabolism of ropinirole. There is thus the potential for inducers or inhibitors of this enzyme to alter the clearance of ropinirole. Therefore, if therapy with a drug known to be a potent inducer or inhibitor of CYP1A2 is stopped or started during treatment with ropinirole, adjustment of the dose of ropinirole may be required).

No products indexed under this heading.

Erythromycin Stearate (In vitro metabolism studies showed that CYP1A2 is the major enzyme responsible for the metabolism of ropinirole. There is thus the potential for inducers or inhibitors of this enzyme to alter the clearance of ropinirole. Therefore, if therapy with a drug known to be a potent inducer or inhibitor of CYP1A2 is stopped or started during treatment with ropinirole, adjustment of the dose of ropinirole may be required).

No products indexed under this heading.

Escitalopram Oxalate (Because of possible additive effects, caution should be advised when patients are taking other sedating medications, alcohol, or other CNS depressants (e.g., benzodiazepines, antipsychotics, antidepressants) in combination with ropinirole). Products include:

Lexapro Oral Suspension ... **1174**
Lexapro Tablets ... **1174**

Estazolam (Sedating medications (such as alcohol or CNS depressants), the presence of sleeping disorders, or other medications that increase plasma levels of ropinirole, may increase the risk of somnlence or falling asleep while engaged in activities of daily living. Because of possible additive effects, caution should be advised when patients are taking other sedating medications, alcohol, or other CNS depressants (e.g., benzodiazepines, antipsychotics, antidepressants) in combination with ropinirole).

No products indexed under this heading.

Estradiol (Population pharmacokinetic analysis revealed that higher doses of estrogens (usually associated with hormone replacement therapy) reduced the oral clearance of ropinirole by approximately 35%. Dosage adjustment is not needed for initiating ropinirole in patients on estrogen therapy because patients are individually titrated with ropinirole to tolerance or adequate effect. If estrogen therapy is stopped or started during treatment with ropinirole, then adjustment of the dose of ropinirole may be required). Products include:

Activella Tablets ... **2347**
Angeliq Tablets ... **751**
Climara Transdermal System ... **763**
Climara Pro Transdermal System ... **768**
Divigel ... **3167**
Vagifem Tablets ... **2375**

Estrogens, Conjugated (Population pharmacokinetic analysis revealed that higher doses of estrogens (usually associated with hormone replacement therapy) reduced the oral clearance of ropinirole by approximately 35%. Dosage adjustment is not needed for initiating ropinirole in patients on estrogen therapy because patients are individually titrated with ropinirole to tolerance or adequate effect. If estrogen therapy is stopped or started during treatment with ropinirole, then adjustment of the dose of ropinirole may be required). Products include:

Premarin Intravenous ... **3217**
Premarin Tablets ... **3221**
Premarin Vaginal Cream ... **3228**
Premphase Tablets ... **3232**
Prempro Tablets ... **3232**

Estrogens, Esterified (Population pharmacokinetic analysis revealed that higher doses of estrogens (usually associated with hormone replacement therapy) reduced the oral clearance of ropinirole by approximately 35%. Dosage adjustment is not needed for initiating ropinirole in patients on estrogen therapy because patients are individually titrated with ropinirole to tolerance or adequate effect. If estrogen therapy is stopped or started during treatment with ropinirole, then adjustment of the dose of ropinirole may be required). Products include:

Estratest Tablets ... **3043**
Estratest H.S. Tablets ... **3043**

Estropipate (Population pharmacokinetic analysis revealed that higher doses of estrogens (usually associated with hormone replacement therapy) reduced the oral clearance of ropinirole by approximately 35%. Dosage adjustment is not needed for initiating ropinirole in patients on estrogen therapy because patients are individually titrated with ropinirole to tolerance or adequate effect. If estrogen therapy is stopped or started during treatment with ropinirole, then adjustment of the dose of ropinirole may be required).

No products indexed under this heading.

Ethanol (Sedating medications (such as alcohol or CNS depressants), the presence of sleeping disorders, or other medications that increase plasma levels of ropinirole, may increase the risk of somnolence or falling asleep while engaged in activities of daily living. Because of possible additive effects, caution should be advised when patients are taking other sedating medications, alcohol, or other CNS depressants (e.g., benzodiazepines, antipsychotics, antidepressants) in combination with ropinirole).

No products indexed under this heading.

Ethchlorvynol (Sedating medications (such as alcohol or CNS depressants), the presence of sleeping disorders, or other medications that increase plasma levels of ropinirole, may increase the risk of somnlence or falling asleep while engaged in activities of daily living. Because of possible additive effects, caution should be advised when patients are taking other sedating medications, alcohol, or other CNS depressants (e.g., benzodiazepines, antipsychotics, antidepressants) in combination with ropinirole).

No products indexed under this heading.

Ethinamate (Sedating medications (such as alcohol or CNS depressants), the presence of sleeping disorders, or other medications that increase plasma levels of ropinirole, may increase the risk of somnlence or falling asleep while engaged in activities of daily living. Because of possible additive effects, caution should be advised when patients are taking other sedating medications, alcohol, or other CNS depressants (e.g., benzodiazepines, antipsychotics, antidepressants) in combination with ropinirole).

No products indexed under this heading.

Ethinyl Estradiol (Population pharmacokinetic analysis revealed that higher doses of estrogens (usually associated with hormone replacement therapy) reduced the oral clearance of ropinirole by approximately 35%. Dosage adjustment is not needed for initiating ropinirole in patients on estrogen therapy because patients are individually titrated with ropinirole to tolerance or adequate effect. If estrogen therapy is stopped or started during treatment with ropinirole, then adjustment of the dose of ropinirole may be required). Products include:

Lybrel Tablets ... **3204**
Mircette Tablets ... **1034**
NuvaRing ... **2897**
Ortho-Cyclen/Ortho Tri-Cyclen ... **2449**
Ortho Evra Transdermal System ... **2437**
Ortho Tri-Cyclen Lo Tablets ... **2458**
Seasonique Tablets ... **1046**
Yaz Tablets ... **805**

Ethyl Alcohol (Sedating medications (such as alcohol or CNS depressants), the presence of sleeping disorders, or other medications that increase plasma levels of ropinirole, may increase the risk of somnolence or falling asleep while engaged in activities of daily living. Because of possible additive effects, caution should be advised when patients are taking other sedating medications, alcohol, or other CNS depressants (e.g., benzodiazepines, antipsychotics, antidepressants) in combination with ropinirole).

No products indexed under this heading.

Fentanyl (Sedating medications (such as alcohol or CNS depressants), the presence of sleeping disorders, or other medications that increase plasma levels of ropinirole, may increase the risk of somnlence or falling asleep while engaged in activities of daily living. Because of possible additive effects, caution should be advised when patients are taking other sedating medications, alcohol, or other CNS depressants (e.g., benzodiazepines, antipsychotics, antidepressants) in combination with ropinirole). Products include:

Duragesic Transdermal System ... **2405**
Ionsys Transdermal System ... **2410**

Fentanyl Citrate (Sedating medications (such as alcohol or CNS depressants), the presence of sleeping disorders, or other medications that increase plasma levels of ropinirole, may increase the risk of somnlence or falling asleep while engaged in activities of daily living. Because of possible additive effects, caution should be advised when patients are taking other sedating medications; alcohol, or other CNS depressants (e.g., benzodiazepines, antipsychotics, antidepressants) in combination with ropinirole). Products include:

Actiq ... **959**
Fentora Tablets ... **968**

Fluoxetine Hydrochloride (Because of possible additive effects, caution should be advised when patients are taking other sedating medications, alcohol, or other CNS depressants (e.g., benzodiazepines, antipsychotics, antidepressants) in combination with ropinirole). Products include:

Prozac Weekly Capsules ... **1852**
Prozac Pulvules and Liquid ... **1852**
Symbyax Capsules ... **1871**

Fluphenazine Decanoate (Sedating medications (such as alcohol or CNS depressants), the presence of sleeping disorders, or other medications that increase plasma levels of ropinirole, may increase the risk of somnlence or falling asleep while engaged in activities of daily living. Because of possible additive effects, caution should be advised when patients are taking other sedating medications, alcohol, or other CNS depressants (e.g., benzodiazepines, antipsychotics, antidepressants) in combination with ropinirole).

No products indexed under this heading.

Fluphenazine Enanthate (Sedating medications (such as alcohol or CNS depressants), the presence of sleeping disorders, or other medications that increase plasma levels of ropinirole, may increase the risk of somnlence or falling asleep while engaged in activities of daily living. Because of possible additive effects, caution should be advised when patients are taking other sedating medications, alcohol, or other CNS depressants (e.g., benzodiazepines, antipsychotics, antidepressants) in combination with ropinirole).

No products indexed under this heading.

Fluphenazine Hydrochloride (Sedating medications (such as alcohol or CNS depressants), the presence of sleeping disorders, or other medications that increase plasma levels of ropinirole, may increase the risk of somnlence or falling asleep while engaged in activities of daily living. Because of possible additive effects, caution should be advised when patients are taking other sedating medications, alcohol, or other CNS depressants (e.g., benzodiazepines, antipsychotics, antidepressants) in combination with ropinirole).

No products indexed under this heading.

Flurazepam Hydrochloride (Sedating medications (such as alcohol or CNS depressants), the presence of sleeping disorders, or other medications that increase plasma levels of ropinirole, may increase the risk of somnlence or falling asleep while engaged in activities of daily living. Because of possible additive effects, caution should be advised when patients are taking other sedating medications, alcohol, or other CNS depressants (e.g., benzodiazepines, antipsychotics, antidepressants) in combination with

ropinirole).
No products indexed under this heading.

Fluvoxamine (In vitro metabolism studies showed that CYP1A2 is the major enzyme responsible for the metabolism of ropinirole. There is thus the potential for inducers or inhibitors of this enzyme to alter the clearance of ropinirole. Therefore, if therapy with a drug known to be a potent inducer or inhibitor of CYP1A2 is stopped or started during treatment with ropinirole, adjustment of the dose of ropinirole may be required).
No products indexed under this heading.

Fluvoxamine Maleate (In vitro metabolism studies showed that CYP1A2 is the major enzyme responsible for the metabolism of ropinirole. There is thus the potential for inducers or inhibitors of this enzyme to alter the clearance of ropinirole. Therefore, if therapy with a drug known to be a potent inducer or inhibitor of CYP1A2 is stopped or started during treatment with ropinirole, adjustment of the dose of ropinirole may be required). Products include:
Luvox CR Extended-Release Capsules 1759

Gatifloxacin (In vitro metabolism studies showed that CYP1A2 is the major enzyme responsible for the metabolism of ropinirole. There is thus the potential for inducers or inhibitors of this enzyme to alter the clearance of ropinirole. Therefore, if therapy with a drug known to be a potent inducer or inhibitor of CYP1A2 is stopped or started during treatment with ropinirole, adjustment of the dose of ropinirole may be required).
No products indexed under this heading.

Gemifloxacin Mesylate (In vitro metabolism studies showed that CYP1A2 is the major enzyme responsible for the metabolism of ropinirole. There is thus the potential for inducers or inhibitors of this enzyme to alter the clearance of ropinirole. Therefore, if therapy with a drug known to be a potent inducer or inhibitor of CYP1A2 is stopped or started during treatment with ropinirole, adjustment of the dose of ropinirole may be required).
No products indexed under this heading.

Glutethimide (Sedating medications (such as alcohol or CNS depressants), the presence of sleeping disorders, or other medications that increase plasma levels of ropinirole, may increase the risk of somnlence or falling asleep while engaged in activities of daily living. Because of possible additive effects, caution should be advised when patients are taking other sedating medications, alcohol, or other CNS depressants (e.g., benzodiazepines, antipsychotics, antidepressants) in combination with ropinirole).
No products indexed under this heading.

Grepafloxacin Hydrochloride (In vitro metabolism studies showed that CYP1A2 is the major enzyme responsible for the metabolism of ropinirole. There is thus the potential for inducers or inhibitors of this enzyme to alter the clearance of ropinirole. Therefore, if therapy with a drug known to be a potent inducer or inhibitor of CYP1A2 is stopped or started during treatment with ropinirole, adjustment of the dose of ropinirole may be required).
No products indexed under this heading.

Halazepam (Because of possible additive effects, caution should be advised when patients are taking other sedating medications, alcohol, or other CNS depressants (e.g., benzodiazepines, antipsychotics, antidepressants) in combination with ropinirole).
No products indexed under this heading.

Haloperidol (Sedating medications (such as alcohol or CNS depressants), the presence of sleeping disorders, or other medications that increase plasma levels of ropinirole, may increase the risk of somnlence or falling asleep while engaged in activities of daily living. Because of possible additive effects, caution should be advised when patients are taking other sedating medications, alcohol, or other CNS depressants (e.g., benzodiazepines, antipsychotics, antidepressants) in combination with ropinirole).
No products indexed under this heading.

Haloperidol Decanoate (Sedating medications (such as alcohol or CNS depressants), the presence of sleeping disorders, or other medications that increase plasma levels of ropinirole, may increase the risk of somnlence or falling asleep while engaged in activities of daily living. Because of possible additive effects, caution should be advised when patients are taking other sedating medications, alcohol, or other CNS depressants (e.g., benzodiazepines, antipsychotics, antidepressants) in combination with ropinirole).
No products indexed under this heading.

Hydrocodone Bitartrate (Sedating medications (such as alcohol or CNS depressants), the presence of sleeping disorders, or other medications that increase plasma levels of ropinirole, may increase the risk of somnlence or falling asleep while engaged in activities of daily living. Because of possible additive effects, caution should be advised when patients are taking other sedating medications, alcohol, or other CNS depressants (e.g., benzodiazepines, antipsychotics, antidepressants) in combination with ropinirole). Products include:
Lortab 5/500 Tablets 3143
Lortab 7.5/500 Tablets 3144
Lortab 10/500 Tablets 3144
Vicodin Tablets 529
Vicodin ES Tablets 530
Vicodin HP Tablets 531
Vicoprofen Tablets 533
Zydone Tablets 1132

Hydrocodone Polistirex (Sedating medications (such as alcohol or CNS depressants), the presence of sleeping disorders, or other medications that increase plasma levels of ropinirole, may increase the risk of somnlence or falling asleep while engaged in activities of daily living. Because of possible additive effects, caution should be advised when patients are taking other sedating medications, alcohol, or other CNS depressants (e.g., benzodiazepines, antipsychotics, antidepressants) in combination with ropinirole). Products include:
Tussionex Pennkinetic Extended-Release Suspension 3154

Hydromorphone Hydrochloride (Sedating medications (such as alcohol or CNS depressants), the presence of sleeping disorders, or other medications that increase plasma levels of ropinirole, may increase the risk of somnlence or falling asleep while engaged in activities of daily living. Because of possible additive effects, caution should be advised when patients are taking other sedating medications, alcohol, or other CNS depressants (e.g., benzodiazepines, antipsychotics, antidepressants) in combination with ropinirole).
No products indexed under this heading.

Hydroxyzine Hydrochloride (Sedating medications (such as alcohol or CNS depressants), the presence of sleeping disorders, or other medications that increase plasma levels of ropinirole, may increase the risk of somnlence or falling asleep while engaged in activities of daily living. Because of possible additive effects, caution should be advised when patients are taking other sedating medications, alcohol, or other CNS depressants (e.g., benzodiazepines, antipsychotics, antidepressants) in combination with ropinirole).
No products indexed under this heading.

Hypericum (In vitro metabolism studies showed that CYP1A2 is the major enzyme responsible for the metabolism of ropinirole. There is thus the potential for inducers or inhibitors of this enzyme to alter the clearance of ropinirole. Therefore, if therapy with a drug known to be a potent inducer or inhibitor of CYP1A2 is stopped or started during treatment with ropinirole, adjustment of the dose of ropinirole may be required). Products include:
Satieté Tablets .... ▣640

Imipramine Hydrochloride (Because of possible additive effects, caution should be advised when patients are taking other sedating medications, alcohol, or other CNS depressants (e.g., benzodiazepines, antipsychotics, antidepressants) in combination with ropinirole).
No products indexed under this heading.

Imipramine Pamoate (Because of possible additive effects, caution should be advised when patients are taking other sedating medications, alcohol, or other CNS depressants (e.g., benzodiazepines, antipsychotics, antidepressants) in combination with ropinirole).
No products indexed under this heading.

Insulin (In vitro metabolism studies showed that CYP1A2 is the major enzyme responsible for the metabolism of ropinirole. There is thus the potential for inducers or inhibitors of this enzyme to alter the clearance of ropinirole. Therefore, if therapy with a drug known to be a potent inducer or inhibitor of CYP1A2 is stopped or started during treatment with ropinirole, adjustment of the dose of ropinirole may be required).
No products indexed under this heading.

Isocarboxazid (Because of possible additive effects, caution should be advised when patients are taking other sedating medications, alcohol, or other CNS depressants (e.g., benzodiazepines, antipsychotics, antidepressants) in combination with ropinirole). Products include:
Marplan Tablets 3177

Isoflurane (Sedating medications (such as alcohol or CNS depressants), the presence of sleeping disorders, or other medications that increase plasma levels of ropinirole, may increase the risk of somnlence or falling asleep while engaged in activities of daily living. Because of possible additive effects, caution should be advised when patients are taking other sedating medications, alcohol, or other CNS depressants (e.g., benzodiazepines, antipsychotics, antidepressants) in combination with ropinirole).
No products indexed under this heading.

Isoniazid (In vitro metabolism studies showed that CYP1A2 is the major enzyme responsible for the metabolism of ropinirole. There is thus the potential for inducers or inhibitors of this enzyme to alter the clearance of ropinirole. Therefore, if therapy with a drug known to be a potent inducer or inhibitor of CYP1A2 is stopped or started during treatment with ropinirole, adjustment of the dose of ropinirole may be required).
No products indexed under this heading.

Ketamine Hydrochloride (Sedating medications (such as alcohol or CNS depressants), the presence of sleeping disorders, or other medications that increase plasma levels of ropinirole, may increase the risk of somnlence or falling asleep while engaged in activities of daily living. Because of possible additive effects, caution should be advised when patients are taking other sedating medications, alcohol, or other CNS depressants (e.g., benzodiazepines, antipsychotics, antidepressants) in combination with ropinirole).
No products indexed under this heading.

Ketoconazole (In vitro metabolism studies showed that CYP1A2 is the major enzyme responsible for the metabolism of ropinirole. There is thus the potential for inducers or inhibitors of this enzyme to alter the clearance of ropinirole. Therefore, if therapy with a drug known to be a potent inducer or inhibitor of CYP1A2 is stopped or started during treatment with ropinirole, adjustment of the dose of ropinirole may be required). Products include:
Extina Foam, 2% 3057
Nizoral A-D Shampoo 1901

Lansoprazole (In vitro metabolism studies showed that CYP1A2 is the major enzyme responsible for the metabolism of ropinirole. There is thus the potential for inducers or inhibitors of this enzyme to alter the clearance of ropinirole. Therefore, if therapy with a drug known to be a potent inducer or inhibitor of CYP1A2 is stopped or started during treatment with ropinirole, adjustment of the dose of ropinirole may be

required).
No products indexed under this heading.

Levodopa (Co-administration of carbidopa+L-dopa (Sinemet) with immediate-release ropinirole had no effect on the steady-state pharmacokinetics of ropinirole. Oral administration of immediate-release ropinirole increased mean steady-state Cmax of L-dope by 20%, but its AUC was unaffected). Products include:
Stalevo Tablets **2309**

Levofloxacin (In vitro metabolism studies showed that CYP1A2 is the major enzyme responsible for the metabolism of ropinirole. There is thus the potential for inducers or inhibitors of this enzyme to alter the clearance of ropinirole. Therefore, if therapy with a drug known to be a potent inducer or inhibitor of CYP1A2 is stopped or started during treatment with ropinirole, adjustment of the dose of ropinirole may be required). Products include:
Iquix Ophthalmic Solution **3183**
Levaquin **2416**
Levaquin in 5% Dextrose Injection **2416**
Quixin Ophthalmic Solution **3184**

Levomethadyl Acetate Hydrochloride (Sedating medications (such as alcohol or CNS depressants), the presence of sleeping disorders, or other medications that increase plasma levels of ropinirole, may increase the risk of somnlence or falling asleep while engaged in activities of daily living. Because of possible additive effects, caution should be advised when patients are taking other sedating medications, alcohol, or other CNS depressants (e.g., benzodiazepines, antipsychotics, antidepressants) in combination with ropinirole).
No products indexed under this heading.

Levonorgestrel (In vitro metabolism studies showed that CYP1A2 is the major enzyme responsible for the metabolism of ropinirole. There is thus the potential for inducers or inhibitors of this enzyme to alter the clearance of ropinirole. Therefore, if therapy with a drug known to be a potent inducer or inhibitor of CYP1A2 is stopped or started during treatment with ropinirole, adjustment of the dose of ropinirole may be required). Products include:
Climara Pro Transdermal System **768**
Lybrel Tablets **3204**
Mirena Intrauterine System **779**
Plan B Tablets **1044**
Seasonique Tablets **1046**

Levorphanol Tartrate (Sedating medications (such as alcohol or CNS depressants), the presence of sleeping disorders, or other medications that increase plasma levels of ropinirole, may increase the risk of somnlence or falling asleep while engaged in activities of daily living. Because of possible additive effects, caution should be advised when patients are taking other sedating medications, alcohol, or other CNS depressants (e.g., benzodiazepines, antipsychotics, antidepressants) in combination with ropinirole).
No products indexed under this heading.

Lithium Carbonate (Because of possible additive effects, caution should be advised when patients are taking other sedating medications, alcohol, or other CNS depressants (e.g., benzodiazepines, antipsychotics, antidepressants) in combination with ropinirole).
No products indexed under this heading.

Lithium Citrate (Because of possible additive effects, caution should be advised when patients are taking other sedating medications, alcohol, or other CNS depressants (e.g., benzodiazepines, antipsychotics, antidepressants) in combination with ropinirole).
No products indexed under this heading.

Lomefloxacin Hydrochloride (In vitro metabolism studies showed that CYP1A2 is the major enzyme responsible for the metabolism of ropinirole. There is thus the potential for inducers or inhibitors of this enzyme to alter the clearance of ropinirole. Therefore, if therapy with a drug known to be a potent inducer or inhibitor of CYP1A2 is stopped or started during treatment with ropinirole, adjustment of the dose of ropinirole may be required).
No products indexed under this heading.

Lorazepam (Sedating medications (such as alcohol or CNS depressants), the presence of sleeping disorders, or other medications that increase plasma levels of ropinirole, may increase the risk of somnlence or falling asleep while engaged in activities of daily living. Because of possible additive effects, caution should be advised when patients are taking other sedating medications, alcohol, or other CNS depressants (e.g., benzodiazepines, antipsychotics, antidepressants) in combination with ropinirole).
No products indexed under this heading.

Loxapine Hydrochloride (Sedating medications (such as alcohol or CNS depressants), the presence of sleeping disorders, or other medications that increase plasma levels of ropinirole, may increase the risk of somnlence or falling asleep while engaged in activities of daily living. Because of possible additive effects, caution should be advised when patients are taking other sedating medications, alcohol, or other CNS depressants (e.g., benzodiazepines, antipsychotics, antidepressants) in combination with ropinirole).
No products indexed under this heading.

Loxapine Succinate (Sedating medications (such as alcohol or CNS depressants), the presence of sleeping disorders, or other medications that increase plasma levels of ropinirole, may increase the risk of somnlence or falling asleep while engaged in activities of daily living. Because of possible additive effects, caution should be advised when patients are taking other sedating medications, alcohol, or other CNS depressants (e.g., benzodiazepines, antipsychotics, antidepressants) in combination with ropinirole).
No products indexed under this heading.

Maprotiline Hydrochloride (Because of possible additive effects, caution should be advised when patients are taking other sedating medications, alcohol, or other CNS depressants (e.g., benzodiazepines, antipsychotics, antidepressants) in combination with ropinirole).
No products indexed under this heading.

Meperidine Hydrochloride (Sedating medications (such as alcohol or CNS depressants), the presence of sleeping disorders, or other medications that increase plasma levels of ropinirole, may increase the risk of somnlence or falling asleep while engaged in activities of daily living. Because of possible additive effects, caution should be advised when patients are taking other sedating medications, alcohol, or other CNS depressants (e.g., benzodiazepines, antipsychotics, antidepressants) in combination with ropinirole).
No products indexed under this heading.

Mephobarbital (Sedating medications (such as alcohol or CNS depressants), the presence of sleeping disorders, or other medications that increase plasma levels of ropinirole, may increase the risk of somnlence or falling asleep while engaged in activities of daily living. Because of possible additive effects, caution should be advised when patients are taking other sedating medications, alcohol, or other CNS depressants (e.g., benzodiazepines, antipsychotics, antidepressants) in combination with ropinirole).
No products indexed under this heading.

Meprobamate (Sedating medications (such as alcohol or CNS depressants), the presence of sleeping disorders, or other medications that increase plasma levels of ropinirole, may increase the risk of somnlence or falling asleep while engaged in activities of daily living. Because of possible additive effects, caution should be advised when patients are taking other sedating medications, alcohol, or other CNS depressants (e.g., benzodiazepines, antipsychotics, antidepressants) in combination with ropinirole).
No products indexed under this heading.

Mesoridazine Besylate (Sedating medications (such as alcohol or CNS depressants), the presence of sleeping disorders, or other medications that increase plasma levels of ropinirole, may increase the risk of somnlence or falling asleep while engaged in activities of daily living. Because of possible additive effects, caution should be advised when patients are taking other sedating medications, alcohol, or other CNS depressants (e.g., benzodiazepines, antipsychotics, antidepressants) in combination with ropinirole).
No products indexed under this heading.

Mestranol (In vitro metabolism studies showed that CYP1A2 is the major enzyme responsible for the metabolism of ropinirole. There is thus the potential for inducers or inhibitors of this enzyme to alter the clearance of ropinirole. Therefore, if therapy with a drug known to be a potent inducer or inhibitor of CYP1A2 is stopped or started during treatment with ropinirole, adjustment of the dose of ropinirole may be required).
No products indexed under this heading.

Methadone Hydrochloride (Sedating medications (such as alcohol or CNS depressants), the presence of sleeping disorders, or other medications that increase plasma levels of ropinirole, may increase the risk of somnlence or falling asleep while engaged in activities of daily living. Because of possible additive effects, caution should be advised when patients are taking other sedating medications, alcohol, or other CNS depressants (e.g., benzodiazepines, antipsychotics, antidepressants) in combination with ropinirole).
No products indexed under this heading.

Methohexital Sodium (Sedating medications (such as alcohol or CNS depressants), the presence of sleeping disorders, or other medications that increase plasma levels of ropinirole, may increase the risk of somnlence or falling asleep while engaged in activities of daily living. Because of possible additive effects, caution should be advised when patients are taking other sedating medications, alcohol, or other CNS depressants (e.g., benzodiazepines, antipsychotics, antidepressants) in combination with ropinirole).
No products indexed under this heading.

Methotrimeprazine (Sedating medications (such as alcohol or CNS depressants), the presence of sleeping disorders, or other medications that increase plasma levels of ropinirole, may increase the risk of somnlence or falling asleep while engaged in activities of daily living. Because of possible additive effects, caution should be advised when patients are taking other sedating medications, alcohol, or other CNS depressants (e.g., benzodiazepines, antipsychotics, antidepressants) in combination with ropinirole).
No products indexed under this heading.

Methoxsalen (In vitro metabolism studies showed that CYP1A2 is the major enzyme responsible for the metabolism of ropinirole. There is thus the potential for inducers or inhibitors of this enzyme to alter the clearance of ropinirole. Therefore, if therapy with a drug known to be a potent inducer or inhibitor of CYP1A2 is stopped or started during treatment with ropinirole, adjustment of the dose of ropinirole may be required).
No products indexed under this heading.

Methoxyflurane (Sedating medications (such as alcohol or CNS depressants), the presence of sleeping disorders, or other medications that increase plasma levels of ropinirole, may increase the risk of somnlence or falling asleep while engaged in activities of daily living. Because of possible additive effects, caution should be advised when patients are taking other sedating medications, alcohol, or other CNS depressants (e.g., benzodiazepines, antipsychotics, antidepressants) in combination

with ropinirole).
No products indexed under this heading.

Metoclopramide Hydrochloride (Since ropinirole is a dopamine agonist, it is possible that dopamine antagonists such as neuroleptics (e.g., phenothiazines, butyrophenones, thioxanthenes) or metoclopramide hydrochloride may diminish the effectiveness of ropinirole. Patients with a history or presence of major psychotic disorders should be treated with dopamine agonists only if the potential benefits outweigh the risks).
No products indexed under this heading.

Mexiletine Hydrochloride (In vitro metabolism studies showed that CYP1A2 is the major enzyme responsible for the metabolism of ropinirole. There is thus the potential for inducers or inhibitors of this enzyme to alter the clearance of ropinirole. Therefore, if therapy with a drug known to be a potent inducer or inhibitor of CYP1A2 is stopped or started during treatment with ropinirole, adjustment of the dose of ropinirole may be required).
No products indexed under this heading.

Mibefradil Dihydrochloride (In vitro metabolism studies showed that CYP1A2 is the major enzyme responsible for the metabolism of ropinirole. There is thus the potential for inducers or inhibitors of this enzyme to alter the clearance of ropinirole. Therefore, if therapy with a drug known to be a potent inducer or inhibitor of CYP1A2 is stopped or started during treatment with ropinirole, adjustment of the dose of ropinirole may be required).
No products indexed under this heading.

Midazolam Hydrochloride (Sedating medications (such as alcohol or CNS depressants), the presence of sleeping disorders, or other medications that increase plasma levels of ropinirole, may increase the risk of somnlence or falling asleep while engaged in activities of daily living. Because of possible additive effects, caution should be advised when patients are taking other sedating medications, alcohol, or other CNS depressants (e.g., benzodiazepines, antipsychotics, antidepressants) in combination with ropinirole).
No products indexed under this heading.

Mirtazapine (Because of possible additive effects, caution should be advised when patients are taking other sedating medications, alcohol, or other CNS depressants (e.g., benzodiazepines, antipsychotics, antidepressants) in combination with ropinirole). Products include:
Remeron Tablets 2924
RemeronSolTab Tablets 2927

Molindone Hydrochloride (Sedating medications (such as alcohol or CNS depressants), the presence of sleeping disorders, or other medications that increase plasma levels of ropinirole, may increase the risk of somnlence or falling asleep while engaged in activities of daily living. Because of possible additive effects, caution should be advised when patients are taking other sedating medications, alcohol, or other CNS depressants (e.g., benzodiazepines, antipsychotics, antidepressants) in combination with ropinirole).
Products include:
Moban Tablets 1116

Morphine Sulfate (Sedating medications (such as alcohol or CNS depressants), the presence of sleeping disorders, or other medications that increase plasma levels of ropinirole, may increase the risk of somnlence or falling asleep while engaged in activities of daily living. Because of possible additive effects, caution should be advised when patients are taking other sedating medications, alcohol, or other CNS depressants (e.g., benzodiazepines, antipsychotics, antidepressants) in combination with ropinirole). Products include:
Avinza Capsules 1772
DepoDur Injection 1095
MS Contin Tablets 2585

Moxifloxacin Hydrochloride (In vitro metabolism studies showed that CYP1A2 is the major enzyme responsible for the metabolism of ropinirole. There is thus the potential for inducers or inhibitors of this enzyme to alter the clearance of ropinirole. Therefore, if therapy with a drug known to be a potent inducer or inhibitor of CYP1A2 is stopped or started during treatment with ropinirole, adjustment of the dose of ropinirole may be required). Products include:
Avelox 2803
Vigamox Ophthalmic Solution 548

Nafcillin Sodium (In vitro metabolism studies showed that CYP1A2 is the major enzyme responsible for the metabolism of ropinirole. There is thus the potential for inducers or inhibitors of this enzyme to alter the clearance of ropinirole. Therefore, if therapy with a drug known to be a potent inducer or inhibitor of CYP1A2 is stopped or started during treatment with ropinirole, adjustment of the dose of ropinirole may be required).
No products indexed under this heading.

Nalidixic Acid (In vitro metabolism studies showed that CYP1A2 is the major enzyme responsible for the metabolism of ropinirole. There is thus the potential for inducers or inhibitors of this enzyme to alter the clearance of ropinirole. Therefore, if therapy with a drug known to be a potent inducer or inhibitor of CYP1A2 is stopped or started during treatment with ropinirole, adjustment of the dose of ropinirole may be required).
No products indexed under this heading.

Nefazodone Hydrochloride (Because of possible additive effects, caution should be advised when patients are taking other sedating medications, alcohol, or other CNS depressants (e.g., benzodiazepines, antipsychotics, antidepressants) in combination with ropinirole).
No products indexed under this heading.

Nicotine (In vitro metabolism studies showed that CYP1A2 is the major enzyme responsible for the metabolism of ropinirole. There is thus the potential for inducers or inhibitors of this enzyme to alter the clearance of ropinirole. Therefore, if therapy with a drug known to be a potent inducer or inhibitor of CYP1A2 is stopped or started during treatment with ropinirole, adjustment of the dose of ropinirole may be required).
No products indexed under this heading.

Nicotine Polacrilex (In vitro metabolism studies showed that CYP1A2 is the major enzyme responsible for the metabolism of ropinirole. There is thus the potential for inducers or inhibitors of this enzyme to alter the clearance of ropinirole. Therefore, if therapy with a drug known to be a potent inducer or inhibitor of CYP1A2 is stopped or started during treatment with ropinirole, adjustment of the dose of ropinirole may be required).
No products indexed under this heading.

Nicotine Salicylate (In vitro metabolism studies showed that CYP1A2 is the major enzyme responsible for the metabolism of ropinirole. There is thus the potential for inducers or inhibitors of this enzyme to alter the clearance of ropinirole. Therefore, if therapy with a drug known to be a potent inducer or inhibitor of CYP1A2 is stopped or started during treatment with ropinirole, adjustment of the dose of ropinirole may be required).
No products indexed under this heading.

Nicotine Sulfate (In vitro metabolism studies showed that CYP1A2 is the major enzyme responsible for the metabolism of ropinirole. There is thus the potential for inducers or inhibitors of this enzyme to alter the clearance of ropinirole. Therefore, if therapy with a drug known to be a potent inducer or inhibitor of CYP1A2 is stopped or started during treatment with ropinirole, adjustment of the dose of ropinirole may be required).
No products indexed under this heading.

Norethindrone (In vitro metabolism studies showed that CYP1A2 is the major enzyme responsible for the metabolism of ropinirole. There is thus the potential for inducers or inhibitors of this enzyme to alter the clearance of ropinirole. Therefore, if therapy with a drug known to be a potent inducer or inhibitor of CYP1A2 is stopped or started during treatment with ropinirole, adjustment of the dose of ropinirole may be required). Products include:
Ortho Micronor Tablets 2446

Norfloxacin (In vitro metabolism studies showed that CYP1A2 is the major enzyme responsible for the metabolism of ropinirole. There is thus the potential for inducers or inhibitors of this enzyme to alter the clearance of ropinirole. Therefore, if therapy with a drug known to be a potent inducer or inhibitor of CYP1A2 is stopped or started during treatment with ropinirole, adjustment of the dose of ropinirole may be required). Products include:
Noroxin Tablets 2069

Norgestrel (In vitro metabolism studies showed that CYP1A2 is the major enzyme responsible for the metabolism of ropinirole. There is thus the potential for inducers or inhibitors of this enzyme to alter the clearance of ropinirole. Therefore, if therapy with a drug known to be a potent inducer or inhibitor of CYP1A2 is stopped or started during treatment with ropinirole, adjustment of the dose of ropinirole may be required).
No products indexed under this heading.

Nortriptyline Hydrochloride (Because of possible additive effects, caution should be advised when patients are taking other sedating medications, alcohol, or other CNS depressants (e.g., benzodiazepines, antipsychotics, antidepressants) in combination with ropinirole).
No products indexed under this heading.

Ofloxacin (In vitro metabolism studies showed that CYP1A2 is the major enzyme responsible for the metabolism of ropinirole. There is thus the potential for inducers or inhibitors of this enzyme to alter the clearance of ropinirole. Therefore, if therapy with a drug known to be a potent inducer or inhibitor of CYP1A2 is stopped or started during treatment with ropinirole, adjustment of the dose of ropinirole may be required). Products include:
Ofloxacin Ophthalmic Solution 0.3% .... ⊙243

Olanzapine (Sedating medications (such as alcohol or CNS depressants), the presence of sleeping disorders, or other medications that increase plasma levels of ropinirole, may increase the risk of somnlence or falling asleep while engaged in activities of daily living. Because of possible additive effects, caution should be advised when patients are taking other sedating medications, alcohol, or other CNS depressants (e.g., benzodiazepines, antipsychotics, antidepressants) in combination with ropinirole). Products include:
Symbyax Capsules 1871
Zyprexa Tablets 1883
Zyprexa IntraMuscular 1883
Zyprexa ZYDIS Orally Disintegrating Tablets 1883

Omeprazole (In vitro metabolism studies showed that CYP1A2 is the major enzyme responsible for the metabolism of ropinirole. There is thus the potential for inducers or inhibitors of this enzyme to alter the clearance of ropinirole. Therefore, if therapy with a drug known to be a potent inducer or inhibitor of CYP1A2 is stopped or started during treatment with ropinirole, adjustment of the dose of ropinirole may be required).
No products indexed under this heading.

Oxazepam (Sedating medications (such as alcohol or CNS depressants), the presence of sleeping disorders, or other medications that increase plasma levels of ropinirole, may increase the risk of somnlence or falling asleep while engaged in activities of daily living. Because of possible additive effects, caution should be advised when patients are taking other sedating medications, alcohol, or other CNS depressants (e.g., benzodiazepines, antipsychotics, antidepressants) in combination with ropinirole).
No products indexed under this heading.

Oxycodone Hydrochloride (Sedating medications (such as alcohol or CNS depressants), the presence of sleeping disorders, or other medications that increase plasma

levels of ropinirole, may increase the risk of somnlence or falling asleep while engaged in activities of daily living. Because of possible additive effects, caution should be advised when patients are taking other sedating medications, alcohol, or other CNS depressants (e.g., benzodiazepines, antipsychotics, antidepressants) in combination with ropinirole). Products include:

OxyContin Tablets **2589**
OxyIR Capsules **2593**
Percocet Tablets **1127**
Percodan Tablets **1130**

Paliperidone (Because of possible additive effects, caution should be advised when patients are taking other sedating medications, alcohol, or other CNS depressants (e.g., benzodiazepines, antipsychotics, antidepressants) in combination with ropinirole). Products include:

Invega Extended-Release Tablets **1748**

Paroxetine Hydrochloride (Because of possible additive effects, caution should be advised when patients are taking other sedating medications, alcohol, or other CNS depressants (e.g., benzodiazepines, antipsychotics, antidepressants) in combination with ropinirole). Products include:

Paxil **1535**
Paxil CR Controlled-Release Tablets **1544**

Pentobarbital Sodium (Sedating medications (such as alcohol or CNS depressants), the presence of sleeping disorders, or other medications that increase plasma levels of ropinirole, may increase the risk of somnlence or falling asleep while engaged in activities of daily living. Because of possible additive effects, caution should be advised when patients are taking other sedating medications, alcohol, or other CNS depressants (e.g., benzodiazepines, antipsychotics, antidepressants) in combination with ropinirole). Products include:

Nembutal Sodium Solution, USP **2494**

Perphenazine (Sedating medications (such as alcohol or CNS depressants), the presence of sleeping disorders, or other medications that increase plasma levels of ropinirole, may increase the risk of somnlence or falling asleep while engaged in activities of daily living. Because of possible additive effects, caution should be advised when patients are taking other sedating medications, alcohol, or other CNS depressants (e.g., benzodiazepines, antipsychotics, antidepressants) in combination with ropinirole).

No products indexed under this heading.

Phenelzine Sulfate (Because of possible additive effects, caution should be advised when patients are taking other sedating medications, alcohol, or other CNS depressants (e.g., benzodiazepines, antipsychotics, antidepressants) in combination with ropinirole).

No products indexed under this heading.

Phenobarbital (Sedating medications (such as alcohol or CNS depressants), the presence of sleeping disorders, or other medications that increase plasma levels of ropinirole, may increase the risk of somnlence or falling asleep while engaged in activities of daily living. Because of possible additive effects, caution should be advised when patients are taking other sedating medications, alcohol, or other CNS depressants (e.g., benzodiazepines, antipsychotics, antidepressants) in combination with ropinirole). Products include:

Donnatal Extentabs **2507**

Phenytoin (In vitro metabolism studies showed that CYP1A2 is the major enzyme responsible for the metabolism of ropinirole. There is thus the potential for inducers or inhibitors of this enzyme to alter the clearance of ropinirole. Therefore, if therapy with a drug known to be a potent inducer or inhibitor of CYP1A2 is stopped or started during treatment with ropinirole, adjustment of the dose of ropinirole may be required).

No products indexed under this heading.

Phenytoin Sodium (In vitro metabolism studies showed that CYP1A2 is the major enzyme responsible for the metabolism of ropinirole. There is thus the potential for inducers or inhibitors of this enzyme to alter the clearance of ropinirole. Therefore, if therapy with a drug known to be a potent inducer or inhibitor of CYP1A2 is stopped or started during treatment with ropinirole, adjustment of the dose of ropinirole may be required). Products include:

Phenytek Capsules **2192**

Polyestradiol Phosphate (Population pharmacokinetic analysis revealed that higher doses of estrogens (usually associated with hormone replacement therapy) reduced the oral clearance of ropinirole by approximately 35%. Dosage adjustment is not needed for initiating ropinirole in patients on estrogen therapy because patients are individually titrated with ropinirole to tolerance or adequate effect. If estrogen therapy is stopped or started during treatment with ropinirole, then adjustment of the dose of ropinirole may be required).

No products indexed under this heading.

Prazepam (Sedating medications (such as alcohol or CNS depressants), the presence of sleeping disorders, or other medications that increase plasma levels of ropinirole, may increase the risk of somnlence or falling asleep while engaged in activities of daily living. Because of possible additive effects, caution should be advised when patients are taking other sedating medications, alcohol, or other CNS depressants (e.g., benzodiazepines, antipsychotics, antidepressants) in combination with ropinirole).

No products indexed under this heading.

Primidone (In vitro metabolism studies showed that CYP1A2 is the major enzyme responsible for the metabolism of ropinirole. There is thus the potential for inducers or inhibitors of this enzyme to alter the clearance of ropinirole. Therefore, if therapy with a drug known to be a potent inducer or inhibitor of CYP1A2 is stopped or started during treatment with ropinirole, adjustment of the dose of ropinirole may be required).

No products indexed under this heading.

Prochlorperazine (Sedating medications (such as alcohol or CNS depressants), the presence of sleeping disorders, or other medications that increase plasma levels of ropinirole, may increase the risk of somnlence or falling asleep while engaged in activities of daily living. Because of possible additive effects, caution should be advised when patients are taking other sedating medications, alcohol, or other CNS depressants (e.g., benzodiazepines, antipsychotics, antidepressants) in combination with ropinirole).

No products indexed under this heading.

Promethazine Hydrochloride (Sedating medications (such as alcohol or CNS depressants), the presence of sleeping disorders, or other medications that increase plasma levels of ropinirole, may increase the risk of somnlence or falling asleep while engaged in activities of daily living. Because of possible additive effects, caution should be advised when patients are taking other sedating medications, alcohol, or other CNS depressants (e.g., benzodiazepines, antipsychotics, antidepressants) in combination with ropinirole).

No products indexed under this heading.

Propofol (Sedating medications (such as alcohol or CNS depressants), the presence of sleeping disorders, or other medications that increase plasma levels of ropinirole, may increase the risk of somnlence or falling asleep while engaged in activities of daily living. Because of possible additive effects, caution should be advised when patients are taking other sedating medications, alcohol, or other CNS depressants (e.g., benzodiazepines, antipsychotics, antidepressants) in combination with ropinirole).

No products indexed under this heading.

Propoxyphene Hydrochloride (Sedating medications (such as alcohol or CNS depressants), the presence of sleeping disorders, or other medications that increase plasma levels of ropinirole, may increase the risk of somnlence or falling asleep while engaged in activities of daily living. Because of possible additive effects, caution should be advised when patients are taking other sedating medications, alcohol, or other CNS depressants (e.g., benzodiazepines, antipsychotics, antidepressants) in combination with ropinirole).

No products indexed under this heading.

Propoxyphene Napsylate (Sedating medications (such as alcohol or CNS depressants), the presence of sleeping disorders, or other medications that increase plasma levels of ropinirole, may increase the risk of somnlence or falling asleep while engaged in activities of daily living. Because of possible additive effects, caution should be advised when patients are taking other sedating medications, alcohol, or other CNS depressants (e.g., benzodiazepines, antipsychotics, antidepressants) in combination with ropinirole).

No products indexed under this heading.

Protriptyline Hydrochloride (Because of possible additive effects, caution should be advised when patients are taking other sedating medications, alcohol, or other CNS depressants (e.g., benzodiazepines, antipsychotics, antidepressants) in combination with ropinirole).

No products indexed under this heading.

Quazepam (Sedating medications (such as alcohol or CNS depressants), the presence of sleeping disorders, or other medications that increase plasma levels of ropinirole, may increase the risk of somnlence or falling asleep while engaged in activities of daily living. Because of possible additive effects, caution should be advised when patients are taking other sedating medications, alcohol, or other CNS depressants (e.g., benzodiazepines, antipsychotics, antidepressants) in combination with ropinirole).

No products indexed under this heading.

Quetiapine Fumarate (Sedating medications (such as alcohol or CNS depressants), the presence of sleeping disorders, or other medications that increase plasma levels of ropinirole, may increase the risk of somnlence or falling asleep while engaged in activities of daily living. Because of possible additive effects, caution should be advised when patients are taking other sedating medications, alcohol, or other CNS depressants (e.g., benzodiazepines, antipsychotics, antidepressants) in combination with ropinirole).

No products indexed under this heading.

Quinestrol (Population pharmacokinetic analysis revealed that higher doses of estrogens (usually associated with hormone replacement therapy) reduced the oral clearance of ropinirole by approximately 35%. Dosage adjustment is not needed for initiating ropinirole in patients on estrogen therapy because patients are individually titrated with ropinirole to tolerance or adequate effect. If estrogen therapy is stopped or started during treatment with ropinirole, then adjustment of the dose of ropinirole may be required).

No products indexed under this heading.

Ranitidine Hydrochloride (In vitro metabolism studies showed that CYP1A2 is the major enzyme responsible for the metabolism of ropinirole. There is thus the potential for inducers or inhibitors of this enzyme to alter the clearance of ropinirole. Therefore, if therapy with a drug known to be a potent inducer or inhibitor of CYP1A2 is stopped or started during treatment with ropinirole, adjustment of the dose of ropinirole may be required). Products include:

Zantac 75 Tablets **603**
Zantac **1670**
Zantac Injection **1666**
Zantac Injection Pharmacy Bulk Package **1668**
Maximum Strength Zantac 150 Tablets **603**
Maximum Strength Zantac 150 Cool Mint Tablets **603**

Remifentanil Hydrochloride (Sedating medications (such as alcohol or CNS depressants), the pres-

ence of sleeping disorders, or other medications that increase plasma levels of ropinirole, may increase the risk of somnlence or falling asleep while engaged in activities of daily living. Because of possible additive effects, caution should be advised when patients are taking other sedating medications, alcohol, or other CNS depressants (e.g., benzodiazepines, antipsychotics, antidepressants) in combination with ropinirole).

No products indexed under this heading.

Rifampicin (In vitro metabolism studies showed that CYP1A2 is the major enzyme responsible for the metabolism of ropinirole. There is thus the potential for inducers or inhibitors of this enzyme to alter the clearance of ropinirole. Therefore, if therapy with a drug known to be a potent inducer or inhibitor of CYP1A2 is stopped or started during treatment with ropinirole, adjustment of the dose of ropinirole may be required).

No products indexed under this heading.

Rifampin (In vitro metabolism studies showed that CYP1A2 is the major enzyme responsible for the metabolism of ropinirole. There is thus the potential for inducers or inhibitors of this enzyme to alter the clearance of ropinirole. Therefore, if therapy with a drug known to be a potent inducer or inhibitor of CYP1A2 is stopped or started during treatment with ropinirole, adjustment of the dose of ropinirole may be required).

No products indexed under this heading.

Risperidone (Sedating medications (such as alcohol or CNS depressants), the presence of sleeping disorders, or other medications that increase plasma levels of ropinirole, may increase the risk of somnlence or falling asleep while engaged in activities of daily living. Because of possible additive effects, caution should be advised when patients are taking other sedating medications, alcohol, or other CNS depressants (e.g., benzodiazepines, antipsychotics, antidepressants) in combination with ropinirole). Products include:

Risperdal Consta Long-Acting Injection 1753

Ritonavir (In vitro metabolism studies showed that CYP1A2 is the major enzyme responsible for the metabolism of ropinirole. There is thus the potential for inducers or inhibitors of this enzyme to alter the clearance of ropinirole. Therefore, if therapy with a drug known to be a potent inducer or inhibitor of CYP1A2 is stopped or started during treatment with ropinirole, adjustment of the dose of ropinirole may be required). Products include:

Kaletra 452
Norvir 489

Secobarbital Sodium (Sedating medications (such as alcohol or CNS depressants), the presence of sleeping disorders, or other medications that increase plasma levels of ropinirole, may increase the risk of somnlence or falling asleep while engaged in activities of daily living. Because of possible additive effects, caution should be advised when patients are taking other sedating medications, alcohol, or other CNS depressants (e.g., benzodiazepines, antipsychotics, antidepressants) in combination with ropinirole).

No products indexed under this heading.

Selegiline (Because of possible additive effects, caution should be advised when patients are taking other sedating medications, alcohol, or other CNS depressants (e.g., benzodiazepines, antipsychotics, antidepressants) in combination with ropinirole). Products include:

Emsam Transdermal System 905

Selegiline Hydrochloride (Because of possible additive effects, caution should be advised when patients are taking other sedating medications, alcohol, or other CNS depressants (e.g., benzodiazepines, antipsychotics, antidepressants) in combination with ropinirole). Products include:

Eldepryl Capsules 3052

Sertraline Hydrochloride (Because of possible additive effects, caution should be advised when patients are taking other sedating medications, alcohol, or other CNS depressants (e.g., benzodiazepines, antipsychotics, antidepressants) in combination with ropinirole).

No products indexed under this heading.

Sevoflurane (Sedating medications (such as alcohol or CNS depressants), the presence of sleeping disorders, or other medications that increase plasma levels of ropinirole, may increase the risk of somnlence or falling asleep while engaged in activities of daily living. Because of possible additive effects, caution should be advised when patients are taking other sedating medications, alcohol, or other CNS depressants (e.g., benzodiazepines, antipsychotics, antidepressants) in combination with ropinirole). Products include:

Ultane Liquid for Inhalation 524

Sildenafil Citrate (In vitro metabolism studies showed that CYP1A2 is the major enzyme responsible for the metabolism of ropinirole. There is thus the potential for inducers or inhibitors of this enzyme to alter the clearance of ropinirole. Therefore, if therapy with a drug known to be a potent inducer or inhibitor of CYP1A2 is stopped or started during treatment with ropinirole, adjustment of the dose of ropinirole may be required).

No products indexed under this heading.

Sodium Oxybate (Sedating medications (such as alcohol or CNS depressants), the presence of sleeping disorders, or other medications that increase plasma levels of ropinirole, may increase the risk of somnlence or falling asleep while engaged in activities of daily living. Because of possible additive effects, caution should be advised when patients are taking other sedating medications, alcohol, or other CNS depressants (e.g., benzodiazepines, antipsychotics, antidepressants) in combination with ropinirole). Products include:

Xyrem Oral Solution 1766

Sparfloxacin (In vitro metabolism studies showed that CYP1A2 is the major enzyme responsible for the metabolism of ropinirole. There is thus the potential for inducers or inhibitors of this enzyme to alter the clearance of ropinirole. Therefore, if therapy with a drug known to be a potent inducer or inhibitor of CYP1A2 is stopped or started during treatment with ropinirole, adjustment of the dose of ropinirole may be required).

No products indexed under this heading.

Sufentanil Citrate (Sedating medications (such as alcohol or CNS depressants), the presence of sleeping disorders, or other medications that increase plasma levels of ropinirole, may increase the risk of somnlence or falling asleep while engaged in activities of daily living. Because of possible additive effects, caution should be advised when patients are taking other sedating medications, alcohol, or other CNS depressants (e.g., benzodiazepines, antipsychotics, antidepressants) in combination with ropinirole).

No products indexed under this heading.

Tacrine Hydrochloride (In vitro metabolism studies showed that CYP1A2 is the major enzyme responsible for the metabolism of ropinirole. There is thus the potential for inducers or inhibitors of this enzyme to alter the clearance of ropinirole. Therefore, if therapy with a drug known to be a potent inducer or inhibitor of CYP1A2 is stopped or started during treatment with ropinirole, adjustment of the dose of ropinirole may be required).

No products indexed under this heading.

Temazepam (Sedating medications (such as alcohol or CNS depressants), the presence of sleeping disorders, or other medications that increase plasma levels of ropinirole, may increase the risk of somnlence or falling asleep while engaged in activities of daily living. Because of possible additive effects, caution should be advised when patients are taking other sedating medications, alcohol, or other CNS depressants (e.g., benzodiazepines, antipsychotics, antidepressants) in combination with ropinirole).

No products indexed under this heading.

Thiamylal Sodium (Sedating medications (such as alcohol or CNS depressants), the presence of sleeping disorders, or other medications that increase plasma levels of ropinirole, may increase the risk of somnlence or falling asleep while engaged in activities of daily living. Because of possible additive effects, caution should be advised when patients are taking other sedating medications, alcohol, or other CNS depressants (e.g., benzodiazepines, antipsychotics, antidepressants) in combination with ropinirole).

No products indexed under this heading.

Thioridazine Hydrochloride (Sedating medications (such as alcohol or CNS depressants), the presence of sleeping disorders, or other medications that increase plasma levels of ropinirole, may increase the risk of somnlence or falling asleep while engaged in activities of daily living. Because of possible additive effects, caution should be advised when patients are taking other sedating medications, alcohol, or other CNS depressants (e.g., benzodiazepines, antipsychotics, antidepressants) in combination with ropinirole). Products include:

Thioridazine Hydrochloride Tablets 2195

Thiothixene (Sedating medications (such as alcohol or CNS depressants), the presence of sleeping disorders, or other medications that increase plasma levels of ropinirole, may increase the risk of somnlence or falling asleep while engaged in activities of daily living. Because of possible additive effects, caution should be advised when patients are taking other sedating medications, alcohol, or other CNS depressants (e.g., benzodiazepines, antipsychotics, antidepressants) in combination with ropinirole). Products include:

Thiothixene Capsules 2197

Ticlopidine Hydrochloride (In vitro metabolism studies showed that CYP1A2 is the major enzyme responsible for the metabolism of ropinirole. There is thus the potential for inducers or inhibitors of this enzyme to alter the clearance of ropinirole. Therefore, if therapy with a drug known to be a potent inducer or inhibitor of CYP1A2 is stopped or started during treatment with ropinirole, adjustment of the dose of ropinirole may be required).

No products indexed under this heading.

Tobacco (Cigarette smoking is expected to increase the clearance of ropinirole since CYP1A2 is known to be induced by smoking. In one study in patients with restless legs syndrome, cigarette smokers had an approximate 30% lower Cmax and a 38% lower AUC than nonsmokers, when those parameters were normalized for dose).

No products indexed under this heading.

Tranylcypromine Sulfate (Because of possible additive effects, caution should be advised when patients are taking other sedating medications, alcohol, or other CNS depressants (e.g., benzodiazepines, antipsychotics, antidepressants) in combination with ropinirole). Products include:

Parnate Tablets 1532

Trazodone Hydrochloride (Because of possible additive effects, caution should be advised when patients are taking other sedating medications, alcohol, or other CNS depressants (e.g., benzodiazepines, antipsychotics, antidepressants) in combination with ropinirole).

No products indexed under this heading.

Triazolam (Sedating medications (such as alcohol or CNS depressants), the presence of sleeping disorders, or other medications that increase plasma levels of ropinirole, may increase the risk of somnlence or falling asleep while engaged in activities of daily living. Because of possible additive effects, caution should be advised when patients are taking other sedating medications, alcohol, or other CNS depressants (e.g., benzodiazepines, antipsychotics, antidepressants) in combination with ropinirole).

No products indexed under this heading.

Trifluoperazine Hydrochloride (Sedating medications (such as alco-

hol or CNS depressants), the presence of sleeping disorders, or other medications that increase plasma levels of ropinirole, may increase the risk of somnlence or falling asleep while engaged in activities of daily living. Because of possible additive effects, caution should be advised when patients are taking other sedating medications, alcohol, or other CNS depressants (e.g., benzodiazepines, antipsychotics, antidepressants) in combination with ropinirole).
No products indexed under this heading.

Trimipramine Maleate (Because of possible additive effects, caution should be advised when patients are taking other sedating medications, alcohol, or other CNS depressants (e.g., benzodiazepines, antipsychotics, antidepressants) in combination with ropinirole).
No products indexed under this heading.

Troleandomycin (In vitro metabolism studies showed that CYP1A2 is the major enzyme responsible for the metabolism of ropinirole. There is thus the potential for inducers or inhibitors of this enzyme to alter the clearance of ropinirole. Therefore, if therapy with a drug known to be a potent inducer or inhibitor of CYP1A2 is stopped or started during treatment with ropinirole, adjustment of the dose of ropinirole may be required).
No products indexed under this heading.

Trovafloxacin Mesylate (In vitro metabolism studies showed that CYP1A2 is the major enzyme responsible for the metabolism of ropinirole. There is thus the potential for inducers or inhibitors of this enzyme to alter the clearance of ropinirole. Therefore, if therapy with a drug known to be a potent inducer or inhibitor of CYP1A2 is stopped or started during treatment with ropinirole, adjustment of the dose of ropinirole may be required).
No products indexed under this heading.

Vardenafil Hydrochloride (In vitro metabolism studies showed that CYP1A2 is the major enzyme responsible for the metabolism of ropinirole. There is thus the potential for inducers or inhibitors of this enzyme to alter the clearance of ropinirole. Therefore, if therapy with a drug known to be a potent inducer or inhibitor of CYP1A2 is stopped or started during treatment with ropinirole, adjustment of the dose of ropinirole may be required). Products include:
Levitra Tablets 2876

Venlafaxine Hydrochloride (Because of possible additive effects, caution should be advised when patients are taking other sedating medications, alcohol, or other CNS depressants (e.g., benzodiazepines, antipsychotics, antidepressants) in combination with ropinirole). Products include:
Effexor XR Extended-Release Capsules 3195
Venlafaxine Hydrochloride Tablets ... 2199

Zaleplon (Sedating medications (such as alcohol or CNS depressants), the presence of sleeping disorders, or other medications that increase plasma levels of ropinirole, may increase the risk of somnlence or falling asleep while engaged in activities of daily living. Because of possible additive effects, caution should be advised when patients are taking other sedating medications, alcohol, or other CNS depressants (e.g., benzodiazepines, antipsychotics, antidepressants) in combination with ropinirole).
No products indexed under this heading.

Zileuton (In vitro metabolism studies showed that CYP1A2 is the major enzyme responsible for the metabolism of ropinirole. There is thus the potential for inducers or inhibitors of this enzyme to alter the clearance of ropinirole. Therefore, if therapy with a drug known to be a potent inducer or inhibitor of CYP1A2 is stopped or started during treatment with ropinirole, adjustment of the dose of ropinirole may be required).
No products indexed under this heading.

Ziprasidone Hydrochloride (Sedating medications (such as alcohol or CNS depressants), the presence of sleeping disorders, or other medications that increase plasma levels of ropinirole, may increase the risk of somnlence or falling asleep while engaged in activities of daily living. Because of possible additive effects, caution should be advised when patients are taking other sedating medications, alcohol, or other CNS depressants (e.g., benzodiazepines, antipsychotics, antidepressants) in combination with ropinirole). Products include:
Geodon Capsules 2520

Zolpidem Tartrate (Sedating medications (such as alcohol or CNS depressants), the presence of sleeping disorders, or other medications that increase plasma levels of ropinirole, may increase the risk of somnlence or falling asleep while engaged in activities of daily living. Because of possible additive effects, caution should be advised when patients are taking other sedating medications, alcohol, or other CNS depressants (e.g., benzodiazepines, antipsychotics, antidepressants) in combination with ropinirole). Products include:
Ambien Tablets 2692
Ambien CR Tablets 2696

Food Interactions

Alcohol (Sedating medications (such as alcohol or CNS depressants), the presence of sleeping disorders, or other medications that increase plasma levels of ropinirole, may increase the risk of somnolence or falling asleep while engaged in activities of daily living. Because of possible additive effects, caution should be advised when patients are taking other sedating medications, alcohol, or other CNS depressants (e.g., benzodiazepines, antipsychotics, antidepressants) in combination with ropinirole).

Broccoli (In vitro metabolism studies showed that CYP1A2 is the major enzyme responsible for the metabolism of ropinirole. There is thus the potential for inducers or inhibitors of this enzyme to alter the clearance of ropinirole. Therefore, if therapy with a drug known to be a potent inducer or inhibitor of CYP1A2 is stopped or started during treatment with ropinirole, adjustment of the dose of ropinirole may be required).

Brussel Sprouts (In vitro metabolism studies showed that CYP1A2 is the major enzyme responsible for the metabolism of ropinirole. There is thus the potential for inducers or inhibitors of this enzyme to alter the clearance of ropinirole. Therefore, if therapy with a drug known to be a potent inducer or inhibitor of CYP1A2 is stopped or started during treatment with ropinirole, adjustment of the dose of ropinirole may be required).

Charbroiled Food (In vitro metabolism studies showed that CYP1A2 is the major enzyme responsible for the metabolism of ropinirole. There is thus the potential for inducers or inhibitors of this enzyme to alter the clearance of ropinirole. Therefore, if therapy with a drug known to be a potent inducer or inhibitor of CYP1A2 is stopped or started during treatment with ropinirole, adjustment of the dose of ropinirole may be required).

Food, unspecified (Food does not affect the extent of absorption of ropinirole, although its Tmax is increased by two and a half hours and its Cmax is decreased by approximately 25% when the drug is taken with a high-fat meal).

Grapefruit Juice (In vitro metabolism studies showed that CYP1A2 is the major enzyme responsible for the metabolism of ropinirole. There is thus the potential for inducers or inhibitors of this enzyme to alter the clearance of ropinirole. Therefore, if therapy with a drug known to be a potent inducer or inhibitor of CYP1A2 is stopped or started during treatment with ropinirole, adjustment of the dose of ropinirole may be required).

REQUIP XL TABLETS

(Ropinirole Hydrochloride) 1568
May interact with benzodiazepines, butyrophenones, central nervous system depressants, cytochrome p450 1a2 inducers (selected), cytochrome p450 1a2 inhibitors (selected), antidepressant drugs, dopamine D2 antagonists, estrogens, phenothiazines, psychotropics, and certain other agents. Compounds in these categories include:

Alatrofloxacin Mesylate (In vitro metabolism studies showed that CYP1A2 is the major enzyme responsible for the metabolism of ropinirole. There is thus the potential for inducers or inhibitors of this enzyme to alter the clearance of ropinirole. Therefore, if therapy with a drug known to be a potent inducer or inhibitor of CYP1A2 is stopped or started during treatment with ropinirole, adjustment of the dose of ropinirole may be required).
No products indexed under this heading.

Alfentanil Hydrochloride (Sedating medications (such as alcohol or CNS depressants), the presence of sleeping disorders, or other medications that increase plasma levels of ropinirole, may increase the risk of somnolence or falling asleep while engaged in activities of daily living. Because of possible additive effects, caution should be advised when patients are taking other sedating medications, alcohol, or other CNS depressants (e.g., benzodiazepines, antipsychotics, antidepressants) in combination with ropinirole).
No products indexed under this heading.

Alprazolam (Sedating medications (such as alcohol or CNS depressants), the presence of sleeping disorders, or other medications that increase plasma levels of ropinirole, may increase the risk of somnlence or falling asleep while engaged in activities of daily living. Because of possible additive effects, caution should be advised when patients are taking other sedating medications, alcohol, or other CNS depressants (e.g., benzodiazepines, antipsychotics, antidepressants) in combination with ropinirole).
No products indexed under this heading.

Amiodarone Hydrochloride (In vitro metabolism studies showed that CYP1A2 is the major enzyme responsible for the metabolism of ropinirole. There is thus the potential for inducers or inhibitors of this enzyme to alter the clearance of ropinirole. Therefore, if therapy with a drug known to be a potent inducer or inhibitor of CYP1A2 is stopped or started during treatment with ropinirole, adjustment of the dose of ropinirole may be required).
No products indexed under this heading.

Amitriptyline Hydrochloride (Because of possible additive effects, caution should be advised when patients are taking other sedating medications, alcohol, or other CNS depressants (e.g., benzodiazepines, antipsychotics, antidepressants) in combination with ropinirole).
No products indexed under this heading.

Amoxapine (Because of possible additive effects, caution should be advised when patients are taking other sedating medications, alcohol, or other CNS depressants (e.g., benzodiazepines, antipsychotics, antidepressants) in combination with ropinirole).
No products indexed under this heading.

Anastrozole (In vitro metabolism studies showed that CYP1A2 is the major enzyme responsible for the metabolism of ropinirole. There is thus the potential for inducers or inhibitors of this enzyme to alter the clearance of ropinirole. Therefore, if therapy with a drug known to be a potent inducer or inhibitor of CYP1A2 is stopped or started during treatment with ropinirole, adjustment of the dose of ropinirole may be required). Products include:
Arimidex Tablets 672

Aprobarbital (Sedating medications (such as alcohol or CNS depressants), the presence of sleeping disorders, or other medications that increase plasma levels of ropinirole, may increase the risk of somnlence or falling asleep while engaged in activities of daily living. Because of possible additive effects, caution should be advised when patients are taking other sedating medications, alcohol, or other CNS depressants (e.g., benzodiazepines, antipsychotics, antidepressants) in combination with ropinirole).
No products indexed under this heading.

Buprenorphine Hydrochloride (Sedating medications (such as alcohol or CNS depressants), the presence of sleeping disorders, or other medications that increase plasma levels of ropinirole, may increase the

risk of somnlence or falling asleep while engaged in activities of daily living. Because of possible additive effects, caution should be advised when patients are taking other sedating medications, alcohol, or other CNS depressants (e.g., benzodiazepines, antipsychotics, antidepressants) in combination with ropinirole). Products include:

Suboxone Tablets 2601
Subutex Tablets 2601

Bupropion Hydrochloride (Because of possible additive effects, caution should be advised when patients are taking other sedating medications, alcohol, or other CNS depressants (e.g., benzodiazepines, antipsychotics, antidepressants) in combination with ropinirole). Products include:

Wellbutrin Tablets 1648
Wellbutrin SR Sustained-Release Tablets 1653
Wellbutrin XL Extended-Release Tablets 1659
Zyban Sustained-Release Tablets 1692

Buspirone Hydrochloride (Sedating medications (such as alcohol or CNS depressants), the presence of sleeping disorders, or other medications that increase plasma levels of ropinirole, may increase the risk of somnlence or falling asleep while engaged in activities of daily living. Because of possible additive effects, caution should be advised when patients are taking other sedating medications, alcohol, or other CNS depressants (e.g., benzodiazepines, antipsychotics, antidepressants) in combination with ropinirole).

No products indexed under this heading.

Butabarbital (Sedating medications (such as alcohol or CNS depressants), the presence of sleeping disorders, or other medications that increase plasma levels of ropinirole, may increase the risk of somnlence or falling asleep while engaged in activities of daily living. Because of possible additive effects, caution should be advised when patients are taking other sedating medications, alcohol, or other CNS depressants (e.g., benzodiazepines, antipsychotics, antidepressants) in combination with ropinirole).

No products indexed under this heading.

Butalbital (Sedating medications (such as alcohol or CNS depressants), the presence of sleeping disorders, or other medications that increase plasma levels of ropinirole, may increase the risk of somnlence or falling asleep while engaged in activities of daily living. Because of possible additive effects, caution should be advised when patients are taking other sedating medications, alcohol, or other CNS depressants (e.g., benzodiazepines, antipsychotics, antidepressants) in combination with ropinirole).

No products indexed under this heading.

Carbamazepine (In vitro metabolism studies showed that CYP1A2 is the major enzyme responsible for the metabolism of ropinirole. There is thus the potential for inducers or inhibitors of this enzyme to alter the clearance of ropinirole. Therefore, if therapy with a drug known to be a potent inducer or inhibitor of CYP1A2 is stopped or started during treatment with ropinirole, adjustment of the dose of ropinirole may be required). Products include:

Carbatrol Capsules 3019
Equetro Extended-Release Capsules 3174

Chlordiazepoxide (Sedating medications (such as alcohol or CNS depressants), the presence of sleeping disorders, or other medications that increase plasma levels of ropinirole, may increase the risk of somnlence or falling asleep while engaged in activities of daily living. Because of possible additive effects, caution should be advised when patients are taking other sedating medications, alcohol, or other CNS depressants (e.g., benzodiazepines, antipsychotics, antidepressants) in combination with ropinirole).

No products indexed under this heading.

Chlordiazepoxide Hydrochloride (Sedating medications (such as alcohol or CNS depressants), the presence of sleeping disorders, or other medications that increase plasma levels of ropinirole, may increase the risk of somnlence or falling asleep while engaged in activities of daily living. Because of possible additive effects, caution should be advised when patients are taking other sedating medications, alcohol, or other CNS depressants (e.g., benzodiazepines, antipsychotics, antidepressants) in combination with ropinirole).

No products indexed under this heading.

Chlorotrianisene (Population pharmacokinetic analysis revealed that higher doses of estrogens (usually associated with hormone replacement therapy) reduced the oral clearance of ropinirole by approximately 35%. Dosage adjustment is not needed for initiating ropinirole inpatients on estrogen therapy because patients are individually titrated with ropinirole to tolerance or adequate effect. If estrogen therapy is stopped or started during treatment with ropinirole, then adjustment of the dose of ropinirole may be required).

No products indexed under this heading.

Chlorpromazine (Sedating medications (such as alcohol or CNS depressants), the presence of sleeping disorders, or other medications that increase plasma levels of ropinirole, may increase the risk of somnlence or falling asleep while engaged in activities of daily living. Because of possible additive effects, caution should be advised when patients are taking other sedating medications, alcohol, or other CNS depressants (e.g., benzodiazepines, antipsychotics, antidepressants) in combination with ropinirole).

No products indexed under this heading.

Chlorpromazine Hydrochloride (Sedating medications (such as alcohol or CNS depressants), the presence of sleeping disorders, or other medications that increase plasma levels of ropinirole, may increase the risk of somnlence or falling asleep while engaged in activities of daily living. Because of possible additive effects, caution should be advised when patients are taking other sedating medications, alcohol, or other CNS depressants (e.g., benzodiazepines, antipsychotics, antidepressants) in combination with ropinirole).

No products indexed under this heading.

Chlorprothixene (Sedating medications (such as alcohol or CNS depressants), the presence of sleeping disorders, or other medications that increase plasma levels of ropinirole, may increase the risk of somnlence or falling asleep while engaged in activities of daily living. Because of possible additive effects, caution should be advised when patients are taking other sedating medications, alcohol, or other CNS depressants (e.g., benzodiazepines, antipsychotics, antidepressants) in combination with ropinirole).

No products indexed under this heading.

Chlorprothixene Hydrochloride (Sedating medications (such as alcohol or CNS depressants), the presence of sleeping disorders, or other medications that increase plasma levels of ropinirole, may increase the risk of somnlence or falling asleep while engaged in activities of daily living. Because of possible additive effects, caution should be advised when patients are taking other sedating medications, alcohol, or other CNS depressants (e.g., benzodiazepines, antipsychotics, antidepressants) in combination with ropinirole).

No products indexed under this heading.

Chlorprothixene Lactate (Sedating medications (such as alcohol or CNS depressants), the presence of sleeping disorders, or other medications that increase plasma levels of ropinirole, may increase the risk of somnlence or falling asleep while engaged in activities of daily living. Because of possible additive effects, caution should be advised when patients are taking other sedating medications, alcohol, or other CNS depressants (e.g., benzodiazepines, antipsychotics, antidepressants) in combination with ropinirole).

No products indexed under this heading.

Cimetidine (In vitro metabolism studies showed that CYP1A2 is the major enzyme responsible for the metabolism of ropinirole. There is thus the potential for inducers or inhibitors of this enzyme to alter the clearance of ropinirole. Therefore, if therapy with a drug known to be a potent inducer or inhibitor of CYP1A2 is stopped or started during treatment with ropinirole, adjustment of the dose of ropinirole may be required).

No products indexed under this heading.

Cimetidine Hydrochloride (In vitro metabolism studies showed that CYP1A2 is the major enzyme responsible for the metabolism of ropinirole. There is thus the potential for inducers or inhibitors of this enzyme to alter the clearance of ropinirole. Therefore, if therapy with a drug known to be a potent inducer or inhibitor of CYP1A2 is stopped or started during treatment with ropinirole, adjustment of the dose of ropinirole may be required).

No products indexed under this heading.

Ciprofloxacin (In vitro metabolism studies showed that CYP1A2 is the major enzyme responsible for the metabolism of ropinirole. There is thus the potential for inducers or inhibitors of this enzyme to alter the clearance of ropinirole. Therefore, if therapy with a drug known to be a potent inducer or inhibitor of CYP1A2 is stopped or started during treatment with ropinirole, adjustment of the dose of ropinirole may be required. Co-administration of ciprofloxacin, an inhibitor of CYP1A2, with immediate-release ropinirole increased the AUC of ropinirole by 84% on average and Cmax by 60%). Products include:

Cipro I.V. 2817
Cipro Oral Suspension 2810
Cipro XR Tablets 2823
Ciprodex Otic Suspension 541

Ciprofloxacin Hydrochloride (In vitro metabolism studies showed that CYP1A2 is the major enzyme responsible for the metabolism of ropinirole. There is thus the potential for inducers or inhibitors of this enzyme to alter the clearance of ropinirole. Therefore, if therapy with a drug known to be a potent inducer or inhibitor of CYP1A2 is stopped or started during treatment with ropinirole, adjustment of the dose of ropinirole may be required. Co-administration of ciprofloxacin, an inhibitor of CYP1A2, with immediate-release ropinirole increased the AUC of ropinirole by 84% on average and Cmax by 60%). Products include:

Cipro Tablets 2810

Citalopram Hydrobromide (Because of possible additive effects, caution should be advised when patients are taking other sedating medications, alcohol, or other CNS depressants (e.g., benzodiazepines, antipsychotics, antidepressants) in combination with ropinirole). Products include:

Celexa 1160

Clarithromycin (In vitro metabolism studies showed that CYP1A2 is the major enzyme responsible for the metabolism of ropinirole. There is thus the potential for inducers or inhibitors of this enzyme to alter the clearance of ropinirole. Therefore, if therapy with a drug known to be a potent inducer or inhibitor of CYP1A2 is stopped or started during treatment with ropinirole, adjustment of the dose of ropinirole may be required). Products include:

Biaxin/Biaxin XL 411

Clorazepate Dipotassium (Sedating medications (such as alcohol or CNS depressants), the presence of sleeping disorders, or other medications that increase plasma levels of ropinirole, may increase the risk of somnlence or falling asleep while engaged in activities of daily living. Because of possible additive effects, caution should be advised when patients are taking other sedating medications, alcohol, or other CNS depressants (e.g., benzodiazepines, antipsychotics, antidepressants) in combination with ropinirole).

No products indexed under this heading.

Clozapine (Sedating medications (such as alcohol or CNS depressants), the presence of sleeping disorders, or other medications that increase plasma levels of ropinirole, may increase the risk of somnlence

or falling asleep while engaged in activities of daily living. Because of possible additive effects, caution should be advised when patients are taking other sedating medications, alcohol, or other CNS depressants (e.g., benzodiazepines, antipsychotics, antidepressants) in combination with ropinirole).
No products indexed under this heading.

Codeine Phosphate (Sedating medications (such as alcohol or CNS depressants), the presence of sleeping disorders, or other medications that increase plasma levels of ropinirole, may increase the risk of somnlence or falling asleep while engaged in activities of daily living. Because of possible additive effects, caution should be advised when patients are taking other sedating medications, alcohol, or other CNS depressants (e.g., benzodiazepines, antipsychotics, antidepressants) in combination with ropinirole). Products include:
Tylenol with Codeine Tablets **2427**

Desflurane (Sedating medications (such as alcohol or CNS depressants), the presence of sleeping disorders, or other medications that increase plasma levels of ropinirole, may increase the risk of somnlence or falling asleep while engaged in activities of daily living. Because of possible additive effects, caution should be advised when patients are taking other sedating medications, alcohol, or other CNS depressants (e.g., benzodiazepines, antipsychotics, antidepressants) in combination with ropinirole).
No products indexed under this heading.

Desipramine Hydrochloride (Because of possible additive effects, caution should be advised when patients are taking other sedating medications, alcohol, or other CNS depressants (e.g., benzodiazepines, antipsychotics, antidepressants) in combination with ropinirole).
No products indexed under this heading.

Desogestrel (In vitro metabolism studies showed that CYP1A2 is the major enzyme responsible for the metabolism of ropinirole. There is thus the potential for inducers or inhibitors of this enzyme to alter the clearance of ropinirole. Therefore, if therapy with a drug known to be a potent inducer or inhibitor of CYP1A2 is stopped or started during treatment with ropinirole, adjustment of the dose of ropinirole may be required). Products include:
Mircette Tablets **1034**

Dezocine (Sedating medications (such as alcohol or CNS depressants), the presence of sleeping disorders, or other medications that increase plasma levels of ropinirole, may increase the risk of somnlence or falling asleep while engaged in activities of daily living. Because of possible additive effects, caution should be advised when patients are taking other sedating medications, alcohol, or other CNS depressants (e.g., benzodiazepines, antipsychotics, antidepressants) in combination with ropinirole).
No products indexed under this heading.

Diazepam (Sedating medications (such as alcohol or CNS depressants), the presence of sleeping disorders, or other medications that increase plasma levels of ropinirole, may increase the risk of somnlence or falling asleep while engaged in activities of daily living. Because of possible additive effects, caution should be advised when patients are taking other sedating medications, alcohol, or other CNS depressants (e.g., benzodiazepines, antipsychotics, antidepressants) in combination with ropinirole). Products include:
Valium Tablets **2658**

Dienestrol (Population pharmacokinetic analysis revealed that higher doses of estrogens (usually associated with hormone replacement therapy) reduced the oral clearance of ropinirole by approximately 35%. Dosage adjustment is not needed for initiating ropinirole inpatients on estrogen therapy because patients are individually titrated with ropinirole to tolerance or adequate effect. If estrogen therapy is stopped or started during treatment with ropinirole, then adjustment of the dose of ropinirole may be required).
No products indexed under this heading.

Diethylstilbestrol (Population pharmacokinetic analysis revealed that higher doses of estrogens (usually associated with hormone replacement therapy) reduced the oral clearance of ropinirole by approximately 35%. Dosage adjustment is not needed for initiating ropinirole inpatients on estrogen therapy because patients are individually titrated with ropinirole to tolerance or adequate effect. If estrogen therapy is stopped or started during treatment with ropinirole, then adjustment of the dose of ropinirole may be required).
No products indexed under this heading.

Diltiazem Hydrochloride (In vitro metabolism studies showed that CYP1A2 is the major enzyme responsible for the metabolism of ropinirole. There is thus the potential for inducers or inhibitors of this enzyme to alter the clearance of ropinirole. Therefore, if therapy with a drug known to be a potent inducer or inhibitor of CYP1A2 is stopped or started during treatment with ropinirole, adjustment of the dose of ropinirole may be required). Products include:
Cardizem LA Extended Release Tablets **421**

Diltiazem Maleate (In vitro metabolism studies showed that CYP1A2 is the major enzyme responsible for the metabolism of ropinirole. There is thus the potential for inducers or inhibitors of this enzyme to alter the clearance of ropinirole. Therefore, if therapy with a drug known to be a potent inducer or inhibitor of CYP1A2 is stopped or started during treatment with ropinirole, adjustment of the dose of ropinirole may be required).
No products indexed under this heading.

Doxepin Hydrochloride (Because of possible additive effects, caution should be advised when patients are taking other sedating medications, alcohol, or other CNS depressants (e.g., benzodiazepines, antipsychotics, antidepressants) in combination with ropinirole).
No products indexed under this heading.

Droperidol (Sedating medications (such as alcohol or CNS depressants), the presence of sleeping disorders, or other medications that increase plasma levels of ropinirole, may increase the risk of somnlence or falling asleep while engaged in activities of daily living. Because of possible additive effects, caution should be advised when patients are taking other sedating medications, alcohol, or other CNS depressants (e.g., benzodiazepines, antipsychotics, antidepressants) in combination with ropinirole).
No products indexed under this heading.

Enflurane (Sedating medications (such as alcohol or CNS depressants), the presence of sleeping disorders, or other medications that increase plasma levels of ropinirole, may increase the risk of somnlence or falling asleep while engaged in activities of daily living. Because of possible additive effects, caution should be advised when patients are taking other sedating medications, alcohol, or other CNS depressants (e.g., benzodiazepines, antipsychotics, antidepressants) in combination with ropinirole).
No products indexed under this heading.

Enoxacin (In vitro metabolism studies showed that CYP1A2 is the major enzyme responsible for the metabolism of ropinirole. There is thus the potential for inducers or inhibitors of this enzyme to alter the clearance of ropinirole. Therefore, if therapy with a drug known to be a potent inducer or inhibitor of CYP1A2 is stopped or started during treatment with ropinirole, adjustment of the dose of ropinirole may be required).
No products indexed under this heading.

Erythromycin (In vitro metabolism studies showed that CYP1A2 is the major enzyme responsible for the metabolism of ropinirole. There is thus the potential for inducers or inhibitors of this enzyme to alter the clearance of ropinirole. Therefore, if therapy with a drug known to be a potent inducer or inhibitor of CYP1A2 is stopped or started during treatment with ropinirole, adjustment of the dose of ropinirole may be required).
No products indexed under this heading.

Erythromycin Estolate (In vitro metabolism studies showed that CYP1A2 is the major enzyme responsible for the metabolism of ropinirole. There is thus the potential for inducers or inhibitors of this enzyme to alter the clearance of ropinirole. Therefore, if therapy with a drug known to be a potent inducer or inhibitor of CYP1A2 is stopped or started during treatment with ropinirole, adjustment of the dose of ropinirole may be required).
No products indexed under this heading.

Erythromycin Ethylsuccinate (In vitro metabolism studies showed that CYP1A2 is the major enzyme responsible for the metabolism of ropinirole. There is thus the potential for inducers or inhibitors of this enzyme to alter the clearance of ropinirole. Therefore, if therapy with a drug known to be a potent inducer or inhibitor of CYP1A2 is stopped or started during treatment with ropinirole, adjustment of the dose of ropinirole may be required). Products include:
E.E.S. **433**
EryPed **431**

Erythromycin Gluceptate (In vitro metabolism studies showed that CYP1A2 is the major enzyme responsible for the metabolism of ropinirole. There is thus the potential for inducers or inhibitors of this enzyme to alter the clearance of ropinirole. Therefore, if therapy with a drug known to be a potent inducer or inhibitor of CYP1A2 is stopped or started during treatment with ropinirole, adjustment of the dose of ropinirole may be required).
No products indexed under this heading.

Erythromycin Lactobionate (In vitro metabolism studies showed that CYP1A2 is the major enzyme responsible for the metabolism of ropinirole. There is thus the potential for inducers or inhibitors of this enzyme to alter the clearance of ropinirole. Therefore, if therapy with a drug known to be a potent inducer or inhibitor of CYP1A2 is stopped or started during treatment with ropinirole, adjustment of the dose of ropinirole may be required).
No products indexed under this heading.

Erythromycin Stearate (In vitro metabolism studies showed that CYP1A2 is the major enzyme responsible for the metabolism of ropinirole. There is thus the potential for inducers or inhibitors of this enzyme to alter the clearance of ropinirole. Therefore, if therapy with a drug known to be a potent inducer or inhibitor of CYP1A2 is stopped or started during treatment with ropinirole, adjustment of the dose of ropinirole may be required).
No products indexed under this heading.

Escitalopram Oxalate (Because of possible additive effects, caution should be advised when patients are taking other sedating medications, alcohol, or other CNS depressants (e.g., benzodiazepines, antipsychotics, antidepressants) in combination with ropinirole). Products include:
Lexapro Oral Suspension **1174**
Lexapro Tablets **1174**

Estazolam (Sedating medications (such as alcohol or CNS depressants), the presence of sleeping disorders, or other medications that increase plasma levels of ropinirole, may increase the risk of somnlence or falling asleep while engaged in activities of daily living. Because of possible additive effects, caution should be advised when patients are taking other sedating medications, alcohol, or other CNS depressants (e.g., benzodiazepines, antipsychotics, antidepressants) in combination with ropinirole).
No products indexed under this heading.

Estradiol (Population pharmacokinetic analysis revealed that higher doses of estrogens (usually associated with hormone replacement therapy) reduced the oral clearance of ropinirole by approximately 35%. Dosage adjustment is not needed for initiating ropinirole inpatients on estrogen therapy because patients are individually titrated with ropinirole

to tolerance or adequate effect. If estrogen therapy is stopped or started during treatment with ropinirole, then adjustment of the dose of ropinirole may be required). Products include:

Activella Tablets ... 2347
Angeliq Tablets ... 751
Climara Transdermal System ... 763
Climara Pro Transdermal System ... 768
Divigel ... 3167
Vagifem Tablets ... 2375

Estrogens, Conjugated (Population pharmacokinetic analysis revealed that higher doses of estrogens (usually associated with hormone replacement therapy) reduced the oral clearance of ropinirole by approximately 35%. Dosage adjustment is not needed for initiating ropinirole inpatients on estrogen therapy because patients are individually titrated with ropinirole to tolerance or adequate effect. If estrogen therapy is stopped or started during treatment with ropinirole, then adjustment of the dose of ropinirole may be required). Products include:

Premarin Intravenous ... 3217
Premarin Tablets ... 3221
Premarin Vaginal Cream ... 3228
Premphase Tablets ... 3232
Prempro Tablets ... 3232

Estrogens, Esterified (Population pharmacokinetic analysis revealed that higher doses of estrogens (usually associated with hormone replacement therapy) reduced the oral clearance of ropinirole by approximately 35%. Dosage adjustment is not needed for initiating ropinirole inpatients on estrogen therapy because patients are individually titrated with ropinirole to tolerance or adequate effect. If estrogen therapy is stopped or started during treatment with ropinirole, then adjustment of the dose of ropinirole may be required). Products include:

Estratest Tablets ... 3043
Estratest H.S. Tablets ... 3043

Estropipate (Population pharmacokinetic analysis revealed that higher doses of estrogens (usually associated with hormone replacement therapy) reduced the oral clearance of ropinirole by approximately 35%. Dosage adjustment is not needed for initiating ropinirole inpatients on estrogen therapy because patients are individually titrated with ropinirole to tolerance or adequate effect. If estrogen therapy is stopped or started during treatment with ropinirole, then adjustment of the dose of ropinirole may be required).

No products indexed under this heading.

Ethanol (Sedating medications (such as alcohol or CNS depressants), the presence of sleeping disorders, or other medications that increase plasma levels of ropinirole, may increase the risk of somnolence or falling asleep while engaged in activities of daily living. Because of possible additive effects, caution should be advised when patients are taking other sedating medications, alcohol, or other CNS depressants (e.g., benzodiazepines, antipsychotics, antidepressants) in combination with ropinirole).

No products indexed under this heading.

Ethchlorvynol (Sedating medications (such as alcohol or CNS depressants), the presence of sleeping disorders, or other medications that increase plasma levels of ropinirole, may increase the risk of somnlence or falling asleep while engaged in activities of daily living. Because of possible additive effects, caution should be advised when patients are taking other sedating medications, alcohol, or other CNS depressants (e.g., benzodiazepines, antipsychotics, antidepressants) in combination with ropinirole).

No products indexed under this heading.

Ethinamate (Sedating medications (such as alcohol or CNS depressants), the presence of sleeping disorders, or other medications that increase plasma levels of ropinirole, may increase the risk of somnlence or falling asleep while engaged in activities of daily living. Because of possible additive effects, caution should be advised when patients are taking other sedating medications, alcohol, or other CNS depressants (e.g., benzodiazepines, antipsychotics, antidepressants) in combination with ropinirole).

No products indexed under this heading.

Ethinyl Estradiol (Population pharmacokinetic analysis revealed that higher doses of estrogens (usually associated with hormone replacement therapy) reduced the oral clearance of ropinirole by approximately 35%. Dosage adjustment is not needed for initiating ropinirole inpatients on estrogen therapy because patients are individually titrated with ropinirole to tolerance or adequate effect. If estrogen therapy is stopped or started during treatment with ropinirole, then adjustment of the dose of ropinirole may be required). Products include:

Lybrel Tablets ... 3204
Mircette Tablets ... 1034
NuvaRing ... 2897
Ortho-Cyclen/Ortho Tri-Cyclen ... 2449
Ortho Evra Transdermal System ... 2437
Ortho Tri-Cyclen Lo Tablets ... 2458
Seasonique Tablets ... 1046
Yaz Tablets ... 805

Ethyl Alcohol (Sedating medications (such as alcohol or CNS depressants), the presence of sleeping disorders, or other medications that increase plasma levels of ropinirole, may increase the risk of somnolence or falling asleep while engaged in activities of daily living. Because of possible additive effects, caution should be advised when patients are taking other sedating medications, alcohol, or other CNS depressants (e.g., benzodiazepines, antipsychotics, antidepressants) in combination with ropinirole).

No products indexed under this heading.

Fentanyl (Sedating medications (such as alcohol or CNS depressants), the presence of sleeping disorders, or other medications that increase plasma levels of ropinirole, may increase the risk of somnlence or falling asleep while engaged in activities of daily living. Because of possible additive effects, caution should be advised when patients are taking other sedating medications, alcohol, or other CNS depressants (e.g., benzodiazepines, antipsychotics, antidepressants) in combination with ropinirole). Products include:

Duragesic Transdermal System ... 2405
Ionsys Transdermal System ... 2410

Fentanyl Citrate (Sedating medications (such as alcohol or CNS depressants), the presence of sleeping disorders, or other medications that increase plasma levels of ropinirole, may increase the risk of somnlence or falling asleep while engaged in activities of daily living. Because of possible additive effects, caution should be advised when patients are taking other sedating medications, alcohol, or other CNS depressants (e.g., benzodiazepines, antipsychotics, antidepressants) in combination with ropinirole). Products include:

Actiq ... 959
Fentora Tablets ... 968

Fluoxetine Hydrochloride (Because of possible additive effects, caution should be advised when patients are taking other sedating medications, alcohol, or other CNS depressants (e.g., benzodiazepines, antipsychotics, antidepressants) in combination with ropinirole). Products include:

Prozac Weekly Capsules ... 1852
Prozac Pulvules and Liquid ... 1852
Symbyax Capsules ... 1871

Fluphenazine Decanoate (Sedating medications (such as alcohol or CNS depressants), the presence of sleeping disorders, or other medications that increase plasma levels of ropinirole, may increase the risk of somnlence or falling asleep while engaged in activities of daily living. Because of possible additive effects, caution should be advised when patients are taking other sedating medications, alcohol, or other CNS depressants (e.g., benzodiazepines, antipsychotics, antidepressants) in combination with ropinirole).

No products indexed under this heading.

Fluphenazine Enanthate (Sedating medications (such as alcohol or CNS depressants), the presence of sleeping disorders, or other medications that increase plasma levels of ropinirole, may increase the risk of somnlence or falling asleep while engaged in activities of daily living. Because of possible additive effects, caution should be advised when patients are taking other sedating medications, alcohol, or other CNS depressants (e.g., benzodiazepines, antipsychotics, antidepressants) in combination with ropinirole).

No products indexed under this heading.

Fluphenazine Hydrochloride (Sedating medications (such as alcohol or CNS depressants), the presence of sleeping disorders, or other medications that increase plasma levels of ropinirole, may increase the risk of somnlence or falling asleep while engaged in activities of daily living. Because of possible additive effects, caution should be advised when patients are taking other sedating medications, alcohol, or other CNS depressants (e.g., benzodiazepines, antipsychotics, antidepressants) in combination with ropinirole).

No products indexed under this heading.

Flurazepam Hydrochloride (Sedating medications (such as alcohol or CNS depressants), the presence of sleeping disorders, or other medications that increase plasma levels of ropinirole, may increase the risk of somnlence or falling asleep while engaged in activities of daily living. Because of possible additive effects, caution should be advised when patients are taking other sedating medications, alcohol, or other CNS depressants (e.g., benzodiazepines, antipsychotics, antidepressants) in combination with ropinirole).

No products indexed under this heading.

Fluvoxamine (In vitro metabolism studies showed that CYP1A2 is the major enzyme responsible for the metabolism of ropinirole. There is thus the potential for inducers or inhibitors of this enzyme to alter the clearance of ropinirole. Therefore, if therapy with a drug known to be a potent inducer or inhibitor of CYP1A2 is stopped or started during treatment with ropinirole, adjustment of the dose of ropinirole may be required).

No products indexed under this heading.

Fluvoxamine Maleate (In vitro metabolism studies showed that CYP1A2 is the major enzyme responsible for the metabolism of ropinirole. There is thus the potential for inducers or inhibitors of this enzyme to alter the clearance of ropinirole. Therefore, if therapy with a drug known to be a potent inducer or inhibitor of CYP1A2 is stopped or started during treatment with ropinirole, adjustment of the dose of ropinirole may be required). Products include:

Luvox CR Extended-Release Capsules ... 1759

Gatifloxacin (In vitro metabolism studies showed that CYP1A2 is the major enzyme responsible for the metabolism of ropinirole. There is thus the potential for inducers or inhibitors of this enzyme to alter the clearance of ropinirole. Therefore, if therapy with a drug known to be a potent inducer or inhibitor of CYP1A2 is stopped or started during treatment with ropinirole, adjustment of the dose of ropinirole may be required).

No products indexed under this heading.

Gemifloxacin Mesylate (In vitro metabolism studies showed that CYP1A2 is the major enzyme responsible for the metabolism of ropinirole. There is thus the potential for inducers or inhibitors of this enzyme to alter the clearance of ropinirole. Therefore, if therapy with a drug known to be a potent inducer or inhibitor of CYP1A2 is stopped or started during treatment with ropinirole, adjustment of the dose of ropinirole may be required).

No products indexed under this heading.

Glutethimide (Sedating medications (such as alcohol or CNS depressants), the presence of sleeping disorders, or other medications that increase plasma levels of ropinirole, may increase the risk of somnlence or falling asleep while engaged in activities of daily living. Because of possible additive effects, caution should be advised when patients are taking other sedating medications, alcohol, or other CNS depressants (e.g., benzodiazepines, antipsychotics, antidepressants) in combination

with ropinirole).
No products indexed under this heading.

Grepafloxacin Hydrochloride (In vitro metabolism studies showed that CYP1A2 is the major enzyme responsible for the metabolism of ropinirole. There is thus the potential for inducers or inhibitors of this enzyme to alter the clearance of ropinirole. Therefore, if therapy with a drug known to be a potent inducer or inhibitor of CYP1A2 is stopped or started during treatment with ropinirole, adjustment of the dose of ropinirole may be required).
No products indexed under this heading.

Halazepam (Because of possible additive effects, caution should be advised when patients are taking other sedating medications, alcohol, or other CNS depressants (e.g., benzodiazepines, antipsychotics, antidepressants) in combination with ropinirole).
No products indexed under this heading.

Haloperidol (Sedating medications (such as alcohol or CNS depressants), the presence of sleeping disorders, or other medications that increase plasma levels of ropinirole, may increase the risk of somnlence or falling asleep while engaged in activities of daily living. Because of possible additive effects, caution should be advised when patients are taking other sedating medications, alcohol, or other CNS depressants (e.g., benzodiazepines, antipsychotics, antidepressants) in combination with ropinirole).
No products indexed under this heading.

Haloperidol Decanoate (Sedating medications (such as alcohol or CNS depressants), the presence of sleeping disorders, or other medications that increase plasma levels of ropinirole, may increase the risk of somnlence or falling asleep while engaged in activities of daily living. Because of possible additive effects, caution should be advised when patients are taking other sedating medications, alcohol, or other CNS depressants (e.g., benzodiazepines, antipsychotics, antidepressants) in combination with ropinirole).
No products indexed under this heading.

Hydrocodone Bitartrate (Sedating medications (such as alcohol or CNS depressants), the presence of sleeping disorders, or other medications that increase plasma levels of ropinirole, may increase the risk of somnlence or falling asleep while engaged in activities of daily living. Because of possible additive effects, caution should be advised when patients are taking other sedating medications, alcohol, or other CNS depressants (e.g., benzodiazepines, antipsychotics, antidepressants) in combination with ropinirole). Products include:

Lortab 5/500 Tablets **3143**
Lortab 7.5/500 Tablets **3144**
Lortab 10/500 Tablets **3144**
Vicodin Tablets **529**
Vicodin ES Tablets **530**
Vicodin HP Tablets **531**
Vicoprofen Tablets **533**
Zydone Tablets **1132**

Hydrocodone Polistirex (Sedating medications (such as alcohol or CNS depressants), the presence of sleeping disorders, or other medications that increase plasma levels of ropinirole, may increase the risk of somnlence or falling asleep while engaged in activities of daily living. Because of possible additive effects, caution should be advised when patients are taking other sedating medications, alcohol, or other CNS depressants (e.g., benzodiazepines, antipsychotics, antidepressants) in combination with ropinirole). Products include:

Tussionex Pennkinetic Extended-Release Suspension **3154**

Hydromorphone Hydrochloride (Sedating medications (such as alcohol or CNS depressants), the presence of sleeping disorders, or other medications that increase plasma levels of ropinirole, may increase the risk of somnlence or falling asleep while engaged in activities of daily living. Because of possible additive effects, caution should be advised when patients are taking other sedating medications, alcohol, or other CNS depressants (e.g., benzodiazepines, antipsychotics, antidepressants) in combination with ropinirole).
No products indexed under this heading.

Hydroxyzine Hydrochloride (Sedating medications (such as alcohol or CNS depressants), the presence of sleeping disorders, or other medications that increase plasma levels of ropinirole, may increase the risk of somnlence or falling asleep while engaged in activities of daily living. Because of possible additive effects, caution should be advised when patients are taking other sedating medications, alcohol, or other CNS depressants (e.g., benzodiazepines, antipsychotics, antidepressants) in combination with ropinirole).
No products indexed under this heading.

Hypericum (In vitro metabolism studies showed that CYP1A2 is the major enzyme responsible for the metabolism of ropinirole. There is thus the potential for inducers or inhibitors of this enzyme to alter the clearance of ropinirole. Therefore, if therapy with a drug known to be a potent inducer or inhibitor of CYP1A2 is stopped or started during treatment with ropinirole, adjustment of the dose of ropinirole may be required). Products include:

Satieté Tablets **640**

Imipramine Hydrochloride (Because of possible additive effects, caution should be advised when patients are taking other sedating medications, alcohol, or other CNS depressants (e.g., benzodiazepines, antipsychotics, antidepressants) in combination with ropinirole).
No products indexed under this heading.

Imipramine Pamoate (Because of possible additive effects, caution should be advised when patients are taking other sedating medications, alcohol, or other CNS depressants (e.g., benzodiazepines, antipsychotics, antidepressants) in combination with ropinirole).
No products indexed under this heading.

Insulin (In vitro metabolism studies showed that CYP1A2 is the major enzyme responsible for the metabolism of ropinirole. There is thus the potential for inducers or inhibitors of this enzyme to alter the clearance of ropinirole. Therefore, if therapy with a drug known to be a potent inducer or inhibitor of CYP1A2 is stopped or started during treatment with ropinirole, adjustment of the dose of ropinirole may be required).
No products indexed under this heading.

Isocarboxazid (Because of possible additive effects, caution should be advised when patients are taking other sedating medications, alcohol, or other CNS depressants (e.g., benzodiazepines, antipsychotics, antidepressants) in combination with ropinirole). Products include:

Marplan Tablets **3177**

Isoflurane (Sedating medications (such as alcohol or CNS depressants), the presence of sleeping disorders, or other medications that increase plasma levels of ropinirole, may increase the risk of somnlence or falling asleep while engaged in activities of daily living. Because of possible additive effects, caution should be advised when patients are taking other sedating medications, alcohol, or other CNS depressants (e.g., benzodiazepines, antipsychotics, antidepressants) in combination with ropinirole).
No products indexed under this heading.

Isoniazid (In vitro metabolism studies showed that CYP1A2 is the major enzyme responsible for the metabolism of ropinirole. There is thus the potential for inducers or inhibitors of this enzyme to alter the clearance of ropinirole. Therefore, if therapy with a drug known to be a potent inducer or inhibitor of CYP1A2 is stopped or started during treatment with ropinirole, adjustment of the dose of ropinirole may be required).
No products indexed under this heading.

Ketamine Hydrochloride (Sedating medications (such as alcohol or CNS depressants), the presence of sleeping disorders, or other medications that increase plasma levels of ropinirole, may increase the risk of somnlence or falling asleep while engaged in activities of daily living. Because of possible additive effects, caution should be advised when patients are taking other sedating medications, alcohol, or other CNS depressants (e.g., benzodiazepines, antipsychotics, antidepressants) in combination with ropinirole).
No products indexed under this heading.

Ketoconazole (In vitro metabolism studies showed that CYP1A2 is the major enzyme responsible for the metabolism of ropinirole. There is thus the potential for inducers or inhibitors of this enzyme to alter the clearance of ropinirole. Therefore, if therapy with a drug known to be a potent inducer or inhibitor of CYP1A2 is stopped or started during treatment with ropinirole, adjustment of the dose of ropinirole may be required). Products include:

Extina Foam, 2% **3057**
Nizoral A-D Shampoo **1901**

Lansoprazole (In vitro metabolism studies showed that CYP1A2 is the major enzyme responsible for the metabolism of ropinirole. There is thus the potential for inducers or inhibitors of this enzyme to alter the clearance of ropinirole. Therefore, if therapy with a drug known to be a potent inducer or inhibitor of CYP1A2 is stopped or started during treatment with ropinirole, adjustment of the dose of ropinirole may be required).
No products indexed under this heading.

Levodopa (Co-administration of carbidopa+L-dopa (Sinemet) with immediate-release ropinirole had no effect on the steady-state pharmacokinetics of ropinirole. Oral administration of immediate-release ropinirole increased mean steady-state Cmax of L-dope by 20%, but its AUC was unaffected). Products include:

Stalevo Tablets **2309**

Levofloxacin (In vitro metabolism studies showed that CYP1A2 is the major enzyme responsible for the metabolism of ropinirole. There is thus the potential for inducers or inhibitors of this enzyme to alter the clearance of ropinirole. Therefore, if therapy with a drug known to be a potent inducer or inhibitor of CYP1A2 is stopped or started during treatment with ropinirole, adjustment of the dose of ropinirole may be required). Products include:

Iquix Ophthalmic Solution **3183**
Levaquin **2416**
Levaquin in 5% Dextrose Injection **2416**
Quixin Ophthalmic Solution **3184**

Levomethadyl Acetate Hydrochloride (Sedating medications (such as alcohol or CNS depressants), the presence of sleeping disorders, or other medications that increase plasma levels of ropinirole, may increase the risk of somnlence or falling asleep while engaged in activities of daily living. Because of possible additive effects, caution should be advised when patients are taking other sedating medications, alcohol, or other CNS depressants (e.g., benzodiazepines, antipsychotics, antidepressants) in combination with ropinirole).
No products indexed under this heading.

Levonorgestrel (In vitro metabolism studies showed that CYP1A2 is the major enzyme responsible for the metabolism of ropinirole. There is thus the potential for inducers or inhibitors of this enzyme to alter the clearance of ropinirole. Therefore, if therapy with a drug known to be a potent inducer or inhibitor of CYP1A2 is stopped or started during treatment with ropinirole, adjustment of the dose of ropinirole may be required). Products include:

Climara Pro Transdermal System **768**
Lybrel Tablets **3204**
Mirena Intrauterine System **779**
Plan B Tablets **1044**
Seasonique Tablets **1046**

Levorphanol Tartrate (Sedating medications (such as alcohol or CNS depressants), the presence of sleeping disorders, or other medications that increase plasma levels of ropinirole, may increase the risk of somnlence or falling asleep while engaged in activities of daily living. Because of possible additive effects, caution should be advised when patients are taking other sedating medications, alcohol, or other CNS depressants (e.g., benzodiazepines, antipsychotics, antidepressants) in combination

with ropinirole).
No products indexed under this heading.

Lithium Carbonate (Because of possible additive effects, caution should be advised when patients are taking other sedating medications, alcohol, or other CNS depressants (e.g., benzodiazepines, antipsychotics, antidepressants) in combination with ropinirole).
No products indexed under this heading.

Lithium Citrate (Because of possible additive effects, caution should be advised when patients are taking other sedating medications, alcohol, or other CNS depressants (e.g., benzodiazepines, antipsychotics, antidepressants) in combination with ropinirole).
No products indexed under this heading.

Lomefloxacin Hydrochloride (In vitro metabolism studies showed that CYP1A2 is the major enzyme responsible for the metabolism of ropinirole. There is thus the potential for inducers or inhibitors of this enzyme to alter the clearance of ropinirole. Therefore, if therapy with a drug known to be a potent inducer or inhibitor of CYP1A2 is stopped or started during treatment with ropinirole, adjustment of the dose of ropinirole may be required).
No products indexed under this heading.

Lorazepam (Sedating medications (such as alcohol or CNS depressants), the presence of sleeping disorders, or other medications that increase plasma levels of ropinirole, may increase the risk of somnlence or falling asleep while engaged in activities of daily living. Because of possible additive effects, caution should be advised when patients are taking other sedating medications, alcohol, or other CNS depressants (e.g., benzodiazepines, antipsychotics, antidepressants) in combination with ropinirole).
No products indexed under this heading.

Loxapine Hydrochloride (Sedating medications (such as alcohol or CNS depressants), the presence of sleeping disorders, or other medications that increase plasma levels of ropinirole, may increase the risk of somnlence or falling asleep while engaged in activities of daily living. Because of possible additive effects, caution should be advised when patients are taking other sedating medications, alcohol, or other CNS depressants (e.g., benzodiazepines, antipsychotics, antidepressants) in combination with ropinirole).
No products indexed under this heading.

Loxapine Succinate (Sedating medications (such as alcohol or CNS depressants), the presence of sleeping disorders, or other medications that increase plasma levels of ropinirole, may increase the risk of somnlence or falling asleep while engaged in activities of daily living. Because of possible additive effects, caution should be advised when patients are taking other sedating medications, alcohol, or other CNS depressants (e.g., benzodiazepines, antipsychotics, antidepressants) in combination with ropinirole).
No products indexed under this heading.

Maprotiline Hydrochloride (Because of possible additive effects, caution should be advised when patients are taking other sedating medications, alcohol, or other CNS depressants (e.g., benzodiazepines, antipsychotics, antidepressants) in combination with ropinirole).
No products indexed under this heading.

Meperidine Hydrochloride (Sedating medications (such as alcohol or CNS depressants), the presence of sleeping disorders, or other medications that increase plasma levels of ropinirole, may increase the risk of somnlence or falling asleep while engaged in activities of daily living. Because of possible additive effects, caution should be advised when patients are taking other sedating medications, alcohol, or other CNS depressants (e.g., benzodiazepines, antipsychotics, antidepressants) in combination with ropinirole).
No products indexed under this heading.

Mephobarbital (Sedating medications (such as alcohol or CNS depressants), the presence of sleeping disorders, or other medications that increase plasma levels of ropinirole, may increase the risk of somnlence or falling asleep while engaged in activities of daily living. Because of possible additive effects, caution should be advised when patients are taking other sedating medications, alcohol, or other CNS depressants (e.g., benzodiazepines, antipsychotics, antidepressants) in combination with ropinirole).
No products indexed under this heading.

Meprobamate (Sedating medications (such as alcohol or CNS depressants), the presence of sleeping disorders, or other medications that increase plasma levels of ropinirole, may increase the risk of somnlence or falling asleep while engaged in activities of daily living. Because of possible additive effects, caution should be advised when patients are taking other sedating medications, alcohol, or other CNS depressants (e.g., benzodiazepines, antipsychotics, antidepressants) in combination with ropinirole).
No products indexed under this heading.

Mesoridazine Besylate (Sedating medications (such as alcohol or CNS depressants), the presence of sleeping disorders, or other medications that increase plasma levels of ropinirole, may increase the risk of somnlence or falling asleep while engaged in activities of daily living. Because of possible additive effects, caution should be advised when patients are taking other sedating medications, alcohol, or other CNS depressants (e.g., benzodiazepines, antipsychotics, antidepressants) in combination with ropinirole).
No products indexed under this heading.

Mestranol (In vitro metabolism studies showed that CYP1A2 is the major enzyme responsible for the metabolism of ropinirole. There is thus the potential for inducers or inhibitors of this enzyme to alter the clearance of ropinirole. Therefore, if therapy with a drug known to be a potent inducer or inhibitor of CYP1A2 is stopped or started during treatment with ropinirole, adjustment of the dose of ropinirole may be required).
No products indexed under this heading.

Methadone Hydrochloride (Sedating medications (such as alcohol or CNS depressants), the presence of sleeping disorders, or other medications that increase plasma levels of ropinirole, may increase the risk of somnlence or falling asleep while engaged in activities of daily living. Because of possible additive effects, caution should be advised when patients are taking other sedating medications, alcohol, or other CNS depressants (e.g., benzodiazepines, antipsychotics, antidepressants) in combination with ropinirole).
No products indexed under this heading.

Methohexital Sodium (Sedating medications (such as alcohol or CNS depressants), the presence of sleeping disorders, or other medications that increase plasma levels of ropinirole, may increase the risk of somnlence or falling asleep while engaged in activities of daily living. Because of possible additive effects, caution should be advised when patients are taking other sedating medications, alcohol, or other CNS depressants (e.g., benzodiazepines, antipsychotics, antidepressants) in combination with ropinirole).
No products indexed under this heading.

Methotrimeprazine (Sedating medications (such as alcohol or CNS depressants), the presence of sleeping disorders, or other medications that increase plasma levels of ropinirole, may increase the risk of somnlence or falling asleep while engaged in activities of daily living. Because of possible additive effects, caution should be advised when patients are taking other sedating medications, alcohol, or other CNS depressants (e.g., benzodiazepines, antipsychotics, antidepressants) in combination with ropinirole).
No products indexed under this heading.

Methoxsalen (In vitro metabolism studies showed that CYP1A2 is the major enzyme responsible for the metabolism of ropinirole. There is thus the potential for inducers or inhibitors of this enzyme to alter the clearance of ropinirole. Therefore, if therapy with a drug known to be a potent inducer or inhibitor of CYP1A2 is stopped or started during treatment with ropinirole, adjustment of the dose of ropinirole may be required).
No products indexed under this heading.

Methoxyflurane (Sedating medications (such as alcohol or CNS depressants), the presence of sleeping disorders, or other medications that increase plasma levels of ropinirole, may increase the risk of somnlence or falling asleep while engaged in activities of daily living. Because of possible additive effects, caution should be advised when patients are taking other sedating medications, alcohol, or other CNS depressants (e.g., benzodiazepines, antipsychotics, antidepressants) in combination with ropinirole).
No products indexed under this heading.

Metoclopramide Hydrochloride (Since ropinirole is a dopamine agonist, it is possible that dopamine antagonists such as neuroleptics (e.g., phenothiazines, butyrophenones, thioxanthenes) or metoclopramide hydrochloride may diminish the effectiveness of ropinirole. Patients with a history or presence of major psychotic disorders should be treated with dopamine agonists only if the potential benefits outweigh the risks).
No products indexed under this heading.

Mexiletine Hydrochloride (In vitro metabolism studies showed that CYP1A2 is the major enzyme responsible for the metabolism of ropinirole. There is thus the potential for inducers or inhibitors of this enzyme to alter the clearance of ropinirole. Therefore, if therapy with a drug known to be a potent inducer or inhibitor of CYP1A2 is stopped or started during treatment with ropinirole, adjustment of the dose of ropinirole may be required).
No products indexed under this heading.

Mibefradil Dihydrochloride (In vitro metabolism studies showed that CYP1A2 is the major enzyme responsible for the metabolism of ropinirole. There is thus the potential for inducers or inhibitors of this enzyme to alter the clearance of ropinirole. Therefore, if therapy with a drug known to be a potent inducer or inhibitor of CYP1A2 is stopped or started during treatment with ropinirole, adjustment of the dose of ropinirole may be required).
No products indexed under this heading.

Midazolam Hydrochloride (Sedating medications (such as alcohol or CNS depressants), the presence of sleeping disorders, or other medications that increase plasma levels of ropinirole, may increase the risk of somnlence or falling asleep while engaged in activities of daily living. Because of possible additive effects, caution should be advised when patients are taking other sedating medications, alcohol, or other CNS depressants (e.g., benzodiazepines, antipsychotics, antidepressants) in combination with ropinirole).
No products indexed under this heading.

Mirtazapine (Because of possible additive effects, caution should be advised when patients are taking other sedating medications, alcohol, or other CNS depressants (e.g., benzodiazepines, antipsychotics, antidepressants) in combination with ropinirole). Products include:

Remeron Tablets 2924
RemeronSolTab Tablets 2927

Molindone Hydrochloride (Sedating medications (such as alcohol or CNS depressants), the presence of sleeping disorders, or other medications that increase plasma levels of ropinirole, may increase the risk of somnlence or falling asleep while engaged in activities of daily living. Because of possible additive effects, caution should be advised when

patients are taking other sedating medications, alcohol, or other CNS depressants (e.g., benzodiazepines, antipsychotics, antidepressants) in combination with ropinirole).
Products include:
Moban Tablets 1116

Morphine Sulfate (Sedating medications (such as alcohol or CNS depressants), the presence of sleeping disorders, or other medications that increase plasma levels of ropinirole, may increase the risk of somnlence or falling asleep while engaged in activities of daily living. Because of possible additive effects, caution should be advised when patients are taking other sedating medications, alcohol, or other CNS depressants (e.g., benzodiazepines, antipsychotics, antidepressants) in combination with ropinirole). Products include:
Avinza Capsules 1772
DepoDur Injection 1095
MS Contin Tablets 2585

Moxifloxacin Hydrochloride (In vitro metabolism studies showed that CYP1A2 is the major enzyme responsible for the metabolism of ropinirole. There is thus the potential for inducers or inhibitors of this enzyme to alter the clearance of ropinirole. Therefore, if therapy with a drug known to be a potent inducer or inhibitor of CYP1A2 is stopped or started during treatment with ropinirole, adjustment of the dose of ropinirole may be required). Products include:
Avelox 2803
Vigamox Ophthalmic Solution 548

Nafcillin Sodium (In vitro metabolism studies showed that CYP1A2 is the major enzyme responsible for the metabolism of ropinirole. There is thus the potential for inducers or inhibitors of this enzyme to alter the clearance of ropinirole. Therefore, if therapy with a drug known to be a potent inducer or inhibitor of CYP1A2 is stopped or started during treatment with ropinirole, adjustment of the dose of ropinirole may be required).
No products indexed under this heading.

Nalidixic Acid (In vitro metabolism studies showed that CYP1A2 is the major enzyme responsible for the metabolism of ropinirole. There is thus the potential for inducers or inhibitors of this enzyme to alter the clearance of ropinirole. Therefore, if therapy with a drug known to be a potent inducer or inhibitor of CYP1A2 is stopped or started during treatment with ropinirole, adjustment of the dose of ropinirole may be required).
No products indexed under this heading.

Nefazodone Hydrochloride (Because of possible additive effects, caution should be advised when patients are taking other sedating medications, alcohol, or other CNS depressants (e.g., benzodiazepines, antipsychotics, antidepressants) in combination with ropinirole).
No products indexed under this heading.

Nicotine (In vitro metabolism studies showed that CYP1A2 is the major enzyme responsible for the metabolism of ropinirole. There is thus the potential for inducers or inhibitors of this enzyme to alter the clearance of ropinirole. Therefore, if therapy with a drug known to be a potent inducer or inhibitor of CYP1A2 is stopped or started during treatment with ropinirole, adjustment of the dose of ropinirole may be required).
No products indexed under this heading.

Nicotine Polacrilex (In vitro metabolism studies showed that CYP1A2 is the major enzyme responsible for the metabolism of ropinirole. There is thus the potential for inducers or inhibitors of this enzyme to alter the clearance of ropinirole. Therefore, if therapy with a drug known to be a potent inducer or inhibitor of CYP1A2 is stopped or started during treatment with ropinirole, adjustment of the dose of ropinirole may be required).
No products indexed under this heading.

Nicotine Salicylate (In vitro metabolism studies showed that CYP1A2 is the major enzyme responsible for the metabolism of ropinirole. There is thus the potential for inducers or inhibitors of this enzyme to alter the clearance of ropinirole. Therefore, if therapy with a drug known to be a potent inducer or inhibitor of CYP1A2 is stopped or started during treatment with ropinirole, adjustment of the dose of ropinirole may be required).
No products indexed under this heading.

Nicotine Sulfate (In vitro metabolism studies showed that CYP1A2 is the major enzyme responsible for the metabolism of ropinirole. There is thus the potential for inducers or inhibitors of this enzyme to alter the clearance of ropinirole. Therefore, if therapy with a drug known to be a potent inducer or inhibitor of CYP1A2 is stopped or started during treatment with ropinirole, adjustment of the dose of ropinirole may be required).
No products indexed under this heading.

Norethindrone (In vitro metabolism studies showed that CYP1A2 is the major enzyme responsible for the metabolism of ropinirole. There is thus the potential for inducers or inhibitors of this enzyme to alter the clearance of ropinirole. Therefore, if therapy with a drug known to be a potent inducer or inhibitor of CYP1A2 is stopped or started during treatment with ropinirole, adjustment of the dose of ropinirole may be required). Products include:
Ortho Micronor Tablets 2446

Norfloxacin (In vitro metabolism studies showed that CYP1A2 is the major enzyme responsible for the metabolism of ropinirole. There is thus the potential for inducers or inhibitors of this enzyme to alter the clearance of ropinirole. Therefore, if therapy with a drug known to be a potent inducer or inhibitor of CYP1A2 is stopped or started during treatment with ropinirole, adjustment of the dose of ropinirole may be required). Products include:
Noroxin Tablets 2069

Norgestrel (In vitro metabolism studies showed that CYP1A2 is the major enzyme responsible for the metabolism of ropinirole. There is thus the potential for inducers or inhibitors of this enzyme to alter the clearance of ropinirole. Therefore, if therapy with a drug known to be a potent inducer or inhibitor of CYP1A2 is stopped or started during treatment with ropinirole, adjustment of the dose of ropinirole may be required).
No products indexed under this heading.

Nortriptyline Hydrochloride (Because of possible additive effects, caution should be advised when patients are taking other sedating medications, alcohol, or other CNS depressants (e.g., benzodiazepines, antipsychotics, antidepressants) in combination with ropinirole).
No products indexed under this heading.

Ofloxacin (In vitro metabolism studies showed that CYP1A2 is the major enzyme responsible for the metabolism of ropinirole. There is thus the potential for inducers or inhibitors of this enzyme to alter the clearance of ropinirole. Therefore, if therapy with a drug known to be a potent inducer or inhibitor of CYP1A2 is stopped or started during treatment with ropinirole, adjustment of the dose of ropinirole may be required). Products include:
Ofloxacin Ophthalmic Solution 0.3% .... ⊙243

Olanzapine (Sedating medications (such as alcohol or CNS depressants), the presence of sleeping disorders, or other medications that increase plasma levels of ropinirole, may increase the risk of somnlence or falling asleep while engaged in activities of daily living. Because of possible additive effects, caution should be advised when patients are taking other sedating medications, alcohol, or other CNS depressants (e.g., benzodiazepines, antipsychotics, antidepressants) in combination with ropinirole). Products include:
Symbyax Capsules 1871
Zyprexa Tablets 1883
Zyprexa IntraMuscular 1883
Zyprexa ZYDIS Orally Disintegrating Tablets 1883

Omeprazole (In vitro metabolism studies showed that CYP1A2 is the major enzyme responsible for the metabolism of ropinirole. There is thus the potential for inducers or inhibitors of this enzyme to alter the clearance of ropinirole. Therefore, if therapy with a drug known to be a potent inducer or inhibitor of CYP1A2 is stopped or started during treatment with ropinirole, adjustment of the dose of ropinirole may be required).
No products indexed under this heading.

Oxazepam (Sedating medications (such as alcohol or CNS depressants), the presence of sleeping disorders, or other medications that increase plasma levels of ropinirole, may increase the risk of somnlence or falling asleep while engaged in activities of daily living. Because of possible additive effects, caution should be advised when patients are taking other sedating medications, alcohol, or other CNS depressants (e.g., benzodiazepines, antipsychotics, antidepressants) in combination with ropinirole).
No products indexed under this heading.

Oxycodone Hydrochloride (Sedating medications (such as alcohol or CNS depressants), the presence of sleeping disorders, or other medications that increase plasma levels of ropinirole, may increase the risk of somnlence or falling asleep while engaged in activities of daily living. Because of possible additive effects, caution should be advised when patients are taking other sedating medications, alcohol, or other CNS depressants (e.g., benzodiazepines, antipsychotics, antidepressants) in combination with ropinirole). Products include:
OxyContin Tablets 2589
OxyIR Capsules 2593
Percocet Tablets 1127
Percodan Tablets 1130

Paliperidone (Because of possible additive effects, caution should be advised when patients are taking other sedating medications, alcohol, or other CNS depressants (e.g., benzodiazepines, antipsychotics, antidepressants) in combination with ropinirole). Products include:
Invega Extended-Release Tablets 1748

Paroxetine Hydrochloride (Because of possible additive effects, caution should be advised when patients are taking other sedating medications, alcohol, or other CNS depressants (e.g., benzodiazepines, antipsychotics, antidepressants) in combination with ropinirole). Products include:
Paxil 1535
Paxil CR Controlled-Release Tablets 1544

Pentobarbital Sodium (Sedating medications (such as alcohol or CNS depressants), the presence of sleeping disorders, or other medications that increase plasma levels of ropinirole, may increase the risk of somnlence or falling asleep while engaged in activities of daily living. Because of possible additive effects, caution should be advised when patients are taking other sedating medications, alcohol, or other CNS depressants (e.g., benzodiazepines, antipsychotics, antidepressants) in combination with ropinirole). Products include:
Nembutal Sodium Solution, USP 2494

Perphenazine (Sedating medications (such as alcohol or CNS depressants), the presence of sleeping disorders, or other medications that increase plasma levels of ropinirole, may increase the risk of somnlence or falling asleep while engaged in activities of daily living. Because of possible additive effects, caution should be advised when patients are taking other sedating medications, alcohol, or other CNS depressants (e.g., benzodiazepines, antipsychotics, antidepressants) in combination with ropinirole).
No products indexed under this heading.

Phenelzine Sulfate (Because of possible additive effects, caution should be advised when patients are taking other sedating medications, alcohol, or other CNS depressants (e.g., benzodiazepines, antipsychotics, antidepressants) in combination with ropinirole).
No products indexed under this heading.

Phenobarbital (Sedating medications (such as alcohol or CNS depressants), the presence of sleeping disorders, or other medications that increase plasma levels of ropinirole, may increase the risk of somnlence or falling asleep while engaged in activities of daily living. Because of possible additive effects, caution should be advised when patients are taking other sedating medications, alcohol, or other CNS depressants (e.g., benzodiazepines, antipsychotics, antidepressants) in combination with ropinirole). Products include:

Donnatal Extentabs 2507

Phenytoin (In vitro metabolism studies showed that CYP1A2 is the major enzyme responsible for the metabolism of ropinirole. There is thus the potential for inducers or inhibitors of this enzyme to alter the clearance of ropinirole. Therefore, if therapy with a drug known to be a potent inducer or inhibitor of CYP1A2 is stopped or started during treatment with ropinirole, adjustment of the dose of ropinirole may be required).

No products indexed under this heading.

Phenytoin Sodium (In vitro metabolism studies showed that CYP1A2 is the major enzyme responsible for the metabolism of ropinirole. There is thus the potential for inducers or inhibitors of this enzyme to alter the clearance of ropinirole. Therefore, if therapy with a drug known to be a potent inducer or inhibitor of CYP1A2 is stopped or started during treatment with ropinirole, adjustment of the dose of ropinirole may be required). Products include:

Phenytek Capsules 2192

Polyestradiol Phosphate (Population pharmacokinetic analysis revealed that higher doses of estrogens (usually associated with hormone replacement therapy) reduced the oral clearance of ropinirole by approximately 35%. Dosage adjustment is not needed for initiating ropinirole inpatients on estrogen therapy because patients are individually titrated with ropinirole to tolerance or adequate effect. If estrogen therapy is stopped or started during treatment with ropinirole, then adjustment of the dose of ropinirole may be required).

No products indexed under this heading.

Prazepam (Sedating medications (such as alcohol or CNS depressants), the presence of sleeping disorders, or other medications that increase plasma levels of ropinirole, may increase the risk of somnlence or falling asleep while engaged in activities of daily living. Because of possible additive effects, caution should be advised when patients are taking other sedating medications, alcohol, or other CNS depressants (e.g., benzodiazepines, antipsychotics, antidepressants) in combination with ropinirole).

No products indexed under this heading.

Primidone (In vitro metabolism studies showed that CYP1A2 is the major enzyme responsible for the metabolism of ropinirole. There is thus the potential for inducers or inhibitors of this enzyme to alter the clearance of ropinirole. Therefore, if therapy with a drug known to be a potent inducer or inhibitor of CYP1A2 is stopped or started during treatment with ropinirole, adjustment of the dose of ropinirole may be required).

No products indexed under this heading.

Prochlorperazine (Sedating medications (such as alcohol or CNS depressants), the presence of sleeping disorders, or other medications that increase plasma levels of ropinirole, may increase the risk of somnlence or falling asleep while engaged in activities of daily living. Because of possible additive effects, caution should be advised when patients are taking other sedating medications, alcohol, or other CNS depressants (e.g., benzodiazepines, antipsychotics, antidepressants) in combination with ropinirole).

No products indexed under this heading.

Promethazine Hydrochloride (Sedating medications (such as alcohol or CNS depressants), the presence of sleeping disorders, or other medications that increase plasma levels of ropinirole, may increase the risk of somnlence or falling asleep while engaged in activities of daily living. Because of possible additive effects, caution should be advised when patients are taking other sedating medications, alcohol, or other CNS depressants (e.g., benzodiazepines, antipsychotics, antidepressants) in combination with ropinirole).

No products indexed under this heading.

Propofol (Sedating medications (such as alcohol or CNS depressants), the presence of sleeping disorders, or other medications that increase plasma levels of ropinirole, may increase the risk of somnlence or falling asleep while engaged in activities of daily living. Because of possible additive effects, caution should be advised when patients are taking other sedating medications, alcohol, or other CNS depressants (e.g., benzodiazepines, antipsychotics, antidepressants) in combination with ropinirole).

No products indexed under this heading.

Propoxyphene Hydrochloride (Sedating medications (such as alcohol or CNS depressants), the presence of sleeping disorders, or other medications that increase plasma levels of ropinirole, may increase the risk of somnlence or falling asleep while engaged in activities of daily living. Because of possible additive effects, caution should be advised when patients are taking other sedating medications, alcohol, or other CNS depressants (e.g., benzodiazepines, antipsychotics, antidepressants) in combination with ropinirole).

No products indexed under this heading.

Propoxyphene Napsylate (Sedating medications (such as alcohol or CNS depressants), the presence of sleeping disorders, or other medications that increase plasma levels of ropinirole, may increase the risk of somnlence or falling asleep while engaged in activities of daily living. Because of possible additive effects, caution should be advised when patients are taking other sedating medications, alcohol, or other CNS depressants (e.g., benzodiazepines, antipsychotics, antidepressants) in combination with ropinirole).

No products indexed under this heading.

Protriptyline Hydrochloride (Because of possible additive effects, caution should be advised when patients are taking other sedating medications, alcohol, or other CNS depressants (e.g., benzodiazepines, antipsychotics, antidepressants) in combination with ropinirole).

No products indexed under this heading.

Quazepam (Sedating medications (such as alcohol or CNS depressants), the presence of sleeping disorders, or other medications that increase plasma levels of ropinirole, may increase the risk of somnlence or falling asleep while engaged in activities of daily living. Because of possible additive effects, caution should be advised when patients are taking other sedating medications, alcohol, or other CNS depressants (e.g., benzodiazepines, antipsychotics, antidepressants) in combination with ropinirole).

No products indexed under this heading.

Quetiapine Fumarate (Sedating medications (such as alcohol or CNS depressants), the presence of sleeping disorders, or other medications that increase plasma levels of ropinirole, may increase the risk of somnlence or falling asleep while engaged in activities of daily living. Because of possible additive effects, caution should be advised when patients are taking other sedating medications, alcohol, or other CNS depressants (e.g., benzodiazepines, antipsychotics, antidepressants) in combination with ropinirole).

No products indexed under this heading.

Quinestrol (Population pharmacokinetic analysis revealed that higher doses of estrogens (usually associated with hormone replacement therapy) reduced the oral clearance of ropinirole by approximately 35%. Dosage adjustment is not needed for initiating ropinirole inpatients on estrogen therapy because patients are individually titrated with ropinirole to tolerance or adequate effect. If estrogen therapy is stopped or started during treatment with ropinirole, then adjustment of the dose of ropinirole may be required).

No products indexed under this heading.

Ranitidine Hydrochloride (In vitro metabolism studies showed that CYP1A2 is the major enzyme responsible for the metabolism of ropinirole. There is thus the potential for inducers or inhibitors of this enzyme to alter the clearance of ropinirole. Therefore, if therapy with a drug known to be a potent inducer or inhibitor of CYP1A2 is stopped or started during treatment with ropinirole, adjustment of the dose of ropinirole may be required). Products include:

Zantac 75 Tablets .... ▣ 603
Zantac 1670
Zantac Injection 1666
Zantac Injection Pharmacy Bulk Package 1668
Maximum Strength Zantac 150 Tablets .... ▣ 603
Maximum Strength Zantac 150 Cool Mint Tablets .... ▣ 603

Remifentanil Hydrochloride (Sedating medications (such as alcohol or CNS depressants), the presence of sleeping disorders, or other medications that increase plasma levels of ropinirole, may increase the risk of somnlence or falling asleep while engaged in activities of daily living. Because of possible additive effects, caution should be advised when patients are taking other sedating medications, alcohol, or other CNS depressants (e.g., benzodiazepines, antipsychotics, antidepressants) in combination with ropinirole).

No products indexed under this heading.

Rifampicin (In vitro metabolism studies showed that CYP1A2 is the major enzyme responsible for the metabolism of ropinirole. There is thus the potential for inducers or inhibitors of this enzyme to alter the clearance of ropinirole. Therefore, if therapy with a drug known to be a potent inducer or inhibitor of CYP1A2 is stopped or started during treatment with ropinirole, adjustment of the dose of ropinirole may be required).

No products indexed under this heading.

Rifampin (In vitro metabolism studies showed that CYP1A2 is the major enzyme responsible for the metabolism of ropinirole. There is thus the potential for inducers or inhibitors of this enzyme to alter the clearance of ropinirole. Therefore, if therapy with a drug known to be a potent inducer or inhibitor of CYP1A2 is stopped or started during treatment with ropinirole, adjustment of the dose of ropinirole may be required).

No products indexed under this heading.

Risperidone (Sedating medications (such as alcohol or CNS depressants), the presence of sleeping disorders, or other medications that increase plasma levels of ropinirole, may increase the risk of somnlence or falling asleep while engaged in activities of daily living. Because of possible additive effects, caution should be advised when patients are taking other sedating medications, alcohol, or other CNS depressants (e.g., benzodiazepines, antipsychotics, antidepressants) in combination with ropinirole). Products include:

Risperdal Consta Long-Acting Injection 1753

Ritonavir (In vitro metabolism studies showed that CYP1A2 is the major enzyme responsible for the metabolism of ropinirole. There is thus the potential for inducers or inhibitors of this enzyme to alter the clearance of ropinirole. Therefore, if therapy with a drug known to be a potent inducer or inhibitor of CYP1A2 is stopped or started during treatment with ropinirole, adjustment of the dose of ropinirole may be required). Products include:

Kaletra 452
Norvir 489

Secobarbital Sodium (Sedating medications (such as alcohol or CNS depressants), the presence of sleeping disorders, or other medications that increase plasma levels of ropinirole, may increase the risk of somnlence or falling asleep while engaged in activities of daily living. Because of possible additive effects, caution should be advised when patients are taking other sedating medications, alcohol, or other CNS depressants

(e.g., benzodiazepines, antipsychotics, antidepressants) in combination with ropinirole).
No products indexed under this heading.

Selegiline (Because of possible additive effects, caution should be advised when patients are taking other sedating medications, alcohol, or other CNS depressants (e.g., benzodiazepines, antipsychotics, antidepressants) in combination with ropinirole). Products include:
Emsam Transdermal System 905

Selegiline Hydrochloride (Because of possible additive effects, caution should be advised when patients are taking other sedating medications, alcohol, or other CNS depressants (e.g., benzodiazepines, antipsychotics, antidepressants) in combination with ropinirole). Products include:
Eldepryl Capsules 3052

Sertraline Hydrochloride (Because of possible additive effects, caution should be advised when patients are taking other sedating medications, alcohol, or other CNS depressants (e.g., benzodiazepines, antipsychotics, antidepressants) in combination with ropinirole).
No products indexed under this heading.

Sevoflurane (Sedating medications (such as alcohol or CNS depressants), the presence of sleeping disorders, or other medications that increase plasma levels of ropinirole, may increase the risk of somnlence or falling asleep while engaged in activities of daily living. Because of possible additive effects, caution should be advised when patients are taking other sedating medications, alcohol, or other CNS depressants (e.g., benzodiazepines, antipsychotics, antidepressants) in combination with ropinirole). Products include:
Ultane Liquid for Inhalation 524

Sildenafil Citrate (In vitro metabolism studies showed that CYP1A2 is the major enzyme responsible for the metabolism of ropinirole. There is thus the potential for inducers or inhibitors of this enzyme to alter the clearance of ropinirole. Therefore, if therapy with a drug known to be a potent inducer or inhibitor of CYP1A2 is stopped or started during treatment with ropinirole, adjustment of the dose of ropinirole may be required).
No products indexed under this heading.

Sodium Oxybate (Sedating medications (such as alcohol or CNS depressants), the presence of sleeping disorders, or other medications that increase plasma levels of ropinirole, may increase the risk of somnlence or falling asleep while engaged in activities of daily living. Because of possible additive effects, caution should be advised when patients are taking other sedating medications, alcohol, or other CNS depressants (e.g., benzodiazepines, antipsychotics, antidepressants) in combination with ropinirole). Products include:
Xyrem Oral Solution 1766

Sparfloxacin (In vitro metabolism studies showed that CYP1A2 is the major enzyme responsible for the metabolism of ropinirole. There is thus the potential for inducers or inhibitors of this enzyme to alter the clearance of ropinirole. Therefore, if therapy with a drug known to be a potent inducer or inhibitor of CYP1A2 is stopped or started during treatment with ropinirole, adjustment of the dose of ropinirole may be required).
No products indexed under this heading.

Sufentanil Citrate (Sedating medications (such as alcohol or CNS depressants), the presence of sleeping disorders, or other medications that increase plasma levels of ropinirole, may increase the risk of somnlence or falling asleep while engaged in activities of daily living. Because of possible additive effects, caution should be advised when patients are taking other sedating medications, alcohol, or other CNS depressants (e.g., benzodiazepines, antipsychotics, antidepressants) in combination with ropinirole).
No products indexed under this heading.

Tacrine Hydrochloride (In vitro metabolism studies showed that CYP1A2 is the major enzyme responsible for the metabolism of ropinirole. There is thus the potential for inducers or inhibitors of this enzyme to alter the clearance of ropinirole. Therefore, if therapy with a drug known to be a potent inducer or inhibitor of CYP1A2 is stopped or started during treatment with ropinirole, adjustment of the dose of ropinirole may be required).
No products indexed under this heading.

Temazepam (Sedating medications (such as alcohol or CNS depressants), the presence of sleeping disorders, or other medications that increase plasma levels of ropinirole, may increase the risk of somnlence or falling asleep while engaged in activities of daily living. Because of possible additive effects, caution should be advised when patients are taking other sedating medications, alcohol, or other CNS depressants (e.g., benzodiazepines, antipsychotics, antidepressants) in combination with ropinirole).
No products indexed under this heading.

Thiamylal Sodium (Sedating medications (such as alcohol or CNS depressants), the presence of sleeping disorders, or other medications that increase plasma levels of ropinirole, may increase the risk of somnlence or falling asleep while engaged in activities of daily living. Because of possible additive effects, caution should be advised when patients are taking other sedating medications, alcohol, or other CNS depressants (e.g., benzodiazepines, antipsychotics, antidepressants) in combination with ropinirole).
No products indexed under this heading.

Thioridazine Hydrochloride (Sedating medications (such as alcohol or CNS depressants), the presence of sleeping disorders, or other medications that increase plasma levels of ropinirole, may increase the risk of somnlence or falling asleep while engaged in activities of daily living. Because of possible additive effects, caution should be advised when patients are taking other sedating medications, alcohol, or other CNS depressants (e.g., benzodiazepines, antipsychotics, antidepressants) in combination with ropinirole). Products include:
Thioridazine Hydrochloride Tablets 2195

Thiothixene (Sedating medications (such as alcohol or CNS depressants), the presence of sleeping disorders, or other medications that increase plasma levels of ropinirole, may increase the risk of somnlence or falling asleep while engaged in activities of daily living. Because of possible additive effects, caution should be advised when patients are taking other sedating medications, alcohol, or other CNS depressants (e.g., benzodiazepines, antipsychotics, antidepressants) in combination with ropinirole). Products include:
Thiothixene Capsules 2197

Ticlopidine Hydrochloride (In vitro metabolism studies showed that CYP1A2 is the major enzyme responsible for the metabolism of ropinirole. There is thus the potential for inducers or inhibitors of this enzyme to alter the clearance of ropinirole. Therefore, if therapy with a drug known to be a potent inducer or inhibitor of CYP1A2 is stopped or started during treatment with ropinirole, adjustment of the dose of ropinirole may be required).
No products indexed under this heading.

Tobacco (Cigarette smoking is expected to increase the clearance of ropinirole since CYP1A2 is known to be induced by smoking. In one study in patients with restless legs syndrome, cigarette smokers had an approximate 30% lower Cmax and a 38% lower AUC than nonsmokers, when those parameters were normalized for dose).
No products indexed under this heading.

Tranylcypromine Sulfate (Because of possible additive effects, caution should be advised when patients are taking other sedating medications, alcohol, or other CNS depressants (e.g., benzodiazepines, antipsychotics, antidepressants) in combination with ropinirole). Products include:
Parnate Tablets 1532

Trazodone Hydrochloride (Because of possible additive effects, caution should be advised when patients are taking other sedating medications, alcohol, or other CNS depressants (e.g., benzodiazepines, antipsychotics, antidepressants) in combination with ropinirole).
No products indexed under this heading.

Triazolam (Sedating medications (such as alcohol or CNS depressants), the presence of sleeping disorders, or other medications that increase plasma levels of ropinirole, may increase the risk of somnlence or falling asleep while engaged in activities of daily living. Because of possible additive effects, caution should be advised when patients are taking other sedating medications, alcohol, or other CNS depressants (e.g., benzodiazepines, antipsychotics, antidepressants) in combination with ropinirole).
No products indexed under this heading.

Trifluoperazine Hydrochloride (Sedating medications (such as alcohol or CNS depressants), the presence of sleeping disorders, or other medications that increase plasma levels of ropinirole, may increase the risk of somnlence or falling asleep while engaged in activities of daily living. Because of possible additive effects, caution should be advised when patients are taking other sedating medications, alcohol, or other CNS depressants (e.g., benzodiazepines, antipsychotics, antidepressants) in combination with ropinirole).
No products indexed under this heading.

Trimipramine Maleate (Because of possible additive effects, caution should be advised when patients are taking other sedating medications, alcohol, or other CNS depressants (e.g., benzodiazepines, antipsychotics, antidepressants) in combination with ropinirole).
No products indexed under this heading.

Troleandomycin (In vitro metabolism studies showed that CYP1A2 is the major enzyme responsible for the metabolism of ropinirole. There is thus the potential for inducers or inhibitors of this enzyme to alter the clearance of ropinirole. Therefore, if therapy with a drug known to be a potent inducer or inhibitor of CYP1A2 is stopped or started during treatment with ropinirole, adjustment of the dose of ropinirole may be required).
No products indexed under this heading.

Trovafloxacin Mesylate (In vitro metabolism studies showed that CYP1A2 is the major enzyme responsible for the metabolism of ropinirole. There is thus the potential for inducers or inhibitors of this enzyme to alter the clearance of ropinirole. Therefore, if therapy with a drug known to be a potent inducer or inhibitor of CYP1A2 is stopped or started during treatment with ropinirole, adjustment of the dose of ropinirole may be required).
No products indexed under this heading.

Vardenafil Hydrochloride (In vitro metabolism studies showed that CYP1A2 is the major enzyme responsible for the metabolism of ropinirole. There is thus the potential for inducers or inhibitors of this enzyme to alter the clearance of ropinirole. Therefore, if therapy with a drug known to be a potent inducer or inhibitor of CYP1A2 is stopped or started during treatment with ropinirole, adjustment of the dose of ropinirole may be required). Products include:
Levitra Tablets 2876

Venlafaxine Hydrochloride (Because of possible additive effects, caution should be advised when patients are taking other sedating medications, alcohol, or other CNS depressants (e.g., benzodiazepines, antipsychotics, antidepressants) in combination with ropinirole). Products include:
Effexor XR Extended-Release Capsules 3195
Venlafaxine Hydrochloride Tablets ... 2199

Zaleplon (Sedating medications (such as alcohol or CNS depressants), the presence of sleeping disorders, or other medications that increase plasma levels of ropinirole,

may increase the risk of somnlence or falling asleep while engaged in activities of daily living. Because of possible additive effects, caution should be advised when patients are taking other sedating medications, alcohol, or other CNS depressants (e.g., benzodiazepines, antipsychotics, antidepressants) in combination with ropinirole).

No products indexed under this heading.

Zileuton (In vitro metabolism studies showed that CYP1A2 is the major enzyme responsible for the metabolism of ropinirole. There is thus the potential for inducers or inhibitors of this enzyme to alter the clearance of ropinirole. Therefore, if therapy with a drug known to be a potent inducer or inhibitor of CYP1A2 is stopped or started during treatment with ropinirole, adjustment of the dose of ropinirole may be required).

No products indexed under this heading.

Ziprasidone Hydrochloride (Sedating medications (such as alcohol or CNS depressants), the presence of sleeping disorders, or other medications that increase plasma levels of ropinirole, may increase the risk of somnlence or falling asleep while engaged in activities of daily living. Because of possible additive effects, caution should be advised when patients are taking other sedating medications, alcohol, or other CNS depressants (e.g., benzodiazepines, antipsychotics, antidepressants) in combination with ropinirole). Products include:

Geodon Capsules 2520

Zolpidem Tartrate (Sedating medications (such as alcohol or CNS depressants), the presence of sleeping disorders, or other medications that increase plasma levels of ropinirole, may increase the risk of somnlence or falling asleep while engaged in activities of daily living. Because of possible additive effects, caution should be advised when patients are taking other sedating medications, alcohol, or other CNS depressants (e.g., benzodiazepines, antipsychotics, antidepressants) in combination with ropinirole). Products include:

Ambien Tablets 2692
Ambien CR Tablets 2696

Food Interactions

Alcohol (Sedating medications (such as alcohol or CNS depressants), the presence of sleeping disorders, or other medications that increase plasma levels of ropinirole, may increase the risk of somnolence or falling asleep while engaged in activities of daily living. Because of possible additive effects, caution should be advised when patients are taking other sedating medications, alcohol, or other CNS depressants (e.g., benzodiazepines, antipsychotics, antidepressants) in combination with ropinirole).

Broccoli (In vitro metabolism studies showed that CYP1A2 is the major enzyme responsible for the metabolism of ropinirole. There is thus the potential for inducers or inhibitors of this enzyme to alter the clearance of ropinirole. Therefore, if therapy with a drug known to be a potent inducer or inhibitor of CYP1A2 is stopped or started during treatment with ropinirole, adjustment of the dose of ropinirole may be required).

Brussel Sprouts (In vitro metabolism studies showed that CYP1A2 is the major enzyme responsible for the metabolism of ropinirole. There is thus the potential for inducers or inhibitors of this enzyme to alter the clearance of ropinirole. Therefore, if therapy with a drug known to be a potent inducer or inhibitor of CYP1A2 is stopped or started during treatment with ropinirole, adjustment of the dose of ropinirole may be required).

Charbroiled Food (In vitro metabolism studies showed that CYP1A2 is the major enzyme responsible for the metabolism of ropinirole. There is thus the potential for inducers or inhibitors of this enzyme to alter the clearance of ropinirole. Therefore, if therapy with a drug known to be a potent inducer or inhibitor of CYP1A2 is stopped or started during treatment with ropinirole, adjustment of the dose of ropinirole may be required).

Food, unspecified (In a single-dose study, administration of ropinirole to healthy volunteers with food (eg, high-fat meal) increased AUC by approximately 30% and Cmax by approximately 44%, compared with dosing under fasted conditions. In a repeat-dose study in patients with Parkinson's disease, food (eg, high-fat meal) increased AUC by approximately 20% and Cmax by approximately 44%; Tmax was prolonged by 3 hours (median prolongation) compared with dosing under fasted conditions).

Grapefruit Juice (In vitro metabolism studies showed that CYP1A2 is the major enzyme responsible for the metabolism of ropinirole. There is thus the potential for inducers or inhibitors of this enzyme to alter the clearance of ropinirole. Therefore, if therapy with a drug known to be a potent inducer or inhibitor of CYP1A2 is stopped or started during treatment with ropinirole, adjustment of the dose of ropinirole may be required).

RESTASIS OPHTHALMIC EMULSION

(Cyclosporine) 557
None cited in PDR database.

RETROVIR CAPSULES

(Zidovudine) 1574
May interact with cytotoxic drugs, Interferon alpha, phenytoin, valproate, and certain other agents. Compounds in these categories include:

Atovaquone (Co-administration results in increased AUC of zidovudine; routine dose modification of zidovudine is not warranted). Products include:

Malarone Pediatric Tablets 1521
Malarone Tablets 1521
Mepron Suspension 1526

Bleomycin Sulfate (Co-administration with cytotoxic agents may increase the hematologic toxicity of zidovudine).

No products indexed under this heading.

Bone Marrow Suppressants, unspecified (May increase the hematologic toxicity of zidovudine).

No products indexed under this heading.

Cyclophosphamide (Co-administration with cytotoxic agents may increase the hematologic toxicity of zidovudine).

No products indexed under this heading.

Daunorubicin Hydrochloride (Co-administration with cytotoxic agents may increase the hematologic toxicity of zidovudine).

No products indexed under this heading.

Divalproex Sodium (Co-administration results in increased AUC of zidovudine by 80%; routine dose modification of zidovudine is not warranted unless patient is experiencing pronounced anemia or other severe zidovudine-associated events). Products include:

Depakote ER Tablets 423

Doxorubicin Hydrochloride (Concomitant use should be avoided since an antagonistic relationship has been demonstrated).

No products indexed under this heading.

Epirubicin Hydrochloride (Co-administration with cytotoxic agents may increase the hematologic toxicity of zidovudine).

No products indexed under this heading.

Fluconazole (Co-administration results in increased AUC of zidovudine by 74%; routine dose modification of zidovudine is not warranted unless patient is experiencing pronounced anemia or other severe zidovudine-associated events).

No products indexed under this heading.

Fluorouracil (Co-administration with cytotoxic agents may increase the hematologic toxicity of zidovudine). Products include:

Carac Cream 0.5% 2722

Fosphenytoin Sodium (Co-administration has resulted in low phenytoin levels in some patients and a high level in one case; a 30% decrease in oral zidovudine clearance was observed with phenytoin).

No products indexed under this heading.

Ganciclovir Sodium (May increase the hematologic toxicity of zidovudine).

No products indexed under this heading.

Hydroxyurea (Co-administration with cytotoxic agents may increase the hematologic toxicity of zidovudine).

No products indexed under this heading.

Interferon alfa-2a, Recombinant (Hepatic decompensation (some fatal) has occurred in HIV/HCV co-infected patients receiving combination antiretroviral therapy for HIV and interferon alfa and ribavirin. Patients receiving interferon alfa with or without ribavirin and zidovudine shouldbe closely monitored for treatment-associated toxicities, especially neutropenia, anemia and hepatic decompensation. Discontinuation of zidovudine should be considered as medically appropriate. Dose reduction or discontinuation of interferon alfa, ribavirin or both should also be considered if worsening of clinical toxicities are observed, including hepatic decompensation (e.g., Childs Pugh greater than 6)).

No products indexed under this heading.

Interferon alfa-2b, Recombinant (Hepatic decompensation (some fatal) has occurred in HIV/HCV co-infected patients receiving combination antiretroviral therapy for HIV and interferon alfa and ribavirin. Patients receiving interferon alfa with or without ribavirin and zidovudine shouldbe closely monitored for treatment-associated toxicities, especially neutropenia, anemia and hepatic decompensation. Discontinuation of zidovudine should be considered as medically appropriate. Dose reduction or discontinuation of interferon alfa, ribavirin or both should also be considered if worsening of clinical toxicities are observed, including hepatic decompensation (e.g., Childs Pugh greater than 6)). Products include:

Intron A for Injection 2859

Interferon alfa-N3 (Human Leukocyte Derived) (Hepatic decompensation (some fatal) has occurred in HIV/HCV co-infected patients receiving combination antiretroviral therapy for HIV and interferon alfa and ribavirin. Patients receiving interferon alfa with or without ribavirin and zidovudine shouldbe closely monitored for treatment-associated toxicities, especially neutropenia, anemia and hepatic decompensation. Discontinuation of zidovudine should be considered as medically appropriate. Dose reduction or discontinuation of interferon alfa, ribavirin or both should also be considered if worsening of clinical toxicities are observed, including hepatic decompensation (e.g., Childs Pugh greater than 6)). Products include:

Alferon N Injection 1726

Methadone Hydrochloride (Co-administration results in increased AUC of zidovudine; routine dose modification of zidovudine is not warranted).

No products indexed under this heading.

Methotrexate Sodium (Co-administration with cytotoxic agents may increase the hematologic toxicity of zidovudine).

No products indexed under this heading.

Mitotane (Co-administration with cytotoxic agents may increase the hematologic toxicity of zidovudine).

No products indexed under this heading.

Mitoxantrone Hydrochloride (Co-administration with cytotoxic agents may increase the hematologic toxicity of zidovudine). Products include:

Novantrone for Injection Concentrate 1100

Nelfinavir Mesylate (Co-administration results in decreased AUC of zidovudine; routine dose modification of zidovudine is not warranted).

No products indexed under this heading.

Peginterferon Alfa-2b (May increase the hematologic toxicity of zidovudine). Products include:

PegIntron Powder for Injection 2903

Phenytoin (Co-administration has resulted in low phenytoin levels in some patients and a high level in one case; a 30% decrease in oral zidovudine clearance was observed with phenytoin).

No products indexed under this heading.

Phenytoin Sodium (Co-administration has resulted in low phenytoin levels in some patients and a high level in one case; a 30%

decrease in oral zidovudine clearance was observed with phenytoin). Products include:
Phenytek Capsules 2192

Probenecid (Co-administration results in increased AUC of zidovudine by 106%; routine dose modification of zidovudine is not warranted unless patient is experiencing pronounced anemia or other severe zidovudine-associated events).
No products indexed under this heading.

Procarbazine Hydrochloride (Co-administration with cytotoxic agents may increase the hematologic toxicity of zidovudine).
No products indexed under this heading.

Ribavirin (Antagonizes the in vitro antiviral activity of zidovudine against HIV; concomitant use should be avoided). Products include:
Rebetol 2917

Rifampin (Co-administration results in decreased AUC of zidovudine; routine dose modification of zidovudine is not warranted).
No products indexed under this heading.

Ritonavir (Co-administration results in decreased AUC of zidovudine; routine dose modification of zidovudine is not warranted). Products include:
Kaletra 452
Norvir 489

Stavudine (Concomitant use should be avoided since an antagonistic relationship has been demonstrated in vitro).
No products indexed under this heading.

Tamoxifen Citrate (Co-administration with cytotoxic agents may increase the hematologic toxicity of zidovudine).
No products indexed under this heading.

Valproate Sodium (Co-administration results in increased AUC of zidovudine by 80%; routine dose modification of zidovudine is not warranted unless patient is experiencing pronounced anemia or other severe zidovudine-associated events).
No products indexed under this heading.

Valproic Acid (Co-administration results in increased AUC of zidovudine by 80%; routine dose modification of zidovudine is not warranted unless patient is experiencing pronounced anemia or other severe zidovudine-associated events).
No products indexed under this heading.

Vincristine Sulfate (Co-administration with cytotoxic agents may increase the hematologic toxicity of zidovudine).
No products indexed under this heading.

RETROVIR IV INFUSION

(Zidovudine) 1579
See Retrovir Capsules

RETROVIR SYRUP

(Zidovudine) 1574
See Retrovir Capsules

RETROVIR TABLETS

(Zidovudine) 1574
See Retrovir Capsules

REYATAZ CAPSULES

(Atazanavir Sulfate) 3299
May interact with antacids, cytochrome p450 1a2 substrates (selected), cytochrome p450 2c9 substrates (selected), cytochrome p450 3a inducers (selected), cytochrome p450 3a inhibitors (selected), ergot-containing drugs, histamine H_2-receptor antagonists, immunosuppressive agents, oral contraceptives, protease inhibitors, proton pump inhibitor, tricyclic antidepressants, and certain other agents. Compounds in these categories include:

Acarbose (Atazanavir sulfate competitively inhibits CYP1A2 and CYP2C9. There is a potential drug-drug interaction between atazanavir sulfate and CYP1A2 or CYP2C9 substrates). Products include:
Precose Tablets 792

Acetaminophen (Atazanavir sulfate competitively inhibits CYP1A2 and CYP2C9. There is a potential drug-drug interaction between atazanavir sulfate and CYP1A2 or CYP2C9 substrates). Products include:
Benadryl Allergy & Cold Kapgels 1895
Benadryl Allergy & Sinus Headache Kapgels 1895
Benadryl Severe Allergy & Sinus Headache Caplets 1897
Lortab 5/500 Tablets 3143
Lortab 7.5/500 Tablets 3144
Lortab 10/500 Tablets 3144
Percocet Tablets 1127
Sinutab Sinus Caplets 1905
Sudafed PE Cold & Cough Caplets 1907
Sudafed PE Nighttime Cold Caplets 1907
Sudafed PE Severe Cold Caplets 1908
Sudafed PE Sinus Headache Caplets 1908
Regular Strength Tylenol Tablets 1915
Tylenol 8 Hour Extended Release Caplets 1915
Extra Strength Tylenol Caplets, Cool Caplets, and EZ Tabs 1915
Extra Strength Tylenol Adult Rapid Blast Liquid 1915
Extra Strength Tylenol PM Caplets, Geltabs, Liquid, and Rapid Release Gels 1915
Extra Strength Tylenol Rapid Release Gels 1915
Tylenol with Codeine Tablets 2427
Tylenol Allergy Multi-Symptom Caplets with Cool Burst and Rapid Release Gelcaps 1916
Tylenol Allergy Multi-Symptom Nighttime Caplets with Cool Burst 1916
Tylenol Severe Allergy Caplets 1916
Tylenol Arthritis Pain Extended Release Geltabs/Caplets 1915
Tylenol Chest Congestion Caplets with Cool Burst 1910
Tylenol Chest Congestion Liquid with Cool Burst 1910
Children's Tylenol Plus Cold Suspension Liquid 1912
Children's Tylenol Plus Cold & Allergy Suspension Liquid 1914
Children's Tylenol Plus Cough & Runny Nose Suspension Liquid 1912
Children's Tylenol Plus Cough & Sore Throat Suspension Liquid 1912
Children's Tylenol Plus Flu Suspension Liquid 1914
Children's Tylenol Suspension Liquid 1909
Children's Tylenol Meltaways 1909
Children's Tylenol Plus Multi-Symptom Cold Suspension Liquid 1912
Tylenol Cold Severe Congestion Daytime Caplets with Cool Burst 1912
Tylenol Cold Head Congestion Daytime Caplets with Cool Burst 1910
Tylenol Cold Head Congestion Nighttime Caplets with Cool Burst 1910
Tylenol Cold Head Congestion Severe Daytime Caplets with Cool Burst 1910
Tylenol Cold Multi-Symptom Daytime Caplets with Cool Burst and Rapid Release Gels 1913
Tylenol Cold Multi-Symptom Daytime Liquid with Citrus Burst ... 1913
Tylenol Cold Multi-Symptom Nighttime Caplets with Cool Burst 1913
Tylenol Cold Multi-Symptom Nighttime Liquid with Cool Burst ... 1913
Tylenol Cold Multi-Symptom Severe Caplets with Cool Burst 1913
Tylenol Cold Multi-Symptom Severe Daytime Liquid with Citrus Burst 1913
Tylenol Cough & Sore Throat Daytime Liquid with Cool Burst...... 1918
Tylenol Cough & Sore Throat Nighttime Liquid with Cool Burst ... 1918
Concentrated Tylenol Infants' Drops 1909
Jr. Tylenol Meltaways 1909
Tylenol Sinus Congestion & Pain Daytime Caplets with Cool Burst and Gelcaps 1917
Tylenol Sinus Congestion & Pain Nighttime Caplets with Cool Burst 1917
Tylenol Sinus Congestion & Pain Severe Caplets with Cool Burst..... 1917
Tylenol Sinus Severe Congestion Caplets with Cool Burst 1917
Tylenol Sore Throat Daytime Liquid with Cool Burst 1918
Tylenol Sore Throat Nighttime Liquid with Cool Burst 1918
Women's Tylenol Menstrual Relief Caplets 1919
Vicks DayQuil Cold & Flu Multi-Symptom Relief 616
Vicks DayQuil LiquiCaps 2567
Vicks DayQuil Liquid 2567
Vicks DayQuil Multi-Symptom Cold/Flu Relief 2567
Vicks NyQuil Cold & Flu Multi-Symptom Relief 617
Vicks NyQuil LiquiCaps 2567
Vicks NyQuil Liquid 2567
Vicks NyQuil Multi-Symptom Cold/Flu Relief 2567
Vicodin Tablets 529
Vicodin ES Tablets 530
Vicodin HP Tablets 531
Zydone Tablets 1132

Alatrofloxacin Mesylate (Atazanavir sulfate competitively inhibits CYP1A2 and CYP2C9. There is a potential drug-drug interaction between atazanavir sulfate and CYP1A2 or CYP2C9 substrates).
No products indexed under this heading.

Allium sativum (Drugs that induce CYP3A activity may increase the clearance of atazanavir sulfate, resulting in lowered plasma concentrations).
No products indexed under this heading.

Aluminum Carbonate (Reduced plasma concentrations of atazanavir are expected if antacids, including buffered medications, are administered with atazanavir sulfate. Atazanavir sulfate should be administered 2 hours before or 1 hour after these medications).
No products indexed under this heading.

Aluminum Hydroxide (Reduced plasma concentrations of atazanavir are expected if antacids, including buffered medications, are administered with atazanavir sulfate. Atazanavir sulfate should be administered 2 hours before or 1 hour after these medications).
No products indexed under this heading.

Amiodarone Hydrochloride (Co-administration with atazanavir sulfate has the potential to produce serious and/or life-threatening adverse events and has not been studied. Caution is warranted and therapeutic concentration monitoring of these drugs is recommended if they are used concomitantly with atazanavir sulfate).
No products indexed under this heading.

Amitriptyline Hydrochloride (Atazanavir sulfate competitively inhibits CYP1A2 and CYP2C9. There is a potential drug-drug interaction between atazanavir sulfate and CYP1A2 or CYP2C9 substrates).
No products indexed under this heading.

Amoxapine (Atazanavir sulfate competitively inhibits CYP1A2 and CYP2C9. There is a potential drug-drug interaction between atazanavir sulfate and CYP1A2 or CYP2C9 substrates).
No products indexed under this heading.

Amprenavir (Co-administration of atazanavir sulfate/ritonavir and other protease inhibitors would be expected to increase exposure to the other protease inhibitors; co-administration is not recommended).
No products indexed under this heading.

Anagrelide Hydrochloride (Atazanavir sulfate competitively inhibits CYP1A2 and CYP2C9. There is a potential drug-drug interaction between atazanavir sulfate and CYP1A2 or CYP2C9 substrates). Products include:
Agrylin Capsules 3017

Aprepitant (Drugs that induce CYP3A activity may increase the clearance of atazanavir sulfate, resulting in lowered plasma concentrations). Products include:
Emend Capsules 1992

Atorvastatin Calcium (The risk of myopathy, including rhabdomyolysis, may be increased when protease inhibitors, including atazanavir sulfate, are used in combination with atorvastatin. Caution should be exercised). Products include:
Lipitor Tablets 2501

Azathioprine (Therapeutic concentration monitoring is recommended for immunosuppressant agents when co-administered with atazanavir sulfate).
No products indexed under this heading.

Basiliximab (Therapeutic concentration monitoring is recommended for immunosuppressant agents when co-administered with atazanavir sulfate). Products include:
Simulect for Injection 2306

Bepridil Hydrochloride (Co-administration with atazanavir sulfate has the potential to produce serious and/or life-threatening adverse events and has not been studied. Caution is warranted and therapeutic concentration monitoring of these drugs is recommended if they are used concomitantly with atazanavir sulfate).
No products indexed under this heading.

Caffeine (Atazanavir sulfate competitively inhibits CYP1A2 and CYP2C9. There is a potential drug-

IMPORTANT NOTE: Always consult each drug listing in the patient's regimen for possible interactions.

drug interaction between atazanavir sulfate and CYP1A2 or CYP2C9 substrates). Products include:
BioLean Free Tablets 635
BioLean II Tablets 635
Winrgy Dietary Supplement 642

Caffeine Anhydrous (Atazanavir sulfate competitively inhibits CYP1A2 and CYP2C9. There is a potential drug-drug interaction between atazanavir sulfate and CYP1A2 or CYP2C9 substrates).
No products indexed under this heading.

Candesartan Cilexetil (Atazanavir sulfate competitively inhibits CYP1A2 and CYP2C9. There is a potential drug-drug interaction between atazanavir sulfate and CYP1A2 or CYP2C9 substrates). Products include:
Atacand Tablets 639
Atacand HCT 642

Carbamazepine (Atazanavir sulfate competitively inhibits CYP1A2 and CYP2C9. There is a potential drug-drug interaction between atazanavir sulfate and CYP1A2 or CYP2C9 substrates). Products include:
Carbatrol Capsules 3019
Equetro Extended-Release Capsules 3174

Carvedilol (Atazanavir sulfate competitively inhibits CYP1A2 and CYP2C9. There is a potential drug-drug interaction between atazanavir sulfate and CYP1A2 or CYP2C9 substrates). Products include:
Coreg Tablets 1387

Celecoxib (Atazanavir sulfate competitively inhibits CYP1A2 and CYP2C9. There is a potential drug-drug interaction between atazanavir sulfate and CYP1A2 or CYP2C9 substrates). Products include:
Celebrex Capsules 2979

Chlordiazepoxide (Atazanavir sulfate competitively inhibits CYP1A2 and CYP2C9. There is a potential drug-drug interaction between atazanavir sulfate and CYP1A2 or CYP2C9 substrates).
No products indexed under this heading.

Chlordiazepoxide Hydrochloride (Atazanavir sulfate competitively inhibits CYP1A2 and CYP2C9. There is a potential drug-drug interaction between atazanavir sulfate and CYP1A2 or CYP2C9 substrates).
No products indexed under this heading.

Chlorpropamide (Atazanavir sulfate competitively inhibits CYP1A2 and CYP2C9. There is a potential drug-drug interaction between atazanavir sulfate and CYP1A2 or CYP2C9 substrates).
No products indexed under this heading.

Cimetidine (Reduced plasma concentrations of atazanavir are expected if H2-receptor antagonists are administered with atazanavir sulfate. This may result in loss of therapeutic effect and development of resistance. To lessen the effect of H2-receptor antagonists on atazanavir exposure, it is recommended that an H2-receptor antagonist and atazanavir sulfate be administered as far apart as possible, preferably 12 hours apart).
No products indexed under this heading.

Cimetidine Hydrochloride (Reduced plasma concentrations of atazanavir are expected if H2-receptor antagonists are administered with atazanavir sulfate. This may result in loss of therapeutic effect and development of resistance. To lessen the effect of H2-receptor antagonists on atazanavir exposure, it is recommended that an H2-receptor antagonist and atazanavir sulfate be administered as far apart as possible, preferably 12 hours apart).
No products indexed under this heading.

Ciprofloxacin (Atazanavir sulfate competitively inhibits CYP1A2 and CYP2C9. There is a potential drug-drug interaction between atazanavir sulfate and CYP1A2 or CYP2C9 substrates). Products include:
Cipro I.V. 2817
Cipro Oral Suspension 2810
Cipro XR Tablets 2823
Ciprodex Otic Suspension 541

Ciprofloxacin Hydrochloride (Atazanavir sulfate competitively inhibits CYP1A2 and CYP2C9. There is a potential drug-drug interaction between atazanavir sulfate and CYP1A2 or CYP2C9 substrates). Products include:
Cipro Tablets 2810

Cisapride (Contraindicated due to potential for serious and/or life-threatening reactions such as cardiac arrhythmias).
No products indexed under this heading.

Clarithromycin (Increased concentrations of clarithromycin may cause QTc prolongations; therefore, a dose reduction of clarithromycin by 50% should be considered when it is co-administered with atazanavir sulfate. In addition, concentrations of the active metabolite 14-OH clarithromycin are significantly reduced; consider alternative therapy for indications other than infections due to Mycobacterium Avium Complex). Products include:
Biaxin/Biaxin XL 411

Clomipramine Hydrochloride (Atazanavir sulfate competitively inhibits CYP1A2 and CYP2C9. There is a potential drug-drug interaction between atazanavir sulfate and CYP1A2 or CYP2C9 substrates).
No products indexed under this heading.

Clopidogrel Bisulfate (Atazanavir sulfate competitively inhibits CYP1A2 and CYP2C9. There is a potential drug-drug interaction between atazanavir sulfate and CYP1A2 or CYP2C9 substrates). Products include:
Plavix Tablets 926
Plavix Tablets 2767

Clozapine (Atazanavir sulfate competitively inhibits CYP1A2 and CYP2C9. There is a potential drug-drug interaction between atazanavir sulfate and CYP1A2 or CYP2C9 substrates).
No products indexed under this heading.

Cyclobenzaprine (Atazanavir sulfate competitively inhibits CYP1A2 and CYP2C9. There is a potential drug-drug interaction between atazanavir sulfate and CYP1A2 or CYP2C9 substrates).
No products indexed under this heading.

Cyclobenzaprine Hydrochloride (Atazanavir sulfate competitively inhibits CYP1A2 and CYP2C9. There is a potential drug-drug interaction between atazanavir sulfate and CYP1A2 or CYP2C9 substrates). Products include:
Amrix Capsules 966

Cyclosporine (Therapeutic concentration monitoring is recommended for immunosuppressant agents when co-administered with atazanavir sulfate). Products include:
Gengraf Capsules 435
Neoral Oral Solution 2280
Neoral Soft Gelatin Capsules 2280
Restasis Ophthalmic Emulsion 557
Sandimmune 2296

Darunavir (Co-administration of atazanavir sulfate/ritonavir and other protease inhibitors would be expected to increase exposure to the other protease inhibitors; co-administration is not recommended).
No products indexed under this heading.

Delavirdine Mesylate (Co-administration of atazanavir sulfate and other drugs that inhibit CYP3A may increase atazanavir sulfate plasma concentrations).
No products indexed under this heading.

Desipramine Hydrochloride (Atazanavir sulfate competitively inhibits CYP1A2 and CYP2C9. There is a potential drug-drug interaction between atazanavir sulfate and CYP1A2 or CYP2C9 substrates).
No products indexed under this heading.

Desogestrel (Because contraceptive steriod concentrations may be altered when atazanavir sulfate or atazanavir sulfate/ritonavir is co-administered with oral contraceptives or with the contraceptive patch, alternate methods of non-hormonal contraception are recommended). Products include:
Mircette Tablets 1034

Dexamethasone (Drugs that induce CYP3A activity may increase the clearance of atazanavir sulfate, resulting in lowered plasma concentrations). Products include:
Ciprodex Otic Suspension 541

Dextromethorphan (Atazanavir sulfate competitively inhibits CYP1A2 and CYP2C9. There is a potential drug-drug interaction between atazanavir sulfate and CYP1A2 or CYP2C9 substrates).
No products indexed under this heading.

Diazepam (Atazanavir sulfate competitively inhibits CYP1A2 and CYP2C9. There is a potential drug-drug interaction between atazanavir sulfate and CYP1A2 or CYP2C9 substrates). Products include:
Valium Tablets 2658

Diclofenac Potassium (Atazanavir sulfate competitively inhibits CYP1A2 and CYP2C9. There is a potential drug-drug interaction between atazanavir sulfate and CYP1A2 or CYP2C9 substrates).
No products indexed under this heading.

Diclofenac Sodium (Atazanavir sulfate competitively inhibits CYP1A2 and CYP2C9. There is a potential drug-drug interaction between atazanavir sulfate and CYP1A2 or CYP2C9 substrates). Products include:
Diclofenac Sodium Ophthalmic Solution ..... ⊙240
Voltaren Ophthalmic Solution 2336
Voltaren Tablets 2334
Voltaren-XR Tablets 2337

Didanosine (Presumably due to the increase in gastric pH caused by buffers in the didanosine buffered tablets, exposure to atazanavir sulfate was markedly decreased. Atazanavir sulfate should be given 2 hours before or 1 hour after didanosine buffered formulations. Didanosine EC capsules and atazanavir should also be given at different times).
No products indexed under this heading.

Dihydroergotamine Mesylate (Contraindicated due to potential for serious and/or life-threatening events such as acute ergot toxicity characterized by peripheral vasospasm and ischemia of the extremities and other tissues).
No products indexed under this heading.

Diltiazem Hydrochloride (Concomitant administration may lead to increased levels of diltiazem and desacetyl-diltiazem; therefore, caution is warranted and dose reduction of diltiazem by 50% should be considered. ECG monitoring is also recommended). Products include:
Cardizem LA Extended Release Tablets 421

Diltiazem Maleate (Atazanavir sulfate competitively inhibits CYP1A2 and CYP2C9. There is a potential drug-drug interaction between atazanavir sulfate and CYP1A2 or CYP2C9 substrates).
No products indexed under this heading.

Doxepin Hydrochloride (Atazanavir sulfate competitively inhibits CYP1A2 and CYP2C9. There is a potential drug-drug interaction between atazanavir sulfate and CYP1A2 or CYP2C9 substrates).
No products indexed under this heading.

Dronabinol (Atazanavir sulfate competitively inhibits CYP1A2 and CYP2C9. There is a potential drug-drug interaction between atazanavir sulfate and CYP1A2 or CYP2C9 substrates). Products include:
Marinol Capsules 3163

Efavirenz (If atazanavir sulfate is to be co-administered with efavirenz, which decreases atazanavir exposure, it is recommended that atazanavir sulfate 300mg with ritonavir 100mg be co-administered with efavirenz 600mg, as this combination results in atazanavir exposure that approximates the mean exposure to atazanavir produced by 400mg of atazanavir sulfate alone. Atazanavir sulfate without ritonavir should not be co-administered with efavirenz). Products include:
Atripla Tablets 938
Sustiva Capsules 930
Sustiva Tablets 930

Enoxacin (Atazanavir sulfate competitively inhibits CYP1A2 and CYP2C9. There is a potential drug-drug interaction between atazanavir sulfate and CYP1A2 or CYP2C9 substrates).
No products indexed under this heading.

Eprosartan Mesylate (Atazanavir sulfate competitively inhibits CYP1A2 and CYP2C9. There is a potential drug-drug interaction between atazanavir sulfate and CYP1A2 or CYP2C9 substrates). Products include:

Teveten Tablets 515
Teveten HCT Tablets 517

Ergonovine Maleate (Contraindicated due to potential for serious and/or life-threatening events such as acute ergot toxicity characterized by peripheral vasospasm and ischemia of the extremities and other tissues).
No products indexed under this heading.

Ergotamine Tartrate (Contraindicated due to potential for serious and/or life-threatening events such as acute ergot toxicity characterized by peripheral vasospasm and ischemia of the extremities and other tissues).
No products indexed under this heading.

Erythromycin (Atazanavir sulfate competitively inhibits CYP1A2 and CYP2C9. There is a potential drug-drug interaction between atazanavir sulfate and CYP1A2 or CYP2C9 substrates).
No products indexed under this heading.

Erythromycin Estolate (Atazanavir sulfate competitively inhibits CYP1A2 and CYP2C9. There is a potential drug-drug interaction between atazanavir sulfate and CYP1A2 or CYP2C9 substrates).
No products indexed under this heading.

Erythromycin Ethylsuccinate (Atazanavir sulfate competitively inhibits CYP1A2 and CYP2C9. There is a potential drug-drug interaction between atazanavir sulfate and CYP1A2 or CYP2C9 substrates). Products include:
E.E.S. 433
EryPed 431

Erythromycin Gluceptate (Atazanavir sulfate competitively inhibits CYP1A2 and CYP2C9. There is a potential drug-drug interaction between atazanavir sulfate and CYP1A2 or CYP2C9 substrates).
No products indexed under this heading.

Erythromycin Lactobionate (Atazanavir sulfate competitively inhibits CYP1A2 and CYP2C9. There is a potential drug-drug interaction between atazanavir sulfate and CYP1A2 or CYP2C9 substrates).
No products indexed under this heading.

Erythromycin Stearate (Atazanavir sulfate competitively inhibits CYP1A2 and CYP2C9. There is a potential drug-drug interaction between atazanavir sulfate and CYP1A2 or CYP2C9 substrates).
No products indexed under this heading.

Esomeprazole Magnesium (Concomitant use of atazanavir sulfate and proton-pump inhibitors is not recommended. Co-administration of atazanavir sulfate with proton-pump inhibitors is expected to substantially decrease atazanavir sulfate plasma concentrations and reduce its therapeutic effect). Products include:
Nexium Delayed-Release Capsules 645
Nexium Delayed-Release Oral Suspension 645

Estradiol (Atazanavir sulfate competitively inhibits CYP1A2 and CYP2C9. There is a potential drug-drug interaction between atazanavir sulfate and CYP1A2 or CYP2C9 substrates). Products include:
Activella Tablets 2347
Angeliq Tablets 751
Climara Transdermal System 763
Climara Pro Transdermal System 768
Divigel 3167
Vagifem Tablets 2375

Estradiol Benzoate (Atazanavir sulfate competitively inhibits CYP1A2 and CYP2C9. There is a potential drug-drug interaction between atazanavir sulfate and CYP1A2 or CYP2C9 substrates).
No products indexed under this heading.

Estradiol Cypionate (Atazanavir sulfate competitively inhibits CYP1A2 and CYP2C9. There is a potential drug-drug interaction between atazanavir sulfate and CYP1A2 or CYP2C9 substrates).
No products indexed under this heading.

Ethinyl Estradiol (Because contraceptive steriod concentrations may be altered when atazanavir sulfate or atazanavir sulfate/ritonavir is co-administered with oral contraceptives or with the contraceptive patch, alternate methods of non-hormonal contraception are recommended). Products include:
Lybrel Tablets 3204
Mircette Tablets 1034
NuvaRing 2897
Ortho-Cyclen/Ortho Tri-Cyclen 2449
Ortho Evra Transdermal System 2437
Ortho Tri-Cyclen Lo Tablets 2458
Seasonique Tablets 1046
Yaz Tablets 805

Ethosuximide (Drugs that induce CYP3A activity may increase the clearance of atazanavir sulfate, resulting in lowered plasma concentrations).
No products indexed under this heading.

Ethynodiol Diacetate (Because contraceptive steriod concentrations may be altered when atazanavir sulfate or atazanavir sulfate/ritonavir is co-administered with oral contraceptives or with the contraceptive patch, alternate methods of non-hormonal contraception are recommended).
No products indexed under this heading.

Etodolac (Atazanavir sulfate competitively inhibits CYP1A2 and CYP2C9. There is a potential drug-drug interaction between atazanavir sulfate and CYP1A2 or CYP2C9 substrates).
No products indexed under this heading.

Famotidine (Reduced plasma concentrations of atazanavir are expected if H2-receptor antagonists are administered with atazanavir sulfate. This may result in loss of therapeutic effect and development of resistance. To lessen the effect of H2-receptor antagonists on atazanavir exposure, it is recommended that an H2-receptor antagonist and atazanavir sulfate be administered as far apart as possible, preferably 12 hours apart). Products include:
Pepcid Tablets 2075
Original Strength Pepcid AC Gelcaps 1771
Original Strength Pepcid AC Tablets 1771
Maximum Strength Pepcid AC Tablets 1771
Pepcid Complete Chewable Tablets 1771

Felodipine (Caution is warranted. Dose titration of the calcium channel blocker should be considered. ECG monitoring is recommended).
No products indexed under this heading.

Fenoprofen Calcium (Atazanavir sulfate competitively inhibits CYP1A2 and CYP2C9. There is a potential drug-drug interaction between atazanavir sulfate and CYP1A2 or CYP2C9 substrates). Products include:
Nalfon Capsules 2508

Fluconazole (Co-administration of atazanavir sulfate and other drugs that inhibit CYP3A may increase atazanavir sulfate plasma concentrations).
No products indexed under this heading.

Fluoxetine (Co-administration of atazanavir sulfate and other drugs that inhibit CYP3A may increase atazanavir sulfate plasma concentrations).
No products indexed under this heading.

Fluoxetine Hydrochloride (Atazanavir sulfate competitively inhibits CYP1A2 and CYP2C9. There is a potential drug-drug interaction between atazanavir sulfate and CYP1A2 or CYP2C9 substrates). Products include:
Prozac Weekly Capsules 1852
Prozac Pulvules and Liquid 1852
Symbyax Capsules 1871

Flurbiprofen (Atazanavir sulfate competitively inhibits CYP1A2 and CYP2C9. There is a potential drug-drug interaction between atazanavir sulfate and CYP1A2 or CYP2C9 substrates).
No products indexed under this heading.

Flurbiprofen Sodium (Atazanavir sulfate competitively inhibits CYP1A2 and CYP2C9. There is a potential drug-drug interaction between atazanavir sulfate and CYP1A2 or CYP2C9 substrates).
No products indexed under this heading.

Flutamide (Atazanavir sulfate competitively inhibits CYP1A2 and CYP2C9. There is a potential drug-drug interaction between atazanavir sulfate and CYP1A2 or CYP2C9 substrates).
No products indexed under this heading.

Fluticasone Propionate (A study has shown that ritonavir significantly increases plasma fluticasone propionate exposures, resulting in significantly decreased serum cortisol concentrations. Concomitant use of atazanavir with ritonavir and fluticasone propionate is expected to produce the same effects. Systemic corticosteroid effects, including Cushing's syndrome and adrenal suppression have been reported during postmarketing use in patients receiving ritonavir and inhaled or intranasally administered fluticasone propionate. Therefore, co-administration of fluticasone propionate and atazanavir/ritonavir is not recommended unless the potential benefit to the patient outweighs the risk of systemic corticosteroid side effects). Products include:
Advair Diskus 100/50 1276
Advair Diskus 250/50 1276
Advair Diskus 500/50 1276
Advair HFA 45/21 Inhalation Aerosol 1288
Advair HFA 115/21 Inhalation Aerosol 1288
Advair HFA 230/21 Inhalation Aerosol 1288
Flonase Nasal Spray 1431
Flovent Diskus 50 mcg 1435

Fluticasone Propionate HFA (A study has shown that ritonavir significantly increases plasma fluticasone propionate exposures, resulting in significantly decreased serum cortisol concentrations. Concomitant use of atazanavir with ritonavir and fluticasone propionate is expected to produce the same effects. Systemic corticosteroid effects, including Cushing's syndrome and adrenal suppression have been reported during postmarketing use in patients receiving ritonavir and inhaled or intranasally administered fluticasone propionate. Therefore, co-administration of fluticasone propionate and atazanavir/ritonavir is not recommended unless the potential benefit to the patient outweighs the risk of systemic corticosteroid side effects). Products include:
Flovent HFA 1440

Fluvastatin Sodium (Atazanavir sulfate competitively inhibits CYP1A2 and CYP2C9. There is a potential drug-drug interaction between atazanavir sulfate and CYP1A2 or CYP2C9 substrates). Products include:
Lescol Capsules 2268
Lescol XL Tablets 2268

Fluvoxamine Maleate (Atazanavir sulfate competitively inhibits CYP1A2 and CYP2C9. There is a potential drug-drug interaction between atazanavir sulfate and CYP1A2 or CYP2C9 substrates). Products include:
Luvox CR Extended-Release Capsules 1759

Fosamprenavir Calcium (Co-administration of atazanavir sulfate/ritonavir and other protease inhibitors would be expected to increase exposure to the other protease inhibitors; co-administration is not recommended). Products include:
Lexiva Oral Suspension 1510
Lexiva Tablets 1510

Glimepiride (Atazanavir sulfate competitively inhibits CYP1A2 and CYP2C9. There is a potential drug-drug interaction between atazanavir sulfate and CYP1A2 or CYP2C9 substrates). Products include:
Avandaryl Tablets 1344
Duetact Tablets 3085

Glipizide (Atazanavir sulfate competitively inhibits CYP1A2 and CYP2C9. There is a potential drug-drug interaction between atazanavir sulfate and CYP1A2 or CYP2C9 substrates).
No products indexed under this heading.

Grepafloxacin Hydrochloride (Atazanavir sulfate competitively inhibits CYP1A2 and CYP2C9. There is a potential drug-drug interaction between atazanavir sulfate and CYP1A2 or CYP2C9 substrates).
No products indexed under this heading.

Haloperidol (Atazanavir sulfate competitively inhibits CYP1A2 and CYP2C9. There is a potential drug-drug interaction between atazanavir sulfate and CYP1A2 or CYP2C9 substrates).
No products indexed under this heading.

Haloperidol Decanoate (Atazanavir sulfate competitively inhibits CYP1A2 and CYP2C9. There is a potential drug-drug interaction between atazanavir sulfate and CYP1A2 or CYP2C9 substrates).
No products indexed under this heading.

Haloperidol Lactate (Atazanavir sulfate competitively inhibits CYP1A2 and CYP2C9. There is a potential drug-drug interaction between atazanavir sulfate and CYP1A2 or CYP2C9 substrates).
No products indexed under this heading.

Hypericum Perforatum (Concomitant use of atazanavir sulfate and St. John's Wort, or products containing St. John's Wort, is not recommended. Co-administration of protease inhibitors with St. John's Wort is expected to substantially decrease concentrations of the protease inhibitor and may result in suboptimal levels of atazanavir sulfate and lead to loss of virologic response and possible resistance to atazanavir sulfate or to the class of protease inhibitors).
No products indexed under this heading.

Ibuprofen (Atazanavir sulfate competitively inhibits CYP1A2 and CYP2C9. There is a potential drug-drug interaction between atazanavir sulfate and CYP1A2 or CYP2C9 substrates). Products include:
Motrin IB Tablets and Caplets 1900
Children's Motrin Oral Suspension ... 1901
Children's Motrin Non-Staining Dye-Free Oral Suspension............ 1901
Children's Motrin Cold Oral Suspension 1899
Infants' Motrin Concentrated Drops.. 1901
Infants' Motrin Non-Staining Dye-Free Concentrated Drops....... 1901
Junior Strength Motrin Caplets and Chewable Tablets.................. 1901
Vicoprofen Tablets 533

Imipramine Hydrochloride (Atazanavir sulfate competitively inhibits CYP1A2 and CYP2C9. There is a potential drug-drug interaction between atazanavir sulfate and CYP1A2 or CYP2C9 substrates).
No products indexed under this heading.

Imipramine Pamoate (Atazanavir sulfate competitively inhibits CYP1A2 and CYP2C9. There is a potential drug-drug interaction between atazanavir sulfate and CYP1A2 or CYP2C9 substrates).
No products indexed under this heading.

Indinavir Sulfate (Both atazanavir sulfate and indinavir are associated with indirect hyperbilirubinemia. Co-administration is contraindicated). Products include:
Crixivan Capsules 1979

Indomethacin (Atazanavir sulfate competitively inhibits CYP1A2 and CYP2C9. There is a potential drug-drug interaction between atazanavir sulfate and CYP1A2 or CYP2C9 substrates). Products include:
Indocin 2024

Indomethacin Sodium Trihydrate (Atazanavir sulfate competitively inhibits CYP1A2 and CYP2C9. There is a potential drug-drug interaction between atazanavir sulfate and CYP1A2 or CYP2C9 substrates). Products include:
Indocin I.V. 2489

Irbesartan (Atazanavir sulfate competitively inhibits CYP1A2 and CYP2C9. There is a potential drug-drug interaction between atazanavir sulfate and CYP1A2 or CYP2C9 substrates). Products include:
Avalide Tablets 892
Avalide Tablets 2713
Avapro Tablets 897
Avapro Tablets 2718

Irinotecan Hydrochloride (Atazanavir inhibits UGT and may interfere with the metabolism of irinotecan, resulting in increased irinotecan toxicity. Co-administration with atazanavir is contraindicated).
No products indexed under this heading.

Isoniazid (Co-administration of atazanavir sulfate and other drugs that inhibit CYP3A may increase atazanavir sulfate plasma concentrations).
No products indexed under this heading.

Itraconazole (Due to the effect of ritonavir on ketoconazole, high doses of ketoconazole and itraconazole (greater than 200 mg/day) should be used cautiously with atazanavir sulfate/ritonavir).
No products indexed under this heading.

Ketoconazole (Due to the effect of ritonavir on ketoconazole, high doses of ketoconazole and itraconazole (greater than 200 mg/day) should be used cautiously with atazanavir sulfate/ritonavir). Products include:
Extina Foam, 2% 3057
Nizoral A-D Shampoo 1901

Ketoprofen (Atazanavir sulfate competitively inhibits CYP1A2 and CYP2C9. There is a potential drug-drug interaction between atazanavir sulfate and CYP1A2 or CYP2C9 substrates).
No products indexed under this heading.

Ketorolac Tromethamine (Atazanavir sulfate competitively inhibits CYP1A2 and CYP2C9. There is a potential drug-drug interaction between atazanavir sulfate and CYP1A2 or CYP2C9 substrates).
No products indexed under this heading.

Lansoprazole (Concomitant use of atazanavir sulfate and proton-pump inhibitors is not recommended. Co-administration of atazanavir sulfate with proton-pump inhibitors is expected to substantially decrease atazanavir sulfate plasma concentrations and reduce its therapeutic effect).
No products indexed under this heading.

Levobupivacaine Hydrochloride (Atazanavir sulfate competitively inhibits CYP1A2 and CYP2C9. There is a potential drug-drug interaction between atazanavir sulfate and CYP1A2 or CYP2C9 substrates).
No products indexed under this heading.

Levonorgestrel (Because contraceptive steriod concentrations may be altered when atazanavir sulfate or atazanavir sulfate/ritonavir is co-administered with oral contraceptives or with the contraceptive patch, alternate methods of non-hormonal contraception are recommended). Products include:
Climara Pro Transdermal System 768
Lybrel Tablets 3204
Mirena Intrauterine System 779
Plan B Tablets 1044
Seasonique Tablets 1046

Lidocaine (Co-administration with atazanavir sulfate has the potential to produce serious and/or life-threatening adverse events and has not been studied. Caution is warranted and therapeutic concentration monitoring of these drugs is recommended if they are used concomitantly with atazanavir sulfate). Products include:
Lidoderm Patch 1114

Lidocaine Hydrochloride (Co-administration with atazanavir sulfate has the potential to produce serious and/or life-threatening adverse events and has not been studied. Caution is warranted and therapeutic concentration monitoring of these drugs is recommended if they are used concomitantly with atazanavir sulfate).
No products indexed under this heading.

Lomefloxacin Hydrochloride (Atazanavir sulfate competitively inhibits CYP1A2 and CYP2C9. There is a potential drug-drug interaction between atazanavir sulfate and CYP1A2 or CYP2C9 substrates).
No products indexed under this heading.

Lopinavir (Co-administration of atazanavir sulfate/ritonavir and other protease inhibitors would be expected to increase exposure to the other protease inhibitors; co-administration is not recommended). Products include:
Kaletra 452

Losartan Potassium (Atazanavir sulfate competitively inhibits CYP1A2 and CYP2C9. There is a potential drug-drug interaction between atazanavir sulfate and CYP1A2 or CYP2C9 substrates). Products include:
Cozaar Tablets 1973

Lovastatin (Concomitant use of atazanavir sulfate with lovastatin is not recommended. Caution should be exercised if HIV protease inhibitors, including atazanavir sulfate, are used concurrently with other HMG-CoA reductase inhibitors that are also metabolized by theCYP3A4 pathway. The risk of myopathy, including rhabdomyolysis, may be increased when HIV protease inhibitors, including atazanavir sulfate, are used in combination with these drugs). Products include:
Advicor Tablets 402
Mevacor Tablets 2063

Magaldrate (Reduced plasma concentrations of atazanavir are expected if antacids, including buffered medications, are administered with atazanavir sulfate. Atazanavir sulfate should be administered 2 hours before or 1 hour after these medications).
No products indexed under this heading.

Magnesium Hydroxide (Reduced plasma concentrations of atazanavir are expected if antacids, including buffered medications, are administered with atazanavir sulfate. Atazanavir sulfate should be administered 2 hours before or 1 hour after these medications). Products include:
Fleet Pedia-Lax Chewable Tablets 1145
Pepcid Complete Chewable Tablets 1771
Extra Strength Rolaids Freshmint Tablets 1903
Rolaids Multi-Symptom Berry Tablets 1903
Rolaids Original Peppermint Tablets 1903

Magnesium Oxide (Reduced plasma concentrations of atazanavir are expected if antacids, including buffered medications, are administered with atazanavir sulfate. Atazanavir sulfate should be administered 2 hours before or 1 hour after these medications). Products include:
Beelith Tablets 813

Maprotiline Hydrochloride (Atazanavir sulfate competitively inhibits CYP1A2 and CYP2C9. There is a potential drug-drug interaction between atazanavir sulfate and CYP1A2 or CYP2C9 substrates).
No products indexed under this heading.

Meclofenamate Sodium (Atazanavir sulfate competitively inhibits CYP1A2 and CYP2C9. There is a potential drug-drug interaction between atazanavir sulfate and CYP1A2 or CYP2C9 substrates).
No products indexed under this heading.

Mefenamic Acid (Atazanavir sulfate competitively inhibits CYP1A2 and CYP2C9. There is a potential drug-drug interaction between atazanavir sulfate and CYP1A2 or CYP2C9 substrates).
No products indexed under this heading.

Meloxicam (Atazanavir sulfate competitively inhibits CYP1A2 and CYP2C9. There is a potential drug-drug interaction between atazanavir sulfate and CYP1A2 or CYP2C9 substrates). Products include:
Mobic Oral Suspension 863
Mobic Tablets 863

Mestranol (Because contraceptive steriod concentrations may be altered when atazanavir sulfate or atazanavir sulfate/ritonavir is co-administered with oral contraceptives or with the contraceptive patch, alternate methods of non-hormonal contraception are recommended).
No products indexed under this heading.

Metformin Hydrochloride (Atazanavir sulfate competitively inhibits CYP1A2 and CYP2C9. There is a potential drug-drug interaction between atazanavir sulfate and CYP1A2 or CYP2C9 substrates). Products include:
ActoPlus Met Tablets 3071
Avandamet Tablets 1336
Janumet Tablets 2041
PrandiMet Tablets 2967

Methadone Hydrochloride (Atazanavir sulfate competitively inhibits CYP1A2 and CYP2C9. There is a potential drug-drug interaction between atazanavir sulfate and CYP1A2 or CYP2C9 substrates).
No products indexed under this heading.

Methylergonovine Maleate (Contraindicated due to potential for serious and/or life-threatening events such as acute ergot toxicity characterized by peripheral vasospasm and ischemia of the extremities and other tissues).
No products indexed under this heading.

Methysergide Maleate (Contraindicated due to potential for serious and/or life-threatening events such as acute ergot toxicity characterized by peripheral vasospasm and ischemia of the extremities and other tissues).
No products indexed under this heading.

Metronidazole (Co-administration of atazanavir sulfate and other drugs that inhibit CYP3A may increase atazanavir sulfate plasma concentrations). Products include:
Pylera Capsules 714

Metronidazole Benzoate (Co-administration of atazanavir sulfate and other drugs that inhibit CYP3A may increase atazanavir sulfate plasma concentrations).
No products indexed under this heading.

Metronidazole Hydrochloride (Co-administration of atazanavir sulfate and other drugs that inhibit CYP3A may increase atazanavir sulfate plasma concentrations).
No products indexed under this heading.

Mexiletine Hydrochloride (Atazanavir sulfate competitively inhibits CYP1A2 and CYP2C9. There is a potential drug-drug interaction between atazanavir sulfate and CYP1A2 or CYP2C9 substrates).
No products indexed under this heading.

Miconazole (Co-administration of atazanavir sulfate and other drugs that inhibit CYP3A may increase atazanavir sulfate plasma concentrations).
No products indexed under this heading.

Midazolam Hydrochloride (Contraindicated due to potential for serious and/or life-threatening events, such as prolonged or increased sedation or respiratory depression).
No products indexed under this heading.

Miglitol (Atazanavir sulfate competitively inhibits CYP1A2 and CYP2C9. There is a potential drug-drug interaction between atazanavir sulfate and CYP1A2 or CYP2C9 substrates).
No products indexed under this heading.

Mirtazapine (Atazanavir sulfate competitively inhibits CYP1A2 and CYP2C9. There is a potential drug-drug interaction between atazanavir sulfate and CYP1A2 or CYP2C9 substrates). Products include:
Remeron Tablets 2924
RemeronSolTab Tablets 2927

Modafinil (Drugs that induce CYP3A activity may increase the clearance of atazanavir sulfate, resulting in lowered plasma concentrations). Products include:
Provigil Tablets 977

Montelukast Sodium (Atazanavir sulfate competitively inhibits CYP1A2 and CYP2C9. There is a potential drug-drug interaction between atazanavir sulfate and CYP1A2 or CYP2C9 substrates). Products include:
Singulair 2114

Moxifloxacin Hydrochloride (Atazanavir sulfate competitively inhibits CYP1A2 and CYP2C9. There is a potential drug-drug interaction between atazanavir sulfate and CYP1A2 or CYP2C9 substrates). Products include:
Avelox 2803
Vigamox Ophthalmic Solution 548

Muromonab-CD3 (Therapeutic concentration monitoring is recommended for immunosuppressant agents when co-administered with atazanavir sulfate). Products include:
Orthoclone OKT3 Sterile Solution 2387

Mycophenolate Mofetil (Therapeutic concentration monitoring is recommended for immunosuppressant agents when co-administered with atazanavir sulfate). Products include:
CellCept Capsules 2622
CellCept Oral Suspension 2622
CellCept Tablets 2622

Nabumetone (Atazanavir sulfate competitively inhibits CYP1A2 and CYP2C9. There is a potential drug-drug interaction between atazanavir sulfate and CYP1A2 or CYP2C9 substrates).
No products indexed under this heading.

Nafcillin Sodium (Atazanavir sulfate competitively inhibits CYP1A2 and CYP2C9. There is a potential drug-drug interaction between atazanavir sulfate and CYP1A2 or CYP2C9 substrates).
No products indexed under this heading.

Naproxen (Atazanavir sulfate competitively inhibits CYP1A2 and CYP2C9. There is a potential drug-drug interaction between atazanavir sulfate and CYP1A2 or CYP2C9 substrates). Products include:
EC-Naprosyn Delayed-Release Tablets 2632
Naprosyn Suspension 2632
Naprosyn Tablets 2632

Naproxen Sodium (Atazanavir sulfate competitively inhibits CYP1A2 and CYP2C9. There is a potential drug-drug interaction between atazanavir sulfate and CYP1A2 or CYP2C9 substrates). Products include:
Anaprox Tablets 2632
Anaprox DS Tablets 2632
Treximet Tablets 1616

Nateglinide (Atazanavir sulfate competitively inhibits CYP1A2 and CYP2C9. There is a potential drug-drug interaction between atazanavir sulfate and CYP1A2 or CYP2C9 substrates). Products include:
Starlix Tablets 2314

Nefazodone Hydrochloride (Co-administration of atazanavir sulfate and other drugs that inhibit CYP3A may increase atazanavir sulfate plasma concentrations).
No products indexed under this heading.

Nelfinavir Mesylate (Co-administration of atazanavir sulfate/ritonavir and other protease inhibitors would be expected to increase exposure to the other protease inhibitors; co-administration is not recommended).
No products indexed under this heading.

Nevirapine (Nevirapine, an inducer of CYP3A, is expected to decrease atazanavir sulfate exposure. In the absence of data, co-administration is not recommended). Products include:
Viramune Oral Suspension 873
Viramune Tablets 873

Nicardipine Hydrochloride (Caution is warranted. Dose titration of the calcium channel blocker should be considered. ECG monitoring is recommended). Products include:
Cardene I.V. 1093

Nicotine Polacrilex (Atazanavir sulfate competitively inhibits CYP1A2 and CYP2C9. There is a potential drug-drug interaction between atazanavir sulfate and CYP1A2 or CYP2C9 substrates).
No products indexed under this heading.

Nicotine Salicylate (Atazanavir sulfate competitively inhibits CYP1A2 and CYP2C9. There is a potential drug-drug interaction between atazanavir sulfate and CYP1A2 or CYP2C9 substrates).
No products indexed under this heading.

Nicotine Sulfate (Atazanavir sulfate competitively inhibits CYP1A2 and CYP2C9. There is a potential drug-drug interaction between atazanavir sulfate and CYP1A2 or CYP2C9 substrates).
No products indexed under this heading.

Nifedipine (Caution is warranted. Dose titration of the calcium channel blocker should be considered. ECG monitoring is recommended).
No products indexed under this heading.

Nizatidine (Reduced plasma concentrations of atazanavir are expected if H2-receptor antagonists are administered with atazanavir sulfate. This may result in loss of therapeutic effect and development of resistance. To lessen the effect of H2-receptor antagonists on atazanavir exposure, it is recommended that an H2-receptor antagonist and atazanavir sulfate be administered as far apart as possible, preferably 12 hours apart). Products include:
Axid Capsules 1364

Norethindrone (Because contraceptive steriod concentrations may be altered when atazanavir sulfate or atazanavir sulfate/ritonavir is co-administered with oral contraceptives or with the contraceptive patch, alternate methods of non-hormonal contraception are recommended). Products include:
Ortho Micronor Tablets 2446

Norethindrone Acetate (Atazanavir sulfate competitively inhibits CYP1A2 and CYP2C9. There is a potential drug-drug interaction between atazanavir sulfate and CYP1A2 or CYP2C9 substrates). Products include:
Activella Tablets 2347

Norethynodrel (Because contraceptive steriod concentrations may be altered when atazanavir sulfate or atazanavir sulfate/ritonavir is co-administered with oral contraceptives or with the contraceptive patch, alternate methods of non-hormonal contraception are recommended).
No products indexed under this heading.

Norfloxacin (Atazanavir sulfate competitively inhibits CYP1A2 and CYP2C9. There is a potential drug-drug interaction between atazanavir sulfate and CYP1A2 or CYP2C9 substrates). Products include:
Noroxin Tablets 2069

Norgestimate (Because contraceptive steriod concentrations may be altered when atazanavir sulfate or atazanavir sulfate/ritonavir is co-administered with oral contraceptives or with the contraceptive patch, alternate methods of non-hormonal contraception are recommended). Products include:
Ortho-Cyclen/Ortho Tri-Cyclen 2449
Ortho Tri-Cyclen Lo Tablets 2458

Norgestrel (Because contraceptive steriod concentrations may be altered when atazanavir sulfate or atazanavir sulfate/ritonavir is co-administered with oral contraceptives or with the contraceptive patch, alternate methods of non-hormonal contraception are recommended).
No products indexed under this heading.

Nortriptyline Hydrochloride (Atazanavir sulfate competitively inhibits CYP1A2 and CYP2C9. There is a potential drug-drug interaction between atazanavir sulfate and CYP1A2 or CYP2C9 substrates).
No products indexed under this heading.

Ofloxacin (Atazanavir sulfate competitively inhibits CYP1A2 and CYP2C9. There is a potential drug-drug interaction between atazanavir sulfate and CYP1A2 or CYP2C9 substrates). Products include:
Ofloxacin Ophthalmic Solution 0.3% .... ⊙243

Olanzapine (Atazanavir sulfate competitively inhibits CYP1A2 and CYP2C9. There is a potential drug-drug interaction between atazanavir sulfate and CYP1A2 or CYP2C9 substrates). Products include:
Symbyax Capsules 1871
Zyprexa Tablets 1883
Zyprexa IntraMuscular 1883
Zyprexa ZYDIS Orally Disintegrating Tablets 1883

Omeprazole (Concomitant use of atazanavir sulfate and proton-pump inhibitors is not recommended. Co-administration of atazanavir sulfate with proton-pump inhibitors is expected to substantially decrease atazanavir sulfate plasma concentrations and reduce its therapeutic effect).
No products indexed under this heading.

Ondansetron (Atazanavir sulfate competitively inhibits CYP1A2 and CYP2C9. There is a potential drug-drug interaction between atazanavir sulfate and CYP1A2 or CYP2C9 substrates). Products include:
Zofran ODT Orally Disintegrating Tablets 1687

Ondansetron Hydrochloride (Atazanavir sulfate competitively inhibits CYP1A2 and CYP2C9. There is a potential drug-drug interaction between atazanavir sulfate and CYP1A2 or CYP2C9 substrates). Products include:
Zofran Injection 1682
Zofran 1687

Oxaprozin (Atazanavir sulfate competitively inhibits CYP1A2 and CYP2C9. There is a potential drug-drug interaction between atazanavir sulfate and CYP1A2 or CYP2C9 substrates).
No products indexed under this heading.

Pantoprazole Sodium (Concomitant use of atazanavir sulfate and proton-pump inhibitors is not recommended. Co-administration of atazanavir sulfate with proton-pump inhibitors is expected to substantially decrease atazanavir sulfate plasma concentrations and reduce its therapeutic effect). Products include:
Protonix for Delayed-Release Oral Suspension 3254
Protonix Delayed-Release Tablets 3254
Protonix I.V. 3257

Paroxetine Hydrochloride (Co-administration of atazanavir sulfate and other drugs that inhibit CYP3A may increase atazanavir sulfate plasma concentrations). Products include:
Paxil 1535
Paxil CR Controlled-Release Tablets 1544

Phenobarbital (Drugs that induce CYP3A activity may increase the clearance of atazanavir sulfate, resulting in lowered plasma concentrations). Products include:
Donnatal Extentabs 2507

Phenobarbital Sodium (Atazanavir sulfate competitively inhibits CYP1A2 and CYP2C9. There is a potential drug-drug interaction between atazanavir sulfate and CYP1A2 or CYP2C9 substrates).
No products indexed under this heading.

Phenylbutazone (Atazanavir sulfate competitively inhibits CYP1A2 and CYP2C9. There is a potential drug-drug interaction between atazanavir sulfate and CYP1A2 or CYP2C9 substrates).
No products indexed under this heading.

Phenytoin (Atazanavir sulfate competitively inhibits CYP1A2 and CYP2C9. There is a potential drug-drug interaction between atazanavir sulfate and CYP1A2 or CYP2C9 substrates).
No products indexed under this heading.

Phenytoin Sodium (Atazanavir sulfate competitively inhibits CYP1A2 and CYP2C9. There is a potential drug-drug interaction between atazanavir sulfate and CYP1A2 or CYP2C9 substrates). Products include:
Phenytek Capsules 2192

Pimozide (Contraindicated due to potential for serious and/or life-threatening reactions, such as cardiac arrhythmias).
No products indexed under this heading.

Pioglitazone Hydrochloride (Atazanavir sulfate competitively inhibits CYP1A2 and CYP2C9. There is a potential drug-drug interaction between atazanavir sulfate and CYP1A2 or CYP2C9 substrates). Products include:
ActoPlus Met Tablets 3071
Actos Tablets 3077
Duetact Tablets 3085

Piroxicam (Atazanavir sulfate competitively inhibits CYP1A2 and CYP2C9. There is a potential drug-drug interaction between atazanavir sulfate and CYP1A2 or CYP2C9 substrates).
No products indexed under this heading.

Propafenone Hydrochloride (Atazanavir sulfate competitively inhibits CYP1A2 and CYP2C9. There is a potential drug-drug interaction between atazanavir sulfate and CYP1A2 or CYP2C9 substrates). Products include:
Rythmol Tablets 1586
Rythmol SR Capsules 1590

Propranolol Hydrochloride (Atazanavir sulfate competitively inhibits CYP1A2 and CYP2C9. There is a potential drug-drug interaction between atazanavir sulfate and CYP1A2 or CYP2C9 substrates). Products include:
InnoPran XL Extended Release Capsules 1484

Protriptyline Hydrochloride (Atazanavir sulfate competitively inhibits CYP1A2 and CYP2C9. There is a potential drug-drug interaction between atazanavir sulfate and CYP1A2 or CYP2C9 substrates).
No products indexed under this heading.

Quinidine (Co-administration with atazanavir sulfate has the potential to produce serious and/or life-threatening adverse events and has not been studied. Caution is warranted and therapeutic concentration monitoring of these drugs is recommended if they are used concomitantly with atazanavir sulfate).
No products indexed under this heading.

Quinidine Gluconate (Co-administration with atazanavir sulfate has the potential to produce serious and/or life-threatening adverse events and has not been studied. Caution is warranted and therapeutic concentration monitoring of these drugs is recommended if they are used concomitantly with atazanavir sulfate).
No products indexed under this heading.

Quinidine Hydrochloride (Co-administration with atazanavir sulfate has the potential to produce serious and/or life-threatening adverse events and has not been studied. Concentration monitoring of these drugs is recommended if they are used concomitantly with atazanavir sulfate).
No products indexed under this heading.

Quinidine Polygalacturonate (Co-administration with atazanavir sulfate has the potential to produce serious and/or life-threatening adverse events and has not been studied. Caution is warranted and therapeutic concentration monitoring of these drugs is recommended if they are used concomitantly with atazanavir sulfate).
No products indexed under this heading.

Quinidine Sulfate (Co-administration with atazanavir sulfate has the potential to produce serious and/or life-threatening adverse events and has not been studied. Caution is warranted and therapeutic concentration monitoring of these drugs is recommended if they are used concomitantly with atazanavir sulfate).
No products indexed under this heading.

Quinine (Co-administration of atazanavir sulfate and other drugs that inhibit CYP3A may increase atazanavir sulfate plasma concentrations).
No products indexed under this heading.

Quinine Sulfate (Co-administration of atazanavir sulfate and other drugs that inhibit CYP3A may increase atazanavir sulfate plasma concentrations).
No products indexed under this heading.

Rabeprazole Sodium (Concomitant use of atazanavir sulfate and proton-pump inhibitors is not recommended. Co-administration of atazanavir sulfate with proton-pump inhibitors is expected to substantially decrease atazanavir sulfate plasma concentrations and reduce its therapeutic effect). Products include:
Aciphex Tablets 1053

Ranitidine Bismuth Citrate (Reduced plasma concentrations of atazanavir are expected if H2-receptor antagonists are administered with atazanavir sulfate. This may result in loss of therapeutic effect and development of resistance. To lessen the effect of H2-receptor antagonists on atazanavir exposure, it is recommended that an H2-receptor antagonist and atazanavir sulfate be administered as far apart as possible, preferably 12 hours apart).
No products indexed under this heading.

Ranitidine Hydrochloride (Reduced plasma concentrations of atazanavir are expected if H2-receptor antagonists are administered with atazanavir sulfate. This may result in loss of therapeutic effect and development of resistance. To lessen the effect of H2-receptor antagonists on atazanavir exposure, it is recommended that an H2-receptor antagonist and atazanavir sulfate be administered as far apart as possible, preferably 12 hours apart). Products include:
Zantac 75 Tablets ..... ■603
Zantac 1670
Zantac Injection 1666
Zantac Injection Pharmacy Bulk Package 1668
Maximum Strength Zantac 150 Tablets ..... ■603
Maximum Strength Zantac 150 Cool Mint Tablets ..... ■603

Repaglinide (Atazanavir sulfate competitively inhibits CYP1A2 and CYP2C9. There is a potential drug-drug interaction between atazanavir sulfate and CYP1A2 or CYP2C9 substrates). Products include:
PrandiMet Tablets 2967
Prandin Tablets 2971

Rifabutin (A rifabutin dose reduction of up to 75% (e.g., 150mg every other day or three times a week) is recommended).
No products indexed under this heading.

Rifampicin (Drugs that induce CYP3A activity may increase the clearance of atazanavir sulfate, resulting in lowered plasma concentrations).
No products indexed under this heading.

Rifampin (Co-administration of atazanavir sulfate and drugs that induce CYP3A, such as rifampin, may decrease atazanavir plasma concentrations and reduce its therapeutic effect. Rifampin decreases plasma concentrations and AUC of most protease inhibitors by about 90%. This may result in loss of theraputic effect and development of resistance. Co-administration is contraindicated).
No products indexed under this heading.

Rifapentine (Drugs that induce CYP3A activity may increase the clearance of atazanavir sulfate, resulting in lowered plasma concentrations).
No products indexed under this heading.

Riluzole (Atazanavir sulfate competitively inhibits CYP1A2 and CYP2C9. There is a potential drug-drug interaction between atazanavir sulfate and CYP1A2 or CYP2C9 substrates). Products include:
Rilutek Tablets 2771

Ritonavir (If atazanavir sulfate is co-administered with ritonavir, it is recommended that atazanavir sulfate 300 mg once daily be given with ritonavir 100 mg once daily with food). Products include:
Kaletra 452
Norvir 489

Rofecoxib (Atazanavir sulfate competitively inhibits CYP1A2 and CYP2C9. There is a potential drug-drug interaction between atazanavir sulfate and CYP1A2 or CYP2C9 substrates).
No products indexed under this heading.

Ropinirole Hydrochloride (Atazanavir sulfate competitively inhibits CYP1A2 and CYP2C9. There is a potential drug-drug interaction between atazanavir sulfate and CYP1A2 or CYP2C9 substrates). Products include:
Requip Tablets 1561
Requip XL Tablets 1568

Ropivacaine Hydrochloride (Atazanavir sulfate competitively inhibits CYP1A2 and CYP2C9. There is a potential drug-drug interaction between atazanavir sulfate and CYP1A2 or CYP2C9 substrates).
No products indexed under this heading.

Rosiglitazone Maleate (Atazanavir sulfate competitively inhibits CYP1A2 and CYP2C9. There is a potential drug-drug interaction between atazanavir sulfate and CYP1A2 or CYP2C9 substrates). Products include:
Avandamet Tablets 1336
Avandaryl Tablets 1344
Avandia Tablets 1351

Saquinavir (Saquinavir 1200 mg co-administered with atazanavir sulfate 400 mg and tenofovir 300 mg (all given once daily) plus nucleoside analogue reverse transcriptase inhibitors did not provide adequate efficacy).
No products indexed under this heading.

Saquinavir Mesylate (Saquinavir 1200 mg co-administered with atazanavir sulfate 400 mg and tenofovir 300 mg (all given once daily) plus nucleoside analogue reverse transcriptase inhibitors did not provide adequate efficacy).
No products indexed under this heading.

Sertraline Hydrochloride (Co-administration of atazanavir sulfate and other drugs that inhibit CYP3A may increase atazanavir sulfate plasma concentrations).
No products indexed under this heading.

Sildenafil Citrate (Co-administration may result in an increase in PDE5 inhibitor-associated adverse events, including hypertension, visual changes, and priapism. Use sildenafil with caution at reduced doses of 25 mg every 48 hours with increased monitoring for adverse events).
No products indexed under this heading.

Simvastatin (Concomitant use of atazanavir sulfate with simvastatin is not recommended. Caution should be exercised if HIV protease inhibitors, including atazanavir sulfate, are used concurrently with other HMG-CoA reductase inhibitors that are also metabolized by the CYP3A4 pathway. The risk of myopathy, including rhabdomyolysis, may be increased when HIV protease inhibitors, including atazanavir sulfate, are used in combination with these drugs). Products include:
Simcor Tablets ... 502
Vytorin 10/10 Tablets ... 2149
Vytorin 10/10 Tablets ... 2939
Vytorin 10/20 Tablets ... 2149
Vytorin 10/20 Tablets ... 2939
Vytorin 10/40 Tablets ... 2149
Vytorin 10/40 Tablets ... 2939
Vytorin 10/80 Tablets ... 2149
Vytorin 10/80 Tablets ... 2939
Zocor Tablets ... 2136

Sirolimus (Therapeutic concentration monitoring is recommended for immunosuppressant agents when co-administered with atazanavir sulfate). Products include:
Rapamune ... 3260

Sodium Bicarbonate (Reduced plasma concentrations of atazanavir are expected if antacids, including buffered medications, are administered with atazanavir sulfate. Atazanavir sulfate should be administered 2 hours before or 1 hour after these medications). Products include:
Ceo-Two Laxative Suppository ... 815

Sulfamethoxazole (Atazanavir sulfate competitively inhibits CYP1A2 and CYP2C9. There is a potential drug-drug interaction between atazanavir sulfate and CYP1A2 or CYP2C9 substrates).
No products indexed under this heading.

Sulindac (Atazanavir sulfate competitively inhibits CYP1A2 and CYP2C9. There is a potential drug-drug interaction between atazanavir sulfate and CYP1A2 or CYP2C9 substrates). Products include:
Clinoril Tablets ... 1962

Suprofen (Atazanavir sulfate competitively inhibits CYP1A2 and CYP2C9. There is a potential drug-drug interaction between atazanavir sulfate and CYP1A2 or CYP2C9 substrates).
No products indexed under this heading.

Tacrine Hydrochloride (Atazanavir sulfate competitively inhibits CYP1A2 and CYP2C9. There is a potential drug-drug interaction between atazanavir sulfate and CYP1A2 or CYP2C9 substrates).
No products indexed under this heading.

Tacrolimus (Therapeutic concentration monitoring is recommended for immunosuppressant agents when co-administered with atazanavir sulfate). Products include:
Prograf Capsules and Injection ... 622
Protopic Ointment ... 628

Tadalafil (Co-administration may result in an increase in PDE5 inhibitor-associated adverse events, including hypertension, visual changes, and priapism. Use tadalafil with caution at reduced doses of 10 mg every 72 hours with increased monitoring of adverse events). Products include:
Cialis Tablets ... 1792

Tamoxifen Citrate (Atazanavir sulfate competitively inhibits CYP1A2 and CYP2C9. There is a potential drug-drug interaction between atazanavir sulfate and CYP1A2 or CYP2C9 substrates).
No products indexed under this heading.

Telmisartan (Atazanavir sulfate competitively inhibits CYP1A2 and CYP2C9. There is a potential drug-drug interaction between atazanavir sulfate and CYP1A2 or CYP2C9 substrates). Products include:
Micardis Tablets ... 852
Micardis HCT Tablets ... 854

Tenofovir Disoproxil Fumarate (Tenofovir may decrease the AUC and Cmin of atazanavir sulfate, while atazanavir sulfate increases tenofovir concentrations. It is recommended to administer tenofovir 300 mg with atazanavir sulfate 300 mg and ritonavir 100 mg as a single dose). Products include:
Atripla Tablets ... 938
Truvada Tablets ... 1262
Viread Tablets ... 1268

Theophylline (Atazanavir sulfate competitively inhibits CYP1A2 and CYP2C9. There is a potential drug-drug interaction between atazanavir sulfate and CYP1A2 or CYP2C9 substrates).
No products indexed under this heading.

Theophylline Anhydrous (Atazanavir sulfate competitively inhibits CYP1A2 and CYP2C9. There is a potential drug-drug interaction between atazanavir sulfate and CYP1A2 or CYP2C9 substrates). Products include:
Uniphyl Tablets ... 2595

Theophylline Calcium Salicylate (Atazanavir sulfate competitively inhibits CYP1A2 and CYP2C9. There is a potential drug-drug interaction between atazanavir sulfate and CYP1A2 or CYP2C9 substrates).
No products indexed under this heading.

Theophylline Dihydroxypropyl (Glyceryl) (Atazanavir sulfate competitively inhibits CYP1A2 and CYP2C9. There is a potential drug-drug interaction between atazanavir sulfate and CYP1A2 or CYP2C9 substrates).
No products indexed under this heading.

Theophylline Ethylenediamine (Atazanavir sulfate competitively inhibits CYP1A2 and CYP2C9. There is a potential drug-drug interaction between atazanavir sulfate and CYP1A2 or CYP2C9 substrates).
No products indexed under this heading.

Tipranavir (Co-administration of atazanavir sulfate/ritonavir and other protease inhibitors would be expected to increase exposure to the other protease inhibitors; co-administration is not recommended). Products include:
Aptivus Capsules ... 823
Aptivus Oral Solution ... 823

Tolazamide (Atazanavir sulfate competitively inhibits CYP1A2 and CYP2C9. There is a potential drug-drug interaction between atazanavir sulfate and CYP1A2 or CYP2C9 substrates).
No products indexed under this heading.

Tolbutamide (Atazanavir sulfate competitively inhibits CYP1A2 and CYP2C9. There is a potential drug-drug interaction between atazanavir sulfate and CYP1A2 or CYP2C9 substrates).
No products indexed under this heading.

Tolbutamide Sodium (Atazanavir sulfate competitively inhibits CYP1A2 and CYP2C9. There is a potential drug-drug interaction between atazanavir sulfate and CYP1A2 or CYP2C9 substrates).
No products indexed under this heading.

Tolmetin Sodium (Atazanavir sulfate competitively inhibits CYP1A2 and CYP2C9. There is a potential drug-drug interaction between atazanavir sulfate and CYP1A2 or CYP2C9 substrates).
No products indexed under this heading.

Torsemide (Atazanavir sulfate competitively inhibits CYP1A2 and CYP2C9. There is a potential drug-drug interaction between atazanavir sulfate and CYP1A2 or CYP2C9 substrates). Products include:
Demadex Injection ... 2630
Demadex Tablets ... 2630

Trazodone Hydrochloride (Concomitant use will increase plasma concentration of trazodone).
No products indexed under this heading.

Triazolam (Contraindicated due to potential for serious and/or life-threatening events, such as prolonged or increased sedation or respiratory depression).
No products indexed under this heading.

Trimethaphan Camsylate (Atazanavir sulfate competitively inhibits CYP1A2 and CYP2C9. There is a potential drug-drug interaction between atazanavir sulfate and CYP1A2 or CYP2C9 substrates).
No products indexed under this heading.

Trimipramine Maleate (Atazanavir sulfate competitively inhibits CYP1A2 and CYP2C9. There is a potential drug-drug interaction between atazanavir sulfate and CYP1A2 or CYP2C9 substrates).
No products indexed under this heading.

Troglitazone (Atazanavir sulfate competitively inhibits CYP1A2 and CYP2C9. There is a potential drug-drug interaction between atazanavir sulfate and CYP1A2 or CYP2C9 substrates).
No products indexed under this heading.

Troleandomycin (Co-administration of atazanavir sulfate and other drugs that inhibit CYP3A may increase atazanavir sulfate plasma concentrations).
No products indexed under this heading.

Trovafloxacin Mesylate (Atazanavir sulfate competitively inhibits CYP1A2 and CYP2C9. There is a potential drug-drug interaction between atazanavir sulfate and CYP1A2 or CYP2C9 substrates).
No products indexed under this heading.

Valdecoxib (Atazanavir sulfate competitively inhibits CYP1A2 and CYP2C9. There is a potential drug-drug interaction between atazanavir sulfate and CYP1A2 or CYP2C9 substrates).
No products indexed under this heading.

Valsartan (Atazanavir sulfate competitively inhibits CYP1A2 and CYP2C9. There is a potential drug-drug interaction between atazanavir sulfate and CYP1A2 or CYP2C9 substrates). Products include:
Diovan Tablets ... 2212
Diovan HCT Tablets ... 2216
Exforge Tablets ... 2238

Vardenafil Hydrochloride (Co-administration may result in an increase in PDE5 inhibitor-associated adverse events, including hypertension, visual changes, and priapism. Use vardenafil with caution at reduced doses of no more than 2.5 mg every 72 hours with increased monitoring of adverse events). Products include:
Levitra Tablets ... 2876

Venlafaxine Hydrochloride (Co-administration of atazanavir sulfate and other drugs that inhibit CYP3A may increase atazanavir sulfate plasma concentrations). Products include:
Effexor XR Extended-Release Capsules ... 3195
Venlafaxine Hydrochloride Tablets ... 2199

Verapamil Hydrochloride (Caution is warranted. Dose titration of the calcium channel blocker should be considered. ECG monitoring is recommended). Products include:
Tarka Tablets ... 511

Voriconazole (Voriconazole with ritonavir 400 mg every 12 hours decreased voriconazole steady state AUC by 82%; therefore, voriconazole should not be co-administered with atazanavir sulfate/ritonavir. Co-administration of voriconazole with atazanavir sulfate (without ritonavir) may increase atazanavir sulfate concentrations; however, no data are available).
No products indexed under this heading.

Warfarin Sodium (Atazanavir sulfate competitively inhibits CYP1A2 and CYP2C9. There is a potential drug-drug interaction between atazanavir sulfate and CYP1A2 or CYP2C9 substrates).
No products indexed under this heading.

Zafirlukast (Atazanavir sulfate competitively inhibits CYP1A2 and CYP2C9. There is a potential drug-drug interaction between atazanavir sulfate and CYP1A2 or CYP2C9 substrates). Products include:
Accolate Tablets 669

Zileuton (Atazanavir sulfate competitively inhibits CYP1A2 and CYP2C9. There is a potential drug-drug interaction between atazanavir sulfate and CYP1A2 or CYP2C9 substrates).
No products indexed under this heading.

Zolmitriptan (Atazanavir sulfate competitively inhibits CYP1A2 and CYP2C9. There is a potential drug-drug interaction between atazanavir sulfate and CYP1A2 or CYP2C9 substrates). Products include:
Zomig Tablets 694
Zomig Nasal Spray 689
Zomig-ZMT Tablets 694

Food Interactions

Grapefruit (Co-administration of atazanavir sulfate and other drugs that inhibit CYP3A may increase atazanavir sulfate plasma concentrations).

RILUTEK TABLETS

(Riluzole) 2771
May interact with quinolones, xanthines, and certain other agents. Compounds in these categories include:

Alatrofloxacin Mesylate (Potential inhibitors of CYP1A2, such as quinolones, could decrease the rate of riluzole elimination).
No products indexed under this heading.

Allopurinol (Riluzole induces hepatic injury; ALS patients on concomitant hepatotoxic drugs, such as allopurinol, were excluded in the clinical trials; if such combination is used, practitioner should exercise caution).
No products indexed under this heading.

Aminophylline (Potential inhibitors of CYP1A2, such as theophylline, could decrease the rate of riluzole elimination).
No products indexed under this heading.

Amitriptyline Hydrochloride (Potential inhibitors of CYP1A2, such as amitriptyline, could decrease the rate of riluzole elimination).
No products indexed under this heading.

Caffeine (Potential inhibitors of CYP1A2, such as caffeine, could decrease the rate of riluzole elimination). Products include:
BioLean Free Tablets .... ▣635
BioLean II Tablets .... ▣635
Winrgy Dietary Supplement .... ▣642

Ciprofloxacin (Potential inhibitors of CYP1A2, such as quinolones, could decrease the rate of riluzole elimination). Products include:
Cipro I.V. 2817
Cipro Oral Suspension 2810
Cipro XR Tablets 2823
Ciprodex Otic Suspension 541

Ciprofloxacin Hydrochloride (Potential inhibitors of CYP1A2, such as quinolones, could decrease the rate of riluzole elimination). Products include:
Cipro Tablets 2810

Dyphylline (Potential inhibitors of CYP1A2, such as theophylline, could decrease the rate of riluzole elimination).
No products indexed under this heading.

Enoxacin (Potential inhibitors of CYP1A2, such as quinolones, could decrease the rate of riluzole elimination).
No products indexed under this heading.

Grepafloxacin Hydrochloride (Potential inhibitors of CYP1A2, such as quinolones, could decrease the rate of riluzole elimination).
No products indexed under this heading.

Lomefloxacin Hydrochloride (Potential inhibitors of CYP1A2, such as quinolones, could decrease the rate of riluzole elimination).
No products indexed under this heading.

Methyldopa (Riluzole induces hepatic injury; ALS patients on concomitant hepatotoxic drugs, such as methyldopa, were excluded in the clinical trials; if such combination is used, practitioner should exercise caution).
No products indexed under this heading.

Moxifloxacin Hydrochloride (Potential inhibitors of CYP1A2, such as quinolones, could decrease the rate of riluzole elimination). Products include:
Avelox 2803
Vigamox Ophthalmic Solution 548

Norfloxacin (Potential inhibitors of CYP1A2, such as quinolones, could decrease the rate of riluzole elimination). Products include:
Noroxin Tablets 2069

Ofloxacin (Potential inhibitors of CYP1A2, such as quinolones, could decrease the rate of riluzole elimination). Products include:
Ofloxacin Ophthalmic Solution 0.3% .... ⊙243

Omeprazole (Potential inducers of CYP1A2, such as theophylline, could increase the rate of riluzole elimination).
No products indexed under this heading.

Phenacetin (Potential inhibitors of CYP1A2, such as phenacetin, could decrease the rate of riluzole elimination).
No products indexed under this heading.

Rifampin (Potential inducers of CYP1A2, such as theophylline, could increase the rate of riluzole elimination).
No products indexed under this heading.

Sulfasalazine (Riluzole induces hepatic injury; ALS patients on concomitant hepatotoxic drugs, such as sulfasalazine, were excluded in the clinical trials; if such combination is used, practitioner should exercise caution).
No products indexed under this heading.

Tacrine Hydrochloride (CYP1A2 is the principal isoenzyme involved in the initial oxidative metabolism of riluzole; potential interaction may occur when co-administered with other agents, such as tacrine, which are also metabolized primarily by CYP1A2).
No products indexed under this heading.

Theophylline (Potential inhibitors of CYP1A2, such as theophylline, could decrease the rate of riluzole elimination).
No products indexed under this heading.

Theophylline Anhydrous (Potential inhibitors of CYP1A2, such as theophylline, could decrease the rate of riluzole elimination). Products include:
Uniphyl Tablets 2595

Theophylline Calcium Salicylate (Potential inhibitors of CYP1A2, such as theophylline, could decrease the rate of riluzole elimination).
No products indexed under this heading.

Theophylline Dihydroxypropyl (Glyceryl) (Potential inhibitors of CYP1A2, such as theophylline, could decrease the rate of riluzole elimination).
No products indexed under this heading.

Theophylline Ethylenediamine (Potential inhibitors of CYP1A2, such as theophylline, could decrease the rate of riluzole elimination).
No products indexed under this heading.

Theophylline Sodium Glycinate (Potential inhibitors of CYP1A2, such as theophylline, could decrease the rate of riluzole elimination).
No products indexed under this heading.

Trovafloxacin Mesylate (Potential inhibitors of CYP1A2, such as quinolones, could decrease the rate of riluzole elimination).
No products indexed under this heading.

Food Interactions

Alcohol (Alcohol may increase the risk of hepatotoxicity; patients on riluzole should be discouraged from drinking excessive amounts of alcohol).

Diet, high-lipid (Co-administration with high-fat meal decreases absorption, reduces AUC by about 20% and peak blood levels by about 45%).

Food, charcoal-broiled (Potential inducers of CYP1A2, such as charcoal-broiled food, could increase the rate of riluzole elimination).

RISPERDAL CONSTA LONG-ACTING INJECTION

(Risperidone) 1753
May interact with antihypertensives, central nervous system depressants, central nervous system stimulants, cytochrome p450 2d6 inhibitors (selected), cytochrome p450 3a4 inducers (selected), dopamine agonists, hepatic microsomal enzyme inducers, and certain other agents. Compounds in these categories include:

Acebutolol Hydrochloride (Because of its potential for inducing hypotension, risperidone may enhance the hypotensive effects of other therapeutic agents with this potential).
No products indexed under this heading.

Alfentanil Hydrochloride (Given the primary CNS effects of risperidone, caution should be used if taken in combination with other centrally-acting drugs).
No products indexed under this heading.

Aliskiren (Because of its potential for inducing hypotension, risperidone may enhance the hypotensive effects of other therapeutic agents with this potential). Products include:
Tekturna Tablets 2321
Tekturna HCT Tablets 2324

Allium sativum (Co-administration of know CYP3A4 enzyme inducers (e.g., phenytoin, rifampin, and phenobarbital) with risperidone may cause decreases in the combined plasma concentrations of ripseridone and 9-hydroxyrisperidone, which could lead to decreased efficacy of Risperdal Consta treatment. At the initiation of therapy with known CYP3A4 hepatic enzyme inducers, patients should be closely monitored during the first 4-8 weeks, since the dose of Risperdal Consta may need to be adjusted. A dose increase, or additionaloral risperidone, may need to be considered. On discontinuation of CYP3A4 hepatic enzyme inducers, the dosage of Risperdal Consta should be re-evaluated and, if necessary, decreased).
No products indexed under this heading.

Alprazolam (Given the primary CNS effects of risperidone, caution should be used if taken in combination with other centrally-acting drugs).
No products indexed under this heading.

Amiodarone Hydrochloride (Risperidone is metabolized to 9-hydroxyrisperidone by CYP2D6. Drug interactions that reduce the metabolism of risperidone to 9-hydroxyrisperidone would increase the plasma concentrations of risperidone and lower the concentrations of 9-hydroxyrisperidone).
No products indexed under this heading.

Amitriptyline Hydrochloride (Risperidone is metabolized to 9-hydroxyrisperidone by CYP2D6. Drug interactions that reduce the metabolism of risperidone to 9-hydroxyrisperidone would increase the plasma concentrations of risperidone and lower the concentrations of 9-hydroxyrisperidone).
No products indexed under this heading.

Amlodipine Besylate (Because of its potential for inducing hypotension, risperidone may enhance the hypotensive effects of other therapeutic agents with this potential). Products include:
Azor Tablets 1005
Exforge Tablets 2238

Amoxapine (Risperidone is metabolized to 9-hydroxyrisperidone by CYP2D6. Drug interactions that reduce the metabolism of risperidone to 9-hydroxyrisperidone would increase the plasma concentrations of risperidone and lower the concentrations of 9-hydroxyrisperidone).
No products indexed under this heading.

Amphetamine Resins (Given the primary CNS effects of risperdone, caution should be taken with other centrally-acting drugs).
No products indexed under this heading.

Aprepitant (Co-administration of know CYP3A4 enzyme inducers (e.g., phenytoin, rifampin, and phenobarbital) with risperidone may cause decreases in the combined plasma concentrations of ripseridone and 9-hydroxyrisperidone, which could lead to decreased efficacy of Risperdal Consta treatment. At the initiation of therapy with known CYP3A4 hepatic enzyme inducers, patients should be closely monitored during the first 4-8 weeks, since the dose of Risperdal Consta may need to be adjusted. A dose increase, or additionaloral risperidone, may need to be considered. On discontinuation of CYP3A4 hepatic enzyme inducers, the dosage of Risperdal Consta should be re-evaluated and, if necessary, decreased). Products include:
Emend Capsules 1992

Aprobarbital (Given the primary CNS effects of risperidone, caution should be used if taken in combination with other centrally-acting drugs).
No products indexed under this heading.

Atenolol (Because of its potential for inducing hypotension, risperidone may enhance the hypotensive effects of other therapeutic agents with this potential).
No products indexed under this heading.

Benazepril Hydrochloride (Because of its potential for inducing hypotension, risperidone may enhance the hypotensive effects of other therapeutic agents with this potential).
No products indexed under this heading.

Bendroflumethiazide (Because of its potential for inducing hypotension, risperidone may enhance the hypotensive effects of other therapeutic agents with this potential).
No products indexed under this heading.

Betamethasone Acetate (Co-administration of know CYP3A4 enzyme inducers (e.g., phenytoin, rifampin, and phenobarbital) with risperidone may cause decreases in the combined plasma concentrations of ripseridone and 9-hydroxyrisperidone, which could lead to decreased efficacy of Risperdal Consta treatment. At the initiation of therapy with known CYP3A4 hepatic enzyme inducers, patients should be closely monitored during the first 4-8 weeks, since the dose of Risperdal Consta may need to be adjusted. A dose increase, or additionaloral risperidone, may need to be considered. On discontinuation of CYP3A4 hepatic enzyme inducers, the dosage of Risperdal Consta should be re-evaluated and, if necessary, decreased).
No products indexed under this heading.

Betamethasone Sodium Phosphate (Co-administration of know CYP3A4 enzyme inducers (e.g., phenytoin, rifampin, and phenobarbital) with risperidone may cause decreases in the combined plasma concentrations of ripseridone and 9-hydroxyrisperidone, which could lead to decreased efficacy of Risperdal Consta treatment. At the initiation of therapy with known CYP3A4 hepatic enzyme inducers, patients should be closely monitored during the first 4-8 weeks, since the dose of Risperdal Consta may need to be adjusted. A dose increase, or additionaloral risperidone, may need to be considered. On discontinuation of CYP3A4 hepatic enzyme inducers, the dosage of Risperdal Consta should be re-evaluated and, if necessary, decreased).
No products indexed under this heading.

Betaxolol Hydrochloride (Because of its potential for inducing hypotension, risperidone may enhance the hypotensive effects of other therapeutic agents with this potential).
No products indexed under this heading.

Bisoprolol Fumarate (Because of its potential for inducing hypotension, risperidone may enhance the hypotensive effects of other therapeutic agents with this potential).
No products indexed under this heading.

Bromocriptine Mesylate (Risperidone may antagonize the effect of dopamine agonists).
No products indexed under this heading.

Buprenorphine Hydrochloride (Given the primary CNS effects of risperidone, caution should be used if taken in combination with other centrally-acting drugs). Products include:
Suboxone Tablets 2601
Subutex Tablets 2601

Bupropion Hydrochloride (Risperidone is metabolized to 9-hydroxyrisperidone by CYP2D6. Drug interactions that reduce the metabolism of risperidone to 9-hydroxyrisperidone would increase the plasma concentrations of risperidone and lower the concentrations of 9-hydroxyrisperidone). Products include:
Wellbutrin Tablets 1648
Wellbutrin SR Sustained-Release Tablets 1653
Wellbutrin XL Extended-Release Tablets 1659
Zyban Sustained-Release Tablets 1692

Buspirone Hydrochloride (Given the primary CNS effects of risperidone, caution should be used if taken in combination with other centrally-acting drugs).
No products indexed under this heading.

Butabarbital (Given the primary CNS effects of risperidone, caution should be used if taken in combination with other centrally-acting drugs).
No products indexed under this heading.

Butalbital (Given the primary CNS effects of risperidone, caution should be used if taken in combination with other centrally-acting drugs).
No products indexed under this heading.

Candesartan Cilexetil (Because of its potential for inducing hypotension, risperidone may enhance the hypotensive effects of other therapeutic agents with this potential). Products include:
Atacand Tablets 639
Atacand HCT 642

Captopril (Because of its potential for inducing hypotension, risperidone may enhance the hypotensive effects of other therapeutic agents with this potential). Products include:
Captopril Tablets 2182

Carbamazepine (During co-administration, the plasma concentrations of risperidone and its pharmacologically active metabolite, 9-hydroxyrisperidone, were decreased by about 50%. Plasma concentrations of carbamazepine did not appear to be affected. At initiation of therapy with carbamazepine, patients should be closely monitored during the first 4-8 weeks, since the dose of Risperdal Consta may need to be adjusted. A dose increase, or additional oral risperidone, may be considered. On discontinuation of carbamazepine, the dosage of Risperdal Consta should be re-evaluated and, if necessary, decreased). Products include:
Carbatrol Capsules 3019
Equetro Extended-Release Capsules 3174

Carteolol Hydrochloride (Because of its potential for inducing hypotension, risperidone may enhance the hypotensive effects of other therapeutic agents with this potential).
No products indexed under this heading.

Celecoxib (Risperidone is metabolized to 9-hydroxyrisperidone by CYP2D6. Drug interactions that reduce the metabolism of risperidone to 9-hydroxyrisperidone would increase the plasma concentrations of risperidone and lower the concentrations of 9-hydroxyrisperidone). Products include:
Celebrex Capsules 2979

Chlordiazepoxide (Given the primary CNS effects of risperidone, caution should be used if taken in combination with other centrally-acting drugs).
No products indexed under this heading.

Chlordiazepoxide Hydrochloride (Given the primary CNS effects of risperidone, caution should be used if taken in combination with other centrally-acting drugs).
No products indexed under this heading.

Chloroquine Hydrochloride (Risperidone is metabolized to 9-hydroxyrisperidone by CYP2D6. Drug interactions that reduce the metabolism of risperidone to 9-hydroxyrisperidone would increase the plasma concentrations of risperidone and lower the concentrations of 9-hydroxyrisperidone).
No products indexed under this heading.

Chloroquine Phosphate (Risperidone is metabolized to 9-hydroxyrisperidone by CYP2D6. Drug interactions that reduce the metabolism of risperidone to 9-hydroxyrisperidone would increase the plasma concentrations of risperidone and lower the concentrations of 9-hydroxyrisperidone).
No products indexed under this heading.

Chlorothiazide (Because of its potential for inducing hypotension, risperidone may enhance the hypotensive effects of other therapeutic agents with this potential).
No products indexed under this heading.

Chlorothiazide Sodium (Because of its potential for inducing hypotension, risperidone may enhance the hypotensive effects of other therapeutic agents with this potential). Products include:
Intravenous Sodium Diuril 2490

Chlorpheniramine (Risperidone is metabolized to 9-hydroxyrisperidone by CYP2D6. Drug interactions that reduce the metabolism of risperidone to 9-hydroxyrisperidone would increase the plasma concentrations of risperidone and lower the concentrations of 9-hydroxyrisperidone).
No products indexed under this heading.

Chlorpheniramine Maleate (Risperidone is metabolized to 9-hydroxyrisperidone by CYP2D6. Drug interactions that reduce the metabolism of risperidone to 9-hydroxyrisperidone would increase the plasma concentrations of risperidone and lower the concentrations of 9-hydroxyrisperidone). Products include:
Actifed Cold & Allergy Tablets 1895
Sudafed PE Sinus & Allergy Tablets 1908
Tylenol Allergy Multi-Symptom Caplets with Cool Burst and Rapid Release Gelcaps 1916
Children's Tylenol Plus Cold Suspension Liquid 1912
Children's Tylenol Plus Cough & Runny Nose Suspension Liquid 1912
Children's Tylenol Plus Flu Suspension Liquid 1914
Children's Tylenol Plus Multi-Symptom Cold Suspension Liquid 1912
Tylenol Cold Head Congestion Nighttime Caplets with Cool Burst 1910
Tylenol Cold Multi-Symptom Nighttime Caplets with Cool Burst 1913
Tylenol Sinus Congestion & Pain Nighttime Caplets with Cool Burst 1917

Chlorpheniramine Polistirex (Risperidone is metabolized to 9-hydroxyrisperidone by CYP2D6. Drug interactions that reduce the metabolism of risperidone to 9-hydroxyrisperidone would increase the plasma concentrations of risperidone and lower the concentrations of 9-hydroxyrisperidone). Products include:
Tussionex Pennkinetic Extended-Release Suspension 3154

Chlorpheniramine Tannate (Risperidone is metabolized to 9-hydroxyrisperidone by CYP2D6. Drug interactions that reduce the metabolism of risperidone to 9-hydroxyrisperidone would increase the plasma concentrations of risperidone and lower the concentrations of 9-hydroxyrisperidone).
No products indexed under this heading.

Chlorpromazine (Given the primary CNS effects of risperidone, caution should be used if taken in combination with other centrally-acting drugs).
No products indexed under this heading.

Chlorpromazine Hydrochloride (Given the primary CNS effects of risperidone, caution should be used if taken in combination with other centrally-acting drugs).
No products indexed under this heading.

Chlorpropamide (Co-administration of known enzyme inducers (e.g., phenytoin, rifampin and phenobarbital) with risperidone may cause decreases in the combined plasma concentrations of risperidone and 9-hydroxyrisperidone, which could lead to decreased efficacy. The dose of risperidone may need to be adjusted accordingly, particularly during the initiation or discontinuation of therapy with enzyme inducers).
No products indexed under this heading.

Chlorprothixene (Given the primary CNS effects of risperidone, caution should be used if taken in combination with other centrally-acting drugs).
No products indexed under this heading.

Chlorprothixene Hydrochloride (Given the primary CNS effects of risperidone, caution should be used if taken in combination with other centrally-acting drugs).
No products indexed under this heading.

Chlorprothixene Lactate (Given the primary CNS effects of risperidone, caution should be used if taken in combination with other centrally-acting drugs).
No products indexed under this heading.

Chlorthalidone (Because of its potential for inducing hypotension, risperidone may enhance the hypotensive effects of other therapeutic agents with this potential). Products include:
Clorpres Tablets 2185

Cimetidine (Cimetidine increased the bioavailability of risperidone by 64%. However, cimetidine did not affect the AUC of the active moiety).
No products indexed under this heading.

Cimetidine Hydrochloride (Cimetidine increased the bioavailability of risperidone by 64%. However, cimetidine did not affect the AUC of the active moiety).
No products indexed under this heading.

Ciprofloxacin Hydrochloride (Co-administration of know CYP3A4 enzyme inducers (e.g., phenytoin, rifampin, and phenobarbital) with risperidone may cause decreases in the combined plasma concentrations of ripseridone and 9-hydroxyrisperidone, which could lead to decreased efficacy of Risperdal Consta treatment. At the initiation of therapy with known CYP3A4 hepatic enzyme inducers, patients should be closely monitored during the first 4-8 weeks, since the dose of Risperdal Consta may need to be adjusted. A dose increase, or additionaloral risperidone, may need to be considered. On discontinuation of CYP3A4 hepatic enzyme inducers, the dosage of Risperdal Consta should be re-evaluated and, if necessary, decreased). Products include:
Cipro Tablets 2810

Cisplatin (Co-administration of know CYP3A4 enzyme inducers (e.g., phenytoin, rifampin, and phenobarbital) with risperidone may cause decreases in the combined plasma concentrations of ripseridone and 9-hydroxyrisperidone, which could lead to decreased efficacy of Risperdal Consta treatment. At the initiation of therapy with known CYP3A4 hepatic enzyme inducers, patients should be closely monitored during the first 4-8 weeks, since the dose of Risperdal Consta may need to be adjusted. A dose increase, or additionaloral risperidone, may need to be considered. On discontinuation of CYP3A4 hepatic enzyme inducers, the dosage of Risperdal Consta should be re-evaluated and, if necessary, decreased).
No products indexed under this heading.

Citalopram Hydrobromide (Risperidone is metabolized to 9-hydroxyrisperidone by CYP2D6. Drug interactions that reduce the metabolism of risperidone to 9-hydroxyrisperidone would increase the plasma concentrations of risperidone and lower the concentrations of 9-hydroxyrisperidone). Products include:
Celexa 1160

Clomipramine Hydrochloride (Risperidone is metabolized to 9-hydroxyrisperidone by CYP2D6. Drug interactions that reduce the metabolism of risperidone to 9-hydroxyrisperidone would increase the plasma concentrations of risperidone and lower the concentrations of 9-hydroxyrisperidone).
No products indexed under this heading.

Clonidine (Because of its potential for inducing hypotension, risperidone may enhance the hypotensive effects of other therapeutic agents with this potential). Products include:
Catapres-TTS 842

Clonidine Hydrochloride (Because of its potential for inducing hypotension, risperidone may enhance the hypotensive effects of other therapeutic agents with this potential). Products include:
Catapres Tablets 841
Clorpres Tablets 2185

Clorazepate Dipotassium (Given the primary CNS effects of risperidone, caution should be used if taken in combination with other centrally-acting drugs).
No products indexed under this heading.

Clozapine (Chronic administration of clozapine with risperidone may decrease the clearance of risperidone).
No products indexed under this heading.

CNS-Active Drugs, unspecified (Given the primary CNS effects of risperidone, caution should be taken if used with centrally-acting drugs).
No products indexed under this heading.

Cocaine Hydrochloride (Risperidone is metabolized to 9-hydroxyrisperidone by CYP2D6. Drug interactions that reduce the metabolism of risperidone to 9-hydroxyrisperidone would increase the plasma concentrations of risperidone and lower the concentrations of 9-hydroxyrisperidone).
No products indexed under this heading.

Codeine Phosphate (Given the primary CNS effects of risperidone, caution should be used if taken in combination with other centrally-acting drugs). Products include:
Tylenol with Codeine Tablets 2427

Cortisone Acetate (Co-administration of know CYP3A4 enzyme inducers (e.g., phenytoin, rifampin, and phenobarbital) with risperidone may cause decreases in the combined plasma concentrations of ripseridone and 9-hydroxyrisperidone, which could lead to decreased efficacy of Risperdal Consta treatment. At the initiation of therapy with known CYP3A4 hepatic enzyme inducers, patients should be closely monitored during the first 4-8 weeks, since the dose of Risperdal Consta may need to be adjusted. A dose increase, or additionaloral risperidone, may need to be considered. On discontinuation of CYP3A4 hepatic enzyme inducers, the dosage of Risperdal Consta should be re-evaluated and, if necessary, decreased).
No products indexed under this heading.

Deserpidine (Because of its potential for inducing hypotension, risperidone may enhance the hypotensive effects of other therapeutic agents with this potential).
No products indexed under this heading.

Desflurane (Given the primary CNS effects of risperidone, caution should be used if taken in combination with other centrally-acting drugs).
No products indexed under this heading.

Desipramine Hydrochloride (Risperidone is metabolized to 9-hydroxyrisperidone by CYP2D6. Drug interactions that reduce the metabolism of risperidone to 9-hydroxyrisperidone would increase the plasma concentrations of risperidone and lower the concentrations of 9-hydroxyrisperidone).
No products indexed under this heading.

Dexamethasone (Co-administration of know CYP3A4 enzyme inducers (e.g., phenytoin, rifampin, and phenobarbital) with risperidone may cause decreases in the combined plasma concentrations of ripseridone and 9-hydroxyrisperidone, which could lead to decreased efficacy of Risperdal Consta treatment. At the initiation of therapy with known CYP3A4 hepatic enzyme inducers, patients should be closely monitored during the first 4-8 weeks, since the dose of Risperdal Consta may need to be adjusted. A dose increase, or additionaloral risperidone, may need to be considered. On discontinuation of CYP3A4 hepatic enzyme inducers, the dosage of Risperdal Consta should be re-evaluated and, if necessary, decreased). Products include:
Ciprodex Otic Suspension 541

Dexamethasone Acetate (Co-administration of know CYP3A4 enzyme inducers (e.g., phenytoin, rifampin, and phenobarbital) with risperidone may cause decreases in the combined plasma concentrations of ripseridone and 9-hydroxyrisperidone, which could lead to decreased efficacy of Risperdal Consta treatment. At the initiation of therapy with known CYP3A4 hepatic enzyme inducers, patients should be closely monitored during the first 4-8 weeks, since the dose of Risperdal Consta may need to be adjusted. A dose increase, or additionaloral risperidone, may need to be considered. On discontinuation of CYP3A4 hepatic enzyme inducers, the dosage of Risperdal Consta should be re-evaluated and, if necessary, decreased).
No products indexed under this heading.

Dexamethasone Sodium Phosphate (Co-administration of know CYP3A4 enzyme inducers (e.g., phenytoin, rifampin, and phenobarbital) with risperidone may cause decreases in the combined plasma concentrations of ripseridone and 9-hydroxyrisperidone, which could lead to decreased efficacy of Risperdal Consta treatment. At the initiation of therapy with known CYP3A4 hepatic enzyme inducers, patients should be closely monitored during the first 4-8 weeks, since the dose of Risperdal Consta may need to be adjusted. A dose increase, or additionaloral risperidone, may need to be considered. On discontinuation of CYP3A4 hepatic enzyme inducers, the dosage of Risperdal Consta should be re-evaluated and, if necessary, decreased).
No products indexed under this heading.

Dextroamphetamine Sulfate (Given the primary CNS effects of risperdone, caution should be taken with other centrally-acting drugs). Products include:
Adderall XR Capsules 3012
Dexedrine 1401

Dezocine (Given the primary CNS effects of risperidone, caution should be used if taken in combination with other centrally-acting drugs).
No products indexed under this heading.

Diazepam (Given the primary CNS effects of risperidone, caution should be used if taken in combination with other centrally-acting drugs). Products include:
Valium Tablets 2658

Diazoxide (Because of its potential for inducing hypotension, risperidone may enhance the hypotensive effects of other therapeutic agents with this potential). Products include:
Proglycem Capsules 1185
Proglycem Suspension 1185

Diltiazem Hydrochloride (Because of its potential for inducing hypotension, risperidone may enhance the hypotensive effects of other therapeutic agents with this potential). Products include:
Cardizem LA Extended Release Tablets 421

Diphenhydramine (Risperidone is metabolized to 9-hydroxyrisperidone by CYP2D6. Drug interactions that reduce the metabolism of risperidone to 9-hydroxyrisperidone would increase the plasma concentrations of risperidone and lower the concentrations of 9-hydroxyrisperidone).
No products indexed under this heading.

Diphenhydramine Hydrochloride (Risperidone is metabolized to 9-hydroxyrisperidone by CYP2D6. Drug interactions that reduce the metabolism of risperidone to 9-hydroxyrisperidone would increase the plasma concentrations of risperidone and lower the concentrations of 9-hydroxyrisperidone). Products include:
Benadryl Allergy & Cold Kapgels **1895**
Benadryl Allergy & Sinus Headache Kapgels **1895**
Benadryl Severe Allergy & Sinus Headache Caplets **1897**
Benadryl Dye-Free Allergy Liqui-gels Softgels **1897**
Benadryl Allergy Kapgels **1895**
Benadryl Allergy Quick Dissolve Strips **1896**
Benadryl Allergy Ultratab Tablets **1896**
Children's Benadryl Dye-Free Allergy Liquid **1897**
Children's Benadryl Allergy Fastmelts **1897**
Children's Benadryl Allergy Liquid **1898**
Children's Benadryl Allergy Perfect Measure **1896**
Children's Benadryl-D Allergy & Sinus Liquid **1896**
Benadryl-D Allergy & Sinus Tablet **1896**
PediaCare Children's Allergy & Cold Liquid **1902**
PediaCare Children's Allergy Liquid **1902**
Simply Sleep Caplets **1905**
Sudafed PE Nighttime Cold Caplets **1907**
Sudafed PE Severe Cold Caplets **1908**
Extra Strength Tylenol PM Caplets, Geltabs, Liquid, and Rapid Release Gels **1915**
Tylenol Allergy Multi-Symptom Nighttime Caplets with Cool Burst **1916**
Tylenol Severe Allergy Caplets **1916**
Children's Tylenol Plus Cold & Allergy Suspension Liquid **1914**
Tylenol Sore Throat Nighttime Liquid with Cool Burst **1918**

Divalproex Sodium (Repeated oral doses of risperidone (4 mg QD) did not affect the pre-dose or average plasma concentrations and exposure (AUC) of valproate (1000 mg/day in three divided doses) compared to placebo (n=21). However, there was a 20% increase of valproate peak plasma concentration (Cmax) after concomitant administration of risperidone). Products include:
Depakote ER Tablets **423**

Dopamine Hydrochloride (Risperidone may antagonize the effect of dopamine agonists).
No products indexed under this heading.

Doxazosin Mesylate (Because of its potential for inducing hypotension, risperidone may enhance the hypotensive effects of other therapeutic agents with this potential).
No products indexed under this heading.

Doxepin Hydrochloride (Risperidone is metabolized to 9-hydroxyrisperidone by CYP2D6. Drug interactions that reduce the metabolism of risperidone to 9-hydroxyrisperidone would increase the plasma concentrations of risperidone and lower the concentrations of 9-hydroxyrisperidone).
No products indexed under this heading.

Doxorubicin Hydrochloride (Co-administration of know CYP3A4 enzyme inducers (e.g., phenytoin, rifampin, and phenobarbital) with risperidone may cause decreases in the combined plasma concentrations of ripseridone and 9-hydroxyrisperidone, which could lead to decreased efficacy of Risperdal Consta treatment. At the initiation of therapy with known CYP3A4 hepatic enzyme inducers, patients should be closely monitored during the first 4-8 weeks, since the dose of Risperdal Consta may need to be adjusted. A dose increase, or additionaloral risperidone, may need to be considered. On discontinuation of CYP3A4 hepatic enzyme inducers, the dosage of Risperdal Consta should be re-evaluated and, if necessary, decreased).
No products indexed under this heading.

Droperidol (Given the primary CNS effects of risperidone, caution should be used if taken in combination with other centrally-acting drugs).
No products indexed under this heading.

Efavirenz (Co-administration of know CYP3A4 enzyme inducers (e.g., phenytoin, rifampin, and phenobarbital) with risperidone may cause decreases in the combined plasma concentrations of ripseridone and 9-hydroxyrisperidone, which could lead to decreased efficacy of Risperdal Consta treatment. At the initiation of therapy with known CYP3A4 hepatic enzyme inducers, patients should be closely monitored during the first 4-8 weeks, since the dose of Risperdal Consta may need to be adjusted. A dose increase, or additionaloral risperidone, may need to be considered. On discontinuation of CYP3A4 hepatic enzyme inducers, the dosage of Risperdal Consta should be re-evaluated and, if necessary, decreased). Products include:
Atripla Tablets **938**
Sustiva Capsules **930**
Sustiva Tablets **930**

Enalapril Maleate (Because of its potential for inducing hypotension, risperidone may enhance the hypotensive effects of other therapeutic agents with this potential).
No products indexed under this heading.

Enalaprilat (Because of its potential for inducing hypotension, risperidone may enhance the hypotensive effects of other therapeutic agents with this potential).
No products indexed under this heading.

Enflurane (Given the primary CNS effects of risperidone, caution should be used if taken in combination with other centrally-acting drugs).
No products indexed under this heading.

Eprosartan Mesylate (Because of its potential for inducing hypotension, risperidone may enhance the hypotensive effects of other therapeutic agents with this potential). Products include:
Teveten Tablets **515**
Teveten HCT Tablets **517**

Escitalopram Oxalate (Risperidone is metabolized to 9-hydroxyrisperidone by CYP2D6. Drug interactions that reduce the metabolism of risperidone to 9-hydroxyrisperidone would increase the plasma concentrations of risperidone and lower the concentrations of 9-hydroxyrisperidone). Products include:
Lexapro Oral Suspension **1174**
Lexapro Tablets **1174**

Esmolol Hydrochloride (Because of its potential for inducing hypotension, risperidone may enhance the hypotensive effects of other therapeutic agents with this potential).
No products indexed under this heading.

Estazolam (Given the primary CNS effects of risperidone, caution should be used if taken in combination with other centrally-acting drugs).
No products indexed under this heading.

Ethanol (Given the primary CNS effects of risperidone, caution should be used if taken in combination with other centrally-acting drugs).
No products indexed under this heading.

Ethchlorvynol (Given the primary CNS effects of risperidone, caution should be used if taken in combination with other centrally-acting drugs).
No products indexed under this heading.

Ethinamate (Given the primary CNS effects of risperidone, caution should be used if taken in combination with other centrally-acting drugs).
No products indexed under this heading.

Ethosuximide (Co-administration of know CYP3A4 enzyme inducers (e.g., phenytoin, rifampin, and phenobarbital) with risperidone may cause decreases in the combined plasma concentrations of ripseridone and 9-hydroxyrisperidone, which could lead to decreased efficacy of Risperdal Consta treatment. At the initiation of therapy with known CYP3A4 hepatic enzyme inducers, patients should be closely monitored during the first 4-8 weeks, since the dose of Risperdal Consta may need to be adjusted. A dose increase, or additionaloral risperidone, may need to be considered. On discontinuation of CYP3A4 hepatic enzyme inducers, the dosage of Risperdal Consta should be re-evaluated and, if necessary, decreased).
No products indexed under this heading.

Ethyl Alcohol (Given the primary CNS effects of risperidone, caution should be used if taken in combination with other centrally-acting drugs).
No products indexed under this heading.

Felbamate (Co-administration of know CYP3A4 enzyme inducers (e.g., phenytoin, rifampin, and phenobarbital) with risperidone may cause decreases in the combined plasma concentrations of ripseridone and 9-hydroxyrisperidone, which could lead to decreased efficacy of Risperdal Consta treatment. At the initiation of therapy with known CYP3A4 hepatic enzyme inducers, patients should be closely monitored during the first 4-8 weeks, since the dose of Risperdal Consta may need to be adjusted. A dose increase, or additionaloral risperidone, may need to be considered. On discontinuation of CYP3A4 hepatic enzyme inducers, the dosage of Risperdal Consta should be re-evaluated and, if necessary, decreased).
No products indexed under this heading.

Felodipine (Because of its potential for inducing hypotension, risperidone may enhance the hypotensive effects of other therapeutic agents with this potential).
No products indexed under this heading.

Fentanyl (Given the primary CNS effects of risperidone, caution should be used if taken in combination with other centrally-acting drugs). Products include:
Duragesic Transdermal System **2405**
Ionsys Transdermal System **2410**

Fentanyl Citrate (Given the primary CNS effects of risperidone, caution should be used if taken in combination with other centrally-acting drugs). Products include:
Actiq **959**
Fentora Tablets **968**

Fludrocortisone Acetate (Co-administration of know CYP3A4 enzyme inducers (e.g., phenytoin, rifampin, and phenobarbital) with risperidone may cause decreases in the combined plasma concentrations of ripseridone and 9-hydroxyrisperidone, which could lead to decreased efficacy of Risperdal Consta treatment. At the initiation of therapy with known CYP3A4 hepatic enzyme inducers, patients should be closely monitored during the first 4-8 weeks, since the dose of Risperdal Consta may need to be adjusted. A dose increase, or additionaloral risperidone, may need to be considered. On discontinuation of CYP3A4 hepatic enzyme inducers, the dosage of Risperdal Consta should be re-evaluated and, if necessary, decreased).
No products indexed under this heading.

Fluoxetine (Fluoxetine (20 mg QD), a CYP2D6 inhibitor, has been shown to increase the plasma concentration of risperidone 2.5-2.8 fold. Fluoxetine did not affect the plasma concentration of 9-hydroxyrisperidone. When concomitant fluoxetine is initiated or discontinued, the dose of Risperdal Consta should be re-evaluated. When initiation of fluoxetine is considered, patients may be placed on a lower dose of Risperdal Consta between 2-4 weeks before the planned start of fluoxetine therapy to adjust for the expected increase in plasma concentrations of risperidone).
No products indexed under this heading.

Fluoxetine Hydrochloride (Fluoxetine (20 mg QD), a CYP2D6 inhibitor, has been shown to increase the plasma concentration of risperidone 2.5-2.8 fold. Fluoxetine did not affect the plasma concentration of 9-hydroxyrisperidone. When concomitant fluoxetine is initiated or discontinued, the dose of Risperdal Consta should be re-evaluated. When initiation of fluoxetine is considered, patients may be placed on a lower dose of Risperdal Consta between 2-4 weeks before the planned start of fluoxetine therapy to adjust for the expected increase in plasma concentrations of risperidone). Products include:

Prozac Weekly Capsules 1852
Prozac Pulvules and Liquid 1852
Symbyax Capsules 1871

Fluphenazine Decanoate (Given the primary CNS effects of risperidone, caution should be used if taken in combination with other centrally-acting drugs).
No products indexed under this heading.

Fluphenazine Enanthate (Given the primary CNS effects of risperidone, caution should be used if taken in combination with other centrally-acting drugs).
No products indexed under this heading.

Fluphenazine Hydrochloride (Given the primary CNS effects of risperidone, caution should be used if taken in combination with other centrally-acting drugs).
No products indexed under this heading.

Flurazepam Hydrochloride (Given the primary CNS effects of risperidone, caution should be used if taken in combination with other centrally-acting drugs).
No products indexed under this heading.

Fluvoxamine Maleate (Risperidone is metabolized to 9-hydroxyrisperidone by CYP2D6. Drug interactions that reduce the metabolism of risperidone to 9-hydroxyrisperidone would increase the plasma concentrations of risperidone and lower the concentrations of 9-hydroxyrisperidone). Products include:

Luvox CR Extended-Release Capsules 1759

Fosinopril Sodium (Because of its potential for inducing hypotension, risperidone may enhance the hypotensive effects of other therapeutic agents with this potential).
No products indexed under this heading.

Fosphenytoin Sodium (Co-administration of know CYP3A4 enzyme inducers (e.g., phenytoin, rifampin, and phenobarbital) with risperidone may cause decreases in the combined plasma concentrations of ripseridone and 9-hydroxyrisperidone, which could lead to decreased efficacy of Risperdal Consta treatment. At the initiation of therapy with known CYP3A4 hepatic enzyme inducers, patients should be closely monitored during the first 4-8 weeks, since the dose of Risperdal Consta may need to be adjusted. A dose increase, or additionaloral risperidone, may need to be considered. On discontinuation of CYP3A4 hepatic enzyme inducers, the dosage of Risperdal Consta should be re-evaluated and, if necessary, decreased).
No products indexed under this heading.

Furosemide (In 2 of 4 placebo-controlled trials in elderly patients with dementia-related psychosis, a higher incidence of mortality was observed in patients treated with furosemide plus oral risperidone when compared to patients treated with oral risperidone alone or with oral placebo plus furosemide. No pathological mechanism has been identified to explain this finding, and no consistent pattern for cause of death was observed. An increase of mortality in elderly patients with dementia-related psychosis was seen with the use of oral risperidone regardless of concomitant use with furosemide). Products include:

Furosemide Tablets 2186

Garlic Extract (Co-administration of know CYP3A4 enzyme inducers (e.g., phenytoin, rifampin, and phenobarbital) with risperidone may cause decreases in the combined plasma concentrations of ripseridone and 9-hydroxyrisperidone, which could lead to decreased efficacy of Risperdal Consta treatment. At the initiation of therapy with known CYP3A4 hepatic enzyme inducers, patients should be closely monitored during the first 4-8 weeks, since the dose of Risperdal Consta may need to be adjusted. A dose increase, or additionaloral risperidone, may need to be considered. On discontinuation of CYP3A4 hepatic enzyme inducers, the dosage of Risperdal Consta should be re-evaluated and, if necessary, decreased).
No products indexed under this heading.

Garlic Oil (Co-administration of know CYP3A4 enzyme inducers (e.g., phenytoin, rifampin, and phenobarbital) with risperidone may cause decreases in the combined plasma concentrations of ripseridone and 9-hydroxyrisperidone, which could lead to decreased efficacy of Risperdal Consta treatment. At the initiation of therapy with known CYP3A4 hepatic enzyme inducers, patients should be closely monitored during the first 4-8 weeks, since the dose of Risperdal Consta may need to be adjusted. A dose increase, or additionaloral risperidone, may need to be considered. On discontinuation of CYP3A4 hepatic enzyme inducers, the dosage of Risperdal Consta should be re-evaluated and, if necessary, decreased).
No products indexed under this heading.

Glipizide (Co-administration of known enzyme inducers (e.g., phenytoin, rifampin and phenobarbital) with risperidone may cause decreases in the combined plasma concentrations of risperidone and 9-hydroxyrisperidone, which could lead to decreased efficacy. The dose of risperidone may need to be adjusted accordingly, particularly during the initiation or discontinuation of therapy with enzyme inducers).
No products indexed under this heading.

Glutethimide (Given the primary CNS effects of risperidone, caution should be used if taken in combination with other centrally-acting drugs).
No products indexed under this heading.

Glyburide (Co-administration of known enzyme inducers (e.g., phenytoin, rifampin and phenobarbital) with risperidone may cause decreases in the combined plasma concentrations of risperidone and 9-hydroxyrisperidone, which could lead to decreased efficacy. The dose of risperidone may need to be adjusted accordingly, particularly during the initiation or discontinuation of therapy with enzyme inducers).
No products indexed under this heading.

Guanabenz Acetate (Because of its potential for inducing hypotension, risperidone may enhance the hypotensive effects of other therapeutic agents with this potential).
No products indexed under this heading.

Guanethidine Monosulfate (Because of its potential for inducing hypotension, risperidone may enhance the hypotensive effects of other therapeutic agents with this potential).
No products indexed under this heading.

Halofantrine Hydrochloride (Risperidone is metabolized to 9-hydroxyrisperidone by CYP2D6. Drug interactions that reduce the metabolism of risperidone to 9-hydroxyrisperidone would increase the plasma concentrations of risperidone and lower the concentrations of 9-hydroxyrisperidone).
No products indexed under this heading.

Haloperidol (Given the primary CNS effects of risperidone, caution should be used if taken in combination with other centrally-acting drugs).
No products indexed under this heading.

Haloperidol Decanoate (Given the primary CNS effects of risperidone, caution should be used if taken in combination with other centrally-acting drugs).
No products indexed under this heading.

Hydralazine Hydrochloride (Because of its potential for inducing hypotension, risperidone may enhance the hypotensive effects of other therapeutic agents with this potential).
No products indexed under this heading.

Hydrochlorothiazide (Because of its potential for inducing hypotension, risperidone may enhance the hypotensive effects of other therapeutic agents with this potential). Products include:

Atacand HCT 642
Avalide Tablets 892
Avalide Tablets 2713
Benicar HCT Tablets 1010
Diovan HCT Tablets 2216
Dyazide Capsules 1405
Micardis HCT Tablets 854
Prinzide Tablets 2092
Tekturna HCT Tablets 2324
Teveten HCT Tablets 517

Hydrocodone Bitartrate (Given the primary CNS effects of risperidone, caution should be used if taken in combination with other centrally-acting drugs). Products include:

Lortab 5/500 Tablets 3143
Lortab 7.5/500 Tablets 3144
Lortab 10/500 Tablets 3144
Vicodin Tablets 529
Vicodin ES Tablets 530
Vicodin HP Tablets 531
Vicoprofen Tablets 533
Zydone Tablets 1132

Hydrocodone Polistirex (Given the primary CNS effects of risperidone, caution should be used if taken in combination with other centrally-acting drugs). Products include:

Tussionex Pennkinetic Extended-Release Suspension 3154

Hydrocortisone (Co-administration of know CYP3A4 enzyme inducers (e.g., phenytoin, rifampin, and phenobarbital) with risperidone may cause decreases in the combined plasma concentrations of ripseridone and 9-hydroxyrisperidone, which could lead to decreased efficacy of Risperdal Consta treatment. At the initiation of therapy with known CYP3A4 hepatic enzyme inducers, patients should be closely monitored during the first 4-8 weeks, since the dose of Risperdal Consta may need to be adjusted. A dose increase, or additionaloral risperidone, may need to be considered. On discontinuation of CYP3A4 hepatic enzyme inducers, the dosage of Risperdal Consta should be re-evaluated and, if necessary, decreased).
No products indexed under this heading.

Hydrocortisone Acetate (Co-administration of know CYP3A4 enzyme inducers (e.g., phenytoin, rifampin, and phenobarbital) with risperidone may cause decreases in the combined plasma concentrations of ripseridone and 9-hydroxyrisperidone, which could lead to decreased efficacy of Risperdal Consta treatment. At the initiation of therapy with known CYP3A4 hepatic enzyme inducers, patients should be closely monitored during the first 4-8 weeks, since the dose of Risperdal Consta may need to be adjusted. A dose increase, or additionaloral risperidone, may need to be considered. On discontinuation of CYP3A4 hepatic enzyme inducers, the dosage of Risperdal Consta should be re-evaluated and, if necessary, decreased). Products include:

Analpram-HC 1140
Pramosone 1141

Hydrocortisone Butyrate (Co-administration of know CYP3A4 enzyme inducers (e.g., phenytoin, rifampin, and phenobarbital) with risperidone may cause decreases in the combined plasma concentrations of ripseridone and 9-hydroxyrisperidone, which could lead to decreased efficacy of Risperdal Consta treatment. At the initiation of therapy with known CYP3A4 hepatic enzyme inducers, patients should be closely monitored during the first 4-8 weeks, since the dose of Risperdal Consta may need to be adjusted. A dose increase, or additionaloral risperidone, may need to be considered. On discontinuation of

CYP3A4 hepatic enzyme inducers, the dosage of Risperdal Consta should be re-evaluated and, if necessary, decreased).

No products indexed under this heading.

Hydrocortisone Cypionate (Co-administration of know CYP3A4 enzyme inducers (e.g., phenytoin, rifampin, and phenobarbital) with risperidone may cause decreases in the combined plasma concentrations of ripseridone and 9-hydroxyrisperidone, which could lead to decreased efficacy of Risperdal Consta treatment. At the initiation of therapy with known CYP3A4 hepatic enzyme inducers, patients should be closely monitored during the first 4-8 weeks, since the dose of Risperdal Consta may need to be adjusted. A dose increase, or additionaloral risperidone, may need to be considered. On discontinuation of CYP3A4 hepatic enzyme inducers, the dosage of Risperdal Consta should be re-evaluated and, if necessary, decreased).

No products indexed under this heading.

Hydrocortisone Hemisuccinate (Co-administration of know CYP3A4 enzyme inducers (e.g., phenytoin, rifampin, and phenobarbital) with risperidone may cause decreases in the combined plasma concentrations of ripseridone and 9-hydroxyrisperidone, which could lead to decreased efficacy of Risperdal Consta treatment. At the initiation of therapy with known CYP3A4 hepatic enzyme inducers, patients should be closely monitored during the first 4-8 weeks, since the dose of Risperdal Consta may need to be adjusted. A dose increase, or additionaloral risperidone, may need to be considered. On discontinuation of CYP3A4 hepatic enzyme inducers, the dosage of Risperdal Consta should be re-evaluated and, if necessary, decreased).

No products indexed under this heading.

Hydrocortisone Probutate (Co-administration of know CYP3A4 enzyme inducers (e.g., phenytoin, rifampin, and phenobarbital) with risperidone may cause decreases in the combined plasma concentrations of ripseridone and 9-hydroxyrisperidone, which could lead to decreased efficacy of Risperdal Consta treatment. At the initiation of therapy with known CYP3A4 hepatic enzyme inducers, patients should be closely monitored during the first 4-8 weeks, since the dose of Risperdal Consta may need to be adjusted. A dose increase, or additionaloral risperidone, may need to be considered. On discontinuation of CYP3A4 hepatic enzyme inducers, the dosage of Risperdal Consta should be re-evaluated and, if necessary, decreased).

No products indexed under this heading.

Hydrocortisone Sodium Phosphate (Co-administration of know CYP3A4 enzyme inducers (e.g., phenytoin, rifampin, and phenobarbital) with risperidone may cause decreases in the combined plasma concentrations of ripseridone and 9-hydroxyrisperidone, which could lead to decreased efficacy of Risperdal Consta treatment. At the initiation of therapy with known CYP3A4 hepatic enzyme inducers, patients should be closely monitored during the first 4-8 weeks, since the dose of Risperdal Consta may need to be adjusted. A dose increase, or additionaloral risperidone, may need to be considered. On discontinuation of CYP3A4 hepatic enzyme inducers, the dosage of Risperdal Consta should be re-evaluated and, if necessary, decreased).

No products indexed under this heading.

Hydrocortisone Sodium Succinate (Co-administration of know CYP3A4 enzyme inducers (e.g., phenytoin, rifampin, and phenobarbital) with risperidone may cause decreases in the combined plasma concentrations of ripseridone and 9-hydroxyrisperidone, which could lead to decreased efficacy of Risperdal Consta treatment. At the initiation of therapy with known CYP3A4 hepatic enzyme inducers, patients should be closely monitored during the first 4-8 weeks, since the dose of Risperdal Consta may need to be adjusted. A dose increase, or additionaloral risperidone, may need to be considered. On discontinuation of CYP3A4 hepatic enzyme inducers, the dosage of Risperdal Consta should be re-evaluated and, if necessary, decreased).

No products indexed under this heading.

Hydrocortisone Valerate (Co-administration of know CYP3A4 enzyme inducers (e.g., phenytoin, rifampin, and phenobarbital) with risperidone may cause decreases in the combined plasma concentrations of ripseridone and 9-hydroxyrisperidone, which could lead to decreased efficacy of Risperdal Consta treatment. At the initiation of therapy with known CYP3A4 hepatic enzyme inducers, patients should be closely monitored during the first 4-8 weeks, since the dose of Risperdal Consta may need to be adjusted. A dose increase, or additionaloral risperidone, may need to be considered. On discontinuation of CYP3A4 hepatic enzyme inducers, the dosage of Risperdal Consta should be re-evaluated and, if necessary, decreased).

No products indexed under this heading.

Hydroflumethiazide (Because of its potential for inducing hypotension, risperidone may enhance the hypotensive effects of other therapeutic agents with this potential).

No products indexed under this heading.

Hydromorphone Hydrochloride (Given the primary CNS effects of risperidone, caution should be used if taken in combination with other centrally-acting drugs).

No products indexed under this heading.

Hydroxychloroquine Sulfate (Risperidone is metabolized to 9-hydroxyrisperidone by CYP2D6. Drug interactions that reduce the metabolism of risperidone to 9-hydroxyrisperidone would increase the plasma concentrations of risperidone and lower the concentrations of 9-hydroxyrisperidone).

No products indexed under this heading.

Hydroxyzine Hydrochloride (Given the primary CNS effects of risperidone, caution should be used if taken in combination with other centrally-acting drugs).

No products indexed under this heading.

Hypericum (Co-administration of know CYP3A4 enzyme inducers (e.g., phenytoin, rifampin, and phenobarbital) with risperidone may cause decreases in the combined plasma concentrations of ripseridone and 9-hydroxyrisperidone, which could lead to decreased efficacy of Risperdal Consta treatment. At the initiation of therapy with known CYP3A4 hepatic enzyme inducers, patients should be closely monitored during the first 4-8 weeks, since the dose of Risperdal Consta may need to be adjusted. A dose increase, or additionaloral risperidone, may need to be considered. On discontinuation of CYP3A4 hepatic enzyme inducers, the dosage of Risperdal Consta should be re-evaluated and, if necessary, decreased). Products include:

Satieté Tablets 640

Hypericum Perforatum (Co-administration of know CYP3A4 enzyme inducers (e.g., phenytoin, rifampin, and phenobarbital) with risperidone may cause decreases in the combined plasma concentrations of ripseridone and 9-hydroxyrisperidone, which could lead to decreased efficacy of Risperdal Consta treatment. At the initiation of therapy with known CYP3A4 hepatic enzyme inducers, patients should be closely monitored during the first 4-8 weeks, since the dose of Risperdal Consta may need to be adjusted. A dose increase, or additionaloral risperidone, may need to be considered. On discontinuation of CYP3A4 hepatic enzyme inducers, the dosage of Risperdal Consta should be re-evaluated and, if necessary, decreased).

No products indexed under this heading.

Imatinib Mesylate (Risperidone is metabolized to 9-hydroxyrisperidone by CYP2D6. Drug interactions that reduce the metabolism of risperidone to 9-hydroxyrisperidone would increase the plasma concentrations of risperidone and lower the concentrations of 9-hydroxyrisperidone). Products include:

Gleevec Tablets 2255

Imipramine Hydrochloride (Risperidone is metabolized to 9-hydroxyrisperidone by CYP2D6. Drug interactions that reduce the metabolism of risperidone to 9-hydroxyrisperidone would increase the plasma concentrations of risperidone and lower the concentrations of 9-hydroxyrisperidone).

No products indexed under this heading.

Imipramine Pamoate (Risperidone is metabolized to 9-hydroxyrisperidone by CYP2D6. Drug interactions that reduce the metabolism of risperidone to 9-hydroxyrisperidone would increase the plasma concentrations of risperidone and lower the concentrations of 9-hydroxyrisperidone).

No products indexed under this heading.

Indapamide (Because of its potential for inducing hypotension, risperidone may enhance the hypotensive effects of other therapeutic agents with this potential). Products include:

Indapamide Tablets 2188

Irbesartan (Because of its potential for inducing hypotension, risperidone may enhance the hypotensive effects of other therapeutic agents with this potential). Products include:

Avalide Tablets 892
Avalide Tablets 2713
Avapro Tablets 897
Avapro Tablets 2718

Isoflurane (Given the primary CNS effects of risperidone, caution should be used if taken in combination with other centrally-acting drugs).

No products indexed under this heading.

Isradipine (Because of its potential for inducing hypotension, risperidone may enhance the hypotensive effects of other therapeutic agents with this potential). Products include:

DynaCirc CR Controlled Release Tablets 1407

Ketamine Hydrochloride (Given the primary CNS effects of risperidone, caution should be used if taken in combination with other centrally-acting drugs).

No products indexed under this heading.

Labetalol Hydrochloride (Because of its potential for inducing hypotension, risperidone may enhance the hypotensive effects of other therapeutic agents with this potential).

No products indexed under this heading.

Levodopa (Risperidone may antagonize the effect of levodopa). Products include:

Stalevo Tablets 2309

Levomethadyl Acetate Hydrochloride (Given the primary CNS effects of risperidone, caution should be used if taken in combination with other centrally-acting drugs).

No products indexed under this heading.

Levorphanol Tartrate (Given the primary CNS effects of risperidone, caution should be used if taken in combination with other centrally-acting drugs).

No products indexed under this heading.

Lisinopril (Because of its potential for inducing hypotension, risperidone may enhance the hypotensive effects of other therapeutic agents with this potential). Products include:

Prinivil Tablets 2087
Prinzide Tablets 2092

Lorazepam (Given the primary CNS effects of risperidone, caution should be used if taken in combination with other centrally-acting drugs).

No products indexed under this heading.

Losartan Potassium (Because of its potential for inducing hypotension, risperidone may enhance the hypotensive effects of other therapeutic agents with this potential). Products include:

Cozaar Tablets 1973

Loxapine Hydrochloride (Given the primary CNS effects of risperidone, caution should be used if taken in combination with other centrally-acting drugs).
No products indexed under this heading.

Loxapine Succinate (Given the primary CNS effects of risperidone, caution should be used if taken in combination with other centrally-acting drugs).
No products indexed under this heading.

Maprotiline Hydrochloride (Risperidone is metabolized to 9-hydroxyrisperidone by CYP2D6. Drug interactions that reduce the metabolism of risperidone to 9-hydroxyrisperidone would increase the plasma concentrations of risperidone and lower the concentrations of 9-hydroxyrisperidone).
No products indexed under this heading.

Mecamylamine Hydrochloride (Because of its potential for inducing hypotension, risperidone may enhance the hypotensive effects of other therapeutic agents with this potential).
No products indexed under this heading.

Meperidine Hydrochloride (Given the primary CNS effects of risperidone, caution should be used if taken in combination with other centrally-acting drugs).
No products indexed under this heading.

Mephenytoin (Co-administration of know CYP3A4 enzyme inducers (e.g., phenytoin, rifampin, and phenobarbital) with risperidone may cause decreases in the combined plasma concentrations of ripseridone and 9-hydroxyrisperidone, which could lead to decreased efficacy of Risperdal Consta treatment. At the initiation of therapy with known CYP3A4 hepatic enzyme inducers, patients should be closely monitored during the first 4-8 weeks, since the dose of Risperdal Consta may need to be adjusted. A dose increase, or additionaloral risperidone, may need to be considered. On discontinuation of CYP3A4 hepatic enzyme inducers, the dosage of Risperdal Consta should be re-evaluated and, if necessary, decreased).
No products indexed under this heading.

Mephobarbital (Given the primary CNS effects of risperidone, caution should be used if taken in combination with other centrally-acting drugs).
No products indexed under this heading.

Meprobamate (Given the primary CNS effects of risperidone, caution should be used if taken in combination with other centrally-acting drugs).
No products indexed under this heading.

Mesoridazine Besylate (Given the primary CNS effects of risperidone, caution should be used if taken in combination with other centrally-acting drugs).
No products indexed under this heading.

Methadone Hydrochloride (Given the primary CNS effects of risperidone, caution should be used if taken in combination with other centrally-acting drugs).
No products indexed under this heading.

Methamphetamine Hydrochloride (Given the primary CNS effects of risperdone, caution should be taken with other centrally-acting drugs).
No products indexed under this heading.

Methohexital Sodium (Given the primary CNS effects of risperidone, caution should be used if taken in combination with other centrally-acting drugs).
No products indexed under this heading.

Methotrimeprazine (Given the primary CNS effects of risperidone, caution should be used if taken in combination with other centrally-acting drugs).
No products indexed under this heading.

Methoxyflurane (Given the primary CNS effects of risperidone, caution should be used if taken in combination with other centrally-acting drugs).
No products indexed under this heading.

Methsuximide (Co-administration of know CYP3A4 enzyme inducers (e.g., phenytoin, rifampin, and phenobarbital) with risperidone may cause decreases in the combined plasma concentrations of ripseridone and 9-hydroxyrisperidone, which could lead to decreased efficacy of Risperdal Consta treatment. At the initiation of therapy with known CYP3A4 hepatic enzyme inducers, patients should be closely monitored during the first 4-8 weeks, since the dose of Risperdal Consta may need to be adjusted. A dose increase, or additionaloral risperidone, may need to be considered. On discontinuation of CYP3A4 hepatic enzyme inducers, the dosage of Risperdal Consta should be re-evaluated and, if necessary, decreased).
No products indexed under this heading.

Methyclothiazide (Because of its potential for inducing hypotension, risperidone may enhance the hypotensive effects of other therapeutic agents with this potential).
No products indexed under this heading.

Methyldopa (Because of its potential for inducing hypotension, risperidone may enhance the hypotensive effects of other therapeutic agents with this potential).
No products indexed under this heading.

Methyldopate Hydrochloride (Because of its potential for inducing hypotension, risperidone may enhance the hypotensive effects of other therapeutic agents with this potential).
No products indexed under this heading.

Methylphenidate (Given the primary CNS effects of risperdone, caution should be taken with other centrally-acting drugs). Products include:
Daytrana Transdermal Patch 3022

Methylphenidate Hydrochloride (Given the primary CNS effects of risperdone, caution should be taken with other centrally-acting drugs). Products include:
Concerta Extended-Release Tablets 1925
Metadate CD Capsules 3146

Methylprednisolone (Co-administration of know CYP3A4 enzyme inducers (e.g., phenytoin, rifampin, and phenobarbital) with risperidone may cause decreases in the combined plasma concentrations of ripseridone and 9-hydroxyrisperidone, which could lead to decreased efficacy of Risperdal Consta treatment. At the initiation of therapy with known CYP3A4 hepatic enzyme inducers, patients should be closely monitored during the first 4-8 weeks, since the dose of Risperdal Consta may need to be adjusted. A dose increase, or additionaloral risperidone, may need to be considered. On discontinuation of CYP3A4 hepatic enzyme inducers, the dosage of Risperdal Consta should be re-evaluated and, if necessary, decreased).
No products indexed under this heading.

Methylprednisolone Acetate (Co-administration of know CYP3A4 enzyme inducers (e.g., phenytoin, rifampin, and phenobarbital) with risperidone may cause decreases in the combined plasma concentrations of ripseridone and 9-hydroxyrisperidone, which could lead to decreased efficacy of Risperdal Consta treatment. At the initiation of therapy with known CYP3A4 hepatic enzyme inducers, patients should be closely monitored during the first 4-8 weeks, since the dose of Risperdal Consta may need to be adjusted. A dose increase, or additionaloral risperidone, may need to be considered. On discontinuation of CYP3A4 hepatic enzyme inducers, the dosage of Risperdal Consta should be re-evaluated and, if necessary, decreased).
No products indexed under this heading.

Methylprednisolone Sodium Succinate (Co-administration of know CYP3A4 enzyme inducers (e.g., phenytoin, rifampin, and phenobarbital) with risperidone may cause decreases in the combined plasma concentrations of ripseridone and 9-hydroxyrisperidone, which could lead to decreased efficacy of Risperdal Consta treatment. At the initiation of therapy with known CYP3A4 hepatic enzyme inducers, patients should be closely monitored during the first 4-8 weeks, since the dose of Risperdal Consta may need to be adjusted. A dose increase, or additionaloral risperidone, may need to be considered. On discontinuation of CYP3A4 hepatic enzyme inducers, the dosage of Risperdal Consta should be re-evaluated and, if necessary, decreased).
No products indexed under this heading.

Metolazone (Because of its potential for inducing hypotension, risperidone may enhance the hypotensive effects of other therapeutic agents with this potential).
No products indexed under this heading.

Metoprolol Succinate (Because of its potential for inducing hypotension, risperidone may enhance the hypotensive effects of other therapeutic agents with this potential). Products include:
Toprol-XL Tablets 666

Metoprolol Tartrate (Because of its potential for inducing hypotension, risperidone may enhance the hypotensive effects of other therapeutic agents with this potential).
No products indexed under this heading.

Metyrosine (Because of its potential for inducing hypotension, risperidone may enhance the hypotensive effects of other therapeutic agents with this potential). Products include:
Demser Capsules 1989

Mibefradil Dihydrochloride (Because of its potential for inducing hypotension, risperidone may enhance the hypotensive effects of other therapeutic agents with this potential).
No products indexed under this heading.

Midazolam Hydrochloride (Given the primary CNS effects of risperidone, caution should be used if taken in combination with other centrally-acting drugs).
No products indexed under this heading.

Minoxidil (Because of its potential for inducing hypotension, risperidone may enhance the hypotensive effects of other therapeutic agents with this potential).
No products indexed under this heading.

Moclobemide (Risperidone is metabolized to 9-hydroxyrisperidone by CYP2D6. Drug interactions that reduce the metabolism of risperidone to 9-hydroxyrisperidone would increase the plasma concentrations of risperidone and lower the concentrations of 9-hydroxyrisperidone).
No products indexed under this heading.

Modafinil (Co-administration of know CYP3A4 enzyme inducers (e.g., phenytoin, rifampin, and phenobarbital) with risperidone may cause decreases in the combined plasma concentrations of ripseridone and 9-hydroxyrisperidone, which could lead to decreased efficacy of Risperdal Consta treatment. At the initiation of therapy with known CYP3A4 hepatic enzyme inducers, patients should be closely monitored during the first 4-8 weeks, since the dose of Risperdal Consta may need to be adjusted. A dose increase, or additionaloral risperidone, may need to be considered. On discontinuation of CYP3A4 hepatic enzyme inducers, the dosage of Risperdal Consta should be re-evaluated and, if necessary, decreased). Products include:
Provigil Tablets 977

Moexipril Hydrochloride (Because of its potential for inducing hypotension, risperidone may enhance the hypotensive effects of other therapeutic agents with this potential).
No products indexed under this heading.

Molindone Hydrochloride (Given the primary CNS effects of risperidone, caution should be used if

taken in combination with other centrally-acting drugs). Products include:
Moban Tablets ... 1116

Morphine Sulfate (Given the primary CNS effects of risperidone, caution should be used if taken in combination with other centrally-acting drugs). Products include:
Avinza Capsules ... 1772
DepoDur Injection ... 1095
MS Contin Tablets ... 2585

Nadolol (Because of its potential for inducing hypotension, risperidone may enhance the hypotensive effects of other therapeutic agents with this potential). Products include:
Nadolol Tablets ... 2191

Nebivolol (Because of its potential for inducing hypotension, risperidone may enhance the hypotensive effects of other therapeutic agents with this potential). Products include:
Bystolic Tablets ... 1155

Nevirapine (Co-administration of know CYP3A4 enzyme inducers (e.g., phenytoin, rifampin, and phenobarbital) with risperidone may cause decreases in the combined plasma concentrations of ripseridone and 9-hydroxyrisperidone, which could lead to decreased efficacy of Risperdal Consta treatment. At the initiation of therapy with known CYP3A4 hepatic enzyme inducers, patients should be closely monitored during the first 4-8 weeks, since the dose of Risperdal Consta may need to be adjusted. A dose increase, or additionaloral risperidone, may need to be considered. On discontinuation of CYP3A4 hepatic enzyme inducers, the dosage of Risperdal Consta should be re-evaluated and, if necessary, decreased). Products include:
Viramune Oral Suspension ... 873
Viramune Tablets ... 873

Nicardipine Hydrochloride (Because of its potential for inducing hypotension, risperidone may enhance the hypotensive effects of other therapeutic agents with this potential). Products include:
Cardene I.V. ... 1093

Nifedipine (Because of its potential for inducing hypotension, risperidone may enhance the hypotensive effects of other therapeutic agents with this potential).
No products indexed under this heading.

Nisoldipine (Because of its potential for inducing hypotension, risperidone may enhance the hypotensive effects of other therapeutic agents with this potential). Products include:
Sular Extended Release Tablets ... 2975

Nitroglycerin (Because of its potential for inducing hypotension, risperidone may enhance the hypotensive effects of other therapeutic agents with this potential). Products include:
Nitro-Dur Transdermal Infusion System ... 2887
Nitrolingual Pumpspray ... 2965

Nortriptyline Hydrochloride (Risperidone is metabolized to 9-hydroxyrisperidone by CYP2D6. Drug interactions that reduce the metabolism of risperidone to 9-hydroxyrisperidone would increase the plasma concentrations of risperidone and lower the concentrations of 9-hydroxyrisperidone).
No products indexed under this heading.

Olanzapine (Given the primary CNS effects of risperidone, caution should be used if taken in combination with other centrally-acting drugs). Products include:
Symbyax Capsules ... 1871
Zyprexa Tablets ... 1883
Zyprexa IntraMuscular ... 1883
Zyprexa ZYDIS Orally Disintegrating Tablets ... 1883

Oxazepam (Given the primary CNS effects of risperidone, caution should be used if taken in combination with other centrally-acting drugs).
No products indexed under this heading.

Oxcarbazepine (Co-administration of know CYP3A4 enzyme inducers (e.g., phenytoin, rifampin, and phenobarbital) with risperidone may cause decreases in the combined plasma concentrations of ripseridone and 9-hydroxyrisperidone, which could lead to decreased efficacy of Risperdal Consta treatment. At the initiation of therapy with known CYP3A4 hepatic enzyme inducers, patients should be closely monitored during the first 4-8 weeks, since the dose of Risperdal Consta may need to be adjusted. A dose increase, or additionaloral risperidone, may need to be considered. On discontinuation of CYP3A4 hepatic enzyme inducers, the dosage of Risperdal Consta should be re-evaluated and, if necessary, decreased).
No products indexed under this heading.

Oxycodone Hydrochloride (Given the primary CNS effects of risperidone, caution should be used if taken in combination with other centrally-acting drugs). Products include:
OxyContin Tablets ... 2589
OxyIR Capsules ... 2593
Percocet Tablets ... 1127
Percodan Tablets ... 1130

Paroxetine Hydrochloride (Paroxetine (20mg QD), a CYP2D6, has been shown to increase the plasma concentration of risperidone 3-9 fold. Paroxetine lowered the concentration of 9-hydroxyrisperidone by about 10%. When concomitant paroxetine is initiated or discontinued, the dose of Risperdal Consta should be re-evaluated. When initiation of paroxetine is considered, patients may be placed on a lower dose of Risperdal Consta between 2-4 weeks before the planned start of paroxetine therapy to adjust for the expected increase in plasma concentrations of risperidone). Products include:
Paxil ... 1535
Paxil CR Controlled-Release Tablets ... 1544

Paroxetine Mesylate (Paroxetine (20mg QD), a CYP2D6, has been shown to increase the plasma concentration of risperidone 3-9 fold. Paroxetine lowered the concentration of 9-hydroxyrisperidone by about 10%. When concomitant paroxetine is initiated or discontinued, the doseof Risperdal Consta should be re-evaluated. When initiation of paroxetine is considered, patients may be placed on a lower dose of Risperdal Consta between 2-4 weeks before the planned start of paroxetine therapy to adjust for the expected increase in plasma concentrations of risperidone).
No products indexed under this heading.

Pemoline (Given the primary CNS effects of risperdone, caution should be taken with other centrally-acting drugs).
No products indexed under this heading.

Penbutolol Sulfate (Because of its potential for inducing hypotension, risperidone may enhance the hypotensive effects of other therapeutic agents with this potential).
No products indexed under this heading.

Pentobarbital Sodium (Given the primary CNS effects of risperidone, caution should be used if taken in combination with other centrally-acting drugs). Products include:
Nembutal Sodium Solution, USP ... 2494

Pergolide Mesylate (Risperidone may antagonize the effect of dopamine agonists).
No products indexed under this heading.

Perindopril Erbumine (Because of its potential for inducing hypotension, risperidone may enhance the hypotensive effects of other therapeutic agents with this potential). Products include:
Aceon Tablets (2 mg, 4 mg, 8 mg) ... 3038

Perphenazine (Given the primary CNS effects of risperidone, caution should be used if taken in combination with other centrally-acting drugs).
No products indexed under this heading.

Phenobarbital (Co-administration of know CYP3A4 enzyme inducers (e.g., phenytoin, rifampin, and phenobarbital) with risperidone may cause decreases in the combined plasma concentrations of ripseridone and 9-hydroxyrisperidone, which could lead to decreased efficacy of Risperdal Consta treatment. At the initiation of therapy with known CYP3A4 hepatic enzyme inducers, patients should be closely monitored during the first 4-8 weeks, since the dose of Risperdal Consta may need to be adjusted. A dose increase, or additionaloral risperidone, may need to be considered. On discontinuation of CYP3A4 hepatic enzyme inducers, the dosage of Risperdal Consta should be re-evaluated and, if necessary, decreased). Products include:
Donnatal Extentabs ... 2507

Phenobarbital Sodium (Co-administration of know CYP3A4 enzyme inducers (e.g., phenytoin, rifampin, and phenobarbital) with risperidone may cause decreases in the combined plasma concentrations of ripseridone and 9-hydroxyrisperidone, which could lead to decreased efficacy of Risperdal Consta treatment. At the initiation of therapy with known CYP3A4 hepatic enzyme inducers, patients should be closely monitored during the first 4-8 weeks, since the dose of Risperdal Consta may need to be adjusted. A dose increase, or additionaloral risperidone, may need to be considered. On discontinuation of CYP3A4 hepatic enzyme inducers, the dosage of Risperdal Consta should be re-evaluated and, if necessary, decreased).
No products indexed under this heading.

Phenoxybenzamine Hydrochloride (Because of its potential for inducing hypotension, risperidone may enhance the hypotensive effects of other therapeutic agents with this potential). Products include:
Dibenzyline Capsules ... 3188

Phentolamine Mesylate (Because of its potential for inducing hypotension, risperidone may enhance the hypotensive effects of other therapeutic agents with this potential).
No products indexed under this heading.

Phenylbutazone (Co-administration of known enzyme inducers (e.g., phenytoin, rifampin and phenobarbital) with risperidone may cause decreases in the combined plasma concentrations of risperidone and 9-hydroxyrisperidone, which could lead to decreased efficacy. The dose of risperidone may need to be adjusted accordingly, particularly during the initiation or discontinuation of therapy with enzyme inducers).
No products indexed under this heading.

Phenytoin (Co-administration of know CYP3A4 enzyme inducers (e.g., phenytoin, rifampin, and phenobarbital) with risperidone may cause decreases in the combined plasma concentrations of ripseridone and 9-hydroxyrisperidone, which could lead to decreased efficacy of Risperdal Consta treatment. At the initiation of therapy with known CYP3A4 hepatic enzyme inducers, patients should be closely monitored during the first 4-8 weeks, since the dose of Risperdal Consta may need to be adjusted. A dose increase, or additionaloral risperidone, may need to be considered. On discontinuation of CYP3A4 hepatic enzyme inducers, the dosage of Risperdal Consta should be re-evaluated and, if necessary, decreased).
No products indexed under this heading.

Phenytoin Sodium (Co-administration of know CYP3A4 enzyme inducers (e.g., phenytoin, rifampin, and phenobarbital) with risperidone may cause decreases in the combined plasma concentrations of ripseridone and 9-hydroxyrisperidone, which could lead to decreased efficacy of Risperdal Consta treatment. At the initiation of therapy with known CYP3A4 hepatic enzyme inducers, patients should be closely monitored during the first 4-8 weeks, since the dose of Risperdal Consta may need to be adjusted. A dose increase, or additionaloral risperidone, may need to be considered. On discontinuation of CYP3A4 hepatic enzyme inducers, the dosage of Risperdal Consta should be re-evaluated and, if necessary, decreased). Products include:
Phenytek Capsules ... 2192

Pindolol (Because of its potential for inducing hypotension, risperidone may enhance the hypotensive effects of other therapeutic agents with this potential).
No products indexed under this heading.

Polythiazide (Because of its potential for inducing hypotension, risperidone may enhance the hypotensive effects of other therapeutic agents with this potential).
No products indexed under this heading.

Pramipexole Dihydrochloride (Risperidone may antagonize the effect of dopamine agonists). Products include:
Mirapex Tablets 857

Prazepam (Given the primary CNS effects of risperidone, caution should be used if taken in combination with other centrally-acting drugs).
No products indexed under this heading.

Prazosin Hydrochloride (Because of its potential for inducing hypotension, risperidone may enhance the hypotensive effects of other therapeutic agents with this potential).
No products indexed under this heading.

Prednisolone Acetate (Co-administration of know CYP3A4 enzyme inducers (e.g., phenytoin, rifampin, and phenobarbital) with risperidone may cause decreases in the combined plasma concentrations of ripseridone and 9-hydroxyrisperidone, which could lead to decreased efficacy of Risperdal Consta treatment. At the initiation of therapy with known CYP3A4 hepatic enzyme inducers, patients should be closely monitored during the first 4-8 weeks, since the dose of Risperdal Consta may need to be adjusted. A dose increase, or additionaloral risperidone, may need to be considered. On discontinuation of CYP3A4 hepatic enzyme inducers, the dosage of Risperdal Consta should be re-evaluated and, if necessary, decreased). Products include:
Pred Forte Ophthalmic Suspension .... ⊙227
Pred Mild Ophthalmic Suspension .... ⊙230
Pred-G Ophthalmic Ointment .... ⊙229
Pred-G Ophthalmic Suspension ...... ⊙228

Prednisolone Sodium Phosphate (Co-administration of know CYP3A4 enzyme inducers (e.g., phenytoin, rifampin, and phenobarbital) with risperidone may cause decreases in the combined plasma concentrations of ripseridone and 9-hydroxyrisperidone, which could lead to decreased efficacy of Risperdal Consta treatment. At the initiation of therapy with known CYP3A4 hepatic enzyme inducers, patients should be closely monitored during the first 4-8 weeks, since the dose of Risperdal Consta may need to be adjusted. A dose increase, or additionaloral risperidone, may need to be considered. On discontinuation of CYP3A4 hepatic enzyme inducers, the dosage of Risperdal Consta should be re-evaluated and, if necessary, decreased).
No products indexed under this heading.

Prednisolone Tebutate (Co-administration of know CYP3A4 enzyme inducers (e.g., phenytoin, rifampin, and phenobarbital) with risperidone may cause decreases in the combined plasma concentrations of ripseridone and 9-hydroxyrisperidone, which could lead to decreased efficacy of Risperdal Consta treatment. At the initiation of therapy with known CYP3A4 hepatic enzyme inducers, patients should be closely monitored during the first 4-8 weeks, since the dose of Risperdal Consta may need to be adjusted. A dose increase, or additionaloral risperidone, may need to be considered. On discontinuation of CYP3A4 hepatic enzyme inducers, the dosage of Risperdal Consta should be re-evaluated and, if necessary, decreased).
No products indexed under this heading.

Prednisone (Co-administration of know CYP3A4 enzyme inducers (e.g., phenytoin, rifampin, and phenobarbital) with risperidone may cause decreases in the combined plasma concentrations of ripseridone and 9-hydroxyrisperidone, which could lead to decreased efficacy of Risperdal Consta treatment. At the initiation of therapy with known CYP3A4 hepatic enzyme inducers, patients should be closely monitored during the first 4-8 weeks, since the dose of Risperdal Consta may need to be adjusted. A dose increase, or additionaloral risperidone, may need to be considered. On discontinuation of CYP3A4 hepatic enzyme inducers, the dosage of Risperdal Consta should be re-evaluated and, if necessary, decreased).
No products indexed under this heading.

Primidone (Co-administration of know CYP3A4 enzyme inducers (e.g., phenytoin, rifampin, and phenobarbital) with risperidone may cause decreases in the combined plasma concentrations of ripseridone and 9-hydroxyrisperidone, which could lead to decreased efficacy of Risperdal Consta treatment. At the initiation of therapy with known CYP3A4 hepatic enzyme inducers, patients should be closely monitored during the first 4-8 weeks, since the dose of Risperdal Consta may need to be adjusted. A dose increase, or additionaloral risperidone, may need to be considered. On discontinuation of CYP3A4 hepatic enzyme inducers, the dosage of Risperdal Consta should be re-evaluated and, if necessary, decreased).
No products indexed under this heading.

Prochlorperazine (Given the primary CNS effects of risperidone, caution should be used if taken in combination with other centrally-acting drugs).
No products indexed under this heading.

Promethazine Hydrochloride (Given the primary CNS effects of risperidone, caution should be used if taken in combination with other centrally-acting drugs).
No products indexed under this heading.

Propafenone Hydrochloride (Risperidone is metabolized to 9-hydroxyrisperidone by CYP2D6. Drug interactions that reduce the metabolism of risperidone to 9-hydroxyrisperidone would increase the plasma concentrations of risperidone and lower the concentrations of 9-hydroxyrisperidone). Products include:
Rythmol Tablets 1586
Rythmol SR Capsules 1590

Propofol (Given the primary CNS effects of risperidone, caution should be used if taken in combination with other centrally-acting drugs).
No products indexed under this heading.

Propoxyphene Hydrochloride (Given the primary CNS effects of risperidone, caution should be used if taken in combination with other centrally-acting drugs).
No products indexed under this heading.

Propoxyphene Napsylate (Given the primary CNS effects of risperidone, caution should be used if taken in combination with other centrally-acting drugs).
No products indexed under this heading.

Propranolol Hydrochloride (Because of its potential for inducing hypotension, risperidone may enhance the hypotensive effects of other therapeutic agents with this potential). Products include:
InnoPran XL Extended Release Capsules 1484

Protriptyline Hydrochloride (Risperidone is metabolized to 9-hydroxyrisperidone by CYP2D6. Drug interactions that reduce the metabolism of risperidone to 9-hydroxyrisperidone would increase the plasma concentrations of risperidone and lower the concentrations of 9-hydroxyrisperidone).
No products indexed under this heading.

Quazepam (Given the primary CNS effects of risperidone, caution should be used if taken in combination with other centrally-acting drugs).
No products indexed under this heading.

Quetiapine Fumarate (Given the primary CNS effects of risperidone, caution should be used if taken in combination with other centrally-acting drugs).
No products indexed under this heading.

Quinacrine Hydrochloride (Risperidone is metabolized to 9-hydroxyrisperidone by CYP2D6. Drug interactions that reduce the metabolism of risperidone to 9-hydroxyrisperidone would increase the plasma concentrations of risperidone and lower the concentrations of 9-hydroxyrisperidone).
No products indexed under this heading.

Quinapril Hydrochloride (Because of its potential for inducing hypotension, risperidone may enhance the hypotensive effects of other therapeutic agents with this potential).
No products indexed under this heading.

Quinidine Gluconate (Risperidone is metabolized to 9-hydroxyrisperidone by CYP2D6. Drug interactions that reduce the metabolism of risperidone to 9-hydroxyrisperidone would increase the plasma concentrations of risperidone and lower the concentrations of 9-hydroxyrisperidone).
No products indexed under this heading.

Quinidine Hydrochloride (Risperidone is metabolized to 9-hydroxyrisperidone by CYP2D6. Drug interactions that reduce the metabolism of risperidone to 9-hydroxyrisperidone would increase the plasma concentrations of risperidone and lower the concentrations of 9-hydroxyrisperidone).
No products indexed under this heading.

Quinidine Polygalacturonate (Risperidone is metabolized to 9-hydroxyrisperidone by CYP2D6. Drug interactions that reduce the metabolism of risperidone to 9-hydroxyrisperidone would increase the plasma concentrations of risperidone and lower the concentrations of 9-hydroxyrisperidone).
No products indexed under this heading.

Quinidine Sulfate (Risperidone is metabolized to 9-hydroxyrisperidone by CYP2D6. Drug interactions that reduce the metabolism of risperidone to 9-hydroxyrisperidone would increase the plasma concentrations of risperidone and lower the concentrations of 9-hydroxyrisperidone).
No products indexed under this heading.

Ramipril (Because of its potential for inducing hypotension, risperidone may enhance the hypotensive effects of other therapeutic agents with this potential).
No products indexed under this heading.

Ranitidine Bismuth Citrate (Cimetidine increased the bioavailability of risperidone, but only marginally increased the plasma concentration of the active anti-psychotic fraction).
No products indexed under this heading.

Ranitidine Hydrochloride (Ranitidine increased the bioavailability of risperidone by 26%. Ranitidine increased the AUC of the active moiety by 20%). Products include:
Zantac 75 Tablets .... ▣603
Zantac 1670
Zantac Injection 1666
Zantac Injection Pharmacy Bulk Package 1668
Maximum Strength Zantac 150 Tablets .... ▣603
Maximum Strength Zantac 150 Cool Mint Tablets .... ▣603

Rauwolfia Serpentina (Because of its potential for inducing hypotension, risperidone may enhance the hypotensive effects of other therapeutic agents with this potential).
No products indexed under this heading.

Remifentanil Hydrochloride (Given the primary CNS effects of risperidone, caution should be used if taken in combination with other centrally-acting drugs).
No products indexed under this heading.

Rescinnamine (Because of its potential for inducing hypotension, risperidone may enhance the hypotensive effects of other therapeutic agents with this potential).
No products indexed under this heading.

Reserpine (Because of its potential for inducing hypotension, risperidone may enhance the hypotensive effects of other therapeutic agents with this potential).
No products indexed under this heading.

Rifabutin (Co-administration of know CYP3A4 enzyme inducers (e.g., phenytoin, rifampin, and phenobarbital) with risperidone may cause decreases in the combined plasma concentrations of ripseridone and 9-hydroxyrisperidone, which could lead to decreased efficacy of Risperdal Consta treatment. At the initiation of therapy with known CYP3A4 hepatic enzyme inducers, patients should be closely monitored during the first 4-8 weeks, since the dose of Risperdal Consta may need to be adjusted. A dose increase, or additionaloral risperidone, may need to be considered. On discontinuation of CYP3A4 hepatic enzyme inducers, the dosage of Risperdal Consta should be re-evaluated and, if necessary, decreased).
No products indexed under this heading.

Rifampicin (Co-administration of know CYP3A4 enzyme inducers (e.g., phenytoin, rifampin, and phenobarbital) with risperidone may cause decreases in the combined plasma concentrations of ripseridone and 9-hydroxyrisperidone, which could lead to decreased efficacy of Risperdal Consta treatment. At the initiation of therapy with known CYP3A4 hepatic enzyme inducers, patients should be closely monitored during the first 4-8 weeks, since the dose of Risperdal Consta may need to be adjusted. A dose increase, or additionaloral risperidone, may need to be considered. On discontinuation of CYP3A4 hepatic enzyme inducers, the dosage of Risperdal Consta should be re-evaluated and, if necessary, decreased).
No products indexed under this heading.

Rifampin (Co-administration of know CYP3A4 enzyme inducers (e.g., phenytoin, rifampin, and phenobarbital) with risperidone may cause decreases in the combined plasma concentrations of ripseridone and 9-hydroxyrisperidone, which could lead to decreased efficacy of Risperdal Consta treatment. At the initiation of therapy with known CYP3A4 hepatic enzyme inducers, patients should be closely monitored during the first 4-8 weeks, since the dose of Risperdal Consta may need to be adjusted. A dose increase, or additionaloral risperidone, may need to be considered. On discontinuation of CYP3A4 hepatic enzyme inducers, the dosage of Risperdal Consta should be re-evaluated and, if necessary, decreased).
No products indexed under this heading.

Rifapentine (Co-administration of know CYP3A4 enzyme inducers (e.g., phenytoin, rifampin, and phenobarbital) with risperidone may cause decreases in the combined plasma concentrations of ripseridone and 9-hydroxyrisperidone, which could lead to decreased efficacy of Risperdal Consta treatment. At the initiation of therapy with known CYP3A4 hepatic enzyme inducers, patients should be closely monitored during the first 4-8 weeks, since the dose of Risperdal Consta may need to be adjusted. A dose increase, or additionaloral risperidone, may need to be considered. On discontinuation of CYP3A4 hepatic enzyme inducers, the dosage of Risperdal Consta should be re-evaluated and, if necessary, decreased).
No products indexed under this heading.

Ritonavir (Risperidone is metabolized to 9-hydroxyrisperidone by CYP2D6. Drug interactions that reduce the metabolism of risperidone to 9-hydroxyrisperidone would increase the plasma concentrations of risperidone and lower the concentrations of 9-hydroxyrisperidone). Products include:
Kaletra **452**
Norvir **489**

Ropinirole Hydrochloride (Risperidone may antagonize the effect of dopamine agonists). Products include:
Requip Tablets **1561**
Requip XL Tablets **1568**

Secobarbital Sodium (Given the primary CNS effects of risperidone, caution should be used if taken in combination with other centrally-acting drugs).
No products indexed under this heading.

Sertraline Hydrochloride (Risperidone is metabolized to 9-hydroxyrisperidone by CYP2D6. Drug interactions that reduce the metabolism of risperidone to 9-hydroxyrisperidone would increase the plasma concentrations of risperidone and lower the concentrations of 9-hydroxyrisperidone).
No products indexed under this heading.

Sevoflurane (Given the primary CNS effects of risperidone, caution should be used if taken in combination with other centrally-acting drugs). Products include:
Ultane Liquid for Inhalation **524**

Sildenafil Citrate (Risperidone is metabolized to 9-hydroxyrisperidone by CYP2D6. Drug interactions that reduce the metabolism of risperidone to 9-hydroxyrisperidone would increase the plasma concentrations of risperidone and lower the concentrations of 9-hydroxyrisperidone).
No products indexed under this heading.

Sodium Nitroprusside (Because of its potential for inducing hypotension, risperidone may enhance the hypotensive effects of other therapeutic agents with this potential).
No products indexed under this heading.

Sodium Oxybate (Given the primary CNS effects of risperidone, caution should be used if taken in combination with other centrally-acting drugs). Products include:
Xyrem Oral Solution **1766**

Sotalol Hydrochloride (Because of its potential for inducing hypotension, risperidone may enhance the hypotensive effects of other therapeutic agents with this potential).
No products indexed under this heading.

Spirapril Hydrochloride (Because of its potential for inducing hypotension, risperidone may enhance the hypotensive effects of other therapeutic agents with this potential).
No products indexed under this heading.

Sufentanil Citrate (Given the primary CNS effects of risperidone, caution should be used if taken in combination with other centrally-acting drugs).
No products indexed under this heading.

Sulfinpyrazone (Co-administration of know CYP3A4 enzyme inducers (e.g., phenytoin, rifampin, and phenobarbital) with risperidone may cause decreases in the combined plasma concentrations of ripseridone and 9-hydroxyrisperidone, which could lead to decreased efficacy of Risperdal Consta treatment. At the initiation of therapy with known CYP3A4 hepatic enzyme inducers, patients should be closely monitored during the first 4-8 weeks, since the dose of Risperdal Consta may need to be adjusted. A dose increase, or additionaloral risperidone, may need to be considered. On discontinuation of CYP3A4 hepatic enzyme inducers, the dosage of Risperdal Consta should be re-evaluated and, if necessary, decreased).
No products indexed under this heading.

Telmisartan (Because of its potential for inducing hypotension, risperidone may enhance the hypotensive effects of other therapeutic agents with this potential). Products include:
Micardis Tablets **852**
Micardis HCT Tablets **854**

Temazepam (Given the primary CNS effects of risperidone, caution should be used if taken in combination with other centrally-acting drugs).
No products indexed under this heading.

Terazosin Hydrochloride (Because of its potential for inducing hypotension, risperidone may enhance the hypotensive effects of other therapeutic agents with this potential).
No products indexed under this heading.

Terbinafine Hydrochloride (Risperidone is metabolized to 9-hydroxyrisperidone by CYP2D6. Drug interactions that reduce the metabolism of risperidone to 9-hydroxyrisperidone would increase the plasma concentrations of risperidone and lower the concentrations of 9-hydroxyrisperidone). Products include:
Lamisil Oral Granules **2264**
Lamisil Tablets **2266**

Theophylline (Co-administration of know CYP3A4 enzyme inducers (e.g., phenytoin, rifampin, and phenobarbital) with risperidone may cause decreases in the combined plasma concentrations of ripseridone and 9-hydroxyrisperidone, which could lead to decreased efficacy of Risperdal Consta treatment. At the initiation of therapy with known CYP3A4 hepatic enzyme inducers, patients should be closely monitored during the first 4-8 weeks, since the dose of Risperdal Consta may need to be adjusted. A dose increase, or additionaloral risperidone, may need to be considered. On discontinuation of CYP3A4 hepatic enzyme inducers, the dosage of Risperdal Consta should be re-evaluated and, if necessary, decreased).
No products indexed under this heading.

Theophylline Anhydrous (Co-administration of know CYP3A4 enzyme inducers (e.g., phenytoin, rifampin, and phenobarbital) with risperidone may cause decreases in the combined plasma concentrations of ripseridone and 9-hydroxyrisperidone, which could lead to decreased efficacy of Risperdal Consta treatment. At the initiation of therapy with known CYP3A4 hepatic enzyme inducers, patients should be closely monitored during the first 4-8 weeks, since the dose of Risperdal Consta may need to be adjusted. A dose increase, or additionaloral risperidone, may need to be considered. On discontinuation of CYP3A4 hepatic enzyme inducers, the dosage of Risperdal Consta should be re-evaluated and, if necessary, decreased). Products include:
Uniphyl Tablets **2595**

Theophylline Calcium Salicylate (Co-administration of know CYP3A4 enzyme inducers (e.g., phenytoin, rifampin, and phenobarbital) with risperidone may cause decreases in the combined plasma concentrations of ripseridone and 9-hydroxyrisperidone, which could lead to decreased efficacy of Risperdal Consta treatment. At the initiation of therapy with known CYP3A4 hepatic enzyme inducers, patients should be closely monitored during the first 4-8 weeks, since the dose of Risperdal Consta may need to be adjusted. A dose increase, or additionaloral risperidone, may need to be considered. On discontinuation of CYP3A4 hepatic enzyme inducers, the dosage of Risperdal Consta should be re-evaluated and, if necessary, decreased).
No products indexed under this heading.

Theophylline Dihydroxypropyl (Glyceryl) (Co-administration of know CYP3A4 enzyme inducers (e.g., phenytoin, rifampin, and phenobarbital) with risperidone may cause decreases in the combined plasma concentrations of ripseridone and 9-hydroxyrisperidone, which could lead to decreased efficacy of Risperdal Consta treatment. At the initiation of therapy with known CYP3A4 hepatic enzyme inducers, patients should be closely monitored during the first 4-8 weeks, since the dose of Risperdal Consta may need to be adjusted. A dose increase, or additionaloral risperidone, may need to be considered. On discontinuation of CYP3A4 hepatic enzyme inducers, the dosage of Risperdal Consta should be re-evaluated and, if necessary, decreased).
No products indexed under this heading.

Theophylline Ethylenediamine (Co-administration of know CYP3A4 enzyme inducers (e.g., phenytoin, rifampin, and phenobarbital) with risperidone may cause decreases in the combined plasma concentrations of ripseridone and 9-hydroxyrisperidone, which could lead to decreased efficacy of Risperdal Consta treatment. At the initiation of therapy with known CYP3A4 hepatic enzyme inducers, patients should be closely monitored during

the first 4-8 weeks, since the dose of Risperdal Consta may need to be adjusted. A dose increase, or additionaloral risperidone, may need to be considered. On discontinuation of CYP3A4 hepatic enzyme inducers, the dosage of Risperdal Consta should be re-evaluated and, if necessary, decreased).
No products indexed under this heading.

Thiamylal Sodium (Given the primary CNS effects of risperidone, caution should be used if taken in combination with other centrally-acting drugs).
No products indexed under this heading.

Thioridazine Hydrochloride (Given the primary CNS effects of risperidone, caution should be used if taken in combination with other centrally-acting drugs). Products include:
Thioridazine Hydrochloride Tablets 2195

Thiothixene (Given the primary CNS effects of risperidone, caution should be used if taken in combination with other centrally-acting drugs). Products include:
Thiothixene Capsules 2197

Timolol Maleate (Because of its potential for inducing hypotension, risperidone may enhance the hypotensive effects of other therapeutic agents with this potential). Products include:
Combigan Ophthalmic Solution 553
Cosopt Sterile Ophthalmic Solution 1969
Timoptic Sterile Ophthalmic Solution 2121
Timoptic in Ocudose 2124
Timoptic-XE Sterile Ophthalmic Gel Forming Solution 2125

Tolazamide (Co-administration of known enzyme inducers (e.g., phenytoin, rifampin and phenobarbital) with risperidone may cause decreases in the combined plasma concentrations of risperidone and 9-hydroxyrisperidone, which could lead to decreased efficacy. The dose of risperidone may need to be adjusted accordingly, particularly during the initiation or discontinuation of therapy with enzyme inducers).
No products indexed under this heading.

Tolbutamide (Co-administration of known enzyme inducers (e.g., phenytoin, rifampin and phenobarbital) with risperidone may cause decreases in the combined plasma concentrations of risperidone and 9-hydroxyrisperidone, which could lead to decreased efficacy. The dose of risperidone may need to be adjusted accordingly, particularly during the initiation or discontinuation of therapy with enzyme inducers).
No products indexed under this heading.

Torsemide (Because of its potential for inducing hypotension, risperidone may enhance the hypotensive effects of other therapeutic agents with this potential). Products include:
Demadex Injection 2630
Demadex Tablets 2630

Trandolapril (Because of its potential for inducing hypotension, risperidone may enhance the hypotensive effects of other therapeutic agents with this potential). Products include:
Mavik Tablets 472
Tarka Tablets 511

Triamcinolone (Co-administration of know CYP3A4 enzyme inducers (e.g., phenytoin, rifampin, and phenobarbital) with risperidone may cause decreases in the combined plasma concentrations of ripseridone and 9-hydroxyrisperidone, which could lead to decreased efficacy of Risperdal Consta treatment. At the initiation of therapy with known CYP3A4 hepatic enzyme inducers, patients should be closely monitored during the first 4-8 weeks, since the dose of Risperdal Consta may need to be adjusted. A dose increase, or additionaloral risperidone, may need to be considered. On discontinuation of CYP3A4 hepatic enzyme inducers, the dosage of Risperdal Consta should be re-evaluated and, if necessary, decreased).
No products indexed under this heading.

Triamcinolone Acetonide (Co-administration of know CYP3A4 enzyme inducers (e.g., phenytoin, rifampin, and phenobarbital) with risperidone may cause decreases in the combined plasma concentrations of ripseridone and 9-hydroxyrisperidone, which could lead to decreased efficacy of Risperdal Consta treatment. At the initiation of therapy with known CYP3A4 hepatic enzyme inducers, patients should be closely monitored during the first 4-8 weeks, since the dose of Risperdal Consta may need to be adjusted. A dose increase, or additionaloral risperidone, may need to be considered. On discontinuation of CYP3A4 hepatic enzyme inducers, the dosage of Risperdal Consta should be re-evaluated and, if necessary, decreased). Products include:
Azmacort Inhalation Aerosol 407
Nasacort AQ Nasal Spray 2765
Triesence Injectable Suspension .... ⊙ 209

Triamcinolone Diacetate (Co-administration of know CYP3A4 enzyme inducers (e.g., phenytoin, rifampin, and phenobarbital) with risperidone may cause decreases in the combined plasma concentrations of ripseridone and 9-hydroxyrisperidone, which could lead to decreased efficacy of Risperdal Consta treatment. At the initiation of therapy with known CYP3A4 hepatic enzyme inducers, patients should be closely monitored during the first 4-8 weeks, since the dose of Risperdal Consta may need to be adjusted. A dose increase, or additionaloral risperidone, may need to be considered. On discontinuation of CYP3A4 hepatic enzyme inducers, the dosage of Risperdal Consta should be re-evaluated and, if necessary, decreased).
No products indexed under this heading.

Triamcinolone Hexacetonide (Co-administration of know CYP3A4 enzyme inducers (e.g., phenytoin, rifampin, and phenobarbital) with risperidone may cause decreases in the combined plasma concentrations of ripseridone and 9-hydroxyrisperidone, which could lead to decreased efficacy of Risperdal Consta treatment. At the initiation of therapy with known CYP3A4 hepatic enzyme inducers, patients should be closely monitored during the first 4-8 weeks, since the dose of Risperdal Consta may need to be adjusted. A dose increase, or additionaloral risperidone, may need to be considered. On discontinuation of CYP3A4 hepatic enzyme inducers, the dosage of Risperdal Consta should be re-evaluated and, if necessary, decreased).
No products indexed under this heading.

Triazolam (Given the primary CNS effects of risperidone, caution should be used if taken in combination with other centrally-acting drugs).
No products indexed under this heading.

Trifluoperazine Hydrochloride (Given the primary CNS effects of risperidone, caution should be used if taken in combination with other centrally-acting drugs).
No products indexed under this heading.

Trimethaphan Camsylate (Because of its potential for inducing hypotension, risperidone may enhance the hypotensive effects of other therapeutic agents with this potential).
No products indexed under this heading.

Trimipramine Maleate (Risperidone is metabolized to 9-hydroxyrisperidone by CYP2D6. Drug interactions that reduce the metabolism of risperidone to 9-hydroxyrisperidone would increase the plasma concentrations of risperidone and lower the concentrations of 9-hydroxyrisperidone).
No products indexed under this heading.

Troglitazone (Co-administration of know CYP3A4 enzyme inducers (e.g., phenytoin, rifampin, and phenobarbital) with risperidone may cause decreases in the combined plasma concentrations of ripseridone and 9-hydroxyrisperidone, which could lead to decreased efficacy of Risperdal Consta treatment. At the initiation of therapy with known CYP3A4 hepatic enzyme inducers, patients should be closely monitored during the first 4-8 weeks, since the dose of Risperdal Consta may need to be adjusted. A dose increase, or additionaloral risperidone, may need to be considered. On discontinuation of CYP3A4 hepatic enzyme inducers, the dosage of Risperdal Consta should be re-evaluated and, if necessary, decreased).
No products indexed under this heading.

Valproate Sodium (Repeated oral doses of risperidone (4mg QD) did not affect the pre-dose or average plasma concentrations exposure (AUC) of valproate (1000 mg/day in three divided doses) compared to placebo (n=21). However, there was a 20% increase of valproate peak plasma concentration (Cmax) after concomitant administration of risperidone).
No products indexed under this heading.

Valproic Acid (Repeated oral doses of risperidone (4 mg QD) did not affect the pre-dose or average plasma concentrations and exposure (AUC) of valproate (1000 mg/day in three divided doses) compared to placebo (n=21). However, there was a 20% increase of valproate peak plasma concentration (Cmax) after concomitant administration of risperidone).
No products indexed under this heading.

Valsartan (Because of its potential for inducing hypotension, risperidone may enhance the hypotensive effects of other therapeutic agents with this potential). Products include:
Diovan Tablets 2212
Diovan HCT Tablets 2216
Exforge Tablets 2238

Vardenafil Hydrochloride (Risperidone is metabolized to 9-hydroxyrisperidone by CYP2D6. Drug interactions that reduce the metabolism of risperidone to 9-hydroxyrisperidone would increase the plasma concentrations of risperidone and lower the concentrations of 9-hydroxyrisperidone). Products include:
Levitra Tablets 2876

Verapamil Hydrochloride (Because of its potential for inducing hypotension, risperidone may enhance the hypotensive effects of other therapeutic agents with this potential). Products include:
Tarka Tablets 511

Zaleplon (Given the primary CNS effects of risperidone, caution should be used if taken in combination with other centrally-acting drugs).
No products indexed under this heading.

Ziprasidone Hydrochloride (Given the primary CNS effects of risperidone, caution should be used if taken in combination with other centrally-acting drugs). Products include:
Geodon Capsules 2520

Zolpidem Tartrate (Given the primary CNS effects of risperidone, caution should be used if taken in combination with other centrally-acting drugs). Products include:
Ambien Tablets 2692
Ambien CR Tablets 2696

Food Interactions

Alcohol (Caution should be used when risperidone is taken in combination with alcohol).

RITUXAN I.V.

(Rituximab) 1223
May interact with vaccines, live. Compounds in these categories include:

BCG Vaccine (Vaccination with live virus vaccines is not recommended).
No products indexed under this heading.

Influenza Vaccine, Live Attenuated (Vaccination with live virus vaccines is not recommended).
No products indexed under this heading.

Influenza Virus Vaccine Live, Intranasal (Vaccination with live virus vaccines is not recommended). Products include:
FluMist Vaccine 1945

Measles, Mumps, Rubella and Varicella Virus Vaccine Live (Vac-

cination with live virus vaccines is not recommended). Products include:
ProQuad 2099

Measles, Mumps & Rubella Virus Vaccine, Live (Vaccination with live virus vaccines is not recommended). Products include:
M-M-R II 2054

Measles & Rubella Virus Vaccine Live (Vaccination with live virus vaccines is not recommended).
No products indexed under this heading.

Measles Virus Vaccine Live (Vaccination with live virus vaccines is not recommended). Products include:
Attenuvax 1951

Mumps Virus Vaccine, Live (Vaccination with live virus vaccines is not recommended). Products include:
Mumpsvax 2068

Poliovirus Vaccine, Live, Oral, Trivalent, Types 1,2,3 (Sabin) (Vaccination with live virus vaccines is not recommended).
No products indexed under this heading.

Rotavirus Vaccine, Live, Oral, Tetravalent (Vaccination with live virus vaccines is not recommended).
No products indexed under this heading.

Rubella & Mumps Virus Vaccine Live (Vaccination with live virus vaccines is not recommended).
No products indexed under this heading.

Rubella Virus Vaccine Live (Vaccination with live virus vaccines is not recommended). Products include:
Meruvax II 2061

Smallpox Vaccine (Vaccination with live virus vaccines is not recommended).
No products indexed under this heading.

Typhoid Vaccine (Vaccination with live virus vaccines is not recommended).
No products indexed under this heading.

Varicella Virus Vaccine Live (Vaccination with live virus vaccines is not recommended). Products include:
Varivax 2133

Yellow Fever Vaccine (Vaccination with live virus vaccines is not recommended).
No products indexed under this heading.

Zoster Vaccine Live (Vaccination with live virus vaccines is not recommended). Products include:
Zostavax Injection 2145

ROCALTROL CAPSULES

(Calcitriol) 1150

May interact with calcium preparations, corticosteroids, cardiac glycosides, magnesium-containing antacids, phenytoin, phosphate-binding agents, and thiazides. Compounds in these categories include:

Antacids, magnesium-containing (Magnesium-containing preparations (e.g., antacids) may cause hypermagnesemia and should therefore not be taken during therapy with calcitriol by patients on chronic renal dialysis).
No products indexed under this heading.

Bendroflumethiazide (Thiazides are known to induce hypercalcemia by the reduction of calcium excretion in urine. Some reports have shown that the concomitant administration of thiazides with calcitriol causes hypercalcemia. Therefore, precaution should be taken when co-administration is necessary).
No products indexed under this heading.

Betamethasone Acetate (A relationship of functional antagonism exists between vitamin D analogues, which promote calcium absorption, and corticosteroids, which inhibit calcium absorption).
No products indexed under this heading.

Betamethasone Sodium Phosphate (A relationship of functional antagonism exists between vitamin D analogues, which promote calcium absorption, and corticosteroids, which inhibit calcium absorption).
No products indexed under this heading.

Budesonide (A relationship of functional antagonism exists between vitamin D analogues, which promote calcium absorption, and corticosteroids, which inhibit calcium absorption). Products include:
Pulmicort Flexhaler 654
Symbicort 80/4.5 Inhalation Aerosol 659
Symbicort 160/4.5 Inhalation Aerosol 659

Calcium (Uncontrolled intake of additional calcium-containing preparations should be avoided). Products include:
Phyto-Vite Tablets 639
Vibe Liquid Multi-Nutrient Supplement 626

Calcium, intravenous (Uncontrolled intake of additional calcium-containing preparations should be avoided).
No products indexed under this heading.

Calcium (Oyster Shell) (Uncontrolled intake of additional calcium-containing preparations should be avoided).
No products indexed under this heading.

Calcium Acetate (Uncontrolled intake of additional calcium-containing preparations should be avoided). Products include:
PhosLo GelCaps 1184

Calcium Ascorbate (Uncontrolled intake of additional calcium-containing preparations should be avoided).
No products indexed under this heading.

Calcium Carbaspirin (Uncontrolled intake of additional calcium-containing preparations should be avoided).
No products indexed under this heading.

Calcium Carbonate (Uncontrolled intake of additional calcium-containing preparations should be avoided). Products include:
Accelerator Tablets 634
Actonel with Calcium Tablets 2574
BioLean II Tablets 635
Calcet Triple Calcium + Vitamin D Tablets 629
D-Cal Chewable Caplets 624
Elixir Capsules 636
Pepcid Complete Chewable Tablets 1771
Extra Strength Rolaids Plus Gas Relief Tropical Fruit Softchews 1903
Extra Strength Rolaids Softchews Vanilla Creme 1903
Extra Strength Rolaids Freshmint Tablets 1903
Rolaids Multi-Symptom Berry Tablets 1903
Rolaids Original Peppermint Tablets 1903

Calcium Carbonate, Precipitated (Uncontrolled intake of additional calcium-containing preparations should be avoided).
No products indexed under this heading.

Calcium Caseinate (Uncontrolled intake of additional calcium-containing preparations should be avoided).
No products indexed under this heading.

Calcium Chloride (Uncontrolled intake of additional calcium-containing preparations should be avoided).
No products indexed under this heading.

Calcium Citrate (Uncontrolled intake of additional calcium-containing preparations should be avoided). Products include:
Active Calcium Tablets 3173
CitraNatal DHA Tablets 2175
CitraNatal 90 DHA Tablets 2175

Calcium Glubionate (Uncontrolled intake of additional calcium-containing preparations should be avoided).
No products indexed under this heading.

Calcium Gluconate (Uncontrolled intake of additional calcium-containing preparations should be avoided). Products include:
Calcet Triple Calcium + Vitamin D Tablets 629

Calcium Lactate (Uncontrolled intake of additional calcium-containing preparations should be avoided). Products include:
Calcet Triple Calcium + Vitamin D Tablets 629

Calcium Phosphate (Uncontrolled intake of additional calcium-containing preparations should be avoided).
No products indexed under this heading.

Calcium Phosphate, Dibasic (Uncontrolled intake of additional calcium-containing preparations should be avoided). Products include:
Accelerator Tablets 634

Calcium Phosphate, Tribasic (Uncontrolled intake of additional calcium-containing preparations should be avoided).
No products indexed under this heading.

Calcium Phosphorus Preparations (Uncontrolled intake of additional calcium-containing preparations should be avoided).
No products indexed under this heading.

Calcium Polycarbophil (Uncontrolled intake of additional calcium-containing preparations should be avoided).
No products indexed under this heading.

Calcium Salts (Uncontrolled intake of additional calcium-containing preparations should be avoided).
No products indexed under this heading.

Chlorothiazide (Thiazides are known to induce hypercalcemia by the reduction of calcium excretion in urine. Some reports have shown that the concomitant administration of thiazides with calcitriol causes hypercalcemia. Therefore, precaution should be taken when co-administration is necessary).
No products indexed under this heading.

Chlorothiazide Sodium (Thiazides are known to induce hypercalcemia by the reduction of calcium excretion in urine. Some reports have shown that the concomitant administration of thiazides with calcitriol causes hypercalcemia. Therefore, precaution should be taken when co-administration is necessary). Products include:
Intravenous Sodium Diuril 2490

Cholestyramine (Cholestryramine has been reported to reduce intestinal absorption of fat-soluble vitamins; as such it may impair intestinal absorption of calcitriol).
No products indexed under this heading.

Ciclesonide (A relationship of functional antagonism exists between vitamin D analogues, which promote calcium absorption, and corticosteroids, which inhibit calcium absorption). Products include:
Alvesco Inhalation Aerosol 2985
Omnaris Nasal Spray 2998

Cortisone Acetate (A relationship of functional antagonism exists between vitamin D analogues, which promote calcium absorption, and corticosteroids, which inhibit calcium absorption).
No products indexed under this heading.

Deslanoside (Calcitriol dosage must be determined with care in patients undergoing treamtent with digitalis, as hypercalcemia in such patients may precipitate cardiac arrhythmias).
No products indexed under this heading.

Dexamethasone (A relationship of functional antagonism exists between vitamin D analogues, which promote calcium absorption, and corticosteroids, which inhibit calcium absorption). Products include:
Ciprodex Otic Suspension 541

Dexamethasone Acetate (A relationship of functional antagonism exists between vitamin D analogues, which promote calcium absorption, and corticosteroids, which inhibit calcium absorption).
No products indexed under this heading.

Dexamethasone Sodium Phosphate (A relationship of functional antagonism exists between vitamin D analogues, which promote calcium absorption, and corticosteroids, which inhibit calcium absorption).
No products indexed under this heading.

Digitalis Glycoside Preparations (Calcitriol dosage must be determined with care in patients undergoing treamtent with digitalis, as hypercalcemia in such patients may precipitate cardiac arrhythmias).
No products indexed under this heading.

IMPORTANT NOTE: Always consult each drug listing in the patient's regimen for possible interactions.

Digitoxin (Calcitriol dosage must be determined with care in patients undergoing treamtent with digitalis, as hypercalcemia in such patients may precipitate cardiac arrhythmias).

No products indexed under this heading.

Digoxin (Calcitriol dosage must be determined with care in patients undergoing treamtent with digitalis, as hypercalcemia in such patients may precipitate cardiac arrhythmias). Products include:

- Lanoxin Injection 1498
- Lanoxin Injection Pediatric 1502
- Lanoxin Tablets 1505

Fludrocortisone Acetate (A relationship of functional antagonism exists between vitamin D analogues, which promote calcium absorption, and corticosteroids, which inhibit calcium absorption).

No products indexed under this heading.

Flunisolide (A relationship of functional antagonism exists between vitamin D analogues, which promote calcium absorption, and corticosteroids, which inhibit calcium absorption). Products include:

- Aerobid/Aerobid-M 1153

Fluticasone Propionate (A relationship of functional antagonism exists between vitamin D analogues, which promote calcium absorption, and corticosteroids, which inhibit calcium absorption). Products include:

- Advair Diskus 100/50 1276
- Advair Diskus 250/50 1276
- Advair Diskus 500/50 1276
- Advair HFA 45/21 Inhalation Aerosol 1288
- Advair HFA 115/21 Inhalation Aerosol 1288
- Advair HFA 230/21 Inhalation Aerosol 1288
- Flonase Nasal Spray 1431
- Flovent Diskus 50 mcg 1435

Fluticasone Propionate HFA (A relationship of functional antagonism exists between vitamin D analogues, which promote calcium absorption, and corticosteroids, which inhibit calcium absorption). Products include:

- Flovent HFA 1440

Fosphenytoin Sodium (The coadministration of phenytoin will not affect plasma concentrations of calcitriol, but may reduce endogenous plasma levels of 25(OH)D3 by accelerating metabolism. Since blood level of calcitriol will be reduced, higher doses of calcitriol may be necessary if these drugs are administered simultaneously).

No products indexed under this heading.

Hydrochlorothiazide (Thiazides are known to induce hypercalcemia by the reduction of calcium excretion in urine. Some reports have shown that the concomitant administration of thiazides with calcitriol causes hypercalcemia. Therefore, precaution should be taken when coadministration is necessary). Products include:

- Atacand HCT 642
- Avalide Tablets 892
- Avalide Tablets 2713
- Benicar HCT Tablets 1010
- Diovan HCT Tablets 2216
- Dyazide Capsules 1405
- Micardis HCT Tablets 854
- Prinzide Tablets 2092
- Tekturna HCT Tablets 2324
- Teveten HCT Tablets 517

Hydrocortisone (A relationship of functional antagonism exists between vitamin D analogues, which promote calcium absorption, and corticosteroids, which inhibit calcium absorption).

No products indexed under this heading.

Hydrocortisone Acetate (A relationship of functional antagonism exists between vitamin D analogues, which promote calcium absorption, and corticosteroids, which inhibit calcium absorption). Products include:

- Analpram-HC 1140
- Pramosone 1141

Hydrocortisone Sodium Phosphate (A relationship of functional antagonism exists between vitamin D analogues, which promote calcium absorption, and corticosteroids, which inhibit calcium absorption).

No products indexed under this heading.

Hydrocortisone Sodium Succinate (A relationship of functional antagonism exists between vitamin D analogues, which promote calcium absorption, and corticosteroids, which inhibit calcium absorption).

No products indexed under this heading.

Hydroflumethiazide (Thiazides are known to induce hypercalcemia by the reduction of calcium excretion in urine. Some reports have shown that the concomitant administration of thiazides with calcitriol causes hypercalcemia. Therefore, precaution should be taken when coadministration is necessary).

No products indexed under this heading.

Ketoconazole (Ketoconazole may inhibit both synthetic and catabolic enzymes of calcitriol. Reductions in serum endogenous calcitriol concentrations have been observed following the administation of 300 mg/day to 1200 mg/day ketoconazole for a week to healthy men. However, in vivo dug interaction studies of ketoconazole with calcitriol have not been investigated). Products include:

- Extina Foam, 2% 3057
- Nizoral A-D Shampoo 1901

Lanthanum Carbonate (Since calcitriol has an effect on phosphate transport in the intestine, kidneys and bones, the dosage of phosphate-binding agents must be adjusted in accordance with the serum phosphate concentration). Products include:

- Fosrenol Chewable Tablets 3027

Laxatives, magnesium-containing (Magnesium-containing preparations may cause hypermagnesemia and should therefore not be taken during therapy with calcitriol by patients on chronic renal dialysis).

No products indexed under this heading.

Magaldrate (Magnesium-containing preparations (e.g., antacids) may cause hypermagnesemia and should therefore not be taken during therapy with calcitriol by patients on chronic renal dialysis).

No products indexed under this heading.

Magnesium (Magnesium-containing preparations may cause hypermagnesemia and should therefore not be taken during therapy with calcitriol by patients on chronic renal dialysis). Products include:

- Protector Capsules .... ■639
- Vibe Liquid Multi-Nutrient Supplement .... ■626

Magnesium Carbonate (Magnesium-containing preparations may cause hypermagnesemia and should therefore not be taken during therapy with calcitriol by patients on chronic renal dialysis).

No products indexed under this heading.

Magnesium Chloride (Magnesium-containing preparations may cause hypermagnesemia and should therefore not be taken during therapy with calcitriol by patients on chronic renal dialysis).

No products indexed under this heading.

Magnesium Citrate (Magnesium-containing preparations may cause hypermagnesemia and should therefore not be taken during therapy with calcitriol by patients on chronic renal dialysis).

No products indexed under this heading.

Magnesium Gluconate (Magnesium-containing preparations may cause hypermagnesemia and should therefore not be taken during therapy with calcitriol by patients on chronic renal dialysis).

No products indexed under this heading.

Magnesium Hydroxide (Magnesium-containing preparations may cause hypermagnesemia and should therefore not be taken during therapy with calcitriol by patients on chronic renal dialysis). Products include:

- Fleet Pedia-Lax Chewable Tablets 1145
- Pepcid Complete Chewable Tablets 1771
- Extra Strength Rolaids Freshmint Tablets 1903
- Rolaids Multi-Symptom Berry Tablets 1903
- Rolaids Original Peppermint Tablets 1903

Magnesium Lactate (Magnesium-containing preparations may cause hypermagnesemia and should therefore not be taken during therapy with calcitriol by patients on chronic renal dialysis).

No products indexed under this heading.

Magnesium Oxide (Magnesium-containing preparations may cause hypermagnesemia and should therefore not be taken during therapy with calcitriol by patients on chronic renal dialysis). Products include:

- Beelith Tablets 813

Magnesium Salicylate (Magnesium-containing preparations may cause hypermagnesemia and should therefore not be taken during therapy with calcitriol by patients on chronic renal dialysis).

No products indexed under this heading.

Magnesium Salicylate Tetrahydrate (Magnesium-containing preparations may cause hypermagnesemia and should therefore not be taken during therapy with calcitriol by patients on chronic renal dialysis).

No products indexed under this heading.

Magnesium Salts (Magnesium-containing preparations may cause hypermagnesemia and should therefore not be taken during therapy with calcitriol by patients on chronic renal dialysis).

No products indexed under this heading.

Magnesium Sulfate (Magnesium-containing preparations may cause hypermagnesemia and should therefore not be taken during therapy with calcitriol by patients on chronic renal dialysis).

No products indexed under this heading.

Magnesium Trisilicate (Magnesium-containing preparations may cause hypermagnesemia and should therefore not be taken during therapy with calcitriol by patients on chronic renal dialysis).

No products indexed under this heading.

Methyclothiazide (Thiazides are known to induce hypercalcemia by the reduction of calcium excretion in urine. Some reports have shown that the concomitant administration of thiazides with calcitriol causes hypercalcemia. Therefore, precaution should be taken when coadministration is necessary).

No products indexed under this heading.

Methylprednisolone Acetate (A relationship of functional antagonism exists between vitamin D analogues, which promote calcium absorption, and corticosteroids, which inhibit calcium absorption).

No products indexed under this heading.

Methylprednisolone Sodium Succinate (A relationship of functional antagonism exists between vitamin D analogues, which promote calcium absorption, and corticosteroids, which inhibit calcium absorption).

No products indexed under this heading.

Mometasone Furoate (A relationship of functional antagonism exists between vitamin D analogues, which promote calcium absorption, and corticosteroids, which inhibit calcium absorption). Products include:

- Asmanex Twisthaler 2797
- Elocon Cream 0.1% 2840
- Elocon Lotion 0.1% 2841
- Elocon Ointment 0.1% 2842

Mometasone Furoate Monohydrate (A relationship of functional antagonism exists between vitamin D analogues, which promote calcium absorption, and corticosteroids, which inhibit calcium absorption). Products include:

- Nasonex Nasal Spray 2883

Phenobarbital (The coadministration of phenobarbital will not affect plasma concentrations of calcitriol, but may reduce endogenous plasma levels of 25(OH)D3 by accelerating metabolism. Since blood level of calcitriol will be reduced, higher doses of calcitriol may be necessary if these drugs are administered simultaneously). Products include:

- Donnatal Extentabs 2507

Phenobarbital Sodium (The co-administration of phenobarbital will not affect plasma concentrations of calcitrol, but may reduce endogenous plasma levels of 25(OH)D3 by accelerating metabolism. Since blood level of calcitriol will be reduced, higher doses of calcitriol may benecessary if these drugs are administered simultaneously).
No products indexed under this heading.

Phenytoin (The co-administration of phenytoin will not affect plasma concentrations of calcitriol, but may reduce endogenous plasma levels of 25(OH)D3 by accelerating metabolism. Since blood level of calcitriol will be reduced, higher doses of calcitriol may be necessary if these drugs are administered simultaneously).
No products indexed under this heading.

Phenytoin Sodium (The co-administration of phenytoin will not affect plasma concentrations of calcitriol, but may reduce endogenous plasma levels of 25(OH)D3 by accelerating metabolism. Since blood level of calcitriol will be reduced, higher doses of calcitriol may be necessary if these drugs are administered simultaneously). Products include:
Phenytek Capsules ... **2192**

Polythiazide (Thiazides are known to induce hypercalcemia by the reduction of calcium excretion in urine. Some reports have shown that the concomitant administration of thiazides with calcitriol causes hypercalcemia. Therefore, precaution should be taken when co-administration is necessary).
No products indexed under this heading.

Prednisolone Acetate (A relationship of functional antagonism exists between vitamin D analogues, which promote calcium absorption, and corticosteroids, which inhibit calcium absorption). Products include:
Pred Forte Ophthalmic Suspension ... ⊙**227**
Pred Mild Ophthalmic Suspension ... ⊙**230**
Pred-G Ophthalmic Ointment ... ⊙**229**
Pred-G Ophthalmic Suspension ... ⊙**228**

Prednisolone Sodium Phosphate (A relationship of functional antagonism exists between vitamin D analogues, which promote calcium absorption, and corticosteroids, which inhibit calcium absorption).
No products indexed under this heading.

Prednisolone Tebutate (A relationship of functional antagonism exists between vitamin D analogues, which promote calcium absorption, and corticosteroids, which inhibit calcium absorption).
No products indexed under this heading.

Prednisone (A relationship of functional antagonism exists between vitamin D analogues, which promote calcium absorption, and corticosteroids, which inhibit calcium absorption).
No products indexed under this heading.

Sevelamer Hydrochloride (Since calcitriol has an effect on phosphate transport in the intestine, kidneys and bones, the dosage of phosphate-binding agents must be adjusted in accordance with the serum phosphate concentration).
No products indexed under this heading.

Triamcinolone (A relationship of functional antagonism exists between vitamin D analogues, which promote calcium absorption, and corticosteroids, which inhibit calcium absorption).
No products indexed under this heading.

Triamcinolone Acetonide (A relationship of functional antagonism exists between vitamin D analogues, which promote calcium absorption, and corticosteroids, which inhibit calcium absorption). Products include:
Azmacort Inhalation Aerosol ... **407**
Nasacort AQ Nasal Spray ... **2765**
Triesence Injectable Suspension ... ⊙**209**

Triamcinolone Diacetate (A relationship of functional antagonism exists between vitamin D analogues, which promote calcium absorption, and corticosteroids, which inhibit calcium absorption).
No products indexed under this heading.

Triamcinolone Hexacetonide (A relationship of functional antagonism exists between vitamin D analogues, which promote calcium absorption, and corticosteroids, which inhibit calcium absorption).
No products indexed under this heading.

Vitamin D (Since calcitriol is the most potent active metabolite of vitamin D3, pharmacological doses of vitamin D and its derivatives should be withheld during treatment with calcitriol to avoid possible additive effects of hypercalcemia). Products include:
Active Calcium Tablets ... **3173**
D-Cal Chewable Caplets ... ▣**624**
Norwegian Cod Liver Oil ... **949**

ROCALTROL ORAL SOLUTION
(Calcitriol) ... **1150**
See Rocaltrol Capsules

ROCEPHIN INJECTABLE VIALS, ADD-VANTAGE, GALAXY, BULK
(Ceftriaxone Sodium) ... **2642**
May interact with calcium preparations. Compounds in these categories include:

Calcium Carbonate (Avoid co-administration with calcium-containing IV solutions in neonates because of risk of precipitation of ceftriaxone-calcium salt. There are no reports to date of intravascular or pulmonary precipitations in patients, other than neonates, treated with ceftriaxone and calcium-containing IV solutions. However, the theoretical possibility exists for an interaction between ceftriaxone and IV calcium-containing solutions in patients other than neonates. Therefore, ceftriaxone sodium and calcium-containing solutions, should not be mixed or co-administered to any patient irrespective of age, even via different infusion lines at different sites. Administration within 48 hours of each other in any patient). Products include:
Accelerator Tablets ... ▣**634**
Actonel with Calcium Tablets ... **2574**
BioLean II Tablets ... ▣**635**
Calcet Triple Calcium + Vitamin D Tablets ... ▣**629**
D-Cal Chewable Caplets ... ▣**624**
Elixir Capsules ... ▣**636**
Pepcid Complete Chewable Tablets ... **1771**
Extra Strength Rolaids Plus Gas Relief Tropical Fruit Softchews ... **1903**
Extra Strength Rolaids Softchews Vanilla Creme ... **1903**
Extra Strength Rolaids Freshmint Tablets ... **1903**
Rolaids Multi-Symptom Berry Tablets ... **1903**
Rolaids Original Peppermint Tablets ... **1903**

Calcium Chloride (Avoid co-administration with calcium-containing IV solutions in neonates because of risk of precipitation of ceftriaxone-calcium salt. There are no reports to date of intravascular or pulmonary precipitations in patients, other than neonates, treated with ceftriaxone and calcium-containing IV solutions. However, the theoretical possibility exists for an interaction between ceftriaxone and IV calcium-containing solutions in patients other than neonates. Therefore, ceftriaxone sodium and calcium-containing solutions, should not be mixed or co-administered to any patient irrespective of age, even via different infusion lines at different sites. Administration within 48 hours of each other in any patient).
No products indexed under this heading.

Calcium Citrate (Avoid co-administration with calcium-containing IV solutions in neonates because of risk of precipitation of ceftriaxone-calcium salt. There are no reports to date of intravascular or pulmonary precipitations in patients, other than neonates, treated with ceftriaxone and calcium-containing IV solutions. However, the theoretical possibility exists for an interaction between ceftriaxone and IV calcium-containing solutions in patients other than neonates. Therefore, ceftriaxone sodium and calcium-containing solutions, should not be mixed or co-administered to any patient irrespective of age, even via different infusion lines at different sites. Administration within 48 hours of each other in any patient). Products include:
Active Calcium Tablets ... **3173**
CitraNatal DHA Tablets ... **2175**
CitraNatal 90 DHA Tablets ... **2175**

Calcium Glubionate (Avoid co-administration with calcium-containing IV solutions in neonates because of risk of precipitation of ceftriaxone-calcium salt. There are no reports to date of intravascular or pulmonary precipitations in patients, other than neonates, treated with ceftriaxone and calcium-containing IV solutions. However, the theoretical possibility exists for an interaction between ceftriaxone and IV calcium-containing solutions in patients other than neonates. Therefore, ceftriaxone sodium and calcium-containing solutions, should not be mixed or co-administered to any patient irrespective of age, even via different infusion lines at different sites. Administration within 48 hours of each other in any patient).
No products indexed under this heading.

EXTRA STRENGTH ROLAIDS PLUS GAS RELIEF TROPICAL FRUIT SOFTCHEWS
(Calcium Carbonate, Simethicone) ... **1903**
May interact with:

Drugs, Oral, unspecified (Antacids may interact with certain prescription drugs).
No products indexed under this heading.

EXTRA STRENGTH ROLAIDS SOFTCHEWS VANILLA CREME
(Calcium Carbonate) ... **1903**
May interact with:

Drugs, Oral, unspecified (Antacids may interact with certain prescription drugs).
No products indexed under this heading.

EXTRA STRENGTH ROLAIDS FRESHMINT TABLETS
(Calcium Carbonate, Magnesium Hydroxide) ... **1903**
May interact with:

Drugs, Oral, unspecified (Antacids may interact with certain prescription drugs).
No products indexed under this heading.

ROLAIDS MULTI-SYMPTOM BERRY TABLETS
(Calcium Carbonate, Magnesium Hydroxide, Simethicone) ... **1903**
May interact with:

Prescription Drugs, unspecified (Antacids may interact with certain prescription drugs).
No products indexed under this heading.

ROLAIDS ORIGINAL PEPPERMINT TABLETS
(Calcium Carbonate, Magnesium Hydroxide) ... **1903**
May interact with:

Drugs, Oral, unspecified (Antacids may interact with certain unspecified prescription drugs).
No products indexed under this heading.

ROMAZICON INJECTION
(Flumazenil) ... **2646**
May interact with antidepressant drugs, neuromuscular blocking agents, and certain other agents. Compounds in these categories include:

Amitriptyline Hydrochloride (Toxic effects of cyclic antidepressant may emerge with the reversal of the benzodiazepine effect).
No products indexed under this heading.

Amoxapine (Toxic effects of cyclic antidepressants may emerge with the reversal of the benzodiazepine effect).
No products indexed under this heading.

Atracurium Besylate (Romazicon should not be used until the effects of neuromuscular blockade have been fully reversed).
No products indexed under this heading.

Bupropion Hydrochloride (Toxic effects of cyclic antidepressants may emerge with the reversal of the benzodiazepine effect). Products include:
Wellbutrin Tablets 1648
Wellbutrin SR Sustained-Release Tablets 1653
Wellbutrin XL Extended-Release Tablets 1659
Zyban Sustained-Release Tablets 1692

Cisatracurium Besylate (Romazicon should not be used until the effects of neuromuscular blockade have been fully reversed). Products include:
Nimbex Injection 484

Citalopram Hydrobromide (Toxic effects of cyclic antidepressants may emerge with the reversal of the benzodiazepine effect). Products include:
Celexa 1160

Desipramine Hydrochloride (Toxic effects of cyclic antidepressants may emerge with the reversal of the benzodiazepine effect).
No products indexed under this heading.

Doxacurium Chloride (Romazicon should not be used until the effects of neuromuscular blockade have been fully reversed).
No products indexed under this heading.

Doxepin Hydrochloride (Toxic effects of cyclic antidepressants may emerge with the reversal of the benzodiazepine effect).
No products indexed under this heading.

Escitalopram Oxalate (Toxic effects of cyclic antidepressants may emerge with the reversal of the benzodiazepine effect). Products include:
Lexapro Oral Suspension 1174
Lexapro Tablets 1174

Fluoxetine Hydrochloride (Toxic effects of cyclic antidepressants may emerge with the reversal of the benzodiazepine effect). Products include:
Prozac Weekly Capsules 1852
Prozac Pulvules and Liquid 1852
Symbyax Capsules 1871

Imipramine Hydrochloride (Toxic effects of cyclic antidepressants may emerge with the reversal of the benzodiazepine effect).
No products indexed under this heading.

Imipramine Pamoate (Toxic effects of cyclic antidepressants may emerge with the reversal of the benzodiazepine effect).
No products indexed under this heading.

Isocarboxazid (Toxic effects of cyclic antidepressants may emerge with the reversal of the benzodiazepine effect). Products include:
Marplan Tablets 3177

Maprotiline Hydrochloride (Toxic effects of cyclic antidepressants may emerge with the reversal of the benzodiazepine effect).
No products indexed under this heading.

Metocurine Iodide (Romazicon should not be used until the effects of neuromuscular blockade have been fully reversed).
No products indexed under this heading.

Mirtazapine (Toxic effects of cyclic antidepressants may emerge with the reversal of the benzodiazepine effect). Products include:
Remeron Tablets 2924
RemeronSolTab Tablets 2927

Mivacurium Chloride (Romazicon should not be used until the effects of neuromuscular blockade have been fully reversed).
No products indexed under this heading.

Nefazodone Hydrochloride (Toxic effects of cyclic antidepressants may emerge with the reversal of the benzodiazepine effect).
No products indexed under this heading.

Nortriptyline Hydrochloride (Toxic effects of cyclic antidepressants may emerge with the reversal of the benzodiazepine effect).
No products indexed under this heading.

Pancuronium Bromide (Romazicon should not be used until the effects of neuromuscular blockade have been fully reversed).
No products indexed under this heading.

Paroxetine Hydrochloride (Toxic effects of cyclic antidepressants may emerge with the reversal of the benzodiazepine effect). Products include:
Paxil 1535
Paxil CR Controlled-Release Tablets 1544

Phenelzine Sulfate (Toxic effects of cyclic antidepressants may emerge with the reversal of the benzodiazepine effect).
No products indexed under this heading.

Protriptyline Hydrochloride (Toxic effects of cyclic antidepressants may emerge with the reversal of the benzodiazepine effect).
No products indexed under this heading.

Rapacuronium Bromide (Romazicon should not be used until the effects of neuromuscular blockade have been fully reversed).
No products indexed under this heading.

Rocuronium Bromide (Romazicon should not be used until the effects of neuromuscular blockade have been fully reversed). Products include:
Zemuron Injection 2947

Selegiline (Toxic effects of cyclic antidepressants may emerge with the reversal of the benzodiazepine effect). Products include:
Emsam Transdermal System 905

Selegiline Hydrochloride (Toxic effects of cyclic antidepressants may emerge with the reversal of the benzodiazepine effect). Products include:
Eldepryl Capsules 3052

Sertraline Hydrochloride (Toxic effects of cyclic antidepressants may emerge with the reversal of the benzodiazepine effect).
No products indexed under this heading.

Succinylcholine Chloride (Romazicon should not be used until the effects of neuromuscular blockade have been fully reversed).
No products indexed under this heading.

Tranylcypromine Sulfate (Toxic effects of cyclic antidepressants may emerge with the reversal of the benzodiazepine effect). Products include:
Parnate Tablets 1532

Trazodone Hydrochloride (Toxic effects of cyclic antidepressants may emerge with the reversal of the benzodiazepine effect).
No products indexed under this heading.

Trimipramine Maleate (Toxic effects of cyclic antidepressants may emerge with the reversal of the benzodiazepine effect).
No products indexed under this heading.

Vecuronium Bromide (Romazicon should not be used until the effects of neuromuscular blockade have been fully reversed).
No products indexed under this heading.

Venlafaxine Hydrochloride (Toxic effects of cyclic antidepressants may emerge with the reversal of the benzodiazepine effect). Products include:
Effexor XR Extended-Release Capsules 3195
Venlafaxine Hydrochloride Tablets 2199

Food Interactions

Food, unspecified (Ingestion of food during an IV infusion results in a 50% increase in clearance).

ROSAC WASH
(Sodium Sulfacetamide) 3062
None cited in PDR database.

ROTARIX ORAL SUSPENSION
(Rotavirus Vaccine, Live, Oral) 1582
May interact with alkylating agents, antimetabolites, corticosteroids, cytotoxic drugs, immunosuppressive agents, and certain other agents. Compounds in these categories include:

Azathioprine (Immunosuppressive therapies may reduce the immune response to Rotarix).
No products indexed under this heading.

Basiliximab (Immunosuppressive therapies may reduce the immune response to Rotarix). Products include:
Simulect for Injection 2306

Betamethasone Acetate (Corticosteroids (used in greater than physiologic doses) may reduce the immune response to Rotarix).
No products indexed under this heading.

Betamethasone Sodium Phosphate (Corticosteroids (used in greater than physiologic doses) may reduce the immune response to Rotarix).
No products indexed under this heading.

Bleomycin Sulfate (Immunosuppressive therapies, including cytotoxic drugs, may reduce the immune response to Rotarix).
No products indexed under this heading.

Budesonide (Corticosteroids (used in greater than physiologic doses) may reduce the immune response to Rotarix). Products include:
Pulmicort Flexhaler 654
Symbicort 80/4.5 Inhalation Aerosol 659
Symbicort 160/4.5 Inhalation Aerosol 659

Busulfan (Immunosuppressive therapies, including alkylating agents, may reduce the immune response to Rotarix). Products include:
Busulfex Injection 2477
Myleran Tablets 1530

Capecitabine (Immunosuppressive therapies, including antimetabolites, may reduce the immune response to Rotarix). Products include:
Xeloda Tablets 2662

Carmustine (BCNU) (Immunosuppressive therapies, including alkylating agents, may reduce the immune response to Rotarix).
No products indexed under this heading.

Chlorambucil (Immunosuppressive therapies, including alkylating agents, may reduce the immune response to Rotarix). Products include:
Leukeran Tablets 1508

Ciclesonide (Corticosteroids (used in greater than physiologic doses) may reduce the immune response to Rotarix). Products include:
Alvesco Inhalation Aerosol 2985
Omnaris Nasal Spray 2998

Cladribine (Immunosuppressive therapies, including antimetabolites, may reduce the immune response to Rotarix). Products include:
Leustatin Injection 2384

Cortisone Acetate (Corticosteroids (used in greater than physiologic doses) may reduce the immune response to Rotarix).
No products indexed under this heading.

Cyclophosphamide (Immunosuppressive therapies, including alkylating agents, may reduce the immune response to Rotarix).
No products indexed under this heading.

Cyclosporine (Immunosuppressive therapies may reduce the immune response to Rotarix). Products include:
Gengraf Capsules 435
Neoral Oral Solution 2280
Neoral Soft Gelatin Capsules 2280
Restasis Ophthalmic Emulsion 557
Sandimmune 2296

Cytarabine (Immunosuppressive therapies, including antimetabolites, may reduce the immune response to Rotarix).
No products indexed under this heading.

Dacarbazine (Immunosuppressive therapies, including alkylating agents, may reduce the immune response to Rotarix).
No products indexed under this heading.

Daunorubicin Hydrochloride (Immunosuppressive therapies, including cytotoxic drugs, may reduce the immune response to Rotarix).
No products indexed under this heading.

Dexamethasone (Corticosteroids (used in greater than physiologic doses) may reduce the immune response to Rotarix). Products include:

Ciprodex Otic Suspension 541

Dexamethasone Acetate (Corticosteroids (used in greater than physiologic doses) may reduce the immune response to Rotarix).
No products indexed under this heading.

Dexamethasone Sodium Phosphate (Corticosteroids (used in greater than physiologic doses) may reduce the immune response to Rotarix).
No products indexed under this heading.

Doxorubicin Hydrochloride (Immunosuppressive therapies, including cytotoxic drugs, may reduce the immune response to Rotarix).
No products indexed under this heading.

Epirubicin Hydrochloride (Immunosuppressive therapies, including cytotoxic drugs, may reduce the immune response to Rotarix).
No products indexed under this heading.

Floxuridine (Immunosuppressive therapies, including antimetabolites, may reduce the immune response to Rotarix).
No products indexed under this heading.

Fludarabine Phosphate (Immunosuppressive therapies, including antimetabolites, may reduce the immune response to Rotarix).
No products indexed under this heading.

Fludrocortisone Acetate (Corticosteroids (used in greater than physiologic doses) may reduce the immune response to Rotarix).
No products indexed under this heading.

Flunisolide (Corticosteroids (used in greater than physiologic doses) may reduce the immune response to Rotarix). Products include:
Aerobid/Aerobid-M 1153

Fluorouracil (Immunosuppressive therapies, including antimetabolites, may reduce the immune response to Rotarix). Products include:
Carac Cream 0.5% 2722

Fluticasone Propionate (Corticosteroids (used in greater than physiologic doses) may reduce the immune response to Rotarix). Products include:
Advair Diskus 100/50 1276
Advair Diskus 250/50 1276
Advair Diskus 500/50 1276
Advair HFA 45/21 Inhalation Aerosol 1288
Advair HFA 115/21 Inhalation Aerosol 1288
Advair HFA 230/21 Inhalation Aerosol 1288
Flonase Nasal Spray 1431
Flovent Diskus 50 mcg 1435

Fluticasone Propionate HFA (Corticosteroids (used in greater than physiologic doses) may reduce the immune response to Rotarix). Products include:
Flovent HFA 1440

Gemcitabine Hydrochloride (Immunosuppressive therapies, including antimetabolites, may reduce the immune response to Rotarix). Products include:
Gemzar for Injection 1820

Hydrocortisone (Corticosteroids (used in greater than physiologic doses) may reduce the immune response to Rotarix).
No products indexed under this heading.

Hydrocortisone Acetate (Corticosteroids (used in greater than physiologic doses) may reduce the immune response to Rotarix). Products include:
Analpram-HC 1140
Pramosone 1141

Hydrocortisone Sodium Phosphate (Corticosteroids (used in greater than physiologic doses) may reduce the immune response to Rotarix).
No products indexed under this heading.

Hydrocortisone Sodium Succinate (Corticosteroids (used in greater than physiologic doses) may reduce the immune response to Rotarix).
No products indexed under this heading.

Hydroxyurea (Immunosuppressive therapies, including cytotoxic drugs, may reduce the immune response to Rotarix).
No products indexed under this heading.

Lomustine (CCNU) (Immunosuppressive therapies, including alkylating agents, may reduce the immune response to Rotarix).
No products indexed under this heading.

Mechlorethamine Hydrochloride (Immunosuppressive therapies, including alkylating agents, may reduce the immune response to Rotarix). Products include:
Mustargen for Injection 2492

Melphalan (Immunosuppressive therapies, including alkylating agents, may reduce the immune response to Rotarix).
No products indexed under this heading.

Mercaptopurine (Immunosuppressive therapies, including antimetabolites, may reduce the immune response to Rotarix).
No products indexed under this heading.

Methotrexate (Immunosuppressive therapies, including antimetabolites, may reduce the immune response to Rotarix).
No products indexed under this heading.

Methotrexate Sodium (Immunosuppressive therapies, including cytotoxic drugs, may reduce the immune response to Rotarix).
No products indexed under this heading.

Methylprednisolone Acetate (Corticosteroids (used in greater than physiologic doses) may reduce the immune response to Rotarix).
No products indexed under this heading.

Methylprednisolone Sodium Succinate (Corticosteroids (used in greater than physiologic doses) may reduce the immune response to Rotarix).
No products indexed under this heading.

Mitotane (Immunosuppressive therapies, including cytotoxic drugs, may reduce the immune response to Rotarix).
No products indexed under this heading.

Mitoxantrone Hydrochloride (Immunosuppressive therapies, including cytotoxic drugs, may reduce the immune response to Rotarix). Products include:
Novantrone for Injection Concentrate 1100

Mometasone Furoate (Corticosteroids (used in greater than physiologic doses) may reduce the immune response to Rotarix). Products include:
Asmanex Twisthaler 2797
Elocon Cream 0.1% 2840
Elocon Lotion 0.1% 2841
Elocon Ointment 0.1% 2842

Mometasone Furoate Monohydrate (Corticosteroids (used in greater than physiologic doses) may reduce the immune response to Rotarix). Products include:
Nasonex Nasal Spray 2883

Muromonab-CD3 (Immunosuppressive therapies may reduce the immune response to Rotarix). Products include:
Orthoclone OKT3 Sterile Solution 2387

Mycophenolate Mofetil (Immunosuppressive therapies may reduce the immune response to Rotarix). Products include:
CellCept Capsules 2622
CellCept Oral Suspension 2622
CellCept Tablets 2622

Pentostatin (Immunosuppressive therapies, including antimetabolites, may reduce the immune response to Rotarix).
No products indexed under this heading.

Prednisolone Acetate (Corticosteroids (used in greater than physiologic doses) may reduce the immune response to Rotarix). Products include:
Pred Forte Ophthalmic Suspension .... ⊙227
Pred Mild Ophthalmic Suspension .... ⊙230
Pred-G Ophthalmic Ointment .... ⊙229
Pred-G Ophthalmic Suspension ...... ⊙228

Prednisolone Sodium Phosphate (Corticosteroids (used in greater than physiologic doses) may reduce the immune response to Rotarix).
No products indexed under this heading.

Prednisolone Tebutate (Corticosteroids (used in greater than physiologic doses) may reduce the immune response to Rotarix).
No products indexed under this heading.

Prednisone (Corticosteroids (used in greater than physiologic doses) may reduce the immune response to Rotarix).
No products indexed under this heading.

Procarbazine Hydrochloride (Immunosuppressive therapies, including cytotoxic drugs, may reduce the immune response to Rotarix).
No products indexed under this heading.

Radiation (Immunosuppressive therapies, including irradiation, may reduce the immune response to Rotarix).
No products indexed under this heading.

Sirolimus (Immunosuppressive therapies may reduce the immune response to Rotarix). Products include:
Rapamune 3260

Tacrolimus (Immunosuppressive therapies may reduce the immune response to Rotarix). Products include:
Prograf Capsules and Injection 622
Protopic Ointment 628

Tamoxifen Citrate (Immunosuppressive therapies, including cytotoxic drugs, may reduce the immune response to Rotarix).
No products indexed under this heading.

Thioguanine (Immunosuppressive therapies, including antimetabolites, may reduce the immune response to Rotarix). Products include:
Tabloid Tablets 1601

Thiotepa (Immunosuppressive therapies, including alkylating agents, may reduce the immune response to Rotarix).
No products indexed under this heading.

Triamcinolone (Corticosteroids (used in greater than physiologic doses) may reduce the immune response to Rotarix).
No products indexed under this heading.

Triamcinolone Acetonide (Corticosteroids (used in greater than physiologic doses) may reduce the immune response to Rotarix). Products include:
Azmacort Inhalation Aerosol 407
Nasacort AQ Nasal Spray 2765
Triesence Injectable Suspension .... ⊙209

Triamcinolone Diacetate (Corticosteroids (used in greater than physiologic doses) may reduce the immune response to Rotarix).
No products indexed under this heading.

Triamcinolone Hexacetonide (Corticosteroids (used in greater than physiologic doses) may reduce the immune response to Rotarix).
No products indexed under this heading.

Vincristine Sulfate (Immunosuppressive therapies, including cytotoxic drugs, may reduce the immune response to Rotarix).
No products indexed under this heading.

ROTATEQ

(Rotavirus vaccine, live, oral, pentavalent)...................................... 2110
May interact with alkylating agents, antimetabolites, corticosteroids, and cytotoxic drugs. Compounds in these categories include:

Betamethasone Acetate (Immunosuppressive therapies including corticosteroids (used in greater than physiologic doses) may reduce the immune response to vaccines).
No products indexed under this heading.

Betamethasone Sodium Phosphate (Immunosuppressive therapies including corticosteroids (used in greater than physiologic doses) may reduce the immune response to vaccines).
No products indexed under this heading.

Bleomycin Sulfate (Immunosuppressive therapies including cytotoxic drugs may reduce the immune response to vaccines).
No products indexed under this heading.

Budesonide (Immunosuppressive therapies including corticosteroids

(used in greater than physiologic doses) may reduce the immune response to vaccines). Products include:
Pulmicort Flexhaler 654
Symbicort 80/4.5 Inhalation Aerosol.. 659
Symbicort 160/4.5 Inhalation Aerosol.. 659

Busulfan (Immunosuppressive therapies including alkylating agents may reduce the immune response to vaccines). Products include:
Busulfex Injection 2477
Myleran Tablets 1530

Capecitabine (Immunosuppresive therapies including antimetabolites may reduce the immune response to vaccines). Products include:
Xeloda Tablets 2662

Carmustine (BCNU) (Immunosuppressive therapies including alkylating agents may reduce the immune response to vaccines).
No products indexed under this heading.

Chlorambucil (Immunosuppressive therapies including alkylating agents may reduce the immune response to vaccines). Products include:
Leukeran Tablets 1508

Ciclesonide (Immunosuppressive therapies including corticosteroids (used in greater than physiologic doses) may reduce the immune response to vaccines). Products include:
Alvesco Inhalation Aerosol 2985
Omnaris Nasal Spray 2998

Cladribine (Immunosuppresive therapies including antimetabolites may reduce the immune response to vaccines). Products include:
Leustatin Injection 2384

Cortisone Acetate (Immunosuppressive therapies including corticosteroids (used in greater than physiologic doses) may reduce the immune response to vaccines).
No products indexed under this heading.

Cyclophosphamide (Immunosuppressive therapies including alkylating agents may reduce the immune response to vaccines).
No products indexed under this heading.

Cytarabine (Immunosuppresive therapies including antimetabolites may reduce the immune response to vaccines).
No products indexed under this heading.

Dacarbazine (Immunosuppressive therapies including alkylating agents may reduce the immune response to vaccines).
No products indexed under this heading.

Daunorubicin Hydrochloride (Immunosuppressive therapies including cytotoxic drugs may reduce the immune response to vaccines).
No products indexed under this heading.

Dexamethasone (Immunosuppressive therapies including corticosteroids (used in greater than physiologic doses) may reduce the immune response to vaccines). Products include:
Ciprodex Otic Suspension 541

Dexamethasone Acetate (Immunosuppressive therapies including corticosteroids (used in greater than physiologic doses) may reduce the immune response to vaccines).
No products indexed under this heading.

Dexamethasone Sodium Phosphate (Immunosuppressive therapies including corticosteroids (used in greater than physiologic doses) may reduce the immune response to vaccines).
No products indexed under this heading.

Doxorubicin Hydrochloride (Immunosuppressive therapies including cytotoxic drugs may reduce the immune response to vaccines).
No products indexed under this heading.

Epirubicin Hydrochloride (Immunosuppressive therapies including cytotoxic drugs may reduce the immune response to vaccines).
No products indexed under this heading.

Floxuridine (Immunosuppresive therapies including antimetabolites may reduce the immune response to vaccines).
No products indexed under this heading.

Fludarabine Phosphate (Immunosuppresive therapies including antimetabolites may reduce the immune response to vaccines).
No products indexed under this heading.

Fludrocortisone Acetate (Immunosuppressive therapies including corticosteroids (used in greater than physiologic doses) may reduce the immune response to vaccines).
No products indexed under this heading.

Flunisolide (Immunosuppressive therapies including corticosteroids (used in greater than physiologic doses) may reduce the immune response to vaccines). Products include:
Aerobid/Aerobid-M 1153

Fluorouracil (Immunosuppresive therapies including antimetabolites may reduce the immune response to vaccines). Products include:
Carac Cream 0.5% 2722

Fluticasone Propionate (Immunosuppressive therapies including corticosteroids (used in greater than physiologic doses) may reduce the immune response to vaccines). Products include:
Advair Diskus 100/50 1276
Advair Diskus 250/50 1276
Advair Diskus 500/50 1276
Advair HFA 45/21 Inhalation Aerosol.. 1288
Advair HFA 115/21 Inhalation Aerosol.. 1288
Advair HFA 230/21 Inhalation Aerosol.. 1288
Flonase Nasal Spray 1431
Flovent Diskus 50 mcg 1435

Fluticasone Propionate HFA (Immunosuppressive therapies including corticosteroids (used in greater than physiologic doses) may reduce the immune response to vaccines). Products include:
Flovent HFA 1440

Gemcitabine Hydrochloride (Immunosuppresive therapies including antimetabolites may reduce the immune response to vaccines). Products include:
Gemzar for Injection 1820

Hydrocortisone (Immunosuppressive therapies including corticosteroids (used in greater than physiologic doses) may reduce the immune response to vaccines).
No products indexed under this heading.

Hydrocortisone Acetate (Immunosuppressive therapies including corticosteroids (used in greater than physiologic doses) may reduce the immune response to vaccines). Products include:
Analpram-HC 1140
Pramosone 1141

Hydrocortisone Sodium Phosphate (Immunosuppressive therapies including corticosteroids (used in greater than physiologic doses) may reduce the immune response to vaccines).
No products indexed under this heading.

Hydrocortisone Sodium Succinate (Immunosuppressive therapies including corticosteroids (used in greater than physiologic doses) may reduce the immune response to vaccines).
No products indexed under this heading.

Hydroxyurea (Immunosuppressive therapies including cytotoxic drugs may reduce the immune response to vaccines).
No products indexed under this heading.

Lomustine (CCNU) (Immunosuppressive therapies including alkylating agents may reduce the immune response to vaccines).
No products indexed under this heading.

Mechlorethamine Hydrochloride (Immunosuppressive therapies including alkylating agents may reduce the immune response to vaccines). Products include:
Mustargen for Injection 2492

Melphalan (Immunosuppressive therapies including alkylating agents may reduce the immune response to vaccines).
No products indexed under this heading.

Mercaptopurine (Immunosuppressive therapies including antimetabolites may reduce the immune response to vaccines).
No products indexed under this heading.

Methotrexate (Immunosuppresive therapies including antimetabolites may reduce the immune response to vaccines).
No products indexed under this heading.

Methotrexate Sodium (Immunosuppressive therapies including cytotoxic drugs may reduce the immune response to vaccines).
No products indexed under this heading.

Methylprednisolone Acetate (Immunosuppressive therapies including corticosteroids (used in greater than physiologic doses) may reduce the immune response to vaccines).
No products indexed under this heading.

Methylprednisolone Sodium Succinate (Immunosuppressive therapies including corticosteroids (used in greater than physiologic doses) may reduce the immune response to vaccines).
No products indexed under this heading.

Mitotane (Immunosuppressive therapies including cytotoxic drugs may reduce the immune response to vaccines).
No products indexed under this heading.

Mitoxantrone Hydrochloride (Immunosuppressive therapies including cytotoxic drugs may reduce the immune response to vaccines). Products include:
Novantrone for Injection Concentrate 1100

Mometasone Furoate (Immunosuppressive therapies including corticosteroids (used in greater than physiologic doses) may reduce the immune response to vaccines). Products include:
Asmanex Twisthaler 2797
Elocon Cream 0.1% 2840
Elocon Lotion 0.1% 2841
Elocon Ointment 0.1% 2842

Mometasone Furoate Monohydrate (Immunosuppressive therapies including corticosteroids (used in greater than physiologic doses) may reduce the immune response to vaccines). Products include:
Nasonex Nasal Spray 2883

Pentostatin (Immunosuppresive therapies including antimetabolites may reduce the immune response to vaccines).
No products indexed under this heading.

Prednisolone Acetate (Immunosuppressive therapies including corticosteroids (used in greater than physiologic doses) may reduce the immune response to vaccines). Products include:
Pred Forte Ophthalmic Suspension .... ⊙227
Pred Mild Ophthalmic Suspension .... ⊙230
Pred-G Ophthalmic Ointment .... ⊙229
Pred-G Ophthalmic Suspension ...... ⊙228

Prednisolone Sodium Phosphate (Immunosuppressive therapies including corticosteroids (used in greater than physiologic doses) may reduce the immune response to vaccines).
No products indexed under this heading.

Prednisolone Tebutate (Immunosuppressive therapies including corticosteroids (used in greater than physiologic doses) may reduce the immune response to vaccines).
No products indexed under this heading.

Prednisone (Immunosuppressive therapies including corticosteroids (used in greater than physiologic doses) may reduce the immune response to vaccines).
No products indexed under this heading.

Procarbazine Hydrochloride (Immunosuppressive therapies including cytotoxic drugs may reduce the immune response to vaccines).
No products indexed under this heading.

Tamoxifen Citrate (Immunosuppressive therapies including cytotoxic drugs may reduce the immune response to vaccines).
No products indexed under this heading.

Thioguanine (Immunosuppresive therapies including antimetabolites may reduce the immune response to vaccines). Products include:
Tabloid Tablets 1601

Thiotepa (Immunosuppressive therapies including alkylating agents may reduce the immune response to vaccines).
No products indexed under this heading.

Triamcinolone (Immunosuppressive therapies including corticosteroids (used in greater than physiologic doses) may reduce the immune response to vaccines).
No products indexed under this heading.

Triamcinolone Acetonide (Immunosuppressive therapies including corticosteroids (used in greater than physiologic doses) may reduce the immune response to vaccines).
Products include:
Azmacort Inhalation Aerosol 407
Nasacort AQ Nasal Spray 2765
Triesence Injectable Suspension .... ⊙209

Triamcinolone Diacetate (Immunosuppressive therapies including corticosteroids (used in greater than physiologic doses) may reduce the immune response to vaccines).
No products indexed under this heading.

Triamcinolone Hexacetonide (Immunosuppressive therapies including corticosteroids (used in greater than physiologic doses) may reduce the immune response to vaccines).
No products indexed under this heading.

Vincristine Sulfate (Immunosuppressive therapies including cytotoxic drugs may reduce the immune response to vaccines).
No products indexed under this heading.

ROZEREM TABLETS

(Ramelteon) 3091
May interact with cytochrome p450 1a2 inducers (selected), cytochrome p450 1a2 inhibitors (selected), cytochrome p450 2c8 inducers (selected), cytochrome p450 2c9 inducers (selected), cytochrome p450 2c9 inhibitors (selected), cytochrome p450 2d6 inducers (selected), cytochrome p450 3a4 inducers (selected), cytochrome p450 3a4 inhibitors (selected), cytochrome p450 3a inducers (selected), and certain other agents. Compounds in these categories include:

Acetazolamide (Ramelteon should be administered with caution in subjects taking strong CYP2C9 inhibitors such as fluconazole).
No products indexed under this heading.

Alatrofloxacin Mesylate (Ramelteon should be administered with caution in subjects taking strong CYP2C9 inhibitors such as fluconazole).
No products indexed under this heading.

Allium sativum (Efficacy may be reduced when ramelteon is used in combination with strong CYP enzyme inducers such as rifampin).
No products indexed under this heading.

Amiodarone Hydrochloride (Ramelteon should be administered with caution in subjects taking strong CYP2C9 inhibitors such as fluconazole).
No products indexed under this heading.

Amprenavir (Ramelteon should be administered with caution in subjects taking strong CYP2C9 inhibitors such as fluconazole).
No products indexed under this heading.

Anastrozole (Ramelteon should be administered with caution in subjects taking strong CYP2C9 inhibitors such as fluconazole). Products include:
Arimidex Tablets 672

Aprepitant (Ramelteon should be administered with caution in subjects taking strong CYP2C9 inhibitors such as fluconazole). Products include:
Emend Capsules 1992

Atazanavir (Ramelteon should be administered with caution in subjects taking strong CYP2C9 inhibitors such as fluconazole).
No products indexed under this heading.

Atazanavir Sulfate (Ramelteon should be administered with caution in subjects taking strong CYP2C9 inhibitors such as fluconazole).
Products include:
Reyataz Capsules 3299

Bendroflumethiazide (Ramelteon should be administered with caution in subjects taking strong CYP2C9 inhibitors such as fluconazole).
No products indexed under this heading.

Betamethasone Acetate (Efficacy may be reduced when ramelteon is used in combination with strong CYP enzyme inducers such as rifampin).
No products indexed under this heading.

Betamethasone Sodium Phosphate (Efficacy may be reduced when ramelteon is used in combination with strong CYP enzyme inducers such as rifampin).
No products indexed under this heading.

Carbamazepine (Efficacy may be reduced when ramelteon is used in combination with strong CYP enzyme inducers such as rifampin).
Products include:
Carbatrol Capsules 3019
Equetro Extended-Release Capsules 3174

Chloramphenicol (Ramelteon should be administered with caution in subjects taking strong CYP2C9 inhibitors such as fluconazole).
No products indexed under this heading.

Chlorothiazide (Ramelteon should be administered with caution in subjects taking strong CYP2C9 inhibitors such as fluconazole).
No products indexed under this heading.

Chlorothiazide Sodium (Ramelteon should be administered with caution in subjects taking strong CYP2C9 inhibitors such as fluconazole). Products include:
Intravenous Sodium Diuril 2490

Chlorpropamide (Ramelteon should be administered with caution in subjects taking strong CYP2C9 inhibitors such as fluconazole).
No products indexed under this heading.

Cimetidine (Ramelteon should be administered with caution in subjects taking strong CYP2C9 inhibitors such as fluconazole).
No products indexed under this heading.

Cimetidine Hydrochloride (Ramelteon should be administered with caution in subjects taking strong CYP2C9 inhibitors such as fluconazole).
No products indexed under this heading.

Ciprofloxacin (Ramelteon should be administered with caution in subjects taking strong CYP2C9 inhibitors such as fluconazole). Products include:
Cipro I.V. 2817
Cipro Oral Suspension 2810
Cipro XR Tablets 2823
Ciprodex Otic Suspension 541

Ciprofloxacin Hydrochloride (Ramelteon should be administered with caution in subjects taking strong CYP2C9 inhibitors such as fluconazole). Products include:
Cipro Tablets 2810

Cisplatin (Efficacy may be reduced when ramelteon is used in combination with strong CYP enzyme inducers such as rifampin).
No products indexed under this heading.

Citalopram Hydrobromide (Efficacy may be reduced when ramelteon is used in combination with strong CYP enzyme inducers such as rifampin). Products include:
Celexa 1160

Clarithromycin (Ramelteon should be administered with caution in subjects taking strong CYP2C9 inhibitors such as fluconazole). Products include:
Biaxin/Biaxin XL 411

Clopidogrel Hydrogen Sulfate (Ramelteon should be administered with caution in subjects taking strong CYP2C9 inhibitors such as fluconazole).
No products indexed under this heading.

Clotrimazole (Ramelteon should be administered with caution in subjects taking strong CYP2C9 inhibitors such as fluconazole). Products include:
Lotrisone 2881

Cortisone Acetate (Efficacy may be reduced when ramelteon is used in combination with strong CYP enzyme inducers such as rifampin).
No products indexed under this heading.

Cyclosporine (Ramelteon should be administered with caution in subjects taking strong CYP2C9 inhibitors such as fluconazole). Products include:
Gengraf Capsules 435
Neoral Oral Solution 2280
Neoral Soft Gelatin Capsules 2280
Restasis Ophthalmic Emulsion 557
Sandimmune 2296

Dalfopristin (Ramelteon should be administered with caution in subjects taking strong CYP2C9 inhibitors such as fluconazole).
No products indexed under this heading.

Danazol (Ramelteon should be administered with caution in subjects taking strong CYP2C9 inhibitors such as fluconazole).
No products indexed under this heading.

Delavirdine Mesylate (Ramelteon should be administered with caution in subjects taking strong CYP2C9 inhibitors such as fluconazole).
No products indexed under this heading.

Desogestrel (Ramelteon should be administered with caution in subjects taking strong CYP2C9 inhibitors such as fluconazole). Products include:
Mircette Tablets 1034

Dexamethasone (Efficacy may be reduced when ramelteon is used in combination with strong CYP enzyme inducers such as rifampin).
Products include:
Ciprodex Otic Suspension 541

Dexamethasone Acetate (Efficacy may be reduced when ramelteon is used in combination with strong CYP enzyme inducers such as rifampin).
No products indexed under this heading.

Dexamethasone Sodium Phosphate (Efficacy may be reduced when ramelteon is used in combination with strong CYP enzyme inducers such as rifampin).
No products indexed under this heading.

Diclofenac Potassium (Ramelteon should be administered with caution in subjects taking strong CYP2C9 inhibitors such as fluconazole).
No products indexed under this heading.

Diclofenac Sodium (Ramelteon should be administered with caution in subjects taking strong CYP2C9 inhibitors such as fluconazole).
Products include:
Diclofenac Sodium Ophthalmic Solution .... ⊙240
Voltaren Ophthalmic Solution 2336
Voltaren Tablets 2334
Voltaren-XR Tablets 2337

Diltiazem Hydrochloride (Ramelteon should be administered with caution in subjects taking strong CYP2C9 inhibitors such as fluconazole). Products include:
Cardizem LA Extended Release Tablets 421

Diltiazem Maleate (Ramelteon should be administered with caution in subjects taking strong CYP2C9 inhibitors such as fluconazole).
No products indexed under this heading.

Disulfiram (Ramelteon should be administered with caution in subjects taking strong CYP2C9 inhibitors such as fluconazole).
No products indexed under this heading.

Doxorubicin Hydrochloride (Efficacy may be reduced when ramelteon is used in combination with strong CYP enzyme inducers such as rifampin).
No products indexed under this heading.

Efavirenz (Ramelteon should be administered with caution in subjects taking strong CYP2C9 inhibitors such as fluconazole). Products include:

Atripla Tablets ... 938
Sustiva Capsules ... 930
Sustiva Tablets ... 930

Enoxacin (Ramelteon should be administered with caution in subjects taking strong CYP2C9 inhibitors such as fluconazole).
No products indexed under this heading.

Erythromycin (Ramelteon should be administered with caution in subjects taking strong CYP2C9 inhibitors such as fluconazole).
No products indexed under this heading.

Erythromycin Estolate (Ramelteon should be administered with caution in subjects taking strong CYP2C9 inhibitors such as fluconazole).
No products indexed under this heading.

Erythromycin Ethylsuccinate (Ramelteon should be administered with caution in subjects taking strong CYP2C9 inhibitors such as fluconazole). Products include:

E.E.S. ... 433
EryPed ... 431

Erythromycin Gluceptate (Ramelteon should be administered with caution in subjects taking strong CYP2C9 inhibitors such as fluconazole).
No products indexed under this heading.

Erythromycin Lactobionate (Ramelteon should be administered with caution in subjects taking strong CYP2C9 inhibitors such as fluconazole).
No products indexed under this heading.

Erythromycin Stearate (Ramelteon should be administered with caution in subjects taking strong CYP2C9 inhibitors such as fluconazole).
No products indexed under this heading.

Esomeprazole Magnesium (Ramelteon should be administered with caution in subjects taking strong CYP2C9 inhibitors such as fluconazole). Products include:

Nexium Delayed-Release Capsules ... 645
Nexium Delayed-Release Oral Suspension ... 645

Ethanol (Efficacy may be reduced when ramelteon is used in combination with strong CYP enzyme inducers such as rifampin).
No products indexed under this heading.

Ethinyl Estradiol (Ramelteon should be administered with caution in subjects taking strong CYP2C9 inhibitors such as fluconazole). Products include:

Lybrel Tablets ... 3204
Mircette Tablets ... 1034
NuvaRing ... 2897
Ortho-Cyclen/Ortho Tri-Cyclen ... 2449
Ortho Evra Transdermal System ... 2437
Ortho Tri-Cyclen Lo Tablets ... 2458
Seasonique Tablets ... 1046
Yaz Tablets ... 805

Ethosuximide (Efficacy may be reduced when ramelteon is used in combination with strong CYP enzyme inducers such as rifampin).
No products indexed under this heading.

Felbamate (Efficacy may be reduced when ramelteon is used in combination with strong CYP enzyme inducers such as rifampin).
No products indexed under this heading.

Fenofibrate (Ramelteon should be administered with caution in subjects taking strong CYP2C9 inhibitors such as fluconazole). Products include:

Fenoglide Tablets ... 2960
Tricor Tablets ... 520

Fluconazole (The total and peak systemic exposure (AUC 0-inf and Cmax) of ramelteon after a single 16 mg dose of ramelteon was increased by approximately 150% when administered with fluconazole. Similar increases were also seen in M-II exposure. Ramelteon should be administered with caution in subjects taking strong CYP2C9 inhibitors such as fluconazole).
No products indexed under this heading.

Fludrocortisone Acetate (Efficacy may be reduced when ramelteon is used in combination with strong CYP enzyme inducers such as rifampin).
No products indexed under this heading.

Fluorouracil (Ramelteon should be administered with caution in subjects taking strong CYP2C9 inhibitors such as fluconazole). Products include:

Carac Cream 0.5% ... 2722

Fluoxetine (Ramelteon should be administered with caution in subjects taking strong CYP2C9 inhibitors such as fluconazole).
No products indexed under this heading.

Fluoxetine Hydrochloride (Ramelteon should be administered with caution in subjects taking strong CYP2C9 inhibitors such as fluconazole). Products include:

Prozac Weekly Capsules ... 1852
Prozac Pulvules and Liquid ... 1852
Symbyax Capsules ... 1871

Flurbiprofen (Ramelteon should be administered with caution in subjects taking strong CYP2C9 inhibitors such as fluconazole).
No products indexed under this heading.

Flurbiprofen Sodium (Ramelteon should be administered with caution in subjects taking strong CYP2C9 inhibitors such as fluconazole).
No products indexed under this heading.

Fluvastatin Sodium (Ramelteon should be administered with caution in subjects taking strong CYP2C9 inhibitors such as fluconazole). Products include:

Lescol Capsules ... 2268
Lescol XL Tablets ... 2268

Fluvoxamine (When fluvoxamine 100 mg twice daily was administered for 3 days prior to single-dose co-administration of ramelteon 16 mg and fluvoxamine, the AUC 0-inf for ramelteon increased approximately 190-fold, and the Cmax increased approximately 70-fold, compared to ramelteon administered alone. Ramelteon should not be used in combination with fluvoxamine. Other less potent CYP1A2 inhibitors have not been adequately studied. Ramelteon should be administered with caution to patients taking less strong CYP1A2 inhibitors).
No products indexed under this heading.

Fluvoxamine Maleate (Ramelteon should be administered with caution in subjects taking strong CYP2C9 inhibitors such as fluconazole). Products include:

Luvox CR Extended-Release Capsules ... 1759

Fosamprenavir Calcium (Ramelteon should be administered with caution in subjects taking strong CYP2C9 inhibitors such as fluconazole). Products include:

Lexiva Oral Suspension ... 1510
Lexiva Tablets ... 1510

Fosphenytoin Sodium (Efficacy may be reduced when ramelteon is used in combination with strong CYP enzyme inducers such as rifampin).
No products indexed under this heading.

Garlic Extract (Efficacy may be reduced when ramelteon is used in combination with strong CYP enzyme inducers such as rifampin).
No products indexed under this heading.

Garlic Oil (Efficacy may be reduced when ramelteon is used in combination with strong CYP enzyme inducers such as rifampin).
No products indexed under this heading.

Gatifloxacin (Ramelteon should be administered with caution in subjects taking strong CYP2C9 inhibitors such as fluconazole).
No products indexed under this heading.

Gemfibrozil (Ramelteon should be administered with caution in subjects taking strong CYP2C9 inhibitors such as fluconazole).
No products indexed under this heading.

Gemifloxacin Mesylate (Ramelteon should be administered with caution in subjects taking strong CYP2C9 inhibitors such as fluconazole).
No products indexed under this heading.

Glipizide (Ramelteon should be administered with caution in subjects taking strong CYP2C9 inhibitors such as fluconazole).
No products indexed under this heading.

Glyburide (Ramelteon should be administered with caution in subjects taking strong CYP2C9 inhibitors such as fluconazole).
No products indexed under this heading.

Grepafloxacin Hydrochloride (Ramelteon should be administered with caution in subjects taking strong CYP2C9 inhibitors such as fluconazole).
No products indexed under this heading.

Hydrochlorothiazide (Ramelteon should be administered with caution in subjects taking strong CYP2C9 inhibitors such as fluconazole). Products include:

Atacand HCT ... 642
Avalide Tablets ... 892
Avalide Tablets ... 2713
Benicar HCT Tablets ... 1010
Diovan HCT Tablets ... 2216
Dyazide Capsules ... 1405
Micardis HCT Tablets ... 854
Prinzide Tablets ... 2092
Tekturna HCT Tablets ... 2324
Teveten HCT Tablets ... 517

Hydrocortisone (Efficacy may be reduced when ramelteon is used in combination with strong CYP enzyme inducers such as rifampin).
No products indexed under this heading.

Hydrocortisone Acetate (Efficacy may be reduced when ramelteon is used in combination with strong CYP enzyme inducers such as rifampin). Products include:

Analpram-HC ... 1140
Pramosone ... 1141

Hydrocortisone Butyrate (Efficacy may be reduced when ramelteon is used in combination with strong CYP enzyme inducers such as rifampin).
No products indexed under this heading.

Hydrocortisone Cypionate (Efficacy may be reduced when ramelteon is used in combination with strong CYP enzyme inducers such as rifampin).
No products indexed under this heading.

Hydrocortisone Hemisuccinate (Efficacy may be reduced when ramelteon is used in combination with strong CYP enzyme inducers such as rifampin).
No products indexed under this heading.

Hydrocortisone Probutate (Efficacy may be reduced when ramelteon is used in combination with strong CYP enzyme inducers such as rifampin).
No products indexed under this heading.

Hydrocortisone Sodium Phosphate (Efficacy may be reduced when ramelteon is used in combination with strong CYP enzyme inducers such as rifampin).
No products indexed under this heading.

Hydrocortisone Sodium Succinate (Efficacy may be reduced when ramelteon is used in combination with strong CYP enzyme inducers such as rifampin).
No products indexed under this heading.

Hydrocortisone Valerate (Efficacy may be reduced when ramelteon is used in combination with strong CYP enzyme inducers such as rifampin).
No products indexed under this heading.

Hydroflumethiazide (Ramelteon should be administered with caution in subjects taking strong CYP2C9 inhibitors such as fluconazole).
No products indexed under this heading.

Hypericum (Efficacy may be reduced when ramelteon is used in combination with strong CYP enzyme inducers such as rifampin). Products include:

Satieté Tablets ... ▣640

Hypericum Perforatum (Efficacy may be reduced when ramelteon is used in combination with strong CYP enzyme inducers such as rifampin).
No products indexed under this heading.

Imatinib Mesylate (Ramelteon should be administered with caution in subjects taking strong CYP2C9 inhibitors such as fluconazole). Products include:
Gleevec Tablets 2255

Indinavir Sulfate (Ramelteon should be administered with caution in subjects taking strong CYP2C9 inhibitors such as fluconazole). Products include:
Crixivan Capsules 1979

Insulin (Efficacy may be reduced when ramelteon is used in combination with strong CYP enzyme inducers such as rifampin).
No products indexed under this heading.

Isoniazid (Ramelteon should be administered with caution in subjects taking strong CYP2C9 inhibitors such as fluconazole).
No products indexed under this heading.

Itraconazole (Ramelteon should be administered with caution in subjects taking strong CYP2C9 inhibitors such as fluconazole).
No products indexed under this heading.

Ketoconazole (The AUC 0-inf and Cmax of ramelteon increased by approximately 84% and 36%, respectively, when a single 16 mg dose of ramelteon was administered on the fourth day of ketoconazole 200 mg twice daily administration, compared to administration of rameIteonalone. Similar increases were seen in M-II pharmacokinetic variables. Ramelteon should be administered with caution in subjects taking strong CYP3A4 inhibitors such as ketoconazole). Products include:
Extina Foam, 2% 3057
Nizoral A-D Shampoo 1901

Ketoprofen (Ramelteon should be administered with caution in subjects taking strong CYP2C9 inhibitors such as fluconazole).
No products indexed under this heading.

Lansoprazole (Efficacy may be reduced when ramelteon is used in combination with strong CYP enzyme inducers such as rifampin).
No products indexed under this heading.

Leflunomide (Ramelteon should be administered with caution in subjects taking strong CYP2C9 inhibitors such as fluconazole).
No products indexed under this heading.

Levofloxacin (Ramelteon should be administered with caution in subjects taking strong CYP2C9 inhibitors such as fluconazole). Products include:
Iquix Ophthalmic Solution 3183
Levaquin 2416
Levaquin in 5% Dextrose Injection 2416
Quixin Ophthalmic Solution 3184

Levonorgestrel (Ramelteon should be administered with caution in subjects taking strong CYP2C9 inhibitors such as fluconazole). Products include:
Climara Pro Transdermal System 768
Lybrel Tablets 3204
Mirena Intrauterine System 779
Plan B Tablets 1044
Seasonique Tablets 1046

Lomefloxacin Hydrochloride (Ramelteon should be administered with caution in subjects taking strong CYP2C9 inhibitors such as fluconazole).
No products indexed under this heading.

Lopinavir (Ramelteon should be administered with caution in subjects taking strong CYP2C9 inhibitors such as fluconazole). Products include:
Kaletra 452

Loratadine (Ramelteon should be administered with caution in subjects taking strong CYP2C9 inhibitors such as fluconazole).
No products indexed under this heading.

Lovastatin (Ramelteon should be administered with caution in subjects taking strong CYP2C9 inhibitors such as fluconazole). Products include:
Advicor Tablets 402
Mevacor Tablets 2063

Mephenytoin (Efficacy may be reduced when ramelteon is used in combination with strong CYP enzyme inducers such as rifampin).
No products indexed under this heading.

Mestranol (Ramelteon should be administered with caution in subjects taking strong CYP2C9 inhibitors such as fluconazole).
No products indexed under this heading.

Methoxsalen (Ramelteon should be administered with caution in subjects taking strong CYP2C9 inhibitors such as fluconazole).
No products indexed under this heading.

Methsuximide (Efficacy may be reduced when ramelteon is used in combination with strong CYP enzyme inducers such as rifampin).
No products indexed under this heading.

Methyclothiazide (Ramelteon should be administered with caution in subjects taking strong CYP2C9 inhibitors such as fluconazole).
No products indexed under this heading.

Methylprednisolone (Efficacy may be reduced when ramelteon is used in combination with strong CYP enzyme inducers such as rifampin).
No products indexed under this heading.

Methylprednisolone Acetate (Efficacy may be reduced when ramelteon is used in combination with strong CYP enzyme inducers such as rifampin).
No products indexed under this heading.

Methylprednisolone Sodium Succinate (Efficacy may be reduced when ramelteon is used in combination with strong CYP enzyme inducers such as rifampin).
No products indexed under this heading.

Metronidazole (Ramelteon should be administered with caution in subjects taking strong CYP2C9 inhibitors such as fluconazole). Products include:
Pylera Capsules 714

Metronidazole Benzoate (Ramelteon should be administered with caution in subjects taking strong CYP2C9 inhibitors such as fluconazole).
No products indexed under this heading.

Metronidazole Hydrochloride (Ramelteon should be administered with caution in subjects taking strong CYP2C9 inhibitors such as fluconazole).
No products indexed under this heading.

Mexiletine Hydrochloride (Ramelteon should be administered with caution in subjects taking strong CYP2C9 inhibitors such as fluconazole).
No products indexed under this heading.

Mibefradil Dihydrochloride (Ramelteon should be administered with caution in subjects taking strong CYP2C9 inhibitors such as fluconazole).
No products indexed under this heading.

Miconazole (Ramelteon should be administered with caution in subjects taking strong CYP2C9 inhibitors such as fluconazole).
No products indexed under this heading.

Miconazole Nitrate (Ramelteon should be administered with caution in subjects taking strong CYP2C9 inhibitors such as fluconazole).
No products indexed under this heading.

Modafinil (Ramelteon should be administered with caution in subjects taking strong CYP2C9 inhibitors such as fluconazole). Products include:
Provigil Tablets 977

Moxifloxacin Hydrochloride (Ramelteon should be administered with caution in subjects taking strong CYP2C9 inhibitors such as fluconazole). Products include:
Avelox 2803
Vigamox Ophthalmic Solution 548

Nafcillin Sodium (Efficacy may be reduced when ramelteon is used in combination with strong CYP enzyme inducers such as rifampin).
No products indexed under this heading.

Nalidixic Acid (Ramelteon should be administered with caution in subjects taking strong CYP2C9 inhibitors such as fluconazole).
No products indexed under this heading.

Nefazodone Hydrochloride (Ramelteon should be administered with caution in subjects taking strong CYP2C9 inhibitors such as fluconazole).
No products indexed under this heading.

Nelfinavir Mesylate (Ramelteon should be administered with caution in subjects taking strong CYP2C9 inhibitors such as fluconazole).
No products indexed under this heading.

Nevirapine (Ramelteon should be administered with caution in subjects taking strong CYP2C9 inhibitors such as fluconazole). Products include:
Viramune Oral Suspension 873
Viramune Tablets 873

Niacinamide (Ramelteon should be administered with caution in subjects taking strong CYP2C9 inhibitors such as fluconazole). Products include:
BioLean Free Tablets 635

Nicotinamide (Ramelteon should be administered with caution in subjects taking strong CYP2C9 inhibitors such as fluconazole).
No products indexed under this heading.

Nicotine (Efficacy may be reduced when ramelteon is used in combination with strong CYP enzyme inducers such as rifampin).
No products indexed under this heading.

Nicotine Polacrilex (Efficacy may be reduced when ramelteon is used in combination with strong CYP enzyme inducers such as rifampin).
No products indexed under this heading.

Nicotine Salicylate (Efficacy may be reduced when ramelteon is used in combination with strong CYP enzyme inducers such as rifampin).
No products indexed under this heading.

Nicotine Sulfate (Efficacy may be reduced when ramelteon is used in combination with strong CYP enzyme inducers such as rifampin).
No products indexed under this heading.

Nifedipine (Ramelteon should be administered with caution in subjects taking strong CYP2C9 inhibitors such as fluconazole).
No products indexed under this heading.

Norethindrone (Ramelteon should be administered with caution in subjects taking strong CYP2C9 inhibitors such as fluconazole). Products include:
Ortho Micronor Tablets 2446

Norfloxacin (Ramelteon should be administered with caution in subjects taking strong CYP2C9 inhibitors such as fluconazole). Products include:
Noroxin Tablets 2069

Norgestrel (Ramelteon should be administered with caution in subjects taking strong CYP2C9 inhibitors such as fluconazole).
No products indexed under this heading.

Ofloxacin (Ramelteon should be administered with caution in subjects taking strong CYP2C9 inhibitors such as fluconazole). Products include:
Ofloxacin Ophthalmic Solution 0.3% .... ⊙ 243

Omeprazole (Ramelteon should be administered with caution in subjects taking strong CYP2C9 inhibitors such as fluconazole).
No products indexed under this heading.

Oxcarbazepine (Efficacy may be reduced when ramelteon is used in combination with strong CYP enzyme inducers such as rifampin).
No products indexed under this heading.

Oxiconazole Nitrate (Ramelteon should be administered with caution in subjects taking strong CYP2C9 inhibitors such as fluconazole).
No products indexed under this heading.

Paroxetine Hydrochloride (Ramelteon should be administered

with caution in subjects taking strong CYP2C9 inhibitors such as fluconazole). Products include:
Paxil 1535
Paxil CR Controlled-Release Tablets 1544

Phenobarbital (Efficacy may be reduced when ramelteon is used in combination with strong CYP enzyme inducers such as rifampin). Products include:
Donnatal Extentabs 2507

Phenobarbital Sodium (Efficacy may be reduced when ramelteon is used in combination with strong CYP enzyme inducers such as rifampin).
No products indexed under this heading.

Phenylbutazone (Ramelteon should be administered with caution in subjects taking strong CYP2C9 inhibitors such as fluconazole).
No products indexed under this heading.

Phenytoin (Efficacy may be reduced when ramelteon is used in combination with strong CYP enzyme inducers such as rifampin).
No products indexed under this heading.

Phenytoin Sodium (Efficacy may be reduced when ramelteon is used in combination with strong CYP enzyme inducers such as rifampin). Products include:
Phenytek Capsules 2192

Polythiazide (Ramelteon should be administered with caution in subjects taking strong CYP2C9 inhibitors such as fluconazole).
No products indexed under this heading.

Prednisolone Acetate (Efficacy may be reduced when ramelteon is used in combination with strong CYP enzyme inducers such as rifampin). Products include:
Pred Forte Ophthalmic Suspension .... ⊙227
Pred Mild Ophthalmic Suspension .... ⊙230
Pred-G Ophthalmic Ointment .... ⊙229
Pred-G Ophthalmic Suspension .... ⊙228

Prednisolone Sodium Phosphate (Efficacy may be reduced when ramelteon is used in combination with strong CYP enzyme inducers such as rifampin).
No products indexed under this heading.

Prednisolone Tebutate (Efficacy may be reduced when ramelteon is used in combination with strong CYP enzyme inducers such as rifampin).
No products indexed under this heading.

Prednisone (Efficacy may be reduced when ramelteon is used in combination with strong CYP enzyme inducers such as rifampin).
No products indexed under this heading.

Primidone (Efficacy may be reduced when ramelteon is used in combination with strong CYP enzyme inducers such as rifampin).
No products indexed under this heading.

Propoxyphene Hydrochloride (Ramelteon should be administered with caution in subjects taking strong CYP2C9 inhibitors such as fluconazole).
No products indexed under this heading.

Propoxyphene Napsylate (Ramelteon should be administered with caution in subjects taking strong CYP2C9 inhibitors such as fluconazole).
No products indexed under this heading.

Quinidine (Ramelteon should be administered with caution in subjects taking strong CYP2C9 inhibitors such as fluconazole).
No products indexed under this heading.

Quinidine Hydrochloride (Ramelteon should be administered with caution in subjects taking strong CYP2C9 inhibitors such as fluconazole).
No products indexed under this heading.

Quinidine Polygalacturonate (Ramelteon should be administered with caution in subjects taking strong CYP2C9 inhibitors such as fluconazole).
No products indexed under this heading.

Quinidine Sulfate (Ramelteon should be administered with caution in subjects taking strong CYP2C9 inhibitors such as fluconazole).
No products indexed under this heading.

Quinine (Ramelteon should be administered with caution in subjects taking strong CYP2C9 inhibitors such as fluconazole).
No products indexed under this heading.

Quinine Sulfate (Ramelteon should be administered with caution in subjects taking strong CYP2C9 inhibitors such as fluconazole).
No products indexed under this heading.

Quinupristin (Ramelteon should be administered with caution in subjects taking strong CYP2C9 inhibitors such as fluconazole).
No products indexed under this heading.

Ranitidine Bismuth Citrate (Ramelteon should be administered with caution in subjects taking strong CYP2C9 inhibitors such as fluconazole).
No products indexed under this heading.

Ranitidine Hydrochloride (Ramelteon should be administered with caution in subjects taking strong CYP2C9 inhibitors such as fluconazole). Products include:
Zantac 75 Tablets .... ▣603
Zantac 1670
Zantac Injection 1666
Zantac Injection Pharmacy Bulk Package 1668
Maximum Strength Zantac 150 Tablets .... ▣603
Maximum Strength Zantac 150 Cool Mint Tablets .... ▣603

Rifabutin (Efficacy may be reduced when ramelteon is used in combination with strong CYP enzyme inducers such as rifampin).
No products indexed under this heading.

Rifampicin (Efficacy may be reduced when ramelteon is used in combination with strong CYP enzyme inducers such as rifampin).
No products indexed under this heading.

Rifampin (Administration of rifampin 600 mg once daily for 11 days resulted in a mean decrease of approximately 80% (40% to 90%) in total exposure to ramelteon and metabolite M-II, (both AUC 0-inf and Cmax) after a single 32 mg dose of ramelteon. Efficacy may be reduced when ramelteon is used in combination with strong CYP enzyme inducers such as rifampin).
No products indexed under this heading.

Rifapentine (Efficacy may be reduced when ramelteon is used in combination with strong CYP enzyme inducers such as rifampin).
No products indexed under this heading.

Ritonavir (Ramelteon should be administered with caution in subjects taking strong CYP2C9 inhibitors such as fluconazole). Products include:
Kaletra 452
Norvir 489

Saquinavir (Ramelteon should be administered with caution in subjects taking strong CYP2C9 inhibitors such as fluconazole).
No products indexed under this heading.

Saquinavir Mesylate (Ramelteon should be administered with caution in subjects taking strong CYP2C9 inhibitors such as fluconazole).
No products indexed under this heading.

Secobarbital Sodium (Efficacy may be reduced when ramelteon is used in combination with strong CYP enzyme inducers such as rifampin).
No products indexed under this heading.

Sertraline Hydrochloride (Ramelteon should be administered with caution in subjects taking strong CYP2C9 inhibitors such as fluconazole).
No products indexed under this heading.

Sildenafil Citrate (Ramelteon should be administered with caution in subjects taking strong CYP2C9 inhibitors such as fluconazole).
No products indexed under this heading.

Sparfloxacin (Ramelteon should be administered with caution in subjects taking strong CYP2C9 inhibitors such as fluconazole).
No products indexed under this heading.

Sulfacytine (Ramelteon should be administered with caution in subjects taking strong CYP2C9 inhibitors such as fluconazole).
No products indexed under this heading.

Sulfamethizole (Ramelteon should be administered with caution in subjects taking strong CYP2C9 inhibitors such as fluconazole).
No products indexed under this heading.

Sulfamethoxazole (Ramelteon should be administered with caution in subjects taking strong CYP2C9 inhibitors such as fluconazole).
No products indexed under this heading.

Sulfasalazine (Ramelteon should be administered with caution in subjects taking strong CYP2C9 inhibitors such as fluconazole).
No products indexed under this heading.

Sulfinpyrazone (Ramelteon should be administered with caution in subjects taking strong CYP2C9 inhibitors such as fluconazole).
No products indexed under this heading.

Sulfisoxazole Acetyl (Ramelteon should be administered with caution in subjects taking strong CYP2C9 inhibitors such as fluconazole).
No products indexed under this heading.

Sulfisoxazole Diolamine (Ramelteon should be administered with caution in subjects taking strong CYP2C9 inhibitors such as fluconazole).
No products indexed under this heading.

Tacrine Hydrochloride (Ramelteon should be administered with caution in subjects taking strong CYP2C9 inhibitors such as fluconazole).
No products indexed under this heading.

Telithromycin (Ramelteon should be administered with caution in subjects taking strong CYP2C9 inhibitors such as fluconazole). Products include:
Ketek Tablets 2744

Terconazole (Ramelteon should be administered with caution in subjects taking strong CYP2C9 inhibitors such as fluconazole).
No products indexed under this heading.

Theophylline (Efficacy may be reduced when ramelteon is used in combination with strong CYP enzyme inducers such as rifampin).
No products indexed under this heading.

Theophylline Anhydrous (Efficacy may be reduced when ramelteon is used in combination with strong CYP enzyme inducers such as rifampin). Products include:
Uniphyl Tablets 2595

Theophylline Calcium Salicylate (Efficacy may be reduced when ramelteon is used in combination with strong CYP enzyme inducers such as rifampin).
No products indexed under this heading.

Theophylline Dihydroxypropyl (Glyceryl) (Efficacy may be reduced when ramelteon is used in combination with strong CYP enzyme inducers such as rifampin).
No products indexed under this heading.

Theophylline Ethylenediamine (Efficacy may be reduced when ramelteon is used in combination with strong CYP enzyme inducers such as rifampin).
No products indexed under this heading.

Ticlopidine Hydrochloride (Ramelteon should be administered with caution in subjects taking strong CYP2C9 inhibitors such as fluconazole).
No products indexed under this heading.

Tobacco (Efficacy may be reduced when ramelteon is used in combination with strong CYP enzyme inducers such as rifampin).
No products indexed under this heading.

Tolazamide (Ramelteon should be administered with caution in subjects taking strong CYP2C9 inhibitors such as fluconazole).
No products indexed under this heading.

Tolbutamide (Ramelteon should be administered with caution in subjects taking strong CYP2C9 inhibitors such as fluconazole).
No products indexed under this heading.

Tolbutamide Sodium (Ramelteon should be administered with caution in subjects taking strong CYP2C9 inhibitors such as fluconazole).
No products indexed under this heading.

Triamcinolone (Efficacy may be reduced when ramelteon is used in combination with strong CYP enzyme inducers such as rifampin).
No products indexed under this heading.

Triamcinolone Acetonide (Efficacy may be reduced when ramelteon is used in combination with strong CYP enzyme inducers such as rifampin). Products include:
Azmacort Inhalation Aerosol 407
Nasacort AQ Nasal Spray 2765
Triesence Injectable Suspension .... ⊙209

Triamcinolone Diacetate (Efficacy may be reduced when ramelteon is used in combination with strong CYP enzyme inducers such as rifampin).
No products indexed under this heading.

Triamcinolone Hexacetonide (Efficacy may be reduced when ramelteon is used in combination with strong CYP enzyme inducers such as rifampin).
No products indexed under this heading.

Troglitazone (Ramelteon should be administered with caution in subjects taking strong CYP2C9 inhibitors such as fluconazole).
No products indexed under this heading.

Troleandomycin (Ramelteon should be administered with caution in subjects taking strong CYP2C9 inhibitors such as fluconazole).
No products indexed under this heading.

Trovafloxacin Mesylate (Ramelteon should be administered with caution in subjects taking strong CYP2C9 inhibitors such as fluconazole).
No products indexed under this heading.

Valproate Sodium (Ramelteon should be administered with caution in subjects taking strong CYP2C9 inhibitors such as fluconazole).
No products indexed under this heading.

Vardenafil Hydrochloride (Ramelteon should be administered with caution in subjects taking strong CYP2C9 inhibitors such as fluconazole). Products include:
Levitra Tablets 2876

Verapamil Hydrochloride (Ramelteon should be administered with caution in subjects taking strong CYP2C9 inhibitors such as fluconazole). Products include:
Tarka Tablets 511

Voriconazole (Ramelteon should be administered with caution in subjects taking strong CYP2C9 inhibitors such as fluconazole).
No products indexed under this heading.

Zafirlukast (Ramelteon should be administered with caution in subjects taking strong CYP2C9 inhibitors such as fluconazole). Products include:
Accolate Tablets 669

Zileuton (Ramelteon should be administered with caution in subjects taking strong CYP2C9 inhibitors such as fluconazole).
No products indexed under this heading.

Food Interactions

Alcohol (With single-dose, daytime co-administration of ramelteon 32 mg and alcohol (0.6 g/kg), there were no clinically meaningful or statistically significant effects on peak or total exposure to ramelteon. However, an additive effect was seen on some measures of psychomotor performance (ie. the Digit Symbol Substitution Test, the Psychomotor Vigilance Task Test, and a Visual Analog Scale of sedation) at some post-dose time points. No additive effect was seen on the Delayed Word Recognition Test. Because alcohol by itself impairs performance, and the intended effect of ramelteon is to promote sleep, patients should be cautioned not to consume alcohol when using ramelteon).

Broccoli (Efficacy may be reduced when ramelteon is used in combination with strong CYP enzyme inducers such as rifampin).

Brussel Sprouts (Efficacy may be reduced when ramelteon is used in combination with strong CYP enzyme inducers such as rifampin).

Charbroiled Food (Efficacy may be reduced when ramelteon is used in combination with strong CYP enzyme inducers such as rifampin).

Grapefruit (Ramelteon should be administered with caution in subjects taking strong CYP2C9 inhibitors such as fluconazole).

Grapefruit Juice (Ramelteon should be administered with caution in subjects taking strong CYP2C9 inhibitors such as fluconazole).

RYTHMOL TABLETS

(Propafenone Hydrochloride) 1586
May interact with beta blockers, cytochrome p450 1a2 inhibitors (selected), cytochrome p450 2d6 inhibitors (selected), cytochrome p450 2d6 substrates (selected), cytochrome p450 3a4 inhibitors (selected), erythromycin, quinidine, and certain other agents. Compounds in these categories include:

Acebutolol Hydrochloride (Concomitant use of propafenone and propranolol in healthy subjects increased propranolol plasma concentrations at steady state by 113%. In 4 patients, administration of metoprolol with propafenone increased the metoprolol plasma concentrations at steady state by 100% to 400%. The pharmacokinetics of propafenone was not affected by the co-administration of either propranolol or metoprolol. In clinical trials using propafenone immediate release tablets, patients who were receiving beta-blockers concurrently did not experience an increased incidence of side effects).
No products indexed under this heading.

Acetazolamide (Propafenone is metabolized by CYP3A4. Drugs that inhibit CYP3A4 can be expected to cause increased plasma levels of propafenone. Appropriate monitoring is recommended when propafenone is used together with such drugs).
No products indexed under this heading.

Alatrofloxacin Mesylate (Propafenone is metabolized by CYP1A2. Drugs that inhibit CYP1A2 can be expected to cause increased plasma levels of propafenone. Appropriate monitoring is recommended when propafenone is used together with such drugs).
No products indexed under this heading.

Amiodarone Hydrochloride (Concomitant administration of propafenone and amiodarone can affect conduction and repolarization and is not recommended).
No products indexed under this heading.

Amitriptyline Hydrochloride (Propafenone is metabolized by CYP2D6 (major pathway). Drugs that inhibit CYP2D6 can be expected to cause increased plasma levels of propafenone. Appropriate monitoring is recommended when propafenone is used together with such drugs).
No products indexed under this heading.

Amoxapine (Propafenone is metabolized by CYP2D6 (major pathway). Drugs that inhibit CYP2D6 can be expected to cause increased plasma levels of propafenone. Appropriate monitoring is recommended when propafenone is used together with such drugs).
No products indexed under this heading.

Amphetamine Aspartate (Propafenone is an inhibitor of CYP2D6. Co-administration of propafenone with drugs metabolized by CYP2D6 might lead to increased plasma concentrations of these drugs). Products include:
Adderall XR Capsules 3012

Amphetamine Aspartate Monohydrate (Propafenone is an inhibitor of CYP2D6. Co-administration of propafenone with drugs metabolized by CYP2D6 might lead to increased plasma concentrations of these drugs).
No products indexed under this heading.

Amphetamine Sulfate (Propafenone is an inhibitor of CYP2D6. Co-administration of propafenone with drugs metabolized by CYP2D6 might lead to increased plasma concentrations of these drugs). Products include:
Adderall XR Capsules 3012

Amprenavir (Propafenone is metabolized by CYP3A4. Drugs that inhibit CYP3A4 can be expected to cause increased plasma levels of propafenone. Appropriate monitoring is recommended when propafenone is used together with such drugs).
No products indexed under this heading.

Anastrozole (Propafenone is metabolized by CYP1A2. Drugs that inhibit CYP1A2 can be expected to cause increased plasma levels of propafenone. Appropriate monitoring is recommended when propafenone is used together with such drugs). Products include:
Arimidex Tablets 672

Aprepitant (Propafenone is metabolized by CYP3A4. Drugs that inhibit CYP3A4 can be expected to cause increased plasma levels of propafenone. Appropriate monitoring is recommended when propafenone is used together with such drugs). Products include:
Emend Capsules 1992

Atazanavir (Propafenone is metabolized by CYP3A4. Drugs that inhibit CYP3A4 can be expected to cause increased plasma levels of propafenone. Appropriate monitoring is recommended when propafenone is used together with such drugs). .
No products indexed under this heading.

Atazanavir Sulfate (Propafenone is metabolized by CYP3A4. Drugs that inhibit CYP3A4 can be expected to cause increased plasma levels of propafenone. Appropriate monitoring is recommended when propafenone is used together with such drugs). Products include:
Reyataz Capsules 3299

Atenolol (Concomitant use of propafenone and propranolol in healthy subjects increased propranolol plasma concentrations at steady state by 113%. In 4 patients, administration of metoprolol with propafenone increased the metoprolol plasma concentrations at steady state by 100% to 400%. The pharmacokinetics of propafenone was not affected by the co-administration of either propranolol or metoprolol. In clinical trials using propafenone immediate release tablets, patients who were receiving beta-blockers concurrently did not experience an increased incidence of side effects).
No products indexed under this heading.

Atomoxetine Hydrochloride (Propafenone is an inhibitor of CYP2D6. Co-administration of propafenone with drugs metabolized by CYP2D6 might lead to increased plasma concentrations of these drugs). Products include:
Strattera Capsules 1864

Betaxolol Hydrochloride (Concomitant use of propafenone and propranolol in healthy subjects increased propranolol plasma concentrations at steady state by 113%. In 4 patients, administration of metoprolol with propafenone increased the metoprolol plasma concentrations at steady state by 100% to 400%. The pharmacokinetics of propafenone was not affected by the co-administration of either propranolol or metoprolol. In clinical trials using propafenone immediate release tablets, patients who were receiving beta-blockers concurrently did not experience an increased incidence of side effects).
No products indexed under this heading.

Bisoprolol Fumarate (Concomitant use of propafenone and propranolol in healthy subjects increased propranolol plasma concentrations at steady state by 113%. In 4 patients, administration of metoprolol with propafenone increased the metoprolol plasma concentrations at steady state by 100% to 400%. The

pharmacokinetics of propafenone was not affected by the co-administration of either propranolol or metoprolol. In clinical trials using propafenone immediate release tablets, patients who were receiving beta-blockers concurrently did not experience an increased incidence of side effects).
No products indexed under this heading.

Bupropion Hydrochloride (Propafenone is metabolized by CYP2D6 (major pathway). Drugs that inhibit CYP2D6 can be expected to cause increased plasma levels of propafenone. Appropriate monitoring is recommended when propafenone is used together with such drugs).
Products include:
Wellbutrin Tablets **1648**
Wellbutrin SR Sustained-Release Tablets **1653**
Wellbutrin XL Extended-Release Tablets **1659**
Zyban Sustained-Release Tablets **1692**

Captopril (Propafenone is an inhibitor of CYP2D6. Co-administration of propafenone with drugs metabolized by CYP2D6 might lead to increased plasma concentrations of these drugs). Products include:
Captopril Tablets **2182**

Carteolol Hydrochloride (Concomitant use of propafenone and propranolol in healthy subjects increased propranolol plasma concentrations at steady state by 113%. In 4 patients, administration of metoprolol with propafenone increased the metoprolol plasma concentrations at steady state by 100% to 400%. The pharmacokinetics of propafenone was not affected by the co-administration of either propranolol or metoprolol. In clinical trials using propafenone immediate release tablets, patients who were receiving beta-blockers concurrently did not experience an increased incidence of side effects).
No products indexed under this heading.

Carvedilol (Propafenone is an inhibitor of CYP2D6. Co-administration of propafenone with drugs metabolized by CYP2D6 might lead to increased plasma concentrations of these drugs). Products include:
Coreg Tablets **1387**

Celecoxib (Propafenone is metabolized by CYP2D6 (major pathway). Drugs that inhibit CYP2D6 can be expected to cause increased plasma levels of propafenone. Appropriate monitoring is recommended when propafenone is used together with such drugs). Products include:
Celebrex Capsules **2979**

Cevimeline Hydrochloride (Propafenone is an inhibitor of CYP2D6. Co-administration of propafenone with drugs metabolized by CYP2D6 might lead to increased plasma concentrations of these drugs).
Products include:
Evoxac Capsules **1013**

Chloroquine Hydrochloride (Propafenone is metabolized by CYP2D6 (major pathway). Drugs that inhibit CYP2D6 can be expected to cause increased plasma levels of propafenone. Appropriate monitoring is recommended when propafenone is used together with such drugs).
No products indexed under this heading.

Chloroquine Phosphate (Propafenone is metabolized by CYP2D6 (major pathway). Drugs that inhibit CYP2D6 can be expected to cause increased plasma levels of propafenone. Appropriate monitoring is recommended when propafenone is used together with such drugs).
No products indexed under this heading.

Chlorpheniramine (Propafenone is metabolized by CYP2D6 (major pathway). Drugs that inhibit CYP2D6 can be expected to cause increased plasma levels of propafenone. Appropriate monitoring is recommended when propafenone is used together with such drugs).
No products indexed under this heading.

Chlorpheniramine Maleate (Propafenone is metabolized by CYP2D6 (major pathway). Drugs that inhibit CYP2D6 can be expected to cause increased plasma levels of propafenone. Appropriate monitoring is recommended when propafenone is used together with such drugs).
Products include:
Actifed Cold & Allergy Tablets **1895**
Sudafed PE Sinus & Allergy Tablets **1908**
Tylenol Allergy Multi-Symptom Caplets with Cool Burst and Rapid Release Gelcaps **1916**
Children's Tylenol Plus Cold Suspension Liquid **1912**
Children's Tylenol Plus Cough & Runny Nose Suspension Liquid **1912**
Children's Tylenol Plus Flu Suspension Liquid **1914**
Children's Tylenol Plus Multi-Symptom Cold Suspension Liquid **1912**
Tylenol Cold Head Congestion Nighttime Caplets with Cool Burst **1910**
Tylenol Cold Multi-Symptom Nighttime Caplets with Cool Burst **1913**
Tylenol Sinus Congestion & Pain Nighttime Caplets with Cool Burst **1917**

Chlorpheniramine Polistirex (Propafenone is metabolized by CYP2D6 (major pathway). Drugs that inhibit CYP2D6 can be expected to cause increased plasma levels of propafenone. Appropriate monitoring is recommended when propafenone is used together with such drugs).
Products include:
Tussionex Pennkinetic Extended-Release Suspension **3154**

Chlorpheniramine Tannate (Propafenone is metabolized by CYP2D6 (major pathway). Drugs that inhibit CYP2D6 can be expected to cause increased plasma levels of propafenone. Appropriate monitoring is recommended when propafenone is used together with such drugs).
No products indexed under this heading.

Chlorpromazine (Propafenone is an inhibitor of CYP2D6. Co-administration of propafenone with drugs metabolized by CYP2D6 might lead to increased plasma concentrations of these drugs).
No products indexed under this heading.

Chlorpromazine Hydrochloride (Propafenone is an inhibitor of CYP2D6. Co-administration of propafenone with drugs metabolized by CYP2D6 might lead to increased plasma concentrations of these drugs).
No products indexed under this heading.

Chlorpropamide (Propafenone is an inhibitor of CYP2D6. Co-administration of propafenone with drugs metabolized by CYP2D6 might lead to increased plasma concentrations of these drugs).
No products indexed under this heading.

Cimetidine (Concomitant administration of propafenone immediate release tablets and cimetidine in 12 healthy subjects resulted in a 20% increase in steady-state plasma concentrations of propafenone).
No products indexed under this heading.

Cimetidine Hydrochloride (Concomitant administration of propafenone immediate release tablets and cimetidine in 12 healthy subjects resulted in a 20% increase in steady-state plasma concentrations of propafenone).
No products indexed under this heading.

Ciprofloxacin (Propafenone is metabolized by CYP1A2. Drugs that inhibit CYP1A2 can be expected to cause increased plasma levels of propafenone. Appropriate monitoring is recommended when propafenone is used together with such drugs).
Products include:
Cipro I.V. **2817**
Cipro Oral Suspension **2810**
Cipro XR Tablets **2823**
Ciprodex Otic Suspension **541**

Ciprofloxacin Hydrochloride (Propafenone is metabolized by CYP1A2. Drugs that inhibit CYP1A2 can be expected to cause increased plasma levels of propafenone. Appropriate monitoring is recommended when propafenone is used together with such drugs). Products include:
Cipro Tablets **2810**

Citalopram Hydrobromide (Propafenone is metabolized by CYP2D6 (major pathway). Drugs that inhibit CYP2D6 can be expected to cause increased plasma levels of propafenone. Appropriate monitoring is recommended when propafenone is used together with such drugs).
Products include:
Celexa **1160**

Clarithromycin (Propafenone is metabolized by CYP1A2. Drugs that inhibit CYP1A2 can be expected to cause increased plasma levels of propafenone. Appropriate monitoring is recommended when propafenone is used together with such drugs).
Products include:
Biaxin/Biaxin XL **411**

Clomipramine Hydrochloride (Propafenone is metabolized by CYP2D6 (major pathway). Drugs that inhibit CYP2D6 can be expected to cause increased plasma levels of propafenone. Appropriate monitoring is recommended when propafenone is used together with such drugs).
No products indexed under this heading.

Clotrimazole (Propafenone is metabolized by CYP3A4. Drugs that inhibit CYP3A4 can be expected to cause increased plasma levels of propafenone. Appropriate monitoring is recommended when propafenone is used together with such drugs).
Products include:
Lotrisone **2881**

Clozapine (Propafenone is an inhibitor of CYP2D6. Co-administration of propafenone with drugs metabolized by CYP2D6 might lead to increased plasma concentrations of these drugs).
No products indexed under this heading.

Cocaine Hydrochloride (Propafenone is metabolized by CYP2D6 (major pathway). Drugs that inhibit CYP2D6 can be expected to cause increased plasma levels of propafenone. Appropriate monitoring is recommended when propafenone is used together with such drugs).
No products indexed under this heading.

Codeine Phosphate (Propafenone is an inhibitor of CYP2D6. Co-administration of propafenone with drugs metabolized by CYP2D6 might lead to increased plasma concentrations of these drugs). Products include:
Tylenol with Codeine Tablets **2427**

Codeine Sulfate (Propafenone is an inhibitor of CYP2D6. Co-administration of propafenone with drugs metabolized by CYP2D6 might lead to increased plasma concentrations of these drugs).
No products indexed under this heading.

Cyclobenzaprine Hydrochloride (Propafenone is an inhibitor of CYP2D6. Co-administration of propafenone with drugs metabolized by CYP2D6 might lead to increased plasma concentrations of these drugs). Products include:
Amrix Capsules **966**

Cyclosporine (Propafenone is metabolized by CYP3A4. Drugs that inhibit CYP3A4 can be expected to cause increased plasma levels of propafenone. Appropriate monitoring is recommended when propafenone is used together with such drugs).
Products include:
Gengraf Capsules **435**
Neoral Oral Solution **2280**
Neoral Soft Gelatin Capsules **2280**
Restasis Ophthalmic Emulsion **557**
Sandimmune **2296**

Dalfopristin (Propafenone is metabolized by CYP3A4. Drugs that inhibit CYP3A4 can be expected to cause increased plasma levels of propafenone. Appropriate monitoring is recommended when propafenone is used together with such drugs).
No products indexed under this heading.

Danazol (Propafenone is metabolized by CYP3A4. Drugs that inhibit CYP3A4 can be expected to cause increased plasma levels of propafenone. Appropriate monitoring is recommended when propafenone is used together with such drugs).
No products indexed under this heading.

Delavirdine Mesylate (Propafenone is metabolized by CYP3A4. Drugs that inhibit CYP3A4 can be expected to cause increased plasma levels of propafenone. Appropriate monitoring is recommended when propafenone is used together with such drugs).
No products indexed under this heading.

Desipramine Hydrochloride (Co-administration of drugs which are metabolized and inhibited by CYP2D6 such as desipramine, may lead to increased levels of propafenone and desipramine. Appropriate monitoring is recommended when propafenone is used together with desipramine).
No products indexed under this heading.

Desogestrel (Propafenone is metabolized by CYP1A2. Drugs that inhibit CYP1A2 can be expected to cause increased plasma levels of propafenone. Appropriate monitoring is recommended when propafenone is used together with such drugs). Products include:
Mircette Tablets 1034

Dexfenfluramine Hydrochloride (Propafenone is an inhibitor of CYP2D6. Co-administration of propafenone with drugs metabolized by CYP2D6 might lead to increased plasma concentrations of these drugs).
No products indexed under this heading.

Dextromethorphan Hydrobromide (Propafenone is an inhibitor of CYP2D6. Co-administration of propafenone with drugs metabolized by CYP2D6 might lead to increased plasma concentrations of these drugs). Products include:
PediaCare Children's Liquid Multi-Symptom Cold 1902
PediaCare Children's Long-Acting Cough 1902
Children's Sudafed PE Cold & Cough Liquid 1907
Sudafed PE Cold & Cough Caplets 1907
Children's Tylenol Plus Cough & Runny Nose Suspension Liquid 1912
Children's Tylenol Plus Cough & Sore Throat Suspension Liquid 1912
Children's Tylenol Plus Flu Suspension Liquid 1914
Children's Tylenol Plus Multi-Symptom Cold Suspension Liquid 1912
Tylenol Cold Severe Congestion Daytime Caplets with Cool Burst 1912
Tylenol Cold Head Congestion Daytime Caplets with Cool Burst 1910
Tylenol Cold Head Congestion Nighttime Caplets with Cool Burst 1910
Tylenol Cold Head Congestion Severe Daytime Caplets with Cool Burst 1910
Tylenol Cold Multi-Symptom Daytime Caplets with Cool Burst and Rapid Release Gels 1913
Tylenol Cold Multi-Symptom Daytime Liquid with Citrus Burst 1913
Tylenol Cold Multi-Symptom Nighttime Caplets with Cool Burst 1913
Tylenol Cold Multi-Symptom Nighttime Liquid with Cool Burst 1913
Tylenol Cold Multi-Symptom Severe Caplets with Cool Burst 1913
Tylenol Cold Multi-Symptom Severe Daytime Liquid with Citrus Burst 1913
Tylenol Cough & Sore Throat Daytime Liquid with Cool Burst 1918
Tylenol Cough & Sore Throat Nighttime Liquid with Cool Burst 1918
Vicks DayQuil Cold & Flu Multi-Symptom Relief 616
Vicks DayQuil LiquiCaps 2567
Vicks DayQuil Liquid 2567
Vicks DayQuil Multi-Symptom Cold/Flu Relief 2567
Vicks NyQuil Cold & Flu Multi-Symptom Relief 617
Vicks NyQuil LiquiCaps 2567
Vicks NyQuil Liquid 2567
Vicks NyQuil Multi-Symptom Cold/Flu Relief 2567

Dextromethorphan Polistirex (Propafenone is an inhibitor of CYP2D6. Co-administration of propafenone with drugs metabolized by CYP2D6 might lead to increased plasma concentrations of these drugs).
No products indexed under this heading.

Digoxin (Concomitant use of propafenone and digoxin increased steady-state serum digoxin exposure (AUC) in patients by 60% to 270%, and decreased the clearance of digoxin by 31% to 67%. Plasma digoxin levels of patients receiving propafenone should be monitored and digoxin dosage adjusted as needed). Products include:
Lanoxin Injection 1498
Lanoxin Injection Pediatric 1502
Lanoxin Tablets 1505

Diltiazem Hydrochloride (Propafenone is metabolized by CYP3A4. Drugs that inhibit CYP3A4 can be expected to cause increased plasma levels of propafenone. Appropriate monitoring is recommended when propafenone is used together with such drugs). Products include:
Cardizem LA Extended Release Tablets 421

Diltiazem Maleate (Propafenone is metabolized by CYP3A4. Drugs that inhibit CYP3A4 can be expected to cause increased plasma levels of propafenone. Appropriate monitoring is recommended when propafenone is used together with such drugs).
No products indexed under this heading.

Diphenhydramine (Propafenone is metabolized by CYP2D6 (major pathway). Drugs that inhibit CYP2D6 can be expected to cause increased plasma levels of propafenone. Appropriate monitoring is recommended when propafenone is used together with such drugs).
No products indexed under this heading.

Diphenhydramine Hydrochloride (Propafenone is metabolized by CYP2D6 (major pathway). Drugs that inhibit CYP2D6 can be expected to cause increased plasma levels of propafenone. Appropriate monitoring is recommended when propafenone is used together with such drugs). Products include:
Benadryl Allergy & Cold Kapgels 1895
Benadryl Allergy & Sinus Headache Kapgels 1895
Benadryl Severe Allergy & Sinus Headache Caplets 1897
Benadryl Dye-Free Allergy Liqui-gels Softgels 1897
Benadryl Allergy Kapgels 1895
Benadryl Allergy Quick Dissolve Strips 1896
Benadryl Allergy Ultratab Tablets 1896
Children's Benadryl Dye-Free Allergy Liquid 1897
Children's Benadryl Allergy Fastmelts 1897
Children's Benadryl Allergy Liquid 1898
Children's Benadryl Allergy Perfect Measure 1896
Children's Benadryl-D Allergy & Sinus Liquid 1896
Benadryl-D Allergy & Sinus Tablet 1896
PediaCare Children's Allergy & Cold Liquid 1902
PediaCare Children's Allergy Liquid 1902
Simply Sleep Caplets 1905
Sudafed PE Nighttime Cold Caplets 1907
Sudafed PE Severe Cold Caplets 1908
Extra Strength Tylenol PM Caplets, Geltabs, Liquid, and Rapid Release Gels 1915
Tylenol Allergy Multi-Symptom Nighttime Caplets with Cool Burst 1916
Tylenol Severe Allergy Caplets 1916
Children's Tylenol Plus Cold & Allergy Suspension Liquid 1914
Tylenol Sore Throat Nighttime Liquid with Cool Burst 1918

Dolasetron Mesylate (Propafenone is an inhibitor of CYP2D6. Co-administration of propafenone with drugs metabolized by CYP2D6 might lead to increased plasma concentrations of these drugs). Products include:
Anzemet Injection 2701
Anzemet Tablets 2704

Donepezil Hydrochloride (Propafenone is an inhibitor of CYP2D6. Co-administration of propafenone with drugs metabolized by CYP2D6 might lead to increased plasma concentrations of these drugs). Products include:
Aricept Tablets 1062
Aricept ODT Tablets 1062

Doxepin Hydrochloride (Propafenone is metabolized by CYP2D6 (major pathway). Drugs that inhibit CYP2D6 can be expected to cause increased plasma levels of propafenone. Appropriate monitoring is recommended when propafenone is used together with such drugs).
No products indexed under this heading.

Efavirenz (Propafenone is metabolized by CYP3A4. Drugs that inhibit CYP3A4 can be expected to cause increased plasma levels of propafenone. Appropriate monitoring is recommended when propafenone is used together with such drugs). Products include:
Atripla Tablets 938
Sustiva Capsules 930
Sustiva Tablets 930

Encainide Hydrochloride (Propafenone is an inhibitor of CYP2D6. Co-administration of propafenone with drugs metabolized by CYP2D6 might lead to increased plasma concentrations of these drugs).
No products indexed under this heading.

Enoxacin (Propafenone is metabolized by CYP1A2. Drugs that inhibit CYP1A2 can be expected to cause increased plasma levels of propafenone. Appropriate monitoring is recommended when propafenone is used together with such drugs).
No products indexed under this heading.

Erythromycin (Propafenone is metabolized by CYP3A4. Drugs that inhibit CYP3A4 (such as erythromycin), can be expected to cause increased plasma levels of propafenone. Appropriate monitoring is recommended when propafenone is used together with such drugs).
No products indexed under this heading.

Erythromycin Estolate (Propafenone is metabolized by CYP3A4. Drugs that inhibit CYP3A4 (such as erythromycin), can be expected to cause increased plasma levels of propafenone. Appropriate monitoring is recommended when propafenone is used together with such drugs).
No products indexed under this heading.

Erythromycin Ethylsuccinate (Propafenone is metabolized by CYP3A4. Drugs that inhibit CYP3A4 (such as erythromycin), can be expected to cause increased plasma levels of propafenone. Appropriate monitoring is recommended when propafenone is used together with such drugs). Products include:
E.E.S. 433
EryPed 431

Erythromycin Gluceptate (Propafenone is metabolized by CYP3A4. Drugs that inhibit CYP3A4 (such as erythromycin), can be expected to cause increased plasma levels of propafenone. Appropriate monitoring is recommended when propafenone is used together with such drugs).
No products indexed under this heading.

Erythromycin Lactobionate (Propafenone is metabolized by CYP3A4. Drugs that inhibit CYP3A4 (such as erythromycin), can be expected to cause increased plasma levels of propafenone. Appropriate monitoring is recommended when propafenone is used together with such drugs).
No products indexed under this heading.

Erythromycin Stearate (Propafenone is metabolized by CYP3A4. Drugs that inhibit CYP3A4 (such as erythromycin), can be expected to cause increased plasma levels of propafenone. Appropriate monitoring is recommended when propafenone is used together with such drugs).
No products indexed under this heading.

Escitalopram Oxalate (Propafenone is metabolized by CYP2D6 (major pathway). Drugs that inhibit CYP2D6 can be expected to cause increased plasma levels of propafenone. Appropriate monitoring is recommended when propafenone is used together with such drugs). Products include:
Lexapro Oral Suspension 1174
Lexapro Tablets 1174

Esmolol Hydrochloride (Concomitant use of propafenone and propranolol in healthy subjects increased propranolol plasma concentrations at steady state by 113%. In 4 patients, administration of metoprolol with propafenone increased the metoprolol plasma concentrations at steady state by 100% to 400%. The pharmacokinetics of propafenone was not affected by the co-administration of either propranolol or metoprolol. In clinical trials using propafenone immediate release tablets, patients who were receiving beta-blockers concurrently did not experience an increased incidence of side effects).
No products indexed under this heading.

Esomeprazole Magnesium (Propafenone is metabolized by CYP3A4. Drugs that inhibit CYP3A4 can be expected to cause increased plasma levels of propafenone. Appropriate monitoring is recommended when propafenone is used together with such drugs). Products include:
Nexium Delayed-Release Capsules 645
Nexium Delayed-Release Oral Suspension 645

Ethinyl Estradiol (Propafenone is metabolized by CYP1A2. Drugs that inhibit CYP1A2 can be expected to cause increased plasma levels of

propafenone. Appropriate monitoring is recommended when propafenone is used together with such drugs). Products include:

Lybrel Tablets **3204**
Mircette Tablets **1034**
NuvaRing **2897**
Ortho-Cyclen/Ortho Tri-Cyclen **2449**
Ortho Evra Transdermal System **2437**
Ortho Tri-Cyclen Lo Tablets **2458**
Seasonique Tablets **1046**
Yaz Tablets **805**

Fentanyl (Propafenone is an inhibitor of CYP2D6. Co-administration of propafenone with drugs metabolized by CYP2D6 might lead to increased plasma concentrations of these drugs). Products include:

Duragesic Transdermal System **2405**
Ionsys Transdermal System **2410**

Fentanyl Citrate (Propafenone is an inhibitor of CYP2D6. Co-administration of propafenone with drugs metabolized by CYP2D6 might lead to increased plasma concentrations of these drugs). Products include:

Actiq **959**
Fentora Tablets **968**

Flecainide Acetate (Propafenone is an inhibitor of CYP2D6. Co-administration of propafenone with drugs metabolized by CYP2D6 might lead to increased plasma concentrations of these drugs).

No products indexed under this heading.

Fluconazole (Propafenone is metabolized by CYP3A4. Drugs that inhibit CYP3A4 can be expected to cause increased plasma levels of propafenone. Appropriate monitoring is recommended when propafenone is used together with such drugs).

No products indexed under this heading.

Fluoxetine (Concomitant administration of propafenone and fluoxetine in extensive metabolizers increased the S propafenone Cmax and AUC by 39% and 50%, respectively, and the R propafenone Cmax and AUC by 71% and 50%, respectively).

No products indexed under this heading.

Fluoxetine Hydrochloride (Concomitant administration of propafenone and fluoxetine in extensive metabolizers increased the S propafenone Cmax and AUC by 39% and 50%, respectively, and the R propafenone Cmax and AUC by 71% and 50%, respectively). Products include:

Prozac Weekly Capsules **1852**
Prozac Pulvules and Liquid **1852**
Symbyax Capsules **1871**

Fluphenazine Decanoate (Propafenone is metabolized by CYP2D6 (major pathway). Drugs that inhibit CYP2D6 can be expected to cause increased plasma levels of propafenone. Appropriate monitoring is recommended when propafenone is used together with such drugs).

No products indexed under this heading.

Fluphenazine Enanthate (Propafenone is metabolized by CYP2D6 (major pathway). Drugs that inhibit CYP2D6 can be expected to cause increased plasma levels of propafenone. Appropriate monitoring is recommended when propafenone is used together with such drugs).

No products indexed under this heading.

Fluphenazine Hydrochloride (Propafenone is metabolized by CYP2D6 (major pathway). Drugs that inhibit CYP2D6 can be expected to cause increased plasma levels of propafenone. Appropriate monitoring is recommended when propafenone is used together with such drugs).

No products indexed under this heading.

Fluvoxamine (Propafenone is metabolized by CYP1A2. Drugs that inhibit CYP1A2 can be expected to cause increased plasma levels of propafenone. Appropriate monitoring is recommended when propafenone is used together with such drugs).

No products indexed under this heading.

Fluvoxamine Maleate (Propafenone is metabolized by CYP2D6 (major pathway). Drugs that inhibit CYP2D6 can be expected to cause increased plasma levels of propafenone. Appropriate monitoring is recommended when propafenone is used together with such drugs). Products include:

Luvox CR Extended-Release Capsules **1759**

Formoterol Fumarate (Propafenone is an inhibitor of CYP2D6. Co-administration of propafenone with drugs metabolized by CYP2D6 might lead to increased plasma concentrations of these drugs). Products include:

Foradil Aerolizer **2849**
Perforomist Inhalation Solution **1025**

Fosamprenavir Calcium (Propafenone is metabolized by CYP3A4. Drugs that inhibit CYP3A4 can be expected to cause increased plasma levels of propafenone. Appropriate monitoring is recommended when propafenone is used together with such drugs). Products include:

Lexiva Oral Suspension **1510**
Lexiva Tablets **1510**

Galantamine Hydrobromide (Propafenone is an inhibitor of CYP2D6. Co-administration of propafenone with drugs metabolized by CYP2D6 might lead to increased plasma concentrations of these drugs).

No products indexed under this heading.

Gatifloxacin (Propafenone is metabolized by CYP1A2. Drugs that inhibit CYP1A2 can be expected to cause increased plasma levels of propafenone. Appropriate monitoring is recommended when propafenone is used together with such drugs).

No products indexed under this heading.

Gemifloxacin Mesylate (Propafenone is metabolized by CYP1A2. Drugs that inhibit CYP1A2 can be expected to cause increased plasma levels of propafenone. Appropriate monitoring is recommended when propafenone is used together with such drugs).

No products indexed under this heading.

Grepafloxacin Hydrochloride (Propafenone is metabolized by CYP1A2. Drugs that inhibit CYP1A2 can be expected to cause increased plasma levels of propafenone. Appropriate monitoring is recommended when propafenone is used together with such drugs).

No products indexed under this heading.

Halofantrine Hydrochloride (Propafenone is metabolized by CYP2D6 (major pathway). Drugs that inhibit CYP2D6 can be expected to cause increased plasma levels of propafenone. Appropriate monitoring is recommended when propafenone is used together with such drugs).

No products indexed under this heading.

Haloperidol (Propafenone is an inhibitor of CYP2D6. Co-administration of propafenone with drugs metabolized by CYP2D6 (such as haloperidol) might lead to increased plasma levels of haloperidol).

No products indexed under this heading.

Haloperidol Decanoate (Propafenone is an inhibitor of CYP2D6. Co-administration of propafenone with drugs metabolized by CYP2D6 (such as haloperidol) might lead to increased plasma levels of haloperidol).

No products indexed under this heading.

Haloperidol Lactate (Propafenone is an inhibitor of CYP2D6. Co-administration of propafenone with drugs metabolized by CYP2D6 (such as haloperidol) might lead to increased plasma levels of haloperidol).

No products indexed under this heading.

Hydrocodone Bitartrate (Propafenone is an inhibitor of CYP2D6. Co-administration of propafenone with drugs metabolized by CYP2D6 might lead to increased plasma concentrations of these drugs). Products include:

Lortab 5/500 Tablets **3143**
Lortab 7.5/500 Tablets **3144**
Lortab 10/500 Tablets **3144**
Vicodin Tablets **529**
Vicodin ES Tablets **530**
Vicodin HP Tablets **531**
Vicoprofen Tablets **533**
Zydone Tablets **1132**

Hydroxychloroquine Sulfate (Propafenone is metabolized by CYP2D6 (major pathway). Drugs that inhibit CYP2D6 can be expected to cause increased plasma levels of propafenone. Appropriate monitoring is recommended when propafenone is used together with such drugs).

No products indexed under this heading.

Imatinib Mesylate (Propafenone is metabolized by CYP2D6 (major pathway). Drugs that inhibit CYP2D6 can be expected to cause increased plasma levels of propafenone. Appropriate monitoring is recommended when propafenone is used together with such drugs). Products include:

Gleevec Tablets **2255**

Imipramine Hydrochloride (Propafenone is metabolized by CYP2D6. Co-administration of propafenone with drugs metabolized by CYP2D6 (such as imipramine) might lead to increased plasma concentrations of imipramine).

No products indexed under this heading.

Imipramine Pamoate (Propafenone is metabolized by CYP2D6. Co-administration of propafenone with drugs metabolized by CYP2D6 (such as imipramine) might lead to increased plasma concentrations of imipramine).

No products indexed under this heading.

Indinavir Sulfate (Propafenone is metabolized by CYP3A4. Drugs that inhibit CYP3A4 can be expected to cause increased plasma levels of propafenone. Appropriate monitoring is recommended when propafenone is used together with such drugs). Products include:

Crixivan Capsules **1979**

Indoramin Hydrochloride (Propafenone is an inhibitor of CYP2D6. Co-administration of propafenone with drugs metabolized by CYP2D6 might lead to increased plasma concentrations of these drugs).

No products indexed under this heading.

Isoniazid (Propafenone is metabolized by CYP1A2. Drugs that inhibit CYP1A2 can be expected to cause increased plasma levels of propafenone. Appropriate monitoring is recommended when propafenone is used together with such drugs).

No products indexed under this heading.

Itraconazole (Propafenone is metabolized by CYP3A4. Drugs that inhibit CYP3A4 can be expected to cause increased plasma levels of propafenone. Appropriate monitoring is recommended when propafenone is used together with such drugs).

No products indexed under this heading.

Ketoconazole (Propafenone is metabolized by CYP3A4. Drugs that inhibit CYP3A4 (such as ketoconazole) can be expected to cause increased plasma levels of propafenone. Appropriate monitoring is recommended when propafenone is used together with such drugs). Products include:

Extina Foam, 2% **3057**
Nizoral A-D Shampoo **1901**

Labetalol Hydrochloride (Concomitant use of propafenone and propranolol in healthy subjects increased propranolol plasma concentrations at steady state by 113%. In 4 patients, administration of metoprolol with propafenone increased the metoprolol plasma concentrations at steady state by 100% to 400%. The pharmacokinetics of propafenone was not affected by the co-administration of either propranolol or metoprolol. In clinical trials using propafenone immediate release tablets, patients who were receiving beta-blockers concurrently did not experience an increased incidence of side effects).

No products indexed under this heading.

Levobunolol Hydrochloride (Concomitant use of propafenone and propranolol in healthy subjects increased propranolol plasma concentrations at steady state by 113%. In 4 patients, administration of metoprolol with propafenone increased the metoprolol plasma concentrations at steady state by 100% to 400%. The pharmacokinetics of propafenone was not affected by the co-administration of either propranolol or metoprolol. In clinical trials using propafenone immediate release tablets, patients who were receiving beta-blockers concurrently did not experience an increased incidence of side effects).

No products indexed under this heading.

Levofloxacin (Propafenone is metabolized by CYP1A2. Drugs that inhibit CYP1A2 can be expected to cause increased plasma levels of propafenone. Appropriate monitoring is recommended when propafenone is used together with such drugs). Products include:

Iquix Ophthalmic Solution 3183
Levaquin 2416
Levaquin in 5% Dextrose Injection 2416
Quixin Ophthalmic Solution 3184

Levonorgestrel (Propafenone is metabolized by CYP1A2. Drugs that inhibit CYP1A2 can be expected to cause increased plasma levels of propafenone. Appropriate monitoring is recommended when propafenone is used together with such drugs). Products include:

Climara Pro Transdermal System 768
Lybrel Tablets 3204
Mirena Intrauterine System 779
Plan B Tablets 1044
Seasonique Tablets 1046

Lidocaine (No significant effects on the pharmacokinetics of propafenone or lidocaine have been seen following their concomitant use in patients. However, concomitant use of propafenone and lidocaine have been reported to increase the risks of central nervous system side effects of lidocaine). Products include:

Lidoderm Patch 1114

Lidocaine Base (No significant effects on the pharmacokinetics of propafenone or lidocaine have been seen following their concomitant use in patients. However, concomitant use of propafenone and lidocaine have been reported to increase the risks of central nervous system side effects of lidocaine).

No products indexed under this heading.

Lidocaine Hydrochloride (No significant effects on the pharmacokinetics of propafenone or lidocaine have been seen following their concomitant use in patients. However, concomitant use of propafenone and lidocaine have been reported to increase the risks of central nervous system side effects of lidocaine).

No products indexed under this heading.

Lomefloxacin Hydrochloride (Propafenone is metabolized by CYP1A2. Drugs that inhibit CYP1A2 can be expected to cause increased plasma levels of propafenone. Appropriate monitoring is recommended when propafenone is used together with such drugs).

No products indexed under this heading.

Lopinavir (Propafenone is metabolized by CYP3A4. Drugs that inhibit CYP3A4 can be expected to cause increased plasma levels of propafenone. Appropriate monitoring is recommended when propafenone is used together with such drugs). Products include:

Kaletra 452

Loratadine (Propafenone is metabolized by CYP3A4. Drugs that inhibit CYP3A4 can be expected to cause increased plasma levels of propafenone. Appropriate monitoring is recommended when propafenone is used together with such drugs).

No products indexed under this heading.

Maprotiline Hydrochloride (Propafenone is metabolized by CYP2D6 (major pathway). Drugs that inhibit CYP2D6 can be expected to cause increased plasma levels of propafenone. Appropriate monitoring is recommended when propafenone is used together with such drugs).

No products indexed under this heading.

Meperidine Hydrochloride (Propafenone is an inhibitor of CYP2D6. Co-administration of propafenone with drugs metabolized by CYP2D6 might lead to increased plasma concentrations of these drugs).

No products indexed under this heading.

Mestranol (Propafenone is metabolized by CYP1A2. Drugs that inhibit CYP1A2 can be expected to cause increased plasma levels of propafenone. Appropriate monitoring is recommended when propafenone is used together with such drugs).

No products indexed under this heading.

Methadone Hydrochloride (Propafenone is metabolized by CYP2D6 (major pathway). Drugs that inhibit CYP2D6 can be expected to cause increased plasma levels of propafenone. Appropriate monitoring is recommended when propafenone is used together with such drugs).

No products indexed under this heading.

Methamphetamine Hydrochloride (Propafenone is an inhibitor of CYP2D6. Co-administration of propafenone with drugs metabolized by CYP2D6 might lead to increased plasma concentrations of these drugs).

No products indexed under this heading.

Methoxsalen (Propafenone is metabolized by CYP1A2. Drugs that inhibit CYP1A2 can be expected to cause increased plasma levels of propafenone. Appropriate monitoring is recommended when propafenone is used together with such drugs).

No products indexed under this heading.

Metipranolol Hydrochloride (Concomitant use of propafenone and propranolol in healthy subjects increased propranolol plasma concentrations at steady state by 113%. In 4 patients, administration of metoprolol with propafenone increased the metoprolol plasma concentrations at steady state by 100% to 400%. The pharmacokinetics of propafenone was not affected by the co-administration of either propranolol or metoprolol. In clinical trials using propafenone immediate release tablets, patients who were receiving beta-blockers concurrently did not experience an increased incidence of side effects).

No products indexed under this heading.

Metoprolol Succinate (In 4 patients, administration of metoprolol with propafenone increased the metoprolol plasma concentrations at steady state by 100% to 400%. The pharmacokinetics of propafenone was not affected by the co-administration of metoprolol. In clinical trials using propafenone immediate release tablets, patients who were receiving beta-blockers concurrently did not experience an increased incidence of side effects). Products include:

Toprol-XL Tablets 666

Metoprolol Tartrate (In 4 patients, administration of metoprolol with propafenone increased the metoprolol plasma concentrations at steady state by 100% to 400%. The pharmacokinetics of propafenone was not affected by the co-administration of metoprolol. In clinical trials using propafenone immediate release tablets, patients who were receiving beta-blockers concurrently did not experience an increased incidence of side effects).

No products indexed under this heading.

Metronidazole (Propafenone is metabolized by CYP3A4. Drugs that inhibit CYP3A4 can be expected to cause increased plasma levels of propafenone. Appropriate monitoring is recommended when propafenone is used together with such drugs). Products include:

Pylera Capsules 714

Metronidazole Benzoate (Propafenone is metabolized by CYP3A4. Drugs that inhibit CYP3A4 can be expected to cause increased plasma levels of propafenone. Appropriate monitoring is recommended when propafenone is used together with such drugs).

No products indexed under this heading.

Metronidazole Hydrochloride (Propafenone is metabolized by CYP3A4. Drugs that inhibit CYP3A4 can be expected to cause increased plasma levels of propafenone. Appropriate monitoring is recommended when propafenone is used together with such drugs).

No products indexed under this heading.

Metronidazole Sodium (Propafenone is metabolized by CYP3A4. Drugs that inhibit CYP3A4 can be expected to cause increased plasma levels of propafenone. Appropriate monitoring is recommended when propafenone is used together with such drugs).

No products indexed under this heading.

Mexiletine Hydrochloride (Propafenone is metabolized by CYP1A2. Drugs that inhibit CYP1A2 can be expected to cause increased plasma levels of propafenone. Appropriate monitoring is recommended when propafenone is used together with such drugs).

No products indexed under this heading.

Mibefradil Dihydrochloride (Propafenone is metabolized by CYP2D6 (major pathway). Drugs that inhibit CYP2D6 can be expected to cause increased plasma levels of propafenone. Appropriate monitoring is recommended when propafenone is used together with such drugs).

No products indexed under this heading.

Miconazole (Propafenone is metabolized by CYP3A4. Drugs that inhibit CYP3A4 can be expected to cause increased plasma levels of propafenone. Appropriate monitoring is recommended when propafenone is used together with such drugs).

No products indexed under this heading.

Miconazole Nitrate (Propafenone is metabolized by CYP3A4. Drugs that inhibit CYP3A4 can be expected to cause increased plasma levels of propafenone. Appropriate monitoring is recommended when propafenone is used together with such drugs).

No products indexed under this heading.

Mirtazapine (Propafenone is an inhibitor of CYP2D6. Co-administration of propafenone with drugs metabolized by CYP2D6 might lead to increased plasma concentrations of these drugs). Products include:

Remeron Tablets 2924
RemeronSolTab Tablets 2927

Moclobemide (Propafenone is metabolized by CYP2D6 (major pathway). Drugs that inhibit CYP2D6 can be expected to cause increased plasma levels of propafenone. Appropriate monitoring is recommended when propafenone is used together with such drugs).

No products indexed under this heading.

Morphine Sulfate (Propafenone is an inhibitor of CYP2D6. Co-administration of propafenone with drugs metabolized by CYP2D6 might lead to increased plasma concentrations of these drugs). Products include:

Avinza Capsules 1772
DepoDur Injection 1095
MS Contin Tablets 2585

Moxifloxacin Hydrochloride (Propafenone is metabolized by CYP1A2. Drugs that inhibit CYP1A2 can be expected to cause increased plasma levels of propafenone. Appropriate monitoring is recommended when propafenone is used together with such drugs). Products include:

Avelox 2803
Vigamox Ophthalmic Solution 548

Nadolol (Concomitant use of propafenone and propranolol in healthy subjects increased propranolol plasma concentrations at steady state by 113%. In 4 patients, administration of metoprolol with propafenone increased the metoprolol plasma concentrations at steady state by 100% to 400%. The pharmacokinetics of propafenone was not affected by the co-administration of either propranolol or metoprolol. In clinical trials using propafenone immediate release tablets, patients who were receiving beta-blockers concurrently did not experience an increased incidence of side effects). Products include:

Nadolol Tablets 2191

Nalidixic Acid (Propafenone is metabolized by CYP1A2. Drugs that inhibit CYP1A2 can be expected to cause increased plasma levels of propafenone. Appropriate monitoring is recommended when propafenone is used together with such drugs).

No products indexed under this heading.

Nebivolol (Concomitant use of propafenone and propranolol in healthy subjects increased propranolol plas-

ma concentrations at steady state by 113%. In 4 patients, administration of metoprolol with propafenone increased the metoprolol plasma concentrations at steady state by 100% to 400%. The pharmacokinetics of propafenone was not affected by the co-administration of either propranolol or metoprolol. In clinical trials using propafenone immediate release tablets, patients who were receiving beta-blockers concurrently did not experience an increased incidence of side effects). Products include:

Bystolic Tablets **1155**

Nefazodone Hydrochloride (Propafenone is metabolized by CYP3A4. Drugs that inhibit CYP3A4 can be expected to cause increased plasma levels of propafenone. Appropriate monitoring is recommended when propafenone is used together with such drugs).

No products indexed under this heading.

Nelfinavir Mesylate (Propafenone is metabolized by CYP3A4. Drugs that inhibit CYP3A4 can be expected to cause increased plasma levels of propafenone. Appropriate monitoring is recommended when propafenone is used together with such drugs).

No products indexed under this heading.

Nevirapine (Propafenone is metabolized by CYP3A4. Drugs that inhibit CYP3A4 can be expected to cause increased plasma levels of propafenone. Appropriate monitoring is recommended when propafenone is used together with such drugs). Products include:

Viramune Oral Suspension **873**
Viramune Tablets **873**

Niacinamide (Propafenone is metabolized by CYP3A4. Drugs that inhibit CYP3A4 can be expected to cause increased plasma levels of propafenone. Appropriate monitoring is recommended when propafenone is used together with such drugs). Products include:

BioLean Free Tablets .... ▣**635**

Nicotinamide (Propafenone is metabolized by CYP3A4. Drugs that inhibit CYP3A4 can be expected to cause increased plasma levels of propafenone. Appropriate monitoring is recommended when propafenone is used together with such drugs).

No products indexed under this heading.

Nifedipine (Propafenone is metabolized by CYP3A4. Drugs that inhibit CYP3A4 can be expected to cause increased plasma levels of propafenone. Appropriate monitoring is recommended when propafenone is used together with such drugs).

No products indexed under this heading.

Norethindrone (Propafenone is metabolized by CYP1A2. Drugs that inhibit CYP1A2 can be expected to cause increased plasma levels of propafenone. Appropriate monitoring is recommended when propafenone is used together with such drugs). Products include:

Ortho Micronor Tablets **2446**

Norfloxacin (Propafenone is metabolized by CYP1A2. Drugs that inhibit CYP1A2 can be expected to cause increased plasma levels of propafenone. Appropriate monitoring is recommended when propafenone is used together with such drugs). Products include:

Noroxin Tablets **2069**

Norgestrel (Propafenone is metabolized by CYP1A2. Drugs that inhibit CYP1A2 can be expected to cause increased plasma levels of propafenone. Appropriate monitoring is recommended when propafenone is used together with such drugs).

No products indexed under this heading.

Nortriptyline Hydrochloride (Propafenone is metabolized by CYP2D6 (major pathway). Drugs that inhibit CYP2D6 can be expected to cause increased plasma levels of propafenone. Appropriate monitoring is recommended when propafenone is used together with such drugs).

No products indexed under this heading.

Ofloxacin (Propafenone is metabolized by CYP1A2. Drugs that inhibit CYP1A2 can be expected to cause increased plasma levels of propafenone. Appropriate monitoring is recommended when propafenone is used together with such drugs). Products include:

Ofloxacin Ophthalmic Solution 0.3% .... ⊙**243**

Olanzapine (Propafenone is an inhibitor of CYP2D6. Co-administration of propafenone with drugs metabolized by CYP2D6 might lead to increased plasma concentrations of these drugs). Products include:

Symbyax Capsules **1871**
Zyprexa Tablets **1883**
Zyprexa IntraMuscular **1883**
Zyprexa ZYDIS Orally Disintegrating Tablets **1883**

Omeprazole (Propafenone is metabolized by CYP1A2. Drugs that inhibit CYP1A2 can be expected to cause increased plasma levels of propafenone. Appropriate monitoring is recommended when propafenone is used together with such drugs).

No products indexed under this heading.

Ondansetron (Propafenone is an inhibitor of CYP2D6. Co-administration of propafenone with drugs metabolized by CYP2D6 might lead to increased plasma concentrations of these drugs). Products include:

Zofran ODT Orally Disintegrating Tablets **1687**

Ondansetron Hydrochloride (Propafenone is an inhibitor of CYP2D6. Co-administration of propafenone with drugs metabolized by CYP2D6 might lead to increased plasma concentrations of these drugs). Products include:

Zofran Injection **1682**
Zofran **1687**

Orlistat (Orlistat may limit the fraction of propafenone available for absorption. In post-marketing reports, abrupt cessation of orlistat in patients stabilized on propafenone has resulted in severe adverse events including convulsions, atrioventricular block and acute circulatory failure). Products include:

Xenical Capsules **2672**

Oxycodone Hydrochloride (Propafenone is an inhibitor of CYP2D6. Co-administration of propafenone with drugs metabolized by CYP2D6 might lead to increased plasma concentrations of these drugs). Products include:

OxyContin Tablets **2589**
OxyIR Capsules **2593**
Percocet Tablets **1127**
Percodan Tablets **1130**

Paclitaxel (Propafenone is an inhibitor of CYP2D6. Co-administration of propafenone with drugs metabolized by CYP2D6 might lead to increased plasma concentrations of these drugs).

No products indexed under this heading.

Paroxetine (Propafenone is metabolized by CYP2D6 (major pathway). Drugs that inhibit CYP2D6 (such as paroxetine), can be expected to cause increased plasma levels of propafenone. Appropriate monitoring is recommended when propafenone is used together with such drugs).

No products indexed under this heading.

Paroxetine Hydrochloride (Propafenone is metabolized by CYP2D6 (major pathway). Drugs that inhibit CYP2D6 (such as paroxetine), can be expected to cause increased plasma levels of propafenone. Appropriate monitoring is recommended when propafenone is used together with such drugs). Products include:

Paxil **1535**
Paxil CR Controlled-Release Tablets **1544**

Paroxetine Mesylate (Propafenone is metabolized by CYP2D6 (major pathway). Drugs that inhibit CYP2D6 (such as paroxetine), can be expected to cause increased plasma levels of propafenone. Appropriate monitoring is recommended when propafenone is used together with such drugs).

No products indexed under this heading.

Penbutolol Sulfate (Concomitant use of propafenone and propranolol in healthy subjects increased propranolol plasma concentrations at steady state by 113%. In 4 patients, administration of metoprolol with propafenone increased the metoprolol plasma concentrations at steady state by 100% to 400%. The pharmacokinetics of propafenone was not affected by the co-administration of either propranolol or metoprolol. In clinical trials using propafenone immediate release tablets, patients who were receiving beta-blockers concurrently did not experience an increased incidence of side effects).

No products indexed under this heading.

Perphenazine (Propafenone is metabolized by CYP2D6 (major pathway). Drugs that inhibit CYP2D6 can be expected to cause increased plasma levels of propafenone. Appropriate monitoring is recommended when propafenone is used together with such drugs).

No products indexed under this heading.

Pindolol (Concomitant use of propafenone and propranolol in healthy subjects increased propranolol plasma concentrations at steady state by 113%. In 4 patients, administration of metoprolol with propafenone increased the metoprolol plasma concentrations at steady state by 100% to 400%. The pharmacokinetics of propafenone was not affected by the co-administration of either propranolol or metoprolol. In clinical trials using propafenone immediate release tablets, patients who were receiving beta-blockers concurrently did not experience an increased incidence of side effects).

No products indexed under this heading.

Propoxyphene Hydrochloride (Propafenone is metabolized by CYP2D6 (major pathway). Drugs that inhibit CYP2D6 can be expected to cause increased plasma levels of propafenone. Appropriate monitoring is recommended when propafenone is used together with such drugs).

No products indexed under this heading.

Propoxyphene Napsylate (Propafenone is metabolized by CYP2D6 (major pathway). Drugs that inhibit CYP2D6 can be expected to cause increased plasma levels of propafenone. Appropriate monitoring is recommended when propafenone is used together with such drugs).

No products indexed under this heading.

Propranolol (Concomitant use of propafenone and propranolol in healthy subjects increased propranolol plasma concentrations at steady state by 113%. The pharmacokinetics of propafenone was not affected by the co-administration of propranolol. In clinical trials using propafenone immediate release tablets, patients who were receiving beta-blockers concurrently did not experience an increased incidence of side effects).

No products indexed under this heading.

Propranolol Hydrochloride (Concomitant use of propafenone and propranolol in healthy subjects increased propranolol plasma concentrations at steady state by 113%. The pharmacokinetics of propafenone was not affected by the co-administration of propranolol. In clinical trials using propafenone immediate release tablets, patients who were receiving beta-blockers concurrently did not experience an increased incidence of side effects). Products include:

InnoPran XL Extended Release Capsules **1484**

Protriptyline Hydrochloride (Propafenone is metabolized by CYP2D6 (major pathway). Drugs that inhibit CYP2D6 can be expected to cause increased plasma levels of propafenone. Appropriate monitoring is recommended when propafenone is used together with such drugs).

No products indexed under this heading.

Quetiapine Fumarate (Propafenone is an inhibitor of CYP2D6. Co-administration of propafenone with drugs metabolized by CYP2D6 might lead to increased plasma concentrations of these drugs).

No products indexed under this heading.

Quinacrine Hydrochloride (Propafenone is metabolized by CYP2D6 (major pathway). Drugs that inhibit CYP2D6 can be expected to cause increased plasma levels of propafenone. Appropriate monitoring is recommended when propafenone is used together with such drugs).

No products indexed under this heading.

Quinidine (Small doses of quinidine completely inhibit the CYP2D6 hydroxylation metabolic pathways, making all patients, in effect, slow metabolizers. Concomitant administration of quinidine (50 mg TID) with 150 mg immediate release propafenone TID decreased the clearance of propafenone by 60% in extensive metabolizers (EM), making them poor metabolizers (PM). Steady-state plasma concentrations increased by more than 2-fold for propafenone, and decreased 50% for 5-OH-propafenone. A 100 mg dose of quinidine increased steady-state concentrations of propafenone 3-fold. Concomitant use of propafenone and quinidine is not recommended).

No products indexed under this heading.

Quinidine Gluconate (Small doses of quinidine completely inhibit the CYP2D6 hydroxylation metabolic pathways, making all patients, in effect, slow metabolizers. Concomitant administration of quinidine (50 mg TID) with 150 mg immediate release propafenone TID decreased the clearance of propafenone by 60% in extensive metabolizers (EM), making them poor metabolizers (PM). Steady-state plasma concentrations increased by more than 2-fold for propafenone, and decreased 50% for 5-OH-propafenone. A 100 mg dose of quinidine increased steady-state concentrations of propafenone 3-fold. Concomitant use of propafenone and quinidine is not recommended).

No products indexed under this heading.

Quinidine Hydrochloride (Small doses of quinidine completely inhibit the CYP2D6 hydroxylation metabolic pathways, making all patients, in effect, slow metabolizers. Concomitant administration of quinidine (50 mg TID) with 150 mg immediate release propafenone TID decreased the clearance of propafenone by 60% in extensive metabolizers (EM), making them poor metabolizers (PM). Steady-state plasma concentrations increased by more than 2-fold for propafenone, and decreased 50% for 5-OH-propafenone. A 100 mg dose of quinidine increased steady-state concentrations of propafenone 3-fold. Concomitant use of propafenone and quinidine is not recommended).

No products indexed under this heading.

Quinidine Polygalacturonate (Small doses of quinidine completely inhibit the CYP2D6 hydroxylation metabolic pathways, making all patients, in effect, slow metabolizers. Concomitant administration of quinidine (50 mg TID) with 150 mg immediate release propafenone TID decreased the clearance of propafenone by 60% in extensive metabolizers (EM), making them poor metabolizers (PM). Steady-state plasma concentrations increased by more than 2-fold for propafenone, and decreased 50% for 5-OH-propafenone. A 100 mg dose of quinidine increased steady-state concentrations of propafenone 3-fold. Concomitant use of propafenone and quinidine is not recommended).

No products indexed under this heading.

Quinidine Sulfate (Small doses of quinidine completely inhibit the CYP2D6 hydroxylation metabolic pathways, making all patients, in effect, slow metabolizers. Concomitant administration of quinidine (50 mg TID) with 150 mg immediate release propafenone TID decreased the clearance of propafenone by 60% in extensive metabolizers (EM), making them poor metabolizers (PM). Steady-state plasma concentrations increased by more than 2-fold for propafenone, and decreased 50% for 5-OH-propafenone. A 100 mg dose of quinidine increased steady-state concentrations of propafenone 3-fold. Concomitant use of propafenone and quinidine is not recommended).

No products indexed under this heading.

Quinine (Propafenone is metabolized by CYP3A4. Drugs that inhibit CYP3A4 can be expected to cause increased plasma levels of propafenone. Appropriate monitoring is recommended when propafenone is used together with such drugs).

No products indexed under this heading.

Quinine Sulfate (Propafenone is metabolized by CYP3A4. Drugs that inhibit CYP3A4 can be expected to cause increased plasma levels of propafenone. Appropriate monitoring is recommended when propafenone is used together with such drugs).

No products indexed under this heading.

Quinupristin (Propafenone is metabolized by CYP3A4. Drugs that inhibit CYP3A4 can be expected to cause increased plasma levels of propafenone. Appropriate monitoring is recommended when propafenone is used together with such drugs).

No products indexed under this heading.

Ranitidine Bismuth Citrate (Propafenone is metabolized by CYP2D6 (major pathway). Drugs that inhibit CYP2D6 can be expected to cause increased plasma levels of propafenone. Appropriate monitoring is recommended when propafenone is used together with such drugs).

No products indexed under this heading.

Ranitidine Hydrochloride (Propafenone is metabolized by CYP2D6 (major pathway). Drugs that inhibit CYP2D6 can be expected to cause increased plasma levels of propafenone. Appropriate monitoring is recommended when propafenone is used together with such drugs). Products include:

Zantac 75 Tablets 603
Zantac **1670**
Zantac Injection **1666**
Zantac Injection Pharmacy Bulk Package **1668**
Maximum Strength Zantac 150 Tablets 603
Maximum Strength Zantac 150 Cool Mint Tablets 603

Rifampin (Concomitant administration of rifampin and propafenone in extensive metabolizers decreased the plasma concentrations of propafenone by 67% with a corresponding decrease of 5OH-propafenone by 65%. The concentrations of norpropafenone increased by 30%. In poor metabolizers, there was a 50% decrease in propafenone plasma concentrations and an increase in the AUC and Cmax of norpropafenone by 74% and 20%, respectively. Urinary excretion of propafenone and its metabolites decreased significantly. Similar results were noted in elderly patients: Both the AUC and Cmax of propafenone decreased by 84%, with a corresponding decrease in AUC and Cmax of 5OH-propafenone by 69% and 57%).

No products indexed under this heading.

Risperidone (Propafenone is an inhibitor of CYP2D6. Co-administration of propafenone with drugs metabolized by CYP2D6 might lead to increased plasma concentrations of these drugs). Products include:

Risperdal Consta Long-Acting Injection **1753**

Ritonavir (Propafenone is metabolized by CYP2D6 (major pathway) and CYP3A4. Drugs that inhibit CYP2D6 and CYP3A4 (such as ritonavir), can be expected to cause increased plasma levels of propafenone. Appropriate monitoring is recommended when propafenone is used together with such drugs). Products include:

Kaletra **452**
Norvir **489**

Saquinavir (Propafenone is metabolized by CYP3A4. Drugs that inhibit CYP3A4 (such as saquinavir), can be expected to cause increased plasma levels of propafenone. Appropriate monitoring is recommended when propafenone is used together with such drugs).

No products indexed under this heading.

Saquinavir Mesylate (Propafenone is metabolized by CYP3A4. Drugs that inhibit CYP3A4 (such as saquinavir), can be expected to cause increased plasma levels of propafenone. Appropriate monitoring is recommended when propafenone is used together with such drugs).

No products indexed under this heading.

Sertraline Hydrochloride (Propafenone is metabolized by CYP2D6 (major pathway). Drugs that inhibit CYP2D6 (such as sertaline), can be expected to cause increased plasma levels of propafenone. Appropriate monitoring is recommended when propafenone is used together with such drugs).

No products indexed under this heading.

Sildenafil Citrate (Propafenone is metabolized by CYP2D6 (major pathway). Drugs that inhibit CYP2D6 can be expected to cause increased plasma levels of propafenone. Appropriate monitoring is recommended when propafenone is used together with such drugs).

No products indexed under this heading.

Sotalol Hydrochloride (Concomitant use of propafenone and propranolol in healthy subjects increased propranolol plasma concentrations at steady state by 113%. In 4 patients, administration of metoprolol with propafenone increased the metoprolol plasma concentrations at steady state by 100% to 400%. The pharmacokinetics of propafenone was not affected by the co-administration of either propranolol or metoprolol. In clinical trials using propafenone immediate release tablets, patients who were receiving beta-blockers concurrently did not experience an increased incidence of side effects).

No products indexed under this heading.

Sparfloxacin (Propafenone is metabolized by CYP1A2. Drugs that inhibit CYP1A2 can be expected to cause increased plasma levels of propafenone. Appropriate monitoring is recommended when propafenone is used together with such drugs).

No products indexed under this heading.

Tacrine Hydrochloride (Propafenone is metabolized by CYP1A2. Drugs that inhibit CYP1A2 can be expected to cause increased plasma levels of propafenone. Appropriate monitoring is recommended when propafenone is used together with such drugs).

No products indexed under this heading.

Tamoxifen Citrate (Propafenone is an inhibitor of CYP2D6. Co-administration of propafenone with drugs metabolized by CYP2D6 might lead to increased plasma concentrations of these drugs).

No products indexed under this heading.

Telithromycin (Propafenone is metabolized by CYP3A4. Drugs that inhibit CYP3A4 can be expected to cause increased plasma levels of propafenone. Appropriate monitoring is recommended when propafenone is used together with such drugs). Products include:

Ketek Tablets **2744**

Teniposide (Propafenone is an inhibitor of CYP2D6. Co-administration of propafenone with drugs metabolized by CYP2D6 might lead to increased plasma concentrations of these drugs).

No products indexed under this heading.

Terbinafine Hydrochloride (Propafenone is metabolized by CYP2D6 (major pathway). Drugs that inhibit CYP2D6 can be expected to cause increased plasma levels of propafenone. Appropriate monitoring is recommended when propafenone is used together with such drugs). Products include:

Lamisil Oral Granules **2264**
Lamisil Tablets **2266**

Testosterone (Propafenone is an inhibitor of CYP2D6. Co-administration of propafenone with drugs metabolized by CYP2D6 might lead to increased plasma concentrations of these drugs). Products include:

AndroGel **3159**
Testim 1% Gel **701**

Testosterone Cypionate (Propafenone is an inhibitor of CYP2D6. Co-administration of propafenone with drugs metabolized by CYP2D6 might lead to increased plasma concentrations of these drugs).

No products indexed under this heading.

Testosterone Enanthate (Propafenone is an inhibitor of CYP2D6. Co-administration of propafenone with drugs metabolized by CYP2D6

IMPORTANT NOTE: Always consult each drug listing in the patient's regimen for possible interactions.

might lead to increased plasma concentrations of these drugs). Products include:

Delatestryl Injection 1730

Testosterone Propionate (Propafenone is an inhibitor of CYP2D6. Co-administration of propafenone with drugs metabolized by CYP2D6 might lead to increased plasma concentrations of these drugs).

No products indexed under this heading.

Thioridazine (Propafenone is an inhibitor of CYP2D6. Co-administration of propafenone with drugs metabolized by CYP2D6 might lead to increased plasma concentrations of these drugs).

No products indexed under this heading.

Thioridazine Hydrochloride (Propafenone is metabolized by CYP2D6 (major pathway). Drugs that inhibit CYP2D6 can be expected to cause increased plasma levels of propafenone. Appropriate monitoring is recommended when propafenone is used together with such drugs). Products include:

Thioridazine Hydrochloride Tablets 2195

Ticlopidine Hydrochloride (Propafenone is metabolized by CYP1A2. Drugs that inhibit CYP1A2 can be expected to cause increased plasma levels of propafenone. Appropriate monitoring is recommended when propafenone is used together with such drugs).

No products indexed under this heading.

Timolol Hemihydrate (Concomitant use of propafenone and propranolol in healthy subjects increased propranolol plasma concentrations at steady state by 113%. In 4 patients, administration of metoprolol with propafenone increased the metoprolol plasma concentrations at steady state by 100% to 400%. The pharmacokinetics of propafenone was not affected by the co-administration of either propranolol or metoprolol. In clinical trials using propafenone immediate release tablets, patients who were receiving beta-blockers concurrently did not experience an increased incidence of side effects). Products include:

Betimol Ophthalmic Solution 3181

Timolol Maleate (Concomitant use of propafenone and propranolol in healthy subjects increased propranolol plasma concentrations at steady state by 113%. In 4 patients, administration of metoprolol with propafenone increased the metoprolol plasma concentrations at steady state by 100% to 400%. The pharmacokinetics of propafenone was not affected by the co-administration of either propranolol or metoprolol. In clinical trials using propafenone immediate release tablets, patients who were receiving beta-blockers concurrently did not experience an increased incidence of side effects). Products include:

Combigan Ophthalmic Solution 553
Cosopt Sterile Ophthalmic Solution 1969
Timoptic Sterile Ophthalmic Solution 2121
Timoptic in Ocudose 2124
Timoptic-XE Sterile Ophthalmic Gel Forming Solution 2125

Tolterodine Tartrate (Propafenone is an inhibitor of CYP2D6. Co-administration of propafenone with drugs metabolized by CYP2D6 might lead to increased plasma concentrations of these drugs).

No products indexed under this heading.

Tramadol Hydrochloride (Propafenone is an inhibitor of CYP2D6. Co-administration of propafenone with drugs metabolized by CYP2D6 might lead to increased plasma concentrations of these drugs). Products include:

Ultram ER Extended-Release Tablets 2428

Trazodone Hydrochloride (Propafenone is an inhibitor of CYP2D6. Co-administration of propafenone with drugs metabolized by CYP2D6 might lead to increased plasma concentrations of these drugs).

No products indexed under this heading.

Triazolam (Propafenone is an inhibitor of CYP2D6. Co-administration of propafenone with drugs metabolized by CYP2D6 might lead to increased plasma concentrations of these drugs).

No products indexed under this heading.

Trimipramine Maleate (Propafenone is metabolized by CYP2D6 (major pathway). Drugs that inhibit CYP2D6 can be expected to cause increased plasma levels of propafenone. Appropriate monitoring is recommended when propafenone is used together with such drugs).

No products indexed under this heading.

Troglitazone (Propafenone is metabolized by CYP3A4. Drugs that inhibit CYP3A4 can be expected to cause increased plasma levels of propafenone. Appropriate monitoring is recommended when propafenone is used together with such drugs).

No products indexed under this heading.

Troleandomycin (Propafenone is metabolized by CYP1A2. Drugs that inhibit CYP1A2 can be expected to cause increased plasma levels of propafenone. Appropriate monitoring is recommended when propafenone is used together with such drugs).

No products indexed under this heading.

Trovafloxacin Mesylate (Propafenone is metabolized by CYP1A2. Drugs that inhibit CYP1A2 can be expected to cause increased plasma levels of propafenone. Appropriate monitoring is recommended when propafenone is used together with such drugs).

No products indexed under this heading.

Valproate Sodium (Propafenone is metabolized by CYP3A4. Drugs that inhibit CYP3A4 can be expected to cause increased plasma levels of propafenone. Appropriate monitoring is recommended when propafenone is used together with such drugs).

No products indexed under this heading.

Vardenafil Hydrochloride (Propafenone is metabolized by CYP2D6 (major pathway). Drugs that inhibit CYP2D6 can be expected to cause increased plasma levels of propafenone. Appropriate monitoring is recommended when propafenone is used together with such drugs). Products include:

Levitra Tablets 2876

Venlafaxine Hydrochloride (Propafenone is an inhibitor of CYP2D6. Co-administration of propafenone with drugs metabolized by CYP2D6 (such as venlafaxine) might lead to increased plasma levels of venlafaxine). Products include:

Effexor XR Extended-Release Capsules 3195
Venlafaxine Hydrochloride Tablets ... 2199

Verapamil Hydrochloride (Propafenone is metabolized by CYP3A4. Drugs that inhibit CYP3A4 can be expected to cause increased plasma levels of propafenone. Appropriate monitoring is recommended when propafenone is used together with such drugs). Products include:

Tarka Tablets 511

Vinblastine Sulfate (Propafenone is an inhibitor of CYP2D6. Co-administration of propafenone with drugs metabolized by CYP2D6 might lead to increased plasma concentrations of these drugs).

No products indexed under this heading.

Voriconazole (Propafenone is metabolized by CYP3A4. Drugs that inhibit CYP3A4 can be expected to cause increased plasma levels of propafenone. Appropriate monitoring is recommended when propafenone is used together with such drugs).

No products indexed under this heading.

Warfarin Sodium (The concomitant administration of propafenone and warfarin increased warfarin plasma concentrations at steady state by 39% in healthy volunteers and prolonged the prothrombin time in patients taking warfarin. Adjustment of the warfarin dose should be guided by monitoring prothrombin time).

No products indexed under this heading.

Zafirlukast (Propafenone is metabolized by CYP3A4. Drugs that inhibit CYP3A4 can be expected to cause increased plasma levels of propafenone. Appropriate monitoring is recommended when propafenone is used together with such drugs). Products include:

Accolate Tablets 669

Zileuton (Propafenone is metabolized by CYP1A2. Drugs that inhibit CYP1A2 can be expected to cause increased plasma levels of propafenone. Appropriate monitoring is recommended when propafenone is used together with such drugs).

No products indexed under this heading.

Zonisamide (Propafenone is an inhibitor of CYP2D6. Co-administration of propafenone with drugs metabolized by CYP2D6 might lead to increased plasma concentrations of these drugs). Products include:

Zonegran Capsules 1089

Food Interactions

Grapefruit (Propafenone is metabolized by CYP3A4. Drugs that inhibit CYP3A4 can be expected to cause increased plasma levels of propafenone. Appropriate monitoring is recommended when propafenone is used together with such drugs).

Grapefruit Juice (Propafenone is metabolized by CYP3A4. Agents that inhibit CYP3A4 (such as grapefruit juice), can be expected to cause increased plasma levels of propafenone. Appropriate monitoring is recommended when propafenone is used together with such agents).

RYTHMOL SR CAPSULES

(Propafenone Hydrochloride) 1590

May interact with class 1A antiarrhythmics, class III antiarrhythmics, cytochrome p450 1a2 inhibitors (selected), cytochrome p450 2d6 inhibitors (selected), cytochrome p450 3a4 inhibitors (selected), cardiac glycosides, local anesthetics, macrolide antibiotics, drugs that prolong the QT interval, quinidine, xanthines, and certain other agents. Compounds in these categories include:

Acetazolamide (Drugs that inhibit CYP3A4 might lead to increased plasma levels of propafenone; patients should be closely monitored and the propafenone dose adjusted accordingly).

No products indexed under this heading.

Alatrofloxacin Mesylate (Drugs that inhibit CYP1A2 might lead to increased plasma levels of propafenone; patients should be closely monitored and the propafenone dose adjusted accordingly).

No products indexed under this heading.

Alprazolam (The use of propafenone in conjunction with other drugs that prolong the QT interval has not been extensively studied and is not recommended).

No products indexed under this heading.

Aminophylline (Combined therapy may result in an increase in theophylline concentration with the development of theophylline toxicity).

No products indexed under this heading.

Amiodarone Hydrochloride (The use of propafenone in conjunction with other drugs that prolong the QT interval has not been extensively studied and is not recommended).

No products indexed under this heading.

Amitriptyline Hydrochloride (The use of propafenone in conjunction with other drugs that prolong the QT interval has not been extensively studied and is not recommended).

No products indexed under this heading.

Amoxapine (The use of propafenone in conjunction with other drugs that prolong the QT interval has not been extensively studied and is not recommended).

No products indexed under this heading.

Amprenavir (Drugs that inhibit CYP3A4 might lead to increased plasma levels of propafenone; patients should be closely monitored and the propafenone dose adjusted accordingly).

No products indexed under this heading.

Anastrozole (Drugs that inhibit CYP1A2 might lead to increased plasma levels of propafenone; patients should be closely monitored and the propafenone dose adjusted accordingly). Products include:

Arimidex Tablets 672

Aprepitant (Drugs that inhibit CYP3A4 might lead to increased plasma levels of propafenone; patients should be closely monitored and the propafenone dose adjusted accordingly). Products include:
Emend Capsules 1992

Astemizole (The use of propafenone in conjunction with other drugs that prolong the QT interval has not been extensively studied and is not recommended).
No products indexed under this heading.

Atazanavir (Drugs that inhibit CYP3A4 might lead to increased plasma levels of propafenone; patients should be closely monitored and the propafenone dose adjusted accordingly).
No products indexed under this heading.

Atazanavir Sulfate (Drugs that inhibit CYP3A4 might lead to increased plasma levels of propafenone; patients should be closely monitored and the propafenone dose adjusted accordingly). Products include:
Reyataz Capsules 3299

Azithromycin Dihydrate (The use of propafenone in conjunction with other drugs that prolong the QT interval has not been extensively studied and is not recommended).
No products indexed under this heading.

Bepridil Hydrochloride (The use of propafenone in conjunction with other drugs that prolong the QT interval has not been extensively studied and is not recommended).
No products indexed under this heading.

Bretylium Tosylate (The use of propafenone in conjunction with other drugs that prolong the QT interval has not been extensively studied and is not recommended).
No products indexed under this heading.

Bupivacaine Hydrochloride (Concomitant use of local anesthetics may increase the risk of CNS side effects).
No products indexed under this heading.

Bupropion Hydrochloride (Drugs that inhibit CYP2D6 might lead to increased plasma levels of propafenone; patients should be closely monitored and the propafenone dose adjusted accordingly). Products include:
Wellbutrin Tablets 1648
Wellbutrin SR Sustained-Release Tablets 1653
Wellbutrin XL Extended-Release Tablets 1659
Zyban Sustained-Release Tablets 1692

Buspirone Hydrochloride (The use of propafenone in conjunction with other drugs that prolong the QT interval has not been extensively studied and is not recommended).
No products indexed under this heading.

Celecoxib (Drugs that inhibit CYP2D6 might lead to increased plasma levels of propafenone; patients should be closely monitored and the propafenone dose adjusted accordingly). Products include:
Celebrex Capsules 2979

Chlordiazepoxide (The use of propafenone in conjunction with other drugs that prolong the QT interval has not been extensively studied and is not recommended).
No products indexed under this heading.

Chlordiazepoxide Hydrochloride (The use of propafenone in conjunction with other drugs that prolong the QT interval has not been extensively studied and is not recommended).
No products indexed under this heading.

Chloroprocaine Hydrochloride (Concomitant use of local anesthetics may increase the risk of CNS side effects).
No products indexed under this heading.

Chloroquine Hydrochloride (Drugs that inhibit CYP2D6 might lead to increased plasma levels of propafenone; patients should be closely monitored and the propafenone dose adjusted accordingly).
No products indexed under this heading.

Chloroquine Phosphate (Drugs that inhibit CYP2D6 might lead to increased plasma levels of propafenone; patients should be closely monitored and the propafenone dose adjusted accordingly).
No products indexed under this heading.

Chlorpheniramine (Drugs that inhibit CYP2D6 might lead to increased plasma levels of propafenone; patients should be closely monitored and the propafenone dose adjusted accordingly).
No products indexed under this heading.

Chlorpheniramine Maleate (Drugs that inhibit CYP2D6 might lead to increased plasma levels of propafenone; patients should be closely monitored and the propafenone dose adjusted accordingly). Products include:
Actifed Cold & Allergy Tablets 1895
Sudafed PE Sinus & Allergy Tablets 1908
Tylenol Allergy Multi-Symptom Caplets with Cool Burst and Rapid Release Gelcaps 1916
Children's Tylenol Plus Cold Suspension Liquid 1912
Children's Tylenol Plus Cough & Runny Nose Suspension Liquid 1912
Children's Tylenol Plus Flu Suspension Liquid 1914
Children's Tylenol Plus Multi-Symptom Cold Suspension Liquid 1912
Tylenol Cold Head Congestion Nighttime Caplets with Cool Burst 1910
Tylenol Cold Multi-Symptom Nighttime Caplets with Cool Burst 1913
Tylenol Sinus Congestion & Pain Nighttime Caplets with Cool Burst 1917

Chlorpheniramine Polistirex (Drugs that inhibit CYP2D6 might lead to increased plasma levels of propafenone; patients should be closely monitored and the propafenone dose adjusted accordingly). Products include:
Tussionex Pennkinetic Extended-Release Suspension 3154

Chlorpheniramine Tannate (Drugs that inhibit CYP2D6 might lead to increased plasma levels of propafenone; patients should be closely monitored and the propafenone dose adjusted accordingly).
No products indexed under this heading.

Chlorpromazine (The use of propafenone in conjunction with other drugs that prolong the QT interval has not been extensively studied and is not recommended).
No products indexed under this heading.

Chlorpromazine Hydrochloride (The use of propafenone in conjunction with other drugs that prolong the QT interval has not been extensively studied and is not recommended).
No products indexed under this heading.

Chlorprothixene (The use of propafenone in conjunction with other drugs that prolong the QT interval has not been extensively studied and is not recommended).
No products indexed under this heading.

Chlorprothixene Hydrochloride (The use of propafenone in conjunction with other drugs that prolong the QT interval has not been extensively studied and is not recommended).
No products indexed under this heading.

Cimetidine (Increases steady-state plasma concentrations with no detectable changes in electrocardiographic parameters).
No products indexed under this heading.

Cimetidine Hydrochloride (Increases steady-state plasma concentrations with no detectable changes in electrocardiographic parameters).
No products indexed under this heading.

Ciprofloxacin (Drugs that inhibit CYP1A2 might lead to increased plasma levels of propafenone; patients should be closely monitored and the propafenone dose adjusted accordingly). Products include:
Cipro I.V. 2817
Cipro Oral Suspension 2810
Cipro XR Tablets 2823
Ciprodex Otic Suspension 541

Ciprofloxacin Hydrochloride (Drugs that inhibit CYP1A2 might lead to increased plasma levels of propafenone; patients should be closely monitored and the propafenone dose adjusted accordingly). Products include:
Cipro Tablets 2810

Cisapride (The use of propafenone in conjunction with other drugs that prolong the QT interval has not been extensively studied and is not recommended).
No products indexed under this heading.

Citalopram Hydrobromide (Drugs that inhibit CYP2D6 might lead to increased plasma levels of propafenone; patients should be closely monitored and the propafenone dose adjusted accordingly). Products include:
Celexa 1160

Clarithromycin (The use of propafenone in conjunction with other drugs that prolong the QT interval has not been extensively studied and is not recommended). Products include:
Biaxin/Biaxin XL 411

Clomipramine Hydrochloride (The use of propafenone in conjunction with other drugs that prolong the QT interval has not been extensively studied and is not recommended).
No products indexed under this heading.

Clorazepate Dipotassium (The use of propafenone in conjunction with other drugs that prolong the QT interval has not been extensively studied and is not recommended).
No products indexed under this heading.

Clotrimazole (Drugs that inhibit CYP3A4 might lead to increased plasma levels of propafenone; patients should be closely monitored and the propafenone dose adjusted accordingly). Products include:
Lotrisone 2881

Clozapine (The use of propafenone in conjunction with other drugs that prolong the QT interval has not been extensively studied and is not recommended).
No products indexed under this heading.

Cocaine Hydrochloride (Drugs that inhibit CYP2D6 might lead to increased plasma levels of propafenone; patients should be closely monitored and the propafenone dose adjusted accordingly).
No products indexed under this heading.

Cyclosporine (Propafenone therapy may increase levels of cyclosporine). Products include:
Gengraf Capsules 435
Neoral Oral Solution 2280
Neoral Soft Gelatin Capsules 2280
Restasis Ophthalmic Emulsion 557
Sandimmune 2296

Dalfopristin (Drugs that inhibit CYP3A4 might lead to increased plasma levels of propafenone; patients should be closely monitored and the propafenone dose adjusted accordingly).
No products indexed under this heading.

Danazol (Drugs that inhibit CYP3A4 might lead to increased plasma levels of propafenone; patients should be closely monitored and the propafenone dose adjusted accordingly).
No products indexed under this heading.

Delavirdine Mesylate (Drugs that inhibit CYP3A4 might lead to increased plasma levels of propafenone; patients should be closely monitored and the propafenone dose adjusted accordingly).
No products indexed under this heading.

Desipramine Hydrochloride (Coadministration may result in elevated serum desipramine levels).
No products indexed under this heading.

Deslanoside (Potential for elevated digoxin levels; dosage reduction of digitalis may be necessary).
No products indexed under this heading.

IMPORTANT NOTE: Always consult each drug listing in the patient's regimen for possible interactions.

Desogestrel (Drugs that inhibit CYP1A2 might lead to increased plasma levels of propafenone; patients should be closely monitored and the propafenone dose adjusted accordingly). Products include:
Mircette Tablets 1034

Diazepam (The use of propafenone in conjunction with other drugs that prolong the QT interval has not been extensively studied and is not recommended). Products include:
Valium Tablets 2658

Digitalis Glycoside Preparations (Potential for elevated digoxin levels; dosage reduction of digitalis may be necessary).
No products indexed under this heading.

Digitoxin (Potential for elevated digoxin levels; dosage reduction of digitalis may be necessary).
No products indexed under this heading.

Digoxin (Potential for elevated digoxin levels; dosage reduction of digitalis may be necessary). Products include:
Lanoxin Injection 1498
Lanoxin Injection Pediatric 1502
Lanoxin Tablets 1505

Diltiazem Hydrochloride (Drugs that inhibit CYP3A4 might lead to increased plasma levels of propafenone; patients should be closely monitored and the propafenone dose adjusted accordingly). Products include:
Cardizem LA Extended Release Tablets 421

Diltiazem Maleate (Drugs that inhibit CYP3A4 might lead to increased plasma levels of propafenone; patients should be closely monitored and the propafenone dose adjusted accordingly).
No products indexed under this heading.

Diphenhydramine (Drugs that inhibit CYP2D6 might lead to increased plasma levels of propafenone; patients should be closely monitored and the propafenone dose adjusted accordingly).
No products indexed under this heading.

Diphenhydramine Hydrochloride (Drugs that inhibit CYP2D6 might lead to increased plasma levels of propafenone; patients should be closely monitored and the propafenone dose adjusted accordingly). Products include:
Benadryl Allergy & Cold Kapgels 1895
Benadryl Allergy & Sinus Headache Kapgels 1895
Benadryl Severe Allergy & Sinus Headache Caplets 1897
Benadryl Dye-Free Allergy Liqui-gels Softgels 1897
Benadryl Allergy Kapgels 1895
Benadryl Allergy Quick Dissolve Strips 1896
Benadryl Allergy Ultratab Tablets 1896
Children's Benadryl Dye-Free Allergy Liquid 1897
Children's Benadryl Allergy Fastmelts 1897
Children's Benadryl Allergy Liquid 1898
Children's Benadryl Allergy Perfect Measure 1896
Children's Benadryl-D Allergy & Sinus Liquid 1896
Benadryl-D Allergy & Sinus Tablet 1896
PediaCare Children's Allergy & Cold Liquid 1902
PediaCare Children's Allergy Liquid 1902
Simply Sleep Caplets 1905
Sudafed PE Nighttime Cold Caplets 1907
Sudafed PE Severe Cold Caplets 1908
Extra Strength Tylenol PM Caplets, Geltabs, Liquid, and Rapid Release Gels 1915
Tylenol Allergy Multi-Symptom Nighttime Caplets with Cool Burst 1916
Tylenol Severe Allergy Caplets 1916
Children's Tylenol Plus Cold & Allergy Suspension Liquid 1914
Tylenol Sore Throat Nighttime Liquid with Cool Burst 1918

Dirithromycin (The use of propafenone in conjunction with other drugs that prolong the QT interval has not been extensively studied and is not recommended).
No products indexed under this heading.

Disopyramide (Class Ia antiarrythmic agents should be withheld for at least five half-lives prior to dosing with extended release propafenone. The use of propafenone with Class Ia antiarrythmic agents is not recommended).
No products indexed under this heading.

Disopyramide Phosphate (The use of propafenone in conjunction with other drugs that prolong the QT interval has not been extensively studied and is not recommended).
No products indexed under this heading.

Dofetilide (The use of propafenone in conjunction with other drugs that prolong the QT interval has not been extensively studied and is not recommended).
No products indexed under this heading.

Doxepin Hydrochloride (The use of propafenone in conjunction with other drugs that prolong the QT interval has not been extensively studied and is not recommended).
No products indexed under this heading.

Droperidol (The use of propafenone in conjunction with other drugs that prolong the QT interval has not been extensively studied and is not recommended).
No products indexed under this heading.

Dyphylline (Combined therapy may result in an increase in theophylline concentration with the development of theophylline toxicity).
No products indexed under this heading.

Efavirenz (Drugs that inhibit CYP3A4 might lead to increased plasma levels of propafenone; patients should be closely monitored and the propafenone dose adjusted accordingly). Products include:
Atripla Tablets 938
Sustiva Capsules 930
Sustiva Tablets 930

Enoxacin (Drugs that inhibit CYP1A2 might lead to increased plasma levels of propafenone; patients should be closely monitored and the propafenone dose adjusted accordingly).
No products indexed under this heading.

Erythromycin (The use of propafenone in conjunction with other drugs that prolong the QT interval has not been extensively studied and is not recommended).
No products indexed under this heading.

Erythromycin Estolate (The use of propafenone in conjunction with other drugs that prolong the QT interval has not been extensively studied and is not recommended).
No products indexed under this heading.

Erythromycin Ethylsuccinate (The use of propafenone in conjunction with other drugs that prolong the QT interval has not been extensively studied and is not recommended). Products include:
E.E.S. 433
EryPed 431

Erythromycin Gluceptate (The use of propafenone in conjunction with other drugs that prolong the QT interval has not been extensively studied and is not recommended).
No products indexed under this heading.

Erythromycin Lactobionate (The use of propafenone in conjunction with other drugs that prolong the QT interval has not been extensively studied and is not recommended).
No products indexed under this heading.

Erythromycin Stearate (The use of propafenone in conjunction with other drugs that prolong the QT interval has not been extensively studied and is not recommended).
No products indexed under this heading.

Escitalopram Oxalate (Drugs that inhibit CYP2D6 might lead to increased plasma levels of propafenone; patients should be closely monitored and the propafenone dose adjusted accordingly). Products include:
Lexapro Oral Suspension 1174
Lexapro Tablets 1174

Esomeprazole Magnesium (Drugs that inhibit CYP3A4 might lead to increased plasma levels of propafenone; patients should be closely monitored and the propafenone dose adjusted accordingly). Products include:
Nexium Delayed-Release Capsules 645
Nexium Delayed-Release Oral Suspension 645

Ethinyl Estradiol (Drugs that inhibit CYP1A2 might lead to increased plasma levels of propafenone; patients should be closely monitored and the propafenone dose adjusted accordingly). Products include:
Lybrel Tablets 3204
Mircette Tablets 1034
NuvaRing 2897
Ortho-Cyclen/Ortho Tri-Cyclen 2449
Ortho Evra Transdermal System 2437
Ortho Tri-Cyclen Lo Tablets 2458
Seasonique Tablets 1046
Yaz Tablets 805

Etidocaine Hydrochloride (Concomitant use of local anesthetics may increase the risk of CNS side effects).
No products indexed under this heading.

Flecainide Acetate (The use of propafenone in conjunction with other drugs that prolong the QT interval has not been extensively studied and is not recommended).
No products indexed under this heading.

Fluconazole (Drugs that inhibit CYP3A4 might lead to increased plasma levels of propafenone; patients should be closely monitored and the propafenone dose adjusted accordingly).
No products indexed under this heading.

Fluoxetine (Drugs that inhibit CYP2D6 might lead to increased plasma levels of propafenone; patients should be closely monitored and the propafenone dose adjusted accordingly).
No products indexed under this heading.

Fluoxetine Hydrochloride (Drugs that inhibit CYP2D6 might lead to increased plasma levels of propafenone; patients should be closely monitored and the propafenone dose adjusted accordingly). Products include:
Prozac Weekly Capsules 1852
Prozac Pulvules and Liquid 1852
Symbyax Capsules 1871

Fluphenazine Decanoate (The use of propafenone in conjunction with other drugs that prolong the QT interval has not been extensively studied and is not recommended).
No products indexed under this heading.

Fluphenazine Enanthate (The use of propafenone in conjunction with other drugs that prolong the QT interval has not been extensively studied and is not recommended).
No products indexed under this heading.

Fluphenazine Hydrochloride (The use of propafenone in conjunction with other drugs that prolong the QT interval has not been extensively studied and is not recommended).
No products indexed under this heading.

Fluvoxamine (Drugs that inhibit CYP1A2 might lead to increased plasma levels of propafenone; patients should be closely monitored and the propafenone dose adjusted accordingly).
No products indexed under this heading.

Fluvoxamine Maleate (Drugs that inhibit CYP2D6 might lead to increased plasma levels of propafenone; patients should be closely monitored and the propafenone dose adjusted accordingly). Products include:
Luvox CR Extended-Release Capsules 1759

Fosamprenavir Calcium (Drugs that inhibit CYP3A4 might lead to increased plasma levels of propafenone; patients should be closely monitored and the propafenone dose adjusted accordingly). Products include:
Lexiva Oral Suspension 1510
Lexiva Tablets 1510

Gatifloxacin (Drugs that inhibit CYP1A2 might lead to increased plasma levels of propafenone; patients should be closely monitored and the propafenone dose adjusted accordingly).
No products indexed under this heading.

Gemifloxacin Mesylate (Drugs that inhibit CYP1A2 might lead to increased plasma levels of propafenone; patients should be closely monitored and the propafenone dose adjusted accordingly).

No products indexed under this heading.

Grepafloxacin Hydrochloride (Drugs that inhibit CYP1A2 might lead to increased plasma levels of propafenone; patients should be closely monitored and the propafenone dose adjusted accordingly).

No products indexed under this heading.

Halofantrine Hydrochloride (Drugs that inhibit CYP2D6 might lead to increased plasma levels of propafenone; patients should be closely monitored and the propafenone dose adjusted accordingly).

No products indexed under this heading.

Haloperidol (The use of propafenone in conjunction with other drugs that prolong the QT interval has not been extensively studied and is not recommended).

No products indexed under this heading.

Haloperidol Decanoate (The use of propafenone in conjunction with other drugs that prolong the QT interval has not been extensively studied and is not recommended).

No products indexed under this heading.

Hydroxychloroquine Sulfate (Drugs that inhibit CYP2D6 might lead to increased plasma levels of propafenone; patients should be closely monitored and the propafenone dose adjusted accordingly).

No products indexed under this heading.

Hydroxyzine Hydrochloride (The use of propafenone in conjunction with other drugs that prolong the QT interval has not been extensively studied and is not recommended).

No products indexed under this heading.

Imatinib Mesylate (Drugs that inhibit CYP2D6 might lead to increased plasma levels of propafenone; patients should be closely monitored and the propafenone dose adjusted accordingly). Products include:

Gleevec Tablets **2255**

Imipramine Hydrochloride (The use of propafenone in conjunction with other drugs that prolong the QT interval has not been extensively studied and is not recommended).

No products indexed under this heading.

Imipramine Pamoate (The use of propafenone in conjunction with other drugs that prolong the QT interval has not been extensively studied and is not recommended).

No products indexed under this heading.

Indinavir Sulfate (Drugs that inhibit CYP3A4 might lead to increased plasma levels of propafenone; patients should be closely monitored and the propafenone dose adjusted accordingly). Products include:

Crixivan Capsules **1979**

Isocarboxazid (The use of propafenone in conjunction with other drugs that prolong the QT interval has not been extensively studied and is not recommended). Products include:

Marplan Tablets **3177**

Isoniazid (Drugs that inhibit CYP1A2 might lead to increased plasma levels of propafenone; patients should be closely monitored and the propafenone dose adjusted accordingly).

No products indexed under this heading.

Itraconazole (Drugs that inhibit CYP3A4 might lead to increased plasma levels of propafenone; patients should be closely monitored and the propafenone dose adjusted accordingly).

No products indexed under this heading.

Ketoconazole (Drugs that inhibit CYP1A2 might lead to increased plasma levels of propafenone; patients should be closely monitored and the propafenone dose adjusted accordingly). Products include:

Extina Foam, 2% **3057**
Nizoral A-D Shampoo **1901**

Levobupivacaine Hydrochloride (Concomitant use of local anesthetics may increase the risk of CNS side effects).

No products indexed under this heading.

Levofloxacin (Drugs that inhibit CYP1A2 might lead to increased plasma levels of propafenone; patients should be closely monitored and the propafenone dose adjusted accordingly). Products include:

Iquix Ophthalmic Solution **3183**
Levaquin **2416**
Levaquin in 5% Dextrose Injection **2416**
Quixin Ophthalmic Solution **3184**

Levonorgestrel (Drugs that inhibit CYP1A2 might lead to increased plasma levels of propafenone; patients should be closely monitored and the propafenone dose adjusted accordingly). Products include:

Climara Pro Transdermal System **768**
Lybrel Tablets **3204**
Mirena Intrauterine System **779**
Plan B Tablets **1044**
Seasonique Tablets **1046**

Lidocaine Hydrochloride (The use of propafenone in conjunction with other drugs that prolong the QT interval has not been extensively studied and is not recommended).

No products indexed under this heading.

Lithium Carbonate (The use of propafenone in conjunction with other drugs that prolong the QT interval has not been extensively studied and is not recommended).

No products indexed under this heading.

Lithium Citrate (The use of propafenone in conjunction with other drugs that prolong the QT interval has not been extensively studied and is not recommended).

No products indexed under this heading.

Lomefloxacin Hydrochloride (Drugs that inhibit CYP1A2 might lead to increased plasma levels of propafenone; patients should be closely monitored and the propafenone dose adjusted accordingly).

No products indexed under this heading.

Lopinavir (Drugs that inhibit CYP3A4 might lead to increased plasma levels of propafenone; patients should be closely monitored and the propafenone dose adjusted accordingly). Products include:

Kaletra **452**

Loratadine (Drugs that inhibit CYP3A4 might lead to increased plasma levels of propafenone; patients should be closely monitored and the propafenone dose adjusted accordingly).

No products indexed under this heading.

Lorazepam (The use of propafenone in conjunction with other drugs that prolong the QT interval has not been extensively studied and is not recommended).

No products indexed under this heading.

Loxapine Hydrochloride (The use of propafenone in conjunction with other drugs that prolong the QT interval has not been extensively studied and is not recommended).

No products indexed under this heading.

Loxapine Succinate (The use of propafenone in conjunction with other drugs that prolong the QT interval has not been extensively studied and is not recommended).

No products indexed under this heading.

Maprotiline Hydrochloride (The use of propafenone in conjunction with other drugs that prolong the QT interval has not been extensively studied and is not recommended).

No products indexed under this heading.

Mepivacaine Hydrochloride (Concomitant use of local anesthetics may increase the risk of CNS side effects).

No products indexed under this heading.

Meprobamate (The use of propafenone in conjunction with other drugs that prolong the QT interval has not been extensively studied and is not recommended).

No products indexed under this heading.

Mesoridazine Besylate (The use of propafenone in conjunction with other drugs that prolong the QT interval has not been extensively studied and is not recommended).

No products indexed under this heading.

Mestranol (Drugs that inhibit CYP1A2 might lead to increased plasma levels of propafenone; patients should be closely monitored and the propafenone dose adjusted accordingly).

No products indexed under this heading.

Methadone Hydrochloride (Drugs that inhibit CYP2D6 might lead to increased plasma levels of propafenone; patients should be closely monitored and the propafenone dose adjusted accordingly).

No products indexed under this heading.

Methoxsalen (Drugs that inhibit CYP1A2 might lead to increased plasma levels of propafenone; patients should be closely monitored and the propafenone dose adjusted accordingly).

No products indexed under this heading.

Metoprolol Succinate (Co-administration can result in substantial increases in metoprolol concentration and elimination half-life; increased plasma levels of metoprolol could overcome its cardioselectivity). Products include:

Toprol-XL Tablets **666**

Metoprolol Tartrate (Co-administration can result in substantial increases in metoprolol concentration and elimination half-life; increased plasma levels of metoprolol could overcome its cardioselectivity).

No products indexed under this heading.

Metronidazole (Drugs that inhibit CYP3A4 might lead to increased plasma levels of propafenone; patients should be closely monitored and the propafenone dose adjusted accordingly). Products include:

Pylera Capsules **714**

Metronidazole Benzoate (Drugs that inhibit CYP3A4 might lead to increased plasma levels of propafenone; patients should be closely monitored and the propafenone dose adjusted accordingly).

No products indexed under this heading.

Metronidazole Hydrochloride (Drugs that inhibit CYP3A4 might lead to increased plasma levels of propafenone; patients should be closely monitored and the propafenone dose adjusted accordingly).

No products indexed under this heading.

Mexiletine Hydrochloride (The use of propafenone in conjunction with other drugs that prolong the QT interval has not been extensively studied and is not recommended).

No products indexed under this heading.

Mibefradil Dihydrochloride (Drugs that inhibit CYP2D6 might lead to increased plasma levels of propafenone; patients should be closely monitored and the propafenone dose adjusted accordingly).

No products indexed under this heading.

Miconazole (Drugs that inhibit CYP3A4 might lead to increased plasma levels of propafenone; patients should be closely monitored and the propafenone dose adjusted accordingly).

No products indexed under this heading.

Miconazole Nitrate (Drugs that inhibit CYP3A4 might lead to increased plasma levels of propafenone; patients should be closely monitored and the propafenone dose adjusted accordingly).

No products indexed under this heading.

Midazolam Hydrochloride (The use of propafenone in conjunction with other drugs that prolong the QT interval has not been extensively studied and is not recommended).

No products indexed under this heading.

Moclobemide (Drugs that inhibit CYP2D6 might lead to increased plasma levels of propafenone; patients should be closely monitored and the propafenone dose adjusted accordingly).

No products indexed under this heading.

Molindone Hydrochloride (The use of propafenone in conjunction with other drugs that prolong the QT interval has not been extensively studied and is not recommended). Products include:
- Moban Tablets 1116

Moricizine Hydrochloride (Class Ia antiarrythmic agents should be withheld for at least five half-lives prior to dosing with extended release propafenone. The use of propafenone with Class Ia antiarrythmic agents is not recommended).
- No products indexed under this heading.

Moxifloxacin Hydrochloride (Drugs that inhibit CYP1A2 might lead to increased plasma levels of propafenone; patients should be closely monitored and the propafenone dose adjusted accordingly). Products include:
- Avelox 2803
- Vigamox Ophthalmic Solution 548

Nalidixic Acid (Drugs that inhibit CYP1A2 might lead to increased plasma levels of propafenone; patients should be closely monitored and the propafenone dose adjusted accordingly).
- No products indexed under this heading.

Nefazodone Hydrochloride (Drugs that inhibit CYP3A4 might lead to increased plasma levels of propafenone; patients should be closely monitored and the propafenone dose adjusted accordingly).
- No products indexed under this heading.

Nelfinavir Mesylate (Drugs that inhibit CYP3A4 might lead to increased plasma levels of propafenone; patients should be closely monitored and the propafenone dose adjusted accordingly).
- No products indexed under this heading.

Nevirapine (Drugs that inhibit CYP3A4 might lead to increased plasma levels of propafenone; patients should be closely monitored and the propafenone dose adjusted accordingly). Products include:
- Viramune Oral Suspension 873
- Viramune Tablets 873

Niacinamide (Drugs that inhibit CYP3A4 might lead to increased plasma levels of propafenone; patients should be closely monitored and the propafenone dose adjusted accordingly). Products include:
- BioLean Free Tablets .... ▣635

Nicotinamide (Drugs that inhibit CYP3A4 might lead to increased plasma levels of propafenone; patients should be closely monitored and the propafenone dose adjusted accordingly).
- No products indexed under this heading.

Nifedipine (Drugs that inhibit CYP3A4 might lead to increased plasma levels of propafenone; patients should be closely monitored and the propafenone dose adjusted accordingly).
- No products indexed under this heading.

Norethindrone (Drugs that inhibit CYP1A2 might lead to increased plasma levels of propafenone; patients should be closely monitored and the propafenone dose adjusted accordingly). Products include:
- Ortho Micronor Tablets 2446

Norfloxacin (Drugs that inhibit CYP1A2 might lead to increased plasma levels of propafenone; patients should be closely monitored and the propafenone dose adjusted accordingly). Products include:
- Noroxin Tablets 2069

Norgestrel (Drugs that inhibit CYP1A2 might lead to increased plasma levels of propafenone; patients should be closely monitored and the propafenone dose adjusted accordingly).
- No products indexed under this heading.

Nortriptyline Hydrochloride (The use of propafenone in conjunction with other drugs that prolong the QT interval has not been extensively studied and is not recommended).
- No products indexed under this heading.

Ofloxacin (Drugs that inhibit CYP1A2 might lead to increased plasma levels of propafenone; patients should be closely monitored and the propafenone dose adjusted accordingly). Products include:
- Ofloxacin Ophthalmic Solution 0.3% .... ⊙243

Olanzapine (The use of propafenone in conjunction with other drugs that prolong the QT interval has not been extensively studied and is not recommended). Products include:
- Symbyax Capsules 1871
- Zyprexa Tablets 1883
- Zyprexa IntraMuscular 1883
- Zyprexa ZYDIS Orally Disintegrating Tablets 1883

Omeprazole (Drugs that inhibit CYP1A2 might lead to increased plasma levels of propafenone; patients should be closely monitored and the propafenone dose adjusted accordingly).
- No products indexed under this heading.

Oxazepam (The use of propafenone in conjunction with other drugs that prolong the QT interval has not been extensively studied and is not recommended).
- No products indexed under this heading.

Paroxetine Hydrochloride (Drugs that inhibit CYP2D6 might lead to increased plasma levels of propafenone; patients should be closely monitored and the propafenone dose adjusted accordingly). Products include:
- Paxil 1535
- Paxil CR Controlled-Release Tablets 1544

Perphenazine (The use of propafenone in conjunction with other drugs that prolong the QT interval has not been extensively studied and is not recommended).
- No products indexed under this heading.

Phenelzine Sulfate (The use of propafenone in conjunction with other drugs that prolong the QT interval has not been extensively studied and is not recommended).
- No products indexed under this heading.

Prazepam (The use of propafenone in conjunction with other drugs that prolong the QT interval has not been extensively studied and is not recommended).
- No products indexed under this heading.

Procainamide (Class Ia antiarrythmic agents should be withheld for at least five half-lives prior to dosing with extended release propafenone. The use of propafenone with Class Ia antiarrythmic agents is not recommended).
- No products indexed under this heading.

Procainamide Hydrochloride (The use of propafenone in conjunction with other drugs that prolong the QT interval has not been extensively studied and is not recommended).
- No products indexed under this heading.

Procaine Hydrochloride (Concomitant use of local anesthetics may increase the risk of CNS side effects).
- No products indexed under this heading.

Prochlorperazine (The use of propafenone in conjunction with other drugs that prolong the QT interval has not been extensively studied and is not recommended).
- No products indexed under this heading.

Promethazine Hydrochloride (The use of propafenone in conjunction with other drugs that prolong the QT interval has not been extensively studied and is not recommended).
- No products indexed under this heading.

Propoxyphene Hydrochloride (Drugs that inhibit CYP2D6 might lead to increased plasma levels of propafenone; patients should be closely monitored and the propafenone dose adjusted accordingly).
- No products indexed under this heading.

Propoxyphene Napsylate (Drugs that inhibit CYP2D6 might lead to increased plasma levels of propafenone; patients should be closely monitored and the propafenone dose adjusted accordingly).
- No products indexed under this heading.

Propranolol Hydrochloride (Coadministration has resulted in substantial increases in propranolol concentration and elimination half-life). Products include:
- InnoPran XL Extended Release Capsules 1484

Protriptyline Hydrochloride (The use of propafenone in conjunction with other drugs that prolong the QT interval has not been extensively studied and is not recommended).
- No products indexed under this heading.

Quetiapine Fumarate (The use of propafenone in conjunction with other drugs that prolong the QT interval has not been extensively studied and is not recommended).
- No products indexed under this heading.

Quinacrine Hydrochloride (Drugs that inhibit CYP2D6 might lead to increased plasma levels of propafenone; patients should be closely monitored and the propafenone dose adjusted accordingly).
- No products indexed under this heading.

Quinidine (Class Ia antiarrythmic agents should be withheld for at least five half-lives prior to dosing with extended release propafenone. The use of propafenone with Class Ia antiarrythmic agents is not recommended).
- No products indexed under this heading.

Quinidine Gluconate (The use of propafenone in conjunction with other drugs that prolong the QT interval has not been extensively studied and is not recommended).
- No products indexed under this heading.

Quinidine Hydrochloride (Class Ia antiarrythmic agents should be withheld for at least five half-lives prior to dosing with extended release propafenone. The use of propafenone with Class Ia antiarrythmic agents is not recommended).
- No products indexed under this heading.

Quinidine Polygalacturonate (The use of propafenone in conjunction with other drugs that prolong the QT interval has not been extensively studied and is not recommended).
- No products indexed under this heading.

Quinidine Sulfate (The use of propafenone in conjunction with other drugs that prolong the QT interval has not been extensively studied and is not recommended).
- No products indexed under this heading.

Quinine (Drugs that inhibit CYP3A4 might lead to increased plasma levels of propafenone; patients should be closely monitored and the propafenone dose adjusted accordingly).
- No products indexed under this heading.

Quinine Sulfate (Drugs that inhibit CYP3A4 might lead to increased plasma levels of propafenone; patients should be closely monitored and the propafenone dose adjusted accordingly).
- No products indexed under this heading.

Quinupristin (Drugs that inhibit CYP3A4 might lead to increased plasma levels of propafenone; patients should be closely monitored and the propafenone dose adjusted accordingly).
- No products indexed under this heading.

Ranitidine Bismuth Citrate (Drugs that inhibit CYP2D6 might lead to increased plasma levels of propafenone; patients should be closely monitored and the propafenone dose adjusted accordingly).
- No products indexed under this heading.

Ranitidine Hydrochloride (Drugs that inhibit CYP2D6 might lead to increased plasma levels of propafenone; patients should be closely monitored and the propafenone dose adjusted accordingly). Products include:
- Zantac 75 Tablets .... ▣603
- Zantac 1670
- Zantac Injection 1666
- Zantac Injection Pharmacy Bulk Package 1668
- Maximum Strength Zantac 150 Tablets .... ▣603

(▣ Described in PDR® For Nonprescription Drugs)

(⊙ Described in PDR® For Ophthalmic Medicines)

Maximum Strength Zantac 150 Cool Mint Tablets 603

Rifampin (May accelerate the metabolism and decrease the plasma levels and antiarythmic efficacy of propafenone).
No products indexed under this heading.

Risperidone (The use of propafenone in conjunction with other drugs that prolong the QT interval has not been extensively studied and is not recommended). Products include:
Risperdal Consta Long-Acting Injection 1753

Ritonavir (Drugs that inhibit CYP2D6 might lead to increased plasma levels of propafenone; patients should be closely monitored and the propafenone dose adjusted accordingly). Products include:
Kaletra 452
Norvir 489

Saquinavir (Drugs that inhibit CYP3A4 might lead to increased plasma levels of propafenone; patients should be closely monitored and the propafenone dose adjusted accordingly).
No products indexed under this heading.

Saquinavir Mesylate (Drugs that inhibit CYP3A4 might lead to increased plasma levels of propafenone; patients should be closely monitored and the propafenone dose adjusted accordingly).
No products indexed under this heading.

Sertraline Hydrochloride (Drugs that inhibit CYP2D6 might lead to increased plasma levels of propafenone; patients should be closely monitored and the propafenone dose adjusted accordingly).
No products indexed under this heading.

Sildenafil Citrate (Drugs that inhibit CYP2D6 might lead to increased plasma levels of propafenone; patients should be closely monitored and the propafenone dose adjusted accordingly).
No products indexed under this heading.

Sotalol Hydrochloride (Class III antiarrythmic agents should be withheld for at least five half-lives prior to dosing with extended release propafenone. The use of propafenone with Class III antiarrythmic agents is not recommended).
No products indexed under this heading.

Sparfloxacin (Drugs that inhibit CYP1A2 might lead to increased plasma levels of propafenone; patients should be closely monitored and the propafenone dose adjusted accordingly).
No products indexed under this heading.

Tacrine Hydrochloride (Drugs that inhibit CYP1A2 might lead to increased plasma levels of propafenone; patients should be closely monitored and the propafenone dose adjusted accordingly).
No products indexed under this heading.

Telithromycin (Drugs that inhibit CYP3A4 might lead to increased plasma levels of propafenone; patients should be closely monitored and the propafenone dose adjusted accordingly). Products include:
Ketek Tablets 2744

Terbinafine Hydrochloride (Drugs that inhibit CYP2D6 might lead to increased plasma levels of propafenone; patients should be closely monitored and the propafenone dose adjusted accordingly). Products include:
Lamisil Oral Granules 2264
Lamisil Tablets 2266

Tetracaine Hydrochloride (Concomitant use of local anesthetics may increase the risk of CNS side effects).
No products indexed under this heading.

Theophylline (Combined therapy may result in an increase in theophylline concentration with the development of theophylline toxicity).
No products indexed under this heading.

Theophylline Anhydrous (Combined therapy may result in an increase in theophylline concentration with the development of theophylline toxicity). Products include:
Uniphyl Tablets 2595

Theophylline Calcium Salicylate (Combined therapy may result in an increase in theophylline concentration with the development of theophylline toxicity).
No products indexed under this heading.

Theophylline Dihydroxypropyl (Glyceryl) (Combined therapy may result in an increase in theophylline concentration with the development of theophylline toxicity).
No products indexed under this heading.

Theophylline Ethylenediamine (Combined therapy may result in an increase in theophylline concentration with the development of theophylline toxicity).
No products indexed under this heading.

Theophylline Sodium Glycinate (Combined therapy may result in an increase in theophylline concentration with the development of theophylline toxicity).
No products indexed under this heading.

Thioridazine Hydrochloride (The use of propafenone in conjunction with other drugs that prolong the QT interval has not been extensively studied and is not recommended). Products include:
Thioridazine Hydrochloride Tablets 2195

Thiothixene (The use of propafenone in conjunction with other drugs that prolong the QT interval has not been extensively studied and is not recommended). Products include:
Thiothixene Capsules 2197

Ticlopidine Hydrochloride (Drugs that inhibit CYP1A2 might lead to increased plasma levels of propafenone; patients should be closely monitored and the propafenone dose adjusted accordingly).
No products indexed under this heading.

Tocainide Hydrochloride (The use of propafenone in conjunction with other drugs that prolong the QT interval has not been extensively studied and is not recommended).
No products indexed under this heading.

Tranylcypromine Sulfate (The use of propafenone in conjunction with other drugs that prolong the QT interval has not been extensively studied and is not recommended). Products include:
Parnate Tablets 1532

Trifluoperazine Hydrochloride (The use of propafenone in conjunction with other drugs that prolong the QT interval has not been extensively studied and is not recommended).
No products indexed under this heading.

Trimipramine Maleate (The use of propafenone in conjunction with other drugs that prolong the QT interval has not been extensively studied and is not recommended).
No products indexed under this heading.

Troglitazone (Drugs that inhibit CYP3A4 might lead to increased plasma levels of propafenone; patients should be closely monitored and the propafenone dose adjusted accordingly).
No products indexed under this heading.

Troleandomycin (The use of propafenone in conjunction with other drugs that prolong the QT interval has not been extensively studied and is not recommended).
No products indexed under this heading.

Trovafloxacin Mesylate (Drugs that inhibit CYP1A2 might lead to increased plasma levels of propafenone; patients should be closely monitored and the propafenone dose adjusted accordingly).
No products indexed under this heading.

Valproate Sodium (Drugs that inhibit CYP3A4 might lead to increased plasma levels of propafenone; patients should be closely monitored and the propafenone dose adjusted accordingly).
No products indexed under this heading.

Vardenafil Hydrochloride (Drugs that inhibit CYP2D6 might lead to increased plasma levels of propafenone; patients should be closely monitored and the propafenone dose adjusted accordingly). Products include:
Levitra Tablets 2876

Verapamil Hydrochloride (Drugs that inhibit CYP3A4 might lead to increased plasma levels of propafenone; patients should be closely monitored and the propafenone dose adjusted accordingly). Products include:
Tarka Tablets 511

Voriconazole (Drugs that inhibit CYP3A4 might lead to increased plasma levels of propafenone; patients should be closely monitored and the propafenone dose adjusted accordingly).
No products indexed under this heading.

Warfarin Sodium (Increase in mean steady-state plasma levels of warfarin resulting in increased prothrombin time).
No products indexed under this heading.

Zafirlukast (Drugs that inhibit CYP3A4 might lead to increased plasma levels of propafenone; patients should be closely monitored and the propafenone dose adjusted accordingly). Products include:
Accolate Tablets 669

Zileuton (Drugs that inhibit CYP1A2 might lead to increased plasma levels of propafenone; patients should be closely monitored and the propafenone dose adjusted accordingly).
No products indexed under this heading.

Ziprasidone Hydrochloride (The use of propafenone in conjunction with other drugs that prolong the QT interval has not been extensively studied and is not recommended). Products include:
Geodon Capsules 2520

Food Interactions

Food, unspecified (Increased peak blood level and bioavailability in a single dose study).

Grapefruit (Drugs that inhibit CYP3A4 might lead to increased plasma levels of propafenone; patients should be closely monitored and the propafenone dose adjusted accordingly).

Grapefruit Juice (Drugs that inhibit CYP1A2 might lead to increased plasma levels of propafenone; patients should be closely monitored and the propafenone dose adjusted accordingly).

ST. JOSEPH 81 MG ASPIRIN CHEWABLE AND ENTERIC COATED TABLETS

(Aspirin) 1903

May interact with ACE inhibitors, beta blockers, anticoagulants, diuretics, oral hypoglycemic agents, non-steroidal anti-inflammatory agents, phenytoin, valproate, and certain other agents. Compounds in these categories include:

Acarbose (Moderate doses of aspirin may increase the effectiveness of oral hypoglycemic agents leading to hypoglycemia). Products include:
Precose Tablets 792

Acebutolol Hydrochloride (Decreased hypotensive effects of beta-blockers).
No products indexed under this heading.

Acetazolamide (Co-administration can lead to high serum concentrations of acetazolamide and its toxicity).
No products indexed under this heading.

Acetazolamide Sodium (Co-administration can lead to high serum concentrations of acetazolamide and its toxicity).
No products indexed under this heading.

Amiloride Hydrochloride (Diminished effectiveness of diuretics in patients with underlying renal or cardiovascular disease).
No products indexed under this heading.

Anisindione (Patients on anticoagulant therapy are at increased risk of bleeding).
No products indexed under this heading.

Ardeparin Sodium (Patients on anticoagulant therapy are at increased risk of bleeding).
No products indexed under this heading.

Atenolol (Decreased hypotensive effects of beta-blockers).
No products indexed under this heading.

Benazepril Hydrochloride (Co-administration may result in diminished hyponatremic and hypotensive effects of ACE inhibitors).
No products indexed under this heading.

Bendroflumethiazide (Diminished effectiveness of diuretics in patients with underlying renal or cardiovascular disease).
No products indexed under this heading.

Betaxolol Hydrochloride (Decreased hypotensive effects of beta-blockers).
No products indexed under this heading.

Bisoprolol Fumarate (Decreased hypotensive effects of beta-blockers).
No products indexed under this heading.

Bumetanide (Diminished effectiveness of diuretics in patients with underlying renal or cardiovascular disease).
No products indexed under this heading.

Captopril (Co-administration may result in diminished hyponatremic and hypotensive effects of ACE inhibitors). Products include:
Captopril Tablets 2182

Carteolol Hydrochloride (Decreased hypotensive effects of beta-blockers).
No products indexed under this heading.

Celecoxib (Co-administration may increase bleeding or lead to decreased renal function). Products include:
Celebrex Capsules 2979

Chlorothiazide (Diminished effectiveness of diuretics in patients with underlying renal or cardiovascular disease).
No products indexed under this heading.

Chlorothiazide Sodium (Diminished effectiveness of diuretics in patients with underlying renal or cardiovascular disease). Products include:
Intravenous Sodium Diuril 2490

Chlorpropamide (Moderate doses of aspirin may increase the effectiveness of oral hypoglycemic agents leading to hypoglycemia).
No products indexed under this heading.

Chlorthalidone (Diminished effectiveness of diuretics in patients with underlying renal or cardiovascular disease). Products include:
Clorpres Tablets 2185

Dalteparin Sodium (Patients on anticoagulant therapy are at increased risk of bleeding). Products include:
Fragmin Injection 1070

Danaparoid Sodium (Patients on anticoagulant therapy are at increased risk of bleeding).
No products indexed under this heading.

Diclofenac Epolamine (Co-administration may increase bleeding or lead to decreased renal function). Products include:
Flector Patch 561

Diclofenac Potassium (Co-administration may increase bleeding or lead to decreased renal function).
No products indexed under this heading.

Diclofenac Sodium (Co-administration may increase bleeding or lead to decreased renal function). Products include:
Diclofenac Sodium Ophthalmic Solution .... ⊙240
Voltaren Ophthalmic Solution 2336
Voltaren Tablets 2334
Voltaren-XR Tablets 2337

Dicumarol (Patients on anticoagulant therapy are at increased risk of bleeding).
No products indexed under this heading.

Divalproex Sodium (Salicylate can displace protein-bound valproic acid leading to an increase in serum valproic acid levels). Products include:
Depakote ER Tablets 423

Enalapril Maleate (Co-administration may result in diminished hyponatremic and hypotensive effects of ACE inhibitors).
No products indexed under this heading.

Enalaprilat (Co-administration may result in diminished hyponatremic and hypotensive effects of ACE inhibitors).
No products indexed under this heading.

Enoxaparin Sodium (Patients on anticoagulant therapy are at increased risk of bleeding). Products include:
Lovenox Injection 2756

Esmolol Hydrochloride (Decreased hypotensive effects of beta-blockers).
No products indexed under this heading.

Ethacrynic Acid (Diminished effectiveness of diuretics in patients with underlying renal or cardiovascular disease). Products include:
Edecrin Tablets 698

Etodolac (Co-administration may increase bleeding or lead to decreased renal function).
No products indexed under this heading.

Fenoprofen Calcium (Co-administration may increase bleeding or lead to decreased renal function). Products include:
Nalfon Capsules 2508

Flurbiprofen (Co-administration may increase bleeding or lead to decreased renal function).
No products indexed under this heading.

Fondaparinux Sodium (Patients on anticoagulant therapy are at increased risk of bleeding). Products include:
Arixtra Injection 1313

Fosinopril Sodium (Co-administration may result in diminished hyponatremic and hypotensive effects of ACE inhibitors).
No products indexed under this heading.

Fosphenytoin Sodium (Salicylate can displace protein-bound phenytoin leading to a decrease in the total concentration of phenytoin).
No products indexed under this heading.

Furosemide (Diminished effectiveness of diuretics in patients with underlying renal or cardiovascular disease). Products include:
Furosemide Tablets 2186

Glimepiride (Moderate doses of aspirin may increase the effectiveness of oral hypoglycemic agents leading to hypoglycemia). Products include:
Avandaryl Tablets 1344
Duetact Tablets 3085

Glipizide (Moderate doses of aspirin may increase the effectiveness of oral hypoglycemic agents leading to hypoglycemia).
No products indexed under this heading.

Glyburide (Moderate doses of aspirin may increase the effectiveness of oral hypoglycemic agents leading to hypoglycemia).
No products indexed under this heading.

Heparin Calcium (Patients on anticoagulant therapy are at increased risk of bleeding).
No products indexed under this heading.

Heparin Sodium (Aspirin can increase the anticoagulant activity of heparin increasing bleeding risk).
No products indexed under this heading.

Hydrochlorothiazide (Diminished effectiveness of diuretics in patients with underlying renal or cardiovascular disease). Products include:
Atacand HCT 642
Avalide Tablets 892
Avalide Tablets 2713
Benicar HCT Tablets 1010
Diovan HCT Tablets 2216
Dyazide Capsules 1405
Micardis HCT Tablets 854
Prinzide Tablets 2092
Tekturna HCT Tablets 2324
Teveten HCT Tablets 517

Hydroflumethiazide (Diminished effectiveness of diuretics in patients with underlying renal or cardiovascular disease).
No products indexed under this heading.

Ibuprofen (Co-administration may increase bleeding or lead to decreased renal function). Products include:
Motrin IB Tablets and Caplets 1900
Children's Motrin Oral Suspension ... 1901
Children's Motrin Non-Staining Dye-Free Oral Suspension 1901
Children's Motrin Cold Oral Suspension 1899
Infants' Motrin Concentrated Drops 1901
Infants' Motrin Non-Staining Dye-Free Concentrated Drops 1901
Junior Strength Motrin Caplets and Chewable Tablets 1901
Vicoprofen Tablets 533

Indapamide (Diminished effectiveness of diuretics in patients with underlying renal or cardiovascular disease). Products include:
Indapamide Tablets 2188

Indomethacin (Co-administration may increase bleeding or lead to decreased renal function). Products include:
Indocin 2024

Indomethacin Sodium Trihydrate (Co-administration may increase bleeding or lead to decreased renal function). Products include:
Indocin I.V. 2489

Ketoprofen (Co-administration may increase bleeding or lead to decreased renal function).
No products indexed under this heading.

Ketorolac Tromethamine (Co-administration may increase bleeding or lead to decreased renal function).
No products indexed under this heading.

Labetalol Hydrochloride (Decreased hypotensive effects of beta-blockers).
No products indexed under this heading.

Levobunolol Hydrochloride (Decreased hypotensive effects of beta-blockers).
No products indexed under this heading.

Lisinopril (Co-administration may result in diminished hyponatremic and hypotensive effects of ACE inhibitors). Products include:
Prinivil Tablets 2087
Prinzide Tablets 2092

Low Molecular Weight Heparins (Patients on anticoagulant therapy are at increased risk of bleeding).
No products indexed under this heading.

Meclofenamate Sodium (Co-administration may increase bleeding or lead to decreased renal function).
No products indexed under this heading.

Mefenamic Acid (Co-administration may increase bleeding or lead to decreased renal function).
No products indexed under this heading.

Meloxicam (Co-administration may increase bleeding or lead to decreased renal function). Products include:
Mobic Oral Suspension 863
Mobic Tablets 863

Metformin Hydrochloride (Moderate doses of aspirin may increase the effectiveness of oral hypoglycemic agents leading to hypoglycemia). Products include:
ActoPlus Met Tablets 3071
Avandamet Tablets 1336
Janumet Tablets 2041
PrandiMet Tablets 2967

Methotrexate Sodium (Salicylate can inhibit renal clearance of methotrexate leading to bone marrow toxicity, especially in the elderly or renal impaired).
No products indexed under this heading.

Methyclothiazide (Diminished effectiveness of diuretics in patients with underlying renal or cardiovascular disease).
No products indexed under this heading.

Metipranolol Hydrochloride (Decreased hypotensive effects of beta-blockers).
No products indexed under this heading.

Metolazone (Diminished effectiveness of diuretics in patients with underlying renal or cardiovascular disease).
No products indexed under this heading.

Metoprolol Succinate (Decreased hypotensive effects of beta-blockers). Products include:

Toprol-XL Tablets 666

Metoprolol Tartrate (Decreased hypotensive effects of beta-blockers).
No products indexed under this heading.

Miglitol (Moderate doses of aspirin may increase the effectiveness of oral hypoglycemic agents leading to hypoglycemia).
No products indexed under this heading.

Moexipril Hydrochloride (Co-administration may result in diminished hyponatremic and hypotensive effects of ACE inhibitors).
No products indexed under this heading.

Nabumetone (Co-administration may increase bleeding or lead to decreased renal function).
No products indexed under this heading.

Nadolol (Decreased hypotensive effects of beta-blockers). Products include:
Nadolol Tablets 2191

Naproxen (Co-administration may increase bleeding or lead to decreased renal function). Products include:
EC-Naprosyn Delayed-Release Tablets 2632
Naprosyn Suspension 2632
Naprosyn Tablets 2632

Naproxen Sodium (Co-administration may increase bleeding or lead to decreased renal function). Products include:
Anaprox Tablets 2632
Anaprox DS Tablets 2632
Treximet Tablets 1616

Nateglinide (Moderate doses of aspirin may increase the effectiveness of oral hypoglycemic agents leading to hypoglycemia). Products include:
Starlix Tablets 2314

Nebivolol (Decreased hypotensive effects of beta-blockers). Products include:
Bystolic Tablets 1155

Oxaprozin (Co-administration may increase bleeding or lead to decreased renal function).
No products indexed under this heading.

Penbutolol Sulfate (Decreased hypotensive effects of beta-blockers).
No products indexed under this heading.

Perindopril Erbumine (Co-administration may result in diminished hyponatremic and hypotensive effects of ACE inhibitors). Products include:
Aceon Tablets (2 mg, 4 mg, 8 mg) 3038

Phenylbutazone (Co-administration may increase bleeding or lead to decreased renal function).
No products indexed under this heading.

Phenytoin (Salicylate can displace protein-bound phenytoin leading to a decrease in the total concentration of phenytoin).
No products indexed under this heading.

Phenytoin Sodium (Salicylate can displace protein-bound phenytoin leading to a decrease in the total concentration of phenytoin). Products include:
Phenytek Capsules 2192

Pindolol (Decreased hypotensive effects of beta-blockers).
No products indexed under this heading.

Pioglitazone Hydrochloride (Moderate doses of aspirin may increase the effectiveness of oral hypoglycemic agents leading to hypoglycemia). Products include:
ActoPlus Met Tablets 3071
Actos Tablets 3077
Duetact Tablets 3085

Piroxicam (Co-administration may increase bleeding or lead to decreased renal function).
No products indexed under this heading.

Polythiazide (Diminished effectiveness of diuretics in patients with underlying renal or cardiovascular disease).
No products indexed under this heading.

Probenecid (Salicylate antagonizes the uricosuric action of probenecid).
No products indexed under this heading.

Propranolol Hydrochloride (Decreased hypotensive effects of beta-blockers). Products include:
InnoPran XL Extended Release Capsules 1484

Quinapril Hydrochloride (Co-administration may result in diminished hyponatremic and hypotensive effects of ACE inhibitors).
No products indexed under this heading.

Ramipril (Co-administration may result in diminished hyponatremic and hypotensive effects of ACE inhibitors).
No products indexed under this heading.

Repaglinide (Moderate doses of aspirin may increase the effectiveness of oral hypoglycemic agents leading to hypoglycemia). Products include:
PrandiMet Tablets 2967
Prandin Tablets 2971

Rofecoxib (Co-administration may increase bleeding or lead to decreased renal function).
No products indexed under this heading.

Rosiglitazone Maleate (Moderate doses of aspirin may increase the effectiveness of oral hypoglycemic agents leading to hypoglycemia). Products include:
Avandamet Tablets 1336
Avandaryl Tablets 1344
Avandia Tablets 1351

Sitagliptin Phosphate (Moderate doses of aspirin may increase the effectiveness of oral hypoglycemic agents leading to hypoglycemia). Products include:
Janumet Tablets 2041
Januvia Tablets 2048

Sotalol Hydrochloride (Decreased hypotensive effects of beta-blockers).
No products indexed under this heading.

Spirapril Hydrochloride (Co-administration may result in diminished hyponatremic and hypotensive effects of ACE inhibitors).
No products indexed under this heading.

Spironolactone (Diminished effectiveness of diuretics in patients with underlying renal or cardiovascular disease).
No products indexed under this heading.

Sulfinpyrazone (Salicylate antagonizes the uricosuric action of sulfinpyrazone).
No products indexed under this heading.

Sulindac (Co-administration may increase bleeding or lead to decreased renal function). Products include:
Clinoril Tablets 1962

Timolol Hemihydrate (Decreased hypotensive effects of beta-blockers). Products include:
Betimol Ophthalmic Solution 3181

Timolol Maleate (Decreased hypotensive effects of beta-blockers). Products include:
Combigan Ophthalmic Solution 553
Cosopt Sterile Ophthalmic Solution 1969
Timoptic Sterile Ophthalmic Solution 2121
Timoptic in Ocudose 2124
Timoptic-XE Sterile Ophthalmic Gel Forming Solution 2125

Tinzaparin Sodium (Patients on anticoagulant therapy are at increased risk of bleeding).
No products indexed under this heading.

Tolazamide (Moderate doses of aspirin may increase the effectiveness of oral hypoglycemic agents leading to hypoglycemia).
No products indexed under this heading.

Tolbutamide (Moderate doses of aspirin may increase the effectiveness of oral hypoglycemic agents leading to hypoglycemia).
No products indexed under this heading.

Tolmetin Sodium (Co-administration may increase bleeding or lead to decreased renal function).
No products indexed under this heading.

Torsemide (Diminished effectiveness of diuretics in patients with underlying renal or cardiovascular disease). Products include:
Demadex Injection 2630
Demadex Tablets 2630

Trandolapril (Co-administration may result in diminished hyponatremic and hypotensive effects of ACE inhibitors). Products include:
Mavik Tablets 472
Tarka Tablets 511

Triamterene (Diminished effectiveness of diuretics in patients with underlying renal or cardiovascular disease). Products include:
Dyazide Capsules 1405
Dyrenium Capsules 3189

Troglitazone (Moderate doses of aspirin may increase the effectiveness of oral hypoglycemic agents leading to hypoglycemia).
No products indexed under this heading.

Valdecoxib (Co-administration may increase bleeding or lead to decreased renal function).
No products indexed under this heading.

Valproate Sodium (Salicylate can displace protein-bound valproic acid leading to an increase in serum valproic acid levels).
No products indexed under this heading.

Valproic Acid (Salicylate can displace protein-bound valproic acid leading to an increase in serum valproic acid levels).
No products indexed under this heading.

Warfarin Sodium (Aspirin can displace Warfarin from protein binding sites leading to prolongation of both the prothrombin time and the bleeding time).
No products indexed under this heading.

Food Interactions

Alcohol (Chronic heavy alcohol users, 3 or more drinks per day, in combination with analgesic/antipyretic drug products containing aspirin increases the risk of adverse GI events, including stomach bleeding).

SALAGEN TABLETS

(Pilocarpine Hydrochloride) 1082
May interact with anticholinergics, beta blockers, and parasympathomimetics. Compounds in these categories include:

Acebutolol Hydrochloride (Pilocarpine should be administered with caution in patients taking beta adrenergic antagonists because of the possibility of conduction disturbances).
No products indexed under this heading.

Atenolol (Pilocarpine should be administered with caution in patients taking beta adrenergic antagonists because of the possibility of conduction disturbances).
No products indexed under this heading.

Atropine Sulfate (Pilocarpine might antagonize the anticholinergic effects of drugs used concomitantly. These effects should be considered when anticholinergic properties may be contributing to the therapeutic effect of concomitant medication). Products include:
Donnatal Extentabs 2507

Belladonna Alkaloids (Pilocarpine might antagonize the anticholinergic effects of drugs used concomitantly. These effects should be considered when anticholinergic properties may be contributing to the therapeutic effect of concomitant medication). Products include:
Hyland's Teething Tablets 621

Benztropine Mesylate (Pilocarpine might antagonize the anticholinergic effects of drugs used concomitantly. These effects should be considered when anticholinergic properties may be contributing to the therapeutic effect of concomitant medication).
No products indexed under this heading.

Betaxolol Hydrochloride (Pilocarpine should be administered with caution in patients taking beta adrenergic antagonists because of the possibility of conduction disturbances).
No products indexed under this heading.

IMPORTANT NOTE: Always consult each drug listing in the patient's regimen for possible interactions.

Biperiden Hydrochloride (Pilocarpine might antagonize the anticholinergic effects of drugs used concomitantly. These effects should be considered when anticholinergic properties may be contributing to the therapeutic effect of concomitant medication).
No products indexed under this heading.

Bisoprolol Fumarate (Pilocarpine should be administered with caution in patients taking beta adrenergic antagonists because of the possibility of conduction disturbances).
No products indexed under this heading.

Carteolol Hydrochloride (Pilocarpine should be administered with caution in patients taking beta adrenergic antagonists because of the possibility of conduction disturbances).
No products indexed under this heading.

Cevimeline Hydrochloride (Drugs with parasympathomimetic effects administered concurrently with pilocarpine would be expected to result in additive pharmacologic effects).
Products include:
Evoxac Capsules 1013

Clidinium Bromide (Pilocarpine might antagonize the anticholinergic effects of drugs used concomitantly. These effects should be considered when anticholinergic properties may be contributing to the therapeutic effect of concomitant medication).
No products indexed under this heading.

Dicyclomine Hydrochloride (Pilocarpine might antagonize the anticholinergic effects of drugs used concomitantly. These effects should be considered when anticholinergic properties may be contributing to the therapeutic effect of concomitant medication). Products include:
Bentyl Capsules 703
Bentyl Injection 703
Bentyl Syrup 703
Bentyl Tablets 703

Edrophonium Chloride (Drugs with parasympathomimetic effects administered concurrently with pilocarpine would be expected to result in additive pharmacologic effects).
No products indexed under this heading.

Esmolol Hydrochloride (Pilocarpine should be administered with caution in patients taking beta adrenergic antagonists because of the possibility of conduction disturbances).
No products indexed under this heading.

Glycopyrrolate (Pilocarpine might antagonize the anticholinergic effects of drugs used concomitantly. These effects should be considered when anticholinergic properties may be contributing to the therapeutic effect of concomitant medication).
No products indexed under this heading.

Hyoscyamine (Pilocarpine might antagonize the anticholinergic effects of drugs used concomitantly. These effects should be considered when anticholinergic properties may be contributing to the therapeutic effect of concomitant medication).
No products indexed under this heading.

Hyoscyamine Sulfate (Pilocarpine might antagonize the anticholinergic effects of drugs used concomitantly. These effects should be considered when anticholinergic properties may be contributing to the therapeutic effect of concomitant medication).
Products include:
Donnatal Extentabs 2507

Ipratropium Bromide (Pilocarpine might antagonize the anticholinergic effects of drugs used concomitantly. These effects should be considered when anticholinergic properties may be contributing to the therapeutic effect of concomitant medication).
Products include:
Atrovent HFA Inhalation Aerosol 839
Atrovent Nasal Spray 0.03% 834
Atrovent Nasal Spray 0.06% 836
Combivent Inhalation Aerosol 845

Labetalol Hydrochloride (Pilocarpine should be administered with caution in patients taking beta adrenergic antagonists because of the possibility of conduction disturbances).
No products indexed under this heading.

Levobunolol Hydrochloride (Pilocarpine should be administered with caution in patients taking beta adrenergic antagonists because of the possibility of conduction disturbances).
No products indexed under this heading.

Mepenzolate Bromide (Pilocarpine might antagonize the anticholinergic effects of drugs used concomitantly. These effects should be considered when anticholinergic properties may be contributing to the therapeutic effect of concomitant medication).
No products indexed under this heading.

Metipranolol Hydrochloride (Pilocarpine should be administered with caution in patients taking beta adrenergic antagonists because of the possibility of conduction disturbances).
No products indexed under this heading.

Metoprolol Succinate (Pilocarpine should be administered with caution in patients taking beta adrenergic antagonists because of the possibility of conduction disturbances).
Products include:
Toprol-XL Tablets 666

Metoprolol Tartrate (Pilocarpine should be administered with caution in patients taking beta adrenergic antagonists because of the possibility of conduction disturbances).
No products indexed under this heading.

Nadolol (Pilocarpine should be administered with caution in patients taking beta adrenergic antagonists because of the possibility of conduction disturbances). Products include:
Nadolol Tablets 2191

Nebivolol (Pilocarpine should be administered with caution in patients taking beta adrenergic antagonists because of the possibility of conduction disturbances). Products include:
Bystolic Tablets 1155

Neostigmine Bromide (Drugs with parasympathomimetic effects administered concurrently with pilocarpine would be expected to result in additive pharmacologic effects).
No products indexed under this heading.

Neostigmine Methylsulfate (Drugs with parasympathomimetic effects administered concurrently with pilocarpine would be expected to result in additive pharmacologic effects).
No products indexed under this heading.

Oxybutynin Chloride (Pilocarpine might antagonize the anticholinergic effects of drugs used concomitantly. These effects should be considered when anticholinergic properties may be contributing to the therapeutic effect of concomitant medication).
No products indexed under this heading.

Penbutolol Sulfate (Pilocarpine should be administered with caution in patients taking beta adrenergic antagonists because of the possibility of conduction disturbances).
No products indexed under this heading.

Pindolol (Pilocarpine should be administered with caution in patients taking beta adrenergic antagonists because of the possibility of conduction disturbances).
No products indexed under this heading.

Procyclidine Hydrochloride (Pilocarpine might antagonize the anticholinergic effects of drugs used concomitantly. These effects should be considered when anticholinergic properties may be contributing to the therapeutic effect of concomitant medication).
No products indexed under this heading.

Propantheline Bromide (Pilocarpine might antagonize the anticholinergic effects of drugs used concomitantly. These effects should be considered when anticholinergic properties may be contributing to the therapeutic effect of concomitant medication).
No products indexed under this heading.

Propranolol Hydrochloride (Pilocarpine should be administered with caution in patients taking beta adrenergic antagonists because of the possibility of conduction disturbances). Products include:
InnoPran XL Extended Release Capsules 1484

Pyridostigmine Bromide (Drugs with parasympathomimetic effects administered concurrently with pilocarpine would be expected to result in additive pharmacologic effects).
No products indexed under this heading.

Scopolamine (Pilocarpine might antagonize the anticholinergic effects of drugs used concomitantly. These effects should be considered when anticholinergic properties may be contributing to the therapeutic effect of concomitant medication).
Products include:
Transderm Scōp Transdermal Therapeutic System 2206

Scopolamine Hydrobromide (Pilocarpine might antagonize the anticholinergic effects of drugs used concomitantly. These effects should be considered when anticholinergic properties may be contributing to the therapeutic effect of concomitant medication). Products include:
Donnatal Extentabs 2507

Sotalol Hydrochloride (Pilocarpine should be administered with caution in patients taking beta adrenergic antagonists because of the possibility of conduction disturbances).
No products indexed under this heading.

Timolol Hemihydrate (Pilocarpine should be administered with caution in patients taking beta adrenergic antagonists because of the possibility of conduction disturbances).
Products include:
Betimol Ophthalmic Solution 3181

Timolol Maleate (Pilocarpine should be administered with caution in patients taking beta adrenergic antagonists because of the possibility of conduction disturbances).
Products include:
Combigan Ophthalmic Solution 553
Cosopt Sterile Ophthalmic Solution 1969
Timoptic Sterile Ophthalmic Solution 2121
Timoptic in Ocudose 2124
Timoptic-XE Sterile Ophthalmic Gel Forming Solution 2125

Tolterodine Tartrate (Pilocarpine might antagonize the anticholinergic effects of drugs used concomitantly. These effects should be considered when anticholinergic properties may be contributing to the therapeutic effect of concomitant medication).
No products indexed under this heading.

Tridihexethyl Chloride (Pilocarpine might antagonize the anticholinergic effects of drugs used concomitantly. These effects should be considered when anticholinergic properties may be contributing to the therapeutic effect of concomitant medication).
No products indexed under this heading.

Trihexyphenidyl Hydrochloride (Pilocarpine might antagonize the anticholinergic effects of drugs used concomitantly. These effects should be considered when anticholinergic properties may be contributing to the therapeutic effect of concomitant medication).
No products indexed under this heading.

SALONPAS AQUA-PATCH

(Menthol) .... ■610
None cited in PDR database.

SALONPAS ARTHRITIS PAIN PATCHES

(Menthol, Methyl Salicylate) .... ■608
May interact with aspirin-acetylsalicylic acid, anticoagulants, corticosteroids, non-steroidal anti-inflammatory agents, and certain other agents. Compounds in these categories include:

Anisindione (Taking a blood thinning agent (eg, anticoagulants) may increase the chance stomach bleeding).
No products indexed under this heading.

Ardeparin Sodium (Taking a blood thinning agent (eg, anticoagulants) may increase the chance stomach bleeding).
No products indexed under this heading.

Aspirin (Taking other drugs containing aspirin increases the chance of causing stomach bleeding).
Products include:
- Aggrenox Capsules 819
- Bayer Aspirin 750
- Percodan Tablets 1130
- St. Joseph 81 mg Aspirin Chewable and Enteric Coated Tablets 1903

Aspirin, Enteric Coated (Taking other drugs containing aspirin increases the chance of causing stomach bleeding).
No products indexed under this heading.

Aspirin Buffered (Taking other drugs containing aspirin increases the chance of causing stomach bleeding).
No products indexed under this heading.

Betamethasone Acetate (Taking a steroid may increase the chance of stomach bleeding).
No products indexed under this heading.

Betamethasone Sodium Phosphate (Taking a steroid may increase the chance of stomach bleeding).
No products indexed under this heading.

Budesonide (Taking a steroid may increase the chance of stomach bleeding). Products include:
- Pulmicort Flexhaler 654
- Symbicort 80/4.5 Inhalation Aerosol 659
- Symbicort 160/4.5 Inhalation Aerosol 659

Celecoxib (Taking other drugs containing an NSAID (e.g., ibuprofen, naproxen, or others) increases the chance of causing stomach bleeding). Products include:
- Celebrex Capsules 2979

Ciclesonide (Taking a steroid may increase the chance of stomach bleeding). Products include:
- Alvesco Inhalation Aerosol 2985
- Omnaris Nasal Spray 2998

Cortisone Acetate (Taking a steroid may increase the chance of stomach bleeding).
No products indexed under this heading.

Dalteparin Sodium (Taking a blood thinning agent (eg, anticoagulants) may increase the chance stomach bleeding). Products include:
- Fragmin Injection 1070

Danaparoid Sodium (Taking a blood thinning agent (eg, anticoagulants) may increase the chance stomach bleeding).
No products indexed under this heading.

Dexamethasone (Taking a steroid may increase the chance of stomach bleeding). Products include:
- Ciprodex Otic Suspension 541

Dexamethasone Acetate (Taking a steroid may increase the chance of stomach bleeding).
No products indexed under this heading.

Dexamethasone Sodium Phosphate (Taking a steroid may increase the chance of stomach bleeding).
No products indexed under this heading.

Diclofenac Epolamine (Taking other drugs containing an NSAID (e.g., ibuprofen, naproxen, or others) increases the chance of causing stomach bleeding). Products include:
- Flector Patch 561

Diclofenac Potassium (Taking other drugs containing an NSAID (e.g., ibuprofen, naproxen, or others) increases the chance of causing stomach bleeding).
No products indexed under this heading.

Diclofenac Sodium (Taking other drugs containing an NSAID (e.g., ibuprofen, naproxen, or others) increases the chance of causing stomach bleeding). Products include:
- Diclofenac Sodium Ophthalmic Solution ⊙ 240
- Voltaren Ophthalmic Solution 2336
- Voltaren Tablets 2334
- Voltaren-XR Tablets 2337

Dicumarol (Taking a blood thinning agent (eg, anticoagulants) may increase the chance stomach bleeding).
No products indexed under this heading.

Enoxaparin Sodium (Taking a blood thinning agent (eg, anticoagulants) may increase the chance stomach bleeding). Products include:
- Lovenox Injection 2756

Etodolac (Taking other drugs containing an NSAID (e.g., ibuprofen, naproxen, or others) increases the chance of causing stomach bleeding).
No products indexed under this heading.

Fenoprofen Calcium (Taking other drugs containing an NSAID (e.g., ibuprofen, naproxen, or others) increases the chance of causing stomach bleeding). Products include:
- Nalfon Capsules 2508

Fludrocortisone Acetate (Taking a steroid may increase the chance of stomach bleeding).
No products indexed under this heading.

Flunisolide (Taking a steroid may increase the chance of stomach bleeding). Products include:
- Aerobid/Aerobid-M 1153

Flurbiprofen (Taking other drugs containing an NSAID (e.g., ibuprofen, naproxen, or others) increases the chance of causing stomach bleeding).
No products indexed under this heading.

Fluticasone Propionate (Taking a steroid may increase the chance of stomach bleeding). Products include:
- Advair Diskus 100/50 1276
- Advair Diskus 250/50 1276
- Advair Diskus 500/50 1276
- Advair HFA 45/21 Inhalation Aerosol 1288
- Advair HFA 115/21 Inhalation Aerosol 1288
- Advair HFA 230/21 Inhalation Aerosol 1288
- Flonase Nasal Spray 1431
- Flovent Diskus 50 mcg 1435

Fluticasone Propionate HFA (Taking a steroid may increase the chance of stomach bleeding). Products include:
- Flovent HFA 1440

Fondaparinux Sodium (Taking a blood thinning agent (eg, anticoagulants) may increase the chance stomach bleeding). Products include:
- Arixtra Injection 1313

Heparin Calcium (Taking a blood thinning agent (eg, anticoagulants) may increase the chance stomach bleeding).
No products indexed under this heading.

Heparin Sodium (Taking a blood thinning agent (eg, anticoagulants) may increase the chance stomach bleeding).
No products indexed under this heading.

Hydrocortisone (Taking a steroid may increase the chance of stomach bleeding).
No products indexed under this heading.

Hydrocortisone Acetate (Taking a steroid may increase the chance of stomach bleeding). Products include:
- Analpram-HC 1140
- Pramosone 1141

Hydrocortisone Sodium Phosphate (Taking a steroid may increase the chance of stomach bleeding).
No products indexed under this heading.

Hydrocortisone Sodium Succinate (Taking a steroid may increase the chance of stomach bleeding).
No products indexed under this heading.

Ibuprofen (Taking other drugs containing an NSAID (e.g., ibuprofen, naproxen, or others) increases the chance of causing stomach bleeding). Products include:
- Motrin IB Tablets and Caplets 1900
- Children's Motrin Oral Suspension 1901
- Children's Motrin Non-Staining Dye-Free Oral Suspension 1901
- Children's Motrin Cold Oral Suspension 1899
- Infants' Motrin Concentrated Drops 1901
- Infants' Motrin Non-Staining Dye-Free Concentrated Drops 1901
- Junior Strength Motrin Caplets and Chewable Tablets 1901
- Vicoprofen Tablets 533

Indomethacin (Taking other drugs containing an NSAID (e.g., ibuprofen, naproxen, or others) increases the chance of causing stomach bleeding). Products include:
- Indocin 2024

Indomethacin Sodium Trihydrate (Taking other drugs containing an NSAID (e.g., ibuprofen, naproxen, or others) increases the chance of causing stomach bleeding). Products include:
- Indocin I.V. 2489

Ketoprofen (Taking other drugs containing an NSAID (e.g., ibuprofen, naproxen, or others) increases the chance of causing stomach bleeding).
No products indexed under this heading.

Ketorolac Tromethamine (Taking other drugs containing an NSAID (e.g., ibuprofen, naproxen, or others) increases the chance of causing stomach bleeding).
No products indexed under this heading.

Low Molecular Weight Heparins (Taking a blood thinning agent (eg, anticoagulants) may increase the chance stomach bleeding).
No products indexed under this heading.

Meclofenamate Sodium (Taking other drugs containing an NSAID (e.g., ibuprofen, naproxen, or others) increases the chance of causing stomach bleeding).
No products indexed under this heading.

Mefenamic Acid (Taking other drugs containing an NSAID (e.g., ibuprofen, naproxen, or others) increases the chance of causing stomach bleeding).
No products indexed under this heading.

Meloxicam (Taking other drugs containing an NSAID (e.g., ibuprofen, naproxen, or others) increases the chance of causing stomach bleeding). Products include:
- Mobic Oral Suspension 863
- Mobic Tablets 863

Methylprednisolone Acetate (Taking a steroid may increase the chance of stomach bleeding).
No products indexed under this heading.

Methylprednisolone Sodium Succinate (Taking a steroid may increase the chance of stomach bleeding).
No products indexed under this heading.

Mometasone Furoate (Taking a steroid may increase the chance of stomach bleeding). Products include:
- Asmanex Twisthaler 2797
- Elocon Cream 0.1% 2840
- Elocon Lotion 0.1% 2841
- Elocon Ointment 0.1% 2842

Mometasone Furoate Monohydrate (Taking a steroid may increase the chance of stomach bleeding). Products include:
- Nasonex Nasal Spray 2883

Nabumetone (Taking other drugs containing an NSAID (e.g., ibuprofen, naproxen, or others) increases the chance of causing stomach bleeding).
No products indexed under this heading.

Naproxen (Taking other drugs containing an NSAID (e.g., ibuprofen, naproxen, or others) increases the chance of causing stomach bleeding). Products include:
- EC-Naprosyn Delayed-Release Tablets 2632
- Naprosyn Suspension 2632
- Naprosyn Tablets 2632

Naproxen Sodium (Taking other drugs containing an NSAID (e.g., ibuprofen, naproxen, or others) increases the chance of causing stomach bleeding). Products include:
- Anaprox Tablets 2632
- Anaprox DS Tablets 2632
- Treximet Tablets 1616

Oxaprozin (Taking other drugs containing an NSAID (e.g., ibuprofen, naproxen, or others) increases the chance of causing stomach bleeding).
No products indexed under this heading.

IMPORTANT NOTE: Always consult each drug listing in the patient's regimen for possible interactions.

Phenylbutazone (Taking other drugs containing an NSAID (e.g., ibuprofen, naproxen, or others) increases the chance of causing stomach bleeding).
No products indexed under this heading.

Piroxicam (Taking other drugs containing an NSAID (e.g., ibuprofen, naproxen, or others) increases the chance of causing stomach bleeding).
No products indexed under this heading.

Prednisolone Acetate (Taking a steroid may increase the chance of stomach bleeding). Products include:
Pred Forte Ophthalmic Suspension .... ⊙227
Pred Mild Ophthalmic Suspension .... ⊙230
Pred-G Ophthalmic Ointment .... ⊙229
Pred-G Ophthalmic Suspension .... ⊙228

Prednisolone Sodium Phosphate (Taking a steroid may increase the chance of stomach bleeding).
No products indexed under this heading.

Prednisolone Tebutate (Taking a steroid may increase the chance of stomach bleeding).
No products indexed under this heading.

Prednisone (Taking a steroid may increase the chance of stomach bleeding).
No products indexed under this heading.

Rofecoxib (Taking other drugs containing an NSAID (e.g., ibuprofen, naproxen, or others) increases the chance of causing stomach bleeding).
No products indexed under this heading.

Sulindac (Taking other drugs containing an NSAID (e.g., ibuprofen, naproxen, or others) increases the chance of causing stomach bleeding). Products include:
Clinoril Tablets 1962

Tinzaparin Sodium (Taking a blood thinning agent (eg, anticoagulants) may increase the chance stomach bleeding).
No products indexed under this heading.

Tolmetin Sodium (Taking other drugs containing an NSAID (e.g., ibuprofen, naproxen, or others) increases the chance of causing stomach bleeding).
No products indexed under this heading.

Triamcinolone (Taking a steroid may increase the chance of stomach bleeding).
No products indexed under this heading.

Triamcinolone Acetonide (Taking a steroid may increase the chance of stomach bleeding). Products include:
Azmacort Inhalation Aerosol 407
Nasacort AQ Nasal Spray 2765
Triesence Injectable Suspension .... ⊙209

Triamcinolone Diacetate (Taking a steroid may increase the chance of stomach bleeding).
No products indexed under this heading.

Triamcinolone Hexacetonide (Taking a steroid may increase the chance of stomach bleeding).
No products indexed under this heading.

Valdecoxib (Taking other drugs containing an NSAID (e.g., ibuprofen, naproxen, or others) increases the chance of causing stomach bleeding).
No products indexed under this heading.

Warfarin Sodium (Taking a blood thinning agent (eg, anticoagulants) may increase the chance stomach bleeding).
No products indexed under this heading.

Food Interactions

Alcohol (Having 3 or more alcoholic drinks every day while using this product increases the chance of stomach bleeding).

SALONPAS GEL

(Menthol, Methyl Salicylate) .... ▣609
None cited in PDR database.

SALONPAS GEL-PATCH HOT SOOTHING

(Capsicum Extract, Menthol) .... ▣609
None cited in PDR database.

SALONPAS PAIN RELIEF PATCH

(Menthol, Methyl Salicylate) .... ▣608
See Salonpas Arthritis Pain Patches

SALONPAS-HOT PATCH

(Capsicum Extract) .... ▣609
None cited in PDR database.

SANCTURA XR CAPSULES

(Trospium Chloride) 557
May interact with antacids and certain other agents. Compounds in these categories include:

Aluminum Carbonate (A study has shown that 5 individuals demonstrated either an increase or decrease in trospium exposure in presence of antacids. The clinical relevance of these findings is not known).
No products indexed under this heading.

Aluminum Hydroxide (A study has shown that 5 individuals demonstrated either an increase or decrease in trospium exposure in presence of antacids. The clinical relevance of these findings is not known).
No products indexed under this heading.

Magaldrate (A study has shown that 5 individuals demonstrated either an increase or decrease in trospium exposure in presence of antacids. The clinical relevance of these findings is not known).
No products indexed under this heading.

Magnesium Hydroxide (A study has shown that 5 individuals demonstrated either an increase or decrease in trospium exposure in presence of antacids. The clinical relevance of these findings is not known). Products include:
Fleet Pedia-Lax Chewable Tablets 1145
Pepcid Complete Chewable Tablets 1771
Extra Strength Rolaids Freshmint Tablets 1903
Rolaids Multi-Symptom Berry Tablets 1903
Rolaids Original Peppermint Tablets 1903

Magnesium Oxide (A study has shown that 5 individuals demonstrated either an increase or decrease in trospium exposure in presence of antacids. The clinical relevance of these findings is not known). Products include:
Beelith Tablets 813

Sodium Bicarbonate (A study has shown that 5 individuals demonstrated either an increase or decrease in trospium exposure in presence of antacids. The clinical relevance of these findings is not known). Products include:
Ceo-Two Laxative Suppository 815

Food Interactions

Food, unspecified (Administration of trospium immediately after a high fat-content meal reduced the oral bioavailability of trospium chloride by 35% for AUC and by 60% for Cmax. It is recommended that trospium be taken on an empty stomach at least one hour before a meal).

SANDIMMUNE ORAL SOLUTION

(Cyclosporine) 2296
See Sandimmune I.V. Ampuls for Infusion

SANDIMMUNE I.V. AMPULS FOR INFUSION

(Cyclosporine) 2296
May interact with ACE inhibitors, angiotensin-II receptor antagonists, erythromycin, fibrates, HMG-CoA reductase inhibitors, methylprednisolone, non-steroidal anti-inflammatory agents, oral contraceptives, phenytoin, potassium preparations, prednisolone, protease inhibitors, potassium sparing diuretics, vaccines, live, and certain other agents. Compounds in these categories include:

Allopurinol (Increases cyclosporine concentrations).
No products indexed under this heading.

Amiloride Hydrochloride (Cyclosporine may cause hyperkalemia; concurrent use should be avoided).
No products indexed under this heading.

Amiodarone Hydrochloride (Increases cyclosporine concentrations).
No products indexed under this heading.

Amphotericin B (May potentiate renal dysfunction).
No products indexed under this heading.

Amprenavir (The HIV protease inhibitors are known to inhibit CYP450 3A and, thus, could potentially increase the concentrations of cyclosporine).
No products indexed under this heading.

Antibiotics, unspecified (Potential synergies of nephrotoxicity may occur).
No products indexed under this heading.

Atorvastatin Calcium (Cyclosporine may reduce the clearance of HMG-CoA reductase inhibitors (statins). Literature and postmarketing cases of myotoxicity, including muscle pain and weakness, myositis, and rhabdomyolysis have been reported with concomitant administration of cyclosporine and atorvastatin. When concurrently administered with cyclosporine, the dosage of atorvastatin should be reduced. Statin therapy needs to be temporarily withheld or discontinued in patients with signs/symptoms of myopathy or those with risk factors predisposing to severe renal injury). Products include:
Lipitor Tablets 2501

Azapropazon (May potentiate renal dysfunction).
No products indexed under this heading.

Azithromycin (Concomitant azithromycin may increase cyclosporine concentrations). Products include:
AzaSite Ophthalmic Drops 1740

BCG Vaccine (During treatment with cyclosporine, vaccination may be less effective; the use of live vaccines should be avoided).
No products indexed under this heading.

Benazepril Hydrochloride (Caution is required when cyclosporine is co-administered with potassium-sparing drugs, such as angiotensin-converting enzyme inhibitors).
No products indexed under this heading.

Bromocriptine Mesylate (Increases cyclosporine levels; dosage adjustments are essential).
No products indexed under this heading.

Candesartan Cilexetil (Caution is required when cyclosporine is co-administered with potassium-sparing drugs, such as angiotensin II receptor antagonists). Products include:
Atacand Tablets 639
Atacand HCT 642

Captopril (Caution is required when cyclosporine is co-administered with potassium-sparing drugs, such as angiotensin-converting enzyme inhibitors). Products include:
Captopril Tablets 2182

Carbamazepine (Decreases cyclosporine plasma concentrations; dosage adjustments are essential). Products include:
Carbatrol Capsules 3019
Equetro Extended-Release Capsules 3174

Celecoxib (Co-administration with NSAID's, particularly in the setting of dehydration, may potentiate renal dysfunction). Products include:
Celebrex Capsules 2979

Cerivastatin Sodium (Literature and post-marketing cases of myotoxicity, including muscle pain and weakness, myositis, and rhabdomyolysis, have been reported with concomitant administration of cyclosporine with lovastatin, simvastatin, atorvastatin, pravastatin, and rarely, fluvastatin. When concurrently administered with cyclosporine, the dosage of these statins should be reduced according to label recommendations. Statin therapy needs to be temporarily withheld or discontinued in patients with signs and symptoms of myopathy or those with risk factors predisposing to severe renal injury, including renal failure, secondary to rhabomyolysis).
No products indexed under this heading.

Cimetidine (May potentiate renal dysfunction).
No products indexed under this heading.

Cimetidine Hydrochloride (May potentiate renal dysfunction).
No products indexed under this heading.

Ciprofloxacin (Concomitant ciprofloxacin may potentiate renal dysfunction). Products include:
- Cipro I.V. 2817
- Cipro Oral Suspension 2810
- Cipro XR Tablets 2823
- Ciprodex Otic Suspension 541

Ciprofloxacin Hydrochloride (Concomitant ciprofloxacin may potentiate renal dysfunction). Products include:
- Cipro Tablets 2810

Clarithromycin (Concomitant clarithromycin may increase cyclosporine concentrations). Products include:
- Biaxin/Biaxin XL 411

Clofibrate (Concomitant fibric acid derivatives may potentiate renal dysfunction).
No products indexed under this heading.

Colchicine (Co-administration results in increased cyclosporine concentrations and potentiation of renal dysfunction. Cyclosporine may reduce the clearance of colchicine. There are reports on the potential of cyclosporine to enhance the toxic effects of colchicine, such as myopathy and neuropathy, especially in patients with renal dysfunction. If colchicine is used concurrently with cyclosporine, close clinical observation is required).
No products indexed under this heading.

Dalfopristin (Co-administration with substrates that inhibit CYP450 3A, such as dalfopristin, could decrease metabolism and increase cyclosporine concentrations).
No products indexed under this heading.

Danazol (Increases cyclosporine plasma concentrations; dosage adjustments are essential).
No products indexed under this heading.

Darunavir (The HIV protease inhibitors are known to inhibit CYP450 3A and, thus, could potentially increase the concentrations of cyclosporine).
No products indexed under this heading.

Desogestrel (Concomitant oral contraceptives may increase cyclosporine concentrations). Products include:
- Mircette Tablets 1034

Diclofenac Epolamine (Co-administration with NSAID's, particularly in the setting of dehydration, may potentiate renal dysfunction). Products include:
- Flector Patch 561

Diclofenac Potassium (Co-administration with NSAID's, particularly in the setting of dehydration, may potentiate renal dysfunction).
No products indexed under this heading.

Diclofenac Sodium (Co-administration with NSAID's, particularly in the setting of dehydration, may potentiate renal dysfunction). Products include:
- Diclofenac Sodium Ophthalmic Solution .... ⊙ 240
- Voltaren Ophthalmic Solution 2336
- Voltaren Tablets 2334
- Voltaren-XR Tablets 2337

Digoxin (Reduced clearance of digoxin and potential for severe digitalis toxicity. If digoxin is used concurrently with cyclosporine, close clinical observation is required). Products include:
- Lanoxin Injection 1498
- Lanoxin Injection Pediatric 1502
- Lanoxin Tablets 1505

Diltiazem Hydrochloride (Increases cyclosporine plasma concentrations; dosage adjustments are essential). Products include:
- Cardizem LA Extended Release Tablets 421

Enalapril Maleate (Caution is required when cyclosporine is co-administered with potassium-sparing drugs, such as angiotensin-converting enzyme inhibitors).
No products indexed under this heading.

Enalaprilat (Caution is required when cyclosporine is co-administered with potassium-sparing drugs, such as angiotensin-converting enzyme inhibitors).
No products indexed under this heading.

Eprosartan Mesylate (Caution is required when cyclosporine is co-administered with potassium-sparing drugs, such as angiotensin II receptor antagonists). Products include:
- Teveten Tablets 515
- Teveten HCT Tablets 517

Erythromycin (Co-administration with substrates that inhibit CYP450 3A, such as erythromycin, could decrease metabolism and increase cyclosporine concentrations).
No products indexed under this heading.

Erythromycin Estolate (Co-administration with substrates that inhibit CYP450 3A, such as erythromycin, could decrease metabolism and increase cyclosporine concentrations).
No products indexed under this heading.

Erythromycin Ethylsuccinate (Co-administration with substrates that inhibit CYP450 3A, such as erythromycin, could decrease metabolism and increase cyclosporine concentrations). Products include:
- E.E.S. 433
- EryPed 431

Erythromycin Gluceptate (Co-administration with substrates that inhibit CYP450 3A, such as erythromycin, could decrease metabolism and increase cyclosporine concentrations).
No products indexed under this heading.

Erythromycin Lactobionate (Co-administration with substrates that inhibit CYP450 3A, such as erythromycin, could decrease metabolism and increase cyclosporine concentrations).
No products indexed under this heading.

Erythromycin Stearate (Co-administration with substrates that inhibit CYP450 3A, such as erythromycin, could decrease metabolism and increase cyclosporine concentrations).
No products indexed under this heading.

Ethinyl Estradiol (Concomitant oral contraceptives may increase cyclosporine concentrations). Products include:
- Lybrel Tablets 3204
- Mircette Tablets 1034
- NuvaRing 2897
- Ortho-Cyclen/Ortho Tri-Cyclen 2449
- Ortho Evra Transdermal System 2437
- Ortho Tri-Cyclen Lo Tablets 2458
- Seasonique Tablets 1046
- Yaz Tablets 805

Ethynodiol Diacetate (Concomitant oral contraceptives may increase cyclosporine concentrations).
No products indexed under this heading.

Etodolac (Co-administration with NSAID's, particularly in the setting of dehydration, may potentiate renal dysfunction).
No products indexed under this heading.

Fenofibrate (Concomitant fibric acid derivatives may potentiate renal dysfunction). Products include:
- Fenoglide Tablets 2960
- Tricor Tablets 520

Fenoprofen Calcium (Co-administration with NSAID's, particularly in the setting of dehydration, may potentiate renal dysfunction). Products include:
- Nalfon Capsules 2508

Fluconazole (Increases cyclosporine levels; dosage adjustments are essential).
No products indexed under this heading.

Flurbiprofen (Co-administration with NSAID's, particularly in the setting of dehydration, may potentiate renal dysfunction).
No products indexed under this heading.

Fluvastatin Sodium (Cyclosporine may reduce the clearance of HMG-CoA reductase inhibitors (statins). Literature and postmarketing cases of myotoxicity, including muscle pain and weakness, myositis, and rhabdomyolysis have been reported with concomitant administration of cyclosporine and fluvastatin. When concurrently administered with cyclosporine, the dosage of fluvastatin should be reduced. Statin therapy needs to be temporarily withheld or discontinued in patients with signs/symptoms of myopathy or those with risk factors predisposing to severe renal injury). Products include:
- Lescol Capsules 2268
- Lescol XL Tablets 2268

Fosamprenavir Calcium (The HIV protease inhibitors are known to inhibit CYP450 3A and, thus, could potentially increase the concentrations of cyclosporine). Products include:
- Lexiva Oral Suspension 1510
- Lexiva Tablets 1510

Fosinopril Sodium (Caution is required when cyclosporine is co-administered with potassium-sparing drugs, such as angiotensin-converting enzyme inhibitors).
No products indexed under this heading.

Fosphenytoin Sodium (Co-administration with agents that are known to induce CYP450 system, such as phenytoin, will increase hepatic metabolism and decrease cyclosporine levels).
No products indexed under this heading.

Gemfibrozil (Concomitant fibric acid derivatives may potentiate renal dysfunction).
No products indexed under this heading.

Gentamicin Sulfate (May potentiate renal dysfunction). Products include:
- Pred-G Ophthalmic Ointment .... ⊙ 229
- Pred-G Ophthalmic Suspension .... ⊙ 228

Hypericum (Co-administration has been reported to produce a marked reduction in blood cyclosporine concentrations, resulting in subtherapeutic levels, rejection of transplanted organs, and graft loss). Products include:
- Satiété Tablets 640

Ibuprofen (Co-administration with NSAID's, particularly in the setting of dehydration, may potentiate renal dysfunction). Products include:
- Motrin IB Tablets and Caplets 1900
- Children's Motrin Oral Suspension 1901
- Children's Motrin Non-Staining Dye-Free Oral Suspension 1901
- Children's Motrin Cold Oral Suspension 1899
- Infants' Motrin Concentrated Drops 1901
- Infants' Motrin Non-Staining Dye-Free Concentrated Drops 1901
- Junior Strength Motrin Caplets and Chewable Tablets 1901
- Vicoprofen Tablets 533

Imatinib Mesylate (Concomitant imatinib may increase cyclosporine concentrations). Products include:
- Gleevec Tablets 2255

Immune Globulin Intravenous (Human) (Increases susceptibility to infection). Products include:
- Flebogamma 5% DIF 1718
- Gammagard Liquid 730
- Gammagard S/D 734
- Gamunex 3094

Indinavir Sulfate (The HIV protease inhibitors are known to inhibit CYP450 3A and, thus, could potentially increase the concentrations of cyclosporine). Products include:
- Crixivan Capsules 1979

Indomethacin (Co-administration with NSAID's, particularly in the setting of dehydration, may potentiate renal dysfunction). Products include:
- Indocin 2024

Indomethacin Sodium Trihydrate (Co-administration with NSAID's, particularly in the setting of dehydration, may potentiate renal dysfunction). Products include:
- Indocin I.V. 2489

Influenza Vaccine, Live Attenuated (During treatment with cyclosporine, vaccination may be less effective; the use of live vaccines should be avoided).
No products indexed under this heading.

Influenza Virus Vaccine Live, Intranasal (During treatment with cyclosporine, vaccination may be less effective; the use of live vaccines should be avoided). Products include:
- FluMist Vaccine 1945

Irbesartan (Caution is required when cyclosporine is co-administered with potassium-sparing drugs, such as angiotensin II receptor antagonists). Products include:
- Avalide Tablets 892
- Avalide Tablets 2713
- Avapro Tablets 897
- Avapro Tablets 2718

Itraconazole (Increases cyclosporine levels; dosage adjustments are essential).
No products indexed under this heading.

Ketoconazole (May potentiate renal dysfunction; co-administration

with substrates that inhibit CYP450 3A, such as ketoconazole, could decrease metabolism and increase cyclosporine concentrations). Products include:
Extina Foam, 2% 3057
Nizoral A-D Shampoo 1901

Ketoprofen (Co-administration with NSAID's, particularly in the setting of dehydration, may potentiate renal dysfunction).
No products indexed under this heading.

Ketorolac Tromethamine (Co-administration with NSAID's, particularly in the setting of dehydration, may potentiate renal dysfunction).
No products indexed under this heading.

Levonorgestrel (Concomitant oral contraceptives may increase cyclosporine concentrations). Products include:
Climara Pro Transdermal System 768
Lybrel Tablets 3204
Mirena Intrauterine System 779
Plan B Tablets 1044
Seasonique Tablets 1046

Lisinopril (Caution is required when cyclosporine is co-administered with potassium-sparing drugs, such as angiotensin-converting enzyme inhibitors). Products include:
Prinivil Tablets 2087
Prinzide Tablets 2092

Lopinavir (The HIV protease inhibitors are known to inhibit CYP450 3A and, thus, could potentially increase the concentrations of cyclosporine). Products include:
Kaletra 452

Losartan Potassium (Caution is required when cyclosporine is co-administered with potassium-sparing drugs, such as angiotensin II receptor antagonists). Products include:
Cozaar Tablets 1973

Lovastatin (Cyclosporine may reduce the clearance of HMG-CoA reductase inhibitors (statins). Literature and postmarketing cases of myotoxicity, including muscle pain and weakness, myositis, and rhabdomyolysis have been reported with concomitant administration of cyclosporine and lovastatin. When concurrently administered with cyclosporine, the dosage of lovastatin should be reduced. Statin therapy needs to be temporarily withheld or discontinued in patients with signs/symptoms of myopathy or those with risk factors predisposing to severe renal injury). Products include:
Advicor Tablets 402
Mevacor Tablets 2063

Measles, Mumps, Rubella and Varicella Virus Vaccine Live (During treatment with cyclosporine, vaccination may be less effective; the use of live vaccines should be avoided). Products include:
ProQuad 2099

Measles, Mumps & Rubella Virus Vaccine, Live (During treatment with cyclosporine, vaccination may be less effective; the use of live vaccines should be avoided). Products include:
M-M-R II 2054

Measles & Rubella Virus Vaccine Live (During treatment with cyclosporine, vaccination may be less effective; the use of live vaccines should be avoided).
No products indexed under this heading.

Measles Virus Vaccine Live (During treatment with cyclosporine, vaccination may be less effective; the use of live vaccines should be avoided). Products include:
Attenuvax 1951

Meclofenamate Sodium (Co-administration with NSAID's, particularly in the setting of dehydration, may potentiate renal dysfunction).
No products indexed under this heading.

Mefenamic Acid (Co-administration with NSAID's, particularly in the setting of dehydration, may potentiate renal dysfunction).
No products indexed under this heading.

Meloxicam (Co-administration with NSAID's, particularly in the setting of dehydration, may potentiate renal dysfunction). Products include:
Mobic Oral Suspension 863
Mobic Tablets 863

Melphalan (May potentiate renal dysfunction).
No products indexed under this heading.

Mestranol (Concomitant oral contraceptives may increase cyclosporine concentrations).
No products indexed under this heading.

Methotrexate Sodium (Co-administration in rheumatoid arthritis patients has resulted in increased AUC of methotrexate by approximately 30% and concentration of its metabolite decreased by approximately 80%; the clinical significance is not known).
No products indexed under this heading.

Methylprednisolone (Co-administration with agents that are known to inhibit CYP450 system, such as methylprednisolone, will decrease hepatic metabolism and increase cyclosporine levels; convulsions have been reported with concomitant high doses of methylprednisolone).
No products indexed under this heading.

Methylprednisolone Acetate (Co-administration with agents that are known to inhibit CYP450 system, such as methylprednisolone, will decrease hepatic metabolism and increase cyclosporine levels; convulsions have been reported with concomitant high doses of methylprednisolone).
No products indexed under this heading.

Methylprednisolone Sodium Succinate (Co-administration with agents that are known to inhibit CYP450 system, such as methylprednisolone, will decrease hepatic metabolism and increase cyclosporine levels; convulsions have been reported with concomitant high doses of methylprednisolone).
No products indexed under this heading.

Metoclopramide Hydrochloride (Increases cyclosporine levels; dosage adjustments are essential).
No products indexed under this heading.

Moexipril Hydrochloride (Caution is required when cyclosporine is co-administered with potassium-sparing drugs, such as angiotensin-converting enzyme inhibitors).
No products indexed under this heading.

Mumps Virus Vaccine, Live (During treatment with cyclosporine, vaccination may be less effective; the use of live vaccines should be avoided). Products include:
Mumpsvax 2068

Muromonab-CD3 (Increased susceptibility to infection and increased risk for development of lymphomas and malignancies). Products include:
Orthoclone OKT3 Sterile Solution 2387

Nabumetone (Co-administration with NSAID's, particularly in the setting of dehydration, may potentiate renal dysfunction).
No products indexed under this heading.

Nafcillin Sodium (Decreases cyclosporine concentrations).
No products indexed under this heading.

Naproxen (Co-administration with NSAID's, particularly in the setting of dehydration, may potentiate renal dysfunction). Products include:
EC-Naprosyn Delayed-Release Tablets 2632
Naprosyn Suspension 2632
Naprosyn Tablets 2632

Naproxen Sodium (Co-administration with NSAID's, particularly in the setting of dehydration, may potentiate renal dysfunction). Products include:
Anaprox Tablets 2632
Anaprox DS Tablets 2632
Treximet Tablets 1616

Nelfinavir Mesylate (The HIV protease inhibitors are known to inhibit CYP450 3A and, thus, could potentially increase the concentrations of cyclosporine).
No products indexed under this heading.

Nephrotoxic Drugs (Potential synergics of nephrotoxicity).
No products indexed under this heading.

Nicardipine Hydrochloride (Increases cyclosporine plasma concentrations; dosage adjustments are essential). Products include:
Cardene I.V. 1093

Nifedipine (Potential for frequent gingival hyperplasia).
No products indexed under this heading.

Norethindrone (Concomitant oral contraceptives may increase cyclosporine concentrations). Products include:
Ortho Micronor Tablets 2446

Norethynodrel (Concomitant oral contraceptives may increase cyclosporine concentrations).
No products indexed under this heading.

Norgestimate (Concomitant oral contraceptives may increase cyclosporine concentrations). Products include:
Ortho-Cyclen/Ortho Tri-Cyclen 2449
Ortho Tri-Cyclen Lo Tablets 2458

Norgestrel (Concomitant oral contraceptives may increase cyclosporine concentrations).
No products indexed under this heading.

Octreotide Acetate (Decreases cyclosporine concentrations). Products include:
Sandostatin Injection 2300
Sandostatin LAR Depot 2302

Orlistat (Co-administration can result in decreased absorption of cyclosporine; concomitant use should be avoided). Products include:
Xenical Capsules 2672

Oxaprozin (Co-administration with NSAID's, particularly in the setting of dehydration, may potentiate renal dysfunction).
No products indexed under this heading.

Perindopril Erbumine (Caution is required when cyclosporine is co-administered with potassium-sparing drugs, such as angiotensin-converting enzyme inhibitors). Products include:
Aceon Tablets (2 mg, 4 mg, 8 mg) 3038

Phenobarbital (Decreases cyclosporine plasma levels; dosage adjustments are essential). Products include:
Donnatal Extentabs 2507

Phenylbutazone (Co-administration with NSAID's, particularly in the setting of dehydration, may potentiate renal dysfunction).
No products indexed under this heading.

Phenytoin (Co-administration with agents that are known to induce CYP450 system, such as phenytoin, will increase hepatic metabolism and decrease cyclosporine levels).
No products indexed under this heading.

Phenytoin Sodium (Co-administration with agents that are known to induce CYP450 system, such as phenytoin, will increase hepatic metabolism and decrease cyclosporine levels). Products include:
Phenytek Capsules 2192

Piroxicam (Co-administration with NSAID's, particularly in the setting of dehydration, may potentiate renal dysfunction).
No products indexed under this heading.

Poliovirus Vaccine, Live, Oral, Trivalent, Types 1,2,3 (Sabin) (During treatment with cyclosporine, vaccination may be less effective; the use of live vaccines should be avoided).
No products indexed under this heading.

Potassium Acid Phosphate (Caution is required when cyclosporine in co-administered with potassium-containing drugs). Products include:
K-Phos Original (Sodium Free) Tablets 814

Potassium Bicarbonate (Caution is required when cyclosporine in co-administered with potassium-containing drugs).
No products indexed under this heading.

Potassium Chloride (Caution is required when cyclosporine in co-administered with potassium-containing drugs). Products include:

MoviPrep Oral Solution 2679

Potassium Citrate (Caution is required when cyclosporine in co-administered with potassium-containing drugs). Products include:

BioLean Free Tables 635
Urocit-K Tablets 2176

Potassium Gluconate (Caution is required when cyclosporine in co-administered with potassium-containing drugs).

No products indexed under this heading.

Potassium Phosphate (Caution is required when cyclosporine in co-administered with potassium-containing drugs). Products include:

K-Phos Neutral Tablets 813

Pravastatin Sodium (Cyclosporine may reduce the clearance of HMG-CoA reductase inhibitors (statins). Literature and postmarketing cases of myotoxicity, including muscle pain and weakness, myositis, and rhabdomyolysis have been reported with concomitant administration of cyclosporine and pravastatin. When concurrently administered with cyclosporine, the dosage of pravastatin should be reduced. Statin therapy needs to be temporarily withheld or discontinued in patients with signs/symptoms of myopathy or those with risk factors predisposing to severe renal injury).

No products indexed under this heading.

Prednisolone (Co-administration results in reduced clearance of prednisolone).

No products indexed under this heading.

Prednisolone Acetate (Co-administration results in reduced clearance of prednisolone). Products include:

Pred Forte Ophthalmic Suspension .... ⊙227
Pred Mild Ophthalmic Suspension .... ⊙230
Pred-G Ophthalmic Ointment .... ⊙229
Pred-G Ophthalmic Suspension ...... ⊙228

Prednisolone Sodium Phosphate (Co-administration results in reduced clearance of prednisolone).

No products indexed under this heading.

Prednisolone Tebutate (Co-administration results in reduced clearance of prednisolone).

No products indexed under this heading.

Quinapril Hydrochloride (Caution is required when cyclosporine is co-administered with potassium-sparing drugs, such as angiotensin-converting enzyme inhibitors).

No products indexed under this heading.

Quinupristin (Co-administration with substrates that inhibit CYP450 3A, such as quinupristine, could decrease metabolism and increase cyclosporine concentrations).

No products indexed under this heading.

Ramipril (Caution is required when cyclosporine is co-administered with potassium-sparing drugs, such as angiotensin-converting enzyme inhibitors).

No products indexed under this heading.

Ranitidine Hydrochloride (May potentiate renal dysfunction). Products include:

Zantac 75 Tablets 603
Zantac 1670
Zantac Injection 1666
Zantac Injection Pharmacy Bulk Package 1668
Maximum Strength Zantac 150 Tablets..................................... 603
Maximum Strength Zantac 150 Cool Mint Tablets 603

Rifabutin (Rifabutin is known to increase the metabolism of other drugs metabolized by CYP450 system; the interaction between cyclosporine and rifabutin has not been studied; care should be exercised).

No products indexed under this heading.

Rifampin (Decreases cyclosporine plasma levels; dosage adjustments are essential).

No products indexed under this heading.

Ritonavir (The HIV protease inhibitors are known to inhibit CYP450 3A and, thus, could potentially increase the concentrations of cyclosporine). Products include:

Kaletra 452
Norvir 489

Rofecoxib (Co-administration with NSAID's, particularly in the setting of dehydration, may potentiate renal dysfunction).

No products indexed under this heading.

Rosuvastatin Calcium (Literature and post-marketing cases of myotoxicity, including muscle pain and weakness, myositis, and rhabdomyolysis, have been reported with concomitant administration of cyclosporine with lovastatin, simvastatin, atorvastatin, pravastatin, and rarely, fluvastatin. When concurrently administered with cyclosporine, the dosage of these statins should be reduced according to label recommendations. Statin therapy needs to be temporarily withheld or discontinued in patients with signs and symptoms of myopathy or those with risk factors predisposing to severe renal injury, including renal failure, secondary to rhabomyolysis). Products include:

Crestor Tablets 677

Rotavirus Vaccine, Live, Oral, Tetravalent (During treatment with cyclosporine, vaccination may be less effective; the use of live vaccines should be avoided).

No products indexed under this heading.

Rubella & Mumps Virus Vaccine Live (During treatment with cyclosporine, vaccination may be less effective; the use of live vaccines should be avoided).

No products indexed under this heading.

Rubella Virus Vaccine Live (During treatment with cyclosporine, vaccination may be less effective; the use of live vaccines should be avoided). Products include:

Meruvax II 2061

Saquinavir (The HIV protease inhibitors are known to inhibit CYP450 3A and, thus, could potentially increase the concentrations of cyclosporine).

No products indexed under this heading.

Saquinavir Mesylate (The HIV protease inhibitors are known to inhibit CYP450 3A and, thus, could potentially increase the concentrations of cyclosporine).

No products indexed under this heading.

Simvastatin (Cyclosporine may reduce the clearance of HMG-CoA reductase inhibitors (statins). Literature and postmarketing cases of myotoxicity, including muscle pain and weakness, myositis, and rhabdomyolysis have been reported with concomitant administration of cyclosporine and simvastatin. When concurrently administered with cyclosporine, the dosage of simvastatin should be reduced. Statin therapy needs to be temporarily withheld or discontinued in patients with signs/symptoms of myopathy or those with risk factors predisposing to severe renal injury). Products include:

Simcor Tablets 502
Vytorin 10/10 Tablets 2149
Vytorin 10/10 Tablets 2939
Vytorin 10/20 Tablets 2149
Vytorin 10/20 Tablets 2939
Vytorin 10/40 Tablets 2149
Vytorin 10/40 Tablets 2939
Vytorin 10/80 Tablets 2149
Vytorin 10/80 Tablets 2939
Zocor Tablets 2136

Sirolimus (Elevations in serum creatinine were observed in studies using sirolimus in combination with full-dose cyclosporine. The effect is often reversible with cyclosporine dose reduction. Simultaneous co-administration of cyclosproine significantly increases blood levels of sirolimus. To minimize increases in sirolimus blood concentrations, it is recommended that sirolimus be given 4 hours after cyclosporine administration). Products include:

Rapamune 3260

Smallpox Vaccine (During treatment with cyclosporine, vaccination may be less effective; the use of live vaccines should be avoided).

No products indexed under this heading.

Spirapril Hydrochloride (Caution is required when cyclosporine is co-administered with potassium-sparing drugs, such as angiotensin-converting enzyme inhibitors).

No products indexed under this heading.

Spironolactone (Cyclosporine may cause hyperkalemia; concurrent use should be avoided).

No products indexed under this heading.

Sulfamethoxazole (May potentiate renal dysfunction).

No products indexed under this heading.

Sulfinpyrazone (Concomitant sulfinpyrazone may decrease cyclosporine concentrations).

No products indexed under this heading.

Sulindac (Co-administration with NSAID's, particularly in the setting of dehydration, may potentiate renal dysfunction). Products include:

Clinoril Tablets 1962

Tacrolimus (May potentiate renal dysfunction). Products include:

Prograf Capsules and Injection 622
Protopic Ointment 628

Telmisartan (Caution is required when cyclosporine is co-administered with potassium-sparing drugs, such as angiotensin II receptor antagonists). Products include:

Micardis Tablets 852
Micardis HCT Tablets 854

Terbinafine Hydrochloride (Concomitant terbinafine may decrease cyclosporine concentrations). Products include:

Lamisil Oral Granules 2264
Lamisil Tablets 2266

Ticlopidine Hydrochloride (Decreases cyclosporine concentrations).

No products indexed under this heading.

Tipranavir (The HIV protease inhibitors are known to inhibit CYP450 3A and, thus, could potentially increase the concentrations of cyclosporine). Products include:

Aptivus Capsules 823
Aptivus Oral Solution 823

Tobramycin (May potentiate renal dysfunction). Products include:

Zylet Ophthalmic Suspension .... ⊙247

Tobramycin Sulfate (May potentiate renal dysfunction).

No products indexed under this heading.

Tolmetin Sodium (Co-administration with NSAID's, particularly in the setting of dehydration, may potentiate renal dysfunction).

No products indexed under this heading.

Trandolapril (Caution is required when cyclosporine is co-administered with potassium-sparing drugs, such as angiotensin-converting enzyme inhibitors). Products include:

Mavik Tablets 472
Tarka Tablets 511

Triamterene (Cyclosporine may cause hyperkalemia; concurrent use should be avoided). Products include:

Dyazide Capsules 1405
Dyrenium Capsules 3189

Trimethoprim (May potentiate renal dysfunction).

No products indexed under this heading.

Typhoid Vaccine (During treatment with cyclosporine, vaccination may be less effective; the use of live vaccines should be avoided).

No products indexed under this heading.

Valdecoxib (Co-administration with NSAID's, particularly in the setting of dehydration, may potentiate renal dysfunction).

No products indexed under this heading.

Valsartan (Caution is required when cyclosporine is co-administered with potassium-sparing drugs, such as angiotensin II receptor antagonists). Products include:

Diovan Tablets 2212
Diovan HCT Tablets 2216
Exforge Tablets 2238

Vancomycin Hydrochloride (May potentiate renal dysfunction).

No products indexed under this heading.

Varicella Virus Vaccine Live (During treatment with cyclosporine, vaccination may be less effective; the use of live vaccines should be avoided). Products include:

Varivax 2133

Verapamil Hydrochloride (Increases cyclosporine levels; dosage adjustments are essential). Products include:
Tarka Tablets 511

Yellow Fever Vaccine (During treatment with cyclosporine, vaccination may be less effective; the use of live vaccines should be avoided).
No products indexed under this heading.

Zoster Vaccine Live (During treatment with cyclosporine, vaccination may be less effective; the use of live vaccines should be avoided).
Products include:
Zostavax Injection 2145

Food Interactions

Grapefruit (Co-administration results in increased blood concentrations of cyclosporine; concurrent use should be avoided).

Grapefruit Juice (Co-administration results in increased blood concentrations of cyclosporine; concurrent use should be avoided).

SANDIMMUNE SOFT GELATIN CAPSULES

(Cyclosporine) 2296
See Sandimmune I.V. Ampuls for Infusion

SANDOSTATIN INJECTION

(Octreotide Acetate) 2300
See Sandostatin LAR Depot

SANDOSTATIN LAR DEPOT

(Octreotide Acetate) 2302
May interact with beta blockers, cytochrome p450 3a4 substrates (selected), oral hypoglycemic agents, insulin, drugs which undergo biotransformation by cytochrome p-450 mixed function oxidase, quinidine, and certain other agents. Compounds in these categories include:

Acarbose (Octreotide inhibits the secretion of insulin and glucagon. Therefore, blood glucose levels should be monitored when octreotide is initiated or when the dose is altered and antidiabetic treatment should be adjusted accordingly).
Products include:
Precose Tablets 792

Acebutolol Hydrochloride (Concomitant administration of bradycardia inducing drugs (e.g., beta blockers) may have an additive effect on the reduction of heart rate associated with octreotide. Dose adjustment of concomitant medication may be necessary).
No products indexed under this heading.

Acetaminophen (Limited published data indicate that somatostatin analogs may decrease the metabolic clearance of compounds known to be metabolized by cytochrome P450 enzymes, which may be due to the suppression of growth hormone).
Products include:
Benadryl Allergy & Cold Kapgels 1895
Benadryl Allergy & Sinus Headache Kapgels 1895
Benadryl Severe Allergy & Sinus Headache Caplets 1897
Lortab 5/500 Tablets 3143
Lortab 7.5/500 Tablets 3144
Lortab 10/500 Tablets 3144
Percocet Tablets 1127
Sinutab Sinus Caplets 1905
Sudafed PE Cold & Cough Caplets 1907
Sudafed PE Nighttime Cold Caplets 1907
Sudafed PE Severe Cold Caplets 1908
Sudafed PE Sinus Headache Caplets 1908
Regular Strength Tylenol Tablets 1915
Tylenol 8 Hour Extended Release Caplets 1915
Extra Strength Tylenol Caplets, Cool Caplets, and EZ Tabs 1915
Extra Strength Tylenol Adult Rapid Blast Liquid 1915
Extra Strength Tylenol PM Caplets, Geltabs, Liquid, and Rapid Release Gels 1915
Extra Strength Tylenol Rapid Release Gels 1915
Tylenol with Codeine Tablets 2427
Tylenol Allergy Multi-Symptom Caplets with Cool Burst and Rapid Release Gelcaps 1916
Tylenol Allergy Multi-Symptom Nighttime Caplets with Cool Burst 1916
Tylenol Severe Allergy Caplets 1916
Tylenol Arthritis Pain Extended Release Geltabs/Caplets 1915
Tylenol Chest Congestion Caplets with Cool Burst 1910
Tylenol Chest Congestion Liquid with Cool Burst 1910
Children's Tylenol Plus Cold Suspension Liquid 1912
Children's Tylenol Plus Cold & Allergy Suspension Liquid 1914
Children's Tylenol Plus Cough & Runny Nose Suspension Liquid 1912
Children's Tylenol Plus Cough & Sore Throat Suspension Liquid 1912
Children's Tylenol Plus Flu Suspension Liquid 1914
Children's Tylenol Suspension Liquid 1909
Children's Tylenol Meltaways 1909
Children's Tylenol Plus Multi-Symptom Cold Suspension Liquid 1912
Tylenol Cold Severe Congestion Daytime Caplets with Cool Burst 1912
Tylenol Cold Head Congestion Daytime Caplets with Cool Burst 1910
Tylenol Cold Head Congestion Nighttime Caplets with Cool Burst 1910
Tylenol Cold Head Congestion Severe Daytime Caplets with Cool Burst 1910
Tylenol Cold Multi-Symptom Daytime Caplets with Cool Burst and Rapid Release Gels 1913
Tylenol Cold Multi-Symptom Daytime Liquid with Citrus Burst 1913
Tylenol Cold Multi-Symptom Nighttime Caplets with Cool Burst 1913
Tylenol Cold Multi-Symptom Nighttime Liquid with Cool Burst 1913
Tylenol Cold Multi-Symptom Severe Caplets with Cool Burst 1913
Tylenol Cold Multi-Symptom Severe Daytime Liquid with Citrus Burst 1913
Tylenol Cough & Sore Throat Daytime Liquid with Cool Burst 1918
Tylenol Cough & Sore Throat Nighttime Liquid with Cool Burst 1918
Concentrated Tylenol Infants' Drops 1909
Jr. Tylenol Meltaways 1909
Tylenol Sinus Congestion & Pain Daytime Caplets with Cool Burst and Gelcaps 1917
Tylenol Sinus Congestion & Pain Nighttime Caplets with Cool Burst 1917
Tylenol Sinus Congestion & Pain Severe Caplets with Cool Burst 1917
Tylenol Sinus Severe Congestion Caplets with Cool Burst 1917
Tylenol Sore Throat Daytime Liquid with Cool Burst 1918
Tylenol Sore Throat Nighttime Liquid with Cool Burst 1918
Women's Tylenol Menstrual Relief Caplets 1919
Vicks DayQuil Cold & Flu Multi-Symptom Relief .... ■ 616
Vicks DayQuil LiquiCaps 2567
Vicks DayQuil Liquid 2567
Vicks DayQuil Multi-Symptom Cold/Flu Relief 2567
Vicks NyQuil Cold & Flu Multi-Symptom Relief .... ■ 617
Vicks NyQuil LiquiCaps 2567
Vicks NyQuil Liquid 2567
Vicks NyQuil Multi-Symptom Cold/Flu Relief 2567
Vicodin Tablets 529
Vicodin ES Tablets 530
Vicodin HP Tablets 531
Zydone Tablets 1132

Alatrofloxacin Mesylate (Limited published data indicate that somatostatin analogs may decrease the metabolic clearance of compounds known to be metabolized by cytochrome P450 enzymes, which may be due to the suppression of growth hormone).
No products indexed under this heading.

Alfentanil Hydrochloride (Limited published data indicate that somatostatin analogs may decrease the metabolic clearance of compounds known to be metabolized by cytochrome P450 enzymes, which may be due to the suppression of growth hormone. Since it cannot be excluded that octreotide may have this effect, other drugs mainly metabolized by CYP3A4 and which have a low therapeutic index (e.g., quinidine, terfenadine) should therefore be used with caution).
No products indexed under this heading.

Alprazolam (Limited published data indicate that somatostatin analogs may decrease the metabolic clearance of compounds known to be metabolized by cytochrome P450 enzymes, which may be due to the suppression of growth hormone. Since it cannot be excluded that octreotide may have this effect, other drugs mainly metabolized by CYP3A4 and which have a low therapeutic index (e.g., quinidine, terfenadine) should therefore be used with caution).
No products indexed under this heading.

Aminophylline (Limited published data indicate that somatostatin analogs may decrease the metabolic clearance of compounds known to be metabolized by cytochrome P450 enzymes, which may be due to the suppression of growth hormone).
No products indexed under this heading.

Amiodarone Hydrochloride (Limited published data indicate that somatostatin analogs may decrease the metabolic clearance of compounds known to be metabolized by cytochrome P450 enzymes, which may be due to the suppression of growth hormone. Since it cannot be excluded that octreotide may have this effect, other drugs mainly metabolized by CYP3A4 and which have a low therapeutic index (e.g., quinidine, terfenadine) should therefore be used with caution).
No products indexed under this heading.

Amitriptyline Hydrochloride (Limited published data indicate that somatostatin analogs may decrease the metabolic clearance of compounds known to be metabolized by cytochrome P450 enzymes, which may be due to the suppression of growth hormone. Since it cannot be excluded that octreotide may have this effect, other drugs mainly metabolized by CYP3A4 and which have a low therapeutic index (e.g., quinidine, terfenadine) should therefore be used with caution).
No products indexed under this heading.

Amlodipine Besylate (Limited published data indicate that somatostatin analogs may decrease the metabolic clearance of compounds known to be metabolized by cytochrome P450 enzymes, which may be due to the suppression of growth hormone. Since it cannot be excluded that octreotide may have this effect, other drugs mainly metabolized by CYP3A4 and which have a low therapeutic index (e.g., quinidine, terfenadine) should therefore be used with caution). Products include:
Azor Tablets 1005
Exforge Tablets 2238

Amoxapine (Limited published data indicate that somatostatin analogs may decrease the metabolic clearance of compounds known to be metabolized by cytochrome P450 enzymes, which may be due to the suppression of growth hormone).
No products indexed under this heading.

Amphetamine Aspartate (Limited published data indicate that somatostatin analogs may decrease the metabolic clearance of compounds known to be metabolized by cytochrome P450 enzymes, which may be due to the suppression of growth hormone). Products include:
Adderall XR Capsules 3012

Amphetamine Aspartate Monohydrate (Limited published data indicate that somatostatin analogs may decrease the metabolic clearance of compounds known to be metabolized by cytochrome P450 enzymes, which may be due to the suppression of growth hormone).
No products indexed under this heading.

Amphetamine Sulfate (Limited published data indicate that somatostatin analogs may decrease the metabolic clearance of compounds known to be metabolized by cytochrome P450 enzymes, which may be due to the suppression of growth hormone). Products include:
Adderall XR Capsules 3012

Aprepitant (Limited published data indicate that somatostatin analogs may decrease the metabolic clearance of compounds known to be metabolized by cytochrome P450 enzymes, which may be due to the suppression of growth hormone. Since it cannot be excluded that octreotide may have this effect, other drugs mainly metabolized by CYP3A4 and which have a low therapeutic index (e.g., quinidine, terfenadine) should therefore be used with caution). Products include:
Emend Capsules 1992

Astemizole (Limited published data indicate that somatostatin analogs may decrease the metabolic clearance of compounds known to be metabolized by cytochrome P450 enzymes, which may be due to the suppression of growth hormone.

Since it cannot be excluded that octreotide may have this effect, other drugs mainly metabolized by CYP3A4 and which have a low therapeutic index (e.g., quinidine, terfenadine) should therefore be used with caution).
No products indexed under this heading.

Atenolol (Concomitant administration of bradycardia inducing drugs (e.g., beta blockers) may have an additive effect on the reduction of heart rate associated with octreotide. Dose adjustment of concomitant medication may be necessary).
No products indexed under this heading.

Atomoxetine Hydrochloride (Limited published data indicate that somatostatin analogs may decrease the metabolic clearance of compounds known to be metabolized by cytochrome P450 enzymes, which may be due to the suppression of growth hormone). Products include:
Strattera Capsules 1864

Atorvastatin Calcium (Limited published data indicate that somatostatin analogs may decrease the metabolic clearance of compounds known to be metabolized by cytochrome P450 enzymes, which may be due to the suppression of growth hormone. Since it cannot be excluded that octreotide may have this effect, other drugs mainly metabolized by CYP3A4 and which have a low therapeutic index (e.g., quinidine, terfenadine) should therefore be used with caution). Products include:
Lipitor Tables 2501

Belladonna Ergotamine (Limited published data indicate that somatostatin analogs may decrease the metabolic clearance of compounds known to be metabolized by cytochrome P450 enzymes, which may be due to the suppression of growth hormone. Since it cannot be excluded that octreotide may have this effect, other drugs mainly metabolized by CYP3A4 and which have a low therapeutic index (e.g., quinidine, terfenadine) should therefore be used with caution).
No products indexed under this heading.

Benzphetamine Hydrochloride (Limited published data indicate that somatostatin analogs may decrease the metabolic clearance of compounds known to be metabolized by cytochrome P450 enzymes, which may be due to the suppression of growth hormone).
No products indexed under this heading.

Betaxolol Hydrochloride (Concomitant administration of bradycardia inducing drugs (e.g., beta blockers) may have an additive effect on the reduction of heart rate associated with octreotide. Dose adjustment of concomitant medication may be necessary).
No products indexed under this heading.

Bisoprolol Fumarate (Concomitant administration of bradycardia inducing drugs (e.g., beta blockers) may have an additive effect on the reduction of heart rate associated with octreotide. Dose adjustment of concomitant medication may be necessary).
No products indexed under this heading.

Bromocriptine Mesylate (Concomitant administration of octreotide and bromocriptine increases the availability of bromocriptine).
No products indexed under this heading.

Buspirone Hydrochloride (Limited published data indicate that somatostatin analogs may decrease the metabolic clearance of compounds known to be metabolized by cytochrome P450 enzymes, which may be due to the suppression of growth hormone. Since it cannot be excluded that octreotide may have this effect, other drugs mainly metabolized by CYP3A4 and which have a low therapeutic index (e.g., quinidine, terfenadine) should therefore be used with caution).
No products indexed under this heading.

Busulfan (Limited published data indicate that somatostatin analogs may decrease the metabolic clearance of compounds known to be metabolized by cytochrome P450 enzymes, which may be due to the suppression of growth hormone. Since it cannot be excluded that octreotide may have this effect, other drugs mainly metabolized by CYP3A4 and which have a low therapeutic index (e.g., quinidine, terfenadine) should therefore be used with caution). Products include:
Busulfex Injection 2477
Myleran Tablets 1530

Caffeine (Limited published data indicate that somatostatin analogs may decrease the metabolic clearance of compounds known to be metabolized by cytochrome P450 enzymes, which may be due to the suppression of growth hormone). Products include:
BioLean Free Tablets 635
BioLean II Tablets 635
Winrgy Dietary Supplement 642

Caffeine Anhydrous (Limited published data indicate that somatostatin analogs may decrease the metabolic clearance of compounds known to be metabolized by cytochrome P450 enzymes, which may be due to the suppression of growth hormone).
No products indexed under this heading.

Caffeine Citrate (Limited published data indicate that somatostatin analogs may decrease the metabolic clearance of compounds known to be metabolized by cytochrome P450 enzymes, which may be due to the suppression of growth hormone).
No products indexed under this heading.

Candesartan Cilexetil (Limited published data indicate that somatostatin analogs may decrease the metabolic clearance of compounds known to be metabolized by cytochrome P450 enzymes, which may be due to the suppression of growth hormone). Products include:
Atacand Tablets 639
Atacand HCT 642

Captopril (Limited published data indicate that somatostatin analogs may decrease the metabolic clearance of compounds known to be metabolized by cytochrome P450 enzymes, which may be due to the suppression of growth hormone). Products include:
Captopril Tablets 2182

Carbamazepine (Limited published data indicate that somatostatin analogs may decrease the metabolic clearance of compounds known to be metabolized by cytochrome P450 enzymes, which may be due to the suppression of growth hormone. Since it cannot be excluded that octreotide may have this effect, other drugs mainly metabolized by CYP3A4 and which have a low therapeutic index (e.g., quinidine, terfenadine) should therefore be used with caution). Products include:
Carbatrol Capsules 3019
Equetro Extended-Release Capsules 3174

Carisoprodol (Limited published data indicate that somatostatin analogs may decrease the metabolic clearance of compounds known to be metabolized by cytochrome P450 enzymes, which may be due to the suppression of growth hormone). Products include:
Soma Tablets 1931

Carteolol Hydrochloride (Concomitant administration of bradycardia inducing drugs (e.g., beta blockers) may have an additive effect on the reduction of heart rate associated with octreotide. Dose adjustment of concomitant medication may be necessary).
No products indexed under this heading.

Carvedilol (Limited published data indicate that somatostatin analogs may decrease the metabolic clearance of compounds known to be metabolized by cytochrome P450 enzymes, which may be due to the suppression of growth hormone). Products include:
Coreg Tablets 1387

Celecoxib (Limited published data indicate that somatostatin analogs may decrease the metabolic clearance of compounds known to be metabolized by cytochrome P450 enzymes, which may be due to the suppression of growth hormone). Products include:
Celebrex Capsules 2979

Cerivastatin Sodium (Limited published data indicate that somatostatin analogs may decrease the metabolic clearance of compounds known to be metabolized by cytochrome P450 enzymes, which may be due to the suppression of growth hormone. Since it cannot be excluded that octreotide may have this effect, other drugs mainly metabolized by CYP3A4 and which have a low therapeutic index (e.g., quinidine, terfenadine) should therefore be used with caution).
No products indexed under this heading.

Cevimeline Hydrochloride (Limited published data indicate that somatostatin analogs may decrease the metabolic clearance of compounds known to be metabolized by cytochrome P450 enzymes, which may be due to the suppression of growth hormone). Products include:
Evoxac Capsules 1013

Chlordiazepoxide (Limited published data indicate that somatostatin analogs may decrease the metabolic clearance of compounds known to be metabolized by cytochrome P450 enzymes, which may be due to the suppression of growth hormone).
No products indexed under this heading.

Chlordiazepoxide Hydrochloride (Limited published data indicate that somatostatin analogs may decrease the metabolic clearance of compounds known to be metabolized by cytochrome P450 enzymes, which may be due to the suppression of growth hormone).
No products indexed under this heading.

Chlorpheniramine (Limited published data indicate that somatostatin analogs may decrease the metabolic clearance of compounds known to be metabolized by cytochrome P450 enzymes, which may be due to the suppression of growth hormone. Since it cannot be excluded that octreotide may have this effect, other drugs mainly metabolized by CYP3A4 and which have a low therapeutic index (e.g., quinidine, terfenadine) should therefore be used with caution).
No products indexed under this heading.

Chlorpheniramine Maleate (Limited published data indicate that somatostatin analogs may decrease the metabolic clearance of compounds known to be metabolized by cytochrome P450 enzymes, which may be due to the suppression of growth hormone. Since it cannot be excluded that octreotide may have this effect, other drugs mainly metabolized by CYP3A4 and which have a low therapeutic index (e.g., quinidine, terfenadine) should therefore be used with caution). Products include:
Actifed Cold & Allergy Tablets 1895
Sudafed PE Sinus & Allergy Tablets 1908
Tylenol Allergy Multi-Symptom Caplets with Cool Burst and Rapid Release Gelcaps 1916
Children's Tylenol Plus Cold Suspension Liquid 1912
Children's Tylenol Plus Cough & Runny Nose Suspension Liquid 1912
Children's Tylenol Plus Flu Suspension Liquid 1914
Children's Tylenol Plus Multi-Symptom Cold Suspension Liquid 1912
Tylenol Cold Head Congestion Nighttime Caplets with Cool Burst 1910
Tylenol Cold Multi-Symptom Nighttime Caplets with Cool Burst 1913
Tylenol Sinus Congestion & Pain Nighttime Caplets with Cool Burst 1917

Chlorpheniramine Polistirex (Limited published data indicate that somatostatin analogs may decrease the metabolic clearance of compounds known to be metabolized by cytochrome P450 enzymes, which may be due to the suppression of growth hormone. Since it cannot be excluded that octreotide may have this effect, other drugs mainly metabolized by CYP3A4 and which have a low therapeutic index (e.g., quinidine, terfenadine) should therefore be used with caution). Products include:

Tussionex Pennkinetic Extended-Release Suspension 3154

Chlorpheniramine Tannate (Limited published data indicate that somatostatin analogs may decrease the metabolic clearance of compounds known to be metabolized by cytochrome P450 enzymes, which may be due to the suppression of growth hormone. Since it cannot be excluded that octreotide may have this effect, other drugs mainly metabolized by CYP3A4 and which have a low therapeutic index (e.g., quinidine, terfenadine) should therefore be used with caution).

No products indexed under this heading.

Chlorpromazine (Limited published data indicate that somatostatin analogs may decrease the metabolic clearance of compounds known to be metabolized by cytochrome P450 enzymes, which may be due to the suppression of growth hormone).

No products indexed under this heading.

Chlorpromazine Hydrochloride (Limited published data indicate that somatostatin analogs may decrease the metabolic clearance of compounds known to be metabolized by cytochrome P450 enzymes, which may be due to the suppression of growth hormone).

No products indexed under this heading.

Chlorpropamide (Octreotide inhibits the secretion of insulin and glucagon. Therefore, blood glucose levels should be monitored when octreotide is initiated or when the dose is altered and antidiabetic treatment should be adjusted accordingly).

No products indexed under this heading.

Cilostazol (Limited published data indicate that somatostatin analogs may decrease the metabolic clearance of compounds known to be metabolized by cytochrome P450 enzymes, which may be due to the suppression of growth hormone). Products include:

Pletal Tablets 2481

Cimetidine Hydrochloride (Limited published data indicate that somatostatin analogs may decrease the metabolic clearance of compounds known to be metabolized by cytochrome P450 enzymes, which may be due to the suppression of growth hormone).

No products indexed under this heading.

Ciprofloxacin (Limited published data indicate that somatostatin analogs may decrease the metabolic clearance of compounds known to be metabolized by cytochrome P450 enzymes, which may be due to the suppression of growth hormone). Products include:

Cipro I.V. 2817
Cipro Oral Suspension 2810
Cipro XR Tablets 2823
Ciprodex Otic Suspension 541

Ciprofloxacin Hydrochloride (Limited published data indicate that somatostatin analogs may decrease the metabolic clearance of compounds known to be metabolized by cytochrome P450 enzymes, which may be due to the suppression of growth hormone). Products include:

Cipro Tablets 2810

Cisapride (Limited published data indicate that somatostatin analogs may decrease the metabolic clearance of compounds known to be metabolized by cytochrome P450 enzymes, which may be due to the suppression of growth hormone. Since it cannot be excluded that octreotide may have this effect, other drugs mainly metabolized by CYP3A4 and which have a low therapeutic index (e.g., quinidine, terfenadine) should therefore be used with caution).

No products indexed under this heading.

Citalopram Hydrobromide (Limited published data indicate that somatostatin analogs may decrease the metabolic clearance of compounds known to be metabolized by cytochrome P450 enzymes, which may be due to the suppression of growth hormone). Products include:

Celexa 1160

Clarithromycin (Limited published data indicate that somatostatin analogs may decrease the metabolic clearance of compounds known to be metabolized by cytochrome P450 enzymes, which may be due to the suppression of growth hormone. Since it cannot be excluded that octreotide may have this effect, other drugs mainly metabolized by CYP3A4 and which have a low therapeutic index (e.g., quinidine, terfenadine) should therefore be used with caution). Products include:

Biaxin/Biaxin XL 411

Clomipramine Hydrochloride (Limited published data indicate that somatostatin analogs may decrease the metabolic clearance of compounds known to be metabolized by cytochrome P450 enzymes, which may be due to the suppression of growth hormone).

No products indexed under this heading.

Clopidogrel Hydrogen Sulfate (Limited published data indicate that somatostatin analogs may decrease the metabolic clearance of compounds known to be metabolized by cytochrome P450 enzymes, which may be due to the suppression of growth hormone).

No products indexed under this heading.

Clozapine (Limited published data indicate that somatostatin analogs may decrease the metabolic clearance of compounds known to be metabolized by cytochrome P450 enzymes, which may be due to the suppression of growth hormone).

No products indexed under this heading.

Codeine Phosphate (Limited published data indicate that somatostatin analogs may decrease the metabolic clearance of compounds known to be metabolized by cytochrome P450 enzymes, which may be due to the suppression of growth hormone). Products include:

Tylenol with Codeine Tablets 2427

Codeine Sulfate (Limited published data indicate that somatostatin analogs may decrease the metabolic clearance of compounds known to be metabolized by cytochrome P450 enzymes, which may be due to the suppression of growth hormone).

No products indexed under this heading.

Cyclobenzaprine (Limited published data indicate that somatostatin analogs may decrease the metabolic clearance of compounds known to be metabolized by cytochrome P450 enzymes, which may be due to the suppression of growth hormone).

No products indexed under this heading.

Cyclobenzaprine Hydrochloride (Limited published data indicate that somatostatin analogs may decrease the metabolic clearance of compounds known to be metabolized by cytochrome P450 enzymes, which may be due to the suppression of growth hormone). Products include:

Amrix Capsules 966

Cyclophosphamide (Limited published data indicate that somatostatin analogs may decrease the metabolic clearance of compounds known to be metabolized by cytochrome P450 enzymes, which may be due to the suppression of growth hormone).

No products indexed under this heading.

Cyclosporine (Concomitant administration of octreotide injection with cyclosporine may decrease blood levels of cyclosporine and result in transplant rejection). Products include:

Gengraf Capsules 435
Neoral Oral Solution 2280
Neoral Soft Gelatin Capsules 2280
Restasis Ophthalmic Emulsion 557
Sandimmune 2296

Desipramine Hydrochloride (Limited published data indicate that somatostatin analogs may decrease the metabolic clearance of compounds known to be metabolized by cytochrome P450 enzymes, which may be due to the suppression of growth hormone).

No products indexed under this heading.

Desogestrel (Limited published data indicate that somatostatin analogs may decrease the metabolic clearance of compounds known to be metabolized by cytochrome P450 enzymes, which may be due to the suppression of growth hormone. Since it cannot be excluded that octreotide may have this effect, other drugs mainly metabolized by CYP3A4 and which have a low therapeutic index (e.g., quinidine, terfenadine) should therefore be used with caution). Products include:

Mircette Tablets 1034

Dexamethasone (Limited published data indicate that somatostatin analogs may decrease the metabolic clearance of compounds known to be metabolized by cytochrome P450 enzymes, which may be due to the suppression of growth hormone). Products include:

Ciprodex Otic Suspension 541

Dexamethasone Acetate (Limited published data indicate that somatostatin analogs may decrease the metabolic clearance of compounds known to be metabolized by cytochrome P450 enzymes, which may be due to the suppression of growth hormone).

No products indexed under this heading.

Dexamethasone Phosphate (Limited published data indicate that somatostatin analogs may decrease the metabolic clearance of compounds known to be metabolized by cytochrome P450 enzymes, which may be due to the suppression of growth hormone).

No products indexed under this heading.

Dexamethasone Sodium (Limited published data indicate that somatostatin analogs may decrease the metabolic clearance of compounds known to be metabolized by cytochrome P450 enzymes, which may be due to the suppression of growth hormone).

No products indexed under this heading.

Dexamethasone Sodium Phosphate (Limited published data indicate that somatostatin analogs may decrease the metabolic clearance of compounds known to be metabolized by cytochrome P450 enzymes, which may be due to the suppression of growth hormone).

No products indexed under this heading.

Dexfenfluramine Hydrochloride (Limited published data indicate that somatostatin analogs may decrease the metabolic clearance of compounds known to be metabolized by cytochrome P450 enzymes, which may be due to the suppression of growth hormone).

No products indexed under this heading.

Dextromethorphan (Limited published data indicate that somatostatin analogs may decrease the metabolic clearance of compounds known to be metabolized by cytochrome P450 enzymes, which may be due to the suppression of growth hormone).

No products indexed under this heading.

Dextromethorphan Hydrobromide (Limited published data indicate that somatostatin analogs may decrease the metabolic clearance of compounds known to be metabolized by cytochrome P450 enzymes, which may be due to the suppression of growth hormone). Products include:

PediaCare Children's Liquid Multi-Symptom Cold 1902
PediaCare Children's Long-Acting Cough 1902
Children's Sudafed PE Cold & Cough Liquid 1907
Sudafed PE Cold & Cough Caplets 1907
Children's Tylenol Plus Cough & Runny Nose Suspension Liquid 1912
Children's Tylenol Plus Cough & Sore Throat Suspension Liquid 1912
Children's Tylenol Plus Flu Suspension Liquid 1914
Children's Tylenol Plus Multi-Symptom Cold Suspension Liquid 1912
Tylenol Cold Severe Congestion Daytime Caplets with Cool Burst 1912

Tylenol Cold Head Congestion Daytime Caplets with Cool Burst 1910
Tylenol Cold Head Congestion Nighttime Caplets with Cool Burst 1910
Tylenol Cold Head Congestion Severe Daytime Caplets with Cool Burst 1910
Tylenol Cold Multi-Symptom Daytime Caplets with Cool Burst and Rapid Release Gels 1913
Tylenol Cold Multi-Symptom Daytime Liquid with Citrus Burst ... 1913
Tylenol Cold Multi-Symptom Nighttime Caplets with Cool Burst 1913
Tylenol Cold Multi-Symptom Nighttime Liquid with Cool Burst ... 1913
Tylenol Cold Multi-Symptom Severe Caplets with Cool Burst 1913
Tylenol Cold Multi-Symptom Severe Daytime Liquid with Citrus Burst 1913
Tylenol Cough & Sore Throat Daytime Liquid with Cool Burst 1918
Tylenol Cough & Sore Throat Nighttime Liquid with Cool Burst ... 1918
Vicks DayQuil Cold & Flu Multi-Symptom Relief .... ▣616
Vicks DayQuil LiquiCaps 2567
Vicks DayQuil Liquid 2567
Vicks DayQuil Multi-Symptom Cold/Flu Relief 2567
Vicks NyQuil Cold & Flu Multi-Symptom Relief .... ▣617
Vicks NyQuil LiquiCaps 2567
Vicks NyQuil Liquid 2567
Vicks NyQuil Multi-Symptom Cold/Flu Relief 2567

Dextromethorphan Polistirex (Limited published data indicate that somatostatin analogs may decrease the metabolic clearance of compounds known to be metabolized by cytochrome P450 enzymes, which may be due to the suppression of growth hormone).
No products indexed under this heading.

Diazepam (Limited published data indicate that somatostatin analogs may decrease the metabolic clearance of compounds known to be metabolized by cytochrome P450 enzymes, which may be due to the suppression of growth hormone. Since it cannot be excluded that octreotide may have this effect, other drugs mainly metabolized by CYP3A4 and which have a low therapeutic index (e.g., quinidine, terfenadine) should therefore be used with caution). Products include:
Valium Tablets 2658

Diclofenac Potassium (Limited published data indicate that somatostatin analogs may decrease the metabolic clearance of compounds known to be metabolized by cytochrome P450 enzymes, which may be due to the suppression of growth hormone).
No products indexed under this heading.

Diclofenac Sodium (Limited published data indicate that somatostatin analogs may decrease the metabolic clearance of compounds known to be metabolized by cytochrome P450 enzymes, which may be due to the suppression of growth hormone). Products include:
Diclofenac Sodium Ophthalmic Solution .... ⊙240
Voltaren Ophthalmic Solution 2336
Voltaren Tablets 2334
Voltaren-XR Tablets 2337

Dihydroergotamine Mesylate (Limited published data indicate that somatostatin analogs may decrease the metabolic clearance of compounds known to be metabolized by cytochrome P450 enzymes, which may be due to the suppression of growth hormone. Since it cannot be excluded that octreotide may have this effect, other drugs mainly metabolized by CYP3A4 and which have a low therapeutic index (e.g., quinidine, terfenadine) should therefore be used with caution).
No products indexed under this heading.

Diltiazem Hydrochloride (Limited published data indicate that somatostatin analogs may decrease the metabolic clearance of compounds known to be metabolized by cytochrome P450 enzymes, which may be due to the suppression of growth hormone. Since it cannot be excluded that octreotide may have this effect, other drugs mainly metabolized by CYP3A4 and which have a low therapeutic index (e.g., quinidine, terfenadine) should therefore be used with caution). Products include:
Cardizem LA Extended Release Tablets 421

Diltiazem Maleate (Limited published data indicate that somatostatin analogs may decrease the metabolic clearance of compounds known to be metabolized by cytochrome P450 enzymes, which may be due to the suppression of growth hormone. Since it cannot be excluded that octreotide may have this effect, other drugs mainly metabolized by CYP3A4 and which have a low therapeutic index (e.g., quinidine, terfenadine) should therefore be used with caution).
No products indexed under this heading.

Disopyramide (Limited published data indicate that somatostatin analogs may decrease the metabolic clearance of compounds known to be metabolized by cytochrome P450 enzymes, which may be due to the suppression of growth hormone. Since it cannot be excluded that octreotide may have this effect, other drugs mainly metabolized by CYP3A4 and which have a low therapeutic index (e.g., quinidine, terfenadine) should therefore be used with caution).
No products indexed under this heading.

Disopyramide Phosphate (Limited published data indicate that somatostatin analogs may decrease the metabolic clearance of compounds known to be metabolized by cytochrome P450 enzymes, which may be due to the suppression of growth hormone. Since it cannot be excluded that octreotide may have this effect, other drugs mainly metabolized by CYP3A4 and which have a low therapeutic index (e.g., quinidine, terfenadine) should therefore be used with caution).
No products indexed under this heading.

Disulfiram (Limited published data indicate that somatostatin analogs may decrease the metabolic clearance of compounds known to be metabolized by cytochrome P450 enzymes, which may be due to the suppression of growth hormone. Since it cannot be excluded that octreotide may have this effect, other drugs mainly metabolized by CYP3A4 and which have a low therapeutic index (e.g., quinidine, terfenadine) should therefore be used with caution).
No products indexed under this heading.

Divalproex Sodium (Limited published data indicate that somatostatin analogs may decrease the metabolic clearance of compounds known to be metabolized by cytochrome P450 enzymes, which may be due to the suppression of growth hormone). Products include:
Depakote ER Tablets 423

Docetaxel (Limited published data indicate that somatostatin analogs may decrease the metabolic clearance of compounds known to be metabolized by cytochrome P450 enzymes, which may be due to the suppression of growth hormone). Products include:
Taxotere Injection Concentrate 2773

Dolasetron Mesylate (Limited published data indicate that somatostatin analogs may decrease the metabolic clearance of compounds known to be metabolized by cytochrome P450 enzymes, which may be due to the suppression of growth hormone). Products include:
Anzemet Injection 2701
Anzemet Tablets 2704

Donepezil Hydrochloride (Limited published data indicate that somatostatin analogs may decrease the metabolic clearance of compounds known to be metabolized by cytochrome P450 enzymes, which may be due to the suppression of growth hormone). Products include:
Aricept Tablets 1062
Aricept ODT Tablets 1062

Doxepin Hydrochloride (Limited published data indicate that somatostatin analogs may decrease the metabolic clearance of compounds known to be metabolized by cytochrome P450 enzymes, which may be due to the suppression of growth hormone).
No products indexed under this heading.

Doxorubicin Hydrochloride (Limited published data indicate that somatostatin analogs may decrease the metabolic clearance of compounds known to be metabolized by cytochrome P450 enzymes, which may be due to the suppression of growth hormone. Since it cannot be excluded that octreotide may have this effect, other drugs mainly metabolized by CYP3A4 and which have a low therapeutic index (e.g., quinidine, terfenadine) should therefore be used with caution).
No products indexed under this heading.

Dronabinol (Limited published data indicate that somatostatin analogs may decrease the metabolic clearance of compounds known to be metabolized by cytochrome P450 enzymes, which may be due to the suppression of growth hormone. Since it cannot be excluded that octreotide may have this effect, other drugs mainly metabolized by CYP3A4 and which have a low therapeutic index (e.g., quinidine, terfenadine) should therefore be used with caution). Products include:
Marinol Capsules 3163

Drugs, Oral, unspecified (Octreotide has been associated with alterations in nutrient absorption, so it may have an effect on absorption of orally administered drugs).
No products indexed under this heading.

Drugs that Undergo Biotransformation by Cytochrome P-450 Mixed Function Oxidase (Limited published data indicate that somatostatin analogs may decrease the metabolic clearance of compounds known to be metabolized by cytochrome P450 enzymes, which may be due to the suppression of growth hormone).
No products indexed under this heading.

Dyphylline (Limited published data indicate that somatostatin analogs may decrease the metabolic clearance of compounds known to be metabolized by cytochrome P450 enzymes, which may be due to the suppression of growth hormone).
No products indexed under this heading.

Encainide Hydrochloride (Limited published data indicate that somatostatin analogs may decrease the metabolic clearance of compounds known to be metabolized by cytochrome P450 enzymes, which may be due to the suppression of growth hormone).
No products indexed under this heading.

Enoxacin (Limited published data indicate that somatostatin analogs may decrease the metabolic clearance of compounds known to be metabolized by cytochrome P450 enzymes, which may be due to the suppression of growth hormone).
No products indexed under this heading.

Eprosartan Mesylate (Limited published data indicate that somatostatin analogs may decrease the metabolic clearance of compounds known to be metabolized by cytochrome P450 enzymes, which may be due to the suppression of growth hormone). Products include:
Teveten Tablets 515
Teveten HCT Tablets 517

Ergotamine Tartrate (Limited published data indicate that somatostatin analogs may decrease the metabolic clearance of compounds known to be metabolized by cytochrome P450 enzymes, which may be due to the suppression of growth hormone. Since it cannot be excluded that octreotide may have this effect, other drugs mainly metabolized by CYP3A4 and which have a low therapeutic index (e.g., quinidine, terfenadine) should therefore be used with caution).
No products indexed under this heading.

Erythromycin (Limited published data indicate that somatostatin analogs may decrease the metabolic clearance of compounds known to be metabolized by cytochrome P450 enzymes, which may be due to the suppression of growth hormone. Since it cannot be excluded that octreotide may have this effect, other drugs mainly metabolized by CYP3A4 and which have a low therapeutic index (e.g., quinidine, terfenadine) should therefore be used with

caution).
No products indexed under this heading.

Erythromycin Estolate (Limited published data indicate that somatostatin analogs may decrease the metabolic clearance of compounds known to be metabolized by cytochrome P450 enzymes, which may be due to the suppression of growth hormone. Since it cannot be excluded that octreotide may have this effect, other drugs mainly metabolized by CYP3A4 and which have a low therapeutic index (e.g., quinidine, terfenadine) should therefore be used with caution).
No products indexed under this heading.

Erythromycin Ethylsuccinate (Limited published data indicate that somatostatin analogs may decrease the metabolic clearance of compounds known to be metabolized by cytochrome P450 enzymes, which may be due to the suppression of growth hormone. Since it cannot be excluded that octreotide may have this effect, other drugs mainly metabolized by CYP3A4 and which have a low therapeutic index (e.g., quinidine, terfenadine) should therefore be used with caution). Products include:
E.E.S. 433
EryPed 431

Erythromycin Gluceptate (Limited published data indicate that somatostatin analogs may decrease the metabolic clearance of compounds known to be metabolized by cytochrome P450 enzymes, which may be due to the suppression of growth hormone. Since it cannot be excluded that octreotide may have this effect, other drugs mainly metabolized by CYP3A4 and which have a low therapeutic index (e.g., quinidine, terfenadine) should therefore be used with caution).
No products indexed under this heading.

Erythromycin Lactobionate (Limited published data indicate that somatostatin analogs may decrease the metabolic clearance of compounds known to be metabolized by cytochrome P450 enzymes, which may be due to the suppression of growth hormone. Since it cannot be excluded that octreotide may have this effect, other drugs mainly metabolized by CYP3A4 and which have a low therapeutic index (e.g., quinidine, terfenadine) should therefore be used with caution).
No products indexed under this heading.

Erythromycin Stearate (Limited published data indicate that somatostatin analogs may decrease the metabolic clearance of compounds known to be metabolized by cytochrome P450 enzymes, which may be due to the suppression of growth hormone. Since it cannot be excluded that octreotide may have this effect, other drugs mainly metabolized by CYP3A4 and which have a low therapeutic index (e.g., quinidine, terfenadine) should therefore be used with caution).
No products indexed under this heading.

Esmolol Hydrochloride (Concomitant administration of bradycardia inducing drugs (e.g., beta blockers) may have an additive effect on the reduction of heart rate associated with octreotide. Dose adjustment of concomitant medication may be necessary).
No products indexed under this heading.

Esomeprazole Magnesium (Limited published data indicate that somatostatin analogs may decrease the metabolic clearance of compounds known to be metabolized by cytochrome P450 enzymes, which may be due to the suppression of growth hormone). Products include:
Nexium Delayed-Release Capsules 645
Nexium Delayed-Release Oral Suspension 645

Estradiol (Limited published data indicate that somatostatin analogs may decrease the metabolic clearance of compounds known to be metabolized by cytochrome P450 enzymes, which may be due to the suppression of growth hormone. Since it cannot be excluded that octreotide may have this effect, other drugs mainly metabolized by CYP3A4 and which have a low therapeutic index (e.g., quinidine, terfenadine) should therefore be used with caution). Products include:
Activella Tablets 2347
Angeliq Tablets 751
Climara Transdermal System 763
Climara Pro Transdermal System 768
Divigel 3167
Vagifem Tablets 2375

Estradiol Benzoate (Limited published data indicate that somatostatin analogs may decrease the metabolic clearance of compounds known to be metabolized by cytochrome P450 enzymes, which may be due to the suppression of growth hormone. Since it cannot be excluded that octreotide may have this effect, other drugs mainly metabolized by CYP3A4 and which have a low therapeutic index (e.g., quinidine, terfenadine) should therefore be used with caution).
No products indexed under this heading.

Estradiol Cypionate (Limited published data indicate that somatostatin analogs may decrease the metabolic clearance of compounds known to be metabolized by cytochrome P450 enzymes, which may be due to the suppression of growth hormone. Since it cannot be excluded that octreotide may have this effect, other drugs mainly metabolized by CYP3A4 and which have a low therapeutic index (e.g., quinidine, terfenadine) should therefore be used with caution).
No products indexed under this heading.

Estradiol Valerate (Limited published data indicate that somatostatin analogs may decrease the metabolic clearance of compounds known to be metabolized by cytochrome P450 enzymes, which may be due to the suppression of growth hormone. Since it cannot be excluded that octreotide may have this effect, other drugs mainly metabolized by CYP3A4 and which have a low therapeutic index (e.g., quinidine, terfenadine) should therefore be used with caution).
No products indexed under this heading.

Estrogen (Limited published data indicate that somatostatin analogs may decrease the metabolic clearance of compounds known to be metabolized by cytochrome P450 enzymes, which may be due to the suppression of growth hormone).
No products indexed under this heading.

Estrogens, Conjugated (Limited published data indicate that somatostatin analogs may decrease the metabolic clearance of compounds known to be metabolized by cytochrome P450 enzymes, which may be due to the suppression of growth hormone). Products include:
Premarin Intravenous 3217
Premarin Tablets 3221
Premarin Vaginal Cream 3228
Premphase Tablets 3232
Prempro Tablets 3232

Estrogens, Conjugated, Synthetic A (Limited published data indicate that somatostatin analogs may decrease the metabolic clearance of compounds known to be metabolized by cytochrome P450 enzymes, which may be due to the suppression of growth hormone).
No products indexed under this heading.

Estrogens, Esterified (Limited published data indicate that somatostatin analogs may decrease the metabolic clearance of compounds known to be metabolized by cytochrome P450 enzymes, which may be due to the suppression of growth hormone). Products include:
Estratest Tablets 3043
Estratest H.S. Tablets 3043

Ethinyl Estradiol (Limited published data indicate that somatostatin analogs may decrease the metabolic clearance of compounds known to be metabolized by cytochrome P450 enzymes, which may be due to the suppression of growth hormone. Since it cannot be excluded that octreotide may have this effect, other drugs mainly metabolized by CYP3A4 and which have a low therapeutic index (e.g., quinidine, terfenadine) should therefore be used with caution). Products include:
Lybrel Tablets 3204
Mircette Tablets 1034
NuvaRing 2897
Ortho-Cyclen/Ortho Tri-Cyclen 2449
Ortho Evra Transdermal System 2437
Ortho Tri-Cyclen Lo Tablets 2458
Seasonique Tablets 1046
Yaz Tablets 805

Ethosuximide (Limited published data indicate that somatostatin analogs may decrease the metabolic clearance of compounds known to be metabolized by cytochrome P450 enzymes, which may be due to the suppression of growth hormone. Since it cannot be excluded that octreotide may have this effect, other drugs mainly metabolized by CYP3A4 and which have a low therapeutic index (e.g., quinidine, terfenadine) should therefore be used with caution).
No products indexed under this heading.

Ethotoin (Limited published data indicate that somatostatin analogs may decrease the metabolic clearance of compounds known to be metabolized by cytochrome P450 enzymes, which may be due to the suppression of growth hormone).
No products indexed under this heading.

Ethynodiol Diacetate (Limited published data indicate that somatostatin analogs may decrease the metabolic clearance of compounds known to be metabolized by cytochrome P450 enzymes, which may be due to the suppression of growth hormone. Since it cannot be excluded that octreotide may have this effect, other drugs mainly metabolized by CYP3A4 and which have a low therapeutic index (e.g., quinidine, terfenadine) should therefore be used with caution).
No products indexed under this heading.

Etodolac (Limited published data indicate that somatostatin analogs may decrease the metabolic clearance of compounds known to be metabolized by cytochrome P450 enzymes, which may be due to the suppression of growth hormone).
No products indexed under this heading.

Etoposide (Limited published data indicate that somatostatin analogs may decrease the metabolic clearance of compounds known to be metabolized by cytochrome P450 enzymes, which may be due to the suppression of growth hormone. Since it cannot be excluded that octreotide may have this effect, other drugs mainly metabolized by CYP3A4 and which have a low therapeutic index (e.g., quinidine, terfenadine) should therefore be used with caution).
No products indexed under this heading.

Etoposide Phosphate (Limited published data indicate that somatostatin analogs may decrease the metabolic clearance of compounds known to be metabolized by cytochrome P450 enzymes, which may be due to the suppression of growth hormone. Since it cannot be excluded that octreotide may have this effect, other drugs mainly metabolized by CYP3A4 and which have a low therapeutic index (e.g., quinidine, terfenadine) should therefore be used with caution).
No products indexed under this heading.

Felbamate (Limited published data indicate that somatostatin analogs may decrease the metabolic clearance of compounds known to be metabolized by cytochrome P450 enzymes, which may be due to the suppression of growth hormone).
No products indexed under this heading.

Felodipine (Limited published data indicate that somatostatin analogs may decrease the metabolic clearance of compounds known to be metabolized by cytochrome P450 enzymes, which may be due to the suppression of growth hormone. Since it cannot be excluded that octreotide may have this effect, other drugs mainly metabolized by CYP3A4 and which have a low therapeutic index (e.g., quinidine, terfenadine) should therefore be used with

caution).
No products indexed under this heading.

Fenoprofen Calcium (Limited published data indicate that somatostatin analogs may decrease the metabolic clearance of compounds known to be metabolized by cytochrome P450 enzymes, which may be due to the suppression of growth hormone). Products include:
Nalfon Capsules 2508

Fentanyl (Limited published data indicate that somatostatin analogs may decrease the metabolic clearance of compounds known to be metabolized by cytochrome P450 enzymes, which may be due to the suppression of growth hormone. Since it cannot be excluded that octreotide may have this effect, other drugs mainly metabolized by CYP3A4 and which have a low therapeutic index (e.g., quinidine, terfenadine) should therefore be used with caution). Products include:
Duragesic Transdermal System 2405
Ionsys Transdermal System 2410

Fentanyl Citrate (Limited published data indicate that somatostatin analogs may decrease the metabolic clearance of compounds known to be metabolized by cytochrome P450 enzymes, which may be due to the suppression of growth hormone. Since it cannot be excluded that octreotide may have this effect, other drugs mainly metabolized by CYP3A4 and which have a low therapeutic index (e.g., quinidine, terfenadine) should therefore be used with caution). Products include:
Actiq 959
Fentora Tablets 968

Flecainide Acetate (Limited published data indicate that somatostatin analogs may decrease the metabolic clearance of compounds known to be metabolized by cytochrome P450 enzymes, which may be due to the suppression of growth hormone).
No products indexed under this heading.

Fluoxetine (Limited published data indicate that somatostatin analogs may decrease the metabolic clearance of compounds known to be metabolized by cytochrome P450 enzymes, which may be due to the suppression of growth hormone).
No products indexed under this heading.

Fluoxetine Hydrochloride (Limited published data indicate that somatostatin analogs may decrease the metabolic clearance of compounds known to be metabolized by cytochrome P450 enzymes, which may be due to the suppression of growth hormone). Products include:
Prozac Weekly Capsules 1852
Prozac Pulvules and Liquid 1852
Symbyax Capsules 1871

Fluphenazine Decanoate (Limited published data indicate that somatostatin analogs may decrease the metabolic clearance of compounds known to be metabolized by cytochrome P450 enzymes, which may be due to the suppression of growth hormone).
No products indexed under this heading.

Fluphenazine Enanthate (Limited published data indicate that somatostatin analogs may decrease the metabolic clearance of compounds known to be metabolized by cytochrome P450 enzymes, which may be due to the suppression of growth hormone).
No products indexed under this heading.

Fluphenazine Hydrochloride (Limited published data indicate that somatostatin analogs may decrease the metabolic clearance of compounds known to be metabolized by cytochrome P450 enzymes, which may be due to the suppression of growth hormone).
No products indexed under this heading.

Flurbiprofen (Limited published data indicate that somatostatin analogs may decrease the metabolic clearance of compounds known to be metabolized by cytochrome P450 enzymes, which may be due to the suppression of growth hormone).
No products indexed under this heading.

Flurbiprofen Sodium (Limited published data indicate that somatostatin analogs may decrease the metabolic clearance of compounds known to be metabolized by cytochrome P450 enzymes, which may be due to the suppression of growth hormone).
No products indexed under this heading.

Flutamide (Limited published data indicate that somatostatin analogs may decrease the metabolic clearance of compounds known to be metabolized by cytochrome P450 enzymes, which may be due to the suppression of growth hormone).
No products indexed under this heading.

Fluticasone Propionate (Limited published data indicate that somatostatin analogs may decrease the metabolic clearance of compounds known to be metabolized by cytochrome P450 enzymes, which may be due to the suppression of growth hormone). Products include:
Advair Diskus 100/50 1276
Advair Diskus 250/50 1276
Advair Diskus 500/50 1276
Advair HFA 45/21 Inhalation Aerosol 1288
Advair HFA 115/21 Inhalation Aerosol 1288
Advair HFA 230/21 Inhalation Aerosol 1288
Flonase Nasal Spray 1431
Flovent Diskus 50 mcg 1435

Fluvastatin Sodium (Limited published data indicate that somatostatin analogs may decrease the metabolic clearance of compounds known to be metabolized by cytochrome P450 enzymes, which may be due to the suppression of growth hormone). Products include:
Lescol Capsules 2268
Lescol XL Tablets 2268

Fluvoxamine Maleate (Limited published data indicate that somatostatin analogs may decrease the metabolic clearance of compounds known to be metabolized by cytochrome P450 enzymes, which may be due to the suppression of growth hormone). Products include:
Luvox CR Extended-Release Capsules 1759

Formoterol Fumarate (Limited published data indicate that somatostatin analogs may decrease the metabolic clearance of compounds known to be metabolized by cytochrome P450 enzymes, which may be due to the suppression of growth hormone). Products include:
Foradil Aerolizer 2849
Perforomist Inhalation Solution 1025

Fosphenytoin (Limited published data indicate that somatostatin analogs may decrease the metabolic clearance of compounds known to be metabolized by cytochrome P450 enzymes, which may be due to the suppression of growth hormone).
No products indexed under this heading.

Fosphenytoin Sodium (Limited published data indicate that somatostatin analogs may decrease the metabolic clearance of compounds known to be metabolized by cytochrome P450 enzymes, which may be due to the suppression of growth hormone).
No products indexed under this heading.

Gabapentin (Limited published data indicate that somatostatin analogs may decrease the metabolic clearance of compounds known to be metabolized by cytochrome P450 enzymes, which may be due to the suppression of growth hormone).
No products indexed under this heading.

Galantamine Hydrobromide (Limited published data indicate that somatostatin analogs may decrease the metabolic clearance of compounds known to be metabolized by cytochrome P450 enzymes, which may be due to the suppression of growth hormone).
No products indexed under this heading.

Glimepiride (Octreotide inhibits the secretion of insulin and glucagon. Therefore, blood glucose levels should be monitored when octreotide is initiated or when the dose is altered and antidiabetic treatment should be adjusted accordingly). Products include:
Avandaryl Tablets 1344
Duetact Tablets 3085

Glipizide (Octreotide inhibits the secretion of insulin and glucagon. Therefore, blood glucose levels should be monitored when octreotide is initiated or when the dose is altered and antidiabetic treatment should be adjusted accordingly).
No products indexed under this heading.

Glyburide (Octreotide inhibits the secretion of insulin and glucagon. Therefore, blood glucose levels should be monitored when octreotide is initiated or when the dose is altered and antidiabetic treatment should be adjusted accordingly).
No products indexed under this heading.

Grepafloxacin Hydrochloride (Limited published data indicate that somatostatin analogs may decrease the metabolic clearance of compounds known to be metabolized by cytochrome P450 enzymes, which may be due to the suppression of growth hormone).
No products indexed under this heading.

Haloperidol (Limited published data indicate that somatostatin analogs may decrease the metabolic clearance of compounds known to be metabolized by cytochrome P450 enzymes, which may be due to the suppression of growth hormone. Since it cannot be excluded that octreotide may have this effect, other drugs mainly metabolized by CYP3A4 and which have a low therapeutic index (e.g., quinidine, terfenadine) should therefore be used with caution).
No products indexed under this heading.

Haloperidol Decanoate (Limited published data indicate that somatostatin analogs may decrease the metabolic clearance of compounds known to be metabolized by cytochrome P450 enzymes, which may be due to the suppression of growth hormone. Since it cannot be excluded that octreotide may have this effect, other drugs mainly metabolized by CYP3A4 and which have a low therapeutic index (e.g., quinidine, terfenadine) should therefore be used with caution).
No products indexed under this heading.

Haloperidol Lactate (Limited published data indicate that somatostatin analogs may decrease the metabolic clearance of compounds known to be metabolized by cytochrome P450 enzymes, which may be due to the suppression of growth hormone. Since it cannot be excluded that octreotide may have this effect, other drugs mainly metabolized by CYP3A4 and which have a low therapeutic index (e.g., quinidine, terfenadine) should therefore be used with caution).
No products indexed under this heading.

Hydrocodone Bitartrate (Limited published data indicate that somatostatin analogs may decrease the metabolic clearance of compounds known to be metabolized by cytochrome P450 enzymes, which may be due to the suppression of growth hormone). Products include:
Lortab 5/500 Tablets 3143
Lortab 7.5/500 Tablets 3144
Lortab 10/500 Tablets 3144
Vicodin Tablets 529
Vicodin ES Tablets 530
Vicodin HP Tablets 531
Vicoprofen Tablets 533
Zydone Tablets 1132

Ibuprofen (Limited published data indicate that somatostatin analogs may decrease the metabolic clearance of compounds known to be metabolized by cytochrome P450 enzymes, which may be due to the suppression of growth hormone). Products include:
Motrin IB Tablets and Caplets 1900
Children's Motrin Oral Suspension ... 1901
Children's Motrin Non-Staining Dye-Free Oral Suspension 1901
Children's Motrin Cold Oral Suspension 1899
Infants' Motrin Concentrated Drops 1901
Infants' Motrin Non-Staining Dye-Free Concentrated Drops 1901
Junior Strength Motrin Caplets and Chewable Tablets 1901
Vicoprofen Tablets 533

Imipramine Hydrochloride (Limited published data indicate that somatostatin analogs may decrease the metabolic clearance of compounds known to be metabolized by cytochrome P450 enzymes, which may be due to the suppression of growth hormone).
No products indexed under this heading.

Imipramine Pamoate (Limited published data indicate that somatostatin analogs may decrease the metabolic clearance of compounds known to be metabolized by cytochrome P450 enzymes, which may be due to the suppression of growth hormone).
No products indexed under this heading.

Indinavir Sulfate (Limited published data indicate that somatostatin analogs may decrease the metabolic clearance of compounds known to be metabolized by cytochrome P450 enzymes, which may be due to the suppression of growth hormone. Since it cannot be excluded that octreotide may have this effect, other drugs mainly metabolized by CYP3A4 and which have a low therapeutic index (e.g., quinidine, terfenadine) should therefore be used with caution). Products include:
Crixivan Capsules 1979

Indomethacin (Limited published data indicate that somatostatin analogs may decrease the metabolic clearance of compounds known to be metabolized by cytochrome P450 enzymes, which may be due to the suppression of growth hormone). Products include:
Indocin 2024

Indomethacin Sodium Trihydrate (Limited published data indicate that somatostatin analogs may decrease the metabolic clearance of compounds known to be metabolized by cytochrome P450 enzymes, which may be due to the suppression of growth hormone). Products include:
Indocin I.V. 2489

Indoramin Hydrochloride (Limited published data indicate that somatostatin analogs may decrease the metabolic clearance of compounds known to be metabolized by cytochrome P450 enzymes, which may be due to the suppression of growth hormone).
No products indexed under this heading.

Insulin (Octreotide inhibits the secretion of insulin and glucagon. Therefore, blood glucose levels should be monitored when octreotide is initiated or when the dose is altered and antidiabetic treatment should be adjusted accordingly).
No products indexed under this heading.

Insulin, Human, Zinc Suspension (Octreotide inhibits the secretion of insulin and glucagon. Therefore, blood glucose levels should be monitored when octreotide is initiated or when the dose is altered and antidiabetic treatment should be adjusted accordingly).
No products indexed under this heading.

Insulin, Human (rDNA origin) (Octreotide inhibits the secretion of insulin and glucagon. Therefore, blood glucose levels should be monitored when octreotide is initiated or when the dose is altered and antidiabetic treatment should be adjusted accordingly). Products include:
Exubera Inhalation Powder 2515

Insulin, Human NPH (Octreotide inhibits the secretion of insulin and glucagon. Therefore, blood glucose levels should be monitored when octreotide is initiated or when the dose is altered and antidiabetic treatment should be adjusted accordingly). Products include:
Humulin N Vial 1846

Insulin, Human Regular (Octreotide inhibits the secretion of insulin and glucagon. Therefore, blood glucose levels should be monitored when octreotide is initiated or when the dose is altered and antidiabetic treatment should be adjusted accordingly). Products include:
Humulin R 1849
Humulin R (U-500) 1850

Insulin, Human Regular and Human NPH Mixture (Octreotide inhibits the secretion of insulin and glucagon. Therefore, blood glucose levels should be monitored when octreotide is initiated or when the dose is altered and antidiabetic treatment should be adjusted accordingly). Products include:
Humulin 50/50, 100 Units 1843
Humulin 70/30 Vial 1844

Insulin, NPH (Octreotide inhibits the secretion of insulin and glucagon. Therefore, blood glucose levels should be monitored when octreotide is initiated or when the dose is altered and antidiabetic treatment should be adjusted accordingly).
No products indexed under this heading.

Insulin, Regular (Octreotide inhibits the secretion of insulin and glucagon. Therefore, blood glucose levels should be monitored when octreotide is initiated or when the dose is altered and antidiabetic treatment should be adjusted accordingly).
No products indexed under this heading.

Insulin, Regular and NPH mixture (Octreotide inhibits the secretion of insulin and glucagon. Therefore, blood glucose levels should be monitored when octreotide is initiated or when the dose is altered and antidiabetic treatment should be adjusted accordingly).
No products indexed under this heading.

Insulin, Zinc Crystals (Octreotide inhibits the secretion of insulin and glucagon. Therefore, blood glucose levels should be monitored when octreotide is initiated or when the dose is altered and antidiabetic treatment should be adjusted accordingly).
No products indexed under this heading.

Insulin, Zinc Suspension (Octreotide inhibits the secretion of insulin and glucagon. Therefore, blood glucose levels should be monitored when octreotide is initiated or when the dose is altered and antidiabetic treatment should be adjusted accordingly).
No products indexed under this heading.

Insulin Aspart (Octreotide inhibits the secretion of insulin and glucagon. Therefore, blood glucose levels should be monitored when octreotide is initiated or when the dose is altered and antidiabetic treatment should be adjusted accordingly).
No products indexed under this heading.

Insulin Aspart, Human (Octreotide inhibits the secretion of insulin and glucagon. Therefore, blood glucose levels should be monitored when octreotide is initiated or when the dose is altered and antidiabetic treatment should be adjusted accordingly). Products include:
NovoLog Mix 70/30 2364

Insulin Aspart, Human Regular (Octreotide inhibits the secretion of insulin and glucagon. Therefore, blood glucose levels should be monitored when octreotide is initiated or when the dose is altered and antidiabetic treatment should be adjusted accordingly). Products include:
NovoLog Injection 2359

Insulin Aspart Protamine, Human (Octreotide inhibits the secretion of insulin and glucagon. Therefore, blood glucose levels should be monitored when octreotide is initiated or when the dose is altered and antidiabetic treatment should be adjusted accordingly). Products include:
NovoLog Mix 70/30 2364

Insulin Detemir (rDNA Origin) (Octreotide inhibits the secretion of insulin and glucagon. Therefore, blood glucose levels should be monitored when octreotide is initiated or when the dose is altered and antidiabetic treatment should be adjusted accordingly). Products include:
Levemir Injection 2352

Insulin glargine (Octreotide inhibits the secretion of insulin and glucagon. Therefore, blood glucose levels should be monitored when octreotide is initiated or when the dose is altered and antidiabetic treatment should be adjusted accordingly). Products include:
Lantus Injection 2749

Insulin Glulisine (Octreotide inhibits the secretion of insulin and glucagon. Therefore, blood glucose levels should be monitored when octreotide is initiated or when the dose is altered and antidiabetic treatment should be adjusted accordingly). Products include:
Apidra Injection 2706

Insulin Lispro, Human (Octreotide inhibits the secretion of insulin and glucagon. Therefore, blood glucose levels should be monitored when octreotide is initiated or when the dose is altered and antidiabetic treatment should be adjusted accordingly). Products include:
Humalog-Pen and KwikPen 1829
Humalog Mix 50/50-Pen and KwikPen 1833
Humalog Mix 75/25-Pen and KwikPen 1835

Insulin Lispro Protamine, Human (Octreotide inhibits the secretion of insulin and glucagon. Therefore, blood glucose levels should be monitored when octreotide is initiated or when the dose is altered and antidiabetic treatment should be adjusted accordingly). Products include:
Humalog Mix 50/50-Pen and KwikPen 1833
Humalog Mix 75/25-Pen and KwikPen 1835

Irbesartan (Limited published data indicate that somatostatin analogs may decrease the metabolic clearance of compounds known to be metabolized by cytochrome P450 enzymes, which may be due to the suppression of growth hormone). Products include:
Avalide Tablets 892
Avalide Tablets 2713
Avapro Tablets 897
Avapro Tablets 2718

Isotretinoin (Limited published data indicate that somatostatin analogs may decrease the metabolic clearance of compounds known to be metabolized by cytochrome P450 enzymes, which may be due to the suppression of growth hormone). Products include:
Accutane Capsules 2607

Isradipine (Limited published data indicate that somatostatin analogs may decrease the metabolic clearance of compounds known to be metabolized by cytochrome P450 enzymes, which may be due to the suppression of growth hormone. Since it cannot be excluded that octreotide may have this effect, other drugs mainly metabolized by CYP3A4 and which have a low therapeutic index (e.g., quinidine, terfenadine) should therefore be used with caution). Products include:
DynaCirc CR Controlled Release Tablets 1407

Itraconazole (Limited published data indicate that somatostatin analogs may decrease the metabolic clearance of compounds known to be metabolized by cytochrome P450 enzymes, which may be due to the suppression of growth hormone. Since it cannot be excluded that octreotide may have this effect, other drugs mainly metabolized by CYP3A4 and which have a low therapeutic index (e.g., quinidine, terfenadine) should therefore be used with caution).
No products indexed under this heading.

Ixabepilone (Limited published data indicate that somatostatin analogs may decrease the metabolic clearance of compounds known to be metabolized by cytochrome P450 enzymes, which may be due to the suppression of growth hormone. Since it cannot be excluded that octreotide may have this effect, other drugs mainly metabolized by CYP3A4 and which have a low therapeutic index (e.g., quinidine, terfenadine) should therefore be used with caution). Products include:
Ixempra Kit for Injection 915

Ketoconazole (Limited published data indicate that somatostatin analogs may decrease the metabolic clearance of compounds known to be metabolized by cytochrome P450 enzymes, which may be due to the suppression of growth hormone. Since it cannot be excluded that octreotide may have this effect, other drugs mainly metabolized by CYP3A4 and which have a low therapeutic index (e.g., quinidine, terfenadine) should therefore be used with caution). Products include:
Extina Foam, 2% 3057
Nizoral A-D Shampoo 1901

Ketoprofen (Limited published data indicate that somatostatin analogs may decrease the metabolic clearance of compounds known to be metabolized by cytochrome P450 enzymes, which may be due to the suppression of growth hormone).
No products indexed under this heading.

Ketorolac Tromethamine (Limited published data indicate that somatostatin analogs may decrease the metabolic clearance of compounds known to be metabolized by cytochrome P450 enzymes, which may be due to the suppression of growth hormone).
No products indexed under this heading.

Labetalol Hydrochloride (Concomitant administration of bradycardia inducing drugs (e.g., beta blockers) may have an additive effect on the reduction of heart rate associated with octreotide. Dose adjustment of concomitant medication may be necessary).
No products indexed under this heading.

Lamotrigine (Limited published data indicate that somatostatin analogs may decrease the metabolic clearance of compounds known to be metabolized by cytochrome P450 enzymes, which may be due to the suppression of growth hormone). Products include:
Lamictal 1488

Lansoprazole (Limited published data indicate that somatostatin analogs may decrease the metabolic clearance of compounds known to be metabolized by cytochrome P450 enzymes, which may be due to the suppression of growth hormone).
No products indexed under this heading.

Levetiracetam (Limited published data indicate that somatostatin analogs may decrease the metabolic clearance of compounds known to be metabolized by cytochrome P450 enzymes, which may be due to the suppression of growth hormone). Products include:
Keppra Injection 3137
Keppra Oral Solution 3131
Keppra Tablets 3131

Levobunolol Hydrochloride (Concomitant administration of bradycardia inducing drugs (e.g., beta blockers) may have an additive effect on the reduction of heart rate associated with octreotide. Dose adjustment of concomitant medication may be necessary).
No products indexed under this heading.

Levobupivacaine Hydrochloride (Limited published data indicate that somatostatin analogs may decrease the metabolic clearance of compounds known to be metabolized by cytochrome P450 enzymes, which may be due to the suppression of growth hormone).
No products indexed under this heading.

Levonorgestrel (Limited published data indicate that somatostatin analogs may decrease the metabolic clearance of compounds known to be metabolized by cytochrome P450 enzymes, which may be due to the suppression of growth hormone. Since it cannot be excluded that octreotide may have this effect, other drugs mainly metabolized by CYP3A4 and which have a low therapeutic index (e.g., quinidine, terfenadine) should therefore be used with caution). Products include:
Climara Pro Transdermal System 768
Lybrel Tablets 3204
Mirena Intrauterine System 779
Plan B Tablets 1044
Seasonique Tablets 1046

Lidocaine (Limited published data indicate that somatostatin analogs may decrease the metabolic clearance of compounds known to be metabolized by cytochrome P450 enzymes, which may be due to the suppression of growth hormone. Since it cannot be excluded that octreotide may have this effect, other drugs mainly metabolized by CYP3A4 and which have a low therapeutic index (e.g., quinidine, terfenadine) should therefore be used with caution). Products include:
Lidoderm Patch 1114

Lidocaine Base (Limited published data indicate that somatostatin analogs may decrease the metabolic clearance of compounds known to be metabolized by cytochrome P450 enzymes, which may be due to the suppression of growth hormone).
No products indexed under this heading.

Lidocaine Hydrochloride (Limited published data indicate that somatostatin analogs may decrease the metabolic clearance of compounds known to be metabolized by cytochrome P450 enzymes, which may be due to the suppression of growth hormone. Since it cannot be excluded that octreotide may have this effect, other drugs mainly metabolized by CYP3A4 and which have a low therapeutic index (e.g., quinidine, terfenadine) should therefore be used with caution).
No products indexed under this heading.

Lomefloxacin Hydrochloride (Limited published data indicate that somatostatin analogs may decrease the metabolic clearance of compounds known to be metabolized by cytochrome P450 enzymes, which may be due to the suppression of growth hormone).
No products indexed under this heading.

Losartan Potassium (Limited published data indicate that somatostatin analogs may decrease the metabolic clearance of compounds known to be metabolized by cytochrome P450 enzymes, which may be due to the suppression of growth hormone). Products include:
Cozaar Tablets 1973

Lovastatin (Limited published data indicate that somatostatin analogs may decrease the metabolic clearance of compounds known to be metabolized by cytochrome P450 enzymes, which may be due to the suppression of growth hormone. Since it cannot be excluded that octreotide may have this effect, other drugs mainly metabolized by CYP3A4 and which have a low therapeutic index (e.g., quinidine, terfenadine) should therefore be used with caution). Products include:
Advicor Tablets 402
Mevacor Tablets 2063

Maprotiline Hydrochloride (Limited published data indicate that somatostatin analogs may decrease the metabolic clearance of compounds known to be metabolized by cytochrome P450 enzymes, which may be due to the suppression of growth hormone).
No products indexed under this heading.

Meclofenamate Sodium (Limited published data indicate that somatostatin analogs may decrease the metabolic clearance of compounds known to be metabolized by cytochrome P450 enzymes, which may be due to the suppression of growth hormone).
No products indexed under this heading.

Mefenamic Acid (Limited published data indicate that somatostatin analogs may decrease the metabolic clearance of compounds known to be metabolized by cytochrome P450 enzymes, which may be due to the suppression of growth hormone).
No products indexed under this heading.

Meloxicam (Limited published data indicate that somatostatin analogs may decrease the metabolic clearance of compounds known to be metabolized by cytochrome P450 enzymes, which may be due to the suppression of growth hormone). Products include:
Mobic Oral Suspension 863
Mobic Tablets 863

Meperidine Hydrochloride (Limited published data indicate that somatostatin analogs may decrease the metabolic clearance of compounds known to be metabolized by cytochrome P450 enzymes, which may be due to the suppression of growth hormone).
No products indexed under this heading.

Mephenytoin (Limited published data indicate that somatostatin analogs may decrease the metabolic clearance of compounds known to be metabolized by cytochrome P450 enzymes, which may be due to the suppression of growth hormone).
No products indexed under this heading.

Mephobarbital (Limited published data indicate that somatostatin analogs may decrease the metabolic clearance of compounds known to be metabolized by cytochrome P450 enzymes, which may be due to the suppression of growth hormone).
No products indexed under this heading.

Meprobamate (Limited published data indicate that somatostatin analogs may decrease the metabolic clearance of compounds known to be metabolized by cytochrome P450 enzymes, which may be due to the suppression of growth hormone).
No products indexed under this heading.

Mestranol (Limited published data indicate that somatostatin analogs may decrease the metabolic clearance of compounds known to be metabolized by cytochrome P450 enzymes, which may be due to the suppression of growth hormone. Since it cannot be excluded that octreotide may have this effect, other drugs mainly metabolized by CYP3A4 and which have a low therapeutic index (e.g., quinidine, terfenadine) should therefore be used with caution).
No products indexed under this heading.

Metformin Hydrochloride (Octreotide inhibits the secretion of insulin and glucagon. Therefore, blood glucose levels should be monitored when octreotide is initiated or when the dose is altered and antidiabetic treatment should be adjusted accordingly). Products include:
ActoPlus Met Tablets 3071
Avandamet Tablets 1336
Janumet Tablets 2041
PrandiMet Tablets 2967

Methadone Hydrochloride (Limited published data indicate that somatostatin analogs may decrease the metabolic clearance of compounds known to be metabolized by cytochrome P450 enzymes, which may be due to the suppression of growth hormone. Since it cannot be excluded that octreotide may have this effect, other drugs mainly metabolized by CYP3A4 and which have a low therapeutic index (e.g., quinidine, terfenadine) should therefore be used with caution).
No products indexed under this heading.

Methamphetamine Hydrochloride (Limited published data indicate that somatostatin analogs may decrease the metabolic clearance of compounds known to be metabolized by cytochrome P450 enzymes, which may be due to the suppression of growth hormone).
No products indexed under this heading.

Methsuximide (Limited published data indicate that somatostatin analogs may decrease the metabolic clearance of compounds known to be metabolized by cytochrome P450 enzymes, which may be due to the suppression of growth hormone).
No products indexed under this heading.

Metipranolol Hydrochloride (Concomitant administration of bradycardia inducing drugs (e.g., beta blockers) may have an additive effect on the reduction of heart rate associated with octreotide. Dose adjustment of concomitant medication may be necessary).
No products indexed under this heading.

Metoprolol Succinate (Concomitant administration of bradycardia inducing drugs (e.g., beta blockers) may have an additive effect on the reduction of heart rate associated with octreotide. Dose adjustment of concomitant medication may be necessary). Products include:
Toprol-XL Tablets 666

Metoprolol Tartrate (Concomitant administration of bradycardia inducing drugs (e.g., beta blockers) may have an additive effect on the reduction of heart rate associated with octreotide. Dose adjustment of concomitant medication may be necessary).
No products indexed under this heading.

Mexiletine Hydrochloride (Limited published data indicate that somatostatin analogs may decrease the metabolic clearance of compounds known to be metabolized by cytochrome P450 enzymes, which may be due to the suppression of growth hormone).
No products indexed under this heading.

Midazolam Hydrochloride (Limited published data indicate that somatostatin analogs may decrease the metabolic clearance of compounds known to be metabolized by cytochrome P450 enzymes, which may be due to the suppression of growth hormone. Since it cannot be excluded that octreotide may have this effect, other drugs mainly metabolized by CYP3A4 and which have a low therapeutic index (e.g., quinidine, terfenadine) should therefore be used with caution).
No products indexed under this heading.

Miglitol (Octreotide inhibits the secretion of insulin and glucagon. Therefore, blood glucose levels should be monitored when octreotide is initiated or when the dose is altered and antidiabetic treatment should be adjusted accordingly).
No products indexed under this heading.

Mirtazapine (Limited published data indicate that somatostatin analogs may decrease the metabolic clearance of compounds known to be metabolized by cytochrome P450 enzymes, which may be due to the suppression of growth hormone). Products include:
Remeron Tablets ... 2924
RemeronSolTab Tablets ... 2927

Montelukast Sodium (Limited published data indicate that somatostatin analogs may decrease the metabolic clearance of compounds known to be metabolized by cytochrome P450 enzymes, which may be due to the suppression of growth hormone). Products include:
Singulair ... 2114

Morphine Sulfate (Limited published data indicate that somatostatin analogs may decrease the metabolic clearance of compounds known to be metabolized by cytochrome P450 enzymes, which may be due to the suppression of growth hormone). Products include:
Avinza Capsules ... 1772
DepoDur Injection ... 1095
MS Contin Tablets ... 2585

Moxifloxacin Hydrochloride (Limited published data indicate that somatostatin analogs may decrease the metabolic clearance of compounds known to be metabolized by cytochrome P450 enzymes, which may be due to the suppression of growth hormone). Products include:
Avelox ... 2803
Vigamox Ophthalmic Solution ... 548

Nabumetone (Limited published data indicate that somatostatin analogs may decrease the metabolic clearance of compounds known to be metabolized by cytochrome P450 enzymes, which may be due to the suppression of growth hormone).
No products indexed under this heading.

Nadolol (Concomitant administration of bradycardia inducing drugs (e.g., beta blockers) may have an additive effect on the reduction of heart rate associated with octreotide. Dose adjustment of concomitant medication may be necessary). Products include:
Nadolol Tablets ... 2191

Nafcillin Sodium (Limited published data indicate that somatostatin analogs may decrease the metabolic clearance of compounds known to be metabolized by cytochrome P450 enzymes, which may be due to the suppression of growth hormone).
No products indexed under this heading.

Naproxen (Limited published data indicate that somatostatin analogs may decrease the metabolic clearance of compounds known to be metabolized by cytochrome P450 enzymes, which may be due to the suppression of growth hormone). Products include:
EC-Naprosyn Delayed-Release Tablets ... 2632
Naprosyn Suspension ... 2632
Naprosyn Tablets ... 2632

Naproxen Sodium (Limited published data indicate that somatostatin analogs may decrease the metabolic clearance of compounds known to be metabolized by cytochrome P450 enzymes, which may be due to the suppression of growth hormone). Products include:
Anaprox Tablets ... 2632
Anaprox DS Tablets ... 2632
Treximet Tablets ... 1616

Nateglinide (Octreotide inhibits the secretion of insulin and glucagon. Therefore, blood glucose levels should be monitored when octreotide is initiated or when the dose is altered and antidiabetic treatment should be adjusted accordingly). Products include:
Starlix Tablets ... 2314

Nebivolol (Concomitant administration of bradycardia inducing drugs (e.g., beta blockers) may have an additive effect on the reduction of heart rate associated with octreotide. Dose adjustment of concomitant medication may be necessary). Products include:
Bystolic Tablets ... 1155

Nefazodone Hydrochloride (Limited published data indicate that somatostatin analogs may decrease the metabolic clearance of compounds known to be metabolized by cytochrome P450 enzymes, which may be due to the suppression of growth hormone. Since it cannot be excluded that octreotide may have this effect, other drugs mainly metabolized by CYP3A4 and which have a low therapeutic index (e.g., quinidine, terfenadine) should therefore be used with caution).
No products indexed under this heading.

Nelfinavir Mesylate (Limited published data indicate that somatostatin analogs may decrease the metabolic clearance of compounds known to be metabolized by cytochrome P450 enzymes, which may be due to the suppression of growth hormone. Since it cannot be excluded that octreotide may have this effect, other drugs mainly metabolized by CYP3A4 and which have a low therapeutic index (e.g., quinidine, terfenadine) should therefore be used with caution).
No products indexed under this heading.

Nicardipine (Limited published data indicate that somatostatin analogs may decrease the metabolic clearance of compounds known to be metabolized by cytochrome P450 enzymes, which may be due to the suppression of growth hormone).
No products indexed under this heading.

Nicardipine Hydrochloride (Limited published data indicate that somatostatin analogs may decrease the metabolic clearance of compounds known to be metabolized by cytochrome P450 enzymes, which may be due to the suppression of growth hormone. Since it cannot be excluded that octreotide may have this effect, other drugs mainly metabolized by CYP3A4 and which have a low therapeutic index (e.g., quinidine, terfenadine) should therefore be used with caution). Products include:
Cardene I.V. ... 1093

Nicotine Polacrilex (Limited published data indicate that somatostatin analogs may decrease the metabolic clearance of compounds known to be metabolized by cytochrome P450 enzymes, which may be due to the suppression of growth hormone).
No products indexed under this heading.

Nicotine Salicylate (Limited published data indicate that somatostatin analogs may decrease the metabolic clearance of compounds known to be metabolized by cytochrome P450 enzymes, which may be due to the suppression of growth hormone).
No products indexed under this heading.

Nicotine Sulfate (Limited published data indicate that somatostatin analogs may decrease the metabolic clearance of compounds known to be metabolized by cytochrome P450 enzymes, which may be due to the suppression of growth hormone).
No products indexed under this heading.

Nifedipine (Limited published data indicate that somatostatin analogs may decrease the metabolic clearance of compounds known to be metabolized by cytochrome P450 enzymes, which may be due to the suppression of growth hormone. Since it cannot be excluded that octreotide may have this effect, other drugs mainly metabolized by CYP3A4 and which have a low therapeutic index (e.g., quinidine, terfenadine) should therefore be used with caution).
No products indexed under this heading.

Nilutamide (Limited published data indicate that somatostatin analogs may decrease the metabolic clearance of compounds known to be metabolized by cytochrome P450 enzymes, which may be due to the suppression of growth hormone).
No products indexed under this heading.

Nimodipine (Limited published data indicate that somatostatin analogs may decrease the metabolic clearance of compounds known to be metabolized by cytochrome P450 enzymes, which may be due to the suppression of growth hormone. Since it cannot be excluded that octreotide may have this effect, other drugs mainly metabolized by CYP3A4 and which have a low therapeutic index (e.g., quinidine, terfenadine) should therefore be used with caution). Products include:
Nimotop Capsules ... 790

Nisoldipine (Limited published data indicate that somatostatin analogs may decrease the metabolic clearance of compounds known to be metabolized by cytochrome P450 enzymes, which may be due to the suppression of growth hormone. Since it cannot be excluded that octreotide may have this effect, other drugs mainly metabolized by CYP3A4 and which have a low therapeutic index (e.g., quinidine, terfenadine) should therefore be used with caution). Products include:
Sular Extended Release Tablets ... 2975

Nitrendipine (Limited published data indicate that somatostatin analogs may decrease the metabolic clearance of compounds known to be metabolized by cytochrome P450 enzymes, which may be due to the suppression of growth hormone. Since it cannot be excluded that octreotide may have this effect, other drugs mainly metabolized by CYP3A4 and which have a low therapeutic index (e.g., quinidine, terfenadine) should therefore be used with caution).
No products indexed under this heading.

Norethindrone (Limited published data indicate that somatostatin analogs may decrease the metabolic clearance of compounds known to be metabolized by cytochrome P450 enzymes, which may be due to the suppression of growth hormone. Since it cannot be excluded that octreotide may have this effect, other drugs mainly metabolized by CYP3A4 and which have a low therapeutic index (e.g., quinidine, terfenadine) should therefore be used with caution). Products include:
Ortho Micronor Tablets ... 2446

Norethindrone Acetate (Limited published data indicate that somatostatin analogs may decrease the metabolic clearance of compounds known to be metabolized by cytochrome P450 enzymes, which may be due to the suppression of growth hormone. Since it cannot be excluded that octreotide may have this effect, other drugs mainly metabolized by CYP3A4 and which have a low therapeutic index (e.g., quinidine, terfenadine) should therefore be used with caution). Products include:
Activella Tablets ... 2347

Norfloxacin (Limited published data indicate that somatostatin analogs may decrease the metabolic clearance of compounds known to be metabolized by cytochrome P450 enzymes, which may be due to the suppression of growth hormone). Products include:
Noroxin Tablets ... 2069

Norgestrel (Limited published data indicate that somatostatin analogs may decrease the metabolic clearance of compounds known to be metabolized by cytochrome P450 enzymes, which may be due to the suppression of growth hormone. Since it cannot be excluded that octreotide may have this effect, other drugs mainly metabolized by

CYP3A4 and which have a low therapeutic index (e.g., quinidine, terfenadine) should therefore be used with caution).
No products indexed under this heading.

Nortriptyline Hydrochloride (Limited published data indicate that somatostatin analogs may decrease the metabolic clearance of compounds known to be metabolized by cytochrome P450 enzymes, which may be due to the suppression of growth hormone).
No products indexed under this heading.

Ofloxacin (Limited published data indicate that somatostatin analogs may decrease the metabolic clearance of compounds known to be metabolized by cytochrome P450 enzymes, which may be due to the suppression of growth hormone). Products include:
Ofloxacin Ophthalmic Solution 0.3% .... ⊙**243**

Olanzapine (Limited published data indicate that somatostatin analogs may decrease the metabolic clearance of compounds known to be metabolized by cytochrome P450 enzymes, which may be due to the suppression of growth hormone). Products include:
Symbyax Capsules **1871**
Zyprexa Tablets **1883**
Zyprexa IntraMuscular **1883**
Zyprexa ZYDIS Orally Disintegrating Tablets **1883**

Omeprazole (Limited published data indicate that somatostatin analogs may decrease the metabolic clearance of compounds known to be metabolized by cytochrome P450 enzymes, which may be due to the suppression of growth hormone).
No products indexed under this heading.

Ondansetron (Limited published data indicate that somatostatin analogs may decrease the metabolic clearance of compounds known to be metabolized by cytochrome P450 enzymes, which may be due to the suppression of growth hormone. Since it cannot be excluded that octreotide may have this effect, other drugs mainly metabolized by CYP3A4 and which have a low therapeutic index (e.g., quinidine, terfenadine) should therefore be used with caution). Products include:
Zofran ODT Orally Disintegrating Tablets **1687**

Ondansetron Hydrochloride (Limited published data indicate that somatostatin analogs may decrease the metabolic clearance of compounds known to be metabolized by cytochrome P450 enzymes, which may be due to the suppression of growth hormone. Since it cannot be excluded that octreotide may have this effect, other drugs mainly metabolized by CYP3A4 and which have a low therapeutic index (e.g., quinidine, terfenadine) should therefore be used with caution). Products include:
Zofran Injection **1682**
Zofran **1687**

Oxaprozin (Limited published data indicate that somatostatin analogs may decrease the metabolic clearance of compounds known to be metabolized by cytochrome P450 enzymes, which may be due to the suppression of growth hormone).
No products indexed under this heading.

Oxcarbazepine (Limited published data indicate that somatostatin analogs may decrease the metabolic clearance of compounds known to be metabolized by cytochrome P450 enzymes, which may be due to the suppression of growth hormone).
No products indexed under this heading.

Oxycodone Hydrochloride (Limited published data indicate that somatostatin analogs may decrease the metabolic clearance of compounds known to be metabolized by cytochrome P450 enzymes, which may be due to the suppression of growth hormone). Products include:
OxyContin Tablets **2589**
OxyIR Capsules **2593**
Percocet Tablets **1127**
Percodan Tablets **1130**

Paclitaxel (Limited published data indicate that somatostatin analogs may decrease the metabolic clearance of compounds known to be metabolized by cytochrome P450 enzymes, which may be due to the suppression of growth hormone. Since it cannot be excluded that octreotide may have this effect, other drugs mainly metabolized by CYP3A4 and which have a low therapeutic index (e.g., quinidine, terfenadine) should therefore be used with caution).
No products indexed under this heading.

Pantoprazole Sodium (Limited published data indicate that somatostatin analogs may decrease the metabolic clearance of compounds known to be metabolized by cytochrome P450 enzymes, which may be due to the suppression of growth hormone). Products include:
Protonix for Delayed-Release Oral Suspension **3254**
Protonix Delayed-Release Tablets **3254**
Protonix I.V. **3257**

Paramethadione (Limited published data indicate that somatostatin analogs may decrease the metabolic clearance of compounds known to be metabolized by cytochrome P450 enzymes, which may be due to the suppression of growth hormone).
No products indexed under this heading.

Paroxetine Hydrochloride (Limited published data indicate that somatostatin analogs may decrease the metabolic clearance of compounds known to be metabolized by cytochrome P450 enzymes, which may be due to the suppression of growth hormone). Products include:
Paxil **1535**
Paxil CR Controlled-Release Tablets **1544**

Penbutolol Sulfate (Concomitant administration of bradycardia inducing drugs (e.g., beta blockers) may have an additive effect on the reduction of heart rate associated with octreotide. Dose adjustment of concomitant medication may be necessary).
No products indexed under this heading.

Pentamidine Isethionate (Limited published data indicate that somatostatin analogs may decrease the metabolic clearance of compounds known to be metabolized by cytochrome P450 enzymes, which may be due to the suppression of growth hormone).
No products indexed under this heading.

Phenacemide (Limited published data indicate that somatostatin analogs may decrease the metabolic clearance of compounds known to be metabolized by cytochrome P450 enzymes, which may be due to the suppression of growth hormone).
No products indexed under this heading.

Phenobarbital (Limited published data indicate that somatostatin analogs may decrease the metabolic clearance of compounds known to be metabolized by cytochrome P450 enzymes, which may be due to the suppression of growth hormone). Products include:
Donnatal Extentabs **2507**

Phenobarbital Sodium (Limited published data indicate that somatostatin analogs may decrease the metabolic clearance of compounds known to be metabolized by cytochrome P450 enzymes, which may be due to the suppression of growth hormone).
No products indexed under this heading.

Phensuximide (Limited published data indicate that somatostatin analogs may decrease the metabolic clearance of compounds known to be metabolized by cytochrome P450 enzymes, which may be due to the suppression of growth hormone).
No products indexed under this heading.

Phenylbutazone (Limited published data indicate that somatostatin analogs may decrease the metabolic clearance of compounds known to be metabolized by cytochrome P450 enzymes, which may be due to the suppression of growth hormone).
No products indexed under this heading.

Phenytoin (Limited published data indicate that somatostatin analogs may decrease the metabolic clearance of compounds known to be metabolized by cytochrome P450 enzymes, which may be due to the suppression of growth hormone).
No products indexed under this heading.

Phenytoin Sodium (Limited published data indicate that somatostatin analogs may decrease the metabolic clearance of compounds known to be metabolized by cytochrome P450 enzymes, which may be due to the suppression of growth hormone). Products include:
Phenytek Capsules **2192**

Pimozide (Limited published data indicate that somatostatin analogs may decrease the metabolic clearance of compounds known to be metabolized by cytochrome P450 enzymes, which may be due to the suppression of growth hormone. Since it cannot be excluded that octreotide may have this effect, other drugs mainly metabolized by CYP3A4 and which have a low therapeutic index (e.g., quinidine, terfenadine) should therefore be used with caution).
No products indexed under this heading.

Pindolol (Concomitant administration of bradycardia inducing drugs (e.g., beta blockers) may have an additive effect on the reduction of heart rate associated with octreotide. Dose adjustment of concomitant medication may be necessary).
No products indexed under this heading.

Pioglitazone Hydrochloride (Octreotide inhibits the secretion of insulin and glucagon. Therefore, blood glucose levels should be monitored when octreotide is initiated or when the dose is altered and antidiabetic treatment should be adjusted accordingly). Products include:
ActoPlus Met Tablets **3071**
Actos Tablets **3077**
Duetact Tablets **3085**

Piroxicam (Limited published data indicate that somatostatin analogs may decrease the metabolic clearance of compounds known to be metabolized by cytochrome P450 enzymes, which may be due to the suppression of growth hormone).
No products indexed under this heading.

Polyestradiol Phosphate (Limited published data indicate that somatostatin analogs may decrease the metabolic clearance of compounds known to be metabolized by cytochrome P450 enzymes, which may be due to the suppression of growth hormone. Since it cannot be excluded that octreotide may have this effect, other drugs mainly metabolized by CYP3A4 and which have a low therapeutic index (e.g., quinidine, terfenadine) should therefore be used with caution).
No products indexed under this heading.

Primidone (Limited published data indicate that somatostatin analogs may decrease the metabolic clearance of compounds known to be metabolized by cytochrome P450 enzymes, which may be due to the suppression of growth hormone).
No products indexed under this heading.

Progesterone (Limited published data indicate that somatostatin analogs may decrease the metabolic clearance of compounds known to be metabolized by cytochrome P450 enzymes, which may be due to the suppression of growth hormone). Products include:
Crinone 4% Gel **992**
Crinone 8% Gel **992**
Prometrium Capsules (100 mg, 200 mg) **3047**

Proguanil Hydrochloride (Limited published data indicate that somatostatin analogs may decrease the metabolic clearance of compounds known to be metabolized by cytochrome P450 enzymes, which may be due to the suppression of growth hormone). Products include:
Malarone Pediatric Tablets **1521**
Malarone Tablets **1521**

Propafenone Hydrochloride (Limited published data indicate that somatostatin analogs may decrease the metabolic clearance of compounds known to be metabolized by cytochrome P450 enzymes, which may be due to the suppression of growth hormone). Products include:
Rythmol Tablets **1586**
Rythmol SR Capsules **1590**

Propoxyphene Hydrochloride (Limited published data indicate that somatostatin analogs may decrease the metabolic clearance of compounds known to be metabolized by cytochrome P450 enzymes, which may be due to the suppression of growth hormone).
No products indexed under this heading.

Propoxyphene Napsylate (Limited published data indicate that somatostatin analogs may decrease the metabolic clearance of compounds known to be metabolized by cytochrome P450 enzymes, which may be due to the suppression of growth hormone).
No products indexed under this heading.

Propranolol Hydrochloride (Concomitant administration of bradycardia inducing drugs (e.g., beta blockers) may have an additive effect on the reduction of heart rate associated with octreotide. Dose adjustment of concomitant medication may be necessary). Products include:
InnoPran XL Extended Release Capsules 1484

Protriptyline Hydrochloride (Limited published data indicate that somatostatin analogs may decrease the metabolic clearance of compounds known to be metabolized by cytochrome P450 enzymes, which may be due to the suppression of growth hormone).
No products indexed under this heading.

Quetiapine Fumarate (Limited published data indicate that somatostatin analogs may decrease the metabolic clearance of compounds known to be metabolized by cytochrome P450 enzymes, which may be due to the suppression of growth hormone).
No products indexed under this heading.

Quinidine (Limited published data indicate that somatostatin analogs may decrease the metabolic clearance of compounds known to be metabolized by cytochrome P450 enzymes, which may be due to the suppression of growth hormone. Since it cannot be excluded that octreotide may have this effect, other drugs mainly metabolized by CYP3A4 and which have a low therapeutic index such as quinidine, should therefore be used with caution).
No products indexed under this heading.

Quinidine Gluconate (Limited published data indicate that somatostatin analogs may decrease the metabolic clearance of compounds known to be metabolized by cytochrome P450 enzymes, which may be due to the suppression of growth hormone. Since it cannot be excluded that octreotide may have this effect, other drugs mainly metabolized by CYP3A4 and which have a low therapeutic index such as quinidine, should therefore be used with caution).
No products indexed under this heading.

Quinidine Hydrochloride (Limited published data indicate that somatostatin analogs may decrease the metabolic clearance of compounds known to be metabolized by cytochrome P450 enzymes, which may be due to the suppression of growth hormone. Since it cannot be excluded that octreotide may have this effect, other drugs mainly metabolized by CYP3A4 and which have a low therapeutic index such as quinidine, should therefore be used with caution).
No products indexed under this heading.

Quinidine Polygalacturonate (Limited published data indicate that somatostatin analogs may decrease the metabolic clearance of compounds known to be metabolized by cytochrome P450 enzymes, which may be due to the suppression of growth hormone. Since it cannot be excluded that octreotide may have this effect, other drugs mainly metabolized by CYP3A4 and which have a low therapeutic index such as quinidine, should therefore be used with caution).
No products indexed under this heading.

Quinidine Sulfate (Limited published data indicate that somatostatin analogs may decrease the metabolic clearance of compounds known to be metabolized by cytochrome P450 enzymes, which may be due to the suppression of growth hormone. Since it cannot be excluded that octreotide may have this effect, other drugs mainly metabolized by CYP3A4 and which have a low therapeutic index such as quinidine, should therefore be used with caution).
No products indexed under this heading.

Quinine (Limited published data indicate that somatostatin analogs may decrease the metabolic clearance of compounds known to be metabolized by cytochrome P450 enzymes, which may be due to the suppression of growth hormone).
No products indexed under this heading.

Quinine Sulfate (Limited published data indicate that somatostatin analogs may decrease the metabolic clearance of compounds known to be metabolized by cytochrome P450 enzymes, which may be due to the suppression of growth hormone).
No products indexed under this heading.

Rabeprazole Sodium (Limited published data indicate that somatostatin analogs may decrease the metabolic clearance of compounds known to be metabolized by cytochrome P450 enzymes, which may be due to the suppression of growth hormone). Products include:
Aciphex Tablets 1053

Repaglinide (Octreotide inhibits the secretion of insulin and glucagon. Therefore, blood glucose levels should be monitored when octreotide is initiated or when the dose is altered and antidiabetic treatment should be adjusted accordingly). Products include:
PrandiMet Tablets 2967
Prandin Tablets 2971

Rifabutin (Limited published data indicate that somatostatin analogs may decrease the metabolic clearance of compounds known to be metabolized by cytochrome P450 enzymes, which may be due to the suppression of growth hormone. Since it cannot be excluded that octreotide may have this effect, other drugs mainly metabolized by CYP3A4 and which have a low therapeutic index (e.g., quinidine, terfenadine) should therefore be used with caution).
No products indexed under this heading.

Riluzole (Limited published data indicate that somatostatin analogs may decrease the metabolic clearance of compounds known to be metabolized by cytochrome P450 enzymes, which may be due to the suppression of growth hormone). Products include:
Rilutek Tablets 2771

Risperidone (Limited published data indicate that somatostatin analogs may decrease the metabolic clearance of compounds known to be metabolized by cytochrome P450 enzymes, which may be due to the suppression of growth hormone). Products include:
Risperdal Consta Long-Acting Injection 1753

Ritonavir (Limited published data indicate that somatostatin analogs may decrease the metabolic clearance of compounds known to be metabolized by cytochrome P450 enzymes, which may be due to the suppression of growth hormone. Since it cannot be excluded that octreotide may have this effect, other drugs mainly metabolized by CYP3A4 and which have a low therapeutic index (e.g., quinidine, terfenadine) should therefore be used with caution). Products include:
Kaletra 452
Norvir 489

Rofecoxib (Limited published data indicate that somatostatin analogs may decrease the metabolic clearance of compounds known to be metabolized by cytochrome P450 enzymes, which may be due to the suppression of growth hormone).
No products indexed under this heading.

Ropinirole Hydrochloride (Limited published data indicate that somatostatin analogs may decrease the metabolic clearance of compounds known to be metabolized by cytochrome P450 enzymes, which may be due to the suppression of growth hormone). Products include:
Requip Tablets 1561
Requip XL Tablets 1568

Ropivacaine Hydrochloride (Limited published data indicate that somatostatin analogs may decrease the metabolic clearance of compounds known to be metabolized by cytochrome P450 enzymes, which may be due to the suppression of growth hormone).
No products indexed under this heading.

Rosiglitazone Maleate (Octreotide inhibits the secretion of insulin and glucagon. Therefore, blood glucose levels should be monitored when octreotide is initiated or when the dose is altered and antidiabetic treatment should be adjusted accordingly). Products include:
Avandamet Tablets 1336
Avandaryl Tablets 1344
Avandia Tablets 1351

Saquinavir (Limited published data indicate that somatostatin analogs may decrease the metabolic clearance of compounds known to be metabolized by cytochrome P450 enzymes, which may be due to the suppression of growth hormone. Since it cannot be excluded that octreotide may have this effect, other drugs mainly metabolized by CYP3A4 and which have a low therapeutic index (e.g., quinidine, terfenadine) should therefore be used with caution).
No products indexed under this heading.

Saquinavir Mesylate (Limited published data indicate that somatostatin analogs may decrease the metabolic clearance of compounds known to be metabolized by cytochrome P450 enzymes, which may be due to the suppression of growth hormone. Since it cannot be excluded that octreotide may have this effect, other drugs mainly metabolized by CYP3A4 and which have a low therapeutic index (e.g., quinidine, terfenadine) should therefore be used with caution).
No products indexed under this heading.

Sertraline Hydrochloride (Limited published data indicate that somatostatin analogs may decrease the metabolic clearance of compounds known to be metabolized by cytochrome P450 enzymes, which may be due to the suppression of growth hormone. Since it cannot be excluded that octreotide may have this effect, other drugs mainly metabolized by CYP3A4 and which have a low therapeutic index (e.g., quinidine, terfenadine) should therefore be used with caution).
No products indexed under this heading.

Sildenafil Citrate (Limited published data indicate that somatostatin analogs may decrease the metabolic clearance of compounds known to be metabolized by cytochrome P450 enzymes, which may be due to the suppression of growth hormone. Since it cannot be excluded that octreotide may have this effect, other drugs mainly metabolized by CYP3A4 and which have a low therapeutic index (e.g., quinidine, terfenadine) should therefore be used with caution).
No products indexed under this heading.

Simvastatin (Limited published data indicate that somatostatin analogs may decrease the metabolic clearance of compounds known to be metabolized by cytochrome P450 enzymes, which may be due to the suppression of growth hormone. Since it cannot be excluded that octreotide may have this effect, other drugs mainly metabolized by CYP3A4 and which have a low therapeutic index (e.g., quinidine, terfenadine) should therefore be used with caution). Products include:
Simcor Tablets 502
Vytorin 10/10 Tablets 2149
Vytorin 10/10 Tablets 2939
Vytorin 10/20 Tablets 2149
Vytorin 10/20 Tablets 2939
Vytorin 10/40 Tablets 2149
Vytorin 10/40 Tablets 2939
Vytorin 10/80 Tablets 2149
Vytorin 10/80 Tablets 2939
Zocor Tablets 2136

Sirolimus (Limited published data indicate that somatostatin analogs may decrease the metabolic clearance of compounds known to be

metabolized by cytochrome P450 enzymes, which may be due to the suppression of growth hormone. Since it cannot be excluded that octreotide may have this effect, other drugs mainly metabolized by CYP3A4 and which have a low therapeutic index (e.g., quinidine, terfenadine) should therefore be used with caution). Products include:

Rapamune **3260**

Sitagliptin Phosphate (Octreotide inhibits the secretion of insulin and glucagon. Therefore, blood glucose levels should be monitored when octreotide is initiated or when the dose is altered and antidiabetic treatment should be adjusted accordingly). Products include:

Janumet Tablets **2041**
Januvia Tablets **2048**

Sotalol Hydrochloride (Concomitant administration of bradycardia inducing drugs (e.g., beta blockers) may have an additive effect on the reduction of heart rate associated with octreotide. Dose adjustment of concomitant medication may be necessary).

No products indexed under this heading.

Sulfamethoxazole (Limited published data indicate that somatostatin analogs may decrease the metabolic clearance of compounds known to be metabolized by cytochrome P450 enzymes, which may be due to the suppression of growth hormone).

No products indexed under this heading.

Sulindac (Limited published data indicate that somatostatin analogs may decrease the metabolic clearance of compounds known to be metabolized by cytochrome P450 enzymes, which may be due to the suppression of growth hormone). Products include:

Clinoril Tablets **1962**

Suprofen (Limited published data indicate that somatostatin analogs may decrease the metabolic clearance of compounds known to be metabolized by cytochrome P450 enzymes, which may be due to the suppression of growth hormone).

No products indexed under this heading.

Tacrine Hydrochloride (Limited published data indicate that somatostatin analogs may decrease the metabolic clearance of compounds known to be metabolized by cytochrome P450 enzymes, which may be due to the suppression of growth hormone).

No products indexed under this heading.

Tacrolimus (Limited published data indicate that somatostatin analogs may decrease the metabolic clearance of compounds known to be metabolized by cytochrome P450 enzymes, which may be due to the suppression of growth hormone. Since it cannot be excluded that octreotide may have this effect, other drugs mainly metabolized by CYP3A4 and which have a low therapeutic index (e.g., quinidine, terfenadine) should therefore be used with caution). Products include:

Prograf Capsules and Injection **622**
Protopic Ointment **628**

Tadalafil (Limited published data indicate that somatostatin analogs may decrease the metabolic clearance of compounds known to be metabolized by cytochrome P450 enzymes, which may be due to the suppression of growth hormone. Since it cannot be excluded that octreotide may have this effect, other drugs mainly metabolized by CYP3A4 and which have a low therapeutic index (e.g., quinidine, terfenadine) should therefore be used with caution). Products include:

Cialis Tablets **1792**

Tamoxifen Citrate (Limited published data indicate that somatostatin analogs may decrease the metabolic clearance of compounds known to be metabolized by cytochrome P450 enzymes, which may be due to the suppression of growth hormone. Since it cannot be excluded that octreotide may have this effect, other drugs mainly metabolized by CYP3A4 and which have a low therapeutic index (e.g., quinidine, terfenadine) should therefore be used with caution).

No products indexed under this heading.

Telmisartan (Limited published data indicate that somatostatin analogs may decrease the metabolic clearance of compounds known to be metabolized by cytochrome P450 enzymes, which may be due to the suppression of growth hormone). Products include:

Micardis Tablets **852**
Micardis HCT Tablets **854**

Teniposide (Limited published data indicate that somatostatin analogs may decrease the metabolic clearance of compounds known to be metabolized by cytochrome P450 enzymes, which may be due to the suppression of growth hormone).

No products indexed under this heading.

Terfenadine (Limited published data indicate that somatostatin analogs may decrease the metabolic clearance of compounds known to be metabolized by cytochrome P450 enzymes, which may be due to the suppression of growth hormone. Since it cannot be excluded that octreotide may have this effect, other drugs mainly metabolized by CYP3A4 and which have a low therapeutic index such as terfenadine, should therefore be used with caution).

No products indexed under this heading.

Testosterone (Limited published data indicate that somatostatin analogs may decrease the metabolic clearance of compounds known to be metabolized by cytochrome P450 enzymes, which may be due to the suppression of growth hormone). Products include:

AndroGel **3159**
Testim 1% Gel **701**

Testosterone Cypionate (Limited published data indicate that somatostatin analogs may decrease the metabolic clearance of compounds known to be metabolized by cytochrome P450 enzymes, which may be due to the suppression of growth hormone).

No products indexed under this heading.

Testosterone Enanthate (Limited published data indicate that somatostatin analogs may decrease the metabolic clearance of compounds known to be metabolized by cytochrome P450 enzymes, which may be due to the suppression of growth hormone). Products include:

Delatestryl Injection **1730**

Testosterone Propionate (Limited published data indicate that somatostatin analogs may decrease the metabolic clearance of compounds known to be metabolized by cytochrome P450 enzymes, which may be due to the suppression of growth hormone).

No products indexed under this heading.

Theophylline (Limited published data indicate that somatostatin analogs may decrease the metabolic clearance of compounds known to be metabolized by cytochrome P450 enzymes, which may be due to the suppression of growth hormone).

No products indexed under this heading.

Theophylline Anhydrous (Limited published data indicate that somatostatin analogs may decrease the metabolic clearance of compounds known to be metabolized by cytochrome P450 enzymes, which may be due to the suppression of growth hormone). Products include:

Uniphyl Tablets **2595**

Theophylline Sodium Glycinate (Limited published data indicate that somatostatin analogs may decrease the metabolic clearance of compounds known to be metabolized by cytochrome P450 enzymes, which may be due to the suppression of growth hormone).

No products indexed under this heading.

Thioridazine (Limited published data indicate that somatostatin analogs may decrease the metabolic clearance of compounds known to be metabolized by cytochrome P450 enzymes, which may be due to the suppression of growth hormone).

No products indexed under this heading.

Thioridazine Hydrochloride (Limited published data indicate that somatostatin analogs may decrease the metabolic clearance of compounds known to be metabolized by cytochrome P450 enzymes, which may be due to the suppression of growth hormone). Products include:

Thioridazine Hydrochloride Tablets **2195**

Tiagabine Hydrochloride (Limited published data indicate that somatostatin analogs may decrease the metabolic clearance of compounds known to be metabolized by cytochrome P450 enzymes, which may be due to the suppression of growth hormone. Since it cannot be excluded that octreotide may have this effect, other drugs mainly metabolized by CYP3A4 and which have a low therapeutic index (e.g., quinidine, terfenadine) should therefore be used with caution). Products include:

Gabitril Tablets **973**

Timolol Hemihydrate (Concomitant administration of bradycardia inducing drugs (e.g., beta blockers) may have an additive effect on the reduction of heart rate associated with octreotide. Dose adjustment of concomitant medication may be necessary). Products include:

Betimol Ophthalmic Solution **3181**

Timolol Maleate (Concomitant administration of bradycardia inducing drugs (e.g., beta blockers) may have an additive effect on the reduction of heart rate associated with octreotide. Dose adjustment of concomitant medication may be necessary). Products include:

Combigan Ophthalmic Solution **553**
Cosopt Sterile Ophthalmic Solution **1969**
Timoptic Sterile Ophthalmic Solution **2121**
Timoptic in Ocudose **2124**
Timoptic-XE Sterile Ophthalmic Gel Forming Solution **2125**

Tolazamide (Octreotide inhibits the secretion of insulin and glucagon. Therefore, blood glucose levels should be monitored when octreotide is initiated or when the dose is altered and antidiabetic treatment should be adjusted accordingly).

No products indexed under this heading.

Tolbutamide (Octreotide inhibits the secretion of insulin and glucagon. Therefore, blood glucose levels should be monitored when octreotide is initiated or when the dose is altered and antidiabetic treatment should be adjusted accordingly).

No products indexed under this heading.

Tolbutamide Sodium (Limited published data indicate that somatostatin analogs may decrease the metabolic clearance of compounds known to be metabolized by cytochrome P450 enzymes, which may be due to the suppression of growth hormone).

No products indexed under this heading.

Tolmetin Sodium (Limited published data indicate that somatostatin analogs may decrease the metabolic clearance of compounds known to be metabolized by cytochrome P450 enzymes, which may be due to the suppression of growth hormone).

No products indexed under this heading.

Tolterodine Tartrate (Limited published data indicate that somatostatin analogs may decrease the metabolic clearance of compounds known to be metabolized by cytochrome P450 enzymes, which may be due to the suppression of growth hormone. Since it cannot be excluded that octreotide may have this effect, other drugs mainly metabolized by CYP3A4 and which have a low therapeutic index (e.g., quinidine, terfenadine) should therefore be used with caution).

No products indexed under this heading.

Topiramate (Limited published data indicate that somatostatin analogs may decrease the metabolic clearance of compounds known to be metabolized by cytochrome P450 enzymes, which may be due to the suppression of growth hormone).

No products indexed under this heading.

Torsemide (Limited published data indicate that somatostatin analogs may decrease the metabolic clearance of compounds known to be metabolized by cytochrome P450 enzymes, which may be due to the suppression of growth hormone). Products include:

Demadex Injection **2630**

Demadex Tablets 2630

Tramadol Hydrochloride (Limited published data indicate that somatostatin analogs may decrease the metabolic clearance of compounds known to be metabolized by cytochrome P450 enzymes, which may be due to the suppression of growth hormone). Products include:

Ultram ER Extended-Release Tablets 2428

Trazodone Hydrochloride (Limited published data indicate that somatostatin analogs may decrease the metabolic clearance of compounds known to be metabolized by cytochrome P450 enzymes, which may be due to the suppression of growth hormone. Since it cannot be excluded that octreotide may have this effect, other drugs mainly metabolized by CYP3A4 and which have a low therapeutic index (e.g., quinidine, terfenadine) should therefore be used with caution).

No products indexed under this heading.

Tretinoin (Limited published data indicate that somatostatin analogs may decrease the metabolic clearance of compounds known to be metabolized by cytochrome P450 enzymes, which may be due to the suppression of growth hormone). Products include:

Vesanoid Capsules 2660
Ziana Gel 1942

Triazolam (Limited published data indicate that somatostatin analogs may decrease the metabolic clearance of compounds known to be metabolized by cytochrome P450 enzymes, which may be due to the suppression of growth hormone. Since it cannot be excluded that octreotide may have this effect, other drugs mainly metabolized by CYP3A4 and which have a low therapeutic index (e.g., quinidine, terfenadine) should therefore be used with caution).

No products indexed under this heading.

Trimethadione (Limited published data indicate that somatostatin analogs may decrease the metabolic clearance of compounds known to be metabolized by cytochrome P450 enzymes, which may be due to the suppression of growth hormone).

No products indexed under this heading.

Trimethaphan Camsylate (Limited published data indicate that somatostatin analogs may decrease the metabolic clearance of compounds known to be metabolized by cytochrome P450 enzymes, which may be due to the suppression of growth hormone).

No products indexed under this heading.

Trimipramine Maleate (Limited published data indicate that somatostatin analogs may decrease the metabolic clearance of compounds known to be metabolized by cytochrome P450 enzymes, which may be due to the suppression of growth hormone).

No products indexed under this heading.

Troglitazone (Octreotide inhibits the secretion of insulin and glucagon. Therefore, blood glucose levels should be monitored when octreotide is initiated or when the dose is altered and antidiabetic treatment should be adjusted accordingly).

No products indexed under this heading.

Trovafloxacin Mesylate (Limited published data indicate that somatostatin analogs may decrease the metabolic clearance of compounds known to be metabolized by cytochrome P450 enzymes, which may be due to the suppression of growth hormone).

No products indexed under this heading.

Valdecoxib (Limited published data indicate that somatostatin analogs may decrease the metabolic clearance of compounds known to be metabolized by cytochrome P450 enzymes, which may be due to the suppression of growth hormone).

No products indexed under this heading.

Valproate Sodium (Limited published data indicate that somatostatin analogs may decrease the metabolic clearance of compounds known to be metabolized by cytochrome P450 enzymes, which may be due to the suppression of growth hormone).

No products indexed under this heading.

Valproic Acid (Limited published data indicate that somatostatin analogs may decrease the metabolic clearance of compounds known to be metabolized by cytochrome P450 enzymes, which may be due to the suppression of growth hormone).

No products indexed under this heading.

Valsartan (Limited published data indicate that somatostatin analogs may decrease the metabolic clearance of compounds known to be metabolized by cytochrome P450 enzymes, which may be due to the suppression of growth hormone). Products include:

Diovan Tablets 2212
Diovan HCT Tablets 2216
Exforge Tablets 2238

Vardenafil Hydrochloride (Limited published data indicate that somatostatin analogs may decrease the metabolic clearance of compounds known to be metabolized by cytochrome P450 enzymes, which may be due to the suppression of growth hormone. Since it cannot be excluded that octreotide may have this effect, other drugs mainly metabolized by CYP3A4 and which have a low therapeutic index (e.g., quinidine, terfenadine) should therefore be used with caution). Products include:

Levitra Tablets 2876

Venlafaxine Hydrochloride (Limited published data indicate that somatostatin analogs may decrease the metabolic clearance of compounds known to be metabolized by cytochrome P450 enzymes, which may be due to the suppression of growth hormone). Products include:

Effexor XR Extended-Release Capsules.. 3195
Venlafaxine Hydrochloride Tablets ... 2199

Verapamil Hydrochloride (Limited published data indicate that somatostatin analogs may decrease the metabolic clearance of compounds known to be metabolized by cytochrome P450 enzymes, which may be due to the suppression of growth hormone. Since it cannot be excluded that octreotide may have this effect, other drugs mainly metabolized by CYP3A4 and which have a low therapeutic index (e.g., quinidine, terfenadine) should therefore be used with caution). Products include:

Tarka Tablets 511

Vinblastine Sulfate (Limited published data indicate that somatostatin analogs may decrease the metabolic clearance of compounds known to be metabolized by cytochrome P450 enzymes, which may be due to the suppression of growth hormone. Since it cannot be excluded that octreotide may have this effect, other drugs mainly metabolized by CYP3A4 and which have a low therapeutic index (e.g., quinidine, terfenadine) should therefore be used with caution).

No products indexed under this heading.

Vincristine Sulfate (Limited published data indicate that somatostatin analogs may decrease the metabolic clearance of compounds known to be metabolized by cytochrome P450 enzymes, which may be due to the suppression of growth hormone. Since it cannot be excluded that octreotide may have this effect, other drugs mainly metabolized by CYP3A4 and which have a low therapeutic index (e.g., quinidine, terfenadine) should therefore be used with caution).

No products indexed under this heading.

Vitamin A (Limited published data indicate that somatostatin analogs may decrease the metabolic clearance of compounds known to be metabolized by cytochrome P450 enzymes, which may be due to the suppression of growth hormone). Products include:

Norwegian Cod Liver Oil 949

Vitamin A Acetate (Limited published data indicate that somatostatin analogs may decrease the metabolic clearance of compounds known to be metabolized by cytochrome P450 enzymes, which may be due to the suppression of growth hormone).

No products indexed under this heading.

Voriconazole (Limited published data indicate that somatostatin analogs may decrease the metabolic clearance of compounds known to be metabolized by cytochrome P450 enzymes, which may be due to the suppression of growth hormone).

No products indexed under this heading.

Warfarin Sodium (Limited published data indicate that somatostatin analogs may decrease the metabolic clearance of compounds known to be metabolized by cytochrome P450 enzymes, which may be due to the suppression of growth hormone. Since it cannot be excluded that octreotide may have this effect, other drugs mainly metabolized by CYP3A4 and which have a low therapeutic index (e.g., quinidine, terfenadine) should therefore be used with caution).

No products indexed under this heading.

Zafirlukast (Limited published data indicate that somatostatin analogs may decrease the metabolic clearance of compounds known to be metabolized by cytochrome P450 enzymes, which may be due to the suppression of growth hormone). Products include:

Accolate Tablets 669

Zileuton (Limited published data indicate that somatostatin analogs may decrease the metabolic clearance of compounds known to be metabolized by cytochrome P450 enzymes, which may be due to the suppression of growth hormone).

No products indexed under this heading.

Zolmitriptan (Limited published data indicate that somatostatin analogs may decrease the metabolic clearance of compounds known to be metabolized by cytochrome P450 enzymes, which may be due to the suppression of growth hormone). Products include:

Zomig Tablets 694
Zomig Nasal Spray 689
Zomig-ZMT Tablets 694

Zonisamide (Limited published data indicate that somatostatin analogs may decrease the metabolic clearance of compounds known to be metabolized by cytochrome P450 enzymes, which may be due to the suppression of growth hormone). Products include:

Zonegran Capsules 1089

Zopiclone (Limited published data indicate that somatostatin analogs may decrease the metabolic clearance of compounds known to be metabolized by cytochrome P450 enzymes, which may be due to the suppression of growth hormone).

No products indexed under this heading.

SANTYL COLLAGENASE OINTMENT

(Collagenase) 1724

May interact with:

Antiseptics (The enzymatic activity of collagenase is adversely affected by heavy metal ions which are in some antiseptics. When use of such agents is suspected, the site should be cleaned by repeated washing with normal saline before applying collagenase).

No products indexed under this heading.

Cortisone Acetate (Chronic concurrent use may result in systemic manifestations of hypersensitivity to collagenase).

No products indexed under this heading.

Soap (The enzymatic activity of collagenase is adversely affected by certain detergents. When use of such agents is suspected, the site should be cleaned by repeated washing with normal saline before applying collagenase).

No products indexed under this heading.

SATIETE TABLETS

(Amino Acid Preparations, Folic Acid, Ginkgo biloba, Herbals with Vitamins & Minerals, Hypericum)....... 640

May interact with anorexiants, monoamine oxidase inhibitors, selective serotonin reuptake inhibitors, and tricyclic antidepressants. Compounds in these categories include:

Amitriptyline Hydrochloride (Concurrent use with tricyclic antidepressants is not recommended without medical supervision).
No products indexed under this heading.

Amoxapine (Concurrent use with tricyclic antidepressants is not recommended without medical supervision).
No products indexed under this heading.

Amphetamine Resins (Concurrent use with prescription diet drugs is not recommended without medical supervision).
No products indexed under this heading.

Benzphetamine Hydrochloride (Concurrent use with prescription diet drugs is not recommended without medical supervision).
No products indexed under this heading.

Citalopram Hydrobromide (Concurrent use with SSRI antidepressants is not recommended without medical supervision). Products include:
Celexa **1160**

Clomipramine Hydrochloride (Concurrent use with tricyclic antidepressants is not recommended without medical supervision).
No products indexed under this heading.

Desipramine Hydrochloride (Concurrent use with tricyclic antidepressants is not recommended without medical supervision).
No products indexed under this heading.

Dextroamphetamine Sulfate (Concurrent use with prescription diet drugs is not recommended without medical supervision). Products include:
Adderall XR Capsules **3012**
Dexedrine **1401**

Diethylpropion Hydrochloride (Concurrent use with prescription diet drugs is not recommended without medical supervision).
No products indexed under this heading.

Doxepin Hydrochloride (Concurrent use with tricyclic antidepressants is not recommended without medical supervision).
No products indexed under this heading.

Escitalopram Oxalate (Concurrent use with SSRI antidepressants is not recommended without medical supervision). Products include:
Lexapro Oral Suspension **1174**
Lexapro Tablets **1174**

Fenfluramine Hydrochloride (Concurrent use with prescription diet drugs is not recommended without medical supervision).
No products indexed under this heading.

Fluoxetine (Concurrent use with SSRI antidepressants is not recommended without medical supervision).
No products indexed under this heading.

Fluoxetine Hydrochloride (Concurrent use with SSRI antidepressants is not recommended without medical supervision). Products include:
Prozac Weekly Capsules **1852**
Prozac Pulvules and Liquid **1852**
Symbyax Capsules **1871**

Fluvoxamine Maleate (Concurrent use with SSRI antidepressants is not recommended without medical supervision). Products include:
Luvox CR Extended-Release Capsules **1759**

Imipramine Hydrochloride (Concurrent use with tricyclic antidepressants is not recommended without medical supervision).
No products indexed under this heading.

Imipramine Pamoate (Concurrent use with tricyclic antidepressants is not recommended without medical supervision).
No products indexed under this heading.

Isocarboxazid (Concurrent use with MAO inhibitors is not recommended without medical supervision). Products include:
Marplan Tablets **3177**

Maprotiline Hydrochloride (Concurrent use with tricyclic antidepressants is not recommended without medical supervision).
No products indexed under this heading.

Mazindol (Concurrent use with prescription diet drugs is not recommended without medical supervision).
No products indexed under this heading.

Methamphetamine Hydrochloride (Concurrent use with prescription diet drugs is not recommended without medical supervision).
No products indexed under this heading.

Moclobemide (Concurrent use with MAO inhibitors is not recommended without medical supervision).
No products indexed under this heading.

Nortriptyline Hydrochloride (Concurrent use with tricyclic antidepressants is not recommended without medical supervision).
No products indexed under this heading.

Pargyline Hydrochloride (Concurrent use with MAO inhibitors is not recommended without medical supervision).
No products indexed under this heading.

Paroxetine Hydrochloride (Concurrent use with SSRI antidepressants is not recommended without medical supervision). Products include:
Paxil **1535**
Paxil CR Controlled-Release Tablets **1544**

Phendimetrazine Tartrate (Concurrent use with prescription diet drugs is not recommended without medical supervision).
No products indexed under this heading.

Phenelzine Sulfate (Concurrent use with MAO inhibitors is not recommended without medical supervision).
No products indexed under this heading.

Phenmetrazine Hydrochloride (Concurrent use with prescription diet drugs is not recommended without medical supervision).
No products indexed under this heading.

Procarbazine Hydrochloride (Concurrent use with MAO inhibitors is not recommended without medical supervision).
No products indexed under this heading.

Protriptyline Hydrochloride (Concurrent use with tricyclic antidepressants is not recommended without medical supervision).
No products indexed under this heading.

Rasagiline Mesylate (Concurrent use with MAO inhibitors is not recommended without medical supervision). Products include:
Azilect Tablets **3106**

Selegiline (Concurrent use with MAO inhibitors is not recommended without medical supervision). Products include:
Emsam Transdermal System **905**

Selegiline Hydrochloride (Concurrent use with MAO inhibitors is not recommended without medical supervision). Products include:
Eldepryl Capsules **3052**

Sertraline Hydrochloride (Concurrent use with SSRI antidepressants is not recommended without medical supervision).
No products indexed under this heading.

Sibutramine Hydrochloride Monohydrate (Concurrent use with prescription diet drugs is not recommended without medical supervision). Products include:
Meridia Capsules **475**

Tranylcypromine Sulfate (Concurrent use with MAO inhibitors is not recommended without medical supervision). Products include:
Parnate Tablets **1532**

Trimipramine Maleate (Concurrent use with tricyclic antidepressants is not recommended without medical supervision).
No products indexed under this heading.

SEASONIQUE TABLETS

(Ethinyl Estradiol, Levonorgestrel) **1046**

May interact with certain other agents. Compounds in these categories include:

Acetaminophen (Acetaminophen may increase plasma ethinyl estradiol levels, possibly by inhibition of conjugation. Decreased plasma concentrations of acetaminophen have been noted when co-administered with combination oral contraceptives). Products include:
Benadryl Allergy & Cold Kapgels **1895**
Benadryl Allergy & Sinus Headache Kapgels **1895**
Benadryl Severe Allergy & Sinus Headache Caplets **1897**
Lortab 5/500 Tablets **3143**
Lortab 7.5/500 Tablets **3144**
Lortab 10/500 Tablets **3144**
Percocet Tablets **1127**
Sinutab Sinus Caplets **1905**
Sudafed PE Cold & Cough Caplets **1907**
Sudafed PE Nighttime Cold Caplets **1907**
Sudafed PE Severe Cold Caplets **1908**
Sudafed PE Sinus Headache Caplets **1908**
Regular Strength Tylenol Tablets **1915**
Tylenol 8 Hour Extended Release Caplets **1915**
Extra Strength Tylenol Caplets, Cool Caplets, and EZ Tabs **1915**
Extra Strength Tylenol Adult Rapid Blast Liquid **1915**
Extra Strength Tylenol PM Caplets, Geltabs, Liquid, and Rapid Release Gels **1915**
Extra Strength Tylenol Rapid Release Gels **1915**
Tylenol with Codeine Tablets **2427**
Tylenol Allergy Multi-Symptom Caplets with Cool Burst and Rapid Release Gelcaps **1916**
Tylenol Allergy Multi-Symptom Nighttime Caplets with Cool Burst **1916**
Tylenol Severe Allergy Caplets **1916**
Tylenol Arthritis Pain Extended Release Geltabs/Caplets **1915**
Tylenol Chest Congestion Caplets with Cool Burst **1910**
Tylenol Chest Congestion Liquid with Cool Burst **1910**
Children's Tylenol Plus Cold Suspension Liquid **1912**
Children's Tylenol Plus Cold & Allergy Suspension Liquid **1914**
Children's Tylenol Plus Cough & Runny Nose Suspension Liquid **1912**
Children's Tylenol Plus Cough & Sore Throat Suspension Liquid **1912**
Children's Tylenol Plus Flu Suspension Liquid **1914**
Children's Tylenol Suspension Liquid **1909**
Children's Tylenol Meltaways **1909**
Children's Tylenol Plus Multi-Symptom Cold Suspension Liquid **1912**
Tylenol Cold Severe Congestion Daytime Caplets with Cool Burst **1912**
Tylenol Cold Head Congestion Daytime Caplets with Cool Burst **1910**
Tylenol Cold Head Congestion Nighttime Caplets with Cool Burst **1910**
Tylenol Cold Head Congestion Severe Daytime Caplets with Cool Burst **1910**
Tylenol Cold Multi-Symptom Daytime Caplets with Cool Burst and Rapid Release Gels **1913**
Tylenol Cold Multi-Symptom Daytime Liquid with Citrus Burst ... **1913**
Tylenol Cold Multi-Symptom Nighttime Caplets with Cool Burst **1913**
Tylenol Cold Multi-Symptom Nighttime Liquid with Cool Burst ... **1913**
Tylenol Cold Multi-Symptom Severe Caplets with Cool Burst **1913**
Tylenol Cold Multi-Symptom Severe Daytime Liquid with Citrus Burst **1913**
Tylenol Cough & Sore Throat Daytime Liquid with Cool Burst **1918**
Tylenol Cough & Sore Throat Nighttime Liquid with Cool Burst ... **1918**
Concentrated Tylenol Infants' Drops **1909**
Jr. Tylenol Meltaways **1909**
Tylenol Sinus Congestion & Pain Daytime Caplets with Cool Burst and Gelcaps **1917**
Tylenol Sinus Congestion & Pain Nighttime Caplets with Cool Burst **1917**
Tylenol Sinus Congestion & Pain Severe Caplets with Cool Burst **1917**
Tylenol Sinus Severe Congestion Caplets with Cool Burst **1917**
Tylenol Sore Throat Daytime Liquid with Cool Burst **1918**
Tylenol Sore Throat Nighttime Liquid with Cool Burst **1918**

Women's Tylenol Menstrual Relief Caplets.......... 1919
Vicks DayQuil Cold & Flu Multi-Symptom Relief.......... ▣616
Vicks DayQuil LiquiCaps.......... 2567
Vicks DayQuil Liquid.......... 2567
Vicks DayQuil Multi-Symptom Cold/Flu Relief.......... 2567
Vicks NyQuil Cold & Flu Multi-Symptom Relief.......... ▣617
Vicks NyQuil LiquiCaps.......... 2567
Vicks NyQuil Liquid.......... 2567
Vicks NyQuil Multi-Symptom Cold/Flu Relief.......... 2567
Vicodin Tablets.......... 529
Vicodin ES Tablets.......... 530
Vicodin HP Tablets.......... 531
Zydone Tablets.......... 1132

Acetazolamide (CYP3A4 inhibitors may increase plasma ethinyl estradiol levels).
No products indexed under this heading.

Amiodarone Hydrochloride (CYP3A4 inhibitors may increase plasma ethinyl estradiol levels).
No products indexed under this heading.

Ampicillin (Several cases of contraceptive failure and breakthrough bleeding have been reported in the literature with concomitant administration of antibiotics, such as ampicillin; however, clinical pharmacology studies investigating drug interactions between combined oral contraceptives and these antibiotics have reported inconsistent results).
No products indexed under this heading.

Ampicillin Sodium (Several cases of contraceptive failure and breakthrough bleeding have been reported in the literature with concomitant administration of antibiotics, such as ampicillin; however, clinical pharmacology studies investigating drug interactions between combined oral contraceptives and these antibiotics have reported inconsistent results).
No products indexed under this heading.

Ampicillin Trihydrate (Several cases of contraceptive failure and breakthrough bleeding have been reported in the literature with concomitant administration of antibiotics, such as ampicillin; however, clinical pharmacology studies investigating drug interactions between combined oral contraceptives and these antibiotics have reported inconsistent results).
No products indexed under this heading.

Amprenavir (Several protease inhibitors have been studied with co-administration of oral combination hormonal contraceptives with significant changes (increase and decrease) in the plasma levels of the estrogen and progestin being noted in some cases).
No products indexed under this heading.

Anastrozole (CYP3A4 inhibitors may increase plasma ethinyl estradiol levels). Products include:
Arimidex Tablets.......... 672

Aprepitant (CYP3A4 inhibitors may increase plasma ethinyl estradiol levels). Products include:
Emend Capsules.......... 1992

Aprobarbital (Contraceptive effectivness may be reduced when hormonal contraceptives are co-administered with drugs that increase the metabolism of contraceptive steroids, such as barbiturates).
No products indexed under this heading.

Ascorbic Acid (Ascorbic acid may increase plasma ethinyl estradiol levels, possibly by inhibition of conjugation).
No products indexed under this heading.

Aspirin (Increased clearance of salicylic acid due to induction of conjugation has been noted when co-administered with combination oral contraceptives). Products include:
Aggrenox Capsules.......... 819
Bayer Aspirin.......... 750
Percodan Tablets.......... 1130
St. Joseph 81 mg Aspirin Chewable and Enteric Coated Tablets.......... 1903

Aspirin, Enteric Coated (Increased clearance of salicylic acid due to induction of conjugation has been noted when co-administered with combination oral contraceptives).
No products indexed under this heading.

Aspirin Buffered (Increased clearance of salicylic acid due to induction of conjugation has been noted when co-administered with combination oral contraceptives).
No products indexed under this heading.

Atazanavir (CYP3A4 inhibitors may increase plasma ethinyl estradiol levels).
No products indexed under this heading.

Atazanavir Sulfate (CYP3A4 inhibitors may increase plasma ethinyl estradiol levels). Products include:
Reyataz Capsules.......... 3299

Atorvastatin Calcium (Co-administration of atorvastatin and certain combination oral contraceptives containing ethinyl estradiol increase AUC values for ethinyl estradiol by approximately 20%). Products include:
Lipitor Tablets.......... 2501

Butabarbital (Contraceptive effectivness may be reduced when hormonal contraceptives are co-administered with drugs that increase the metabolism of contraceptive steroids, such as barbiturates).
No products indexed under this heading.

Butalbital (Contraceptive effectivness may be reduced when hormonal contraceptives are co-administered with drugs that increase the metabolism of contraceptive steroids, such as barbiturates).
No products indexed under this heading.

Carbamazepine (Contraceptive effectiveness may be reduced when hormonal contraceptives are co-administered with drugs that increase the metabolism of contraceptive steroids, such as carbamazepine). Products include:
Carbatrol Capsules.......... 3019
Equetro Extended-Release Capsules.......... 3174

Choline Magnesium Trisalicylate (Increased clearance of salicylic acid due to induction of conjugation has been noted when co-administered with combination oral contraceptives).
No products indexed under this heading.

Cimetidine (CYP3A4 inhibitors may increase plasma ethinyl estradiol levels).
No products indexed under this heading.

Cimetidine Hydrochloride (CYP3A4 inhibitors may increase plasma ethinyl estradiol levels).
No products indexed under this heading.

Ciprofloxacin (CYP3A4 inhibitors may increase plasma ethinyl estradiol levels). Products include:
Cipro I.V... 2817
Cipro Oral Suspension.......... 2810
Cipro XR Tablets.......... 2823
Ciprodex Otic Suspension.......... 541

Clarithromycin (CYP3A4 inhibitors may increase plasma ethinyl estradiol levels). Products include:
Biaxin/Biaxin XL.......... 411

Clotrimazole (CYP3A4 inhibitors may increase plasma ethinyl estradiol levels). Products include:
Lotrisone.......... 2881

Cyclosporine (Combination hormonal contraceptives containing some synthetic estrogens (e.g. ethinyl estradiol) may inhibit the metabolism of other compounds. Increased plasma concentrations of cyclosporine have been reported with concomitant administration of combination oral contraceptives). Products include:
Gengraf Capsules.......... 435
Neoral Oral Solution.......... 2280
Neoral Soft Gelatin Capsules.......... 2280
Restasis Ophthalmic Emulsion.......... 557
Sandimmune.......... 2296

Dalfopristin (CYP3A4 inhibitors may increase plasma ethinyl estradiol levels).
No products indexed under this heading.

Danazol (CYP3A4 inhibitors may increase plasma ethinyl estradiol levels).
No products indexed under this heading.

Darunavir (Several protease inhibitors have been studied with co-administration of oral combination hormonal contraceptives with significant changes (increase and decrease) in the plasma levels of the estrogen and progestin being noted in some cases).
No products indexed under this heading.

Delavirdine Mesylate (CYP3A4 inhibitors may increase plasma ethinyl estradiol levels).
No products indexed under this heading.

Demeclocycline Hydrochloride (Several cases of contraceptive failure and breakthrough bleeding have been reported in the literature concomitant administration of antibiotics, such as tetracyclines; however, clinical pharmacology studies investigating drug interactions between combined oral contraceptives and these antibiotics have reported inconsistent results).
No products indexed under this heading.

Diflunisal (Increased clearance of salicylic acid due to induction of conjugation has been noted when co-administered with combination oral contraceptives).
No products indexed under this heading.

Diltiazem Hydrochloride (CYP3A4 inhibitors may increase plasma ethinyl estradiol levels). Products include:
Cardizem LA Extended Release Tablets.......... 421

Diltiazem Maleate (CYP3A4 inhibitors may increase plasma ethinyl estradiol levels).
No products indexed under this heading.

Doxycycline Calcium (Several cases of contraceptive failure and breakthrough bleeding have been reported in the literature concomitant administration of antibiotics, such as tetracyclines; however, clinical pharmacology studies investigating drug interactions between combined oral contraceptives and these antibiotics have reported inconsistent results).
No products indexed under this heading.

Doxycycline Hyclate (Several cases of contraceptive failure and breakthrough bleeding have been reported in the literature concomitant administration of antibiotics, such as tetracyclines; however, clinical pharmacology studies investigating drug interactions between combined oral contraceptives and these antibiotics have reported inconsistent results).
No products indexed under this heading.

Doxycycline Monohydrate (Several cases of contraceptive failure and breakthrough bleeding have been reported in the literature concomitant administration of antibiotics, such as tetracyclines; however, clinical pharmacology studies investigating drug interactions between combined oral contraceptives and these antibiotics have reported inconsistent results).
No products indexed under this heading.

Efavirenz (CYP3A4 inhibitors may increase plasma ethinyl estradiol levels). Products include:
Atripla Tablets.......... 938
Sustiva Capsules.......... 930
Sustiva Tablets.......... 930

Erythromycin (CYP3A4 inhibitors may increase plasma ethinyl estradiol levels).
No products indexed under this heading.

Erythromycin Estolate (CYP3A4 inhibitors may increase plasma ethinyl estradiol levels).
No products indexed under this heading.

Erythromycin Ethylsuccinate (CYP3A4 inhibitors may increase plasma ethinyl estradiol levels). Products include:
E.E.S... 433
EryPed.......... 431

Erythromycin Gluceptate (CYP3A4 inhibitors may increase plasma ethinyl estradiol levels).
No products indexed under this heading.

Erythromycin Lactobionate (CYP3A4 inhibitors may increase plasma ethinyl estradiol levels).
No products indexed under this heading.

Erythromycin Stearate (CYP3A4 inhibitors may increase plasma ethinyl estradiol levels).
No products indexed under this heading.

Esomeprazole Magnesium (CYP3A4 inhibitors may increase plasma ethinyl estradiol levels). Products include:
Nexium Delayed-Release Capsules 645
Nexium Delayed-Release Oral Suspension 645

Felbamate (Contraceptive effectiveness may be reduced when hormonal contraceptives are co-administered with drugs that increase the metabolism of contraceptive steroids, such as felbamate).
No products indexed under this heading.

Fluconazole (CYP3A4 inhibitors may increase plasma ethinyl estradiol levels).
No products indexed under this heading.

Fluoxetine (CYP3A4 inhibitors may increase plasma ethinyl estradiol levels).
No products indexed under this heading.

Fluoxetine Hydrochloride (CYP3A4 inhibitors may increase plasma ethinyl estradiol levels). Products include:
Prozac Weekly Capsules 1852
Prozac Pulvules and Liquid 1852
Symbyax Capsules 1871

Fluvoxamine Maleate (CYP3A4 inhibitors may increase plasma ethinyl estradiol levels). Products include:
Luvox CR Extended-Release Capsules 1759

Fosamprenavir Calcium (Several protease inhibitors have been studied with co-administration of oral combination hormonal contraceptives with significant changes (increase and decrease) in the plasma levels of the estrogen and progestin being noted in some cases). Products include:
Lexiva Oral Suspension 1510
Lexiva Tablets 1510

Fosphenytoin Sodium (Contraceptive effectivness may be reduced when hormonal contraceptives are co-administered with drugs that increase the metabolism of contraceptive steroids, such as phenytoin).
No products indexed under this heading.

Griseofulvin (Contraceptive effectiveness may be reduced when hormonal contraceptives are co-administered with drugs that increase the metabolism of contraceptive steroids, such as griseofulvin). Products include:
Gris-PEG Tablets 2507

Hypericum (Herbal products containing St. John's Wort (hypericum perforatum) may induce hepatic enzymes (cytochrome p450) and p-glycoprotein transporter and may reduce the effectiveness of contraceptive steroids. This may also result in breakthrough bleeding). Products include:
Satieté Tablets 640

Hypericum Perforatum (Herbal products containing St. John's Wort (hypericum perforatum) may induce hepatic enzymes (cytochrome p450) and p-glycoprotein transporter and may reduce the effectiveness of contraceptive steroids. This may also result in breakthrough bleeding).
No products indexed under this heading.

Indinavir Sulfate (Several protease inhibitors have been studied with co-administration of oral combination hormonal contraceptives with significant changes (increase and decrease) in the plasma levels of the estrogen and progestin being noted in some cases). Products include:
Crixivan Capsules 1979

Isoniazid (CYP3A4 inhibitors may increase plasma ethinyl estradiol levels).
No products indexed under this heading.

Itraconazole (CYP3A4 inhibitors may increase plasma ethinyl estradiol levels).
No products indexed under this heading.

Ketoconazole (CYP3A4 inhibitors may increase plasma ethinyl estradiol levels). Products include:
Extina Foam, 2% 3057
Nizoral A-D Shampoo 1901

Lopinavir (Several protease inhibitors have been studied with co-administration of oral combination hormonal contraceptives with significant changes (increase and decrease) in the plasma levels of the estrogen and progestin being noted in some cases). Products include:
Kaletra 452

Loratadine (CYP3A4 inhibitors may increase plasma ethinyl estradiol levels).
No products indexed under this heading.

Magnesium Salicylate (Increased clearance of salicylic acid due to induction of conjugation has been noted when co-administered with combination oral contraceptives).
No products indexed under this heading.

Mephobarbital (Contraceptive effectivness may be reduced when hormonal contraceptives are co-administered with drugs that increase the metabolism of contraceptive steroids, such as barbiturates).
No products indexed under this heading.

Methacycline Hydrochloride (Several cases of contraceptive failure and breakthrough bleeding have been reported in the literature concomitant administration of antibiotics, such as tetracyclines; however, clinical pharmacology studies investigating drug interactions between combined oral contraceptives and these antibiotics have reported inconsistent results).
No products indexed under this heading.

Metronidazole (CYP3A4 inhibitors may increase plasma ethinyl estradiol levels). Products include:
Pylera Capsules 714

Metronidazole Benzoate (CYP3A4 inhibitors may increase plasma ethinyl estradiol levels).
No products indexed under this heading.

Metronidazole Hydrochloride (CYP3A4 inhibitors may increase plasma ethinyl estradiol levels).
No products indexed under this heading.

Miconazole (CYP3A4 inhibitors may increase plasma ethinyl estradiol levels).
No products indexed under this heading.

Miconazole Nitrate (CYP3A4 inhibitors may increase plasma ethinyl estradiol levels).
No products indexed under this heading.

Minocycline Hydrochloride (Several cases of contraceptive failure and breakthrough bleeding have been reported in the literature concomitant administration of antibiotics, such as tetracyclines; however, clinical pharmacology studies investigating drug interactions between combined oral contraceptives and these antibiotics have reported inconsistent results). Products include:
Solodyn Extended Release Tablets 1938

Nefazodone Hydrochloride (CYP3A4 inhibitors may increase plasma ethinyl estradiol levels).
No products indexed under this heading.

Nelfinavir Mesylate (Several protease inhibitors have been studied with co-administration of oral combination hormonal contraceptives with significant changes (increase and decrease) in the plasma levels of the estrogen and progestin being noted in some cases).
No products indexed under this heading.

Nevirapine (CYP3A4 inhibitors may increase plasma ethinyl estradiol levels). Products include:
Viramune Oral Suspension 873
Viramune Tablets 873

Niacinamide (CYP3A4 inhibitors may increase plasma ethinyl estradiol levels). Products include:
BioLean Free Tablets 635

Nicotinamide (CYP3A4 inhibitors may increase plasma ethinyl estradiol levels).
No products indexed under this heading.

Nifedipine (CYP3A4 inhibitors may increase plasma ethinyl estradiol levels).
No products indexed under this heading.

Norfloxacin (CYP3A4 inhibitors may increase plasma ethinyl estradiol levels). Products include:
Noroxin Tablets 2069

Omeprazole (CYP3A4 inhibitors may increase plasma ethinyl estradiol levels).
No products indexed under this heading.

Oxcarbazepine (Contraceptive effectiveness may be reduced when hormonal contraceptives are co-administered with drugs that increase the metabolism of contraceptive steroids, such as oxcarbazepine).
No products indexed under this heading.

Oxytetracycline Hydrochloride (Several cases of contraceptive failure and breakthrough bleeding have been reported in the literature concomitant administration of antibiotics, such as tetracyclines; however, clinical pharmacology studies investigating drug interactions between combined oral contraceptives and these antibiotics have reported inconsistent results).
No products indexed under this heading.

Paroxetine Hydrochloride (CYP3A4 inhibitors may increase plasma ethinyl estradiol levels). Products include:
Paxil 1535
Paxil CR Controlled-Release Tablets 1544

Pentobarbital Sodium (Contraceptive effectivness may be reduced when hormonal contraceptives are co-administered with drugs that increase the metabolism of contraceptive steroids, such as barbiturates). Products include:
Nembutal Sodium Solution, USP 2494

Phenobarbital (Contraceptive effectivness may be reduced when hormonal contraceptives are co-administered with drugs that increase the metabolism of contraceptive steroids, such as barbiturates). Products include:
Donnatal Extentabs 2507

Phenytoin (Contraceptive effectivness may be reduced when hormonal contraceptives are co-administered with drugs that increase the metabolism of contraceptive steroids, such as phenytoin).
No products indexed under this heading.

Phenytoin Sodium (Contraceptive effectivness may be reduced when hormonal contraceptives are co-administered with drugs that increase the metabolism of contraceptive steroids, such as phenytoin). Products include:
Phenytek Capsules 2192

Prednisolone (Combination hormonal contraceptives containing some synthetic estrogens (e.g. ethinyl estradiol) may inhibit the metabolism of other compounds. Increased plasma concentrations of prednisolone have been reported with concomitant adminstration of combination oral contraceptives).
No products indexed under this heading.

Prednisolone Acetate (Combination hormonal contraceptives containing some synthetic estrogens (e.g. ethinyl estradiol) may inhibit the metabolism of other compounds. Increased plasma concentrations of prednisolone have been reported with concomitant adminstration of combination oral contraceptives). Products include:
Pred Forte Ophthalmic Suspension .... ⊙ 227
Pred Mild Ophthalmic Suspension .... ⊙ 230
Pred-G Ophthalmic Ointment .... ⊙ 229
Pred-G Ophthalmic Suspension .... ⊙ 228

Prednisolone Sodium Phosphate (Combination hormonal contraceptives containing some synthetic estrogens (e.g. ethinyl estradiol) may inhibit the metabolism of other compounds. Increased plasma concentrations of prednisolone have been reported with concomitant adminstration of combination oral contraceptives).
No products indexed under this heading.

Prednisolone Tebutate (Combination hormonal contraceptives containing some synthetic estrogens (e.g. ethinyl estradiol) may inhibit the metabolism of other compounds. Increased plasma concentrations of prednisolone have been reported with concomitant adminstration of combination oral contraceptives).
No products indexed under this heading.

Propoxyphene Hydrochloride (CYP3A4 inhibitors may increase plasma ethinyl estradiol levels).
No products indexed under this heading.

Propoxyphene Napsylate (CYP3A4 inhibitors may increase plasma ethinyl estradiol levels).
No products indexed under this heading.

Quinidine (CYP3A4 inhibitors may increase plasma ethinyl estradiol levels).
No products indexed under this heading.

Quinidine Hydrochloride (CYP3A4 inhibitors may increase plasma ethinyl estradiol levels).
No products indexed under this heading.

Quinidine Polygalacturonate (CYP3A4 inhibitors may increase plasma ethinyl estradiol levels).
No products indexed under this heading.

Quinidine Sulfate (CYP3A4 inhibitors may increase plasma ethinyl estradiol levels).
No products indexed under this heading.

Quinine (CYP3A4 inhibitors may increase plasma ethinyl estradiol levels).
No products indexed under this heading.

Quinine Sulfate (CYP3A4 inhibitors may increase plasma ethinyl estradiol levels).
No products indexed under this heading.

Quinupristin (CYP3A4 inhibitors may increase plasma ethinyl estradiol levels).
No products indexed under this heading.

Ranitidine Bismuth Citrate (CYP3A4 inhibitors may increase plasma ethinyl estradiol levels).
No products indexed under this heading.

Ranitidine Hydrochloride (CYP3A4 inhibitors may increase plasma ethinyl estradiol levels). Products include:
- Zantac 75 Tablets .... ▣ 603
- Zantac 1670
- Zantac Injection 1666
- Zantac Injection Pharmacy Bulk Package 1668
- Maximum Strength Zantac 150 Tablets .... ▣ 603
- Maximum Strength Zantac 150 Cool Mint Tablets .... ▣ 603

Rifampin (Contraceptive effectiveness may be reduced when hormonal contraceptives are co-administered with drugs that increase the metabolism of contraceptive steroids, such as rifampin).
No products indexed under this heading.

Ritonavir (Several protease inhibitors have been studied with co-administration of oral combination hormonal contraceptives with significant changes (increase and decrease) in the plasma levels of the estrogen and progestin being noted in some cases). Products include:
- Kaletra 452
- Norvir 489

Salsalate (Increased clearance of salicylic acid due to induction of conjugation has been noted when co-administered with combination oral contraceptives).
No products indexed under this heading.

Saquinavir (Several protease inhibitors have been studied with co-administration of oral combination hormonal contraceptives with significant changes (increase and decrease) in the plasma levels of the estrogen and progestin being noted in some cases).
No products indexed under this heading.

Saquinavir Mesylate (Several protease inhibitors have been studied with co-administration of oral combination hormonal contraceptives with significant changes (increase and decrease) in the plasma levels of the estrogen and progestin being noted in some cases).
No products indexed under this heading.

Secobarbital Sodium (Contraceptive effectivness may be reduced when hormonal contraceptives are co-administered with drugs that increase the metabolism of contraceptive steroids, such as barbiturates).
No products indexed under this heading.

Sertraline Hydrochloride (CYP3A4 inhibitors may increase plasma ethinyl estradiol levels).
No products indexed under this heading.

Sildenafil Citrate (CYP3A4 inhibitors may increase plasma ethinyl estradiol levels).
No products indexed under this heading.

Telithromycin (CYP3A4 inhibitors may increase plasma ethinyl estradiol levels). Products include:
- Ketek Tablets 2744

Temazepam (Increased clearance of temazepam due to induction of conjugation has been noted when co-administered with combination oral contraceptives).
No products indexed under this heading.

Tetracycline Hydrochloride (Several cases of contraceptive failure and breakthrough bleeding have been reported in the literature concomitant administration of antibiotics, such as tetracyclines; however, clinical pharmacology studies investigating drug interactions between combined oral contraceptives and these antibiotics have reported inconsistent results). Products include:
- Pylera Capsules 714

Theophylline (Combination hormonal contraceptives containing some synthetic estrogens (e.g. ethinyl estradiol) may inhibit the metabolism of other compounds. Increased plasma concentrations of theophylline have been reported with concomitant administration of combination oral contraceptives).
No products indexed under this heading.

Theophylline Anhydrous (Combination hormonal contraceptives containing some synthetic estrogens (e.g. ethinyl estradiol) may inhibit the metabolism of other compounds. Increased plasma concentrations of theophylline have been reported with concomitant administration of combination oral contraceptives). Products include:
- Uniphyl Tablets 2595

Theophylline Calcium Salicylate (Combination hormonal contraceptives containing some synthetic estrogens (e.g. ethinyl estradiol) may inhibit the metabolism of other compounds. Increased plasma concentrations of theophylline have been reported with concomitant administration of combination oral contraceptives).
No products indexed under this heading.

Theophylline Dihydroxypropyl (Glyceryl) (Combination hormonal contraceptives containing some synthetic estrogens (e.g. ethinyl estradiol) may inhibit the metabolism of other compounds. Increased plasma concentrations of theophylline have been reported with concomitant administration of combination oral contraceptives).
No products indexed under this heading.

Theophylline Ethylenediamine (Combination hormonal contraceptives containing some synthetic estrogens (e.g. ethinyl estradiol) may inhibit the metabolism of other compounds. Increased plasma concentrations of theophylline have been reported with concomitant administration of combination oral contraceptives).
No products indexed under this heading.

Theophylline Sodium Glycinate (Combination hormonal contraceptives containing some synthetic estrogens (e.g. ethinyl estradiol) may inhibit the metabolism of other compounds. Increased plasma concentrations of theophylline have been reported with concomitant administration of combination oral contraceptives).
No products indexed under this heading.

Thiamylal Sodium (Contraceptive effectivness may be reduced when hormonal contraceptives are co-administered with drugs that increase the metabolism of contraceptive steroids, such as barbiturates).
No products indexed under this heading.

Tipranavir (Several protease inhibitors have been studied with co-administration of oral combination hormonal contraceptives with significant changes (increase and decrease) in the plasma levels of the estrogen and progestin being noted in some cases). Products include:
- Aptivus Capsules 823
- Aptivus Oral Solution 823

Topiramate (Contraceptive effectiveness may be reduced when hormonal contraceptives are co-administered with drugs that increase the metabolism of contraceptive steroids, such as topiramate).
No products indexed under this heading.

Troglitazone (CYP3A4 inhibitors may increase plasma ethinyl estradiol levels).
No products indexed under this heading.

Troleandomycin (CYP3A4 inhibitors may increase plasma ethinyl estradiol levels).
No products indexed under this heading.

Valproate Sodium (CYP3A4 inhibitors may increase plasma ethinyl estradiol levels).
No products indexed under this heading.

Vardenafil Hydrochloride (CYP3A4 inhibitors may increase plasma ethinyl estradiol levels). Products include:
- Levitra Tablets 2876

Verapamil Hydrochloride (CYP3A4 inhibitors may increase plasma ethinyl estradiol levels). Products include:
- Tarka Tablets 511

Vitamin C (Ascorbic acid may increase plasma ethinyl estradiol levels, possibly by inhibition of conjugation). Products include:
- Bausch & Lomb Ocuvite Adult 50+ Vitamin and Mineral Supplement .... ⊙ 237
- Comax Dietary Supplement 995
- Ferralet 90 Tablets 2175
- Glaucofit Dietary Supplement 995
- Glauma Dietary Supplement 995
- MoviPrep Oral Solution 2679
- Procosa II Tablets 3174
- Proflavanol 90 Tablets 3174
- Tonox Dietary Supplement 995
- Vibe Liquid Multi-Nutrient Supplement .... ▣ 626

Voriconazole (CYP3A4 inhibitors may increase plasma ethinyl estradiol levels).
No products indexed under this heading.

Zafirlukast (CYP3A4 inhibitors may increase plasma ethinyl estradiol levels). Products include:
- Accolate Tablets 669

Zileuton (CYP3A4 inhibitors may increase plasma ethinyl estradiol levels).
No products indexed under this heading.

Food Interactions

Grapefruit (CYP3A4 inhibitors may increase plasma ethinyl estradiol levels).

Grapefruit Juice (CYP3A4 inhibitors may increase plasma ethinyl estradiol levels).

SELZENTRY TABLETS

(Maraviroc) 2534

May interact with:

Hypericum Perforatum (Concomitant use of maraviroc and St. John's wort (hypericum perforatum) or products containing St. John's wort is not recommended. Co-administration of maraviroc with St. John's wort is expected to substantially decrease maraviroc concentrations and may result in suboptimal

levels of maraviroc and lead to loss of virologic response and possible resistance to maraviroc).
No products indexed under this heading.

SEN-SEI-RO LIQUID GOLD
(Dietary Supplement) 1785
None cited in PDR database.

SEN-SEI-RO LIQUID ROYAL
(Dietary Supplement) 1785
None cited in PDR database.

SEN-SEI-RO POWDER GOLD
(Dietary Supplement) 1786
None cited in PDR database.

SENSIPAR TABLETS
(Cinacalcet Hydrochloride) 594
May interact with cytochrome p450 2d6 substrates (selected), cytochrome p450 3a inhibitors (selected), and certain other agents. Compounds in these categories include:

Amiodarone Hydrochloride (Since cinacalcet hydrochloride is metabolized in part by CYP3A4, dose adjustment of cinacalcet hydrochloride may be required and PTH and serum calcium concentrations closely monitored if a patient initiates or discontinues therapy with a strong CYP3A4 inhibitor).
No products indexed under this heading.

Amitriptyline Hydrochloride (Administration of 25mg or 100mg cinacalcet with 50mg amitriptyline increased amitriptyline exposure and nortriptyline (active metabolite) exposure by approximately 20% in CYP2D6 extensive metabolizers. Cinacalcet hydrochloride is a strong in vitro inhibitor of CYP2D6. Therefore, dose adjustments of concomitant medications that are predominantly metabolized by CYP2D6 and have a narrow therapeutic index may be required).
No products indexed under this heading.

Amphetamine Aspartate (Cinacalcet hydrochloride is a strong in vitro inhibitor of CYP2D6. Therefore, dose adjustments of concomitant medications that are predominantly metabolized by CYP2D6 and have a narrow therapeutic index may be required). Products include:
Adderall XR Capsules 3012

Amphetamine Aspartate Monohydrate (Cinacalcet hydrochloride is a strong in vitro inhibitor of CYP2D6. Therefore, dose adjustments of concomitant medications that are predominantly metabolized by CYP2D6 and have a narrow therapeutic index may be required).
No products indexed under this heading.

Amphetamine Sulfate (Cinacalcet hydrochloride is a strong in vitro inhibitor of CYP2D6. Therefore, dose adjustments of concomitant medications that are predominantly metabolized by CYP2D6 and have a narrow therapeutic index may be required). Products include:
Adderall XR Capsules 3012

Amprenavir (Since cinacalcet hydrochloride is metabolized in part by CYP3A4, dose adjustment of cinacalcet hydrochloride may be required and PTH and serum calcium concentrations closely monitored if a patient initiates or discontinues therapy with a strong CYP3A4 inhibitor).
No products indexed under this heading.

Aprepitant (Since cinacalcet hydrochloride is metabolized in part by CYP3A4, dose adjustment of cinacalcet hydrochloride may be required and PTH and serum calcium concentrations closely monitored if a patient initiates or discontinues therapy with a strong CYP3A4 inhibitor). Products include:
Emend Capsules 1992

Atomoxetine Hydrochloride (Cinacalcet hydrochloride is a strong in vitro inhibitor of CYP2D6. Therefore, dose adjustments of concomitant medications that are predominantly metabolized by CYP2D6 and have a narrow therapeutic index may be required). Products include:
Strattera Capsules 1864

Bisoprolol Fumarate (Cinacalcet hydrochloride is a strong in vitro inhibitor of CYP2D6. Therefore, dose adjustments of concomitant medications that are predominantly metabolized by CYP2D6 and have a narrow therapeutic index may be required).
No products indexed under this heading.

Captopril (Cinacalcet hydrochloride is a strong in vitro inhibitor of CYP2D6. Therefore, dose adjustments of concomitant medications that are predominantly metabolized by CYP2D6 and have a narrow therapeutic index may be required). Products include:
Captopril Tablets 2182

Carvedilol (Cinacalcet hydrochloride is a strong in vitro inhibitor of CYP2D6. Therefore, dose adjustments of concomitant medications that are predominantly metabolized by CYP2D6 and have a narrow therapeutic index may be required). Products include:
Coreg Tablets 1387

Cevimeline Hydrochloride (Cinacalcet hydrochloride is a strong in vitro inhibitor of CYP2D6. Therefore, dose adjustments of concomitant medications that are predominantly metabolized by CYP2D6 and have a narrow therapeutic index may be required). Products include:
Evoxac Capsules 1013

Chlorpromazine (Cinacalcet hydrochloride is a strong in vitro inhibitor of CYP2D6. Therefore, dose adjustments of concomitant medications that are predominantly metabolized by CYP2D6 and have a narrow therapeutic index may be required).
No products indexed under this heading.

Chlorpromazine Hydrochloride (Cinacalcet hydrochloride is a strong in vitro inhibitor of CYP2D6. Therefore, dose adjustments of concomitant medications that are predominantly metabolized by CYP2D6 and have a narrow therapeutic index may be required).
No products indexed under this heading.

Chlorpropamide (Cinacalcet hydrochloride is a strong in vitro inhibitor of CYP2D6. Therefore, dose adjustments of concomitant medications that are predominantly metabolized by CYP2D6 and have a narrow therapeutic index may be required).
No products indexed under this heading.

Cimetidine (Since cinacalcet hydrochloride is metabolized in part by CYP3A4, dose adjustment of cinacalcet hydrochloride may be required and PTH and serum calcium concentrations closely monitored if a patient initiates or discontinues therapy with a strong CYP3A4 inhibitor).
No products indexed under this heading.

Cimetidine Hydrochloride (Since cinacalcet hydrochloride is metabolized in part by CYP3A4, dose adjustment of cinacalcet hydrochloride may be required and PTH and serum calcium concentrations closely monitored if a patient initiates or discontinues therapy with a strong CYP3A4 inhibitor).
No products indexed under this heading.

Ciprofloxacin (Since cinacalcet hydrochloride is metabolized in part by CYP3A4, dose adjustment of cinacalcet hydrochloride may be required and PTH and serum calcium concentrations closely monitored if a patient initiates or discontinues therapy with a strong CYP3A4 inhibitor). Products include:
Cipro I.V. 2817
Cipro Oral Suspension 2810
Cipro XR Tablets 2823
Ciprodex Otic Suspension 541

Ciprofloxacin Hydrochloride (Since cinacalcet hydrochloride is metabolized in part by CYP3A4, dose adjustment of cinacalcet hydrochloride may be required and PTH and serum calcium concentrations closely monitored if a patient initiates or discontinues therapy with a strong CYP3A4 inhibitor). Products include:
Cipro Tablets 2810

Clarithromycin (Since cinacalcet hydrochloride is metabolized in part by CYP3A4, dose adjustment of cinacalcet hydrochloride may be required and PTH and serum calcium concentrations closely monitored if a patient initiates or discontinues therapy with a strong CYP3A4 inhibitor). Products include:
Biaxin/Biaxin XL 411

Clomipramine Hydrochloride (Cinacalcet hydrochloride is a strong in vitro inhibitor of CYP2D6. Therefore, dose adjustments of concomitant medications that are predominantly metabolized by CYP2D6 and have a narrow therapeutic index may be required).
No products indexed under this heading.

Clozapine (Cinacalcet hydrochloride is a strong in vitro inhibitor of CYP2D6. Therefore, dose adjustments of concomitant medications that are predominantly metabolized by CYP2D6 and have a narrow therapeutic index may be required).
No products indexed under this heading.

Codeine Phosphate (Cinacalcet hydrochloride is a strong in vitro inhibitor of CYP2D6. Therefore, dose adjustments of concomitant medications that are predominantly metabolized by CYP2D6 and have a narrow therapeutic index may be required). Products include:
Tylenol with Codeine Tablets 2427

Codeine Sulfate (Cinacalcet hydrochloride is a strong in vitro inhibitor of CYP2D6. Therefore, dose adjustments of concomitant medications that are predominantly metabolized by CYP2D6 and have a narrow therapeutic index may be required).
No products indexed under this heading.

Cyclobenzaprine Hydrochloride (Cinacalcet hydrochloride is a strong in vitro inhibitor of CYP2D6. Therefore, dose adjustments of concomitant medications that are predominantly metabolized by CYP2D6 and have a narrow therapeutic index may be required). Products include:
Amrix Capsules 966

Cyclosporine (Since cinacalcet hydrochloride is metabolized in part by CYP3A4, dose adjustment of cinacalcet hydrochloride may be required and PTH and serum calcium concentrations closely monitored if a patient initiates or discontinues therapy with a strong CYP3A4 inhibitor). Products include:
Gengraf Capsules 435
Neoral Oral Solution 2280
Neoral Soft Gelatin Capsules 2280
Restasis Ophthalmic Emulsion 557
Sandimmune 2296

Delavirdine Mesylate (Since cinacalcet hydrochloride is metabolized in part by CYP3A4, dose adjustment of cinacalcet hydrochloride may be required and PTH and serum calcium concentrations closely monitored if a patient initiates or discontinues therapy with a strong CYP3A4 inhibitor).
No products indexed under this heading.

Desipramine Hydrochloride (Cinacalcet hydrochloride is a strong in vitro inhibitor of CYP2D6. Therefore, dose adjustments of concomitant medications that are predominantly metabolized by CYP2D6 and have a narrow therapeutic index may be required. Concurrent administration of cinacalcet (90 mg) with desipramine (50 mg) increased the exposure of desipramine by 3.6 fold in CYP2D6 extensive metabolizers).
No products indexed under this heading.

Dexfenfluramine Hydrochloride (Cinacalcet hydrochloride is a strong in vitro inhibitor of CYP2D6. Therefore, dose adjustments of concomitant medications that are predominantly metabolized by CYP2D6 and have a narrow therapeutic index may be required).
No products indexed under this heading.

Dextromethorphan Hydrobromide (Cinacalcet hydrochloride is a strong in vitro inhibitor of CYP2D6. Therefore, dose adjustments of concomitant medications that are predominantly metabolized by CYP2D6 and have a narrow therapeutic index may be required). Products include:
PediaCare Children's Liquid Multi-Symptom Cold..................... 1902
PediaCare Children's Long-Acting Cough 1902
Children's Sudafed PE Cold & Cough Liquid 1907
Sudafed PE Cold & Cough Caplets... 1907
Children's Tylenol Plus Cough & Runny Nose Suspension Liquid..... 1912

IMPORTANT NOTE: Always consult each drug listing in the patient's regimen for possible interactions.

Children's Tylenol Plus Cough & Sore Throat Suspension Liquid 1912
Children's Tylenol Plus Flu Suspension Liquid 1914
Children's Tylenol Plus Multi-Symptom Cold Suspension Liquid 1912
Tylenol Cold Severe Congestion Daytime Caplets with Cool Burst 1912
Tylenol Cold Head Congestion Daytime Caplets with Cool Burst 1910
Tylenol Cold Head Congestion Nighttime Caplets with Cool Burst 1910
Tylenol Cold Head Congestion Severe Daytime Caplets with Cool Burst 1910
Tylenol Cold Multi-Symptom Daytime Caplets with Cool Burst and Rapid Release Gels 1913
Tylenol Cold Multi-Symptom Daytime Liquid with Citrus Burst 1913
Tylenol Cold Multi-Symptom Nighttime Caplets with Cool Burst 1913
Tylenol Cold Multi-Symptom Nighttime Liquid with Cool Burst 1913
Tylenol Cold Multi-Symptom Severe Caplets with Cool Burst 1913
Tylenol Cold Multi-Symptom Severe Daytime Liquid with Citrus Burst 1913
Tylenol Cough & Sore Throat Daytime Liquid with Cool Burst 1918
Tylenol Cough & Sore Throat Nighttime Liquid with Cool Burst 1918
Vicks DayQuil Cold & Flu Multi-Symptom Relief ..... ▣616
Vicks DayQuil LiquiCaps 2567
Vicks DayQuil Liquid 2567
Vicks DayQuil Multi-Symptom Cold/Flu Relief 2567
Vicks NyQuil Cold & Flu Multi-Symptom Relief ..... ▣617
Vicks NyQuil LiquiCaps 2567
Vicks NyQuil Liquid 2567
Vicks NyQuil Multi-Symptom Cold/Flu Relief 2567

Dextromethorphan Polistirex (Cinacalcet hydrochloride is a strong in vitro inhibitor of CYP2D6. Therefore, dose adjustments of concomitant medications that are predominantly metabolized by CYP2D6 and have a narrow therapeutic index may be required).
No products indexed under this heading.

Diltiazem Hydrochloride (Since cinacalcet hydrochloride is metabolized in part by CYP3A4, dose adjustment of cinacalcet hydrochloride may be required and PTH and serum calcium concentrations closely monitored if a patient initiates or discontinues therapy with a strong CYP3A4 inhibitor). Products include:
Cardizem LA Extended Release Tablets 421

Diltiazem Maleate (Since cinacalcet hydrochloride is metabolized in part by CYP3A4, dose adjustment of cinacalcet hydrochloride may be required and PTH and serum calcium concentrations closely monitored if a patient initiates or discontinues therapy with a strong CYP3A4 inhibitor).
No products indexed under this heading.

Dolasetron Mesylate (Cinacalcet hydrochloride is a strong in vitro inhibitor of CYP2D6. Therefore, dose adjustments of concomitant medications that are predominantly metabolized by CYP2D6 and have a narrow therapeutic index may be required). Products include:
Anzemet Injection 2701
Anzemet Tablets 2704

Donepezil Hydrochloride (Cinacalcet hydrochloride is a strong in vitro inhibitor of CYP2D6. Therefore, dose adjustments of concomitant medications that are predominantly metabolized by CYP2D6 and have a narrow therapeutic index may be required). Products include:
Aricept Tablets 1062
Aricept ODT Tablets 1062

Doxepin Hydrochloride (Cinacalcet hydrochloride is a strong in vitro inhibitor of CYP2D6. Therefore, dose adjustments of concomitant medications that are predominantly metabolized by CYP2D6 and have a narrow therapeutic index may be required).
No products indexed under this heading.

Efavirenz (Since cinacalcet hydrochloride is metabolized in part by CYP3A4, dose adjustment of cinacalcet hydrochloride may be required and PTH and serum calcium concentrations closely monitored if a patient initiates or discontinues therapy with a strong CYP3A4 inhibitor). Products include:
Atripla Tablets 938
Sustiva Capsules 930
Sustiva Tablets 930

Encainide Hydrochloride (Cinacalcet hydrochloride is a strong in vitro inhibitor of CYP2D6. Therefore, dose adjustments of concomitant medications that are predominantly metabolized by CYP2D6 and have a narrow therapeutic index may be required).
No products indexed under this heading.

Erythromycin (Since cinacalcet hydrochloride is metabolized in part by CYP3A4, dose adjustment of cinacalcet hydrochloride may be required and PTH and serum calcium concentrations closely monitored if a patient initiates or discontinues therapy with a strong CYP3A4 inhibitor).
No products indexed under this heading.

Fentanyl (Cinacalcet hydrochloride is a strong in vitro inhibitor of CYP2D6. Therefore, dose adjustments of concomitant medications that are predominantly metabolized by CYP2D6 and have a narrow therapeutic index may be required). Products include:
Duragesic Transdermal System 2405
Ionsys Transdermal System 2410

Fentanyl Citrate (Cinacalcet hydrochloride is a strong in vitro inhibitor of CYP2D6. Therefore, dose adjustments of concomitant medications that are predominantly metabolized by CYP2D6 and have a narrow therapeutic index may be required). Products include:
Actiq 959
Fentora Tablets 968

Flecainide Acetate (Cinacalcet hydrochloride is a strong in vitro inhibitor of CYP2D6. Therefore, dose adjustments of concomitant medications that are predominantly metabolized by CYP2D6 and have a narrow therapeutic index may be required).
No products indexed under this heading.

Fluconazole (Since cinacalcet hydrochloride is metabolized in part by CYP3A4, dose adjustment of cinacalcet hydrochloride may be required and PTH and serum calcium concentrations closely monitored if a patient initiates or discontinues therapy with a strong CYP3A4 inhibitor).
No products indexed under this heading.

Fluoxetine (Cinacalcet hydrochloride is a strong in vitro inhibitor of CYP2D6. Therefore, dose adjustments of concomitant medications that are predominantly metabolized by CYP2D6 and have a narrow therapeutic index may be required).
No products indexed under this heading.

Fluoxetine Hydrochloride (Cinacalcet hydrochloride is a strong in vitro inhibitor of CYP2D6. Therefore, dose adjustments of concomitant medications that are predominantly metabolized by CYP2D6 and have a narrow therapeutic index may be required). Products include:
Prozac Weekly Capsules 1852
Prozac Pulvules and Liquid 1852
Symbyax Capsules 1871

Fluphenazine Decanoate (Cinacalcet hydrochloride is a strong in vitro inhibitor of CYP2D6. Therefore, dose adjustments of concomitant medications that are predominantly metabolized by CYP2D6 and have a narrow therapeutic index may be required).
No products indexed under this heading.

Fluphenazine Enanthate (Cinacalcet hydrochloride is a strong in vitro inhibitor of CYP2D6. Therefore, dose adjustments of concomitant medications that are predominantly metabolized by CYP2D6 and have a narrow therapeutic index may be required).
No products indexed under this heading.

Fluphenazine Hydrochloride (Cinacalcet hydrochloride is a strong in vitro inhibitor of CYP2D6. Therefore, dose adjustments of concomitant medications that are predominantly metabolized by CYP2D6 and have a narrow therapeutic index may be required).
No products indexed under this heading.

Fluvoxamine Maleate (Cinacalcet hydrochloride is a strong in vitro inhibitor of CYP2D6. Therefore, dose adjustments of concomitant medications that are predominantly metabolized by CYP2D6 and have a narrow therapeutic index may be required). Products include:
Luvox CR Extended-Release Capsules 1759

Formoterol Fumarate (Cinacalcet hydrochloride is a strong in vitro inhibitor of CYP2D6. Therefore, dose adjustments of concomitant medications that are predominantly metabolized by CYP2D6 and have a narrow therapeutic index may be required). Products include:
Foradil Aerolizer 2849
Perforomist Inhalation Solution 1025

Galantamine Hydrobromide (Cinacalcet hydrochloride is a strong in vitro inhibitor of CYP2D6. Therefore, dose adjustments of concomitant medications that are predominantly metabolized by CYP2D6 and have a narrow therapeutic index may be required).
No products indexed under this heading.

Haloperidol (Cinacalcet hydrochloride is a strong in vitro inhibitor of CYP2D6. Therefore, dose adjustments of concomitant medications that are predominantly metabolized by CYP2D6 and have a narrow therapeutic index may be required).
No products indexed under this heading.

Haloperidol Decanoate (Cinacalcet hydrochloride is a strong in vitro inhibitor of CYP2D6. Therefore, dose adjustments of concomitant medications that are predominantly metabolized by CYP2D6 and have a narrow therapeutic index may be required).
No products indexed under this heading.

Hydrocodone Bitartrate (Cinacalcet hydrochloride is a strong in vitro inhibitor of CYP2D6. Therefore, dose adjustments of concomitant medications that are predominantly metabolized by CYP2D6 and have a narrow therapeutic index may be required). Products include:
Lortab 5/500 Tablets 3143
Lortab 7.5/500 Tablets 3144
Lortab 10/500 Tablets 3144
Vicodin Tablets 529
Vicodin ES Tablets 530
Vicodin HP Tablets 531
Vicoprofen Tablets 533
Zydone Tablets 1132

Imipramine Hydrochloride (Cinacalcet hydrochloride is a strong in vitro inhibitor of CYP2D6. Therefore, dose adjustments of concomitant medications that are predominantly metabolized by CYP2D6 and have a narrow therapeutic index may be required).
No products indexed under this heading.

Imipramine Pamoate (Cinacalcet hydrochloride is a strong in vitro inhibitor of CYP2D6. Therefore, dose adjustments of concomitant medications that are predominantly metabolized by CYP2D6 and have a narrow therapeutic index may be required).
No products indexed under this heading.

Indinavir Sulfate (Since cinacalcet hydrochloride is metabolized in part by CYP3A4, dose adjustment of cinacalcet hydrochloride may be required and PTH and serum calcium concentrations closely monitored if a patient initiates or discontinues therapy with a strong CYP3A4 inhibitor). Products include:
Crixivan Capsules 1979

Indoramin Hydrochloride (Cinacalcet hydrochloride is a strong in vitro inhibitor of CYP2D6. Therefore, dose adjustments of concomitant medications that are predominantly metabolized by CYP2D6 and have a narrow therapeutic index may be required).
No products indexed under this heading.

Isoniazid (Since cinacalcet hydrochloride is metabolized in part by CYP3A4, dose adjustment of cinacalcet hydrochloride may be required and PTH and serum calcium concentrations closely monitored if a patient initiates or discontinues therapy with a strong CYP3A4 inhibitor).
No products indexed under this heading.

Itraconazole (Since cinacalcet hydrochloride is metabolized in part by CYP3A4, dose adjustment of cinacalcet hydrochloride may be required and PTH and serum calcium concentrations closely monitored if a patient initiates or discontinues therapy with a strong CYP3A4 inhibitor).
No products indexed under this heading.

Ketoconazole (Co-administration of ketoconazole, a strong inhibitor of CYP3A4, increased cinacalcet exposure following a single 90 mg dose

of cinacalcet hydrochloride by 2.3 fold. Since cinacalcet hydrochloride is metabolized in part by CYP3A4, dose adjustment of cinacalcet hydrochloride may be required and PTH and serum calcium concentrations closely monitored if a patient initiates or discontinues therapy with a strong CYP3A4 inhibitor). Products include:

Extina Foam, 2% 3057
Nizoral A-D Shampoo 1901

Labetalol Hydrochloride (Cinacalcet hydrochloride is a strong in vitro inhibitor of CYP2D6. Therefore, dose adjustments of concomitant medications that are predominantly metabolized by CYP2D6 and have a narrow therapeutic index may be required).
No products indexed under this heading.

Lidocaine (Cinacalcet hydrochloride is a strong in vitro inhibitor of CYP2D6. Therefore, dose adjustments of concomitant medications that are predominantly metabolized by CYP2D6 and have a narrow therapeutic index may be required). Products include:

Lidoderm Patch 1114

Lidocaine Hydrochloride (Cinacalcet hydrochloride is a strong in vitro inhibitor of CYP2D6. Therefore, dose adjustments of concomitant medications that are predominantly metabolized by CYP2D6 and have a narrow therapeutic index may be required).
No products indexed under this heading.

Lopinavir (Since cinacalcet hydrochloride is metabolized in part by CYP3A4, dose adjustment of cinacalcet hydrochloride may be required and PTH and serum calcium concentrations closely monitored if a patient initiates or discontinues therapy with a strong CYP3A4 inhibitor). Products include:

Kaletra 452

Maprotiline Hydrochloride (Cinacalcet hydrochloride is a strong in vitro inhibitor of CYP2D6. Therefore, dose adjustments of concomitant medications that are predominantly metabolized by CYP2D6 and have a narrow therapeutic index may be required).
No products indexed under this heading.

Meperidine Hydrochloride (Cinacalcet hydrochloride is a strong in vitro inhibitor of CYP2D6. Therefore, dose adjustments of concomitant medications that are predominantly metabolized by CYP2D6 and have a narrow therapeutic index may be required).
No products indexed under this heading.

Methadone Hydrochloride (Cinacalcet hydrochloride is a strong in vitro inhibitor of CYP2D6. Therefore, dose adjustments of concomitant medications that are predominantly metabolized by CYP2D6 and have a narrow therapeutic index may be required).
No products indexed under this heading.

Methamphetamine Hydrochloride (Cinacalcet hydrochloride is a strong in vitro inhibitor of CYP2D6. Therefore, dose adjustments of concomitant medications that are predominantly metabolized by CYP2D6 and have a narrow therapeutic index may be required).
No products indexed under this heading.

Metoprolol Succinate (Cinacalcet hydrochloride is a strong in vitro inhibitor of CYP2D6. Therefore, dose adjustments of concomitant medications that are predominantly metabolized by CYP2D6 and have a narrow therapeutic index may be required). Products include:

Toprol-XL Tablets 666

Metoprolol Tartrate (Cinacalcet hydrochloride is a strong in vitro inhibitor of CYP2D6. Therefore, dose adjustments of concomitant medications that are predominantly metabolized by CYP2D6 and have a narrow therapeutic index may be required).
No products indexed under this heading.

Metronidazole (Since cinacalcet hydrochloride is metabolized in part by CYP3A4, dose adjustment of cinacalcet hydrochloride may be required and PTH and serum calcium concentrations closely monitored if a patient initiates or discontinues therapy with a strong CYP3A4 inhibitor). Products include:

Pylera Capsules 714

Metronidazole Benzoate (Since cinacalcet hydrochloride is metabolized in part by CYP3A4, dose adjustment of cinacalcet hydrochloride may be required and PTH and serum calcium concentrations closely monitored if a patient initiates or discontinues therapy with a strong CYP3A4 inhibitor).
No products indexed under this heading.

Metronidazole Hydrochloride (Since cinacalcet hydrochloride is metabolized in part by CYP3A4, dose adjustment of cinacalcet hydrochloride may be required and PTH and serum calcium concentrations closely monitored if a patient initiates or discontinues therapy with a strong CYP3A4 inhibitor).
No products indexed under this heading.

Mexiletine Hydrochloride (Cinacalcet hydrochloride is a strong in vitro inhibitor of CYP2D6. Therefore, dose adjustments of concomitant medications that are predominantly metabolized by CYP2D6 and have a narrow therapeutic index may be required).
No products indexed under this heading.

Miconazole (Since cinacalcet hydrochloride is metabolized in part by CYP3A4, dose adjustment of cinacalcet hydrochloride may be required and PTH and serum calcium concentrations closely monitored if a patient initiates or discontinues therapy with a strong CYP3A4 inhibitor).
No products indexed under this heading.

Mirtazapine (Cinacalcet hydrochloride is a strong in vitro inhibitor of CYP2D6. Therefore, dose adjustments of concomitant medications that are predominantly metabolized by CYP2D6 and have a narrow therapeutic index may be required). Products include:

Remeron Tablets 2924
RemeronSolTab Tablets 2927

Morphine Sulfate (Cinacalcet hydrochloride is a strong in vitro inhibitor of CYP2D6. Therefore, dose adjustments of concomitant medications that are predominantly metabolized by CYP2D6 and have a narrow therapeutic index may be required). Products include:

Avinza Capsules 1772
DepoDur Injection 1095
MS Contin Tablets 2585

Nefazodone Hydrochloride (Since cinacalcet hydrochloride is metabolized in part by CYP3A4, dose adjustment of cinacalcet hydrochloride may be required and PTH and serum calcium concentrations closely monitored if a patient initiates or discontinues therapy with a strong CYP3A4 inhibitor).
No products indexed under this heading.

Nelfinavir Mesylate (Cinacalcet hydrochloride is a strong in vitro inhibitor of CYP2D6. Therefore, dose adjustments of concomitant medications that are predominantly metabolized by CYP2D6 and have a narrow therapeutic index may be required).
No products indexed under this heading.

Nifedipine (Since cinacalcet hydrochloride is metabolized in part by CYP3A4, dose adjustment of cinacalcet hydrochloride may be required and PTH and serum calcium concentrations closely monitored if a patient initiates or discontinues therapy with a strong CYP3A4 inhibitor).
No products indexed under this heading.

Norfloxacin (Since cinacalcet hydrochloride is metabolized in part by CYP3A4, dose adjustment of cinacalcet hydrochloride may be required and PTH and serum calcium concentrations closely monitored if a patient initiates or discontinues therapy with a strong CYP3A4 inhibitor). Products include:

Noroxin Tablets 2069

Nortriptyline Hydrochloride (Cinacalcet hydrochloride is a strong in vitro inhibitor of CYP2D6. Therefore, dose adjustments of concomitant medications that are predominantly metabolized by CYP2D6 and have a narrow therapeutic index may be required).
No products indexed under this heading.

Olanzapine (Cinacalcet hydrochloride is a strong in vitro inhibitor of CYP2D6. Therefore, dose adjustments of concomitant medications that are predominantly metabolized by CYP2D6 and have a narrow therapeutic index may be required). Products include:

Symbyax Capsules 1871
Zyprexa Tablets 1883
Zyprexa IntraMuscular 1883
Zyprexa ZYDIS Orally Disintegrating Tablets 1883

Omeprazole (Cinacalcet hydrochloride is a strong in vitro inhibitor of CYP2D6. Therefore, dose adjustments of concomitant medications that are predominantly metabolized by CYP2D6 and have a narrow therapeutic index may be required).
No products indexed under this heading.

Ondansetron (Cinacalcet hydrochloride is a strong in vitro inhibitor of CYP2D6. Therefore, dose adjustments of concomitant medications that are predominantly metabolized by CYP2D6 and have a narrow therapeutic index may be required). Products include:

Zofran ODT Orally Disintegrating Tablets 1687

Ondansetron Hydrochloride (Cinacalcet hydrochloride is a strong in vitro inhibitor of CYP2D6. Therefore, dose adjustments of concomitant medications that are predominantly metabolized by CYP2D6 and have a narrow therapeutic index may be required). Products include:

Zofran Injection 1682
Zofran 1687

Oxycodone Hydrochloride (Cinacalcet hydrochloride is a strong in vitro inhibitor of CYP2D6. Therefore, dose adjustments of concomitant medications that are predominantly metabolized by CYP2D6 and have a narrow therapeutic index may be required). Products include:

OxyContin Tablets 2589
OxyIR Capsules 2593
Percocet Tablets 1127
Percodan Tablets 1130

Paclitaxel (Cinacalcet hydrochloride is a strong in vitro inhibitor of CYP2D6. Therefore, dose adjustments of concomitant medications that are predominantly metabolized by CYP2D6 and have a narrow therapeutic index may be required).
No products indexed under this heading.

Paroxetine Hydrochloride (Cinacalcet hydrochloride is a strong in vitro inhibitor of CYP2D6. Therefore, dose adjustments of concomitant medications that are predominantly metabolized by CYP2D6 and have a narrow therapeutic index may be required). Products include:

Paxil 1535
Paxil CR Controlled-Release Tablets 1544

Pindolol (Cinacalcet hydrochloride is a strong in vitro inhibitor of CYP2D6. Therefore, dose adjustments of concomitant medications that are predominantly metabolized by CYP2D6 and have a narrow therapeutic index may be required).
No products indexed under this heading.

Propafenone Hydrochloride (Cinacalcet hydrochloride is a strong in vitro inhibitor of CYP2D6. Therefore, dose adjustments of concomitant medications that are predominantly metabolized by CYP2D6 and have a narrow therapeutic index may be required). Products include:

Rythmol Tablets 1586
Rythmol SR Capsules 1590

Propoxyphene Hydrochloride (Cinacalcet hydrochloride is a strong in vitro inhibitor of CYP2D6. Therefore, dose adjustments of concomitant medications that are predominantly metabolized by CYP2D6 and have a narrow therapeutic index may be required).
No products indexed under this heading.

Propoxyphene Napsylate (Cinacalcet hydrochloride is a strong in vitro inhibitor of CYP2D6. Therefore, dose adjustments of concomitant medications that are predominantly metabolized by CYP2D6 and have a narrow therapeutic index may be required).
No products indexed under this heading.

Propranolol Hydrochloride (Cinacalcet hydrochloride is a strong in vitro inhibitor of CYP2D6. Therefore, dose adjustments of concomitant medications that are predominantly

metabolized by CYP2D6 and have a narrow therapeutic index may be required). Products include:
InnoPran XL Extended Release Capsules 1484

Quetiapine Fumarate (Cinacalcet hydrochloride is a strong in vitro inhibitor of CYP2D6. Therefore, dose adjustments of concomitant medications that are predominantly metabolized by CYP2D6 and have a narrow therapeutic index may be required).
No products indexed under this heading.

Quinidine Gluconate (Cinacalcet hydrochloride is a strong in vitro inhibitor of CYP2D6. Therefore, dose adjustments of concomitant medications that are predominantly metabolized by CYP2D6 and have a narrow therapeutic index may be required).
No products indexed under this heading.

Quinidine Hydrochloride (Cinacalcet hydrochloride is a strong in vitro inhibitor of CYP2D6. Therefore, dose adjustments of concomitant medications that are predominantly metabolized by CYP2D6 and have a narrow therapeutic index may be required).
No products indexed under this heading.

Quinidine Polygalacturonate (Cinacalcet hydrochloride is a strong in vitro inhibitor of CYP2D6. Therefore, dose adjustments of concomitant medications that are predominantly metabolized by CYP2D6 and have a narrow therapeutic index may be required).
No products indexed under this heading.

Quinidine Sulfate (Cinacalcet hydrochloride is a strong in vitro inhibitor of CYP2D6. Therefore, dose adjustments of concomitant medications that are predominantly metabolized by CYP2D6 and have a narrow therapeutic index may be required).
No products indexed under this heading.

Quinine (Since cinacalcet hydrochloride is metabolized in part by CYP3A4, dose adjustment of cinacalcet hydrochloride may be required and PTH and serum calcium concentrations closely monitored if a patient initiates or discontinues therapy with a strong CYP3A4 inhibitor).
No products indexed under this heading.

Quinine Sulfate (Since cinacalcet hydrochloride is metabolized in part by CYP3A4, dose adjustment of cinacalcet hydrochloride may be required and PTH and serum calcium concentrations closely monitored if a patient initiates or discontinues therapy with a strong CYP3A4 inhibitor).
No products indexed under this heading.

Risperidone (Cinacalcet hydrochloride is a strong in vitro inhibitor of CYP2D6. Therefore, dose adjustments of concomitant medications that are predominantly metabolized by CYP2D6 and have a narrow therapeutic index may be required). Products include:
Risperdal Consta Long-Acting Injection 1753

Ritonavir (Cinacalcet hydrochloride is a strong in vitro inhibitor of CYP2D6. Therefore, dose adjustments of concomitant medications that are predominantly metabolized by CYP2D6 and have a narrow therapeutic index may be required). Products include:
Kaletra 452
Norvir 489

Saquinavir (Since cinacalcet hydrochloride is metabolized in part by CYP3A4, dose adjustment of cinacalcet hydrochloride may be required and PTH and serum calcium concentrations closely monitored if a patient initiates or discontinues therapy with a strong CYP3A4 inhibitor).
No products indexed under this heading.

Saquinavir Mesylate (Since cinacalcet hydrochloride is metabolized in part by CYP3A4, dose adjustment of cinacalcet hydrochloride may be required and PTH and serum calcium concentrations closely monitored if a patient initiates or discontinues therapy with a strong CYP3A4 inhibitor).
No products indexed under this heading.

Sertraline Hydrochloride (Since cinacalcet hydrochloride is metabolized in part by CYP3A4, dose adjustment of cinacalcet hydrochloride may be required and PTH and serum calcium concentrations closely monitored if a patient initiates or discontinues therapy with a strong CYP3A4 inhibitor).
No products indexed under this heading.

Tamoxifen Citrate (Cinacalcet hydrochloride is a strong in vitro inhibitor of CYP2D6. Therefore, dose adjustments of concomitant medications that are predominantly metabolized by CYP2D6 and have a narrow therapeutic index may be required).
No products indexed under this heading.

Teniposide (Cinacalcet hydrochloride is a strong in vitro inhibitor of CYP2D6. Therefore, dose adjustments of concomitant medications that are predominantly metabolized by CYP2D6 and have a narrow therapeutic index may be required).
No products indexed under this heading.

Testosterone (Cinacalcet hydrochloride is a strong in vitro inhibitor of CYP2D6. Therefore, dose adjustments of concomitant medications that are predominantly metabolized by CYP2D6 and have a narrow therapeutic index may be required). Products include:
AndroGel 3159
Testim 1% Gel 701

Testosterone Cypionate (Cinacalcet hydrochloride is a strong in vitro inhibitor of CYP2D6. Therefore, dose adjustments of concomitant medications that are predominantly metabolized by CYP2D6 and have a narrow therapeutic index may be required).
No products indexed under this heading.

Testosterone Enanthate (Cinacalcet hydrochloride is a strong in vitro inhibitor of CYP2D6. Therefore, dose adjustments of concomitant medications that are predominantly metabolized by CYP2D6 and have a narrow therapeutic index may be required). Products include:
Delatestryl Injection 1730

Testosterone Propionate (Cinacalcet hydrochloride is a strong in vitro inhibitor of CYP2D6. Therefore, dose adjustments of concomitant medications that are predominantly metabolized by CYP2D6 and have a narrow therapeutic index may be required).
No products indexed under this heading.

Thioridazine (Cinacalcet hydrochloride is a strong in vitro inhibitor of CYP2D6. Therefore, dose adjustments of concomitant medications that are predominantly metabolized by CYP2D6 and have a narrow therapeutic index may be required).
No products indexed under this heading.

Thioridazine Hydrochloride (Cinacalcet hydrochloride is a strong in vitro inhibitor of CYP2D6. Therefore, dose adjustments of concomitant medications that are predominantly metabolized by CYP2D6 and have a narrow therapeutic index may be required). Products include:
Thioridazine Hydrochloride Tablets 2195

Timolol Maleate (Cinacalcet hydrochloride is a strong in vitro inhibitor of CYP2D6. Therefore, dose adjustments of concomitant medications that are predominantly metabolized by CYP2D6 and have a narrow therapeutic index may be required). Products include:
Combigan Ophthalmic Solution 553
Cosopt Sterile Ophthalmic Solution 1969
Timoptic Sterile Ophthalmic Solution 2121
Timoptic in Ocudose 2124
Timoptic-XE Sterile Ophthalmic Gel Forming Solution 2125

Tolterodine Tartrate (Cinacalcet hydrochloride is a strong in vitro inhibitor of CYP2D6. Therefore, dose adjustments of concomitant medications that are predominantly metabolized by CYP2D6 and have a narrow therapeutic index may be required).
No products indexed under this heading.

Tramadol Hydrochloride (Cinacalcet hydrochloride is a strong in vitro inhibitor of CYP2D6. Therefore, dose adjustments of concomitant medications that are predominantly metabolized by CYP2D6 and have a narrow therapeutic index may be required). Products include:
Ultram ER Extended-Release Tablets 2428

Trazodone Hydrochloride (Cinacalcet hydrochloride is a strong in vitro inhibitor of CYP2D6. Therefore, dose adjustments of concomitant medications that are predominantly metabolized by CYP2D6 and have a narrow therapeutic index may be required).
No products indexed under this heading.

Triazolam (Cinacalcet hydrochloride is a strong in vitro inhibitor of CYP2D6. Therefore, dose adjustments of concomitant medications that are predominantly metabolized by CYP2D6 and have a narrow therapeutic index may be required).
No products indexed under this heading.

Trimipramine Maleate (Cinacalcet hydrochloride is a strong in vitro inhibitor of CYP2D6. Therefore, dose adjustments of concomitant medications that are predominantly metabolized by CYP2D6 and have a narrow therapeutic index may be required).
No products indexed under this heading.

Troleandomycin (Since cinacalcet hydrochloride is metabolized in part by CYP3A4, dose adjustment of cinacalcet hydrochloride may be required and PTH and serum calcium concentrations closely monitored if a patient initiates or discontinues therapy with a strong CYP3A4 inhibitor).
No products indexed under this heading.

Venlafaxine Hydrochloride (Cinacalcet hydrochloride is a strong in vitro inhibitor of CYP2D6. Therefore, dose adjustments of concomitant medications that are predominantly metabolized by CYP2D6 and have a narrow therapeutic index may be required). Products include:
Effexor XR Extended-Release Capsules 3195
Venlafaxine Hydrochloride Tablets 2199

Verapamil Hydrochloride (Since cinacalcet hydrochloride is metabolized in part by CYP3A4, dose adjustment of cinacalcet hydrochloride may be required and PTH and serum calcium concentrations closely monitored if a patient initiates or discontinues therapy with a strong CYP3A4 inhibitor). Products include:
Tarka Tablets 511

Vinblastine Sulfate (Cinacalcet hydrochloride is a strong in vitro inhibitor of CYP2D6. Therefore, dose adjustments of concomitant medications that are predominantly metabolized by CYP2D6 and have a narrow therapeutic index may be required).
No products indexed under this heading.

Voriconazole (Since cinacalcet hydrochloride is metabolized in part by CYP3A4, dose adjustment of cinacalcet hydrochloride may be required and PTH and serum calcium concentrations closely monitored if a patient initiates or discontinues therapy with a strong CYP3A4 inhibitor).
No products indexed under this heading.

Zafirlukast (Since cinacalcet hydrochloride is metabolized in part by CYP3A4, dose adjustment of cinacalcet hydrochloride may be required and PTH and serum calcium concentrations closely monitored if a patient initiates or discontinues therapy with a strong CYP3A4 inhibitor). Products include:
Accolate Tablets 669

Zileuton (Since cinacalcet hydrochloride is metabolized in part by CYP3A4, dose adjustment of cinacalcet hydrochloride may be required and PTH and serum calcium concentrations closely monitored if a patient initiates or discontinues therapy with a strong CYP3A4 inhibitor).
No products indexed under this heading.

Zonisamide (Cinacalcet hydrochloride is a strong in vitro inhibitor of CYP2D6. Therefore, dose adjustments of concomitant medications that are predominantly metabolized by CYP2D6 and have a narrow therapeutic index may be required). Products include:

Food Interactions

Grapefruit (Since cinacalcet hydrochloride is metabolized in part by CYP3A4, dose adjustment of cinacalcet hydrochloride may be required and PTH and serum calcium concentrations closely monitored if a patient initiates or discontinues therapy with a strong CYP3A4 inhibitor).

SEREVENT DISKUS

May interact with beta blockers, cytochrome p450 3a4 inhibitors (selected), monoamine oxidase inhibitors, nonpotassium-sparing diuretics, and tricyclic antidepressants. Compounds in these categories include:

Acebutolol Hydrochloride (Beta-adrenergic blockers may produce severe bronchospasm in asthmatic patients, however, beta blockers do not block the pulmonary effect of beta-agonists).
No products indexed under this heading.

Acetazolamide (Co-administration of salmeterol and a strong CYP3A4 inhibitor ketoconazole resulted in a significant increase in plasma salmeterol exposure as determined by a 16-fold increase in AUC mainly due to increased bioavailability of swallowed portion of the dose. Although there was no statistical effect on the mean QTc, co-administration of salmeterol and ketoconazole was associated with more frequent increases in QTc duration compared with salmeterol and placebo administration. Due to the potential increased risk of cardiovascular adverse events, the concomitant use of salmeterol with strong CYP3A4 inhibitors, (eg, ketoconazole, ritonavir, atazanavir, clarithromycin, indinavir, itraconazole, nefazodone, nelfinavir, saquinavir, telithromycin) is not recommended).
No products indexed under this heading.

Amiodarone Hydrochloride (Co-administration of salmeterol and a strong CYP3A4 inhibitor ketoconazole resulted in a significant increase in plasma salmeterol exposure as determined by a 16-fold increase in AUC mainly due to increased bioavailability of swallowed portion of the dose. Although there was no statistical effect on the mean QTc, co-administration of salmeterol and ketoconazole was associated with more frequent increases in QTc duration compared with salmeterol and placebo administration. Due to the potential increased risk of cardiovascular adverse events, the concomitant use of salmeterol with strong CYP3A4 inhibitors, (eg, ketoconazole, ritonavir, atazanavir, clarithromycin, indinavir, itraconazole, nefazodone, nelfinavir, saquinavir, telithromycin) is not recommended).
No products indexed under this heading.

Amitriptyline Hydrochloride (The action of salmeterol on the vascular system may be potentiated by tricyclic antidepressant).
No products indexed under this heading.

Amoxapine (The action of salmeterol on the vascular system may be potentiated by tricyclic antidepressant).
No products indexed under this heading.

Amprenavir (Co-administration of salmeterol and a strong CYP3A4 inhibitor ketoconazole resulted in a significant increase in plasma salmeterol exposure as determined by a 16-fold increase in AUC mainly due to increased bioavailability of swallowed portion of the dose. Although there was no statistical effect on the mean QTc, co-administration of salmeterol and ketoconazole was associated with more frequent increases in QTc duration compared with salmeterol and placebo administration. Due to the potential increased risk of cardiovascular adverse events, the concomitant use of salmeterol with strong CYP3A4 inhibitors, (eg, ketoconazole, ritonavir, atazanavir, clarithromycin, indinavir, itraconazole, nefazodone, nelfinavir, saquinavir, telithromycin) is not recommended).
No products indexed under this heading.

Anastrozole (Co-administration of salmeterol and a strong CYP3A4 inhibitor ketoconazole resulted in a significant increase in plasma salmeterol exposure as determined by a 16-fold increase in AUC mainly due to increased bioavailability of swallowed portion of the dose. Although there was no statistical effect on the mean QTc, co-administration of salmeterol and ketoconazole was associated with more frequent increases in QTc duration compared with salmeterol and placebo administration. Due to the potential increased risk of cardiovascular adverse events, the concomitant use of salmeterol with strong CYP3A4 inhibitors, (eg, ketoconazole, ritonavir, atazanavir, clarithromycin, indinavir, itraconazole, nefazodone, nelfinavir, saquinavir, telithromycin) is not recommended). Products include:

Aprepitant (Co-administration of salmeterol and a strong CYP3A4 inhibitor ketoconazole resulted in a significant increase in plasma salmeterol exposure as determined by a 16-fold increase in AUC mainly due to increased bioavailability of swallowed portion of the dose. Although there was no statistical effect on the mean QTc, co-administration of salmeterol and ketoconazole was associated with more frequent increases in QTc duration compared with salmeterol and placebo administration. Due to the potential increased risk of cardiovascular adverse events, the concomitant use of salmeterol with strong CYP3A4 inhibitors, (eg, ketoconazole, ritonavir, atazanavir, clarithromycin, indinavir, itraconazole, nefazodone, nelfinavir, saquinavir, telithromycin) is not recommended). Products include:

Atazanavir (Co-administration of salmeterol and a strong CYP3A4 inhibitor ketoconazole resulted in a significant increase in plasma salmeterol exposure as determined by a 16-fold increase in AUC mainly due to increased bioavailability of swallowed portion of the dose. Although there was no statistical effect on the mean QTc, co-administration of salmeterol and ketoconazole was associated with more frequent increases in QTc duration compared with salmeterol and placebo administration. Due to the potential increased risk of cardiovascular adverse events, the concomitant use of salmeterol with strong CYP3A4 inhibitors, (eg, ketoconazole, ritonavir, atazanavir, clarithromycin, indinavir, itraconazole, nefazodone, nelfinavir, saquinavir, telithromycin) is not recommended).
No products indexed under this heading.

Atazanavir Sulfate (Co-administration of salmeterol and a strong CYP3A4 inhibitor ketoconazole resulted in a significant increase in plasma salmeterol exposure as determined by a 16-fold increase in AUC mainly due to increased bioavailability of swallowed portion of the dose. Although there was no statistical effect on the mean QTc, co-administration of salmeterol and ketoconazole was associated with more frequent increases in QTc duration compared with salmeterol and placebo administration. Due to the potential increased risk of cardiovascular adverse events, the concomitant use of salmeterol with strong CYP3A4 inhibitors, (eg, ketoconazole, ritonavir, atazanavir, clarithromycin, indinavir, itraconazole, nefazodone, nelfinavir, saquinavir, telithromycin) is not recommended). Products include:

Atenolol (Beta-adrenergic blockers may produce severe bronchospasm in asthmatic patients, however, beta blockers do not block the pulmonary effect of beta-agonists).
No products indexed under this heading.

Bendroflumethiazide (The ECG changes and/or hypokalemia that may result from the administration of nonpotassium-sparing diuretics can be acutely worsened by beta-agonists, especially when the recommended dose of beta-agonist is exceeded).
No products indexed under this heading.

Betaxolol Hydrochloride (Beta-adrenergic blockers may produce severe bronchospasm in asthmatic patients, however, beta blockers do not block the pulmonary effect of beta-agonists).
No products indexed under this heading.

Bisoprolol Fumarate (Beta-adrenergic blockers may produce severe bronchospasm in asthmatic patients, however, beta blockers do not block the pulmonary effect of beta-agonists).
No products indexed under this heading.

Bumetanide (The ECG changes and/or hypokalemia that may result from the administration of nonpotassium-sparing diuretics can be acutely worsened by beta-agonists, especially when the recommended dose of beta-agonist is exceeded).
No products indexed under this heading.

Carteolol Hydrochloride (Beta-adrenergic blockers may produce severe bronchospasm in asthmatic patients, however, beta blockers do not block the pulmonary effect of beta-agonists).
No products indexed under this heading.

Chlorothiazide (The ECG changes and/or hypokalemia that may result from the administration of nonpotassium-sparing diuretics can be acutely worsened by beta-agonists, especially when the recommended dose of beta-agonist is exceeded).
No products indexed under this heading.

Chlorothiazide Sodium (The ECG changes and/or hypokalemia that may result from the administration of nonpotassium-sparing diuretics can be acutely worsened by beta-agonists, especially when the recommended dose of beta-agonist is exceeded). Products include:

Cimetidine (Co-administration of salmeterol and a strong CYP3A4 inhibitor ketoconazole resulted in a significant increase in plasma salmeterol exposure as determined by a 16-fold increase in AUC mainly due to increased bioavailability of swallowed portion of the dose. Although there was no statistical effect on the mean QTc, co-administration of salmeterol and ketoconazole was associated with more frequent increases in QTc duration compared with salmeterol and placebo administration. Due to the potential increased risk of cardiovascular adverse events, the concomitant use of salmeterol with strong CYP3A4 inhibitors, (eg, ketoconazole, ritonavir, atazanavir, clarithromycin, indinavir, itraconazole, nefazodone, nelfinavir, saquinavir, telithromycin) is not recommended).
No products indexed under this heading.

Cimetidine Hydrochloride (Co-administration of salmeterol and a strong CYP3A4 inhibitor ketoconazole resulted in a significant increase in plasma salmeterol exposure as determined by a 16-fold increase in AUC mainly due to increased bioavailability of swallowed portion of the dose. Although there was no statistical effect on the mean QTc, co-administration of salmeterol and ketoconazole was associated with more frequent increases in QTc duration compared with salmeterol and placebo administration. Due to the potential increased risk of cardiovascular adverse events, the concomitant use of salmeterol with strong CYP3A4 inhibitors, (eg, ketoconazole, ritonavir, atazanavir, clarithromycin, indinavir, itraconazole, nefazodone, nelfinavir, saquinavir, telithromycin) is not recommended).
No products indexed under this heading.

Ciprofloxacin (Co-administration of salmeterol and a strong CYP3A4 inhibitor ketoconazole resulted in a significant increase in plasma salmeterol exposure as determined by a 16-fold increase in AUC mainly due to increased bioavailability of swallowed portion of the dose. Although there was no statistical effect on the mean QTc, co-administration of salmeterol and ketoconazole was associated with more frequent increases in QTc duration compared with salmeterol and placebo administration. Due to the potential increased risk of cardiovascular adverse events, the concomitant use of salmeterol with strong CYP3A4 inhibitors, (eg, ketoconazole, ritonavir, atazanavir, clarithromycin, indinavir, itraconazole, nefazodone, nelfinavir, saquinavir, telithromycin) is not recommended). Products include:

Cipro I.V. 2817
Cipro Oral Suspension 2810
Cipro XR Tablets 2823
Ciprodex Otic Suspension 541

Clarithromycin (Co-administration of salmeterol and a strong CYP3A4 inhibitor ketoconazole resulted in a significant increase in plasma salmeterol exposure as determined by a 16-fold increase in AUC mainly due to increased bioavailability of swallowed portion of the dose. Although there was no statistical effect on the mean QTc, co-administration of salmeterol and ketoconazole was associated with more frequent increases in QTc duration compared with salmeterol and placebo administration. Due to the potential increased risk of cardiovascular adverse events, the concomitant use of salmeterol with strong CYP3A4 inhibitors, (eg, ketoconazole, ritonavir, atazanavir, clarithromycin, indinavir, itraconazole, nefazodone, nelfinavir, saquinavir, telithromycin) is not recommended). Products include:

Biaxin/Biaxin XL 411

Clomipramine Hydrochloride (The action of salmeterol on the vascular system may be potentiated by tricyclic antidepressant).

No products indexed under this heading.

Clotrimazole (Co-administration of salmeterol and a strong CYP3A4 inhibitor ketoconazole resulted in a significant increase in plasma salmeterol exposure as determined by a 16-fold increase in AUC mainly due to increased bioavailability of swallowed portion of the dose. Although there was no statistical effect on the mean QTc, co-administration of salmeterol and ketoconazole was associated with more frequent increases in QTc duration compared with salmeterol and placebo administration. Due to the potential increased risk of cardiovascular adverse events, the concomitant use of salmeterol with strong CYP3A4 inhibitors, (eg, ketoconazole, ritonavir, atazanavir, clarithromycin, indinavir, itraconazole, nefazodone, nelfinavir, saquinavir, telithromycin) is not recommended). Products include:

Lotrisone 2881

Cyclosporine (Co-administration of salmeterol and a strong CYP3A4 inhibitor ketoconazole resulted in a significant increase in plasma salmeterol exposure as determined by a 16-fold increase in AUC mainly due to increased bioavailability of swallowed portion of the dose. Although there was no statistical effect on the mean QTc, co-administration of salmeterol and ketoconazole was associated with more frequent increases in QTc duration compared with salmeterol and placebo administration. Due to the potential increased risk of cardiovascular adverse events, the concomitant use of salmeterol with strong CYP3A4 inhibitors, (eg, ketoconazole, ritonavir, atazanavir, clarithromycin, indinavir, itraconazole, nefazodone, nelfinavir, saquinavir, telithromycin) is not recommended). Products include:

Gengraf Capsules 435
Neoral Oral Solution 2280
Neoral Soft Gelatin Capsules 2280
Restasis Ophthalmic Emulsion 557
Sandimmune 2296

Dalfopristin (Co-administration of salmeterol and a strong CYP3A4 inhibitor ketoconazole resulted in a significant increase in plasma salmeterol exposure as determined by a 16-fold increase in AUC mainly due to increased bioavailability of swallowed portion of the dose. Although there was no statistical effect on the mean QTc, co-administration of salmeterol and ketoconazole was associated with more frequent increases in QTc duration compared with salmeterol and placebo administration. Due to the potential increased risk of cardiovascular adverse events, the concomitant use of salmeterol with strong CYP3A4 inhibitors, (eg, ketoconazole, ritonavir, atazanavir, clarithromycin, indinavir, itraconazole, nefazodone, nelfinavir, saquinavir, telithromycin) is not recommended).

No products indexed under this heading.

Danazol (Co-administration of salmeterol and a strong CYP3A4 inhibitor ketoconazole resulted in a significant increase in plasma salmeterol exposure as determined by a 16-fold increase in AUC mainly due to increased bioavailability of swallowed portion of the dose. Although there was no statistical effect on the mean QTc, co-administration of salmeterol and ketoconazole was associated with more frequent increases in QTc duration compared with salmeterol and placebo administration. Due to the potential increased risk of cardiovascular adverse events, the concomitant use of salmeterol with strong CYP3A4 inhibitors, (eg, ketoconazole, ritonavir, atazanavir, clarithromycin, indinavir, itraconazole, nefazodone, nelfinavir, saquinavir, telithromycin) is not recommended).

No products indexed under this heading.

Delavirdine Mesylate (Co-administration of salmeterol and a strong CYP3A4 inhibitor ketoconazole resulted in a significant increase in plasma salmeterol exposure as determined by a 16-fold increase in AUC mainly due to increased bioavailability of swallowed portion of the dose. Although there was no statistical effect on the mean QTc, co-administration of salmeterol and ketoconazole was associated with more frequent increases in QTc duration compared with salmeterol and placebo administration. Due to the potential increased risk of cardiovascular adverse events, the concomitant use of salmeterol with strong CYP3A4 inhibitors, (eg, ketoconazole, ritonavir, atazanavir, clarithromycin, indinavir, itraconazole, nefazodone, nelfinavir, saquinavir, telithromycin) is not recommended).

No products indexed under this heading.

Desipramine Hydrochloride (The action of salmeterol on the vascular system may be potentiated by tricyclic antidepressant).

No products indexed under this heading.

Diltiazem Hydrochloride (Co-administration of salmeterol and a strong CYP3A4 inhibitor ketoconazole resulted in a significant increase in plasma salmeterol exposure as determined by a 16-fold increase in AUC mainly due to increased bioavailability of swallowed portion of the dose. Although there was no statistical effect on the mean QTc, co-administration of salmeterol and ketoconazole was associated with more frequent increases in QTc duration compared with salmeterol and placebo administration. Due to the potential increased risk of cardiovascular adverse events, the concomitant use of salmeterol with strong CYP3A4 inhibitors, (eg, ketoconazole, ritonavir, atazanavir, clarithromycin, indinavir, itraconazole, nefazodone, nelfinavir, saquinavir, telithromycin) is not recommended). Products include:

Cardizem LA Extended Release Tablets 421

Diltiazem Maleate (Co-administration of salmeterol and a strong CYP3A4 inhibitor ketoconazole resulted in a significant increase in plasma salmeterol exposure as determined by a 16-fold increase in AUC mainly due to increased bioavailability of swallowed portion of the dose. Although there was no statistical effect on the mean QTc, co-administration of salmeterol and ketoconazole was associated with more frequent increases in QTc duration compared with salmeterol and placebo administration. Due to the potential increased risk of cardiovascular adverse events, the concomitant use of salmeterol with strong CYP3A4 inhibitors, (eg, ketoconazole, ritonavir, atazanavir, clarithromycin, indinavir, itraconazole, nefazodone, nelfinavir, saquinavir, telithromycin) is not recommended).

No products indexed under this heading.

Doxepin Hydrochloride (The action of salmeterol on the vascular system may be potentiated by tricyclic antidepressant).

No products indexed under this heading.

Efavirenz (Co-administration of salmeterol and a strong CYP3A4 inhibitor ketoconazole resulted in a significant increase in plasma salmeterol exposure as determined by a 16-fold increase in AUC mainly due to increased bioavailability of swallowed portion of the dose. Although there was no statistical effect on the mean QTc, co-administration of salmeterol and ketoconazole was associated with more frequent increases in QTc duration compared with salmeterol and placebo administration. Due to the potential increased risk of cardiovascular adverse events, the concomitant use of salmeterol with strong CYP3A4 inhibitors, (eg, ketoconazole, ritonavir, atazanavir, clarithromycin, indinavir, itraconazole, nefazodone, nelfinavir, saquinavir, telithromycin) is not recommended). Products include:

Atripla Tablets 938
Sustiva Capsules 930
Sustiva Tablets 930

Erythromycin (Co-administration of salmeterol and a strong CYP3A4 inhibitor ketoconazole resulted in a significant increase in plasma salmeterol exposure as determined by a 16-fold increase in AUC mainly due to increased bioavailability of swallowed portion of the dose. Although there was no statistical effect on the mean QTc, co-administration of salmeterol and ketoconazole was associated with more frequent increases in QTc duration compared with salmeterol and placebo administration. Due to the potential increased risk of cardiovascular adverse events, the concomitant use of salmeterol with strong CYP3A4 inhibitors, (eg, ketoconazole, ritonavir, atazanavir, clarithromycin, indinavir, itraconazole, nefazodone, nelfinavir, saquinavir, telithromycin) is not recommended).

No products indexed under this heading.

Erythromycin Estolate (Co-administration of salmeterol and a strong CYP3A4 inhibitor ketoconazole resulted in a significant increase in plasma salmeterol exposure as determined by a 16-fold increase in AUC mainly due to increased bioavailability of swallowed portion of the dose. Although there was no statistical effect on the mean QTc, co-administration of salmeterol and ketoconazole was associated with more frequent increases in QTc duration compared with salmeterol and placebo administration. Due to the potential increased risk of cardiovascular adverse events, the concomitant use of salmeterol with strong CYP3A4 inhibitors, (eg, ketoconazole, ritonavir, atazanavir, clarithromycin, indinavir, itraconazole, nefazodone, nelfinavir, saquinavir, telithromycin) is not recommended).

No products indexed under this heading.

Erythromycin Ethylsuccinate (Co-administration of salmeterol and a strong CYP3A4 inhibitor ketoconazole resulted in a significant increase in plasma salmeterol exposure as determined by a 16-fold increase in AUC mainly due to increased bioavailability of swallowed portion of the dose. Although there was no statistical effect on the mean QTc, co-administration of salmeterol and ketoconazole was associated with more frequent increases in QTc duration compared with salmeterol and placebo administration. Due to the potential increased risk of cardiovascular adverse events, the concomitant use of salmeterol with strong CYP3A4 inhibitors, (eg, ketoconazole, ritonavir, atazanavir, clarithromycin, indinavir, itraconazole, nefazodone, nelfinavir, saquinavir, telithromycin) is not recommended). Products include:

E.E.S. 433
EryPed 431

Erythromycin Gluceptate (Co-administration of salmeterol and a strong CYP3A4 inhibitor ketoconazole resulted in a significant increase in plasma salmeterol exposure as determined by a 16-fold increase in AUC mainly due to increased bioavailability of swallowed portion of the dose. Although there was no statistical effect on the mean QTc, co-administration of salmeterol and

ketoconazole was associated with more frequent increases in QTc duration compared with salmeterol and placebo administration. Due to the potential increased risk of cardiovascular adverse events, the concomitant use of salmeterol with strong CYP3A4 inhibitors, (eg, ketoconazole, ritonavir, atazanavir, clarithromycin, indinavir, itraconazole, nefazodone, nelfinavir, saquinavir, telithromycin) is not recommended).

No products indexed under this heading.

Erythromycin Lactobionate (Co-administration of salmeterol and a strong CYP3A4 inhibitor ketoconazole resulted in a significant increase in plasma salmeterol exposure as determined by a 16-fold increase in AUC mainly due to increased bioavailability of swallowed portion of the dose. Although there was no statistical effect on the mean QTc, co-administration of salmeterol and ketoconazole was associated with more frequent increases in QTc duration compared with salmeterol and placebo administration. Due to the potential increased risk of cardiovascular adverse events, the concomitant use of salmeterol with strong CYP3A4 inhibitors, (eg, ketoconazole, ritonavir, atazanavir, clarithromycin, indinavir, itraconazole, nefazodone, nelfinavir, saquinavir, telithromycin) is not recommended).

No products indexed under this heading.

Erythromycin Stearate (Co-administration of salmeterol and a strong CYP3A4 inhibitor ketoconazole resulted in a significant increase in plasma salmeterol exposure as determined by a 16-fold increase in AUC mainly due to increased bioavailability of swallowed portion of the dose. Although there was no statistical effect on the mean QTc, co-administration of salmeterol and ketoconazole was associated with more frequent increases in QTc duration compared with salmeterol and placebo administration. Due to the potential increased risk of cardiovascular adverse events, the concomitant use of salmeterol with strong CYP3A4 inhibitors, (eg, ketoconazole, ritonavir, atazanavir, clarithromycin, indinavir, itraconazole, nefazodone, nelfinavir, saquinavir, telithromycin) is not recommended).

No products indexed under this heading.

Esmolol Hydrochloride (Beta-adrenergic blockers may produce severe bronchospasm in asthmatic patients, however, beta blockers do not block the pulmonary effect of beta-agonists).

No products indexed under this heading.

Esomeprazole Magnesium (Co-administration of salmeterol and a strong CYP3A4 inhibitor ketoconazole resulted in a significant increase in plasma salmeterol exposure as determined by a 16-fold increase in AUC mainly due to increased bioavailability of swallowed portion of the dose. Although there was no statistical effect on the mean QTc, co-administration of salmeterol and ketoconazole was associated with more frequent increases in QTc duration compared with salmeterol and placebo administration. Due to the potential increased risk of cardiovascular adverse events, the concomitant use of salmeterol with strong CYP3A4 inhibitors, (eg, ketoconazole, ritonavir, atazanavir, clarithromycin, indinavir, itraconazole, nefazodone, nelfinavir, saquinavir, telithromycin) is not recommended). Products include:

Nexium Delayed-Release Capsules 645
Nexium Delayed-Release Oral Suspension 645

Ethacrynic Acid (The ECG changes and/or hypokalemia that may result from the administration of nonpotassium-sparing diuretics can be acutely worsened by beta-agonists, especially when the recommended dose of beta-agonist is exceeded). Products include:

Edecrin Tablets 698

Fluconazole (Co-administration of salmeterol and a strong CYP3A4 inhibitor ketoconazole resulted in a significant increase in plasma salmeterol exposure as determined by a 16-fold increase in AUC mainly due to increased bioavailability of swallowed portion of the dose. Although there was no statistical effect on the mean QTc, co-administration of salmeterol and ketoconazole was associated with more frequent increases in QTc duration compared with salmeterol and placebo administration. Due to the potential increased risk of cardiovascular adverse events, the concomitant use of salmeterol with strong CYP3A4 inhibitors, (eg, ketoconazole, ritonavir, atazanavir, clarithromycin, indinavir, itraconazole, nefazodone, nelfinavir, saquinavir, telithromycin) is not recommended).

No products indexed under this heading.

Fluoxetine (Co-administration of salmeterol and a strong CYP3A4 inhibitor ketoconazole resulted in a significant increase in plasma salmeterol exposure as determined by a 16-fold increase in AUC mainly due to increased bioavailability of swallowed portion of the dose. Although there was no statistical effect on the mean QTc, co-administration of salmeterol and ketoconazole was associated with more frequent increases in QTc duration compared with salmeterol and placebo administration. Due to the potential increased risk of cardiovascular adverse events, the concomitant use of salmeterol with strong CYP3A4 inhibitors, (eg, ketoconazole, ritonavir, atazanavir, clarithromycin, indinavir, itraconazole, nefazodone, nelfinavir, saquinavir, telithromycin) is not recommended).

No products indexed under this heading.

Fluoxetine Hydrochloride (Co-administration of salmeterol and a strong CYP3A4 inhibitor ketoconazole resulted in a significant increase in plasma salmeterol exposure as determined by a 16-fold increase in AUC mainly due to increased bioavailability of swallowed portion of the dose. Although there was no statistical effect on the mean QTc, co-administration of salmeterol and ketoconazole was associated with more frequent increases in QTc duration compared with salmeterol and placebo administration. Due to the potential increased risk of cardiovascular adverse events, the concomitant use of salmeterol with strong CYP3A4 inhibitors, (eg, ketoconazole, ritonavir, atazanavir, clarithromycin, indinavir, itraconazole, nefazodone, nelfinavir, saquinavir, telithromycin) is not recommended). Products include:

Prozac Weekly Capsules 1852
Prozac Pulvules and Liquid 1852
Symbyax Capsules 1871

Fluvoxamine Maleate (Co-administration of salmeterol and a strong CYP3A4 inhibitor ketoconazole resulted in a significant increase in plasma salmeterol exposure as determined by a 16-fold increase in AUC mainly due to increased bioavailability of swallowed portion of the dose. Although there was no statistical effect on the mean QTc, co-administration of salmeterol and ketoconazole was associated with more frequent increases in QTc duration compared with salmeterol and placebo administration. Due to the potential increased risk of cardiovascular adverse events, the concomitant use of salmeterol with strong CYP3A4 inhibitors, (eg, ketoconazole, ritonavir, atazanavir, clarithromycin, indinavir, itraconazole, nefazodone, nelfinavir, saquinavir, telithromycin) is not recommended). Products include:

Luvox CR Extended-Release Capsules 1759

Fosamprenavir Calcium (Co-administration of salmeterol and a strong CYP3A4 inhibitor ketoconazole resulted in a significant increase in plasma salmeterol exposure as determined by a 16-fold increase in AUC mainly due to increased bioavailability of swallowed portion of the dose. Although there was no statistical effect on the mean QTc, co-administration of salmeterol and ketoconazole was associated with more frequent increases in QTc duration compared with salmeterol and placebo administration. Due to the potential increased risk of cardiovascular adverse events, the concomitant use of salmeterol with strong CYP3A4 inhibitors, (eg, ketoconazole, ritonavir, atazanavir, clarithromycin, indinavir, itraconazole, nefazodone, nelfinavir, saquinavir, telithromycin) is not recommended). Products include:

Lexiva Oral Suspension 1510
Lexiva Tablets 1510

Furosemide (The ECG changes and/or hypokalemia that may result from the administration of nonpotassium-sparing diuretics can be acutely worsened by beta-agonists, especially when the recommended dose of beta-agonist is exceeded). Products include:

Furosemide Tablets 2186

Hydrochlorothiazide (The ECG changes and/or hypokalemia that may result from the administration of nonpotassium-sparing diuretics can be acutely worsened by beta-agonists, especially when the recommended dose of beta-agonist is exceeded). Products include:

Atacand HCT 642
Avalide Tablets 892
Avalide Tablets 2713
Benicar HCT Tablets 1010
Diovan HCT Tablets 2216
Dyazide Capsules 1405
Micardis HCT Tablets 854
Prinzide Tablets 2092
Tekturna HCT Tablets 2324
Teveten HCT Tablets 517

Hydroflumethiazide (The ECG changes and/or hypokalemia that may result from the administration of nonpotassium-sparing diuretics can be acutely worsened by beta-agonists, especially when the recommended dose of beta-agonist is exceeded).

No products indexed under this heading.

Imipramine Hydrochloride (The action of salmeterol on the vascular system may be potentiated by tricyclic antidepressant).

No products indexed under this heading.

Imipramine Pamoate (The action of salmeterol on the vascular system may be potentiated by tricyclic antidepressant).

No products indexed under this heading.

Indinavir Sulfate (Co-administration of salmeterol and a strong CYP3A4 inhibitor ketoconazole resulted in a significant increase in plasma salmeterol exposure as determined by a 16-fold increase in AUC mainly due to increased bioavailability of swallowed portion of the dose. Although there was no statistical effect on the mean QTc, co-administration of salmeterol and ketoconazole was associated with more frequent increases in QTc duration compared with salmeterol and placebo administration. Due to the potential increased risk of cardiovascular adverse events, the concomitant use of salmeterol with strong CYP3A4 inhibitors, (eg, ketoconazole, ritonavir, atazanavir, clarithromycin, indinavir, itraconazole, nefazodone, nelfinavir, saquinavir, telithromycin) is not recommended). Products include:

Crixivan Capsules 1979

Isocarboxazid (The action of salmeterol on the vascular system may be potentiated by a MAO inhibitor). Products include:

Marplan Tablets 3177

Isoniazid (Co-administration of salmeterol and a strong CYP3A4 inhibitor ketoconazole resulted in a significant increase in plasma salmeterol exposure as determined by a 16-fold increase in AUC mainly due to increased bioavailability of swallowed portion of the dose. Although there was no statistical effect on the mean QTc, co-administration of salmeterol and ketoconazole was associated with more frequent increases in QTc duration compared with salmeterol and placebo administration. Due to the potential increased risk of cardiovascular adverse events, the concomitant use of salmeterol with strong CYP3A4 inhibitors, (eg, ketoconazole, ritonavir, atazanavir, clarithromycin, indinavir, itraconazole, nefazodone, nelfinavir, saquinavir, telithromycin) is not recommended).

No products indexed under this heading.

Itraconazole (Co-administration of salmeterol and a strong CYP3A4 inhibitor ketoconazole resulted in a significant increase in plasma salmeterol exposure as determined by a 16-fold increase in AUC mainly due to increased bioavailability of swallowed portion of the dose. Although there was no statistical effect on the mean QTc, co-administration of salmeterol and ketoconazole was asso-

ciated with more frequent increases in QTc duration compared with salmeterol and placebo administration. Due to the potential increased risk of cardiovascular adverse events, the concomitant use of salmeterol with strong CYP3A4 inhibitors, (eg, ketoconazole, ritonavir, atazanavir, clarithromycin, indinavir, itraconazole, nefazodone, nelfinavir, saquinavir, telithromycin) is not recommended).
No products indexed under this heading.

Ketoconazole (Co-administration of salmeterol and a strong CYP3A4 inhibitor ketoconazole resulted in a significant increase in plasma salmeterol exposure as determined by a 16-fold increase in AUC mainly due to increased bioavailability of swallowed portion of the dose. Although there was no statistical effect on the mean QTc, co-administration of salmeterol and ketoconazole was associated with more frequent increases in QTc duration compared with salmeterol and placebo administration. Due to the potential increased risk of cardiovascular adverse events, the concomitant use of salmeterol with strong CYP3A4 inhibitors, (eg, ketoconazole) is not recommended). Products include:
Extina Foam, 2% 3057
Nizoral A-D Shampoo 1901

Labetalol Hydrochloride (Beta-adrenergic blockers may produce severe bronchospasm in asthmatic patients, however, beta blockers do not block the pulmonary effect of beta-agonists).
No products indexed under this heading.

Levobunolol Hydrochloride (Beta-adrenergic blockers may produce severe bronchospasm in asthmatic patients, however, beta blockers do not block the pulmonary effect of beta-agonists).
No products indexed under this heading.

Lopinavir (Co-administration of salmeterol and a strong CYP3A4 inhibitor ketoconazole resulted in a significant increase in plasma salmeterol exposure as determined by a 16-fold increase in AUC mainly due to increased bioavailability of swallowed portion of the dose. Although there was no statistical effect on the mean QTc, co-administration of salmeterol and ketoconazole was associated with more frequent increases in QTc duration compared with salmeterol and placebo administration. Due to the potential increased risk of cardiovascular adverse events, the concomitant use of salmeterol with strong CYP3A4 inhibitors, (eg, ketoconazole, ritonavir, atazanavir, clarithromycin, indinavir, itraconazole, nefazodone, nelfinavir, saquinavir, telithromycin) is not recommended). Products include:
Kaletra 452

Loratadine (Co-administration of salmeterol and a strong CYP3A4 inhibitor ketoconazole resulted in a significant increase in plasma salmeterol exposure as determined by a 16-fold increase in AUC mainly due to increased bioavailability of swallowed portion of the dose. Although there was no statistical effect on the mean QTc, co-administration of salmeterol and ketoconazole was associated with more frequent increases in QTc duration compared with salmeterol and placebo administration. Due to the potential increased risk of cardiovascular adverse events, the concomitant use of salmeterol with strong CYP3A4 inhibitors, (eg, ketoconazole, ritonavir, atazanavir, clarithromycin, indinavir, itraconazole, nefazodone, nelfinavir, saquinavir, telithromycin) is not recommended).
No products indexed under this heading.

Maprotiline Hydrochloride (The action of salmeterol on the vascular system may be potentiated by tricyclic antidepressant).
No products indexed under this heading.

Methyclothiazide (The ECG changes and/or hypokalemia that may result from the administration of nonpotassium-sparing diuretics can be acutely worsened by beta-agonists, especially when the recommended dose of beta-agonist is exceeded).
No products indexed under this heading.

Metipranolol Hydrochloride (Beta-adrenergic blockers may produce severe bronchospasm in asthmatic patients, however, beta blockers do not block the pulmonary effect of beta-agonists).
No products indexed under this heading.

Metoprolol Succinate (Beta-adrenergic blockers may produce severe bronchospasm in asthmatic patients, however, beta blockers do not block the pulmonary effect of beta-agonists). Products include:
Toprol-XL Tablets 666

Metoprolol Tartrate (Beta-adrenergic blockers may produce severe bronchospasm in asthmatic patients, however, beta blockers do not block the pulmonary effect of beta-agonists).
No products indexed under this heading.

Metronidazole (Co-administration of salmeterol and a strong CYP3A4 inhibitor ketoconazole resulted in a significant increase in plasma salmeterol exposure as determined by a 16-fold increase in AUC mainly due to increased bioavailability of swallowed portion of the dose. Although there was no statistical effect on the mean QTc, co-administration of salmeterol and ketoconazole was associated with more frequent increases in QTc duration compared with salmeterol and placebo administration. Due to the potential increased risk of cardiovascular adverse events, the concomitant use of salmeterol with strong CYP3A4 inhibitors, (eg, ketoconazole, ritonavir, atazanavir, clarithromycin, indinavir, itraconazole, nefazodone, nelfinavir, saquinavir, telithromycin) is not recommended). Products include:
Pylera Capsules 714

Metronidazole Benzoate (Co-administration of salmeterol and a strong CYP3A4 inhibitor ketoconazole resulted in a significant increase in plasma salmeterol exposure as determined by a 16-fold increase in AUC mainly due to increased bioavailability of swallowed portion of the dose. Although there was no statistical effect on the mean QTc, co-administration of salmeterol and ketoconazole was associated with more frequent increases in QTc duration compared with salmeterol and placebo administration. Due to the potential increased risk of cardiovascular adverse events, the concomitant use of salmeterol with strong CYP3A4 inhibitors, (eg, ketoconazole, ritonavir, atazanavir, clarithromycin, indinavir, itraconazole, nefazodone, nelfinavir, saquinavir, telithromycin) is not recommended).
No products indexed under this heading.

Metronidazole Hydrochloride (Co-administration of salmeterol and a strong CYP3A4 inhibitor ketoconazole resulted in a significant increase in plasma salmeterol exposure as determined by a 16-fold increase in AUC mainly due to increased bioavailability of swallowed portion of the dose. Although there was no statistical effect on the mean QTc, co-administration of salmeterol and ketoconazole was associated with more frequent increases in QTc duration compared with salmeterol and placebo administration. Due to the potential increased risk of cardiovascular adverse events, the concomitant use of salmeterol with strong CYP3A4 inhibitors, (eg, ketoconazole, ritonavir, atazanavir, clarithromycin, indinavir, itraconazole, nefazodone, nelfinavir, saquinavir, telithromycin) is not recommended).
No products indexed under this heading.

Metronidazole Sodium (Co-administration of salmeterol and a strong CYP3A4 inhibitor ketoconazole resulted in a significant increase in plasma salmeterol exposure as determined by a 16-fold increase in AUC mainly due to increased bioavailability of swallowed portion of the dose. Although there was no statistical effect on the mean QTc, co-administration of salmeterol and ketoconazole was associated with more frequent increases in QTc duration compared with salmeterol and placebo administration. Due to the potential increased risk of cardiovascular adverse events, the concomitant use of salmeterol with strong CYP3A4 inhibitors, (eg, ketoconazole, ritonavir, atazanavir, clarithromycin, indinavir, itraconazole, nefazodone, nelfinavir, saquinavir, telithromycin) is not recommended).
No products indexed under this heading.

Miconazole (Co-administration of salmeterol and a strong CYP3A4 inhibitor ketoconazole resulted in a significant increase in plasma salmeterol exposure as determined by a 16-fold increase in AUC mainly due to increased bioavailability of swallowed portion of the dose. Although there was no statistical effect on the mean QTc, co-administration of salmeterol and ketoconazole was associated with more frequent increases in QTc duration compared with salmeterol and placebo administration. Due to the potential increased risk of cardiovascular adverse events, the concomitant use of salmeterol with strong CYP3A4 inhibitors, (eg, ketoconazole, ritonavir, atazanavir, clarithromycin, indinavir, itraconazole, nefazodone, nelfinavir, saquinavir, telithromycin) is not recommended).
No products indexed under this heading.

Miconazole Nitrate (Co-administration of salmeterol and a strong CYP3A4 inhibitor ketoconazole resulted in a significant increase in plasma salmeterol exposure as determined by a 16-fold increase in AUC mainly due to increased bioavailability of swallowed portion of the dose. Although there was no statistical effect on the mean QTc, co-administration of salmeterol and ketoconazole was associated with more frequent increases in QTc duration compared with salmeterol and placebo administration. Due to the potential increased risk of cardiovascular adverse events, the concomitant use of salmeterol with strong CYP3A4 inhibitors, (eg, ketoconazole, ritonavir, atazanavir, clarithromycin, indinavir, itraconazole, nefazodone, nelfinavir, saquinavir, telithromycin) is not recommended).
No products indexed under this heading.

Moclobemide (The action of salmeterol on the vascular system may be potentiated by a MAO inhibitor).
No products indexed under this heading.

Nadolol (Beta-adrenergic blockers may produce severe bronchospasm in asthmatic patients, however, beta blockers do not block the pulmonary effect of beta-agonists). Products include:
Nadolol Tablets 2191

Nebivolol (Beta-adrenergic blockers may produce severe bronchospasm in asthmatic patients, however, beta blockers do not block the pulmonary effect of beta-agonists). Products include:
Bystolic Tablets 1155

Nefazodone Hydrochloride (Co-administration of salmeterol and a strong CYP3A4 inhibitor ketoconazole resulted in a significant increase in plasma salmeterol exposure as determined by a 16-fold increase in AUC mainly due to increased bioavailability of swallowed portion of the dose. Although there was no statistical effect on the mean QTc, co-administration of salmeterol and ketoconazole was associated with more frequent increases in QTc duration compared with salmeterol and placebo administration. Due to the potential increased risk of cardiovascular adverse events, the concomitant use of salmeterol with strong CYP3A4 inhibitors, (eg, ketoconazole, ritonavir, atazanavir, clarithromycin, indinavir, itraconazole, nefazodone, nelfinavir, saquinavir, telithromycin) is not recommended).
No products indexed under this heading.

Nelfinavir Mesylate (Co-administration of salmeterol and a strong CYP3A4 inhibitor ketoconazole resulted in a significant increase in plasma salmeterol exposure as determined by a 16-fold increase in AUC mainly due to increased bioavailability of swallowed portion of the dose. Although there was no statistical effect on the mean QTc, co-administration of salmeterol and ketoconazole was associated with more frequent increases in QTc duration compared with salmeterol and placebo administration. Due to the potential increased risk of cardiovas-

cular adverse events, the concomitant use of salmeterol with strong CYP3A4 inhibitors, (eg, ketoconazole, ritonavir, atazanavir, clarithromycin, indinavir, itraconazole, nefazodone, nelfinavir, saquinavir, telithromycin) is not recommended).

No products indexed under this heading.

Nevirapine (Co-administration of salmeterol and a strong CYP3A4 inhibitor ketoconazole resulted in a significant increase in plasma salmeterol exposure as determined by a 16-fold increase in AUC mainly due to increased bioavailability of swallowed portion of the dose. Although there was no statistical effect on the mean QTc, co-administration of salmeterol and ketoconazole was associated with more frequent increases in QTc duration compared with salmeterol and placebo administration. Due to the potential increased risk of cardiovascular adverse events, the concomitant use of salmeterol with strong CYP3A4 inhibitors, (eg, ketoconazole, ritonavir, atazanavir, clarithromycin, indinavir, itraconazole, nefazodone, nelfinavir, saquinavir, telithromycin) is not recommended). Products include:

Viramune Oral Suspension **873**
Viramune Tablets **873**

Niacinamide (Co-administration of salmeterol and a strong CYP3A4 inhibitor ketoconazole resulted in a significant increase in plasma salmeterol exposure as determined by a 16-fold increase in AUC mainly due to increased bioavailability of swallowed portion of the dose. Although there was no statistical effect on the mean QTc, co-administration of salmeterol and ketoconazole was associated with more frequent increases in QTc duration compared with salmeterol and placebo administration. Due to the potential increased risk of cardiovascular adverse events, the concomitant use of salmeterol with strong CYP3A4 inhibitors, (eg, ketoconazole, ritonavir, atazanavir, clarithromycin, indinavir, itraconazole, nefazodone, nelfinavir, saquinavir, telithromycin) is not recommended). Products include:

BioLean Free Tablets **635**

Nicotinamide (Co-administration of salmeterol and a strong CYP3A4 inhibitor ketoconazole resulted in a significant increase in plasma salmeterol exposure as determined by a 16-fold increase in AUC mainly due to increased bioavailability of swallowed portion of the dose. Although there was no statistical effect on the mean QTc, co-administration of salmeterol and ketoconazole was associated with more frequent increases in QTc duration compared with salmeterol and placebo administration. Due to the potential increased risk of cardiovascular adverse events, the concomitant use of salmeterol with strong CYP3A4 inhibitors, (eg, ketoconazole, ritonavir, atazanavir, clarithromycin, indinavir, itraconazole, nefazodone, nelfinavir, saquinavir, telithromycin) is not recommended).

No products indexed under this heading.

Nifedipine (Co-administration of salmeterol and a strong CYP3A4 inhibitor ketoconazole resulted in a significant increase in plasma salmeterol exposure as determined by a 16-fold increase in AUC mainly due to increased bioavailability of swallowed portion of the dose. Although there was no statistical effect on the mean QTc, co-administration of salmeterol and ketoconazole was associated with more frequent increases in QTc duration compared with salmeterol and placebo administration. Due to the potential increased risk of cardiovascular adverse events, the concomitant use of salmeterol with strong CYP3A4 inhibitors, (eg, ketoconazole, ritonavir, atazanavir, clarithromycin, indinavir, itraconazole, nefazodone, nelfinavir, saquinavir, telithromycin) is not recommended).

No products indexed under this heading.

Norfloxacin (Co-administration of salmeterol and a strong CYP3A4 inhibitor ketoconazole resulted in a significant increase in plasma salmeterol exposure as determined by a 16-fold increase in AUC mainly due to increased bioavailability of swallowed portion of the dose. Although there was no statistical effect on the mean QTc, co-administration of salmeterol and ketoconazole was associated with more frequent increases in QTc duration compared with salmeterol and placebo administration. Due to the potential increased risk of cardiovascular adverse events, the concomitant use of salmeterol with strong CYP3A4 inhibitors, (eg, ketoconazole, ritonavir, atazanavir, clarithromycin, indinavir, itraconazole, nefazodone, nelfinavir, saquinavir, telithromycin) is not recommended). Products include:

Noroxin Tablets **2069**

Nortriptyline Hydrochloride (The action of salmeterol on the vascular system may be potentiated by tricyclic antidepressant).

No products indexed under this heading.

Omeprazole (Co-administration of salmeterol and a strong CYP3A4 inhibitor ketoconazole resulted in a significant increase in plasma salmeterol exposure as determined by a 16-fold increase in AUC mainly due to increased bioavailability of swallowed portion of the dose. Although there was no statistical effect on the mean QTc, co-administration of salmeterol and ketoconazole was associated with more frequent increases in QTc duration compared with salmeterol and placebo administration. Due to the potential increased risk of cardiovascular adverse events, the concomitant use of salmeterol with strong CYP3A4 inhibitors, (eg, ketoconazole, ritonavir, atazanavir, clarithromycin, indinavir, itraconazole, nefazodone, nelfinavir, saquinavir, telithromycin) is not recommended).

No products indexed under this heading.

Pargyline Hydrochloride (The action of salmeterol on the vascular system may be potentiated by a MAO inhibitor).

No products indexed under this heading.

Paroxetine Hydrochloride (Co-administration of salmeterol and a strong CYP3A4 inhibitor ketoconazole resulted in a significant increase in plasma salmeterol exposure as determined by a 16-fold increase in AUC mainly due to increased bioavailability of swallowed portion of the dose. Although there was no statistical effect on the mean QTc, co-administration of salmeterol and ketoconazole was associated with more frequent increases in QTc duration compared with salmeterol and placebo administration. Due to the potential increased risk of cardiovascular adverse events, the concomitant use of salmeterol with strong CYP3A4 inhibitors, (eg, ketoconazole, ritonavir, atazanavir, clarithromycin, indinavir, itraconazole, nefazodone, nelfinavir, saquinavir, telithromycin) is not recommended). Products include:

Paxil **1535**
Paxil CR Controlled-Release Tablets **1544**

Penbutolol Sulfate (Beta-adrenergic blockers may produce severe bronchospasm in asthmatic patients, however, beta blockers do not block the pulmonary effect of beta-agonists).

No products indexed under this heading.

Phenelzine Sulfate (The action of salmeterol on the vascular system may be potentiated by a MAO inhibitor).

No products indexed under this heading.

Pindolol (Beta-adrenergic blockers may produce severe bronchospasm in asthmatic patients, however, beta blockers do not block the pulmonary effect of beta-agonists).

No products indexed under this heading.

Polythiazide (The ECG changes and/or hypokalemia that may result from the administration of nonpotassium-sparing diuretics can be acutely worsened by beta-agonists, especially when the recommended dose of beta-agonist is exceeded).

No products indexed under this heading.

Procarbazine Hydrochloride (The action of salmeterol on the vascular system may be potentiated by a MAO inhibitor).

No products indexed under this heading.

Propoxyphene Hydrochloride (Co-administration of salmeterol and a strong CYP3A4 inhibitor ketoconazole resulted in a significant increase in plasma salmeterol exposure as determined by a 16-fold increase in AUC mainly due to increased bioavailability of swallowed portion of the dose. Although there was no statistical effect on the mean QTc, co-administration of salmeterol and ketoconazole was associated with more frequent increases in QTc duration compared with salmeterol and placebo administration. Due to the potential increased risk of cardiovascular adverse events, the concomitant use of salmeterol with strong CYP3A4 inhibitors, (eg, ketoconazole, ritonavir, atazanavir, clarithromycin, indinavir, itraconazole, nefazodone, nelfinavir, saquinavir, telithromycin) is not recommended).

No products indexed under this heading.

Propoxyphene Napsylate (Co-administration of salmeterol and a strong CYP3A4 inhibitor ketoconazole resulted in a significant increase in plasma salmeterol exposure as determined by a 16-fold increase in AUC mainly due to increased bioavailability of swallowed portion of the dose. Although there was no statistical effect on the mean QTc, co-administration of salmeterol and ketoconazole was associated with more frequent increases in QTc duration compared with salmeterol and placebo administration. Due to the potential increased risk of cardiovascular adverse events, the concomitant use of salmeterol with strong CYP3A4 inhibitors, (eg, ketoconazole, ritonavir, atazanavir, clarithromycin, indinavir, itraconazole, nefazodone, nelfinavir, saquinavir, telithromycin) is not recommended).

No products indexed under this heading.

Propranolol Hydrochloride (Beta-adrenergic blockers may produce severe bronchospasm in asthmatic patients, however, beta blockers do not block the pulmonary effect of beta-agonists). Products include:

InnoPran XL Extended Release Capsules **1484**

Protriptyline Hydrochloride (The action of salmeterol on the vascular system may be potentiated by tricyclic antidepressant).

No products indexed under this heading.

Quinidine (Co-administration of salmeterol and a strong CYP3A4 inhibitor ketoconazole resulted in a significant increase in plasma salmeterol exposure as determined by a 16-fold increase in AUC mainly due to increased bioavailability of swallowed portion of the dose. Although there was no statistical effect on the mean QTc, co-administration of salmeterol and ketoconazole was associated with more frequent increases in QTc duration compared with salmeterol and placebo administration. Due to the potential increased risk of cardiovascular adverse events, the concomitant use of salmeterol with strong CYP3A4 inhibitors, (eg, ketoconazole, ritonavir, atazanavir, clarithromycin, indinavir, itraconazole, nefazodone, nelfinavir, saquinavir, telithromycin) is not recommended).

No products indexed under this heading.

Quinidine Hydrochloride (Co-administration of salmeterol and a strong CYP3A4 inhibitor ketoconazole resulted in a significant increase in plasma salmeterol exposure as determined by a 16-fold increase in AUC mainly due to increased bioavailability of swallowed portion of the dose. Although there was no statistical effect on the mean QTc, co-administration of salmeterol and ketoconazole was associated with more frequent increases in QTc duration compared with salmeterol and placebo administration. Due to the potential increased risk of cardiovascular adverse events, the concomitant use of salmeterol with strong CYP3A4 inhibitors, (eg, ketoconazole, ritonavir, atazanavir, clarithromycin, indinavir, itraconazole, nefazodone, nelfinavir, saquinavir, telithromycin) is not recommended).

No products indexed under this heading.

Quinidine Polygalacturonate (Co-administration of salmeterol and a strong CYP3A4 inhibitor ketoconazole resulted in a significant increase

in plasma salmeterol exposure as determined by a 16-fold increase in AUC mainly due to increased bioavailability of swallowed portion of the dose. Although there was no statistical effect on the mean QTc, co-administration of salmeterol and ketoconazole was associated with more frequent increases in QTc duration compared with salmeterol and placebo administration. Due to the potential increased risk of cardiovascular adverse events, the concomitant use of salmeterol with strong CYP3A4 inhibitors, (eg, ketoconazole, ritonavir, atazanavir, clarithromycin, indinavir, itraconazole, nefazodone, nelfinavir, saquinavir, telithromycin) is not recommended).

No products indexed under this heading.

Quinidine Sulfate (Co-administration of salmeterol and a strong CYP3A4 inhibitor ketoconazole resulted in a significant increase in plasma salmeterol exposure as determined by a 16-fold increase in AUC mainly due to increased bioavailability of swallowed portion of the dose. Although there was no statistical effect on the mean QTc, co-administration of salmeterol and ketoconazole was associated with more frequent increases in QTc duration compared with salmeterol and placebo administration. Due to the potential increased risk of cardiovascular adverse events, the concomitant use of salmeterol with strong CYP3A4 inhibitors, (eg, ketoconazole, ritonavir, atazanavir, clarithromycin, indinavir, itraconazole, nefazodone, nelfinavir, saquinavir, telithromycin) is not recommended).

No products indexed under this heading.

Quinine (Co-administration of salmeterol and a strong CYP3A4 inhibitor ketoconazole resulted in a significant increase in plasma salmeterol exposure as determined by a 16-fold increase in AUC mainly due to increased bioavailability of swallowed portion of the dose. Although there was no statistical effect on the mean QTc, co-administration of salmeterol and ketoconazole was associated with more frequent increases in QTc duration compared with salmeterol and placebo administration. Due to the potential increased risk of cardiovascular adverse events, the concomitant use of salmeterol with strong CYP3A4 inhibitors, (eg, ketoconazole, ritonavir, atazanavir, clarithromycin, indinavir, itraconazole, nefazodone, nelfinavir, saquinavir, telithromycin) is not recommended).

No products indexed under this heading.

Quinine Sulfate (Co-administration of salmeterol and a strong CYP3A4 inhibitor ketoconazole resulted in a significant increase in plasma salmeterol exposure as determined by a 16-fold increase in AUC mainly due to increased bioavailability of swallowed portion of the dose. Although there was no statistical effect on the mean QTc, co-administration of salmeterol and ketoconazole was associated with more frequent increases in QTc duration compared with salmeterol and placebo administration. Due to the potential increased risk of cardiovascular adverse events, the concomitant use of salmeterol with strong CYP3A4 inhibitors, (eg, ketoconazole, ritonavir, atazanavir, clarithromycin, indinavir, itraconazole, nefazodone, nelfinavir, saquinavir, telithromycin) is not recommended).

No products indexed under this heading.

Quinupristin (Co-administration of salmeterol and a strong CYP3A4 inhibitor ketoconazole resulted in a significant increase in plasma salmeterol exposure as determined by a 16-fold increase in AUC mainly due to increased bioavailability of swallowed portion of the dose. Although there was no statistical effect on the mean QTc, co-administration of salmeterol and ketoconazole was associated with more frequent increases in QTc duration compared with salmeterol and placebo administration. Due to the potential increased risk of cardiovascular adverse events, the concomitant use of salmeterol with strong CYP3A4 inhibitors, (eg, ketoconazole, ritonavir, atazanavir, clarithromycin, indinavir, itraconazole, nefazodone, nelfinavir, saquinavir, telithromycin) is not recommended).

No products indexed under this heading.

Ranitidine Bismuth Citrate (Co-administration of salmeterol and a strong CYP3A4 inhibitor ketoconazole resulted in a significant increase in plasma salmeterol exposure as determined by a 16-fold increase in AUC mainly due to increased bioavailability of swallowed portion of the dose. Although there was no statistical effect on the mean QTc, co-administration of salmeterol and ketoconazole was associated with more frequent increases in QTc duration compared with salmeterol and placebo administration. Due to the potential increased risk of cardiovascular adverse events, the concomitant use of salmeterol with strong CYP3A4 inhibitors, (eg, ketoconazole, ritonavir, atazanavir, clarithromycin, indinavir, itraconazole, nefazodone, nelfinavir, saquinavir, telithromycin) is not recommended).

No products indexed under this heading.

Ranitidine Hydrochloride (Co-administration of salmeterol and a strong CYP3A4 inhibitor ketoconazole resulted in a significant increase in plasma salmeterol exposure as determined by a 16-fold increase in AUC mainly due to increased bioavailability of swallowed portion of the dose. Although there was no statistical effect on the mean QTc, co-administration of salmeterol and ketoconazole was associated with more frequent increases in QTc duration compared with salmeterol and placebo administration. Due to the potential increased risk of cardiovascular adverse events, the concomitant use of salmeterol with strong CYP3A4 inhibitors, (eg, ketoconazole, ritonavir, atazanavir, clarithromycin, indinavir, itraconazole, nefazodone, nelfinavir, saquinavir, telithromycin) is not recommended). Products include:

Zantac 75 Tablets .... ▣ 603
Zantac 1670
Zantac Injection 1666
Zantac Injection Pharmacy Bulk Package 1668
Maximum Strength Zantac 150 Tablets .... ▣ 603
Maximum Strength Zantac 150 Cool Mint Tablets .... ▣ 603

Rasagiline Mesylate (The action of salmeterol on the vascular system may be potentiated by a MAO inhibitor). Products include:

Azilect Tablets 3106

Ritonavir (Co-administration of salmeterol and a strong CYP3A4 inhibitor ketoconazole resulted in a significant increase in plasma salmeterol exposure as determined by a 16-fold increase in AUC mainly due to increased bioavailability of swallowed portion of the dose. Although there was no statistical effect on the mean QTc, co-administration of salmeterol and ketoconazole was associated with more frequent increases in QTc duration compared with salmeterol and placebo administration. Due to the potential increased risk of cardiovascular adverse events, the concomitant use of salmeterol with strong CYP3A4 inhibitors, (eg, ketoconazole, ritonavir, atazanavir, clarithromycin, indinavir, itraconazole, nefazodone, nelfinavir, saquinavir, telithromycin) is not recommended). Products include:

Kaletra 452
Norvir 489

Saquinavir (Co-administration of salmeterol and a strong CYP3A4 inhibitor ketoconazole resulted in a significant increase in plasma salmeterol exposure as determined by a 16-fold increase in AUC mainly due to increased bioavailability of swallowed portion of the dose. Although there was no statistical effect on the mean QTc, co-administration of salmeterol and ketoconazole was associated with more frequent increases in QTc duration compared with salmeterol and placebo administration. Due to the potential increased risk of cardiovascular adverse events, the concomitant use of salmeterol with strong CYP3A4 inhibitors, (eg, ketoconazole, ritonavir, atazanavir, clarithromycin, indinavir, itraconazole, nefazodone, nelfinavir, saquinavir, telithromycin) is not recommended).

No products indexed under this heading.

Saquinavir Mesylate (Co-administration of salmeterol and a strong CYP3A4 inhibitor ketoconazole resulted in a significant increase in plasma salmeterol exposure as determined by a 16-fold increase in AUC mainly due to increased bioavailability of swallowed portion of the dose. Although there was no statistical effect on the mean QTc, co-administration of salmeterol and ketoconazole was associated with more frequent increases in QTc duration compared with salmeterol and placebo administration. Due to the potential increased risk of cardiovascular adverse events, the concomitant use of salmeterol with strong CYP3A4 inhibitors, (eg, ketoconazole, ritonavir, atazanavir, clarithromycin, indinavir, itraconazole, nefazodone, nelfinavir, saquinavir, telithromycin) is not recommended).

No products indexed under this heading.

Selegiline (The action of salmeterol on the vascular system may be potentiated by a MAO inhibitor). Products include:

Emsam Transdermal System 905

Selegiline Hydrochloride (The action of salmeterol on the vascular system may be potentiated by a MAO inhibitor). Products include:

Eldepryl Capsules 3052

Sertraline Hydrochloride (Co-administration of salmeterol and a strong CYP3A4 inhibitor ketoconazole resulted in a significant increase in plasma salmeterol exposure as determined by a 16-fold increase in AUC mainly due to increased bioavailability of swallowed portion of the dose. Although there was no statistical effect on the mean QTc, co-administration of salmeterol and ketoconazole was associated with more frequent increases in QTc duration compared with salmeterol and placebo administration. Due to the potential increased risk of cardiovascular adverse events, the concomitant use of salmeterol with strong CYP3A4 inhibitors, (eg, ketoconazole, ritonavir, atazanavir, clarithromycin, indinavir, itraconazole, nefazodone, nelfinavir, saquinavir, telithromycin) is not recommended).

No products indexed under this heading.

Sildenafil Citrate (Co-administration of salmeterol and a strong CYP3A4 inhibitor ketoconazole resulted in a significant increase in plasma salmeterol exposure as determined by a 16-fold increase in AUC mainly due to increased bioavailability of swallowed portion of the dose. Although there was no statistical effect on the mean QTc, co-administration of salmeterol and ketoconazole was associated with more frequent increases in QTc duration compared with salmeterol and placebo administration. Due to the potential increased risk of cardiovascular adverse events, the concomitant use of salmeterol with strong CYP3A4 inhibitors, (eg, ketoconazole, ritonavir, atazanavir, clarithromycin, indinavir, itraconazole, nefazodone, nelfinavir, saquinavir, telithromycin) is not recommended).

No products indexed under this heading.

Sotalol Hydrochloride (Beta-adrenergic blockers may produce severe bronchospasm in asthmatic patients, however, beta blockers do not block the pulmonary effect of beta-agonists).

No products indexed under this heading.

Telithromycin (Co-administration of salmeterol and a strong CYP3A4 inhibitor ketoconazole resulted in a significant increase in plasma salmeterol exposure as determined by a 16-fold increase in AUC mainly due to increased bioavailability of swallowed portion of the dose. Although there was no statistical effect on the mean QTc, co-administration of salmeterol and ketoconazole was associated with more frequent increases in QTc duration compared with salmeterol and placebo administration. Due to the potential increased risk of cardiovascular adverse events, the concomitant use of salmeterol with strong CYP3A4 inhibitors, (eg, ketoconazole, ritonavir, atazanavir, clarithromycin, indinavir, itraconazole, nefazodone, nelfinavir, saquinavir, telithromycin) is not recommended). Products include:

Ketek Tablets 2744

Timolol Hemihydrate (Beta-adrenergic blockers may produce severe bronchospasm in asthmatic patients, however, beta blockers do not block the pulmonary effect of beta-agonists). Products include:

Betimol Ophthalmic Solution **3181**

Timolol Maleate (Beta-adrenergic blockers may produce severe bronchospasm in asthmatic patients, however, beta blockers do not block the pulmonary effect of beta-agonists). Products include:

Combigan Ophthalmic Solution **553**
Cosopt Sterile Ophthalmic Solution **1969**
Timoptic Sterile Ophthalmic Solution **2121**
Timoptic in Ocudose **2124**
Timoptic-XE Sterile Ophthalmic Gel Forming Solution **2125**

Torsemide (The ECG changes and/or hypokalemia that may result from the administration of nonpotassium-sparing diuretics can be acutely worsened by beta-agonists, especially when the recommended dose of beta-agonist is exceeded). Products include:

Demadex Injection **2630**
Demadex Tablets **2630**

Tranylcypromine Sulfate (The action of salmeterol on the vascular system may be potentiated by a MAO inhibitor). Products include:

Parnate Tablets **1532**

Trimipramine Maleate (The action of salmeterol on the vascular system may be potentiated by tricyclic antidepressant).

No products indexed under this heading.

Troglitazone (Co-administration of salmeterol and a strong CYP3A4 inhibitor ketoconazole resulted in a significant increase in plasma salmeterol exposure as determined by a 16-fold increase in AUC mainly due to increased bioavailability of swallowed portion of the dose. Although there was no statistical effect on the mean QTc, co-administration of salmeterol and ketoconazole was associated with more frequent increases in QTc duration compared with salmeterol and placebo administration. Due to the potential increased risk of cardiovascular adverse events, the concomitant use of salmeterol with strong CYP3A4 inhibitors, (eg, ketoconazole, ritonavir, atazanavir, clarithromycin, indinavir, itraconazole, nefazodone, nelfinavir, saquinavir, telithromycin) is not recommended).

No products indexed under this heading.

Troleandomycin (Co-administration of salmeterol and a strong CYP3A4 inhibitor ketoconazole resulted in a significant increase in plasma salmeterol exposure as determined by a 16-fold increase in AUC mainly due to increased bioavailability of swallowed portion of the dose. Although there was no statistical effect on the mean QTc, co-administration of salmeterol and ketoconazole was associated with more frequent increases in QTc duration compared with salmeterol and placebo administration. Due to the potential increased risk of cardiovascular adverse events, the concomitant use of salmeterol with strong CYP3A4 inhibitors, (eg, ketoconazole, ritonavir, atazanavir, clarithromycin, indinavir, itraconazole, nefazodone, nelfinavir, saquinavir, telithromycin) is not recommended).

No products indexed under this heading.

Valproate Sodium (Co-administration of salmeterol and a strong CYP3A4 inhibitor ketoconazole resulted in a significant increase in plasma salmeterol exposure as determined by a 16-fold increase in AUC mainly due to increased bioavailability of swallowed portion of the dose. Although there was no statistical effect on the mean QTc, co-administration of salmeterol and ketoconazole was associated with more frequent increases in QTc duration compared with salmeterol and placebo administration. Due to the potential increased risk of cardiovascular adverse events, the concomitant use of salmeterol with strong CYP3A4 inhibitors, (eg, ketoconazole, ritonavir, atazanavir, clarithromycin, indinavir, itraconazole, nefazodone, nelfinavir, saquinavir, telithromycin) is not recommended).

No products indexed under this heading.

Vardenafil Hydrochloride (Co-administration of salmeterol and a strong CYP3A4 inhibitor ketoconazole resulted in a significant increase in plasma salmeterol exposure as determined by a 16-fold increase in AUC mainly due to increased bioavailability of swallowed portion of the dose. Although there was no statistical effect on the mean QTc, co-administration of salmeterol and ketoconazole was associated with more frequent increases in QTc duration compared with salmeterol and placebo administration. Due to the potential increased risk of cardiovascular adverse events, the concomitant use of salmeterol with strong CYP3A4 inhibitors, (eg, ketoconazole, ritonavir, atazanavir, clarithromycin, indinavir, itraconazole, nefazodone, nelfinavir, saquinavir, telithromycin) is not recommended). Products include:

Levitra Tablets **2876**

Verapamil Hydrochloride (Co-administration of salmeterol and a strong CYP3A4 inhibitor ketoconazole resulted in a significant increase in plasma salmeterol exposure as determined by a 16-fold increase in AUC mainly due to increased bioavailability of swallowed portion of the dose. Although there was no statistical effect on the mean QTc, co-administration of salmeterol and ketoconazole was associated with more frequent increases in QTc duration compared with salmeterol and placebo administration. Due to the potential increased risk of cardiovascular adverse events, the concomitant use of salmeterol with strong CYP3A4 inhibitors, (eg, ketoconazole, ritonavir, atazanavir, clarithromycin, indinavir, itraconazole, nefazodone, nelfinavir, saquinavir, telithromycin) is not recommended). Products include:

Tarka Tablets **511**

Voriconazole (Co-administration of salmeterol and a strong CYP3A4 inhibitor ketoconazole resulted in a significant increase in plasma salmeterol exposure as determined by a 16-fold increase in AUC mainly due to increased bioavailability of swallowed portion of the dose. Although there was no statistical effect on the mean QTc, co-administration of salmeterol and ketoconazole was associated with more frequent increases in QTc duration compared with salmeterol and placebo administration. Due to the potential increased risk of cardiovascular adverse events, the concomitant use of salmeterol with strong CYP3A4 inhibitors, (eg, ketoconazole, ritonavir, atazanavir, clarithromycin, indinavir, itraconazole, nefazodone, nelfinavir, saquinavir, telithromycin) is not recommended).

No products indexed under this heading.

Zafirlukast (Co-administration of salmeterol and a strong CYP3A4 inhibitor ketoconazole resulted in a significant increase in plasma salmeterol exposure as determined by a 16-fold increase in AUC mainly due to increased bioavailability of swallowed portion of the dose. Although there was no statistical effect on the mean QTc, co-administration of salmeterol and ketoconazole was associated with more frequent increases in QTc duration compared with salmeterol and placebo administration. Due to the potential increased risk of cardiovascular adverse events, the concomitant use of salmeterol with strong CYP3A4 inhibitors, (eg, ketoconazole, ritonavir, atazanavir, clarithromycin, indinavir, itraconazole, nefazodone, nelfinavir, saquinavir, telithromycin) is not recommended). Products include:

Accolate Tablets **669**

Zileuton (Co-administration of salmeterol and a strong CYP3A4 inhibitor ketoconazole resulted in a significant increase in plasma salmeterol exposure as determined by a 16-fold increase in AUC mainly due to increased bioavailability of swallowed portion of the dose. Although there was no statistical effect on the mean QTc, co-administration of salmeterol and ketoconazole was associated with more frequent increases in QTc duration compared with salmeterol and placebo administration. Due to the potential increased risk of cardiovascular adverse events, the concomitant use of salmeterol with strong CYP3A4 inhibitors, (eg, ketoconazole, ritonavir, atazanavir, clarithromycin, indinavir, itraconazole, nefazodone, nelfinavir, saquinavir, telithromycin) is not recommended).

No products indexed under this heading.

Food Interactions

Grapefruit (Co-administration of salmeterol and a strong CYP3A4 inhibitor ketoconazole resulted in a significant increase in plasma salmeterol exposure as determined by a 16-fold increase in AUC mainly due to increased bioavailability of swallowed portion of the dose. Although there was no statistical effect on the mean QTc, co-administration of salmeterol and ketoconazole was associated with more frequent increases in QTc duration compared with salmeterol and placebo administration. Due to the potential increased risk of cardiovascular adverse events, the concomitant use of salmeterol with strong CYP3A4 inhibitors, (eg, ketoconazole, ritonavir, atazanavir, clarithromycin, indinavir, itraconazole, nefazodone, nelfinavir, saquinavir, telithromycin) is not recommended).

Grapefruit Juice (Co-administration of salmeterol and a strong CYP3A4 inhibitor ketoconazole resulted in a significant increase in plasma salmeterol exposure as determined by a 16-fold increase in AUC mainly due to increased bioavailability of swallowed portion of the dose. Although there was no statistical effect on the mean QTc, co-administration of salmeterol and ketoconazole was associated with more frequent increases in QTc duration compared with salmeterol and placebo administration. Due to the potential increased risk of cardiovascular adverse events, the concomitant use of salmeterol with strong CYP3A4 inhibitors, (eg, ketoconazole, ritonavir, atazanavir, clarithromycin, indinavir, itraconazole, nefazodone, nelfinavir, saquinavir, telithromycin) is not recommended).

SEROMYCIN CAPSULES

(Cycloserine) **1864**

May interact with antituberculosis drugs and certain other agents. Compounds in these categories include:

Aminosalicylic Acid (Co-administration has been associated with a few instances of vitamin B_{12} and/or folic acid deficiency, megaloblastic anemia, and sideroblastic anemia). Products include:

Paser Granules **1747**

p-Aminosalicylic Acid (Co-administration has been associated with a few instances of vitamin B_{12} and/or folic acid deficiency, megaloblastic anemia, and sideroblastic anemia).

No products indexed under this heading.

Ethambutol Hydrochloride (Co-administration has been associated with a few instances of vitamin B_{12}2 and/or folic acid deficiency, megaloblastic anemia, and sideroblastic anemia).

No products indexed under this heading.

Ethionamide (Co-administration has been reported to potentiate neurotoxic side effects).

No products indexed under this heading.

Isoniazid (Co-administration may result in increased incidence of CNS effects, such as dizziness or drowsiness).

No products indexed under this heading.

Pyrazinamide (Co-administration has been associated with a few instances of vitamin B_{12} and/or folic acid deficiency, megaloblastic anemia, and sideroblastic anemia).

No products indexed under this heading.

Rifampin (Co-administration has been associated with a few instances of vitamin B_{12} and/or folic acid deficiency, megaloblastic anemia, and sideroblastic anemia).

No products indexed under this heading.

Rifapentine (Co-administration has been associated with a few instances of vitamin B_{12} and/or folic acid deficiency, megaloblastic anemia, and sideroblastic anemia).

No products indexed under this heading.

Food Interactions

Alcohol (Concurrent use increases the possibility and risk of epileptic episodes).

SIMCOR TABLETS
(Niacin, Simvastatin) 502
May interact with antihypertensives, aspirin-acetylsalicylic acid, bile acid sequestering agents, oral anticoagulants, cytochrome p450 3a4 inhibitors (selected), fibrates, and certain other agents. Compounds in these categories include:

Acebutolol Hydrochloride (Niacin may potentiate the effects of ganglionic blocking agents and vasoactive drugs resulting in postural hypotension).
No products indexed under this heading.

Acetazolamide (Potent inhibitors of CYP3A4 increase the risk of myopathy by reducing the elimination of simvastatin. Hence when simvastatin is used with a potent inhibitor of CYP3A4, elevated plasma levels of HMG-CoA reductase inhibitory activity can increase the riskof myopathy and rhabdomyolysis, particularly with higher doses of simvastatin. Concomitant use of drugs labeled as potent inhibitors of CYP3A4 should be avoided unless the benefits of combined therapy outweigh the increased risk. If treatment with itraconazole, ketoconazole, erythromycin, clarithromycin or telithromycin is unavoidable, therapy with Simcor should be suspended during the course of treatment).
No products indexed under this heading.

Aliskiren (Niacin may potentiate the effects of ganglionic blocking agents and vasoactive drugs resulting in postural hypotension). Products include:
Tekturna Tablets 2321
Tekturna HCT Tablets 2324

Amiodarone Hydrochloride (The risk of myopathy/rhabdomyolysis is increased by concomitant administration of amiodarone or verapamil with higher doses of simvastatin. Combination with Simcor should be limited to the 20 mg once daily dose of simvastatin).
No products indexed under this heading.

Amlodipine Besylate (Niacin may potentiate the effects of ganglionic blocking agents and vasoactive drugs resulting in postural hypotension). Products include:
Azor Tablets 1005
Exforge Tablets 2238

Amprenavir (Potent inhibitors of CYP3A4 increase the risk of myopathy by reducing the elimination of simvastatin. Hence when simvastatin is used with a potent inhibitor of CYP3A4, elevated plasma levels of HMG-CoA reductase inhibitory activity can increase the riskof myopathy and rhabdomyolysis, particularly with higher doses of simvastatin. Concomitant use of drugs labeled as potent inhibitors of CYP3A4 should be avoided unless the benefits of combined therapy outweigh the increased risk. If treatment with itraconazole, ketoconazole, erythromycin, clarithromycin or telithromycin is unavoidable, therapy with Simcor should be suspended during the course of treatment).
No products indexed under this heading.

Anastrozole (Potent inhibitors of CYP3A4 increase the risk of myopathy by reducing the elimination of simvastatin. Hence when simvastatin is used with a potent inhibitor of CYP3A4, elevated plasma levels of HMG-CoA reductase inhibitory activity can increase the riskof myopathy and rhabdomyolysis, particularly with higher doses of simvastatin. Concomitant use of drugs labeled as potent inhibitors of CYP3A4 should be avoided unless the benefits of combined therapy outweigh the increased risk. If treatment with itraconazole, ketoconazole, erythromycin, clarithromycin or telithromycin is unavoidable, therapy with Simcor should be suspended during the course of treatment). Products include:
Arimidex Tablets 672

Anisindione (Co-administration prolongs INR. Achieve stable INR prior to starting Simcor. Monitor INR frequently until stable upon initiation or alteration of Simcor therapy).
No products indexed under this heading.

Aprepitant (Potent inhibitors of CYP3A4 increase the risk of myopathy by reducing the elimination of simvastatin. Hence when simvastatin is used with a potent inhibitor of CYP3A4, elevated plasma levels of HMG-CoA reductase inhibitory activity can increase the riskof myopathy and rhabdomyolysis, particularly with higher doses of simvastatin. Concomitant use of drugs labeled as potent inhibitors of CYP3A4 should be avoided unless the benefits of combined therapy outweigh the increased risk. If treatment with itraconazole, ketoconazole, erythromycin, clarithromycin or telithromycin is unavoidable, therapy with Simcor should be suspended during the course of treatment). Products include:
Emend Capsules 1992

Aspirin (Concomitant use of aspirin may decrease the metabolic clearance of niacin. The clinical relevance of this finding is unclear). Products include:
Aggrenox Capsules 819
Bayer Aspirin 750
Percodan Tablets 1130
St. Joseph 81 mg Aspirin Chewable and Enteric Coated Tablets 1903

Aspirin, Enteric Coated (Concomitant use of aspirin may decrease the metabolic clearance of niacin. The clinical relevance of this finding is unclear).
No products indexed under this heading.

Aspirin Buffered (Concomitant use of aspirin may decrease the metabolic clearance of niacin. The clinical relevance of this finding is unclear).
No products indexed under this heading.

Atazanavir (Potent inhibitors of CYP3A4 increase the risk of myopathy by reducing the elimination of simvastatin. Hence when simvastatin is used with a potent inhibitor of CYP3A4, elevated plasma levels of HMG-CoA reductase inhibitory activity can increase the riskof myopathy and rhabdomyolysis, particularly with higher doses of simvastatin. Concomitant use of drugs labeled as potent inhibitors of CYP3A4 should be avoided unless the benefits of combined therapy outweigh the increased risk. If treatment with itraconazole, ketoconazole, erythromycin, clarithromycin or telithromycin is unavoidable, therapy with Simcor should be suspended during the course of treatment).
No products indexed under this heading.

Atazanavir Sulfate (Potent inhibitors of CYP3A4 increase the risk of myopathy by reducing the elimination of simvastatin. Hence when simvastatin is used with a potent inhibitor of CYP3A4, elevated plasma levels of HMG-CoA reductase inhibitory activity can increase the riskof myopathy and rhabdomyolysis, particularly with higher doses of simvastatin. Concomitant use of drugs labeled as potent inhibitors of CYP3A4 should be avoided unless the benefits of combined therapy outweigh the increased risk. If treatment with itraconazole, ketoconazole, erythromycin, clarithromycin or telithromycin is unavoidable, therapy with Simcor should be suspended during the course of treatment). Products include:
Reyataz Capsules 3299

Atenolol (Niacin may potentiate the effects of ganglionic blocking agents and vasoactive drugs resulting in postural hypotension).
No products indexed under this heading.

Benazepril Hydrochloride (Niacin may potentiate the effects of ganglionic blocking agents and vasoactive drugs resulting in postural hypotension).
No products indexed under this heading.

Bendroflumethiazide (Niacin may potentiate the effects of ganglionic blocking agents and vasoactive drugs resulting in postural hypotension).
No products indexed under this heading.

Betaxolol Hydrochloride (Niacin may potentiate the effects of ganglionic blocking agents and vasoactive drugs resulting in postural hypotension).
No products indexed under this heading.

Bisoprolol Fumarate (Niacin may potentiate the effects of ganglionic blocking agents and vasoactive drugs resulting in postural hypotension).
No products indexed under this heading.

Candesartan Cilexetil (Niacin may potentiate the effects of ganglionic blocking agents and vasoactive drugs resulting in postural hypotension). Products include:
Atacand Tablets 639
Atacand HCT 642

Captopril (Niacin may potentiate the effects of ganglionic blocking agents and vasoactive drugs resulting in postural hypotension). Products include:
Captopril Tablets 2182

Carteolol Hydrochloride (Niacin may potentiate the effects of ganglionic blocking agents and vasoactive drugs resulting in postural hypotension).
No products indexed under this heading.

Chlorothiazide (Niacin may potentiate the effects of ganglionic blocking agents and vasoactive drugs resulting in postural hypotension).
No products indexed under this heading.

Chlorothiazide Sodium (Niacin may potentiate the effects of ganglionic blocking agents and vasoactive drugs resulting in postural hypotension). Products include:
Intravenous Sodium Diuril 2490

Chlorthalidone (Niacin may potentiate the effects of ganglionic blocking agents and vasoactive drugs resulting in postural hypotension). Products include:
Clorpres Tablets 2185

Cholestyramine (An in vitro study was carried out investigating the niacin-binding capacity of colestipol and cholestyramine. About 98% of available niacin was bound to colestipol, with 10% to 30% binding to cholestyramine. These results suggest that 4 to 6 hours, or as great an interval as possible, should elapse between the ingestion of bile acid-binding resins and the administration of Simcor).
No products indexed under this heading.

Cimetidine (Potent inhibitors of CYP3A4 increase the risk of myopathy by reducing the elimination of simvastatin. Hence when simvastatin is used with a potent inhibitor of CYP3A4, elevated plasma levels of HMG-CoA reductase inhibitory activity can increase the riskof myopathy and rhabdomyolysis, particularly with higher doses of simvastatin. Concomitant use of drugs labeled as potent inhibitors of CYP3A4 should be avoided unless the benefits of combined therapy outweigh the increased risk. If treatment with itraconazole, ketoconazole, erythromycin, clarithromycin or telithromycin is unavoidable, therapy with Simcor should be suspended during the course of treatment).
No products indexed under this heading.

Cimetidine Hydrochloride (Potent inhibitors of CYP3A4 increase the risk of myopathy by reducing the elimination of simvastatin. Hence when simvastatin is used with a potent inhibitor of CYP3A4, elevated plasma levels of HMG-CoA reductase inhibitory activity can increase the riskof myopathy and rhabdomyolysis, particularly with higher doses of simvastatin. Concomitant use of drugs labeled as potent inhibitors of CYP3A4 should be avoided unless the benefits of combined therapy outweigh the increased risk. If treatment with itraconazole, ketoconazole, erythromycin, clarithromycin or telithromycin is unavoidable, therapy with Simcor should be suspended during the course of treatment).
No products indexed under this heading.

Ciprofloxacin (Potent inhibitors of CYP3A4 increase the risk of myopathy by reducing the elimination of simvastatin. Hence when simvastatin is used with a potent inhibitor of CYP3A4, elevated plasma levels of HMG-CoA reductase inhibitory activity can increase the riskof myopathy and rhabdomyolysis, particularly with higher doses of simvastatin. Concomitant use of drugs labeled as potent inhibitors of CYP3A4 should be avoided unless the benefits of combined therapy outweigh the increased risk. If treatment with itraconazole, ketoconazole, erythromycin, clarithromycin or telithromycin is unavoidable, therapy with Simcor

should be suspended during the course of treatment). Products include:
Cipro I.V. 2817
Cipro Oral Suspension 2810
Cipro XR Tablets 2823
Ciprodex Otic Suspension 541

Clarithromycin (Potent inhibitors of CYP3A4 increase the risk of myopathy by reducing the elimination of simvastatin. Hence when simvastatin is used with a potent inhibitor of CYP3A4, elevated plasma levels of HMG-CoA reductase inhibitory activity can increase the riskof myopathy and rhabdomyolysis, particularly with higher doses of simvastatin. Concomitant use of drugs labeled as potent inhibitors of CYP3A4 should be avoided unless the benefits of combined therapy outweigh the increased risk. If treatment with itraconazole, ketoconazole, erythromycin, clarithromycin or telithromycin is unavoidable, therapy with Simcor should be suspended during the course of treatment). Products include:
Biaxin/Biaxin XL 411

Clofibrate (Co-administration of gemfibrozil (600 mg bid for 3 days) with simvastatin (40 mg daily) resulted in clinically significant increases in simvastatin acid AUC (185%) and peak plasma concentration (Cmax, 112%), possibly due to inhibition of simvastatin acid glucuronidation by gemfibrozil. The increase in simvastatin exposure increases the risk of myopathy when co-administered with gemfibrozil. The combined use of Simcor with gemfibrozil should be avoided. The risk of myopathy also increases to a lesser extent when simvastatin is used in combination with other fibrates. Combination therapy with Simcor should be avoided).
No products indexed under this heading.

Clonidine (Niacin may potentiate the effects of ganglionic blocking agents and vasoactive drugs resulting in postural hypotension). Products include:
Catapres-TTS 842

Clonidine Hydrochloride (Niacin may potentiate the effects of ganglionic blocking agents and vasoactive drugs resulting in postural hypotension). Products include:
Catapres Tablets 841
Clorpres Tablets 2185

Clotrimazole (Potent inhibitors of CYP3A4 increase the risk of myopathy by reducing the elimination of simvastatin. Hence when simvastatin is used with a potent inhibitor of CYP3A4, elevated plasma levels of HMG-CoA reductase inhibitory activity can increase the riskof myopathy and rhabdomyolysis, particularly with higher doses of simvastatin. Concomitant use of drugs labeled as potent inhibitors of CYP3A4 should be avoided unless the benefits of combined therapy outweigh the increased risk. If treatment with itraconazole, ketoconazole, erythromycin, clarithromycin or telithromycin is unavoidable, therapy with Simcor should be suspended during the course of treatment). Products include:
Lotrisone 2881

Colesevelam Hydrochloride (An in vitro study was carried out investigating the niacin-binding capacity of colestipol and cholestyramine. About 98% of available niacin was bound to colestipol, with 10% to 30% binding to cholestyramine. These results suggest that 4 to 6 hours, or as great an interval as possible, should elapse between the ingestion of bile acid-binding resins and the administration of Simcor). Products include:
WelChol Tablets 1015

Colestipol Hydrochloride (An in vitro study was carried out investigating the niacin-binding capacity of colestipol and cholestyramine. About 98% of available niacin was bound to colestipol, with 10% to 30% binding to cholestyramine. These results suggest that 4 to 6 hours, or as great an interval as possible, should elapse between the ingestion of bile acid-binding resins and the administration of Simcor).
No products indexed under this heading.

Cyclosporine (Although the mechanism is not fully understood, cyclosporine has been shown to increase the AUC of HMG-CoA reductase inhibitors. The increase in AUC for simvastatin acid is presumably due, in part, to inhibition of CYP3A4. The risk of myopathy/rhabdomyolysis is increased by concomitant administration of cyclosporine or danazol particularly with higher doses of simvastatin. Co-administration with Simcor should be avoided). Products include:
Gengraf Capsules 435
Neoral Oral Solution 2280
Neoral Soft Gelatin Capsules 2280
Restasis Ophthalmic Emulsion 557
Sandimmune 2296

Dalfopristin (Potent inhibitors of CYP3A4 increase the risk of myopathy by reducing the elimination of simvastatin. Hence when simvastatin is used with a potent inhibitor of CYP3A4, elevated plasma levels of HMG-CoA reductase inhibitory activity can increase the riskof myopathy and rhabdomyolysis, particularly with higher doses of simvastatin. Concomitant use of drugs labeled as potent inhibitors of CYP3A4 should be avoided unless the benefits of combined therapy outweigh the increased risk. If treatment with itraconazole, ketoconazole, erythromycin, clarithromycin or telithromycin is unavoidable, therapy with Simcor should be suspended during the course of treatment).
No products indexed under this heading.

Danazol (Although the mechanism is not fully understood, cyclosporine has been shown to increase the AUC of HMG-CoA reductase inhibitors. The increase in AUC for simvastatin acid is presumably due, in part, to inhibition of CYP3A4. The risk of myopathy/rhabdomyolysis is increased by concomitant administration of cyclosporine or danazol particularly with higher doses of simvastatin. Co-administration with Simcor should be avoided).
No products indexed under this heading.

Delavirdine Mesylate (Potent inhibitors of CYP3A4 increase the risk of myopathy by reducing the elimination of simvastatin. Hence when simvastatin is used with a potent inhibitor of CYP3A4, elevated plasma levels of HMG-CoA reductase inhibitory activity can increase the riskof myopathy and rhabdomyolysis, particularly with higher doses of simvastatin. Concomitant use of drugs labeled as potent inhibitors of CYP3A4 should be avoided unless the benefits of combined therapy outweigh the increased risk. If treatment with itraconazole, ketoconazole, erythromycin, clarithromycin or telithromycin is unavoidable, therapy with Simcor should be suspended during the course of treatment).
No products indexed under this heading.

Deserpidine (Niacin may potentiate the effects of ganglionic blocking agents and vasoactive drugs resulting in postural hypotension).
No products indexed under this heading.

Diazoxide (Niacin may potentiate the effects of ganglionic blocking agents and vasoactive drugs resulting in postural hypotension). Products include:
Proglycem Capsules 1185
Proglycem Suspension 1185

Dicumarol (Co-administration prolongs INR. Achieve stable INR prior to starting Simcor. Monitor INR frequently until stable upon initiation or alteration of Simcor therapy).
No products indexed under this heading.

Digoxin (Concomitant administration of a single dose of digoxin in healthy male volunteers receiving simvastatin resulted in a slight elevation (less than 0.3 ng/mL) in digoxin concentrations in plasma (as measured by a radioimmunoassay) compared to concomitant administration of placebo and digoxin. Patients taking digoxin should be monitored appropriately when Simcor is initiated). Products include:
Lanoxin Injection 1498
Lanoxin Injection Pediatric 1502
Lanoxin Tablets 1505

Diltiazem Hydrochloride (Niacin may potentiate the effects of ganglionic blocking agents and vasoactive drugs resulting in postural hypotension). Products include:
Cardizem LA Extended Release Tablets 421

Diltiazem Maleate (Potent inhibitors of CYP3A4 increase the risk of myopathy by reducing the elimination of simvastatin. Hence when simvastatin is used with a potent inhibitor of CYP3A4, elevated plasma levels of HMG-CoA reductase inhibitory activity can increase the riskof myopathy and rhabdomyolysis, particularly with higher doses of simvastatin. Concomitant use of drugs labeled as potent inhibitors of CYP3A4 should be avoided unless the benefits of combined therapy outweigh the increased risk. If treatment with itraconazole, ketoconazole, erythromycin, clarithromycin or telithromycin is unavoidable, therapy with Simcor should be suspended during the course of treatment).
No products indexed under this heading.

Doxazosin Mesylate (Niacin may potentiate the effects of ganglionic blocking agents and vasoactive drugs resulting in postural hypotension).
No products indexed under this heading.

Efavirenz (Potent inhibitors of CYP3A4 increase the risk of myopathy by reducing the elimination of simvastatin. Hence when simvastatin is used with a potent inhibitor of CYP3A4, elevated plasma levels of HMG-CoA reductase inhibitory activity can increase the riskof myopathy and rhabdomyolysis, particularly with higher doses of simvastatin. Concomitant use of drugs labeled as potent inhibitors of CYP3A4 should be avoided unless the benefits of combined therapy outweigh the increased risk. If treatment with itraconazole, ketoconazole, erythromycin, clarithromycin or telithromycin is unavoidable, therapy with Simcor should be suspended during the course of treatment). Products include:
Atripla Tablets 938
Sustiva Capsules 930
Sustiva Tablets 930

Enalapril Maleate (Niacin may potentiate the effects of ganglionic blocking agents and vasoactive drugs resulting in postural hypotension).
No products indexed under this heading.

Enalaprilat (Niacin may potentiate the effects of ganglionic blocking agents and vasoactive drugs resulting in postural hypotension).
No products indexed under this heading.

Eprosartan Mesylate (Niacin may potentiate the effects of ganglionic blocking agents and vasoactive drugs resulting in postural hypotension). Products include:
Teveten Tablets 515
Teveten HCT Tablets 517

Erythromycin (Potent inhibitors of CYP3A4 increase the risk of myopathy by reducing the elimination of simvastatin. Hence when simvastatin is used with a potent inhibitor of CYP3A4, elevated plasma levels of HMG-CoA reductase inhibitory activity can increase the riskof myopathy and rhabdomyolysis, particularly with higher doses of simvastatin. Concomitant use of drugs labeled as potent inhibitors of CYP3A4 should be avoided unless the benefits of combined therapy outweigh the increased risk. If treatment with itraconazole, ketoconazole, erythromycin, clarithromycin or telithromycin is unavoidable, therapy with Simcor should be suspended during the course of treatment).
No products indexed under this heading.

Erythromycin Estolate (Potent inhibitors of CYP3A4 increase the risk of myopathy by reducing the elimination of simvastatin. Hence when simvastatin is used with a potent inhibitor of CYP3A4, elevated plasma levels of HMG-CoA reductase inhibitory activity can increase the riskof myopathy and rhabdomyolysis, particularly with higher doses of simvastatin. Concomitant use of drugs labeled as potent inhibitors of CYP3A4 should be avoided unless the benefits of combined therapy outweigh the increased risk. If treatment with itraconazole, ketoconazole, erythromycin, clarithromycin or telithromycin is unavoidable, therapy with Simcor should be suspended during the course of treatment).
No products indexed under this heading.

Erythromycin Ethylsuccinate (Potent inhibitors of CYP3A4 increase the risk of myopathy by reducing the elimination of simvasta-

tin. Hence when simvastatin is used with a potent inhibitor of CYP3A4, elevated plasma levels of HMG-CoA reductase inhibitory activity can increase the riskof myopathy and rhabdomyolysis, particularly with higher doses of simvastatin. Concomitant use of drugs labeled as potent inhibitors of CYP3A4 should be avoided unless the benefits of combined therapy outweigh the increased risk. If treatment with itraconazole, ketoconazole, erythromycin, clarithromycin or telithromycin is unavoidable, therapy with Simcor should be suspended during the course of treatment). Products include:

E.E.S. 433
EryPed 431

Erythromycin Gluceptate (Potent inhibitors of CYP3A4 increase the risk of myopathy by reducing the elimination of simvastatin. Hence when simvastatin is used with a potent inhibitor of CYP3A4, elevated plasma levels of HMG-CoA reductase inhibitory activity can increase the riskof myopathy and rhabdomyolysis, particularly with higher doses of simvastatin. Concomitant use of drugs labeled as potent inhibitors of CYP3A4 should be avoided unless the benefits of combined therapy outweigh the increased risk. If treatment with itraconazole, ketoconazole, erythromycin, clarithromycin or telithromycin is unavoidable, therapy with Simcor should be suspended during the course of treatment).

No products indexed under this heading.

Erythromycin Lactobionate (Potent inhibitors of CYP3A4 increase the risk of myopathy by reducing the elimination of simvastatin. Hence when simvastatin is used with a potent inhibitor of CYP3A4, elevated plasma levels of HMG-CoA reductase inhibitory activity can increase the riskof myopathy and rhabdomyolysis, particularly with higher doses of simvastatin. Concomitant use of drugs labeled as potent inhibitors of CYP3A4 should be avoided unless the benefits of combined therapy outweigh the increased risk. If treatment with itraconazole, ketoconazole, erythromycin, clarithromycin or telithromycin is unavoidable, therapy with Simcor should be suspended during the course of treatment).

No products indexed under this heading.

Erythromycin Stearate (Potent inhibitors of CYP3A4 increase the risk of myopathy by reducing the elimination of simvastatin. Hence when simvastatin is used with a potent inhibitor of CYP3A4, elevated plasma levels of HMG-CoA reductase inhibitory activity can increase the riskof myopathy and rhabdomyolysis, particularly with higher doses of simvastatin. Concomitant use of drugs labeled as potent inhibitors of CYP3A4 should be avoided unless the benefits of combined therapy outweigh the increased risk. If treatment with itraconazole, ketoconazole, erythromycin, clarithromycin or telithromycin is unavoidable, therapy with Simcor should be suspended during the course of treatment).

No products indexed under this heading.

Esmolol Hydrochloride (Niacin may potentiate the effects of ganglionic blocking agents and vasoactive drugs resulting in postural hypotension).

No products indexed under this heading.

Esomeprazole Magnesium (Potent inhibitors of CYP3A4 increase the risk of myopathy by reducing the elimination of simvastatin. Hence when simvastatin is used with a potent inhibitor of CYP3A4, elevated plasma levels of HMG-CoA reductase inhibitory activity can increase the riskof myopathy and rhabdomyolysis, particularly with higher doses of simvastatin. Concomitant use of drugs labeled as potent inhibitors of CYP3A4 should be avoided unless the benefits of combined therapy outweigh the increased risk. If treatment with itraconazole, ketoconazole, erythromycin, clarithromycin or telithromycin is unavoidable, therapy with Simcor should be suspended during the course of treatment). Products include:

Nexium Delayed-Release Capsules 645
Nexium Delayed-Release Oral Suspension 645

Felodipine (Niacin may potentiate the effects of ganglionic blocking agents and vasoactive drugs resulting in postural hypotension).

No products indexed under this heading.

Fenofibrate (Co-administration of gemfibrozil (600 mg bid for 3 days) with simvastatin (40 mg daily) resulted in clinically significant increases in simvastatin acid AUC (185%) and peak plasma concentration (Cmax, 112%), possibly due to inhibition of simvastatin acid glucuronidation by gemfibrozil. The increase in simvastatin exposure increases the risk of myopathy when co-administered with gemfibrozil. The combined use of Simcor with gemfibrozil should be avoided. The risk of myopathy also increases to a lesser extent when simvastatin is used in combination with other fibrates. Combination therapy with Simcor should be avoided). Products include:

Fenoglide Tablets 2960
Tricor Tablets 520

Fluconazole (Potent inhibitors of CYP3A4 increase the risk of myopathy by reducing the elimination of simvastatin. Hence when simvastatin is used with a potent inhibitor of CYP3A4, elevated plasma levels of HMG-CoA reductase inhibitory activity can increase the riskof myopathy and rhabdomyolysis, particularly with higher doses of simvastatin. Concomitant use of drugs labeled as potent inhibitors of CYP3A4 should be avoided unless the benefits of combined therapy outweigh the increased risk. If treatment with itraconazole, ketoconazole, erythromycin, clarithromycin or telithromycin is unavoidable, therapy with Simcor should be suspended during the course of treatment).

No products indexed under this heading.

Fluoxetine (Potent inhibitors of CYP3A4 increase the risk of myopathy by reducing the elimination of simvastatin. Hence when simvastatin is used with a potent inhibitor of CYP3A4, elevated plasma levels of HMG-CoA reductase inhibitory activity can increase the riskof myopathy and rhabdomyolysis, particularly with higher doses of simvastatin. Concomitant use of drugs labeled as potent inhibitors of CYP3A4 should be avoided unless the benefits of combined therapy outweigh the increased risk. If treatment with itraconazole, ketoconazole, erythromycin, clarithromycin or telithromycin is unavoidable, therapy with Simcor should be suspended during the course of treatment).

No products indexed under this heading.

Fluoxetine Hydrochloride (Potent inhibitors of CYP3A4 increase the risk of myopathy by reducing the elimination of simvastatin. Hence when simvastatin is used with a potent inhibitor of CYP3A4, elevated plasma levels of HMG-CoA reductase inhibitory activity can increase the riskof myopathy and rhabdomyolysis, particularly with higher doses of simvastatin. Concomitant use of drugs labeled as potent inhibitors of CYP3A4 should be avoided unless the benefits of combined therapy outweigh the increased risk. If treatment with itraconazole, ketoconazole, erythromycin, clarithromycin or telithromycin is unavoidable, therapy with Simcor should be suspended during the course of treatment). Products include:

Prozac Weekly Capsules 1852
Prozac Pulvules and Liquid 1852
Symbyax Capsules 1871

Fluvoxamine Maleate (Potent inhibitors of CYP3A4 increase the risk of myopathy by reducing the elimination of simvastatin. Hence when simvastatin is used with a potent inhibitor of CYP3A4, elevated plasma levels of HMG-CoA reductase inhibitory activity can increase the riskof myopathy and rhabdomyolysis, particularly with higher doses of simvastatin. Concomitant use of drugs labeled as potent inhibitors of CYP3A4 should be avoided unless the benefits of combined therapy outweigh the increased risk. If treatment with itraconazole, ketoconazole, erythromycin, clarithromycin or telithromycin is unavoidable, therapy with Simcor should be suspended during the course of treatment). Products include:

Luvox CR Extended-Release Capsules 1759

Fosamprenavir Calcium (Potent inhibitors of CYP3A4 increase the risk of myopathy by reducing the elimination of simvastatin. Hence when simvastatin is used with a potent inhibitor of CYP3A4, elevated plasma levels of HMG-CoA reductase inhibitory activity can increase the riskof myopathy and rhabdomyolysis, particularly with higher doses of simvastatin. Concomitant use of drugs labeled as potent inhibitors of CYP3A4 should be avoided unless the benefits of combined therapy outweigh the increased risk. If treatment with itraconazole, ketoconazole, erythromycin, clarithromycin or telithromycin is unavoidable, therapy with Simcor should be suspended during the course of treatment). Products include:

Lexiva Oral Suspension 1510
Lexiva Tablets 1510

Fosinopril Sodium (Niacin may potentiate the effects of ganglionic blocking agents and vasoactive drugs resulting in postural hypotension).

No products indexed under this heading.

Furosemide (Niacin may potentiate the effects of ganglionic blocking agents and vasoactive drugs resulting in postural hypotension). Products include:

Furosemide Tablets 2186

Gemfibrozil (Co-administration of gemfibrozil (600 mg twice daily for 3 days) with simvastatin (40 mg daily) resulted in clinically significant increases in simvastatin acid AUC (185%) and peak plasma concentration (C, 112%), possibly due to inhibition of simvastatin acid glucuronidation by gemfibrozil. The increase in simvastatin exposure increases the risk of myopathy when co-administered with gemfibrozil. The combined use of SIMCOR with gemfibrozil should be avoided).

No products indexed under this heading.

Guanabenz Acetate (Niacin may potentiate the effects of ganglionic blocking agents and vasoactive drugs resulting in postural hypotension).

No products indexed under this heading.

Guanethidine Monosulfate (Niacin may potentiate the effects of ganglionic blocking agents and vasoactive drugs resulting in postural hypotension).

No products indexed under this heading.

Hydralazine Hydrochloride (Niacin may potentiate the effects of ganglionic blocking agents and vasoactive drugs resulting in postural hypotension).

No products indexed under this heading.

Hydrochlorothiazide (Niacin may potentiate the effects of ganglionic blocking agents and vasoactive drugs resulting in postural hypotension). Products include:

Atacand HCT 642
Avalide Tablets 892
Avalide Tablets 2713
Benicar HCT Tablets 1010
Diovan HCT Tablets 2216
Dyazide Capsules 1405
Micardis HCT Tablets 854
Prinzide Tablets 2092
Tekturna HCT Tablets 2324
Teveten HCT Tablets 517

Hydroflumethiazide (Niacin may potentiate the effects of ganglionic blocking agents and vasoactive drugs resulting in postural hypotension).

No products indexed under this heading.

Indapamide (Niacin may potentiate the effects of ganglionic blocking agents and vasoactive drugs resulting in postural hypotension). Products include:

Indapamide Tablets 2188

Indinavir Sulfate (Potent inhibitors of CYP3A4 increase the risk of myopathy by reducing the elimination of simvastatin. Hence when simvastatin is used with a potent inhibitor of CYP3A4, elevated plasma levels of HMG-CoA reductase inhibitory activity can increase the riskof myopathy and rhabdomyolysis, particularly with higher doses of simvastatin. Concomitant use of drugs labeled as potent inhibitors of CYP3A4 should be avoided unless the benefits of combined therapy outweigh the increased risk. If treatment with itraconazole, ketoconazole, erythromycin, clarithromycin or telithromycin is unavoidable, therapy with Simcor should be suspended during the course of treatment). Products include:

Crixivan Capsules 1979

Irbesartan (Niacin may potentiate the effects of ganglionic blocking agents and vasoactive drugs resulting in postural hypotension). Products include:

Avalide Tablets 892
Avalide Tablets 2713
Avapro Tablets 897
Avapro Tablets 2718

Isoniazid (Potent inhibitors of CYP3A4 increase the risk of myopathy by reducing the elimination of simvastatin. Hence when simvastatin is used with a potent inhibitor of CYP3A4, elevated plasma levels of HMG-CoA reductase inhibitory activity can increase the riskof myopathy and rhabdomyolysis, particularly with higher doses of simvastatin. Concomitant use of drugs labeled as potent inhibitors of CYP3A4 should be avoided unless the benefits of combined therapy outweigh the increased risk. If treatment with itraconazole, ketoconazole, erythromycin, clarithromycin or telithromycin is unavoidable, therapy with Simcor should be suspended during the course of treatment).

No products indexed under this heading.

Isradipine (Niacin may potentiate the effects of ganglionic blocking agents and vasoactive drugs resulting in postural hypotension). Products include:

DynaCirc CR Controlled Release Tablets 1407

Itraconazole (Potent inhibitors of CYP3A4 increase the risk of myopathy by reducing the elimination of simvastatin. Hence when simvastatin is used with a potent inhibitor of CYP3A4, elevated plasma levels of HMG-CoA reductase inhibitory activity can increase the riskof myopathy and rhabdomyolysis, particularly with higher doses of simvastatin. Concomitant use of drugs labeled as potent inhibitors of CYP3A4 should be avoided unless the benefits of combined therapy outweigh the increased risk. If treatment with itraconazole, ketoconazole, erythromycin, clarithromycin or telithromycin is unavoidable, therapy with Simcor should be suspended during the course of treatment).

No products indexed under this heading.

Ketoconazole (Potent inhibitors of CYP3A4 increase the risk of myopathy by reducing the elimination of simvastatin. Hence when simvastatin is used with a potent inhibitor of CYP3A4, elevated plasma levels of HMG-CoA reductase inhibitory activity can increase the riskof myopathy and rhabdomyolysis, particularly with higher doses of simvastatin. Concomitant use of drugs labeled as potent inhibitors of CYP3A4 should be avoided unless the benefits of combined therapy outweigh the increased risk. If treatment with itraconazole, ketoconazole, erythromycin, clarithromycin or telithromycin is unavoidable, therapy with Simcor should be suspended during the course of treatment). Products include:

Extina Foam, 2% 3057
Nizoral A-D Shampoo 1901

Labetalol Hydrochloride (Niacin may potentiate the effects of ganglionic blocking agents and vasoactive drugs resulting in postural hypotension).

No products indexed under this heading.

Lisinopril (Niacin may potentiate the effects of ganglionic blocking agents and vasoactive drugs resulting in postural hypotension). Products include:

Prinivil Tablets 2087
Prinzide Tablets 2092

Lopinavir (Potent inhibitors of CYP3A4 increase the risk of myopathy by reducing the elimination of simvastatin. Hence when simvastatin is used with a potent inhibitor of CYP3A4, elevated plasma levels of HMG-CoA reductase inhibitory activity can increase the riskof myopathy and rhabdomyolysis, particularly with higher doses of simvastatin. Concomitant use of drugs labeled as potent inhibitors of CYP3A4 should be avoided unless the benefits of combined therapy outweigh the increased risk. If treatment with itraconazole, ketoconazole, erythromycin, clarithromycin or telithromycin is unavoidable, therapy with Simcor should be suspended during the course of treatment). Products include:

Kaletra 452

Loratadine (Potent inhibitors of CYP3A4 increase the risk of myopathy by reducing the elimination of simvastatin. Hence when simvastatin is used with a potent inhibitor of CYP3A4, elevated plasma levels of HMG-CoA reductase inhibitory activity can increase the riskof myopathy and rhabdomyolysis, particularly with higher doses of simvastatin. Concomitant use of drugs labeled as potent inhibitors of CYP3A4 should be avoided unless the benefits of combined therapy outweigh the increased risk. If treatment with itraconazole, ketoconazole, erythromycin, clarithromycin or telithromycin is unavoidable, therapy with Simcor should be suspended during the course of treatment).

No products indexed under this heading.

Losartan Potassium (Niacin may potentiate the effects of ganglionic blocking agents and vasoactive drugs resulting in postural hypotension). Products include:

Cozaar Tablets 1973

Mecamylamine Hydrochloride (Niacin may potentiate the effects of ganglionic blocking agents and vasoactive drugs resulting in postural hypotension).

No products indexed under this heading.

Methyclothiazide (Niacin may potentiate the effects of ganglionic blocking agents and vasoactive drugs resulting in postural hypotension).

No products indexed under this heading.

Methyldopa (Niacin may potentiate the effects of ganglionic blocking agents and vasoactive drugs resulting in postural hypotension).

No products indexed under this heading.

Methyldopate Hydrochloride (Niacin may potentiate the effects of ganglionic blocking agents and vasoactive drugs resulting in postural hypotension).

No products indexed under this heading.

Metolazone (Niacin may potentiate the effects of ganglionic blocking agents and vasoactive drugs resulting in postural hypotension).

No products indexed under this heading.

Metoprolol Succinate (Niacin may potentiate the effects of ganglionic blocking agents and vasoactive drugs resulting in postural hypotension). Products include:

Toprol-XL Tablets 666

Metoprolol Tartrate (Niacin may potentiate the effects of ganglionic blocking agents and vasoactive drugs resulting in postural hypotension).

No products indexed under this heading.

Metronidazole (Potent inhibitors of CYP3A4 increase the risk of myopathy by reducing the elimination of simvastatin. Hence when simvastatin is used with a potent inhibitor of CYP3A4, elevated plasma levels of HMG-CoA reductase inhibitory activity can increase the riskof myopathy and rhabdomyolysis, particularly with higher doses of simvastatin. Concomitant use of drugs labeled as potent inhibitors of CYP3A4 should be avoided unless the benefits of combined therapy outweigh the increased risk. If treatment with itraconazole, ketoconazole, erythromycin, clarithromycin or telithromycin is unavoidable, therapy with Simcor should be suspended during the course of treatment). Products include:

Pylera Capsules 714

Metronidazole Benzoate (Potent inhibitors of CYP3A4 increase the risk of myopathy by reducing the elimination of simvastatin. Hence when simvastatin is used with a potent inhibitor of CYP3A4, elevated plasma levels of HMG-CoA reductase inhibitory activity can increase the riskof myopathy and rhabdomyolysis, particularly with higher doses of simvastatin. Concomitant use of drugs labeled as potent inhibitors of CYP3A4 should be avoided unless the benefits of combined therapy outweigh the increased risk. If treatment with itraconazole, ketoconazole, erythromycin, clarithromycin or telithromycin is unavoidable, therapy with Simcor should be suspended during the course of treatment).

No products indexed under this heading.

Metronidazole Hydrochloride (Potent inhibitors of CYP3A4 increase the risk of myopathy by reducing the elimination of simvastatin. Hence when simvastatin is used with a potent inhibitor of CYP3A4, elevated plasma levels of HMG-CoA reductase inhibitory activity can increase the riskof myopathy and rhabdomyolysis, particularly with higher doses of simvastatin. Concomitant use of drugs labeled as potent inhibitors of CYP3A4 should be avoided unless the benefits of combined therapy outweigh the increased risk. If treatment with itraconazole, ketoconazole, erythromycin, clarithromycin or telithromycin is unavoidable, therapy with Simcor should be suspended during the course of treatment).

No products indexed under this heading.

Metronidazole Sodium (Potent inhibitors of CYP3A4 increase the risk of myopathy by reducing the elimination of simvastatin. Hence when simvastatin is used with a potent inhibitor of CYP3A4, elevated plasma levels of HMG-CoA reductase inhibitory activity can increase the riskof myopathy and rhabdomyolysis, particularly with higher doses of simvastatin. Concomitant use of drugs labeled as potent inhibitors of CYP3A4 should be avoided unless the benefits of combined therapy outweigh the increased risk. If treatment with itraconazole, ketoconazole, erythromycin, clarithromycin or telithromycin is unavoidable, therapy with Simcor should be suspended during the course of treatment).

No products indexed under this heading.

Metyrosine (Niacin may potentiate the effects of ganglionic blocking agents and vasoactive drugs resulting in postural hypotension). Products include:

Demser Capsules 1989

Mibefradil Dihydrochloride (Niacin may potentiate the effects of ganglionic blocking agents and vasoactive drugs resulting in postural hypotension).

No products indexed under this heading.

Miconazole (Potent inhibitors of CYP3A4 increase the risk of myopathy by reducing the elimination of simvastatin. Hence when simvastatin is used with a potent inhibitor of CYP3A4, elevated plasma levels of HMG-CoA reductase inhibitory activity can increase the riskof myopathy and rhabdomyolysis, particularly with higher doses of simvastatin. Concomitant use of drugs labeled as potent inhibitors of CYP3A4 should be avoided unless the benefits of combined therapy outweigh the increased risk. If treatment with itraconazole, ketoconazole, erythromycin, clarithromycin or telithromycin is unavoidable, therapy with Simcor should be suspended during the course of treatment).

No products indexed under this heading.

Miconazole Nitrate (Potent inhibitors of CYP3A4 increase the risk of myopathy by reducing the elimination of simvastatin. Hence when simvastatin is used with a potent inhibitor of CYP3A4, elevated plasma levels of HMG-CoA reductase inhibitory activity can increase the riskof myopathy and rhabdomyolysis, particularly with higher doses of simvastatin. Concomitant use of drugs labeled as potent inhibitors of CYP3A4 should be avoided unless the benefits of combined therapy outweigh the increased risk. If treatment with itraconazole, ketoconazole, erythromycin, clarithromycin or telithromycin is unavoidable, therapy with Simcor should be suspended

during the course of treatment).
No products indexed under this heading.

Minoxidil (Niacin may potentiate the effects of ganglionic blocking agents and vasoactive drugs resulting in postural hypotension).
No products indexed under this heading.

Moexipril Hydrochloride (Niacin may potentiate the effects of ganglionic blocking agents and vasoactive drugs resulting in postural hypotension).
No products indexed under this heading.

Multivitamins with Minerals (Nutritional supplements containing large doses of niacin or related compounds may potentiate the adverse effects of Simcor). Products include:
CitraNatal DHA Tablets 2175
CitraNatal 90 DHA Tablets 2175

Nadolol (Niacin may potentiate the effects of ganglionic blocking agents and vasoactive drugs resulting in postural hypotension). Products include:
Nadolol Tablets 2191

Nebivolol (Niacin may potentiate the effects of ganglionic blocking agents and vasoactive drugs resulting in postural hypotension). Products include:
Bystolic Tablets 1155

Nefazodone Hydrochloride (Potent inhibitors of CYP3A4 increase the risk of myopathy by reducing the elimination of simvastatin. Hence when simvastatin is used with a potent inhibitor of CYP3A4, elevated plasma levels of HMG-CoA reductase inhibitory activity can increase the riskof myopathy and rhabdomyolysis, particularly with higher doses of simvastatin. Concomitant use of drugs labeled as potent inhibitors of CYP3A4 should be avoided unless the benefits of combined therapy outweigh the increased risk. If treatment with itraconazole, ketoconazole, erythromycin, clarithromycin or telithromycin is unavoidable, therapy with Simcor should be suspended during the course of treatment).
No products indexed under this heading.

Nelfinavir Mesylate (Potent inhibitors of CYP3A4 increase the risk of myopathy by reducing the elimination of simvastatin. Hence when simvastatin is used with a potent inhibitor of CYP3A4, elevated plasma levels of HMG-CoA reductase inhibitory activity can increase the riskof myopathy and rhabdomyolysis, particularly with higher doses of simvastatin. Concomitant use of drugs labeled as potent inhibitors of CYP3A4 should be avoided unless the benefits of combined therapy outweigh the increased risk. If treatment with itraconazole, ketoconazole, erythromycin, clarithromycin or telithromycin is unavoidable, therapy with Simcor should be suspended during the course of treatment).
No products indexed under this heading.

Nevirapine (Potent inhibitors of CYP3A4 increase the risk of myopathy by reducing the elimination of simvastatin. Hence when simvastatin is used with a potent inhibitor of CYP3A4, elevated plasma levels of HMG-CoA reductase inhibitory activity can increase the riskof myopathy and rhabdomyolysis, particularly with higher doses of simvastatin. Concomitant use of drugs labeled as potent inhibitors of CYP3A4 should be avoided unless the benefits of combined therapy outweigh the increased risk. If treatment with itraconazole, ketoconazole, erythromycin, clarithromycin or telithromycin is unavoidable, therapy with Simcor should be suspended during the course of treatment). Products include:
Viramune Oral Suspension 873
Viramune Tablets 873

Niacinamide (Potent inhibitors of CYP3A4 increase the risk of myopathy by reducing the elimination of simvastatin. Hence when simvastatin is used with a potent inhibitor of CYP3A4, elevated plasma levels of HMG-CoA reductase inhibitory activity can increase the riskof myopathy and rhabdomyolysis, particularly with higher doses of simvastatin. Concomitant use of drugs labeled as potent inhibitors of CYP3A4 should be avoided unless the benefits of combined therapy outweigh the increased risk. If treatment with itraconazole, ketoconazole, erythromycin, clarithromycin or telithromycin is unavoidable, therapy with Simcor should be suspended during the course of treatment). Products include:
BioLean Free Tablets .... ▣635

Nicardipine Hydrochloride (Niacin may potentiate the effects of ganglionic blocking agents and vasoactive drugs resulting in postural hypotension). Products include:
Cardene I.V. 1093

Nicotinamide (Potent inhibitors of CYP3A4 increase the risk of myopathy by reducing the elimination of simvastatin. Hence when simvastatin is used with a potent inhibitor of CYP3A4, elevated plasma levels of HMG-CoA reductase inhibitory activity can increase the riskof myopathy and rhabdomyolysis, particularly with higher doses of simvastatin. Concomitant use of drugs labeled as potent inhibitors of CYP3A4 should be avoided unless the benefits of combined therapy outweigh the increased risk. If treatment with itraconazole, ketoconazole, erythromycin, clarithromycin or telithromycin is unavoidable, therapy with Simcor should be suspended during the course of treatment).
No products indexed under this heading.

Nifedipine (Niacin may potentiate the effects of ganglionic blocking agents and vasoactive drugs resulting in postural hypotension).
No products indexed under this heading.

Nisoldipine (Niacin may potentiate the effects of ganglionic blocking agents and vasoactive drugs resulting in postural hypotension). Products include:
Sular Extended Release Tablets 2975

Nitroglycerin (Niacin may potentiate the effects of ganglionic blocking agents and vasoactive drugs resulting in postural hypotension). Products include:
Nitro-Dur Transdermal Infusion System....................................... 2887
Nitrolingual Pumpspray 2965

Norfloxacin (Potent inhibitors of CYP3A4 increase the risk of myopathy by reducing the elimination of simvastatin. Hence when simvastatin is used with a potent inhibitor of CYP3A4, elevated plasma levels of HMG-CoA reductase inhibitory activity can increase the riskof myopathy and rhabdomyolysis, particularly with higher doses of simvastatin. Concomitant use of drugs labeled as potent inhibitors of CYP3A4 should be avoided unless the benefits of combined therapy outweigh the increased risk. If treatment with itraconazole, ketoconazole, erythromycin, clarithromycin or telithromycin is unavoidable, therapy with Simcor should be suspended during the course of treatment). Products include:
Noroxin Tablets 2069

Nutritional Supplement (Nutritional supplements containing large doses of niacin or related compounds may potentiate the adverse effects of Simcor).
No products indexed under this heading.

Omeprazole (Potent inhibitors of CYP3A4 increase the risk of myopathy by reducing the elimination of simvastatin. Hence when simvastatin is used with a potent inhibitor of CYP3A4, elevated plasma levels of HMG-CoA reductase inhibitory activity can increase the riskof myopathy and rhabdomyolysis, particularly with higher doses of simvastatin. Concomitant use of drugs labeled as potent inhibitors of CYP3A4 should be avoided unless the benefits of combined therapy outweigh the increased risk. If treatment with itraconazole, ketoconazole, erythromycin, clarithromycin or telithromycin is unavoidable, therapy with Simcor should be suspended during the course of treatment).
No products indexed under this heading.

Paroxetine Hydrochloride (Potent inhibitors of CYP3A4 increase the risk of myopathy by reducing the elimination of simvastatin. Hence when simvastatin is used with a potent inhibitor of CYP3A4, elevated plasma levels of HMG-CoA reductase inhibitory activity can increase the riskof myopathy and rhabdomyolysis, particularly with higher doses of simvastatin. Concomitant use of drugs labeled as potent inhibitors of CYP3A4 should be avoided unless the benefits of combined therapy outweigh the increased risk. If treatment with itraconazole, ketoconazole, erythromycin, clarithromycin or telithromycin is unavoidable, therapy with Simcor should be suspended during the course of treatment). Products include:
Paxil 1535
Paxil CR Controlled-Release Tablets... 1544

Penbutolol Sulfate (Niacin may potentiate the effects of ganglionic blocking agents and vasoactive drugs resulting in postural hypotension).
No products indexed under this heading.

Perindopril Erbumine (Niacin may potentiate the effects of ganglionic blocking agents and vasoactive drugs resulting in postural hypotension). Products include:
Aceon Tablets (2 mg, 4 mg, 8 mg)... 3038

Phenoxybenzamine Hydrochloride (Niacin may potentiate the effects of ganglionic blocking agents and vasoactive drugs resulting in postural hypotension). Products include:
Dibenzyline Capsules 3188

Phentolamine Mesylate (Niacin may potentiate the effects of ganglionic blocking agents and vasoactive drugs resulting in postural hypotension).
No products indexed under this heading.

Pindolol (Niacin may potentiate the effects of ganglionic blocking agents and vasoactive drugs resulting in postural hypotension).
No products indexed under this heading.

Polythiazide (Niacin may potentiate the effects of ganglionic blocking agents and vasoactive drugs resulting in postural hypotension).
No products indexed under this heading.

Prazosin Hydrochloride (Niacin may potentiate the effects of ganglionic blocking agents and vasoactive drugs resulting in postural hypotension).
No products indexed under this heading.

Propoxyphene Hydrochloride (Potent inhibitors of CYP3A4 increase the risk of myopathy by reducing the elimination of simvastatin. Hence when simvastatin is used with a potent inhibitor of CYP3A4, elevated plasma levels of HMG-CoA reductase inhibitory activity can increase the riskof myopathy and rhabdomyolysis, particularly with higher doses of simvastatin. Concomitant use of drugs labeled as potent inhibitors of CYP3A4 should be avoided unless the benefits of combined therapy outweigh the increased risk. If treatment with itraconazole, ketoconazole, erythromycin, clarithromycin or telithromycin is unavoidable, therapy with Simcor should be suspended during the course of treatment).
No products indexed under this heading.

Propoxyphene Napsylate (Potent inhibitors of CYP3A4 increase the risk of myopathy by reducing the elimination of simvastatin. Hence when simvastatin is used with a potent inhibitor of CYP3A4, elevated plasma levels of HMG-CoA reductase inhibitory activity can increase the riskof myopathy and rhabdomyolysis, particularly with higher doses of simvastatin. Concomitant use of drugs labeled as potent inhibitors of CYP3A4 should be avoided unless the benefits of combined therapy outweigh the increased risk. If treatment with itraconazole, ketoconazole, erythromycin, clarithromycin or telithromycin is unavoidable, therapy with Simcor should be suspended during the course of treatment).
No products indexed under this heading.

Propranolol Hydrochloride (In healthy male volunteers there was a significant decrease in mean Cmax, but no change in AUC, for simvastatin total and active inhibitors with concomitant administration of single doses of simvastatin and propranolol. The clinical relevance of this finding is unclear. The pharmacokinetics

of the enantiomers of propranolol were not affected). Products include:
InnoPran XL Extended Release Capsules 1484

Quinapril Hydrochloride (Niacin may potentiate the effects of ganglionic blocking agents and vasoactive drugs resulting in postural hypotension).
No products indexed under this heading.

Quinidine (Potent inhibitors of CYP3A4 increase the risk of myopathy by reducing the elimination of simvastatin. Hence when simvastatin is used with a potent inhibitor of CYP3A4, elevated plasma levels of HMG-CoA reductase inhibitory activity can increase the riskof myopathy and rhabdomyolysis, particularly with higher doses of simvastatin. Concomitant use of drugs labeled as potent inhibitors of CYP3A4 should be avoided unless the benefits of combined therapy outweigh the increased risk. If treatment with itraconazole, ketoconazole, erythromycin, clarithromycin or telithromycin is unavoidable, therapy with Simcor should be suspended during the course of treatment).
No products indexed under this heading.

Quinidine Hydrochloride (Potent inhibitors of CYP3A4 increase the risk of myopathy by reducing the elimination of simvastatin. Hence when simvastatin is used with a potent inhibitor of CYP3A4, elevated plasma levels of HMG-CoA reductase inhibitory activity can increase the riskof myopathy and rhabdomyolysis, particularly with higher doses of simvastatin. Concomitant use of drugs labeled as potent inhibitors of CYP3A4 should be avoided unless the benefits of combined therapy outweigh the increased risk. If treatment with itraconazole, ketoconazole, erythromycin, clarithromycin or telithromycin is unavoidable, therapy with Simcor should be suspended during the course of treatment).
No products indexed under this heading.

Quinidine Polygalacturonate (Potent inhibitors of CYP3A4 increase the risk of myopathy by reducing the elimination of simvastatin. Hence when simvastatin is used with a potent inhibitor of CYP3A4, elevated plasma levels of HMG-CoA reductase inhibitory activity can increase the riskof myopathy and rhabdomyolysis, particularly with higher doses of simvastatin. Concomitant use of drugs labeled as potent inhibitors of CYP3A4 should be avoided unless the benefits of combined therapy outweigh the increased risk. If treatment with itraconazole, ketoconazole, erythromycin, clarithromycin or telithromycin is unavoidable, therapy with Simcor should be suspended during the course of treatment).
No products indexed under this heading.

Quinidine Sulfate (Potent inhibitors of CYP3A4 increase the risk of myopathy by reducing the elimination of simvastatin. Hence when simvastatin is used with a potent inhibitor of CYP3A4, elevated plasma levels of HMG-CoA reductase inhibitory activity can increase the riskof myopathy and rhabdomyolysis, particularly with higher doses of simvastatin. Concomitant use of drugs labeled as potent inhibitors of CYP3A4 should be avoided unless the benefits of combined therapy outweigh the increased risk. If treatment with itraconazole, ketoconazole, erythromycin, clarithromycin or telithromycin is unavoidable, therapy with Simcor should be suspended during the course of treatment).
No products indexed under this heading.

Quinine (Potent inhibitors of CYP3A4 increase the risk of myopathy by reducing the elimination of simvastatin. Hence when simvastatin is used with a potent inhibitor of CYP3A4, elevated plasma levels of HMG-CoA reductase inhibitory activity can increase the riskof myopathy and rhabdomyolysis, particularly with higher doses of simvastatin. Concomitant use of drugs labeled as potent inhibitors of CYP3A4 should be avoided unless the benefits of combined therapy outweigh the increased risk. If treatment with itraconazole, ketoconazole, erythromycin, clarithromycin or telithromycin is unavoidable, therapy with Simcor should be suspended during the course of treatment).
No products indexed under this heading.

Quinine Sulfate (Potent inhibitors of CYP3A4 increase the risk of myopathy by reducing the elimination of simvastatin. Hence when simvastatin is used with a potent inhibitor of CYP3A4, elevated plasma levels of HMG-CoA reductase inhibitory activity can increase the riskof myopathy and rhabdomyolysis, particularly with higher doses of simvastatin. Concomitant use of drugs labeled as potent inhibitors of CYP3A4 should be avoided unless the benefits of combined therapy outweigh the increased risk. If treatment with itraconazole, ketoconazole, erythromycin, clarithromycin or telithromycin is unavoidable, therapy with Simcor should be suspended during the course of treatment).
No products indexed under this heading.

Quinupristin (Potent inhibitors of CYP3A4 increase the risk of myopathy by reducing the elimination of simvastatin. Hence when simvastatin is used with a potent inhibitor of CYP3A4, elevated plasma levels of HMG-CoA reductase inhibitory activity can increase the riskof myopathy and rhabdomyolysis, particularly with higher doses of simvastatin. Concomitant use of drugs labeled as potent inhibitors of CYP3A4 should be avoided unless the benefits of combined therapy outweigh the increased risk. If treatment with itraconazole, ketoconazole, erythromycin, clarithromycin or telithromycin is unavoidable, therapy with Simcor should be suspended during the course of treatment).
No products indexed under this heading.

Ramipril (Niacin may potentiate the effects of ganglionic blocking agents and vasoactive drugs resulting in postural hypotension).
No products indexed under this heading.

Ranitidine Bismuth Citrate (Potent inhibitors of CYP3A4 increase the risk of myopathy by reducing the elimination of simvastatin. Hence when simvastatin is used with a potent inhibitor of CYP3A4, elevated plasma levels of HMG-CoA reductase inhibitory activity can increase the riskof myopathy and rhabdomyolysis, particularly with higher doses of simvastatin. Concomitant use of drugs labeled as potent inhibitors of CYP3A4 should be avoided unless the benefits of combined therapy outweigh the increased risk. If treatment with itraconazole, ketoconazole, erythromycin, clarithromycin or telithromycin is unavoidable, therapy with Simcor should be suspended during the course of treatment).
No products indexed under this heading.

Ranitidine Hydrochloride (Potent inhibitors of CYP3A4 increase the risk of myopathy by reducing the elimination of simvastatin. Hence when simvastatin is used with a potent inhibitor of CYP3A4, elevated plasma levels of HMG-CoA reductase inhibitory activity can increase the riskof myopathy and rhabdomyolysis, particularly with higher doses of simvastatin. Concomitant use of drugs labeled as potent inhibitors of CYP3A4 should be avoided unless the benefits of combined therapy outweigh the increased risk. If treatment with itraconazole, ketoconazole, erythromycin, clarithromycin or telithromycin is unavoidable, therapy with Simcor should be suspended during the course of treatment). Products include:
Zantac 75 Tablets .... ▣603
Zantac 1670
Zantac Injection 1666
Zantac Injection Pharmacy Bulk Package 1668
Maximum Strength Zantac 150 Tablets .... ▣603
Maximum Strength Zantac 150 Cool Mint Tablets .... ▣603

Rauwolfia Serpentina (Niacin may potentiate the effects of ganglionic blocking agents and vasoactive drugs resulting in postural hypotension).
No products indexed under this heading.

Rescinnamine (Niacin may potentiate the effects of ganglionic blocking agents and vasoactive drugs resulting in postural hypotension).
No products indexed under this heading.

Reserpine (Niacin may potentiate the effects of ganglionic blocking agents and vasoactive drugs resulting in postural hypotension).
No products indexed under this heading.

Ritonavir (Potent inhibitors of CYP3A4 increase the risk of myopathy by reducing the elimination of simvastatin. Hence when simvastatin is used with a potent inhibitor of CYP3A4, elevated plasma levels of HMG-CoA reductase inhibitory activity can increase the riskof myopathy and rhabdomyolysis, particularly with higher doses of simvastatin. Concomitant use of drugs labeled as potent inhibitors of CYP3A4 should be avoided unless the benefits of combined therapy outweigh the increased risk. If treatment with itraconazole, ketoconazole, erythromycin, clarithromycin or telithromycin is unavoidable, therapy with Simcor should be suspended during the course of treatment). Products include:
Kaletra 452
Norvir 489

Saquinavir (Potent inhibitors of CYP3A4 increase the risk of myopathy by reducing the elimination of simvastatin. Hence when simvastatin is used with a potent inhibitor of CYP3A4, elevated plasma levels of HMG-CoA reductase inhibitory activity can increase the riskof myopathy and rhabdomyolysis, particularly with higher doses of simvastatin. Concomitant use of drugs labeled as potent inhibitors of CYP3A4 should be avoided unless the benefits of combined therapy outweigh the increased risk. If treatment with itraconazole, ketoconazole, erythromycin, clarithromycin or telithromycin is unavoidable, therapy with Simcor should be suspended during the course of treatment).
No products indexed under this heading.

Saquinavir Mesylate (Potent inhibitors of CYP3A4 increase the risk of myopathy by reducing the elimination of simvastatin. Hence when simvastatin is used with a potent inhibitor of CYP3A4, elevated plasma levels of HMG-CoA reductase inhibitory activity can increase the riskof myopathy and rhabdomyolysis, particularly with higher doses of simvastatin. Concomitant use of drugs labeled as potent inhibitors of CYP3A4 should be avoided unless the benefits of combined therapy outweigh the increased risk. If treatment with itraconazole, ketoconazole, erythromycin, clarithromycin or telithromycin is unavoidable, therapy with Simcor should be suspended during the course of treatment).
No products indexed under this heading.

Sertraline Hydrochloride (Potent inhibitors of CYP3A4 increase the risk of myopathy by reducing the elimination of simvastatin. Hence when simvastatin is used with a potent inhibitor of CYP3A4, elevated plasma levels of HMG-CoA reductase inhibitory activity can increase the riskof myopathy and rhabdomyolysis, particularly with higher doses of simvastatin. Concomitant use of drugs labeled as potent inhibitors of CYP3A4 should be avoided unless the benefits of combined therapy outweigh the increased risk. If treatment with itraconazole, ketoconazole, erythromycin, clarithromycin or telithromycin is unavoidable, therapy with Simcor should be suspended during the course of treatment).
No products indexed under this heading.

Sildenafil Citrate (Potent inhibitors of CYP3A4 increase the risk of myopathy by reducing the elimination of simvastatin. Hence when simvastatin is used with a potent inhibitor of CYP3A4, elevated plasma levels of HMG-CoA reductase inhibitory activity can increase the riskof myopathy and rhabdomyolysis, particularly with higher doses of simvastatin. Concomitant use of drugs labeled as potent inhibitors of CYP3A4 should be avoided unless the benefits of combined therapy outweigh the increased risk. If treatment with itraconazole, ketoconazole, erythromycin, clarithromycin or telithromycin is unavoidable, therapy with Simcor should be suspended

during the course of treatment).
No products indexed under this heading.

Sodium Nitroprusside (Niacin may potentiate the effects of ganglionic blocking agents and vasoactive drugs resulting in postural hypotension).
No products indexed under this heading.

Sotalol Hydrochloride (Niacin may potentiate the effects of ganglionic blocking agents and vasoactive drugs resulting in postural hypotension).
No products indexed under this heading.

Spirapril Hydrochloride (Niacin may potentiate the effects of ganglionic blocking agents and vasoactive drugs resulting in postural hypotension).
No products indexed under this heading.

Telithromycin (Potent inhibitors of CYP3A4 increase the risk of myopathy by reducing the elimination of simvastatin. Hence when simvastatin is used with a potent inhibitor of CYP3A4, elevated plasma levels of HMG-CoA reductase inhibitory activity can increase the riskof myopathy and rhabdomyolysis, particularly with higher doses of simvastatin. Concomitant use of drugs labeled as potent inhibitors of CYP3A4 should be avoided unless the benefits of combined therapy outweigh the increased risk. If treatment with itraconazole, ketoconazole, erythromycin, clarithromycin or telithromycin is unavoidable, therapy with Simcor should be suspended during the course of treatment). Products include:
Ketek Tablets 2744

Telmisartan (Niacin may potentiate the effects of ganglionic blocking agents and vasoactive drugs resulting in postural hypotension).
Products include:
Micardis Tablets 852
Micardis HCT Tablets 854

Terazosin Hydrochloride (Niacin may potentiate the effects of ganglionic blocking agents and vasoactive drugs resulting in postural hypotension).
No products indexed under this heading.

Timolol Maleate (Niacin may potentiate the effects of ganglionic blocking agents and vasoactive drugs resulting in postural hypotension). Products include:
Combigan Ophthalmic Solution 553
Cosopt Sterile Ophthalmic Solution 1969
Timoptic Sterile Ophthalmic Solution 2121
Timoptic in Ocudose 2124
Timoptic-XE Sterile Ophthalmic Gel Forming Solution 2125

Torsemide (Niacin may potentiate the effects of ganglionic blocking agents and vasoactive drugs resulting in postural hypotension).
Products include:
Demadex Injection 2630
Demadex Tablets 2630

Trandolapril (Niacin may potentiate the effects of ganglionic blocking agents and vasoactive drugs resulting in postural hypotension).
Products include:
Mavik Tablets 472
Tarka Tablets 511

Trimethaphan Camsylate (Niacin may potentiate the effects of ganglionic blocking agents and vasoactive drugs resulting in postural hypotension).
No products indexed under this heading.

Troglitazone (Potent inhibitors of CYP3A4 increase the risk of myopathy by reducing the elimination of simvastatin. Hence when simvastatin is used with a potent inhibitor of CYP3A4, elevated plasma levels of HMG-CoA reductase inhibitory activity can increase the riskof myopathy and rhabdomyolysis, particularly with higher doses of simvastatin. Concomitant use of drugs labeled as potent inhibitors of CYP3A4 should be avoided unless the benefits of combined therapy outweigh the increased risk. If treatment with itraconazole, ketoconazole, erythromycin, clarithromycin or telithromycin is unavoidable, therapy with Simcor should be suspended during the course of treatment).
No products indexed under this heading.

Troleandomycin (Potent inhibitors of CYP3A4 increase the risk of myopathy by reducing the elimination of simvastatin. Hence when simvastatin is used with a potent inhibitor of CYP3A4, elevated plasma levels of HMG-CoA reductase inhibitory activity can increase the riskof myopathy and rhabdomyolysis, particularly with higher doses of simvastatin. Concomitant use of drugs labeled as potent inhibitors of CYP3A4 should be avoided unless the benefits of combined therapy outweigh the increased risk. If treatment with itraconazole, ketoconazole, erythromycin, clarithromycin or telithromycin is unavoidable, therapy with Simcor should be suspended during the course of treatment).
No products indexed under this heading.

Valproate Sodium (Potent inhibitors of CYP3A4 increase the risk of myopathy by reducing the elimination of simvastatin. Hence when simvastatin is used with a potent inhibitor of CYP3A4, elevated plasma levels of HMG-CoA reductase inhibitory activity can increase the riskof myopathy and rhabdomyolysis, particularly with higher doses of simvastatin. Concomitant use of drugs labeled as potent inhibitors of CYP3A4 should be avoided unless the benefits of combined therapy outweigh the increased risk. If treatment with itraconazole, ketoconazole, erythromycin, clarithromycin or telithromycin is unavoidable, therapy with Simcor should be suspended during the course of treatment).
No products indexed under this heading.

Valsartan (Niacin may potentiate the effects of ganglionic blocking agents and vasoactive drugs resulting in postural hypotension).
Products include:
Diovan Tablets 2212
Diovan HCT Tablets 2216
Exforge Tablets 2238

Vardenafil Hydrochloride (Potent inhibitors of CYP3A4 increase the risk of myopathy by reducing the elimination of simvastatin. Hence when simvastatin is used with a potent inhibitor of CYP3A4, elevated plasma levels of HMG-CoA reductase inhibitory activity can increase the riskof myopathy and rhabdomyolysis, particularly with higher doses of simvastatin. Concomitant use of drugs labeled as potent inhibitors of CYP3A4 should be avoided unless the benefits of combined therapy outweigh the increased risk. If treatment with itraconazole, ketoconazole, erythromycin, clarithromycin or telithromycin is unavoidable, therapy with Simcor should be suspended during the course of treatment).
Products include:
Levitra Tablets 2876

Verapamil Hydrochloride (The risk of myopathy/rhabdomyolysis is increased by concomitant administration of amiodarone or verapamil with higher doses of simvastatin. Combination with Simcor should be limited to the 20 mg once daily dose of simvastatin). Products include:
Tarka Tablets 511

Vitamin B Complex (Nutritional supplements containing large doses of niacin or related compounds may potentiate the adverse effects of simvastatin).
No products indexed under this heading.

Vitamin B Complex With Vitamin C (Nutritional supplements containing large doses of niacin or related compounds may potentiate the adverse effects of simvastatin).
No products indexed under this heading.

Vitamins, Multiple (Nutritional supplements containing large doses of niacin or related compounds may potentiate the adverse effects of Simcor). Products include:
Bausch & Lomb Ocuvite DF Vitamin Supplement .... ⊙ 238
Mega Antioxidant Tablets 3174
Vibe Liquid Multi-Nutrient Supplement .... ▣ 626

Voriconazole (Potent inhibitors of CYP3A4 increase the risk of myopathy by reducing the elimination of simvastatin. Hence when simvastatin is used with a potent inhibitor of CYP3A4, elevated plasma levels of HMG-CoA reductase inhibitory activity can increase the riskof myopathy and rhabdomyolysis, particularly with higher doses of simvastatin. Concomitant use of drugs labeled as potent inhibitors of CYP3A4 should be avoided unless the benefits of combined therapy outweigh the increased risk. If treatment with itraconazole, ketoconazole, erythromycin, clarithromycin or telithromycin is unavoidable, therapy with Simcor should be suspended during the course of treatment).
No products indexed under this heading.

Warfarin Sodium (Coadministration prolongs INR. Achieve stable INR prior to starting Simcor. Monitor INR frequently until stable upon initiation or alteration of Simcor therapy).
No products indexed under this heading.

Zafirlukast (Potent inhibitors of CYP3A4 increase the risk of myopathy by reducing the elimination of simvastatin. Hence when simvastatin is used with a potent inhibitor of CYP3A4, elevated plasma levels of HMG-CoA reductase inhibitory activity can increase the riskof myopathy and rhabdomyolysis, particularly with higher doses of simvastatin. Concomitant use of drugs labeled as potent inhibitors of CYP3A4 should be avoided unless the benefits of combined therapy outweigh the increased risk. If treatment with itraconazole, ketoconazole, erythromycin, clarithromycin or telithromycin is unavoidable, therapy with Simcor should be suspended during the course of treatment). Products include:
Accolate Tablets 669

Zileuton (Potent inhibitors of CYP3A4 increase the risk of myopathy by reducing the elimination of simvastatin. Hence when simvastatin is used with a potent inhibitor of CYP3A4, elevated plasma levels of HMG-CoA reductase inhibitory activity can increase the riskof myopathy and rhabdomyolysis, particularly with higher doses of simvastatin. Concomitant use of drugs labeled as potent inhibitors of CYP3A4 should be avoided unless the benefits of combined therapy outweigh the increased risk. If treatment with itraconazole, ketoconazole, erythromycin, clarithromycin or telithromycin is unavoidable, therapy with Simcor should be suspended during the course of treatment).
No products indexed under this heading.

Food Interactions

Grapefruit (Potent inhibitors of CYP3A4 increase the risk of myopathy by reducing the elimination of simvastatin. Hence when simvastatin is used with a potent inhibitor of CYP3A4, elevated plasma levels of HMG-CoA reductase inhibitory activity can increase the riskof myopathy and rhabdomyolysis, particularly with higher doses of simvastatin. Concomitant use of drugs labeled as potent inhibitors of CYP3A4 should be avoided unless the benefits of combined therapy outweigh the increased risk. If treatment with itraconazole, ketoconazole, erythromycin, clarithromycin or telithromycin is unavoidable, therapy with Simcor should be suspended during the course of treatment).

Grapefruit Juice (Potent inhibitors of CYP3A4 increase the risk of myopathy by reducing the elimination of simvastatin. Hence when simvastatin is used with a potent inhibitor of CYP3A4, elevated plasma levels of HMG-CoA reductase inhibitory activity can increase the riskof myopathy and rhabdomyolysis, particularly with higher doses of simvastatin. Concomitant use of drugs labeled as potent inhibitors of CYP3A4 should be avoided unless the benefits of combined therapy outweigh the increased risk. If treatment with itraconazole, ketoconazole, erythromycin, clarithromycin or telithromycin is unavoidable, therapy with Simcor should be suspended during the course of treatment).

SIMPLY SLEEP CAPLETS

(Diphenhydramine Hydrochloride) 1905
May interact with hypnotics and sedatives, tranquilizers, and certain other agents. Compounds in these categories include:

Alprazolam (Diphenhydramine is an antihistamine with sedative properties; concurrent use should be avoided).
No products indexed under this heading.

Buspirone Hydrochloride (Diphenhydramine is an antihistamine with sedative properties; concurrent use should be avoided).
No products indexed under this heading.

Butabarbital (Diphenhydramine is an antihistamine with sedative properties; concurrent use should be avoided).
No products indexed under this heading.

Butabarbital Sodium (Diphenhydramine is an antihistamine with sedative properties; concurrent use should be avoided).
No products indexed under this heading.

Chloral Hydrate (Diphenhydramine is an antihistamine with sedative properties; concurrent use should be avoided).
No products indexed under this heading.

Chlordiazepoxide (Diphenhydramine is an antihistamine with sedative properties; concurrent use should be avoided).
No products indexed under this heading.

Chlordiazepoxide Hydrochloride (Diphenhydramine is an antihistamine with sedative properties; concurrent use should be avoided).
No products indexed under this heading.

Chlorpromazine (Diphenhydramine is an antihistamine with sedative properties; concurrent use should be avoided).
No products indexed under this heading.

Chlorpromazine Hydrochloride (Diphenhydramine is an antihistamine with sedative properties; concurrent use should be avoided).
No products indexed under this heading.

Chlorprothixene (Diphenhydramine is an antihistamine with sedative properties; concurrent use should be avoided).
No products indexed under this heading.

Chlorprothixene Hydrochloride (Diphenhydramine is an antihistamine with sedative properties; concurrent use should be avoided).
No products indexed under this heading.

Clorazepate Dipotassium (Diphenhydramine is an antihistamine with sedative properties; concurrent use should be avoided).
No products indexed under this heading.

Diazepam (Diphenhydramine is an antihistamine with sedative properties; concurrent use should be avoided). Products include:
Valium Tablets 2658

Droperidol (Diphenhydramine is an antihistamine with sedative properties; concurrent use should be avoided).
No products indexed under this heading.

Estazolam (Diphenhydramine is an antihistamine with sedative properties; concurrent use should be avoided).
No products indexed under this heading.

Ethchlorvynol (Diphenhydramine is an antihistamine with sedative properties; concurrent use should be avoided).
No products indexed under this heading.

Ethinamate (Diphenhydramine is an antihistamine with sedative properties; concurrent use should be avoided).
No products indexed under this heading.

Fluphenazine Decanoate (Diphenhydramine is an antihistamine with sedative properties; concurrent use should be avoided).
No products indexed under this heading.

Fluphenazine Enanthate (Diphenhydramine is an antihistamine with sedative properties; concurrent use should be avoided).
No products indexed under this heading.

Fluphenazine Hydrochloride (Diphenhydramine is an antihistamine with sedative properties; concurrent use should be avoided).
No products indexed under this heading.

Flurazepam Hydrochloride (Diphenhydramine is an antihistamine with sedative properties; concurrent use should be avoided).
No products indexed under this heading.

Glutethimide (Diphenhydramine is an antihistamine with sedative properties; concurrent use should be avoided).
No products indexed under this heading.

Haloperidol (Diphenhydramine is an antihistamine with sedative properties; concurrent use should be avoided).
No products indexed under this heading.

Haloperidol Decanoate (Diphenhydramine is an antihistamine with sedative properties; concurrent use should be avoided).
No products indexed under this heading.

Hydroxyzine Hydrochloride (Diphenhydramine is an antihistamine with sedative properties; concurrent use should be avoided).
No products indexed under this heading.

Lorazepam (Diphenhydramine is an antihistamine with sedative properties; concurrent use should be avoided).
No products indexed under this heading.

Loxapine Hydrochloride (Diphenhydramine is an antihistamine with sedative properties; concurrent use should be avoided).
No products indexed under this heading.

Loxapine Succinate (Diphenhydramine is an antihistamine with sedative properties; concurrent use should be avoided).
No products indexed under this heading.

Meprobamate (Diphenhydramine is an antihistamine with sedative properties; concurrent use should be avoided).
No products indexed under this heading.

Mesoridazine Besylate (Diphenhydramine is an antihistamine with sedative properties; concurrent use should be avoided).
No products indexed under this heading.

Midazolam Hydrochloride (Diphenhydramine is an antihistamine with sedative properties; concurrent use should be avoided).
No products indexed under this heading.

Molindone Hydrochloride (Diphenhydramine is an antihistamine with sedative properties; concurrent use should be avoided). Products include:
Moban Tablets 1116

Oxazepam (Diphenhydramine is an antihistamine with sedative properties; concurrent use should be avoided).
No products indexed under this heading.

Perphenazine (Diphenhydramine is an antihistamine with sedative properties; concurrent use should be avoided).
No products indexed under this heading.

Prazepam (Diphenhydramine is an antihistamine with sedative properties; concurrent use should be avoided).
No products indexed under this heading.

Prochlorperazine (Diphenhydramine is an antihistamine with sedative properties; concurrent use should be avoided).
No products indexed under this heading.

Promethazine Hydrochloride (Diphenhydramine is an antihistamine with sedative properties; concurrent use should be avoided).
No products indexed under this heading.

Propofol (Diphenhydramine is an antihistamine with sedative properties; concurrent use should be avoided).
No products indexed under this heading.

Quazepam (Diphenhydramine is an antihistamine with sedative properties; concurrent use should be avoided).
No products indexed under this heading.

Ramelteon (Diphenhydramine is an antihistamine with sedative properties; concurrent use should be avoided). Products include:
Rozerem Tablets 3091

Secobarbital Sodium (Diphenhydramine is an antihistamine with sedative properties; concurrent use should be avoided).
No products indexed under this heading.

Sodium Butabarbital (Diphenhydramine is an antihistamine with sedative properties; concurrent use should be avoided).
No products indexed under this heading.

Temazepam (Diphenhydramine is an antihistamine with sedative properties; concurrent use should be avoided).
No products indexed under this heading.

Thioridazine Hydrochloride (Diphenhydramine is an antihistamine with sedative properties; concurrent use should be avoided). Products include:
Thioridazine Hydrochloride Tablets 2195

Thiothixene (Diphenhydramine is an antihistamine with sedative properties; concurrent use should be avoided). Products include:
Thiothixene Capsules 2197

Triazolam (Diphenhydramine is an antihistamine with sedative properties; concurrent use should be avoided).
No products indexed under this heading.

Trifluoperazine Hydrochloride (Diphenhydramine is an antihistamine with sedative properties; concurrent use should be avoided).
No products indexed under this heading.

Zaleplon (Diphenhydramine is an antihistamine with sedative properties; concurrent use should be avoided).
No products indexed under this heading.

Zolpidem Tartrate (Diphenhydramine is an antihistamine with sedative properties; concurrent use should be avoided). Products include:
Ambien Tablets 2692
Ambien CR Tablets 2696

Food Interactions

Alcohol (Diphenhydramine is an antihistamine with sedative properties; concurrent use with alcoholic beverages should be avoided).

SIMPLY SOOTHING SALINE DROPS
(Sodium Chloride) 1905
None cited in PDR database.

SIMPLY SOOTHING SALINE SPRAY
(Sodium Chloride) 1905
None cited in PDR database.

SIMULECT FOR INJECTION
(Basiliximab) 2306
None cited in PDR database.

SINGULAIR TABLETS
(Montelukast Sodium) 2114
May interact with cytochrome p450 2c8 substrates (selected) and certain other agents. Compounds in these categories include:

Amiodarone Hydrochloride (Montelukast is a potent inhibitor of P450 2C8, but no in vivo drug interaction studies have been conducted between montelukast and cytochrome P450 2C8 substrates. Caution should be exercised when concomitantly administering a cytochrome P450 2C8 substrate).
No products indexed under this heading.

Amitriptyline Hydrochloride (Montelukast is a potent inhibitor of P450 2C8, but no in vivo drug interaction studies have been conducted between montelukast and cytochrome P450 2C8 substrates. Caution should be exercised when concomitantly administering a cytochrome P450 2C8 substrate).
No products indexed under this heading.

Amoxapine (Montelukast is a potent inhibitor of P450 2C8, but no in vivo drug interaction studies have been conducted between montelukast and cytochrome P450 2C8 substrates. Caution should be exercised when concomitantly administering a cytochrome P450 2C8 substrate).
No products indexed under this heading.

Benzphetamine Hydrochloride (Montelukast is a potent inhibitor of P450 2C8, but no in vivo drug interaction studies have been conducted between montelukast and cytochrome P450 2C8 substrates. Caution should be exercised when concomitantly administering a cytochrome P450 2C8 substrate).
No products indexed under this heading.

Carbamazepine (Montelukast is a potent inhibitor of P450 2C8, but no in vivo drug interaction studies have been conducted between montelukast and cytochrome P450 2C8 substrates. Caution should be exercised when concomitantly administering a cytochrome P450 2C8 substrate). Products include:
Carbatrol Capsules **3019**
Equetro Extended-Release Capsules **3174**

Clomipramine Hydrochloride (Montelukast is a potent inhibitor of P450 2C8, but no in vivo drug interaction studies have been conducted between montelukast and cytochrome P450 2C8 substrates. Caution should be exercised when concomitantly administering a cytochrome P450 2C8 substrate).
No products indexed under this heading.

Desipramine Hydrochloride (Montelukast is a potent inhibitor of P450 2C8, but no in vivo drug interaction studies have been conducted between montelukast and cytochrome P450 2C8 substrates. Caution should be exercised when concomitantly administering a cytochrome P450 2C8 substrate).
No products indexed under this heading.

Diazepam (Montelukast is a potent inhibitor of P450 2C8, but no in vivo drug interaction studies have been conducted between montelukast and cytochrome P450 2C8 substrates. Caution should be exercised when concomitantly administering a cytochrome P450 2C8 substrate).
Products include:
Valium Tablets **2658**

Diclofenac Potassium (Montelukast is a potent inhibitor of P450 2C8, but no in vivo drug interaction studies have been conducted between montelukast and cytochrome P450 2C8 substrates. Caution should be exercised when concomitantly administering a cytochrome P450 2C8 substrate).
No products indexed under this heading.

Diclofenac Sodium (Montelukast is a potent inhibitor of P450 2C8, but no in vivo drug interaction studies have been conducted between montelukast and cytochrome P450 2C8 substrates. Caution should be exercised when concomitantly administering a cytochrome P450 2C8 substrate). Products include:
Diclofenac Sodium Ophthalmic Solution .... ⊙**240**
Voltaren Ophthalmic Solution **2336**
Voltaren Tablets **2334**
Voltaren-XR Tablets **2337**

Docetaxel (Montelukast is a potent inhibitor of P450 2C8, but no in vivo drug interaction studies have been conducted between montelukast and cytochrome P450 2C8 substrates. Caution should be exercised when concomitantly administering a cytochrome P450 2C8 substrate).
Products include:
Taxotere Injection Concentrate **2773**

Doxepin Hydrochloride (Montelukast is a potent inhibitor of P450 2C8, but no in vivo drug interaction studies have been conducted between montelukast and cytochrome P450 2C8 substrates. Caution should be exercised when concomitantly administering a cytochrome P450 2C8 substrate).
No products indexed under this heading.

Fluvastatin Sodium (Montelukast is a potent inhibitor of P450 2C8, but no in vivo drug interaction studies have been conducted between montelukast and cytochrome P450 2C8 substrates. Caution should be exercised when concomitantly administering a cytochrome P450 2C8 substrate). Products include:
Lescol Capsules **2268**
Lescol XL Tablets **2268**

Imipramine Hydrochloride (Montelukast is a potent inhibitor of P450 2C8, but no in vivo drug interaction studies have been conducted between montelukast and cytochrome P450 2C8 substrates. Caution should be exercised when concomitantly administering a cytochrome P450 2C8 substrate).
No products indexed under this heading.

Imipramine Pamoate (Montelukast is a potent inhibitor of P450 2C8, but no in vivo drug interaction studies have been conducted between montelukast and cytochrome P450 2C8 substrates. Caution should be exercised when concomitantly administering a cytochrome P450 2C8 substrate).
No products indexed under this heading.

Isotretinoin (Montelukast is a potent inhibitor of P450 2C8, but no in vivo drug interaction studies have been conducted between montelukast and cytochrome P450 2C8 substrates. Caution should be exercised when concomitantly administering a cytochrome P450 2C8 substrate). Products include:
Accutane Capsules **2607**

Maprotiline Hydrochloride (Montelukast is a potent inhibitor of P450 2C8, but no in vivo drug interaction studies have been conducted between montelukast and cytochrome P450 2C8 substrates. Caution should be exercised when concomitantly administering a cytochrome P450 2C8 substrate).
No products indexed under this heading.

Mephobarbital (Montelukast is a potent inhibitor of P450 2C8, but no in vivo drug interaction studies have been conducted between montelukast and cytochrome P450 2C8 substrates. Caution should be exercised when concomitantly administering a cytochrome P450 2C8 substrate).
No products indexed under this heading.

Nortriptyline Hydrochloride (Montelukast is a potent inhibitor of P450 2C8, but no in vivo drug interaction studies have been conducted between montelukast and cytochrome P450 2C8 substrates. Caution should be exercised when concomitantly administering a cytochrome P450 2C8 substrate).
No products indexed under this heading.

Omeprazole (Montelukast is a potent inhibitor of P450 2C8, but no in vivo drug interaction studies have been conducted between montelukast and cytochrome P450 2C8 substrates. Caution should be exercised when concomitantly administering a cytochrome P450 2C8 substrate).
No products indexed under this heading.

Paclitaxel (Montelukast is a potent inhibitor of P450 2C8, but no in vivo drug interaction studies have been conducted between montelukast and cytochrome P450 2C8 substrates. Caution should be exercised when concomitantly administering a cytochrome P450 2C8 substrate).
No products indexed under this heading.

Phenobarbital (Induces hepatic metabolism and decreases the AUC of montelukast approximately 40%; no dosage adjustment for Singulair is recommended). Products include:
Donnatal Extentabs **2507**

Phenytoin (Montelukast is a potent inhibitor of P450 2C8, but no in vivo drug interaction studies have been conducted between montelukast and cytochrome P450 2C8 substrates. Caution should be exercised when concomitantly administering a cytochrome P450 2C8 substrate).
No products indexed under this heading.

Phenytoin Sodium (Montelukast is a potent inhibitor of P450 2C8, but no in vivo drug interaction studies have been conducted between montelukast and cytochrome P450 2C8 substrates. Caution should be exercised when concomitantly administering a cytochrome P450 2C8 substrate). Products include:
Phenytek Capsules **2192**

Pioglitazone Hydrochloride (Montelukast is a potent inhibitor of P450 2C8, but no in vivo drug interaction studies have been conducted between montelukast and cytochrome P450 2C8 substrates. Caution should be exercised when concomitantly administering a cytochrome P450 2C8 substrate).
Products include:
ActoPlus Met Tablets **3071**
Actos Tablets **3077**
Duetact Tablets **3085**

Protriptyline Hydrochloride (Montelukast is a potent inhibitor of P450 2C8, but no in vivo drug interaction studies have been conducted between montelukast and cytochrome P450 2C8 substrates. Caution should be exercised when concomitantly administering a cytochrome P450 2C8 substrate).
No products indexed under this heading.

Repaglinide (Montelukast is a potent inhibitor of P450 2C8, but no in vivo drug interaction studies have been conducted between montelukast and cytochrome P450 2C8 substrates. Caution should be exercised when concomitantly administering a cytochrome P450 2C8 substrate). Products include:
PrandiMet Tablets **2967**
Prandin Tablets **2971**

Rifampin (Co-administration with CYP450 enzyme inducers, such as rifampin, may alter metabolism of montelukast; it is reasonable to employ appropriate clinical monitoring).
No products indexed under this heading.

Rosiglitazone Maleate (Montelukast is a potent inhibitor of P450 2C8, but no in vivo drug interaction studies have been conducted between montelukast and cytochrome P450 2C8 substrates. Caution should be exercised when concomitantly administering a cytochrome P450 2C8 substrate).
Products include:
Avandamet Tablets **1336**
Avandaryl Tablets **1344**
Avandia Tablets **1351**

Rosiglitazone/Metformin (Montelukast is a potent inhibitor of P450 2C8, but no in vivo drug interaction studies have been conducted between montelukast and cytochrome P450 2C8 substrates. Caution should be exercised when concomitantly administering a cytochrome P450 2C8 substrate).
No products indexed under this heading.

Tolbutamide (Montelukast is a potent inhibitor of P450 2C8, but no in vivo drug interaction studies have been conducted between montelukast and cytochrome P450 2C8 substrates. Caution should be exercised when concomitantly administering a cytochrome P450 2C8 substrate).
No products indexed under this heading.

Tolbutamide Sodium (Montelukast is a potent inhibitor of P450 2C8, but no in vivo drug interaction studies have been conducted between montelukast and cytochrome P450 2C8 substrates. Caution should be exercised when concomitantly administering a cytochrome P450 2C8 substrate).
No products indexed under this heading.

Tretinoin (Montelukast is a potent inhibitor of P450 2C8, but no in vivo drug interaction studies have been conducted between montelukast and cytochrome P450 2C8 substrates. Caution should be exercised when concomitantly administering a cytochrome P450 2C8 substrate).
Products include:
Vesanoid Capsules **2660**
Ziana Gel **1942**

Trimipramine Maleate (Montelukast is a potent inhibitor of P450 2C8, but no in vivo drug interaction studies have been conducted between montelukast and cytochrome P450 2C8 substrates. Caution should be exercised when concomitantly administering a cytochrome P450 2C8 substrate).
No products indexed under this heading.

Verapamil Hydrochloride (Montelukast is a potent inhibitor of P450 2C8, but no in vivo drug interaction studies have been conducted between montelukast and cytochrome P450 2C8 substrates. Caution should be exercised when concomitantly administering a cytochrome P450 2C8 substrate).
Products include:
Tarka Tablets 511

Vitamin A (Montelukast is a potent inhibitor of P450 2C8, but no in vivo drug interaction studies have been conducted between montelukast and cytochrome P450 2C8 substrates. Caution should be exercised when concomitantly administering a cytochrome P450 2C8 substrate).
Products include:
Norwegian Cod Liver Oil 949

Vitamin A Acetate (Montelukast is a potent inhibitor of P450 2C8, but no in vivo drug interaction studies have been conducted between montelukast and cytochrome P450 2C8 substrates. Caution should be exercised when concomitantly administering a cytochrome P450 2C8 substrate).
No products indexed under this heading.

Warfarin Sodium (Montelukast is a potent inhibitor of P450 2C8, but no in vivo drug interaction studies have been conducted between montelukast and cytochrome P450 2C8 substrates. Caution should be exercised when concomitantly administering a cytochrome P450 2C8 substrate).
No products indexed under this heading.

Zopiclone (Montelukast is a potent inhibitor of P450 2C8, but no in vivo drug interaction studies have been conducted between montelukast and cytochrome P450 2C8 substrates. Caution should be exercised when concomitantly administering a cytochrome P450 2C8 substrate).
No products indexed under this heading.

SINGULAIR CHEWABLE TABLETS
(Montelukast Sodium) 2114
See Singulair Tablets

SINGULAIR ORAL GRANULES
(Montelukast Sodium) 2114
See Singulair Tablets

SINUTAB NON-DRYING CAPLETS
(Guaifenesin, Phenylephrine Hydrochloride) 1905
May interact with monoamine oxidase inhibitors and certain other agents. Compounds in these categories include:

Isocarboxazid (Concurrent and/or sequential use with MAO inhibitors is not recommended). Products include:
Marplan Tablets 3177

Moclobemide (Concurrent and/or sequential use with MAO inhibitors is not recommended).
No products indexed under this heading.

Pargyline Hydrochloride (Concurrent and/or sequential use with MAO inhibitors is not recommended).
No products indexed under this heading.

Phenelzine Sulfate (Concurrent and/or sequential use with MAO inhibitors is not recommended).
No products indexed under this heading.

Procarbazine Hydrochloride (Concurrent and/or sequential use with MAO inhibitors is not recommended).
No products indexed under this heading.

Rasagiline Mesylate (Concurrent and/or sequential use with MAO inhibitors is not recommended).
Products include:
Azilect Tablets 3106

Selegiline (Concurrent and/or sequential use with MAO inhibitors is not recommended). Products include:
Emsam Transdermal System 905

Selegiline Hydrochloride (Concurrent and/or sequential use with MAO inhibitors is not recommended).
Products include:
Eldepryl Capsules 3052

Tranylcypromine Sulfate (Concurrent and/or sequential use with MAO inhibitors is not recommended).
Products include:
Parnate Tablets 1532

Food Interactions

Alcohol (Patients consuming 3 or more alcohol-containing drinks per day should consult physician for advice on when and how they should take this product).

SINUTAB SINUS CAPLETS
(Acetaminophen, Phenylephrine Hydrochloride) 1905
May interact with monoamine oxidase inhibitors and certain other agents. Compounds in these categories include:

Isocarboxazid (Concurrent and/or sequential use with MAO inhibitors is not recommended). Products include:
Marplan Tablets 3177

Moclobemide (Concurrent and/or sequential use with MAO inhibitors is not recommended).
No products indexed under this heading.

Pargyline Hydrochloride (Concurrent and/or sequential use with MAO inhibitors is not recommended).
No products indexed under this heading.

Phenelzine Sulfate (Concurrent and/or sequential use with MAO inhibitors is not recommended).
No products indexed under this heading.

Procarbazine Hydrochloride (Concurrent and/or sequential use with MAO inhibitors is not recommended).
No products indexed under this heading.

Rasagiline Mesylate (Concurrent and/or sequential use with MAO inhibitors is not recommended).
Products include:
Azilect Tablets 3106

Selegiline (Concurrent and/or sequential use with MAO inhibitors is not recommended). Products include:
Emsam Transdermal System 905

Selegiline Hydrochloride (Concurrent and/or sequential use with MAO inhibitors is not recommended).
Products include:
Eldepryl Capsules 3052

Tranylcypromine Sulfate (Concurrent and/or sequential use with MAO inhibitors is not recommended).
Products include:
Parnate Tablets 1532

Food Interactions

Alcohol (Patients consuming 3 or more alcohol-containing drinks per day should consult physician for advice on when and how they should take this product).

SKELAXIN TABLETS
(Metaxalone) 1784
May interact with barbiturates, central nervous system depressants, and certain other agents. Compounds in these categories include:

Alfentanil Hydrochloride (Skelaxin may enhance the effects of alcohol, barbiturates and other CNS depressants).
No products indexed under this heading.

Alprazolam (Skelaxin may enhance the effects of alcohol, barbiturates and other CNS depressants).
No products indexed under this heading.

Aprobarbital (Skelaxin may enhance the effects of alcohol, barbiturates and other CNS depressants).
No products indexed under this heading.

Buprenorphine Hydrochloride (Skelaxin may enhance the effects of alcohol, barbiturates and other CNS depressants). Products include:
Suboxone Tablets 2601
Subutex Tablets 2601

Buspirone Hydrochloride (Skelaxin may enhance the effects of alcohol, barbiturates and other CNS depressants).
No products indexed under this heading.

Butabarbital (Skelaxin may enhance the effects of alcohol, barbiturates and other CNS depressants).
No products indexed under this heading.

Butalbital (Skelaxin may enhance the effects of alcohol, barbiturates and other CNS depressants).
No products indexed under this heading.

Chlordiazepoxide (Skelaxin may enhance the effects of alcohol, barbiturates and other CNS depressants).
No products indexed under this heading.

Chlordiazepoxide Hydrochloride (Skelaxin may enhance the effects of alcohol, barbiturates and other CNS depressants).
No products indexed under this heading.

Chlorpromazine (Skelaxin may enhance the effects of alcohol, barbiturates and other CNS depressants).
No products indexed under this heading.

Chlorpromazine Hydrochloride (Skelaxin may enhance the effects of alcohol, barbiturates and other CNS depressants).
No products indexed under this heading.

Chlorprothixene (Skelaxin may enhance the effects of alcohol, barbiturates and other CNS depressants).
No products indexed under this heading.

Chlorprothixene Hydrochloride (Skelaxin may enhance the effects of alcohol, barbiturates and other CNS depressants).
No products indexed under this heading.

Chlorprothixene Lactate (Skelaxin may enhance the effects of alcohol, barbiturates and other CNS depressants).
No products indexed under this heading.

Clorazepate Dipotassium (Skelaxin may enhance the effects of alcohol, barbiturates and other CNS depressants).
No products indexed under this heading.

Clozapine (Skelaxin may enhance the effects of alcohol, barbiturates and other CNS depressants).
No products indexed under this heading.

Codeine Phosphate (Skelaxin may enhance the effects of alcohol, barbiturates and other CNS depressants). Products include:
Tylenol with Codeine Tablets 2427

Desflurane (Skelaxin may enhance the effects of alcohol, barbiturates and other CNS depressants).
No products indexed under this heading.

Dezocine (Skelaxin may enhance the effects of alcohol, barbiturates and other CNS depressants).
No products indexed under this heading.

Diazepam (Skelaxin may enhance the effects of alcohol, barbiturates and other CNS depressants).
Products include:
Valium Tablets 2658

Droperidol (Skelaxin may enhance the effects of alcohol, barbiturates and other CNS depressants).
No products indexed under this heading.

Enflurane (Skelaxin may enhance the effects of alcohol, barbiturates and other CNS depressants).
No products indexed under this heading.

Estazolam (Skelaxin may enhance the effects of alcohol, barbiturates and other CNS depressants).
No products indexed under this heading.

Ethanol (Skelaxin may enhance the effects of alcohol, barbiturates and other CNS depressants).
No products indexed under this heading.

Ethchlorvynol (Skelaxin may enhance the effects of alcohol, barbiturates and other CNS depressants).
No products indexed under this heading.

Ethinamate (Skelaxin may enhance the effects of alcohol, barbiturates and other CNS depressants).
No products indexed under this heading.

Ethyl Alcohol (Skelaxin may enhance the effects of alcohol, barbiturates and other CNS depressants).
No products indexed under this heading.

Fentanyl (Skelaxin may enhance the effects of alcohol, barbiturates and other CNS depressants). Products include:
Duragesic Transdermal System 2405
Ionsys Transdermal System 2410

Fentanyl Citrate (Skelaxin may enhance the effects of alcohol, barbiturates and other CNS depressants). Products include:
Actiq 959
Fentora Tablets 968

Fluphenazine Decanoate (Skelaxin may enhance the effects of alcohol, barbiturates and other CNS depressants).
No products indexed under this heading.

Fluphenazine Enanthate (Skelaxin may enhance the effects of alcohol, barbiturates and other CNS depressants).
No products indexed under this heading.

Fluphenazine Hydrochloride (Skelaxin may enhance the effects of alcohol, barbiturates and other CNS depressants).
No products indexed under this heading.

Flurazepam Hydrochloride (Skelaxin may enhance the effects of alcohol, barbiturates and other CNS depressants).
No products indexed under this heading.

Glutethimide (Skelaxin may enhance the effects of alcohol, barbiturates and other CNS depressants).
No products indexed under this heading.

Haloperidol (Skelaxin may enhance the effects of alcohol, barbiturates and other CNS depressants).
No products indexed under this heading.

Haloperidol Decanoate (Skelaxin may enhance the effects of alcohol, barbiturates and other CNS depressants).
No products indexed under this heading.

Hydrocodone Bitartrate (Skelaxin may enhance the effects of alcohol, barbiturates and other CNS depressants). Products include:
Lortab 5/500 Tablets 3143
Lortab 7.5/500 Tablets 3144
Lortab 10/500 Tablets 3144
Vicodin Tablets 529
Vicodin ES Tablets 530
Vicodin HP Tablets 531
Vicoprofen Tablets 533
Zydone Tablets 1132

Hydrocodone Polistirex (Skelaxin may enhance the effects of alcohol, barbiturates and other CNS depressants). Products include:
Tussionex Pennkinetic Extended-Release Suspension 3154

Hydromorphone Hydrochloride (Skelaxin may enhance the effects of alcohol, barbiturates and other CNS depressants).
No products indexed under this heading.

Hydroxyzine Hydrochloride (Skelaxin may enhance the effects of alcohol, barbiturates and other CNS depressants).
No products indexed under this heading.

Isoflurane (Skelaxin may enhance the effects of alcohol, barbiturates and other CNS depressants).
No products indexed under this heading.

Ketamine Hydrochloride (Skelaxin may enhance the effects of alcohol, barbiturates and other CNS depressants).
No products indexed under this heading.

Levomethadyl Acetate Hydrochloride (Skelaxin may enhance the effects of alcohol, barbiturates and other CNS depressants).
No products indexed under this heading.

Levorphanol Tartrate (Skelaxin may enhance the effects of alcohol, barbiturates and other CNS depressants).
No products indexed under this heading.

Lorazepam (Skelaxin may enhance the effects of alcohol, barbiturates and other CNS depressants).
No products indexed under this heading.

Loxapine Hydrochloride (Skelaxin may enhance the effects of alcohol, barbiturates and other CNS depressants).
No products indexed under this heading.

Loxapine Succinate (Skelaxin may enhance the effects of alcohol, barbiturates and other CNS depressants).
No products indexed under this heading.

Meperidine Hydrochloride (Skelaxin may enhance the effects of alcohol, barbiturates and other CNS depressants).
No products indexed under this heading.

Mephobarbital (Skelaxin may enhance the effects of alcohol, barbiturates and other CNS depressants).
No products indexed under this heading.

Meprobamate (Skelaxin may enhance the effects of alcohol, barbiturates and other CNS depressants).
No products indexed under this heading.

Mesoridazine Besylate (Skelaxin may enhance the effects of alcohol, barbiturates and other CNS depressants).
No products indexed under this heading.

Methadone Hydrochloride (Skelaxin may enhance the effects of alcohol, barbiturates and other CNS depressants).
No products indexed under this heading.

Methohexital Sodium (Skelaxin may enhance the effects of alcohol, barbiturates and other CNS depressants).
No products indexed under this heading.

Methotrimeprazine (Skelaxin may enhance the effects of alcohol, barbiturates and other CNS depressants).
No products indexed under this heading.

Methoxyflurane (Skelaxin may enhance the effects of alcohol, barbiturates and other CNS depressants).
No products indexed under this heading.

Midazolam Hydrochloride (Skelaxin may enhance the effects of alcohol, barbiturates and other CNS depressants).
No products indexed under this heading.

Molindone Hydrochloride (Skelaxin may enhance the effects of alcohol, barbiturates and other CNS depressants). Products include:
Moban Tablets 1116

Morphine Sulfate (Skelaxin may enhance the effects of alcohol, barbiturates and other CNS depressants). Products include:
Avinza Capsules 1772
DepoDur Injection 1095
MS Contin Tablets 2585

Olanzapine (Skelaxin may enhance the effects of alcohol, barbiturates and other CNS depressants). Products include:
Symbyax Capsules 1871
Zyprexa Tablets 1883
Zyprexa IntraMuscular 1883
Zyprexa ZYDIS Orally Disintegrating Tablets 1883

Oxazepam (Skelaxin may enhance the effects of alcohol, barbiturates and other CNS depressants).
No products indexed under this heading.

Oxycodone Hydrochloride (Skelaxin may enhance the effects of alcohol, barbiturates and other CNS depressants). Products include:
OxyContin Tablets 2589
OxyIR Capsules 2593
Percocet Tablets 1127
Percodan Tablets 1130

Pentobarbital Sodium (Skelaxin may enhance the effects of alcohol, barbiturates and other CNS depressants). Products include:
Nembutal Sodium Solution, USP 2494

Perphenazine (Skelaxin may enhance the effects of alcohol, barbiturates and other CNS depressants).
No products indexed under this heading.

Phenobarbital (Skelaxin may enhance the effects of alcohol, barbiturates and other CNS depressants). Products include:
Donnatal Extentabs 2507

Prazepam (Skelaxin may enhance the effects of alcohol, barbiturates and other CNS depressants).
No products indexed under this heading.

Prochlorperazine (Skelaxin may enhance the effects of alcohol, barbiturates and other CNS depressants).
No products indexed under this heading.

Promethazine Hydrochloride (Skelaxin may enhance the effects of alcohol, barbiturates and other CNS depressants).
No products indexed under this heading.

Propofol (Skelaxin may enhance the effects of alcohol, barbiturates and other CNS depressants).
No products indexed under this heading.

Propoxyphene Hydrochloride (Skelaxin may enhance the effects of alcohol, barbiturates and other CNS depressants).
No products indexed under this heading.

Propoxyphene Napsylate (Skelaxin may enhance the effects of alcohol, barbiturates and other CNS depressants).
No products indexed under this heading.

Quazepam (Skelaxin may enhance the effects of alcohol, barbiturates and other CNS depressants).
No products indexed under this heading.

Quetiapine Fumarate (Skelaxin may enhance the effects of alcohol, barbiturates and other CNS depressants).
No products indexed under this heading.

Remifentanil Hydrochloride (Skelaxin may enhance the effects of alcohol, barbiturates and other CNS depressants).
No products indexed under this heading.

Risperidone (Skelaxin may enhance the effects of alcohol, barbiturates and other CNS depressants). Products include:
Risperdal Consta Long-Acting Injection 1753

Secobarbital Sodium (Skelaxin may enhance the effects of alcohol, barbiturates and other CNS depressants).
No products indexed under this heading.

Sevoflurane (Skelaxin may enhance the effects of alcohol, barbiturates and other CNS depressants). Products include:
Ultane Liquid for Inhalation 524

Sodium Oxybate (Skelaxin may enhance the effects of alcohol, barbiturates and other CNS depressants). Products include:
Xyrem Oral Solution 1766

Sufentanil Citrate (Skelaxin may enhance the effects of alcohol, barbiturates and other CNS depressants).
No products indexed under this heading.

Temazepam (Skelaxin may enhance the effects of alcohol, barbiturates and other CNS depressants).
No products indexed under this heading.

Thiamylal Sodium (Skelaxin may enhance the effects of alcohol, barbiturates and other CNS depressants).
No products indexed under this heading.

Thioridazine Hydrochloride (Skelaxin may enhance the effects of alcohol, barbiturates and other CNS depressants). Products include:
Thioridazine Hydrochloride Tablets 2195

Thiothixene (Skelaxin may enhance the effects of alcohol, barbiturates and other CNS depressants). Products include:
Thiothixene Capsules 2197

Triazolam (Skelaxin may enhance the effects of alcohol, barbiturates and other CNS depressants).
No products indexed under this heading.

Trifluoperazine Hydrochloride (Skelaxin may enhance the effects of alcohol, barbiturates and other CNS depressants).
No products indexed under this heading.

Zaleplon (Skelaxin may enhance the effects of alcohol, barbiturates and other CNS depressants).
No products indexed under this heading.

Ziprasidone Hydrochloride (Skelaxin may enhance the effects of alcohol, barbiturates and other CNS depressants). Products include:
Geodon Capsules 2520

Zolpidem Tartrate (Skelaxin may enhance the effects of alcohol, barbiturates and other CNS depressants). Products include:
Ambien Tablets 2692
Ambien CR Tablets 2696

Food Interactions

Alcohol (Skelaxin may enhance the effects of alcohol, barbiturates and other CNS depressants).

Food, unspecified (Taking metaxalone with food may enhance general CNS depression, especially in the elderly).

SLEEP-TITE CAPLETS

(Herbals with Minerals) 640
May interact with monoamine oxidase inhibitors and certain other agents. Compounds in these categories include:

Isocarboxazid (Concurrent use with monoamine oxidase inhibitors is not recommended). Products include:
Marplan Tablets 3177

Moclobemide (Concurrent use with monoamine oxidase inhibitors is not recommended).
No products indexed under this heading.

Pargyline Hydrochloride (Concurrent use with monoamine oxidase inhibitors is not recommended).
No products indexed under this heading.

Phenelzine Sulfate (Concurrent use with monoamine oxidase inhibitors is not recommended).
No products indexed under this heading.

Procarbazine Hydrochloride (Concurrent use with monoamine oxidase inhibitors is not recommended).
No products indexed under this heading.

Rasagiline Mesylate (Concurrent use with monoamine oxidase inhibitors is not recommended). Products include:
Azilect Tablets 3106

Selegiline (Concurrent use with monoamine oxidase inhibitors is not recommended). Products include:
Emsam Transdermal System 905

Selegiline Hydrochloride (Concurrent use with monoamine oxidase inhibitors is not recommended). Products include:
Eldepryl Capsules 3052

Tranylcypromine Sulfate (Concurrent use with monoamine oxidase inhibitors is not recommended). Products include:
Parnate Tablets 1532

Food Interactions

Alcohol (Concurrent use is not recommended).

SMILE'S PRID SALVE

(Homeopathic Formulations) 620
None cited in PDR database.

SNORESTOP EXTINGUISHER 120 ORAL SPRAY

(Homeopathic Formulations) 607
None cited in PDR database.

SNORESTOP MAXIMUM STRENGTH CHEWABLE TABLETS

(Homeopathic Formulations) 607
None cited in PDR database.

SOLODYN EXTENDED RELEASE TABLETS

(Minocycline Hydrochloride) 1938
May interact with antacids containing aluminum, calcium and magnesium, oral anticoagulants, iron containing oral preparations, oral contraceptives, penicillins, and certain other agents. Compounds in these categories include:

Aluminum Carbonate (Absorption of tetracyclines is impaired by antacids containing aluminum, calcium or magnesium).
No products indexed under this heading.

Aluminum Hydroxide (Absorption of tetracyclines is impaired by antacids containing aluminum, calcium or magnesium).
No products indexed under this heading.

5-Amino-Salicylic Acid (Since bacteriostatic drugs may interfere with bactericidal action of penicillin, it is advisable to avoid giving tetracycline-class drugs in conjunction with penicillin).
No products indexed under this heading.

Amoxicillin (Since bacteriostatic drugs may interfere with bactericidal action of penicillin, it is advisable to avoid giving tetracycline-class drugs in conjunction with penicillin). Products include:
Amoxil Capsules 1305
Amoxil Chewable Tablets 1305
Amoxil Pediatric Drops for Oral Suspension 1305
Amoxil Powder for Oral Suspension 1305
Amoxil Tablets 1305
Augmentin 1323
Augmentin Tablets 1327
Augmentin XR Extended Release Tablets 1333
Augmentin ES-600 Powder for Oral Suspension 1329
Moxatag Tablets 2165

Amoxicillin Trihydrate (Since bacteriostatic drugs may interfere with bactericidal action of penicillin, it is advisable to avoid giving tetracycline-class drugs in conjunction with penicillin).
No products indexed under this heading.

Ampicillin (Since bacteriostatic drugs may interfere with bactericidal action of penicillin, it is advisable to avoid giving tetracycline-class drugs in conjunction with penicillin).
No products indexed under this heading.

Ampicillin Sodium (Since bacteriostatic drugs may interfere with bactericidal action of penicillin, it is advisable to avoid giving tetracycline-class drugs in conjunction with penicillin).
No products indexed under this heading.

Ampicillin Trihydrate (Since bacteriostatic drugs may interfere with bactericidal action of penicillin, it is advisable to avoid giving tetracycline-class drugs in conjunction with penicillin).
No products indexed under this heading.

Anisindione (Because tetracyclines have been shown to depress plasma prothrombin activity, patients who are on anticoagulant therapy may require downward adjustment of their anticoagulant dosage).
No products indexed under this heading.

Azlocillin Sodium (Since bacteriostatic drugs may interfere with bactericidal action of penicillin, it is advisable to avoid giving tetracycline-class drugs in conjunction with penicillin).
No products indexed under this heading.

Bacampicillin Hydrochloride (Since bacteriostatic drugs may interfere with bactericidal action of penicillin, it is advisable to avoid giving tetracycline-class drugs in conjunction with penicillin).
No products indexed under this heading.

Carbenicillin Disodium (Since bacteriostatic drugs may interfere with bactericidal action of penicillin, it is advisable to avoid giving tetracycline-class drugs in conjunction with penicillin).
No products indexed under this heading.

Carbenicillin Indanyl Sodium (Since bacteriostatic drugs may interfere with bactericidal action of penicillin, it is advisable to avoid giving tetracycline-class drugs in conjunction with penicillin).
No products indexed under this heading.

Desogestrel (To avoid contraceptive failure, female patients are advised to use a second form of contraceptive during treatment with minocyline). Products include:
Mircette Tablets 1034

Dicloxacillin Sodium (Since bacteriostatic drugs may interfere with bactericidal action of penicillin, it is advisable to avoid giving tetracycline-class drugs in conjunction with penicillin).
No products indexed under this heading.

Dicumarol (Because tetracyclines have been shown to depress plasma prothrombin activity, patients who are on anticoagulant therapy may require downward adjustment of their anticoagulant dosage).
No products indexed under this heading.

Ethinyl Estradiol (To avoid contraceptive failure, female patients are advised to use a second form of contraceptive during treatment with minocyline). Products include:
Lybrel Tablets 3204
Mircette Tablets 1034
NuvaRing 2897
Ortho-Cyclen/Ortho Tri-Cyclen 2449
Ortho Evra Transdermal System 2437
Ortho Tri-Cyclen Lo Tablets 2458
Seasonique Tablets 1046
Yaz Tablets 805

Ethynodiol Diacetate (To avoid contraceptive failure, female patients are advised to use a second form of contraceptive during treatment with minocyline).
No products indexed under this heading.

Ferrous Fumarate (Absorption of tetracyclines is impaired by iron-containing preparations).
No products indexed under this heading.

Ferrous Gluconate (Absorption of tetracyclines is impaired by iron-containing preparations). Products include:
CitraNatal DHA Tablets 2175

Ferrous Sulfate (Absorption of tetracyclines is impaired by iron-containing preparations).
No products indexed under this heading.

Iron (Absorption of tetracyclines is impaired by iron-containing preparations). Products include:
Phyto-Vite Tablets 639

Levonorgestrel (To avoid contraceptive failure, female patients are advised to use a second form of contraceptive during treatment with minocyline). Products include:
Climara Pro Transdermal System 768
Lybrel Tablets 3204
Mirena Intrauterine System 779
Plan B Tablets 1044
Seasonique Tablets 1046

Magaldrate (Absorption of tetracyclines is impaired by antacids containing aluminum, calcium or magnesium).
No products indexed under this heading.

Magnesium Hydroxide (Absorption of tetracyclines is impaired by antacids containing aluminum, calcium or magnesium). Products include:
Fleet Pedia-Lax Chewable Tablets 1145
Pepcid Complete Chewable Tablets 1771
Extra Strength Rolaids Freshmint Tablets 1903
Rolaids Multi-Symptom Berry Tablets 1903
Rolaids Original Peppermint Tablets 1903

Magnesium Oxide (Absorption of tetracyclines is impaired by antacids containing aluminum, calcium or magnesium). Products include:
Beelith Tablets 813

Mestranol (To avoid contraceptive failure, female patients are advised to use a second form of contraceptive during treatment with minocyline).
No products indexed under this heading.

Methoxyflurane (The concurrent use of tetracyclines and methoxyflurane has been reported to result in fatal renal toxicity).
No products indexed under this heading.

Mezlocillin Sodium (Since bacteriostatic drugs may interfere with bactericidal action of penicillin, it is advisable to avoid giving tetracycline-class drugs in conjunction with penicillin).
No products indexed under this heading.

Nafcillin Sodium (Since bacteriostatic drugs may interfere with bactericidal action of penicillin, it is advisable to avoid giving tetracycline-class drugs in conjunction with penicillin).
No products indexed under this heading.

Norethindrone (To avoid contraceptive failure, female patients are advised to use a second form of contraceptive during treatment with minocyline). Products include:
Ortho Micronor Tablets 2446

Norethynodrel (To avoid contraceptive failure, female patients are advised to use a second form of contraceptive during treatment with minocyline).
No products indexed under this heading.

Norgestimate (To avoid contraceptive failure, female patients are advised to use a second form of contraceptive during treatment with minocyline). Products include:
Ortho-Cyclen/Ortho Tri-Cyclen 2449
Ortho Tri-Cyclen Lo Tablets 2458

Norgestrel (To avoid contraceptive failure, female patients are advised to use a second form of contraceptive during treatment with minocyline).
No products indexed under this heading.

Penicillin G Benzathine (Since bacteriostatic drugs may interfere with bactericidal action of penicillin, it is advisable to avoid giving tetracycline-class drugs in conjunction with penicillin). Products include:
Bicillin C-R Injectable Suspension 1775
Bicillin L-A Injection 1777

Penicillin G Potassium (Since bacteriostatic drugs may interfere with bactericidal action of penicillin, it is advisable to avoid giving tetracycline-class drugs in conjunction with penicillin).
No products indexed under this heading.

Penicillin G Procaine (Since bacteriostatic drugs may interfere with bactericidal action of penicillin, it is advisable to avoid giving tetracycline-class drugs in conjunction with penicillin). Products include:
Bicillin C-R Injectable Suspension 1775
Bicillin L-A Injection 1777

Penicillin G Sodium (Since bacteriostatic drugs may interfere with bactericidal action of penicillin, it is advisable to avoid giving tetracycline-class drugs in conjunction with penicillin).
No products indexed under this heading.

Penicillin V Potassium (Since bacteriostatic drugs may interfere with bactericidal action of penicillin, it is advisable to avoid giving tetracycline-class drugs in conjunction with penicillin).
No products indexed under this heading.

Polysaccharide Iron Complex (Absorption of tetracyclines is impaired by iron-containing preparations). Products include:
Nu-Iron 150 Capsules 2165

Ticarcillin Disodium (Since bacteriostatic drugs may interfere with bactericidal action of penicillin, it is advisable to avoid giving tetracycline-class drugs in conjunction with penicillin). Products include:
Timentin ADD-Vantage 1606
Timentin Injection Galaxy Container 1609
Timentin IV Infusion 1603
Timentin Pharmacy Bulk Package 1613

Warfarin Sodium (Because tetracyclines have been shown to depress plasma prothrombin activity, patients who are on anticoagulant therapy may require downward adjustment of their anticoagulant dosage).
No products indexed under this heading.

SOMA TABLETS

(Carisoprodol) 1931
May interact with aspirin-acetylsalicylic acid, benzodiazepines, central nervous system depressants, cytochrome p450 2c19 inducers (selected), cytochrome p450 2c19 inhibitors (selected), narcotic analgesics, tricyclic antidepressants, and certain other agents. Compounds in these categories include:

Alfentanil Hydrochloride (The sedative effects of carisoprodol and other CNS depressants may be additive. Therefore, caution should be exercised with patients who take more than one CNS depressant simultaneously).
No products indexed under this heading.

Alprazolam (The sedative effects of carisoprodol and other CNS depressants may be additive. Therefore, caution should be exercised with patients who take more than one CNS depressant simultaneously).
No products indexed under this heading.

Amitriptyline Hydrochloride (The sedative effects of carisoprodol and other CNS depressants (eg, tricyclic antidepressants) may be additive. Therefore, caution should be exercised with patients who take more than one CNS depressant simultaneously).
No products indexed under this heading.

Amoxapine (The sedative effects of carisoprodol and other CNS depressants (eg, tricyclic antidepressants) may be additive. Therefore, caution should be exercised with patients who take more than one CNS depressant simultaneously).
No products indexed under this heading.

Aprobarbital (The sedative effects of carisoprodol and other CNS depressants may be additive. Therefore, caution should be exercised with patients who take more than one CNS depressant simultaneously).
No products indexed under this heading.

Aspirin (Carisoprodol is metabolized in the liver by CYP2C19 to form meprobamate. Low dose aspirin showed induction effects on CYP2C19. Co-administration of CYP2C19 inducers with carisoprodol could result in decreased exposure of carisoprodol and increased exposure of meprobamate. The full pharmacological impact of these potential alterations of exposures in terms of either efficacy or safety of carisoprodol is unknown). Products include:
Aggrenox Capsules 819
Bayer Aspirin 750
Percodan Tablets 1130
St. Joseph 81 mg Aspirin Chewable and Enteric Coated Tablets 1903

Aspirin, Enteric Coated (Carisoprodol is metabolized in the liver by CYP2C19 to form meprobamate. Low dose aspirin showed induction effects on CYP2C19. Co-administration of CYP2C19 inducers with carisoprodol could result in decreased exposure of carisoprodol and increased exposure of meprobamate. The full pharmacological impact of these potential alterations of exposures in terms of either efficacy or safety of carisoprodol is unknown).
No products indexed under this heading.

Aspirin Buffered (Carisoprodol is metabolized in the liver by CYP2C19 to form meprobamate. Low dose aspirin showed induction effects on CYP2C19. Co-administration of CYP2C19 inducers with carisoprodol could result in decreased exposure of carisoprodol and increased exposure of meprobamate. The full pharmacological impact of these potential alterations of exposures in terms of either efficacy or safety of carisoprodol is unknown).
No products indexed under this heading.

Buprenorphine Hydrochloride (The sedative effects of carisoprodol and other CNS depressants may be additive. Therefore, caution should be exercised with patients who take more than one CNS depressant simultaneously). Products include:
Suboxone Tablets 2601
Subutex Tablets 2601

Buspirone Hydrochloride (The sedative effects of carisoprodol and other CNS depressants may be additive. Therefore, caution should be exercised with patients who take more than one CNS depressant simultaneously).
No products indexed under this heading.

Butabarbital (The sedative effects of carisoprodol and other CNS depressants may be additive. Therefore, caution should be exercised with patients who take more than one CNS depressant simultaneously).
No products indexed under this heading.

Butalbital (The sedative effects of carisoprodol and other CNS depressants may be additive. Therefore, caution should be exercised with patients who take more than one CNS depressant simultaneously).
No products indexed under this heading.

Carbamazepine (Carisoprodol is metabolized in the liver by CYP2C19 to form meprobamate. Co-administration of CYP2C19 inducers with carisoprodol could result in decreased exposure of carisoprodol and increased exposure of meprobamate. The full pharmacological impact of these potential alterations of exposures in terms of either efficacy or safety of carisoprodol is unknown). Products include:
Carbatrol Capsules 3019
Equetro Extended-Release Capsules 3174

Chlordiazepoxide (The sedative effects of carisoprodol and other CNS depressants may be additive. Therefore, caution should be exercised with patients who take more than one CNS depressant simultaneously).
No products indexed under this heading.

Chlordiazepoxide Hydrochloride (The sedative effects of carisoprodol and other CNS depressants may be additive. Therefore, caution should be exercised with patients who take more than one CNS depressant simultaneously).
No products indexed under this heading.

Chlorpromazine (The sedative effects of carisoprodol and other CNS depressants may be additive. Therefore, caution should be exercised with patients who take more than one CNS depressant simultaneously).
No products indexed under this heading.

Chlorpromazine Hydrochloride (The sedative effects of carisoprodol and other CNS depressants may be additive. Therefore, caution should be exercised with patients who take more than one CNS depressant simultaneously).
No products indexed under this heading.

Chlorprothixene (The sedative effects of carisoprodol and other CNS depressants may be additive. Therefore, caution should be exercised with patients who take more than one CNS depressant simultaneously).
No products indexed under this heading.

Chlorprothixene Hydrochloride (The sedative effects of carisoprodol and other CNS depressants may be additive. Therefore, caution should be exercised with patients who take more than one CNS depressant simultaneously).
No products indexed under this heading.

Chlorprothixene Lactate (The sedative effects of carisoprodol and other CNS depressants may be additive. Therefore, caution should be exercised with patients who take more than one CNS depressant simultaneously).
No products indexed under this heading.

Cimetidine (Carisoprodol is metabolized in the liver by CYP2C19 to form meprobamate. Co-administration of CYP2C19 inhibitors with carisoprodol could result in increased exposure of carisoprodol and decreased exposure of meprobamate. The full pharmacological impactof these potential alterations of exposures in terms of either efficacy or safety of carisoprodol is unknown).
No products indexed under this heading.

Cimetidine Hydrochloride (Carisoprodol is metabolized in the liver by CYP2C19 to form meprobamate. Co-administration of CYP2C19 inhibitors with carisoprodol could result in increased exposure of carisoprodol and decreased exposure of meprobamate. The full pharmacological impactof these potential alterations of exposures in terms of either efficacy or safety of carisoprodol is unknown).
No products indexed under this heading.

Citalopram Hydrobromide (Carisoprodol is metabolized in the liver by CYP2C19 to form meprobamate. Co-administration of CYP2C19 inhibitors with carisoprodol could result in increased exposure of carisoprodol and decreased exposure of meprobamate. The full pharmacological impactof these potential alterations of exposures in terms of either efficacy or safety of carisoprodol is unknown). Products include:
Celexa 1160

Clomipramine Hydrochloride (The sedative effects of carisoprodol and other CNS depressants (eg, tricyclic antidepressants) may be additive. Therefore, caution should be exercised with patients who take more than one CNS depressant simultaneously).
No products indexed under this heading.

Clorazepate Dipotassium (The sedative effects of carisoprodol and other CNS depressants may be additive. Therefore, caution should be exercised with patients who take more than one CNS depressant simultaneously).
No products indexed under this heading.

Clozapine (The sedative effects of carisoprodol and other CNS depressants may be additive. Therefore, caution should be exercised with patients who take more than one CNS depressant simultaneously).
No products indexed under this heading.

Codeine Phosphate (The sedative effects of carisoprodol and other CNS depressants may be additive. Therefore, caution should be exercised with patients who take more than one CNS depressant simultaneously). Products include:
Tylenol with Codeine Tablets 2427

Delavirdine Mesylate (Carisoprodol is metabolized in the liver by CYP2C19 to form meprobamate. Co-administration of CYP2C19 inhibitors with carisoprodol could result in increased exposure of carisoprodol and decreased exposure of meprobamate. The full pharmacological impactof these potential alterations of exposures in terms of either efficacy or safety of carisoprodol is unknown).
No products indexed under this heading.

Desflurane (The sedative effects of carisoprodol and other CNS depressants may be additive. Therefore, caution should be exercised with patients who take more than one CNS depressant simultaneously).
No products indexed under this heading.

Desipramine Hydrochloride (The sedative effects of carisoprodol and other CNS depressants (eg, tricyclic antidepressants) may be additive. Therefore, caution should be exercised with patients who take more than one CNS depressant simultaneously).
No products indexed under this heading.

Desogestrel (Carisoprodol is metabolized in the liver by CYP2C19 to form meprobamate. Co-administration of CYP2C19 inhibitors with carisoprodol could result in increased exposure of carisoprodol and decreased exposure of meprobamate. The full pharmacological impactof these potential alterations of exposures in terms of either efficacy or safety of carisoprodol is unknown). Products include:
Mircette Tablets 1034

Dezocine (The sedative effects of carisoprodol and other CNS depressants may be additive. Therefore, caution should be exercised with patients who take more than one CNS depressant simultaneously).
No products indexed under this heading.

Diazepam (The sedative effects of carisoprodol and other CNS depressants may be additive. Therefore, caution should be exercised with patients who take more than one CNS depressant simultaneously). Products include:
Valium Tablets 2658

Doxepin Hydrochloride (The sedative effects of carisoprodol and other CNS depressants (eg, tricyclic antidepressants) may be additive. Therefore, caution should be exercised with patients who take more than one CNS depressant simultaneously).
No products indexed under this heading.

Droperidol (The sedative effects of carisoprodol and other CNS depressants may be additive. Therefore, caution should be exercised with patients who take more than one CNS depressant simultaneously).
No products indexed under this heading.

Efavirenz (Carisoprodol is metabolized in the liver by CYP2C19 to form meprobamate. Co-administration of CYP2C19 inhibitors with carisoprodol could result in increased exposure of carisoprodol and decreased exposure of meprobamate. The full pharmacological impactof these potential alterations of exposures in terms of either efficacy or safety of carisoprodol is unknown). Products include:
Atripla Tablets 938
Sustiva Capsules 930
Sustiva Tablets 930

Enflurane (The sedative effects of carisoprodol and other CNS depressants may be additive. Therefore, caution should be exercised with patients who take more than one CNS depressant simultaneously).
No products indexed under this heading.

Estazolam (The sedative effects of carisoprodol and other CNS depressants may be additive. Therefore, caution should be exercised with patients who take more than one CNS depressant simultaneously).
No products indexed under this heading.

Ethanol (The sedative effects of carisoprodol and other CNS depressants (eg, alcohol) may be additive. Therefore, caution should be exercised with patients who take more than one CNS depressant simultaneously)..
No products indexed under this heading.

Ethchlorvynol (The sedative effects of carisoprodol and other CNS depressants may be additive. Therefore, caution should be exercised with patients who take more than one CNS depressant simultaneously).
No products indexed under this heading.

Ethinamate (The sedative effects of carisoprodol and other CNS depressants may be additive. Therefore, caution should be exercised with patients who take more than one CNS depressant simultaneously).
No products indexed under this heading.

Ethinyl Estradiol (Carisoprodol is metabolized in the liver by CYP2C19 to form meprobamate. Co-administration of CYP2C19 inhibitors with carisoprodol could result in increased exposure of carisoprodol and decreased exposure of meprobamate. The full pharmacological impactof these potential alterations of exposures in terms of either efficacy or safety of carisoprodol is unknown). Products include:
Lybrel Tablets 3204
Mircette Tablets 1034
NuvaRing 2897
Ortho-Cyclen/Ortho Tri-Cyclen 2449
Ortho Evra Transdermal System 2437
Ortho Tri-Cyclen Lo Tablets 2458
Seasonique Tablets 1046
Yaz Tablets 805

Ethyl Alcohol (The sedative effects of carisoprodol and other CNS depressants (eg, alcohol) may be additive. Therefore, caution should be exercised with patients who take more than one CNS depressant simultaneously).
No products indexed under this heading.

Ethynodiol Diacetate (Carisoprodol is metabolized in the liver by CYP2C19 to form meprobamate. Co-administration of CYP2C19 inhibitors with carisoprodol could result in increased exposure of carisoprodol and decreased exposure of meprobamate. The full pharmacological impactof these potential alterations of exposures in terms of either efficacy or safety of carisoprodol is unknown).
No products indexed under this heading.

Felbamate (Carisoprodol is metabolized in the liver by CYP2C19 to form meprobamate. Co-administration of CYP2C19 inhibitors with carisoprodol could result in increased exposure of carisoprodol and decreased exposure of meprobamate. The full pharmacological impactof these potential alterations of exposures in terms of either efficacy or safety of carisoprodol is unknown).
No products indexed under this heading.

Fentanyl (The sedative effects of carisoprodol and other CNS depressants may be additive. Therefore, caution should be exercised with patients who take more than one CNS depressant simultaneously). Products include:
Duragesic Transdermal System 2405
Ionsys Transdermal System 2410

Fentanyl Citrate (The sedative effects of carisoprodol and other CNS depressants may be additive. Therefore, caution should be exercised with patients who take more than one CNS depressant simultaneously). Products include:
Actiq 959
Fentora Tablets 968

Fluoxetine (Carisoprodol is metabolized in the liver by CYP2C19 to form meprobamate. Co-administration of CYP2C19 inhibitors with carisoprodol could result in increased exposure of carisoprodol and decreased exposure of meprobamate. The full pharmacological impactof these potential alterations of exposures in terms of either efficacy or safety of carisoprodol is unknown).
No products indexed under this heading.

Fluoxetine Hydrochloride (Carisoprodol is metabolized in the liver by CYP2C19 to form meprobamate. Co-administration of CYP2C19 inhibitors with carisoprodol could result in increased exposure of carisoprodol and decreased exposure of meprobamate. The full pharmacological impactof these potential alterations of exposures in terms of either efficacy or safety of carisoprodol is unknown). Products include:
Prozac Weekly Capsules 1852
Prozac Pulvules and Liquid 1852
Symbyax Capsules 1871

Fluphenazine Decanoate (The sedative effects of carisoprodol and other CNS depressants may be additive. Therefore, caution should be exercised with patients who take more than one CNS depressant simultaneously).
No products indexed under this heading.

Fluphenazine Enanthate (The sedative effects of carisoprodol and other CNS depressants may be additive. Therefore, caution should be exercised with patients who take more than one CNS depressant simultaneously).
No products indexed under this heading.

Fluphenazine Hydrochloride (The sedative effects of carisoprodol and other CNS depressants may be additive. Therefore, caution should be exercised with patients who take more than one CNS depressant simultaneously).
No products indexed under this heading.

Flurazepam Hydrochloride (The sedative effects of carisoprodol and other CNS depressants may be additive. Therefore, caution should be exercised with patients who take more than one CNS depressant simultaneously).
No products indexed under this heading.

Fluvastatin Sodium (Carisoprodol is metabolized in the liver by CYP2C19 to form meprobamate. Co-administration of CYP2C19 inhibitors with carisoprodol could result in increased exposure of carisoprodol and decreased exposure of meprobamate. The full pharmacological impactof these potential alterations of exposures in terms of either efficacy or safety of carisoprodol is unknown). Products include:
Lescol Capsules 2268
Lescol XL Tablets 2268

Fluvoxamine (Carisoprodol is metabolized in the liver by CYP2C19 to form meprobamate. Co-administration of CYP2C19 inhibitors, such as fluvoxamine, with carisoprodol could result in increased exposure of carisoprodol and decreased exposure of meprobamate. The full pharmacological impact of these potential alterations of exposures in terms of either efficacy or safety of carisoprodol is unknown).
No products indexed under this heading.

Fluvoxamine Maleate (Carisoprodol is metabolized in the liver by CYP2C19 to form meprobamate. Co-administration of CYP2C19 inhibitors, such as fluvoxamine, with carisoprodol could result in increased exposure of carisoprodol and decreased exposure of meprobamate. The full pharmacological impact of these potential alterations of exposures in terms of either efficacy or safety of carisoprodol is unknown). Products include:
Luvox CR Extended-Release Capsules 1759

Glutethimide (The sedative effects of carisoprodol and other CNS depressants may be additive. Therefore, caution should be exercised with patients who take more than one CNS depressant simultaneously).
No products indexed under this heading.

Halazepam (The sedative effects of carisoprodol and other CNS depressants (eg, benzodiazepines) may be additive. Therefore, caution should be exercised with patients who take more than one CNS depressant simultaneously).
No products indexed under this heading.

Haloperidol (The sedative effects of carisoprodol and other CNS depressants may be additive. Therefore, caution should be exercised with patients who take more than one CNS depressant simultaneously).
No products indexed under this heading.

Haloperidol Decanoate (The sedative effects of carisoprodol and other CNS depressants may be additive. Therefore, caution should be exercised with patients who take more than one CNS depressant simultaneously).
No products indexed under this heading.

Hydrocodone Bitartrate (The sedative effects of carisoprodol and other CNS depressants may be additive. Therefore, caution should be exercised with patients who take more than one CNS depressant simultaneously). Products include:
Lortab 5/500 Tablets 3143
Lortab 7.5/500 Tablets 3144
Lortab 10/500 Tablets 3144
Vicodin Tablets 529
Vicodin ES Tablets 530
Vicodin HP Tablets 531
Vicoprofen Tablets 533
Zydone Tablets 1132

Hydrocodone Polistirex (The sedative effects of carisoprodol and other CNS depressants may be additive. Therefore, caution should be exercised with patients who take more than one CNS depressant simultaneously). Products include:
Tussionex Pennkinetic Extended-Release Suspension 3154

Hydromorphone Hydrochloride (The sedative effects of carisoprodol and other CNS depressants may be additive. Therefore, caution should be exercised with patients who take more than one CNS depressant simultaneously).
No products indexed under this heading.

Hydroxyzine Hydrochloride (The sedative effects of carisoprodol and other CNS depressants may be additive. Therefore, caution should be exercised with patients who take more than one CNS depressant simultaneously).
No products indexed under this heading.

Hypericum (Carisoprodol is metabolized in the liver by CYP2C19 to form meprobamate. Co-administration of CYP2C19 inducers, such as St. John's Wort, with carisoprodol could result in decreased exposure of carisoprodol and increased exposure of meprobamate. The full pharmacological impact of these potential alterations of exposures in terms of either efficacy or safety of carisoprodol is unknown). Products include:
Satieté Tablets .... ▣ 640

Imipramine Hydrochloride (The sedative effects of carisoprodol and other CNS depressants (eg, tricyclic antidepressants) may be additive. Therefore, caution should be exercised with patients who take more than one CNS depressant simultaneously).
No products indexed under this heading.

Imipramine Pamoate (The sedative effects of carisoprodol and other CNS depressants (eg, tricyclic antidepressants) may be additive. Therefore, caution should be exercised with patients who take more than one CNS depressant simultaneously).
No products indexed under this heading.

Indomethacin (Carisoprodol is metabolized in the liver by CYP2C19 to form meprobamate. Co-administration of CYP2C19 inhibitors with carisoprodol could result in increased exposure of carisoprodol and decreased exposure of meprobamate. The full pharmacological impactof these potential alterations of exposures in terms of either efficacy or safety of carisoprodol is unknown). Products include:
Indocin 2024

Indomethacin Sodium Trihydrate (Carisoprodol is metabolized in the liver by CYP2C19 to form meprobamate. Co-administration of CYP2C19 inhibitors with carisoprodol could result in increased exposure of carisoprodol and decreased exposure of meprobamate. The full pharmacological impactof these potential alterations of exposures in terms of either efficacy or safety of carisoprodol is unknown). Products include:
Indocin I.V. 2489

Isoflurane (The sedative effects of carisoprodol and other CNS depressants may be additive. Therefore, caution should be exercised with patients who take more than one CNS depressant simultaneously).
No products indexed under this heading.

Isoniazid (Carisoprodol is metabolized in the liver by CYP2C19 to form meprobamate. Co-administration of CYP2C19 inhibitors with carisoprodol could result in increased exposure of carisoprodol and decreased exposure of meprobamate. The full pharmacological impactof these potential alterations of exposures in terms of either efficacy or safety of carisoprodol is unknown).
No products indexed under this heading.

Ketamine Hydrochloride (The sedative effects of carisoprodol and other CNS depressants may be additive. Therefore, caution should be exercised with patients who take more than one CNS depressant simultaneously).
No products indexed under this heading.

Ketoconazole (Carisoprodol is metabolized in the liver by CYP2C19 to form meprobamate. Co-administration of CYP2C19 inhibitors with carisoprodol could result in increased exposure of carisoprodol and decreased exposure of meprobamate. The full pharmacological impactof these potential alterations of exposures in terms of either efficacy or safety of carisoprodol is unknown). Products include:
Extina Foam, 2% 3057
Nizoral A-D Shampoo 1901

Lansoprazole (Carisoprodol is metabolized in the liver by CYP2C19 to form meprobamate. Co-administration of CYP2C19 inhibitors with carisoprodol could result in increased exposure of carisoprodol and decreased exposure of meprobamate. The full pharmacological impactof these potential alterations of exposures in terms of either efficacy or safety of carisoprodol is unknown).
No products indexed under this heading.

Letrozole (Carisoprodol is metabolized in the liver by CYP2C19 to form meprobamate. Co-administration of CYP2C19 inhibitors with carisoprodol could result in increased exposure of carisoprodol and decreased exposure of meprobamate. The full pharmacological impactof these potential alterations of exposures in terms of either efficacy or safety of carisoprodol is unknown). Products include:
Femara Tablets 2246

Levomethadyl Acetate Hydrochloride (The sedative effects of carisoprodol and other CNS depressants may be additive. Therefore, caution should be exercised with patients who take more than one CNS depressant simultaneously).
No products indexed under this heading.

Levonorgestrel (Carisoprodol is metabolized in the liver by CYP2C19 to form meprobamate. Co-administration of CYP2C19 inhibitors with carisoprodol could result in increased exposure of carisoprodol and decreased exposure of meprobamate. The full pharmacological impactof these potential alterations of exposures in terms of either efficacy or safety of carisoprodol is unknown). Products include:
Climara Pro Transdermal System 768
Lybrel Tablets 3204
Mirena Intrauterine System 779
Plan B Tablets 1044
Seasonique Tablets 1046

Levorphanol Tartrate (The sedative effects of carisoprodol and other CNS depressants may be additive. Therefore, caution should be exercised with patients who take more than one CNS depressant simultaneously).
No products indexed under this heading.

Lorazepam (The sedative effects of carisoprodol and other CNS depressants may be additive. Therefore, caution should be exercised with patients who take more than one CNS depressant simultaneously).
No products indexed under this heading.

Loxapine Hydrochloride (The sedative effects of carisoprodol and other CNS depressants may be additive. Therefore, caution should be exercised with patients who take more than one CNS depressant simultaneously).
No products indexed under this heading.

Loxapine Succinate (The sedative effects of carisoprodol and other CNS depressants may be additive. Therefore, caution should be exercised with patients who take more than one CNS depressant simultaneously).
No products indexed under this heading.

Maprotiline Hydrochloride (The sedative effects of carisoprodol and other CNS depressants (eg, tricyclic antidepressants) may be additive. Therefore, caution should be exercised with patients who take more than one CNS depressant simultaneously).
No products indexed under this heading.

Meperidine Hydrochloride (The sedative effects of carisoprodol and other CNS depressants may be additive. Therefore, caution should be exercised with patients who take more than one CNS depressant simultaneously).
No products indexed under this heading.

Mephobarbital (The sedative effects of carisoprodol and other CNS depressants may be additive. Therefore, caution should be exercised with patients who take more than one CNS depressant simultaneously).
No products indexed under this heading.

Meprobamate (Concomitant use of carisoprodol and meprobamate, a metabolite of carisoprodol, is not recommended).
No products indexed under this heading.

Mesoridazine Besylate (The sedative effects of carisoprodol and other CNS depressants may be additive. Therefore, caution should be exercised with patients who take more than one CNS depressant simultaneously).
No products indexed under this heading.

Mestranol (Carisoprodol is metabolized in the liver by CYP2C19 to form meprobamate. Co-administration of CYP2C19 inhibitors with carisoprodol could result in increased exposure of carisoprodol and decreased exposure of meprobamate. The full pharmacological impactof these potential alterations of exposures in terms of either efficacy or safety of carisoprodol is unknown).
No products indexed under this heading.

Methadone Hydrochloride (The sedative effects of carisoprodol and other CNS depressants may be additive. Therefore, caution should be exercised with patients who take more than one CNS depressant simultaneously).
No products indexed under this heading.

Methohexital Sodium (The sedative effects of carisoprodol and other CNS depressants may be additive. Therefore, caution should be exercised with patients who take more than one CNS depressant simultaneously).
No products indexed under this heading.

Methotrimeprazine (The sedative effects of carisoprodol and other CNS depressants may be additive. Therefore, caution should be exercised with patients who take more than one CNS depressant simultaneously).
No products indexed under this heading.

Methoxyflurane (The sedative effects of carisoprodol and other CNS depressants may be additive. Therefore, caution should be exercised with patients who take more than one CNS depressant simultaneously).
No products indexed under this heading.

Midazolam Hydrochloride (The sedative effects of carisoprodol and other CNS depressants may be additive. Therefore, caution should be exercised with patients who take more than one CNS depressant simultaneously).
No products indexed under this heading.

Modafinil (Carisoprodol is metabolized in the liver by CYP2C19 to form meprobamate. Co-administration of CYP2C19 inhibitors with carisoprodol could result in increased exposure of carisoprodol and decreased exposure of meprobamate. The full pharmacological impactof these potential alterations of exposures in terms of either efficacy or safety of carisoprodol is unknown). Products include:
Provigil Tablets **977**

Molindone Hydrochloride (The sedative effects of carisoprodol and other CNS depressants may be additive. Therefore, caution should be exercised with patients who take more than one CNS depressant simultaneously). Products include:
Moban Tablets **1116**

Morphine Sulfate (The sedative effects of carisoprodol and other CNS depressants may be additive. Therefore, caution should be exercised with patients who take more than one CNS depressant simultaneously). Products include:
Avinza Capsules **1772**
DepoDur Injection **1095**
MS Contin Tablets **2585**

Norethindrone (Carisoprodol is metabolized in the liver by CYP2C19 to form meprobamate. Co-administration of CYP2C19 inhibitors with carisoprodol could result in increased exposure of carisoprodol and decreased exposure of meprobamate. The full pharmacological impactof these potential alterations of exposures in terms of either efficacy or safety of carisoprodol is unknown). Products include:
Ortho Micronor Tablets **2446**

Norethindrone Acetate (Carisoprodol is metabolized in the liver by CYP2C19 to form meprobamate. Co-administration of CYP2C19 inducers with carisoprodol could result in decreased exposure of carisoprodol and increased exposure of meprobamate. The full pharmacological impact of these potential alterations of exposures in terms of either efficacy or safety of carisoprodol is unknown). Products include:
Activella Tablets **2347**

Norethynodrel (Carisoprodol is metabolized in the liver by CYP2C19 to form meprobamate. Co-administration of CYP2C19 inhibitors with carisoprodol could result in increased exposure of carisoprodol and decreased exposure of meprobamate. The full pharmacological impactof these potential alterations of exposures in terms of either efficacy or safety of carisoprodol is unknown).
No products indexed under this heading.

Norgestimate (Carisoprodol is metabolized in the liver by CYP2C19 to form meprobamate. Co-administration of CYP2C19 inhibitors with carisoprodol could result in increased exposure of carisoprodol and decreased exposure of meprobamate. The full pharmacological impactof these potential alterations of exposures in terms of either efficacy or safety of carisoprodol is unknown). Products include:
Ortho-Cyclen/Ortho Tri-Cyclen **2449**
Ortho Tri-Cyclen Lo Tablets **2458**

Norgestrel (Carisoprodol is metabolized in the liver by CYP2C19 to form meprobamate. Co-administration of CYP2C19 inhibitors with carisoprodol could result in increased exposure of carisoprodol and decreased exposure of meprobamate. The full pharmacological impactof these potential alterations of exposures in terms of either efficacy or safety of carisoprodol is unknown).
No products indexed under this heading.

Nortriptyline Hydrochloride (The sedative effects of carisoprodol and other CNS depressants (eg, tricyclic antidepressants) may be additive. Therefore, caution should be exercised with patients who take more than one CNS depressant simultaneously).
No products indexed under this heading.

Olanzapine (The sedative effects of carisoprodol and other CNS depressants may be additive. Therefore, caution should be exercised with patients who take more than one CNS depressant simultaneously). Products include:
Symbyax Capsules **1871**
Zyprexa Tablets **1883**
Zyprexa IntraMuscular **1883**
Zyprexa ZYDIS Orally Disintegrating Tablets **1883**

Omeprazole (Carisoprodol is metabolized in the liver by CYP2C19 to form meprobamate. Co-administration of CYP2C19 inhibitors, such as omeprazole, with carisoprodol could result in increased exposure of carisoprodol and decreased exposure of meprobamate. The full pharmacological impact of these potential alterations of exposures in terms of either efficacy or safety of carisoprodol is unknown).
No products indexed under this heading.

Omeprazole Magnesium (Carisoprodol is metabolized in the liver by CYP2C19 to form meprobamate. Co-administration of CYP2C19 inhibitors, such as omeprazole, with carisoprodol could result in increased exposure of carisoprodol and decreased exposure of meprobamate. The full pharmacological impact of these potential alterations of exposures in terms of either efficacy or safety of carisoprodol is unknown). Products include:
Prilosec OTC Tablets **2565**

Oxazepam (The sedative effects of carisoprodol and other CNS depressants may be additive. Therefore, caution should be exercised with patients who take more than one CNS depressant simultaneously).
No products indexed under this heading.

Oxcarbazepine (Carisoprodol is metabolized in the liver by CYP2C19 to form meprobamate. Co-administration of CYP2C19 inhibitors with carisoprodol could result in increased exposure of carisoprodol and decreased exposure of meprobamate. The full pharmacological impactof these potential alterations of exposures in terms of either efficacy or safety of carisoprodol is unknown).
No products indexed under this heading.

Oxycodone Hydrochloride (The sedative effects of carisoprodol and other CNS depressants may be additive. Therefore, caution should be exercised with patients who take more than one CNS depressant simultaneously). Products include:
OxyContin Tablets **2589**
OxyIR Capsules **2593**
Percocet Tablets **1127**
Percodan Tablets **1130**

Paroxetine Hydrochloride (Carisoprodol is metabolized in the liver by CYP2C19 to form meprobamate. Co-administration of CYP2C19 inhibitors with carisoprodol could result in increased exposure of carisoprodol and decreased exposure of meprobamate. The full pharmacological impactof these potential alterations of exposures in terms of either efficacy or safety of carisoprodol is unknown). Products include:
Paxil **1535**
Paxil CR Controlled-Release Tablets **1544**

Pentobarbital Sodium (The sedative effects of carisoprodol and other CNS depressants may be additive. Therefore, caution should be exercised with patients who take more than one CNS depressant simultaneously). Products include:
Nembutal Sodium Solution, USP **2494**

Perphenazine (The sedative effects of carisoprodol and other CNS depressants may be additive. Therefore, caution should be exercised with patients who take more than one CNS depressant simultaneously).
No products indexed under this heading.

Phenobarbital (The sedative effects of carisoprodol and other CNS depressants may be additive. Therefore, caution should be exercised with patients who take more than one CNS depressant simultaneously). Products include:
Donnatal Extentabs **2507**

Phenobarbital Sodium (Carisoprodol is metabolized in the liver by CYP2C19 to form meprobamate. Co-administration of CYP2C19 inducers with carisoprodol could result in decreased exposure of carisoprodol and increased exposure of meprobamate. The full pharmacological impact of these potential alterations of exposures in terms of either efficacy or safety of carisoprodol is unknown).
No products indexed under this heading.

Phenytoin (Carisoprodol is metabolized in the liver by CYP2C19 to form meprobamate. Co-administration of CYP2C19 inducers with carisoprodol could result in decreased exposure of carisoprodol and increased exposure of meprobamate. The full pharmacological impact of these potential alterations of exposures in terms of either efficacy or safety of carisoprodol is unknown).
No products indexed under this heading.

Phenytoin Sodium (Carisoprodol is metabolized in the liver by CYP2C19 to form meprobamate. Co-administration of CYP2C19 inducers with carisoprodol could result in decreased exposure of carisoprodol and increased exposure of meprobamate. The full pharmacological impact of these potential alterations

of exposures in terms of either efficacy or safety of carisoprodol is unknown). Products include:
Phenytek Capsules 2192

Prazepam (The sedative effects of carisoprodol and other CNS depressants may be additive. Therefore, caution should be exercised with patients who take more than one CNS depressant simultaneously).
No products indexed under this heading.

Prednisone (Carisoprodol is metabolized in the liver by CYP2C19 to form meprobamate. Co-administration of CYP2C19 inducers with carisoprodol could result in decreased exposure of carisoprodol and increased exposure of meprobamate. The full pharmacological impact of these potential alterations of exposures in terms of either efficacy or safety of carisoprodol is unknown).
No products indexed under this heading.

Prochlorperazine (The sedative effects of carisoprodol and other CNS depressants may be additive. Therefore, caution should be exercised with patients who take more than one CNS depressant simultaneously).
No products indexed under this heading.

Promethazine Hydrochloride (The sedative effects of carisoprodol and other CNS depressants may be additive. Therefore, caution should be exercised with patients who take more than one CNS depressant simultaneously).
No products indexed under this heading.

Propofol (The sedative effects of carisoprodol and other CNS depressants may be additive. Therefore, caution should be exercised with patients who take more than one CNS depressant simultaneously).
No products indexed under this heading.

Propoxyphene Hydrochloride (The sedative effects of carisoprodol and other CNS depressants may be additive. Therefore, caution should be exercised with patients who take more than one CNS depressant simultaneously).
No products indexed under this heading.

Propoxyphene Napsylate (The sedative effects of carisoprodol and other CNS depressants may be additive. Therefore, caution should be exercised with patients who take more than one CNS depressant simultaneously).
No products indexed under this heading.

Protriptyline Hydrochloride (The sedative effects of carisoprodol and other CNS depressants (eg, tricyclic antidepressants) may be additive. Therefore, caution should be exercised with patients who take more than one CNS depressant simultaneously).
No products indexed under this heading.

Quazepam (The sedative effects of carisoprodol and other CNS depressants may be additive. Therefore, caution should be exercised with patients who take more than one CNS depressant simultaneously).
No products indexed under this heading.

Quetiapine Fumarate (The sedative effects of carisoprodol and other CNS depressants may be additive. Therefore, caution should be exercised with patients who take more than one CNS depressant simultaneously).
No products indexed under this heading.

Remifentanil Hydrochloride (The sedative effects of carisoprodol and other CNS depressants may be additive. Therefore, caution should be exercised with patients who take more than one CNS depressant simultaneously).
No products indexed under this heading.

Rifampin (Carisoprodol is metabolized in the liver by CYP2C19 to form meprobamate. Co-administration of CYP2C19 inducers, such as rifampin, with carisoprodol could result in decreased exposure of carisoprodol and increased exposure of meprobamate. The full pharmacological impact of these potential alterations of exposures in terms of either efficacy or safety of carisoprodol is unknown).
No products indexed under this heading.

Risperidone (The sedative effects of carisoprodol and other CNS depressants may be additive. Therefore, caution should be exercised with patients who take more than one CNS depressant simultaneously). Products include:
Risperdal Consta Long-Acting Injection 1753

Ritonavir (Carisoprodol is metabolized in the liver by CYP2C19 to form meprobamate. Co-administration of CYP2C19 inhibitors with carisoprodol could result in increased exposure of carisoprodol and decreased exposure of meprobamate. The full pharmacological impactof these potential alterations of exposures in terms of either efficacy or safety of carisoprodol is unknown). Products include:
Kaletra 452
Norvir 489

Secobarbital Sodium (The sedative effects of carisoprodol and other CNS depressants may be additive. Therefore, caution should be exercised with patients who take more than one CNS depressant simultaneously).
No products indexed under this heading.

Sertraline Hydrochloride (Carisoprodol is metabolized in the liver by CYP2C19 to form meprobamate. Co-administration of CYP2C19 inhibitors with carisoprodol could result in increased exposure of carisoprodol and decreased exposure of meprobamate. The full pharmacological impactof these potential alterations of exposures in terms of either efficacy or safety of carisoprodol is unknown).
No products indexed under this heading.

Sevoflurane (The sedative effects of carisoprodol and other CNS depressants may be additive. Therefore, caution should be exercised with patients who take more than one CNS depressant simultaneously). Products include:
Ultane Liquid for Inhalation 524

Sildenafil Citrate (Carisoprodol is metabolized in the liver by CYP2C19 to form meprobamate. Co-administration of CYP2C19 inhibitors with carisoprodol could result in increased exposure of carisoprodol and decreased exposure of meprobamate. The full pharmacological impactof these potential alterations of exposures in terms of either efficacy or safety of carisoprodol is unknown).
No products indexed under this heading.

Sodium Oxybate (The sedative effects of carisoprodol and other CNS depressants may be additive. Therefore, caution should be exercised with patients who take more than one CNS depressant simultaneously). Products include:
Xyrem Oral Solution 1766

Sufentanil Citrate (The sedative effects of carisoprodol and other CNS depressants may be additive. Therefore, caution should be exercised with patients who take more than one CNS depressant simultaneously).
No products indexed under this heading.

Sulfaphenazole (Carisoprodol is metabolized in the liver by CYP2C19 to form meprobamate. Co-administration of CYP2C19 inhibitors with carisoprodol could result in increased exposure of carisoprodol and decreased exposure of meprobamate. The full pharmacological impactof these potential alterations of exposures in terms of either efficacy or safety of carisoprodol is unknown).
No products indexed under this heading.

Telmisartan (Carisoprodol is metabolized in the liver by CYP2C19 to form meprobamate. Co-administration of CYP2C19 inhibitors with carisoprodol could result in increased exposure of carisoprodol and decreased exposure of meprobamate. The full pharmacological impactof these potential alterations of exposures in terms of either efficacy or safety of carisoprodol is unknown). Products include:
Micardis Tablets 852
Micardis HCT Tablets 854

Temazepam (The sedative effects of carisoprodol and other CNS depressants may be additive. Therefore, caution should be exercised with patients who take more than one CNS depressant simultaneously).
No products indexed under this heading.

Thiamylal Sodium (The sedative effects of carisoprodol and other CNS depressants may be additive. Therefore, caution should be exercised with patients who take more than one CNS depressant simultaneously).
No products indexed under this heading.

Thioridazine Hydrochloride (The sedative effects of carisoprodol and other CNS depressants may be additive. Therefore, caution should be exercised with patients who take more than one CNS depressant simultaneously). Products include:
Thioridazine Hydrochloride Tablets 2195

Thiothixene (The sedative effects of carisoprodol and other CNS depressants may be additive. Therefore, caution should be exercised with patients who take more than one CNS depressant simultaneously). Products include:
Thiothixene Capsules 2197

Ticlopidine Hydrochloride (Carisoprodol is metabolized in the liver by CYP2C19 to form meprobamate. Co-administration of CYP2C19 inhibitors with carisoprodol could result in increased exposure of carisoprodol and decreased exposure of meprobamate. The full pharmacological impactof these potential alterations of exposures in terms of either efficacy or safety of carisoprodol is unknown).
No products indexed under this heading.

Tolbutamide (Carisoprodol is metabolized in the liver by CYP2C19 to form meprobamate. Co-administration of CYP2C19 inhibitors with carisoprodol could result in increased exposure of carisoprodol and decreased exposure of meprobamate. The full pharmacological impactof these potential alterations of exposures in terms of either efficacy or safety of carisoprodol is unknown).
No products indexed under this heading.

Tolbutamide Sodium (Carisoprodol is metabolized in the liver by CYP2C19 to form meprobamate. Co-administration of CYP2C19 inhibitors with carisoprodol could result in increased exposure of carisoprodol and decreased exposure of meprobamate. The full pharmacological impactof these potential alterations of exposures in terms of either efficacy or safety of carisoprodol is unknown).
No products indexed under this heading.

Topiramate (Carisoprodol is metabolized in the liver by CYP2C19 to form meprobamate. Co-administration of CYP2C19 inhibitors with carisoprodol could result in increased exposure of carisoprodol and decreased exposure of meprobamate. The full pharmacological impactof these potential alterations of exposures in terms of either efficacy or safety of carisoprodol is unknown).
No products indexed under this heading.

Triazolam (The sedative effects of carisoprodol and other CNS depressants may be additive. Therefore, caution should be exercised with patients who take more than one CNS depressant simultaneously).
No products indexed under this heading.

Trifluoperazine Hydrochloride (The sedative effects of carisoprodol and other CNS depressants may be additive. Therefore, caution should be exercised with patients who take more than one CNS depressant simultaneously).
No products indexed under this heading.

Trimipramine Maleate (The sedative effects of carisoprodol and other CNS depressants (eg, tricyclic antidepressants) may be additive. Therefore, caution should be exercised with patients who take more than one CNS depressant simultaneously).

No products indexed under this heading.

Vardenafil Hydrochloride (Carisoprodol is metabolized in the liver by CYP2C19 to form meprobamate. Co-administration of CYP2C19 inhibitors with carisoprodol could result in increased exposure of carisoprodol and decreased exposure of meprobamate. The full pharmacological impactof these potential alterations of exposures in terms of either efficacy or safety of carisoprodol is unknown). Products include:

Levitra Tablets **2876**

Voriconazole (Carisoprodol is metabolized in the liver by CYP2C19 to form meprobamate. Co-administration of CYP2C19 inhibitors with carisoprodol could result in increased exposure of carisoprodol and decreased exposure of meprobamate. The full pharmacological impactof these potential alterations of exposures in terms of either efficacy or safety of carisoprodol is unknown).

No products indexed under this heading.

Zaleplon (The sedative effects of carisoprodol and other CNS depressants may be additive. Therefore, caution should be exercised with patients who take more than one CNS depressant simultaneously).

No products indexed under this heading.

Ziprasidone Hydrochloride (The sedative effects of carisoprodol and other CNS depressants may be additive. Therefore, caution should be exercised with patients who take more than one CNS depressant simultaneously). Products include:

Geodon Capsules **2520**

Zolpidem Tartrate (The sedative effects of carisoprodol and other CNS depressants may be additive. Therefore, caution should be exercised with patients who take more than one CNS depressant simultaneously). Products include:

Ambien Tablets **2692**
Ambien CR Tablets **2696**

Food Interactions

Alcohol (The sedative effects of carisoprodol and other CNS depressants (eg, alcohol) may be additive. Therefore, caution should be exercised with patients who take more than one CNS depressant simultaneously).

SOMATULINE DEPOT INJECTION

(Lanreotide) **3102**

May interact with beta blockers, cytochrome p450 3a4 substrates (selected), oral hypoglycemic agents, insulin, and certain other agents. Compounds in these categories include:

Acarbose (Lanreotide inhibits the secretion of insulin and glucagon. Therefore, blood glucose levels should be monitored when lanreotide treatment is initiated or when the dose is altered and antidiabetic treatment should be adjusted accordingly). Products include:

Precose Tablets **792**

Acebutolol Hydrochloride (Concomitant administration of bradycardia-inducing drugs may have an additive effect on the reduction of heart rate associated with lanreotide. Dose adjustments of concomitant medication may be necessary).

No products indexed under this heading.

Alfentanil Hydrochloride (The limited published data available indicate that somatostatin analogs may decrease the metabolic clearance of compounds known to be metabolized by the cytochrome P450 enzymes, which may be due to the suppression of growth hormone. Since it cannot be excluded that lanreotide may have this effect, other drugs mainly metabolized by CYP3A4 and which have a low therapeutic index should therefore be used with caution. Drugs metabolized by the liver may be metabolized more slowly during lanreotide treatment and dose reductions of the concomitantly administered medications should be considered).

No products indexed under this heading.

Alprazolam (The limited published data available indicate that somatostatin analogs may decrease the metabolic clearance of compounds known to be metabolized by the cytochrome P450 enzymes, which may be due to the suppression of growth hormone. Since it cannot be excluded that lanreotide may have this effect, other drugs mainly metabolized by CYP3A4 and which have a low therapeutic index should therefore be used with caution. Drugs metabolized by the liver may be metabolized more slowly during lanreotide treatment and dose reductions of the concomitantly administered medications should be considered).

No products indexed under this heading.

Amiodarone Hydrochloride (The limited published data available indicate that somatostatin analogs may decrease the metabolic clearance of compounds known to be metabolized by the cytochrome P450 enzymes, which may be due to the suppression of growth hormone. Since it cannot be excluded that lanreotide may have this effect, other drugs mainly metabolized by CYP3A4 and which have a low therapeutic index should therefore be used with caution. Drugs metabolized by the liver may be metabolized more slowly during lanreotide treatment and dose reductions of the concomitantly administered medications should be considered).

No products indexed under this heading.

Amitriptyline Hydrochloride (The limited published data available indicate that somatostatin analogs may decrease the metabolic clearance of compounds known to be metabolized by the cytochrome P450 enzymes, which may be due to the suppression of growth hormone. Since it cannot be excluded that lanreotide may have this effect, other drugs mainly metabolized by CYP3A4 and which have a low therapeutic index should therefore be used with caution. Drugs metabolized by the liver may be metabolized more slowly during lanreotide treatment and dose reductions of the concomitantly administered medications should be considered).

No products indexed under this heading.

Amlodipine Besylate (The limited published data available indicate that somatostatin analogs may decrease the metabolic clearance of compounds known to be metabolized by the cytochrome P450 enzymes, which may be due to the suppression of growth hormone. Since it cannot be excluded that lanreotide may have this effect, other drugs mainly metabolized by CYP3A4 and which have a low therapeutic index should therefore be used with caution. Drugs metabolized by the liver may be metabolized more slowly during lanreotide treatment and dose reductions of the concomitantly administered medications should be considered). Products include:

Azor Tablets **1005**
Exforge Tablets **2238**

Aprepitant (The limited published data available indicate that somatostatin analogs may decrease the metabolic clearance of compounds known to be metabolized by the cytochrome P450 enzymes, which may be due to the suppression of growth hormone. Since it cannot be excluded that lanreotide may have this effect, other drugs mainly metabolized by CYP3A4 and which have a low therapeutic index should therefore be used with caution. Drugs metabolized by the liver may be metabolized more slowly during lanreotide treatment and dose reductions of the concomitantly administered medications should be considered). Products include:

Emend Capsules **1992**

Astemizole (The limited published data available indicate that somatostatin analogs may decrease the metabolic clearance of compounds known to be metabolized by the cytochrome P450 enzymes, which may be due to the suppression of growth hormone. Since it cannot be excluded that lanreotide may have this effect, other drugs mainly metabolized by CYP3A4 and which have a low therapeutic index should therefore be used with caution. Drugs metabolized by the liver may be metabolized more slowly during lanreotide treatment and dose reductions of the concomitantly administered medications should be considered).

No products indexed under this heading.

Atenolol (Concomitant administration of bradycardia-inducing drugs may have an additive effect on the reduction of heart rate associated with lanreotide. Dose adjustments of concomitant medication may be necessary).

No products indexed under this heading.

Atorvastatin Calcium (The limited published data available indicate that somatostatin analogs may decrease the metabolic clearance of compounds known to be metabolized by the cytochrome P450 enzymes, which may be due to the suppression of growth hormone. Since it cannot be excluded that lanreotide may have this effect, other drugs mainly metabolized by CYP3A4 and which have a low therapeutic index should therefore be used with caution. Drugs metabolized by the liver may be metabolized more slowly during lanreotide treatment and dose reductions of the concomitantly administered medications should be considered). Products include:

Lipitor Tablets **2501**

Belladonna Ergotamine (The limited published data available indicate that somatostatin analogs may decrease the metabolic clearance of compounds known to be metabolized by the cytochrome P450 enzymes, which may be due to the suppression of growth hormone. Since it cannot be excluded that lanreotide may have this effect, other drugs mainly metabolized by CYP3A4 and which have a low therapeutic index should therefore be used with caution. Drugs metabolized by the liver may be metabolized more slowly during lanreotide treatment and dose reductions of the concomitantly administered medications should be considered).

No products indexed under this heading.

Betaxolol Hydrochloride (Concomitant administration of bradycardia-inducing drugs may have an additive effect on the reduction of heart rate associated with lanreotide. Dose adjustments of concomitant medication may be necessary).

No products indexed under this heading.

Bisoprolol Fumarate (Concomitant administration of bradycardia-inducing drugs may have an additive effect on the reduction of heart rate associated with lanreotide. Dose adjustments of concomitant medication may be necessary).

No products indexed under this heading.

Bromocriptine Mesylate (Limited published data indicate that concomitant administration of a somatostatin analog and bromocriptine may increase the availability of bromocriptine).

No products indexed under this heading.

Buspirone Hydrochloride (The limited published data available indicate that somatostatin analogs may decrease the metabolic clearance of compounds known to be metabolized by the cytochrome P450 enzymes, which may be due to the suppression of growth hormone. Since it cannot be excluded that lanreotide may have this effect, other drugs mainly metabolized by CYP3A4 and which have a low therapeutic index should therefore be used with caution. Drugs metabolized by the liver may be metabolized more slowly during lanreotide treatment and dose reductions of the concomitantly administered medications should be considered).

No products indexed under this heading.

Busulfan (The limited published data available indicate that somatostatin analogs may decrease the metabolic clearance of compounds known to be metabolized by the cytochrome P450 enzymes, which may be due to the suppression of growth hormone. Since it cannot be excluded that lanreotide may have this effect, other drugs mainly metabolized by CYP3A4 and which have a low therapeutic index should therefore be used with caution. Drugs metabolized by the liver may be metabolized more slowly during lanreotide treatment and dose reductions of the concomitantly administered medications should be considered). Products include:

Busulfex Injection 2477
Myleran Tablets 1530

Carbamazepine (The limited published data available indicate that somatostatin analogs may decrease the metabolic clearance of compounds known to be metabolized by the cytochrome P450 enzymes, which may be due to the suppression of growth hormone. Since it cannot be excluded that lanreotide may have this effect, other drugs mainly metabolized by CYP3A4 and which have a low therapeutic index should therefore be used with caution. Drugs metabolized by the liver may be metabolized more slowly during lanreotide treatment and dose reductions of the concomitantly administered medications should be considered). Products include:

Carbatrol Capsules 3019
Equetro Extended-Release Capsules 3174

Carteolol Hydrochloride (Concomitant administration of bradycardia-inducing drugs may have an additive effect on the reduction of heart rate associated with lanreotide. Dose adjustments of concomitant medication may be necessary).

No products indexed under this heading.

Cerivastatin Sodium (The limited published data available indicate that somatostatin analogs may decrease the metabolic clearance of compounds known to be metabolized by the cytochrome P450 enzymes, which may be due to the suppression of growth hormone. Since it cannot be excluded that lanreotide may have this effect, other drugs mainly metabolized by CYP3A4 and which have a low therapeutic index should therefore be used with caution. Drugs metabolized by the liver may be metabolized more slowly during lanreotide treatment and dose reductions of the concomitantly administered medications should be considered).

No products indexed under this heading.

Chlorpheniramine (The limited published data available indicate that somatostatin analogs may decrease the metabolic clearance of compounds known to be metabolized by the cytochrome P450 enzymes, which may be due to the suppression of growth hormone. Since it cannot be excluded that lanreotide may have this effect, other drugs mainly metabolized by CYP3A4 and which have a low therapeutic index should therefore be used with caution. Drugs metabolized by the liver may be metabolized more slowly during lanreotide treatment and dose reductions of the concomitantly administered medications should be considered).

No products indexed under this heading.

Chlorpheniramine Maleate (The limited published data available indicate that somatostatin analogs may decrease the metabolic clearance of compounds known to be metabolized by the cytochrome P450 enzymes, which may be due to the suppression of growth hormone. Since it cannot be excluded that lanreotide may have this effect, other drugs mainly metabolized by CYP3A4 and which have a low therapeutic index should therefore be used with caution. Drugs metabolized by the liver may be metabolized more slowly during lanreotide treatment and dose reductions of the concomitantly administered medications should be considered). Products include:

Actifed Cold & Allergy Tablets 1895
Sudafed PE Sinus & Allergy Tablets 1908
Tylenol Allergy Multi-Symptom Caplets with Cool Burst and Rapid Release Gelcaps 1916
Children's Tylenol Plus Cold Suspension Liquid 1912
Children's Tylenol Plus Cough & Runny Nose Suspension Liquid 1912
Children's Tylenol Plus Flu Suspension Liquid 1914
Children's Tylenol Plus Multi-Symptom Cold Suspension Liquid 1912
Tylenol Cold Head Congestion Nighttime Caplets with Cool Burst 1910
Tylenol Cold Multi-Symptom Nighttime Caplets with Cool Burst 1913
Tylenol Sinus Congestion & Pain Nighttime Caplets with Cool Burst 1917

Chlorpheniramine Polistirex (The limited published data available indicate that somatostatin analogs may decrease the metabolic clearance of compounds known to be metabolized by the cytochrome P450 enzymes, which may be due to the suppression of growth hormone. Since it cannot be excluded that lanreotide may have this effect, other drugs mainly metabolized by CYP3A4 and which have a low therapeutic index should therefore be used with caution. Drugs metabolized by the liver may be metabolized more slowly during lanreotide treatment and dose reductions of the concomitantly administered medications should be considered). Products include:

Tussionex Pennkinetic Extended-Release Suspension 3154

Chlorpheniramine Tannate (The limited published data available indicate that somatostatin analogs may decrease the metabolic clearance of compounds known to be metabolized by the cytochrome P450 enzymes, which may be due to the suppression of growth hormone. Since it cannot be excluded that lanreotide may have this effect, other drugs mainly metabolized by CYP3A4 and which have a low therapeutic index should therefore be used with caution. Drugs metabolized by the liver may be metabolized more slowly during lanreotide treatment and dose reductions of the concomitantly administered medications should be considered).

No products indexed under this heading.

Chlorpropamide (Lanreotide inhibits the secretion of insulin and glucagon. Therefore, blood glucose levels should be monitored when lanreotide treatment is initiated or when the dose is altered and antidiabetic treatment should be adjusted accordingly).

No products indexed under this heading.

Cisapride (The limited published data available indicate that somatostatin analogs may decrease the metabolic clearance of compounds known to be metabolized by the cytochrome P450 enzymes, which may be due to the suppression of growth hormone. Since it cannot be excluded that lanreotide may have this effect, other drugs mainly metabolized by CYP3A4 and which have a low therapeutic index should therefore be used with caution. Drugs metabolized by the liver may be metabolized more slowly during lanreotide treatment and dose reductions of the concomitantly administered medications should be considered).

No products indexed under this heading.

Clarithromycin (The limited published data available indicate that somatostatin analogs may decrease the metabolic clearance of compounds known to be metabolized by the cytochrome P450 enzymes, which may be due to the suppression of growth hormone. Since it cannot be excluded that lanreotide may have this effect, other drugs mainly metabolized by CYP3A4 and which have a low therapeutic index should therefore be used with caution. Drugs metabolized by the liver may be metabolized more slowly during lanreotide treatment and dose reductions of the concomitantly administered medications should be considered). Products include:

Biaxin/Biaxin XL 411

Cyclosporine (Concomitant administration of cyclosporine with lanreotide may decrease the relative bioavailability of cyclosporine and, therefore, may necessitate adjustment of cyclosporine dose to maintain therapeutic levels). Products include:

Gengraf Capsules 435
Neoral Oral Solution 2280
Neoral Soft Gelatin Capsules 2280
Restasis Ophthalmic Emulsion 557
Sandimmune 2296

Desogestrel (The limited published data available indicate that somatostatin analogs may decrease the metabolic clearance of compounds known to be metabolized by the cytochrome P450 enzymes, which may be due to the suppression of growth hormone. Since it cannot be excluded that lanreotide may have this effect, other drugs mainly metabolized by CYP3A4 and which have a low therapeutic index should therefore be used with caution. Drugs metabolized by the liver may be metabolized more slowly during lanreotide treatment and dose reductions of the concomitantly administered medications should be considered). Products include:

Mircette Tablets 1034

Diazepam (The limited published data available indicate that somatostatin analogs may decrease the metabolic clearance of compounds known to be metabolized by the cytochrome P450 enzymes, which may be due to the suppression of growth hormone. Since it cannot be excluded that lanreotide may have this effect, other drugs mainly metabolized by CYP3A4 and which have a low therapeutic index should therefore be used with caution. Drugs metabolized by the liver may be metabolized more slowly during lanreotide treatment and dose reductions of the concomitantly administered medications should be considered). Products include:

Valium Tablets 2658

Dihydroergotamine Mesylate (The limited published data available indicate that somatostatin analogs may decrease the metabolic clearance of compounds known to be metabolized by the cytochrome P450 enzymes, which may be due to the suppression of growth hormone. Since it cannot be excluded that lanreotide may have this effect, other drugs mainly metabolized by CYP3A4 and which have a low therapeutic index should therefore be used with caution. Drugs metabolized by the liver may be metabolized more slowly during lanreotide treatment and dose reductions of the concomitantly administered medications should be considered).

No products indexed under this heading.

Diltiazem Hydrochloride (The limited published data available indicate that somatostatin analogs may decrease the metabolic clearance of compounds known to be metabolized by the cytochrome P450 enzymes, which may be due to the suppression of growth hormone. Since it cannot be excluded that lanreotide may have this effect, other drugs mainly metabolized by CYP3A4 and which have a low therapeutic index should therefore be used with caution. Drugs metabolized by the liver may be metabolized more slowly during lanreotide treatment and dose reductions of the concomitantly administered medications should be considered). Products include:

Cardizem LA Extended Release Tablets 421

Diltiazem Maleate (The limited published data available indicate that somatostatin analogs may decrease the metabolic clearance of compounds known to be metabolized by the cytochrome P450 enzymes, which may be due to the suppression of growth hormone. Since it cannot be excluded that lanreotide may have this effect, other drugs mainly metabolized by CYP3A4 and which have a low therapeutic index should therefore be used with caution. Drugs metabolized by the liver may be metabolized more slowly during lanreotide treatment and dose reductions of the concomitantly administered medications should be considered).

No products indexed under this heading.

Disopyramide (The limited published data available indicate that somatostatin analogs may decrease the metabolic clearance of compounds known to be metabolized by the cytochrome P450 enzymes, which may be due to the suppression of growth hormone. Since it

cannot be excluded that lanreotide may have this effect, other drugs mainly metabolized by CYP3A4 and which have a low therapeutic index should therefore be used with caution. Drugs metabolized by the liver may be metabolized more slowly during lanreotide treatment and dose reductions of the concomitantly administered medications should be considered).

No products indexed under this heading.

Disopyramide Phosphate (The limited published data available indicate that somatostatin analogs may decrease the metabolic clearance of compounds known to be metabolized by the cytochrome P450 enzymes, which may be due to the suppression of growth hormone. Since it cannot be excluded that lanreotide may have this effect, other drugs mainly metabolized by CYP3A4 and which have a low therapeutic index should therefore be used with caution. Drugs metabolized by the liver may be metabolized more slowly during lanreotide treatment and dose reductions of the concomitantly administered medications should be considered).

No products indexed under this heading.

Disulfiram (The limited published data available indicate that somatostatin analogs may decrease the metabolic clearance of compounds known to be metabolized by the cytochrome P450 enzymes, which may be due to the suppression of growth hormone. Since it cannot be excluded that lanreotide may have this effect, other drugs mainly metabolized by CYP3A4 and which have a low therapeutic index should therefore be used with caution. Drugs metabolized by the liver may be metabolized more slowly during lanreotide treatment and dose reductions of the concomitantly administered medications should be considered).

No products indexed under this heading.

Doxorubicin Hydrochloride (The limited published data available indicate that somatostatin analogs may decrease the metabolic clearance of compounds known to be metabolized by the cytochrome P450 enzymes, which may be due to the suppression of growth hormone. Since it cannot be excluded that lanreotide may have this effect, other drugs mainly metabolized by CYP3A4 and which have a low therapeutic index should therefore be used with caution. Drugs metabolized by the liver may be metabolized more slowly during lanreotide treatment and dose reductions of the concomitantly administered medications should be considered).

No products indexed under this heading.

Dronabinol (The limited published data available indicate that somatostatin analogs may decrease the metabolic clearance of compounds known to be metabolized by the cytochrome P450 enzymes, which may be due to the suppression of growth hormone. Since it cannot be excluded that lanreotide may have this effect, other drugs mainly metabolized by CYP3A4 and which have a low therapeutic index should therefore be used with caution. Drugs metabolized by the liver may be metabolized more slowly during lanreotide treatment and dose reductions of the concomitantly administered medications should be considered). Products include:

Marinol Capsules **3163**

Ergotamine Tartrate (The limited published data available indicate that somatostatin analogs may decrease the metabolic clearance of compounds known to be metabolized by the cytochrome P450 enzymes, which may be due to the suppression of growth hormone. Since it cannot be excluded that lanreotide may have this effect, other drugs mainly metabolized by CYP3A4 and which have a low therapeutic index should therefore be used with caution. Drugs metabolized by the liver may be metabolized more slowly during lanreotide treatment and dose reductions of the concomitantly administered medications should be considered).

No products indexed under this heading.

Erythromycin (The limited published data available indicate that somatostatin analogs may decrease the metabolic clearance of compounds known to be metabolized by the cytochrome P450 enzymes, which may be due to the suppression of growth hormone. Since it cannot be excluded that lanreotide may have this effect, other drugs mainly metabolized by CYP3A4 and which have a low therapeutic index should therefore be used with caution. Drugs metabolized by the liver may be metabolized more slowly during lanreotide treatment and dose reductions of the concomitantly administered medications should be considered).

No products indexed under this heading.

Erythromycin Estolate (The limited published data available indicate that somatostatin analogs may decrease the metabolic clearance of compounds known to be metabolized by the cytochrome P450 enzymes, which may be due to the suppression of growth hormone. Since it cannot be excluded that lanreotide may have this effect, other drugs mainly metabolized by CYP3A4 and which have a low therapeutic index should therefore be used with caution. Drugs metabolized by the liver may be metabolized more slowly during lanreotide treatment and dose reductions of the concomitantly administered medications should be considered).

No products indexed under this heading.

Erythromycin Ethylsuccinate (The limited published data available indicate that somatostatin analogs may decrease the metabolic clearance of compounds known to be metabolized by the cytochrome P450 enzymes, which may be due to the suppression of growth hormone. Since it cannot be excluded that lanreotide may have this effect, other drugs mainly metabolized by CYP3A4 and which have a low therapeutic index should therefore be used with caution. Drugs metabolized by the liver may be metabolized more slowly during lanreotide treatment and dose reductions of the concomitantly administered medications should be considered). Products include:

E.E.S. **433**
EryPed **431**

Erythromycin Gluceptate (The limited published data available indicate that somatostatin analogs may decrease the metabolic clearance of compounds known to be metabolized by the cytochrome P450 enzymes, which may be due to the suppression of growth hormone. Since it cannot be excluded that lanreotide may have this effect, other drugs mainly metabolized by CYP3A4 and which have a low therapeutic index should therefore be used with caution. Drugs metabolized by the liver may be metabolized more slowly during lanreotide treatment and dose reductions of the concomitantly administered medications should be considered).

No products indexed under this heading.

Erythromycin Lactobionate (The limited published data available indicate that somatostatin analogs may decrease the metabolic clearance of compounds known to be metabolized by the cytochrome P450 enzymes, which may be due to the suppression of growth hormone. Since it cannot be excluded that lanreotide may have this effect, other drugs mainly metabolized by CYP3A4 and which have a low therapeutic index should therefore be used with caution. Drugs metabolized by the liver may be metabolized more slowly during lanreotide treatment and dose reductions of the concomitantly administered medications should be considered).

No products indexed under this heading.

Erythromycin Stearate (The limited published data available indicate that somatostatin analogs may decrease the metabolic clearance of compounds known to be metabolized by the cytochrome P450 enzymes, which may be due to the suppression of growth hormone. Since it cannot be excluded that lanreotide may have this effect, other drugs mainly metabolized by CYP3A4 and which have a low therapeutic index should therefore be used with caution. Drugs metabolized by the liver may be metabolized more slowly during lanreotide treatment and dose reductions of the concomitantly administered medications should be considered).

No products indexed under this heading.

Esmolol Hydrochloride (Concomitant administration of bradycardia-inducing drugs may have an additive effect on the reduction of heart rate associated with lanreotide. Dose adjustments of concomitant medication may be necessary).

No products indexed under this heading.

Estradiol (The limited published data available indicate that somatostatin analogs may decrease the metabolic clearance of compounds known to be metabolized by the cytochrome P450 enzymes, which may be due to the suppression of growth hormone. Since it cannot be excluded that lanreotide may have this effect, other drugs mainly metabolized by CYP3A4 and which have a low therapeutic index should therefore be used with caution. Drugs metabolized by the liver may be metabolized more slowly during lanreotide treatment and dose reductions of the concomitantly administered medications should be considered). Products include:

Activella Tablets **2347**
Angeliq Tablets **751**
Climara Transdermal System **763**
Climara Pro Transdermal System **768**
Divigel **3167**
Vagifem Tablets **2375**

Estradiol Benzoate (The limited published data available indicate that somatostatin analogs may decrease the metabolic clearance of compounds known to be metabolized by the cytochrome P450 enzymes, which may be due to the suppression of growth hormone. Since it cannot be excluded that lanreotide may have this effect, other drugs mainly metabolized by CYP3A4 and which have a low therapeutic index should therefore be used with caution. Drugs metabolized by the liver may be metabolized more slowly during lanreotide treatment and dose reductions of the concomitantly administered medications should be considered).

No products indexed under this heading.

Estradiol Cypionate (The limited published data available indicate that somatostatin analogs may decrease the metabolic clearance of compounds known to be metabolized by the cytochrome P450 enzymes, which may be due to the suppression of growth hormone. Since it cannot be excluded that lanreotide may have this effect, other drugs mainly metabolized by CYP3A4 and which have a low therapeutic index should therefore be used with caution. Drugs metabolized by the liver may be metabolized more slowly during lanreotide treatment and dose reductions of the concomitantly administered medications should be considered).

No products indexed under this heading.

Estradiol Valerate (The limited published data available indicate that somatostatin analogs may decrease the metabolic clearance of compounds known to be metabolized by the cytochrome P450 enzymes, which may be due to the suppression of growth hormone. Since it cannot be excluded that lanreotide may have this effect, other drugs mainly metabolized by CYP3A4 and which have a low therapeutic index should therefore be used with caution. Drugs metabolized by the liver may be metabolized more slowly during lanreotide treatment and dose reductions of the concomitantly administered medications should be considered).

No products indexed under this heading.

Ethinyl Estradiol (The limited published data available indicate that somatostatin analogs may decrease the metabolic clearance of compounds known to be metabolized by the cytochrome P450 enzymes, which may be due to the suppression of growth hormone. Since it cannot be excluded that lanreotide may have this effect, other drugs mainly metabolized by CYP3A4 and

which have a low therapeutic index should therefore be used with caution. Drugs metabolized by the liver may be metabolized more slowly during lanreotide treatment and dose reductions of the concomitantly administered medications should be considered). Products include:

Lybrel Tablets 3204
Mircette Tablets 1034
NuvaRing 2897
Ortho-Cyclen/Ortho Tri-Cyclen 2449
Ortho Evra Transdermal System 2437
Ortho Tri-Cyclen Lo Tablets 2458
Seasonique Tablets 1046
Yaz Tablets 805

Ethosuximide (The limited published data available indicate that somatostatin analogs may decrease the metabolic clearance of compounds known to be metabolized by the cytochrome P450 enzymes, which may be due to the suppression of growth hormone. Since it cannot be excluded that lanreotide may have this effect, other drugs mainly metabolized by CYP3A4 and which have a low therapeutic index should therefore be used with caution. Drugs metabolized by the liver may be metabolized more slowly during lanreotide treatment and dose reductions of the concomitantly administered medications should be considered).
No products indexed under this heading.

Ethynodiol Diacetate (The limited published data available indicate that somatostatin analogs may decrease the metabolic clearance of compounds known to be metabolized by the cytochrome P450 enzymes, which may be due to the suppression of growth hormone. Since it cannot be excluded that lanreotide may have this effect, other drugs mainly metabolized by CYP3A4 and which have a low therapeutic index should therefore be used with caution. Drugs metabolized by the liver may be metabolized more slowly during lanreotide treatment and dose reductions of the concomitantly administered medications should be considered).
No products indexed under this heading.

Etoposide (The limited published data available indicate that somatostatin analogs may decrease the metabolic clearance of compounds known to be metabolized by the cytochrome P450 enzymes, which may be due to the suppression of growth hormone. Since it cannot be excluded that lanreotide may have this effect, other drugs mainly metabolized by CYP3A4 and which have a low therapeutic index should therefore be used with caution. Drugs metabolized by the liver may be metabolized more slowly during lanreotide treatment and dose reductions of the concomitantly administered medications should be considered).
No products indexed under this heading.

Etoposide Phosphate (The limited published data available indicate that somatostatin analogs may decrease the metabolic clearance of compounds known to be metabolized by the cytochrome P450 enzymes, which may be due to the suppression of growth hormone. Since it cannot be excluded that lanreotide may have this effect, other drugs mainly metabolized by CYP3A4 and which have a low therapeutic index should therefore be used with caution. Drugs metabolized by the liver may be metabolized more slowly during lanreotide treatment and dose reductions of the concomitantly administered medications should be considered).
No products indexed under this heading.

Felodipine (The limited published data available indicate that somatostatin analogs may decrease the metabolic clearance of compounds known to be metabolized by the cytochrome P450 enzymes, which may be due to the suppression of growth hormone. Since it cannot be excluded that lanreotide may have this effect, other drugs mainly metabolized by CYP3A4 and which have a low therapeutic index should therefore be used with caution. Drugs metabolized by the liver may be metabolized more slowly during lanreotide treatment and dose reductions of the concomitantly administered medications should be considered).
No products indexed under this heading.

Fentanyl (The limited published data available indicate that somatostatin analogs may decrease the metabolic clearance of compounds known to be metabolized by the cytochrome P450 enzymes, which may be due to the suppression of growth hormone. Since it cannot be excluded that lanreotide may have this effect, other drugs mainly metabolized by CYP3A4 and which have a low therapeutic index should therefore be used with caution. Drugs metabolized by the liver may be metabolized more slowly during lanreotide treatment and dose reductions of the concomitantly administered medications should be considered). Products include:

Duragesic Transdermal System 2405
Ionsys Transdermal System 2410

Fentanyl Citrate (The limited published data available indicate that somatostatin analogs may decrease the metabolic clearance of compounds known to be metabolized by the cytochrome P450 enzymes, which may be due to the suppression of growth hormone. Since it cannot be excluded that lanreotide may have this effect, other drugs mainly metabolized by CYP3A4 and which have a low therapeutic index should therefore be used with caution. Drugs metabolized by the liver may be metabolized more slowly during lanreotide treatment and dose reductions of the concomitantly administered medications should be considered). Products include:

Actiq 959
Fentora Tablets 968

Glimepiride (Lanreotide inhibits the secretion of insulin and glucagon. Therefore, blood glucose levels should be monitored when lanreotide treatment is initiated or when the dose is altered and antidiabetic treatment should be adjusted accordingly). Products include:

Avandaryl Tablets 1344
Duetact Tablets 3085

Glipizide (Lanreotide inhibits the secretion of insulin and glucagon. Therefore, blood glucose levels should be monitored when lanreotide treatment is initiated or when the dose is altered and antidiabetic treatment should be adjusted accordingly).
No products indexed under this heading.

Glyburide (Lanreotide inhibits the secretion of insulin and glucagon. Therefore, blood glucose levels should be monitored when lanreotide treatment is initiated or when the dose is altered and antidiabetic treatment should be adjusted accordingly).
No products indexed under this heading.

Haloperidol (The limited published data available indicate that somatostatin analogs may decrease the metabolic clearance of compounds known to be metabolized by the cytochrome P450 enzymes, which may be due to the suppression of growth hormone. Since it cannot be excluded that lanreotide may have this effect, other drugs mainly metabolized by CYP3A4 and which have a low therapeutic index should therefore be used with caution. Drugs metabolized by the liver may be metabolized more slowly during lanreotide treatment and dose reductions of the concomitantly administered medications should be considered).
No products indexed under this heading.

Haloperidol Decanoate (The limited published data available indicate that somatostatin analogs may decrease the metabolic clearance of compounds known to be metabolized by the cytochrome P450 enzymes, which may be due to the suppression of growth hormone. Since it cannot be excluded that lanreotide may have this effect, other drugs mainly metabolized by CYP3A4 and which have a low therapeutic index should therefore be used with caution. Drugs metabolized by the liver may be metabolized more slowly during lanreotide treatment and dose reductions of the concomitantly administered medications should be considered).
No products indexed under this heading.

Haloperidol Lactate (The limited published data available indicate that somatostatin analogs may decrease the metabolic clearance of compounds known to be metabolized by the cytochrome P450 enzymes, which may be due to the suppression of growth hormone. Since it cannot be excluded that lanreotide may have this effect, other drugs mainly metabolized by CYP3A4 and which have a low therapeutic index should therefore be used with caution. Drugs metabolized by the liver may be metabolized more slowly during lanreotide treatment and dose reductions of the concomitantly administered medications should be considered).
No products indexed under this heading.

Indinavir Sulfate (The limited published data available indicate that somatostatin analogs may decrease the metabolic clearance of compounds known to be metabolized by the cytochrome P450 enzymes, which may be due to the suppression of growth hormone. Since it cannot be excluded that lanreotide may have this effect, other drugs mainly metabolized by CYP3A4 and which have a low therapeutic index should therefore be used with caution. Drugs metabolized by the liver may be metabolized more slowly during lanreotide treatment and dose reductions of the concomitantly administered medications should be considered). Products include:

Crixivan Capsules 1979

Insulin (Lanreotide inhibits the secretion of insulin and glucagon. Therefore, blood glucose levels should be monitored when lanreotide treatment is initiated or when the dose is altered and antidiabetic treatment should be adjusted accordingly).
No products indexed under this heading.

Insulin, Human, Zinc Suspension (Lanreotide inhibits the secretion of insulin and glucagon. Therefore, blood glucose levels should be monitored when lanreotide treatment is initiated or when the dose is altered and antidiabetic treatment should be adjusted accordingly).
No products indexed under this heading.

Insulin, Human (rDNA origin) (Lanreotide inhibits the secretion of insulin and glucagon. Therefore, blood glucose levels should be monitored when lanreotide treatment is initiated or when the dose is altered and antidiabetic treatment should be adjusted accordingly). Products include:

Exubera Inhalation Powder 2515

Insulin, Human NPH (Lanreotide inhibits the secretion of insulin and glucagon. Therefore, blood glucose levels should be monitored when lanreotide treatment is initiated or when the dose is altered and antidiabetic treatment should be adjusted accordingly). Products include:

Humulin N Vial 1846

Insulin, Human Regular (Lanreotide inhibits the secretion of insulin and glucagon. Therefore, blood glucose levels should be monitored when lanreotide treatment is initiated or when the dose is altered and antidiabetic treatment should be adjusted accordingly). Products include:

Humulin R 1849
Humulin R (U-500) 1850

Insulin, Human Regular and Human NPH Mixture (Lanreotide inhibits the secretion of insulin and glucagon. Therefore, blood glucose levels should be monitored when lanreotide treatment is initiated or when the dose is altered and antidiabetic treatment should be adjusted accordingly). Products include:

Humulin 50/50, 100 Units 1843
Humulin 70/30 Vial 1844

Insulin, NPH (Lanreotide inhibits the secretion of insulin and glucagon. Therefore, blood glucose levels should be monitored when lanreotide treatment is initiated or when the dose is altered and antidiabetic treatment should be adjusted accordingly).
No products indexed under this heading.

Insulin, Regular (Lanreotide inhibits the secretion of insulin and glucagon. Therefore, blood glucose levels should be monitored when lanreotide treatment is initiated or when the dose is altered and antidiabetic treatment should be adjusted accordingly).

No products indexed under this heading.

Insulin, Regular and NPH mixture (Lanreotide inhibits the secretion of insulin and glucagon. Therefore, blood glucose levels should be monitored when lanreotide treatment is initiated or when the dose is altered and antidiabetic treatment should be adjusted accordingly).

No products indexed under this heading.

Insulin, Zinc Crystals (Lanreotide inhibits the secretion of insulin and glucagon. Therefore, blood glucose levels should be monitored when lanreotide treatment is initiated or when the dose is altered and antidiabetic treatment should be adjusted accordingly).

No products indexed under this heading.

Insulin, Zinc Suspension (Lanreotide inhibits the secretion of insulin and glucagon. Therefore, blood glucose levels should be monitored when lanreotide treatment is initiated or when the dose is altered and antidiabetic treatment should be adjusted accordingly).

No products indexed under this heading.

Insulin Aspart (Lanreotide inhibits the secretion of insulin and glucagon. Therefore, blood glucose levels should be monitored when lanreotide treatment is initiated or when the dose is altered and antidiabetic treatment should be adjusted accordingly).

No products indexed under this heading.

Insulin Aspart, Human (Lanreotide inhibits the secretion of insulin and glucagon. Therefore, blood glucose levels should be monitored when lanreotide treatment is initiated or when the dose is altered and antidiabetic treatment should be adjusted accordingly). Products include:

NovoLog Mix 70/30 2364

Insulin Aspart, Human Regular (Lanreotide inhibits the secretion of insulin and glucagon. Therefore, blood glucose levels should be monitored when lanreotide treatment is initiated or when the dose is altered and antidiabetic treatment should be adjusted accordingly). Products include:

NovoLog Injection 2359

Insulin Aspart Protamine, Human (Lanreotide inhibits the secretion of insulin and glucagon. Therefore, blood glucose levels should be monitored when lanreotide treatment is initiated or when the dose is altered and antidiabetic treatment should be adjusted accordingly). Products include:

NovoLog Mix 70/30 2364

Insulin Detemir (rDNA Origin) (Lanreotide inhibits the secretion of insulin and glucagon. Therefore, blood glucose levels should be monitored when lanreotide treatment is initiated or when the dose is altered and antidiabetic treatment should be adjusted accordingly). Products include:

Levemir Injection 2352

Insulin glargine (Lanreotide inhibits the secretion of insulin and glucagon. Therefore, blood glucose levels should be monitored when lanreotide treatment is initiated or when the dose is altered and antidiabetic treatment should be adjusted accordingly). Products include:

Lantus Injection 2749

Insulin Glulisine (Lanreotide inhibits the secretion of insulin and glucagon. Therefore, blood glucose levels should be monitored when lanreotide treatment is initiated or when the dose is altered and antidiabetic treatment should be adjusted accordingly). Products include:

Apidra Injection 2706

Insulin Lispro, Human (Lanreotide inhibits the secretion of insulin and glucagon. Therefore, blood glucose levels should be monitored when lanreotide treatment is initiated or when the dose is altered and antidiabetic treatment should be adjusted accordingly). Products include:

Humalog-Pen and KwikPen 1829
Humalog Mix 50/50-Pen and KwikPen 1833
Humalog Mix 75/25-Pen and KwikPen 1835

Insulin Lispro Protamine, Human (Lanreotide inhibits the secretion of insulin and glucagon. Therefore, blood glucose levels should be monitored when lanreotide treatment is initiated or when the dose is altered and antidiabetic treatment should be adjusted accordingly). Products include:

Humalog Mix 50/50-Pen and KwikPen 1833
Humalog Mix 75/25-Pen and KwikPen 1835

Isradipine (The limited published data available indicate that somatostatin analogs may decrease the metabolic clearance of compounds known to be metabolized by the cytochrome P450 enzymes, which may be due to the suppression of growth hormone. Since it cannot be excluded that lanreotide may have this effect, other drugs mainly metabolized by CYP3A4 and which have a low therapeutic index should therefore be used with caution. Drugs metabolized by the liver may be metabolized more slowly during lanreotide treatment and dose reductions of the concomitantly administered medications should be considered). Products include:

DynaCirc CR Controlled Release Tablets 1407

Itraconazole (The limited published data available indicate that somatostatin analogs may decrease the metabolic clearance of compounds known to be metabolized by the cytochrome P450 enzymes, which may be due to the suppression of growth hormone. Since it cannot be excluded that lanreotide may have this effect, other drugs mainly metabolized by CYP3A4 and which have a low therapeutic index should therefore be used with caution. Drugs metabolized by the liver may be metabolized more slowly during lanreotide treatment and dose reductions of the concomitantly administered medications should be considered).

No products indexed under this heading.

Ixabepilone (The limited published data available indicate that somatostatin analogs may decrease the metabolic clearance of compounds known to be metabolized by the cytochrome P450 enzymes, which may be due to the suppression of growth hormone. Since it cannot be excluded that lanreotide may have this effect, other drugs mainly metabolized by CYP3A4 and which have a low therapeutic index should therefore be used with caution. Drugs metabolized by the liver may be metabolized more slowly during lanreotide treatment and dose reductions of the concomitantly administered medications should be considered). Products include:

Ixempra Kit for Injection 915

Ketoconazole (The limited published data available indicate that somatostatin analogs may decrease the metabolic clearance of compounds known to be metabolized by the cytochrome P450 enzymes, which may be due to the suppression of growth hormone. Since it cannot be excluded that lanreotide may have this effect, other drugs mainly metabolized by CYP3A4 and which have a low therapeutic index should therefore be used with caution. Drugs metabolized by the liver may be metabolized more slowly during lanreotide treatment and dose reductions of the concomitantly administered medications should be considered). Products include:

Extina Foam, 2% 3057
Nizoral A-D Shampoo 1901

Labetalol Hydrochloride (Concomitant administration of bradycardia-inducing drugs may have an additive effect on the reduction of heart rate associated with lanreotide. Dose adjustments of concomitant medication may be necessary).

No products indexed under this heading.

Levobunolol Hydrochloride (Concomitant administration of bradycardia-inducing drugs may have an additive effect on the reduction of heart rate associated with lanreotide. Dose adjustments of concomitant medication may be necessary).

No products indexed under this heading.

Levonorgestrel (The limited published data available indicate that somatostatin analogs may decrease the metabolic clearance of compounds known to be metabolized by the cytochrome P450 enzymes, which may be due to the suppression of growth hormone. Since it cannot be excluded that lanreotide may have this effect, other drugs mainly metabolized by CYP3A4 and which have a low therapeutic index should therefore be used with caution. Drugs metabolized by the liver may be metabolized more slowly during lanreotide treatment and dose reductions of the concomitantly administered medications should be considered). Products include:

Climara Pro Transdermal System 768
Lybrel Tablets 3204
Mirena Intrauterine System 779
Plan B Tablets 1044
Seasonique Tablets 1046

Lidocaine (The limited published data available indicate that somatostatin analogs may decrease the metabolic clearance of compounds known to be metabolized by the cytochrome P450 enzymes, which may be due to the suppression of growth hormone. Since it cannot be excluded that lanreotide may have this effect, other drugs mainly metabolized by CYP3A4 and which have a low therapeutic index should therefore be used with caution. Drugs metabolized by the liver may be metabolized more slowly during lanreotide treatment and dose reductions of the concomitantly administered medications should be considered). Products include:

Lidoderm Patch 1114

Lidocaine Hydrochloride (The limited published data available indicate that somatostatin analogs may decrease the metabolic clearance of compounds known to be metabolized by the cytochrome P450 enzymes, which may be due to the suppression of growth hormone. Since it cannot be excluded that lanreotide may have this effect, other drugs mainly metabolized by CYP3A4 and which have a low therapeutic index should therefore be used with caution. Drugs metabolized by the liver may be metabolized more slowly during lanreotide treatment and dose reductions of the concomitantly administered medications should be considered).

No products indexed under this heading.

Lovastatin (The limited published data available indicate that somatostatin analogs may decrease the metabolic clearance of compounds known to be metabolized by the cytochrome P450 enzymes, which may be due to the suppression of growth hormone. Since it cannot be excluded that lanreotide may have this effect, other drugs mainly metabolized by CYP3A4 and which have a low therapeutic index should therefore be used with caution. Drugs metabolized by the liver may be metabolized more slowly during lanreotide treatment and dose reductions of the concomitantly administered medications should be considered). Products include:

Advicor Tablets 402
Mevacor Tablets 2063

Mestranol (The limited published data available indicate that somatostatin analogs may decrease the metabolic clearance of compounds known to be metabolized by the cytochrome P450 enzymes, which may be due to the suppression of growth hormone. Since it cannot be excluded that lanreotide may have this effect, other drugs mainly metabolized by CYP3A4 and which have a low therapeutic index should therefore be used with caution. Drugs metabolized by the liver may be metabolized more slowly during lanreotide treatment and dose reductions of the concomitantly administered medications should be considered).

No products indexed under this heading.

Metformin Hydrochloride (Lanreotide inhibits the secretion of insulin and glucagon. Therefore, blood glucose levels should be monitored when lanreotide treatment is initiated

or when the dose is altered and antidiabetic treatment should be adjusted accordingly). Products include:
ActoPlus Met Tablets 3071
Avandamet Tablets 1336
Janumet Tablets 2041
PrandiMet Tablets 2967

Methadone Hydrochloride (The limited published data available indicate that somatostatin analogs may decrease the metabolic clearance of compounds known to be metabolized by the cytochrome P450 enzymes, which may be due to the suppression of growth hormone. Since it cannot be excluded that lanreotide may have this effect, other drugs mainly metabolized by CYP3A4 and which have a low therapeutic index should therefore be used with caution. Drugs metabolized by the liver may be metabolized more slowly during lanreotide treatment and dose reductions of the concomitantly administered medications should be considered).
No products indexed under this heading.

Metipranolol Hydrochloride (Concomitant administration of bradycardia-inducing drugs may have an additive effect on the reduction of heart rate associated with lanreotide. Dose adjustments of concomitant medication may be necessary).
No products indexed under this heading.

Metoprolol Succinate (Concomitant administration of bradycardia-inducing drugs may have an additive effect on the reduction of heart rate associated with lanreotide. Dose adjustments of concomitant medication may be necessary). Products include:
Toprol-XL Tablets 666

Metoprolol Tartrate (Concomitant administration of bradycardia-inducing drugs may have an additive effect on the reduction of heart rate associated with lanreotide. Dose adjustments of concomitant medication may be necessary).
No products indexed under this heading.

Midazolam Hydrochloride (The limited published data available indicate that somatostatin analogs may decrease the metabolic clearance of compounds known to be metabolized by the cytochrome P450 enzymes, which may be due to the suppression of growth hormone. Since it cannot be excluded that lanreotide may have this effect, other drugs mainly metabolized by CYP3A4 and which have a low therapeutic index should therefore be used with caution. Drugs metabolized by the liver may be metabolized more slowly during lanreotide treatment and dose reductions of the concomitantly administered medications should be considered).
No products indexed under this heading.

Miglitol (Lanreotide inhibits the secretion of insulin and glucagon. Therefore, blood glucose levels should be monitored when lanreotide treatment is initiated or when the dose is altered and antidiabetic treatment should be adjusted accordingly).
No products indexed under this heading.

Nadolol (Concomitant administration of bradycardia-inducing drugs may have an additive effect on the reduction of heart rate associated with lanreotide. Dose adjustments of concomitant medication may be necessary). Products include:
Nadolol Tablets 2191

Nateglinide (Lanreotide inhibits the secretion of insulin and glucagon. Therefore, blood glucose levels should be monitored when lanreotide treatment is initiated or when the dose is altered and antidiabetic treatment should be adjusted accordingly). Products include:
Starlix Tablets 2314

Nebivolol (Concomitant administration of bradycardia-inducing drugs may have an additive effect on the reduction of heart rate associated with lanreotide. Dose adjustments of concomitant medication may be necessary). Products include:
Bystolic Tablets 1155

Nefazodone Hydrochloride (The limited published data available indicate that somatostatin analogs may decrease the metabolic clearance of compounds known to be metabolized by the cytochrome P450 enzymes, which may be due to the suppression of growth hormone. Since it cannot be excluded that lanreotide may have this effect, other drugs mainly metabolized by CYP3A4 and which have a low therapeutic index should therefore be used with caution. Drugs metabolized by the liver may be metabolized more slowly during lanreotide treatment and dose reductions of the concomitantly administered medications should be considered).
No products indexed under this heading.

Nelfinavir Mesylate (The limited published data available indicate that somatostatin analogs may decrease the metabolic clearance of compounds known to be metabolized by the cytochrome P450 enzymes, which may be due to the suppression of growth hormone. Since it cannot be excluded that lanreotide may have this effect, other drugs mainly metabolized by CYP3A4 and which have a low therapeutic index should therefore be used with caution. Drugs metabolized by the liver may be metabolized more slowly during lanreotide treatment and dose reductions of the concomitantly administered medications should be considered).
No products indexed under this heading.

Nicardipine Hydrochloride (The limited published data available indicate that somatostatin analogs may decrease the metabolic clearance of compounds known to be metabolized by the cytochrome P450 enzymes, which may be due to the suppression of growth hormone. Since it cannot be excluded that lanreotide may have this effect, other drugs mainly metabolized by CYP3A4 and which have a low therapeutic index should therefore be used with caution. Drugs metabolized by the liver may be metabolized more slowly during lanreotide treatment and dose reductions of the concomitantly administered medications should be considered). Products include:
Cardene I.V. 1093

Nifedipine (The limited published data available indicate that somatostatin analogs may decrease the metabolic clearance of compounds known to be metabolized by the cytochrome P450 enzymes, which may be due to the suppression of growth hormone. Since it cannot be excluded that lanreotide may have this effect, other drugs mainly metabolized by CYP3A4 and which have a low therapeutic index should therefore be used with caution. Drugs metabolized by the liver may be metabolized more slowly during lanreotide treatment and dose reductions of the concomitantly administered medications should be considered).
No products indexed under this heading.

Nimodipine (The limited published data available indicate that somatostatin analogs may decrease the metabolic clearance of compounds known to be metabolized by the cytochrome P450 enzymes, which may be due to the suppression of growth hormone. Since it cannot be excluded that lanreotide may have this effect, other drugs mainly metabolized by CYP3A4 and which have a low therapeutic index should therefore be used with caution. Drugs metabolized by the liver may be metabolized more slowly during lanreotide treatment and dose reductions of the concomitantly administered medications should be considered). Products include:
Nimotop Capsules 790

Nisoldipine (The limited published data available indicate that somatostatin analogs may decrease the metabolic clearance of compounds known to be metabolized by the cytochrome P450 enzymes, which may be due to the suppression of growth hormone. Since it cannot be excluded that lanreotide may have this effect, other drugs mainly metabolized by CYP3A4 and which have a low therapeutic index should therefore be used with caution. Drugs metabolized by the liver may be metabolized more slowly during lanreotide treatment and dose reductions of the concomitantly administered medications should be considered). Products include:
Sular Extended Release Tablets 2975

Nitrendipine (The limited published data available indicate that somatostatin analogs may decrease the metabolic clearance of compounds known to be metabolized by the cytochrome P450 enzymes, which may be due to the suppression of growth hormone. Since it cannot be excluded that lanreotide may have this effect, other drugs mainly metabolized by CYP3A4 and which have a low therapeutic index should therefore be used with caution. Drugs metabolized by the liver may be metabolized more slowly during lanreotide treatment and dose reductions of the concomitantly administered medications should be considered).
No products indexed under this heading.

Norethindrone (The limited published data available indicate that somatostatin analogs may decrease the metabolic clearance of compounds known to be metabolized by the cytochrome P450 enzymes, which may be due to the suppression of growth hormone. Since it cannot be excluded that lanreotide may have this effect, other drugs mainly metabolized by CYP3A4 and which have a low therapeutic index should therefore be used with caution. Drugs metabolized by the liver may be metabolized more slowly during lanreotide treatment and dose reductions of the concomitantly administered medications should be considered). Products include:
Ortho Micronor Tablets 2446

Norethindrone Acetate (The limited published data available indicate that somatostatin analogs may decrease the metabolic clearance of compounds known to be metabolized by the cytochrome P450 enzymes, which may be due to the suppression of growth hormone. Since it cannot be excluded that lanreotide may have this effect, other drugs mainly metabolized by CYP3A4 and which have a low therapeutic index should therefore be used with caution. Drugs metabolized by the liver may be metabolized more slowly during lanreotide treatment and dose reductions of the concomitantly administered medications should be considered). Products include:
Activella Tablets 2347

Norgestrel (The limited published data available indicate that somatostatin analogs may decrease the metabolic clearance of compounds known to be metabolized by the cytochrome P450 enzymes, which may be due to the suppression of growth hormone. Since it cannot be excluded that lanreotide may have this effect, other drugs mainly metabolized by CYP3A4 and which have a low therapeutic index should therefore be used with caution. Drugs metabolized by the liver may be metabolized more slowly during lanreotide treatment and dose reductions of the concomitantly administered medications should be considered).
No products indexed under this heading.

Ondansetron (The limited published data available indicate that somatostatin analogs may decrease the metabolic clearance of compounds known to be metabolized by the cytochrome P450 enzymes, which may be due to the suppression of growth hormone. Since it cannot be excluded that lanreotide may have this effect, other drugs mainly metabolized by CYP3A4 and which have a low therapeutic index should therefore be used with caution. Drugs metabolized by the liver may be metabolized more slowly during lanreotide treatment and dose reductions of the concomitantly administered medications should be considered). Products include:
Zofran ODT Orally Disintegrating Tablets 1687

Ondansetron Hydrochloride (The limited published data available indicate that somatostatin analogs may decrease the metabolic clearance of compounds known to be metabolized by the cytochrome P450 enzymes, which may be due to the suppression of growth hormone. Since it cannot be excluded that lanreotide may have this effect, other drugs mainly metabolized by

CYP3A4 and which have a low therapeutic index should therefore be used with caution. Drugs metabolized by the liver may be metabolized more slowly during lanreotide treatment and dose reductions of the concomitantly administered medications should be considered).
Products include:
Zofran Injection 1682
Zofran 1687

Paclitaxel (The limited published data available indicate that somatostatin analogs may decrease the metabolic clearance of compounds known to be metabolized by the cytochrome P450 enzymes, which may be due to the suppression of growth hormone. Since it cannot be excluded that lanreotide may have this effect, other drugs mainly metabolized by CYP3A4 and which have a low therapeutic index should therefore be used with caution. Drugs metabolized by the liver may be metabolized more slowly during lanreotide treatment and dose reductions of the concomitantly administered medications should be considered).
No products indexed under this heading.

Penbutolol Sulfate (Concomitant administration of bradycardia-inducing drugs may have an additive effect on the reduction of heart rate associated with lanreotide. Dose adjustments of concomitant medication may be necessary).
No products indexed under this heading.

Pimozide (The limited published data available indicate that somatostatin analogs may decrease the metabolic clearance of compounds known to be metabolized by the cytochrome P450 enzymes, which may be due to the suppression of growth hormone. Since it cannot be excluded that lanreotide may have this effect, other drugs mainly metabolized by CYP3A4 and which have a low therapeutic index should therefore be used with caution. Drugs metabolized by the liver may be metabolized more slowly during lanreotide treatment and dose reductions of the concomitantly administered medications should be considered).
No products indexed under this heading.

Pindolol (Concomitant administration of bradycardia-inducing drugs may have an additive effect on the reduction of heart rate associated with lanreotide. Dose adjustments of concomitant medication may be necessary).
No products indexed under this heading.

Pioglitazone Hydrochloride (Lanreotide inhibits the secretion of insulin and glucagon. Therefore, blood glucose levels should be monitored when lanreotide treatment is initiated or when the dose is altered and antidiabetic treatment should be adjusted accordingly). Products include:
ActoPlus Met Tablets 3071
Actos Tablets 3077
Duetact Tablets 3085

Polyestradiol Phosphate (The limited published data available indicate that somatostatin analogs may decrease the metabolic clearance of compounds known to be metabolized by the cytochrome P450 enzymes, which may be due to the suppression of growth hormone. Since it cannot be excluded that lanreotide may have this effect, other drugs mainly metabolized by CYP3A4 and which have a low therapeutic index should therefore be used with caution. Drugs metabolized by the liver may be metabolized more slowly during lanreotide treatment and dose reductions of the concomitantly administered medications should be considered).
No products indexed under this heading.

Propranolol Hydrochloride (Concomitant administration of bradycardia-inducing drugs may have an additive effect on the reduction of heart rate associated with lanreotide. Dose adjustments of concomitant medication may be necessary). Products include:
InnoPran XL Extended Release Capsules 1484

Quinidine Gluconate (The limited published data available indicate that somatostatin analogs may decrease the metabolic clearance of compounds known to be metabolized by the cytochrome P450 enzymes, which may be due to the suppression of growth hormone. Since it cannot be excluded that lanreotide may have this effect, other drugs mainly metabolized by CYP3A4 and which have a low therapeutic index should therefore be used with caution. Drugs metabolized by the liver may be metabolized more slowly during lanreotide treatment and dose reductions of the concomitantly administered medications should be considered).
No products indexed under this heading.

Quinidine Polygalacturonate (The limited published data available indicate that somatostatin analogs may decrease the metabolic clearance of compounds known to be metabolized by the cytochrome P450 enzymes, which may be due to the suppression of growth hormone. Since it cannot be excluded that lanreotide may have this effect, other drugs mainly metabolized by CYP3A4 and which have a low therapeutic index should therefore be used with caution. Drugs metabolized by the liver may be metabolized more slowly during lanreotide treatment and dose reductions of the concomitantly administered medications should be considered).
No products indexed under this heading.

Quinidine Sulfate (The limited published data available indicate that somatostatin analogs may decrease the metabolic clearance of compounds known to be metabolized by the cytochrome P450 enzymes, which may be due to the suppression of growth hormone. Since it cannot be excluded that lanreotide may have this effect, other drugs mainly metabolized by CYP3A4 and which have a low therapeutic index should therefore be used with caution. Drugs metabolized by the liver may be metabolized more slowly during lanreotide treatment and dose reductions of the concomitantly administered medications should be considered).
No products indexed under this heading.

Repaglinide (Lanreotide inhibits the secretion of insulin and glucagon. Therefore, blood glucose levels should be monitored when lanreotide treatment is initiated or when the dose is altered and antidiabetic treatment should be adjusted accordingly). Products include:
PrandiMet Tablets 2967
Prandin Tablets 2971

Rifabutin (The limited published data available indicate that somatostatin analogs may decrease the metabolic clearance of compounds known to be metabolized by the cytochrome P450 enzymes, which may be due to the suppression of growth hormone. Since it cannot be excluded that lanreotide may have this effect, other drugs mainly metabolized by CYP3A4 and which have a low therapeutic index should therefore be used with caution. Drugs metabolized by the liver may be metabolized more slowly during lanreotide treatment and dose reductions of the concomitantly administered medications should be considered).
No products indexed under this heading.

Ritonavir (The limited published data available indicate that somatostatin analogs may decrease the metabolic clearance of compounds known to be metabolized by the cytochrome P450 enzymes, which may be due to the suppression of growth hormone. Since it cannot be excluded that lanreotide may have this effect, other drugs mainly metabolized by CYP3A4 and which have a low therapeutic index should therefore be used with caution. Drugs metabolized by the liver may be metabolized more slowly during lanreotide treatment and dose reductions of the concomitantly administered medications should be considered). Products include:
Kaletra 452
Norvir 489

Rosiglitazone Maleate (Lanreotide inhibits the secretion of insulin and glucagon. Therefore, blood glucose levels should be monitored when lanreotide treatment is initiated or when the dose is altered and antidiabetic treatment should be adjusted accordingly). Products include:
Avandamet Tablets 1336
Avandaryl Tablets 1344
Avandia Tablets 1351

Saquinavir (The limited published data available indicate that somatostatin analogs may decrease the metabolic clearance of compounds known to be metabolized by the cytochrome P450 enzymes, which may be due to the suppression of growth hormone. Since it cannot be excluded that lanreotide may have this effect, other drugs mainly metabolized by CYP3A4 and which have a low therapeutic index should therefore be used with caution. Drugs metabolized by the liver may be metabolized more slowly during lanreotide treatment and dose reductions of the concomitantly administered medications should be considered).
No products indexed under this heading.

Saquinavir Mesylate (The limited published data available indicate that somatostatin analogs may decrease the metabolic clearance of compounds known to be metabolized by the cytochrome P450 enzymes, which may be due to the suppression of growth hormone. Since it cannot be excluded that lanreotide may have this effect, other drugs mainly metabolized by CYP3A4 and which have a low therapeutic index should therefore be used with caution. Drugs metabolized by the liver may be metabolized more slowly during lanreotide treatment and dose reductions of the concomitantly administered medications should be considered).
No products indexed under this heading.

Sertraline Hydrochloride (The limited published data available indicate that somatostatin analogs may decrease the metabolic clearance of compounds known to be metabolized by the cytochrome P450 enzymes, which may be due to the suppression of growth hormone. Since it cannot be excluded that lanreotide may have this effect, other drugs mainly metabolized by CYP3A4 and which have a low therapeutic index should therefore be used with caution. Drugs metabolized by the liver may be metabolized more slowly during lanreotide treatment and dose reductions of the concomitantly administered medications should be considered).
No products indexed under this heading.

Sildenafil Citrate (The limited published data available indicate that somatostatin analogs may decrease the metabolic clearance of compounds known to be metabolized by the cytochrome P450 enzymes, which may be due to the suppression of growth hormone. Since it cannot be excluded that lanreotide may have this effect, other drugs mainly metabolized by CYP3A4 and which have a low therapeutic index should therefore be used with caution. Drugs metabolized by the liver may be metabolized more slowly during lanreotide treatment and dose reductions of the concomitantly administered medications should be considered).
No products indexed under this heading.

Simvastatin (The limited published data available indicate that somatostatin analogs may decrease the metabolic clearance of compounds known to be metabolized by the cytochrome P450 enzymes, which may be due to the suppression of growth hormone. Since it cannot be excluded that lanreotide may have this effect, other drugs mainly metabolized by CYP3A4 and which have a low therapeutic index should therefore be used with caution. Drugs metabolized by the liver may be metabolized more slowly during lanreotide treatment and dose reductions of the concomitantly administered medications should be considered). Products include:
Simcor Tablets 502
Vytorin 10/10 Tablets 2149
Vytorin 10/10 Tablets 2939
Vytorin 10/20 Tablets 2149
Vytorin 10/20 Tablets 2939
Vytorin 10/40 Tablets 2149
Vytorin 10/40 Tablets 2939
Vytorin 10/80 Tablets 2149
Vytorin 10/80 Tablets 2939
Zocor Tablets 2136

Sirolimus (The limited published data available indicate that somatostatin analogs may decrease the metabolic clearance of compounds known to be metabolized by the cytochrome P450 enzymes, which may be due to the suppression of growth hormone. Since it cannot be excluded that lanreotide may have this effect, other drugs mainly metabolized by CYP3A4 and which have a low therapeutic index should therefore be used with caution. Drugs metabolized by the liver may be metabolized more slowly during lanreotide treatment and dose reductions of the concomitantly administered medications should be considered). Products include:

Rapamune 3260

Sitagliptin Phosphate (Lanreotide inhibits the secretion of insulin and glucagon. Therefore, blood glucose levels should be monitored when lanreotide treatment is initiated or when the dose is altered and antidiabetic treatment should be adjusted accordingly). Products include:

Janumet Tablets 2041
Januvia Tablets 2048

Sotalol Hydrochloride (Concomitant administration of bradycardia-inducing drugs may have an additive effect on the reduction of heart rate associated with lanreotide. Dose adjustments of concomitant medication may be necessary).

No products indexed under this heading.

Tacrolimus (The limited published data available indicate that somatostatin analogs may decrease the metabolic clearance of compounds known to be metabolized by the cytochrome P450 enzymes, which may be due to the suppression of growth hormone. Since it cannot be excluded that lanreotide may have this effect, other drugs mainly metabolized by CYP3A4 and which have a low therapeutic index should therefore be used with caution. Drugs metabolized by the liver may be metabolized more slowly during lanreotide treatment and dose reductions of the concomitantly administered medications should be considered). Products include:

Prograf Capsules and Injection 622
Protopic Ointment 628

Tadalafil (The limited published data available indicate that somatostatin analogs may decrease the metabolic clearance of compounds known to be metabolized by the cytochrome P450 enzymes, which may be due to the suppression of growth hormone. Since it cannot be excluded that lanreotide may have this effect, other drugs mainly metabolized by CYP3A4 and which have a low therapeutic index should therefore be used with caution. Drugs metabolized by the liver may be metabolized more slowly during lanreotide treatment and dose reductions of the concomitantly administered medications should be considered). Products include:

Cialis Tablets 1792

Tamoxifen Citrate (The limited published data available indicate that somatostatin analogs may decrease the metabolic clearance of compounds known to be metabolized by the cytochrome P450 enzymes, which may be due to the suppression of growth hormone. Since it cannot be excluded that lanreotide may have this effect, other drugs mainly metabolized by CYP3A4 and which have a low therapeutic index should therefore be used with caution. Drugs metabolized by the liver may be metabolized more slowly during lanreotide treatment and dose reductions of the concomitantly administered medications should be considered).

No products indexed under this heading.

Tiagabine Hydrochloride (The limited published data available indicate that somatostatin analogs may decrease the metabolic clearance of compounds known to be metabolized by the cytochrome P450 enzymes, which may be due to the suppression of growth hormone. Since it cannot be excluded that lanreotide may have this effect, other drugs mainly metabolized by CYP3A4 and which have a low therapeutic index should therefore be used with caution. Drugs metabolized by the liver may be metabolized more slowly during lanreotide treatment and dose reductions of the concomitantly administered medications should be considered). Products include:

Gabitril Tablets 973

Timolol Hemihydrate (Concomitant administration of bradycardia-inducing drugs may have an additive effect on the reduction of heart rate associated with lanreotide. Dose adjustments of concomitant medication may be necessary). Products include:

Betimol Ophthalmic Solution 3181

Timolol Maleate (Concomitant administration of bradycardia-inducing drugs may have an additive effect on the reduction of heart rate associated with lanreotide. Dose adjustments of concomitant medication may be necessary). Products include:

Combigan Ophthalmic Solution 553
Cosopt Sterile Ophthalmic Solution 1969
Timoptic Sterile Ophthalmic Solution 2121
Timoptic in Ocudose 2124
Timoptic-XE Sterile Ophthalmic Gel Forming Solution 2125

Tolazamide (Lanreotide inhibits the secretion of insulin and glucagon. Therefore, blood glucose levels should be monitored when lanreotide treatment is initiated or when the dose is altered and antidiabetic treatment should be adjusted accordingly).

No products indexed under this heading.

Tolbutamide (Lanreotide inhibits the secretion of insulin and glucagon. Therefore, blood glucose levels should be monitored when lanreotide treatment is initiated or when the dose is altered and antidiabetic treatment should be adjusted accordingly).

No products indexed under this heading.

Tolterodine Tartrate (The limited published data available indicate that somatostatin analogs may decrease the metabolic clearance of compounds known to be metabolized by the cytochrome P450 enzymes, which may be due to the suppression of growth hormone. Since it cannot be excluded that lanreotide may have this effect, other drugs mainly metabolized by CYP3A4 and which have a low therapeutic index should therefore be used with caution. Drugs metabolized by the liver may be metabolized more slowly during lanreotide treatment and dose reductions of the concomitantly administered medications should be considered).

No products indexed under this heading.

Trazodone Hydrochloride (The limited published data available indicate that somatostatin analogs may decrease the metabolic clearance of compounds known to be metabolized by the cytochrome P450 enzymes, which may be due to the suppression of growth hormone. Since it cannot be excluded that lanreotide may have this effect, other drugs mainly metabolized by CYP3A4 and which have a low therapeutic index should therefore be used with caution. Drugs metabolized by the liver may be metabolized more slowly during lanreotide treatment and dose reductions of the concomitantly administered medications should be considered).

No products indexed under this heading.

Triazolam (The limited published data available indicate that somatostatin analogs may decrease the metabolic clearance of compounds known to be metabolized by the cytochrome P450 enzymes, which may be due to the suppression of growth hormone. Since it cannot be excluded that lanreotide may have this effect, other drugs mainly metabolized by CYP3A4 and which have a low therapeutic index should therefore be used with caution. Drugs metabolized by the liver may be metabolized more slowly during lanreotide treatment and dose reductions of the concomitantly administered medications should be considered).

No products indexed under this heading.

Troglitazone (Lanreotide inhibits the secretion of insulin and glucagon. Therefore, blood glucose levels should be monitored when lanreotide treatment is initiated or when the dose is altered and antidiabetic treatment should be adjusted accordingly).

No products indexed under this heading.

Vardenafil Hydrochloride (The limited published data available indicate that somatostatin analogs may decrease the metabolic clearance of compounds known to be metabolized by the cytochrome P450 enzymes, which may be due to the suppression of growth hormone. Since it cannot be excluded that lanreotide may have this effect, other drugs mainly metabolized by CYP3A4 and which have a low therapeutic index should therefore be used with caution. Drugs metabolized by the liver may be metabolized more slowly during lanreotide treatment and dose reductions of the concomitantly administered medications should be considered). Products include:

Levitra Tablets 2876

Verapamil Hydrochloride (The limited published data available indicate that somatostatin analogs may decrease the metabolic clearance of compounds known to be metabolized by the cytochrome P450 enzymes, which may be due to the suppression of growth hormone. Since it cannot be excluded that lanreotide may have this effect, other drugs mainly metabolized by CYP3A4 and which have a low therapeutic index should therefore be used with caution. Drugs metabolized by the liver may be metabolized more slowly during lanreotide treatment and dose reductions of the concomitantly administered medications should be considered). Products include:

Tarka Tablets 511

Vinblastine Sulfate (The limited published data available indicate that somatostatin analogs may decrease the metabolic clearance of compounds known to be metabolized by the cytochrome P450 enzymes, which may be due to the suppression of growth hormone. Since it cannot be excluded that lanreotide may have this effect, other drugs mainly metabolized by CYP3A4 and which have a low therapeutic index should therefore be used with caution. Drugs metabolized by the liver may be metabolized more slowly during lanreotide treatment and dose reductions of the concomitantly administered medications should be considered).

No products indexed under this heading.

Vincristine Sulfate (The limited published data available indicate that somatostatin analogs may decrease the metabolic clearance of compounds known to be metabolized by the cytochrome P450 enzymes, which may be due to the suppression of growth hormone. Since it cannot be excluded that lanreotide may have this effect, other drugs mainly metabolized by CYP3A4 and which have a low therapeutic index should therefore be used with caution. Drugs metabolized by the liver may be metabolized more slowly during lanreotide treatment and dose reductions of the concomitantly administered medications should be considered).

No products indexed under this heading.

Warfarin Sodium (The limited published data available indicate that somatostatin analogs may decrease the metabolic clearance of compounds known to be metabolized by the cytochrome P450 enzymes, which may be due to the suppression of growth hormone. Since it cannot be excluded that lanreotide may have this effect, other drugs mainly metabolized by CYP3A4 and which have a low therapeutic index should therefore be used with caution. Drugs metabolized by the liver may be metabolized more slowly during lanreotide treatment and dose reductions of the concomitantly administered medications should be considered).

No products indexed under this heading.

SON FORMULA TABLETS

(Amino Acid Preparations) 1745

None cited in PDR database.

SOOTHE LUBRICANT EYE DROPS

(Glycerin, Propylene Glycol) .... ⊙246

None cited in PDR database.

SOOTHE XP EYE DROPS

(Mineral Oil) .... ⊙246

None cited in PDR database.

SORIATANE CAPSULES

(Acitretin) 3062

May interact with tetracyclines and certain other agents. Compounds in these categories include:

Demeclocycline Hydrochloride (Since both Soriatane and tetracyclines can cause increases in intracranial pressure, their combined use is contraindicated).

No products indexed under this heading.

Doxycycline Calcium (Since both Soriatane and tetracyclines can cause increases in intracranial pressure, their combined use is contraindicated).

No products indexed under this heading.

Doxycycline Hyclate (Since both Soriatane and tetracyclines can cause increases in intracranial pressure, their combined use is contraindicated).

No products indexed under this heading.

Doxycycline Monohydrate (Since both Soriatane and tetracyclines can cause increases in intracranial pressure, their combined use is contraindicated).

No products indexed under this heading.

Glibenclamide (Acitretin treatment potentiated the blood glucose lowering affect of glibenclamide in 3 of the 7 male volunteers).

No products indexed under this heading.

Methacycline Hydrochloride (Since both Soriatane and tetracyclines can cause increases in intracranial pressure, their combined use is contraindicated).

No products indexed under this heading.

Methotrexate (An increased risk of hepatitis has been reported to result from combined use of methotrexate and etretinate).

No products indexed under this heading.

Minocycline Hydrochloride (Since both Soriatane and tetracyclines can cause increases in intracranial pressure, their combined use is contraindicated). Products include:

Solodyn Extended Release Tablets 1938

Oxytetracycline Hydrochloride (Since both Soriatane and tetracyclines can cause increases in intracranial pressure, their combined use is contraindicated).

No products indexed under this heading.

Phenytoin (If acitretin is given concurrently with phenytoin, the protein binding of phenytoin may be reduced).

No products indexed under this heading.

Tetracycline Hydrochloride (Since both Soriatane and tetracyclines can cause increases in intracranial pressure, their combined use is contraindicated). Products include:

Pylera Capsules 714

Vitamin A (Concomitant administration of vitamin A and/or other oral retinoids with acitretin must be avoided because of the risk of hypervitaminosis A). Products include:

Norwegian Cod Liver Oil 949

Food Interactions

Alcohol (Clinical evidence has shown that etretinate can be formed with concurrent ingestion of acitretin and ethanol).

SPIRIVA HANDIHALER

(Tiotropium bromide) 870

May interact with anticholinergics and certain other agents. Compounds in these categories include:

Atropine Sulfate (Co-administration of tiotropium with other anticholinergic-containing drugs (e.g., ipratropium) has not been studied and is therefore not recommended). Products include:

Donnatal Extentabs 2507

Belladonna Alkaloids (Co-administration of tiotropium with other anticholinergic-containing drugs (e.g., ipratropium) has not been studied and is therefore not recommended). Products include:

Hyland's Teething Tablets .... ■621

Benztropine Mesylate (Co-administration of tiotropium with other anticholinergic-containing drugs (e.g., ipratropium) has not been studied and is therefore not recommended).

No products indexed under this heading.

Biperiden Hydrochloride (Co-administration of tiotropium with other anticholinergic-containing drugs (e.g., ipratropium) has not been studied and is therefore not recommended).

No products indexed under this heading.

Cimetidine (Concomitant administration of cimetidine with tiotropium resulted in a 20% increase in the AUC_{0-4h}, a 28% increase in the renal clearance of tiotropium and no significant change in the Cmax and amount excreted in urine over 96 hours. Therefore, no clinically significant interaction occurred between tiotropium and cimetidine).

No products indexed under this heading.

Cimetidine Hydrochloride (Concomitant administration of cimetidine with tiotropium resulted in a 20% increase in the AUC0-4h, a 28% increase in the renal clearance of tiotropium and no significant change in the Cmax and amount excreted in urine over 96 hours. Therefore, no clinically significant interaction occurred between tiotropium and cimetidine).

No products indexed under this heading.

Clidinium Bromide (Co-administration of tiotropium with other anticholinergic-containing drugs (e.g., ipratropium) has not been studied and is therefore not recommended).

No products indexed under this heading.

Dicyclomine Hydrochloride (Co-administration of tiotropium with other anticholinergic-containing drugs (e.g., ipratropium) has not been studied and is therefore not recommended). Products include:

Bentyl Capsules 703
Bentyl Injection 703
Bentyl Syrup 703
Bentyl Tablets 703

Glycopyrrolate (Co-administration of tiotropium with other anticholinergic-containing drugs (e.g., ipratropium) has not been studied and is therefore not recommended).

No products indexed under this heading.

Hyoscyamine (Co-administration of tiotropium with other anticholinergic-containing drugs (e.g., ipratropium) has not been studied and is therefore not recommended).

No products indexed under this heading.

Hyoscyamine Sulfate (Co-administration of tiotropium with other anticholinergic-containing drugs (e.g., ipratropium) has not been studied and is therefore not recommended). Products include:

Donnatal Extentabs 2507

Ipratropium Bromide (Co-administration of tiotropium with other anticholinergic-containing drugs (e.g., ipratropium) has not been studied and is therefore not recommended). Products include:

Atrovent HFA Inhalation Aerosol 839
Atrovent Nasal Spray 0.03% 834
Atrovent Nasal Spray 0.06% 836
Combivent Inhalation Aerosol 845

Mepenzolate Bromide (Co-administration of tiotropium with other anticholinergic-containing drugs (e.g., ipratropium) has not been studied and is therefore not recommended).

No products indexed under this heading.

Oxybutynin Chloride (Co-administration of tiotropium with other anticholinergic-containing drugs (e.g., ipratropium) has not been studied and is therefore not recommended).

No products indexed under this heading.

Procyclidine Hydrochloride (Co-administration of tiotropium with other anticholinergic-containing drugs (e.g., ipratropium) has not been studied and is therefore not recommended).

No products indexed under this heading.

Propantheline Bromide (Co-administration of tiotropium with other anticholinergic-containing drugs (e.g., ipratropium) has not been studied and is therefore not recommended).

No products indexed under this heading.

Scopolamine (Co-administration of tiotropium with other anticholinergic-containing drugs (e.g., ipratropium) has not been studied and is therefore not recommended). Products include:

Transderm Scōp Transdermal Therapeutic System 2206

Scopolamine Hydrobromide (Co-administration of tiotropium with other anticholinergic-containing drugs (e.g., ipratropium) has not been studied and is therefore not recommended). Products include:

Donnatal Extentabs 2507

Tolterodine Tartrate (Co-administration of tiotropium with other anticholinergic-containing drugs (e.g., ipratropium) has not been studied and is therefore not recommended).

No products indexed under this heading.

Tridihexethyl Chloride (Co-administration of tiotropium with other anticholinergic-containing drugs (e.g., ipratropium) has not been studied and is therefore not recommended).

No products indexed under this heading.

Trihexyphenidyl Hydrochloride (Co-administration of tiotropium with other anticholinergic-containing drugs (e.g., ipratropium) has not been studied and is therefore not recommended).

No products indexed under this heading.

STALEVO TABLETS

(Carbidopa, Entacapone, Levodopa) 2309

May interact with antihypertensives, drugs metabolized by Catechol-O-methytransferase, dopamine D2 antagonists, iron containing oral preparations, monoamine oxidase inhibitors, tricyclic antidepressants, and certain other agents. Compounds in these categories include:

Acebutolol Hydrochloride (Symptomatic postural hypotension has occurred when carbidopa-levodopa was added to the treatment of a patient receiving antihypertensive drugs).

No products indexed under this heading.

Aliskiren (Symptomatic postural hypotension has occurred when carbidopa-levodopa was added to the treatment of a patient receiving antihypertensive drugs). Products include:

Tekturna Tablets 2321
Tekturna HCT Tablets 2324

Amitriptyline Hydrochloride (There have been rare reports of adverse reactions, including hypertension and dyskinesia, resulting from the concomitant use of tricylic antidepressants and carbidopa-levodopa).

No products indexed under this heading.

Amlodipine Besylate (Symptomatic postural hypotension has occurred when carbidopa-levodopa was added to the treatment of a patient receiving antihypertensive drugs). Products include:

Azor Tablets 1005
Exforge Tablets 2238

Amoxapine (There have been rare reports of adverse reactions, including hypertension and dyskinesia, resulting from the concomitant use of tricylic antidepressants and carbidopa-levodopa).

No products indexed under this heading.

Ampicillin (As most entacapone excretion is via the bile, caution should be exercised when drugs known to interfere with biliary excretion, glucuronidation, and intestinal beta-glucuronidase are given concurrently with entacapone).

No products indexed under this heading.

Ampicillin Sodium (As most entacapone excretion is via the bile, caution should be exercised when drugs known to interfere with biliary excretion, glucuronidation, and intestinal beta-glucuronidase are given concurrently with entacapone).
No products indexed under this heading.

Ampicillin Trihydrate (As most entacapone excretion is via the bile, caution should be exercised when drugs known to interfere with biliary excretion, glucuronidation, and intestinal beta-glucuronidase are given concurrently with entacapone).
No products indexed under this heading.

Apomorphine (Drugs known to be metabolized by COMT should be administered with caution in patients receiving entacapone regardless of the route of administration (including inhalation), as their interaction may result in increased heart rates, possibly arrhythmias, and excessive changes in blood pressure).
No products indexed under this heading.

Atenolol (Symptomatic postural hypotension has occurred when carbidopa-levodopa was added to the treatment of a patient receiving antihypertensive drugs).
No products indexed under this heading.

Bacampicillin Hydrochloride (As most entacapone excretion is via the bile, caution should be exercised when drugs known to interfere with biliary excretion, glucuronidation, and intestinal beta-glucuronidase are given concurrently with entacapone).
No products indexed under this heading.

Benazepril Hydrochloride (Symptomatic postural hypotension has occurred when carbidopa-levodopa was added to the treatment of a patient receiving antihypertensive drugs).
No products indexed under this heading.

Bendroflumethiazide (Symptomatic postural hypotension has occurred when carbidopa-levodopa was added to the treatment of a patient receiving antihypertensive drugs).
No products indexed under this heading.

Betaxolol Hydrochloride (Symptomatic postural hypotension has occurred when carbidopa-levodopa was added to the treatment of a patient receiving antihypertensive drugs).
No products indexed under this heading.

Bisoprolol Fumarate (Symptomatic postural hypotension has occurred when carbidopa-levodopa was added to the treatment of a patient receiving antihypertensive drugs).
No products indexed under this heading.

Bitolterol Mesylate (Drugs known to be metabolized by COMT should be administered with caution in patients receiving entacapone regardless of the route of administration (including inhalation), as their interaction may result in increased heart rates, possibly arrhythmias, and excessive changes in blood pressure).
No products indexed under this heading.

Candesartan Cilexetil (Symptomatic postural hypotension has occurred when carbidopa-levodopa was added to the treatment of a patient receiving antihypertensive drugs). Products include:
Atacand Tablets **639**
Atacand HCT **642**

Captopril (Symptomatic postural hypotension has occurred when carbidopa-levodopa was added to the treatment of a patient receiving antihypertensive drugs). Products include:
Captopril Tablets **2182**

Carteolol Hydrochloride (Symptomatic postural hypotension has occurred when carbidopa-levodopa was added to the treatment of a patient receiving antihypertensive drugs).
No products indexed under this heading.

Chloramphenicol (As most entacapone excretion is via the bile, caution should be exercised when drugs known to interfere with biliary excretion, glucuronidation, and intestinal beta-glucuronidase are given concurrently with entacapone).
No products indexed under this heading.

Chloramphenicol Palmitate (As most entacapone excretion is via the bile, caution should be exercised when drugs known to interfere with biliary excretion, glucuronidation, and intestinal beta-glucuronidase are given concurrently with entacapone).
No products indexed under this heading.

Chloramphenicol Sodium Succinate (As most entacapone excretion is via the bile, caution should be exercised when drugs known to interfere with biliary excretion, glucuronidation, and intestinal beta-glucuronidase are given concurrently with entacapone).
No products indexed under this heading.

Chlorothiazide (Symptomatic postural hypotension has occurred when carbidopa-levodopa was added to the treatment of a patient receiving antihypertensive drugs).
No products indexed under this heading.

Chlorothiazide Sodium (Symptomatic postural hypotension has occurred when carbidopa-levodopa was added to the treatment of a patient receiving antihypertensive drugs). Products include:
Intravenous Sodium Diuril **2490**

Chlorpromazine (Dopamine D2 receptor antagonists may reduce the therapeutic effects of levodopa).
No products indexed under this heading.

Chlorpromazine Hydrochloride (Dopamine D2 receptor antagonists may reduce the therapeutic effects of levodopa).
No products indexed under this heading.

Chlorprothixene (Dopamine D2 receptor antagonists may reduce the therapeutic effects of levodopa).
No products indexed under this heading.

Chlorprothixene Hydrochloride (Dopamine D2 receptor antagonists may reduce the therapeutic effects of levodopa).
No products indexed under this heading.

Chlorthalidone (Symptomatic postural hypotension has occurred when carbidopa-levodopa was added to the treatment of a patient receiving antihypertensive drugs). Products include:
Clorpres Tablets **2185**

Cholestyramine (As most entacapone excretion is via the bile, caution should be exercised when drugs known to interfere with biliary excretion, glucuronidation, and intestinal beta-glucuronidase are given concurrently with entacapone).
No products indexed under this heading.

Clomipramine Hydrochloride (There have been rare reports of adverse reactions, including hypertension and dyskinesia, resulting from the concomitant use of tricylic antidepressants and carbidopa-levodopa).
No products indexed under this heading.

Clonidine (Symptomatic postural hypotension has occurred when carbidopa-levodopa was added to the treatment of a patient receiving antihypertensive drugs). Products include:
Catapres-TTS **842**

Clonidine Hydrochloride (Symptomatic postural hypotension has occurred when carbidopa-levodopa was added to the treatment of a patient receiving antihypertensive drugs). Products include:
Catapres Tablets **841**
Clorpres Tablets **2185**

Deserpidine (Symptomatic postural hypotension has occurred when carbidopa-levodopa was added to the treatment of a patient receiving antihypertensive drugs).
No products indexed under this heading.

Desipramine Hydrochloride (There have been rare reports of adverse reactions, including hypertension and dyskinesia, resulting from the concomitant use of tricylic antidepressants and carbidopa-levodopa).
No products indexed under this heading.

Diazoxide (Symptomatic postural hypotension has occurred when carbidopa-levodopa was added to the treatment of a patient receiving antihypertensive drugs). Products include:
Proglycem Capsules **1185**
Proglycem Suspension **1185**

Diltiazem Hydrochloride (Symptomatic postural hypotension has occurred when carbidopa-levodopa was added to the treatment of a patient receiving antihypertensive drugs). Products include:
Cardizem LA Extended Release Tablets **421**

Dobutamine Hydrochloride (Drugs known to be metabolized by COMT should be administered with caution in patients receiving entacapone regardless of the route of administration (including inhalation), as their interaction may result in increased heart rates, possibly arrhythmias, and excessive changes in blood pressure).
No products indexed under this heading.

Dopamine Hydrochloride (Drugs known to be metabolized by COMT should be administered with caution in patients receiving entacapone regardless of the route of administration (including inhalation), as their interaction may result in increased heart rates, possibly arrhythmias, and excessive changes in blood pressure).
No products indexed under this heading.

Doxazosin Mesylate (Symptomatic postural hypotension has occurred when carbidopa-levodopa was added to the treatment of a patient receiving antihypertensive drugs).
No products indexed under this heading.

Doxepin Hydrochloride (There have been rare reports of adverse reactions, including hypertension and dyskinesia, resulting from the concomitant use of tricylic antidepressants and carbidopa-levodopa).
No products indexed under this heading.

Enalapril Maleate (Symptomatic postural hypotension has occurred when carbidopa-levodopa was added to the treatment of a patient receiving antihypertensive drugs).
No products indexed under this heading.

Enalaprilat (Symptomatic postural hypotension has occurred when carbidopa-levodopa was added to the treatment of a patient receiving antihypertensive drugs).
No products indexed under this heading.

Epinephrine (Drugs known to be metabolized by COMT should be administered with caution in patients receiving entacapone regardless of the route of administration (including inhalation), as their interaction may result in increased heart rates, possibly arrhythmias, and excessive changes in blood pressure). Products include:
EpiPen **1024**

Epinephrine Bitartrate (Drugs known to be metabolized by COMT should be administered with caution in patients receiving entacapone regardless of the route of administration (including inhalation), as their interaction may result in increased heart rates, possibly arrhythmias, and excessive changes in blood pressure).
No products indexed under this heading.

Epinephrine Hydrochloride (Drugs known to be metabolized by COMT should be administered with caution in patients receiving entacapone regardless of the route of administration (including inhalation), as their interaction may result in increased heart rates, possibly arrhythmias, and excessive changes in blood pressure).
No products indexed under this heading.

Eprosartan Mesylate (Symptomatic postural hypotension has occurred when carbidopa-levodopa was added to the treatment of a patient receiving antihypertensive drugs). Products include:
Teveten Tablets **515**
Teveten HCT Tablets **517**

Erythromycin (As most entacapone excretion is via the bile, caution should be exercised when drugs known to interfere with biliary excretion, glucuronidation, and intestinal beta-glucuronidase are given concurrently with entacapone).
No products indexed under this heading.

Erythromycin Enteric Coated Tablets (As most entacapone excretion is via the bile, caution should be exercised when drugs known to interfere with biliary excretion, glucuronidation, and intestinal beta-glucuronidase are given concurrently with entacapone).
No products indexed under this heading.

Erythromycin Estolate (As most entacapone excretion is via the bile, caution should be exercised when drugs known to interfere with biliary excretion, glucuronidation, and intestinal beta-glucuronidase are given concurrently with entacapone).
No products indexed under this heading.

Erythromycin Ethylsuccinate (As most entacapone excretion is via the bile, caution should be exercised when drugs known to interfere with biliary excretion, glucuronidation, and intestinal beta-glucuronidase are given concurrently with entacapone). Products include:
E.E.S. **433**
EryPed **431**

Erythromycin Gluceptate (As most entacapone excretion is via the bile, caution should be exercised when drugs known to interfere with biliary excretion, glucuronidation, and intestinal beta-glucuronidase are given concurrently with entacapone).
No products indexed under this heading.

Erythromycin Lactobionate (As most entacapone excretion is via the bile, caution should be exercised when drugs known to interfere with biliary excretion, glucuronidation, and intestinal beta-glucuronidase are given concurrently with entacapone).
No products indexed under this heading.

Erythromycin Stearate (As most entacapone excretion is via the bile, caution should be exercised when drugs known to interfere with biliary excretion, glucuronidation, and intestinal beta-glucuronidase are given concurrently with entacapone).
No products indexed under this heading.

Esmolol Hydrochloride (Symptomatic postural hypotension has occurred when carbidopa-levodopa was added to the treatment of a patient receiving antihypertensive drugs).
No products indexed under this heading.

Ethylpapaverine Hydrochloride (The beneficial effects of levodopa in Parkinson's disease have been reported to be reversed by papaverine).
No products indexed under this heading.

Felodipine (Symptomatic postural hypotension has occurred when carbidopa-levodopa was added to the treatment of a patient receiving antihypertensive drugs).
No products indexed under this heading.

Ferrous Fumarate (Iron salts may reduce the bioavailability of levodopa, carbidopa and entacapone).
No products indexed under this heading.

Ferrous Gluconate (Iron salts may reduce the bioavailability of levodopa, carbidopa and entacapone). Products include:
CitraNatal DHA Tablets **2175**

Ferrous Sulfate (Iron salts may reduce the bioavailability of levodopa, carbidopa and entacapone).
No products indexed under this heading.

Fluphenazine Decanoate (Dopamine D2 receptor antagonists may reduce the therapeutic effects of levodopa).
No products indexed under this heading.

Fluphenazine Enanthate (Dopamine D2 receptor antagonists may reduce the therapeutic effects of levodopa).
No products indexed under this heading.

Fluphenazine Hydrochloride (Dopamine D2 receptor antagonists may reduce the therapeutic effects of levodopa).
No products indexed under this heading.

Fosinopril Sodium (Symptomatic postural hypotension has occurred when carbidopa-levodopa was added to the treatment of a patient receiving antihypertensive drugs).
No products indexed under this heading.

Fosphenytoin (The beneficial effects of levodopa in Parkinson's disease have been reported to be reversed by phenytoin).
No products indexed under this heading.

Fosphenytoin Sodium (The beneficial effects of levodopa in Parkinson's disease have been reported to be reversed by phenytoin).
No products indexed under this heading.

Furosemide (Symptomatic postural hypotension has occurred when carbidopa-levodopa was added to the treatment of a patient receiving antihypertensive drugs). Products include:
Furosemide Tablets **2186**

Guanabenz Acetate (Symptomatic postural hypotension has occurred when carbidopa-levodopa was added to the treatment of a patient receiving antihypertensive drugs).
No products indexed under this heading.

Guanethidine Monosulfate (Symptomatic postural hypotension has occurred when carbidopa-levodopa was added to the treatment of a patient receiving antihypertensive drugs).
No products indexed under this heading.

Haloperidol (Dopamine D2 receptor antagonists may reduce the therapeutic effects of levodopa).
No products indexed under this heading.

Haloperidol Decanoate (Dopamine D2 receptor antagonists may reduce the therapeutic effects of levodopa).
No products indexed under this heading.

Hydralazine Hydrochloride (Symptomatic postural hypotension has occurred when carbidopa-levodopa was added to the treatment of a patient receiving antihypertensive drugs).
No products indexed under this heading.

Hydrochlorothiazide (Symptomatic postural hypotension has occurred when carbidopa-levodopa was added to the treatment of a patient receiving antihypertensive drugs). Products include:
Atacand HCT **642**
Avalide Tablets **892**
Avalide Tablets **2713**
Benicar HCT Tablets **1010**
Diovan HCT Tablets **2216**
Dyazide Capsules **1405**
Micardis HCT Tablets **854**
Prinzide Tablets **2092**
Tekturna HCT Tablets **2324**
Teveten HCT Tablets **517**

Hydroflumethiazide (Symptomatic postural hypotension has occurred when carbidopa-levodopa was added to the treatment of a patient receiving antihypertensive drugs).
No products indexed under this heading.

Imipramine Hydrochloride (There have been rare reports of adverse reactions, including hypertension and dyskinesia, resulting from the concomitant use of tricyclic antidepressants and carbidopa-levodopa).
No products indexed under this heading.

Imipramine Pamoate (There have been rare reports of adverse reactions, including hypertension and dyskinesia, resulting from the concomitant use of tricylic antidepressants and carbidopa-levodopa).
No products indexed under this heading.

Indapamide (Symptomatic postural hypotension has occurred when carbidopa-levodopa was added to the treatment of a patient receiving antihypertensive drugs). Products include:
Indapamide Tablets **2188**

Irbesartan (Symptomatic postural hypotension has occurred when carbidopa-levodopa was added to the treatment of a patient receiving antihypertensive drugs). Products include:
Avalide Tablets **892**
Avalide Tablets **2713**
Avapro Tablets **897**
Avapro Tablets **2718**

Iron (Iron salts may reduce the bioavailability of levodopa, carbidopa and entacapone). Products include:
Phyto-Vite Tablets **639**

Isocarboxazid (Nonselective monoamine oxidase (MAO) inhibitors are contraindicated for use with Stalevo). Products include:
Marplan Tablets **3177**

Isoetharine (Drugs known to be metabolized by COMT should be administered with caution in patients receiving entacapone regardless of the route of administration (including inhalation), as their interaction may result in increased heart rates, possibly arrhythmias, and excessive changes in blood pressure).
No products indexed under this heading.

Isoniazid (Isoniazid may reduce the therapeutic effects of levodopa).
No products indexed under this heading.

Isoproterenol Hydrochloride (Drugs known to be metabolized by COMT should be administered with caution in patients receiving entacapone regardless of the route of administration (including inhalation), as their interaction may result in increased heart rates, possibly arrhythmias, and excessive changes in blood pressure).
No products indexed under this heading.

Isoproterenol Sulfate (Drugs known to be metabolized by COMT should be administered with caution in patients receiving entacapone regardless of the route of administration (including inhalation), as their interaction may result in increased heart rates, possibly arrhythmias, and excessive changes in blood pressure).
No products indexed under this heading.

Isradipine (Symptomatic postural hypotension has occurred when carbidopa-levodopa was added to the treatment of a patient receiving antihypertensive drugs). Products include:
DynaCirc CR Controlled Release Tablets **1407**

Labetalol Hydrochloride (Symptomatic postural hypotension has occurred when carbidopa-levodopa was added to the treatment of a patient receiving antihypertensive drugs).
No products indexed under this heading.

Lisinopril (Symptomatic postural hypotension has occurred when carbidopa-levodopa was added to the treatment of a patient receiving antihypertensive drugs). Products include:
Prinivil Tablets **2087**
Prinzide Tablets **2092**

Losartan Potassium (Symptomatic postural hypotension has occurred when carbidopa-levodopa was added to the treatment of a patient receiving antihypertensive drugs). Products include:
Cozaar Tablets **1973**

Loxapine Hydrochloride (Dopamine D2 receptor antagonists may reduce the therapeutic effects of levodopa).
No products indexed under this heading.

Loxapine Succinate (Dopamine D2 receptor antagonists may reduce the therapeutic effects of levodopa).
No products indexed under this heading.

Maprotiline Hydrochloride (There have been rare reports of adverse reactions, including hypertension and dyskinesia, resulting from the concomitant use of tricylic antidepressants and carbidopa-levodopa).
No products indexed under this heading.

Mecamylamine Hydrochloride (Symptomatic postural hypotension has occurred when carbidopa-levodopa was added to the treatment of a patient receiving antihypertensive drugs).
No products indexed under this heading.

Mephenytoin (The beneficial effects of levodopa in Parkinson's disease have been reported to be reversed by phenytoin).
No products indexed under this heading.

Mesoridazine Besylate (Dopamine D2 receptor antagonists may reduce the therapeutic effects of levodopa).
No products indexed under this heading.

Methotrimeprazine (Dopamine D2 receptor antagonists may reduce the therapeutic effects of levodopa).
No products indexed under this heading.

Methyclothiazide (Symptomatic postural hypotension has occurred when carbidopa-levodopa was added to the treatment of a patient receiving antihypertensive drugs).
No products indexed under this heading.

Methyldopa (Drugs known to be metabolized by COMT should be administered with caution in patients receiving entacapone regardless of the route of administration (including inhalation), as their interaction may result in increased heart rates, possibly arrhythmias, and excessive changes in blood pressure).
No products indexed under this heading.

Methyldopate Hydrochloride (Symptomatic postural hypotension has occurred when carbidopa-levodopa was added to the treatment of a patient receiving antihypertensive drugs).
No products indexed under this heading.

Metoclopramide Hydrochloride (Although metoclopramide may increase the bioavailability of levodopa by increasing gastric emptying, metoclopramide may also adversely affect disease control by its dopamine receptor antagonistic properties).
No products indexed under this heading.

Metolazone (Symptomatic postural hypotension has occurred when carbidopa-levodopa was added to the treatment of a patient receiving antihypertensive drugs).
No products indexed under this heading.

Metoprolol Succinate (Symptomatic postural hypotension has occurred when carbidopa-levodopa was added to the treatment of a patient receiving antihypertensive drugs). Products include:
Toprol-XL Tablets 666

Metoprolol Tartrate (Symptomatic postural hypotension has occurred when carbidopa-levodopa was added to the treatment of a patient receiving antihypertensive drugs).
No products indexed under this heading.

Metyrosine (Symptomatic postural hypotension has occurred when carbidopa-levodopa was added to the treatment of a patient receiving antihypertensive drugs). Products include:
Demser Capsules 1989

Mibefradil Dihydrochloride (Symptomatic postural hypotension has occurred when carbidopa-levodopa was added to the treatment of a patient receiving antihypertensive drugs).
No products indexed under this heading.

Minoxidil (Symptomatic postural hypotension has occurred when carbidopa-levodopa was added to the treatment of a patient receiving antihypertensive drugs).
No products indexed under this heading.

Moclobemide (Nonselective monoamine oxidase (MAO) inhibitors are contraindicated for use with Stalevo).
No products indexed under this heading.

Moexipril Hydrochloride (Symptomatic postural hypotension has occurred when carbidopa-levodopa was added to the treatment of a patient receiving antihypertensive drugs).
No products indexed under this heading.

Molindone Hydrochloride (Dopamine D2 receptor antagonists may reduce the therapeutic effects of levodopa). Products include:
Moban Tablets 1116

Nadolol (Symptomatic postural hypotension has occurred when carbidopa-levodopa was added to the treatment of a patient receiving antihypertensive drugs). Products include:
Nadolol Tablets 2191

Nebivolol (Symptomatic postural hypotension has occurred when carbidopa-levodopa was added to the treatment of a patient receiving antihypertensive drugs). Products include:
Bystolic Tablets 1155

Nicardipine Hydrochloride (Symptomatic postural hypotension has occurred when carbidopa-levodopa was added to the treatment of a patient receiving antihypertensive drugs). Products include:
Cardene I.V. 1093

Nifedipine (Symptomatic postural hypotension has occurred when carbidopa-levodopa was added to the treatment of a patient receiving antihypertensive drugs).
No products indexed under this heading.

Nisoldipine (Symptomatic postural hypotension has occurred when carbidopa-levodopa was added to the treatment of a patient receiving antihypertensive drugs). Products include:
Sular Extended Release Tablets 2975

Nitroglycerin (Symptomatic postural hypotension has occurred when carbidopa-levodopa was added to the treatment of a patient receiving antihypertensive drugs). Products include:
Nitro-Dur Transdermal Infusion System 2887
Nitrolingual Pumpspray 2965

Norepinephrine Bitartrate (Drugs known to be metabolized by COMT should be administered with caution in patients receiving entacapone regardless of the route of administration (including inhalation), as their interaction may result in increased heart rates, possibly arrhythmias, and excessive changes in blood pressure).
No products indexed under this heading.

Nortriptyline Hydrochloride (There have been rare reports of adverse reactions, including hypertension and dyskinesia, resulting from the concomitant use of tricylic antidepressants and carbidopa-levodopa).
No products indexed under this heading.

Papaverine (The beneficial effects of levodopa in Parkinson's disease have been reported to be reversed by papaverine).
No products indexed under this heading.

Papaverine Hydrochloride (The beneficial effects of levodopa in Parkinson's disease have been reported to be reversed by papaverine).
No products indexed under this heading.

Pargyline Hydrochloride (Nonselective monoamine oxidase (MAO) inhibitors are contraindicated for use with Stalevo).
No products indexed under this heading.

Penbutolol Sulfate (Symptomatic postural hypotension has occurred when carbidopa-levodopa was added to the treatment of a patient receiving antihypertensive drugs).
No products indexed under this heading.

Perindopril Erbumine (Symptomatic postural hypotension has occurred when carbidopa-levodopa was added to the treatment of a patient receiving antihypertensive drugs). Products include:
Aceon Tablets (2 mg, 4 mg, 8 mg) 3038

Perphenazine (Dopamine D2 receptor antagonists may reduce the therapeutic effects of levodopa).
No products indexed under this heading.

Phenelzine Sulfate (Nonselective monoamine oxidase (MAO) inhibitors are contraindicated for use with Stalevo).
No products indexed under this heading.

Phenoxybenzamine Hydrochloride (Symptomatic postural hypotension has occurred when carbidopa-levodopa was added to the treatment of a patient receiving antihypertensive drugs). Products include:
Dibenzyline Capsules 3188

Phentolamine Mesylate (Symptomatic postural hypotension has occurred when carbidopa-levodopa was added to the treatment of a patient receiving antihypertensive drugs).
No products indexed under this heading.

Phenytoin (The beneficial effects of levodopa in Parkinson's disease have been reported to be reversed by phenytoin).
No products indexed under this heading.

Phenytoin Sodium (The beneficial effects of levodopa in Parkinson's disease have been reported to be reversed by phenytoin). Products include:
Phenytek Capsules 2192

Pindolol (Symptomatic postural hypotension has occurred when carbidopa-levodopa was added to the treatment of a patient receiving antihypertensive drugs).
No products indexed under this heading.

Polysaccharide Iron Complex (Iron salts may reduce the bioavailability of levodopa, carbidopa and entacapone). Products include:
Nu-Iron 150 Capsules 2165

Polythiazide (Symptomatic postural hypotension has occurred when carbidopa-levodopa was added to the treatment of a patient receiving antihypertensive drugs).
No products indexed under this heading.

Prazosin Hydrochloride (Symptomatic postural hypotension has occurred when carbidopa-levodopa was added to the treatment of a patient receiving antihypertensive drugs).
No products indexed under this heading.

Probenecid (As most entacapone excretion is via the bile, caution should be exercised when drugs known to interfere with biliary excretion, glucuronidation, and intestinal beta-glucuronidase are given concurrently with entacapone).
No products indexed under this heading.

Procarbazine Hydrochloride (Nonselective monoamine oxidase (MAO) inhibitors are contraindicated for use with Stalevo).
No products indexed under this heading.

Prochlorperazine (Dopamine D2 receptor antagonists may reduce the therapeutic effects of levodopa).
No products indexed under this heading.

Promethazine Hydrochloride (Dopamine D2 receptor antagonists may reduce the therapeutic effects of levodopa).
No products indexed under this heading.

Propranolol Hydrochloride (Symptomatic postural hypotension has occurred when carbidopa-levodopa was added to the treatment of a patient receiving antihypertensive drugs). Products include:
InnoPran XL Extended Release Capsules 1484

Protriptyline Hydrochloride (There have been rare reports of adverse reactions, including hypertension and dyskinesia, resulting from the concomitant use of tricylic antidepressants and carbidopa-levodopa).
No products indexed under this heading.

Quetiapine Fumarate (Dopamine D2 receptor antagonists may reduce the therapeutic effects of levodopa).
No products indexed under this heading.

Quinapril Hydrochloride (Symptomatic postural hypotension has occurred when carbidopa-levodopa was added to the treatment of a patient receiving antihypertensive drugs).
No products indexed under this heading.

Ramipril (Symptomatic postural hypotension has occurred when carbidopa-levodopa was added to the treatment of a patient receiving antihypertensive drugs).
No products indexed under this heading.

Rasagiline Mesylate (Nonselective monoamine oxidase (MAO) inhibitors are contraindicated for use with Stalevo). Products include:
Azilect Tablets ... 3106

Rauwolfia Serpentina (Symptomatic postural hypotension has occurred when carbidopa-levodopa was added to the treatment of a patient receiving antihypertensive drugs).
No products indexed under this heading.

Rescinnamine (Symptomatic postural hypotension has occurred when carbidopa-levodopa was added to the treatment of a patient receiving antihypertensive drugs).
No products indexed under this heading.

Reserpine (Symptomatic postural hypotension has occurred when carbidopa-levodopa was added to the treatment of a patient receiving antihypertensive drugs).
No products indexed under this heading.

Rifampicin (As most entacapone excretion is via the bile, caution should be exercised when drugs known to interfere with biliary excretion, glucuronidation, and intestinal beta-glucuronidase are given concurrently with entacapone).
No products indexed under this heading.

Risperidone (Dopamine D2 receptor antagonists may reduce the therapeutic effects of levodopa).
Products include:
Risperdal Consta Long-Acting Injection ... 1753

Selegiline (Nonselective monoamine oxidase (MAO) inhibitors are contraindicated for use with Stalevo). Products include:
Emsam Transdermal System ... 905

Selegiline Hydrochloride (Nonselective monoamine oxidase (MAO) inhibitors are contraindicated for use with Stalevo). Products include:
Eldepryl Capsules ... 3052

Sodium Nitroprusside (Symptomatic postural hypotension has occurred when carbidopa-levodopa was added to the treatment of a patient receiving antihypertensive drugs).
No products indexed under this heading.

Sotalol Hydrochloride (Symptomatic postural hypotension has occurred when carbidopa-levodopa was added to the treatment of a patient receiving antihypertensive drugs).
No products indexed under this heading.

Spirapril Hydrochloride (Symptomatic postural hypotension has occurred when carbidopa-levodopa was added to the treatment of a patient receiving antihypertensive drugs).
No products indexed under this heading.

Telmisartan (Symptomatic postural hypotension has occurred when carbidopa-levodopa was added to the treatment of a patient receiving antihypertensive drugs). Products include:
Micardis Tablets ... 852
Micardis HCT Tablets ... 854

Terazosin Hydrochloride (Symptomatic postural hypotension has occurred when carbidopa-levodopa was added to the treatment of a patient receiving antihypertensive drugs).
No products indexed under this heading.

Thioridazine Hydrochloride (Dopamine D2 receptor antagonists may reduce the therapeutic effects of levodopa). Products include:
Thioridazine Hydrochloride Tablets ... 2195

Thiothixene (Dopamine D2 receptor antagonists may reduce the therapeutic effects of levodopa).
Products include:
Thiothixene Capsules ... 2197

Timolol Maleate (Symptomatic postural hypotension has occurred when carbidopa-levodopa was added to the treatment of a patient receiving antihypertensive drugs).
Products include:
Combigan Ophthalmic Solution ... 553
Cosopt Sterile Ophthalmic Solution ... 1969
Timoptic Sterile Ophthalmic Solution ... 2121
Timoptic in Ocudose ... 2124
Timoptic-XE Sterile Ophthalmic Gel Forming Solution ... 2125

Torsemide (Symptomatic postural hypotension has occurred when carbidopa-levodopa was added to the treatment of a patient receiving antihypertensive drugs). Products include:
Demadex Injection ... 2630
Demadex Tablets ... 2630

Trandolapril (Symptomatic postural hypotension has occurred when carbidopa-levodopa was added to the treatment of a patient receiving antihypertensive drugs). Products include:
Mavik Tablets ... 472
Tarka Tablets ... 511

Tranylcypromine Sulfate (Nonselective monoamine oxidase (MAO) inhibitors are contraindicated for use with Stalevo). Products include:
Parnate Tablets ... 1532

Trifluoperazine Hydrochloride (Dopamine D2 receptor antagonists may reduce the therapeutic effects of levodopa).
No products indexed under this heading.

Trimethaphan Camsylate (Symptomatic postural hypotension has occurred when carbidopa-levodopa was added to the treatment of a patient receiving antihypertensive drugs).
No products indexed under this heading.

Trimipramine Maleate (There have been rare reports of adverse reactions, including hypertension and dyskinesia, resulting from the concomitant use of tricylic antidepressants and carbidopa-levodopa).
No products indexed under this heading.

Valsartan (Symptomatic postural hypotension has occurred when carbidopa-levodopa was added to the treatment of a patient receiving antihypertensive drugs). Products include:
Diovan Tablets ... 2212
Diovan HCT Tablets ... 2216
Exforge Tablets ... 2238

Verapamil Hydrochloride (Symptomatic postural hypotension has occurred when carbidopa-levodopa was added to the treatment of a patient receiving antihypertensive drugs). Products include:
Tarka Tablets ... 511

STARLIX TABLETS

(Nateglinide) ... 2314
May interact with nonspecific beta-blockers, corticosteroids, monoamine oxidase inhibitors, non-steroidal anti-inflammatory agents, salicylates, sympathomimetics, thiazides, thyroid preparations, and certain other agents. Compounds in these categories include:

Albuterol (Certain drugs including sympathomimetics may reduce the hypoglycemic action of nateglinide. When sympathomimetics are administered to or withdrawn from patients receiving nateglinide, the patient should be observed closely for changes in glycemic control).
No products indexed under this heading.

Albuterol Sulfate (Certain drugs including sympathomimetics may reduce the hypoglycemic action of nateglinide. When sympathomimetics are administered to or withdrawn from patients receiving nateglinide, the patient should be observed closely for changes in glycemic control). Products include:
Combivent Inhalation Aerosol ... 845
ProAir HFA Inhalation Aerosol ... 3113
Proventil HFA Inhalation Aerosol ... 2914
Ventolin HFA Inhalation Aerosol ... 1638

Aspirin (Certain drugs including salicylates may potentiate the hypoglycemic action of nateglinide).
Products include:
Aggrenox Capsules ... 819
Bayer Aspirin ... 750
Percodan Tablets ... 1130
St. Joseph 81 mg Aspirin Chewable and Enteric Coated Tablets ... 1903

Aspirin, Enteric Coated (Certain drugs including salicylates may potentiate the hypoglycemic action of nateglinide).
No products indexed under this heading.

Aspirin Buffered (Certain drugs including salicylates may potentiate the hypoglycemic action of nateglinide).
No products indexed under this heading.

Bendroflumethiazide (Certain drugs including thiazides may reduce the hypoglycemic action of nateglinide. When thiazides are administered to or withdrawn from patients receiving nateglinide, the patient should be observed closely for changes in glycemic control).
No products indexed under this heading.

Betamethasone Acetate (Certain drugs including corticosteroids may reduce the hypoglycemic action of nateglinide. When corticosteroids are administered to or withdrawn from patients receiving nateglinide, the patient should be observed closely for changes in glycemic control).
No products indexed under this heading.

Betamethasone Sodium Phosphate (Certain drugs including corticosteroids may reduce the hypoglycemic action of nateglinide. When corticosteroids are administered to or withdrawn from patients receiving nateglinide, the patient should be observed closely for changes in glycemic control).
No products indexed under this heading.

Budesonide (Certain drugs including corticosteroids may reduce the hypoglycemic action of nateglinide. When corticosteroids are administered to or withdrawn from patients receiving nateglinide, the patient should be observed closely for changes in glycemic control).
Products include:
Pulmicort Flexhaler ... 654
Symbicort 80/4.5 Inhalation Aerosol ... 659
Symbicort 160/4.5 Inhalation Aerosol ... 659

Celecoxib (Certain drugs including nonsteroidal anti-inflammatory agents (NSAIDs) may potentiate the hypoglycemic action of nateglinide).
Products include:
Celebrex Capsules ... 2979

Chlorothiazide (Certain drugs including thiazides may reduce the hypoglycemic action of nateglinide. When thiazides are administered to or withdrawn from patients receiving nateglinide, the patient should be observed closely for changes in glycemic control).
No products indexed under this heading.

Chlorothiazide Sodium (Certain drugs including thiazides may reduce the hypoglycemic action of nateglinide. When thiazides are administered to or withdrawn from patients receiving nateglinide, the patient should be observed closely for changes in glycemic control).
Products include:
Intravenous Sodium Diuril ... 2490

Choline Magnesium Trisalicylate (Certain drugs including salicylates may potentiate the hypoglycemic action of nateglinide).
No products indexed under this heading.

Ciclesonide (Certain drugs including corticosteroids may reduce the hypoglycemic action of nateglinide. When corticosteroids are administered to or withdrawn from patients receiving nateglinide, the patient should be observed closely for changes in glycemic control).
Products include:

Alvesco Inhalation Aerosol 2985
Omnaris Nasal Spray 2998

Cortisone Acetate (Certain drugs including corticosteroids may reduce the hypoglycemic action of nateglinide. When corticosteroids are administered to or withdrawn from patients receiving nateglinide, the patient should be observed closely for changes in glycemic control).
No products indexed under this heading.

Dexamethasone (Certain drugs including corticosteroids may reduce the hypoglycemic action of nateglinide. When corticosteroids are administered to or withdrawn from patients receiving nateglinide, the patient should be observed closely for changes in glycemic control). Products include:
Ciprodex Otic Suspension 541

Dexamethasone Acetate (Certain drugs including corticosteroids may reduce the hypoglycemic action of nateglinide. When corticosteroids are administered to or withdrawn from patients receiving nateglinide, the patient should be observed closely for changes in glycemic control).
No products indexed under this heading.

Dexamethasone Sodium Phosphate (Certain drugs including corticosteroids may reduce the hypoglycemic action of nateglinide. When corticosteroids are administered to or withdrawn from patients receiving nateglinide, the patient should be observed closely for changes in glycemic control).
No products indexed under this heading.

Diclofenac Epolamine (Certain drugs including nonsteroidal anti-inflammatory agents (NSAIDs) may potentiate the hypoglycemic action of nateglinide). Products include:
Flector Patch 561

Diclofenac Potassium (Certain drugs including nonsteroidal anti-inflammatory agents (NSAIDs) may potentiate the hypoglycemic action of nateglinide).
No products indexed under this heading.

Diclofenac Sodium (Certain drugs including nonsteroidal anti-inflammatory agents (NSAIDs) may potentiate the hypoglycemic action of nateglinide). Products include:
Diclofenac Sodium Ophthalmic Solution.................................. ⊙ 240
Voltaren Ophthalmic Solution 2336
Voltaren Tablets 2334
Voltaren-XR Tablets 2337

Diflunisal (Certain drugs including salicylates may potentiate the hypoglycemic action of nateglinide).
No products indexed under this heading.

Dobutamine Hydrochloride (Certain drugs including sympathomimetics may reduce the hypoglycemic action of nateglinide. When sympathomimetics are administered to or withdrawn from patients receiving nateglinide, the patient should be observed closely for changes in glycemic control).
No products indexed under this heading.

Dopamine Hydrochloride (Certain drugs including sympathomimetics may reduce the hypoglycemic action of nateglinide. When sympathomimetics are administered to or withdrawn from patients receiving nateglinide, the patient should be observed closely for changes in glycemic control).
No products indexed under this heading.

Ephedrine Hydrochloride (Certain drugs including sympathomimetics may reduce the hypoglycemic action of nateglinide. When sympathomimetics are administered to or withdrawn from patients receiving nateglinide, the patient should be observed closely for changes in glycemic control).
No products indexed under this heading.

Ephedrine Sulfate (Certain drugs including sympathomimetics may reduce the hypoglycemic action of nateglinide. When sympathomimetics are administered to or withdrawn from patients receiving nateglinide, the patient should be observed closely for changes in glycemic control).
No products indexed under this heading.

Ephedrine Tannate (Certain drugs including sympathomimetics may reduce the hypoglycemic action of nateglinide. When sympathomimetics are administered to or withdrawn from patients receiving nateglinide, the patient should be observed closely for changes in glycemic control).
No products indexed under this heading.

Epinephrine (Certain drugs including sympathomimetics may reduce the hypoglycemic action of nateglinide. When sympathomimetics are administered to or withdrawn from patients receiving nateglinide, the patient should be observed closely for changes in glycemic control). Products include:
EpiPen 1024

Epinephrine Bitartrate (Certain drugs including sympathomimetics may reduce the hypoglycemic action of nateglinide. When sympathomimetics are administered to or withdrawn from patients receiving nateglinide, the patient should be observed closely for changes in glycemic control).
No products indexed under this heading.

Epinephrine Hydrochloride (Certain drugs including sympathomimetics may reduce the hypoglycemic action of nateglinide. When sympathomimetics are administered to or withdrawn from patients receiving nateglinide, the patient should be observed closely for changes in glycemic control).
No products indexed under this heading.

Etodolac (Certain drugs including nonsteroidal anti-inflammatory agents (NSAIDs) may potentiate the hypoglycemic action of nateglinide).
No products indexed under this heading.

Fenoprofen Calcium (Certain drugs including nonsteroidal anti-inflammatory agents (NSAIDs) may potentiate the hypoglycemic action of nateglinide). Products include:
Nalfon Capsules 2508

Fludrocortisone Acetate (Certain drugs including corticosteroids may reduce the hypoglycemic action of nateglinide. When corticosteroids are administered to or withdrawn from patients receiving nateglinide, the patient should be observed closely for changes in glycemic control).
No products indexed under this heading.

Flunisolide (Certain drugs including corticosteroids may reduce the hypoglycemic action of nateglinide. When corticosteroids are administered to or withdrawn from patients receiving nateglinide, the patient should be observed closely for changes in glycemic control). Products include:
Aerobid/Aerobid-M 1153

Flurbiprofen (Certain drugs including nonsteroidal anti-inflammatory agents (NSAIDs) may potentiate the hypoglycemic action of nateglinide).
No products indexed under this heading.

Fluticasone Propionate (Certain drugs including corticosteroids may reduce the hypoglycemic action of nateglinide. When corticosteroids are administered to or withdrawn from patients receiving nateglinide, the patient should be observed closely for changes in glycemic control). Products include:
Advair Diskus 100/50 1276
Advair Diskus 250/50 1276
Advair Diskus 500/50 1276
Advair HFA 45/21 Inhalation Aerosol.. 1288
Advair HFA 115/21 Inhalation Aerosol.. 1288
Advair HFA 230/21 Inhalation Aerosol.. 1288
Flonase Nasal Spray 1431
Flovent Diskus 50 mcg 1435

Fluticasone Propionate HFA (Certain drugs including corticosteroids may reduce the hypoglycemic action of nateglinide. When corticosteroids are administered to or withdrawn from patients receiving nateglinide, the patient should be observed closely for changes in glycemic control). Products include:
Flovent HFA 1440

Hydrochlorothiazide (Certain drugs including thiazides may reduce the hypoglycemic action of nateglinide. When thiazides are administered to or withdrawn from patients receiving nateglinide, the patient should be observed closely for changes in glycemic control). Products include:
Atacand HCT 642
Avalide Tablets 892
Avalide Tablets 2713
Benicar HCT Tablets 1010
Diovan HCT Tablets 2216
Dyazide Capsules 1405
Micardis HCT Tablets 854
Prinzide Tablets 2092
Tekturna HCT Tablets 2324
Teveten HCT Tablets 517

Hydrocortisone (Certain drugs including corticosteroids may reduce the hypoglycemic action of nateglinide. When corticosteroids are administered to or withdrawn from patients receiving nateglinide, the patient should be observed closely for changes in glycemic control).
No products indexed under this heading.

Hydrocortisone Acetate (Certain drugs including corticosteroids may reduce the hypoglycemic action of nateglinide. When corticosteroids are administered to or withdrawn from patients receiving nateglinide, the patient should be observed closely for changes in glycemic control). Products include:
Analpram-HC 1140
Pramosone 1141

Hydrocortisone Sodium Phosphate (Certain drugs including corticosteroids may reduce the hypoglycemic action of nateglinide. When corticosteroids are administered to or withdrawn from patients receiving nateglinide, the patient should be observed closely for changes in glycemic control).
No products indexed under this heading.

Hydrocortisone Sodium Succinate (Certain drugs including corticosteroids may reduce the hypoglycemic action of nateglinide. When corticosteroids are administered to or withdrawn from patients receiving nateglinide, the patient should be observed closely for changes in glycemic control).
No products indexed under this heading.

Hydroflumethiazide (Certain drugs including thiazides may reduce the hypoglycemic action of nateglinide. When thiazides are administered to or withdrawn from patients receiving nateglinide, the patient should be observed closely for changes in glycemic control).
No products indexed under this heading.

Ibuprofen (Certain drugs including nonsteroidal anti-inflammatory agents (NSAIDs) may potentiate the hypoglycemic action of nateglinide). Products include:
Motrin IB Tablets and Caplets 1900
Children's Motrin Oral Suspension ... 1901
Children's Motrin Non-Staining Dye-Free Oral Suspension............ 1901
Children's Motrin Cold Oral Suspension 1899
Infants' Motrin Concentrated Drops.. 1901
Infants' Motrin Non-Staining Dye-Free Concentrated Drops....... 1901
Junior Strength Motrin Caplets and Chewable Tablets.................. 1901
Vicoprofen Tablets 533

Indomethacin (Certain drugs including nonsteroidal anti-inflammatory agents (NSAIDs) may potentiate the hypoglycemic action of nateglinide). Products include:
Indocin 2024

Indomethacin Sodium Trihydrate (Certain drugs including nonsteroidal anti-inflammatory agents (NSAIDs) may potentiate the hypoglycemic action of nateglinide). Products include:
Indocin I.V. 2489

Isocarboxazid (Certain drugs including monoamine oxidase inhibitors may potentiate the hypoglycemic action of nateglinide). Products include:
Marplan Tablets 3177

Isoproterenol Hydrochloride (Certain drugs including sympathomimetics may reduce the hypoglycemic action of nateglinide. When sympathomimetics are administered to or withdrawn from patients receiving nateglinide, the patient should be observed closely for changes in glycemic control).
No products indexed under this heading.

Isoproterenol Sulfate (Certain drugs including sympathomimetics may reduce the hypoglycemic action of nateglinide. When sympathomimetics are administered to or withdrawn from patients receiving nateglinide, the patient should be observed closely for changes in glycemic control).
No products indexed under this heading.

Ketoprofen (Certain drugs including nonsteroidal anti-inflammatory agents (NSAIDs) may potentiate the hypoglycemic action of nateglinide).
No products indexed under this heading.

Ketorolac Tromethamine (Certain drugs including nonsteroidal anti-inflammatory agents (NSAIDs) may potentiate the hypoglycemic action of nateglinide).
No products indexed under this heading.

Labetalol Hydrochloride (Certain drugs including non-selective beta adrenergic blocking agents may potentiate the hypoglycemic action of nateglinide).
No products indexed under this heading.

Levalbuterol Hydrochloride (Certain drugs including sympathomimetics may reduce the hypoglycemic action of nateglinide. When sympathomimetics are administered to or withdrawn from patients receiving nateglinide, the patient should be observed closely for changes in glycemic control). Products include:
Xopenex Inhalation Solution 3001
Xopenex Inhalation Solution Concentrate 3005

Levothyroxine Sodium (Certain drugs including thyroid products may reduce the hypoglycemic action of nateglinide. When thyroid products are administered to or withdrawn from patients receiving nateglinide, the patient should be observed closely for changes in glycemic control). Products include:
Levothroid Tablets 1170
Levoxyl Tablets 1780
Synthroid Tablets 507

Liothyronine Sodium (Certain drugs including thyroid products may reduce the hypoglycemic action of nateglinide. When thyroid products are administered to or withdrawn from patients receiving nateglinide, the patient should be observed closely for changes in glycemic control). Products include:
Cytomel Tablets 1778

Liotrix (Certain drugs including thyroid products may reduce the hypoglycemic action of nateglinide. When thyroid products are administered to or withdrawn from patients receiving nateglinide, the patient should be observed closely for changes in glycemic control).
No products indexed under this heading.

Magnesium Salicylate (Certain drugs including salicylates may potentiate the hypoglycemic action of nateglinide).
No products indexed under this heading.

Meclofenamate Sodium (Certain drugs including nonsteroidal anti-inflammatory agents (NSAIDs) may potentiate the hypoglycemic action of nateglinide).
No products indexed under this heading.

Mefenamic Acid (Certain drugs including nonsteroidal anti-inflammatory agents (NSAIDs) may potentiate the hypoglycemic action of nateglinide).
No products indexed under this heading.

Meloxicam (Certain drugs including nonsteroidal anti-inflammatory agents (NSAIDs) may potentiate the hypoglycemic action of nateglinide). Products include:
Mobic Oral Suspension 863
Mobic Tablets 863

Metaproterenol Sulfate (Certain drugs including sympathomimetics may reduce the hypoglycemic action of nateglinide. When sympathomimetics are administered to or withdrawn from patients receiving nateglinide, the patient should be observed closely for changes in glycemic control).
No products indexed under this heading.

Metaraminol Bitartrate (Certain drugs including sympathomimetics may reduce the hypoglycemic action of nateglinide. When sympathomimetics are administered to or withdrawn from patients receiving nateglinide, the patient should be observed closely for changes in glycemic control).
No products indexed under this heading.

Methoxamine Hydrochloride (Certain drugs including sympathomimetics may reduce the hypoglycemic action of nateglinide. When sympathomimetics are administered to or withdrawn from patients receiving nateglinide, the patient should be observed closely for changes in glycemic control).
No products indexed under this heading.

Methyclothiazide (Certain drugs including thiazides may reduce the hypoglycemic action of nateglinide. When thiazides are administered to or withdrawn from patients receiving nateglinide, the patient should be observed closely for changes in glycemic control).
No products indexed under this heading.

Methylprednisolone Acetate (Certain drugs including corticosteroids may reduce the hypoglycemic action of nateglinide. When corticosteroids are administered to or withdrawn from patients receiving nateglinide, the patient should be observed closely for changes in glycemic control).
No products indexed under this heading.

Methylprednisolone Sodium Succinate (Certain drugs including corticosteroids may reduce the hypoglycemic action of nateglinide. When corticosteroids are administered to or withdrawn from patients receiving nateglinide, the patient should be observed closely for changes in glycemic control).
No products indexed under this heading.

Moclobemide (Certain drugs including monoamine oxidase inhibitors may potentiate the hypoglycemic action of nateglinide).
No products indexed under this heading.

Mometasone Furoate (Certain drugs including corticosteroids may reduce the hypoglycemic action of nateglinide. When corticosteroids are administered to or withdrawn from patients receiving nateglinide, the patient should be observed closely for changes in glycemic control). Products include:
Asmanex Twisthaler 2797
Elocon Cream 0.1% 2840
Elocon Lotion 0.1% 2841
Elocon Ointment 0.1% 2842

Mometasone Furoate Monohydrate (Certain drugs including corticosteroids may reduce the hypoglycemic action of nateglinide. When corticosteroids are administered to or withdrawn from patients receiving nateglinide, the patient should be observed closely for changes in glycemic control). Products include:
Nasonex Nasal Spray 2883

Nabumetone (Certain drugs including nonsteroidal anti-inflammatory agents (NSAIDs) may potentiate the hypoglycemic action of nateglinide).
No products indexed under this heading.

Nadolol (Certain drugs including non-selective beta adrenergic blocking agents may potentiate the hypoglycemic action of nateglinide). Products include:
Nadolol Tablets 2191

Naproxen (Certain drugs including nonsteroidal anti-inflammatory agents (NSAIDs) may potentiate the hypoglycemic action of nateglinide). Products include:
EC-Naprosyn Delayed-Release Tablets 2632
Naprosyn Suspension 2632
Naprosyn Tablets 2632

Naproxen Sodium (Certain drugs including nonsteroidal anti-inflammatory agents (NSAIDs) may potentiate the hypoglycemic action of nateglinide). Products include:
Anaprox Tablets 2632
Anaprox DS Tablets 2632
Treximet Tablets 1616

Norepinephrine Bitartrate (Certain drugs including sympathomimetics may reduce the hypoglycemic action of nateglinide. When sympathomimetics are administered to or withdrawn from patients receiving nateglinide, the patient should be observed closely for changes in glycemic control).
No products indexed under this heading.

Oxaprozin (Certain drugs including nonsteroidal anti-inflammatory agents (NSAIDs) may potentiate the hypoglycemic action of nateglinide).
No products indexed under this heading.

Pargyline Hydrochloride (Certain drugs including monoamine oxidase inhibitors may potentiate the hypoglycemic action of nateglinide).
No products indexed under this heading.

Phenelzine Sulfate (Certain drugs including monoamine oxidase inhibitors may potentiate the hypoglycemic action of nateglinide).
No products indexed under this heading.

Phenylbutazone (Certain drugs including nonsteroidal anti-inflammatory agents (NSAIDs) may potentiate the hypoglycemic action of nateglinide).
No products indexed under this heading.

Phenylephrine Bitartrate (Certain drugs including sympathomimetics may reduce the hypoglycemic action of nateglinide. When sympathomimetics are administered to or withdrawn from patients receiving nateglinide, the patient should be observed closely for changes in glycemic control).
No products indexed under this heading.

Phenylephrine Hydrochloride (Certain drugs including sympathomimetics may reduce the hypoglycemic action of nateglinide. When sympathomimetics are administered to or withdrawn from patients receiving nateglinide, the patient should be observed closely for changes in glycemic control). Products include:
Actifed Cold & Allergy Tablets 1895
Benadryl Allergy & Cold Kapgels 1895
Benadryl Allergy & Sinus Headache Kapgels 1895
Benadryl Severe Allergy & Sinus Headache Caplets 1897
Children's Benadryl-D Allergy & Sinus Liquid 1896
Benadryl-D Allergy & Sinus Tablet 1896
PediaCare Children's Allergy & Cold Liquid 1902
PediaCare Children's Decongestant Liquid 1902
PediaCare Children's Liquid Multi-Symptom Cold 1902
Sinutab Non-Drying Caplets 1905
Sinutab Sinus Caplets 1905
Children's Sudafed PE Cold & Cough Liquid 1907
Children's Sudafed PE Nasal Decongestant Liquid 1906
Sudafed PE Cold & Cough Caplets 1907
Sudafed PE Nasal Decongestant Tablets 1907
Sudafed PE Nighttime Cold Caplets 1907
Sudafed PE Non-Drying Sinus Caplets 1908
Sudafed PE Severe Cold Caplets 1908
Sudafed PE Sinus & Allergy Tablets 1908
Sudafed PE Sinus Headache Caplets 1908
Tylenol Allergy Multi-Symptom Caplets with Cool Burst and Rapid Release Gelcaps 1916
Tylenol Allergy Multi-Symptom Nighttime Caplets with Cool Burst 1916
Children's Tylenol Plus Cold Suspension Liquid 1912
Children's Tylenol Plus Cold & Allergy Suspension Liquid 1914
Children's Tylenol Plus Flu Suspension Liquid 1914
Children's Tylenol Plus Multi-Symptom Cold Suspension Liquid 1912
Tylenol Cold Head Congestion Daytime Caplets with Cool Burst 1910
Tylenol Cold Head Congestion Nighttime Caplets with Cool Burst 1910
Tylenol Cold Head Congestion Severe Daytime Caplets with Cool Burst 1910
Tylenol Cold Multi-Symptom Daytime Caplets with Cool Burst and Rapid Release Gels 1913
Tylenol Cold Multi-Symptom Daytime Liquid with Citrus Burst 1913
Tylenol Cold Multi-Symptom Nighttime Caplets with Cool Burst 1913
Tylenol Cold Multi-Symptom Nighttime Liquid with Cool Burst 1913
Tylenol Cold Multi-Symptom Severe Caplets with Cool Burst 1913
Tylenol Cold Multi-Symptom Severe Daytime Liquid with Citrus Burst 1913
Tylenol Sinus Congestion & Pain Daytime Caplets with Cool Burst and Gelcaps 1917

Tylenol Sinus Congestion & Pain Nighttime Caplets with Cool Burst 1917
Tylenol Sinus Congestion & Pain Severe Caplets with Cool Burst 1917
Vicks DayQuil Cold & Flu Multi-Symptom Relief .... ▣616
Vicks DayQuil LiquiCaps 2567
Vicks DayQuil Liquid 2567
Vicks DayQuil Multi-Symptom Cold/Flu Relief 2567

Phenylephrine Tannate (Certain drugs including sympathomimetics may reduce the hypoglycemic action of nateglinide. When sympathomimetics are administered to or withdrawn from patients receiving nateglinide, the patient should be observed closely for changes in glycemic control).
No products indexed under this heading.

Phenylpropanolamine Hydrochloride (Certain drugs including sympathomimetics may reduce the hypoglycemic action of nateglinide. When sympathomimetics are administered to or withdrawn from patients receiving nateglinide, the patient should be observed closely for changes in glycemic control).
No products indexed under this heading.

Pindolol (Certain drugs including non-selective beta adrenergic blocking agents may potentiate the hypoglycemic action of nateglinide).
No products indexed under this heading.

Pirbuterol Acetate (Certain drugs including sympathomimetics may reduce the hypoglycemic action of nateglinide. When sympathomimetics are administered to or withdrawn from patients receiving nateglinide, the patient should be observed closely for changes in glycemic control). Products include:
Maxair Autohaler 1705

Piroxicam (Certain drugs including nonsteroidal anti-inflammatory agents (NSAIDs) may potentiate the hypoglycemic action of nateglinide).
No products indexed under this heading.

Polythiazide (Certain drugs including thiazides may reduce the hypoglycemic action of nateglinide. When thiazides are administered to or withdrawn from patients receiving nateglinide, the patient should be observed closely for changes in glycemic control).
No products indexed under this heading.

Prednisolone Acetate (Certain drugs including corticosteroids may reduce the hypoglycemic action of nateglinide. When corticosteroids are administered to or withdrawn from patients receiving nateglinide, the patient should be observed closely for changes in glycemic control). Products include:
Pred Forte Ophthalmic Suspension .... ⊙227
Pred Mild Ophthalmic Suspension .... ⊙230
Pred-G Ophthalmic Ointment .... ⊙229
Pred-G Ophthalmic Suspension .... ⊙228

Prednisolone Sodium Phosphate (Certain drugs including corticosteroids may reduce the hypoglycemic action of nateglinide. When corticosteroids are administered to or withdrawn from patients receiving nateglinide, the patient should be observed closely for changes in glycemic control).
No products indexed under this heading.

Prednisolone Tebutate (Certain drugs including corticosteroids may reduce the hypoglycemic action of nateglinide. When corticosteroids are administered to or withdrawn from patients receiving nateglinide, the patient should be observed closely for changes in glycemic control).
No products indexed under this heading.

Prednisone (Certain drugs including corticosteroids may reduce the hypoglycemic action of nateglinide. When corticosteroids are administered to or withdrawn from patients receiving nateglinide, the patient should be observed closely for changes in glycemic control).
No products indexed under this heading.

Procarbazine Hydrochloride (Certain drugs including monoamine oxidase inhibitors may potentiate the hypoglycemic action of nateglinide).
No products indexed under this heading.

Propranolol Hydrochloride (Certain drugs including non-selective beta adrenergic blocking agents may potentiate the hypoglycemic action of nateglinide). Products include:
InnoPran XL Extended Release Capsules 1484

Pseudoephedrine Hydrochloride (Certain drugs including sympathomimetics may reduce the hypoglycemic action of nateglinide. When sympathomimetics are administered to or withdrawn from patients receiving nateglinide, the patient should be observed closely for changes in glycemic control). Products include:
Allegra-D 12 Hour Extended-Release Tablets 2687
Allegra-D 24 Hour Extended-Release Tablets 2690
Children's Motrin Cold Oral Suspension 1899
Sudafed 12 Hour Nasal Decongestant Non-Drowsy Caplets 1909
Sudafed 24 Hour Non-Drowsy Nasal Decongestant Tablets 1906
Children's Sudafed Nasal Decongestant Liquid 1906
Sudafed Nasal Decongestant Tablets 1906
Tylenol Cold Severe Congestion Daytime Caplets with Cool Burst 1912
Tylenol Sinus Severe Congestion Caplets with Cool Burst 1917
Vicks NyQuil LiquiCaps 2567
Vicks NyQuil Liquid 2567
Vicks NyQuil Multi-Symptom Cold/Flu Relief 2567
Zyrtec-D 12 Hour Extended Release Tablets 1923
Zyrtec-D Allergy & Congestion Extended-Release Tablets 1923

Pseudoephedrine Sulfate (Certain drugs including sympathomimetics may reduce the hypoglycemic action of nateglinide. When sympathomimetics are administered to or withdrawn from patients receiving nateglinide, the patient should be observed closely for changes in glycemic control). Products include:
Clarinex-D 12-Hour Extended-Release Tablets 2831
Clarinex-D 24-Hour Extended-Release Tablets 2834

Rasagiline Mesylate (Certain drugs including monoamine oxidase inhibitors may potentiate the hypoglycemic action of nateglinide). Products include:
Azilect Tablets 3106

Rofecoxib (Certain drugs including nonsteroidal anti-inflammatory agents (NSAIDs) may potentiate the hypoglycemic action of nateglinide).
No products indexed under this heading.

Salmeterol Xinafoate (Certain drugs including sympathomimetics may reduce the hypoglycemic action of nateglinide. When sympathomimetics are administered to or withdrawn from patients receiving nateglinide, the patient should be observed closely for changes in glycemic control). Products include:
Advair Diskus 100/50 1276
Advair Diskus 250/50 1276
Advair Diskus 500/50 1276
Advair HFA 45/21 Inhalation Aerosol 1288
Advair HFA 115/21 Inhalation Aerosol 1288
Advair HFA 230/21 Inhalation Aerosol 1288
Serevent Diskus 1594

Salsalate (Certain drugs including salicylates may potentiate the hypoglycemic action of nateglinide).
No products indexed under this heading.

Selegiline (Certain drugs including monoamine oxidase inhibitors may potentiate the hypoglycemic action of nateglinide). Products include:
Emsam Transdermal System 905

Selegiline Hydrochloride (Certain drugs including monoamine oxidase inhibitors may potentiate the hypoglycemic action of nateglinide). Products include:
Eldepryl Capsules 3052

Sulindac (Certain drugs including nonsteroidal anti-inflammatory agents (NSAIDs) may potentiate the hypoglycemic action of nateglinide). Products include:
Clinoril Tablets 1962

Terbutaline Sulfate (Certain drugs including sympathomimetics may reduce the hypoglycemic action of nateglinide. When sympathomimetics are administered to or withdrawn from patients receiving nateglinide, the patient should be observed closely for changes in glycemic control).
No products indexed under this heading.

Thyroglobulin (Certain drugs including thyroid products may reduce the hypoglycemic action of nateglinide. When thyroid products are administered to or withdrawn from patients receiving nateglinide, the patient should be observed closely for changes in glycemic control).
No products indexed under this heading.

Thyroid (Certain drugs including thyroid products may reduce the hypoglycemic action of nateglinide. When thyroid products are administered to or withdrawn from patients receiving nateglinide, the patient should be observed closely for changes in glycemic control). Products include:
Naturethroid Tablets 2605

Thyroxine (Certain drugs including thyroid products may reduce the hypoglycemic action of nateglinide. When thyroid products are administered to or withdrawn from patients receiving nateglinide, the patient should be observed closely for changes in glycemic control).
No products indexed under this heading.

Thyroxine Sodium (Certain drugs including thyroid products may reduce the hypoglycemic action of nateglinide. When thyroid products are administered to or withdrawn from patients receiving nateglinide, the patient should be observed closely for changes in glycemic control).
No products indexed under this heading.

Timolol Maleate (Certain drugs including non-selective beta adrenergic blocking agents may potentiate the hypoglycemic action of nateglinide). Products include:
Combigan Ophthalmic Solution 553
Cosopt Sterile Ophthalmic Solution 1969
Timoptic Sterile Ophthalmic Solution 2121
Timoptic in Ocudose 2124
Timoptic-XE Sterile Ophthalmic Gel Forming Solution 2125

Tolbutamide (Nateglinide is a potential inhibitor of the CYP2C9 isoenzyme in vivo as indicated by its ability to inhibit the in vitro metabolism of tolbutamide).
No products indexed under this heading.

Tolbutamide Sodium (Nateglinide is a potential inhibitor of the CYP2C9 isoenzyme in vivo as indicated by its ability to inhibit the in vitro metabolism of tolbutamide).
No products indexed under this heading.

Tolmetin Sodium (Certain drugs including nonsteroidal anti-inflammatory agents (NSAIDs) may potentiate the hypoglycemic action of nateglinide).
No products indexed under this heading.

Tranylcypromine Sulfate (Certain drugs including monoamine oxidase inhibitors may potentiate the hypoglycemic action of nateglinide). Products include:
Parnate Tablets 1532

Triamcinolone (Certain drugs including corticosteroids may reduce the hypoglycemic action of nateglinide. When corticosteroids are administered to or withdrawn from patients receiving nateglinide, the patient should be observed closely for changes in glycemic control).
No products indexed under this heading.

Triamcinolone Acetonide (Certain drugs including corticosteroids may reduce the hypoglycemic action of nateglinide. When corticosteroids are administered to or withdrawn from patients receiving nateglinide, the patient should be observed closely for changes in glycemic control). Products include:
Azmacort Inhalation Aerosol 407
Nasacort AQ Nasal Spray 2765
Triesence Injectable Suspension .... ⊙209

Triamcinolone Diacetate (Certain drugs including corticosteroids may reduce the hypoglycemic action of nateglinide. When corticosteroids are administered to or withdrawn from patients receiving nateglinide, the patient should be observed closely for changes in glycemic control).
No products indexed under this heading.

Triamcinolone Hexacetonide (Certain drugs including corticosteroids may reduce the hypoglycemic action of nateglinide. When corticosteroids are administered to or withdrawn from patients receiving nateglinide, the patient should be observed closely for changes in glycemic control).
No products indexed under this heading.

Valdecoxib (Certain drugs including nonsteroidal anti-inflammatory agents (NSAIDs) may potentiate the hypoglycemic action of nateglinide).
No products indexed under this heading.

Food Interactions

Food, unspecified (The pharmacokinetics of nateglinide were not affected by the composition of a meal (high protein, fat, or carbohydrate). However, peak plasma levels were significantly reduced when nateglinide was administered 10 minutes prior to a liquid meal).

STRATTERA CAPSULES

(Atomoxetine Hydrochloride) 1864

May interact with beta-adrenergic stimulating agents, cytochrome p450 2d6 inhibitors (selected), monoamine oxidase inhibitors, vasopressors, and certain other agents. Compounds in these categories include:

Albuterol (Atomoxetine hydrochloride should be administered with caution to patients being treated with systemically-administered (oral or intravenous) albuterol (or other beta2 agonists) because the action of albuterol on the cardiovascular system can be potentiated resulting in increases in heart rate and blood pressure. Albuterol (600 mcg IV over 2 hours) increases heart rate and blood pressure).
No products indexed under this heading.

Albuterol Sulfate (Atomoxetine hydrochloride should be administered with caution to patients being treated with systemically-administered (oral or intravenous) albuterol (or other beta2 agonists) because the action of albuterol on the cardiovascular system can be potentiated resulting in increases in heart rate and blood pressure. Albuterol (600 mcg IV over 2 hours) increases heart rate and blood pressure). Products include:
- Combivent Inhalation Aerosol 845
- ProAir HFA Inhalation Aerosol 3113
- Proventil HFA Inhalation Aerosol 2914
- Ventolin HFA Inhalation Aerosol 1638

Amiodarone Hydrochloride (Atomoxetine is primarily metabolized by the CYP2D6 pathway to 4-hydroxyatomoxetine. Dosage adjustment of atomoxetine hydrochloride may be necessary when co-administered with potent CYP2D6 inhibitors (e.g., paroxetine, fluoxetine, and quinidine)).
No products indexed under this heading.

Amitriptyline Hydrochloride (Atomoxetine is primarily metabolized by the CYP2D6 pathway to 4-hydroxyatomoxetine. Dosage adjustment of atomoxetine hydrochloride may be necessary when co-administered with potent CYP2D6 inhibitors (e.g., paroxetine, fluoxetine, and quinidine)).
No products indexed under this heading.

Amoxapine (Atomoxetine is primarily metabolized by the CYP2D6 pathway to 4-hydroxyatomoxetine. Dosage adjustment of atomoxetine hydrochloride may be necessary when co-administered with potent CYP2D6 inhibitors (e.g., paroxetine, fluoxetine, and quinidine)).
No products indexed under this heading.

Bitolterol Mesylate (Atomoxetine hydrochloride should be administered with caution to patients being treated with systemically-administered (oral or intravenous) albuterol (or other beta2 agonists) because the action of albuterol on the cardiovascular system can be potentiated resulting in increases in heart rate and blood pressure. Albuterol (600 mcg IV over 2 hours) increases heart rate and blood pressure).
No products indexed under this heading.

Bupropion Hydrochloride (Atomoxetine is primarily metabolized by the CYP2D6 pathway to 4-hydroxyatomoxetine. Dosage adjustment of atomoxetine hydrochloride may be necessary when co-administered with potent CYP2D6 inhibitors (e.g., paroxetine, fluoxetine, and quinidine)). Products include:
- Wellbutrin Tablets 1648
- Wellbutrin SR Sustained-Release Tablets 1653
- Wellbutrin XL Extended-Release Tablets 1659
- Zyban Sustained-Release Tablets 1692

Celecoxib (Atomoxetine is primarily metabolized by the CYP2D6 pathway to 4-hydroxyatomoxetine. Dosage adjustment of atomoxetine hydrochloride may be necessary when co-administered with potent CYP2D6 inhibitors (e.g., paroxetine, fluoxetine, and quinidine)). Products include:
- Celebrex Capsules 2979

Chloroquine Hydrochloride (Atomoxetine is primarily metabolized by the CYP2D6 pathway to 4-hydroxyatomoxetine. Dosage adjustment of atomoxetine hydrochloride may be necessary when co-administered with potent CYP2D6 inhibitors (e.g., paroxetine, fluoxetine, and quinidine)).
No products indexed under this heading.

Chloroquine Phosphate (Atomoxetine is primarily metabolized by the CYP2D6 pathway to 4-hydroxyatomoxetine. Dosage adjustment of atomoxetine hydrochloride may be necessary when co-administered with potent CYP2D6 inhibitors (e.g., paroxetine, fluoxetine, and quinidine)).
No products indexed under this heading.

Chlorpheniramine (Atomoxetine is primarily metabolized by the CYP2D6 pathway to 4-hydroxyatomoxetine. Dosage adjustment of atomoxetine hydrochloride may be necessary when co-administered with potent CYP2D6 inhibitors (e.g., paroxetine, fluoxetine, and quinidine)).
No products indexed under this heading.

Chlorpheniramine Maleate (Atomoxetine is primarily metabolized by the CYP2D6 pathway to 4-hydroxyatomoxetine. Dosage adjustment of atomoxetine hydrochloride may be necessary when co-administered with potent CYP2D6 inhibitors (e.g., paroxetine, fluoxetine, and quinidine)). Products include:
- Actifed Cold & Allergy Tablets 1895
- Sudafed PE Sinus & Allergy Tablets 1908
- Tylenol Allergy Multi-Symptom Caplets with Cool Burst and Rapid Release Gelcaps 1916
- Children's Tylenol Plus Cold Suspension Liquid 1912
- Children's Tylenol Plus Cough & Runny Nose Suspension Liquid 1912
- Children's Tylenol Plus Flu Suspension Liquid 1914
- Children's Tylenol Plus Multi-Symptom Cold Suspension Liquid 1912
- Tylenol Cold Head Congestion Nighttime Caplets with Cool Burst 1910
- Tylenol Cold Multi-Symptom Nighttime Caplets with Cool Burst 1913
- Tylenol Sinus Congestion & Pain Nighttime Caplets with Cool Burst 1917

Chlorpheniramine Polistirex (Atomoxetine is primarily metabolized by the CYP2D6 pathway to 4-hydroxyatomoxetine. Dosage adjustment of atomoxetine hydrochloride may be necessary when co-administered with potent CYP2D6 inhibitors (e.g., paroxetine, fluoxetine, and quinidine)). Products include:
- Tussionex Pennkinetic Extended-Release Suspension 3154

Chlorpheniramine Tannate (Atomoxetine is primarily metabolized by the CYP2D6 pathway to 4-hydroxyatomoxetine. Dosage adjustment of atomoxetine hydrochloride may be necessary when co-administered with potent CYP2D6 inhibitors (e.g., paroxetine, fluoxetine, and quinidine)).
No products indexed under this heading.

Cimetidine (Atomoxetine is primarily metabolized by the CYP2D6 pathway to 4-hydroxyatomoxetine. Dosage adjustment of atomoxetine hydrochloride may be necessary when co-administered with potent CYP2D6 inhibitors (e.g., paroxetine, fluoxetine, and quinidine)).
No products indexed under this heading.

Cimetidine Hydrochloride (Atomoxetine is primarily metabolized by the CYP2D6 pathway to 4-hydroxyatomoxetine. Dosage adjustment of atomoxetine hydrochloride may be necessary when co-administered with potent CYP2D6 inhibitors (e.g., paroxetine, fluoxetine, and quinidine)).
No products indexed under this heading.

Citalopram Hydrobromide (Atomoxetine is primarily metabolized by the CYP2D6 pathway to 4-hydroxyatomoxetine. Dosage adjustment of atomoxetine hydrochloride may be necessary when co-administered with potent CYP2D6 inhibitors (e.g., paroxetine, fluoxetine, and quinidine)). Products include:
- Celexa 1160

Clomipramine Hydrochloride (Atomoxetine is primarily metabolized by the CYP2D6 pathway to 4-hydroxyatomoxetine. Dosage adjustment of atomoxetine hydrochloride may be necessary when co-administered with potent CYP2D6 inhibitors (e.g., paroxetine, fluoxetine, and quinidine)).
No products indexed under this heading.

Cocaine Hydrochloride (Atomoxetine is primarily metabolized by the CYP2D6 pathway to 4-hydroxyatomoxetine. Dosage adjustment of atomoxetine hydrochloride may be necessary when co-administered with potent CYP2D6 inhibitors (e.g., paroxetine, fluoxetine, and quinidine)).
No products indexed under this heading.

Desipramine Hydrochloride (Atomoxetine is primarily metabolized by the CYP2D6 pathway to 4-hydroxyatomoxetine. Dosage adjustment of atomoxetine hydrochloride may be necessary when co-administered with potent CYP2D6 inhibitors (e.g., paroxetine, fluoxetine, and quinidine)).
No products indexed under this heading.

Diphenhydramine (Atomoxetine is primarily metabolized by the CYP2D6 pathway to 4-hydroxyatomoxetine. Dosage adjustment of atomoxetine hydrochloride may be necessary when co-administered with potent CYP2D6 inhibitors (e.g., paroxetine, fluoxetine, and quinidine)).
No products indexed under this heading.

Diphenhydramine Hydrochloride (Atomoxetine is primarily metabolized by the CYP2D6 pathway to 4-hydroxyatomoxetine. Dosage adjustment of atomoxetine hydrochloride may be necessary when co-administered with potent CYP2D6 inhibitors (e.g., paroxetine, fluoxetine, and quinidine)). Products include:
- Benadryl Allergy & Cold Kapgels 1895
- Benadryl Allergy & Sinus Headache Kapgels 1895
- Benadryl Severe Allergy & Sinus Headache Caplets 1897
- Benadryl Dye-Free Allergy Liqui-gels Softgels 1897
- Benadryl Allergy Kapgels 1895
- Benadryl Allergy Quick Dissolve Strips 1896
- Benadryl Allergy Ultratab Tablets 1896
- Children's Benadryl Dye-Free Allergy Liquid 1897
- Children's Benadryl Allergy Fastmelts 1897
- Children's Benadryl Allergy Liquid 1898
- Children's Benadryl Allergy Perfect Measure 1896
- Children's Benadryl-D Allergy & Sinus Liquid 1896
- Benadryl-D Allergy & Sinus Tablet 1896
- PediaCare Children's Allergy & Cold Liquid 1902
- PediaCare Children's Allergy Liquid 1902

Simply Sleep Caplets 1905
Sudafed PE Nighttime Cold Caplets.. 1907
Sudafed PE Severe Cold Caplets..... 1908
Extra Strength Tylenol PM Caplets, Geltabs, Liquid, and Rapid Release Gels...................... 1915
Tylenol Allergy Multi-Symptom Nighttime Caplets with Cool Burst.. 1916
Tylenol Severe Allergy Caplets......... 1916
Children's Tylenol Plus Cold & Allergy Suspension Liquid............. 1914
Tylenol Sore Throat Nighttime Liquid with Cool Burst................... 1918

Dobutamine (Atomoxetine hydrochloride should be administered with caution to patients being treated with systemically-administered (oral or intravenous) albuterol (or other beta2 agonists) because the action of albuterol on the cardiovascular system can be potentiated resulting in increases in heart rate and blood pressure. Albuterol (600 mcg IV over 2 hours) increases heart rate and blood pressure).
No products indexed under this heading.

Dobutamine Hydrochloride (Atomoxetine hydrochloride should be administered with caution to patients being treated with systemically-administered (oral or intravenous) albuterol (or other beta2 agonists) because the action of albuterol on the cardiovascular system can be potentiated resulting in increases in heart rate and blood pressure. Albuterol (600 mcg IV over 2 hours) increases heart rate and blood pressure).
No products indexed under this heading.

Dopamine Hydrochloride (Because of possible effects on blood pressure, atomoxetine hydrochloride should be used cautiously with pressor agents (e.g., dopamine, dobutamine)).
No products indexed under this heading.

Doxepin Hydrochloride (Atomoxetine is primarily metabolized by the CYP2D6 pathway to 4-hydroxyatomoxetine. Dosage adjustment of atomoxetine hydrochloride may be necessary when co-administered with potent CYP2D6 inhibitors (e.g., paroxetine, fluoxetine, and quinidine)).
No products indexed under this heading.

Ephedrine Hydrochloride (Atomoxetine hydrochloride should be administered with caution to patients being treated with systemically-administered (oral or intravenous) albuterol (or other beta2 agonists) because the action of albuterol on the cardiovascular system can be potentiated resulting in increases in heart rate and blood pressure. Albuterol (600 mcg IV over 2 hours) increases heart rate and blood pressure).
No products indexed under this heading.

Ephedrine Sulfate (Atomoxetine HCl should be administered with caution to patients being treated with systemically-administered (oral or intravenous) albuterol (or other beta2 agonists) because the action of albuterol on the cardiovascular system can be potentiated resulting in increases in heart rate and blood pressure. Because of possible effects on blood pressure, atomoxetine hydrochloride should be use cautiously with pressor agents).
No products indexed under this heading.

Ephedrine Tannate (Atomoxetine hydrochloride should be administered with caution to patients being treated with systemically-administered (oral or intravenous) albuterol (or other beta2 agonists) because the action of albuterol on the cardiovascular system can be potentiated resulting in increases in heart rate and blood pressure. Albuterol (600 mcg IV over 2 hours) increases heart rate and blood pressure).
No products indexed under this heading.

Epinephrine (Atomoxetine hydrochloride should be administered with caution to patients being treated with systemically-administered (oral or intravenous) albuterol (or other beta2 agonists) because the action of albuterol on the cardiovascular system can be potentiated resulting in increases in heart rate and blood pressure. Albuterol (600 mcg IV over 2 hours) increases heart rate and blood pressure). Products include:

EpiPen 1024

Epinephrine Bitartrate (Because of possible effects on blood pressure, atomoxetine hydrochloride should be used cautiously with pressor agents (e.g., dopamine, dobutamine)).
No products indexed under this heading.

Epinephrine Hydrochloride (Atomoxetine hydrochloride should be administered with caution to patients being treated with systemically-administered (oral or intravenous) albuterol (or other beta2 agonists) because the action of albuterol on the cardiovascular system can be potentiated resulting in increases in heart rate and blood pressure. Albuterol (600 mcg IV over 2 hours) increases heart rate and blood pressure).
No products indexed under this heading.

Escitalopram Oxalate (Atomoxetine is primarily metabolized by the CYP2D6 pathway to 4-hydroxyatomoxetine. Dosage adjustment of atomoxetine hydrochloride may be necessary when co-administered with potent CYP2D6 inhibitors (e.g., paroxetine, fluoxetine, and quinidine)). Products include:

Lexapro Oral Suspension 1174
Lexapro Tablets 1174

Fluoxetine (Atomoxetine is primarily metabolized by the CYP2D6 pathway to 4-hydroxyatomoxetine. Dosage adjustment of atomoxetine hydrochloride may be necessary when co-administered with potent CYP2D6 inhibitors (e.g., paroxetine, fluoxetine, and quinidine)).
No products indexed under this heading.

Fluoxetine Hydrochloride (Atomoxetine is primarily metabolized by the CYP2D6 pathway to 4-hydroxyatomoxetine. Dosage adjustment of atomoxetine hydrochloride may be necessary when co-administered with potent CYP2D6 inhibitors (e.g., paroxetine, fluoxetine, and quinidine)). Products include:

Prozac Weekly Capsules 1852
Prozac Pulvules and Liquid 1852
Symbyax Capsules 1871

Fluphenazine Decanoate (Atomoxetine is primarily metabolized by the CYP2D6 pathway to 4-hydroxyatomoxetine. Dosage adjustment of atomoxetine hydrochloride may be necessary when co-administered with potent CYP2D6 inhibitors (e.g., paroxetine, fluoxetine, and quinidine)).
No products indexed under this heading.

Fluphenazine Enanthate (Atomoxetine is primarily metabolized by the CYP2D6 pathway to 4-hydroxyatomoxetine. Dosage adjustment of atomoxetine hydrochloride may be necessary when co-administered with potent CYP2D6 inhibitors (e.g., paroxetine, fluoxetine, and quinidine)).
No products indexed under this heading.

Fluphenazine Hydrochloride (Atomoxetine is primarily metabolized by the CYP2D6 pathway to 4-hydroxyatomoxetine. Dosage adjustment of atomoxetine hydrochloride may be necessary when co-administered with potent CYP2D6 inhibitors (e.g., paroxetine, fluoxetine, and quinidine)).
No products indexed under this heading.

Fluvoxamine Maleate (Atomoxetine is primarily metabolized by the CYP2D6 pathway to 4-hydroxyatomoxetine. Dosage adjustment of atomoxetine hydrochloride may be necessary when co-administered with potent CYP2D6 inhibitors (e.g., paroxetine, fluoxetine, and quinidine)). Products include:

Luvox CR Extended-Release Capsules...................................... 1759

Halofantrine Hydrochloride (Atomoxetine is primarily metabolized by the CYP2D6 pathway to 4-hydroxyatomoxetine. Dosage adjustment of atomoxetine hydrochloride may be necessary when co-administered with potent CYP2D6 inhibitors (e.g., paroxetine, fluoxetine, and quinidine)).
No products indexed under this heading.

Haloperidol (Atomoxetine is primarily metabolized by the CYP2D6 pathway to 4-hydroxyatomoxetine. Dosage adjustment of atomoxetine hydrochloride may be necessary when co-administered with potent CYP2D6 inhibitors (e.g., paroxetine, fluoxetine, and quinidine)).
No products indexed under this heading.

Haloperidol Decanoate (Atomoxetine is primarily metabolized by the CYP2D6 pathway to 4-hydroxyatomoxetine. Dosage adjustment of atomoxetine hydrochloride may be necessary when co-administered with potent CYP2D6 inhibitors (e.g., paroxetine, fluoxetine, and quinidine)).
No products indexed under this heading.

Hydroxychloroquine Sulfate (Atomoxetine is primarily metabolized by the CYP2D6 pathway to 4-hydroxyatomoxetine. Dosage adjustment of atomoxetine hydrochloride may be necessary when co-administered with potent CYP2D6 inhibitors (e.g., paroxetine, fluoxetine, and quinidine)).
No products indexed under this heading.

Imatinib Mesylate (Atomoxetine is primarily metabolized by the CYP2D6 pathway to 4-hydroxyatomoxetine. Dosage adjustment of atomoxetine hydrochloride may be necessary when co-administered with potent CYP2D6 inhibitors (e.g., paroxetine, fluoxetine, and quinidine)). Products include:

Gleevec Tablets 2255

Imipramine Hydrochloride (Atomoxetine is primarily metabolized by the CYP2D6 pathway to 4-hydroxyatomoxetine. Dosage adjustment of atomoxetine hydrochloride may be necessary when co-administered with potent CYP2D6 inhibitors (e.g., paroxetine, fluoxetine, and quinidine)).
No products indexed under this heading.

Imipramine Pamoate (Atomoxetine is primarily metabolized by the CYP2D6 pathway to 4-hydroxyatomoxetine. Dosage adjustment of atomoxetine hydrochloride may be necessary when co-administered with potent CYP2D6 inhibitors (e.g., paroxetine, fluoxetine, and quinidine)).
No products indexed under this heading.

Isocarboxazid (Atomoxetine hydrochloride should not be taken with an MAOI, or within 2 weeks after discontinuing an MAOI. Treatment with an MAOI should not be initiated within 2 weeks after discontinuing atomoxetine hydrochloride. With other drugs that affect brain monoamine concentrations, there have been reports of serious, sometimes fatal reactions (including hyperthermia, rigidity, myoclonus, autonomic instability with possible rapid fluctuations of vital signs, and mental status changes that include extreme agitation progressing to delirium and coma) when taken in combination with an MAOI. Some cases presented with features resembling neuroleptic malignant syndrome. Such reactions may occur when these drugs are given concurrently or in close proximity). Products include:

Marplan Tablets 3177

Isoetharine (Atomoxetine hydrochloride should be administered with caution to patients being treated with systemically-administered (oral or intravenous) albuterol (or other beta2 agonists) because the action of albuterol on the cardiovascular system can be potentiated resulting in increases in heart rate and blood pressure. Albuterol (600 mcg IV over 2 hours) increases heart rate and blood pressure).
No products indexed under this heading.

Isoproterenol Hydrochloride (Atomoxetine hydrochloride should be administered with caution to patients being treated with systemically-administered (oral or intravenous) albuterol (or other beta2 agonists) because the action of albuterol on the cardiovascular system can be potentiated resulting in increases in heart rate and blood pressure. Albuterol (600 mcg IV over 2 hours) increases heart rate and blood pressure).

No products indexed under this heading.

Isoproterenol Sulfate (Atomoxetine hydrochloride should be administered with caution to patients being treated with systemically-administered (oral or intravenous) albuterol (or other beta2 agonists) because the action of albuterol on the cardiovascular system can be potentiated resulting in increases in heart rate and blood pressure. Albuterol (600 mcg IV over 2 hours) increases heart rate and blood pressure).

No products indexed under this heading.

Levalbuterol Hydrochloride (Atomoxetine hydrochloride should be administered with caution to patients being treated with systemically-administered (oral or intravenous) albuterol (or other beta2 agonists) because the action of albuterol on the cardiovascular system can be potentiated resulting in increases in heart rate and blood pressure. Albuterol (600 mcg IV over 2 hours) increases heart rate and blood pressure). Products include:

Xopenex Inhalation Solution 3001
Xopenex Inhalation Solution Concentrate 3005

Maprotiline Hydrochloride (Atomoxetine is primarily metabolized by the CYP2D6 pathway to 4-hydroxyatomoxetine. Dosage adjustment of atomoxetine hydrochloride may be necessary when co-administered with potent CYP2D6 inhibitors (e.g., paroxetine, fluoxetine, and quinidine)).

No products indexed under this heading.

Mephentermine Sulfate (Because of possible effects on blood pressure, atomoxetine hydrochloride should be used cautiously with pressor agents (e.g., dopamine, dobutamine)).

No products indexed under this heading.

Metaproterenol Sulfate (Atomoxetine hydrochloride should be administered with caution to patients being treated with systemically-administered (oral or intravenous) albuterol (or other beta2 agonists) because the action of albuterol on the cardiovascular system can be potentiated resulting in increases in heart rate and blood pressure. Albuterol (600 mcg IV over 2 hours) increases heart rate and blood pressure).

No products indexed under this heading.

Metaraminol Bitartrate (Because of possible effects on blood pressure, atomoxetine hydrochloride should be used cautiously with pressor agents (e.g., dopamine, dobutamine)).

No products indexed under this heading.

Methadone Hydrochloride (Atomoxetine is primarily metabolized by the CYP2D6 pathway to 4-hydroxyatomoxetine. Dosage adjustment of atomoxetine hydrochloride may be necessary when co-administered with potent CYP2D6 inhibitors (e.g., paroxetine, fluoxetine, and quinidine)).

No products indexed under this heading.

Methoxamine Hydrochloride (Because of possible effects on blood pressure, atomoxetine hydrochloride should be used cautiously with pressor agents (e.g., dopamine, dobutamine)).

No products indexed under this heading.

Mibefradil Dihydrochloride (Atomoxetine is primarily metabolized by the CYP2D6 pathway to 4-hydroxyatomoxetine. Dosage adjustment of atomoxetine hydrochloride may be necessary when co-administered with potent CYP2D6 inhibitors (e.g., paroxetine, fluoxetine, and quinidine)).

No products indexed under this heading.

Moclobemide (Atomoxetine hydrochloride should not be taken with an MAOI, or within 2 weeks after discontinuing an MAOI. Treatment with an MAOI should not be initiated within 2 weeks after discontinuing atomoxetine hydrochloride. With other drugs that affect brain monoamine concentrations, there have been reports of serious, sometimes fatal reactions (including hyperthermia, rigidity, myoclonus, autonomic instability with possible rapid fluctuations of vital signs, and mental status changes that include extreme agitation progressing to delirium and coma) when taken in combination with an MAOI. Some cases presented with features resembling neuroleptic malignant syndrome. Such reactions may occur when these drugs are given concurrently or in close proximity).

No products indexed under this heading.

Norepinephrine Bitartrate (Because of possible effects on blood pressure, atomoxetine hydrochloride should be used cautiously with pressor agents (e.g., dopamine, dobutamine)).

No products indexed under this heading.

Nortriptyline Hydrochloride (Atomoxetine is primarily metabolized by the CYP2D6 pathway to 4-hydroxyatomoxetine. Dosage adjustment of atomoxetine hydrochloride may be necessary when co-administered with potent CYP2D6 inhibitors (e.g., paroxetine, fluoxetine, and quinidine)).

No products indexed under this heading.

Pargyline Hydrochloride (Atomoxetine hydrochloride should not be taken with an MAOI, or within 2 weeks after discontinuing an MAOI. Treatment with an MAOI should not be initiated within 2 weeks after discontinuing atomoxetine hydrochloride. With other drugs that affect brain monoamine concentrations, there have been reports of serious, sometimes fatal reactions (including hyperthermia, rigidity, myoclonus, autonomic instability with possible rapid fluctuations of vital signs, and mental status changes that include extreme agitation progressing to delirium and coma) when taken in combination with an MAOI. Some cases presented with features resembling neuroleptic malignant syndrome. Such reactions may occur when these drugs are given concurrently or in close proximity).

No products indexed under this heading.

Paroxetine Hydrochloride (Atomoxetine is primarily metabolized by the CYP2D6 pathway to 4-hydroxyatomoxetine. Dosage adjustment of atomoxetine hydrochloride may be necessary when co-administered with potent CYP2D6 inhibitors (e.g., paroxetine, fluoxetine, and quinidine)). Products include:

Paxil 1535
Paxil CR Controlled-Release Tablets 1544

Perphenazine (Atomoxetine is primarily metabolized by the CYP2D6 pathway to 4-hydroxyatomoxetine. Dosage adjustment of atomoxetine hydrochloride may be necessary when co-administered with potent CYP2D6 inhibitors (e.g., paroxetine, fluoxetine, and quinidine)).

No products indexed under this heading.

Phenelzine Sulfate (Atomoxetine hydrochloride should not be taken with an MAOI, or within 2 weeks after discontinuing an MAOI. Treatment with an MAOI should not be initiated within 2 weeks after discontinuing atomoxetine hydrochloride. With other drugs that affect brain monoamine concentrations, there have been reports of serious, sometimes fatal reactions (including hyperthermia, rigidity, myoclonus, autonomic instability with possible rapid fluctuations of vital signs, and mental status changes that include extreme agitation progressing to delirium and coma) when taken in combination with an MAOI. Some cases presented with features resembling neuroleptic malignant syndrome. Such reactions may occur when these drugs are given concurrently or in close proximity).

No products indexed under this heading.

Phenylephrine Hydrochloride (Because of possible effects on blood pressure, atomoxetine hydrochloride should be used cautiously with pressor agents (e.g., dopamine, dobutamine)). Products include:

Actifed Cold & Allergy Tablets 1895
Benadryl Allergy & Cold Kapgels 1895
Benadryl Allergy & Sinus Headache Kapgels 1895
Benadryl Severe Allergy & Sinus Headache Caplets 1897
Children's Benadryl-D Allergy & Sinus Liquid 1896
Benadryl-D Allergy & Sinus Tablet 1896
PediaCare Children's Allergy & Cold Liquid 1902
PediaCare Children's Decongestant Liquid 1902
PediaCare Children's Liquid Multi-Symptom Cold 1902
Sinutab Non-Drying Caplets 1905
Sinutab Sinus Caplets 1905
Children's Sudafed PE Cold & Cough Liquid 1907
Children's Sudafed PE Nasal Decongestant Liquid 1906
Sudafed PE Cold & Cough Caplets 1907
Sudafed PE Nasal Decongestant Tablets 1907
Sudafed PE Nighttime Cold Caplets 1907
Sudafed PE Non-Drying Sinus Caplets 1908
Sudafed PE Severe Cold Caplets 1908
Sudafed PE Sinus & Allergy Tablets 1908
Sudafed PE Sinus Headache Caplets 1908
Tylenol Allergy Multi-Symptom Caplets with Cool Burst and Rapid Release Gelcaps 1916
Tylenol Allergy Multi-Symptom Nighttime Caplets with Cool Burst 1916
Children's Tylenol Plus Cold Suspension Liquid 1912
Children's Tylenol Plus Cold & Allergy Suspension Liquid 1914
Children's Tylenol Plus Flu Suspension Liquid 1914
Children's Tylenol Plus Multi-Symptom Cold Suspension Liquid 1912
Tylenol Cold Head Congestion Daytime Caplets with Cool Burst 1910
Tylenol Cold Head Congestion Nighttime Caplets with Cool Burst 1910
Tylenol Cold Head Congestion Severe Daytime Caplets with Cool Burst 1910
Tylenol Cold Multi-Symptom Daytime Caplets with Cool Burst and Rapid Release Gels 1913
Tylenol Cold Multi-Symptom Daytime Liquid with Citrus Burst 1913
Tylenol Cold Multi-Symptom Nighttime Caplets with Cool Burst 1913
Tylenol Cold Multi-Symptom Nighttime Liquid with Cool Burst 1913
Tylenol Cold Multi-Symptom Severe Caplets with Cool Burst 1913
Tylenol Cold Multi-Symptom Severe Daytime Liquid with Citrus Burst 1913
Tylenol Sinus Congestion & Pain Daytime Caplets with Cool Burst and Gelcaps 1917
Tylenol Sinus Congestion & Pain Nighttime Caplets with Cool Burst 1917
Tylenol Sinus Congestion & Pain Severe Caplets with Cool Burst 1917
Vicks DayQuil Cold & Flu Multi-Symptom Relief 616
Vicks DayQuil LiquiCaps 2567
Vicks DayQuil Liquid 2567
Vicks DayQuil Multi-Symptom Cold/Flu Relief 2567

Pirbuterol Acetate (Atomoxetine hydrochloride should be administered with caution to patients being treated with systemically-administered (oral or intravenous) albuterol (or other beta2 agonists) because the action of albuterol on the cardiovascular system can be potentiated resulting in increases in heart rate and blood pressure. Albuterol (600 mcg IV over 2 hours) increases heart rate and blood pressure). Products include:

Maxair Autohaler 1705

Procarbazine Hydrochloride (Atomoxetine hydrochloride should not be taken with an MAOI, or within 2 weeks after discontinuing an MAOI. Treatment with an MAOI should not be initiated within 2 weeks after discontinuing atomoxetine hydrochloride. With other drugs that affect brain monoamine concentrations, there have been reports of serious, sometimes fatal reactions (including hyperthermia, rigidity, myoclonus, autonomic instability with possible rapid fluctuations of vital signs, and mental status changes that include extreme agitation progressing to delirium and coma) when taken in combination with an MAOI. Some cases presented with features resembling neuroleptic malignant syndrome. Such reactions may occur when these drugs are given concurrently or in close proximity).

No products indexed under this heading.

Propafenone Hydrochloride (Atomoxetine is primarily metabolized by the CYP2D6 pathway to 4-hydroxyatomoxetine. Dosage adjustment of atomoxetine hydrochloride may be necessary when co-administered with potent CYP2D6 inhibitors (e.g., paroxetine, fluoxetine, and quinidine)). Products include:

Rythmol Tablets 1586
Rythmol SR Capsules 1590

Propoxyphene Hydrochloride (Atomoxetine is primarily metabolized by the CYP2D6 pathway to 4-hydroxyatomoxetine. Dosage adjustment of atomoxetine hydrochloride may be necessary when co-administered with potent CYP2D6 inhibitors (e.g., paroxetine, fluoxetine, and quinidine)).

No products indexed under this heading.

Propoxyphene Napsylate (Atomoxetine is primarily metabolized by the CYP2D6 pathway to 4-hydroxyatomoxetine. Dosage adjustment of atomoxetine hydrochloride may be necessary when co-administered with potent CYP2D6 inhibitors (e.g., paroxetine, fluoxetine, and quinidine)).

No products indexed under this heading.

Protriptyline Hydrochloride (Atomoxetine is primarily metabolized by the CYP2D6 pathway to 4-hydroxyatomoxetine. Dosage adjustment of atomoxetine hydrochloride may be necessary when co-administered with potent CYP2D6 inhibitors (e.g., paroxetine, fluoxetine, and quinidine)).

No products indexed under this heading.

Quinacrine Hydrochloride (Atomoxetine is primarily metabolized by the CYP2D6 pathway to 4-hydroxyatomoxetine. Dosage adjustment of atomoxetine hydrochloride may be necessary when co-administered with potent CYP2D6 inhibitors (e.g., paroxetine, fluoxetine, and quinidine)).

No products indexed under this heading.

Quinidine (Atomoxetine is primarily metabolized by the CYP2D6 pathway to 4-hydroxyatomoxetine. Dosage adjustment of atomoxetine hydrochloride may be necessary when co-administered with potent CYP2D6 inhibitors (e.g., quinidine)).

No products indexed under this heading.

Quinidine Gluconate (Atomoxetine is primarily metabolized by the CYP2D6 pathway to 4-hydroxyatomoxetine. Dosage adjustment of atomoxetine hydrochloride may be necessary when co-administered with potent CYP2D6 inhibitors (e.g., paroxetine, fluoxetine, and quinidine)).

No products indexed under this heading.

Quinidine Hydrochloride (Atomoxetine is primarily metabolized by the CYP2D6 pathway to 4-hydroxyatomoxetine. Dosage adjustment of atomoxetine hydrochloride may be necessary when co-administered with potent CYP2D6 inhibitors (e.g., paroxetine, fluoxetine, and quinidine)).

No products indexed under this heading.

Quinidine Polygalacturonate (Atomoxetine is primarily metabolized by the CYP2D6 pathway to 4-hydroxyatomoxetine. Dosage adjustment of atomoxetine hydrochloride may be necessary when co-administered with potent CYP2D6 inhibitors (e.g., paroxetine, fluoxetine, and quinidine)).

No products indexed under this heading.

Quinidine Sulfate (Atomoxetine is primarily metabolized by the CYP2D6 pathway to 4-hydroxyatomoxetine. Dosage adjustment of atomoxetine hydrochloride may be necessary when co-administered with potent CYP2D6 inhibitors (e.g., paroxetine, fluoxetine, and quinidine)).

No products indexed under this heading.

Ranitidine Bismuth Citrate (Atomoxetine is primarily metabolized by the CYP2D6 pathway to 4-hydroxyatomoxetine. Dosage adjustment of atomoxetine hydrochloride may be necessary when co-administered with potent CYP2D6 inhibitors (e.g., paroxetine, fluoxetine, and quinidine)).

No products indexed under this heading.

Ranitidine Hydrochloride (Atomoxetine is primarily metabolized by the CYP2D6 pathway to 4-hydroxyatomoxetine. Dosage adjustment of atomoxetine hydrochloride may be necessary when co-administered with potent CYP2D6 inhibitors (e.g., paroxetine, fluoxetine, and quinidine)). Products include:

Zantac 75 Tablets .... ▣603
Zantac 1670
Zantac Injection 1666
Zantac Injection Pharmacy Bulk Package 1668
Maximum Strength Zantac 150 Tablets .... ▣603
Maximum Strength Zantac 150 Cool Mint Tablets .... ▣603

Rasagiline Mesylate (Atomoxetine hydrochloride should not be taken with an MAOI, or within 2 weeks after discontinuing an MAOI. Treatment with an MAOI should not be initiated within 2 weeks after discontinuing atomoxetine hydrochloride. With other drugs that affect brain monoamine concentrations, there have been reports of serious, sometimes fatal reactions (including hyperthermia, rigidity, myoclonus, autonomic instability with possible rapid fluctuations of vital signs, and mental status changes that include extreme agitation progressing to delirium and coma) when taken in combination with an MAOI. Some cases presented with features resembling neuroleptic malignant syndrome. Such reactions may occur when these drugs are given concurrently or in close proximity). Products include:

Azilect Tablets 3106

Ritonavir (Atomoxetine is primarily metabolized by the CYP2D6 pathway to 4-hydroxyatomoxetine. Dosage adjustment of atomoxetine hydrochloride may be necessary when co-administered with potent CYP2D6 inhibitors (e.g., paroxetine, fluoxetine, and quinidine)). Products include:

Kaletra 452
Norvir 489

Salmeterol Xinafoate (Atomoxetine hydrochloride should be administered with caution to patients being treated with systemically-administered (oral or intravenous) albuterol (or other beta2 agonists) because the action of albuterol on the cardiovascular system can be potentiated resulting in increases in heart rate and blood pressure. Albuterol (600 mcg IV over 2 hours) increases heart rate and blood pressure). Products include:

Advair Diskus 100/50 1276
Advair Diskus 250/50 1276
Advair Diskus 500/50 1276
Advair HFA 45/21 Inhalation Aerosol 1288
Advair HFA 115/21 Inhalation Aerosol 1288
Advair HFA 230/21 Inhalation Aerosol 1288
Serevent Diskus 1594

Selegiline (Atomoxetine hydrochloride should not be taken with an MAOI, or within 2 weeks after discontinuing an MAOI. Treatment with an MAOI should not be initiated within 2 weeks after discontinuing atomoxetine hydrochloride. With other drugs that affect brain monoamine concentrations, there have been reports of serious, sometimes fatal reactions (including hyperthermia, rigidity, myoclonus, autonomic instability with possible rapid fluctuations of vital signs, and mental status changes that include extreme agitation progressing to delirium and coma) when taken in combination with an MAOI. Some cases presented with features resembling neuroleptic malignant syndrome. Such reactions may occur when these drugs are given concurrently or in close proximity). Products include:

Emsam Transdermal System 905

Selegiline Hydrochloride (Atomoxetine hydrochloride should not be taken with an MAOI, or within 2 weeks after discontinuing an MAOI. Treatment with an MAOI should not be initiated within 2 weeks after discontinuing atomoxetine hydrochloride. With other drugs that affect brain monoamine concentrations, there have been reports of serious, sometimes fatal reactions (including hyperthermia, rigidity, myoclonus, autonomic instability with possible rapid fluctuations of vital signs, and mental status changes that include extreme agitation progressing to delirium and coma) when taken in combination with an MAOI. Some cases presented with features resembling neuroleptic malignant syndrome. Such reactions may occur when these drugs are given concurrently or in close proximity). Products include:

Eldepryl Capsules 3052

Sertraline Hydrochloride (Atomoxetine is primarily metabolized by the CYP2D6 pathway to 4-hydroxyatomoxetine. Dosage adjustment of atomoxetine hydrochloride may be necessary when co-administered with potent CYP2D6 inhibitors (e.g., paroxetine, fluoxetine, and quinidine)).

No products indexed under this heading.

Sildenafil Citrate (Atomoxetine is primarily metabolized by the CYP2D6 pathway to 4-hydroxyatomoxetine. Dosage adjustment of atomoxetine hydrochloride may be necessary when co-administered with potent CYP2D6 inhibitors (e.g., paroxetine, fluoxetine, and quinidine)).

No products indexed under this heading.

Terbinafine Hydrochloride (Atomoxetine is primarily metabolized by the CYP2D6 pathway to 4-hydroxyatomoxetine. Dosage adjustment of atomoxetine hydrochloride may be necessary when co-administered with potent CYP2D6 inhibitors (e.g., paroxetine, fluoxetine, and quinidine)). Products include:

Lamisil Oral Granules 2264
Lamisil Tablets 2266

Terbutaline Sulfate (Atomoxetine hydrochloride should be administered with caution to patients being treated with systemically-administered (oral or intravenous) albuterol (or other beta2 agonists) because the action of albuterol on the cardiovascular system can be potentiated resulting in increases in heart rate and blood pressure. Albuterol (600 mcg IV over 2 hours) increases heart rate and blood pressure).

No products indexed under this heading.

Thioridazine Hydrochloride (Atomoxetine is primarily metabolized by the CYP2D6 pathway to 4-hydroxyatomoxetine. Dosage adjustment of atomoxetine hydrochloride may be necessary when co-administered with potent CYP2D6 inhibitors (e.g., paroxetine, fluoxetine, and quinidine)). Products include:

Thioridazine Hydrochloride Tablets 2195

Tranylcypromine Sulfate (Atomoxetine hydrochloride should not be taken with an MAOI, or within 2 weeks after discontinuing an MAOI. Treatment with an MAOI should not be initiated within 2 weeks after discontinuing atomoxetine hydrochloride. With other drugs that affect brain monoamine concentrations, there have been reports of serious, sometimes fatal reactions (including hyperthermia, rigidity, myoclonus, autonomic instability with possible rapid fluctuations of vital signs, and mental status changes that include extreme agitation progressing to delirium and coma) when taken in combination with an MAOI. Some cases presented with features resembling neuroleptic malignant syndrome. Such reactions may occur when these drugs are given concurrently or in close proximity). Products include:

Parnate Tablets 1532

Trimipramine Maleate (Atomoxetine is primarily metabolized by the CYP2D6 pathway to 4-hydroxyatomoxetine. Dosage adjustment of atomoxetine hydrochloride may be necessary when co-administered with potent CYP2D6 inhibitors (e.g., paroxetine, fluoxetine, and quinidine)).
No products indexed under this heading.

Vardenafil Hydrochloride (Atomoxetine is primarily metabolized by the CYP2D6 pathway to 4-hydroxyatomoxetine. Dosage adjustment of atomoxetine hydrochloride may be necessary when co-administered with potent CYP2D6 inhibitors (e.g., paroxetine, fluoxetine, and quinidine)). Products include:
Levitra Tablets 2876

STROMECTOL TABLETS

(Ivermectin) 2120
May interact with:

Warfarin Sodium (Very rare post-marketing reports of increased INR (International Normalized Ratio) have been reported when ivermectin was co-administered with warfarin).
No products indexed under this heading.

SUBOXONE TABLETS

(Buprenorphine Hydrochloride, Naloxone Hydrochloride).................... 2601
May interact with cytochrome p450 3a4 inhibitors (selected). Compounds in these categories include:

Acetazolamide (Buprenorphine is metabolized to norbuprenorphine by cytochrome CYP3A4. Because CYP3A4 inhibitors may increase plasma concentrations of buprenorphine, patients already on CYP3A4 inhibitors should have their dose of Subutex or Subuxone adjusted).
No products indexed under this heading.

Amiodarone Hydrochloride (Buprenorphine is metabolized to norbuprenorphine by cytochrome CYP3A4. Because CYP3A4 inhibitors may increase plasma concentrations of buprenorphine, patients already on CYP3A4 inhibitors should have their dose of Subutex or Subuxone adjusted).
No products indexed under this heading.

Amprenavir (Buprenorphine is metabolized to norbuprenorphine by cytochrome CYP3A4. Because CYP3A4 inhibitors may increase plasma concentrations of buprenorphine, patients already on CYP3A4 inhibitors should have their dose of Subutex or Subuxone adjusted).
No products indexed under this heading.

Anastrozole (Buprenorphine is metabolized to norbuprenorphine by cytochrome CYP3A4. Because CYP3A4 inhibitors may increase plasma concentrations of buprenorphine, patients already on CYP3A4 inhibitors should have their dose of Subutex or Subuxone adjusted). Products include:
Arimidex Tablets 672

Aprepitant (Buprenorphine is metabolized to norbuprenorphine by cytochrome CYP3A4. Because CYP3A4 inhibitors may increase plasma concentrations of buprenorphine, patients already on CYP3A4 inhibitors should have their dose of Subutex or Subuxone adjusted). Products include:
Emend Capsules 1992

Atazanavir (Buprenorphine is metabolized to norbuprenorphine by cytochrome CYP3A4. Because CYP3A4 inhibitors may increase plasma concentrations of buprenorphine, patients already on CYP3A4 inhibitors should have their dose of Subutex or Subuxone adjusted).
No products indexed under this heading.

Atazanavir Sulfate (Buprenorphine is metabolized to norbuprenorphine by cytochrome CYP3A4. Because CYP3A4 inhibitors may increase plasma concentrations of buprenorphine, patients already on CYP3A4 inhibitors should have their dose of Subutex or Subuxone adjusted). Products include:
Reyataz Capsules 3299

Cimetidine (Buprenorphine is metabolized to norbuprenorphine by cytochrome CYP3A4. Because CYP3A4 inhibitors may increase plasma concentrations of buprenorphine, patients already on CYP3A4 inhibitors should have their dose of Subutex or Subuxone adjusted).
No products indexed under this heading.

Cimetidine Hydrochloride (Buprenorphine is metabolized to norbuprenorphine by cytochrome CYP3A4. Because CYP3A4 inhibitors may increase plasma concentrations of buprenorphine, patients already on CYP3A4 inhibitors should have their dose of Subutex or Subuxone adjusted).
No products indexed under this heading.

Ciprofloxacin (Buprenorphine is metabolized to norbuprenorphine by cytochrome CYP3A4. Because CYP3A4 inhibitors may increase plasma concentrations of buprenorphine, patients already on CYP3A4 inhibitors should have their dose of Subutex or Subuxone adjusted). Products include:
Cipro I.V. 2817
Cipro Oral Suspension 2810
Cipro XR Tablets 2823
Ciprodex Otic Suspension 541

Clarithromycin (Buprenorphine is metabolized to norbuprenorphine by cytochrome CYP3A4. Because CYP3A4 inhibitors may increase plasma concentrations of buprenorphine, patients already on CYP3A4 inhibitors should have their dose of Subutex or Subuxone adjusted). Products include:
Biaxin/Biaxin XL 411

Clotrimazole (Buprenorphine is metabolized to norbuprenorphine by cytochrome CYP3A4. Because CYP3A4 inhibitors may increase plasma concentrations of buprenorphine, patients already on CYP3A4 inhibitors should have their dose of Subutex or Subuxone adjusted). Products include:
Lotrisone 2881

Cyclosporine (Buprenorphine is metabolized to norbuprenorphine by cytochrome CYP3A4. Because CYP3A4 inhibitors may increase plasma concentrations of buprenorphine, patients already on CYP3A4 inhibitors should have their dose of Subutex or Subuxone adjusted). Products include:
Gengraf Capsules 435
Neoral Oral Solution 2280
Neoral Soft Gelatin Capsules 2280
Restasis Ophthalmic Emulsion 557
Sandimmune 2296

Dalfopristin (Buprenorphine is metabolized to norbuprenorphine by cytochrome CYP3A4. Because CYP3A4 inhibitors may increase plasma concentrations of buprenorphine, patients already on CYP3A4 inhibitors should have their dose of Subutex or Subuxone adjusted).
No products indexed under this heading.

Danazol (Buprenorphine is metabolized to norbuprenorphine by cytochrome CYP3A4. Because CYP3A4 inhibitors may increase plasma concentrations of buprenorphine, patients already on CYP3A4 inhibitors should have their dose of Subutex or Subuxone adjusted).
No products indexed under this heading.

Delavirdine Mesylate (Buprenorphine is metabolized to norbuprenorphine by cytochrome CYP3A4. Because CYP3A4 inhibitors may increase plasma concentrations of buprenorphine, patients already on CYP3A4 inhibitors should have their dose of Subutex or Subuxone adjusted).
No products indexed under this heading.

Diltiazem Hydrochloride (Buprenorphine is metabolized to norbuprenorphine by cytochrome CYP3A4. Because CYP3A4 inhibitors may increase plasma concentrations of buprenorphine, patients already on CYP3A4 inhibitors should have their dose of Subutex or Subuxone adjusted). Products include:
Cardizem LA Extended Release Tablets 421

Diltiazem Maleate (Buprenorphine is metabolized to norbuprenorphine by cytochrome CYP3A4. Because CYP3A4 inhibitors may increase plasma concentrations of buprenorphine, patients already on CYP3A4 inhibitors should have their dose of Subutex or Subuxone adjusted).
No products indexed under this heading.

Efavirenz (Buprenorphine is metabolized to norbuprenorphine by cytochrome CYP3A4. Because CYP3A4 inhibitors may increase plasma concentrations of buprenorphine, patients already on CYP3A4 inhibitors should have their dose of Subutex or Subuxone adjusted). Products include:
Atripla Tablets 938
Sustiva Capsules 930
Sustiva Tablets 930

Erythromycin (Buprenorphine is metabolized to norbuprenorphine by cytochrome CYP3A4. Because CYP3A4 inhibitors may increase plasma concentrations of buprenorphine, patients already on CYP3A4 inhibitors should have their dose of Subutex or Subuxone adjusted).
No products indexed under this heading.

Erythromycin Estolate (Buprenorphine is metabolized to norbuprenorphine by cytochrome CYP3A4. Because CYP3A4 inhibitors may increase plasma concentrations of buprenorphine, patients already on CYP3A4 inhibitors should have their dose of Subutex or Subuxone adjusted).
No products indexed under this heading.

Erythromycin Ethylsuccinate (Buprenorphine is metabolized to norbuprenorphine by cytochrome CYP3A4. Because CYP3A4 inhibitors may increase plasma concentrations of buprenorphine, patients already on CYP3A4 inhibitors should have their dose of Subutex or Subuxone adjusted). Products include:
E.E.S. 433
EryPed 431

Erythromycin Gluceptate (Buprenorphine is metabolized to norbuprenorphine by cytochrome CYP3A4. Because CYP3A4 inhibitors may increase plasma concentrations of buprenorphine, patients already on CYP3A4 inhibitors should have their dose of Subutex or Subuxone adjusted).
No products indexed under this heading.

Erythromycin Lactobionate (Buprenorphine is metabolized to norbuprenorphine by cytochrome CYP3A4. Because CYP3A4 inhibitors may increase plasma concentrations of buprenorphine, patients already on CYP3A4 inhibitors should have their dose of Subutex or Subuxone adjusted).
No products indexed under this heading.

Erythromycin Stearate (Buprenorphine is metabolized to norbuprenorphine by cytochrome CYP3A4. Because CYP3A4 inhibitors may increase plasma concentrations of buprenorphine, patients already on CYP3A4 inhibitors should have their dose of Subutex or Subuxone adjusted).
No products indexed under this heading.

Esomeprazole Magnesium (Buprenorphine is metabolized to norbuprenorphine by cytochrome CYP3A4. Because CYP3A4 inhibitors may increase plasma concentrations of buprenorphine, patients already on CYP3A4 inhibitors should have their dose of Subutex or Subuxone adjusted). Products include:
Nexium Delayed-Release Capsules 645
Nexium Delayed-Release Oral Suspension................................. 645

Fluconazole (Buprenorphine is metabolized to norbuprenorphine by cytochrome CYP3A4. Because CYP3A4 inhibitors may increase plasma concentrations of buprenorphine, patients already on CYP3A4 inhibitors should have their dose of Subutex or Subuxone adjusted).
No products indexed under this heading.

Fluoxetine (Buprenorphine is metabolized to norbuprenorphine by cytochrome CYP3A4. Because CYP3A4 inhibitors may increase plasma concentrations of buprenorphine, patients already on CYP3A4 inhibitors should have their dose of Subutex or Subuxone adjusted).
No products indexed under this heading.

Fluoxetine Hydrochloride (Buprenorphine is metabolized to norbuprenorphine by cytochrome CYP3A4. Because CYP3A4 inhibitors may increase plasma concentrations of buprenorphine, patients already on CYP3A4 inhibitors should have their dose of Subutex or Suboxone adjusted). Products include:
- Prozac Weekly Capsules **1852**
- Prozac Pulvules and Liquid **1852**
- Symbyax Capsules **1871**

Fluvoxamine Maleate (Buprenorphine is metabolized to norbuprenorphine by cytochrome CYP3A4. Because CYP3A4 inhibitors may increase plasma concentrations of buprenorphine, patients already on CYP3A4 inhibitors should have their dose of Subutex or Suboxone adjusted). Products include:
- Luvox CR Extended-Release Capsules **1759**

Fosamprenavir Calcium (Buprenorphine is metabolized to norbuprenorphine by cytochrome CYP3A4. Because CYP3A4 inhibitors may increase plasma concentrations of buprenorphine, patients already on CYP3A4 inhibitors should have their dose of Subutex or Suboxone adjusted). Products include:
- Lexiva Oral Suspension **1510**
- Lexiva Tablets **1510**

Indinavir Sulfate (Buprenorphine is metabolized to norbuprenorphine by cytochrome CYP3A4. Because CYP3A4 inhibitors may increase plasma concentrations of buprenorphine, patients already on CYP3A4 inhibitors should have their dose of Subutex or Suboxone adjusted). Products include:
- Crixivan Capsules **1979**

Isoniazid (Buprenorphine is metabolized to norbuprenorphine by cytochrome CYP3A4. Because CYP3A4 inhibitors may increase plasma concentrations of buprenorphine, patients already on CYP3A4 inhibitors should have their dose of Subutex or Suboxone adjusted).
No products indexed under this heading.

Itraconazole (Buprenorphine is metabolized to norbuprenorphine by cytochrome CYP3A4. Because CYP3A4 inhibitors may increase plasma concentrations of buprenorphine, patients already on CYP3A4 inhibitors should have their dose of Subutex or Suboxone adjusted).
No products indexed under this heading.

Ketoconazole (Buprenorphine is metabolized to norbuprenorphine by cytochrome CYP3A4. Because CYP3A4 inhibitors may increase plasma concentrations of buprenorphine, patients already on CYP3A4 inhibitors should have their dose of Subutex or Suboxone adjusted). Products include:
- Extina Foam, 2% **3057**
- Nizoral A-D Shampoo **1901**

Lopinavir (Buprenorphine is metabolized to norbuprenorphine by cytochrome CYP3A4. Because CYP3A4 inhibitors may increase plasma concentrations of buprenorphine, patients already on CYP3A4 inhibitors should have their dose of Subutex or Suboxone adjusted). Products include:
- Kaletra **452**

Loratadine (Buprenorphine is metabolized to norbuprenorphine by cytochrome CYP3A4. Because CYP3A4 inhibitors may increase plasma concentrations of buprenorphine, patients already on CYP3A4 inhibitors should have their dose of Subutex or Suboxone adjusted).
No products indexed under this heading.

Metronidazole (Buprenorphine is metabolized to norbuprenorphine by cytochrome CYP3A4. Because CYP3A4 inhibitors may increase plasma concentrations of buprenorphine, patients already on CYP3A4 inhibitors should have their dose of Subutex or Suboxone adjusted). Products include:
- Pylera Capsules **714**

Metronidazole Benzoate (Buprenorphine is metabolized to norbuprenorphine by cytochrome CYP3A4. Because CYP3A4 inhibitors may increase plasma concentrations of buprenorphine, patients already on CYP3A4 inhibitors should have their dose of Subutex or Suboxone adjusted).
No products indexed under this heading.

Metronidazole Hydrochloride (Buprenorphine is metabolized to norbuprenorphine by cytochrome CYP3A4. Because CYP3A4 inhibitors may increase plasma concentrations of buprenorphine, patients already on CYP3A4 inhibitors should have their dose of Subutex or Suboxone adjusted).
No products indexed under this heading.

Miconazole (Buprenorphine is metabolized to norbuprenorphine by cytochrome CYP3A4. Because CYP3A4 inhibitors may increase plasma concentrations of buprenorphine, patients already on CYP3A4 inhibitors should have their dose of Subutex or Suboxone adjusted).
No products indexed under this heading.

Miconazole Nitrate (Buprenorphine is metabolized to norbuprenorphine by cytochrome CYP3A4. Because CYP3A4 inhibitors may increase plasma concentrations of buprenorphine, patients already on CYP3A4 inhibitors should have their dose of Subutex or Suboxone adjusted).
No products indexed under this heading.

Nefazodone Hydrochloride (Buprenorphine is metabolized to norbuprenorphine by cytochrome CYP3A4. Because CYP3A4 inhibitors may increase plasma concentrations of buprenorphine, patients already on CYP3A4 inhibitors should have their dose of Subutex or Suboxone adjusted).
No products indexed under this heading.

Nelfinavir Mesylate (Buprenorphine is metabolized to norbuprenorphine by cytochrome CYP3A4. Because CYP3A4 inhibitors may increase plasma concentrations of buprenorphine, patients already on CYP3A4 inhibitors should have their dose of Subutex or Suboxone adjusted).
No products indexed under this heading.

Nevirapine (Buprenorphine is metabolized to norbuprenorphine by cytochrome CYP3A4. Because CYP3A4 inhibitors may increase plasma concentrations of buprenorphine, patients already on CYP3A4 inhibitors should have their dose of Subutex or Suboxone adjusted). Products include:
- Viramune Oral Suspension **873**
- Viramune Tablets **873**

Niacinamide (Buprenorphine is metabolized to norbuprenorphine by cytochrome CYP3A4. Because CYP3A4 inhibitors may increase plasma concentrations of buprenorphine, patients already on CYP3A4 inhibitors should have their dose of Subutex or Suboxone adjusted). Products include:
- BioLean Free Tablets .... ▣ **635**

Nicotinamide (Buprenorphine is metabolized to norbuprenorphine by cytochrome CYP3A4. Because CYP3A4 inhibitors may increase plasma concentrations of buprenorphine, patients already on CYP3A4 inhibitors should have their dose of Subutex or Suboxone adjusted).
No products indexed under this heading.

Nifedipine (Buprenorphine is metabolized to norbuprenorphine by cytochrome CYP3A4. Because CYP3A4 inhibitors may increase plasma concentrations of buprenorphine, patients already on CYP3A4 inhibitors should have their dose of Subutex or Suboxone adjusted).
No products indexed under this heading.

Norfloxacin (Buprenorphine is metabolized to norbuprenorphine by cytochrome CYP3A4. Because CYP3A4 inhibitors may increase plasma concentrations of buprenorphine, patients already on CYP3A4 inhibitors should have their dose of Subutex or Suboxone adjusted). Products include:
- Noroxin Tablets **2069**

Omeprazole (Buprenorphine is metabolized to norbuprenorphine by cytochrome CYP3A4. Because CYP3A4 inhibitors may increase plasma concentrations of buprenorphine, patients already on CYP3A4 inhibitors should have their dose of Subutex or Suboxone adjusted).
No products indexed under this heading.

Paroxetine Hydrochloride (Buprenorphine is metabolized to norbuprenorphine by cytochrome CYP3A4. Because CYP3A4 inhibitors may increase plasma concentrations of buprenorphine, patients already on CYP3A4 inhibitors should have their dose of Subutex or Suboxone adjusted). Products include:
- Paxil **1535**
- Paxil CR Controlled-Release Tablets **1544**

Propoxyphene Hydrochloride (Buprenorphine is metabolized to norbuprenorphine by cytochrome CYP3A4. Because CYP3A4 inhibitors may increase plasma concentrations of buprenorphine, patients already on CYP3A4 inhibitors should have their dose of Subutex or Suboxone adjusted).
No products indexed under this heading.

Propoxyphene Napsylate (Buprenorphine is metabolized to norbuprenorphine by cytochrome CYP3A4. Because CYP3A4 inhibitors may increase plasma concentrations of buprenorphine, patients already on CYP3A4 inhibitors should have their dose of Subutex or Suboxone adjusted).
No products indexed under this heading.

Quinidine (Buprenorphine is metabolized to norbuprenorphine by cytochrome CYP3A4. Because CYP3A4 inhibitors may increase plasma concentrations of buprenorphine, patients already on CYP3A4 inhibitors should have their dose of Subutex or Suboxone adjusted).
No products indexed under this heading.

Quinidine Hydrochloride (Buprenorphine is metabolized to norbuprenorphine by cytochrome CYP3A4. Because CYP3A4 inhibitors may increase plasma concentrations of buprenorphine, patients already on CYP3A4 inhibitors should have their dose of Subutex or Suboxone adjusted).
No products indexed under this heading.

Quinidine Polygalacturonate (Buprenorphine is metabolized to norbuprenorphine by cytochrome CYP3A4. Because CYP3A4 inhibitors may increase plasma concentrations of buprenorphine, patients already on CYP3A4 inhibitors should have their dose of Subutex or Suboxone adjusted).
No products indexed under this heading.

Quinidine Sulfate (Buprenorphine is metabolized to norbuprenorphine by cytochrome CYP3A4. Because CYP3A4 inhibitors may increase plasma concentrations of buprenorphine, patients already on CYP3A4 inhibitors should have their dose of Subutex or Suboxone adjusted).
No products indexed under this heading.

Quinine (Buprenorphine is metabolized to norbuprenorphine by cytochrome CYP3A4. Because CYP3A4 inhibitors may increase plasma concentrations of buprenorphine, patients already on CYP3A4 inhibitors should have their dose of Subutex or Suboxone adjusted).
No products indexed under this heading.

Quinine Sulfate (Buprenorphine is metabolized to norbuprenorphine by cytochrome CYP3A4. Because CYP3A4 inhibitors may increase plasma concentrations of buprenorphine, patients already on CYP3A4 inhibitors should have their dose of Subutex or Suboxone adjusted).
No products indexed under this heading.

Quinupristin (Buprenorphine is metabolized to norbuprenorphine by cytochrome CYP3A4. Because CYP3A4 inhibitors may increase plasma concentrations of buprenorphine, patients already on CYP3A4 inhibitors should have their dose of Subutex or Suboxone adjusted).
No products indexed under this heading.

Ranitidine Bismuth Citrate (Buprenorphine is metabolized to norbuprenorphine by cytochrome CYP3A4. Because CYP3A4 inhibitors may increase plasma concentrations of buprenorphine, patients already on CYP3A4 inhibitors should have their dose of Subutex or Subuxone adjusted).

No products indexed under this heading.

Ranitidine Hydrochloride (Buprenorphine is metabolized to norbuprenorphine by cytochrome CYP3A4. Because CYP3A4 inhibitors may increase plasma concentrations of buprenorphine, patients already on CYP3A4 inhibitors should have their dose of Subutex or Subuxone adjusted). Products include:

Zantac 75 Tablets 603
Zantac 1670
Zantac Injection 1666
Zantac Injection Pharmacy Bulk Package 1668
Maximum Strength Zantac 150 Tablets 603
Maximum Strength Zantac 150 Cool Mint Tablets 603

Ritonavir (Buprenorphine is metabolized to norbuprenorphine by cytochrome CYP3A4. Because CYP3A4 inhibitors may increase plasma concentrations of buprenorphine, patients already on CYP3A4 inhibitors should have their dose of Subutex or Subuxone adjusted). Products include:

Kaletra 452
Norvir 489

Saquinavir (Buprenorphine is metabolized to norbuprenorphine by cytochrome CYP3A4. Because CYP3A4 inhibitors may increase plasma concentrations of buprenorphine, patients already on CYP3A4 inhibitors should have their dose of Subutex or Subuxone adjusted).

No products indexed under this heading.

Saquinavir Mesylate (Buprenorphine is metabolized to norbuprenorphine by cytochrome CYP3A4. Because CYP3A4 inhibitors may increase plasma concentrations of buprenorphine, patients already on CYP3A4 inhibitors should have their dose of Subutex or Subuxone adjusted).

No products indexed under this heading.

Sertraline Hydrochloride (Buprenorphine is metabolized to norbuprenorphine by cytochrome CYP3A4. Because CYP3A4 inhibitors may increase plasma concentrations of buprenorphine, patients already on CYP3A4 inhibitors should have their dose of Subutex or Subuxone adjusted).

No products indexed under this heading.

Sildenafil Citrate (Buprenorphine is metabolized to norbuprenorphine by cytochrome CYP3A4. Because CYP3A4 inhibitors may increase plasma concentrations of buprenorphine, patients already on CYP3A4 inhibitors should have their dose of Subutex or Subuxone adjusted).

No products indexed under this heading.

Telithromycin (Buprenorphine is metabolized to norbuprenorphine by cytochrome CYP3A4. Because CYP3A4 inhibitors may increase plasma concentrations of buprenorphine, patients already on CYP3A4 inhibitors should have their dose of Subutex or Subuxone adjusted). Products include:

Ketek Tablets 2744

Troglitazone (Buprenorphine is metabolized to norbuprenorphine by cytochrome CYP3A4. Because CYP3A4 inhibitors may increase plasma concentrations of buprenorphine, patients already on CYP3A4 inhibitors should have their dose of Subutex or Subuxone adjusted).

No products indexed under this heading.

Troleandomycin (Buprenorphine is metabolized to norbuprenorphine by cytochrome CYP3A4. Because CYP3A4 inhibitors may increase plasma concentrations of buprenorphine, patients already on CYP3A4 inhibitors should have their dose of Subutex or Subuxone adjusted).

No products indexed under this heading.

Valproate Sodium (Buprenorphine is metabolized to norbuprenorphine by cytochrome CYP3A4. Because CYP3A4 inhibitors may increase plasma concentrations of buprenorphine, patients already on CYP3A4 inhibitors should have their dose of Subutex or Subuxone adjusted).

No products indexed under this heading.

Vardenafil Hydrochloride (Buprenorphine is metabolized to norbuprenorphine by cytochrome CYP3A4. Because CYP3A4 inhibitors may increase plasma concentrations of buprenorphine, patients already on CYP3A4 inhibitors should have their dose of Subutex or Subuxone adjusted). Products include:

Levitra Tablets 2876

Verapamil Hydrochloride (Buprenorphine is metabolized to norbuprenorphine by cytochrome CYP3A4. Because CYP3A4 inhibitors may increase plasma concentrations of buprenorphine, patients already on CYP3A4 inhibitors should have their dose of Subutex or Subuxone adjusted). Products include:

Tarka Tablets 511

Voriconazole (Buprenorphine is metabolized to norbuprenorphine by cytochrome CYP3A4. Because CYP3A4 inhibitors may increase plasma concentrations of buprenorphine, patients already on CYP3A4 inhibitors should have their dose of Subutex or Subuxone adjusted).

No products indexed under this heading.

Zafirlukast (Buprenorphine is metabolized to norbuprenorphine by cytochrome CYP3A4. Because CYP3A4 inhibitors may increase plasma concentrations of buprenorphine, patients already on CYP3A4 inhibitors should have their dose of Subutex or Subuxone adjusted). Products include:

Accolate Tablets 669

Zileuton (Buprenorphine is metabolized to norbuprenorphine by cytochrome CYP3A4. Because CYP3A4 inhibitors may increase plasma concentrations of buprenorphine, patients already on CYP3A4 inhibitors should have their dose of Subutex or Subuxone adjusted).

No products indexed under this heading.

Food Interactions

Grapefruit (Buprenorphine is metabolized to norbuprenorphine by cytochrome CYP3A4. Because CYP3A4 inhibitors may increase plasma concentrations of buprenorphine, patients already on CYP3A4 inhibitors should have their dose of Subutex or Subuxone adjusted).

Grapefruit Juice (Buprenorphine is metabolized to norbuprenorphine by cytochrome CYP3A4. Because CYP3A4 inhibitors may increase plasma concentrations of buprenorphine, patients already on CYP3A4 inhibitors should have their dose of Subutex or Subuxone adjusted).

SUBUTEX TABLETS

(Buprenorphine Hydrochloride) 2601

May interact with cytochrome p450 3a4 inhibitors (selected). Compounds in these categories include:

Acetazolamide (Buprenorphine is metabolized to norbuprenorphine by cytochrome CYP3A4. Because CYP3A4 inhibitors may increase plasma concentrations of buprenorphine, patients already on CYP3A4 inhibitors should have their dose of Subutex or Subuxone adjusted).

No products indexed under this heading.

Amiodarone Hydrochloride (Buprenorphine is metabolized to norbuprenorphine by cytochrome CYP3A4. Because CYP3A4 inhibitors may increase plasma concentrations of buprenorphine, patients already on CYP3A4 inhibitors should have their dose of Subutex or Subuxone adjusted).

No products indexed under this heading.

Amprenavir (Buprenorphine is metabolized to norbuprenorphine by cytochrome CYP3A4. Because CYP3A4 inhibitors may increase plasma concentrations of buprenorphine, patients already on CYP3A4 inhibitors should have their dose of Subutex or Subuxone adjusted).

No products indexed under this heading.

Anastrozole (Buprenorphine is metabolized to norbuprenorphine by cytochrome CYP3A4. Because CYP3A4 inhibitors may increase plasma concentrations of buprenorphine, patients already on CYP3A4 inhibitors should have their dose of Subutex or Subuxone adjusted). Products include:

Arimidex Tablets 672

Aprepitant (Buprenorphine is metabolized to norbuprenorphine by cytochrome CYP3A4. Because CYP3A4 inhibitors may increase plasma concentrations of buprenorphine, patients already on CYP3A4 inhibitors should have their dose of Subutex or Subuxone adjusted). Products include:

Emend Capsules 1992

Atazanavir (Buprenorphine is metabolized to norbuprenorphine by cytochrome CYP3A4. Because CYP3A4 inhibitors may increase plasma concentrations of buprenorphine, patients already on CYP3A4 inhibitors should have their dose of Subutex or Subuxone adjusted).

No products indexed under this heading.

Atazanavir Sulfate (Buprenorphine is metabolized to norbuprenorphine by cytochrome CYP3A4. Because CYP3A4 inhibitors may increase plasma concentrations of buprenorphine, patients already on CYP3A4 inhibitors should have their dose of Subutex or Subuxone adjusted). Products include:

Reyataz Capsules 3299

Cimetidine (Buprenorphine is metabolized to norbuprenorphine by cytochrome CYP3A4. Because CYP3A4 inhibitors may increase plasma concentrations of buprenorphine, patients already on CYP3A4 inhibitors should have their dose of Subutex or Subuxone adjusted).

No products indexed under this heading.

Cimetidine Hydrochloride (Buprenorphine is metabolized to norbuprenorphine by cytochrome CYP3A4. Because CYP3A4 inhibitors may increase plasma concentrations of buprenorphine, patients already on CYP3A4 inhibitors should have their dose of Subutex or Subuxone adjusted).

No products indexed under this heading.

Ciprofloxacin (Buprenorphine is metabolized to norbuprenorphine by cytochrome CYP3A4. Because CYP3A4 inhibitors may increase plasma concentrations of buprenorphine, patients already on CYP3A4 inhibitors should have their dose of Subutex or Subuxone adjusted). Products include:

Cipro I.V. 2817
Cipro Oral Suspension 2810
Cipro XR Tablets 2823
Ciprodex Otic Suspension 541

Clarithromycin (Buprenorphine is metabolized to norbuprenorphine by cytochrome CYP3A4. Because CYP3A4 inhibitors may increase plasma concentrations of buprenorphine, patients already on CYP3A4 inhibitors should have their dose of Subutex or Subuxone adjusted). Products include:

Biaxin/Biaxin XL 411

Clotrimazole (Buprenorphine is metabolized to norbuprenorphine by cytochrome CYP3A4. Because CYP3A4 inhibitors may increase plasma concentrations of buprenorphine, patients already on CYP3A4 inhibitors should have their dose of Subutex or Subuxone adjusted). Products include:

Lotrisone 2881

Cyclosporine (Buprenorphine is metabolized to norbuprenorphine by cytochrome CYP3A4. Because CYP3A4 inhibitors may increase plasma concentrations of buprenorphine, patients already on CYP3A4 inhibitors should have their dose of Subutex or Subuxone adjusted). Products include:

Gengraf Capsules 435
Neoral Oral Solution 2280
Neoral Soft Gelatin Capsules 2280
Restasis Ophthalmic Emulsion 557
Sandimmune 2296

Dalfopristin (Buprenorphine is metabolized to norbuprenorphine by cytochrome CYP3A4. Because CYP3A4 inhibitors may increase plasma concentrations of buprenorphine, patients already on CYP3A4 inhibitors should have their dose of Subutex or Subuxone adjusted).

No products indexed under this heading.

Danazol (Buprenorphine is metabolized to norbuprenorphine by cytochrome CYP3A4. Because CYP3A4 inhibitors may increase plasma concentrations of buprenorphine, patients already on CYP3A4 inhibitors should have their dose of Subutex or Suboxone adjusted).
No products indexed under this heading.

Delavirdine Mesylate (Buprenorphine is metabolized to norbuprenorphine by cytochrome CYP3A4. Because CYP3A4 inhibitors may increase plasma concentrations of buprenorphine, patients already on CYP3A4 inhibitors should have their dose of Subutex or Suboxone adjusted).
No products indexed under this heading.

Diltiazem Hydrochloride (Buprenorphine is metabolized to norbuprenorphine by cytochrome CYP3A4. Because CYP3A4 inhibitors may increase plasma concentrations of buprenorphine, patients already on CYP3A4 inhibitors should have their dose of Subutex or Suboxone adjusted). Products include:
Cardizem LA Extended Release Tablets 421

Diltiazem Maleate (Buprenorphine is metabolized to norbuprenorphine by cytochrome CYP3A4. Because CYP3A4 inhibitors may increase plasma concentrations of buprenorphine, patients already on CYP3A4 inhibitors should have their dose of Subutex or Suboxone adjusted).
No products indexed under this heading.

Efavirenz (Buprenorphine is metabolized to norbuprenorphine by cytochrome CYP3A4. Because CYP3A4 inhibitors may increase plasma concentrations of buprenorphine, patients already on CYP3A4 inhibitors should have their dose of Subutex or Suboxone adjusted). Products include:
Atripla Tablets 938
Sustiva Capsules 930
Sustiva Tablets 930

Erythromycin (Buprenorphine is metabolized to norbuprenorphine by cytochrome CYP3A4. Because CYP3A4 inhibitors may increase plasma concentrations of buprenorphine, patients already on CYP3A4 inhibitors should have their dose of Subutex or Suboxone adjusted).
No products indexed under this heading.

Erythromycin Estolate (Buprenorphine is metabolized to norbuprenorphine by cytochrome CYP3A4. Because CYP3A4 inhibitors may increase plasma concentrations of buprenorphine, patients already on CYP3A4 inhibitors should have their dose of Subutex or Suboxone adjusted).
No products indexed under this heading.

Erythromycin Ethylsuccinate (Buprenorphine is metabolized to norbuprenorphine by cytochrome CYP3A4. Because CYP3A4 inhibitors may increase plasma concentrations of buprenorphine, patients already on CYP3A4 inhibitors should have their dose of Subutex or Suboxone adjusted). Products include:
E.E.S. 433
EryPed 431

Erythromycin Gluceptate (Buprenorphine is metabolized to norbuprenorphine by cytochrome CYP3A4. Because CYP3A4 inhibitors may increase plasma concentrations of buprenorphine, patients already on CYP3A4 inhibitors should have their dose of Subutex or Suboxone adjusted).
No products indexed under this heading.

Erythromycin Lactobionate (Buprenorphine is metabolized to norbuprenorphine by cytochrome CYP3A4. Because CYP3A4 inhibitors may increase plasma concentrations of buprenorphine, patients already on CYP3A4 inhibitors should have their dose of Subutex or Suboxone adjusted).
No products indexed under this heading.

Erythromycin Stearate (Buprenorphine is metabolized to norbuprenorphine by cytochrome CYP3A4. Because CYP3A4 inhibitors may increase plasma concentrations of buprenorphine, patients already on CYP3A4 inhibitors should have their dose of Subutex or Suboxone adjusted).
No products indexed under this heading.

Esomeprazole Magnesium (Buprenorphine is metabolized to norbuprenorphine by cytochrome CYP3A4. Because CYP3A4 inhibitors may increase plasma concentrations of buprenorphine, patients already on CYP3A4 inhibitors should have their dose of Subutex or Suboxone adjusted). Products include:
Nexium Delayed-Release Capsules 645
Nexium Delayed-Release Oral Suspension 645

Fluconazole (Buprenorphine is metabolized to norbuprenorphine by cytochrome CYP3A4. Because CYP3A4 inhibitors may increase plasma concentrations of buprenorphine, patients already on CYP3A4 inhibitors should have their dose of Subutex or Suboxone adjusted).
No products indexed under this heading.

Fluoxetine (Buprenorphine is metabolized to norbuprenorphine by cytochrome CYP3A4. Because CYP3A4 inhibitors may increase plasma concentrations of buprenorphine, patients already on CYP3A4 inhibitors should have their dose of Subutex or Suboxone adjusted).
No products indexed under this heading.

Fluoxetine Hydrochloride (Buprenorphine is metabolized to norbuprenorphine by cytochrome CYP3A4. Because CYP3A4 inhibitors may increase plasma concentrations of buprenorphine, patients already on CYP3A4 inhibitors should have their dose of Subutex or Suboxone adjusted). Products include:
Prozac Weekly Capsules 1852
Prozac Pulvules and Liquid 1852
Symbyax Capsules 1871

Fluvoxamine Maleate (Buprenorphine is metabolized to norbuprenorphine by cytochrome CYP3A4. Because CYP3A4 inhibitors may increase plasma concentrations of buprenorphine, patients already on CYP3A4 inhibitors should have their dose of Subutex or Suboxone adjusted). Products include:
Luvox CR Extended-Release Capsules 1759

Fosamprenavir Calcium (Buprenorphine is metabolized to norbuprenorphine by cytochrome CYP3A4. Because CYP3A4 inhibitors may increase plasma concentrations of buprenorphine, patients already on CYP3A4 inhibitors should have their dose of Subutex or Suboxone adjusted). Products include:
Lexiva Oral Suspension 1510
Lexiva Tablets 1510

Indinavir Sulfate (Buprenorphine is metabolized to norbuprenorphine by cytochrome CYP3A4. Because CYP3A4 inhibitors may increase plasma concentrations of buprenorphine, patients already on CYP3A4 inhibitors should have their dose of Subutex or Suboxone adjusted). Products include:
Crixivan Capsules 1979

Isoniazid (Buprenorphine is metabolized to norbuprenorphine by cytochrome CYP3A4. Because CYP3A4 inhibitors may increase plasma concentrations of buprenorphine, patients already on CYP3A4 inhibitors should have their dose of Subutex or Suboxone adjusted).
No products indexed under this heading.

Itraconazole (Buprenorphine is metabolized to norbuprenorphine by cytochrome CYP3A4. Because CYP3A4 inhibitors may increase plasma concentrations of buprenorphine, patients already on CYP3A4 inhibitors should have their dose of Subutex or Suboxone adjusted).
No products indexed under this heading.

Ketoconazole (Buprenorphine is metabolized to norbuprenorphine by cytochrome CYP3A4. Because CYP3A4 inhibitors may increase plasma concentrations of buprenorphine, patients already on CYP3A4 inhibitors should have their dose of Subutex or Suboxone adjusted). Products include:
Extina Foam, 2% 3057
Nizoral A-D Shampoo 1901

Lopinavir (Buprenorphine is metabolized to norbuprenorphine by cytochrome CYP3A4. Because CYP3A4 inhibitors may increase plasma concentrations of buprenorphine, patients already on CYP3A4 inhibitors should have their dose of Subutex or Suboxone adjusted). Products include:
Kaletra 452

Loratadine (Buprenorphine is metabolized to norbuprenorphine by cytochrome CYP3A4. Because CYP3A4 inhibitors may increase plasma concentrations of buprenorphine, patients already on CYP3A4 inhibitors should have their dose of Subutex or Suboxone adjusted).
No products indexed under this heading.

Metronidazole (Buprenorphine is metabolized to norbuprenorphine by cytochrome CYP3A4. Because CYP3A4 inhibitors may increase plasma concentrations of buprenorphine, patients already on CYP3A4 inhibitors should have their dose of Subutex or Suboxone adjusted). Products include:
Pylera Capsules 714

Metronidazole Benzoate (Buprenorphine is metabolized to norbuprenorphine by cytochrome CYP3A4. Because CYP3A4 inhibitors may increase plasma concentrations of buprenorphine, patients already on CYP3A4 inhibitors should have their dose of Subutex or Suboxone adjusted).
No products indexed under this heading.

Metronidazole Hydrochloride (Buprenorphine is metabolized to norbuprenorphine by cytochrome CYP3A4. Because CYP3A4 inhibitors may increase plasma concentrations of buprenorphine, patients already on CYP3A4 inhibitors should have their dose of Subutex or Suboxone adjusted).
No products indexed under this heading.

Miconazole (Buprenorphine is metabolized to norbuprenorphine by cytochrome CYP3A4. Because CYP3A4 inhibitors may increase plasma concentrations of buprenorphine, patients already on CYP3A4 inhibitors should have their dose of Subutex or Suboxone adjusted).
No products indexed under this heading.

Miconazole Nitrate (Buprenorphine is metabolized to norbuprenorphine by cytochrome CYP3A4. Because CYP3A4 inhibitors may increase plasma concentrations of buprenorphine, patients already on CYP3A4 inhibitors should have their dose of Subutex or Suboxone adjusted).
No products indexed under this heading.

Nefazodone Hydrochloride (Buprenorphine is metabolized to norbuprenorphine by cytochrome CYP3A4. Because CYP3A4 inhibitors may increase plasma concentrations of buprenorphine, patients already on CYP3A4 inhibitors should have their dose of Subutex or Suboxone adjusted).
No products indexed under this heading.

Nelfinavir Mesylate (Buprenorphine is metabolized to norbuprenorphine by cytochrome CYP3A4. Because CYP3A4 inhibitors may increase plasma concentrations of buprenorphine, patients already on CYP3A4 inhibitors should have their dose of Subutex or Suboxone adjusted).
No products indexed under this heading.

Nevirapine (Buprenorphine is metabolized to norbuprenorphine by cytochrome CYP3A4. Because CYP3A4 inhibitors may increase plasma concentrations of buprenorphine, patients already on CYP3A4 inhibitors should have their dose of Subutex or Suboxone adjusted). Products include:
Viramune Oral Suspension 873
Viramune Tablets 873

Niacinamide (Buprenorphine is metabolized to norbuprenorphine by cytochrome CYP3A4. Because CYP3A4 inhibitors may increase plasma concentrations of buprenorphine, patients already on CYP3A4 inhibitors should have their dose of Subutex or Suboxone adjusted). Products include:
BioLean Free Tablets .... ■635

Nicotinamide (Buprenorphine is metabolized to norbuprenorphine by cytochrome CYP3A4. Because CYP3A4 inhibitors may increase plasma concentrations of buprenorphine, patients already on CYP3A4 inhibitors should have their dose of Subutex or Subuxone adjusted).
No products indexed under this heading.

Nifedipine (Buprenorphine is metabolized to norbuprenorphine by cytochrome CYP3A4. Because CYP3A4 inhibitors may increase plasma concentrations of buprenorphine, patients already on CYP3A4 inhibitors should have their dose of Subutex or Subuxone adjusted).
No products indexed under this heading.

Norfloxacin (Buprenorphine is metabolized to norbuprenorphine by cytochrome CYP3A4. Because CYP3A4 inhibitors may increase plasma concentrations of buprenorphine, patients already on CYP3A4 inhibitors should have their dose of Subutex or Subuxone adjusted). Products include:
Noroxin Tablets 2069

Omeprazole (Buprenorphine is metabolized to norbuprenorphine by cytochrome CYP3A4. Because CYP3A4 inhibitors may increase plasma concentrations of buprenorphine, patients already on CYP3A4 inhibitors should have their dose of Subutex or Subuxone adjusted).
No products indexed under this heading.

Paroxetine Hydrochloride (Buprenorphine is metabolized to norbuprenorphine by cytochrome CYP3A4. Because CYP3A4 inhibitors may increase plasma concentrations of buprenorphine, patients already on CYP3A4 inhibitors should have their dose of Subutex or Subuxone adjusted). Products include:
Paxil 1535
Paxil CR Controlled-Release Tablets 1544

Propoxyphene Hydrochloride (Buprenorphine is metabolized to norbuprenorphine by cytochrome CYP3A4. Because CYP3A4 inhibitors may increase plasma concentrations of buprenorphine, patients already on CYP3A4 inhibitors should have their dose of Subutex or Subuxone adjusted).
No products indexed under this heading.

Propoxyphene Napsylate (Buprenorphine is metabolized to norbuprenorphine by cytochrome CYP3A4. Because CYP3A4 inhibitors may increase plasma concentrations of buprenorphine, patients already on CYP3A4 inhibitors should have their dose of Subutex or Subuxone adjusted).
No products indexed under this heading.

Quinidine (Buprenorphine is metabolized to norbuprenorphine by cytochrome CYP3A4. Because CYP3A4 inhibitors may increase plasma concentrations of buprenorphine, patients already on CYP3A4 inhibitors should have their dose of Subutex or Subuxone adjusted).
No products indexed under this heading.

Quinidine Hydrochloride (Buprenorphine is metabolized to norbuprenorphine by cytochrome CYP3A4. Because CYP3A4 inhibitors may increase plasma concentrations of buprenorphine, patients already on CYP3A4 inhibitors should have their dose of Subutex or Subuxone adjusted).
No products indexed under this heading.

Quinidine Polygalacturonate (Buprenorphine is metabolized to norbuprenorphine by cytochrome CYP3A4. Because CYP3A4 inhibitors may increase plasma concentrations of buprenorphine, patients already on CYP3A4 inhibitors should have their dose of Subutex or Subuxone adjusted).
No products indexed under this heading.

Quinidine Sulfate (Buprenorphine is metabolized to norbuprenorphine by cytochrome CYP3A4. Because CYP3A4 inhibitors may increase plasma concentrations of buprenorphine, patients already on CYP3A4 inhibitors should have their dose of Subutex or Subuxone adjusted).
No products indexed under this heading.

Quinine (Buprenorphine is metabolized to norbuprenorphine by cytochrome CYP3A4. Because CYP3A4 inhibitors may increase plasma concentrations of buprenorphine, patients already on CYP3A4 inhibitors should have their dose of Subutex or Subuxone adjusted).
No products indexed under this heading.

Quinine Sulfate (Buprenorphine is metabolized to norbuprenorphine by cytochrome CYP3A4. Because CYP3A4 inhibitors may increase plasma concentrations of buprenorphine, patients already on CYP3A4 inhibitors should have their dose of Subutex or Subuxone adjusted).
No products indexed under this heading.

Quinupristin (Buprenorphine is metabolized to norbuprenorphine by cytochrome CYP3A4. Because CYP3A4 inhibitors may increase plasma concentrations of buprenorphine, patients already on CYP3A4 inhibitors should have their dose of Subutex or Subuxone adjusted).
No products indexed under this heading.

Ranitidine Bismuth Citrate (Buprenorphine is metabolized to norbuprenorphine by cytochrome CYP3A4. Because CYP3A4 inhibitors may increase plasma concentrations of buprenorphine, patients already on CYP3A4 inhibitors should have their dose of Subutex or Subuxone adjusted).
No products indexed under this heading.

Ranitidine Hydrochloride (Buprenorphine is metabolized to norbuprenorphine by cytochrome CYP3A4. Because CYP3A4 inhibitors may increase plasma concentrations of buprenorphine, patients already on CYP3A4 inhibitors should have their dose of Subutex or Subuxone adjusted). Products include:
Zantac 75 Tablets 603
Zantac 1670
Zantac Injection 1666
Zantac Injection Pharmacy Bulk Package 1668
Maximum Strength Zantac 150 Tablets 603
Maximum Strength Zantac 150 Cool Mint Tablets 603

Ritonavir (Buprenorphine is metabolized to norbuprenorphine by cytochrome CYP3A4. Because CYP3A4 inhibitors may increase plasma concentrations of buprenorphine, patients already on CYP3A4 inhibitors should have their dose of Subutex or Subuxone adjusted). Products include:
Kaletra 452
Norvir 489

Saquinavir (Buprenorphine is metabolized to norbuprenorphine by cytochrome CYP3A4. Because CYP3A4 inhibitors may increase plasma concentrations of buprenorphine, patients already on CYP3A4 inhibitors should have their dose of Subutex or Subuxone adjusted).
No products indexed under this heading.

Saquinavir Mesylate (Buprenorphine is metabolized to norbuprenorphine by cytochrome CYP3A4. Because CYP3A4 inhibitors may increase plasma concentrations of buprenorphine, patients already on CYP3A4 inhibitors should have their dose of Subutex or Subuxone adjusted).
No products indexed under this heading.

Sertraline Hydrochloride (Buprenorphine is metabolized to norbuprenorphine by cytochrome CYP3A4. Because CYP3A4 inhibitors may increase plasma concentrations of buprenorphine, patients already on CYP3A4 inhibitors should have their dose of Subutex or Subuxone adjusted).
No products indexed under this heading.

Sildenafil Citrate (Buprenorphine is metabolized to norbuprenorphine by cytochrome CYP3A4. Because CYP3A4 inhibitors may increase plasma concentrations of buprenorphine, patients already on CYP3A4 inhibitors should have their dose of Subutex or Subuxone adjusted).
No products indexed under this heading.

Telithromycin (Buprenorphine is metabolized to norbuprenorphine by cytochrome CYP3A4. Because CYP3A4 inhibitors may increase plasma concentrations of buprenorphine, patients already on CYP3A4 inhibitors should have their dose of Subutex or Subuxone adjusted). Products include:
Ketek Tablets 2744

Troglitazone (Buprenorphine is metabolized to norbuprenorphine by cytochrome CYP3A4. Because CYP3A4 inhibitors may increase plasma concentrations of buprenorphine, patients already on CYP3A4 inhibitors should have their dose of Subutex or Subuxone adjusted).
No products indexed under this heading.

Troleandomycin (Buprenorphine is metabolized to norbuprenorphine by cytochrome CYP3A4. Because CYP3A4 inhibitors may increase plasma concentrations of buprenorphine, patients already on CYP3A4 inhibitors should have their dose of Subutex or Subuxone adjusted).
No products indexed under this heading.

Valproate Sodium (Buprenorphine is metabolized to norbuprenorphine by cytochrome CYP3A4. Because CYP3A4 inhibitors may increase plasma concentrations of buprenorphine, patients already on CYP3A4 inhibitors should have their dose of Subutex or Subuxone adjusted).
No products indexed under this heading.

Vardenafil Hydrochloride (Buprenorphine is metabolized to norbuprenorphine by cytochrome CYP3A4. Because CYP3A4 inhibitors may increase plasma concentrations of buprenorphine, patients already on CYP3A4 inhibitors should have their dose of Subutex or Subuxone adjusted). Products include:
Levitra Tablets 2876

Verapamil Hydrochloride (Buprenorphine is metabolized to norbuprenorphine by cytochrome CYP3A4. Because CYP3A4 inhibitors may increase plasma concentrations of buprenorphine, patients already on CYP3A4 inhibitors should have their dose of Subutex or Subuxone adjusted). Products include:
Tarka Tablets 511

Voriconazole (Buprenorphine is metabolized to norbuprenorphine by cytochrome CYP3A4. Because CYP3A4 inhibitors may increase plasma concentrations of buprenorphine, patients already on CYP3A4 inhibitors should have their dose of Subutex or Subuxone adjusted).
No products indexed under this heading.

Zafirlukast (Buprenorphine is metabolized to norbuprenorphine by cytochrome CYP3A4. Because CYP3A4 inhibitors may increase plasma concentrations of buprenorphine, patients already on CYP3A4 inhibitors should have their dose of Subutex or Subuxone adjusted). Products include:
Accolate Tablets 669

Zileuton (Buprenorphine is metabolized to norbuprenorphine by cytochrome CYP3A4. Because CYP3A4 inhibitors may increase plasma concentrations of buprenorphine, patients already on CYP3A4 inhibitors should have their dose of Subutex or Subuxone adjusted).
No products indexed under this heading.

Food Interactions

Grapefruit (Buprenorphine is metabolized to norbuprenorphine by cytochrome CYP3A4. Because CYP3A4 inhibitors may increase plasma concentrations of buprenorphine, patients already on CYP3A4 inhibitors should have their dose of Subutex or Subuxone adjusted).

Grapefruit Juice (Buprenorphine is metabolized to norbuprenorphine by cytochrome CYP3A4. Because CYP3A4 inhibitors may increase plasma concentrations of buprenorphine, patients already on CYP3A4 inhibitors should have their dose of Subutex or Subuxone adjusted).

SUDAFED 12 HOUR NASAL DECONGESTANT NON-DROWSY CAPLETS

(Pseudoephedrine Hydrochloride) 1909
See Sudafed Nasal Decongestant Tablets

IMPORTANT NOTE: Always consult each drug listing in the patient's regimen for possible interactions.

SUDAFED 24 HOUR NON-DROWSY NASAL DECONGESTANT TABLETS
(Pseudoephedrine Hydrochloride) 1906
See Sudafed Nasal Decongestant Tablets

CHILDREN'S SUDAFED NASAL DECONGESTANT LIQUID
(Pseudoephedrine Hydrochloride) 1906
See Sudafed Nasal Decongestant Tablets

CHILDREN'S SUDAFED PE COLD & COUGH LIQUID
(Dextromethorphan Hydrobromide, Phenylephrine Hydrochloride) 1907
May interact with monoamine oxidase inhibitors. Compounds in these categories include:

Isocarboxazid (Concurrent and/or sequential use with MAO inhibitors is not recommended). Products include:
Marplan Tablets 3177
Moclobemide (Concurrent and/or sequential use with MAO inhibitors is not recommended).
No products indexed under this heading.
Pargyline Hydrochloride (Concurrent and/or sequential use with MAO inhibitors is not recommended).
No products indexed under this heading.
Phenelzine Sulfate (Concurrent and/or sequential use with MAO inhibitors is not recommended).
No products indexed under this heading.
Procarbazine Hydrochloride (Concurrent and/or sequential use with MAO inhibitors is not recommended).
No products indexed under this heading.
Rasagiline Mesylate (Concurrent and/or sequential use with MAO inhibitors is not recommended). Products include:
Azilect Tablets 3106
Selegiline (Concurrent and/or sequential use with MAO inhibitors is not recommended). Products include:
Emsam Transdermal System 905
Selegiline Hydrochloride (Concurrent and/or sequential use with MAO inhibitors is not recommended). Products include:
Eldepryl Capsules 3052
Tranylcypromine Sulfate (Concurrent and/or sequential use with MAO inhibitors is not recommended). Products include:
Parnate Tablets 1532

CHILDREN'S SUDAFED PE NASAL DECONGESTANT LIQUID
(Phenylephrine Hydrochloride) 1906
May interact with monoamine oxidase inhibitors. Compounds in these categories include:

Isocarboxazid (Concurrent and/or sequential use with MAO inhibitors is not recommended). Products include:
Marplan Tablets 3177
Moclobemide (Concurrent and/or sequential use with MAO inhibitors is not recommended).
No products indexed under this heading.
Pargyline Hydrochloride (Concurrent and/or sequential use with MAO inhibitors is not recommended).
No products indexed under this heading.
Phenelzine Sulfate (Concurrent and/or sequential use with MAO inhibitors is not recommended).
No products indexed under this heading.
Procarbazine Hydrochloride (Concurrent and/or sequential use with MAO inhibitors is not recommended).
No products indexed under this heading.
Rasagiline Mesylate (Concurrent and/or sequential use with MAO inhibitors is not recommended). Products include:
Azilect Tablets 3106
Selegiline (Concurrent and/or sequential use with MAO inhibitors is not recommended). Products include:
Emsam Transdermal System 905
Selegiline Hydrochloride (Concurrent and/or sequential use with MAO inhibitors is not recommended). Products include:
Eldepryl Capsules 3052
Tranylcypromine Sulfate (Concurrent and/or sequential use with MAO inhibitors is not recommended). Products include:
Parnate Tablets 1532

SUDAFED NASAL DECONGESTANT TABLETS
(Pseudoephedrine Hydrochloride) 1906
May interact with monoamine oxidase inhibitors. Compounds in these categories include:

Isocarboxazid (Concurrent and/or sequential use with MAO inhibitors is not recommended). Products include:
Marplan Tablets 3177
Moclobemide (Concurrent and/or sequential use with MAO inhibitors is not recommended).
No products indexed under this heading.
Pargyline Hydrochloride (Concurrent and/or sequential use with MAO inhibitors is not recommended).
No products indexed under this heading.
Phenelzine Sulfate (Concurrent and/or sequential use with MAO inhibitors is not recommended).
No products indexed under this heading.
Procarbazine Hydrochloride (Concurrent and/or sequential use with MAO inhibitors is not recommended).
No products indexed under this heading.
Rasagiline Mesylate (Concurrent and/or sequential use with MAO inhibitors is not recommended). Products include:
Azilect Tablets 3106
Selegiline (Concurrent and/or sequential use with MAO inhibitors is not recommended). Products include:
Emsam Transdermal System 905
Selegiline Hydrochloride (Concurrent and/or sequential use with MAO inhibitors is not recommended). Products include:
Eldepryl Capsules 3052
Tranylcypromine Sulfate (Concurrent and/or sequential use with MAO inhibitors is not recommended). Products include:
Parnate Tablets 1532

SUDAFED OM SINUS COLD MOISTURIZING NASAL SPRAY
(Oxymetazoline Hydrochloride) 1906
None cited in PDR database.

SUDAFED OM SINUS CONGESTION MOISTURIZING NASAL SPRAY
(Oxymetazoline Hydrochloride) 1906
None cited in PDR database.

SUDAFED PE COLD & COUGH CAPLETS
(Acetaminophen, Dextromethorphan Hydrobromide, Guaifenesin, Phenylephrine Hydrochloride)................................. 1907
May interact with monoamine oxidase inhibitors. Compounds in these categories include:

Isocarboxazid (Concurrent and/or sequential use with MAO inhibitors is not recommended). Products include:
Marplan Tablets 3177
Moclobemide (Concurrent and/or sequential use with MAO inhibitors is not recommended).
No products indexed under this heading.
Pargyline Hydrochloride (Concurrent and/or sequential use with MAO inhibitors is not recommended).
No products indexed under this heading.
Phenelzine Sulfate (Concurrent and/or sequential use with MAO inhibitors is not recommended).
No products indexed under this heading.
Procarbazine Hydrochloride (Concurrent and/or sequential use with MAO inhibitors is not recommended).
No products indexed under this heading.
Rasagiline Mesylate (Concurrent and/or sequential use with MAO inhibitors is not recommended). Products include:
Azilect Tablets 3106
Selegiline (Concurrent and/or sequential use with MAO inhibitors is not recommended). Products include:
Emsam Transdermal System 905
Selegiline Hydrochloride (Concurrent and/or sequential use with MAO inhibitors is not recommended). Products include:
Eldepryl Capsules 3052
Tranylcypromine Sulfate (Concurrent and/or sequential use with MAO inhibitors is not recommended). Products include:
Parnate Tablets 1532

SUDAFED PE NASAL DECONGESTANT TABLETS
(Phenylephrine Hydrochloride) 1907
See Sudafed Nasal Decongestant Tablets

SUDAFED PE NIGHTTIME COLD CAPLETS
(Acetaminophen, Diphenhydramine Hydrochloride, Phenylephrine Hydrochloride)................................. 1907
See Sudafed PE Severe Cold Caplets

SUDAFED PE NON-DRYING SINUS CAPLETS
(Guaifenesin, Phenylephrine Hydrochloride)................................. 1908
May interact with monoamine oxidase inhibitors. Compounds in these categories include:

Isocarboxazid (Concurrent and/or sequential use with MAO inhibitors is not recommended). Products include:
Marplan Tablets 3177
Moclobemide (Concurrent and/or sequential use with MAO inhibitors is not recommended).
No products indexed under this heading.
Pargyline Hydrochloride (Concurrent and/or sequential use with MAO inhibitors is not recommended).
No products indexed under this heading.
Phenelzine Sulfate (Concurrent and/or sequential use with MAO inhibitors is not recommended).
No products indexed under this heading.
Procarbazine Hydrochloride (Concurrent and/or sequential use with MAO inhibitors is not recommended).
No products indexed under this heading.
Rasagiline Mesylate (Concurrent and/or sequential use with MAO inhibitors is not recommended). Products include:
Azilect Tablets 3106
Selegiline (Concurrent and/or sequential use with MAO inhibitors is not recommended). Products include:
Emsam Transdermal System 905
Selegiline Hydrochloride (Concurrent and/or sequential use with MAO inhibitors is not recommended). Products include:
Eldepryl Capsules 3052
Tranylcypromine Sulfate (Concurrent and/or sequential use with MAO inhibitors is not recommended). Products include:
Parnate Tablets 1532

SUDAFED PE SEVERE COLD CAPLETS
(Acetaminophen, Diphenhydramine Hydrochloride, Phenylephrine Hydrochloride)................................. 1908
May interact with hypnotics and sedatives, monoamine oxidase inhibitors, tranquilizers, and certain other agents. Compounds in these categories include:

Alprazolam (Concurrent use may increase drowsiness effect).
No products indexed under this heading.
Buspirone Hydrochloride (Concurrent use may increase drowsiness effect).
No products indexed under this heading.
Butabarbital (Concurrent use may increase drowsiness effect).
No products indexed under this heading.

Butabarbital Sodium (Concurrent use may increase drowsiness effect).
No products indexed under this heading.

Chloral Hydrate (Concurrent use may increase drowsiness effect).
No products indexed under this heading.

Chlordiazepoxide (Concurrent use may increase drowsiness effect).
No products indexed under this heading.

Chlordiazepoxide Hydrochloride (Concurrent use may increase drowsiness effect).
No products indexed under this heading.

Chlorpromazine (Concurrent use may increase drowsiness effect).
No products indexed under this heading.

Chlorpromazine Hydrochloride (Concurrent use may increase drowsiness effect).
No products indexed under this heading.

Chlorprothixene (Concurrent use may increase drowsiness effect).
No products indexed under this heading.

Chlorprothixene Hydrochloride (Concurrent use may increase drowsiness effect).
No products indexed under this heading.

Clorazepate Dipotassium (Concurrent use may increase drowsiness effect).
No products indexed under this heading.

Diazepam (Concurrent use may increase drowsiness effect). Products include:
Valium Tablets 2658

Droperidol (Concurrent use may increase drowsiness effect).
No products indexed under this heading.

Estazolam (Concurrent use may increase drowsiness effect).
No products indexed under this heading.

Ethchlorvynol (Concurrent use may increase drowsiness effect).
No products indexed under this heading.

Ethinamate (Concurrent use may increase drowsiness effect).
No products indexed under this heading.

Fluphenazine Decanoate (Concurrent use may increase drowsiness effect).
No products indexed under this heading.

Fluphenazine Enanthate (Concurrent use may increase drowsiness effect).
No products indexed under this heading.

Fluphenazine Hydrochloride (Concurrent use may increase drowsiness effect).
No products indexed under this heading.

Flurazepam Hydrochloride (Concurrent use may increase drowsiness effect).
No products indexed under this heading.

Glutethimide (Concurrent use may increase drowsiness effect).
No products indexed under this heading.

Haloperidol (Concurrent use may increase drowsiness effect).
No products indexed under this heading.

Haloperidol Decanoate (Concurrent use may increase drowsiness effect).
No products indexed under this heading.

Hydroxyzine Hydrochloride (Concurrent use may increase drowsiness effect).
No products indexed under this heading.

Isocarboxazid (Concurrent and/or sequential use with MAO inhibitors is not recommended). Products include:
Marplan Tablets 3177

Lorazepam (Concurrent use may increase drowsiness effect).
No products indexed under this heading.

Loxapine Hydrochloride (Concurrent use may increase drowsiness effect).
No products indexed under this heading.

Loxapine Succinate (Concurrent use may increase drowsiness effect).
No products indexed under this heading.

Meprobamate (Concurrent use may increase drowsiness effect).
No products indexed under this heading.

Mesoridazine Besylate (Concurrent use may increase drowsiness effect).
No products indexed under this heading.

Moclobemide (Concurrent and/or sequential use with MAO inhibitors is not recommended).
No products indexed under this heading.

Molindone Hydrochloride (Concurrent use may increase drowsiness effect). Products include:
Moban Tablets 1116

Oxazepam (Concurrent use may increase drowsiness effect).
No products indexed under this heading.

Pargyline Hydrochloride (Concurrent and/or sequential use with MAO inhibitors is not recommended).
No products indexed under this heading.

Perphenazine (Concurrent use may increase drowsiness effect).
No products indexed under this heading.

Phenelzine Sulfate (Concurrent and/or sequential use with MAO inhibitors is not recommended).
No products indexed under this heading.

Prazepam (Concurrent use may increase drowsiness effect).
No products indexed under this heading.

Procarbazine Hydrochloride (Concurrent and/or sequential use with MAO inhibitors is not recommended).
No products indexed under this heading.

Prochlorperazine (Concurrent use may increase drowsiness effect).
No products indexed under this heading.

Promethazine Hydrochloride (Concurrent use may increase drowsiness effect).
No products indexed under this heading.

Ramelteon (Concurrent use may increase drowsiness effect). Products include:
Rozerem Tablets 3091

Rasagiline Mesylate (Concurrent and/or sequential use with MAO inhibitors is not recommended). Products include:
Azilect Tablets 3106

Selegiline (Concurrent and/or sequential use with MAO inhibitors is not recommended). Products include:
Emsam Transdermal System 905

Selegiline Hydrochloride (Concurrent and/or sequential use with MAO inhibitors is not recommended). Products include:
Eldepryl Capsules 3052

Thioridazine Hydrochloride (Concurrent use may increase drowsiness effect). Products include:
Thioridazine Hydrochloride Tablets 2195

Thiothixene (Concurrent use may increase drowsiness effect). Products include:
Thiothixene Capsules 2197

Tranylcypromine Sulfate (Concurrent and/or sequential use with MAO inhibitors is not recommended). Products include:
Parnate Tablets 1532

Trifluoperazine Hydrochloride (Concurrent use may increase drowsiness effect).
No products indexed under this heading.

Food Interactions

Alcohol (Chronic heavy alcohol abusers, 3 or more drinks per day, should consult their physicians for advice on when and how they should take pain relievers/fever reducers including acetaminophen. Acetaminophen may cause liver damage).

SUDAFED PE SINUS & ALLERGY TABLETS

(Chlorpheniramine Maleate, Phenylephrine Hydrochloride) 1908
May interact with hypnotics and sedatives, monoamine oxidase inhibitors, tranquilizers, and certain other agents. Compounds in these categories include:

Alprazolam (Concomitant use may cause increased drowsiness).
No products indexed under this heading.

Buspirone Hydrochloride (Concomitant use may cause increased drowsiness).
No products indexed under this heading.

Butabarbital (Concomitant use may cause increased drowsiness).
No products indexed under this heading.

Butabarbital Sodium (Concomitant use may cause increased drowsiness).
No products indexed under this heading.

Chloral Hydrate (Concomitant use may cause increased drowsiness).
No products indexed under this heading.

Chlordiazepoxide (Concomitant use may cause increased drowsiness).
No products indexed under this heading.

Chlordiazepoxide Hydrochloride (Concomitant use may cause increased drowsiness).
No products indexed under this heading.

Chlorpromazine (Concomitant use may cause increased drowsiness).
No products indexed under this heading.

Chlorpromazine Hydrochloride (Concomitant use may cause increased drowsiness).
No products indexed under this heading.

Chlorprothixene (Concomitant use may cause increased drowsiness).
No products indexed under this heading.

Chlorprothixene Hydrochloride (Concomitant use may cause increased drowsiness).
No products indexed under this heading.

Clorazepate Dipotassium (Concomitant use may cause increased drowsiness).
No products indexed under this heading.

Diazepam (Concomitant use may cause increased drowsiness). Products include:
Valium Tablets 2658

Droperidol (Concomitant use may cause increased drowsiness).
No products indexed under this heading.

Estazolam (Concomitant use may cause increased drowsiness).
No products indexed under this heading.

Ethchlorvynol (Concomitant use may cause increased drowsiness).
No products indexed under this heading.

Ethinamate (Concomitant use may cause increased drowsiness).
No products indexed under this heading.

Fluphenazine Decanoate (Concomitant use may cause increased drowsiness).
No products indexed under this heading.

Fluphenazine Enanthate (Concomitant use may cause increased drowsiness).
No products indexed under this heading.

Fluphenazine Hydrochloride (Concomitant use may cause increased drowsiness).
No products indexed under this heading.

Flurazepam Hydrochloride (Concomitant use may cause increased drowsiness).
No products indexed under this heading.

Glutethimide (Concomitant use may cause increased drowsiness).
No products indexed under this heading.

Haloperidol (Concomitant use may cause increased drowsiness).
No products indexed under this heading.

Haloperidol Decanoate (Concomitant use may cause increased drowsiness).
No products indexed under this heading.

Hydroxyzine Hydrochloride (Concomitant use may cause increased drowsiness).
No products indexed under this heading.

Isocarboxazid (Phenylephrine should not be taken concomitantly with MAO inhibitors, or for two weeks after stopping MAO inhibitor). Products include:
Marplan Tablets 3177

Lorazepam (Concomitant use may cause increased drowsiness).
No products indexed under this heading.

Midazolam Hydrochloride (Concomitant use may cause increased drowsiness).
No products indexed under this heading.

Moclobemide (Phenylephrine should not be taken concomitantly with MAO inhibitors, or for two weeks after stopping MAO inhibitor).
No products indexed under this heading.

Pargyline Hydrochloride (Phenylephrine should not be taken concomitantly with MAO inhibitors, or for two weeks after stopping MAO inhibitor).
No products indexed under this heading.

Phenelzine Sulfate (Phenylephrine should not be taken concomitantly with MAO inhibitors, or for two weeks after stopping MAO inhibitor).
No products indexed under this heading.

Procarbazine Hydrochloride (Phenylephrine should not be taken concomitantly with MAO inhibitors, or for two weeks after stopping MAO inhibitor).
No products indexed under this heading.

Propofol (Concomitant use may cause increased drowsiness).
No products indexed under this heading.

Quazepam (Concomitant use may cause increased drowsiness).
No products indexed under this heading.

Ramelteon (Concomitant use may cause increased drowsiness). Products include:
Rozerem Tablets 3091

Rasagiline Mesylate (Phenylephrine should not be taken concomitantly with MAO inhibitors, or for two weeks after stopping MAO inhibitor). Products include:
Azilect Tablets 3106

Secobarbital Sodium (Concomitant use may cause increased drowsiness).
No products indexed under this heading.

Selegiline (Phenylephrine should not be taken concomitantly with MAO inhibitors, or for two weeks after stopping MAO inhibitor). Products include:
Emsam Transdermal System 905

Selegiline Hydrochloride (Phenylephrine should not be taken concomitantly with MAO inhibitors, or for two weeks after stopping MAO inhibitor). Products include:
Eldepryl Capsules 3052

Sodium Butabarbital (Concomitant use may cause increased drowsiness).
No products indexed under this heading.

Temazepam (Concomitant use may cause increased drowsiness).
No products indexed under this heading.

Tranylcypromine Sulfate (Phenylephrine should not be taken concomitantly with MAO inhibitors, or for two weeks after stopping MAO inhibitor). Products include:
Parnate Tablets 1532

Triazolam (Concomitant use may cause increased drowsiness).
No products indexed under this heading.

Zaleplon (Concomitant use may cause increased drowsiness).
No products indexed under this heading.

Zolpidem Tartrate (Concomitant use may cause increased drowsiness). Products include:
Ambien Tablets 2692
Ambien CR Tablets 2696

Food Interactions

Alcohol (Concomitant use may cause increased drowsiness).

SUDAFED PE SINUS HEADACHE CAPLETS

(Acetaminophen, Phenylephrine Hydrochloride).................................. 1908
May interact with monoamine oxidase inhibitors and certain other agents. Compounds in these categories include:

Isocarboxazid (Concurrent and/or sequential use with MAO inhibitors is not recommended). Products include:
Marplan Tablets 3177

Moclobemide (Concurrent and/or sequential use with MAO inhibitors is not recommended).
No products indexed under this heading.

Pargyline Hydrochloride (Concurrent and/or sequential use with MAO inhibitors is not recommended).
No products indexed under this heading.

Phenelzine Sulfate (Concurrent and/or sequential use with MAO inhibitors is not recommended).
No products indexed under this heading.

Procarbazine Hydrochloride (Concurrent and/or sequential use with MAO inhibitors is not recommended).
No products indexed under this heading.

Rasagiline Mesylate (Concurrent and/or sequential use with MAO inhibitors is not recommended). Products include:
Azilect Tablets 3106

Selegiline (Concurrent and/or sequential use with MAO inhibitors is not recommended). Products include:
Emsam Transdermal System 905

Selegiline Hydrochloride (Concurrent and/or sequential use with MAO inhibitors is not recommended). Products include:
Eldepryl Capsules 3052

Tranylcypromine Sulfate (Concurrent and/or sequential use with MAO inhibitors is not recommended). Products include:
Parnate Tablets 1532

Food Interactions

Alcohol (Chronic heavy alcohol abusers, 3 or more drinks per day, should consult their physicians for advice on when and how they should take pain relievers/fever reducers including acetaminophen. Acetaminophen may cause liver damage).

SULAR EXTENDED RELEASE TABLETS

(Nisoldipine) 2975
May interact with dexamethasone, phenytoin, quinidine, and certain other agents. Compounds in these categories include:

Atenolol (Greater blood pressure effect of Sular with concomitant use).
No products indexed under this heading.

Carbamazepine (Co-administration of nisoldipine with known CYP3A4 inducer, such as carbamazepine, should be avoided because of possible reduced nisoldipine plasma concentrations). Products include:
Carbatrol Capsules 3019
Equetro Extended-Release Capsules 3174

Cimetidine (Concomitant use increases nisoldipine AUC and Cmax by 30% to 45%).
No products indexed under this heading.

Cimetidine Hydrochloride (Concomitant use increases nisoldipine AUC and Cmax by 30% to 45%).
No products indexed under this heading.

Dexamethasone (Co-administration of nisoldipine with known CYP3A4 inducer, such as dexamethasone, should be avoided because of possible reduced nisoldipine plasma concentrations). Products include:
Ciprodex Otic Suspension 541

Dexamethasone Acetate (Co-administration of nisoldipine with known CYP3A4 inducer, such as dexamethasone, should be avoided because of possible reduced nisoldipine plasma concentrations).
No products indexed under this heading.

Dexamethasone Sodium Phosphate (Co-administration of nisoldipine with known CYP3A4 inducer, such as dexamethasone, should be avoided because of possible reduced nisoldipine plasma concentrations).
No products indexed under this heading.

Fat (A pronounced food-effect is observed when nislodipine is administered with a high-fat meal resulting in an increased peak concentration (Cmax) of up to 245%. Total exposure (AUC) is decreased by 22%. As a result, nislodipine should be taken on an empty stomach (1 hour before or 2 hours after a meal)).
No products indexed under this heading.

Fosphenytoin Sodium (Co-administration in epileptic patients has resulted in reduced nisoldipine plasma concentrations to undetectable levels).
No products indexed under this heading.

Phenobarbital (Co-administration of nisoldipine with known CYP3A4 inducer, such as phenobarbital, should be avoided because of possible reduced nisoldipine plasma concentrations). Products include:
Donnatal Extentabs 2507

Phenytoin (Co-administration in epileptic patients has resulted in reduced nisoldipine plasma concentrations to undetectable levels).
No products indexed under this heading.

Phenytoin Sodium (Co-administration in epileptic patients has resulted in reduced nisoldipine plasma concentrations to undetectable levels). Products include:
Phenytek Capsules 2192

Propranolol Hydrochloride (Propanolol attenuates the heart rate increase following the administration of immediate-release nisoldipine). Products include:
InnoPran XL Extended Release Capsules 1484

Quinidine (May decrease the bioavailability (AUC) of nisoldipine by 26%, but not the peak concentration; clinical significance is not known).
No products indexed under this heading.

Quinidine Gluconate (May decrease the bioavailability (AUC) of nisoldipine by 26%, but not the peak concentration; clinical significance is not known).
No products indexed under this heading.

Quinidine Hydrochloride (May decrease the bioavailability (AUC) of nisoldipine by 26%, but not the peak concentration; clinical significance is not known).
No products indexed under this heading.

Quinidine Polygalacturonate (May decrease the bioavailability (AUC) of nisoldipine by 26%, but not the peak concentration; clinical significance is not known).
No products indexed under this heading.

Quinidine Sulfate (May decrease the bioavailability (AUC) of nisoldipine by 26%, but not the peak concentration; clinical significance is not known).
No products indexed under this heading.

Ranitidine Hydrochloride (Concomitant use decreases AUC by 15% to 20%). Products include:
Zantac 75 Tablets .... ▣ 603
Zantac 1670
Zantac Injection 1666
Zantac Injection Pharmacy Bulk Package 1668
Maximum Strength Zantac 150 Tablets .... ▣ 603
Maximum Strength Zantac 150 Cool Mint Tablets .... ▣ 603

Rifampin (Co-administration of nisoldipine with known CYP3A4 inducer, such as rifampin, should be avoided because of possible reduced nisoldipine plasma concentrations).
No products indexed under this heading.

Food Interactions

Diet, high-lipid (Food with a high fat content has a pronounced effect on the release of nisoldipine resulting in a significant increase in peak concentration (Cmax) by up to 300%; concomitant intake of high-fat meal should be avoided).

Food, unspecified (A pronounced food-effect is observed when nislodipine is administered with a high-fat meal resulting in an increased peak concentration (Cmax) of up to 245%. Total exposure (AUC) is decreased by 22%. As a result, nislodipine should be taken on an empty stomach (1 hour before or 2 hours after a meal)).

SULFAMYLON CREAM

(Mafenide Acetate) **2194**
None cited in PDR database.

SULFAMYLON FOR 5% TOPICAL SOLUTION

(Mafenide Acetate) **2194**
None cited in PDR database.

SUPPRELIN LA IMPLANT

(Histrelin Acetate) **1731**
None cited in PDR database.

SUPRAX FOR ORAL SUSPENSION

(Cefixime) **1891**
May interact with anticoagulants and certain other agents. Compounds in these categories include:

Anisindione (Increased prothrombin time, with or without clinical bleeding, has been reported when cefixime is administered concomitantly).
No products indexed under this heading.

Ardeparin Sodium (Increased prothrombin time, with or without clinical bleeding, has been reported when cefixime is administered concomitantly).
No products indexed under this heading.

Carbamazepine (Elevated carbamazepine levels have been reported in postmarketing experience when cefixime is administered concomitantly. Drug monitoring may be of assistance in detecting alterations in carbamazepine plasma concentrations). Products include:
Carbatrol Capsules **3019**
Equetro Extended-Release Capsules **3174**

Dalteparin Sodium (Increased prothrombin time, with or without clinical bleeding, has been reported when cefixime is administered concomitantly). Products include:
Fragmin Injection **1070**

Danaparoid Sodium (Increased prothrombin time, with or without clinical bleeding, has been reported when cefixime is administered concomitantly).
No products indexed under this heading.

Dicumarol (Increased prothrombin time, with or without clinical bleeding, has been reported when cefixime is administered concomitantly).
No products indexed under this heading.

Enoxaparin Sodium (Increased prothrombin time, with or without clinical bleeding, has been reported when cefixime is administered concomitantly). Products include:
Lovenox Injection **2756**

Fondaparinux Sodium (Increased prothrombin time, with or without clinical bleeding, has been reported when cefixime is administered concomitantly). Products include:
Arixtra Injection **1313**

Heparin Calcium (Increased prothrombin time, with or without clinical bleeding, has been reported when cefixime is administered concomitantly).
No products indexed under this heading.

Heparin Sodium (Increased prothrombin time, with or without clinical bleeding, has been reported when cefixime is administered concomitantly).
No products indexed under this heading.

Low Molecular Weight Heparins (Increased prothrombin time, with or without clinical bleeding, has been reported when cefixime is administered concomitantly).
No products indexed under this heading.

Tinzaparin Sodium (Increased prothrombin time, with or without clinical bleeding, has been reported when cefixime is administered concomitantly).
No products indexed under this heading.

Warfarin Sodium (Increased prothrombin time, with or without clinical bleeding, has been reported when cefixime is administered concomitantly).
No products indexed under this heading.

Food Interactions

Food, unspecified (Cefixime, given orally, is about 40% to 50% absorbed whether administered with or without food; however, time to maximal absorption is increased approximately 0.8 hours when administered with food).

SUPRAX TABLETS

(Cefixime) **1891**
See Suprax for Oral Suspension

SURE2ENDURE TABLETS

(Glucosamine Hydrochloride, Herbals with Vitamins & Minerals)...... **641**
None cited in PDR database.

SUSTIVA CAPSULES

(Efavirenz) **930**
May interact with calcium channel blockers, central nervous system depressants, ergot-containing drugs, HMG-CoA reductase inhibitors, phenytoin, and certain other agents. Compounds in these categories include:

Alfentanil Hydrochloride (Potential for additive central nervous system effects when Sustiva is used concomitantly with other CNS depressants).
No products indexed under this heading.

Alprazolam (Potential for additive central nervous system effects when Sustiva is used concomitantly with other CNS depressants).
No products indexed under this heading.

Amlodipine Besylate (No data is available on the potential interactions of efavirenz with other calcium channel blockers that are substrates of CYP3A4 enzyme. The potential exists for reduction in plasma concentrations of the calcium channel blocker. Dose adjustments shouldbe guided by clinical response. Concomitant use of calcium channel blockers such as bepridil is contraindicated due to the potential for serious and/or life threatening reactions such as cardiac arrhythmias). Products include:
Azor Tablets **1005**
Exforge Tablets **2238**

Amprenavir (Efavirenz has the potential to decrease serum concentrations of amprenavir).
No products indexed under this heading.

Aprobarbital (Potential for additive central nervous system effects when Sustiva is used concomitantly with other CNS depressants).
No products indexed under this heading.

Astemizole (Efavirenz has been shown *in vivo* to induce CYP3A4, other compounds that are substrates of CYP3A4, such as astemizole, may have decreased plasma concentrations when co-administered; *in vitro* efavirenz inhibits 3A4, co-administration with the drugs primarily metabolized by this isoenzyme, such as astemizole, may result in altered plasma concentrations of astemizole; concurrent use should be avoided).
No products indexed under this heading.

Atazanavir (Co-administration has resulted in decreases in atazanavir Cmax (59%) and AUC (74%)).
No products indexed under this heading.

Atorvastatin Calcium (Concomitant use of HMG-CoA reductase inhibitors such as atorvastatin, pravastatin, and simvastatin with efavirenz leads to decreased HMG-CoA reductase inhibitors plasma concentrations). Products include:
Lipitor Tablets **2501**

Azithromycin Dihydrate (Co-administration has resulted in increases in azithromycin Cmax (22%) with no change in AUC; no dosage adjustment is necessary).
No products indexed under this heading.

Bepridil Hydrochloride (No data is available on the potential interactions of efavirenz with other calcium channel blockers that are substrates of CYP3A4 enzyme. The potential exists for reduction in plasma concentrations of the calcium channel blocker. Dose adjustments shouldbe guided by clinical response. Concomitant use of calcium channel blockers such as bepridil is contraindicated due to the potential for serious and/or life threatening reactions such as cardiac arrhythmias).
No products indexed under this heading.

Buprenorphine Hydrochloride (Potential for additive central nervous system effects when Sustiva is used concomitantly with other CNS depressants). Products include:
Suboxone Tablets **2601**
Subutex Tablets **2601**

Buspirone Hydrochloride (Potential for additive central nervous system effects when Sustiva is used concomitantly with other CNS depressants).
No products indexed under this heading.

Butabarbital (Potential for additive central nervous system effects when Sustiva is used concomitantly with other CNS depressants).
No products indexed under this heading.

Butalbital (Potential for additive central nervous system effects when Sustiva is used concomitantly with other CNS depressants).
No products indexed under this heading.

Carbamazepine (Potential for reduction in anticonvulsant and/or efavirenz plasma levels). Products include:
Carbatrol Capsules **3019**
Equetro Extended-Release Capsules **3174**

Cerivastatin Sodium (Concomitant use of HMG-CoA reductase inhibitors such as atorvastatin, pravastatin, and simvastatin with efavirenz leads to decreased HMG-CoA reductase inhibitors plasma concentrations).
No products indexed under this heading.

Chlordiazepoxide (Potential for additive central nervous system effects when Sustiva is used concomitantly with other CNS depressants).
No products indexed under this heading.

Chlordiazepoxide Hydrochloride (Potential for additive central nervous system effects when Sustiva is used concomitantly with other CNS depressants).
No products indexed under this heading.

Chlorpromazine (Potential for additive central nervous system effects when Sustiva is used concomitantly with other CNS depressants).
No products indexed under this heading.

Chlorpromazine Hydrochloride (Potential for additive central nervous system effects when Sustiva is used concomitantly with other CNS depressants).
No products indexed under this heading.

Chlorprothixene (Potential for additive central nervous system effects when Sustiva is used concomitantly with other CNS depressants).
No products indexed under this heading.

Chlorprothixene Hydrochloride (Potential for additive central nervous system effects when Sustiva is used concomitantly with other CNS depressants).
No products indexed under this heading.

Chlorprothixene Lactate (Potential for additive central nervous system effects when Sustiva is used concomitantly with other CNS depressants).
No products indexed under this heading.

Cisapride (Efavirenz has been shown *in vivo* to induce CYP3A4, other compounds that are substrates of CYP3A4, such as cisapride, may have decreased plasma concentrations when co-administered; *in vitro* efavirenz inhibits 3A4, co-administration with the drugs primarily metabolized by this isoenzyme, such as cisapride, may

result in altered plasma concentrations of cisapride; concurrent use should be avoided).
No products indexed under this heading.

Clarithromycin (Decreased plasma concentration of clarithromycin and increased 14-OH metabolite concentration; clinical significance is not known). Products include:
Biaxin/Biaxin XL ... 411

Clorazepate Dipotassium (Potential for additive central nervous system effects when Sustiva is used concomitantly with other CNS depressants).
No products indexed under this heading.

Clozapine (Potential for additive central nervous system effects when Sustiva is used concomitantly with other CNS depressants).
No products indexed under this heading.

Codeine Phosphate (Potential for additive central nervous system effects when Sustiva is used concomitantly with other CNS depressants). Products include:
Tylenol with Codeine Tablets ... 2427

Desflurane (Potential for additive central nervous system effects when Sustiva is used concomitantly with other CNS depressants).
No products indexed under this heading.

Dezocine (Potential for additive central nervous system effects when Sustiva is used concomitantly with other CNS depressants).
No products indexed under this heading.

Diazepam (Potential for additive central nervous system effects when Sustiva is used concomitantly with other CNS depressants). Products include:
Valium Tablets ... 2658

Dihydroergotamine Mesylate (Efavirenz has been shown *in vivo* to induce CYP3A4, other compounds that are substrates of CYP3A4, such as ergot derivatives, may have decreased plasma concentrations when co-administered; *in vitro* efavirenz inhibits 3A4, co-administration with the drugs primarily metabolized by this isoenzyme, such as ergot derivatives, may result in altered plasma concentrations of ergot derivatives; concurrent use should be avoided).
No products indexed under this heading.

Diltiazem Hydrochloride (No data is available on the potential interactions of efavirenz with other calcium channel blockers that are substrates of CYP3A4 enzyme. The potential exists for reduction in plasma concentrations of the calcium channel blocker. Dose adjustments shouldbe guided by clinical response. Concomitant use of calcium channel blockers such as bepridil is contraindicated due to the potential for serious and/or life threatening reactions such as cardiac arrhythmias). Products include:
Cardizem LA Extended Release Tablets ... 421

Droperidol (Potential for additive central nervous system effects when Sustiva is used concomitantly with other CNS depressants).
No products indexed under this heading.

Enflurane (Potential for additive central nervous system effects when Sustiva is used concomitantly with other CNS depressants).
No products indexed under this heading.

Ergonovine Maleate (Efavirenz has been shown *in vivo* to induce CYP3A4, other compounds that are substrates of CYP3A4, such as ergot derivatives, may have decreased plasma concentrations when co-administered; *in vitro* efavirenz inhibits 3A4, co-administration with the drugs primarily metabolized by this isoenzyme, such as ergot derivatives, may result in altered plasma concentrations of ergot derivatives; concurrent use should be avoided).
No products indexed under this heading.

Ergotamine Tartrate (Efavirenz has been shown *in vivo* to induce CYP3A4, other compounds that are substrates of CYP3A4, such as ergot derivatives, may have decreased plasma concentrations when co-administered; *in vitro* efavirenz inhibits 3A4, co-administration with the drugs primarily metabolized by this isoenzyme, such as ergot derivatives, may result in altered plasma concentrations of ergot derivatives; concurrent use should be avoided).
No products indexed under this heading.

Estazolam (Potential for additive central nervous system effects when Sustiva is used concomitantly with other CNS depressants).
No products indexed under this heading.

Ethanol (Potential for additive central nervous system effects when Sustiva is used concomitantly with other CNS depressants).
No products indexed under this heading.

Ethchlorvynol (Potential for additive central nervous system effects when Sustiva is used concomitantly with other CNS depressants).
No products indexed under this heading.

Ethinamate (Potential for additive central nervous system effects when Sustiva is used concomitantly with other CNS depressants).
No products indexed under this heading.

Ethinyl Estradiol (Co-administration has resulted in increased AUC for ethinyl estradiol; there was no effect on efavirenz AUC or Cmax; clinical significance is unknown). Products include:
Lybrel Tablets ... 3204
Mircette Tablets ... 1034
NuvaRing ... 2897
Ortho-Cyclen/Ortho Tri-Cyclen ... 2449
Ortho Evra Transdermal System ... 2437
Ortho Tri-Cyclen Lo Tablets ... 2458
Seasonique Tablets ... 1046
Yaz Tablets ... 805

Ethyl Alcohol (Potential for additive central nervous system effects when Sustiva is used concomitantly with other CNS depressants).
No products indexed under this heading.

Felodipine (No data is available on the potential interactions of efavirenz with other calcium channel blockers that are substrates of CYP3A4 enzyme. The potential exists for reduction in plasma concentrations of the calcium channel blocker. Dose adjustments shouldbe guided by clinical response. Concomitant use of calcium channel blockers such as bepridil is contraindicated due to the potential for serious and/or life threatening reactions such as cardiac arrhythmias).
No products indexed under this heading.

Fentanyl (Potential for additive central nervous system effects when Sustiva is used concomitantly with other CNS depressants). Products include:
Duragesic Transdermal System ... 2405
Ionsys Transdermal System ... 2410

Fentanyl Citrate (Potential for additive central nervous system effects when Sustiva is used concomitantly with other CNS depressants). Products include:
Actiq ... 959
Fentora Tablets ... 968

Fluconazole (Co-administration has resulted in increase in 16% AUC for efavirenz; there was no change in fluconazole Cmax or AUC).
No products indexed under this heading.

Fluphenazine Decanoate (Potential for additive central nervous system effects when Sustiva is used concomitantly with other CNS depressants).
No products indexed under this heading.

Fluphenazine Enanthate (Potential for additive central nervous system effects when Sustiva is used concomitantly with other CNS depressants).
No products indexed under this heading.

Fluphenazine Hydrochloride (Potential for additive central nervous system effects when Sustiva is used concomitantly with other CNS depressants).
No products indexed under this heading.

Flurazepam Hydrochloride (Potential for additive central nervous system effects when Sustiva is used concomitantly with other CNS depressants).
No products indexed under this heading.

Fluvastatin Sodium (Concomitant use of HMG-CoA reductase inhibitors such as atorvastatin, pravastatin, and simvastatin with efavirenz leads to decreased HMG-CoA reductase inhibitors plasma concentrations). Products include:
Lescol Capsules ... 2268
Lescol XL Tablets ... 2268

Fosphenytoin Sodium (Potential for reduction in anticonvulsant and/or efavirenz plasma levels).
No products indexed under this heading.

Glutethimide (Potential for additive central nervous system effects when Sustiva is used concomitantly with other CNS depressants).
No products indexed under this heading.

Haloperidol (Potential for additive central nervous system effects when Sustiva is used concomitantly with other CNS depressants).
No products indexed under this heading.

Haloperidol Decanoate (Potential for additive central nervous system effects when Sustiva is used concomitantly with other CNS depressants).
No products indexed under this heading.

Hydrocodone Bitartrate (Potential for additive central nervous system effects when Sustiva is used concomitantly with other CNS depressants). Products include:
Lortab 5/500 Tablets ... 3143
Lortab 7.5/500 Tablets ... 3144
Lortab 10/500 Tablets ... 3144
Vicodin Tablets ... 529
Vicodin ES Tablets ... 530
Vicodin HP Tablets ... 531
Vicoprofen Tablets ... 533
Zydone Tablets ... 1132

Hydrocodone Polistirex (Potential for additive central nervous system effects when Sustiva is used concomitantly with other CNS depressants). Products include:
Tussionex Pennkinetic Extended-Release Suspension ... 3154

Hydromorphone Hydrochloride (Potential for additive central nervous system effects when Sustiva is used concomitantly with other CNS depressants).
No products indexed under this heading.

Hydroxyzine Hydrochloride (Potential for additive central nervous system effects when Sustiva is used concomitantly with other CNS depressants).
No products indexed under this heading.

Hypericum (St. John's Wort is expected to substantially decrease plasma levels of efavirenz; concurrent use is not recommended). Products include:
Satieté Tablets ... ▣ 640

Indinavir Sulfate (Decreased plasma concentration of indinavir; indinavir dose should be increased). Products include:
Crixivan Capsules ... 1979

Isoflurane (Potential for additive central nervous system effects when Sustiva is used concomitantly with other CNS depressants).
No products indexed under this heading.

Isradipine (No data is available on the potential interactions of efavirenz with other calcium channel blockers that are substrates of CYP3A4 enzyme. The potential exists for reduction in plasma concentrations of the calcium channel blocker. Dose adjustments shouldbe guided by clinical response. Concomitant use of calcium channel blockers such as bepridil is contraindicated due to the potential for serious and/or life threatening reactions such as cardiac arrhythmias). Products include:
DynaCirc CR Controlled Release Tablets ... 1407

Itraconazole (Potential for decreased itraconazole concentrations. Since no dose recommendation for itraconazole can be made, alternative antifungal treatment should be considered).
No products indexed under this heading.

Ketamine Hydrochloride (Potential for additive central nervous system effects when Sustiva is used concomitantly with other CNS depressants).
No products indexed under this heading.

Ketoconazole (Potential for decreased ketoconazole concentrations). Products include:
Extina Foam, 2% ... 3057
Nizoral A-D Shampoo ... 1901

Levomethadyl Acetate Hydrochloride (Potential for additive central nervous system effects when Sustiva is used concomitantly with other CNS depressants).
No products indexed under this heading.

Levorphanol Tartrate (Potential for additive central nervous system effects when Sustiva is used concomitantly with other CNS depressants).
No products indexed under this heading.

Lorazepam (Potential for additive central nervous system effects when Sustiva is used concomitantly with other CNS depressants).
No products indexed under this heading.

Lovastatin (Concomitant use of HMG-CoA reductase inhibitors such as atorvastatin, pravastatin, and simvastatin with efavirenz leads to decreased HMG-CoA reductase inhibitors plasma concentrations). Products include:
Advicor Tablets ... 402
Mevacor Tablets ... 2063

Loxapine Hydrochloride (Potential for additive central nervous system effects when Sustiva is used concomitantly with other CNS depressants).
No products indexed under this heading.

Loxapine Succinate (Potential for additive central nervous system effects when Sustiva is used concomitantly with other CNS depressants).
No products indexed under this heading.

Meperidine Hydrochloride (Potential for additive central nervous system effects when Sustiva is used concomitantly with other CNS depressants).
No products indexed under this heading.

Mephobarbital (Potential for additive central nervous system effects when Sustiva is used concomitantly with other CNS depressants).
No products indexed under this heading.

Meprobamate (Potential for additive central nervous system effects when Sustiva is used concomitantly with other CNS depressants).
No products indexed under this heading.

Mesoridazine Besylate (Potential for additive central nervous system effects when Sustiva is used concomitantly with other CNS depressants).
No products indexed under this heading.

Methadone Hydrochloride (Decreased plasma concentration of methadone; methadone dose may need to be increased).
No products indexed under this heading.

Methohexital Sodium (Potential for additive central nervous system effects when Sustiva is used concomitantly with other CNS depressants).
No products indexed under this heading.

Methotrimeprazine (Potential for additive central nervous system effects when Sustiva is used concomitantly with other CNS depressants).
No products indexed under this heading.

Methoxyflurane (Potential for additive central nervous system effects when Sustiva is used concomitantly with other CNS depressants).
No products indexed under this heading.

Methylergonovine Maleate (Efavirenz has been shown *in vivo* to induce CYP3A4, other compounds that are substrates of CYP3A4, such as ergot derivatives, may have decreased plasma concentrations when co-administered; *in vitro* efavirenz inhibits 3A4, co-administration with the drugs primarily metabolized by this isoenzyme, such as ergot derivatives, may result in altered plasma concentrations of ergot derivatives; concurrent use should be avoided).
No products indexed under this heading.

Methysergide Maleate (Efavirenz has been shown *in vivo* to induce CYP3A4, other compounds that are substrates of CYP3A4, such as ergot derivatives, may have decreased plasma concentrations when co-administered; *in vitro* efavirenz inhibits 3A4, co-administration with the drugs primarily metabolized by this isoenzyme, such as ergot derivatives, may result in altered plasma concentrations of ergot derivatives; concurrent use should be avoided).
No products indexed under this heading.

Mibefradil Dihydrochloride (No data is available on the potential interactions of efavirenz with other calcium channel blockers that are substrates of CYP3A4 enzyme. The potential exists for reduction in plasma concentrations of the calcium channel blocker. Dose adjustments shouldbe guided by clinical response. Concomitant use of calcium channel blockers such as bepridil is contraindicated due to the potential for serious and/or life threatening reactions such as cardiac arrhythmias).
No products indexed under this heading.

Midazolam Hydrochloride (Efavirenz has been shown *in vivo* to induce CYP3A4, other compounds that are substrates of CYP3A4, such as midazolam, may have decreased plasma concentrations when co-administered; *in vitro* efavirenz inhibits 3A4, co-administration with the drugs primarily metabolized by this isoenzyme, such as midazolam, may result in altered plasma concentrations of midazolam; concurrent use should be avoided).
No products indexed under this heading.

Molindone Hydrochloride (Potential for additive central nervous system effects when Sustiva is used concomitantly with other CNS depressants). Products include:
Moban Tablets ... 1116

Morphine Sulfate (Potential for additive central nervous system effects when Sustiva is used concomitantly with other CNS depressants). Products include:
Avinza Capsules ... 1772
DepoDur Injection ... 1095
MS Contin Tablets ... 2585

Nelfinavir Mesylate (Co-administration in uninfected individuals has resulted in increases in AUC (20%) and Cmax (21%) for nelfinavir; no dose adjustment is necessary).
No products indexed under this heading.

Nicardipine Hydrochloride (No data is available on the potential interactions of efavirenz with other calcium channel blockers that are substrates of CYP3A4 enzyme. The potential exists for reduction in plasma concentrations of the calcium channel blocker. Dose adjustments shouldbe guided by clinical response. Concomitant use of calcium channel blockers such as bepridil is contraindicated due to the potential for serious and/or life threatening reactions such as cardiac arrhythmias). Products include:
Cardene I.V. ... 1093

Nifedipine (No data is available on the potential interactions of efavirenz with other calcium channel blockers that are substrates of CYP3A4 enzyme. The potential exists for reduction in plasma concentrations of the calcium channel blocker. Dose adjustments shouldbe guided by clinical response. Concomitant use of calcium channel blockers such as bepridil is contraindicated due to the potential for serious and/or life threatening reactions such as cardiac arrhythmias).
No products indexed under this heading.

Nimodipine (No data is available on the potential interactions of efavirenz with other calcium channel blockers that are substrates of CYP3A4 enzyme. The potential exists for reduction in plasma concentrations of the calcium channel blocker. Dose adjustments shouldbe guided by clinical response. Concomitant use of calcium channel blockers such as bepridil is contraindicated due to the potential for serious and/or life threatening reactions such as cardiac arrhythmias). Products include:
Nimotop Capsules ... 790

Nisoldipine (No data is available on the potential interactions of efavirenz with other calcium channel blockers that are substrates of CYP3A4 enzyme. The potential exists for reduction in plasma concentrations of the calcium channel blocker. Dose adjustments shouldbe guided by clinical response. Concomitant use of calcium channel blockers such as bepridil is contraindicated due to the potential for serious and/or life threatening reactions such as cardiac arrhythmias). Products include:
Sular Extended Release Tablets ... 2975

Olanzapine (Potential for additive central nervous system effects when Sustiva is used concomitantly with other CNS depressants). Products include:
Symbyax Capsules ... 1871
Zyprexa Tablets ... 1883
Zyprexa IntraMuscular ... 1883
Zyprexa ZYDIS Orally Disintegrating Tablets ... 1883

Oxazepam (Potential for additive central nervous system effects when Sustiva is used concomitantly with other CNS depressants).
No products indexed under this heading.

Oxycodone Hydrochloride (Potential for additive central nervous system effects when Sustiva is used concomitantly with other CNS depressants). Products include:
OxyContin Tablets ... 2589
OxyIR Capsules ... 2593
Percocet Tablets ... 1127
Percodan Tablets ... 1130

Pentobarbital Sodium (Potential for additive central nervous system effects when Sustiva is used concomitantly with other CNS depressants). Products include:
Nembutal Sodium Solution, USP ... 2494

Perphenazine (Potential for additive central nervous system effects when Sustiva is used concomitantly with other CNS depressants).
No products indexed under this heading.

Phenobarbital (Potential for reduction in anticonvulsant and/or efavirenz plasma levels). Products include:
Donnatal Extentabs ... 2507

Phenytoin (Potential for reduction in anticonvulsant and/or efavirenz plasma levels).
No products indexed under this heading.

Phenytoin Sodium (Potential for reduction in anticonvulsant and/or efavirenz plasma levels). Products include:
Phenytek Capsules ... 2192

Pimozide (Concomitant use of neuroleptic drugs with efavirenz is contraindicated due to the potential for serious and/or life-threatening reactions such as cardiac arrhythmias).
No products indexed under this heading.

Pravastatin Sodium (Concomitant use of HMG-CoA reductase inhibitors such as atorvastatin, pravastatin, and simvastatin with efavirenz leads to decreased HMG-CoA reductase inhibitors plasma concentrations).
No products indexed under this heading.

Prazepam (Potential for additive central nervous system effects when Sustiva is used concomitantly with other CNS depressants).
No products indexed under this heading.

Prochlorperazine (Potential for additive central nervous system effects when Sustiva is used concomitantly with other CNS depressants).
No products indexed under this heading.

Promethazine Hydrochloride (Potential for additive central nervous system effects when Sustiva is used concomitantly with other CNS depressants).
No products indexed under this heading.

Propofol (Potential for additive central nervous system effects when Sustiva is used concomitantly with other CNS depressants).
No products indexed under this heading.

Propoxyphene Hydrochloride (Potential for additive central nervous system effects when Sustiva is used concomitantly with other CNS depressants).
No products indexed under this heading.

Propoxyphene Napsylate (Potential for additive central nervous system effects when Sustiva is used concomitantly with other CNS depressants).
No products indexed under this heading.

Quazepam (Potential for additive central nervous system effects when Sustiva is used concomitantly with other CNS depressants).
No products indexed under this heading.

Quetiapine Fumarate (Potential for additive central nervous system effects when Sustiva is used concomitantly with other CNS depressants).
No products indexed under this heading.

Remifentanil Hydrochloride (Potential for additive central nervous system effects when Sustiva is used concomitantly with other CNS depressants).
No products indexed under this heading.

Rifabutin (Decreased plasma concentration of rifabutin; rifabutin dose should be increased by 50%).
No products indexed under this heading.

Rifampin (Co-administration has resulted in decreased efavirenz plasma concentrations; clinical significance is unknown).
No products indexed under this heading.

Risperidone (Potential for additive central nervous system effects when Sustiva is used concomitantly with other CNS depressants). Products include:
Risperdal Consta Long-Acting Injection **1753**

Ritonavir (Co-administration has resulted in increases in AUC for each drug by 20%; the combination was associated with a higher frequency of adverse clinical experiences including dizziness, nausea, paresthesia, and laboratory abnormalities (elevated liver enzymes)). Products include:
Kaletra **452**
Norvir **489**

Rosuvastatin Calcium (Concomitant use of HMG-CoA reductase inhibitors such as atorvastatin, pravastatin, and simvastatin with efavirenz leads to decreased HMG-CoA reductase inhibitors plasma concentrations). Products include:
Crestor Tablets **677**

Saquinavir (Co-administration with saquinavir soft gelatin capsule has resulted in decreases in AUC (62%) and Cmax (50%) for saquinavir; saquinavir should not be used as sole protease inhibitor in combination with Sustiva).
No products indexed under this heading.

Saquinavir Mesylate (Co-administration with saquinavir soft gelatin capsule has resulted in decreases in AUC (62%) and Cmax (50%) for saquinavir; saquinavir should not be used as sole protease inhibitor in combination with Sustiva).
No products indexed under this heading.

Secobarbital Sodium (Potential for additive central nervous system effects when Sustiva is used concomitantly with other CNS depressants).
No products indexed under this heading.

Sevoflurane (Potential for additive central nervous system effects when Sustiva is used concomitantly with other CNS depressants). Products include:
Ultane Liquid for Inhalation **524**

Simvastatin (Concomitant use of HMG-CoA reductase inhibitors such as atorvastatin, pravastatin, and simvastatin with efavirenz leads to decreased HMG-CoA reductase inhibitors plasma concentrations). Products include:
Simcor Tablets **502**
Vytorin 10/10 Tablets **2149**
Vytorin 10/10 Tablets **2939**
Vytorin 10/20 Tablets **2149**
Vytorin 10/20 Tablets **2939**
Vytorin 10/40 Tablets **2149**
Vytorin 10/40 Tablets **2939**
Vytorin 10/80 Tablets **2149**
Vytorin 10/80 Tablets **2939**
Zocor Tablets **2136**

Sodium Oxybate (Potential for additive central nervous system effects when Sustiva is used concomitantly with other CNS depressants). Products include:
Xyrem Oral Solution **1766**

Sufentanil Citrate (Potential for additive central nervous system effects when Sustiva is used concomitantly with other CNS depressants).
No products indexed under this heading.

Temazepam (Potential for additive central nervous system effects when Sustiva is used concomitantly with other CNS depressants).
No products indexed under this heading.

Thiamylal Sodium (Potential for additive central nervous system effects when Sustiva is used concomitantly with other CNS depressants).
No products indexed under this heading.

Thioridazine Hydrochloride (Potential for additive central nervous system effects when Sustiva is used concomitantly with other CNS depressants). Products include:
Thioridazine Hydrochloride Tablets **2195**

Thiothixene (Potential for additive central nervous system effects when Sustiva is used concomitantly with other CNS depressants). Products include:
Thiothixene Capsules **2197**

Triazolam (Efavirenz has been shown *in vivo* to induce CYP3A4, other compounds that are substrates of CYP3A4, such as triazolam, may have decreased plasma concentrations when co-administered; *in vitro* efavirenz inhibits 3A4, co-administration with the drugs primarily metabolized by this isoenzyme, such as triazolam, may result in altered plasma concentrations of triazolam; concurrent use should be avoided).
No products indexed under this heading.

Trifluoperazine Hydrochloride (Potential for additive central nervous system effects when Sustiva is used concomitantly with other CNS depressants).
No products indexed under this heading.

Verapamil Hydrochloride (No data is available on the potential interactions of efavirenz with other calcium channel blockers that are substrates of CYP3A4 enzyme. The potential exists for reduction in plasma concentrations of the calcium channel blocker. Dose adjustments shouldbe guided by clinical response. Concomitant use of calcium channel blockers such as bepridil is contraindicated due to the potential for serious and/or life threatening reactions such as cardiac arrhythmias). Products include:
Tarka Tablets **511**

Voriconazole (Co-administration has resulted in increases in voriconazole Cmax (38%) and AUC (44%); efavirenz will significantly decrease voriconazole concentration, therefore, co-administration is contraindicated).
No products indexed under this heading.

Warfarin Sodium (Co-administration may result in increased or decreased plasma concentrations and effects of warfarin).
No products indexed under this heading.

Zaleplon (Potential for additive central nervous system effects when Sustiva is used concomitantly with other CNS depressants).
No products indexed under this heading.

Ziprasidone Hydrochloride (Potential for additive central nervous system effects when Sustiva is used concomitantly with other CNS depressants). Products include:
Geodon Capsules **2520**

Zolpidem Tartrate (Potential for additive central nervous system effects when Sustiva is used concomitantly with other CNS depressants). Products include:
Ambien Tablets **2692**
Ambien CR Tablets **2696**

Food Interactions

Alcohol (Potential for additive central nervous system effects when Sustiva is used concomitantly with alcohol).

Food, unspecified (High fat meal may increase the absorption of Sustiva and should be avoided; it can be taken with or without meals of normal composition).

SUSTIVA TABLETS

(Efavirenz) **930**
See Sustiva Capsules

SUTENT CAPSULES

(Sunitinib malate) **2540**
May interact with antiarrhythmics, cytochrome p450 3a4 inducers (selected), cytochrome p450 3a4 inhibitors, potent, and certain other agents. Compounds in these categories include:

Acebutolol Hydrochloride (Sunitinib has been shown to prolong QT interval in a dose dependent manner: caution is advised in patients taking sunitinib and antiarrhythmics concomittantly).
No products indexed under this heading.

Adenosine (Sunitinib has been shown to prolong QT interval in a dose dependent manner: caution is advised in patients taking sunitinib and antiarrhythmics concomittantly). Products include:
Adenocard IV Injection **603**
Adenoscan **605**

Allium sativum (Concurrent administration of sunitinib with CYP3A4 inducers (e.g., rifampin) may decrease plasma sunitinib concentrations. Dose increase of sunitinib to 87.5 mg daily should be considered with co-administration).
No products indexed under this heading.

Amiodarone Hydrochloride (Sunitinib has been shown to prolong QT interval in a dose dependent manner: caution is advised in patients taking sunitinib and antiarrhythmics concomittantly).
No products indexed under this heading.

Amprenavir (Concurrent administration of sunitinib with strong CYP3A4 inhibitors (e.g., ketoconazole) may increase sunitinib plasma concentrations. Dose reduction of sunitinib to 37.5 mg daily is recommended with co-administration).
No products indexed under this heading.

Aprepitant (Concurrent administration of sunitinib with CYP3A4 inducers (e.g., rifampin) may decrease plasma sunitinib concentrations. Dose increase of sunitinib to 87.5 mg daily should be considered with co-administration). Products include:
Emend Capsules **1992**

Atazanavir (Concurrent administration of sunitinib with strong CYP3A4 inhibitors (e.g., ketoconazole) may increase sunitinib plasma concentrations. Dose reduction of sunitinib to 37.5 mg daily is recommended with co-administration).
No products indexed under this heading.

Atazanavir Sulfate (Concurrent administration of sunitinib with strong CYP3A4 inhibitors (e.g., ketoconazole) may increase sunitinib plasma concentrations. Dose reduction of sunitinib to 37.5 mg daily is recommended with co-administration). Products include:
Reyataz Capsules **3299**

Betamethasone Acetate (Concurrent administration of sunitinib with CYP3A4 inducers (e.g., rifampin) may decrease plasma sunitinib concentrations. Dose increase of sunitinib to 87.5 mg daily should be considered with co-administration).
No products indexed under this heading.

Betamethasone Sodium Phosphate (Concurrent administration of sunitinib with CYP3A4 inducers (e.g., rifampin) may decrease plasma sunitinib concentrations. Dose increase of sunitinib to 87.5 mg daily should be considered with co-administration).
No products indexed under this heading.

Bretylium Tosylate (Sunitinib has been shown to prolong QT interval in a dose dependent manner: caution is advised in patients taking sunitinib and antiarrhythmics concomittantly).
No products indexed under this heading.

Carbamazepine (Concurrent administration of sunitinib with CYP3A4 inducers (e.g., rifampin) may decrease plasma sunitinib concentrations. Dose increase of sunitinib to 87.5 mg daily should be considered with co-administration). Products include:
Carbatrol Capsules 3019
Equetro Extended-Release Capsules.. 3174

Ciprofloxacin Hydrochloride (Concurrent administration of sunitinib with CYP3A4 inducers (e.g., rifampin) may decrease plasma sunitinib concentrations. Dose increase of sunitinib to 87.5 mg daily should be considered with co-administration). Products include:
Cipro Tablets 2810

Cisplatin (Concurrent administration of sunitinib with CYP3A4 inducers (e.g., rifampin) may decrease plasma sunitinib concentrations. Dose increase of sunitinib to 87.5 mg daily should be considered with co-administration).
No products indexed under this heading.

Clarithromycin (Concurrent administration of sunitinib with strong CYP3A4 inhibitors (e.g., ketoconazole) may increase sunitinib plasma concentrations. Dose reduction of sunitinib to 37.5 mg daily is recommended with co-administration). Products include:
Biaxin/Biaxin XL 411

Cortisone Acetate (Concurrent administration of sunitinib with CYP3A4 inducers (e.g., rifampin) may decrease plasma sunitinib concentrations. Dose increase of sunitinib to 87.5 mg daily should be considered with co-administration).
No products indexed under this heading.

Delavirdine Mesylate (Concurrent administration of sunitinib with strong CYP3A4 inhibitors (e.g., ketoconazole) may increase sunitinib plasma concentrations. Dose reduction of sunitinib to 37.5 mg daily is recommended with co-administration).
No products indexed under this heading.

Delavirine (Concurrent administration of sunitinib with strong CYP3A4 inhibitors (e.g., ketoconazole) may increase sunitinib plasma concentrations. Dose reduction of sunitinib to 37.5 mg daily is recommended with co-administration).
No products indexed under this heading.

Dexamethasone (Concurrent administration of sunitinib with CYP3A4 inducers (e.g., rifampin) may decrease plasma sunitinib concentrations. Dose increase of sunitinib to 87.5 mg daily should be considered with co-administration). Products include:
Ciprodex Otic Suspension 541

Dexamethasone Acetate (Concurrent administration of sunitinib with CYP3A4 inducers (e.g., rifampin) may decrease plasma sunitinib concentrations. Dose increase of sunitinib to 87.5 mg daily should be considered with co-administration).
No products indexed under this heading.

Dexamethasone Sodium Phosphate (Concurrent administration of sunitinib with CYP3A4 inducers (e.g., rifampin) may decrease plasma sunitinib concentrations. Dose increase of sunitinib to 87.5 mg daily should be considered with co-administration).
No products indexed under this heading.

Disopyramide Phosphate (Sunitinib has been shown to prolong QT interval in a dose dependent manner: caution is advised in patients taking sunitinib and antiarrhythmics concomittantly).
No products indexed under this heading.

Dofetilide (Sunitinib has been shown to prolong QT interval in a dose dependent manner: caution is advised in patients taking sunitinib and antiarrhythmics concomittantly).
No products indexed under this heading.

Doxorubicin Hydrochloride (Concurrent administration of sunitinib with CYP3A4 inducers (e.g., rifampin) may decrease plasma sunitinib concentrations. Dose increase of sunitinib to 87.5 mg daily should be considered with co-administration).
No products indexed under this heading.

Efavirenz (Concurrent administration of sunitinib with CYP3A4 inducers (e.g., rifampin) may decrease plasma sunitinib concentrations. Dose increase of sunitinib to 87.5 mg daily should be considered with co-administration). Products include:
Atripla Tablets 938
Sustiva Capsules 930
Sustiva Tablets 930

Ethosuximide (Concurrent administration of sunitinib with CYP3A4 inducers (e.g., rifampin) may decrease plasma sunitinib concentrations. Dose increase of sunitinib to 87.5 mg daily should be considered with co-administration).
No products indexed under this heading.

Felbamate (Concurrent administration of sunitinib with CYP3A4 inducers (e.g., rifampin) may decrease plasma sunitinib concentrations. Dose increase of sunitinib to 87.5 mg daily should be considered with co-administration).
No products indexed under this heading.

Flecainide Acetate (Sunitinib has been shown to prolong QT interval in a dose dependent manner: caution is advised in patients taking sunitinib and antiarrhythmics concomittantly).
No products indexed under this heading.

Fludrocortisone Acetate (Concurrent administration of sunitinib with CYP3A4 inducers (e.g., rifampin) may decrease plasma sunitinib concentrations. Dose increase of sunitinib to 87.5 mg daily should be considered with co-administration).
No products indexed under this heading.

Fosamprenavir Calcium (Concurrent administration of sunitinib with strong CYP3A4 inhibitors (e.g., ketoconazole) may increase sunitinib plasma concentrations. Dose reduction of sunitinib to 37.5 mg daily is recommended with co-administration). Products include:
Lexiva Oral Suspension 1510
Lexiva Tablets 1510

Fosphenytoin Sodium (Concurrent administration of sunitinib with CYP3A4 inducers (e.g., rifampin) may decrease plasma sunitinib concentrations. Dose increase of sunitinib to 87.5 mg daily should be considered with co-administration).
No products indexed under this heading.

Garlic Extract (Concurrent administration of sunitinib with CYP3A4 inducers (e.g., rifampin) may decrease plasma sunitinib concentrations. Dose increase of sunitinib to 87.5 mg daily should be considered with co-administration).
No products indexed under this heading.

Garlic Oil (Concurrent administration of sunitinib with CYP3A4 inducers (e.g., rifampin) may decrease plasma sunitinib concentrations. Dose increase of sunitinib to 87.5 mg daily should be considered with co-administration).
No products indexed under this heading.

Hydrocortisone (Concurrent administration of sunitinib with CYP3A4 inducers (e.g., rifampin) may decrease plasma sunitinib concentrations. Dose increase of sunitinib to 87.5 mg daily should be considered with co-administration).
No products indexed under this heading.

Hydrocortisone Acetate (Concurrent administration of sunitinib with CYP3A4 inducers (e.g., rifampin) may decrease plasma sunitinib concentrations. Dose increase of sunitinib to 87.5 mg daily should be considered with co-administration). Products include:
Analpram-HC 1140
Pramosone 1141

Hydrocortisone Butyrate (Concurrent administration of sunitinib with CYP3A4 inducers (e.g., rifampin) may decrease plasma sunitinib concentrations. Dose increase of sunitinib to 87.5 mg daily should be considered with co-administration).
No products indexed under this heading.

Hydrocortisone Cypionate (Concurrent administration of sunitinib with CYP3A4 inducers (e.g., rifampin) may decrease plasma sunitinib concentrations. Dose increase of sunitinib to 87.5 mg daily should be considered with co-administration).
No products indexed under this heading.

Hydrocortisone Hemisuccinate (Concurrent administration of sunitinib with CYP3A4 inducers (e.g., rifampin) may decrease plasma sunitinib concentrations. Dose increase of sunitinib to 87.5 mg daily should be considered with co-administration).
No products indexed under this heading.

Hydrocortisone Probutate (Concurrent administration of sunitinib with CYP3A4 inducers (e.g., rifampin) may decrease plasma sunitinib concentrations. Dose increase of sunitinib to 87.5 mg daily should be considered with co-administration).
No products indexed under this heading.

Hydrocortisone Sodium Phosphate (Concurrent administration of sunitinib with CYP3A4 inducers (e.g., rifampin) may decrease plasma sunitinib concentrations. Dose increase of sunitinib to 87.5 mg daily should be considered with co-administration).
No products indexed under this heading.

Hydrocortisone Sodium Succinate (Concurrent administration of sunitinib with CYP3A4 inducers (e.g., rifampin) may decrease plasma sunitinib concentrations. Dose increase of sunitinib to 87.5 mg daily should be considered with co-administration).
No products indexed under this heading.

Hydrocortisone Valerate (Concurrent administration of sunitinib with CYP3A4 inducers (e.g., rifampin) may decrease plasma sunitinib concentrations. Dose increase of sunitinib to 87.5 mg daily should be considered with co-administration).
No products indexed under this heading.

Hypericum (Co-administration of St. John's wort with sunitinib may decrease plasma concentrations of sunitinib unpredictably. Avoid concurrent administration of St. John's wort with sunitinib). Products include:
Satieté Tablets 640

Hypericum Perforatum (Co-administration of St. John's wort with sunitinib may decrease plasma concentrations of sunitinib unpredictably. Avoid concurrent administration of St. John's wort with sunitinib).
No products indexed under this heading.

Indinavir Sulfate (Concurrent administration of sunitinib with strong CYP3A4 inhibitors (e.g., ketoconazole) may increase sunitinib plasma concentrations. Dose reduction of sunitinib to 37.5 mg daily is recommended with co-administration). Products include:
Crixivan Capsules 1979

Itraconazole (Concurrent administration of sunitinib with strong CYP3A4 inhibitors (e.g., ketoconazole) may increase sunitinib plasma concentrations. Dose reduction of sunitinib to 37.5 mg daily is recommended with co-administration).
No products indexed under this heading.

Ketoconazole (Concurrent administration of sunitinib with strong CYP3A4 inhibitors (e.g., ketoconazole) may increase sunitinib plasma concentrations. Dose reduction of

sunitinib to 37.5 mg daily is recommended with co-administration). Products include:
Extina Foam, 2% 3057
Nizoral A-D Shampoo 1901

Lidocaine Hydrochloride (Sunitinib has been shown to prolong QT interval in a dose dependent manner: caution is advised in patients taking sunitinib and antiarrhythmics concomittantly).
No products indexed under this heading.

Lopinavir (Concurrent administration of sunitinib with strong CYP3A4 inhibitors (e.g., ketoconazole) may increase sunitinib plasma concentrations. Dose reduction of sunitinib to 37.5 mg daily is recommended with co-administration). Products include:
Kaletra 452

Mephenytoin (Concurrent administration of sunitinib with CYP3A4 inducers (e.g., rifampin) may decrease plasma sunitinib concentrations. Dose increase of sunitinib to 87.5 mg daily should be considered with co-administration).
No products indexed under this heading.

Methsuximide (Concurrent administration of sunitinib with CYP3A4 inducers (e.g., rifampin) may decrease plasma sunitinib concentrations. Dose increase of sunitinib to 87.5 mg daily should be considered with co-administration).
No products indexed under this heading.

Methylprednisolone (Concurrent administration of sunitinib with CYP3A4 inducers (e.g., rifampin) may decrease plasma sunitinib concentrations. Dose increase of sunitinib to 87.5 mg daily should be considered with co-administration).
No products indexed under this heading.

Methylprednisolone Acetate (Concurrent administration of sunitinib with CYP3A4 inducers (e.g., rifampin) may decrease plasma sunitinib concentrations. Dose increase of sunitinib to 87.5 mg daily should be considered with co-administration).
No products indexed under this heading.

Methylprednisolone Sodium Succinate (Concurrent administration of sunitinib with CYP3A4 inducers (e.g., rifampin) may decrease plasma sunitinib concentrations. Dose increase of sunitinib to 87.5 mg daily should be considered with co-administration).
No products indexed under this heading.

Mexiletine Hydrochloride (Sunitinib has been shown to prolong QT interval in a dose dependent manner: caution is advised in patients taking sunitinib and antiarrhythmics concomittantly).
No products indexed under this heading.

Modafinil (Concurrent administration of sunitinib with CYP3A4 inducers (e.g., rifampin) may decrease plasma sunitinib concentrations. Dose increase of sunitinib to 87.5 mg daily should be considered with co-administration). Products include:
Provigil Tablets 977

Moricizine Hydrochloride (Sunitinib has been shown to prolong QT interval in a dose dependent manner: caution is advised in patients taking sunitinib and antiarrhythmics concomittantly).
No products indexed under this heading.

Nefazodone Hydrochloride (Concurrent administration of sunitinib with strong CYP3A4 inhibitors (e.g., ketoconazole) may increase sunitinib plasma concentrations. Dose reduction of sunitinib to 37.5 mg daily is recommended with co-administration).
No products indexed under this heading.

Nelfinavir Mesylate (Concurrent administration of sunitinib with strong CYP3A4 inhibitors (e.g., ketoconazole) may increase sunitinib plasma concentrations. Dose reduction of sunitinib to 37.5 mg daily is recommended with co-administration).
No products indexed under this heading.

Nevirapine (Concurrent administration of sunitinib with CYP3A4 inducers (e.g., rifampin) may decrease plasma sunitinib concentrations. Dose increase of sunitinib to 87.5 mg daily should be considered with co-administration). Products include:
Viramune Oral Suspension 873
Viramune Tablets 873

Oxcarbazepine (Concurrent administration of sunitinib with CYP3A4 inducers (e.g., rifampin) may decrease plasma sunitinib concentrations. Dose increase of sunitinib to 87.5 mg daily should be considered with co-administration).
No products indexed under this heading.

Phenobarbital (Concurrent administration of sunitinib with CYP3A4 inducers (e.g., rifampin) may decrease plasma sunitinib concentrations. Dose increase of sunitinib to 87.5 mg daily should be considered with co-administration). Products include:
Donnatal Extentabs 2507

Phenobarbital Sodium (Concurrent administration of sunitinib with CYP3A4 inducers (e.g., rifampin) may decrease plasma sunitinib concentrations. Dose increase of sunitinib to 87.5 mg daily should be considered with co-administration).
No products indexed under this heading.

Phenytoin (Concurrent administration of sunitinib with CYP3A4 inducers (e.g., rifampin) may decrease plasma sunitinib concentrations. Dose increase of sunitinib to 87.5 mg daily should be considered with co-administration).
No products indexed under this heading.

Phenytoin Sodium (Concurrent administration of sunitinib with CYP3A4 inducers (e.g., rifampin) may decrease plasma sunitinib concentrations. Dose increase of sunitinib to 87.5 mg daily should be considered with co-administration). Products include:
Phenytek Capsules 2192

Prednisolone Acetate (Concurrent administration of sunitinib with CYP3A4 inducers (e.g., rifampin) may decrease plasma sunitinib concentrations. Dose increase of sunitinib to 87.5 mg daily should be considered with co-administration). Products include:
Pred Forte Ophthalmic Suspension .... ⊙ 227
Pred Mild Ophthalmic Suspension .... ⊙ 230
Pred-G Ophthalmic Ointment .... ⊙ 229
Pred-G Ophthalmic Suspension .... ⊙ 228

Prednisolone Sodium Phosphate (Concurrent administration of sunitinib with CYP3A4 inducers (e.g., rifampin) may decrease plasma sunitinib concentrations. Dose increase of sunitinib to 87.5 mg daily should be considered with co-administration).
No products indexed under this heading.

Prednisolone Tebutate (Concurrent administration of sunitinib with CYP3A4 inducers (e.g., rifampin) may decrease plasma sunitinib concentrations. Dose increase of sunitinib to 87.5 mg daily should be considered with co-administration).
No products indexed under this heading.

Prednisone (Concurrent administration of sunitinib with CYP3A4 inducers (e.g., rifampin) may decrease plasma sunitinib concentrations. Dose increase of sunitinib to 87.5 mg daily should be considered with co-administration).
No products indexed under this heading.

Primidone (Concurrent administration of sunitinib with CYP3A4 inducers (e.g., rifampin) may decrease plasma sunitinib concentrations. Dose increase of sunitinib to 87.5 mg daily should be considered with co-administration).
No products indexed under this heading.

Procainamide Hydrochloride (Sunitinib has been shown to prolong QT interval in a dose dependent manner: caution is advised in patients taking sunitinib and antiarrhythmics concomittantly).
No products indexed under this heading.

Propafenone Hydrochloride (Sunitinib has been shown to prolong QT interval in a dose dependent manner: caution is advised in patients taking sunitinib and antiarrhythmics concomittantly). Products include:
Rythmol Tablets 1586
Rythmol SR Capsules 1590

Propranolol Hydrochloride (Sunitinib has been shown to prolong QT interval in a dose dependent manner: caution is advised in patients taking sunitinib and antiarrhythmics concomittantly). Products include:
InnoPran XL Extended Release Capsules 1484

Quinidine Gluconate (Sunitinib has been shown to prolong QT interval in a dose dependent manner: caution is advised in patients taking sunitinib and antiarrhythmics concomittantly).
No products indexed under this heading.

Quinidine Polygalacturonate (Sunitinib has been shown to prolong QT interval in a dose dependent manner: caution is advised in patients taking sunitinib and antiarrhythmics concomittantly).
No products indexed under this heading.

Quinidine Sulfate (Sunitinib has been shown to prolong QT interval in a dose dependent manner: caution is advised in patients taking sunitinib and antiarrhythmics concomittantly).
No products indexed under this heading.

Rifabutin (Concurrent administration of sunitinib with CYP3A4 inducers (e.g., rifampin) may decrease plasma sunitinib concentrations. Dose increase of sunitinib to 87.5 mg daily should be considered with co-administration).
No products indexed under this heading.

Rifampicin (Concurrent administration of sunitinib with CYP3A4 inducers (e.g., rifampin) may decrease plasma sunitinib concentrations. Dose increase of sunitinib to 87.5 mg daily should be considered with co-administration).
No products indexed under this heading.

Rifampin (Concurrent administration of sunitinib with CYP3A4 inducers (e.g., rifampin) may decrease plasma sunitinib concentrations. Dose increase of sunitinib to 87.5 mg daily should be considered with co-administration).
No products indexed under this heading.

Rifapentine (Concurrent administration of sunitinib with CYP3A4 inducers (e.g., rifampin) may decrease plasma sunitinib concentrations. Dose increase of sunitinib to 87.5 mg daily should be considered with co-administration).
No products indexed under this heading.

Ritonavir (Concurrent administration of sunitinib with strong CYP3A4 inhibitors (e.g., ketoconazole) may increase sunitinib plasma concentrations. Dose reduction of sunitinib to 37.5 mg daily is recommended with co-administration). Products include:
Kaletra 452
Norvir 489

Saquinavir (Concurrent administration of sunitinib with strong CYP3A4 inhibitors (e.g., ketoconazole) may increase sunitinib plasma concentrations. Dose reduction of sunitinib to 37.5 mg daily is recommended with co-administration).
No products indexed under this heading.

Saquinavir Mesylate (Concurrent administration of sunitinib with strong CYP3A4 inhibitors (e.g., ketoconazole) may increase sunitinib plasma concentrations. Dose reduction of sunitinib to 37.5 mg daily is recommended with co-administration).
No products indexed under this heading.

Sotalol Hydrochloride (Sunitinib has been shown to prolong QT interval in a dose dependent manner: caution is advised in patients taking sunitinib and antiarrhythmics concomittantly).
No products indexed under this heading.

Sulfinpyrazone (Concurrent administration of sunitinib with CYP3A4 inducers (e.g., rifampin) may decrease plasma sunitinib concentrations. Dose increase of sunitinib to 87.5 mg daily should be considered with co-administration).
No products indexed under this heading.

Telithromycin (Concurrent administration of sunitinib with strong CYP3A4 inhibitors (e.g., ketoconazole) may increase sunitinib plasma concentrations. Dose reduction of sunitinib to 37.5 mg daily is recommended with co-administration). Products include:
Ketek Tablets 2744

Theophylline (Concurrent administration of sunitinib with CYP3A4 inducers (e.g., rifampin) may decrease plasma sunitinib concentrations. Dose increase of sunitinib to 87.5 mg daily should be considered with co-administration).
No products indexed under this heading.

Theophylline Anhydrous (Concurrent administration of sunitinib with CYP3A4 inducers (e.g., rifampin) may decrease plasma sunitinib concentrations. Dose increase of sunitinib to 87.5 mg daily should be considered with co-administration). Products include:
Uniphyl Tablets 2595

Theophylline Calcium Salicylate (Concurrent administration of sunitinib with CYP3A4 inducers (e.g., rifampin) may decrease plasma sunitinib concentrations. Dose increase of sunitinib to 87.5 mg daily should be considered with co-administration).
No products indexed under this heading.

Theophylline Dihydroxypropyl (Glyceryl) (Concurrent administration of sunitinib with CYP3A4 inducers (e.g., rifampin) may decrease plasma sunitinib concentrations. Dose increase of sunitinib to 87.5 mg daily should be considered with co-administration).
No products indexed under this heading.

Theophylline Ethylenediamine (Concurrent administration of sunitinib with CYP3A4 inducers (e.g., rifampin) may decrease plasma sunitinib concentrations. Dose increase of sunitinib to 87.5 mg daily should be considered with co-administration).
No products indexed under this heading.

Tocainide Hydrochloride (Sunitinib has been shown to prolong QT interval in a dose dependent manner: caution is advised in patients taking sunitinib and antiarrhythmics concomittantly).
No products indexed under this heading.

Triamcinolone (Concurrent administration of sunitinib with CYP3A4 inducers (e.g., rifampin) may decrease plasma sunitinib concentrations. Dose increase of sunitinib to 87.5 mg daily should be considered with co-administration).
No products indexed under this heading.

Triamcinolone Acetonide (Concurrent administration of sunitinib with CYP3A4 inducers (e.g., rifampin) may decrease plasma sunitinib concentrations. Dose increase of sunitinib to 87.5 mg daily should be considered with co-administration). Products include:
Azmacort Inhalation Aerosol 407
Nasacort AQ Nasal Spray 2765
Triesence Injectable Suspension .... ⊙209

Triamcinolone Diacetate (Concurrent administration of sunitinib with CYP3A4 inducers (e.g., rifampin) may decrease plasma sunitinib concentrations. Dose increase of sunitinib to 87.5 mg daily should be considered with co-administration).
No products indexed under this heading.

Triamcinolone Hexacetonide (Concurrent administration of sunitinib with CYP3A4 inducers (e.g., rifampin) may decrease plasma sunitinib concentrations. Dose increase of sunitinib to 87.5 mg daily should be considered with co-administration).
No products indexed under this heading.

Troglitazone (Concurrent administration of sunitinib with CYP3A4 inducers (e.g., rifampin) may decrease plasma sunitinib concentrations. Dose increase of sunitinib to 87.5 mg daily should be considered with co-administration).
No products indexed under this heading.

Troleandomycin (Concurrent administration of sunitinib with strong CYP3A4 inhibitors (e.g., ketoconazole) may increase sunitinib plasma concentrations. Dose reduction of sunitinib to 37.5 mg daily is recommended with co-administration).
No products indexed under this heading.

Verapamil Hydrochloride (Sunitinib has been shown to prolong QT interval in a dose dependent manner: caution is advised in patients taking sunitinib and antiarrhythmics concomittantly). Products include:
Tarka Tablets 511

Voriconazole (Concurrent administration of sunitinib with strong CYP3A4 inhibitors (e.g., ketoconazole) may increase sunitinib plasma concentrations. Dose reduction of sunitinib to 37.5 mg daily is recommended with co-administration).
No products indexed under this heading.

Food Interactions

Grapefruit (Grapefruit may increase plasma concentrations of sunitinib maleate).

Grapefruit Juice (Grapefruit may increase plasma concentrations of sunitinib maleate).

SYMBICORT 80/4.5 INHALATION AEROSOL

(Budesonide, Formoterol fumarate dihydrate).. 659

May interact with beta blockers, cytochrome p450 3a4 inhibitors (selected), diuretics, monoamine oxidase inhibitors, tricyclic antidepressants, and certain other agents. Compounds in these categories include:

Acebutolol Hydrochloride (Beta-blockers (including eye drops) may not only block the pulmonary effect of beta-agonists (e.g., formoterol- a component of Symbicort), but may produce severe bronchospasm in asthma patients).
No products indexed under this heading.

Acetazolamide (Concomitant administration of CYP3A4 inhibitors (e.g., itraconazole, clarithromycin, erythromycin, etc.) may inhibit the metabolism of, and increase the systemic exposure to, budesonide. Caution should be exercised with co-administration of Symbicort with potent CYP3A4 inhibitors).
No products indexed under this heading.

Amiloride Hydrochloride (The ECG changes and/or hypokalemia that may result from the administration of nonpotassium-sparing diuretics (e.g., loop or thiazide diuretics) can be acutely worsened by beta-agonists, especially when the recommended dose of the beta-agonist is exceeded. Caution is advised with co-administration of Symbicort with nonpotassium-sparing diuretics).
No products indexed under this heading.

Amiodarone Hydrochloride (Concomitant administration of CYP3A4 inhibitors (e.g., itraconazole, clarithromycin, erythromycin, etc.) may inhibit the metabolism of, and increase the systemic exposure to, budesonide. Caution should be exercised with co-administration of Symbicort with potent CYP3A4 inhibitors).
No products indexed under this heading.

Amitriptyline Hydrochloride (Symbicort should be administered with caution to patients treated with TCAs, or within 2 weeks of discontinuation of TCAs, since these agents may potentiate formoterol action on the vascular system).
No products indexed under this heading.

Amoxapine (Symbicort should be administered with caution to patients treated with TCAs, or within 2 weeks of discontinuation of TCAs, since these agents may potentiate formoterol action on the vascular system).
No products indexed under this heading.

Amprenavir (Concomitant administration of CYP3A4 inhibitors (e.g., itraconazole, clarithromycin, erythromycin, etc.) may inhibit the metabolism of, and increase the systemic exposure to, budesonide. Caution should be exercised with co-administration of Symbicort with potent CYP3A4 inhibitors).
No products indexed under this heading.

Anastrozole (Concomitant administration of CYP3A4 inhibitors (e.g., itraconazole, clarithromycin, erythromycin, etc.) may inhibit the metabolism of, and increase the systemic exposure to, budesonide. Caution should be exercised with co-administration of Symbicort with potent CYP3A4 inhibitors). Products include:
Arimidex Tablets 672

Aprepitant (Concomitant administration of CYP3A4 inhibitors (e.g., itraconazole, clarithromycin, erythromycin, etc.) may inhibit the metabolism of, and increase the systemic exposure to, budesonide. Caution should be exercised with co-administration of Symbicort with potent CYP3A4 inhibitors). Products include:
Emend Capsules 1992

Atazanavir (Concomitant administration of CYP3A4 inhibitors (e.g., itraconazole, clarithromycin, erythromycin, etc.) may inhibit the metabolism of, and increase the systemic exposure to, budesonide. Caution should be exercised with co-administration of Symbicort with potent CYP3A4 inhibitors).
No products indexed under this heading.

Atazanavir Sulfate (Concomitant administration of CYP3A4 inhibitors (e.g., itraconazole, clarithromycin, erythromycin, etc.) may inhibit the metabolism of, and increase the systemic exposure to, budesonide. Caution should be exercised with co-administration of Symbicort with potent CYP3A4 inhibitors). Products include:
Reyataz Capsules 3299

Atenolol (Beta-blockers (including eye drops) may not only block the pulmonary effect of beta-agonists (e.g., formoterol- a component of Symbicort), but may produce severe bronchospasm in asthma patients).
No products indexed under this heading.

Bendroflumethiazide (The ECG changes and/or hypokalemia that may result from the administration of nonpotassium-sparing diuretics (e.g., loop or thiazide diuretics) can be acutely worsened by beta-agonists, especially when the recommended dose of the beta-agonist is exceeded. Caution is advised with co-administration of Symbicort with nonpotassium-sparing diuretics).
No products indexed under this heading.

Betaxolol Hydrochloride (Beta-blockers (including eye drops) may not only block the pulmonary effect of beta-agonists (e.g., formoterol- a component of Symbicort), but may produce severe bronchospasm in asthma patients).
No products indexed under this heading.

Bisoprolol Fumarate (Beta-blockers (including eye drops) may not only block the pulmonary effect of beta-agonists (e.g., formoterol- a component of Symbicort), but may produce severe bronchospasm in asthma patients).
No products indexed under this heading.

Bumetanide (The ECG changes and/or hypokalemia that may result from the administration of nonpotassium-sparing diuretics (e.g., loop or thiazide diuretics) can be acutely worsened by beta-agonists, especially when the recommended dose of the beta-agonist is exceeded. Caution is advised with co-administration of Symbicort with nonpotassium-sparing diuretics).
No products indexed under this heading.

Carteolol Hydrochloride (Beta-blockers (including eye drops) may not only block the pulmonary effect of beta-agonists (e.g., formoterol- a component of Symbicort), but may produce severe bronchospasm in asthma patients).
No products indexed under this heading.

Chlorothiazide (The ECG changes and/or hypokalemia that may result from the administration of nonpotassium-sparing diuretics (e.g., loop or thiazide diuretics) can be acutely worsened by beta-agonists, especially when the recommended dose of the beta-agonist is exceeded. Caution is advised with co-administration of Symbicort with nonpotassium-sparing diuretics).
No products indexed under this heading.

Chlorothiazide Sodium (The ECG changes and/or hypokalemia that may result from the administration of nonpotassium-sparing diuretics (e.g., loop or thiazide diuretics) can be acutely worsened by beta-agonists, especially when the recommended dose of the beta-agonist is exceeded. Caution is advised with co-administration of Symbicort with nonpotassium-sparing diuretics). Products include:
Intravenous Sodium Diuril 2490

Chlorthalidone (The ECG changes and/or hypokalemia that may result from the administration of nonpotassium-sparing diuretics (e.g., loop or thiazide diuretics) can be acutely worsened by beta-agonists, especially when the recommended dose of the beta-agonist is exceeded. Caution is advised with co-administration of Symbicort with nonpotassium-sparing diuretics). Products include:
Clorpres Tablets 2185

Cimetidine (Concomitant administration of CYP3A4 inhibitors (e.g., itraconazole, clarithromycin, erythromycin, etc.) may inhibit the metabolism of, and increase the systemic exposure to, budesonide. Caution should be exercised with co-administration of Symbicort with potent CYP3A4 inhibitors).
No products indexed under this heading.

Cimetidine Hydrochloride (Concomitant administration of CYP3A4 inhibitors (e.g., itraconazole, clarithromycin, erythromycin, etc.) may inhibit the metabolism of, and increase the systemic exposure to, budesonide. Caution should be exercised with co-administration of Symbicort with potent CYP3A4 inhibitors).
No products indexed under this heading.

Ciprofloxacin (Concomitant administration of CYP3A4 inhibitors (e.g., itraconazole, clarithromycin, erythromycin, etc.) may inhibit the metabolism of, and increase the systemic exposure to, budesonide. Caution should be exercised with co-administration of Symbicort with potent CYP3A4 inhibitors). Products include:
Cipro I.V. 2817
Cipro Oral Suspension 2810
Cipro XR Tablets 2823
Ciprodex Otic Suspension 541

Clarithromycin (Concomitant administration of CYP3A4 inhibitors (e.g., itraconazole, clarithromycin, erythromycin, etc.) may inhibit the metabolism of, and increase the systemic exposure to, budesonide. Caution should be exercised with co-administration of Symbicort with potent CYP3A4 inhibitors). Products include:
Biaxin/Biaxin XL 411

Clomipramine Hydrochloride (Symbicort should be administered with caution to patients treated with TCAs, or within 2 weeks of discontinuation of TCAs, since these agents may potentiate formoterol action on the vascular system).
No products indexed under this heading.

Clotrimazole (Concomitant administration of CYP3A4 inhibitors (e.g., itraconazole, clarithromycin, erythromycin, etc.) may inhibit the metabolism of, and increase the systemic exposure to, budesonide. Caution should be exercised with co-administration of Symbicort with potent CYP3A4 inhibitors). Products include:
Lotrisone 2881

Cyclosporine (Concomitant administration of CYP3A4 inhibitors (e.g., itraconazole, clarithromycin, erythromycin, etc.) may inhibit the metabolism of, and increase the systemic exposure to, budesonide. Caution should be exercised with co-administration of Symbicort with potent CYP3A4 inhibitors). Products include:
Gengraf Capsules 435
Neoral Oral Solution 2280
Neoral Soft Gelatin Capsules 2280
Restasis Ophthalmic Emulsion 557
Sandimmune 2296

Dalfopristin (Concomitant administration of CYP3A4 inhibitors (e.g., itraconazole, clarithromycin, erythromycin, etc.) may inhibit the metabolism of, and increase the systemic exposure to, budesonide. Caution should be exercised with co-administration of Symbicort with potent CYP3A4 inhibitors).
No products indexed under this heading.

Danazol (Concomitant administration of CYP3A4 inhibitors (e.g., itraconazole, clarithromycin, erythromycin, etc.) may inhibit the metabolism of, and increase the systemic exposure to, budesonide. Caution should be exercised with co-administration of Symbicort with potent CYP3A4 inhibitors).
No products indexed under this heading.

Delavirdine Mesylate (Concomitant administration of CYP3A4 inhibitors (e.g., itraconazole, clarithromycin, erythromycin, etc.) may inhibit the metabolism of, and increase the systemic exposure to, budesonide. Caution should be exercised with co-administration of Symbicort with potent CYP3A4 inhibitors).
No products indexed under this heading.

Desipramine Hydrochloride (Symbicort should be administered with caution to patients treated with TCAs, or within 2 weeks of discontinuation of TCAs, since these agents may potentiate formoterol action on the vascular system).
No products indexed under this heading.

Diltiazem Hydrochloride (Concomitant administration of CYP3A4 inhibitors (e.g., itraconazole, clarithromycin, erythromycin, etc.) may inhibit the metabolism of, and increase the systemic exposure to, budesonide. Caution should be exercised with co-administration of Symbicort with potent CYP3A4 inhibitors). Products include:
Cardizem LA Extended Release Tablets 421

Diltiazem Maleate (Concomitant administration of CYP3A4 inhibitors (e.g., itraconazole, clarithromycin, erythromycin, etc.) may inhibit the metabolism of, and increase the systemic exposure to, budesonide. Caution should be exercised with co-administration of Symbicort with potent CYP3A4 inhibitors).
No products indexed under this heading.

Doxepin Hydrochloride (Symbicort should be administered with caution to patients treated with TCAs, or within 2 weeks of discontinuation of TCAs, since these agents may potentiate formoterol action on the vascular system).
No products indexed under this heading.

Efavirenz (Concomitant administration of CYP3A4 inhibitors (e.g., itraconazole, clarithromycin, erythromycin, etc.) may inhibit the metabolism of, and increase the systemic exposure to, budesonide. Caution should be exercised with co-administration of Symbicort with potent CYP3A4 inhibitors). Products include:
Atripla Tablets 938
Sustiva Capsules 930
Sustiva Tablets 930

Erythromycin (Concomitant administration of CYP3A4 inhibitors (e.g., itraconazole, clarithromycin, erythromycin, etc.) may inhibit the metabolism of, and increase the systemic exposure to, budesonide. Caution should be exercised with co-administration of Symbicort with potent CYP3A4 inhibitors).
No products indexed under this heading.

Erythromycin Estolate (Concomitant administration of CYP3A4 inhibitors (e.g., itraconazole, clarithromycin, erythromycin, etc.) may inhibit the metabolism of, and increase the systemic exposure to, budesonide. Caution should be exercised with co-administration of Symbicort with potent CYP3A4 inhibitors).
No products indexed under this heading.

Erythromycin Ethylsuccinate (Concomitant administration of CYP3A4 inhibitors (e.g., itraconazole, clarithromycin, erythromycin, etc.) may inhibit the metabolism of, and increase the systemic exposure to, budesonide. Caution should be exercised with co-administration of Symbicort with potent CYP3A4 inhibitors). Products include:
E.E.S. 433
EryPed 431

Erythromycin Gluceptate (Concomitant administration of CYP3A4 inhibitors (e.g., itraconazole, clarithromycin, erythromycin, etc.) may inhibit the metabolism of, and increase the systemic exposure to, budesonide. Caution should be exercised with co-administration of Symbicort with potent CYP3A4 inhibitors).
No products indexed under this heading.

Erythromycin Lactobionate (Concomitant administration of CYP3A4 inhibitors (e.g., itraconazole, clarithromycin, erythromycin, etc.) may inhibit the metabolism of, and increase the systemic exposure to, budesonide. Caution should be exercised with co-administration of Symbicort with potent CYP3A4 inhibitors).
No products indexed under this heading.

Erythromycin Stearate (Concomitant administration of CYP3A4 inhibitors (e.g., itraconazole, clarithromycin, erythromycin, etc.) may inhibit the metabolism of, and increase the systemic exposure to, budesonide. Caution should be exercised with co-administration of Symbicort with potent CYP3A4 inhibitors).
No products indexed under this heading.

Esmolol Hydrochloride (Beta-blockers (including eye drops) may not only block the pulmonary effect of beta-agonists (e.g., formoterol- a component of Symbicort), but may produce severe bronchospasm in asthma patients).
No products indexed under this heading.

Esomeprazole Magnesium (Concomitant administration of CYP3A4 inhibitors (e.g., itraconazole, clarithromycin, erythromycin, etc.) may inhibit the metabolism of, and increase the systemic exposure to, budesonide. Caution should be exercised with co-administration of Symbicort with potent CYP3A4 inhibitors). Products include:
Nexium Delayed-Release Capsules 645
Nexium Delayed-Release Oral Suspension 645

Ethacrynic Acid (The ECG changes and/or hypokalemia that may result from the administration of nonpotassium-sparing diuretics (e.g., loop or thiazide diuretics) can be acutely worsened by beta-agonists, especially when the recommended dose of the beta-agonist is exceeded. Caution is advised with co-administration of Symbicort with nonpotassium-sparing diuretics). Products include:
Edecrin Tablets 698

Fluconazole (Concomitant administration of CYP3A4 inhibitors (e.g., itraconazole, clarithromycin, erythromycin, etc.) may inhibit the metabolism of, and increase the systemic exposure to, budesonide. Caution should be exercised with co-administration of Symbicort with potent CYP3A4 inhibitors).
No products indexed under this heading.

Fluoxetine (Concomitant administration of CYP3A4 inhibitors (e.g., itraconazole, clarithromycin, erythromycin, etc.) may inhibit the metabolism of, and increase the systemic exposure to, budesonide. Caution should be exercised with co-administration of Symbicort with potent CYP3A4 inhibitors).
No products indexed under this heading.

Fluoxetine Hydrochloride (Concomitant administration of CYP3A4 inhibitors (e.g., itraconazole, clarithromycin, erythromycin, etc.) may inhibit the metabolism of, and increase the systemic exposure to, budesonide. Caution should be exer-

cised with co-administration of Symbicort with potent CYP3A4 inhibitors). Products include:
Prozac Weekly Capsules 1852
Prozac Pulvules and Liquid 1852
Symbyax Capsules 1871

Fluvoxamine Maleate (Concomitant administration of CYP3A4 inhibitors (e.g., itraconazole, clarithromycin, erythromycin, etc.) may inhibit the metabolism of, and increase the systemic exposure to, budesonide. Caution should be exercised with co-administration of Symbicort with potent CYP3A4 inhibitors). Products include:
Luvox CR Extended-Release Capsules 1759

Fosamprenavir Calcium (Concomitant administration of CYP3A4 inhibitors (e.g., itraconazole, clarithromycin, erythromycin, etc.) may inhibit the metabolism of, and increase the systemic exposure to, budesonide. Caution should be exercised with co-administration of Symbicort with potent CYP3A4 inhibitors). Products include:
Lexiva Oral Suspension 1510
Lexiva Tablets 1510

Furosemide (The ECG changes and/or hypokalemia that may result from the administration of nonpotassium-sparing diuretics (e.g., loop or thiazide diuretics) can be acutely worsened by beta-agonists, especially when the recommended dose of the beta-agonist is exceeded. Caution is advised with co-administration of Symbicort with nonpotassium-sparing diuretics). Products include:
Furosemide Tablets 2186

Hydrochlorothiazide (The ECG changes and/or hypokalemia that may result from the administration of nonpotassium-sparing diuretics (e.g., loop or thiazide diuretics) can be acutely worsened by beta-agonists, especially when the recommended dose of the beta-agonist is exceeded. Caution is advised with co-administration of Symbicort with nonpotassium-sparing diuretics). Products include:
Atacand HCT 642
Avalide Tablets 892
Avalide Tablets 2713
Benicar HCT Tablets 1010
Diovan HCT Tablets 2216
Dyazide Capsules 1405
Micardis HCT Tablets 854
Prinzide Tablets 2092
Tekturna HCT Tablets 2324
Teveten HCT Tablets 517

Hydroflumethiazide (The ECG changes and/or hypokalemia that may result from the administration of nonpotassium-sparing diuretics (e.g., loop or thiazide diuretics) can be acutely worsened by beta-agonists, especially when the recommended dose of the beta-agonist is exceeded. Caution is advised with co-administration of Symbicort with nonpotassium-sparing diuretics).
No products indexed under this heading.

Imipramine Hydrochloride (Symbicort should be administered with caution to patients treated with TCAs, or within 2 weeks of discontinuation of TCAs, since these agents may potentiate formoterol action on the vascular system).
No products indexed under this heading.

Imipramine Pamoate (Symbicort should be administered with caution to patients treated with TCAs, or within 2 weeks of discontinuation of TCAs, since these agents may potentiate formoterol action on the vascular system).
No products indexed under this heading.

Indapamide (The ECG changes and/or hypokalemia that may result from the administration of nonpotassium-sparing diuretics (e.g., loop or thiazide diuretics) can be acutely worsened by beta-agonists, especially when the recommended dose of the beta-agonist is exceeded. Caution is advised with co-administration of Symbicort with nonpotassium-sparing diuretics). Products include:
Indapamide Tablets 2188

Indinavir Sulfate (Concomitant administration of CYP3A4 inhibitors (e.g., itraconazole, clarithromycin, erythromycin, etc.) may inhibit the metabolism of, and increase the systemic exposure to, budesonide. Caution should be exercised with co-administration of Symbicort with potent CYP3A4 inhibitors). Products include:
Crixivan Capsules 1979

Isocarboxazid (Symbicort should be administered with caution to patients treated with MAOIs, or within 2 weeks of discontinuation of MAOIs, since these agents may potentiate formoterol action on the vascular system). Products include:
Marplan Tablets 3177

Isoniazid (Concomitant administration of CYP3A4 inhibitors (e.g., itraconazole, clarithromycin, erythromycin, etc.) may inhibit the metabolism of, and increase the systemic exposure to, budesonide. Caution should be exercised with co-administration of Symbicort with potent CYP3A4 inhibitors).
No products indexed under this heading.

Itraconazole (Concomitant administration of CYP3A4 inhibitors (e.g., itraconazole, clarithromycin, erythromycin, etc.) may inhibit the metabolism of, and increase the systemic exposure to, budesonide. Caution should be exercised with co-administration of Symbicort with potent CYP3A4 inhibitors).
No products indexed under this heading.

Ketoconazole (Co-administration of ketoconazole and Symbicort increases the mean plasma concentration of orally administered budesonide. Caution should be excercised when considering co-administration of Symbicort with long-term ketoconazole). Products include:
Extina Foam, 2% 3057
Nizoral A-D Shampoo 1901

Labetalol Hydrochloride (Beta-blockers (including eye drops) may not only block the pulmonary effect of beta-agonists (e.g., formoterol- a component of Symbicort), but may produce severe bronchospasm in asthma patients).
No products indexed under this heading.

Levobunolol Hydrochloride (Beta-blockers (including eye drops) may not only block the pulmonary effect of beta-agonists (e.g., formoterol- a component of Symbicort), but may produce severe bronchospasm in asthma patients).
No products indexed under this heading.

Lopinavir (Concomitant administration of CYP3A4 inhibitors (e.g., itraconazole, clarithromycin, erythromycin, etc.) may inhibit the metabolism of, and increase the systemic exposure to, budesonide. Caution should be exercised with co-administration of Symbicort with potent CYP3A4 inhibitors). Products include:
Kaletra 452

Loratadine (Concomitant administration of CYP3A4 inhibitors (e.g., itraconazole, clarithromycin, erythromycin, etc.) may inhibit the metabolism of, and increase the systemic exposure to, budesonide. Caution should be exercised with co-administration of Symbicort with potent CYP3A4 inhibitors).
No products indexed under this heading.

Maprotiline Hydrochloride (Symbicort should be administered with caution to patients treated with TCAs, or within 2 weeks of discontinuation of TCAs, since these agents may potentiate formoterol action on the vascular system).
No products indexed under this heading.

Methyclothiazide (The ECG changes and/or hypokalemia that may result from the administration of nonpotassium-sparing diuretics (e.g., loop or thiazide diuretics) can be acutely worsened by beta-agonists, especially when the recommended dose of the beta-agonist is exceeded. Caution is advised with co-administration of Symbicort with nonpotassium-sparing diuretics).
No products indexed under this heading.

Metipranolol Hydrochloride (Beta-blockers (including eye drops) may not only block the pulmonary effect of beta-agonists (e.g., formoterol- a component of Symbicort), but may produce severe bronchospasm in asthma patients).
No products indexed under this heading.

Metolazone (The ECG changes and/or hypokalemia that may result from the administration of nonpotassium-sparing diuretics (e.g., loop or thiazide diuretics) can be acutely worsened by beta-agonists, especially when the recommended dose of the beta-agonist is exceeded. Caution is advised with co-administration of Symbicort with nonpotassium-sparing diuretics).
No products indexed under this heading.

Metoprolol Succinate (Beta-blockers (including eye drops) may not only block the pulmonary effect of beta-agonists (e.g., formoterol- a component of Symbicort), but may produce severe bronchospasm in asthma patients). Products include:
Toprol-XL Tablets 666

Metoprolol Tartrate (Beta-blockers (including eye drops) may not only block the pulmonary effect of beta-agonists (e.g., formoterol- a component of Symbicort), but may produce severe bronchospasm in asthma patients).
No products indexed under this heading.

Metronidazole (Concomitant administration of CYP3A4 inhibitors (e.g., itraconazole, clarithromycin, erythromycin, etc.) may inhibit the metabolism of, and increase the systemic exposure to, budesonide. Caution should be exercised with co-administration of Symbicort with potent CYP3A4 inhibitors). Products include:
Pylera Capsules 714

Metronidazole Benzoate (Concomitant administration of CYP3A4 inhibitors (e.g., itraconazole, clarithromycin, erythromycin, etc.) may inhibit the metabolism of, and increase the systemic exposure to, budesonide. Caution should be exercised with co-administration of Symbicort with potent CYP3A4 inhibitors).
No products indexed under this heading.

Metronidazole Hydrochloride (Concomitant administration of CYP3A4 inhibitors (e.g., itraconazole, clarithromycin, erythromycin, etc.) may inhibit the metabolism of, and increase the systemic exposure to, budesonide. Caution should be exercised with co-administration of Symbicort with potent CYP3A4 inhibitors).
No products indexed under this heading.

Metronidazole Sodium (Concomitant administration of CYP3A4 inhibitors (e.g., itraconazole, clarithromycin, erythromycin, etc.) may inhibit the metabolism of, and increase the systemic exposure to, budesonide. Caution should be exercised with co-administration of Symbicort with potent CYP3A4 inhibitors).
No products indexed under this heading.

Miconazole (Concomitant administration of CYP3A4 inhibitors (e.g., itraconazole, clarithromycin, erythromycin, etc.) may inhibit the metabolism of, and increase the systemic exposure to, budesonide. Caution should be exercised with co-administration of Symbicort with potent CYP3A4 inhibitors).
No products indexed under this heading.

Miconazole Nitrate (Concomitant administration of CYP3A4 inhibitors (e.g., itraconazole, clarithromycin, erythromycin, etc.) may inhibit the metabolism of, and increase the systemic exposure to, budesonide. Caution should be exercised with co-administration of Symbicort with potent CYP3A4 inhibitors).
No products indexed under this heading.

Moclobemide (Symbicort should be administered with caution to patients treated with MAOIs, or within 2 weeks of discontinuation of MAOIs, since these agents may potentiate formoterol action on the vascular system).
No products indexed under this heading.

Nadolol (Beta-blockers (including eye drops) may not only block the

pulmonary effect of beta-agonists (e.g., formoterol- a component of Symbicort), but may produce severe bronchospasm in asthma patients). Products include:

Nadolol Tablets 2191

Nebivolol (Beta-blockers (including eye drops) may not only block the pulmonary effect of beta-agonists (e.g., formoterol- a component of Symbicort), but may produce severe bronchospasm in asthma patients). Products include:

Bystolic Tablets 1155

Nefazodone Hydrochloride (Concomitant administration of CYP3A4 inhibitors (e.g., itraconazole, clarithromycin, erythromycin, etc.) may inhibit the metabolism of, and increase the systemic exposure to, budesonide. Caution should be exercised with co-administration of Symbicort with potent CYP3A4 inhibitors).

No products indexed under this heading.

Nelfinavir Mesylate (Concomitant administration of CYP3A4 inhibitors (e.g., itraconazole, clarithromycin, erythromycin, etc.) may inhibit the metabolism of, and increase the systemic exposure to, budesonide. Caution should be exercised with co-administration of Symbicort with potent CYP3A4 inhibitors).

No products indexed under this heading.

Nevirapine (Concomitant administration of CYP3A4 inhibitors (e.g., itraconazole, clarithromycin, erythromycin, etc.) may inhibit the metabolism of, and increase the systemic exposure to, budesonide. Caution should be exercised with co-administration of Symbicort with potent CYP3A4 inhibitors). Products include:

Viramune Oral Suspension 873

Viramune Tablets 873

Niacinamide (Concomitant administration of CYP3A4 inhibitors (e.g., itraconazole, clarithromycin, erythromycin, etc.) may inhibit the metabolism of, and increase the systemic exposure to, budesonide. Caution should be exercised with co-administration of Symbicort with potent CYP3A4 inhibitors). Products include:

BioLean Free Tablets .... ▣635

Nicotinamide (Concomitant administration of CYP3A4 inhibitors (e.g., itraconazole, clarithromycin, erythromycin, etc.) may inhibit the metabolism of, and increase the systemic exposure to, budesonide. Caution should be exercised with co-administration of Symbicort with potent CYP3A4 inhibitors).

No products indexed under this heading.

Nifedipine (Concomitant administration of CYP3A4 inhibitors (e.g., itraconazole, clarithromycin, erythromycin, etc.) may inhibit the metabolism of, and increase the systemic exposure to, budesonide. Caution should be exercised with co-administration of Symbicort with potent CYP3A4 inhibitors).

No products indexed under this heading.

Norfloxacin (Concomitant administration of CYP3A4 inhibitors (e.g., itraconazole, clarithromycin, erythromycin, etc.) may inhibit the metabolism of, and increase the systemic exposure to, budesonide. Caution should be exercised with co-administration of Symbicort with potent CYP3A4 inhibitors). Products include:

Noroxin Tablets 2069

Nortriptyline Hydrochloride (Symbicort should be administered with caution to patients treated with TCAs, or within 2 weeks of discontinuation of TCAs, since these agents may potentiate formoterol action on the vascular system).

No products indexed under this heading.

Omeprazole (Concomitant administration of CYP3A4 inhibitors (e.g., itraconazole, clarithromycin, erythromycin, etc.) may inhibit the metabolism of, and increase the systemic exposure to, budesonide. Caution should be exercised with co-administration of Symbicort with potent CYP3A4 inhibitors).

No products indexed under this heading.

Pargyline Hydrochloride (Symbicort should be administered with caution to patients treated with MAOIs, or within 2 weeks of discontinuation of MAOIs, since these agents may potentiate formoterol action on the vascular system).

No products indexed under this heading.

Paroxetine Hydrochloride (Concomitant administration of CYP3A4 inhibitors (e.g., itraconazole, clarithromycin, erythromycin, etc.) may inhibit the metabolism of, and increase the systemic exposure to, budesonide. Caution should be exercised with co-administration of Symbicort with potent CYP3A4 inhibitors). Products include:

Paxil 1535

Paxil CR Controlled-Release Tablets 1544

Penbutolol Sulfate (Beta-blockers (including eye drops) may not only block the pulmonary effect of beta-agonists (e.g., formoterol- a component of Symbicort), but may produce severe bronchospasm in asthma patients).

No products indexed under this heading.

Phenelzine Sulfate (Symbicort should be administered with caution to patients treated with MAOIs, or within 2 weeks of discontinuation of MAOIs, since these agents may potentiate formoterol action on the vascular system).

No products indexed under this heading.

Pindolol (Beta-blockers (including eye drops) may not only block the pulmonary effect of beta-agonists (e.g., formoterol- a component of Symbicort), but may produce severe bronchospasm in asthma patients).

No products indexed under this heading.

Polythiazide (The ECG changes and/or hypokalemia that may result from the administration of nonpotassium-sparing diuretics (e.g., loop or thiazide diuretics) can be acutely worsened by beta-agonists, especially when the recommended dose of the beta-agonist is exceeded. Caution is advised with co-administration of Symbicort with nonpotassium-sparing diuretics).

No products indexed under this heading.

Procarbazine Hydrochloride (Symbicort should be administered with caution to patients treated with MAOIs, or within 2 weeks of discontinuation of MAOIs, since these agents may potentiate formoterol action on the vascular system).

No products indexed under this heading.

Propoxyphene Hydrochloride (Concomitant administration of CYP3A4 inhibitors (e.g., itraconazole, clarithromycin, erythromycin, etc.) may inhibit the metabolism of, and increase the systemic exposure to, budesonide. Caution should be exercised with co-administration of Symbicort with potent CYP3A4 inhibitors).

No products indexed under this heading.

Propoxyphene Napsylate (Concomitant administration of CYP3A4 inhibitors (e.g., itraconazole, clarithromycin, erythromycin, etc.) may inhibit the metabolism of, and increase the systemic exposure to, budesonide. Caution should be exercised with co-administration of Symbicort with potent CYP3A4 inhibitors).

No products indexed under this heading.

Propranolol Hydrochloride (Beta-blockers (including eye drops) may not only block the pulmonary effect of beta-agonists (e.g., formoterol- a component of Symbicort), but may produce severe bronchospasm in asthma patients). Products include:

InnoPran XL Extended Release Capsules 1484

Protriptyline Hydrochloride (Symbicort should be administered with caution to patients treated with TCAs, or within 2 weeks of discontinuation of TCAs, since these agents may potentiate formoterol action on the vascular system).

No products indexed under this heading.

Quinidine (Concomitant administration of CYP3A4 inhibitors (e.g., itraconazole, clarithromycin, erythromycin, etc.) may inhibit the metabolism of, and increase the systemic exposure to, budesonide. Caution should be exercised with co-administration of Symbicort with potent CYP3A4 inhibitors).

No products indexed under this heading.

Quinidine Hydrochloride (Concomitant administration of CYP3A4 inhibitors (e.g., itraconazole, clarithromycin, erythromycin, etc.) may inhibit the metabolism of, and increase the systemic exposure to, budesonide. Caution should be exercised with co-administration of Symbicort with potent CYP3A4 inhibitors).

No products indexed under this heading.

Quinidine Polygalacturonate (Concomitant administration of CYP3A4 inhibitors (e.g., itraconazole, clarithromycin, erythromycin, etc.) may inhibit the metabolism of, and increase the systemic exposure to, budesonide. Caution should be exercised with co-administration of Symbicort with potent CYP3A4 inhibitors).

No products indexed under this heading.

Quinidine Sulfate (Concomitant administration of CYP3A4 inhibitors (e.g., itraconazole, clarithromycin, erythromycin, etc.) may inhibit the metabolism of, and increase the systemic exposure to, budesonide. Caution should be exercised with co-administration of Symbicort with potent CYP3A4 inhibitors).

No products indexed under this heading.

Quinine (Concomitant administration of CYP3A4 inhibitors (e.g., itraconazole, clarithromycin, erythromycin, etc.) may inhibit the metabolism of, and increase the systemic exposure to, budesonide. Caution should be exercised with co-administration of Symbicort with potent CYP3A4 inhibitors).

No products indexed under this heading.

Quinine Sulfate (Concomitant administration of CYP3A4 inhibitors (e.g., itraconazole, clarithromycin, erythromycin, etc.) may inhibit the metabolism of, and increase the systemic exposure to, budesonide. Caution should be exercised with co-administration of Symbicort with potent CYP3A4 inhibitors).

No products indexed under this heading.

Quinupristin (Concomitant administration of CYP3A4 inhibitors (e.g., itraconazole, clarithromycin, erythromycin, etc.) may inhibit the metabolism of, and increase the systemic exposure to, budesonide. Caution should be exercised with co-administration of Symbicort with potent CYP3A4 inhibitors).

No products indexed under this heading.

Ranitidine Bismuth Citrate (Concomitant administration of CYP3A4 inhibitors (e.g., itraconazole, clarithromycin, erythromycin, etc.) may inhibit the metabolism of, and increase the systemic exposure to, budesonide. Caution should be exercised with co-administration of Symbicort with potent CYP3A4 inhibitors).

No products indexed under this heading.

Ranitidine Hydrochloride (Concomitant administration of CYP3A4 inhibitors (e.g., itraconazole, clarithromycin, erythromycin, etc.) may inhibit the metabolism of, and increase the systemic exposure to, budesonide. Caution should be exercised with co-administration of Symbicort with potent CYP3A4 inhibitors). Products include:

Zantac 75 Tablets .... ▣603

Zantac 1670

Zantac Injection 1666

Zantac Injection Pharmacy Bulk Package 1668

Maximum Strength Zantac 150 Tablets .... ▣603

Maximum Strength Zantac 150 Cool Mint Tablets .... ▣603

Rasagiline Mesylate (Symbicort should be administered with caution to patients treated with MAOIs, or within 2 weeks of discontinuation of MAOIs, since these agents may potentiate formoterol action on the vascular system). Products include:

Azilect Tablets 3106

Ritonavir (Concomitant administration of CYP3A4 inhibitors (e.g., itraconazole, clarithromycin, erythromycin, etc.) may inhibit the metabolism of, and increase the systemic expo-

sure to, budesonide. Caution should be exercised with co-administration of Symbicort with potent CYP3A4 inhibitors). Products include:

Kaletra 452
Norvir 489

Saquinavir (Concomitant administration of CYP3A4 inhibitors (e.g., itraconazole, clarithromycin, erythromycin, etc.) may inhibit the metabolism of, and increase the systemic exposure to, budesonide. Caution should be exercised with co-administration of Symbicort with potent CYP3A4 inhibitors).

No products indexed under this heading.

Saquinavir Mesylate (Concomitant administration of CYP3A4 inhibitors (e.g., itraconazole, clarithromycin, erythromycin, etc.) may inhibit the metabolism of, and increase the systemic exposure to, budesonide. Caution should be exercised with co-administration of Symbicort with potent CYP3A4 inhibitors).

No products indexed under this heading.

Selegiline (Symbicort should be administered with caution to patients treated with MAOIs, or within 2 weeks of discontinuation of MAOIs, since these agents may potentiate formoterol action on the vascular system). Products include:

Emsam Transdermal System 905

Selegiline Hydrochloride (Symbicort should be administered with caution to patients treated with MAOIs, or within 2 weeks of discontinuation of MAOIs, since these agents may potentiate formoterol action on the vascular system). Products include:

Eldepryl Capsules 3052

Sertraline Hydrochloride (Concomitant administration of CYP3A4 inhibitors (e.g., itraconazole, clarithromycin, erythromycin, etc.) may inhibit the metabolism of, and increase the systemic exposure to, budesonide. Caution should be exercised with co-administration of Symbicort with potent CYP3A4 inhibitors).

No products indexed under this heading.

Sildenafil Citrate (Concomitant administration of CYP3A4 inhibitors (e.g., itraconazole, clarithromycin, erythromycin, etc.) may inhibit the metabolism of, and increase the systemic exposure to, budesonide. Caution should be exercised with co-administration of Symbicort with potent CYP3A4 inhibitors).

No products indexed under this heading.

Sotalol Hydrochloride (Beta-blockers (including eye drops) may not only block the pulmonary effect of beta-agonists (e.g., formoterol- a component of Symbicort), but may produce severe bronchospasm in asthma patients).

No products indexed under this heading.

Spironolactone (The ECG changes and/or hypokalemia that may result from the administration of nonpotassium-sparing diuretics (e.g., loop or thiazide diuretics) can be acutely worsened by beta-agonists, especially when the recommended dose of the beta-agonist is exceeded. Caution is advised with co-administration of Symbicort with nonpotassium-sparing diuretics).

No products indexed under this heading.

Telithromycin (Concomitant administration of CYP3A4 inhibitors (e.g., itraconazole, clarithromycin, erythromycin, etc.) may inhibit the metabolism of, and increase the systemic exposure to, budesonide. Caution should be exercised with co-administration of Symbicort with potent CYP3A4 inhibitors). Products include:

Ketek Tablets 2744

Timolol Hemihydrate (Beta-blockers (including eye drops) may not only block the pulmonary effect of beta-agonists (e.g., formoterol- a component of Symbicort), but may produce severe bronchospasm in asthma patients). Products include:

Betimol Ophthalmic Solution 3181

Timolol Maleate (Beta-blockers (including eye drops) may not only block the pulmonary effect of beta-agonists (e.g., formoterol- a component of Symbicort), but may produce severe bronchospasm in asthma patients). Products include:

Combigan Ophthalmic Solution 553
Cosopt Sterile Ophthalmic Solution....................................... 1969
Timoptic Sterile Ophthalmic Solution....................................... 2121
Timoptic in Ocudose 2124
Timoptic-XE Sterile Ophthalmic Gel Forming Solution 2125

Torsemide (The ECG changes and/or hypokalemia that may result from the administration of nonpotassium-sparing diuretics (e.g., loop or thiazide diuretics) can be acutely worsened by beta-agonists, especially when the recommended dose of the beta-agonist is exceeded. Caution is advised with co-administration of Symbicort with nonpotassium-sparing diuretics). Products include:

Demadex Injection 2630
Demadex Tablets 2630

Tranylcypromine Sulfate (Symbicort should be administered with caution to patients treated with MAOIs, or within 2 weeks of discontinuation of MAOIs, since these agents may potentiate formoterol action on the vascular system). Products include:

Parnate Tablets 1532

Triamterene (The ECG changes and/or hypokalemia that may result from the administration of nonpotassium-sparing diuretics (e.g., loop or thiazide diuretics) can be acutely worsened by beta-agonists, especially when the recommended dose of the beta-agonist is exceeded. Caution is advised with co-administration of Symbicort with nonpotassium-sparing diuretics). Products include:

Dyazide Capsules 1405
Dyrenium Capsules 3189

Trimipramine Maleate (Symbicort should be administered with caution to patients treated with TCAs, or within 2 weeks of discontinuation of TCAs, since these agents may potentiate formoterol action on the vascular system).

No products indexed under this heading.

Troglitazone (Concomitant administration of CYP3A4 inhibitors (e.g., itraconazole, clarithromycin, erythromycin, etc.) may inhibit the metabolism of, and increase the systemic exposure to, budesonide. Caution should be exercised with co-administration of Symbicort with potent CYP3A4 inhibitors).

No products indexed under this heading.

Troleandomycin (Concomitant administration of CYP3A4 inhibitors (e.g., itraconazole, clarithromycin, erythromycin, etc.) may inhibit the metabolism of, and increase the systemic exposure to, budesonide. Caution should be exercised with co-administration of Symbicort with potent CYP3A4 inhibitors).

No products indexed under this heading.

Valproate Sodium (Concomitant administration of CYP3A4 inhibitors (e.g., itraconazole, clarithromycin, erythromycin, etc.) may inhibit the metabolism of, and increase the systemic exposure to, budesonide. Caution should be exercised with co-administration of Symbicort with potent CYP3A4 inhibitors).

No products indexed under this heading.

Vardenafil Hydrochloride (Concomitant administration of CYP3A4 inhibitors (e.g., itraconazole, clarithromycin, erythromycin, etc.) may inhibit the metabolism of, and increase the systemic exposure to, budesonide. Caution should be exercised with co-administration of Symbicort with potent CYP3A4 inhibitors). Products include:

Levitra Tablets 2876

Verapamil Hydrochloride (Concomitant administration of CYP3A4 inhibitors (e.g., itraconazole, clarithromycin, erythromycin, etc.) may inhibit the metabolism of, and increase the systemic exposure to, budesonide. Caution should be exercised with co-administration of Symbicort with potent CYP3A4 inhibitors). Products include:

Tarka Tablets 511

Voriconazole (Concomitant administration of CYP3A4 inhibitors (e.g., itraconazole, clarithromycin, erythromycin, etc.) may inhibit the metabolism of, and increase the systemic exposure to, budesonide. Caution should be exercised with co-administration of Symbicort with potent CYP3A4 inhibitors).

No products indexed under this heading.

Zafirlukast (Concomitant administration of CYP3A4 inhibitors (e.g., itraconazole, clarithromycin, erythromycin, etc.) may inhibit the metabolism of, and increase the systemic exposure to, budesonide. Caution should be exercised with co-administration of Symbicort with potent CYP3A4 inhibitors). Products include:

Accolate Tablets 669

Zileuton (Concomitant administration of CYP3A4 inhibitors (e.g., itraconazole, clarithromycin, erythromycin, etc.) may inhibit the metabolism of, and increase the systemic exposure to, budesonide. Caution should be exercised with co-administration of Symbicort with potent CYP3A4 inhibitors).

No products indexed under this heading.

Food Interactions

Grapefruit (Concomitant administration of CYP3A4 inhibitors (e.g., itraconazole, clarithromycin, erythromycin, etc.) may inhibit the metabolism of, and increase the systemic exposure to, budesonide. Caution should be exercised with co-administration of Symbicort with potent CYP3A4 inhibitors).

Grapefruit Juice (Concomitant administration of CYP3A4 inhibitors (e.g., itraconazole, clarithromycin, erythromycin, etc.) may inhibit the metabolism of, and increase the systemic exposure to, budesonide. Caution should be exercised with co-administration of Symbicort with potent CYP3A4 inhibitors).

SYMBICORT 160/4.5 INHALATION AEROSOL

(Budesonide, Formoterol fumarate dihydrate).. 659

See Symbicort 80/4.5 Inhalation Aerosol

SYMBYAX CAPSULES

(Fluoxetine Hydrochloride, Olanzapine).. 1871

May interact with antihypertensives, cytochrome p450 1a2 inducers (selected), cytochrome p450 2d6 substrates (selected), diuretics, dopamine agonists, monoamine oxidase inhibitors, non-steroidal anti-inflammatory agents, phenytoin, highly protein bound drugs (selected), serotoninergic agents, Serotonin and Norepinephrine Reuptake Inhibitors, selective serotonin reuptake inhibitors, tricyclic antidepressants, triptans, and certain other agents. Compounds in these categories include:

5-hydroxytryptophan (Five patients receiving fluoxetine in combination with tryptophan experienced adverse reactions, including agitation, restlessness, and gastrointestinal distress).

No products indexed under this heading.

Acebutolol Hydrochloride (Because of the potential for olanzapine to induce hypotension, Symbyax may enhance the effects of certain antihypertensive agents).

No products indexed under this heading.

Aliskiren (Because of the potential for olanzapine to induce hypotension, Symbyax may enhance the effects of certain antihypertensive agents). Products include:

Tekturna Tablets 2321
Tekturna HCT Tablets 2324

Almotriptan Malate (If concomitant treatment of sertraline with a triptan is clinically warranted, careful observation of the patient is advised, particularly during treatment initiation and dose increases). Products include:

Axert Tablets 2431

Alprazolam (Co-administration of alprazolam and fluoxetine resulted in increased alprazolam plasma concentrations and in further psychomotor performance decrement due to increased alprazolam levels).
No products indexed under this heading.

Amiloride Hydrochloride (Hyponatremia may occur as a result of treatment with SSRIs and SNRIs, including Symbyax. In many cases, this hyponatremia appears to be the result of the syndrome of inappropriate antidiuretic hormone secretion (SIADH). Cases with serum sodium lower than 110 mmol/L have been reported and appeared to be reversible when Symbyax was discontinued. Elderly patients may be at greater risk of developing hyponatremia with SSRIs and SNRIs. Also, patients taking diuretics or who are otherwise volume depleted may be at greater risk. Discontinuation of Symbyax should be considered in patients with symptomatic hyponatremia and appropriate medical intervention should be instituted).
No products indexed under this heading.

Amiodarone Hydrochloride (Because fluoxetine is tightly bound to plasma protein, the administration of fluoxetine to a patient taking another drug that is tightly bound to protein may cause a shift in plasma concentrations potentially resulting in an adverse effect. Conversely, adverse effects may result from displacement of protein-bound fluoxetine by other tightly bound drugs).
No products indexed under this heading.

Amitriptyline Hydrochloride (In two fluoxetine studies, previously stable plasma levels of imipramine and desipramine have increased >2- to 10-fold when fluoxetine has been administered in combination. This influence may persist for three weeks or longer after fluoxetine is discontinued. Thus, the dose of TCA may need to be reduced and plasma TCA concentrations may need to be monitored temporarily when Symbyax is co-administered or has been recently discontinued).
No products indexed under this heading.

Amlodipine Besylate (Because of the potential for olanzapine to induce hypotension, Symbyax may enhance the effects of certain antihypertensive agents). Products include:
Azor Tablets 1005
Exforge Tablets 2238

Amoxapine (In two fluoxetine studies, previously stable plasma levels of imipramine and desipramine have increased >2- to 10-fold when fluoxetine has been administered in combination. This influence may persist for three weeks or longer after fluoxetine is discontinued. Thus, the dose of TCA may need to be reduced and plasma TCA concentrations may need to be monitored temporarily when Symbyax is co-administered or has been recently discontinued).
No products indexed under this heading.

Amphetamine Aspartate (Fluoxetine, like other agents that are metabolized by CYP2D6, inhibits the activity of this isoenzyme. Therapy with medications that are predominately metabolized by the CYP2D6 system and have a relatively narrow therapeutic index should be initiated at the low end of the dose range if the patient is receiving fluoxetine concurrently or has taken it in the previous five weeks. If fluoxetine is added to the treatment regimen of a patient already receiving a drug metabolized by CYP2D6, the need for a decreased dose of the original medication should be considered). Products include:
Adderall XR Capsules 3012

Amphetamine Aspartate Monohydrate (Fluoxetine, like other agents that are metabolized by CYP2D6, inhibits the activity of this isoenzyme. Therapy with medications that are predominately metabolized by the CYP2D6 system and have a relatively narrow therapeutic index should be initiated at the low end of the dose range if the patient is receiving fluoxetine concurrently or has taken it in the previous five weeks. If fluoxetine is added to the treatment regimen of a patient already receiving a drug metabolized by CYP2D6, the need for a decreased dose of the original medication should be considered).
No products indexed under this heading.

Amphetamine Sulfate (Fluoxetine, like other agents that are metabolized by CYP2D6, inhibits the activity of this isoenzyme. Therapy with medications that are predominately metabolized by the CYP2D6 system and have a relatively narrow therapeutic index should be initiated at the low end of the dose range if the patient is receiving fluoxetine concurrently or has taken it in the previous five weeks. If fluoxetine is added to the treatment regimen of a patient already receiving a drug metabolized by CYP2D6, the need for a decreased dose of the original medication should be considered). Products include:
Adderall XR Capsules 3012

Aspirin (Serotonin release by platelets plays an important role in hemostasis. Studies have demonstrated an association between the use of psychotropic drugs that interfere with serotonin reuptake and the occurrence of upper gastrointestinal bleeding. These studies have also shown that concurrent use of aspirin potentiated the risk of bleeding. Therefore, patients should be cautioned about the use of aspirin concurrently with Symbyax). Products include:
Aggrenox Capsules 819
Bayer Aspirin 750
Percodan Tablets 1130
St. Joseph 81 mg Aspirin Chewable and Enteric Coated Tablets 1903

Aspirin, Enteric Coated (Serotonin release by platelets plays an important role in hemostasis. Studies have demonstrated an association between the use of psychotropic drugs that interfere with serotonin reuptake and the occurrence of upper gastrointestinal bleeding. These studies have also shown that concurrent use of aspirin potentiated the risk of bleeding. Therefore, patients should be cautioned about the use of aspirin concurrently with Symbyax).
No products indexed under this heading.

Aspirin Buffered (Serotonin release by platelets plays an important role in hemostasis. Studies have demonstrated an association between the use of psychotropic drugs that interfere with serotonin reuptake and the occurrence of upper gastrointestinal bleeding. These studies have also shown that concurrent use of aspirin potentiated the risk of bleeding. Therefore, patients should be cautioned about the use of aspirin concurrently with Symbyax).
No products indexed under this heading.

Atenolol (Because of the potential for olanzapine to induce hypotension, Symbyax may enhance the effects of certain antihypertensive agents).
No products indexed under this heading.

Atomoxetine Hydrochloride (Fluoxetine, like other agents that are metabolized by CYP2D6, inhibits the activity of this isoenzyme. Therapy with medications that are predominately metabolized by the CYP2D6 system and have a relatively narrow therapeutic index should be initiated at the low end of the dose range if the patient is receiving fluoxetine concurrently or has taken it in the previous five weeks. If fluoxetine is added to the treatment regimen of a patient already receiving a drug metabolized by CYP2D6, the need for a decreased dose of the original medication should be considered). Products include:
Strattera Capsules 1864

Atovaquone (Because fluoxetine is tightly bound to plasma protein, the administration of fluoxetine to a patient taking another drug that is tightly bound to protein may cause a shift in plasma concentrations potentially resulting in an adverse effect. Conversely, adverse effects may result from displacement of protein-bound fluoxetine by other tightly bound drugs). Products include:
Malarone Pediatric Tablets 1521
Malarone Tablets 1521
Mepron Suspension 1526

Benazepril Hydrochloride (Because of the potential for olanzapine to induce hypotension, Symbyax may enhance the effects of certain antihypertensive agents).
No products indexed under this heading.

Bendroflumethiazide (Because of the potential for olanzapine to induce hypotension, Symbyax may enhance the effects of certain antihypertensive agents).
No products indexed under this heading.

Betaxolol Hydrochloride (Because of the potential for olanzapine to induce hypotension, Symbyax may enhance the effects of certain antihypertensive agents).
No products indexed under this heading.

Bisoprolol Fumarate (Because of the potential for olanzapine to induce hypotension, Symbyax may enhance the effects of certain antihypertensive agents).
No products indexed under this heading.

Bromocriptine Mesylate (The olanzapine component of Symbyax may antagonize the effects of levodopa and dopamine agonists).
No products indexed under this heading.

Bumetanide (Hyponatremia may occur as a result of treatment with SSRIs and SNRIs, including Symbyax. In many cases, this hyponatremia appears to be the result of the syndrome of inappropriate antidiuretic hormone secretion (SIADH). Cases with serum sodium lower than 110 mmol/L have been reported and appeared to be reversible when Symbyax was discontinued. Elderly patients may be at greater risk of developing hyponatremia with SSRIs and SNRIs. Also, patients taking diuretics or who are otherwise volume depleted may be at greater risk. Discontinuation of Symbyax should be considered in patients with symptomatic hyponatremia and appropriate medical intervention should be instituted).
No products indexed under this heading.

Candesartan Cilexetil (Because of the potential for olanzapine to induce hypotension, Symbyax may enhance the effects of certain antihypertensive agents). Products include:
Atacand Tablets 639
Atacand HCT 642

Captopril (Because of the potential for olanzapine to induce hypotension, Symbyax may enhance the effects of certain antihypertensive agents). Products include:
Captopril Tablets 2182

Carbamazepine (Carbamazepine therapy (200 mg bid) causes an approximate 50% increase in the clearance of olanzapine; higher daily doses of carbamazepine may cause an even greater increase in olanzapine clearance. Patients on stable dose of carbamazepine have developed elevated plasma anticonvulsant concentrations and clinical anticonvulsant toxicity following initiation of concomitant fluoxetine treatment). Products include:
Carbatrol Capsules 3019
Equetro Extended-Release Capsules 3174

Carteolol Hydrochloride (Because of the potential for olanzapine to induce hypotension, Symbyax may enhance the effects of certain antihypertensive agents).
No products indexed under this heading.

Carvedilol (Fluoxetine, like other agents that are metabolized by CYP2D6, inhibits the activity of this isoenzyme. Therapy with medications that are predominately metabolized by the CYP2D6 system and have a relatively narrow therapeutic index should be initiated at the low end of the dose range if the patient is receiving fluoxetine concurrently or has taken it in the previous five weeks. If fluoxetine is added to the treatment regimen of a patient already receiving a drug metabolized by CYP2D6, the need for a decreased dose of the original medication should be considered). Products include:
Coreg Tablets 1387

Cefonicid Sodium (Because fluoxetine is tightly bound to plasma protein, the administration of fluoxetine to a patient taking another drug that is tightly bound to protein may cause a shift in plasma concentrations potentially resulting in an adverse effect. Conversely, adverse effects may result from displacement of protein-bound fluoxetine by other tightly bound drugs).
No products indexed under this heading.

Celecoxib (Serotonin release by platelets plays an important role in hemostasis. Studies have demonstrated an association between the use of psychotropic drugs that interfere with serotonin reuptake and the occurrence of upper gastrointestinal bleeding. These studies have also shown that concurrent use of an NSAID potentiated the risk of bleeding. Therefore, patients should be cautioned about the use of NSAIDs concurrently with Symbyax).
Products include:
Celebrex Capsules **2979**

Cevimeline Hydrochloride (Fluoxetine, like other agents that are metabolized by CYP2D6, inhibits the activity of this isoenzyme. Therapy with medications that are predominately metabolized by the CYP2D6 system and have a relatively narrow therapeutic index should be initiated at the low end of the dose range if the patient is receiving fluoxetine concurrently or has taken it in the previous five weeks. If fluoxetine is added to the treatment regimen of a patient already receiving a drug metabolized by CYP2D6, the need for a decreased dose of the original medication should be considered).
Products include:
Evoxac Capsules **1013**

Chlordiazepoxide (Because fluoxetine is tightly bound to plasma protein, the administration of fluoxetine to a patient taking another drug that is tightly bound to protein may cause a shift in plasma concentrations potentially resulting in an adverse effect. Conversely, adverse effects may result from displacement of protein-bound fluoxetine by other tightly bound drugs).
No products indexed under this heading.

Chlordiazepoxide Hydrochloride (Because fluoxetine is tightly bound to plasma protein, the administration of fluoxetine to a patient taking another drug that is tightly bound to protein may cause a shift in plasma concentrations potentially resulting in an adverse effect. Conversely, adverse effects may result from displacement of protein-bound fluoxetine by other tightly bound drugs).
No products indexed under this heading.

Chlorothiazide (Because of the potential for olanzapine to induce hypotension, Symbyax may enhance the effects of certain antihypertensive agents).
No products indexed under this heading.

Chlorothiazide Sodium (Because of the potential for olanzapine to induce hypotension, Symbyax may enhance the effects of certain antihypertensive agents). Products include:
Intravenous Sodium Diuril **2490**

Chlorpromazine (Because fluoxetine is tightly bound to plasma protein, the administration of fluoxetine to a patient taking another drug that is tightly bound to protein may cause a shift in plasma concentrations potentially resulting in an adverse effect. Conversely, adverse effects may result from displacement of protein-bound fluoxetine by other tightly bound drugs).
No products indexed under this heading.

Chlorpromazine Hydrochloride (Because fluoxetine is tightly bound to plasma protein, the administration of fluoxetine to a patient taking another drug that is tightly bound to protein may cause a shift in plasma concentrations potentially resulting in an adverse effect. Conversely, adverse effects may result from displacement of protein-bound fluoxetine by other tightly bound drugs).
No products indexed under this heading.

Chlorpropamide (Fluoxetine, like other agents that are metabolized by CYP2D6, inhibits the activity of this isoenzyme. Therapy with medications that are predominately metabolized by the CYP2D6 system and have a relatively narrow therapeutic index should be initiated at the low end of the dose range if the patient is receiving fluoxetine concurrently or has taken it in the previous five weeks. If fluoxetine is added to the treatment regimen of a patient already receiving a drug metabolized by CYP2D6, the need for a decreased dose of the original medication should be considered).
No products indexed under this heading.

Chlorthalidone (Because of the potential for olanzapine to induce hypotension, Symbyax may enhance the effects of certain antihypertensive agents). Products include:
Clorpres Tablets **2185**

Citalopram Hydrobromide (Based on the mechanism of action of SNRIs and SSRIs and the potential for serotonin syndrome, caution is advised when sertraline is co-administered with other drugs that may effect the serotonergic neurotransmitter systems). Products include:
Celexa **1160**

Clomipramine Hydrochloride (In two fluoxetine studies, previously stable plasma levels of imipramine and desipramine have increased >2- to 10-fold when fluoxetine has been administered in combination. This influence may persist for three weeks or longer after fluoxetine is discontinued. Thus, the dose of TCA may need to be reduced and plasma TCA concentrations may need to be monitored temporarily when Symbyax is co-administered or has been recently discontinued).
No products indexed under this heading.

Clonidine (Because of the potential for olanzapine to induce hypotension, Symbyax may enhance the effects of certain antihypertensive agents). Products include:
Catapres-TTS **842**

Clonidine Hydrochloride (Because of the potential for olanzapine to induce hypotension, Symbyax may enhance the effects of certain antihypertensive agents). Products include:
Catapres Tablets **841**
Clorpres Tablets **2185**

Clozapine (Elevation of blood levels of clozapine has been observed in patients receiving concomitant fluoxetine).
No products indexed under this heading.

Codeine Phosphate (Fluoxetine, like other agents that are metabolized by CYP2D6, inhibits the activity of this isoenzyme. Therapy with medications that are predominately metabolized by the CYP2D6 system and have a relatively narrow therapeutic index should be initiated at the low end of the dose range if the patient is receiving fluoxetine concurrently or has taken it in the previous five weeks. If fluoxetine is added to the treatment regimen of a patient already receiving a drug metabolized by CYP2D6, the need for a decreased dose of the original medication should be considered).
Products include:
Tylenol with Codeine Tablets **2427**

Codeine Sulfate (Fluoxetine, like other agents that are metabolized by CYP2D6, inhibits the activity of this isoenzyme. Therapy with medications that are predominately metabolized by the CYP2D6 system and have a relatively narrow therapeutic index should be initiated at the low end of the dose range if the patient is receiving fluoxetine concurrently or has taken it in the previous five weeks. If fluoxetine is added to the treatment regimen of a patient already receiving a drug metabolized by CYP2D6, the need for a decreased dose of the original medication should be considered).
No products indexed under this heading.

Cyclobenzaprine Hydrochloride (Fluoxetine, like other agents that are metabolized by CYP2D6, inhibits the activity of this isoenzyme. Therapy with medications that are predominately metabolized by the CYP2D6 system and have a relatively narrow therapeutic index should be initiated at the low end of the dose range if the patient is receiving fluoxetine concurrently or has taken it in the previous five weeks. If fluoxetine is added to the treatment regimen of a patient already receiving a drug metabolized by CYP2D6, the need for a decreased dose of the original medication should be considered).
Products include:
Amrix Capsules **966**

Cyclosporine (Because fluoxetine is tightly bound to plasma protein, the administration of fluoxetine to a patient taking another drug that is tightly bound to protein may cause a shift in plasma concentrations potentially resulting in an adverse effect. Conversely, adverse effects may result from displacement of protein-bound fluoxetine by other tightly bound drugs). Products include:
Gengraf Capsules **435**
Neoral Oral Solution **2280**
Neoral Soft Gelatin Capsules **2280**
Restasis Ophthalmic Emulsion **557**
Sandimmune **2296**

Deserpidine (Because of the potential for olanzapine to induce hypotension, Symbyax may enhance the effects of certain antihypertensive agents).
No products indexed under this heading.

Desipramine Hydrochloride (In two fluoxetine studies, previously stable plasma levels of imipramine and desipramine have increased >2- to 10-fold when fluoxetine has been administered in combination. This influence may persist for three weeks or longer after fluoxetine is discontinued. Thus, the dose of TCA may need to be reduced and plasma TCA concentrations may need to be monitored temporarily when Symbyax is co-administered or has been recently discontinued).
No products indexed under this heading.

Desvenlafaxine Succinate (Based on the mechanism of action of SNRIs and SSRIs and the potential for serotonin syndrome, caution is advised when sertraline is co-administered with other drugs that may effect the serotonergic neurotransmitter systems). Products include:
Pristiq Extended-Release Tablets **3247**

Dexfenfluramine Hydrochloride (Fluoxetine, like other agents that are metabolized by CYP2D6, inhibits the activity of this isoenzyme. Therapy with medications that are predominately metabolized by the CYP2D6 system and have a relatively narrow therapeutic index should be initiated at the low end of the dose range if the patient is receiving fluoxetine concurrently or has taken it in the previous five weeks. If fluoxetine is added to the treatment regimen of a patient already receiving a drug metabolized by CYP2D6, the need for a decreased dose of the original medication should be considered).
No products indexed under this heading.

Dextromethorphan Hydrobromide (Fluoxetine, like other agents that are metabolized by CYP2D6, inhibits the activity of this isoenzyme. Therapy with medications that are predominately metabolized by the CYP2D6 system and have a relatively narrow therapeutic index should be initiated at the low end of the dose range if the patient is receiving fluoxetine concurrently or has taken it in the previous five weeks. If fluoxetine is added to the treatment regimen of a patient already receiving a drug metabolized by CYP2D6, the need for a decreased dose of the original medication should be considered).
Products include:
PediaCare Children's Liquid Multi-Symptom Cold **1902**
PediaCare Children's Long-Acting Cough **1902**
Children's Sudafed PE Cold & Cough Liquid **1907**
Sudafed PE Cold & Cough Caplets **1907**
Children's Tylenol Plus Cough & Runny Nose Suspension Liquid **1912**
Children's Tylenol Plus Cough & Sore Throat Suspension Liquid **1912**
Children's Tylenol Plus Flu Suspension Liquid **1914**
Children's Tylenol Plus Multi-Symptom Cold Suspension Liquid **1912**
Tylenol Cold Severe Congestion Daytime Caplets with Cool Burst **1912**

Tylenol Cold Head Congestion Daytime Caplets with Cool Burst 1910
Tylenol Cold Head Congestion Nighttime Caplets with Cool Burst 1910
Tylenol Cold Head Congestion Severe Daytime Caplets with Cool Burst 1910
Tylenol Cold Multi-Symptom Daytime Caplets with Cool Burst and Rapid Release Gels 1913
Tylenol Cold Multi-Symptom Daytime Liquid with Citrus Burst 1913
Tylenol Cold Multi-Symptom Nighttime Caplets with Cool Burst 1913
Tylenol Cold Multi-Symptom Nighttime Liquid with Cool Burst 1913
Tylenol Cold Multi-Symptom Severe Caplets with Cool Burst 1913
Tylenol Cold Multi-Symptom Severe Daytime Liquid with Citrus Burst 1913
Tylenol Cough & Sore Throat Daytime Liquid with Cool Burst 1918
Tylenol Cough & Sore Throat Nighttime Liquid with Cool Burst 1918
Vicks DayQuil Cold & Flu Multi-Symptom Relief .... ■616
Vicks DayQuil LiquiCaps 2567
Vicks DayQuil Liquid 2567
Vicks DayQuil Multi-Symptom Cold/Flu Relief 2567
Vicks NyQuil Cold & Flu Multi-Symptom Relief .... ■617
Vicks NyQuil LiquiCaps 2567
Vicks NyQuil Liquid 2567
Vicks NyQuil Multi-Symptom Cold/Flu Relief 2567

Dextromethorphan Polistirex (Fluoxetine, like other agents that are metabolized by CYP2D6, inhibits the activity of this isoenzyme. Therapy with medications that are predominately metabolized by the CYP2D6 system and have a relatively narrow therapeutic index should be initiated at the low end of the dose range if the patient is receiving fluoxetine concurrently or has taken it in the previous five weeks. If fluoxetine is added to the treatment regimen of a patient already receiving a drug metabolized by CYP2D6, the need for a decreased dose of the original medication should be considered).
No products indexed under this heading.

Diazepam (The co-administration of diazepam with olanzapine may potentiate the orthostatic hypotension observed with olanzapine). Products include:
Valium Tablets 2658

Diazoxide (Because of the potential for olanzapine to induce hypotension, Symbyax may enhance the effects of certain antihypertensive agents). Products include:
Proglycem Capsules 1185
Proglycem Suspension 1185

Diclofenac Epolamine (Serotonin release by platelets plays an important role in hemostasis. Studies have demonstrated an association between the use of psychotropic drugs that interfere with serotonin reuptake and the occurrence of upper gastrointestinal bleeding. These studies have also shown that concurrent use of an NSAID potentiated the risk of bleeding. Therefore, patients should be cautioned about the use of NSAIDs concurrently with Symbyax). Products include:
Flector Patch 561

Diclofenac Potassium (Serotonin release by platelets plays an important role in hemostasis. Studies have demonstrated an association between the use of psychotropic drugs that interfere with serotonin reuptake and the occurrence of upper gastrointestinal bleeding. These studies have also shown that concurrent use of an NSAID potentiated the risk of bleeding. Therefore, patients should be cautioned about the use of NSAIDs concurrently with Symbyax).
No products indexed under this heading.

Diclofenac Sodium (Serotonin release by platelets plays an important role in hemostasis. Studies have demonstrated an association between the use of psychotropic drugs that interfere with serotonin reuptake and the occurrence of upper gastrointestinal bleeding. These studies have also shown that concurrent use of an NSAID potentiated the risk of bleeding. Therefore, patients should be cautioned about the use of NSAIDs concurrently with Symbyax). Products include:
Diclofenac Sodium Ophthalmic Solution .... ⊙240
Voltaren Ophthalmic Solution 2336
Voltaren Tablets 2334
Voltaren-XR Tablets 2337

Diltiazem Hydrochloride (Because of the potential for olanzapine to induce hypotension, Symbyax may enhance the effects of certain antihypertensive agents). Products include:
Cardizem LA Extended Release Tablets 421

Diltiazem Maleate (Agents that induce CYP1A2 or glucuronyl transferase enzymes may cause an increase in olanzapine concentration).
No products indexed under this heading.

Dipyridamole (Because fluoxetine is tightly bound to plasma protein, the administration of fluoxetine to a patient taking another drug that is tightly bound to protein may cause a shift in plasma concentrations potentially resulting in an adverse effect. Conversely, adverse effects may result from displacement of protein-bound fluoxetine by other tightly bound drugs). Products include:
Aggrenox Capsules 819
Persantine Tablets 869

Dolasetron Mesylate (Fluoxetine, like other agents that are metabolized by CYP2D6, inhibits the activity of this isoenzyme. Therapy with medications that are predominately metabolized by the CYP2D6 system and have a relatively narrow therapeutic index should be initiated at the low end of the dose range if the patient is receiving fluoxetine concurrently or has taken it in the previous five weeks. If fluoxetine is added to the treatment regimen of a patient already receiving a drug metabolized by CYP2D6, the need for a decreased dose of the original medication should be considered). Products include:
Anzemet Injection 2701
Anzemet Tablets 2704

Donepezil Hydrochloride (Fluoxetine, like other agents that are metabolized by CYP2D6, inhibits the activity of this isoenzyme. Therapy with medications that are predominately metabolized by the CYP2D6 system and have a relatively narrow therapeutic index should be initiated at the low end of the dose range if the patient is receiving fluoxetine concurrently or has taken it in the previous five weeks. If fluoxetine is added to the treatment regimen of a patient already receiving a drug metabolized by CYP2D6, the need for a decreased dose of the original medication should be considered). Products include:
Aricept Tablets 1062
Aricept ODT Tablets 1062

Dopamine Hydrochloride (The olanzapine component of Symbyax may antagonize the effects of levodopa and dopamine agonists).
No products indexed under this heading.

Doxazosin Mesylate (Because of the potential for olanzapine to induce hypotension, Symbyax may enhance the effects of certain antihypertensive agents).
No products indexed under this heading.

Doxepin Hydrochloride (In two fluoxetine studies, previously stable plasma levels of imipramine and desipramine have increased >2- to 10-fold when fluoxetine has been administered in combination. This influence may persist for three weeks or longer after fluoxetine is discontinued. Thus, the dose of TCA may need to be reduced and plasma TCA concentrations may need to be monitored temporarily when Symbyax is co-administered or has been recently discontinued).
No products indexed under this heading.

Duloxetine Hydrochloride (Based on the mechanism of action of SNRIs and SSRIs and the potential for serotonin syndrome, caution is advised when sertraline is co-administered with other drugs that may effect the serotonergic neurotransmitter systems). Products include:
Cymbalta Delayed-Release Capsules 1801

Eletriptan Hydrobromide (If concomitant treatment of sertraline with a triptan is clinically warranted, careful observation of the patient is advised, particularly during treatment initiation and dose increases).
No products indexed under this heading.

Enalapril Maleate (Because of the potential for olanzapine to induce hypotension, Symbyax may enhance the effects of certain antihypertensive agents).
No products indexed under this heading.

Enalaprilat (Because of the potential for olanzapine to induce hypotension, Symbyax may enhance the effects of certain antihypertensive agents).
No products indexed under this heading.

Encainide Hydrochloride (Fluoxetine, like other agents that are metabolized by CYP2D6, inhibits the activity of this isoenzyme. Therapy with medications that are predominately metabolized by the CYP2D6 system and have a relatively narrow therapeutic index should be initiated at the low end of the dose range if the patient is receiving fluoxetine concurrently or has taken it in the previous five weeks. If fluoxetine is added to the treatment regimen of a patient already receiving a drug metabolized by CYP2D6, the need for a decreased dose of the original medication should be considered).
No products indexed under this heading.

Eprosartan Mesylate (Because of the potential for olanzapine to induce hypotension, Symbyax may enhance the effects of certain antihypertensive agents). Products include:
Teveten Tablets 515
Teveten HCT Tablets 517

Erythromycin (Agents that induce CYP1A2 or glucuronyl transferase enzymes may cause an increase in olanzapine concentration).
No products indexed under this heading.

Erythromycin Estolate (Agents that induce CYP1A2 or glucuronyl transferase enzymes may cause an increase in olanzapine concentration).
No products indexed under this heading.

Erythromycin Ethylsuccinate (Agents that induce CYP1A2 or glucuronyl transferase enzymes may cause an increase in olanzapine concentration). Products include:
E.E.S. 433
EryPed 431

Erythromycin Gluceptate (Agents that induce CYP1A2 or glucuronyl transferase enzymes may cause an increase in olanzapine concentration).
No products indexed under this heading.

Erythromycin Lactobionate (Agents that induce CYP1A2 or glucuronyl transferase enzymes may cause an increase in olanzapine concentration).
No products indexed under this heading.

Erythromycin Stearate (Agents that induce CYP1A2 or glucuronyl transferase enzymes may cause an increase in olanzapine concentration).
No products indexed under this heading.

Escitalopram Oxalate (Based on the mechanism of action of SNRIs and SSRIs and the potential for serotonin syndrome, caution is advised when sertraline is co-administered with other drugs that may effect the serotonergic neurotransmitter systems). Products include:
Lexapro Oral Suspension 1174
Lexapro Tablets 1174

Esmolol Hydrochloride (Because of the potential for olanzapine to induce hypotension, Symbyax may enhance the effects of certain antihypertensive agents).
No products indexed under this heading.

Ethacrynic Acid (Hyponatremia may occur as a result of treatment with SSRIs and SNRIs, including Symbyax. In many cases, this hyponatremia appears to be the result of the syndrome of inappropriate antidiuretic hormone secretion (SIADH). Cases with serum sodium lower than 110 mmol/L have been reported and appeared to be reversible when Symbyax was discontinued. Elderly patients may be at greater risk of developing hyponatremia with SSRIs and SNRIs. Also, patients taking diuretics or who are otherwise volume depleted may be at greater risk. Discontinuation of Symbyax should be considered in patients with symptomatic hyponatremia and

appropriate medical intervention should be instituted). Products include:
Edecrin Tablets 698

Ethanol (Alcohol may potentiate the orthostatic effect of olanzapine, increasing the risk of orthostatic hypotension. Therefore, patients should be advised to avoid alcohol while taking Symbyax).
No products indexed under this heading.

Ethyl Alcohol (Alcohol may potentiate the orthostatic effect of olanzapine, increasing the risk of orthostatic hypotension. Therefore, patients should be advised to avoid alcohol while taking Symbyax).
No products indexed under this heading.

Etodolac (Serotonin release by platelets plays an important role in hemostasis. Studies have demonstrated an association between the use of psychotropic drugs that interfere with serotonin reuptake and the occurrence of upper gastrointestinal bleeding. These studies have also shown that concurrent use of an NSAID potentiated the risk of bleeding. Therefore, patients should be cautioned about the use of NSAIDs concurrently with Symbyax).
No products indexed under this heading.

Felodipine (Because of the potential for olanzapine to induce hypotension, Symbyax may enhance the effects of certain antihypertensive agents).
No products indexed under this heading.

Fenoprofen Calcium (Serotonin release by platelets plays an important role in hemostasis. Studies have demonstrated an association between the use of psychotropic drugs that interfere with serotonin reuptake and the occurrence of upper gastrointestinal bleeding. These studies have also shown that concurrent use of an NSAID potentiated the risk of bleeding. Therefore, patients should be cautioned about the use of NSAIDs concurrently with Symbyax). Products include:
Nalfon Capsules 2508

Fentanyl (Fluoxetine, like other agents that are metabolized by CYP2D6, inhibits the activity of this isoenzyme. Therapy with medications that are predominately metabolized by the CYP2D6 system and have a relatively narrow therapeutic index should be initiated at the low end of the dose range if the patient is receiving fluoxetine concurrently or has taken it in the previous five weeks. If fluoxetine is added to the treatment regimen of a patient already receiving a drug metabolized by CYP2D6, the need for a decreased dose of the original medication should be considered). Products include:
Duragesic Transdermal System 2405
Ionsys Transdermal System 2410

Fentanyl Citrate (Fluoxetine, like other agents that are metabolized by CYP2D6, inhibits the activity of this isoenzyme. Therapy with medications that are predominately metabolized by the CYP2D6 system and have a relatively narrow therapeutic index should be initiated at the low end of the dose range if the patient is receiving fluoxetine concurrently or has taken it in the previous five weeks. If fluoxetine is added to the treatment regimen of a patient already receiving a drug metabolized by CYP2D6, the need for a decreased dose of the original medication should be considered). Products include:
Actiq 959
Fentora Tablets 968

Flecainide Acetate (Fluoxetine, like other agents that are metabolized by CYP2D6, inhibits the activity of this isoenzyme. Therapy with medications that are predominately metabolized by the CYP2D6 system and have a relatively narrow therapeutic index should be initiated at the low end of the dose range if the patient is receiving fluoxetine concurrently or has taken it in the previous five weeks. If fluoxetine is added to the treatment regimen of a patient already receiving a drug metabolized by CYP2D6, the need for a decreased dose of the original medication should be considered).
No products indexed under this heading.

Fluoxetine (Based on the mechanism of action of SNRIs and SSRIs and the potential for serotonin syndrome, caution is advised when sertraline is co-administered with other drugs that may effect the serotonergic neurotransmitter systems).
No products indexed under this heading.

Fluphenazine Decanoate (Fluoxetine, like other agents that are metabolized by CYP2D6, inhibits the activity of this isoenzyme. Therapy with medications that are predominately metabolized by the CYP2D6 system and have a relatively narrow therapeutic index should be initiated at the low end of the dose range if the patient is receiving fluoxetine concurrently or has taken it in the previous five weeks. If fluoxetine is added to the treatment regimen of a patient already receiving a drug metabolized by CYP2D6, the need for a decreased dose of the original medication should be considered).
No products indexed under this heading.

Fluphenazine Enanthate (Fluoxetine, like other agents that are metabolized by CYP2D6, inhibits the activity of this isoenzyme. Therapy with medications that are predominately metabolized by the CYP2D6 system and have a relatively narrow therapeutic index should be initiated at the low end of the dose range if the patient is receiving fluoxetine concurrently or has taken it in the previous five weeks. If fluoxetine is added to the treatment regimen of a patient already receiving a drug metabolized by CYP2D6, the need for a decreased dose of the original medication should be considered).
No products indexed under this heading.

Fluphenazine Hydrochloride (Fluoxetine, like other agents that are metabolized by CYP2D6, inhibits the activity of this isoenzyme. Therapy with medications that are predominately metabolized by the CYP2D6 system and have a relatively narrow therapeutic index should be initiated at the low end of the dose range if the patient is receiving fluoxetine concurrently or has taken it in the previous five weeks. If fluoxetine is added to the treatment regimen of a patient already receiving a drug metabolized by CYP2D6, the need for a decreased dose of the original medication should be considered).
No products indexed under this heading.

Flurazepam Hydrochloride (Because fluoxetine is tightly bound to plasma protein, the administration of fluoxetine to a patient taking another drug that is tightly bound to protein may cause a shift in plasma concentrations potentially resulting in an adverse effect. Conversely, adverse effects may result from displacement of protein-bound fluoxetine by other tightly bound drugs).
No products indexed under this heading.

Flurbiprofen (Serotonin release by platelets plays an important role in hemostasis. Studies have demonstrated an association between the use of psychotropic drugs that interfere with serotonin reuptake and the occurrence of upper gastrointestinal bleeding. These studies have also shown that concurrent use of an NSAID potentiated the risk of bleeding. Therefore, patients should be cautioned about the use of NSAIDs concurrently with Symbyax).
No products indexed under this heading.

Fluvoxamine (Fluvoxamine, a CYP1A2 inhibitor, decreases the clearance of olanzapine. This results in a mean increase in olanzapine Cmax and AUC following fluvoxamine administration. Lower doses of the olanzapine component of Symbyax should be considered in patients receiving concomitant treatment with fluvoxamine).
No products indexed under this heading.

Fluvoxamine Maleate (Fluvoxamine, a CYP1A2 inhibitor, decreases the clearance of olanzapine. This results in a mean increase in olanzapine Cmax and AUC following fluvoxamine administration. Lower doses of the olanzapine component of Symbyax should be considered in patients receiving concomitant treatment with fluvoxamine). Products include:
Luvox CR Extended-Release Capsules..................................... 1759

Formoterol Fumarate (Fluoxetine, like other agents that are metabolized by CYP2D6, inhibits the activity of this isoenzyme. Therapy with medications that are predominately metabolized by the CYP2D6 system and have a relatively narrow therapeutic index should be initiated at the low end of the dose range if the patient is receiving fluoxetine concurrently or has taken it in the previous five weeks. If fluoxetine is added to the treatment regimen of a patient already receiving a drug metabolized by CYP2D6, the need for a decreased dose of the original medication should be considered). Products include:
Foradil Aerolizer 2849
Perforomist Inhalation Solution 1025

Fosinopril Sodium (Because of the potential for olanzapine to induce hypotension, Symbyax may enhance the effects of certain antihypertensive agents).
No products indexed under this heading.

Fosphenytoin Sodium (Patients on stable doses of phenytoin have developed elevated plasma levels of phenytoin with clinical pheytoin toxicity following initiation of concomitant fluoxetine).
No products indexed under this heading.

Frovatriptan Succinate (If concomitant treatment of sertraline with a triptan is clinically warranted, careful observation of the patient is advised, particularly during treatment initiation and dose increases). Products include:
Frova Tablets 1111

Furosemide (Because of the potential for olanzapine to induce hypotension, Symbyax may enhance the effects of certain antihypertensive agents). Products include:
Furosemide Tablets 2186

Galantamine Hydrobromide (Fluoxetine, like other agents that are metabolized by CYP2D6, inhibits the activity of this isoenzyme. Therapy with medications that are predominately metabolized by the CYP2D6 system and have a relatively narrow therapeutic index should be initiated at the low end of the dose range if the patient is receiving fluoxetine concurrently or has taken it in the previous five weeks. If fluoxetine is added to the treatment regimen of a patient already receiving a drug metabolized by CYP2D6, the need for a decreased dose of the original medication should be considered).
No products indexed under this heading.

Glipizide (Because fluoxetine is tightly bound to plasma protein, the administration of fluoxetine to a patient taking another drug that is tightly bound to protein may cause a shift in plasma concentrations potentially resulting in an adverse effect. Conversely, adverse effects may result from displacement of protein-bound fluoxetine by other tightly bound drugs).
No products indexed under this heading.

Guanabenz Acetate (Because of the potential for olanzapine to induce hypotension, Symbyax may enhance the effects of certain antihypertensive agents).
No products indexed under this heading.

Guanethidine Monosulfate (Because of the potential for olanzapine to induce hypotension, Symbyax may enhance the effects of certain antihypertensive agents).
No products indexed under this heading.

Haloperidol (Elevation of blood levels of haloperidol has been observed in patients receiving concomitant fluoxetine).
No products indexed under this heading.

Haloperidol Decanoate (Elevation of blood levels of haloperidol has been observed in patients receiving concomitant fluoxetine).
No products indexed under this heading.

Haloperidol Lactate (Elevation of blood levels of haloperidol have been observed in patients receiving concomitant fluoxetine).
No products indexed under this heading.

Hydralazine Hydrochloride (Because of the potential for olanzapine to induce hypotension, Symbyax may enhance the effects of certain antihypertensive agents).
No products indexed under this heading.

Hydrochlorothiazide (Because of the potential for olanzapine to induce hypotension, Symbyax may enhance the effects of certain antihypertensive agents). Products include:
Atacand HCT ... 642
Avalide Tablets ... 892
Avalide Tablets ... 2713
Benicar HCT Tablets ... 1010
Diovan HCT Tablets ... 2216
Dyazide Capsules ... 1405
Micardis HCT Tablets ... 854
Prinzide Tablets ... 2092
Tekturna HCT Tablets ... 2324
Teveten HCT Tablets ... 517

Hydrocodone Bitartrate (Fluoxetine, like other agents that are metabolized by CYP2D6, inhibits the activity of this isoenzyme. Therapy with medications that are predominately metabolized by the CYP2D6 system and have a relatively narrow therapeutic index should be initiated at the low end of the dose range if the patient is receiving fluoxetine concurrently or has taken it in the previous five weeks. If fluoxetine is added to the treatment regimen of a patient already receiving a drug metabolized by CYP2D6, the need for a decreased dose of the original medication should be considered). Products include:
Lortab 5/500 Tablets ... 3143
Lortab 7.5/500 Tablets ... 3144
Lortab 10/500 Tablets ... 3144
Vicodin Tablets ... 529
Vicodin ES Tablets ... 530
Vicodin HP Tablets ... 531
Vicoprofen Tablets ... 533
Zydone Tablets ... 1132

Hydroflumethiazide (Because of the potential for olanzapine to induce hypotension, Symbyax may enhance the effects of certain antihypertensive agents).
No products indexed under this heading.

Hypericum (Agents that induce CYP1A2 or glucuronyl transferase enzymes may cause an increase in olanzapine concentration). Products include:
Satieté Tablets ... ▣ 640

Ibuprofen (Serotonin release by platelets plays an important role in hemostasis. Studies have demonstrated an association between the use of psychotropic drugs that interfere with serotonin reuptake and the occurrence of upper gastrointestinal bleeding. These studies have also shown that concurrent use of an NSAID potentiated the risk of bleeding. Therefore, patients should be cautioned about the use of NSAIDs concurrently with Symbyax). Products include:
Motrin IB Tablets and Caplets ... 1900
Children's Motrin Oral Suspension ... 1901
Children's Motrin Non-Staining Dye-Free Oral Suspension ... 1901
Children's Motrin Cold Oral Suspension ... 1899
Infants' Motrin Concentrated Drops ... 1901
Infants' Motrin Non-Staining Dye-Free Concentrated Drops ... 1901
Junior Strength Motrin Caplets and Chewable Tablets ... 1901
Vicoprofen Tablets ... 533

Imipramine Hydrochloride (In two fluoxetine studies, previously stable plasma levels of imipramine and desipramine have increased >2- to 10-fold when fluoxetine has been administered in combination. This influence may persist for three weeks or longer after fluoxetine is discontinued. Thus, the dose of TCA may need to be reduced and plasma TCA concentrations may need to be monitored temporarily when Symbyax is co-administered or has been recently discontinued).
No products indexed under this heading.

Imipramine Pamoate (In two fluoxetine studies, previously stable plasma levels of imipramine and desipramine have increased >2- to 10-fold when fluoxetine has been administered in combination. This influence may persist for three weeks or longer after fluoxetine is discontinued. Thus, the dose of TCA may need to be reduced and plasma TCA concentrations may need to be monitored temporarily when Symbyax is co-administered or has been recently discontinued).
No products indexed under this heading.

Indapamide (Because of the potential for olanzapine to induce hypotension, Symbyax may enhance the effects of certain antihypertensive agents). Products include:
Indapamide Tablets ... 2188

Indomethacin (Serotonin release by platelets plays an important role in hemostasis. Studies have demonstrated an association between the use of psychotropic drugs that interfere with serotonin reuptake and the occurrence of upper gastrointestinal bleeding. These studies have also shown that concurrent use of an NSAID potentiated the risk of bleeding. Therefore, patients should be cautioned about the use of NSAIDs concurrently with Symbyax). Products include:
Indocin ... 2024

Indomethacin Sodium Trihydrate (Serotonin release by platelets plays an important role in hemostasis. Studies have demonstrated an association between the use of psychotropic drugs that interfere with serotonin reuptake and the occurrence of upper gastrointestinal bleeding. These studies have also shown that concurrent use of an NSAID potentiated the risk of bleeding. Therefore, patients should be cautioned about the use of NSAIDs concurrently with Symbyax). Products include:
Indocin I.V. ... 2489

Indoramin Hydrochloride (Fluoxetine, like other agents that are metabolized by CYP2D6, inhibits the activity of this isoenzyme. Therapy with medications that are predominately metabolized by the CYP2D6 system and have a relatively narrow therapeutic index should be initiated at the low end of the dose range if the patient is receiving fluoxetine concurrently or has taken it in the previous five weeks. If fluoxetine is added to the treatment regimen of a patient already receiving a drug metabolized by CYP2D6, the need for a decreased dose of the original medication should be considered).
No products indexed under this heading.

Insulin (Agents that induce CYP1A2 or glucuronyl transferase enzymes may cause an increase in olanzapine concentration).
No products indexed under this heading.

Irbesartan (Because of the potential for olanzapine to induce hypotension, Symbyax may enhance the effects of certain antihypertensive agents). Products include:
Avalide Tablets ... 892
Avalide Tablets ... 2713
Avapro Tablets ... 897
Avapro Tablets ... 2718

Isocarboxazid (Concomitant use in patients taking MAO inhibitors is contraindicated. There have been reports of serious, sometimes fatal, reactions in patients receiving, or who have recently discontinued, fluoxetine and are then started on an MAO inhibitor. Therefore, Symbyax should not be used in combination with, or within a minimum of 14 days of discontinuing, MAO inhibitors). Products include:
Marplan Tablets ... 3177

Isradipine (Because of the potential for olanzapine to induce hypotension, Symbyax may enhance the effects of certain antihypertensive agents). Products include:
DynaCirc CR Controlled Release Tablets ... 1407

Ketoprofen (Serotonin release by platelets plays an important role in hemostasis. Studies have demonstrated an association between the use of psychotropic drugs that interfere with serotonin reuptake and the occurrence of upper gastrointestinal bleeding. These studies have also shown that concurrent use of an NSAID potentiated the risk of bleeding. Therefore, patients should be cautioned about the use of NSAIDs concurrently with Symbyax).
No products indexed under this heading.

Ketorolac Tromethamine (Serotonin release by platelets plays an important role in hemostasis. Studies have demonstrated an association between the use of psychotropic drugs that interfere with serotonin reuptake and the occurrence of upper gastrointestinal bleeding. These studies have also shown that concurrent use of an NSAID potentiated the risk of bleeding. Therefore, patients should be cautioned about the use of NSAIDs concurrently with Symbyax).
No products indexed under this heading.

Labetalol Hydrochloride (Because of the potential for olanzapine to induce hypotension, Symbyax may enhance the effects of certain antihypertensive agents).
No products indexed under this heading.

Lansoprazole (Agents that induce CYP1A2 or glucuronyl transferase enzymes may cause an increase in olanzapine concentration).
No products indexed under this heading.

Levodopa (The olanzapine component of Symbyax may antagonize the effects of levodopa and dopamine agonists). Products include:
Stalevo Tablets ... 2309

Lidocaine (Fluoxetine, like other agents that are metabolized by CYP2D6, inhibits the activity of this isoenzyme. Therapy with medications that are predominately metabolized by the CYP2D6 system and have a relatively narrow therapeutic index should be initiated at the low end of the dose range if the patient is receiving fluoxetine concurrently or has taken it in the previous five weeks. If fluoxetine is added to the treatment regimen of a patient already receiving a drug metabolized by CYP2D6, the need for a decreased dose of the original medication should be considered). Products include:
Lidoderm Patch ... 1114

Lidocaine Hydrochloride (Fluoxetine, like other agents that are metabolized by CYP2D6, inhibits the activity of this isoenzyme. Therapy with medications that are predominately metabolized by the CYP2D6 system and have a relatively narrow therapeutic index should be initiated at the low end of the dose range if the patient is receiving fluoxetine concurrently or has taken it in the previous five weeks. If fluoxetine is added to the treatment regimen of a patient already receiving a drug metabolized by CYP2D6, the need for a decreased dose of the original medication should be considered).
No products indexed under this heading.

Lisinopril (Because of the potential for olanzapine to induce hypotension, Symbyax may enhance the effects of certain antihypertensive agents). Products include:
Prinivil Tablets ... 2087
Prinzide Tablets ... 2092

Lithium (There have been reports of both increased and decreased lithium levels when lithium was used concomitantly with fluoxetine. Cases of lithium toxicity and increased serotonergic effects have been reported. Lithium levels should be monitored in patients taking Symbyax concomitantly with lithium).
No products indexed under this heading.

Lithium Carbonate (There have been reports of both increased and decreased lithium levels when lithium was used concomitantly with fluoxetine. Cases of lithium toxicity and increased serotonergic effects have been reported. Lithium levels should be monitored in patients taking Symbyax concomitantly with lithium).
No products indexed under this heading.

Lithium Citrate (There have been reports of both increased and decreased lithium levels when lithium was used concomitantly with fluoxetine. Cases of lithium toxicity and increased serotonergic effects have been reported. Lithium levels should be monitored in patients taking Symbyax concomitantly with lithium).
No products indexed under this heading.

Losartan Potassium (Because of the potential for olanzapine to induce hypotension, Symbyax may enhance the effects of certain antihypertensive agents). Products include:
Cozaar Tablets ... 1973

Maprotiline Hydrochloride (In two fluoxetine studies, previously stable plasma levels of imipramine and desipramine have increased >2- to 10-fold when fluoxetine has been administered in combination. This influence may persist for three

weeks or longer after fluoxetine is discontinued. Thus, the dose of TCA may need to be reduced and plasma TCA concentrations may need to be monitored temporarily when Symbyax is co-administered or has been recently discontinued).
No products indexed under this heading.

Mecamylamine Hydrochloride (Because of the potential for olanzapine to induce hypotension, Symbyax may enhance the effects of certain antihypertensive agents).
No products indexed under this heading.

Meclofenamate Sodium (Serotonin release by platelets plays an important role in hemostasis. Studies have demonstrated an association between the use of psychotropic drugs that interfere with serotonin reuptake and the occurrence of upper gastrointestinal bleeding. These studies have also shown that concurrent use of an NSAID potentiated the risk of bleeding. Therefore, patients should be cautioned about the use of NSAIDs concurrently with Symbyax).
No products indexed under this heading.

Mefenamic Acid (Serotonin release by platelets plays an important role in hemostasis. Studies have demonstrated an association between the use of psychotropic drugs that interfere with serotonin reuptake and the occurrence of upper gastrointestinal bleeding. These studies have also shown that concurrent use of an NSAID potentiated the risk of bleeding. Therefore, patients should be cautioned about the use of NSAIDs concurrently with Symbyax).
No products indexed under this heading.

Meloxicam (Serotonin release by platelets plays an important role in hemostasis. Studies have demonstrated an association between the use of psychotropic drugs that interfere with serotonin reuptake and the occurrence of upper gastrointestinal bleeding. These studies have also shown that concurrent use of an NSAID potentiated the risk of bleeding. Therefore, patients should be cautioned about the use of NSAIDs concurrently with Symbyax).
Products include:
Mobic Oral Suspension 863
Mobic Tablets 863

Meperidine Hydrochloride (Fluoxetine, like other agents that are metabolized by CYP2D6, inhibits the activity of this isoenzyme. Therapy with medications that are predominately metabolized by the CYP2D6 system and have a relatively narrow therapeutic index should be initiated at the low end of the dose range if the patient is receiving fluoxetine concurrently or has taken it in the previous five weeks. If fluoxetine is added to the treatment regimen of a patient already receiving a drug metabolized by CYP2D6, the need for a decreased dose of the original medication should be considered).
No products indexed under this heading.

Methadone Hydrochloride (Fluoxetine, like other agents that are metabolized by CYP2D6, inhibits the activity of this isoenzyme. Therapy with medications that are predominately metabolized by the CYP2D6 system and have a relatively narrow therapeutic index should be initiated at the low end of the dose range if the patient is receiving fluoxetine concurrently or has taken it in the previous five weeks. If fluoxetine is added to the treatment regimen of a patient already receiving a drug metabolized by CYP2D6, the need for a decreased dose of the original medication should be considered).
No products indexed under this heading.

Methamphetamine Hydrochloride (Fluoxetine, like other agents that are metabolized by CYP2D6, inhibits the activity of this isoenzyme. Therapy with medications that are predominately metabolized by the CYP2D6 system and have a relatively narrow therapeutic index should be initiated at the low end of the dose range if the patient is receiving fluoxetine concurrently or has taken it in the previous five weeks. If fluoxetine is added to the treatment regimen of a patient already receiving a drug metabolized by CYP2D6, the need for a decreased dose of the original medication should be considered).
No products indexed under this heading.

Methyclothiazide (Because of the potential for olanzapine to induce hypotension, Symbyax may enhance the effects of certain antihypertensive agents).
No products indexed under this heading.

Methyldopa (Because of the potential for olanzapine to induce hypotension, Symbyax may enhance the effects of certain antihypertensive agents).
No products indexed under this heading.

Methyldopate Hydrochloride (Because of the potential for olanzapine to induce hypotension, Symbyax may enhance the effects of certain antihypertensive agents).
No products indexed under this heading.

Metolazone (Because of the potential for olanzapine to induce hypotension, Symbyax may enhance the effects of certain antihypertensive agents).
No products indexed under this heading.

Metoprolol Succinate (Because of the potential for olanzapine to induce hypotension, Symbyax may enhance the effects of certain antihypertensive agents). Products include:
Toprol-XL Tablets 666

Metoprolol Tartrate (Because of the potential for olanzapine to induce hypotension, Symbyax may enhance the effects of certain antihypertensive agents).
No products indexed under this heading.

Metyrosine (Because of the potential for olanzapine to induce hypotension, Symbyax may enhance the effects of certain antihypertensive agents). Products include:
Demser Capsules 1989

Mexiletine Hydrochloride (Fluoxetine, like other agents that are metabolized by CYP2D6, inhibits the activity of this isoenzyme. Therapy with medications that are predominately metabolized by the CYP2D6 system and have a relatively narrow therapeutic index should be initiated at the low end of the dose range if the patient is receiving fluoxetine concurrently or has taken it in the previous five weeks. If fluoxetine is added to the treatment regimen of a patient already receiving a drug metabolized by CYP2D6, the need for a decreased dose of the original medication should be considered).
No products indexed under this heading.

Mibefradil Dihydrochloride (Because of the potential for olanzapine to induce hypotension, Symbyax may enhance the effects of certain antihypertensive agents).
No products indexed under this heading.

Midazolam Hydrochloride (Because fluoxetine is tightly bound to plasma protein, the administration of fluoxetine to a patient taking another drug that is tightly bound to protein may cause a shift in plasma concentrations potentially resulting in an adverse effect. Conversely, adverse effects may result from displacement of protein-bound fluoxetine by other tightly bound drugs).
No products indexed under this heading.

Minoxidil (Because of the potential for olanzapine to induce hypotension, Symbyax may enhance the effects of certain antihypertensive agents).
No products indexed under this heading.

Mirtazapine (Fluoxetine, like other agents that are metabolized by CYP2D6, inhibits the activity of this isoenzyme. Therapy with medications that are predominately metabolized by the CYP2D6 system and have a relatively narrow therapeutic index should be initiated at the low end of the dose range if the patient is receiving fluoxetine concurrently or has taken it in the previous five weeks. If fluoxetine is added to the treatment regimen of a patient already receiving a drug metabolized by CYP2D6, the need for a decreased dose of the original medication should be considered).
Products include:
Remeron Tablets 2924
RemeronSolTab Tablets 2927

Moclobemide (Concomitant use in patients taking MAO inhibitors is contraindicated. There have been reports of serious, sometimes fatal, reactions in patients receiving, or who have recently discontinued, fluoxetine and are then started on an MAO inhibitor. Therefore, Symbyax should not be used in combination with, or within a minimum of 14 days of discontinuing, MAO inhibitors).
No products indexed under this heading.

Moexipril Hydrochloride (Because of the potential for olanzapine to induce hypotension, Symbyax may enhance the effects of certain antihypertensive agents).
No products indexed under this heading.

Morphine Sulfate (Fluoxetine, like other agents that are metabolized by CYP2D6, inhibits the activity of this isoenzyme. Therapy with medications that are predominately metabolized by the CYP2D6 system and have a relatively narrow therapeutic index should be initiated at the low end of the dose range if the patient is receiving fluoxetine concurrently or has taken it in the previous five weeks. If fluoxetine is added to the treatment regimen of a patient already receiving a drug metabolized by CYP2D6, the need for a decreased dose of the original medication should be considered).
Products include:
Avinza Capsules 1772
DepoDur Injection 1095
MS Contin Tablets 2585

Nabumetone (Serotonin release by platelets plays an important role in hemostasis. Studies have demonstrated an association between the use of psychotropic drugs that interfere with serotonin reuptake and the occurrence of upper gastrointestinal bleeding. These studies have also shown that concurrent use of an NSAID potentiated the risk of bleeding. Therefore, patients should be cautioned about the use of NSAIDs concurrently with Symbyax).
No products indexed under this heading.

Nadolol (Because of the potential for olanzapine to induce hypotension, Symbyax may enhance the effects of certain antihypertensive agents). Products include:
Nadolol Tablets 2191

Nafcillin Sodium (Agents that induce CYP1A2 or glucuronyl transferase enzymes may cause an increase in olanzapine concentration).
No products indexed under this heading.

Naproxen (Serotonin release by platelets plays an important role in hemostasis. Studies have demonstrated an association between the use of psychotropic drugs that interfere with serotonin reuptake and the occurrence of upper gastrointestinal bleeding. These studies have also shown that concurrent use of an NSAID potentiated the risk of bleeding. Therefore, patients should be cautioned about the use of NSAIDs concurrently with Symbyax).
Products include:
EC-Naprosyn Delayed-Release Tablets 2632
Naprosyn Suspension 2632
Naprosyn Tablets 2632

Naproxen Sodium (Serotonin release by platelets plays an important role in hemostasis. Studies have demonstrated an association between the use of psychotropic drugs that interfere with serotonin reuptake and the occurrence of upper gastrointestinal bleeding. These studies have also shown that concurrent use of an NSAID potentiated the risk of bleeding. Therefore, patients should be cautioned about the use of NSAIDs concurrently with Symbyax). Products include:
Anaprox Tablets 2632
Anaprox DS Tablets 2632
Treximet Tablets 1616

Naratriptan Hydrochloride (If concomitant treatment of sertraline with a triptan is clinically warranted, careful observation of the patient is advised, particularly during treatment initiation and dose increases).
Products include:
Amerge Tablets 1301

Nebivolol (Because of the potential for olanzapine to induce hypoten-

sion, Symbyax may enhance the effects of certain antihypertensive agents). Products include:
Bystolic Tablets 1155

Nefazodone Hydrochloride (Based on the mechanism of action of SNRIs and SSRIs and the potential for serotonin syndrome, caution is advised when sertraline is co-administered with other drugs that may effect the serotonergic neuro-transmitter systems).
No products indexed under this heading.

Nelfinavir Mesylate (Fluoxetine, like other agents that are metabolized by CYP2D6, inhibits the activity of this isoenzyme. Therapy with medications that are predominately metabolized by the CYP2D6 system and have a relatively narrow therapeutic index should be initiated at the low end of the dose range if the patient is receiving fluoxetine concurrently or has taken it in the previous five weeks. If fluoxetine is added to the treatment regimen of a patient already receiving a drug metabolized by CYP2D6, the need for a decreased dose of the original medication should be considered).
No products indexed under this heading.

Nicardipine Hydrochloride (Because of the potential for olanzapine to induce hypotension, Symbyax may enhance the effects of certain antihypertensive agents).
Products include:
Cardene I.V. 1093

Nicotine (Agents that induce CYP1A2 or glucuronyl transferase enzymes may cause an increase in olanzapine concentration).
No products indexed under this heading.

Nicotine Polacrilex (Agents that induce CYP1A2 or glucuronyl transferase enzymes may cause an increase in olanzapine concentration).
No products indexed under this heading.

Nicotine Salicylate (Agents that induce CYP1A2 or glucuronyl transferase enzymes may cause an increase in olanzapine concentration).
No products indexed under this heading.

Nicotine Sulfate (Agents that induce CYP1A2 or glucuronyl transferase enzymes may cause an increase in olanzapine concentration).
No products indexed under this heading.

Nifedipine (Because of the potential for olanzapine to induce hypotension, Symbyax may enhance the effects of certain antihypertensive agents).
No products indexed under this heading.

Nisoldipine (Because of the potential for olanzapine to induce hypotension, Symbyax may enhance the effects of certain antihypertensive agents). Products include:
Sular Extended Release Tablets 2975

Nitroglycerin (Because of the potential for olanzapine to induce hypotension, Symbyax may enhance the effects of certain antihypertensive agents). Products include:
Nitro-Dur Transdermal Infusion System.. 2887
Nitrolingual Pumpspray 2965

Nortriptyline Hydrochloride (In two fluoxetine studies, previously stable plasma levels of imipramine and desipramine have increased >2- to 10-fold when fluoxetine has been administered in combination. This influence may persist for three weeks or longer after fluoxetine is discontinued. Thus, the dose of TCA may need to be reduced and plasma TCA concentrations may need to be monitored temporarily when Symbyax is co-administered or has been recently discontinued).
No products indexed under this heading.

Omeprazole (Agents that induce CYP1A2 or glucuronyl transferase enzymes may cause an increase in olanzapine concentration).
No products indexed under this heading.

Ondansetron (Fluoxetine, like other agents that are metabolized by CYP2D6, inhibits the activity of this isoenzyme. Therapy with medications that are predominately metabolized by the CYP2D6 system and have a relatively narrow therapeutic index should be initiated at the low end of the dose range if the patient is receiving fluoxetine concurrently or has taken it in the previous five weeks. If fluoxetine is added to the treatment regimen of a patient already receiving a drug metabolized by CYP2D6, the need for a decreased dose of the original medication should be considered).
Products include:
Zofran ODT Orally Disintegrating Tablets.. 1687

Ondansetron Hydrochloride (Fluoxetine, like other agents that are metabolized by CYP2D6, inhibits the activity of this isoenzyme. Therapy with medications that are predominately metabolized by the CYP2D6 system and have a relatively narrow therapeutic index should be initiated at the low end of the dose range if the patient is receiving fluoxetine concurrently or has taken it in the previous five weeks. If fluoxetine is added to the treatment regimen of a patient already receiving a drug metabolized by CYP2D6, the need for a decreased dose of the original medication should be considered).
Products include:
Zofran Injection 1682
Zofran 1687

Oxaprozin (Serotonin release by platelets plays an important role in hemostasis. Studies have demonstrated an association between the use of psychotropic drugs that interfere with serotonin reuptake and the occurrence of upper gastrointestinal bleeding. These studies have also shown that concurrent use of an NSAID potentiated the risk of bleeding. Therefore, patients should be cautioned about the use of NSAIDs concurrently with Symbyax).
No products indexed under this heading.

Oxazepam (Because fluoxetine is tightly bound to plasma protein, the administration of fluoxetine to a patient taking another drug that is tightly bound to protein may cause a shift in plasma concentrations potentially resulting in an adverse effect. Conversely, adverse effects may result from displacement of protein-bound fluoxetine by other tightly bound drugs).
No products indexed under this heading.

Oxycodone Hydrochloride (Fluoxetine, like other agents that are metabolized by CYP2D6, inhibits the activity of this isoenzyme. Therapy with medications that are predominately metabolized by the CYP2D6 system and have a relatively narrow therapeutic index should be initiated at the low end of the dose range if the patient is receiving fluoxetine concurrently or has taken it in the previous five weeks. If fluoxetine is added to the treatment regimen of a patient already receiving a drug metabolized by CYP2D6, the need for a decreased dose of the original medication should be considered).
Products include:
OxyContin Tablets 2589
OxyIR Capsules 2593
Percocet Tablets 1127
Percodan Tablets 1130

Paclitaxel (Fluoxetine, like other agents that are metabolized by CYP2D6, inhibits the activity of this isoenzyme. Therapy with medications that are predominately metabolized by the CYP2D6 system and have a relatively narrow therapeutic index should be initiated at the low end of the dose range if the patient is receiving fluoxetine concurrently or has taken it in the previous five weeks. If fluoxetine is added to the treatment regimen of a patient already receiving a drug metabolized by CYP2D6, the need for a decreased dose of the original medication should be considered).
No products indexed under this heading.

Pargyline Hydrochloride (Concomitant use in patients taking MAO inhibitors is contraindicated. There have been reports of serious, sometimes fatal, reactions in patients receiving, or who have recently discontinued, fluoxetine and are then started on an MAO inhibitor. Therefore, Symbyax should not be used in combination with, or within a minimum of 14 days of discontinuing, MAO inhibitors).
No products indexed under this heading.

Paroxetine Hydrochloride (Based on the mechanism of action of SNRIs and SSRIs and the potential for serotonin syndrome, caution is advised when sertraline is co-administered with other drugs that may effect the serotonergic neurotransmitter systems). Products include:
Paxil 1535
Paxil CR Controlled-Release Tablets.. 1544

Penbutolol Sulfate (Because of the potential for olanzapine to induce hypotension, Symbyax may enhance the effects of certain antihypertensive agents).
No products indexed under this heading.

Pergolide Mesylate (The olanzapine component of Symbyax may antagonize the effects of levodopa and dopamine agonists).
No products indexed under this heading.

Perindopril Erbumine (Because of the potential for olanzapine to induce hypotension, Symbyax may enhance the effects of certain antihypertensive agents). Products include:
Aceon Tablets (2 mg, 4 mg, 8 mg)... 3038

Phenelzine Sulfate (Concomitant use in patients taking MAO inhibitors is contraindicated. There have been reports of serious, sometimes fatal, reactions in patients receiving, or who have recently discontinued, fluoxetine and are then started on an MAO inhibitor. Therefore, Symbyax should not be used in combination with, or within a minimum of 14 days of discontinuing, MAO inhibitors).
No products indexed under this heading.

Phenobarbital (Agents that induce CYP1A2 or glucuronyl transferase enzymes may cause an increase in olanzapine concentration). Products include:
Donnatal Extentabs 2507

Phenoxybenzamine Hydrochloride (Because of the potential for olanzapine to induce hypotension, Symbyax may enhance the effects of certain antihypertensive agents).
Products include:
Dibenzyline Capsules 3188

Phentolamine Mesylate (Because of the potential for olanzapine to induce hypotension, Symbyax may enhance the effects of certain antihypertensive agents).
No products indexed under this heading.

Phenylbutazone (Serotonin release by platelets plays an important role in hemostasis. Studies have demonstrated an association between the use of psychotropic drugs that interfere with serotonin reuptake and the occurrence of upper gastrointestinal bleeding. These studies have also shown that concurrent use of an NSAID potentiated the risk of bleeding. Therefore, patients should be cautioned about the use of NSAIDs concurrently with Symbyax).
No products indexed under this heading.

Phenytoin (Patients on stable doses of phenytoin have developed elevated plasma levels of phenytoin with clinical pheytoin toxicity following initiation of concomitant fluoxetine).
No products indexed under this heading.

Phenytoin Sodium (Patients on stable doses of phenytoin have developed elevated plasma levels of phenytoin with clinical pheytoin toxicity following initiation of concomitant fluoxetine). Products include:
Phenytek Capsules 2192

Pimozide (Concomitant use in patients taking pimozide is contraindicated).
No products indexed under this heading.

Pindolol (Because of the potential for olanzapine to induce hypotension, Symbyax may enhance the effects of certain antihypertensive agents).
No products indexed under this heading.

Piroxicam (Serotonin release by platelets plays an important role in hemostasis. Studies have demonstrated an association between the use of psychotropic drugs that interfere with serotonin reuptake and the occurrence of upper gastrointestinal bleeding. These studies have also shown that concurrent use of an NSAID potentiated the risk of bleeding. Therefore, patients should be cautioned about the use of NSAIDs concurrently with Symbyax).
No products indexed under this heading.

Polythiazide (Because of the potential for olanzapine to induce hypotension, Symbyax may enhance the effects of certain antihypertensive agents).
No products indexed under this heading.

Pramipexole Dihydrochloride (The olanzapine component of Symbyax may antagonize the effects of levodopa and dopamine agonists). Products include:
Mirapex Tablets 857

Prazosin Hydrochloride (Because of the potential for olanzapine to induce hypotension, Symbyax may enhance the effects of certain antihypertensive agents).
No products indexed under this heading.

Primidone (Agents that induce CYP1A2 or glucuronyl transferase enzymes may cause an increase in olanzapine concentration).
No products indexed under this heading.

Procarbazine Hydrochloride (Concomitant use in patients taking MAO inhibitors is contraindicated. There have been reports of serious, sometimes fatal, reactions in patients receiving, or who have recently discontinued, fluoxetine and are then started on an MAO inhibitor. Therefore, Symbyax should not be used in combination with, or within a minimum of 14 days of discontinuing, MAO inhibitors).
No products indexed under this heading.

Propafenone Hydrochloride (Fluoxetine, like other agents that are metabolized by CYP2D6, inhibits the activity of this isoenzyme. Therapy with medications that are predominately metabolized by the CYP2D6 system and have a relatively narrow therapeutic index should be initiated at the low end of the dose range if the patient is receiving fluoxetine concurrently or has taken it in the previous five weeks. If fluoxetine is added to the treatment regimen of a patient already receiving a drug metabolized by CYP2D6, the need for a decreased dose of the original medication should be considered). Products include:
Rythmol Tablets 1586
Rythmol SR Capsules 1590

Propoxyphene Hydrochloride (Fluoxetine, like other agents that are metabolized by CYP2D6, inhibits the activity of this isoenzyme. Therapy with medications that are predominately metabolized by the CYP2D6 system and have a relatively narrow therapeutic index should be initiated at the low end of the dose range if the patient is receiving fluoxetine concurrently or has taken it in the previous five weeks. If fluoxetine is added to the treatment regimen of a patient already receiving a drug metabolized by CYP2D6, the need for a decreased dose of the original medication should be considered).
No products indexed under this heading.

Propoxyphene Napsylate (Fluoxetine, like other agents that are metabolized by CYP2D6, inhibits the activity of this isoenzyme. Therapy with medications that are predominately metabolized by the CYP2D6 system and have a relatively narrow therapeutic index should be initiated at the low end of the dose range if the patient is receiving fluoxetine concurrently or has taken it in the previous five weeks. If fluoxetine is added to the treatment regimen of a patient already receiving a drug metabolized by CYP2D6, the need for a decreased dose of the original medication should be considered).
No products indexed under this heading.

Propranolol Hydrochloride (Because of the potential for olanzapine to induce hypotension, Symbyax may enhance the effects of certain antihypertensive agents). Products include:
InnoPran XL Extended Release Capsules.................................... 1484

Protriptyline Hydrochloride (In two fluoxetine studies, previously stable plasma levels of imipramine and desipramine have increased >2- to 10-fold when fluoxetine has been administered in combination. This influence may persist for three weeks or longer after fluoxetine is discontinued. Thus, the dose of TCA may need to be reduced and plasma TCA concentrations may need to be monitored temporarily when Symbyax is co-administered or has been recently discontinued).
No products indexed under this heading.

Quetiapine Fumarate (Fluoxetine, like other agents that are metabolized by CYP2D6, inhibits the activity of this isoenzyme. Therapy with medications that are predominately metabolized by the CYP2D6 system and have a relatively narrow therapeutic index should be initiated at the low end of the dose range if the patient is receiving fluoxetine concurrently or has taken it in the previous five weeks. If fluoxetine is added to the treatment regimen of a patient already receiving a drug metabolized by CYP2D6, the need for a decreased dose of the original medication should be considered).
No products indexed under this heading.

Quinapril Hydrochloride (Because of the potential for olanzapine to induce hypotension, Symbyax may enhance the effects of certain antihypertensive agents).
No products indexed under this heading.

Quinidine Gluconate (Fluoxetine, like other agents that are metabolized by CYP2D6, inhibits the activity of this isoenzyme. Therapy with medications that are predominately metabolized by the CYP2D6 system and have a relatively narrow therapeutic index should be initiated at the low end of the dose range if the patient is receiving fluoxetine concurrently or has taken it in the previous five weeks. If fluoxetine is added to the treatment regimen of a patient already receiving a drug metabolized by CYP2D6, the need for a decreased dose of the original medication should be considered).
No products indexed under this heading.

Quinidine Hydrochloride (Fluoxetine, like other agents that are metabolized by CYP2D6, inhibits the activity of this isoenzyme. Therapy with medications that are predominately metabolized by the CYP2D6 system and have a relatively narrow therapeutic index should be initiated at the low end of the dose range if the patient is receiving fluoxetine concurrently or has taken it in the previous five weeks. If fluoxetine is added to the treatment regimen of a patient already receiving a drug metabolized by CYP2D6, the need for a decreased dose of the original medication should be considered).
No products indexed under this heading.

Quinidine Polygalacturonate (Fluoxetine, like other agents that are metabolized by CYP2D6, inhibits the activity of this isoenzyme. Therapy with medications that are predominately metabolized by the CYP2D6 system and have a relatively narrow therapeutic index should be initiated at the low end of the dose range if the patient is receiving fluoxetine concurrently or has taken it in the previous five weeks. If fluoxetine is added to the treatment regimen of a patient already receiving a drug metabolized by CYP2D6, the need for a decreased dose of the original medication should be considered).
No products indexed under this heading.

Quinidine Sulfate (Fluoxetine, like other agents that are metabolized by CYP2D6, inhibits the activity of this isoenzyme. Therapy with medications that are predominately metabolized by the CYP2D6 system and have a relatively narrow therapeutic index should be initiated at the low end of the dose range if the patient is receiving fluoxetine concurrently or has taken it in the previous five weeks. If fluoxetine is added to the treatment regimen of a patient already receiving a drug metabolized by CYP2D6, the need for a decreased dose of the original medication should be considered).
No products indexed under this heading.

Ramipril (Because of the potential for olanzapine to induce hypotension, Symbyax may enhance the effects of certain antihypertensive agents).
No products indexed under this heading.

Rasagiline Mesylate (Concomitant use in patients taking MAO inhibitors is contraindicated. There have been reports of serious, sometimes fatal, reactions in patients receiving, or who have recently discontinued, fluoxetine and are then started on an MAO inhibitor. Therefore, Symbyax should not be used in combination with, or within a minimum of 14 days of discontinuing, MAO inhibitors). Products include:
Azilect Tablets 3106

Rauwolfia Serpentina (Because of the potential for olanzapine to induce hypotension, Symbyax may enhance the effects of certain antihypertensive agents).
No products indexed under this heading.

Rescinnamine (Because of the potential for olanzapine to induce hypotension, Symbyax may enhance the effects of certain antihypertensive agents).
No products indexed under this heading.

Reserpine (Because of the potential for olanzapine to induce hypotension, Symbyax may enhance the effects of certain antihypertensive agents).
No products indexed under this heading.

Rifampicin (Agents that induce CYP1A2 or glucuronyl transferase enzymes may cause an increase in olanzapine concentration).
No products indexed under this heading.

Rifampin (Agents that induce CYP1A2 or glucuronyl transferase enzymes may cause an increase in olanzapine concentration).
No products indexed under this heading.

Risperidone (Fluoxetine, like other agents that are metabolized by CYP2D6, inhibits the activity of this isoenzyme. Therapy with medications that are predominately metabolized by the CYP2D6 system and have a relatively narrow therapeutic index should be initiated at the low end of the dose range if the patient is receiving fluoxetine concurrently or has taken it in the previous five weeks. If fluoxetine is added to the treatment regimen of a patient already receiving a drug metabolized by CYP2D6, the need for a decreased dose of the original medication should be considered). Products include:
Risperdal Consta Long-Acting Injection 1753

Ritonavir (Agents that induce CYP1A2 or glucuronyl transferase enzymes may cause an increase in olanzapine concentration). Products include:
Kaletra 452
Norvir 489

Rizatriptan Benzoate (If concomitant treatment of sertraline with a triptan is clinically warranted, careful observation of the patient is advised, particularly during treatment initiation and dose increases). Products include:
Maxalt Tablets 2056
Maxalt-MLT Orally Disintegrating Tablets 2056

Rofecoxib (Serotonin release by platelets plays an important role in hemostasis. Studies have demonstrated an association between the use of psychotropic drugs that interfere with serotonin reuptake and the occurrence of upper gastrointestinal bleeding. These studies have also shown that concurrent use of an NSAID potentiated the risk of bleeding. Therefore, patients should be cautioned about the use of NSAIDs

concurrently with Symbyax).
No products indexed under this heading.

Ropinirole Hydrochloride (The olanzapine component of Symbyax may antagonize the effects of levodopa and dopamine agonists). Products include:
Requip Tablets ... 1561
Requip XL Tablets ... 1568

Selegiline (Concomitant use in patients taking MAO inhibitors is contraindicated. There have been reports of serious, sometimes fatal, reactions in patients receiving, or who have recently discontinued, fluoxetine and are then started on an MAO inhibitor. Therefore, Symbyax should not be used in combination with, or within a minimum of 14 days of discontinuing, MAO inhibitors). Products include:
Emsam Transdermal System ... 905

Selegiline Hydrochloride (Concomitant use in patients taking MAO inhibitors is contraindicated. There have been reports of serious, sometimes fatal, reactions in patients receiving, or who have recently discontinued, fluoxetine and are then started on an MAO inhibitor. Therefore, Symbyax should not be used in combination with, or within a minimum of 14 days of discontinuing, MAO inhibitors). Products include:
Eldepryl Capsules ... 3052

Sertraline Hydrochloride (Based on the mechanism of action of SNRIs and SSRIs and the potential for serotonin syndrome, caution is advised when sertraline is co-administered with other drugs that may effect the serotonergic neurotransmitter systems).
No products indexed under this heading.

Sodium Nitroprusside (Because of the potential for olanzapine to induce hypotension, Symbyax may enhance the effects of certain antihypertensive agents).
No products indexed under this heading.

Sotalol Hydrochloride (Because of the potential for olanzapine to induce hypotension, Symbyax may enhance the effects of certain antihypertensive agents).
No products indexed under this heading.

Spirapril Hydrochloride (Because of the potential for olanzapine to induce hypotension, Symbyax may enhance the effects of certain antihypertensive agents).
No products indexed under this heading.

Spironolactone (Hyponatremia may occur as a result of treatment with SSRIs and SNRIs, including Symbyax. In many cases, this hyponatremia appears to be the result of the syndrome of inappropriate antidiuretic hormone secretion (SIADH). Cases with serum sodium lower than 110 mmol/L have been reported and appeared to be reversible when Symbyax was discontinued. Elderly patients may be at greater risk of developing hyponatremia with SSRIs and SNRIs. Also, patients taking diuretics or who are otherwise volume depleted may be at greater risk. Discontinuation of Symbyax should be considered in patients with symptomatic hyponatremia and appropriate medical intervention should be instituted).
No products indexed under this heading.

Sulindac (Serotonin release by platelets plays an important role in hemostasis. Studies have demonstrated an association between the use of psychotropic drugs that interfere with serotonin reuptake and the occurrence of upper gastrointestinal bleeding. These studies have also shown that concurrent use of an NSAID potentiated the risk of bleeding. Therefore, patients should be cautioned about the use of NSAIDs concurrently with Symbyax). Products include:
Clinoril Tablets ... 1962

Sumatriptan (There have been rare postmarketing reports describing patients with weakness, hyperreflexia, and incoordination following the use of an SSRI and sumatriptan. If concomitant treatment with sumatriptan and an SSRI is clinically warranted, appropriate observation of the patient is advised). Products include:
Imitrex Nasal Spray ... 1470

Sumatriptan Succinate (There have been rare postmarketing reports describing patients with weakness, hyperreflexia, and incoordination following the use of an SSRI and sumatriptan. If concomitant treatment with sumatriptan and an SSRI is clinically warranted, appropriate observation of the patient is advised). Products include:
Imitrex Injection ... 1465
Imitrex Tablets ... 1474
Treximet Tablets ... 1616

Tamoxifen Citrate (Fluoxetine, like other agents that are metabolized by CYP2D6, inhibits the activity of this isoenzyme. Therapy with medications that are predominately metabolized by the CYP2D6 system and have a relatively narrow therapeutic index should be initiated at the low end of the dose range if the patient is receiving fluoxetine concurrently or has taken it in the previous five weeks. If fluoxetine is added to the treatment regimen of a patient already receiving a drug metabolized by CYP2D6, the need for a decreased dose of the original medication should be considered).
No products indexed under this heading.

Telmisartan (Because of the potential for olanzapine to induce hypotension, Symbyax may enhance the effects of certain antihypertensive agents). Products include:
Micardis Tablets ... 852
Micardis HCT Tablets ... 854

Temazepam (Because fluoxetine is tightly bound to plasma protein, the administration of fluoxetine to a patient taking another drug that is tightly bound to protein may cause a shift in plasma concentrations potentially resulting in an adverse effect. Conversely, adverse effects may result from displacement of protein-bound fluoxetine by other tightly bound drugs).
No products indexed under this heading.

Teniposide (Fluoxetine, like other agents that are metabolized by CYP2D6, inhibits the activity of this isoenzyme. Therapy with medications that are predominately metabolized by the CYP2D6 system and have a relatively narrow therapeutic index should be initiated at the low end of the dose range if the patient is receiving fluoxetine concurrently or has taken it in the previous five weeks. If fluoxetine is added to the treatment regimen of a patient already receiving a drug metabolized by CYP2D6, the need for a decreased dose of the original medication should be considered).
No products indexed under this heading.

Terazosin Hydrochloride (Because of the potential for olanzapine to induce hypotension, Symbyax may enhance the effects of certain antihypertensive agents).
No products indexed under this heading.

Testosterone (Fluoxetine, like other agents that are metabolized by CYP2D6, inhibits the activity of this isoenzyme. Therapy with medications that are predominately metabolized by the CYP2D6 system and have a relatively narrow therapeutic index should be initiated at the low end of the dose range if the patient is receiving fluoxetine concurrently or has taken it in the previous five weeks. If fluoxetine is added to the treatment regimen of a patient already receiving a drug metabolized by CYP2D6, the need for a decreased dose of the original medication should be considered). Products include:
AndroGel ... 3159
Testim 1% Gel ... 701

Testosterone Cypionate (Fluoxetine, like other agents that are metabolized by CYP2D6, inhibits the activity of this isoenzyme. Therapy with medications that are predominately metabolized by the CYP2D6 system and have a relatively narrow therapeutic index should be initiated at the low end of the dose range if the patient is receiving fluoxetine concurrently or has taken it in the previous five weeks. If fluoxetine is added to the treatment regimen of a patient already receiving a drug metabolized by CYP2D6, the need for a decreased dose of the original medication should be considered).
No products indexed under this heading.

Testosterone Enanthate (Fluoxetine, like other agents that are metabolized by CYP2D6, inhibits the activity of this isoenzyme. Therapy with medications that are predominately metabolized by the CYP2D6 system and have a relatively narrow therapeutic index should be initiated at the low end of the dose range if the patient is receiving fluoxetine concurrently or has taken it in the previous five weeks. If fluoxetine is added to the treatment regimen of a patient already receiving a drug metabolized by CYP2D6, the need for a decreased dose of the original medication should be considered). Products include:
Delatestryl Injection ... 1730

Testosterone Propionate (Fluoxetine, like other agents that are metabolized by CYP2D6, inhibits the activity of this isoenzyme. Therapy with medications that are predominately metabolized by the CYP2D6 system and have a relatively narrow therapeutic index should be initiated at the low end of the dose range if the patient is receiving fluoxetine concurrently or has taken it in the previous five weeks. If fluoxetine is added to the treatment regimen of a patient already receiving a drug metabolized by CYP2D6, the need for a decreased dose of the original medication should be considered).
No products indexed under this heading.

Thioridazine (Concomitant use in patients taking Thioridazine is contraindicated. Thioridazine should not be administered with Symbyax or administered within a minimum of 5 weeks after discontinuation of Symbyax).
No products indexed under this heading.

Thioridazine Hydrochloride (Concomitant use in patients taking Thioridazine is contraindicated. Thioridazine should not be administered with Symbyax or administered within a minimum of 5 weeks after discontinuation of Symbyax). Products include:
Thioridazine Hydrochloride Tablets ... 2195

Timolol Maleate (Because of the potential for olanzapine to induce hypotension, Symbyax may enhance the effects of certain antihypertensive agents). Products include:
Combigan Ophthalmic Solution ... 553
Cosopt Sterile Ophthalmic Solution ... 1969
Timoptic Sterile Ophthalmic Solution ... 2121
Timoptic in Ocudose ... 2124
Timoptic-XE Sterile Ophthalmic Gel Forming Solution ... 2125

Tobacco (Agents that induce CYP1A2 or glucuronyl transferase enzymes may cause an increase in olanzapine concentration).
No products indexed under this heading.

Tolbutamide (Because fluoxetine is tightly bound to plasma protein, the administration of fluoxetine to a patient taking another drug that is tightly bound to protein may cause a shift in plasma concentrations potentially resulting in an adverse effect. Conversely, adverse effects may result from displacement of protein-bound fluoxetine by other tightly bound drugs).
No products indexed under this heading.

Tolmetin Sodium (Serotonin release by platelets plays an important role in hemostasis. Studies have demonstrated an association between the use of psychotropic drugs that interfere with serotonin reuptake and the occurrence of upper gastrointestinal bleeding. These studies have also shown that concurrent use of an NSAID potentiated the risk of bleeding. Therefore, patients should be cautioned about the use of NSAIDs concurrently with Symbyax).
No products indexed under this heading.

Tolterodine Tartrate (Fluoxetine, like other agents that are metabolized by CYP2D6, inhibits the activity of this isoenzyme. Therapy with medications that are predominately metabolized by the CYP2D6 system and have a relatively narrow therapeutic index should be initiated at the low end of the dose range if the patient is receiving fluoxetine concurrently or has taken it in the previous five weeks. If fluoxetine is added to the treatment regimen of a patient

already receiving a drug metabolized by CYP2D6, the need for a decreased dose of the original medication should be considered).

No products indexed under this heading.

Torsemide (Because of the potential for olanzapine to induce hypotension, Symbyax may enhance the effects of certain antihypertensive agents). Products include:

Demadex Injection 2630
Demadex Tablets 2630

Tramadol Hydrochloride (Based on the mechanism of action of SNRIs and SSRIs and the potential for serotonin syndrome, caution is advised when sertraline is co-administered with other drugs that may effect the serotonergic neurotransmitter systems, such as tramadol). Products include:

Ultram ER Extended-Release Tablets 2428

Trandolapril (Because of the potential for olanzapine to induce hypotension, Symbyax may enhance the effects of certain antihypertensive agents). Products include:

Mavik Tablets 472
Tarka Tablets 511

Tranylcypromine Sulfate (Concomitant use in patients taking MAO inhibitors is contraindicated. There have been reports of serious, sometimes fatal, reactions in patients receiving, or who have recently discontinued, fluoxetine and are then started on an MAO inhibitor. Therefore, Symbyax should not be used in combination with, or within a minimum of 14 days of discontinuing, MAO inhibitors). Products include:

Parnate Tablets 1532

Trazodone Hydrochloride (Fluoxetine, like other agents that are metabolized by CYP2D6, inhibits the activity of this isoenzyme. Therapy with medications that are predominately metabolized by the CYP2D6 system and have a relatively narrow therapeutic index should be initiated at the low end of the dose range if the patient is receiving fluoxetine concurrently or has taken it in the previous five weeks. If fluoxetine is added to the treatment regimen of a patient already receiving a drug metabolized by CYP2D6, the need for a decreased dose of the original medication should be considered).

No products indexed under this heading.

Triamterene (Hyponatremia may occur as a result of treatment with SSRIs and SNRIs, including Symbyax. In many cases, this hyponatremia appears to be the result of the syndrome of inappropriate antidiuretic hormone secretion (SIADH). Cases with serum sodium lower than 110 mmol/L have been reported and appeared to be reversible when Symbyax was discontinued. Elderly patients may be at greater risk of developing hyponatremia with SSRIs and SNRIs. Also, patients taking diuretics or who are otherwise volume depleted may be at greater risk. Discontinuation of Symbyax should be considered in patients with symptomatic hyponatremia and appropriate medical intervention should be instituted). Products include:

Dyazide Capsules 1405
Dyrenium Capsules 3189

Triazolam (Fluoxetine, like other agents that are metabolized by CYP2D6, inhibits the activity of this isoenzyme. Therapy with medications that are predominately metabolized by the CYP2D6 system and have a relatively narrow therapeutic index should be initiated at the low end of the dose range if the patient is receiving fluoxetine concurrently or has taken it in the previous five weeks. If fluoxetine is added to the treatment regimen of a patient already receiving a drug metabolized by CYP2D6, the need for a decreased dose of the original medication should be considered).

No products indexed under this heading.

Trimethaphan Camsylate (Because of the potential for olanzapine to induce hypotension, Symbyax may enhance the effects of certain antihypertensive agents).

No products indexed under this heading.

Trimipramine Maleate (In two fluoxetine studies, previously stable plasma levels of imipramine and desipramine have increased >2- to 10-fold when fluoxetine has been administered in combination. This influence may persist for three weeks or longer after fluoxetine is discontinued. Thus, the dose of TCA may need to be reduced and plasma TCA concentrations may need to be monitored temporarily when Symbyax is co-administered or has been recently discontinued).

No products indexed under this heading.

L-Tryptophan (Five patients receiving fluoxetine in combination with tryptophan experienced adverse reactions, including agitation, restlessness, and gastrointestinal distress. Concomitant use of Symbyax with serotonin precursors, such as tryptophan, is not recommended).

No products indexed under this heading.

Valdecoxib (Serotonin release by platelets plays an important role in hemostasis. Studies have demonstrated an association between the use of psychotropic drugs that interfere with serotonin reuptake and the occurrence of upper gastrointestinal bleeding. These studies have also shown that concurrent use of an NSAID potentiated the risk of bleeding. Therefore, patients should be cautioned about the use of NSAIDs concurrently with Symbyax).

No products indexed under this heading.

Valsartan (Because of the potential for olanzapine to induce hypotension, Symbyax may enhance the effects of certain antihypertensive agents). Products include:

Diovan Tablets 2212
Diovan HCT Tablets 2216
Exforge Tablets 2238

Venlafaxine Hydrochloride (Based on the mechanism of action of SNRIs and SSRIs and the potential for serotonin syndrome, caution is advised when sertraline is co-administered with other drugs that may effect the serotonergic neurotransmitter systems). Products include:

Effexor XR Extended-Release Capsules 3195
Venlafaxine Hydrochloride Tablets ... 2199

Verapamil Hydrochloride (Because of the potential for olanzapine to induce hypotension, Symbyax may enhance the effects of certain antihypertensive agents). Products include:

Tarka Tablets 511

Vinblastine Sulfate (Fluoxetine, like other agents that are metabolized by CYP2D6, inhibits the activity of this isoenzyme. Therapy with medications that are predominately metabolized by the CYP2D6 system and have a relatively narrow therapeutic index should be initiated at the low end of the dose range if the patient is receiving fluoxetine concurrently or has taken it in the previous five weeks. If fluoxetine is added to the treatment regimen of a patient already receiving a drug metabolized by CYP2D6, the need for a decreased dose of the original medication should be considered).

No products indexed under this heading.

Warfarin Sodium (Altered anticoagulant effects, including increased bleeding, have been reported when SSRIs or SNRIs are co-administered with warfarin. Patients receiving warfarin therapy should receive careful coagulation monitoring when Symbyax is initiated or stopped).

No products indexed under this heading.

Zolmitriptan (If concomitant treatment of sertraline with a triptan is clinically warranted, careful observation of the patient is advised, particularly during treatment initiation and dose increases). Products include:

Zomig Tablets 694
Zomig Nasal Spray 689
Zomig-ZMT Tablets 694

Zonisamide (Fluoxetine, like other agents that are metabolized by CYP2D6, inhibits the activity of this isoenzyme. Therapy with medications that are predominately metabolized by the CYP2D6 system and have a relatively narrow therapeutic index should be initiated at the low end of the dose range if the patient is receiving fluoxetine concurrently or has taken it in the previous five weeks. If fluoxetine is added to the treatment regimen of a patient already receiving a drug metabolized by CYP2D6, the need for a decreased dose of the original medication should be considered). Products include:

Zonegran Capsules 1089

Food Interactions

Alcohol (Alcohol may potentiate the orthostatic effect of olanzapine, increasing the risk of orthostatic hypotension. Therefore, patients should be advised to avoid alcohol while taking Symbyax).

Broccoli (Agents that induce CYP1A2 or glucuronyl transferase enzymes may cause an increase in olanzapine concentration).

Brussel Sprouts (Agents that induce CYP1A2 or glucuronyl transferase enzymes may cause an increase in olanzapine concentration).

Charbroiled Food (Agents that induce CYP1A2 or glucuronyl transferase enzymes may cause an increase in olanzapine concentration).

SYNAGIS INTRAMUSCULAR SOLUTION

(Palivizumab) 1948
None cited in PDR database.

SYNERGYDEFENSE CAPSULES

(Herbals, Multiple) 625
None cited in PDR database.

SYNTHROID TABLETS

(Levothyroxine Sodium) 507
May interact with androgens, antithyroid agents, beta blockers, oral anticoagulants, cytokines, dopamine agonists, estrogens, glucocorticoids, cardiac glycosides, hepatic microsomal enzyme inducers, oral hypoglycemic agents, insulin, lithium preparations, phenytoin, radiographic iodinated contrast media, salicylates, sulfonamides, sulfonylureas, sympathomimetics, thiazides, tricyclic antidepressants, xanthines, and certain other agents. Compounds in these categories include:

Acarbose (Requirements of oral antidiabetic agents may be reduced in hypothyroid patients with diabetes and may be subsequently increased with initiation of thyroid hormone therapy). Products include:

Precose Tablets 792

Acebutolol Hydrochloride (Alters thyroid hormone or TSH levels; actions of some beta blockers may be impaired when hypothyroid patients become euthyroid).

No products indexed under this heading.

Albuterol (Possible increased risk of coronary insufficiency in patients with coronary artery disease).

No products indexed under this heading.

Albuterol Sulfate (Possible increased risk of coronary insufficiency in patients with coronary artery disease). Products include:

Combivent Inhalation Aerosol 845
ProAir HFA Inhalation Aerosol 3113
Proventil HFA Inhalation Aerosol 2914
Ventolin HFA Inhalation Aerosol 1638

Aldesleukin (Cytokines have been reported to induce both hyperthyroidism or hypothyroidism; dosage adjustment may be necessary). Products include:

Proleukin for Injection 2287

Aluminum Hydroxide (Binds and decreases absorption of levothyroxine sodium from the gastrointestinal tract).

No products indexed under this heading.

Aminoglutethimide (Alters thyroid hormone or TSH levels).

No products indexed under this heading.

Aminophylline (Theophylline clearance may be decreased in hypothyroid patients and return toward normal when euthyroid state is achieved).

No products indexed under this heading.

p-Aminosalicylic Acid (Alters thyroid hormone or TSH levels).

No products indexed under this heading.

Amiodarone Hydrochloride (Amiodarone therapy alone can cause hypothyroidism or hyperthyroidism).

No products indexed under this heading.

Amitriptyline Hydrochloride (Concurrent use may increase the therapeutic and toxic effects of both drugs; onset of action of tricyclics may be accelerated).
No products indexed under this heading.

Amoxapine (Concurrent use may increase the therapeutic and toxic effects of both drugs; onset of action of tricyclics may be accelerated).
No products indexed under this heading.

Anisindione (The hypoprothrombinemic effect of anticoagulants may be potentiated).
No products indexed under this heading.

Asparaginase (May inhibit levothyroxine sodium binding to serum proteins or alter the concentrations of serum proteins). Products include:
Elspar for Injection ... 1990
Elspar for Injection ... 2488

Aspirin (May inhibit levothyroxine sodium binding to serum proteins or alter the concentrations of serum proteins). Products include:
Aggrenox Capsules ... 819
Bayer Aspirin ... 750
Percodan Tablets ... 1130
St. Joseph 81 mg Aspirin Chewable and Enteric Coated Tablets ... 1903

Aspirin, Enteric Coated (May inhibit levothyroxine sodium binding to serum proteins or alter the concentrations of serum proteins).
No products indexed under this heading.

Aspirin Buffered (May inhibit levothyroxine sodium binding to serum proteins or alter the concentrations of serum proteins).
No products indexed under this heading.

Atenolol (Alters thyroid hormone or TSH levels; actions of some beta blockers may be impaired when hypothyroid patients become euthyroid).
No products indexed under this heading.

Bendroflumethiazide (Alters thyroid hormone or TSH levels).
No products indexed under this heading.

Betamethasone Acetate (May inhibit levothyroxine sodium binding to serum proteins or alter the concentrations of serum proteins).
No products indexed under this heading.

Betamethasone Sodium Phosphate (May inhibit levothyroxine sodium binding to serum proteins or alter the concentrations of serum proteins).
No products indexed under this heading.

Betaxolol Hydrochloride (Alters thyroid hormone or TSH levels; actions of some beta blockers may be impaired when hypothyroid patients become euthyroid).
No products indexed under this heading.

Bisoprolol Fumarate (Alters thyroid hormone or TSH levels; actions of some beta blockers may be impaired when hypothyroid patients become euthyroid).
No products indexed under this heading.

Bromocriptine Mesylate (Alters thyroid hormone or TSH levels).
No products indexed under this heading.

Carbamazepine (Alters thyroid hormone or TSH levels). Products include:
Carbatrol Capsules ... 3019
Equetro Extended-Release Capsules ... 3174

Carteolol Hydrochloride (Alters thyroid hormone or TSH levels; actions of some beta blockers may be impaired when hypothyroid patients become euthyroid).
No products indexed under this heading.

Chloral Hydrate (Alters thyroid hormone or TSH levels).
No products indexed under this heading.

Chlorothiazide (Alters thyroid hormone or TSH levels).
No products indexed under this heading.

Chlorothiazide Sodium (Alters thyroid hormone or TSH levels). Products include:
Intravenous Sodium Diuril ... 2490

Chlorotrianisene (Estrogens or estrogen-containing compounds may inhibit levothyroxine sodium binding to serum proteins or alter the concentrations of serum proteins).
No products indexed under this heading.

Chlorpropamide (Alters thyroid hormone or TSH levels).
No products indexed under this heading.

Cholestyramine (Binds and decreases absorption of levothyroxine sodium from the gastrointestinal tract).
No products indexed under this heading.

Choline Magnesium Trisalicylate (May inhibit levothyroxine sodium binding to serum proteins or alter the concentrations of serum proteins).
No products indexed under this heading.

Clofibrate (May inhibit levothyroxine sodium binding to serum proteins or alter the concentrations of serum proteins).
No products indexed under this heading.

Clomipramine Hydrochloride (Concurrent use may increase the therapeutic and toxic effects of both drugs; onset of action of tricyclics may be accelerated).
No products indexed under this heading.

Colestipol Hydrochloride (Binds and decreases absorption of levothyroxine sodium from the gastrointestinal tract).
No products indexed under this heading.

Cortisone Acetate (May inhibit levothyroxine sodium binding to serum proteins or alter the concentrations of serum proteins).
No products indexed under this heading.

Desipramine Hydrochloride (Concurrent use may increase the therapeutic and toxic effects of both drugs; onset of action of tricyclics may be accelerated).
No products indexed under this heading.

Deslanoside (Therapeutic effects of digitalis glycosides may be reduced; serum digitalis levels may be decreased in hyperthyroidism or when a hypothyroid patient becomes euthyroid).
No products indexed under this heading.

Dexamethasone (May inhibit levothyroxine sodium binding to serum proteins or alter the concentrations of serum proteins). Products include:
Ciprodex Otic Suspension ... 541

Dexamethasone Acetate (May inhibit levothyroxine sodium binding to serum proteins or alter the concentrations of serum proteins).
No products indexed under this heading.

Dexamethasone Sodium Phosphate (May inhibit levothyroxine sodium binding to serum proteins or alter the concentrations of serum proteins).
No products indexed under this heading.

Diatrizoate Meglumine (Alters thyroid hormone or TSH levels).
No products indexed under this heading.

Diatrizoate Sodium (Alters thyroid hormone or TSH levels).
No products indexed under this heading.

Diazepam (Alters thyroid hormone or TSH levels). Products include:
Valium Tablets ... 2658

Dicumarol (The hypoprothrombinemic effect of anticoagulants may be potentiated).
No products indexed under this heading.

Dienestrol (Estrogens or estrogen-containing compounds may inhibit levothyroxine sodium binding to serum proteins or alter the concentrations of serum proteins).
No products indexed under this heading.

Diethylstilbestrol (Estrogens or estrogen-containing compounds may inhibit levothyroxine sodium binding to serum proteins or alter the concentrations of serum proteins).
No products indexed under this heading.

Diflunisal (May inhibit levothyroxine sodium binding to serum proteins or alter the concentrations of serum proteins).
No products indexed under this heading.

Digitalis Glycoside Preparations (Therapeutic effects of digitalis glycosides may be reduced; serum digitalis levels may be decreased in hyperthyroidism or when a hypothyroid patient becomes euthyroid).
No products indexed under this heading.

Digitoxin (Therapeutic effects of digitalis glycosides may be reduced; serum digitalis levels may be decreased in hyperthyroidism or when a hypothyroid patient becomes euthyroid).
No products indexed under this heading.

Digoxin (Therapeutic effects of digitalis glycosides may be reduced; serum digitalis levels may be decreased in hyperthyroidism or when a hypothyroid patient becomes euthyroid). Products include:
Lanoxin Injection ... 1498
Lanoxin Injection Pediatric ... 1502
Lanoxin Tablets ... 1505

Dobutamine Hydrochloride (Possible increased risk of coronary insufficiency in patients with coronary artery disease).
No products indexed under this heading.

Dopamine Hydrochloride (Alters thyroid hormone or TSH levels).
No products indexed under this heading.

Doxepin Hydrochloride (Concurrent use may increase the therapeutic and toxic effects of both drugs; onset of action of tricyclics may be accelerated).
No products indexed under this heading.

Dyphylline (Theophylline clearance may be decreased in hypothyroid patients and return toward normal when euthyroid state is achieved).
No products indexed under this heading.

Ephedrine Hydrochloride (Possible increased risk of coronary insufficiency in patients with coronary artery disease).
No products indexed under this heading.

Ephedrine Sulfate (Possible increased risk of coronary insufficiency in patients with coronary artery disease).
No products indexed under this heading.

Ephedrine Tannate (Possible increased risk of coronary insufficiency in patients with coronary artery disease).
No products indexed under this heading.

Epinephrine (Possible increased risk of coronary insufficiency in patients with coronary artery disease). Products include:
EpiPen ... 1024

Epinephrine Bitartrate (Possible increased risk of coronary insufficiency in patients with coronary artery disease).
No products indexed under this heading.

Epinephrine Hydrochloride (Possible increased risk of coronary insufficiency in patients with coronary artery disease).
No products indexed under this heading.

Esmolol Hydrochloride (Alters thyroid hormone or TSH levels; actions of some beta blockers may be impaired when hypothyroid patients become euthyroid).
No products indexed under this heading.

Estradiol (Estrogens or estrogen-containing compounds may inhibit levothyroxine sodium binding to serum proteins or alter the concentrations of serum proteins). Products include:
Activella Tablets ... 2347
Angeliq Tablets ... 751
Climara Transdermal System ... 763
Climara Pro Transdermal System ... 768
Divigel ... 3167
Vagifem Tablets ... 2375

Estrogens, Conjugated (Estrogens or estrogen-containing compounds may inhibit levothyroxine sodium binding to serum proteins or alter the concentrations of serum proteins). Products include:
Premarin Intravenous ... 3217
Premarin Tablets ... 3221

Premarin Vaginal Cream 3228
Premphase Tablets 3232
Prempro Tablets 3232

Estrogens, Esterified (Estrogens or estrogen-containing compounds may inhibit levothyroxine sodium binding to serum proteins or alter the concentrations of serum proteins). Products include:
Estratest Tablets 3043
Estratest H.S. Tablets 3043

Estropipate (Estrogens or estrogen-containing compounds may inhibit levothyroxine sodium binding to serum proteins or alter the concentrations of serum proteins).
No products indexed under this heading.

Ethanol (Alters thyroid hormone or TSH levels).
No products indexed under this heading.

Ethinyl Estradiol (Estrogens or estrogen-containing compounds may inhibit levothyroxine sodium binding to serum proteins or alter the concentrations of serum proteins). Products include:
Lybrel Tablets 3204
Mircette Tablets 1034
NuvaRing 2897
Ortho-Cyclen/Ortho Tri-Cyclen 2449
Ortho Evra Transdermal System 2437
Ortho Tri-Cyclen Lo Tablets 2458
Seasonique Tablets 1046
Yaz Tablets 805

Ethiodized Oil (Alters thyroid hormone or TSH levels).
No products indexed under this heading.

Ethionamide (Alters thyroid hormone or TSH levels).
No products indexed under this heading.

Ferrous Sulfate (Binds and decreases absorption of levothyroxine sodium from the gastrointestinal tract).
No products indexed under this heading.

Fludrocortisone Acetate (May inhibit levothyroxine sodium binding to serum proteins or alter the concentrations of serum proteins).
No products indexed under this heading.

Fluorouracil (May inhibit levothyroxine sodium binding to serum proteins or alter the concentrations of serum proteins). Products include:
Carac Cream 0.5% 2722

Fluoxymesterone (May inhibit levothyroxine sodium binding to serum proteins or alter the concentrations of serum proteins; alters TSH or thyroid hormone levels).
No products indexed under this heading.

Fosphenytoin Sodium (Alters thyroid hormone or TSH levels).
No products indexed under this heading.

Furosemide (May inhibit levothyroxine sodium binding to serum proteins or alter the concentrations of serum proteins). Products include:
Furosemide Tablets 2186

Gadopentetate Dimeglumine (Alters thyroid hormone or TSH levels).
No products indexed under this heading.

Glimepiride (Alters thyroid hormone or TSH levels; requirements of oral antidiabetic agents may be reduced in hypothyroid patients with diabetes and may be subsequently increased with initiation of thyroid hormone therapy). Products include:
Avandaryl Tablets 1344
Duetact Tablets 3085

Glipizide (Alters thyroid hormone or TSH levels).
No products indexed under this heading.

Glyburide (Alters thyroid hormone or TSH levels).
No products indexed under this heading.

Heparin Sodium (Alters thyroid hormone or TSH levels).
No products indexed under this heading.

Hydrochlorothiazide (Alters thyroid hormone or TSH levels). Products include:
Atacand HCT 642
Avalide Tablets 892
Avalide Tablets 2713
Benicar HCT Tablets 1010
Diovan HCT Tablets 2216
Dyazide Capsules 1405
Micardis HCT Tablets 854
Prinzide Tablets 2092
Tekturna HCT Tablets 2324
Teveten HCT Tablets 517

Hydrocortisone (May inhibit levothyroxine sodium binding to serum proteins or alter the concentrations of serum proteins).
No products indexed under this heading.

Hydrocortisone Acetate (May inhibit levothyroxine sodium binding to serum proteins or alter the concentrations of serum proteins). Products include:
Analpram-HC 1140
Pramosone 1141

Hydrocortisone Sodium Phosphate (May inhibit levothyroxine sodium binding to serum proteins or alter the concentrations of serum proteins).
No products indexed under this heading.

Hydrocortisone Sodium Succinate (May inhibit levothyroxine sodium binding to serum proteins or alter the concentrations of serum proteins).
No products indexed under this heading.

Hydroflumethiazide (Alters thyroid hormone or TSH levels).
No products indexed under this heading.

Imipramine Hydrochloride (Concurrent use may increase the therapeutic and toxic effects of both drugs; onset of action of tricyclics may be accelerated).
No products indexed under this heading.

Imipramine Pamoate (Concurrent use may increase the therapeutic and toxic effects of both drugs; onset of action of tricyclics may be accelerated).
No products indexed under this heading.

Insulin (Requirements of insulin may be reduced in hypothyroid patients with diabetes and may be subsequently increased with initiation of thyroid hormone therapy).
No products indexed under this heading.

Insulin, Human, Zinc Suspension (Requirements of insulin may be reduced in hypothyroid patients with diabetes and may be subsequently increased with initiation of thyroid hormone therapy).
No products indexed under this heading.

Insulin, Human (rDNA origin) (Requirements of insulin may be reduced in hypothyroid patients with diabetes and may be subsequently increased with initiation of thyroid hormone therapy). Products include:
Exubera Inhalation Powder 2515

Insulin, Human NPH (Requirements of insulin may be reduced in hypothyroid patients with diabetes and may be subsequently increased with initiation of thyroid hormone therapy). Products include:
Humulin N Vial 1846

Insulin, Human Regular (Requirements of insulin may be reduced in hypothyroid patients with diabetes and may be subsequently increased with initiation of thyroid hormone therapy). Products include:
Humulin R 1849
Humulin R (U-500) 1850

Insulin, Human Regular and Human NPH Mixture (Requirements of insulin may be reduced in hypothyroid patients with diabetes and may be subsequently increased with initiation of thyroid hormone therapy). Products include:
Humulin 50/50, 100 Units 1843
Humulin 70/30 Vial 1844

Insulin, NPH (Requirements of insulin may be reduced in hypothyroid patients with diabetes and may be subsequently increased with initiation of thyroid hormone therapy).
No products indexed under this heading.

Insulin, Regular (Requirements of insulin may be reduced in hypothyroid patients with diabetes and may be subsequently increased with initiation of thyroid hormone therapy).
No products indexed under this heading.

Insulin, Regular and NPH mixture (Requirements of insulin may be reduced in hypothyroid patients with diabetes and may be subsequently increased with initiation of thyroid hormone therapy).
No products indexed under this heading.

Insulin, Zinc Crystals (Requirements of insulin may be reduced in hypothyroid patients with diabetes and may be subsequently increased with initiation of thyroid hormone therapy).
No products indexed under this heading.

Insulin, Zinc Suspension (Requirements of insulin may be reduced in hypothyroid patients with diabetes and may be subsequently increased with initiation of thyroid hormone therapy).
No products indexed under this heading.

Insulin Aspart (Requirements of insulin may be reduced in hypothyroid patients with diabetes and may be subsequently increased with initiation of thyroid hormone therapy).
No products indexed under this heading.

Insulin Aspart, Human (Requirements of insulin may be reduced in hypothyroid patients with diabetes and may be subsequently increased with initiation of thyroid hormone therapy). Products include:
NovoLog Mix 70/30 2364

Insulin Aspart, Human Regular (Requirements of insulin may be reduced in hypothyroid patients with diabetes and may be subsequently increased with initiation of thyroid hormone therapy). Products include:
NovoLog Injection 2359

Insulin Aspart Protamine, Human (Requirements of insulin may be reduced in hypothyroid patients with diabetes and may be subsequently increased with initiation of thyroid hormone therapy). Products include:
NovoLog Mix 70/30 2364

Insulin Detemir (rDNA Origin) (Requirements of insulin may be reduced in hypothyroid patients with diabetes and may be subsequently increased with initiation of thyroid hormone therapy). Products include:
Levemir Injection 2352

Insulin glargine (Requirements of insulin may be reduced in hypothyroid patients with diabetes and may be subsequently increased with initiation of thyroid hormone therapy). Products include:
Lantus Injection 2749

Insulin Glulisine (Requirements of insulin may be reduced in hypothyroid patients with diabetes and may be subsequently increased with initiation of thyroid hormone therapy). Products include:
Apidra Injection 2706

Insulin Lispro, Human (Requirements of insulin may be reduced in hypothyroid patients with diabetes and may be subsequently increased with initiation of thyroid hormone therapy). Products include:
Humalog-Pen and KwikPen 1829
Humalog Mix 50/50-Pen and KwikPen 1833
Humalog Mix 75/25-Pen and KwikPen 1835

Insulin Lispro Protamine, Human (Requirements of insulin may be reduced in hypothyroid patients with diabetes and may be subsequently increased with initiation of thyroid hormone therapy). Products include:
Humalog Mix 50/50-Pen and KwikPen 1833
Humalog Mix 75/25-Pen and KwikPen 1835

Interferon alfa-2a, Recombinant (Cytokines have been reported to induce both hyperthyroidism or hypothyroidism; dosage adjustment may be necessary).
No products indexed under this heading.

Interferon alfa-2b, Recombinant (Cytokines have been reported to induce both hyperthyroidism or hypothyroidism; dosage adjustment may be necessary). Products include:
Intron A for Injection 2859

Interferon alfa-N3 (Human Leukocyte Derived) (Cytokines have been reported to induce both hyperthyroidism or hypothyroidism; dosage adjustment may be necessary). Products include:
Alferon N Injection 1726

Interferon Beta-1b (Cytokines have been reported to induce both hyperthyroidism or hypothyroidism; dosage adjustment may be necessary). Products include:

Betaseron for SC Injection 756

Interferon Gamma-1B (Cytokines have been reported to induce both hyperthyroidism or hypothyroidism; dosage adjustment may be necessary). Products include:

Actimmune 1743

Iodamide Meglumine (Alters thyroid hormone or TSH levels).

No products indexed under this heading.

Iodinated Glycerol (Alters thyroid hormone or TSH levels).

No products indexed under this heading.

Iodine, radiolabeled (Uptake of radiolabeled ions may be decreased).

No products indexed under this heading.

Iohexol (Alters thyroid hormone or TSH levels).

No products indexed under this heading.

Iopamidol (Alters thyroid hormone or TSH levels).

No products indexed under this heading.

Iopanoic Acid (Alters thyroid hormone or TSH levels).

No products indexed under this heading.

Iothalamate Meglumine (Alters thyroid hormone or TSH levels).

No products indexed under this heading.

Ioxaglate Meglumine (Alters thyroid hormone or TSH levels).

No products indexed under this heading.

Ioxaglate Sodium (Alters thyroid hormone or TSH levels).

No products indexed under this heading.

Isoproterenol Hydrochloride (Possible increased risk of coronary insufficiency in patients with coronary artery disease).

No products indexed under this heading.

Isoproterenol Sulfate (Possible increased risk of coronary insufficiency in patients with coronary artery disease).

No products indexed under this heading.

Ketamine Hydrochloride (Coadministration produces marked hypertension and tachycardia).

No products indexed under this heading.

Labetalol Hydrochloride (Alters thyroid hormone or TSH levels; actions of some beta blockers may be impaired when hypothyroid patients become euthyroid).

No products indexed under this heading.

Levalbuterol Hydrochloride (Possible increased risk of coronary insufficiency in patients with coronary artery disease). Products include:

Xopenex Inhalation Solution 3001

Xopenex Inhalation Solution Concentrate 3005

Levobunolol Hydrochloride (Alters thyroid hormone or TSH levels; actions of some beta blockers may be impaired when hypothyroid patients become euthyroid).

No products indexed under this heading.

Levodopa (Alters thyroid hormone or TSH levels). Products include:

Stalevo Tablets 2309

Lithium (Blocks the TSH-mediated release of T4 and T3; thyroid function should therefore be carefully monitored during lithium initiation, stablization, and maintenence; if hypothyroidism occurs during lithium treatment, a higher than usual Synthroid dose may be required).

No products indexed under this heading.

Lithium Carbonate (Blocks the TSH-mediated release of T4 and T3; thyroid function should therefore be carefully monitored during lithium initiation, stablization, and maintenence; if hypothyroidism occurs during lithium treatment, a higher than usual Synthroid dose may be required).

No products indexed under this heading.

Lithium Citrate (Blocks the TSH-mediated release of T4 and T3; thyroid function should therefore be carefully monitored during lithium initiation, stablization, and maintenence; if hypothyroidism occurs during lithium treatment, a higher than usual Synthroid dose may be required).

No products indexed under this heading.

Lovastatin (Alters thyroid hormone or TSH levels). Products include:

Advicor Tablets 402

Mevacor Tablets 2063

Magnesium Salicylate (May inhibit levothyroxine sodium binding to serum proteins or alter the concentrations of serum proteins).

No products indexed under this heading.

Maprotiline Hydrochloride (Risk of cardiac arrhythmias may increase).

No products indexed under this heading.

Meclofenamate Sodium (Meclofenamic acid may inhibit levothyroxine sodium binding to serum proteins or alter the concentrations of serum proteins).

No products indexed under this heading.

Mefenamic Acid (May inhibit levothyroxine sodium binding to serum proteins or alter the concentrations of serum proteins).

No products indexed under this heading.

Mercaptopurine (Alters thyroid hormone or TSH levels).

No products indexed under this heading.

Metaproterenol Sulfate (Possible increased risk of coronary insufficiency in patients with coronary artery disease).

No products indexed under this heading.

Metaraminol Bitartrate (Possible increased risk of coronary insufficiency in patients with coronary artery disease).

No products indexed under this heading.

Metformin Hydrochloride (Requirements of oral antidiabetic agents may be reduced in hypothyroid patients with diabetes and may be subsequently increased with initiation of thyroid hormone therapy). Products include:

ActoPlus Met Tablets 3071

Avandamet Tablets 1336

Janumet Tablets 2041

PrandiMet Tablets 2967

Methadone Hydrochloride (May inhibit levothyroxine sodium binding to serum proteins or alter the concentrations of serum proteins).

No products indexed under this heading.

Methimazole (Alters thyroid hormone or TSH levels).

No products indexed under this heading.

Methoxamine Hydrochloride (Possible increased risk of coronary insufficiency in patients with coronary artery disease).

No products indexed under this heading.

Methyclothiazide (Alters thyroid hormone or TSH levels).

No products indexed under this heading.

Methylprednisolone Acetate (May inhibit levothyroxine sodium binding to serum proteins or alter the concentrations of serum proteins).

No products indexed under this heading.

Methylprednisolone Sodium Succinate (May inhibit levothyroxine sodium binding to serum proteins or alter the concentrations of serum proteins).

No products indexed under this heading.

Methyltestosterone (May inhibit levothyroxine sodium binding to serum proteins or alter the concentrations of serum proteins; alters TSH or thyroid hormone levels). Products include:

Estratest Tablets 3043

Estratest H.S. Tablets 3043

Metipranolol Hydrochloride (Alters thyroid hormone or TSH levels; actions of some beta blockers may be impaired when hypothyroid patients become euthyroid).

No products indexed under this heading.

Metoclopramide Hydrochloride (Alters thyroid hormone or TSH levels).

No products indexed under this heading.

Metoprolol Succinate (Alters thyroid hormone or TSH levels; actions of some beta blockers may be impaired when hypothyroid patients become euthyroid). Products include:

Toprol-XL Tablets 666

Metoprolol Tartrate (Alters thyroid hormone or TSH levels; actions of some beta blockers may be impaired when hypothyroid patients become euthyroid).

No products indexed under this heading.

Miglitol (Requirements of oral antidiabetic agents may be reduced in hypothyroid patients with diabetes and may be subsequently increased with initiation of thyroid hormone therapy).

No products indexed under this heading.

Mitotane (Alters thyroid hormone or TSH levels).

No products indexed under this heading.

Nadolol (Alters thyroid hormone or TSH levels; actions of some beta blockers may be impaired when hypothyroid patients become euthyroid). Products include:

Nadolol Tablets 2191

Nateglinide (Requirements of oral antidiabetic agents may be reduced in hypothyroid patients with diabetes and may be subsequently increased with initiation of thyroid hormone therapy). Products include:

Starlix Tablets 2314

Nebivolol (Alters thyroid hormone or TSH levels; actions of some beta blockers may be impaired when hypothyroid patients become euthyroid). Products include:

Bystolic Tablets 1155

Norepinephrine Bitartrate (Possible increased risk of coronary insufficiency in patients with coronary artery disease).

No products indexed under this heading.

Nortriptyline Hydrochloride (Concurrent use may increase the therapeutic and toxic effects of both drugs; onset of action of tricyclics may be accelerated).

No products indexed under this heading.

Octreotide Acetate (Alters thyroid hormone or TSH levels). Products include:

Sandostatin Injection 2300

Sandostatin LAR Depot 2302

Orlistat (Concurrent use may reduce the efficacy of levothyroxine by binding and delaying or preventing absorption, potentially resulting in hypothyroidism. Patients treated concomitantly with orlistat and levothyroxine should be monitored for changes in thyroid function). Products include:

Xenical Capsules 2672

Oxandrolone (May inhibit levothyroxine sodium binding to serum proteins or alter the concentrations of serum proteins; alters TSH or thyroid hormone levels).

No products indexed under this heading.

Oxymetholone (May inhibit levothyroxine sodium binding to serum proteins or alter the concentrations of serum proteins; alters TSH or thyroid hormone levels).

No products indexed under this heading.

Penbutolol Sulfate (Alters thyroid hormone or TSH levels; actions of some beta blockers may be impaired when hypothyroid patients become euthyroid).

No products indexed under this heading.

Pergolide Mesylate (Alters thyroid hormone or TSH levels).

No products indexed under this heading.

Perphenazine (May inhibit levothyroxine sodium binding to serum proteins or alter the concentrations of serum proteins).

No products indexed under this heading.

Phenobarbital (Alters thyroid hormone or TSH levels). Products include:

Donnatal Extentabs 2507

Phenylbutazone (May inhibit levothyroxine sodium binding to serum proteins or alter the concentrations of serum proteins; alters thyroid hormone or TSH levels).

No products indexed under this heading.

Phenylephrine Bitartrate (Possible increased risk of coronary insufficiency in patients with coronary artery disease).
No products indexed under this heading.

Phenylephrine Hydrochloride (Possible increased risk of coronary insufficiency in patients with coronary artery disease). Products include:
- Actifed Cold & Allergy Tablets **1895**
- Benadryl Allergy & Cold Kapgels **1895**
- Benadryl Allergy & Sinus Headache Kapgels **1895**
- Benadryl Severe Allergy & Sinus Headache Caplets **1897**
- Children's Benadryl-D Allergy & Sinus Liquid **1896**
- Benadryl-D Allergy & Sinus Tablet **1896**
- PediaCare Children's Allergy & Cold Liquid **1902**
- PediaCare Children's Decongestant Liquid **1902**
- PediaCare Children's Liquid Multi-Symptom Cold **1902**
- Sinutab Non-Drying Caplets **1905**
- Sinutab Sinus Caplets **1905**
- Children's Sudafed PE Cold & Cough Liquid **1907**
- Children's Sudafed PE Nasal Decongestant Liquid **1906**
- Sudafed PE Cold & Cough Caplets **1907**
- Sudafed PE Nasal Decongestant Tablets **1907**
- Sudafed PE Nighttime Cold Caplets **1907**
- Sudafed PE Non-Drying Sinus Caplets **1908**
- Sudafed PE Severe Cold Caplets **1908**
- Sudafed PE Sinus & Allergy Tablets **1908**
- Sudafed PE Sinus Headache Caplets **1908**
- Tylenol Allergy Multi-Symptom Caplets with Cool Burst and Rapid Release Gelcaps **1916**
- Tylenol Allergy Multi-Symptom Nighttime Caplets with Cool Burst **1916**
- Children's Tylenol Plus Cold Suspension Liquid **1912**
- Children's Tylenol Plus Cold & Allergy Suspension Liquid **1914**
- Children's Tylenol Plus Flu Suspension Liquid **1914**
- Children's Tylenol Plus Multi-Symptom Cold Suspension Liquid **1912**
- Tylenol Cold Head Congestion Daytime Caplets with Cool Burst **1910**
- Tylenol Cold Head Congestion Nighttime Caplets with Cool Burst **1910**
- Tylenol Cold Head Congestion Severe Daytime Caplets with Cool Burst **1910**
- Tylenol Cold Multi-Symptom Daytime Caplets with Cool Burst and Rapid Release Gels **1913**
- Tylenol Cold Multi-Symptom Daytime Liquid with Citrus Burst ... **1913**
- Tylenol Cold Multi-Symptom Nighttime Caplets with Cool Burst **1913**
- Tylenol Cold Multi-Symptom Nighttime Liquid with Cool Burst ... **1913**
- Tylenol Cold Multi-Symptom Severe Caplets with Cool Burst **1913**
- Tylenol Cold Multi-Symptom Severe Daytime Liquid with Citrus Burst **1913**
- Tylenol Sinus Congestion & Pain Daytime Caplets with Cool Burst and Gelcaps **1917**
- Tylenol Sinus Congestion & Pain Nighttime Caplets with Cool Burst **1917**
- Tylenol Sinus Congestion & Pain Severe Caplets with Cool Burst **1917**
- Vicks DayQuil Cold & Flu Multi-Symptom Relief .... **▣616**
- Vicks DayQuil LiquiCaps **2567**
- Vicks DayQuil Liquid **2567**
- Vicks DayQuil Multi-Symptom Cold/Flu Relief **2567**

Phenylephrine Tannate (Possible increased risk of coronary insufficiency in patients with coronary artery disease).
No products indexed under this heading.

Phenylpropanolamine Hydrochloride (Possible increased risk of coronary insufficiency in patients with coronary artery disease).
No products indexed under this heading.

Phenytoin (May inhibit levothyroxine sodium binding to serum proteins or alter the concentrations of serum proteins; alters thyroid hormone or TSH levels).
No products indexed under this heading.

Phenytoin Sodium (May inhibit levothyroxine sodium binding to serum proteins or alter the concentrations of serum proteins; alters thyroid hormone or TSH levels). Products include:
- Phenytek Capsules **2192**

Pindolol (Alters thyroid hormone or TSH levels; actions of some beta blockers may be impaired when hypothyroid patients become euthyroid).
No products indexed under this heading.

Pioglitazone Hydrochloride (Requirements of oral antidiabetic agents may be reduced in hypothyroid patients with diabetes and may be subsequently increased with initiation of thyroid hormone therapy). Products include:
- ActoPlus Met Tablets **3071**
- Actos Tablets **3077**
- Duetact Tablets **3085**

Pirbuterol Acetate (Possible increased risk of coronary insufficiency in patients with coronary artery disease). Products include:
- Maxair Autohaler **1705**

Polyestradiol Phosphate (Estrogens or estrogen-containing compounds may inhibit levothyroxine sodium binding to serum proteins or alter the concentrations of serum proteins).
No products indexed under this heading.

Polythiazide (Alters thyroid hormone or TSH levels).
No products indexed under this heading.

Pramipexole Dihydrochloride (Alters thyroid hormone or TSH levels). Products include:
- Mirapex Tablets **857**

Prednisolone Acetate (May inhibit levothyroxine sodium binding to serum proteins or alter the concentrations of serum proteins). Products include:
- Pred Forte Ophthalmic Suspension .... **⊙227**
- Pred Mild Ophthalmic Suspension .... **⊙230**
- Pred-G Ophthalmic Ointment .... **⊙229**
- Pred-G Ophthalmic Suspension ...... **⊙228**

Prednisolone Sodium Phosphate (May inhibit levothyroxine sodium binding to serum proteins or alter the concentrations of serum proteins).
No products indexed under this heading.

Prednisolone Tebutate (May inhibit levothyroxine sodium binding to serum proteins or alter the concentrations of serum proteins).
No products indexed under this heading.

Prednisone (May inhibit levothyroxine sodium binding to serum proteins or alter the concentrations of serum proteins).
No products indexed under this heading.

Propranolol Hydrochloride (Alters thyroid hormone or TSH levels; actions of some beta blockers may be impaired when hypothyroid patients become euthyroid). Products include:
- InnoPran XL Extended Release Capsules **1484**

Propylthiouracil (Concurrent use may decrease thyroid hormone secretion, which may result in hypothyroidism).
No products indexed under this heading.

Protriptyline Hydrochloride (Concurrent use may increase the therapeutic and toxic effects of both drugs; onset of action of tricyclics may be accelerated).
No products indexed under this heading.

Pseudoephedrine Hydrochloride (Possible increased risk of coronary insufficiency in patients with coronary artery disease). Products include:
- Allegra-D 12 Hour Extended-Release Tablets **2687**
- Allegra-D 24 Hour Extended-Release Tablets **2690**
- Children's Motrin Cold Oral Suspension **1899**
- Sudafed 12 Hour Nasal Decongestant Non-Drowsy Caplets **1909**
- Sudafed 24 Hour Non-Drowsy Nasal Decongestant Tablets **1906**
- Children's Sudafed Nasal Decongestant Liquid **1906**
- Sudafed Nasal Decongestant Tablets **1906**
- Tylenol Cold Severe Congestion Daytime Caplets with Cool Burst **1912**
- Tylenol Sinus Severe Congestion Caplets with Cool Burst **1917**
- Vicks NyQuil LiquiCaps **2567**
- Vicks NyQuil Liquid **2567**
- Vicks NyQuil Multi-Symptom Cold/Flu Relief **2567**
- Zyrtec-D 12 Hour Extended Release Tablets **1923**
- Zyrtec-D Allergy & Congestion Extended-Release Tablets **1923**

Pseudoephedrine Sulfate (Possible increased risk of coronary insufficiency in patients with coronary artery disease). Products include:
- Clarinex-D 12-Hour Extended-Release Tablets **2831**
- Clarinex-D 24-Hour Extended-Release Tablets **2834**

Quinestrol (Estrogens or estrogen-containing compounds may inhibit levothyroxine sodium binding to serum proteins or alter the concentrations of serum proteins).
No products indexed under this heading.

Repaglinide (Requirements of oral antidiabetic agents may be reduced in hypothyroid patients with diabetes and may be subsequently increased with initiation of thyroid hormone therapy). Products include:
- PrandiMet Tablets **2967**
- Prandin Tablets **2971**

Resorcinol (Alters thyroid hormone or TSH levels).
No products indexed under this heading.

Rifampin (Alters thyroid hormone or TSH levels).
No products indexed under this heading.

Rifapentine (Alters thyroid hormone or TSH levels).
No products indexed under this heading.

Ropinirole Hydrochloride (Alters thyroid hormone or TSH levels). Products include:
- Requip Tablets **1561**
- Requip XL Tablets **1568**

Rosiglitazone Maleate (Requirements of oral antidiabetic agents may be reduced in hypothyroid patients with diabetes and may be subsequently increased with initiation of thyroid hormone therapy). Products include:
- Avandamet Tablets **1336**
- Avandaryl Tablets **1344**
- Avandia Tablets **1351**

Salmeterol Xinafoate (Possible increased risk of coronary insufficiency in patients with coronary artery disease). Products include:
- Advair Diskus 100/50 .... **1276**
- Advair Diskus 250/50 .... **1276**
- Advair Diskus 500/50 .... **1276**
- Advair HFA 45/21 Inhalation Aerosol **1288**
- Advair HFA 115/21 Inhalation Aerosol **1288**
- Advair HFA 230/21 Inhalation Aerosol **1288**
- Serevent Diskus **1594**

Salsalate (May inhibit levothyroxine sodium binding to serum proteins or alter the concentrations of serum proteins).
No products indexed under this heading.

Sitagliptin Phosphate (Requirements of oral antidiabetic agents may be reduced in hypothyroid patients with diabetes and may be subsequently increased with initiation of thyroid hormone therapy). Products include:
- Janumet Tablets **2041**
- Januvia Tablets **2048**

Sodium Iodide I 123 (Uptake of radiolabeled ions may be decreased).
No products indexed under this heading.

Sodium Iodide I 131 (Uptake of radiolabeled ions may be decreased).
No products indexed under this heading.

Sodium Nitroprusside (Alters thyroid hormone or TSH levels).
No products indexed under this heading.

Sodium Pertechnetate (Alters thyroid hormone or TSH levels).
No products indexed under this heading.

Sodium Polystyrene Sulfonate (Binds and decreases absorption of levothyroxine sodium from the gastrointestinal tract).
No products indexed under this heading.

Somatrem (Excessive concurrent use of thyroid hormone may accelerate epiphyseal closure; untreated hypothyroidism may interfere with the growth response to somatrem).
No products indexed under this heading.

Somatropin (Excessive concurrent use of thyroid hormone may accelerate epiphyseal closure; untreated hypothyroidism may interfere with the growth response to somatrem). Products include:
- Genotropin Lyophilized Powder **2547**
- Humatrope Vials and Cartridges **1838**
- Nutropin for Injection **1208**
- Nutropin AQ Injection **1212**
- Nutropin AQ NuSpin Injection **1212**
- Nutropin AQ Pen **1212**
- Nutropin AQ Pen Cartridge **1212**

Sotalol Hydrochloride (Alters thyroid hormone or TSH levels; actions of some beta blockers may be impaired when hypothyroid patients become euthyroid).
No products indexed under this heading.

Stanozolol (May inhibit levothyroxine sodium binding to serum proteins or alter the concentrations of serum proteins; alters TSH or thyroid hormone levels).
No products indexed under this heading.

Sucralfate (Binds and decreases absorption of levothyroxine sodium from the gastrointestinal tract). Products include:
- Carafate Suspension **706**
- Carafate Tablets **707**

Sulfacytine (Alters thyroid hormone or TSH levels).
No products indexed under this heading.

Sulfamethizole (Alters thyroid hormone or TSH levels).
No products indexed under this heading.

Sulfamethoxazole (Alters thyroid hormone or TSH levels).
No products indexed under this heading.

Sulfasalazine (Alters thyroid hormone or TSH levels).
No products indexed under this heading.

Sulfinpyrazone (Alters thyroid hormone or TSH levels).
No products indexed under this heading.

Sulfisoxazole Acetyl (Alters thyroid hormone or TSH levels).
No products indexed under this heading.

Sulfisoxazole Diolamine (Alters thyroid hormone or TSH levels).
No products indexed under this heading.

Tamoxifen Citrate (May inhibit levothyroxine sodium binding to serum proteins or alter the concentrations of serum proteins).
No products indexed under this heading.

Terbutaline Sulfate (Possible increased risk of coronary insufficiency in patients with coronary artery disease).
No products indexed under this heading.

Theophylline (Theophylline clearance may be decreased in hypothyroid patients and return toward normal when euthyroid state is achieved).
No products indexed under this heading.

Theophylline Anhydrous (Theophylline clearance may be decreased in hypothyroid patients and return toward normal when euthyroid state is achieved). Products include:
- Uniphyl Tablets **2595**

Theophylline Calcium Salicylate (Theophylline clearance may be decreased in hypothyroid patients and return toward normal when euthyroid state is achieved).
No products indexed under this heading.

Theophylline Dihydroxypropyl (Glyceryl) (Theophylline clearance may be decreased in hypothyroid patients and return toward normal when euthyroid state is achieved).
No products indexed under this heading.

Theophylline Ethylenediamine (Theophylline clearance may be decreased in hypothyroid patients and return toward normal when euthyroid state is achieved).
No products indexed under this heading.

Theophylline Sodium Glycinate (Theophylline clearance may be decreased in hypothyroid patients and return toward normal when euthyroid state is achieved).
No products indexed under this heading.

Timolol Hemihydrate (Alters thyroid hormone or TSH levels; actions of some beta blockers may be impaired when hypothyroid patients become euthyroid). Products include:
- Betimol Ophthalmic Solution **3181**

Timolol Maleate (Alters thyroid hormone or TSH levels; actions of some beta blockers may be impaired when hypothyroid patients become euthyroid). Products include:
- Combigan Ophthalmic Solution **553**
- Cosopt Sterile Ophthalmic Solution **1969**
- Timoptic Sterile Ophthalmic Solution **2121**
- Timoptic in Ocudose **2124**
- Timoptic-XE Sterile Ophthalmic Gel Forming Solution **2125**

Tolazamide (Alters thyroid hormone or TSH levels).
No products indexed under this heading.

Tolbutamide (Alters thyroid hormone or TSH levels).
No products indexed under this heading.

Triamcinolone (May inhibit levothyroxine sodium binding to serum proteins or alter the concentrations of serum proteins).
No products indexed under this heading.

Triamcinolone Acetonide (May inhibit levothyroxine sodium binding to serum proteins or alter the concentrations of serum proteins). Products include:
- Azmacort Inhalation Aerosol **407**
- Nasacort AQ Nasal Spray **2765**
- Triesence Injectable Suspension .... ⊙ **209**

Triamcinolone Diacetate (May inhibit levothyroxine sodium binding to serum proteins or alter the concentrations of serum proteins).
No products indexed under this heading.

Triamcinolone Hexacetonide (May inhibit levothyroxine sodium binding to serum proteins or alter the concentrations of serum proteins).
No products indexed under this heading.

Trimipramine Maleate (Concurrent use may increase the therapeutic and toxic effects of both drugs; onset of action of tricyclics may be accelerated).
No products indexed under this heading.

Troglitazone (Requirements of oral antidiabetic agents may be reduced in hypothyroid patients with diabetes and may be subsequently increased with initiation of thyroid hormone therapy).
No products indexed under this heading.

Tyropanoate Sodium (Alters thyroid hormone or TSH levels).
No products indexed under this heading.

Warfarin Sodium (The hypoprothrombinemic effect of anticoagulants may be potentiated).
No products indexed under this heading.

Food Interactions

Soybean Formula, Children's (Binds and decreases absorption of levothyroxine sodium from the gastrointestinal tract).

SYSTANE ULTRA LUBRICATING EYE DROPS
(Polyethylene Glycol, Propylene Glycol).. ⊙ **207**
None cited in PDR database.

SYSTANE ULTRA LUBRICATING EYE DROPS
(Polyethylene Glycol, Propylene Glycol).. **547**
None cited in PDR database.

TABLOID TABLETS
(Thioguanine) **1601**
May interact with cytotoxic drugs, drugs that inhibit thiopurine methyltransferase (TPMT), and certain other agents. Compounds in these categories include:

Bleomycin Sulfate (Combination therapy may produce hepatic disease).
No products indexed under this heading.

Busulfan (Potential for esophageal varices associated with abnormal liver function tests). Products include:
- Busulfex Injection **2477**
- Myleran Tablets **1530**

Cyclophosphamide (Combination therapy may produce hepatic disease).
No products indexed under this heading.

Daunorubicin Hydrochloride (Combination therapy may produce hepatic disease).
No products indexed under this heading.

Doxorubicin Hydrochloride (Combination therapy may produce hepatic disease).
No products indexed under this heading.

Epirubicin Hydrochloride (Combination therapy may produce hepatic disease).
No products indexed under this heading.

Fluorouracil (Combination therapy may produce hepatic disease). Products include:
- Carac Cream 0.5% **2722**

Hydroxyurea (Combination therapy may produce hepatic disease).
No products indexed under this heading.

Mercaptopurine (Complete cross-resistance).
No products indexed under this heading.

Mesalamine (Individuals with inherited deficiency of the enzyme TPMT are unusually sensitive to the myelosuppressive effects of mercaptopurine and are prone to developing rapid bone marrow suppression; co-administration with drugs that inhibit TPMT could exacerbate this toxicity). Products include:
- Asacol Delayed-Release Tablets **2579**
- Canasa Rectal Suppositories **705**
- Lialda Tablets **3029**
- Pentasa Capsules **3030**

Mesalazine (Individuals with inherited deficiency of the enzyme TPMT are unusually sensitive to the myelosuppressive effects of mercaptopurine and are prone to developing rapid bone marrow suppression; co-administration with drugs that inhibit TPMT could exacerbate this toxicity).
No products indexed under this heading.

Methotrexate Sodium (Combination therapy may produce hepatic disease).
No products indexed under this heading.

Mitotane (Combination therapy may produce hepatic disease).
No products indexed under this heading.

Mitoxantrone Hydrochloride (Combination therapy may produce hepatic disease). Products include:
- Novantrone for Injection Concentrate **1100**

Olsalazine Sodium (Individuals with inherited deficiency of the enzyme TPMT are unusually sensitive to the myelosuppressive effects of mercaptopurine and are prone to developing rapid bone marrow suppression; co-administration with drugs that inhibit TPMT could exacerbate this toxicity).
No products indexed under this heading.

Procarbazine Hydrochloride (Combination therapy may produce hepatic disease).
No products indexed under this heading.

Sulphasalazine (Individuals with inherited deficiency of the enzyme TPMT are unusually sensitive to the myelosuppressive effects of mercaptopurine and are prone to developing rapid bone marrow suppression; co-administration with drugs that inhibit TPMT could exacerbate this toxicity).
No products indexed under this heading.

Tamoxifen Citrate (Combination therapy may produce hepatic disease).
No products indexed under this heading.

Vincristine Sulfate (Combination therapy may produce hepatic disease).
No products indexed under this heading.

TAHITIAN NONI LEAF SERUM SOOTHING GEL
(Herbal Medicines, unspecified) .... ▣ **632**
None cited in PDR database.

TAHITIAN NONI LIQUID

(Dietary Supplement) 633
None cited in PDR database.

TAHITIAN NONI SEED OIL

(Herbal Medicines, unspecified) 634
None cited in PDR database.

TAMIFLU CAPSULES

(Oseltamivir Phosphate) **2649**
May interact with:

Influenza Vaccine, Live Attenuated (The concomitant use of oseltamivir phosphate with live attenuated influenza vaccine (LAIV) intranasal has not been evaluated. However, because of the potential for interference between these products, LAIV, should not be administered within 2 weeks before or 48 hours after administration of oseltamivir phosphate, unless medically indicated. The concern about possible interferences arises from the potential for antiviral drugs to inhibit replication of live vaccine virus. Trivalent inactivated influenza vaccine can be administered at any time relative to use of oseltamivir phosphate).
No products indexed under this heading.

Probenecid (Co-administration with probenecid results in an approximate two-fold increase in exposure to oseltamivir due to a decrease in active anionic tubular secretion in the kidneys; no dose adjustments are required due to the safety margin of oseltamivir).
No products indexed under this heading.

TAMIFLU ORAL SUSPENSION

(Oseltamivir Phosphate) **2649**
See Tamiflu Capsules

TARCEVA TABLETS

(Erlotinib) **1228**
May interact with cytochrome p450 3a4 inducers (selected), cytochrome p450 3a4 inhibitors (selected), and certain other agents. Compounds in these categories include:

Acetazolamide (Caution when administering or taking erlotinib with strong CYP3A4 inhibitors such as atazanavir, clarithromycin, indinavir, itraconazole, nefazodone, nelfinavir, ritonavir, saquinavir, telithromycin, troleandomycin, and voriconazole).
No products indexed under this heading.

Allium sativum (Pre-treatment with the CYP3A4 inducer rifampicin decreased erlotinib AUC by about 2/3 to 4/5. Alternate treatments lacking CYP3A4 inducing activity should be considered. If an alternative treatment is unavailable, an increase in the dose of erlotinib should be considered as tolerated at two week intervals while monitoring the patient's safety. If the erlotinib dose is adjusted upward, the dose will need to be reduced upon discontinuation of rifampicin or other CYP3A4 inducers).
No products indexed under this heading.

Amiodarone Hydrochloride (Caution when administering or taking erlotinib with strong CYP3A4 inhibitors such as atazanavir, clarithromycin, indinavir, itraconazole, nefazodone, nelfinavir, ritonavir, saquinavir, telithromycin, troleandomycin, and voriconazole).
No products indexed under this heading.

Amprenavir (Caution when administering or taking erlotinib with strong CYP3A4 inhibitors such as atazanavir, clarithromycin, indinavir, itraconazole, nefazodone, nelfinavir, ritonavir, saquinavir, telithromycin, troleandomycin, and voriconazole).
No products indexed under this heading.

Anastrozole (Caution when administering or taking erlotinib with strong CYP3A4 inhibitors such as atazanavir, clarithromycin, indinavir, itraconazole, nefazodone, nelfinavir, ritonavir, saquinavir, telithromycin, troleandomycin, and voriconazole). Products include:
Arimidex Tablets **672**

Aprepitant (Caution when administering or taking erlotinib with strong CYP3A4 inhibitors such as atazanavir, clarithromycin, indinavir, itraconazole, nefazodone, nelfinavir, ritonavir, saquinavir, telithromycin, troleandomycin, and voriconazole). Products include:
Emend Capsules **1992**

Atazanavir (Co-treatment with the potent CYP3A4 inhibitor ketoconazole increases erlotinib AUC by 2/3. Caution should be used when administering or taking erlotinib with ketoconazole and other strong CYP3A4 inhibitors such as atazanavir).
No products indexed under this heading.

Atazanavir Sulfate (Co-treatment with the potent CYP3A4 inhibitor ketoconazole increases erlotinib AUC by 2/3. Caution should be used when administering or taking erlotinib with ketoconazole and other strong CYP3A4 inhibitors such as atazanavir). Products include:
Reyataz Capsules **3299**

Betamethasone Acetate (Pre-treatment with the CYP3A4 inducer rifampicin decreased erlotinib AUC by about 2/3 to 4/5. Alternate treatments lacking CYP3A4 inducing activity should be considered. If an alternative treatment is unavailable, an increase in the dose of erlotinib should be considered as tolerated at two week intervals while monitoring the patient's safety. If the erlotinib dose is adjusted upward, the dose will need to be reduced upon discontinuation of rifampicin or other CYP3A4 inducers).
No products indexed under this heading.

Betamethasone Sodium Phosphate (Pre-treatment with the CYP3A4 inducer rifampicin decreased erlotinib AUC by about 2/3 to 4/5. Alternate treatments lacking CYP3A4 inducing activity should be considered. If an alternative treatment is unavailable, an increase in the dose of erlotinib should be considered as tolerated at two week intervals while monitoring the patient's safety. If the erlotinib dose is adjusted upward, the dose will need to be reduced upon discontinuation of rifampicin or other CYP3A4 inducers).
No products indexed under this heading.

Carbamazepine (Pre-treatment with the CYP3A4 inducer rifampicin decreased erlotinib AUC by about 2/3 to 4/5. Alternate treatments lacking CYP3A4 inducing activity should be considered. If an alternative treatment is unavailable, an increase in the dose of erlotinib should be considered as tolerated at two week intervals while monitoring the patient's safety. If the erlotinib dose is adjusted upward, the dose will need to be reduced upon discontinuation of rifampicin or other CYP3A4 inducers). Products include:
Carbatrol Capsules **3019**
Equetro Extended-Release Capsules **3174**

Cimetidine (Caution when administering or taking erlotinib with strong CYP3A4 inhibitors such as atazanavir, clarithromycin, indinavir, itraconazole, nefazodone, nelfinavir, ritonavir, saquinavir, telithromycin, troleandomycin, and voriconazole).
No products indexed under this heading.

Cimetidine Hydrochloride (Caution when administering or taking erlotinib with strong CYP3A4 inhibitors such as atazanavir, clarithromycin, indinavir, itraconazole, nefazodone, nelfinavir, ritonavir, saquinavir, telithromycin, troleandomycin, and voriconazole).
No products indexed under this heading.

Ciprofloxacin (Caution when administering or taking erlotinib with strong CYP3A4 inhibitors such as atazanavir, clarithromycin, indinavir, itraconazole, nefazodone, nelfinavir, ritonavir, saquinavir, telithromycin, troleandomycin, and voriconazole). Products include:
Cipro I.V. **2817**
Cipro Oral Suspension **2810**
Cipro XR Tablets **2823**
Ciprodex Otic Suspension **541**

Ciprofloxacin Hydrochloride (Pre-treatment with the CYP3A4 inducer rifampicin decreased erlotinib AUC by about 2/3 to 4/5. Alternate treatments lacking CYP3A4 inducing activity should be considered. If an alternative treatment is unavailable, an increase in the dose of erlotinib should be considered as tolerated at two week intervals while monitoring the patient's safety. If the erlotinib dose is adjusted upward, the dose will need to be reduced upon discontinuation of rifampicin or other CYP3A4 inducers). Products include:
Cipro Tablets **2810**

Cisplatin (Pre-treatment with the CYP3A4 inducer rifampicin decreased erlotinib AUC by about 2/3 to 4/5. Alternate treatments lacking CYP3A4 inducing activity should be considered. If an alternative treatment is unavailable, an increase in the dose of erlotinib should be considered as tolerated at two week intervals while monitoring the patient's safety. If the erlotinib dose is adjusted upward, the dose will need to be reduced upon discontinuation of rifampicin or other CYP3A4 inducers).
No products indexed under this heading.

Clarithromycin (Co-treatment with the potent CYP3A4 inhibitor ketoconazole increases erlotinib AUC by 2/3. Caution should be used when administering or taking erlotinib with ketoconazole and other strong CYP3A4 inhibitors such as clarithromycin). Products include:
Biaxin/Biaxin XL **411**

Clotrimazole (Caution when administering or taking erlotinib with strong CYP3A4 inhibitors such as atazanavir, clarithromycin, indinavir, itraconazole, nefazodone, nelfinavir, ritonavir, saquinavir, telithromycin, troleandomycin, and voriconazole). Products include:
Lotrisone **2881**

Cortisone Acetate (Pre-treatment with the CYP3A4 inducer rifampicin decreased erlotinib AUC by about 2/3 to 4/5. Alternate treatments lacking CYP3A4 inducing activity should be considered. If an alternative treatment is unavailable, an increase in the dose of erlotinib should be considered as tolerated at two week intervals while monitoring the patient's safety. If the erlotinib dose is adjusted upward, the dose will need to be reduced upon discontinuation of rifampicin or other CYP3A4 inducers).
No products indexed under this heading.

Cyclosporine (Caution when administering or taking erlotinib with strong CYP3A4 inhibitors such as atazanavir, clarithromycin, indinavir, itraconazole, nefazodone, nelfinavir, ritonavir, saquinavir, telithromycin, troleandomycin, and voriconazole). Products include:
Gengraf Capsules **435**
Neoral Oral Solution **2280**
Neoral Soft Gelatin Capsules **2280**
Restasis Ophthalmic Emulsion **557**
Sandimmune **2296**

Dalfopristin (Caution when administering or taking erlotinib with strong CYP3A4 inhibitors such as atazanavir, clarithromycin, indinavir, itraconazole, nefazodone, nelfinavir, ritonavir, saquinavir, telithromycin, troleandomycin, and voriconazole).
No products indexed under this heading.

Danazol (Caution when administering or taking erlotinib with strong CYP3A4 inhibitors such as atazanavir, clarithromycin, indinavir, itraconazole, nefazodone, nelfinavir, ritonavir, saquinavir, telithromycin, troleandomycin, and voriconazole).
No products indexed under this heading.

Delavirdine Mesylate (Caution when administering or taking erlotinib with strong CYP3A4 inhibitors such as atazanavir, clarithromycin, indinavir, itraconazole, nefazodone, nelfinavir, ritonavir, saquinavir, telithromycin, troleandomycin, and voriconazole).
No products indexed under this heading.

Dexamethasone (Pre-treatment with the CYP3A4 inducer rifampicin decreased erlotinib AUC by about 2/3 to 4/5. Alternate treatments lacking CYP3A4 inducing activity should be considered. If an alternative treatment is unavailable, an increase in the dose of erlotinib should be considered as tolerated at two week intervals while monitoring the patient's safety. If the erlotinib dose is adjusted upward, the dose will need to be reduced upon discon-

tinuation of rifampicin or other CYP3A4 inducers). Products include:
Ciprodex Otic Suspension 541

Dexamethasone Acetate (Pre-treatment with the CYP3A4 inducer rifampicin decreased erlotinib AUC by about 2/3 to 4/5. Alternate treatments lacking CYP3A4 inducing activity should be considered. If an alternative treatment is unavailable, an increase in the dose of erlotinib should be considered as tolerated at two week intervals while monitoring the patient's safety. If the erlotinib dose is adjusted upward, the dose will need to be reduced upon discontinuation of rifampicin or other CYP3A4 inducers).
No products indexed under this heading.

Dexamethasone Sodium Phosphate (Pre-treatment with the CYP3A4 inducer rifampicin decreased erlotinib AUC by about 2/3 to 4/5. Alternate treatments lacking CYP3A4 inducing activity should be considered. If an alternative treatment is unavailable, an increase in the dose of erlotinib should be considered as tolerated at two week intervals while monitoring the patient's safety. If the erlotinib dose is adjusted upward, the dose will need to be reduced upon discontinuation of rifampicin or other CYP3A4 inducers).
No products indexed under this heading.

Diltiazem Hydrochloride (Caution when administering or taking erlotinib with strong CYP3A4 inhibitors such as atazanavir, clarithromycin, indinavir, itraconazole, nefazodone, nelfinavir, ritonavir, saquinavir, telithromycin, troleandomycin, and voriconazole). Products include:
Cardizem LA Extended Release Tablets 421

Diltiazem Maleate (Caution when administering or taking erlotinib with strong CYP3A4 inhibitors such as atazanavir, clarithromycin, indinavir, itraconazole, nefazodone, nelfinavir, ritonavir, saquinavir, telithromycin, troleandomycin, and voriconazole).
No products indexed under this heading.

Doxorubicin Hydrochloride (Pre-treatment with the CYP3A4 inducer rifampicin decreased erlotinib AUC by about 2/3 to 4/5. Alternate treatments lacking CYP3A4 inducing activity should be considered. If an alternative treatment is unavailable, an increase in the dose of erlotinib should be considered as tolerated at two week intervals while monitoring the patient's safety. If the erlotinib dose is adjusted upward, the dose will need to be reduced upon discontinuation of rifampicin or other CYP3A4 inducers).
No products indexed under this heading.

Efavirenz (Caution when administering or taking erlotinib with strong CYP3A4 inhibitors such as atazanavir, clarithromycin, indinavir, itraconazole, nefazodone, nelfinavir, ritonavir, saquinavir, telithromycin, troleandomycin, and voriconazole). Products include:
Atripla Tablets 938
Sustiva Capsules 930
Sustiva Tablets 930

Erythromycin (Caution when administering or taking erlotinib with strong CYP3A4 inhibitors such as atazanavir, clarithromycin, indinavir, itraconazole, nefazodone, nelfinavir, ritonavir, saquinavir, telithromycin, troleandomycin, and voriconazole).
No products indexed under this heading.

Erythromycin Estolate (Caution when administering or taking erlotinib with strong CYP3A4 inhibitors such as atazanavir, clarithromycin, indinavir, itraconazole, nefazodone, nelfinavir, ritonavir, saquinavir, telithromycin, troleandomycin, and voriconazole).
No products indexed under this heading.

Erythromycin Ethylsuccinate (Caution when administering or taking erlotinib with strong CYP3A4 inhibitors such as atazanavir, clarithromycin, indinavir, itraconazole, nefazodone, nelfinavir, ritonavir, saquinavir, telithromycin, troleandomycin, and voriconazole). Products include:
E.E.S. 433
EryPed 431

Erythromycin Gluceptate (Caution when administering or taking erlotinib with strong CYP3A4 inhibitors such as atazanavir, clarithromycin, indinavir, itraconazole, nefazodone, nelfinavir, ritonavir, saquinavir, telithromycin, troleandomycin, and voriconazole).
No products indexed under this heading.

Erythromycin Lactobionate (Caution when administering or taking erlotinib with strong CYP3A4 inhibitors such as atazanavir, clarithromycin, indinavir, itraconazole, nefazodone, nelfinavir, ritonavir, saquinavir, telithromycin, troleandomycin, and voriconazole).
No products indexed under this heading.

Erythromycin Stearate (Caution when administering or taking erlotinib with strong CYP3A4 inhibitors such as atazanavir, clarithromycin, indinavir, itraconazole, nefazodone, nelfinavir, ritonavir, saquinavir, telithromycin, troleandomycin, and voriconazole).
No products indexed under this heading.

Esomeprazole Magnesium (Caution when administering or taking erlotinib with strong CYP3A4 inhibitors such as atazanavir, clarithromycin, indinavir, itraconazole, nefazodone, nelfinavir, ritonavir, saquinavir, telithromycin, troleandomycin, and voriconazole). Products include:
Nexium Delayed-Release Capsules 645
Nexium Delayed-Release Oral Suspension................................ 645

Ethosuximide (Pre-treatment with the CYP3A4 inducer rifampicin decreased erlotinib AUC by about 2/3 to 4/5. Alternate treatments lacking CYP3A4 inducing activity should be considered. If an alternative treatment is unavailable, an increase in the dose of erlotinib should be considered as tolerated at two week intervals while monitoring the patient's safety. If the erlotinib dose is adjusted upward, the dose will need to be reduced upon discontinuation of rifampicin or other CYP3A4 inducers).
No products indexed under this heading.

Felbamate (Pre-treatment with the CYP3A4 inducer rifampicin decreased erlotinib AUC by about 2/3 to 4/5. Alternate treatments lacking CYP3A4 inducing activity should be considered. If an alternative treatment is unavailable, an increase in the dose of erlotinib should be considered as tolerated at two week intervals while monitoring the patient's safety. If the erlotinib dose is adjusted upward, the dose will need to be reduced upon discontinuation of rifampicin or other CYP3A4 inducers).
No products indexed under this heading.

Fluconazole (Caution when administering or taking erlotinib with strong CYP3A4 inhibitors such as atazanavir, clarithromycin, indinavir, itraconazole, nefazodone, nelfinavir, ritonavir, saquinavir, telithromycin, troleandomycin, and voriconazole).
No products indexed under this heading.

Fludrocortisone Acetate (Pre-treatment with the CYP3A4 inducer rifampicin decreased erlotinib AUC by about 2/3 to 4/5. Alternate treatments lacking CYP3A4 inducing activity should be considered. If an alternative treatment is unavailable, an increase in the dose of erlotinib should be considered as tolerated at two week intervals while monitoring the patient's safety. If the erlotinib dose is adjusted upward, the dose will need to be reduced upon discontinuation of rifampicin or other CYP3A4 inducers).
No products indexed under this heading.

Fluoxetine (Caution when administering or taking erlotinib with strong CYP3A4 inhibitors such as atazanavir, clarithromycin, indinavir, itraconazole, nefazodone, nelfinavir, ritonavir, saquinavir, telithromycin, troleandomycin, and voriconazole).
No products indexed under this heading.

Fluoxetine Hydrochloride (Caution when administering or taking erlotinib with strong CYP3A4 inhibitors such as atazanavir, clarithromycin, indinavir, itraconazole, nefazodone, nelfinavir, ritonavir, saquinavir, telithromycin, troleandomycin, and voriconazole). Products include:
Prozac Weekly Capsules 1852
Prozac Pulvules and Liquid 1852
Symbyax Capsules 1871

Fluvoxamine Maleate (Caution when administering or taking erlotinib with strong CYP3A4 inhibitors such as atazanavir, clarithromycin, indinavir, itraconazole, nefazodone, nelfinavir, ritonavir, saquinavir, telithromycin, troleandomycin, and voriconazole). Products include:
Luvox CR Extended-Release Capsules.................................. 1759

Fosamprenavir Calcium (Caution when administering or taking erlotinib with strong CYP3A4 inhibitors such as atazanavir, clarithromycin, indinavir, itraconazole, nefazodone, nelfinavir, ritonavir, saquinavir, telithromycin, troleandomycin, and voriconazole). Products include:
Lexiva Oral Suspension 1510
Lexiva Tablets 1510

Fosphenytoin Sodium (Pre-treatment with the CYP3A4 inducer rifampicin decreased erlotinib AUC by about 2/3 to 4/5. Alternate treatments lacking CYP3A4 inducing activity should be considered. If an alternative treatment is unavailable, an increase in the dose of erlotinib should be considered as tolerated at two week intervals while monitoring the patient's safety. If the erlotinib dose is adjusted upward, the dose will need to be reduced upon discontinuation of rifampicin or other CYP3A4 inducers).
No products indexed under this heading.

Garlic Extract (Pre-treatment with the CYP3A4 inducer rifampicin decreased erlotinib AUC by about 2/3 to 4/5. Alternate treatments lacking CYP3A4 inducing activity should be considered. If an alternative treatment is unavailable, an increase in the dose of erlotinib should be considered as tolerated at two week intervals while monitoring the patient's safety. If the erlotinib dose is adjusted upward, the dose will need to be reduced upon discontinuation of rifampicin or other CYP3A4 inducers).
No products indexed under this heading.

Garlic Oil (Pre-treatment with the CYP3A4 inducer rifampicin decreased erlotinib AUC by about 2/3 to 4/5. Alternate treatments lacking CYP3A4 inducing activity should be considered. If an alternative treatment is unavailable, an increase in the dose of erlotinib should be considered as tolerated at two week intervals while monitoring the patient's safety. If the erlotinib dose is adjusted upward, the dose will need to be reduced upon discontinuation of rifampicin or other CYP3A4 inducers).
No products indexed under this heading.

Hydrocortisone (Pre-treatment with the CYP3A4 inducer rifampicin decreased erlotinib AUC by about 2/3 to 4/5. Alternate treatments lacking CYP3A4 inducing activity should be considered. If an alternative treatment is unavailable, an increase in the dose of erlotinib should be considered as tolerated at two week intervals while monitoring the patient's safety. If the erlotinib dose is adjusted upward, the dose will need to be reduced upon discontinuation of rifampicin or other CYP3A4 inducers).
No products indexed under this heading.

Hydrocortisone Acetate (Pre-treatment with the CYP3A4 inducer rifampicin decreased erlotinib AUC by about 2/3 to 4/5. Alternate treatments lacking CYP3A4 inducing activity should be considered. If an alternative treatment is unavailable, an increase in the dose of erlotinib should be considered as tolerated at two week intervals while monitoring the patient's safety. If the erlotinib dose is adjusted upward, the dose will need to be reduced upon discontinuation of rifampicin or other CYP3A4 inducers). Products include:
Analpram-HC 1140
Pramosone 1141

Hydrocortisone Butyrate (Pre-treatment with the CYP3A4 inducer rifampicin decreased erlotinib AUC

by about 2/3 to 4/5. Alternate treatments lacking CYP3A4 inducing activity should be considered. If an alternative treatment is unavailable, an increase in the dose of erlotinib should be considered as tolerated at two week intervals while monitoring the patient's safety. If the erlotinib dose is adjusted upward, the dose will need to be reduced upon discontinuation of rifampicin or other CYP3A4 inducers).
No products indexed under this heading.

Hydrocortisone Cypionate (Pre-treatment with the CYP3A4 inducer rifampicin decreased erlotinib AUC by about 2/3 to 4/5. Alternate treatments lacking CYP3A4 inducing activity should be considered. If an alternative treatment is unavailable, an increase in the dose of erlotinib should be considered as tolerated at two week intervals while monitoring the patient's safety. If the erlotinib dose is adjusted upward, the dose will need to be reduced upon discontinuation of rifampicin or other CYP3A4 inducers).
No products indexed under this heading.

Hydrocortisone Hemisuccinate (Pre-treatment with the CYP3A4 inducer rifampicin decreased erlotinib AUC by about 2/3 to 4/5. Alternate treatments lacking CYP3A4 inducing activity should be considered. If an alternative treatment is unavailable, an increase in the dose of erlotinib should be considered as tolerated at two week intervals while monitoring the patient's safety. If the erlotinib dose is adjusted upward, the dose will need to be reduced upon discontinuation of rifampicin or other CYP3A4 inducers).
No products indexed under this heading.

Hydrocortisone Probutate (Pre-treatment with the CYP3A4 inducer rifampicin decreased erlotinib AUC by about 2/3 to 4/5. Alternate treatments lacking CYP3A4 inducing activity should be considered. If an alternative treatment is unavailable, an increase in the dose of erlotinib should be considered as tolerated at two week intervals while monitoring the patient's safety. If the erlotinib dose is adjusted upward, the dose will need to be reduced upon discontinuation of rifampicin or other CYP3A4 inducers).
No products indexed under this heading.

Hydrocortisone Sodium Phosphate (Pre-treatment with the CYP3A4 inducer rifampicin decreased erlotinib AUC by about 2/3 to 4/5. Alternate treatments lacking CYP3A4 inducing activity should be considered. If an alternative treatment is unavailable, an increase in the dose of erlotinib should be considered as tolerated at two week intervals while monitoring the patient's safety. If the erlotinib dose is adjusted upward, the dose will need to be reduced upon discontinuation of rifampicin or other CYP3A4 inducers).
No products indexed under this heading.

Hydrocortisone Sodium Succinate (Pre-treatment with the CYP3A4 inducer rifampicin decreased erlotinib AUC by about 2/3 to 4/5. Alternate treatments lacking CYP3A4 inducing activity should be considered. If an alternative treatment is unavailable, an increase in the dose of erlotinib should be considered as tolerated at two week intervals while monitoring the patient's safety. If the erlotinib dose is adjusted upward, the dose will need to be reduced upon discontinuation of rifampicin or other CYP3A4 inducers).
No products indexed under this heading.

Hydrocortisone Valerate (Pre-treatment with the CYP3A4 inducer rifampicin decreased erlotinib AUC by about 2/3 to 4/5. Alternate treatments lacking CYP3A4 inducing activity should be considered. If an alternative treatment is unavailable, an increase in the dose of erlotinib should be considered as tolerated at two week intervals while monitoring the patient's safety. If the erlotinib dose is adjusted upward, the dose will need to be reduced upon discontinuation of rifampicin or other CYP3A4 inducers).
No products indexed under this heading.

Hypericum (Pre-treatment with the CYP3A4 inducer rifampicin decreased erlotinib AUC by about 2/3 to 4/5. Alternate treatments lacking CYP3A4 inducing activity should be considered. If an alternative treatment is unavailable, an increase in the dose of erlotinib should be considered as tolerated at two week intervals while monitoring the patient's safety. If the erlotinib dose is adjusted upward, the dose will need to be reduced upon discontinuation of rifampicin or other CYP3A4 inducers). Products include:
Satieté Tablets .... ▣ 640

Hypericum Perforatum (Pre-treatment with the CYP3A4 inducer rifampicin decreased erlotinib AUC by about 2/3 to 4/5. Alternate treatments lacking CYP3A4 inducing activity should be considered. If an alternative treatment is unavailable, an increase in the dose of erlotinib should be considered as tolerated at two week intervals while monitoring the patient's safety. If the erlotinib dose is adjusted upward, the dose will need to be reduced upon discontinuation of rifampicin or other CYP3A4 inducers).
No products indexed under this heading.

Indinavir Sulfate (Co-treatment with the potent CYP3A4 inhibitor ketoconazole increases erlotinib AUC by 2/3. Caution should be used when administering or taking erlotinib with ketoconazole and other strong CYP3A4 inhibitors such as indinavir). Products include:
Crixivan Capsules 1979

Isoniazid (Caution when administering or taking erlotinib with strong CYP3A4 inhibitors such as atazanavir, clarithromycin, indinavir, itraconazole, nefazodone, nelfinavir, ritonavir, saquinavir, telithromycin, troleandomycin, and voriconazole).
No products indexed under this heading.

Itraconazole (Co-treatment with the potent CYP3A4 inhibitor ketoconazole increases erlotinib AUC by 2/3. Caution should be used when administering or taking erlotinib with ketoconazole and other strong CYP3A4 inhibitors such as itraconazole).
No products indexed under this heading.

Ketoconazole (Co-treatment with the potent CYP3A4 inhibitor ketoconazole increases erlotinib AUC by 2/3. Caution should be used when administering or taking erlotinib with ketoconazole and other strong CYP3A4 inhibitors). Products include:
Extina Foam, 2% 3057
Nizoral A-D Shampoo 1901

Lopinavir (Caution when administering or taking erlotinib with strong CYP3A4 inhibitors such as atazanavir, clarithromycin, indinavir, itraconazole, nefazodone, nelfinavir, ritonavir, saquinavir, telithromycin, troleandomycin, and voriconazole). Products include:
Kaletra 452

Loratadine (Caution when administering or taking erlotinib with strong CYP3A4 inhibitors such as atazanavir, clarithromycin, indinavir, itraconazole, nefazodone, nelfinavir, ritonavir, saquinavir, telithromycin, troleandomycin, and voriconazole).
No products indexed under this heading.

Mephenytoin (Pre-treatment with the CYP3A4 inducer rifampicin decreased erlotinib AUC by about 2/3 to 4/5. Alternate treatments lacking CYP3A4 inducing activity should be considered. If an alternative treatment is unavailable, an increase in the dose of erlotinib should be considered as tolerated at two week intervals while monitoring the patient's safety. If the erlotinib dose is adjusted upward, the dose will need to be reduced upon discontinuation of rifampicin or other CYP3A4 inducers).
No products indexed under this heading.

Methsuximide (Pre-treatment with the CYP3A4 inducer rifampicin decreased erlotinib AUC by about 2/3 to 4/5. Alternate treatments lacking CYP3A4 inducing activity should be considered. If an alternative treatment is unavailable, an increase in the dose of erlotinib should be considered as tolerated at two week intervals while monitoring the patient's safety. If the erlotinib dose is adjusted upward, the dose will need to be reduced upon discontinuation of rifampicin or other CYP3A4 inducers).
No products indexed under this heading.

Methylprednisolone (Pre-treatment with the CYP3A4 inducer rifampicin decreased erlotinib AUC by about 2/3 to 4/5. Alternate treatments lacking CYP3A4 inducing activity should be considered. If an alternative treatment is unavailable, an increase in the dose of erlotinib should be considered as tolerated at two week intervals while monitoring the patient's safety. If the erlotinib dose is adjusted upward, the dose will need to be reduced upon discontinuation of rifampicin or other CYP3A4 inducers).
No products indexed under this heading.

Methylprednisolone Acetate (Pre-treatment with the CYP3A4 inducer rifampicin decreased erlotinib AUC by about 2/3 to 4/5. Alternate treatments lacking CYP3A4 inducing activity should be considered. If an alternative treatment is unavailable, an increase in the dose of erlotinib should be considered as tolerated at two week intervals while monitoring the patient's safety. If the erlotinib dose is adjusted upward, the dose will need to be reduced upon discontinuation of rifampicin or other CYP3A4 inducers).
No products indexed under this heading.

Methylprednisolone Sodium Succinate (Pre-treatment with the CYP3A4 inducer rifampicin decreased erlotinib AUC by about 2/3 to 4/5. Alternate treatments lacking CYP3A4 inducing activity should be considered. If an alternative treatment is unavailable, an increase in the dose of erlotinib should be considered as tolerated at two week intervals while monitoring the patient's safety. If the erlotinib dose is adjusted upward, the dose will need to be reduced upon discontinuation of rifampicin or other CYP3A4 inducers).
No products indexed under this heading.

Metronidazole (Caution when administering or taking erlotinib with strong CYP3A4 inhibitors such as atazanavir, clarithromycin, indinavir, itraconazole, nefazodone, nelfinavir, ritonavir, saquinavir, telithromycin, troleandomycin, and voriconazole). Products include:
Pylera Capsules 714

Metronidazole Benzoate (Caution when administering or taking erlotinib with strong CYP3A4 inhibitors such as atazanavir, clarithromycin, indinavir, itraconazole, nefazodone, nelfinavir, ritonavir, saquinavir, telithromycin, troleandomycin, and voriconazole).
No products indexed under this heading.

Metronidazole Hydrochloride (Caution when administering or taking erlotinib with strong CYP3A4 inhibitors such as atazanavir, clarithromycin, indinavir, itraconazole, nefazodone, nelfinavir, ritonavir, saquinavir, telithromycin, troleandomycin, and voriconazole).
No products indexed under this heading.

Miconazole (Caution when administering or taking erlotinib with strong CYP3A4 inhibitors such as atazanavir, clarithromycin, indinavir, itraconazole, nefazodone, nelfinavir, ritonavir, saquinavir, telithromycin, troleandomycin, and voriconazole).
No products indexed under this heading.

Miconazole Nitrate (Caution when administering or taking erlotinib with strong CYP3A4 inhibitors such as atazanavir, clarithromycin, indinavir, itraconazole, nefazodone, nelfinavir, ritonavir, saquinavir, telithromycin, troleandomycin, and voriconazole).
No products indexed under this heading.

Modafinil (Pre-treatment with the CYP3A4 inducer rifampicin decreased erlotinib AUC by about 2/3 to 4/5. Alternate treatments lacking CYP3A4 inducing activity should be considered. If an alternative treatment is unavailable, an increase in the dose of erlotinib should be considered as tolerated at two week intervals while monitoring the patient's safety. If the erlotinib dose is adjusted upward, the dose will need to be reduced upon discontinuation of rifampicin or other CYP3A4 inducers). Products include:

Provigil Tablets ... 977

Nefazodone Hydrochloride (Co-treatment with the potent CYP3A4 inhibitor ketoconazole increases erlotinib AUC by 2/3. Caution should be used when administering or taking erlotinib with ketoconazole and other strong CYP3A4 inhibitors such as nefazodone).
No products indexed under this heading.

Nelfinavir Mesylate (Co-treatment with the potent CYP3A4 inhibitor ketoconazole increases erlotinib AUC by 2/3. Caution should be used when administering or taking erlotinib with ketoconazole and other strong CYP3A4 inhibitors such as nelfinavir).
No products indexed under this heading.

Nevirapine (Caution when administering or taking erlotinib with strong CYP3A4 inhibitors such as atazanavir, clarithromycin, indinavir, itraconazole, nefazodone, nelfinavir, ritonavir, saquinavir, telithromycin, troleandomycin, and voriconazole). Products include:
Viramune Oral Suspension ... 873
Viramune Tablets ... 873

Niacinamide (Caution when administering or taking erlotinib with strong CYP3A4 inhibitors such as atazanavir, clarithromycin, indinavir, itraconazole, nefazodone, nelfinavir, ritonavir, saquinavir, telithromycin, troleandomycin, and voriconazole). Products include:
BioLean Free Tablets ... ▣635

Nicotinamide (Caution when administering or taking erlotinib with strong CYP3A4 inhibitors such as atazanavir, clarithromycin, indinavir, itraconazole, nefazodone, nelfinavir, ritonavir, saquinavir, telithromycin, troleandomycin, and voriconazole).
No products indexed under this heading.

Nifedipine (Caution when administering or taking erlotinib with strong CYP3A4 inhibitors such as atazanavir, clarithromycin, indinavir, itraconazole, nefazodone, nelfinavir, ritonavir, saquinavir, telithromycin, troleandomycin, and voriconazole).
No products indexed under this heading.

Norfloxacin (Caution when administering or taking erlotinib with strong CYP3A4 inhibitors such as atazanavir, clarithromycin, indinavir, itraconazole, nefazodone, nelfinavir, ritonavir, saquinavir, telithromycin, troleandomycin, and voriconazole). Products include:
Noroxin Tablets ... 2069

Omeprazole (Caution when administering or taking erlotinib with strong CYP3A4 inhibitors such as atazanavir, clarithromycin, indinavir, itraconazole, nefazodone, nelfinavir, ritonavir, saquinavir, telithromycin, troleandomycin, and voriconazole).
No products indexed under this heading.

Oxcarbazepine (Pre-treatment with the CYP3A4 inducer rifampicin decreased erlotinib AUC by about 2/3 to 4/5. Alternate treatments lacking CYP3A4 inducing activity should be considered. If an alternative treatment is unavailable, an increase in the dose of erlotinib should be considered as tolerated at two week intervals while monitoring the patient's safety. If the erlotinib dose is adjusted upward, the dose will need to be reduced upon discontinuation of rifampicin or other CYP3A4 inducers).
No products indexed under this heading.

Paroxetine Hydrochloride (Caution when administering or taking erlotinib with strong CYP3A4 inhibitors such as atazanavir, clarithromycin, indinavir, itraconazole, nefazodone, nelfinavir, ritonavir, saquinavir, telithromycin, troleandomycin, and voriconazole). Products include:
Paxil ... 1535
Paxil CR Controlled-Release Tablets ... 1544

Phenobarbital (Pre-treatment with the CYP3A4 inducer rifampicin decreased erlotinib AUC by about 2/3 to 4/5. Alternate treatments lacking CYP3A4 inducing activity should be considered. If an alternative treatment is unavailable, an increase in the dose of erlotinib should be considered as tolerated at two week intervals while monitoring the patient's safety. If the erlotinib dose is adjusted upward, the dose will need to be reduced upon discontinuation of rifampicin or other CYP3A4 inducers). Products include:
Donnatal Extentabs ... 2507

Phenobarbital Sodium (Pre-treatment with the CYP3A4 inducer rifampicin decreased erlotinib AUC by about 2/3 to 4/5. Alternate treatments lacking CYP3A4 inducing activity should be considered. If an alternative treatment is unavailable, an increase in the dose of erlotinib should be considered as tolerated at two week intervals while monitoring the patient's safety. If the erlotinib dose is adjusted upward, the dose will need to be reduced upon discontinuation of rifampicin or other CYP3A4 inducers).
No products indexed under this heading.

Phenytoin (Pre-treatment with the CYP3A4 inducer rifampicin decreased erlotinib AUC by about 2/3 to 4/5. Alternate treatments lacking CYP3A4 inducing activity should be considered. If an alternative treatment is unavailable, an increase in the dose of erlotinib should be considered as tolerated at two week intervals while monitoring the patient's safety. If the erlotinib dose is adjusted upward, the dose will need to be reduced upon discontinuation of rifampicin or other CYP3A4 inducers).
No products indexed under this heading.

Phenytoin Sodium (Pre-treatment with the CYP3A4 inducer rifampicin decreased erlotinib AUC by about 2/3 to 4/5. Alternate treatments lacking CYP3A4 inducing activity should be considered. If an alternative treatment is unavailable, an increase in the dose of erlotinib should be considered as tolerated at two week intervals while monitoring the patient's safety. If the erlotinib dose is adjusted upward, the dose will need to be reduced upon discontinuation of rifampicin or other CYP3A4 inducers). Products include:
Phenytek Capsules ... 2192

Prednisolone Acetate (Pre-treatment with the CYP3A4 inducer rifampicin decreased erlotinib AUC by about 2/3 to 4/5. Alternate treatments lacking CYP3A4 inducing activity should be considered. If an alternative treatment is unavailable, an increase in the dose of erlotinib should be considered as tolerated at two week intervals while monitoring the patient's safety. If the erlotinib dose is adjusted upward, the dose will need to be reduced upon discontinuation of rifampicin or other CYP3A4 inducers). Products include:
Pred Forte Ophthalmic Suspension ... ⊙227
Pred Mild Ophthalmic Suspension ... ⊙230
Pred-G Ophthalmic Ointment ... ⊙229
Pred-G Ophthalmic Suspension ... ⊙228

Prednisolone Sodium Phosphate (Pre-treatment with the CYP3A4 inducer rifampicin decreased erlotinib AUC by about 2/3 to 4/5. Alternate treatments lacking CYP3A4 inducing activity should be considered. If an alternative treatment is unavailable, an increase in the dose of erlotinib should be considered as tolerated at two week intervals while monitoring the patient's safety. If the erlotinib dose is adjusted upward, the dose will need to be reduced upon discontinuation of rifampicin or other CYP3A4 inducers).
No products indexed under this heading.

Prednisolone Tebutate (Pre-treatment with the CYP3A4 inducer rifampicin decreased erlotinib AUC by about 2/3 to 4/5. Alternate treatments lacking CYP3A4 inducing activity should be considered. If an alternative treatment is unavailable, an increase in the dose of erlotinib should be considered as tolerated at two week intervals while monitoring the patient's safety. If the erlotinib dose is adjusted upward, the dose will need to be reduced upon discontinuation of rifampicin or other CYP3A4 inducers).
No products indexed under this heading.

Prednisone (Pre-treatment with the CYP3A4 inducer rifampicin decreased erlotinib AUC by about 2/3 to 4/5. Alternate treatments lacking CYP3A4 inducing activity should be considered. If an alternative treatment is unavailable, an increase in the dose of erlotinib should be considered as tolerated at two week intervals while monitoring the patient's safety. If the erlotinib dose is adjusted upward, the dose will need to be reduced upon discontinuation of rifampicin or other CYP3A4 inducers).
No products indexed under this heading.

Primidone (Pre-treatment with the CYP3A4 inducer rifampicin decreased erlotinib AUC by about 2/3 to 4/5. Alternate treatments lacking CYP3A4 inducing activity should be considered. If an alternative treatment is unavailable, an increase in the dose of erlotinib should be considered as tolerated at two week intervals while monitoring the patient's safety. If the erlotinib dose is adjusted upward, the dose will need to be reduced upon discontinuation of rifampicin or other CYP3A4 inducers).
No products indexed under this heading.

Propoxyphene Hydrochloride (Caution when administering or taking erlotinib with strong CYP3A4 inhibitors such as atazanavir, clarithromycin, indinavir, itraconazole, nefazodone, nelfinavir, ritonavir, saquinavir, telithromycin, troleandomycin, and voriconazole).
No products indexed under this heading.

Propoxyphene Napsylate (Caution when administering or taking erlotinib with strong CYP3A4 inhibitors such as atazanavir, clarithromycin, indinavir, itraconazole, nefazodone, nelfinavir, ritonavir, saquinavir, telithromycin, troleandomycin, and voriconazole).
No products indexed under this heading.

Quinidine (Caution when administering or taking erlotinib with strong CYP3A4 inhibitors such as atazanavir, clarithromycin, indinavir, itraconazole, nefazodone, nelfinavir, ritonavir, saquinavir, telithromycin, troleandomycin, and voriconazole).
No products indexed under this heading.

Quinidine Hydrochloride (Caution when administering or taking erlotinib with strong CYP3A4 inhibitors such as atazanavir, clarithromycin, indinavir, itraconazole, nefazodone, nelfinavir, ritonavir, saquinavir, telithromycin, troleandomycin, and voriconazole).
No products indexed under this heading.

Quinidine Polygalacturonate (Caution when administering or taking erlotinib with strong CYP3A4 inhibitors such as atazanavir, clarithromycin, indinavir, itraconazole, nefazodone, nelfinavir, ritonavir, saquinavir, telithromycin, troleandomycin, and voriconazole).
No products indexed under this heading.

Quinidine Sulfate (Caution when administering or taking erlotinib with strong CYP3A4 inhibitors such as atazanavir, clarithromycin, indinavir, itraconazole, nefazodone, nelfinavir, ritonavir, saquinavir, telithromycin, troleandomycin, and voriconazole).
No products indexed under this heading.

Quinine (Caution when administering or taking erlotinib with strong CYP3A4 inhibitors such as atazanavir, clarithromycin, indinavir, itraconazole, nefazodone, nelfinavir, ritonavir, saquinavir, telithromycin, troleandomycin, and voriconazole).
No products indexed under this heading.

Quinine Sulfate (Caution when administering or taking erlotinib with strong CYP3A4 inhibitors such as atazanavir, clarithromycin, indinavir, itraconazole, nefazodone, nelfinavir, ritonavir, saquinavir, telithromycin, troleandomycin, and voriconazole).
No products indexed under this heading.

Quinupristin (Caution when administering or taking erlotinib with strong CYP3A4 inhibitors such as atazanavir, clarithromycin, indinavir, itraconazole, nefazodone, nelfinavir, ritonavir, saquinavir, telithromycin, troleandomycin, and voriconazole).
No products indexed under this heading.

Ranitidine Bismuth Citrate (Caution when administering or taking erlotinib with strong CYP3A4 inhibitors such as atazanavir, clarithromycin, indinavir, itraconazole, nefazodone, nelfinavir, ritonavir, saquinavir, telithromycin, troleandomycin, and voriconazole).
No products indexed under this heading.

Ranitidine Hydrochloride (Caution when administering or taking erlotinib with strong CYP3A4 inhibitors such as atazanavir, clarithromycin, indinavir, itraconazole, nefazodone, nelfinavir, ritonavir, saquinavir, telithromycin, troleandomycin, and voriconazole). Products include:
Zantac 75 Tablets .... ▣**603**
Zantac **1670**
Zantac Injection **1666**
Zantac Injection Pharmacy Bulk Package **1668**
Maximum Strength Zantac 150 Tablets.. ▣**603**
Maximum Strength Zantac 150 Cool Mint Tablets .... ▣**603**

Rifabutin (Pre-treatment with the CYP3A4 inducer rifampicin decreased erlotinib AUC by about 2/3 to 4/5. Alternate treatments lacking CYP3A4 inducing activity should be considered. If an alternative treatment is unavailable, an increase in the dose of erlotinib should be considered as tolerated at two week intervals while monitoring the patient's safety. If the erlotinib dose is adjusted upward, the dose will need to be reduced upon discontinuation of rifampicin or other CYP3A4 inducers).
No products indexed under this heading.

Rifampicin (Pre-treatment with the CYP3A4 inducer rifampicin decreased erlotinib AUC by about 2/3 to 4/5. Alternate treatments lacking CYP3A4 inducing activity should be considered. If an alternative treatment is unavailable, an increase in the dose of erlotinib should be considered as tolerated at two week intervals while monitoring the patient's safety. If the erlotinib dose is adjusted upward, the dose will need to be reduced upon discontinuation of rifampicin or other CYP3A4 inducers).
No products indexed under this heading.

Rifampin (Pre-treatment with the CYP3A4 inducer rifampicin decreased erlotinib AUC by about 2/3 to 4/5. Alternate treatments lacking CYP3A4 inducing activity should be considered. If an alternative treatment is unavailable, an increase in the dose of erlotinib should be considered as tolerated at two week intervals while monitoring the patient's safety. If the erlotinib dose is adjusted upward, the dose will need to be reduced upon discontinuation of rifampicin or other CYP3A4 inducers).
No products indexed under this heading.

Rifapentine (Pre-treatment with the CYP3A4 inducer rifampicin decreased erlotinib AUC by about 2/3 to 4/5. Alternate treatments lacking CYP3A4 inducing activity should be considered. If an alternative treatment is unavailable, an increase in the dose of erlotinib should be considered as tolerated at two week intervals while monitoring the patient's safety. If the erlotinib dose is adjusted upward, the dose will need to be reduced upon discontinuation of rifampicin or other CYP3A4 inducers).
No products indexed under this heading.

Ritonavir (Co-treatment with the potent CYP3A4 inhibitor ketoconazole increases erlotinib AUC by 2/3. Caution should be used when administering or taking erlotinib with ketoconazole and other strong CYP3A4 inhibitors such as ritonavir). Products include:
Kaletra **452**
Norvir **489**

Saquinavir (Co-treatment with the potent CYP3A4 inhibitor ketoconazole increases erlotinib AUC by 2/3. Caution should be used when administering or taking erlotinib with ketoconazole and other strong CYP3A4 inhibitors such as saquinavir).
No products indexed under this heading.

Saquinavir Mesylate (Co-treatment with the potent CYP3A4 inhibitor ketoconazole increases erlotinib AUC by 2/3. Caution should be used when administering or taking erlotinib with ketoconazole and other strong CYP3A4 inhibitors such as saquinavir).
No products indexed under this heading.

Sertraline Hydrochloride (Caution when administering or taking erlotinib with strong CYP3A4 inhibitors such as atazanavir, clarithromycin, indinavir, itraconazole, nefazodone, nelfinavir, ritonavir, saquinavir, telithromycin, troleandomycin, and voriconazole).
No products indexed under this heading.

Sildenafil Citrate (Caution when administering or taking erlotinib with strong CYP3A4 inhibitors such as atazanavir, clarithromycin, indinavir, itraconazole, nefazodone, nelfinavir, ritonavir, saquinavir, telithromycin, troleandomycin, and voriconazole).
No products indexed under this heading.

Sulfinpyrazone (Pre-treatment with the CYP3A4 inducer rifampicin decreased erlotinib AUC by about 2/3 to 4/5. Alternate treatments lacking CYP3A4 inducing activity should be considered. If an alternative treatment is unavailable, an increase in the dose of erlotinib should be considered as tolerated at two week intervals while monitoring the patient's safety. If the erlotinib dose is adjusted upward, the dose will need to be reduced upon discontinuation of rifampicin or other CYP3A4 inducers).
No products indexed under this heading.

Telithromycin (Co-treatment with the potent CYP3A4 inhibitor ketoconazole increases erlotinib AUC by 2/3. Caution should be used when administering or taking erlotinib with ketoconazole and other strong CYP3A4 inhibitors such as telithromycin). Products include:
Ketek Tablets **2744**

Theophylline (Pre-treatment with the CYP3A4 inducer rifampicin decreased erlotinib AUC by about 2/3 to 4/5. Alternate treatments lacking CYP3A4 inducing activity should be considered. If an alternative treatment is unavailable, an increase in the dose of erlotinib should be considered as tolerated at two week intervals while monitoring the patient's safety. If the erlotinib dose is adjusted upward, the dose will need to be reduced upon discontinuation of rifampicin or other CYP3A4 inducers).
No products indexed under this heading.

Theophylline Anhydrous (Pre-treatment with the CYP3A4 inducer rifampicin decreased erlotinib AUC by about 2/3 to 4/5. Alternate treatments lacking CYP3A4 inducing activity should be considered. If an alternative treatment is unavailable, an increase in the dose of erlotinib should be considered as tolerated at two week intervals while monitoring the patient's safety. If the erlotinib dose is adjusted upward, the dose will need to be reduced upon discontinuation of rifampicin or other CYP3A4 inducers). Products include:
Uniphyl Tablets **2595**

Theophylline Calcium Salicylate (Pre-treatment with the CYP3A4 inducer rifampicin decreased erlotinib AUC by about 2/3 to 4/5. Alternate treatments lacking CYP3A4 inducing activity should be considered. If an alternative treatment is unavailable, an increase in the dose of erlotinib should be considered as tolerated at two week intervals while monitoring the patient's safety. If the erlotinib dose is adjusted upward, the dose will need to be reduced upon discontinuation of rifampicin or other CYP3A4 inducers).
No products indexed under this heading.

Theophylline Dihydroxypropyl (Glyceryl) (Pre-treatment with the CYP3A4 inducer rifampicin decreased erlotinib AUC by about 2/3 to 4/5. Alternate treatments lacking CYP3A4 inducing activity should be considered. If an alternative treatment is unavailable, an increase in the dose of erlotinib should be considered as tolerated at two week intervals while monitoring the patient's safety. If the erlotinib dose is adjusted upward, the dose will need to be reduced upon discontinuation of rifampicin or other CYP3A4 inducers).
No products indexed under this heading.

Theophylline Ethylenediamine (Pre-treatment with the CYP3A4 inducer rifampicin decreased erlotinib AUC by about 2/3 to 4/5. Alternate treatments lacking CYP3A4 inducing activity should be considered. If an alternative treatment is unavailable, an increase in the dose of erlotinib should be considered as tolerated at two week intervals while monitoring the patient's safety. If the erlotinib dose is adjusted upward, the dose will need to be reduced upon discontinuation of rifampicin or other CYP3A4 inducers).
No products indexed under this heading.

Triamcinolone (Pre-treatment with the CYP3A4 inducer rifampicin decreased erlotinib AUC by about 2/3 to 4/5. Alternate treatments lacking CYP3A4 inducing activity should be considered. If an alternative treatment is unavailable, an increase in the dose of erlotinib should be considered as tolerated at two week intervals while monitoring the patient's safety. If the erlotinib dose is adjusted upward, the dose will need to be reduced upon discontinuation of rifampicin or other CYP3A4 inducers).
No products indexed under this heading.

Triamcinolone Acetonide (Pre-treatment with the CYP3A4 inducer rifampicin decreased erlotinib AUC by about 2/3 to 4/5. Alternate treatments lacking CYP3A4 inducing activity should be considered. If an alternative treatment is unavailable, an increase in the dose of erlotinib should be considered as tolerated at two week intervals while monitoring the patient's safety. If the erlotinib dose is adjusted upward, the dose will need to be reduced upon discontinuation of rifampicin or other CYP3A4 inducers). Products include:
Azmacort Inhalation Aerosol **407**
Nasacort AQ Nasal Spray **2765**
Triesence Injectable Suspension .... ⊙**209**

Triamcinolone Diacetate (Pre-treatment with the CYP3A4 inducer rifampicin decreased erlotinib AUC by about 2/3 to 4/5. Alternate treatments lacking CYP3A4 inducing activity should be considered. If an alternative treatment is unavailable, an increase in the dose of erlotinib should be considered as tolerated at two week intervals while monitoring the patient's safety. If the erlotinib dose is adjusted upward, the dose will need to be reduced upon discontinuation of rifampicin or other CYP3A4 inducers).
No products indexed under this heading.

Triamcinolone Hexacetonide (Pre-treatment with the CYP3A4 inducer rifampicin decreased erlotinib AUC by about 2/3 to 4/5. Alternate treatments lacking CYP3A4 inducing activity should be considered. If an alternative treatment is unavailable, an increase in the dose of erlotinib should be considered as tolerated at two week intervals while monitoring the patient's safety. If the erlotinib dose is adjusted upward, the dose will need to be reduced upon discontinuation of rifampicin or other CYP3A4 inducers).
No products indexed under this heading.

Troglitazone (Caution when administering or taking erlotinib with strong CYP3A4 inhibitors such as atazanavir, clarithromycin, indinavir, itraconazole, nefazodone, nelfinavir, ritonavir, saquinavir, telithromycin, troleandomycin, and voriconazole).
No products indexed under this heading.

Troleandomycin (Co-treatment with the potent CYP3A4 inhibitor ketoconazole increases erlotinib AUC by 2/3. Caution should be used when administering or taking erlotinib with ketoconazole and other strong CYP3A4 inhibitors such as troleandomycin).
No products indexed under this heading.

Valproate Sodium (Caution when administering or taking erlotinib with strong CYP3A4 inhibitors such as atazanavir, clarithromycin, indinavir, itraconazole, nefazodone, nelfinavir, ritonavir, saquinavir, telithromycin, troleandomycin, and voriconazole).
No products indexed under this heading.

Vardenafil Hydrochloride (Caution when administering or taking erlotinib with strong CYP3A4 inhibitors such as atazanavir, clarithromycin, indinavir, itraconazole, nefazodone, nelfinavir, ritonavir, saquinavir, telithromycin, troleandomycin, and voriconazole). Products include:
Levitra Tablets 2876

Verapamil Hydrochloride (Caution when administering or taking erlotinib with strong CYP3A4 inhibitors such as atazanavir, clarithromycin, indinavir, itraconazole, nefazodone, nelfinavir, ritonavir, saquinavir, telithromycin, troleandomycin, and voriconazole). Products include:
Tarka Tablets 511

Voriconazole (Co-treatment with the potent CYP3A4 inhibitor ketoconazole increases erlotinib AUC by 2/3. Caution should be used when administering or taking erlotinib with ketoconazole and other strong CYP3A4 inhibitors such as voriconazole).
No products indexed under this heading.

Zafirlukast (Caution when administering or taking erlotinib with strong CYP3A4 inhibitors such as atazanavir, clarithromycin, indinavir, itraconazole, nefazodone, nelfinavir, ritonavir, saquinavir, telithromycin, troleandomycin, and voriconazole). Products include:
Accolate Tablets 669

Zileuton (Caution when administering or taking erlotinib with strong CYP3A4 inhibitors such as atazanavir, clarithromycin, indinavir, itraconazole, nefazodone, nelfinavir, ritonavir, saquinavir, telithromycin, troleandomycin, and voriconazole).
No products indexed under this heading.

Food Interactions

Grapefruit (Caution when administering or taking erlotinib with strong CYP3A4 inhibitors such as atazanavir, clarithromycin, indinavir, itraconazole, nefazodone, nelfinavir, ritonavir, saquinavir, telithromycin, troleandomycin, and voriconazole).

Grapefruit Juice (Caution when administering or taking erlotinib with strong CYP3A4 inhibitors such as atazanavir, clarithromycin, indinavir, itraconazole, nefazodone, nelfinavir, ritonavir, saquinavir, telithromycin, troleandomycin, and voriconazole).

TARGRETIN CAPSULES

(Bexarotene) 1084

May interact with erythromycin, oral hypoglycemic agents, insulin, oral contraceptives, phenytoin, protease inhibitors, and certain other agents. Compounds in these categories include:

Acarbose (Bexarotene could enhance the action of hypoglycemic agents resulting in hypoglycemia). Products include:
Precose Tablets 792

Amiodarone Hydrochloride (Bexarotene is metabolized by CYP4503A4; co-administration with inhibitors of CYP4503A4, such as amiodarone, would be expected to lead to an increase in plasma bexarotene concentrations).
No products indexed under this heading.

Amprenavir (Bexarotene is metabolized by CYP4503A4; co-administration with inhibitors of CYP4503A4, such as protease inhibitors, would be expected to lead to an increase in plasma bexarotene concentrations).
No products indexed under this heading.

Carbamazepine (Bexarotene is metabolized by CYP4503A4; co-administration with inducers of CYP4503A4, such as carbamazepine, may cause a reduction in plasma bexarotene concentrations). Products include:
Carbatrol Capsules 3019
Equetro Extended-Release Capsules 3174

Chlorpropamide (Bexarotene could enhance the action of hypoglycemic agents resulting in hypoglycemia).
No products indexed under this heading.

Darunavir (Bexarotene is metabolized by CYP4503A4; co-administration with inhibitors of CYP4503A4, such as protease inhibitors, would be expected to lead to an increase in plasma bexarotene concentrations).
No products indexed under this heading.

Desogestrel (Bexarotene may theoretically increase the rate of metabolism and reduce plasma concentrations of other substrates metabolized by CYP4503A4, including hormonal contraceptives; it is strongly recommended that two reliable forms of contraception be used concurrently, one of which should be non-hormonal). Products include:
Mircette Tablets 1034

Erythromycin (Bexarotene is metabolized by CYP4503A4; co-administration with inhibitors of CYP4503A4, such as erythromycin, would be expected to lead to an increase in plasma bexarotene concentrations).
No products indexed under this heading.

Erythromycin Estolate (Bexarotene is metabolized by CYP4503A4; co-administration with inhibitors of CYP4503A4, such as erythromycin, would be expected to lead to an increase in plasma bexarotene concentrations).
No products indexed under this heading.

Erythromycin Ethylsuccinate (Bexarotene is metabolized by CYP4503A4; co-administration with inhibitors of CYP4503A4, such as erythromycin, would be expected to lead to an increase in plasma bexarotene concentrations). Products include:
E.E.S. 433
EryPed 431

Erythromycin Gluceptate (Bexarotene is metabolized by CYP4503A4; co-administration with inhibitors of CYP4503A4, such as erythromycin, would be expected to lead to an increase in plasma bexarotene concentrations).
No products indexed under this heading.

Erythromycin Lactobionate (Bexarotene is metabolized by CYP4503A4; co-administration with inhibitors of CYP4503A4, such as erythromycin, would be expected to lead to an increase in plasma bexarotene concentrations).
No products indexed under this heading.

Erythromycin Stearate (Bexarotene is metabolized by CYP4503A4; co-administration with inhibitors of CYP4503A4, such as erythromycin, would be expected to lead to an increase in plasma bexarotene concentrations).
No products indexed under this heading.

Ethinyl Estradiol (Bexarotene may theoretically increase the rate of metabolism and reduce plasma concentrations of other substrates metabolized by CYP4503A4, including hormonal contraceptives; it is strongly recommended that two reliable forms of contraception be used concurrently, one of which should be non-hormonal). Products include:
Lybrel Tablets 3204
Mircette Tablets 1034
NuvaRing 2897
Ortho-Cyclen/Ortho Tri-Cyclen 2449
Ortho Evra Transdermal System 2437
Ortho Tri-Cyclen Lo Tablets 2458
Seasonique Tablets 1046
Yaz Tablets 805

Ethynodiol Diacetate (Bexarotene may theoretically increase the rate of metabolism and reduce plasma concentrations of other substrates metabolized by CYP4503A4, including hormonal contraceptives; it is strongly recommended that two reliable forms of contraception be used concurrently, one of which should be non-hormonal).
No products indexed under this heading.

Fosamprenavir Calcium (Bexarotene is metabolized by CYP4503A4; co-administration with inhibitors of CYP4503A4, such as protease inhibitors, would be expected to lead to an increase in plasma bexarotene concentrations). Products include:
Lexiva Oral Suspension 1510
Lexiva Tablets 1510

Fosphenytoin Sodium (Bexarotene is metabolized by CYP4503A4; co-administration with inducers of CYP4503A4, such as phenytoin, may cause a reduction in plasma bexarotene concentrations).
No products indexed under this heading.

Gemfibrozil (Co-administration has resulted in substantial increases in plasma bexarotene concentrations; concomitant administration is not recommended).
No products indexed under this heading.

Glimepiride (Bexarotene could enhance the action of hypoglycemic agents resulting in hypoglycemia). Products include:
Avandaryl Tablets 1344
Duetact Tablets 3085

Glipizide (Bexarotene could enhance the action of hypoglycemic agents resulting in hypoglycemia).
No products indexed under this heading.

Glyburide (Bexarotene could enhance the action of hypoglycemic agents resulting in hypoglycemia).
No products indexed under this heading.

Hypericum (Bexarotene is metabolized by CYP4503A4; co-administration with inducers of CYP4503A4, such as St. John's Wort, may cause a reduction in plasma bexarotene concentrations). Products include:
Satieté Tablets .... ■ 640

Indinavir Sulfate (Bexarotene is metabolized by CYP4503A4; co-administration with inhibitors of CYP4503A4, such as protease inhibitors, would be expected to lead to an increase in plasma bexarotene concentrations). Products include:
Crixivan Capsules 1979

Insulin (Bexarotene could enhance the action of insulin resulting in hypoglycemia).
No products indexed under this heading.

Insulin, Human, Zinc Suspension (Bexarotene could enhance the action of insulin resulting in hypoglycemia).
No products indexed under this heading.

Insulin, Human (rDNA origin) (Bexarotene could enhance the action of insulin resulting in hypoglycemia). Products include:
Exubera Inhalation Powder 2515

Insulin, Human NPH (Bexarotene could enhance the action of insulin resulting in hypoglycemia). Products include:
Humulin N Vial 1846

Insulin, Human Regular (Bexarotene could enhance the action of insulin resulting in hypoglycemia). Products include:
Humulin R 1849
Humulin R (U-500) 1850

Insulin, Human Regular and Human NPH Mixture (Bexarotene could enhance the action of insulin resulting in hypoglycemia). Products include:
Humulin 50/50, 100 Units 1843
Humulin 70/30 Vial 1844

Insulin, NPH (Bexarotene could enhance the action of insulin resulting in hypoglycemia).
No products indexed under this heading.

Insulin, Regular (Bexarotene could enhance the action of insulin resulting in hypoglycemia).
No products indexed under this heading.

Insulin, Regular and NPH mixture (Bexarotene could enhance the action of insulin resulting in hypoglycemia).
No products indexed under this heading.

Insulin, Zinc Crystals (Bexarotene could enhance the action of insulin resulting in hypoglycemia).
No products indexed under this heading.

Insulin, Zinc Suspension (Bexarotene could enhance the action of insulin resulting in hypoglycemia).
No products indexed under this heading.

Insulin Aspart (Bexarotene could enhance the action of insulin resulting in hypoglycemia).
No products indexed under this heading.

Insulin Aspart, Human (Bexarotene could enhance the action of insulin resulting in hypoglycemia). Products include:
NovoLog Mix 70/30 2364

Insulin Aspart, Human Regular (Bexarotene could enhance the action of insulin resulting in hypoglycemia). Products include:
NovoLog Injection 2359

Insulin Aspart Protamine, Human (Bexarotene could enhance the action of insulin resulting in hypoglycemia). Products include:
NovoLog Mix 70/30 2364

Insulin Detemir (rDNA Origin) (Bexarotene could enhance the action of insulin resulting in hypoglycemia). Products include:
Levemir Injection 2352

Insulin glargine (Bexarotene could enhance the action of insulin resulting in hypoglycemia). Products include:
Lantus Injection 2749

Insulin Glulisine (Bexarotene could enhance the action of insulin resulting in hypoglycemia). Products include:
Apidra Injection 2706

Insulin Lispro, Human (Bexarotene could enhance the action of insulin resulting in hypoglycemia). Products include:
Humalog-Pen and KwikPen 1829
Humalog Mix 50/50-Pen and KwikPen 1833
Humalog Mix 75/25-Pen and KwikPen 1835

Insulin Lispro Protamine, Human (Bexarotene could enhance the action of insulin resulting in hypoglycemia). Products include:
Humalog Mix 50/50-Pen and KwikPen 1833
Humalog Mix 75/25-Pen and KwikPen 1835

Itraconazole (Bexarotene is metabolized by CYP4503A4; co-administration with inhibitors of CYP4503A4, such as itraconazole, would be expected to lead to an increase in plasma bexarotene concentrations).
No products indexed under this heading.

Ketoconazole (Bexarotene is metabolized by CYP4503A4; co-administration with inhibitors of CYP4503A4, such as ketoconazole, would be expected to lead to an increase in plasma concentrations). Products include:
Extina Foam, 2% 3057
Nizoral A-D Shampoo 1901

Levonorgestrel (Bexarotene may theoretically increase the rate of metabolism and reduce plasma concentrations of other substrates metabolized by CYP4503A4, including hormonal contraceptives; it is strongly recommended that two reliable forms of contraception be used concurrently, one of which should be non-hormonal). Products include:
Climara Pro Transdermal System 768
Lybrel Tablets 3204
Mirena Intrauterine System 779
Plan B Tablets 1044
Seasonique Tablets 1046

Lopinavir (Bexarotene is metabolized by CYP4503A4; co-administration with inhibitors of CYP4503A4, such as protease inhibitors, would be expected to lead to an increase in plasma bexarotene concentrations). Products include:
Kaletra 452

Mestranol (Bexarotene may theoretically increase the rate of metabolism and reduce plasma concentrations of other substrates metabolized by CYP4503A4, including hormonal contraceptives; it is strongly recommended that two reliable forms of contraception be used concurrently, one of which should be non-hormonal).
No products indexed under this heading.

Metformin Hydrochloride (Bexarotene could enhance the action of hypoglycemic agents resulting in hypoglycemia). Products include:
ActoPlus Met Tablets 3071
Avandamet Tablets 1336
Janumet Tablets 2041
PrandiMet Tablets 2967

Miglitol (Bexarotene could enhance the action of hypoglycemic agents resulting in hypoglycemia).
No products indexed under this heading.

Nateglinide (Bexarotene could enhance the action of hypoglycemic agents resulting in hypoglycemia). Products include:
Starlix Tablets 2314

Nefazodone Hydrochloride (Bexarotene is metabolized by CYP4503A4; co-administration with inhibitors of CYP4503A4, such as nefazodone, would be expected to lead to an increase in plasma bexarotene concentrations).
No products indexed under this heading.

Nelfinavir Mesylate (Bexarotene is metabolized by CYP4503A4; co-administration with inhibitors of CYP4503A4, such as protease inhibitors, would be expected to lead to an increase in plasma bexarotene concentrations).
No products indexed under this heading.

Norethindrone (Bexarotene may theoretically increase the rate of metabolism and reduce plasma concentrations of other substrates metabolized by CYP4503A4, including hormonal contraceptives; it is strongly recommended that two reliable forms of contraception be used concurrently, one of which should be non-hormonal). Products include:
Ortho Micronor Tablets 2446

Norethynodrel (Bexarotene may theoretically increase the rate of metabolism and reduce plasma concentrations of other substrates metabolized by CYP4503A4, including hormonal contraceptives; it is strongly recommended that two reliable forms of contraception be used concurrently, one of which should be non-hormonal).
No products indexed under this heading.

Norgestimate (Bexarotene may theoretically increase the rate of metabolism and reduce plasma concentrations of other substrates metabolized by CYP4503A4, including hormonal contraceptives; it is strongly recommended that two reliable forms of contraception be used concurrently, one of which should be non-hormonal). Products include:
Ortho-Cyclen/Ortho Tri-Cyclen 2449
Ortho Tri-Cyclen Lo Tablets 2458

Norgestrel (Bexarotene may theoretically increase the rate of metabolism and reduce plasma concentrations of other substrates metabolized by CYP4503A4, including hormonal contraceptives; it is strongly recommended that two reliable forms of contraception be used concurrently, one of which should be non-hormonal).
No products indexed under this heading.

Phenobarbital (Bexarotene is metabolized by CYP4503A4; co-administration with inducers of CYP4503A4, such as phenobarbital, may cause a reduction in plasma bexarotene concentrations). Products include:
Donnatal Extentabs 2507

Phenytoin (Bexarotene is metabolized by CYP4503A4; co-administration with inducers of CYP4503A4, such as phenytoin, may cause a reduction in plasma bexarotene concentrations).
No products indexed under this heading.

Phenytoin Sodium (Bexarotene is metabolized by CYP4503A4; co-administration with inducers of CYP4503A4, such as phenytoin, may cause a reduction in plasma bexarotene concentrations). Products include:
Phenytek Capsules 2192

Pioglitazone Hydrochloride (Bexarotene could enhance the action of hypoglycemic agents resulting in hypoglycemia). Products include:
ActoPlus Met Tablets 3071
Actos Tablets 3077
Duetact Tablets 3085

Repaglinide (Bexarotene could enhance the action of hypoglycemic agents resulting in hypoglycemia). Products include:
PrandiMet Tablets 2967
Prandin Tablets 2971

Rifampin (Bexarotene is metabolized by CYP4503A4; co-administration with inducers of CYP4503A4, such as rifampin, may cause a reduction in plasma bexarotene concentrations).
No products indexed under this heading.

Ritonavir (Bexarotene is metabolized by CYP4503A4; co-administration with inhibitors of CYP4503A4, such as protease inhibitors, would be expected to lead to an increase in plasma bexarotene concentrations). Products include:
Kaletra 452
Norvir 489

Rosiglitazone Maleate (Bexarotene could enhance the action of hypoglycemic agents resulting in hypoglycemia). Products include:
Avandamet Tablets 1336
Avandaryl Tablets 1344
Avandia Tablets 1351

Saquinavir (Bexarotene is metabolized by CYP4503A4; co-administration with inhibitors of CYP4503A4, such as protease inhibitors, would be expected to lead to an increase in plasma bexarotene concentrations).
No products indexed under this heading.

Saquinavir Mesylate (Bexarotene is metabolized by CYP4503A4; co-administration with inhibitors of CYP4503A4, such as protease inhibitors, would be expected to lead to an increase in plasma bexarotene concentrations).
No products indexed under this heading.

Sitagliptin Phosphate (Bexarotene could enhance the action of hypoglycemic agents resulting in hypoglycemia). Products include:
Janumet Tablets 2041
Januvia Tablets 2048

Tamoxifen Citrate (Co-administration has resulted in a modest decrease in plasma concentrations of tamoxifen).
No products indexed under this heading.

Tipranavir (Bexarotene is metabolized by CYP4503A4; co-administration with inhibitors of CYP4503A4, such as protease inhibitors, would be expected to lead to an increase in plasma bexarotene concentrations). Products include:
Aptivus Capsules 823
Aptivus Oral Solution 823

Tolazamide (Bexarotene could enhance the action of hypoglycemic agents resulting in hypoglycemia).
No products indexed under this heading.

Tolbutamide (Bexarotene could enhance the action of hypoglycemic agents resulting in hypoglycemia).
No products indexed under this heading.

Troglitazone (Bexarotene could enhance the action of hypoglycemic agents resulting in hypoglycemia).
No products indexed under this heading.

Vitamin A (Potential for additive toxic effects because of the relationship of bexarotene to vitamin A; patients should be advised to limit their vitamin A intake). Products include:
Norwegian Cod Liver Oil 949

Food Interactions

Food, unspecified (Co-administration with a fat-containing meal has resulted in higher plasma bexarotene AUC and Cmax values; because safety and efficacy data are based upon administration with food, it is recommended that Targretin capsules be administered with or immediately following a meal).

Grapefruit Juice (Bexarotene is metabolized by CYP403A4; co-administration with inhibitors of CYP4503A4, such as grapefruit juice, would be expected to lead to an increase in plasma bexarotene concentrations).

TARGRETIN GEL 1%

(Bexarotene) 1088

May interact with cytochrome p450 3a4 inducers (selected), cytochrome p450 3a4 inhibitors (selected), erythromycin, oral contraceptives, and certain other agents. Compounds in these categories include:

Acetazolamide (Drugs that affect levels of activity of cytochrome P450 3A4 may potentially affect the disposition of bexarotene).
No products indexed under this heading.

Allium sativum (Drugs that affect levels of activity of cytochrome P450 3A4 may potentially affect the disposition of bexarotene).
No products indexed under this heading.

Amiodarone Hydrochloride (Drugs that affect levels of activity of cytochrome P450 3A4 may potentially affect the disposition of bexarotene).
No products indexed under this heading.

Amprenavir (Drugs that affect levels of activity of cytochrome P450 3A4 may potentially affect the disposition of bexarotene).
No products indexed under this heading.

Anastrozole (Drugs that affect levels of activity of cytochrome P450 3A4 may potentially affect the disposition of bexarotene). Products include:
Arimidex Tablets **672**

Aprepitant (Drugs that affect levels of activity of cytochrome P450 3A4 may potentially affect the disposition of bexarotene). Products include:
Emend Capsules **1992**

Atazanavir (Drugs that affect levels of activity of cytochrome P450 3A4 may potentially affect the disposition of bexarotene).
No products indexed under this heading.

Atazanavir Sulfate (Drugs that affect levels of activity of cytochrome P450 3A4 may potentially affect the disposition of bexarotene). Products include:
Reyataz Capsules **3299**

Betamethasone Acetate (Drugs that affect levels of activity of cytochrome P450 3A4 may potentially affect the disposition of bexarotene).
No products indexed under this heading.

Betamethasone Sodium Phosphate (Drugs that affect levels of activity of cytochrome P450 3A4 may potentially affect the disposition of bexarotene).
No products indexed under this heading.

Carbamazepine (Drugs that affect levels of activity of cytochrome P450 3A4 may potentially affect the disposition of bexarotene). Products include:
Carbatrol Capsules **3019**
Equetro Extended-Release Capsules **3174**

Cimetidine (Drugs that affect levels of activity of cytochrome P450 3A4 may potentially affect the disposition of bexarotene).
No products indexed under this heading.

Cimetidine Hydrochloride (Drugs that affect levels of activity of cytochrome P450 3A4 may potentially affect the disposition of bexarotene).
No products indexed under this heading.

Ciprofloxacin (Drugs that affect levels of activity of cytochrome P450 3A4 may potentially affect the disposition of bexarotene). Products include:
Cipro I.V. **2817**
Cipro Oral Suspension **2810**
Cipro XR Tablets **2823**
Ciprodex Otic Suspension **541**

Ciprofloxacin Hydrochloride (Drugs that affect levels of activity of cytochrome P450 3A4 may potentially affect the disposition of bexarotene). Products include:
Cipro Tablets **2810**

Cisplatin (Drugs that affect levels of activity of cytochrome P450 3A4 may potentially affect the disposition of bexarotene).
No products indexed under this heading.

Clarithromycin (Drugs that affect levels of activity of cytochrome P450 3A4 may potentially affect the disposition of bexarotene). Products include:
Biaxin/Biaxin XL **411**

Clotrimazole (Drugs that affect levels of activity of cytochrome P450 3A4 may potentially affect the disposition of bexarotene). Products include:
Lotrisone **2881**

Cortisone Acetate (Drugs that affect levels of activity of cytochrome P450 3A4 may potentially affect the disposition of bexarotene).
No products indexed under this heading.

Cyclosporine (Drugs that affect levels of activity of cytochrome P450 3A4 may potentially affect the disposition of bexarotene). Products include:
Gengraf Capsules **435**
Neoral Oral Solution **2280**
Neoral Soft Gelatin Capsules **2280**
Restasis Ophthalmic Emulsion **557**
Sandimmune **2296**

Dalfopristin (Drugs that affect levels of activity of cytochrome P450 3A4 may potentially affect the disposition of bexarotene).
No products indexed under this heading.

Danazol (Drugs that affect levels of activity of cytochrome P450 3A4 may potentially affect the disposition of bexarotene).
No products indexed under this heading.

Delavirdine Mesylate (Drugs that affect levels of activity of cytochrome P450 3A4 may potentially affect the disposition of bexarotene).
No products indexed under this heading.

Desogestrel (Effective contraception must be used for one month prior to initiation of therapy, during therapy, and for at least one month following discontinuation of therapy; it is recommended that two reliable forms of contraception be used simultaneously unless abstinence is the chosen method). Products include:
Mircette Tablets **1034**

Dexamethasone (Drugs that affect levels of activity of cytochrome P450 3A4 may potentially affect the disposition of bexarotene). Products include:
Ciprodex Otic Suspension **541**

Dexamethasone Acetate (Drugs that affect levels of activity of cytochrome P450 3A4 may potentially affect the disposition of bexarotene).
No products indexed under this heading.

Dexamethasone Sodium Phosphate (Drugs that affect levels of activity of cytochrome P450 3A4 may potentially affect the disposition of bexarotene).
No products indexed under this heading.

Diltiazem Hydrochloride (Drugs that affect levels of activity of cytochrome P450 3A4 may potentially affect the disposition of bexarotene). Products include:
Cardizem LA Extended Release Tablets **421**

Diltiazem Maleate (Drugs that affect levels of activity of cytochrome P450 3A4 may potentially affect the disposition of bexarotene).
No products indexed under this heading.

Doxorubicin Hydrochloride (Drugs that affect levels of activity of cytochrome P450 3A4 may potentially affect the disposition of bexarotene).
No products indexed under this heading.

Efavirenz (Drugs that affect levels of activity of cytochrome P450 3A4 may potentially affect the disposition of bexarotene). Products include:
Atripla Tablets **938**
Sustiva Capsules **930**
Sustiva Tablets **930**

Erythromycin (Bexarotene is metabolized by CYP4503A4; co-administration with inhibitors of CYP4503A4, such as erythromycin, would be expected to lead to an increase in plasma bexarotene concentrations).
No products indexed under this heading.

Erythromycin Estolate (Bexarotene is metabolized by CYP4503A4; co-administration with inhibitors of CYP4503A4, such as erythromycin, would be expected to lead to an increase in plasma bexarotene concentrations).
No products indexed under this heading.

Erythromycin Ethylsuccinate (Bexarotene is metabolized by CYP4503A4; co-administration with inhibitors of CYP4503A4, such as erythromycin, would be expected to lead to an increase in plasma bexarotene concentrations). Products include:
E.E.S. **433**
EryPed **431**

Erythromycin Gluceptate (Bexarotene is metabolized by CYP4503A4; co-administration with inhibitors of CYP4503A4, such as erythromycin, would be expected to lead to an increase in plasma bexarotene concentrations).
No products indexed under this heading.

Erythromycin Lactobionate (Bexarotene is metabolized by CYP4503A4; co-administration with inhibitors of CYP4503A4, such as erythromycin, would be expected to lead to an increase in plasma bexarotene concentrations).
No products indexed under this heading.

Erythromycin Stearate (Bexarotene is metabolized by CYP4503A4; co-administration with inhibitors of CYP4503A4, such as erythromycin, would be expected to lead to an increase in plasma bexarotene concentrations).
No products indexed under this heading.

Esomeprazole Magnesium (Drugs that affect levels of activity of cytochrome P450 3A4 may potentially affect the disposition of bexarotene). Products include:
Nexium Delayed-Release Capsules **645**
Nexium Delayed-Release Oral Suspension **645**

Ethinyl Estradiol (Effective contraception must be used for one month prior to initiation of therapy, during therapy, and for at least one month following discontinuation of therapy; it is recommended that two reliable forms of contraception be used simultaneously unless abstinence is the chosen method). Products include:
Lybrel Tablets **3204**
Mircette Tablets **1034**
NuvaRing **2897**
Ortho-Cyclen/Ortho Tri-Cyclen **2449**
Ortho Evra Transdermal System **2437**
Ortho Tri-Cyclen Lo Tablets **2458**
Seasonique Tablets **1046**
Yaz Tablets **805**

Ethosuximide (Drugs that affect levels of activity of cytochrome P450 3A4 may potentially affect the disposition of bexarotene).
No products indexed under this heading.

Ethynodiol Diacetate (Effective contraception must be used for one month prior to initiation of therapy, during therapy, and for at least one month following discontinuation of therapy; it is recommended that two reliable forms of contraception be used simultaneously unless abstinence is the chosen method).
No products indexed under this heading.

Felbamate (Drugs that affect levels of activity of cytochrome P450 3A4 may potentially affect the disposition of bexarotene).
No products indexed under this heading.

Fluconazole (Drugs that affect levels of activity of cytochrome P450 3A4 may potentially affect the disposition of bexarotene).
No products indexed under this heading.

Fludrocortisone Acetate (Drugs that affect levels of activity of cytochrome P450 3A4 may potentially affect the disposition of bexarotene).
No products indexed under this heading.

Fluoxetine (Drugs that affect levels of activity of cytochrome P450 3A4 may potentially affect the disposition of bexarotene).
No products indexed under this heading.

Fluoxetine Hydrochloride (Drugs that affect levels of activity of cytochrome P450 3A4 may potentially affect the disposition of bexarotene). Products include:
Prozac Weekly Capsules **1852**
Prozac Pulvules and Liquid **1852**
Symbyax Capsules **1871**

Fluvoxamine Maleate (Drugs that affect levels of activity of cytochrome P450 3A4 may potentially affect the disposition of bexarotene). Products include:
Luvox CR Extended-Release Capsules **1759**

Fosamprenavir Calcium (Drugs that affect levels of activity of cytochrome P450 3A4 may potentially affect the disposition of bexarotene). Products include:
Lexiva Oral Suspension **1510**
Lexiva Tablets **1510**

Fosphenytoin Sodium (Drugs that affect levels of activity of cytochrome P450 3A4 may potentially affect the disposition of bexarotene).
No products indexed under this heading.

Garlic Extract (Drugs that affect levels of activity of cytochrome P450 3A4 may potentially affect the disposition of bexarotene).
No products indexed under this heading.

Garlic Oil (Drugs that affect levels of activity of cytochrome P450 3A4 may potentially affect the disposition of bexarotene).
No products indexed under this heading.

Gemfibrozil (Concomitant gemfibrozil was associated with increased bexarotene concentrations following oral administration of bexarotene).
No products indexed under this heading.

Hydrocortisone (Drugs that affect levels of activity of cytochrome P450 3A4 may potentially affect the disposition of bexarotene).
No products indexed under this heading.

Hydrocortisone Acetate (Drugs that affect levels of activity of cytochrome P450 3A4 may potentially affect the disposition of bexarotene). Products include:
Analpram-HC **1140**
Pramosone **1141**

Hydrocortisone Butyrate (Drugs that affect levels of activity of cytochrome P450 3A4 may potentially affect the disposition of bexarotene).
No products indexed under this heading.

Hydrocortisone Cypionate (Drugs that affect levels of activity of cytochrome P450 3A4 may potentially affect the disposition of bexarotene).
No products indexed under this heading.

Hydrocortisone Hemisuccinate (Drugs that affect levels of activity of cytochrome P450 3A4 may potentially affect the disposition of bexarotene).
No products indexed under this heading.

Hydrocortisone Probutate (Drugs that affect levels of activity of cytochrome P450 3A4 may potentially affect the disposition of bexarotene).
No products indexed under this heading.

Hydrocortisone Sodium Phosphate (Drugs that affect levels of activity of cytochrome P450 3A4 may potentially affect the disposition of bexarotene).
No products indexed under this heading.

Hydrocortisone Sodium Succinate (Drugs that affect levels of activity of cytochrome P450 3A4 may potentially affect the disposition of bexarotene).
No products indexed under this heading.

Hydrocortisone Valerate (Drugs that affect levels of activity of cytochrome P450 3A4 may potentially affect the disposition of bexarotene).
No products indexed under this heading.

Hypericum (Drugs that affect levels of activity of cytochrome P450 3A4 may potentially affect the disposition of bexarotene). Products include:
Satieté Tablets **640**

Hypericum Perforatum (Drugs that affect levels of activity of cytochrome P450 3A4 may potentially affect the disposition of bexarotene).
No products indexed under this heading.

Indinavir Sulfate (Drugs that affect levels of activity of cytochrome P450 3A4 may potentially affect the disposition of bexarotene). Products include:
Crixivan Capsules **1979**

Isoniazid (Drugs that affect levels of activity of cytochrome P450 3A4 may potentially affect the disposition of bexarotene).
No products indexed under this heading.

Itraconazole (Bexarotene is metabolized by CYP4503A4; coadministration with inhibitors of CYP4503A4, such as itraconazole, could lead to an increase in plasma bexarotene concentrations).
No products indexed under this heading.

Ketoconazole (Bexarotene is metabolized vy CYP4503A4; coadministration with inhibitors of CYP4503A4, such as keoconazole, could lead to an increase in plasma concentrations). Products include:
Extina Foam, 2% **3057**
Nizoral A-D Shampoo **1901**

Levonorgestrel (Effective contraception must be used for one month prior to initiation of therapy, during therapy, and for at least one month following discontinuation of therapy; it is recommended that two reliable forms of contraception be used simultaneously unless abstinence is the chosen method). Products include:
Climara Pro Transdermal System **768**
Lybrel Tablets **3204**
Mirena Intrauterine System **779**
Plan B Tablets **1044**
Seasonique Tablets **1046**

Lopinavir (Drugs that affect levels of activity of cytochrome P450 3A4 may potentially affect the disposition of bexarotene). Products include:
Kaletra **452**

Loratadine (Drugs that affect levels of activity of cytochrome P450 3A4 may potentially affect the disposition of bexarotene).
No products indexed under this heading.

Mephenytoin (Drugs that affect levels of activity of cytochrome P450 3A4 may potentially affect the disposition of bexarotene).
No products indexed under this heading.

Mestranol (Effective contraception must be used for one month prior to initiation of therapy, during therapy, and for at least one month following discontinuation of therapy; it is recommended that two reliable forms of contraception be used simultaneously unless abstinence is the chosen method).
No products indexed under this heading.

Methsuximide (Drugs that affect levels of activity of cytochrome P450 3A4 may potentially affect the disposition of bexarotene).
No products indexed under this heading.

Methylprednisolone (Drugs that affect levels of activity of cytochrome P450 3A4 may potentially affect the disposition of bexarotene).
No products indexed under this heading.

Methylprednisolone Acetate (Drugs that affect levels of activity of cytochrome P450 3A4 may potentially affect the disposition of bexarotene).
No products indexed under this heading.

Methylprednisolone Sodium Succinate (Drugs that affect levels of activity of cytochrome P450 3A4 may potentially affect the disposition of bexarotene).
No products indexed under this heading.

Metronidazole (Drugs that affect levels of activity of cytochrome P450 3A4 may potentially affect the disposition of bexarotene). Products include:
Pylera Capsules **714**

Metronidazole Benzoate (Drugs that affect levels of activity of cytochrome P450 3A4 may potentially affect the disposition of bexarotene).
No products indexed under this heading.

Metronidazole Hydrochloride (Drugs that affect levels of activity of cytochrome P450 3A4 may potentially affect the disposition of bexarotene).
No products indexed under this heading.

Miconazole (Drugs that affect levels of activity of cytochrome P450 3A4 may potentially affect the disposition of bexarotene).
No products indexed under this heading.

Miconazole Nitrate (Drugs that affect levels of activity of cytochrome P450 3A4 may potentially affect the disposition of bexarotene).
No products indexed under this heading.

Modafinil (Drugs that affect levels of activity of cytochrome P450 3A4 may potentially affect the disposition of bexarotene). Products include:
Provigil Tablets **977**

Nefazodone Hydrochloride (Drugs that affect levels of activity of cytochrome P450 3A4 may potentially affect the disposition of bexarotene).
No products indexed under this heading.

Nelfinavir Mesylate (Drugs that affect levels of activity of cytochrome P450 3A4 may potentially affect the disposition of bexarotene).
No products indexed under this heading.

Nevirapine (Drugs that affect levels of activity of cytochrome P450 3A4 may potentially affect the disposition of bexarotene). Products include:
Viramune Oral Suspension **873**
Viramune Tablets **873**

Niacinamide (Drugs that affect levels of activity of cytochrome P450 3A4 may potentially affect the disposition of bexarotene). Products include:
BioLean Free Tablets **635**

Nicotinamide (Drugs that affect levels of activity of cytochrome P450 3A4 may potentially affect the disposition of bexarotene).
No products indexed under this heading.

Nifedipine (Drugs that affect levels of activity of cytochrome P450 3A4 may potentially affect the disposition of bexarotene).
No products indexed under this heading.

Norethindrone (Effective contraception must be used for one month prior to initiation of therapy, during therapy, and for at least one month following discontinuation of therapy; it is recommended that two reliable forms of contraception be used simultaneously unless abstinence is the chosen method). Products include:
Ortho Micronor Tablets **2446**

Norethynodrel (Effective contraception must be used for one month prior to initiation of therapy, during therapy, and for at least one month following discontinuation of therapy; it is recommended that two reliable forms of contraception be used simultaneously unless abstinence is the chosen method).
No products indexed under this heading.

Norfloxacin (Drugs that affect levels of activity of cytochrome P450 3A4 may potentially affect the disposition of bexarotene). Products include:
Noroxin Tablets **2069**

Norgestimate (Effective contraception must be used for one month prior to initiation of therapy, during therapy, and for at least one month following discontinuation of therapy; it is recommended that two reliable forms of contraception be used simultaneously unless abstinence is the chosen method). Products include:
Ortho-Cyclen/Ortho Tri-Cyclen **2449**
Ortho Tri-Cyclen Lo Tablets **2458**

Norgestrel (Effective contraception must be used for one month prior to initiation of therapy, during therapy, and for at least one month following discontinuation of therapy; it is recommended that two reliable forms of contraception be used simultaneously unless abstinence is the chosen method).
No products indexed under this heading.

Omeprazole (Drugs that affect levels of activity of cytochrome P450 3A4 may potentially affect the disposition of bexarotene).
No products indexed under this heading.

Oxcarbazepine (Drugs that affect levels of activity of cytochrome P450 3A4 may potentially affect the disposition of bexarotene).
No products indexed under this heading.

Paroxetine Hydrochloride (Drugs that affect levels of activity of cytochrome P450 3A4 may potentially affect the disposition of bexarotene). Products include:
Paxil **1535**
Paxil CR Controlled-Release Tablets **1544**

Phenobarbital (Drugs that affect levels of activity of cytochrome

P450 3A4 may potentially affect the disposition of bexarotene). Products include:

Donnatal Extentabs 2507

Phenobarbital Sodium (Drugs that affect levels of activity of cytochrome P450 3A4 may potentially affect the disposition of bexarotene).

No products indexed under this heading.

Phenytoin (Drugs that affect levels of activity of cytochrome P450 3A4 may potentially affect the disposition of bexarotene).

No products indexed under this heading.

Phenytoin Sodium (Drugs that affect levels of activity of cytochrome P450 3A4 may potentially affect the disposition of bexarotene). Products include:

Phenytek Capsules 2192

Prednisolone Acetate (Drugs that affect levels of activity of cytochrome P450 3A4 may potentially affect the disposition of bexarotene). Products include:

Pred Forte Ophthalmic Suspension .... ⊙ 227
Pred Mild Ophthalmic Suspension .... ⊙ 230
Pred-G Ophthalmic Ointment .... ⊙ 229
Pred-G Ophthalmic Suspension ...... ⊙ 228

Prednisolone Sodium Phosphate (Drugs that affect levels of activity of cytochrome P450 3A4 may potentially affect the disposition of bexarotene).

No products indexed under this heading.

Prednisolone Tebutate (Drugs that affect levels of activity of cytochrome P450 3A4 may potentially affect the disposition of bexarotene).

No products indexed under this heading.

Prednisone (Drugs that affect levels of activity of cytochrome P450 3A4 may potentially affect the disposition of bexarotene).

No products indexed under this heading.

Primidone (Drugs that affect levels of activity of cytochrome P450 3A4 may potentially affect the disposition of bexarotene).

No products indexed under this heading.

Propoxyphene Hydrochloride (Drugs that affect levels of activity of cytochrome P450 3A4 may potentially affect the disposition of bexarotene).

No products indexed under this heading.

Propoxyphene Napsylate (Drugs that affect levels of activity of cytochrome P450 3A4 may potentially affect the disposition of bexarotene).

No products indexed under this heading.

Quinidine (Drugs that affect levels of activity of cytochrome P450 3A4 may potentially affect the disposition of bexarotene).

No products indexed under this heading.

Quinidine Hydrochloride (Drugs that affect levels of activity of cytochrome P450 3A4 may potentially affect the disposition of bexarotene).

No products indexed under this heading.

Quinidine Polygalacturonate (Drugs that affect levels of activity of cytochrome P450 3A4 may potentially affect the disposition of bexarotene).

No products indexed under this heading.

Quinidine Sulfate (Drugs that affect levels of activity of cytochrome P450 3A4 may potentially affect the disposition of bexarotene).

No products indexed under this heading.

Quinine (Drugs that affect levels of activity of cytochrome P450 3A4 may potentially affect the disposition of bexarotene).

No products indexed under this heading.

Quinine Sulfate (Drugs that affect levels of activity of cytochrome P450 3A4 may potentially affect the disposition of bexarotene).

No products indexed under this heading.

Quinupristin (Drugs that affect levels of activity of cytochrome P450 3A4 may potentially affect the disposition of bexarotene).

No products indexed under this heading.

Ranitidine Bismuth Citrate (Drugs that affect levels of activity of cytochrome P450 3A4 may potentially affect the disposition of bexarotene).

No products indexed under this heading.

Ranitidine Hydrochloride (Drugs that affect levels of activity of cytochrome P450 3A4 may potentially affect the disposition of bexarotene). Products include:

Zantac 75 Tablets .... ▣ 603
Zantac 1670
Zantac Injection 1666
Zantac Injection Pharmacy Bulk Package 1668
Maximum Strength Zantac 150 Tablets .... ▣ 603
Maximum Strength Zantac 150 Cool Mint Tablets .... ▣ 603

Rifabutin (Drugs that affect levels of activity of cytochrome P450 3A4 may potentially affect the disposition of bexarotene).

No products indexed under this heading.

Rifampicin (Drugs that affect levels of activity of cytochrome P450 3A4 may potentially affect the disposition of bexarotene).

No products indexed under this heading.

Rifampin (Drugs that affect levels of activity of cytochrome P450 3A4 may potentially affect the disposition of bexarotene).

No products indexed under this heading.

Rifapentine (Drugs that affect levels of activity of cytochrome P450 3A4 may potentially affect the disposition of bexarotene).

No products indexed under this heading.

Ritonavir (Drugs that affect levels of activity of cytochrome P450 3A4 may potentially affect the disposition of bexarotene). Products include:

Kaletra 452
Norvir 489

Saquinavir (Drugs that affect levels of activity of cytochrome P450 3A4 may potentially affect the disposition of bexarotene).

No products indexed under this heading.

Saquinavir Mesylate (Drugs that affect levels of activity of cytochrome P450 3A4 may potentially affect the disposition of bexarotene).

No products indexed under this heading.

Sertraline Hydrochloride (Drugs that affect levels of activity of cytochrome P450 3A4 may potentially affect the disposition of bexarotene).

No products indexed under this heading.

Sildenafil Citrate (Drugs that affect levels of activity of cytochrome P450 3A4 may potentially affect the disposition of bexarotene).

No products indexed under this heading.

Sulfinpyrazone (Drugs that affect levels of activity of cytochrome P450 3A4 may potentially affect the disposition of bexarotene).

No products indexed under this heading.

Telithromycin (Drugs that affect levels of activity of cytochrome P450 3A4 may potentially affect the disposition of bexarotene). Products include:

Ketek Tablets 2744

Theophylline (Drugs that affect levels of activity of cytochrome P450 3A4 may potentially affect the disposition of bexarotene).

No products indexed under this heading.

Theophylline Anhydrous (Drugs that affect levels of activity of cytochrome P450 3A4 may potentially affect the disposition of bexarotene). Products include:

Uniphyl Tablets 2595

Theophylline Calcium Salicylate (Drugs that affect levels of activity of cytochrome P450 3A4 may potentially affect the disposition of bexarotene).

No products indexed under this heading.

Theophylline Dihydroxypropyl (Glyceryl) (Drugs that affect levels of activity of cytochrome P450 3A4 may potentially affect the disposition of bexarotene).

No products indexed under this heading.

Theophylline Ethylenediamine (Drugs that affect levels of activity of cytochrome P450 3A4 may potentially affect the disposition of bexarotene).

No products indexed under this heading.

Triamcinolone (Drugs that affect levels of activity of cytochrome P450 3A4 may potentially affect the disposition of bexarotene).

No products indexed under this heading.

Triamcinolone Acetonide (Drugs that affect levels of activity of cytochrome P450 3A4 may potentially affect the disposition of bexarotene). Products include:

Azmacort Inhalation Aerosol 407
Nasacort AQ Nasal Spray 2765
Triesence Injectable Suspension .... ⊙ 209

Triamcinolone Diacetate (Drugs that affect levels of activity of cytochrome P450 3A4 may potentially affect the disposition of bexarotene).

No products indexed under this heading.

Triamcinolone Hexacetonide (Drugs that affect levels of activity of cytochrome P450 3A4 may potentially affect the disposition of bexarotene).

No products indexed under this heading.

Troglitazone (Drugs that affect levels of activity of cytochrome P450 3A4 may potentially affect the disposition of bexarotene).

No products indexed under this heading.

Troleandomycin (Drugs that affect levels of activity of cytochrome P450 3A4 may potentially affect the disposition of bexarotene).

No products indexed under this heading.

Valproate Sodium (Drugs that affect levels of activity of cytochrome P450 3A4 may potentially affect the disposition of bexarotene).

No products indexed under this heading.

Vardenafil Hydrochloride (Drugs that affect levels of activity of cytochrome P450 3A4 may potentially affect the disposition of bexarotene). Products include:

Levitra Tablets 2876

Verapamil Hydrochloride (Drugs that affect levels of activity of cytochrome P450 3A4 may potentially affect the disposition of bexarotene). Products include:

Tarka Tablets 511

Vitamin A (Potential for additive toxic effects because of the relationship of bexarotene to vitamin A; patients should be advised to limit their vitamin A intake). Products include:

Norwegian Cod Liver Oil 949

Voriconazole (Drugs that affect levels of activity of cytochrome P450 3A4 may potentially affect the disposition of bexarotene).

No products indexed under this heading.

Zafirlukast (Drugs that affect levels of activity of cytochrome P450 3A4 may potentially affect the disposition of bexarotene). Products include:

Accolate Tablets 669

Zileuton (Drugs that affect levels of activity of cytochrome P450 3A4 may potentially affect the disposition of bexarotene).

No products indexed under this heading.

Food Interactions

Grapefruit (Bexarotene is metabolized by CYP4503A4; co-administration with inhibitors of CYP4503A4, such as grapefruit juice, could lead to an increase in plasma bexarotene concentrations).

Grapefruit Juice (Bexarotene is metabolized by CYP4503A4; co-administration with inhibitors of CYP4503A4, such as grapefruit juice, could lead to an increase in plasma bexarotene concentrations).

TARKA TABLETS
(Trandolapril, Verapamil Hydrochloride)........................ 511
May interact with beta blockers, diuretics, cardiac glycosides, inhalant anesthetics, lithium preparations, neuromuscular blocking agents, potassium preparations, potassium sparing diuretics, quinidine, xanthines, and certain other agents. Compounds in these categories include:

Acebutolol Hydrochloride (Co-administration of beta blockers and verapamil may result in additive effects on heart rate, atrioventricular conduction, and/or cardiac contractility).
No products indexed under this heading.

Amiloride Hydrochloride (Increased risk of hyperkalemia; patients on diuretics, especially those on recently instituted diuretic therapy, may occasionally experience an excessive reduction of blood pressure after initiation of therapy with Tarka).
No products indexed under this heading.

Aminophylline (Verapamil may inhibit the clearance and increase the plasma levels of theophylline).
No products indexed under this heading.

Atenolol (Co-administration of beta blockers and verapamil may result in additive effects on heart rate, atrioventricular conduction, and/or cardiac contractility).
No products indexed under this heading.

Atracurium Besylate (Verapamil may potentiate the activity of neuromuscular blocking agents).
No products indexed under this heading.

Bendroflumethiazide (Patients on diuretics, especially those on recently instituted diuretic therapy, may occasionally experience an excessive reduction of blood pressure after initiation of therapy with Tarka).
No products indexed under this heading.

Betaxolol Hydrochloride (Co-administration of beta blockers and verapamil may result in additive effects on heart rate, atrioventricular conduction, and/or cardiac contractility).
No products indexed under this heading.

Bisoprolol Fumarate (Co-administration of beta blockers and verapamil may result in additive effects on heart rate, atrioventricular conduction, and/or cardiac contractility).
No products indexed under this heading.

Bumetanide (Patients on diuretics, especially those on recently instituted diuretic therapy, may occasionally experience an excessive reduction of blood pressure after initiation of therapy with Tarka).
No products indexed under this heading.

Carbamazepine (Combined therapy of verapamil and carbamazepine may increase carbamazepine concentrations resulting in side effects such as diplopia, ataxia, and headache). Products include:
Carbatrol Capsules 3019
Equetro Extended-Release Capsules 3174

Carteolol Hydrochloride (Co-administration of beta blockers and verapamil may result in additive effects on heart rate, atrioventricular conduction, and/or cardiac contractility).
No products indexed under this heading.

Chlorothiazide (Patients on diuretics, especially those on recently instituted diuretic therapy, may occasionally experience an excessive reduction of blood pressure after initiation of therapy with Tarka).
No products indexed under this heading.

Chlorothiazide Sodium (Patients on diuretics, especially those on recently instituted diuretic therapy, may occasionally experience an excessive reduction of blood pressure after initiation of therapy with Tarka). Products include:
Intravenous Sodium Diuril 2490

Chlorthalidone (Patients on diuretics, especially those on recently instituted diuretic therapy, may occasionally experience an excessive reduction of blood pressure after initiation of therapy with Tarka). Products include:
Clorpres Tablets 2185

Cimetidine (Variable results on clearance have been obtained in acute studies during concomitant therapy; clearance of verapamil may be reduced or unchanged).
No products indexed under this heading.

Cimetidine Hydrochloride (Variable results on clearance have been obtained in acute studies during concomitant therapy; clearance of verapamil may be reduced or unchanged).
No products indexed under this heading.

Cisatracurium Besylate (Verapamil may potentiate the activity of neuromuscular blocking agents). Products include:
Nimbex Injection 484

Cyclosporine (Increased serum levels of cyclosporine). Products include:
Gengraf Capsules 435
Neoral Oral Solution 2280
Neoral Soft Gelatin Capsules 2280
Restasis Ophthalmic Emulsion 557
Sandimmune 2296

Desflurane (Potential for excessive cardiovascular depression).
No products indexed under this heading.

Deslanoside (Chronic verapamil therapy can increase serum digoxin levels by 50% to 75% during the first week, and this can result in digoxin toxicity; patient should be carefully monitored to avoid over- or under-digitalization).
No products indexed under this heading.

Digitalis Glycoside Preparations (Chronic verapamil therapy can increase serum digoxin levels by 50% to 75% during the first week, and this can result in digoxin toxicity; patient should be carefully monitored to avoid over- or under-digitalization).
No products indexed under this heading.

Digitoxin (Chronic verapamil therapy can increase serum digoxin levels by 50% to 75% during the first week, and this can result in digoxin toxicity; patient should be carefully monitored to avoid over- or under-digitalization).
No products indexed under this heading.

Digoxin (Chronic verapamil therapy can increase serum digoxin levels by 50% to 75% during the first week, and this can result in digoxin toxicity; patient should be carefully monitored to avoid over- or under-digitalization). Products include:
Lanoxin Injection 1498
Lanoxin Injection Pediatric 1502
Lanoxin Tablets 1505

Doxacurium Chloride (Verapamil may potentiate the activity of neuromuscular blocking agents).
No products indexed under this heading.

Dyphylline (Verapamil may inhibit the clearance and increase the plasma levels of theophylline).
No products indexed under this heading.

Enflurane (Potential for excessive cardiovascular depression).
No products indexed under this heading.

Esmolol Hydrochloride (Co-administration of beta blockers and verapamil may result in additive effects on heart rate, atrioventricular conduction, and/or cardiac contractility).
No products indexed under this heading.

Ethacrynic Acid (Patients on diuretics, especially those on recently instituted diuretic therapy, may occasionally experience an excessive reduction of blood pressure after initiation of therapy with Tarka). Products include:
Edecrin Tablets 698

Flecainide Acetate (Concomitant use may result in additive effects on myocardial contractility, AV conduction and repolarization; concurrent use of flecainide and verapamil may result in additive inotropic effect and prolongation of atrioventricular conduction).
No products indexed under this heading.

Furosemide (Patients on diuretics, especially those on recently instituted diuretic therapy, may occasionally experience an excessive reduction of blood pressure after initiation of therapy with Tarka). Products include:
Furosemide Tablets 2186

Halothane (Potential for excessive cardiovascular depression).
No products indexed under this heading.

Hydrochlorothiazide (Patients on diuretics, especially those on recently instituted diuretic therapy, may occasionally experience an excessive reduction of blood pressure after initiation of therapy with Tarka). Products include:
Atacand HCT 642
Avalide Tablets 892
Avalide Tablets 2713
Benicar HCT Tablets 1010
Diovan HCT Tablets 2216
Dyazide Capsules 1405
Micardis HCT Tablets 854
Prinzide Tablets 2092
Tekturna HCT Tablets 2324
Teveten HCT Tablets 517

Hydroflumethiazide (Patients on diuretics, especially those on recently instituted diuretic therapy, may occasionally experience an excessive reduction of blood pressure after initiation of therapy with Tarka).
No products indexed under this heading.

Indapamide (Patients on diuretics, especially those on recently instituted diuretic therapy, may occasionally experience an excessive reduction of blood pressure after initiation of therapy with Tarka). Products include:
Indapamide Tablets 2188

Isoflurane (Potential for excessive cardiovascular depression).
No products indexed under this heading.

Labetalol Hydrochloride (Co-administration of beta blockers and verapamil may result in additive effects on heart rate, atrioventricular conduction, and/or cardiac contractility).
No products indexed under this heading.

Levobunolol Hydrochloride (Co-administration of beta blockers and verapamil may result in additive effects on heart rate, atrioventricular conduction, and/or cardiac contractility).
No products indexed under this heading.

Lithium (Co-administration results in increased sensitivity to the effects of lithium (neurotoxicity) with either no change or increase in serum lithium levels; increased lithium levels have been reported in patients receiving lithium and ACE inhibitor).
No products indexed under this heading.

Lithium Carbonate (Co-administration results in increased sensitivity to the effects of lithium (neurotoxicity) with either no change or increase in serum lithium levels; increased lithium levels have been reported in patients receiving lithium and ACE inhibitor).
No products indexed under this heading.

Lithium Citrate (Co-administration results in increased sensitivity to the effects of lithium (neurotoxicity) with either no change or increase in serum lithium levels; increased lithium levels have been reported in patients receiving lithium and ACE inhibitor).
No products indexed under this heading.

Methoxyflurane (Potential for excessive cardiovascular depression).
No products indexed under this heading.

Methyclothiazide (Patients on diuretics, especially those on recently instituted diuretic therapy, may occasionally experience an excessive reduction of blood pressure after initiation of therapy with Tarka).
No products indexed under this heading.

Metipranolol Hydrochloride (Co-administration of beta blockers and verapamil may result in additive effects on heart rate, atrioventricular conduction, and/or cardiac contractility).
No products indexed under this heading.

IMPORTANT NOTE: Always consult each drug listing in the patient's regimen for possible interactions.

Metocurine Iodide (Verapamil may potentiate the activity of neuromuscular blocking agents).
No products indexed under this heading.

Metolazone (Patients on diuretics, especially those on recently instituted diuretic therapy, may occasionally experience an excessive reduction of blood pressure after initiation of therapy with Tarka).
No products indexed under this heading.

Metoprolol Succinate (Co-administration of beta blockers and verapamil may result in additive effects on heart rate, atrioventricular conduction, and/or cardiac contractility). Products include:
Toprol-XL Tablets 666

Metoprolol Tartrate (Co-administration of beta blockers and verapamil may result in additive effects on heart rate, atrioventricular conduction, and/or cardiac contractility).
No products indexed under this heading.

Mivacurium Chloride (Verapamil may potentiate the activity of neuromuscular blocking agents).
No products indexed under this heading.

Nadolol (Co-administration of beta blockers and verapamil may result in additive effects on heart rate, atrioventricular conduction, and/or cardiac contractility). Products include:
Nadolol Tablets 2191

Nebivolol (Co-administration of beta blockers and verapamil may result in additive effects on heart rate, atrioventricular conduction, and/or cardiac contractility). Products include:
Bystolic Tablets 1155

Pancuronium Bromide (Verapamil may potentiate the activity of neuromuscular blocking agents).
No products indexed under this heading.

Penbutolol Sulfate (Co-administration of beta blockers and verapamil may result in additive effects on heart rate, atrioventricular conduction, and/or cardiac contractility).
No products indexed under this heading.

Phenobarbital (May increase verapamil clearance). Products include:
Donnatal Extentabs 2507

Pindolol (Co-administration of beta blockers and verapamil may result in additive effects on heart rate, atrioventricular conduction, and/or cardiac contractility).
No products indexed under this heading.

Polythiazide (Patients on diuretics, especially those on recently instituted diuretic therapy, may occasionally experience an excessive reduction of blood pressure after initiation of therapy with Tarka).
No products indexed under this heading.

Potassium Acid Phosphate (Increased risk of hyperkalemia). Products include:
K-Phos Original (Sodium Free) Tablets 814

Potassium Bicarbonate (Increased risk of hyperkalemia).
No products indexed under this heading.

Potassium Chloride (Increased risk of hyperkalemia). Products include:
MoviPrep Oral Solution 2679

Potassium Citrate (Increased risk of hyperkalemia). Products include:
BioLean Free Tablets .... ▣635
Urocit-K Tablets 2176

Potassium Gluconate (Increased risk of hyperkalemia).
No products indexed under this heading.

Potassium Phosphate (Increased risk of hyperkalemia). Products include:
K-Phos Neutral Tablets 813

Propranolol Hydrochloride (Co-administration of beta blockers and verapamil may result in additive effects on heart rate, atrioventricular conduction, and/or cardiac contractility). Products include:
InnoPran XL Extended Release Capsules 1484

Quinidine (Concomitant use of verapamil and quinidine has resulted in significant hypotension and/or increased quinidine levels during verapamil therapy).
No products indexed under this heading.

Quinidine Gluconate (Concomitant use of verapamil and quinidine has resulted in significant hypotension and/or increased quinidine levels during verapamil therapy).
No products indexed under this heading.

Quinidine Hydrochloride (Concomitant use of verapamil and quinidine has resulted in significant hypotension and/or increased quinidine levels during verapamil therapy).
No products indexed under this heading.

Quinidine Polygalacturonate (Concomitant use of verapamil and quinidine has resulted in significant hypotension and/or increased quinidine levels during verapamil therapy).
No products indexed under this heading.

Quinidine Sulfate (Concomitant use of verapamil and quinidine has resulted in significant hypotension and/or increased quinidine levels during verapamil therapy).
No products indexed under this heading.

Rapacuronium Bromide (Verapamil may potentiate the activity of neuromuscular blocking agents).
No products indexed under this heading.

Rifampin (May markedly reduce oral verapamil bioavailability).
No products indexed under this heading.

Rocuronium Bromide (Verapamil may potentiate the activity of neuromuscular blocking agents). Products include:
Zemuron Injection 2947

Sotalol Hydrochloride (Co-administration of beta blockers and verapamil may result in additive effects on heart rate, atrioventricular conduction, and/or cardiac contractility).
No products indexed under this heading.

Spironolactone (Increased risk of hyperkalemia; patients on diuretics, especially those on recently instituted diuretic therapy, may occasionally experience an excessive reduction of blood pressure after initiation of therapy with Tarka).
No products indexed under this heading.

Succinylcholine Chloride (Verapamil may potentiate the activity of neuromuscular blocking agents).
No products indexed under this heading.

Theophylline (Verapamil may inhibit the clearance and increase the plasma levels of theophylline).
No products indexed under this heading.

Theophylline Anhydrous (Verapamil may inhibit the clearance and increase the plasma levels of theophylline). Products include:
Uniphyl Tablets 2595

Theophylline Calcium Salicylate (Verapamil may inhibit the clearance and increase the plasma levels of theophylline).
No products indexed under this heading.

Theophylline Dihydroxypropyl (Glyceryl) (Verapamil may inhibit the clearance and increase the plasma levels of theophylline).
No products indexed under this heading.

Theophylline Ethylenediamine (Verapamil may inhibit the clearance and increase the plasma levels of theophylline).
No products indexed under this heading.

Theophylline Sodium Glycinate (Verapamil may inhibit the clearance and increase the plasma levels of theophylline).
No products indexed under this heading.

Timolol Hemihydrate (Concomitant use of timolol eye drops and verapamil has resulted in asymptomatic bradycardia with wandering atrial pacemaker). Products include:
Betimol Ophthalmic Solution 3181

Timolol Maleate (Concomitant use of timolol eye drops and verapamil has resulted in asymptomatic bradycardia with wandering atrial pacemaker). Products include:
Combigan Ophthalmic Solution 553
Cosopt Sterile Ophthalmic Solution 1969
Timoptic Sterile Ophthalmic Solution 2121
Timoptic in Ocudose 2124
Timoptic-XE Sterile Ophthalmic Gel Forming Solution 2125

Torsemide (Patients on diuretics, especially those on recently instituted diuretic therapy, may occasionally experience an excessive reduction of blood pressure after initiation of therapy with Tarka). Products include:
Demadex Injection 2630
Demadex Tablets 2630

Triamterene (Increased risk of hyperkalemia; patients on diuretics, especially those on recently instituted diuretic therapy, may occasionally experience an excessive reduction of blood pressure after initiation of therapy with Tarka). Products include:
Dyazide Capsules 1405
Dyrenium Capsules 3189

Vecuronium Bromide (Verapamil may potentiate the activity of neuromuscular blocking agents).
No products indexed under this heading.

Food Interactions

Food, unspecified (Co-administration with food decreases verapamil bioavailability and the time to peak plasma concentration is delayed; bioavailability of trandolapril is not altered; Tarka should be administered with food).

TASIGNA CAPSULES

(Nilotinib) 2316
May interact with cytochrome p450 2c8 substrates (selected), cytochrome p450 2c9 substrates (selected), cytochrome p450 2d6 substrates (selected), cytochrome p450 3a4 inducers (selected), cytochrome p450 3a4 inhibitors, potent, cytochrome p450 3a4 substrates (selected), dexamethasone, P-glycoprotein inhibitors, P-glycoprotein substrates, phenytoin, drugs that prolong the QT interval, and certain other agents. Compounds in these categories include:

Acarbose (Nilotinib is a competitive inhibitor of CYP2C9, potentially increasing the concentration of drugs eliminated by CYP2C9. Caution should be exercised when co-administering nilotinib with substrates for CYP2C9 that have a narrow therapeutic index. Studies also suggest that nilotinib may induce CYP2B6, CYP2C8 and CYP2C9, and thereby has the potential to decrease the concentrations of drugs which are eliminated by these enzymes). Products include:
Precose Tablets 792

Alfentanil Hydrochloride (Nilotinib is a competitive inhibitor of CYP3A4 which may potentially increase the concentration of drugs eliminated by CYP3A4. Caution should be exercised when co-administering nilotinib with substrates for CYP3A4 that have a narrow therapeutic index).
No products indexed under this heading.

Allium sativum (The concomitant use of strong CYP3A4 inducers should be avoided. If patients must be co-administered a strong CYP3A4 inducer, the dose of nilotinib may need to be increased, depending on patient tolerability. If the strong inducer is discontinued, the nilotinib dose should be reduced to the indicated dose).
No products indexed under this heading.

Alprazolam (The administration of nilotinib with agents that prolong the QT interval should be avoided. Should treatment with any of these agents be required, it is recommended that therapy with nilotinib be interrupted. If interruption of treatment with nilotinib is not possible, patients who require treatment with a drug that prolongs the QT interval should be closely monitored for prolongation of the QT interval).
No products indexed under this heading.

Ambrisentan (Nilotinib inhibits human P-glycoprotein. If nilotinib is administered with drugs that are substrates of Pgp, increased concentrations of the substrate drug are likely, and caution should be exercised). Products include:

Letairis Tablets 1258

Amiodarone Hydrochloride (The administration of nilotinib with agents that prolong the QT interval should be avoided. Should treatment with any of these agents be required, it is recommended that therapy with nilotinib be interrupted. If interruption of treatment with nilotinib is not possible, patients who require treatment with a drug that prolongs the QT interval should be closely monitored for prolongation of the QT interval).
No products indexed under this heading.

Amitriptyline Hydrochloride (The administration of nilotinib with agents that prolong the QT interval should be avoided. Should treatment with any of these agents be required, it is recommended that therapy with nilotinib be interrupted. If interruption of treatment with nilotinib is not possible, patients who require treatment with a drug that prolongs the QT interval should be closely monitored for prolongation of the QT interval).
No products indexed under this heading.

Amlodipine Besylate (Nilotinib is a substrate of the efflux transporter P-glycoprotein (Pgp, ABCB1). If nilotinib is administered with drugs that inhibit Pgp, increased concentrations of nilotinib are likely, and caution should be exercised). Products include:
Azor Tablets 1005
Exforge Tablets 2238

Amoxapine (The administration of nilotinib with agents that prolong the QT interval should be avoided. Should treatment with any of these agents be required, it is recommended that therapy with nilotinib be interrupted. If interruption of treatment with nilotinib is not possible, patients who require treatment with a drug that prolongs the QT interval should be closely monitored for prolongation of the QT interval).
No products indexed under this heading.

Amphetamine Aspartate (Nilotinib is a competitive inhibitor of CYP2D6, potentially increasing the concentration of drugs eliminated by CYP2D6. Caution should be exercised when co-administering nilotinib with substrates for CYP2D6 that have a narrow therapeutic index). Products include:
Adderall XR Capsules 3012

Amphetamine Aspartate Monohydrate (Nilotinib is a competitive inhibitor of CYP2D6, potentially increasing the concentration of drugs eliminated by CYP2D6. Caution should be exercised when co-administering nilotinib with substrates for CYP2D6 that have a narrow therapeutic index).
No products indexed under this heading.

Amphetamine Sulfate (Nilotinib is a competitive inhibitor of CYP2D6, potentially increasing the concentration of drugs eliminated by CYP2D6. Caution should be exercised when co-administering nilotinib with substrates for CYP2D6 that have a narrow therapeutic index). Products include:
Adderall XR Capsules 3012

Amprenavir (The concomitant use of strong CYP3A4 inhibitors should be avoided. Should treatment with any of these agents be required, it is recommended that therapy with nilotinib be interrupted. If patients must be co-administered a strong CYP3A4 inhibitor, based on pharmacokinetic studies, 400 mg once daily is predicted to adjust the nilotinib AUC to the AUC observed without inhibitors. However, there are no clinical data with this dose adjustment in patients receiving strong CYP3A4 inhibitors. If the strong inhibitor is discontinued, a washout period should be allowed before the nilotinib dose is adjusted upward to the indicated dose. Close monitoring for prolongation of the QT interval is indicated for patients who cannot avoid strong CYP3A4 inhibitors).
No products indexed under this heading.

Aprepitant (The concomitant use of strong CYP3A4 inducers should be avoided. If patients must be co-administered a strong CYP3A4 inducer, the dose of nilotinib may need to be increased, depending on patient tolerability. If the strong inducer is discontinued, the nilotinib dose should be reduced to the indicated dose). Products include:
Emend Capsules 1992

Astemizole (The administration of nilotinib with agents that prolong the QT interval should be avoided. Should treatment with any of these agents be required, it is recommended that therapy with nilotinib be interrupted. If interruption of treatment with nilotinib is not possible, patients who require treatment with a drug that prolongs the QT interval should be closely monitored for prolongation of the QT interval).
No products indexed under this heading.

Atazanavir (The concomitant use of strong CYP3A4 inhibitors such as atazanavir should be avoided. If treatment is required, it is recommended that therapy with nilotinib be interrupted. If patients must be co-administered a strong CYP3A4 inhibitor, based on pharmacokinetic studies, 400 mg q.d. is predicted to adjust the nilotinib AUC to the AUC observed without inhibitors. However, there are no clinical data with this dose adjustment in patients receiving strong CYP3A4 inhibitors. If the strong inhibitor is discontinued, a washout period should be allowed before the nilotinib dose is adjusted upward to the indicated dose. Close monitoring for prolongation of the QT interval is indicated for patients who cannot avoid strong CYP3A4 inhibitors).
No products indexed under this heading.

Atazanavir Sulfate (The concomitant use of strong CYP3A4 inhibitors such as atazanavir should be avoided. If treatment is required, it is recommended that therapy with nilotinib be interrupted. If patients must be co-administered a strong CYP3A4 inhibitor, based on pharmacokinetic studies, 400 mg q.d. is predicted to adjust the nilotinib AUC to the AUC observed without inhibitors. However, there are no clinical data with this dose adjustment in patients receiving strong CYP3A4 inhibitors. If the strong inhibitor is discontinued, a washout period should be allowed before the nilotinib dose is adjusted upward to the indicated dose. Close monitoring for prolongation of the QT interval is indicated for patients who cannot avoid strong CYP3A4 inhibitors). Products include:
Reyataz Capsules 3299

Atenolol (Nilotinib is a substrate of the efflux transporter P-glycoprotein (Pgp, ABCB1). If nilotinib is administered with drugs that inhibit Pgp, increased concentrations of nilotinib are likely, and caution should be exercised).
No products indexed under this heading.

Atomoxetine Hydrochloride (Nilotinib is a competitive inhibitor of CYP2D6, potentially increasing the concentration of drugs eliminated by CYP2D6. Caution should be exercised when co-administering nilotinib with substrates for CYP2D6 that have a narrow therapeutic index). Products include:
Strattera Capsules 1864

Atorvastatin Calcium (Nilotinib is a substrate of the efflux transporter P-glycoprotein (Pgp, ABCB1). If nilotinib is administered with drugs that inhibit Pgp, increased concentrations of nilotinib are likely, and caution should be exercised). Products include:
Lipitor Tablets 2501

Azithromycin Dihydrate (Nilotinib is a substrate of the efflux transporter P-glycoprotein (Pgp, ABCB1). If nilotinib is administered with drugs that inhibit Pgp, increased concentrations of nilotinib are likely, and caution should be exercised).
No products indexed under this heading.

Belladonna Ergotamine (Nilotinib is a competitive inhibitor of CYP3A4 which may potentially increase the concentration of drugs eliminated by CYP3A4. Caution should be exercised when co-administering nilotinib with substrates for CYP3A4 that have a narrow therapeutic index).
No products indexed under this heading.

Benzphetamine Hydrochloride (Nilotinib is a competitive inhibitor of CYP2C8, potentially increasing the concentration of drugs eliminated by CYP2C8. Caution should be exercised when co-administering nilotinib with substrates for CYP2C8 that have a narrow therapeutic index. Studies also suggest that nilotinib may induce CYP2B6, CYP2C8 and CYP2C9, and thereby has the potential to decrease the concentrations of drugs which are eliminated by these enzymes).
No products indexed under this heading.

Betamethasone Acetate (The concomitant use of strong CYP3A4 inducers should be avoided. If patients must be co-administered a strong CYP3A4 inducer, the dose of nilotinib may need to be increased, depending on patient tolerability. If the strong inducer is discontinued, the nilotinib dose should be reduced to the indicated dose).
No products indexed under this heading.

Betamethasone Sodium Phosphate (The concomitant use of strong CYP3A4 inducers should be avoided. If patients must be co-administered a strong CYP3A4 inducer, the dose of nilotinib may need to be increased, depending on patient tolerability. If the strong inducer is discontinued, the nilotinib dose should be reduced to the indicated dose).
No products indexed under this heading.

Bisoprolol Fumarate (Nilotinib is a competitive inhibitor of CYP2D6, potentially increasing the concentration of drugs eliminated by CYP2D6. Caution should be exercised when co-administering nilotinib with substrates for CYP2D6 that have a narrow therapeutic index).
No products indexed under this heading.

Bretylium Tosylate (The administration of nilotinib with agents that prolong the QT interval should be avoided. Should treatment with any of these agents be required, it is recommended that therapy with nilotinib be interrupted. If interruption of treatment with nilotinib is not possible, patients who require treatment with a drug that prolongs the QT interval should be closely monitored for prolongation of the QT interval).
No products indexed under this heading.

Buspirone Hydrochloride (The administration of nilotinib with agents that prolong the QT interval should be avoided. Should treatment with any of these agents be required, it is recommended that therapy with nilotinib be interrupted. If interruption of treatment with nilotinib is not possible, patients who require treatment with a drug that prolongs the QT interval should be closely monitored for prolongation of the QT interval).
No products indexed under this heading.

Busulfan (Nilotinib is a competitive inhibitor of CYP3A4 which may potentially increase the concentration of drugs eliminated by CYP3A4. Caution should be exercised when co-administering nilotinib with substrates for CYP3A4 that have a narrow therapeutic index). Products include:
Busulfex Injection 2477
Myleran Tablets 1530

Candesartan Cilexetil (Nilotinib is a competitive inhibitor of CYP2C9, potentially increasing the concentration of drugs eliminated by CYP2C9. Caution should be exercised when co-administering nilotinib with substrates for CYP2C9 that have a narrow therapeutic index. Studies also suggest that nilotinib may induce CYP2B6, CYP2C8 and CYP2C9, and thereby has the potential to decrease the concentrations of drugs which are eliminated by these enzymes). Products include:
Atacand Tablets 639
Atacand HCT 642

Captopril (Nilotinib is a competitive inhibitor of CYP2D6, potentially increasing the concentration of drugs eliminated by CYP2D6. Caution should be exercised when co-administering nilotinib with substrates for CYP2D6 that have a narrow therapeutic index). Products include:

Captopril Tablets 2182

Carbamazepine (The concomitant use of strong CYP3A4 inducers such as carbamazepine should be avoided. If patients must be co-administered a strong CYP3A4 inducer, the dose of nilotinib may need to be increased, depending on patient tolerability. If the strong inducer is discontinued, the nilotinib dose should be reduced to the indicated dose). Products include:

Carbatrol Capsules 3019
Equetro Extended-Release Capsules 3174

Carvedilol (Nilotinib is a competitive inhibitor of CYP2C9, potentially increasing the concentration of drugs eliminated by CYP2C9. Caution should be exercised when co-administering nilotinib with substrates for CYP2C9 that have a narrow therapeutic index. Studies also suggest that nilotinib may induce CYP2B6, CYP2C8 and CYP2C9, and thereby has the potential to decrease the concentrations of drugs which are eliminated by these enzymes). Products include:

Coreg Tablets 1387

Celecoxib (Nilotinib is a competitive inhibitor of CYP2C9, potentially increasing the concentration of drugs eliminated by CYP2C9. Caution should be exercised when co-administering nilotinib with substrates for CYP2C9 that have a narrow therapeutic index. Studies also suggest that nilotinib may induce CYP2B6, CYP2C8 and CYP2C9, and thereby has the potential to decrease the concentrations of drugs which are eliminated by these enzymes). Products include:

Celebrex Capsules 2979

Cerivastatin Sodium (Nilotinib is a competitive inhibitor of CYP3A4 which may potentially increase the concentration of drugs eliminated by CYP3A4. Caution should be exercised when co-administering nilotinib with substrates for CYP3A4 that have a narrow therapeutic index).

No products indexed under this heading.

Cevimeline Hydrochloride (Nilotinib is a competitive inhibitor of CYP2D6, potentially increasing the concentration of drugs eliminated by CYP2D6. Caution should be exercised when co-administering nilotinib with substrates for CYP2D6 that have a narrow therapeutic index). Products include:

Evoxac Capsules 1013

Chlordiazepoxide (The administration of nilotinib with agents that prolong the QT interval should be avoided. Should treatment with any of these agents be required, it is recommended that therapy with nilotinib be interrupted. If interruption of treatment with nilotinib is not possible, patients who require treatment with a drug that prolongs the QT interval should be closely monitored for prolongation of the QT interval).

No products indexed under this heading.

Chlordiazepoxide Hydrochloride (The administration of nilotinib with agents that prolong the QT interval should be avoided. Should treatment with any of these agents be required, it is recommended that therapy with nilotinib be interrupted. If interruption of treatment with nilotinib is not possible, patients who require treatment with a drug that prolongs the QT interval should be closely monitored for prolongation of the QT interval).

No products indexed under this heading.

Chlorpheniramine (Nilotinib is a competitive inhibitor of CYP3A4 which may potentially increase the concentration of drugs eliminated by CYP3A4. Caution should be exercised when co-administering nilotinib with substrates for CYP3A4 that have a narrow therapeutic index).

No products indexed under this heading.

Chlorpheniramine Maleate (Nilotinib is a competitive inhibitor of CYP3A4 which may potentially increase the concentration of drugs eliminated by CYP3A4. Caution should be exercised when co-administering nilotinib with substrates for CYP3A4 that have a narrow therapeutic index). Products include:

Actifed Cold & Allergy Tablets 1895
Sudafed PE Sinus & Allergy Tablets 1908
Tylenol Allergy Multi-Symptom Caplets with Cool Burst and Rapid Release Gelcaps 1916
Children's Tylenol Plus Cold Suspension Liquid 1912
Children's Tylenol Plus Cough & Runny Nose Suspension Liquid 1912
Children's Tylenol Plus Flu Suspension Liquid 1914
Children's Tylenol Plus Multi-Symptom Cold Suspension Liquid 1912
Tylenol Cold Head Congestion Nighttime Caplets with Cool Burst 1910
Tylenol Cold Multi-Symptom Nighttime Caplets with Cool Burst 1913
Tylenol Sinus Congestion & Pain Nighttime Caplets with Cool Burst 1917

Chlorpheniramine Polistirex (Nilotinib is a competitive inhibitor of CYP3A4 which may potentially increase the concentration of drugs eliminated by CYP3A4. Caution should be exercised when co-administering nilotinib with substrates for CYP3A4 that have a narrow therapeutic index). Products include:

Tussionex Pennkinetic Extended-Release Suspension 3154

Chlorpheniramine Tannate (Nilotinib is a competitive inhibitor of CYP3A4 which may potentially increase the concentration of drugs eliminated by CYP3A4. Caution should be exercised when co-administering nilotinib with substrates for CYP3A4 that have a narrow therapeutic index).

No products indexed under this heading.

Chlorpromazine (The administration of nilotinib with agents that prolong the QT interval should be avoided. Should treatment with any of these agents be required, it is recommended that therapy with nilotinib be interrupted. If interruption of treatment with nilotinib is not possible, patients who require treatment with a drug that prolongs the QT interval should be closely monitored for prolongation of the QT interval).

No products indexed under this heading.

Chlorpromazine Hydrochloride (The administration of nilotinib with agents that prolong the QT interval should be avoided. Should treatment with any of these agents be required, it is recommended that therapy with nilotinib be interrupted. If interruption of treatment with nilotinib is not possible, patients who require treatment with a drug that prolongs the QT interval should be closely monitored for prolongation of the QT interval).

No products indexed under this heading.

Chlorpropamide (Nilotinib is a competitive inhibitor of CYP2C9, potentially increasing the concentration of drugs eliminated by CYP2C9. Caution should be exercised when co-administering nilotinib with substrates for CYP2C9 that have a narrow therapeutic index. Studies also suggest that nilotinib may induce CYP2B6, CYP2C8 and CYP2C9, and thereby has the potential to decrease the concentrations of drugs which are eliminated by these enzymes).

No products indexed under this heading.

Chlorprothixene (The administration of nilotinib with agents that prolong the QT interval should be avoided. Should treatment with any of these agents be required, it is recommended that therapy with nilotinib be interrupted. If interruption of treatment with nilotinib is not possible, patients who require treatment with a drug that prolongs the QT interval should be closely monitored for prolongation of the QT interval).

No products indexed under this heading.

Chlorprothixene Hydrochloride (The administration of nilotinib with agents that prolong the QT interval should be avoided. Should treatment with any of these agents be required, it is recommended that therapy with nilotinib be interrupted. If interruption of treatment with nilotinib is not possible, patients who require treatment with a drug that prolongs the QT interval should be closely monitored for prolongation of the QT interval).

No products indexed under this heading.

Ciprofloxacin Hydrochloride (The concomitant use of strong CYP3A4 inducers should be avoided. If patients must be co-administered a strong CYP3A4 inducer, the dose of nilotinib may need to be increased, depending on patient tolerability. If the strong inducer is discontinued, the nilotinib dose should be reduced to the indicated dose). Products include:

Cipro Tablets 2810

Cisapride (Nilotinib is a competitive inhibitor of CYP3A4 which may potentially increase the concentration of drugs eliminated by CYP3A4. Caution should be exercised when co-administering nilotinib with substrates for CYP3A4 that have a narrow therapeutic index).

No products indexed under this heading.

Cisplatin (The concomitant use of strong CYP3A4 inducers should be avoided. If patients must be co-administered a strong CYP3A4 inducer, the dose of nilotinib may need to be increased, depending on patient tolerability. If the strong inducer is discontinued, the nilotinib dose should be reduced to the indicated dose).

No products indexed under this heading.

Clarithromycin (The concomitant use of strong CYP3A4 inhibitors such as clarithromycin should be avoided. If treatment is required, it is recommended that therapy with nilotinib be interrupted. If patients must be co-administered a strong CYP3A4 inhibitor, based on pharmacokinetic studies, 400 mg q.d. is predicted to adjust the nilotinib AUC to the AUC observed without inhibitors. However, there are no clinical data with this dose adjustment in patients receiving strong CYP3A4 inhibitors. If the strong inhibitor is discontinued, a washout period should be allowed before the nilotinib dose is adjusted upward to the indicated dose. Close monitoring for prolongation of the QT interval is indicated for patients who cannot avoid strong CYP3A4 inhibitors). Products include:

Biaxin/Biaxin XL 411

Clomipramine Hydrochloride (The administration of nilotinib with agents that prolong the QT interval should be avoided. Should treatment with any of these agents be required, it is recommended that therapy with nilotinib be interrupted. If interruption of treatment with nilotinib is not possible, patients who require treatment with a drug that prolongs the QT interval should be closely monitored for prolongation of the QT interval).

No products indexed under this heading.

Clorazepate Dipotassium (The administration of nilotinib with agents that prolong the QT interval should be avoided. Should treatment with any of these agents be required, it is recommended that therapy with nilotinib be interrupted. If interruption of treatment with nilotinib is not possible, patients who require treatment with a drug that prolongs the QT interval should be closely monitored for prolongation of the QT interval).

No products indexed under this heading.

Clozapine (The administration of nilotinib with agents that prolong the QT interval should be avoided. Should treatment with any of these agents be required, it is recommended that therapy with nilotinib be interrupted. If interruption of treatment with nilotinib is not possible, patients who require treatment with a drug that prolongs the QT interval should be closely monitored for prolongation of the QT interval).

No products indexed under this heading.

Codeine Phosphate (Nilotinib is a competitive inhibitor of CYP2D6, potentially increasing the concentration of drugs eliminated by CYP2D6. Caution should be exercised when co-administering nilotinib with substrates for CYP2D6 that have a narrow therapeutic index). Products include:

Tylenol with Codeine Tablets 2427

Codeine Sulfate (Nilotinib is a competitive inhibitor of CYP2D6, potentially increasing the concentration of drugs eliminated by CYP2D6. Caution should be exercised when co-administering nilotinib with substrates for CYP2D6 that have a narrow therapeutic index).

No products indexed under this heading.

Cortisone Acetate (The concomitant use of strong CYP3A4 inducers should be avoided. If patients must be co-administered a strong CYP3A4 inducer, the dose of nilotinib may need to be increased, depending on patient tolerability. If the strong inducer is discontinued, the nilotinib dose should be reduced to the indicated dose).

No products indexed under this heading.

Cyclobenzaprine Hydrochloride (Nilotinib is a competitive inhibitor of CYP2D6, potentially increasing the concentration of drugs eliminated by CYP2D6. Caution should be exercised when co-administering nilotinib with substrates for CYP2D6 that have a narrow therapeutic index). Products include:

Amrix Capsules 966

Cyclosporine (Nilotinib is a substrate of the efflux transporter P-glycoprotein (Pgp, ABCB1). If nilotinib is administered with drugs that inhibit Pgp, increased concentrations of nilotinib are likely, and caution should be exercised). Products include:

Gengraf Capsules 435
Neoral Oral Solution 2280
Neoral Soft Gelatin Capsules 2280
Restasis Ophthalmic Emulsion 557
Sandimmune 2296

Delavirdine Mesylate (The concomitant use of strong CYP3A4 inhibitors should be avoided. Should treatment with any of these agents be required, it is recommended that therapy with nilotinib be interrupted. If patients must be co-administered a strong CYP3A4 inhibitor, based on pharmacokinetic studies, 400 mg once daily is predicted to adjust the nilotinib AUC to the AUC observed without inhibitors. However, there are no clinical data with this dose adjustment in patients receiving strong CYP3A4 inhibitors. If the strong inhibitor is discontinued, a washout period should be allowed before the nilotinib dose is adjusted upward to the indicated dose. Close monitoring for prolongation of the QT interval is indicated for patients who cannot avoid strong CYP3A4 inhibitors).

No products indexed under this heading.

Delavirine (The concomitant use of strong CYP3A4 inhibitors should be avoided. Should treatment with any of these agents be required, it is recommended that therapy with nilotinib be interrupted. If patients must be co-administered a strong CYP3A4 inhibitor, based on pharmacokinetic studies, 400 mg once daily is predicted to adjust the nilotinib AUC to the AUC observed without inhibitors. However, there are no clinical data with this dose adjustment in patients receiving strong CYP3A4 inhibitors. If the strong inhibitor is discontinued, a washout period should be allowed before the nilotinib dose is adjusted upward to the indicated dose. Close monitoring for prolongation of the QT interval is indicated for patients who cannot avoid strong CYP3A4 inhibitors).

No products indexed under this heading.

Desipramine Hydrochloride (The administration of nilotinib with agents that prolong the QT interval should be avoided. Should treatment with any of these agents be required, it is recommended that therapy with nilotinib be interrupted. If interruption of treatment with nilotinib is not possible, patients who require treatment with a drug that prolongs the QT interval should be closely monitored for prolongation of the QT interval).

No products indexed under this heading.

Desogestrel (Nilotinib is a competitive inhibitor of CYP3A4 which may potentially increase the concentration of drugs eliminated by CYP3A4. Caution should be exercised when co-administering nilotinib with substrates for CYP3A4 that have a narrow therapeutic index). Products include:

Mircette Tablets 1034

Dexamethasone (The concomitant use of strong CYP3A4 inducers such as dexamethasone should be avoided. If patients must be co-administered a strong CYP3A4 inducer, the dose of nilotinib may need to be increased, depending on patient tolerability. If the strong inducer is discontinued, the nilotinib dose should be reduced to the indicated dose). Products include:

Ciprodex Otic Suspension 541

Dexamethasone Acetate (The concomitant use of strong CYP3A4 inducers such as dexamethasone should be avoided. If patients must be co-administered a strong CYP3A4 inducer, the dose of nilotinib may need to be increased, depending on patient tolerability. If the strong inducer is discontinued, the nilotinib dose should be reduced to the indicated dose).

No products indexed under this heading.

Dexamethasone Sodium Phosphate (The concomitant use of strong CYP3A4 inducers such as dexamethasone should be avoided. If patients must be co-administered a strong CYP3A4 inducer, the dose of nilotinib may need to be increased, depending on patient tolerability. If the strong inducer is discontinued, the nilotinib dose should be reduced to the indicated dose).

No products indexed under this heading.

Dexfenfluramine Hydrochloride (Nilotinib is a competitive inhibitor of CYP2D6, potentially increasing the concentration of drugs eliminated by CYP2D6. Caution should be exercised when co-administering nilotinib with substrates for CYP2D6 that have a narrow therapeutic index).

No products indexed under this heading.

Dextromethorphan (Nilotinib is a competitive inhibitor of CYP2C9, potentially increasing the concentration of drugs eliminated by CYP2C9. Caution should be exercised when co-administering nilotinib with substrates for CYP2C9 that have a narrow therapeutic index. Studies also suggest that nilotinib may induce CYP2B6, CYP2C8 and CYP2C9, and thereby has the potential to decrease the concentrations of drugs which are eliminated by these enzymes).

No products indexed under this heading.

Dextromethorphan Hydrobromide (Nilotinib is a competitive inhibitor of CYP2D6, potentially increasing the concentration of drugs eliminated by CYP2D6. Caution should be exercised when co-administering nilotinib with substrates for CYP2D6 that have a narrow therapeutic index). Products include:

PediaCare Children's Liquid Multi-Symptom Cold.................... 1902
PediaCare Children's Long-Acting Cough 1902
Children's Sudafed PE Cold & Cough Liquid 1907
Sudafed PE Cold & Cough Caplets.. 1907
Children's Tylenol Plus Cough & Runny Nose Suspension Liquid..... 1912
Children's Tylenol Plus Cough & Sore Throat Suspension Liquid..... 1912
Children's Tylenol Plus Flu Suspension Liquid 1914
Children's Tylenol Plus Multi-Symptom Cold Suspension Liquid 1912
Tylenol Cold Severe Congestion Daytime Caplets with Cool Burst.. 1912
Tylenol Cold Head Congestion Daytime Caplets with Cool Burst.. 1910
Tylenol Cold Head Congestion Nighttime Caplets with Cool Burst.. 1910
Tylenol Cold Head Congestion Severe Daytime Caplets with Cool Burst.. 1910
Tylenol Cold Multi-Symptom Daytime Caplets with Cool Burst and Rapid Release Gels....... 1913
Tylenol Cold Multi-Symptom Daytime Liquid with Citrus Burst... 1913
Tylenol Cold Multi-Symptom Nighttime Caplets with Cool Burst.. 1913
Tylenol Cold Multi-Symptom Nighttime Liquid with Cool Burst... 1913
Tylenol Cold Multi-Symptom Severe Caplets with Cool Burst..... 1913
Tylenol Cold Multi-Symptom Severe Daytime Liquid with Citrus Burst................................ 1913
Tylenol Cough & Sore Throat Daytime Liquid with Cool Burst...... 1918
Tylenol Cough & Sore Throat Nighttime Liquid with Cool Burst... 1918
Vicks DayQuil Cold & Flu Multi-Symptom Relief 616
Vicks DayQuil LiquiCaps 2567
Vicks DayQuil Liquid 2567
Vicks DayQuil Multi-Symptom Cold/Flu Relief............................ 2567
Vicks NyQuil Cold & Flu Multi-Symptom Relief 617
Vicks NyQuil LiquiCaps 2567
Vicks NyQuil Liquid 2567
Vicks NyQuil Multi-Symptom Cold/Flu Relief............................ 2567

Dextromethorphan Polistirex (Nilotinib is a competitive inhibitor of CYP2D6, potentially increasing the concentration of drugs eliminated by CYP2D6. Caution should be exercised when co-administering nilotinib with substrates for CYP2D6 that have a narrow therapeutic index).

No products indexed under this heading.

Diazepam (The administration of nilotinib with agents that prolong the QT interval should be avoided. Should treatment with any of these agents be required, it is recommended that therapy with nilotinib be interrupted. If interruption of treatment with nilotinib is not possible, patients who require treatment with a drug that prolongs the QT interval should be closely monitored for prolongation of the QT interval). Products include:

Valium Tablets 2658

Diclofenac Potassium (Nilotinib is a competitive inhibitor of CYP2C8, potentially increasing the concentration of drugs eliminated by CYP2C8. Caution should be exercised when co-administering nilotinib with substrates for CYP2C8 that have a narrow therapeutic index. Studies also suggest that nilotinib may induce CYP2B6, CYP2C8 and CYP2C9, and thereby has the potential to decrease the concentrations of drugs which are eliminated by these enzymes).

No products indexed under this heading.

Diclofenac Sodium (Nilotinib is a competitive inhibitor of CYP2C8, potentially increasing the concentration of drugs eliminated by CYP2C8. Caution should be exercised when co-administering nilotinib with substrates for CYP2C8 that have a narrow therapeutic index. Studies also suggest that nilotinib may induce CYP2B6, CYP2C8 and CYP2C9, and thereby has the potential to decrease the concentrations of drugs which are eliminated by these enzymes). Products include:

Diclofenac Sodium Ophthalmic Solution..................................... ⊙240
Voltaren Ophthalmic Solution 2336
Voltaren Tablets 2334
Voltaren-XR Tablets 2337

Digoxin (Nilotinib is a substrate of the efflux transporter P-glycoprotein (Pgp, ABCB1). If nilotinib is administered with drugs that inhibit Pgp, increased concentrations of nilotinib are likely, and caution should be exercised). Products include:

Lanoxin Injection 1498
Lanoxin Injection Pediatric 1502
Lanoxin Tablets 1505

Digoxin Immune Fab (Ovine) (Nilotinib inhibits human P-glycoprotein. If nilotinib is administered with drugs that are substrates of Pgp, increased concentrations of the substrate drug are likely, and caution should be exercised). Products include:

Digibind for Injection 1403

Dihydroergotamine Mesylate (Nilotinib is a competitive inhibitor of CYP3A4 which may potentially increase the concentration of drugs eliminated by CYP3A4. Caution should be exercised when co-administering nilotinib with substrates for CYP3A4 that have a narrow therapeutic index).

No products indexed under this heading.

Diltiazem Hydrochloride (Nilotinib is a substrate of the efflux transporter P-glycoprotein (Pgp, ABCB1). If nilotinib is administered with drugs that inhibit Pgp, increased concentrations of nilotinib are likely, and caution should be exercised). Products include:

Cardizem LA Extended Release Tablets 421

Diltiazem Maleate (Nilotinib is a substrate of the efflux transporter P-glycoprotein (Pgp, ABCB1). If nilotinib is administered with drugs that inhibit Pgp, increased concentrations of nilotinib are likely, and caution should be exercised).

No products indexed under this heading.

Dirithromycin (Nilotinib is a substrate of the efflux transporter P-glycoprotein (Pgp, ABCB1). If nilotinib is administered with drugs that inhibit Pgp, increased concentrations of nilotinib are likely, and caution should be exercised).

No products indexed under this heading.

Disopyramide (Nilotinib is a competitive inhibitor of CYP3A4 which may potentially increase the concentration of drugs eliminated by CYP3A4. Caution should be exercised when co-administering nilotinib with substrates for CYP3A4 that have a narrow therapeutic index).

No products indexed under this heading.

Disopyramide Phosphate (The administration of nilotinib with agents that prolong the QT interval should be avoided. Should treatment with any of these agents be required, it is recommended that therapy with nilotinib be interrupted. If interruption of treatment with nilotinib is not possible, patients who require treatment with a drug that prolongs the QT interval should be closely monitored for prolongation of the QT interval).

No products indexed under this heading.

Disulfiram (Nilotinib is a competitive inhibitor of CYP3A4 which may potentially increase the concentration of drugs eliminated by CYP3A4. Caution should be exercised when co-administering nilotinib with substrates for CYP3A4 that have a narrow therapeutic index).

No products indexed under this heading.

Docetaxel (Nilotinib is a competitive inhibitor of CYP2C8, potentially increasing the concentration of drugs eliminated by CYP2C8. Caution should be exercised when co-administering nilotinib with substrates for CYP2C8 that have a narrow therapeutic index. Studies also suggest that nilotinib may induce CYP2B6, CYP2C8 and CYP2C9, and thereby has the potential to decrease the concentrations of drugs which are eliminated by these enzymes). Products include:

Taxotere Injection Concentrate **2773**

Dofetilide (The administration of nilotinib with agents that prolong the QT interval should be avoided. Should treatment with any of these agents be required, it is recommended that therapy with nilotinib be interrupted. If interruption of treatment with nilotinib is not possible, patients who require treatment with a drug that prolongs the QT interval should be closely monitored for prolongation of the QT interval).

No products indexed under this heading.

Dolasetron Mesylate (Nilotinib is a competitive inhibitor of CYP2D6, potentially increasing the concentration of drugs eliminated by CYP2D6. Caution should be exercised when co-administering nilotinib with substrates for CYP2D6 that have a narrow therapeutic index). Products include:

Anzemet Injection **2701**
Anzemet Tablets **2704**

Donepezil Hydrochloride (Nilotinib is a competitive inhibitor of CYP2D6, potentially increasing the concentration of drugs eliminated by CYP2D6. Caution should be exercised when co-administering nilotinib with substrates for CYP2D6 that have a narrow therapeutic index). Products include:

Aricept Tablets **1062**
Aricept ODT Tablets **1062**

Doxepin Hydrochloride (The administration of nilotinib with agents that prolong the QT interval should be avoided. Should treatment with any of these agents be required, it is recommended that therapy with nilotinib be interrupted. If interruption of treatment with nilotinib is not possible, patients who require treatment with a drug that prolongs the QT interval should be closely monitored for prolongation of the QT interval).

No products indexed under this heading.

Doxorubicin Hydrochloride (The concomitant use of strong CYP3A4 inducers should be avoided. If patients must be co-administered a strong CYP3A4 inducer, the dose of nilotinib may need to be increased, depending on patient tolerability. If the strong inducer is discontinued, the nilotinib dose should be reduced to the indicated dose).

No products indexed under this heading.

Dronabinol (Nilotinib is a competitive inhibitor of CYP3A4 which may potentially increase the concentration of drugs eliminated by CYP3A4. Caution should be exercised when co-administering nilotinib with substrates for CYP3A4 that have a narrow therapeutic index). Products include:

Marinol Capsules **3163**

Droperidol (The administration of nilotinib with agents that prolong the QT interval should be avoided. Should treatment with any of these agents be required, it is recommended that therapy with nilotinib be interrupted. If interruption of treatment with nilotinib is not possible, patients who require treatment with a drug that prolongs the QT interval should be closely monitored for prolongation of the QT interval).

No products indexed under this heading.

Efavirenz (The concomitant use of strong CYP3A4 inducers should be avoided. If patients must be co-administered a strong CYP3A4 inducer, the dose of nilotinib may need to be increased, depending on patient tolerability. If the strong inducer is discontinued, the nilotinib dose should be reduced to the indicated dose). Products include:

Atripla Tablets **938**
Sustiva Capsules **930**
Sustiva Tablets **930**

Elacridar (Nilotinib is a substrate of the efflux transporter P-glycoprotein (Pgp, ABCB1). If nilotinib is administered with drugs that inhibit Pgp, increased concentrations of nilotinib are likely, and caution should be exercised).

No products indexed under this heading.

Encainide Hydrochloride (Nilotinib is a competitive inhibitor of CYP2D6, potentially increasing the concentration of drugs eliminated by CYP2D6. Caution should be exercised when co-administering nilotinib with substrates for CYP2D6 that have a narrow therapeutic index).

No products indexed under this heading.

Eprosartan Mesylate (Nilotinib is a competitive inhibitor of CYP2C9, potentially increasing the concentration of drugs eliminated by CYP2C9. Caution should be exercised when co-administering nilotinib with substrates for CYP2C9 that have a narrow therapeutic index. Studies also suggest that nilotinib may induce CYP2B6, CYP2C8 and CYP2C9, and thereby has the potential to decrease the concentrations of drugs which are eliminated by these enzymes). Products include:

Teveten Tablets **515**
Teveten HCT Tablets **517**

Ergotamine Tartrate (Nilotinib is a competitive inhibitor of CYP3A4 which may potentially increase the concentration of drugs eliminated by CYP3A4. Caution should be exercised when co-administering nilotinib with substrates for CYP3A4 that have a narrow therapeutic index).

No products indexed under this heading.

Erythromycin (The administration of nilotinib with agents that prolong the QT interval should be avoided. Should treatment with any of these agents be required, it is recommended that therapy with nilotinib be interrupted. If interruption of treatment with nilotinib is not possible, patients who require treatment with a drug that prolongs the QT interval should be closely monitored for prolongation of the QT interval).

No products indexed under this heading.

Erythromycin Estolate (The administration of nilotinib with agents that prolong the QT interval should be avoided. Should treatment with any of these agents be required, it is recommended that therapy with nilotinib be interrupted. If interruption of treatment with nilotinib is not possible, patients who require treatment with a drug that prolongs the QT interval should be closely monitored for prolongation of the QT interval).

No products indexed under this heading.

Erythromycin Ethylsuccinate (The administration of nilotinib with agents that prolong the QT interval should be avoided. Should treatment with any of these agents be required, it is recommended that therapy with nilotinib be interrupted. If interruption of treatment with nilotinib is not possible, patients who require treatment with a drug that prolongs the QT interval should be closely monitored for prolongation of the QT interval). Products include:

E.E.S. **433**
EryPed **431**

Erythromycin Gluceptate (The administration of nilotinib with agents that prolong the QT interval should be avoided. Should treatment with any of these agents be required, it is recommended that therapy with nilotinib be interrupted. If interruption of treatment with nilotinib is not possible, patients who require treatment with a drug that prolongs the QT interval should be closely monitored for prolongation of the QT interval).

No products indexed under this heading.

Erythromycin Lactobionate (The administration of nilotinib with agents that prolong the QT interval should be avoided. Should treatment with any of these agents be required, it is recommended that therapy with nilotinib be interrupted. If interruption of treatment with nilotinib is not possible, patients who require treatment with a drug that prolongs the QT interval should be closely monitored for prolongation of the QT interval).

No products indexed under this heading.

Erythromycin Stearate (The administration of nilotinib with agents that prolong the QT interval should be avoided. Should treatment with any of these agents be required, it is recommended that therapy with nilotinib be interrupted. If interruption of treatment with nilotinib is not possible, patients who require treatment with a drug that prolongs the QT interval should be closely monitored for prolongation of the QT interval).

No products indexed under this heading.

Estradiol (Nilotinib is a competitive inhibitor of CYP3A4 which may potentially increase the concentration of drugs eliminated by CYP3A4. Caution should be exercised when co-administering nilotinib with substrates for CYP3A4 that have a narrow therapeutic index). Products include:

Activella Tablets **2347**
Angeliq Tablets **751**
Climara Transdermal System **763**
Climara Pro Transdermal System **768**
Divigel **3167**
Vagifem Tablets **2375**

Estradiol Benzoate (Nilotinib is a competitive inhibitor of CYP3A4 which may potentially increase the concentration of drugs eliminated by CYP3A4. Caution should be exercised when co-administering nilotinib with substrates for CYP3A4 that have a narrow therapeutic index).

No products indexed under this heading.

Estradiol Cypionate (Nilotinib is a competitive inhibitor of CYP3A4 which may potentially increase the concentration of drugs eliminated by CYP3A4. Caution should be exercised when co-administering nilotinib with substrates for CYP3A4 that have a narrow therapeutic index).

No products indexed under this heading.

Estradiol Valerate (Nilotinib is a competitive inhibitor of CYP3A4 which may potentially increase the concentration of drugs eliminated by CYP3A4. Caution should be exercised when co-administering nilotinib with substrates for CYP3A4 that have a narrow therapeutic index).
No products indexed under this heading.

Ethinyl Estradiol (Nilotinib is a competitive inhibitor of CYP3A4 which may potentially increase the concentration of drugs eliminated by CYP3A4. Caution should be exercised when co-administering nilotinib with substrates for CYP3A4 that have a narrow therapeutic index). Products include:
Lybrel Tablets 3204
Mircette Tablets 1034
NuvaRing 2897
Ortho-Cyclen/Ortho Tri-Cyclen 2449
Ortho Evra Transdermal System 2437
Ortho Tri-Cyclen Lo Tablets 2458
Seasonique Tablets 1046
Yaz Tablets 805

Ethosuximide (The concomitant use of strong CYP3A4 inducers should be avoided. If patients must be co-administered a strong CYP3A4 inducer, the dose of nilotinib may need to be increased, depending on patient tolerability. If the strong inducer is discontinued, the nilotinib dose should be reduced to the indicated dose).
No products indexed under this heading.

Ethynodiol Diacetate (Nilotinib is a competitive inhibitor of CYP3A4 which may potentially increase the concentration of drugs eliminated by CYP3A4. Caution should be exercised when co-administering nilotinib with substrates for CYP3A4 that have a narrow therapeutic index).
No products indexed under this heading.

Etodolac (Nilotinib is a competitive inhibitor of CYP2C9, potentially increasing the concentration of drugs eliminated by CYP2C9. Caution should be exercised when co-administering nilotinib with substrates for CYP2C9 that have a narrow therapeutic index. Studies also suggest that nilotinib may induce CYP2B6, CYP2C8 and CYP2C9, and thereby has the potential to decrease the concentrations of drugs which are eliminated by these enzymes).
No products indexed under this heading.

Etoposide (Nilotinib is a competitive inhibitor of CYP3A4 which may potentially increase the concentration of drugs eliminated by CYP3A4. Caution should be exercised when co-administering nilotinib with substrates for CYP3A4 that have a narrow therapeutic index).
No products indexed under this heading.

Etoposide Phosphate (Nilotinib is a competitive inhibitor of CYP3A4 which may potentially increase the concentration of drugs eliminated by CYP3A4. Caution should be exercised when co-administering nilotinib with substrates for CYP3A4 that have a narrow therapeutic index).
No products indexed under this heading.

Felbamate (The concomitant use of strong CYP3A4 inducers should be avoided. If patients must be co-administered a strong CYP3A4 inducer, the dose of nilotinib may need to be increased, depending on patient tolerability. If the strong inducer is discontinued, the nilotinib dose should be reduced to the indicated dose).
No products indexed under this heading.

Felodipine (Nilotinib is a competitive inhibitor of CYP3A4 which may potentially increase the concentration of drugs eliminated by CYP3A4. Caution should be exercised when co-administering nilotinib with substrates for CYP3A4 that have a narrow therapeutic index).
No products indexed under this heading.

Fenoprofen Calcium (Nilotinib is a competitive inhibitor of CYP2C9, potentially increasing the concentration of drugs eliminated by CYP2C9. Caution should be exercised when co-administering nilotinib with substrates for CYP2C9 that have a narrow therapeutic index. Studies also suggest that nilotinib may induce CYP2B6, CYP2C8 and CYP2C9, and thereby has the potential to decrease the concentrations of drugs which are eliminated by these enzymes). Products include:
Nalfon Capsules 2508

Fentanyl (Nilotinib is a competitive inhibitor of CYP3A4 which may potentially increase the concentration of drugs eliminated by CYP3A4. Caution should be exercised when co-administering nilotinib with substrates for CYP3A4 that have a narrow therapeutic index). Products include:
Duragesic Transdermal System 2405
Ionsys Transdermal System 2410

Fentanyl Citrate (Nilotinib is a competitive inhibitor of CYP3A4 which may potentially increase the concentration of drugs eliminated by CYP3A4. Caution should be exercised when co-administering nilotinib with substrates for CYP3A4 that have a narrow therapeutic index). Products include:
Actiq 959
Fentora Tablets 968

Flecainide Acetate (The administration of nilotinib with agents that prolong the QT interval should be avoided. Should treatment with any of these agents be required, it is recommended that therapy with nilotinib be interrupted. If interruption of treatment with nilotinib is not possible, patients who require treatment with a drug that prolongs the QT interval should be closely monitored for prolongation of the QT interval).
No products indexed under this heading.

Fludrocortisone Acetate (The concomitant use of strong CYP3A4 inducers should be avoided. If patients must be co-administered a strong CYP3A4 inducer, the dose of nilotinib may need to be increased, depending on patient tolerability. If the strong inducer is discontinued, the nilotinib dose should be reduced to the indicated dose).
No products indexed under this heading.

Fluoxetine (Nilotinib is a competitive inhibitor of CYP2D6, potentially increasing the concentration of drugs eliminated by CYP2D6. Caution should be exercised when co-administering nilotinib with substrates for CYP2D6 that have a narrow therapeutic index).
No products indexed under this heading.

Fluoxetine Hydrochloride (Nilotinib is a competitive inhibitor of CYP2C9, potentially increasing the concentration of drugs eliminated by CYP2C9. Caution should be exercised when co-administering nilotinib with substrates for CYP2C9 that have a narrow therapeutic index. Studies also suggest that nilotinib may induce CYP2B6, CYP2C8 and CYP2C9, and thereby has the potential to decrease the concentrations of drugs which are eliminated by these enzymes). Products include:
Prozac Weekly Capsules 1852
Prozac Pulvules and Liquid 1852
Symbyax Capsules 1871

Fluphenazine Decanoate (The administration of nilotinib with agents that prolong the QT interval should be avoided. Should treatment with any of these agents be required, it is recommended that therapy with nilotinib be interrupted. If interruption of treatment with nilotinib is not possible, patients who require treatment with a drug that prolongs the QT interval should be closely monitored for prolongation of the QT interval).
No products indexed under this heading.

Fluphenazine Enanthate (The administration of nilotinib with agents that prolong the QT interval should be avoided. Should treatment with any of these agents be required, it is recommended that therapy with nilotinib be interrupted. If interruption of treatment with nilotinib is not possible, patients who require treatment with a drug that prolongs the QT interval should be closely monitored for prolongation of the QT interval).
No products indexed under this heading.

Fluphenazine Hydrochloride (The administration of nilotinib with agents that prolong the QT interval should be avoided. Should treatment with any of these agents be required, it is recommended that therapy with nilotinib be interrupted. If interruption of treatment with nilotinib is not possible, patients who require treatment with a drug that prolongs the QT interval should be closely monitored for prolongation of the QT interval).
No products indexed under this heading.

Flurbiprofen (Nilotinib is a competitive inhibitor of CYP2C9, potentially increasing the concentration of drugs eliminated by CYP2C9. Caution should be exercised when co-administering nilotinib with substrates for CYP2C9 that have a narrow therapeutic index. Studies also suggest that nilotinib may induce CYP2B6, CYP2C8 and CYP2C9, and thereby has the potential to decrease the concentrations of drugs which are eliminated by these enzymes).
No products indexed under this heading.

Flurbiprofen Sodium (Nilotinib is a competitive inhibitor of CYP2C9, potentially increasing the concentration of drugs eliminated by CYP2C9. Caution should be exercised when co-administering nilotinib with substrates for CYP2C9 that have a narrow therapeutic index. Studies also suggest that nilotinib may induce CYP2B6, CYP2C8 and CYP2C9, and thereby has the potential to decrease the concentrations of drugs which are eliminated by these enzymes).
No products indexed under this heading.

Fluvastatin Sodium (Nilotinib is a competitive inhibitor of CYP2C8, potentially increasing the concentration of drugs eliminated by CYP2C8. Caution should be exercised when co-administering nilotinib with substrates for CYP2C8 that have a narrow therapeutic index. Studies also suggest that nilotinib may induce CYP2B6, CYP2C8 and CYP2C9, and thereby has the potential to decrease the concentrations of drugs which are eliminated by these enzymes). Products include:
Lescol Capsules 2268
Lescol XL Tablets 2268

Fluvoxamine Maleate (Nilotinib is a competitive inhibitor of CYP2D6, potentially increasing the concentration of drugs eliminated by CYP2D6. Caution should be exercised when co-administering nilotinib with substrates for CYP2D6 that have a narrow therapeutic index). Products include:
Luvox CR Extended-Release Capsules 1759

Formoterol Fumarate (Nilotinib is a competitive inhibitor of CYP2D6, potentially increasing the concentration of drugs eliminated by CYP2D6. Caution should be exercised when co-administering nilotinib with substrates for CYP2D6 that have a narrow therapeutic index). Products include:
Foradil Aerolizer 2849
Perforomist Inhalation Solution 1025

Fosamprenavir Calcium (The concomitant use of strong CYP3A4 inhibitors should be avoided. Should treatment with any of these agents be required, it is recommended that therapy with nilotinib be interrupted. If patients must be co-administered a strong CYP3A4 inhibitor, based on pharmacokinetic studies, 400 mg once daily is predicted to adjust the nilotinib AUC to the AUC observed without inhibitors. However, there are no clinical data with this dose adjustment in patients receiving strong CYP3A4 inhibitors. If the strong inhibitor is discontinued, a washout period should be allowed before the nilotinib dose is adjusted upward to the indicated dose. Close monitoring for prolongation of the QT interval is indicated for patients who cannot avoid strong CYP3A4 inhibitors). Products include:
Lexiva Oral Suspension 1510
Lexiva Tablets 1510

Fosphenytoin Sodium (The concomitant use of strong CYP3A4 inducers such as phenytoin should be avoided. If patients must be co-administered a strong CYP3A4 inducer, the dose of nilotinib may need to be increased, depending on patient tolerability. If the strong inducer is discontinued, the nilotinib dose should be reduced to the indicated dose).
No products indexed under this heading.

Galantamine Hydrobromide (Nilotinib is a competitive inhibitor of CYP2D6, potentially increasing the concentration of drugs eliminated by CYP2D6. Caution should be exercised when co-administering nilotinib with substrates for CYP2D6 that have a narrow therapeutic index).
No products indexed under this heading.

Garlic Extract (The concomitant use of strong CYP3A4 inducers should be avoided. If patients must be co-administered a strong CYP3A4 inducer, the dose of nilotinib may need to be increased, depending on patient tolerability. If the strong inducer is discontinued, the nilotinib dose should be reduced to the indicated dose).
No products indexed under this heading.

Garlic Oil (The concomitant use of strong CYP3A4 inducers should be avoided. If patients must be co-administered a strong CYP3A4 inducer, the dose of nilotinib may need to be increased, depending on patient tolerability. If the strong inducer is discontinued, the nilotinib dose should be reduced to the indicated dose).
No products indexed under this heading.

Glimepiride (Nilotinib is a competitive inhibitor of CYP2C9, potentially increasing the concentration of drugs eliminated by CYP2C9. Caution should be exercised when co-administering nilotinib with substrates for CYP2C9 that have a narrow therapeutic index. Studies also suggest that nilotinib may induce CYP2B6, CYP2C8 and CYP2C9, and thereby has the potential to decrease the concentrations of drugs which are eliminated by these enzymes). Products include:
Avandaryl Tablets 1344
Duetact Tablets 3085

Glipizide (Nilotinib is a competitive inhibitor of CYP2C9, potentially increasing the concentration of drugs eliminated by CYP2C9. Caution should be exercised when co-administering nilotinib with substrates for CYP2C9 that have a narrow therapeutic index. Studies also suggest that nilotinib may induce CYP2B6, CYP2C8 and CYP2C9, and thereby has the potential to decrease the concentrations of drugs which are eliminated by these enzymes).
No products indexed under this heading.

Haloperidol (The administration of nilotinib with agents that prolong the QT interval should be avoided. Should treatment with any of these agents be required, it is recommended that therapy with nilotinib be interrupted. If interruption of treatment with nilotinib is not possible, patients who require treatment with a drug that prolongs the QT interval should be closely monitored for prolongation of the QT interval).
No products indexed under this heading.

Haloperidol Decanoate (The administration of nilotinib with agents that prolong the QT interval should be avoided. Should treatment with any of these agents be required, it is recommended that therapy with nilotinib be interrupted. If interruption of treatment with nilotinib is not possible, patients who require treatment with a drug that prolongs the QT interval should be closely monitored for prolongation of the QT interval).
No products indexed under this heading.

Haloperidol Lactate (Nilotinib is a competitive inhibitor of CYP3A4 which may potentially increase the concentration of drugs eliminated by CYP3A4. Caution should be exercised when co-administering nilotinib with substrates for CYP3A4 that have a narrow therapeutic index).
No products indexed under this heading.

Hydrocodone Bitartrate (Nilotinib is a competitive inhibitor of CYP2D6, potentially increasing the concentration of drugs eliminated by CYP2D6. Caution should be exercised when co-administering nilotinib with substrates for CYP2D6 that have a narrow therapeutic index). Products include:
Lortab 5/500 Tablets 3143
Lortab 7.5/500 Tablets 3144
Lortab 10/500 Tablets 3144
Vicodin Tablets 529
Vicodin ES Tablets 530
Vicodin HP Tablets 531
Vicoprofen Tablets 533
Zydone Tablets 1132

Hydrocortisone (The concomitant use of strong CYP3A4 inducers should be avoided. If patients must be co-administered a strong CYP3A4 inducer, the dose of nilotinib may need to be increased, depending on patient tolerability. If the strong inducer is discontinued, the nilotinib dose should be reduced to the indicated dose).
No products indexed under this heading.

Hydrocortisone Acetate (The concomitant use of strong CYP3A4 inducers should be avoided. If patients must be co-administered a strong CYP3A4 inducer, the dose of nilotinib may need to be increased, depending on patient tolerability. If the strong inducer is discontinued, the nilotinib dose should be reduced to the indicated dose). Products include:
Analpram-HC 1140
Pramosone 1141

Hydrocortisone Butyrate (The concomitant use of strong CYP3A4 inducers should be avoided. If patients must be co-administered a strong CYP3A4 inducer, the dose of nilotinib may need to be increased, depending on patient tolerability. If the strong inducer is discontinued, the nilotinib dose should be reduced to the indicated dose).
No products indexed under this heading.

Hydrocortisone Cypionate (The concomitant use of strong CYP3A4 inducers should be avoided. If patients must be co-administered a strong CYP3A4 inducer, the dose of nilotinib may need to be increased, depending on patient tolerability. If the strong inducer is discontinued, the nilotinib dose should be reduced to the indicated dose).
No products indexed under this heading.

Hydrocortisone Hemisuccinate (The concomitant use of strong CYP3A4 inducers should be avoided. If patients must be co-administered a strong CYP3A4 inducer, the dose of nilotinib may need to be increased, depending on patient tolerability. If the strong inducer is discontinued, the nilotinib dose should be reduced to the indicated dose).
No products indexed under this heading.

Hydrocortisone Probutate (The concomitant use of strong CYP3A4 inducers should be avoided. If patients must be co-administered a strong CYP3A4 inducer, the dose of nilotinib may need to be increased, depending on patient tolerability. If the strong inducer is discontinued, the nilotinib dose should be reduced to the indicated dose).
No products indexed under this heading.

Hydrocortisone Sodium Phosphate (The concomitant use of strong CYP3A4 inducers should be avoided. If patients must be co-administered a strong CYP3A4 inducer, the dose of nilotinib may need to be increased, depending on patient tolerability. If the strong inducer is discontinued, the nilotinib dose should be reduced to the indicated dose).
No products indexed under this heading.

Hydrocortisone Sodium Succinate (The concomitant use of strong CYP3A4 inducers should be avoided. If patients must be co-administered a strong CYP3A4 inducer, the dose of nilotinib may need to be increased, depending on patient tolerability. If the strong inducer is discontinued, the nilotinib dose should be reduced to the indicated dose).
No products indexed under this heading.

Hydrocortisone Valerate (The concomitant use of strong CYP3A4 inducers should be avoided. If patients must be co-administered a strong CYP3A4 inducer, the dose of nilotinib may need to be increased, depending on patient tolerability. If the strong inducer is discontinued, the nilotinib dose should be reduced to the indicated dose).
No products indexed under this heading.

Hydroxyzine Hydrochloride (The administration of nilotinib with agents that prolong the QT interval should be avoided. Should treatment with any of these agents be required, it is recommended that therapy with nilotinib be interrupted. If interruption of treatment with nilotinib is not possible, patients who require treatment with a drug that prolongs the QT interval should be closely monitored for prolongation of the QT interval).
No products indexed under this heading.

Hypericum (Concomitant use with St. John's Wort should be avoided). Products include:
Satieté Tablets .... ▣ 640

Hypericum Perforatum (The concomitant use of strong CYP3A4 inducers should be avoided. If patients must be co-administered a strong CYP3A4 inducer, the dose of nilotinib may need to be increased, depending on patient tolerability. If the strong inducer is discontinued, the nilotinib dose should be reduced to the indicated dose).
No products indexed under this heading.

Ibuprofen (Nilotinib is a competitive inhibitor of CYP2C9, potentially increasing the concentration of drugs eliminated by CYP2C9. Caution should be exercised when co-administering nilotinib with substrates for CYP2C9 that have a narrow therapeutic index. Studies also suggest that nilotinib may induce CYP2B6, CYP2C8 and CYP2C9, and thereby has the potential to decrease the concentrations of drugs which are eliminated by these enzymes). Products include:
Motrin IB Tablets and Caplets 1900
Children's Motrin Oral Suspension ... 1901
Children's Motrin Non-Staining Dye-Free Oral Suspension 1901
Children's Motrin Cold Oral Suspension 1899
Infants' Motrin Concentrated Drops 1901
Infants' Motrin Non-Staining Dye-Free Concentrated Drops 1901
Junior Strength Motrin Caplets and Chewable Tablets 1901
Vicoprofen Tablets 533

Imipramine Hydrochloride (The administration of nilotinib with agents that prolong the QT interval should be avoided. Should treatment with any of these agents be required, it is recommended that therapy with nilotinib be interrupted. If interruption of treatment with nilotinib is not possible, patients who require treatment with a drug that prolongs the QT interval should be closely monitored for prolongation of the QT interval).
No products indexed under this heading.

Imipramine Pamoate (The administration of nilotinib with agents that prolong the QT interval should be avoided. Should treatment with any of these agents be required, it is recommended that therapy with nilotinib be interrupted. If interruption of treatment with nilotinib is not possible, patients who require treatment with a drug that prolongs the QT interval should be closely monitored for prolongation of the QT interval).
No products indexed under this heading.

Indinavir Sulfate (The concomitant use of strong CYP3A4 inhibitors such as indinavir should be avoided. If treatment is required, it is recommended that therapy with nilotinib be interrupted. If patients must be co-administered a strong CYP3A4 inhibitor, based on pharmacokinetic studies, 400 mg q.d. is predicted to adjust the nilotinib AUC to the AUC observed without inhibitors. However, there are no clinical data with this dose adjustment in patients receiving strong CYP3A4 inhibitors. If the strong inhibitor is discontinued, a washout period should be allowed before the nilotinib dose is adjusted

upward to the indicated dose. Close monitoring for prolongation of the QT interval is indicated for patients who cannot avoid strong CYP3A4 inhibitors). Products include:

Crixivan Capsules 1979

Indomethacin (Nilotinib is a competitive inhibitor of CYP2C9, potentially increasing the concentration of drugs eliminated by CYP2C9. Caution should be exercised when co-administering nilotinib with substrates for CYP2C9 that have a narrow therapeutic index. Studies also suggest that nilotinib may induce CYP2B6, CYP2C8 and CYP2C9, and thereby has the potential to decrease the concentrations of drugs which are eliminated by these enzymes). Products include:

Indocin 2024

Indomethacin Sodium Trihydrate (Nilotinib is a competitive inhibitor of CYP2C9, potentially increasing the concentration of drugs eliminated by CYP2C9. Caution should be exercised when co-administering nilotinib with substrates for CYP2C9 that have a narrow therapeutic index. Studies also suggest that nilotinib may induce CYP2B6, CYP2C8 and CYP2C9, and thereby has the potential to decrease the concentrations of drugs which are eliminated by these enzymes). Products include:

Indocin I.V. 2489

Indoramin Hydrochloride (Nilotinib is a competitive inhibitor of CYP2D6, potentially increasing the concentration of drugs eliminated by CYP2D6. Caution should be exercised when co-administering nilotinib with substrates for CYP2D6 that have a narrow therapeutic index).

No products indexed under this heading.

Irbesartan (Nilotinib is a competitive inhibitor of CYP2C9, potentially increasing the concentration of drugs eliminated by CYP2C9. Caution should be exercised when co-administering nilotinib with substrates for CYP2C9 that have a narrow therapeutic index. Studies also suggest that nilotinib may induce CYP2B6, CYP2C8 and CYP2C9, and thereby has the potential to decrease the concentrations of drugs which are eliminated by these enzymes). Products include:

Avalide Tablets 892
Avalide Tablets 2713
Avapro Tablets 897
Avapro Tablets 2718

Isocarboxazid (The administration of nilotinib with agents that prolong the QT interval should be avoided. Should treatment with any of these agents be required, it is recommended that therapy with nilotinib be interrupted. If interruption of treatment with nilotinib is not possible, patients who require treatment with a drug that prolongs the QT interval should be closely monitored for prolongation of the QT interval). Products include:

Marplan Tablets 3177

Isotretinoin (Nilotinib is a competitive inhibitor of CYP2C8, potentially increasing the concentration of drugs eliminated by CYP2C8. Caution should be exercised when co-administering nilotinib with substrates for CYP2C8 that have a narrow therapeutic index. Studies also suggest that nilotinib may induce CYP2B6, CYP2C8 and CYP2C9, and thereby has the potential to decrease the concentrations of drugs which are eliminated by these enzymes). Products include:

Accutane Capsules 2607

Isradipine (Nilotinib is a competitive inhibitor of CYP3A4 which may potentially increase the concentration of drugs eliminated by CYP3A4. Caution should be exercised when co-administering nilotinib with substrates for CYP3A4 that have a narrow therapeutic index). Products include:

DynaCirc CR Controlled Release Tablets 1407

Itraconazole (The concomitant use of strong CYP3A4 inhibitors such as itraconazole should be avoided. If treatment is required, it is recommended that therapy with nilotinib be interrupted. If patients must be co-administered a strong CYP3A4 inhibitor, based on pharmacokinetic studies, 400 mg q.d. is predicted to adjust the nilotinib AUC to the AUC observed without inhibitors. However, there are no clinical data with this dose adjustment in patients receiving strong CYP3A4 inhibitors. If the strong inhibitor is discontinued, a washout period should be allowed before the nilotinib dose is adjusted upward to the indicated dose. Close monitoring for prolongation of the QT interval is indicated for patients who cannot avoid strong CYP3A4 inhibitors).

No products indexed under this heading.

Ixabepilone (Nilotinib is a competitive inhibitor of CYP3A4 which may potentially increase the concentration of drugs eliminated by CYP3A4. Caution should be exercised when co-administering nilotinib with substrates for CYP3A4 that have a narrow therapeutic index). Products include:

Ixempra Kit for Injection 915

Ketoconazole (The concomitant use of strong CYP3A4 inhibitors such as ketoconazole should be avoided. If treatment is required, it is recommended that therapy with nilotinib be interrupted. If patients must be co-administered a strong CYP3A4 inhibitor, based on pharmacokinetic studies, 400 mg q.d. is predicted to adjust the nilotinib AUC to the AUC observed without inhibitors. However, there are no clinical data with this dose adjustment in patients receiving strong CYP3A4 inhibitors. If the strong inhibitor is discontinued, a washout period should be allowed before the nilotinib dose is adjusted upward to the indicated dose. Close monitoring for prolongation of the QT interval is indicated for patients who cannot avoid strong CYP3A4 inhibitors). Products include:

Extina Foam, 2% 3057
Nizoral A-D Shampoo 1901

Ketoprofen (Nilotinib is a competitive inhibitor of CYP2C9, potentially increasing the concentration of drugs eliminated by CYP2C9. Caution should be exercised when co-administering nilotinib with substrates for CYP2C9 that have a narrow therapeutic index. Studies also suggest that nilotinib may induce CYP2B6, CYP2C8 and CYP2C9, and thereby has the potential to decrease the concentrations of drugs which are eliminated by these enzymes).

No products indexed under this heading.

Ketorolac Tromethamine (Nilotinib is a competitive inhibitor of CYP2C9, potentially increasing the concentration of drugs eliminated by CYP2C9. Caution should be exercised when co-administering nilotinib with substrates for CYP2C9 that have a narrow therapeutic index. Studies also suggest that nilotinib may induce CYP2B6, CYP2C8 and CYP2C9, and thereby has the potential to decrease the concentrations of drugs which are eliminated by these enzymes).

No products indexed under this heading.

Labetalol Hydrochloride (Nilotinib is a competitive inhibitor of CYP2D6, potentially increasing the concentration of drugs eliminated by CYP2D6. Caution should be exercised when co-administering nilotinib with substrates for CYP2D6 that have a narrow therapeutic index).

No products indexed under this heading.

Lansoprazole (Nilotinib is a competitive inhibitor of CYP2C9, potentially increasing the concentration of drugs eliminated by CYP2C9. Caution should be exercised when co-administering nilotinib with substrates for CYP2C9 that have a narrow therapeutic index. Studies also suggest that nilotinib may induce CYP2B6, CYP2C8 and CYP2C9, and thereby has the potential to decrease the concentrations of drugs which are eliminated by these enzymes).

No products indexed under this heading.

Lapatinib (Nilotinib inhibits human P-glycoprotein. If nilotinib is administered with drugs that are substrates of Pgp, increased concentrations of the substrate drug are likely, and caution should be exercised). Products include:

Tykerb Tablets 1631

Levonorgestrel (Nilotinib is a competitive inhibitor of CYP3A4 which may potentially increase the concentration of drugs eliminated by CYP3A4. Caution should be exercised when co-administering nilotinib with substrates for CYP3A4 that have a narrow therapeutic index). Products include:

Climara Pro Transdermal System 768
Lybrel Tablets 3204
Mirena Intrauterine System 779
Plan B Tablets 1044
Seasonique Tablets 1046

Lidocaine (Nilotinib is a competitive inhibitor of CYP3A4 which may potentially increase the concentration of drugs eliminated by CYP3A4. Caution should be exercised when co-administering nilotinib with substrates for CYP3A4 that have a narrow therapeutic index). Products include:

Lidoderm Patch 1114

Lidocaine Hydrochloride (The administration of nilotinib with agents that prolong the QT interval should be avoided. Should treatment with any of these agents be required, it is recommended that therapy with nilotinib be interrupted. If interruption of treatment with nilotinib is not possible, patients who require treatment with a drug that prolongs the QT interval should be closely monitored for prolongation of the QT interval).

No products indexed under this heading.

Lithium Carbonate (The administration of nilotinib with agents that prolong the QT interval should be avoided. Should treatment with any of these agents be required, it is recommended that therapy with nilotinib be interrupted. If interruption of treatment with nilotinib is not possible, patients who require treatment with a drug that prolongs the QT interval should be closely monitored for prolongation of the QT interval).

No products indexed under this heading.

Lithium Citrate (The administration of nilotinib with agents that prolong the QT interval should be avoided. Should treatment with any of these agents be required, it is recommended that therapy with nilotinib be interrupted. If interruption of treatment with nilotinib is not possible, patients who require treatment with a drug that prolongs the QT interval should be closely monitored for prolongation of the QT interval).

No products indexed under this heading.

Lopinavir (The concomitant use of strong CYP3A4 inhibitors should be avoided. Should treatment with any of these agents be required, it is recommended that therapy with nilotinib be interrupted. If patients must be co-administered a strong CYP3A4 inhibitor, based on pharmacokinetic studies, 400 mg once daily is predicted to adjust the nilotinib AUC to the AUC observed without inhibitors. However, there are no clinical data with this dose adjustment in patients receiving strong CYP3A4 inhibitors. If the strong inhibitor is discontinued, a washout period should be allowed before the nilotinib dose is adjusted upward to the indicated dose. Close monitoring for prolongation of the QT interval is indicated for patients who cannot avoid strong CYP3A4 inhibitors). Products include:

Kaletra 452

Lorazepam (The administration of nilotinib with agents that prolong the QT interval should be avoided. Should treatment with any of these agents be required, it is recommended that therapy with nilotinib be interrupted. If interruption of treatment with nilotinib is not possible, patients who require treatment with a drug that prolongs the QT interval should be closely monitored for prolongation of the QT interval).

No products indexed under this heading.

Losartan Potassium (Nilotinib is a competitive inhibitor of CYP2C9, potentially increasing the concentration of drugs eliminated by CYP2C9. Caution should be exercised when co-administering nilotinib with substrates for CYP2C9 that have a narrow therapeutic index. Studies also suggest that nilotinib may induce CYP2B6, CYP2C8 and CYP2C9, and thereby has the potential to decrease the concentrations of drugs which are eliminated by these enzymes). Products include:

Cozaar Tablets 1973

Lovastatin (Nilotinib inhibits human P-glycoprotein. If nilotinib is administered with drugs that are substrates of Pgp, increased concentrations of the substrate drug are likely, and caution should be exercised). Products include:

Advicor Tablets **402**
Mevacor Tablets **2063**

Loxapine Hydrochloride (The administration of nilotinib with agents that prolong the QT interval should be avoided. Should treatment with any of these agents be required, it is recommended that therapy with nilotinib be interrupted. If interruption of treatment with nilotinib is not possible, patients who require treatment with a drug that prolongs the QT interval should be closely monitored for prolongation of the QT interval).
No products indexed under this heading.

Loxapine Succinate (The administration of nilotinib with agents that prolong the QT interval should be avoided. Should treatment with any of these agents be required, it is recommended that therapy with nilotinib be interrupted. If interruption of treatment with nilotinib is not possible, patients who require treatment with a drug that prolongs the QT interval should be closely monitored for prolongation of the QT interval).
No products indexed under this heading.

Maprotiline Hydrochloride (The administration of nilotinib with agents that prolong the QT interval should be avoided. Should treatment with any of these agents be required, it is recommended that therapy with nilotinib be interrupted. If interruption of treatment with nilotinib is not possible, patients who require treatment with a drug that prolongs the QT interval should be closely monitored for prolongation of the QT interval).
No products indexed under this heading.

Maraviroc (Nilotinib inhibits human P-glycoprotein. If nilotinib is administered with drugs that are substrates of Pgp, increased concentrations of the substrate drug are likely, and caution should be exercised). Products include:

Selzentry Tablets **2534**

Meclofenamate Sodium (Nilotinib is a competitive inhibitor of CYP2C9, potentially increasing the concentration of drugs eliminated by CYP2C9. Caution should be exercised when co-administering nilotinib with substrates for CYP2C9 that have a narrow therapeutic index. Studies also suggest that nilotinib may induce CYP2B6, CYP2C8 and CYP2C9, and thereby has the potential to decrease the concentrations of drugs which are eliminated by these enzymes).
No products indexed under this heading.

Mefenamic Acid (Nilotinib is a competitive inhibitor of CYP2C9, potentially increasing the concentration of drugs eliminated by CYP2C9. Caution should be exercised when co-administering nilotinib with substrates for CYP2C9 that have a narrow therapeutic index. Studies also suggest that nilotinib may induce CYP2B6, CYP2C8 and CYP2C9, and thereby has the potential to decrease the concentrations of drugs which are eliminated by these enzymes).
No products indexed under this heading.

Meloxicam (Nilotinib is a competitive inhibitor of CYP2C9, potentially increasing the concentration of drugs eliminated by CYP2C9. Caution should be exercised when co-administering nilotinib with substrates for CYP2C9 that have a narrow therapeutic index. Studies also suggest that nilotinib may induce CYP2B6, CYP2C8 and CYP2C9, and thereby has the potential to decrease the concentrations of drugs which are eliminated by these enzymes). Products include:

Mobic Oral Suspension **863**
Mobic Tablets **863**

Meperidine Hydrochloride (Nilotinib is a competitive inhibitor of CYP2D6, potentially increasing the concentration of drugs eliminated by CYP2D6. Caution should be exercised when co-administering nilotinib with substrates for CYP2D6 that have a narrow therapeutic index).
No products indexed under this heading.

Mephenytoin (The concomitant use of strong CYP3A4 inducers should be avoided. If patients must be co-administered a strong CYP3A4 inducer, the dose of nilotinib may need to be increased, depending on patient tolerability. If the strong inducer is discontinued, the nilotinib dose should be reduced to the indicated dose).
No products indexed under this heading.

Mephobarbital (Nilotinib is a competitive inhibitor of CYP2C8, potentially increasing the concentration of drugs eliminated by CYP2C8. Caution should be exercised when co-administering nilotinib with substrates for CYP2C8 that have a narrow therapeutic index. Studies also suggest that nilotinib may induce CYP2B6, CYP2C8 and CYP2C9, and thereby has the potential to decrease the concentrations of drugs which are eliminated by these enzymes).
No products indexed under this heading.

Meprobamate (The administration of nilotinib with agents that prolong the QT interval should be avoided. Should treatment with any of these agents be required, it is recommended that therapy with nilotinib be interrupted. If interruption of treatment with nilotinib is not possible, patients who require treatment with a drug that prolongs the QT interval should be closely monitored for prolongation of the QT interval).
No products indexed under this heading.

Mesoridazine Besylate (The administration of nilotinib with agents that prolong the QT interval should be avoided. Should treatment with any of these agents be required, it is recommended that therapy with nilotinib be interrupted. If interruption of treatment with nilotinib is not possible, patients who require treatment with a drug that prolongs the QT interval should be closely monitored for prolongation of the QT interval).
No products indexed under this heading.

Mestranol (Nilotinib is a competitive inhibitor of CYP3A4 which may potentially increase the concentration of drugs eliminated by CYP3A4. Caution should be exercised when co-administering nilotinib with substrates for CYP3A4 that have a narrow therapeutic index).
No products indexed under this heading.

Metformin Hydrochloride (Nilotinib is a competitive inhibitor of CYP2C9, potentially increasing the concentration of drugs eliminated by CYP2C9. Caution should be exercised when co-administering nilotinib with substrates for CYP2C9 that have a narrow therapeutic index. Studies also suggest that nilotinib may induce CYP2B6, CYP2C8 and CYP2C9, and thereby has the potential to decrease the concentrations of drugs which are eliminated by these enzymes). Products include:

ActoPlus Met Tablets **3071**
Avandamet Tablets **1336**
Janumet Tablets **2041**
PrandiMet Tablets **2967**

Methadone Hydrochloride (Nilotinib is a competitive inhibitor of CYP3A4 which may potentially increase the concentration of drugs eliminated by CYP3A4. Caution should be exercised when co-administering nilotinib with substrates for CYP3A4 that have a narrow therapeutic index).
No products indexed under this heading.

Methamphetamine Hydrochloride (Nilotinib is a competitive inhibitor of CYP2D6, potentially increasing the concentration of drugs eliminated by CYP2D6. Caution should be exercised when co-administering nilotinib with substrates for CYP2D6 that have a narrow therapeutic index).
No products indexed under this heading.

Methsuximide (The concomitant use of strong CYP3A4 inducers should be avoided. If patients must be co-administered a strong CYP3A4 inducer, the dose of nilotinib may need to be increased, depending on patient tolerability. If the strong inducer is discontinued, the nilotinib dose should be reduced to the indicated dose).
No products indexed under this heading.

Methylprednisolone (The concomitant use of strong CYP3A4 inducers should be avoided. If patients must be co-administered a strong CYP3A4 inducer, the dose of nilotinib may need to be increased, depending on patient tolerability. If the strong inducer is discontinued, the nilotinib dose should be reduced to the indicated dose).
No products indexed under this heading.

Methylprednisolone Acetate (The concomitant use of strong CYP3A4 inducers should be avoided. If patients must be co-administered a strong CYP3A4 inducer, the dose of nilotinib may need to be increased, depending on patient tolerability. If the strong inducer is discontinued, the nilotinib dose should be reduced to the indicated dose).
No products indexed under this heading.

Methylprednisolone Sodium Succinate (The concomitant use of strong CYP3A4 inducers should be avoided. If patients must be co-administered a strong CYP3A4 inducer, the dose of nilotinib may need to be increased, depending on patient tolerability. If the strong inducer is discontinued, the nilotinib dose should be reduced to the indicated dose).
No products indexed under this heading.

Metoprolol Succinate (Nilotinib is a competitive inhibitor of CYP2D6, potentially increasing the concentration of drugs eliminated by CYP2D6. Caution should be exercised when co-administering nilotinib with substrates for CYP2D6 that have a narrow therapeutic index). Products include:

Toprol-XL Tablets **666**

Metoprolol Tartrate (Nilotinib is a competitive inhibitor of CYP2D6, potentially increasing the concentration of drugs eliminated by CYP2D6. Caution should be exercised when co-administering nilotinib with substrates for CYP2D6 that have a narrow therapeutic index).
No products indexed under this heading.

Mexiletine Hydrochloride (The administration of nilotinib with agents that prolong the QT interval should be avoided. Should treatment with any of these agents be required, it is recommended that therapy with nilotinib be interrupted. If interruption of treatment with nilotinib is not possible, patients who require treatment with a drug that prolongs the QT interval should be closely monitored for prolongation of the QT interval).
No products indexed under this heading.

Mibefradil Dihydrochloride (Nilotinib is a substrate of the efflux transporter P-glycoprotein (Pgp, ABCB1). If nilotinib is administered with drugs that inhibit Pgp, increased concentrations of nilotinib are likely, and caution should be exercised).
No products indexed under this heading.

Midazolam Hydrochloride (Single-dose administration of nilotinib with midazolam (a CYP3A4 substrate) to healthy subjects increased midazolam exposure by 30%).
No products indexed under this heading.

Miglitol (Nilotinib is a competitive inhibitor of CYP2C9, potentially increasing the concentration of drugs eliminated by CYP2C9. Caution should be exercised when co-administering nilotinib with substrates for CYP2C9 that have a narrow therapeutic index. Studies also suggest that nilotinib may induce CYP2B6, CYP2C8 and CYP2C9, and thereby has the potential to decrease the concentrations of drugs which are eliminated by these enzymes).
No products indexed under this heading.

Mirtazapine (Nilotinib is a competitive inhibitor of CYP2C9, potentially increasing the concentration of drugs eliminated by CYP2C9. Caution should be exercised when co-administering nilotinib with substrates for CYP2C9 that have a

narrow therapeutic index. Studies also suggest that nilotinib may induce CYP2B6, CYP2C8 and CYP2C9, and thereby has the potential to decrease the concentrations of drugs which are eliminated by these enzymes). Products include:
Remeron Tablets **2924**
RemeronSolTab Tablets **2927**

Modafinil (The concomitant use of strong CYP3A4 inducers should be avoided. If patients must be co-administered a strong CYP3A4 inducer, the dose of nilotinib may need to be increased, depending on patient tolerability. If the strong inducer is discontinued, the nilotinib dose should be reduced to the indicated dose). Products include:
Provigil Tablets **977**

Molindone Hydrochloride (The administration of nilotinib with agents that prolong the QT interval should be avoided. Should treatment with any of these agents be required, it is recommended that therapy with nilotinib be interrupted. If interruption of treatment with nilotinib is not possible, patients who require treatment with a drug that prolongs the QT interval should be closely monitored for prolongation of the QT interval). Products include:
Moban Tablets **1116**

Montelukast Sodium (Nilotinib is a competitive inhibitor of CYP2C9, potentially increasing the concentration of drugs eliminated by CYP2C9. Caution should be exercised when co-administering nilotinib with substrates for CYP2C9 that have a narrow therapeutic index. Studies also suggest that nilotinib may induce CYP2B6, CYP2C8 and CYP2C9, and thereby has the potential to decrease the concentrations of drugs which are eliminated by these enzymes). Products include:
Singulair **2114**

Morphine Sulfate (Nilotinib is a competitive inhibitor of CYP2D6, potentially increasing the concentration of drugs eliminated by CYP2D6. Caution should be exercised when co-administering nilotinib with substrates for CYP2D6 that have a narrow therapeutic index). Products include:
Avinza Capsules **1772**
DepoDur Injection **1095**
MS Contin Tablets **2585**

Nabumetone (Nilotinib is a competitive inhibitor of CYP2C9, potentially increasing the concentration of drugs eliminated by CYP2C9. Caution should be exercised when co-administering nilotinib with substrates for CYP2C9 that have a narrow therapeutic index. Studies also suggest that nilotinib may induce CYP2B6, CYP2C8 and CYP2C9, and thereby has the potential to decrease the concentrations of drugs which are eliminated by these enzymes).
No products indexed under this heading.

Naproxen (Nilotinib is a competitive inhibitor of CYP2C9, potentially increasing the concentration of drugs eliminated by CYP2C9. Caution should be exercised when co-administering nilotinib with substrates for CYP2C9 that have a narrow therapeutic index. Studies also suggest that nilotinib may induce CYP2B6, CYP2C8 and CYP2C9, and thereby has the potential to decrease the concentrations of drugs which are eliminated by these enzymes). Products include:
EC-Naprosyn Delayed-Release Tablets **2632**
Naprosyn Suspension **2632**
Naprosyn Tablets **2632**

Naproxen Sodium (Nilotinib is a competitive inhibitor of CYP2C9, potentially increasing the concentration of drugs eliminated by CYP2C9. Caution should be exercised when co-administering nilotinib with substrates for CYP2C9 that have a narrow therapeutic index. Studies also suggest that nilotinib may induce CYP2B6, CYP2C8 and CYP2C9, and thereby has the potential to decrease the concentrations of drugs which are eliminated by these enzymes). Products include:
Anaprox Tablets **2632**
Anaprox DS Tablets **2632**
Treximet Tablets **1616**

Nateglinide (Nilotinib is a competitive inhibitor of CYP2C9, potentially increasing the concentration of drugs eliminated by CYP2C9. Caution should be exercised when co-administering nilotinib with substrates for CYP2C9 that have a narrow therapeutic index. Studies also suggest that nilotinib may induce CYP2B6, CYP2C8 and CYP2C9, and thereby has the potential to decrease the concentrations of drugs which are eliminated by these enzymes). Products include:
Starlix Tablets **2314**

Nefazodone Hydrochloride (The concomitant use of strong CYP3A4 inhibitors such as nefazodone should be avoided. If treatment is required, it is recommended that therapy with nilotinib be interrupted. If patients must be co-administered a strong CYP3A4 inhibitor, based on pharmacokinetic studies, 400 mg q.d. is predicted to adjust the nilotinib AUC to the AUC observed without inhibitors. However, there are no clinical data with this dose adjustment in patients receiving strong CYP3A4 inhibitors. If the strong inhibitor is discontinued, a washout period should be allowed before the nilotinib dose is adjusted upward to the indicated dose. Close monitoring for prolongation of the QT interval is indicated for patients who cannot avoid strong CYP3A4 inhibitors).
No products indexed under this heading.

Nelfinavir Mesylate (The concomitant use of strong CYP3A4 inhibitors such as neflinavir should be avoided. If treatment is required, it is recommended that therapy with nilotinib be interrupted. If patients must be co-administered a strong CYP3A4 inhibitor, based on pharmacokinetic studies, 400 mg q.d. is predicted to adjust the nilotinib AUC to the AUC observed without inhibitors. However, there are no clinical data with this dose adjustment in patients receiving strong CYP3A4 inhibitors. If the strong inhibitor is discontinued, a washout period should be allowed before the nilotinib dose is adjusted upward to the indicated dose. Close monitoring for prolongation of the QT interval is indicated for patients who cannot avoid strong CYP3A4 inhibitors).
No products indexed under this heading.

Nevirapine (The concomitant use of strong CYP3A4 inducers should be avoided. If patients must be co-administered a strong CYP3A4 inducer, the dose of nilotinib may need to be increased, depending on patient tolerability. If the strong inducer is discontinued, the nilotinib dose should be reduced to the indicated dose). Products include:
Viramune Oral Suspension **873**
Viramune Tablets **873**

Nicardipine Hydrochloride (Nilotinib is a competitive inhibitor of CYP3A4 which may potentially increase the concentration of drugs eliminated by CYP3A4. Caution should be exercised when co-administering nilotinib with substrates for CYP3A4 that have a narrow therapeutic index). Products include:
Cardene I.V. **1093**

Nifedipine (Nilotinib is a competitive inhibitor of CYP3A4 which may potentially increase the concentration of drugs eliminated by CYP3A4. Caution should be exercised when co-administering nilotinib with substrates for CYP3A4 that have a narrow therapeutic index).
No products indexed under this heading.

Nimodipine (Nilotinib is a competitive inhibitor of CYP3A4 which may potentially increase the concentration of drugs eliminated by CYP3A4. Caution should be exercised when co-administering nilotinib with substrates for CYP3A4 that have a narrow therapeutic index). Products include:
Nimotop Capsules **790**

Nisoldipine (Nilotinib is a competitive inhibitor of CYP3A4 which may potentially increase the concentration of drugs eliminated by CYP3A4. Caution should be exercised when co-administering nilotinib with substrates for CYP3A4 that have a narrow therapeutic index). Products include:
Sular Extended Release Tablets **2975**

Nitrendipine (Nilotinib is a competitive inhibitor of CYP3A4 which may potentially increase the concentration of drugs eliminated by CYP3A4. Caution should be exercised when co-administering nilotinib with substrates for CYP3A4 that have a narrow therapeutic index).
No products indexed under this heading.

Norethindrone (Nilotinib is a competitive inhibitor of CYP3A4 which may potentially increase the concentration of drugs eliminated by CYP3A4. Caution should be exercised when co-administering nilotinib with substrates for CYP3A4 that have a narrow therapeutic index). Products include:
Ortho Micronor Tablets **2446**

Norethindrone Acetate (Nilotinib is a competitive inhibitor of CYP3A4 which may potentially increase the concentration of drugs eliminated by CYP3A4. Caution should be exercised when co-administering nilotinib with substrates for CYP3A4 that have a narrow therapeutic index). Products include:
Activella Tablets **2347**

Norgestrel (Nilotinib is a competitive inhibitor of CYP3A4 which may potentially increase the concentration of drugs eliminated by CYP3A4. Caution should be exercised when co-administering nilotinib with substrates for CYP3A4 that have a narrow therapeutic index).
No products indexed under this heading.

Nortriptyline Hydrochloride (The administration of nilotinib with agents that prolong the QT interval should be avoided. Should treatment with any of these agents be required, it is recommended that therapy with nilotinib be interrupted. If interruption of treatment with nilotinib is not possible, patients who require treatment with a drug that prolongs the QT interval should be closely monitored for prolongation of the QT interval).
No products indexed under this heading.

Olanzapine (The administration of nilotinib with agents that prolong the QT interval should be avoided. Should treatment with any of these agents be required, it is recommended that therapy with nilotinib be interrupted. If interruption of treatment with nilotinib is not possible, patients who require treatment with a drug that prolongs the QT interval should be closely monitored for prolongation of the QT interval). Products include:
Symbyax Capsules **1871**
Zyprexa Tablets **1883**
Zyprexa IntraMuscular **1883**
Zyprexa ZYDIS Orally Disintegrating Tablets **1883**

Omeprazole (Nilotinib is a competitive inhibitor of CYP2C8, potentially increasing the concentration of drugs eliminated by CYP2C8. Caution should be exercised when co-administering nilotinib with substrates for CYP2C8 that have a narrow therapeutic index. Studies also suggest that nilotinib may induce CYP2B6, CYP2C8 and CYP2C9, and thereby has the potential to decrease the concentrations of drugs which are eliminated by these enzymes).
No products indexed under this heading.

Ondansetron (Nilotinib is a competitive inhibitor of CYP3A4 which may potentially increase the concentration of drugs eliminated by CYP3A4. Caution should be exercised when co-administering nilotinib with substrates for CYP3A4 that have a narrow therapeutic index). Products include:
Zofran ODT Orally Disintegrating Tablets **1687**

Ondansetron Hydrochloride (Nilotinib is a competitive inhibitor of CYP3A4 which may potentially increase the concentration of drugs eliminated by CYP3A4. Caution should be exercised when co-administering nilotinib with substrates for CYP3A4 that have a narrow therapeutic index). Products include:
Zofran Injection **1682**
Zofran **1687**

Oxaprozin (Nilotinib is a competitive inhibitor of CYP2C9, potentially increasing the concentration of drugs eliminated by CYP2C9. Caution should be exercised when co-administering nilotinib with sub-

strates for CYP2C9 that have a narrow therapeutic index. Studies also suggest that nilotinib may induce CYP2B6, CYP2C8 and CYP2C9, and thereby has the potential to decrease the concentrations of drugs which are eliminated by these enzymes).
No products indexed under this heading.

Oxazepam (The administration of nilotinib with agents that prolong the QT interval should be avoided. Should treatment with any of these agents be required, it is recommended that therapy with nilotinib be interrupted. If interruption of treatment with nilotinib is not possible, patients who require treatment with a drug that prolongs the QT interval should be closely monitored for prolongation of the QT interval).
No products indexed under this heading.

Oxcarbazepine (The concomitant use of strong CYP3A4 inducers should be avoided. If patients must be co-administered a strong CYP3A4 inducer, the dose of nilotinib may need to be increased, depending on patient tolerability. If the strong inducer is discontinued, the nilotinib dose should be reduced to the indicated dose).
No products indexed under this heading.

Oxycodone Hydrochloride (Nilotinib is a competitive inhibitor of CYP2D6, potentially increasing the concentration of drugs eliminated by CYP2D6. Caution should be exercised when co-administering nilotinib with substrates for CYP2D6 that have a narrow therapeutic index). Products include:
OxyContin Tablets 2589
OxyIR Capsules 2593
Percocet Tablets 1127
Percodan Tablets 1130

Paclitaxel (Nilotinib is a competitive inhibitor of CYP3A4 which may potentially increase the concentration of drugs eliminated by CYP3A4. Caution should be exercised when co-administering nilotinib with substrates for CYP3A4 that have a narrow therapeutic index).
No products indexed under this heading.

Paroxetine Hydrochloride (Nilotinib is a competitive inhibitor of CYP2D6, potentially increasing the concentration of drugs eliminated by CYP2D6. Caution should be exercised when co-administering nilotinib with substrates for CYP2D6 that have a narrow therapeutic index). Products include:
Paxil 1535
Paxil CR Controlled-Release Tablets 1544

Perphenazine (The administration of nilotinib with agents that prolong the QT interval should be avoided. Should treatment with any of these agents be required, it is recommended that therapy with nilotinib be interrupted. If interruption of treatment with nilotinib is not possible, patients who require treatment with a drug that prolongs the QT interval should be closely monitored for prolongation of the QT interval).
No products indexed under this heading.

Phenelzine Sulfate (The administration of nilotinib with agents that prolong the QT interval should be avoided. Should treatment with any of these agents be required, it is recommended that therapy with nilotinib be interrupted. If interruption of treatment with nilotinib is not possible, patients who require treatment with a drug that prolongs the QT interval should be closely monitored for prolongation of the QT interval).
No products indexed under this heading.

Phenobarbital (The concomitant use of strong CYP3A4 inducers such as phenobarbital should be avoided. If patients must be co-administered a strong CYP3A4 inducer, the dose of nilotinib may need to be increased, depending on patient tolerability. If the strong inducer is discontinued, the nilotinib dose should be reduced to the indicated dose). Products include:
Donnatal Extentabs 2507

Phenobarbital Sodium (The concomitant use of strong CYP3A4 inducers such as phenobarbital should be avoided. If patients must be co-administered a strong CYP3A4 inducer, the dose of nilotinib may need to be increased, depending on patient tolerability. If the strong inducer is discontinued, the nilotinib dose should be reduced to the indicated dose).
No products indexed under this heading.

Phenylbutazone (Nilotinib is a competitive inhibitor of CYP2C9, potentially increasing the concentration of drugs eliminated by CYP2C9. Caution should be exercised when co-administering nilotinib with substrates for CYP2C9 that have a narrow therapeutic index. Studies also suggest that nilotinib may induce CYP2B6, CYP2C8 and CYP2C9, and thereby has the potential to decrease the concentrations of drugs which are eliminated by these enzymes).
No products indexed under this heading.

Phenytoin (The concomitant use of strong CYP3A4 inducers such as phenytoin should be avoided. If patients must be co-administered a strong CYP3A4 inducer, the dose of nilotinib may need to be increased, depending on patient tolerability. If the strong inducer is discontinued, the nilotinib dose should be reduced to the indicated dose).
No products indexed under this heading.

Phenytoin Sodium (The concomitant use of strong CYP3A4 inducers such as phenytoin should be avoided. If patients must be co-administered a strong CYP3A4 inducer, the dose of nilotinib may need to be increased, depending on patient tolerability. If the strong inducer is discontinued, the nilotinib dose should be reduced to the indicated dose). Products include:
Phenytek Capsules 2192

Pimozide (Nilotinib is a competitive inhibitor of CYP3A4 which may potentially increase the concentration of drugs eliminated by CYP3A4. Caution should be exercised when co-administering nilotinib with substrates for CYP3A4 that have a narrow therapeutic index).
No products indexed under this heading.

Pindolol (Nilotinib is a competitive inhibitor of CYP2D6, potentially increasing the concentration of drugs eliminated by CYP2D6. Caution should be exercised when co-administering nilotinib with substrates for CYP2D6 that have a narrow therapeutic index).
No products indexed under this heading.

Pioglitazone Hydrochloride (Nilotinib is a competitive inhibitor of CYP2C8, potentially increasing the concentration of drugs eliminated by CYP2C8. Caution should be exercised when co-administering nilotinib with substrates for CYP2C8 that have a narrow therapeutic index. Studies also suggest that nilotinib may induce CYP2B6, CYP2C8 and CYP2C9, and thereby has the potential to decrease the concentrations of drugs which are eliminated by these enzymes). Products include:
ActoPlus Met Tablets 3071
Actos Tablets 3077
Duetact Tablets 3085

Piroxicam (Nilotinib is a competitive inhibitor of CYP2C9, potentially increasing the concentration of drugs eliminated by CYP2C9. Caution should be exercised when co-administering nilotinib with substrates for CYP2C9 that have a narrow therapeutic index. Studies also suggest that nilotinib may induce CYP2B6, CYP2C8 and CYP2C9, and thereby has the potential to decrease the concentrations of drugs which are eliminated by these enzymes).
No products indexed under this heading.

Polyestradiol Phosphate (Nilotinib is a competitive inhibitor of CYP3A4 which may potentially increase the concentration of drugs eliminated by CYP3A4. Caution should be exercised when co-administering nilotinib with substrates for CYP3A4 that have a narrow therapeutic index).
No products indexed under this heading.

Posaconazole (Nilotinib inhibits human P-glycoprotein. If nilotinib is administered with drugs that are substrates of Pgp, increased concentrations of the substrate drug are likely, and caution should be exercised). Products include:
Noxafil Oral Suspension 2889

Prazepam (The administration of nilotinib with agents that prolong the QT interval should be avoided. Should treatment with any of these agents be required, it is recommended that therapy with nilotinib be interrupted. If interruption of treatment with nilotinib is not possible, patients who require treatment with a drug that prolongs the QT interval should be closely monitored for prolongation of the QT interval).
No products indexed under this heading.

Prednisolone Acetate (The concomitant use of strong CYP3A4 inducers should be avoided. If patients must be co-administered a strong CYP3A4 inducer, the dose of nilotinib may need to be increased, depending on patient tolerability. If the strong inducer is discontinued, the nilotinib dose should be reduced to the indicated dose). Products include:
Pred Forte Ophthalmic Suspension .... ⊙ 227
Pred Mild Ophthalmic Suspension .... ⊙ 230
Pred-G Ophthalmic Ointment .... ⊙ 229
Pred-G Ophthalmic Suspension .... ⊙ 228

Prednisolone Sodium Phosphate (The concomitant use of strong CYP3A4 inducers should be avoided. If patients must be co-administered a strong CYP3A4 inducer, the dose of nilotinib may need to be increased, depending on patient tolerability. If the strong inducer is discontinued, the nilotinib dose should be reduced to the indicated dose).
No products indexed under this heading.

Prednisolone Tebutate (The concomitant use of strong CYP3A4 inducers should be avoided. If patients must be co-administered a strong CYP3A4 inducer, the dose of nilotinib may need to be increased, depending on patient tolerability. If the strong inducer is discontinued, the nilotinib dose should be reduced to the indicated dose).
No products indexed under this heading.

Prednisone (The concomitant use of strong CYP3A4 inducers should be avoided. If patients must be co-administered a strong CYP3A4 inducer, the dose of nilotinib may need to be increased, depending on patient tolerability. If the strong inducer is discontinued, the nilotinib dose should be reduced to the indicated dose).
No products indexed under this heading.

Primidone (The concomitant use of strong CYP3A4 inducers should be avoided. If patients must be co-administered a strong CYP3A4 inducer, the dose of nilotinib may need to be increased, depending on patient tolerability. If the strong inducer is discontinued, the nilotinib dose should be reduced to the indicated dose).
No products indexed under this heading.

Procainamide Hydrochloride (The administration of nilotinib with agents that prolong the QT interval should be avoided. Should treatment with any of these agents be required, it is recommended that therapy with nilotinib be interrupted. If interruption of treatment with nilotinib is not possible, patients who require treatment with a drug that prolongs the QT interval should be closely monitored for prolongation of the QT interval).
No products indexed under this heading.

Prochlorperazine (The administration of nilotinib with agents that prolong the QT interval should be avoided. Should treatment with any of these agents be required, it is recommended that therapy with nilotinib be interrupted. If interruption of treatment with nilotinib is not possible, patients who require treatment with a drug that prolongs the QT interval should be closely monitored for prolongation of the QT interval).
No products indexed under this heading.

Promethazine Hydrochloride (The administration of nilotinib with agents that prolong the QT interval should be avoided. Should treatment with any of these agents be

required, it is recommended that therapy with nilotinib be interrupted. If interruption of treatment with nilotinib is not possible, patients who require treatment with a drug that prolongs the QT interval should be closely monitored for prolongation of the QT interval).
No products indexed under this heading.

Propafenone Hydrochloride (The administration of nilotinib with agents that prolong the QT interval should be avoided. Should treatment with any of these agents be required, it is recommended that therapy with nilotinib be interrupted. If interruption of treatment with nilotinib is not possible, patients who require treatment with a drug that prolongs the QT interval should be closely monitored for prolongation of the QT interval). Products include:
Rythmol Tablets 1586
Rythmol SR Capsules 1590

Propoxyphene Hydrochloride (Nilotinib is a competitive inhibitor of CYP2D6, potentially increasing the concentration of drugs eliminated by CYP2D6. Caution should be exercised when co-administering nilotinib with substrates for CYP2D6 that have a narrow therapeutic index).
No products indexed under this heading.

Propoxyphene Napsylate (Nilotinib is a competitive inhibitor of CYP2D6, potentially increasing the concentration of drugs eliminated by CYP2D6. Caution should be exercised when co-administering nilotinib with substrates for CYP2D6 that have a narrow therapeutic index).
No products indexed under this heading.

Propranolol Hydrochloride (Nilotinib is a competitive inhibitor of CYP2D6, potentially increasing the concentration of drugs eliminated by CYP2D6. Caution should be exercised when co-administering nilotinib with substrates for CYP2D6 that have a narrow therapeutic index). Products include:
InnoPran XL Extended Release Capsules 1484

Protriptyline Hydrochloride (The administration of nilotinib with agents that prolong the QT interval should be avoided. Should treatment with any of these agents be required, it is recommended that therapy with nilotinib be interrupted. If interruption of treatment with nilotinib is not possible, patients who require treatment with a drug that prolongs the QT interval should be closely monitored for prolongation of the QT interval).
No products indexed under this heading.

Quetiapine Fumarate (The administration of nilotinib with agents that prolong the QT interval should be avoided. Should treatment with any of these agents be required, it is recommended that therapy with nilotinib be interrupted. If interruption of treatment with nilotinib is not possible, patients who require treatment with a drug that prolongs the QT interval should be closely monitored for prolongation of the QT interval).
No products indexed under this heading.

Quinidine (Nilotinib is a substrate of the efflux transporter P-glycoprotein (Pgp, ABCB1). If nilotinib is administered with drugs that inhibit Pgp, increased concentrations of nilotinib are likely, and caution should be exercised).
No products indexed under this heading.

Quinidine Gluconate (The administration of nilotinib with agents that prolong the QT interval should be avoided. Should treatment with any of these agents be required, it is recommended that therapy with nilotinib be interrupted. If interruption of treatment with nilotinib is not possible, patients who require treatment with a drug that prolongs the QT interval should be closely monitored for prolongation of the QT interval).
No products indexed under this heading.

Quinidine Hydrochloride (Nilotinib is a substrate of the efflux transporter P-glycoprotein (Pgp, ABCB1). If nilotinib is administered with drugs that inhibit Pgp, increased concentrations of nilotinib are likely, and caution should be exercised).
No products indexed under this heading.

Quinidine Polygalacturonate (The administration of nilotinib with agents that prolong the QT interval should be avoided. Should treatment with any of these agents be required, it is recommended that therapy with nilotinib be interrupted. If interruption of treatment with nilotinib is not possible, patients who require treatment with a drug that prolongs the QT interval should be closely monitored for prolongation of the QT interval).
No products indexed under this heading.

Quinidine Sulfate (The administration of nilotinib with agents that prolong the QT interval should be avoided. Should treatment with any of these agents be required, it is recommended that therapy with nilotinib be interrupted. If interruption of treatment with nilotinib is not possible, patients who require treatment with a drug that prolongs the QT interval should be closely monitored for prolongation of the QT interval).
No products indexed under this heading.

Ranolazine (Nilotinib inhibits human P-glycoprotein. If nilotinib is administered with drugs that are substrates of Pgp, increased concentrations of the substrate drug are likely, and caution should be exercised).
No products indexed under this heading.

Repaglinide (Nilotinib is a competitive inhibitor of CYP2C8, potentially increasing the concentration of drugs eliminated by CYP2C8. Caution should be exercised when co-administering nilotinib with substrates for CYP2C8 that have a narrow therapeutic index. Studies also suggest that nilotinib may induce CYP2B6, CYP2C8 and CYP2C9, and thereby has the potential to decrease the concentrations of drugs which are eliminated by these enzymes). Products include:
PrandiMet Tablets 2967
Prandin Tablets 2971

Rifabutin (The concomitant use of strong CYP3A4 inducers such as rifabutin should be avoided. If patients must be co-administered a strong CYP3A4 inducer, the dose of nilotinib may need to be increased, depending on patient tolerability. If the strong inducer is discontinued, the nilotinib dose should be reduced to the indicated dose).
No products indexed under this heading.

Rifampicin (In healthy subjects receiving the CYP3A4 inducer, rifampicin, at 600 mg daily for 12 days, systemic exposure (AUC) to nilotinib was decreased by approximately 80%).
No products indexed under this heading.

Rifampin (The concomitant use of strong CYP3A4 inducers such as rifampin should be avoided. If patients must be co-administered a strong CYP3A4 inducer, the dose of nilotinib may need to be increased, depending on patient tolerability. If the strong inducer is discontinued, the nilotinib dose should be reduced to the indicated dose).
No products indexed under this heading.

Rifapentine (The concomitant use of strong CYP3A4 inducers such as rifapentine should be avoided. If patients must be co-administered a strong CYP3A4 inducer, the dose of nilotinib may need to be increased, depending on patient tolerability. If the strong inducer is discontinued, the nilotinib dose should be reduced to the indicated dose).
No products indexed under this heading.

Risperidone (The administration of nilotinib with agents that prolong the QT interval should be avoided. Should treatment with any of these agents be required, it is recommended that therapy with nilotinib be interrupted. If interruption of treatment with nilotinib is not possible, patients who require treatment with a drug that prolongs the QT interval should be closely monitored for prolongation of the QT interval). Products include:
Risperdal Consta Long-Acting Injection 1753

Ritonavir (The concomitant use of strong CYP3A4 inhibitors such as ritonavir should be avoided. If treatment is required, it is recommended that therapy with nilotinib be interrupted. If patients must be co-administered a strong CYP3A4 inhibitor, based on pharmacokinetic studies, 400 mg q.d. is predicted to adjust the nilotinib AUC to the AUC observed without inhibitors. However, there are no clinical data with this dose adjustment in patients receiving strong CYP3A4 inhibitors. If the strong inhibitor is discontinued, a washout period should be allowed before the nilotinib dose is adjusted upward to the indicated dose. Close monitoring for prolongation of the QT interval is indicated for patients who cannot avoid strong CYP3A4 inhibitors). Products include:
Kaletra 452
Norvir 489

Rofecoxib (Nilotinib is a competitive inhibitor of CYP2C9, potentially increasing the concentration of drugs eliminated by CYP2C9. Caution should be exercised when co-administering nilotinib with substrates for CYP2C9 that have a narrow therapeutic index. Studies also suggest that nilotinib may induce CYP2B6, CYP2C8 and CYP2C9, and thereby has the potential to decrease the concentrations of drugs which are eliminated by these enzymes).
No products indexed under this heading.

Rosiglitazone Maleate (Nilotinib is a competitive inhibitor of CYP2C8, potentially increasing the concentration of drugs eliminated by CYP2C8. Caution should be exercised when co-administering nilotinib with substrates for CYP2C8 that have a narrow therapeutic index. Studies also suggest that nilotinib may induce CYP2B6, CYP2C8 and CYP2C9, and thereby has the potential to decrease the concentrations of drugs which are eliminated by these enzymes). Products include:
Avandamet Tablets 1336
Avandaryl Tablets 1344
Avandia Tablets 1351

Rosiglitazone/Metformin (Nilotinib is a competitive inhibitor of CYP2C8, potentially increasing the concentration of drugs eliminated by CYP2C8. Caution should be exercised when co-administering nilotinib with substrates for CYP2C8 that have a narrow therapeutic index. Studies also suggest that nilotinib may induce CYP2B6, CYP2C8 and CYP2C9, and thereby has the potential to decrease the concentrations of drugs which are eliminated by these enzymes).
No products indexed under this heading.

Saquinavir (The concomitant use of strong CYP3A4 inhibitors such as saquinavir should be avoided. If treatment is required, it is recommended that therapy with nilotinib be interrupted. If patients must be co-administered a strong CYP3A4 inhibitor, based on pharmacokinetic studies, 400 mg q.d. is predicted to adjust the nilotinib AUC to the AUC observed without inhibitors. However, there are no clinical data with this dose adjustment in patients receiving strong CYP3A4 inhibitors. If the strong inhibitor is discontinued, a washout period should be allowed before the nilotinib dose is adjusted upward to the indicated dose. Close monitoring for prolongation of the QT interval is indicated for patients who cannot avoid strong CYP3A4 inhibitors).
No products indexed under this heading.

Saquinavir Mesylate (The concomitant use of strong CYP3A4 inhibitors such as saquinavir should be avoided. If treatment is required, it is recommended that therapy with nilotinib be interrupted. If patients must be co-administered a strong CYP3A4 inhibitor, based on pharmacokinetic studies, 400 mg q.d. is predicted to adjust the nilotinib AUC to the AUC observed without inhibitors. However, there are no clinical data with this dose adjustment in patients receiving strong CYP3A4 inhibitors. If the strong inhibitor is discontinued, a washout period should be allowed before the nilotinib dose is adjusted upward to the indicated dose. Close monitoring for prolongation of the QT interval is

indicated for patients who cannot avoid strong CYP3A4 inhibitors).
No products indexed under this heading.

Sertraline Hydrochloride (Nilotinib is a competitive inhibitor of CYP3A4 which may potentially increase the concentration of drugs eliminated by CYP3A4. Caution should be exercised when co-administering nilotinib with substrates for CYP3A4 that have a narrow therapeutic index).
No products indexed under this heading.

Sildenafil Citrate (Nilotinib is a competitive inhibitor of CYP3A4 which may potentially increase the concentration of drugs eliminated by CYP3A4. Caution should be exercised when co-administering nilotinib with substrates for CYP3A4 that have a narrow therapeutic index).
No products indexed under this heading.

Simvastatin (Nilotinib inhibits human P-glycoprotein. If nilotinib is administered with drugs that are substrates of Pgp, increased concentrations of the substrate drug are likely, and caution should be exercised). Products include:
Simcor Tablets ... 502
Vytorin 10/10 Tablets ... 2149
Vytorin 10/10 Tablets ... 2939
Vytorin 10/20 Tablets ... 2149
Vytorin 10/20 Tablets ... 2939
Vytorin 10/40 Tablets ... 2149
Vytorin 10/40 Tablets ... 2939
Vytorin 10/80 Tablets ... 2149
Vytorin 10/80 Tablets ... 2939
Zocor Tablets ... 2136

Sirolimus (Nilotinib inhibits human P-glycoprotein. If nilotinib is administered with drugs that are substrates of Pgp, increased concentrations of the substrate drug are likely, and caution should be exercised). Products include:
Rapamune ... 3260

Sitagliptin Phosphate (Nilotinib inhibits human P-glycoprotein. If nilotinib is administered with drugs that are substrates of Pgp, increased concentrations of the substrate drug are likely, and caution should be exercised). Products include:
Janumet Tablets ... 2041
Januvia Tablets ... 2048

Sulfamethoxazole (Nilotinib is a competitive inhibitor of CYP2C9, potentially increasing the concentration of drugs eliminated by CYP2C9. Caution should be exercised when co-administering nilotinib with substrates for CYP2C9 that have a narrow therapeutic index. Studies also suggest that nilotinib may induce CYP2B6, CYP2C8 and CYP2C9, and thereby has the potential to decrease the concentrations of drugs which are eliminated by these enzymes).
No products indexed under this heading.

Sulfinpyrazone (The concomitant use of strong CYP3A4 inducers should be avoided. If patients must be co-administered a strong CYP3A4 inducer, the dose of nilotinib may need to be increased, depending on patient tolerability. If the strong inducer is discontinued, the nilotinib dose should be reduced to the indicated dose).
No products indexed under this heading.

Sulindac (Nilotinib is a competitive inhibitor of CYP2C9, potentially increasing the concentration of drugs eliminated by CYP2C9. Caution should be exercised when co-administering nilotinib with substrates for CYP2C9 that have a narrow therapeutic index. Studies also suggest that nilotinib may induce CYP2B6, CYP2C8 and CYP2C9, and thereby has the potential to decrease the concentrations of drugs which are eliminated by these enzymes). Products include:
Clinoril Tablets ... 1962

Suprofen (Nilotinib is a competitive inhibitor of CYP2C9, potentially increasing the concentration of drugs eliminated by CYP2C9. Caution should be exercised when co-administering nilotinib with substrates for CYP2C9 that have a narrow therapeutic index. Studies also suggest that nilotinib may induce CYP2B6, CYP2C8 and CYP2C9, and thereby has the potential to decrease the concentrations of drugs which are eliminated by these enzymes).
No products indexed under this heading.

Tacrolimus (Nilotinib is a competitive inhibitor of CYP3A4 which may potentially increase the concentration of drugs eliminated by CYP3A4. Caution should be exercised when co-administering nilotinib with substrates for CYP3A4 that have a narrow therapeutic index). Products include:
Prograf Capsules and Injection ... 622
Protopic Ointment ... 628

Tadalafil (Nilotinib is a competitive inhibitor of CYP3A4 which may potentially increase the concentration of drugs eliminated by CYP3A4. Caution should be exercised when co-administering nilotinib with substrates for CYP3A4 that have a narrow therapeutic index). Products include:
Cialis Tablets ... 1792

Tamoxifen Citrate (Nilotinib is a competitive inhibitor of CYP3A4 which may potentially increase the concentration of drugs eliminated by CYP3A4. Caution should be exercised when co-administering nilotinib with substrates for CYP3A4 that have a narrow therapeutic index).
No products indexed under this heading.

Telithromycin (The concomitant use of strong CYP3A4 inhibitors such as telithromycin should be avoided. If treatment is required, it is recommended that therapy with nilotinib be interrupted. If patients must be co-administered a strong CYP3A4 inhibitor, based on pharmacokinetic studies, 400 mg q.d. is predicted to adjust the nilotinib AUC to the AUC observed without inhibitors. However, there are no clinical data with this dose adjustment in patients receiving strong CYP3A4 inhibitors. If the strong inhibitor is discontinued, a washout period should be allowed before the nilotinib dose is adjusted upward to the indicated dose. Close monitoring for prolongation of the QT interval is indicated for patients who cannot avoid strong CYP3A4 inhibitors). Products include:
Ketek Tablets ... 2744

Telmisartan (Nilotinib is a competitive inhibitor of CYP2C9, potentially increasing the concentration of drugs eliminated by CYP2C9. Caution should be exercised when co-administering nilotinib with substrates for CYP2C9 that have a narrow therapeutic index. Studies also suggest that nilotinib may induce CYP2B6, CYP2C8 and CYP2C9, and thereby has the potential to decrease the concentrations of drugs which are eliminated by these enzymes). Products include:
Micardis Tablets ... 852
Micardis HCT Tablets ... 854

Temsirolimus (Nilotinib inhibits human P-glycoprotein. If nilotinib is administered with drugs that are substrates of Pgp, increased concentrations of the substrate drug are likely, and caution should be exercised). Products include:
Torisel Injection ... 3272

Teniposide (Nilotinib is a competitive inhibitor of CYP2D6, potentially increasing the concentration of drugs eliminated by CYP2D6. Caution should be exercised when co-administering nilotinib with substrates for CYP2D6 that have a narrow therapeutic index).
No products indexed under this heading.

Testosterone (Nilotinib is a competitive inhibitor of CYP2D6, potentially increasing the concentration of drugs eliminated by CYP2D6. Caution should be exercised when co-administering nilotinib with substrates for CYP2D6 that have a narrow therapeutic index). Products include:
AndroGel ... 3159
Testim 1% Gel ... 701

Testosterone Cypionate (Nilotinib is a competitive inhibitor of CYP2D6, potentially increasing the concentration of drugs eliminated by CYP2D6. Caution should be exercised when co-administering nilotinib with substrates for CYP2D6 that have a narrow therapeutic index).
No products indexed under this heading.

Testosterone Enanthate (Nilotinib is a competitive inhibitor of CYP2D6, potentially increasing the concentration of drugs eliminated by CYP2D6. Caution should be exercised when co-administering nilotinib with substrates for CYP2D6 that have a narrow therapeutic index). Products include:
Delatestryl Injection ... 1730

Testosterone Propionate (Nilotinib is a competitive inhibitor of CYP2D6, potentially increasing the concentration of drugs eliminated by CYP2D6. Caution should be exercised when co-administering nilotinib with substrates for CYP2D6 that have a narrow therapeutic index).
No products indexed under this heading.

Theophylline (The concomitant use of strong CYP3A4 inducers should be avoided. If patients must be co-administered a strong CYP3A4 inducer, the dose of nilotinib may need to be increased, depending on patient tolerability. If the strong inducer is discontinued, the nilotinib dose should be reduced to the indicated dose).
No products indexed under this heading.

Theophylline Anhydrous (The concomitant use of strong CYP3A4 inducers should be avoided. If patients must be co-administered a strong CYP3A4 inducer, the dose of nilotinib may need to be increased, depending on patient tolerability. If the strong inducer is discontinued, the nilotinib dose should be reduced to the indicated dose). Products include:
Uniphyl Tablets ... 2595

Theophylline Calcium Salicylate (The concomitant use of strong CYP3A4 inducers should be avoided. If patients must be co-administered a strong CYP3A4 inducer, the dose of nilotinib may need to be increased, depending on patient tolerability. If the strong inducer is discontinued, the nilotinib dose should be reduced to the indicated dose).
No products indexed under this heading.

Theophylline Dihydroxypropyl (Glyceryl) (The concomitant use of strong CYP3A4 inducers should be avoided. If patients must be co-administered a strong CYP3A4 inducer, the dose of nilotinib may need to be increased, depending on patient tolerability. If the strong inducer is discontinued, the nilotinib dose should be reduced to the indicated dose).
No products indexed under this heading.

Theophylline Ethylenediamine (The concomitant use of strong CYP3A4 inducers should be avoided. If patients must be co-administered a strong CYP3A4 inducer, the dose of nilotinib may need to be increased, depending on patient tolerability. If the strong inducer is discontinued, the nilotinib dose should be reduced to the indicated dose).
No products indexed under this heading.

Thioridazine (Nilotinib is a competitive inhibitor of CYP2D6, potentially increasing the concentration of drugs eliminated by CYP2D6. Caution should be exercised when co-administering nilotinib with substrates for CYP2D6 that have a narrow therapeutic index).
No products indexed under this heading.

Thioridazine Hydrochloride (The administration of nilotinib with agents that prolong the QT interval should be avoided. Should treatment with any of these agents be required, it is recommended that therapy with nilotinib be interrupted. If interruption of treatment with nilotinib is not possible, patients who require treatment with a drug that prolongs the QT interval should be closely monitored for prolongation of the QT interval). Products include:
Thioridazine Hydrochloride Tablets ... 2195

Thiothixene (The administration of nilotinib with agents that prolong the QT interval should be avoided. Should treatment with any of these agents be required, it is recommended that therapy with nilotinib be interrupted. If interruption of treatment with nilotinib is not possible, patients who require treatment with a drug that prolongs the QT interval should be closely monitored for prolongation of the QT interval). Products include:
Thiothixene Capsules ... 2197

Tiagabine Hydrochloride (Nilotinib is a competitive inhibitor of CYP3A4 which may potentially increase the concentration of drugs

eliminated by CYP3A4. Caution should be exercised when co-administering nilotinib with substrates for CYP3A4 that have a narrow therapeutic index). Products include:

Gabitril Tablets 973

Timolol Maleate (Nilotinib is a competitive inhibitor of CYP2D6, potentially increasing the concentration of drugs eliminated by CYP2D6. Caution should be exercised when co-administering nilotinib with substrates for CYP2D6 that have a narrow therapeutic index). Products include:

Combigan Ophthalmic Solution 553
Cosopt Sterile Ophthalmic Solution 1969
Timoptic Sterile Ophthalmic Solution 2121
Timoptic in Ocudose 2124
Timoptic-XE Sterile Ophthalmic Gel Forming Solution 2125

Tipranavir (Nilotinib inhibits human P-glycoprotein. If nilotinib is administered with drugs that are substrates of Pgp, increased concentrations of the substrate drug are likely, and caution should be exercised). Products include:

Aptivus Capsules 823
Aptivus Oral Solution 823

Tocainide Hydrochloride (The administration of nilotinib with agents that prolong the QT interval should be avoided. Should treatment with any of these agents be required, it is recommended that therapy with nilotinib be interrupted. If interruption of treatment with nilotinib is not possible, patients who require treatment with a drug that prolongs the QT interval should be closely monitored for prolongation of the QT interval).

No products indexed under this heading.

Tolazamide (Nilotinib is a competitive inhibitor of CYP2C9, potentially increasing the concentration of drugs eliminated by CYP2C9. Caution should be exercised when co-administering nilotinib with substrates for CYP2C9 that have a narrow therapeutic index. Studies also suggest that nilotinib may induce CYP2B6, CYP2C8 and CYP2C9, and thereby has the potential to decrease the concentrations of drugs which are eliminated by these enzymes).

No products indexed under this heading.

Tolbutamide (Nilotinib is a competitive inhibitor of CYP2C8, potentially increasing the concentration of drugs eliminated by CYP2C8. Caution should be exercised when co-administering nilotinib with substrates for CYP2C8 that have a narrow therapeutic index. Studies also suggest that nilotinib may induce CYP2B6, CYP2C8 and CYP2C9, and thereby has the potential to decrease the concentrations of drugs which are eliminated by these enzymes).

No products indexed under this heading.

Tolbutamide Sodium (Nilotinib is a competitive inhibitor of CYP2C8, potentially increasing the concentration of drugs eliminated by CYP2C8. Caution should be exercised when co-administering nilotinib with substrates for CYP2C8 that have a narrow therapeutic index. Studies also suggest that nilotinib may induce CYP2B6, CYP2C8 and CYP2C9, and thereby has the potential to decrease the concentrations of drugs which are eliminated by these enzymes).

No products indexed under this heading.

Tolmetin Sodium (Nilotinib is a competitive inhibitor of CYP2C9, potentially increasing the concentration of drugs eliminated by CYP2C9. Caution should be exercised when co-administering nilotinib with substrates for CYP2C9 that have a narrow therapeutic index. Studies also suggest that nilotinib may induce CYP2B6, CYP2C8 and CYP2C9, and thereby has the potential to decrease the concentrations of drugs which are eliminated by these enzymes).

No products indexed under this heading.

Tolterodine Tartrate (Nilotinib is a competitive inhibitor of CYP3A4 which may potentially increase the concentration of drugs eliminated by CYP3A4. Caution should be exercised when co-administering nilotinib with substrates for CYP3A4 that have a narrow therapeutic index).

No products indexed under this heading.

Torsemide (Nilotinib is a competitive inhibitor of CYP2C9, potentially increasing the concentration of drugs eliminated by CYP2C9. Caution should be exercised when co-administering nilotinib with substrates for CYP2C9 that have a narrow therapeutic index. Studies also suggest that nilotinib may induce CYP2B6, CYP2C8 and CYP2C9, and thereby has the potential to decrease the concentrations of drugs which are eliminated by these enzymes). Products include:

Demadex Injection 2630
Demadex Tablets 2630

Tramadol Hydrochloride (Nilotinib is a competitive inhibitor of CYP2D6, potentially increasing the concentration of drugs eliminated by CYP2D6. Caution should be exercised when co-administering nilotinib with substrates for CYP2D6 that have a narrow therapeutic index). Products include:

Ultram ER Extended-Release Tablets 2428

Tranylcypromine Sulfate (The administration of nilotinib with agents that prolong the QT interval should be avoided. Should treatment with any of these agents be required, it is recommended that therapy with nilotinib be interrupted. If interruption of treatment with nilotinib is not possible, patients who require treatment with a drug that prolongs the QT interval should be closely monitored for prolongation of the QT interval). Products include:

Parnate Tablets 1532

Trazodone Hydrochloride (Nilotinib is a competitive inhibitor of CYP3A4 which may potentially increase the concentration of drugs eliminated by CYP3A4. Caution should be exercised when co-administering nilotinib with substrates for CYP3A4 that have a narrow therapeutic index).

No products indexed under this heading.

Tretinoin (Nilotinib is a competitive inhibitor of CYP2C8, potentially increasing the concentration of drugs eliminated by CYP2C8. Caution should be exercised when co-administering nilotinib with substrates for CYP2C8 that have a narrow therapeutic index. Studies also suggest that nilotinib may induce CYP2B6, CYP2C8 and CYP2C9, and thereby has the potential to decrease the concentrations of drugs which are eliminated by these enzymes). Products include:

Vesanoid Capsules 2660
Ziana Gel 1942

Triamcinolone (The concomitant use of strong CYP3A4 inducers should be avoided. If patients must be co-administered a strong CYP3A4 inducer, the dose of nilotinib may need to be increased, depending on patient tolerability. If the strong inducer is discontinued, the nilotinib dose should be reduced to the indicated dose).

No products indexed under this heading.

Triamcinolone Acetonide (The concomitant use of strong CYP3A4 inducers should be avoided. If patients must be co-administered a strong CYP3A4 inducer, the dose of nilotinib may need to be increased, depending on patient tolerability. If the strong inducer is discontinued, the nilotinib dose should be reduced to the indicated dose). Products include:

Azmacort Inhalation Aerosol 407
Nasacort AQ Nasal Spray 2765
Triesence Injectable Suspension .... ⊙209

Triamcinolone Diacetate (The concomitant use of strong CYP3A4 inducers should be avoided. If patients must be co-administered a strong CYP3A4 inducer, the dose of nilotinib may need to be increased, depending on patient tolerability. If the strong inducer is discontinued, the nilotinib dose should be reduced to the indicated dose).

No products indexed under this heading.

Triamcinolone Hexacetonide (The concomitant use of strong CYP3A4 inducers should be avoided. If patients must be co-administered a strong CYP3A4 inducer, the dose of nilotinib may need to be increased, depending on patient tolerability. If the strong inducer is discontinued, the nilotinib dose should be reduced to the indicated dose).

No products indexed under this heading.

Triazolam (Nilotinib is a competitive inhibitor of CYP3A4 which may potentially increase the concentration of drugs eliminated by CYP3A4. Caution should be exercised when co-administering nilotinib with substrates for CYP3A4 that have a narrow therapeutic index).

No products indexed under this heading.

Trifluoperazine Hydrochloride (The administration of nilotinib with agents that prolong the QT interval should be avoided. Should treatment with any of these agents be required, it is recommended that therapy with nilotinib be interrupted. If interruption of treatment with nilotinib is not possible, patients who require treatment with a drug that prolongs the QT interval should be closely monitored for prolongation of the QT interval).

No products indexed under this heading.

Trimipramine Maleate (The administration of nilotinib with agents that prolong the QT interval should be avoided. Should treatment with any of these agents be required, it is recommended that therapy with nilotinib be interrupted. If interruption of treatment with nilotinib is not possible, patients who require treatment with a drug that prolongs the QT interval should be closely monitored for prolongation of the QT interval).

No products indexed under this heading.

Troglitazone (The concomitant use of strong CYP3A4 inducers should be avoided. If patients must be co-administered a strong CYP3A4 inducer, the dose of nilotinib may need to be increased, depending on patient tolerability. If the strong inducer is discontinued, the nilotinib dose should be reduced to the indicated dose).

No products indexed under this heading.

Troleandomycin (Nilotinib is a substrate of the efflux transporter P-glycoprotein (Pgp, ABCB1). If nilotinib is administered with drugs that inhibit Pgp, increased concentrations of nilotinib are likely, and caution should be exercised).

No products indexed under this heading.

Valdecoxib (Nilotinib is a competitive inhibitor of CYP2C9, potentially increasing the concentration of drugs eliminated by CYP2C9. Caution should be exercised when co-administering nilotinib with substrates for CYP2C9 that have a narrow therapeutic index. Studies also suggest that nilotinib may induce CYP2B6, CYP2C8 and CYP2C9, and thereby has the potential to decrease the concentrations of drugs which are eliminated by these enzymes).

No products indexed under this heading.

Valsartan (Nilotinib is a competitive inhibitor of CYP2C9, potentially increasing the concentration of drugs eliminated by CYP2C9. Caution should be exercised when co-administering nilotinib with substrates for CYP2C9 that have a narrow therapeutic index. Studies also suggest that nilotinib may induce CYP2B6, CYP2C8 and CYP2C9, and thereby has the potential to decrease the concentrations of drugs which are eliminated by these enzymes). Products include:

Diovan Tablets 2212
Diovan HCT Tablets 2216
Exforge Tablets 2238

Vardenafil Hydrochloride (Nilotinib is a competitive inhibitor of CYP3A4 which may potentially increase the concentration of drugs eliminated by CYP3A4. Caution should be exercised when co-administering nilotinib with substrates for CYP3A4 that have a narrow therapeutic index). Products include:

Levitra Tablets 2876

Venlafaxine Hydrochloride (Nilotinib is a competitive inhibitor of CYP2D6, potentially increasing the concentration of drugs eliminated by CYP2D6. Caution should be exercised when co-administering nilotinib

with substrates for CYP2D6 that have a narrow therapeutic index). Products include:

Effexor XR Extended-Release Capsules 3195
Venlafaxine Hydrochloride Tablets ... 2199

Verapamil Hydrochloride (Nilotinib is a substrate of the efflux transporter P-glycoprotein (Pgp, ABCB1). If nilotinib is administered with drugs that inhibit Pgp, increased concentrations of nilotinib are likely, and caution should be exercised). Products include:

Tarka Tablets 511

Vinblastine Sulfate (Nilotinib inhibits human P-glycoprotein. If nilotinib is administered with drugs that are substrates of Pgp, increased concentrations of the substrate drug are likely, and caution should be exercised).

No products indexed under this heading.

Vincristine Sulfate (Nilotinib is a competitive inhibitor of CYP3A4 which may potentially increase the concentration of drugs eliminated by CYP3A4. Caution should be exercised when co-administering nilotinib with substrates for CYP3A4 that have a narrow therapeutic index).

No products indexed under this heading.

Vitamin A (Nilotinib is a competitive inhibitor of CYP2C8, potentially increasing the concentration of drugs eliminated by CYP2C8. Caution should be exercised when co-administering nilotinib with substrates for CYP2C8 that have a narrow therapeutic index. Studies also suggest that nilotinib may induce CYP2B6, CYP2C8 and CYP2C9, and thereby has the potential to decrease the concentrations of drugs which are eliminated by these enzymes). Products include:

Norwegian Cod Liver Oil 949

Vitamin A Acetate (Nilotinib is a competitive inhibitor of CYP2C8, potentially increasing the concentration of drugs eliminated by CYP2C8. Caution should be exercised when co-administering nilotinib with substrates for CYP2C8 that have a narrow therapeutic index. Studies also suggest that nilotinib may induce CYP2B6, CYP2C8 and CYP2C9, and thereby has the potential to decrease the concentrations of drugs which are eliminated by these enzymes).

No products indexed under this heading.

Voriconazole (The concomitant use of strong CYP3A4 inhibitors such as voriconazole should be avoided. If treatment is required, it is recommended that therapy with nilotinib be interrupted. If patients must be co-administered a strong CYP3A4 inhibitor, based on pharmacokinetic studies, 400 mg q.d. is predicted to adjust the nilotinib AUC to the AUC observed without inhibitors. However, there are no clinical data with this dose adjustment in patients receiving strong CYP3A4 inhibitors. If the strong inhibitor is discontinued, a washout period should be allowed before the nilotinib dose is adjusted upward to the indicated dose. Close monitoring for prolongation of the QT interval is indicated for patients who cannot avoid strong CYP3A4 inhibitors).

No products indexed under this heading.

Warfarin Sodium (Since warfarin is metabolized by CYP2C9 and CYP3A4, it should be avoided if possible).

No products indexed under this heading.

Zafirlukast (Nilotinib is a competitive inhibitor of CYP2C9, potentially increasing the concentration of drugs eliminated by CYP2C9. Caution should be exercised when co-administering nilotinib with substrates for CYP2C9 that have a narrow therapeutic index. Studies also suggest that nilotinib may induce CYP2B6, CYP2C8 and CYP2C9, and thereby has the potential to decrease the concentrations of drugs which are eliminated by these enzymes). Products include:

Accolate Tablets 669

Zileuton (Nilotinib is a competitive inhibitor of CYP2C9, potentially increasing the concentration of drugs eliminated by CYP2C9. Caution should be exercised when co-administering nilotinib with substrates for CYP2C9 that have a narrow therapeutic index. Studies also suggest that nilotinib may induce CYP2B6, CYP2C8 and CYP2C9, and thereby has the potential to decrease the concentrations of drugs which are eliminated by these enzymes).

No products indexed under this heading.

Ziprasidone Hydrochloride (The administration of nilotinib with agents that prolong the QT interval should be avoided. Should treatment with any of these agents be required, it is recommended that therapy with nilotinib be interrupted. If interruption of treatment with nilotinib is not possible, patients who require treatment with a drug that prolongs the QT interval should be closely monitored for prolongation of the QT interval). Products include:

Geodon Capsules 2520

Zonisamide (Nilotinib is a competitive inhibitor of CYP2D6, potentially increasing the concentration of drugs eliminated by CYP2D6. Caution should be exercised when co-administering nilotinib with substrates for CYP2D6 that have a narrow therapeutic index). Products include:

Zonegran Capsules 1089

Zopiclone (Nilotinib is a competitive inhibitor of CYP2C8, potentially increasing the concentration of drugs eliminated by CYP2C8. Caution should be exercised when co-administering nilotinib with substrates for CYP2C8 that have a narrow therapeutic index. Studies also suggest that nilotinib may induce CYP2B6, CYP2C8 and CYP2C9, and thereby has the potential to decrease the concentrations of drugs which are eliminated by these enzymes).

No products indexed under this heading.

Food Interactions

Food, unspecified (The bioavailability of nilotinib is increased with food. Nilotinib should not be taken with food. No food should be taken at least 2 hours before and at least one hour after the dose is taken).

Grapefruit (Grapefruit products may increase serum concentrations of nilotinib and should be avoided).

Grapefruit Juice (Grapefruit products may increase serum concentrations of nilotinib and should be avoided).

TAXOTERE INJECTION CONCENTRATE

(Docetaxel) 2773

May interact with cytochrome p450 3a4 inducers (selected), cytochrome p450 3a4 inhibitors (selected), cytochrome p450 3a4 substrates (selected), erythromycin, and certain other agents. Compounds in these categories include:

Acetazolamide (The metabolism of docetaxel may be modified by the concomitant administration of compounds that inhibit cytochrome P450 3A4. Caution should be exercised with these drugs when treating patients receiving docetaxel as there is a potential for a significant reaction).

No products indexed under this heading.

Alfentanil Hydrochloride (The metabolism of docetaxel may be modified by the concomitant administration of compounds that are metabolized by cytochrome P450 3A4. Caution should be exercised with these drugs when treating patients receiving docetaxel as there is a potential for a significant reaction).

No products indexed under this heading.

Allium sativum (The metabolism of docetaxel may be modified by the concomitant administration of compounds that induce cytochrome P450 3A4. Caution should be exercised with these drugs when treating patients receiving docetaxel as there is a potential for a significant reaction).

No products indexed under this heading.

Alprazolam (The metabolism of docetaxel may be modified by the concomitant administration of compounds that are metabolized by cytochrome P450 3A4. Caution should be exercised with these drugs when treating patients receiving docetaxel as there is a potential for a significant reaction).

No products indexed under this heading.

Amiodarone Hydrochloride (The metabolism of docetaxel may be modified by the concomitant administration of compounds that inhibit cytochrome P450 3A4. Caution should be exercised with these drugs when treating patients receiving docetaxel as there is a potential for a significant reaction).

No products indexed under this heading.

Amitriptyline Hydrochloride (The metabolism of docetaxel may be modified by the concomitant administration of compounds that are metabolized by cytochrome P450 3A4. Caution should be exercised with these drugs when treating patients receiving docetaxel as there is a potential for a significant reaction).

No products indexed under this heading.

Amlodipine Besylate (The metabolism of docetaxel may be modified by the concomitant administration of compounds that are metabolized by cytochrome P450 3A4. Caution should be exercised with these drugs when treating patients receiving docetaxel as there is a potential for a significant reaction). Products include:

Azor Tablets 1005
Exforge Tablets 2238

Amprenavir (The metabolism of docetaxel may be modified by the concomitant administration of compounds that inhibit cytochrome P450 3A4. Caution should be exercised with these drugs when treating patients receiving docetaxel as there is a potential for a significant reaction).

No products indexed under this heading.

Anastrozole (The metabolism of docetaxel may be modified by the concomitant administration of compounds that inhibit cytochrome P450 3A4. Caution should be exercised with these drugs when treating patients receiving docetaxel as there is a potential for a significant reaction). Products include:

Arimidex Tablets 672

Aprepitant (The metabolism of docetaxel may be modified by the concomitant administration of compounds that induce cytochrome P450 3A4. Caution should be exercised with these drugs when treating patients receiving docetaxel as there is a potential for a significant reaction). Products include:

Emend Capsules 1992

Astemizole (The metabolism of docetaxel may be modified by the concomitant administration of compounds that are metabolized by cytochrome P450 3A4. Caution should be exercised with these drugs when treating patients receiving docetaxel as there is a potential for a significant reaction).

No products indexed under this heading.

Atazanavir (The metabolism of docetaxel may be modified by the concomitant administration of compounds that inhibit cytochrome P450 3A4. Caution should be exercised with these drugs when treating patients receiving docetaxel as there is a potential for a significant reaction).

No products indexed under this heading.

Atazanavir Sulfate (The metabolism of docetaxel may be modified by the concomitant administration of compounds that inhibit cytochrome P450 3A4. Caution should be exercised with these drugs when treating patients receiving docetaxel as there is a potential for a significant reaction). Products include:

Reyataz Capsules 3299

Atorvastatin Calcium (The metabolism of docetaxel may be modified by the concomitant administration of compounds that are metabolized by cytochrome P450 3A4. Caution should be exercised with these drugs when treating patients receiving docetaxel as there is a potential for a significant reaction). Products include:

Lipitor Tablets 2501

Belladonna Ergotamine (The metabolism of docetaxel may be modified by the concomitant administration of compounds that are metabolized by cytochrome P450 3A4. Caution should be exercised with these drugs when treating patients receiving docetaxel as there is a potential for a significant reaction).
No products indexed under this heading.

Betamethasone Acetate (The metabolism of docetaxel may be modified by the concomitant administration of compounds that induce cytochrome P450 3A4. Caution should be exercised with these drugs when treating patients receiving docetaxel as there is a potential for a significant reaction).
No products indexed under this heading.

Betamethasone Sodium Phosphate (The metabolism of docetaxel may be modified by the concomitant administration of compounds that induce cytochrome P450 3A4. Caution should be exercised with these drugs when treating patients receiving docetaxel as there is a potential for a significant reaction).
No products indexed under this heading.

Buspirone Hydrochloride (The metabolism of docetaxel may be modified by the concomitant administration of compounds that are metabolized by cytochrome P450 3A4. Caution should be exercised with these drugs when treating patients receiving docetaxel as there is a potential for a significant reaction).
No products indexed under this heading.

Busulfan (The metabolism of docetaxel may be modified by the concomitant administration of compounds that are metabolized by cytochrome P450 3A4. Caution should be exercised with these drugs when treating patients receiving docetaxel as there is a potential for a significant reaction). Products include:
Busulfex Injection 2477
Myleran Tablets 1530

Carbamazepine (The metabolism of docetaxel may be modified by the concomitant administration of compounds that induce cytochrome P450 3A4. Caution should be exercised with these drugs when treating patients receiving docetaxel as there is a potential for a significant reaction). Products include:
Carbatrol Capsules 3019
Equetro Extended-Release Capsules 3174

Cerivastatin Sodium (The metabolism of docetaxel may be modified by the concomitant administration of compounds that are metabolized by cytochrome P450 3A4. Caution should be exercised with these drugs when treating patients receiving docetaxel as there is a potential for a significant reaction).
No products indexed under this heading.

Chlorpheniramine (The metabolism of docetaxel may be modified by the concomitant administration of compounds that are metabolized by cytochrome P450 3A4. Caution should be exercised with these drugs when treating patients receiving docetaxel as there is a potential for a significant reaction).
No products indexed under this heading.

Chlorpheniramine Maleate (The metabolism of docetaxel may be modified by the concomitant administration of compounds that are metabolized by cytochrome P450 3A4. Caution should be exercised with these drugs when treating patients receiving docetaxel as there is a potential for a significant reaction). Products include:
Actifed Cold & Allergy Tablets 1895
Sudafed PE Sinus & Allergy Tablets 1908
Tylenol Allergy Multi-Symptom Caplets with Cool Burst and Rapid Release Gelcaps 1916
Children's Tylenol Plus Cold Suspension Liquid 1912
Children's Tylenol Plus Cough & Runny Nose Suspension Liquid 1912
Children's Tylenol Plus Flu Suspension Liquid 1914
Children's Tylenol Plus Multi-Symptom Cold Suspension Liquid 1912
Tylenol Cold Head Congestion Nighttime Caplets with Cool Burst 1910
Tylenol Cold Multi-Symptom Nighttime Caplets with Cool Burst 1913
Tylenol Sinus Congestion & Pain Nighttime Caplets with Cool Burst 1917

Chlorpheniramine Polistirex (The metabolism of docetaxel may be modified by the concomitant administration of compounds that are metabolized by cytochrome P450 3A4. Caution should be exercised with these drugs when treating patients receiving docetaxel as there is a potential for a significant reaction). Products include:
Tussionex Pennkinetic Extended-Release Suspension 3154

Chlorpheniramine Tannate (The metabolism of docetaxel may be modified by the concomitant administration of compounds that are metabolized by cytochrome P450 3A4. Caution should be exercised with these drugs when treating patients receiving docetaxel as there is a potential for a significant reaction).
No products indexed under this heading.

Cimetidine (The metabolism of docetaxel may be modified by the concomitant administration of compounds that inhibit cytochrome P450 3A4. Caution should be exercised with these drugs when treating patients receiving docetaxel as there is a potential for a significant reaction).
No products indexed under this heading.

Cimetidine Hydrochloride (The metabolism of docetaxel may be modified by the concomitant administration of compounds that inhibit cytochrome P450 3A4. Caution should be exercised with these drugs when treating patients receiving docetaxel as there is a potential for a significant reaction).
No products indexed under this heading.

Ciprofloxacin (The metabolism of docetaxel may be modified by the concomitant administration of compounds that inhibit cytochrome P450 3A4. Caution should be exercised with these drugs when treating patients receiving docetaxel as there is a potential for a significant reaction). Products include:
Cipro I.V. 2817
Cipro Oral Suspension 2810
Cipro XR Tablets 2823
Ciprodex Otic Suspension 541

Ciprofloxacin Hydrochloride (The metabolism of docetaxel may be modified by the concomitant administration of compounds that induce cytochrome P450 3A4. Caution should be exercised with these drugs when treating patients receiving docetaxel as there is a potential for a significant reaction). Products include:
Cipro Tablets 2810

Cisapride (The metabolism of docetaxel may be modified by the concomitant administration of compounds that are metabolized by cytochrome P450 3A4. Caution should be exercised with these drugs when treating patients receiving docetaxel as there is a potential for a significant reaction).
No products indexed under this heading.

Cisplatin (The metabolism of docetaxel may be modified by the concomitant administration of compounds that induce cytochrome P450 3A4. Caution should be exercised with these drugs when treating patients receiving docetaxel as there is a potential for a significant reaction).
No products indexed under this heading.

Clarithromycin (The metabolism of docetaxel may be modified by the concomitant administration of compounds that inhibit cytochrome P450 3A4. Caution should be exercised with these drugs when treating patients receiving docetaxel as there is a potential for a significant reaction). Products include:
Biaxin/Biaxin XL 411

Clotrimazole (The metabolism of docetaxel may be modified by the concomitant administration of compounds that inhibit cytochrome P450 3A4. Caution should be exercised with these drugs when treating patients receiving docetaxel as there is a potential for a significant reaction). Products include:
Lotrisone 2881

Cortisone Acetate (The metabolism of docetaxel may be modified by the concomitant administration of compounds that induce cytochrome P450 3A4. Caution should be exercised with these drugs when treating patients receiving docetaxel as there is a potential for a significant reaction).
No products indexed under this heading.

Cyclosporine (The metabolism of docetaxel may be modified by the concomitant administration of compounds that induce, inhibit, or are metabolized by cytochrome P450 3A4, such as cyclosporine. Caution should be exercised with cyclosporine when treating patients receiving docetaxel as there is a potential for a significant reaction). Products include:
Gengraf Capsules 435
Neoral Oral Solution 2280
Neoral Soft Gelatin Capsules 2280
Restasis Ophthalmic Emulsion 557
Sandimmune 2296

Dalfopristin (The metabolism of docetaxel may be modified by the concomitant administration of compounds that inhibit cytochrome P450 3A4. Caution should be exercised with these drugs when treating patients receiving docetaxel as there is a potential for a significant reaction).
No products indexed under this heading.

Danazol (The metabolism of docetaxel may be modified by the concomitant administration of compounds that inhibit cytochrome P450 3A4. Caution should be exercised with these drugs when treating patients receiving docetaxel as there is a potential for a significant reaction).
No products indexed under this heading.

Delavirdine Mesylate (The metabolism of docetaxel may be modified by the concomitant administration of compounds that inhibit cytochrome P450 3A4. Caution should be exercised with these drugs when treating patients receiving docetaxel as there is a potential for a significant reaction).
No products indexed under this heading.

Desogestrel (The metabolism of docetaxel may be modified by the concomitant administration of compounds that are metabolized by cytochrome P450 3A4. Caution should be exercised with these drugs when treating patients receiving docetaxel as there is a potential for a significant reaction). Products include:
Mircette Tablets 1034

Dexamethasone (The metabolism of docetaxel may be modified by the concomitant administration of compounds that induce cytochrome P450 3A4. Caution should be exercised with these drugs when treating patients receiving docetaxel as there is a potential for a significant reaction). Products include:
Ciprodex Otic Suspension 541

Dexamethasone Acetate (The metabolism of docetaxel may be modified by the concomitant administration of compounds that induce cytochrome P450 3A4. Caution should be exercised with these drugs when treating patients receiving docetaxel as there is a potential for a significant reaction).
No products indexed under this heading.

Dexamethasone Sodium Phosphate (The metabolism of docetaxel may be modified by the concomitant administration of compounds that induce cytochrome P450 3A4. Caution should be exercised with these drugs when treating patients receiving docetaxel as there is a potential for a significant reaction).
No products indexed under this heading.

Diazepam (The metabolism of docetaxel may be modified by the concomitant administration of compounds that are metabolized by cytochrome P450 3A4. Caution should be exercised with these drugs when treating patients receiving docetaxel as there is a potential for a significant reaction). Products include:

Valium Tablets 2658

Dihydroergotamine Mesylate (The metabolism of docetaxel may be modified by the concomitant administration of compounds that are metabolized by cytochrome P450 3A4. Caution should be exercised with these drugs when treating patients receiving docetaxel as there is a potential for a significant reaction).

No products indexed under this heading.

Diltiazem Hydrochloride (The metabolism of docetaxel may be modified by the concomitant administration of compounds that inhibit cytochrome P450 3A4. Caution should be exercised with these drugs when treating patients receiving docetaxel as there is a potential for a significant reaction). Products include:

Cardizem LA Extended Release Tablets 421

Diltiazem Maleate (The metabolism of docetaxel may be modified by the concomitant administration of compounds that inhibit cytochrome P450 3A4. Caution should be exercised with these drugs when treating patients receiving docetaxel as there is a potential for a significant reaction).

No products indexed under this heading.

Disopyramide (The metabolism of docetaxel may be modified by the concomitant administration of compounds that are metabolized by cytochrome P450 3A4. Caution should be exercised with these drugs when treating patients receiving docetaxel as there is a potential for a significant reaction).

No products indexed under this heading.

Disopyramide Phosphate (The metabolism of docetaxel may be modified by the concomitant administration of compounds that are metabolized by cytochrome P450 3A4. Caution should be exercised with these drugs when treating patients receiving docetaxel as there is a potential for a significant reaction).

No products indexed under this heading.

Disulfiram (The metabolism of docetaxel may be modified by the concomitant administration of compounds that are metabolized by cytochrome P450 3A4. Caution should be exercised with these drugs when treating patients receiving docetaxel as there is a potential for a significant reaction).

No products indexed under this heading.

Doxorubicin Hydrochloride (The metabolism of docetaxel may be modified by the concomitant administration of compounds that induce cytochrome P450 3A4. Caution should be exercised with these drugs when treating patients receiving docetaxel as there is a potential for a significant reaction).

No products indexed under this heading.

Dronabinol (The metabolism of docetaxel may be modified by the concomitant administration of compounds that are metabolized by cytochrome P450 3A4. Caution should be exercised with these drugs when treating patients receiving docetaxel as there is a potential for a significant reaction). Products include:

Marinol Capsules 3163

Efavirenz (The metabolism of docetaxel may be modified by the concomitant administration of compounds that induce cytochrome P450 3A4. Caution should be exercised with these drugs when treating patients receiving docetaxel as there is a potential for a significant reaction). Products include:

Atripla Tablets 938
Sustiva Capsules 930
Sustiva Tablets 930

Ergotamine Tartrate (The metabolism of docetaxel may be modified by the concomitant administration of compounds that are metabolized by cytochrome P450 3A4. Caution should be exercised with these drugs when treating patients receiving docetaxel as there is a potential for a significant reaction).

No products indexed under this heading.

Erythromycin (The metabolism of docetaxel may be modified by the concomitant administration of compounds that induce, inhibit, or are metabolized by cytochrome P450 3A4, such as erythromycin. Caution should be exercised with erythromycin when treating patients receiving docetaxel as there is a potential for a significant reaction).

No products indexed under this heading.

Erythromycin Estolate (The metabolism of docetaxel may be modified by the concomitant administration of compounds that induce, inhibit, or are metabolized by cytochrome P450 3A4, such as erythromycin. Caution should be exercised with erythromycin when treating patients receiving docetaxel as there is a potential for a significant reaction).

No products indexed under this heading.

Erythromycin Ethylsuccinate (The metabolism of docetaxel may be modified by the concomitant administration of compounds that induce, inhibit, or are metabolized by cytochrome P450 3A4, such as erythromycin. Caution should be exercised with erythromycin when treating patients receiving docetaxel as there is a potential for a significant reaction). Products include:

E.E.S. 433
EryPed 431

Erythromycin Gluceptate (The metabolism of docetaxel may be modified by the concomitant administration of compounds that induce, inhibit, or are metabolized by cytochrome P450 3A4, such as erythromycin. Caution should be exercised with erythromycin when treating patients receiving docetaxel as there is a potential for a significant reaction).

No products indexed under this heading.

Erythromycin Lactobionate (The metabolism of docetaxel may be modified by the concomitant administration of compounds that induce, inhibit, or are metabolized by cytochrome P450 3A4, such as erythromycin. Caution should be exercised with erythromycin when treating patients receiving docetaxel as there is a potential for a significant reaction).

No products indexed under this heading.

Erythromycin Stearate (The metabolism of docetaxel may be modified by the concomitant administration of compounds that induce, inhibit, or are metabolized by cytochrome P450 3A4, such as erythromycin. Caution should be exercised with erythromycin when treating patients receiving docetaxel as there is a potential for a significant reaction).

No products indexed under this heading.

Esomeprazole Magnesium (The metabolism of docetaxel may be modified by the concomitant administration of compounds that inhibit cytochrome P450 3A4. Caution should be exercised with these drugs when treating patients receiving docetaxel as there is a potential for a significant reaction). Products include:

Nexium Delayed-Release Capsules 645
Nexium Delayed-Release Oral Suspension 645

Estradiol (The metabolism of docetaxel may be modified by the concomitant administration of compounds that are metabolized by cytochrome P450 3A4. Caution should be exercised with these drugs when treating patients receiving docetaxel as there is a potential for a significant reaction). Products include:

Activella Tablets 2347
Angeliq Tablets 751
Climara Transdermal System 763
Climara Pro Transdermal System 768
Divigel 3167
Vagifem Tablets 2375

Estradiol Benzoate (The metabolism of docetaxel may be modified by the concomitant administration of compounds that are metabolized by cytochrome P450 3A4. Caution should be exercised with these drugs when treating patients receiving docetaxel as there is a potential for a significant reaction).

No products indexed under this heading.

Estradiol Cypionate (The metabolism of docetaxel may be modified by the concomitant administration of compounds that are metabolized by cytochrome P450 3A4. Caution should be exercised with these drugs when treating patients receiving docetaxel as there is a potential for a significant reaction).

No products indexed under this heading.

Estradiol Valerate (The metabolism of docetaxel may be modified by the concomitant administration of compounds that are metabolized by cytochrome P450 3A4. Caution should be exercised with these drugs when treating patients receiving docetaxel as there is a potential for a significant reaction).

No products indexed under this heading.

Ethinyl Estradiol (The metabolism of docetaxel may be modified by the concomitant administration of compounds that are metabolized by cytochrome P450 3A4. Caution should be exercised with these drugs when treating patients receiving docetaxel as there is a potential for a significant reaction). Products include:

Lybrel Tablets 3204
Mircette Tablets 1034
NuvaRing 2897
Ortho-Cyclen/Ortho Tri-Cyclen 2449
Ortho Evra Transdermal System 2437
Ortho Tri-Cyclen Lo Tablets 2458
Seasonique Tablets 1046
Yaz Tablets 805

Ethosuximide (The metabolism of docetaxel may be modified by the concomitant administration of compounds that induce cytochrome P450 3A4. Caution should be exercised with these drugs when treating patients receiving docetaxel as there is a potential for a significant reaction).

No products indexed under this heading.

Ethynodiol Diacetate (The metabolism of docetaxel may be modified by the concomitant administration of compounds that are metabolized by cytochrome P450 3A4. Caution should be exercised with these drugs when treating patients receiving docetaxel as there is a potential for a significant reaction).

No products indexed under this heading.

Etoposide (The metabolism of docetaxel may be modified by the concomitant administration of compounds that are metabolized by cytochrome P450 3A4. Caution should be exercised with these drugs when treating patients receiving docetaxel as there is a potential for a significant reaction).

No products indexed under this heading.

Etoposide Phosphate (The metabolism of docetaxel may be modified by the concomitant administration of compounds that are metabolized by cytochrome P450 3A4. Caution should be exercised with these drugs when treating patients receiving docetaxel as there is a potential for a significant reaction).

No products indexed under this heading.

Felbamate (The metabolism of docetaxel may be modified by the concomitant administration of compounds that induce cytochrome P450 3A4. Caution should be exercised with these drugs when treating patients receiving docetaxel as there is a potential for a significant reaction).

No products indexed under this heading.

Felodipine (The metabolism of docetaxel may be modified by the concomitant administration of compounds that are metabolized by cytochrome P450 3A4. Caution should be exercised with these drugs when treating patients receiving docetaxel as there is a potential for a significant reaction).

No products indexed under this heading.

Fentanyl (The metabolism of docetaxel may be modified by the concomitant administration of compounds that are metabolized by cytochrome P450 3A4. Caution

should be exercised with these drugs when treating patients receiving docetaxel as there is a potential for a significant reaction). Products include:

Duragesic Transdermal System 2405
Ionsys Transdermal System 2410

Fentanyl Citrate (The metabolism of docetaxel may be modified by the concomitant administration of compounds that are metabolized by cytochrome P450 3A4. Caution should be exercised with these drugs when treating patients receiving docetaxel as there is a potential for a significant reaction). Products include:

Actiq 959
Fentora Tablets 968

Fluconazole (The metabolism of docetaxel may be modified by the concomitant administration of compounds that inhibit cytochrome P450 3A4. Caution should be exercised with these drugs when treating patients receiving docetaxel as there is a potential for a significant reaction).

No products indexed under this heading.

Fludrocortisone Acetate (The metabolism of docetaxel may be modified by the concomitant administration of compounds that induce cytochrome P450 3A4. Caution should be exercised with these drugs when treating patients receiving docetaxel as there is a potential for a significant reaction).

No products indexed under this heading.

Fluoxetine (The metabolism of docetaxel may be modified by the concomitant administration of compounds that inhibit cytochrome P450 3A4. Caution should be exercised with these drugs when treating patients receiving docetaxel as there is a potential for a significant reaction).

No products indexed under this heading.

Fluoxetine Hydrochloride (The metabolism of docetaxel may be modified by the concomitant administration of compounds that inhibit cytochrome P450 3A4. Caution should be exercised with these drugs when treating patients receiving docetaxel as there is a potential for a significant reaction). Products include:

Prozac Weekly Capsules 1852
Prozac Pulvules and Liquid 1852
Symbyax Capsules 1871

Fluvoxamine Maleate (The metabolism of docetaxel may be modified by the concomitant administration of compounds that inhibit cytochrome P450 3A4. Caution should be exercised with these drugs when treating patients receiving docetaxel as there is a potential for a significant reaction). Products include:

Luvox CR Extended-Release Capsules.................................... 1759

Fosamprenavir Calcium (The metabolism of docetaxel may be modified by the concomitant administration of compounds that inhibit cytochrome P450 3A4. Caution should be exercised with these drugs when treating patients receiving docetaxel as there is a potential for a significant reaction). Products include:

Lexiva Oral Suspension 1510
Lexiva Tablets 1510

Fosphenytoin Sodium (The metabolism of docetaxel may be modified by the concomitant administration of compounds that induce cytochrome P450 3A4. Caution should be exercised with these drugs when treating patients receiving docetaxel as there is a potential for a significant reaction).

No products indexed under this heading.

Garlic Extract (The metabolism of docetaxel may be modified by the concomitant administration of compounds that induce cytochrome P450 3A4. Caution should be exercised with these drugs when treating patients receiving docetaxel as there is a potential for a significant reaction).

No products indexed under this heading.

Garlic Oil (The metabolism of docetaxel may be modified by the concomitant administration of compounds that induce cytochrome P450 3A4. Caution should be exercised with these drugs when treating patients receiving docetaxel as there is a potential for a significant reaction).

No products indexed under this heading.

Haloperidol (The metabolism of docetaxel may be modified by the concomitant administration of compounds that are metabolized by cytochrome P450 3A4. Caution should be exercised with these drugs when treating patients receiving docetaxel as there is a potential for a significant reaction).

No products indexed under this heading.

Haloperidol Decanoate (The metabolism of docetaxel may be modified by the concomitant administration of compounds that are metabolized by cytochrome P450 3A4. Caution should be exercised with these drugs when treating patients receiving docetaxel as there is a potential for a significant reaction).

No products indexed under this heading.

Haloperidol Lactate (The metabolism of docetaxel may be modified by the concomitant administration of compounds that are metabolized by cytochrome P450 3A4. Caution should be exercised with these drugs when treating patients receiving docetaxel as there is a potential for a significant reaction).

No products indexed under this heading.

Hydrocortisone (The metabolism of docetaxel may be modified by the concomitant administration of compounds that induce cytochrome P450 3A4. Caution should be exercised with these drugs when treating patients receiving docetaxel as there is a potential for a significant reaction).

No products indexed under this heading.

Hydrocortisone Acetate (The metabolism of docetaxel may be modified by the concomitant administration of compounds that induce cytochrome P450 3A4. Caution should be exercised with these drugs when treating patients receiving docetaxel as there is a potential for a significant reaction). Products include:

Analpram-HC 1140
Pramosone 1141

Hydrocortisone Butyrate (The metabolism of docetaxel may be modified by the concomitant administration of compounds that induce cytochrome P450 3A4. Caution should be exercised with these drugs when treating patients receiving docetaxel as there is a potential for a significant reaction).

No products indexed under this heading.

Hydrocortisone Cypionate (The metabolism of docetaxel may be modified by the concomitant administration of compounds that induce cytochrome P450 3A4. Caution should be exercised with these drugs when treating patients receiving docetaxel as there is a potential for a significant reaction).

No products indexed under this heading.

Hydrocortisone Hemisuccinate (The metabolism of docetaxel may be modified by the concomitant administration of compounds that induce cytochrome P450 3A4. Caution should be exercised with these drugs when treating patients receiving docetaxel as there is a potential for a significant reaction).

No products indexed under this heading.

Hydrocortisone Probutate (The metabolism of docetaxel may be modified by the concomitant administration of compounds that induce cytochrome P450 3A4. Caution should be exercised with these drugs when treating patients receiving docetaxel as there is a potential for a significant reaction).

No products indexed under this heading.

Hydrocortisone Sodium Phosphate (The metabolism of docetaxel may be modified by the concomitant administration of compounds that induce cytochrome P450 3A4. Caution should be exercised with these drugs when treating patients receiving docetaxel as there is a potential for a significant reaction).

No products indexed under this heading.

Hydrocortisone Sodium Succinate (The metabolism of docetaxel may be modified by the concomitant administration of compounds that induce cytochrome P450 3A4. Caution should be exercised with these drugs when treating patients receiving docetaxel as there is a potential for a significant reaction).

No products indexed under this heading.

Hydrocortisone Valerate (The metabolism of docetaxel may be modified by the concomitant administration of compounds that induce cytochrome P450 3A4. Caution should be exercised with these drugs when treating patients receiving docetaxel as there is a potential for a significant reaction).

No products indexed under this heading.

Hypericum (The metabolism of docetaxel may be modified by the concomitant administration of compounds that induce cytochrome P450 3A4. Caution should be exercised with these drugs when treating patients receiving docetaxel as there is a potential for a significant reaction). Products include:

Satieté Tablets 640

Hypericum Perforatum (The metabolism of docetaxel may be modified by the concomitant administration of compounds that induce cytochrome P450 3A4. Caution should be exercised with these drugs when treating patients receiving docetaxel as there is a potential for a significant reaction).

No products indexed under this heading.

Indinavir Sulfate (The metabolism of docetaxel may be modified by the concomitant administration of compounds that inhibit cytochrome P450 3A4. Caution should be exercised with these drugs when treating patients receiving docetaxel as there is a potential for a significant reaction). Products include:

Crixivan Capsules 1979

Isoniazid (The metabolism of docetaxel may be modified by the concomitant administration of compounds that inhibit cytochrome P450 3A4. Caution should be exercised with these drugs when treating patients receiving docetaxel as there is a potential for a significant reaction).

No products indexed under this heading.

Isradipine (The metabolism of docetaxel may be modified by the concomitant administration of compounds that are metabolized by cytochrome P450 3A4. Caution should be exercised with these drugs when treating patients receiving docetaxel as there is a potential for a significant reaction). Products include:

DynaCirc CR Controlled Release Tablets....................................... 1407

Itraconazole (The metabolism of docetaxel may be modified by the concomitant administration of compounds that inhibit cytochrome P450 3A4. Caution should be exercised with these drugs when treating patients receiving docetaxel as there is a potential for a significant reaction).

No products indexed under this heading.

Ixabepilone (The metabolism of docetaxel may be modified by the concomitant administration of compounds that are metabolized by cytochrome P450 3A4. Caution should be exercised with these drugs when treating patients receiving docetaxel as there is a potential for a significant reaction). Products include:

Ixempra Kit for Injection 915

Ketoconazole (The metabolism of docetaxel may be modified by the concomitant administration of compounds that induce, inhibit, or are metabolized by cytochrome P450 3A4, such as ketoconazole. Caution should be exercised with ketoconazole when treating patients receiving docetaxel as there is a potential for a significant reaction). Products include:

Extina Foam, 2% 3057
Nizoral A-D Shampoo 1901

Levonorgestrel (The metabolism of docetaxel may be modified by the concomitant administration of compounds that are metabolized by cytochrome P450 3A4. Caution should be exercised with these drugs when treating patients receiving docetaxel as there is a potential for a significant reaction). Products include:

Climara Pro Transdermal System **768**
Lybrel Tablets **3204**
Mirena Intrauterine System **779**
Plan B Tablets **1044**
Seasonique Tablets **1046**

Lidocaine (The metabolism of docetaxel may be modified by the concomitant administration of compounds that are metabolized by cytochrome P450 3A4. Caution should be exercised with these drugs when treating patients receiving docetaxel as there is a potential for a significant reaction). Products include:
Lidoderm Patch **1114**

Lidocaine Hydrochloride (The metabolism of docetaxel may be modified by the concomitant administration of compounds that are metabolized by cytochrome P450 3A4. Caution should be exercised with these drugs when treating patients receiving docetaxel as there is a potential for a significant reaction).
No products indexed under this heading.

Lopinavir (The metabolism of docetaxel may be modified by the concomitant administration of compounds that inhibit cytochrome P450 3A4. Caution should be exercised with these drugs when treating patients receiving docetaxel as there is a potential for a significant reaction). Products include:
Kaletra **452**

Loratadine (The metabolism of docetaxel may be modified by the concomitant administration of compounds that inhibit cytochrome P450 3A4. Caution should be exercised with these drugs when treating patients receiving docetaxel as there is a potential for a significant reaction).
No products indexed under this heading.

Lovastatin (The metabolism of docetaxel may be modified by the concomitant administration of compounds that are metabolized by cytochrome P450 3A4. Caution should be exercised with these drugs when treating patients receiving docetaxel as there is a potential for a significant reaction). Products include:
Advicor Tablets **402**
Mevacor Tablets **2063**

Mephenytoin (The metabolism of docetaxel may be modified by the concomitant administration of compounds that induce cytochrome P450 3A4. Caution should be exercised with these drugs when treating patients receiving docetaxel as there is a potential for a significant reaction).
No products indexed under this heading.

Mestranol (The metabolism of docetaxel may be modified by the concomitant administration of compounds that are metabolized by cytochrome P450 3A4. Caution should be exercised with these drugs when treating patients receiving docetaxel as there is a potential for a significant reaction).
No products indexed under this heading.

Methadone Hydrochloride (The metabolism of docetaxel may be modified by the concomitant administration of compounds that are metabolized by cytochrome P450 3A4. Caution should be exercised with these drugs when treating patients receiving docetaxel as there is a potential for a significant reaction).
No products indexed under this heading.

Methsuximide (The metabolism of docetaxel may be modified by the concomitant administration of compounds that induce cytochrome P450 3A4. Caution should be exercised with these drugs when treating patients receiving docetaxel as there is a potential for a significant reaction).
No products indexed under this heading.

Methylprednisolone (The metabolism of docetaxel may be modified by the concomitant administration of compounds that induce cytochrome P450 3A4. Caution should be exercised with these drugs when treating patients receiving docetaxel as there is a potential for a significant reaction).
No products indexed under this heading.

Methylprednisolone Acetate (The metabolism of docetaxel may be modified by the concomitant administration of compounds that induce cytochrome P450 3A4. Caution should be exercised with these drugs when treating patients receiving docetaxel as there is a potential for a significant reaction).
No products indexed under this heading.

Methylprednisolone Sodium Succinate (The metabolism of docetaxel may be modified by the concomitant administration of compounds that induce cytochrome P450 3A4. Caution should be exercised with these drugs when treating patients receiving docetaxel as there is a potential for a significant reaction).
No products indexed under this heading.

Metronidazole (The metabolism of docetaxel may be modified by the concomitant administration of compounds that inhibit cytochrome P450 3A4. Caution should be exercised with these drugs when treating patients receiving docetaxel as there is a potential for a significant reaction). Products include:
Pylera Capsules **714**

Metronidazole Benzoate (The metabolism of docetaxel may be modified by the concomitant administration of compounds that inhibit cytochrome P450 3A4. Caution should be exercised with these drugs when treating patients receiving docetaxel as there is a potential for a significant reaction).
No products indexed under this heading.

Metronidazole Hydrochloride (The metabolism of docetaxel may be modified by the concomitant administration of compounds that inhibit cytochrome P450 3A4. Caution should be exercised with these drugs when treating patients receiving docetaxel as there is a potential for a significant reaction).
No products indexed under this heading.

Metronidazole Sodium (The metabolism of docetaxel may be modified by the concomitant administration of compounds that inhibit cytochrome P450 3A4. Caution should be exercised with these drugs when treating patients receiving docetaxel as there is a potential for a significant reaction).
No products indexed under this heading.

Miconazole (The metabolism of docetaxel may be modified by the concomitant administration of compounds that inhibit cytochrome P450 3A4. Caution should be exercised with these drugs when treating patients receiving docetaxel as there is a potential for a significant reaction).
No products indexed under this heading.

Miconazole Nitrate (The metabolism of docetaxel may be modified by the concomitant administration of compounds that inhibit cytochrome P450 3A4. Caution should be exercised with these drugs when treating patients receiving docetaxel as there is a potential for a significant reaction).
No products indexed under this heading.

Midazolam Hydrochloride (The metabolism of docetaxel may be modified by the concomitant administration of compounds that are metabolized by cytochrome P450 3A4. Caution should be exercised with these drugs when treating patients receiving docetaxel as there is a potential for a significant reaction).
No products indexed under this heading.

Modafinil (The metabolism of docetaxel may be modified by the concomitant administration of compounds that induce cytochrome P450 3A4. Caution should be exercised with these drugs when treating patients receiving docetaxel as there is a potential for a significant reaction). Products include:
Provigil Tablets **977**

Nefazodone Hydrochloride (The metabolism of docetaxel may be modified by the concomitant administration of compounds that inhibit cytochrome P450 3A4. Caution should be exercised with these drugs when treating patients receiving docetaxel as there is a potential for a significant reaction).
No products indexed under this heading.

Nelfinavir Mesylate (The metabolism of docetaxel may be modified by the concomitant administration of compounds that inhibit cytochrome P450 3A4. Caution should be exercised with these drugs when treating patients receiving docetaxel as there is a potential for a significant reaction).
No products indexed under this heading.

Nevirapine (The metabolism of docetaxel may be modified by the concomitant administration of compounds that induce cytochrome P450 3A4. Caution should be exercised with these drugs when treating patients receiving docetaxel as there is a potential for a significant reaction). Products include:
Viramune Oral Suspension **873**
Viramune Tablets **873**

Niacinamide (The metabolism of docetaxel may be modified by the concomitant administration of compounds that inhibit cytochrome P450 3A4. Caution should be exercised with these drugs when treating patients receiving docetaxel as there is a potential for a significant reaction). Products include:
BioLean Free Tablets .... ▣**635**

Nicardipine Hydrochloride (The metabolism of docetaxel may be modified by the concomitant administration of compounds that are metabolized by cytochrome P450 3A4. Caution should be exercised with these drugs when treating patients receiving docetaxel as there is a potential for a significant reaction). Products include:
Cardene I.V. **1093**

Nicotinamide (The metabolism of docetaxel may be modified by the concomitant administration of compounds that inhibit cytochrome P450 3A4. Caution should be exercised with these drugs when treating patients receiving docetaxel as there is a potential for a significant reaction).
No products indexed under this heading.

Nifedipine (The metabolism of docetaxel may be modified by the concomitant administration of compounds that inhibit cytochrome P450 3A4. Caution should be exercised with these drugs when treating patients receiving docetaxel as there is a potential for a significant reaction).
No products indexed under this heading.

Nimodipine (The metabolism of docetaxel may be modified by the concomitant administration of compounds that are metabolized by cytochrome P450 3A4. Caution should be exercised with these drugs when treating patients receiving docetaxel as there is a potential for a significant reaction). Products include:
Nimotop Capsules **790**

Nisoldipine (The metabolism of docetaxel may be modified by the concomitant administration of compounds that are metabolized by cytochrome P450 3A4. Caution should be exercised with these drugs when treating patients receiving docetaxel as there is a potential for a significant reaction). Products include:
Sular Extended Release Tablets **2975**

Nitrendipine (The metabolism of docetaxel may be modified by the concomitant administration of compounds that are metabolized by cytochrome P450 3A4. Caution should be exercised with these drugs when treating patients receiving docetaxel as there is a potential for a significant reaction).
No products indexed under this heading.

Norethindrone (The metabolism of docetaxel may be modified by the concomitant administration of compounds that are metabolized by cytochrome P450 3A4. Caution should be exercised with these drugs when treating patients receiving docetaxel as there is a potential for a significant reaction). Products include:
Ortho Micronor Tablets **2446**

Norethindrone Acetate (The metabolism of docetaxel may be modified by the concomitant administration of compounds that are metabolized by cytochrome P450 3A4. Caution should be exercised with these drugs when treating patients receiving docetaxel as there is a potential for a significant reaction). Products include:

Activella Tablets 2347

Norfloxacin (The metabolism of docetaxel may be modified by the concomitant administration of compounds that inhibit cytochrome P450 3A4. Caution should be exercised with these drugs when treating patients receiving docetaxel as there is a potential for a significant reaction). Products include:

Noroxin Tablets 2069

Norgestrel (The metabolism of docetaxel may be modified by the concomitant administration of compounds that are metabolized by cytochrome P450 3A4. Caution should be exercised with these drugs when treating patients receiving docetaxel as there is a potential for a significant reaction).

No products indexed under this heading.

Omeprazole (The metabolism of docetaxel may be modified by the concomitant administration of compounds that inhibit cytochrome P450 3A4. Caution should be exercised with these drugs when treating patients receiving docetaxel as there is a potential for a significant reaction).

No products indexed under this heading.

Ondansetron (The metabolism of docetaxel may be modified by the concomitant administration of compounds that are metabolized by cytochrome P450 3A4. Caution should be exercised with these drugs when treating patients receiving docetaxel as there is a potential for a significant reaction). Products include:

Zofran ODT Orally Disintegrating Tablets 1687

Ondansetron Hydrochloride (The metabolism of docetaxel may be modified by the concomitant administration of compounds that are metabolized by cytochrome P450 3A4. Caution should be exercised with these drugs when treating patients receiving docetaxel as there is a potential for a significant reaction). Products include:

Zofran Injection 1682
Zofran 1687

Oxcarbazepine (The metabolism of docetaxel may be modified by the concomitant administration of compounds that induce cytochrome P450 3A4. Caution should be exercised with these drugs when treating patients receiving docetaxel as there is a potential for a significant reaction).

No products indexed under this heading.

Paclitaxel (The metabolism of docetaxel may be modified by the concomitant administration of compounds that are metabolized by cytochrome P450 3A4. Caution should be exercised with these drugs when treating patients receiving docetaxel as there is a potential for a significant reaction).

No products indexed under this heading.

Paroxetine Hydrochloride (The metabolism of docetaxel may be modified by the concomitant administration of compounds that inhibit cytochrome P450 3A4. Caution should be exercised with these drugs when treating patients receiving docetaxel as there is a potential for a significant reaction). Products include:

Paxil 1535
Paxil CR Controlled-Release Tablets 1544

Phenobarbital (The metabolism of docetaxel may be modified by the concomitant administration of compounds that induce cytochrome P450 3A4. Caution should be exercised with these drugs when treating patients receiving docetaxel as there is a potential for a significant reaction). Products include:

Donnatal Extentabs 2507

Phenobarbital Sodium (The metabolism of docetaxel may be modified by the concomitant administration of compounds that induce cytochrome P450 3A4. Caution should be exercised with these drugs when treating patients receiving docetaxel as there is a potential for a significant reaction).

No products indexed under this heading.

Phenytoin (The metabolism of docetaxel may be modified by the concomitant administration of compounds that induce cytochrome P450 3A4. Caution should be exercised with these drugs when treating patients receiving docetaxel as there is a potential for a significant reaction).

No products indexed under this heading.

Phenytoin Sodium (The metabolism of docetaxel may be modified by the concomitant administration of compounds that induce cytochrome P450 3A4. Caution should be exercised with these drugs when treating patients receiving docetaxel as there is a potential for a significant reaction). Products include:

Phenytek Capsules 2192

Pimozide (The metabolism of docetaxel may be modified by the concomitant administration of compounds that are metabolized by cytochrome P450 3A4. Caution should be exercised with these drugs when treating patients receiving docetaxel as there is a potential for a significant reaction).

No products indexed under this heading.

Polyestradiol Phosphate (The metabolism of docetaxel may be modified by the concomitant administration of compounds that are metabolized by cytochrome P450 3A4. Caution should be exercised with these drugs when treating patients receiving docetaxel as there is a potential for a significant reaction).

No products indexed under this heading.

Prednisolone Acetate (The metabolism of docetaxel may be modified by the concomitant administration of compounds that induce cytochrome P450 3A4. Caution should be exercised with these drugs when treating patients receiving docetaxel as there is a potential for a significant reaction). Products include:

Pred Forte Ophthalmic Suspension .... ⊙227
Pred Mild Ophthalmic Suspension .... ⊙230
Pred-G Ophthalmic Ointment .... ⊙229
Pred-G Ophthalmic Suspension .... ⊙228

Prednisolone Sodium Phosphate (The metabolism of docetaxel may be modified by the concomitant administration of compounds that induce cytochrome P450 3A4. Caution should be exercised with these drugs when treating patients receiving docetaxel as there is a potential for a significant reaction).

No products indexed under this heading.

Prednisolone Tebutate (The metabolism of docetaxel may be modified by the concomitant administration of compounds that induce cytochrome P450 3A4. Caution should be exercised with these drugs when treating patients receiving docetaxel as there is a potential for a significant reaction).

No products indexed under this heading.

Prednisone (The metabolism of docetaxel may be modified by the concomitant administration of compounds that induce cytochrome P450 3A4. Caution should be exercised with these drugs when treating patients receiving docetaxel as there is a potential for a significant reaction).

No products indexed under this heading.

Primidone (The metabolism of docetaxel may be modified by the concomitant administration of compounds that induce cytochrome P450 3A4. Caution should be exercised with these drugs when treating patients receiving docetaxel as there is a potential for a significant reaction).

No products indexed under this heading.

Propoxyphene Hydrochloride (The metabolism of docetaxel may be modified by the concomitant administration of compounds that inhibit cytochrome P450 3A4. Caution should be exercised with these drugs when treating patients receiving docetaxel as there is a potential for a significant reaction).

No products indexed under this heading.

Propoxyphene Napsylate (The metabolism of docetaxel may be modified by the concomitant administration of compounds that inhibit cytochrome P450 3A4. Caution should be exercised with these drugs when treating patients receiving docetaxel as there is a potential for a significant reaction).

No products indexed under this heading.

Quinidine (The metabolism of docetaxel may be modified by the concomitant administration of compounds that inhibit cytochrome P450 3A4. Caution should be exercised with these drugs when treating patients receiving docetaxel as there is a potential for a significant reaction).

No products indexed under this heading.

Quinidine Gluconate (The metabolism of docetaxel may be modified by the concomitant administration of compounds that are metabolized by cytochrome P450 3A4. Caution should be exercised with these drugs when treating patients receiving docetaxel as there is a potential for a significant reaction).

No products indexed under this heading.

Quinidine Hydrochloride (The metabolism of docetaxel may be modified by the concomitant administration of compounds that inhibit cytochrome P450 3A4. Caution should be exercised with these drugs when treating patients receiving docetaxel as there is a potential for a significant reaction).

No products indexed under this heading.

Quinidine Polygalacturonate (The metabolism of docetaxel may be modified by the concomitant administration of compounds that inhibit cytochrome P450 3A4. Caution should be exercised with these drugs when treating patients receiving docetaxel as there is a potential for a significant reaction).

No products indexed under this heading.

Quinidine Sulfate (The metabolism of docetaxel may be modified by the concomitant administration of compounds that inhibit cytochrome P450 3A4. Caution should be exercised with these drugs when treating patients receiving docetaxel as there is a potential for a significant reaction).

No products indexed under this heading.

Quinine (The metabolism of docetaxel may be modified by the concomitant administration of compounds that inhibit cytochrome P450 3A4. Caution should be exercised with these drugs when treating patients receiving docetaxel as there is a potential for a significant reaction).

No products indexed under this heading.

Quinine Sulfate (The metabolism of docetaxel may be modified by the concomitant administration of compounds that inhibit cytochrome P450 3A4. Caution should be exercised with these drugs when treating patients receiving docetaxel as there is a potential for a significant reaction).

No products indexed under this heading.

Quinupristin (The metabolism of docetaxel may be modified by the concomitant administration of compounds that inhibit cytochrome P450 3A4. Caution should be exercised with these drugs when treating patients receiving docetaxel as there is a potential for a significant reaction).

No products indexed under this heading.

Ranitidine Bismuth Citrate (The metabolism of docetaxel may be modified by the concomitant administration of compounds that inhibit cytochrome P450 3A4. Caution should be exercised with these drugs when treating patients receiving docetaxel as there is a potential for a significant reaction).

No products indexed under this heading.

Ranitidine Hydrochloride (The metabolism of docetaxel may be modified by the concomitant administration of compounds that inhibit cytochrome P450 3A4. Caution should be exercised with these drugs when treating patients receiving docetaxel as there is a potential for a significant reaction). Products include:

- Zantac 75 Tablets .... ▣603
- Zantac 1670
- Zantac Injection 1666
- Zantac Injection Pharmacy Bulk Package 1668
- Maximum Strength Zantac 150 Tablets .... ▣603
- Maximum Strength Zantac 150 Cool Mint Tablets .... ▣603

Rifabutin (The metabolism of docetaxel may be modified by the concomitant administration of compounds that induce cytochrome P450 3A4. Caution should be exercised with these drugs when treating patients receiving docetaxel as there is a potential for a significant reaction).

No products indexed under this heading.

Rifampicin (The metabolism of docetaxel may be modified by the concomitant administration of compounds that induce cytochrome P450 3A4. Caution should be exercised with these drugs when treating patients receiving docetaxel as there is a potential for a significant reaction).

No products indexed under this heading.

Rifampin (The metabolism of docetaxel may be modified by the concomitant administration of compounds that induce cytochrome P450 3A4. Caution should be exercised with these drugs when treating patients receiving docetaxel as there is a potential for a significant reaction).

No products indexed under this heading.

Rifapentine (The metabolism of docetaxel may be modified by the concomitant administration of compounds that induce cytochrome P450 3A4. Caution should be exercised with these drugs when treating patients receiving docetaxel as there is a potential for a significant reaction).

No products indexed under this heading.

Ritonavir (The metabolism of docetaxel may be modified by the concomitant administration of compounds that inhibit cytochrome P450 3A4. Caution should be exercised with these drugs when treating patients receiving docetaxel as there is a potential for a significant reaction). Products include:

- Kaletra 452
- Norvir 489

Saquinavir (The metabolism of docetaxel may be modified by the concomitant administration of compounds that inhibit cytochrome P450 3A4. Caution should be exercised with these drugs when treating patients receiving docetaxel as there is a potential for a significant reaction).

No products indexed under this heading.

Saquinavir Mesylate (The metabolism of docetaxel may be modified by the concomitant administration of compounds that inhibit cytochrome P450 3A4. Caution should be exercised with these drugs when treating patients receiving docetaxel as there is a potential for a significant reaction).

No products indexed under this heading.

Sertraline Hydrochloride (The metabolism of docetaxel may be modified by the concomitant administration of compounds that inhibit cytochrome P450 3A4. Caution should be exercised with these drugs when treating patients receiving docetaxel as there is a potential for a significant reaction).

No products indexed under this heading.

Sildenafil Citrate (The metabolism of docetaxel may be modified by the concomitant administration of compounds that inhibit cytochrome P450 3A4. Caution should be exercised with these drugs when treating patients receiving docetaxel as there is a potential for a significant reaction).

No products indexed under this heading.

Simvastatin (The metabolism of docetaxel may be modified by the concomitant administration of compounds that are metabolized by cytochrome P450 3A4. Caution should be exercised with these drugs when treating patients receiving docetaxel as there is a potential for a significant reaction). Products include:

- Simcor Tablets 502
- Vytorin 10/10 Tablets 2149
- Vytorin 10/10 Tablets 2939
- Vytorin 10/20 Tablets 2149
- Vytorin 10/20 Tablets 2939
- Vytorin 10/40 Tablets 2149
- Vytorin 10/40 Tablets 2939
- Vytorin 10/80 Tablets 2149
- Vytorin 10/80 Tablets 2939
- Zocor Tablets 2136

Sirolimus (The metabolism of docetaxel may be modified by the concomitant administration of compounds that are metabolized by cytochrome P450 3A4. Caution should be exercised with these drugs when treating patients receiving docetaxel as there is a potential for a significant reaction). Products include:

- Rapamune 3260

Sulfinpyrazone (The metabolism of docetaxel may be modified by the concomitant administration of compounds that induce cytochrome P450 3A4. Caution should be exercised with these drugs when treating patients receiving docetaxel as there is a potential for a significant reaction).

No products indexed under this heading.

Tacrolimus (The metabolism of docetaxel may be modified by the concomitant administration of compounds that are metabolized by cytochrome P450 3A4. Caution should be exercised with these drugs when treating patients receiving docetaxel as there is a potential for a significant reaction). Products include:

- Prograf Capsules and Injection 622
- Protopic Ointment 628

Tadalafil (The metabolism of docetaxel may be modified by the concomitant administration of compounds that are metabolized by cytochrome P450 3A4. Caution should be exercised with these drugs when treating patients receiving docetaxel as there is a potential for a significant reaction). Products include:

- Cialis Tablets 1792

Tamoxifen Citrate (The metabolism of docetaxel may be modified by the concomitant administration of compounds that are metabolized by cytochrome P450 3A4. Caution should be exercised with these drugs when treating patients receiving docetaxel as there is a potential for a significant reaction).

No products indexed under this heading.

Telithromycin (The metabolism of docetaxel may be modified by the concomitant administration of compounds that inhibit cytochrome P450 3A4. Caution should be exercised with these drugs when treating patients receiving docetaxel as there is a potential for a significant reaction). Products include:

- Ketek Tablets 2744

Terfenadine (The metabolism of docetaxel may be modified by the concomitant administration of compounds that induce, inhibit, or are metabolized by cytochrome P450 3A4, such as terfenadine. Caution should be exercised with terfenadine when treating patients receiving docetaxel as there is a potential for a significant reaction).

No products indexed under this heading.

Theophylline (The metabolism of docetaxel may be modified by the concomitant administration of compounds that induce cytochrome P450 3A4. Caution should be exercised with these drugs when treating patients receiving docetaxel as there is a potential for a significant reaction).

No products indexed under this heading.

Theophylline Anhydrous (The metabolism of docetaxel may be modified by the concomitant administration of compounds that induce cytochrome P450 3A4. Caution should be exercised with these drugs when treating patients receiving docetaxel as there is a potential for a significant reaction). Products include:

- Uniphyl Tablets 2595

Theophylline Calcium Salicylate (The metabolism of docetaxel may be modified by the concomitant administration of compounds that induce cytochrome P450 3A4. Caution should be exercised with these drugs when treating patients receiving docetaxel as there is a potential for a significant reaction).

No products indexed under this heading.

Theophylline Dihydroxypropyl (Glyceryl) (The metabolism of docetaxel may be modified by the concomitant administration of compounds that induce cytochrome P450 3A4. Caution should be exercised with these drugs when treating patients receiving docetaxel as there is a potential for a significant reaction).

No products indexed under this heading.

Theophylline Ethylenediamine (The metabolism of docetaxel may be modified by the concomitant administration of compounds that induce cytochrome P450 3A4. Caution should be exercised with these drugs when treating patients receiving docetaxel as there is a potential for a significant reaction).

No products indexed under this heading.

Tiagabine Hydrochloride (The metabolism of docetaxel may be modified by the concomitant administration of compounds that are metabolized by cytochrome P450 3A4. Caution should be exercised with these drugs when treating patients receiving docetaxel as there is a potential for a significant reaction). Products include:

- Gabitril Tablets 973

Tolterodine Tartrate (The metabolism of docetaxel may be modified by the concomitant administration of compounds that are metabolized by cytochrome P450 3A4. Caution should be exercised with these drugs when treating patients receiving docetaxel as there is a potential for a significant reaction).

No products indexed under this heading.

Trazodone Hydrochloride (The metabolism of docetaxel may be modified by the concomitant administration of compounds that are metabolized by cytochrome P450 3A4. Caution should be exercised with these drugs when treating patients receiving docetaxel as there is a potential for a significant reaction).

No products indexed under this heading.

Triamcinolone (The metabolism of docetaxel may be modified by the concomitant administration of compounds that induce cytochrome P450 3A4. Caution should be exercised with these drugs when treating patients receiving docetaxel as there is a potential for a significant reaction).

No products indexed under this heading.

Triamcinolone Acetonide (The metabolism of docetaxel may be modified by the concomitant administration of compounds that induce cytochrome P450 3A4. Caution should be exercised with these drugs when treating patients receiving docetaxel as there is a potential for a significant reaction). Products include:

- Azmacort Inhalation Aerosol 407
- Nasacort AQ Nasal Spray 2765
- Triesence Injectable Suspension .... ⊙209

Triamcinolone Diacetate (The metabolism of docetaxel may be modified by the concomitant administration of compounds that induce cytochrome P450 3A4. Caution should be exercised with these drugs when treating patients receiving docetaxel as there is a potential for a significant reaction).

No products indexed under this heading.

Triamcinolone Hexacetonide (The metabolism of docetaxel may be modified by the concomitant administration of compounds that induce cytochrome P450 3A4. Caution should be exercised with these drugs when treating patients receiving docetaxel as there is a potential for a significant reaction).
No products indexed under this heading.

Triazolam (The metabolism of docetaxel may be modified by the concomitant administration of compounds that are metabolized by cytochrome P450 3A4. Caution should be exercised with these drugs when treating patients receiving docetaxel as there is a potential for a significant reaction).
No products indexed under this heading.

Troglitazone (The metabolism of docetaxel may be modified by the concomitant administration of compounds that induce cytochrome P450 3A4. Caution should be exercised with these drugs when treating patients receiving docetaxel as there is a potential for a significant reaction).
No products indexed under this heading.

Troleandomycin (The metabolism of docetaxel may be modified by the concomitant administration of compounds that induce, inhibit, or are metabolized by cytochrome P450 3A4, such as troleandomycin. Caution should be exercised with troleandomycin when treating patients receiving docetaxel as there is a potential for a significant reaction).
No products indexed under this heading.

Valproate Sodium (The metabolism of docetaxel may be modified by the concomitant administration of compounds that inhibit cytochrome P450 3A4. Caution should be exercised with these drugs when treating patients receiving docetaxel as there is a potential for a significant reaction).
No products indexed under this heading.

Vardenafil Hydrochloride (The metabolism of docetaxel may be modified by the concomitant administration of compounds that inhibit cytochrome P450 3A4. Caution should be exercised with these drugs when treating patients receiving docetaxel as there is a potential for a significant reaction). Products include:
Levitra Tablets ... 2876

Verapamil Hydrochloride (The metabolism of docetaxel may be modified by the concomitant administration of compounds that inhibit cytochrome P450 3A4. Caution should be exercised with these drugs when treating patients receiving docetaxel as there is a potential for a significant reaction). Products include:
Tarka Tablets ... 511

Vinblastine Sulfate (The metabolism of docetaxel may be modified by the concomitant administration of compounds that are metabolized by cytochrome P450 3A4. Caution should be exercised with these drugs when treating patients receiving docetaxel as there is a potential for a significant reaction).
No products indexed under this heading.

Vincristine Sulfate (The metabolism of docetaxel may be modified by the concomitant administration of compounds that are metabolized by cytochrome P450 3A4. Caution should be exercised with these drugs when treating patients receiving docetaxel as there is a potential for a significant reaction).
No products indexed under this heading.

Voriconazole (The metabolism of docetaxel may be modified by the concomitant administration of compounds that inhibit cytochrome P450 3A4. Caution should be exercised with these drugs when treating patients receiving docetaxel as there is a potential for a significant reaction).
No products indexed under this heading.

Warfarin Sodium (The metabolism of docetaxel may be modified by the concomitant administration of compounds that are metabolized by cytochrome P450 3A4. Caution should be exercised with these drugs when treating patients receiving docetaxel as there is a potential for a significant reaction).
No products indexed under this heading.

Zafirlukast (The metabolism of docetaxel may be modified by the concomitant administration of compounds that inhibit cytochrome P450 3A4. Caution should be exercised with these drugs when treating patients receiving docetaxel as there is a potential for a significant reaction). Products include:
Accolate Tablets ... 669

Zileuton (The metabolism of docetaxel may be modified by the concomitant administration of compounds that inhibit cytochrome P450 3A4. Caution should be exercised with these drugs when treating patients receiving docetaxel as there is a potential for a significant reaction).
No products indexed under this heading.

Food Interactions

Grapefruit (The metabolism of docetaxel may be modified by the concomitant administration of compounds that inhibit cytochrome P450 3A4. Caution should be exercised with these drugs when treating patients receiving docetaxel as there is a potential for a significant reaction).

Grapefruit Juice (The metabolism of docetaxel may be modified by the concomitant administration of compounds that inhibit cytochrome P450 3A4. Caution should be exercised with these drugs when treating patients receiving docetaxel as there is a potential for a significant reaction).

TĒGREEN 97 CAPSULES

(Camellia sinensis) ... 2561
May interact with oral anticoagulants. Compounds in these categories include:

Anisindione (Concurrent use with anticoagulants requires consultation with a physician).
No products indexed under this heading.

Dicumarol (Concurrent use with anticoagulants requires consultation with a physician).
No products indexed under this heading.

Warfarin Sodium (Concurrent use with anticoagulants requires consultation with a physician).
No products indexed under this heading.

TEKTURNA TABLETS

(Aliskiren) ... 2321
May interact with:

Atorvastatin Calcium (Co-administration of atorvastatin, a potent Pgp inhibitor, resulted in about a 50% increase in aliskiren Cmax and AUC after multiple dosing). Products include:
Lipitor Tablets ... 2501

Cyclosporine (When aliskiren was given with cyclosporine, the blood concentrations of aliskiren were significantly increased. Concomitant use of aliskiren with cyclosporine is not recommended). Products include:
Gengraf Capsules ... 435
Neoral Oral Solution ... 2280
Neoral Soft Gelatin Capsules ... 2280
Restasis Ophthalmic Emulsion ... 557
Sandimmune ... 2296

Furosemide (Concomitant use leads to a significant decrease in furosemide blood concentrations. Patients using furosemide could find its effect diminished after starting aliskiren). Products include:
Furosemide Tablets ... 2186

Irbesartan (Co-administration of irbesartan reduced aliskiren Cmax up to 50% after multiple dosing). Products include:
Avalide Tablets ... 892
Avalide Tablets ... 2713
Avapro Tablets ... 897
Avapro Tablets ... 2718

Ketoconazole (Co-administration of 200 mg twice-daily ketoconazole, a potent Pgp inhibitor, with aliskiren resulted in an approximate 80% increase in plasma levels of aliskiren). Products include:
Extina Foam, 2% ... 3057
Nizoral A-D Shampoo ... 1901

TEKTURNA HCT TABLETS

(Aliskiren, Hydrochlorothiazide) ... 2324
May interact with antihypertensives, barbiturates, corticosteroids, oral hypoglycemic agents, insulin, lithium preparations, narcotic analgesics, nondepolarizing neuromuscular blocking agents, non-steroidal anti-inflammatory agents, P-glycoprotein inhibitors, potassium preparations, potassium sparing diuretics, and certain other agents. Compounds in these categories include:

Acarbose (Concurrent use may require dosage adjustment of the antidiabetic drug). Products include:
Precose Tablets ... 792

Acebutolol Hydrochloride (Concurrent use with other antihypertensives may cause an additive effect or potentiation).
No products indexed under this heading.

ACTH (Intensified electrolyte depletion, particularly hypokalemia with concurrent use).
No products indexed under this heading.

Alfentanil Hydrochloride (Potentiation of orthostatic hypotension may occur with concurrent use).
No products indexed under this heading.

Amiloride Hydrochloride (Based on experience with the use of other substances that affect the renin-angiotensin system (RAS), concomitant use of Tekturna HCT with potassium-sparing diuretics may lead to increases in serum potassium. If concomitant use is considered necessary, caution should be exercised).
No products indexed under this heading.

Amlodipine Besylate (Concurrent use with other antihypertensives may cause an additive effect or potentiation). Products include:
Azor Tablets ... 1005
Exforge Tablets ... 2238

Aprobarbital (Potentiation of orthostatic hypotension may occur with concurrent use).
No products indexed under this heading.

Atenolol (Concurrent use with other antihypertensives may cause an additive effect or potentiation).
No products indexed under this heading.

Atorvastatin Calcium (Co-administration of atorvastatin resulted in about a 50% increase in aliskiren Cmax and AUC after multiple dosing). Products include:
Lipitor Tablets ... 2501

Atracurium Besylate (Concurrent use may increase the responsiveness to the muscle relaxant).
No products indexed under this heading.

Azithromycin Dihydrate (Pgp (MDR1/Mdr1a/1b) was found to be the major efflux system involved in absorption and disposition of aliskiren in preclinical studies. The potential for drug interactions at the Pgp site will likely depend on the degree of inhibition of this transporter).
No products indexed under this heading.

Benazepril Hydrochloride (Concurrent use with other antihypertensives may cause an additive effect or potentiation).
No products indexed under this heading.

Bendroflumethiazide (Concurrent use with other antihypertensives may cause an additive effect or potentiation).
No products indexed under this heading.

Betamethasone Acetate (Intensified electrolyte depletion, particularly hypokalemia with concurrent use).
No products indexed under this heading.

Betamethasone Sodium Phosphate (Intensified electrolyte depletion, particularly hypokalemia with concurrent use).
No products indexed under this heading.

Betaxolol Hydrochloride (Concurrent use with other antihypertensives may cause an additive effect or potentiation).
No products indexed under this heading.

Bisoprolol Fumarate (Concurrent use with other antihypertensives may cause an additive effect or potentiation).
No products indexed under this heading.

Budesonide (Intensified electrolyte depletion, particularly hypokalemia with concurrent use). Products include:
Pulmicort Flexhaler ... 654
Symbicort 80/4.5 Inhalation Aerosol ... 659
Symbicort 160/4.5 Inhalation Aerosol ... 659

Buprenorphine Hydrochloride (Potentiation of orthostatic hypotension may occur with concurrent use). Products include:
Suboxone Tablets ... 2601
Subutex Tablets ... 2601

Butabarbital (Potentiation of orthostatic hypotension may occur with concurrent use).
No products indexed under this heading.

Butalbital (Potentiation of orthostatic hypotension may occur with concurrent use).
No products indexed under this heading.

Candesartan Cilexetil (Concurrent use with other antihypertensives may cause an additive effect or potentiation). Products include:
Atacand Tablets ... 639
Atacand HCT ... 642

Captopril (Concurrent use with other antihypertensives may cause an additive effect or potentiation). Products include:
Captopril Tablets ... 2182

Carteolol Hydrochloride (Concurrent use with other antihypertensives may cause an additive effect or potentiation).
No products indexed under this heading.

Celecoxib (In some patients, the administration of a nonsteroidal anti-inflammatory agent can reduce the diuretic, natriuretic, and antihypertensive effects of thiazide diuretics. Therefore, when Tekturna HCT and nonsteroidal anti-inflammatory agents are used concomitantly, the patient should be observed closely to determine if the desired effect of the diuretic is obtained). Products include:
Celebrex Capsules ... 2979

Chlorothiazide (Concurrent use with other antihypertensives may cause an additive effect or potentiation).
No products indexed under this heading.

Chlorothiazide Sodium (Concurrent use with other antihypertensives may cause an additive effect or potentiation). Products include:
Intravenous Sodium Diuril ... 2490

Chlorpropamide (Concurrent use may require dosage adjustment of the antidiabetic drug).
No products indexed under this heading.

Chlorthalidone (Concurrent use with other antihypertensives may cause an additive effect or potentiation). Products include:
Clorpres Tablets ... 2185

Cholestyramine (Absorption of hydrochlorothiazide is impaired in the presence of anionic exchange resins. Single doses of cholestyramine bind the hydrochlorothiazide and reduce its absorption from the gastrointestinal tract by up to 85%).
No products indexed under this heading.

Ciclesonide (Intensified electrolyte depletion, particularly hypokalemia with concurrent use). Products include:
Alvesco Inhalation Aerosol ... 2985
Omnaris Nasal Spray ... 2998

Cisatracurium Besylate (Concurrent use may increase the responsiveness to the muscle relaxant). Products include:
Nimbex Injection ... 484

Clarithromycin (Pgp (MDR1/Mdr1a/1b) was found to be the major efflux system involved in absorption and disposition of aliskiren in preclinical studies. The potential for drug interactions at the Pgp site will likely depend on the degree of inhibition of this transporter). Products include:
Biaxin/Biaxin XL ... 411

Clonidine (Concurrent use with other antihypertensives may cause an additive effect or potentiation). Products include:
Catapres-TTS ... 842

Clonidine Hydrochloride (Concurrent use with other antihypertensives may cause an additive effect or potentiation). Products include:
Catapres Tablets ... 841
Clorpres Tablets ... 2185

Codeine Phosphate (Potentiation of orthostatic hypotension may occur with concurrent use). Products include:
Tylenol with Codeine Tablets ... 2427

Colestipol (Absorption of hydrochlorothiazide is impaired in the presence of anionic exchange resins. Single doses of colestipol resins bind the hydrochlorothiazide and reduce its absorption from the gastrointestinal tract by up to 43%).
No products indexed under this heading.

Colestipol Hydrochloride (Absorption of hydrochlorothiazide is impaired in the presence of anionic exchange resins. Single doses of colestipol resins bind the hydrochlorothiazide and reduce its absorption from the gastrointestinal tract by up to 43%).
No products indexed under this heading.

Cortisone Acetate (Intensified electrolyte depletion, particularly hypokalemia with concurrent use).
No products indexed under this heading.

Cyclosporine (Co-administration of 200 mg and 600 mg cyclosporine, a potent Pgp inhibitor, with 75 mg aliskiren resulted in an approximate 2.5-fold increase in Cmax and 5-fold increase in AUC of aliskiren. Concomitant use of aliskiren with cyclosporine is not recommended). Products include:
Gengraf Capsules ... 435
Neoral Oral Solution ... 2280
Neoral Soft Gelatin Capsules ... 2280
Restasis Ophthalmic Emulsion ... 557
Sandimmune ... 2296

Deserpidine (Concurrent use with other antihypertensives may cause an additive effect or potentiation).
No products indexed under this heading.

Dexamethasone (Intensified electrolyte depletion, particularly hypokalemia with concurrent use). Products include:
Ciprodex Otic Suspension ... 541

Dexamethasone Acetate (Intensified electrolyte depletion, particularly hypokalemia with concurrent use).
No products indexed under this heading.

Dexamethasone Sodium Phosphate (Intensified electrolyte depletion, particularly hypokalemia with concurrent use).
No products indexed under this heading.

Dezocine (Potentiation of orthostatic hypotension may occur with concurrent use).
No products indexed under this heading.

Diazoxide (Concurrent use with other antihypertensives may cause an additive effect or potentiation). Products include:
Proglycem Capsules ... 1185
Proglycem Suspension ... 1185

Diclofenac Epolamine (In some patients, the administration of a nonsteroidal anti-inflammatory agent can reduce the diuretic, natriuretic, and antihypertensive effects of thiazide diuretics. Therefore, when Tekturna HCT and nonsteroidal anti-inflammatory agents are used concomitantly, the patient should be observed closely to determine if the desired effect of the diuretic is obtained). Products include:
Flector Patch ... 561

Diclofenac Potassium (In some patients, the administration of a nonsteroidal anti-inflammatory agent can reduce the diuretic, natriuretic, and antihypertensive effects of thiazide diuretics. Therefore, when Tekturna HCT and nonsteroidal anti-inflammatory agents are used concomitantly, the patient should be observed closely to determine if the desired effect of the diuretic is obtained).
No products indexed under this heading.

Diclofenac Sodium (In some patients, the administration of a nonsteroidal anti-inflammatory agent can reduce the diuretic, natriuretic, and antihypertensive effects of thiazide diuretics. Therefore, when Tekturna HCT and nonsteroidal anti-inflammatory agents are used concomitantly, the patient should be observed closely to determine if the desired effect of the diuretic is obtained). Products include:
Diclofenac Sodium Ophthalmic Solution ... ⊙240
Voltaren Ophthalmic Solution ... 2336
Voltaren Tablets ... 2334
Voltaren-XR Tablets ... 2337

Digoxin (Pgp (MDR1/Mdr1a/1b) was found to be the major efflux system involved in absorption and disposition of aliskiren in preclinical studies. The potential for drug interactions at the Pgp site will likely depend on the degree of inhibition of this transporter). Products include:
Lanoxin Injection ... 1498
Lanoxin Injection Pediatric ... 1502
Lanoxin Tablets ... 1505

Diltiazem Hydrochloride (Concurrent use with other antihypertensives may cause an additive effect or potentiation). Products include:
Cardizem LA Extended Release Tablets ... 421

Diltiazem Maleate (Pgp (MDR1/Mdr1a/1b) was found to be the major efflux system involved in absorption and disposition of aliskiren in preclinical studies. The potential for drug interactions at the Pgp site will likely depend on the degree of inhibition of this transporter).
No products indexed under this heading.

Dirithromycin (Pgp (MDR1/Mdr1a/1b) was found to be the major efflux system involved in absorption and disposition of aliskiren in preclinical studies. The potential for drug interactions at the Pgp site will likely depend on the degree of inhibition of this transporter).
No products indexed under this heading.

Doxazosin Mesylate (Concurrent use with other antihypertensives may cause an additive effect or potentiation).
No products indexed under this heading.

Elacridar (Pgp (MDR1/Mdr1a/1b) was found to be the major efflux system involved in absorption and disposition of aliskiren in preclinical studies. The potential for drug interactions at the Pgp site will likely depend on the degree of inhibition of this transporter).
No products indexed under this heading.

Enalapril Maleate (Concurrent use with other antihypertensives may cause an additive effect or potentiation).
No products indexed under this heading.

Enalaprilat (Concurrent use with other antihypertensives may cause an additive effect or potentiation).
No products indexed under this heading.

Eprosartan Mesylate (Concurrent use with other antihypertensives may cause an additive effect or potentiation). Products include:
Teveten Tablets ... 515
Teveten HCT Tablets ... 517

Erythromycin (Pgp (MDR1/Mdr1a/1b) was found to be the major efflux system involved in absorption and disposition of aliskiren in preclinical studies. The potential for drug interactions at the Pgp site will likely depend on the degree of inhibition of this transporter).
No products indexed under this heading.

Erythromycin Estolate (Pgp (MDR1/Mdr1a/1b) was found to be the major efflux system involved in absorption and disposition of aliskiren in preclinical studies. The potential for drug interactions at the Pgp site will likely depend on the degree of inhibition of this transporter).
No products indexed under this heading.

Erythromycin Ethylsuccinate (Pgp (MDR1/Mdr1a/1b) was found to be the major efflux system involved in absorption and disposition of aliskiren in preclinical studies. The potential for drug interactions at the Pgp site will likely depend on the degree of inhibition of this transporter). Products include:
E.E.S. ... 433
EryPed ... 431

Erythromycin Gluceptate (Pgp (MDR1/Mdr1a/1b) was found to be the major efflux system involved in absorption and disposition of aliskiren in preclinical studies. The potential for drug interactions at the Pgp site will likely depend on the degree of inhibition of this transporter).
No products indexed under this heading.

Erythromycin Stearate (Pgp (MDR1/Mdr1a/1b) was found to be the major efflux system involved in absorption and disposition of aliskiren in preclinical studies. The potential for drug interactions at the Pgp site will likely depend on the degree of inhibition of this transporter).
No products indexed under this heading.

Esmolol Hydrochloride (Concurrent use with other antihypertensives may cause an additive effect or potentiation).
No products indexed under this heading.

Ethanol (Potentiation of orthostatic hypotension may occur with concurrent use).
No products indexed under this heading.

Ethyl Alcohol (Potentiation of orthostatic hypotension may occur with concurrent use).
No products indexed under this heading.

Etodolac (In some patients, the administration of a nonsteroidal anti-inflammatory agent can reduce the diuretic, natriuretic, and antihypertensive effects of thiazide diuretics. Therefore, when Tekturna HCT and nonsteroidal anti-inflammatory agents are used concomitantly, the patient should be observed closely to determine if the desired effect of the diuretic is obtained).
No products indexed under this heading.

Felodipine (Concurrent use with other antihypertensives may cause an additive effect or potentiation).
No products indexed under this heading.

Fenoprofen Calcium (In some patients, the administration of a nonsteroidal anti-inflammatory agent can reduce the diuretic, natriuretic, and antihypertensive effects of thiazide diuretics. Therefore, when Tekturna HCT and nonsteroidal anti-inflammatory agents are used concomitantly, the patient should be observed closely to determine if the desired effect of the diuretic is obtained). Products include:
Nalfon Capsules **2508**

Fentanyl (Potentiation of orthostatic hypotension may occur with concurrent use). Products include:
Duragesic Transdermal System **2405**
Ionsys Transdermal System **2410**

Fentanyl Citrate (Potentiation of orthostatic hypotension may occur with concurrent use). Products include:
Actiq **959**
Fentora Tablets **968**

Fludrocortisone Acetate (Intensified electrolyte depletion, particularly hypokalemia with concurrent use).
No products indexed under this heading.

Flunisolide (Intensified electrolyte depletion, particularly hypokalemia with concurrent use). Products include:
Aerobid/Aerobid-M **1153**

Flurbiprofen (In some patients, the administration of a nonsteroidal anti-inflammatory agent can reduce the diuretic, natriuretic, and antihypertensive effects of thiazide diuretics. Therefore, when Tekturna HCT and nonsteroidal anti-inflammatory agents are used concomitantly, the patient should be observed closely to determine if the desired effect of the diuretic is obtained).
No products indexed under this heading.

Fluticasone Propionate (Intensified electrolyte depletion, particularly hypokalemia with concurrent use). Products include:
Advair Diskus 100/50 .... **1276**
Advair Diskus 250/50 .... **1276**
Advair Diskus 500/50 .... **1276**
Advair HFA 45/21 Inhalation Aerosol **1288**
Advair HFA 115/21 Inhalation Aerosol **1288**
Advair HFA 230/21 Inhalation Aerosol **1288**
Flonase Nasal Spray **1431**
Flovent Diskus 50 mcg **1435**

Fluticasone Propionate HFA (Intensified electrolyte depletion, particularly hypokalemia with concurrent use). Products include:
Flovent HFA **1440**

Fosinopril Sodium (Concurrent use with other antihypertensives may cause an additive effect or potentiation).
No products indexed under this heading.

Furosemide (When aliskiren was co-administered with furosemide, the AUC and Cmax of furosemide were reduced by about 30% and 50%, respectively. Patients receiving furosemide could find its effect diminished after starting aliskiren). Products include:
Furosemide Tablets **2186**

Glimepiride (Concurrent use may require dosage adjustment of the antidiabetic drug). Products include:
Avandaryl Tablets **1344**
Duetact Tablets **3085**

Glipizide (Concurrent use may require dosage adjustment of the antidiabetic drug).
No products indexed under this heading.

Glyburide (Concurrent use may require dosage adjustment of the antidiabetic drug).
No products indexed under this heading.

Guanabenz Acetate (Concurrent use with other antihypertensives may cause an additive effect or potentiation).
No products indexed under this heading.

Guanethidine Monosulfate (Concurrent use with other antihypertensives may cause an additive effect or potentiation).
No products indexed under this heading.

Hydralazine Hydrochloride (Concurrent use with other antihypertensives may cause an additive effect or potentiation).
No products indexed under this heading.

Hydrocodone Bitartrate (Potentiation of orthostatic hypotension may occur with concurrent use). Products include:
Lortab 5/500 Tablets **3143**
Lortab 7.5/500 Tablets **3144**
Lortab 10/500 Tablets **3144**
Vicodin Tablets **529**
Vicodin ES Tablets **530**
Vicodin HP Tablets **531**
Vicoprofen Tablets **533**
Zydone Tablets **1132**

Hydrocodone Polistirex (Potentiation of orthostatic hypotension may occur with concurrent use). Products include:
Tussionex Pennkinetic Extended-Release Suspension **3154**

Hydrocortisone (Intensified electrolyte depletion, particularly hypokalemia with concurrent use).
No products indexed under this heading.

Hydrocortisone Acetate (Intensified electrolyte depletion, particularly hypokalemia with concurrent use). Products include:
Analpram-HC **1140**
Pramosone **1141**

Hydrocortisone Sodium Phosphate (Intensified electrolyte depletion, particularly hypokalemia with concurrent use).
No products indexed under this heading.

Hydrocortisone Sodium Succinate (Intensified electrolyte depletion, particularly hypokalemia with concurrent use).
No products indexed under this heading.

Hydroflumethiazide (Concurrent use with other antihypertensives may cause an additive effect or potentiation).
No products indexed under this heading.

Hydromorphone Hydrochloride (Potentiation of orthostatic hypotension may occur with concurrent use).
No products indexed under this heading.

Ibuprofen (In some patients, the administration of a nonsteroidal anti-inflammatory agent can reduce the diuretic, natriuretic, and antihypertensive effects of thiazide diuretics. Therefore, when Tekturna HCT and nonsteroidal anti-inflammatory agents are used concomitantly, the patient should be observed closely to determine if the desired effect of the diuretic is obtained). Products include:
Motrin IB Tablets and Caplets **1900**
Children's Motrin Oral Suspension ... **1901**
Children's Motrin Non-Staining Dye-Free Oral Suspension **1901**
Children's Motrin Cold Oral Suspension **1899**
Infants' Motrin Concentrated Drops **1901**
Infants' Motrin Non-Staining Dye-Free Concentrated Drops **1901**
Junior Strength Motrin Caplets and Chewable Tablets **1901**
Vicoprofen Tablets **533**

Indapamide (Concurrent use with other antihypertensives may cause an additive effect or potentiation). Products include:
Indapamide Tablets **2188**

Indomethacin (In some patients, the administration of a nonsteroidal anti-inflammatory agent can reduce the diuretic, natriuretic, and antihypertensive effects of thiazide diuretics. Therefore, when Tekturna HCT and nonsteroidal anti-inflammatory agents are used concomitantly, the patient should be observed closely to determine if the desired effect of the diuretic is obtained). Products include:
Indocin **2024**

Indomethacin Sodium Trihydrate (In some patients, the administration of a nonsteroidal anti-inflammatory agent can reduce the diuretic, natriuretic, and antihypertensive effects of thiazide diuretics. Therefore, when Tekturna HCT and nonsteroidal anti-inflammatory agents are used concomitantly, the patient should be observed closely to determine if the desired effect of the diuretic is obtained). Products include:
Indocin I.V. **2489**

Insulin (Concurrent use may require dosage adjustment of the antidiabetic drug).
No products indexed under this heading.

Insulin, Human, Zinc Suspension (Concurrent use may require dosage adjustment of the antidiabetic drug).
No products indexed under this heading.

Insulin, Human (rDNA origin) (Concurrent use may require dosage adjustment of the antidiabetic drug). Products include:
Exubera Inhalation Powder **2515**

Insulin, Human NPH (Concurrent use may require dosage adjustment of the antidiabetic drug). Products include:
Humulin N Vial **1846**

Insulin, Human Regular (Concurrent use may require dosage adjustment of the antidiabetic drug). Products include:
Humulin R **1849**
Humulin R (U-500) **1850**

Insulin, Human Regular and Human NPH Mixture (Concurrent use may require dosage adjustment of the antidiabetic drug). Products include:
Humulin 50/50, 100 Units **1843**
Humulin 70/30 Vial **1844**

Insulin, NPH (Concurrent use may require dosage adjustment of the antidiabetic drug).
No products indexed under this heading.

Insulin, Regular (Concurrent use may require dosage adjustment of the antidiabetic drug).
No products indexed under this heading.

Insulin, Regular and NPH mixture (Concurrent use may require dosage adjustment of the antidiabetic drug).
No products indexed under this heading.

Insulin, Zinc Crystals (Concurrent use may require dosage adjustment of the antidiabetic drug).
No products indexed under this heading.

Insulin, Zinc Suspension (Concurrent use may require dosage adjustment of the antidiabetic drug).
No products indexed under this heading.

Insulin Aspart (Concurrent use may require dosage adjustment of the antidiabetic drug).
No products indexed under this heading.

Insulin Aspart, Human (Concurrent use may require dosage adjustment of the antidiabetic drug). Products include:
NovoLog Mix 70/30 2364

Insulin Aspart, Human Regular (Concurrent use may require dosage adjustment of the antidiabetic drug). Products include:
NovoLog Injection 2359

Insulin Aspart Protamine, Human (Concurrent use may require dosage adjustment of the antidiabetic drug). Products include:
NovoLog Mix 70/30 2364

Insulin Detemir (rDNA Origin) (Concurrent use may require dosage adjustment of the antidiabetic drug). Products include:
Levemir Injection 2352

Insulin glargine (Concurrent use may require dosage adjustment of the antidiabetic drug). Products include:
Lantus Injection 2749

Insulin Glulisine (Concurrent use may require dosage adjustment of the antidiabetic drug). Products include:
Apidra Injection 2706

Insulin Lispro, Human (Concurrent use may require dosage adjustment of the antidiabetic drug). Products include:
Humalog-Pen and KwikPen 1829
Humalog Mix 50/50-Pen and KwikPen 1833
Humalog Mix 75/25-Pen and KwikPen 1835

Insulin Lispro Protamine, Human (Concurrent use may require dosage adjustment of the antidiabetic drug). Products include:
Humalog Mix 50/50-Pen and KwikPen 1833
Humalog Mix 75/25-Pen and KwikPen 1835

Irbesartan (Co-administration of irbesartan reduced aliskiren Cmax up to 50% after multiple dosing). Products include:
Avalide Tablets 892
Avalide Tablets 2713
Avapro Tablets 897
Avapro Tablets 2718

Isradipine (Concurrent use with other antihypertensives may cause an additive effect or potentiation). Products include:
DynaCirc CR Controlled Release Tablets 1407

Itraconazole (Pgp (MDR1/Mdr1a/1b) was found to be the major efflux system involved in absorption and disposition of aliskiren in preclinical studies. The potential for drug interactions at the Pgp site will likely depend on the degree of inhibition of this transporter).
No products indexed under this heading.

Ketoconazole (Co-administration of 200 mg twice-daily ketoconazole, a potent Pgp inhibitor, with aliskiren resulted in an approximate 80% increase in plasma levels of aliskiren. A 400 mg once-daily dose was not studied, but would be expected to increase aliskiren blood levels further). Products include:
Extina Foam, 2% 3057
Nizoral A-D Shampoo 1901

Ketoprofen (In some patients, the administration of a nonsteroidal anti-inflammatory agent can reduce the diuretic, natriuretic, and antihypertensive effects of thiazide diuretics. Therefore, when Tekturna HCT and nonsteroidal anti-inflammatory agents are used concomitantly, the patient should be observed closely to determine if the desired effect of the diuretic is obtained).
No products indexed under this heading.

Ketorolac Tromethamine (In some patients, the administration of a nonsteroidal anti-inflammatory agent can reduce the diuretic, natriuretic, and antihypertensive effects of thiazide diuretics. Therefore, when Tekturna HCT and nonsteroidal anti-inflammatory agents are used concomitantly, the patient should be observed closely to determine if the desired effect of the diuretic is obtained).
No products indexed under this heading.

Labetalol Hydrochloride (Concurrent use with other antihypertensives may cause an additive effect or potentiation).
No products indexed under this heading.

Levorphanol Tartrate (Potentiation of orthostatic hypotension may occur with concurrent use).
No products indexed under this heading.

Lisinopril (Concurrent use with other antihypertensives may cause an additive effect or potentiation). Products include:
Prinivil Tablets 2087
Prinzide Tablets 2092

Lithium (Diuretic agents reduce the renal clearance of lithium and increase the risk of lithium toxicity. Concurrent use should generally be avoided).
No products indexed under this heading.

Lithium Carbonate (Diuretic agents reduce the renal clearance of lithium and increase the risk of lithium toxicity. Concurrent use should generally be avoided).
No products indexed under this heading.

Lithium Citrate (Diuretic agents reduce the renal clearance of lithium and increase the risk of lithium toxicity. Concurrent use should generally be avoided).
No products indexed under this heading.

Losartan Potassium (Concurrent use with other antihypertensives may cause an additive effect or potentiation). Products include:
Cozaar Tablets 1973

Mecamylamine Hydrochloride (Concurrent use with other antihypertensives may cause an additive effect or potentiation).
No products indexed under this heading.

Meclofenamate Sodium (In some patients, the administration of a nonsteroidal anti-inflammatory agent can reduce the diuretic, natriuretic, and antihypertensive effects of thiazide diuretics. Therefore, when Tekturna HCT and nonsteroidal anti-inflammatory agents are used concomitantly, the patient should be observed closely to determine if the desired effect of the diuretic is obtained).
No products indexed under this heading.

Mefenamic Acid (In some patients, the administration of a nonsteroidal anti-inflammatory agent can reduce the diuretic, natriuretic, and antihypertensive effects of thiazide diuretics. Therefore, when Tekturna HCT and nonsteroidal anti-inflammatory agents are used concomitantly, the patient should be observed closely to determine if the desired effect of the diuretic is obtained).
No products indexed under this heading.

Meloxicam (In some patients, the administration of a nonsteroidal anti-inflammatory agent can reduce the diuretic, natriuretic, and antihypertensive effects of thiazide diuretics. Therefore, when Tekturna HCT and nonsteroidal anti-inflammatory agents are used concomitantly, the patient should be observed closely to determine if the desired effect of the diuretic is obtained). Products include:
Mobic Oral Suspension 863
Mobic Tablets 863

Meperidine Hydrochloride (Potentiation of orthostatic hypotension may occur with concurrent use).
No products indexed under this heading.

Mephobarbital (Potentiation of orthostatic hypotension may occur with concurrent use).
No products indexed under this heading.

Metformin Hydrochloride (Concurrent use may require dosage adjustment of the antidiabetic drug). Products include:
ActoPlus Met Tablets 3071
Avandamet Tablets 1336
Janumet Tablets 2041
PrandiMet Tablets 2967

Methadone Hydrochloride (Potentiation of orthostatic hypotension may occur with concurrent use).
No products indexed under this heading.

Methyclothiazide (Concurrent use with other antihypertensives may cause an additive effect or potentiation).
No products indexed under this heading.

Methyldopa (Concurrent use with other antihypertensives may cause an additive effect or potentiation).
No products indexed under this heading.

Methyldopate Hydrochloride (Concurrent use with other antihypertensives may cause an additive effect or potentiation).
No products indexed under this heading.

Methylprednisolone Acetate (Intensified electrolyte depletion, particularly hypokalemia with concurrent use).
No products indexed under this heading.

Methylprednisolone Sodium Succinate (Intensified electrolyte depletion, particularly hypokalemia with concurrent use).
No products indexed under this heading.

Metocurine Iodide (Concurrent use may increase the responsiveness to the muscle relaxant).
No products indexed under this heading.

Metolazone (Concurrent use with other antihypertensives may cause an additive effect or potentiation).
No products indexed under this heading.

Metoprolol Succinate (Concurrent use with other antihypertensives may cause an additive effect or potentiation). Products include:
Toprol-XL Tablets 666

Metoprolol Tartrate (Concurrent use with other antihypertensives may cause an additive effect or potentiation).
No products indexed under this heading.

Metyrosine (Concurrent use with other antihypertensives may cause an additive effect or potentiation). Products include:
Demser Capsules 1989

Mibefradil Dihydrochloride (Concurrent use with other antihypertensives may cause an additive effect or potentiation).
No products indexed under this heading.

Miglitol (Concurrent use may require dosage adjustment of the antidiabetic drug).
No products indexed under this heading.

Minoxidil (Concurrent use with other antihypertensives may cause an additive effect or potentiation).
No products indexed under this heading.

Mivacurium Chloride (Concurrent use may increase the responsiveness to the muscle relaxant).
No products indexed under this heading.

Moexipril Hydrochloride (Concurrent use with other antihypertensives may cause an additive effect or potentiation).
No products indexed under this heading.

Mometasone Furoate (Intensified electrolyte depletion, particularly hypokalemia with concurrent use). Products include:
Asmanex Twisthaler 2797
Elocon Cream 0.1% 2840
Elocon Lotion 0.1% 2841
Elocon Ointment 0.1% 2842

Mometasone Furoate Monohydrate (Intensified electrolyte depletion, particularly hypokalemia with concurrent use). Products include:
Nasonex Nasal Spray 2883

Morphine Sulfate (Potentiation of orthostatic hypotension may occur with concurrent use). Products include:
Avinza Capsules 1772
DepoDur Injection 1095
MS Contin Tablets 2585

Nabumetone (In some patients, the administration of a nonsteroidal anti-inflammatory agent can reduce the diuretic, natriuretic, and antihypertensive effects of thiazide diuretics. Therefore, when Tekturna HCT and nonsteroidal anti-inflammatory agents are used concomitantly, the patient should be observed closely to determine if the desired effect of the diuretic is obtained).
No products indexed under this heading.

Nadolol (Concurrent use with other antihypertensives may cause an additive effect or potentiation). Products include:
Nadolol Tablets **2191**

Naproxen (In some patients, the administration of a nonsteroidal anti-inflammatory agent can reduce the diuretic, natriuretic, and antihypertensive effects of thiazide diuretics. Therefore, when Tekturna HCT and nonsteroidal anti-inflammatory agents are used concomitantly, the patient should be observed closely to determine if the desired effect of the diuretic is obtained). Products include:
EC-Naprosyn Delayed-Release Tablets **2632**
Naprosyn Suspension **2632**
Naprosyn Tablets **2632**

Naproxen Sodium (In some patients, the administration of a nonsteroidal anti-inflammatory agent can reduce the diuretic, natriuretic, and antihypertensive effects of thiazide diuretics. Therefore, when Tekturna HCT and nonsteroidal anti-inflammatory agents are used concomitantly, the patient should be observed closely to determine if the desired effect of the diuretic is obtained). Products include:
Anaprox Tablets **2632**
Anaprox DS Tablets **2632**
Treximet Tablets **1616**

Nateglinide (Concurrent use may require dosage adjustment of the antidiabetic drug). Products include:
Starlix Tablets **2314**

Nebivolol (Concurrent use with other antihypertensives may cause an additive effect or potentiation). Products include:
Bystolic Tablets **1155**

Nicardipine Hydrochloride (Concurrent use with other antihypertensives may cause an additive effect or potentiation). Products include:
Cardene I.V. **1093**

Nifedipine (Concurrent use with other antihypertensives may cause an additive effect or potentiation).
No products indexed under this heading.

Nisoldipine (Concurrent use with other antihypertensives may cause an additive effect or potentiation). Products include:
Sular Extended Release Tablets **2975**

Nitroglycerin (Concurrent use with other antihypertensives may cause an additive effect or potentiation). Products include:
Nitro-Dur Transdermal Infusion System **2887**
Nitrolingual Pumpspray **2965**

Norepinephrine Bitartrate (Possible decreased response to pressor amines, but not sufficient to preclude their use).
No products indexed under this heading.

Norepinephrine Hydrochloride (Possible decreased response to pressor amines, but not sufficient to preclude their use).
No products indexed under this heading.

Oxaprozin (In some patients, the administration of a nonsteroidal anti-inflammatory agent can reduce the diuretic, natriuretic, and antihypertensive effects of thiazide diuretics. Therefore, when Tekturna HCT and nonsteroidal anti-inflammatory agents are used concomitantly, the patient should be observed closely to determine if the desired effect of the diuretic is obtained).
No products indexed under this heading.

Oxycodone Hydrochloride (Potentiation of orthostatic hypotension may occur with concurrent use). Products include:
OxyContin Tablets **2589**
OxyIR Capsules **2593**
Percocet Tablets **1127**
Percodan Tablets **1130**

Pancuronium Bromide (Concurrent use may increase the responsiveness to the muscle relaxant).
No products indexed under this heading.

Penbutolol Sulfate (Concurrent use with other antihypertensives may cause an additive effect or potentiation).
No products indexed under this heading.

Pentobarbital Sodium (Potentiation of orthostatic hypotension may occur with concurrent use). Products include:
Nembutal Sodium Solution, USP **2494**

Perindopril Erbumine (Concurrent use with other antihypertensives may cause an additive effect or potentiation). Products include:
Aceon Tablets (2 mg, 4 mg, 8 mg) **3038**

Phenobarbital (Potentiation of orthostatic hypotension may occur with concurrent use). Products include:
Donnatal Extentabs **2507**

Phenoxybenzamine Hydrochloride (Concurrent use with other antihypertensives may cause an additive effect or potentiation). Products include:
Dibenzyline Capsules **3188**

Phentolamine Mesylate (Concurrent use with other antihypertensives may cause an additive effect or potentiation).
No products indexed under this heading.

Phenylbutazone (In some patients, the administration of a nonsteroidal anti-inflammatory agent can reduce the diuretic, natriuretic, and antihypertensive effects of thiazide diuretics. Therefore, when Tekturna HCT and nonsteroidal anti-inflammatory agents are used concomitantly, the patient should be observed closely to determine if the desired effect of the diuretic is obtained).
No products indexed under this heading.

Pindolol (Concurrent use with other antihypertensives may cause an additive effect or potentiation).
No products indexed under this heading.

Pioglitazone Hydrochloride (Concurrent use may require dosage adjustment of the antidiabetic drug). Products include:
ActoPlus Met Tablets **3071**
Actos Tablets **3077**
Duetact Tablets **3085**

Piroxicam (In some patients, the administration of a nonsteroidal anti-inflammatory agent can reduce the diuretic, natriuretic, and antihypertensive effects of thiazide diuretics. Therefore, when Tekturna HCT and nonsteroidal anti-inflammatory agents are used concomitantly, the patient should be observed closely to determine if the desired effect of the diuretic is obtained).
No products indexed under this heading.

Polythiazide (Concurrent use with other antihypertensives may cause an additive effect or potentiation).
No products indexed under this heading.

Potassium Acid Phosphate (Based on experience with the use of other substances that affect the renin-angiotensin system (RAS), concomitant use of Tekturna HCT with potassium supplements or salt substitutes containing potassium, or other drugs that increase potassium may lead to increases in serum potassium. If concomitant use is considered necessary, caution should be exercised). Products include:
K-Phos Original (Sodium Free) Tablets **814**

Potassium Bicarbonate (Based on experience with the use of other substances that affect the renin-angiotensin system (RAS), concomitant use of Tekturna HCT with potassium supplements or salt substitutes containing potassium, or other drugs that increase potassium may lead to increases in serum potassium. If concomitant use is considered necessary, caution should be exercised).
No products indexed under this heading.

Potassium Chloride (Based on experience with the use of other substances that affect the renin-angiotensin system (RAS), concomitant use of Tekturna HCT with potassium supplements or salt substitutes containing potassium, or other drugs that increase potassium may lead to increases in serum potassium. If concomitant use is considered necessary, caution should be exercised). Products include:
MoviPrep Oral Solution **2679**

Potassium Citrate (Based on experience with the use of other substances that affect the renin-angiotensin system (RAS), concomitant use of Tekturna HCT with potassium supplements or salt substitutes containing potassium, or other drugs that increase potassium may lead to increases in serum potassium. If concomitant use is considered necessary, caution should be exercised). Products include:
BioLean Free Tablets **635**
Urocit-K Tablets **2176**

Potassium Gluconate (Based on experience with the use of other substances that affect the renin-angiotensin system (RAS), concomitant use of Tekturna HCT with potassium supplements or salt substitutes containing potassium, or other drugs that increase potassium may lead to increases in serum potassium. If concomitant use is considered necessary, caution should be exercised).
No products indexed under this heading.

Potassium Phosphate (Based on experience with the use of other substances that affect the renin-angiotensin system (RAS), concomitant use of Tekturna HCT with potassium supplements or salt substitutes containing potassium, or other drugs that increase potassium may lead to increases in serum potassium. If concomitant use is considered necessary, caution should be exercised). Products include:
K-Phos Neutral Tablets **813**

Prazosin Hydrochloride (Concurrent use with other antihypertensives may cause an additive effect or potentiation).
No products indexed under this heading.

Prednisolone Acetate (Intensified electrolyte depletion, particularly hypokalemia with concurrent use). Products include:
Pred Forte Ophthalmic Suspension .... ⊙ **227**
Pred Mild Ophthalmic Suspension .... ⊙ **230**
Pred-G Ophthalmic Ointment .... ⊙ **229**
Pred-G Ophthalmic Suspension .... ⊙ **228**

Prednisolone Sodium Phosphate (Intensified electrolyte depletion, particularly hypokalemia with concurrent use).
No products indexed under this heading.

Prednisolone Tebutate (Intensified electrolyte depletion, particularly hypokalemia with concurrent use).
No products indexed under this heading.

Prednisone (Intensified electrolyte depletion, particularly hypokalemia with concurrent use).
No products indexed under this heading.

Propoxyphene Hydrochloride (Potentiation of orthostatic hypotension may occur with concurrent use).
No products indexed under this heading.

Propoxyphene Napsylate (Potentiation of orthostatic hypotension may occur with concurrent use).
No products indexed under this heading.

Propranolol Hydrochloride (Concurrent use with other antihypertensives may cause an additive effect or potentiation). Products include:
InnoPran XL Extended Release Capsules **1484**

Quinapril Hydrochloride (Concurrent use with other antihypertensives may cause an additive effect or potentiation).
No products indexed under this heading.

Quinidine (Pgp (MDR1/Mdr1a/1b) was found to be the major efflux system involved in absorption and disposition of aliskiren in preclinical studies. The potential for drug interactions at the Pgp site will likely depend on the degree of inhibition of this transporter).
No products indexed under this heading.

Quinidine Gluconate (Pgp (MDR1/Mdr1a/1b) was found to be the major efflux system involved in absorption and disposition of aliskiren in preclinical studies. The potential for drug interactions at the Pgp site will likely depend on the degree of inhibition of this transporter).
No products indexed under this heading.

Quinidine Hydrochloride (Pgp (MDR1/Mdr1a/1b) was found to be the major efflux system involved in absorption and disposition of aliskiren in preclinical studies. The potential for drug interactions at the Pgp site will likely depend on the degree of inhibition of this transporter).
No products indexed under this heading.

Quinidine Polygalacturonate (Pgp (MDR1/Mdr1a/1b) was found to be the major efflux system involved in absorption and dispositi-on of aliskiren in preclinical studies. The potential for drug interactions at the Pgp site will likely depend on the degree of inhibition of this transporter).
No products indexed under this heading.

Quinidine Sulfate (Pgp (MDR1/Mdr1a/1b) was found to be the major efflux system involved in absorption and disposition of aliskiren in preclinical studies. The potential for drug interactions at the Pgp site will likely depend on the degree of inhibition of this transporter).
No products indexed under this heading.

Ramipril (Concurrent use with other antihypertensives may cause an additive effect or potentiation).
No products indexed under this heading.

Rapacuronium Bromide (Concurrent use may increase the responsiveness to the muscle relaxant).
No products indexed under this heading.

Rauwolfia Serpentina (Concurrent use with other antihypertensives may cause an additive effect or potentiation).
No products indexed under this heading.

Remifentanil Hydrochloride (Potentiation of orthostatic hypotension may occur with concurrent use).
No products indexed under this heading.

Repaglinide (Concurrent use may require dosage adjustment of the antidiabetic drug). Products include:
PrandiMet Tablets 2967
Prandin Tablets 2971

Rescinnamine (Concurrent use with other antihypertensives may cause an additive effect or potentiation).
No products indexed under this heading.

Reserpine (Concurrent use with other antihypertensives may cause an additive effect or potentiation).
No products indexed under this heading.

Rocuronium Bromide (Concurrent use may increase the responsiveness to the muscle relaxant). Products include:
Zemuron Injection 2947

Rofecoxib (In some patients, the administration of a nonsteroidal anti-inflammatory agent can reduce the diuretic, natriuretic, and antihypertensive effects of thiazide diuretics. Therefore, when Tekturna HCT and nonsteroidal anti-inflammatory agents are used concomitantly, the patient should be observed closely to determine if the desired effect of the diuretic is obtained).
No products indexed under this heading.

Rosiglitazone Maleate (Concurrent use may require dosage adjustment of the antidiabetic drug). Products include:
Avandamet Tablets 1336
Avandaryl Tablets 1344
Avandia Tablets 1351

Secobarbital Sodium (Potentiation of orthostatic hypotension may occur with concurrent use).
No products indexed under this heading.

Sitagliptin Phosphate (Concurrent use may require dosage adjustment of the antidiabetic drug). Products include:
Janumet Tablets 2041
Januvia Tablets 2048

Sodium Nitroprusside (Concurrent use with other antihypertensives may cause an additive effect or potentiation).
No products indexed under this heading.

Sotalol Hydrochloride (Concurrent use with other antihypertensives may cause an additive effect or potentiation).
No products indexed under this heading.

Spirapril Hydrochloride (Concurrent use with other antihypertensives may cause an additive effect or potentiation).
No products indexed under this heading.

Spironolactone (Based on experience with the use of other substances that affect the renin-angiotensin system (RAS), concomitant use of Tekturna HCT with potassium-sparing diuretics may lead to increases in serum potassium. If concomitant use is considered necessary, caution should be exercised).
No products indexed under this heading.

Sufentanil Citrate (Potentiation of orthostatic hypotension may occur with concurrent use).
No products indexed under this heading.

Sulindac (In some patients, the administration of a nonsteroidal anti-inflammatory agent can reduce the diuretic, natriuretic, and antihypertensive effects of thiazide diuretics. Therefore, when Tekturna HCT and nonsteroidal anti-inflammatory agents are used concomitantly, the patient should be observed closely to determine if the desired effect of the diuretic is obtained). Products include:
Clinoril Tablets 1962

Telmisartan (Concurrent use with other antihypertensives may cause an additive effect or potentiation). Products include:
Micardis Tablets 852
Micardis HCT Tablets 854

Terazosin Hydrochloride (Concurrent use with other antihypertensives may cause an additive effect or potentiation).
No products indexed under this heading.

Thiamylal Sodium (Potentiation of orthostatic hypotension may occur with concurrent use).
No products indexed under this heading.

Timolol Maleate (Concurrent use with other antihypertensives may cause an additive effect or potentiation). Products include:
Combigan Ophthalmic Solution 553
Cosopt Sterile Ophthalmic Solution 1969
Timoptic Sterile Ophthalmic Solution 2121
Timoptic in Ocudose 2124
Timoptic-XE Sterile Ophthalmic Gel Forming Solution 2125

Tolazamide (Concurrent use may require dosage adjustment of the antidiabetic drug).
No products indexed under this heading.

Tolbutamide (Concurrent use may require dosage adjustment of the antidiabetic drug).
No products indexed under this heading.

Tolmetin Sodium (In some patients, the administration of a nonsteroidal anti-inflammatory agent can reduce the diuretic, natriuretic, and antihypertensive effects of thiazide diuretics. Therefore, when Tekturna HCT and nonsteroidal anti-inflammatory agents are used concomitantly, the patient should be observed closely to determine if the desired effect of the diuretic is obtained).
No products indexed under this heading.

Torsemide (Concurrent use with other antihypertensives may cause an additive effect or potentiation). Products include:
Demadex Injection 2630
Demadex Tablets 2630

Trandolapril (Concurrent use with other antihypertensives may cause an additive effect or potentiation). Products include:
Mavik Tablets 472
Tarka Tablets 511

Triamcinolone (Intensified electrolyte depletion, particularly hypokalemia with concurrent use).
No products indexed under this heading.

Triamcinolone Acetonide (Intensified electrolyte depletion, particularly hypokalemia with concurrent use). Products include:
Azmacort Inhalation Aerosol 407
Nasacort AQ Nasal Spray 2765
Triesence Injectable Suspension .... ⊙209

Triamcinolone Diacetate (Intensified electrolyte depletion, particularly hypokalemia with concurrent use).
No products indexed under this heading.

Triamcinolone Hexacetonide (Intensified electrolyte depletion, particularly hypokalemia with concurrent use).
No products indexed under this heading.

Triamterene (Based on experience with the use of other substances that affect the renin-angiotensin system (RAS), concomitant use of Tekturna HCT with potassium-sparing diuretics may lead to increases in serum potassium. If concomitant use is considered necessary, caution should be exercised). Products include:
Dyazide Capsules 1405
Dyrenium Capsules 3189

Trimethaphan Camsylate (Concurrent use with other antihypertensives may cause an additive effect or potentiation).
No products indexed under this heading.

Troglitazone (Concurrent use may require dosage adjustment of the antidiabetic drug).
No products indexed under this heading.

Troleandomycin (Pgp (MDR1/Mdr1a/1b) was found to be the major efflux system involved in absorption and disposition of aliskiren in preclinical studies. The potential for drug interactions at the Pgp site will likely depend on the degree of inhibition of this transporter).
No products indexed under this heading.

Tubocurarine Chloride (Concurrent use may increase the responsiveness to tubocurarine).
No products indexed under this heading.

Valdecoxib (In some patients, the administration of a nonsteroidal anti-inflammatory agent can reduce the diuretic, natriuretic, and antihypertensive effects of thiazide diuretics. Therefore, when Tekturna HCT and nonsteroidal anti-inflammatory agents are used concomitantly, the patient should be observed closely to determine if the desired effect of the diuretic is obtained).
No products indexed under this heading.

Valsartan (Concurrent use with other antihypertensives may cause an additive effect or potentiation). Products include:
Diovan Tablets 2212
Diovan HCT Tablets 2216
Exforge Tablets 2238

Vecuronium Bromide (Concurrent use may increase the responsiveness to the muscle relaxant).
No products indexed under this heading.

Verapamil Hydrochloride (Concurrent use with other antihypertensives may cause an additive effect or potentiation). Products include:
Tarka Tablets 511

Food Interactions

Alcohol (Potentiation of orthostatic hypotension may occur with concurrent use).

TEMODAR CAPSULES

(Temozolomide) 2931
May interact with valproate. Compounds in these categories include:

Divalproex Sodium (Co-administration with valproic acid

decreases oral clearance of temozolomide by about 5%; the clinical implication of this effect is not known). Products include:

Depakote ER Tablets 423

Valproate Sodium (Co-administration with valproic acid decreases oral clearance of temozolomide by about 5%; the clinical implication of this effect is not known).

No products indexed under this heading.

Valproic Acid (Co-administration with valproic acid decreases oral clearance of temozolomide by about 5%; the clinical implication of this effect is not known).

No products indexed under this heading.

TESSALON CAPSULES

(Benzonatate) 1183

None cited in PDR database.

TESSALON PERLES

(Benzonatate) 1183

None cited in PDR database.

TESTIM 1% GEL

(Testosterone) 701

May interact with corticosteroids, insulin, and certain other agents. Compounds in these categories include:

ACTH (Co-administration of testosterone with ACTH may enhance edema formation).

No products indexed under this heading.

Betamethasone Acetate (Co-administration of testosterone with corticosteroids may enhance edema formation).

No products indexed under this heading.

Betamethasone Sodium Phosphate (Co-administration of testosterone with corticosteroids may enhance edema formation).

No products indexed under this heading.

Budesonide (Co-administration of testosterone with corticosteroids may enhance edema formation). Products include:

Pulmicort Flexhaler 654
Symbicort 80/4.5 Inhalation Aerosol... 659
Symbicort 160/4.5 Inhalation Aerosol... 659

Ciclesonide (Co-administration of testosterone with corticosteroids may enhance edema formation). Products include:

Alvesco Inhalation Aerosol 2985
Omnaris Nasal Spray 2998

Cortisone Acetate (Co-administration of testosterone with corticosteroids may enhance edema formation).

No products indexed under this heading.

Dexamethasone (Co-administration of testosterone with corticosteroids may enhance edema formation). Products include:

Ciprodex Otic Suspension 541

Dexamethasone Acetate (Co-administration of testosterone with corticosteroids may enhance edema formation).

No products indexed under this heading.

Dexamethasone Sodium Phosphate (Co-administration of testosterone with corticosteroids may enhance edema formation).

No products indexed under this heading.

Fludrocortisone Acetate (Co-administration of testosterone with corticosteroids may enhance edema formation).

No products indexed under this heading.

Flunisolide (Co-administration of testosterone with corticosteroids may enhance edema formation). Products include:

Aerobid/Aerobid-M 1153

Fluticasone Propionate (Co-administration of testosterone with corticosteroids may enhance edema formation). Products include:

Advair Diskus 100/50 1276
Advair Diskus 250/50 1276
Advair Diskus 500/50 1276
Advair HFA 45/21 Inhalation Aerosol... 1288
Advair HFA 115/21 Inhalation Aerosol... 1288
Advair HFA 230/21 Inhalation Aerosol... 1288
Flonase Nasal Spray 1431
Flovent Diskus 50 mcg 1435

Fluticasone Propionate HFA (Co-administration of testosterone with corticosteroids may enhance edema formation). Products include:

Flovent HFA 1440

Hydrocortisone (Co-administration of testosterone with corticosteroids may enhance edema formation).

No products indexed under this heading.

Hydrocortisone Acetate (Co-administration of testosterone with corticosteroids may enhance edema formation). Products include:

Analpram-HC 1140
Pramosone 1141

Hydrocortisone Sodium Phosphate (Co-administration of testosterone with corticosteroids may enhance edema formation).

No products indexed under this heading.

Hydrocortisone Sodium Succinate (Co-administration of testosterone with corticosteroids may enhance edema formation).

No products indexed under this heading.

Insulin (In diabetic patients, the metabolic effects of androgens may decrease blood glucose and, therefore, insulin requirements).

No products indexed under this heading.

Insulin, Human, Zinc Suspension (In diabetic patients, the metabolic effects of androgens may decrease blood glucose and, therefore, insulin requirements).

No products indexed under this heading.

Insulin, Human (rDNA origin) (In diabetic patients, the metabolic effects of androgens may decrease blood glucose and, therefore, insulin requirements). Products include:

Exubera Inhalation Powder 2515

Insulin, Human NPH (In diabetic patients, the metabolic effects of androgens may decrease blood glucose and, therefore, insulin requirements). Products include:

Humulin N Vial 1846

Insulin, Human Regular (In diabetic patients, the metabolic effects of androgens may decrease blood glucose and, therefore, insulin requirements). Products include:

Humulin R 1849
Humulin R (U-500) 1850

Insulin, Human Regular and Human NPH Mixture (In diabetic patients, the metabolic effects of androgens may decrease blood glucose and, therefore, insulin requirements). Products include:

Humulin 50/50, 100 Units 1843
Humulin 70/30 Vial 1844

Insulin, NPH (In diabetic patients, the metabolic effects of androgens may decrease blood glucose and, therefore, insulin requirements).

No products indexed under this heading.

Insulin, Regular (In diabetic patients, the metabolic effects of androgens may decrease blood glucose and, therefore, insulin requirements).

No products indexed under this heading.

Insulin, Regular and NPH mixture (In diabetic patients, the metabolic effects of androgens may decrease blood glucose and, therefore, insulin requirements).

No products indexed under this heading.

Insulin, Zinc Crystals (In diabetic patients, the metabolic effects of androgens may decrease blood glucose and, therefore, insulin requirements).

No products indexed under this heading.

Insulin, Zinc Suspension (In diabetic patients, the metabolic effects of androgens may decrease blood glucose and, therefore, insulin requirements).

No products indexed under this heading.

Insulin Aspart (In diabetic patients, the metabolic effects of androgens may decrease blood glucose and, therefore, insulin requirements).

No products indexed under this heading.

Insulin Aspart, Human (In diabetic patients, the metabolic effects of androgens may decrease blood glucose and, therefore, insulin requirements). Products include:

NovoLog Mix 70/30 2364

Insulin Aspart, Human Regular (In diabetic patients, the metabolic effects of androgens may decrease blood glucose and, therefore, insulin requirements). Products include:

NovoLog Injection 2359

Insulin Aspart Protamine, Human (In diabetic patients, the metabolic effects of androgens may decrease blood glucose and, therefore, insulin requirements). Products include:

NovoLog Mix 70/30 2364

Insulin Detemir (rDNA Origin) (In diabetic patients, the metabolic effects of androgens may decrease blood glucose and, therefore, insulin requirements). Products include:

Levemir Injection 2352

Insulin glargine (In diabetic patients, the metabolic effects of androgens may decrease blood glucose and, therefore, insulin requirements). Products include:

Lantus Injection 2749

Insulin Glulisine (In diabetic patients, the metabolic effects of androgens may decrease blood glucose and, therefore, insulin requirements). Products include:

Apidra Injection 2706

Insulin Lispro, Human (In diabetic patients, the metabolic effects of androgens may decrease blood glucose and, therefore, insulin requirements). Products include:

Humalog-Pen and KwikPen 1829
Humalog Mix 50/50-Pen and KwikPen... 1833
Humalog Mix 75/25-Pen and KwikPen... 1835

Insulin Lispro Protamine, Human (In diabetic patients, the metabolic effects of androgens may decrease blood glucose and, therefore, insulin requirements). Products include:

Humalog Mix 50/50-Pen and KwikPen... 1833
Humalog Mix 75/25-Pen and KwikPen... 1835

Methylprednisolone Acetate (Co-administration of testosterone with corticosteroids may enhance edema formation).

No products indexed under this heading.

Methylprednisolone Sodium Succinate (Co-administration of testosterone with corticosteroids may enhance edema formation).

No products indexed under this heading.

Mometasone Furoate (Co-administration of testosterone with corticosteroids may enhance edema formation). Products include:

Asmanex Twisthaler 2797
Elocon Cream 0.1% 2840
Elocon Lotion 0.1% 2841
Elocon Ointment 0.1% 2842

Mometasone Furoate Monohydrate (Co-administration of testosterone with corticosteroids may enhance edema formation). Products include:

Nasonex Nasal Spray 2883

Oxyphenbutazone (Co-administration of androgens and oxyphenbutazone may result in elevated serum levels of oxyphenbutazone).

No products indexed under this heading.

Prednisolone Acetate (Co-administration of testosterone with corticosteroids may enhance edema formation). Products include:

Pred Forte Ophthalmic Suspension.................................. ⊙ 227
Pred Mild Ophthalmic Suspension.................................. ⊙ 230
Pred-G Ophthalmic Ointment .... ⊙ 229
Pred-G Ophthalmic Suspension ...... ⊙ 228

Prednisolone Sodium Phosphate (Co-administration of testosterone with corticosteroids may enhance edema formation).

No products indexed under this heading.

Prednisolone Tebutate (Co-administration of testosterone with corticosteroids may enhance edema formation).

No products indexed under this heading.

Prednisone (Co-administration of testosterone with corticosteroids may enhance edema formation).

No products indexed under this heading.

Propranolol Hydrochloride (Co-administration of injectable testosterone cypionate has resulted in an increased clearance of propranolol). Products include:

InnoPran XL Extended Release Capsules 1484

Triamcinolone (Co-administration of testosterone with corticosteroids may enhance edema formation).
No products indexed under this heading.

Triamcinolone Acetonide (Co-administration of testosterone with corticosteroids may enhance edema formation). Products include:
Azmacort Inhalation Aerosol 407
Nasacort AQ Nasal Spray 2765
Triesence Injectable Suspension .... ⊙209

Triamcinolone Diacetate (Co-administration of testosterone with corticosteroids may enhance edema formation).
No products indexed under this heading.

Triamcinolone Hexacetonide (Co-administration of testosterone with corticosteroids may enhance edema formation).
No products indexed under this heading.

TEVETEN TABLETS

(Eprosartan Mesylate) 515

Food Interactions

Food, unspecified (Co-administration with food delays absorption and causes variable changes in Cmax and AUC values which do not appear clinically important).

TEVETEN HCT TABLETS

(Eprosartan Mesylate, Hydrochlorothiazide) 517
May interact with antihypertensives, barbiturates, corticosteroids, cardiac glycosides, oral hypoglycemic agents, insulin, lithium preparations, narcotic analgesics, nondepolarizing neuromuscular blocking agents, nonsteroidal anti-inflammatory agents, potassium preparations, potassium sparing diuretics, and certain other agents. Compounds in these categories include:

Acarbose (Hyperglycemia may occur with thiazide diuretics; oral hypoglycemic dosage may need to be adjusted). Products include:
Precose Tablets 792

Acebutolol Hydrochloride (Co-administration of thiazides with other antihypertensive agents may lead to additive effects or potentiation).
No products indexed under this heading.

ACTH (Intensifies the electrolyte balance, particularly hypokalemia).
No products indexed under this heading.

Alfentanil Hydrochloride (Narcotics may potentiate orthostatic hypotension).
No products indexed under this heading.

Aliskiren (Co-administration of thiazides with other antihypertensive agents may lead to additive effects or potentiation). Products include:
Tekturna Tablets 2321
Tekturna HCT Tablets 2324

Amiloride Hydrochloride (Concomitant use of potassium sparing diuretics with eprosartan may lead to hyperkalemia).
No products indexed under this heading.

Amlodipine Besylate (Co-administration of thiazides with other antihypertensive agents may lead to additive effects or potentiation). Products include:
Azor Tablets 1005
Exforge Tablets 2238

Aprobarbital (Barbiturates may potentiate orthostatic hypotension).
No products indexed under this heading.

Atenolol (Co-administration of thiazides with other antihypertensive agents may lead to additive effects or potentiation).
No products indexed under this heading.

Atracurium Besylate (Possible increased responsiveness to muscle relaxants).
No products indexed under this heading.

Benazepril Hydrochloride (Co-administration of thiazides with other antihypertensive agents may lead to additive effects or potentiation).
No products indexed under this heading.

Bendroflumethiazide (Co-administration of thiazides with other antihypertensive agents may lead to additive effects or potentiation).
No products indexed under this heading.

Betamethasone Acetate (Corticosteroids intensify the electrolyte imbalance, particularly hypokalemia).
No products indexed under this heading.

Betamethasone Sodium Phosphate (Corticosteroids intensify the electrolyte imbalance, particularly hypokalemia).
No products indexed under this heading.

Betaxolol Hydrochloride (Co-administration of thiazides with other antihypertensive agents may lead to additive effects or potentiation).
No products indexed under this heading.

Bisoprolol Fumarate (Co-administration of thiazides with other antihypertensive agents may lead to additive effects or potentiation).
No products indexed under this heading.

Budesonide (Corticosteroids intensify the electrolyte imbalance, particularly hypokalemia). Products include:
Pulmicort Flexhaler 654
Symbicort 80/4.5 Inhalation Aerosol 659
Symbicort 160/4.5 Inhalation Aerosol 659

Buprenorphine Hydrochloride (Narcotics may potentiate orthostatic hypotension). Products include:
Suboxone Tablets 2601
Subutex Tablets 2601

Butabarbital (Barbiturates may potentiate orthostatic hypotension).
No products indexed under this heading.

Butalbital (Barbiturates may potentiate orthostatic hypotension).
No products indexed under this heading.

Candesartan Cilexetil (Co-administration of thiazides with other antihypertensive agents may lead to additive effects or potentiation). Products include:
Atacand Tablets 639
Atacand HCT 642

Captopril (Co-administration of thiazides with other antihypertensive agents may lead to additive effects or potentiation). Products include:
Captopril Tablets 2182

Carteolol Hydrochloride (Co-administration of thiazides with other antihypertensive agents may lead to additive effects or potentiation).
No products indexed under this heading.

Celecoxib (Nonsteroidal anti-inflammatory agents can reduce the natriuretic, diuretic, and antihypertensive effects). Products include:
Celebrex Capsules 2979

Chlorothiazide (Co-administration of thiazides with other antihypertensive agents may lead to additive effects or potentiation).
No products indexed under this heading.

Chlorothiazide Sodium (Co-administration of thiazides with other antihypertensive agents may lead to additive effects or potentiation). Products include:
Intravenous Sodium Diuril 2490

Chlorpropamide (Hyperglycemia may occur with thiazide diuretics; oral hypoglycemic dosage may need to be adjusted).
No products indexed under this heading.

Chlorthalidone (Co-administration of thiazides with other antihypertensive agents may lead to additive effects or potentiation). Products include:
Clorpres Tablets 2185

Cholestyramine (Binds hydrochlorothiazide and reduces its absorption from gastrointestinal tract by 85%).
No products indexed under this heading.

Ciclesonide (Corticosteroids intensify the electrolyte imbalance, particularly hypokalemia). Products include:
Alvesco Inhalation Aerosol 2985
Omnaris Nasal Spray 2998

Cisatracurium Besylate (Possible increased responsiveness to muscle relaxants). Products include:
Nimbex Injection 484

Clonidine (Co-administration of thiazides with other antihypertensive agents may lead to additive effects or potentiation). Products include:
Catapres-TTS 842

Clonidine Hydrochloride (Co-administration of thiazides with other antihypertensive agents may lead to additive effects or potentiation). Products include:
Catapres Tablets 841
Clorpres Tablets 2185

Codeine Phosphate (Narcotics may potentiate orthostatic hypotension). Products include:
Tylenol with Codeine Tablets 2427

Colestipol Hydrochloride (Binds hydrochlorothiazide and reduces its absorption from gastrointestinal tract by 43%).
No products indexed under this heading.

Cortisone Acetate (Corticosteroids intensify the electrolyte imbalance, particularly hypokalemia).
No products indexed under this heading.

Deserpidine (Co-administration of thiazides with other antihypertensive agents may lead to additive effects or potentiation).
No products indexed under this heading.

Deslanoside (Thiazide-induced hypokalemia may cause cardiac arrhythmias and may also sensitize or exaggerate response of the heart to the toxic effects of digitalis).
No products indexed under this heading.

Dexamethasone (Corticosteroids intensify the electrolyte imbalance, particularly hypokalemia). Products include:
Ciprodex Otic Suspension 541

Dexamethasone Acetate (Corticosteroids intensify the electrolyte imbalance, particularly hypokalemia).
No products indexed under this heading.

Dexamethasone Sodium Phosphate (Corticosteroids intensify the electrolyte imbalance, particularly hypokalemia).
No products indexed under this heading.

Dezocine (Narcotics may potentiate orthostatic hypotension).
No products indexed under this heading.

Diazoxide (Co-administration of thiazides with other antihypertensive agents may lead to additive effects or potentiation). Products include:
Proglycem Capsules 1185
Proglycem Suspension 1185

Diclofenac Epolamine (Nonsteroidal anti-inflammatory agents can reduce the natriuretic, diuretic, and antihypertensive effects). Products include:
Flector Patch 561

Diclofenac Potassium (Nonsteroidal anti-inflammatory agents can reduce the natriuretic, diuretic, and antihypertensive effects).
No products indexed under this heading.

Diclofenac Sodium (Nonsteroidal anti-inflammatory agents can reduce the natriuretic, diuretic, and antihypertensive effects). Products include:
Diclofenac Sodium Ophthalmic Solution .... ⊙240
Voltaren Ophthalmic Solution 2336
Voltaren Tablets 2334
Voltaren-XR Tablets 2337

Digitalis Glycoside Preparations (Thiazide-induced hypokalemia may cause cardiac arrhythmias and may also sensitize or exaggerate response of the heart to the toxic effects of digitalis).
No products indexed under this heading.

Digitoxin (Thiazide-induced hypokalemia may cause cardiac arrhythmias and may also sensitize or exaggerate response of the heart to the toxic effects of digitalis).
No products indexed under this heading.

Digoxin (Thiazide-induced hypokalemia may cause cardiac arrhythmias and may also sensitize or exaggerate response of the heart to the toxic effects of digitalis). Products include:
Lanoxin Injection 1498
Lanoxin Injection Pediatric 1502
Lanoxin Tablets 1505

Diltiazem Hydrochloride (Co-administration of thiazides with other antihypertensive agents may lead to additive effects or potentiation). Products include:
Cardizem LA Extended Release Tablets 421

Doxazosin Mesylate (Co-administration of thiazides with other antihypertensive agents may lead to additive effects or potentiation).
No products indexed under this heading.

Enalapril Maleate (Co-administration of thiazides with other antihypertensive agents may lead to additive effects or potentiation).
No products indexed under this heading.

Enalaprilat (Co-administration of thiazides with other antihypertensive agents may lead to additive effects or potentiation).
No products indexed under this heading.

Esmolol Hydrochloride (Co-administration of thiazides with other antihypertensive agents may lead to additive effects or potentiation).
No products indexed under this heading.

Etodolac (Nonsteroidal anti-inflammatory agents can reduce the natriuretic, diuretic, and antihypertensive effects).
No products indexed under this heading.

Felodipine (Co-administration of thiazides with other antihypertensive agents may lead to additive effects or potentiation).
No products indexed under this heading.

Fenoprofen Calcium (Nonsteroidal anti-inflammatory agents can reduce the natriuretic, diuretic, and antihypertensive effects). Products include:
Nalfon Capsules 2508

Fentanyl (Narcotics may potentiate orthostatic hypotension). Products include:
Duragesic Transdermal System 2405
Ionsys Transdermal System 2410

Fentanyl Citrate (Narcotics may potentiate orthostatic hypotension). Products include:
Actiq 959
Fentora Tablets 968

Fludrocortisone Acetate (Corticosteroids intensify the electrolyte imbalance, particularly hypokalemia).
No products indexed under this heading.

Flunisolide (Corticosteroids intensify the electrolyte imbalance, particularly hypokalemia). Products include:
Aerobid/Aerobid-M 1153

Flurbiprofen (Nonsteroidal anti-inflammatory agents can reduce the natriuretic, diuretic, and antihypertensive effects).
No products indexed under this heading.

Fluticasone Propionate (Corticosteroids intensify the electrolyte imbalance, particularly hypokalemia). Products include:
Advair Diskus 100/50 1276
Advair Diskus 250/50 1276
Advair Diskus 500/50 1276
Advair HFA 45/21 Inhalation Aerosol............ 1288
Advair HFA 115/21 Inhalation Aerosol............ 1288
Advair HFA 230/21 Inhalation Aerosol............ 1288
Flonase Nasal Spray 1431
Flovent Diskus 50 mcg 1435

Fluticasone Propionate HFA (Corticosteroids intensify the electrolyte imbalance, particularly hypokalemia). Products include:
Flovent HFA 1440

Fosinopril Sodium (Co-administration of thiazides with other antihypertensive agents may lead to additive effects or potentiation).
No products indexed under this heading.

Furosemide (Co-administration of thiazides with other antihypertensive agents may lead to additive effects or potentiation). Products include:
Furosemide Tablets 2186

Glimepiride (Hyperglycemia may occur with thiazide diuretics; oral hypoglycemic dosage may need to be adjusted). Products include:
Avandaryl Tablets 1344
Duetact Tablets 3085

Glipizide (Hyperglycemia may occur with thiazide diuretics; oral hypoglycemic dosage may need to be adjusted).
No products indexed under this heading.

Glyburide (Hyperglycemia may occur with thiazide diuretics; oral hypoglycemic dosage may need to be adjusted).
No products indexed under this heading.

Guanabenz Acetate (Co-administration of thiazides with other antihypertensive agents may lead to additive effects or potentiation).
No products indexed under this heading.

Guanethidine Monosulfate (Co-administration of thiazides with other antihypertensive agents may lead to additive effects or potentiation).
No products indexed under this heading.

Hydralazine Hydrochloride (Co-administration of thiazides with other antihypertensive agents may lead to additive effects or potentiation).
No products indexed under this heading.

Hydrocodone Bitartrate (Narcotics may potentiate orthostatic hypotension). Products include:
Lortab 5/500 Tablets 3143
Lortab 7.5/500 Tablets 3144
Lortab 10/500 Tablets 3144
Vicodin Tablets 529
Vicodin ES Tablets 530
Vicodin HP Tablets 531
Vicoprofen Tablets 533
Zydone Tablets 1132

Hydrocodone Polistirex (Narcotics may potentiate orthostatic hypotension). Products include:
Tussionex Pennkinetic Extended-Release Suspension...... 3154

Hydrocortisone (Corticosteroids intensify the electrolyte imbalance, particularly hypokalemia).
No products indexed under this heading.

Hydrocortisone Acetate (Corticosteroids intensify the electrolyte imbalance, particularly hypokalemia). Products include:
Analpram-HC 1140
Pramosone 1141

Hydrocortisone Sodium Phosphate (Corticosteroids intensify the electrolyte imbalance, particularly hypokalemia).
No products indexed under this heading.

Hydrocortisone Sodium Succinate (Corticosteroids intensify the electrolyte imbalance, particularly hypokalemia).
No products indexed under this heading.

Hydroflumethiazide (Co-administration of thiazides with other antihypertensive agents may lead to additive effects or potentiation).
No products indexed under this heading.

Hydromorphone Hydrochloride (Narcotics may potentiate orthostatic hypotension).
No products indexed under this heading.

Ibuprofen (Nonsteroidal anti-inflammatory agents can reduce the natriuretic, diuretic, and antihypertensive effects). Products include:
Motrin IB Tablets and Caplets 1900
Children's Motrin Oral Suspension ... 1901
Children's Motrin Non-Staining Dye-Free Oral Suspension............ 1901
Children's Motrin Cold Oral Suspension 1899
Infants' Motrin Concentrated Drops............ 1901
Infants' Motrin Non-Staining Dye-Free Concentrated Drops....... 1901
Junior Strength Motrin Caplets and Chewable Tablets............ 1901
Vicoprofen Tablets 533

Indapamide (Co-administration of thiazides with other antihypertensive agents may lead to additive effects or potentiation). Products include:
Indapamide Tablets 2188

Indomethacin (Nonsteroidal anti-inflammatory agents can reduce the natriuretic, diuretic, and antihypertensive effects). Products include:
Indocin 2024

Indomethacin Sodium Trihydrate (Nonsteroidal anti-inflammatory agents can reduce the natriuretic, diuretic, and antihypertensive effects). Products include:
Indocin I.V. 2489

Insulin (Hyperglycemia may occur with thiazide diuretics; insulin dosage may need to be adjusted).
No products indexed under this heading.

Insulin, Human, Zinc Suspension (Hyperglycemia may occur with thiazide diuretics; insulin dosage may need to be adjusted).
No products indexed under this heading.

Insulin, Human (rDNA origin) (Hyperglycemia may occur with thiazide diuretics; insulin dosage may need to be adjusted). Products include:
Exubera Inhalation Powder 2515

Insulin, Human NPH (Hyperglycemia may occur with thiazide diuretics; insulin dosage may need to be adjusted). Products include:
Humulin N Vial 1846

Insulin, Human Regular (Hyperglycemia may occur with thiazide diuretics; insulin dosage may need to be adjusted). Products include:
Humulin R............ 1849
Humulin R (U-500) 1850

Insulin, Human Regular and Human NPH Mixture (Hyperglycemia may occur with thiazide diuretics; insulin dosage may need to be adjusted). Products include:
Humulin 50/50, 100 Units 1843
Humulin 70/30 Vial 1844

Insulin, NPH (Hyperglycemia may occur with thiazide diuretics; insulin dosage may need to be adjusted).
No products indexed under this heading.

Insulin, Regular (Hyperglycemia may occur with thiazide diuretics; insulin dosage may need to be adjusted).
No products indexed under this heading.

Insulin, Regular and NPH mixture (Hyperglycemia may occur with thiazide diuretics; insulin dosage may need to be adjusted).
No products indexed under this heading.

Insulin, Zinc Crystals (Hyperglycemia may occur with thiazide diuretics; insulin dosage may need to be adjusted).
No products indexed under this heading.

Insulin, Zinc Suspension (Hyperglycemia may occur with thiazide diuretics; insulin dosage may need to be adjusted).
No products indexed under this heading.

Insulin Aspart (Hyperglycemia may occur with thiazide diuretics; insulin dosage may need to be adjusted).
No products indexed under this heading.

Insulin Aspart, Human (Hyperglycemia may occur with thiazide diuretics; insulin dosage may need to be adjusted). Products include:
NovoLog Mix 70/30 2364

Insulin Aspart, Human Regular (Hyperglycemia may occur with thiazide diuretics; insulin dosage may need to be adjusted). Products include:
NovoLog Injection 2359

Insulin Aspart Protamine, Human (Hyperglycemia may occur with thiazide diuretics; insulin dosage may need to be adjusted). Products include:
NovoLog Mix 70/30 2364

Insulin Detemir (rDNA Origin) (Hyperglycemia may occur with thiazide diuretics; insulin dosage may need to be adjusted). Products include:
Levemir Injection 2352

Insulin glargine (Hyperglycemia may occur with thiazide diuretics; insulin dosage may need to be adjusted). Products include:
Lantus Injection 2749

Insulin Glulisine (Hyperglycemia may occur with thiazide diuretics; insulin dosage may need to be adjusted). Products include:
Apidra Injection 2706

Insulin Lispro, Human (Hyperglycemia may occur with thiazide diuretics; insulin dosage may need to be adjusted). Products include:
Humalog-Pen and KwikPen 1829
Humalog Mix 50/50-Pen and KwikPen............ 1833
Humalog Mix 75/25-Pen and KwikPen............ 1835

Insulin Lispro Protamine, Human (Hyperglycemia may occur with thiazide diuretics; insulin dosage may need to be adjusted). Products include:
Humalog Mix 50/50-Pen and KwikPen............ 1833
Humalog Mix 75/25-Pen and KwikPen............ 1835

Irbesartan (Co-administration of thiazides with other antihypertensive agents may lead to additive effects or potentiation). Products include:
Avalide Tablets 892
Avalide Tablets 2713
Avapro Tablets 897

Avapro Tablets ... 2718

Isradipine (Co-administration of thiazides with other antihypertensive agents may lead to additive effects or potentiation). Products include:

DynaCirc CR Controlled Release Tablets ... 1407

Ketoprofen (Nonsteroidal anti-inflammatory agents can reduce the natriuretic, diuretic, and antihypertensive effects).

No products indexed under this heading.

Ketorolac Tromethamine (Nonsteroidal anti-inflammatory agents can reduce the natriuretic, diuretic, and antihypertensive effects).

No products indexed under this heading.

Labetalol Hydrochloride (Co-administration of thiazides with other antihypertensive agents may lead to additive effects or potentiation).

No products indexed under this heading.

Levorphanol Tartrate (Narcotics may potentiate orthostatic hypotension).

No products indexed under this heading.

Lisinopril (Co-administration of thiazides with other antihypertensive agents may lead to additive effects or potentiation). Products include:

Prinivil Tablets ... 2087
Prinzide Tablets ... 2092

Lithium (Diuretics reduce the renal clearance of lithium and add a high risk of lithium toxicity).

No products indexed under this heading.

Lithium Carbonate (Diuretics reduce the renal clearance of lithium and add a high risk of lithium toxicity).

No products indexed under this heading.

Lithium Citrate (Diuretics reduce the renal clearance of lithium and add a high risk of lithium toxicity).

No products indexed under this heading.

Losartan Potassium (Co-administration of thiazides with other antihypertensive agents may lead to additive effects or potentiation). Products include:

Cozaar Tablets ... 1973

Mecamylamine Hydrochloride (Co-administration of thiazides with other antihypertensive agents may lead to additive effects or potentiation).

No products indexed under this heading.

Meclofenamate Sodium (Nonsteroidal anti-inflammatory agents can reduce the natriuretic, diuretic, and antihypertensive effects).

No products indexed under this heading.

Mefenamic Acid (Nonsteroidal anti-inflammatory agents can reduce the natriuretic, diuretic, and antihypertensive effects).

No products indexed under this heading.

Meloxicam (Nonsteroidal anti-inflammatory agents can reduce the natriuretic, diuretic, and antihypertensive effects). Products include:

Mobic Oral Suspension ... 863
Mobic Tablets ... 863

Meperidine Hydrochloride (Narcotics may potentiate orthostatic hypotension).

No products indexed under this heading.

Mephobarbital (Barbiturates may potentiate orthostatic hypotension).

No products indexed under this heading.

Metformin Hydrochloride (Hyperglycemia may occur with thiazide diuretics; oral hypoglycemic dosage may need to be adjusted). Products include:

ActoPlus Met Tablets ... 3071
Avandamet Tablets ... 1336
Janumet Tablets ... 2041
PrandiMet Tablets ... 2967

Methadone Hydrochloride (Narcotics may potentiate orthostatic hypotension).

No products indexed under this heading.

Methyclothiazide (Co-administration of thiazides with other antihypertensive agents may lead to additive effects or potentiation).

No products indexed under this heading.

Methyldopa (Co-administration of thiazides with other antihypertensive agents may lead to additive effects or potentiation).

No products indexed under this heading.

Methyldopate Hydrochloride (Co-administration of thiazides with other antihypertensive agents may lead to additive effects or potentiation).

No products indexed under this heading.

Methylprednisolone Acetate (Corticosteroids intensify the electrolyte imbalance, particularly hypokalemia).

No products indexed under this heading.

Methylprednisolone Sodium Succinate (Corticosteroids intensify the electrolyte imbalance, particularly hypokalemia).

No products indexed under this heading.

Metocurine Iodide (Possible increased responsiveness to muscle relaxants).

No products indexed under this heading.

Metolazone (Co-administration of thiazides with other antihypertensive agents may lead to additive effects or potentiation).

No products indexed under this heading.

Metoprolol Succinate (Co-administration of thiazides with other antihypertensive agents may lead to additive effects or potentiation). Products include:

Toprol-XL Tablets ... 666

Metoprolol Tartrate (Co-administration of thiazides with other antihypertensive agents may lead to additive effects or potentiation).

No products indexed under this heading.

Metyrosine (Co-administration of thiazides with other antihypertensive agents may lead to additive effects or potentiation). Products include:

Demser Capsules ... 1989

Mibefradil Dihydrochloride (Co-administration of thiazides with other antihypertensive agents may lead to additive effects or potentiation).

No products indexed under this heading.

Miglitol (Hyperglycemia may occur with thiazide diuretics; oral hypoglycemic dosage may need to be adjusted).

No products indexed under this heading.

Minoxidil (Co-administration of thiazides with other antihypertensive agents may lead to additive effects or potentiation).

No products indexed under this heading.

Mivacurium Chloride (Possible increased responsiveness to muscle relaxants).

No products indexed under this heading.

Moexipril Hydrochloride (Co-administration of thiazides with other antihypertensive agents may lead to additive effects or potentiation).

No products indexed under this heading.

Mometasone Furoate (Corticosteroids intensify the electrolyte imbalance, particularly hypokalemia). Products include:

Asmanex Twisthaler ... 2797
Elocon Cream 0.1% ... 2840
Elocon Lotion 0.1% ... 2841
Elocon Ointment 0.1% ... 2842

Mometasone Furoate Monohydrate (Corticosteroids intensify the electrolyte imbalance, particularly hypokalemia). Products include:

Nasonex Nasal Spray ... 2883

Morphine Sulfate (Narcotics may potentiate orthostatic hypotension). Products include:

Avinza Capsules ... 1772
DepoDur Injection ... 1095
MS Contin Tablets ... 2585

Nabumetone (Nonsteroidal anti-inflammatory agents can reduce the natriuretic, diuretic, and antihypertensive effects).

No products indexed under this heading.

Nadolol (Co-administration of thiazides with other antihypertensive agents may lead to additive effects or potentiation). Products include:

Nadolol Tablets ... 2191

Naproxen (Nonsteroidal anti-inflammatory agents can reduce the natriuretic, diuretic, and antihypertensive effects). Products include:

EC-Naprosyn Delayed-Release Tablets ... 2632
Naprosyn Suspension ... 2632
Naprosyn Tablets ... 2632

Naproxen Sodium (Nonsteroidal anti-inflammatory agents can reduce the natriuretic, diuretic, and antihypertensive effects). Products include:

Anaprox Tablets ... 2632
Anaprox DS Tablets ... 2632
Treximet Tablets ... 1616

Nateglinide (Hyperglycemia may occur with thiazide diuretics; oral hypoglycemic dosage may need to be adjusted). Products include:

Starlix Tablets ... 2314

Nebivolol (Co-administration of thiazides with other antihypertensive agents may lead to additive effects or potentiation). Products include:

Bystolic Tablets ... 1155

Nicardipine Hydrochloride (Co-administration of thiazides with other antihypertensive agents may lead to additive effects or potentiation). Products include:

Cardene I.V. ... 1093

Nifedipine (Co-administration of thiazides with other antihypertensive agents may lead to additive effects or potentiation).

No products indexed under this heading.

Nisoldipine (Co-administration of thiazides with other antihypertensive agents may lead to additive effects or potentiation). Products include:

Sular Extended Release Tablets ... 2975

Nitroglycerin (Co-administration of thiazides with other antihypertensive agents may lead to additive effects or potentiation). Products include:

Nitro-Dur Transdermal Infusion System ... 2887
Nitrolingual Pumpspray ... 2965

Norepinephrine Bitartrate (Possible decreased response to pressor amines).

No products indexed under this heading.

Oxaprozin (Nonsteroidal anti-inflammatory agents can reduce the natriuretic, diuretic, and antihypertensive effects).

No products indexed under this heading.

Oxycodone Hydrochloride (Narcotics may potentiate orthostatic hypotension). Products include:

OxyContin Tablets ... 2589
OxyIR Capsules ... 2593
Percocet Tablets ... 1127
Percodan Tablets ... 1130

Pancuronium Bromide (Possible increased responsiveness to muscle relaxants).

No products indexed under this heading.

Penbutolol Sulfate (Co-administration of thiazides with other antihypertensive agents may lead to additive effects or potentiation).

No products indexed under this heading.

Pentobarbital Sodium (Barbiturates may potentiate orthostatic hypotension). Products include:

Nembutal Sodium Solution, USP ... 2494

Perindopril Erbumine (Co-administration of thiazides with other antihypertensive agents may lead to additive effects or potentiation). Products include:

Aceon Tablets (2 mg, 4 mg, 8 mg) ... 3038

Phenobarbital (Barbiturates may potentiate orthostatic hypotension). Products include:

Donnatal Extentabs ... 2507

Phenoxybenzamine Hydrochloride (Co-administration of thiazides with other antihypertensive agents may lead to additive effects or potentiation). Products include:

Dibenzyline Capsules ... 3188

Phentolamine Mesylate (Co-administration of thiazides with other antihypertensive agents may lead to additive effects or potentiation).

No products indexed under this heading.

Phenylbutazone (Nonsteroidal anti-inflammatory agents can reduce the natriuretic, diuretic, and antihypertensive effects).

No products indexed under this heading.

Pindolol (Co-administration of thiazides with other antihypertensive agents may lead to additive effects or potentiation).
No products indexed under this heading.

Pioglitazone Hydrochloride (Hyperglycemia may occur with thiazide diuretics; oral hypoglycemic dosage may need to be adjusted). Products include:
- ActoPlus Met Tablets **3071**
- Actos Tablets **3077**
- Duetact Tablets **3085**

Piroxicam (Nonsteroidal anti-inflammatory agents can reduce the natriuretic, diuretic, and antihypertensive effects).
No products indexed under this heading.

Polythiazide (Co-administration of thiazides with other antihypertensive agents may lead to additive effects or potentiation).
No products indexed under this heading.

Potassium Acid Phosphate (Concomitant use of potassium supplements with eprosartan may lead to hyperkalemia). Products include:
- K-Phos Original (Sodium Free) Tablets **814**

Potassium Bicarbonate (Concomitant use of potassium supplements with eprosartan may lead to hyperkalemia).
No products indexed under this heading.

Potassium Chloride (Concomitant use of potassium supplements with eprosartan may lead to hyperkalemia). Products include:
- MoviPrep Oral Solution **2679**

Potassium Citrate (Concomitant use of potassium supplements with eprosartan may lead to hyperkalemia). Products include:
- BioLean Free Tablets **635**
- Urocit-K Tablets **2176**

Potassium Gluconate (Concomitant use of potassium supplements with eprosartan may lead to hyperkalemia).
No products indexed under this heading.

Potassium Phosphate (Concomitant use of potassium supplements with eprosartan may lead to hyperkalemia). Products include:
- K-Phos Neutral Tablets **813**

Prazosin Hydrochloride (Co-administration of thiazides with other antihypertensive agents may lead to additive effects or potentiation).
No products indexed under this heading.

Prednisolone Acetate (Corticosteroids intensify the electrolyte imbalance, particularly hypokalemia). Products include:
- Pred Forte Ophthalmic Suspension ...... ⊙ **227**
- Pred Mild Ophthalmic Suspension ...... ⊙ **230**
- Pred-G Ophthalmic Ointment ...... ⊙ **229**
- Pred-G Ophthalmic Suspension ...... ⊙ **228**

Prednisolone Sodium Phosphate (Corticosteroids intensify the electrolyte imbalance, particularly hypokalemia).
No products indexed under this heading.

Prednisolone Tebutate (Corticosteroids intensify the electrolyte imbalance, particularly hypokalemia).
No products indexed under this heading.

Prednisone (Corticosteroids intensify the electrolyte imbalance, particularly hypokalemia).
No products indexed under this heading.

Propoxyphene Hydrochloride (Narcotics may potentiate orthostatic hypotension).
No products indexed under this heading.

Propoxyphene Napsylate (Narcotics may potentiate orthostatic hypotension).
No products indexed under this heading.

Propranolol Hydrochloride (Co-administration of thiazides with other antihypertensive agents may lead to additive effects or potentiation). Products include:
- InnoPran XL Extended Release Capsules **1484**

Quinapril Hydrochloride (Co-administration of thiazides with other antihypertensive agents may lead to additive effects or potentiation).
No products indexed under this heading.

Ramipril (Co-administration of thiazides with other antihypertensive agents may lead to additive effects or potentiation).
No products indexed under this heading.

Rapacuronium Bromide (Possible increased responsiveness to muscle relaxants).
No products indexed under this heading.

Rauwolfia Serpentina (Co-administration of thiazides with other antihypertensive agents may lead to additive effects or potentiation).
No products indexed under this heading.

Remifentanil Hydrochloride (Narcotics may potentiate orthostatic hypotension).
No products indexed under this heading.

Repaglinide (Hyperglycemia may occur with thiazide diuretics; oral hypoglycemic dosage may need to be adjusted). Products include:
- PrandiMet Tablets **2967**
- Prandin Tablets **2971**

Rescinnamine (Co-administration of thiazides with other antihypertensive agents may lead to additive effects or potentiation).
No products indexed under this heading.

Reserpine (Co-administration of thiazides with other antihypertensive agents may lead to additive effects or potentiation).
No products indexed under this heading.

Rocuronium Bromide (Possible increased responsiveness to muscle relaxants). Products include:
- Zemuron Injection **2947**

Rofecoxib (Nonsteroidal anti-inflammatory agents can reduce the natriuretic, diuretic, and antihypertensive effects).
No products indexed under this heading.

Rosiglitazone Maleate (Hyperglycemia may occur with thiazide diuretics; oral hypoglycemic dosage may need to be adjusted). Products include:
- Avandamet Tablets **1336**
- Avandaryl Tablets **1344**
- Avandia Tablets **1351**

Secobarbital Sodium (Barbiturates may potentiate orthostatic hypotension).
No products indexed under this heading.

Sitagliptin Phosphate (Hyperglycemia may occur with thiazide diuretics; oral hypoglycemic dosage may need to be adjusted). Products include:
- Janumet Tablets **2041**
- Januvia Tablets **2048**

Sodium Nitroprusside (Co-administration of thiazides with other antihypertensive agents may lead to additive effects or potentiation).
No products indexed under this heading.

Sotalol Hydrochloride (Co-administration of thiazides with other antihypertensive agents may lead to additive effects or potentiation).
No products indexed under this heading.

Spirapril Hydrochloride (Co-administration of thiazides with other antihypertensive agents may lead to additive effects or potentiation).
No products indexed under this heading.

Spironolactone (Concomitant use of potassium sparing diuretics with eprosartan may lead to hyperkalemia).
No products indexed under this heading.

Sufentanil Citrate (Narcotics may potentiate orthostatic hypotension).
No products indexed under this heading.

Sulindac (Nonsteroidal anti-inflammatory agents can reduce the natriuretic, diuretic, and antihypertensive effects). Products include:
- Clinoril Tablets **1962**

Telmisartan (Co-administration of thiazides with other antihypertensive agents may lead to additive effects or potentiation). Products include:
- Micardis Tablets **852**
- Micardis HCT Tablets **854**

Terazosin Hydrochloride (Co-administration of thiazides with other antihypertensive agents may lead to additive effects or potentiation).
No products indexed under this heading.

Thiamylal Sodium (Barbiturates may potentiate orthostatic hypotension).
No products indexed under this heading.

Timolol Maleate (Co-administration of thiazides with other antihypertensive agents may lead to additive effects or potentiation). Products include:
- Combigan Ophthalmic Solution **553**
- Cosopt Sterile Ophthalmic Solution **1969**
- Timoptic Sterile Ophthalmic Solution **2121**
- Timoptic in Ocudose **2124**
- Timoptic-XE Sterile Ophthalmic Gel Forming Solution **2125**

Tolazamide (Hyperglycemia may occur with thiazide diuretics; oral hypoglycemic dosage may need to be adjusted).
No products indexed under this heading.

Tolbutamide (Hyperglycemia may occur with thiazide diuretics; oral hypoglycemic dosage may need to be adjusted).
No products indexed under this heading.

Tolmetin Sodium (Nonsteroidal anti-inflammatory agents can reduce the natriuretic, diuretic, and antihypertensive effects).
No products indexed under this heading.

Torsemide (Co-administration of thiazides with other antihypertensive agents may lead to additive effects or potentiation). Products include:
- Demadex Injection **2630**
- Demadex Tablets **2630**

Trandolapril (Co-administration of thiazides with other antihypertensive agents may lead to additive effects or potentiation). Products include:
- Mavik Tablets **472**
- Tarka Tablets **511**

Triamcinolone (Corticosteroids intensify the electrolyte imbalance, particularly hypokalemia).
No products indexed under this heading.

Triamcinolone Acetonide (Corticosteroids intensify the electrolyte imbalance, particularly hypokalemia). Products include:
- Azmacort Inhalation Aerosol **407**
- Nasacort AQ Nasal Spray **2765**
- Triesence Injectable Suspension ...... ⊙ **209**

Triamcinolone Diacetate (Corticosteroids intensify the electrolyte imbalance, particularly hypokalemia).
No products indexed under this heading.

Triamcinolone Hexacetonide (Corticosteroids intensify the electrolyte imbalance, particularly hypokalemia).
No products indexed under this heading.

Triamterene (Concomitant use of potassium sparing diuretics with eprosartan may lead to hyperkalemia). Products include:
- Dyazide Capsules **1405**
- Dyrenium Capsules **3189**

Trimethaphan Camsylate (Co-administration of thiazides with other antihypertensive agents may lead to additive effects or potentiation).
No products indexed under this heading.

Troglitazone (Hyperglycemia may occur with thiazide diuretics; oral hypoglycemic dosage may need to be adjusted).
No products indexed under this heading.

Tubocurarine Chloride (Possible increased responsiveness to muscle relaxant).
No products indexed under this heading.

Valdecoxib (Nonsteroidal anti-inflammatory agents can reduce the natriuretic, diuretic, and antihypertensive effects).
No products indexed under this heading.

Valsartan (Co-administration of thiazides with other antihypertensive agents may lead to additive effects or potentiation). Products include:
- Diovan Tablets **2212**
- Diovan HCT Tablets **2216**
- Exforge Tablets **2238**

Vecuronium Bromide (Possible increased responsiveness to muscle relaxants).
No products indexed under this heading.

Verapamil Hydrochloride (Co-administration of thiazides with other antihypertensive agents may lead to additive effects or potentiation). Products include:

Tarka Tablets ... 511

Food Interactions

Alcohol (May potentiate orthostatic hypotension).

TEV-TROPIN FOR INJECTION

(Somatropin (rDNA Origin)) ... 1187

May interact with glucocorticoids and drugs which undergo biotransformation by cytochrome p-450 mixed function oxidase. Compounds in these categories include:

Acarbose (Somatropin administration may alter the clearance of compounds known to be metabolized by CYP450). Products include:
- Precose Tablets ... 792

Acetaminophen (Somatropin administration may alter the clearance of compounds known to be metabolized by CYP450). Products include:
- Benadryl Allergy & Cold Kapgels ... 1895
- Benadryl Allergy & Sinus Headache Kapgels ... 1895
- Benadryl Severe Allergy & Sinus Headache Caplets ... 1897
- Lortab 5/500 Tablets ... 3143
- Lortab 7.5/500 Tablets ... 3144
- Lortab 10/500 Tablets ... 3144
- Percocet Tablets ... 1127
- Sinutab Sinus Caplets ... 1905
- Sudafed PE Cold & Cough Caplets ... 1907
- Sudafed PE Nighttime Cold Caplets ... 1907
- Sudafed PE Severe Cold Caplets ... 1908
- Sudafed PE Sinus Headache Caplets ... 1908
- Regular Strength Tylenol Tablets ... 1915
- Tylenol 8 Hour Extended Release Caplets ... 1915
- Extra Strength Tylenol Caplets, Cool Caplets, and EZ Tabs ... 1915
- Extra Strength Tylenol Adult Rapid Blast Liquid ... 1915
- Extra Strength Tylenol PM Caplets, Geltabs, Liquid, and Rapid Release Gels ... 1915
- Extra Strength Tylenol Rapid Release Gels ... 1915
- Tylenol with Codeine Tablets ... 2427
- Tylenol Allergy Multi-Symptom Caplets with Cool Burst and Rapid Release Gelcaps ... 1916
- Tylenol Allergy Multi-Symptom Nighttime Caplets with Cool Burst ... 1916
- Tylenol Severe Allergy Caplets ... 1916
- Tylenol Arthritis Pain Extended Release Geltabs/Caplets ... 1915
- Tylenol Chest Congestion Caplets with Cool Burst ... 1910
- Tylenol Chest Congestion Liquid with Cool Burst ... 1910
- Children's Tylenol Plus Cold Suspension Liquid ... 1912
- Children's Tylenol Plus Cold & Allergy Suspension Liquid ... 1914
- Children's Tylenol Plus Cough & Runny Nose Suspension Liquid ... 1912
- Children's Tylenol Plus Cough & Sore Throat Suspension Liquid ... 1912
- Children's Tylenol Plus Flu Suspension Liquid ... 1914
- Children's Tylenol Suspension Liquid ... 1909
- Children's Tylenol Meltaways ... 1909
- Children's Tylenol Plus Multi-Symptom Cold Suspension Liquid ... 1912
- Tylenol Cold Severe Congestion Daytime Caplets with Cool Burst ... 1912
- Tylenol Cold Head Congestion Daytime Caplets with Cool Burst ... 1910
- Tylenol Cold Head Congestion Nighttime Caplets with Cool Burst ... 1910
- Tylenol Cold Head Congestion Severe Daytime Caplets with Cool Burst ... 1910
- Tylenol Cold Multi-Symptom Daytime Caplets with Cool Burst and Rapid Release Gels ... 1913
- Tylenol Cold Multi-Symptom Daytime Liquid with Citrus Burst ... 1913
- Tylenol Cold Multi-Symptom Nighttime Caplets with Cool Burst ... 1913
- Tylenol Cold Multi-Symptom Nighttime Liquid with Cool Burst ... 1913
- Tylenol Cold Multi-Symptom Severe Caplets with Cool Burst ... 1913
- Tylenol Cold Multi-Symptom Severe Daytime Liquid with Citrus Burst ... 1913
- Tylenol Cough & Sore Throat Daytime Liquid with Cool Burst ... 1918
- Tylenol Cough & Sore Throat Nighttime Liquid with Cool Burst ... 1918
- Concentrated Tylenol Infants' Drops ... 1909
- Jr. Tylenol Meltaways ... 1909
- Tylenol Sinus Congestion & Pain Daytime Caplets with Cool Burst and Gelcaps ... 1917
- Tylenol Sinus Congestion & Pain Nighttime Caplets with Cool Burst ... 1917
- Tylenol Sinus Congestion & Pain Severe Caplets with Cool Burst ... 1917
- Tylenol Sinus Severe Congestion Caplets with Cool Burst ... 1917
- Tylenol Sore Throat Daytime Liquid with Cool Burst ... 1918
- Tylenol Sore Throat Nighttime Liquid with Cool Burst ... 1918
- Women's Tylenol Menstrual Relief Caplets ... 1919
- Vicks DayQuil Cold & Flu Multi-Symptom Relief ... ■616
- Vicks DayQuil LiquiCaps ... 2567
- Vicks DayQuil Liquid ... 2567
- Vicks DayQuil Multi-Symptom Cold/Flu Relief ... 2567
- Vicks NyQuil Cold & Flu Multi-Symptom Relief ... ■617
- Vicks NyQuil LiquiCaps ... 2567
- Vicks NyQuil Liquid ... 2567
- Vicks NyQuil Multi-Symptom Cold/Flu Relief ... 2567
- Vicodin Tablets ... 529
- Vicodin ES Tablets ... 530
- Vicodin HP Tablets ... 531
- Zydone Tablets ... 1132

Alatrofloxacin Mesylate (Somatropin administration may alter the clearance of compounds known to be metabolized by CYP450).
No products indexed under this heading.

Alfentanil Hydrochloride (Somatropin administration may alter the clearance of compounds known to be metabolized by CYP450).
No products indexed under this heading.

Alprazolam (Somatropin administration may alter the clearance of compounds known to be metabolized by CYP450).
No products indexed under this heading.

Aminophylline (Somatropin administration may alter the clearance of compounds known to be metabolized by CYP450).
No products indexed under this heading.

Amiodarone Hydrochloride (Somatropin administration may alter the clearance of compounds known to be metabolized by CYP450).
No products indexed under this heading.

Amitriptyline Hydrochloride (Somatropin administration may alter the clearance of compounds known to be metabolized by CYP450).
No products indexed under this heading.

Amlodipine Besylate (Somatropin administration may alter the clearance of compounds known to be metabolized by CYP450). Products include:
- Azor Tablets ... 1005
- Exforge Tablets ... 2238

Amoxapine (Somatropin administration may alter the clearance of compounds known to be metabolized by CYP450).
No products indexed under this heading.

Amphetamine Aspartate (Somatropin administration may alter the clearance of compounds known to be metabolized by CYP450). Products include:
- Adderall XR Capsules ... 3012

Amphetamine Sulfate (Somatropin administration may alter the clearance of compounds known to be metabolized by CYP450). Products include:
- Adderall XR Capsules ... 3012

Aprepitant (Somatropin administration may alter the clearance of compounds known to be metabolized by CYP450). Products include:
- Emend Capsules ... 1992

Astemizole (Somatropin administration may alter the clearance of compounds known to be metabolized by CYP450).
No products indexed under this heading.

Atorvastatin Calcium (Somatropin administration may alter the clearance of compounds known to be metabolized by CYP450). Products include:
- Lipitor Tablets ... 2501

Belladonna Ergotamine (Somatropin administration may alter the clearance of compounds known to be metabolized by CYP450).
No products indexed under this heading.

Benzphetamine Hydrochloride (Somatropin administration may alter the clearance of compounds known to be metabolized by CYP450).
No products indexed under this heading.

Betamethasone Acetate (Glucocorticoid therapy may inhibit the growth-promoting effect of human growth hormone. Patients with co-existing ACTH deficiency should have their glucocorticoid replacement dose carefully adjusted to avoid an inhibitory effect on growth).
No products indexed under this heading.

Betamethasone Sodium Phosphate (Glucocorticoid therapy may inhibit the growth-promoting effect of human growth hormone. Patients with co-existing ACTH deficiency should have their glucocorticoid replacement dose carefully adjusted to avoid an inhibitory effect on growth).
No products indexed under this heading.

Bisoprolol Fumarate (Somatropin administration may alter the clearance of compounds known to be metabolized by CYP450).
No products indexed under this heading.

Buspirone Hydrochloride (Somatropin administration may alter the clearance of compounds known to be metabolized by CYP450).
No products indexed under this heading.

Busulfan (Somatropin administration may alter the clearance of compounds known to be metabolized by CYP450). Products include:
- Busulfex Injection ... 2477
- Myleran Tablets ... 1530

Caffeine (Somatropin administration may alter the clearance of compounds known to be metabolized by CYP450). Products include:
- BioLean Free Tablets ... ■635
- BioLean II Tablets ... ■635
- Winrgy Dietary Supplement ... ■642

Caffeine Anhydrous (Somatropin administration may alter the clearance of compounds known to be metabolized by CYP450).
No products indexed under this heading.

Caffeine Citrate (Somatropin administration may alter the clearance of compounds known to be metabolized by CYP450).
No products indexed under this heading.

Captopril (Somatropin administration may alter the clearance of compounds known to be metabolized by CYP450). Products include:
- Captopril Tablets ... 2182

Carbamazepine (Somatropin administration may alter the clearance of compounds known to be metabolized by CYP450). Products include:
- Carbatrol Capsules ... 3019
- Equetro Extended-Release Capsules ... 3174

Carisoprodol (Somatropin administration may alter the clearance of compounds known to be metabolized by CYP450). Products include:
- Soma Tablets ... 1931

Chlordiazepoxide (Somatropin administration may alter the clearance of compounds known to be metabolized by CYP450).
No products indexed under this heading.

Chlordiazepoxide Hydrochloride (Somatropin administration may alter the clearance of compounds known to be metabolized by CYP450).
No products indexed under this heading.

Chlorpheniramine (Somatropin administration may alter the clearance of compounds known to be metabolized by CYP450).
No products indexed under this heading.

Chlorpheniramine Maleate (Somatropin administration may alter the clearance of compounds known to be metabolized by CYP450). Products include:
- Actifed Cold & Allergy Tablets ... 1895
- Sudafed PE Sinus & Allergy Tablets ... 1908
- Tylenol Allergy Multi-Symptom Caplets with Cool Burst and Rapid Release Gelcaps ... 1916
- Children's Tylenol Plus Cold Suspension Liquid ... 1912
- Children's Tylenol Plus Cough & Runny Nose Suspension Liquid ... 1912
- Children's Tylenol Plus Flu Suspension Liquid ... 1914
- Children's Tylenol Plus Multi-Symptom Cold Suspension Liquid ... 1912
- Tylenol Cold Head Congestion Nighttime Caplets with Cool Burst ... 1910
- Tylenol Cold Multi-Symptom Nighttime Caplets with Cool Burst ... 1913

Tylenol Sinus Congestion & Pain Nighttime Caplets with Cool Burst 1917

Chlorpheniramine Polistirex (Somatropin administration may alter the clearance of compounds known to be metabolized by CYP450). Products include:

Tussionex Pennkinetic Extended-Release Suspension 3154

Chlorpheniramine Tannate (Somatropin administration may alter the clearance of compounds known to be metabolized by CYP450).

No products indexed under this heading.

Chlorpromazine (Somatropin administration may alter the clearance of compounds known to be metabolized by CYP450).

No products indexed under this heading.

Chlorpromazine Hydrochloride (Somatropin administration may alter the clearance of compounds known to be metabolized by CYP450).

No products indexed under this heading.

Chlorpropamide (Somatropin administration may alter the clearance of compounds known to be metabolized by CYP450).

No products indexed under this heading.

Cimetidine Hydrochloride (Somatropin administration may alter the clearance of compounds known to be metabolized by CYP450).

No products indexed under this heading.

Ciprofloxacin (Somatropin administration may alter the clearance of compounds known to be metabolized by CYP450). Products include:

Cipro I.V. 2817
Cipro Oral Suspension 2810
Cipro XR Tablets 2823
Ciprodex Otic Suspension 541

Ciprofloxacin Hydrochloride (Somatropin administration may alter the clearance of compounds known to be metabolized by CYP450). Products include:

Cipro Tablets 2810

Cisapride (Somatropin administration may alter the clearance of compounds known to be metabolized by CYP450).

No products indexed under this heading.

Clarithromycin (Somatropin administration may alter the clearance of compounds known to be metabolized by CYP450). Products include:

Biaxin/Biaxin XL 411

Clomipramine Hydrochloride (Somatropin administration may alter the clearance of compounds known to be metabolized by CYP450).

No products indexed under this heading.

Clozapine (Somatropin administration may alter the clearance of compounds known to be metabolized by CYP450).

No products indexed under this heading.

Codeine Phosphate (Somatropin administration may alter the clearance of compounds known to be metabolized by CYP450). Products include:

Tylenol with Codeine Tablets 2427

Codeine Sulfate (Somatropin administration may alter the clearance of compounds known to be metabolized by CYP450).

No products indexed under this heading.

Cortisone Acetate (Glucocorticoid therapy may inhibit the growth-promoting effect of human growth hormone. Patients with co-existing ACTH deficiency should have their glucocorticoid replacement dose carefully adjusted to avoid an inhibitory effect on growth).

No products indexed under this heading.

Cyclobenzaprine Hydrochloride (Somatropin administration may alter the clearance of compounds known to be metabolized by CYP450). Products include:

Amrix Capsules 966

Cyclophosphamide (Somatropin administration may alter the clearance of compounds known to be metabolized by CYP450).

No products indexed under this heading.

Cyclosporine (Somatropin administration may alter the clearance of compounds known to be metabolized by CYP450). Products include:

Gengraf Capsules 435
Neoral Oral Solution 2280
Neoral Soft Gelatin Capsules 2280
Restasis Ophthalmic Emulsion 557
Sandimmune 2296

Desipramine Hydrochloride (Somatropin administration may alter the clearance of compounds known to be metabolized by CYP450).

No products indexed under this heading.

Desogestrel (Somatropin administration may alter the clearance of compounds known to be metabolized by CYP450). Products include:

Mircette Tablets 1034

Dexamethasone (Glucocorticoid therapy may inhibit the growth-promoting effect of human growth hormone. Patients with co-existing ACTH deficiency should have their glucocorticoid replacement dose carefully adjusted to avoid an inhibitory effect on growth). Products include:

Ciprodex Otic Suspension 541

Dexamethasone Acetate (Glucocorticoid therapy may inhibit the growth-promoting effect of human growth hormone. Patients with co-existing ACTH deficiency should have their glucocorticoid replacement dose carefully adjusted to avoid an inhibitory effect on growth).

No products indexed under this heading.

Dexamethasone Sodium Phosphate (Glucocorticoid therapy may inhibit the growth-promoting effect of human growth hormone. Patients with co-existing ACTH deficiency should have their glucocorticoid replacement dose carefully adjusted to avoid an inhibitory effect on growth).

No products indexed under this heading.

Estrogen (Somatropin administration may alter the clearance of compounds known to be metabolized by CYP450).

No products indexed under this heading.

Fludrocortisone Acetate (Glucocorticoid therapy may inhibit the growth-promoting effect of human growth hormone. Patients with co-existing ACTH deficiency should have their glucocorticoid replacement dose carefully adjusted to avoid an inhibitory effect on growth).

No products indexed under this heading.

Galantamine Hydrobromide (Somatropin administration may alter the clearance of compounds known to be metabolized by CYP450).

No products indexed under this heading.

Hydrocortisone (Glucocorticoid therapy may inhibit the growth-promoting effect of human growth hormone. Patients with co-existing ACTH deficiency should have their glucocorticoid replacement dose carefully adjusted to avoid an inhibitory effect on growth).

No products indexed under this heading.

Hydrocortisone Acetate (Glucocorticoid therapy may inhibit the growth-promoting effect of human growth hormone. Patients with co-existing ACTH deficiency should have their glucocorticoid replacement dose carefully adjusted to avoid an inhibitory effect on growth). Products include:

Analpram-HC 1140
Pramosone 1141

Hydrocortisone Sodium Phosphate (Glucocorticoid therapy may inhibit the growth-promoting effect of human growth hormone. Patients with co-existing ACTH deficiency should have their glucocorticoid replacement dose carefully adjusted to avoid an inhibitory effect on growth).

No products indexed under this heading.

Hydrocortisone Sodium Succinate (Glucocorticoid therapy may inhibit the growth-promoting effect of human growth hormone. Patients with co-existing ACTH deficiency should have their glucocorticoid replacement dose carefully adjusted to avoid an inhibitory effect on growth).

No products indexed under this heading.

Methylprednisolone Acetate (Glucocorticoid therapy may inhibit the growth-promoting effect of human growth hormone. Patients with co-existing ACTH deficiency should have their glucocorticoid replacement dose carefully adjusted to avoid an inhibitory effect on growth).

No products indexed under this heading.

Methylprednisolone Sodium Succinate (Glucocorticoid therapy may inhibit the growth-promoting effect of human growth hormone. Patients with co-existing ACTH deficiency should have their glucocorticoid replacement dose carefully adjusted to avoid an inhibitory effect on growth).

No products indexed under this heading.

Ondansetron (Somatropin administration may alter the clearance of compounds known to be metabolized by CYP450). Products include:

Zofran ODT Orally Disintegrating Tablets 1687

Prednisolone Acetate (Glucocorticoid therapy may inhibit the growth-promoting effect of human growth hormone. Patients with co-existing ACTH deficiency should have their glucocorticoid replacement dose carefully adjusted to avoid an inhibitory effect on growth). Products include:

Pred Forte Ophthalmic Suspension .... ⊙ 227
Pred Mild Ophthalmic Suspension .... ⊙ 230
Pred-G Ophthalmic Ointment .... ⊙ 229
Pred-G Ophthalmic Suspension .... ⊙ 228

Prednisolone Sodium Phosphate (Glucocorticoid therapy may inhibit the growth-promoting effect of human growth hormone. Patients with co-existing ACTH deficiency should have their glucocorticoid replacement dose carefully adjusted to avoid an inhibitory effect on growth).

No products indexed under this heading.

Prednisolone Tebutate (Glucocorticoid therapy may inhibit the growth-promoting effect of human growth hormone. Patients with co-existing ACTH deficiency should have their glucocorticoid replacement dose carefully adjusted to avoid an inhibitory effect on growth).

No products indexed under this heading.

Prednisone (Glucocorticoid therapy may inhibit the growth-promoting effect of human growth hormone. Patients with co-existing ACTH deficiency should have their glucocorticoid replacement dose carefully adjusted to avoid an inhibitory effect on growth).

No products indexed under this heading.

Tiagabine Hydrochloride (Somatropin administration may alter the clearance of compounds known to be metabolized by CYP450). Products include:

Gabitril Tablets 973

Triamcinolone (Glucocorticoid therapy may inhibit the growth-promoting effect of human growth hormone. Patients with co-existing ACTH deficiency should have their glucocorticoid replacement dose carefully adjusted to avoid an inhibitory effect on growth).

No products indexed under this heading.

Triamcinolone Acetonide (Glucocorticoid therapy may inhibit the growth-promoting effect of human growth hormone. Patients with co-existing ACTH deficiency should have their glucocorticoid replacement dose carefully adjusted to avoid an inhibitory effect on growth). Products include:

Azmacort Inhalation Aerosol 407
Nasacort AQ Nasal Spray 2765
Triesence Injectable Suspension .... ⊙ 209

Triamcinolone Diacetate (Glucocorticoid therapy may inhibit the growth-promoting effect of human growth hormone. Patients with co-existing ACTH deficiency should have their glucocorticoid replacement dose carefully adjusted to avoid an inhibitory effect on growth).

No products indexed under this heading.

IMPORTANT NOTE: Always consult each drug listing in the patient's regimen for possible interactions.

Triamcinolone Hexacetonide (Glucocorticoid therapy may inhibit the growth-promoting effect of human growth hormone. Patients with co-existing ACTH deficiency should have their glucocorticoid replacement dose carefully adjusted to avoid an inhibitory effect on growth).
No products indexed under this heading.

Voriconazole (Somatropin administration may alter the clearance of compounds known to be metabolized by CYP450).
No products indexed under this heading.

THERA-GESIC CREME

(Menthol, Methyl Salicylate) .... ▣610
None cited in PDR database.

THERMACARE THERAPEUTIC HEAT WRAPS

(Device) 2566
None cited in PDR database.

THIORIDAZINE HYDROCHLORIDE TABLETS

(Thioridazine Hydrochloride) 2195
May interact with central nervous system depressants, erythromycin, potassium-depleting diuretics, quinidine, and certain other agents. Compounds in these categories include:

Alfentanil Hydrochloride (Thioridazine is capable of potentiating CNS depressants).
No products indexed under this heading.

Alprazolam (Thioridazine is capable of potentiating CNS depressants).
No products indexed under this heading.

Amiodarone Hydrochloride (Thioridazine has been shown to prolong QTc interval in a dose-related manner; drugs with this potential have been associated with Torsade de pointes-type arrhythmias and sudden death; co-administration with other drugs that are known to prolong QTc interval is contraindicated).
No products indexed under this heading.

Aprobarbital (Thioridazine is capable of potentiating CNS depressants).
No products indexed under this heading.

Arsenic Trioxide (Thioridazine has been shown to prolong QTc interval in a dose-related manner; drugs with this potential have been associated with torsade de pointes-type arrhythmias and sudden death; co-administration with other drugs that are known to prolong QTc interval is contraindicated). Products include:
Trisenox Injection 986

Atropine Sulfate (Thioridazine is capable of potentiating atropine). Products include:
Donnatal Extentabs 2507

Bendroflumethiazide (Hypokalemia may result from diuretic therapy and this may increase the risk of QT prolongation and arrhythmias; co-administration may increase the risk of serious, potentially fatal, cardiac arrhythmias).
No products indexed under this heading.

Bepridil Hydrochloride (Thioridazine has been shown to prolong QTc interval in a dose-related manner; drugs with this potential have been associated with torsade de pointes-type arrhythmias and sudden death; co-administration with other drugs that are known to prolong QTc interval is contraindicated).
No products indexed under this heading.

Bumetanide (Hypokalemia may result from diuretic therapy and this may increase the risk of QT prolongation and arrhythmias; co-administration may increase the risk of serious, potentially fatal, cardiac arrhythmias).
No products indexed under this heading.

Buprenorphine Hydrochloride (Thioridazine is capable of potentiating CNS depressants). Products include:
Suboxone Tablets 2601
Subutex Tablets 2601

Buspirone Hydrochloride (Thioridazine is capable of potentiating CNS depressants).
No products indexed under this heading.

Butabarbital (Thioridazine is capable of potentiating CNS depressants).
No products indexed under this heading.

Butalbital (Thioridazine is capable of potentiating CNS depressants).
No products indexed under this heading.

Chlordiazepoxide (Thioridazine is capable of potentiating CNS depressants).
No products indexed under this heading.

Chlordiazepoxide Hydrochloride (Thioridazine is capable of potentiating CNS depressants).
No products indexed under this heading.

Chlorothiazide (Hypokalemia may result from diuretic therapy and this may increase the risk of QT prolongation and arrhythmias; co-administration may increase the risk of serious, potentially fatal, cardiac arrhythmias).
No products indexed under this heading.

Chlorothiazide Sodium (Hypokalemia may result from diuretic therapy and this may increase the risk of QT prolongation and arrhythmias; co-administration may increase the risk of serious, potentially fatal, cardiac arrhythmias). Products include:
Intravenous Sodium Diuril 2490

Chlorpromazine (Thioridazine is capable of potentiating CNS depressants).
No products indexed under this heading.

Chlorpromazine Hydrochloride (Thioridazine is capable of potentiating CNS depressants).
No products indexed under this heading.

Chlorprothixene (Thioridazine is capable of potentiating CNS depressants).
No products indexed under this heading.

Chlorprothixene Hydrochloride (Thioridazine is capable of potentiating CNS depressants).
No products indexed under this heading.

Chlorprothixene Lactate (Thioridazine is capable of potentiating CNS depressants).
No products indexed under this heading.

Clorazepate Dipotassium (Thioridazine is capable of potentiating CNS depressants).
No products indexed under this heading.

Clozapine (Thioridazine is capable of potentiating CNS depressants).
No products indexed under this heading.

Codeine Phosphate (Thioridazine is capable of potentiating CNS depressants). Products include:
Tylenol with Codeine Tablets 2427

Desflurane (Thioridazine is capable of potentiating CNS depressants).
No products indexed under this heading.

Desipramine Hydrochloride (Thioridazine has been shown to prolong QTc interval in a dose-related manner; drugs with this potential have been associated with torsade de pointes-type arrhythmias and sudden death; co-administration with other drugs that are known to prolong QTc interval is contraindicated).
No products indexed under this heading.

Dezocine (Thioridazine is capable of potentiating CNS depressants).
No products indexed under this heading.

Diazepam (Thioridazine is capable of potentiating CNS depressants). Products include:
Valium Tablets 2658

Disopyramide Phosphate (Thioridazine has been shown to prolong QTc interval in a dose-related manner; drugs with this potential have been associated with torsade de pointes-type arrhythmias and sudden death; co-administration with other drugs that are known to prolong QTc interval is contraindicated).
No products indexed under this heading.

Dofetilide (Thioridazine has been shown to prolong QTc interval in a dose-related manner; drugs with this potential have been associated with Torsade de pointes-type arrhythmias and sudden death; co-administration with other drugs that are known to prolong QTc interval is contraindicated).
No products indexed under this heading.

Dolasetron Mesylate (Thioridazine has been shown to prolong QTc interval in a dose-related manner; drugs with this potential have been associated with Torsade de pointes-type arrhythmias and sudden death; co-administration with other drugs that are known to prolong QTc interval is contraindicated). Products include:
Anzemet Injection 2701
Anzemet Tablets 2704

Droperidol (Thioridazine has been shown to prolong QTc interval in a dose-related manner; drugs with this potential have been associated with torsade de pointes-type arrhythmias and sudden death; co-administration with other drugs that are known to prolong QTc interval is contraindicated).
No products indexed under this heading.

Enflurane (Thioridazine is capable of potentiating CNS depressants).
No products indexed under this heading.

Epinephrine (Thioridazine causes orthostatic hypotension, especially in female patients; use of epinephrine should be avoided in view of the fact that phenothiazines may induce a reversed epinephrine effect). Products include:
EpiPen 1024

Epinephrine Hydrochloride (Thioridazine causes orthostatic hypotension, especially in female patients; use of epinephrine should be avoided in view of the fact that phenothiazines may induce a reversed epinephrine effect).
No products indexed under this heading.

Erythromycin (Thioridazine has been shown to prolong QTc interval in a dose-related manner; drugs with this potential have been associated with torsade de pointes-type arrhythmias and sudden death; co-administration with other drugs that are known to prolong QTc interval is contraindicated).
No products indexed under this heading.

Erythromycin Estolate (Thioridazine has been shown to prolong QTc interval in a dose-related manner; drugs with this potential have been associated with torsade de pointes-type arrhythmias and sudden death; co-administration with other drugs that are known to prolong QTc interval is contraindicated).
No products indexed under this heading.

Erythromycin Ethylsuccinate (Thioridazine has been shown to prolong QTc interval in a dose-related manner; drugs with this potential have been associated with torsade de pointes-type arrhythmias and sudden death; co-administration with other drugs that are known to prolong QTc interval is contraindicated). Products include:
E.E.S. 433
EryPed 431

Erythromycin Gluceptate (Thioridazine has been shown to prolong QTc interval in a dose-related manner; drugs with this potential have been associated with torsade de pointes-type arrhythmias and sudden death; co-administration with other drugs that are known to prolong QTc interval is contraindicated).
No products indexed under this heading.

Erythromycin Lactobionate (Thioridazine has been shown to prolong QTc interval in a dose-related manner; drugs with this potential have been associated with torsade de pointes-type arrhythmias and sudden death; co-administration with other drugs that are known to prolong QTc interval is contraindicated).
No products indexed under this heading.

Erythromycin Stearate (Thioridazine has been shown to prolong QTc interval in a dose-related manner; drugs with this potential have been associated with torsade de pointes-type arrhythmias and sudden death; co-administration with other drugs that are known to prolong QTc interval is contraindicated).
No products indexed under this heading.

Estazolam (Thioridazine is capable of potentiating CNS depressants).
No products indexed under this heading.

Ethacrynic Acid (Hypokalemia may result from diuretic therapy and this may increase the risk of QT prolongation and arrhythmias; co-administration may increase the risk of serious, potentially fatal, cardiac arrhythmias). Products include:
Edecrin Tablets **698**

Ethanol (Thioridazine is capable of potentiating CNS depressants).
No products indexed under this heading.

Ethchlorvynol (Thioridazine is capable of potentiating CNS depressants).
No products indexed under this heading.

Ethinamate (Thioridazine is capable of potentiating CNS depressants).
No products indexed under this heading.

Ethyl Alcohol (Thioridazine is capable of potentiating CNS depressants).
No products indexed under this heading.

Fentanyl (Thioridazine is capable of potentiating CNS depressants). Products include:
Duragesic Transdermal System **2405**
Ionsys Transdermal System **2410**

Fentanyl Citrate (Thioridazine is capable of potentiating CNS depressants). Products include:
Actiq **959**
Fentora Tablets **968**

Flecainide Acetate (Thioridazine has been shown to prolong QTc interval in a dose-related manner; drugs with this potential have been associated with Torsade de pointes-type arrhythmias and sudden death; co-administration with other drugs that are known to prolong QTc interval is contraindicated).
No products indexed under this heading.

Fluoxetine Hydrochloride (Co-administration with drugs that inhibit CYP450 2D6 isoenzyme will appreciably inhibit metabolism of thioridazine and resulting elevated levels of thioridazine would be expected to augment the prolongation of QTc interval and may increase the risk of serious, potentially fatal, cardiac arrhythmias; concurrent use is contraindicated). Products include:
Prozac Weekly Capsules **1852**
Prozac Pulvules and Liquid **1852**
Symbyax Capsules **1871**

Fluphenazine Decanoate (Thioridazine is capable of potentiating CNS depressants).
No products indexed under this heading.

Fluphenazine Enanthate (Thioridazine is capable of potentiating CNS depressants).
No products indexed under this heading.

Fluphenazine Hydrochloride (Thioridazine is capable of potentiating CNS depressants).
No products indexed under this heading.

Flurazepam Hydrochloride (Thioridazine is capable of potentiating CNS depressants).
No products indexed under this heading.

Fluvoxamine Maleate (Co-administration with drugs that inhibit CYP450 2D6 isoenzyme will appreciably inhibit metabolism of thioridazine and resulting elevated levels of thioridazine would be expected to augment the prolongation of QTc interval and may increase the risk of serious, potentially fatal, cardiac arrhythmias; concurrent use is contraindicated). Products include:
Luvox CR Extended-Release Capsules **1759**

Furosemide (Hypokalemia may result from diuretic therapy and this may increase the risk of QT prolongation and arrhythmias; co-administration may increase the risk of serious, potentially fatal, cardiac arrhythmias). Products include:
Furosemide Tablets **2186**

Gatifloxacin (Thioridazine has been shown to prolong QTc interval in a dose-related manner; drugs with this potential have been associated with torsade de pointes-type arrhythmias and sudden death; co-administration with other drugs that are known to prolong QTc interval is contraindicated).
No products indexed under this heading.

Glutethimide (Thioridazine is capable of potentiating CNS depressants).
No products indexed under this heading.

Halofantrine (Thioridazine has been shown to prolong QTc interval in a dose-related manner; drugs with this potential have been associated with Torsade de pointes-type arrhythmias and sudden death; co-administration with other drugs that are known to prolong QTc interval is contraindicated).
No products indexed under this heading.

Haloperidol (Thioridazine is capable of potentiating CNS depressants).
No products indexed under this heading.

Haloperidol Decanoate (Thioridazine is capable of potentiating CNS depressants).
No products indexed under this heading.

Hydrochlorothiazide (Hypokalemia may result from diuretic therapy and this may increase the risk of QT prolongation and arrhythmias; co-administration may increase the risk of serious, potentially fatal, cardiac arrhythmias). Products include:
Atacand HCT **642**
Avalide Tablets **892**
Avalide Tablets **2713**
Benicar HCT Tablets **1010**
Diovan HCT Tablets **2216**
Dyazide Capsules **1405**
Micardis HCT Tablets **854**
Prinzide Tablets **2092**
Tekturna HCT Tablets **2324**
Teveten HCT Tablets **517**

Hydrocodone Bitartrate (Thioridazine is capable of potentiating CNS depressants). Products include:
Lortab 5/500 Tablets **3143**
Lortab 7.5/500 Tablets **3144**
Lortab 10/500 Tablets **3144**
Vicodin Tablets **529**
Vicodin ES Tablets **530**
Vicodin HP Tablets **531**
Vicoprofen Tablets **533**
Zydone Tablets **1132**

Hydrocodone Polistirex (Thioridazine is capable of potentiating CNS depressants). Products include:
Tussionex Pennkinetic Extended-Release Suspension **3154**

Hydroflumethiazide (Hypokalemia may result from diuretic therapy and this may increase the risk of QT prolongation and arrhythmias; co-administration may increase the risk of serious, potentially fatal, cardiac arrhythmias).
No products indexed under this heading.

Hydromorphone Hydrochloride (Thioridazine is capable of potentiating CNS depressants).
No products indexed under this heading.

Hydroxyzine Hydrochloride (Thioridazine is capable of potentiating CNS depressants).
No products indexed under this heading.

Ibutilide Fumarate (Thioridazine has been shown to prolong QTc interval in a dose-related manner; drugs with this potential have been associated with torsade de pointes-type arrhythmias and sudden death; co-administration with other drugs that are known to prolong QTc interval is contraindicated).
No products indexed under this heading.

Isoflurane (Thioridazine is capable of potentiating CNS depressants).
No products indexed under this heading.

Ketamine Hydrochloride (Thioridazine is capable of potentiating CNS depressants).
No products indexed under this heading.

Levomethadyl Acetate Hydrochloride (Thioridazine has been shown to prolong QTc interval in a dose-related manner; drugs with this potential have been associated with torsade de pointes-type arrhythmias and sudden death; co-administration with other drugs that are known to prolong QTc interval is contraindicated).
No products indexed under this heading.

Levorphanol Tartrate (Thioridazine is capable of potentiating CNS depressants).
No products indexed under this heading.

Lorazepam (Thioridazine is capable of potentiating CNS depressants).
No products indexed under this heading.

Loxapine Hydrochloride (Thioridazine is capable of potentiating CNS depressants).
No products indexed under this heading.

Loxapine Succinate (Thioridazine is capable of potentiating CNS depressants).
No products indexed under this heading.

Mefloquine Hydrochloride (Thioridazine has been shown to prolong QTc interval in a dose-related manner; drugs with this potential have been associated with Torsade de pointes-type arrhythmias and sudden death; co-administration with other drugs that are known to prolong QTc interval is contraindicated).
No products indexed under this heading.

Meperidine Hydrochloride (Thioridazine is capable of potentiating CNS depressants).
No products indexed under this heading.

Mephobarbital (Thioridazine is capable of potentiating CNS depressants).
No products indexed under this heading.

Meprobamate (Thioridazine is capable of potentiating CNS depressants).
No products indexed under this heading.

Mesoridazine Besylate (Thioridazine is capable of potentiating CNS depressants).
No products indexed under this heading.

Methadone Hydrochloride (Thioridazine is capable of potentiating CNS depressants).
No products indexed under this heading.

Methohexital Sodium (Thioridazine is capable of potentiating CNS depressants).
No products indexed under this heading.

Methotrimeprazine (Thioridazine is capable of potentiating CNS depressants).
No products indexed under this heading.

Methoxyflurane (Thioridazine is capable of potentiating CNS depressants).
No products indexed under this heading.

Methyclothiazide (Hypokalemia may result from diuretic therapy and this may increase the risk of QT prolongation and arrhythmias; co-administration may increase the risk of serious, potentially fatal, cardiac arrhythmias).
No products indexed under this heading.

Midazolam Hydrochloride (Thioridazine is capable of potentiating CNS depressants).
No products indexed under this heading.

Molindone Hydrochloride (Thioridazine is capable of potentiating CNS depressants). Products include:
Moban Tablets **1116**

Morphine Sulfate (Thioridazine is capable of potentiating CNS depressants). Products include:
Avinza Capsules **1772**
DepoDur Injection **1095**
MS Contin Tablets **2585**

Moxifloxacin Hydrochloride (Thioridazine has been shown to prolong QTc interval in a dose-related manner; drugs with this potential have been associated with torsade de pointes-type arrhythmias and sudden death; co-administration with other drugs that are known to prolong QTc interval is contraindicated). Products include:
Avelox **2803**
Vigamox Ophthalmic Solution **548**

Olanzapine (Thioridazine is capable of potentiating CNS depressants). Products include:
Symbyax Capsules **1871**
Zyprexa Tablets **1883**
Zyprexa IntraMuscular **1883**
Zyprexa ZYDIS Orally Disintegrating Tablets **1883**

Oxazepam (Thioridazine is capable of potentiating CNS depressants).
No products indexed under this heading.

Oxycodone Hydrochloride (Thioridazine is capable of potentiating CNS depressants). Products include:
OxyContin Tablets 2589
OxyIR Capsules 2593
Percocet Tablets 1127
Percodan Tablets 1130

Paroxetine Hydrochloride (Co-administration with drugs that inhibit CYP450 2D6 isoenzyme will appreciably inhibit metabolism of thioridazine and resulting elevated levels of thioridazine would be expected to augment the prolongation of QTc interval and may increase the risk of serious, potentially fatal, cardiac arrhythmias; concurrent use is contraindicated). Products include:
Paxil 1535
Paxil CR Controlled-Release Tablets 1544

Pentamidine Isethionate (Thioridazine has been shown to prolong QTc interval in a dose-related manner; drugs with this potential have been associated with torsade de pointes-type arrhythmias and sudden death; co-administration with other drugs that are known to prolong QTc interval is contraindicated).
No products indexed under this heading.

Pentobarbital Sodium (Thioridazine is capable of potentiating CNS depressants). Products include:
Nembutal Sodium Solution, USP 2494

Perphenazine (Thioridazine is capable of potentiating CNS depressants).
No products indexed under this heading.

Phenobarbital (Thioridazine is capable of potentiating CNS depressants). Products include:
Donnatal Extentabs 2507

Pimozide (Thioridazine has been shown to prolong QTc interval in a dose-related manner; drugs with this potential have been associated with torsade de pointes-type arrhythmias and sudden death; co-administration with other drugs that are known to prolong QTc interval is contraindicated).
No products indexed under this heading.

Pindolol (Co-administration with drugs that inhibit CYP450 2D6 isoenzyme will appreciably inhibit metabolism of thioridazine and resulting elevated levels of thioridazine would be expected to augment the prolongation of QTc interval and may increase the risk of serious, potentially fatal, cardiac arrhythmias; concurrent use is contraindicated).
No products indexed under this heading.

Polythiazide (Hypokalemia may result from diuretic therapy and this may increase the risk of QT prolongation and arrhythmias; co-administration may increase the risk of serious, potentially fatal, cardiac arrhythmias).
No products indexed under this heading.

Prazepam (Thioridazine is capable of potentiating CNS depressants).
No products indexed under this heading.

Procainamide Hydrochloride (Thioridazine has been shown to prolong QTc interval in a dose-related manner; drugs with this potential have been associated with torsade de pointes-type arrhythmias and sudden death; co-administration with other drugs that are known to prolong QTc interval is contraindicated).
No products indexed under this heading.

Prochlorperazine (Thioridazine is capable of potentiating CNS depressants).
No products indexed under this heading.

Promethazine Hydrochloride (Thioridazine is capable of potentiating CNS depressants).
No products indexed under this heading.

Propofol (Thioridazine is capable of potentiating CNS depressants).
No products indexed under this heading.

Propoxyphene Hydrochloride (Thioridazine is capable of potentiating CNS depressants).
No products indexed under this heading.

Propoxyphene Napsylate (Thioridazine is capable of potentiating CNS depressants).
No products indexed under this heading.

Propranolol Hydrochloride (Co-administration with drugs that inhibit CYP450 2D6 isoenzyme will appreciably inhibit metabolism of thioridazine and resulting elevated levels of thioridazine would be expected to augment the prolongation of QTc interval and may increase the risk of serious, potentially fatal, cardiac arrhythmias; concurrent use is contraindicated). Products include:
InnoPran XL Extended Release Capsules 1484

Quazepam (Thioridazine is capable of potentiating CNS depressants).
No products indexed under this heading.

Quetiapine Fumarate (Thioridazine is capable of potentiating CNS depressants).
No products indexed under this heading.

Quinidine (Thioridazine has been shown to prolong QTc interval in a dose-related manner; drugs with this potential have been associated with torsade de pointes-type arrhythmias and sudden death; co-administration with other drugs that are known to prolong QTc interval is contraindicated).
No products indexed under this heading.

Quinidine Gluconate (Thioridazine has been shown to prolong QTc interval in a dose-related manner; drugs with this potential have been associated with torsade de pointes-type arrhythmias and sudden death; co-administration with other drugs that are known to prolong QTc interval is contraindicated).
No products indexed under this heading.

Quinidine Hydrochloride (Thioridazine has been shown to prolong QTc interval in a dose-related manner; drugs with this potential have been associated with torsade de pointes-type arrhythmias and sudden death; co-administration with other drugs that are known to prolong QTc interval is contraindicated).
No products indexed under this heading.

Quinidine Polygalacturonate (Thioridazine has been shown to prolong QTc interval in a dose-related manner; drugs with this potential have been associated with torsade de pointes-type arrhythmias and sudden death; co-administration with other drugs that are known to prolong QTc interval is contraindicated).
No products indexed under this heading.

Quinidine Sulfate (Thioridazine has been shown to prolong QTc interval in a dose-related manner; drugs with this potential have been associated with torsade de pointes-type arrhythmias and sudden death; co-administration with other drugs that are known to prolong QTc interval is contraindicated).
No products indexed under this heading.

Remifentanil Hydrochloride (Thioridazine is capable of potentiating CNS depressants).
No products indexed under this heading.

Risperidone (Thioridazine is capable of potentiating CNS depressants). Products include:
Risperdal Consta Long-Acting Injection 1753

Secobarbital Sodium (Thioridazine is capable of potentiating CNS depressants).
No products indexed under this heading.

Sevoflurane (Thioridazine is capable of potentiating CNS depressants). Products include:
Ultane Liquid for Inhalation 524

Sotalol Hydrochloride (Thioridazine has been shown to prolong QTc interval in a dose-related manner; drugs with this potential have been associated with torsade de pointes-type arrhythmias and sudden death; co-administration with other drugs that are known to prolong QTc interval is contraindicated).
No products indexed under this heading.

Sparfloxacin (Thioridazine has been shown to prolong QTc interval in a dose-related manner; drugs with this potential have been associated with torsade de pointes-type arrhythmias and sudden death; co-administration with other drugs that are known to prolong QTc interval is contraindicated).
No products indexed under this heading.

Sufentanil Citrate (Thioridazine is capable of potentiating CNS depressants).
No products indexed under this heading.

Tacrolimus (Thioridazine has been shown to prolong QTc interval in a dose-related manner; drugs with this potential have been associated with torsade de pointes-type arrhythmias and sudden death; co-administration with other drugs that are known to prolong QTc interval is contraindicated). Products include:
Prograf Capsules and Injection 622
Protopic Ointment 628

Temazepam (Thioridazine is capable of potentiating CNS depressants).
No products indexed under this heading.

Thiamylal Sodium (Thioridazine is capable of potentiating CNS depressants).
No products indexed under this heading.

Thiothixene (Thioridazine is capable of potentiating CNS depressants). Products include:
Thiothixene Capsules 2197

Torsemide (Hypokalemia may result from diuretic therapy and this may increase the risk of QT prolongation and arrhythmias; co-administration may increase the risk of serious, potentially fatal, cardiac arrhythmias). Products include:
Demadex Injection 2630
Demadex Tablets 2630

Triazolam (Thioridazine is capable of potentiating CNS depressants).
No products indexed under this heading.

Trifluoperazine Hydrochloride (Thioridazine is capable of potentiating CNS depressants).
No products indexed under this heading.

Zaleplon (Thioridazine is capable of potentiating CNS depressants).
No products indexed under this heading.

Ziprasidone Hydrochloride (Thioridazine has been shown to prolong QTc interval in a dose-related manner; drugs with this potential have been associated with torsade de pointes-type arrhythmias and sudden death; co-administration with other drugs that are known to prolong QTc interval is contraindicated). Products include:
Geodon Capsules 2520

Ziprasidone Mesylate (Thioridazine has been shown to prolong QTc interval in a dose-related manner; drugs with this potential have been associated with torsade de pointes-type arrhythmias and sudden death; co-administration with other drugs that are known to prolong QTc interval is contraindicated). Products include:
Geodon for Injection 2520

Zolpidem Tartrate (Thioridazine is capable of potentiating CNS depressants). Products include:
Ambien Tablets 2692
Ambien CR Tablets 2696

Food Interactions

Alcohol (Thioridazine is capable of potentiating CNS depressants).

THIOTHIXENE CAPSULES

(Thiothixene) 2197

May interact with belladona products, central nervous system depressants, and certain other agents. Compounds in these categories include:

Alfentanil Hydrochloride (As with the case of other CNS-acting drugs, patients receiving thiothixene should be cautioned about the possible additive effects (which may include hypotension) with CNS depressants).
No products indexed under this heading.

Alprazolam (As with the case of other CNS-acting drugs, patients receiving thiothixene should be cautioned about the possible additive effects (which may include hypotension) with CNS depressants).
No products indexed under this heading.

Aprobarbital (As with the case of other CNS-acting drugs, patients receiving thiothixene should be cautioned about the possible additive effects (which may include hypotension) with CNS depressants).
No products indexed under this heading.

Atropine Sulfate (Through exhibiting rather weak anticholinergic properties, thiothixene should be used with caution in patients who are receiving atropine or related drugs). Products include:
Donnatal Extentabs 2507

Belladonna Alkaloids (Through exhibiting rather weak anticholinergic properties, thiothixene should be used with caution in patients who are receiving atropine or related drugs). Products include:
Hyland's Teething Tablets .... ▣ 621

Buprenorphine Hydrochloride (As with the case of other CNS-acting drugs, patients receiving thiothixene should be cautioned about the possible additive effects (which may include hypotension) with CNS depressants). Products include:
Suboxone Tablets 2601
Subutex Tablets 2601

Buspirone Hydrochloride (As with the case of other CNS-acting drugs, patients receiving thiothixene should be cautioned about the possible additive effects (which may include hypotension) with CNS depressants).
No products indexed under this heading.

Butabarbital (As with the case of other CNS-acting drugs, patients receiving thiothixene should be cautioned about the possible additive effects (which may include hypotension) with CNS depressants).
No products indexed under this heading.

Butalbital (As with the case of other CNS-acting drugs, patients receiving thiothixene should be cautioned about the possible additive effects (which may include hypotension) with CNS depressants).
No products indexed under this heading.

Chlordiazepoxide (As with the case of other CNS-acting drugs, patients receiving thiothixene should be cautioned about the possible additive effects (which may include hypotension) with CNS depressants).
No products indexed under this heading.

Chlordiazepoxide Hydrochloride (As with the case of other CNS-acting drugs, patients receiving thiothixene should be cautioned about the possible additive effects (which may include hypotension) with CNS depressants).
No products indexed under this heading.

Chlorpromazine (As with the case of other CNS-acting drugs, patients receiving thiothixene should be cautioned about the possible additive effects (which may include hypotension) with CNS depressants).
No products indexed under this heading.

Chlorpromazine Hydrochloride (As with the case of other CNS-acting drugs, patients receiving thiothixene should be cautioned about the possible additive effects (which may include hypotension) with CNS depressants).
No products indexed under this heading.

Chlorprothixene (As with the case of other CNS-acting drugs, patients receiving thiothixene should be cautioned about the possible additive effects (which may include hypotension) with CNS depressants).
No products indexed under this heading.

Chlorprothixene Hydrochloride (As with the case of other CNS-acting drugs, patients receiving thiothixene should be cautioned about the possible additive effects (which may include hypotension) with CNS depressants).
No products indexed under this heading.

Chlorprothixene Lactate (As with the case of other CNS-acting drugs, patients receiving thiothixene should be cautioned about the possible additive effects (which may include hypotension) with CNS depressants).
No products indexed under this heading.

Clorazepate Dipotassium (As with the case of other CNS-acting drugs, patients receiving thiothixene should be cautioned about the possible additive effects (which may include hypotension) with CNS depressants).
No products indexed under this heading.

Clozapine (As with the case of other CNS-acting drugs, patients receiving thiothixene should be cautioned about the possible additive effects (which may include hypotension) with CNS depressants).
No products indexed under this heading.

Codeine Phosphate (As with the case of other CNS-acting drugs, patients receiving thiothixene should be cautioned about the possible additive effects (which may include hypotension) with CNS depressants). Products include:
Tylenol with Codeine Tablets 2427

Desflurane (As with the case of other CNS-acting drugs, patients receiving thiothixene should be cautioned about the possible additive effects (which may include hypotension) with CNS depressants).
No products indexed under this heading.

Dezocine (As with the case of other CNS-acting drugs, patients receiving thiothixene should be cautioned about the possible additive effects (which may include hypotension) with CNS depressants).
No products indexed under this heading.

Diazepam (As with the case of other CNS-acting drugs, patients receiving thiothixene should be cautioned about the possible additive effects (which may include hypotension) with CNS depressants). Products include:
Valium Tablets 2658

Droperidol (As with the case of other CNS-acting drugs, patients receiving thiothixene should be cautioned about the possible additive effects (which may include hypotension) with CNS depressants).
No products indexed under this heading.

Enflurane (As with the case of other CNS-acting drugs, patients receiving thiothixene should be cautioned about the possible additive effects (which may include hypotension) with CNS depressants).
No products indexed under this heading.

Estazolam (As with the case of other CNS-acting drugs, patients receiving thiothixene should be cautioned about the possible additive effects (which may include hypotension) with CNS depressants).
No products indexed under this heading.

Ethanol (As with the case of other CNS-acting drugs, patients receiving thiothixene should be cautioned about the possible additive effects (which may include hypotension) with alcohol).
No products indexed under this heading.

Ethchlorvynol (As with the case of other CNS-acting drugs, patients receiving thiothixene should be cautioned about the possible additive effects (which may include hypotension) with CNS depressants).
No products indexed under this heading.

Ethinamate (As with the case of other CNS-acting drugs, patients receiving thiothixene should be cautioned about the possible additive effects (which may include hypotension) with CNS depressants).
No products indexed under this heading.

Ethyl Alcohol (As with the case of other CNS-acting drugs, patients receiving thiothixene should be cautioned about the possible additive effects (which may include hypotension) with alcohol).
No products indexed under this heading.

Fentanyl (As with the case of other CNS-acting drugs, patients receiving thiothixene should be cautioned about the possible additive effects (which may include hypotension) with CNS depressants). Products include:
Duragesic Transdermal System 2405
Ionsys Transdermal System 2410

Fentanyl Citrate (As with the case of other CNS-acting drugs, patients receiving thiothixene should be cautioned about the possible additive effects (which may include hypotension) with CNS depressants). Products include:
Actiq 959
Fentora Tablets 968

Fluphenazine Decanoate (As with the case of other CNS-acting drugs, patients receiving thiothixene should be cautioned about the possible additive effects (which may include hypotension) with CNS depressants).
No products indexed under this heading.

Fluphenazine Enanthate (As with the case of other CNS-acting drugs, patients receiving thiothixene should be cautioned about the possible additive effects (which may include hypotension) with CNS depressants).
No products indexed under this heading.

Fluphenazine Hydrochloride (As with the case of other CNS-acting drugs, patients receiving thiothixene should be cautioned about the possible additive effects (which may include hypotension) with CNS depressants).
No products indexed under this heading.

Flurazepam Hydrochloride (As with the case of other CNS-acting drugs, patients receiving thiothixene should be cautioned about the possible additive effects (which may include hypotension) with CNS depressants).
No products indexed under this heading.

Glutethimide (As with the case of other CNS-acting drugs, patients receiving thiothixene should be cautioned about the possible additive effects (which may include hypotension) with CNS depressants).
No products indexed under this heading.

Haloperidol (As with the case of other CNS-acting drugs, patients receiving thiothixene should be cautioned about the possible additive effects (which may include hypotension) with CNS depressants).
No products indexed under this heading.

Haloperidol Decanoate (As with the case of other CNS-acting drugs, patients receiving thiothixene should be cautioned about the possible additive effects (which may include hypotension) with CNS depressants).
No products indexed under this heading.

Hydrocodone Bitartrate (As with the case of other CNS-acting drugs, patients receiving thiothixene should be cautioned about the possible additive effects (which may include hypotension) with CNS depressants). Products include:
Lortab 5/500 Tablets 3143
Lortab 7.5/500 Tablets 3144
Lortab 10/500 Tablets 3144
Vicodin Tablets 529
Vicodin ES Tablets 530
Vicodin HP Tablets 531
Vicoprofen Tablets 533
Zydone Tablets 1132

Hydrocodone Polistirex (As with the case of other CNS-acting drugs, patients receiving thiothixene should be cautioned about the possible additive effects (which may include hypotension) with CNS depressants). Products include:
Tussionex Pennkinetic
Extended-Release Suspension 3154

Hydromorphone Hydrochloride (As with the case of other CNS-acting drugs, patients receiving thiothixene should be cautioned about the possible additive effects (which may include hypotension) with CNS depressants).
No products indexed under this heading.

IMPORTANT NOTE: Always consult each drug listing in the patient's regimen for possible interactions.

Hydroxyzine Hydrochloride (As with the case of other CNS-acting drugs, patients receiving thiothixene should be cautioned about the possible additive effects (which may include hypotension) with CNS depressants).
No products indexed under this heading.

Hyoscyamine (Through exhibiting rather weak anticholinergic properties, thiothixene should be used with caution in patients who are receiving atropine or related drugs).
No products indexed under this heading.

Hyoscyamine Sulfate (Through exhibiting rather weak anticholinergic properties, thiothixene should be used with caution in patients who are receiving atropine or related drugs).
Products include:
Donnatal Extentabs 2507

Isoflurane (As with the case of other CNS-acting drugs, patients receiving thiothixene should be cautioned about the possible additive effects (which may include hypotension) with CNS depressants).
No products indexed under this heading.

Ketamine Hydrochloride (As with the case of other CNS-acting drugs, patients receiving thiothixene should be cautioned about the possible additive effects (which may include hypotension) with CNS depressants).
No products indexed under this heading.

Levomethadyl Acetate Hydrochloride (As with the case of other CNS-acting drugs, patients receiving thiothixene should be cautioned about the possible additive effects (which may include hypotension) with CNS depressants).
No products indexed under this heading.

Levorphanol Tartrate (As with the case of other CNS-acting drugs, patients receiving thiothixene should be cautioned about the possible additive effects (which may include hypotension) with CNS depressants).
No products indexed under this heading.

Lorazepam (As with the case of other CNS-acting drugs, patients receiving thiothixene should be cautioned about the possible additive effects (which may include hypotension) with CNS depressants).
No products indexed under this heading.

Loxapine Hydrochloride (As with the case of other CNS-acting drugs, patients receiving thiothixene should be cautioned about the possible additive effects (which may include hypotension) with CNS depressants).
No products indexed under this heading.

Loxapine Succinate (As with the case of other CNS-acting drugs, patients receiving thiothixene should be cautioned about the possible additive effects (which may include hypotension) with CNS depressants).
No products indexed under this heading.

Meperidine Hydrochloride (As with the case of other CNS-acting drugs, patients receiving thiothixene should be cautioned about the possible additive effects (which may include hypotension) with CNS depressants).
No products indexed under this heading.

Mephobarbital (As with the case of other CNS-acting drugs, patients receiving thiothixene should be cautioned about the possible additive effects (which may include hypotension) with CNS depressants).
No products indexed under this heading.

Meprobamate (As with the case of other CNS-acting drugs, patients receiving thiothixene should be cautioned about the possible additive effects (which may include hypotension) with CNS depressants).
No products indexed under this heading.

Mesoridazine Besylate (As with the case of other CNS-acting drugs, patients receiving thiothixene should be cautioned about the possible additive effects (which may include hypotension) with CNS depressants).
No products indexed under this heading.

Methadone Hydrochloride (As with the case of other CNS-acting drugs, patients receiving thiothixene should be cautioned about the possible additive effects (which may include hypotension) with CNS depressants).
No products indexed under this heading.

Methohexital Sodium (As with the case of other CNS-acting drugs, patients receiving thiothixene should be cautioned about the possible additive effects (which may include hypotension) with CNS depressants).
No products indexed under this heading.

Methotrimeprazine (As with the case of other CNS-acting drugs, patients receiving thiothixene should be cautioned about the possible additive effects (which may include hypotension) with CNS depressants).
No products indexed under this heading.

Methoxyflurane (As with the case of other CNS-acting drugs, patients receiving thiothixene should be cautioned about the possible additive effects (which may include hypotension) with CNS depressants).
No products indexed under this heading.

Midazolam Hydrochloride (As with the case of other CNS-acting drugs, patients receiving thiothixene should be cautioned about the possible additive effects (which may include hypotension) with CNS depressants).
No products indexed under this heading.

Molindone Hydrochloride (As with the case of other CNS-acting drugs, patients receiving thiothixene should be cautioned about the possible additive effects (which may include hypotension) with CNS depressants).
Products include:
Moban Tablets 1116

Morphine Sulfate (As with the case of other CNS-acting drugs, patients receiving thiothixene should be cautioned about the possible additive effects (which may include hypotension) with CNS depressants).
Products include:
Avinza Capsules 1772
DepoDur Injection 1095
MS Contin Tablets 2585

Olanzapine (As with the case of other CNS-acting drugs, patients receiving thiothixene should be cautioned about the possible additive effects (which may include hypotension) with CNS depressants).
Products include:
Symbyax Capsules 1871
Zyprexa Tablets 1883
Zyprexa IntraMuscular 1883
Zyprexa ZYDIS Orally Disintegrating Tablets 1883

Oxazepam (As with the case of other CNS-acting drugs, patients receiving thiothixene should be cautioned about the possible additive effects (which may include hypotension) with CNS depressants).
No products indexed under this heading.

Oxycodone Hydrochloride (As with the case of other CNS-acting drugs, patients receiving thiothixene should be cautioned about the possible additive effects (which may include hypotension) with CNS depressants). Products include:
OxyContin Tablets 2589
OxyIR Capsules 2593
Percocet Tablets 1127
Percodan Tablets 1130

Pentobarbital Sodium (As with the case of other CNS-acting drugs, patients receiving thiothixene should be cautioned about the possible additive effects (which may include hypotension) with CNS depressants).
Products include:
Nembutal Sodium Solution, USP 2494

Perphenazine (As with the case of other CNS-acting drugs, patients receiving thiothixene should be cautioned about the possible additive effects (which may include hypotension) with CNS depressants).
No products indexed under this heading.

Phenobarbital (As with the case of other CNS-acting drugs, patients receiving thiothixene should be cautioned about the possible additive effects (which may include hypotension) with CNS depressants).
Products include:
Donnatal Extentabs 2507

Prazepam (As with the case of other CNS-acting drugs, patients receiving thiothixene should be cautioned about the possible additive effects (which may include hypotension) with CNS depressants).
No products indexed under this heading.

Prochlorperazine (As with the case of other CNS-acting drugs, patients receiving thiothixene should be cautioned about the possible additive effects (which may include hypotension) with CNS depressants).
No products indexed under this heading.

Promethazine Hydrochloride (As with the case of other CNS-acting drugs, patients receiving thiothixene should be cautioned about the possible additive effects (which may include hypotension) with CNS depressants).
No products indexed under this heading.

Propofol (As with the case of other CNS-acting drugs, patients receiving thiothixene should be cautioned about the possible additive effects (which may include hypotension) with CNS depressants).
No products indexed under this heading.

Propoxyphene Hydrochloride (As with the case of other CNS-acting drugs, patients receiving thiothixene should be cautioned about the possible additive effects (which may include hypotension) with CNS depressants).
No products indexed under this heading.

Propoxyphene Napsylate (As with the case of other CNS-acting drugs, patients receiving thiothixene should be cautioned about the possible additive effects (which may include hypotension) with CNS depressants).
No products indexed under this heading.

Quazepam (As with the case of other CNS-acting drugs, patients receiving thiothixene should be cautioned about the possible additive effects (which may include hypotension) with CNS depressants).
No products indexed under this heading.

Quetiapine Fumarate (As with the case of other CNS-acting drugs, patients receiving thiothixene should be cautioned about the possible additive effects (which may include hypotension) with CNS depressants).
No products indexed under this heading.

Remifentanil Hydrochloride (As with the case of other CNS-acting drugs, patients receiving thiothixene should be cautioned about the possible additive effects (which may include hypotension) with CNS depressants).
No products indexed under this heading.

Risperidone (As with the case of other CNS-acting drugs, patients receiving thiothixene should be cautioned about the possible additive effects (which may include hypotension) with CNS depressants).
Products include:
Risperdal Consta Long-Acting Injection 1753

Scopolamine (Through exhibiting rather weak anticholinergic properties, thiothixene should be used with caution in patients who are receiving atropine or related drugs). Products include:
Transderm Scōp Transdermal Therapeutic System 2206

Scopolamine Hydrobromide (Through exhibiting rather weak anticholinergic properties, thiothixene should be used with caution in patients who are receiving atropine or related drugs). Products include:
Donnatal Extentabs 2507

Secobarbital Sodium (As with the case of other CNS-acting drugs, patients receiving thiothixene should be cautioned about the possible additive effects (which may include hypotension) with CNS depressants).
No products indexed under this heading.

Sevoflurane (As with the case of other CNS-acting drugs, patients receiving thiothixene should be cautioned about the possible additive

effects (which may include hypotension) with CNS depressants). Products include:

Ultane Liquid for Inhalation 524

Sodium Oxybate (As with the case of other CNS-acting drugs, patients receiving thiothixene should be cautioned about the possible additive effects (which may include hypotension) with CNS depressants). Products include:

Xyrem Oral Solution 1766

Sufentanil Citrate (As with the case of other CNS-acting drugs, patients receiving thiothixene should be cautioned about the possible additive effects (which may include hypotension) with CNS depressants).

No products indexed under this heading.

Temazepam (As with the case of other CNS-acting drugs, patients receiving thiothixene should be cautioned about the possible additive effects (which may include hypotension) with CNS depressants).

No products indexed under this heading.

Thiamylal Sodium (As with the case of other CNS-acting drugs, patients receiving thiothixene should be cautioned about the possible additive effects (which may include hypotension) with CNS depressants).

No products indexed under this heading.

Thioridazine Hydrochloride (As with the case of other CNS-acting drugs, patients receiving thiothixene should be cautioned about the possible additive effects (which may include hypotension) with CNS depressants). Products include:

Thioridazine Hydrochloride Tablets 2195

Triazolam (As with the case of other CNS-acting drugs, patients receiving thiothixene should be cautioned about the possible additive effects (which may include hypotension) with CNS depressants).

No products indexed under this heading.

Trifluoperazine Hydrochloride (As with the case of other CNS-acting drugs, patients receiving thiothixene should be cautioned about the possible additive effects (which may include hypotension) with CNS depressants).

No products indexed under this heading.

Zaleplon (As with the case of other CNS-acting drugs, patients receiving thiothixene should be cautioned about the possible additive effects (which may include hypotension) with CNS depressants).

No products indexed under this heading.

Ziprasidone Hydrochloride (As with the case of other CNS-acting drugs, patients receiving thiothixene should be cautioned about the possible additive effects (which may include hypotension) with CNS depressants). Products include:

Geodon Capsules 2520

Zolpidem Tartrate (As with the case of other CNS-acting drugs, patients receiving thiothixene should be cautioned about the possible additive effects (which may include hypotension) with CNS depressants). Products include:

Ambien Tablets 2692

Ambien CR Tablets 2696

Food Interactions

Alcohol (As with the case of other CNS-acting drugs, patients receiving thiothixene should be cautioned about the possible additive effects (which may include hypotension) with alcohol).

THYROGEN FOR INJECTION

(Thyrotropin alfa) 1244

None cited in PDR database.

TICE BCG

(BCG, Live (Intravesical)) 2936

May interact with aminoglycosides, azole antifungals, bacteriostatic antibiotics, beta-lactams antibiotics, corticosteroids, cytotoxic drugs, doxycycline, erythromycin, fluoroquinolone antibiotics, immunosuppressive agents, macrolide antibiotics, penicillins, antituberculosis drugs, and tetracyclines. Compounds in these categories include:

Alatrofloxacin Mesylate (Antimicrobial therapy for other infections may interfere with the effectiveness of BCG, live).

No products indexed under this heading.

Amikacin Sulfate (Antimicrobial therapy for other infections may interfere with the effectiveness of BCG, live).

No products indexed under this heading.

5-Amino-Salicylic Acid (Antimicrobial therapy for other infections may interfere with the effectiveness of BCG, live).

No products indexed under this heading.

Aminosalicylic Acid (Antituberculosis drugs (e.g., isoniazid) should not be used to prevent or treat the local, irritative toxicities of BCG, live). Products include:

Paser Granules 1747

p-Aminosalicylic Acid (Antituberculosis drugs (e.g., isoniazid) should not be used to prevent or treat the local, irritative toxicities of BCG, live).

No products indexed under this heading.

Amoxicillin (Antimicrobial therapy for other infections may interfere with the effectiveness of BCG, live). Products include:

Amoxil Capsules 1305

Amoxil Chewable Tablets 1305

Amoxil Pediatric Drops for Oral Suspension 1305

Amoxil Powder for Oral Suspension 1305

Amoxil Tablets 1305

Augmentin 1323

Augmentin Tablets 1327

Augmentin XR Extended Release Tablets 1333

Augmentin ES-600 Powder for Oral Suspension 1329

Moxatag Tablets 2165

Amoxicillin Trihydrate (Antimicrobial therapy for other infections may interfere with the effectiveness of BCG, live).

No products indexed under this heading.

Ampicillin (Antimicrobial therapy for other infections may interfere with the effectiveness of BCG, live).

No products indexed under this heading.

Ampicillin Sodium (Antimicrobial therapy for other infections may interfere with the effectiveness of BCG, live).

No products indexed under this heading.

Ampicillin Trihydrate (Antimicrobial therapy for other infections may interfere with the effectiveness of BCG, live).

No products indexed under this heading.

Azathioprine (BCG, live should not be used in immunosuppressed patients or persons with congenital or acquired immune deficiencies, whether due to concurrent disease (e.g., AIDS, leukemia, lymphoma), cancer therapy (e.g., cytotoxic drugs, radiation), or immunosuppressive therapy (e.g., corticosteroids)).

No products indexed under this heading.

Azithromycin Dihydrate (Antimicrobial therapy for other infections may interfere with the effectiveness of BCG, live).

No products indexed under this heading.

Azlocillin Sodium (Antimicrobial therapy for other infections may interfere with the effectiveness of BCG, live).

No products indexed under this heading.

Aztreonam (Antimicrobial therapy for other infections may interfere with the effectiveness of BCG, live).

No products indexed under this heading.

Bacampicillin Hydrochloride (Antimicrobial therapy for other infections may interfere with the effectiveness of BCG, live).

No products indexed under this heading.

Basiliximab (BCG, live should not be used in immunosuppressed patients or persons with congenital or acquired immune deficiencies, whether due to concurrent disease (e.g., AIDS, leukemia, lymphoma), cancer therapy (e.g., cytotoxic drugs, radiation), or immunosuppressive therapy (e.g., corticosteroids)). Products include:

Simulect for Injection 2306

Betamethasone Acetate (BCG, live should not be used in immunosuppressed patients or persons with congenital or acquired immune deficiencies, whether due to concurrent disease (e.g., AIDS, leukemia, lymphoma), cancer therapy (e.g., cytotoxic drugs, radiation), or immunosuppressive therapy (e.g., corticosteroids)).

No products indexed under this heading.

Betamethasone Sodium Phosphate (BCG, live should not be used in immunosuppressed patients or persons with congenital or acquired immune deficiencies, whether due to concurrent disease (e.g., AIDS, leukemia, lymphoma), cancer therapy (e.g., cytotoxic drugs, radiation), or immunosuppressive therapy (e.g., corticosteroids)).

No products indexed under this heading.

Bleomycin Sulfate (BCG, live should not be used in immunosuppressed patients or persons with congenital or acquired immune deficiencies, whether due to concurrent disease (e.g., AIDS, leukemia, lymphoma), cancer therapy (e.g., cytotoxic drugs, radiation), or immunosuppressive therapy (e.g., corticosteroids)).

No products indexed under this heading.

Budesonide (BCG, live should not be used in immunosuppressed patients or persons with congenital or acquired immune deficiencies, whether due to concurrent disease (e.g., AIDS, leukemia, lymphoma), cancer therapy (e.g., cytotoxic drugs, radiation), or immunosuppressive therapy (e.g., corticosteroids)). Products include:

Pulmicort Flexhaler 654

Symbicort 80/4.5 Inhalation Aerosol 659

Symbicort 160/4.5 Inhalation Aerosol 659

Carbenicillin Disodium (Antimicrobial therapy for other infections may interfere with the effectiveness of BCG, live).

No products indexed under this heading.

Carbenicillin Indanyl Sodium (Antimicrobial therapy for other infections may interfere with the effectiveness of BCG, live).

No products indexed under this heading.

Cefaclor (Antimicrobial therapy for other infections may interfere with the effectiveness of BCG, live).

No products indexed under this heading.

Cefadroxil (Antimicrobial therapy for other infections may interfere with the effectiveness of BCG, live).

No products indexed under this heading.

Cefamandole Nafate (Antimicrobial therapy for other infections may interfere with the effectiveness of BCG, live).

No products indexed under this heading.

Cefazolin Sodium (Antimicrobial therapy for other infections may interfere with the effectiveness of BCG, live).

No products indexed under this heading.

Cefixime (Antimicrobial therapy for other infections may interfere with the effectiveness of BCG, live). Products include:

Suprax for Oral Suspension 1891

Suprax Tablets 1891

Cefmetazole Sodium (Antimicrobial therapy for other infections may interfere with the effectiveness of BCG, live).

No products indexed under this heading.

Cefonicid Sodium (Antimicrobial therapy for other infections may interfere with the effectiveness of BCG, live).

No products indexed under this heading.

Cefoperazone Sodium (Antimicrobial therapy for other infections may interfere with the effectiveness of BCG, live).

No products indexed under this heading.

Ceforanide (Antimicrobial therapy for other infections may interfere with the effectiveness of BCG, live).
No products indexed under this heading.

Cefotaxime Sodium (Antimicrobial therapy for other infections may interfere with the effectiveness of BCG, live).
No products indexed under this heading.

Cefotetan (Antimicrobial therapy for other infections may interfere with the effectiveness of BCG, live).
No products indexed under this heading.

Cefoxitin Sodium (Antimicrobial therapy for other infections may interfere with the effectiveness of BCG, live).
No products indexed under this heading.

Cefpodoxime Proxetil (Antimicrobial therapy for other infections may interfere with the effectiveness of BCG, live).
No products indexed under this heading.

Cefprozil (Antimicrobial therapy for other infections may interfere with the effectiveness of BCG, live).
No products indexed under this heading.

Ceftazidime (Antimicrobial therapy for other infections may interfere with the effectiveness of BCG, live). Products include:
Fortaz 1450

Ceftizoxime Sodium (Antimicrobial therapy for other infections may interfere with the effectiveness of BCG, live).
No products indexed under this heading.

Ceftriaxone Sodium (Antimicrobial therapy for other infections may interfere with the effectiveness of BCG, live). Products include:
Rocephin Injectable Vials, ADD-Vantage, Galaxy, Bulk 2642

Cefuroxime Axetil (Antimicrobial therapy for other infections may interfere with the effectiveness of BCG, live). Products include:
Ceftin 1380

Cefuroxime Sodium (Antimicrobial therapy for other infections may interfere with the effectiveness of BCG, live).
No products indexed under this heading.

Cephalexin (Antimicrobial therapy for other infections may interfere with the effectiveness of BCG, live).
No products indexed under this heading.

Cephalothin Sodium (Antimicrobial therapy for other infections may interfere with the effectiveness of BCG, live).
No products indexed under this heading.

Cephapirin Sodium (Antimicrobial therapy for other infections may interfere with the effectiveness of BCG, live).
No products indexed under this heading.

Cephradine (Antimicrobial therapy for other infections may interfere with the effectiveness of BCG, live).
No products indexed under this heading.

Chloramphenicol (Antimicrobial therapy for other infections may interfere with the effectiveness of BCG, live).
No products indexed under this heading.

Chloramphenicol Palmitate (Antimicrobial therapy for other infections may interfere with the effectiveness of BCG, live).
No products indexed under this heading.

Chloramphenicol Sodium Succinate (Antimicrobial therapy for other infections may interfere with the effectiveness of BCG, live).
No products indexed under this heading.

Ciclesonide (BCG, live should not be used in immunosuppressed patients or persons with congenital or acquired immune deficiencies, whether due to concurrent disease (e.g., AIDS, leukemia, lymphoma), cancer therapy (e.g., cytotoxic drugs, radiation), or immunosuppressive therapy (e.g., corticosteroids)). Products include:
Alvesco Inhalation Aerosol 2985
Omnaris Nasal Spray 2998

Cilastatin Sodium (Antimicrobial therapy for other infections may interfere with the effectiveness of BCG, live). Products include:
Primaxin I.M. 2080
Primaxin I.V. 2083

Ciprofloxacin (Antimicrobial therapy for other infections may interfere with the effectiveness of BCG, live). Products include:
Cipro I.V. 2817
Cipro Oral Suspension 2810
Cipro XR Tablets 2823
Ciprodex Otic Suspension 541

Ciprofloxacin Hydrochloride (Antimicrobial therapy for other infections may interfere with the effectiveness of BCG, live). Products include:
Cipro Tablets 2810

Clarithromycin (Antimicrobial therapy for other infections may interfere with the effectiveness of BCG, live). Products include:
Biaxin/Biaxin XL 411

Clotrimazole (Antimicrobial therapy for other infections may interfere with the effectiveness of BCG, live). Products include:
Lotrisone 2881

Cortisone Acetate (BCG, live should not be used in immunosuppressed patients or persons with congenital or acquired immune deficiencies, whether due to concurrent disease (e.g., AIDS, leukemia, lymphoma), cancer therapy (e.g., cytotoxic drugs, radiation), or immunosuppressive therapy (e.g., corticosteroids)).
No products indexed under this heading.

Cyclophosphamide (BCG, live should not be used in immunosuppressed patients or persons with congenital or acquired immune deficiencies, whether due to concurrent disease (e.g., AIDS, leukemia, lymphoma), cancer therapy (e.g., cytotoxic drugs, radiation), or immunosuppressive therapy (e.g., corticosteroids)).
No products indexed under this heading.

Cycloserine (Antituberculosis drugs (e.g., isoniazid) should not be used to prevent or treat the local, irritative toxicities of BCG, live). Products include:
Seromycin Capsules 1864

Cyclosporine (BCG, live should not be used in immunosuppressed patients or persons with congenital or acquired immune deficiencies, whether due to concurrent disease (e.g., AIDS, leukemia, lymphoma), cancer therapy (e.g., cytotoxic drugs, radiation), or immunosuppressive therapy (e.g., corticosteroids)). Products include:
Gengraf Capsules 435
Neoral Oral Solution 2280
Neoral Soft Gelatin Capsules 2280
Restasis Ophthalmic Emulsion 557
Sandimmune 2296

Daunorubicin Hydrochloride (BCG, live should not be used in immunosuppressed patients or persons with congenital or acquired immune deficiencies, whether due to concurrent disease (e.g., AIDS, leukemia, lymphoma), cancer therapy (e.g., cytotoxic drugs, radiation), or immunosuppressive therapy (e.g., corticosteroids)).
No products indexed under this heading.

Demeclocycline Hydrochloride (Antimicrobial therapy for other infections may interfere with the effectiveness of BCG, live).
No products indexed under this heading.

Dexamethasone (BCG, live should not be used in immunosuppressed patients or persons with congenital or acquired immune deficiencies, whether due to concurrent disease (e.g., AIDS, leukemia, lymphoma), cancer therapy (e.g., cytotoxic drugs, radiation), or immunosuppressive therapy (e.g., corticosteroids)). Products include:
Ciprodex Otic Suspension 541

Dexamethasone Acetate (BCG, live should not be used in immunosuppressed patients or persons with congenital or acquired immune deficiencies, whether due to concurrent disease (e.g., AIDS, leukemia, lymphoma), cancer therapy (e.g., cytotoxic drugs, radiation), or immunosuppressive therapy (e.g., corticosteroids)).
No products indexed under this heading.

Dexamethasone Sodium Phosphate (BCG, live should not be used in immunosuppressed patients or persons with congenital or acquired immune deficiencies, whether due to concurrent disease (e.g., AIDS, leukemia, lymphoma), cancer therapy (e.g., cytotoxic drugs, radiation), or immunosuppressive therapy (e.g., corticosteroids)).
No products indexed under this heading.

Dicloxacillin Sodium (Antimicrobial therapy for other infections may interfere with the effectiveness of BCG, live).
No products indexed under this heading.

Dirithromycin (Antimicrobial therapy for other infections may interfere with the effectiveness of BCG, live).
No products indexed under this heading.

Doxorubicin Hydrochloride (BCG, live should not be used in immunosuppressed patients or persons with congenital or acquired immune deficiencies, whether due to concurrent disease (e.g., AIDS, leukemia, lymphoma), cancer therapy (e.g., cytotoxic drugs, radiation), or immunosuppressive therapy (e.g., corticosteroids)).
No products indexed under this heading.

Doxycycline Calcium (Antimicrobial therapy for other infections may interfere with the effectiveness of BCG, live).
No products indexed under this heading.

Doxycycline Hyclate (Antimicrobial therapy for other infections may interfere with the effectiveness of BCG, live).
No products indexed under this heading.

Doxycycline Monohydrate (Antimicrobial therapy for other infections may interfere with the effectiveness of BCG, live).
No products indexed under this heading.

Enoxacin (Antimicrobial therapy for other infections may interfere with the effectiveness of BCG, live).
No products indexed under this heading.

Epirubicin Hydrochloride (BCG, live should not be used in immunosuppressed patients or persons with congenital or acquired immune deficiencies, whether due to concurrent disease (e.g., AIDS, leukemia, lymphoma), cancer therapy (e.g., cytotoxic drugs, radiation), or immunosuppressive therapy (e.g., corticosteroids)).
No products indexed under this heading.

Erythromycin (Antimicrobial therapy for other infections may interfere with the effectiveness of BCG, live).
No products indexed under this heading.

Erythromycin Estolate (Antimicrobial therapy for other infections may interfere with the effectiveness of BCG, live).
No products indexed under this heading.

Erythromycin Ethylsuccinate (Antimicrobial therapy for other infections may interfere with the effectiveness of BCG, live). Products include:
E.E.S. 433
EryPed 431

Erythromycin Gluceptate (Antimicrobial therapy for other infections may interfere with the effectiveness of BCG, live).
No products indexed under this heading.

Erythromycin Lactobionate (Antimicrobial therapy for other infections may interfere with the effectiveness of BCG, live).
No products indexed under this heading.

Erythromycin Stearate (Antimicrobial therapy for other infections may interfere with the effectiveness of BCG, live).
No products indexed under this heading.

Ethambutol Hydrochloride (Antituberculosis drugs (e.g., isoniazid) should not be used to prevent or treat the local, irritative toxicities of BCG, live).
No products indexed under this heading.

Fluconazole (Antimicrobial therapy for other infections may interfere with the effectiveness of BCG, live).
No products indexed under this heading.

Fludrocortisone Acetate (BCG, live should not be used in immunosuppressed patients or persons with congenital or acquired immune deficiencies, whether due to concurrent disease (e.g., AIDS, leukemia, lymphoma), cancer therapy (e.g., cytotoxic drugs, radiation), or immunosuppressive therapy (e.g., corticosteroids)).
No products indexed under this heading.

Flunisolide (BCG, live should not be used in immunosuppressed patients or persons with congenital or acquired immune deficiencies, whether due to concurrent disease (e.g., AIDS, leukemia, lymphoma), cancer therapy (e.g., cytotoxic drugs, radiation), or immunosuppressive therapy (e.g., corticosteroids)). Products include:
Aerobid/Aerobid-M **1153**

Fluorouracil (BCG, live should not be used in immunosuppressed patients or persons with congenital or acquired immune deficiencies, whether due to concurrent disease (e.g., AIDS, leukemia, lymphoma), cancer therapy (e.g., cytotoxic drugs, radiation), or immunosuppressive therapy (e.g., corticosteroids)). Products include:
Carac Cream 0.5% **2722**

Fluticasone Propionate (BCG, live should not be used in immunosuppressed patients or persons with congenital or acquired immune deficiencies, whether due to concurrent disease (e.g., AIDS, leukemia, lymphoma), cancer therapy (e.g., cytotoxic drugs, radiation), or immunosuppressive therapy (e.g., corticosteroids)). Products include:
Advair Diskus 100/50 .... **1276**
Advair Diskus 250/50 .... **1276**
Advair Diskus 500/50 .... **1276**
Advair HFA 45/21 Inhalation Aerosol **1288**
Advair HFA 115/21 Inhalation Aerosol **1288**
Advair HFA 230/21 Inhalation Aerosol **1288**
Flonase Nasal Spray **1431**
Flovent Diskus 50 mcg **1435**

Fluticasone Propionate HFA (BCG, live should not be used in immunosuppressed patients or persons with congenital or acquired immune deficiencies, whether due to concurrent disease (e.g., AIDS, leukemia, lymphoma), cancer therapy (e.g., cytotoxic drugs, radiation), or immunosuppressive therapy (e.g., corticosteroids)). Products include:
Flovent HFA **1440**

Gatifloxacin (Antimicrobial therapy for other infections may interfere with the effectiveness of BCG, live).
No products indexed under this heading.

Gentamicin Sulfate (Antimicrobial therapy for other infections may interfere with the effectiveness of BCG, live). Products include:
Pred-G Ophthalmic Ointment .... ⊙ **229**
Pred-G Ophthalmic Suspension .... ⊙ **228**

Grepafloxacin Hydrochloride (Antimicrobial therapy for other infections may interfere with the effectiveness of BCG, live).
No products indexed under this heading.

Hydrocortisone (BCG, live should not be used in immunosuppressed patients or persons with congenital or acquired immune deficiencies, whether due to concurrent disease (e.g., AIDS, leukemia, lymphoma), cancer therapy (e.g., cytotoxic drugs, radiation), or immunosuppressive therapy (e.g., corticosteroids)).
No products indexed under this heading.

Hydrocortisone Acetate (BCG, live should not be used in immunosuppressed patients or persons with congenital or acquired immune deficiencies, whether due to concurrent disease (e.g., AIDS, leukemia, lymphoma), cancer therapy (e.g., cytotoxic drugs, radiation), or immunosuppressive therapy (e.g., corticosteroids)). Products include:
Analpram-HC **1140**
Pramosone **1141**

Hydrocortisone Sodium Phosphate (BCG, live should not be used in immunosuppressed patients or persons with congenital or acquired immune deficiencies, whether due to concurrent disease (e.g., AIDS, leukemia, lymphoma), cancer therapy (e.g., cytotoxic drugs, radiation), or immunosuppressive therapy (e.g., corticosteroids)).
No products indexed under this heading.

Hydrocortisone Sodium Succinate (BCG, live should not be used in immunosuppressed patients or persons with congenital or acquired immune deficiencies, whether due to concurrent disease (e.g., AIDS, leukemia, lymphoma), cancer therapy (e.g., cytotoxic drugs, radiation), or immunosuppressive therapy (e.g., corticosteroids)).
No products indexed under this heading.

Hydroxyurea (BCG, live should not be used in immunosuppressed patients or persons with congenital or acquired immune deficiencies, whether due to concurrent disease (e.g., AIDS, leukemia, lymphoma), cancer therapy (e.g., cytotoxic drugs, radiation), or immunosuppressive therapy (e.g., corticosteroids)).
No products indexed under this heading.

Imipenem (Antimicrobial therapy for other infections may interfere with the effectiveness of BCG, live). Products include:
Primaxin I.M. **2080**
Primaxin I.V. **2083**

Isoniazid (Antituberculosis drugs (e.g., isoniazid) should not be used to prevent or treat the local, irritative toxicities of BCG, live).
No products indexed under this heading.

Itraconazole (Antimicrobial therapy for other infections may interfere with the effectiveness of BCG, live).
No products indexed under this heading.

Kanamycin Sulfate (Antimicrobial therapy for other infections may interfere with the effectiveness of BCG, live).
No products indexed under this heading.

Ketoconazole (Antimicrobial therapy for other infections may interfere with the effectiveness of BCG, live). Products include:
Extina Foam, 2% **3057**
Nizoral A-D Shampoo **1901**

Levofloxacin (Antimicrobial therapy for other infections may interfere with the effectiveness of BCG, live). Products include:
Iquix Ophthalmic Solution **3183**
Levaquin **2416**
Levaquin in 5% Dextrose Injection **2416**
Quixin Ophthalmic Solution **3184**

Lomefloxacin Hydrochloride (Antimicrobial therapy for other infections may interfere with the effectiveness of BCG, live).
No products indexed under this heading.

Loracarbef (Antimicrobial therapy for other infections may interfere with the effectiveness of BCG, live).
No products indexed under this heading.

Methacycline Hydrochloride (Antimicrobial therapy for other infections may interfere with the effectiveness of BCG, live).
No products indexed under this heading.

Methotrexate Sodium (BCG, live should not be used in immunosuppressed patients or persons with congenital or acquired immune deficiencies, whether due to concurrent disease (e.g., AIDS, leukemia, lymphoma), cancer therapy (e.g., cytotoxic drugs, radiation), or immunosuppressive therapy (e.g., corticosteroids)).
No products indexed under this heading.

Methylprednisolone Acetate (BCG, live should not be used in immunosuppressed patients or persons with congenital or acquired immune deficiencies, whether due to concurrent disease (e.g., AIDS, leukemia, lymphoma), cancer therapy (e.g., cytotoxic drugs, radiation), or immunosuppressive therapy (e.g., corticosteroids)).
No products indexed under this heading.

Methylprednisolone Sodium Succinate (BCG, live should not be used in immunosuppressed patients or persons with congenital or acquired immune deficiencies, whether due to concurrent disease (e.g., AIDS, leukemia, lymphoma), cancer therapy (e.g., cytotoxic drugs, radiation), or immunosuppressive therapy (e.g., corticosteroids)).
No products indexed under this heading.

Mezlocillin Sodium (Antimicrobial therapy for other infections may interfere with the effectiveness of BCG, live).
No products indexed under this heading.

Miconazole (Antimicrobial therapy for other infections may interfere with the effectiveness of BCG, live).
No products indexed under this heading.

Minocycline Hydrochloride (Antimicrobial therapy for other infections may interfere with the effectiveness of BCG, live). Products include:
Solodyn Extended Release Tablets **1938**

Mitotane (BCG, live should not be used in immunosuppressed patients or persons with congenital or acquired immune deficiencies, whether due to concurrent disease (e.g., AIDS, leukemia, lymphoma), cancer therapy (e.g., cytotoxic drugs, radiation), or immunosuppressive therapy (e.g., corticosteroids)).
No products indexed under this heading.

Mitoxantrone Hydrochloride (BCG, live should not be used in immunosuppressed patients or persons with congenital or acquired immune deficiencies, whether due to concurrent disease (e.g., AIDS, leukemia, lymphoma), cancer therapy (e.g., cytotoxic drugs, radiation), or immunosuppressive therapy (e.g., corticosteroids)). Products include:
Novantrone for Injection Concentrate **1100**

Mometasone Furoate (BCG, live should not be used in immunosuppressed patients or persons with congenital or acquired immune deficiencies, whether due to concurrent disease (e.g., AIDS, leukemia, lymphoma), cancer therapy (e.g., cytotoxic drugs, radiation), or immunosuppressive therapy (e.g., corticosteroids)). Products include:
Asmanex Twisthaler **2797**
Elocon Cream 0.1% **2840**
Elocon Lotion 0.1% **2841**
Elocon Ointment 0.1% **2842**

Mometasone Furoate Monohydrate (BCG, live should not be used in immunosuppressed patients or persons with congenital or acquired immune deficiencies, whether due to concurrent disease (e.g., AIDS, leukemia, lymphoma), cancer therapy (e.g., cytotoxic drugs, radiation), or immunosuppressive therapy (e.g., corticosteroids)). Products include:
Nasonex Nasal Spray **2883**

Moxifloxacin Hydrochloride (Antimicrobial therapy for other infections may interfere with the effectiveness of BCG, live). Products include:
Avelox **2803**
Vigamox Ophthalmic Solution **548**

Muromonab-CD3 (BCG, live should not be used in immunosuppressed patients or persons with congenital or acquired immune deficiencies, whether due to concurrent disease (e.g., AIDS, leukemia, lymphoma), cancer therapy (e.g., cytotoxic drugs, radiation), or immunosuppressive therapy (e.g., corticosteroids)). Products include:
Orthoclone OKT3 Sterile Solution **2387**

Mycophenolate Mofetil (BCG, live should not be used in immunosuppressed patients or persons with congenital or acquired immune deficiencies, whether due to concurrent disease (e.g., AIDS, leukemia, lymphoma), cancer therapy (e.g., cytotoxic drugs, radiation), or immunosuppressive therapy (e.g., corticosteroids)). Products include:
CellCept Capsules **2622**
CellCept Oral Suspension **2622**
CellCept Tablets **2622**

Nafcillin Sodium (Antimicrobial therapy for other infections may interfere with the effectiveness of BCG, live).
No products indexed under this heading.

Norfloxacin (Antimicrobial therapy for other infections may interfere with the effectiveness of BCG, live). Products include:
Noroxin Tablets 2069

Ofloxacin (Antimicrobial therapy for other infections may interfere with the effectiveness of BCG, live). Products include:
Ofloxacin Ophthalmic Solution 0.3% .... ⊙243

Oxiconazole Nitrate (Antimicrobial therapy for other infections may interfere with the effectiveness of BCG, live).
No products indexed under this heading.

Oxytetracycline Hydrochloride (Antimicrobial therapy for other infections may interfere with the effectiveness of BCG, live).
No products indexed under this heading.

Penicillin G Benzathine (Antimicrobial therapy for other infections may interfere with the effectiveness of BCG, live). Products include:
Bicillin C-R Injectable Suspension 1775
Bicillin L-A Injection 1777

Penicillin G Potassium (Antimicrobial therapy for other infections may interfere with the effectiveness of BCG, live).
No products indexed under this heading.

Penicillin G Procaine (Antimicrobial therapy for other infections may interfere with the effectiveness of BCG, live). Products include:
Bicillin C-R Injectable Suspension 1775
Bicillin L-A Injection 1777

Penicillin G Sodium (Antimicrobial therapy for other infections may interfere with the effectiveness of BCG, live).
No products indexed under this heading.

Penicillin V Potassium (Antimicrobial therapy for other infections may interfere with the effectiveness of BCG, live).
No products indexed under this heading.

Posaconazole (Antimicrobial therapy for other infections may interfere with the effectiveness of BCG, live). Products include:
Noxafil Oral Suspension 2889

Prednisolone Acetate (BCG, live should not be used in immunosuppressed patients or persons with congenital or acquired immune deficiencies, whether due to concurrent disease (e.g., AIDS, leukemia, lymphoma), cancer therapy (e.g., cytotoxic drugs, radiation), or immunosuppressive therapy (e.g., corticosteroids)). Products include:
Pred Forte Ophthalmic Suspension .... ⊙227
Pred Mild Ophthalmic Suspension .... ⊙230
Pred-G Ophthalmic Ointment .... ⊙229
Pred-G Ophthalmic Suspension .... ⊙228

Prednisolone Sodium Phosphate (BCG, live should not be used in immunosuppressed patients or persons with congenital or acquired immune deficiencies, whether due to concurrent disease (e.g., AIDS, leukemia, lymphoma), cancer therapy (e.g., cytotoxic drugs, radiation), or immunosuppressive therapy (e.g., corticosteroids)).
No products indexed under this heading.

Prednisolone Tebutate (BCG, live should not be used in immunosuppressed patients or persons with congenital or acquired immune deficiencies, whether due to concurrent disease (e.g., AIDS, leukemia, lymphoma), cancer therapy (e.g., cytotoxic drugs, radiation), or immunosuppressive therapy (e.g., corticosteroids)).
No products indexed under this heading.

Prednisone (BCG, live should not be used in immunosuppressed patients or persons with congenital or acquired immune deficiencies, whether due to concurrent disease (e.g., AIDS, leukemia, lymphoma), cancer therapy (e.g., cytotoxic drugs, radiation), or immunosuppressive therapy (e.g., corticosteroids)).
No products indexed under this heading.

Procarbazine Hydrochloride (BCG, live should not be used in immunosuppressed patients or persons with congenital or acquired immune deficiencies, whether due to concurrent disease (e.g., AIDS, leukemia, lymphoma), cancer therapy (e.g., cytotoxic drugs, radiation), or immunosuppressive therapy (e.g., corticosteroids)).
No products indexed under this heading.

Pyrazinamide (Antituberculosis drugs (e.g., isoniazid) should not be used to prevent or treat the local, irritative toxicities of BCG, live).
No products indexed under this heading.

Rifampin (Antituberculosis drugs (e.g., isoniazid) should not be used to prevent or treat the local, irritative toxicities of BCG, live).
No products indexed under this heading.

Rifapentine (Antituberculosis drugs (e.g., isoniazid) should not be used to prevent or treat the local, irritative toxicities of BCG, live).
No products indexed under this heading.

Sirolimus (BCG, live should not be used in immunosuppressed patients or persons with congenital or acquired immune deficiencies, whether due to concurrent disease (e.g., AIDS, leukemia, lymphoma), cancer therapy (e.g., cytotoxic drugs, radiation), or immunosuppressive therapy (e.g., corticosteroids)). Products include:
Rapamune 3260

Streptomycin Sulfate (Antimicrobial therapy for other infections may interfere with the effectiveness of BCG, live).
No products indexed under this heading.

Sulfamethizole (Antimicrobial therapy for other infections may interfere with the effectiveness of BCG, live).
No products indexed under this heading.

Sulfamethoxazole (Antimicrobial therapy for other infections may interfere with the effectiveness of BCG, live).
No products indexed under this heading.

Sulfisoxazole Acetyl (Antimicrobial therapy for other infections may interfere with the effectiveness of BCG, live).
No products indexed under this heading.

Tacrolimus (BCG, live should not be used in immunosuppressed patients or persons with congenital or acquired immune deficiencies, whether due to concurrent disease (e.g., AIDS, leukemia, lymphoma), cancer therapy (e.g., cytotoxic drugs, radiation), or immunosuppressive therapy (e.g., corticosteroids)). Products include:
Prograf Capsules and Injection 622
Protopic Ointment 628

Tamoxifen Citrate (BCG, live should not be used in immunosuppressed patients or persons with congenital or acquired immune deficiencies, whether due to concurrent disease (e.g., AIDS, leukemia, lymphoma), cancer therapy (e.g., cytotoxic drugs, radiation), or immunosuppressive therapy (e.g., corticosteroids)).
No products indexed under this heading.

Terconazole (Antimicrobial therapy for other infections may interfere with the effectiveness of BCG, live).
No products indexed under this heading.

Tetracycline Hydrochloride (Antimicrobial therapy for other infections may interfere with the effectiveness of BCG, live). Products include:
Pylera Capsules 714

Ticarcillin Disodium (Antimicrobial therapy for other infections may interfere with the effectiveness of BCG, live). Products include:
Timentin ADD-Vantage 1606
Timentin Injection Galaxy Container 1609
Timentin IV Infusion 1603
Timentin Pharmacy Bulk Package 1613

Tobramycin (Antimicrobial therapy for other infections may interfere with the effectiveness of BCG, live). Products include:
Zylet Ophthalmic Suspension .... ⊙247

Tobramycin Sulfate (Antimicrobial therapy for other infections may interfere with the effectiveness of BCG, live).
No products indexed under this heading.

Triamcinolone (BCG, live should not be used in immunosuppressed patients or persons with congenital or acquired immune deficiencies, whether due to concurrent disease (e.g., AIDS, leukemia, lymphoma), cancer therapy (e.g., cytotoxic drugs, radiation), or immunosuppressive therapy (e.g., corticosteroids)).
No products indexed under this heading.

Triamcinolone Acetonide (BCG, live should not be used in immunosuppressed patients or persons with congenital or acquired immune deficiencies, whether due to concurrent disease (e.g., AIDS, leukemia, lymphoma), cancer therapy (e.g., cytotoxic drugs, radiation), or immunosuppressive therapy (e.g., corticosteroids)). Products include:
Azmacort Inhalation Aerosol 407
Nasacort AQ Nasal Spray 2765
Triesence Injectable Suspension .... ⊙209

Triamcinolone Diacetate (BCG, live should not be used in immunosuppressed patients or persons with congenital or acquired immune deficiencies, whether due to concurrent disease (e.g., AIDS, leukemia, lymphoma), cancer therapy (e.g., cytotoxic drugs, radiation), or immunosuppressive therapy (e.g., corticosteroids)).
No products indexed under this heading.

Triamcinolone Hexacetonide (BCG, live should not be used in immunosuppressed patients or persons with congenital or acquired immune deficiencies, whether due to concurrent disease (e.g., AIDS, leukemia, lymphoma), cancer therapy (e.g., cytotoxic drugs, radiation), or immunosuppressive therapy (e.g., corticosteroids)).
No products indexed under this heading.

Troleandomycin (Antimicrobial therapy for other infections may interfere with the effectiveness of BCG, live).
No products indexed under this heading.

Trovafloxacin Mesylate (Antimicrobial therapy for other infections may interfere with the effectiveness of BCG, live).
No products indexed under this heading.

Vincristine Sulfate (BCG, live should not be used in immunosuppressed patients or persons with congenital or acquired immune deficiencies, whether due to concurrent disease (e.g., AIDS, leukemia, lymphoma), cancer therapy (e.g., cytotoxic drugs, radiation), or immunosuppressive therapy (e.g., corticosteroids)).
No products indexed under this heading.

Voriconazole (Antimicrobial therapy for other infections may interfere with the effectiveness of BCG, live).
No products indexed under this heading.

TIMENTIN ADD-VANTAGE

(Clavulanate Potassium, Ticarcillin Disodium) 1606
See Timentin IV Infusion

TIMENTIN INJECTION GALAXY CONTAINER

(Clavulanate Potassium, Ticarcillin Disodium) 1609
See Timentin IV Infusion

TIMENTIN IV INFUSION

(Clavulanate Potassium, Ticarcillin Disodium) 1603
May interact with aminoglycosides, oral contraceptives, and certain other agents. Compounds in these categories include:

Amikacin Sulfate (The mixing of Timentin with an aminoglycoside in solutions for parental administration can result in substantial inactivation of the aminoglycoside).
No products indexed under this heading.

Desogestrel (Timentin may affect the gut flora, leading to lower estrogen reabsorption and reduced efficacy of combined oral estrogen/progesterone contraceptives). Products include:

Mircette Tablets 1034

Ethinyl Estradiol (Timentin may affect the gut flora, leading to lower estrogen reabsorption and reduced efficacy of combined oral estrogen/progesterone contraceptives). Products include:

Lybrel Tablets 3204
Mircette Tablets 1034
NuvaRing 2897
Ortho-Cyclen/Ortho Tri-Cyclen 2449
Ortho Evra Transdermal System 2437
Ortho Tri-Cyclen Lo Tablets 2458
Seasonique Tablets 1046
Yaz Tablets 805

Ethynodiol Diacetate (Timentin may affect the gut flora, leading to lower estrogen reabsorption and reduced efficacy of combined oral estrogen/progesterone contraceptives).

No products indexed under this heading.

Gentamicin Sulfate (The mixing of Timentin with an aminoglycoside in solutions for parenteral administration can result in substantial inactivation of the aminoglycoside). Products include:

Pred-G Ophthalmic Ointment .... ⊙229
Pred-G Ophthalmic Suspension .... ⊙228

Kanamycin Sulfate (The mixing of Timentin with an aminoglycoside in solutions for parenteral administration can result in substantial inactivation of the aminoglycoside).

No products indexed under this heading.

Levonorgestrel (Timentin may affect the gut flora, leading to lower estrogen reabsorption and reduced efficacy of combined oral estrogen/progesterone contraceptives). Products include:

Climara Pro Transdermal System 768
Lybrel Tablets 3204
Mirena Intrauterine System 779
Plan B Tablets 1044
Seasonique Tablets 1046

Mestranol (Timentin may affect the gut flora, leading to lower estrogen reabsorption and reduced efficacy of combined oral estrogen/progesterone contraceptives).

No products indexed under this heading.

Norethindrone (Timentin may affect the gut flora, leading to lower estrogen reabsorption and reduced efficacy of combined oral estrogen/progesterone contraceptives). Products include:

Ortho Micronor Tablets 2446

Norethynodrel (Timentin may affect the gut flora, leading to lower estrogen reabsorption and reduced efficacy of combined oral estrogen/progesterone contraceptives).

No products indexed under this heading.

Norgestimate (Timentin may affect the gut flora, leading to lower estrogen reabsorption and reduced efficacy of combined oral estrogen/progesterone contraceptives). Products include:

Ortho-Cyclen/Ortho Tri-Cyclen 2449
Ortho Tri-Cyclen Lo Tablets 2458

Norgestrel (Timentin may affect the gut flora, leading to lower estrogen reabsorption and reduced efficacy of combined oral estrogen/progesterone contraceptives).

No products indexed under this heading.

Probenecid (Interferes with the renal tubular secretion of ticarcillin, thereby increasing serum concentrations and prolonged serum half-life of the antibiotic).

No products indexed under this heading.

Streptomycin Sulfate (The mixing of Timentin with an aminoglycoside in solutions for parental administration can result in substantial inactivation of the aminoglycoside).

No products indexed under this heading.

Tobramycin (The mixing of Timentin with an aminoglycoside in solutions for parental administration can result in substantial inactivation of the aminoglycoside). Products include:

Zylet Ophthalmic Suspension .... ⊙247

Tobramycin Sulfate (The mixing of Timentin with an aminoglycoside in solutions for parental administration can result in substantial inactivation of the aminoglycoside).

No products indexed under this heading.

TIMENTIN PHARMACY BULK PACKAGE

(Clavulanate Potassium, Ticarcillin Disodium) 1613

See Timentin IV Infusion

TIMOPTIC STERILE OPHTHALMIC SOLUTION

(Timolol Maleate) 2121

See Timoptic in Ocudose

TIMOPTIC IN OCUDOSE

(Timolol Maleate) 2124

May interact with beta blockers, catecholamine depleting drugs, calcium channel blockers, cardiac glycosides, oral hypoglycemic agents, insulin, quinidine, and certain other agents. Compounds in these categories include:

Acarbose (Beta blocking agents, usually systemic, may mask the sign and symptoms of acute hypoglycemia). Products include:

Precose Tablets 792

Acebutolol Hydrochloride (Concurrent use with systemic beta blocker may have additive effects of beta blockade, both systemic and on intraocular pressure).

No products indexed under this heading.

Amlodipine Besylate (Possible atrioventricular conduction disturbances, left ventricular failure, or hypotension when used concurrently). Products include:

Azor Tablets 1005
Exforge Tablets 2238

Atenolol (Concurrent use with systemic beta blocker may have additive effects of beta blockade, both systemic and on intraocular pressure).

No products indexed under this heading.

Bepridil Hydrochloride (Possible atrioventricular conduction disturbances, left ventricular failure, or hypotension when used concurrently).

No products indexed under this heading.

Betaxolol Hydrochloride (Concurrent use with systemic beta blocker may have additive effects of beta blockade, both systemic and on intraocular pressure; concurrent use of two topical beta blockers is not recommended).

No products indexed under this heading.

Bisoprolol Fumarate (Concurrent use with systemic beta blocker may have additive effects of beta blockade, both systemic and on intraocular pressure).

No products indexed under this heading.

Carteolol Hydrochloride (Concurrent use with systemic beta blocker may have additive effects of beta blockade, both systemic and on intraocular pressure; concurrent use of two topical beta blockers is not recommended).

No products indexed under this heading.

Chlorpropamide (Beta blocking agents, usually systemic, may mask the sign and symptoms of acute hypoglycemia).

No products indexed under this heading.

Clonidine (Oral beta-adrenergic blocking agents may exacerbate the rebound hypertension which can follow the withdrawal of clonidine; there have been no reports of exacerbation of rebound hypertension with ophthalmic timolol). Products include:

Catapres-TTS 842

Clonidine Hydrochloride (Oral beta-adrenergic blocking agents may exacerbate the rebound hypertension which can follow the withdrawal of clonidine; there have been no reports of exacerbation of rebound hypertension with ophthalmic timolol). Products include:

Catapres Tablets 841
Clorpres Tablets 2185

Deserpidine (Possible additive effects and the production of hypotension and/or bradycardia).

No products indexed under this heading.

Deslanoside (Co-administration with digitalis and calcium antagonists may have additive effects in prolonging atrioventricular conduction time).

No products indexed under this heading.

Digitalis Glycoside Preparations (Co-administration with digitalis and calcium antagonists may have additive effects in prolonging atrioventricular conduction time).

No products indexed under this heading.

Digitoxin (Co-administration with digitalis and calcium antagonists may have additive effects in prolonging atrioventricular conduction time).

No products indexed under this heading.

Digoxin (Co-administration with digitalis and calcium antagonists may have additive effects in prolonging atrioventricular conduction time). Products include:

Lanoxin Injection 1498
Lanoxin Injection Pediatric 1502
Lanoxin Tablets 1505

Diltiazem Hydrochloride (Possible atrioventricular conduction disturbances, left ventricular failure, or hypotension when used concurrently). Products include:

Cardizem LA Extended Release Tablets 421

Epinephrine (Patients with a history of atopy or anaphylactic reactions to a variety of allergens may be unresponsive to the usual dose of injectable epinephrine used to treat allergic reactions). Products include:

EpiPen 1024

Epinephrine Bitartrate (Patients with a history of atopy or anaphylactic reactions to a variety of allergens may be unresponsive to the usual dose of injectable epinephrine used to treat allergic reactions).

No products indexed under this heading.

Esmolol Hydrochloride (Concurrent use with systemic beta blocker may have additive effects of beta blockade, both systemic and on intraocular pressure).

No products indexed under this heading.

Felodipine (Possible atrioventricular conduction disturbances, left ventricular failure, or hypotension when used concurrently).

No products indexed under this heading.

Glimepiride (Beta blocking agents, usually systemic, may mask the sign and symptoms of acute hypoglycemia). Products include:

Avandaryl Tablets 1344
Duetact Tablets 3085

Glipizide (Beta blocking agents, usually systemic, may mask the sign and symptoms of acute hypoglycemia).

No products indexed under this heading.

Glyburide (Beta blocking agents, usually systemic, may mask the sign and symptoms of acute hypoglycemia).

No products indexed under this heading.

Guanethidine Monosulfate (Possible additive effects and the production of hypotension and/or bradycardia).

No products indexed under this heading.

Insulin (Beta blocking agents, usually systemic, may mask the sign and symptoms of acute hypoglycemia).

No products indexed under this heading.

Insulin, Human, Zinc Suspension (Beta blocking agents, usually systemic, may mask the sign and symptoms of acute hypoglycemia).

No products indexed under this heading.

Insulin, Human (rDNA origin) (Beta blocking agents, usually systemic, may mask the sign and symptoms of acute hypoglycemia). Products include:

Exubera Inhalation Powder 2515

Insulin, Human NPH (Beta blocking agents, usually systemic, may mask the sign and symptoms of acute hypoglycemia). Products include:

Humulin N Vial 1846

Insulin, Human Regular (Beta blocking agents, usually systemic,

may mask the sign and symptoms of acute hypoglycemia). Products include:
Humulin R 1849
Humulin R (U-500) 1850

Insulin, Human Regular and Human NPH Mixture (Beta blocking agents, usually systemic, may mask the sign and symptoms of acute hypoglycemia). Products include:
Humulin 50/50, 100 Units 1843
Humulin 70/30 Vial 1844

Insulin, NPH (Beta blocking agents, usually systemic, may mask the sign and symptoms of acute hypoglycemia).
No products indexed under this heading.

Insulin, Regular (Beta blocking agents, usually systemic, may mask the sign and symptoms of acute hypoglycemia).
No products indexed under this heading.

Insulin, Regular and NPH mixture (Beta blocking agents, usually systemic, may mask the sign and symptoms of acute hypoglycemia).
No products indexed under this heading.

Insulin, Zinc Crystals (Beta blocking agents, usually systemic, may mask the sign and symptoms of acute hypoglycemia).
No products indexed under this heading.

Insulin, Zinc Suspension (Beta blocking agents, usually systemic, may mask the sign and symptoms of acute hypoglycemia).
No products indexed under this heading.

Insulin Aspart (Beta blocking agents, usually systemic, may mask the sign and symptoms of acute hypoglycemia).
No products indexed under this heading.

Insulin Aspart, Human (Beta blocking agents, usually systemic, may mask the sign and symptoms of acute hypoglycemia). Products include:
NovoLog Mix 70/30 2364

Insulin Aspart, Human Regular (Beta blocking agents, usually systemic, may mask the sign and symptoms of acute hypoglycemia). Products include:
NovoLog Injection 2359

Insulin Aspart Protamine, Human (Beta blocking agents, usually systemic, may mask the sign and symptoms of acute hypoglycemia). Products include:
NovoLog Mix 70/30 2364

Insulin Detemir (rDNA Origin) (Beta blocking agents, usually systemic, may mask the sign and symptoms of acute hypoglycemia). Products include:
Levemir Injection 2352

Insulin glargine (Beta blocking agents, usually systemic, may mask the sign and symptoms of acute hypoglycemia). Products include:
Lantus Injection 2749

Insulin Glulisine (Beta blocking agents, usually systemic, may mask the sign and symptoms of acute hypoglycemia). Products include:
Apidra Injection 2706

Insulin Lispro, Human (Beta blocking agents, usually systemic, may mask the sign and symptoms of acute hypoglycemia). Products include:
Humalog-Pen and KwikPen 1829
Humalog Mix 50/50-Pen and KwikPen 1833
Humalog Mix 75/25-Pen and KwikPen 1835

Insulin Lispro Protamine, Human (Beta blocking agents, usually systemic, may mask the sign and symptoms of acute hypoglycemia). Products include:
Humalog Mix 50/50-Pen and KwikPen 1833
Humalog Mix 75/25-Pen and KwikPen 1835

Isradipine (Possible atrioventricular conduction disturbances, left ventricular failure, or hypotension when used concurrently). Products include:
DynaCirc CR Controlled Release Tablets 1407

Labetalol Hydrochloride (Concurrent use with systemic beta blocker may have additive effects of beta blockade, both systemic and on intraocular pressure).
No products indexed under this heading.

Levobunolol Hydrochloride (Concurrent use of two topical beta blockers is not recommended).
No products indexed under this heading.

Metformin Hydrochloride (Beta blocking agents, usually systemic, may mask the sign and symptoms of acute hypoglycemia). Products include:
ActoPlus Met Tablets 3071
Avandamet Tablets 1336
Janumet Tablets 2041
PrandiMet Tablets 2967

Metipranolol Hydrochloride (Concurrent use of two topical beta blockers is not recommended).
No products indexed under this heading.

Metoprolol Succinate (Concurrent use with systemic beta blocker may have additive effects of beta blockade, both systemic and on intraocular pressure). Products include:
Toprol-XL Tablets 666

Metoprolol Tartrate (Concurrent use with systemic beta blocker may have additive effects of beta blockade, both systemic and on intraocular pressure).
No products indexed under this heading.

Mibefradil Dihydrochloride (Possible atrioventricular conduction disturbances, left ventricular failure, or hypotension when used concurrently).
No products indexed under this heading.

Miglitol (Beta blocking agents, usually systemic, may mask the sign and symptoms of acute hypoglycemia).
No products indexed under this heading.

Nadolol (Concurrent use with systemic beta blocker may have additive effects of beta blockade, both systemic and on intraocular pressure). Products include:
Nadolol Tablets 2191

Nateglinide (Beta blocking agents, usually systemic, may mask the sign and symptoms of acute hypoglycemia). Products include:
Starlix Tablets 2314

Nebivolol (Concurrent use with systemic beta blocker may have additive effects of beta blockade, both systemic and on intraocular pressure). Products include:
Bystolic Tablets 1155

Nicardipine Hydrochloride (Possible atrioventricular conduction disturbances, left ventricular failure, or hypotension when used concurrently). Products include:
Cardene I.V. 1093

Nifedipine (Possible atrioventricular conduction disturbances, left ventricular failure, or hypotension when used concurrently).
No products indexed under this heading.

Nimodipine (Possible atrioventricular conduction disturbances, left ventricular failure, or hypotension when used concurrently). Products include:
Nimotop Capsules 790

Nisoldipine (Possible atrioventricular conduction disturbances, left ventricular failure, or hypotension when used concurrently). Products include:
Sular Extended Release Tablets 2975

Penbutolol Sulfate (Concurrent use with systemic beta blocker may have additive effects of beta blockade, both systemic and on intraocular pressure).
No products indexed under this heading.

Pindolol (Concurrent use with systemic beta blocker may have additive effects of beta blockade, both systemic and on intraocular pressure).
No products indexed under this heading.

Pioglitazone Hydrochloride (Beta blocking agents, usually systemic, may mask the sign and symptoms of acute hypoglycemia). Products include:
ActoPlus Met Tablets 3071
Actos Tablets 3077
Duetact Tablets 3085

Propranolol Hydrochloride (Concurrent use with systemic beta blocker may have additive effects of beta blockade, both systemic and on intraocular pressure). Products include:
InnoPran XL Extended Release Capsules 1484

Quinidine (Co-administration has resulted in potentiated systemic beta-blockade, e.g., decreased heart rate).
No products indexed under this heading.

Quinidine Gluconate (Co-administration has resulted in potentiated systemic beta-blockade, e.g., decreased heart rate).
No products indexed under this heading.

Quinidine Hydrochloride (Co-administration has resulted in potentiated systemic beta-blockade, e.g., decreased heart rate).
No products indexed under this heading.

Quinidine Polygalacturonate (Co-administration has resulted in potentiated systemic beta-blockade, e.g., decreased heart rate).
No products indexed under this heading.

Quinidine Sulfate (Co-administration has resulted in potentiated systemic beta-blockade, e.g., decreased heart rate).
No products indexed under this heading.

Rauwolfia Serpentina (Possible additive effects and the production of hypotension and/or bradycardia).
No products indexed under this heading.

Repaglinide (Beta blocking agents, usually systemic, may mask the sign and symptoms of acute hypoglycemia). Products include:
PrandiMet Tablets 2967
Prandin Tablets 2971

Rescinnamine (Possible additive effects and the production of hypotension and/or bradycardia).
No products indexed under this heading.

Reserpine (Possible additive effects and the production of hypotension and/or bradycardia).
No products indexed under this heading.

Rosiglitazone Maleate (Beta blocking agents, usually systemic, may mask the sign and symptoms of acute hypoglycemia). Products include:
Avandamet Tablets 1336
Avandaryl Tablets 1344
Avandia Tablets 1351

Sitagliptin Phosphate (Beta blocking agents, usually systemic, may mask the sign and symptoms of acute hypoglycemia). Products include:
Janumet Tablets 2041
Januvia Tablets 2048

Sotalol Hydrochloride (Concurrent use with systemic beta blocker may have additive effects of beta blockade, both systemic and on intraocular pressure).
No products indexed under this heading.

Timolol Hemihydrate (Concurrent use of two topical beta blockers is not recommended). Products include:
Betimol Ophthalmic Solution 3181

Tolazamide (Beta blocking agents, usually systemic, may mask the sign and symptoms of acute hypoglycemia).
No products indexed under this heading.

Tolbutamide (Beta blocking agents, usually systemic, may mask the sign and symptoms of acute hypoglycemia).
No products indexed under this heading.

Troglitazone (Beta blocking agents, usually systemic, may mask the sign and symptoms of acute hypoglycemia).
No products indexed under this heading.

Verapamil Hydrochloride (Possible atrioventricular conduction disturbances, left ventricular failure, or hypotension when used concurrently). Products include:
Tarka Tablets 511

TIMOPTIC-XE STERILE OPHTHALMIC GEL FORMING SOLUTION

(Timolol Maleate) 2125
See Timoptic in Ocudose

TNKASE
(Tenecteplase) 1233
May interact with anticoagulants, platelet inhibitors, vitamin K antagonists, and certain other agents. Compounds in these categories include:

Abciximab (Drugs that alter platelet function, such as abciximab, may increase the risk of bleeding if administered prior to or after tenecteplase therapy). Products include:
ReoPro Vials 1860

Anisindione (Anticoagulants may increase the risk of bleeding if administered prior to, during, or after tenecteplase therapy).
No products indexed under this heading.

Ardeparin Sodium (Anticoagulants may increase the risk of bleeding if administered prior to, during, or after tenecteplase therapy).
No products indexed under this heading.

Aspirin (Drugs that alter platelet function, such as aspirin, may increase the risk of bleeding if administered prior to or after tenecteplase therapy). Products include:
Aggrenox Capsules 819
Bayer Aspirin 750
Percodan Tablets 1130
St. Joseph 81 mg Aspirin Chewable and Enteric Coated Tablets 1903

Aspirin, Enteric Coated (Drugs that alter platelet function may increase the risk of bleeding if administered prior to, during, or after tenecteplase therapy).
No products indexed under this heading.

Aspirin Buffered (Drugs that alter platelet function may increase the risk of bleeding if administered prior to, during, or after tenecteplase therapy).
No products indexed under this heading.

Azlocillin Sodium (Drugs that alter platelet function may increase the risk of bleeding if administered prior to, during, or after tenecteplase therapy).
No products indexed under this heading.

Carbenicillin Indanyl Sodium (Drugs that alter platelet function may increase the risk of bleeding if administered prior to, during, or after tenecteplase therapy).
No products indexed under this heading.

Choline Magnesium Trisalicylate (Drugs that alter platelet function may increase the risk of bleeding if administered prior to, during, or after tenecteplase therapy).
No products indexed under this heading.

Clopidogrel Bisulfate (Drugs that alter platelet function, such as clopidogrel, may increase the risk of bleeding if administered prior to or after tenecteplase therapy). Products include:
Plavix Tablets 926
Plavix Tablets 2767

Dalteparin Sodium (Anticoagulants may increase the risk of bleeding if administered prior to, during, or after tenecteplase therapy). Products include:
Fragmin Injection 1070

Danaparoid Sodium (Anticoagulants may increase the risk of bleeding if administered prior to, during, or after tenecteplase therapy).
No products indexed under this heading.

Diclofenac Potassium (Drugs that alter platelet function may increase the risk of bleeding if administered prior to, during, or after tenecteplase therapy).
No products indexed under this heading.

Diclofenac Sodium (Drugs that alter platelet function may increase the risk of bleeding if administered prior to, during, or after tenecteplase therapy). Products include:
Diclofenac Sodium Ophthalmic Solution .... ⊙240
Voltaren Ophthalmic Solution 2336
Voltaren Tablets 2334
Voltaren-XR Tablets 2337

Dicumarol (Co-administration increases the risk of bleeding).
No products indexed under this heading.

Diflunisal (Drugs that alter platelet function may increase the risk of bleeding if administered prior to, during, or after tenecteplase therapy).
No products indexed under this heading.

Dipyridamole (Drugs that alter platelet function, such as dipyridamole, may increase the risk of bleeding if administered prior to or after tenecteplase therapy). Products include:
Aggrenox Capsules 819
Persantine Tablets 869

Enoxaparin Sodium (Anticoagulants may increase the risk of bleeding if administered prior to, during, or after tenecteplase therapy). Products include:
Lovenox Injection 2756

Epitifibatide (Drugs that alter platelet function, such as epitifibatide, may increase the risk of bleeding if administered prior to or after tenecteplase therapy).
No products indexed under this heading.

Fenoprofen Calcium (Drugs that alter platelet function may increase the risk of bleeding if administered prior to, during, or after tenecteplase therapy). Products include:
Nalfon Capsules 2508

Flurbiprofen (Drugs that alter platelet function may increase the risk of bleeding if administered prior to, during, or after tenecteplase therapy).
No products indexed under this heading.

Fondaparinux Sodium (Anticoagulants may increase the risk of bleeding if administered prior to, during, or after tenecteplase therapy). Products include:
Arixtra Injection 1313

Heparin Calcium (Anticoagulants may increase the risk of bleeding if administered prior to, during, or after tenecteplase therapy).
No products indexed under this heading.

Heparin Sodium (Anticoagulants may increase the risk of bleeding if administered prior to, during, or after tenecteplase therapy).
No products indexed under this heading.

Ibuprofen (Drugs that alter platelet function may increase the risk of bleeding if administered prior to, during, or after tenecteplase therapy). Products include:
Motrin IB Tablets and Caplets 1900
Children's Motrin Oral Suspension ... 1901
Children's Motrin Non-Staining Dye-Free Oral Suspension 1901
Children's Motrin Cold Oral Suspension 1899
Infants' Motrin Concentrated Drops 1901
Infants' Motrin Non-Staining Dye-Free Concentrated Drops 1901
Junior Strength Motrin Caplets and Chewable Tablets 1901
Vicoprofen Tablets 533

Indomethacin (Drugs that alter platelet function may increase the risk of bleeding if administered prior to, during, or after tenecteplase therapy). Products include:
Indocin 2024

Indomethacin Sodium Trihydrate (Drugs that alter platelet function may increase the risk of bleeding if administered prior to, during, or after tenecteplase therapy). Products include:
Indocin I.V. 2489

Ketoprofen (Drugs that alter platelet function may increase the risk of bleeding if administered prior to, during, or after tenecteplase therapy).
No products indexed under this heading.

Low Molecular Weight Heparins (Anticoagulants may increase the risk of bleeding if administered prior to, during, or after tenecteplase therapy).
No products indexed under this heading.

Magnesium Salicylate (Drugs that alter platelet function may increase the risk of bleeding if administered prior to, during, or after tenecteplase therapy).
No products indexed under this heading.

Meclofenamate Sodium (Drugs that alter platelet function may increase the risk of bleeding if administered prior to, during, or after tenecteplase therapy).
No products indexed under this heading.

Mefenamic Acid (Drugs that alter platelet function may increase the risk of bleeding if administered prior to, during, or after tenecteplase therapy).
No products indexed under this heading.

Mezlocillin Sodium (Drugs that alter platelet function may increase the risk of bleeding if administered prior to, during, or after tenecteplase therapy).
No products indexed under this heading.

Nafcillin Sodium (Drugs that alter platelet function may increase the risk of bleeding if administered prior to, during, or after tenecteplase therapy).
No products indexed under this heading.

Naproxen (Drugs that alter platelet function may increase the risk of bleeding if administered prior to, during, or after tenecteplase therapy). Products include:
EC-Naprosyn Delayed-Release Tablets 2632
Naprosyn Suspension 2632
Naprosyn Tablets 2632

Naproxen Sodium (Drugs that alter platelet function may increase the risk of bleeding if administered prior to, during, or after tenecteplase therapy). Products include:
Anaprox Tablets 2632
Anaprox DS Tablets 2632
Treximet Tablets 1616

Penicillin G Benzathine (Drugs that alter platelet function may increase the risk of bleeding if administered prior to, during, or after tenecteplase therapy). Products include:
Bicillin C-R Injectable Suspension 1775
Bicillin L-A Injection 1777

Penicillin G Procaine (Drugs that alter platelet function may increase the risk of bleeding if administered prior to, during, or after tenecteplase therapy). Products include:
Bicillin C-R Injectable Suspension 1775
Bicillin L-A Injection 1777

Phenylbutazone (Drugs that alter platelet function may increase the risk of bleeding if administered prior to, during, or after tenecteplase therapy).
No products indexed under this heading.

Piroxicam (Drugs that alter platelet function may increase the risk of bleeding if administered prior to, during, or after tenecteplase therapy).
No products indexed under this heading.

Salsalate (Drugs that alter platelet function may increase the risk of bleeding if administered prior to, during, or after tenecteplase therapy).
No products indexed under this heading.

Sulindac (Drugs that alter platelet function may increase the risk of bleeding if administered prior to, during, or after tenecteplase therapy). Products include:
Clinoril Tablets 1962

Ticarcillin Disodium (Drugs that alter platelet function may increase the risk of bleeding if administered prior to, during, or after tenecteplase therapy). Products include:
Timentin ADD-Vantage 1606
Timentin Injection Galaxy Container 1609
Timentin IV Infusion 1603
Timentin Pharmacy Bulk Package 1613

Ticlopidine Hydrochloride (Drugs that alter platelet function, such as ticlopidine, may increase the risk of bleeding if administered prior to or after tenecteplase therapy).
No products indexed under this heading.

Tinzaparin Sodium (Anticoagulants may increase the risk of bleeding if administered prior to, during, or after tenecteplase therapy).
No products indexed under this heading.

Tirofiban Hydrochloride (Drugs that alter platelet function, such as tirofiban, may increase the risk of bleeding if administered prior to or after tenecteplase therapy).
No products indexed under this heading.

Tolmetin Sodium (Drugs that alter platelet function may increase the risk of bleeding if administered prior to, during, or after tenecteplase therapy).
No products indexed under this heading.

Warfarin Sodium (Co-administration increases the risk of bleeding).
No products indexed under this heading.

TOFIPAN DIETARY SUPPLEMENT
(Dehydroepiandrosterone, Herbal Medicines, unspecified, Vitex agnus-castus) 995
None cited in PDR database.

TOFIPAN-Z DIETARY SUPPLEMENT
(Dehydroepiandrosterone, Herbal Medicines, unspecified, Vitex agnus-castus) 995
None cited in PDR database.

TONOX DIETARY SUPPLEMENT
(Alpha Lipoic Acid, Lutein, Peptidase, Rutoside, Selenium, Vitamin B_{12}, Vitamin C, Vitamin E, Zeaxanthin, Zinc) 995
None cited in PDR database.

TOPRICIN PAIN RELIEF AND HEALING CREAM
(Homeopathic Formulations) .... ▣621
None cited in PDR database.

TOPROL-XL TABLETS
(Metoprolol Succinate) 666
May interact with catecholamine depleting drugs, cytochrome p450 2d6 inhibitors (selected), cardiac glycosides, monoamine oxidase inhibitors, and certain other agents. Compounds in these categories include:

Amiodarone Hydrochloride (Co-administration of metoprolol with drugs that inhibit CYP2D6 is likely to increase metoprolol concentration; this increase in plasma concentration would decrease the cardioselectivity of metoprolol).
No products indexed under this heading.

Amitriptyline Hydrochloride (Co-administration of metoprolol with drugs that inhibit CYP2D6 is likely to increase metoprolol concentration; this increase in plasma concentration would decrease the cardioselectivity of metoprolol).
No products indexed under this heading.

Amoxapine (Co-administration of metoprolol with drugs that inhibit CYP2D6 is likely to increase metoprolol concentration; this increase in plasma concentration would decrease the cardioselectivity of metoprolol).
No products indexed under this heading.

Bupropion Hydrochloride (Co-administration of metoprolol with drugs that inhibit CYP2D6 is likely to increase metoprolol concentration; this increase in plasma concentration would decrease the cardioselectivity of metoprolol). Products include:
- Wellbutrin Tablets 1648
- Wellbutrin SR Sustained-Release Tablets 1653
- Wellbutrin XL Extended-Release Tablets 1659
- Zyban Sustained-Release Tablets 1692

Celecoxib (Co-administration of metoprolol with drugs that inhibit CYP2D6 is likely to increase metoprolol concentration; this increase in plasma concentration would decrease the cardioselectivity of metoprolol). Products include:
- Celebrex Capsules 2979

Chloroquine Hydrochloride (Co-administration of metoprolol with drugs that inhibit CYP2D6 is likely to increase metoprolol concentration; this increase in plasma concentration would decrease the cardioselectivity of metoprolol).
No products indexed under this heading.

Chloroquine Phosphate (Co-administration of metoprolol with drugs that inhibit CYP2D6 is likely to increase metoprolol concentration; this increase in plasma concentration would decrease the cardioselectivity of metoprolol).
No products indexed under this heading.

Chlorpheniramine (Co-administration of metoprolol with drugs that inhibit CYP2D6 is likely to increase metoprolol concentration; this increase in plasma concentration would decrease the cardioselectivity of metoprolol).
No products indexed under this heading.

Chlorpheniramine Maleate (Co-administration of metoprolol with drugs that inhibit CYP2D6 is likely to increase metoprolol concentration; this increase in plasma concentration would decrease the cardioselectivity of metoprolol). Products include:
- Actifed Cold & Allergy Tablets 1895
- Sudafed PE Sinus & Allergy Tablets 1908
- Tylenol Allergy Multi-Symptom Caplets with Cool Burst and Rapid Release Gelcaps 1916
- Children's Tylenol Plus Cold Suspension Liquid 1912
- Children's Tylenol Plus Cough & Runny Nose Suspension Liquid 1912
- Children's Tylenol Plus Flu Suspension Liquid 1914
- Children's Tylenol Plus Multi-Symptom Cold Suspension Liquid 1912
- Tylenol Cold Head Congestion Nighttime Caplets with Cool Burst 1910
- Tylenol Cold Multi-Symptom Nighttime Caplets with Cool Burst 1913
- Tylenol Sinus Congestion & Pain Nighttime Caplets with Cool Burst 1917

Chlorpheniramine Polistirex (Co-administration of metoprolol with drugs that inhibit CYP2D6 is likely to increase metoprolol concentration; this increase in plasma concentration would decrease the cardioselectivity of metoprolol). Products include:
- Tussionex Pennkinetic Extended-Release Suspension 3154

Chlorpheniramine Tannate (Co-administration of metoprolol with drugs that inhibit CYP2D6 is likely to increase metoprolol concentration; this increase in plasma concentration would decrease the cardioselectivity of metoprolol).
No products indexed under this heading.

Cimetidine (Co-administration of metoprolol with drugs that inhibit CYP2D6 is likely to increase metoprolol concentration; this increase in plasma concentration would decrease the cardioselectivity of metoprolol).
No products indexed under this heading.

Cimetidine Hydrochloride (Co-administration of metoprolol with drugs that inhibit CYP2D6 is likely to increase metoprolol concentration; this increase in plasma concentration would decrease the cardioselectivity of metoprolol).
No products indexed under this heading.

Citalopram Hydrobromide (Co-administration of metoprolol with drugs that inhibit CYP2D6 is likely to increase metoprolol concentration; this increase in plasma concentration would decrease the cardioselectivity of metoprolol). Products include:
- Celexa 1160

Clomipramine Hydrochloride (Co-administration of metoprolol with drugs that inhibit CYP2D6 is likely to increase metoprolol concentration; this increase in plasma concentration would decrease the cardioselectivity of metoprolol).
No products indexed under this heading.

Clonidine (Beta-blockers may exacerbate the rebound hypertension which can follow the withdrawal of clonidine. If co-administered, withdraw beta-blockers several days before the gradual withdrawal of clonidine. If replacing clonidine by beta-blocker therapy, delay start of beta-blockers for several days after clonidine administration has stopped). Products include:
- Catapres-TTS 842

Cocaine Hydrochloride (Co-administration of metoprolol with drugs that inhibit CYP2D6 is likely to increase metoprolol concentration; this increase in plasma concentration would decrease the cardioselectivity of metoprolol).
No products indexed under this heading.

Deserpidine (Catecholamine-depleting drugs may have an additive effect when given with beta-blocking agents; monitor closely for signs of hypotension or marked bradycardia).
No products indexed under this heading.

Desipramine Hydrochloride (Co-administration of metoprolol with drugs that inhibit CYP2D6 is likely to increase metoprolol concentration; this increase in plasma concentration would decrease the cardioselectivity of metoprolol).
No products indexed under this heading.

Deslanoside (Both digitalis glycosides and beta-blockers slow atrioventricular conduction and decrease heart rate. Concomitant use can increase the risk of bradycardia).
No products indexed under this heading.

Digitalis Glycoside Preparations (Both digitalis glycosides and beta-blockers slow atrioventricular conduction and decrease heart rate. Concomitant use can increase the risk of bradycardia).
No products indexed under this heading.

Digitoxin (Both digitalis glycosides and beta-blockers slow atrioventricular conduction and decrease heart rate. Concomitant use can increase the risk of bradycardia).
No products indexed under this heading.

Digoxin (Both digitalis glycosides and beta-blockers slow atrioventricular conduction and decrease heart rate. Concomitant use can increase the risk of bradycardia). Products include:
- Lanoxin Injection 1498
- Lanoxin Injection Pediatric 1502
- Lanoxin Tablets 1505

Diltiazem Hydrochloride (Because of significant inotropic and chronotropic effects in patients treated with beta-blockers and calcium-channel blockers of the diltiazem type, caution should be exercised in patients treated with these agents concomitantly). Products include:
- Cardizem LA Extended Release Tablets 421

Diphenhydramine (Co-administration of metoprolol with drugs that inhibit CYP2D6 is likely to increase metoprolol concentration; this increase in plasma concentration would decrease the cardioselectivity of metoprolol).
No products indexed under this heading.

Diphenhydramine Hydrochloride (Co-administration of metoprolol with drugs that inhibit CYP2D6 is likely to increase metoprolol concentration; this increase in plasma concentration would decrease the cardioselectivity of metoprolol). Products include:
- Benadryl Allergy & Cold Kapgels 1895
- Benadryl Allergy & Sinus Headache Kapgels 1895
- Benadryl Severe Allergy & Sinus Headache Caplets 1897
- Benadryl Dye-Free Allergy Liqui-gels Softgels 1897
- Benadryl Allergy Kapgels 1895
- Benadryl Allergy Quick Dissolve Strips 1896
- Benadryl Allergy Ultratab Tablets 1896
- Children's Benadryl Dye-Free Allergy Liquid 1897
- Children's Benadryl Allergy Fastmelts 1897
- Children's Benadryl Allergy Liquid 1898
- Children's Benadryl Allergy Perfect Measure 1896
- Children's Benadryl-D Allergy & Sinus Liquid 1896
- Benadryl-D Allergy & Sinus Tablet 1896
- PediaCare Children's Allergy & Cold Liquid 1902
- PediaCare Children's Allergy Liquid 1902
- Simply Sleep Caplets 1905
- Sudafed PE Nighttime Cold Caplets 1907
- Sudafed PE Severe Cold Caplets 1908
- Extra Strength Tylenol PM Caplets, Geltabs, Liquid, and Rapid Release Gels 1915
- Tylenol Allergy Multi-Symptom Nighttime Caplets with Cool Burst 1916
- Tylenol Severe Allergy Caplets 1916
- Children's Tylenol Plus Cold & Allergy Suspension Liquid 1914
- Tylenol Sore Throat Nighttime Liquid with Cool Burst 1918

Doxepin Hydrochloride (Co-administration of metoprolol with drugs that inhibit CYP2D6 is likely to increase metoprolol concentration; this increase in plasma concentration would decrease the cardioselectivity of metoprolol).
No products indexed under this heading.

Epinephrine Hydrochloride (Potential unresponsiveness to the usual dose of epinephrine to treat allergic reactions in certain patients).
No products indexed under this heading.

Escitalopram Oxalate (Co-administration of metoprolol with drugs that inhibit CYP2D6 is likely to increase metoprolol concentration; this increase in plasma concentration would decrease the cardioselectivity of metoprolol). Products include:

Lexapro Oral Suspension 1174
Lexapro Tablets 1174

Fluoxetine (Co-administration of metoprolol with drugs that inhibit CYP2D6 is likely to increase metoprolol concentration; this increase in plasma concentration would decrease the cardioselectivity of metoprolol).

No products indexed under this heading.

Fluoxetine Hydrochloride (Co-administration with drugs that inhibit CYP2D6, such as fluoxetine, are likely to increase metoprolol concentrations; these increases in plasma concentration would decrease the cardioselectivity of metoprolol). Products include:

Prozac Weekly Capsules 1852
Prozac Pulvules and Liquid 1852
Symbyax Capsules 1871

Fluphenazine Decanoate (Co-administration of metoprolol with drugs that inhibit CYP2D6 is likely to increase metoprolol concentration; this increase in plasma concentration would decrease the cardioselectivity of metoprolol).

No products indexed under this heading.

Fluphenazine Enanthate (Co-administration of metoprolol with drugs that inhibit CYP2D6 is likely to increase metoprolol concentration; this increase in plasma concentration would decrease the cardioselectivity of metoprolol).

No products indexed under this heading.

Fluphenazine Hydrochloride (Co-administration of metoprolol with drugs that inhibit CYP2D6 is likely to increase metoprolol concentration; this increase in plasma concentration would decrease the cardioselectivity of metoprolol).

No products indexed under this heading.

Fluvoxamine Maleate (Co-administration of metoprolol with drugs that inhibit CYP2D6 is likely to increase metoprolol concentration; this increase in plasma concentration would decrease the cardioselectivity of metoprolol). Products include:

Luvox CR Extended-Release Capsules 1759

Guanethidine Monosulfate (Catecholamine-depleting drugs may have an additive effect when given with beta-blocking agents; monitor closely for signs of hypotension or marked bradycardia).

No products indexed under this heading.

Halofantrine Hydrochloride (Co-administration of metoprolol with drugs that inhibit CYP2D6 is likely to increase metoprolol concentration; this increase in plasma concentration would decrease the cardioselectivity of metoprolol).

No products indexed under this heading.

Haloperidol (Co-administration of metoprolol with drugs that inhibit CYP2D6 is likely to increase metoprolol concentration; this increase in plasma concentration would decrease the cardioselectivity of metoprolol).

No products indexed under this heading.

Haloperidol Decanoate (Co-administration of metoprolol with drugs that inhibit CYP2D6 is likely to increase metoprolol concentration; this increase in plasma concentration would decrease the cardioselectivity of metoprolol).

No products indexed under this heading.

Hydroxychloroquine Sulfate (Co-administration of metoprolol with drugs that inhibit CYP2D6 is likely to increase metoprolol concentration; this increase in plasma concentration would decrease the cardioselectivity of metoprolol).

No products indexed under this heading.

Imatinib Mesylate (Co-administration of metoprolol with drugs that inhibit CYP2D6 is likely to increase metoprolol concentration; this increase in plasma concentration would decrease the cardioselectivity of metoprolol). Products include:

Gleevec Tablets 2255

Imipramine Hydrochloride (Co-administration of metoprolol with drugs that inhibit CYP2D6 is likely to increase metoprolol concentration; this increase in plasma concentration would decrease the cardioselectivity of metoprolol).

No products indexed under this heading.

Imipramine Pamoate (Co-administration of metoprolol with drugs that inhibit CYP2D6 is likely to increase metoprolol concentration; this increase in plasma concentration would decrease the cardioselectivity of metoprolol).

No products indexed under this heading.

Isocarboxazid (Catecholamine-depleting drugs may have an additive effect when given with beta-blocking agents; monitor closely for signs of hypotension or marked bradycardia). Products include:

Marplan Tablets 3177

Maprotiline Hydrochloride (Co-administration of metoprolol with drugs that inhibit CYP2D6 is likely to increase metoprolol concentration; this increase in plasma concentration would decrease the cardioselectivity of metoprolol).

No products indexed under this heading.

Methadone Hydrochloride (Co-administration of metoprolol with drugs that inhibit CYP2D6 is likely to increase metoprolol concentration; this increase in plasma concentration would decrease the cardioselectivity of metoprolol).

No products indexed under this heading.

Mibefradil Dihydrochloride (Co-administration of metoprolol with drugs that inhibit CYP2D6 is likely to increase metoprolol concentration; this increase in plasma concentration would decrease the cardioselectivity of metoprolol).

No products indexed under this heading.

Moclobemide (Catecholamine-depleting drugs may have an additive effect when given with beta-blocking agents; monitor closely for signs of hypotension or marked bradycardia).

No products indexed under this heading.

Nortriptyline Hydrochloride (Co-administration of metoprolol with drugs that inhibit CYP2D6 is likely to increase metoprolol concentration; this increase in plasma concentration would decrease the cardioselectivity of metoprolol).

No products indexed under this heading.

Pargyline Hydrochloride (Catecholamine-depleting drugs may have an additive effect when given with beta-blocking agents; monitor closely for signs of hypotension or marked bradycardia).

No products indexed under this heading.

Paroxetine Hydrochloride (Co-administration with drugs that inhibit CYP2D6, such as paroxetine, are likely to increase metoprolol concentrations; these increases in plasma concentration would decrease the cardioselectivity of metoprolol). Products include:

Paxil 1535
Paxil CR Controlled-Release Tablets 1544

Perphenazine (Co-administration of metoprolol with drugs that inhibit CYP2D6 is likely to increase metoprolol concentration; this increase in plasma concentration would decrease the cardioselectivity of metoprolol).

No products indexed under this heading.

Phenelzine Sulfate (Catecholamine-depleting drugs may have an additive effect when given with beta-blocking agents; monitor closely for signs of hypotension or marked bradycardia).

No products indexed under this heading.

Procarbazine Hydrochloride (Catecholamine-depleting drugs may have an additive effect when given with beta-blocking agents; monitor closely for signs of hypotension or marked bradycardia).

No products indexed under this heading.

Propafenone Hydrochloride (Co-administration with drugs that inhibit CYP2D6, such as propafenone, are likely to increase metoprolol concentrations; these increases in plasma concentration would decrease the cardioselectivity of metoprolol). Products include:

Rythmol Tablets 1586
Rythmol SR Capsules 1590

Propoxyphene Hydrochloride (Co-administration of metoprolol with drugs that inhibit CYP2D6 is likely to increase metoprolol concentration; this increase in plasma concentration would decrease the cardioselectivity of metoprolol).

No products indexed under this heading.

Propoxyphene Napsylate (Co-administration of metoprolol with drugs that inhibit CYP2D6 is likely to increase metoprolol concentration; this increase in plasma concentration would decrease the cardioselectivity of metoprolol).

No products indexed under this heading.

Protriptyline Hydrochloride (Co-administration of metoprolol with drugs that inhibit CYP2D6 is likely to increase metoprolol concentration; this increase in plasma concentration would decrease the cardioselectivity of metoprolol).

No products indexed under this heading.

Quinacrine Hydrochloride (Co-administration of metoprolol with drugs that inhibit CYP2D6 is likely to increase metoprolol concentration; this increase in plasma concentration would decrease the cardioselectivity of metoprolol).

No products indexed under this heading.

Quinidine Gluconate (Co-administration of metoprolol with drugs that inhibit CYP2D6 is likely to increase metoprolol concentration; this increase in plasma concentration would decrease the cardioselectivity of metoprolol).

No products indexed under this heading.

Quinidine Hydrochloride (Co-administration of metoprolol with drugs that inhibit CYP2D6 is likely to increase metoprolol concentration; this increase in plasma concentration would decrease the cardioselectivity of metoprolol).

No products indexed under this heading.

Quinidine Polygalacturonate (Co-administration of metoprolol with drugs that inhibit CYP2D6 is likely to increase metoprolol concentration; this increase in plasma concentration would decrease the cardioselectivity of metoprolol).

No products indexed under this heading.

Quinidine Sulfate (Co-administration of metoprolol with drugs that inhibit CYP2D6 is likely to increase metoprolol concentration; this increase in plasma concentration would decrease the cardioselectivity of metoprolol).

No products indexed under this heading.

Ranitidine Bismuth Citrate (Co-administration of metoprolol with drugs that inhibit CYP2D6 is likely to increase metoprolol concentration; this increase in plasma concentration would decrease the cardioselectivity of metoprolol).

No products indexed under this heading.

Ranitidine Hydrochloride (Co-administration of metoprolol with drugs that inhibit CYP2D6 is likely to increase metoprolol concentration; this increase in plasma concentra-

tion would decrease the cardioselectivity of metoprolol). Products include:

Zantac 75 Tablets .... ▣603
Zantac 1670
Zantac Injection 1666
Zantac Injection Pharmacy Bulk Package 1668
Maximum Strength Zantac 150 Tablets .... ▣603
Maximum Strength Zantac 150 Cool Mint Tablets .... ▣603

Rasagiline Mesylate (Catecholamine-depleting drugs may have an additive effect when given with beta-blocking agents; monitor closely for signs of hypotension or marked bradycardia). Products include:

Azilect Tablets 3106

Rauwolfia Serpentina (Catecholamine-depleting drugs may have an additive effect when given with beta-blocking agents; monitor closely for signs of hypotension or marked bradycardia).

No products indexed under this heading.

Rescinnamine (Catecholamine-depleting drugs may have an additive effect when given with beta-blocking agents; monitor closely for signs of hypotension or marked bradycardia).

No products indexed under this heading.

Reserpine (Catecholamine-depleting drugs may have an additive effect when given with beta-blocking agents; monitor closely for signs of hypotension or marked bradycardia).

No products indexed under this heading.

Ritonavir (Co-administration of metoprolol with drugs that inhibit CYP2D6 is likely to increase metoprolol concentration; this increase in plasma concentration would decrease the cardioselectivity of metoprolol). Products include:

Kaletra 452
Norvir 489

Selegiline (Catecholamine-depleting drugs may have an additive effect when given with beta-blocking agents; monitor closely for signs of hypotension or marked bradycardia). Products include:

Emsam Transdermal System 905

Selegiline Hydrochloride (Catecholamine-depleting drugs may have an additive effect when given with beta-blocking agents; monitor closely for signs of hypotension or marked bradycardia). Products include:

Eldepryl Capsules 3052

Sertraline Hydrochloride (Co-administration of metoprolol with drugs that inhibit CYP2D6 is likely to increase metoprolol concentration; this increase in plasma concentration would decrease the cardioselectivity of metoprolol).

No products indexed under this heading.

Sildenafil Citrate (Co-administration of metoprolol with drugs that inhibit CYP2D6 is likely to increase metoprolol concentration; this increase in plasma concentration would decrease the cardioselectivity of metoprolol).

No products indexed under this heading.

Terbinafine Hydrochloride (Co-administration of metoprolol with drugs that inhibit CYP2D6 is likely to increase metoprolol concentration; this increase in plasma concentration would decrease the cardioselectivity of metoprolol). Products include:

Lamisil Oral Granules 2264
Lamisil Tablets 2266

Thioridazine Hydrochloride (Co-administration of metoprolol with drugs that inhibit CYP2D6 is likely to increase metoprolol concentration; this increase in plasma concentration would decrease the cardioselectivity of metoprolol). Products include:

Thioridazine Hydrochloride Tablets 2195

Tranylcypromine Sulfate (Catecholamine-depleting drugs may have an additive effect when given with beta-blocking agents; monitor closely for signs of hypotension or marked bradycardia). Products include:

Parnate Tablets 1532

Trimipramine Maleate (Co-administration of metoprolol with drugs that inhibit CYP2D6 is likely to increase metoprolol concentration; this increase in plasma concentration would decrease the cardioselectivity of metoprolol).

No products indexed under this heading.

Vardenafil Hydrochloride (Co-administration of metoprolol with drugs that inhibit CYP2D6 is likely to increase metoprolol concentration; this increase in plasma concentration would decrease the cardioselectivity of metoprolol). Products include:

Levitra Tablets 2876

Verapamil Hydrochloride (Because of significant inotropic and chronotropic effects in patients treated with beta-blockers and calcium-channel blockers of the verapamil type, caution should be exercised in patients treated with these agents concomitantly). Products include:

Tarka Tablets 511

TORISEL INJECTION

(Temsirolimus) 3272

May interact with cytochrome p450 2d6 substrates (selected), cytochrome p450 3a4 inducers (selected), cytochrome p450 3a4 inhibitors, potent, vaccines, live, and certain other agents. Compounds in these categories include:

Allium sativum (The concomitant use of strong CYP3A4 inducers should be avoided. If patients must be co-administered a strong CYP3A4 inducer, based on pharmacokinetic studies, a Torisel dose increase from 25mg/week up to 50mg/week should be considered. This dose of Torisel is predicted to adjust the AUC to the range observed without inducers. However, there are no clinical data with this dose adjustment in patients receiving strong CYP3A4 inducers. If the strong inducer is discontinued, the temsirolimus dose should be returned to the dose used prior to initiation of the strong CYP3A4 inducer).

No products indexed under this heading.

Amitriptyline Hydrochloride (The concentration of desipramin, a CYP2D6 substrate, was unaffected when 25mg of Torisel was co-administered. No clinically significant effect is anticipated when temsirolimus is co-administered with agents that are metabolized by CYP2D6 or CYP3A4).

No products indexed under this heading.

Amphetamine Aspartate (The concentration of desipramin, a CYP2D6 substrate, was unaffected when 25mg of Torisel was co-administered. No clinically significant effect is anticipated when temsirolimus is co-administered with agents that are metabolized by CYP2D6 or CYP3A4). Products include:

Adderall XR Capsules 3012

Amphetamine Aspartate Monohydrate (The concentration of desipramin, a CYP2D6 substrate, was unaffected when 25mg of Torisel was co-administered. No clinically significant effect is anticipated when temsirolimus is co-administered with agents that are metabolized by CYP2D6 or CYP3A4).

No products indexed under this heading.

Amphetamine Sulfate (The concentration of desipramin, a CYP2D6 substrate, was unaffected when 25mg of Torisel was co-administered. No clinically significant effect is anticipated when temsirolimus is co-administered with agents that are metabolized by CYP2D6 or CYP3A4). Products include:

Adderall XR Capsules 3012

Amprenavir (The concomitant use of strong CYP3A4 inhibitors should be avoided. If patients must be co-administered a strong CYP3A4 inhibitor, based on pharmacokinetic studies, a Torisel dose reduction to 12.5mg/week should be considered. This dose is predicted to adjust the AUC to the range observed without inhibitors. However, there are no clinical data with this dose adjustment in patients receiving strong CYP3A4 inhibitors. If strong inhibitor is discontimued, a washout period of approximately 1 week should be allowed before the Torisel dose is adjusted back to the dose used prior to initiation of the strong CYP3A4 inhibitor).

No products indexed under this heading.

Aprepitant (The concomitant use of strong CYP3A4 inducers should be avoided. If patients must be co-administered a strong CYP3A4 inducer, based on pharmacokinetic studies, a Torisel dose increase from 25mg/week up to 50mg/week should be considered. This dose of Torisel is predicted to adjust the AUC to the range observed without inducers. However, there are no clinical data with this dose adjustment in patients receiving strong CYP3A4 inducers. If the strong inducer is discontinued, the temsirolimus dose should be returned to the dose used prior to initiation of the strong CYP3A4 inducer). Products include:

Emend Capsules 1992

Atazanavir (The concomitant use of strong CYP3A4 inhibitors should be avoided. If patients must be co-administered a strong CYP3A4 inhibitor, based on pharmacokinetic studies, a Torisel dose reduction to 12.5mg/week should be considered. This dose is predicted to adjust the AUC to the range observed without inhibitors. However, there are no clinical data with this dose adjustment in patients receiving strong CYP3A4 inhibitors. If strong inhibitor is discontimued, a washout period of approximately 1 week should be allowed before the Torisel dose is adjusted back to the dose used prior to initiation of the strong CYP3A4 inhibitor).

No products indexed under this heading.

Atazanavir Sulfate (The concomitant use of strong CYP3A4 inhibitors should be avoided. If patients must be co-administered a strong CYP3A4 inhibitor, based on pharmacokinetic studies, a Torisel dose reduction to 12.5mg/week should be considered. This dose is predicted to adjust the AUC to the range observed without inhibitors. However, there are no clinical data with this dose adjustment in patients receiving strong CYP3A4 inhibitors. If strong inhibitor is discontimued, a washout period of approximately 1 week should be allowed before the Torisel dose is adjusted back to the dose used prior to initiation of the strong CYP3A4 inhibitor). Products include:

Reyataz Capsules 3299

Atomoxetine Hydrochloride (The concentration of desipramin, a CYP2D6 substrate, was unaffected when 25mg of Torisel was co-administered. No clinically significant effect is anticipated when temsirolimus is co-administered with agents that are metabolized by CYP2D6 or CYP3A4). Products include:

Strattera Capsules 1864

BCG Vaccine (The use of live vaccines and close contact with those who have received live vaccines should be avoided).

No products indexed under this heading.

Betamethasone Acetate (The concomitant use of strong CYP3A4 inducers should be avoided. If patients must be co-administered a strong CYP3A4 inducer, based on pharmacokinetic studies, a Torisel dose increase from 25mg/week up to 50mg/week should be considered. This dose of Torisel is predicted to adjust the AUC to the range observed without inducers. However, there are no clinical data with this dose adjustment in patients receiving strong CYP3A4 inducers. If the strong inducer is discontinued, the temsirolimus dose should be returned to the dose used prior to initiation of the strong CYP3A4 inducer).

No products indexed under this heading.

Betamethasone Sodium Phosphate (The concomitant use of strong CYP3A4 inducers should be avoided. If patients must be co-administered a strong CYP3A4 inducer, based on pharmacokinetic studies, a Torisel dose increase from 25mg/week up to 50mg/week should be considered. This dose of Torisel is predicted to adjust the AUC to the range observed without inducers. However, there are no clinical data with this dose adjustment in patients receiving strong CYP3A4

inducers. If the strong inducer is discontinued, the temsirolimus dose should be returned to the dose used prior to initiation of the strong CYP3A4 inducer).
No products indexed under this heading.

Bisoprolol Fumarate (The concentration of desipramin, a CYP2D6 substrate, was unaffected when 25mg of Torisel was co-administered. No clinically significant effect is anticipated when temsirolimus is co-administered with agents that are metabolized by CYP2D6 or CYP3A4).
No products indexed under this heading.

Captopril (The concentration of desipramin, a CYP2D6 substrate, was unaffected when 25mg of Torisel was co-administered. No clinically significant effect is anticipated when temsirolimus is co-administered with agents that are metabolized by CYP2D6 or CYP3A4). Products include:
Captopril Tablets **2182**

Carbamazepine (The concomitant use of strong CYP3A4 inducers should be avoided. If patients must be co-administered a strong CYP3A4 inducer, based on pharmacokinetic studies, a Torisel dose increase from 25mg/week up to 50mg/week should be considered. This dose of Torisel is predicted to adjust the AUC to the range observed without inducers. However, there are no clinical data with this dose adjustment in patients receiving strong CYP3A4 inducers. If the strong inducer is discontinued, the temsirolimus dose should be returned to the dose used prior to initiation of the strong CYP3A4 inducer). Products include:
Carbatrol Capsules **3019**
Equetro Extended-Release Capsules **3174**

Carvedilol (The concentration of desipramin, a CYP2D6 substrate, was unaffected when 25mg of Torisel was co-administered. No clinically significant effect is anticipated when temsirolimus is co-administered with agents that are metabolized by CYP2D6 or CYP3A4). Products include:
Coreg Tablets **1387**

Cevimeline Hydrochloride (The concentration of desipramin, a CYP2D6 substrate, was unaffected when 25mg of Torisel was co-administered. No clinically significant effect is anticipated when temsirolimus is co-administered with agents that are metabolized by CYP2D6 or CYP3A4). Products include:
Evoxac Capsules **1013**

Chlorpromazine (The concentration of desipramin, a CYP2D6 substrate, was unaffected when 25mg of Torisel was co-administered. No clinically significant effect is anticipated when temsirolimus is co-administered with agents that are metabolized by CYP2D6 or CYP3A4).
No products indexed under this heading.

Chlorpromazine Hydrochloride (The concentration of desipramin, a CYP2D6 substrate, was unaffected when 25mg of Torisel was co-administered. No clinically significant effect is anticipated when temsirolimus is co-administered with agents that are metabolized by CYP2D6 or CYP3A4).
No products indexed under this heading.

Chlorpropamide (The concentration of desipramin, a CYP2D6 substrate, was unaffected when 25mg of Torisel was co-administered. No clinically significant effect is anticipated when temsirolimus is co-administered with agents that are metabolized by CYP2D6 or CYP3A4).
No products indexed under this heading.

Ciprofloxacin Hydrochloride (The concomitant use of strong CYP3A4 inducers should be avoided. If patients must be co-administered a strong CYP3A4 inducer, based on pharmacokinetic studies, a Torisel dose increase from 25mg/week up to 50mg/week should be considered. This dose of Torisel is predicted to adjust the AUC to the range observed without inducers. However, there are no clinical data with this dose adjustment in patients receiving strong CYP3A4 inducers. If the strong inducer is discontinued, the temsirolimus dose should be returned to the dose used prior to initiation of the strong CYP3A4 inducer). Products include:
Cipro Tablets **2810**

Cisplatin (The concomitant use of strong CYP3A4 inducers should be avoided. If patients must be co-administered a strong CYP3A4 inducer, based on pharmacokinetic studies, a Torisel dose increase from 25mg/week up to 50mg/week should be considered. This dose of Torisel is predicted to adjust the AUC to the range observed without inducers. However, there are no clinical data with this dose adjustment in patients receiving strong CYP3A4 inducers. If the strong inducer is discontinued, the temsirolimus dose should be returned to the dose used prior to initiation of the strong CYP3A4 inducer).
No products indexed under this heading.

Clarithromycin (The concomitant use of strong CYP3A4 inhibitors should be avoided. If patients must be co-administered a strong CYP3A4 inhibitor, based on pharmacokinetic studies, a Torisel dose reduction to 12.5mg/week should be considered. This dose is predicted to adjust the AUC to the range observed without inhibitors. However, there are no clinical data with this dose adjustment in patients receiving strong CYP3A4 inhibitors. If strong inhibitor is discontimued, a washout period of approximately 1 week should be allowed before the Torisel dose is adjusted back to the dose used prior to initiation of the strong CYP3A4 inhibitor). Products include:
Biaxin/Biaxin XL **411**

Clomipramine Hydrochloride (The concentration of desipramin, a CYP2D6 substrate, was unaffected when 25mg of Torisel was co-administered. No clinically significant effect is anticipated when temsirolimus is co-administered with agents that are metabolized by CYP2D6 or CYP3A4).
No products indexed under this heading.

Clozapine (The concentration of desipramin, a CYP2D6 substrate, was unaffected when 25mg of Torisel was co-administered. No clinically significant effect is anticipated when temsirolimus is co-administered with agents that are metabolized by CYP2D6 or CYP3A4).
No products indexed under this heading.

Codeine Phosphate (The concentration of desipramin, a CYP2D6 substrate, was unaffected when 25mg of Torisel was co-administered. No clinically significant effect is anticipated when temsirolimus is co-administered with agents that are metabolized by CYP2D6 or CYP3A4). Products include:
Tylenol with Codeine Tablets **2427**

Codeine Sulfate (The concentration of desipramin, a CYP2D6 substrate, was unaffected when 25mg of Torisel was co-administered. No clinically significant effect is anticipated when temsirolimus is co-administered with agents that are metabolized by CYP2D6 or CYP3A4).
No products indexed under this heading.

Cortisone Acetate (The concomitant use of strong CYP3A4 inducers should be avoided. If patients must be co-administered a strong CYP3A4 inducer, based on pharmacokinetic studies, a Torisel dose increase from 25mg/week up to 50mg/week should be considered. This dose of Torisel is predicted to adjust the AUC to the range observed without inducers. However, there are no clinical data with this dose adjustment in patients receiving strong CYP3A4 inducers. If the strong inducer is discontinued, the temsirolimus dose should be returned to the dose used prior to initiation of the strong CYP3A4 inducer).
No products indexed under this heading.

Cyclobenzaprine Hydrochloride (The concentration of desipramin, a CYP2D6 substrate, was unaffected when 25mg of Torisel was co-administered. No clinically significant effect is anticipated when temsirolimus is co-administered with agents that are metabolized by CYP2D6 or CYP3A4). Products include:
Amrix Capsules **966**

Delavirdine Mesylate (The concomitant use of strong CYP3A4 inhibitors should be avoided. If patients must be co-administered a strong CYP3A4 inhibitor, based on pharmacokinetic studies, a Torisel dose reduction to 12.5mg/week should be considered. This dose is predicted to adjust the AUC to the range observed without inhibitors. However, there are no clinical data with this dose adjustment in patients receiving strong CYP3A4 inhibitors. If strong inhibitor is discontimued, a washout period of approximately 1 week should be allowed before the Torisel dose is adjusted back to the dose used prior to initiation of the strong CYP3A4 inhibitor).
No products indexed under this heading.

Delavirine (The concomitant use of strong CYP3A4 inhibitors should be avoided. If patients must be co-administered a strong CYP3A4 inhibitor, based on pharmacokinetic studies, a Torisel dose reduction to 12.5mg/week should be considered. This dose is predicted to adjust the AUC to the range observed without inhibitors. However, there are no clinical data with this dose adjustment in patients receiving strong CYP3A4 inhibitors. If strong inhibitor is discontimued, a washout period of approximately 1 week should be allowed before the Torisel dose is adjusted back to the dose used prior to initiation of the strong CYP3A4 inhibitor).
No products indexed under this heading.

Desipramine Hydrochloride (The concentration of desipramin, a CYP2D6 substrate, was unaffected when 25mg of Torisel was co-administered. No clinically significant effect is anticipated when temsirolimus is co-administered with agents that are metabolized by CYP2D6 or CYP3A4).
No products indexed under this heading.

Dexamethasone (The concomitant use of strong CYP3A4 inducers should be avoided. If patients must be co-administered a strong CYP3A4 inducer, based on pharmacokinetic studies, a Torisel dose increase from 25mg/week up to 50mg/week should be considered. This dose of Torisel is predicted to adjust the AUC to the range observed without inducers. However, there are no clinical data with this dose adjustment in patients receiving strong CYP3A4 inducers. If the strong inducer is discontinued, the temsirolimus dose should be returned to the dose used prior to initiation of the strong CYP3A4 inducer). Products include:
Ciprodex Otic Suspension **541**

Dexamethasone Acetate (The concomitant use of strong CYP3A4 inducers should be avoided. If patients must be co-administered a strong CYP3A4 inducer, based on pharmacokinetic studies, a Torisel dose increase from 25mg/week up to 50mg/week should be considered. This dose of Torisel is predicted to adjust the AUC to the range observed without inducers. However, there are no clinical data with this dose adjustment in patients receiving strong CYP3A4 inducers. If the strong inducer is discontinued, the temsirolimus dose should be returned to the dose used prior to initiation of the strong CYP3A4 inducer).
No products indexed under this heading.

Dexamethasone Sodium Phosphate (The concomitant use of strong CYP3A4 inducers should be avoided. If patients must be co-administered a strong CYP3A4 inducer, based on pharmacokinetic studies, a Torisel dose increase from 25mg/week up to 50mg/week should be considered. This dose of

Torisel is predicted to adjust the AUC to the range observed without inducers. However, there are no clinical data with this dose adjustment in patients receiving strong CYP3A4 inducers. If the strong inducer is discontinued, the temsirolimus dose should be returned to the dose used prior to initiation of the strong CYP3A4 inducer).

No products indexed under this heading.

Dexfenfluramine Hydrochloride (The concentration of desipramin, a CYP2D6 substrate, was unaffected when 25mg of Torisel was co-administered. No clinically significant effect is anticipated when temsirolimus is co-administered with agents that are metabolized by CYP2D6 or CYP3A4).

No products indexed under this heading.

Dextromethorphan Hydrobromide (The concentration of desipramin, a CYP2D6 substrate, was unaffected when 25mg of Torisel was co-administered. No clinically significant effect is anticipated when temsirolimus is co-administered with agents that are metabolized by CYP2D6 or CYP3A4). Products include:

PediaCare Children's Liquid Multi-Symptom Cold 1902
PediaCare Children's Long-Acting Cough 1902
Children's Sudafed PE Cold & Cough Liquid 1907
Sudafed PE Cold & Cough Caplets 1907
Children's Tylenol Plus Cough & Runny Nose Suspension Liquid 1912
Children's Tylenol Plus Cough & Sore Throat Suspension Liquid 1912
Children's Tylenol Plus Flu Suspension Liquid 1914
Children's Tylenol Plus Multi-Symptom Cold Suspension Liquid 1912
Tylenol Cold Severe Congestion Daytime Caplets with Cool Burst 1912
Tylenol Cold Head Congestion Daytime Caplets with Cool Burst 1910
Tylenol Cold Head Congestion Nighttime Caplets with Cool Burst 1910
Tylenol Cold Head Congestion Severe Daytime Caplets with Cool Burst 1910
Tylenol Cold Multi-Symptom Daytime Caplets with Cool Burst and Rapid Release Gels 1913
Tylenol Cold Multi-Symptom Daytime Liquid with Citrus Burst 1913
Tylenol Cold Multi-Symptom Nighttime Caplets with Cool Burst 1913
Tylenol Cold Multi-Symptom Nighttime Liquid with Cool Burst 1913
Tylenol Cold Multi-Symptom Severe Caplets with Cool Burst 1913
Tylenol Cold Multi-Symptom Severe Daytime Liquid with Citrus Burst 1913
Tylenol Cough & Sore Throat Daytime Liquid with Cool Burst 1918
Tylenol Cough & Sore Throat Nighttime Liquid with Cool Burst 1918
Vicks DayQuil Cold & Flu Multi-Symptom Relief ..... ■□616
Vicks DayQuil LiquiCaps 2567
Vicks DayQuil Liquid 2567
Vicks DayQuil Multi-Symptom Cold/Flu Relief 2567
Vicks NyQuil Cold & Flu Multi-Symptom Relief ..... ■□617
Vicks NyQuil LiquiCaps 2567
Vicks NyQuil Liquid 2567
Vicks NyQuil Multi-Symptom Cold/Flu Relief 2567

Dextromethorphan Polistirex (The concentration of desipramin, a CYP2D6 substrate, was unaffected when 25mg of Torisel was co-administered. No clinically significant effect is anticipated when temsirolimus is co-administered with agents that are metabolized by CYP2D6 or CYP3A4).

No products indexed under this heading.

Dolasetron Mesylate (The concentration of desipramin, a CYP2D6 substrate, was unaffected when 25mg of Torisel was co-administered. No clinically significant effect is anticipated when temsirolimus is co-administered with agents that are metabolized by CYP2D6 or CYP3A4). Products include:

Anzemet Injection 2701
Anzemet Tablets 2704

Donepezil Hydrochloride (The concentration of desipramin, a CYP2D6 substrate, was unaffected when 25mg of Torisel was co-administered. No clinically significant effect is anticipated when temsirolimus is co-administered with agents that are metabolized by CYP2D6 or CYP3A4). Products include:

Aricept Tablets 1062
Aricept ODT Tablets 1062

Doxepin Hydrochloride (The concentration of desipramin, a CYP2D6 substrate, was unaffected when 25mg of Torisel was co-administered. No clinically significant effect is anticipated when temsirolimus is co-administered with agents that are metabolized by CYP2D6 or CYP3A4).

No products indexed under this heading.

Doxorubicin Hydrochloride (The concomitant use of strong CYP3A4 inducers should be avoided. If patients must be co-administered a strong CYP3A4 inducer, based on pharmacokinetic studies, a Torisel dose increase from 25mg/week up to 50mg/week should be considered. This dose of Torisel is predicted to adjust the AUC to the range observed without inducers. However, there are no clinical data with this dose adjustment in patients receiving strong CYP3A4 inducers. If the strong inducer is discontinued, the temsirolimus dose should be returned to the dose used prior to initiation of the strong CYP3A4 inducer).

No products indexed under this heading.

Efavirenz (The concomitant use of strong CYP3A4 inducers should be avoided. If patients must be co-administered a strong CYP3A4 inducer, based on pharmacokinetic studies, a Torisel dose increase from 25mg/week up to 50mg/week should be considered. This dose of Torisel is predicted to adjust the AUC to the range observed without inducers. However, there are no clinical data with this dose adjustment in patients receiving strong CYP3A4 inducers. If the strong inducer is discontinued, the temsirolimus dose should be returned to the dose used prior to initiation of the strong CYP3A4 inducer). Products include:

Atripla Tablets 938
Sustiva Capsules 930
Sustiva Tablets 930

Encainide Hydrochloride (The concentration of desipramin, a CYP2D6 substrate, was unaffected when 25mg of Torisel was co-administered. No clinically significant effect is anticipated when temsirolimus is co-administered with agents that are metabolized by CYP2D6 or CYP3A4).

No products indexed under this heading.

Ethosuximide (The concomitant use of strong CYP3A4 inducers should be avoided. If patients must be co-administered a strong CYP3A4 inducer, based on pharmacokinetic studies, a Torisel dose increase from 25mg/week up to 50mg/week should be considered. This dose of Torisel is predicted to adjust the AUC to the range observed without inducers. However, there are no clinical data with this dose adjustment in patients receiving strong CYP3A4 inducers. If the strong inducer is discontinued, the temsirolimus dose should be returned to the dose used prior to initiation of the strong CYP3A4 inducer).

No products indexed under this heading.

Felbamate (The concomitant use of strong CYP3A4 inducers should be avoided. If patients must be co-administered a strong CYP3A4 inducer, based on pharmacokinetic studies, a Torisel dose increase from 25mg/week up to 50mg/week should be considered. This dose of Torisel is predicted to adjust the AUC to the range observed without inducers. However, there are no clinical data with this dose adjustment in patients receiving strong CYP3A4 inducers. If the strong inducer is discontinued, the temsirolimus dose should be returned to the dose used prior to initiation of the strong CYP3A4 inducer).

No products indexed under this heading.

Fentanyl (The concentration of desipramin, a CYP2D6 substrate, was unaffected when 25mg of Torisel was co-administered. No clinically significant effect is anticipated when temsirolimus is co-administered with agents that are metabolized by CYP2D6 or CYP3A4). Products include:

Duragesic Transdermal System 2405
Ionsys Transdermal System 2410

Fentanyl Citrate (The concentration of desipramin, a CYP2D6 substrate, was unaffected when 25mg of Torisel was co-administered. No clinically significant effect is anticipated when temsirolimus is co-administered with agents that are metabolized by CYP2D6 or CYP3A4). Products include:

Actiq 959
Fentora Tablets 968

Flecainide Acetate (The concentration of desipramin, a CYP2D6 substrate, was unaffected when 25mg of Torisel was co-administered. No clinically significant effect is anticipated when temsirolimus is co-administered with agents that are metabolized by CYP2D6 or CYP3A4).

No products indexed under this heading.

Fludrocortisone Acetate (The concomitant use of strong CYP3A4 inducers should be avoided. If patients must be co-administered a strong CYP3A4 inducer, based on pharmacokinetic studies, a Torisel dose increase from 25mg/week up to 50mg/week should be considered. This dose of Torisel is predicted to adjust the AUC to the range observed without inducers. However, there are no clinical data with this dose adjustment in patients receiving strong CYP3A4 inducers. If the strong inducer is discontinued, the temsirolimus dose should be returned to the dose used prior to initiation of the strong CYP3A4 inducer).

No products indexed under this heading.

Fluoxetine (The concentration of desipramin, a CYP2D6 substrate, was unaffected when 25mg of Torisel was co-administered. No clinically significant effect is anticipated when temsirolimus is co-administered with agents that are metabolized by CYP2D6 or CYP3A4).

No products indexed under this heading.

Fluoxetine Hydrochloride (The concentration of desipramin, a CYP2D6 substrate, was unaffected when 25mg of Torisel was co-administered. No clinically significant effect is anticipated when temsirolimus is co-administered with agents that are metabolized by CYP2D6 or CYP3A4). Products include:

Prozac Weekly Capsules 1852
Prozac Pulvules and Liquid 1852
Symbyax Capsules 1871

Fluphenazine Decanoate (The concentration of desipramin, a CYP2D6 substrate, was unaffected when 25mg of Torisel was co-administered. No clinically significant effect is anticipated when temsirolimus is co-administered with agents that are metabolized by CYP2D6 or CYP3A4).

No products indexed under this heading.

Fluphenazine Enanthate (The concentration of desipramin, a CYP2D6 substrate, was unaffected when 25mg of Torisel was co-administered. No clinically significant effect is anticipated when temsirolimus is co-administered with agents that are metabolized by CYP2D6 or CYP3A4).

No products indexed under this heading.

Fluphenazine Hydrochloride (The concentration of desipramin, a CYP2D6 substrate, was unaffected when 25mg of Torisel was co-administered. No clinically significant effect is anticipated when temsirolimus is co-administered with agents that are metabolized by CYP2D6 or CYP3A4).

No products indexed under this heading.

Fluvoxamine Maleate (The concentration of desipramin, a CYP2D6 substrate, was unaffected when 25mg of Torisel was co-administered. No clinically significant effect is anticipated when temsirolimus is co-administered with agents that are metabolized by CYP2D6 or CYP3A4). Products include:

Luvox CR Extended-Release Capsules 1759

Formoterol Fumarate (The concentration of desipramin, a CYP2D6 substrate, was unaffected when 25mg of Torisel was co-administered. No clinically significant effect is anticipated when temsirolimus is co-administered with agents that are metabolized by CYP2D6 or CYP3A4). Products include:

Foradil Aerolizer 2849
Perforomist Inhalation Solution 1025

Fosamprenavir Calcium (The concomitant use of strong CYP3A4 inhibitors should be avoided. If patients must be co-administered a strong CYP3A4 inhibitor, based on pharmacokinetic studies, a Torisel dose reduction to 12.5mg/week should be considered. This dose is predicted to adjust the AUC to the range observed without inhibitors. However, there are no clinical data with this dose adjustment in patients receiving strong CYP3A4 inhibitors. If strong inhibitor is discontimued, a washout period of approximately 1 week should be allowed before the Torisel dose is adjusted back to the dose used prior to initiation of the strong CYP3A4 inhibitor). Products include:

Lexiva Oral Suspension 1510
Lexiva Tablets 1510

Fosphenytoin Sodium (The concomitant use of strong CYP3A4 inducers should be avoided. If patients must be co-administered a strong CYP3A4 inducer, based on pharmacokinetic studies, a Torisel dose increase from 25mg/week up to 50mg/week should be considered. This dose of Torisel is predicted to adjust the AUC to the range observed without inducers. However, there are no clinical data with this dose adjustment in patients receiving strong CYP3A4 inducers. If the strong inducer is discontinued, the temsirolimus dose should be returned to the dose used prior to initiation of the strong CYP3A4 inducer).

No products indexed under this heading.

Galantamine Hydrobromide (The concentration of desipramin, a CYP2D6 substrate, was unaffected when 25mg of Torisel was co-administered. No clinically significant effect is anticipated when temsirolimus is co-administered with agents that are metabolized by CYP2D6 or CYP3A4).

No products indexed under this heading.

Garlic Extract (The concomitant use of strong CYP3A4 inducers should be avoided. If patients must be co-administered a strong CYP3A4 inducer, based on pharmacokinetic studies, a Torisel dose increase from 25mg/week up to 50mg/week should be considered. This dose of Torisel is predicted to adjust the AUC to the range observed without inducers. However, there are no clinical data with this dose adjustment in patients receiving strong CYP3A4 inducers. If the strong inducer is discontinued, the temsirolimus dose should be returned to the dose used prior to initiation of the strong CYP3A4 inducer).

No products indexed under this heading.

Garlic Oil (The concomitant use of strong CYP3A4 inducers should be avoided. If patients must be co-administered a strong CYP3A4 inducer, based on pharmacokinetic studies, a Torisel dose increase from 25mg/week up to 50mg/week should be considered. This dose of Torisel is predicted to adjust the AUC to the range observed without inducers. However, there are no clinical data with this dose adjustment in patients receiving strong CYP3A4 inducers. If the strong inducer is discontinued, the temsirolimus dose should be returned to the dose used prior to initiation of the strong CYP3A4 inducer).

No products indexed under this heading.

Haloperidol (The concentration of desipramin, a CYP2D6 substrate, was unaffected when 25mg of Torisel was co-administered. No clinically significant effect is anticipated when temsirolimus is co-administered with agents that are metabolized by CYP2D6 or CYP3A4).

No products indexed under this heading.

Haloperidol Decanoate (The concentration of desipramin, a CYP2D6 substrate, was unaffected when 25mg of Torisel was co-administered. No clinically significant effect is anticipated when temsirolimus is co-administered with agents that are metabolized by CYP2D6 or CYP3A4).

No products indexed under this heading.

Hydrocodone Bitartrate (The concentration of desipramin, a CYP2D6 substrate, was unaffected when 25mg of Torisel was co-administered. No clinically significant effect is anticipated when temsirolimus is co-administered with agents that are metabolized by CYP2D6 or CYP3A4). Products include:

Lortab 5/500 Tablets 3143
Lortab 7.5/500 Tablets 3144
Lortab 10/500 Tablets 3144
Vicodin Tablets 529
Vicodin ES Tablets 530
Vicodin HP Tablets 531
Vicoprofen Tablets 533
Zydone Tablets 1132

Hydrocortisone (The concomitant use of strong CYP3A4 inducers should be avoided. If patients must be co-administered a strong CYP3A4 inducer, based on pharmacokinetic studies, a Torisel dose increase from 25mg/week up to 50mg/week should be considered. This dose of Torisel is predicted to adjust the AUC to the range observed without inducers. However, there are no clinical data with this dose adjustment in patients receiving strong CYP3A4 inducers. If the strong inducer is discontinued, the temsirolimus dose should be returned to the dose used prior to initiation of the strong CYP3A4 inducer).

No products indexed under this heading.

Hydrocortisone Acetate (The concomitant use of strong CYP3A4 inducers should be avoided. If patients must be co-administered a strong CYP3A4 inducer, based on pharmacokinetic studies, a Torisel dose increase from 25mg/week up to 50mg/week should be considered. This dose of Torisel is predicted to adjust the AUC to the range observed without inducers. However, there are no clinical data with this dose adjustment in patients receiving strong CYP3A4 inducers. If the strong inducer is discontinued, the temsirolimus dose should be returned to the dose used prior to initiation of the strong CYP3A4 inducer). Products include:

Analpram-HC 1140
Pramosone 1141

Hydrocortisone Butyrate (The concomitant use of strong CYP3A4 inducers should be avoided. If patients must be co-administered a strong CYP3A4 inducer, based on pharmacokinetic studies, a Torisel dose increase from 25mg/week up to 50mg/week should be considered. This dose of Torisel is predicted to adjust the AUC to the range observed without inducers. However, there are no clinical data with this dose adjustment in patients receiving strong CYP3A4 inducers. If the strong inducer is discontinued, the temsirolimus dose should be returned to the dose used prior to initiation of the strong CYP3A4 inducer).

No products indexed under this heading.

Hydrocortisone Cypionate (The concomitant use of strong CYP3A4 inducers should be avoided. If patients must be co-administered a strong CYP3A4 inducer, based on pharmacokinetic studies, a Torisel dose increase from 25mg/week up to 50mg/week should be considered. This dose of Torisel is predicted to adjust the AUC to the range observed without inducers. However, there are no clinical data with this dose adjustment in patients receiving strong CYP3A4 inducers. If the strong inducer is discontinued, the temsirolimus dose should be returned to the dose used prior to initiation of the strong CYP3A4 inducer).

No products indexed under this heading.

Hydrocortisone Hemisuccinate (The concomitant use of strong CYP3A4 inducers should be avoided. If patients must be co-administered a strong CYP3A4 inducer, based on pharmacokinetic studies, a Torisel dose increase from 25mg/week up to 50mg/week should be considered. This dose of Torisel is predicted to adjust the AUC to the range observed without inducers. However, there are no clinical data with this dose adjustment in patients receiving strong CYP3A4 inducers. If the strong inducer is discontinued, the temsirolimus dose should be returned to the dose used prior to initiation of the strong CYP3A4 inducer).

No products indexed under this heading.

Hydrocortisone Probutate (The concomitant use of strong CYP3A4 inducers should be avoided. If patients must be co-administered a strong CYP3A4 inducer, based on pharmacokinetic studies, a Torisel dose increase from 25mg/week up to 50mg/week should be considered. This dose of Torisel is predicted to adjust the AUC to the range observed without inducers. However, there are no clinical data with this dose adjustment in patients receiving strong CYP3A4 inducers. If the strong inducer is discontinued, the temsirolimus dose should be returned to the dose used prior to initiation of the strong CYP3A4 inducer).

No products indexed under this heading.

Hydrocortisone Sodium Phosphate (The concomitant use of strong CYP3A4 inducers should be avoided. If patients must be co-administered a strong CYP3A4 inducer, based on pharmacokinetic studies, a Torisel dose increase from 25mg/week up to 50mg/week should be considered. This dose of Torisel is predicted to adjust the AUC to the range observed without inducers. However, there are no clinical data with this dose adjustment in patients receiving strong CYP3A4 inducers. If the strong inducer is discontinued, the temsirolimus dose should be returned to the dose used prior to initiation of the strong CYP3A4 inducer).

No products indexed under this heading.

Hydrocortisone Sodium Succinate (The concomitant use of strong CYP3A4 inducers should be avoided. If patients must be co-administered a strong CYP3A4 inducer, based on pharmacokinetic studies, a Torisel dose increase from 25mg/week up to 50mg/week should be considered. This dose of Torisel is predicted to adjust the AUC to the range observed without inducers. However, there are no clinical data with this dose adjustment in patients receiving strong CYP3A4 inducers. If the strong inducer is discontinued, the temsirolimus dose should be returned to the dose used prior to initiation of the strong CYP3A4 inducer).

No products indexed under this heading.

Hydrocortisone Valerate (The concomitant use of strong CYP3A4 inducers should be avoided. If patients must be co-administered a strong CYP3A4 inducer, based on pharmacokinetic studies, a Torisel dose increase from 25mg/week up to 50mg/week should be considered. This dose of Torisel is predicted to adjust the AUC to the range observed without inducers. However, there are no clinical data with this dose adjustment in patients receiving strong CYP3A4 inducers. If the strong inducer is discontinued, the temsirolimus dose should be returned to the dose used prior to initiation of the strong CYP3A4 inducer).

No products indexed under this heading.

Hypericum (The concomitant use of strong CYP3A4 inducers should be avoided. If patients must be co-administered a strong CYP3A4 inducer, based on pharmacokinetic studies, a Torisel dose increase from 25mg/week up to 50mg/week should be considered. This dose of Torisel is predicted to adjust the AUC to the range observed without inducers. However, there are no clinical data with this dose adjustment in patients receiving strong CYP3A4 inducers. If the strong inducer is discontinued, the temsirolimus dose should be returned to the dose used prior to initiation of the strong CYP3A4 inducer). Products include:

Satieté Tablets 640

Hypericum Perforatum (May decrease Torisel plasma concentration unpredictably).
No products indexed under this heading.

Imipramine Hydrochloride (The concentration of desipramin, a CYP2D6 substrate, was unaffected when 25mg of Torisel was co-administered. No clinically significant effect is anticipated when temsirolimus is co-administered with agents that are metabolized by CYP2D6 or CYP3A4).
No products indexed under this heading.

Imipramine Pamoate (The concentration of desipramin, a CYP2D6 substrate, was unaffected when 25mg of Torisel was co-administered. No clinically significant effect is anticipated when temsirolimus is co-administered with agents that are metabolized by CYP2D6 or CYP3A4).
No products indexed under this heading.

Indinavir Sulfate (The concomitant use of strong CYP3A4 inhibitors should be avoided. If patients must be co-administered a strong CYP3A4 inhibitor, based on pharmacokinetic studies, a Torisel dose reduction to 12.5mg/week should be considered. This dose is predicted to adjust the AUC to the range observed without inhibitors. However, there are no clinical data with this dose adjustment in patients receiving strong CYP3A4 inhibitors. If strong inhibitor is discontimued, a washout period of approximately 1 week should be allowed before the Torisel dose is adjusted back to the dose used prior to initiation of the strong CYP3A4 inhibitor). Products include:
Crixivan Capsules 1979

Indoramin Hydrochloride (The concentration of desipramin, a CYP2D6 substrate, was unaffected when 25mg of Torisel was co-administered. No clinically significant effect is anticipated when temsirolimus is co-administered with agents that are metabolized by CYP2D6 or CYP3A4).
No products indexed under this heading.

Influenza Vaccine, Live Attenuated (The use of live vaccines and close contact with those who have received live vaccines should be avoided).
No products indexed under this heading.

Influenza Virus Vaccine Live, Intranasal (The use of live vaccines and close contact with those who have received live vaccines should be avoided). Products include:
FluMist Vaccine 1945

Itraconazole (The concomitant use of strong CYP3A4 inhibitors should be avoided. If patients must be co-administered a strong CYP3A4 inhibitor, based on pharmacokinetic studies, a Torisel dose reduction to 12.5mg/week should be considered. This dose is predicted to adjust the AUC to the range observed without inhibitors. However, there are no clinical data with this dose adjustment in patients receiving strong CYP3A4 inhibitors. If strong inhibitor is discontimued, a washout period of approximately 1 week should be allowed before the Torisel dose is adjusted back to the dose used prior to initiation of the strong CYP3A4 inhibitor).
No products indexed under this heading.

Ketoconazole (The concomitant use of strong CYP3A4 inhibitors should be avoided. If patients must be co-administered a strong CYP3A4 inhibitor, based on pharmacokinetic studies, a Torisel dose reduction to 12.5mg/week should be considered. This dose is predicted to adjust the AUC to the range observed without inhibitors. However, there are no clinical data with this dose adjustment in patients receiving strong CYP3A4 inhibitors. If strong inhibitor is discontimued, a washout period of approximately 1 week should be allowed before the Torisel dose is adjusted back to the dose used prior to initiation of the strong CYP3A4 inhibitor). Products include:
Extina Foam, 2% 3057
Nizoral A-D Shampoo 1901

Labetalol Hydrochloride (The concentration of desipramin, a CYP2D6 substrate, was unaffected when 25mg of Torisel was co-administered. No clinically significant effect is anticipated when temsirolimus is co-administered with agents that are metabolized by CYP2D6 or CYP3A4).
No products indexed under this heading.

Lidocaine (The concentration of desipramin, a CYP2D6 substrate, was unaffected when 25mg of Torisel was co-administered. No clinically significant effect is anticipated when temsirolimus is co-administered with agents that are metabolized by CYP2D6 or CYP3A4). Products include:
Lidoderm Patch 1114

Lidocaine Hydrochloride (The concentration of desipramin, a CYP2D6 substrate, was unaffected when 25mg of Torisel was co-administered. No clinically significant effect is anticipated when temsirolimus is co-administered with agents that are metabolized by CYP2D6 or CYP3A4).
No products indexed under this heading.

Lopinavir (The concomitant use of strong CYP3A4 inhibitors should be avoided. If patients must be co-administered a strong CYP3A4 inhibitor, based on pharmacokinetic studies, a Torisel dose reduction to 12.5mg/week should be considered. This dose is predicted to adjust the AUC to the range observed without inhibitors. However, there are no clinical data with this dose adjustment in patients receiving strong CYP3A4 inhibitors. If strong inhibitor is discontimued, a washout period of approximately 1 week should be allowed before the Torisel dose is adjusted back to the dose used prior to initiation of the strong CYP3A4 inhibitor). Products include:
Kaletra 452

Maprotiline Hydrochloride (The concentration of desipramin, a CYP2D6 substrate, was unaffected when 25mg of Torisel was co-administered. No clinically significant effect is anticipated when temsirolimus is co-administered with agents that are metabolized by CYP2D6 or CYP3A4).
No products indexed under this heading.

Measles, Mumps, Rubella and Varicella Virus Vaccine Live (The use of live vaccines and close contact with those who have received live vaccines should be avoided). Products include:
ProQuad 2099

Measles, Mumps & Rubella Virus Vaccine, Live (The use of live vaccines and close contact with those who have received live vaccines should be avoided). Products include:
M-M-R II 2054

Measles & Rubella Virus Vaccine Live (The use of live vaccines and close contact with those who have received live vaccines should be avoided).
No products indexed under this heading.

Measles Virus Vaccine Live (The use of live vaccines and close contact with those who have received live vaccines should be avoided). Products include:
Attenuvax 1951

Meperidine Hydrochloride (The concentration of desipramin, a CYP2D6 substrate, was unaffected when 25mg of Torisel was co-administered. No clinically significant effect is anticipated when temsirolimus is co-administered with agents that are metabolized by CYP2D6 or CYP3A4).
No products indexed under this heading.

Mephenytoin (The concomitant use of strong CYP3A4 inducers should be avoided. If patients must be co-administered a strong CYP3A4 inducer, based on pharmacokinetic studies, a Torisel dose increase from 25mg/week up to 50mg/week should be considered. This dose of Torisel is predicted to adjust the AUC to the range observed without inducers. However, there are no clinical data with this dose adjustment in patients receiving strong CYP3A4 inducers. If the strong inducer is discontinued, the temsirolimus dose should be returned to the dose used prior to initiation of the strong CYP3A4 inducer).
No products indexed under this heading.

Methadone Hydrochloride (The concentration of desipramin, a CYP2D6 substrate, was unaffected when 25mg of Torisel was co-administered. No clinically significant effect is anticipated when temsirolimus is co-administered with agents that are metabolized by CYP2D6 or CYP3A4).
No products indexed under this heading.

Methamphetamine Hydrochloride (The concentration of desipramin, a CYP2D6 substrate, was unaffected when 25mg of Torisel was co-administered. No clinically significant effect is anticipated when temsirolimus is co-administered with agents that are metabolized by CYP2D6 or CYP3A4).
No products indexed under this heading.

Methsuximide (The concomitant use of strong CYP3A4 inducers should be avoided. If patients must be co-administered a strong CYP3A4 inducer, based on pharmacokinetic studies, a Torisel dose increase from 25mg/week up to 50mg/week should be considered. This dose of Torisel is predicted to adjust the AUC to the range observed without inducers. However, there are no clinical data with this dose adjustment in patients receiving strong CYP3A4 inducers. If the strong inducer is discontinued, the temsirolimus dose should be returned to the dose used prior to initiation of the strong CYP3A4 inducer).
No products indexed under this heading.

Methylprednisolone (The concomitant use of strong CYP3A4 inducers should be avoided. If patients must be co-administered a strong CYP3A4 inducer, based on pharmacokinetic studies, a Torisel dose increase from 25mg/week up to 50mg/week should be considered. This dose of Torisel is predicted to adjust the AUC to the range observed without inducers. However, there are no clinical data with this dose adjustment in patients receiving strong CYP3A4 inducers. If the strong inducer is discontinued, the temsirolimus dose should be returned to the dose used prior to initiation of the strong CYP3A4 inducer).
No products indexed under this heading.

Methylprednisolone Acetate (The concomitant use of strong CYP3A4 inducers should be avoided. If patients must be co-administered a strong CYP3A4 inducer, based on pharmacokinetic studies, a Torisel dose increase from 25mg/week up to 50mg/week should be considered. This dose of Torisel is predicted to adjust the AUC to the range observed without inducers. However, there are no clinical data with this dose adjustment in patients receiving strong CYP3A4 inducers. If the strong inducer is discontinued, the temsirolimus dose should be returned to the dose used prior to initiation of the strong CYP3A4 inducer).
No products indexed under this heading.

Methylprednisolone Sodium Succinate (The concomitant use of strong CYP3A4 inducers should be avoided. If patients must be co-administered a strong CYP3A4 inducer, based on pharmacokinetic studies, a Torisel dose increase from 25mg/week up to 50mg/week should be considered. This dose of Torisel is predicted to adjust the AUC to the range observed without inducers. However, there are no clinical data with this dose adjustment in patients receiving strong CYP3A4 inducers. If the strong inducer is

discontinued, the temsirolimus dose should be returned to the dose used prior to initiation of the strong CYP3A4 inducer).

No products indexed under this heading.

Metoprolol Succinate (The concentration of desipramin, a CYP2D6 substrate, was unaffected when 25mg of Torisel was co-administered. No clinically significant effect is anticipated when temsirolimus is co-administered with agents that are metabolized by CYP2D6 or CYP3A4). Products include:

Toprol-XL Tablets **666**

Metoprolol Tartrate (The concentration of desipramin, a CYP2D6 substrate, was unaffected when 25mg of Torisel was co-administered. No clinically significant effect is anticipated when temsirolimus is co-administered with agents that are metabolized by CYP2D6 or CYP3A4).

No products indexed under this heading.

Mexiletine Hydrochloride (The concentration of desipramin, a CYP2D6 substrate, was unaffected when 25mg of Torisel was co-administered. No clinically significant effect is anticipated when temsirolimus is co-administered with agents that are metabolized by CYP2D6 or CYP3A4).

No products indexed under this heading.

Mirtazapine (The concentration of desipramin, a CYP2D6 substrate, was unaffected when 25mg of Torisel was co-administered. No clinically significant effect is anticipated when temsirolimus is co-administered with agents that are metabolized by CYP2D6 or CYP3A4). Products include:

Remeron Tablets **2924**
RemeronSolTab Tablets **2927**

Modafinil (The concomitant use of strong CYP3A4 inducers should be avoided. If patients must be co-administered a strong CYP3A4 inducer, based on pharmacokinetic studies, a Torisel dose increase from 25mg/week up to 50mg/week should be considered. This dose of Torisel is predicted to adjust the AUC to the range observed without inducers. However, there are no clinical data with this dose adjustment in patients receiving strong CYP3A4 inducers. If the strong inducer is discontinued, the temsirolimus dose should be returned to the dose used prior to initiation of the strong CYP3A4 inducer). Products include:

Provigil Tablets **977**

Morphine Sulfate (The concentration of desipramin, a CYP2D6 substrate, was unaffected when 25mg of Torisel was co-administered. No clinically significant effect is anticipated when temsirolimus is co-administered with agents that are metabolized by CYP2D6 or CYP3A4). Products include:

Avinza Capsules **1772**
DepoDur Injection **1095**
MS Contin Tablets **2585**

Mumps Virus Vaccine, Live (The use of live vaccines and close contact with those who have received live vaccines should be avoided). Products include:

Mumpsvax **2068**

Nefazodone Hydrochloride (The concomitant use of strong CYP3A4 inhibitors should be avoided. If patients must be co-administered a strong CYP3A4 inhibitor, based on pharmacokinetic studies, a Torisel dose reduction to 12.5mg/week should be considered. This dose is predicted to adjust the AUC to the range observed without inhibitors. However, there are no clinical data with this dose adjustment in patients receiving strong CYP3A4 inhibitors. If strong inhibitor is discontimued, a washout period of approximately 1 week should be allowed before the Torisel dose is adjusted back to the dose used prior to initiation of the strong CYP3A4 inhibitor).

No products indexed under this heading.

Nelfinavir Mesylate (The concomitant use of strong CYP3A4 inhibitors should be avoided. If patients must be co-administered a strong CYP3A4 inhibitor, based on pharmacokinetic studies, a Torisel dose reduction to 12.5mg/week should be considered. This dose is predicted to adjust the AUC to the range observed without inhibitors. However, there are no clinical data with this dose adjustment in patients receiving strong CYP3A4 inhibitors. If strong inhibitor is discontimued, a washout period of approximately 1 week should be allowed before the Torisel dose is adjusted back to the dose used prior to initiation of the strong CYP3A4 inhibitor).

No products indexed under this heading.

Nevirapine (The concomitant use of strong CYP3A4 inducers should be avoided. If patients must be co-administered a strong CYP3A4 inducer, based on pharmacokinetic studies, a Torisel dose increase from 25mg/week up to 50mg/week should be considered. This dose of Torisel is predicted to adjust the AUC to the range observed without inducers. However, there are no clinical data with this dose adjustment in patients receiving strong CYP3A4 inducers. If the strong inducer is discontinued, the temsirolimus dose should be returned to the dose used prior to initiation of the strong CYP3A4 inducer). Products include:

Viramune Oral Suspension **873**
Viramune Tablets **873**

Nortriptyline Hydrochloride (The concentration of desipramin, a CYP2D6 substrate, was unaffected when 25mg of Torisel was co-administered. No clinically significant effect is anticipated when temsirolimus is co-administered with agents that are metabolized by CYP2D6 or CYP3A4).

No products indexed under this heading.

Olanzapine (The concentration of desipramin, a CYP2D6 substrate, was unaffected when 25mg of Torisel was co-administered. No clinically significant effect is anticipated when temsirolimus is co-administered with agents that are metabolized by CYP2D6 or CYP3A4). Products include:

Symbyax Capsules **1871**
Zyprexa Tablets **1883**
Zyprexa IntraMuscular **1883**
Zyprexa ZYDIS Orally Disintegrating Tablets **1883**

Omeprazole (The concentration of desipramin, a CYP2D6 substrate, was unaffected when 25mg of Torisel was co-administered. No clinically significant effect is anticipated when temsirolimus is co-administered with agents that are metabolized by CYP2D6 or CYP3A4).

No products indexed under this heading.

Ondansetron (The concentration of desipramin, a CYP2D6 substrate, was unaffected when 25mg of Torisel was co-administered. No clinically significant effect is anticipated when temsirolimus is co-administered with agents that are metabolized by CYP2D6 or CYP3A4). Products include:

Zofran ODT Orally Disintegrating Tablets **1687**

Ondansetron Hydrochloride (The concentration of desipramin, a CYP2D6 substrate, was unaffected when 25mg of Torisel was co-administered. No clinically significant effect is anticipated when temsirolimus is co-administered with agents that are metabolized by CYP2D6 or CYP3A4). Products include:

Zofran Injection **1682**
Zofran **1687**

Oxcarbazepine (The concomitant use of strong CYP3A4 inducers should be avoided. If patients must be co-administered a strong CYP3A4 inducer, based on pharmacokinetic studies, a Torisel dose increase from 25mg/week up to 50mg/week should be considered. This dose of Torisel is predicted to adjust the AUC to the range observed without inducers. However, there are no clinical data with this dose adjustment in patients receiving strong CYP3A4 inducers. If the strong inducer is discontinued, the temsirolimus dose should be returned to the dose used prior to initiation of the strong CYP3A4 inducer).

No products indexed under this heading.

Oxycodone Hydrochloride (The concentration of desipramin, a CYP2D6 substrate, was unaffected when 25mg of Torisel was co-administered. No clinically significant effect is anticipated when temsirolimus is co-administered with agents that are metabolized by CYP2D6 or CYP3A4). Products include:

OxyContin Tablets **2589**
OxyIR Capsules **2593**
Percocet Tablets **1127**
Percodan Tablets **1130**

Paclitaxel (The concentration of desipramin, a CYP2D6 substrate, was unaffected when 25mg of Torisel was co-administered. No clinically significant effect is anticipated when temsirolimus is co-administered with agents that are metabolized by CYP2D6 or CYP3A4).

No products indexed under this heading.

Paroxetine Hydrochloride (The concentration of desipramin, a CYP2D6 substrate, was unaffected when 25mg of Torisel was co-administered. No clinically significant effect is anticipated when temsirolimus is co-administered with agents that are metabolized by CYP2D6 or CYP3A4). Products include:

Paxil **1535**
Paxil CR Controlled-Release Tablets **1544**

Phenobarbital (The concomitant use of strong CYP3A4 inducers should be avoided. If patients must be co-administered a strong CYP3A4 inducer, based on pharmacokinetic studies, a Torisel dose increase from 25mg/week up to 50mg/week should be considered. This dose of Torisel is predicted to adjust the AUC to the range observed without inducers. However, there are no clinical data with this dose adjustment in patients receiving strong CYP3A4 inducers. If the strong inducer is discontinued, the temsirolimus dose should be returned to the dose used prior to initiation of the strong CYP3A4 inducer). Products include:

Donnatal Extentabs **2507**

Phenobarbital Sodium (The concomitant use of strong CYP3A4 inducers should be avoided. If patients must be co-administered a strong CYP3A4 inducer, based on pharmacokinetic studies, a Torisel dose increase from 25mg/week up to 50mg/week should be considered. This dose of Torisel is predicted to adjust the AUC to the range observed without inducers. However, there are no clinical data with this dose adjustment in patients receiving strong CYP3A4 inducers. If the strong inducer is discontinued, the temsirolimus dose should be returned to the dose used prior to initiation of the strong CYP3A4 inducer).

No products indexed under this heading.

Phenytoin (The concomitant use of strong CYP3A4 inducers should be avoided. If patients must be co-administered a strong CYP3A4 inducer, based on pharmacokinetic studies, a Torisel dose increase from 25mg/week up to 50mg/week should be considered. This dose of Torisel is predicted to adjust the AUC to the range observed without inducers. However, there are no clinical data with this dose adjustment in patients receiving strong CYP3A4 inducers. If the strong inducer is discontinued, the temsirolimus dose should be returned to the dose used prior to initiation of the strong CYP3A4 inducer).

No products indexed under this heading.

Phenytoin Sodium (The concomitant use of strong CYP3A4 inducers should be avoided. If patients must be co-administered a strong CYP3A4 inducer, based on pharmacokinetic studies, a Torisel dose increase from 25mg/week up to 50mg/week should be considered. This dose of Torisel is predicted to adjust the AUC to the range observed without inducers. However, there are no clinical data with this dose adjustment in patients receiving strong CYP3A4 inducers. If the strong inducer is discontinued, the temsirolimus dose should be returned to the dose used prior to initiation of the strong CYP3A4 inducer). Products include:

Phenytek Capsules **2192**

Pindolol (The concentration of desipramin, a CYP2D6 substrate, was unaffected when 25mg of Torisel was co-administered. No clinically significant effect is anticipated when temsirolimus is co-administered with agents that are metabolized by CYP2D6 or CYP3A4).

No products indexed under this heading.

Poliovirus Vaccine, Live, Oral, Trivalent, Types 1,2,3 (Sabin) (The use of live vaccines and close contact with those who have received live vaccines should be avoided).

No products indexed under this heading.

Prednisolone Acetate (The concomitant use of strong CYP3A4 inducers should be avoided. If patients must be co-administered a strong CYP3A4 inducer, based on pharmacokinetic studies, a Torisel dose increase from 25mg/week up to 50mg/week should be considered. This dose of Torisel is predicted to adjust the AUC to the range observed without inducers. However, there are no clinical data with this dose adjustment in patients receiving strong CYP3A4 inducers. If the strong inducer is discontinued, the temsirolimus dose should be returned to the dose used prior to initiation of the strong CYP3A4 inducer). Products include:

Pred Forte Ophthalmic Suspension ⊙ 227
Pred Mild Ophthalmic Suspension ⊙ 230
Pred-G Ophthalmic Ointment ⊙ 229
Pred-G Ophthalmic Suspension ⊙ 228

Prednisolone Sodium Phosphate (The concomitant use of strong CYP3A4 inducers should be avoided. If patients must be co-administered a strong CYP3A4 inducer, based on pharmacokinetic studies, a Torisel dose increase from 25mg/week up to 50mg/week should be considered. This dose of Torisel is predicted to adjust the AUC to the range observed without inducers. However, there are no clinical data with this dose adjustment in patients receiving strong CYP3A4 inducers. If the strong inducer is discontinued, the temsirolimus dose should be returned to the dose used prior to initiation of the strong CYP3A4 inducer).

No products indexed under this heading.

Prednisolone Tebutate (The concomitant use of strong CYP3A4 inducers should be avoided. If patients must be co-administered a strong CYP3A4 inducer, based on pharmacokinetic studies, a Torisel dose increase from 25mg/week up to 50mg/week should be considered. This dose of Torisel is predicted to adjust the AUC to the range observed without inducers. However, there are no clinical data with this dose adjustment in patients receiving strong CYP3A4 inducers. If the strong inducer is discontinued, the temsirolimus dose should be returned to the dose used prior to initiation of the strong CYP3A4 inducer).

No products indexed under this heading.

Prednisone (The concomitant use of strong CYP3A4 inducers should be avoided. If patients must be co-administered a strong CYP3A4 inducer, based on pharmacokinetic studies, a Torisel dose increase from 25mg/week up to 50mg/week should be considered. This dose of Torisel is predicted to adjust the AUC to the range observed without inducers. However, there are no clinical data with this dose adjustment in patients receiving strong CYP3A4 inducers. If the strong inducer is discontinued, the temsirolimus dose should be returned to the dose used prior to initiation of the strong CYP3A4 inducer).

No products indexed under this heading.

Primidone (The concomitant use of strong CYP3A4 inducers should be avoided. If patients must be co-administered a strong CYP3A4 inducer, based on pharmacokinetic studies, a Torisel dose increase from 25mg/week up to 50mg/week should be considered. This dose of Torisel is predicted to adjust the AUC to the range observed without inducers. However, there are no clinical data with this dose adjustment in patients receiving strong CYP3A4 inducers. If the strong inducer is discontinued, the temsirolimus dose should be returned to the dose used prior to initiation of the strong CYP3A4 inducer).

No products indexed under this heading.

Propafenone Hydrochloride (The concentration of desipramin, a CYP2D6 substrate, was unaffected when 25mg of Torisel was co-administered. No clinically significant effect is anticipated when temsirolimus is co-administered with agents that are metabolized by CYP2D6 or CYP3A4). Products include:

Rythmol Tablets 1586
Rythmol SR Capsules 1590

Propoxyphene Hydrochloride (The concentration of desipramin, a CYP2D6 substrate, was unaffected when 25mg of Torisel was co-administered. No clinically significant effect is anticipated when temsirolimus is co-administered with agents that are metabolized by CYP2D6 or CYP3A4).

No products indexed under this heading.

Propoxyphene Napsylate (The concentration of desipramin, a CYP2D6 substrate, was unaffected when 25mg of Torisel was co-administered. No clinically significant effect is anticipated when temsirolimus is co-administered with agents that are metabolized by CYP2D6 or CYP3A4).

No products indexed under this heading.

Propranolol Hydrochloride (The concentration of desipramin, a CYP2D6 substrate, was unaffected when 25mg of Torisel was co-administered. No clinically significant effect is anticipated when temsirolimus is co-administered with agents that are metabolized by CYP2D6 or CYP3A4). Products include:

InnoPran XL Extended Release Capsules 1484

Quetiapine Fumarate (The concentration of desipramin, a CYP2D6 substrate, was unaffected when 25mg of Torisel was co-administered. No clinically significant effect is anticipated when temsirolimus is co-administered with agents that are metabolized by CYP2D6 or CYP3A4).

No products indexed under this heading.

Quinidine Gluconate (The concentration of desipramin, a CYP2D6 substrate, was unaffected when 25mg of Torisel was co-administered. No clinically significant effect is anticipated when temsirolimus is co-administered with agents that are metabolized by CYP2D6 or CYP3A4).

No products indexed under this heading.

Quinidine Hydrochloride (The concentration of desipramin, a CYP2D6 substrate, was unaffected when 25mg of Torisel was co-administered. No clinically significant effect is anticipated when temsirolimus is co-administered with agents that are metabolized by CYP2D6 or CYP3A4).

No products indexed under this heading.

Quinidine Polygalacturonate (The concentration of desipramin, a CYP2D6 substrate, was unaffected when 25mg of Torisel was co-administered. No clinically significant effect is anticipated when temsirolimus is co-administered with agents that are metabolized by CYP2D6 or CYP3A4).

No products indexed under this heading.

Quinidine Sulfate (The concentration of desipramin, a CYP2D6 substrate, was unaffected when 25mg of Torisel was co-administered. No clinically significant effect is anticipated when temsirolimus is co-administered with agents that are metabolized by CYP2D6 or CYP3A4).

No products indexed under this heading.

Rifabutin (The concomitant use of strong CYP3A4 inducers should be avoided. If patients must be co-administered a strong CYP3A4 inducer, based on pharmacokinetic studies, a Torisel dose increase from 25mg/week up to 50mg/week should be considered. This dose of Torisel is predicted to adjust the AUC to the range observed without inducers. However, there are no clinical data with this dose adjustment in patients receiving strong CYP3A4 inducers. If the strong inducer is discontinued, the temsirolimus dose should be returned to the dose used prior to initiation of the strong CYP3A4 inducer).

No products indexed under this heading.

Rifampicin (The concomitant use of strong CYP3A4 inducers should be avoided. If patients must be co-administered a strong CYP3A4 inducer, based on pharmacokinetic studies, a Torisel dose increase from 25mg/week up to 50mg/week should be considered. This dose of Torisel is predicted to adjust the AUC to the range observed without inducers. However, there are no clinical data with this dose adjustment in patients receiving strong CYP3A4 inducers. If the strong inducer is discontinued, the temsirolimus dose should be returned to the dose used prior to initiation of the strong CYP3A4 inducer).

No products indexed under this heading.

Rifampin (The concomitant use of strong CYP3A4 inducers should be avoided. If patients must be co-administered a strong CYP3A4 inducer, based on pharmacokinetic studies, a Torisel dose increase from 25mg/week up to 50mg/week should be considered. This dose of Torisel is predicted to adjust the AUC to the range observed without inducers. However, there are no clinical data with this dose adjustment in patients receiving strong CYP3A4 inducers. If the strong inducer is discontinued, the temsirolimus dose should be returned to the dose used prior to initiation of the strong CYP3A4 inducer).

No products indexed under this heading.

Rifapentine (The concomitant use of strong CYP3A4 inducers should be avoided. If patients must be co-administered a strong CYP3A4 inducer, based on pharmacokinetic studies, a Torisel dose increase from 25mg/week up to 50mg/week should be considered. This dose of Torisel is predicted to adjust the AUC to the range observed without inducers. However, there are no clinical data with this dose adjustment in patients receiving strong CYP3A4 inducers. If the strong inducer is discontinued, the temsirolimus dose should be returned to the dose used prior to initiation of the strong CYP3A4 inducer).

No products indexed under this heading.

Risperidone (The concentration of desipramin, a CYP2D6 substrate, was unaffected when 25mg of Torisel was co-administered. No clinically significant effect is anticipated when temsirolimus is co-administered with agents that are metabolized by CYP2D6 or CYP3A4). Products include:

Risperdal Consta Long-Acting Injection 1753

Ritonavir (The concomitant use of strong CYP3A4 inhibitors should be avoided. If patients must be co-administered a strong CYP3A4 inhibitor, based on pharmacokinetic studies, a Torisel dose reduction to 12.5mg/week should be considered. This dose is predicted to adjust the AUC to the range observed without inhibitors. However, there are no clinical data with this dose adjustment in patients receiving strong CYP3A4 inhibitors. If strong inhibitor is discontimued, a washout period of approximately 1 week should be allowed before the Torisel dose is adjusted back to the dose used prior to initiation of the strong CYP3A4 inhibitor). Products include:

Kaletra 452
Norvir 489

Rotavirus Vaccine, Live, Oral, Tetravalent (The use of live vaccines and close contact with those who have received live vaccines should be avoided).

No products indexed under this heading.

Rubella & Mumps Virus Vaccine Live (The use of live vaccines and close contact with those who have received live vaccines should be avoided).
No products indexed under this heading.

Rubella Virus Vaccine Live (The use of live vaccines and close contact with those who have received live vaccines should be avoided). Products include:
Meruvax II 2061

Saquinavir (The concomitant use of strong CYP3A4 inhibitors should be avoided. If patients must be co-administered a strong CYP3A4 inhibitor, based on pharmacokinetic studies, a Torisel dose reduction to 12.5mg/week should be considered. This dose is predicted to adjust the AUC to the range observed without inhibitors. However, there are no clinical data with this dose adjustment in patients receiving strong CYP3A4 inhibitors. If strong inhibitor is discontimued, a washout period of approximately 1 week should be allowed before the Torisel dose is adjusted back to the dose used prior to initiation of the strong CYP3A4 inhibitor).
No products indexed under this heading.

Saquinavir Mesylate (The concomitant use of strong CYP3A4 inhibitors should be avoided. If patients must be co-administered a strong CYP3A4 inhibitor, based on pharmacokinetic studies, a Torisel dose reduction to 12.5mg/week should be considered. This dose is predicted to adjust the AUC to the range observed without inhibitors. However, there are no clinical data with this dose adjustment in patients receiving strong CYP3A4 inhibitors. If strong inhibitor is discontimued, a washout period of approximately 1 week should be allowed before the Torisel dose is adjusted back to the dose used prior to initiation of the strong CYP3A4 inhibitor).
No products indexed under this heading.

Smallpox Vaccine (The use of live vaccines and close contact with those who have received live vaccines should be avoided).
No products indexed under this heading.

Sulfinpyrazone (The concomitant use of strong CYP3A4 inducers should be avoided. If patients must be co-administered a strong CYP3A4 inducer, based on pharmacokinetic studies, a Torisel dose increase from 25mg/week up to 50mg/week should be considered. This dose of Torisel is predicted to adjust the AUC to the range observed without inducers. However, there are no clinical data with this dose adjustment in patients receiving strong CYP3A4 inducers. If the strong inducer is discontinued, the temsirolimus dose should be returned to the dose used prior to initiation of the strong CYP3A4 inducer).
No products indexed under this heading.

Sunitinib (The combination of Torisel and sunitinib resulted in dose-limiting toxicity).
No products indexed under this heading.

Tamoxifen Citrate (The concentration of desipramin, a CYP2D6 substrate, was unaffected when 25mg of Torisel was co-administered. No clinically significant effect is anticipated when temsirolimus is co-administered with agents that are metabolized by CYP2D6 or CYP3A4).
No products indexed under this heading.

Telithromycin (The concomitant use of strong CYP3A4 inhibitors should be avoided. If patients must be co-administered a strong CYP3A4 inhibitor, based on pharmacokinetic studies, a Torisel dose reduction to 12.5mg/week should be considered. This dose is predicted to adjust the AUC to the range observed without inhibitors. However, there are no clinical data with this dose adjustment in patients receiving strong CYP3A4 inhibitors. If strong inhibitor is discontimued, a washout period of approximately 1 week should be allowed before the Torisel dose is adjusted back to the dose used prior to initiation of the strong CYP3A4 inhibitor). Products include:
Ketek Tablets 2744

Teniposide (The concentration of desipramin, a CYP2D6 substrate, was unaffected when 25mg of Torisel was co-administered. No clinically significant effect is anticipated when temsirolimus is co-administered with agents that are metabolized by CYP2D6 or CYP3A4).
No products indexed under this heading.

Testosterone (The concentration of desipramin, a CYP2D6 substrate, was unaffected when 25mg of Torisel was co-administered. No clinically significant effect is anticipated when temsirolimus is co-administered with agents that are metabolized by CYP2D6 or CYP3A4). Products include:
AndroGel 3159
Testim 1% Gel 701

Testosterone Cypionate (The concentration of desipramin, a CYP2D6 substrate, was unaffected when 25mg of Torisel was co-administered. No clinically significant effect is anticipated when temsirolimus is co-administered with agents that are metabolized by CYP2D6 or CYP3A4).
No products indexed under this heading.

Testosterone Enanthate (The concentration of desipramin, a CYP2D6 substrate, was unaffected when 25mg of Torisel was co-administered. No clinically significant effect is anticipated when temsirolimus is co-administered with agents that are metabolized by CYP2D6 or CYP3A4). Products include:
Delatestryl Injection 1730

Testosterone Propionate (The concentration of desipramin, a CYP2D6 substrate, was unaffected when 25mg of Torisel was co-administered. No clinically significant effect is anticipated when temsirolimus is co-administered with agents that are metabolized by CYP2D6 or CYP3A4).
No products indexed under this heading.

Theophylline (The concomitant use of strong CYP3A4 inducers should be avoided. If patients must be co-administered a strong CYP3A4 inducer, based on pharmacokinetic studies, a Torisel dose increase from 25mg/week up to 50mg/week should be considered. This dose of Torisel is predicted to adjust the AUC to the range observed without inducers. However, there are no clinical data with this dose adjustment in patients receiving strong CYP3A4 inducers. If the strong inducer is discontinued, the temsirolimus dose should be returned to the dose used prior to initiation of the strong CYP3A4 inducer).
No products indexed under this heading.

Theophylline Anhydrous (The concomitant use of strong CYP3A4 inducers should be avoided. If patients must be co-administered a strong CYP3A4 inducer, based on pharmacokinetic studies, a Torisel dose increase from 25mg/week up to 50mg/week should be considered. This dose of Torisel is predicted to adjust the AUC to the range observed without inducers. However, there are no clinical data with this dose adjustment in patients receiving strong CYP3A4 inducers. If the strong inducer is discontinued, the temsirolimus dose should be returned to the dose used prior to initiation of the strong CYP3A4 inducer). Products include:
Uniphyl Tablets 2595

Theophylline Calcium Salicylate (The concomitant use of strong CYP3A4 inducers should be avoided. If patients must be co-administered a strong CYP3A4 inducer, based on pharmacokinetic studies, a Torisel dose increase from 25mg/week up to 50mg/week should be considered. This dose of Torisel is predicted to adjust the AUC to the range observed without inducers. However, there are no clinical data with this dose adjustment in patients receiving strong CYP3A4 inducers. If the strong inducer is discontinued, the temsirolimus dose should be returned to the dose used prior to initiation of the strong CYP3A4 inducer).
No products indexed under this heading.

Theophylline Dihydroxypropyl (Glyceryl) (The concomitant use of strong CYP3A4 inducers should be avoided. If patients must be co-administered a strong CYP3A4 inducer, based on pharmacokinetic studies, a Torisel dose increase from 25mg/week up to 50mg/week should be considered. This dose of Torisel is predicted to adjust the AUC to the range observed without inducers. However, there are no clinical data with this dose adjustment in patients receiving strong CYP3A4 inducers. If the strong inducer is discontinued, the temsirolimus dose should be returned to the dose used prior to initiation of the strong CYP3A4 inducer).
No products indexed under this heading.

Theophylline Ethylenediamine (The concomitant use of strong CYP3A4 inducers should be avoided. If patients must be co-administered a strong CYP3A4 inducer, based on pharmacokinetic studies, a Torisel dose increase from 25mg/week up to 50mg/week should be considered. This dose of Torisel is predicted to adjust the AUC to the range observed without inducers. However, there are no clinical data with this dose adjustment in patients receiving strong CYP3A4 inducers. If the strong inducer is discontinued, the temsirolimus dose should be returned to the dose used prior to initiation of the strong CYP3A4 inducer).
No products indexed under this heading.

Thioridazine (The concentration of desipramin, a CYP2D6 substrate, was unaffected when 25mg of Torisel was co-administered. No clinically significant effect is anticipated when temsirolimus is co-administered with agents that are metabolized by CYP2D6 or CYP3A4).
No products indexed under this heading.

Thioridazine Hydrochloride (The concentration of desipramin, a CYP2D6 substrate, was unaffected when 25mg of Torisel was co-administered. No clinically significant effect is anticipated when temsirolimus is co-administered with agents that are metabolized by CYP2D6 or CYP3A4). Products include:
Thioridazine Hydrochloride Tablets 2195

Timolol Maleate (The concentration of desipramin, a CYP2D6 substrate, was unaffected when 25mg of Torisel was co-administered. No clinically significant effect is anticipated when temsirolimus is co-administered with agents that are metabolized by CYP2D6 or CYP3A4). Products include:
Combigan Ophthalmic Solution 553
Cosopt Sterile Ophthalmic Solution 1969
Timoptic Sterile Ophthalmic Solution 2121
Timoptic in Ocudose 2124
Timoptic-XE Sterile Ophthalmic Gel Forming Solution 2125

Tolterodine Tartrate (The concentration of desipramin, a CYP2D6 substrate, was unaffected when 25mg of Torisel was co-administered. No clinically significant effect is anticipated when temsirolimus is co-administered with agents that are metabolized by CYP2D6 or CYP3A4).
No products indexed under this heading.

Tramadol Hydrochloride (The concentration of desipramin, a CYP2D6 substrate, was unaffected when 25mg of Torisel was co-administered. No clinically significant effect is anticipated when temsirolimus is co-administered with agents that are metabolized by CYP2D6 or CYP3A4). Products include:
Ultram ER Extended-Release Tablets 2428

Trazodone Hydrochloride (The concentration of desipramin, a CYP2D6 substrate, was unaffected when 25mg of Torisel was co-administered. No clinically significant effect is anticipated when temsirolimus is co-administered with agents that are metabolized by CYP2D6 or CYP3A4).
No products indexed under this heading.

Triamcinolone (The concomitant use of strong CYP3A4 inducers should be avoided. If patients must

be co-administered a strong CYP3A4 inducer, based on pharmacokinetic studies, a Torisel dose increase from 25mg/week up to 50mg/week should be considered. This dose of Torisel is predicted to adjust the AUC to the range observed without inducers. However, there are no clinical data with this dose adjustment in patients receiving strong CYP3A4 inducers. If the strong inducer is discontinued, the temsirolimus dose should be returned to the dose used prior to initiation of the strong CYP3A4 inducer).
No products indexed under this heading.

Triamcinolone Acetonide (The concomitant use of strong CYP3A4 inducers should be avoided. If patients must be co-administered a strong CYP3A4 inducer, based on pharmacokinetic studies, a Torisel dose increase from 25mg/week up to 50mg/week should be considered. This dose of Torisel is predicted to adjust the AUC to the range observed without inducers. However, there are no clinical data with this dose adjustment in patients receiving strong CYP3A4 inducers. If the strong inducer is discontinued, the temsirolimus dose should be returned to the dose used prior to initiation of the strong CYP3A4 inducer). Products include:
Azmacort Inhalation Aerosol **407**
Nasacort AQ Nasal Spray **2765**
Triesence Injectable Suspension .... ⊙**209**

Triamcinolone Diacetate (The concomitant use of strong CYP3A4 inducers should be avoided. If patients must be co-administered a strong CYP3A4 inducer, based on pharmacokinetic studies, a Torisel dose increase from 25mg/week up to 50mg/week should be considered. This dose of Torisel is predicted to adjust the AUC to the range observed without inducers. However, there are no clinical data with this dose adjustment in patients receiving strong CYP3A4 inducers. If the strong inducer is discontinued, the temsirolimus dose should be returned to the dose used prior to initiation of the strong CYP3A4 inducer).
No products indexed under this heading.

Triamcinolone Hexacetonide (The concomitant use of strong CYP3A4 inducers should be avoided. If patients must be co-administered a strong CYP3A4 inducer, based on pharmacokinetic studies, a Torisel dose increase from 25mg/week up to 50mg/week should be considered. This dose of Torisel is predicted to adjust the AUC to the range observed without inducers. However, there are no clinical data with this dose adjustment in patients receiving strong CYP3A4 inducers. If the strong inducer is discontinued, the temsirolimus dose should be returned to the dose used prior to initiation of the strong CYP3A4 inducer).
No products indexed under this heading.

Triazolam (The concentration of desipramin, a CYP2D6 substrate, was unaffected when 25mg of Torisel was co-administered. No clinically significant effect is anticipated when temsirolimus is co-administered with agents that are metabolized by CYP2D6 or CYP3A4).
No products indexed under this heading.

Trimipramine Maleate (The concentration of desipramin, a CYP2D6 substrate, was unaffected when 25mg of Torisel was co-administered. No clinically significant effect is anticipated when temsirolimus is co-administered with agents that are metabolized by CYP2D6 or CYP3A4).
No products indexed under this heading.

Troglitazone (The concomitant use of strong CYP3A4 inducers should be avoided. If patients must be co-administered a strong CYP3A4 inducer, based on pharmacokinetic studies, a Torisel dose increase from 25mg/week up to 50mg/week should be considered. This dose of Torisel is predicted to adjust the AUC to the range observed without inducers. However, there are no clinical data with this dose adjustment in patients receiving strong CYP3A4 inducers. If the strong inducer is discontinued, the temsirolimus dose should be returned to the dose used prior to initiation of the strong CYP3A4 inducer).
No products indexed under this heading.

Troleandomycin (The concomitant use of strong CYP3A4 inhibitors should be avoided. If patients must be co-administered a strong CYP3A4 inhibitor, based on pharmacokinetic studies, a Torisel dose reduction to 12.5mg/week should be considered. This dose is predicted to adjust the AUC to the range observed without inhibitors. However, there are no clinical data with this dose adjustment in patients receiving strong CYP3A4 inhibitors. If strong inhibitor is discontimued, a washout period of approximately 1 week should be allowed before the Torisel dose is adjusted back to the dose used prior to initiation of the strong CYP3A4 inhibitor).
No products indexed under this heading.

Typhoid Vaccine (The use of live vaccines and close contact with those who have received live vaccines should be avoided).
No products indexed under this heading.

Varicella Virus Vaccine Live (The use of live vaccines and close contact with those who have received live vaccines should be avoided). Products include:
Varivax **2133**

Venlafaxine Hydrochloride (The concentration of desipramin, a CYP2D6 substrate, was unaffected when 25mg of Torisel was co-administered. No clinically significant effect is anticipated when temsirolimus is co-administered with agents that are metabolized by CYP2D6 or CYP3A4). Products include:
Effexor XR Extended-Release Capsules.. **3195**
Venlafaxine Hydrochloride Tablets ... **2199**

Vinblastine Sulfate (The concentration of desipramin, a CYP2D6 substrate, was unaffected when 25mg of Torisel was co-administered. No clinically significant effect is anticipated when temsirolimus is co-administered with agents that are metabolized by CYP2D6 or CYP3A4).
No products indexed under this heading.

Voriconazole (The concomitant use of strong CYP3A4 inhibitors should be avoided. If patients must be co-administered a strong CYP3A4 inhibitor, based on pharmacokinetic studies, a Torisel dose reduction to 12.5mg/week should be considered. This dose is predicted to adjust the AUC to the range observed without inhibitors. However, there are no clinical data with this dose adjustment in patients receiving strong CYP3A4 inhibitors. If strong inhibitor is discontinued, a washout period of approximately 1 week should be allowed before the Torisel dose is adjusted back to the dose used prior to initiation of the strong CYP3A4 inhibitor).
No products indexed under this heading.

Yellow Fever Vaccine (The use of live vaccines and close contact with those who have received live vaccines should be avoided).
No products indexed under this heading.

Zonisamide (The concentration of desipramin, a CYP2D6 substrate, was unaffected when 25mg of Torisel was co-administered. No clinically significant effect is anticipated when temsirolimus is co-administered with agents that are metabolized by CYP2D6 or CYP3A4). Products include:
Zonegran Capsules **1089**

Zoster Vaccine Live (The use of live vaccines and close contact with those who have received live vaccines should be avoided). Products include:
Zostavax Injection **2145**

Food Interactions

Grapefruit Juice (May increase plasma concentrations of sirolimus (a major metabolite of temsirolimus) and should be avoided).

TRACLEER TABLETS

(Bosentan) **3289**
May interact with cytochrome p450 2c9 inhibitors (selected), cytochrome p450 3a4 inhibitors (selected), oral contraceptives, statins that are metabolized by CYP3A4, and certain other agents. Compounds in these categories include:

Acetazolamide (Co-administration of both a CYP2C9 inhibitor and a CYP3A4 inhibitor with bosentan will likely lead to large increases in plasma concentrations of bosentan and is not recommended).
No products indexed under this heading.

Amiodarone Hydrochloride (Co-administration of both a CYP2C9 inhibitor and a CYP3A4 inhibitor with bosentan will likely lead to large increases in plasma concentrations of bosentan and is not recommended).
No products indexed under this heading.

Amprenavir (Co-administration of both a CYP2C9 inhibitor and a CYP3A4 inhibitor with bosentan will likely lead to large increases in plasma concentrations of bosentan and is not recommended).
No products indexed under this heading.

Anastrozole (Co-administration of both a CYP2C9 inhibitor and a CYP3A4 inhibitor with bosentan will likely lead to large increases in plasma concentrations of bosentan and is not recommended). Products include:
Arimidex Tablets **672**

Aprepitant (Co-administration of both a CYP2C9 inhibitor and a CYP3A4 inhibitor with bosentan will likely lead to large increases in plasma concentrations of bosentan and is not recommended). Products include:
Emend Capsules **1992**

Atazanavir (Co-administration of both a CYP2C9 inhibitor and a CYP3A4 inhibitor with bosentan will likely lead to large increases in plasma concentrations of bosentan and is not recommended).
No products indexed under this heading.

Atazanavir Sulfate (Co-administration of both a CYP2C9 inhibitor and a CYP3A4 inhibitor with bosentan will likely lead to large increases in plasma concentrations of bosentan and is not recommended). Products include:
Reyataz Capsules **3299**

Atorvastatin Calcium (Bosentan is expected to reduce plasma concentrations of statins that have significant metabolism by CYP3A4, such as atorvastatin). Products include:
Lipitor Tablets **2501**

Bendroflumethiazide (Co-administration of both a CYP2C9 inhibitor and a CYP3A4 inhibitor with bosentan will likely lead to large increases in plasma concentrations of bosentan and is not recommended).
No products indexed under this heading.

Chloramphenicol (Co-administration of both a CYP2C9 inhibitor and a CYP3A4 inhibitor with bosentan will likely lead to large increases in plasma concentrations of bosentan and is not recommended).
No products indexed under this heading.

Chlorothiazide (Co-administration of both a CYP2C9 inhibitor and a CYP3A4 inhibitor with bosentan will likely lead to large increases in plasma concentrations of bosentan and is not recommended).
No products indexed under this heading.

Chlorothiazide Sodium (Co-administration of both a CYP2C9 inhibitor and a CYP3A4 inhibitor with bosentan will likely lead to large increases in plasma concentrations of bosentan and is not recommended). Products include:
Intravenous Sodium Diuril **2490**

Chlorpropamide (Co-administration of both a CYP2C9 inhibitor and a CYP3A4 inhibitor with bosentan will likely lead to large increases in plasma concentrations of bosentan and is not recommended).

No products indexed under this heading.

Cimetidine (Co-administration of both a CYP2C9 inhibitor and a CYP3A4 inhibitor with bosentan will likely lead to large increases in plasma concentrations of bosentan and is not recommended).

No products indexed under this heading.

Cimetidine Hydrochloride (Co-administration of both a CYP2C9 inhibitor and a CYP3A4 inhibitor with bosentan will likely lead to large increases in plasma concentrations of bosentan and is not recommended).

No products indexed under this heading.

Ciprofloxacin (Co-administration of both a CYP2C9 inhibitor and a CYP3A4 inhibitor with bosentan will likely lead to large increases in plasma concentrations of bosentan and is not recommended). Products include:

Cipro I.V. **2817**
Cipro Oral Suspension **2810**
Cipro XR Tablets **2823**
Ciprodex Otic Suspension **541**

Clarithromycin (Co-administration of both a CYP2C9 inhibitor and a CYP3A4 inhibitor with bosentan will likely lead to large increases in plasma concentrations of bosentan and is not recommended). Products include:

Biaxin/Biaxin XL **411**

Clopidogrel Hydrogen Sulfate (Co-administration of both a CYP2C9 inhibitor and a CYP3A4 inhibitor with bosentan will likely lead to large increases in plasma concentrations of bosentan and is not recommended).

No products indexed under this heading.

Clotrimazole (Co-administration of both a CYP2C9 inhibitor and a CYP3A4 inhibitor with bosentan will likely lead to large increases in plasma concentrations of bosentan and is not recommended). Products include:

Lotrisone **2881**

Cyclosporine (Co-administration has resulted in markedly increased plasma concentrations of bosentan; concurrent use is contraindicated). Products include:

Gengraf Capsules **435**
Neoral Oral Solution **2280**
Neoral Soft Gelatin Capsules **2280**
Restasis Ophthalmic Emulsion **557**
Sandimmune **2296**

Dalfopristin (Co-administration of both a CYP2C9 inhibitor and a CYP3A4 inhibitor with bosentan will likely lead to large increases in plasma concentrations of bosentan and is not recommended).

No products indexed under this heading.

Danazol (Co-administration of both a CYP2C9 inhibitor and a CYP3A4 inhibitor with bosentan will likely lead to large increases in plasma concentrations of bosentan and is not recommended).

No products indexed under this heading.

Delavirdine Mesylate (Co-administration of both a CYP2C9 inhibitor and a CYP3A4 inhibitor with bosentan will likely lead to large increases in plasma concentrations of bosentan and is not recommended).

No products indexed under this heading.

Desogestrel (Co-administration increases the possibility of failure of contraception. Women should practice additional methods of contraception). Products include:

Mircette Tablets **1034**

Diclofenac Potassium (Co-administration of both a CYP2C9 inhibitor and a CYP3A4 inhibitor with bosentan will likely lead to large increases in plasma concentrations of bosentan and is not recommended).

No products indexed under this heading.

Diclofenac Sodium (Co-administration of both a CYP2C9 inhibitor and a CYP3A4 inhibitor with bosentan will likely lead to large increases in plasma concentrations of bosentan and is not recommended). Products include:

Diclofenac Sodium Ophthalmic Solution .... ⊙**240**
Voltaren Ophthalmic Solution **2336**
Voltaren Tablets **2334**
Voltaren-XR Tablets **2337**

Diltiazem Hydrochloride (Co-administration of both a CYP2C9 inhibitor and a CYP3A4 inhibitor with bosentan will likely lead to large increases in plasma concentrations of bosentan and is not recommended). Products include:

Cardizem LA Extended Release Tablets **421**

Diltiazem Maleate (Co-administration of both a CYP2C9 inhibitor and a CYP3A4 inhibitor with bosentan will likely lead to large increases in plasma concentrations of bosentan and is not recommended).

No products indexed under this heading.

Disulfiram (Co-administration of both a CYP2C9 inhibitor and a CYP3A4 inhibitor with bosentan will likely lead to large increases in plasma concentrations of bosentan and is not recommended).

No products indexed under this heading.

Efavirenz (Co-administration of both a CYP2C9 inhibitor and a CYP3A4 inhibitor with bosentan will likely lead to large increases in plasma concentrations of bosentan and is not recommended). Products include:

Atripla Tablets **938**
Sustiva Capsules **930**
Sustiva Tablets **930**

Erythromycin (Co-administration of both a CYP2C9 inhibitor and a CYP3A4 inhibitor with bosentan will likely lead to large increases in plasma concentrations of bosentan and is not recommended).

No products indexed under this heading.

Erythromycin Estolate (Co-administration of both a CYP2C9 inhibitor and a CYP3A4 inhibitor with bosentan will likely lead to large increases in plasma concentrations of bosentan and is not recommended).

No products indexed under this heading.

Erythromycin Ethylsuccinate (Co-administration of both a CYP2C9 inhibitor and a CYP3A4 inhibitor with bosentan will likely lead to large increases in plasma concentrations of bosentan and is not recommended). Products include:

E.E.S. **433**
EryPed **431**

Erythromycin Gluceptate (Co-administration of both a CYP2C9 inhibitor and a CYP3A4 inhibitor with bosentan will likely lead to large increases in plasma concentrations of bosentan and is not recommended).

No products indexed under this heading.

Erythromycin Lactobionate (Co-administration of both a CYP2C9 inhibitor and a CYP3A4 inhibitor with bosentan will likely lead to large increases in plasma concentrations of bosentan and is not recommended).

No products indexed under this heading.

Erythromycin Stearate (Co-administration of both a CYP2C9 inhibitor and a CYP3A4 inhibitor with bosentan will likely lead to large increases in plasma concentrations of bosentan and is not recommended).

No products indexed under this heading.

Esomeprazole Magnesium (Co-administration of both a CYP2C9 inhibitor and a CYP3A4 inhibitor with bosentan will likely lead to large increases in plasma concentrations of bosentan and is not recommended). Products include:

Nexium Delayed-Release Capsules **645**
Nexium Delayed-Release Oral Suspension **645**

Ethinyl Estradiol (Co-administration increases the possibility of failure of contraception. Women should practice additional methods of contraception). Products include:

Lybrel Tablets **3204**
Mircette Tablets **1034**
NuvaRing **2897**
Ortho-Cyclen/Ortho Tri-Cyclen **2449**
Ortho Evra Transdermal System **2437**
Ortho Tri-Cyclen Lo Tablets **2458**
Seasonique Tablets **1046**
Yaz Tablets **805**

Ethynodiol Diacetate (Co-administration increases the possibility of failure of contraception. Women should practice additional methods of contraception).

No products indexed under this heading.

Fenofibrate (Co-administration of both a CYP2C9 inhibitor and a CYP3A4 inhibitor with bosentan will likely lead to large increases in plasma concentrations of bosentan and is not recommended). Products include:

Fenoglide Tablets **2960**
Tricor Tablets **520**

Fluconazole (Co-administration of both a CYP2C9 inhibitor and a CYP3A4 inhibitor with bosentan will likely lead to large increases in plasma concentrations of bosentan and is not recommended).

No products indexed under this heading.

Fluorouracil (Co-administration of both a CYP2C9 inhibitor and a CYP3A4 inhibitor with bosentan will likely lead to large increases in plasma concentrations of bosentan and is not recommended). Products include:

Carac Cream 0.5% **2722**

Fluoxetine (Co-administration of both a CYP2C9 inhibitor and a CYP3A4 inhibitor with bosentan will likely lead to large increases in plasma concentrations of bosentan and is not recommended).

No products indexed under this heading.

Fluoxetine Hydrochloride (Co-administration of both a CYP2C9 inhibitor and a CYP3A4 inhibitor with bosentan will likely lead to large increases in plasma concentrations of bosentan and is not recommended). Products include:

Prozac Weekly Capsules **1852**
Prozac Pulvules and Liquid **1852**
Symbyax Capsules **1871**

Flurbiprofen (Co-administration of both a CYP2C9 inhibitor and a CYP3A4 inhibitor with bosentan will likely lead to large increases in plasma concentrations of bosentan and is not recommended).

No products indexed under this heading.

Flurbiprofen Sodium (Co-administration of both a CYP2C9 inhibitor and a CYP3A4 inhibitor with bosentan will likely lead to large increases in plasma concentrations of bosentan and is not recommended).

No products indexed under this heading.

Fluvastatin Sodium (Co-administration of both a CYP2C9 inhibitor and a CYP3A4 inhibitor with bosentan will likely lead to large increases in plasma concentrations of bosentan and is not recommended). Products include:

Lescol Capsules **2268**
Lescol XL Tablets **2268**

Fluvoxamine Maleate (Co-administration of both a CYP2C9 inhibitor and a CYP3A4 inhibitor with bosentan will likely lead to large increases in plasma concentrations of bosentan and is not recommended). Products include:

Luvox CR Extended-Release Capsules **1759**

Fosamprenavir Calcium (Co-administration of both a CYP2C9 inhibitor and a CYP3A4 inhibitor with bosentan will likely lead to large increases in plasma concentrations of bosentan and is not recommended). Products include:

Lexiva Oral Suspension **1510**
Lexiva Tablets **1510**

Gemfibrozil (Co-administration of both a CYP2C9 inhibitor and a CYP3A4 inhibitor with bosentan will likely lead to large increases in plasma concentrations of bosentan and is not recommended).
No products indexed under this heading.

Glipizide (Co-administration of both a CYP2C9 inhibitor and a CYP3A4 inhibitor with bosentan will likely lead to large increases in plasma concentrations of bosentan and is not recommended).
No products indexed under this heading.

Glyburide (Co-administration increases the risk of liver enzyme elevation; concurrent use is contraindicated).
No products indexed under this heading.

Hydrochlorothiazide (Co-administration of both a CYP2C9 inhibitor and a CYP3A4 inhibitor with bosentan will likely lead to large increases in plasma concentrations of bosentan and is not recommended). Products include:
Atacand HCT ... 642
Avalide Tablets ... 892
Avalide Tablets ... 2713
Benicar HCT Tablets ... 1010
Diovan HCT Tablets ... 2216
Dyazide Capsules ... 1405
Micardis HCT Tablets ... 854
Prinzide Tablets ... 2092
Tekturna HCT Tablets ... 2324
Teveten HCT Tablets ... 517

Hydroflumethiazide (Co-administration of both a CYP2C9 inhibitor and a CYP3A4 inhibitor with bosentan will likely lead to large increases in plasma concentrations of bosentan and is not recommended).
No products indexed under this heading.

Imatinib Mesylate (Co-administration of both a CYP2C9 inhibitor and a CYP3A4 inhibitor with bosentan will likely lead to large increases in plasma concentrations of bosentan and is not recommended). Products include:
Gleevec Tablets ... 2255

Indinavir Sulfate (Co-administration of both a CYP2C9 inhibitor and a CYP3A4 inhibitor with bosentan will likely lead to large increases in plasma concentrations of bosentan and is not recommended). Products include:
Crixivan Capsules ... 1979

Isoniazid (Co-administration of both a CYP2C9 inhibitor and a CYP3A4 inhibitor with bosentan will likely lead to large increases in plasma concentrations of bosentan and is not recommended).
No products indexed under this heading.

Itraconazole (Co-administration of both a CYP2C9 inhibitor and a CYP3A4 inhibitor with bosentan will likely lead to large increases in plasma concentrations of bosentan and is not recommended).
No products indexed under this heading.

Ketoconazole (Co-administration increases the plasma concentrations of bosentan by approximately two-fold). Products include:
Extina Foam, 2% ... 3057
Nizoral A-D Shampoo ... 1901

Ketoprofen (Co-administration of both a CYP2C9 inhibitor and a CYP3A4 inhibitor with bosentan will likely lead to large increases in plasma concentrations of bosentan and is not recommended).
No products indexed under this heading.

Leflunomide (Co-administration of both a CYP2C9 inhibitor and a CYP3A4 inhibitor with bosentan will likely lead to large increases in plasma concentrations of bosentan and is not recommended).
No products indexed under this heading.

Levonorgestrel (Co-administration increases the possibility of failure of contraception. Women should practice additional methods of contraception). Products include:
Climara Pro Transdermal System ... 768
Lybrel Tablets ... 3204
Mirena Intrauterine System ... 779
Plan B Tablets ... 1044
Seasonique Tablets ... 1046

Lopinavir (Co-administration of both a CYP2C9 inhibitor and a CYP3A4 inhibitor with bosentan will likely lead to large increases in plasma concentrations of bosentan and is not recommended). Products include:
Kaletra ... 452

Loratadine (Co-administration of both a CYP2C9 inhibitor and a CYP3A4 inhibitor with bosentan will likely lead to large increases in plasma concentrations of bosentan and is not recommended).
No products indexed under this heading.

Lovastatin (Bosentan is expected to reduce plasma concentrations of statins that have significant metabolism by CYP3A4, such as lovastatin). Products include:
Advicor Tablets ... 402
Mevacor Tablets ... 2063

Mestranol (Co-administration increases the possibility of failure of contraception. Women should practice additional methods of contraception).
No products indexed under this heading.

Methyclothiazide (Co-administration of both a CYP2C9 inhibitor and a CYP3A4 inhibitor with bosentan will likely lead to large increases in plasma concentrations of bosentan and is not recommended).
No products indexed under this heading.

Metronidazole (Co-administration of both a CYP2C9 inhibitor and a CYP3A4 inhibitor with bosentan will likely lead to large increases in plasma concentrations of bosentan and is not recommended). Products include:
Pylera Capsules ... 714

Metronidazole Benzoate (Co-administration of both a CYP2C9 inhibitor and a CYP3A4 inhibitor with bosentan will likely lead to large increases in plasma concentrations of bosentan and is not recommended).
No products indexed under this heading.

Metronidazole Hydrochloride (Co-administration of both a CYP2C9 inhibitor and a CYP3A4 inhibitor with bosentan will likely lead to large increases in plasma concentrations of bosentan and is not recommended).
No products indexed under this heading.

Miconazole (Co-administration of both a CYP2C9 inhibitor and a CYP3A4 inhibitor with bosentan will likely lead to large increases in plasma concentrations of bosentan and is not recommended).
No products indexed under this heading.

Miconazole Nitrate (Co-administration of both a CYP2C9 inhibitor and a CYP3A4 inhibitor with bosentan will likely lead to large increases in plasma concentrations of bosentan and is not recommended).
No products indexed under this heading.

Modafinil (Co-administration of both a CYP2C9 inhibitor and a CYP3A4 inhibitor with bosentan will likely lead to large increases in plasma concentrations of bosentan and is not recommended). Products include:
Provigil Tablets ... 977

Nefazodone Hydrochloride (Co-administration of both a CYP2C9 inhibitor and a CYP3A4 inhibitor with bosentan will likely lead to large increases in plasma concentrations of bosentan and is not recommended).
No products indexed under this heading.

Nelfinavir Mesylate (Co-administration of both a CYP2C9 inhibitor and a CYP3A4 inhibitor with bosentan will likely lead to large increases in plasma concentrations of bosentan and is not recommended).
No products indexed under this heading.

Nevirapine (Co-administration of both a CYP2C9 inhibitor and a CYP3A4 inhibitor with bosentan will likely lead to large increases in plasma concentrations of bosentan and is not recommended). Products include:
Viramune Oral Suspension ... 873
Viramune Tablets ... 873

Niacinamide (Co-administration of both a CYP2C9 inhibitor and a CYP3A4 inhibitor with bosentan will likely lead to large increases in plasma concentrations of bosentan and is not recommended). Products include:
BioLean Free Tablets ... ▣ 635

Nicotinamide (Co-administration of both a CYP2C9 inhibitor and a CYP3A4 inhibitor with bosentan will likely lead to large increases in plasma concentrations of bosentan and is not recommended).
No products indexed under this heading.

Nifedipine (Co-administration of both a CYP2C9 inhibitor and a CYP3A4 inhibitor with bosentan will likely lead to large increases in plasma concentrations of bosentan and is not recommended).
No products indexed under this heading.

Norethindrone (Co-administration increases the possibility of failure of contraception. Women should practice additional methods of contraception). Products include:
Ortho Micronor Tablets ... 2446

Norethynodrel (Co-administration increases the possibility of failure of contraception. Women should practice additional methods of contraception).
No products indexed under this heading.

Norfloxacin (Co-administration of both a CYP2C9 inhibitor and a CYP3A4 inhibitor with bosentan will likely lead to large increases in plasma concentrations of bosentan and is not recommended). Products include:
Noroxin Tablets ... 2069

Norgestimate (Co-administration increases the possibility of failure of contraception. Women should practice additional methods of contraception). Products include:
Ortho-Cyclen/Ortho Tri-Cyclen ... 2449
Ortho Tri-Cyclen Lo Tablets ... 2458

Norgestrel (Co-administration increases the possibility of failure of contraception. Women should practice additional methods of contraception).
No products indexed under this heading.

Omeprazole (Co-administration of both a CYP2C9 inhibitor and a CYP3A4 inhibitor with bosentan will likely lead to large increases in plasma concentrations of bosentan and is not recommended).
No products indexed under this heading.

Oxiconazole Nitrate (Co-administration of both a CYP2C9 inhibitor and a CYP3A4 inhibitor with bosentan will likely lead to large increases in plasma concentrations of bosentan and is not recommended).
No products indexed under this heading.

Paroxetine Hydrochloride (Co-administration of both a CYP2C9 inhibitor and a CYP3A4 inhibitor with bosentan will likely lead to large increases in plasma concentrations of bosentan and is not recommended). Products include:
Paxil ... 1535
Paxil CR Controlled-Release Tablets ... 1544

Phenylbutazone (Co-administration of both a CYP2C9 inhibitor and a CYP3A4 inhibitor with bosentan will likely lead to large increases in plasma concentrations of bosentan and is not recommended).
No products indexed under this heading.

Polythiazide (Co-administration of both a CYP2C9 inhibitor and a CYP3A4 inhibitor with bosentan will likely lead to large increases in plasma concentrations of bosentan and is not recommended).
No products indexed under this heading.

Propoxyphene Hydrochloride (Co-administration of both a CYP2C9 inhibitor and a CYP3A4 inhibitor with bosentan will likely lead to large increases in plasma concentrations of bosentan and is not recommended).
No products indexed under this heading.

Propoxyphene Napsylate (Co-administration of both a CYP2C9 inhibitor and a CYP3A4 inhibitor with bosentan will likely lead to large increases in plasma concentrations of bosentan and is not recommended).
No products indexed under this heading.

Quinidine (Co-administration of both a CYP2C9 inhibitor and a CYP3A4 inhibitor with bosentan will likely lead to large increases in plasma concentrations of bosentan and is not recommended).
No products indexed under this heading.

Quinidine Hydrochloride (Co-administration of both a CYP2C9 inhibitor and a CYP3A4 inhibitor with bosentan will likely lead to large increases in plasma concentrations of bosentan and is not recommended).
No products indexed under this heading.

Quinidine Polygalacturonate (Co-administration of both a CYP2C9 inhibitor and a CYP3A4 inhibitor with bosentan will likely lead to large increases in plasma concentrations of bosentan and is not recommended).
No products indexed under this heading.

Quinidine Sulfate (Co-administration of both a CYP2C9 inhibitor and a CYP3A4 inhibitor with bosentan will likely lead to large increases in plasma concentrations of bosentan and is not recommended).
No products indexed under this heading.

Quinine (Co-administration of both a CYP2C9 inhibitor and a CYP3A4 inhibitor with bosentan will likely lead to large increases in plasma concentrations of bosentan and is not recommended).
No products indexed under this heading.

Quinine Sulfate (Co-administration of both a CYP2C9 inhibitor and a CYP3A4 inhibitor with bosentan will likely lead to large increases in plasma concentrations of bosentan and is not recommended).
No products indexed under this heading.

Quinupristin (Co-administration of both a CYP2C9 inhibitor and a CYP3A4 inhibitor with bosentan will likely lead to large increases in plasma concentrations of bosentan and is not recommended).
No products indexed under this heading.

Ranitidine Bismuth Citrate (Co-administration of both a CYP2C9 inhibitor and a CYP3A4 inhibitor with bosentan will likely lead to large increases in plasma concentrations of bosentan and is not recommended).
No products indexed under this heading.

Ranitidine Hydrochloride (Co-administration of both a CYP2C9 inhibitor and a CYP3A4 inhibitor with bosentan will likely lead to large increases in plasma concentrations of bosentan and is not recommended). Products include:
Zantac 75 Tablets 603
Zantac 1670
Zantac Injection 1666
Zantac Injection Pharmacy Bulk Package 1668
Maximum Strength Zantac 150 Tablets 603
Maximum Strength Zantac 150 Cool Mint Tablets 603

Rifampicin (Co-administration of bosentan and rifampicin in normal volunteers resulted in a mean 6-fold increase in bosentan trough levels after the first concomitant dose, but about 60% decrease in bosentan levels at steady-state. The effect of bosentan on rifampicin levels has not been assessed. When consideration of the potential benefits and known and unknown risks leads to concomitant use, measure LFTs weekly for the first 4 weeks before reverting to normal monitoring).
No products indexed under this heading.

Ritonavir (Co-administration of both a CYP2C9 inhibitor and a CYP3A4 inhibitor with bosentan will likely lead to large increases in plasma concentrations of bosentan and is not recommended). Products include:
Kaletra 452
Norvir 489

Saquinavir (Co-administration of both a CYP2C9 inhibitor and a CYP3A4 inhibitor with bosentan will likely lead to large increases in plasma concentrations of bosentan and is not recommended).
No products indexed under this heading.

Saquinavir Mesylate (Co-administration of both a CYP2C9 inhibitor and a CYP3A4 inhibitor with bosentan will likely lead to large increases in plasma concentrations of bosentan and is not recommended).
No products indexed under this heading.

Sertraline Hydrochloride (Co-administration of both a CYP2C9 inhibitor and a CYP3A4 inhibitor with bosentan will likely lead to large increases in plasma concentrations of bosentan and is not recommended).
No products indexed under this heading.

Sildenafil Citrate (In healthy subjects, co-administration of multiple doses of 125mg twice daily bosentan and 80mg three times daily sildenafil resulted in a reduction of sildenafil plasma concentrations by 50%. A dose adjustment of neither drug is necessary. This recommendation holds true when sildenafil is used for the treatment of pulmonary arterial hypertension or erectile dysfunction).
No products indexed under this heading.

Simvastatin (Co-administration decreases plasma concentrations of simvastatin and its active metabolite by 50%). Products include:
Simcor Tablets 502
Vytorin 10/10 Tablets 2149
Vytorin 10/10 Tablets 2939
Vytorin 10/20 Tablets 2149
Vytorin 10/20 Tablets 2939
Vytorin 10/40 Tablets 2149
Vytorin 10/40 Tablets 2939
Vytorin 10/80 Tablets 2149
Vytorin 10/80 Tablets 2939
Zocor Tablets 2136

Sulfacytine (Co-administration of both a CYP2C9 inhibitor and a CYP3A4 inhibitor with bosentan will likely lead to large increases in plasma concentrations of bosentan and is not recommended).
No products indexed under this heading.

Sulfamethizole (Co-administration of both a CYP2C9 inhibitor and a CYP3A4 inhibitor with bosentan will likely lead to large increases in plasma concentrations of bosentan and is not recommended).
No products indexed under this heading.

Sulfamethoxazole (Co-administration of both a CYP2C9 inhibitor and a CYP3A4 inhibitor with bosentan will likely lead to large increases in plasma concentrations of bosentan and is not recommended).
No products indexed under this heading.

Sulfasalazine (Co-administration of both a CYP2C9 inhibitor and a CYP3A4 inhibitor with bosentan will likely lead to large increases in plasma concentrations of bosentan and is not recommended).
No products indexed under this heading.

Sulfinpyrazone (Co-administration of both a CYP2C9 inhibitor and a CYP3A4 inhibitor with bosentan will likely lead to large increases in plasma concentrations of bosentan and is not recommended).
No products indexed under this heading.

Sulfisoxazole Acetyl (Co-administration of both a CYP2C9 inhibitor and a CYP3A4 inhibitor with bosentan will likely lead to large increases in plasma concentrations of bosentan and is not recommended).
No products indexed under this heading.

Sulfisoxazole Diolamine (Co-administration of both a CYP2C9 inhibitor and a CYP3A4 inhibitor with bosentan will likely lead to large increases in plasma concentrations of bosentan and is not recommended).
No products indexed under this heading.

Tacrolimus (Caution should be exercised if tacrolimus and bosentan are used together). Products include:
Prograf Capsules and Injection 622
Protopic Ointment 628

Telithromycin (Co-administration of both a CYP2C9 inhibitor and a CYP3A4 inhibitor with bosentan will likely lead to large increases in plasma concentrations of bosentan and is not recommended). Products include:
Ketek Tablets 2744

Terconazole (Co-administration of both a CYP2C9 inhibitor and a CYP3A4 inhibitor with bosentan will likely lead to large increases in plasma concentrations of bosentan and is not recommended).
No products indexed under this heading.

Ticlopidine Hydrochloride (Co-administration of both a CYP2C9 inhibitor and a CYP3A4 inhibitor with bosentan will likely lead to large increases in plasma concentrations of bosentan and is not recommended).
No products indexed under this heading.

Tolazamide (Co-administration of both a CYP2C9 inhibitor and a CYP3A4 inhibitor with bosentan will likely lead to large increases in plasma concentrations of bosentan and is not recommended).
No products indexed under this heading.

Tolbutamide (Co-administration of both a CYP2C9 inhibitor and a CYP3A4 inhibitor with bosentan will likely lead to large increases in plasma concentrations of bosentan and is not recommended).
No products indexed under this heading.

Tolbutamide Sodium (Co-administration of both a CYP2C9 inhibitor and a CYP3A4 inhibitor with bosentan will likely lead to large increases in plasma concentrations of bosentan and is not recommended).
No products indexed under this heading.

Troglitazone (Co-administration of both a CYP2C9 inhibitor and a CYP3A4 inhibitor with bosentan will likely lead to large increases in plasma concentrations of bosentan and is not recommended).
No products indexed under this heading.

Troleandomycin (Co-administration of both a CYP2C9 inhibitor and a CYP3A4 inhibitor with bosentan will likely lead to large increases in plasma concentrations of bosentan and is not recommended).
No products indexed under this heading.

Valproate Sodium (Co-administration of both a CYP2C9 inhibitor and a CYP3A4 inhibitor with bosentan will likely lead to large increases in plasma concentrations of bosentan and is not recommended).
No products indexed under this heading.

Vardenafil Hydrochloride (Co-administration of both a CYP2C9 inhibitor and a CYP3A4 inhibitor with bosentan will likely lead to large increases in plasma concentrations of bosentan and is not recommended). Products include:
Levitra Tablets 2876

Verapamil Hydrochloride (Co-administration of both a CYP2C9 inhibitor and a CYP3A4 inhibitor with bosentan will likely lead to large increases in plasma concentrations of bosentan and is not recommended). Products include:
Tarka Tablets 511

Voriconazole (Co-administration of both a CYP2C9 inhibitor and a CYP3A4 inhibitor with bosentan will likely lead to large increases in plasma concentrations of bosentan and is not recommended).
No products indexed under this heading.

Zafirlukast (Co-administration of both a CYP2C9 inhibitor and a CYP3A4 inhibitor with bosentan will likely lead to large increases in plas-

IMPORTANT NOTE: Always consult each drug listing in the patient's regimen for possible interactions.

ma concentrations of bosentan and is not recommended). Products include:

Accolate Tablets 669

Zileuton (Co-administration of both a CYP2C9 inhibitor and a CYP3A4 inhibitor with bosentan will likely lead to large increases in plasma concentrations of bosentan and is not recommended).

No products indexed under this heading.

Food Interactions

Grapefruit (Co-administration of both a CYP2C9 inhibitor and a CYP3A4 inhibitor with bosentan will likely lead to large increases in plasma concentrations of bosentan and is not recommended).

Grapefruit Juice (Co-administration of both a CYP2C9 inhibitor and a CYP3A4 inhibitor with bosentan will likely lead to large increases in plasma concentrations of bosentan and is not recommended).

TRANQUILITY CAPSULES

(Amino Acid Preparations, Herbals with Vitamins & Minerals, Soy-containing dietary supplements, Valeriana officinalis)..... ▣ 641

None cited in PDR database.

TRANSDERM SCOP TRANSDERMAL THERAPEUTIC SYSTEM

(Scopolamine) 2206

May interact with anticholinergics, antihistamines, central nervous system depressants, hypnotics and sedatives, muscle relaxants, tranquilizers, tricyclic antidepressants, and certain other agents. Compounds in these categories include:

Acrivastine (Antihistamines have anticholinergic properties and co-administration may result in additive effects).

No products indexed under this heading.

Alfentanil Hydrochloride (Scopolamine is an anticholinergic agent and causes certain CNS effects, such as drowsiness and dizziness, and hence it should be used with care in patients on concomitant therapy).

No products indexed under this heading.

Alprazolam (Scopolamine is an anticholinergic agent and causes certain CNS effects, such as drowsiness and dizziness, and hence it should be used with care in patients on concomitant therapy).

No products indexed under this heading.

Amitriptyline Hydrochloride (Tricyclic antidepressants have anticholinergic properties and co-administration may result in additive effects).

No products indexed under this heading.

Amoxapine (Tricyclic antidepressants have anticholinergic properties and co-administration may result in additive effects).

No products indexed under this heading.

Aprobarbital (Scopolamine is an anticholinergic agent and causes certain CNS effects, such as drowsiness and dizziness, and hence it should be used with care in patients on concomitant therapy).

No products indexed under this heading.

Astemizole (Antihistamines have anticholinergic properties and co-administration may result in additive effects).

No products indexed under this heading.

Atracurium Besylate (Co-administration may result in addititve anticholinergic effects).

No products indexed under this heading.

Atropine Sulfate (Co-administration may result in additive anticholinergic effects). Products include:

Donnatal Extentabs 2507

Azatadine Maleate (Antihistamines have anticholinergic properties and co-administration may result in additive effects).

No products indexed under this heading.

Baclofen (Co-administration may result in addititve anticholinergic effects).

No products indexed under this heading.

Belladonna Alkaloids (Co-administration may result in additive anticholinergic effects). Products include:

Hyland's Teething Tablets .... ▣ 621

Benztropine Mesylate (Co-administration may result in additive anticholinergic effects).

No products indexed under this heading.

Biperiden Hydrochloride (Co-administration may result in additive anticholinergic effects).

No products indexed under this heading.

Bromodiphenhydramine Hydrochloride (Antihistamines have anticholinergic properties and co-administration may result in additive effects).

No products indexed under this heading.

Brompheniramine Maleate (Antihistamines have anticholinergic properties and co-administration may result in additive effects).

No products indexed under this heading.

Buprenorphine Hydrochloride (Scopolamine is an anticholinergic agent and causes certain CNS effects, such as drowsiness and dizziness, and hence it should be used with care in patients on concomitant therapy). Products include:

Suboxone Tablets 2601
Subutex Tablets 2601

Buspirone Hydrochloride (Scopolamine is an anticholinergic agent and causes certain CNS effects, such as drowsiness and dizziness, and hence it should be used with care in patients on concomitant therapy).

No products indexed under this heading.

Butabarbital (Scopolamine is an anticholinergic agent and causes certain CNS effects, such as drowsiness and dizziness, and hence it should be used with care in patients on concomitant therapy).

No products indexed under this heading.

Butabarbital Sodium (Scopolamine is an anticholinergic agent and causes certain CNS effects, such as drowsiness and dizziness, and hence it should be used with care in patients on concomitant therapy).

No products indexed under this heading.

Butalbital (Scopolamine is an anticholinergic agent and causes certain CNS effects, such as drowsiness and dizziness, and hence it should be used with care in patients on concomitant therapy).

No products indexed under this heading.

Carisoprodol (Co-administration may result in addititve anticholinergic effects). Products include:

Soma Tablets 1931

Cetirizine Hydrochloride (Antihistamines have anticholinergic properties and co-administration may result in additive effects). Products include:

Zyrtec Allergy Tablets 1919
Zyrtec Chewable Tablets 1920
Children's Zyrtec Allergy Chewable Tablets 1922
Children's Zyrtec Allergy Syrup 1920
Children's Zyrtec Hives Relief Syrup 1920
Zyrtec Syrup 1920
Zyrtec Tablets 1920
Zyrtec-D 12 Hour Extended Release Tablets 1923
Zyrtec-D Allergy & Congestion Extended-Release Tablets 1923

Chloral Hydrate (Scopolamine is an anticholinergic agent and causes certain CNS effects, such as drowsiness and dizziness, and hence it should be used with care in patients on concomitant therapy).

No products indexed under this heading.

Chlordiazepoxide (Scopolamine is an anticholinergic agent and causes certain CNS effects, such as drowsiness and dizziness, and hence it should be used with care in patients on concomitant therapy).

No products indexed under this heading.

Chlordiazepoxide Hydrochloride (Scopolamine is an anticholinergic agent and causes certain CNS effects, such as drowsiness and dizziness, and hence it should be used with care in patients on concomitant therapy).

No products indexed under this heading.

Chlorpheniramine Maleate (Antihistamines have anticholinergic properties and co-administration may result in additive effects). Products include:

Actifed Cold & Allergy Tablets 1895
Sudafed PE Sinus & Allergy Tablets 1908
Tylenol Allergy Multi-Symptom Caplets with Cool Burst and Rapid Release Gelcaps 1916
Children's Tylenol Plus Cold Suspension Liquid 1912
Children's Tylenol Plus Cough & Runny Nose Suspension Liquid 1912
Children's Tylenol Plus Flu Suspension Liquid 1914
Children's Tylenol Plus Multi-Symptom Cold Suspension Liquid 1912
Tylenol Cold Head Congestion Nighttime Caplets with Cool Burst 1910
Tylenol Cold Multi-Symptom Nighttime Caplets with Cool Burst 1913
Tylenol Sinus Congestion & Pain Nighttime Caplets with Cool Burst 1917

Chlorpheniramine Polistirex (Antihistamines have anticholinergic properties and co-administration may result in additive effects). Products include:

Tussionex Pennkinetic Extended-Release Suspension 3154

Chlorpheniramine Tannate (Antihistamines have anticholinergic properties and co-administration may result in additive effects).

No products indexed under this heading.

Chlorpromazine (Scopolamine is an anticholinergic agent and causes certain CNS effects, such as drowsiness and dizziness, and hence it should be used with care in patients on concomitant therapy).

No products indexed under this heading.

Chlorpromazine Hydrochloride (Scopolamine is an anticholinergic agent and causes certain CNS effects, such as drowsiness and dizziness, and hence it should be used with care in patients on concomitant therapy).

No products indexed under this heading.

Chlorprothixene (Scopolamine is an anticholinergic agent and causes certain CNS effects, such as drowsiness and dizziness, and hence it should be used with care in patients on concomitant therapy).

No products indexed under this heading.

Chlorprothixene Hydrochloride (Scopolamine is an anticholinergic agent and causes certain CNS effects, such as drowsiness and dizziness, and hence it should be used with care in patients on concomitant therapy).

No products indexed under this heading.

Chlorprothixene Lactate (Scopolamine is an anticholinergic agent and causes certain CNS effects, such as drowsiness and dizziness, and hence it should be used with care in patients on concomitant therapy).

No products indexed under this heading.

Chlorzoxazone (Co-administration may result in addititve anticholinergic effects).

No products indexed under this heading.

Cisatracurium Besylate (Co-administration may result in addititve anticholinergic effects). Products include:

Nimbex Injection 484

Clemastine Fumarate (Antihistamines have anticholinergic properties and co-administration may result in additive effects).

No products indexed under this heading.

Clidinium Bromide (Co-administration may result in additive anticholinergic effects).

No products indexed under this heading.

Clomipramine Hydrochloride (Tricyclic antidepressants have anticholinergic properties and co-administration may result in additive effects).

No products indexed under this heading.

Clorazepate Dipotassium (Scopolamine is an anticholinergic agent and causes certain CNS effects, such as drowsiness and dizziness, and hence it should be used with care in patients on concomitant therapy).

No products indexed under this heading.

Clozapine (Scopolamine is an anticholinergic agent and causes certain CNS effects, such as drowsiness and dizziness, and hence it should be used with care in patients on concomitant therapy).
No products indexed under this heading.

Codeine Phosphate (Scopolamine is an anticholinergic agent and causes certain CNS effects, such as drowsiness and dizziness, and hence it should be used with care in patients on concomitant therapy).
Products include:
Tylenol with Codeine Tablets ... 2427

Cyclobenzaprine Hydrochloride (Co-administration may result in additive anticholinergic effects).
Products include:
Amrix Capsules ... 966

Cyproheptadine Hydrochloride (Antihistamines have anticholinergic properties and co-administration may result in additive effects).
No products indexed under this heading.

Dantrolene Sodium (Co-administration may result in additive anticholinergic effects). Products include:
Dantrium Capsules ... 2580
Dantrium Intravenous ... 2582

Desflurane (Scopolamine is an anticholinergic agent and causes certain CNS effects, such as drowsiness and dizziness, and hence it should be used with care in patients on concomitant therapy).
No products indexed under this heading.

Desipramine Hydrochloride (Tricyclic antidepressants have anticholinergic properties and co-administration may result in additive effects).
No products indexed under this heading.

Dexchlorpheniramine Maleate (Antihistamines have anticholinergic properties and co-administration may result in additive effects).
No products indexed under this heading.

Dezocine (Scopolamine is an anticholinergic agent and causes certain CNS effects, such as drowsiness and dizziness, and hence it should be used with care in patients on concomitant therapy).
No products indexed under this heading.

Diazepam (Scopolamine is an anticholinergic agent and causes certain CNS effects, such as drowsiness and dizziness, and hence it should be used with care in patients on concomitant therapy). Products include:
Valium Tablets ... 2658

Dicyclomine Hydrochloride (Co-administration may result in additive anticholinergic effects). Products include:
Bentyl Capsules ... 703
Bentyl Injection ... 703
Bentyl Syrup ... 703
Bentyl Tablets ... 703

Diphenhydramine Citrate (Antihistamines have anticholinergic properties and co-administration may result in additive effects).
No products indexed under this heading.

Diphenhydramine Hydrochloride (Antihistamines have anticholinergic properties and co-administration may result in additive effects).
Products include:
Benadryl Allergy & Cold Kapgels ... 1895
Benadryl Allergy & Sinus Headache Kapgels ... 1895
Benadryl Severe Allergy & Sinus Headache Caplets ... 1897
Benadryl Dye-Free Allergy Liqui-gels Softgels ... 1897
Benadryl Allergy Kapgels ... 1895
Benadryl Allergy Quick Dissolve Strips ... 1896
Benadryl Allergy Ultratab Tablets ... 1896
Children's Benadryl Dye-Free Allergy Liquid ... 1897
Children's Benadryl Allergy Fastmelts ... 1897
Children's Benadryl Allergy Liquid ... 1898
Children's Benadryl Allergy Perfect Measure ... 1896
Children's Benadryl-D Allergy & Sinus Liquid ... 1896
Benadryl-D Allergy & Sinus Tablet ... 1896
PediaCare Children's Allergy & Cold Liquid ... 1902
PediaCare Children's Allergy Liquid ... 1902
Simply Sleep Caplets ... 1905
Sudafed PE Nighttime Cold Caplets ... 1907
Sudafed PE Severe Cold Caplets ... 1908
Extra Strength Tylenol PM Caplets, Geltabs, Liquid, and Rapid Release Gels ... 1915
Tylenol Allergy Multi-Symptom Nighttime Caplets with Cool Burst ... 1916
Tylenol Severe Allergy Caplets ... 1916
Children's Tylenol Plus Cold & Allergy Suspension Liquid ... 1914
Tylenol Sore Throat Nighttime Liquid with Cool Burst ... 1918

Diphenylpyraline Hydrochloride (Antihistamines have anticholinergic properties and co-administration may result in additive effects).
No products indexed under this heading.

Doxacurium Chloride (Co-administration may result in additive anticholinergic effects).
No products indexed under this heading.

Doxepin Hydrochloride (Tricyclic antidepressants have anticholinergic properties and co-administration may result in additive effects).
No products indexed under this heading.

Droperidol (Scopolamine is an anticholinergic agent and causes certain CNS effects, such as drowsiness and dizziness, and hence it should be used with care in patients on concomitant therapy).
No products indexed under this heading.

Enflurane (Scopolamine is an anticholinergic agent and causes certain CNS effects, such as drowsiness and dizziness, and hence it should be used with care in patients on concomitant therapy).
No products indexed under this heading.

Estazolam (Scopolamine is an anticholinergic agent and causes certain CNS effects, such as drowsiness and dizziness, and hence it should be used with care in patients on concomitant therapy).
No products indexed under this heading.

Ethanol (Scopolamine is an anticholinergic agent and causes certain CNS effects, such as drowsiness and dizziness, and hence it should be used with care in patients on concomitant therapy).
No products indexed under this heading.

Ethchlorvynol (Scopolamine is an anticholinergic agent and causes certain CNS effects, such as drowsiness and dizziness, and hence it should be used with care in patients on concomitant therapy).
No products indexed under this heading.

Ethinamate (Scopolamine is an anticholinergic agent and causes certain CNS effects, such as drowsiness and dizziness, and hence it should be used with care in patients on concomitant therapy).
No products indexed under this heading.

Ethyl Alcohol (Scopolamine is an anticholinergic agent and causes certain CNS effects, such as drowsiness and dizziness, and hence it should be used with care in patients on concomitant therapy).
No products indexed under this heading.

Fentanyl (Scopolamine is an anticholinergic agent and causes certain CNS effects, such as drowsiness and dizziness, and hence it should be used with care in patients on concomitant therapy). Products include:
Duragesic Transdermal System ... 2405
Ionsys Transdermal System ... 2410

Fentanyl Citrate (Scopolamine is an anticholinergic agent and causes certain CNS effects, such as drowsiness and dizziness, and hence it should be used with care in patients on concomitant therapy). Products include:
Actiq ... 959
Fentora Tablets ... 968

Fexofenadine Hydrochloride (Antihistamines have anticholinergic properties and co-administration may result in additive effects).
Products include:
Allegra Oral Solution ... 2684
Allegra Tablets ... 2684
Allegra-D 12 Hour Extended-Release Tablets ... 2687
Allegra-D 24 Hour Extended-Release Tablets ... 2690

Fluphenazine Decanoate (Scopolamine is an anticholinergic agent and causes certain CNS effects, such as drowsiness and dizziness, and hence it should be used with care in patients on concomitant therapy).
No products indexed under this heading.

Fluphenazine Enanthate (Scopolamine is an anticholinergic agent and causes certain CNS effects, such as drowsiness and dizziness, and hence it should be used with care in patients on concomitant therapy).
No products indexed under this heading.

Fluphenazine Hydrochloride (Scopolamine is an anticholinergic agent and causes certain CNS effects, such as drowsiness and dizziness, and hence it should be used with care in patients on concomitant therapy).
No products indexed under this heading.

Flurazepam Hydrochloride (Scopolamine is an anticholinergic agent and causes certain CNS effects, such as drowsiness and dizziness, and hence it should be used with care in patients on concomitant therapy).
No products indexed under this heading.

Glutethimide (Scopolamine is an anticholinergic agent and causes certain CNS effects, such as drowsiness and dizziness, and hence it should be used with care in patients on concomitant therapy).
No products indexed under this heading.

Glycopyrrolate (Co-administration may result in additive anticholinergic effects).
No products indexed under this heading.

Haloperidol (Scopolamine is an anticholinergic agent and causes certain CNS effects, such as drowsiness and dizziness, and hence it should be used with care in patients on concomitant therapy).
No products indexed under this heading.

Haloperidol Decanoate (Scopolamine is an anticholinergic agent and causes certain CNS effects, such as drowsiness and dizziness, and hence it should be used with care in patients on concomitant therapy).
No products indexed under this heading.

Hydrocodone Bitartrate (Scopolamine is an anticholinergic agent and causes certain CNS effects, such as drowsiness and dizziness, and hence it should be used with care in patients on concomitant therapy).
Products include:
Lortab 5/500 Tablets ... 3143
Lortab 7.5/500 Tablets ... 3144
Lortab 10/500 Tablets ... 3144
Vicodin Tablets ... 529
Vicodin ES Tablets ... 530
Vicodin HP Tablets ... 531
Vicoprofen Tablets ... 533
Zydone Tablets ... 1132

Hydrocodone Polistirex (Scopolamine is an anticholinergic agent and causes certain CNS effects, such as drowsiness and dizziness, and hence it should be used with care in patients on concomitant therapy).
Products include:
Tussionex Pennkinetic Extended-Release Suspension ... 3154

Hydromorphone Hydrochloride (Scopolamine is an anticholinergic agent and causes certain CNS effects, such as drowsiness and dizziness, and hence it should be used with care in patients on concomitant therapy).
No products indexed under this heading.

Hydroxyzine Hydrochloride (Scopolamine is an anticholinergic agent and causes certain CNS effects, such as drowsiness and dizziness, and hence it should be used with care in patients on concomitant therapy).
No products indexed under this heading.

Hyoscyamine (Co-administration may result in additive anticholinergic effects).
No products indexed under this heading.

Hyoscyamine Sulfate (Co-administration may result in additive anticholinergic effects). Products include:

Donnatal Extentabs 2507

Imipramine Hydrochloride (Tricyclic antidepressants have anticholinergic properties and co-administration may result in additive effects).

No products indexed under this heading.

Imipramine Pamoate (Tricyclic antidepressants have anticholinergic properties and co-administration may result in additive effects).

No products indexed under this heading.

Ipratropium Bromide (Co-administration may result in additive anticholinergic effects). Products include:

Atrovent HFA Inhalation Aerosol 839
Atrovent Nasal Spray 0.03% 834
Atrovent Nasal Spray 0.06% 836
Combivent Inhalation Aerosol 845

Isoflurane (Scopolamine is an anticholinergic agent and causes certain CNS effects, such as drowsiness and dizziness, and hence it should be used with care in patients on concomitant therapy).

No products indexed under this heading.

Ketamine Hydrochloride (Scopolamine is an anticholinergic agent and causes certain CNS effects, such as drowsiness and dizziness, and hence it should be used with care in patients on concomitant therapy).

No products indexed under this heading.

Levomethadyl Acetate Hydrochloride (Scopolamine is an anticholinergic agent and causes certain CNS effects, such as drowsiness and dizziness, and hence it should be used with care in patients on concomitant therapy).

No products indexed under this heading.

Levorphanol Tartrate (Scopolamine is an anticholinergic agent and causes certain CNS effects, such as drowsiness and dizziness, and hence it should be used with care in patients on concomitant therapy).

No products indexed under this heading.

Loratadine (Antihistamines have anticholinergic properties and co-administration may result in additive effects).

No products indexed under this heading.

Lorazepam (Scopolamine is an anticholinergic agent and causes certain CNS effects, such as drowsiness and dizziness, and hence it should be used with care in patients on concomitant therapy).

No products indexed under this heading.

Loxapine Hydrochloride (Scopolamine is an anticholinergic agent and causes certain CNS effects, such as drowsiness and dizziness, and hence it should be used with care in patients on concomitant therapy).

No products indexed under this heading.

Loxapine Succinate (Scopolamine is an anticholinergic agent and causes certain CNS effects, such as drowsiness and dizziness, and hence it should be used with care in patients on concomitant therapy).

No products indexed under this heading.

Maprotiline Hydrochloride (Tricyclic antidepressants have anticholinergic properties and co-administration may result in additive effects).

No products indexed under this heading.

Meclizine Hydrochloride (Antihistamines have anticholinergic properties and co-administration may result in additive effects). Products include:

Dramamine Less Drowsy Tablets 1898

Mepenzolate Bromide (Co-administration may result in additive anticholinergic effects).

No products indexed under this heading.

Meperidine Hydrochloride (Scopolamine is an anticholinergic agent and causes certain CNS effects, such as drowsiness and dizziness, and hence it should be used with care in patients on concomitant therapy).

No products indexed under this heading.

Mephobarbital (Scopolamine is an anticholinergic agent and causes certain CNS effects, such as drowsiness and dizziness, and hence it should be used with care in patients on concomitant therapy).

No products indexed under this heading.

Meprobamate (Scopolamine is an anticholinergic agent and causes certain CNS effects, such as drowsiness and dizziness, and hence it should be used with care in patients on concomitant therapy).

No products indexed under this heading.

Mesoridazine Besylate (Scopolamine is an anticholinergic agent and causes certain CNS effects, such as drowsiness and dizziness, and hence it should be used with care in patients on concomitant therapy).

No products indexed under this heading.

Metaxalone (Co-administration may result in additive anticholinergic effects). Products include:

Skelaxin Tablets 1784

Methadone Hydrochloride (Scopolamine is an anticholinergic agent and causes certain CNS effects, such as drowsiness and dizziness, and hence it should be used with care in patients on concomitant therapy).

No products indexed under this heading.

Methdilazine Hydrochloride (Antihistamines have anticholinergic properties and co-administration may result in additive effects).

No products indexed under this heading.

Methocarbamol (Co-administration may result in additive anticholinergic effects).

No products indexed under this heading.

Methohexital Sodium (Scopolamine is an anticholinergic agent and causes certain CNS effects, such as drowsiness and dizziness, and hence it should be used with care in patients on concomitant therapy).

No products indexed under this heading.

Methotrimeprazine (Scopolamine is an anticholinergic agent and causes certain CNS effects, such as drowsiness and dizziness, and hence it should be used with care in patients on concomitant therapy).

No products indexed under this heading.

Methoxyflurane (Scopolamine is an anticholinergic agent and causes certain CNS effects, such as drowsiness and dizziness, and hence it should be used with care in patients on concomitant therapy).

No products indexed under this heading.

Metocurine Iodide (Co-administration may result in addititve anticholinergic effects).

No products indexed under this heading.

Midazolam Hydrochloride (Scopolamine is an anticholinergic agent and causes certain CNS effects, such as drowsiness and dizziness, and hence it should be used with care in patients on concomitant therapy).

No products indexed under this heading.

Mivacurium Chloride (Co-administration may result in addititve anticholinergic effects).

No products indexed under this heading.

Molindone Hydrochloride (Scopolamine is an anticholinergic agent and causes certain CNS effects, such as drowsiness and dizziness, and hence it should be used with care in patients on concomitant therapy). Products include:

Moban Tablets 1116

Morphine Sulfate (Scopolamine is an anticholinergic agent and causes certain CNS effects, such as drowsiness and dizziness, and hence it should be used with care in patients on concomitant therapy). Products include:

Avinza Capsules 1772
DepoDur Injection 1095
MS Contin Tablets 2585

Nortriptyline Hydrochloride (Tricyclic antidepressants have anticholinergic properties and co-administration may result in additive effects).

No products indexed under this heading.

Olanzapine (Scopolamine is an anticholinergic agent and causes certain CNS effects, such as drowsiness and dizziness, and hence it should be used with care in patients on concomitant therapy). Products include:

Symbyax Capsules 1871
Zyprexa Tablets 1883
Zyprexa IntraMuscular 1883
Zyprexa ZYDIS Orally Disintegrating Tablets 1883

Oral Medications, unspecified (The absorption of oral medications may be decreased during the concurrent use of scopolamine because of decreased gastric motility and delayed gastric emptying).

No products indexed under this heading.

Orphenadrine Citrate (Co-administration may result in addititve anticholinergic effects).

No products indexed under this heading.

Oxazepam (Scopolamine is an anticholinergic agent and causes certain CNS effects, such as drowsiness and dizziness, and hence it should be used with care in patients on concomitant therapy).

No products indexed under this heading.

Oxybutynin Chloride (Co-administration may result in additive anticholinergic effects).

No products indexed under this heading.

Oxycodone Hydrochloride (Scopolamine is an anticholinergic agent and causes certain CNS effects, such as drowsiness and dizziness, and hence it should be used with care in patients on concomitant therapy). Products include:

OxyContin Tablets 2589
OxyIR Capsules 2593
Percocet Tablets 1127
Percodan Tablets 1130

Pancuronium Bromide (Co-administration may result in addititve anticholinergic effects).

No products indexed under this heading.

Pentobarbital Sodium (Scopolamine is an anticholinergic agent and causes certain CNS effects, such as drowsiness and dizziness, and hence it should be used with care in patients on concomitant therapy). Products include:

Nembutal Sodium Solution, USP 2494

Perphenazine (Scopolamine is an anticholinergic agent and causes certain CNS effects, such as drowsiness and dizziness, and hence it should be used with care in patients on concomitant therapy).

No products indexed under this heading.

Phenobarbital (Scopolamine is an anticholinergic agent and causes certain CNS effects, such as drowsiness and dizziness, and hence it should be used with care in patients on concomitant therapy). Products include:

Donnatal Extentabs 2507

Prazepam (Scopolamine is an anticholinergic agent and causes certain CNS effects, such as drowsiness and dizziness, and hence it should be used with care in patients on concomitant therapy).

No products indexed under this heading.

Prochlorperazine (Scopolamine is an anticholinergic agent and causes certain CNS effects, such as drowsiness and dizziness, and hence it should be used with care in patients on concomitant therapy).

No products indexed under this heading.

Procyclidine Hydrochloride (Co-administration may result in additive anticholinergic effects).

No products indexed under this heading.

Promethazine Hydrochloride (Antihistamines have anticholinergic properties and co-administration may result in additive effects).
No products indexed under this heading.

Propantheline Bromide (Co-administration may result in additive anticholinergic effects).
No products indexed under this heading.

Propofol (Scopolamine is an anticholinergic agent and causes certain CNS effects, such as drowsiness and dizziness, and hence it should be used with care in patients on concomitant therapy).
No products indexed under this heading.

Propoxyphene Hydrochloride (Scopolamine is an anticholinergic agent and causes certain CNS effects, such as drowsiness and dizziness, and hence it should be used with care in patients on concomitant therapy).
No products indexed under this heading.

Propoxyphene Napsylate (Scopolamine is an anticholinergic agent and causes certain CNS effects, such as drowsiness and dizziness, and hence it should be used with care in patients on concomitant therapy).
No products indexed under this heading.

Protriptyline Hydrochloride (Tricyclic antidepressants have anticholinergic properties and co-administration may result in additive effects).
No products indexed under this heading.

Pyrilamine Maleate (Antihistamines have anticholinergic properties and co-administration may result in additive effects).
No products indexed under this heading.

Pyrilamine Tannate (Antihistamines have anticholinergic properties and co-administration may result in additive effects).
No products indexed under this heading.

Quazepam (Scopolamine is an anticholinergic agent and causes certain CNS effects, such as drowsiness and dizziness, and hence it should be used with care in patients on concomitant therapy).
No products indexed under this heading.

Quetiapine Fumarate (Scopolamine is an anticholinergic agent and causes certain CNS effects, such as drowsiness and dizziness, and hence it should be used with care in patients on concomitant therapy).
No products indexed under this heading.

Ramelteon (Scopolamine is an anticholinergic agent and causes certain CNS effects, such as drowsiness and dizziness, and hence it should be used with care in patients on concomitant therapy). Products include:
Rozerem Tablets 3091

Rapacuronium Bromide (Co-administration may result in addititve anticholinergic effects).
No products indexed under this heading.

Remifentanil Hydrochloride (Scopolamine is an anticholinergic agent and causes certain CNS effects, such as drowsiness and dizziness, and hence it should be used with care in patients on concomitant therapy).
No products indexed under this heading.

Risperidone (Scopolamine is an anticholinergic agent and causes certain CNS effects, such as drowsiness and dizziness, and hence it should be used with care in patients on concomitant therapy). Products include:
Risperdal Consta Long-Acting Injection 1753

Rocuronium Bromide (Co-administration may result in addititve anticholinergic effects). Products include:
Zemuron Injection 2947

Scopolamine Hydrobromide (Co-administration may result in additive anticholinergic effects). Products include:
Donnatal Extentabs 2507

Secobarbital Sodium (Scopolamine is an anticholinergic agent and causes certain CNS effects, such as drowsiness and dizziness, and hence it should be used with care in patients on concomitant therapy).
No products indexed under this heading.

Sevoflurane (Scopolamine is an anticholinergic agent and causes certain CNS effects, such as drowsiness and dizziness, and hence it should be used with care in patients on concomitant therapy). Products include:
Ultane Liquid for Inhalation 524

Sodium Butabarbital (Scopolamine is an anticholinergic agent and causes certain CNS effects, such as drowsiness and dizziness, and hence it should be used with care in patients on concomitant therapy).
No products indexed under this heading.

Sodium Oxybate (Scopolamine is an anticholinergic agent and causes certain CNS effects, such as drowsiness and dizziness, and hence it should be used with care in patients on concomitant therapy). Products include:
Xyrem Oral Solution 1766

Succinylcholine Chloride (Co-administration may result in addititve anticholinergic effects).
No products indexed under this heading.

Sufentanil Citrate (Scopolamine is an anticholinergic agent and causes certain CNS effects, such as drowsiness and dizziness, and hence it should be used with care in patients on concomitant therapy).
No products indexed under this heading.

Temazepam (Scopolamine is an anticholinergic agent and causes certain CNS effects, such as drowsiness and dizziness, and hence it should be used with care in patients on concomitant therapy).
No products indexed under this heading.

Terfenadine (Antihistamines have anticholinergic properties and co-administration may result in additive effects).
No products indexed under this heading.

Thiamylal Sodium (Scopolamine is an anticholinergic agent and causes certain CNS effects, such as drowsiness and dizziness, and hence it should be used with care in patients on concomitant therapy).
No products indexed under this heading.

Thioridazine Hydrochloride (Scopolamine is an anticholinergic agent and causes certain CNS effects, such as drowsiness and dizziness, and hence it should be used with care in patients on concomitant therapy). Products include:
Thioridazine Hydrochloride Tablets 2195

Thiothixene (Scopolamine is an anticholinergic agent and causes certain CNS effects, such as drowsiness and dizziness, and hence it should be used with care in patients on concomitant therapy). Products include:
Thiothixene Capsules 2197

Tolterodine Tartrate (Co-administration may result in additive anticholinergic effects).
No products indexed under this heading.

Triazolam (Scopolamine is an anticholinergic agent and causes certain CNS effects, such as drowsiness and dizziness, and hence it should be used with care in patients on concomitant therapy).
No products indexed under this heading.

Tridihexethyl Chloride (Co-administration may result in additive anticholinergic effects).
No products indexed under this heading.

Trifluoperazine Hydrochloride (Scopolamine is an anticholinergic agent and causes certain CNS effects, such as drowsiness and dizziness, and hence it should be used with care in patients on concomitant therapy).
No products indexed under this heading.

Trihexyphenidyl Hydrochloride (Co-administration may result in additive anticholinergic effects).
No products indexed under this heading.

Trimeprazine Tartrate (Antihistamines have anticholinergic properties and co-administration may result in additive effects).
No products indexed under this heading.

Trimipramine Maleate (Tricyclic antidepressants have anticholinergic properties and co-administration may result in additive effects).
No products indexed under this heading.

Tripelennamine Hydrochloride (Antihistamines have anticholinergic properties and co-administration may result in additive effects).
No products indexed under this heading.

Triprolidine Hydrochloride (Antihistamines have anticholinergic properties and co-administration may result in additive effects).
No products indexed under this heading.

Vecuronium Bromide (Co-administration may result in addititve anticholinergic effects).
No products indexed under this heading.

Zaleplon (Scopolamine is an anticholinergic agent and causes certain CNS effects, such as drowsiness and dizziness, and hence it should be used with care in patients on concomitant therapy).
No products indexed under this heading.

Ziprasidone Hydrochloride (Scopolamine is an anticholinergic agent and causes certain CNS effects, such as drowsiness and dizziness, and hence it should be used with care in patients on concomitant therapy). Products include:
Geodon Capsules **2520**

Zolpidem Tartrate (Scopolamine is an anticholinergic agent and causes certain CNS effects, such as drowsiness and dizziness, and hence it should be used with care in patients on concomitant therapy). Products include:
Ambien Tablets **2692**
Ambien CR Tablets **2696**

Food Interactions

Alcohol (Scopolamine is an anticholinergic agent and causes certain CNS effects, such as drowsiness and dizziness, and hence it should be used with care in patients on concomitant therapy).

4LIFE TRANSFER FACTOR PLUS TRI-FACTOR FORMULA

(Colostrum, Polysaccharides, Transfer factor)................................ 628
None cited in PDR database.

TRASYLOL INJECTION

(Aprotinin) **799**
May interact with fibrinolytic agents and certain other agents. Compounds in these categories include:

Alteplase (Aprotinin may inhibit the effects of fibrinolytic agents). Products include:
Activase I.V. **1188**
Cathflo Activase **1198**

Anistreplase (Aprotinin may inhibit the effects of fibrinolytic agents).
No products indexed under this heading.

Captopril (Aprotinin may block the acute hypotensive effects of captopril). Products include:
Captopril Tablets **2182**

Heparin Sodium (Aprotinin, in the presence of heparin, has been found to prolong the activated clotting time (ACT) as measured by surface activation methods).
No products indexed under this heading.

Streptokinase (Aprotinin may inhibit the effects of fibrinolytic agents).
No products indexed under this heading.

Urokinase (Aprotinin may inhibit the effects of fibrinolytic agents).
No products indexed under this heading.

TRAUMEEL INJECTION SOLUTION

(Homeopathic Formulations) **1725**
None cited in PDR database.

TRAVATAN Z OPHTHALMIC SOLUTION

(Travoprost) **547**
None cited in PDR database.

IMPORTANT NOTE: Always consult each drug listing in the patient's regimen for possible interactions.

TREANDA FOR INJECTION
(Bendamustine Hydrochloride) **983**
May interact with cytochrome p450 1a2 inducers (selected) and cytochrome p450 1a2 inhibitors (selected). Compounds in these categories include:

Alatrofloxacin Mesylate (Inhibitors of CYP1A2 (e.g., fluvoxamine, ciprofloxacin) have potential to increase plasma concentrations of bendamustine and decrease plasma concentrations of active metabolites. Caution should be used, or alternative treatments considered if concomitant treatment with CYP1A2 inhibitors is needed).
No products indexed under this heading.

Amiodarone Hydrochloride (Inhibitors of CYP1A2 (e.g., fluvoxamine, ciprofloxacin) have potential to increase plasma concentrations of bendamustine and decrease plasma concentrations of active metabolites. Caution should be used, or alternative treatments considered if concomitant treatment with CYP1A2 inhibitors is needed).
No products indexed under this heading.

Anastrozole (Inhibitors of CYP1A2 (e.g., fluvoxamine, ciprofloxacin) have potential to increase plasma concentrations of bendamustine and decrease plasma concentrations of active metabolites. Caution should be used, or alternative treatments considered if concomitant treatment with CYP1A2 inhibitors is needed). Products include:
Arimidex Tablets **672**

Carbamazepine (Inducers of CYP1A2 (e.g., omeprazole, smoking) have potential to decrease plasma concentrations of bendamustine and increase plasma concentrations of its active metabolites. Caution should be used, or alternative treatments considered if concomitant treatment with CYP1A2 inducers is needed). Products include:
Carbatrol Capsules **3019**
Equetro Extended-Release Capsules................................. **3174**

Cimetidine (Inhibitors of CYP1A2 (e.g., fluvoxamine, ciprofloxacin) have potential to increase plasma concentrations of bendamustine and decrease plasma concentrations of active metabolites. Caution should be used, or alternative treatments considered if concomitant treatment with CYP1A2 inhibitors is needed).
No products indexed under this heading.

Cimetidine Hydrochloride (Inhibitors of CYP1A2 (e.g., fluvoxamine, ciprofloxacin) have potential to increase plasma concentrations of bendamustine and decrease plasma concentrations of active metabolites. Caution should be used, or alternative treatments considered if concomitant treatment with CYP1A2 inhibitors is needed).
No products indexed under this heading.

Ciprofloxacin (Inhibitors of CYP1A2 (e.g., fluvoxamine, ciprofloxacin) have potential to increase plasma concentrations of bendamustine and decrease plasma concentrations of active metabolites. Caution should be used, or alternative treatments considered if concomitant treatment with CYP1A2 inhibitors is needed). Products include:
Cipro I.V. **2817**
Cipro Oral Suspension **2810**
Cipro XR Tablets **2823**
Ciprodex Otic Suspension **541**

Ciprofloxacin Hydrochloride (Inhibitors of CYP1A2 (e.g., fluvoxamine, ciprofloxacin) have potential to increase plasma concentrations of bendamustine and decrease plasma concentrations of active metabolites. Caution should be used, or alternative treatments considered if concomitant treatment with CYP1A2 inhibitors is needed). Products include:
Cipro Tablets **2810**

Clarithromycin (Inhibitors of CYP1A2 (e.g., fluvoxamine, ciprofloxacin) have potential to increase plasma concentrations of bendamustine and decrease plasma concentrations of active metabolites. Caution should be used, or alternative treatments considered if concomitant treatment with CYP1A2 inhibitors is needed). Products include:
Biaxin/Biaxin XL **411**

Desogestrel (Inhibitors of CYP1A2 (e.g., fluvoxamine, ciprofloxacin) have potential to increase plasma concentrations of bendamustine and decrease plasma concentrations of active metabolites. Caution should be used, or alternative treatments considered if concomitant treatment with CYP1A2 inhibitors is needed). Products include:
Mircette Tablets **1034**

Diltiazem Hydrochloride (Inducers of CYP1A2 (e.g., omeprazole, smoking) have potential to decrease plasma concentrations of bendamustine and increase plasma concentrations of its active metabolites. Caution should be used, or alternative treatments considered if concomitant treatment with CYP1A2 inducers is needed). Products include:
Cardizem LA Extended Release Tablets **421**

Enoxacin (Inhibitors of CYP1A2 (e.g., fluvoxamine, ciprofloxacin) have potential to increase plasma concentrations of bendamustine and decrease plasma concentrations of active metabolites. Caution should be used, or alternative treatments considered if concomitant treatment with CYP1A2 inhibitors is needed).
No products indexed under this heading.

Erythromycin (Inducers of CYP1A2 (e.g., omeprazole, smoking) have potential to decrease plasma concentrations of bendamustine and increase plasma concentrations of its active metabolites. Caution should be used, or alternative treatments considered if concomitant treatment with CYP1A2 inducers is needed).
No products indexed under this heading.

Erythromycin Estolate (Inducers of CYP1A2 (e.g., omeprazole, smoking) have potential to decrease plasma concentrations of bendamustine and increase plasma concentrations of its active metabolites. Caution should be used, or alternative treatments considered if concomitant treatment with CYP1A2 inducers is needed).
No products indexed under this heading.

Erythromycin Ethylsuccinate (Inducers of CYP1A2 (e.g., omeprazole, smoking) have potential to decrease plasma concentrations of bendamustine and increase plasma concentrations of its active metabolites. Caution should be used, or alternative treatments considered if concomitant treatment with CYP1A2 inducers is needed). Products include:
E.E.S. **433**
EryPed **431**

Erythromycin Gluceptate (Inducers of CYP1A2 (e.g., omeprazole, smoking) have potential to decrease plasma concentrations of bendamustine and increase plasma concentrations of its active metabolites. Caution should be used, or alternative treatments considered if concomitant treatment with CYP1A2 inducers is needed).
No products indexed under this heading.

Erythromycin Lactobionate (Inducers of CYP1A2 (e.g., omeprazole, smoking) have potential to decrease plasma concentrations of bendamustine and increase plasma concentrations of its active metabolites. Caution should be used, or alternative treatments considered if concomitant treatment with CYP1A2 inducers is needed).
No products indexed under this heading.

Erythromycin Stearate (Inducers of CYP1A2 (e.g., omeprazole, smoking) have potential to decrease plasma concentrations of bendamustine and increase plasma concentrations of its active metabolites. Caution should be used, or alternative treatments considered if concomitant treatment with CYP1A2 inducers is needed).
No products indexed under this heading.

Ethinyl Estradiol (Inhibitors of CYP1A2 (e.g., fluvoxamine, ciprofloxacin) have potential to increase plasma concentrations of bendamustine and decrease plasma concentrations of active metabolites. Caution should be used, or alternative treatments considered if concomitant treatment with CYP1A2 inhibitors is needed). Products include:
Lybrel Tablets **3204**
Mircette Tablets **1034**
NuvaRing **2897**
Ortho-Cyclen/Ortho Tri-Cyclen **2449**
Ortho Evra Transdermal System **2437**
Ortho Tri-Cyclen Lo Tablets **2458**
Seasonique Tablets **1046**
Yaz Tablets **805**

Fluvoxamine (Inhibitors of CYP1A2 (e.g., fluvoxamine, ciprofloxacin) have potential to increase plasma concentrations of bendamustine and decrease plasma concentrations of active metabolites. Caution should be used, or alternative treatments considered if concomitant treatment with CYP1A2 inhibitors is needed).
No products indexed under this heading.

Fluvoxamine Maleate (Inhibitors of CYP1A2 (e.g., fluvoxamine, ciprofloxacin) have potential to increase plasma concentrations of bendamustine and decrease plasma concentrations of active metabolites. Caution should be used, or alternative treatments considered if concomitant treatment with CYP1A2 inhibitors is needed). Products include:
Luvox CR Extended-Release Capsules.. **1759**

Gatifloxacin (Inhibitors of CYP1A2 (e.g., fluvoxamine, ciprofloxacin) have potential to increase plasma concentrations of bendamustine and decrease plasma concentrations of active metabolites. Caution should be used, or alternative treatments considered if concomitant treatment with CYP1A2 inhibitors is needed).
No products indexed under this heading.

Gemifloxacin Mesylate (Inhibitors of CYP1A2 (e.g., fluvoxamine, ciprofloxacin) have potential to increase plasma concentrations of bendamustine and decrease plasma concentrations of active metabolites. Caution should be used, or alternative treatments considered if concomitant treatment with CYP1A2 inhibitors is needed).
No products indexed under this heading.

Grepafloxacin Hydrochloride (Inhibitors of CYP1A2 (e.g., fluvoxamine, ciprofloxacin) have potential to increase plasma concentrations of bendamustine and decrease plasma concentrations of active metabolites. Caution should be used, or alternative treatments considered if concomitant treatment with CYP1A2 inhibitors is needed).
No products indexed under this heading.

Isoniazid (Inhibitors of CYP1A2 (e.g., fluvoxamine, ciprofloxacin) have potential to increase plasma concentrations of bendamustine and decrease plasma concentrations of active metabolites. Caution should be used, or alternative treatments considered if concomitant treatment with CYP1A2 inhibitors is needed).
No products indexed under this heading.

Ketoconazole (Inhibitors of CYP1A2 (e.g., fluvoxamine, ciprofloxacin) have potential to increase plasma concentrations of bendamustine and decrease plasma concentrations of active metabolites. Caution should be used, or alternative treatments considered if concomitant treatment with CYP1A2 inhibitors is needed). Products include:
Extina Foam, 2% **3057**
Nizoral A-D Shampoo **1901**

Levofloxacin (Inhibitors of CYP1A2 (e.g., fluvoxamine, ciprofloxacin) have potential to increase plasma concentrations of bendamustine and decrease plasma concentrations of active metabolites. Caution should be used, or alternative treatments considered if concomitant treatment with CYP1A2 inhibitors is needed). Products include:
Iquix Ophthalmic Solution **3183**
Levaquin **2416**
Levaquin in 5% Dextrose Injection **2416**
Quixin Ophthalmic Solution **3184**

Levonorgestrel (Inhibitors of CYP1A2 (e.g., fluvoxamine, ciprofloxacin) have potential to increase plasma concentrations of bendamustine and decrease plasma concentrations of active metabolites. Caution should be used, or alternative treatments considered if concomitant treatment with CYP1A2 inhibitors is needed). Products include:
Climara Pro Transdermal System **768**
Lybrel Tablets **3204**
Mirena Intrauterine System **779**
Plan B Tablets **1044**
Seasonique Tablets **1046**

Lomefloxacin Hydrochloride (Inhibitors of CYP1A2 (e.g., fluvoxamine, ciprofloxacin) have potential to increase plasma concentrations of bendamustine and decrease plasma concentrations of active metabolites. Caution should be used, or alternative treatments considered if concomitant treatment with CYP1A2 inhibitors is needed).
No products indexed under this heading.

Mestranol (Inhibitors of CYP1A2 (e.g., fluvoxamine, ciprofloxacin) have potential to increase plasma concentrations of bendamustine and decrease plasma concentrations of active metabolites. Caution should be used, or alternative treatments considered if concomitant treatment with CYP1A2 inhibitors is needed).
No products indexed under this heading.

Methoxsalen (Inhibitors of CYP1A2 (e.g., fluvoxamine, ciprofloxacin) have potential to increase plasma concentrations of bendamustine and decrease plasma concentrations of active metabolites. Caution should be used, or alternative treatments considered if concomitant treatment with CYP1A2 inhibitors is needed).
No products indexed under this heading.

Mexiletine Hydrochloride (Inhibitors of CYP1A2 (e.g., fluvoxamine, ciprofloxacin) have potential to increase plasma concentrations of bendamustine and decrease plasma concentrations of active metabolites. Caution should be used, or alternative treatments considered if concomitant treatment with CYP1A2 inhibitors is needed).
No products indexed under this heading.

Mibefradil Dihydrochloride (Inhibitors of CYP1A2 (e.g., fluvoxamine, ciprofloxacin) have potential to increase plasma concentrations of bendamustine and decrease plasma concentrations of active metabolites. Caution should be used, or alternative treatments considered if concomitant treatment with CYP1A2 inhibitors is needed).
No products indexed under this heading.

Moxifloxacin Hydrochloride (Inhibitors of CYP1A2 (e.g., fluvoxamine, ciprofloxacin) have potential to increase plasma concentrations of bendamustine and decrease plasma concentrations of active metabolites. Caution should be used, or alternative treatments considered if concomitant treatment with CYP1A2 inhibitors is needed). Products include:
Avelox 2803
Vigamox Ophthalmic Solution 548

Nalidixic Acid (Inhibitors of CYP1A2 (e.g., fluvoxamine, ciprofloxacin) have potential to increase plasma concentrations of bendamustine and decrease plasma concentrations of active metabolites. Caution should be used, or alternative treatments considered if concomitant treatment with CYP1A2 inhibitors is needed).
No products indexed under this heading.

Nicotine Salicylate (Inducers of CYP1A2 (e.g., omeprazole, smoking) have potential to decrease plasma concentrations of bendamustine and increase plasma concentrations of its active metabolites. Caution should be used, or alternative treatments considered if concomitant treatment with CYP1A2 inducers is needed).
No products indexed under this heading.

Norethindrone (Inhibitors of CYP1A2 (e.g., fluvoxamine, ciprofloxacin) have potential to increase plasma concentrations of bendamustine and decrease plasma concentrations of active metabolites. Caution should be used, or alternative treatments considered if concomitant treatment with CYP1A2 inhibitors is needed). Products include:
Ortho Micronor Tablets 2446

Norfloxacin (Inhibitors of CYP1A2 (e.g., fluvoxamine, ciprofloxacin) have potential to increase plasma concentrations of bendamustine and decrease plasma concentrations of active metabolites. Caution should be used, or alternative treatments considered if concomitant treatment with CYP1A2 inhibitors is needed). Products include:
Noroxin Tablets 2069

Norgestrel (Inhibitors of CYP1A2 (e.g., fluvoxamine, ciprofloxacin) have potential to increase plasma concentrations of bendamustine and decrease plasma concentrations of active metabolites. Caution should be used, or alternative treatments considered if concomitant treatment with CYP1A2 inhibitors is needed).
No products indexed under this heading.

Ofloxacin (Inhibitors of CYP1A2 (e.g., fluvoxamine, ciprofloxacin) have potential to increase plasma concentrations of bendamustine and decrease plasma concentrations of active metabolites. Caution should be used, or alternative treatments considered if concomitant treatment with CYP1A2 inhibitors is needed). Products include:
Ofloxacin Ophthalmic Solution 0.3% .... ⊙ 243

Omeprazole (Inhibitors of CYP1A2 (e.g., fluvoxamine, ciprofloxacin) have potential to increase plasma concentrations of bendamustine and decrease plasma concentrations of active metabolites. Caution should be used, or alternative treatments considered if concomitant treatment with CYP1A2 inhibitors is needed).
No products indexed under this heading.

Paroxetine Hydrochloride (Inhibitors of CYP1A2 (e.g., fluvoxamine, ciprofloxacin) have potential to increase plasma concentrations of bendamustine and decrease plasma concentrations of active metabolites. Caution should be used, or alternative treatments considered if concomitant treatment with CYP1A2 inhibitors is needed). Products include:
Paxil 1535
Paxil CR Controlled-Release Tablets 1544

Ranitidine Hydrochloride (Inhibitors of CYP1A2 (e.g., fluvoxamine, ciprofloxacin) have potential to increase plasma concentrations of bendamustine and decrease plasma concentrations of active metabolites. Caution should be used, or alternative treatments considered if concomitant treatment with CYP1A2 inhibitors is needed). Products include:
Zantac 75 Tablets 603
Zantac 1670
Zantac Injection 1666
Zantac Injection Pharmacy Bulk Package 1668
Maximum Strength Zantac 150 Tablets 603
Maximum Strength Zantac 150 Cool Mint Tablets 603

Rifampicin (Inducers of CYP1A2 (e.g., omeprazole, smoking) have potential to decrease plasma concentrations of bendamustine and increase plasma concentrations of its active metabolites. Caution should be used, or alternative treatments considered if concomitant treatment with CYP1A2 inducers is needed).
No products indexed under this heading.

Ritonavir (Inhibitors of CYP1A2 (e.g., fluvoxamine, ciprofloxacin) have potential to increase plasma concentrations of bendamustine and decrease plasma concentrations of active metabolites. Caution should be used, or alternative treatments considered if concomitant treatment with CYP1A2 inhibitors is needed). Products include:
Kaletra 452
Norvir 489

Sildenafil Citrate (Inhibitors of CYP1A2 (e.g., fluvoxamine, ciprofloxacin) have potential to increase plasma concentrations of bendamustine and decrease plasma concentrations of active metabolites. Caution should be used, or alternative treatments considered if concomitant treatment with CYP1A2 inhibitors is needed).
No products indexed under this heading.

Sparfloxacin (Inhibitors of CYP1A2 (e.g., fluvoxamine, ciprofloxacin) have potential to increase plasma concentrations of bendamustine and decrease plasma concentrations of active metabolites. Caution should be used, or alternative treatments considered if concomitant treatment with CYP1A2 inhibitors is needed).
No products indexed under this heading.

Tacrine Hydrochloride (Inhibitors of CYP1A2 (e.g., fluvoxamine, ciprofloxacin) have potential to increase plasma concentrations of bendamustine and decrease plasma concentrations of active metabolites. Caution should be used, or alternative treatments considered if concomitant treatment with CYP1A2 inhibitors is needed).
No products indexed under this heading.

Ticlopidine Hydrochloride (Inhibitors of CYP1A2 (e.g., fluvoxamine, ciprofloxacin) have potential to increase plasma concentrations of bendamustine and decrease plasma concentrations of active metabolites. Caution should be used, or alternative treatments considered if concomitant treatment with CYP1A2 inhibitors is needed).
No products indexed under this heading.

Troleandomycin (Inhibitors of CYP1A2 (e.g., fluvoxamine, ciprofloxacin) have potential to increase plasma concentrations of bendamustine and decrease plasma concentrations of active metabolites. Caution should be used, or alternative treatments considered if concomitant treatment with CYP1A2 inhibitors is needed).
No products indexed under this heading.

Trovafloxacin Mesylate (Inhibitors of CYP1A2 (e.g., fluvoxamine, ciprofloxacin) have potential to increase plasma concentrations of bendamustine and decrease plasma concentrations of active metabolites. Caution should be used, or alternative treatments considered if concomitant treatment with CYP1A2 inhibitors is needed).
No products indexed under this heading.

Vardenafil Hydrochloride (Inhibitors of CYP1A2 (e.g., fluvoxamine, ciprofloxacin) have potential to increase plasma concentrations of bendamustine and decrease plasma concentrations of active metabolites. Caution should be used, or alternative treatments considered if concomitant treatment with CYP1A2 inhibitors is needed). Products include:
Levitra Tablets 2876

Zileuton (Inhibitors of CYP1A2 (e.g., fluvoxamine, ciprofloxacin) have potential to increase plasma concentrations of bendamustine and decrease plasma concentrations of active metabolites. Caution should be used, or alternative treatments considered if concomitant treatment with CYP1A2 inhibitors is needed).
No products indexed under this heading.

Food Interactions

Broccoli (Inducers of CYP1A2 (e.g., omeprazole, smoking) have potential to decrease plasma concentrations of bendamustine and increase plasma concentrations of its active metabolites. Caution should be used, or alternative treatments considered if concomitant treatment with CYP1A2 inducers is needed).

Grapefruit Juice (Inhibitors of CYP1A2 (e.g., fluvoxamine, ciprofloxacin) have potential to increase plasma concentrations of bendamustine and decrease plasma concentrations of active metabolites. Caution should be used, or alternative treatments considered if concomitant treatment with CYP1A2 inhibitors is needed).

TREXIMET TABLETS

(Naproxen Sodium, Sumatriptan Succinate) 1616

May interact with aspirin-acetylsalicylic acid, beta blockers, ergot-containing drugs, lithium preparations, monoamine oxidase inhibitors, Serotonin and Norepinephrine Reuptake Inhibitors, selective serotonin reuptake inhibitors, triptans, and certain other agents. Compounds in these categories include:

Acebutolol Hydrochloride (Naproxen and other NSAIDs can reduce the antihypertensive effect of propranolol and other beta blockers).
No products indexed under this heading.

Almotriptan Malate (Cases of life-threatening serotonin syndrome

have been reported during combined use of triptans with Treximet). Products include:
Axert Tablets 2431

Aspirin (When naproxen is administered with aspirin/ aspirin-acetylsalicylic acid, its protein binding is reduced, although the clearance of free naproxen is not altered. The clinical significance of this interaction is not known, however, as with other NSAID-containing products, concomitant administration of Treximet and aspirin/ aspirin-acetylsalicylic acid is not generally recommended because of the potential of increased adverse side effects). Products include:
Aggrenox Capsules 819
Bayer Aspirin 750
Percodan Tablets 1130
St. Joseph 81 mg Aspirin Chewable and Enteric Coated Tablets 1903

Aspirin, Enteric Coated (When naproxen is administered with aspirin/aspirin-acetylsalicylic acid, its protein binding is reduced, although the clearance of free naproxen is not altered. The clinical significance of this interaction is not known, however, as with other NSAID-containing products, concomitant administration of Treximet and aspirin/aspirin-acetylsalicylic acid is not generally recommended because of the potential of increased adverse side effects).
No products indexed under this heading.

Aspirin Buffered (When naproxen is administered with aspirin/ aspirin-acetylsalicylic acid, its protein binding is reduced, although the clearance of free naproxen is not altered. The clinical significance of this interaction is not known, however, as with other NSAID-containing products, concomitant administration of Treximet and aspirin/ aspirin-acetylsalicylic acid is not generally recommended because of the potential of increased adverse side effects).
No products indexed under this heading.

Atenolol (Naproxen and other NSAIDs can reduce the antihypertensive effect of propranolol and other beta blockers).
No products indexed under this heading.

Betaxolol Hydrochloride (Naproxen and other NSAIDs can reduce the antihypertensive effect of propranolol and other beta blockers).
No products indexed under this heading.

Bisoprolol Fumarate (Naproxen and other NSAIDs can reduce the antihypertensive effect of propranolol and other beta blockers).
No products indexed under this heading.

Carteolol Hydrochloride (Naproxen and other NSAIDs can reduce the antihypertensive effect of propranolol and other beta blockers).
No products indexed under this heading.

Citalopram Hydrobromide (Cases of life-threatening serotonin syndrome have been reported during combined use of selective serotonin reuptake inhibitors with Treximet). Products include:
Celexa 1160

Desvenlafaxine Succinate (Cases of life-threatening serotonin syndrome have been reported during combined use of serotonin and norepinephrine reuptake inhibitors with Treximet). Products include:
Pristiq Extended-Release Tablets 3247

Dihydroergotamine Mesylate (Ergot-containing drugs may cause prolonged vasospastic reactions. The use of ergot-type or ergot-containing medications (e.g., dihydroergotamine, methysergide) and Treximet within 24 hours of each other should be avoided).
No products indexed under this heading.

Duloxetine Hydrochloride (Cases of life-threatening serotonin syndrome have been reported during combined use of serotonin and norepinephrine reuptake inhibitors with Treximet). Products include:
Cymbalta Delayed-Release Capsules 1801

Eletriptan Hydrobromide (Cases of life-threatening serotonin syndrome have been reported during combined use of triptans with Treximet).
No products indexed under this heading.

Ergonovine Maleate (Ergot-containing drugs may cause prolonged vasospastic reactions. The use of ergot-type or ergot-containing medications (e.g., dihydroergotamine, methysergide) and Treximet within 24 hours of each other should be avoided).
No products indexed under this heading.

Ergotamine Tartrate (Ergot-containing drugs may cause prolonged vasospastic reactions. The use of ergot-type or ergot-containing medications (e.g., dihydroergotamine, methysergide) and Treximet within 24 hours of each other should be avoided).
No products indexed under this heading.

Escitalopram Oxalate (Cases of life-threatening serotonin syndrome have been reported during combined use of selective serotonin reuptake inhibitors with Treximet). Products include:
Lexapro Oral Suspension 1174
Lexapro Tablets 1174

Esmolol Hydrochloride (Naproxen and other NSAIDs can reduce the antihypertensive effect of propranolol and other beta blockers).
No products indexed under this heading.

Fluoxetine (Cases of life-threatening serotonin syndrome have been reported during combined use of selective serotonin reuptake inhibitors with Treximet).
No products indexed under this heading.

Fluoxetine Hydrochloride (Cases of life-threatening serotonin syndrome have been reported during combined use of selective serotonin reuptake inhibitors with Treximet). Products include:
Prozac Weekly Capsules 1852
Prozac Pulvules and Liquid 1852
Symbyax Capsules 1871

Fluvoxamine Maleate (Cases of life-threatening serotonin syndrome have been reported during combined use of selective serotonin reuptake inhibitors with Treximet). Products include:
Luvox CR Extended-Release Capsules 1759

Frovatriptan Succinate (Cases of life-threatening serotonin syndrome have been reported during combined use of triptans with Treximet). Products include:
Frova Tablets 1111

Furosemide (Studies and postmarketing observations have shown that NSAIDs can reduce the natriuretic effect of furosemide and thiazides in some patients. During concomitant therapy with NSAIDs, the patient should be observed closely for signs of renal failure, as well as to assure diuretic efficacy). Products include:
Furosemide Tablets 2186

Isocarboxazid (The use of Treximet in patients receiving monoamine oxidase inhibitors is contraindicated. MAIOs reduce sumatriptan clearance, significantly increasing systemic exposure). Products include:
Marplan Tablets 3177

Labetalol Hydrochloride (Naproxen and other NSAIDs can reduce the antihypertensive effect of propranolol and other beta blockers).
No products indexed under this heading.

Levobunolol Hydrochloride (Naproxen and other NSAIDs can reduce the antihypertensive effect of propranolol and other beta blockers).
No products indexed under this heading.

Lithium (NSAIDs have produced an elevation of plasma lithium levels and a reduction in renal lithium clearance. The mean minimum lithium concentration increased 15% and the renal clearance was decreased by approximately 20%. These effects have been attributed to inhibition of renal prostaglandin synthesis by the NSAID. When Treximet and lithium are administered concurrently, patients should be observed carefully for signs of lithium toxicity).
No products indexed under this heading.

Lithium Carbonate (NSAIDs have produced an elevation of plasma lithium levels and a reduction in renal lithium clearance. The mean minimum lithium concentration increased 15% and the renal clearance was decreased by approximately 20%. These effects have been attributed to inhibition of renal prostaglandin synthesis by the NSAID. When Treximet and lithium are administered concurrently, patients should be observed carefully for signs of lithium toxicity).
No products indexed under this heading.

Lithium Citrate (NSAIDs have produced an elevation of plasma lithium levels and a reduction in renal lithium clearance. The mean minimum lithium concentration increased 15% and the renal clearance was decreased by approximately 20%. These effects have been attributed to inhibition of renal prostaglandin synthesis by the NSAID. When Treximet and lithium are administered concurrently, patients should be observed carefully for signs of lithium toxicity).
No products indexed under this heading.

Methotrexate Sodium (Caution should be used if Treximet is administered concomitantly with methotrexate. Concomitant administration of some NSAIDs with high-dose methotrexate therapy has been reported to elevate and prolong serum methotrexate levels, resulting in deaths from severe hematologic and gastrointestinal toxicity).
No products indexed under this heading.

Methylergonovine Maleate (Ergot-containing drugs may cause prolonged vasospastic reactions. The use of ergot-type or ergot-containing medications (e.g., dihydroergotamine, methysergide) and Treximet within 24 hours of each other should be avoided).
No products indexed under this heading.

Methysergide Maleate (Ergot-containing drugs may cause prolonged vasospastic reactions. The use of ergot-type or ergot-containing medications (e.g., dihydroergotamine, methysergide) and Treximet within 24 hours of each other should be avoided).
No products indexed under this heading.

Metipranolol Hydrochloride (Naproxen and other NSAIDs can reduce the antihypertensive effect of propranolol and other beta blockers).
No products indexed under this heading.

Metoprolol Succinate (Naproxen and other NSAIDs can reduce the antihypertensive effect of propranolol and other beta blockers). Products include:
Toprol-XL Tablets 666

Metoprolol Tartrate (Naproxen and other NSAIDs can reduce the antihypertensive effect of propranolol and other beta blockers).
No products indexed under this heading.

Moclobemide (The use of Treximet in patients receiving monoamine oxidase inhibitors is contraindicated. MAIOs reduce sumatriptan clearance, significantly increasing systemic exposure).
No products indexed under this heading.

Nadolol (Naproxen and other NSAIDs can reduce the antihypertensive effect of propranolol and other beta blockers). Products include:
Nadolol Tablets 2191

Naratriptan Hydrochloride (Cases of life-threatening serotonin syndrome have been reported during combined use of triptans with Treximet). Products include:
Amerge Tablets 1301

Nebivolol (Naproxen and other NSAIDs can reduce the antihypertensive effect of propranolol and other beta blockers). Products include:
Bystolic Tablets 1155

Nefazodone Hydrochloride (Cases of life-threatening serotonin syndrome have been reported during combined use of serotonin and norepinephrine reuptake inhibitors with Treximet).
No products indexed under this heading.

Pargyline Hydrochloride (The use of Treximet in patients receiving monoamine oxidase inhibitors is contraindicated. MAIOs reduce sumatriptan clearance, significantly increasing systemic exposure).
No products indexed under this heading.

Paroxetine Hydrochloride (Cases of life-threatening serotonin syndrome have been reported during combined use of selective serotonin reuptake inhibitors with Treximet). Products include:
Paxil ... 1535
Paxil CR Controlled-Release Tablets ... 1544

Penbutolol Sulfate (Naproxen and other NSAIDs can reduce the antihypertensive effect of propranolol and other beta blockers).
No products indexed under this heading.

Phenelzine Sulfate (The use of Treximet in patients receiving monoamine oxidase inhibitors is contraindicated. MAIOs reduce sumatriptan clearance, significantly increasing systemic exposure).
No products indexed under this heading.

Pindolol (Naproxen and other NSAIDs can reduce the antihypertensive effect of propranolol and other beta blockers).
No products indexed under this heading.

Probenecid (Concurrent use of probenecid with Treximet increases naproxen anion plasma levels and extends its plasma half-life significantly).
No products indexed under this heading.

Procarbazine Hydrochloride (The use of Treximet in patients receiving monoamine oxidase inhibitors is contraindicated. MAIOs reduce sumatriptan clearance, significantly increasing systemic exposure).
No products indexed under this heading.

Propranolol Hydrochloride (Naproxen and other NSAIDs can reduce the antihypertensive effect of propranolol and other beta-blockers). Products include:
InnoPran XL Extended Release Capsules ... 1484

Rasagiline Mesylate (The use of Treximet in patients receiving monoamine oxidase inhibitors is contraindicated. MAIOs reduce sumatriptan clearance, significantly increasing systemic exposure). Products include:
Azilect Tablets ... 3106

Rizatriptan Benzoate (Cases of life-threatening serotonin syndrome have been reported during combined use of triptans with Treximet). Products include:
Maxalt Tablets ... 2056
Maxalt-MLT Orally Disintegrating Tablets ... 2056

Selegiline (The use of Treximet in patients receiving monoamine oxidase inhibitors is contraindicated. MAIOs reduce sumatriptan clearance, significantly increasing systemic exposure). Products include:
Emsam Transdermal System ... 905

Selegiline Hydrochloride (The use of Treximet in patients receiving monoamine oxidase inhibitors is contraindicated. MAIOs reduce sumatriptan clearance, significantly increasing systemic exposure). Products include:
Eldepryl Capsules ... 3052

Sertraline Hydrochloride (Cases of life-threatening serotonin syndrome have been reported during combined use of selective serotonin reuptake inhibitors with Treximet).
No products indexed under this heading.

Sotalol Hydrochloride (Naproxen and other NSAIDs can reduce the antihypertensive effect of propranolol and other beta blockers).
No products indexed under this heading.

Sumatriptan (Cases of life-threatening serotonin syndrome have been reported during combined use of triptans with Treximet). Products include:
Imitrex Nasal Spray ... 1470

Timolol Hemihydrate (Naproxen and other NSAIDs can reduce the antihypertensive effect of propranolol and other beta blockers). Products include:
Betimol Ophthalmic Solution ... 3181

Timolol Maleate (Naproxen and other NSAIDs can reduce the antihypertensive effect of propranolol and other beta blockers). Products include:
Combigan Ophthalmic Solution ... 553
Cosopt Sterile Ophthalmic Solution ... 1969
Timoptic Sterile Ophthalmic Solution ... 2121
Timoptic in Ocudose ... 2124
Timoptic-XE Sterile Ophthalmic Gel Forming Solution ... 2125

Tranylcypromine Sulfate (The use of Treximet in patients receiving monoamine oxidase inhibitors is contraindicated. MAIOs reduce sumatriptan clearance, significantly increasing systemic exposure). Products include:
Parnate Tablets ... 1532

Venlafaxine Hydrochloride (Cases of life-threatening serotonin syndrome have been reported during combined use of serotonin and norepinephrine reuptake inhibitors with Treximet). Products include:
Effexor XR Extended-Release Capsules ... 3195
Venlafaxine Hydrochloride Tablets ... 2199

Warfarin Sodium (The effects of warfarin and NSAIDs on gastrointestinal bleeding are synergistic, such that patients taking both drugs have a higher risk of serious gastrointestinal bleeding than patients taking each drug alone).
No products indexed under this heading.

Zolmitriptan (Cases of life-threatening serotonin syndrome have been reported during combined use of triptans with Treximet). Products include:
Zomig Tablets ... 694
Zomig Nasal Spray ... 689
Zomig-ZMT Tablets ... 694

TRICOR TABLETS

(Fenofibrate) ... 520
May interact with bile acid sequestering agents, oral anticoagulants, HMG-CoA reductase inhibitors, immunosuppressive agents, nephrotoxic agents, and certain other agents. Compounds in these categories include:

Abacavir Sulfate (The benefits and risks of using fenofibrate tablets with immunosuppressants and other potentially nephrotoxic agents should be carefully considered and the lowest effective dose employed). Products include:
Epzicom Tablets ... 1422
Trizivir Tablets ... 1622
Ziagen ... 1673

Acyclovir (The benefits and risks of using fenofibrate tablets with immunosuppressants and other potentially nephrotoxic agents should be carefully considered and the lowest effective dose employed). Products include:
Zovirax ... 1690
Zovirax Cream ... 817
Zovirax Ointment ... 819

Acyclovir Sodium (The benefits and risks of using fenofibrate tablets with immunosuppressants and other potentially nephrotoxic agents should be carefully considered and the lowest effective dose employed).
No products indexed under this heading.

Alatrofloxacin Mesylate (The benefits and risks of using fenofibrate tablets with immunosuppressants and other potentially nephrotoxic agents should be carefully considered and the lowest effective dose employed).
No products indexed under this heading.

Aldesleukin (The benefits and risks of using fenofibrate tablets with immunosuppressants and other potentially nephrotoxic agents should be carefully considered and the lowest effective dose employed). Products include:
Proleukin for Injection ... 2287

Amikacin Sulfate (The benefits and risks of using fenofibrate tablets with immunosuppressants and other potentially nephrotoxic agents should be carefully considered and the lowest effective dose employed).
No products indexed under this heading.

Amoxicillin (The benefits and risks of using fenofibrate tablets with immunosuppressants and other potentially nephrotoxic agents should be carefully considered and the lowest effective dose employed). Products include:
Amoxil Capsules ... 1305
Amoxil Chewable Tablets ... 1305
Amoxil Pediatric Drops for Oral Suspension ... 1305
Amoxil Powder for Oral Suspension ... 1305
Amoxil Tablets ... 1305
Augmentin ... 1323
Augmentin Tablets ... 1327
Augmentin XR Extended Release Tablets ... 1333
Augmentin ES-600 Powder for Oral Suspension ... 1329
Moxatag Tablets ... 2165

Amoxicillin Trihydrate (The benefits and risks of using fenofibrate tablets with immunosuppressants and other potentially nephrotoxic agents should be carefully considered and the lowest effective dose employed).
No products indexed under this heading.

Amphotericin B (The benefits and risks of using fenofibrate tablets with immunosuppressants and other potentially nephrotoxic agents should be carefully considered and the lowest effective dose employed).
No products indexed under this heading.

Amphotericin B, liposomal (The benefits and risks of using fenofibrate tablets with immunosuppressants and other potentially nephrotoxic agents should be carefully considered and the lowest effective dose employed). Products include:
AmBisome for Injection ... 606

Amphotericin B Cholesteryl Sulfate (The benefits and risks of using fenofibrate tablets with immunosuppressants and other potentially nephrotoxic agents should be carefully considered and the lowest effective dose employed).
No products indexed under this heading.

Amphotericin B Lipid Complex (The benefits and risks of using fenofibrate tablets with immunosuppressants and other potentially nephrotoxic agents should be carefully considered and the lowest effective dose employed). Products include:
Abelcet Injection ... 1134

Ampicillin (The benefits and risks of using fenofibrate tablets with immunosuppressants and other potentially nephrotoxic agents should be carefully considered and the lowest effective dose employed).
No products indexed under this heading.

Ampicillin Sodium (The benefits and risks of using fenofibrate tablets with immunosuppressants and other potentially nephrotoxic agents should be carefully considered and the lowest effective dose employed).
No products indexed under this heading.

Ampicillin Trihydrate (The benefits and risks of using fenofibrate tablets with immunosuppressants and other potentially nephrotoxic agents should be carefully considered and the lowest effective dose employed).
No products indexed under this heading.

Amprenavir (The benefits and risks of using fenofibrate tablets with immunosuppressants and other potentially nephrotoxic agents should be carefully considered and the lowest effective dose employed).
No products indexed under this heading.

Anisindione (Caution should be exercised when anticoagulants are given in conjunction with fenofibrate because of the potentiation of coumarin-type anticoagulants in prolonging the PT/INR. The dosage of the anticoagulant should be reduced to maintain the PT/INR at the desired level to prevent bleeding complications. Frequent PT/INR determinations are advisable until it has been definitely determined that the PT/INR has stabilized).
No products indexed under this heading.

Aspirin (The benefits and risks of using fenofibrate tablets with immunosuppressants and other potentially nephrotoxic agents should be care-

fully considered and the lowest effective dose employed). Products include:

Aggrenox Capsules 819
Bayer Aspirin 750
Percodan Tablets 1130
St. Joseph 81 mg Aspirin Chewable and Enteric Coated Tablets 1903

Atazanavir (The benefits and risks of using fenofibrate tablets with immunosuppressants and other potentially nephrotoxic agents should be carefully considered and the lowest effective dose employed).
No products indexed under this heading.

Atorvastatin Calcium (Co-administration of fibric acid derivatives and HMG-CoA reductase inhibitors has been associated with rhabdomyolysis, markedly elevated creatine kinase levels and myoglobulinuria, leading in a high proportion of cases to acute renal failure; the combined use should be avoided unless the benefit of further alterations in lipid levels is likely to outweigh the increased risk of this combination). Products include:

Lipitor Tablets 2501

Azathioprine (The benefits and risks of using fenofibrate tablets with immunosuppressants and other potentially nephrotoxic agents should be carefully considered and the lowest effective dose employed).
No products indexed under this heading.

Azithromycin Dihydrate (The benefits and risks of using fenofibrate tablets with immunosuppressants and other potentially nephrotoxic agents should be carefully considered and the lowest effective dose employed).
No products indexed under this heading.

Azlocillin Sodium (The benefits and risks of using fenofibrate tablets with immunosuppressants and other potentially nephrotoxic agents should be carefully considered and the lowest effective dose employed).
No products indexed under this heading.

Aztreonam (The benefits and risks of using fenofibrate tablets with immunosuppressants and other potentially nephrotoxic agents should be carefully considered and the lowest effective dose employed).
No products indexed under this heading.

Bacampicillin Hydrochloride (The benefits and risks of using fenofibrate tablets with immunosuppressants and other potentially nephrotoxic agents should be carefully considered and the lowest effective dose employed).
No products indexed under this heading.

Balsalazide Disodium (The benefits and risks of using fenofibrate tablets with immunosuppressants and other potentially nephrotoxic agents should be carefully considered and the lowest effective dose employed).
No products indexed under this heading.

Basiliximab (The benefits and risks of using fenofibrate tablets with immunosuppressants and other potentially nephrotoxic agents should be carefully considered and the lowest effective dose employed). Products include:

Simulect for Injection 2306

Benazepril Hydrochloride (The benefits and risks of using fenofibrate tablets with immunosuppressants and other potentially nephrotoxic agents should be carefully considered and the lowest effective dose employed).
No products indexed under this heading.

Bendroflumethiazide (The benefits and risks of using fenofibrate tablets with immunosuppressants and other potentially nephrotoxic agents should be carefully considered and the lowest effective dose employed).
No products indexed under this heading.

Caffeine (The benefits and risks of using fenofibrate tablets with immunosuppressants and other potentially nephrotoxic agents should be carefully considered and the lowest effective dose employed). Products include:

BioLean Free Tablets .... ▣635
BioLean II Tablets .... ▣635
Winrgy Dietary Supplement .... ▣642

Captopril (The benefits and risks of using fenofibrate tablets with immunosuppressants and other potentially nephrotoxic agents should be carefully considered and the lowest effective dose employed). Products include:

Captopril Tablets 2182

Carbenicillin Disodium (The benefits and risks of using fenofibrate tablets with immunosuppressants and other potentially nephrotoxic agents should be carefully considered and the lowest effective dose employed).
No products indexed under this heading.

Carbenicillin Indanyl Sodium (The benefits and risks of using fenofibrate tablets with immunosuppressants and other potentially nephrotoxic agents should be carefully considered and the lowest effective dose employed).
No products indexed under this heading.

Carboplatin (The benefits and risks of using fenofibrate tablets with immunosuppressants and other potentially nephrotoxic agents should be carefully considered and the lowest effective dose employed).
No products indexed under this heading.

Carmustine (BCNU) (The benefits and risks of using fenofibrate tablets with immunosuppressants and other potentially nephrotoxic agents should be carefully considered and the lowest effective dose employed).
No products indexed under this heading.

Cefaclor (The benefits and risks of using fenofibrate tablets with immunosuppressants and other potentially nephrotoxic agents should be carefully considered and the lowest effective dose employed).
No products indexed under this heading.

Cefadroxil (The benefits and risks of using fenofibrate tablets with immunosuppressants and other potentially nephrotoxic agents should be carefully considered and the lowest effective dose employed).
No products indexed under this heading.

Cefamandole Nafate (The benefits and risks of using fenofibrate tablets with immunosuppressants and other potentially nephrotoxic agents should be carefully considered and the lowest effective dose employed).
No products indexed under this heading.

Cefazolin Sodium (The benefits and risks of using fenofibrate tablets with immunosuppressants and other potentially nephrotoxic agents should be carefully considered and the lowest effective dose employed).
No products indexed under this heading.

Cefdinir (The benefits and risks of using fenofibrate tablets with immunosuppressants and other potentially nephrotoxic agents should be carefully considered and the lowest effective dose employed). Products include:

Omnicef Capsules 497
Omnicef for Oral Suspension 497

Cefepime Hydrochloride (The benefits and risks of using fenofibrate tablets with immunosuppressants and other potentially nephrotoxic agents should be carefully considered and the lowest effective dose employed).
No products indexed under this heading.

Cefixime (The benefits and risks of using fenofibrate tablets with immunosuppressants and other potentially nephrotoxic agents should be carefully considered and the lowest effective dose employed). Products include:

Suprax for Oral Suspension 1891
Suprax Tablets 1891

Cefmetazole Sodium (The benefits and risks of using fenofibrate tablets with immunosuppressants and other potentially nephrotoxic agents should be carefully considered and the lowest effective dose employed).
No products indexed under this heading.

Cefonicid Sodium (The benefits and risks of using fenofibrate tablets with immunosuppressants and other potentially nephrotoxic agents should be carefully considered and the lowest effective dose employed).
No products indexed under this heading.

Cefoperazone Sodium (The benefits and risks of using fenofibrate tablets with immunosuppressants and other potentially nephrotoxic agents should be carefully considered and the lowest effective dose employed).
No products indexed under this heading.

Ceforanide (The benefits and risks of using fenofibrate tablets with immunosuppressants and other potentially nephrotoxic agents should be carefully considered and the lowest effective dose employed).
No products indexed under this heading.

Cefotaxime Sodium (The benefits and risks of using fenofibrate tablets with immunosuppressants and other potentially nephrotoxic agents should be carefully considered and the lowest effective dose employed).
No products indexed under this heading.

Cefotetan (The benefits and risks of using fenofibrate tablets with immunosuppressants and other potentially nephrotoxic agents should be carefully considered and the lowest effective dose employed).
No products indexed under this heading.

Cefoxitin Sodium (The benefits and risks of using fenofibrate tablets with immunosuppressants and other potentially nephrotoxic agents should be carefully considered and the lowest effective dose employed).
No products indexed under this heading.

Cefpodoxime Proxetil (The benefits and risks of using fenofibrate tablets with immunosuppressants and other potentially nephrotoxic agents should be carefully considered and the lowest effective dose employed).
No products indexed under this heading.

Cefprozil (The benefits and risks of using fenofibrate tablets with immunosuppressants and other potentially nephrotoxic agents should be carefully considered and the lowest effective dose employed).
No products indexed under this heading.

Ceftazidime (The benefits and risks of using fenofibrate tablets with immunosuppressants and other potentially nephrotoxic agents should be carefully considered and the lowest effective dose employed). Products include:

Fortaz 1450

Ceftizoxime Sodium (The benefits and risks of using fenofibrate tablets with immunosuppressants and other potentially nephrotoxic agents should be carefully considered and the lowest effective dose employed).
No products indexed under this heading.

Ceftriaxone Sodium (The benefits and risks of using fenofibrate tablets with immunosuppressants and other potentially nephrotoxic agents should be carefully considered and the lowest effective dose employed). Products include:

Rocephin Injectable Vials, ADD-Vantage, Galaxy, Bulk 2642

Cefuroxime Axetil (The benefits and risks of using fenofibrate tablets with immunosuppressants and other potentially nephrotoxic agents should be carefully considered and the lowest effective dose employed). Products include:

Ceftin 1380

Cefuroxime Sodium (The benefits and risks of using fenofibrate tablets with immunosuppressants and other potentially nephrotoxic agents should be carefully considered and the lowest effective dose employed).
No products indexed under this heading.

Celecoxib (The benefits and risks of using fenofibrate tablets with immunosuppressants and other potentially nephrotoxic agents

should be carefully considered and the lowest effective dose employed). Products include:

Celebrex Capsules **2979**

Cephalexin (The benefits and risks of using fenofibrate tablets with immunosuppressants and other potentially nephrotoxic agents should be carefully considered and the lowest effective dose employed).

No products indexed under this heading.

Cephalothin Sodium (The benefits and risks of using fenofibrate tablets with immunosuppressants and other potentially nephrotoxic agents should be carefully considered and the lowest effective dose employed).

No products indexed under this heading.

Cephapirin Sodium (The benefits and risks of using fenofibrate tablets with immunosuppressants and other potentially nephrotoxic agents should be carefully considered and the lowest effective dose employed).

No products indexed under this heading.

Cephradine (The benefits and risks of using fenofibrate tablets with immunosuppressants and other potentially nephrotoxic agents should be carefully considered and the lowest effective dose employed).

No products indexed under this heading.

Cerivastatin Sodium (Co-administration of fibric acid derivatives and HMG-CoA reductase inhibitors has been associated with rhabdomyolysis, markedly elevated creatine kinase levels and myoglobulinuria, leading in a high proportion of cases to acute renal failure; the combined use should be avoided unless the benefit of further alterations in lipid levels is likely to outweigh the increased risk of this combination).

No products indexed under this heading.

Chlorothiazide (The benefits and risks of using fenofibrate tablets with immunosuppressants and other potentially nephrotoxic agents should be carefully considered and the lowest effective dose employed).

No products indexed under this heading.

Chlorothiazide Sodium (The benefits and risks of using fenofibrate tablets with immunosuppressants and other potentially nephrotoxic agents should be carefully considered and the lowest effective dose employed). Products include:

Intravenous Sodium Diuril **2490**

Chlorpropamide (The benefits and risks of using fenofibrate tablets with immunosuppressants and other potentially nephrotoxic agents should be carefully considered and the lowest effective dose employed).

No products indexed under this heading.

Cholestyramine (Bile acid sequestrants may bind fenofibrate; fenofibrate should be taken at least 1 hour before or 4-6 hours after a bile acid binding resin to avoid impeding its absorption).

No products indexed under this heading.

Cidofovir (The benefits and risks of using fenofibrate tablets with immunosuppressants and other potentially nephrotoxic agents should be carefully considered and the lowest effective dose employed).

No products indexed under this heading.

Cilastatin Sodium (The benefits and risks of using fenofibrate tablets with immunosuppressants and other potentially nephrotoxic agents should be carefully considered and the lowest effective dose employed). Products include:

Primaxin I.M. **2080**
Primaxin I.V. **2083**

Cimetidine (The benefits and risks of using fenofibrate tablets with immunosuppressants and other potentially nephrotoxic agents should be carefully considered and the lowest effective dose employed).

No products indexed under this heading.

Cimetidine Hydrochloride (The benefits and risks of using fenofibrate tablets with immunosuppressants and other potentially nephrotoxic agents should be carefully considered and the lowest effective dose employed).

No products indexed under this heading.

Cisplatin (The benefits and risks of using fenofibrate tablets with immunosuppressants and other potentially nephrotoxic agents should be carefully considered and the lowest effective dose employed).

No products indexed under this heading.

Cladribine (The benefits and risks of using fenofibrate tablets with immunosuppressants and other potentially nephrotoxic agents should be carefully considered and the lowest effective dose employed). Products include:

Leustatin Injection **2384**

Clozapine (The benefits and risks of using fenofibrate tablets with immunosuppressants and other potentially nephrotoxic agents should be carefully considered and the lowest effective dose employed).

No products indexed under this heading.

Colesevelam Hydrochloride (Bile acid sequestrants may bind fenofibrate; fenofibrate should be taken at least 1 hour before or 4-6 hours after a bile acid binding resin to avoid impeding its absorption). Products include:

WelChol Tablets **1015**

Colestipol Hydrochloride (Bile acid sequestrants may bind fenofibrate; fenofibrate should be taken at least 1 hour before or 4-6 hours after a bile acid binding resin to avoid impeding its absorption).

No products indexed under this heading.

Colistimethate Sodium (The benefits and risks of using fenofibrate tablets with immunosuppressants and other potentially nephrotoxic agents should be carefully considered and the lowest effective dose employed).

No products indexed under this heading.

Colistin Sulfate (The benefits and risks of using fenofibrate tablets with immunosuppressants and other potentially nephrotoxic agents should be carefully considered and the lowest effective dose employed).

No products indexed under this heading.

Cyclophosphamide (The benefits and risks of using fenofibrate tablets with immunosuppressants and other potentially nephrotoxic agents should be carefully considered and the lowest effective dose employed).

No products indexed under this heading.

Cyclosporine (Because cyclosporine can produce nephrotoxicity with decreases in creatinine clearance and rises in serum creatinine, and because renal excretion is the primary elimination route of fibrate drugs including fenofibrate, there is a risk that an interaction will lead to deterioration. The benefits and risks of using fenofibrate tablets with immunosuppressants and other potentially nephrotoxic agents should be carefully considered and the lowest effective dose employed). Products include:

Gengraf Capsules **435**
Neoral Oral Solution **2280**
Neoral Soft Gelatin Capsules **2280**
Restasis Ophthalmic Emulsion **557**
Sandimmune **2296**

Cytarabine (The benefits and risks of using fenofibrate tablets with immunosuppressants and other potentially nephrotoxic agents should be carefully considered and the lowest effective dose employed).

No products indexed under this heading.

Cytarabine Liposome (The benefits and risks of using fenofibrate tablets with immunosuppressants and other potentially nephrotoxic agents should be carefully considered and the lowest effective dose employed). Products include:

DepoCyt Injection **1136**

Delavirdine Mesylate (The benefits and risks of using fenofibrate tablets with immunosuppressants and other potentially nephrotoxic agents should be carefully considered and the lowest effective dose employed).

No products indexed under this heading.

Diatrizoate Meglumine (The benefits and risks of using fenofibrate tablets with immunosuppressants and other potentially nephrotoxic agents should be carefully considered and the lowest effective dose employed).

No products indexed under this heading.

Diatrizoate Sodium (The benefits and risks of using fenofibrate tablets with immunosuppressants and other potentially nephrotoxic agents should be carefully considered and the lowest effective dose employed).

No products indexed under this heading.

Diclofenac Potassium (The benefits and risks of using fenofibrate tablets with immunosuppressants and other potentially nephrotoxic agents should be carefully considered and the lowest effective dose employed).

No products indexed under this heading.

Diclofenac Sodium (The benefits and risks of using fenofibrate tablets with immunosuppressants and other potentially nephrotoxic agents should be carefully considered and the lowest effective dose employed). Products include:

Diclofenac Sodium Ophthalmic Solution.. ⊙ **240**
Voltaren Ophthalmic Solution **2336**
Voltaren Tablets **2334**
Voltaren-XR Tablets **2337**

Dicloxacillin Sodium (The benefits and risks of using fenofibrate tablets with immunosuppressants and other potentially nephrotoxic agents should be carefully considered and the lowest effective dose employed).

No products indexed under this heading.

Dicumarol (Caution should be exercised when anticoagulants are given in conjunction with fenofibrate because of the potentiation of coumarin-type anticoagulants in prolonging the PT/INR. The dosage of the anticoagulant should be reduced to maintain the PT/INR at the desired level to prevent bleeding complications. Frequent PT/INR determinations are advisable until it has been definitely determined that the PT/INR has stabilized).

No products indexed under this heading.

Didanosine (The benefits and risks of using fenofibrate tablets with immunosuppressants and other potentially nephrotoxic agents should be carefully considered and the lowest effective dose employed).

No products indexed under this heading.

Efavirenz (The benefits and risks of using fenofibrate tablets with immunosuppressants and other potentially nephrotoxic agents should be carefully considered and the lowest effective dose employed). Products include:

Atripla Tablets **938**
Sustiva Capsules **930**
Sustiva Tablets **930**

Emtricitabine (The benefits and risks of using fenofibrate tablets with immunosuppressants and other potentially nephrotoxic agents should be carefully considered and the lowest effective dose employed). Products include:

Atripla Tablets **938**
Emtriva Capsules **1246**
Emtriva Oral Solution **1246**
Truvada Tablets **1262**

Enalapril Maleate (The benefits and risks of using fenofibrate tablets with immunosuppressants and other potentially nephrotoxic agents should be carefully considered and the lowest effective dose employed).

No products indexed under this heading.

Enalaprilat (The benefits and risks of using fenofibrate tablets with immunosuppressants and other potentially nephrotoxic agents should be carefully considered and the lowest effective dose employed).

No products indexed under this heading.

Enfuvirtide (The benefits and risks of using fenofibrate tablets with immunosuppressants and other potentially nephrotoxic agents should be carefully considered and the lowest effective dose employed).

No products indexed under this heading.

Ethiodized Oil (The benefits and risks of using fenofibrate tablets with immunosuppressants and other potentially nephrotoxic agents should be carefully considered and the lowest effective dose employed).
No products indexed under this heading.

Etodolac (The benefits and risks of using fenofibrate tablets with immunosuppressants and other potentially nephrotoxic agents should be carefully considered and the lowest effective dose employed).
No products indexed under this heading.

Fenoprofen Calcium (The benefits and risks of using fenofibrate tablets with immunosuppressants and other potentially nephrotoxic agents should be carefully considered and the lowest effective dose employed). Products include:
Nalfon Capsules 2508

Filgrastim (The benefits and risks of using fenofibrate tablets with immunosuppressants and other potentially nephrotoxic agents should be carefully considered and the lowest effective dose employed). Products include:
Neupogen for Injection 589

Fluorouracil (The benefits and risks of using fenofibrate tablets with immunosuppressants and other potentially nephrotoxic agents should be carefully considered and the lowest effective dose employed). Products include:
Carac Cream 0.5% 2722

Flurbiprofen (The benefits and risks of using fenofibrate tablets with immunosuppressants and other potentially nephrotoxic agents should be carefully considered and the lowest effective dose employed).
No products indexed under this heading.

Fluvastatin Sodium (Co-administration of fibric acid derivatives and HMG-CoA reductase inhibitors has been associated with rhabdomyolysis, markedly elevated creatine kinase levels and myoglobulinuria, leading in a high proportion of cases to acute renal failure; the combined use should be avoided unless the benefit of further alterations in lipid levels is likely to outweigh the increased risk of this combination). Products include:
Lescol Capsules 2268
Lescol XL Tablets 2268

Foscarnet Sodium (The benefits and risks of using fenofibrate tablets with immunosuppressants and other potentially nephrotoxic agents should be carefully considered and the lowest effective dose employed).
No products indexed under this heading.

Fosinopril Sodium (The benefits and risks of using fenofibrate tablets with immunosuppressants and other potentially nephrotoxic agents should be carefully considered and the lowest effective dose employed).
No products indexed under this heading.

Furosemide (The benefits and risks of using fenofibrate tablets with immunosuppressants and other potentially nephrotoxic agents should be carefully considered and the lowest effective dose employed). Products include:
Furosemide Tablets 2186

Gadopentetate Dimeglumine (The benefits and risks of using fenofibrate tablets with immunosuppressants and other potentially nephrotoxic agents should be carefully considered and the lowest effective dose employed).
No products indexed under this heading.

Gentamicin (The benefits and risks of using fenofibrate tablets with immunosuppressants and other potentially nephrotoxic agents should be carefully considered and the lowest effective dose employed).
No products indexed under this heading.

Gentamicin Sulfate (The benefits and risks of using fenofibrate tablets with immunosuppressants and other potentially nephrotoxic agents should be carefully considered and the lowest effective dose employed). Products include:
Pred-G Ophthalmic Ointment .... ⊙229
Pred-G Ophthalmic Suspension .... ⊙228

Glipizide (The benefits and risks of using fenofibrate tablets with immunosuppressants and other potentially nephrotoxic agents should be carefully considered and the lowest effective dose employed).
No products indexed under this heading.

Globulin, Immune (Human) (The benefits and risks of using fenofibrate tablets with immunosuppressants and other potentially nephrotoxic agents should be carefully considered and the lowest effective dose employed). Products include:
Flebogamma 5% 1715

Glyburide (The benefits and risks of using fenofibrate tablets with immunosuppressants and other potentially nephrotoxic agents should be carefully considered and the lowest effective dose employed).
No products indexed under this heading.

Gold Therapy (The benefits and risks of using fenofibrate tablets with immunosuppressants and other potentially nephrotoxic agents should be carefully considered and the lowest effective dose employed).
No products indexed under this heading.

HMG-CoA Reductase Inhibitors (The benefits and risks of using fenofibrate tablets with immunosuppressants and other potentially nephrotoxic agents should be carefully considered and the lowest effective dose employed).
No products indexed under this heading.

Hydrochlorothiazide (The benefits and risks of using fenofibrate tablets with immunosuppressants and other potentially nephrotoxic agents should be carefully considered and the lowest effective dose employed). Products include:
Atacand HCT 642
Avalide Tablets 892
Avalide Tablets 2713
Benicar HCT Tablets 1010
Diovan HCT Tablets 2216
Dyazide Capsules 1405
Micardis HCT Tablets 854
Prinzide Tablets 2092
Tekturna HCT Tablets 2324
Teveten HCT Tablets 517

Hydroflumethiazide (The benefits and risks of using fenofibrate tablets with immunosuppressants and other potentially nephrotoxic agents should be carefully considered and the lowest effective dose employed).
No products indexed under this heading.

Ibuprofen (The benefits and risks of using fenofibrate tablets with immunosuppressants and other potentially nephrotoxic agents should be carefully considered and the lowest effective dose employed). Products include:
Motrin IB Tablets and Caplets 1900
Children's Motrin Oral Suspension ... 1901
Children's Motrin Non-Staining Dye-Free Oral Suspension 1901
Children's Motrin Cold Oral Suspension 1899
Infants' Motrin Concentrated Drops 1901
Infants' Motrin Non-Staining Dye-Free Concentrated Drops 1901
Junior Strength Motrin Caplets and Chewable Tablets 1901
Vicoprofen Tablets 533

Idarubicin Hydrochloride (The benefits and risks of using fenofibrate tablets with immunosuppressants and other potentially nephrotoxic agents should be carefully considered and the lowest effective dose employed).
No products indexed under this heading.

Ifosfamide (The benefits and risks of using fenofibrate tablets with immunosuppressants and other potentially nephrotoxic agents should be carefully considered and the lowest effective dose employed).
No products indexed under this heading.

Imipenem (The benefits and risks of using fenofibrate tablets with immunosuppressants and other potentially nephrotoxic agents should be carefully considered and the lowest effective dose employed). Products include:
Primaxin I.M. 2080
Primaxin I.V. 2083

Immune Globulin Intravenous (Human) (The benefits and risks of using fenofibrate tablets with immunosuppressants and other potentially nephrotoxic agents should be carefully considered and the lowest effective dose employed). Products include:
Flebogamma 5% DIF 1718
Gammagard Liquid 730
Gammagard S/D 734
Gamunex 3094

Indinavir Sulfate (The benefits and risks of using fenofibrate tablets with immunosuppressants and other potentially nephrotoxic agents should be carefully considered and the lowest effective dose employed). Products include:
Crixivan Capsules 1979

Indomethacin (The benefits and risks of using fenofibrate tablets with immunosuppressants and other potentially nephrotoxic agents should be carefully considered and the lowest effective dose employed). Products include:
Indocin 2024

Indomethacin Sodium Trihydrate (The benefits and risks of using fenofibrate tablets with immunosuppressants and other potentially nephrotoxic agents should be carefully considered and the lowest effective dose employed). Products include:
Indocin I.V. 2489

Interferon Beta-1b (The benefits and risks of using fenofibrate tablets with immunosuppressants and other potentially nephrotoxic agents should be carefully considered and the lowest effective dose employed). Products include:
Betaseron for SC Injection 756

Interleuken-2 (The benefits and risks of using fenofibrate tablets with immunosuppressants and other potentially nephrotoxic agents should be carefully considered and the lowest effective dose employed).
No products indexed under this heading.

Iodamide Meglumine (The benefits and risks of using fenofibrate tablets with immunosuppressants and other potentially nephrotoxic agents should be carefully considered and the lowest effective dose employed).
No products indexed under this heading.

Iohexol (The benefits and risks of using fenofibrate tablets with immunosuppressants and other potentially nephrotoxic agents should be carefully considered and the lowest effective dose employed).
No products indexed under this heading.

Iopamidol (The benefits and risks of using fenofibrate tablets with immunosuppressants and other potentially nephrotoxic agents should be carefully considered and the lowest effective dose employed).
No products indexed under this heading.

Iopanoic Acid (The benefits and risks of using fenofibrate tablets with immunosuppressants and other potentially nephrotoxic agents should be carefully considered and the lowest effective dose employed).
No products indexed under this heading.

Iothalamate Meglumine (The benefits and risks of using fenofibrate tablets with immunosuppressants and other potentially nephrotoxic agents should be carefully considered and the lowest effective dose employed).
No products indexed under this heading.

Ioxaglate Meglumine (The benefits and risks of using fenofibrate tablets with immunosuppressants and other potentially nephrotoxic agents should be carefully considered and the lowest effective dose employed).
No products indexed under this heading.

Ioxaglate Sodium (The benefits and risks of using fenofibrate tablets with immunosuppressants and other potentially nephrotoxic agents should be carefully considered and the lowest effective dose employed).
No products indexed under this heading.

Kanamycin Sulfate (The benefits and risks of using fenofibrate tablets with immunosuppressants and other potentially nephrotoxic agents should be carefully considered and the lowest effective dose employed).
No products indexed under this heading.

Ketoprofen (The benefits and risks of using fenofibrate tablets with immunosuppressants and other potentially nephrotoxic agents should be carefully considered and the lowest effective dose employed).
No products indexed under this heading.

Ketorolac Tromethamine (The benefits and risks of using fenofibrate tablets with immunosuppressants and other potentially nephrotoxic agents should be carefully considered and the lowest effective dose employed).
No products indexed under this heading.

Lamium album (The benefits and risks of using fenofibrate tablets with immunosuppressants and other potentially nephrotoxic agents should be carefully considered and the lowest effective dose employed).
No products indexed under this heading.

Lisinopril (The benefits and risks of using fenofibrate tablets with immunosuppressants and other potentially nephrotoxic agents should be carefully considered and the lowest effective dose employed). Products include:
Prinivil Tablets 2087
Prinzide Tablets 2092

Lithium (The benefits and risks of using fenofibrate tablets with immunosuppressants and other potentially nephrotoxic agents should be carefully considered and the lowest effective dose employed).
No products indexed under this heading.

Lithium Carbonate (The benefits and risks of using fenofibrate tablets with immunosuppressants and other potentially nephrotoxic agents should be carefully considered and the lowest effective dose employed).
No products indexed under this heading.

Lithium Citrate (The benefits and risks of using fenofibrate tablets with immunosuppressants and other potentially nephrotoxic agents should be carefully considered and the lowest effective dose employed).
No products indexed under this heading.

Lopinavir (The benefits and risks of using fenofibrate tablets with immunosuppressants and other potentially nephrotoxic agents should be carefully considered and the lowest effective dose employed). Products include:
Kaletra 452

Loracarbef (The benefits and risks of using fenofibrate tablets with immunosuppressants and other potentially nephrotoxic agents should be carefully considered and the lowest effective dose employed).
No products indexed under this heading.

Lovastatin (Co-administration of fibric acid derivatives and HMG-CoA reductase inhibitors has been associated with rhabdomyolysis, markedly elevated creatine kinase levels and myoglobulinuria, leading in a high proportion of cases to acute renal failure; the combined use should be avoided unless the benefit of further alterations in lipid levels is likely to outweigh the increased risk of this combination). Products include:
Advicor Tablets 402
Mevacor Tablets 2063

Meclofenamate Sodium (The benefits and risks of using fenofibrate tablets with immunosuppressants and other potentially nephrotoxic agents should be carefully considered and the lowest effective dose employed).
No products indexed under this heading.

Mefenamic Acid (The benefits and risks of using fenofibrate tablets with immunosuppressants and other potentially nephrotoxic agents should be carefully considered and the lowest effective dose employed).
No products indexed under this heading.

Meloxicam (The benefits and risks of using fenofibrate tablets with immunosuppressants and other potentially nephrotoxic agents should be carefully considered and the lowest effective dose employed). Products include:
Mobic Oral Suspension 863
Mobic Tablets 863

Melphalan Hydrochloride (The benefits and risks of using fenofibrate tablets with immunosuppressants and other potentially nephrotoxic agents should be carefully considered and the lowest effective dose employed).
No products indexed under this heading.

Mesalamine (The benefits and risks of using fenofibrate tablets with immunosuppressants and other potentially nephrotoxic agents should be carefully considered and the lowest effective dose employed). Products include:
Asacol Delayed-Release Tablets 2579
Canasa Rectal Suppositories 705
Lialda Tablets 3029
Pentasa Capsules 3030

Methimazole (The benefits and risks of using fenofibrate tablets with immunosuppressants and other potentially nephrotoxic agents should be carefully considered and the lowest effective dose employed).
No products indexed under this heading.

Methotrexate (The benefits and risks of using fenofibrate tablets with immunosuppressants and other potentially nephrotoxic agents should be carefully considered and the lowest effective dose employed).
No products indexed under this heading.

Methotrexate Sodium (The benefits and risks of using fenofibrate tablets with immunosuppressants and other potentially nephrotoxic agents should be carefully considered and the lowest effective dose employed).
No products indexed under this heading.

Methyclothiazide (The benefits and risks of using fenofibrate tablets with immunosuppressants and other potentially nephrotoxic agents should be carefully considered and the lowest effective dose employed).
No products indexed under this heading.

Mezlocillin Sodium (The benefits and risks of using fenofibrate tablets with immunosuppressants and other potentially nephrotoxic agents should be carefully considered and the lowest effective dose employed).
No products indexed under this heading.

Minocycline Hydrochloride (The benefits and risks of using fenofibrate tablets with immunosuppressants and other potentially nephrotoxic agents should be carefully considered and the lowest effective dose employed). Products include:
Solodyn Extended Release Tablets 1938

Mitomycin (Mitomycin-C) (The benefits and risks of using fenofibrate tablets with immunosuppressants and other potentially nephrotoxic agents should be carefully considered and the lowest effective dose employed).
No products indexed under this heading.

Moexipril Hydrochloride (The benefits and risks of using fenofibrate tablets with immunosuppressants and other potentially nephrotoxic agents should be carefully considered and the lowest effective dose employed).
No products indexed under this heading.

Muromonab-CD3 (The benefits and risks of using fenofibrate tablets with immunosuppressants and other potentially nephrotoxic agents should be carefully considered and the lowest effective dose employed). Products include:
Orthoclone OKT3 Sterile Solution 2387

Mycophenolate Mofetil (The benefits and risks of using fenofibrate tablets with immunosuppressants and other potentially nephrotoxic agents should be carefully considered and the lowest effective dose employed). Products include:
CellCept Capsules 2622
CellCept Oral Suspension 2622
CellCept Tablets 2622

Nabumetone (The benefits and risks of using fenofibrate tablets with immunosuppressants and other potentially nephrotoxic agents should be carefully considered and the lowest effective dose employed).
No products indexed under this heading.

Nafcillin Sodium (The benefits and risks of using fenofibrate tablets with immunosuppressants and other potentially nephrotoxic agents should be carefully considered and the lowest effective dose employed).
No products indexed under this heading.

Naproxen (The benefits and risks of using fenofibrate tablets with immunosuppressants and other potentially nephrotoxic agents should be carefully considered and the lowest effective dose employed). Products include:
EC-Naprosyn Delayed-Release Tablets 2632
Naprosyn Suspension 2632
Naprosyn Tablets 2632

Naproxen Sodium (The benefits and risks of using fenofibrate tablets with immunosuppressants and other potentially nephrotoxic agents should be carefully considered and the lowest effective dose employed). Products include:
Anaprox Tablets 2632
Anaprox DS Tablets 2632
Treximet Tablets 1616

Nelfinavir Mesylate (The benefits and risks of using fenofibrate tablets with immunosuppressants and other potentially nephrotoxic agents should be carefully considered and the lowest effective dose employed).
No products indexed under this heading.

Neomycin (The benefits and risks of using fenofibrate tablets with immunosuppressants and other potentially nephrotoxic agents should be carefully considered and the lowest effective dose employed).
No products indexed under this heading.

Neomycin, oral (The benefits and risks of using fenofibrate tablets with immunosuppressants and other potentially nephrotoxic agents should be carefully considered and the lowest effective dose employed).
No products indexed under this heading.

Neomycin Sulfate (The benefits and risks of using fenofibrate tablets with immunosuppressants and other potentially nephrotoxic agents should be carefully considered and the lowest effective dose employed). Products include:
Neosporin Ophthalmic Solution Sterile .... ⊙ 252

Nevirapine (The benefits and risks of using fenofibrate tablets with immunosuppressants and other potentially nephrotoxic agents should be carefully considered and the lowest effective dose employed). Products include:
Viramune Oral Suspension 873
Viramune Tablets 873

Norfloxacin (The benefits and risks of using fenofibrate tablets with immunosuppressants and other potentially nephrotoxic agents should be carefully considered and the lowest effective dose employed). Products include:
Noroxin Tablets 2069

Olsalazine Sodium (The benefits and risks of using fenofibrate tablets with immunosuppressants and other potentially nephrotoxic agents should be carefully considered and the lowest effective dose employed).
No products indexed under this heading.

Omeprazole (The benefits and risks of using fenofibrate tablets with immunosuppressants and other potentially nephrotoxic agents should be carefully considered and the lowest effective dose employed).
No products indexed under this heading.

Oxaprozin (The benefits and risks of using fenofibrate tablets with immunosuppressants and other potentially nephrotoxic agents should be carefully considered and the lowest effective dose employed).
No products indexed under this heading.

Pamidronate Disodium (The benefits and risks of using fenofibrate tablets with immunosuppressants and other potentially nephrotoxic agents should be carefully considered and the lowest effective dose employed).
No products indexed under this heading.

Paroxetine Hydrochloride (The benefits and risks of using fenofibrate tablets with immunosuppressants and other potentially nephrotoxic agents should be carefully considered and the lowest effective dose employed). Products include:
Paxil 1535
Paxil CR Controlled-Release Tablets 1544

Penicillamine (The benefits and risks of using fenofibrate tablets with immunosuppressants and other potentially nephrotoxic agents should be carefully considered and the lowest effective dose employed). Products include:
Cuprimine Capsules 1986

Penicillin G Benzathine (The benefits and risks of using fenofibrate tablets with immunosuppressants and other potentially nephrotoxic agents should be carefully considered and the lowest effective dose employed). Products include:
Bicillin C-R Injectable Suspension 1775
Bicillin L-A Injection 1777

Penicillin G Potassium (The benefits and risks of using fenofibrate tablets with immunosuppressants and other potentially nephrotoxic agents should be carefully considered and the lowest effective dose employed).
No products indexed under this heading.

Penicillin G Procaine (The benefits and risks of using fenofibrate tablets with immunosuppressants and other potentially nephrotoxic agents should be carefully considered and the lowest effective dose employed). Products include:
Bicillin C-R Injectable Suspension 1775
Bicillin L-A Injection 1777

Penicillin G Sodium (The benefits and risks of using fenofibrate tablets with immunosuppressants and other potentially nephrotoxic agents should be carefully considered and the lowest effective dose employed).
No products indexed under this heading.

Penicillin V Potassium (The benefits and risks of using fenofibrate tablets with immunosuppressants and other potentially nephrotoxic agents should be carefully considered and the lowest effective dose employed).
No products indexed under this heading.

Pentamidine Isethionate (The benefits and risks of using fenofibrate tablets with immunosuppressants and other potentially nephrotoxic agents should be carefully considered and the lowest effective dose employed).
No products indexed under this heading.

Perindopril Erbumine (The benefits and risks of using fenofibrate tablets with immunosuppressants and other potentially nephrotoxic agents should be carefully considered and the lowest effective dose employed). Products include:
Aceon Tablets (2 mg, 4 mg, 8 mg) 3038

Phenylbutazone (The benefits and risks of using fenofibrate tablets with immunosuppressants and other potentially nephrotoxic agents should be carefully considered and the lowest effective dose employed).
No products indexed under this heading.

Piroxicam (The benefits and risks of using fenofibrate tablets with immunosuppressants and other potentially nephrotoxic agents should be carefully considered and the lowest effective dose employed).
No products indexed under this heading.

Plicamycin (The benefits and risks of using fenofibrate tablets with immunosuppressants and other potentially nephrotoxic agents should be carefully considered and the lowest effective dose employed).
No products indexed under this heading.

Polymyxin (The benefits and risks of using fenofibrate tablets with immunosuppressants and other potentially nephrotoxic agents should be carefully considered and the lowest effective dose employed).
No products indexed under this heading.

Polymyxin B Sulfate (The benefits and risks of using fenofibrate tablets with immunosuppressants and other potentially nephrotoxic agents should be carefully considered and the lowest effective dose employed). Products include:
Neosporin Ophthalmic Solution Sterile .... ⊙252

Polythiazide (The benefits and risks of using fenofibrate tablets with immunosuppressants and other potentially nephrotoxic agents should be carefully considered and the lowest effective dose employed).
No products indexed under this heading.

Pravastatin Sodium (Co-administration of fibric acid derivatives and HMG-CoA reductase inhibitors has been associated with rhabdomyolysis, markedly elevated creatine kinase levels and myoglobulinuria, leading in a high proportion of cases to acute renal failure; the combined use should be avoided unless the benefit of further alterations in lipid levels is likely to outweigh the increased risk of this combination).
No products indexed under this heading.

Probenecid (The benefits and risks of using fenofibrate tablets with immunosuppressants and other potentially nephrotoxic agents should be carefully considered and the lowest effective dose employed).
No products indexed under this heading.

Quinapril Hydrochloride (The benefits and risks of using fenofibrate tablets with immunosuppressants and other potentially nephrotoxic agents should be carefully considered and the lowest effective dose employed).
No products indexed under this heading.

Rabeprazole Sodium (The benefits and risks of using fenofibrate tablets with immunosuppressants and other potentially nephrotoxic agents should be carefully considered and the lowest effective dose employed). Products include:
Aciphex Tablets 1053

Ramipril (The benefits and risks of using fenofibrate tablets with immunosuppressants and other potentially nephrotoxic agents should be carefully considered and the lowest effective dose employed).
No products indexed under this heading.

Rifampin (The benefits and risks of using fenofibrate tablets with immunosuppressants and other potentially nephrotoxic agents should be carefully considered and the lowest effective dose employed).
No products indexed under this heading.

Riluzole (The benefits and risks of using fenofibrate tablets with immunosuppressants and other potentially nephrotoxic agents should be carefully considered and the lowest effective dose employed). Products include:
Rilutek Tablets 2771

Ritonavir (The benefits and risks of using fenofibrate tablets with immunosuppressants and other potentially nephrotoxic agents should be carefully considered and the lowest effective dose employed). Products include:
Kaletra 452
Norvir 489

Rofecoxib (The benefits and risks of using fenofibrate tablets with immunosuppressants and other potentially nephrotoxic agents should be carefully considered and the lowest effective dose employed).
No products indexed under this heading.

Rosuvastatin Calcium (Co-administration of fibric acid derivatives and HMG-CoA reductase inhibitors has been associated with rhabdomyolysis, markedly elevated creatine kinase levels and myoglobulinuria, leading in a high proportion of cases to acute renal failure; the combined use should be avoided unless the benefit of further alterations in lipid levels is likely to outweigh the increased risk of this combination). Products include:
Crestor Tablets 677

Saquinavir (The benefits and risks of using fenofibrate tablets with immunosuppressants and other potentially nephrotoxic agents should be carefully considered and the lowest effective dose employed).
No products indexed under this heading.

Sibutramine Hydrochloride Monohydrate (The benefits and risks of using fenofibrate tablets with immunosuppressants and other potentially nephrotoxic agents should be carefully considered and the lowest effective dose employed). Products include:
Meridia Capsules 475

Simvastatin (Co-administration of fibric acid derivatives and HMG-CoA reductase inhibitors has been associated with rhabdomyolysis, markedly elevated creatine kinase levels and myoglobulinuria, leading in a high proportion of cases to acute renal failure; the combined use should be avoided unless the benefit of further alterations in lipid levels is likely to outweigh the increased risk of this combination). Products include:
Simcor Tablets 502
Vytorin 10/10 Tablets 2149
Vytorin 10/10 Tablets 2939
Vytorin 10/20 Tablets 2149
Vytorin 10/20 Tablets 2939
Vytorin 10/40 Tablets 2149
Vytorin 10/40 Tablets 2939
Vytorin 10/80 Tablets 2149
Vytorin 10/80 Tablets 2939
Zocor Tablets 2136

Sirolimus (The benefits and risks of using fenofibrate tablets with immunosuppressants and other potentially nephrotoxic agents should be carefully considered and the lowest effective dose employed). Products include:
Rapamune 3260

Spirapril Hydrochloride (The benefits and risks of using fenofibrate tablets with immunosuppressants and other potentially nephrotoxic agents should be carefully considered and the lowest effective dose employed).
No products indexed under this heading.

Stavudine (The benefits and risks of using fenofibrate tablets with immunosuppressants and other potentially nephrotoxic agents should be carefully considered and the lowest effective dose employed).
No products indexed under this heading.

Streptomycin Sulfate (The benefits and risks of using fenofibrate tablets with immunosuppressants and other potentially nephrotoxic agents should be carefully considered and the lowest effective dose employed).
No products indexed under this heading.

Streptozocin (The benefits and risks of using fenofibrate tablets with immunosuppressants and other potentially nephrotoxic agents should be carefully considered and the lowest effective dose employed).
No products indexed under this heading.

Sulfacytine (The benefits and risks of using fenofibrate tablets with immunosuppressants and other potentially nephrotoxic agents should be carefully considered and the lowest effective dose employed).
No products indexed under this heading.

Sulfamethizole (The benefits and risks of using fenofibrate tablets with immunosuppressants and other potentially nephrotoxic agents should be carefully considered and the lowest effective dose employed).
No products indexed under this heading.

Sulfamethoxazole (The benefits and risks of using fenofibrate tablets with immunosuppressants and other potentially nephrotoxic agents should be carefully considered and the lowest effective dose employed).
No products indexed under this heading.

Sulfasalazine (The benefits and risks of using fenofibrate tablets with immunosuppressants and other potentially nephrotoxic agents should be carefully considered and the lowest effective dose employed).
No products indexed under this heading.

Sulfinpyrazone (The benefits and risks of using fenofibrate tablets with immunosuppressants and other potentially nephrotoxic agents should be carefully considered and the lowest effective dose employed).
No products indexed under this heading.

Sulfisoxazole Acetyl (The benefits and risks of using fenofibrate tablets with immunosuppressants and other potentially nephrotoxic agents should be carefully considered and the lowest effective dose employed).
No products indexed under this heading.

Sulfisoxazole Diolamine (The benefits and risks of using fenofibrate tablets with immunosuppressants and other potentially nephrotoxic agents should be carefully considered and the lowest effective dose employed).
No products indexed under this heading.

Sulindac (The benefits and risks of using fenofibrate tablets with immunosuppressants and other potentially nephrotoxic agents should be carefully considered and the lowest effective dose employed). Products include:
Clinoril Tablets 1962

Tacrolimus (The benefits and risks of using fenofibrate tablets with immunosuppressants and other potentially nephrotoxic agents should be carefully considered and the lowest effective dose employed). Products include:
Prograf Capsules and Injection 622
Protopic Ointment 628

Tenofovir Disoproxil Fumarate (The benefits and risks of using fenofibrate tablets with immunosuppressants and other potentially nephrotoxic agents should be carefully considered and the lowest effective dose employed). Products include:
Atripla Tablets 938
Truvada Tablets 1262
Viread Tablets 1268

Thioguanine (The benefits and risks of using fenofibrate tablets with immunosuppressants and other potentially nephrotoxic agents should be carefully considered and the lowest effective dose employed). Products include:
Tabloid Tablets 1601

Ticarcillin Disodium (The benefits and risks of using fenofibrate tablets with immunosuppressants and other potentially nephrotoxic agents should be carefully considered and the lowest effective dose employed). Products include:
Timentin ADD-Vantage 1606
Timentin Injection Galaxy Container 1609
Timentin IV Infusion 1603
Timentin Pharmacy Bulk Package 1613

Tobramycin (The benefits and risks of using fenofibrate tablets with immunosuppressants and other potentially nephrotoxic agents should be carefully considered and the lowest effective dose employed). Products include:
Zylet Ophthalmic Suspension .... ⊙247

Tobramycin Sulfate (The benefits and risks of using fenofibrate tablets with immunosuppressants and other potentially nephrotoxic agents should be carefully considered and the lowest effective dose employed).
No products indexed under this heading.

Tolazamide (The benefits and risks of using fenofibrate tablets with immunosuppressants and other potentially nephrotoxic agents should be carefully considered and the lowest effective dose employed).
No products indexed under this heading.

Tolbutamide (The benefits and risks of using fenofibrate tablets with immunosuppressants and other potentially nephrotoxic agents should be carefully considered and the lowest effective dose employed).
No products indexed under this heading.

Tolmetin Sodium (The benefits and risks of using fenofibrate tablets with immunosuppressants and other potentially nephrotoxic agents should be carefully considered and the lowest effective dose employed).
No products indexed under this heading.

Trandolapril (The benefits and risks of using fenofibrate tablets with immunosuppressants and other potentially nephrotoxic agents should be carefully considered and the lowest effective dose employed). Products include:
Mavik Tablets 472
Tarka Tablets 511

Triamterene (The benefits and risks of using fenofibrate tablets with immunosuppressants and other potentially nephrotoxic agents should be carefully considered and the lowest effective dose employed). Products include:
Dyazide Capsules 1405
Dyrenium Capsules 3189

Trimethadione (The benefits and risks of using fenofibrate tablets with immunosuppressants and other potentially nephrotoxic agents should be carefully considered and the lowest effective dose employed).
No products indexed under this heading.

Trovafloxacin Mesylate (The benefits and risks of using fenofibrate tablets with immunosuppressants and other potentially nephrotoxic agents should be carefully considered and the lowest effective dose employed).
No products indexed under this heading.

Tyropanoate Sodium (The benefits and risks of using fenofibrate tablets with immunosuppressants and other potentially nephrotoxic agents should be carefully considered and the lowest effective dose employed).
No products indexed under this heading.

Valacyclovir Hydrochloride (The benefits and risks of using fenofibrate tablets with immunosuppressants and other potentially nephrotoxic agents should be carefully considered and the lowest effective dose employed). Products include:
Valtrex Caplets 1635

Valdecoxib (The benefits and risks of using fenofibrate tablets with immunosuppressants and other potentially nephrotoxic agents should be carefully considered and the lowest effective dose employed).
No products indexed under this heading.

Vancomycin Hydrochloride (The benefits and risks of using fenofibrate tablets with immunosuppressants and other potentially nephrotoxic agents should be carefully considered and the lowest effective dose employed).
No products indexed under this heading.

Voriconazole (The benefits and risks of using fenofibrate tablets with immunosuppressants and other potentially nephrotoxic agents should be carefully considered and the lowest effective dose employed).
No products indexed under this heading.

Warfarin Sodium (Caution should be exercised when anticoagulants are given in conjunction with fenofibrate because of the potentiation of coumarin-type anticoagulants in prolonging the PT/INR. The dosage of the anticoagulant should be reduced to maintain the PT/INR at the desired level to prevent bleeding complications. Frequent PT/INR determinations are advisable until it has been definitely determined that the PT/INR has stabilized).
No products indexed under this heading.

Zalcitabine (The benefits and risks of using fenofibrate tablets with immunosuppressants and other potentially nephrotoxic agents should be carefully considered and the lowest effective dose employed).
No products indexed under this heading.

Zidovudine (The benefits and risks of using fenofibrate tablets with immunosuppressants and other potentially nephrotoxic agents should be carefully considered and the lowest effective dose employed). Products include:
Combivir Tablets 1384
Retrovir 1574
Retrovir IV Infusion 1579
Trizivir Tablets 1622

Zoledronic acid (The benefits and risks of using fenofibrate tablets with immunosuppressants and other potentially nephrotoxic agents should be carefully considered and the lowest effective dose employed). Products include:
Reclast Injection 2291
Zometa for Intravenous Infusion 2341

Food Interactions

Food, unspecified (The absorption of fenofibrate is increased when administered with food; Tricor should be given with meals).

TRIESENCE INJECTABLE SUSPENSION

(Triamcinolone Acetonide) .... ⊙209
May interact with anticholinesterase drugs, barbiturates, anticoagulants, cytochrome p450 3a4 inducers (selected), cytochrome p450 3a4 inhibitors (selected), estrogens, oral hypoglycemic agents, insulin, macrolide antibiotics, non-steroidal anti-inflammatory agents, potassium-depleting corticosteroids, potassium-depleting diuretics, antituberculosis drugs, killed/inactivated vaccines, and certain other agents. Compounds in these categories include:

Acarbose (Because corticosteroids may increase blood glucose concentrations, dosage adjustments of antidiabetic agents may be required). Products include:
Precose Tablets 792

Acetazolamide (Ketoconazole has been reported to decrease the metabolism of certain corticosteroids by up to 60% leading to an increased risk of corticosteroid side effects).
No products indexed under this heading.

Allium sativum (Drugs such as barbiturates, phenytoin, ephedrine, and rifampin, which induce hepatic microsomal drug metabolizing enzyme activity may enhance metabolism of corticosteroid and require that the dosage of corticosteroid be increased).
No products indexed under this heading.

Aminosalicylic Acid (Serum concentrations of isoniazid may be decreased). Products include:
Paser Granules 1747

p-Aminosalicylic Acid (Serum concentrations of isoniazid may be decreased).
No products indexed under this heading.

Amiodarone Hydrochloride (Ketoconazole has been reported to decrease the metabolism of certain corticosteroids by up to 60% leading to an increased risk of corticosteroid side effects).
No products indexed under this heading.

Amphotericin B (There have been cases reported in which concomitant use of Amphotericin B and hydrocortisone was followed by cardiac enlargement and congestive heart failure. See Potassium depleting agents).
No products indexed under this heading.

Amprenavir (Ketoconazole has been reported to decrease the metabolism of certain corticosteroids by up to 60% leading to an increased risk of corticosteroid side effects).
No products indexed under this heading.

Anastrozole (Ketoconazole has been reported to decrease the metabolism of certain corticosteroids by up to 60% leading to an increased risk of corticosteroid side effects). Products include:
Arimidex Tablets 672

Anisindione (Co-administration of corticosteroids and warfarin usually results in inhibition of response to warfarin, although there have been some conflicting reports. Therefore, coagulation indices should be monitored frequently to maintain the desired anticoagulant effect).
No products indexed under this heading.

Aprepitant (Drugs such as barbiturates, phenytoin, ephedrine, and rifampin, which induce hepatic microsomal drug metabolizing enzyme activity may enhance metabolism of corticosteroid and require that the dosage of corticosteroid be increased). Products include:
Emend Capsules 1992

Aprobarbital (Drugs which induce hepatic microsomal drug metabolizing enzyme activity may enhance metabolism of corticosteroid and require that the dosage of corticosteroid be increased).
No products indexed under this heading.

Ardeparin Sodium (Co-administration of corticosteroids and warfarin usually results in inhibition of response to warfarin, although there have been some conflicting reports. Therefore, coagulation indices should be monitored frequently to maintain the desired anticoagulant effect).
No products indexed under this heading.

Atazanavir (Ketoconazole has been reported to decrease the metabolism of certain corticosteroids by up to 60% leading to an increased risk of corticosteroid side effects).
No products indexed under this heading.

Atazanavir Sulfate (Ketoconazole has been reported to decrease the metabolism of certain corticosteroids by up to 60% leading to an increased risk of corticosteroid side effects). Products include:
Reyataz Capsules 3299

Azithromycin Dihydrate (Ketoconazole has been reported to decrease the metabolism of certain corticosteroids by up to 60% leading to an increased risk of corticosteroid side effects).
No products indexed under this heading.

Bendroflumethiazide (When corticosteroids are administered concomitantly with potassium-depleting agents, patients should be observed closely for development of hypokalemia).
No products indexed under this heading.

Betamethasone Acetate (When corticosteroids are administered concomitantly with potassium-depleting agents, patients should be observed closely for development of hypokalemia).
No products indexed under this heading.

Betamethasone Sodium Phosphate (When corticosteroids are administered concomitantly with potassium-depleting agents, patients should be observed closely for development of hypokalemia).
No products indexed under this heading.

Bumetanide (When corticosteroids are administered concomitantly with potassium-depleting agents, patients should be observed closely for development of hypokalemia).
No products indexed under this heading.

Butabarbital (Drugs which induce hepatic microsomal drug metabolizing enzyme activity may enhance metabolism of corticosteroid and require that the dosage of corticosteroid be increased).
No products indexed under this heading.

Butalbital (Drugs which induce hepatic microsomal drug metabolizing enzyme activity may enhance metabolism of corticosteroid and require that the dosage of corticosteroid be increased).
No products indexed under this heading.

Carbamazepine (Drugs such as barbiturates, phenytoin, ephedrine, and rifampin, which induce hepatic microsomal drug metabolizing enzyme activity may enhance metabolism of corticosteroid and require that the dosage of corticosteroid be increased). Products include:
Carbatrol Capsules 3019
Equetro Extended-Release Capsules 3174

Celecoxib (Concomitant use of aspirin or other non-steroidal anti-inflammatory agents and corticosteroids increases the risk of gastrointestinal side effects. Aspirin should be used cautiously in conjunction with corticosteroids in hypoprothrombinemia. The clearance of salicylates may be increased with concurrent use of corticosteroids). Products include:
Celebrex Capsules 2979

Chlorothiazide (When corticosteroids are administered concomitantly with potassium-depleting agents, patients should be observed closely for development of hypokalemia).
No products indexed under this heading.

Chlorothiazide Sodium (When corticosteroids are administered concomitantly with potassium-depleting agents, patients should be observed closely for development of hypokalemia). Products include:
Intravenous Sodium Diuril 2490

Chlorotrianisene (Estrogens may decrease the hepatic metabolism of certain corticosteroids thereby increasing their effect).
No products indexed under this heading.

Chlorpropamide (Because corticosteroids may increase blood glucose concentrations, dosage adjustments of antidiabetic agents may be required).
No products indexed under this heading.

Cholestyramine (Cholestyramine may increase the clearance of corticosteroids).
No products indexed under this heading.

Cimetidine (Ketoconazole has been reported to decrease the metabolism of certain corticosteroids by up to 60% leading to an increased risk of corticosteroid side effects).
No products indexed under this heading.

Cimetidine Hydrochloride (Ketoconazole has been reported to decrease the metabolism of certain corticosteroids by up to 60% leading to an increased risk of corticosteroid side effects).
No products indexed under this heading.

Ciprofloxacin (Ketoconazole has been reported to decrease the metabolism of certain corticosteroids by up to 60% leading to an increased risk of corticosteroid side effects). Products include:
Cipro I.V. 2817
Cipro Oral Suspension 2810
Cipro XR Tablets 2823
Ciprodex Otic Suspension 541

Ciprofloxacin Hydrochloride (Drugs such as barbiturates, phenytoin, ephedrine, and rifampin, which induce hepatic microsomal drug metabolizing enzyme activity may enhance metabolism of corticosteroid and require that the dosage of corticosteroid be increased). Products include:
Cipro Tablets 2810

Cisplatin (Drugs such as barbiturates, phenytoin, ephedrine, and rifampin, which induce hepatic microsomal drug metabolizing enzyme activity may enhance metabolism of corticosteroid and require that the dosage of corticosteroid be increased).
No products indexed under this heading.

Clarithromycin (Ketoconazole has been reported to decrease the metabolism of certain corticosteroids by up to 60% leading to an increased risk of corticosteroid side effects). Products include:
Biaxin/Biaxin XL 411

Clotrimazole (Ketoconazole has been reported to decrease the metabolism of certain corticosteroids by up to 60% leading to an increased risk of corticosteroid side effects). Products include:
Lotrisone 2881

Cortisone Acetate (When corticosteroids are administered concomitantly with potassium-depleting agents, patients should be observed closely for development of hypokalemia).
No products indexed under this heading.

Cycloserine (Serum concentrations of isoniazid may be decreased). Products include:
Seromycin Capsules 1864

Cyclosporine (Increased activity of both cyclosporine and corticosteroids may occur when the two are used concurrently. Convulsions have been reported with concurrent use). Products include:
Gengraf Capsules 435
Neoral Oral Solution 2280
Neoral Soft Gelatin Capsules 2280
Restasis Ophthalmic Emulsion 557
Sandimmune 2296

Dalfopristin (Ketoconazole has been reported to decrease the metabolism of certain corticosteroids by up to 60% leading to an increased risk of corticosteroid side effects).
No products indexed under this heading.

Dalteparin Sodium (Co-administration of corticosteroids and warfarin usually results in inhibition of response to warfarin, although there have been some conflicting reports. Therefore, coagulation indices should be monitored frequently to maintain the desired anticoagulant effect). Products include:
Fragmin Injection 1070

Danaparoid Sodium (Co-administration of corticosteroids and warfarin usually results in inhibition of response to warfarin, although there have been some conflicting reports. Therefore, coagulation indices should be monitored frequently to maintain the desired anticoagulant effect).
No products indexed under this heading.

Danazol (Ketoconazole has been reported to decrease the metabolism of certain corticosteroids by up to 60% leading to an increased risk of corticosteroid side effects).
No products indexed under this heading.

Delavirdine Mesylate (Ketoconazole has been reported to decrease the metabolism of certain corticosteroids by up to 60% leading to an increased risk of corticosteroid side effects).
No products indexed under this heading.

Dexamethasone (When corticosteroids are administered concomitantly with potassium-depleting agents, patients should be observed closely for development of hypokalemia). Products include:
Ciprodex Otic Suspension 541

Dexamethasone Acetate (When corticosteroids are administered concomitantly with potassium-depleting agents, patients should be observed closely for development of hypokalemia).
No products indexed under this heading.

Dexamethasone Sodium Phosphate (When corticosteroids are administered concomitantly with potassium-depleting agents, patients should be observed closely for development of hypokalemia).
No products indexed under this heading.

Diclofenac Epolamine (Concomitant use of aspirin or other non-steroidal anti-inflammatory agents and corticosteroids increases the risk of gastrointestinal side effects. Aspirin should be used cautiously in conjunction with corticosteroids in hypoprothrombinemia. The clearance of salicylates may be increased with concurrent use of corticosteroids). Products include:
Flector Patch 561

Diclofenac Potassium (Concomitant use of aspirin or other non-steroidal anti-inflammatory agents and corticosteroids increases the risk of gastrointestinal side effects. Aspirin should be used cautiously in conjunction with corticosteroids in hypoprothrombinemia. The clearance of salicylates may be increased with concurrent use of corticosteroids).
No products indexed under this heading.

Diclofenac Sodium (Concomitant use of aspirin or other non-steroidal anti-inflammatory agents and corticosteroids increases the risk of gastrointestinal side effects. Aspirin should be used cautiously in conjunction with corticosteroids in hypoprothrombinemia. The clearance of salicylates may be increased with concurrent use of corticosteroids). Products include:
Diclofenac Sodium Ophthalmic Solution .... ⊙240
Voltaren Ophthalmic Solution 2336
Voltaren Tablets 2334
Voltaren-XR Tablets 2337

Dicumarol (Co-administration of corticosteroids and warfarin usually results in inhibition of response to warfarin, although there have been some conflicting reports. Therefore, coagulation indices should be monitored frequently to maintain the desired anticoagulant effect).
No products indexed under this heading.

Dienestrol (Estrogens may decrease the hepatic metabolism of certain corticosteroids thereby increasing their effect).
No products indexed under this heading.

Diethylstilbestrol (Estrogens may decrease the hepatic metabolism of certain corticosteroids thereby increasing their effect).
No products indexed under this heading.

Digitalis Glycoside Preparations (Patients on digitalis glycosides may be at increased risk of arrhythmias due to hypokalemia).
No products indexed under this heading.

Diltiazem Hydrochloride (Ketoconazole has been reported to decrease the metabolism of certain corticosteroids by up to 60% leading to an increased risk of corticosteroid side effects). Products include:
Cardizem LA Extended Release Tablets 421

Diltiazem Maleate (Ketoconazole has been reported to decrease the metabolism of certain corticosteroids by up to 60% leading to an increased risk of corticosteroid side effects).
No products indexed under this heading.

Diphtheria & Tetanus Toxoids and Acellular Pertussis Vaccine Adsorbed, Hepatitis B (recombinant) and Inactivated Poliovirus Vaccine Combined (Due to inhibition of antibody response, patients on prolonged corticosteroid therapy may exhibit a diminished response to toxoids and live or inactivated vaccines. Corticosteroids may also potentiate the replication of some organisms contained in live attenuated vaccines).
No products indexed under this heading.

Dirithromycin (Ketoconazole has been reported to decrease the metabolism of certain corticosteroids by up to 60% leading to an increased risk of corticosteroid side effects).
No products indexed under this heading.

Donepezil Hydrochloride (Concomitant use of anticholinesterase agents and corticosteroids may produce severe weakness in patients with myasthenia gravis. If possible, anticholinesterase agents should be withdrawn at least 24 hours before initiating corticosteroid therapy). Products include:
Aricept Tablets 1062
Aricept ODT Tablets 1062

Doxorubicin Hydrochloride (Drugs such as barbiturates, phenytoin, ephedrine, and rifampin, which induce hepatic microsomal drug metabolizing enzyme activity may enhance metabolism of corticosteroid and require that the dosage of corticosteroid be increased).
No products indexed under this heading.

Efavirenz (Drugs such as barbiturates, phenytoin, ephedrine, and rifampin, which induce hepatic microsomal drug metabolizing enzyme activity may enhance metabolism of corticosteroid and require that the dosage of corticosteroid be increased). Products include:
Atripla Tablets 938
Sustiva Capsules 930
Sustiva Tablets 930

Enoxaparin Sodium (Co-administration of corticosteroids and warfarin usually results in inhibition of response to warfarin, although there have been some conflicting reports. Therefore, coagulation indices should be monitored frequently to maintain the desired anticoagulant effect). Products include:
Lovenox Injection 2756

Ephedrine Hydrochloride (Drugs such as barbiturates, phenytoin, ephedrine, and rifampin, which induce hepatic microsomal drug metabolizing enzyme activity may enhance metabolism of corticosteroid and require that the dosage of corticosteroid be increased).
No products indexed under this heading.

Ephedrine Sulfate (Drugs such as barbiturates, phenytoin, ephedrine, and rifampin, which induce hepatic microsomal drug metabolizing enzyme activity may enhance metabolism of corticosteroid and require that the dosage of corticosteroid be increased).
No products indexed under this heading.

Ephedrine Tannate (Drugs such as barbiturates, phenytoin, ephedrine, and rifampin, which induce hepatic microsomal drug metabolizing enzyme activity may enhance metabolism of corticosteroid and require that the dosage of corticosteroid be increased).
No products indexed under this heading.

Erythromycin (Ketoconazole has been reported to decrease the metabolism of certain corticosteroids by up to 60% leading to an increased risk of corticosteroid side effects).
No products indexed under this heading.

Erythromycin Estolate (Ketoconazole has been reported to decrease the metabolism of certain corticosteroids by up to 60% leading to an increased risk of corticosteroid side effects).
No products indexed under this heading.

Erythromycin Ethylsuccinate (Ketoconazole has been reported to decrease the metabolism of certain corticosteroids by up to 60% leading to an increased risk of corticosteroid side effects). Products include:
E.E.S. 433
EryPed 431

Erythromycin Gluceptate (Ketoconazole has been reported to decrease the metabolism of certain corticosteroids by up to 60% leading to an increased risk of corticosteroid side effects).
No products indexed under this heading.

Erythromycin Lactobionate (Ketoconazole has been reported to decrease the metabolism of certain corticosteroids by up to 60% leading to an increased risk of corticosteroid side effects).
No products indexed under this heading.

Erythromycin Stearate (Ketoconazole has been reported to decrease the metabolism of certain corticosteroids by up to 60% leading to an increased risk of corticosteroid side effects).
No products indexed under this heading.

Esomeprazole Magnesium (Ketoconazole has been reported to decrease the metabolism of certain corticosteroids by up to 60% leading to an increased risk of corticosteroid side effects). Products include:
Nexium Delayed-Release Capsules 645
Nexium Delayed-Release Oral Suspension 645

Estradiol (Estrogens may decrease the hepatic metabolism of certain corticosteroids thereby increasing their effect). Products include:
Activella Tablets 2347
Angeliq Tablets 751
Climara Transdermal System 763
Climara Pro Transdermal System 768
Divigel 3167
Vagifem Tablets 2375

Estrogens, Conjugated (Estrogens may decrease the hepatic metabolism of certain corticosteroids thereby increasing their effect). Products include:
Premarin Intravenous 3217
Premarin Tablets 3221
Premarin Vaginal Cream 3228
Premphase Tablets 3232
Prempro Tablets 3232

Estrogens, Esterified (Estrogens may decrease the hepatic metabolism of certain corticosteroids thereby increasing their effect). Products include:
Estratest Tablets 3043
Estratest H.S. Tablets 3043

Estropipate (Estrogens may decrease the hepatic metabolism of certain corticosteroids thereby increasing their effect).
No products indexed under this heading.

Ethacrynic Acid (When corticosteroids are administered concomitantly with potassium-depleting agents, patients should be observed closely for development of hypokalemia). Products include:
Edecrin Tablets 698

Ethambutol Hydrochloride (Serum concentrations of isoniazid may be decreased).
No products indexed under this heading.

Ethinyl Estradiol (Estrogens may decrease the hepatic metabolism of certain corticosteroids thereby increasing their effect). Products include:
Lybrel Tablets 3204
Mircette Tablets 1034
NuvaRing 2897
Ortho-Cyclen/Ortho Tri-Cyclen 2449
Ortho Evra Transdermal System 2437
Ortho Tri-Cyclen Lo Tablets 2458
Seasonique Tablets 1046
Yaz Tablets 805

Ethosuximide (Drugs such as barbiturates, phenytoin, ephedrine, and rifampin, which induce hepatic microsomal drug metabolizing enzyme activity may enhance metabolism of corticosteroid and require that the dosage of corticosteroid be increased).
No products indexed under this heading.

Etodolac (Concomitant use of aspirin or other non-steroidal anti-inflammatory agents and corticosteroids increases the risk of gastrointestinal side effects. Aspirin should be used cautiously in conjunction with corticosteroids in hypoprothrombinemia. The clearance of salicylates may be increased with concurrent use of corticosteroids).
No products indexed under this heading.

Felbamate (Drugs such as barbiturates, phenytoin, ephedrine, and rifampin, which induce hepatic microsomal drug metabolizing enzyme activity may enhance metabolism of corticosteroid and require that the dosage of corticosteroid be increased).
No products indexed under this heading.

Fenoprofen Calcium (Concomitant use of aspirin or other non-steroidal anti-inflammatory agents and corticosteroids increases the risk of gastrointestinal side effects. Aspirin should be used cautiously in conjunction with corticosteroids in hypoprothrombinemia. The clearance of salicylates may be increased with concurrent use of corticosteroids). Products include:
Nalfon Capsules 2508

Fluconazole (Ketoconazole has been reported to decrease the metabolism of certain corticosteroids by up to 60% leading to an increased risk of corticosteroid side effects).
No products indexed under this heading.

Fludrocortisone Acetate (Drugs such as barbiturates, phenytoin, ephedrine, and rifampin, which induce hepatic microsomal drug metabolizing enzyme activity may enhance metabolism of corticosteroid and require that the dosage of corticosteroid be increased).
No products indexed under this heading.

Fluoxetine (Ketoconazole has been reported to decrease the metabolism of certain corticosteroids by up to 60% leading to an increased risk of corticosteroid side effects).
No products indexed under this heading.

Fluoxetine Hydrochloride (Ketoconazole has been reported to decrease the metabolism of certain corticosteroids by up to 60% leading to an increased risk of corticosteroid side effects). Products include:
Prozac Weekly Capsules 1852
Prozac Pulvules and Liquid 1852
Symbyax Capsules 1871

Flurbiprofen (Concomitant use of aspirin or other non-steroidal anti-inflammatory agents and corticosteroids increases the risk of gastrointestinal side effects. Aspirin should be used cautiously in conjunction with corticosteroids in hypoprothrombinemia. The clearance of salicylates may be increased with concurrent use of corticosteroids).
No products indexed under this heading.

Fluvoxamine Maleate (Ketoconazole has been reported to decrease the metabolism of certain corticosteroids by up to 60% leading to an increased risk of corticosteroid side effects). Products include:

Luvox CR Extended-Release Capsules ... 1759

Fondaparinux Sodium (Co-administration of corticosteroids and warfarin usually results in inhibition of response to warfarin, although there have been some conflicting reports. Therefore, coagulation indices should be monitored frequently to maintain the desired anticoagulant effect). Products include:

Arixtra Injection ... 1313

Fosamprenavir Calcium (Ketoconazole has been reported to decrease the metabolism of certain corticosteroids by up to 60% leading to an increased risk of corticosteroid side effects). Products include:

Lexiva Oral Suspension ... 1510
Lexiva Tablets ... 1510

Fosphenytoin Sodium (Drugs such as barbiturates, phenytoin, ephedrine, and rifampin, which induce hepatic microsomal drug metabolizing enzyme activity may enhance metabolism of corticosteroid and require that the dosage of corticosteroid be increased).

No products indexed under this heading.

Furosemide (When corticosteroids are administered concomitantly with potassium-depleting agents, patients should be observed closely for development of hypokalemia). Products include:

Furosemide Tablets ... 2186

Galantamine Hydrobromide (Concomitant use of anticholinesterase agents and corticosteroids may produce severe weakness in patients with myasthenia gravis. If possible, anticholinesterase agents should be withdrawn at least 24 hours before initiating corticosteroid therapy).

No products indexed under this heading.

Garlic Extract (Drugs such as barbiturates, phenytoin, ephedrine, and rifampin, which induce hepatic microsomal drug metabolizing enzyme activity may enhance metabolism of corticosteroid and require that the dosage of corticosteroid be increased).

No products indexed under this heading.

Garlic Oil (Drugs such as barbiturates, phenytoin, ephedrine, and rifampin, which induce hepatic microsomal drug metabolizing enzyme activity may enhance metabolism of corticosteroid and require that the dosage of corticosteroid be increased).

No products indexed under this heading.

Glimepiride (Because corticosteroids may increase blood glucose concentrations, dosage adjustments of antidiabetic agents may be required). Products include:

Avandaryl Tablets ... 1344
Duetact Tablets ... 3085

Glipizide (Because corticosteroids may increase blood glucose concentrations, dosage adjustments of antidiabetic agents may be required).

No products indexed under this heading.

Glyburide (Because corticosteroids may increase blood glucose concentrations, dosage adjustments of antidiabetic agents may be required).

No products indexed under this heading.

Heparin Calcium (Co-administration of corticosteroids and warfarin usually results in inhibition of response to warfarin, although there have been some conflicting reports. Therefore, coagulation indices should be monitored frequently to maintain the desired anticoagulant effect).

No products indexed under this heading.

Heparin Sodium (Co-administration of corticosteroids and warfarin usually results in inhibition of response to warfarin, although there have been some conflicting reports. Therefore, coagulation indices should be monitored frequently to maintain the desired anticoagulant effect).

No products indexed under this heading.

Hepatitis A Vaccine, Inactivated (Due to inhibition of antibody response, patients on prolonged corticosteroid therapy may exhibit a diminished response to toxoids and live or inactivated vaccines. Corticosteroids may also potentiate the replication of some organisms contained in live attenuated vaccines). Products include:

Havrix Injection Vaccine ... 1454
Twinrix Vaccine ... 1628
Vaqta ... 2130

Hydrochlorothiazide (When corticosteroids are administered concomitantly with potassium-depleting agents, patients should be observed closely for development of hypokalemia). Products include:

Atacand HCT ... 642
Avalide Tablets ... 892
Avalide Tablets ... 2713
Benicar HCT Tablets ... 1010
Diovan HCT Tablets ... 2216
Dyazide Capsules ... 1405
Micardis HCT Tablets ... 854
Prinzide Tablets ... 2092
Tekturna HCT Tablets ... 2324
Teveten HCT Tablets ... 517

Hydrocortisone (When corticosteroids are administered concomitantly with potassium-depleting agents, patients should be observed closely for development of hypokalemia).

No products indexed under this heading.

Hydrocortisone Acetate (When corticosteroids are administered concomitantly with potassium-depleting agents, patients should be observed closely for development of hypokalemia). Products include:

Analpram-HC ... 1140
Pramosone ... 1141

Hydrocortisone Butyrate (Drugs such as barbiturates, phenytoin, ephedrine, and rifampin, which induce hepatic microsomal drug metabolizing enzyme activity may enhance metabolism of corticosteroid and require that the dosage of corticosteroid be increased).

No products indexed under this heading.

Hydrocortisone Cypionate (Drugs such as barbiturates, phenytoin, ephedrine, and rifampin, which induce hepatic microsomal drug metabolizing enzyme activity may enhance metabolism of corticosteroid and require that the dosage of corticosteroid be increased).

No products indexed under this heading.

Hydrocortisone Hemisuccinate (Drugs such as barbiturates, phenytoin, ephedrine, and rifampin, which induce hepatic microsomal drug metabolizing enzyme activity may enhance metabolism of corticosteroid and require that the dosage of corticosteroid be increased).

No products indexed under this heading.

Hydrocortisone Probutate (Drugs such as barbiturates, phenytoin, ephedrine, and rifampin, which induce hepatic microsomal drug metabolizing enzyme activity may enhance metabolism of corticosteroid and require that the dosage of corticosteroid be increased).

No products indexed under this heading.

Hydrocortisone Sodium Phosphate (When corticosteroids are administered concomitantly with potassium-depleting agents, patients should be observed closely for development of hypokalemia).

No products indexed under this heading.

Hydrocortisone Sodium Succinate (When corticosteroids are administered concomitantly with potassium-depleting agents, patients should be observed closely for development of hypokalemia).

No products indexed under this heading.

Hydrocortisone Valerate (Drugs such as barbiturates, phenytoin, ephedrine, and rifampin, which induce hepatic microsomal drug metabolizing enzyme activity may enhance metabolism of corticosteroid and require that the dosage of corticosteroid be increased).

No products indexed under this heading.

Hydroflumethiazide (When corticosteroids are administered concomitantly with potassium-depleting agents, patients should be observed closely for development of hypokalemia).

No products indexed under this heading.

Hypericum (Drugs such as barbiturates, phenytoin, ephedrine, and rifampin, which induce hepatic microsomal drug metabolizing enzyme activity may enhance metabolism of corticosteroid and require that the dosage of corticosteroid be increased). Products include:

Satieté Tablets ... ▣ 640

Hypericum Perforatum (Drugs such as barbiturates, phenytoin, ephedrine, and rifampin, which induce hepatic microsomal drug metabolizing enzyme activity may enhance metabolism of corticosteroid and require that the dosage of corticosteroid be increased).

No products indexed under this heading.

Ibuprofen (Concomitant use of aspirin or other non-steroidal anti-inflammatory agents and corticosteroids increases the risk of gastrointestinal side effects. Aspirin should be used cautiously in conjunction with corticosteroids in hypoprothrombinemia. The clearance of salicylates may be increased with concurrent use of corticosteroids). Products include:

Motrin IB Tablets and Caplets ... 1900
Children's Motrin Oral Suspension ... 1901
Children's Motrin Non-Staining Dye-Free Oral Suspension ... 1901
Children's Motrin Cold Oral Suspension ... 1899
Infants' Motrin Concentrated Drops ... 1901
Infants' Motrin Non-Staining Dye-Free Concentrated Drops ... 1901
Junior Strength Motrin Caplets and Chewable Tablets ... 1901
Vicoprofen Tablets ... 533

Indinavir Sulfate (Ketoconazole has been reported to decrease the metabolism of certain corticosteroids by up to 60% leading to an increased risk of corticosteroid side effects). Products include:

Crixivan Capsules ... 1979

Indomethacin (Concomitant use of aspirin or other non-steroidal anti-inflammatory agents and corticosteroids increases the risk of gastrointestinal side effects. Aspirin should be used cautiously in conjunction with corticosteroids in hypoprothrombinemia. The clearance of salicylates may be increased with concurrent use of corticosteroids). Products include:

Indocin ... 2024

Indomethacin Sodium Trihydrate (Concomitant use of aspirin or other non-steroidal anti-inflammatory agents and corticosteroids increases the risk of gastrointestinal side effects. Aspirin should be used cautiously in conjunction with corticosteroids in hypoprothrombinemia. The clearance of salicylates may be increased with concurrent use of corticosteroids). Products include:

Indocin I.V. ... 2489

Influenza Virus Vaccine (Due to inhibition of antibody response, patients on prolonged corticosteroid therapy may exhibit a diminished response to toxoids and live or inactivated vaccines. Corticosteroids may also potentiate the replication of some organisms contained in live attenuated vaccines). Products include:

Fluarix Vaccine ... 1446
Flulaval Injection Vaccine ... 1448

Insulin (Because corticosteroids may increase blood glucose concentrations, dosage adjustments of antidiabetic agents may be required).

No products indexed under this heading.

Insulin, Human, Zinc Suspension (Because corticosteroids may increase blood glucose concentrations, dosage adjustments of antidiabetic agents may be required).

No products indexed under this heading.

Insulin, Human (rDNA origin) (Because corticosteroids may increase blood glucose concentrations, dosage adjustments of antidiabetic agents may be required). Products include:

Exubera Inhalation Powder ... 2515

Insulin, Human NPH (Because corticosteroids may increase blood glucose concentrations, dosage adjustments of antidiabetic agents may be required). Products include:

Humulin N Vial ... 1846

Insulin, Human Regular (Because corticosteroids may increase blood glucose concentrations, dosage adjustments of antidiabetic agents may be required). Products include:

Humulin R ... 1849
Humulin R (U-500) ... 1850

Insulin, Human Regular and Human NPH Mixture (Because corticosteroids may increase blood

Miconazole Nitrate (Ketoconazole has been reported to decrease the metabolism of certain corticosteroids by up to 60% leading to an increased risk of corticosteroid side effects).
No products indexed under this heading.

Miglitol (Because corticosteroids may increase blood glucose concentrations, dosage adjustments of antidiabetic agents may be required).
No products indexed under this heading.

Modafinil (Drugs such as barbiturates, phenytoin, ephedrine, and rifampin, which induce hepatic microsomal drug metabolizing enzyme activity may enhance metabolism of corticosteroid and require that the dosage of corticosteroid be increased). Products include:
Provigil Tablets 977

Nabumetone (Concomitant use of aspirin or other non-steroidal anti-inflammatory agents and corticosteroids increases the risk of gastrointestinal side effects. Aspirin should be used cautiously in conjunction with corticosteroids in hypoprothrombinemia. The clearance of salicylates may be increased with concurrent use of corticosteroids).
No products indexed under this heading.

Naproxen (Concomitant use of aspirin or other non-steroidal anti-inflammatory agents and corticosteroids increases the risk of gastrointestinal side effects. Aspirin should be used cautiously in conjunction with corticosteroids in hypoprothrombinemia. The clearance of salicylates may be increased with concurrent use of corticosteroids). Products include:
EC-Naprosyn Delayed-Release Tablets 2632
Naprosyn Suspension 2632
Naprosyn Tablets 2632

Naproxen Sodium (Concomitant use of aspirin or other non-steroidal anti-inflammatory agents and corticosteroids increases the risk of gastrointestinal side effects. Aspirin should be used cautiously in conjunction with corticosteroids in hypoprothrombinemia. The clearance of salicylates may be increased with concurrent use of corticosteroids). Products include:
Anaprox Tablets 2632
Anaprox DS Tablets 2632
Treximet Tablets 1616

Nateglinide (Because corticosteroids may increase blood glucose concentrations, dosage adjustments of antidiabetic agents may be required). Products include:
Starlix Tablets 2314

Nefazodone Hydrochloride (Ketoconazole has been reported to decrease the metabolism of certain corticosteroids by up to 60% leading to an increased risk of corticosteroid side effects).
No products indexed under this heading.

Nelfinavir Mesylate (Ketoconazole has been reported to decrease the metabolism of certain corticosteroids by up to 60% leading to an increased risk of corticosteroid side effects).
No products indexed under this heading.

Neostigmine Bromide (Concomitant use of anticholinesterase agents and corticosteroids may produce severe weakness in patients with myasthenia gravis. If possible, anticholinesterase agents should be withdrawn at least 24 hours before initiating corticosteroid therapy).
No products indexed under this heading.

Neostigmine Methylsulfate (Concomitant use of anticholinesterase agents and corticosteroids may produce severe weakness in patients with myasthenia gravis. If possible, anticholinesterase agents should be withdrawn at least 24 hours before initiating corticosteroid therapy).
No products indexed under this heading.

Nevirapine (Drugs such as barbiturates, phenytoin, ephedrine, and rifampin, which induce hepatic microsomal drug metabolizing enzyme activity may enhance metabolism of corticosteroid and require that the dosage of corticosteroid be increased). Products include:
Viramune Oral Suspension 873
Viramune Tablets 873

Niacinamide (Ketoconazole has been reported to decrease the metabolism of certain corticosteroids by up to 60% leading to an increased risk of corticosteroid side effects). Products include:
BioLean Free Tablets .... ▣635

Nicotinamide (Ketoconazole has been reported to decrease the metabolism of certain corticosteroids by up to 60% leading to an increased risk of corticosteroid side effects).
No products indexed under this heading.

Nifedipine (Ketoconazole has been reported to decrease the metabolism of certain corticosteroids by up to 60% leading to an increased risk of corticosteroid side effects).
No products indexed under this heading.

Norfloxacin (Ketoconazole has been reported to decrease the metabolism of certain corticosteroids by up to 60% leading to an increased risk of corticosteroid side effects). Products include:
Noroxin Tablets 2069

Omeprazole (Ketoconazole has been reported to decrease the metabolism of certain corticosteroids by up to 60% leading to an increased risk of corticosteroid side effects).
No products indexed under this heading.

Oxaprozin (Concomitant use of aspirin or other non-steroidal anti-inflammatory agents and corticosteroids increases the risk of gastrointestinal side effects. Aspirin should be used cautiously in conjunction with corticosteroids in hypoprothrombinemia. The clearance of salicylates may be increased with concurrent use of corticosteroids).
No products indexed under this heading.

Oxcarbazepine (Drugs such as barbiturates, phenytoin, ephedrine, and rifampin, which induce hepatic microsomal drug metabolizing enzyme activity may enhance metabolism of corticosteroid and require that the dosage of corticosteroid be increased).
No products indexed under this heading.

Paroxetine Hydrochloride (Ketoconazole has been reported to decrease the metabolism of certain corticosteroids by up to 60% leading to an increased risk of corticosteroid side effects). Products include:
Paxil 1535
Paxil CR Controlled-Release Tablets 1544

Pentobarbital Sodium (Drugs which induce hepatic microsomal drug metabolizing enzyme activity may enhance metabolism of corticosteroid and require that the dosage of corticosteroid be increased). Products include:
Nembutal Sodium Solution, USP 2494

Phenobarbital (Drugs which induce hepatic microsomal drug metabolizing enzyme activity may enhance metabolism of corticosteroid and require that the dosage of corticosteroid be increased). Products include:
Donnatal Extentabs 2507

Phenobarbital Sodium (Drugs such as barbiturates, phenytoin, ephedrine, and rifampin, which induce hepatic microsomal drug metabolizing enzyme activity may enhance metabolism of corticosteroid and require that the dosage of corticosteroid be increased).
No products indexed under this heading.

Phenylbutazone (Concomitant use of aspirin or other non-steroidal anti-inflammatory agents and corticosteroids increases the risk of gastrointestinal side effects. Aspirin should be used cautiously in conjunction with corticosteroids in hypoprothrombinemia. The clearance of salicylates may be increased with concurrent use of corticosteroids).
No products indexed under this heading.

Phenytoin (Drugs such as barbiturates, phenytoin, ephedrine, and rifampin, which induce hepatic microsomal drug metabolizing enzyme activity may enhance metabolism of corticosteroid and require that the dosage of corticosteroid be increased).
No products indexed under this heading.

Phenytoin Sodium (Drugs such as barbiturates, phenytoin, ephedrine, and rifampin, which induce hepatic microsomal drug metabolizing enzyme activity may enhance metabolism of corticosteroid and require that the dosage of corticosteroid be increased). Products include:
Phenytek Capsules 2192

Pioglitazone Hydrochloride (Because corticosteroids may increase blood glucose concentrations, dosage adjustments of antidiabetic agents may be required). Products include:
ActoPlus Met Tablets 3071
Actos Tablets 3077
Duetact Tablets 3085

Piroxicam (Concomitant use of aspirin or other non-steroidal anti-inflammatory agents and corticosteroids increases the risk of gastrointestinal side effects. Aspirin should be used cautiously in conjunction with corticosteroids in hypoprothrombinemia. The clearance of salicylates may be increased with concurrent use of corticosteroids).
No products indexed under this heading.

Poliovirus Vaccine Inactivated (Due to inhibition of antibody response, patients on prolonged corticosteroid therapy may exhibit a diminished response to toxoids and live or inactivated vaccines. Corticosteroids may also potentiate the replication of some organisms contained in live attenuated vaccines). Products include:
Pediarix Vaccine 1552

Polyestradiol Phosphate (Estrogens may decrease the hepatic metabolism of certain corticosteroids thereby increasing their effect).
No products indexed under this heading.

Polythiazide (When corticosteroids are administered concomitantly with potassium-depleting agents, patients should be observed closely for development of hypokalemia).
No products indexed under this heading.

Prednisolone Acetate (When corticosteroids are administered concomitantly with potassium-depleting agents, patients should be observed closely for development of hypokalemia). Products include:
Pred Forte Ophthalmic Suspension .... ⊙227
Pred Mild Ophthalmic Suspension .... ⊙230
Pred-G Ophthalmic Ointment .... ⊙229
Pred-G Ophthalmic Suspension .... ⊙228

Prednisolone Sodium Phosphate (When corticosteroids are administered concomitantly with potassium-depleting agents, patients should be observed closely for development of hypokalemia).
No products indexed under this heading.

Prednisolone Tebutate (When corticosteroids are administered concomitantly with potassium-depleting agents, patients should be observed closely for development of hypokalemia).
No products indexed under this heading.

Prednisone (When corticosteroids are administered concomitantly with potassium-depleting agents, patients should be observed closely for development of hypokalemia).
No products indexed under this heading.

Primidone (Drugs such as barbiturates, phenytoin, ephedrine, and rifampin, which induce hepatic microsomal drug metabolizing enzyme activity may enhance metabolism of corticosteroid and require that the dosage of corticosteroid be increased).
No products indexed under this heading.

Propoxyphene Hydrochloride (Ketoconazole has been reported to decrease the metabolism of certain corticosteroids by up to 60% leading to an increased risk of corticosteroid side effects).
No products indexed under this heading.

Propoxyphene Napsylate (Ketoconazole has been reported to decrease the metabolism of certain corticosteroids by up to 60% leading to an increased risk of corticosteroid side effects).
No products indexed under this heading.

Pyrazinamide (Serum concentrations of isoniazid may be decreased).
No products indexed under this heading.

Pyridostigmine Bromide (Concomitant use of anticholinesterase agents and corticosteroids may produce severe weakness in patients with myasthenia gravis. If possible, anticholinesterase agents should be withdrawn at least 24 hours before initiating corticosteroid therapy).
No products indexed under this heading.

Quinestrol (Estrogens may decrease the hepatic metabolism of certain corticosteroids thereby increasing their effect).
No products indexed under this heading.

Quinidine (Ketoconazole has been reported to decrease the metabolism of certain corticosteroids by up to 60% leading to an increased risk of corticosteroid side effects).
No products indexed under this heading.

Quinidine Hydrochloride (Ketoconazole has been reported to decrease the metabolism of certain corticosteroids by up to 60% leading to an increased risk of corticosteroid side effects).
No products indexed under this heading.

Quinidine Polygalacturonate (Ketoconazole has been reported to decrease the metabolism of certain corticosteroids by up to 60% leading to an increased risk of corticosteroid side effects).
No products indexed under this heading.

Quinidine Sulfate (Ketoconazole has been reported to decrease the metabolism of certain corticosteroids by up to 60% leading to an increased risk of corticosteroid side effects).
No products indexed under this heading.

Quinine (Ketoconazole has been reported to decrease the metabolism of certain corticosteroids by up to 60% leading to an increased risk of corticosteroid side effects).
No products indexed under this heading.

Quinine Sulfate (Ketoconazole has been reported to decrease the metabolism of certain corticosteroids by up to 60% leading to an increased risk of corticosteroid side effects).
No products indexed under this heading.

Quinupristin (Ketoconazole has been reported to decrease the metabolism of certain corticosteroids by up to 60% leading to an increased risk of corticosteroid side effects).
No products indexed under this heading.

Ranitidine Bismuth Citrate (Ketoconazole has been reported to decrease the metabolism of certain corticosteroids by up to 60% leading to an increased risk of corticosteroid side effects).
No products indexed under this heading.

Ranitidine Hydrochloride (Ketoconazole has been reported to decrease the metabolism of certain corticosteroids by up to 60% leading to an increased risk of corticosteroid side effects). Products include:
Zantac 75 Tablets 603
Zantac **1670**
Zantac Injection **1666**
Zantac Injection Pharmacy Bulk Package **1668**
Maximum Strength Zantac 150 Tablets 603
Maximum Strength Zantac 150 Cool Mint Tablets 603

Repaglinide (Because corticosteroids may increase blood glucose concentrations, dosage adjustments of antidiabetic agents may be required). Products include:
PrandiMet Tablets **2967**
Prandin Tablets **2971**

Rifabutin (Drugs such as barbiturates, phenytoin, ephedrine, and rifampin, which induce hepatic microsomal drug metabolizing enzyme activity may enhance metabolism of corticosteroid and require that the dosage of corticosteroid be increased).
No products indexed under this heading.

Rifampicin (Drugs such as barbiturates, phenytoin, ephedrine, and rifampin, which induce hepatic microsomal drug metabolizing enzyme activity may enhance metabolism of corticosteroid and require that the dosage of corticosteroid be increased).
No products indexed under this heading.

Rifampin (Drugs such as barbiturates, phenytoin, ephedrine, and rifampin, which induce hepatic microsomal drug metabolizing enzyme activity may enhance metabolism of corticosteroid and require that the dosage of corticosteroid be increased).
No products indexed under this heading.

Rifapentine (Serum concentrations of isoniazid may be decreased).
No products indexed under this heading.

Ritonavir (Ketoconazole has been reported to decrease the metabolism of certain corticosteroids by up to 60% leading to an increased risk of corticosteroid side effects). Products include:
Kaletra **452**
Norvir **489**

Rivastigmine Tartrate (Concomitant use of anticholinesterase agents and corticosteroids may produce severe weakness in patients with myasthenia gravis. If possible, anticholinesterase agents should be withdrawn at least 24 hours before initiating corticosteroid therapy). Products include:
Exelon Capsules **2229**
Exelon Oral Solution **2229**
Exelon Patch **2233**

Rofecoxib (Concomitant use of aspirin or other non-steroidal anti-inflammatory agents and corticosteroids increases the risk of gastrointestinal side effects. Aspirin should be used cautiously in conjunction with corticosteroids in hypoprothrombinemia. The clearance of salicylates may be increased with concurrent use of corticosteroids).
No products indexed under this heading.

Rosiglitazone Maleate (Because corticosteroids may increase blood glucose concentrations, dosage adjustments of antidiabetic agents may be required). Products include:
Avandamet Tablets **1336**
Avandaryl Tablets **1344**
Avandia Tablets **1351**

Saquinavir (Ketoconazole has been reported to decrease the metabolism of certain corticosteroids by up to 60% leading to an increased risk of corticosteroid side effects).
No products indexed under this heading.

Saquinavir Mesylate (Ketoconazole has been reported to decrease the metabolism of certain corticosteroids by up to 60% leading to an increased risk of corticosteroid side effects).
No products indexed under this heading.

Secobarbital Sodium (Drugs which induce hepatic microsomal drug metabolizing enzyme activity may enhance metabolism of corticosteroid and require that the dosage of corticosteroid be increased).
No products indexed under this heading.

Sertraline Hydrochloride (Ketoconazole has been reported to decrease the metabolism of certain corticosteroids by up to 60% leading to an increased risk of corticosteroid side effects).
No products indexed under this heading.

Sildenafil Citrate (Ketoconazole has been reported to decrease the metabolism of certain corticosteroids by up to 60% leading to an increased risk of corticosteroid side effects).
No products indexed under this heading.

Sitagliptin Phosphate (Because corticosteroids may increase blood glucose concentrations, dosage adjustments of antidiabetic agents may be required). Products include:
Janumet Tablets **2041**
Januvia Tablets **2048**

Sulfinpyrazone (Drugs such as barbiturates, phenytoin, ephedrine, and rifampin, which induce hepatic microsomal drug metabolizing enzyme activity may enhance metabolism of corticosteroid and require that the dosage of corticosteroid be increased).
No products indexed under this heading.

Sulindac (Concomitant use of aspirin or other non-steroidal anti-inflammatory agents and corticosteroids increases the risk of gastrointestinal side effects. Aspirin should be used cautiously in conjunction with corticosteroids in hypoprothrombinemia. The clearance of salicylates may be increased with concurrent use of corticosteroids). Products include:
Clinoril Tablets **1962**

Tacrine Hydrochloride (Concomitant use of anticholinesterase agents and corticosteroids may produce severe weakness in patients with myasthenia gravis. If possible, anticholinesterase agents should be withdrawn at least 24 hours before initiating corticosteroid therapy).
No products indexed under this heading.

Telithromycin (Ketoconazole has been reported to decrease the metabolism of certain corticosteroids by up to 60% leading to an increased risk of corticosteroid side effects). Products include:
Ketek Tablets **2744**

Theophylline (Drugs such as barbiturates, phenytoin, ephedrine, and rifampin, which induce hepatic microsomal drug metabolizing enzyme activity may enhance metabolism of corticosteroid and require that the dosage of corticosteroid be increased).
No products indexed under this heading.

Theophylline Anhydrous (Drugs such as barbiturates, phenytoin, ephedrine, and rifampin, which induce hepatic microsomal drug metabolizing enzyme activity may enhance metabolism of corticosteroid and require that the dosage of corticosteroid be increased). Products include:
Uniphyl Tablets **2595**

Theophylline Calcium Salicylate (Drugs such as barbiturates, phenytoin, ephedrine, and rifampin, which induce hepatic microsomal drug metabolizing enzyme activity may enhance metabolism of corticosteroid and require that the dosage of corticosteroid be increased).
No products indexed under this heading.

Theophylline Dihydroxypropyl (Glyceryl) (Drugs such as barbiturates, phenytoin, ephedrine, and rifampin, which induce hepatic microsomal drug metabolizing enzyme activity may enhance metabolism of corticosteroid and require that the dosage of corticosteroid be increased).
No products indexed under this heading.

Theophylline Ethylenediamine (Drugs such as barbiturates, phenytoin, ephedrine, and rifampin, which induce hepatic microsomal drug metabolizing enzyme activity may enhance metabolism of corticosteroid and require that the dosage of corticosteroid be increased).
No products indexed under this heading.

Thiamylal Sodium (Drugs which induce hepatic microsomal drug metabolizing enzyme activity may enhance metabolism of corticosteroid and require that the dosage of corticosteroid be increased).
No products indexed under this heading.

Tinzaparin Sodium (Co-administration of corticosteroids and warfarin usually results in inhibition of response to warfarin, although there have been some conflicting reports. Therefore, coagulation indices should be monitored frequently to maintain the desired anticoagulant effect).
No products indexed under this heading.

Tolazamide (Because corticosteroids may increase blood glucose concentrations, dosage adjustments of antidiabetic agents may be required).
No products indexed under this heading.

Tolbutamide (Because corticosteroids may increase blood glucose concentrations, dosage adjustments of antidiabetic agents may be required).
No products indexed under this heading.

Tolmetin Sodium (Concomitant use of aspirin or other non-steroidal anti-inflammatory agents and corticosteroids increases the risk of gastrointestinal side effects. Aspirin should be used cautiously in conjunction with corticosteroids in hypoprothrombinemia. The clearance of salicylates may be increased with concurrent use of corticosteroids).
No products indexed under this heading.

Torsemide (When corticosteroids are administered concomitantly with potassium-depleting agents, patients should be observed closely for development of hypokalemia).
Products include:
Demadex Injection 2630
Demadex Tablets 2630

Triamcinolone (When corticosteroids are administered concomitantly with potassium-depleting agents, patients should be observed closely for development of hypokalemia).
No products indexed under this heading.

Triamcinolone Diacetate (When corticosteroids are administered concomitantly with potassium-depleting agents, patients should be observed closely for development of hypokalemia).
No products indexed under this heading.

Triamcinolone Hexacetonide (When corticosteroids are administered concomitantly with potassium-depleting agents, patients should be observed closely for development of hypokalemia).
No products indexed under this heading.

Troglitazone (Because corticosteroids may increase blood glucose concentrations, dosage adjustments of antidiabetic agents may be required).
No products indexed under this heading.

Troleandomycin (Ketoconazole has been reported to decrease the metabolism of certain corticosteroids by up to 60% leading to an increased risk of corticosteroid side effects).
No products indexed under this heading.

Valdecoxib (Concomitant use of aspirin or other non-steroidal anti-inflammatory agents and corticosteroids increases the risk of gastrointestinal side effects. Aspirin should be used cautiously in conjunction with corticosteroids in hypoprothrombinemia. The clearance of salicylates may be increased with concurrent use of corticosteroids).
No products indexed under this heading.

Valproate Sodium (Ketoconazole has been reported to decrease the metabolism of certain corticosteroids by up to 60% leading to an increased risk of corticosteroid side effects).
No products indexed under this heading.

Vardenafil Hydrochloride (Ketoconazole has been reported to decrease the metabolism of certain corticosteroids by up to 60% leading to an increased risk of corticosteroid side effects). Products include:
Levitra Tablets 2876

Verapamil Hydrochloride (Ketoconazole has been reported to decrease the metabolism of certain corticosteroids by up to 60% leading to an increased risk of corticosteroid side effects). Products include:
Tarka Tablets 511

Voriconazole (Ketoconazole has been reported to decrease the metabolism of certain corticosteroids by up to 60% leading to an increased risk of corticosteroid side effects).
No products indexed under this heading.

Warfarin Sodium (Co-administration of corticosteroids and warfarin usually results in inhibition of response to warfarin, although there have been some conflicting reports. Therefore, coagulation indices should be monitored frequently to maintain the desired anticoagulant effect).
No products indexed under this heading.

Zafirlukast (Ketoconazole has been reported to decrease the metabolism of certain corticosteroids by up to 60% leading to an increased risk of corticosteroid side effects).
Products include:
Accolate Tablets 669

Zileuton (Ketoconazole has been reported to decrease the metabolism of certain corticosteroids by up to 60% leading to an increased risk of corticosteroid side effects).
No products indexed under this heading.

Food Interactions

Grapefruit (Ketoconazole has been reported to decrease the metabolism of certain corticosteroids by up to 60% leading to an increased risk of corticosteroid side effects).

Grapefruit Juice (Ketoconazole has been reported to decrease the metabolism of certain corticosteroids by up to 60% leading to an increased risk of corticosteroid side effects).

TRISENOX INJECTION

(Arsenic Trioxide) 986
May interact with potassium-depleting diuretics, quinidine, and certain other agents. Compounds in these categories include:

Amiodarone Hydrochloride (Arsenic trioxide can cause QT interval prolongation and complete AV block; QT prolongation can lead to torsade de pointes-type ventricular arrhythmias, which can be fatal; co-administration with other drugs that can prolong the QT interval, such as certain anti-arrhythmics, increases the risk and extent of QT prolongation).
No products indexed under this heading.

Amphotericin B (Arsenic trioxide can cause QT interval prolongation and complete AV block; QT prolongation can lead to torsade de pointes-type ventricular arrhythmias, which can be fatal; co-administration with other drugs that can prolong the QT interval, such as amphotericin B, increases the risk and extent of QT prolongation).
No products indexed under this heading.

Bendroflumethiazide (Arsenic trioxide can cause QT interval prolongation and complete AV block; QT prolongation can lead to torsade de pointes-type ventricular arrhythmias, which can be fatal; co-administration with other drugs that cause hypokalemia or hypomagnesemia resulting in prolongation of the QT interval, such as potassium-wasting diuretics, increases the risk and extent of QT prolongation).
No products indexed under this heading.

Bumetanide (Arsenic trioxide can cause QT interval prolongation and complete AV block; QT prolongation can lead to torsade de pointes-type ventricular arrhythmias, which can be fatal; co-administration with other drugs that cause hypokalemia or hypomagnesemia resulting in prolongation of the QT interval, such as potassium-wasting diuretics, increases the risk and extent of QT prolongation).
No products indexed under this heading.

Chlorothiazide (Arsenic trioxide can cause QT interval prolongation and complete AV block; QT prolongation can lead to torsade de pointes-type ventricular arrhythmias, which can be fatal; co-administration with other drugs that cause hypokalemia or hypomagnesemia resulting in prolongation of the QT interval, such as potassium-wasting diuretics, increases the risk and extent of QT prolongation).
No products indexed under this heading.

Chlorothiazide Sodium (Arsenic trioxide can cause QT interval prolongation and complete AV block; QT prolongation can lead to torsade de pointes-type ventricular arrhythmias, which can be fatal; co-administration with other drugs that cause hypokalemia or hypomagnesemia resulting in prolongation of the QT interval, such as potassium-wasting diuretics, increases the risk and extent of QT prolongation). Products include:
Intravenous Sodium Diuril 2490

Ethacrynic Acid (Arsenic trioxide can cause QT interval prolongation and complete AV block; QT prolongation can lead to torsade de pointes-type ventricular arrhythmias, which can be fatal; co-administration with other drugs that cause hypokalemia or hypomagnesemia resulting in prolongation of the QT interval, such as potassium-wasting diuretics, increases the risk and extent of QT prolongation). Products include:
Edecrin Tablets 698

Furosemide (Arsenic trioxide can cause QT interval prolongation and complete AV block; QT prolongation can lead to torsade de pointes-type ventricular arrhythmias, which can be fatal; co-administration with other drugs that cause hypokalemia or hypomagnesemia resulting in prolongation of the QT interval, such as potassium-wasting diuretics, increases the risk and extent of QT prolongation). Products include:
Furosemide Tablets 2186

Hydrochlorothiazide (Arsenic trioxide can cause QT interval prolongation and complete AV block; QT prolongation can lead to torsade de pointes-type ventricular arrhythmias, which can be fatal; co-administration with other drugs that cause hypokalemia or hypomagnesemia resulting in prolongation of the QT interval, such as potassium-wasting diuretics, increases the risk and extent of QT prolongation). Products include:
Atacand HCT 642
Avalide Tablets 892
Avalide Tablets 2713
Benicar HCT Tablets 1010
Diovan HCT Tablets 2216
Dyazide Capsules 1405
Micardis HCT Tablets 854
Prinzide Tablets 2092
Tekturna HCT Tablets 2324
Teveten HCT Tablets 517

Hydroflumethiazide (Arsenic trioxide can cause QT interval prolongation and complete AV block; QT prolongation can lead to torsade de pointes-type ventricular arrhythmias, which can be fatal; co-administration with other drugs that cause hypokalemia or hypomagnesemia resulting in prolongation of the QT interval, such as potassium-wasting diuretics, increases the risk and extent of QT prolongation).
No products indexed under this heading.

Methyclothiazide (Arsenic trioxide can cause QT interval prolongation and complete AV block; QT prolongation can lead to torsade de pointes-type ventricular arrhythmias, which can be fatal; co-administration with other drugs that cause hypokalemia or hypomagnesemia resulting in prolongation of the QT interval, such as potassium-wasting diuretics, increases the risk and extent of QT prolongation).
No products indexed under this heading.

Polythiazide (Arsenic trioxide can cause QT interval prolongation and complete AV block; QT prolongation can lead to torsade de pointes-type ventricular arrhythmias, which can be fatal; co-administration with other drugs that cause hypokalemia or hypomagnesemia resulting in prolongation of the QT interval, such as potassium-wasting diuretics, increases the risk and extent of QT

prolongation).
No products indexed under this heading.

Procainamide Hydrochloride (Arsenic trioxide can cause QT interval prolongation and complete AV block; QT prolongation can lead to torsade de pointes-type ventricular arrhythmias, which can be fatal; co-administration with other drugs that can prolong the QT interval, such as certain antiarrhythmics, increases the risk and extent of QT prolongation).
No products indexed under this heading.

Quinidine (Arsenic trioxide can cause QT interval prolongation and complete AV block; QT prolongation can lead to torsade de pointes-type ventricular arrhythmias, which can be fatal; co-administration with other drugs that can prolong the QT interval, such as certain anti-arrhythmic quinidine, increases the risk and extent of QT prolongation).
No products indexed under this heading.

Quinidine Gluconate (Arsenic trioxide can cause QT interval prolongation and complete AV block; QT prolongation can lead to torsade de pointes-type ventricular arrhythmias, which can be fatal; co-administration with other drugs that can prolong the QT interval, such as certain anti-arrhythmic quinidine, increases the risk and extent of QT prolongation).
No products indexed under this heading.

Quinidine Hydrochloride (Arsenic trioxide can cause QT interval prolongation and complete AV block; QT prolongation can lead to torsade de pointes-type ventricular arrhythmias, which can be fatal; co-administration with other drugs that can prolong the QT interval, such as certain anti-arrhythmic quinidine, increases the risk and extent of QT prolongation).
No products indexed under this heading.

Quinidine Polygalacturonate (Arsenic trioxide can cause QT interval prolongation and complete AV block; QT prolongation can lead to torsade de pointes-type ventricular arrhythmias, which can be fatal; co-administration with other drugs that can prolong the QT interval, such as certain anti-arrhythmic quinidine, increases the risk and extent of QT prolongation).
No products indexed under this heading.

Quinidine Sulfate (Arsenic trioxide can cause QT interval prolongation and complete AV block; QT prolongation can lead to torsade de pointes-type ventricular arrhythmias, which can be fatal; co-administration with other drugs that can prolong the QT interval, such as certain anti-arrhythmic quinidine, increases the risk and extent of QT prolongation).
No products indexed under this heading.

Sotalol Hydrochloride (Arsenic trioxide can cause QT interval prolongation and complete AV block; QT prolongation can lead to torsade de pointes-type ventricular arrhythmias, which can be fatal; co-administration with other drugs that can prolong the QT interval, such as certain anti-arrhythmics, increases the risk and extent of QT prolongation).
No products indexed under this heading.

Thioridazine Hydrochloride (Arsenic trioxide can cause QT interval prolongation and complete AV block; QT prolongation can lead to torsade de pointes-type ventricular arrhythmias, which can be fatal; co-administration with other drugs that can prolong the QT interval, such as thioridazine, increases the risk and extent of QT prolongation). Products include:
Thioridazine Hydrochloride Tablets 2195

Torsemide (Arsenic trioxide can cause QT interval prolongation and complete AV block; QT prolongation can lead to torsade de pointes-type ventricular arrhythmias, which can be fatal; co-administration with other drugs that cause hypokalemia or hypomagnesemia resulting in prolongation of the QT interval, such as potassium-wasting diuretics, increases the risk and extent of QT prolongation). Products include:
Demadex Injection 2630
Demadex Tablets 2630

TRIZIVIR TABLETS

(Abacavir Sulfate, Lamivudine, Zidovudine) 1622
May interact with cytotoxic drugs, valproate, and certain other agents. Compounds in these categories include:

Atovaquone (Co-administration may alter zidovudine blood concentrations; routine dose modification is not warranted). Products include:
Malarone Pediatric Tablets 1521
Malarone Tablets 1521
Mepron Suspension 1526

Bleomycin Sulfate (Co-administration with cytotoxic agents may increase the hematologic toxicity of zidovudine).
No products indexed under this heading.

Cyclophosphamide (Co-administration with cytotoxic agents may increase the hematologic toxicity of zidovudine).
No products indexed under this heading.

Daunorubicin Hydrochloride (Co-administration with cytotoxic agents may increase the hematologic toxicity of zidovudine).
No products indexed under this heading.

Divalproex Sodium (Co-administration may alter zidovudine blood concentrations; routine dose modification is not warranted). Products include:
Depakote ER Tablets 423

Doxorubicin Hydrochloride (Co-administration with cytotoxic agents may increase the hematologic toxicity of zidovudine).
No products indexed under this heading.

Emtricitabine (Trizivir should not be administered concomitantly with emtricitabine). Products include:
Atripla Tablets 938
Emtriva Capsules 1246
Emtriva Oral Solution 1246
Truvada Tablets 1262

Epirubicin Hydrochloride (Co-administration with cytotoxic agents may increase the hematologic toxicity of zidovudine).
No products indexed under this heading.

Fluconazole (Co-administration may alter zidovudine blood concentrations; routine dose modification is not warranted).
No products indexed under this heading.

Fluorouracil (Co-administration with cytotoxic agents may increase the hematologic toxicity of zidovudine). Products include:
Carac Cream 0.5% 2722

Ganciclovir (Co-administration may increase the hematologic toxicity of zidovudine).
No products indexed under this heading.

Ganciclovir Sodium (Co-administration may increase the hematologic toxicity of zidovudine).
No products indexed under this heading.

Hydroxyurea (Co-administration with cytotoxic agents may increase the hematologic toxicity of zidovudine).
No products indexed under this heading.

Interferon alfa-2a, Recombinant (Hepatic decompensation (some fatal) has occurred in HIV/HCV co-infected patients receiving combination antiretroviral for HIV and interferon alfa and ribavirin. Patients receiving interferon alfa with or without ribavirin and Trizivir should be closely monitored for treatment-associated toxicities, especially hepatic decompensation, neutropenia and anemia. Discontinuation of Trizivir should be considered as medically appropriate. Dose reduction or discontinuation of interferon, alfa, ribavirin or both should also be considered if worsening clinical toxicities are observed, including hepatic decompensation (e.g., Childs Pugh greater than 6)).
No products indexed under this heading.

Interferon alfa-N3 (Human Leukocyte Derived) (Hepatic decompensation (some fatal) has occurred in HIV/HCV co-infected patients receiving combination antiretroviral for HIV and interferon alfa and ribavirin. Patients receiving interferon alfa with or without ribavirin and Trizivir should be closely monitored for treatment-associated toxicities, especially hepatic decompensation, neutropenia and anemia. Discontinuation of Trizivir should be considered as medically appropriate. Dose reduction or discontinuation of interferon, alfa, ribavirin or both should also be considered if worsening clinical toxicities are observed, including hepatic decompensation (e.g., Childs Pugh greater than 6)). Products include:
Alferon N Injection 1726

Methadone Hydrochloride (Co-administration may alter zidovudine blood concentrations; routine dose modification is not warranted).
No products indexed under this heading.

Methotrexate Sodium (Co-administration with cytotoxic agents may increase the hematologic toxicity of zidovudine).
No products indexed under this heading.

Mitotane (Co-administration with cytotoxic agents may increase the hematologic toxicity of zidovudine).
No products indexed under this heading.

Mitoxantrone Hydrochloride (Co-administration with cytotoxic agents may increase the hematologic toxicity of zidovudine). Products include:
Novantrone for Injection Concentrate 1100

Nelfinavir Mesylate (Co-administration may alter lamivudine and zidovudine blood concentrations; routine dose modification is not warranted).
No products indexed under this heading.

Probenecid (Co-administration may alter zidovudine blood concentrations; routine dose modification is not warranted).
No products indexed under this heading.

Procarbazine Hydrochloride (Co-administration with cytotoxic agents may increase the hematologic toxicity of zidovudine).
No products indexed under this heading.

Ribavirin (Co-administration of zidovudine with ribavirin should be avoided since an antagonistic relationship has been demonstrated in vitro). Products include:
Rebetol 2917

Ritonavir (Co-administration may alter zidovudine blood concentrations; routine dose modification is not warranted). Products include:
Kaletra 452
Norvir 489

Stavudine (Co-administration of zidovudine with stavudine should be avoided since an antagonistic relationship has been demonstrated in vitro).
No products indexed under this heading.

Sulfamethoxazole (Co-administration with trimethoprim/sulfamethoxazole may alter lamivudine blood concentrations; routine dose modification is not warranted).
No products indexed under this heading.

Tamoxifen Citrate (Co-administration with cytotoxic agents may increase the hematologic toxicity of zidovudine).
No products indexed under this heading.

Trimethoprim (Co-administration with trimethoprim/sulfamethoxazole may alter lamivudine blood concentrations; routine dose modification is not warranted).
No products indexed under this heading.

Valproate Sodium (Co-administration may alter zidovudine blood concentrations; routine dose modification is not warranted).
No products indexed under this heading.

Valproic Acid (Co-administration may alter zidovudine blood concentrations; routine dose modification is not warranted).
No products indexed under this heading.

Vincristine Sulfate (Co-administration with cytotoxic agents may increase the hematologic toxicity of zidovudine).
No products indexed under this heading.

Zalacitabine (Lamivudine and zalcitabine may inhibit the intracellular phosphorylation of one another; co-administration is not recommended).
No products indexed under this heading.

Food Interactions

Alcohol (Concurrent use decreases the elimination of abacavir causing an increase in overall exposure).

TRUSOPT STERILE OPHTHALMIC SOLUTION

(Dorzolamide Hydrochloride) 2128
May interact with carbonic anhydrase inhibitors and certain other agents. Compounds in these categories include:

Acetazolamide (Potential for an additive effect on the known systemic effects of carbonic anhydrase inhibition in patients receiving a systemic carbonic anhydrase inhibitor and Trusopt).
No products indexed under this heading.

Acetazolamide Sodium (Potential for an additive effect on the known systemic effects of carbonic anhydrase inhibition in patients receiving a systemic carbonic anhydrase inhibitor and Trusopt).
No products indexed under this heading.

Aspirin (Potential for acid-base and electrolyte disturbances with concomitant use; these disturbances have been reported with oral agent and have not been reported during clinical trials with Trusopt). Products include:
Aggrenox Capsules 819
Bayer Aspirin 750
Percodan Tablets 1130
St. Joseph 81 mg Aspirin Chewable and Enteric Coated Tablets 1903

Dichlorphenamide (Potential for an additive effect on the known systemic effects of carbonic anhydrase inhibition in patients receiving a systemic carbonic anhydrase inhibitor and Trusopt).
No products indexed under this heading.

Methazolamide (Potential for an additive effect on the known systemic effects of carbonic anhydrase inhibition in patients receiving a systemic carbonic anhydrase inhibitor and Trusopt).
No products indexed under this heading.

TRUVADA TABLETS

(Emtricitabine, Tenofovir Disoproxil Fumarate)... 1262
May interact with cationic drugs that are eliminated by renal tubular, nephrotoxic agents, and certain other agents. Compounds in these categories include:

Abacavir Sulfate (Drugs that decrease renal function may increase concentrations of emtricitabine and/or tenofovir. Truvada should be avoided with concurrent or recent use of a nephrotoxic agent). Products include:
Epzicom Tablets 1422
Trizivir Tablets 1622
Ziagen 1673

Acyclovir (Emtricitabine and tenofovir are primarily excreted by the kidneys by a combination of glomerular filtration and active tubular secretion. No drug-drug interactions due to competition for renal excretion have been observed; however, co-administration of Truvada with drugs that are eliminated by active tubular secretion may increase concentrations of emtricitabine, tenofovir, and/or the co-administered drug. Some examples include, but are not limited, to acyclovir, adefovir dipivoxil, cidofovir, ganciclovir, valacyclovir, and valganciclovir. Drugs that decrease renal function may increase concentrations of emtricitabine and/or tenofovir). Products include:
Zovirax 1690
Zovirax Cream 817
Zovirax Ointment 819

Acyclovir Sodium (Emtricitabine and tenofovir are primarily excreted by the kidneys by a combination of glomerular filtration and active tubular secretion. No drug-drug interactions due to competition for renal excretion have been observed; however, co-administration of Truvada with drugs that are eliminated by active tubular secretion may increase concentrations of emtricitabine, tenofovir, and/or the co-administered drug. Some examples include, but are not limited, to acyclovir, adefovir dipivoxil, cidofovir, ganciclovir, valacyclovir, and valganciclovir. Drugs that decrease renal function may increase concentrations of emtricitabine and/or tenofovir).
No products indexed under this heading.

Adefovir dipivoxil (Emtricitabine and tenofovir are primarily excreted by the kidneys by a combination of glomerular filtration and active tubular secretion. No drug-drug interactions due to competition for renal excretion have been observed; however, co-administration of Truvada with drugs that are eliminated by active tubular secretion may increase concentrations of emtricitabine, tenofovir, and/or the co-administered drug. Some examples include, but are not limited, to acyclovir, adefovir dipivoxil, cidofovir, ganciclovir, valacyclovir, and valganciclovir. Drugs that decrease renal function may increase concentrations of emtricitabine and/or tenofovir). Products include:
Hepsera Tablets 1253

Alatrofloxacin Mesylate (Drugs that decrease renal function may increase concentrations of emtricitabine and/or tenofovir. Truvada should be avoided with concurrent or recent use of a nephrotoxic agent).
No products indexed under this heading.

Aldesleukin (Drugs that decrease renal function may increase concentrations of emtricitabine and/or tenofovir. Truvada should be avoided with concurrent or recent use of a nephrotoxic agent). Products include:
Proleukin for Injection 2287

Amikacin Sulfate (Drugs that decrease renal function may increase concentrations of emtricitabine and/or tenofovir. Truvada should be avoided with concurrent or recent use of a nephrotoxic agent).
No products indexed under this heading.

Amiloride Hydrochloride (Emtricitabine and tenofovir are primarily excreted by the kidneys by a combination of glomerular filtration and active tubular secretion. No drug-drug interactions due to competition for renal excretion have been observed; however, co-administration of Truvada with drugs that are eliminated by active tubular secretion may increase concentrations of emtricitabine, tenofovir, and/or the co-administered drug).
No products indexed under this heading.

Amoxicillin (Drugs that decrease renal function may increase concentrations of emtricitabine and/or tenofovir. Truvada should be avoided with concurrent or recent use of a nephrotoxic agent). Products include:
Amoxil Capsules 1305
Amoxil Chewable Tablets 1305
Amoxil Pediatric Drops for Oral Suspension 1305
Amoxil Powder for Oral Suspension 1305
Amoxil Tablets 1305
Augmentin 1323
Augmentin Tablets 1327
Augmentin XR Extended Release Tablets 1333
Augmentin ES-600 Powder for Oral Suspension 1329
Moxatag Tablets 2165

Amoxicillin Trihydrate (Drugs that decrease renal function may increase concentrations of emtricitabine and/or tenofovir. Truvada should be avoided with concurrent or recent use of a nephrotoxic agent).
No products indexed under this heading.

Amphotericin B (Drugs that decrease renal function may increase concentrations of emtricitabine and/or tenofovir. Truvada should be avoided with concurrent or recent use of a nephrotoxic agent).
No products indexed under this heading.

Amphotericin B, liposomal (Drugs that decrease renal function may increase concentrations of emtricitabine and/or tenofovir. Truvada should be avoided with concurrent or recent use of a nephrotoxic agent). Products include:
AmBisome for Injection 606

Amphotericin B Cholesteryl Sulfate (Drugs that decrease renal function may increase concentrations of emtricitabine and/or tenofovir. Truvada should be avoided with concurrent or recent use of a nephrotoxic agent).
No products indexed under this heading.

Amphotericin B Lipid Complex (Drugs that decrease renal function may increase concentrations of emtricitabine and/or tenofovir. Truvada should be avoided with concurrent or recent use of a nephrotoxic agent). Products include:
Abelcet Injection 1134

Ampicillin (Drugs that decrease renal function may increase concentrations of emtricitabine and/or tenofovir. Truvada should be avoided with concurrent or recent use of a nephrotoxic agent).
No products indexed under this heading.

Ampicillin Sodium (Drugs that decrease renal function may increase concentrations of emtricitabine and/or tenofovir. Truvada should be avoided with concurrent or recent use of a nephrotoxic agent).
No products indexed under this heading.

Ampicillin Trihydrate (Drugs that decrease renal function may increase concentrations of emtricitabine and/or tenofovir. Truvada should be avoided with concurrent or recent use of a nephrotoxic agent).
No products indexed under this heading.

Amprenavir (Drugs that decrease renal function may increase concentrations of emtricitabine and/or tenofovir. Truvada should be avoided with concurrent or recent use of a nephrotoxic agent).
No products indexed under this heading.

Aspirin (Drugs that decrease renal function may increase concentrations of emtricitabine and/or tenofovir. Truvada should be avoided with concurrent or recent use of a nephrotoxic agent). Products include:
Aggrenox Capsules 819
Bayer Aspirin 750
Percodan Tablets 1130
St. Joseph 81 mg Aspirin Chewable and Enteric Coated Tablets 1903

Atazanavir (Co-administration decreases atazanavir concentrations and increases tenofovir concentrations. Use atazanavir with Truvada only with ritonavir; monitor for evidence of tenofovir toxicity).
No products indexed under this heading.

Atazanavir Sulfate (Co-administration decreases atazanavir concentrations and increases tenofovir concentrations. Use atazanavir with Truvada only with ritonavir; monitor for evidence of tenofovir toxicity). Products include:
Reyataz Capsules 3299

Atorvastatin Calcium (Drugs that decrease renal function may increase concentrations of emtricitabine and/or tenofovir. Truvada should be avoided with concurrent or recent use of a nephrotoxic agent). Products include:
Lipitor Tablets 2501

Azithromycin Dihydrate (Drugs that decrease renal function may increase concentrations of emtricitabine and/or tenofovir. Truvada should be avoided with concurrent or recent use of a nephrotoxic agent).
No products indexed under this heading.

Azlocillin Sodium (Drugs that decrease renal function may increase concentrations of emtricitabine and/or tenofovir. Truvada should be avoided with concurrent or recent use of a nephrotoxic agent).
No products indexed under this heading.

Aztreonam (Drugs that decrease renal function may increase concentrations of emtricitabine and/or tenofovir. Truvada should be avoided with concurrent or recent use of a nephrotoxic agent).
No products indexed under this heading.

Bacampicillin Hydrochloride (Drugs that decrease renal function may increase concentrations of emtricitabine and/or tenofovir. Truvada should be avoided with concurrent or recent use of a nephrotoxic agent).
No products indexed under this heading.

Balsalazide Disodium (Drugs that decrease renal function may increase concentrations of emtricitabine and/or tenofovir. Truvada should be avoided with concurrent or recent use of a nephrotoxic agent).
No products indexed under this heading.

Benazepril Hydrochloride (Drugs that decrease renal function may increase concentrations of emtricitabine and/or tenofovir. Truvada should be avoided with concurrent or recent use of a nephrotoxic agent).
No products indexed under this heading.

Bendroflumethiazide (Drugs that decrease renal function may increase concentrations of emtricitabine and/or tenofovir. Truvada should be avoided with concurrent or recent use of a nephrotoxic agent).
No products indexed under this heading.

Caffeine (Drugs that decrease renal function may increase concentrations of emtricitabine and/or tenofovir. Truvada should be avoided with concurrent or recent use of a nephrotoxic agent). Products include:
BioLean Free Tablets 635
BioLean II Tablets 635
Winrgy Dietary Supplement 642

Captopril (Drugs that decrease renal function may increase concentrations of emtricitabine and/or tenofovir. Truvada should be avoided with concurrent or recent use of a nephrotoxic agent). Products include:
Captopril Tablets 2182

Carbenicillin Disodium (Drugs that decrease renal function may increase concentrations of emtricitabine and/or tenofovir. Truvada should be avoided with concurrent or recent use of a nephrotoxic agent).
No products indexed under this heading.

Carbenicillin Indanyl Sodium (Drugs that decrease renal function may increase concentrations of emtricitabine and/or tenofovir. Truvada should be avoided with concurrent or recent use of a nephrotoxic agent).
No products indexed under this heading.

Carboplatin (Drugs that decrease renal function may increase concentrations of emtricitabine and/or tenofovir. Truvada should be avoided with concurrent or recent use of a nephrotoxic agent).
No products indexed under this heading.

Carmustine (BCNU) (Drugs that decrease renal function may increase concentrations of emtricitabine and/or tenofovir. Truvada should be avoided with concurrent or recent use of a nephrotoxic agent).
No products indexed under this heading.

Cefaclor (Drugs that decrease renal function may increase concentrations of emtricitabine and/or tenofovir. Truvada should be avoided with concurrent or recent use of a nephrotoxic agent).
No products indexed under this heading.

Cefadroxil (Drugs that decrease renal function may increase concentrations of emtricitabine and/or tenofovir. Truvada should be avoided with concurrent or recent use of a nephrotoxic agent).
No products indexed under this heading.

Cefamandole Nafate (Drugs that decrease renal function may increase concentrations of emtricitabine and/or tenofovir. Truvada should be avoided with concurrent or recent use of a nephrotoxic agent).
No products indexed under this heading.

Cefazolin Sodium (Drugs that decrease renal function may increase concentrations of emtricitabine and/or tenofovir. Truvada should be avoided with concurrent or recent use of a nephrotoxic agent).
No products indexed under this heading.

Cefdinir (Drugs that decrease renal function may increase concentrations of emtricitabine and/or tenofovir. Truvada should be avoided with concurrent or recent use of a nephrotoxic agent). Products include:
Omnicef Capsules 497
Omnicef for Oral Suspension 497

Cefepime Hydrochloride (Drugs that decrease renal function may increase concentrations of emtricitabine and/or tenofovir. Truvada should be avoided with concurrent or recent use of a nephrotoxic agent).
No products indexed under this heading.

Cefixime (Drugs that decrease renal function may increase concentrations of emtricitabine and/or tenofovir. Truvada should be avoided with concurrent or recent use of a nephrotoxic agent). Products include:
Suprax for Oral Suspension 1891
Suprax Tablets 1891

Cefmetazole Sodium (Drugs that decrease renal function may increase concentrations of emtricitabine and/or tenofovir. Truvada should be avoided with concurrent or recent use of a nephrotoxic agent).
No products indexed under this heading.

Cefonicid Sodium (Drugs that decrease renal function may increase concentrations of emtricitabine and/or tenofovir. Truvada should be avoided with concurrent or recent use of a nephrotoxic agent).
No products indexed under this heading.

Cefoperazone Sodium (Drugs that decrease renal function may increase concentrations of emtricitabine and/or tenofovir. Truvada should be avoided with concurrent or recent use of a nephrotoxic agent).
No products indexed under this heading.

Ceforanide (Drugs that decrease renal function may increase concentrations of emtricitabine and/or tenofovir. Truvada should be avoided with concurrent or recent use of a nephrotoxic agent).
No products indexed under this heading.

Cefotaxime Sodium (Drugs that decrease renal function may increase concentrations of emtricitabine and/or tenofovir. Truvada should be avoided with concurrent or recent use of a nephrotoxic agent).
No products indexed under this heading.

Cefotetan (Drugs that decrease renal function may increase concentrations of emtricitabine and/or tenofovir. Truvada should be avoided with concurrent or recent use of a nephrotoxic agent).
No products indexed under this heading.

Cefoxitin Sodium (Drugs that decrease renal function may increase concentrations of emtricitabine and/or tenofovir. Truvada should be avoided with concurrent or recent use of a nephrotoxic agent).
No products indexed under this heading.

Cefpodoxime Proxetil (Drugs that decrease renal function may increase concentrations of emtricitabine and/or tenofovir. Truvada should be avoided with concurrent or recent use of a nephrotoxic agent).
No products indexed under this heading.

Cefprozil (Drugs that decrease renal function may increase concentrations of emtricitabine and/or tenofovir. Truvada should be avoided with concurrent or recent use of a nephrotoxic agent).
No products indexed under this heading.

Ceftazidime (Drugs that decrease renal function may increase concentrations of emtricitabine and/or tenofovir. Truvada should be avoided with concurrent or recent use of a nephrotoxic agent). Products include:
Fortaz 1450

Ceftizoxime Sodium (Drugs that decrease renal function may increase concentrations of emtricitabine and/or tenofovir. Truvada should be avoided with concurrent or recent use of a nephrotoxic agent).
No products indexed under this heading.

Ceftriaxone Sodium (Drugs that decrease renal function may increase concentrations of emtricitabine and/or tenofovir. Truvada should be avoided with concurrent or recent use of a nephrotoxic agent). Products include:
Rocephin Injectable Vials, ADD-Vantage, Galaxy, Bulk........... 2642

Cefuroxime Axetil (Drugs that decrease renal function may increase concentrations of emtricitabine and/or tenofovir. Truvada should be avoided with concurrent or recent use of a nephrotoxic agent). Products include:
Ceftin 1380

Cefuroxime Sodium (Drugs that decrease renal function may increase concentrations of emtricitabine and/or tenofovir. Truvada should be avoided with concurrent or recent use of a nephrotoxic agent).
No products indexed under this heading.

Celecoxib (Drugs that decrease renal function may increase concentrations of emtricitabine and/or tenofovir. Truvada should be avoided with concurrent or recent use of a nephrotoxic agent). Products include:
Celebrex Capsules 2979

Cephalexin (Drugs that decrease renal function may increase concentrations of emtricitabine and/or tenofovir. Truvada should be avoided with concurrent or recent use of a nephrotoxic agent).
No products indexed under this heading.

Cephalothin Sodium (Drugs that decrease renal function may increase concentrations of emtricitabine and/or tenofovir. Truvada should be avoided with concurrent or recent use of a nephrotoxic agent).
No products indexed under this heading.

Cephapirin Sodium (Drugs that decrease renal function may increase concentrations of emtricitabine and/or tenofovir. Truvada should be avoided with concurrent or recent use of a nephrotoxic agent).
No products indexed under this heading.

Cephradine (Drugs that decrease renal function may increase concentrations of emtricitabine and/or tenofovir. Truvada should be avoided with concurrent or recent use of a nephrotoxic agent).
No products indexed under this heading.

Cerivastatin Sodium (Drugs that decrease renal function may increase concentrations of emtricitabine and/or tenofovir. Truvada should be avoided with concurrent or recent use of a nephrotoxic agent).
No products indexed under this heading.

Chlorothiazide (Drugs that decrease renal function may increase concentrations of emtricitabine and/or tenofovir. Truvada should be avoided with concurrent or recent use of a nephrotoxic agent).
No products indexed under this heading.

Chlorothiazide Sodium (Drugs that decrease renal function may increase concentrations of emtricitabine and/or tenofovir. Truvada should be avoided with concurrent or recent use of a nephrotoxic agent). Products include:
Intravenous Sodium Diuril 2490

Chlorpropamide (Drugs that decrease renal function may increase concentrations of emtricitabine and/or tenofovir. Truvada should be avoided with concurrent or recent use of a nephrotoxic agent).
No products indexed under this heading.

Cidofovir (Emtricitabine and tenofovir are primarily excreted by the kidneys by a combination of glomerular filtration and active tubular secretion. No drug-drug interactions due to competition for renal excretion have been observed; however, co-administration of Truvada with

drugs that are eliminated by active tubular secretion may increase concentrations of emtricitabine, tenofovir, and/or the co-administered drug. Some examples include, but are not limited, to acyclovir, adefovir dipivoxil, cidofovir, ganciclovir, valacyclovir, and valganciclovir. Drugs that decrease renal function may increase concentrations of emtricitabine and/or tenofovir).
No products indexed under this heading.

Cilastatin Sodium (Drugs that decrease renal function may increase concentrations of emtricitabine and/or tenofovir. Truvada should be avoided with concurrent or recent use of a nephrotoxic agent). Products include:
Primaxin I.M. ... **2080**
Primaxin I.V. ... **2083**

Cimetidine (Drugs that decrease renal function may increase concentrations of emtricitabine and/or tenofovir. Truvada should be avoided with concurrent or recent use of a nephrotoxic agent).
No products indexed under this heading.

Cimetidine Hydrochloride (Drugs that decrease renal function may increase concentrations of emtricitabine and/or tenofovir. Truvada should be avoided with concurrent or recent use of a nephrotoxic agent).
No products indexed under this heading.

Cisplatin (Drugs that decrease renal function may increase concentrations of emtricitabine and/or tenofovir. Truvada should be avoided with concurrent or recent use of a nephrotoxic agent).
No products indexed under this heading.

Cladribine (Drugs that decrease renal function may increase concentrations of emtricitabine and/or tenofovir. Truvada should be avoided with concurrent or recent use of a nephrotoxic agent). Products include:
Leustatin Injection ... **2384**

Clozapine (Drugs that decrease renal function may increase concentrations of emtricitabine and/or tenofovir. Truvada should be avoided with concurrent or recent use of a nephrotoxic agent).
No products indexed under this heading.

Colistimethate Sodium (Drugs that decrease renal function may increase concentrations of emtricitabine and/or tenofovir. Truvada should be avoided with concurrent or recent use of a nephrotoxic agent).
No products indexed under this heading.

Colistin Sulfate (Drugs that decrease renal function may increase concentrations of emtricitabine and/or tenofovir. Truvada should be avoided with concurrent or recent use of a nephrotoxic agent).
No products indexed under this heading.

Cyclophosphamide (Drugs that decrease renal function may increase concentrations of emtricitabine and/or tenofovir. Truvada should be avoided with concurrent or recent use of a nephrotoxic agent).
No products indexed under this heading.

Cyclosporine (Drugs that decrease renal function may increase concentrations of emtricitabine and/or tenofovir. Truvada should be avoided with concurrent or recent use of a nephrotoxic agent). Products include:
Gengraf Capsules ... **435**
Neoral Oral Solution ... **2280**
Neoral Soft Gelatin Capsules ... **2280**
Restasis Ophthalmic Emulsion ... **557**
Sandimmune ... **2296**

Cytarabine (Drugs that decrease renal function may increase concentrations of emtricitabine and/or tenofovir. Truvada should be avoided with concurrent or recent use of a nephrotoxic agent).
No products indexed under this heading.

Cytarabine Liposome (Drugs that decrease renal function may increase concentrations of emtricitabine and/or tenofovir. Truvada should be avoided with concurrent or recent use of a nephrotoxic agent). Products include:
DepoCyt Injection ... **1136**

Delavirdine Mesylate (Drugs that decrease renal function may increase concentrations of emtricitabine and/or tenofovir. Truvada should be avoided with concurrent or recent use of a nephrotoxic agent).
No products indexed under this heading.

Diatrizoate Meglumine (Drugs that decrease renal function may increase concentrations of emtricitabine and/or tenofovir. Truvada should be avoided with concurrent or recent use of a nephrotoxic agent).
No products indexed under this heading.

Diatrizoate Sodium (Drugs that decrease renal function may increase concentrations of emtricitabine and/or tenofovir. Truvada should be avoided with concurrent or recent use of a nephrotoxic agent).
No products indexed under this heading.

Diclofenac Potassium (Drugs that decrease renal function may increase concentrations of emtricitabine and/or tenofovir. Truvada should be avoided with concurrent or recent use of a nephrotoxic agent).
No products indexed under this heading.

Diclofenac Sodium (Drugs that decrease renal function may increase concentrations of emtricitabine and/or tenofovir. Truvada should be avoided with concurrent or recent use of a nephrotoxic agent). Products include:
Diclofenac Sodium Ophthalmic Solution ... ⊙**240**
Voltaren Ophthalmic Solution ... **2336**
Voltaren Tablets ... **2334**
Voltaren-XR Tablets ... **2337**

Dicloxacillin Sodium (Drugs that decrease renal function may increase concentrations of emtricitabine and/or tenofovir. Truvada should be avoided with concurrent or recent use of a nephrotoxic agent).
No products indexed under this heading.

Didanosine (Tenofovir disoproxil fumarate increases didanosine concentrations. Use with caution and monitor for evidence of didanosine toxicity (eg, pancreatitis, neuropathy) when co-administered. Consider dose reduction or discontinuation of didanosine if warranted).
No products indexed under this heading.

Digoxin (Emtricitabine and tenofovir are primarily excreted by the kidneys by a combination of glomerular filtration and active tubular secretion. No drug-drug interactions due to competition for renal excretion have been observed; however, co-administration of Truvada with drugs that are eliminated by active tubular secretion may increase concentrations of emtricitabine, tenofovir, and/or the co-administered drug). Products include:
Lanoxin Injection ... **1498**
Lanoxin Injection Pediatric ... **1502**
Lanoxin Tablets ... **1505**

Efavirenz (Drugs that decrease renal function may increase concentrations of emtricitabine and/or tenofovir. Truvada should be avoided with concurrent or recent use of a nephrotoxic agent). Products include:
Atripla Tablets ... **938**
Sustiva Capsules ... **930**
Sustiva Tablets ... **930**

Enalapril Maleate (Drugs that decrease renal function may increase concentrations of emtricitabine and/or tenofovir. Truvada should be avoided with concurrent or recent use of a nephrotoxic agent).
No products indexed under this heading.

Enalaprilat (Drugs that decrease renal function may increase concentrations of emtricitabine and/or tenofovir. Truvada should be avoided with concurrent or recent use of a nephrotoxic agent).
No products indexed under this heading.

Enfuvirtide (Drugs that decrease renal function may increase concentrations of emtricitabine and/or tenofovir. Truvada should be avoided with concurrent or recent use of a nephrotoxic agent).
No products indexed under this heading.

Ethiodized Oil (Drugs that decrease renal function may increase concentrations of emtricitabine and/or tenofovir. Truvada should be avoided with concurrent or recent use of a nephrotoxic agent).
No products indexed under this heading.

Etodolac (Drugs that decrease renal function may increase concentrations of emtricitabine and/or tenofovir. Truvada should be avoided with concurrent or recent use of a nephrotoxic agent).
No products indexed under this heading.

Fenoprofen Calcium (Drugs that decrease renal function may increase concentrations of emtricitabine and/or tenofovir. Truvada should be avoided with concurrent or recent use of a nephrotoxic agent). Products include:
Nalfon Capsules ... **2508**

Filgrastim (Drugs that decrease renal function may increase concentrations of emtricitabine and/or tenofovir. Truvada should be avoided with concurrent or recent use of a nephrotoxic agent). Products include:
Neupogen for Injection ... **589**

Fluorouracil (Drugs that decrease renal function may increase concentrations of emtricitabine and/or tenofovir. Truvada should be avoided with concurrent or recent use of a nephrotoxic agent). Products include:
Carac Cream 0.5% ... **2722**

Flurbiprofen (Drugs that decrease renal function may increase concentrations of emtricitabine and/or tenofovir. Truvada should be avoided with concurrent or recent use of a nephrotoxic agent).
No products indexed under this heading.

Fluvastatin Sodium (Drugs that decrease renal function may increase concentrations of emtricitabine and/or tenofovir. Truvada should be avoided with concurrent or recent use of a nephrotoxic agent). Products include:
Lescol Capsules ... **2268**
Lescol XL Tablets ... **2268**

Foscarnet Sodium (Drugs that decrease renal function may increase concentrations of emtricitabine and/or tenofovir. Truvada should be avoided with concurrent or recent use of a nephrotoxic agent).
No products indexed under this heading.

Fosinopril Sodium (Drugs that decrease renal function may increase concentrations of emtricitabine and/or tenofovir. Truvada should be avoided with concurrent or recent use of a nephrotoxic agent).
No products indexed under this heading.

Furosemide (Drugs that decrease renal function may increase concentrations of emtricitabine and/or tenofovir. Truvada should be avoided with concurrent or recent use of a nephrotoxic agent). Products include:
Furosemide Tablets ... **2186**

Gadopentetate Dimeglumine (Drugs that decrease renal function may increase concentrations of emtricitabine and/or tenofovir. Truvada should be avoided with concurrent or recent use of a nephrotoxic agent).
No products indexed under this heading.

Ganciclovir (Emtricitabine and tenofovir are primarily excreted by the kidneys by a combination of glomerular filtration and active tubular secretion. No drug-drug interactions due to competition for renal excretion have been observed; however, co-administration of Truvada with drugs that are eliminated by active tubular secretion may increase concentrations of emtricitabine, tenofovir, and/or the co-administered drug. Some examples include, but are not limited, to acyclovir, adefovir dipivoxil, cidofovir, ganciclovir, valacyclovir, and valganciclovir. Drugs that decrease renal function may increase concentrations of emtricitabine and/or tenofovir).
No products indexed under this heading.

Ganciclovir Sodium (Emtricitabine and tenofovir are primarily excreted by the kidneys by a combination of glomerular filtration and active tubular secretion. No drug-drug interactions due to competition for renal excretion have been observed; however, co-administration of Truvada with drugs that are eliminated by active tubular secretion may increase concentrations of emtricitabine, tenofovir, and/or the co-administered drug. Some examples include, but are not limited, to acyclovir, adefovir dipivoxil, cidofovir, ganciclovir, valacyclovir, and valganciclovir. Drugs that decrease renal function may increase concentra-

tions of emtricitabine and/or tenofovir).
No products indexed under this heading.

Gentamicin (Drugs that decrease renal function may increase concentrations of emtricitabine and/or tenofovir. Truvada should be avoided with concurrent or recent use of a nephrotoxic agent).
No products indexed under this heading.

Gentamicin Sulfate (Drugs that decrease renal function may increase concentrations of emtricitabine and/or tenofovir. Truvada should be avoided with concurrent or recent use of a nephrotoxic agent). Products include:
Pred-G Ophthalmic Ointment .... ⊙229
Pred-G Ophthalmic Suspension ...... ⊙228

Glipizide (Drugs that decrease renal function may increase concentrations of emtricitabine and/or tenofovir. Truvada should be avoided with concurrent or recent use of a nephrotoxic agent).
No products indexed under this heading.

Globulin, Immune (Human) (Drugs that decrease renal function may increase concentrations of emtricitabine and/or tenofovir. Truvada should be avoided with concurrent or recent use of a nephrotoxic agent). Products include:
Flebogamma 5% 1715

Glyburide (Drugs that decrease renal function may increase concentrations of emtricitabine and/or tenofovir. Truvada should be avoided with concurrent or recent use of a nephrotoxic agent).
No products indexed under this heading.

Gold Therapy (Drugs that decrease renal function may increase concentrations of emtricitabine and/or tenofovir. Truvada should be avoided with concurrent or recent use of a nephrotoxic agent).
No products indexed under this heading.

HMG-CoA Reductase Inhibitors (Drugs that decrease renal function may increase concentrations of emtricitabine and/or tenofovir. Truvada should be avoided with concurrent or recent use of a nephrotoxic agent).
No products indexed under this heading.

Hydrochlorothiazide (Drugs that decrease renal function may increase concentrations of emtricitabine and/or tenofovir. Truvada should be avoided with concurrent or recent use of a nephrotoxic agent). Products include:
Atacand HCT 642
Avalide Tablets 892
Avalide Tablets 2713
Benicar HCT Tablets 1010
Diovan HCT Tablets 2216
Dyazide Capsules 1405
Micardis HCT Tablets 854
Prinzide Tablets 2092
Tekturna HCT Tablets 2324
Teveten HCT Tablets 517

Hydroflumethiazide (Drugs that decrease renal function may increase concentrations of emtricitabine and/or tenofovir. Truvada should be avoided with concurrent or recent use of a nephrotoxic agent).
No products indexed under this heading.

Ibuprofen (Drugs that decrease renal function may increase concentrations of emtricitabine and/or tenofovir. Truvada should be avoided with concurrent or recent use of a nephrotoxic agent). Products include:
Motrin IB Tablets and Caplets 1900
Children's Motrin Oral Suspension ... 1901
Children's Motrin Non-Staining Dye-Free Oral Suspension............ 1901
Children's Motrin Cold Oral Suspension................................ 1899
Infants' Motrin Concentrated Drops.. 1901
Infants' Motrin Non-Staining Dye-Free Concentrated Drops....... 1901
Junior Strength Motrin Caplets and Chewable Tablets.................. 1901
Vicoprofen Tablets 533

Idarubicin Hydrochloride (Drugs that decrease renal function may increase concentrations of emtricitabine and/or tenofovir. Truvada should be avoided with concurrent or recent use of a nephrotoxic agent).
No products indexed under this heading.

Ifosfamide (Drugs that decrease renal function may increase concentrations of emtricitabine and/or tenofovir. Truvada should be avoided with concurrent or recent use of a nephrotoxic agent).
No products indexed under this heading.

Imipenem (Drugs that decrease renal function may increase concentrations of emtricitabine and/or tenofovir. Truvada should be avoided with concurrent or recent use of a nephrotoxic agent). Products include:
Primaxin I.M. 2080
Primaxin I.V. 2083

Immune Globulin Intravenous (Human) (Drugs that decrease renal function may increase concentrations of emtricitabine and/or tenofovir. Truvada should be avoided with concurrent or recent use of a nephrotoxic agent). Products include:
Flebogamma 5% DIF 1718
Gammagard Liquid 730
Gammagard S/D 734
Gamunex 3094

Indinavir Sulfate (Drugs that decrease renal function may increase concentrations of emtricitabine and/or tenofovir. Truvada should be avoided with concurrent or recent use of a nephrotoxic agent). Products include:
Crixivan Capsules 1979

Indomethacin (Drugs that decrease renal function may increase concentrations of emtricitabine and/or tenofovir. Truvada should be avoided with concurrent or recent use of a nephrotoxic agent). Products include:
Indocin 2024

Indomethacin Sodium Trihydrate (Drugs that decrease renal function may increase concentrations of emtricitabine and/or tenofovir. Truvada should be avoided with concurrent or recent use of a nephrotoxic agent). Products include:
Indocin I.V. 2489

Interferon Beta-1b (Drugs that decrease renal function may increase concentrations of emtricitabine and/or tenofovir. Truvada should be avoided with concurrent or recent use of a nephrotoxic agent). Products include:
Betaseron for SC Injection 756

Interleuken-2 (Drugs that decrease renal function may increase concentrations of emtricitabine and/or tenofovir. Truvada should be avoided with concurrent or recent use of a nephrotoxic agent).
No products indexed under this heading.

Iodamide Meglumine (Drugs that decrease renal function may increase concentrations of emtricitabine and/or tenofovir. Truvada should be avoided with concurrent or recent use of a nephrotoxic agent).
No products indexed under this heading.

Iohexol (Drugs that decrease renal function may increase concentrations of emtricitabine and/or tenofovir. Truvada should be avoided with concurrent or recent use of a nephrotoxic agent).
No products indexed under this heading.

Iopamidol (Drugs that decrease renal function may increase concentrations of emtricitabine and/or tenofovir. Truvada should be avoided with concurrent or recent use of a nephrotoxic agent).
No products indexed under this heading.

Iopanoic Acid (Drugs that decrease renal function may increase concentrations of emtricitabine and/or tenofovir. Truvada should be avoided with concurrent or recent use of a nephrotoxic agent).
No products indexed under this heading.

Iothalamate Meglumine (Drugs that decrease renal function may increase concentrations of emtricitabine and/or tenofovir. Truvada should be avoided with concurrent or recent use of a nephrotoxic agent).
No products indexed under this heading.

Ioxaglate Meglumine (Drugs that decrease renal function may increase concentrations of emtricitabine and/or tenofovir. Truvada should be avoided with concurrent or recent use of a nephrotoxic agent).
No products indexed under this heading.

Ioxaglate Sodium (Drugs that decrease renal function may increase concentrations of emtricitabine and/or tenofovir. Truvada should be avoided with concurrent or recent use of a nephrotoxic agent).
No products indexed under this heading.

Kanamycin Sulfate (Drugs that decrease renal function may increase concentrations of emtricitabine and/or tenofovir. Truvada should be avoided with concurrent or recent use of a nephrotoxic agent).
No products indexed under this heading.

Ketoprofen (Drugs that decrease renal function may increase concentrations of emtricitabine and/or tenofovir. Truvada should be avoided with concurrent or recent use of a nephrotoxic agent).
No products indexed under this heading.

Ketorolac Tromethamine (Drugs that decrease renal function may increase concentrations of emtricitabine and/or tenofovir. Truvada should be avoided with concurrent or recent use of a nephrotoxic agent).
No products indexed under this heading.

Lamium album (Drugs that decrease renal function may increase concentrations of emtricitabine and/or tenofovir. Truvada should be avoided with concurrent or recent use of a nephrotoxic agent).
No products indexed under this heading.

Lamivudine (Due to similarities between emtricitabine and lamivudine, Truvada should not be co-administered with other drugs containing lamivudine). Products include:
Combivir Tablets 1384
Epivir 1412
Epivir-HBV 1417
Epzicom Tablets 1422
Trizivir Tablets 1622

Lisinopril (Drugs that decrease renal function may increase concentrations of emtricitabine and/or tenofovir. Truvada should be avoided with concurrent or recent use of a nephrotoxic agent). Products include:
Prinivil Tablets 2087
Prinzide Tablets 2092

Lithium (Drugs that decrease renal function may increase concentrations of emtricitabine and/or tenofovir. Truvada should be avoided with concurrent or recent use of a nephrotoxic agent).
No products indexed under this heading.

Lithium Carbonate (Drugs that decrease renal function may increase concentrations of emtricitabine and/or tenofovir. Truvada should be avoided with concurrent or recent use of a nephrotoxic agent).
No products indexed under this heading.

Lithium Citrate (Drugs that decrease renal function may increase concentrations of emtricitabine and/or tenofovir. Truvada should be avoided with concurrent or recent use of a nephrotoxic agent).
No products indexed under this heading.

Lopinavir (Co-administration increases tenofovir concentrations. Monitor for evidence of tenofovir toxicity). Products include:
Kaletra 452

Loracarbef (Drugs that decrease renal function may increase concentrations of emtricitabine and/or tenofovir. Truvada should be avoided with concurrent or recent use of a nephrotoxic agent).
No products indexed under this heading.

Lovastatin (Drugs that decrease renal function may increase concentrations of emtricitabine and/or tenofovir. Truvada should be avoided with concurrent or recent use of a nephrotoxic agent). Products include:
Advicor Tablets 402
Mevacor Tablets 2063

Meclofenamate Sodium (Drugs that decrease renal function may increase concentrations of emtricitabine and/or tenofovir. Truvada should be avoided with concurrent or recent use of a nephrotoxic agent).
No products indexed under this heading.

IMPORTANT NOTE: Always consult each drug listing in the patient's regimen for possible interactions.

Mefenamic Acid (Drugs that decrease renal function may increase concentrations of emtricitabine and/or tenofovir. Truvada should be avoided with concurrent or recent use of a nephrotoxic agent).
No products indexed under this heading.

Meloxicam (Drugs that decrease renal function may increase concentrations of emtricitabine and/or tenofovir. Truvada should be avoided with concurrent or recent use of a nephrotoxic agent). Products include:
Mobic Oral Suspension 863
Mobic Tablets 863

Melphalan Hydrochloride (Drugs that decrease renal function may increase concentrations of emtricitabine and/or tenofovir. Truvada should be avoided with concurrent or recent use of a nephrotoxic agent).
No products indexed under this heading.

Mesalamine (Drugs that decrease renal function may increase concentrations of emtricitabine and/or tenofovir. Truvada should be avoided with concurrent or recent use of a nephrotoxic agent). Products include:
Asacol Delayed-Release Tablets 2579
Canasa Rectal Suppositories 705
Lialda Tablets 3029
Pentasa Capsules 3030

Methimazole (Drugs that decrease renal function may increase concentrations of emtricitabine and/or tenofovir. Truvada should be avoided with concurrent or recent use of a nephrotoxic agent).
No products indexed under this heading.

Methotrexate (Drugs that decrease renal function may increase concentrations of emtricitabine and/or tenofovir. Truvada should be avoided with concurrent or recent use of a nephrotoxic agent).
No products indexed under this heading.

Methotrexate Sodium (Drugs that decrease renal function may increase concentrations of emtricitabine and/or tenofovir. Truvada should be avoided with concurrent or recent use of a nephrotoxic agent).
No products indexed under this heading.

Methyclothiazide (Drugs that decrease renal function may increase concentrations of emtricitabine and/or tenofovir. Truvada should be avoided with concurrent or recent use of a nephrotoxic agent).
No products indexed under this heading.

Mezlocillin Sodium (Drugs that decrease renal function may increase concentrations of emtricitabine and/or tenofovir. Truvada should be avoided with concurrent or recent use of a nephrotoxic agent).
No products indexed under this heading.

Minocycline Hydrochloride (Drugs that decrease renal function may increase concentrations of emtricitabine and/or tenofovir. Truvada should be avoided with concurrent or recent use of a nephrotoxic agent). Products include:
Solodyn Extended Release Tablets 1938

Mitomycin (Mitomycin-C) (Drugs that decrease renal function may increase concentrations of emtricitabine and/or tenofovir. Truvada should be avoided with concurrent or recent use of a nephrotoxic agent).
No products indexed under this heading.

Moexipril Hydrochloride (Drugs that decrease renal function may increase concentrations of emtricitabine and/or tenofovir. Truvada should be avoided with concurrent or recent use of a nephrotoxic agent).
No products indexed under this heading.

Morphine Sulfate (Emtricitabine and tenofovir are primarily excreted by the kidneys by a combination of glomerular filtration and active tubular secretion. No drug-drug interactions due to competition for renal excretion have been observed; however, co-administration of Truvada with drugs that are eliminated by active tubular secretion may increase concentrations of emtricitabine, tenofovir, and/or the co-administered drug). Products include:
Avinza Capsules 1772
DepoDur Injection 1095
MS Contin Tablets 2585

Muromonab-CD3 (Drugs that decrease renal function may increase concentrations of emtricitabine and/or tenofovir. Truvada should be avoided with concurrent or recent use of a nephrotoxic agent). Products include:
Orthoclone OKT3 Sterile Solution 2387

Nabumetone (Drugs that decrease renal function may increase concentrations of emtricitabine and/or tenofovir. Truvada should be avoided with concurrent or recent use of a nephrotoxic agent).
No products indexed under this heading.

Nafcillin Sodium (Drugs that decrease renal function may increase concentrations of emtricitabine and/or tenofovir. Truvada should be avoided with concurrent or recent use of a nephrotoxic agent).
No products indexed under this heading.

Naproxen (Drugs that decrease renal function may increase concentrations of emtricitabine and/or tenofovir. Truvada should be avoided with concurrent or recent use of a nephrotoxic agent). Products include:
EC-Naprosyn Delayed-Release Tablets 2632
Naprosyn Suspension 2632
Naprosyn Tablets 2632

Naproxen Sodium (Drugs that decrease renal function may increase concentrations of emtricitabine and/or tenofovir. Truvada should be avoided with concurrent or recent use of a nephrotoxic agent). Products include:
Anaprox Tablets 2632
Anaprox DS Tablets 2632
Treximet Tablets 1616

Nelfinavir Mesylate (Drugs that decrease renal function may increase concentrations of emtricitabine and/or tenofovir. Truvada should be avoided with concurrent or recent use of a nephrotoxic agent).
No products indexed under this heading.

Neomycin (Drugs that decrease renal function may increase concentrations of emtricitabine and/or tenofovir. Truvada should be avoided with concurrent or recent use of a nephrotoxic agent).
No products indexed under this heading.

Neomycin, oral (Drugs that decrease renal function may increase concentrations of emtricitabine and/or tenofovir. Truvada should be avoided with concurrent or recent use of a nephrotoxic agent).
No products indexed under this heading.

Neomycin Sulfate (Drugs that decrease renal function may increase concentrations of emtricitabine and/or tenofovir. Truvada should be avoided with concurrent or recent use of a nephrotoxic agent). Products include:
Neosporin Ophthalmic Solution Sterile .... ⊙252

Nevirapine (Drugs that decrease renal function may increase concentrations of emtricitabine and/or tenofovir. Truvada should be avoided with concurrent or recent use of a nephrotoxic agent). Products include:
Viramune Oral Suspension 873
Viramune Tablets 873

Norfloxacin (Drugs that decrease renal function may increase concentrations of emtricitabine and/or tenofovir. Truvada should be avoided with concurrent or recent use of a nephrotoxic agent). Products include:
Noroxin Tablets 2069

Olsalazine Sodium (Drugs that decrease renal function may increase concentrations of emtricitabine and/or tenofovir. Truvada should be avoided with concurrent or recent use of a nephrotoxic agent).
No products indexed under this heading.

Omeprazole (Drugs that decrease renal function may increase concentrations of emtricitabine and/or tenofovir. Truvada should be avoided with concurrent or recent use of a nephrotoxic agent).
No products indexed under this heading.

Oxaprozin (Drugs that decrease renal function may increase concentrations of emtricitabine and/or tenofovir. Truvada should be avoided with concurrent or recent use of a nephrotoxic agent).
No products indexed under this heading.

Pamidronate Disodium (Drugs that decrease renal function may increase concentrations of emtricitabine and/or tenofovir. Truvada should be avoided with concurrent or recent use of a nephrotoxic agent).
No products indexed under this heading.

Paroxetine Hydrochloride (Drugs that decrease renal function may increase concentrations of emtricitabine and/or tenofovir. Truvada should be avoided with concurrent or recent use of a nephrotoxic agent). Products include:
Paxil 1535
Paxil CR Controlled-Release Tablets 1544

Penicillamine (Drugs that decrease renal function may increase concentrations of emtricitabine and/or tenofovir. Truvada should be avoided with concurrent or recent use of a nephrotoxic agent). Products include:
Cuprimine Capsules 1986

Penicillin G Benzathine (Drugs that decrease renal function may increase concentrations of emtricitabine and/or tenofovir. Truvada should be avoided with concurrent or recent use of a nephrotoxic agent). Products include:
Bicillin C-R Injectable Suspension 1775
Bicillin L-A Injection 1777

Penicillin G Potassium (Drugs that decrease renal function may increase concentrations of emtricitabine and/or tenofovir. Truvada should be avoided with concurrent or recent use of a nephrotoxic agent).
No products indexed under this heading.

Penicillin G Procaine (Drugs that decrease renal function may increase concentrations of emtricitabine and/or tenofovir. Truvada should be avoided with concurrent or recent use of a nephrotoxic agent). Products include:
Bicillin C-R Injectable Suspension 1775
Bicillin L-A Injection 1777

Penicillin G Sodium (Drugs that decrease renal function may increase concentrations of emtricitabine and/or tenofovir. Truvada should be avoided with concurrent or recent use of a nephrotoxic agent).
No products indexed under this heading.

Penicillin V Potassium (Drugs that decrease renal function may increase concentrations of emtricitabine and/or tenofovir. Truvada should be avoided with concurrent or recent use of a nephrotoxic agent).
No products indexed under this heading.

Pentamidine Isethionate (Drugs that decrease renal function may increase concentrations of emtricitabine and/or tenofovir. Truvada should be avoided with concurrent or recent use of a nephrotoxic agent).
No products indexed under this heading.

Perindopril Erbumine (Drugs that decrease renal function may increase concentrations of emtricitabine and/or tenofovir. Truvada should be avoided with concurrent or recent use of a nephrotoxic agent). Products include:
Aceon Tablets (2 mg, 4 mg, 8 mg) 3038

Phenylbutazone (Drugs that decrease renal function may increase concentrations of emtricitabine and/or tenofovir. Truvada should be avoided with concurrent or recent use of a nephrotoxic agent).
No products indexed under this heading.

Piroxicam (Drugs that decrease renal function may increase concentrations of emtricitabine and/or tenofovir. Truvada should be avoided with concurrent or recent use of a nephrotoxic agent).
No products indexed under this heading.

Plicamycin (Drugs that decrease renal function may increase concentrations of emtricitabine and/or tenofovir. Truvada should be avoided with concurrent or recent use of a nephrotoxic agent).
No products indexed under this heading.

Polymyxin (Drugs that decrease renal function may increase concentrations of emtricitabine and/or tenofovir. Truvada should be avoided with concurrent or recent use of a nephrotoxic agent).
No products indexed under this heading.

Polymyxin B Sulfate (Drugs that decrease renal function may increase concentrations of emtricitabine and/or tenofovir. Truvada should be avoided with concurrent or recent use of a nephrotoxic agent). Products include:
Neosporin Ophthalmic Solution Sterile .... ⊙ 252

Polythiazide (Drugs that decrease renal function may increase concentrations of emtricitabine and/or tenofovir. Truvada should be avoided with concurrent or recent use of a nephrotoxic agent).
No products indexed under this heading.

Pravastatin Sodium (Drugs that decrease renal function may increase concentrations of emtricitabine and/or tenofovir. Truvada should be avoided with concurrent or recent use of a nephrotoxic agent).
No products indexed under this heading.

Probenecid (Drugs that decrease renal function may increase concentrations of emtricitabine and/or tenofovir. Truvada should be avoided with concurrent or recent use of a nephrotoxic agent).
No products indexed under this heading.

Procainamide Hydrochloride (Emtricitabine and tenofovir are primarily excreted by the kidneys by a combination of glomerular filtration and active tubular secretion. No drug-drug interactions due to competition for renal excretion have been observed; however, coadministration of Truvada with drugs that are eliminated by active tubular secretion may increase concentrations of emtricitabine, tenofovir, and/or the co-administered drug).
No products indexed under this heading.

Quinapril Hydrochloride (Drugs that decrease renal function may increase concentrations of emtricitabine and/or tenofovir. Truvada should be avoided with concurrent or recent use of a nephrotoxic agent).
No products indexed under this heading.

Quinidine Gluconate (Emtricitabine and tenofovir are primarily excreted by the kidneys by a combination of glomerular filtration and active tubular secretion. No drug-drug interactions due to competition for renal excretion have been observed; however, coadministration of Truvada with drugs that are eliminated by active tubular secretion may increase concentrations of emtricitabine, tenofovir, and/or the co-administered drug).
No products indexed under this heading.

Quinidine Polygalacturonate (Emtricitabine and tenofovir are primarily excreted by the kidneys by a combination of glomerular filtration and active tubular secretion. No drug-drug interactions due to competition for renal excretion have been observed; however, coadministration of Truvada with drugs that are eliminated by active tubular secretion may increase concentrations of emtricitabine, tenofovir, and/or the co-administered drug).
No products indexed under this heading.

Quinidine Sulfate (Emtricitabine and tenofovir are primarily excreted by the kidneys by a combination of glomerular filtration and active tubular secretion. No drug-drug interactions due to competition for renal excretion have been observed; however, co-administration of Truvada with drugs that are eliminated by active tubular secretion may increase concentrations of emtricitabine, tenofovir, and/or the co-administered drug).
No products indexed under this heading.

Quinine Sulfate (Emtricitabine and tenofovir are primarily excreted by the kidneys by a combination of glomerular filtration and active tubular secretion. No drug-drug interactions due to competition for renal excretion have been observed; however, co-administration of Truvada with drugs that are eliminated by active tubular secretion may increase concentrations of emtricitabine, tenofovir, and/or the co-administered drug).
No products indexed under this heading.

Rabeprazole Sodium (Drugs that decrease renal function may increase concentrations of emtricitabine and/or tenofovir. Truvada should be avoided with concurrent or recent use of a nephrotoxic agent). Products include:
Aciphex Tablets 1053

Ramipril (Drugs that decrease renal function may increase concentrations of emtricitabine and/or tenofovir. Truvada should be avoided with concurrent or recent use of a nephrotoxic agent).
No products indexed under this heading.

Ranitidine Hydrochloride (Emtricitabine and tenofovir are primarily excreted by the kidneys by a combination of glomerular filtration and active tubular secretion. No drug-drug interactions due to competition for renal excretion have been observed; however, coadministration of Truvada with drugs that are eliminated by active tubular secretion may increase concentrations of emtricitabine, tenofovir, and/or the co-administered drug). Products include:
Zantac 75 Tablets 603
Zantac 1670
Zantac Injection 1666
Zantac Injection Pharmacy Bulk Package 1668
Maximum Strength Zantac 150 Tablets 603
Maximum Strength Zantac 150 Cool Mint Tablets 603

Rifampin (Drugs that decrease renal function may increase concentrations of emtricitabine and/or tenofovir. Truvada should be avoided with concurrent or recent use of a nephrotoxic agent).
No products indexed under this heading.

Riluzole (Drugs that decrease renal function may increase concentrations of emtricitabine and/or tenofovir. Truvada should be avoided with concurrent or recent use of a nephrotoxic agent). Products include:
Rilutek Tablets 2771

Ritonavir (Co-administration increases tenofovir concentrations. Monitor for evidence of tenofovir toxicity). Products include:
Kaletra 452
Norvir 489

Rofecoxib (Drugs that decrease renal function may increase concentrations of emtricitabine and/or tenofovir. Truvada should be avoided with concurrent or recent use of a nephrotoxic agent).
No products indexed under this heading.

Saquinavir (Co-administration may lead to increased levels of saquinavir).
No products indexed under this heading.

Saquinavir Mesylate (Co-administration may lead to increased lead to increased levels of saquinavir).
No products indexed under this heading.

Sibutramine Hydrochloride Monohydrate (Drugs that decrease renal function may increase concentrations of emtricitabine and/or tenofovir. Truvada should be avoided with concurrent or recent use of a nephrotoxic agent). Products include:
Meridia Capsules 475

Simvastatin (Drugs that decrease renal function may increase concentrations of emtricitabine and/or tenofovir. Truvada should be avoided with concurrent or recent use of a nephrotoxic agent). Products include:
Simcor Tablets 502
Vytorin 10/10 Tablets 2149
Vytorin 10/10 Tablets 2939
Vytorin 10/20 Tablets 2149
Vytorin 10/20 Tablets 2939
Vytorin 10/40 Tablets 2149
Vytorin 10/40 Tablets 2939
Vytorin 10/80 Tablets 2149
Vytorin 10/80 Tablets 2939
Zocor Tablets 2136

Spirapril Hydrochloride (Drugs that decrease renal function may increase concentrations of emtricitabine and/or tenofovir. Truvada should be avoided with concurrent or recent use of a nephrotoxic agent).
No products indexed under this heading.

Stavudine (Drugs that decrease renal function may increase concentrations of emtricitabine and/or tenofovir. Truvada should be avoided with concurrent or recent use of a nephrotoxic agent).
No products indexed under this heading.

Streptomycin Sulfate (Drugs that decrease renal function may increase concentrations of emtricitabine and/or tenofovir. Truvada should be avoided with concurrent or recent use of a nephrotoxic agent).
No products indexed under this heading.

Streptozocin (Drugs that decrease renal function may increase concentrations of emtricitabine and/or tenofovir. Truvada should be avoided with concurrent or recent use of a nephrotoxic agent).
No products indexed under this heading.

Sulfacytine (Drugs that decrease renal function may increase concentrations of emtricitabine and/or tenofovir. Truvada should be avoided with concurrent or recent use of a nephrotoxic agent).
No products indexed under this heading.

Sulfamethizole (Drugs that decrease renal function may increase concentrations of emtricitabine and/or tenofovir. Truvada should be avoided with concurrent or recent use of a nephrotoxic agent).
No products indexed under this heading.

Sulfamethoxazole (Drugs that decrease renal function may increase concentrations of emtricitabine and/or tenofovir. Truvada should be avoided with concurrent or recent use of a nephrotoxic agent).
No products indexed under this heading.

Sulfasalazine (Drugs that decrease renal function may increase concentrations of emtricitabine and/or tenofovir. Truvada should be avoided with concurrent or recent use of a nephrotoxic agent).
No products indexed under this heading.

Sulfinpyrazone (Drugs that decrease renal function may increase concentrations of emtricitabine and/or tenofovir. Truvada should be avoided with concurrent or recent use of a nephrotoxic agent).
No products indexed under this heading.

Sulfisoxazole Acetyl (Drugs that decrease renal function may increase concentrations of emtricitabine and/or tenofovir. Truvada should be avoided with concurrent or recent use of a nephrotoxic agent).
No products indexed under this heading.

Sulfisoxazole Diolamine (Drugs that decrease renal function may increase concentrations of emtricitabine and/or tenofovir. Truvada should be avoided with concurrent or recent use of a nephrotoxic agent).
No products indexed under this heading.

Sulindac (Drugs that decrease renal function may increase concentrations of emtricitabine and/or tenofovir. Truvada should be avoided with concurrent or recent use of a nephrotoxic agent). Products include:
Clinoril Tablets 1962

Tacrolimus (Drugs that decrease renal function may increase concentrations of emtricitabine and/or tenofovir. Truvada should be avoided with concurrent or recent use of a nephrotoxic agent). Products include:
Prograf Capsules and Injection 622
Protopic Ointment 628

Thioguanine (Drugs that decrease renal function may increase concentrations of emtricitabine and/or tenofovir. Truvada should be avoided with concurrent or recent use of a nephrotoxic agent). Products include:
Tabloid Tablets 1601

Ticarcillin Disodium (Drugs that decrease renal function may increase concentrations of emtricitabine and/or tenofovir. Truvada should be avoided with concurrent or recent use of a nephrotoxic agent). Products include:
Timentin ADD-Vantage 1606

Timentin Injection Galaxy Container 1609
Timentin IV Infusion 1603
Timentin Pharmacy Bulk Package 1613

Tobramycin (Drugs that decrease renal function may increase concentrations of emtricitabine and/or tenofovir. Truvada should be avoided with concurrent or recent use of a nephrotoxic agent). Products include:
Zylet Ophthalmic Suspension .... ⊙247

Tobramycin Sulfate (Drugs that decrease renal function may increase concentrations of emtricitabine and/or tenofovir. Truvada should be avoided with concurrent or recent use of a nephrotoxic agent).
No products indexed under this heading.

Tolazamide (Drugs that decrease renal function may increase concentrations of emtricitabine and/or tenofovir. Truvada should be avoided with concurrent or recent use of a nephrotoxic agent).
No products indexed under this heading.

Tolbutamide (Drugs that decrease renal function may increase concentrations of emtricitabine and/or tenofovir. Truvada should be avoided with concurrent or recent use of a nephrotoxic agent).
No products indexed under this heading.

Tolmetin Sodium (Drugs that decrease renal function may increase concentrations of emtricitabine and/or tenofovir. Truvada should be avoided with concurrent or recent use of a nephrotoxic agent).
No products indexed under this heading.

Trandolapril (Drugs that decrease renal function may increase concentrations of emtricitabine and/or tenofovir. Truvada should be avoided with concurrent or recent use of a nephrotoxic agent). Products include:
Mavik Tablets 472
Tarka Tablets 511

Triamterene (Emtricitabine and tenofovir are primarily excreted by the kidneys by a combination of glomerular filtration and active tubular secretion. No drug-drug interactions due to competition for renal excretion have been observed; however, co-administration of Truvada with drugs that are eliminated by active tubular secretion may increase concentrations of emtricitabine, tenofovir, and/or the co-administered drug). Products include:
Dyazide Capsules 1405
Dyrenium Capsules 3189

Trimethadione (Drugs that decrease renal function may increase concentrations of emtricitabine and/or tenofovir. Truvada should be avoided with concurrent or recent use of a nephrotoxic agent).
No products indexed under this heading.

Trimethoprim (Emtricitabine and tenofovir are primarily excreted by the kidneys by a combination of glomerular filtration and active tubular secretion. No drug-drug interactions due to competition for renal excretion have been observed; however, co-administration of Truvada with drugs that are eliminated by active tubular secretion may increase concentrations of emtricitabine, tenofovir, and/or the co-administered drug).
No products indexed under this heading.

Trimethoprim Sulfate (Emtricitabine and tenofovir are primarily excreted by the kidneys by a combination of glomerular filtration and active tubular secretion. No drug-drug interactions due to competition for renal excretion have been observed; however, co-administration of Truvada with drugs that are eliminated by active tubular secretion may increase concentrations of emtricitabine, tenofovir, and/or the co-administered drug).
No products indexed under this heading.

Trovafloxacin Mesylate (Drugs that decrease renal function may increase concentrations of emtricitabine and/or tenofovir. Truvada should be avoided with concurrent or recent use of a nephrotoxic agent).
No products indexed under this heading.

Tyropanoate Sodium (Drugs that decrease renal function may increase concentrations of emtricitabine and/or tenofovir. Truvada should be avoided with concurrent or recent use of a nephrotoxic agent).
No products indexed under this heading.

Valacyclovir Hydrochloride (Emtricitabine and tenofovir are primarily excreted by the kidneys by a combination of glomerular filtration and active tubular secretion. No drug-drug interactions due to competition for renal excretion have been observed; however, co-administration of Truvada with drugs that are eliminated by active tubular secretion may increase concentrations of emtricitabine, tenofovir, and/or the co-administered drug. Some examples include, but are not limited, to acyclovir, adefovir dipivoxil, cidofovir, ganciclovir, valacyclovir, and valganciclovir. Drugs that decrease renal function may increase concentrations of emtricitabine and/or tenofovir). Products include:
Valtrex Caplets 1635

Valdecoxib (Drugs that decrease renal function may increase concentrations of emtricitabine and/or tenofovir. Truvada should be avoided with concurrent or recent use of a nephrotoxic agent).
No products indexed under this heading.

Valganciclovir Hydrochloride (Emtricitabine and tenofovir are primarily excreted by the kidneys by a combination of glomerular filtration and active tubular secretion. No drug-drug interactions due to competition for renal excretion have been observed; however, co-administration of Truvada with drugs that are eliminated by active tubular secretion may increase concentrations of emtricitabine, tenofovir, and/or the co-administered drug. Some examples include, but are not limited, to acyclovir, adefovir dipivoxil, cidofovir, ganciclovir, valacyclovir, and valganciclovir. Drugs that decrease renal function may increase concentrations of emtricitabine and/or tenofovir). Products include:
Valcyte Tablets 2654

Vancomycin Hydrochloride (Emtricitabine and tenofovir are primarily excreted by the kidneys by a combination of glomerular filtration and active tubular secretion. No drug-drug interactions due to competition for renal excretion have been observed; however, co-administration of Truvada with drugs that are eliminated by active tubular secretion may increase concentrations of emtricitabine, tenofovir, and/or the co-administered drug).
No products indexed under this heading.

Voriconazole (Drugs that decrease renal function may increase concentrations of emtricitabine and/or tenofovir. Truvada should be avoided with concurrent or recent use of a nephrotoxic agent).
No products indexed under this heading.

Zalcitabine (Drugs that decrease renal function may increase concentrations of emtricitabine and/or tenofovir. Truvada should be avoided with concurrent or recent use of a nephrotoxic agent).
No products indexed under this heading.

Zidovudine (Co-administration of zidovudine 300 mg twice daily for 7 days and emtricitabine 200 mg once daily for 7 days has resulted in a 17% increase in zidovudine Cmax and 13% increase in zidovudine AUC). Products include:
Combivir Tablets 1384
Retrovir 1574
Retrovir IV Infusion 1579
Trizivir Tablets 1622

Zoledronic acid (Drugs that decrease renal function may increase concentrations of emtricitabine and/or tenofovir. Truvada should be avoided with concurrent or recent use of a nephrotoxic agent). Products include:
Reclast Injection 2291
Zometa for Intravenous Infusion 2341

TUSSIONEX PENNKINETIC EXTENDED-RELEASE SUSPENSION

(Chlorpheniramine Polistirex, Hydrocodone Polistirex) 3154
May interact with anticholinergics, antihistamines, central nervous system depressants, monoamine oxidase inhibitors, tricyclic antidepressants, and certain other agents. Compounds in these categories include:

Acrivastine (Combined therapy may result in additive CNS depression).
No products indexed under this heading.

Alfentanil Hydrochloride (Combined therapy may result in additive CNS depression).
No products indexed under this heading.

Alprazolam (Combined therapy may result in additive CNS depression).
No products indexed under this heading.

Amitriptyline Hydrochloride (Co-administration of hydrocodone with MAO inhibitors may increase the effect of tricyclic antidepressant or hydrocodone).
No products indexed under this heading.

Amoxapine (Co-administration of hydrocodone with MAO inhibitors may increase the effect of tricyclic antidepressant or hydrocodone).
No products indexed under this heading.

Aprobarbital (Combined therapy may result in additive CNS depression).
No products indexed under this heading.

Astemizole (Combined therapy may result in additive CNS depression).
No products indexed under this heading.

Atropine Sulfate (Concurrent use of other anticholinergic agents with hydrocodone may produce paralytic ileus). Products include:
Donnatal Extentabs 2507

Azatadine Maleate (Combined therapy may result in additive CNS depression).
No products indexed under this heading.

Belladonna Alkaloids (Concurrent use of other anticholinergic agents with hydrocodone may produce paralytic ileus). Products include:
Hyland's Teething Tablets .... ▣621

Benztropine Mesylate (Concurrent use of other anticholinergic agents with hydrocodone may produce paralytic ileus).
No products indexed under this heading.

Biperiden Hydrochloride (Concurrent use of other anticholinergic agents with hydrocodone may produce paralytic ileus).
No products indexed under this heading.

Bromodiphenhydramine Hydrochloride (Combined therapy may result in additive CNS depression).
No products indexed under this heading.

Brompheniramine Maleate (Combined therapy may result in additive CNS depression).
No products indexed under this heading.

Buprenorphine Hydrochloride (Combined therapy may result in additive CNS depression). Products include:
Suboxone Tablets 2601
Subutex Tablets 2601

Buspirone Hydrochloride (Combined therapy may result in additive CNS depression).
No products indexed under this heading.

Butabarbital (Combined therapy may result in additive CNS depression).
No products indexed under this heading.

Butalbital (Combined therapy may result in additive CNS depression).
No products indexed under this heading.

Cetirizine Hydrochloride (Combined therapy may result in additive CNS depression). Products include:
Zyrtec Allergy Tablets 1919
Zyrtec Chewable Tablets 1920
Children's Zyrtec Allergy Chewable Tablets 1922
Children's Zyrtec Allergy Syrup 1920
Children's Zyrtec Hives Relief Syrup 1920
Zyrtec Syrup 1920
Zyrtec Tablets 1920
Zyrtec-D 12 Hour Extended Release Tablets 1923

Zyrtec-D Allergy & Congestion Extended-Release Tablets **1923**

Chlordiazepoxide (Combined therapy may result in additive CNS depression).
No products indexed under this heading.

Chlordiazepoxide Hydrochloride (Combined therapy may result in additive CNS depression).
No products indexed under this heading.

Chlorpheniramine Maleate (Combined therapy may result in additive CNS depression). Products include:
Actifed Cold & Allergy Tablets **1895**
Sudafed PE Sinus & Allergy Tablets **1908**
Tylenol Allergy Multi-Symptom Caplets with Cool Burst and Rapid Release Gelcaps **1916**
Children's Tylenol Plus Cold Suspension Liquid **1912**
Children's Tylenol Plus Cough & Runny Nose Suspension Liquid **1912**
Children's Tylenol Plus Flu Suspension Liquid **1914**
Children's Tylenol Plus Multi-Symptom Cold Suspension Liquid **1912**
Tylenol Cold Head Congestion Nighttime Caplets with Cool Burst **1910**
Tylenol Cold Multi-Symptom Nighttime Caplets with Cool Burst **1913**
Tylenol Sinus Congestion & Pain Nighttime Caplets with Cool Burst **1917**

Chlorpheniramine Tannate (Combined therapy may result in additive CNS depression).
No products indexed under this heading.

Chlorpromazine (Combined therapy may result in additive CNS depression).
No products indexed under this heading.

Chlorpromazine Hydrochloride (Combined therapy may result in additive CNS depression).
No products indexed under this heading.

Chlorprothixene (Combined therapy may result in additive CNS depression).
No products indexed under this heading.

Chlorprothixene Hydrochloride (Combined therapy may result in additive CNS depression).
No products indexed under this heading.

Chlorprothixene Lactate (Combined therapy may result in additive CNS depression).
No products indexed under this heading.

Clemastine Fumarate (Combined therapy may result in additive CNS depression).
No products indexed under this heading.

Clidinium Bromide (Concurrent use of other anticholinergic agents with hydrocodone may produce paralytic ileus).
No products indexed under this heading.

Clomipramine Hydrochloride (Co-administration of hydrocodone with MAO inhibitors may increase the effect of tricyclic antidepressant or hydrocodone).
No products indexed under this heading.

Clorazepate Dipotassium (Combined therapy may result in additive CNS depression).
No products indexed under this heading.

Clozapine (Combined therapy may result in additive CNS depression).
No products indexed under this heading.

Codeine Phosphate (Combined therapy may result in additive CNS depression). Products include:
Tylenol with Codeine Tablets **2427**

Cyproheptadine Hydrochloride (Combined therapy may result in additive CNS depression).
No products indexed under this heading.

Desflurane (Combined therapy may result in additive CNS depression).
No products indexed under this heading.

Desipramine Hydrochloride (Co-administration of hydrocodone with MAO inhibitors may increase the effect of tricyclic antidepressant or hydrocodone).
No products indexed under this heading.

Dexchlorpheniramine Maleate (Combined therapy may result in additive CNS depression).
No products indexed under this heading.

Dezocine (Combined therapy may result in additive CNS depression).
No products indexed under this heading.

Diazepam (Combined therapy may result in additive CNS depression). Products include:
Valium Tablets **2658**

Dicyclomine Hydrochloride (Concurrent use of other anticholinergic agents with hydrocodone may produce paralytic ileus). Products include:
Bentyl Capsules **703**
Bentyl Injection **703**
Bentyl Syrup **703**
Bentyl Tablets **703**

Diphenhydramine Citrate (Combined therapy may result in additive CNS depression).
No products indexed under this heading.

Diphenhydramine Hydrochloride (Combined therapy may result in additive CNS depression). Products include:
Benadryl Allergy & Cold Kapgels **1895**
Benadryl Allergy & Sinus Headache Kapgels **1895**
Benadryl Severe Allergy & Sinus Headache Caplets **1897**
Benadryl Dye-Free Allergy Liqui-gels Softgels **1897**
Benadryl Allergy Kapgels **1895**
Benadryl Allergy Quick Dissolve Strips **1896**
Benadryl Allergy Ultratab Tablets **1896**
Children's Benadryl Dye-Free Allergy Liquid **1897**
Children's Benadryl Allergy Fastmelts **1897**
Children's Benadryl Allergy Liquid **1898**
Children's Benadryl Allergy Perfect Measure **1896**
Children's Benadryl-D Allergy & Sinus Liquid **1896**
Benadryl-D Allergy & Sinus Tablet **1896**
PediaCare Children's Allergy & Cold Liquid **1902**
PediaCare Children's Allergy Liquid **1902**
Simply Sleep Caplets **1905**
Sudafed PE Nighttime Cold Caplets **1907**
Sudafed PE Severe Cold Caplets **1908**
Extra Strength Tylenol PM Caplets, Geltabs, Liquid, and Rapid Release Gels **1915**
Tylenol Allergy Multi-Symptom Nighttime Caplets with Cool Burst **1916**
Tylenol Severe Allergy Caplets **1916**
Children's Tylenol Plus Cold & Allergy Suspension Liquid **1914**
Tylenol Sore Throat Nighttime Liquid with Cool Burst **1918**

Diphenylpyraline Hydrochloride (Combined therapy may result in additive CNS depression).
No products indexed under this heading.

Doxepin Hydrochloride (Co-administration of hydrocodone with MAO inhibitors may increase the effect of tricyclic antidepressant or hydrocodone).
No products indexed under this heading.

Droperidol (Combined therapy may result in additive CNS depression).
No products indexed under this heading.

Enflurane (Combined therapy may result in additive CNS depression).
No products indexed under this heading.

Estazolam (Combined therapy may result in additive CNS depression).
No products indexed under this heading.

Ethanol (Combined therapy may result in additive CNS depression).
No products indexed under this heading.

Ethchlorvynol (Combined therapy may result in additive CNS depression).
No products indexed under this heading.

Ethinamate (Combined therapy may result in additive CNS depression).
No products indexed under this heading.

Ethyl Alcohol (Combined therapy may result in additive CNS depression).
No products indexed under this heading.

Fentanyl (Combined therapy may result in additive CNS depression). Products include:
Duragesic Transdermal System **2405**
Ionsys Transdermal System **2410**

Fentanyl Citrate (Combined therapy may result in additive CNS depression). Products include:
Actiq **959**
Fentora Tablets **968**

Fexofenadine Hydrochloride (Combined therapy may result in additive CNS depression). Products include:
Allegra Oral Solution **2684**
Allegra Tablets **2684**
Allegra-D 12 Hour Extended-Release Tablets **2687**
Allegra-D 24 Hour Extended-Release Tablets **2690**

Fluphenazine Decanoate (Combined therapy may result in additive CNS depression).
No products indexed under this heading.

Fluphenazine Enanthate (Combined therapy may result in additive CNS depression).
No products indexed under this heading.

Fluphenazine Hydrochloride (Combined therapy may result in additive CNS depression).
No products indexed under this heading.

Flurazepam Hydrochloride (Combined therapy may result in additive CNS depression).
No products indexed under this heading.

Glutethimide (Combined therapy may result in additive CNS depression).
No products indexed under this heading.

Glycopyrrolate (Concurrent use of other anticholinergic agents with hydrocodone may produce paralytic ileus).
No products indexed under this heading.

Haloperidol (Combined therapy may result in additive CNS depression).
No products indexed under this heading.

Haloperidol Decanoate (Combined therapy may result in additive CNS depression).
No products indexed under this heading.

Hydrocodone Bitartrate (Combined therapy may result in additive CNS depression). Products include:
Lortab 5/500 Tablets **3143**
Lortab 7.5/500 Tablets **3144**
Lortab 10/500 Tablets **3144**
Vicodin Tablets **529**
Vicodin ES Tablets **530**
Vicodin HP Tablets **531**
Vicoprofen Tablets **533**
Zydone Tablets **1132**

Hydromorphone Hydrochloride (Combined therapy may result in additive CNS depression).
No products indexed under this heading.

Hydroxyzine Hydrochloride (Combined therapy may result in additive CNS depression).
No products indexed under this heading.

Hyoscyamine (Concurrent use of other anticholinergic agents with hydrocodone may produce paralytic ileus).
No products indexed under this heading.

Hyoscyamine Sulfate (Concurrent use of other anticholinergic agents with hydrocodone may produce paralytic ileus). Products include:
Donnatal Extentabs **2507**

Imipramine Hydrochloride (Co-administration of hydrocodone with MAO inhibitors may increase the effect of tricyclic antidepressant or hydrocodone).
No products indexed under this heading.

Imipramine Pamoate (Co-administration of hydrocodone with MAO inhibitors may increase the effect of tricyclic antidepressant or hydrocodone).
No products indexed under this heading.

Ipratropium Bromide (Concurrent use of other anticholinergic agents with hydrocodone may produce paralytic ileus). Products include:
Atrovent HFA Inhalation Aerosol **839**
Atrovent Nasal Spray 0.03% **834**
Atrovent Nasal Spray 0.06% **836**
Combivent Inhalation Aerosol **845**

Isocarboxazid (Co-administration of hydrocodone with MAO inhibitors may increase the effect of MAOI or hydrocodone). Products include:
Marplan Tablets 3177

Isoflurane (Combined therapy may result in additive CNS depression).
No products indexed under this heading.

Ketamine Hydrochloride (Combined therapy may result in additive CNS depression).
No products indexed under this heading.

Levomethadyl Acetate Hydrochloride (Combined therapy may result in additive CNS depression).
No products indexed under this heading.

Levorphanol Tartrate (Combined therapy may result in additive CNS depression).
No products indexed under this heading.

Loratadine (Combined therapy may result in additive CNS depression).
No products indexed under this heading.

Lorazepam (Combined therapy may result in additive CNS depression).
No products indexed under this heading.

Loxapine Hydrochloride (Combined therapy may result in additive CNS depression).
No products indexed under this heading.

Loxapine Succinate (Combined therapy may result in additive CNS depression).
No products indexed under this heading.

Maprotiline Hydrochloride (Co-administration of hydrocodone with MAO inhibitors may increase the effect of tricyclic antidepressant or hydrocodone).
No products indexed under this heading.

Mepenzolate Bromide (Concurrent use of other anticholinergic agents with hydrocodone may produce paralytic ileus).
No products indexed under this heading.

Meperidine Hydrochloride (Combined therapy may result in additive CNS depression).
No products indexed under this heading.

Mephobarbital (Combined therapy may result in additive CNS depression).
No products indexed under this heading.

Meprobamate (Combined therapy may result in additive CNS depression).
No products indexed under this heading.

Mesoridazine Besylate (Combined therapy may result in additive CNS depression).
No products indexed under this heading.

Methadone Hydrochloride (Combined therapy may result in additive CNS depression).
No products indexed under this heading.

Methdilazine Hydrochloride (Combined therapy may result in additive CNS depression).
No products indexed under this heading.

Methohexital Sodium (Combined therapy may result in additive CNS depression).
No products indexed under this heading.

Methotrimeprazine (Combined therapy may result in additive CNS depression).
No products indexed under this heading.

Methoxyflurane (Combined therapy may result in additive CNS depression).
No products indexed under this heading.

Midazolam Hydrochloride (Combined therapy may result in additive CNS depression).
No products indexed under this heading.

Moclobemide (Co-administration of hydrocodone with MAO inhibitors may increase the effect of MAOI or hydrocodone).
No products indexed under this heading.

Molindone Hydrochloride (Combined therapy may result in additive CNS depression). Products include:
Moban Tablets 1116

Morphine Sulfate (Combined therapy may result in additive CNS depression). Products include:
Avinza Capsules 1772
DepoDur Injection 1095
MS Contin Tablets 2585

Nortriptyline Hydrochloride (Co-administration of hydrocodone with MAO inhibitors may increase the effect of tricyclic antidepressant or hydrocodone).
No products indexed under this heading.

Olanzapine (Combined therapy may result in additive CNS depression). Products include:
Symbyax Capsules 1871
Zyprexa Tablets 1883
Zyprexa IntraMuscular 1883
Zyprexa ZYDIS Orally Disintegrating Tablets 1883

Oxazepam (Combined therapy may result in additive CNS depression).
No products indexed under this heading.

Oxybutynin Chloride (Concurrent use of other anticholinergic agents with hydrocodone may produce paralytic ileus).
No products indexed under this heading.

Oxycodone Hydrochloride (Combined therapy may result in additive CNS depression). Products include:
OxyContin Tablets 2589
OxyIR Capsules 2593
Percocet Tablets 1127
Percodan Tablets 1130

Pargyline Hydrochloride (Co-administration of hydrocodone with MAO inhibitors may increase the effect of MAOI or hydrocodone).
No products indexed under this heading.

Pentobarbital Sodium (Combined therapy may result in additive CNS depression). Products include:
Nembutal Sodium Solution, USP 2494

Perphenazine (Combined therapy may result in additive CNS depression).
No products indexed under this heading.

Phenelzine Sulfate (Co-administration of hydrocodone with MAO inhibitors may increase the effect of MAOI or hydrocodone).
No products indexed under this heading.

Phenobarbital (Combined therapy may result in additive CNS depression). Products include:
Donnatal Extentabs 2507

Prazepam (Combined therapy may result in additive CNS depression).
No products indexed under this heading.

Procarbazine Hydrochloride (Co-administration of hydrocodone with MAO inhibitors may increase the effect of MAOI or hydrocodone).
No products indexed under this heading.

Prochlorperazine (Combined therapy may result in additive CNS depression).
No products indexed under this heading.

Procyclidine Hydrochloride (Concurrent use of other anticholinergic agents with hydrocodone may produce paralytic ileus).
No products indexed under this heading.

Promethazine Hydrochloride (Combined therapy may result in additive CNS depression).
No products indexed under this heading.

Propantheline Bromide (Concurrent use of other anticholinergic agents with hydrocodone may produce paralytic ileus).
No products indexed under this heading.

Propofol (Combined therapy may result in additive CNS depression).
No products indexed under this heading.

Propoxyphene Hydrochloride (Combined therapy may result in additive CNS depression).
No products indexed under this heading.

Propoxyphene Napsylate (Combined therapy may result in additive CNS depression).
No products indexed under this heading.

Protriptyline Hydrochloride (Co-administration of hydrocodone with MAO inhibitors may increase the effect of tricyclic antidepressant or hydrocodone).
No products indexed under this heading.

Pyrilamine Maleate (Combined therapy may result in additive CNS depression).
No products indexed under this heading.

Pyrilamine Tannate (Combined therapy may result in additive CNS depression).
No products indexed under this heading.

Quazepam (Combined therapy may result in additive CNS depression).
No products indexed under this heading.

Quetiapine Fumarate (Combined therapy may result in additive CNS depression).
No products indexed under this heading.

Rasagiline Mesylate (Co-administration of hydrocodone with MAO inhibitors may increase the effect of MAOI or hydrocodone). Products include:
Azilect Tablets 3106

Remifentanil Hydrochloride (Combined therapy may result in additive CNS depression).
No products indexed under this heading.

Risperidone (Combined therapy may result in additive CNS depression). Products include:
Risperdal Consta Long-Acting Injection 1753

Scopolamine (Concurrent use of other anticholinergic agents with hydrocodone may produce paralytic ileus). Products include:
Transderm Scōp Transdermal Therapeutic System 2206

Scopolamine Hydrobromide (Concurrent use of other anticholinergic agents with hydrocodone may produce paralytic ileus). Products include:
Donnatal Extentabs 2507

Secobarbital Sodium (Combined therapy may result in additive CNS depression).
No products indexed under this heading.

Selegiline (Co-administration of hydrocodone with MAO inhibitors may increase the effect of MAOI or hydrocodone). Products include:
Emsam Transdermal System 905

Selegiline Hydrochloride (Co-administration of hydrocodone with MAO inhibitors may increase the effect of MAOI or hydrocodone). Products include:
Eldepryl Capsules 3052

Sevoflurane (Combined therapy may result in additive CNS depression). Products include:
Ultane Liquid for Inhalation 524

Sodium Oxybate (Combined therapy may result in additive CNS depression). Products include:
Xyrem Oral Solution 1766

Sufentanil Citrate (Combined therapy may result in additive CNS depression).
No products indexed under this heading.

Temazepam (Combined therapy may result in additive CNS depression).
No products indexed under this heading.

Terfenadine (Combined therapy may result in additive CNS depression).
No products indexed under this heading.

Thiamylal Sodium (Combined therapy may result in additive CNS depression).
No products indexed under this heading.

Thioridazine Hydrochloride (Combined therapy may result in additive CNS depression). Products include:
Thioridazine Hydrochloride Tablets 2195

Thiothixene (Combined therapy may result in additive CNS depression). Products include:
Thiothixene Capsules 2197

Tolterodine Tartrate (Concurrent use of other anticholinergic agents with hydrocodone may produce paralytic ileus).
No products indexed under this heading.

Tranylcypromine Sulfate (Co-administration of hydrocodone with

MAO inhibitors may increase the effect of MAOI or hydrocodone). Products include:
Parnate Tablets 1532

Triazolam (Combined therapy may result in additive CNS depression).
No products indexed under this heading.

Tridihexethyl Chloride (Concurrent use of other anticholinergic agents with hydrocodone may produce paralytic ileus).
No products indexed under this heading.

Trifluoperazine Hydrochloride (Combined therapy may result in additive CNS depression).
No products indexed under this heading.

Trihexyphenidyl Hydrochloride (Concurrent use of other anticholinergic agents with hydrocodone may produce paralytic ileus).
No products indexed under this heading.

Trimeprazine Tartrate (Combined therapy may result in additive CNS depression).
No products indexed under this heading.

Trimipramine Maleate (Co-administration of hydrocodone with MAO inhibitors may increase the effect of tricyclic antidepressant or hydrocodone).
No products indexed under this heading.

Tripelennamine Hydrochloride (Combined therapy may result in additive CNS depression).
No products indexed under this heading.

Triprolidine Hydrochloride (Combined therapy may result in additive CNS depression).
No products indexed under this heading.

Zaleplon (Combined therapy may result in additive CNS depression).
No products indexed under this heading.

Ziprasidone Hydrochloride (Combined therapy may result in additive CNS depression). Products include:
Geodon Capsules 2520

Zolpidem Tartrate (Combined therapy may result in additive CNS depression). Products include:
Ambien Tablets 2692
Ambien CR Tablets 2696

Food Interactions

Alcohol (Combined use may result in additive CNS depression).

TWINRIX VACCINE

(Hepatitis A Vaccine, Inactivated, Hepatitis B Vaccine, Recombinant) 1628
None cited in PDR database.

TYGACIL FOR INJECTION

(Tigecycline) 3276
May interact with oral contraceptives and certain other agents. Compounds in these categories include:

Desogestrel (Concurrent use of antibacterial drugs with oral contraceptives may render oral contraceptives less effective). Products include:
Mircette Tablets 1034

Ethinyl Estradiol (Concurrent use of antibacterial drugs with oral contraceptives may render oral contraceptives less effective). Products include:
Lybrel Tablets 3204
Mircette Tablets 1034
NuvaRing 2897
Ortho-Cyclen/Ortho Tri-Cyclen 2449
Ortho Evra Transdermal System 2437
Ortho Tri-Cyclen Lo Tablets 2458
Seasonique Tablets 1046
Yaz Tablets 805

Ethynodiol Diacetate (Concurrent use of antibacterial drugs with oral contraceptives may render oral contraceptives less effective).
No products indexed under this heading.

Levonorgestrel (Concurrent use of antibacterial drugs with oral contraceptives may render oral contraceptives less effective). Products include:
Climara Pro Transdermal System 768
Lybrel Tablets 3204
Mirena Intrauterine System 779
Plan B Tablets 1044
Seasonique Tablets 1046

Mestranol (Concurrent use of antibacterial drugs with oral contraceptives may render oral contraceptives less effective).
No products indexed under this heading.

Norethindrone (Concurrent use of antibacterial drugs with oral contraceptives may render oral contraceptives less effective). Products include:
Ortho Micronor Tablets 2446

Norethynodrel (Concurrent use of antibacterial drugs with oral contraceptives may render oral contraceptives less effective).
No products indexed under this heading.

Norgestimate (Concurrent use of antibacterial drugs with oral contraceptives may render oral contraceptives less effective). Products include:
Ortho-Cyclen/Ortho Tri-Cyclen 2449
Ortho Tri-Cyclen Lo Tablets 2458

Norgestrel (Concurrent use of antibacterial drugs with oral contraceptives may render oral contraceptives less effective).
No products indexed under this heading.

Warfarin Sodium (Prothrombin time or other suitable anticoagulation test should be monitored if tigecycline is administered with warfarin).
No products indexed under this heading.

TYKERB TABLETS

(Lapatinib) 1631
May interact with cytochrome p450 2c8 substrates (selected), cytochrome p450 3a4 inducers (selected), cytochrome p450 3a4 inhibitors, potent, cytochrome p450 3a4 substrates (selected), glycoprotein (GP) IIb/IIIa inhibitors, and certain other agents. Compounds in these categories include:

Abciximab (Lapatinib is a subtrate of the efflux transporter P-glycoprotein (Pgp, ABCB1). If lapatinib is administered with drugs that inhibit Pgp, increased concentrations of lapatinib are likely, and caution should be exercised). Products include:
ReoPro Vials 1860

Alfentanil Hydrochloride (Lapatinib inhibits CYP3A4 in vitro at clinically relevant concentrations. Caution should be exercised and dose reduction of the concomitant substrate drug should be considered when dosing lapatinib concurrently with medications with narrow therapeutic windows that are substrates of CYP3A4).
No products indexed under this heading.

Allium sativum (Lapatinib undergoes extensive metabolism by CYP3A4; concomitant administration of strong inducers of CYP3A4 alter lapatinib concentrations significantly and should be avoided. Dose adjustment of lapatinib should be considered for patients who must receive concomitant strong inducers of CYP3A4 enzymes. Lapatinib inhibits CYP3A4 in vitro at clinically relevant concentrations. Caution should be exercised and dose reduction of the concomitant substrate drug should be considered when dosing lapatinib concurrently with medications with narrow therapeutic windows that are substrates of CYP3A4).
No products indexed under this heading.

Alprazolam (Lapatinib inhibits CYP3A4 in vitro at clinically relevant concentrations. Caution should be exercised and dose reduction of the concomitant substrate drug should be considered when dosing lapatinib concurrently with medications with narrow therapeutic windows that are substrates of CYP3A4).
No products indexed under this heading.

Amiodarone Hydrochloride (Lapatinib inhibits CYP2C8 in vitro at clinically relevant concentrations. Caution should be exercised and dose reduction of the concomitant substrate drug should be considered when dosing lapatinib concurrently with medications with narrow therapeutic windows that are substrates of CYP2C8).
No products indexed under this heading.

Amitriptyline Hydrochloride (Lapatinib inhibits CYP2C8 in vitro at clinically relevant concentrations. Caution should be exercised and dose reduction of the concomitant substrate drug should be considered when dosing lapatinib concurrently with medications with narrow therapeutic windows that are substrates of CYP2C8).
No products indexed under this heading.

Amlodipine Besylate (Lapatinib inhibits CYP3A4 in vitro at clinically relevant concentrations. Caution should be exercised and dose reduction of the concomitant substrate drug should be considered when dosing lapatinib concurrently with medications with narrow therapeutic windows that are substrates of CYP3A4). Products include:
Azor Tablets 1005
Exforge Tablets 2238

Amoxapine (Lapatinib inhibits CYP2C8 in vitro at clinically relevant concentrations. Caution should be exercised and dose reduction of the concomitant substrate drug should be considered when dosing lapatinib concurrently with medications with narrow therapeutic windows that are substrates of CYP2C8).
No products indexed under this heading.

Amprenavir (Lapatinib undergoes extensive metabolism by CYP3A4; concomitant administration of strong inhibitors of CYP3A4 alter lapatinib concentrations significantly and should be avoided. Dose adjustment of lapatinib should be considered for patients who must receive concomitant strong inhibitors of CYP3A4 enzymes. Lapatinib inhibits CYP3A4 in vitro at clinically relevant concentrations. Caution should be exercised and dose reduction of the concomitant substrate drug should be considered when dosing lapatinib concurrently with medications with narrow therapeutic windows that are substrates of CYP3A4).
No products indexed under this heading.

Aprepitant (Lapatinib undergoes extensive metabolism by CYP3A4; concomitant administration of strong inducers of CYP3A4 alter lapatinib concentrations significantly and should be avoided. Dose adjustment of lapatinib should be considered for patients who must receive concomitant strong inducers of CYP3A4 enzymes. Lapatinib inhibits CYP3A4 in vitro at clinically relevant concentrations. Caution should be exercised and dose reduction of the concomitant substrate drug should be considered when dosing lapatinib concurrently with medications with narrow therapeutic windows that are substrates of CYP3A4). Products include:
Emend Capsules 1992

Astemizole (Lapatinib inhibits CYP3A4 in vitro at clinically relevant concentrations. Caution should be exercised and dose reduction of the concomitant substrate drug should be considered when dosing lapatinib concurrently with medications with narrow therapeutic windows that are substrates of CYP3A4).
No products indexed under this heading.

Atazanavir (Lapatinib undergoes extensive metabolism by CYP3A4; concomitant administration of strong inhibitors of CYP3A4 alter lapatinib concentrations significantly and should be avoided. Dose adjustment of lapatinib should be considered for patients who must receive concomitant strong inhibitors of CYP3A4 enzymes. Lapatinib inhibits CYP3A4 in vitro at clinically relevant concentrations. Caution should be exercised and dose reduction of the concomitant substrate drug should be considered when dosing lapatinib concurrently with medications with narrow therapeutic windows that are substrates of CYP3A4).
No products indexed under this heading.

Atazanavir Sulfate (Lapatinib undergoes extensive metabolism by CYP3A4; concomitant administration of strong inhibitors of CYP3A4 alter lapatinib concentrations significantly and should be avoided. Dose adjustment of lapatinib should be considered for patients who must receive concomitant strong inhibitors of CYP3A4 enzymes. Lapatinib inhibits CYP3A4 in vitro at clinically relevant concentrations. Caution should be exercised and dose reduction of the concomitant substrate drug should be considered when dosing lapatinib concurrently with medications with narrow therapeutic windows that are substrates of CYP3A4). Products include:

Reyataz Capsules 3299

Atorvastatin Calcium (Lapatinib inhibits CYP3A4 in vitro at clinically relevant concentrations. Caution should be exercised and dose reduction of the concomitant substrate drug should be considered when dosing lapatinib concurrently with medications with narrow therapeutic windows that are substrates of CYP3A4). Products include:

Lipitor Tablets 2501

Belladonna Ergotamine (Lapatinib inhibits CYP3A4 in vitro at clinically relevant concentrations. Caution should be exercised and dose reduction of the concomitant substrate drug should be considered when dosing lapatinib concurrently with medications with narrow therapeutic windows that are substrates of CYP3A4).

No products indexed under this heading.

Benzphetamine Hydrochloride (Lapatinib inhibits CYP2C8 in vitro at clinically relevant concentrations. Caution should be exercised and dose reduction of the concomitant substrate drug should be considered when dosing lapatinib concurrently with medications with narrow therapeutic windows that are substrates of CYP2C8).

No products indexed under this heading.

Betamethasone Acetate (Lapatinib undergoes extensive metabolism by CYP3A4; concomitant administration of strong inducers of CYP3A4 alter lapatinib concentrations significantly and should be avoided. Dose adjustment of lapatinib should be considered for patients who must receive concomitant strong inducers of CYP3A4 enzymes. Lapatinib inhibits CYP3A4 in vitro at clinically relevant concentrations. Caution should be exercised and dose reduction of the concomitant substrate drug should be considered when dosing lapatinib concurrently with medications with narrow therapeutic windows that are substrates of CYP3A4).

No products indexed under this heading.

Betamethasone Sodium Phosphate (Lapatinib undergoes extensive metabolism by CYP3A4; concomitant administration of strong inducers of CYP3A4 alter lapatinib concentrations significantly and should be avoided. Dose adjustment of lapatinib should be considered for patients who must receive concomitant strong inducers of CYP3A4 enzymes. Lapatinib inhibits CYP3A4 in vitro at clinically relevant concentrations. Caution should be exercised and dose reduction of the concomitant substrate drug should be considered when dosing lapatinib concurrently with medications with narrow therapeutic windows that are substrates of CYP3A4).

No products indexed under this heading.

Buspirone Hydrochloride (Lapatinib inhibits CYP3A4 in vitro at clinically relevant concentrations. Caution should be exercised and dose reduction of the concomitant substrate drug should be considered when dosing lapatinib concurrently with medications with narrow therapeutic windows that are substrates of CYP3A4).

No products indexed under this heading.

Busulfan (Lapatinib inhibits CYP3A4 in vitro at clinically relevant concentrations. Caution should be exercised and dose reduction of the concomitant substrate drug should be considered when dosing lapatinib concurrently with medications with narrow therapeutic windows that are substrates of CYP3A4). Products include:

Busulfex Injection 2477
Myleran Tablets 1530

Carbamazepine (Lapatinib undergoes extensive metabolism by CYP3A4; concomitant administration of strong inducers of CYP3A4 alter lapatinib concentrations significantly and should be avoided. Dose adjustment of lapatinib should be considered for patients who must receive concomitant strong inducers of CYP3A4 enzymes. Lapatinib inhibits CYP3A4 in vitro at clinically relevant concentrations. Caution should be exercised and dose reduction of the concomitant substrate drug should be considered when dosing lapatinib concurrently with medications with narrow therapeutic windows that are substrates of CYP3A4). Products include:

Carbatrol Capsules 3019
Equetro Extended-Release Capsules 3174

Cerivastatin Sodium (Lapatinib inhibits CYP3A4 in vitro at clinically relevant concentrations. Caution should be exercised and dose reduction of the concomitant substrate drug should be considered when dosing lapatinib concurrently with medications with narrow therapeutic windows that are substrates of CYP3A4).

No products indexed under this heading.

Chlorpheniramine (Lapatinib inhibits CYP3A4 in vitro at clinically relevant concentrations. Caution should be exercised and dose reduction of the concomitant substrate drug should be considered when dosing lapatinib concurrently with medications with narrow therapeutic windows that are substrates of CYP3A4).

No products indexed under this heading.

Chlorpheniramine Maleate (Lapatinib inhibits CYP3A4 in vitro at clinically relevant concentrations. Caution should be exercised and dose reduction of the concomitant substrate drug should be considered when dosing lapatinib concurrently with medications with narrow therapeutic windows that are substrates of CYP3A4). Products include:

Actifed Cold & Allergy Tablets 1895
Sudafed PE Sinus & Allergy Tablets 1908
Tylenol Allergy Multi-Symptom Caplets with Cool Burst and Rapid Release Gelcaps 1916
Children's Tylenol Plus Cold Suspension Liquid 1912
Children's Tylenol Plus Cough & Runny Nose Suspension Liquid 1912
Children's Tylenol Plus Flu Suspension Liquid 1914
Children's Tylenol Plus Multi-Symptom Cold Suspension Liquid 1912
Tylenol Cold Head Congestion Nighttime Caplets with Cool Burst... 1910
Tylenol Cold Multi-Symptom Nighttime Caplets with Cool Burst... 1913
Tylenol Sinus Congestion & Pain Nighttime Caplets with Cool Burst... 1917

Chlorpheniramine Polistirex (Lapatinib inhibits CYP3A4 in vitro at clinically relevant concentrations. Caution should be exercised and dose reduction of the concomitant substrate drug should be considered when dosing lapatinib concurrently with medications with narrow therapeutic windows that are substrates of CYP3A4). Products include:

Tussionex Pennkinetic Extended-Release Suspension...... 3154

Chlorpheniramine Tannate (Lapatinib inhibits CYP3A4 in vitro at clinically relevant concentrations. Caution should be exercised and dose reduction of the concomitant substrate drug should be considered when dosing lapatinib concurrently with medications with narrow therapeutic windows that are substrates of CYP3A4).

No products indexed under this heading.

Ciprofloxacin Hydrochloride (Lapatinib undergoes extensive metabolism by CYP3A4; concomitant administration of strong inducers of CYP3A4 alter lapatinib concentrations significantly and should be avoided. Dose adjustment of lapatinib should be considered for patients who must receive concomitant strong inducers of CYP3A4 enzymes. Lapatinib inhibits CYP3A4 in vitro at clinically relevant concentrations. Caution should be exercised and dose reduction of the concomitant substrate drug should be considered when dosing lapatinib concurrently with medications with narrow therapeutic windows that are substrates of CYP3A4). Products include:

Cipro Tablets 2810

Cisapride (Lapatinib inhibits CYP3A4 in vitro at clinically relevant concentrations. Caution should be exercised and dose reduction of the concomitant substrate drug should be considered when dosing lapatinib concurrently with medications with narrow therapeutic windows that are substrates of CYP3A4).

No products indexed under this heading.

Cisplatin (Lapatinib undergoes extensive metabolism by CYP3A4; concomitant administration of strong inducers of CYP3A4 alter lapatinib concentrations significantly and should be avoided. Dose adjustment of lapatinib should be considered for patients who must receive concomitant strong inducers of CYP3A4 enzymes. Lapatinib inhibits CYP3A4 in vitro at clinically relevant concentrations. Caution should be exercised and dose reduction of the concomitant substrate drug should be considered when dosing lapatinib concurrently with medications with narrow therapeutic windows that are substrates of CYP3A4).

No products indexed under this heading.

Clarithromycin (Lapatinib undergoes extensive metabolism by CYP3A4; concomitant administration of strong inhibitors of CYP3A4 alter lapatinib concentrations significantly and should be avoided. Dose adjustment of lapatinib should be considered for patients who must receive concomitant strong inhibitors of CYP3A4 enzymes. Lapatinib inhibits CYP3A4 in vitro at clinically relevant concentrations. Caution should be exercised and dose reduction of the concomitant substrate drug should be considered when dosing lapatinib concurrently with medications with narrow therapeutic windows that are substrates of CYP3A4). Products include:

Biaxin/Biaxin XL 411

Clomipramine Hydrochloride (Lapatinib inhibits CYP2C8 in vitro at clinically relevant concentrations. Caution should be exercised and dose reduction of the concomitant substrate drug should be considered when dosing lapatinib concurrently with medications with narrow therapeutic windows that are substrates of CYP2C8).

No products indexed under this heading.

Cortisone Acetate (Lapatinib undergoes extensive metabolism by CYP3A4; concomitant administration of strong inducers of CYP3A4 alter lapatinib concentrations significantly and should be avoided. Dose adjustment of lapatinib should be considered for patients who must receive concomitant strong inducers of CYP3A4 enzymes. Lapatinib inhibits CYP3A4 in vitro at clinically relevant concentrations. Caution should be exercised and dose reduction of the concomitant substrate drug should be considered when dosing lapatinib concurrently with medications with narrow therapeutic windows that are substrates of CYP3A4).

No products indexed under this heading.

Cyclosporine (Lapatinib inhibits CYP3A4 in vitro at clinically relevant concentrations. Caution should be exercised and dose reduction of the concomitant substrate drug should be considered when dosing lapatinib concurrently with medications with narrow therapeutic windows that are substrates of CYP3A4). Products include:

Gengraf Capsules 435
Neoral Oral Solution 2280
Neoral Soft Gelatin Capsules 2280
Restasis Ophthalmic Emulsion 557
Sandimmune 2296

Delavirdine Mesylate (Lapatinib undergoes extensive metabolism by CYP3A4; concomitant administration of strong inhibitors of CYP3A4 alter lapatinib concentrations significantly and should be avoided. Dose adjustment of lapatinib should be considered for patients who must receive concomitant strong inhibitors of CYP3A4 enzymes. Lapatinib inhibits CYP3A4 in vitro at clinically relevant concentrations. Caution should be exercised and dose reduction of the concomitant substrate drug should

be considered when dosing lapatinib concurrently with medications with narrow therapeutic windows that are substrates of CYP3A4).

No products indexed under this heading.

Delavirine (Lapatinib undergoes extensive metabolism by CYP3A4; concomitant administration of strong inhibitors of CYP3A4 alter lapatinib concentrations significantly and should be avoided. Dose adjustment of lapatinib should be considered for patients who must receive concomitant strong inhibitors of CYP3A4 enzymes. Lapatinib inhibits CYP3A4 in vitro at clinically relevant concentrations. Caution should be exercised and dose reduction of the concomitant substrate drug should be considered when dosing lapatinib concurrently with medications with narrow therapeutic windows that are substrates of CYP3A4).

No products indexed under this heading.

Desipramine Hydrochloride (Lapatinib inhibits CYP2C8 in vitro at clinically relevant concentrations. Caution should be exercised and dose reduction of the concomitant substrate drug should be considered when dosing lapatinib concurrently with medications with narrow therapeutic windows that are substrates of CYP2C8).

No products indexed under this heading.

Desogestrel (Lapatinib inhibits CYP3A4 in vitro at clinically relevant concentrations. Caution should be exercised and dose reduction of the concomitant substrate drug should be considered when dosing lapatinib concurrently with medications with narrow therapeutic windows that are substrates of CYP3A4). Products include:

Mircette Tablets **1034**

Dexamethasone (Lapatinib undergoes extensive metabolism by CYP3A4; concomitant administration of strong inducers of CYP3A4 alter lapatinib concentrations significantly and should be avoided. Dose adjustment of lapatinib should be considered for patients who must receive concomitant strong inducers of CYP3A4 enzymes. Lapatinib inhibits CYP3A4 in vitro at clinically relevant concentrations. Caution should be exercised and dose reduction of the concomitant substrate drug should be considered when dosing lapatinib concurrently with medications with narrow therapeutic windows that are substrates of CYP3A4). Products include:

Ciprodex Otic Suspension **541**

Dexamethasone Acetate (Lapatinib undergoes extensive metabolism by CYP3A4; concomitant administration of strong inducers of CYP3A4 alter lapatinib concentrations significantly and should be avoided. Dose adjustment of lapatinib should be considered for patients who must receive concomitant strong inducers of CYP3A4 enzymes. Lapatinib inhibits CYP3A4 in vitro at clinically relevant concentrations. Caution should be exercised and dose reduction of the concomitant substrate drug should be considered when dosing lapatinib concurrently with medications with narrow therapeutic windows that are substrates of CYP3A4).

No products indexed under this heading.

Dexamethasone Sodium Phosphate (Lapatinib undergoes extensive metabolism by CYP3A4; concomitant administration of strong inducers of CYP3A4 alter lapatinib concentrations significantly and should be avoided. Dose adjustment of lapatinib should be considered for patients who must receive concomitant strong inducers of CYP3A4 enzymes. Lapatinib inhibits CYP3A4 in vitro at clinically relevant concentrations. Caution should be exercised and dose reduction of the concomitant substrate drug should be considered when dosing lapatinib concurrently with medications with narrow therapeutic windows that are substrates of CYP3A4).

No products indexed under this heading.

Diazepam (Lapatinib inhibits CYP2C8 in vitro at clinically relevant concentrations. Caution should be exercised and dose reduction of the concomitant substrate drug should be considered when dosing lapatinib concurrently with medications with narrow therapeutic windows that are substrates of CYP2C8). Products include:

Valium Tablets **2658**

Diclofenac Potassium (Lapatinib inhibits CYP2C8 in vitro at clinically relevant concentrations. Caution should be exercised and dose reduction of the concomitant substrate drug should be considered when dosing lapatinib concurrently with medications with narrow therapeutic windows that are substrates of CYP2C8).

No products indexed under this heading.

Diclofenac Sodium (Lapatinib inhibits CYP2C8 in vitro at clinically relevant concentrations. Caution should be exercised and dose reduction of the concomitant substrate drug should be considered when dosing lapatinib concurrently with medications with narrow therapeutic windows that are substrates of CYP2C8). Products include:

Diclofenac Sodium Ophthalmic Solution .... ⊙ **240**
Voltaren Ophthalmic Solution **2336**
Voltaren Tablets **2334**
Voltaren-XR Tablets **2337**

Dihydroergotamine Mesylate (Lapatinib inhibits CYP3A4 in vitro at clinically relevant concentrations. Caution should be exercised and dose reduction of the concomitant substrate drug should be considered when dosing lapatinib concurrently with medications with narrow therapeutic windows that are substrates of CYP3A4).

No products indexed under this heading.

Diltiazem Hydrochloride (Lapatinib inhibits CYP3A4 in vitro at clinically relevant concentrations. Caution should be exercised and dose reduction of the concomitant substrate drug should be considered when dosing lapatinib concurrently with medications with narrow therapeutic windows that are substrates of CYP3A4). Products include:

Cardizem LA Extended Release Tablets **421**

Diltiazem Maleate (Lapatinib inhibits CYP3A4 in vitro at clinically relevant concentrations. Caution should be exercised and dose reduction of the concomitant substrate drug should be considered when dosing lapatinib concurrently with medications with narrow therapeutic windows that are substrates of CYP3A4).

No products indexed under this heading.

Disopyramide (Lapatinib inhibits CYP3A4 in vitro at clinically relevant concentrations. Caution should be exercised and dose reduction of the concomitant substrate drug should be considered when dosing lapatinib concurrently with medications with narrow therapeutic windows that are substrates of CYP3A4).

No products indexed under this heading.

Disopyramide Phosphate (Lapatinib inhibits CYP3A4 in vitro at clinically relevant concentrations. Caution should be exercised and dose reduction of the concomitant substrate drug should be considered when dosing lapatinib concurrently with medications with narrow therapeutic windows that are substrates of CYP3A4).

No products indexed under this heading.

Disulfiram (Lapatinib inhibits CYP3A4 in vitro at clinically relevant concentrations. Caution should be exercised and dose reduction of the concomitant substrate drug should be considered when dosing lapatinib concurrently with medications with narrow therapeutic windows that are substrates of CYP3A4).

No products indexed under this heading.

Docetaxel (Lapatinib inhibits CYP2C8 in vitro at clinically relevant concentrations. Caution should be exercised and dose reduction of the concomitant substrate drug should be considered when dosing lapatinib concurrently with medications with narrow therapeutic windows that are substrates of CYP2C8). Products include:

Taxotere Injection Concentrate **2773**

Doxepin Hydrochloride (Lapatinib inhibits CYP2C8 in vitro at clinically relevant concentrations. Caution should be exercised and dose reduction of the concomitant substrate drug should be considered when dosing lapatinib concurrently with medications with narrow therapeutic windows that are substrates of CYP2C8).

No products indexed under this heading.

Doxorubicin Hydrochloride (Lapatinib undergoes extensive metabolism by CYP3A4; concomitant administration of strong inducers of CYP3A4 alter lapatinib concentrations significantly and should be avoided. Dose adjustment of lapatinib should be considered for patients who must receive concomitant strong inducers of CYP3A4 enzymes. Lapatinib inhibits CYP3A4 in vitro at clinically relevant concentrations. Caution should be exercised and dose reduction of the concomitant substrate drug should be considered when dosing lapatinib concurrently with medications with narrow therapeutic windows that are substrates of CYP3A4).

No products indexed under this heading.

Dronabinol (Lapatinib inhibits CYP3A4 in vitro at clinically relevant concentrations. Caution should be exercised and dose reduction of the concomitant substrate drug should be considered when dosing lapatinib concurrently with medications with narrow therapeutic windows that are substrates of CYP3A4). Products include:

Marinol Capsules **3163**

Efavirenz (Lapatinib undergoes extensive metabolism by CYP3A4; concomitant administration of strong inducers of CYP3A4 alter lapatinib concentrations significantly and should be avoided. Dose adjustment of lapatinib should be considered for patients who must receive concomitant strong inducers of CYP3A4 enzymes. Lapatinib inhibits CYP3A4 in vitro at clinically relevant concentrations. Caution should be exercised and dose reduction of the concomitant substrate drug should be considered when dosing lapatinib concurrently with medications with narrow therapeutic windows that are substrates of CYP3A4). Products include:

Atripla Tablets **938**
Sustiva Capsules **930**
Sustiva Tablets **930**

Eptifibatide (Lapatinib is a subtrate of the efflux transporter P-glycoprotein (Pgp, ABCB1). If lapatinib is administered with drugs that inhibit Pgp, increased concentrations of lapatinib are likely, and caution should be exercised). Products include:

Integrilin Injection **2855**

Ergotamine Tartrate (Lapatinib inhibits CYP3A4 in vitro at clinically relevant concentrations. Caution should be exercised and dose reduction of the concomitant substrate drug should be considered when dosing lapatinib concurrently with medications with narrow therapeutic windows that are substrates of CYP3A4).

No products indexed under this heading.

Erythromycin (Lapatinib inhibits CYP3A4 in vitro at clinically relevant concentrations. Caution should be exercised and dose reduction of the concomitant substrate drug should be considered when dosing lapatinib concurrently with medications with narrow therapeutic windows that are substrates of CYP3A4).

No products indexed under this heading.

Erythromycin Estolate (Lapatinib inhibits CYP3A4 in vitro at clinically relevant concentrations. Caution should be exercised and dose reduction of the concomitant substrate drug should be considered when dosing lapatinib concurrently with medications with narrow therapeutic windows that are substrates of CYP3A4).

No products indexed under this heading.

Erythromycin Ethylsuccinate (Lapatinib inhibits CYP3A4 in vitro at clinically relevant concentrations. Caution should be exercised and dose reduction of the concomitant substrate drug should be considered when dosing lapatinib concurrently

with medications with narrow therapeutic windows that are substrates of CYP3A4). Products include:
E.E.S. 433
EryPed 431

Erythromycin Gluceptate (Lapatinib inhibits CYP3A4 in vitro at clinically relevant concentrations. Caution should be exercised and dose reduction of the concomitant substrate drug should be considered when dosing lapatinib concurrently with medications with narrow therapeutic windows that are substrates of CYP3A4).
No products indexed under this heading.

Erythromycin Lactobionate (Lapatinib inhibits CYP3A4 in vitro at clinically relevant concentrations. Caution should be exercised and dose reduction of the concomitant substrate drug should be considered when dosing lapatinib concurrently with medications with narrow therapeutic windows that are substrates of CYP3A4).
No products indexed under this heading.

Erythromycin Stearate (Lapatinib inhibits CYP3A4 in vitro at clinically relevant concentrations. Caution should be exercised and dose reduction of the concomitant substrate drug should be considered when dosing lapatinib concurrently with medications with narrow therapeutic windows that are substrates of CYP3A4).
No products indexed under this heading.

Estradiol (Lapatinib inhibits CYP3A4 in vitro at clinically relevant concentrations. Caution should be exercised and dose reduction of the concomitant substrate drug should be considered when dosing lapatinib concurrently with medications with narrow therapeutic windows that are substrates of CYP3A4). Products include:
Activella Tablets 2347
Angeliq Tablets 751
Climara Transdermal System 763
Climara Pro Transdermal System 768
Divigel 3167
Vagifem Tablets 2375

Estradiol Benzoate (Lapatinib inhibits CYP3A4 in vitro at clinically relevant concentrations. Caution should be exercised and dose reduction of the concomitant substrate drug should be considered when dosing lapatinib concurrently with medications with narrow therapeutic windows that are substrates of CYP3A4).
No products indexed under this heading.

Estradiol Cypionate (Lapatinib inhibits CYP3A4 in vitro at clinically relevant concentrations. Caution should be exercised and dose reduction of the concomitant substrate drug should be considered when dosing lapatinib concurrently with medications with narrow therapeutic windows that are substrates of CYP3A4).
No products indexed under this heading.

Estradiol Valerate (Lapatinib inhibits CYP3A4 in vitro at clinically relevant concentrations. Caution should be exercised and dose reduction of the concomitant substrate drug should be considered when dosing lapatinib concurrently with medications with narrow therapeutic windows that are substrates of CYP3A4).
No products indexed under this heading.

Ethinyl Estradiol (Lapatinib inhibits CYP3A4 in vitro at clinically relevant concentrations. Caution should be exercised and dose reduction of the concomitant substrate drug should be considered when dosing lapatinib concurrently with medications with narrow therapeutic windows that are substrates of CYP3A4). Products include:
Lybrel Tablets 3204
Mircette Tablets 1034
NuvaRing 2897
Ortho-Cyclen/Ortho Tri-Cyclen 2449
Ortho Evra Transdermal System 2437
Ortho Tri-Cyclen Lo Tablets 2458
Seasonique Tablets 1046
Yaz Tablets 805

Ethosuximide (Lapatinib undergoes extensive metabolism by CYP3A4; concomitant administration of strong inducers of CYP3A4 alter lapatinib concentrations significantly and should be avoided. Dose adjustment of lapatinib should be considered for patients who must receive concomitant strong inducers of CYP3A4 enzymes. Lapatinib inhibits CYP3A4 in vitro at clinically relevant concentrations. Caution should be exercised and dose reduction of the concomitant substrate drug should be considered when dosing lapatinib concurrently with medications with narrow therapeutic windows that are substrates of CYP3A4).
No products indexed under this heading.

Ethynodiol Diacetate (Lapatinib inhibits CYP3A4 in vitro at clinically relevant concentrations. Caution should be exercised and dose reduction of the concomitant substrate drug should be considered when dosing lapatinib concurrently with medications with narrow therapeutic windows that are substrates of CYP3A4).
No products indexed under this heading.

Etoposide (Lapatinib inhibits CYP3A4 in vitro at clinically relevant concentrations. Caution should be exercised and dose reduction of the concomitant substrate drug should be considered when dosing lapatinib concurrently with medications with narrow therapeutic windows that are substrates of CYP3A4).
No products indexed under this heading.

Etoposide Phosphate (Lapatinib inhibits CYP3A4 in vitro at clinically relevant concentrations. Caution should be exercised and dose reduction of the concomitant substrate drug should be considered when dosing lapatinib concurrently with medications with narrow therapeutic windows that are substrates of CYP3A4).
No products indexed under this heading.

Felbamate (Lapatinib undergoes extensive metabolism by CYP3A4; concomitant administration of strong inducers of CYP3A4 alter lapatinib concentrations significantly and should be avoided. Dose adjustment of lapatinib should be considered for patients who must receive concomitant strong inducers of CYP3A4 enzymes. Lapatinib inhibits CYP3A4 in vitro at clinically relevant concentrations. Caution should be exercised and dose reduction of the concomitant substrate drug should be considered when dosing lapatinib concurrently with medications with narrow therapeutic windows that are substrates of CYP3A4).
No products indexed under this heading.

Felodipine (Lapatinib inhibits CYP3A4 in vitro at clinically relevant concentrations. Caution should be exercised and dose reduction of the concomitant substrate drug should be considered when dosing lapatinib concurrently with medications with narrow therapeutic windows that are substrates of CYP3A4).
No products indexed under this heading.

Fentanyl (Lapatinib inhibits CYP3A4 in vitro at clinically relevant concentrations. Caution should be exercised and dose reduction of the concomitant substrate drug should be considered when dosing lapatinib concurrently with medications with narrow therapeutic windows that are substrates of CYP3A4). Products include:
Duragesic Transdermal System 2405
Ionsys Transdermal System 2410

Fentanyl Citrate (Lapatinib inhibits CYP3A4 in vitro at clinically relevant concentrations. Caution should be exercised and dose reduction of the concomitant substrate drug should be considered when dosing lapatinib concurrently with medications with narrow therapeutic windows that are substrates of CYP3A4). Products include:
Actiq 959
Fentora Tablets 968

Fludrocortisone Acetate (Lapatinib undergoes extensive metabolism by CYP3A4; concomitant administration of strong inducers of CYP3A4 alter lapatinib concentrations significantly and should be avoided. Dose adjustment of lapatinib should be considered for patients who must receive concomitant strong inducers of CYP3A4 enzymes. Lapatinib inhibits CYP3A4 in vitro at clinically relevant concentrations. Caution should be exercised and dose reduction of the concomitant substrate drug should be considered when dosing lapatinib concurrently with medications with narrow therapeutic windows that are substrates of CYP3A4).
No products indexed under this heading.

Fluvastatin Sodium (Lapatinib inhibits CYP2C8 in vitro at clinically relevant concentrations. Caution should be exercised and dose reduction of the concomitant substrate drug should be considered when dosing lapatinib concurrently with medications with narrow therapeutic windows that are substrates of CYP2C8). Products include:
Lescol Capsules 2268
Lescol XL Tablets 2268

Fosamprenavir Calcium (Lapatinib undergoes extensive metabolism by CYP3A4; concomitant administration of strong inhibitors of CYP3A4 alter lapatinib concentrations significantly and should be avoided. Dose adjustment of lapatinib should be considered for patients who must receive concomitant strong inhibitors of CYP3A4 enzymes. Lapatinib inhibits CYP3A4 in vitro at clinically relevant concentrations. Caution should be exercised and dose reduction of the concomitant substrate drug should be considered when dosing lapatinib concurrently with medications with narrow therapeutic windows that are substrates of CYP3A4). Products include:
Lexiva Oral Suspension 1510
Lexiva Tablets 1510

Fosphenytoin Sodium (Lapatinib undergoes extensive metabolism by CYP3A4; concomitant administration of strong inducers of CYP3A4 alter lapatinib concentrations significantly and should be avoided. Dose adjustment of lapatinib should be considered for patients who must receive concomitant strong inducers of CYP3A4 enzymes. Lapatinib inhibits CYP3A4 in vitro at clinically relevant concentrations. Caution should be exercised and dose reduction of the concomitant substrate drug should be considered when dosing lapatinib concurrently with medications with narrow therapeutic windows that are substrates of CYP3A4).
No products indexed under this heading.

Garlic Extract (Lapatinib undergoes extensive metabolism by CYP3A4; concomitant administration of strong inducers of CYP3A4 alter lapatinib concentrations significantly and should be avoided. Dose adjustment of lapatinib should be considered for patients who must receive concomitant strong inducers of CYP3A4 enzymes. Lapatinib inhibits CYP3A4 in vitro at clinically relevant concentrations. Caution should be exercised and dose reduction of the concomitant substrate drug should be considered when dosing lapatinib concurrently with medications with narrow therapeutic windows that are substrates of CYP3A4).
No products indexed under this heading.

Garlic Oil (Lapatinib undergoes extensive metabolism by CYP3A4; concomitant administration of strong inducers of CYP3A4 alter lapatinib concentrations significantly and should be avoided. Dose adjustment of lapatinib should be considered for patients who must receive concomitant strong inducers of CYP3A4 enzymes. Lapatinib inhibits CYP3A4 in vitro at clinically relevant concentrations. Caution should be exercised and dose reduction of the concomitant substrate drug should be considered when dosing lapatinib concurrently with medications with narrow therapeutic windows that are substrates of CYP3A4).
No products indexed under this heading.

Haloperidol (Lapatinib inhibits CYP3A4 in vitro at clinically relevant concentrations. Caution should be exercised and dose reduction of the concomitant substrate drug should be considered when dosing lapatinib concurrently with medications with narrow therapeutic windows that are substrates of CYP3A4).
No products indexed under this heading.

Haloperidol Decanoate (Lapatinib inhibits CYP3A4 in vitro at clinically relevant concentrations. Caution should be exercised and dose reduction of the concomitant substrate drug should be considered when dosing lapatinib concurrently with medications with narrow therapeutic windows that are substrates of CYP3A4).

No products indexed under this heading.

Haloperidol Lactate (Lapatinib inhibits CYP3A4 in vitro at clinically relevant concentrations. Caution should be exercised and dose reduction of the concomitant substrate drug should be considered when dosing lapatinib concurrently with medications with narrow therapeutic windows that are substrates of CYP3A4).

No products indexed under this heading.

Hydrocortisone (Lapatinib undergoes extensive metabolism by CYP3A4; concomitant administration of strong inducers of CYP3A4 alter lapatinib concentrations significantly and should be avoided. Dose adjustment of lapatinib should be considered for patients who must receive concomitant strong inducers of CYP3A4 enzymes. Lapatinib inhibits CYP3A4 in vitro at clinically relevant concentrations. Caution should be exercised and dose reduction of the concomitant substrate drug should be considered when dosing lapatinib concurrently with medications with narrow therapeutic windows that are substrates of CYP3A4).

No products indexed under this heading.

Hydrocortisone Acetate (Lapatinib undergoes extensive metabolism by CYP3A4; concomitant administration of strong inducers of CYP3A4 alter lapatinib concentrations significantly and should be avoided. Dose adjustment of lapatinib should be considered for patients who must receive concomitant strong inducers of CYP3A4 enzymes. Lapatinib inhibits CYP3A4 in vitro at clinically relevant concentrations. Caution should be exercised and dose reduction of the concomitant substrate drug should be considered when dosing lapatinib concurrently with medications with narrow therapeutic windows that are substrates of CYP3A4). Products include:

Analpram-HC 1140
Pramosone 1141

Hydrocortisone Butyrate (Lapatinib undergoes extensive metabolism by CYP3A4; concomitant administration of strong inducers of CYP3A4 alter lapatinib concentrations significantly and should be avoided. Dose adjustment of lapatinib should be considered for patients who must receive concomitant strong inducers of CYP3A4 enzymes. Lapatinib inhibits CYP3A4 in vitro at clinically relevant concentrations. Caution should be exercised and dose reduction of the concomitant substrate drug should be considered when dosing lapatinib concurrently with medications with narrow therapeutic windows that are substrates of CYP3A4).

No products indexed under this heading.

Hydrocortisone Cypionate (Lapatinib undergoes extensive metabolism by CYP3A4; concomitant administration of strong inducers of CYP3A4 alter lapatinib concentrations significantly and should be avoided. Dose adjustment of lapatinib should be considered for patients who must receive concomitant strong inducers of CYP3A4 enzymes. Lapatinib inhibits CYP3A4 in vitro at clinically relevant concentrations. Caution should be exercised and dose reduction of the concomitant substrate drug should be considered when dosing lapatinib concurrently with medications with narrow therapeutic windows that are substrates of CYP3A4).

No products indexed under this heading.

Hydrocortisone Hemisuccinate (Lapatinib undergoes extensive metabolism by CYP3A4; concomitant administration of strong inducers of CYP3A4 alter lapatinib concentrations significantly and should be avoided. Dose adjustment of lapatinib should be considered for patients who must receive concomitant strong inducers of CYP3A4 enzymes. Lapatinib inhibits CYP3A4 in vitro at clinically relevant concentrations. Caution should be exercised and dose reduction of the concomitant substrate drug should be considered when dosing lapatinib concurrently with medications with narrow therapeutic windows that are substrates of CYP3A4).

No products indexed under this heading.

Hydrocortisone Probutate (Lapatinib undergoes extensive metabolism by CYP3A4; concomitant administration of strong inducers of CYP3A4 alter lapatinib concentrations significantly and should be avoided. Dose adjustment of lapatinib should be considered for patients who must receive concomitant strong inducers of CYP3A4 enzymes. Lapatinib inhibits CYP3A4 in vitro at clinically relevant concentrations. Caution should be exercised and dose reduction of the concomitant substrate drug should be considered when dosing lapatinib concurrently with medications with narrow therapeutic windows that are substrates of CYP3A4).

No products indexed under this heading.

Hydrocortisone Sodium Phosphate (Lapatinib undergoes extensive metabolism by CYP3A4; concomitant administration of strong inducers of CYP3A4 alter lapatinib concentrations significantly and should be avoided. Dose adjustment of lapatinib should be considered for patients who must receive concomitant strong inducers of CYP3A4 enzymes. Lapatinib inhibits CYP3A4 in vitro at clinically relevant concentrations. Caution should be exercised and dose reduction of the concomitant substrate drug should be considered when dosing lapatinib concurrently with medications with narrow therapeutic windows that are substrates of CYP3A4).

No products indexed under this heading.

Hydrocortisone Sodium Succinate (Lapatinib undergoes extensive metabolism by CYP3A4; concomitant administration of strong inducers of CYP3A4 alter lapatinib concentrations significantly and should be avoided. Dose adjustment of lapatinib should be considered for patients who must receive concomitant strong inducers of CYP3A4 enzymes. Lapatinib inhibits CYP3A4 in vitro at clinically relevant concentrations. Caution should be exercised and dose reduction of the concomitant substrate drug should be considered when dosing lapatinib concurrently with medications with narrow therapeutic windows that are substrates of CYP3A4).

No products indexed under this heading.

Hydrocortisone Valerate (Lapatinib undergoes extensive metabolism by CYP3A4; concomitant administration of strong inducers of CYP3A4 alter lapatinib concentrations significantly and should be avoided. Dose adjustment of lapatinib should be considered for patients who must receive concomitant strong inducers of CYP3A4 enzymes. Lapatinib inhibits CYP3A4 in vitro at clinically relevant concentrations. Caution should be exercised and dose reduction of the concomitant substrate drug should be considered when dosing lapatinib concurrently with medications with narrow therapeutic windows that are substrates of CYP3A4).

No products indexed under this heading.

Hypericum (Lapatinib undergoes extensive metabolism by CYP3A4; concomitant administration of strong inducers of CYP3A4 alter lapatinib concentrations significantly and should be avoided. Dose adjustment of lapatinib should be considered for patients who must receive concomitant strong inducers of CYP3A4 enzymes. Lapatinib inhibits CYP3A4 in vitro at clinically relevant concentrations. Caution should be exercised and dose reduction of the concomitant substrate drug should be considered when dosing lapatinib concurrently with medications with narrow therapeutic windows that are substrates of CYP3A4). Products include:

Satieté Tablets 640

Hypericum Perforatum (Lapatinib undergoes extensive metabolism by CYP3A4; concomitant administration of strong inducers of CYP3A4 alter lapatinib concentrations significantly and should be avoided. Dose adjustment of lapatinib should be considered for patients who must receive concomitant strong inducers of CYP3A4 enzymes. Lapatinib inhibits CYP3A4 in vitro at clinically relevant concentrations. Caution should be exercised and dose reduction of the concomitant substrate drug should be considered when dosing lapatinib concurrently with medications with narrow therapeutic windows that are substrates of CYP3A4).

No products indexed under this heading.

Imipramine Hydrochloride (Lapatinib inhibits CYP2C8 in vitro at clinically relevant concentrations. Caution should be exercised and dose reduction of the concomitant substrate drug should be considered when dosing lapatinib concurrently with medications with narrow therapeutic windows that are substrates of CYP2C8).

No products indexed under this heading.

Imipramine Pamoate (Lapatinib inhibits CYP2C8 in vitro at clinically relevant concentrations. Caution should be exercised and dose reduction of the concomitant substrate drug should be considered when dosing lapatinib concurrently with medications with narrow therapeutic windows that are substrates of CYP2C8).

No products indexed under this heading.

Indinavir Sulfate (Lapatinib undergoes extensive metabolism by CYP3A4; concomitant administration of strong inhibitors of CYP3A4 alter lapatinib concentrations significantly and should be avoided. Dose adjustment of lapatinib should be considered for patients who must receive concomitant strong inhibitors of CYP3A4 enzymes. Lapatinib inhibits CYP3A4 in vitro at clinically relevant concentrations. Caution should be exercised and dose reduction of the concomitant substrate drug should be considered when dosing lapatinib concurrently with medications with narrow therapeutic windows that are substrates of CYP3A4). Products include:

Crixivan Capsules 1979

Isotretinoin (Lapatinib inhibits CYP2C8 in vitro at clinically relevant concentrations. Caution should be exercised and dose reduction of the concomitant substrate drug should be considered when dosing lapatinib concurrently with medications with narrow therapeutic windows that are substrates of CYP2C8). Products include:

Accutane Capsules 2607

Isradipine (Lapatinib inhibits CYP3A4 in vitro at clinically relevant concentrations. Caution should be exercised and dose reduction of the concomitant substrate drug should be considered when dosing lapatinib concurrently with medications with narrow therapeutic windows that are substrates of CYP3A4). Products include:

DynaCirc CR Controlled Release Tablets 1407

Itraconazole (Lapatinib undergoes extensive metabolism by CYP3A4; concomitant administration of strong inhibitors of CYP3A4 alter lapatinib concentrations significantly and should be avoided. Dose adjustment of lapatinib should be considered for patients who must receive concomitant strong inhibitors of CYP3A4 enzymes. Lapatinib inhibits CYP3A4 in vitro at clinically relevant concentrations. Caution should be exercised and dose reduction of the concomitant substrate drug should be considered when dosing lapatinib concurrently with medications with narrow therapeutic windows that are substrates of CYP3A4).

No products indexed under this heading.

Ixabepilone (Lapatinib inhibits CYP3A4 in vitro at clinically relevant concentrations. Caution should be exercised and dose reduction of the concomitant substrate drug should be considered when dosing lapatinib concurrently with medications with narrow therapeutic windows that are substrates of CYP3A4). Products include:

Ixempra Kit for Injection 915

Ketoconazole (Lapatinib undergoes extensive metabolism by

CYP3A4; concomitant administration of strong inhibitors of CYP3A4 alter lapatinib concentrations significantly and should be avoided. Dose adjustment of lapatinib should be considered for patients who must receive concomitant strong inhibitors of CYP3A4 enzymes. Lapatinib inhibits CYP3A4 in vitro at clinically relevant concentrations. Caution should be exercised and dose reduction of the concomitant substrate drug should be considered when dosing lapatinib concurrently with medications with narrow therapeutic windows that are substrates of CYP3A4). Products include:

Extina Foam, 2% 3057
Nizoral A-D Shampoo 1901

Levonorgestrel (Lapatinib inhibits CYP3A4 in vitro at clinically relevant concentrations. Caution should be exercised and dose reduction of the concomitant substrate drug should be considered when dosing lapatinib concurrently with medications with narrow therapeutic windows that are substrates of CYP3A4). Products include:

Climara Pro Transdermal System 768
Lybrel Tablets 3204
Mirena Intrauterine System 779
Plan B Tablets 1044
Seasonique Tablets 1046

Lidocaine (Lapatinib inhibits CYP3A4 in vitro at clinically relevant concentrations. Caution should be exercised and dose reduction of the concomitant substrate drug should be considered when dosing lapatinib concurrently with medications with narrow therapeutic windows that are substrates of CYP3A4). Products include:

Lidoderm Patch 1114

Lidocaine Hydrochloride (Lapatinib inhibits CYP3A4 in vitro at clinically relevant concentrations. Caution should be exercised and dose reduction of the concomitant substrate drug should be considered when dosing lapatinib concurrently with medications with narrow therapeutic windows that are substrates of CYP3A4).

No products indexed under this heading.

Lopinavir (Lapatinib undergoes extensive metabolism by CYP3A4; concomitant administration of strong inhibitors of CYP3A4 alter lapatinib concentrations significantly and should be avoided. Dose adjustment of lapatinib should be considered for patients who must receive concomitant strong inhibitors of CYP3A4 enzymes. Lapatinib inhibits CYP3A4 in vitro at clinically relevant concentrations. Caution should be exercised and dose reduction of the concomitant substrate drug should be considered when dosing lapatinib concurrently with medications with narrow therapeutic windows that are substrates of CYP3A4). Products include:

Kaletra 452

Lovastatin (Lapatinib inhibits CYP3A4 in vitro at clinically relevant concentrations. Caution should be exercised and dose reduction of the concomitant substrate drug should be considered when dosing lapatinib concurrently with medications with narrow therapeutic windows that are substrates of CYP3A4). Products include:

Advicor Tablets 402
Mevacor Tablets 2063

Maprotiline Hydrochloride (Lapatinib inhibits CYP2C8 in vitro at clinically relevant concentrations. Caution should be exercised and dose reduction of the concomitant substrate drug should be considered when dosing lapatinib concurrently with medications with narrow therapeutic windows that are substrates of CYP2C8).

No products indexed under this heading.

Mephenytoin (Lapatinib undergoes extensive metabolism by CYP3A4; concomitant administration of strong inducers of CYP3A4 alter lapatinib concentrations significantly and should be avoided. Dose adjustment of lapatinib should be considered for patients who must receive concomitant strong inducers of CYP3A4 enzymes. Lapatinib inhibits CYP3A4 in vitro at clinically relevant concentrations. Caution should be exercised and dose reduction of the concomitant substrate drug should be considered when dosing lapatinib concurrently with medications with narrow therapeutic windows that are substrates of CYP3A4).

No products indexed under this heading.

Mephobarbital (Lapatinib inhibits CYP2C8 in vitro at clinically relevant concentrations. Caution should be exercised and dose reduction of the concomitant substrate drug should be considered when dosing lapatinib concurrently with medications with narrow therapeutic windows that are substrates of CYP2C8).

No products indexed under this heading.

Mestranol (Lapatinib inhibits CYP3A4 in vitro at clinically relevant concentrations. Caution should be exercised and dose reduction of the concomitant substrate drug should be considered when dosing lapatinib concurrently with medications with narrow therapeutic windows that are substrates of CYP3A4).

No products indexed under this heading.

Methadone Hydrochloride (Lapatinib inhibits CYP3A4 in vitro at clinically relevant concentrations. Caution should be exercised and dose reduction of the concomitant substrate drug should be considered when dosing lapatinib concurrently with medications with narrow therapeutic windows that are substrates of CYP3A4).

No products indexed under this heading.

Methsuximide (Lapatinib undergoes extensive metabolism by CYP3A4; concomitant administration of strong inducers of CYP3A4 alter lapatinib concentrations significantly and should be avoided. Dose adjustment of lapatinib should be considered for patients who must receive concomitant strong inducers of CYP3A4 enzymes. Lapatinib inhibits CYP3A4 in vitro at clinically relevant concentrations. Caution should be exercised and dose reduction of the concomitant substrate drug should be considered when dosing lapatinib concurrently with medications with narrow therapeutic windows that are substrates of CYP3A4).

No products indexed under this heading.

Methylprednisolone (Lapatinib undergoes extensive metabolism by CYP3A4; concomitant administration of strong inducers of CYP3A4 alter lapatinib concentrations significantly and should be avoided. Dose adjustment of lapatinib should be considered for patients who must receive concomitant strong inducers of CYP3A4 enzymes. Lapatinib inhibits CYP3A4 in vitro at clinically relevant concentrations. Caution should be exercised and dose reduction of the concomitant substrate drug should be considered when dosing lapatinib concurrently with medications with narrow therapeutic windows that are substrates of CYP3A4).

No products indexed under this heading.

Methylprednisolone Acetate (Lapatinib undergoes extensive metabolism by CYP3A4; concomitant administration of strong inducers of CYP3A4 alter lapatinib concentrations significantly and should be avoided. Dose adjustment of lapatinib should be considered for patients who must receive concomitant strong inducers of CYP3A4 enzymes. Lapatinib inhibits CYP3A4 in vitro at clinically relevant concentrations. Caution should be exercised and dose reduction of the concomitant substrate drug should be considered when dosing lapatinib concurrently with medications with narrow therapeutic windows that are substrates of CYP3A4).

No products indexed under this heading.

Methylprednisolone Sodium Succinate (Lapatinib undergoes extensive metabolism by CYP3A4; concomitant administration of strong inducers of CYP3A4 alter lapatinib concentrations significantly and should be avoided. Dose adjustment of lapatinib should be considered for patients who must receive concomitant strong inducers of CYP3A4 enzymes. Lapatinib inhibits CYP3A4 in vitro at clinically relevant concentrations. Caution should be exercised and dose reduction of the concomitant substrate drug should be considered when dosing lapatinib concurrently with medications with narrow therapeutic windows that are substrates of CYP3A4).

No products indexed under this heading.

Midazolam Hydrochloride (Lapatinib inhibits CYP3A4 in vitro at clinically relevant concentrations. Caution should be exercised and dose reduction of the concomitant substrate drug should be considered when dosing lapatinib concurrently with medications with narrow therapeutic windows that are substrates of CYP3A4).

No products indexed under this heading.

Modafinil (Lapatinib undergoes extensive metabolism by CYP3A4; concomitant administration of strong inducers of CYP3A4 alter lapatinib concentrations significantly and should be avoided. Dose adjustment of lapatinib should be considered for patients who must receive concomitant strong inducers of CYP3A4 enzymes. Lapatinib inhibits CYP3A4 in vitro at clinically relevant concentrations. Caution should be exercised and dose reduction of the concomitant substrate drug should be considered when dosing lapatinib concurrently with medications with narrow therapeutic windows that are substrates of CYP3A4). Products include:

Provigil Tablets 977

Nefazodone Hydrochloride (Lapatinib undergoes extensive metabolism by CYP3A4; concomitant administration of strong inhibitors of CYP3A4 alter lapatinib concentrations significantly and should be avoided. Dose adjustment of lapatinib should be considered for patients who must receive concomitant strong inhibitors of CYP3A4 enzymes. Lapatinib inhibits CYP3A4 in vitro at clinically relevant concentrations. Caution should be exercised and dose reduction of the concomitant substrate drug should be considered when dosing lapatinib concurrently with medications with narrow therapeutic windows that are substrates of CYP3A4).

No products indexed under this heading.

Nelfinavir Mesylate (Lapatinib undergoes extensive metabolism by CYP3A4; concomitant administration of strong inhibitors of CYP3A4 alter lapatinib concentrations significantly and should be avoided. Dose adjustment of lapatinib should be considered for patients who must receive concomitant strong inhibitors of CYP3A4 enzymes. Lapatinib inhibits CYP3A4 in vitro at clinically relevant concentrations. Caution should be exercised and dose reduction of the concomitant substrate drug should be considered when dosing lapatinib concurrently with medications with narrow therapeutic windows that are substrates of CYP3A4).

No products indexed under this heading.

Nevirapine (Lapatinib undergoes extensive metabolism by CYP3A4; concomitant administration of strong inducers of CYP3A4 alter lapatinib concentrations significantly and should be avoided. Dose adjustment of lapatinib should be considered for patients who must receive concomitant strong inducers of CYP3A4 enzymes. Lapatinib inhibits CYP3A4 in vitro at clinically relevant concentrations. Caution should be exercised and dose reduction of the concomitant substrate drug should be considered when dosing lapatinib concurrently with medications with narrow therapeutic windows that are substrates of CYP3A4). Products include:

Viramune Oral Suspension 873
Viramune Tablets 873

Nicardipine Hydrochloride (Lapatinib inhibits CYP3A4 in vitro at clinically relevant concentrations. Caution should be exercised and dose reduction of the concomitant substrate drug should be considered when dosing lapatinib concurrently with medications with narrow therapeutic windows that are substrates of CYP3A4). Products include:

Cardene I.V. 1093

Nifedipine (Lapatinib inhibits CYP3A4 in vitro at clinically relevant concentrations. Caution should be exercised and dose reduction of the concomitant substrate drug should be considered when dosing lapatinib concurrently with medications with narrow therapeutic windows that are substrates of CYP3A4).

No products indexed under this heading.

Nimodipine (Lapatinib inhibits CYP3A4 in vitro at clinically relevant concentrations. Caution should be exercised and dose reduction of the concomitant substrate drug should be considered when dosing lapatinib concurrently with medications with narrow therapeutic windows that are substrates of CYP3A4). Products include:

Nimotop Capsules 790

Nisoldipine (Lapatinib inhibits CYP3A4 in vitro at clinically relevant concentrations. Caution should be exercised and dose reduction of the concomitant substrate drug should be considered when dosing lapatinib concurrently with medications with narrow therapeutic windows that are substrates of CYP3A4). Products include:

Sular Extended Release Tablets 2975

Nitrendipine (Lapatinib inhibits CYP3A4 in vitro at clinically relevant concentrations. Caution should be exercised and dose reduction of the concomitant substrate drug should be considered when dosing lapatinib concurrently with medications with narrow therapeutic windows that are substrates of CYP3A4).

No products indexed under this heading.

Norethindrone (Lapatinib inhibits CYP3A4 in vitro at clinically relevant concentrations. Caution should be exercised and dose reduction of the concomitant substrate drug should be considered when dosing lapatinib concurrently with medications with narrow therapeutic windows that are substrates of CYP3A4). Products include:

Ortho Micronor Tablets 2446

Norethindrone Acetate (Lapatinib inhibits CYP3A4 in vitro at clinically relevant concentrations. Caution should be exercised and dose reduction of the concomitant substrate drug should be considered when dosing lapatinib concurrently with medications with narrow therapeutic windows that are substrates of CYP3A4). Products include:

Activella Tablets 2347

Norgestrel (Lapatinib inhibits CYP3A4 in vitro at clinically relevant concentrations. Caution should be exercised and dose reduction of the concomitant substrate drug should be considered when dosing lapatinib concurrently with medications with narrow therapeutic windows that are substrates of CYP3A4).

No products indexed under this heading.

Nortriptyline Hydrochloride (Lapatinib inhibits CYP2C8 in vitro at clinically relevant concentrations. Caution should be exercised and dose reduction of the concomitant substrate drug should be considered when dosing lapatinib concurrently with medications with narrow therapeutic windows that are substrates of CYP2C8).

No products indexed under this heading.

Omeprazole (Lapatinib inhibits CYP2C8 in vitro at clinically relevant concentrations. Caution should be exercised and dose reduction of the concomitant substrate drug should be considered when dosing lapatinib concurrently with medications with narrow therapeutic windows that are substrates of CYP2C8).

No products indexed under this heading.

Ondansetron (Lapatinib inhibits CYP3A4 in vitro at clinically relevant concentrations. Caution should be exercised and dose reduction of the concomitant substrate drug should be considered when dosing lapatinib concurrently with medications with narrow therapeutic windows that are substrates of CYP3A4). Products include:

Zofran ODT Orally Disintegrating Tablets 1687

Ondansetron Hydrochloride (Lapatinib inhibits CYP3A4 in vitro at clinically relevant concentrations. Caution should be exercised and dose reduction of the concomitant substrate drug should be considered when dosing lapatinib concurrently with medications with narrow therapeutic windows that are substrates of CYP3A4). Products include:

Zofran Injection 1682
Zofran 1687

Oxcarbazepine (Lapatinib undergoes extensive metabolism by CYP3A4; concomitant administration of strong inducers of CYP3A4 alter lapatinib concentrations significantly and should be avoided. Dose adjustment of lapatinib should be considered for patients who must receive concomitant strong inducers of CYP3A4 enzymes. Lapatinib inhibits CYP3A4 in vitro at clinically relevant concentrations. Caution should be exercised and dose reduction of the concomitant substrate drug should be considered when dosing lapatinib concurrently with medications with narrow therapeutic windows that are substrates of CYP3A4).

No products indexed under this heading.

Paclitaxel (Lapatinib inhibits CYP2C8 in vitro at clinically relevant concentrations. Caution should be exercised and dose reduction of the concomitant substrate drug should be considered when dosing lapatinib concurrently with medications with narrow therapeutic windows that are substrates of CYP2C8).

No products indexed under this heading.

Phenobarbital (Lapatinib undergoes extensive metabolism by CYP3A4; concomitant administration of strong inducers of CYP3A4 alter lapatinib concentrations significantly and should be avoided. Dose adjustment of lapatinib should be considered for patients who must receive concomitant strong inducers of CYP3A4 enzymes. Lapatinib inhibits CYP3A4 in vitro at clinically relevant concentrations. Caution should be exercised and dose reduction of the concomitant substrate drug should be considered when dosing lapatinib concurrently with medications with narrow therapeutic windows that are substrates of CYP3A4). Products include:

Donnatal Extentabs 2507

Phenobarbital Sodium (Lapatinib undergoes extensive metabolism by CYP3A4; concomitant administration of strong inducers of CYP3A4 alter lapatinib concentrations significantly and should be avoided. Dose adjustment of lapatinib should be considered for patients who must receive concomitant strong inducers of CYP3A4 enzymes. Lapatinib inhibits CYP3A4 in vitro at clinically relevant concentrations. Caution should be exercised and dose reduction of the concomitant substrate drug should be considered when dosing lapatinib concurrently with medications with narrow therapeutic windows that are substrates of CYP3A4).

No products indexed under this heading.

Phenytoin (Lapatinib undergoes extensive metabolism by CYP3A4; concomitant administration of strong inducers of CYP3A4 alter lapatinib concentrations significantly and should be avoided. Dose adjustment of lapatinib should be considered for patients who must receive concomitant strong inducers of CYP3A4 enzymes. Lapatinib inhibits CYP3A4 in vitro at clinically relevant concentrations. Caution should be exercised and dose reduction of the concomitant substrate drug should be considered when dosing lapatinib concurrently with medications with narrow therapeutic windows that are substrates of CYP3A4).

No products indexed under this heading.

Phenytoin Sodium (Lapatinib undergoes extensive metabolism by CYP3A4; concomitant administration of strong inducers of CYP3A4 alter lapatinib concentrations significantly and should be avoided. Dose adjustment of lapatinib should be considered for patients who must receive concomitant strong inducers of CYP3A4 enzymes. Lapatinib inhibits CYP3A4 in vitro at clinically relevant concentrations. Caution should be exercised and dose reduction of the concomitant substrate drug should be considered when dosing lapatinib concurrently with medications with narrow therapeutic windows that are substrates of CYP3A4). Products include:

Phenytek Capsules 2192

Pimozide (Lapatinib inhibits CYP3A4 in vitro at clinically relevant concentrations. Caution should be exercised and dose reduction of the concomitant substrate drug should be considered when dosing lapatinib concurrently with medications with narrow therapeutic windows that are substrates of CYP3A4).

No products indexed under this heading.

Pioglitazone Hydrochloride (Lapatinib inhibits CYP2C8 in vitro at clinically relevant concentrations. Caution should be exercised and dose reduction of the concomitant substrate drug should be considered when dosing lapatinib concurrently with medications with narrow therapeutic windows that are substrates of CYP2C8). Products include:

ActoPlus Met Tablets 3071
Actos Tablets 3077
Duetact Tablets 3085

Polyestradiol Phosphate (Lapatinib inhibits CYP3A4 in vitro at clinically relevant concentrations. Caution should be exercised and dose reduction of the concomitant substrate drug should be considered when dosing lapatinib concurrently with medications with narrow therapeutic windows that are substrates of CYP3A4).

No products indexed under this heading.

Prednisolone Acetate (Lapatinib undergoes extensive metabolism by CYP3A4; concomitant administration of strong inducers of CYP3A4 alter lapatinib concentrations significantly and should be avoided. Dose adjustment of lapatinib should be considered for patients who must receive concomitant strong inducers of CYP3A4 enzymes. Lapatinib inhibits CYP3A4 in vitro at clinically relevant concentrations. Caution should be exercised and dose reduction of the concomitant substrate drug should be considered when dosing lapatinib concurrently with medications with narrow therapeutic windows that are substrates of CYP3A4). Products include:

Pred Forte Ophthalmic Suspension .... ⊙227
Pred Mild Ophthalmic Suspension .... ⊙230
Pred-G Ophthalmic Ointment .... ⊙229
Pred-G Ophthalmic Suspension .... ⊙228

Prednisolone Sodium Phosphate (Lapatinib undergoes extensive metabolism by CYP3A4; concomitant administration of strong inducers of CYP3A4 alter lapatinib concentrations significantly and should be avoided. Dose adjustment of lapatinib should be considered for patients who must receive concomitant strong inducers of CYP3A4 enzymes. Lapatinib inhibits CYP3A4 in vitro at clinically relevant concentrations. Caution should be exercised and dose reduction of the concomitant substrate drug should be considered when dosing lapatinib concurrently with medications with narrow therapeutic windows that are substrates of CYP3A4).

No products indexed under this heading.

Prednisolone Tebutate (Lapatinib undergoes extensive metabolism by CYP3A4; concomitant administration of strong inducers of CYP3A4 alter lapatinib concentrations significantly and should be avoided. Dose adjustment of lapatinib should be considered for patients who must receive concomitant strong inducers of CYP3A4 enzymes. Lapatinib inhibits CYP3A4 in vitro at clinically relevant concentrations. Caution should be exercised and dose reduction of the concomitant substrate drug should be considered when dosing lapatinib concurrently with medications with narrow therapeutic windows that are substrates of CYP3A4).

No products indexed under this heading.

Prednisone (Lapatinib undergoes extensive metabolism by CYP3A4; concomitant administration of strong inducers of CYP3A4 alter lapatinib concentrations significantly and should be avoided. Dose adjustment of lapatinib should be considered for patients who must receive concomitant strong inducers of CYP3A4 enzymes. Lapatinib inhibits CYP3A4 in vitro at clinically relevant concentrations. Caution should be exercised and dose reduction of the concomitant substrate drug should be considered when dosing lapatinib concurrently with medications with narrow therapeutic windows that are substrates of CYP3A4).

No products indexed under this heading.

Primidone (Lapatinib undergoes extensive metabolism by CYP3A4; concomitant administration of strong inducers of CYP3A4 alter lapatinib concentrations significantly and should be avoided. Dose adjustment of lapatinib should be considered for patients who must receive concomi-

tant strong inducers of CYP3A4 enzymes. Lapatinib inhibits CYP3A4 in vitro at clinically relevant concentrations. Caution should be exercised and dose reduction of the concomitant substrate drug should be considered when dosing lapatinib concurrently with medications with narrow therapeutic windows that are substrates of CYP3A4).

No products indexed under this heading.

Protriptyline Hydrochloride (Lapatinib inhibits CYP2C8 in vitro at clinically relevant concentrations. Caution should be exercised and dose reduction of the concomitant substrate drug should be considered when dosing lapatinib concurrently with medications with narrow therapeutic windows that are substrates of CYP2C8).

No products indexed under this heading.

Quinidine Gluconate (Lapatinib inhibits CYP3A4 in vitro at clinically relevant concentrations. Caution should be exercised and dose reduction of the concomitant substrate drug should be considered when dosing lapatinib concurrently with medications with narrow therapeutic windows that are substrates of CYP3A4).

No products indexed under this heading.

Quinidine Polygalacturonate (Lapatinib inhibits CYP3A4 in vitro at clinically relevant concentrations. Caution should be exercised and dose reduction of the concomitant substrate drug should be considered when dosing lapatinib concurrently with medications with narrow therapeutic windows that are substrates of CYP3A4).

No products indexed under this heading.

Quinidine Sulfate (Lapatinib inhibits CYP3A4 in vitro at clinically relevant concentrations. Caution should be exercised and dose reduction of the concomitant substrate drug should be considered when dosing lapatinib concurrently with medications with narrow therapeutic windows that are substrates of CYP3A4).

No products indexed under this heading.

Repaglinide (Lapatinib inhibits CYP2C8 in vitro at clinically relevant concentrations. Caution should be exercised and dose reduction of the concomitant substrate drug should be considered when dosing lapatinib concurrently with medications with narrow therapeutic windows that are substrates of CYP2C8). Products include:

PrandiMet Tablets 2967
Prandin Tablets 2971

Rifabutin (Lapatinib undergoes extensive metabolism by CYP3A4; concomitant administration of strong inducers of CYP3A4 alter lapatinib concentrations significantly and should be avoided. Dose adjustment of lapatinib should be considered for patients who must receive concomitant strong inducers of CYP3A4 enzymes. Lapatinib inhibits CYP3A4 in vitro at clinically relevant concentrations. Caution should be exercised and dose reduction of the concomitant substrate drug should be considered when dosing lapatinib concurrently with medications with narrow therapeutic windows that are substrates of CYP3A4).

No products indexed under this heading.

Rifampicin (Lapatinib undergoes extensive metabolism by CYP3A4; concomitant administration of strong inducers of CYP3A4 alter lapatinib concentrations significantly and should be avoided. Dose adjustment of lapatinib should be considered for patients who must receive concomitant strong inducers of CYP3A4 enzymes. Lapatinib inhibits CYP3A4 in vitro at clinically relevant concentrations. Caution should be exercised and dose reduction of the concomitant substrate drug should be considered when dosing lapatinib concurrently with medications with narrow therapeutic windows that are substrates of CYP3A4).

No products indexed under this heading.

Rifampin (Lapatinib undergoes extensive metabolism by CYP3A4; concomitant administration of strong inducers of CYP3A4 alter lapatinib concentrations significantly and should be avoided. Dose adjustment of lapatinib should be considered for patients who must receive concomitant strong inducers of CYP3A4 enzymes. Lapatinib inhibits CYP3A4 in vitro at clinically relevant concentrations. Caution should be exercised and dose reduction of the concomitant substrate drug should be considered when dosing lapatinib concurrently with medications with narrow therapeutic windows that are substrates of CYP3A4).

No products indexed under this heading.

Rifapentine (Lapatinib undergoes extensive metabolism by CYP3A4; concomitant administration of strong inducers of CYP3A4 alter lapatinib concentrations significantly and should be avoided. Dose adjustment of lapatinib should be considered for patients who must receive concomitant strong inducers of CYP3A4 enzymes. Lapatinib inhibits CYP3A4 in vitro at clinically relevant concentrations. Caution should be exercised and dose reduction of the concomitant substrate drug should be considered when dosing lapatinib concurrently with medications with narrow therapeutic windows that are substrates of CYP3A4).

No products indexed under this heading.

Ritonavir (Lapatinib undergoes extensive metabolism by CYP3A4; concomitant administration of strong inhibitors of CYP3A4 alter lapatinib concentrations significantly and should be avoided. Dose adjustment of lapatinib should be considered for patients who must receive concomitant strong inhibitors of CYP3A4 enzymes. Lapatinib inhibits CYP3A4 in vitro at clinically relevant concentrations. Caution should be exercised and dose reduction of the concomitant substrate drug should be considered when dosing lapatinib concurrently with medications with narrow therapeutic windows that are substrates of CYP3A4). Products include:

Kaletra 452
Norvir 489

Rosiglitazone Maleate (Lapatinib inhibits CYP2C8 in vitro at clinically relevant concentrations. Caution should be exercised and dose reduction of the concomitant substrate drug should be considered when dosing lapatinib concurrently with medications with narrow therapeutic windows that are substrates of CYP2C8). Products include:

Avandamet Tablets 1336
Avandaryl Tablets 1344
Avandia Tablets 1351

Rosiglitazone/Metformin (Lapatinib inhibits CYP2C8 in vitro at clinically relevant concentrations. Caution should be exercised and dose reduction of the concomitant substrate drug should be considered when dosing lapatinib concurrently with medications with narrow therapeutic windows that are substrates of CYP2C8).

No products indexed under this heading.

Saquinavir (Lapatinib undergoes extensive metabolism by CYP3A4; concomitant administration of strong inhibitors of CYP3A4 alter lapatinib concentrations significantly and should be avoided. Dose adjustment of lapatinib should be considered for patients who must receive concomitant strong inhibitors of CYP3A4 enzymes. Lapatinib inhibits CYP3A4 in vitro at clinically relevant concentrations. Caution should be exercised and dose reduction of the concomitant substrate drug should be considered when dosing lapatinib concurrently with medications with narrow therapeutic windows that are substrates of CYP3A4).

No products indexed under this heading.

Saquinavir Mesylate (Lapatinib undergoes extensive metabolism by CYP3A4; concomitant administration of strong inhibitors of CYP3A4 alter lapatinib concentrations significantly and should be avoided. Dose adjustment of lapatinib should be considered for patients who must receive concomitant strong inhibitors of CYP3A4 enzymes. Lapatinib inhibits CYP3A4 in vitro at clinically relevant concentrations. Caution should be exercised and dose reduction of the concomitant substrate drug should be considered when dosing lapatinib concurrently with medications with narrow therapeutic windows that are substrates of CYP3A4).

No products indexed under this heading.

Sertraline Hydrochloride (Lapatinib inhibits CYP3A4 in vitro at clinically relevant concentrations. Caution should be exercised and dose reduction of the concomitant substrate drug should be considered when dosing lapatinib concurrently with medications with narrow therapeutic windows that are substrates of CYP3A4).

No products indexed under this heading.

Sildenafil Citrate (Lapatinib inhibits CYP3A4 in vitro at clinically relevant concentrations. Caution should be exercised and dose reduction of the concomitant substrate drug should be considered when dosing lapatinib concurrently with medications with narrow therapeutic windows that are substrates of CYP3A4).

No products indexed under this heading.

Simvastatin (Lapatinib inhibits CYP3A4 in vitro at clinically relevant concentrations. Caution should be exercised and dose reduction of the concomitant substrate drug should be considered when dosing lapatinib concurrently with medications with narrow therapeutic windows that are substrates of CYP3A4). Products include:

Simcor Tablets 502
Vytorin 10/10 Tablets 2149
Vytorin 10/10 Tablets 2939
Vytorin 10/20 Tablets 2149
Vytorin 10/20 Tablets 2939
Vytorin 10/40 Tablets 2149
Vytorin 10/40 Tablets 2939
Vytorin 10/80 Tablets 2149
Vytorin 10/80 Tablets 2939
Zocor Tablets 2136

Sirolimus (Lapatinib inhibits CYP3A4 in vitro at clinically relevant concentrations. Caution should be exercised and dose reduction of the concomitant substrate drug should be considered when dosing lapatinib concurrently with medications with narrow therapeutic windows that are substrates of CYP3A4). Products include:

Rapamune 3260

Sulfinpyrazone (Lapatinib undergoes extensive metabolism by CYP3A4; concomitant administration of strong inducers of CYP3A4 alter lapatinib concentrations significantly and should be avoided. Dose adjustment of lapatinib should be considered for patients who must receive concomitant strong inducers of CYP3A4 enzymes. Lapatinib inhibits CYP3A4 in vitro at clinically relevant concentrations. Caution should be exercised and dose reduction of the concomitant substrate drug should be considered when dosing lapatinib concurrently with medications with narrow therapeutic windows that are substrates of CYP3A4).

No products indexed under this heading.

Tacrolimus (Lapatinib inhibits CYP3A4 in vitro at clinically relevant concentrations. Caution should be exercised and dose reduction of the concomitant substrate drug should be considered when dosing lapatinib concurrently with medications with narrow therapeutic windows that are substrates of CYP3A4). Products include:

Prograf Capsules and Injection 622
Protopic Ointment 628

Tadalafil (Lapatinib inhibits CYP3A4 in vitro at clinically relevant concentrations. Caution should be exercised and dose reduction of the concomitant substrate drug should be considered when dosing lapatinib concurrently with medications with narrow therapeutic windows that are substrates of CYP3A4). Products include:

Cialis Tablets 1792

Tamoxifen Citrate (Lapatinib inhibits CYP3A4 in vitro at clinically relevant concentrations. Caution should be exercised and dose reduction of the concomitant substrate drug should be considered when dosing lapatinib concurrently with medications with narrow therapeutic windows that are substrates of CYP3A4).

No products indexed under this heading.

Telithromycin (Lapatinib undergoes extensive metabolism by CYP3A4; concomitant administration of strong inhibitors of CYP3A4 alter lapatinib concentrations significantly and

should be avoided. Dose adjustment of lapatinib should be considered for patients who must receive concomitant strong inhibitors of CYP3A4 enzymes. Lapatinib inhibits CYP3A4 in vitro at clinically relevant concentrations. Caution should be exercised and dose reduction of the concomitant substrate drug should be considered when dosing lapatinib concurrently with medications with narrow therapeutic windows that are substrates of CYP3A4). Products include:

Ketek Tablets 2744

Theophylline (Lapatinib undergoes extensive metabolism by CYP3A4; concomitant administration of strong inducers of CYP3A4 alter lapatinib concentrations significantly and should be avoided. Dose adjustment of lapatinib should be considered for patients who must receive concomitant strong inducers of CYP3A4 enzymes. Lapatinib inhibits CYP3A4 in vitro at clinically relevant concentrations. Caution should be exercised and dose reduction of the concomitant substrate drug should be considered when dosing lapatinib concurrently with medications with narrow therapeutic windows that are substrates of CYP3A4).

No products indexed under this heading.

Theophylline Anhydrous (Lapatinib undergoes extensive metabolism by CYP3A4; concomitant administration of strong inducers of CYP3A4 alter lapatinib concentrations significantly and should be avoided. Dose adjustment of lapatinib should be considered for patients who must receive concomitant strong inducers of CYP3A4 enzymes. Lapatinib inhibits CYP3A4 in vitro at clinically relevant concentrations. Caution should be exercised and dose reduction of the concomitant substrate drug should be considered when dosing lapatinib concurrently with medications with narrow therapeutic windows that are substrates of CYP3A4). Products include:

Uniphyl Tablets 2595

Theophylline Calcium Salicylate (Lapatinib undergoes extensive metabolism by CYP3A4; concomitant administration of strong inducers of CYP3A4 alter lapatinib concentrations significantly and should be avoided. Dose adjustment of lapatinib should be considered for patients who must receive concomitant strong inducers of CYP3A4 enzymes. Lapatinib inhibits CYP3A4 in vitro at clinically relevant concentrations. Caution should be exercised and dose reduction of the concomitant substrate drug should be considered when dosing lapatinib concurrently with medications with narrow therapeutic windows that are substrates of CYP3A4).

No products indexed under this heading.

Theophylline Dihydroxypropyl (Glyceryl) (Lapatinib undergoes extensive metabolism by CYP3A4; concomitant administration of strong inducers of CYP3A4 alter lapatinib concentrations significantly and should be avoided. Dose adjustment of lapatinib should be considered for patients who must receive concomitant strong inducers of CYP3A4 enzymes. Lapatinib inhibits CYP3A4 in vitro at clinically relevant concentrations. Caution should be exercised and dose reduction of the concomitant substrate drug should be considered when dosing lapatinib concurrently with medications with narrow therapeutic windows that are substrates of CYP3A4).

No products indexed under this heading.

Theophylline Ethylenediamine (Lapatinib undergoes extensive metabolism by CYP3A4; concomitant administration of strong inducers of CYP3A4 alter lapatinib concentrations significantly and should be avoided. Dose adjustment of lapatinib should be considered for patients who must receive concomitant strong inducers of CYP3A4 enzymes. Lapatinib inhibits CYP3A4 in vitro at clinically relevant concentrations. Caution should be exercised and dose reduction of the concomitant substrate drug should be considered when dosing lapatinib concurrently with medications with narrow therapeutic windows that are substrates of CYP3A4).

No products indexed under this heading.

Tiagabine Hydrochloride (Lapatinib inhibits CYP3A4 in vitro at clinically relevant concentrations. Caution should be exercised and dose reduction of the concomitant substrate drug should be considered when dosing lapatinib concurrently with medications with narrow therapeutic windows that are substrates of CYP3A4). Products include:

Gabitril Tablets 973

Tirofiban Hydrochloride (Lapatinib is a subtrate of the efflux transporter P-glycoprotein (Pgp, ABCB1). If lapatinib is administered with drugs that inhibit Pgp, increased concentrations of lapatinib are likely, and caution should be exercised).

No products indexed under this heading.

Tolbutamide (Lapatinib inhibits CYP2C8 in vitro at clinically relevant concentrations. Caution should be exercised and dose reduction of the concomitant substrate drug should be considered when dosing lapatinib concurrently with medications with narrow therapeutic windows that are substrates of CYP2C8).

No products indexed under this heading.

Tolbutamide Sodium (Lapatinib inhibits CYP2C8 in vitro at clinically relevant concentrations. Caution should be exercised and dose reduction of the concomitant substrate drug should be considered when dosing lapatinib concurrently with medications with narrow therapeutic windows that are substrates of CYP2C8).

No products indexed under this heading.

Tolterodine Tartrate (Lapatinib inhibits CYP3A4 in vitro at clinically relevant concentrations. Caution should be exercised and dose reduction of the concomitant substrate drug should be considered when dosing lapatinib concurrently with medications with narrow therapeutic windows that are substrates of CYP3A4).

No products indexed under this heading.

Trazodone Hydrochloride (Lapatinib inhibits CYP3A4 in vitro at clinically relevant concentrations. Caution should be exercised and dose reduction of the concomitant substrate drug should be considered when dosing lapatinib concurrently with medications with narrow therapeutic windows that are substrates of CYP3A4).

No products indexed under this heading.

Tretinoin (Lapatinib inhibits CYP2C8 in vitro at clinically relevant concentrations. Caution should be exercised and dose reduction of the concomitant substrate drug should be considered when dosing lapatinib concurrently with medications with narrow therapeutic windows that are substrates of CYP2C8). Products include:

Vesanoid Capsules 2660
Ziana Gel 1942

Triamcinolone (Lapatinib undergoes extensive metabolism by CYP3A4; concomitant administration of strong inducers of CYP3A4 alter lapatinib concentrations significantly and should be avoided. Dose adjustment of lapatinib should be considered for patients who must receive concomitant strong inducers of CYP3A4 enzymes. Lapatinib inhibits CYP3A4 in vitro at clinically relevant concentrations. Caution should be exercised and dose reduction of the concomitant substrate drug should be considered when dosing lapatinib concurrently with medications with narrow therapeutic windows that are substrates of CYP3A4).

No products indexed under this heading.

Triamcinolone Acetonide (Lapatinib undergoes extensive metabolism by CYP3A4; concomitant administration of strong inducers of CYP3A4 alter lapatinib concentrations significantly and should be avoided. Dose adjustment of lapatinib should be considered for patients who must receive concomitant strong inducers of CYP3A4 enzymes. Lapatinib inhibits CYP3A4 in vitro at clinically relevant concentrations. Caution should be exercised and dose reduction of the concomitant substrate drug should be considered when dosing lapatinib concurrently with medications with narrow therapeutic windows that are substrates of CYP3A4). Products include:

Azmacort Inhalation Aerosol 407
Nasacort AQ Nasal Spray 2765
Triesence Injectable Suspension .... ⊙209

Triamcinolone Diacetate (Lapatinib undergoes extensive metabolism by CYP3A4; concomitant administration of strong inducers of CYP3A4 alter lapatinib concentrations significantly and should be avoided. Dose adjustment of lapatinib should be considered for patients who must receive concomitant strong inducers of CYP3A4 enzymes. Lapatinib inhibits CYP3A4 in vitro at clinically relevant concentrations. Caution should be exercised and dose reduction of the concomitant substrate drug should be considered when dosing lapatinib concurrently with medications with narrow therapeutic windows that are substrates of CYP3A4).

No products indexed under this heading.

Triamcinolone Hexacetonide (Lapatinib undergoes extensive metabolism by CYP3A4; concomitant administration of strong inducers of CYP3A4 alter lapatinib concentrations significantly and should be avoided. Dose adjustment of lapatinib should be considered for patients who must receive concomitant strong inducers of CYP3A4 enzymes. Lapatinib inhibits CYP3A4 in vitro at clinically relevant concentrations. Caution should be exercised and dose reduction of the concomitant substrate drug should be considered when dosing lapatinib concurrently with medications with narrow therapeutic windows that are substrates of CYP3A4).

No products indexed under this heading.

Triazolam (Lapatinib inhibits CYP3A4 in vitro at clinically relevant concentrations. Caution should be exercised and dose reduction of the concomitant substrate drug should be considered when dosing lapatinib concurrently with medications with narrow therapeutic windows that are substrates of CYP3A4).

No products indexed under this heading.

Trimipramine Maleate (Lapatinib inhibits CYP2C8 in vitro at clinically relevant concentrations. Caution should be exercised and dose reduction of the concomitant substrate drug should be considered when dosing lapatinib concurrently with medications with narrow therapeutic windows that are substrates of CYP2C8).

No products indexed under this heading.

Troglitazone (Lapatinib undergoes extensive metabolism by CYP3A4; concomitant administration of strong inducers of CYP3A4 alter lapatinib concentrations significantly and should be avoided. Dose adjustment of lapatinib should be considered for patients who must receive concomitant strong inducers of CYP3A4 enzymes. Lapatinib inhibits CYP3A4 in vitro at clinically relevant concentrations. Caution should be exercised and dose reduction of the concomitant substrate drug should be considered when dosing lapatinib concurrently with medications with narrow therapeutic windows that are substrates of CYP3A4).

No products indexed under this heading.

Troleandomycin (Lapatinib undergoes extensive metabolism by CYP3A4; concomitant administration of strong inhibitors of CYP3A4 alter lapatinib concentrations significantly and should be avoided. Dose adjustment of lapatinib should be considered for patients who must receive concomitant strong inhibitors of CYP3A4 enzymes. Lapatinib inhibits CYP3A4 in vitro at clinically relevant concentrations. Caution should be exercised and dose reduction of the concomitant substrate drug should be considered when dosing lapatinib concurrently with medications with narrow therapeutic windows that are substrates of CYP3A4).

No products indexed under this heading.

Vardenafil Hydrochloride (Lapatinib inhibits CYP3A4 in vitro at clinically relevant concentrations. Caution should be exercised and dose reduction of the concomitant substrate drug should be considered when dosing lapatinib concurrently with medications with narrow therapeutic windows that are substrates of CYP3A4). Products include:

Levitra Tablets 2876

Verapamil Hydrochloride (Lapatinib inhibits CYP2C8 in vitro at clinically relevant concentrations. Caution should be exercised and dose reduction of the concomitant substrate drug should be considered when dosing lapatinib concurrently with medications with narrow therapeutic windows that are substrates of CYP2C8). Products include:

Tarka Tablets 511

Vinblastine Sulfate (Lapatinib inhibits CYP3A4 in vitro at clinically relevant concentrations. Caution should be exercised and dose reduction of the concomitant substrate drug should be considered when dosing lapatinib concurrently with medications with narrow therapeutic windows that are substrates of CYP3A4).

No products indexed under this heading.

Vincristine Sulfate (Lapatinib inhibits CYP3A4 in vitro at clinically relevant concentrations. Caution should be exercised and dose reduction of the concomitant substrate drug should be considered when dosing lapatinib concurrently with medications with narrow therapeutic windows that are substrates of CYP3A4).

No products indexed under this heading.

Vitamin A (Lapatinib inhibits CYP2C8 in vitro at clinically relevant concentrations. Caution should be exercised and dose reduction of the concomitant substrate drug should be considered when dosing lapatinib concurrently with medications with narrow therapeutic windows that are substrates of CYP2C8). Products include:

Norwegian Cod Liver Oil 949

Vitamin A Acetate (Lapatinib inhibits CYP2C8 in vitro at clinically relevant concentrations. Caution should be exercised and dose reduction of the concomitant substrate drug should be considered when dosing lapatinib concurrently with medications with narrow therapeutic windows that are substrates of CYP2C8).

No products indexed under this heading.

Voriconazole (Lapatinib undergoes extensive metabolism by CYP3A4; concomitant administration of strong inhibitors of CYP3A4 alter lapatinib concentrations significantly and should be avoided. Dose adjustment of lapatinib should be considered for patients who must receive concomitant strong inhibitors of CYP3A4 enzymes. Lapatinib inhibits CYP3A4 in vitro at clinically relevant concentrations. Caution should be exercised and dose reduction of the concomitant substrate drug should be considered when dosing lapatinib concurrently with medications with narrow therapeutic windows that are substrates of CYP3A4).

No products indexed under this heading.

Warfarin Sodium (Lapatinib inhibits CYP2C8 in vitro at clinically relevant concentrations. Caution should be exercised and dose reduction of the concomitant substrate drug should be considered when dosing lapatinib concurrently with medications with narrow therapeutic windows that are substrates of CYP2C8).

No products indexed under this heading.

Zopiclone (Lapatinib inhibits CYP2C8 in vitro at clinically relevant concentrations. Caution should be exercised and dose reduction of the concomitant substrate drug should be considered when dosing lapatinib concurrently with medications with narrow therapeutic windows that are substrates of CYP2C8).

No products indexed under this heading.

Food Interactions

Grapefruit (Grapefruit may also increase plasma concentrations of lapatinib and should be avoided).

Grapefruit Juice (Grapefruit may also increase plasma concentrations of lapatinib and should be avoided).

REGULAR STRENGTH TYLENOL TABLETS

(Acetaminophen) 1915

Food Interactions

Alcohol (Chronic heavy alcohol users, 3 or more drinks per day, should consult their physicians for advice on when and how they should take pain relievers including acetaminophen).

TYLENOL 8 HOUR EXTENDED RELEASE CAPLETS

(Acetaminophen) 1915

See Regular Strength Tylenol Tablets

EXTRA STRENGTH TYLENOL CAPLETS, COOL CAPLETS, AND EZ TABS

(Acetaminophen) 1915

See Regular Strength Tylenol Tablets

EXTRA STRENGTH TYLENOL ADULT RAPID BLAST LIQUID

(Acetaminophen) 1915

See Regular Strength Tylenol Tablets

EXTRA STRENGTH TYLENOL PM CAPLETS, GELTABS, LIQUID, AND RAPID RELEASE GELS

(Acetaminophen, Diphenhydramine Hydrochloride).............................. 1915

May interact with hypnotics and sedatives, tranquilizers, and certain other agents. Compounds in these categories include:

Alprazolam (Concurrent use may increase the drowsiness effect).

No products indexed under this heading.

Buspirone Hydrochloride (Concurrent use may increase the drowsiness effect).

No products indexed under this heading.

Butabarbital (Concurrent use may increase the drowsiness effect).

No products indexed under this heading.

Butabarbital Sodium (Concurrent use may increase the drowsiness effect).

No products indexed under this heading.

Chloral Hydrate (Concurrent use may increase the drowsiness effect).

No products indexed under this heading.

Chlordiazepoxide (Concurrent use may increase the drowsiness effect).

No products indexed under this heading.

Chlordiazepoxide Hydrochloride (Concurrent use may increase the drowsiness effect).

No products indexed under this heading.

Chlorpromazine (Concurrent use may increase the drowsiness effect).

No products indexed under this heading.

Chlorpromazine Hydrochloride (Concurrent use may increase the drowsiness effect).

No products indexed under this heading.

Chlorprothixene (Concurrent use may increase the drowsiness effect).

No products indexed under this heading.

Chlorprothixene Hydrochloride (Concurrent use may increase the drowsiness effect).

No products indexed under this heading.

Clorazepate Dipotassium (Concurrent use may increase the drowsiness effect).

No products indexed under this heading.

Diazepam (Concurrent use may increase the drowsiness effect). Products include:

Valium Tablets 2658

Droperidol (Concurrent use may increase the drowsiness effect).

No products indexed under this heading.

Estazolam (Concurrent use may increase the drowsiness effect).

No products indexed under this heading.

Ethchlorvynol (Concurrent use may increase the drowsiness effect).

No products indexed under this heading.

Ethinamate (Concurrent use may increase the drowsiness effect).

No products indexed under this heading.

Fluphenazine Decanoate (Concurrent use may increase the drowsiness effect).

No products indexed under this heading.

Fluphenazine Enanthate (Concurrent use may increase the drowsiness effect).

No products indexed under this heading.

Fluphenazine Hydrochloride (Concurrent use may increase the drowsiness effect).

No products indexed under this heading.

Flurazepam Hydrochloride (Concurrent use may increase the drowsiness effect).

No products indexed under this heading.

Glutethimide (Concurrent use may increase the drowsiness effect).

No products indexed under this heading.

Haloperidol (Concurrent use may increase the drowsiness effect).

No products indexed under this heading.

Haloperidol Decanoate (Concurrent use may increase the drowsiness effect).

No products indexed under this heading.

Hydroxyzine Hydrochloride (Concurrent use may increase the drowsiness effect).

No products indexed under this heading.

Lorazepam (Concurrent use may increase the drowsiness effect).

No products indexed under this heading.

Loxapine Hydrochloride (Concurrent use may increase the drowsiness effect).

No products indexed under this heading.

Loxapine Succinate (Concurrent use may increase the drowsiness effect).

No products indexed under this heading.

Meprobamate (Concurrent use may increase the drowsiness effect).

No products indexed under this heading.

Mesoridazine Besylate (Concurrent use may increase the drowsiness effect).

No products indexed under this heading.

Midazolam Hydrochloride (Concurrent use may increase the drowsiness effect).

No products indexed under this heading.

Molindone Hydrochloride (Concurrent use may increase the drowsiness effect). Products include:

Moban Tablets 1116

Oxazepam (Concurrent use may increase the drowsiness effect).

No products indexed under this heading.

Perphenazine (Concurrent use may increase the drowsiness effect).

No products indexed under this heading.

Prazepam (Concurrent use may increase the drowsiness effect).

No products indexed under this heading.

Prochlorperazine (Concurrent use may increase the drowsiness effect).

No products indexed under this heading.

Promethazine Hydrochloride (Concurrent use may increase the drowsiness effect).

No products indexed under this heading.

Propofol (Concurrent use may increase the drowsiness effect).

No products indexed under this heading.

Quazepam (Concurrent use may increase the drowsiness effect).

No products indexed under this heading.

Ramelteon (Concurrent use may increase the drowsiness effect). Products include:

Rozerem Tablets 3091

Secobarbital Sodium (Concurrent use may increase the drowsiness effect).

No products indexed under this heading.

Sodium Butabarbital (Concurrent use may increase the drowsiness effect).
No products indexed under this heading.

Temazepam (Concurrent use may increase the drowsiness effect).
No products indexed under this heading.

Thioridazine Hydrochloride (Concurrent use may increase the drowsiness effect). Products include:
Thioridazine Hydrochloride Tablets 2195

Thiothixene (Concurrent use may increase the drowsiness effect). Products include:
Thiothixene Capsules 2197

Triazolam (Concurrent use may increase the drowsiness effect).
No products indexed under this heading.

Trifluoperazine Hydrochloride (Concurrent use may increase the drowsiness effect).
No products indexed under this heading.

Zaleplon (Concurrent use may increase the drowsiness effect).
No products indexed under this heading.

Zolpidem Tartrate (Concurrent use may increase the drowsiness effect). Products include:
Ambien Tablets 2692
Ambien CR Tablets 2696

Food Interactions

Alcohol (Concurrent use may increase drowsiness effect; chronic heavy alcohol abusers, 3 or more drinks per day, may be at increased risk of liver toxicity from excessive acetaminophen use).

EXTRA STRENGTH TYLENOL RAPID RELEASE GELS

(Acetaminophen) 1915
See Regular Strength Tylenol Tablets

TYLENOL WITH CODEINE TABLETS

(Acetaminophen, Codeine Phosphate) 2427
May interact with central nervous system depressants, general anesthetics, hypnotics and sedatives, narcotic analgesics, tranquilizers, and certain other agents. Compounds in these categories include:

Alfentanil Hydrochloride (Concomitant use with other CNS depressants may produce an additive CNS depression and should be avoided).
No products indexed under this heading.

Alprazolam (Concomitant use with other CNS depressants may produce an additive CNS depression and should be avoided).
No products indexed under this heading.

Aprobarbital (Concomitant use with other CNS depressants may produce an additive CNS depression and should be avoided).
No products indexed under this heading.

Buprenorphine Hydrochloride (Concomitant use with other CNS depressants may produce an additive CNS depression and should be avoided). Products include:
Suboxone Tablets 2601
Subutex Tablets 2601

Buspirone Hydrochloride (Concomitant use with other CNS depressants may produce an additive CNS depression and should be avoided).
No products indexed under this heading.

Butabarbital (Concomitant use with other CNS depressants may produce an additive CNS depression and should be avoided).
No products indexed under this heading.

Butabarbital Sodium (Concomitant use may enhance the effects of sedative-hypnotics, causing increased CNS depression).
No products indexed under this heading.

Butalbital (Concomitant use with other CNS depressants may produce an additive CNS depression and should be avoided).
No products indexed under this heading.

Chloral Hydrate (Concomitant use may enhance the effects of sedative-hypnotics, causing increased CNS depression).
No products indexed under this heading.

Chlordiazepoxide (Concomitant use may enhance the effects of tranquilizers such as chlordiazepoxide, causing increased CNS depression).
No products indexed under this heading.

Chlordiazepoxide Hydrochloride (Concomitant use may enhance the effects of tranquilizers such as chlordiazepoxide, causing increased CNS depression).
No products indexed under this heading.

Chlorpromazine (Concomitant use with other CNS depressants may produce an additive CNS depression and should be avoided).
No products indexed under this heading.

Chlorpromazine Hydrochloride (Concomitant use with other CNS depressants may produce an additive CNS depression and should be avoided).
No products indexed under this heading.

Chlorprothixene (Concomitant use with other CNS depressants may produce an additive CNS depression and should be avoided).
No products indexed under this heading.

Chlorprothixene Hydrochloride (Concomitant use with other CNS depressants may produce an additive CNS depression and should be avoided).
No products indexed under this heading.

Chlorprothixene Lactate (Concomitant use with other CNS depressants may produce an additive CNS depression and should be avoided).
No products indexed under this heading.

Clorazepate Dipotassium (Concomitant use with other CNS depressants may produce an additive CNS depression and should be avoided).
No products indexed under this heading.

Clozapine (Concomitant use with other CNS depressants may produce an additive CNS depression and should be avoided).
No products indexed under this heading.

Desflurane (Concomitant use with other CNS depressants may produce an additive CNS depression and should be avoided).
No products indexed under this heading.

Dezocine (Concomitant use with other CNS depressants may produce an additive CNS depression and should be avoided).
No products indexed under this heading.

Diazepam (Concomitant use with other CNS depressants may produce an additive CNS depression and should be avoided). Products include:
Valium Tablets 2658

Droperidol (Concomitant use with other CNS depressants may produce an additive CNS depression and should be avoided).
No products indexed under this heading.

Enflurane (Concomitant use with other CNS depressants may produce an additive CNS depression and should be avoided).
No products indexed under this heading.

Estazolam (Concomitant use with other CNS depressants may produce an additive CNS depression and should be avoided).
No products indexed under this heading.

Ethanol (Concomitant use with alcohol may produce an additive CNS depression and should be avoided).
No products indexed under this heading.

Ethchlorvynol (Concomitant use with other CNS depressants may produce an additive CNS depression and should be avoided).
No products indexed under this heading.

Ethinamate (Concomitant use with other CNS depressants may produce an additive CNS depression and should be avoided).
No products indexed under this heading.

Ethyl Alcohol (Concomitant use with alcohol may produce an additive CNS depression and should be avoided).
No products indexed under this heading.

Fentanyl (Concomitant use with other CNS depressants may produce an additive CNS depression and should be avoided). Products include:
Duragesic Transdermal System 2405
Ionsys Transdermal System 2410

Fentanyl Citrate (Concomitant use with other CNS depressants may produce an additive CNS depression and should be avoided). Products include:
Actiq 959
Fentora Tablets 968

Fluphenazine Decanoate (Concomitant use with other CNS depressants may produce an additive CNS depression and should be avoided).
No products indexed under this heading.

Fluphenazine Enanthate (Concomitant use with other CNS depressants may produce an additive CNS depression and should be avoided).
No products indexed under this heading.

Fluphenazine Hydrochloride (Concomitant use with other CNS depressants may produce an additive CNS depression and should be avoided).
No products indexed under this heading.

Flurazepam Hydrochloride (Concomitant use with other CNS depressants may produce an additive CNS depression and should be avoided).
No products indexed under this heading.

Glutethimide (Concomitant use with other CNS depressants may produce an additive CNS depression and should be avoided).
No products indexed under this heading.

Haloperidol (Concomitant use with other CNS depressants may produce an additive CNS depression and should be avoided).
No products indexed under this heading.

Haloperidol Decanoate (Concomitant use with other CNS depressants may produce an additive CNS depression and should be avoided).
No products indexed under this heading.

Hydrocodone Bitartrate (Concomitant use with other CNS depressants may produce an additive CNS depression and should be avoided). Products include:
Lortab 5/500 Tablets 3143
Lortab 7.5/500 Tablets 3144
Lortab 10/500 Tablets 3144
Vicodin Tablets 529
Vicodin ES Tablets 530
Vicodin HP Tablets 531
Vicoprofen Tablets 533
Zydone Tablets 1132

Hydrocodone Polistirex (Concomitant use with other CNS depressants may produce an additive CNS depression and should be avoided). Products include:
Tussionex Pennkinetic Extended-Release Suspension 3154

Hydromorphone Hydrochloride (Concomitant use with other CNS depressants may produce an additive CNS depression and should be avoided).
No products indexed under this heading.

Hydroxyzine Hydrochloride (Concomitant use with other CNS depressants may produce an additive CNS depression and should be avoided).
No products indexed under this heading.

Isoflurane (Concomitant use with other CNS depressants may produce an additive CNS depression and should be avoided).
No products indexed under this heading.

Ketamine Hydrochloride (Concomitant use with other CNS depressants may produce an additive CNS depression and should be avoided).
No products indexed under this heading.

Levomethadyl Acetate Hydrochloride (Concomitant use with other CNS depressants may produce an additive CNS depression and should be avoided).
No products indexed under this heading.

Levorphanol Tartrate (Concomitant use with other CNS depressants may produce an additive CNS depression and should be avoided).
No products indexed under this heading.

Lorazepam (Concomitant use with other CNS depressants may produce an additive CNS depression and should be avoided).
No products indexed under this heading.

Loxapine Hydrochloride (Concomitant use with other CNS depressants may produce an additive CNS depression and should be avoided).
No products indexed under this heading.

Loxapine Succinate (Concomitant use with other CNS depressants may produce an additive CNS depression and should be avoided).
No products indexed under this heading.

Meperidine Hydrochloride (Concomitant use with other CNS depressants may produce an additive CNS depression and should be avoided).
No products indexed under this heading.

Mephobarbital (Concomitant use with other CNS depressants may produce an additive CNS depression and should be avoided).
No products indexed under this heading.

Meprobamate (Concomitant use with other CNS depressants may produce an additive CNS depression and should be avoided).
No products indexed under this heading.

Mesoridazine Besylate (Concomitant use with other CNS depressants may produce an additive CNS depression and should be avoided).
No products indexed under this heading.

Methadone Hydrochloride (Concomitant use with other CNS depressants may produce an additive CNS depression and should be avoided).
No products indexed under this heading.

Methohexital Sodium (Concomitant use with other CNS depressants may produce an additive CNS depression and should be avoided).
No products indexed under this heading.

Methotrimeprazine (Concomitant use with other CNS depressants may produce an additive CNS depression and should be avoided).
No products indexed under this heading.

Methoxyflurane (Concomitant use with other CNS depressants may produce an additive CNS depression and should be avoided).
No products indexed under this heading.

Midazolam Hydrochloride (Concomitant use with other CNS depressants may produce an additive CNS depression and should be avoided).
No products indexed under this heading.

Molindone Hydrochloride (Concomitant use with other CNS depressants may produce an additive CNS depression and should be avoided). Products include:
Moban Tablets 1116

Morphine Sulfate (Concomitant use with other CNS depressants may produce an additive CNS depression and should be avoided). Products include:
Avinza Capsules 1772
DepoDur Injection 1095
MS Contin Tablets 2585

Olanzapine (Concomitant use with other CNS depressants may produce an additive CNS depression and should be avoided). Products include:
Symbyax Capsules 1871
Zyprexa Tablets 1883
Zyprexa IntraMuscular 1883
Zyprexa ZYDIS Orally Disintegrating Tablets 1883

Oxazepam (Concomitant use with other CNS depressants may produce an additive CNS depression and should be avoided).
No products indexed under this heading.

Oxycodone Hydrochloride (Concomitant use with other CNS depressants may produce an additive CNS depression and should be avoided). Products include:
OxyContin Tablets 2589
OxyIR Capsules 2593
Percocet Tablets 1127
Percodan Tablets 1130

Pentobarbital Sodium (Concomitant use with other CNS depressants may produce an additive CNS depression and should be avoided). Products include:
Nembutal Sodium Solution, USP 2494

Perphenazine (Concomitant use with other CNS depressants may produce an additive CNS depression and should be avoided).
No products indexed under this heading.

Phenobarbital (Concomitant use with other CNS depressants may produce an additive CNS depression and should be avoided). Products include:
Donnatal Extentabs 2507

Prazepam (Concomitant use with other CNS depressants may produce an additive CNS depression and should be avoided).
No products indexed under this heading.

Prochlorperazine (Concomitant use with other CNS depressants may produce an additive CNS depression and should be avoided).
No products indexed under this heading.

Promethazine Hydrochloride (Concomitant use with other CNS depressants may produce an additive CNS depression and should be avoided).
No products indexed under this heading.

Propofol (Concomitant use with other CNS depressants may produce an additive CNS depression and should be avoided).
No products indexed under this heading.

Propoxyphene Hydrochloride (Concomitant use with other CNS depressants may produce an additive CNS depression and should be avoided).
No products indexed under this heading.

Propoxyphene Napsylate (Concomitant use with other CNS depressants may produce an additive CNS depression and should be avoided).
No products indexed under this heading.

Quazepam (Concomitant use with other CNS depressants may produce an additive CNS depression and should be avoided).
No products indexed under this heading.

Quetiapine Fumarate (Concomitant use with other CNS depressants may produce an additive CNS depression and should be avoided).
No products indexed under this heading.

Ramelteon (Concomitant use may enhance the effects of sedative-hypnotics, causing increased CNS depression). Products include:
Rozerem Tablets 3091

Remifentanil Hydrochloride (Concomitant use with other CNS depressants may produce an additive CNS depression and should be avoided).
No products indexed under this heading.

Risperidone (Concomitant use with other CNS depressants may produce an additive CNS depression and should be avoided). Products include:
Risperdal Consta Long-Acting Injection 1753

Secobarbital Sodium (Concomitant use with other CNS depressants may produce an additive CNS depression and should be avoided).
No products indexed under this heading.

Sevoflurane (Concomitant use with other CNS depressants may produce an additive CNS depression and should be avoided). Products include:
Ultane Liquid for Inhalation 524

Sodium Butabarbital (Concomitant use may enhance the effects of sedative-hypnotics, causing increased CNS depression).
No products indexed under this heading.

Sodium Oxybate (Concomitant use with other CNS depressants may produce an additive CNS depression and should be avoided). Products include:
Xyrem Oral Solution 1766

Sufentanil Citrate (Concomitant use with other CNS depressants may produce an additive CNS depression and should be avoided).
No products indexed under this heading.

Temazepam (Concomitant use with other CNS depressants may produce an additive CNS depression and should be avoided).
No products indexed under this heading.

Thiamylal Sodium (Concomitant use with other CNS depressants may produce an additive CNS depression and should be avoided).
No products indexed under this heading.

Thioridazine Hydrochloride (Concomitant use with other CNS depressants may produce an additive CNS depression and should be avoided). Products include:
Thioridazine Hydrochloride Tablets 2195

Thiothixene (Concomitant use with other CNS depressants may produce an additive CNS depression and should be avoided). Products include:
Thiothixene Capsules 2197

Triazolam (Concomitant use with other CNS depressants may produce an additive CNS depression and should be avoided).
No products indexed under this heading.

Trifluoperazine Hydrochloride (Concomitant use with other CNS depressants may produce an additive CNS depression and should be avoided).
No products indexed under this heading.

Zaleplon (Concomitant use with other CNS depressants may produce an additive CNS depression and should be avoided).
No products indexed under this heading.

Ziprasidone Hydrochloride (Concomitant use with other CNS depressants may produce an additive CNS depression and should be avoided). Products include:
Geodon Capsules 2520

Zolpidem Tartrate (Concomitant use with other CNS depressants may produce an additive CNS depression and should be avoided). Products include:
Ambien Tablets 2692
Ambien CR Tablets 2696

Food Interactions

Alcohol (Concomitant use with alcohol may produce an additive CNS depression and should be avoided).

TYLENOL ALLERGY MULTI-SYMPTOM CAPLETS WITH COOL BURST AND RAPID RELEASE GELCAPS

(Acetaminophen, Chlorpheniramine Maleate, Phenylephrine Hydrochloride) 1916
See Tylenol Severe Allergy Caplets

TYLENOL ALLERGY MULTI-SYMPTOM NIGHTTIME CAPLETS WITH COOL BURST

(Acetaminophen, Diphenhydramine Hydrochloride, Phenylephrine Hydrochloride) 1916
See Tylenol Severe Allergy Caplets

TYLENOL SEVERE ALLERGY CAPLETS

(Acetaminophen, Diphenhydramine Hydrochloride) 1916

May interact with hypnotics and sedatives, monoamine oxidase inhibitors, tranquilizers, and certain other agents. Compounds in these categories include:

Alprazolam (Concurrent use may increase drowsiness).
No products indexed under this heading.

Buspirone Hydrochloride (Concurrent use may increase drowsiness).
No products indexed under this heading.

Butabarbital (Concurrent use may increase drowsiness effect).
No products indexed under this heading.

Butabarbital Sodium (Concurrent use may increase drowsiness effect).
No products indexed under this heading.

Chloral Hydrate (Concurrent use may increase drowsiness effect).
No products indexed under this heading.

Chlordiazepoxide (Concurrent use may increase drowsiness).
No products indexed under this heading.

Chlordiazepoxide Hydrochloride (Concurrent use may increase drowsiness).
No products indexed under this heading.

Chlorpromazine (Concurrent use may increase drowsiness).
No products indexed under this heading.

Chlorpromazine Hydrochloride (Concurrent use may increase drowsiness).
No products indexed under this heading.

Chlorprothixene (Concurrent use may increase drowsiness).
No products indexed under this heading.

Chlorprothixene Hydrochloride (Concurrent use may increase drowsiness).
No products indexed under this heading.

Clorazepate Dipotassium (Concurrent use may increase drowsiness).
No products indexed under this heading.

Diazepam (Concurrent use may increase drowsiness). Products include:
Valium Tablets 2658

Droperidol (Concurrent use may increase drowsiness).
No products indexed under this heading.

Estazolam (Concurrent use may increase drowsiness effect).
No products indexed under this heading.

Ethchlorvynol (Concurrent use may increase drowsiness effect).
No products indexed under this heading.

Ethinamate (Concurrent use may increase drowsiness effect).
No products indexed under this heading.

Fluphenazine Decanoate (Concurrent use may increase drowsiness).
No products indexed under this heading.

Fluphenazine Enanthate (Concurrent use may increase drowsiness).
No products indexed under this heading.

Fluphenazine Hydrochloride (Concurrent use may increase drowsiness).
No products indexed under this heading.

Flurazepam Hydrochloride (Concurrent use may increase drowsiness effect).
No products indexed under this heading.

Glutethimide (Concurrent use may increase drowsiness effect).
No products indexed under this heading.

Haloperidol (Concurrent use may increase drowsiness).
No products indexed under this heading.

Haloperidol Decanoate (Concurrent use may increase drowsiness).
No products indexed under this heading.

Hydroxyzine Hydrochloride (Concurrent use may increase drowsiness).
No products indexed under this heading.

Isocarboxazid (Concurrent and/or sequential use with MAO inhibitors is not recommended). Products include:
Marplan Tablets 3177

Lorazepam (Concurrent use may increase drowsiness effect).
No products indexed under this heading.

Loxapine Hydrochloride (Concurrent use may increase drowsiness).
No products indexed under this heading.

Loxapine Succinate (Concurrent use may increase drowsiness).
No products indexed under this heading.

Meprobamate (Concurrent use may increase drowsiness).
No products indexed under this heading.

Mesoridazine Besylate (Concurrent use may increase drowsiness).
No products indexed under this heading.

Midazolam Hydrochloride (Concurrent use may increase drowsiness effect).
No products indexed under this heading.

Moclobemide (Concurrent and/or sequential use with MAO inhibitors is not recommended).
No products indexed under this heading.

Molindone Hydrochloride (Concurrent use may increase drowsiness). Products include:
Moban Tablets 1116

Oxazepam (Concurrent use may increase drowsiness).
No products indexed under this heading.

Pargyline Hydrochloride (Concurrent and/or sequential use with MAO inhibitors is not recommended).
No products indexed under this heading.

Perphenazine (Concurrent use may increase drowsiness).
No products indexed under this heading.

Phenelzine Sulfate (Concurrent and/or sequential use with MAO inhibitors is not recommended).
No products indexed under this heading.

Prazepam (Concurrent use may increase drowsiness).
No products indexed under this heading.

Procarbazine Hydrochloride (Concurrent and/or sequential use with MAO inhibitors is not recommended).
No products indexed under this heading.

Prochlorperazine (Concurrent use may increase drowsiness).
No products indexed under this heading.

Promethazine Hydrochloride (Concurrent use may increase drowsiness).
No products indexed under this heading.

Propofol (Concurrent use may increase drowsiness effect).
No products indexed under this heading.

Quazepam (Concurrent use may increase drowsiness effect).
No products indexed under this heading.

Ramelteon (Concurrent use may increase drowsiness effect). Products include:
Rozerem Tablets 3091

Rasagiline Mesylate (Concurrent and/or sequential use with MAO inhibitors is not recommended). Products include:
Azilect Tablets 3106

Secobarbital Sodium (Concurrent use may increase drowsiness effect).
No products indexed under this heading.

Selegiline (Concurrent and/or sequential use with MAO inhibitors is not recommended). Products include:
Emsam Transdermal System 905

Selegiline Hydrochloride (Concurrent and/or sequential use with MAO inhibitors is not recommended). Products include:
Eldepryl Capsules 3052

Sodium Butabarbital (Concurrent use may increase drowsiness effect).
No products indexed under this heading.

Temazepam (Concurrent use may increase drowsiness effect).
No products indexed under this heading.

Thioridazine Hydrochloride (Concurrent use may increase drowsiness). Products include:
Thioridazine Hydrochloride Tablets 2195

Thiothixene (Concurrent use may increase drowsiness). Products include:
Thiothixene Capsules 2197

Tranylcypromine Sulfate (Concurrent and/or sequential use with MAO inhibitors is not recommended). Products include:
Parnate Tablets 1532

Triazolam (Concurrent use may increase drowsiness effect).
No products indexed under this heading.

Trifluoperazine Hydrochloride (Concurrent use may increase drowsiness).
No products indexed under this heading.

Zaleplon (Concurrent use may increase drowsiness effect).
No products indexed under this heading.

Zolpidem Tartrate (Concurrent use may increase drowsiness effect). Products include:
Ambien Tablets 2692
Ambien CR Tablets 2696

Food Interactions

Alcohol (Concurrent use may increase drowsiness effect; chronic heavy alcohol abusers, 3 or more drinks per day, may be at increased risk of liver toxicity from excessive acetaminophen use).

TYLENOL ARTHRITIS PAIN EXTENDED RELEASE GELTABS/CAPLETS

(Acetaminophen) 1915
See Regular Strength Tylenol Tablets

TYLENOL CHEST CONGESTION CAPLETS WITH COOL BURST

(Acetaminophen, Guaifenesin) 1910

Food Interactions

Alcohol (Concurrent use may increase drowsiness effect; chronic heavy alcohol abusers, 3 or more drinks per day, may be at increased risk of liver toxicity from excessive acetaminophen use).

TYLENOL CHEST CONGESTION LIQUID WITH COOL BURST

(Acetaminophen, Guaifenesin) 1910
See Tylenol Chest Congestion Caplets with Cool Burst

CHILDREN'S TYLENOL PLUS COLD SUSPENSION LIQUID

(Acetaminophen, Chlorpheniramine Maleate, Phenylephrine Hydrochloride)................................ 1912
May interact with hypnotics and sedatives, monoamine oxidase inhibitors, and tranquilizers. Compounds in these categories include:

Alprazolam (Concurrent use may increase drowiness effect).
No products indexed under this heading.

Buspirone Hydrochloride (Concurrent use may increase drowiness effect).
No products indexed under this heading.

Butabarbital (Concurrent use may increase drowiness effect).
No products indexed under this heading.

Butabarbital Sodium (Concurrent use may increase drowsiness effect).
No products indexed under this heading.

Chloral Hydrate (Concurrent use may increase drowiness effect).
No products indexed under this heading.

Chlordiazepoxide (Concurrent use may increase drowiness effect).
No products indexed under this heading.

Chlordiazepoxide Hydrochloride (Concurrent use may increase drowiness effect).
No products indexed under this heading.

Chlorpromazine (Concurrent use may increase drowiness effect).
No products indexed under this heading.

Chlorpromazine Hydrochloride (Concurrent use may increase drowiness effect).
No products indexed under this heading.

Chlorprothixene (Concurrent use may increase drowiness effect).
No products indexed under this heading.

Chlorprothixene Hydrochloride (Concurrent use may increase drowiness effect).
No products indexed under this heading.

Clorazepate Dipotassium (Concurrent use may increase drowiness effect).
No products indexed under this heading.

Diazepam (Concurrent use may increase drowiness effect). Products include:

Lorazepam (Concurrent use may increase drowsiness effect).
No products indexed under this heading.

Loxapine Hydrochloride (Concurrent use may increase drowsiness).
No products indexed under this heading.

Loxapine Succinate (Concurrent use may increase drowsiness).
No products indexed under this heading.

Meprobamate (Concurrent use may increase drowsiness).
No products indexed under this heading.

Mesoridazine Besylate (Concurrent use may increase drowsiness).
No products indexed under this heading.

Midazolam Hydrochloride (Concurrent use may increase drowsiness effect).
No products indexed under this heading.

Moclobemide (Avoid use with monoamine oxidase inhibitors (MAOI) or for two weeks after stopping MAOI drug).
No products indexed under this heading.

Molindone Hydrochloride (Concurrent use may increase drowsiness). Products include:
Moban Tablets 1116

Oxazepam (Concurrent use may increase drowsiness).
No products indexed under this heading.

Pargyline Hydrochloride (Avoid use with monoamine oxidase inhibitors (MAOI) or for two weeks after stopping MAOI drug).
No products indexed under this heading.

Perphenazine (Concurrent use may increase drowsiness).
No products indexed under this heading.

Phenelzine Sulfate (Avoid use with monoamine oxidase inhibitors (MAOI) or for two weeks after stopping MAOI drug).
No products indexed under this heading.

Prazepam (Concurrent use may increase drowsiness).
No products indexed under this heading.

Procarbazine Hydrochloride (Avoid use with monoamine oxidase inhibitors (MAOI) or for two weeks after stopping MAOI drug).
No products indexed under this heading.

Prochlorperazine (Concurrent use may increase drowsiness).
No products indexed under this heading.

Promethazine Hydrochloride (Concurrent use may increase drowsiness).
No products indexed under this heading.

Propofol (Concurrent use may increase drowsiness effect).
No products indexed under this heading.

Quazepam (Concurrent use may increase drowsiness effect).
No products indexed under this heading.

Ramelteon (Concurrent use may increase drowsiness effect). Products include:
Rozerem Tablets 3091

Rasagiline Mesylate (Avoid use with monoamine oxidase inhibitors (MAOI) or for two weeks after stopping MAOI drug). Products include:
Azilect Tablets 3106

Secobarbital Sodium (Concurrent use may increase drowsiness effect).
No products indexed under this heading.

Selegiline (Avoid use with monoamine oxidase inhibitors (MAOI) or for two weeks after stopping MAOI drug). Products include:
Emsam Transdermal System 905

Selegiline Hydrochloride (Avoid use with monoamine oxidase inhibitors (MAOI) or for two weeks after stopping MAOI drug). Products include:
Eldepryl Capsules 3052

Sodium Butabarbital (Concurrent use may increase drowsiness effect).
No products indexed under this heading.

Temazepam (Concurrent use may increase drowsiness effect).
No products indexed under this heading.

Thioridazine Hydrochloride (Concurrent use may increase drowsiness). Products include:
Thioridazine Hydrochloride Tablets 2195

Thiothixene (Concurrent use may increase drowsiness). Products include:
Thiothixene Capsules 2197

Tranylcypromine Sulfate (Avoid use with monoamine oxidase inhibitors (MAOI) or for two weeks after stopping MAOI drug). Products include:
Parnate Tablets 1532

Triazolam (Concurrent use may increase drowsiness effect).
No products indexed under this heading.

Trifluoperazine Hydrochloride (Concurrent use may increase drowsiness).
No products indexed under this heading.

Zaleplon (Concurrent use may increase drowsiness effect).
No products indexed under this heading.

Zolpidem Tartrate (Concurrent use may increase drowsiness effect). Products include:
Ambien Tablets 2692
Ambien CR Tablets 2696

CHILDREN'S TYLENOL PLUS COUGH & RUNNY NOSE SUSPENSION LIQUID

(Acetaminophen, Chlorpheniramine Maleate, Dextromethorphan Hydrobromide) 1912
May interact with hypnotics and sedatives, monoamine oxidase inhibitors, and tranquilizers. Compounds in these categories include:

Alprazolam (Concurrent use may increase drowsiness effect).
No products indexed under this heading.

Buspirone Hydrochloride (Concurrent use may increase drowsiness effect).
No products indexed under this heading.

Butabarbital (Concurrent use may increase drowsiness effect).
No products indexed under this heading.

Butabarbital Sodium (Concurrent use may increase drowsiness effect).
No products indexed under this heading.

Chloral Hydrate (Concurrent use may increase drowsiness effect).
No products indexed under this heading.

Chlordiazepoxide (Concurrent use may increase drowsiness effect).
No products indexed under this heading.

Chlordiazepoxide Hydrochloride (Concurrent use may increase drowsiness effect).
No products indexed under this heading.

Chlorpromazine (Concurrent use may increase drowsiness effect).
No products indexed under this heading.

Chlorpromazine Hydrochloride (Concurrent use may increase drowsiness effect).
No products indexed under this heading.

Chlorprothixene (Concurrent use may increase drowsiness effect).
No products indexed under this heading.

Chlorprothixene Hydrochloride (Concurrent use may increase drowsiness effect).
No products indexed under this heading.

Clorazepate Dipotassium (Concurrent use may increase drowsiness effect).
No products indexed under this heading.

Diazepam (Concurrent use may increase drowsiness effect). Products include:
Valium Tablets 2658

Droperidol (Concurrent use may increase drowsiness effect).
No products indexed under this heading.

Estazolam (Concurrent use may increase drowsiness effect).
No products indexed under this heading.

Ethchlorvynol (Concurrent use may increase drowsiness effect).
No products indexed under this heading.

Ethinamate (Concurrent use may increase drowsiness effect).
No products indexed under this heading.

Fluphenazine Decanoate (Concurrent use may increase drowsiness effect).
No products indexed under this heading.

Fluphenazine Enanthate (Concurrent use may increase drowsiness effect).
No products indexed under this heading.

Fluphenazine Hydrochloride (Concurrent use may increase drowsiness effect).
No products indexed under this heading.

Flurazepam Hydrochloride (Concurrent use may increase drowsiness effect).
No products indexed under this heading.

Glutethimide (Concurrent use may increase drowsiness effect).
No products indexed under this heading.

Haloperidol (Concurrent use may increase drowsiness effect).
No products indexed under this heading.

Haloperidol Decanoate (Concurrent use may increase drowsiness effect).
No products indexed under this heading.

Hydroxyzine Hydrochloride (Concurrent use may increase drowsiness effect).
No products indexed under this heading.

Isocarboxazid (Avoid use with monoamine oxidase inhibitors (MAOI) or for 2 weeks after stopping MAOI drug). Products include:
Marplan Tablets 3177

Lorazepam (Concurrent use may increase drowsiness effect).
No products indexed under this heading.

Loxapine Hydrochloride (Concurrent use may increase drowsiness effect).
No products indexed under this heading.

Loxapine Succinate (Concurrent use may increase drowsiness effect).
No products indexed under this heading.

Meprobamate (Concurrent use may increase drowsiness effect).
No products indexed under this heading.

Mesoridazine Besylate (Concurrent use may increase drowsiness effect).
No products indexed under this heading.

Midazolam Hydrochloride (Concurrent use may increase drowsiness effect).
No products indexed under this heading.

Moclobemide (Avoid use with monoamine oxidase inhibitors (MAOI) or for 2 weeks after stopping MAOI drug).
No products indexed under this heading.

Molindone Hydrochloride (Concurrent use may increase drowsiness effect). Products include:
Moban Tablets 1116

Oxazepam (Concurrent use may increase drowsiness effect).
No products indexed under this heading.

Pargyline Hydrochloride (Avoid use with monoamine oxidase inhibitors (MAOI) or for 2 weeks after stopping MAOI drug).
No products indexed under this heading.

Perphenazine (Concurrent use may increase drowsiness effect).
No products indexed under this heading.

Phenelzine Sulfate (Avoid use with monoamine oxidase inhibitors (MAOI) or for 2 weeks after stopping MAOI drug).
No products indexed under this heading.

Prazepam (Concurrent use may increase drowsiness effect).
No products indexed under this heading.

IMPORTANT NOTE: Always consult each drug listing in the patient's regimen for possible interactions.

Procarbazine Hydrochloride (Avoid use with monoamine oxidase inhibitors (MAOI) or for 2 weeks after stopping MAOI drug).
No products indexed under this heading.

Prochlorperazine (Concurrent use may increase drowsiness effect).
No products indexed under this heading.

Promethazine Hydrochloride (Concurrent use may increase drowsiness effect).
No products indexed under this heading.

Propofol (Concurrent use may increase drowsiness effect).
No products indexed under this heading.

Quazepam (Concurrent use may increase drowsiness effect).
No products indexed under this heading.

Ramelteon (Concurrent use may increase drowsiness effect). Products include:
Rozerem Tablets ... 3091

Rasagiline Mesylate (Avoid use with monoamine oxidase inhibitors (MAOI) or for 2 weeks after stopping MAOI drug). Products include:
Azilect Tablets ... 3106

Secobarbital Sodium (Concurrent use may increase drowsiness effect).
No products indexed under this heading.

Selegiline (Avoid use with monoamine oxidase inhibitors (MAOI) or for 2 weeks after stopping MAOI drug). Products include:
Emsam Transdermal System ... 905

Selegiline Hydrochloride (Avoid use with monoamine oxidase inhibitors (MAOI) or for 2 weeks after stopping MAOI drug). Products include:
Eldepryl Capsules ... 3052

Sodium Butabarbital (Concurrent use may increase drowsiness effect).
No products indexed under this heading.

Temazepam (Concurrent use may increase drowsiness effect).
No products indexed under this heading.

Thioridazine Hydrochloride (Concurrent use may increase drowsiness effect). Products include:
Thioridazine Hydrochloride Tablets ... 2195

Thiothixene (Concurrent use may increase drowsiness effect). Products include:
Thiothixene Capsules ... 2197

Tranylcypromine Sulfate (Avoid use with monoamine oxidase inhibitors (MAOI) or for 2 weeks after stopping MAOI drug). Products include:
Parnate Tablets ... 1532

Triazolam (Concurrent use may increase drowsiness effect).
No products indexed under this heading.

Trifluoperazine Hydrochloride (Concurrent use may increase drowsiness effect).
No products indexed under this heading.

Zaleplon (Concurrent use may increase drowsiness effect).
No products indexed under this heading.

Zolpidem Tartrate (Concurrent use may increase drowsiness effect). Products include:
Ambien Tablets ... 2692
Ambien CR Tablets ... 2696

CHILDREN'S TYLENOL PLUS COUGH & SORE THROAT SUSPENSION LIQUID

(Acetaminophen, Dextromethorphan Hydrobromide) ... 1912
May interact with monoamine oxidase inhibitors. Compounds in these categories include:

Isocarboxazid (Avoid use with monoamine oxidase inhibitors (MAOI) or for 2 weeks after stopping MAOI drug). Products include:
Marplan Tablets ... 3177

Moclobemide (Avoid use with monoamine oxidase inhibitors (MAOI) or for 2 weeks after stopping MAOI drug).
No products indexed under this heading.

Pargyline Hydrochloride (Avoid use with monoamine oxidase inhibitors (MAOI) or for 2 weeks after stopping MAOI drug).
No products indexed under this heading.

Phenelzine Sulfate (Avoid use with monoamine oxidase inhibitors (MAOI) or for 2 weeks after stopping MAOI drug).
No products indexed under this heading.

Procarbazine Hydrochloride (Avoid use with monoamine oxidase inhibitors (MAOI) or for 2 weeks after stopping MAOI drug).
No products indexed under this heading.

Rasagiline Mesylate (Avoid use with monoamine oxidase inhibitors (MAOI) or for 2 weeks after stopping MAOI drug). Products include:
Azilect Tablets ... 3106

Selegiline (Avoid use with monoamine oxidase inhibitors (MAOI) or for 2 weeks after stopping MAOI drug). Products include:
Emsam Transdermal System ... 905

Selegiline Hydrochloride (Avoid use with monoamine oxidase inhibitors (MAOI) or for 2 weeks after stopping MAOI drug). Products include:
Eldepryl Capsules ... 3052

Tranylcypromine Sulfate (Avoid use with monoamine oxidase inhibitors (MAOI) or for 2 weeks after stopping MAOI drug). Products include:
Parnate Tablets ... 1532

CHILDREN'S TYLENOL PLUS FLU SUSPENSION LIQUID

(Acetaminophen, Chlorpheniramine Maleate, Dextromethorphan Hydrobromide, Phenylephrine Hydrochloride) ... 1914
May interact with hypnotics and sedatives, monoamine oxidase inhibitors, tranquilizers, and certain other agents. Compounds in these categories include:

Alprazolam (Concurrent use may increase the drowsiness effect).
No products indexed under this heading.

Buspirone Hydrochloride (Concurrent use may increase the drowsiness effect).
No products indexed under this heading.

Butabarbital (Concurrent use may increase the drowsiness effect).
No products indexed under this heading.

Butabarbital Sodium (Concurrent use may increase the drowsiness effect).
No products indexed under this heading.

Chloral Hydrate (Concurrent use may increase the drowsiness effect).
No products indexed under this heading.

Chlordiazepoxide (Concurrent use may increase the drowsiness effect).
No products indexed under this heading.

Chlordiazepoxide Hydrochloride (Concurrent use may increase the drowsiness effect).
No products indexed under this heading.

Chlorpromazine (Concurrent use may increase the drowsiness effect).
No products indexed under this heading.

Chlorpromazine Hydrochloride (Concurrent use may increase the drowsiness effect).
No products indexed under this heading.

Chlorprothixene (Concurrent use may increase the drowsiness effect).
No products indexed under this heading.

Chlorprothixene Hydrochloride (Concurrent use may increase the drowsiness effect).
No products indexed under this heading.

Clorazepate Dipotassium (Concurrent use may increase the drowsiness effect).
No products indexed under this heading.

Diazepam (Concurrent use may increase the drowsiness effect). Products include:
Valium Tablets ... 2658

Droperidol (Concurrent use may increase the drowsiness effect).
No products indexed under this heading.

Estazolam (Concurrent use may increase the drowsiness effect).
No products indexed under this heading.

Ethchlorvynol (Concurrent use may increase the drowsiness effect).
No products indexed under this heading.

Ethinamate (Concurrent use may increase the drowsiness effect).
No products indexed under this heading.

Fluphenazine Decanoate (Concurrent use may increase the drowsiness effect).
No products indexed under this heading.

Fluphenazine Enanthate (Concurrent use may increase the drowsiness effect).
No products indexed under this heading.

Fluphenazine Hydrochloride (Concurrent use may increase the drowsiness effect).
No products indexed under this heading.

Flurazepam Hydrochloride (Concurrent use may increase the drowsiness effect).
No products indexed under this heading.

Glutethimide (Concurrent use may increase the drowsiness effect).
No products indexed under this heading.

Haloperidol (Concurrent use may increase the drowsiness effect).
No products indexed under this heading.

Haloperidol Decanoate (Concurrent use may increase the drowsiness effect).
No products indexed under this heading.

Hydroxyzine Hydrochloride (Concurrent use may increase the drowsiness effect).
No products indexed under this heading.

Isocarboxazid (Concurrent and/or sequential use with MAO inhibitors is not recommended). Products include:
Marplan Tablets ... 3177

Lorazepam (Concurrent use may increase the drowsiness effect).
No products indexed under this heading.

Loxapine Hydrochloride (Concurrent use may increase the drowsiness effect).
No products indexed under this heading.

Loxapine Succinate (Concurrent use may increase the drowsiness effect).
No products indexed under this heading.

Meprobamate (Concurrent use may increase the drowsiness effect).
No products indexed under this heading.

Mesoridazine Besylate (Concurrent use may increase the drowsiness effect).
No products indexed under this heading.

Midazolam Hydrochloride (Concurrent use may increase the drowsiness effect).
No products indexed under this heading.

Moclobemide (Concurrent and/or sequential use with MAO inhibitors is not recommended).
No products indexed under this heading.

Molindone Hydrochloride (Concurrent use may increase the drowsiness effect). Products include:
Moban Tablets ... 1116

Oxazepam (Concurrent use may increase the drowsiness effect).
No products indexed under this heading.

Pargyline Hydrochloride (Concurrent and/or sequential use with MAO inhibitors is not recommended).
No products indexed under this heading.

Perphenazine (Concurrent use may increase the drowsiness effect).
No products indexed under this heading.

Phenelzine Sulfate (Concurrent and/or sequential use with MAO inhibitors is not recommended).
No products indexed under this heading.

Prazepam (Concurrent use may increase the drowsiness effect).
No products indexed under this heading.

Procarbazine Hydrochloride (Concurrent and/or sequential use with MAO inhibitors is not recommended).
No products indexed under this heading.

Prochlorperazine (Concurrent use may increase the drowsiness effect).
No products indexed under this heading.

Promethazine Hydrochloride (Concurrent use may increase the drowsiness effect).
No products indexed under this heading.

Propofol (Concurrent use may increase the drowsiness effect).
No products indexed under this heading.

Quazepam (Concurrent use may increase the drowsiness effect).
No products indexed under this heading.

Ramelteon (Concurrent use may increase the drowsiness effect).
Products include:
Rozerem Tablets 3091

Rasagiline Mesylate (Concurrent and/or sequential use with MAO inhibitors is not recommended).
Products include:
Azilect Tablets 3106

Secobarbital Sodium (Concurrent use may increase the drowsiness effect).
No products indexed under this heading.

Selegiline (Concurrent and/or sequential use with MAO inhibitors is not recommended). Products include:
Emsam Transdermal System 905

Selegiline Hydrochloride (Concurrent and/or sequential use with MAO inhibitors is not recommended).
Products include:
Eldepryl Capsules 3052

Sodium Butabarbital (Concurrent use may increase the drowsiness effect).
No products indexed under this heading.

Temazepam (Concurrent use may increase the drowsiness effect).
No products indexed under this heading.

Thioridazine Hydrochloride (Concurrent use may increase the drowsiness effect). Products include:
Thioridazine Hydrochloride Tablets 2195

Thiothixene (Concurrent use may increase the drowsiness effect).
Products include:
Thiothixene Capsules 2197

Tranylcypromine Sulfate (Concurrent and/or sequential use with MAO inhibitors is not recommended).
Products include:
Parnate Tablets 1532

Triazolam (Concurrent use may increase the drowsiness effect).
No products indexed under this heading.

Trifluoperazine Hydrochloride (Concurrent use may increase the drowsiness effect).
No products indexed under this heading.

Zaleplon (Concurrent use may increase the drowsiness effect).
No products indexed under this heading.

Zolpidem Tartrate (Concurrent use may increase the drowsiness effect).
Products include:
Ambien Tablets 2692
Ambien CR Tablets 2696

CHILDREN'S TYLENOL SUSPENSION LIQUID

(Acetaminophen) 1909
None cited in PDR database.

CHILDREN'S TYLENOL MELTAWAYS

(Acetaminophen) 1909
None cited in PDR database.

CHILDREN'S TYLENOL PLUS MULTI-SYMPTOM COLD SUSPENSION LIQUID

(Acetaminophen, Chlorpheniramine Maleate, Dextromethorphan Hydrobromide, Phenylephrine Hydrochloride) 1912
See Children's Tylenol Plus Cold Suspension Liquid

TYLENOL COLD SEVERE CONGESTION DAYTIME CAPLETS WITH COOL BURST

(Acetaminophen, Dextromethorphan Hydrobromide, Guaifenesin, Pseudoephedrine Hydrochloride) 1912
May interact with monoamine oxidase inhibitors and certain other agents. Compounds in these categories include:

Isocarboxazid (Concurrent and/or sequential use with MAO inhibitors is not recommended). Products include:
Marplan Tablets 3177

Moclobemide (Concurrent and/or sequential use with MAO inhibitors is not recommended).
No products indexed under this heading.

Pargyline Hydrochloride (Concurrent and/or sequential use with MAO inhibitors is not recommended).
No products indexed under this heading.

Phenelzine Sulfate (Concurrent and/or sequential use with MAO inhibitors is not recommended).
No products indexed under this heading.

Procarbazine Hydrochloride (Concurrent and/or sequential use with MAO inhibitors is not recommended).
No products indexed under this heading.

Rasagiline Mesylate (Concurrent and/or sequential use with MAO inhibitors is not recommended).
Products include:
Azilect Tablets 3106

Selegiline (Concurrent and/or sequential use with MAO inhibitors is not recommended). Products include:
Emsam Transdermal System 905

Selegiline Hydrochloride (Concurrent and/or sequential use with MAO inhibitors is not recommended).
Products include:
Eldepryl Capsules 3052

Tranylcypromine Sulfate (Concurrent and/or sequential use with MAO inhibitors is not recommended).
Products include:
Parnate Tablets 1532

Food Interactions

Alcohol (Chronic heavy alcohol abusers, 3 or more drinks per day, may be at increased risk of liver toxicity from acetaminophen use).

TYLENOL COLD HEAD CONGESTION DAYTIME CAPLETS WITH COOL BURST

(Acetaminophen, Dextromethorphan Hydrobromide, Phenylephrine Hydrochloride) 1910
May interact with monoamine oxidase inhibitors and certain other agents. Compounds in these categories include:

Isocarboxazid (Avoid use with monoamine oxidase inhibitors (MAOIs) or for two weeks after stopping MAOI drug). Products include:
Marplan Tablets 3177

Moclobemide (Avoid use with monoamine oxidase inhibitors (MAOIs) or for two weeks after stopping MAOI drug).
No products indexed under this heading.

Pargyline Hydrochloride (Avoid use with monoamine oxidase inhibitors (MAOIs) or for two weeks after stopping MAOI drug).
No products indexed under this heading.

Phenelzine Sulfate (Avoid use with monoamine oxidase inhibitors (MAOIs) or for two weeks after stopping MAOI drug).
No products indexed under this heading.

Procarbazine Hydrochloride (Avoid use with monoamine oxidase inhibitors (MAOIs) or for two weeks after stopping MAOI drug).
No products indexed under this heading.

Rasagiline Mesylate (Avoid use with monoamine oxidase inhibitors (MAOIs) or for two weeks after stopping MAOI drug). Products include:
Azilect Tablets 3106

Selegiline (Avoid use with monoamine oxidase inhibitors (MAOIs) or for two weeks after stopping MAOI drug). Products include:
Emsam Transdermal System 905

Selegiline Hydrochloride (Avoid use with monoamine oxidase inhibitors (MAOIs) or for two weeks after stopping MAOI drug). Products include:
Eldepryl Capsules 3052

Tranylcypromine Sulfate (Avoid use with monoamine oxidase inhibitors (MAOIs) or for two weeks after stopping MAOI drug). Products include:
Parnate Tablets 1532

Food Interactions

Alcohol (Concurrent use may increase drowsiness effect; chronic heavy alcohol abusers, 3 or more drinks per day, may be at increased risk of liver toxicity from excessive acetaminophen use).

TYLENOL COLD HEAD CONGESTION NIGHTTIME CAPLETS WITH COOL BURST

(Acetaminophen, Chlorpheniramine Maleate, Dextromethorphan Hydrobromide, Phenylephrine Hydrochloride) 1910
May interact with hypnotics and sedatives, monoamine oxidase inhibitors, tranquilizers, and certain other agents. Compounds in these categories include:

Alprazolam (Concurrent use may increase drowsiness).
No products indexed under this heading.

Buspirone Hydrochloride (Concurrent use may increase drowsiness).
No products indexed under this heading.

Butabarbital (Concurrent use may increase drowsiness effect).
No products indexed under this heading.

Butabarbital Sodium (Concurrent use may increase drowsiness effect).
No products indexed under this heading.

Chloral Hydrate (Concurrent use may increase drowsiness effect).
No products indexed under this heading.

Chlordiazepoxide (Concurrent use may increase drowsiness).
No products indexed under this heading.

Chlordiazepoxide Hydrochloride (Concurrent use may increase drowsiness).
No products indexed under this heading.

Chlorpromazine (Concurrent use may increase drowsiness).
No products indexed under this heading.

Chlorpromazine Hydrochloride (Concurrent use may increase drowsiness).
No products indexed under this heading.

Chlorprothixene (Concurrent use may increase drowsiness).
No products indexed under this heading.

Chlorprothixene Hydrochloride (Concurrent use may increase drowsiness).
No products indexed under this heading.

Clorazepate Dipotassium (Concurrent use may increase drowsiness).
No products indexed under this heading.

Diazepam (Concurrent use may increase drowsiness). Products include:
Valium Tablets 2658

Droperidol (Concurrent use may increase drowsiness).
No products indexed under this heading.

Estazolam (Concurrent use may increase drowsiness effect).
No products indexed under this heading.

Ethchlorvynol (Concurrent use may increase drowsiness effect).
No products indexed under this heading.

Ethinamate (Concurrent use may increase drowsiness effect).
No products indexed under this heading.

Fluphenazine Decanoate (Concurrent use may increase drowsiness).
No products indexed under this heading.

Fluphenazine Enanthate (Concurrent use may increase drowsiness).
No products indexed under this heading.

Fluphenazine Hydrochloride (Concurrent use may increase drowsiness).
No products indexed under this heading.

Flurazepam Hydrochloride (Concurrent use may increase drowsiness effect).
No products indexed under this heading.

Glutethimide (Concurrent use may increase drowsiness effect).
No products indexed under this heading.

Haloperidol (Concurrent use may increase drowsiness).
No products indexed under this heading.

Haloperidol Decanoate (Concurrent use may increase drowsiness).
No products indexed under this heading.

Hydroxyzine Hydrochloride (Concurrent use may increase drowsiness).
No products indexed under this heading.

Isocarboxazid (Avoid use with monoamine oxidase inhibitors (MAOIs) or for two weeks after stopping MAOI drug). Products include:
Marplan Tablets 3177

Lorazepam (Concurrent use may increase drowsiness effect).
No products indexed under this heading.

Loxapine Hydrochloride (Concurrent use may increase drowsiness).
No products indexed under this heading.

Loxapine Succinate (Concurrent use may increase drowsiness).
No products indexed under this heading.

Meprobamate (Concurrent use may increase drowsiness).
No products indexed under this heading.

Mesoridazine Besylate (Concurrent use may increase drowsiness).
No products indexed under this heading.

Midazolam Hydrochloride (Concurrent use may increase drowsiness effect).
No products indexed under this heading.

Moclobemide (Avoid use with monoamine oxidase inhibitors (MAOIs) or for two weeks after stopping MAOI drug).
No products indexed under this heading.

Molindone Hydrochloride (Concurrent use may increase drowsiness). Products include:
Moban Tablets 1116

Oxazepam (Concurrent use may increase drowsiness).
No products indexed under this heading.

Pargyline Hydrochloride (Avoid use with monoamine oxidase inhibitors (MAOIs) or for two weeks after stopping MAOI drug).
No products indexed under this heading.

Perphenazine (Concurrent use may increase drowsiness).
No products indexed under this heading.

Phenelzine Sulfate (Avoid use with monoamine oxidase inhibitors (MAOIs) or for two weeks after stopping MAOI drug).
No products indexed under this heading.

Prazepam (Concurrent use may increase drowsiness).
No products indexed under this heading.

Procarbazine Hydrochloride (Avoid use with monoamine oxidase inhibitors (MAOIs) or for two weeks after stopping MAOI drug).
No products indexed under this heading.

Prochlorperazine (Concurrent use may increase drowsiness).
No products indexed under this heading.

Promethazine Hydrochloride (Concurrent use may increase drowsiness).
No products indexed under this heading.

Propofol (Concurrent use may increase drowsiness effect).
No products indexed under this heading.

Quazepam (Concurrent use may increase drowsiness effect).
No products indexed under this heading.

Ramelteon (Concurrent use may increase drowsiness effect). Products include:
Rozerem Tablets 3091

Rasagiline Mesylate (Avoid use with monoamine oxidase inhibitors (MAOIs) or for two weeks after stopping MAOI drug). Products include:
Azilect Tablets 3106

Secobarbital Sodium (Concurrent use may increase drowsiness effect).
No products indexed under this heading.

Selegiline (Avoid use with monoamine oxidase inhibitors (MAOIs) or for two weeks after stopping MAOI drug). Products include:
Emsam Transdermal System 905

Selegiline Hydrochloride (Avoid use with monoamine oxidase inhibitors (MAOIs) or for two weeks after stopping MAOI drug). Products include:
Eldepryl Capsules 3052

Sodium Butabarbital (Concurrent use may increase drowsiness effect).
No products indexed under this heading.

Temazepam (Concurrent use may increase drowsiness effect).
No products indexed under this heading.

Thioridazine Hydrochloride (Concurrent use may increase drowsiness). Products include:
Thioridazine Hydrochloride Tablets 2195

Thiothixene (Concurrent use may increase drowsiness). Products include:
Thiothixene Capsules 2197

Tranylcypromine Sulfate (Avoid use with monoamine oxidase inhibitors (MAOIs) or for two weeks after stopping MAOI drug). Products include:
Parnate Tablets 1532

Triazolam (Concurrent use may increase drowsiness effect).
No products indexed under this heading.

Trifluoperazine Hydrochloride (Concurrent use may increase drowsiness).
No products indexed under this heading.

Zaleplon (Concurrent use may increase drowsiness effect).
No products indexed under this heading.

Zolpidem Tartrate (Concurrent use may increase drowsiness effect). Products include:
Ambien Tablets 2692
Ambien CR Tablets 2696

Food Interactions

Alcohol (Concurrent use may increase drowsiness effect; chronic heavy alcohol abusers, 3 or more drinks per day, may be at increased risk of liver toxicity from excessive acetaminophen use).

TYLENOL COLD HEAD CONGESTION SEVERE DAYTIME CAPLETS WITH COOL BURST

(Acetaminophen, Dextromethorphan Hydrobromide, Guaifenesin, Phenylephrine Hydrochloride).................................. 1910
See Tylenol Cold Head Congestion Daytime Caplets with Cool Burst

TYLENOL COLD MULTI-SYMPTOM DAYTIME CAPLETS WITH COOL BURST AND RAPID RELEASE GELS

(Acetaminophen, Dextromethorphan Hydrobromide, Phenylephrine Hydrochloride)............ 1913
May interact with monoamine oxidase inhibitors and certain other agents. Compounds in these categories include:

Isocarboxazid (Concurrent and/or sequential use with MAO inhibitors is not recommended). Products include:
Marplan Tablets 3177

Moclobemide (Concurrent and/or sequential use with MAO inhibitors is not recommended).
No products indexed under this heading.

Pargyline Hydrochloride (Concurrent and/or sequential use with MAO inhibitors is not recommended).
No products indexed under this heading.

Phenelzine Sulfate (Concurrent and/or sequential use with MAO inhibitors is not recommended).
No products indexed under this heading.

Procarbazine Hydrochloride (Concurrent and/or sequential use with MAO inhibitors is not recommended).
No products indexed under this heading.

Rasagiline Mesylate (Concurrent and/or sequential use with MAO inhibitors is not recommended). Products include:
Azilect Tablets 3106

Selegiline (Concurrent and/or sequential use with MAO inhibitors is not recommended). Products include:
Emsam Transdermal System 905

Selegiline Hydrochloride (Concurrent and/or sequential use with MAO inhibitors is not recommended). Products include:
Eldepryl Capsules 3052

Tranylcypromine Sulfate (Concurrent and/or sequential use with MAO inhibitors is not recommended). Products include:
Parnate Tablets 1532

Food Interactions

Alcohol (Consumption of 3 or more alcoholic drinks every day, need to ask your doctor whether you should take acetaminophen; may be at increased risk of liver toxicity from acetaminophen use).

TYLENOL COLD MULTI-SYMPTOM DAYTIME LIQUID WITH CITRUS BURST

(Acetaminophen, Dextromethorphan Hydrobromide, Phenylephrine Hydrochloride)............ 1913
See Tylenol Cold Multi-Symptom Daytime Caplets with Cool Burst and Rapid Release Gels

TYLENOL COLD MULTI-SYMPTOM NIGHTTIME CAPLETS WITH COOL BURST

(Acetaminophen, Chlorpheniramine Maleate, Dextromethorphan Hydrobromide, Phenylephrine Hydrochloride).................................. 1913
See Tylenol Severe Allergy Caplets

TYLENOL COLD MULTI-SYMPTOM NIGHTTIME LIQUID WITH COOL BURST

(Acetaminophen, Dextromethorphan Hydrobromide, Doxylamine Succinate, Phenylephrine Hydrochloride)............ 1913
See Tylenol Severe Allergy Caplets

TYLENOL COLD MULTI-SYMPTOM SEVERE CAPLETS WITH COOL BURST

(Acetaminophen, Dextromethorphan Hydrobromide, Guaifenesin, Phenylephrine Hydrochloride).................................. 1913
See Tylenol Cold Multi-Symptom Daytime Caplets with Cool Burst and Rapid Release Gels

TYLENOL COLD MULTI-SYMPTOM SEVERE DAYTIME LIQUID WITH CITRUS BURST

(Acetaminophen, Dextromethorphan Hydrobromide, Guaifenesin, Phenylephrine Hydrochloride).................................. 1913
See Tylenol Cold Multi-Symptom Daytime Caplets with Cool Burst and Rapid Release Gels

TYLENOL COUGH & SORE THROAT DAYTIME LIQUID WITH COOL BURST
(Acetaminophen, Dextromethorphan Hydrobromide)...... 1918
May interact with monoamine oxidase inhibitors. Compounds in these categories include:

Isocarboxazid (Avoid concomitant use with a monoamine oxidase inhibitor (MAOI) and for two weeks following discontinuation of a MAOI). Products include:
Marplan Tablets 3177

Moclobemide (Avoid concomitant use with a monoamine oxidase inhibitor (MAOI) and for two weeks following discontinuation of a MAOI).
No products indexed under this heading.

Pargyline Hydrochloride (Avoid concomitant use with a monoamine oxidase inhibitor (MAOI) and for two weeks following discontinuation of a MAOI).
No products indexed under this heading.

Phenelzine Sulfate (Avoid concomitant use with a monoamine oxidase inhibitor (MAOI) and for two weeks following discontinuation of a MAOI).
No products indexed under this heading.

Procarbazine Hydrochloride (Avoid concomitant use with a monoamine oxidase inhibitor (MAOI) and for two weeks following discontinuation of a MAOI).
No products indexed under this heading.

Rasagiline Mesylate (Avoid concomitant use with a monoamine oxidase inhibitor (MAOI) and for two weeks following discontinuation of a MAOI). Products include:
Azilect Tablets 3106

Selegiline (Avoid concomitant use with a monoamine oxidase inhibitor (MAOI) and for two weeks following discontinuation of a MAOI). Products include:
Emsam Transdermal System 905

Selegiline Hydrochloride (Avoid concomitant use with a monoamine oxidase inhibitor (MAOI) and for two weeks following discontinuation of a MAOI). Products include:
Eldepryl Capsules 3052

Tranylcypromine Sulfate (Avoid concomitant use with a monoamine oxidase inhibitor (MAOI) and for two weeks following discontinuation of a MAOI). Products include:
Parnate Tablets 1532

TYLENOL COUGH & SORE THROAT NIGHTTIME LIQUID WITH COOL BURST
(Acetaminophen, Dextromethorphan Hydrobromide, Doxylamine Succinate)....................... 1918
May interact with hypnotics and sedatives, monoamine oxidase inhibitors, tranquilizers, and certain other agents. Compounds in these categories include:

Alprazolam (Concurrent use with tranquilizers may increase drowsiness).
No products indexed under this heading.

Buspirone Hydrochloride (Concurrent use with tranquilizers may increase drowsiness).
No products indexed under this heading.

Butabarbital (Concurrent use with sedatives may increase drowsiness).
No products indexed under this heading.

Butabarbital Sodium (Concurrent use with sedatives may increase drowsiness).
No products indexed under this heading.

Chloral Hydrate (Concurrent use with sedatives may increase drowsiness).
No products indexed under this heading.

Chlordiazepoxide (Concurrent use with tranquilizers may increase drowsiness).
No products indexed under this heading.

Chlordiazepoxide Hydrochloride (Concurrent use with tranquilizers may increase drowsiness).
No products indexed under this heading.

Chlorpromazine (Concurrent use with tranquilizers may increase drowsiness).
No products indexed under this heading.

Chlorpromazine Hydrochloride (Concurrent use with tranquilizers may increase drowsiness).
No products indexed under this heading.

Chlorprothixene (Concurrent use with tranquilizers may increase drowsiness).
No products indexed under this heading.

Chlorprothixene Hydrochloride (Concurrent use with tranquilizers may increase drowsiness).
No products indexed under this heading.

Clorazepate Dipotassium (Concurrent use with tranquilizers may increase drowsiness).
No products indexed under this heading.

Diazepam (Concurrent use with tranquilizers may increase drowsiness). Products include:
Valium Tablets 2658

Droperidol (Concurrent use with tranquilizers may increase drowsiness).
No products indexed under this heading.

Estazolam (Concurrent use with sedatives may increase drowsiness).
No products indexed under this heading.

Ethanol (Concurrent use with alcohol may increase drowsiness. Avoid alcoholic drinks).
No products indexed under this heading.

Ethchlorvynol (Concurrent use with sedatives may increase drowsiness).
No products indexed under this heading.

Ethinamate (Concurrent use with sedatives may increase drowsiness).
No products indexed under this heading.

Ethyl Alcohol (Concurrent use with alcohol may increase drowsiness. Avoid alcoholic drinks).
No products indexed under this heading.

Fluphenazine Decanoate (Concurrent use with tranquilizers may increase drowsiness).
No products indexed under this heading.

Fluphenazine Enanthate (Concurrent use with tranquilizers may increase drowsiness).
No products indexed under this heading.

Fluphenazine Hydrochloride (Concurrent use with tranquilizers may increase drowsiness).
No products indexed under this heading.

Flurazepam Hydrochloride (Concurrent use with sedatives may increase drowsiness).
No products indexed under this heading.

Glutethimide (Concurrent use with sedatives may increase drowsiness).
No products indexed under this heading.

Haloperidol (Concurrent use with tranquilizers may increase drowsiness).
No products indexed under this heading.

Haloperidol Decanoate (Concurrent use with tranquilizers may increase drowsiness).
No products indexed under this heading.

Hydroxyzine Hydrochloride (Concurrent use with tranquilizers may increase drowsiness).
No products indexed under this heading.

Isocarboxazid (Avoid concurrent use with a monoamine oxidase inhibitor (MAOI) and for two weeks after stopping a MAOI). Products include:
Marplan Tablets 3177

Lorazepam (Concurrent use with tranquilizers may increase drowsiness).
No products indexed under this heading.

Loxapine Hydrochloride (Concurrent use with tranquilizers may increase drowsiness).
No products indexed under this heading.

Loxapine Succinate (Concurrent use with tranquilizers may increase drowsiness).
No products indexed under this heading.

Meprobamate (Concurrent use with tranquilizers may increase drowsiness).
No products indexed under this heading.

Mesoridazine Besylate (Concurrent use with tranquilizers may increase drowsiness).
No products indexed under this heading.

Midazolam Hydrochloride (Concurrent use with sedatives may increase drowsiness).
No products indexed under this heading.

Moclobemide (Avoid concurrent use with a monoamine oxidase inhibitor (MAOI) and for two weeks after stopping a MAOI).
No products indexed under this heading.

Molindone Hydrochloride (Concurrent use with tranquilizers may increase drowsiness). Products include:
Moban Tablets 1116

Oxazepam (Concurrent use with tranquilizers may increase drowsiness).
No products indexed under this heading.

Pargyline Hydrochloride (Avoid concurrent use with a monoamine oxidase inhibitor (MAOI) and for two weeks after stopping a MAOI).
No products indexed under this heading.

Perphenazine (Concurrent use with tranquilizers may increase drowsiness).
No products indexed under this heading.

Phenelzine Sulfate (Avoid concurrent use with a monoamine oxidase inhibitor (MAOI) and for two weeks after stopping a MAOI).
No products indexed under this heading.

Prazepam (Concurrent use with tranquilizers may increase drowsiness).
No products indexed under this heading.

Procarbazine Hydrochloride (Avoid concurrent use with a monoamine oxidase inhibitor (MAOI) and for two weeks after stopping a MAOI).
No products indexed under this heading.

Prochlorperazine (Concurrent use with tranquilizers may increase drowsiness).
No products indexed under this heading.

Promethazine Hydrochloride (Concurrent use with tranquilizers may increase drowsiness).
No products indexed under this heading.

Propofol (Concurrent use with sedatives may increase drowsiness).
No products indexed under this heading.

Quazepam (Concurrent use with sedatives may increase drowsiness).
No products indexed under this heading.

Ramelteon (Concurrent use with sedatives may increase drowsiness). Products include:
Rozerem Tablets 3091

Rasagiline Mesylate (Avoid concurrent use with a monoamine oxidase inhibitor (MAOI) and for two weeks after stopping a MAOI). Products include:
Azilect Tablets 3106

Secobarbital Sodium (Concurrent use with sedatives may increase drowsiness).
No products indexed under this heading.

Selegiline (Avoid concurrent use with a monoamine oxidase inhibitor (MAOI) and for two weeks after stopping a MAOI). Products include:
Emsam Transdermal System 905

Selegiline Hydrochloride (Avoid concurrent use with a monoamine oxidase inhibitor (MAOI) and for two weeks after stopping a MAOI). Products include:
Eldepryl Capsules 3052

Sodium Butabarbital (Concurrent use with sedatives may increase drowsiness).
No products indexed under this heading.

IMPORTANT NOTE: Always consult each drug listing in the patient's regimen for possible interactions.

Temazepam (Concurrent use with sedatives may increase drowsiness).
No products indexed under this heading.

Thioridazine Hydrochloride (Concurrent use with tranquilizers may increase drowsiness). Products include:
Thioridazine Hydrochloride Tablets 2195

Thiothixene (Concurrent use with tranquilizers may increase drowsiness). Products include:
Thiothixene Capsules 2197

Tranylcypromine Sulfate (Avoid concurrent use with a monoamine oxidase inhibitor (MAOI) and for two weeks after stopping a MAOI). Products include:
Parnate Tablets 1532

Triazolam (Concurrent use with sedatives may increase drowsiness).
No products indexed under this heading.

Trifluoperazine Hydrochloride (Concurrent use with tranquilizers may increase drowsiness).
No products indexed under this heading.

Zaleplon (Concurrent use with sedatives may increase drowsiness).
No products indexed under this heading.

Zolpidem Tartrate (Concurrent use with sedatives may increase drowsiness). Products include:
Ambien Tablets 2692
Ambien CR Tablets 2696

Food Interactions

Alcohol (Concurrent use with alcohol may increase drowsiness. Avoid alcoholic drinks).

CONCENTRATED TYLENOL INFANTS' DROPS

(Acetaminophen) 1909
None cited in PDR database.

JR. TYLENOL MELTAWAYS

(Acetaminophen) 1909
None cited in PDR database.

TYLENOL SINUS CONGESTION & PAIN DAYTIME CAPLETS WITH COOL BURST AND GELCAPS

(Acetaminophen, Phenylephrine Hydrochloride) 1917
See Tylenol Sinus Severe Congestion Caplets with Cool Burst

TYLENOL SINUS CONGESTION & PAIN NIGHTTIME CAPLETS WITH COOL BURST

(Acetaminophen, Chlorpheniramine Maleate, Phenylephrine Hydrochloride) 1917
May interact with hypnotics and sedatives, monoamine oxidase inhibitors, tranquilizers, and certain other agents. Compounds in these categories include:

Alprazolam (May increase drowsiness effect).
No products indexed under this heading.

Buspirone Hydrochloride (May increase drowsiness effect).
No products indexed under this heading.

Butabarbital (May increase drowsiness effect).
No products indexed under this heading.

Butabarbital Sodium (May increase drowsiness effect).
No products indexed under this heading.

Chloral Hydrate (May increase drowsiness effect).
No products indexed under this heading.

Chlordiazepoxide (May increase drowsiness effect).
No products indexed under this heading.

Chlordiazepoxide Hydrochloride (May increase drowsiness effect).
No products indexed under this heading.

Chlorpromazine (May increase drowsiness effect).
No products indexed under this heading.

Chlorpromazine Hydrochloride (May increase drowsiness effect).
No products indexed under this heading.

Chlorprothixene (May increase drowsiness effect).
No products indexed under this heading.

Chlorprothixene Hydrochloride (May increase drowsiness effect).
No products indexed under this heading.

Clorazepate Dipotassium (May increase drowsiness effect).
No products indexed under this heading.

Diazepam (May increase drowsiness effect). Products include:
Valium Tablets 2658

Droperidol (May increase drowsiness effect).
No products indexed under this heading.

Estazolam (May increase drowsiness effect).
No products indexed under this heading.

Ethchlorvynol (May increase drowsiness effect).
No products indexed under this heading.

Ethinamate (May increase drowsiness effect).
No products indexed under this heading.

Fluphenazine Decanoate (May increase drowsiness effect).
No products indexed under this heading.

Fluphenazine Enanthate (May increase drowsiness effect).
No products indexed under this heading.

Fluphenazine Hydrochloride (May increase drowsiness effect).
No products indexed under this heading.

Flurazepam Hydrochloride (May increase drowsiness effect).
No products indexed under this heading.

Glutethimide (May increase drowsiness effect).
No products indexed under this heading.

Haloperidol (May increase drowsiness effect).
No products indexed under this heading.

Haloperidol Decanoate (May increase drowsiness effect).
No products indexed under this heading.

Hydroxyzine Hydrochloride (May increase drowsiness effect).
No products indexed under this heading.

Isocarboxazid (Avoid use with monoamine oxidase inhibitors (MAOI) or for two weeks after stopping MAOI drug). Products include:
Marplan Tablets 3177

Lorazepam (May increase drowsiness effect).
No products indexed under this heading.

Loxapine Hydrochloride (May increase drowsiness effect).
No products indexed under this heading.

Loxapine Succinate (May increase drowsiness effect).
No products indexed under this heading.

Meprobamate (May increase drowsiness effect).
No products indexed under this heading.

Mesoridazine Besylate (May increase drowsiness effect).
No products indexed under this heading.

Midazolam Hydrochloride (May increase drowsiness effect).
No products indexed under this heading.

Moclobemide (Avoid use with monoamine oxidase inhibitors (MAOI) or for two weeks after stopping MAOI drug).
No products indexed under this heading.

Molindone Hydrochloride (May increase drowsiness effect). Products include:
Moban Tablets 1116

Oxazepam (May increase drowsiness effect).
No products indexed under this heading.

Pargyline Hydrochloride (Avoid use with monoamine oxidase inhibitors (MAOI) or for two weeks after stopping MAOI drug).
No products indexed under this heading.

Perphenazine (May increase drowsiness effect).
No products indexed under this heading.

Phenelzine Sulfate (Avoid use with monoamine oxidase inhibitors (MAOI) or for two weeks after stopping MAOI drug).
No products indexed under this heading.

Prazepam (May increase drowsiness effect).
No products indexed under this heading.

Procarbazine Hydrochloride (Avoid use with monoamine oxidase inhibitors (MAOI) or for two weeks after stopping MAOI drug).
No products indexed under this heading.

Prochlorperazine (May increase drowsiness effect).
No products indexed under this heading.

Promethazine Hydrochloride (May increase drowsiness effect).
No products indexed under this heading.

Propofol (May increase drowsiness effect).
No products indexed under this heading.

Quazepam (May increase drowsiness effect).
No products indexed under this heading.

Ramelteon (May increase drowsiness effect). Products include:
Rozerem Tablets 3091

Rasagiline Mesylate (Avoid use with monoamine oxidase inhibitors (MAOI) or for two weeks after stopping MAOI drug). Products include:
Azilect Tablets 3106

Secobarbital Sodium (May increase drowsiness effect).
No products indexed under this heading.

Selegiline (Avoid use with monoamine oxidase inhibitors (MAOI) or for two weeks after stopping MAOI drug). Products include:
Emsam Transdermal System 905

Selegiline Hydrochloride (Avoid use with monoamine oxidase inhibitors (MAOI) or for two weeks after stopping MAOI drug). Products include:
Eldepryl Capsules 3052

Sodium Butabarbital (May increase drowsiness effect).
No products indexed under this heading.

Temazepam (May increase drowsiness effect).
No products indexed under this heading.

Thioridazine Hydrochloride (May increase drowsiness effect). Products include:
Thioridazine Hydrochloride Tablets 2195

Thiothixene (May increase drowsiness effect). Products include:
Thiothixene Capsules 2197

Tranylcypromine Sulfate (Avoid use with monoamine oxidase inhibitors (MAOI) or for two weeks after stopping MAOI drug). Products include:
Parnate Tablets 1532

Triazolam (May increase drowsiness effect).
No products indexed under this heading.

Trifluoperazine Hydrochloride (May increase drowsiness effect).
No products indexed under this heading.

Zaleplon (May increase drowsiness effect).
No products indexed under this heading.

Zolpidem Tartrate (May increase drowsiness effect). Products include:
Ambien Tablets 2692
Ambien CR Tablets 2696

Food Interactions

Alcohol (May increase drowsiness effect).

TYLENOL SINUS CONGESTION & PAIN SEVERE CAPLETS WITH COOL BURST
(Acetaminophen, Guaifenesin, Phenylephrine Hydrochloride)............ 1917
May interact with monoamine oxidase inhibitors and certain other agents. Compounds in these categories include:

Isocarboxazid (Avoid use with monoamine oxidase inhibitors (MAOI) or for two weeks after stopping MAOI drug). Products include:
Marplan Tablets 3177

Moclobemide (Avoid use with monoamine oxidase inhibitors (MAOI) or for two weeks after stopping MAOI drug).
No products indexed under this heading.

Pargyline Hydrochloride (Avoid use with monoamine oxidase inhibitors (MAOI) or for two weeks after stopping MAOI drug).
No products indexed under this heading.

Phenelzine Sulfate (Avoid use with monoamine oxidase inhibitors (MAOI) or for two weeks after stopping MAOI drug).
No products indexed under this heading.

Procarbazine Hydrochloride (Avoid use with monoamine oxidase inhibitors (MAOI) or for two weeks after stopping MAOI drug).
No products indexed under this heading.

Rasagiline Mesylate (Avoid use with monoamine oxidase inhibitors (MAOI) or for two weeks after stopping MAOI drug). Products include:
Azilect Tablets 3106

Selegiline (Avoid use with monoamine oxidase inhibitors (MAOI) or for two weeks after stopping MAOI drug). Products include:
Emsam Transdermal System 905

Selegiline Hydrochloride (Avoid use with monoamine oxidase inhibitors (MAOI) or for two weeks after stopping MAOI drug). Products include:
Eldepryl Capsules 3052

Tranylcypromine Sulfate (Avoid use with monoamine oxidase inhibitors (MAOI) or for two weeks after stopping MAOI drug). Products include:
Parnate Tablets 1532

Food Interactions

Alcohol (Avoid concurrent use; chronic heavy alcohol abusers, 3 or more drinks per day, may be at increased risk of liver toxicity from acetaminophen use).

TYLENOL SINUS SEVERE CONGESTION CAPLETS WITH COOL BURST
(Acetaminophen, Guaifenesin, Pseudoephedrine Hydrochloride)........ 1917
May interact with monoamine oxidase inhibitors and certain other agents. Compounds in these categories include:

Isocarboxazid (Avoid use with monoamine oxidase inhibitors (MAOI) or for two weeks after stopping MAOI drug). Products include:
Marplan Tablets 3177

Moclobemide (Avoid use with monoamine oxidase inhibitors (MAOI) or for two weeks after stopping MAOI drug).
No products indexed under this heading.

Pargyline Hydrochloride (Avoid use with monoamine oxidase inhibitors (MAOI) or for two weeks after stopping MAOI drug).
No products indexed under this heading.

Phenelzine Sulfate (Avoid use with monoamine oxidase inhibitors (MAOI) or for two weeks after stopping MAOI drug).
No products indexed under this heading.

Procarbazine Hydrochloride (Avoid use with monoamine oxidase inhibitors (MAOI) or for two weeks after stopping MAOI drug).
No products indexed under this heading.

Rasagiline Mesylate (Avoid use with monoamine oxidase inhibitors (MAOI) or for two weeks after stopping MAOI drug). Products include:
Azilect Tablets 3106

Selegiline (Avoid use with monoamine oxidase inhibitors (MAOI) or for two weeks after stopping MAOI drug). Products include:
Emsam Transdermal System 905

Selegiline Hydrochloride (Avoid use with monoamine oxidase inhibitors (MAOI) or for two weeks after stopping MAOI drug). Products include:
Eldepryl Capsules 3052

Tranylcypromine Sulfate (Avoid use with monoamine oxidase inhibitors (MAOI) or for two weeks after stopping MAOI drug). Products include:
Parnate Tablets 1532

Food Interactions

Alcohol (Concurrent use may increase drowsiness effect; chronic heavy alcohol abusers, 3 or more drinks per day, may be at increased risk of liver toxicity from excessive acetaminophen use).

TYLENOL SORE THROAT DAYTIME LIQUID WITH COOL BURST
(Acetaminophen) 1918
None cited in PDR database.

TYLENOL SORE THROAT NIGHTTIME LIQUID WITH COOL BURST
(Acetaminophen, Diphenhydramine Hydrochloride).................................. 1918
May interact with hypnotics and sedatives, tranquilizers, and certain other agents. Compounds in these categories include:

Alprazolam (Concomitant use with tranquilizers may increase drowsiness).
No products indexed under this heading.

Buspirone Hydrochloride (Concomitant use with tranquilizers may increase drowsiness).
No products indexed under this heading.

Butabarbital (Concomitant use with sedatives may increase drowsiness).
No products indexed under this heading.

Butabarbital Sodium (Concomitant use with sedatives may increase drowsiness).
No products indexed under this heading.

Chloral Hydrate (Concomitant use with sedatives may increase drowsiness).
No products indexed under this heading.

Chlordiazepoxide (Concomitant use with tranquilizers may increase drowsiness).
No products indexed under this heading.

Chlordiazepoxide Hydrochloride (Concomitant use with tranquilizers may increase drowsiness).
No products indexed under this heading.

Chlorpromazine (Concomitant use with tranquilizers may increase drowsiness).
No products indexed under this heading.

Chlorpromazine Hydrochloride (Concomitant use with tranquilizers may increase drowsiness).
No products indexed under this heading.

Chlorprothixene (Concomitant use with tranquilizers may increase drowsiness).
No products indexed under this heading.

Chlorprothixene Hydrochloride (Concomitant use with tranquilizers may increase drowsiness).
No products indexed under this heading.

Clorazepate Dipotassium (Concomitant use with tranquilizers may increase drowsiness).
No products indexed under this heading.

Diazepam (Concomitant use with tranquilizers may increase drowsiness). Products include:
Valium Tablets 2658

Droperidol (Concomitant use with tranquilizers may increase drowsiness).
No products indexed under this heading.

Estazolam (Concomitant use with sedatives may increase drowsiness).
No products indexed under this heading.

Ethanol (Concomitant use may increase drowsiness. Avoid alcholic drinks).
No products indexed under this heading.

Ethchlorvynol (Concomitant use with sedatives may increase drowsiness).
No products indexed under this heading.

Ethinamate (Concomitant use with sedatives may increase drowsiness).
No products indexed under this heading.

Ethyl Alcohol (Concomitant use may increase drowsiness. Avoid alcholic drinks).
No products indexed under this heading.

Fluphenazine Decanoate (Concomitant use with tranquilizers may increase drowsiness).
No products indexed under this heading.

Fluphenazine Enanthate (Concomitant use with tranquilizers may increase drowsiness).
No products indexed under this heading.

Fluphenazine Hydrochloride (Concomitant use with tranquilizers may increase drowsiness).
No products indexed under this heading.

Flurazepam Hydrochloride (Concomitant use with sedatives may increase drowsiness).
No products indexed under this heading.

Glutethimide (Concomitant use with sedatives may increase drowsiness).
No products indexed under this heading.

Haloperidol (Concomitant use with tranquilizers may increase drowsiness).
No products indexed under this heading.

Haloperidol Decanoate (Concomitant use with tranquilizers may increase drowsiness).
No products indexed under this heading.

Hydroxyzine Hydrochloride (Concomitant use with tranquilizers may increase drowsiness).
No products indexed under this heading.

Lorazepam (Concomitant use with sedatives may increase drowsiness).
No products indexed under this heading.

Loxapine Hydrochloride (Concomitant use with tranquilizers may increase drowsiness).
No products indexed under this heading.

Loxapine Succinate (Concomitant use with tranquilizers may increase drowsiness).
No products indexed under this heading.

Meprobamate (Concomitant use with tranquilizers may increase drowsiness).
No products indexed under this heading.

Mesoridazine Besylate (Concomitant use with tranquilizers may increase drowsiness).
No products indexed under this heading.

Midazolam Hydrochloride (Concomitant use with sedatives may increase drowsiness).
No products indexed under this heading.

Molindone Hydrochloride (Concomitant use with tranquilizers may increase drowsiness). Products include:
Moban Tablets 1116

Oxazepam (Concomitant use with tranquilizers may increase drowsiness).
No products indexed under this heading.

Perphenazine (Concomitant use with tranquilizers may increase drowsiness).
No products indexed under this heading.

Prazepam (Concomitant use with tranquilizers may increase drowsiness).
No products indexed under this heading.

Prochlorperazine (Concomitant use with tranquilizers may increase drowsiness).
No products indexed under this heading.

Promethazine Hydrochloride (Concomitant use with tranquilizers may increase drowsiness).
No products indexed under this heading.

Propofol (Concomitant use with sedatives may increase drowsiness).
No products indexed under this heading.

Quazepam (Concomitant use with sedatives may increase drowsiness).
No products indexed under this heading.

Ramelteon (Concomitant use with sedatives may increase drowsiness). Products include:
Rozerem Tablets 3091

Secobarbital Sodium (Concomitant use with sedatives may increase drowsiness).
No products indexed under this heading.

Sodium Butabarbital (Concomitant use with sedatives may increase drowsiness).
No products indexed under this heading.

Temazepam (Concomitant use with sedatives may increase drowsiness).
No products indexed under this heading.

Thioridazine Hydrochloride (Concomitant use with tranquilizers may increase drowsiness). Products include:
Thioridazine Hydrochloride Tablets 2195

Thiothixene (Concomitant use with tranquilizers may increase drowsiness). Products include:
Thiothixene Capsules 2197

Triazolam (Concomitant use with sedatives may increase drowsiness).
No products indexed under this heading.

Trifluoperazine Hydrochloride (Concomitant use with tranquilizers may increase drowsiness).
No products indexed under this heading.

Zaleplon (Concomitant use with sedatives may increase drowsiness).
No products indexed under this heading.

Zolpidem Tartrate (Concomitant use with sedatives may increase drowsiness). Products include:
Ambien Tablets 2692
Ambien CR Tablets 2696

Food Interactions

Alcohol (Concomitant use may increase drowsiness. Avoid alcoholic drinks).

WOMEN'S TYLENOL MENSTRUAL RELIEF CAPLETS

(Acetaminophen, Pamabrom) 1919

Food Interactions

Alcohol (Chronic heavy alcohol users, 3 or more drinks per day, should consult their physicians for advice on when and how they should take pain relievers, including acetaminophen. Acetaminophen may cause liver damage).

TYZEKA TABLETS

(Telbivudine) 2328

May interact with nephrotoxic agents. Compounds in these categories include:

Abacavir Sulfate (Because telbivudine is eliminated primarily by renal excretion, co-administration of telbivudine with drugs that alter renal function may alter plasma concentration of telbivudine). Products include:
Epzicom Tablets 1422
Trizivir Tablets 1622
Ziagen 1673

Acyclovir (Because telbivudine is eliminated primarily by renal excretion, co-administration of telbivudine with drugs that alter renal function may alter plasma concentration of telbivudine). Products include:
Zovirax 1690
Zovirax Cream 817
Zovirax Ointment 819

Acyclovir Sodium (Because telbivudine is eliminated primarily by renal excretion, co-administration of telbivudine with drugs that alter renal function may alter plasma concentration of telbivudine).
No products indexed under this heading.

Alatrofloxacin Mesylate (Because telbivudine is eliminated primarily by renal excretion, co-administration of telbivudine with drugs that alter renal function may alter plasma concentration of telbivudine).
No products indexed under this heading.

Aldesleukin (Because telbivudine is eliminated primarily by renal excretion, co-administration of telbivudine with drugs that alter renal function may alter plasma concentration of telbivudine). Products include:
Proleukin for Injection 2287

Amikacin Sulfate (Because telbivudine is eliminated primarily by renal excretion, co-administration of telbivudine with drugs that alter renal function may alter plasma concentration of telbivudine).
No products indexed under this heading.

Amoxicillin (Because telbivudine is eliminated primarily by renal excretion, co-administration of telbivudine with drugs that alter renal function may alter plasma concentration of telbivudine). Products include:
Amoxil Capsules 1305
Amoxil Chewable Tablets 1305
Amoxil Pediatric Drops for Oral Suspension 1305
Amoxil Powder for Oral Suspension 1305
Amoxil Tablets 1305
Augmentin 1323
Augmentin Tablets 1327
Augmentin XR Extended Release Tablets 1333
Augmentin ES-600 Powder for Oral Suspension 1329
Moxatag Tablets 2165

Amoxicillin Trihydrate (Because telbivudine is eliminated primarily by renal excretion, co-administration of telbivudine with drugs that alter renal function may alter plasma concentration of telbivudine).
No products indexed under this heading.

Amphotericin B (Because telbivudine is eliminated primarily by renal excretion, co-administration of telbivudine with drugs that alter renal function may alter plasma concentration of telbivudine).
No products indexed under this heading.

Amphotericin B, liposomal (Because telbivudine is eliminated primarily by renal excretion, co-administration of telbivudine with drugs that alter renal function may alter plasma concentration of telbivudine). Products include:
AmBisome for Injection 606

Amphotericin B Cholesteryl Sulfate (Because telbivudine is eliminated primarily by renal excretion, co-administration of telbivudine with drugs that alter renal function may alter plasma concentration of telbivudine).
No products indexed under this heading.

Amphotericin B Lipid Complex (Because telbivudine is eliminated primarily by renal excretion, co-administration of telbivudine with drugs that alter renal function may alter plasma concentration of telbivudine). Products include:
Abelcet Injection 1134

Ampicillin (Because telbivudine is eliminated primarily by renal excretion, co-administration of telbivudine with drugs that alter renal function may alter plasma concentration of telbivudine).
No products indexed under this heading.

Ampicillin Sodium (Because telbivudine is eliminated primarily by renal excretion, co-administration of telbivudine with drugs that alter renal function may alter plasma concentration of telbivudine).
No products indexed under this heading.

Ampicillin Trihydrate (Because telbivudine is eliminated primarily by renal excretion, co-administration of telbivudine with drugs that alter renal function may alter plasma concentration of telbivudine).
No products indexed under this heading.

Amprenavir (Because telbivudine is eliminated primarily by renal excretion, co-administration of telbivudine with drugs that alter renal function may alter plasma concentration of telbivudine).
No products indexed under this heading.

Aspirin (Because telbivudine is eliminated primarily by renal excretion, co-administration of telbivudine with drugs that alter renal function may alter plasma concentration of telbivudine). Products include:
Aggrenox Capsules 819
Bayer Aspirin 750
Percodan Tablets 1130
St. Joseph 81 mg Aspirin Chewable and Enteric Coated Tablets 1903

Atazanavir (Because telbivudine is eliminated primarily by renal excretion, co-administration of telbivudine with drugs that alter renal function may alter plasma concentration of telbivudine).
No products indexed under this heading.

Atorvastatin Calcium (Because telbivudine is eliminated primarily by renal excretion, co-administration of telbivudine with drugs that alter renal function may alter plasma concentration of telbivudine). Products include:
Lipitor Tablets 2501

Azithromycin Dihydrate (Because telbivudine is eliminated primarily by renal excretion, co-administration of telbivudine with drugs that alter renal function may alter plasma concentration of telbivudine).
No products indexed under this heading.

Azlocillin Sodium (Because telbivudine is eliminated primarily by renal excretion, co-administration of telbivudine with drugs that alter renal function may alter plasma concentration of telbivudine).
No products indexed under this heading.

Aztreonam (Because telbivudine is eliminated primarily by renal excretion, co-administration of telbivudine with drugs that alter renal function may alter plasma concentration of telbivudine).
No products indexed under this heading.

Bacampicillin Hydrochloride (Because telbivudine is eliminated primarily by renal excretion, co-administration of telbivudine with drugs that alter renal function may alter plasma concentration of telbivudine).
No products indexed under this heading.

Balsalazide Disodium (Because telbivudine is eliminated primarily by renal excretion, co-administration of telbivudine with drugs that alter renal function may alter plasma concentration of telbivudine).
No products indexed under this heading.

Benazepril Hydrochloride (Because telbivudine is eliminated primarily by renal excretion, co-administration of telbivudine with drugs that alter renal function may alter plasma concentration of telbivudine).
No products indexed under this heading.

Bendroflumethiazide (Because telbivudine is eliminated primarily by renal excretion, co-administration of telbivudine with drugs that alter renal function may alter plasma concentration of telbivudine).
No products indexed under this heading.

Caffeine (Because telbivudine is eliminated primarily by renal excretion, co-administration of telbivudine with drugs that alter renal function may alter plasma concentration of telbivudine). Products include:
BioLean Free Tablets 635
BioLean II Tablets 635
Winrgy Dietary Supplement 642

Captopril (Because telbivudine is eliminated primarily by renal excretion, co-administration of telbivudine with drugs that alter renal function may alter plasma concentration of telbivudine). Products include:
Captopril Tablets 2182

Carbenicillin Disodium (Because telbivudine is eliminated primarily by renal excretion, co-administration of telbivudine with drugs that alter renal function may alter plasma concentration of telbivudine).
No products indexed under this heading.

Carbenicillin Indanyl Sodium (Because telbivudine is eliminated primarily by renal excretion, co-administration of telbivudine with drugs that alter renal function may alter plasma concentration of telbivudine).
No products indexed under this heading.

Carboplatin (Because telbivudine is eliminated primarily by renal excretion, co-administration of telbivudine with drugs that alter renal function may alter plasma concentration of telbivudine).
No products indexed under this heading.

Carmustine (BCNU) (Because telbivudine is eliminated primarily by renal excretion, co-administration of telbivudine with drugs that alter renal function may alter plasma concentration of telbivudine).
No products indexed under this heading.

Cefaclor (Because telbivudine is eliminated primarily by renal excretion, co-administration of telbivudine with drugs that alter renal function may alter plasma concentration of telbivudine).
No products indexed under this heading.

Cefadroxil (Because telbivudine is eliminated primarily by renal excretion, co-administration of telbivudine with drugs that alter renal function may alter plasma concentration of telbivudine).
No products indexed under this heading.

Cefamandole Nafate (Because telbivudine is eliminated primarily by renal excretion, co-administration of telbivudine with drugs that alter renal function may alter plasma concentration of telbivudine).
No products indexed under this heading.

Cefazolin Sodium (Because telbivudine is eliminated primarily by renal excretion, co-administration of telbivudine with drugs that alter renal function may alter plasma concentration of telbivudine).
No products indexed under this heading.

Cefdinir (Because telbivudine is eliminated primarily by renal excretion, co-administration of telbivudine with drugs that alter renal function may alter plasma concentration of telbivudine). Products include:
Omnicef Capsules 497
Omnicef for Oral Suspension 497

Cefepime Hydrochloride (Because telbivudine is eliminated primarily by renal excretion, co-administration of telbivudine with drugs that alter renal function may alter plasma concentration of telbivudine).
No products indexed under this heading.

Cefixime (Because telbivudine is eliminated primarily by renal excretion, co-administration of telbivudine with drugs that alter renal function may alter plasma concentration of telbivudine). Products include:
Suprax for Oral Suspension 1891
Suprax Tablets 1891

Cefmetazole Sodium (Because telbivudine is eliminated primarily by renal excretion, co-administration of telbivudine with drugs that alter renal function may alter plasma concentration of telbivudine).
No products indexed under this heading.

Cefonicid Sodium (Because telbivudine is eliminated primarily by renal excretion, co-administration of telbivudine with drugs that alter renal function may alter plasma concentration of telbivudine).
No products indexed under this heading.

Cefoperazone Sodium (Because telbivudine is eliminated primarily by renal excretion, co-administration of telbivudine with drugs that alter renal function may alter plasma concentration of telbivudine).
No products indexed under this heading.

Ceforanide (Because telbivudine is eliminated primarily by renal excretion, co-administration of telbivudine with drugs that alter renal function may alter plasma concentration of telbivudine).
No products indexed under this heading.

Cefotaxime Sodium (Because telbivudine is eliminated primarily by renal excretion, co-administration of telbivudine with drugs that alter renal function may alter plasma concentration of telbivudine).
No products indexed under this heading.

Cefotetan (Because telbivudine is eliminated primarily by renal excretion, co-administration of telbivudine with drugs that alter renal function may alter plasma concentration of telbivudine).
No products indexed under this heading.

Cefoxitin Sodium (Because telbivudine is eliminated primarily by renal excretion, co-administration of telbivudine with drugs that alter renal function may alter plasma concentration of telbivudine).
No products indexed under this heading.

Cefpodoxime Proxetil (Because telbivudine is eliminated primarily by renal excretion, co-administration of telbivudine with drugs that alter renal function may alter plasma concentration of telbivudine).
No products indexed under this heading.

Cefprozil (Because telbivudine is eliminated primarily by renal excretion, co-administration of telbivudine with drugs that alter renal function may alter plasma concentration of telbivudine).
No products indexed under this heading.

Ceftazidime (Because telbivudine is eliminated primarily by renal excretion, co-administration of telbivudine with drugs that alter renal function may alter plasma concentration of telbivudine). Products include:
Fortaz 1450

Ceftizoxime Sodium (Because telbivudine is eliminated primarily by renal excretion, co-administration of telbivudine with drugs that alter renal function may alter plasma concentration of telbivudine).
No products indexed under this heading.

Ceftriaxone Sodium (Because telbivudine is eliminated primarily by renal excretion, co-administration of telbivudine with drugs that alter renal function may alter plasma concentration of telbivudine). Products include:
Rocephin Injectable Vials, ADD-Vantage, Galaxy, Bulk........... 2642

Cefuroxime Axetil (Because telbivudine is eliminated primarily by renal excretion, co-administration of telbivudine with drugs that alter renal function may alter plasma concentration of telbivudine). Products include:
Ceftin 1380

Cefuroxime Sodium (Because telbivudine is eliminated primarily by renal excretion, co-administration of telbivudine with drugs that alter renal function may alter plasma concentration of telbivudine).
No products indexed under this heading.

Celecoxib (Because telbivudine is eliminated primarily by renal excretion, co-administration of telbivudine with drugs that alter renal function may alter plasma concentration of telbivudine). Products include:
Celebrex Capsules 2979

Cephalexin (Because telbivudine is eliminated primarily by renal excretion, co-administration of telbivudine with drugs that alter renal function may alter plasma concentration of telbivudine).
No products indexed under this heading.

Cephalothin Sodium (Because telbivudine is eliminated primarily by renal excretion, co-administration of telbivudine with drugs that alter renal function may alter plasma concentration of telbivudine).
No products indexed under this heading.

Cephapirin Sodium (Because telbivudine is eliminated primarily by renal excretion, co-administration of telbivudine with drugs that alter renal function may alter plasma concentration of telbivudine).
No products indexed under this heading.

Cephradine (Because telbivudine is eliminated primarily by renal excretion, co-administration of telbivudine with drugs that alter renal function may alter plasma concentration of telbivudine).
No products indexed under this heading.

Cerivastatin Sodium (Because telbivudine is eliminated primarily by renal excretion, co-administration of telbivudine with drugs that alter renal function may alter plasma concentration of telbivudine).
No products indexed under this heading.

Chlorothiazide (Because telbivudine is eliminated primarily by renal excretion, co-administration of telbivudine with drugs that alter renal function may alter plasma concentration of telbivudine).
No products indexed under this heading.

Chlorothiazide Sodium (Because telbivudine is eliminated primarily by renal excretion, co-administration of telbivudine with drugs that alter renal function may alter plasma concentration of telbivudine). Products include:
Intravenous Sodium Diuril 2490

Chlorpropamide (Because telbivudine is eliminated primarily by renal excretion, co-administration of telbivudine with drugs that alter renal function may alter plasma concentration of telbivudine).
No products indexed under this heading.

Cidofovir (Because telbivudine is eliminated primarily by renal excretion, co-administration of telbivudine with drugs that alter renal function may alter plasma concentration of telbivudine).
No products indexed under this heading.

Cilastatin Sodium (Because telbivudine is eliminated primarily by renal excretion, co-administration of telbivudine with drugs that alter renal function may alter plasma concentration of telbivudine). Products include:
Primaxin I.M. 2080
Primaxin I.V. 2083

Cimetidine (Because telbivudine is eliminated primarily by renal excretion, co-administration of telbivudine with drugs that alter renal function may alter plasma concentration of telbivudine).
No products indexed under this heading.

Cimetidine Hydrochloride (Because telbivudine is eliminated primarily by renal excretion, co-administration of telbivudine with drugs that alter renal function may alter plasma concentration of telbivudine).
No products indexed under this heading.

Cisplatin (Because telbivudine is eliminated primarily by renal excretion, co-administration of telbivudine with drugs that alter renal function may alter plasma concentration of telbivudine).
No products indexed under this heading.

Cladribine (Because telbivudine is eliminated primarily by renal excretion, co-administration of telbivudine with drugs that alter renal function may alter plasma concentration of telbivudine). Products include:
Leustatin Injection 2384

Clozapine (Because telbivudine is eliminated primarily by renal excretion, co-administration of telbivudine with drugs that alter renal function may alter plasma concentration of telbivudine).
No products indexed under this heading.

Colistimethate Sodium (Because telbivudine is eliminated primarily by renal excretion, co-administration of telbivudine with drugs that alter renal function may alter plasma concentration of telbivudine).
No products indexed under this heading.

Colistin Sulfate (Because telbivudine is eliminated primarily by renal excretion, co-administration of telbivudine with drugs that alter renal function may alter plasma concentration of telbivudine).
No products indexed under this heading.

Cyclophosphamide (Because telbivudine is eliminated primarily by renal excretion, co-administration of telbivudine with drugs that alter renal function may alter plasma concentration of telbivudine).
No products indexed under this heading.

Cyclosporine (Because telbivudine is eliminated primarily by renal excretion, co-administration of telbivudine with drugs that alter renal function may alter plasma concentration of telbivudine). Products include:
Gengraf Capsules **435**
Neoral Oral Solution **2280**
Neoral Soft Gelatin Capsules **2280**
Restasis Ophthalmic Emulsion **557**
Sandimmune **2296**

Cytarabine (Because telbivudine is eliminated primarily by renal excretion, co-administration of telbivudine with drugs that alter renal function may alter plasma concentration of telbivudine).
No products indexed under this heading.

Cytarabine Liposome (Because telbivudine is eliminated primarily by renal excretion, co-administration of telbivudine with drugs that alter renal function may alter plasma concentration of telbivudine). Products include:
DepoCyt Injection **1136**

Delavirdine Mesylate (Because telbivudine is eliminated primarily by renal excretion, co-administration of telbivudine with drugs that alter renal function may alter plasma concentration of telbivudine).
No products indexed under this heading.

Diatrizoate Meglumine (Because telbivudine is eliminated primarily by renal excretion, co-administration of telbivudine with drugs that alter renal function may alter plasma concentration of telbivudine).
No products indexed under this heading.

Diatrizoate Sodium (Because telbivudine is eliminated primarily by renal excretion, co-administration of telbivudine with drugs that alter renal function may alter plasma concentration of telbivudine).
No products indexed under this heading.

Diclofenac Potassium (Because telbivudine is eliminated primarily by renal excretion, co-administration of telbivudine with drugs that alter renal function may alter plasma concentration of telbivudine).
No products indexed under this heading.

Diclofenac Sodium (Because telbivudine is eliminated primarily by renal excretion, co-administration of telbivudine with drugs that alter renal function may alter plasma concentration of telbivudine). Products include:
Diclofenac Sodium Ophthalmic Solution .... ⊙**240**
Voltaren Ophthalmic Solution **2336**
Voltaren Tablets **2334**
Voltaren-XR Tablets **2337**

Dicloxacillin Sodium (Because telbivudine is eliminated primarily by renal excretion, co-administration of telbivudine with drugs that alter renal function may alter plasma concentration of telbivudine).
No products indexed under this heading.

Didanosine (Because telbivudine is eliminated primarily by renal excretion, co-administration of telbivudine with drugs that alter renal function may alter plasma concentration of telbivudine).
No products indexed under this heading.

Efavirenz (Because telbivudine is eliminated primarily by renal excretion, co-administration of telbivudine with drugs that alter renal function may alter plasma concentration of telbivudine). Products include:
Atripla Tablets **938**
Sustiva Capsules **930**
Sustiva Tablets **930**

Emtricitabine (Because telbivudine is eliminated primarily by renal excretion, co-administration of telbivudine with drugs that alter renal function may alter plasma concentration of telbivudine). Products include:
Atripla Tablets **938**
Emtriva Capsules **1246**
Emtriva Oral Solution **1246**
Truvada Tablets **1262**

Enalapril Maleate (Because telbivudine is eliminated primarily by renal excretion, co-administration of telbivudine with drugs that alter renal function may alter plasma concentration of telbivudine).
No products indexed under this heading.

Enalaprilat (Because telbivudine is eliminated primarily by renal excretion, co-administration of telbivudine with drugs that alter renal function may alter plasma concentration of telbivudine).
No products indexed under this heading.

Enfuvirtide (Because telbivudine is eliminated primarily by renal excretion, co-administration of telbivudine with drugs that alter renal function may alter plasma concentration of telbivudine).
No products indexed under this heading.

Ethiodized Oil (Because telbivudine is eliminated primarily by renal excretion, co-administration of telbivudine with drugs that alter renal function may alter plasma concentration of telbivudine).
No products indexed under this heading.

Etodolac (Because telbivudine is eliminated primarily by renal excretion, co-administration of telbivudine with drugs that alter renal function may alter plasma concentration of telbivudine).
No products indexed under this heading.

Fenoprofen Calcium (Because telbivudine is eliminated primarily by renal excretion, co-administration of telbivudine with drugs that alter renal function may alter plasma concentration of telbivudine). Products include:
Nalfon Capsules **2508**

Filgrastim (Because telbivudine is eliminated primarily by renal excretion, co-administration of telbivudine with drugs that alter renal function may alter plasma concentration of telbivudine). Products include:
Neupogen for Injection **589**

Fluorouracil (Because telbivudine is eliminated primarily by renal excretion, co-administration of telbivudine with drugs that alter renal function may alter plasma concentration of telbivudine). Products include:
Carac Cream 0.5% **2722**

Flurbiprofen (Because telbivudine is eliminated primarily by renal excretion, co-administration of telbivudine with drugs that alter renal function may alter plasma concentration of telbivudine).
No products indexed under this heading.

Fluvastatin Sodium (Because telbivudine is eliminated primarily by renal excretion, co-administration of telbivudine with drugs that alter renal function may alter plasma concentration of telbivudine). Products include:
Lescol Capsules **2268**
Lescol XL Tablets **2268**

Foscarnet Sodium (Because telbivudine is eliminated primarily by renal excretion, co-administration of telbivudine with drugs that alter renal function may alter plasma concentration of telbivudine).
No products indexed under this heading.

Fosinopril Sodium (Because telbivudine is eliminated primarily by renal excretion, co-administration of telbivudine with drugs that alter renal function may alter plasma concentration of telbivudine).
No products indexed under this heading.

Furosemide (Because telbivudine is eliminated primarily by renal excretion, co-administration of telbivudine with drugs that alter renal function may alter plasma concentration of telbivudine). Products include:
Furosemide Tablets **2186**

Gadopentetate Dimeglumine (Because telbivudine is eliminated primarily by renal excretion, co-administration of telbivudine with drugs that alter renal function may alter plasma concentration of telbivudine).
No products indexed under this heading.

Gentamicin (Because telbivudine is eliminated primarily by renal excretion, co-administration of telbivudine with drugs that alter renal function may alter plasma concentration of telbivudine).
No products indexed under this heading.

Gentamicin Sulfate (Because telbivudine is eliminated primarily by renal excretion, co-administration of telbivudine with drugs that alter renal function may alter plasma concentration of telbivudine). Products include:
Pred-G Ophthalmic Ointment .... ⊙**229**
Pred-G Ophthalmic Suspension .... ⊙**228**

Glipizide (Because telbivudine is eliminated primarily by renal excretion, co-administration of telbivudine with drugs that alter renal function may alter plasma concentration of telbivudine).
No products indexed under this heading.

Globulin, Immune (Human) (Because telbivudine is eliminated primarily by renal excretion, co-administration of telbivudine with drugs that alter renal function may alter plasma concentration of telbivudine). Products include:
Flebogamma 5% **1715**

Glyburide (Because telbivudine is eliminated primarily by renal excretion, co-administration of telbivudine with drugs that alter renal function may alter plasma concentration of telbivudine).
No products indexed under this heading.

Gold Therapy (Because telbivudine is eliminated primarily by renal excretion, co-administration of telbivudine with drugs that alter renal function may alter plasma concentration of telbivudine).
No products indexed under this heading.

HMG-CoA Reductase Inhibitors (Because telbivudine is eliminated primarily by renal excretion, co-administration of telbivudine with drugs that alter renal function may alter plasma concentration of telbivudine).
No products indexed under this heading.

Hydrochlorothiazide (Because telbivudine is eliminated primarily by renal excretion, co-administration of telbivudine with drugs that alter renal function may alter plasma concentration of telbivudine). Products include:
Atacand HCT **642**
Avalide Tablets **892**
Avalide Tablets **2713**
Benicar HCT Tablets **1010**
Diovan HCT Tablets **2216**
Dyazide Capsules **1405**
Micardis HCT Tablets **854**
Prinzide Tablets **2092**
Tekturna HCT Tablets **2324**
Teveten HCT Tablets **517**

Hydroflumethiazide (Because telbivudine is eliminated primarily by renal excretion, co-administration of telbivudine with drugs that alter renal function may alter plasma concentration of telbivudine).
No products indexed under this heading.

Ibuprofen (Because telbivudine is eliminated primarily by renal excretion, co-administration of telbivudine with drugs that alter renal function may alter plasma concentration of telbivudine). Products include:
Motrin IB Tablets and Caplets **1900**
Children's Motrin Oral Suspension **1901**
Children's Motrin Non-Staining Dye-Free Oral Suspension **1901**
Children's Motrin Cold Oral Suspension **1899**
Infants' Motrin Concentrated Drops **1901**
Infants' Motrin Non-Staining Dye-Free Concentrated Drops **1901**
Junior Strength Motrin Caplets and Chewable Tablets **1901**
Vicoprofen Tablets **533**

Idarubicin Hydrochloride (Because telbivudine is eliminated primarily by renal excretion, co-administration of telbivudine with drugs that alter renal function may alter plasma concentration of telbivudine).
No products indexed under this heading.

Ifosfamide (Because telbivudine is eliminated primarily by renal excretion, co-administration of telbivudine with drugs that alter renal function may alter plasma concentration of telbivudine).
No products indexed under this heading.

Imipenem (Because telbivudine is eliminated primarily by renal excretion, co-administration of telbivudine

with drugs that alter renal function may alter plasma concentration of telbivudine). Products include:
Primaxin I.M. 2080
Primaxin I.V. 2083

Immune Globulin Intravenous (Human) (Because telbivudine is eliminated primarily by renal excretion, co-administration of telbivudine with drugs that alter renal function may alter plasma concentration of telbivudine). Products include:
Flebogamma 5% DIF 1718
Gammagard Liquid 730
Gammagard S/D 734
Gamunex 3094

Indinavir Sulfate (Because telbivudine is eliminated primarily by renal excretion, co-administration of telbivudine with drugs that alter renal function may alter plasma concentration of telbivudine). Products include:
Crixivan Capsules 1979

Indomethacin (Because telbivudine is eliminated primarily by renal excretion, co-administration of telbivudine with drugs that alter renal function may alter plasma concentration of telbivudine). Products include:
Indocin 2024

Indomethacin Sodium Trihydrate (Because telbivudine is eliminated primarily by renal excretion, co-administration of telbivudine with drugs that alter renal function may alter plasma concentration of telbivudine). Products include:
Indocin I.V. 2489

Interferon Beta-1b (Because telbivudine is eliminated primarily by renal excretion, co-administration of telbivudine with drugs that alter renal function may alter plasma concentration of telbivudine). Products include:
Betaseron for SC Injection 756

Interleuken-2 (Because telbivudine is eliminated primarily by renal excretion, co-administration of telbivudine with drugs that alter renal function may alter plasma concentration of telbivudine).
No products indexed under this heading.

Iodamide Meglumine (Because telbivudine is eliminated primarily by renal excretion, co-administration of telbivudine with drugs that alter renal function may alter plasma concentration of telbivudine).
No products indexed under this heading.

Iohexol (Because telbivudine is eliminated primarily by renal excretion, co-administration of telbivudine with drugs that alter renal function may alter plasma concentration of telbivudine).
No products indexed under this heading.

Iopamidol (Because telbivudine is eliminated primarily by renal excretion, co-administration of telbivudine with drugs that alter renal function may alter plasma concentration of telbivudine).
No products indexed under this heading.

Iopanoic Acid (Because telbivudine is eliminated primarily by renal excretion, co-administration of telbivudine with drugs that alter renal function may alter plasma concentration of telbivudine).
No products indexed under this heading.

Iothalamate Meglumine (Because telbivudine is eliminated primarily by renal excretion, co-administration of telbivudine with drugs that alter renal function may alter plasma concentration of telbivudine).
No products indexed under this heading.

Ioxaglate Meglumine (Because telbivudine is eliminated primarily by renal excretion, co-administration of telbivudine with drugs that alter renal function may alter plasma concentration of telbivudine).
No products indexed under this heading.

Ioxaglate Sodium (Because telbivudine is eliminated primarily by renal excretion, co-administration of telbivudine with drugs that alter renal function may alter plasma concentration of telbivudine).
No products indexed under this heading.

Kanamycin Sulfate (Because telbivudine is eliminated primarily by renal excretion, co-administration of telbivudine with drugs that alter renal function may alter plasma concentration of telbivudine).
No products indexed under this heading.

Ketoprofen (Because telbivudine is eliminated primarily by renal excretion, co-administration of telbivudine with drugs that alter renal function may alter plasma concentration of telbivudine).
No products indexed under this heading.

Ketorolac Tromethamine (Because telbivudine is eliminated primarily by renal excretion, co-administration of telbivudine with drugs that alter renal function may alter plasma concentration of telbivudine).
No products indexed under this heading.

Lamium album (Because telbivudine is eliminated primarily by renal excretion, co-administration of telbivudine with drugs that alter renal function may alter plasma concentration of telbivudine).
No products indexed under this heading.

Lisinopril (Because telbivudine is eliminated primarily by renal excretion, co-administration of telbivudine with drugs that alter renal function may alter plasma concentration of telbivudine). Products include:
Prinivil Tablets 2087
Prinzide Tablets 2092

Lithium (Because telbivudine is eliminated primarily by renal excretion, co-administration of telbivudine with drugs that alter renal function may alter plasma concentration of telbivudine).
No products indexed under this heading.

Lithium Carbonate (Because telbivudine is eliminated primarily by renal excretion, co-administration of telbivudine with drugs that alter renal function may alter plasma concentration of telbivudine).
No products indexed under this heading.

Lithium Citrate (Because telbivudine is eliminated primarily by renal excretion, co-administration of telbivudine with drugs that alter renal function may alter plasma concentration of telbivudine).
No products indexed under this heading.

Lopinavir (Because telbivudine is eliminated primarily by renal excretion, co-administration of telbivudine with drugs that alter renal function may alter plasma concentration of telbivudine). Products include:
Kaletra 452

Loracarbef (Because telbivudine is eliminated primarily by renal excretion, co-administration of telbivudine with drugs that alter renal function may alter plasma concentration of telbivudine).
No products indexed under this heading.

Lovastatin (Because telbivudine is eliminated primarily by renal excretion, co-administration of telbivudine with drugs that alter renal function may alter plasma concentration of telbivudine). Products include:
Advicor Tablets 402
Mevacor Tablets 2063

Meclofenamate Sodium (Because telbivudine is eliminated primarily by renal excretion, co-administration of telbivudine with drugs that alter renal function may alter plasma concentration of telbivudine).
No products indexed under this heading.

Mefenamic Acid (Because telbivudine is eliminated primarily by renal excretion, co-administration of telbivudine with drugs that alter renal function may alter plasma concentration of telbivudine).
No products indexed under this heading.

Meloxicam (Because telbivudine is eliminated primarily by renal excretion, co-administration of telbivudine with drugs that alter renal function may alter plasma concentration of telbivudine). Products include:
Mobic Oral Suspension 863
Mobic Tablets 863

Melphalan Hydrochloride (Because telbivudine is eliminated primarily by renal excretion, co-administration of telbivudine with drugs that alter renal function may alter plasma concentration of telbivudine).
No products indexed under this heading.

Mesalamine (Because telbivudine is eliminated primarily by renal excretion, co-administration of telbivudine with drugs that alter renal function may alter plasma concentration of telbivudine). Products include:
Asacol Delayed-Release Tablets 2579
Canasa Rectal Suppositories 705
Lialda Tablets 3029
Pentasa Capsules 3030

Methimazole (Because telbivudine is eliminated primarily by renal excretion, co-administration of telbivudine with drugs that alter renal function may alter plasma concentration of telbivudine).
No products indexed under this heading.

Methotrexate (Because telbivudine is eliminated primarily by renal excretion, co-administration of telbivudine with drugs that alter renal function may alter plasma concentration of telbivudine).
No products indexed under this heading.

Methotrexate Sodium (Because telbivudine is eliminated primarily by renal excretion, co-administration of telbivudine with drugs that alter renal function may alter plasma concentration of telbivudine).
No products indexed under this heading.

Methyclothiazide (Because telbivudine is eliminated primarily by renal excretion, co-administration of telbivudine with drugs that alter renal function may alter plasma concentration of telbivudine).
No products indexed under this heading.

Mezlocillin Sodium (Because telbivudine is eliminated primarily by renal excretion, co-administration of telbivudine with drugs that alter renal function may alter plasma concentration of telbivudine).
No products indexed under this heading.

Minocycline Hydrochloride (Because telbivudine is eliminated primarily by renal excretion, co-administration of telbivudine with drugs that alter renal function may alter plasma concentration of telbivudine). Products include:
Solodyn Extended Release Tablets 1938

Mitomycin (Mitomycin-C) (Because telbivudine is eliminated primarily by renal excretion, co-administration of telbivudine with drugs that alter renal function may alter plasma concentration of telbivudine).
No products indexed under this heading.

Moexipril Hydrochloride (Because telbivudine is eliminated primarily by renal excretion, co-administration of telbivudine with drugs that alter renal function may alter plasma concentration of telbivudine).
No products indexed under this heading.

Muromonab-CD3 (Because telbivudine is eliminated primarily by renal excretion, co-administration of telbivudine with drugs that alter renal function may alter plasma concentration of telbivudine). Products include:
Orthoclone OKT3 Sterile Solution 2387

Nabumetone (Because telbivudine is eliminated primarily by renal excretion, co-administration of telbivudine with drugs that alter renal function may alter plasma concentration of telbivudine).
No products indexed under this heading.

Nafcillin Sodium (Because telbivudine is eliminated primarily by renal excretion, co-administration of telbivudine with drugs that alter renal function may alter plasma concentration of telbivudine).
No products indexed under this heading.

Naproxen (Because telbivudine is eliminated primarily by renal excretion, co-administration of telbivudine

with drugs that alter renal function may alter plasma concentration of telbivudine). Products include:

EC-Naprosyn Delayed-Release Tablets 2632
Naprosyn Suspension 2632
Naprosyn Tablets 2632

Naproxen Sodium (Because telbivudine is eliminated primarily by renal excretion, co-administration of telbivudine with drugs that alter renal function may alter plasma concentration of telbivudine). Products include:

Anaprox Tablets 2632
Anaprox DS Tablets 2632
Treximet Tablets 1616

Nelfinavir Mesylate (Because telbivudine is eliminated primarily by renal excretion, co-administration of telbivudine with drugs that alter renal function may alter plasma concentration of telbivudine).

No products indexed under this heading.

Neomycin (Because telbivudine is eliminated primarily by renal excretion, co-administration of telbivudine with drugs that alter renal function may alter plasma concentration of telbivudine).

No products indexed under this heading.

Neomycin, oral (Because telbivudine is eliminated primarily by renal excretion, co-administration of telbivudine with drugs that alter renal function may alter plasma concentration of telbivudine).

No products indexed under this heading.

Neomycin Sulfate (Because telbivudine is eliminated primarily by renal excretion, co-administration of telbivudine with drugs that alter renal function may alter plasma concentration of telbivudine). Products include:

Neosporin Ophthalmic Solution Sterile .... ⊙252

Nevirapine (Because telbivudine is eliminated primarily by renal excretion, co-administration of telbivudine with drugs that alter renal function may alter plasma concentration of telbivudine). Products include:

Viramune Oral Suspension 873
Viramune Tablets 873

Norfloxacin (Because telbivudine is eliminated primarily by renal excretion, co-administration of telbivudine with drugs that alter renal function may alter plasma concentration of telbivudine). Products include:

Noroxin Tablets 2069

Olsalazine Sodium (Because telbivudine is eliminated primarily by renal excretion, co-administration of telbivudine with drugs that alter renal function may alter plasma concentration of telbivudine).

No products indexed under this heading.

Omeprazole (Because telbivudine is eliminated primarily by renal excretion, co-administration of telbivudine with drugs that alter renal function may alter plasma concentration of telbivudine).

No products indexed under this heading.

Oxaprozin (Because telbivudine is eliminated primarily by renal excretion, co-administration of telbivudine with drugs that alter renal function may alter plasma concentration of telbivudine).

No products indexed under this heading.

Pamidronate Disodium (Because telbivudine is eliminated primarily by renal excretion, co-administration of telbivudine with drugs that alter renal function may alter plasma concentration of telbivudine).

No products indexed under this heading.

Paroxetine Hydrochloride (Because telbivudine is eliminated primarily by renal excretion, co-administration of telbivudine with drugs that alter renal function may alter plasma concentration of telbivudine). Products include:

Paxil 1535
Paxil CR Controlled-Release Tablets 1544

Penicillamine (Because telbivudine is eliminated primarily by renal excretion, co-administration of telbivudine with drugs that alter renal function may alter plasma concentration of telbivudine). Products include:

Cuprimine Capsules 1986

Penicillin G Benzathine (Because telbivudine is eliminated primarily by renal excretion, co-administration of telbivudine with drugs that alter renal function may alter plasma concentration of telbivudine). Products include:

Bicillin C-R Injectable Suspension 1775
Bicillin L-A Injection 1777

Penicillin G Potassium (Because telbivudine is eliminated primarily by renal excretion, co-administration of telbivudine with drugs that alter renal function may alter plasma concentration of telbivudine).

No products indexed under this heading.

Penicillin G Procaine (Because telbivudine is eliminated primarily by renal excretion, co-administration of telbivudine with drugs that alter renal function may alter plasma concentration of telbivudine). Products include:

Bicillin C-R Injectable Suspension 1775
Bicillin L-A Injection 1777

Penicillin G Sodium (Because telbivudine is eliminated primarily by renal excretion, co-administration of telbivudine with drugs that alter renal function may alter plasma concentration of telbivudine).

No products indexed under this heading.

Penicillin V Potassium (Because telbivudine is eliminated primarily by renal excretion, co-administration of telbivudine with drugs that alter renal function may alter plasma concentration of telbivudine).

No products indexed under this heading.

Pentamidine Isethionate (Because telbivudine is eliminated primarily by renal excretion, co-administration of telbivudine with drugs that alter renal function may alter plasma concentration of telbivudine).

No products indexed under this heading.

Perindopril Erbumine (Because telbivudine is eliminated primarily by renal excretion, co-administration of telbivudine with drugs that alter renal function may alter plasma concentration of telbivudine). Products include:

Aceon Tablets (2 mg, 4 mg, 8 mg) 3038

Phenylbutazone (Because telbivudine is eliminated primarily by renal excretion, co-administration of telbivudine with drugs that alter renal function may alter plasma concentration of telbivudine).

No products indexed under this heading.

Piroxicam (Because telbivudine is eliminated primarily by renal excretion, co-administration of telbivudine with drugs that alter renal function may alter plasma concentration of telbivudine).

No products indexed under this heading.

Plicamycin (Because telbivudine is eliminated primarily by renal excretion, co-administration of telbivudine with drugs that alter renal function may alter plasma concentration of telbivudine).

No products indexed under this heading.

Polymyxin (Because telbivudine is eliminated primarily by renal excretion, co-administration of telbivudine with drugs that alter renal function may alter plasma concentration of telbivudine).

No products indexed under this heading.

Polymyxin B Sulfate (Because telbivudine is eliminated primarily by renal excretion, co-administration of telbivudine with drugs that alter renal function may alter plasma concentration of telbivudine). Products include:

Neosporin Ophthalmic Solution Sterile .... ⊙252

Polythiazide (Because telbivudine is eliminated primarily by renal excretion, co-administration of telbivudine with drugs that alter renal function may alter plasma concentration of telbivudine).

No products indexed under this heading.

Pravastatin Sodium (Because telbivudine is eliminated primarily by renal excretion, co-administration of telbivudine with drugs that alter renal function may alter plasma concentration of telbivudine).

No products indexed under this heading.

Probenecid (Because telbivudine is eliminated primarily by renal excretion, co-administration of telbivudine with drugs that alter renal function may alter plasma concentration of telbivudine).

No products indexed under this heading.

Quinapril Hydrochloride (Because telbivudine is eliminated primarily by renal excretion, co-administration of telbivudine with drugs that alter renal function may alter plasma concentration of telbivudine).

No products indexed under this heading.

Rabeprazole Sodium (Because telbivudine is eliminated primarily by renal excretion, co-administration of telbivudine with drugs that alter renal function may alter plasma concentration of telbivudine). Products include:

Aciphex Tablets 1053

Ramipril (Because telbivudine is eliminated primarily by renal excretion, co-administration of telbivudine with drugs that alter renal function may alter plasma concentration of telbivudine).

No products indexed under this heading.

Rifampin (Because telbivudine is eliminated primarily by renal excretion, co-administration of telbivudine with drugs that alter renal function may alter plasma concentration of telbivudine).

No products indexed under this heading.

Riluzole (Because telbivudine is eliminated primarily by renal excretion, co-administration of telbivudine with drugs that alter renal function may alter plasma concentration of telbivudine). Products include:

Rilutek Tablets 2771

Ritonavir (Because telbivudine is eliminated primarily by renal excretion, co-administration of telbivudine with drugs that alter renal function may alter plasma concentration of telbivudine). Products include:

Kaletra 452
Norvir 489

Rofecoxib (Because telbivudine is eliminated primarily by renal excretion, co-administration of telbivudine with drugs that alter renal function may alter plasma concentration of telbivudine).

No products indexed under this heading.

Saquinavir (Because telbivudine is eliminated primarily by renal excretion, co-administration of telbivudine with drugs that alter renal function may alter plasma concentration of telbivudine).

No products indexed under this heading.

Sibutramine Hydrochloride Monohydrate (Because telbivudine is eliminated primarily by renal excretion, co-administration of telbivudine with drugs that alter renal function may alter plasma concentration of telbivudine). Products include:

Meridia Capsules 475

Simvastatin (Because telbivudine is eliminated primarily by renal excretion, co-administration of telbivudine with drugs that alter renal function may alter plasma concentration of telbivudine). Products include:

Simcor Tablets 502
Vytorin 10/10 Tablets 2149
Vytorin 10/10 Tablets 2939
Vytorin 10/20 Tablets 2149
Vytorin 10/20 Tablets 2939
Vytorin 10/40 Tablets 2149
Vytorin 10/40 Tablets 2939
Vytorin 10/80 Tablets 2149
Vytorin 10/80 Tablets 2939
Zocor Tablets 2136

Spirapril Hydrochloride (Because telbivudine is eliminated primarily by renal excretion, co-administration of telbivudine with drugs that alter renal function may alter plasma concentration of telbivudine).

No products indexed under this heading.

Stavudine (Because telbivudine is eliminated primarily by renal excretion, co-administration of telbivudine with drugs that alter renal function may alter plasma concentration of telbivudine).

No products indexed under this heading.

Streptomycin Sulfate (Because telbivudine is eliminated primarily by renal excretion, co-administration of telbivudine with drugs that alter renal function may alter plasma concentration of telbivudine).

No products indexed under this heading.

Streptozocin (Because telbivudine is eliminated primarily by renal excretion, co-administration of telbivudine with drugs that alter renal function may alter plasma concentration of telbivudine).
No products indexed under this heading.

Sulfacytine (Because telbivudine is eliminated primarily by renal excretion, co-administration of telbivudine with drugs that alter renal function may alter plasma concentration of telbivudine).
No products indexed under this heading.

Sulfamethizole (Because telbivudine is eliminated primarily by renal excretion, co-administration of telbivudine with drugs that alter renal function may alter plasma concentration of telbivudine).
No products indexed under this heading.

Sulfamethoxazole (Because telbivudine is eliminated primarily by renal excretion, co-administration of telbivudine with drugs that alter renal function may alter plasma concentration of telbivudine).
No products indexed under this heading.

Sulfasalazine (Because telbivudine is eliminated primarily by renal excretion, co-administration of telbivudine with drugs that alter renal function may alter plasma concentration of telbivudine).
No products indexed under this heading.

Sulfinpyrazone (Because telbivudine is eliminated primarily by renal excretion, co-administration of telbivudine with drugs that alter renal function may alter plasma concentration of telbivudine).
No products indexed under this heading.

Sulfisoxazole Acetyl (Because telbivudine is eliminated primarily by renal excretion, co-administration of telbivudine with drugs that alter renal function may alter plasma concentration of telbivudine).
No products indexed under this heading.

Sulfisoxazole Diolamine (Because telbivudine is eliminated primarily by renal excretion, co-administration of telbivudine with drugs that alter renal function may alter plasma concentration of telbivudine).
No products indexed under this heading.

Sulindac (Because telbivudine is eliminated primarily by renal excretion, co-administration of telbivudine with drugs that alter renal function may alter plasma concentration of telbivudine). Products include:
Clinoril Tablets **1962**

Tacrolimus (Because telbivudine is eliminated primarily by renal excretion, co-administration of telbivudine with drugs that alter renal function may alter plasma concentration of telbivudine). Products include:
Prograf Capsules and Injection **622**
Protopic Ointment **628**

Tenofovir Disoproxil Fumarate (Because telbivudine is eliminated primarily by renal excretion, co-administration of telbivudine with drugs that alter renal function may alter plasma concentration of telbivudine). Products include:
Atripla Tablets **938**
Truvada Tablets **1262**
Viread Tablets **1268**

Thioguanine (Because telbivudine is eliminated primarily by renal excretion, co-administration of telbivudine with drugs that alter renal function may alter plasma concentration of telbivudine). Products include:
Tabloid Tablets **1601**

Ticarcillin Disodium (Because telbivudine is eliminated primarily by renal excretion, co-administration of telbivudine with drugs that alter renal function may alter plasma concentration of telbivudine). Products include:
Timentin ADD-Vantage **1606**
Timentin Injection Galaxy Container **1609**
Timentin IV Infusion **1603**
Timentin Pharmacy Bulk Package **1613**

Tobramycin (Because telbivudine is eliminated primarily by renal excretion, co-administration of telbivudine with drugs that alter renal function may alter plasma concentration of telbivudine). Products include:
Zylet Ophthalmic Suspension .... ⊙ **247**

Tobramycin Sulfate (Because telbivudine is eliminated primarily by renal excretion, co-administration of telbivudine with drugs that alter renal function may alter plasma concentration of telbivudine).
No products indexed under this heading.

Tolazamide (Because telbivudine is eliminated primarily by renal excretion, co-administration of telbivudine with drugs that alter renal function may alter plasma concentration of telbivudine).
No products indexed under this heading.

Tolbutamide (Because telbivudine is eliminated primarily by renal excretion, co-administration of telbivudine with drugs that alter renal function may alter plasma concentration of telbivudine).
No products indexed under this heading.

Tolmetin Sodium (Because telbivudine is eliminated primarily by renal excretion, co-administration of telbivudine with drugs that alter renal function may alter plasma concentration of telbivudine).
No products indexed under this heading.

Trandolapril (Because telbivudine is eliminated primarily by renal excretion, co-administration of telbivudine with drugs that alter renal function may alter plasma concentration of telbivudine). Products include:
Mavik Tablets **472**
Tarka Tablets **511**

Triamterene (Because telbivudine is eliminated primarily by renal excretion, co-administration of telbivudine with drugs that alter renal function may alter plasma concentration of telbivudine). Products include:
Dyazide Capsules **1405**
Dyrenium Capsules **3189**

Trimethadione (Because telbivudine is eliminated primarily by renal excretion, co-administration of telbivudine with drugs that alter renal function may alter plasma concentration of telbivudine).
No products indexed under this heading.

Trovafloxacin Mesylate (Because telbivudine is eliminated primarily by renal excretion, co-administration of telbivudine with drugs that alter renal function may alter plasma concentration of telbivudine).
No products indexed under this heading.

Tyropanoate Sodium (Because telbivudine is eliminated primarily by renal excretion, co-administration of telbivudine with drugs that alter renal function may alter plasma concentration of telbivudine).
No products indexed under this heading.

Valacyclovir Hydrochloride (Because telbivudine is eliminated primarily by renal excretion, co-administration of telbivudine with drugs that alter renal function may alter plasma concentration of telbivudine). Products include:
Valtrex Caplets **1635**

Valdecoxib (Because telbivudine is eliminated primarily by renal excretion, co-administration of telbivudine with drugs that alter renal function may alter plasma concentration of telbivudine).
No products indexed under this heading.

Vancomycin Hydrochloride (Because telbivudine is eliminated primarily by renal excretion, co-administration of telbivudine with drugs that alter renal function may alter plasma concentration of telbivudine).
No products indexed under this heading.

Voriconazole (Because telbivudine is eliminated primarily by renal excretion, co-administration of telbivudine with drugs that alter renal function may alter plasma concentration of telbivudine).
No products indexed under this heading.

Zalcitabine (Because telbivudine is eliminated primarily by renal excretion, co-administration of telbivudine with drugs that alter renal function may alter plasma concentration of telbivudine).
No products indexed under this heading.

Zidovudine (Because telbivudine is eliminated primarily by renal excretion, co-administration of telbivudine with drugs that alter renal function may alter plasma concentration of telbivudine). Products include:
Combivir Tablets **1384**
Retrovir **1574**
Retrovir IV Infusion **1579**
Trizivir Tablets **1622**

Zoledronic acid (Because telbivudine is eliminated primarily by renal excretion, co-administration of telbivudine with drugs that alter renal function may alter plasma concentration of telbivudine). Products include:
Reclast Injection **2291**
Zometa for Intravenous Infusion **2341**

ULTANE LIQUID FOR INHALATION

(Sevoflurane) **524**
May interact with benzodiazepines, narcotic analgesics, nondepolarizing neuromuscular blocking agents, and certain other agents. Compounds in these categories include:

Alfentanil Hydrochloride (Benzodiazepines would be expected to decrease the MAC of sevoflurane in the same manner as with other inhalational anesthetics. Sevoflurane administration is compatible with benzodiazepines and opioids as commonly used in surgical practice).
No products indexed under this heading.

Alprazolam (Benzodiazepines would be expected to decrease the MAC of sevoflurane in the same manner as with other inhalational anesthetics. Sevoflurane administration is compatible with benzodiazepines and opioids as commonly used in surgical practice).
No products indexed under this heading.

Atracurium Besylate (Sevoflurane increases both the intensity and duration of neuromuscular blockade induced by non-depolarizing muscle relaxants. When used to supplement alfentanil-nitrous oxide anesthesia, sevoflurane and isoflurane equally potentiate neuromuscular block induced with pancuronium, vecuronium or atracurium. Among available non-depolarizing agents, only vecuronium, pancuronium and atracurium interactions have been studied during sevoflurane anesthesia. In the absence of specific guidelines: 1) For endotracheal intubation, do not reduce the dose of non-depolarizing muscle relaxants. 2) During maintenance of anesthesia, the required dose of non-depolarizing muscle relaxants is likely to be reduced compared to that during nitrous oxide/opioid anesthesia).
No products indexed under this heading.

Buprenorphine Hydrochloride (Benzodiazepines would be expected to decrease the MAC of sevoflurane in the same manner as with other inhalational anesthetics. Sevoflurane administration is compatible with benzodiazepines and opioids as commonly used in surgical practice). Products include:
Suboxone Tablets **2601**
Subutex Tablets **2601**

Chlordiazepoxide (Benzodiazepines would be expected to decrease the MAC of sevoflurane in the same manner as with other inhalational anesthetics. Sevoflurane administration is compatible with benzodiazepines and opioids as commonly used in surgical practice).
No products indexed under this heading.

Chlordiazepoxide Hydrochloride (Benzodiazepines would be expected to decrease the MAC of sevoflurane in the same manner as with other inhalational anesthetics. Sevoflurane administration is compatible with benzodiazepines and opioids as commonly used in surgical practice).
No products indexed under this heading.

Cisatracurium Besylate (Sevoflurane increases both the intensity and duration of neuromuscular blockade

induced by non-depolarizing muscle relaxants. When used to supplement alfentanil-nitrous oxide anesthesia, sevoflurane and isoflurane equally potentiate neuromuscular block induced with pancuronium, vecuronium or atracurium. Among available non-depolarizing agents, only vecuronium, pancuronium and atracurium interactions have been studied during sevoflurane anesthesia. In the absence of specific guidelines: 1) For endotracheal intubation, do not reduce the dose of non-depolarizing muscle relaxants. 2) During maintenance of anesthesia, the required dose of non-depolarizing muscle relaxants is likely to be reduced compared to that during nitrous oxide/opioid anesthesia). Products include:

Nimbex Injection 484

Clorazepate Dipotassium (Benzodiazepines would be expected to decrease the MAC of sevoflurane in the same manner as with other inhalational anesthetics. Sevoflurane administration is compatible with benzodiazepines and opioids as commonly used in surgical practice).

No products indexed under this heading.

Codeine Phosphate (Benzodiazepines would be expected to decrease the MAC of sevoflurane in the same manner as with other inhalational anesthetics. Sevoflurane administration is compatible with benzodiazepines and opioids as commonly used in surgical practice). Products include:

Tylenol with Codeine Tablets 2427

Dezocine (Benzodiazepines would be expected to decrease the MAC of sevoflurane in the same manner as with other inhalational anesthetics. Sevoflurane administration is compatible with benzodiazepines and opioids as commonly used in surgical practice).

No products indexed under this heading.

Diazepam (Benzodiazepines would be expected to decrease the MAC of sevoflurane in the same manner as with other inhalational anesthetics. Sevoflurane administration is compatible with benzodiazepines and opioids as commonly used in surgical practice). Products include:

Valium Tablets 2658

Estazolam (Benzodiazepines would be expected to decrease the MAC of sevoflurane in the same manner as with other inhalational anesthetics. Sevoflurane administration is compatible with benzodiazepines and opioids as commonly used in surgical practice).

No products indexed under this heading.

Fentanyl (Benzodiazepines would be expected to decrease the MAC of sevoflurane in the same manner as with other inhalational anesthetics. Sevoflurane administration is compatible with benzodiazepines and opioids as commonly used in surgical practice). Products include:

Duragesic Transdermal System 2405
Ionsys Transdermal System 2410

Fentanyl Citrate (Benzodiazepines would be expected to decrease the MAC of sevoflurane in the same manner as with other inhalational anesthetics. Sevoflurane administration is compatible with benzodiazepines and opioids as commonly used in surgical practice). Products include:

Actiq 959
Fentora Tablets 968

Flurazepam Hydrochloride (Benzodiazepines would be expected to decrease the MAC of sevoflurane in the same manner as with other inhalational anesthetics. Sevoflurane administration is compatible with benzodiazepines and opioids as commonly used in surgical practice).

No products indexed under this heading.

Halazepam (Benzodiazepines would be expected to decrease the MAC of sevoflurane in the same manner as with other inhalational anesthetics. Sevoflurane administration is compatible with benzodiazepines and opioids as commonly used in surgical practice).

No products indexed under this heading.

Hydrocodone Bitartrate (Benzodiazepines would be expected to decrease the MAC of sevoflurane in the same manner as with other inhalational anesthetics. Sevoflurane administration is compatible with benzodiazepines and opioids as commonly used in surgical practice). Products include:

Lortab 5/500 Tablets 3143
Lortab 7.5/500 Tablets 3144
Lortab 10/500 Tablets 3144
Vicodin Tablets 529
Vicodin ES Tablets 530
Vicodin HP Tablets 531
Vicoprofen Tablets 533
Zydone Tablets 1132

Hydrocodone Polistirex (Benzodiazepines would be expected to decrease the MAC of sevoflurane in the same manner as with other inhalational anesthetics. Sevoflurane administration is compatible with benzodiazepines and opioids as commonly used in surgical practice). Products include:

Tussionex Pennkinetic Extended-Release Suspension 3154

Hydromorphone Hydrochloride (Benzodiazepines would be expected to decrease the MAC of sevoflurane in the same manner as with other inhalational anesthetics. Sevoflurane administration is compatible with benzodiazepines and opioids as commonly used in surgical practice).

No products indexed under this heading.

Levorphanol Tartrate (Benzodiazepines would be expected to decrease the MAC of sevoflurane in the same manner as with other inhalational anesthetics. Sevoflurane administration is compatible with benzodiazepines and opioids as commonly used in surgical practice).

No products indexed under this heading.

Lorazepam (Benzodiazepines would be expected to decrease the MAC of sevoflurane in the same manner as with other inhalational anesthetics. Sevoflurane administration is compatible with benzodiazepines and opioids as commonly used in surgical practice).

No products indexed under this heading.

Meperidine Hydrochloride (Benzodiazepines would be expected to decrease the MAC of sevoflurane in the same manner as with other inhalational anesthetics. Sevoflurane administration is compatible with benzodiazepines and opioids as commonly used in surgical practice).

No products indexed under this heading.

Methadone Hydrochloride (Benzodiazepines would be expected to decrease the MAC of sevoflurane in the same manner as with other inhalational anesthetics. Sevoflurane administration is compatible with benzodiazepines and opioids as commonly used in surgical practice).

No products indexed under this heading.

Metocurine Iodide (Sevoflurane increases both the intensity and duration of neuromuscular blockade induced by non-depolarizing muscle relaxants. When used to supplement alfentanil-nitrous oxide anesthesia, sevoflurane and isoflurane equally potentiate neuromuscular block induced with pancuronium, vecuronium or atracurium. Among available non-depolarizing agents, only vecuronium, pancuronium and atracurium interactions have been studied during sevoflurane anesthesia. In the absence of specific guidelines: 1) For endotracheal intubation, do not reduce the dose of non-depolarizing muscle relaxants. 2) During maintenance of anesthesia, the required dose of non-depolarizing muscle relaxants is likely to be reduced compared to that during nitrous oxide/opioid anesthesia).

No products indexed under this heading.

Midazolam Hydrochloride (Benzodiazepines would be expected to decrease the MAC of sevoflurane in the same manner as with other inhalational anesthetics. Sevoflurane administration is compatible with benzodiazepines and opioids as commonly used in surgical practice).

No products indexed under this heading.

Mivacurium Chloride (Sevoflurane increases both the intensity and duration of neuromuscular blockade induced by non-depolarizing muscle relaxants. When used to supplement alfentanil-nitrous oxide anesthesia, sevoflurane and isoflurane equally potentiate neuromuscular block induced with pancuronium, vecuronium or atracurium. Among available non-depolarizing agents, only vecuronium, pancuronium and atracurium interactions have been studied during sevoflurane anesthesia. In the absence of specific guidelines: 1) For endotracheal intubation, do not reduce the dose of non-depolarizing muscle relaxants. 2) During maintenance of anesthesia, the required dose of non-depolarizing muscle relaxants is likely to be reduced compared to that during nitrous oxide/opioid anesthesia).

No products indexed under this heading.

Morphine Sulfate (Benzodiazepines would be expected to decrease the MAC of sevoflurane in the same manner as with other inhalational anesthetics. Sevoflurane administration is compatible with benzodiazepines and opioids as commonly used in surgical practice). Products include:

Avinza Capsules 1772
DepoDur Injection 1095
MS Contin Tablets 2585

Nitrous Oxide (As with other halogenated volatile anesthetics, the anesthetic requirement for sevoflurane is decreased when administered in combination with nitrous oxide. Using 50% nitrous oxide, the MAC equivalent dose requirement is reduced approximately 50% in adults and approximately 25% in pediatrics patients).

No products indexed under this heading.

Oxazepam (Benzodiazepines would be expected to decrease the MAC of sevoflurane in the same manner as with other inhalational anesthetics. Sevoflurane administration is compatible with benzodiazepines and opioids as commonly used in surgical practice).

No products indexed under this heading.

Oxycodone Hydrochloride (Benzodiazepines would be expected to decrease the MAC of sevoflurane in the same manner as with other inhalational anesthetics. Sevoflurane administration is compatible with benzodiazepines and opioids as commonly used in surgical practice). Products include:

OxyContin Tablets 2589
OxyIR Capsules 2593
Percocet Tablets 1127
Percodan Tablets 1130

Pancuronium Bromide (Sevoflurane increases both the intensity and duration of neuromuscular blockade induced by non-depolarizing muscle relaxants. When used to supplement alfentanil-nitrous oxide anesthesia, sevoflurane and isoflurane equally potentiate neuromuscular block induced with pancuronium, vecuronium or atracurium. Among available non-depolarizing agents, only vecuronium, pancuronium and atracurium interactions have been studied during sevoflurane anesthesia. In the absence of specific guidelines: 1) For endotracheal intubation, do not reduce the dose of non-depolarizing muscle relaxants. 2) During maintenance of anesthesia, the required dose of non-depolarizing muscle relaxants is likely to be reduced compared to that during nitrous oxide/opioid anesthesia).

No products indexed under this heading.

Prazepam (Benzodiazepines would be expected to decrease the MAC of sevoflurane in the same manner as with other inhalational anesthetics. Sevoflurane administration is compatible with benzodiazepines and opioids as commonly used in surgical practice).

No products indexed under this heading.

Propoxyphene Hydrochloride (Benzodiazepines would be expected to decrease the MAC of sevoflurane in the same manner as with other inhalational anesthetics. Sevoflurane administration is compatible with benzodiazepines and opioids as commonly used in surgical practice).

No products indexed under this heading.

Propoxyphene Napsylate (Benzodiazepines would be expected to decrease the MAC of sevoflurane in the same manner as with other inhalational anesthetics. Sevoflurane administration is compatible with benzodiazepines and opioids as commonly used in surgical practice).
No products indexed under this heading.

Quazepam (Benzodiazepines would be expected to decrease the MAC of sevoflurane in the same manner as with other inhalational anesthetics. Sevoflurane administration is compatible with benzodiazepines and opioids as commonly used in surgical practice).
No products indexed under this heading.

Rapacuronium Bromide (Sevoflurane increases both the intensity and duration of neuromuscular blockade induced by non-depolarizing muscle relaxants. When used to supplement alfentanil-nitrous oxide anesthesia, sevoflurane and isoflurane equally potentiate neuromuscular block induced with pancuronium, vecuronium or atracurium. Among available non-depolarizing agents, only vecuronium, pancuronium and atracurium interactions have been studied during sevoflurane anesthesia. In the absence of specific guidelines: 1) For endotracheal intubation, do not reduce the dose of non-depolarizing muscle relaxants. 2) During maintenance of anesthesia, the required dose of non-depolarizing muscle relaxants is likely to be reduced compared to that during nitrous oxide/opioid anesthesia).
No products indexed under this heading.

Remifentanil Hydrochloride (Benzodiazepines would be expected to decrease the MAC of sevoflurane in the same manner as with other inhalational anesthetics. Sevoflurane administration is compatible with benzodiazepines and opioids as commonly used in surgical practice).
No products indexed under this heading.

Rocuronium Bromide (Sevoflurane increases both the intensity and duration of neuromuscular blockade induced by non-depolarizing muscle relaxants. When used to supplement alfentanil-nitrous oxide anesthesia, sevoflurane and isoflurane equally potentiate neuromuscular block induced with pancuronium, vecuronium or atracurium. Among available non-depolarizing agents, only vecuronium, pancuronium and atracurium interactions have been studied during sevoflurane anesthesia. In the absence of specific guidelines: 1) For endotracheal intubation, do not reduce the dose of non-depolarizing muscle relaxants. 2) During maintenance of anesthesia, the required dose of non-depolarizing muscle relaxants is likely to be reduced compared to that during nitrous oxide/opioid anesthesia). Products include:
Zemuron Injection 2947

Sufentanil Citrate (Benzodiazepines would be expected to decrease the MAC of sevoflurane in the same manner as with other inhalational anesthetics. Sevoflurane administration is compatible with benzodiazepines and opioids as commonly used in surgical practice).
No products indexed under this heading.

Temazepam (Benzodiazepines would be expected to decrease the MAC of sevoflurane in the same manner as with other inhalational anesthetics. Sevoflurane administration is compatible with benzodiazepines and opioids as commonly used in surgical practice).
No products indexed under this heading.

Triazolam (Benzodiazepines would be expected to decrease the MAC of sevoflurane in the same manner as with other inhalational anesthetics. Sevoflurane administration is compatible with benzodiazepines and opioids as commonly used in surgical practice).
No products indexed under this heading.

Vecuronium Bromide (Sevoflurane increases both the intensity and duration of neuromuscular blockade induced by non-depolarizing muscle relaxants. When used to supplement alfentanil-nitrous oxide anesthesia, sevoflurane and isoflurane equally potentiate neuromuscular block induced with pancuronium, vecuronium or atracurium. Among available non-depolarizing agents, only vecuronium, pancuronium and atracurium interactions have been studied during sevoflurane anesthesia. In the absence of specific guidelines: 1) For endotracheal intubation, do not reduce the dose of non-depolarizing muscle relaxants. 2) During maintenance of anesthesia, the required dose of non-depolarizing muscle relaxants is likely to be reduced compared to that during nitrous oxide/opioid anesthesia).
No products indexed under this heading.

ULTRAM ER EXTENDED-RELEASE TABLETS

(Tramadol Hydrochloride) 2428

May interact with anesthetics, central nervous system depressants, cytochrome p450 2d6 inhibitors (selected), cytochrome p450 3a4 inducers (selected), cytochrome p450 3a4 inhibitors (selected), hypnotics and sedatives, monoamine oxidase inhibitors, narcotic analgesics, antipsychotic agents, phenothiazines, psychotropics, quinidine, Serotonin and Norepinephrine Reuptake Inhibitors, selective serotonin reuptake inhibitors, tranquilizers, tricyclic antidepressants, triptans, and certain other agents. Compounds in these categories include:

Acetazolamide (Administration of CYP3A4 inhibitors, such as ketoconazole and erythromycin, with tramadol hydrochloride may effect the metabolism of tramadol leading to altered tramadol exposure).
No products indexed under this heading.

Alfentanil Hydrochloride (Tramadol hydrochloride is contraindicated in acute intoxication with narcotics, opioids, and centrally-acting analgesics. Concomitant use of tramadol increases the seizure risk in patients taking opioids. Tramadol hydrochloride should be used with caution and in reduced dosages when administered to patients receiving CNS depressants, such as opioids or narcotics. Tramadol hydrochloride increases the risk of CNS and respiratory depression. Tramadol may be expected to have additive effects when used in conjunction with other opioids).
No products indexed under this heading.

Allium sativum (Administration of CYP3A4 inducers, such as rifampin or St. John's Wort, with tramadol hydrochloride may effect the metabolism of tramadol leading to altered tramadol exposure).
No products indexed under this heading.

Almotriptan Malate (Concomitant use of tramadol increases the seizure risk in patients taking triptans. Concomitant use of tramadol with triptans increases the risk of adverse events, including seizure and serotonin syndrome. If concomitant treatment of tramadol with a drug affecting the serotonergic neurotransmitter system is clinically warranted, careful observation of the patient is advised, particularly during treatment initiation and dose increases). Products include:
Axert Tablets 2431

Alprazolam (Tramadol hydrochloride is contraindicated in acute intoxication with psychotropic drugs).
No products indexed under this heading.

Amiodarone Hydrochloride (In vitro drug interaction studies in human liver microsomes indicate that concomitant administration with inhibitors of CYP2D6 could result in some inhibition of the metabolism of tramadol).
No products indexed under this heading.

Amitriptyline Hydrochloride (Tramadol hydrochloride is contraindicated in acute intoxication with psychotropic drugs).
No products indexed under this heading.

Amoxapine (Tramadol hydrochloride is contraindicated in acute intoxication with psychotropic drugs).
No products indexed under this heading.

Amprenavir (Administration of CYP3A4 inhibitors, such as ketoconazole and erythromycin, with tramadol hydrochloride may effect the metabolism of tramadol leading to altered tramadol exposure).
No products indexed under this heading.

Anastrozole (Administration of CYP3A4 inhibitors, such as ketoconazole and erythromycin, with tramadol hydrochloride may effect the metabolism of tramadol leading to altered tramadol exposure). Products include:
Arimidex Tablets 672

Aprepitant (Administration of CYP3A4 inhibitors, such as ketoconazole and erythromycin, with tramadol hydrochloride may effect the metabolism of tramadol leading to altered tramadol exposure). Products include:
Emend Capsules 1992

Aprobarbital (Tramadol hydrochloride should be used with caution and in reduced dosages when administered to patients receiving CNS depressants, such as alcohol, opioids, anesthetic agents, narcotics, phenothiazines, tranquilizers, or sedative hypnotics. Tramadol hydrochloride increases the risk of CNS and respiratory depression).
No products indexed under this heading.

Aripiprazole (Administration of tramadol may increase the seizure risk in patients taking neuroleptics or other drugs that reduce the seizure threshold). Products include:
Abilify Injection 881
Abilify Injection 2466
Abilify Oral Solution 881
Abilify Oral Solution 2466
Abilify Discmelt Orally Disintegrating Tablets 881
Abilify Discmelt Orally Disintegrating Tablets 2466
Abilify Tablets 881
Abilify Tablets 2466

Atazanavir (Administration of CYP3A4 inhibitors, such as ketoconazole and erythromycin, with tramadol hydrochloride may effect the metabolism of tramadol leading to altered tramadol exposure).
No products indexed under this heading.

Atazanavir Sulfate (Administration of CYP3A4 inhibitors, such as ketoconazole and erythromycin, with tramadol hydrochloride may effect the metabolism of tramadol leading to altered tramadol exposure). Products include:
Reyataz Capsules 3299

Betamethasone Acetate (Administration of CYP3A4 inducers, such as rifampin or St. John's Wort, with tramadol hydrochloride may effect the metabolism of tramadol leading to altered tramadol exposure).
No products indexed under this heading.

Betamethasone Sodium Phosphate (Administration of CYP3A4 inducers, such as rifampin or St. John's Wort, with tramadol hydrochloride may effect the metabolism of tramadol leading to altered tramadol exposure).
No products indexed under this heading.

Buprenorphine Hydrochloride (Tramadol hydrochloride is contraindicated in acute intoxication with narcotics, opioids, and centrally-acting analgesics. Concomitant use of tramadol increases the seizure risk in patients taking opioids. Tramadol hydrochloride should be used with caution and in reduced dosages when administered to patients receiving CNS depressants, such as opioids or narcotics. Tramadol hydrochloride increases the risk of CNS and respiratory depression. Tramadol may be expected to have additive effects when used in conjunction with other opioids). Products include:
Suboxone Tablets 2601
Subutex Tablets 2601

Bupropion Hydrochloride (In vitro drug interaction studies in human liver microsomes indicate that concomitant administration with inhibitors of CYP2D6 could result in some inhibition of the metabolism of tramadol). Products include:
Wellbutrin Tablets 1648

IMPORTANT NOTE: Always consult each drug listing in the patient's regimen for possible interactions.

Wellbutrin SR Sustained-Release Tablets 1653
Wellbutrin XL Extended-Release Tablets 1659
Zyban Sustained-Release Tablets 1692

Buspirone Hydrochloride (Tramadol hydrochloride is contraindicated in acute intoxication with psychotropic drugs).
No products indexed under this heading.

Butabarbital (Tramadol hydrochloride is contraindicated in acute intoxication with hypnotics. Tramadol hydrochloride should be used with caution and in reduced dosages when administered to patients receiving CNS depressants, such as sedative hypnotics. Tramadol hydrochloride increases the risk of CNS and respiratory depression).
No products indexed under this heading.

Butabarbital Sodium (Tramadol hydrochloride is contraindicated in acute intoxication with hypnotics. Tramadol hydrochloride should be used with caution and in reduced dosages when administered to patients receiving CNS depressants, such as sedative hypnotics. Tramadol hydrochloride increases the risk of CNS and respiratory depression).
No products indexed under this heading.

Butalbital (Tramadol hydrochloride should be used with caution and in reduced dosages when administered to patients receiving CNS depressants, such as alcohol, opioids, anesthetic agents, narcotics, phenothiazines, tranquilizers, or sedative hypnotics. Tramadol hydrochloride increases the risk of CNS and respiratory depression).
No products indexed under this heading.

Carbamazepine (Patients taking carbamazepine, a CYP3A4 inducer, may have a significantly reduced analgesic effect of tramadol. Because carbamazepine increases tramadol metabolism and because of the seizure risk associated with tramadol, concomitant administration of tramadol hydrochloride and carbamazepine is not recommended). Products include:
Carbatrol Capsules 3019
Equetro Extended-Release Capsules 3174

Celecoxib (In vitro drug interaction studies in human liver microsomes indicate that concomitant administration with inhibitors of CYP2D6 could result in some inhibition of the metabolism of tramadol). Products include:
Celebrex Capsules 2979

Chloral Hydrate (Tramadol hydrochloride is contraindicated in acute intoxication with hypnotics. Tramadol hydrochloride should be used with caution and in reduced dosages when administered to patients receiving CNS depressants, such as sedative hypnotics. Tramadol hydrochloride increases the risk of CNS and respiratory depression).
No products indexed under this heading.

Chlordiazepoxide (Tramadol hydrochloride is contraindicated in acute intoxication with psychotropic drugs).
No products indexed under this heading.

Chlordiazepoxide Hydrochloride (Tramadol hydrochloride is contraindicated in acute intoxication with psychotropic drugs).
No products indexed under this heading.

Chloroquine Hydrochloride (In vitro drug interaction studies in human liver microsomes indicate that concomitant administration with inhibitors of CYP2D6 could result in some inhibition of the metabolism of tramadol).
No products indexed under this heading.

Chloroquine Phosphate (In vitro drug interaction studies in human liver microsomes indicate that concomitant administration with inhibitors of CYP2D6 could result in some inhibition of the metabolism of tramadol).
No products indexed under this heading.

Chlorpheniramine (In vitro drug interaction studies in human liver microsomes indicate that concomitant administration with inhibitors of CYP2D6 could result in some inhibition of the metabolism of tramadol).
No products indexed under this heading.

Chlorpheniramine Maleate (In vitro drug interaction studies in human liver microsomes indicate that concomitant administration with inhibitors of CYP2D6 could result in some inhibition of the metabolism of tramadol). Products include:
Actifed Cold & Allergy Tablets 1895
Sudafed PE Sinus & Allergy Tablets 1908
Tylenol Allergy Multi-Symptom Caplets with Cool Burst and Rapid Release Gelcaps 1916
Children's Tylenol Plus Cold Suspension Liquid 1912
Children's Tylenol Plus Cough & Runny Nose Suspension Liquid 1912
Children's Tylenol Plus Flu Suspension Liquid 1914
Children's Tylenol Plus Multi-Symptom Cold Suspension Liquid 1912
Tylenol Cold Head Congestion Nighttime Caplets with Cool Burst 1910
Tylenol Cold Multi-Symptom Nighttime Caplets with Cool Burst 1913
Tylenol Sinus Congestion & Pain Nighttime Caplets with Cool Burst 1917

Chlorpheniramine Polistirex (In vitro drug interaction studies in human liver microsomes indicate that concomitant administration with inhibitors of CYP2D6 could result in some inhibition of the metabolism of tramadol). Products include:
Tussionex Pennkinetic Extended-Release Suspension 3154

Chlorpheniramine Tannate (In vitro drug interaction studies in human liver microsomes indicate that concomitant administration with inhibitors of CYP2D6 could result in some inhibition of the metabolism of tramadol).
No products indexed under this heading.

Chlorpromazine (Tramadol hydrochloride is contraindicated in acute intoxication with psychotropic drugs).
No products indexed under this heading.

Chlorpromazine Hydrochloride (Tramadol hydrochloride is contraindicated in acute intoxication with psychotropic drugs).
No products indexed under this heading.

Chlorprothixene (Tramadol hydrochloride is contraindicated in acute intoxication with psychotropic drugs).
No products indexed under this heading.

Chlorprothixene Hydrochloride (Tramadol hydrochloride is contraindicated in acute intoxication with psychotropic drugs).
No products indexed under this heading.

Chlorprothixene Lactate (Tramadol hydrochloride should be used with caution and in reduced dosages when administered to patients receiving CNS depressants, such as alcohol, opioids, anesthetic agents, narcotics, phenothiazines, tranquilizers, or sedative hypnotics. Tramadol hydrochloride increases the risk of CNS and respiratory depression).
No products indexed under this heading.

Cimetidine (In vitro drug interaction studies in human liver microsomes indicate that concomitant administration with inhibitors of CYP2D6 could result in some inhibition of the metabolism of tramadol).
No products indexed under this heading.

Cimetidine Hydrochloride (In vitro drug interaction studies in human liver microsomes indicate that concomitant administration with inhibitors of CYP2D6 could result in some inhibition of the metabolism of tramadol).
No products indexed under this heading.

Ciprofloxacin (Administration of CYP3A4 inhibitors, such as ketoconazole and erythromycin, with tramadol hydrochloride may effect the metabolism of tramadol leading to altered tramadol exposure). Products include:
Cipro I.V. 2817
Cipro Oral Suspension 2810
Cipro XR Tablets 2823
Ciprodex Otic Suspension 541

Ciprofloxacin Hydrochloride (Administration of CYP3A4 inducers, such as rifampin or St. John's Wort, with tramadol hydrochloride may effect the metabolism of tramadol leading to altered tramadol exposure). Products include:
Cipro Tablets 2810

Cisplatin (Administration of CYP3A4 inducers, such as rifampin or St. John's Wort, with tramadol hydrochloride may effect the metabolism of tramadol leading to altered tramadol exposure).
No products indexed under this heading.

Citalopram Hydrobromide (Concomitant use of tramadol increases the seizure risk in patients taking selective serotonin re-uptake inhibitors. Concomitant use of tramadol with SSRIs increases the risk of adverse events, including seizure and serotonin syndrome). Products include:
Celexa 1160

Clarithromycin (Administration of CYP3A4 inhibitors, such as ketoconazole and erythromycin, with tramadol hydrochloride may effect the metabolism of tramadol leading to altered tramadol exposure). Products include:
Biaxin/Biaxin XL 411

Clomipramine Hydrochloride (Concomitant use of tramadol increases the seizure risk in patients taking tricyclic antidepressants).
No products indexed under this heading.

Clorazepate Dipotassium (Tramadol hydrochloride is contraindicated in acute intoxication with psychotropic drugs).
No products indexed under this heading.

Clotrimazole (Administration of CYP3A4 inhibitors, such as ketoconazole and erythromycin, with tramadol hydrochloride may effect the metabolism of tramadol leading to altered tramadol exposure). Products include:
Lotrisone 2881

Clozapine (Tramadol hydrochloride is contraindicated in acute intoxication with psychotropic drugs).
No products indexed under this heading.

Cocaine Hydrochloride (In vitro drug interaction studies in human liver microsomes indicate that concomitant administration with inhibitors of CYP2D6 could result in some inhibition of the metabolism of tramadol).
No products indexed under this heading.

Codeine Phosphate (Tramadol hydrochloride is contraindicated in acute intoxication with narcotics, opioids, and centrally-acting analgesics. Concomitant use of tramadol increases the seizure risk in patients taking opioids. Tramadol hydrochloride should be used with caution and in reduced dosages when administered to patients receiving CNS depressants, such as opioids or narcotics. Tramadol hydrochloride increases the risk of CNS and respiratory depression. Tramadol may be expected to have additive effects when used in conjunction with other opioids). Products include:
Tylenol with Codeine Tablets 2427

Cortisone Acetate (Administration of CYP3A4 inducers, such as rifampin or St. John's Wort, with tramadol hydrochloride may effect the metabolism of tramadol leading to altered tramadol exposure).
No products indexed under this heading.

Cyclobenzaprine (Concomitant use of tramadol increases the seizure risk in patients taking tricyclic compounds, such as cyclobenzaprine).
No products indexed under this heading.

Cyclobenzaprine Hydrochloride (Concomitant use of tramadol increases the seizure risk in patients taking tricyclic compounds, such as cyclobenzaprine). Products include:
Amrix Capsules 966

Cyclosporine (Administration of CYP3A4 inhibitors, such as ketoconazole and erythromycin, with tramadol hydrochloride may effect the metabolism of tramadol leading to altered tramadol exposure). Products include:
Gengraf Capsules 435

Neoral Oral Solution 2280
Neoral Soft Gelatin Capsules 2280
Restasis Ophthalmic Emulsion 557
Sandimmune 2296

Dalfopristin (Administration of CYP3A4 inhibitors, such as ketoconazole and erythromycin, with tramadol hydrochloride may effect the metabolism of tramadol leading to altered tramadol exposure).
No products indexed under this heading.

Danazol (Administration of CYP3A4 inhibitors, such as ketoconazole and erythromycin, with tramadol hydrochloride may effect the metabolism of tramadol leading to altered tramadol exposure).
No products indexed under this heading.

Delavirdine Mesylate (Administration of CYP3A4 inhibitors, such as ketoconazole and erythromycin, with tramadol hydrochloride may effect the metabolism of tramadol leading to altered tramadol exposure).
No products indexed under this heading.

Desflurane (Tramadol hydrochloride should be used with caution and in reduced dosages when administered to patients receiving CNS depressants, such as alcohol, opioids, anesthetic agents, narcotics, phenothiazines, tranquilizers, or sedative hypnotics. Tramadol hydrochloride increases the risk of CNS and respiratory depression).
No products indexed under this heading.

Desipramine Hydrochloride (Tramadol hydrochloride is contraindicated in acute intoxication with psychotropic drugs).
No products indexed under this heading.

Desvenlafaxine Succinate (Concomitant use of tramadol increases the seizure risk in patients taking serotonin and norepinephrine reuptake inhibitors. Concomitant use of tramadol with SNRIs increases the risk of adverse events, including seizure and serotonin syndrome. If concomitant treatment of tramadol with a drug affecting the serotonergic neurotransmitter system is clinically warranted, careful observation of the patient is advised, particularly during treatment initiation and dose increases). Products include:
Pristiq Extended-Release Tablets 3247

Dexamethasone (Administration of CYP3A4 inducers, such as rifampin or St. John's Wort, with tramadol hydrochloride may effect the metabolism of tramadol leading to altered tramadol exposure). Products include:
Ciprodex Otic Suspension 541

Dexamethasone Acetate (Administration of CYP3A4 inducers, such as rifampin or St. John's Wort, with tramadol hydrochloride may effect the metabolism of tramadol leading to altered tramadol exposure).
No products indexed under this heading.

Dexamethasone Sodium Phosphate (Administration of CYP3A4 inducers, such as rifampin or St. John's Wort, with tramadol hydrochloride may effect the metabolism of tramadol leading to altered tramadol exposure).
No products indexed under this heading.

Dezocine (Tramadol hydrochloride is contraindicated in acute intoxication with narcotics, opioids, and centrally-acting analgesics. Concomitant use of tramadol increases the seizure risk in patients taking opioids. Tramadol hydrochloride should be used with caution and in reduced dosages when administered to patients receiving CNS depressants, such as opioids or narcotics. Tramadol hydrochloride increases the risk of CNS and respiratory depression. Tramadol may be expected to have additive effects when used in conjunction with other opioids).
No products indexed under this heading.

Diazepam (Tramadol hydrochloride is contraindicated in acute intoxication with psychotropic drugs). Products include:
Valium Tablets 2658

Digoxin (Post-marketing surveillance of tramadol has revealed rare reports of digoxin toxicity). Products include:
Lanoxin Injection 1498
Lanoxin Injection Pediatric 1502
Lanoxin Tablets 1505

Diltiazem Hydrochloride (Administration of CYP3A4 inhibitors, such as ketoconazole and erythromycin, with tramadol hydrochloride may effect the metabolism of tramadol leading to altered tramadol exposure). Products include:
Cardizem LA Extended Release Tablets 421

Diltiazem Maleate (Administration of CYP3A4 inhibitors, such as ketoconazole and erythromycin, with tramadol hydrochloride may effect the metabolism of tramadol leading to altered tramadol exposure).
No products indexed under this heading.

Diphenhydramine (In vitro drug interaction studies in human liver microsomes indicate that concomitant administration with inhibitors of CYP2D6 could result in some inhibition of the metabolism of tramadol).
No products indexed under this heading.

Diphenhydramine Hydrochloride (In vitro drug interaction studies in human liver microsomes indicate that concomitant administration with inhibitors of CYP2D6 could result in some inhibition of the metabolism of tramadol). Products include:
Benadryl Allergy & Cold Kapgels 1895
Benadryl Allergy & Sinus Headache Kapgels 1895
Benadryl Severe Allergy & Sinus Headache Caplets 1897
Benadryl Dye-Free Allergy Liqui-gels Softgels 1897
Benadryl Allergy Kapgels 1895
Benadryl Allergy Quick Dissolve Strips 1896
Benadryl Allergy Ultratab Tablets 1896
Children's Benadryl Dye-Free Allergy Liquid 1897
Children's Benadryl Allergy Fastmelts 1897
Children's Benadryl Allergy Liquid 1898
Children's Benadryl Allergy Perfect Measure 1896
Children's Benadryl-D Allergy & Sinus Liquid 1896
Benadryl-D Allergy & Sinus Tablet 1896
PediaCare Children's Allergy & Cold Liquid 1902
PediaCare Children's Allergy Liquid 1902
Simply Sleep Caplets 1905
Sudafed PE Nighttime Cold Caplets 1907
Sudafed PE Severe Cold Caplets 1908
Extra Strength Tylenol PM Caplets, Geltabs, Liquid, and Rapid Release Gels 1915
Tylenol Allergy Multi-Symptom Nighttime Caplets with Cool Burst 1916
Tylenol Severe Allergy Caplets 1916
Children's Tylenol Plus Cold & Allergy Suspension Liquid 1914
Tylenol Sore Throat Nighttime Liquid with Cool Burst 1918

Doxepin Hydrochloride (Tramadol hydrochloride is contraindicated in acute intoxication with psychotropic drugs).
No products indexed under this heading.

Doxorubicin Hydrochloride (Administration of CYP3A4 inducers, such as rifampin or St. John's Wort, with tramadol hydrochloride may effect the metabolism of tramadol leading to altered tramadol exposure).
No products indexed under this heading.

Droperidol (Tramadol hydrochloride is contraindicated in acute intoxication with psychotropic drugs).
No products indexed under this heading.

Duloxetine Hydrochloride (Concomitant use of tramadol increases the seizure risk in patients taking serotonin and norepinephrine reuptake inhibitors. Concomitant use of tramadol with SNRIs increases the risk of adverse events, including seizure and serotonin syndrome. If concomitant treatment of tramadol with a drug affecting the serotonergic neurotransmitter system is clinically warranted, careful observation of the patient is advised, particularly during treatment initiation and dose increases). Products include:
Cymbalta Delayed-Release Capsules 1801

Efavirenz (Administration of CYP3A4 inhibitors, such as ketoconazole and erythromycin, with tramadol hydrochloride may effect the metabolism of tramadol leading to altered tramadol exposure). Products include:
Atripla Tablets 938
Sustiva Capsules 930
Sustiva Tablets 930

Eletriptan Hydrobromide (Concomitant use of tramadol increases the seizure risk in patients taking triptans. Concomitant use of tramadol with triptans increases the risk of adverse events, including seizure and serotonin syndrome. If concomitant treatment of tramadol with a drug affecting the serotonergic neurotransmitter system is clinically warranted, careful observation of the patient is advised, particularly during treatment initiation and dose increases).
No products indexed under this heading.

Enflurane (Tramadol hydrochloride should be used with caution and in reduced dosages when administered to patients receiving CNS depressants, such as alcohol, opioids, anesthetic agents, narcotics, phenothiazines, tranquilizers, or sedative hypnotics. Tramadol hydrochloride increases the risk of CNS and respiratory depression).
No products indexed under this heading.

Erythromycin (Administration of CYP3A4 inhibitors, such as ketoconazole and erythromycin, with tramadol hydrochloride may effect the metabolism of tramadol leading to altered tramadol exposure).
No products indexed under this heading.

Erythromycin Estolate (Administration of CYP3A4 inhibitors, such as ketoconazole and erythromycin, with tramadol hydrochloride may effect the metabolism of tramadol leading to altered tramadol exposure).
No products indexed under this heading.

Erythromycin Ethylsuccinate (Administration of CYP3A4 inhibitors, such as ketoconazole and erythromycin, with tramadol hydrochloride may effect the metabolism of tramadol leading to altered tramadol exposure). Products include:
E.E.S. 433
EryPed 431

Erythromycin Gluceptate (Administration of CYP3A4 inhibitors, such as ketoconazole and erythromycin, with tramadol hydrochloride may effect the metabolism of tramadol leading to altered tramadol exposure).
No products indexed under this heading.

Erythromycin Lactobionate (Administration of CYP3A4 inhibitors, such as ketoconazole and erythromycin, with tramadol hydrochloride may effect the metabolism of tramadol leading to altered tramadol exposure).
No products indexed under this heading.

Erythromycin Stearate (Administration of CYP3A4 inhibitors, such as ketoconazole and erythromycin, with tramadol hydrochloride may effect the metabolism of tramadol leading to altered tramadol exposure).
No products indexed under this heading.

Escitalopram Oxalate (Concomitant use of tramadol increases the seizure risk in patients taking selective serotonin re-uptake inhibitors. Concomitant use of tramadol with SSRIs increases the risk of adverse events, including seizure and serotonin syndrome). Products include:
Lexapro Oral Suspension 1174
Lexapro Tablets 1174

Esomeprazole Magnesium (Administration of CYP3A4 inhibitors, such as ketoconazole and erythromycin, with tramadol hydrochloride may effect the metabolism of tramadol leading to altered tramadol exposure). Products include:
Nexium Delayed-Release Capsules 645
Nexium Delayed-Release Oral Suspension 645

Estazolam (Tramadol hydrochloride is contraindicated in acute intoxication with hypnotics. Tramadol hydrochloride should be used with caution and in reduced dosages when administered to patients receiving CNS depressants, such as sedative hypnotics. Tramadol hydrochloride increases the risk of CNS and respiratory depression).
No products indexed under this heading.

Ethanol (Tramadol hydrochloride should be used with caution and in reduced dosages when administered to patients receiving CNS depressants, such as alcohol, opioids, anesthetic agents, narcotics, phenothiazines, tranquilizers, or sedative hypnotics. Tramadol hydrochloride increases the risk of CNS and respiratory depression).
No products indexed under this heading.

Ethchlorvynol (Tramadol hydrochloride is contraindicated in acute intoxication with hypnotics. Tramadol hydrochloride should be used with caution and in reduced dosages when administered to patients receiving CNS depressants, such as sedative hypnotics. Tramadol hydrochloride increases the risk of CNS and respiratory depression).
No products indexed under this heading.

Ethinamate (Tramadol hydrochloride is contraindicated in acute intoxication with hypnotics. Tramadol hydrochloride should be used with caution and in reduced dosages when administered to patients receiving CNS depressants, such as sedative hypnotics. Tramadol hydrochloride increases the risk of CNS and respiratory depression).
No products indexed under this heading.

Ethosuximide (Administration of CYP3A4 inducers, such as rifampin or St. John's Wort, with tramadol hydrochloride may effect the metabolism of tramadol leading to altered tramadol exposure).
No products indexed under this heading.

Ethyl Alcohol (Tramadol hydrochloride should be used with caution and in reduced dosages when administered to patients receiving CNS depressants, such as alcohol, opioids, anesthetic agents, narcotics, phenothiazines, tranquilizers, or sedative hypnotics. Tramadol hydrochloride increases the risk of CNS and respiratory depression).
No products indexed under this heading.

Felbamate (Administration of CYP3A4 inducers, such as rifampin or St. John's Wort, with tramadol hydrochloride may effect the metabolism of tramadol leading to altered tramadol exposure).
No products indexed under this heading.

Fentanyl (Tramadol hydrochloride is contraindicated in acute intoxication with narcotics, opioids, and centrally-acting analgesics. Concomitant use of tramadol increases the seizure risk in patients taking opioids. Tramadol hydrochloride should be used with caution and in reduced dosages when administered to patients receiving CNS depressants, such as opioids or narcotics. Tramadol hydrochloride increases the risk of CNS and respiratory depression. Tramadol may be expected to have additive effects when used in conjunction with other opioids).
Products include:
Duragesic Transdermal System 2405
Ionsys Transdermal System 2410

Fentanyl Citrate (Tramadol hydrochloride is contraindicated in acute intoxication with narcotics, opioids, and centrally-acting analgesics. Concomitant use of tramadol increases the seizure risk in patients taking opioids. Tramadol hydrochloride should be used with caution and in reduced dosages when administered to patients receiving CNS depressants, such as opioids or narcotics. Tramadol hydrochloride increases the risk of CNS and respiratory depression. Tramadol may be expected to have additive effects when used in conjunction with other opioids). Products include:
Actiq 959
Fentora Tablets 968

Fluconazole (Administration of CYP3A4 inhibitors, such as ketoconazole and erythromycin, with tramadol hydrochloride may effect the metabolism of tramadol leading to altered tramadol exposure).
No products indexed under this heading.

Fludrocortisone Acetate (Administration of CYP3A4 inducers, such as rifampin or St. John's Wort, with tramadol hydrochloride may effect the metabolism of tramadol leading to altered tramadol exposure).
No products indexed under this heading.

Fluoxetine (Concomitant use of tramadol increases the seizure risk in patients taking selective serotonin re-uptake inhibitors. Concomitant use of tramadol with SSRIs increases the risk of adverse events, including seizure and serotonin syndrome).
No products indexed under this heading.

Fluoxetine Hydrochloride (Concomitant use of tramadol increases the seizure risk in patients taking selective serotonin re-uptake inhibitors. Concomitant use of tramadol with SSRIs increases the risk of adverse events, including seizure and serotonin syndrome). Products include:
Prozac Weekly Capsules 1852
Prozac Pulvules and Liquid 1852
Symbyax Capsules 1871

Fluphenazine Decanoate (Tramadol hydrochloride is contraindicated in acute intoxication with psychotropic drugs).
No products indexed under this heading.

Fluphenazine Enanthate (Tramadol hydrochloride is contraindicated in acute intoxication with psychotropic drugs).
No products indexed under this heading.

Fluphenazine Hydrochloride (Tramadol hydrochloride is contraindicated in acute intoxication with psychotropic drugs).
No products indexed under this heading.

Flurazepam Hydrochloride (Tramadol hydrochloride is contraindicated in acute intoxication with hypnotics. Tramadol hydrochloride should be used with caution and in reduced dosages when administered to patients receiving CNS depressants, such as sedative hypnotics. Tramadol hydrochloride increases the risk of CNS and respiratory depression).
No products indexed under this heading.

Fluvoxamine Maleate (Concomitant use of tramadol increases the seizure risk in patients taking selective serotonin re-uptake inhibitors. Concomitant use of tramadol with SSRIs increases the risk of adverse events, including seizure and serotonin syndrome). Products include:
Luvox CR Extended-Release Capsules 1759

Fosamprenavir Calcium (Administration of CYP3A4 inhibitors, such as ketoconazole and erythromycin, with tramadol hydrochloride may effect the metabolism of tramadol leading to altered tramadol exposure).
Products include:
Lexiva Oral Suspension 1510
Lexiva Tablets 1510

Fosphenytoin Sodium (Administration of CYP3A4 inducers, such as rifampin or St. John's Wort, with tramadol hydrochloride may effect the metabolism of tramadol leading to altered tramadol exposure).
No products indexed under this heading.

Frovatriptan Succinate (Concomitant use of tramadol increases the seizure risk in patients taking triptans. Concomitant use of tramadol with triptans increases the risk of adverse events, including seizure and serotonin syndrome. If concomitant treatment of tramadol with a drug affecting the serotonergic neurotransmitter system is clinically warranted, careful observation of the patient is advised, particularly during treatment initiation and dose increases). Products include:
Frova Tablets 1111

Garlic Extract (Administration of CYP3A4 inducers, such as rifampin or St. John's Wort, with tramadol hydrochloride may effect the metabolism of tramadol leading to altered tramadol exposure).
No products indexed under this heading.

Garlic Oil (Administration of CYP3A4 inducers, such as rifampin or St. John's Wort, with tramadol hydrochloride may effect the metabolism of tramadol leading to altered tramadol exposure).
No products indexed under this heading.

Glutethimide (Tramadol hydrochloride is contraindicated in acute intoxication with hypnotics. Tramadol hydrochloride should be used with caution and in reduced dosages when administered to patients receiving CNS depressants, such as sedative hypnotics. Tramadol hydrochloride increases the risk of CNS and respiratory depression).
No products indexed under this heading.

Halofantrine Hydrochloride (In vitro drug interaction studies in human liver microsomes indicate that concomitant administration with inhibitors of CYP2D6 could result in some inhibition of the metabolism of tramadol).
No products indexed under this heading.

Haloperidol (Tramadol hydrochloride is contraindicated in acute intoxication with psychotropic drugs).
No products indexed under this heading.

Haloperidol Decanoate (Tramadol hydrochloride is contraindicated in acute intoxication with psychotropic drugs).
No products indexed under this heading.

Halothane (Tramadol hydrochloride should be used with caution and in reduced dosages when administered to patients receiving CNS depressants, such as anesthetic agents. Tramadol hydrochloride increases the risk of CNS and respiratory depression).
No products indexed under this heading.

Hydrocodone Bitartrate (Tramadol hydrochloride is contraindicated in acute intoxication with narcotics, opioids, and centrally-acting analgesics. Concomitant use of tramadol increases the seizure risk in patients taking opioids. Tramadol hydrochloride should be used with caution and in reduced dosages when administered to patients receiving CNS depressants, such as opioids or narcotics. Tramadol hydrochloride increases the risk of CNS and respiratory depression. Tramadol may be expected to have additive effects when used in conjunction with other opioids). Products include:
Lortab 5/500 Tablets 3143
Lortab 7.5/500 Tablets 3144
Lortab 10/500 Tablets 3144
Vicodin Tablets 529
Vicodin ES Tablets 530
Vicodin HP Tablets 531
Vicoprofen Tablets 533
Zydone Tablets 1132

Hydrocodone Polistirex (Tramadol hydrochloride is contraindicated in acute intoxication with narcotics, opioids, and centrally-acting analgesics. Concomitant use of tramadol increases the seizure risk in patients taking opioids. Tramadol hydrochloride should be used with caution and in reduced dosages when administered to patients receiving CNS depressants, such as opioids or narcotics. Tramadol hydrochloride increases the risk of CNS and respiratory depression. Tramadol may be expected to have additive effects when used in conjunction with other opioids). Products include:
Tussionex Pennkinetic Extended-Release Suspension 3154

Hydrocortisone (Administration of CYP3A4 inducers, such as rifampin or St. John's Wort, with tramadol hydrochloride may effect the metabolism of tramadol leading to altered tramadol exposure).
No products indexed under this heading.

Hydrocortisone Acetate (Administration of CYP3A4 inducers, such as rifampin or St. John's Wort, with tramadol hydrochloride may effect the metabolism of tramadol leading to altered tramadol exposure).
Products include:
Analpram-HC 1140
Pramosone 1141

Hydrocortisone Butyrate (Administration of CYP3A4 inducers, such as rifampin or St. John's Wort, with tramadol hydrochloride may effect the metabolism of tramadol leading to altered tramadol exposure).
No products indexed under this heading.

Hydrocortisone Cypionate (Administration of CYP3A4 inducers, such as rifampin or St. John's Wort, with tramadol hydrochloride may effect the metabolism of tramadol leading to altered tramadol exposure).
No products indexed under this heading.

Hydrocortisone Hemisuccinate (Administration of CYP3A4 inducers, such as rifampin or St. John's Wort, with tramadol hydrochloride may effect the metabolism of tramadol leading to altered tramadol exposure).
No products indexed under this heading.

Hydrocortisone Probutate (Administration of CYP3A4 inducers, such as rifampin or St. John's Wort, with tramadol hydrochloride may effect the metabolism of tramadol leading to altered tramadol exposure).
No products indexed under this heading.

Hydrocortisone Sodium Phosphate (Administration of CYP3A4 inducers, such as rifampin or St. John's Wort, with tramadol hydrochloride may effect the metabolism of tramadol leading to altered tramadol exposure).
No products indexed under this heading.

Hydrocortisone Sodium Succinate (Administration of CYP3A4 inducers, such as rifampin or St. John's Wort, with tramadol hydrochloride may effect the metabolism of tramadol leading to altered tramadol exposure).
No products indexed under this heading.

Hydrocortisone Valerate (Administration of CYP3A4 inducers, such as rifampin or St. John's Wort, with tramadol hydrochloride may effect the metabolism of tramadol leading to altered tramadol exposure).
No products indexed under this heading.

Hydromorphone Hydrochloride (Tramadol hydrochloride is contraindicated in acute intoxication with narcotics, opioids, and centrally-acting analgesics. Concomitant use of tramadol increases the seizure risk in patients taking opioids. Tramadol hydrochloride should be used with caution and in reduced dosages when administered to patients receiving CNS depressants, such as opioids or narcotics. Tramadol hydrochloride increases the risk of CNS and respiratory depression. Tramadol may be expected to have additive effects when used in conjunction with other opioids).
No products indexed under this heading.

Hydroxychloroquine Sulfate (In vitro drug interaction studies in human liver microsomes indicate that concomitant administration with inhibitors of CYP2D6 could result in some inhibition of the metabolism of tramadol).
No products indexed under this heading.

Hydroxyzine Hydrochloride (Tramadol hydrochloride is contraindicated in acute intoxication with psychotropic drugs).
No products indexed under this heading.

Hypericum (Administration of CYP3A4 inducers, such as rifampin or St. John's Wort, with tramadol hydrochloride may effect the metabolism of tramadol leading to altered tramadol exposure). Products include:
Satiété Tablets 640

Hypericum Perforatum (Administration of CYP3A4 inducers, such as rifampin or St. John's Wort, with tramadol hydrochloride may effect the metabolism of tramadol leading to altered tramadol exposure).
No products indexed under this heading.

Imatinib Mesylate (In vitro drug interaction studies in human liver microsomes indicate that concomitant administration with inhibitors of CYP2D6 could result in some inhibition of the metabolism of tramadol). Products include:
Gleevec Tablets 2255

Imipramine Hydrochloride (Tramadol hydrochloride is contraindicated in acute intoxication with psychotropic drugs).
No products indexed under this heading.

Imipramine Pamoate (Tramadol hydrochloride is contraindicated in acute intoxication with psychotropic drugs).
No products indexed under this heading.

Indinavir Sulfate (Administration of CYP3A4 inhibitors, such as ketoconazole and erythromycin, with tramadol hydrochloride may effect the metabolism of tramadol leading to the altered tramadol exposure). Products include:
Crixivan Capsules 1979

Isocarboxazid (Tramadol hydrochloride is contraindicated in acute intoxication with psychotropic drugs). Products include:
Marplan Tablets 3177

Isoflurane (Tramadol hydrochloride should be used with caution and in reduced dosages when administered to patients receiving CNS depressants, such as alcohol, opioids, anesthetic agents, narcotics, phenothiazines, tranquilizers, or sedative hypnotics. Tramadol hydrochloride increases the risk of CNS and respiratory depression).
No products indexed under this heading.

Isoniazid (Administration of CYP3A4 inhibitors, such as ketoconazole and erythromycin, with tramadol hydrochloride may effect the metabolism of tramadol leading to altered tramadol exposure).
No products indexed under this heading.

Itraconazole (Administration of CYP3A4 inhibitors, such as ketoconazole and erythromycin, with tramadol hydrochloride may effect the metabolism of tramadol leading to altered tramadol exposure).
No products indexed under this heading.

Ketamine Hydrochloride (Tramadol hydrochloride should be used with caution and in reduced dosages when administered to patients receiving CNS depressants, such as alcohol, opioids, anesthetic agents, narcotics, phenothiazines, tranquilizers, or sedative hypnotics. Tramadol hydrochloride increases the risk of CNS and respiratory depression).
No products indexed under this heading.

Ketoconazole (Administration of CYP3A4 inhibitors, such as ketoconazole and erythromycin, with tramadol hydrochloride may effect the metabolism of tramadol leading to altered tramadol exposure). Products include:
Extina Foam, 2% 3057
Nizoral A-D Shampoo 1901

Levomethadyl Acetate Hydrochloride (Tramadol hydrochloride should be used with caution and in reduced dosages when administered to patients receiving CNS depressants, such as alcohol, opioids, anesthetic agents, narcotics, phenothiazines, tranquilizers, or sedative hypnotics. Tramadol hydrochloride increases the risk of CNS and respiratory depression).
No products indexed under this heading.

Levorphanol Tartrate (Tramadol hydrochloride is contraindicated in acute intoxication with narcotics, opioids, and centrally-acting analgesics. Concomitant use of tramadol increases the seizure risk in patients taking opioids. Tramadol hydrochloride should be used with caution and in reduced dosages when administered to patients receiving CNS depressants, such as opioids or narcotics. Tramadol hydrochloride increases the risk of CNS and respiratory depression. Tramadol may be expected to have additive effects when used in conjunction with other opioids).
No products indexed under this heading.

Lithium Carbonate (Tramadol hydrochloride is contraindicated in acute intoxication with psychotropic drugs).
No products indexed under this heading.

Lithium Citrate (Tramadol hydrochloride is contraindicated in acute intoxication with psychotropic drugs).
No products indexed under this heading.

Lopinavir (Administration of CYP3A4 inhibitors, such as ketoconazole and erythromycin, with tramadol hydrochloride may effect the metabolism of tramadol leading to altered tramadol exposure). Products include:
Kaletra 452

Loratadine (Administration of CYP3A4 inhibitors, such as ketoconazole and erythromycin, with tramadol hydrochloride may effect the metabolism of tramadol leading to altered tramadol exposure).
No products indexed under this heading.

Lorazepam (Tramadol hydrochloride is contraindicated in acute intoxication with hypnotics. Tramadol hydrochloride should be used with caution and in reduced dosages when administered to patients receiving CNS depressants, such as sedative hypnotics. Tramadol hydrochloride increases the risk of CNS and respiratory depression).
No products indexed under this heading.

Loxapine Hydrochloride (Tramadol hydrochloride is contraindicated in acute intoxication with psychotropic drugs).
No products indexed under this heading.

Loxapine Succinate (Tramadol hydrochloride is contraindicated in acute intoxication with psychotropic drugs).
No products indexed under this heading.

Maprotiline Hydrochloride (Tramadol hydrochloride is contraindicated in acute intoxication with psychotropic drugs).
No products indexed under this heading.

Meperidine Hydrochloride (Tramadol hydrochloride is contraindicated in acute intoxication with narcotics, opioids, and centrally-acting analgesics. Concomitant use of tramadol increases the seizure risk in patients taking opioids. Tramadol hydrochloride should be used with caution and in reduced dosages when administered to patients receiving CNS depressants, such as opioids or narcotics. Tramadol hydrochloride increases the risk of CNS and respiratory depression. Tramadol may be expected to have additive effects when used in conjunction with other opioids).
No products indexed under this heading.

Mephenytoin (Administration of CYP3A4 inducers, such as rifampin or St. John's Wort, with tramadol hydrochloride may effect the metabolism of tramadol leading to altered tramadol exposure).
No products indexed under this heading.

Mephobarbital (Tramadol hydrochloride should be used with caution and in reduced dosages when administered to patients receiving CNS depressants, such as alcohol, opioids, anesthetic agents, narcotics, phenothiazines, tranquilizers, or sedative hypnotics. Tramadol hydrochloride increases the risk of CNS and respiratory depression).
No products indexed under this heading.

Meprobamate (Tramadol hydrochloride is contraindicated in acute intoxication with psychotropic drugs).
No products indexed under this heading.

Mesoridazine Besylate (Tramadol hydrochloride is contraindicated in acute intoxication with psychotropic drugs).
No products indexed under this heading.

Methadone Hydrochloride (Tramadol hydrochloride is contraindicated in acute intoxication with narcotics, opioids, and centrally-acting analgesics. Concomitant use of tramadol increases the seizure risk in patients taking opioids. Tramadol hydrochloride should be used with caution and in reduced dosages when administered to patients receiving CNS depressants, such as opioids or narcotics. Tramadol hydrochloride increases the risk of CNS and respiratory depression. Tramadol may be expected to have additive effects when used in conjunction with other opioids).
No products indexed under this heading.

Methohexital Sodium (Tramadol hydrochloride should be used with caution and in reduced dosages when administered to patients receiving CNS depressants, such as alcohol, opioids, anesthetic agents, narcotics, phenothiazines, tranquilizers, or sedative hypnotics. Tramadol hydrochloride increases the risk of CNS and respiratory depression).
No products indexed under this heading.

Methotrimeprazine (Administration of tramadol may increase the seizure risk in patients taking neuroleptics or other drugs that reduce the seizure threshold).
No products indexed under this heading.

Methoxyflurane (Tramadol hydrochloride should be used with caution and in reduced dosages when administered to patients receiving CNS depressants, such as alcohol, opioids, anesthetic agents, narcotics, phenothiazines, tranquilizers, or sedative hypnotics. Tramadol hydrochloride increases the risk of CNS and respiratory depression).
No products indexed under this heading.

Methsuximide (Administration of CYP3A4 inducers, such as rifampin or St. John's Wort, with tramadol hydrochloride may effect the metabolism of tramadol leading to altered tramadol exposure).
No products indexed under this heading.

Methylprednisolone (Administration of CYP3A4 inducers, such as rifampin or St. John's Wort, with tramadol hydrochloride may effect the metabolism of tramadol leading to altered tramadol exposure).
No products indexed under this heading.

Methylprednisolone Acetate (Administration of CYP3A4 inducers, such as rifampin or St. John's Wort, with tramadol hydrochloride may effect the metabolism of tramadol leading to altered tramadol exposure).
No products indexed under this heading.

Methylprednisolone Sodium Succinate (Administration of CYP3A4 inducers, such as rifampin or St. John's Wort, with tramadol hydrochloride may effect the metabolism of tramadol leading to altered tramadol exposure).
No products indexed under this heading.

Metronidazole (Administration of CYP3A4 inhibitors, such as ketoconazole and erythromycin, with tramadol hydrochloride may effect the metabolism of tramadol leading to altered tramadol exposure).
Products include:
Pylera Capsules 714

Metronidazole Benzoate (Administration of CYP3A4 inhibitors, such as ketoconazole and erythromycin, with tramadol hydrochloride may effect the metabolism of tramadol leading to altered tramadol exposure).
No products indexed under this heading.

Metronidazole Hydrochloride (Administration of CYP3A4 inhibitors, such as ketoconazole and erythromycin, with tramadol hydrochloride may effect the metabolism of tramadol leading to altered tramadol exposure).
No products indexed under this heading.

Metronidazole Sodium (Administration of CYP3A4 inhibitors, such as ketoconazole and erythromycin, with tramadol hydrochloride may effect the metabolism of tramadol leading to altered tramadol exposure).
No products indexed under this heading.

Mibefradil Dihydrochloride (In vitro drug interaction studies in human liver microsomes indicate that concomitant administration with inhibitors of CYP2D6 could result in some inhibition of the metabolism of tramadol).
No products indexed under this heading.

Miconazole (Administration of CYP3A4 inhibitors, such as ketoconazole and erythromycin, with tramadol hydrochloride may effect the metabolism of tramadol leading to altered tramadol exposure).
No products indexed under this heading.

Miconazole Nitrate (Administration of CYP3A4 inhibitors, such as ketoconazole and erythromycin, with tramadol hydrochloride may effect the metabolism of tramadol leading to altered tramadol exposure).
No products indexed under this heading.

Midazolam Hydrochloride (Tramadol hydrochloride is contraindicated in acute intoxication with hypnotics. Tramadol hydrochloride should be used with caution and in reduced dosages when administered to patients receiving CNS depressants, such as sedative hypnotics. Tramadol hydrochloride increases the risk of CNS and respiratory depression).
No products indexed under this heading.

Moclobemide (Administration of tramadol may increase the seizure risk in patients taking monoamine oxidase inhibitors or other drugs that reduce the seizure threshold. Use tramadol with great caution in patients taking MAO inhibitors. Concomitant use of tramadol with MAO inhibitors increases the risk of adverse events, including seizure and serotonin syndrome).
No products indexed under this heading.

Modafinil (Administration of CYP3A4 inducers, such as rifampin or St. John's Wort, with tramadol hydrochloride may effect the metabolism of tramadol leading to altered tramadol exposure). Products include:
Provigil Tablets 977

Molindone Hydrochloride (Tramadol hydrochloride is contraindicated in acute intoxication with psychotropic drugs). Products include:
Moban Tablets 1116

Morphine Sulfate (Tramadol hydrochloride is contraindicated in acute intoxication with narcotics, opioids, and centrally-acting analgesics. Concomitant use of tramadol increases the seizure risk in patients taking opioids. Tramadol hydrochloride should be used with caution and in reduced dosages when administered to patients receiving CNS depressants, such as opioids or narcotics. Tramadol hydrochloride increases the risk of CNS and respiratory depression. Tramadol may be expected to have additive effects when used in conjunction with other opioids). Products include:
Avinza Capsules 1772
DepoDur Injection 1095
MS Contin Tablets 2585

Naratriptan Hydrochloride (Concomitant use of tramadol increases the seizure risk in patients taking triptans. Concomitant use of tramadol with triptans increases the risk of adverse events, including seizure and serotonin syndrome. If concomitant treatment of tramadol with a drug affecting the serotonergic neurotransmitter system is clinically warranted, careful observation of the patient is advised, particularly during treatment initiation and dose increases). Products include:
Amerge Tablets 1301

Nefazodone Hydrochloride (Administration of CYP3A4 inhibitors, such as ketoconazole and erythromycin, with tramadol hydrochloride may effect the metabolism of tramadol leading to altered tramadol exposure).
No products indexed under this heading.

Nelfinavir Mesylate (Administration of CYP3A4 inhibitors, such as ketoconazole and erythromycin, with tramadol hydrochloride may effect the metabolism of tramadol leading to altered tramadol exposure).
No products indexed under this heading.

Nevirapine (Administration of CYP3A4 inhibitors, such as ketoconazole and erythromycin, with tramadol hydrochloride may effect the metabolism of tramadol leading to altered tramadol exposure).
Products include:
Viramune Oral Suspension 873
Viramune Tablets 873

Niacinamide (Administration of CYP3A4 inhibitors, such as ketoconazole and erythromycin, with tramadol hydrochloride may effect the metabolism of tramadol leading to altered tramadol exposure).
Products include:
BioLean Free Tablets .... ▣635

Nicotinamide (Administration of CYP3A4 inhibitors, such as ketoconazole and erythromycin, with tramadol hydrochloride may effect the metabolism of tramadol leading to altered tramadol exposure).
No products indexed under this heading.

Nifedipine (Administration of CYP3A4 inhibitors, such as ketoconazole and erythromycin, with tramadol hydrochloride may effect the metabolism of tramadol leading to altered tramadol exposure).
No products indexed under this heading.

Norfloxacin (Administration of CYP3A4 inhibitors, such as ketoconazole and erythromycin, with tramadol hydrochloride may effect the metabolism of tramadol leading to altered tramadol exposure).
Products include:
Noroxin Tablets 2069

Nortriptyline Hydrochloride (Tramadol hydrochloride is contraindicated in acute intoxication with psychotropic drugs).
No products indexed under this heading.

Olanzapine (Tramadol hydrochloride is contraindicated in acute intoxication with psychotropic drugs).
Products include:
Symbyax Capsules 1871
Zyprexa Tablets 1883
Zyprexa IntraMuscular 1883
Zyprexa ZYDIS Orally Disintegrating Tablets 1883

Omeprazole (Administration of CYP3A4 inhibitors, such as ketoconazole and erythromycin, with tramadol hydrochloride may effect the metabolism of tramadol leading to altered tramadol exposure).
No products indexed under this heading.

Oxazepam (Tramadol hydrochloride is contraindicated in acute intoxication with psychotropic drugs).
No products indexed under this heading.

Oxcarbazepine (Administration of CYP3A4 inducers, such as rifampin or St. John's Wort, with tramadol hydrochloride may effect the metabolism of tramadol leading to altered tramadol exposure).
No products indexed under this heading.

Oxycodone Hydrochloride (Tramadol hydrochloride is contraindicated in acute intoxication with narcotics, opioids, and centrally-acting analgesics. Concomitant use of tramadol increases the seizure risk in patients taking opioids. Tramadol hydrochloride should be used with caution and in reduced dosages when administered to patients receiving CNS depressants, such as opioids or narcotics. Tramadol hydrochloride increases the risk of CNS and respiratory depression. Tramadol may be expected to have additive effects when used in conjunction with other opioids).
Products include:
OxyContin Tablets 2589
OxyIR Capsules 2593
Percocet Tablets 1127
Percodan Tablets 1130

Paliperidone (Tramadol hydrochloride is contraindicated in acute intoxication with psychotropic drugs).
Products include:
Invega Extended-Release Tablets 1748

Pargyline Hydrochloride (Administration of tramadol may increase the seizure risk in patients taking monoamine oxidase inhibitors or other drugs that reduce the seizure threshold. Use tramadol with great caution in patients taking MAO inhibitors. Concomitant use of tramadol with MAO inhibitors increases the risk of adverse events, including seizure and serotonin syndrome).
No products indexed under this heading.

Paroxetine Hydrochloride (Concomitant use of tramadol increases the seizure risk in patients taking selective serotonin re-uptake inhibitors. Concomitant use of tramadol with SSRIs increases the risk of adverse events, including seizure and serotonin syndrome). Products include:
Paxil 1535

Paxil CR Controlled-Release Tablets 1544

Pentobarbital Sodium (Tramadol hydrochloride should be used with caution and in reduced dosages when administered to patients receiving CNS depressants, such as alcohol, opioids, anesthetic agents, narcotics, phenothiazines, tranquilizers, or sedative hypnotics. Tramadol hydrochloride increases the risk of CNS and respiratory depression). Products include:

Nembutal Sodium Solution, USP 2494

Perphenazine (Tramadol hydrochloride is contraindicated in acute intoxication with psychotropic drugs).

No products indexed under this heading.

Phenelzine Sulfate (Tramadol hydrochloride is contraindicated in acute intoxication with psychotropic drugs).

No products indexed under this heading.

Phenobarbital (Tramadol hydrochloride should be used with caution and in reduced dosages when administered to patients receiving CNS depressants, such as alcohol, opioids, anesthetic agents, narcotics, phenothiazines, tranquilizers, or sedative hypnotics. Tramadol hydrochloride increases the risk of CNS and respiratory depression). Products include:

Donnatal Extentabs 2507

Phenobarbital Sodium (Administration of CYP3A4 inducers, such as rifampin or St. John's Wort, with tramadol hydrochloride may effect the metabolism of tramadol leading to altered tramadol exposure).

No products indexed under this heading.

Phenytoin (Administration of CYP3A4 inducers, such as rifampin or St. John's Wort, with tramadol hydrochloride may effect the metabolism of tramadol leading to altered tramadol exposure).

No products indexed under this heading.

Phenytoin Sodium (Administration of CYP3A4 inducers, such as rifampin or St. John's Wort, with tramadol hydrochloride may effect the metabolism of tramadol leading to altered tramadol exposure). Products include:

Phenytek Capsules 2192

Pimozide (Administration of tramadol may increase the seizure risk in patients taking neuroleptics or other drugs that reduce the seizure threshold).

No products indexed under this heading.

Prazepam (Tramadol hydrochloride is contraindicated in acute intoxication with psychotropic drugs).

No products indexed under this heading.

Prednisolone Acetate (Administration of CYP3A4 inducers, such as rifampin or St. John's Wort, with tramadol hydrochloride may effect the metabolism of tramadol leading to altered tramadol exposure). Products include:

Pred Forte Ophthalmic Suspension .... ⊙227
Pred Mild Ophthalmic Suspension .... ⊙230
Pred-G Ophthalmic Ointment .... ⊙229
Pred-G Ophthalmic Suspension ...... ⊙228

Prednisolone Sodium Phosphate (Administration of CYP3A4 inducers, such as rifampin or St. John's Wort, with tramadol hydrochloride may effect the metabolism of tramadol leading to altered tramadol exposure).

No products indexed under this heading.

Prednisolone Tebutate (Administration of CYP3A4 inducers, such as rifampin or St. John's Wort, with tramadol hydrochloride may effect the metabolism of tramadol leading to altered tramadol exposure).

No products indexed under this heading.

Prednisone (Administration of CYP3A4 inducers, such as rifampin or St. John's Wort, with tramadol hydrochloride may effect the metabolism of tramadol leading to altered tramadol exposure).

No products indexed under this heading.

Primidone (Administration of CYP3A4 inducers, such as rifampin or St. John's Wort, with tramadol hydrochloride may effect the metabolism of tramadol leading to altered tramadol exposure).

No products indexed under this heading.

Procarbazine Hydrochloride (Administration of tramadol may increase the seizure risk in patients taking monoamine oxidase inhibitors or other drugs that reduce the seizure threshold. Use tramadol with great caution in patients taking MAO inhibitors. Concomitant use of tramadol with MAO inhibitors increases the risk of adverse events, including seizure and serotonin syndrome).

No products indexed under this heading.

Prochlorperazine (Tramadol hydrochloride is contraindicated in acute intoxication with psychotropic drugs).

No products indexed under this heading.

Promethazine (Concomitant use of tramadol increases the seizure risk in patients taking tricyclic compounds, such as promethazine).

No products indexed under this heading.

Promethazine Hydrochloride (Concomitant use of tramadol increases the seizure risk in patients taking tricyclic compounds, such as promethazine).

No products indexed under this heading.

Propafenone Hydrochloride (In vitro drug interaction studies in human liver microsomes indicate that concomitant administration with inhibitors of CYP2D6 could result in some inhibition of the metabolism of tramadol). Products include:

Rythmol Tablets 1586
Rythmol SR Capsules 1590

Propofol (Tramadol hydrochloride is contraindicated in acute intoxication with hypnotics. Tramadol hydrochloride should be used with caution and in reduced dosages when administered to patients receiving CNS depressants, such as sedative hypnotics. Tramadol hydrochloride increases the risk of CNS and respiratory depression).

No products indexed under this heading.

Propoxyphene Hydrochloride (Tramadol hydrochloride is contraindicated in acute intoxication with narcotics, opioids, and centrally-acting analgesics. Concomitant use of tramadol increases the seizure risk in patients taking opioids. Tramadol hydrochloride should be used with caution and in reduced dosages when administered to patients receiving CNS depressants, such as opioids or narcotics. Tramadol hydrochloride increases the risk of CNS and respiratory depression. Tramadol may be expected to have additive effects when used in conjunction with other opioids).

No products indexed under this heading.

Propoxyphene Napsylate (Tramadol hydrochloride is contraindicated in acute intoxication with narcotics, opioids, and centrally-acting analgesics. Concomitant use of tramadol increases the seizure risk in patients taking opioids. Tramadol hydrochloride should be used with caution and in reduced dosages when administered to patients receiving CNS depressants, such as opioids or narcotics. Tramadol hydrochloride increases the risk of CNS and respiratory depression. Tramadol may be expected to have additive effects when used in conjunction with other opioids).

No products indexed under this heading.

Protriptyline Hydrochloride (Tramadol hydrochloride is contraindicated in acute intoxication with psychotropic drugs).

No products indexed under this heading.

Quazepam (Tramadol hydrochloride is contraindicated in acute intoxication with hypnotics. Tramadol hydrochloride should be used with caution and in reduced dosages when administered to patients receiving CNS depressants, such as sedative hypnotics. Tramadol hydrochloride increases the risk of CNS and respiratory depression).

No products indexed under this heading.

Quetiapine Fumarate (Tramadol hydrochloride is contraindicated in acute intoxication with psychotropic drugs).

No products indexed under this heading.

Quinacrine Hydrochloride (In vitro drug interaction studies in human liver microsomes indicate that concomitant administration with inhibitors of CYP2D6 could result in some inhibition of the metabolism of tramadol).

No products indexed under this heading.

Quinidine (Administration of CYP3A4 inhibitors, such as ketoconazole and erythromycin, with tramadol hydrochloride may effect the metabolism of tramadol leading to altered tramadol exposure).

No products indexed under this heading.

Quinidine Gluconate (In vitro drug interaction studies in human liver microsomes indicate that concomitant administration with inhibitors of CYP2D6 could result in some inhibition of the metabolism of tramadol).

No products indexed under this heading.

Quinidine Hydrochloride (In vitro drug interaction studies in human liver microsomes indicate that concomitant administration with inhibitors of CYP2D6 could result in some inhibition of the metabolism of tramadol).

No products indexed under this heading.

Quinidine Polygalacturonate (In vitro drug interaction studies in human liver microsomes indicate that concomitant administration with inhibitors of CYP2D6 could result in some inhibition of the metabolism of tramadol).

No products indexed under this heading.

Quinidine Sulfate (In vitro drug interaction studies in human liver microsomes indicate that concomitant administration with inhibitors of CYP2D6 could result in some inhibition of the metabolism of tramadol).

No products indexed under this heading.

Quinine (Administration of CYP3A4 inhibitors, such as ketoconazole and erythromycin, with tramadol hydrochloride may effect the metabolism of tramadol leading to altered tramadol exposure).

No products indexed under this heading.

Quinine Sulfate (Administration of CYP3A4 inhibitors, such as ketoconazole and erythromycin, with tramadol hydrochloride may effect the metabolism of tramadol leading to altered tramadol exposure).

No products indexed under this heading.

Quinupristin (Administration of CYP3A4 inhibitors, such as ketoconazole and erythromycin, with tramadol hydrochloride may effect the metabolism of tramadol leading to altered tramadol exposure).

No products indexed under this heading.

Ramelteon (Tramadol hydrochloride is contraindicated in acute intoxication with hypnotics. Tramadol hydrochloride should be used with caution and in reduced dosages when administered to patients receiving CNS depressants, such as sedative hypnotics. Tramadol hydrochloride increases the risk of CNS and respiratory depression). Products include:

Rozerem Tablets 3091

Ranitidine Bismuth Citrate (In vitro drug interaction studies in human liver microsomes indicate that concomitant administration with inhibitors of CYP2D6 could result in some inhibition of the metabolism of tramadol).

No products indexed under this heading.

Ranitidine Hydrochloride (In vitro drug interaction studies in human liver microsomes indicate that concomitant administration with inhibitors of CYP2D6 could result in some inhibition of the metabolism of tramadol). Products include:

Zantac 75 Tablets .... ▣603
Zantac 1670
Zantac Injection 1666
Zantac Injection Pharmacy Bulk Package 1668
Maximum Strength Zantac 150 Tablets .... ▣603
Maximum Strength Zantac 150 Cool Mint Tablets .... ▣603

Rasagiline Mesylate (Administration of tramadol may increase the seizure risk in patients taking monoamine oxidase inhibitors or other drugs that reduce the seizure threshold. Use tramadol with great caution in patients taking MAO inhibitors. Concomitant use of tramadol with MAO inhibitors increases the risk of adverse events, including seizure and serotonin syndrome). Products include:
Azilect Tablets 3106

Remifentanil Hydrochloride (Tramadol hydrochloride is contraindicated in acute intoxication with narcotics, opioids, and centrally-acting analgesics. Concomitant use of tramadol increases the seizure risk in patients taking opioids. Tramadol hydrochloride should be used with caution and in reduced dosages when administered to patients receiving CNS depressants, such as opioids or narcotics. Tramadol hydrochloride increases the risk of CNS and respiratory depression. Tramadol may be expected to have additive effects when used in conjunction with other opioids).
No products indexed under this heading.

Rifabutin (Administration of CYP3A4 inducers, such as rifampin or St. John's Wort, with tramadol hydrochloride may effect the metabolism of tramadol leading to altered tramadol exposure).
No products indexed under this heading.

Rifampicin (Administration of CYP3A4 inducers, such as rifampin or St. John's Wort, with tramadol hydrochloride may effect the metabolism of tramadol leading to altered tramadol exposure).
No products indexed under this heading.

Rifampin (Administration of CYP3A4 inducers, such as rifampin or St. John's Wort, with tramadol hydrochloride may effect the metabolism of tramadol leading to altered tramadol exposure).
No products indexed under this heading.

Rifapentine (Administration of CYP3A4 inducers, such as rifampin or St. John's Wort, with tramadol hydrochloride may effect the metabolism of tramadol leading to altered tramadol exposure).
No products indexed under this heading.

Risperidone (Tramadol hydrochloride is contraindicated in acute intoxication with psychotropic drugs). Products include:
Risperdal Consta Long-Acting Injection 1753

Ritonavir (In vitro drug interaction studies in human liver microsomes indicate that concomitant administration with inhibitors of CYP2D6 could result in some inhibition of the metabolism of tramadol). Products include:
Kaletra 452
Norvir 489

Rizatriptan Benzoate (Concomitant use of tramadol increases the seizure risk in patients taking triptans. Concomitant use of tramadol with triptans increases the risk of adverse events, including seizure and serotonin syndrome. If concomitant treatment of tramadol with a drug affecting the serotonergic neurotransmitter system is clinically warranted, careful observation of the patient is advised, particularly during treatment initiation and dose increases). Products include:
Maxalt Tablets 2056
Maxalt-MLT Orally Disintegrating Tablets 2056

Saquinavir (Administration of CYP3A4 inhibitors, such as ketoconazole and erythromycin, with tramadol hydrochloride may effect the metabolism of tramadol leading to altered tramadol exposure).
No products indexed under this heading.

Saquinavir Mesylate (Administration of CYP3A4 inhibitors, such as ketoconazole and erythromycin, with tramadol hydrochloride may effect the metabolism of tramadol leading to altered tramadol exposure).
No products indexed under this heading.

Secobarbital Sodium (Tramadol hydrochloride is contraindicated in acute intoxication with hypnotics. Tramadol hydrochloride should be used with caution and in reduced dosages when administered to patients receiving CNS depressants, such as sedative hypnotics. Tramadol hydrochloride increases the risk of CNS and respiratory depression).
No products indexed under this heading.

Selegiline (Administration of tramadol may increase the seizure risk in patients taking monoamine oxidase inhibitors or other drugs that reduce the seizure threshold. Use tramadol with great caution in patients taking MAO inhibitors. Concomitant use of tramadol with MAO inhibitors increases the risk of adverse events, including seizure and serotonin syndrome). Products include:
Emsam Transdermal System 905

Selegiline Hydrochloride (Administration of tramadol may increase the seizure risk in patients taking monoamine oxidase inhibitors or other drugs that reduce the seizure threshold. Use tramadol with great caution in patients taking MAO inhibitors. Concomitant use of tramadol with MAO inhibitors increases the risk of adverse events, including seizure and serotonin syndrome). Products include:
Eldepryl Capsules 3052

Sertraline Hydrochloride (Concomitant use of tramadol increases the seizure risk in patients taking selective serotonin re-uptake inhibitors. Concomitant use of tramadol with SSRIs increases the risk of adverse events, including seizure and serotonin syndrome).
No products indexed under this heading.

Sevoflurane (Tramadol hydrochloride should be used with caution and in reduced dosages when administered to patients receiving CNS depressants, such as alcohol, opioids, anesthetic agents, narcotics, phenothiazines, tranquilizers, or sedative hypnotics. Tramadol hydrochloride increases the risk of CNS and respiratory depression). Products include:
Ultane Liquid for Inhalation 524

Sildenafil Citrate (In vitro drug interaction studies in human liver microsomes indicate that concomitant administration with inhibitors of CYP2D6 could result in some inhibition of the metabolism of tramadol).
No products indexed under this heading.

Sodium Butabarbital (Tramadol hydrochloride is contraindicated in acute intoxication with hypnotics. Tramadol hydrochloride should be used with caution and in reduced dosages when administered to patients receiving CNS depressants, such as sedative hypnotics. Tramadol hydrochloride increases the risk of CNS and respiratory depression).
No products indexed under this heading.

Sodium Oxybate (Tramadol hydrochloride should be used with caution and in reduced dosages when administered to patients receiving CNS depressants, such as alcohol, opioids, anesthetic agents, narcotics, phenothiazines, tranquilizers, or sedative hypnotics. Tramadol hydrochloride increases the risk of CNS and respiratory depression). Products include:
Xyrem Oral Solution 1766

Sufentanil Citrate (Tramadol hydrochloride is contraindicated in acute intoxication with narcotics, opioids, and centrally-acting analgesics. Concomitant use of tramadol increases the seizure risk in patients taking opioids. Tramadol hydrochloride should be used with caution and in reduced dosages when administered to patients receiving CNS depressants, such as opioids or narcotics. Tramadol hydrochloride increases the risk of CNS and respiratory depression. Tramadol may be expected to have additive effects when used in conjunction with other opioids).
No products indexed under this heading.

Sulfinpyrazone (Administration of CYP3A4 inducers, such as rifampin or St. John's Wort, with tramadol hydrochloride may effect the metabolism of tramadol leading to altered tramadol exposure).
No products indexed under this heading.

Sumatriptan (Concomitant use of tramadol increases the seizure risk in patients taking triptans. Concomitant use of tramadol with triptans increases the risk of adverse events, including seizure and serotonin syndrome. If concomitant treatment of tramadol with a drug affecting the serotonergic neurotransmitter system is clinically warranted, careful observation of the patient is advised, particularly during treatment initiation and dose increases). Products include:
Imitrex Nasal Spray 1470

Sumatriptan Succinate (Concomitant use of tramadol increases the seizure risk in patients taking triptans. Concomitant use of tramadol with triptans increases the risk of adverse events, including seizure and serotonin syndrome. If concomitant treatment of tramadol with a drug affecting the serotonergic neurotransmitter system is clinically warranted, careful observation of the patient is advised, particularly during treatment initiation and dose increases). Products include:
Imitrex Injection 1465
Imitrex Tablets 1474
Treximet Tablets 1616

Telithromycin (Administration of CYP3A4 inhibitors, such as ketoconazole and erythromycin, with tramadol hydrochloride may effect the metabolism of tramadol leading to altered tramadol exposure). Products include:
Ketek Tablets 2744

Temazepam (Tramadol hydrochloride is contraindicated in acute intoxication with hypnotics. Tramadol hydrochloride should be used with caution and in reduced dosages when administered to patients receiving CNS depressants, such as sedative hypnotics. Tramadol hydrochloride increases the risk of CNS and respiratory depression).
No products indexed under this heading.

Terbinafine Hydrochloride (In vitro drug interaction studies in human liver microsomes indicate that concomitant administration with inhibitors of CYP2D6 could result in some inhibition of the metabolism of tramadol). Products include:
Lamisil Oral Granules 2264
Lamisil Tablets 2266

Theophylline (Administration of CYP3A4 inducers, such as rifampin or St. John's Wort, with tramadol hydrochloride may effect the metabolism of tramadol leading to altered tramadol exposure).
No products indexed under this heading.

Theophylline Anhydrous (Administration of CYP3A4 inducers, such as rifampin or St. John's Wort, with tramadol hydrochloride may effect the metabolism of tramadol leading to altered tramadol exposure). Products include:
Uniphyl Tablets 2595

Theophylline Calcium Salicylate (Administration of CYP3A4 inducers, such as rifampin or St. John's Wort, with tramadol hydrochloride may effect the metabolism of tramadol leading to altered tramadol exposure).
No products indexed under this heading.

Theophylline Dihydroxypropyl (Glyceryl) (Administration of CYP3A4 inducers, such as rifampin or St. John's Wort, with tramadol hydrochloride may effect the metabolism of tramadol leading to altered tramadol exposure).
No products indexed under this heading.

Theophylline Ethylenediamine (Administration of CYP3A4 inducers, such as rifampin or St. John's Wort, with tramadol hydrochloride may effect the metabolism of tramadol leading to altered tramadol exposure).
No products indexed under this heading.

Thiamylal Sodium (Tramadol hydrochloride should be used with caution and in reduced dosages when administered to patients receiving CNS depressants, such as alcohol, opioids, anesthetic agents, narcotics, phenothiazines, tranquilizers, or sedative hypnotics. Tramadol hydrochloride increases the risk of CNS and respiratory depression).
No products indexed under this heading.

Thioridazine Hydrochloride (Tramadol hydrochloride is contraindicated in acute intoxication with psychotropic drugs). Products include:
Thioridazine Hydrochloride Tablets 2195

Thiothixene (Tramadol hydrochloride is contraindicated in acute intoxication with psychotropic drugs). Products include:
Thiothixene Capsules 2197

Tranylcypromine Sulfate (Tramadol hydrochloride is contraindicated in acute intoxication with psychotropic drugs). Products include:
Parnate Tablets 1532

Triamcinolone (Administration of CYP3A4 inducers, such as rifampin or St. John's Wort, with tramadol hydrochloride may effect the metabolism of tramadol leading to altered tramadol exposure).
No products indexed under this heading.

Triamcinolone Acetonide (Administration of CYP3A4 inducers, such as rifampin or St. John's Wort, with tramadol hydrochloride may effect the metabolism of tramadol leading to altered tramadol exposure). Products include:
Azmacort Inhalation Aerosol 407
Nasacort AQ Nasal Spray 2765
Triesence Injectable Suspension .... ⊙ 209

Triamcinolone Diacetate (Administration of CYP3A4 inducers, such as rifampin or St. John's Wort, with tramadol hydrochloride may effect the metabolism of tramadol leading to altered tramadol exposure).
No products indexed under this heading.

Triamcinolone Hexacetonide (Administration of CYP3A4 inducers, such as rifampin or St. John's Wort, with tramadol hydrochloride may effect the metabolism of tramadol leading to altered tramadol exposure).
No products indexed under this heading.

Triazolam (Tramadol hydrochloride is contraindicated in acute intoxication with hypnotics. Tramadol hydrochloride should be used with caution and in reduced dosages when administered to patients receiving CNS depressants, such as sedative hypnotics. Tramadol hydrochloride increases the risk of CNS and respiratory depression).
No products indexed under this heading.

Trifluoperazine Hydrochloride (Tramadol hydrochloride is contraindicated in acute intoxication with psychotropic drugs).
No products indexed under this heading.

Trimipramine Maleate (Tramadol hydrochloride is contraindicated in acute intoxication with psychotropic drugs).
No products indexed under this heading.

Troglitazone (Administration of CYP3A4 inhibitors, such as ketoconazole and erythromycin, with tramadol hydrochloride may effect the metabolism of tramadol leading to altered tramadol exposure).
No products indexed under this heading.

Troleandomycin (Administration of CYP3A4 inhibitors, such as ketoconazole and erythromycin, with tramadol hydrochloride may effect the metabolism of tramadol leading to altered tramadol exposure).
No products indexed under this heading.

Valproate Sodium (Administration of CYP3A4 inhibitors, such as ketoconazole and erythromycin, with tramadol hydrochloride may effect the metabolism of tramadol leading to altered tramadol exposure).
No products indexed under this heading.

Vardenafil Hydrochloride (In vitro drug interaction studies in human liver microsomes indicate that concomitant administration with inhibitors of CYP2D6 could result in some inhibition of the metabolism of tramadol). Products include:
Levitra Tablets 2876

Venlafaxine Hydrochloride (Concomitant use of tramadol increases the seizure risk in patients taking serotonin and norepinephrine reuptake inhibitors. Concomitant use of tramadol with SNRIs increases the risk of adverse events, including seizure and serotonin syndrome. If concomitant treatment of tramadol with a drug affecting the serotonergic neurotransmitter system is clinically warranted, careful observation of the patient is advised, particularly during treatment initiation and dose increases). Products include:
Effexor XR Extended-Release Capsules 3195
Venlafaxine Hydrochloride Tablets ... 2199

Verapamil Hydrochloride (Administration of CYP3A4 inhibitors, such as ketoconazole and erythromycin, with tramadol hydrochloride may effect the metabolism of tramadol leading to altered tramadol exposure). Products include:
Tarka Tablets 511

Voriconazole (Administration of CYP3A4 inhibitors, such as ketoconazole and erythromycin, with tramadol hydrochloride may effect the metabolism of tramadol leading to altered tramadol exposure).
No products indexed under this heading.

Warfarin Sodium (Post-marketing surveillance of tramadol has revealed rare reports of alteration of warfarin effect, including elevation of prothrombin times).
No products indexed under this heading.

Zafirlukast (Administration of CYP3A4 inhibitors, such as ketoconazole and erythromycin, with tramadol hydrochloride may effect the metabolism of tramadol leading to altered tramadol exposure). Products include:
Accolate Tablets 669

Zaleplon (Tramadol hydrochloride is contraindicated in acute intoxication with hypnotics. Tramadol hydrochloride should be used with caution and in reduced dosages when administered to patients receiving CNS depressants, such as sedative hypnotics. Tramadol hydrochloride increases the risk of CNS and respiratory depression).
No products indexed under this heading.

Zileuton (Administration of CYP3A4 inhibitors, such as ketoconazole and erythromycin, with tramadol hydrochloride may effect the metabolism of tramadol leading to altered tramadol exposure).
No products indexed under this heading.

Ziprasidone Hydrochloride (Tramadol hydrochloride is contraindicated in acute intoxication with psychotropic drugs). Products include:
Geodon Capsules 2520

Zolmitriptan (Concomitant use of tramadol increases the seizure risk in patients taking triptans. Concomitant use of tramadol with triptans increases the risk of adverse events, including seizure and serotonin syndrome. If concomitant treatment of tramadol with a drug affecting the serotonergic neurotransmitter system is clinically warranted, careful observation of the patient is advised, particularly during treatment initiation and dose increases). Products include:
Zomig Tablets 694
Zomig Nasal Spray 689
Zomig-ZMT Tablets 694

Zolpidem Tartrate (Tramadol hydrochloride is contraindicated in acute intoxication with hypnotics. Tramadol hydrochloride should be used with caution and in reduced dosages when administered to patients receiving CNS depressants, such as sedative hypnotics. Tramadol hydrochloride increases the risk of CNS and respiratory depression). Products include:
Ambien Tablets 2692
Ambien CR Tablets 2696

Food Interactions

Alcohol (Tramadol hydrochloride is contraindicated in acute intoxication with alcohol. Tramadol hydrochloride should be used with caution and in reduced dosages when administered to patients receiving CNS depressants, such as alcohol. Tramadol may be expected to have additive effects when used in conjunction with alcohol).

Grapefruit (Administration of CYP3A4 inhibitors, such as ketoconazole and erythromycin, with tramadol hydrochloride may effect the metabolism of tramadol leading to altered tramadol exposure).

Grapefruit Juice (Administration of CYP3A4 inhibitors, such as ketoconazole and erythromycin, with tramadol hydrochloride may effect the metabolism of tramadol leading to altered tramadol exposure).

ULTRASE CAPSULES

(Pancrelipase) 718

Food Interactions

Food having a pH greater than 5.5 (Can dissolve the protective coating resulting in early release of enzymes, irritation of oral mucosa, and/or loss of enzyme activity).

ULTRASE MT CAPSULES

(Pancrelipase) 719

Food Interactions

Food having a pH greater than 5.5 (Can dissolve the protective enteric shell).

UNIPHYL TABLETS

(Theophylline Anhydrous) 2595
May interact with erythromycin, lithium preparations, and certain other agents. Compounds in these categories include:

Adenosine (Theophylline blocks adenosine receptors; higher doses of adenosine may be required to achieve desired effect). Products include:
Adenocard IV Injection 603
Adenoscan 605

Allopurinol (Decreases theophylline clearance at allopurinol doses greater than or equal to 600 mg/day).
No products indexed under this heading.

Aminoglutethimide (Increases theophylline clearance by induction of microsomal enzyme).
No products indexed under this heading.

Carbamazepine (Increases theophylline clearance by induction of microsomal enzyme). Products include:
Carbatrol Capsules 3019
Equetro Extended-Release Capsules 3174

Cimetidine (Decreases theophylline clearance by inhibiting cytochrome P450 1A2).
No products indexed under this heading.

Cimetidine Hydrochloride (Decreases theophylline clearance by inhibiting cytochrome P450 1A2).
No products indexed under this heading.

Ciprofloxacin (Decreases theophylline clearance by inhibiting cytochrome P450 1A2). Products include:
Cipro I.V. 2817
Cipro Oral Suspension 2810
Cipro XR Tablets 2823
Ciprodex Otic Suspension 541

Ciprofloxacin Hydrochloride (Decreases theophylline clearance by inhibiting cytochrome P450 1A2). Products include:
Cipro Tablets 2810

Clarithromycin (Decreases theophylline clearance by inhibiting cytochrome P450 3A3). Products include:
Biaxin/Biaxin XL 411

Diazepam (Benzodiazepines increase CNS concentrations of adenosine, a potent CNS depressant, while theophylline blocks adenosine receptors; larger diazepam doses may be required to produce desired level of sedation; discontinuation of theophylline without reduction of diazepam dose may result in respiratory depression). Products include:
Valium Tablets 2658

Disulfiram (Decreases theophylline clearance by inhibiting hydroxylation and demethylation).
No products indexed under this heading.

Enoxacin (Decreases theophylline clearance by inhibiting cytochrome P450 1A2).
No products indexed under this heading.

Ephedrine Hydrochloride (Coadministration results in synergistic CNS effects resulting in increased frequency of nausea, nervousness, and insomnia).
No products indexed under this heading.

Ephedrine Sulfate (Co-administration results in synergistic CNS effects resulting in increased frequency of nausea, nervousness, and insomnia).
No products indexed under this heading.

Ephedrine Tannate (Co-administration results in synergistic CNS effects resulting in increased frequency of nausea, nervousness, and insomnia).
No products indexed under this heading.

Erythromycin (Erythromycin metabolite decreases theophylline clearance by inhibiting cytochrome P450 3A3; decreased erythromycin steady-state serum concentrations).
No products indexed under this heading.

Erythromycin Estolate (Erythromycin metabolite decreases theophylline clearance by inhibiting cytochrome P450 3A3; decreased erythromycin steady-state serum concentrations).
No products indexed under this heading.

Erythromycin Ethylsuccinate (Erythromycin metabolite decreases theophylline clearance by inhibiting cytochrome P450 3A3; decreased erythromycin steady-state serum concentrations). Products include:
E.E.S. 433
EryPed 431

Erythromycin Gluceptate (Erythromycin metabolite decreases theophylline clearance by inhibiting cytochrome P450 3A3; decreased erythromycin steady-state serum concentrations).
No products indexed under this heading.

Erythromycin Lactobionate (Erythromycin metabolite decreases theophylline clearance by inhibiting cytochrome P450 3A3; decreased erythromycin steady-state serum concentrations).
No products indexed under this heading.

Erythromycin Stearate (Erythromycin metabolite decreases theophylline clearance by inhibiting cytochrome P450 3A3; decreased erythromycin steady-state serum concentrations).
No products indexed under this heading.

Ethinyl Estradiol (Estrogen containing oral contraceptives decreases theophylline clearance in dose dependent fashion). Products include:
Lybrel Tablets 3204
Mircette Tablets 1034
NuvaRing 2897
Ortho-Cyclen/Ortho Tri-Cyclen 2449
Ortho Evra Transdermal System 2437
Ortho Tri-Cyclen Lo Tablets 2458
Seasonique Tablets 1046
Yaz Tablets 805

Flurazepam Hydrochloride (Benzodiazepines increase CNS concentrations of adenosine, a potent CNS depressant, while theophylline blocks adenosine receptors; larger flurazepam doses may be required to produce desired level of sedation; discontinuation of theophylline without reduction of flurazepam dose may result in respiratory depression).
No products indexed under this heading.

Fluvoxamine Maleate (Decreases theophylline clearance by inhibiting cytochrome P450 1A2). Products include:
Luvox CR Extended-Release Capsules 1759

Halothane (Halothane sensitizes the myocardium to catecholamines; theophylline increases release of endogenous catecholamines resulting in increased risk of ventricular arrhythmias).
No products indexed under this heading.

Hypericum (Increases theophylline clearance; higher doses of theophylline may be required to achieve desired effect; stopping St. John's Wort may result in theophylline toxicity). Products include:
Satieté Tablets .... ■640

Interferon alfa-2a, Recombinant (Decreases theophylline clearance).
No products indexed under this heading.

Isoproterenol Hydrochloride (Co-administration with intravenous isoproterenol decreases theophylline clearance).
No products indexed under this heading.

Ketamine Hydrochloride (May lower theophylline seizure threshold).
No products indexed under this heading.

Lithium (Theophylline increases renal lithium clearance; increase in lithium dose may be required to achieve a therapeutic serum concentration).
No products indexed under this heading.

Lithium Carbonate (Theophylline increases renal lithium clearance; increase in lithium dose may be required to achieve a therapeutic serum concentration).
No products indexed under this heading.

Lithium Citrate (Theophylline increases renal lithium clearance; increase in lithium dose may be required to achieve a therapeutic serum concentration).
No products indexed under this heading.

Lorazepam (Benzodiazepines increase CNS concentrations of adenosine, a potent CNS depressant, while theophylline blocks adenosine receptors; larger lorazepam doses may be required to produce desired level of sedation; discontinuation of theophylline without reduction of lorazepam dose may result in respiratory depression).
No products indexed under this heading.

Mestranol (Estrogen containing oral contraceptives decreases theophylline clearance in dose dependent fashion).
No products indexed under this heading.

Methotrexate Sodium (Decreases theophylline clearance).
No products indexed under this heading.

Mexiletine Hydrochloride (Decreases theophylline clearance by inhibiting hydroxylation and demethylation).
No products indexed under this heading.

Midazolam Hydrochloride (Benzodiazepines increase CNS concentrations of adenosine, a potent CNS depressant, while theophylline blocks adenosine receptors; larger midazolam doses may be required to produce desired level of sedation; discontinuation of theophylline without reduction of midazolam dose may result in respiratory depression).
No products indexed under this heading.

Moricizine Hydrochloride (Increases theophylline clearance).
No products indexed under this heading.

Pancuronium Bromide (Theophylline may antagonize non-depolarizing neuromuscular blocking effects; possibly due to phosphodiesterase inhibition; larger pancuronium doses may be required to achieve neuromuscular blockade).
No products indexed under this heading.

Pentoxifylline (Decreases theophylline clearance).
No products indexed under this heading.

Phenobarbital (Increases theophylline clearance by induction of microsomal enzyme). Products include:
Donnatal Extentabs 2507

Phenytoin (Phenytoin increases theophylline clearance by increasing microsomal enzyme activity; theophylline decreases phenytoin absorption).
No products indexed under this heading.

Phenytoin Sodium (Phenytoin increases theophylline clearance by increasing microsomal enzyme activity; theophylline decreases phenytoin absorption). Products include:
Phenytek Capsules 2192

Propafenone Hydrochloride (Decreases theophylline clearance). Products include:
Rythmol Tablets 1586
Rythmol SR Capsules 1590

Propranolol Hydrochloride (Decreases theophylline clearance by inhibiting cytochrome P450 1A2). Products include:
InnoPran XL Extended Release Capsules 1484

Rifampin (Increases theophylline clearance by increasing cytochrome P450 1A2 and 3A3 activity).
No products indexed under this heading.

Sulfinpyrazone (Increases theophylline clearance by increasing demethylation and hydroxylation; decreases renal clearance of theophylline).
No products indexed under this heading.

Tacrine Hydrochloride (Decreases theophylline clearance by inhibiting cytochrome P450 1A2 and also increases renal clearance of theophylline).
No products indexed under this heading.

Thiabendazole (Decreases theophylline clearance).
No products indexed under this heading.

Ticlopidine Hydrochloride (Decreases theophylline clearance).
No products indexed under this heading.

Troleandomycin (Decreases theophylline clearance by inhibiting cytochrome P450 3A3).
No products indexed under this heading.

Verapamil Hydrochloride (Decreases theophylline clearance by inhibiting hydroxylation and demethylation). Products include:
Tarka Tablets 511

Food Interactions

Alcohol (Concurrent use with a single dose of alcohol (3mL/kg of whiskey) decreases theophylline clearance for up to 24 hours).

Diet, high-lipid (Co-administration with a standardized high-fat meal results in increased peak plasma concentration and bioavailability; however, a precipitous increase in the rate and extent of absorption was not evident; the dosing should be ideally administered consistently either with or without food).

UROCIT-K TABLETS

(Potassium Citrate) 2176
May interact with anticholinergics and potassium sparing diuretics. Compounds in these categories include:

Amiloride Hydrochloride (Co-administration can produce severe hyperkalemia; concurrent use should be avoided).
No products indexed under this heading.

Atropine Sulfate (Co-administration with drugs that slow gastrointestinal transit time, such as anticholinergics, can be expected to increase the gastrointestinal irritation produced by potassium salts; concurrent use is contraindicated).
Products include:
Donnatal Extentabs 2507

Belladonna Alkaloids (Co-administration with drugs that slow gastrointestinal transit time, such as anticholinergics, can be expected to increase the gastrointestinal irritation produced by potassium salts; concurrent use is contraindicated).
Products include:
Hyland's Teething Tablets .... ■621

Benztropine Mesylate (Co-administration with drugs that slow gastrointestinal transit time, such as anticholinergics, can be expected to increase the gastrointestinal irritation produced by potassium salts; concurrent use is contraindicated).
No products indexed under this heading.

Biperiden Hydrochloride (Co-administration with drugs that slow gastrointestinal transit time, such as anticholinergics, can be expected to increase the gastrointestinal irritation produced by potassium salts; concurrent use is contraindicated).
No products indexed under this heading.

Clidinium Bromide (Co-administration with drugs that slow gastrointestinal transit time, such as anticholinergics, can be expected to increase the gastrointestinal irritation produced by potassium salts; concurrent use is contraindicated).
No products indexed under this heading.

Dicyclomine Hydrochloride (Co-administration with drugs that slow gastrointestinal transit time, such as anticholinergics, can be expected to increase the gastrointestinal irrita-

tion produced by potassium salts; concurrent use is contraindicated). Products include:
Bentyl Capsules ... 703
Bentyl Injection ... 703
Bentyl Syrup ... 703
Bentyl Tablets ... 703

Glycopyrrolate (Co-administration with drugs that slow gastrointestinal transit time, such as anticholinergics, can be expected to increase the gastrointestinal irritation produced by potassium salts; concurrent use is contraindicated).
No products indexed under this heading.

Hyoscyamine (Co-administration with drugs that slow gastrointestinal transit time, such as anticholinergics, can be expected to increase the gastrointestinal irritation produced by potassium salts; concurrent use is contraindicated).
No products indexed under this heading.

Hyoscyamine Sulfate (Co-administration with drugs that slow gastrointestinal transit time, such as anticholinergics, can be expected to increase the gastrointestinal irritation produced by potassium salts; concurrent use is contraindicated). Products include:
Donnatal Extentabs ... 2507

Ipratropium Bromide (Co-administration with drugs that slow gastrointestinal transit time, such as anticholinergics, can be expected to increase the gastrointestinal irritation produced by potassium salts; concurrent use is contraindicated). Products include:
Atrovent HFA Inhalation Aerosol ... 839
Atrovent Nasal Spray 0.03% ... 834
Atrovent Nasal Spray 0.06% ... 836
Combivent Inhalation Aerosol ... 845

Mepenzolate Bromide (Co-administration with drugs that slow gastrointestinal transit time, such as anticholinergics, can be expected to increase the gastrointestinal irritation produced by potassium salts; concurrent use is contraindicated).
No products indexed under this heading.

Oxybutynin Chloride (Co-administration with drugs that slow gastrointestinal transit time, such as anticholinergics, can be expected to increase the gastrointestinal irritation produced by potassium salts; concurrent use is contraindicated).
No products indexed under this heading.

Procyclidine Hydrochloride (Co-administration with drugs that slow gastrointestinal transit time, such as anticholinergics, can be expected to increase the gastrointestinal irritation produced by potassium salts; concurrent use is contraindicated).
No products indexed under this heading.

Propantheline Bromide (Co-administration with drugs that slow gastrointestinal transit time, such as anticholinergics, can be expected to increase the gastrointestinal irritation produced by potassium salts; concurrent use is contraindicated).
No products indexed under this heading.

Scopolamine (Co-administration with drugs that slow gastrointestinal transit time, such as anticholinergics, can be expected to increase the gastrointestinal irritation produced by potassium salts; concurrent use is contraindicated). Products include:
Transderm Scōp Transdermal Therapeutic System ... 2206

Scopolamine Hydrobromide (Co-administration with drugs that slow gastrointestinal transit time, such as anticholinergics, can be expected to increase the gastrointestinal irritation produced by potassium salts; concurrent use is contraindicated). Products include:
Donnatal Extentabs ... 2507

Spironolactone (Co-administration can produce severe hyperkalemia; concurrent use should be avoided).
No products indexed under this heading.

Tolterodine Tartrate (Co-administration with drugs that slow gastrointestinal transit time, such as anticholinergics, can be expected to increase the gastrointestinal irritation produced by potassium salts; concurrent use is contraindicated).
No products indexed under this heading.

Triamterene (Co-administration can produce severe hyperkalemia; concurrent use should be avoided). Products include:
Dyazide Capsules ... 1405
Dyrenium Capsules ... 3189

Tridihexethyl Chloride (Co-administration with drugs that slow gastrointestinal transit time, such as anticholinergics, can be expected to increase the gastrointestinal irritation produced by potassium salts; concurrent use is contraindicated).
No products indexed under this heading.

Trihexyphenidyl Hydrochloride (Co-administration with drugs that slow gastrointestinal transit time, such as anticholinergics, can be expected to increase the gastrointestinal irritation produced by potassium salts; concurrent use is contraindicated).
No products indexed under this heading.

UROQID-ACID NO. 2 TABLETS

(Methenamine Mandelate, Sodium Acid Phosphate) ... 814
May interact with:

Acetazolamide (Reduces the effectiveness of methenamine by causing urine to become alkaline).
No products indexed under this heading.

ACTH (Concurrent use with sodium phosphate may result in hypernatremia).
No products indexed under this heading.

Aluminum Carbonate (Reduces the effectiveness of methenamine by causing urine to become alkaline).
No products indexed under this heading.

Aluminum Hydroxide (Reduces the effectiveness of methenamine by causing urine to become alkaline).
No products indexed under this heading.

Aspirin (Concurrent use may lead to increased serum salicylate levels since excretion of salicylates is reduced in acidic urine). Products include:
Aggrenox Capsules ... 819
Bayer Aspirin ... 750
Percodan Tablets ... 1130
St. Joseph 81 mg Aspirin Chewable and Enteric Coated Tablets ... 1903

Bendroflumethiazide (Reduces the effectiveness of methenamine by causing urine to become alkaline).
No products indexed under this heading.

Betamethasone Acetate (Concurrent use with sodium phosphate may result in hypernatremia).
No products indexed under this heading.

Betamethasone Sodium Phosphate (Concurrent use with sodium phosphate may result in hypernatremia).
No products indexed under this heading.

Chlorothiazide (Reduces the effectiveness of methenamine by causing urine to become alkaline).
No products indexed under this heading.

Chlorothiazide Sodium (Reduces the effectiveness of methenamine by causing urine to become alkaline). Products include:
Intravenous Sodium Diuril ... 2490

Choline Magnesium Trisalicylate (Concurrent use may lead to increased serum salicylate levels since excretion of salicylates is reduced in acidic urine).
No products indexed under this heading.

Cortisone Acetate (Concurrent use with sodium phosphate may result in hypernatremia).
No products indexed under this heading.

Deserpidine (Concurrent use with sodium phosphate may result in hypernatremia).
No products indexed under this heading.

Desoxycorticosterone Acetate (Concurrent use with sodium phosphate may result in hypernatremia).
No products indexed under this heading.

Desoxycorticosterone Pivalate (Concurrent use with sodium phosphate may result in hypernatremia).
No products indexed under this heading.

Dexamethasone (Concurrent use with sodium phosphate may result in hypernatremia). Products include:
Ciprodex Otic Suspension ... 541

Dexamethasone Acetate (Concurrent use with sodium phosphate may result in hypernatremia).
No products indexed under this heading.

Dexamethasone Sodium Phosphate (Concurrent use with sodium phosphate may result in hypernatremia).
No products indexed under this heading.

Diazoxide (Concurrant use with sodium phosphate may result in hypernatremia). Products include:
Proglycem Capsules ... 1185
Proglycem Suspension ... 1185

Dichlorphenamide (Reduces the effectiveness of methenamine by causing urine to become alkaline).
No products indexed under this heading.

Diflunisal (Concurrent use may lead to increased serum salicylate levels since excretion of salicylates is reduced in acidic urine).
No products indexed under this heading.

Fludrocortisone Acetate (Concurrent use with sodium phosphate may result in hypernatremia).
No products indexed under this heading.

Guanethidine Monosulfate (Concurrent use with sodium phosphate may result in hypernatremia).
No products indexed under this heading.

Hydralazine Hydrochloride (Concurrent use with sodium phosphate may result in hypernatremia).
No products indexed under this heading.

Hydrochlorothiazide (Reduces the effectiveness of methenamine by causing urine to become alkaline). Products include:
Atacand HCT ... 642
Avalide Tablets ... 892
Avalide Tablets ... 2713
Benicar HCT Tablets ... 1010
Diovan HCT Tablets ... 2216
Dyazide Capsules ... 1405
Micardis HCT Tablets ... 854
Prinzide Tablets ... 2092
Tekturna HCT Tablets ... 2324
Teveten HCT Tablets ... 517

Hydrocortisone (Concurrent use with sodium phosphate may result in hypernatremia).
No products indexed under this heading.

Hydrocortisone Acetate (Concurrent use with sodium phosphate may result in hypernatremia). Products include:
Analpram-HC ... 1140
Pramosone ... 1141

Hydrocortisone Sodium Phosphate (Concurrent use with sodium phosphate may result in hypernatremia).
No products indexed under this heading.

Hydrocortisone Sodium Succinate (Concurrent use with sodium phosphate may result in hypernatremia).
No products indexed under this heading.

Hydroflumethiazide (Reduces the effectiveness of methenamine by causing urine to become alkaline).
No products indexed under this heading.

Magaldrate (Reduces the effectiveness of methenamine by causing urine to become alkaline).
No products indexed under this heading.

Magnesium Hydroxide (Reduces the effectiveness of methenamine by causing urine to become alkaline). Products include:
Fleet Pedia-Lax Chewable Tablets ... 1145
Pepcid Complete Chewable Tablets ... 1771
Extra Strength Rolaids Freshmint Tablets ... 1903
Rolaids Multi-Symptom Berry Tablets ... 1903
Rolaids Original Peppermint Tablets ... 1903

Magnesium Oxide (Reduces the effectiveness of methenamine by causing urine to become alkaline). Products include:
Beelith Tablets ... 813

Magnesium Salicylate (Concurrent use may lead to increased serum salicylate levels since excretion of salicylates is reduced in acidic urine).
No products indexed under this heading.

Methazolamide (Reduces the effectiveness of methenamine by causing urine to become alkaline).
No products indexed under this heading.

Methyclothiazide (Reduces the effectiveness of methenamine by causing urine to become alkaline).
No products indexed under this heading.

Methyldopa (Concurrent use with sodium phosphate may result in hypernatremia).
No products indexed under this heading.

Methylprednisolone Acetate (Concurrent use with sodium phosphate may result in hypernatremia).
No products indexed under this heading.

Methylprednisolone Sodium Succinate (Concurrent use with sodium phosphate may result in hypernatremia).
No products indexed under this heading.

Polythiazide (Reduces the effectiveness of methenamine by causing urine to become alkaline).
No products indexed under this heading.

Potassium Citrate (Reduces the effectiveness of methenamine by causing urine to become alkaline). Products include:
BioLean Free Tablets .... ▣635
Urocit-K Tablets 2176

Prednisolone Acetate (Concurrent use with sodium phosphate may result in hypernatremia). Products include:
Pred Forte Ophthalmic Suspension .... ⊙227
Pred Mild Ophthalmic Suspension .... ⊙230
Pred-G Ophthalmic Ointment .... ⊙229
Pred-G Ophthalmic Suspension ...... ⊙228

Prednisolone Sodium Phosphate (Concurrent use with sodium phosphate may result in hypernatremia).
No products indexed under this heading.

Prednisolone Tebutate (Concurrent use with sodium phosphate may result in hypernatremia).
No products indexed under this heading.

Prednisone (Concurrent use with sodium phosphate may result in hypernatremia).
No products indexed under this heading.

Rauwolfia Serpentina (Concurrent use with sodium phosphate may result in hypernatremia).
No products indexed under this heading.

Rescinnamine (Concurrent use with sodium phosphate may result in hypernatremia).
No products indexed under this heading.

Reserpine (Concurrent use with sodium phosphate may result in hypernatremia).
No products indexed under this heading.

Salsalate (Concurrent use may lead to increased serum salicylate levels since excretion of salicylates is reduced in acidic urine).
No products indexed under this heading.

Sodium Bicarbonate (Reduces the effectiveness of methenamine by causing urine to become alkaline). Products include:
Ceo-Two Laxative Suppository 815

Sodium Citrate (Reduces the effectiveness of methenamine by causing urine to become alkaline).
No products indexed under this heading.

Sulfamethizole (Concurrent use with sulfamethizole and formaldehyde forms an insoluble precipitate in acid urine and increases the risk of crystaluria).
No products indexed under this heading.

Triamcinolone (Concurrent use with sodium phosphate may result in hypernatremia).
No products indexed under this heading.

Triamcinolone Acetonide (Concurrent use with sodium phosphate may result in hypernatremia). Products include:
Azmacort Inhalation Aerosol 407
Nasacort AQ Nasal Spray 2765
Triesence Injectable Suspension .... ⊙209

Triamcinolone Diacetate (Concurrent use with sodium phosphate may result in hypernatremia).
No products indexed under this heading.

Triamcinolone Hexacetonide (Concurrent use with sodium phosphate may result in hypernatremia).
No products indexed under this heading.

UROXATRAL TABLETS

(Alfuzosin Hydrochloride) 2786
May interact with alpha adrenergic blockers, antihypertensives, cytochrome p450 3a4 inhibitors, potent, nitrates and nitrites, and drugs that prolong the QT interval. Compounds in these categories include:

Acebutolol Hydrochloride (As with other alpha-blockers, there may be an increased risk of hypotension/postural hypotension and syncope when taking afluzosin with antihypertensives concomitantly).
No products indexed under this heading.

Aliskiren (As with other alpha-blockers, there may be an increased risk of hypotension/postural hypotension and syncope when taking afluzosin with antihypertensives concomitantly). Products include:
Tekturna Tablets 2321
Tekturna HCT Tablets 2324

Alprazolam (A postmarketing study evaluating the effect of combining alfuzosin hydrochloride with another drug of comparable QT effect showed an increased effect when compared to either drug alone. Although this study was not designed to make direct statistical comparisons between drugs, the QT increase with both drugs was no more than additive and was lower than that of the active control moxifloxacin. These observations should be considered in clinical decisions when prescribing alfuzosin hydrochloride for patients with a known history of QT prolongation or patients who are taking medications which prolong the QT interval).
No products indexed under this heading.

Amiodarone Hydrochloride (A postmarketing study evaluating the effect of combining alfuzosin hydrochloride with another drug of comparable QT effect showed an increased effect when compared to either drug alone. Although this study was not designed to make direct statistical comparisons between drugs, the QT increase with both drugs was no more than additive and was lower than that of the active control moxifloxacin. These observations should be considered in clinical decisions when prescribing alfuzosin hydrochloride for patients with a known history of QT prolongation or patients who are taking medications which prolong the QT interval).
No products indexed under this heading.

Amitriptyline Hydrochloride (A postmarketing study evaluating the effect of combining alfuzosin hydrochloride with another drug of comparable QT effect showed an increased effect when compared to either drug alone. Although this study was not designed to make direct statistical comparisons between drugs, the QT increase with both drugs was no more than additive and was lower than that of the active control moxifloxacin. These observations should be considered in clinical decisions when prescribing alfuzosin hydrochloride for patients with a known history of QT prolongation or patients who are taking medications which prolong the QT interval).
No products indexed under this heading.

Amlodipine Besylate (As with other alpha-blockers, there may be an increased risk of hypotension/postural hypotension and syncope when taking afluzosin with antihypertensives concomitantly). Products include:
Azor Tablets 1005
Exforge Tablets 2238

Amoxapine (A postmarketing study evaluating the effect of combining alfuzosin hydrochloride with another drug of comparable QT effect showed an increased effect when compared to either drug alone. Although this study was not designed to make direct statistical comparisons between drugs, the QT increase with both drugs was no more than additive and was lower than that of the active control moxifloxacin. These observations should be considered in clinical decisions when prescribing alfuzosin hydrochloride for patients with a known history of QT prolongation or patients who are taking medications which prolong the QT interval).
No products indexed under this heading.

Amprenavir (Uroxatral should not be co-administered with potent CYP3A4 inhibitors such as ketoconazole, itraconazole, and ritonavir, since alfuzosin blood levels are increased).
No products indexed under this heading.

Amyl Nitrite (As with other alpha-blockers, there may be an increased risk of hypotension/postural hypotension and syncope when taking afluzosin with antihypertensives concomitantly. Care should be taken when afluzosin is used in combination with nitrates).
No products indexed under this heading.

Astemizole (A postmarketing study evaluating the effect of combining alfuzosin hydrochloride with another drug of comparable QT effect showed an increased effect when compared to either drug alone. Although this study was not designed to make direct statistical comparisons between drugs, the QT increase with both drugs was no more than additive and was lower than that of the active control moxifloxacin. These observations should be considered in clinical decisions when prescribing alfuzosin hydrochloride for patients with a known history of QT prolongation or patients who are taking medications which prolong the QT interval).
No products indexed under this heading.

Atazanavir (Uroxatral should not be co-administered with potent CYP3A4 inhibitors such as ketoconazole, itraconazole, and ritonavir, since alfuzosin blood levels are increased).
No products indexed under this heading.

Atazanavir Sulfate (Uroxatral should not be co-administered with potent CYP3A4 inhibitors such as ketoconazole, itraconazole, and ritonavir, since alfuzosin blood levels are increased). Products include:
Reyataz Capsules 3299

Atenolol (As with other alpha-blockers, there may be an increased risk of hypotension/postural hypotension and syncope when taking afluzosin with antihypertensives concomitantly).
No products indexed under this heading.

Benazepril Hydrochloride (As with other alpha-blockers, there may be an increased risk of hypotension/postural hypotension and syncope when taking afluzosin with antihypertensives concomitantly).
No products indexed under this heading.

Bendroflumethiazide (As with other alpha-blockers, there may be an increased risk of hypotension/postural hypotension and syncope when taking afluzosin with antihypertensives concomitantly).
No products indexed under this heading.

Betaxolol Hydrochloride (As with other alpha-blockers, there may be an increased risk of hypotension/postural hypotension and syncope when taking afluzosin with antihypertensives concomitantly).
No products indexed under this heading.

Bisoprolol Fumarate (As with other alpha-blockers, there may be an increased risk of hypotension/postural hypotension and syncope when taking afluzosin with antihypertensives concomitantly).
No products indexed under this heading.

Bretylium Tosylate (A postmarketing study evaluating the effect of combining alfuzosin hydrochloride with another drug of comparable QT effect showed an increased effect when compared to either drug alone. Although this study was not designed to make direct statistical comparisons between drugs, the QT increase with both drugs was no more than additive and was lower than that of the active control moxifloxacin. These observations should be considered in clinical decisions when prescribing alfuzosin hydrochloride for patients with a known history of QT prolongation or patients who are taking medications which prolong the QT interval).

No products indexed under this heading.

Buspirone Hydrochloride (A postmarketing study evaluating the effect of combining alfuzosin hydrochloride with another drug of comparable QT effect showed an increased effect when compared to either drug alone. Although this study was not designed to make direct statistical comparisons between drugs, the QT increase with both drugs was no more than additive and was lower than that of the active control moxifloxacin. These observations should be considered in clinical decisions when prescribing alfuzosin hydrochloride for patients with a known history of QT prolongation or patients who are taking medications which prolong the QT interval).

No products indexed under this heading.

Candesartan Cilexetil (As with other alpha-blockers, there may be an increased risk of hypotension/postural hypotension and syncope when taking afluzosin with antihypertensives concomitantly). Products include:

Atacand Tablets 639
Atacand HCT 642

Captopril (As with other alpha-blockers, there may be an increased risk of hypotension/postural hypotension and syncope when taking afluzosin with antihypertensives concomitantly). Products include:

Captopril Tablets 2182

Carteolol Hydrochloride (As with other alpha-blockers, there may be an increased risk of hypotension/postural hypotension and syncope when taking afluzosin with antihypertensives concomitantly).

No products indexed under this heading.

Chlordiazepoxide (A postmarketing study evaluating the effect of combining alfuzosin hydrochloride with another drug of comparable QT effect showed an increased effect when compared to either drug alone. Although this study was not designed to make direct statistical comparisons between drugs, the QT increase with both drugs was no more than additive and was lower than that of the active control moxifloxacin. These observations should be considered in clinical decisions when prescribing alfuzosin hydrochloride for patients with a known history of QT prolongation or patients who are taking medications which prolong the QT interval).

No products indexed under this heading.

Chlordiazepoxide Hydrochloride (A postmarketing study evaluating the effect of combining alfuzosin hydrochloride with another drug of comparable QT effect showed an increased effect when compared to either drug alone. Although this study was not designed to make direct statistical comparisons between drugs, the QT increase with both drugs was no more than additive and was lower than that of the active control moxifloxacin. These observations should be considered in clinical decisions when prescribing alfuzosin hydrochloride for patients with a known history of QT prolongation or patients who are taking medications which prolong the QT interval).

No products indexed under this heading.

Chlorothiazide (As with other alpha-blockers, there may be an increased risk of hypotension/postural hypotension and syncope when taking afluzosin with antihypertensives concomitantly).

No products indexed under this heading.

Chlorothiazide Sodium (As with other alpha-blockers, there may be an increased risk of hypotension/postural hypotension and syncope when taking afluzosin with antihypertensives concomitantly). Products include:

Intravenous Sodium Diuril 2490

Chlorpromazine (A postmarketing study evaluating the effect of combining alfuzosin hydrochloride with another drug of comparable QT effect showed an increased effect when compared to either drug alone. Although this study was not designed to make direct statistical comparisons between drugs, the QT increase with both drugs was no more than additive and was lower than that of the active control moxifloxacin. These observations should be considered in clinical decisions when prescribing alfuzosin hydrochloride for patients with a known history of QT prolongation or patients who are taking medications which prolong the QT interval).

No products indexed under this heading.

Chlorpromazine Hydrochloride (A postmarketing study evaluating the effect of combining alfuzosin hydrochloride with another drug of comparable QT effect showed an increased effect when compared to either drug alone. Although this study was not designed to make direct statistical comparisons between drugs, the QT increase with both drugs was no more than additive and was lower than that of the active control moxifloxacin. These observations should be considered in clinical decisions when prescribing alfuzosin hydrochloride for patients with a known history of QT prolongation or patients who are taking medications which prolong the QT interval).

No products indexed under this heading.

Chlorprothixene (A postmarketing study evaluating the effect of combining alfuzosin hydrochloride with another drug of comparable QT effect showed an increased effect when compared to either drug alone. Although this study was not designed to make direct statistical comparisons between drugs, the QT increase with both drugs was no more than additive and was lower than that of the active control moxifloxacin. These observations should be considered in clinical decisions when prescribing alfuzosin hydrochloride for patients with a known history of QT prolongation or patients who are taking medications which prolong the QT interval).

No products indexed under this heading.

Chlorprothixene Hydrochloride (A postmarketing study evaluating the effect of combining alfuzosin hydrochloride with another drug of comparable QT effect showed an increased effect when compared to either drug alone. Although this study was not designed to make direct statistical comparisons between drugs, the QT increase with both drugs was no more than additive and was lower than that of the active control moxifloxacin. These observations should be considered in clinical decisions when prescribing alfuzosin hydrochloride for patients with a known history of QT prolongation or patients who are taking medications which prolong the QT interval).

No products indexed under this heading.

Chlorthalidone (As with other alpha-blockers, there may be an increased risk of hypotension/postural hypotension and syncope when taking afluzosin with antihypertensives concomitantly). Products include:

Clorpres Tablets 2185

Clarithromycin (Uroxatral should not be co-administered with potent CYP3A4 inhibitors such as ketoconazole, itraconazole, and ritonavir, since alfuzosin blood levels are increased). Products include:

Biaxin/Biaxin XL 411

Clomipramine Hydrochloride (A postmarketing study evaluating the effect of combining alfuzosin hydrochloride with another drug of comparable QT effect showed an increased effect when compared to either drug alone. Although this study was not designed to make direct statistical comparisons between drugs, the QT increase with both drugs was no more than additive and was lower than that of the active control moxifloxacin. These observations should be considered in clinical decisions when prescribing alfuzosin hydrochloride for patients with a known history of QT prolongation or patients who are taking medications which prolong the QT interval).

No products indexed under this heading.

Clonidine (As with other alpha-blockers, there may be an increased risk of hypotension/postural hypotension and syncope when taking afluzosin with antihypertensives concomitantly). Products include:

Catapres-TTS 842

Clonidine Hydrochloride (As with other alpha-blockers, there may be an increased risk of hypotension/postural hypotension and syncope when taking afluzosin with antihypertensives concomitantly). Products include:

Catapres Tablets 841
Clorpres Tablets 2185

Clorazepate Dipotassium (A postmarketing study evaluating the effect of combining alfuzosin hydrochloride with another drug of comparable QT effect showed an increased effect when compared to either drug alone. Although this study was not designed to make direct statistical comparisons between drugs, the QT increase with both drugs was no more than additive and was lower than that of the active control moxifloxacin. These observations should be considered in clinical decisions when prescribing alfuzosin hydrochloride for patients with a known history of QT prolongation or patients who are taking medications which prolong the QT interval).

No products indexed under this heading.

Clozapine (A postmarketing study evaluating the effect of combining alfuzosin hydrochloride with another drug of comparable QT effect showed an increased effect when compared to either drug alone. Although this study was not designed to make direct statistical comparisons between drugs, the QT increase with both drugs was no more than additive and was lower than that of the active control moxifloxacin. These observations should be considered in clinical decisions when prescribing alfuzosin hydrochloride for patients with a known history of QT prolongation or patients who are taking medications which prolong the QT interval).

No products indexed under this heading.

Delavirdine Mesylate (Uroxatral should not be co-administered with potent CYP3A4 inhibitors such as ketoconazole, itraconazole, and ritonavir, since alfuzosin blood levels are increased).

No products indexed under this heading.

Delavirine (Uroxatral should not be co-administered with potent CYP3A4 inhibitors such as ketoconazole, itraconazole, and ritonavir, since alfuzosin blood levels are increased).

No products indexed under this heading.

Deserpidine (As with other alpha-blockers, there may be an increased risk of hypotension/postural hypotension and syncope when taking afluzosin with antihypertensives concomitantly).

No products indexed under this heading.

Desipramine Hydrochloride (A postmarketing study evaluating the effect of combining alfuzosin hydrochloride with another drug of comparable QT effect showed an increased effect when compared to either drug alone. Although this study was not designed to make direct statistical comparisons between drugs, the QT increase with both drugs was no more than additive and was lower than that of the active control moxifloxacin. These observations should be considered in clinical decisions when prescribing alfuzosin hydrochloride for patients with a known history of QT prolongation or patients who are taking medications which prolong the QT interval).

No products indexed under this heading.

Diazepam (A postmarketing study evaluating the effect of combining alfuzosin hydrochloride with another drug of comparable QT effect showed an increased effect when compared to either drug alone. Although this study was not designed to make direct statistical comparisons between drugs, the QT increase with both drugs was no more than additive and was lower than that of the active control moxifloxacin. These observations should be considered in clinical decisions when prescribing alfuzosin hydrochloride for patients with a known history of QT prolongation or patients who are taking medications which prolong the QT interval). Products include:

Valium Tablets 2658

Diazoxide (As with other alpha-blockers, there may be an increased risk of hypotension/postural hypotension and syncope when taking afluzosin with antihypertensives concomitantly). Products include:

Proglycem Capsules 1185
Proglycem Suspension 1185

Diltiazem Hydrochloride (As with other alpha-blockers, there may be an increased risk of hypotension/postural hypotension and syncope when taking afluzosin with antihypertensives concomitantly). Products include:

Cardizem LA Extended Release Tablets 421

Disopyramide Phosphate (A postmarketing study evaluating the effect of combining alfuzosin hydrochloride with another drug of comparable QT effect showed an increased effect when compared to either drug alone. Although this study was not designed to make direct statistical comparisons between drugs, the QT increase with both drugs was no more than additive and was lower than that of the active control moxifloxacin. These observations should be considered in clinical decisions when prescribing alfuzosin hydrochloride for patients with a known history of QT prolongation or patients who are taking medications which prolong the QT interval).

No products indexed under this heading.

Dofetilide (A postmarketing study evaluating the effect of combining alfuzosin hydrochloride with another drug of comparable QT effect showed an increased effect when compared to either drug alone. Although this study was not designed to make direct statistical comparisons between drugs, the QT increase with both drugs was no more than additive and was lower than that of the active control moxifloxacin. These observations should be considered in clinical decisions when prescribing alfuzosin hydrochloride for patients with a known history of QT prolongation or patients who are taking medications which prolong the QT interval).

No products indexed under this heading.

Doxazosin Mesylate (Interactions may be expected; uroxatral should not be used in combination with other alpha-blockers).

No products indexed under this heading.

Doxepin Hydrochloride (A postmarketing study evaluating the effect of combining alfuzosin hydrochloride with another drug of comparable QT effect showed an increased effect when compared to either drug alone. Although this study was not designed to make direct statistical comparisons between drugs, the QT increase with both drugs was no more than additive and was lower than that of the active control moxifloxacin. These observations should be considered in clinical decisions when prescribing alfuzosin hydrochloride for patients with a known history of QT prolongation or patients who are taking medications which prolong the QT interval).

No products indexed under this heading.

Droperidol (A postmarketing study evaluating the effect of combining alfuzosin hydrochloride with another drug of comparable QT effect showed an increased effect when compared to either drug alone. Although this study was not designed to make direct statistical comparisons between drugs, the QT increase with both drugs was no more than additive and was lower than that of the active control moxifloxacin. These observations should be considered in clinical decisions when prescribing alfuzosin hydrochloride for patients with a known history of QT prolongation or patients who are taking medications which prolong the QT interval).

No products indexed under this heading.

Enalapril Maleate (As with other alpha-blockers, there may be an increased risk of hypotension/postural hypotension and syncope when taking afluzosin with antihypertensives concomitantly).

No products indexed under this heading.

Enalaprilat (As with other alpha-blockers, there may be an increased risk of hypotension/postural hypotension and syncope when taking afluzosin with antihypertensives concomitantly).

No products indexed under this heading.

Eprosartan Mesylate (As with other alpha-blockers, there may be an increased risk of hypotension/postural hypotension and syncope when taking afluzosin with antihypertensives concomitantly). Products include:

Teveten Tablets 515
Teveten HCT Tablets 517

Erythrityl Tetranitrate (As with other alpha-blockers, there may be an increased risk of hypotension/postural hypotension and syncope when taking afluzosin with antihypertensives concomitantly. Care should be taken when afluzosin is used in combination with nitrates).

No products indexed under this heading.

Erythromycin (A postmarketing study evaluating the effect of combining alfuzosin hydrochloride with another drug of comparable QT effect showed an increased effect when compared to either drug alone. Although this study was not designed to make direct statistical comparisons between drugs, the QT increase with both drugs was no more than additive and was lower than that of the active control moxifloxacin. These observations should be considered in clinical decisions when prescribing alfuzosin hydrochloride for patients with a known history of QT prolongation or patients who are taking medications which prolong the QT interval).

No products indexed under this heading.

Erythromycin Estolate (A postmarketing study evaluating the effect of combining alfuzosin hydrochloride with another drug of comparable QT effect showed an increased effect when compared to either drug alone. Although this study was not designed to make direct statistical comparisons between drugs, the QT increase with both drugs was no more than additive and was lower than that of the active control moxifloxacin. These observations should be considered in clinical decisions when prescribing alfuzosin hydrochloride for patients with a known history of QT prolongation or patients who are taking medications which prolong the QT interval).

No products indexed under this heading.

Erythromycin Ethylsuccinate (A postmarketing study evaluating the effect of combining alfuzosin hydrochloride with another drug of comparable QT effect showed an increased effect when compared to either drug alone. Although this study was not designed to make direct statistical comparisons between drugs, the QT increase with both drugs was no more than additive and was lower than that of the active control moxifloxacin. These observations should be considered in clinical decisions when prescribing alfuzosin hydrochloride for patients with a known history of QT prolongation or patients who are taking medications which prolong the QT interval). Products include:

E.E.S. 433
EryPed 431

Erythromycin Gluceptate (A postmarketing study evaluating the effect of combining alfuzosin hydrochloride with another drug of comparable QT effect showed an increased effect when compared to either drug alone. Although this study was not designed to make direct statistical comparisons between drugs, the QT increase with both drugs was no more than additive and was lower than that of the active control moxifloxacin. These observations should be considered in clinical decisions when prescribing alfuzosin hydrochloride for patients with a known history of QT prolongation or patients who are taking medications which prolong the QT interval).

No products indexed under this heading.

Erythromycin Lactobionate (A postmarketing study evaluating the effect of combining alfuzosin hydrochloride with another drug of comparable QT effect showed an increased effect when compared to either drug alone. Although this study was not designed to make direct statistical comparisons between drugs, the QT increase with both drugs was no more than additive and was lower than that of the active control moxifloxacin. These observations should be considered in clinical decisions when prescribing alfuzosin hydrochloride for patients with a known history of QT prolongation or patients who are taking medications which prolong the QT interval).

No products indexed under this heading.

Erythromycin Stearate (A postmarketing study evaluating the effect of combining alfuzosin hydrochloride with another drug of comparable QT effect showed an increased effect when compared to either drug alone. Although this study was not designed to make direct statistical comparisons between drugs, the QT increase with both drugs was no more than additive and was lower than that of the active control moxifloxacin. These observations should be considered in clinical decisions when prescribing alfuzosin hydrochloride for patients with a known history of QT prolongation or patients who are taking medications which prolong the QT interval).

No products indexed under this heading.

Esmolol Hydrochloride (As with other alpha-blockers, there may be an increased risk of hypotension/postural hypotension and syncope when taking afluzosin with antihypertensives concomitantly).

No products indexed under this heading.

Felodipine (As with other alpha-blockers, there may be an increased risk of hypotension/postural hypotension and syncope when taking afluzosin with antihypertensives concomitantly).

No products indexed under this heading.

Flecainide Acetate (A postmarketing study evaluating the effect of combining alfuzosin hydrochloride with another drug of comparable QT effect showed an increased effect when compared to either drug alone. Although this study was not designed to make direct statistical comparisons between drugs, the QT increase with both drugs was no more than additive and was lower than that of the active control moxifloxacin. These observations should be considered in clinical decisions when prescribing alfuzosin hydrochloride for patients with a known history of QT prolongation or patients who are taking medications which prolong the QT interval).

No products indexed under this heading.

Fluphenazine Decanoate (A postmarketing study evaluating the effect of combining alfuzosin hydrochloride with another drug of comparable QT effect showed an increased effect when compared to either drug alone. Although this study was not designed to make direct statistical comparisons between drugs, the QT increase with both drugs was no more than additive and was lower than that of the active control moxifloxacin. These observations should be considered in clinical decisions when prescribing alfuzosin hydrochloride for patients with a known history of QT prolongation or patients who are taking medications which prolong the QT interval).

No products indexed under this heading.

Fluphenazine Enanthate (A postmarketing study evaluating the effect of combining alfuzosin hydrochloride with another drug of comparable QT effect showed an increased effect when compared to either drug

alone. Although this study was not designed to make direct statistical comparisons between drugs, the QT increase with both drugs was no more than additive and was lower than that of the active control moxifloxacin. These observations should be considered in clinical decisions when prescribing alfuzosin hydrochloride for patients with a known history of QT prolongation or patients who are taking medications which prolong the QT interval).

No products indexed under this heading.

Fluphenazine Hydrochloride (A postmarketing study evaluating the effect of combining alfuzosin hydrochloride with another drug of comparable QT effect showed an increased effect when compared to either drug alone. Although this study was not designed to make direct statistical comparisons between drugs, the QT increase with both drugs was no more than additive and was lower than that of the active control moxifloxacin. These observations should be considered in clinical decisions when prescribing alfuzosin hydrochloride for patients with a known history of QT prolongation or patients who are taking medications which prolong the QT interval).

No products indexed under this heading.

Fosamprenavir Calcium (Uroxatral should not be co-administered with potent CYP3A4 inhibitors such as ketoconazole, itraconazole, and ritonavir, since alfuzosin blood levels are increased). Products include:

Lexiva Oral Suspension 1510
Lexiva Tablets 1510

Fosinopril Sodium (As with other alpha-blockers, there may be an increased risk of hypotension/ postural hypotension and syncope when taking alfuzosin with antihypertensives concomitantly).

No products indexed under this heading.

Furosemide (As with other alpha-blockers, there may be an increased risk of hypotension/postural hypotension and syncope when taking alfuzosin with antihypertensives concomitantly). Products include:

Furosemide Tablets 2186

Guanabenz Acetate (As with other alpha-blockers, there may be an increased risk of hypotension/ postural hypotension and syncope when taking alfuzosin with antihypertensives concomitantly).

No products indexed under this heading.

Guanethidine Monosulfate (As with other alpha-blockers, there may be an increased risk of hypotension/ postural hypotension and syncope when taking alfuzosin with antihypertensives concomitantly).

No products indexed under this heading.

Haloperidol (A postmarketing study evaluating the effect of combining alfuzosin hydrochloride with another drug of comparable QT effect showed an increased effect when compared to either drug alone. Although this study was not designed to make direct statistical comparisons between drugs, the QT increase with both drugs was no more than additive and was lower than that of the active control moxifloxacin. These observations should be considered in clinical decisions when prescribing alfuzosin hydrochloride for patients with a known history of QT prolongation or patients who are taking medications which prolong the QT interval).

No products indexed under this heading.

Haloperidol Decanoate (A postmarketing study evaluating the effect of combining alfuzosin hydrochloride with another drug of comparable QT effect showed an increased effect when compared to either drug alone. Although this study was not designed to make direct statistical comparisons between drugs, the QT increase with both drugs was no more than additive and was lower than that of the active control moxifloxacin. These observations should be considered in clinical decisions when prescribing alfuzosin hydrochloride for patients with a known history of QT prolongation or patients who are taking medications which prolong the QT interval).

No products indexed under this heading.

Hydralazine Hydrochloride (As with other alpha-blockers, there may be an increased risk of hypotension/ postural hypotension and syncope when taking alfuzosin with antihypertensives concomitantly).

No products indexed under this heading.

Hydrochlorothiazide (As with other alpha-blockers, there may be an increased risk of hypotension/ postural hypotension and syncope when taking alfuzosin with antihypertensives concomitantly). Products include:

Atacand HCT 642
Avalide Tablets 892
Avalide Tablets 2713
Benicar HCT Tablets 1010
Diovan HCT Tablets 2216
Dyazide Capsules 1405
Micardis HCT Tablets 854
Prinzide Tablets 2092
Tekturna HCT Tablets 2324
Teveten HCT Tablets 517

Hydroflumethiazide (As with other alpha-blockers, there may be an increased risk of hypotension/ postural hypotension and syncope when taking alfuzosin with antihypertensives concomitantly).

No products indexed under this heading.

Hydroxyzine Hydrochloride (A postmarketing study evaluating the effect of combining alfuzosin hydrochloride with another drug of comparable QT effect showed an increased effect when compared to either drug alone. Although this study was not designed to make direct statistical comparisons between drugs, the QT increase with both drugs was no more than additive and was lower than that of the active control moxifloxacin. These observations should be considered in clinical decisions when prescribing alfuzosin hydrochloride for patients with a known history of QT prolongation or patients who are taking medications which prolong the QT interval).

No products indexed under this heading.

Imipramine Hydrochloride (A postmarketing study evaluating the effect of combining alfuzosin hydrochloride with another drug of comparable QT effect showed an increased effect when compared to either drug alone. Although this study was not designed to make direct statistical comparisons between drugs, the QT increase with both drugs was no more than additive and was lower than that of the active control moxifloxacin. These observations should be considered in clinical decisions when prescribing alfuzosin hydrochloride for patients with a known history of QT prolongation or patients who are taking medications which prolong the QT interval).

No products indexed under this heading.

Imipramine Pamoate (A postmarketing study evaluating the effect of combining alfuzosin hydrochloride with another drug of comparable QT effect showed an increased effect when compared to either drug alone. Although this study was not designed to make direct statistical comparisons between drugs, the QT increase with both drugs was no more than additive and was lower than that of the active control moxifloxacin. These observations should be considered in clinical decisions when prescribing alfuzosin hydrochloride for patients with a known history of QT prolongation or patients who are taking medications which prolong the QT interval).

No products indexed under this heading.

Indapamide (As with other alpha-blockers, there may be an increased risk of hypotension/postural hypotension and syncope when taking alfuzosin with antihypertensives concomitantly). Products include:

Indapamide Tablets 2188

Indinavir Sulfate (Uroxatral should not be co-administered with potent CYP3A4 inhibitors such as ketoconazole, itraconazole, and ritonavir, since alfuzosin blood levels are increased). Products include:

Crixivan Capsules 1979

Irbesartan (As with other alpha-blockers, there may be an increased risk of hypotension/postural hypotension and syncope when taking alfuzosin with antihypertensives concomitantly). Products include:

Avalide Tablets 892
Avalide Tablets 2713
Avapro Tablets 897
Avapro Tablets 2718

Isocarboxazid (A postmarketing study evaluating the effect of combining alfuzosin hydrochloride with another drug of comparable QT effect showed an increased effect when compared to either drug alone. Although this study was not designed to make direct statistical comparisons between drugs, the QT increase with both drugs was no more than additive and was lower than that of the active control moxifloxacin. These observations should be considered in clinical decisions when prescribing alfuzosin hydrochloride for patients with a known history of QT prolongation or patients who are taking medications which prolong the QT interval). Products include:

Marplan Tablets 3177

Isosorbide Dinitrate (As with other alpha-blockers, there may be an increased risk of hypotension/ postural hypotension and syncope when taking alfuzosin with antihypertensives concomitantly. Care should be taken when alfuzosin is used in combination with nitrates).

No products indexed under this heading.

Isosorbide Mononitrate (As with other alpha-blockers, there may be an increased risk of hypotension/ postural hypotension and syncope when taking alfuzosin with antihypertensives concomitantly. Care should be taken when alfuzosin is used in combination with nitrates).

No products indexed under this heading.

Isradipine (As with other alpha-blockers, there may be an increased risk of hypotension/postural hypotension and syncope when taking alfuzosin with antihypertensives concomitantly). Products include:

DynaCirc CR Controlled Release Tablets 1407

Itraconazole (Uroxatral should not be co-administered with potent CYP3A4 inhibitors such as ketoconazole, itraconazole, and ritonavir, since alfuzosin blood levels are increased).

No products indexed under this heading.

Ketoconazole (Uroxatral should not be co-administered with potent CYP3A4 inhibitors such as ketoconazole, itraconazole, and ritonavir, since alfuzosin blood levels are increased). Products include:

Extina Foam, 2% 3057
Nizoral A-D Shampoo 1901

Labetalol Hydrochloride (As with other alpha-blockers, there may be an increased risk of hypotension/ postural hypotension and syncope when taking alfuzosin with antihypertensives concomitantly).

No products indexed under this heading.

Lidocaine Hydrochloride (A postmarketing study evaluating the effect of combining alfuzosin hydrochloride with another drug of comparable QT effect showed an increased effect when compared to either drug alone. Although this study was not designed to make direct statistical comparisons between drugs, the QT increase with both drugs was no more than additive and was lower than that of the active control moxifloxacin. These observations should be considered in clinical decisions when prescribing alfuzosin hydrochloride for patients with a known history of QT prolongation or patients who are taking medications which prolong the QT interval).

No products indexed under this heading.

Lisinopril (As with other alpha-blockers, there may be an increased risk of hypotension/postural hypotension and syncope when taking alfuzosin with antihypertensives concomitantly). Products include:

Prinivil Tablets 2087
Prinzide Tablets 2092

Lithium Carbonate (A postmarketing study evaluating the effect of combining alfuzosin hydrochloride with another drug of comparable QT effect showed an increased effect when compared to either drug alone.

Although this study was not designed to make direct statistical comparisons between drugs, the QT increase with both drugs was no more than additive and was lower than that of the active control moxifloxacin. These observations should be considered in clinical decisions when prescribing alfuzosin hydrochloride for patients with a known history of QT prolongation or patients who are taking medications which prolong the QT interval).
No products indexed under this heading.

Lithium Citrate (A postmarketing study evaluating the effect of combining alfuzosin hydrochloride with another drug of comparable QT effect showed an increased effect when compared to either drug alone. Although this study was not designed to make direct statistical comparisons between drugs, the QT increase with both drugs was no more than additive and was lower than that of the active control moxifloxacin. These observations should be considered in clinical decisions when prescribing alfuzosin hydrochloride for patients with a known history of QT prolongation or patients who are taking medications which prolong the QT interval).
No products indexed under this heading.

Lopinavir (Uroxatral should not be co-administered with potent CYP3A4 inhibitors such as ketoconazole, itraconazole, and ritonavir, since alfuzosin blood levels are increased). Products include:
Kaletra 452

Lorazepam (A postmarketing study evaluating the effect of combining alfuzosin hydrochloride with another drug of comparable QT effect showed an increased effect when compared to either drug alone. Although this study was not designed to make direct statistical comparisons between drugs, the QT increase with both drugs was no more than additive and was lower than that of the active control moxifloxacin. These observations should be considered in clinical decisions when prescribing alfuzosin hydrochloride for patients with a known history of QT prolongation or patients who are taking medications which prolong the QT interval).
No products indexed under this heading.

Losartan Potassium (As with other alpha-blockers, there may be an increased risk of hypotension/postural hypotension and syncope when taking afluzosin with antihypertensives concomitantly). Products include:
Cozaar Tablets 1973

Loxapine Hydrochloride (A postmarketing study evaluating the effect of combining alfuzosin hydrochloride with another drug of comparable QT effect showed an increased effect when compared to either drug alone. Although this study was not designed to make direct statistical comparisons between drugs, the QT increase with both drugs was no more than additive and was lower than that of the active control moxifloxacin. These observations should be considered in clinical decisions when prescribing alfuzosin hydrochloride for patients with a known history of QT prolongation or patients who are taking medications which prolong the QT interval).
No products indexed under this heading.

Loxapine Succinate (A postmarketing study evaluating the effect of combining alfuzosin hydrochloride with another drug of comparable QT effect showed an increased effect when compared to either drug alone. Although this study was not designed to make direct statistical comparisons between drugs, the QT increase with both drugs was no more than additive and was lower than that of the active control moxifloxacin. These observations should be considered in clinical decisions when prescribing alfuzosin hydrochloride for patients with a known history of QT prolongation or patients who are taking medications which prolong the QT interval).
No products indexed under this heading.

Maprotiline Hydrochloride (A postmarketing study evaluating the effect of combining alfuzosin hydrochloride with another drug of comparable QT effect showed an increased effect when compared to either drug alone. Although this study was not designed to make direct statistical comparisons between drugs, the QT increase with both drugs was no more than additive and was lower than that of the active control moxifloxacin. These observations should be considered in clinical decisions when prescribing alfuzosin hydrochloride for patients with a known history of QT prolongation or patients who are taking medications which prolong the QT interval).
No products indexed under this heading.

Mecamylamine Hydrochloride (As with other alpha-blockers, there may be an increased risk of hypotension/postural hypotension and syncope when taking afluzosin with antihypertensives concomitantly).
No products indexed under this heading.

Meprobamate (A postmarketing study evaluating the effect of combining alfuzosin hydrochloride with another drug of comparable QT effect showed an increased effect when compared to either drug alone. Although this study was not designed to make direct statistical comparisons between drugs, the QT increase with both drugs was no more than additive and was lower than that of the active control moxifloxacin. These observations should be considered in clinical decisions when prescribing alfuzosin hydrochloride for patients with a known history of QT prolongation or patients who are taking medications which prolong the QT interval).
No products indexed under this heading.

Mesoridazine Besylate (A postmarketing study evaluating the effect of combining alfuzosin hydrochloride with another drug of comparable QT effect showed an increased effect when compared to either drug alone. Although this study was not designed to make direct statistical comparisons between drugs, the QT increase with both drugs was no more than additive and was lower than that of the active control moxifloxacin. These observations should be considered in clinical decisions when prescribing alfuzosin hydrochloride for patients with a known history of QT prolongation or patients who are taking medications which prolong the QT interval).
No products indexed under this heading.

Methyclothiazide (As with other alpha-blockers, there may be an increased risk of hypotension/postural hypotension and syncope when taking afluzosin with antihypertensives concomitantly).
No products indexed under this heading.

Methyldopa (As with other alpha-blockers, there may be an increased risk of hypotension/postural hypotension and syncope when taking afluzosin with antihypertensives concomitantly).
No products indexed under this heading.

Methyldopate Hydrochloride (As with other alpha-blockers, there may be an increased risk of hypotension/postural hypotension and syncope when taking afluzosin with antihypertensives concomitantly).
No products indexed under this heading.

Metolazone (As with other alpha-blockers, there may be an increased risk of hypotension/postural hypotension and syncope when taking afluzosin with antihypertensives concomitantly).
No products indexed under this heading.

Metoprolol Succinate (As with other alpha-blockers, there may be an increased risk of hypotension/postural hypotension and syncope when taking afluzosin with antihypertensives concomitantly). Products include:
Toprol-XL Tablets 666

Metoprolol Tartrate (As with other alpha-blockers, there may be an increased risk of hypotension/postural hypotension and syncope when taking afluzosin with antihypertensives concomitantly).
No products indexed under this heading.

Metyrosine (As with other alpha-blockers, there may be an increased risk of hypotension/postural hypotension and syncope when taking afluzosin with antihypertensives concomitantly). Products include:
Demser Capsules 1989

Mexiletine Hydrochloride (A postmarketing study evaluating the effect of combining alfuzosin hydrochloride with another drug of comparable QT effect showed an increased effect when compared to either drug alone. Although this study was not designed to make direct statistical comparisons between drugs, the QT increase with both drugs was no more than additive and was lower than that of the active control moxifloxacin. These observations should be considered in clinical decisions when prescribing alfuzosin hydrochloride for patients with a known history of QT prolongation or patients who are taking medications which prolong the QT interval).
No products indexed under this heading.

Mibefradil Dihydrochloride (As with other alpha-blockers, there may be an increased risk of hypotension/postural hypotension and syncope when taking afluzosin with antihypertensives concomitantly).
No products indexed under this heading.

Midazolam Hydrochloride (A postmarketing study evaluating the effect of combining alfuzosin hydrochloride with another drug of comparable QT effect showed an increased effect when compared to either drug alone. Although this study was not designed to make direct statistical comparisons between drugs, the QT increase with both drugs was no more than additive and was lower than that of the active control moxifloxacin. These observations should be considered in clinical decisions when prescribing alfuzosin hydrochloride for patients with a known history of QT prolongation or patients who are taking medications which prolong the QT interval).
No products indexed under this heading.

Minoxidil (As with other alpha-blockers, there may be an increased risk of hypotension/postural hypotension and syncope when taking afluzosin with antihypertensives concomitantly).
No products indexed under this heading.

Moexipril Hydrochloride (As with other alpha-blockers, there may be an increased risk of hypotension/postural hypotension and syncope when taking afluzosin with antihypertensives concomitantly).
No products indexed under this heading.

Molindone Hydrochloride (A postmarketing study evaluating the effect of combining alfuzosin hydrochloride with another drug of comparable QT effect showed an increased effect when compared to either drug alone. Although this study was not designed to make direct statistical comparisons between drugs, the QT increase with both drugs was no more than additive and was lower than that of the active control moxifloxacin. These observations should be considered in clinical decisions when prescribing alfuzosin hydrochloride for patients with a known history of QT prolongation or patients who are taking medications which prolong the QT interval). Products include:
Moban Tablets 1116

Nadolol (As with other alpha-blockers, there may be an increased risk of hypotension/postural hypotension and syncope when taking afluzosin with antihypertensives concomitantly). Products include:
Nadolol Tablets 2191

Nebivolol (As with other alpha-blockers, there may be an increased risk of hypotension/postural hypotension and syncope when taking afluzosin with antihypertensives concomitantly). Products include:
Bystolic Tablets 1155

Nefazodone Hydrochloride (Uroxatral should not be co-administered with potent CYP3A4 inhibitors such as ketoconazole, itraconazole, and ritonavir, since alfuzosin blood levels are increased).
No products indexed under this heading.

Nelfinavir Mesylate (Uroxatral should not be co-administered with potent CYP3A4 inhibitors such as ketoconazole, itraconazole, and ritonavir, since alfuzosin blood levels are increased).
No products indexed under this heading.

Nicardipine Hydrochloride (As with other alpha-blockers, there may be an increased risk of hypotension/postural hypotension and syncope when taking afluzosin with antihypertensives concomitantly). Products include:
Cardene I.V. **1093**

Nifedipine (As with other alpha-blockers, there may be an increased risk of hypotension/postural hypotension and syncope when taking afluzosin with antihypertensives concomitantly).
No products indexed under this heading.

Nisoldipine (As with other alpha-blockers, there may be an increased risk of hypotension/postural hypotension and syncope when taking afluzosin with antihypertensives concomitantly). Products include:
Sular Extended Release Tablets **2975**

Nitroglycerin (As with other alpha-blockers, there may be an increased risk of hypotension/postural hypotension and syncope when taking afluzosin with antihypertensives concomitantly). Products include:
Nitro-Dur Transdermal Infusion System.. **2887**
Nitrolingual Pumpspray **2965**

Nortriptyline Hydrochloride (A postmarketing study evaluating the effect of combining alfuzosin hydrochloride with another drug of comparable QT effect showed an increased effect when compared to either drug alone. Although this study was not designed to make direct statistical comparisons between drugs, the QT increase with both drugs was no more than additive and was lower than that of the active control moxifloxacin. These observations should be considered in clinical decisions when prescribing alfuzosin hydrochloride for patients with a known history of QT prolongation or patients who are taking medications which prolong the QT interval).
No products indexed under this heading.

Olanzapine (A postmarketing study evaluating the effect of combining alfuzosin hydrochloride with another drug of comparable QT effect showed an increased effect when compared to either drug alone. Although this study was not designed to make direct statistical comparisons between drugs, the QT increase with both drugs was no more than additive and was lower than that of the active control moxifloxacin. These observations should be considered in clinical decisions when prescribing alfuzosin hydrochloride for patients with a known history of QT prolongation or patients who are taking medications which prolong the QT interval). Products include:
Symbyax Capsules **1871**
Zyprexa Tablets **1883**
Zyprexa IntraMuscular **1883**
Zyprexa ZYDIS Orally Disintegrating Tablets.................. **1883**

Oxazepam (A postmarketing study evaluating the effect of combining alfuzosin hydrochloride with another drug of comparable QT effect showed an increased effect when compared to either drug alone. Although this study was not designed to make direct statistical comparisons between drugs, the QT increase with both drugs was no more than additive and was lower than that of the active control moxifloxacin. These observations should be considered in clinical decisions when prescribing alfuzosin hydrochloride for patients with a known history of QT prolongation or patients who are taking medications which prolong the QT interval).
No products indexed under this heading.

Penbutolol Sulfate (As with other alpha-blockers, there may be an increased risk of hypotension/postural hypotension and syncope when taking afluzosin with antihypertensives concomitantly).
No products indexed under this heading.

Pentaerythritol Tetranitrate (As with other alpha-blockers, there may be an increased risk of hypotension/postural hypotension and syncope when taking afluzosin with antihypertensives concomitantly. Care should be taken when afluzosin is used in combination with nitrates).
No products indexed under this heading.

Perindopril Erbumine (As with other alpha-blockers, there may be an increased risk of hypotension/postural hypotension and syncope when taking afluzosin with antihypertensives concomitantly). Products include:
Aceon Tablets (2 mg, 4 mg, 8 mg)... **3038**

Perphenazine (A postmarketing study evaluating the effect of combining alfuzosin hydrochloride with another drug of comparable QT effect showed an increased effect when compared to either drug alone. Although this study was not designed to make direct statistical comparisons between drugs, the QT increase with both drugs was no more than additive and was lower than that of the active control moxifloxacin. These observations should be considered in clinical decisions when prescribing alfuzosin hydrochloride for patients with a known history of QT prolongation or patients who are taking medications which prolong the QT interval).
No products indexed under this heading.

Phenelzine Sulfate (A postmarketing study evaluating the effect of combining alfuzosin hydrochloride with another drug of comparable QT effect showed an increased effect when compared to either drug alone. Although this study was not designed to make direct statistical comparisons between drugs, the QT increase with both drugs was no more than additive and was lower than that of the active control moxifloxacin. These observations should be considered in clinical decisions when prescribing alfuzosin hydrochloride for patients with a known history of QT prolongation or patients who are taking medications which prolong the QT interval).
No products indexed under this heading.

Phenoxybenzamine Hydrochloride (As with other alpha-blockers, there may be an increased risk of hypotension/postural hypotension and syncope when taking afluzosin with antihypertensives concomitantly). Products include:
Dibenzyline Capsules **3188**

Phentolamine Mesylate (As with other alpha-blockers, there may be an increased risk of hypotension/postural hypotension and syncope when taking afluzosin with antihypertensives concomitantly).
No products indexed under this heading.

Pindolol (As with other alpha-blockers, there may be an increased risk of hypotension/postural hypotension and syncope when taking afluzosin with antihypertensives concomitantly).
No products indexed under this heading.

Polythiazide (As with other alpha-blockers, there may be an increased risk of hypotension/postural hypotension and syncope when taking afluzosin with antihypertensives concomitantly).
No products indexed under this heading.

Prazepam (A postmarketing study evaluating the effect of combining alfuzosin hydrochloride with another drug of comparable QT effect showed an increased effect when compared to either drug alone. Although this study was not designed to make direct statistical comparisons between drugs, the QT increase with both drugs was no more than additive and was lower than that of the active control moxifloxacin. These observations should be considered in clinical decisions when prescribing alfuzosin hydrochloride for patients with a known history of QT prolongation or patients who are taking medications which prolong the QT interval).
No products indexed under this heading.

Prazosin Hydrochloride (Interactions may be expected; uroxatral should not be used in combination with other alpha-blockers).
No products indexed under this heading.

Procainamide Hydrochloride (A postmarketing study evaluating the effect of combining alfuzosin hydrochloride with another drug of comparable QT effect showed an increased effect when compared to either drug alone. Although this study was not designed to make direct statistical comparisons between drugs, the QT increase with both drugs was no more than additive and was lower than that of the active control moxifloxacin. These observations should be considered in clinical decisions when prescribing alfuzosin hydrochloride for patients with a known history of QT prolongation or patients who are taking medications which prolong the QT interval).
No products indexed under this heading.

Prochlorperazine (A postmarketing study evaluating the effect of combining alfuzosin hydrochloride with another drug of comparable QT effect showed an increased effect when compared to either drug alone. Although this study was not designed to make direct statistical comparisons between drugs, the QT increase with both drugs was no more than additive and was lower than that of the active control moxifloxacin. These observations should be considered in clinical decisions when prescribing alfuzosin hydrochloride for patients with a known history of QT prolongation or patients who are taking medications which prolong the QT interval).
No products indexed under this heading.

Promethazine Hydrochloride (A postmarketing study evaluating the effect of combining alfuzosin hydrochloride with another drug of comparable QT effect showed an increased effect when compared to either drug alone. Although this study was not designed to make direct statistical comparisons between drugs, the QT increase with both drugs was no more than additive and was lower than that of the active control moxifloxacin. These observations should be considered in clinical decisions when prescribing alfuzosin hydrochloride for patients with a known history of QT prolongation or patients who are taking medications which prolong the QT interval).
No products indexed under this heading.

Propafenone Hydrochloride (A postmarketing study evaluating the effect of combining alfuzosin hydrochloride with another drug of comparable QT effect showed an increased effect when compared to either drug alone. Although this study was not designed to make direct statistical comparisons between drugs, the QT increase with both drugs was no more than additive and was lower than that of the active control moxifloxacin. These observations should be considered in clinical decisions when prescribing alfuzosin hydrochloride for patients with a known history of QT prolongation or patients who are taking medications which prolong the QT interval). Products include:
Rythmol Tablets **1586**
Rythmol SR Capsules **1590**

Propranolol Hydrochloride (As with other alpha-blockers, there may be an increased risk of hypotension/postural hypotension and syncope when taking afluzosin with antihypertensives concomitantly). Products include:
InnoPran XL Extended Release Capsules.................................... **1484**

Protriptyline Hydrochloride (A postmarketing study evaluating the effect of combining alfuzosin hydrochloride with another drug of comparable QT effect showed an increased effect when compared to either drug alone. Although this study was not designed to make direct statistical comparisons between drugs, the QT increase with both drugs was no more than additive and was lower than that of the active control moxifloxacin. These observations should be considered in clinical decisions when prescribing alfuzosin hydrochloride for patients with a known history of QT prolongation or patients who are taking medications which prolong the QT interval).
No products indexed under this heading.

Quetiapine Fumarate (A postmarketing study evaluating the effect of combining alfuzosin hydrochloride with another drug of comparable QT effect showed an increased effect when compared to either drug alone. Although this study was not designed to make direct statistical comparisons between drugs, the QT increase with both drugs was no more than additive and was lower than that of the active control moxifloxacin. These observations should be considered in clinical decisions when prescribing alfuzosin hydrochloride for patients with a known history of QT prolongation or patients who are taking medications which prolong the QT interval).
No products indexed under this heading.

Quinapril Hydrochloride (As with other alpha-blockers, there may be an increased risk of hypotension/postural hypotension and syncope when taking afluzosin with antihypertensives concomitantly).
No products indexed under this heading.

Quinidine Gluconate (A postmarketing study evaluating the effect of combining alfuzosin hydrochloride with another drug of comparable QT effect showed an increased effect when compared to either drug alone. Although this study was not designed to make direct statistical comparisons between drugs, the QT increase with both drugs was no more than additive and was lower than that of the active control moxifloxacin. These observations should be considered in clinical decisions when prescribing alfuzosin hydrochloride for patients with a known history of QT prolongation or patients who are taking medications which prolong the QT interval).
No products indexed under this heading.

Quinidine Polygalacturonate (A postmarketing study evaluating the effect of combining alfuzosin hydrochloride with another drug of comparable QT effect showed an increased effect when compared to either drug alone. Although this study was not designed to make direct statistical comparisons between drugs, the QT increase with both drugs was no more than additive and was lower than that of the active control moxifloxacin. These observations should be considered in clinical decisions when prescribing alfuzosin hydrochloride for patients with a known history of QT prolongation or patients who are taking medications which prolong the QT interval).
No products indexed under this heading.

Quinidine Sulfate (A postmarketing study evaluating the effect of combining alfuzosin hydrochloride with another drug of comparable QT effect showed an increased effect when compared to either drug alone. Although this study was not designed to make direct statistical comparisons between drugs, the QT increase with both drugs was no more than additive and was lower than that of the active control moxifloxacin. These observations should be considered in clinical decisions when prescribing alfuzosin hydrochloride for patients with a known history of QT prolongation or patients who are taking medications which prolong the QT interval).
No products indexed under this heading.

Ramipril (As with other alpha-blockers, there may be an increased risk of hypotension/postural hypotension and syncope when taking afluzosin with antihypertensives concomitantly).
No products indexed under this heading.

Rauwolfia Serpentina (As with other alpha-blockers, there may be an increased risk of hypotension/postural hypotension and syncope when taking afluzosin with antihypertensives concomitantly).
No products indexed under this heading.

Rescinnamine (As with other alpha-blockers, there may be an increased risk of hypotension/postural hypotension and syncope when taking afluzosin with antihypertensives concomitantly).
No products indexed under this heading.

Reserpine (As with other alpha-blockers, there may be an increased risk of hypotension/postural hypotension and syncope when taking afluzosin with antihypertensives concomitantly).
No products indexed under this heading.

Risperidone (A postmarketing study evaluating the effect of combining alfuzosin hydrochloride with another drug of comparable QT effect showed an increased effect when compared to either drug alone. Although this study was not designed to make direct statistical comparisons between drugs, the QT increase with both drugs was no more than additive and was lower than that of the active control moxifloxacin. These observations should be considered in clinical decisions when prescribing alfuzosin hydrochloride for patients with a known history of QT prolongation or patients who are taking medications which prolong the QT interval). Products include:
Risperdal Consta Long-Acting Injection 1753

Ritonavir (Uroxatral should not be co-administered with potent CYP3A4 inhibitors such as ketoconazole, itraconazole, and ritonavir, since alfuzosin blood levels are increased). Products include:
Kaletra 452
Norvir 489

Saquinavir (Uroxatral should not be co-administered with potent CYP3A4 inhibitors such as ketoconazole, itraconazole, and ritonavir, since alfuzosin blood levels are increased).
No products indexed under this heading.

Saquinavir Mesylate (Uroxatral should not be co-administered with potent CYP3A4 inhibitors such as ketoconazole, itraconazole, and ritonavir, since alfuzosin blood levels are increased).
No products indexed under this heading.

Sodium Nitroprusside (As with other alpha-blockers, there may be an increased risk of hypotension/postural hypotension and syncope when taking afluzosin with antihypertensives concomitantly).
No products indexed under this heading.

Sotalol Hydrochloride (As with other alpha-blockers, there may be an increased risk of hypotension/postural hypotension and syncope when taking afluzosin with antihypertensives concomitantly).
No products indexed under this heading.

Spirapril Hydrochloride (As with other alpha-blockers, there may be an increased risk of hypotension/postural hypotension and syncope when taking afluzosin with antihypertensives concomitantly).
No products indexed under this heading.

Tamsulosin Hydrochloride (Interactions may be expected; uroxatral should not be used in combination with other alpha-blockers). Products include:
Flomax Capsules 848

Telithromycin (Uroxatral should not be co-administered with potent CYP3A4 inhibitors such as ketoconazole, itraconazole, and ritonavir, since alfuzosin blood levels are increased). Products include:
Ketek Tablets 2744

Telmisartan (As with other alpha-blockers, there may be an increased risk of hypotension/postural hypotension and syncope when taking afluzosin with antihypertensives concomitantly). Products include:
Micardis Tablets 852
Micardis HCT Tablets 854

Terazosin Hydrochloride (Interactions may be expected; uroxatral should not be used in combination with other alpha-blockers).
No products indexed under this heading.

Thioridazine Hydrochloride (A postmarketing study evaluating the effect of combining alfuzosin hydrochloride with another drug of comparable QT effect showed an increased effect when compared to either drug alone. Although this study was not designed to make direct statistical comparisons between drugs, the QT increase with both drugs was no more than additive and was lower than that of the active control moxifloxacin. These observations should be considered in clinical decisions when prescribing alfuzosin hydrochloride for patients with a known history of QT prolongation or patients who are taking medications which prolong the QT interval). Products include:
Thioridazine Hydrochloride Tablets 2195

Thiothixene (A postmarketing study evaluating the effect of combining alfuzosin hydrochloride with another drug of comparable QT effect showed an increased effect when compared to either drug alone. Although this study was not designed to make direct statistical comparisons between drugs, the QT increase with both drugs was no more than additive and was lower than that of the active control moxifloxacin. These observations should be considered in clinical decisions when prescribing alfuzosin hydrochloride for patients with a known history of QT prolongation or patients who are taking medications which prolong the QT interval). Products include:
Thiothixene Capsules 2197

Timolol Maleate (As with other alpha-blockers, there may be an increased risk of hypotension/postural hypotension and syncope when taking afluzosin with antihypertensives concomitantly). Products include:
Combigan Ophthalmic Solution 553
Cosopt Sterile Ophthalmic Solution 1969
Timoptic Sterile Ophthalmic Solution 2121
Timoptic in Ocudose 2124
Timoptic-XE Sterile Ophthalmic Gel Forming Solution 2125

Tocainide Hydrochloride (A postmarketing study evaluating the effect of combining alfuzosin hydrochloride with another drug of comparable QT effect showed an increased effect when compared to either drug alone. Although this study was not designed to make direct statistical comparisons between drugs, the QT increase with both drugs was no more than additive and was lower than that of the active control moxifloxacin. These observations should be considered in clinical decisions when prescribing alfuzosin hydrochloride for patients with a known history of QT prolongation or patients who are taking medications which prolong the QT interval).
No products indexed under this heading.

Torsemide (As with other alpha-blockers, there may be an increased risk of hypotension/postural hypotension and syncope when taking afluzosin with antihypertensives concomitantly). Products include:
Demadex Injection 2630
Demadex Tablets 2630

Trandolapril (As with other alpha-blockers, there may be an increased risk of hypotension/postural hypotension and syncope when taking afluzosin with antihypertensives concomitantly). Products include:
Mavik Tablets 472
Tarka Tablets 511

Tranylcypromine Sulfate (A postmarketing study evaluating the effect of combining alfuzosin hydrochloride with another drug of comparable QT effect showed an increased effect when compared to either drug alone. Although this study was not designed to make direct statistical comparisons between drugs, the QT increase with both drugs was no more than additive and was lower than that of the active control moxifloxacin. These observations should be considered in clinical decisions when prescribing alfuzosin hydrochloride for patients with a known history of QT prolongation or patients who are taking medications which prolong the QT interval). Products include:
Parnate Tablets 1532

Trifluoperazine Hydrochloride (A postmarketing study evaluating the effect of combining alfuzosin hydrochloride with another drug of comparable QT effect showed an increased effect when compared to either drug alone. Although this study was not designed to make direct statistical

comparisons between drugs, the QT increase with both drugs was no more than additive and was lower than that of the active control moxifloxacin. These observations should be considered in clinical decisions when prescribing alfuzosin hydrochloride for patients with a known history of QT prolongation or patients who are taking medications which prolong the QT interval).
No products indexed under this heading.

Trimethaphan Camsylate (As with other alpha-blockers, there may be an increased risk of hypotension/postural hypotension and syncope when taking afluzosin with antihypertensives concomitantly).
No products indexed under this heading.

Trimipramine Maleate (A postmarketing study evaluating the effect of combining alfuzosin hydrochloride with another drug of comparable QT effect showed an increased effect when compared to either drug alone. Although this study was not designed to make direct statistical comparisons between drugs, the QT increase with both drugs was no more than additive and was lower than that of the active control moxifloxacin. These observations should be considered in clinical decisions when prescribing alfuzosin hydrochloride for patients with a known history of QT prolongation or patients who are taking medications which prolong the QT interval).
No products indexed under this heading.

Troleandomycin (Uroxatral should not be co-administered with potent CYP3A4 inhibitors such as ketoconazole, itraconazole, and ritonavir, since alfuzosin blood levels are increased).
No products indexed under this heading.

Valsartan (As with other alpha-blockers, there may be an increased risk of hypotension/postural hypotension and syncope when taking afluzosin with antihypertensives concomitantly). Products include:
Diovan Tablets 2212
Diovan HCT Tablets 2216
Exforge Tablets 2238

Verapamil Hydrochloride (As with other alpha-blockers, there may be an increased risk of hypotension/postural hypotension and syncope when taking afluzosin with antihypertensives concomitantly). Products include:
Tarka Tablets 511

Voriconazole (Uroxatral should not be co-administered with potent CYP3A4 inhibitors such as ketoconazole, itraconazole, and ritonavir, since alfuzosin blood levels are increased).
No products indexed under this heading.

Ziprasidone Hydrochloride (A postmarketing study evaluating the effect of combining alfuzosin hydrochloride with another drug of comparable QT effect showed an increased effect when compared to either drug alone. Although this study was not designed to make direct statistical comparisons between drugs, the QT increase with both drugs was no more than additive and was lower than that of the active control moxifloxacin. These observations should be considered in clinical decisions when prescribing alfuzosin hydrochloride for patients with a known history of QT prolongation or patients who are taking medications which prolong the QT interval).
Products include:
Geodon Capsules 2520

URSO 250 TABLETS

(Ursodiol) 720
May interact with bile acid sequestering agents, estrogens, lipid-lowering drugs, oral contraceptives, and certain other agents. Compounds in these categories include:

Aluminum Hydroxide (Aluminum-based antacids have been shown to adsorb bile acid in vitro and may be expected to interfere with ursodiol in the same manner as the bile acid sequestering agents).
No products indexed under this heading.

Atorvastatin Calcium (Lipid-lowering drugs increase hepatic cholesterol secretion and encourage cholesterol gallstone formation and hence may counteract the effectiveness of ursodiol). Products include:
Lipitor Tablets 2501

Cerivastatin Sodium (Lipid-lowering drugs increase hepatic cholesterol secretion and encourage cholesterol gallstone formation and hence may counteract the effectiveness of ursodiol).
No products indexed under this heading.

Chlorotrianisene (Estrogens and oral contraceptives increase hepatic cholesterol excretion and encourage cholesterol gallstone formation and hence may counteract the effectiveness of ursodiol).
No products indexed under this heading.

Cholestyramine (Lipid-lowering drugs increase hepatic cholesterol secretion and encourage cholesterol gallstone formation and hence may counteract the effectiveness of ursodiol).
No products indexed under this heading.

Clofibrate (Lipid-lowering drugs increase hepatic cholesterol secretion and encourage cholesterol gallstone formation and hence may counteract the effectiveness of ursodiol).
No products indexed under this heading.

Colesevelam Hydrochloride (Bile sequestering agents may interfere with the action of ursodiol by reducing its absorption). Products include:
WelChol Tablets 1015

Colestipol Hydrochloride (Lipid-lowering drugs increase hepatic cholesterol secretion and encourage cholesterol gallstone formation and hence may counteract the effectiveness of ursodiol).
No products indexed under this heading.

Desogestrel (Estrogens and oral contraceptives increase hepatic cholesterol secretion and encourage cholesterol gallstone formation and hence may counteract the effectiveness of ursodiol). Products include:
Mircette Tablets 1034

Dienestrol (Estrogens and oral contraceptives increase hepatic cholesterol excretion and encourage cholesterol gallstone formation and hence may counteract the effectiveness of ursodiol).
No products indexed under this heading.

Diethylstilbestrol (Estrogens and oral contraceptives increase hepatic cholesterol excretion and encourage cholesterol gallstone formation and hence may counteract the effectiveness of ursodiol).
No products indexed under this heading.

Estradiol (Estrogens and oral contraceptives increase hepatic cholesterol excretion and encourage cholesterol gallstone formation and hence may counteract the effectiveness of ursodiol). Products include:
Activella Tablets 2347
Angeliq Tablets 751
Climara Transdermal System 763
Climara Pro Transdermal System 768
Divigel 3167
Vagifem Tablets 2375

Estrogens, Conjugated (Estrogens and oral contraceptives increase hepatic cholesterol excretion and encourage cholesterol gallstone formation and hence may counteract the effectiveness of ursodiol). Products include:
Premarin Intravenous 3217
Premarin Tablets 3221
Premarin Vaginal Cream 3228
Premphase Tablets 3232
Prempro Tablets 3232

Estrogens, Esterified (Estrogens and oral contraceptives increase hepatic cholesterol excretion and encourage cholesterol gallstone formation and hence may counteract the effectiveness of ursodiol).
Products include:
Estratest Tablets 3043
Estratest H.S. Tablets 3043

Estropipate (Estrogens and oral contraceptives increase hepatic cholesterol excretion and encourage cholesterol gallstone formation and hence may counteract the effectiveness of ursodiol).
No products indexed under this heading.

Ethinyl Estradiol (Estrogens and oral contraceptives increase hepatic cholesterol secretion and encourage cholesterol gallstone formation and hence may counteract the effectiveness of ursodiol). Products include:
Lybrel Tablets 3204
Mircette Tablets 1034
NuvaRing 2897
Ortho-Cyclen/Ortho Tri-Cyclen 2449
Ortho Evra Transdermal System 2437
Ortho Tri-Cyclen Lo Tablets 2458
Seasonique Tablets 1046
Yaz Tablets 805

Ethynodiol Diacetate (Estrogens and oral contraceptives increase hepatic cholesterol secretion and encourage cholesterol gallstone formation and hence may counteract the effectiveness of ursodiol).
No products indexed under this heading.

Fenofibrate (Lipid-lowering drugs increase hepatic cholesterol secretion and encourage cholesterol gallstone formation and hence may counteract the effectiveness of ursodiol). Products include:
Fenoglide Tablets 2960
Tricor Tablets 520

Fluvastatin Sodium (Lipid-lowering drugs increase hepatic cholesterol secretion and encourage cholesterol gallstone formation and hence may counteract the effectiveness of ursodiol). Products include:
Lescol Capsules 2268
Lescol XL Tablets 2268

Gemfibrozil (Lipid-lowering drugs increase hepatic cholesterol secretion and encourage cholesterol gallstone formation and hence may counteract the effectiveness of ursodiol).
No products indexed under this heading.

Levonorgestrel (Estrogens and oral contraceptives increase hepatic cholesterol secretion and encourage cholesterol gallstone formation and hence may counteract the effectiveness of ursodiol). Products include:
Climara Pro Transdermal System 768
Lybrel Tablets 3204
Mirena Intrauterine System 779
Plan B Tablets 1044
Seasonique Tablets 1046

Lovastatin (Lipid-lowering drugs increase hepatic cholesterol secretion and encourage cholesterol gallstone formation and hence may counteract the effectiveness of ursodiol). Products include:
Advicor Tablets 402
Mevacor Tablets 2063

Mestranol (Estrogens and oral contraceptives increase hepatic cholesterol excretion and encourage cholesterol gallstone formation and hence may counteract the effectiveness of ursodiol).
No products indexed under this heading.

Norethindrone (Estrogens and oral contraceptives increase hepatic cholesterol secretion and encourage cholesterol gallstone formation and hence may counteract the effectiveness of ursodiol). Products include:
Ortho Micronor Tablets 2446

Norethynodrel (Estrogens and oral contraceptives increase hepatic cholesterol secretion and encourage cholesterol gallstone formation and hence may counteract the effectiveness of ursodiol).
No products indexed under this heading.

Norgestimate (Estrogens and oral contraceptives increase hepatic cholesterol secretion and encourage cholesterol gallstone formation and hence may counteract the effectiveness of ursodiol). Products include:
Ortho-Cyclen/Ortho Tri-Cyclen 2449
Ortho Tri-Cyclen Lo Tablets 2458

Norgestrel (Estrogens and oral contraceptives increase hepatic cholesterol secretion and encourage cholesterol gallstone formation and hence may counteract the effectiveness of ursodiol).
No products indexed under this heading.

Polyestradiol Phosphate (Estrogens and oral contraceptives increase hepatic cholesterol excretion and encourage cholesterol gallstone formation and hence may counteract the effectiveness of ursodiol).
No products indexed under this heading.

Pravastatin Sodium (Lipid-lowering drugs increase hepatic cholesterol secretion and encourage cholesterol gallstone formation and hence may counteract the effectiveness of ursodiol).
No products indexed under this heading.

Probucol (Lipid-lowering drugs increase hepatic cholesterol secretion and encourage cholesterol gallstone formation and hence may counteract the effectiveness of ursodiol).
No products indexed under this heading.

Quinestrol (Estrogens and oral contraceptives increase hepatic cholesterol excretion and encourage cholesterol gallstone formation and hence may counteract the effectiveness of ursodiol).
No products indexed under this heading.

Simvastatin (Lipid-lowering drugs increase hepatic cholesterol secretion and encourage cholesterol gallstone formation and hence may counteract the effectiveness of ursodiol). Products include:
Simcor Tablets ... 502
Vytorin 10/10 Tablets ... 2149
Vytorin 10/10 Tablets ... 2939
Vytorin 10/20 Tablets ... 2149
Vytorin 10/20 Tablets ... 2939
Vytorin 10/40 Tablets ... 2149
Vytorin 10/40 Tablets ... 2939
Vytorin 10/80 Tablets ... 2149
Vytorin 10/80 Tablets ... 2939
Zocor Tablets ... 2136

URSO FORTE TABLETS
(Ursodiol) ... 720
See Urso 250 Tablets

VAGIFEM TABLETS
(Estradiol) ... 2375
None cited in PDR database.

VALCYTE TABLETS
(Valganciclovir Hydrochloride) ... 2654
May interact with:

Didanosine (Valganciclovir is extensively converted to ganciclovir; co-administration of ganciclovir with didanosine has resulted in decreased AUC of ganciclovir and increased AUC of didanosine; patients should be monitored for didanosine toxicity).
No products indexed under this heading.

Mycophenolate Mofetil (Valganciclovir is extensively converted to ganciclovir; co-administration of ganciclovir with mycophenolate in patients with normal renal function has not resulted in any effect on PK parameters, however, patients with renal impairment should be monitored carefully as levels of metabolites or both drugs may increase). Products include:
CellCept Capsules ... 2622
CellCept Oral Suspension ... 2622
CellCept Tablets ... 2622

Probenecid (Valganciclovir is extensively converted to ganciclovir; co-administration of ganciclovir with probenecid results in increase in AUC of ganciclovir and decrease in ganciclovir renal cleareance; patients on concomitant therapy should be monitored for evidence of ganciclovir toxicity).
No products indexed under this heading.

Trimethoprim (Valganciclovir is extensively converted to ganciclovir; co-administration of ganciclovir with trimethoprim has resulted in decreased renal clearance and increased half-life of ganciclovir and an increase in Cmax of trimethoprim; effects of this interaction are not likely to be clinically significant).
No products indexed under this heading.

Zalcitabine (Valganciclovir is extensively converted to ganciclovir; co-administration of ganciclovir with zalcitabine has resulted in increased AUC of ganciclovir; effects of this interaction are not likely to be clinically significant).
No products indexed under this heading.

Zidovudine (Valganciclovir is extensively converted to ganciclovir; co-administration of ganciclovir with zidovudine has resulted in decreased AUC of ganciclovir and increased AUC of zidovudine; zidovudine and valganciclovir each have the potential to cause neutropenia and anemia; some patients may not tolerate concomitant therapy at full dosage). Products include:
Combivir Tablets ... 1384
Retrovir ... 1574
Retrovir IV Infusion ... 1579
Trizivir Tablets ... 1622

Food Interactions

Food, unspecified (Co-administration with high fat meals has resulted in increased steady-state ganciclovir AUC and Cmax without any prolongation in time to peak plasma concentrations; Valcyte should be administered with food).

VALIUM TABLETS
(Diazepam) ... 2658
May interact with anesthetics, antacids, barbiturates, cytochrome p450 2c19 inhibitors (selected), cytochrome p450 3a4 inhibitors (selected), antidepressant drugs, anticonvulsants, hypnotics and sedatives, monoamine oxidase inhibitors, narcotic analgesics, antipsychotic agents, phenothiazines, sedating antihistamines, and certain other agents. Compounds in these categories include:

Acetazolamide (There is a potentially relevant interaction between diazepam and certain hepatic enzyme inhibitors such as CYP450 3A4. It has been shown that these compounds influence the pharmacokinetics of diazepam and may lead to increased and prolonged sedation).
No products indexed under this heading.

Acrivastine (Careful considerations should be given to the pharmacology of other centrally acting agents (e.g., sedating antihistamines) if used concomitantly with diazepam).
No products indexed under this heading.

Alfentanil Hydrochloride (Careful considerations should be given to the pharmacology of other centrally acting agents (e.g., narcotics) if used concomitantly with diazepam).
No products indexed under this heading.

Aluminum Carbonate (Diazepam peak concentrations are lower when antacids are administered concurrently. The peak concentrations appear to be lower due to a slower rate of absorption, with the time required to achieve peak concentration on average 20 to 25 minutes greater in the presence of antacids).
No products indexed under this heading.

Aluminum Hydroxide (Diazepam peak concentrations are lower when antacids are administered concurrently. The peak concentrations appear to be lower due to a slower rate of absorption, with the time required to achieve peak concentration on average 20 to 25 minutes greater in the presence of antacids).
No products indexed under this heading.

Amiodarone Hydrochloride (There is a potentially relevant interaction between diazepam and certain hepatic enzyme inhibitors such as CYP450 3A4. It has been shown that these compounds influence the pharmacokinetics of diazepam and may lead to increased and prolonged sedation).
No products indexed under this heading.

Amitriptyline Hydrochloride (Careful considerations should be given to the pharmacology of other centrally acting agents (e.g., antidepressants) if used concomitantly with diazepam).
No products indexed under this heading.

Amoxapine (Careful considerations should be given to the pharmacology of other centrally acting agents (e.g., antidepressants) if used concomitantly with diazepam).
No products indexed under this heading.

Amprenavir (There is a potentially relevant interaction between diazepam and certain hepatic enzyme inhibitors such as CYP450 3A4. It has been shown that these compounds influence the pharmacokinetics of diazepam and may lead to increased and prolonged sedation).
No products indexed under this heading.

Anastrozole (There is a potentially relevant interaction between diazepam and certain hepatic enzyme inhibitors such as CYP450 3A4. It has been shown that these compounds influence the pharmacokinetics of diazepam and may lead to increased and prolonged sedation). Products include:
Arimidex Tablets ... 672

Aprepitant (There is a potentially relevant interaction between diazepam and certain hepatic enzyme inhibitors such as CYP450 3A4. It has been shown that these compounds influence the pharmacokinetics of diazepam and may lead to increased and prolonged sedation). Products include:
Emend Capsules ... 1992

Aprobarbital (Careful considerations should be given to the pharmacology of other centrally acting agents (e.g., barbiturates) if used concomitantly with diazepam).
No products indexed under this heading.

Aripiprazole (Careful considerations should be given to the pharmacology of other centrally acting agents (e.g., antipsychotics) if used concomitantly with diazepam). Products include:
Abilify Injection ... 881
Abilify Injection ... 2466
Abilify Oral Solution ... 881
Abilify Oral Solution ... 2466
Abilify Discmelt Orally Disintegrating Tablets ... 881
Abilify Discmelt Orally Disintegrating Tablets ... 2466
Abilify Tablets ... 881
Abilify Tablets ... 2466

Atazanavir (There is a potentially relevant interaction between diazepam and certain hepatic enzyme inhibitors such as CYP450 3A4. It has been shown that these compounds influence the pharmacokinetics of diazepam and may lead to increased and prolonged sedation).
No products indexed under this heading.

Atazanavir Sulfate (There is a potentially relevant interaction between diazepam and certain hepatic enzyme inhibitors such as CYP450 3A4. It has been shown that these compounds influence the pharmacokinetics of diazepam and may lead to increased and prolonged sedation). Products include:
Reyataz Capsules ... 3299

Azatadine Maleate (Careful considerations should be given to the pharmacology of other centrally acting agents (e.g., sedating antihistamines) if used concomitantly with diazepam).
No products indexed under this heading.

Bromodiphenhydramine Hydrochloride (Careful considerations should be given to the pharmacology of other centrally acting agents (e.g., sedating antihistamines) if used concomitantly with diazepam).
No products indexed under this heading.

Brompheniramine Maleate (Careful considerations should be given to the pharmacology of other centrally acting agents (e.g., sedating antihistamines) if used concomitantly with diazepam).
No products indexed under this heading.

Buprenorphine Hydrochloride (Careful considerations should be given to the pharmacology of other centrally acting agents (e.g., narcotics) if used concomitantly with diazepam). Products include:
Suboxone Tablets ... 2601
Subutex Tablets ... 2601

Bupropion Hydrochloride (Careful considerations should be given to the pharmacology of other centrally acting agents (e.g., antidepressants) if used concomitantly with diazepam). Products include:
Wellbutrin Tablets ... 1648
Wellbutrin SR Sustained-Release Tablets ... 1653
Wellbutrin XL Extended-Release Tablets ... 1659
Zyban Sustained-Release Tablets ... 1692

Butabarbital (Careful considerations should be given to the pharmacology of other centrally acting agents (e.g., sedatives and hypnotics) if used concomitantly with diazepam).
No products indexed under this heading.

Butabarbital Sodium (Careful considerations should be given to the pharmacology of other centrally acting agents (e.g., sedatives and hypnotics) if used concomitantly with diazepam).
No products indexed under this heading.

Butalbital (Careful considerations should be given to the pharmacology of other centrally acting agents (e.g., barbiturates) if used concomitantly with diazepam).
No products indexed under this heading.

Carbamazepine (Careful considerations should be given to the pharmacology of other centrally acting agents (e.g., anticonvulsants) if used concomitantly with diazepam).
Products include:
Carbatrol Capsules 3019
Equetro Extended-Release Capsules 3174

Chloral Hydrate (Careful considerations should be given to the pharmacology of other centrally acting agents (e.g., sedatives and hypnotics) if used concomitantly with diazepam).
No products indexed under this heading.

Chlorpheniramine Maleate (Careful considerations should be given to the pharmacology of other centrally acting agents (e.g., sedating antihistamines) if used concomitantly with diazepam). Products include:
Actifed Cold & Allergy Tablets 1895
Sudafed PE Sinus & Allergy Tablets 1908
Tylenol Allergy Multi-Symptom Caplets with Cool Burst and Rapid Release Gelcaps 1916
Children's Tylenol Plus Cold Suspension Liquid 1912
Children's Tylenol Plus Cough & Runny Nose Suspension Liquid..... 1912
Children's Tylenol Plus Flu Suspension Liquid 1914
Children's Tylenol Plus Multi-Symptom Cold Suspension Liquid 1912
Tylenol Cold Head Congestion Nighttime Caplets with Cool Burst........................ 1910
Tylenol Cold Multi-Symptom Nighttime Caplets with Cool Burst........................ 1913
Tylenol Sinus Congestion & Pain Nighttime Caplets with Cool Burst........................ 1917

Chlorpheniramine Polistirex (Careful considerations should be given to the pharmacology of other centrally acting agents (e.g., sedating antihistamines) if used concomitantly with diazepam). Products include:
Tussionex Pennkinetic Extended-Release Suspension...... 3154

Chlorpheniramine Tannate (Careful considerations should be given to the pharmacology of other centrally acting agents (e.g., sedating antihistamines) if used concomitantly with diazepam).
No products indexed under this heading.

Chlorpromazine (Careful considerations should be given to the pharmacology of other centrally acting agents (e.g., phenothiazines) if used concomitantly with diazepam).
No products indexed under this heading.

Chlorpromazine Hydrochloride (Careful considerations should be given to the pharmacology of other centrally acting agents (e.g., phenothiazines) if used concomitantly with diazepam).
No products indexed under this heading.

Chlorprothixene (Careful considerations should be given to the pharmacology of other centrally acting agents (e.g., antipsychotics) if used concomitantly with diazepam).
No products indexed under this heading.

Chlorprothixene Hydrochloride (Careful considerations should be given to the pharmacology of other centrally acting agents (e.g., antipsychotics) if used concomitantly with diazepam).
No products indexed under this heading.

Cimetidine (There is a potentially relevant interaction between diazepam and certain hepatic enzyme inhibitors such as cimetidine. It has been shown that these compounds influence the pharmacokinetics of diazepam and may lead to increased and prolonged sedation).
No products indexed under this heading.

Cimetidine Hydrochloride (There is a potentially relevant interaction between diazepam and certain hepatic enzyme inhibitors such as cimetidine. It has been shown that these compounds influence the pharmacokinetics of diazepam and may lead to increased and prolonged sedation).
No products indexed under this heading.

Ciprofloxacin (There is a potentially relevant interaction between diazepam and certain hepatic enzyme inhibitors such as CYP450 3A4. It has been shown that these compounds influence the pharmacokinetics of diazepam and may lead to increased and prolonged sedation). Products include:
Cipro I.V. 2817
Cipro Oral Suspension 2810
Cipro XR Tablets 2823
Ciprodex Otic Suspension 541

Citalopram Hydrobromide (Careful considerations should be given to the pharmacology of other centrally acting agents (e.g., antidepressants) if used concomitantly with diazepam). Products include:
Celexa 1160

Clarithromycin (There is a potentially relevant interaction between diazepam and certain hepatic enzyme inhibitors such as CYP450 3A4. It has been shown that these compounds influence the pharmacokinetics of diazepam and may lead to increased and prolonged sedation). Products include:
Biaxin/Biaxin XL 411

Clemastine Fumarate (Careful considerations should be given to the pharmacology of other centrally acting agents (e.g., sedating antihistamines) if used concomitantly with diazepam).
No products indexed under this heading.

Clonazepam (Co-administration of diazepam as an adjunct in treating convulsive disorders results in possibility of an increase in the frequency and/or severity of grand mal seizures which may require an increase in the dosage of standard anticonvulsant agent; may potentiate the CNS depression caused by diazepam). Products include:
Klonopin 2639

Clotrimazole (There is a potentially relevant interaction between diazepam and certain hepatic enzyme inhibitors such as CYP450 3A4. It has been shown that these compounds influence the pharmacokinetics of diazepam and may lead to increased and prolonged sedation). Products include:
Lotrisone 2881

Clozapine (Careful considerations should be given to the pharmacology of other centrally acting agents (e.g., antipsychotics) if used concomitantly with diazepam).
No products indexed under this heading.

Codeine Phosphate (Careful considerations should be given to the pharmacology of other centrally acting agents (e.g., narcotics) if used concomitantly with diazepam). Products include:
Tylenol with Codeine Tablets 2427

Cyclosporine (There is a potentially relevant interaction between diazepam and certain hepatic enzyme inhibitors such as CYP450 3A4. It has been shown that these compounds influence the pharmacokinetics of diazepam and may lead to increased and prolonged sedation). Products include:
Gengraf Capsules 435
Neoral Oral Solution 2280
Neoral Soft Gelatin Capsules 2280
Restasis Ophthalmic Emulsion 557
Sandimmune 2296

Cyproheptadine Hydrochloride (Careful considerations should be given to the pharmacology of other centrally acting agents (e.g., sedating antihistamines) if used concomitantly with diazepam).
No products indexed under this heading.

Dalfopristin (There is a potentially relevant interaction between diazepam and certain hepatic enzyme inhibitors such as CYP450 3A4. It has been shown that these compounds influence the pharmacokinetics of diazepam and may lead to increased and prolonged sedation).
No products indexed under this heading.

Danazol (There is a potentially relevant interaction between diazepam and certain hepatic enzyme inhibitors such as CYP450 3A4. It has been shown that these compounds influence the pharmacokinetics of diazepam and may lead to increased and prolonged sedation).
No products indexed under this heading.

Delavirdine Mesylate (There is a potentially relevant interaction between diazepam and certain hepatic enzyme inhibitors such as CYP450 3A4. It has been shown that these compounds influence the pharmacokinetics of diazepam and may lead to increased and prolonged sedation).
No products indexed under this heading.

Desipramine Hydrochloride (Careful considerations should be given to the pharmacology of other centrally acting agents (e.g., antidepressants) if used concomitantly with diazepam).
No products indexed under this heading.

Desogestrel (There is a potentially relevant interaction between diazepam and certain hepatic enzyme inhibitors such as CYP450 2C19. It has been shown that these compounds influence the pharmacokinetics of diazepam and may lead to increased and prolonged sedation). Products include:
Mircette Tablets 1034

Dexchlorpheniramine Maleate (Careful considerations should be given to the pharmacology of other centrally acting agents (e.g., sedating antihistamines) if used concomitantly with diazepam).
No products indexed under this heading.

Dezocine (Careful considerations should be given to the pharmacology of other centrally acting agents (e.g., narcotics) if used concomitantly with diazepam).
No products indexed under this heading.

Diltiazem Hydrochloride (There is a potentially relevant interaction between diazepam and certain hepatic enzyme inhibitors such as CYP450 3A4. It has been shown that these compounds influence the pharmacokinetics of diazepam and may lead to increased and prolonged sedation). Products include:
Cardizem LA Extended Release Tablets 421

Diltiazem Maleate (There is a potentially relevant interaction between diazepam and certain hepatic enzyme inhibitors such as CYP450 3A4. It has been shown that these compounds influence the pharmacokinetics of diazepam and may lead to increased and prolonged sedation).
No products indexed under this heading.

Diphenhydramine Citrate (Careful considerations should be given to the pharmacology of other centrally acting agents (e.g., sedating antihistamines) if used concomitantly with diazepam).
No products indexed under this heading.

Diphenhydramine Hydrochloride (Careful considerations should be given to the pharmacology of other centrally acting agents (e.g., sedating antihistamines) if used concomitantly with diazepam). Products include:
Benadryl Allergy & Cold Kapgels 1895
Benadryl Allergy & Sinus Headache Kapgels 1895
Benadryl Severe Allergy & Sinus Headache Caplets 1897
Benadryl Dye-Free Allergy Liqui-gels Softgels 1897
Benadryl Allergy Kapgels 1895
Benadryl Allergy Quick Dissolve Strips 1896
Benadryl Allergy Ultratab Tablets 1896
Children's Benadryl Dye-Free Allergy Liquid 1897
Children's Benadryl Allergy Fastmelts 1897
Children's Benadryl Allergy Liquid 1898
Children's Benadryl Allergy Perfect Measure 1896

Children's Benadryl-D Allergy & Sinus Liquid 1896
Benadryl-D Allergy & Sinus Tablet 1896
PediaCare Children's Allergy & Cold Liquid 1902
PediaCare Children's Allergy Liquid 1902
Simply Sleep Caplets 1905
Sudafed PE Nighttime Cold Caplets 1907
Sudafed PE Severe Cold Caplets 1908
Extra Strength Tylenol PM Caplets, Geltabs, Liquid, and Rapid Release Gels 1915
Tylenol Allergy Multi-Symptom Nighttime Caplets with Cool Burst 1916
Tylenol Severe Allergy Caplets 1916
Children's Tylenol Plus Cold & Allergy Suspension Liquid 1914
Tylenol Sore Throat Nighttime Liquid with Cool Burst 1918

Diphenylpyraline Hydrochloride (Careful considerations should be given to the pharmacology of other centrally acting agents (e.g., sedating antihistamines) if used concomitantly with diazepam).
No products indexed under this heading.

Divalproex Sodium (Careful considerations should be given to the pharmacology of other centrally acting agents (e.g., anticonvulsants) if used concomitantly with diazepam). Products include:
Depakote ER Tablets 423

Doxepin Hydrochloride (Careful considerations should be given to the pharmacology of other centrally acting agents (e.g., antidepressants) if used concomitantly with diazepam).
No products indexed under this heading.

Efavirenz (There is a potentially relevant interaction between diazepam and certain hepatic enzyme inhibitors such as CYP450 3A4. It has been shown that these compounds influence the pharmacokinetics of diazepam and may lead to increased and prolonged sedation). Products include:
Atripla Tablets 938
Sustiva Capsules 930
Sustiva Tablets 930

Enflurane (Careful considerations should be given to the pharmacology of other centrally acting agents (e.g., anesthetics) if used concomitantly with diazepam).
No products indexed under this heading.

Erythromycin (There is a potentially relevant interaction between diazepam and certain hepatic enzyme inhibitors such as CYP450 3A4. It has been shown that these compounds influence the pharmacokinetics of diazepam and may lead to increased and prolonged sedation).
No products indexed under this heading.

Erythromycin Estolate (There is a potentially relevant interaction between diazepam and certain hepatic enzyme inhibitors such as CYP450 3A4. It has been shown that these compounds influence the pharmacokinetics of diazepam and may lead to increased and prolonged sedation).
No products indexed under this heading.

Erythromycin Ethylsuccinate (There is a potentially relevant interaction between diazepam and certain hepatic enzyme inhibitors such as CYP450 3A4. It has been shown that these compounds influence the pharmacokinetics of diazepam and may lead to increased and prolonged sedation). Products include:
E.E.S. 433
EryPed 431

Erythromycin Gluceptate (There is a potentially relevant interaction between diazepam and certain hepatic enzyme inhibitors such as CYP450 3A4. It has been shown that these compounds influence the pharmacokinetics of diazepam and may lead to increased and prolonged sedation).
No products indexed under this heading.

Erythromycin Lactobionate (There is a potentially relevant interaction between diazepam and certain hepatic enzyme inhibitors such as CYP450 3A4. It has been shown that these compounds influence the pharmacokinetics of diazepam and may lead to increased and prolonged sedation).
No products indexed under this heading.

Erythromycin Stearate (There is a potentially relevant interaction between diazepam and certain hepatic enzyme inhibitors such as CYP450 3A4. It has been shown that these compounds influence the pharmacokinetics of diazepam and may lead to increased and prolonged sedation).
No products indexed under this heading.

Escitalopram Oxalate (Careful considerations should be given to the pharmacology of other centrally acting agents (e.g., antidepressants) if used concomitantly with diazepam). Products include:
Lexapro Oral Suspension 1174
Lexapro Tablets 1174

Esomeprazole Magnesium (There is a potentially relevant interaction between diazepam and certain hepatic enzyme inhibitors such as CYP450 3A4. It has been shown that these compounds influence the pharmacokinetics of diazepam and may lead to increased and prolonged sedation). Products include:
Nexium Delayed-Release Capsules 645
Nexium Delayed-Release Oral Suspension 645

Estazolam (Careful considerations should be given to the pharmacology of other centrally acting agents (e.g., sedatives and hypnotics) if used concomitantly with diazepam).
No products indexed under this heading.

Ethchlorvynol (Careful considerations should be given to the pharmacology of other centrally acting agents (e.g., sedatives and hypnotics) if used concomitantly with diazepam).
No products indexed under this heading.

Ethinamate (Careful considerations should be given to the pharmacology of other centrally acting agents (e.g., sedatives and hypnotics) if used concomitantly with diazepam).
No products indexed under this heading.

Ethinyl Estradiol (There is a potentially relevant interaction between diazepam and certain hepatic enzyme inhibitors such as CYP450 2C19. It has been shown that these compounds influence the pharmacokinetics of diazepam and may lead to increased and prolonged sedation). Products include:
Lybrel Tablets 3204
Mircette Tablets 1034
NuvaRing 2897
Ortho-Cyclen/Ortho Tri-Cyclen 2449
Ortho Evra Transdermal System 2437
Ortho Tri-Cyclen Lo Tablets 2458
Seasonique Tablets 1046
Yaz Tablets 805

Ethosuximide (Careful considerations should be given to the pharmacology of other centrally acting agents (e.g., anticonvulsants) if used concomitantly with diazepam).
No products indexed under this heading.

Ethotoin (Careful considerations should be given to the pharmacology of other centrally acting agents (e.g., anticonvulsants) if used concomitantly with diazepam).
No products indexed under this heading.

Ethyl Alcohol (Concomitant use with alcohol is not recommended due to enhancement of the sedative effect).
No products indexed under this heading.

Ethynodiol Diacetate (There is a potentially relevant interaction between diazepam and certain hepatic enzyme inhibitors such as CYP450 2C19. It has been shown that these compounds influence the pharmacokinetics of diazepam and may lead to increased and prolonged sedation).
No products indexed under this heading.

Felbamate (Careful considerations should be given to the pharmacology of other centrally acting agents (e.g., anticonvulsants) if used concomitantly with diazepam).
No products indexed under this heading.

Fentanyl (Careful considerations should be given to the pharmacology of other centrally acting agents (e.g., narcotics) if used concomitantly with diazepam). Products include:
Duragesic Transdermal System 2405
Ionsys Transdermal System 2410

Fentanyl Citrate (Careful considerations should be given to the pharmacology of other centrally acting agents (e.g., narcotics) if used concomitantly with diazepam). Products include:
Actiq 959
Fentora Tablets 968

Fluconazole (There is a potentially relevant interaction between diazepam and certain hepatic enzyme inhibitors such as CYP450 3A4. It has been shown that these compounds influence the pharmacokinetics of diazepam and may lead to increased and prolonged sedation).
No products indexed under this heading.

Fluoxetine (There is a potentially relevant interaction between diazepam and certain hepatic enzyme inhibitors such as fluoxetine. It has been shown that these compounds influence the pharmacokinetics of diazepam and may lead to increased and prolonged sedation).
No products indexed under this heading.

Fluoxetine Hydrochloride (There is a potentially relevant interaction between diazepam and certain hepatic enzyme inhibitors such as fluoxetine. It has been shown that these compounds influence the pharmacokinetics of diazepam and may lead to increased and prolonged sedation). Products include:
Prozac Weekly Capsules 1852
Prozac Pulvules and Liquid 1852
Symbyax Capsules 1871

Fluphenazine Decanoate (Careful considerations should be given to the pharmacology of other centrally acting agents (e.g., phenothiazines) if used concomitantly with diazepam).
No products indexed under this heading.

Fluphenazine Enanthate (Careful considerations should be given to the pharmacology of other centrally acting agents (e.g., phenothiazines) if used concomitantly with diazepam).
No products indexed under this heading.

Fluphenazine Hydrochloride (Careful considerations should be given to the pharmacology of other centrally acting agents (e.g., phenothiazines) if used concomitantly with diazepam).
No products indexed under this heading.

Flurazepam Hydrochloride (Careful considerations should be given to the pharmacology of other centrally acting agents (e.g., sedatives and hypnotics) if used concomitantly with diazepam).
No products indexed under this heading.

Fluvastatin Sodium (There is a potentially relevant interaction between diazepam and certain hepatic enzyme inhibitors such as CYP450 2C19. It has been shown that these compounds influence the pharmacokinetics of diazepam and may lead to increased and prolonged sedation). Products include:
Lescol Capsules 2268
Lescol XL Tablets 2268

Fluvoxamine (There is a potentially relevant interaction between diazepam and certain hepatic enzyme inhibitors such as fluvoxamine. It has been shown that these compounds influence the pharmacokinetics of diazepam and may lead to increased and prolonged sedation).
No products indexed under this heading.

Fluvoxamine Maleate (There is a potentially relevant interaction between diazepam and certain hepatic enzyme inhibitors such as fluvoxamine. It has been shown that these compounds influence the pharmacokinetics of diazepam and may lead to increased and prolonged sedation). Products include:
Luvox CR Extended-Release Capsules 1759

Fosamprenavir Calcium (There is a potentially relevant interaction between diazepam and certain hepatic enzyme inhibitors such as CYP450 3A4. It has been shown that these compounds influence the pharmacokinetics of diazepam and may lead to increased and prolonged sedation). Products include:
Lexiva Oral Suspension 1510
Lexiva Tablets 1510

Fosphenytoin (Careful considerations should be given to the pharmacology of other centrally acting agents (e.g., anticonvulsants) if used concomitantly with diazepam).
No products indexed under this heading.

Fosphenytoin Sodium (Careful considerations should be given to the pharmacology of other centrally acting agents (e.g., anticonvulsants) if used concomitantly with diazepam).
No products indexed under this heading.

Gabapentin (Careful considerations should be given to the pharmacology of other centrally acting agents (e.g., anticonvulsants) if used concomitantly with diazepam).
No products indexed under this heading.

Glutethimide (Careful considerations should be given to the pharmacology of other centrally acting agents (e.g., sedatives and hypnotics) if used concomitantly with diazepam).
No products indexed under this heading.

Haloperidol (Careful considerations should be given to the pharmacology of other centrally acting agents (e.g., antipsychotics) if used concomitantly with diazepam).
No products indexed under this heading.

Haloperidol Decanoate (Careful considerations should be given to the pharmacology of other centrally acting agents (e.g., antipsychotics) if used concomitantly with diazepam).
No products indexed under this heading.

Halothane (Careful considerations should be given to the pharmacology of other centrally acting agents (e.g., anesthetics) if used concomitantly with diazepam).
No products indexed under this heading.

Hydrocodone Bitartrate (Careful considerations should be given to the pharmacology of other centrally acting agents (e.g., narcotics) if used concomitantly with diazepam).
Products include:
Lortab 5/500 Tablets ... 3143
Lortab 7.5/500 Tablets ... 3144
Lortab 10/500 Tablets ... 3144
Vicodin Tablets ... 529
Vicodin ES Tablets ... 530
Vicodin HP Tablets ... 531
Vicoprofen Tablets ... 533
Zydone Tablets ... 1132

Hydrocodone Polistirex (Careful considerations should be given to the pharmacology of other centrally acting agents (e.g., narcotics) if used concomitantly with diazepam).
Products include:
Tussionex Pennkinetic Extended-Release Suspension ... 3154

Hydromorphone Hydrochloride (Careful considerations should be given to the pharmacology of other centrally acting agents (e.g., narcotics) if used concomitantly with diazepam).
No products indexed under this heading.

Imipramine Hydrochloride (Careful considerations should be given to the pharmacology of other centrally acting agents (e.g., antidepressants) if used concomitantly with diazepam).
No products indexed under this heading.

Imipramine Pamoate (Careful considerations should be given to the pharmacology of other centrally acting agents (e.g., antidepressants) if used concomitantly with diazepam).
No products indexed under this heading.

Indinavir Sulfate (There is a potentially relevant interaction between diazepam and certain hepatic enzyme inhibitors such as CYP450 3A4. It has been shown that these compounds influence the pharmacokinetics of diazepam and may lead to increased and prolonged sedation). Products include:
Crixivan Capsules ... 1979

Indomethacin (There is a potentially relevant interaction between diazepam and certain hepatic enzyme inhibitors such as CYP450 2C19. It has been shown that these compounds influence the pharmacokinetics of diazepam and may lead to increased and prolonged sedation).
Products include:
Indocin ... 2024

Indomethacin Sodium Trihydrate (There is a potentially relevant interaction between diazepam and certain hepatic enzyme inhibitors such as CYP450 2C19. It has been shown that these compounds influence the pharmacokinetics of diazepam and may lead to increased and prolonged sedation). Products include:
Indocin I.V. ... 2489

Isocarboxazid (Careful considerations should be given to the pharmacology of other centrally acting agents (e.g., MAO inhibitors) if used concomitantly with diazepam).
Products include:
Marplan Tablets ... 3177

Isoflurane (Careful considerations should be given to the pharmacology of other centrally acting agents (e.g., anesthetics) if used concomitantly with diazepam).
No products indexed under this heading.

Isoniazid (There is a potentially relevant interaction between diazepam and certain hepatic enzyme inhibitors such as CYP450 3A4. It has been shown that these compounds influence the pharmacokinetics of diazepam and may lead to increased and prolonged sedation).
No products indexed under this heading.

Isopropyl Alcohol (Concomitant use with alcohol is not recommended due to enhancement of the sedative effect).
No products indexed under this heading.

Itraconazole (There is a potentially relevant interaction between diazepam and certain hepatic enzyme inhibitors such as CYP450 3A4. It has been shown that these compounds influence the pharmacokinetics of diazepam and may lead to increased and prolonged sedation).
No products indexed under this heading.

Ketamine Hydrochloride (Careful considerations should be given to the pharmacology of other centrally acting agents (e.g., anesthetics) if used concomitantly with diazepam).
No products indexed under this heading.

Ketoconazole (There is a potentially relevant interaction between diazepam and certain hepatic enzyme inhibitors such as ketoconazole. It has been shown that these compounds influence the pharmacokinetics of diazepam and may lead to increased and prolonged sedation).
Products include:
Extina Foam, 2% ... 3057
Nizoral A-D Shampoo ... 1901

Lamotrigine (Careful considerations should be given to the pharmacology of other centrally acting agents (e.g., anticonvulsants) if used concomitantly with diazepam).
Products include:
Lamictal ... 1488

Lansoprazole (There is a potentially relevant interaction between diazepam and certain hepatic enzyme inhibitors such as CYP450 2C19. It has been shown that these compounds influence the pharmacokinetics of diazepam and may lead to increased and prolonged sedation).
No products indexed under this heading.

Letrozole (There is a potentially relevant interaction between diazepam and certain hepatic enzyme inhibitors such as CYP450 2C19. It has been shown that these compounds influence the pharmacokinetics of diazepam and may lead to increased and prolonged sedation).
Products include:
Femara Tablets ... 2246

Levetiracetam (Careful considerations should be given to the pharmacology of other centrally acting agents (e.g., anticonvulsants) if used concomitantly with diazepam).
Products include:
Keppra Injection ... 3137
Keppra Oral Solution ... 3131
Keppra Tablets ... 3131

Levonorgestrel (There is a potentially relevant interaction between diazepam and certain hepatic enzyme inhibitors such as CYP450 2C19. It has been shown that these compounds influence the pharmacokinetics of diazepam and may lead to increased and prolonged sedation). Products include:
Climara Pro Transdermal System ... 768
Lybrel Tablets ... 3204
Mirena Intrauterine System ... 779
Plan B Tablets ... 1044
Seasonique Tablets ... 1046

Levorphanol Tartrate (Careful considerations should be given to the pharmacology of other centrally acting agents (e.g., narcotics) if used concomitantly with diazepam).
No products indexed under this heading.

Lithium Carbonate (Careful considerations should be given to the pharmacology of other centrally acting agents (e.g., antipsychotics) if used concomitantly with diazepam).
No products indexed under this heading.

Lithium Citrate (Careful considerations should be given to the pharmacology of other centrally acting agents (e.g., antipsychotics) if used concomitantly with diazepam).
No products indexed under this heading.

Lopinavir (There is a potentially relevant interaction between diazepam and certain hepatic enzyme inhibitors such as CYP450 3A4. It has been shown that these compounds influence the pharmacokinetics of diazepam and may lead to increased and prolonged sedation).
Products include:
Kaletra ... 452

Loratadine (There is a potentially relevant interaction between diazepam and certain hepatic enzyme inhibitors such as CYP450 3A4. It has been shown that these compounds influence the pharmacokinetics of diazepam and may lead to increased and prolonged sedation).
No products indexed under this heading.

Lorazepam (Careful considerations should be given to the pharmacology of other centrally acting agents (e.g., sedatives and hypnotics) if used concomitantly with diazepam).
No products indexed under this heading.

Loxapine Hydrochloride (Careful considerations should be given to the pharmacology of other centrally acting agents (e.g., antipsychotics) if used concomitantly with diazepam).
No products indexed under this heading.

Loxapine Succinate (Careful considerations should be given to the pharmacology of other centrally acting agents (e.g., antipsychotics) if used concomitantly with diazepam).
No products indexed under this heading.

Magaldrate (Diazepam peak concentrations are lower when antacids are administered concurrently. The peak concentrations appear to be lower due to a slower rate of absorption, with the time required to achieve peak concentration on average 20 to 25 minutes greater in the presence of antacids).
No products indexed under this heading.

Magnesium Hydroxide (Diazepam peak concentrations are lower when antacids are administered concurrently. The peak concentrations appear to be lower due to a slower rate of absorption, with the time required to achieve peak concentration on average 20 to 25 minutes greater in the presence of antacids).
Products include:
Fleet Pedia-Lax Chewable Tablets ... 1145
Pepcid Complete Chewable Tablets ... 1771
Extra Strength Rolaids Freshmint Tablets ... 1903
Rolaids Multi-Symptom Berry Tablets ... 1903
Rolaids Original Peppermint Tablets ... 1903

Magnesium Oxide (Diazepam peak concentrations are lower when antacids are administered concurrently. The peak concentrations appear to be lower due to a slower rate of absorption, with the time required to achieve peak concentration on average 20 to 25 minutes greater in the presence of antacids).
Products include:

IMPORTANT NOTE: Always consult each drug listing in the patient's regimen for possible interactions.

Beelith Tablets 813

Maprotiline Hydrochloride (Careful considerations should be given to the pharmacology of other centrally acting agents (e.g., antidepressants) if used concomitantly with diazepam).
No products indexed under this heading.

Meperidine Hydrochloride (Careful considerations should be given to the pharmacology of other centrally acting agents (e.g., narcotics) if used concomitantly with diazepam).
No products indexed under this heading.

Mephenytoin (Careful considerations should be given to the pharmacology of other centrally acting agents (e.g., anticonvulsants) if used concomitantly with diazepam).
No products indexed under this heading.

Mephobarbital (Careful considerations should be given to the pharmacology of other centrally acting agents (e.g., barbiturates) if used concomitantly with diazepam).
No products indexed under this heading.

Mesoridazine Besylate (Careful considerations should be given to the pharmacology of other centrally acting agents (e.g., phenothiazines) if used concomitantly with diazepam).
No products indexed under this heading.

Mestranol (There is a potentially relevant interaction between diazepam and certain hepatic enzyme inhibitors such as CYP450 2C19. It has been shown that these compounds influence the pharmacokinetics of diazepam and may lead to increased and prolonged sedation).
No products indexed under this heading.

Methadone Hydrochloride (Careful considerations should be given to the pharmacology of other centrally acting agents (e.g., narcotics) if used concomitantly with diazepam).
No products indexed under this heading.

Methdilazine Hydrochloride (Careful considerations should be given to the pharmacology of other centrally acting agents (e.g., sedating antihistamines) if used concomitantly with diazepam).
No products indexed under this heading.

Methohexital Sodium (Careful considerations should be given to the pharmacology of other centrally acting agents (e.g., anesthetics) if used concomitantly with diazepam).
No products indexed under this heading.

Methotrimeprazine (Careful considerations should be given to the pharmacology of other centrally acting agents (e.g., phenothiazines) if used concomitantly with diazepam).
No products indexed under this heading.

Methsuximide (Careful considerations should be given to the pharmacology of other centrally acting agents (e.g., anticonvulsants) if used concomitantly with diazepam).
No products indexed under this heading.

Metronidazole (There is a potentially relevant interaction between diazepam and certain hepatic enzyme inhibitors such as CYP450 3A4. It has been shown that these compounds influence the pharmacokinetics of diazepam and may lead to increased and prolonged sedation). Products include:
Pylera Capsules 714

Metronidazole Benzoate (There is a potentially relevant interaction between diazepam and certain hepatic enzyme inhibitors such as CYP450 3A4. It has been shown that these compounds influence the pharmacokinetics of diazepam and may lead to increased and prolonged sedation).
No products indexed under this heading.

Metronidazole Hydrochloride (There is a potentially relevant interaction between diazepam and certain hepatic enzyme inhibitors such as CYP450 3A4. It has been shown that these compounds influence the pharmacokinetics of diazepam and may lead to increased and prolonged sedation).
No products indexed under this heading.

Metronidazole Sodium (There is a potentially relevant interaction between diazepam and certain hepatic enzyme inhibitors such as CYP450 3A4. It has been shown that these compounds influence the pharmacokinetics of diazepam and may lead to increased and prolonged sedation).
No products indexed under this heading.

Miconazole (There is a potentially relevant interaction between diazepam and certain hepatic enzyme inhibitors such as CYP450 3A4. It has been shown that these compounds influence the pharmacokinetics of diazepam and may lead to increased and prolonged sedation).
No products indexed under this heading.

Miconazole Nitrate (There is a potentially relevant interaction between diazepam and certain hepatic enzyme inhibitors such as CYP450 3A4. It has been shown that these compounds influence the pharmacokinetics of diazepam and may lead to increased and prolonged sedation).
No products indexed under this heading.

Midazolam Hydrochloride (Careful considerations should be given to the pharmacology of other centrally acting agents (e.g., sedatives and hypnotics) if used concomitantly with diazepam).
No products indexed under this heading.

Mirtazapine (Careful considerations should be given to the pharmacology of other centrally acting agents (e.g., antidepressants) if used concomitantly with diazepam). Products include:
Remeron Tablets 2924
RemeronSolTab Tablets 2927

Moclobemide (Careful considerations should be given to the pharmacology of other centrally acting agents (e.g., MAO inhibitors) if used concomitantly with diazepam).
No products indexed under this heading.

Modafinil (There is a potentially relevant interaction between diazepam and certain hepatic enzyme inhibitors such as CYP450 2C19. It has been shown that these compounds influence the pharmacokinetics of diazepam and may lead to increased and prolonged sedation). Products include:
Provigil Tablets 977

Molindone Hydrochloride (Careful considerations should be given to the pharmacology of other centrally acting agents (e.g., antipsychotics) if used concomitantly with diazepam). Products include:
Moban Tablets 1116

Morphine Sulfate (Careful considerations should be given to the pharmacology of other centrally acting agents (e.g., narcotics) if used concomitantly with diazepam). Products include:
Avinza Capsules 1772
DepoDur Injection 1095
MS Contin Tablets 2585

Nefazodone Hydrochloride (Careful considerations should be given to the pharmacology of other centrally acting agents (e.g., antidepressants) if used concomitantly with diazepam).
No products indexed under this heading.

Nelfinavir Mesylate (There is a potentially relevant interaction between diazepam and certain hepatic enzyme inhibitors such as CYP450 3A4. It has been shown that these compounds influence the pharmacokinetics of diazepam and may lead to increased and prolonged sedation).
No products indexed under this heading.

Nevirapine (There is a potentially relevant interaction between diazepam and certain hepatic enzyme inhibitors such as CYP450 3A4. It has been shown that these compounds influence the pharmacokinetics of diazepam and may lead to increased and prolonged sedation). Products include:
Viramune Oral Suspension 873
Viramune Tablets 873

Niacinamide (There is a potentially relevant interaction between diazepam and certain hepatic enzyme inhibitors such as CYP450 3A4. It has been shown that these compounds influence the pharmacokinetics of diazepam and may lead to increased and prolonged sedation). Products include:
BioLean Free Tablets .... ▣635

Nicotinamide (There is a potentially relevant interaction between diazepam and certain hepatic enzyme inhibitors such as CYP450 3A4. It has been shown that these compounds influence the pharmacokinetics of diazepam and may lead to increased and prolonged sedation).
No products indexed under this heading.

Nifedipine (There is a potentially relevant interaction between diazepam and certain hepatic enzyme inhibitors such as CYP450 3A4. It has been shown that these compounds influence the pharmacokinetics of diazepam and may lead to increased and prolonged sedation).
No products indexed under this heading.

Norethindrone (There is a potentially relevant interaction between diazepam and certain hepatic enzyme inhibitors such as CYP450 2C19. It has been shown that these compounds influence the pharmacokinetics of diazepam and may lead to increased and prolonged sedation). Products include:
Ortho Micronor Tablets 2446

Norethynodrel (There is a potentially relevant interaction between diazepam and certain hepatic enzyme inhibitors such as CYP450 2C19. It has been shown that these compounds influence the pharmacokinetics of diazepam and may lead to increased and prolonged sedation).
No products indexed under this heading.

Norfloxacin (There is a potentially relevant interaction between diazepam and certain hepatic enzyme inhibitors such as CYP450 3A4. It has been shown that these compounds influence the pharmacokinetics of diazepam and may lead to increased and prolonged sedation). Products include:
Noroxin Tablets 2069

Norgestimate (There is a potentially relevant interaction between diazepam and certain hepatic enzyme inhibitors such as CYP450 2C19. It has been shown that these compounds influence the pharmacokinetics of diazepam and may lead to increased and prolonged sedation). Products include:
Ortho-Cyclen/Ortho Tri-Cyclen 2449
Ortho Tri-Cyclen Lo Tablets 2458

Norgestrel (There is a potentially relevant interaction between diazepam and certain hepatic enzyme inhibitors such as CYP450 2C19. It has been shown that these compounds influence the pharmacokinetics of diazepam and may lead to increased and prolonged sedation).
No products indexed under this heading.

Nortriptyline Hydrochloride (Careful considerations should be given to the pharmacology of other centrally acting agents (e.g., antidepressants) if used concomitantly with diazepam).
No products indexed under this heading.

Olanzapine (Careful considerations should be given to the pharmacology of other centrally acting agents (e.g., antipsychotics) if used concomitantly with diazepam). Products include:
Symbyax Capsules 1871
Zyprexa Tablets 1883
Zyprexa IntraMuscular 1883
Zyprexa ZYDIS Orally Disintegrating Tablets 1883

Omeprazole (There is a potentially relevant interaction between diazepam and certain hepatic enzyme inhibitors such as omeprazole. It has been shown that these compounds influence the pharmacokinetics of diazepam and may lead to increased and prolonged sedation).
No products indexed under this heading.

Omeprazole Magnesium (There is a potentially relevant interaction between diazepam and certain hepatic enzyme inhibitors such as omeprazole. It has been shown that these compounds influence the pharmacokinetics of diazepam and may lead to increased and prolonged sedation). Products include:
Prilosec OTC Tablets 2565

Oxcarbazepine (Careful considerations should be given to the pharmacology of other centrally acting agents (e.g., anticonvulsants) if used concomitantly with diazepam).
No products indexed under this heading.

Oxycodone Hydrochloride (Careful considerations should be given to the pharmacology of other centrally acting agents (e.g., narcotics) if used concomitantly with diazepam). Products include:
OxyContin Tablets **2589**
OxyIR Capsules **2593**
Percocet Tablets **1127**
Percodan Tablets **1130**

Paliperidone (Careful considerations should be given to the pharmacology of other centrally acting agents (e.g., antipsychotics) if used concomitantly with diazepam). Products include:
Invega Extended-Release Tablets **1748**

Paramethadione (Careful considerations should be given to the pharmacology of other centrally acting agents (e.g., anticonvulsants) if used concomitantly with diazepam).
No products indexed under this heading.

Pargyline Hydrochloride (Careful considerations should be given to the pharmacology of other centrally acting agents (e.g., MAO inhibitors) if used concomitantly with diazepam).
No products indexed under this heading.

Paroxetine Hydrochloride (Careful considerations should be given to the pharmacology of other centrally acting agents (e.g., antidepressants) if used concomitantly with diazepam). Products include:
Paxil **1535**
Paxil CR Controlled-Release Tablets **1544**

Pentobarbital Sodium (Careful considerations should be given to the pharmacology of other centrally acting agents (e.g., barbiturates) if used concomitantly with diazepam). Products include:
Nembutal Sodium Solution, USP **2494**

Perphenazine (Careful considerations should be given to the pharmacology of other centrally acting agents (e.g., phenothiazines) if used concomitantly with diazepam).
No products indexed under this heading.

Phenacemide (Careful considerations should be given to the pharmacology of other centrally acting agents (e.g., anticonvulsants) if used concomitantly with diazepam).
No products indexed under this heading.

Phenelzine Sulfate (Careful considerations should be given to the pharmacology of other centrally acting agents (e.g., MAO inhibitors) if used concomitantly with diazepam).
No products indexed under this heading.

Phenobarbital (Co-administration of diazepam as an adjunct in treating convulsive disorders results in possibility of an increase in the frequency and/or severity of grand mal seizures which may require an increase in the dosage of standard anticonvulsant agent; may potentiate the CNS depression caused by diazepam). Products include:
Donnatal Extentabs **2507**

Phensuximide (Careful considerations should be given to the pharmacology of other centrally acting agents (e.g., anticonvulsants) if used concomitantly with diazepam).
No products indexed under this heading.

Phenytoin (There have been reports that the metabolic elimination of phenytoin is decreased by diazepam).
No products indexed under this heading.

Phenytoin Sodium (There have been reports that the metabolic elimination of phenytoin is decreased by diazepam). Products include:
Phenytek Capsules **2192**

Pimozide (Careful considerations should be given to the pharmacology of other centrally acting agents (e.g., antipsychotics) if used concomitantly with diazepam).
No products indexed under this heading.

Primidone (Careful considerations should be given to the pharmacology of other centrally acting agents (e.g., anticonvulsants) if used concomitantly with diazepam).
No products indexed under this heading.

Procarbazine Hydrochloride (Careful considerations should be given to the pharmacology of other centrally acting agents (e.g., MAO inhibitors) if used concomitantly with diazepam).
No products indexed under this heading.

Prochlorperazine (Careful considerations should be given to the pharmacology of other centrally acting agents (e.g., phenothiazines) if used concomitantly with diazepam).
No products indexed under this heading.

Promethazine Hydrochloride (Careful considerations should be given to the pharmacology of other centrally acting agents (e.g., phenothiazines) if used concomitantly with diazepam).
No products indexed under this heading.

Propofol (Careful considerations should be given to the pharmacology of other centrally acting agents (e.g., sedatives and hypnotics) if used concomitantly with diazepam).
No products indexed under this heading.

Propoxyphene Hydrochloride (Careful considerations should be given to the pharmacology of other centrally acting agents (e.g., narcotics) if used concomitantly with diazepam).
No products indexed under this heading.

Propoxyphene Napsylate (Careful considerations should be given to the pharmacology of other centrally acting agents (e.g., narcotics) if used concomitantly with diazepam).
No products indexed under this heading.

Protriptyline Hydrochloride (Careful considerations should be given to the pharmacology of other centrally acting agents (e.g., antidepressants) if used concomitantly with diazepam).
No products indexed under this heading.

Pyrilamine Maleate (Careful considerations should be given to the pharmacology of other centrally acting agents (e.g., sedating antihistamines) if used concomitantly with diazepam).
No products indexed under this heading.

Pyrilamine Tannate (Careful considerations should be given to the pharmacology of other centrally acting agents (e.g., sedating antihistamines) if used concomitantly with diazepam).
No products indexed under this heading.

Quazepam (Careful considerations should be given to the pharmacology of other centrally acting agents (e.g., sedatives and hypnotics) if used concomitantly with diazepam).
No products indexed under this heading.

Quetiapine Fumarate (Careful considerations should be given to the pharmacology of other centrally acting agents (e.g., antipsychotics) if used concomitantly with diazepam).
No products indexed under this heading.

Quinidine (There is a potentially relevant interaction between diazepam and certain hepatic enzyme inhibitors such as CYP450 3A4. It has been shown that these compounds influence the pharmacokinetics of diazepam and may lead to increased and prolonged sedation).
No products indexed under this heading.

Quinidine Hydrochloride (There is a potentially relevant interaction between diazepam and certain hepatic enzyme inhibitors such as CYP450 3A4. It has been shown that these compounds influence the pharmacokinetics of diazepam and may lead to increased and prolonged sedation).
No products indexed under this heading.

Quinidine Polygalacturonate (There is a potentially relevant interaction between diazepam and certain hepatic enzyme inhibitors such as CYP450 3A4. It has been shown that these compounds influence the pharmacokinetics of diazepam and may lead to increased and prolonged sedation).
No products indexed under this heading.

Quinidine Sulfate (There is a potentially relevant interaction between diazepam and certain hepatic enzyme inhibitors such as CYP450 3A4. It has been shown that these compounds influence the pharmacokinetics of diazepam and may lead to increased and prolonged sedation).
No products indexed under this heading.

Quinine (There is a potentially relevant interaction between diazepam and certain hepatic enzyme inhibitors such as CYP450 3A4. It has been shown that these compounds influence the pharmacokinetics of diazepam and may lead to increased and prolonged sedation).
No products indexed under this heading.

Quinine Sulfate (There is a potentially relevant interaction between diazepam and certain hepatic enzyme inhibitors such as CYP450 3A4. It has been shown that these compounds influence the pharmacokinetics of diazepam and may lead to increased and prolonged sedation).
No products indexed under this heading.

Quinupristin (There is a potentially relevant interaction between diazepam and certain hepatic enzyme inhibitors such as CYP450 3A4. It has been shown that these compounds influence the pharmacokinetics of diazepam and may lead to increased and prolonged sedation).
No products indexed under this heading.

Ramelteon (Careful considerations should be given to the pharmacology of other centrally acting agents (e.g., sedatives and hypnotics) if used concomitantly with diazepam). Products include:
Rozerem Tablets **3091**

Ranitidine Bismuth Citrate (There is a potentially relevant interaction between diazepam and certain hepatic enzyme inhibitors such as CYP450 3A4. It has been shown that these compounds influence the pharmacokinetics of diazepam and may lead to increased and prolonged sedation).
No products indexed under this heading.

Ranitidine Hydrochloride (There is a potentially relevant interaction between diazepam and certain hepatic enzyme inhibitors such as CYP450 3A4. It has been shown that these compounds influence the pharmacokinetics of diazepam and may lead to increased and prolonged sedation). Products include:
Zantac 75 Tablets **603**
Zantac **1670**
Zantac Injection **1666**
Zantac Injection Pharmacy Bulk Package **1668**
Maximum Strength Zantac 150 Tablets **603**
Maximum Strength Zantac 150 Cool Mint Tablets **603**

Rasagiline Mesylate (Careful considerations should be given to the pharmacology of other centrally acting agents (e.g., MAO inhibitors) if used concomitantly with diazepam). Products include:
Azilect Tablets **3106**

Remifentanil Hydrochloride (Careful considerations should be given to the pharmacology of other centrally acting agents (e.g., narcotics) if used concomitantly with diazepam).
No products indexed under this heading.

Risperidone (Careful considerations should be given to the pharmacology of other centrally acting agents (e.g., antipsychotics) if used concomitantly with diazepam). Products include:
Risperdal Consta Long-Acting Injection **1753**

Ritonavir (There is a potentially relevant interaction between diazepam and certain hepatic enzyme inhibitors such as CYP450 3A4. It has been shown that these compounds influence the pharmacokinetics of diazepam and may lead to increased and prolonged sedation). Products include:

Kaletra 452
Norvir 489

Saquinavir (There is a potentially relevant interaction between diazepam and certain hepatic enzyme inhibitors such as CYP450 3A4. It has been shown that these compounds influence the pharmacokinetics of diazepam and may lead to increased and prolonged sedation).
No products indexed under this heading.

Saquinavir Mesylate (There is a potentially relevant interaction between diazepam and certain hepatic enzyme inhibitors such as CYP450 3A4. It has been shown that these compounds influence the pharmacokinetics of diazepam and may lead to increased and prolonged sedation).
No products indexed under this heading.

Secobarbital Sodium (Careful considerations should be given to the pharmacology of other centrally acting agents (e.g., sedatives and hypnotics) if used concomitantly with diazepam).
No products indexed under this heading.

Selegiline (Careful considerations should be given to the pharmacology of other centrally acting agents (e.g., MAO inhibitors) if used concomitantly with diazepam). Products include:

Emsam Transdermal System 905

Selegiline Hydrochloride (Careful considerations should be given to the pharmacology of other centrally acting agents (e.g., MAO inhibitors) if used concomitantly with diazepam). Products include:

Eldepryl Capsules 3052

Sertraline Hydrochloride (Careful considerations should be given to the pharmacology of other centrally acting agents (e.g., antidepressants) if used concomitantly with diazepam).
No products indexed under this heading.

Sildenafil Citrate (There is a potentially relevant interaction between diazepam and certain hepatic enzyme inhibitors such as CYP450 3A4. It has been shown that these compounds influence the pharmacokinetics of diazepam and may lead to increased and prolonged sedation).
No products indexed under this heading.

Sodium Bicarbonate (Diazepam peak concentrations are lower when antacids are administered concurrently. The peak concentrations appear to be lower due to a slower rate of absorption, with the time required to achieve peak concentration on average 20 to 25 minutes greater in the presence of antacids). Products include:

Ceo-Two Laxative Suppository 815

Sodium Butabarbital (Careful considerations should be given to the pharmacology of other centrally acting agents (e.g., sedatives and hypnotics) if used concomitantly with diazepam).
No products indexed under this heading.

Sufentanil Citrate (Careful considerations should be given to the pharmacology of other centrally acting agents (e.g., narcotics) if used concomitantly with diazepam).
No products indexed under this heading.

Sulfaphenazole (There is a potentially relevant interaction between diazepam and certain hepatic enzyme inhibitors such as CYP450 2C19. It has been shown that these compounds influence the pharmacokinetics of diazepam and may lead to increased and prolonged sedation).
No products indexed under this heading.

Telithromycin (There is a potentially relevant interaction between diazepam and certain hepatic enzyme inhibitors such as CYP450 3A4. It has been shown that these compounds influence the pharmacokinetics of diazepam and may lead to increased and prolonged sedation). Products include:

Ketek Tablets 2744

Telmisartan (There is a potentially relevant interaction between diazepam and certain hepatic enzyme inhibitors such as CYP450 2C19. It has been shown that these compounds influence the pharmacokinetics of diazepam and may lead to increased and prolonged sedation). Products include:

Micardis Tablets 852
Micardis HCT Tablets 854

Temazepam (Careful considerations should be given to the pharmacology of other centrally acting agents (e.g., sedatives and hypnotics) if used concomitantly with diazepam).
No products indexed under this heading.

Thiamylal Sodium (Careful considerations should be given to the pharmacology of other centrally acting agents (e.g., barbiturates) if used concomitantly with diazepam).
No products indexed under this heading.

Thioridazine Hydrochloride (Careful considerations should be given to the pharmacology of other centrally acting agents (e.g., phenothiazines) if used concomitantly with diazepam). Products include:

Thioridazine Hydrochloride Tablets 2195

Thiothixene (Careful considerations should be given to the pharmacology of other centrally acting agents (e.g., antipsychotics) if used concomitantly with diazepam). Products include:

Thiothixene Capsules 2197

Tiagabine Hydrochloride (Careful considerations should be given to the pharmacology of other centrally acting agents (e.g., anticonvulsants) if used concomitantly with diazepam). Products include:

Gabitril Tablets 973

Ticlopidine Hydrochloride (There is a potentially relevant interaction between diazepam and certain hepatic enzyme inhibitors such as CYP450 2C19. It has been shown that these compounds influence the pharmacokinetics of diazepam and may lead to increased and prolonged sedation).
No products indexed under this heading.

Tolbutamide (There is a potentially relevant interaction between diazepam and certain hepatic enzyme inhibitors such as CYP450 2C19. It has been shown that these compounds influence the pharmacokinetics of diazepam and may lead to increased and prolonged sedation).
No products indexed under this heading.

Tolbutamide Sodium (There is a potentially relevant interaction between diazepam and certain hepatic enzyme inhibitors such as CYP450 2C19. It has been shown that these compounds influence the pharmacokinetics of diazepam and may lead to increased and prolonged sedation).
No products indexed under this heading.

Topiramate (Careful considerations should be given to the pharmacology of other centrally acting agents (e.g., anticonvulsants) if used concomitantly with diazepam).
No products indexed under this heading.

Tranylcypromine Sulfate (Careful considerations should be given to the pharmacology of other centrally acting agents (e.g., MAO inhibitors) if used concomitantly with diazepam). Products include:

Parnate Tablets 1532

Trazodone Hydrochloride (Careful considerations should be given to the pharmacology of other centrally acting agents (e.g., antidepressants) if used concomitantly with diazepam).
No products indexed under this heading.

Triazolam (Careful considerations should be given to the pharmacology of other centrally acting agents (e.g., sedatives and hypnotics) if used concomitantly with diazepam).
No products indexed under this heading.

Trifluoperazine Hydrochloride (Careful considerations should be given to the pharmacology of other centrally acting agents (e.g., phenothiazines) if used concomitantly with diazepam).
No products indexed under this heading.

Trimeprazine Tartrate (Careful considerations should be given to the pharmacology of other centrally acting agents (e.g., sedating antihistamines) if used concomitantly with diazepam).
No products indexed under this heading.

Trimethadione (Careful considerations should be given to the pharmacology of other centrally acting agents (e.g., anticonvulsants) if used concomitantly with diazepam).
No products indexed under this heading.

Trimipramine Maleate (Careful considerations should be given to the pharmacology of other centrally acting agents (e.g., antidepressants) if used concomitantly with diazepam).
No products indexed under this heading.

Tripelennamine Hydrochloride (Careful considerations should be given to the pharmacology of other centrally acting agents (e.g., sedating antihistamines) if used concomitantly with diazepam).
No products indexed under this heading.

Triprolidine Hydrochloride (Careful considerations should be given to the pharmacology of other centrally acting agents (e.g., sedating antihistamines) if used concomitantly with diazepam).
No products indexed under this heading.

Troglitazone (There is a potentially relevant interaction between diazepam and certain hepatic enzyme inhibitors such as CYP450 3A4. It has been shown that these compounds influence the pharmacokinetics of diazepam and may lead to increased and prolonged sedation).
No products indexed under this heading.

Troleandomycin (There is a potentially relevant interaction between diazepam and certain hepatic enzyme inhibitors such as CYP450 3A4. It has been shown that these compounds influence the pharmacokinetics of diazepam and may lead to increased and prolonged sedation).
No products indexed under this heading.

Valproate Sodium (Careful considerations should be given to the pharmacology of other centrally acting agents (e.g., anticonvulsants) if used concomitantly with diazepam).
No products indexed under this heading.

Valproic Acid (Careful considerations should be given to the pharmacology of other centrally acting agents (e.g., anticonvulsants) if used concomitantly with diazepam).
No products indexed under this heading.

Vardenafil Hydrochloride (There is a potentially relevant interaction between diazepam and certain hepatic enzyme inhibitors such as CYP450 3A4. It has been shown that these compounds influence the pharmacokinetics of diazepam and may lead to increased and prolonged sedation). Products include:

Levitra Tablets 2876

Venlafaxine Hydrochloride (Careful considerations should be given to the pharmacology of other centrally acting agents (e.g., antidepressants) if used concomitantly with diazepam). Products include:

Effexor XR Extended-Release Capsules 3195
Venlafaxine Hydrochloride Tablets ... 2199

Verapamil Hydrochloride (There is a potentially relevant interaction between diazepam and certain hepatic enzyme inhibitors such as CYP450 3A4. It has been shown that these compounds influence the pharmacokinetics of diazepam and may lead to increased and prolonged sedation). Products include:

Tarka Tablets 511

Voriconazole (There is a potentially relevant interaction between diazepam and certain hepatic enzyme inhibitors such as CYP450 3A4. It has been shown that these compounds influence the pharmacokinetics of diazepam and may lead to increased and prolonged sedation).
No products indexed under this heading.

Zafirlukast (There is a potentially relevant interaction between diazepam and certain hepatic enzyme inhibitors such as CYP450 3A4. It has been shown that these compounds influence the pharmacokinetics of diazepam and may lead to increased and prolonged sedation). Products include:
Accolate Tablets 669

Zaleplon (Careful considerations should be given to the pharmacology of other centrally acting agents (e.g., sedatives and hypnotics) if used concomitantly with diazepam).
No products indexed under this heading.

Zileuton (There is a potentially relevant interaction between diazepam and certain hepatic enzyme inhibitors such as CYP450 3A4. It has been shown that these compounds influence the pharmacokinetics of diazepam and may lead to increased and prolonged sedation).
No products indexed under this heading.

Ziprasidone Hydrochloride (Careful considerations should be given to the pharmacology of other centrally acting agents (e.g., antipsychotics) if used concomitantly with diazepam). Products include:
Geodon Capsules 2520

Zolpidem Tartrate (Careful considerations should be given to the pharmacology of other centrally acting agents (e.g., sedatives and hypnotics) if used concomitantly with diazepam). Products include:
Ambien Tablets 2692
Ambien CR Tablets 2696

Zonisamide (Careful considerations should be given to the pharmacology of other centrally acting agents (e.g., anticonvulsants) if used concomitantly with diazepam). Products include:
Zonegran Capsules 1089

Food Interactions

Alcohol (Concomitant use with alcohol is not recommended due to enhancement of the sedative effect).

Grapefruit (There is a potentially relevant interaction between diazepam and certain hepatic enzyme inhibitors such as CYP450 3A4. It has been shown that these compounds influence the pharmacokinetics of diazepam and may lead to increased and prolonged sedation).

Grapefruit Juice (There is a potentially relevant interaction between diazepam and certain hepatic enzyme inhibitors such as CYP450 3A4. It has been shown that these compounds influence the pharmacokinetics of diazepam and may lead to increased and prolonged sedation).

VALSTAR STERILE SOLUTION FOR INTRAVESICAL INSTILLATION
(Valrubicin) 1735
None cited in PDR database.

VALTREX CAPLETS
(Valacyclovir Hydrochloride) 1635
May interact with:

Cimetidine (Co-administration reduces renal clearance of acyclovir causing an increase in acyclovir AUC and Cmax).
No products indexed under this heading.

Cimetidine Hydrochloride (Co-administration reduces renal clearance of acyclovir causing an increase in acyclovir AUC and Cmax).
No products indexed under this heading.

Probenecid (Co-administration reduces renal clearance of acyclovir causing an increase in acyclovir AUC and Cmax).
No products indexed under this heading.

VANOS CREAM
(Fluocinonide) 1941
None cited in PDR database.

VANTAS
(Histrelin Acetate) 1737
None cited in PDR database.

VAPRISOL
(Conivaptan Hydrochloride) 632
May interact with cytochrome p450 3a4 inhibitors (selected), cytochrome p450 3a4 inhibitors, potent, cytochrome p450 3a4 substrates (selected), and certain other agents. Compounds in these categories include:

Acetazolamide (Conivaptan is a substrate of CYP3A4. Co-administration of conivaptan with CYP3A4 inhibitors could lead to an increase in conivaptan concentrations. Concomitant use of conivaptan with potent CYP3A4 inhibitors is contraindicated).
No products indexed under this heading.

Alfentanil Hydrochloride (Conivaptan is a potent inhibitor of CYP3A4. Conivaptan may increase plasma concentrations of co-administered drugs that are primarily metabolized by CYP3A4).
No products indexed under this heading.

Alprazolam (Conivaptan is a potent inhibitor of CYP3A4. Conivaptan may increase plasma concentrations of co-administered drugs that are primarily metabolized by CYP3A4).
No products indexed under this heading.

Amiodarone Hydrochloride (Conivaptan is a substrate of CYP3A4. Co-administration of conivaptan with CYP3A4 inhibitors could lead to an increase in conivaptan concentrations. Concomitant use of conivaptan with potent CYP3A4 inhibitors is contraindicated).
No products indexed under this heading.

Amitriptyline Hydrochloride (Conivaptan is a potent inhibitor of CYP3A4. Conivaptan may increase plasma concentrations of co-administered drugs that are primarily metabolized by CYP3A4).
No products indexed under this heading.

Amlodipine Besylate (Conivaptan is a potent inhibitor of CYP3A4. Conivaptan may increase plasma concentrations of co-administered drugs that are primarily metabolized by CYP3A4). Products include:
Azor Tablets 1005
Exforge Tablets 2238

Amprenavir (Conivaptan is a substrate of CYP3A4. Co-administration of conivaptan with CYP3A4 inhibitors could lead to an increase in conivaptan concentrations. Concomitant use of conivaptan with potent CYP3A4 inhibitors is contraindicated).
No products indexed under this heading.

Anastrozole (Conivaptan is a substrate of CYP3A4. Co-administration of conivaptan with CYP3A4 inhibitors could lead to an increase in conivaptan concentrations. Concomitant use of conivaptan with potent CYP3A4 inhibitors is contraindicated). Products include:
Arimidex Tablets 672

Aprepitant (Conivaptan is a substrate of CYP3A4. Co-administration of conivaptan with CYP3A4 inhibitors could lead to an increase in conivaptan concentrations. Concomitant use of conivaptan with potent CYP3A4 inhibitors is contraindicated). Products include:
Emend Capsules 1992

Astemizole (Conivaptan is a potent inhibitor of CYP3A4. Conivaptan may increase plasma concentrations of co-administered drugs that are primarily metabolized by CYP3A4).
No products indexed under this heading.

Atazanavir (Conivaptan is a substrate of CYP3A4. Co-administration of conivaptan with CYP3A4 inhibitors could lead to an increase in conivaptan concentrations. Concomitant use of conivaptan with potent CYP3A4 inhibitors is contraindicated).
No products indexed under this heading.

Atazanavir Sulfate (Conivaptan is a substrate of CYP3A4. Co-administration of conivaptan with CYP3A4 inhibitors could lead to an increase in conivaptan concentrations. Concomitant use of conivaptan with potent CYP3A4 inhibitors is contraindicated). Products include:
Reyataz Capsules 3299

Atorvastatin Calcium (Conivaptan is a potent inhibitor of CYP3A4. Conivaptan may increase plasma concentrations of co-administered drugs that are primarily metabolized by CYP3A4). Products include:
Lipitor Tablets 2501

Belladonna Ergotamine (Conivaptan is a potent inhibitor of CYP3A4. Conivaptan may increase plasma concentrations of co-administered drugs that are primarily metabolized by CYP3A4).
No products indexed under this heading.

Buspirone Hydrochloride (Conivaptan is a potent inhibitor of CYP3A4. Conivaptan may increase plasma concentrations of co-administered drugs that are primarily metabolized by CYP3A4).
No products indexed under this heading.

Busulfan (Conivaptan is a potent inhibitor of CYP3A4. Conivaptan may increase plasma concentrations of co-administered drugs that are primarily metabolized by CYP3A4). Products include:
Busulfex Injection 2477
Myleran Tablets 1530

Carbamazepine (Conivaptan is a potent inhibitor of CYP3A4. Conivaptan may increase plasma concentrations of co-administered drugs that are primarily metabolized by CYP3A4). Products include:
Carbatrol Capsules 3019
Equetro Extended-Release Capsules 3174

Cerivastatin Sodium (Conivaptan is a potent inhibitor of CYP3A4. Conivaptan may increase plasma concentrations of co-administered drugs that are primarily metabolized by CYP3A4).
No products indexed under this heading.

Chlorpheniramine (Conivaptan is a potent inhibitor of CYP3A4. Conivaptan may increase plasma concentrations of co-administered drugs that are primarily metabolized by CYP3A4).
No products indexed under this heading.

Chlorpheniramine Maleate (Conivaptan is a potent inhibitor of CYP3A4. Conivaptan may increase plasma concentrations of co-administered drugs that are primarily metabolized by CYP3A4). Products include:
Actifed Cold & Allergy Tablets 1895
Sudafed PE Sinus & Allergy Tablets 1908
Tylenol Allergy Multi-Symptom Caplets with Cool Burst and Rapid Release Gelcaps 1916
Children's Tylenol Plus Cold Suspension Liquid 1912
Children's Tylenol Plus Cough & Runny Nose Suspension Liquid 1912
Children's Tylenol Plus Flu Suspension Liquid 1914
Children's Tylenol Plus Multi-Symptom Cold Suspension Liquid 1912
Tylenol Cold Head Congestion Nighttime Caplets with Cool Burst 1910
Tylenol Cold Multi-Symptom Nighttime Caplets with Cool Burst 1913
Tylenol Sinus Congestion & Pain Nighttime Caplets with Cool Burst 1917

Chlorpheniramine Polistirex (Conivaptan is a potent inhibitor of CYP3A4. Conivaptan may increase plasma concentrations of co-administered drugs that are primarily metabolized by CYP3A4). Products include:
Tussionex Pennkinetic Extended-Release Suspension 3154

Chlorpheniramine Tannate (Conivaptan is a potent inhibitor of CYP3A4. Conivaptan may increase plasma concentrations of co-administered drugs that are primarily metabolized by CYP3A4).
No products indexed under this heading.

Cimetidine (Conivaptan is a substrate of CYP3A4. Co-administration of conivaptan with CYP3A4 inhibitors could lead to an increase in conivaptan concentrations. Concomitant use of conivaptan with potent CYP3A4 inhibitors is contraindicated).
No products indexed under this heading.

Cimetidine Hydrochloride (Conivaptan is a substrate of CYP3A4. Co-administration of conivaptan with CYP3A4 inhibitors could lead to an increase in conivaptan concentrations. Concomitant use of conivaptan with potent CYP3A4 inhibitors is contraindicated).
No products indexed under this heading.

Ciprofloxacin (Conivaptan is a substrate of CYP3A4. Co-administration of conivaptan with CYP3A4 inhibitors could lead to an increase in conivaptan concentrations. Concomitant use of conivaptan with potent CYP3A4 inhibitors is contraindicated).
Products include:
- Cipro I.V. 2817
- Cipro Oral Suspension 2810
- Cipro XR Tablets 2823
- Ciprodex Otic Suspension 541

Cisapride (Conivaptan is a potent inhibitor of CYP3A4. Conivaptan may increase plasma concentrations of co-administered drugs that are primarily metabolized by CYP3A4).
No products indexed under this heading.

Clarithromycin (Conivaptan is a substrate of CYP3A4. Co-administration of conivaptan with CYP3A4 inhibitors could lead to an increase in conivaptan concentrations. Concomitant use of conivaptan with potent CYP3A4 inhibitors is contraindicated). Products include:
- Biaxin/Biaxin XL 411

Clotrimazole (Conivaptan is a substrate of CYP3A4. Co-administration of conivaptan with CYP3A4 inhibitors could lead to an increase in conivaptan concentrations. Concomitant use of conivaptan with potent CYP3A4 inhibitors is contraindicated).
Products include:
- Lotrisone 2881

Cyclosporine (Conivaptan is a substrate of CYP3A4. Co-administration of conivaptan with CYP3A4 inhibitors could lead to an increase in conivaptan concentrations. Concomitant use of conivaptan with potent CYP3A4 inhibitors is contraindicated).
Products include:
- Gengraf Capsules 435
- Neoral Oral Solution 2280
- Neoral Soft Gelatin Capsules 2280
- Restasis Ophthalmic Emulsion 557
- Sandimmune 2296

Dalfopristin (Conivaptan is a substrate of CYP3A4. Co-administration of conivaptan with CYP3A4 inhibitors could lead to an increase in conivaptan concentrations. Concomitant use of conivaptan with potent CYP3A4 inhibitors is contraindicated).
No products indexed under this heading.

Danazol (Conivaptan is a substrate of CYP3A4. Co-administration of conivaptan with CYP3A4 inhibitors could lead to an increase in conivaptan concentrations. Concomitant use of conivaptan with potent CYP3A4 inhibitors is contraindicated).
No products indexed under this heading.

Delavirdine Mesylate (Conivaptan is a substrate of CYP3A4. Co-administration of conivaptan with CYP3A4 inhibitors could lead to an increase in conivaptan concentrations. Concomitant use of conivaptan with potent CYP3A4 inhibitors is contraindicated).
No products indexed under this heading.

Delavirdine Mesylate (Conivaptan is a substrate of CYP3A4. Co-administration of conivaptan with CYP3A4 inhibitors could lead to an increase in conivaptan concentrations. Concomitant use of conivaptan with potent CYP3A4 inhibitors is contraindicated).
No products indexed under this heading.

Delavirine (Conivaptan is a substrate of CYP3A4. Co-administration of conivaptan with CYP3A4 inhibitors could lead to an increase in conivaptan concentrations. Concomitant use of conivaptan with potent CYP3A4 inhibitors is contraindicated).
No products indexed under this heading.

Desogestrel (Conivaptan is a potent inhibitor of CYP3A4. Conivaptan may increase plasma concentrations of co-administered drugs that are primarily metabolized by CYP3A4). Products include:
- Mircette Tablets 1034

Diazepam (Conivaptan is a potent inhibitor of CYP3A4. Conivaptan may increase plasma concentrations of co-administered drugs that are primarily metabolized by CYP3A4).
Products include:
- Valium Tablets 2658

Digoxin (Co-administration of digoxin, a P-glycoprotein substrate, with oral conivaptan resulted in a reduction in clearance and an increase in digoxin Cmax and AUC values. Therefore, co-administration may result in increased digoxin levels).
Products include:
- Lanoxin Injection 1498
- Lanoxin Injection Pediatric 1502
- Lanoxin Tablets 1505

Dihydroergotamine Mesylate (Conivaptan is a potent inhibitor of CYP3A4. Conivaptan may increase plasma concentrations of co-administered drugs that are primarily metabolized by CYP3A4).
No products indexed under this heading.

Diltiazem Hydrochloride (Conivaptan is a substrate of CYP3A4. Co-administration of conivaptan with CYP3A4 inhibitors could lead to an increase in conivaptan concentrations. Concomitant use of conivaptan with potent CYP3A4 inhibitors is contraindicated).
Products include:
- Cardizem LA Extended Release Tablets 421

Diltiazem Maleate (Conivaptan is a substrate of CYP3A4. Co-administration of conivaptan with CYP3A4 inhibitors could lead to an increase in conivaptan concentrations. Concomitant use of conivaptan with potent CYP3A4 inhibitors is contraindicated).
No products indexed under this heading.

Disopyramide (Conivaptan is a potent inhibitor of CYP3A4. Conivaptan may increase plasma concentrations of co-administered drugs that are primarily metabolized by CYP3A4).
No products indexed under this heading.

Disopyramide Phosphate (Conivaptan is a potent inhibitor of CYP3A4. Conivaptan may increase plasma concentrations of co-administered drugs that are primarily metabolized by CYP3A4).
No products indexed under this heading.

Disulfiram (Conivaptan is a potent inhibitor of CYP3A4. Conivaptan may increase plasma concentrations of co-administered drugs that are primarily metabolized by CYP3A4).
No products indexed under this heading.

Doxorubicin Hydrochloride (Conivaptan is a potent inhibitor of CYP3A4. Conivaptan may increase plasma concentrations of co-administered drugs that are primarily metabolized by CYP3A4).
No products indexed under this heading.

Dronabinol (Conivaptan is a potent inhibitor of CYP3A4. Conivaptan may increase plasma concentrations of co-administered drugs that are primarily metabolized by CYP3A4).
Products include:
- Marinol Capsules 3163

Efavirenz (Conivaptan is a substrate of CYP3A4. Co-administration of conivaptan with CYP3A4 inhibitors could lead to an increase in conivaptan concentrations. Concomitant use of conivaptan with potent CYP3A4 inhibitors is contraindicated).
Products include:
- Atripla Tablets 938
- Sustiva Capsules 930
- Sustiva Tablets 930

Ergotamine Tartrate (Conivaptan is a potent inhibitor of CYP3A4. Conivaptan may increase plasma concentrations of co-administered drugs that are primarily metabolized by CYP3A4).
No products indexed under this heading.

Erythromycin (Conivaptan is a substrate of CYP3A4. Co-administration of conivaptan with CYP3A4 inhibitors could lead to an increase in conivaptan concentrations. Concomitant use of conivaptan with potent CYP3A4 inhibitors is contraindicated).
No products indexed under this heading.

Erythromycin Estolate (Conivaptan is a substrate of CYP3A4. Co-administration of conivaptan with CYP3A4 inhibitors could lead to an increase in conivaptan concentrations. Concomitant use of conivaptan with potent CYP3A4 inhibitors is contraindicated).
No products indexed under this heading.

Erythromycin Ethylsuccinate (Conivaptan is a substrate of CYP3A4. Co-administration of conivaptan with CYP3A4 inhibitors could lead to an increase in conivaptan concentrations. Concomitant use of conivaptan with potent CYP3A4 inhibitors is contraindicated).
Products include:
- E.E.S. 433
- EryPed 431

Erythromycin Gluceptate (Conivaptan is a substrate of CYP3A4. Co-administration of conivaptan with CYP3A4 inhibitors could lead to an increase in conivaptan concentrations. Concomitant use of conivaptan with potent CYP3A4 inhibitors is contraindicated).
No products indexed under this heading.

Erythromycin Lactobionate (Conivaptan is a substrate of CYP3A4. Co-administration of conivaptan with CYP3A4 inhibitors could lead to an increase in conivaptan concentrations. Concomitant use of conivaptan with potent CYP3A4 inhibitors is contraindicated).
No products indexed under this heading.

Erythromycin Stearate (Conivaptan is a substrate of CYP3A4. Co-administration of conivaptan with CYP3A4 inhibitors could lead to an increase in conivaptan concentrations. Concomitant use of conivaptan with potent CYP3A4 inhibitors is contraindicated).
No products indexed under this heading.

Esomeprazole Magnesium (Conivaptan is a substrate of CYP3A4. Co-administration of conivaptan with CYP3A4 inhibitors could lead to an increase in conivaptan concentrations. Concomitant use of conivaptan with potent CYP3A4 inhibitors is contraindicated).
Products include:
- Nexium Delayed-Release Capsules 645
- Nexium Delayed-Release Oral Suspension 645

Estradiol (Conivaptan is a potent inhibitor of CYP3A4. Conivaptan may increase plasma concentrations of co-administered drugs that are primarily metabolized by CYP3A4).
Products include:
- Activella Tablets 2347
- Angeliq Tablets 751
- Climara Transdermal System 763
- Climara Pro Transdermal System 768
- Divigel 3167
- Vagifem Tablets 2375

Estradiol Benzoate (Conivaptan is a potent inhibitor of CYP3A4. Conivaptan may increase plasma concentrations of co-administered drugs that are primarily metabolized by CYP3A4).
No products indexed under this heading.

Estradiol Cypionate (Conivaptan is a potent inhibitor of CYP3A4. Conivaptan may increase plasma concentrations of co-administered drugs that are primarily metabolized by CYP3A4).
No products indexed under this heading.

Estradiol Valerate (Conivaptan is a potent inhibitor of CYP3A4. Conivaptan may increase plasma concentrations of co-administered drugs that are primarily metabolized by CYP3A4).
No products indexed under this heading.

Ethinyl Estradiol (Conivaptan is a potent inhibitor of CYP3A4. Conivaptan may increase plasma concentrations of co-administered drugs that are primarily metabolized by CYP3A4). Products include:
- Lybrel Tablets 3204
- Mircette Tablets 1034

NuvaRing 2897
Ortho-Cyclen/Ortho Tri-Cyclen 2449
Ortho Evra Transdermal System 2437
Ortho Tri-Cyclen Lo Tablets 2458
Seasonique Tablets 1046
Yaz Tablets 805

Ethosuximide (Conivaptan is a potent inhibitor of CYP3A4. Conivaptan may increase plasma concentrations of co-administered drugs that are primarily metabolized by CYP3A4).
No products indexed under this heading.

Ethynodiol Diacetate (Conivaptan is a potent inhibitor of CYP3A4. Conivaptan may increase plasma concentrations of co-administered drugs that are primarily metabolized by CYP3A4).
No products indexed under this heading.

Etoposide (Conivaptan is a potent inhibitor of CYP3A4. Conivaptan may increase plasma concentrations of co-administered drugs that are primarily metabolized by CYP3A4).
No products indexed under this heading.

Etoposide Phosphate (Conivaptan is a potent inhibitor of CYP3A4. Conivaptan may increase plasma concentrations of co-administered drugs that are primarily metabolized by CYP3A4).
No products indexed under this heading.

Felodipine (Conivaptan is a potent inhibitor of CYP3A4. Conivaptan may increase plasma concentrations of co-administered drugs that are primarily metabolized by CYP3A4).
No products indexed under this heading.

Fentanyl (Conivaptan is a potent inhibitor of CYP3A4. Conivaptan may increase plasma concentrations of co-administered drugs that are primarily metabolized by CYP3A4). Products include:
Duragesic Transdermal System 2405
Ionsys Transdermal System 2410

Fentanyl Citrate (Conivaptan is a potent inhibitor of CYP3A4. Conivaptan may increase plasma concentrations of co-administered drugs that are primarily metabolized by CYP3A4). Products include:
Actiq 959
Fentora Tablets 968

Fluconazole (Conivaptan is a substrate of CYP3A4. Co-administration of conivaptan with CYP3A4 inhibitors could lead to an increase in conivaptan concentrations. Concomitant use of conivaptan with potent CYP3A4 inhibitors is contraindicated).
No products indexed under this heading.

Fluoxetine (Conivaptan is a substrate of CYP3A4. Co-administration of conivaptan with CYP3A4 inhibitors could lead to an increase in conivaptan concentrations. Concomitant use of conivaptan with potent CYP3A4 inhibitors is contraindicated).
No products indexed under this heading.

Fluoxetine Hydrochloride (Conivaptan is a substrate of CYP3A4. Co-administration of conivaptan with CYP3A4 inhibitors could lead to an increase in conivaptan concentrations. Concomitant use of conivaptan with potent CYP3A4 inhibitors is contraindicated). Products include:
Prozac Weekly Capsules 1852
Prozac Pulvules and Liquid 1852
Symbyax Capsules 1871

Fluvoxamine Maleate (Conivaptan is a substrate of CYP3A4. Co-administration of conivaptan with CYP3A4 inhibitors could lead to an increase in conivaptan concentrations. Concomitant use of conivaptan with potent CYP3A4 inhibitors is contraindicated). Products include:
Luvox CR Extended-Release Capsules 1759

Fosamprenavir Calcium (Conivaptan is a substrate of CYP3A4. Co-administration of conivaptan with CYP3A4 inhibitors could lead to an increase in conivaptan concentrations. Concomitant use of conivaptan with potent CYP3A4 inhibitors is contraindicated). Products include:
Lexiva Oral Suspension 1510
Lexiva Tablets 1510

Haloperidol (Conivaptan is a potent inhibitor of CYP3A4. Conivaptan may increase plasma concentrations of co-administered drugs that are primarily metabolized by CYP3A4).
No products indexed under this heading.

Haloperidol Decanoate (Conivaptan is a potent inhibitor of CYP3A4. Conivaptan may increase plasma concentrations of co-administered drugs that are primarily metabolized by CYP3A4).
No products indexed under this heading.

Haloperidol Lactate (Conivaptan is a potent inhibitor of CYP3A4. Conivaptan may increase plasma concentrations of co-administered drugs that are primarily metabolized by CYP3A4).
No products indexed under this heading.

Indinavir Sulfate (Conivaptan is a substrate of CYP3A4. Co-administration of conivaptan with CYP3A4 inhibitors could lead to an increase in conivaptan concentrations. Concomitant use of conivaptan with potent CYP3A4 inhibitors is contraindicated). Products include:
Crixivan Capsules 1979

Isoniazid (Conivaptan is a substrate of CYP3A4. Co-administration of conivaptan with CYP3A4 inhibitors could lead to an increase in conivaptan concentrations. Concomitant use of conivaptan with potent CYP3A4 inhibitors is contraindicated).
No products indexed under this heading.

Isradipine (Conivaptan is a potent inhibitor of CYP3A4. Conivaptan may increase plasma concentrations of co-administered drugs that are primarily metabolized by CYP3A4). Products include:
DynaCirc CR Controlled Release Tablets 1407

Itraconazole (Conivaptan is a substrate of CYP3A4. Co-administration of conivaptan with CYP3A4 inhibitors could lead to an increase in conivaptan concentrations. Concomitant use of conivaptan with potent CYP3A4 inhibitors is contraindicated).
No products indexed under this heading.

Ixabepilone (Conivaptan is a potent inhibitor of CYP3A4. Conivaptan may increase plasma concentrations of co-administered drugs that are primarily metabolized by CYP3A4). Products include:
Ixempra Kit for Injection 915

Ketoconazole (Conivaptan is a substrate of CYP3A4. Co-administration of conivaptan with CYP3A4 inhibitors could lead to an increase in conivaptan concentrations. Concomitant use of conivaptan with potent CYP3A4 inhibitors is contraindicated). Products include:
Extina Foam, 2% 3057
Nizoral A-D Shampoo 1901

Levonorgestrel (Conivaptan is a potent inhibitor of CYP3A4. Conivaptan may increase plasma concentrations of co-administered drugs that are primarily metabolized by CYP3A4). Products include:
Climara Pro Transdermal System 768
Lybrel Tablets 3204
Mirena Intrauterine System 779
Plan B Tablets 1044
Seasonique Tablets 1046

Lidocaine (Conivaptan is a potent inhibitor of CYP3A4. Conivaptan may increase plasma concentrations of co-administered drugs that are primarily metabolized by CYP3A4). Products include:
Lidoderm Patch 1114

Lidocaine Hydrochloride (Conivaptan is a potent inhibitor of CYP3A4. Conivaptan may increase plasma concentrations of co-administered drugs that are primarily metabolized by CYP3A4).
No products indexed under this heading.

Lopinavir (Conivaptan is a substrate of CYP3A4. Co-administration of conivaptan with CYP3A4 inhibitors could lead to an increase in conivaptan concentrations. Concomitant use of conivaptan with potent CYP3A4 inhibitors is contraindicated). Products include:
Kaletra 452

Loratadine (Conivaptan is a substrate of CYP3A4. Co-administration of conivaptan with CYP3A4 inhibitors could lead to an increase in conivaptan concentrations. Concomitant use of conivaptan with potent CYP3A4 inhibitors is contraindicated).
No products indexed under this heading.

Lovastatin (Conivaptan is a potent inhibitor of CYP3A4. Conivaptan may increase plasma concentrations of co-administered drugs that are primarily metabolized by CYP3A4). Products include:
Advicor Tablets 402
Mevacor Tablets 2063

Mestranol (Conivaptan is a potent inhibitor of CYP3A4. Conivaptan may increase plasma concentrations of co-administered drugs that are primarily metabolized by CYP3A4).
No products indexed under this heading.

Methadone Hydrochloride (Conivaptan is a potent inhibitor of CYP3A4. Conivaptan may increase plasma concentrations of co-administered drugs that are primarily metabolized by CYP3A4).
No products indexed under this heading.

Metronidazole (Conivaptan is a substrate of CYP3A4. Co-administration of conivaptan with CYP3A4 inhibitors could lead to an increase in conivaptan concentrations. Concomitant use of conivaptan with potent CYP3A4 inhibitors is contraindicated). Products include:
Pylera Capsules 714

Metronidazole Benzoate (Conivaptan is a substrate of CYP3A4. Co-administration of conivaptan with CYP3A4 inhibitors could lead to an increase in conivaptan concentrations. Concomitant use of conivaptan with potent CYP3A4 inhibitors is contraindicated).
No products indexed under this heading.

Metronidazole Hydrochloride (Conivaptan is a substrate of CYP3A4. Co-administration of conivaptan with CYP3A4 inhibitors could lead to an increase in conivaptan concentrations. Concomitant use of conivaptan with potent CYP3A4 inhibitors is contraindicated).
No products indexed under this heading.

Miconazole (Conivaptan is a substrate of CYP3A4. Co-administration of conivaptan with CYP3A4 inhibitors could lead to an increase in conivaptan concentrations. Concomitant use of conivaptan with potent CYP3A4 inhibitors is contraindicated).
No products indexed under this heading.

Miconazole Nitrate (Conivaptan is a substrate of CYP3A4. Co-administration of conivaptan with CYP3A4 inhibitors could lead to an increase in conivaptan concentrations. Concomitant use of conivaptan with potent CYP3A4 inhibitors is contraindicated).
No products indexed under this heading.

Midazolam Hydrochloride (Conivaptan is a potent inhibitor of CYP3A4. Conivaptan may increase plasma concentrations of co-administered drugs that are primarily metabolized by CYP3A4).
No products indexed under this heading.

Nefazodone Hydrochloride (Conivaptan is a substrate of CYP3A4. Co-administration of conivaptan with CYP3A4 inhibitors could lead to an increase in conivaptan concentrations. Concomitant use of conivaptan with potent CYP3A4 inhibitors is contraindicated).
No products indexed under this heading.

Nelfinavir Mesylate (Conivaptan is a substrate of CYP3A4. Co-administration of conivaptan with CYP3A4 inhibitors could lead to an increase in conivaptan concentrations. Concomitant use of conivaptan with potent CYP3A4 inhibitors is contraindicated).
No products indexed under this heading.

Nevirapine (Conivaptan is a substrate of CYP3A4. Co-administration of conivaptan with CYP3A4 inhibitors could lead to an increase in conivaptan concentrations. Concomitant use of conivaptan with potent CYP3A4 inhibitors is contraindicated). Products include:
Viramune Oral Suspension 873
Viramune Tablets 873

Niacinamide (Conivaptan is a substrate of CYP3A4. Co-administration of conivaptan with CYP3A4 inhibitors could lead to an increase in conivaptan concentrations. Concomitant use of conivaptan with potent CYP3A4 inhibitors is contraindicated). Products include:
BioLean Free Tablets 635

IMPORTANT NOTE: Always consult each drug listing in the patient's regimen for possible interactions.

Nicardipine Hydrochloride (Conivaptan is a potent inhibitor of CYP3A4. Conivaptan may increase plasma concentrations of co-administered drugs that are primarily metabolized by CYP3A4). Products include:

Cardene I.V. 1093

Nicotinamide (Conivaptan is a substrate of CYP3A4. Co-administration of conivaptan with CYP3A4 inhibitors could lead to an increase in conivaptan concentrations. Concomitant use of conivaptan with potent CYP3A4 inhibitors is contraindicated).

No products indexed under this heading.

Nifedipine (Conivaptan is a substrate of CYP3A4. Co-administration of conivaptan with CYP3A4 inhibitors could lead to an increase in conivaptan concentrations. Concomitant use of conivaptan with potent CYP3A4 inhibitors is contraindicated).

No products indexed under this heading.

Nimodipine (Conivaptan is a potent inhibitor of CYP3A4. Conivaptan may increase plasma concentrations of co-administered drugs that are primarily metabolized by CYP3A4). Products include:

Nimotop Capsules 790

Nisoldipine (Conivaptan is a potent inhibitor of CYP3A4. Conivaptan may increase plasma concentrations of co-administered drugs that are primarily metabolized by CYP3A4). Products include:

Sular Extended Release Tablets 2975

Nitrendipine (Conivaptan is a potent inhibitor of CYP3A4. Conivaptan may increase plasma concentrations of co-administered drugs that are primarily metabolized by CYP3A4).

No products indexed under this heading.

Norethindrone (Conivaptan is a potent inhibitor of CYP3A4. Conivaptan may increase plasma concentrations of co-administered drugs that are primarily metabolized by CYP3A4). Products include:

Ortho Micronor Tablets 2446

Norethindrone Acetate (Conivaptan is a potent inhibitor of CYP3A4. Conivaptan may increase plasma concentrations of co-administered drugs that are primarily metabolized by CYP3A4). Products include:

Activella Tablets 2347

Norfloxacin (Conivaptan is a substrate of CYP3A4. Co-administration of conivaptan with CYP3A4 inhibitors could lead to an increase in conivaptan concentrations. Concomitant use of conivaptan with potent CYP3A4 inhibitors is contraindicated). Products include:

Noroxin Tablets 2069

Norgestrel (Conivaptan is a potent inhibitor of CYP3A4. Conivaptan may increase plasma concentrations of co-administered drugs that are primarily metabolized by CYP3A4).

No products indexed under this heading.

Omeprazole (Conivaptan is a substrate of CYP3A4. Co-administration of conivaptan with CYP3A4 inhibitors could lead to an increase in conivaptan concentrations. Concomitant use of conivaptan with potent CYP3A4 inhibitors is contraindicated).

No products indexed under this heading.

Ondansetron (Conivaptan is a potent inhibitor of CYP3A4. Conivaptan may increase plasma concentrations of co-administered drugs that are primarily metabolized by CYP3A4). Products include:

Zofran ODT Orally Disintegrating Tablets 1687

Ondansetron Hydrochloride (Conivaptan is a potent inhibitor of CYP3A4. Conivaptan may increase plasma concentrations of co-administered drugs that are primarily metabolized by CYP3A4). Products include:

Zofran Injection 1682
Zofran 1687

Paclitaxel (Conivaptan is a potent inhibitor of CYP3A4. Conivaptan may increase plasma concentrations of co-administered drugs that are primarily metabolized by CYP3A4).

No products indexed under this heading.

Paroxetine Hydrochloride (Conivaptan is a substrate of CYP3A4. Co-administration of conivaptan with CYP3A4 inhibitors could lead to an increase in conivaptan concentrations. Concomitant use of conivaptan with potent CYP3A4 inhibitors is contraindicated). Products include:

Paxil 1535
Paxil CR Controlled-Release Tablets 1544

Pimozide (Conivaptan is a potent inhibitor of CYP3A4. Conivaptan may increase plasma concentrations of co-administered drugs that are primarily metabolized by CYP3A4).

No products indexed under this heading.

Polyestradiol Phosphate (Conivaptan is a potent inhibitor of CYP3A4. Conivaptan may increase plasma concentrations of co-administered drugs that are primarily metabolized by CYP3A4).

No products indexed under this heading.

Propoxyphene Hydrochloride (Conivaptan is a substrate of CYP3A4. Co-administration of conivaptan with CYP3A4 inhibitors could lead to an increase in conivaptan concentrations. Concomitant use of conivaptan with potent CYP3A4 inhibitors is contraindicated).

No products indexed under this heading.

Propoxyphene Napsylate (Conivaptan is a substrate of CYP3A4. Co-administration of conivaptan with CYP3A4 inhibitors could lead to an increase in conivaptan concentrations. Concomitant use of conivaptan with potent CYP3A4 inhibitors is contraindicated).

No products indexed under this heading.

Quinidine (Conivaptan is a substrate of CYP3A4. Co-administration of conivaptan with CYP3A4 inhibitors could lead to an increase in conivaptan concentrations. Concomitant use of conivaptan with potent CYP3A4 inhibitors is contraindicated).

No products indexed under this heading.

Quinidine Gluconate (Conivaptan is a potent inhibitor of CYP3A4. Conivaptan may increase plasma concentrations of co-administered drugs that are primarily metabolized by CYP3A4).

No products indexed under this heading.

Quinidine Hydrochloride (Conivaptan is a substrate of CYP3A4. Co-administration of conivaptan with CYP3A4 inhibitors could lead to an increase in conivaptan concentrations. Concomitant use of conivaptan with potent CYP3A4 inhibitors is contraindicated).

No products indexed under this heading.

Quinidine Polygalacturonate (Conivaptan is a substrate of CYP3A4. Co-administration of conivaptan with CYP3A4 inhibitors could lead to an increase in conivaptan concentrations. Concomitant use of conivaptan with potent CYP3A4 inhibitors is contraindicated).

No products indexed under this heading.

Quinidine Sulfate (Conivaptan is a substrate of CYP3A4. Co-administration of conivaptan with CYP3A4 inhibitors could lead to an increase in conivaptan concentrations. Concomitant use of conivaptan with potent CYP3A4 inhibitors is contraindicated).

No products indexed under this heading.

Quinine (Conivaptan is a substrate of CYP3A4. Co-administration of conivaptan with CYP3A4 inhibitors could lead to an increase in conivaptan concentrations. Concomitant use of conivaptan with potent CYP3A4 inhibitors is contraindicated).

No products indexed under this heading.

Quinine Sulfate (Conivaptan is a substrate of CYP3A4. Co-administration of conivaptan with CYP3A4 inhibitors could lead to an increase in conivaptan concentrations. Concomitant use of conivaptan with potent CYP3A4 inhibitors is contraindicated).

No products indexed under this heading.

Quinupristin (Conivaptan is a substrate of CYP3A4. Co-administration of conivaptan with CYP3A4 inhibitors could lead to an increase in conivaptan concentrations. Concomitant use of conivaptan with potent CYP3A4 inhibitors is contraindicated).

No products indexed under this heading.

Ranitidine Bismuth Citrate (Conivaptan is a substrate of CYP3A4. Co-administration of conivaptan with CYP3A4 inhibitors could lead to an increase in conivaptan concentrations. Concomitant use of conivaptan with potent CYP3A4 inhibitors is contraindicated).

No products indexed under this heading.

Ranitidine Hydrochloride (Conivaptan is a substrate of CYP3A4. Co-administration of conivaptan with CYP3A4 inhibitors could lead to an increase in conivaptan concentrations. Concomitant use of conivaptan with potent CYP3A4 inhibitors is contraindicated). Products include:

Zantac 75 Tablets ..... ■ 603
Zantac 1670
Zantac Injection 1666
Zantac Injection Pharmacy Bulk Package 1668
Maximum Strength Zantac 150 Tablets ..... ■ 603
Maximum Strength Zantac 150 Cool Mint Tablets ..... ■ 603

Rifabutin (Conivaptan is a potent inhibitor of CYP3A4. Conivaptan may increase plasma concentrations of co-administered drugs that are primarily metabolized by CYP3A4).

No products indexed under this heading.

Ritonavir (Conivaptan is a substrate of CYP3A4. Co-administration of conivaptan with CYP3A4 inhibitors could lead to an increase in conivaptan concentrations. Concomitant use of conivaptan with potent CYP3A4 inhibitors is contraindicated). Products include:

Kaletra 452
Norvir 489

Saquinavir (Conivaptan is a substrate of CYP3A4. Co-administration of conivaptan with CYP3A4 inhibitors could lead to an increase in conivaptan concentrations. Concomitant use of conivaptan with potent CYP3A4 inhibitors is contraindicated).

No products indexed under this heading.

Saquinavir Mesylate (Conivaptan is a substrate of CYP3A4. Co-administration of conivaptan with CYP3A4 inhibitors could lead to an increase in conivaptan concentrations. Concomitant use of conivaptan with potent CYP3A4 inhibitors is contraindicated).

No products indexed under this heading.

Sertraline Hydrochloride (Conivaptan is a substrate of CYP3A4. Co-administration of conivaptan with CYP3A4 inhibitors could lead to an increase in conivaptan concentrations. Concomitant use of conivaptan with potent CYP3A4 inhibitors is contraindicated).

No products indexed under this heading.

Sildenafil Citrate (Conivaptan is a substrate of CYP3A4. Co-administration of conivaptan with CYP3A4 inhibitors could lead to an increase in conivaptan concentrations. Concomitant use of conivaptan with potent CYP3A4 inhibitors is contraindicated).

No products indexed under this heading.

Simvastatin (Conivaptan is a potent inhibitor of CYP3A4. Conivaptan may increase plasma concentrations of co-administered drugs that are primarily metabolized by CYP3A4). Products include:

Simcor Tablets 502
Vytorin 10/10 Tablets 2149
Vytorin 10/10 Tablets 2939
Vytorin 10/20 Tablets 2149
Vytorin 10/20 Tablets 2939
Vytorin 10/40 Tablets 2149
Vytorin 10/40 Tablets 2939
Vytorin 10/80 Tablets 2149
Vytorin 10/80 Tablets 2939
Zocor Tablets 2136

Sirolimus (Conivaptan is a potent inhibitor of CYP3A4. Conivaptan may increase plasma concentrations of co-administered drugs that are primarily metabolized by CYP3A4). Products include:

Rapamune 3260

Tacrolimus (Conivaptan is a potent inhibitor of CYP3A4. Conivaptan may increase plasma concentrations of co-administered drugs that are primarily metabolized by CYP3A4). Products include:

Prograf Capsules and Injection 622
Protopic Ointment 628

Tadalafil (Conivaptan is a potent inhibitor of CYP3A4. Conivaptan may increase plasma concentrations of co-administered drugs that are primarily metabolized by CYP3A4). Products include:
Cialis Tablets 1792

Tamoxifen Citrate (Conivaptan is a potent inhibitor of CYP3A4. Conivaptan may increase plasma concentrations of co-administered drugs that are primarily metabolized by CYP3A4).
No products indexed under this heading.

Telithromycin (Conivaptan is a substrate of CYP3A4. Co-administration of conivaptan with CYP3A4 inhibitors could lead to an increase in conivaptan concentrations. Concomitant use of conivaptan with potent CYP3A4 inhibitors is contraindicated). Products include:
Ketek Tablets 2744

Tiagabine Hydrochloride (Conivaptan is a potent inhibitor of CYP3A4. Conivaptan may increase plasma concentrations of co-administered drugs that are primarily metabolized by CYP3A4). Products include:
Gabitril Tablets 973

Tolterodine Tartrate (Conivaptan is a potent inhibitor of CYP3A4. Conivaptan may increase plasma concentrations of co-administered drugs that are primarily metabolized by CYP3A4).
No products indexed under this heading.

Trazodone Hydrochloride (Conivaptan is a potent inhibitor of CYP3A4. Conivaptan may increase plasma concentrations of co-administered drugs that are primarily metabolized by CYP3A4).
No products indexed under this heading.

Triazolam (Conivaptan is a potent inhibitor of CYP3A4. Conivaptan may increase plasma concentrations of co-administered drugs that are primarily metabolized by CYP3A4).
No products indexed under this heading.

Troglitazone (Conivaptan is a substrate of CYP3A4. Co-administration of conivaptan with CYP3A4 inhibitors could lead to an increase in conivaptan concentrations. Concomitant use of conivaptan with potent CYP3A4 inhibitors is contraindicated).
No products indexed under this heading.

Troleandomycin (Conivaptan is a substrate of CYP3A4. Co-administration of conivaptan with CYP3A4 inhibitors could lead to an increase in conivaptan concentrations. Concomitant use of conivaptan with potent CYP3A4 inhibitors is contraindicated).
No products indexed under this heading.

Valproate Sodium (Conivaptan is a substrate of CYP3A4. Co-administration of conivaptan with CYP3A4 inhibitors could lead to an increase in conivaptan concentrations. Concomitant use of conivaptan with potent CYP3A4 inhibitors is contraindicated).
No products indexed under this heading.

Vardenafil Hydrochloride (Conivaptan is a substrate of CYP3A4. Co-administration of conivaptan with CYP3A4 inhibitors could lead to an increase in conivaptan concentrations. Concomitant use of conivaptan with potent CYP3A4 inhibitors is contraindicated). Products include:
Levitra Tablets 2876

Verapamil Hydrochloride (Conivaptan is a substrate of CYP3A4. Co-administration of conivaptan with CYP3A4 inhibitors could lead to an increase in conivaptan concentrations. Concomitant use of conivaptan with potent CYP3A4 inhibitors is contraindicated). Products include:
Tarka Tablets 511

Vinblastine Sulfate (Conivaptan is a potent inhibitor of CYP3A4. Conivaptan may increase plasma concentrations of co-administered drugs that are primarily metabolized by CYP3A4).
No products indexed under this heading.

Vincristine Sulfate (Conivaptan is a potent inhibitor of CYP3A4. Conivaptan may increase plasma concentrations of co-administered drugs that are primarily metabolized by CYP3A4).
No products indexed under this heading.

Voriconazole (Conivaptan is a substrate of CYP3A4. Co-administration of conivaptan with CYP3A4 inhibitors could lead to an increase in conivaptan concentrations. Concomitant use of conivaptan with potent CYP3A4 inhibitors is contraindicated).
No products indexed under this heading.

Warfarin Sodium (Conivaptan is a potent inhibitor of CYP3A4. Conivaptan may increase plasma concentrations of co-administered drugs that are primarily metabolized by CYP3A4).
No products indexed under this heading.

Zafirlukast (Conivaptan is a substrate of CYP3A4. Co-administration of conivaptan with CYP3A4 inhibitors could lead to an increase in conivaptan concentrations. Concomitant use of conivaptan with potent CYP3A4 inhibitors is contraindicated). Products include:
Accolate Tablets 669

Zileuton (Conivaptan is a substrate of CYP3A4. Co-administration of conivaptan with CYP3A4 inhibitors could lead to an increase in conivaptan concentrations. Concomitant use of conivaptan with potent CYP3A4 inhibitors is contraindicated).
No products indexed under this heading.

Food Interactions

Grapefruit (Conivaptan is a substrate of CYP3A4. Co-administration of conivaptan with CYP3A4 inhibitors could lead to an increase in conivaptan concentrations. Concomitant use of conivaptan with potent CYP3A4 inhibitors is contraindicated).

Grapefruit Juice (Conivaptan is a substrate of CYP3A4. Co-administration of conivaptan with CYP3A4 inhibitors could lead to an increase in conivaptan concentrations. Concomitant use of conivaptan with potent CYP3A4 inhibitors is contraindicated).

VAQTA

(Hepatitis A Vaccine, Inactivated) 2130
May interact with typhoid vaccine and certain other agents. Compounds in these categories include:

Typhoid Vaccine (Co-administration of Vaqta, typhoid and yellow fever vaccines has resulted in reduced GMTs for hepatitis A compared to Vaqta alone; however, following the receipt of the booster dose of Vaqta the GMTs for hepatits A in these two groups were observed to be comparable).
No products indexed under this heading.

Typhoid Vaccine Live Oral TY21a (Co-administration of Vaqta, typhoid and yellow fever vaccines has resulted in reduced GMTs for hepatitis A compared to Vaqta alone; however, following the receipt of the booster dose of Vaqta the GMTs for hepatits A in these two groups were observed to be comparable).
No products indexed under this heading.

Typhoid Vi Polysaccharide Vaccine (Co-administration of Vaqta, typhoid and yellow fever vaccines has resulted in reduced GMTs for hepatitis A compared to Vaqta alone; however, following the receipt of the booster dose of Vaqta the GMTs for hepatits A in these two groups were observed to be comparable).
No products indexed under this heading.

Yellow Fever Vaccine (Co-administration of Vaqta, typhoid and yellow fever vaccines has resulted in reduced GMTs for hepatitis A compared to Vaqta alone; however, following the receipt of the booster dose of Vaqta the GMTs for hepatits A in these two groups were observed to be comparable).
No products indexed under this heading.

VARIVAX

(Varicella Virus Vaccine Live) 2133
May interact with corticosteroids, salicylates, and certain other agents. Compounds in these categories include:

Aspirin (Vaccine recipients should avoid use of salicylates for 6 weeks after vaccination with Varivax because of the potential for Reye's syndrome). Products include:
Aggrenox Capsules 819
Bayer Aspirin 750
Percodan Tablets 1130
St. Joseph 81 mg Aspirin Chewable and Enteric Coated Tablets 1903

Aspirin, Enteric Coated (Vaccine recipients should avoid use of salicylates for 6 weeks after vaccination with Varivax because of the potential for Reye's syndrome).
No products indexed under this heading.

Aspirin Buffered (Vaccine recipients should avoid use of salicylates for 6 weeks after vaccination with Varivax because of the potential for Reye's syndrome).
No products indexed under this heading.

Azathioprine (Concurrent use in individuals who are on immunosuppressant drugs can result in greater susceptibility to infections; co-administration is contraindicated).
No products indexed under this heading.

Betamethasone Acetate (Co-administration in individuals on immunosuppressant doses of corticosteroids can result in more extensive vaccine-associated rash or disseminated disease).
No products indexed under this heading.

Betamethasone Sodium Phosphate (Co-administration in individuals on immunosuppressant doses of corticosteroids can result in more extensive vaccine-associated rash or disseminated disease).
No products indexed under this heading.

Budesonide (Co-administration in individuals on immunosuppressant doses of corticosteroids can result in more extensive vaccine-associated rash or disseminated disease). Products include:
Pulmicort Flexhaler 654
Symbicort 80/4.5 Inhalation Aerosol 659
Symbicort 160/4.5 Inhalation Aerosol 659

Choline Magnesium Trisalicylate (Vaccine recipients should avoid use of salicylates for 6 weeks after vaccination with Varivax because of the potential for Reye's syndrome).
No products indexed under this heading.

Ciclesonide (Co-administration in individuals on immunosuppressant doses of corticosteroids can result in more extensive vaccine-associated rash or disseminated disease). Products include:
Alvesco Inhalation Aerosol 2985
Omnaris Nasal Spray 2998

Cortisone Acetate (Co-administration in individuals on immunosuppressant doses of corticosteroids can result in more extensive vaccine-associated rash or disseminated disease).
No products indexed under this heading.

Cyclosporine (Concurrent use in individuals who are on immunosuppressant drugs can result in greater susceptibility to infections; co-administration is contraindicated). Products include:
Gengraf Capsules 435
Neoral Oral Solution 2280
Neoral Soft Gelatin Capsules 2280
Restasis Ophthalmic Emulsion 557
Sandimmune 2296

Dexamethasone (Co-administration in individuals on immunosuppressant doses of corticosteroids can result in more extensive vaccine-associated rash or disseminated disease). Products include:
Ciprodex Otic Suspension 541

Dexamethasone Acetate (Co-administration in individuals on immunosuppressant doses of corticosteroids can result in more extensive vaccine-associated rash or disseminated disease).
No products indexed under this heading.

Dexamethasone Sodium Phosphate (Co-administration in individuals on immunosuppressant doses of corticosteroids can result in more extensive vaccine-associated rash or disseminated disease).
No products indexed under this heading.

Diflunisal (Vaccine recipients should avoid use of salicylates for 6 weeks after vaccination with Varivax because of the potential for Reye's syndrome).
No products indexed under this heading.

Fludrocortisone Acetate (Co-administration in individuals on immunosuppressant doses of corticosteroids can result in more extensive vaccine-associated rash or disseminated disease).
No products indexed under this heading.

Flunisolide (Co-administration in individuals on immunosuppressant doses of corticosteroids can result in more extensive vaccine-associated rash or disseminated disease). Products include:
Aerobid/Aerobid-M 1153

Fluticasone Propionate (Co-administration in individuals on immunosuppressant doses of corticosteroids can result in more extensive vaccine-associated rash or disseminated disease). Products include:
Advair Diskus 100/50 1276
Advair Diskus 250/50 1276
Advair Diskus 500/50 1276
Advair HFA 45/21 Inhalation Aerosol.......................... 1288
Advair HFA 115/21 Inhalation Aerosol.......................... 1288
Advair HFA 230/21 Inhalation Aerosol.......................... 1288
Flonase Nasal Spray 1431
Flovent Diskus 50 mcg 1435

Fluticasone Propionate HFA (Co-administration in individuals on immunosuppressant doses of corticosteroids can result in more extensive vaccine-associated rash or disseminated disease). Products include:
Flovent HFA 1440

Globulin, Immune (Human) (Vaccination should be deferred for at least 5 months following immune globulin administration; following administration of Varivax, immune globulin should not be given for 2 months). Products include:
Flebogamma 5% 1715

Hydrocortisone (Co-administration in individuals on immunosuppressant doses of corticosteroids can result in more extensive vaccine-associated rash or disseminated disease).
No products indexed under this heading.

Hydrocortisone Acetate (Co-administration in individuals on immunosuppressant doses of corticosteroids can result in more extensive vaccine-associated rash or disseminated disease). Products include:
Analpram-HC 1140
Pramosone 1141

Hydrocortisone Sodium Phosphate (Co-administration in individuals on immunosuppressant doses of corticosteroids can result in more extensive vaccine-associated rash or disseminated disease).
No products indexed under this heading.

Hydrocortisone Sodium Succinate (Co-administration in individuals on immunosuppressant doses of corticosteroids can result in more extensive vaccine-associated rash or disseminated disease).
No products indexed under this heading.

Magnesium Salicylate (Vaccine recipients should avoid use of salicylates for 6 weeks after vaccination with Varivax because of the potential for Reye's syndrome).
No products indexed under this heading.

Methylprednisolone Acetate (Co-administration in individuals on immunosuppressant doses of corticosteroids can result in more extensive vaccine-associated rash or disseminated disease).
No products indexed under this heading.

Methylprednisolone Sodium Succinate (Co-administration in individuals on immunosuppressant doses of corticosteroids can result in more extensive vaccine-associated rash or disseminated disease).
No products indexed under this heading.

Mometasone Furoate (Co-administration in individuals on immunosuppressant doses of corticosteroids can result in more extensive vaccine-associated rash or disseminated disease). Products include:
Asmanex Twisthaler 2797
Elocon Cream 0.1% 2840
Elocon Lotion 0.1% 2841
Elocon Ointment 0.1% 2842

Mometasone Furoate Monohydrate (Co-administration in individuals on immunosuppressant doses of corticosteroids can result in more extensive vaccine-associated rash or disseminated disease). Products include:
Nasonex Nasal Spray 2883

Muromonab-CD3 (Concurrent use in individuals who are on immunosuppressant drugs can result in greater susceptibility to infections; co-administration is contraindicated). Products include:
Orthoclone OKT3 Sterile Solution 2387

Mycophenolate Mofetil (Concurrent use in individuals who are on immunosuppressant drugs can result in greater susceptibility to infections; co-administration is contraindicated). Products include:
CellCept Capsules 2622
CellCept Oral Suspension 2622
CellCept Tablets 2622

Prednisolone Acetate (Co-administration in individuals on immunosuppressant doses of corticosteroids can result in more extensive vaccine-associated rash or disseminated disease). Products include:
Pred Forte Ophthalmic Suspension .... ⊙227
Pred Mild Ophthalmic Suspension .... ⊙230
Pred-G Ophthalmic Ointment .... ⊙229
Pred-G Ophthalmic Suspension ...... ⊙228

Prednisolone Sodium Phosphate (Co-administration in individuals on immunosuppressant doses of corticosteroids can result in more extensive vaccine-associated rash or disseminated disease).
No products indexed under this heading.

Prednisolone Tebutate (Co-administration in individuals on immunosuppressant doses of corticosteroids can result in more extensive vaccine-associated rash or disseminated disease).
No products indexed under this heading.

Prednisone (Co-administration in individuals on immunosuppressant doses of corticosteroids can result in more extensive vaccine-associated rash or disseminated disease).
No products indexed under this heading.

Salsalate (Vaccine recipients should avoid use of salicylates for 6 weeks after vaccination with Varivax because of the potential for Reye's syndrome).
No products indexed under this heading.

Tacrolimus (Concurrent use in individuals who are on immunosuppressant drugs can result in greater susceptibility to infections; co-administration is contraindicated). Products include:
Prograf Capsules and Injection 622
Protopic Ointment 628

Triamcinolone (Co-administration in individuals on immunosuppressant doses of corticosteroids can result in more extensive vaccine-associated rash or disseminated disease).
No products indexed under this heading.

Triamcinolone Acetonide (Co-administration in individuals on immunosuppressant doses of corticosteroids can result in more extensive vaccine-associated rash or disseminated disease). Products include:
Azmacort Inhalation Aerosol 407
Nasacort AQ Nasal Spray 2765
Triesence Injectable Suspension .... ⊙209

Triamcinolone Diacetate (Co-administration in individuals on immunosuppressant doses of corticosteroids can result in more extensive vaccine-associated rash or disseminated disease).
No products indexed under this heading.

Triamcinolone Hexacetonide (Co-administration in individuals on immunosuppressant doses of corticosteroids can result in more extensive vaccine-associated rash or disseminated disease).
No products indexed under this heading.

VECTIBIX
(Panitumumab) 597
None cited in PDR database.

VELCADE FOR INJECTION
(Bortezomib) 2168
May interact with cytochrome p450 2c19 substrates (selected), cytochrome p450 3a4 inducers (selected), cytochrome p450 3a4 inhibitors (selected), oral hypoglycemic agents, and certain other agents. Compounds in these categories include:

Acarbose (During clinical trials, hypoglycemia and hyperglycemia were reported in diabetic patients receiving oral hypoglycemics. Patients on oral antidiabetic agents receiving bortezomib treatment may require close monitoring of their blood glucose levels and adjustment of the dose of their antidiabetic medication). Products include:
Precose Tablets 792

Acetazolamide (Patients who are concomitantly receiving bortezomib and drugs that are inhibitors or inducers of cytochrome P450 3A4 should be closely monitored for either toxicities or reduced efficacy).
No products indexed under this heading.

Allium sativum (Patients who are concomitantly receiving bortezomib and drugs that are inhibitors or inducers of cytochrome P450 3A4 should be closely monitored for either toxicities or reduced efficacy).
No products indexed under this heading.

Amiodarone Hydrochloride (Patients who are concomitantly receiving bortezomib and drugs that are inhibitors or inducers of cytochrome P450 3A4 should be closely monitored for either toxicities or reduced efficacy).
No products indexed under this heading.

Amitriptyline Hydrochloride (Bortezomib may inhibit 2C19 activity and increase exposure to drugs that are substrates for this enzyme).
No products indexed under this heading.

Amoxapine (Bortezomib may inhibit 2C19 activity and increase exposure to drugs that are substrates for this enzyme).
No products indexed under this heading.

Amprenavir (Patients who are concomitantly receiving bortezomib and drugs that are inhibitors or inducers of cytochrome P450 3A4 should be closely monitored for either toxicities or reduced efficacy).
No products indexed under this heading.

Anastrozole (Patients who are concomitantly receiving bortezomib and drugs that are inhibitors or inducers of cytochrome P450 3A4 should be closely monitored for either toxicities or reduced efficacy). Products include:
Arimidex Tablets 672

Aprepitant (Patients who are concomitantly receiving bortezomib and drugs that are inhibitors or inducers of cytochrome P450 3A4 should be closely monitored for either toxicities or reduced efficacy). Products include:
Emend Capsules 1992

Atazanavir (Patients who are concomitantly receiving bortezomib and drugs that are inhibitors or inducers of cytochrome P450 3A4 should be closely monitored for either toxicities or reduced efficacy).
No products indexed under this heading.

Atazanavir Sulfate (Patients who are concomitantly receiving bortezomib and drugs that are inhibitors or inducers of cytochrome P450 3A4 should be closely monitored for either toxicities or reduced efficacy). Products include:
Reyataz Capsules 3299

Betamethasone Acetate (Patients who are concomitantly receiving bortezomib and drugs that are inhibitors or inducers of cytochrome P450 3A4 should be closely monitored for either toxicities or reduced efficacy).
No products indexed under this heading.

Betamethasone Sodium Phosphate (Patients who are concomitantly receiving bortezomib and drugs that are inhibitors or inducers of cytochrome P450 3A4 should be closely monitored for either toxicities or reduced efficacy).
No products indexed under this heading.

Carbamazepine (Patients who are concomitantly receiving bortezomib and drugs that are inhibitors or inducers of cytochrome P450 3A4 should be closely monitored for either toxicities or reduced efficacy). Products include:
Carbatrol Capsules **3019**
Equetro Extended-Release Capsules **3174**

Carisoprodol (Bortezomib may inhibit 2C19 activity and increase exposure to drugs that are substrates for this enzyme). Products include:
Soma Tablets **1931**

Chlorpropamide (During clinical trials, hypoglycemia and hyperglycemia were reported in diabetic patients receiving oral hypoglycemics. Patients on oral antidiabetic agents receiving bortezomib treatment may require close monitoring of their blood glucose levels and adjustment of the dose of their antidiabetic medication).
No products indexed under this heading.

Cilostazol (Bortezomib may inhibit 2C19 activity and increase exposure to drugs that are substrates for this enzyme). Products include:
Pletal Tablets **2481**

Cimetidine (Patients who are concomitantly receiving bortezomib and drugs that are inhibitors or inducers of cytochrome P450 3A4 should be closely monitored for either toxicities or reduced efficacy).
No products indexed under this heading.

Cimetidine Hydrochloride (Patients who are concomitantly receiving bortezomib and drugs that are inhibitors or inducers of cytochrome P450 3A4 should be closely monitored for either toxicities or reduced efficacy).
No products indexed under this heading.

Ciprofloxacin (Patients who are concomitantly receiving bortezomib and drugs that are inhibitors or inducers of cytochrome P450 3A4 should be closely monitored for either toxicities or reduced efficacy). Products include:
Cipro I.V. **2817**
Cipro Oral Suspension **2810**
Cipro XR Tablets **2823**
Ciprodex Otic Suspension **541**

Ciprofloxacin Hydrochloride (Patients who are concomitantly receiving bortezomib and drugs that are inhibitors or inducers of cytochrome P450 3A4 should be closely monitored for either toxicities or reduced efficacy). Products include:
Cipro Tablets **2810**

Cisplatin (Patients who are concomitantly receiving bortezomib and drugs that are inhibitors or inducers of cytochrome P450 3A4 should be closely monitored for either toxicities or reduced efficacy).
No products indexed under this heading.

Citalopram Hydrobromide (Bortezomib may inhibit 2C19 activity and increase exposure to drugs that are substrates for this enzyme). Products include:
Celexa **1160**

Clarithromycin (Patients who are concomitantly receiving bortezomib and drugs that are inhibitors or inducers of cytochrome P450 3A4 should be closely monitored for either toxicities or reduced efficacy). Products include:
Biaxin/Biaxin XL **411**

Clomipramine Hydrochloride (Bortezomib may inhibit 2C19 activity and increase exposure to drugs that are substrates for this enzyme).
No products indexed under this heading.

Clotrimazole (Patients who are concomitantly receiving bortezomib and drugs that are inhibitors or inducers of cytochrome P450 3A4 should be closely monitored for either toxicities or reduced efficacy). Products include:
Lotrisone **2881**

Cortisone Acetate (Patients who are concomitantly receiving bortezomib and drugs that are inhibitors or inducers of cytochrome P450 3A4 should be closely monitored for either toxicities or reduced efficacy).
No products indexed under this heading.

Cyclophosphamide (Bortezomib may inhibit 2C19 activity and increase exposure to drugs that are substrates for this enzyme).
No products indexed under this heading.

Cyclosporine (Patients who are concomitantly receiving bortezomib and drugs that are inhibitors or inducers of cytochrome P450 3A4 should be closely monitored for either toxicities or reduced efficacy). Products include:
Gengraf Capsules **435**
Neoral Oral Solution **2280**
Neoral Soft Gelatin Capsules **2280**
Restasis Ophthalmic Emulsion **557**
Sandimmune **2296**

Dalfopristin (Patients who are concomitantly receiving bortezomib and drugs that are inhibitors or inducers of cytochrome P450 3A4 should be closely monitored for either toxicities or reduced efficacy).
No products indexed under this heading.

Danazol (Patients who are concomitantly receiving bortezomib and drugs that are inhibitors or inducers of cytochrome P450 3A4 should be closely monitored for either toxicities or reduced efficacy).
No products indexed under this heading.

Delavirdine Mesylate (Patients who are concomitantly receiving bortezomib and drugs that are inhibitors or inducers of cytochrome P450 3A4 should be closely monitored for either toxicities or reduced efficacy).
No products indexed under this heading.

Desipramine Hydrochloride (Bortezomib may inhibit 2C19 activity and increase exposure to drugs that are substrates for this enzyme).
No products indexed under this heading.

Dexamethasone (Patients who are concomitantly receiving bortezomib and drugs that are inhibitors or inducers of cytochrome P450 3A4 should be closely monitored for either toxicities or reduced efficacy). Products include:
Ciprodex Otic Suspension **541**

Dexamethasone Acetate (Patients who are concomitantly receiving bortezomib and drugs that are inhibitors or inducers of cytochrome P450 3A4 should be closely monitored for either toxicities or reduced efficacy).
No products indexed under this heading.

Dexamethasone Sodium Phosphate (Patients who are concomitantly receiving bortezomib and drugs that are inhibitors or inducers of cytochrome P450 3A4 should be closely monitored for either toxicities or reduced efficacy).
No products indexed under this heading.

Dextromethorphan (Bortezomib may inhibit 2C19 activity and increase exposure to drugs that are substrates for this enzyme).
No products indexed under this heading.

Dextromethorphan Hydrobromide (Bortezomib may inhibit 2C19 activity and increase exposure to drugs that are substrates for this enzyme). Products include:
PediaCare Children's Liquid Multi-Symptom Cold **1902**
PediaCare Children's Long-Acting Cough **1902**
Children's Sudafed PE Cold & Cough Liquid **1907**
Sudafed PE Cold & Cough Caplets **1907**
Children's Tylenol Plus Cough & Runny Nose Suspension Liquid **1912**
Children's Tylenol Plus Cough & Sore Throat Suspension Liquid **1912**
Children's Tylenol Plus Flu Suspension Liquid **1914**
Children's Tylenol Plus Multi-Symptom Cold Suspension Liquid **1912**
Tylenol Cold Severe Congestion Daytime Caplets with Cool Burst **1912**
Tylenol Cold Head Congestion Daytime Caplets with Cool Burst **1910**
Tylenol Cold Head Congestion Nighttime Caplets with Cool Burst **1910**
Tylenol Cold Head Congestion Severe Daytime Caplets with Cool Burst **1910**
Tylenol Cold Multi-Symptom Daytime Caplets with Cool Burst and Rapid Release Gels **1913**
Tylenol Cold Multi-Symptom Daytime Liquid with Citrus Burst **1913**
Tylenol Cold Multi-Symptom Nighttime Caplets with Cool Burst **1913**
Tylenol Cold Multi-Symptom Nighttime Liquid with Cool Burst **1913**
Tylenol Cold Multi-Symptom Severe Caplets with Cool Burst **1913**
Tylenol Cold Multi-Symptom Severe Daytime Liquid with Citrus Burst **1913**
Tylenol Cough & Sore Throat Daytime Liquid with Cool Burst **1918**
Tylenol Cough & Sore Throat Nighttime Liquid with Cool Burst **1918**
Vicks DayQuil Cold & Flu Multi-Symptom Relief **616**
Vicks DayQuil LiquiCaps **2567**
Vicks DayQuil Liquid **2567**
Vicks DayQuil Multi-Symptom Cold/Flu Relief **2567**
Vicks NyQuil Cold & Flu Multi-Symptom Relief **617**
Vicks NyQuil LiquiCaps **2567**
Vicks NyQuil Liquid **2567**
Vicks NyQuil Multi-Symptom Cold/Flu Relief **2567**

Diazepam (Bortezomib may inhibit 2C19 activity and increase exposure to drugs that are substrates for this enzyme). Products include:
Valium Tablets **2658**

Diltiazem Hydrochloride (Patients who are concomitantly receiving bortezomib and drugs that are inhibitors or inducers of cytochrome P450 3A4 should be closely monitored for either toxicities or reduced efficacy). Products include:
Cardizem LA Extended Release Tablets **421**

Diltiazem Maleate (Patients who are concomitantly receiving bortezomib and drugs that are inhibitors or inducers of cytochrome P450 3A4 should be closely monitored for either toxicities or reduced efficacy).
No products indexed under this heading.

Divalproex Sodium (Bortezomib may inhibit 2C19 activity and increase exposure to drugs that are substrates for this enzyme). Products include:
Depakote ER Tablets **423**

Doxepin Hydrochloride (Bortezomib may inhibit 2C19 activity and increase exposure to drugs that are substrates for this enzyme).
No products indexed under this heading.

Doxorubicin Hydrochloride (Patients who are concomitantly receiving bortezomib and drugs that are inhibitors or inducers of cytochrome P450 3A4 should be closely monitored for either toxicities or reduced efficacy).
No products indexed under this heading.

Efavirenz (Patients who are concomitantly receiving bortezomib and drugs that are inhibitors or inducers of cytochrome P450 3A4 should be closely monitored for either toxicities or reduced efficacy). Products include:
Atripla Tablets **938**
Sustiva Capsules **930**
Sustiva Tablets **930**

Erythromycin (Patients who are concomitantly receiving bortezomib and drugs that are inhibitors or inducers of cytochrome P450 3A4 should be closely monitored for either toxicities or reduced efficacy).
No products indexed under this heading.

Erythromycin Estolate (Patients who are concomitantly receiving bortezomib and drugs that are inhibitors or inducers of cytochrome P450 3A4 should be closely monitored for either toxicities or reduced efficacy).
No products indexed under this heading.

Erythromycin Ethylsuccinate (Patients who are concomitantly receiving bortezomib and drugs that are inhibitors or inducers of cytochrome P450 3A4 should be closely monitored for either toxicities or reduced efficacy). Products include:

E.E.S. 433
EryPed 431

Erythromycin Gluceptate (Patients who are concomitantly receiving bortezomib and drugs that are inhibitors or inducers of cytochrome P450 3A4 should be closely monitored for either toxicities or reduced efficacy).

No products indexed under this heading.

Erythromycin Lactobionate (Patients who are concomitantly receiving bortezomib and drugs that are inhibitors or inducers of cytochrome P450 3A4 should be closely monitored for either toxicities or reduced efficacy).

No products indexed under this heading.

Erythromycin Stearate (Patients who are concomitantly receiving bortezomib and drugs that are inhibitors or inducers of cytochrome P450 3A4 should be closely monitored for either toxicities or reduced efficacy).

No products indexed under this heading.

Esomeprazole Magnesium (Patients who are concomitantly receiving bortezomib and drugs that are inhibitors or inducers of cytochrome P450 3A4 should be closely monitored for either toxicities or reduced efficacy). Products include:

Nexium Delayed-Release Capsules.................................. 645
Nexium Delayed-Release Oral Suspension.................................. 645

Ethosuximide (Patients who are concomitantly receiving bortezomib and drugs that are inhibitors or inducers of cytochrome P450 3A4 should be closely monitored for either toxicities or reduced efficacy).

No products indexed under this heading.

Ethotoin (Bortezomib may inhibit 2C19 activity and increase exposure to drugs that are substrates for this enzyme).

No products indexed under this heading.

Felbamate (Patients who are concomitantly receiving bortezomib and drugs that are inhibitors or inducers of cytochrome P450 3A4 should be closely monitored for either toxicities or reduced efficacy).

No products indexed under this heading.

Fluconazole (Patients who are concomitantly receiving bortezomib and drugs that are inhibitors or inducers of cytochrome P450 3A4 should be closely monitored for either toxicities or reduced efficacy).

No products indexed under this heading.

Fludrocortisone Acetate (Patients who are concomitantly receiving bortezomib and drugs that are inhibitors or inducers of cytochrome P450 3A4 should be closely monitored for either toxicities or reduced efficacy).

No products indexed under this heading.

Fluoxetine (Patients who are concomitantly receiving bortezomib and drugs that are inhibitors or inducers of cytochrome P450 3A4 should be closely monitored for either toxicities or reduced efficacy).

No products indexed under this heading.

Fluoxetine Hydrochloride (Patients who are concomitantly receiving bortezomib and drugs that are inhibitors or inducers of cytochrome P450 3A4 should be closely monitored for either toxicities or reduced efficacy). Products include:

Prozac Weekly Capsules 1852
Prozac Pulvules and Liquid 1852
Symbyax Capsules 1871

Fluvoxamine Maleate (Patients who are concomitantly receiving bortezomib and drugs that are inhibitors or inducers of cytochrome P450 3A4 should be closely monitored for either toxicities or reduced efficacy). Products include:

Luvox CR Extended-Release Capsules.................................. 1759

Formoterol Fumarate (Bortezomib may inhibit 2C19 activity and increase exposure to drugs that are substrates for this enzyme). Products include:

Foradil Aerolizer 2849
Perforomist Inhalation Solution 1025

Fosamprenavir Calcium (Patients who are concomitantly receiving bortezomib and drugs that are inhibitors or inducers of cytochrome P450 3A4 should be closely monitored for either toxicities or reduced efficacy). Products include:

Lexiva Oral Suspension 1510
Lexiva Tablets 1510

Fosphenytoin (Bortezomib may inhibit 2C19 activity and increase exposure to drugs that are substrates for this enzyme).

No products indexed under this heading.

Fosphenytoin Sodium (Patients who are concomitantly receiving bortezomib and drugs that are inhibitors or inducers of cytochrome P450 3A4 should be closely monitored for either toxicities or reduced efficacy).

No products indexed under this heading.

Gabapentin (Bortezomib may inhibit 2C19 activity and increase exposure to drugs that are substrates for this enzyme).

No products indexed under this heading.

Garlic Extract (Patients who are concomitantly receiving bortezomib and drugs that are inhibitors or inducers of cytochrome P450 3A4 should be closely monitored for either toxicities or reduced efficacy).

No products indexed under this heading.

Garlic Oil (Patients who are concomitantly receiving bortezomib and drugs that are inhibitors or inducers of cytochrome P450 3A4 should be closely monitored for either toxicities or reduced efficacy).

No products indexed under this heading.

Glimepiride (During clinical trials, hypoglycemia and hyperglycemia were reported in diabetic patients receiving oral hypoglycemics. Patients on oral antidiabetic agents receiving bortezomib treatment may require close monitoring of their blood glucose levels and adjustment of the dose of their antidiabetic medication). Products include:

Avandaryl Tablets 1344
Duetact Tablets 3085

Glipizide (During clinical trials, hypoglycemia and hyperglycemia were reported in diabetic patients receiving oral hypoglycemics. Patients on oral antidiabetic agents receiving bortezomib treatment may require close monitoring of their blood glucose levels and adjustment of the dose of their antidiabetic medication).

No products indexed under this heading.

Glyburide (During clinical trials, hypoglycemia and hyperglycemia were reported in diabetic patients receiving oral hypoglycemics. Patients on oral antidiabetic agents receiving bortezomib treatment may require close monitoring of their blood glucose levels and adjustment of the dose of their antidiabetic medication).

No products indexed under this heading.

Hydrocortisone (Patients who are concomitantly receiving bortezomib and drugs that are inhibitors or inducers of cytochrome P450 3A4 should be closely monitored for either toxicities or reduced efficacy).

No products indexed under this heading.

Hydrocortisone Acetate (Patients who are concomitantly receiving bortezomib and drugs that are inhibitors or inducers of cytochrome P450 3A4 should be closely monitored for either toxicities or reduced efficacy). Products include:

Analpram-HC 1140
Pramosone 1141

Hydrocortisone Butyrate (Patients who are concomitantly receiving bortezomib and drugs that are inhibitors or inducers of cytochrome P450 3A4 should be closely monitored for either toxicities or reduced efficacy).

No products indexed under this heading.

Hydrocortisone Cypionate (Patients who are concomitantly receiving bortezomib and drugs that are inhibitors or inducers of cytochrome P450 3A4 should be closely monitored for either toxicities or reduced efficacy).

No products indexed under this heading.

Hydrocortisone Hemisuccinate (Patients who are concomitantly receiving bortezomib and drugs that are inhibitors or inducers of cytochrome P450 3A4 should be closely monitored for either toxicities or reduced efficacy).

No products indexed under this heading.

Hydrocortisone Probutate (Patients who are concomitantly receiving bortezomib and drugs that are inhibitors or inducers of cytochrome P450 3A4 should be closely monitored for either toxicities or reduced efficacy).

No products indexed under this heading.

Hydrocortisone Sodium Phosphate (Patients who are concomitantly receiving bortezomib and drugs that are inhibitors or inducers of cytochrome P450 3A4 should be closely monitored for either toxicities or reduced efficacy).

No products indexed under this heading.

Hydrocortisone Sodium Succinate (Patients who are concomitantly receiving bortezomib and drugs that are inhibitors or inducers of cytochrome P450 3A4 should be closely monitored for either toxicities or reduced efficacy).

No products indexed under this heading.

Hydrocortisone Valerate (Patients who are concomitantly receiving bortezomib and drugs that are inhibitors or inducers of cytochrome P450 3A4 should be closely monitored for either toxicities or reduced efficacy).

No products indexed under this heading.

Hypericum (Patients who are concomitantly receiving bortezomib and drugs that are inhibitors or inducers of cytochrome P450 3A4 should be closely monitored for either toxicities or reduced efficacy). Products include:

Satieté Tablets .... ▣640

Hypericum Perforatum (Patients who are concomitantly receiving bortezomib and drugs that are inhibitors or inducers of cytochrome P450 3A4 should be closely monitored for either toxicities or reduced efficacy).

No products indexed under this heading.

Imipramine Hydrochloride (Bortezomib may inhibit 2C19 activity and increase exposure to drugs that are substrates for this enzyme).

No products indexed under this heading.

Imipramine Pamoate (Bortezomib may inhibit 2C19 activity and increase exposure to drugs that are substrates for this enzyme).

No products indexed under this heading.

Indinavir Sulfate (Patients who are concomitantly receiving bortezomib and drugs that are inhibitors or inducers of cytochrome P450 3A4 should be closely monitored for either toxicities or reduced efficacy). Products include:

Crixivan Capsules 1979

Indomethacin (Bortezomib may inhibit 2C19 activity and increase exposure to drugs that are substrates for this enzyme). Products include:

Indocin 2024

Indomethacin Sodium Trihydrate (Bortezomib may inhibit 2C19 activity and increase exposure to drugs that are substrates for this enzyme). Products include:

Indocin I.V. 2489

Isoniazid (Patients who are concomitantly receiving bortezomib and drugs that are inhibitors or inducers of cytochrome P450 3A4 should be closely monitored for either toxicities or reduced efficacy).

No products indexed under this heading.

Itraconazole (Patients who are concomitantly receiving bortezomib and drugs that are inhibitors or inducers of cytochrome P450 3A4 should be closely monitored for either toxicities or reduced efficacy).
No products indexed under this heading.

Ketoconazole (Co-administration of ketoconazole, a potent CYP3A inhibitor, showed a 35% increase in mean bortezomib AUC, based on data from 12 patients. Therefore, patients should be closely monitored when given bortezomib in combination with potent CYP3A4 inhibitors(e.g., ketoconazole)). Products include:
Extina Foam, 2% **3057**
Nizoral A-D Shampoo **1901**

Lamotrigine (Bortezomib may inhibit 2C19 activity and increase exposure to drugs that are substrates for this enzyme). Products include:
Lamictal **1488**

Lansoprazole (Bortezomib may inhibit 2C19 activity and increase exposure to drugs that are substrates for this enzyme).
No products indexed under this heading.

Levetiracetam (Bortezomib may inhibit 2C19 activity and increase exposure to drugs that are substrates for this enzyme). Products include:
Keppra Injection **3137**
Keppra Oral Solution **3131**
Keppra Tablets **3131**

Lopinavir (Patients who are concomitantly receiving bortezomib and drugs that are inhibitors or inducers of cytochrome P450 3A4 should be closely monitored for either toxicities or reduced efficacy). Products include:
Kaletra **452**

Loratadine (Patients who are concomitantly receiving bortezomib and drugs that are inhibitors or inducers of cytochrome P450 3A4 should be closely monitored for either toxicities or reduced efficacy).
No products indexed under this heading.

Maprotiline Hydrochloride (Bortezomib may inhibit 2C19 activity and increase exposure to drugs that are substrates for this enzyme).
No products indexed under this heading.

Melphalan (Co-administration of melphalan-prednisone on bortezomib showed a 17% increase in mean bortezomib AUC based on data from 21 patients. This increase is unlikely to be clinically relevant).
No products indexed under this heading.

Melphalan Hydrochloride (Co-administration of melphalan-prednisone on bortezomib showed a 17% increase in mean bortezomib AUC based on data from 21 patients. This increase is unlikely to be clinically relevant).
No products indexed under this heading.

Mephenytoin (Patients who are concomitantly receiving bortezomib and drugs that are inhibitors or inducers of cytochrome P450 3A4 should be closely monitored for either toxicities or reduced efficacy).
No products indexed under this heading.

Mephobarbital (Bortezomib may inhibit 2C19 activity and increase exposure to drugs that are substrates for this enzyme).
No products indexed under this heading.

Meprobamate (Bortezomib may inhibit 2C19 activity and increase exposure to drugs that are substrates for this enzyme).
No products indexed under this heading.

Metformin Hydrochloride (During clinical trials, hypoglycemia and hyperglycemia were reported in diabetic patients receiving oral hypoglycemics. Patients on oral antidiabetic agents receiving bortezomib treatment may require close monitoring of their blood glucose levels and adjustment of the dose of their antidiabetic medication). Products include:
ActoPlus Met Tablets **3071**
Avandamet Tablets **1336**
Janumet Tablets **2041**
PrandiMet Tablets **2967**

Methsuximide (Patients who are concomitantly receiving bortezomib and drugs that are inhibitors or inducers of cytochrome P450 3A4 should be closely monitored for either toxicities or reduced efficacy).
No products indexed under this heading.

Methylprednisolone (Patients who are concomitantly receiving bortezomib and drugs that are inhibitors or inducers of cytochrome P450 3A4 should be closely monitored for either toxicities or reduced efficacy).
No products indexed under this heading.

Methylprednisolone Acetate (Patients who are concomitantly receiving bortezomib and drugs that are inhibitors or inducers of cytochrome P450 3A4 should be closely monitored for either toxicities or reduced efficacy).
No products indexed under this heading.

Methylprednisolone Sodium Succinate (Patients who are concomitantly receiving bortezomib and drugs that are inhibitors or inducers of cytochrome P450 3A4 should be closely monitored for either toxicities or reduced efficacy).
No products indexed under this heading.

Metronidazole (Patients who are concomitantly receiving bortezomib and drugs that are inhibitors or inducers of cytochrome P450 3A4 should be closely monitored for either toxicities or reduced efficacy). Products include:
Pylera Capsules **714**

Metronidazole Benzoate (Patients who are concomitantly receiving bortezomib and drugs that are inhibitors or inducers of cytochrome P450 3A4 should be closely monitored for either toxicities or reduced efficacy).
No products indexed under this heading.

Metronidazole Hydrochloride (Patients who are concomitantly receiving bortezomib and drugs that are inhibitors or inducers of cytochrome P450 3A4 should be closely monitored for either toxicities or reduced efficacy).
No products indexed under this heading.

Miconazole (Patients who are concomitantly receiving bortezomib and drugs that are inhibitors or inducers of cytochrome P450 3A4 should be closely monitored for either toxicities or reduced efficacy).
No products indexed under this heading.

Miconazole Nitrate (Patients who are concomitantly receiving bortezomib and drugs that are inhibitors or inducers of cytochrome P450 3A4 should be closely monitored for either toxicities or reduced efficacy).
No products indexed under this heading.

Midazolam Hydrochloride (Bortezomib may inhibit 2C19 activity and increase exposure to drugs that are substrates for this enzyme).
No products indexed under this heading.

Miglitol (During clinical trials, hypoglycemia and hyperglycemia were reported in diabetic patients receiving oral hypoglycemics. Patients on oral antidiabetic agents receiving bortezomib treatment may require close monitoring of their blood glucose levels and adjustment of the dose of their antidiabetic medication).
No products indexed under this heading.

Modafinil (Patients who are concomitantly receiving bortezomib and drugs that are inhibitors or inducers of cytochrome P450 3A4 should be closely monitored for either toxicities or reduced efficacy). Products include:
Provigil Tablets **977**

Nateglinide (During clinical trials, hypoglycemia and hyperglycemia were reported in diabetic patients receiving oral hypoglycemics. Patients on oral antidiabetic agents receiving bortezomib treatment may require close monitoring of their blood glucose levels and adjustment of the dose of their antidiabetic medication). Products include:
Starlix Tablets **2314**

Nefazodone Hydrochloride (Patients who are concomitantly receiving bortezomib and drugs that are inhibitors or inducers of cytochrome P450 3A4 should be closely monitored for either toxicities or reduced efficacy).
No products indexed under this heading.

Nelfinavir Mesylate (Patients who are concomitantly receiving bortezomib and drugs that are inhibitors or inducers of cytochrome P450 3A4 should be closely monitored for either toxicities or reduced efficacy).
No products indexed under this heading.

Nevirapine (Patients who are concomitantly receiving bortezomib and drugs that are inhibitors or inducers of cytochrome P450 3A4 should be closely monitored for either toxicities or reduced efficacy). Products include:
Viramune Oral Suspension **873**
Viramune Tablets **873**

Niacinamide (Patients who are concomitantly receiving bortezomib and drugs that are inhibitors or inducers of cytochrome P450 3A4 should be closely monitored for either toxicities or reduced efficacy). Products include:
BioLean Free Tablets **635**

Nicotinamide (Patients who are concomitantly receiving bortezomib and drugs that are inhibitors or inducers of cytochrome P450 3A4 should be closely monitored for either toxicities or reduced efficacy).
No products indexed under this heading.

Nifedipine (Patients who are concomitantly receiving bortezomib and drugs that are inhibitors or inducers of cytochrome P450 3A4 should be closely monitored for either toxicities or reduced efficacy).
No products indexed under this heading.

Nilutamide (Bortezomib may inhibit 2C19 activity and increase exposure to drugs that are substrates for this enzyme).
No products indexed under this heading.

Norfloxacin (Patients who are concomitantly receiving bortezomib and drugs that are inhibitors or inducers of cytochrome P450 3A4 should be closely monitored for either toxicities or reduced efficacy). Products include:
Noroxin Tablets **2069**

Nortriptyline Hydrochloride (Bortezomib may inhibit 2C19 activity and increase exposure to drugs that are substrates for this enzyme).
No products indexed under this heading.

Omeprazole (Patients who are concomitantly receiving bortezomib and drugs that are inhibitors or inducers of cytochrome P450 3A4 should be closely monitored for either toxicities or reduced efficacy).
No products indexed under this heading.

Oxcarbazepine (Patients who are concomitantly receiving bortezomib and drugs that are inhibitors or inducers of cytochrome P450 3A4 should be closely monitored for either toxicities or reduced efficacy).
No products indexed under this heading.

Pantoprazole Sodium (Bortezomib may inhibit 2C19 activity and increase exposure to drugs that are substrates for this enzyme). Products include:
Protonix for Delayed-Release Oral Suspension **3254**
Protonix Delayed-Release Tablets **3254**
Protonix I.V. **3257**

Paramethadione (Bortezomib may inhibit 2C19 activity and increase exposure to drugs that are substrates for this enzyme).
No products indexed under this heading.

Paroxetine Hydrochloride (Patients who are concomitantly receiving bortezomib and drugs that are inhibitors or inducers of cytochrome P450 3A4 should be closely monitored for either toxicities or reduced efficacy). Products include:
Paxil **1535**
Paxil CR Controlled-Release Tablets **1544**

Pentamidine Isethionate (Bortezomib may inhibit 2C19 activity and increase exposure to drugs that are substrates for this enzyme).
No products indexed under this heading.

IMPORTANT NOTE: Always consult each drug listing in the patient's regimen for possible interactions.

Phenacemide (Bortezomib may inhibit 2C19 activity and increase exposure to drugs that are substrates for this enzyme).
No products indexed under this heading.

Phenobarbital (Patients who are concomitantly receiving bortezomib and drugs that are inhibitors or inducers of cytochrome P450 3A4 should be closely monitored for either toxicities or reduced efficacy). Products include:
Donnatal Extentabs 2507

Phenobarbital Sodium (Patients who are concomitantly receiving bortezomib and drugs that are inhibitors or inducers of cytochrome P450 3A4 should be closely monitored for either toxicities or reduced efficacy).
No products indexed under this heading.

Phensuximide (Bortezomib may inhibit 2C19 activity and increase exposure to drugs that are substrates for this enzyme).
No products indexed under this heading.

Phenytoin (Patients who are concomitantly receiving bortezomib and drugs that are inhibitors or inducers of cytochrome P450 3A4 should be closely monitored for either toxicities or reduced efficacy).
No products indexed under this heading.

Phenytoin Sodium (Patients who are concomitantly receiving bortezomib and drugs that are inhibitors or inducers of cytochrome P450 3A4 should be closely monitored for either toxicities or reduced efficacy). Products include:
Phenytek Capsules 2192

Pioglitazone Hydrochloride (During clinical trials, hypoglycemia and hyperglycemia were reported in diabetic patients receiving oral hypoglycemics. Patients on oral antidiabetic agents receiving bortezomib treatment may require close monitoring of their blood glucose levels and adjustment of the dose of their antidiabetic medication). Products include:
ActoPlus Met Tablets 3071
Actos Tablets 3077
Duetact Tablets 3085

Prednisolone Acetate (Patients who are concomitantly receiving bortezomib and drugs that are inhibitors or inducers of cytochrome P450 3A4 should be closely monitored for either toxicities or reduced efficacy). Products include:
Pred Forte Ophthalmic Suspension .... ⊙227
Pred Mild Ophthalmic Suspension .... ⊙230
Pred-G Ophthalmic Ointment .... ⊙229
Pred-G Ophthalmic Suspension .... ⊙228

Prednisolone Sodium Phosphate (Patients who are concomitantly receiving bortezomib and drugs that are inhibitors or inducers of cytochrome P450 3A4 should be closely monitored for either toxicities or reduced efficacy).
No products indexed under this heading.

Prednisolone Tebutate (Patients who are concomitantly receiving bortezomib and drugs that are inhibitors or inducers of cytochrome P450 3A4 should be closely monitored for either toxicities or reduced efficacy).
No products indexed under this heading.

Prednisone (Co-administration of melphalan-prednisone on bortezomib showed a 17% increase in mean bortezomib AUC based on data from 21 patients. This increase is unlikely to be clinically relevant).
No products indexed under this heading.

Primidone (Patients who are concomitantly receiving bortezomib and drugs that are inhibitors or inducers of cytochrome P450 3A4 should be closely monitored for either toxicities or reduced efficacy).
No products indexed under this heading.

Progesterone (Bortezomib may inhibit 2C19 activity and increase exposure to drugs that are substrates for this enzyme). Products include:
Crinone 4% Gel 992
Crinone 8% Gel 992
Prometrium Capsules (100 mg, 200 mg) 3047

Proguanil Hydrochloride (Bortezomib may inhibit 2C19 activity and increase exposure to drugs that are substrates for this enzyme). Products include:
Malarone Pediatric Tablets 1521
Malarone Tablets 1521

Propoxyphene Hydrochloride (Patients who are concomitantly receiving bortezomib and drugs that are inhibitors or inducers of cytochrome P450 3A4 should be closely monitored for either toxicities or reduced efficacy).
No products indexed under this heading.

Propoxyphene Napsylate (Patients who are concomitantly receiving bortezomib and drugs that are inhibitors or inducers of cytochrome P450 3A4 should be closely monitored for either toxicities or reduced efficacy).
No products indexed under this heading.

Propranolol Hydrochloride (Bortezomib may inhibit 2C19 activity and increase exposure to drugs that are substrates for this enzyme). Products include:
InnoPran XL Extended Release Capsules 1484

Protriptyline Hydrochloride (Bortezomib may inhibit 2C19 activity and increase exposure to drugs that are substrates for this enzyme).
No products indexed under this heading.

Quinidine (Patients who are concomitantly receiving bortezomib and drugs that are inhibitors or inducers of cytochrome P450 3A4 should be closely monitored for either toxicities or reduced efficacy).
No products indexed under this heading.

Quinidine Hydrochloride (Patients who are concomitantly receiving bortezomib and drugs that are inhibitors or inducers of cytochrome P450 3A4 should be closely monitored for either toxicities or reduced efficacy).
No products indexed under this heading.

Quinidine Polygalacturonate (Patients who are concomitantly receiving bortezomib and drugs that are inhibitors or inducers of cytochrome P450 3A4 should be closely monitored for either toxicities or reduced efficacy).
No products indexed under this heading.

Quinidine Sulfate (Patients who are concomitantly receiving bortezomib and drugs that are inhibitors or inducers of cytochrome P450 3A4 should be closely monitored for either toxicities or reduced efficacy).
No products indexed under this heading.

Quinine (Patients who are concomitantly receiving bortezomib and drugs that are inhibitors or inducers of cytochrome P450 3A4 should be closely monitored for either toxicities or reduced efficacy).
No products indexed under this heading.

Quinine Sulfate (Patients who are concomitantly receiving bortezomib and drugs that are inhibitors or inducers of cytochrome P450 3A4 should be closely monitored for either toxicities or reduced efficacy).
No products indexed under this heading.

Quinupristin (Patients who are concomitantly receiving bortezomib and drugs that are inhibitors or inducers of cytochrome P450 3A4 should be closely monitored for either toxicities or reduced efficacy).
No products indexed under this heading.

Rabeprazole Sodium (Bortezomib may inhibit 2C19 activity and increase exposure to drugs that are substrates for this enzyme). Products include:
Aciphex Tablets 1053

Ranitidine Bismuth Citrate (Patients who are concomitantly receiving bortezomib and drugs that are inhibitors or inducers of cytochrome P450 3A4 should be closely monitored for either toxicities or reduced efficacy).
No products indexed under this heading.

Ranitidine Hydrochloride (Patients who are concomitantly receiving bortezomib and drugs that are inhibitors or inducers of cytochrome P450 3A4 should be closely monitored for either toxicities or reduced efficacy). Products include:
Zantac 75 Tablets .... ▣603
Zantac 1670
Zantac Injection 1666
Zantac Injection Pharmacy Bulk Package 1668
Maximum Strength Zantac 150 Tablets .... ▣603
Maximum Strength Zantac 150 Cool Mint Tablets .... ▣603

Repaglinide (During clinical trials, hypoglycemia and hyperglycemia were reported in diabetic patients receiving oral hypoglycemics. Patients on oral antidiabetic agents receiving bortezomib treatment may require close monitoring of their blood glucose levels and adjustment of the dose of their antidiabetic medication). Products include:
PrandiMet Tablets 2967
Prandin Tablets 2971

Rifabutin (Patients who are concomitantly receiving bortezomib and drugs that are inhibitors or inducers of cytochrome P450 3A4 should be closely monitored for either toxicities or reduced efficacy).
No products indexed under this heading.

Rifampicin (Patients who are concomitantly receiving bortezomib and drugs that are inhibitors or inducers of cytochrome P450 3A4 should be closely monitored for either toxicities or reduced efficacy).
No products indexed under this heading.

Rifampin (Patients who are concomitantly receiving bortezomib and drugs that are inhibitors or inducers of cytochrome P450 3A4 should be closely monitored for either toxicities or reduced efficacy).
No products indexed under this heading.

Rifapentine (Patients who are concomitantly receiving bortezomib and drugs that are inhibitors or inducers of cytochrome P450 3A4 should be closely monitored for either toxicities or reduced efficacy).
No products indexed under this heading.

Ritonavir (Patients who are concomitantly receiving bortezomib and drugs that are inhibitors or inducers of cytochrome P450 3A4 should be closely monitored for either toxicities or reduced efficacy). Products include:
Kaletra 452
Norvir 489

Rosiglitazone Maleate (During clinical trials, hypoglycemia and hyperglycemia were reported in diabetic patients receiving oral hypoglycemics. Patients on oral antidiabetic agents receiving bortezomib treatment may require close monitoring of their blood glucose levels and adjustment of the dose of their antidiabetic medication). Products include:
Avandamet Tablets 1336
Avandaryl Tablets 1344
Avandia Tablets 1351

Saquinavir (Patients who are concomitantly receiving bortezomib and drugs that are inhibitors or inducers of cytochrome P450 3A4 should be closely monitored for either toxicities or reduced efficacy).
No products indexed under this heading.

Saquinavir Mesylate (Patients who are concomitantly receiving bortezomib and drugs that are inhibitors or inducers of cytochrome P450 3A4 should be closely monitored for either toxicities or reduced efficacy).
No products indexed under this heading.

Sertraline Hydrochloride (Patients who are concomitantly receiving bortezomib and drugs that are inhibitors or inducers of cytochrome P450 3A4 should be closely monitored for either toxicities or reduced efficacy).
No products indexed under this heading.

Sildenafil Citrate (Patients who are concomitantly receiving bortezomib and drugs that are inhibitors or inducers of cytochrome P450 3A4 should be closely monitored for either toxicities or reduced efficacy).
No products indexed under this heading.

Sitagliptin Phosphate (During clinical trials, hypoglycemia and hyperglycemia were reported in diabetic patients receiving oral hypoglycemics. Patients on oral antidiabetic agents receiving bortezomib treatment may require close monitoring of their blood glucose levels and adjustment of the dose of their antidiabetic medication). Products include:
Janumet Tablets 2041
Januvia Tablets 2048

Sulfinpyrazone (Patients who are concomitantly receiving bortezomib and drugs that are inhibitors or inducers of cytochrome P450 3A4 should be closely monitored for either toxicities or reduced efficacy).
No products indexed under this heading.

Telithromycin (Patients who are concomitantly receiving bortezomib and drugs that are inhibitors or inducers of cytochrome P450 3A4 should be closely monitored for either toxicities or reduced efficacy). Products include:
Ketek Tablets 2744

Teniposide (Bortezomib may inhibit 2C19 activity and increase exposure to drugs that are substrates for this enzyme).
No products indexed under this heading.

Theophylline (Patients who are concomitantly receiving bortezomib and drugs that are inhibitors or inducers of cytochrome P450 3A4 should be closely monitored for either toxicities or reduced efficacy).
No products indexed under this heading.

Theophylline Anhydrous (Patients who are concomitantly receiving bortezomib and drugs that are inhibitors or inducers of cytochrome P450 3A4 should be closely monitored for either toxicities or reduced efficacy). Products include:
Uniphyl Tablets 2595

Theophylline Calcium Salicylate (Patients who are concomitantly receiving bortezomib and drugs that are inhibitors or inducers of cytochrome P450 3A4 should be closely monitored for either toxicities or reduced efficacy).
No products indexed under this heading.

Theophylline Dihydroxypropyl (Glyceryl) (Patients who are concomitantly receiving bortezomib and drugs that are inhibitors or inducers of cytochrome P450 3A4 should be closely monitored for either toxicities or reduced efficacy).
No products indexed under this heading.

Theophylline Ethylenediamine (Patients who are concomitantly receiving bortezomib and drugs that are inhibitors or inducers of cytochrome P450 3A4 should be closely monitored for either toxicities or reduced efficacy).
No products indexed under this heading.

Thioridazine (Bortezomib may inhibit 2C19 activity and increase exposure to drugs that are substrates for this enzyme).
No products indexed under this heading.

Thioridazine Hydrochloride (Bortezomib may inhibit 2C19 activity and increase exposure to drugs that are substrates for this enzyme). Products include:
Thioridazine Hydrochloride Tablets 2195

Tiagabine Hydrochloride (Bortezomib may inhibit 2C19 activity and increase exposure to drugs that are substrates for this enzyme). Products include:
Gabitril Tablets 973

Tolazamide (During clinical trials, hypoglycemia and hyperglycemia were reported in diabetic patients receiving oral hypoglycemics. Patients on oral antidiabetic agents receiving bortezomib treatment may require close monitoring of their blood glucose levels and adjustment of the dose of their antidiabetic medication).
No products indexed under this heading.

Tolbutamide (Bortezomib may inhibit 2C19 activity and increase exposure to drugs that are substrates for this enzyme).
No products indexed under this heading.

Tolbutamide Sodium (Bortezomib may inhibit 2C19 activity and increase exposure to drugs that are substrates for this enzyme).
No products indexed under this heading.

Topiramate (Bortezomib may inhibit 2C19 activity and increase exposure to drugs that are substrates for this enzyme).
No products indexed under this heading.

Triamcinolone (Patients who are concomitantly receiving bortezomib and drugs that are inhibitors or inducers of cytochrome P450 3A4 should be closely monitored for either toxicities or reduced efficacy).
No products indexed under this heading.

Triamcinolone Acetonide (Patients who are concomitantly receiving bortezomib and drugs that are inhibitors or inducers of cytochrome P450 3A4 should be closely monitored for either toxicities or reduced efficacy). Products include:
Azmacort Inhalation Aerosol 407
Nasacort AQ Nasal Spray 2765
Triesence Injectable Suspension .... ⊙ 209

Triamcinolone Diacetate (Patients who are concomitantly receiving bortezomib and drugs that are inhibitors or inducers of cytochrome P450 3A4 should be closely monitored for either toxicities or reduced efficacy).
No products indexed under this heading.

Triamcinolone Hexacetonide (Patients who are concomitantly receiving bortezomib and drugs that are inhibitors or inducers of cytochrome P450 3A4 should be closely monitored for either toxicities or reduced efficacy).
No products indexed under this heading.

Trimethadione (Bortezomib may inhibit 2C19 activity and increase exposure to drugs that are substrates for this enzyme).
No products indexed under this heading.

Trimipramine Maleate (Bortezomib may inhibit 2C19 activity and increase exposure to drugs that are substrates for this enzyme).
No products indexed under this heading.

Troglitazone (Patients who are concomitantly receiving bortezomib and drugs that are inhibitors or inducers of cytochrome P450 3A4 should be closely monitored for either toxicities or reduced efficacy).
No products indexed under this heading.

Troleandomycin (Patients who are concomitantly receiving bortezomib and drugs that are inhibitors or inducers of cytochrome P450 3A4 should be closely monitored for either toxicities or reduced efficacy).
No products indexed under this heading.

Valproate Sodium (Patients who are concomitantly receiving bortezomib and drugs that are inhibitors or inducers of cytochrome P450 3A4 should be closely monitored for either toxicities or reduced efficacy).
No products indexed under this heading.

Valproic Acid (Bortezomib may inhibit 2C19 activity and increase exposure to drugs that are substrates for this enzyme).
No products indexed under this heading.

Vardenafil Hydrochloride (Patients who are concomitantly receiving bortezomib and drugs that are inhibitors or inducers of cytochrome P450 3A4 should be closely monitored for either toxicities or reduced efficacy). Products include:
Levitra Tablets 2876

Verapamil Hydrochloride (Patients who are concomitantly receiving bortezomib and drugs that are inhibitors or inducers of cytochrome P450 3A4 should be closely monitored for either toxicities or reduced efficacy). Products include:
Tarka Tablets 511

Voriconazole (Patients who are concomitantly receiving bortezomib and drugs that are inhibitors or inducers of cytochrome P450 3A4 should be closely monitored for either toxicities or reduced efficacy).
No products indexed under this heading.

Warfarin Sodium (Bortezomib may inhibit 2C19 activity and increase exposure to drugs that are substrates for this enzyme).
No products indexed under this heading.

Zafirlukast (Patients who are concomitantly receiving bortezomib and drugs that are inhibitors or inducers of cytochrome P450 3A4 should be closely monitored for either toxicities or reduced efficacy). Products include:
Accolate Tablets 669

Zileuton (Patients who are concomitantly receiving bortezomib and drugs that are inhibitors or inducers of cytochrome P450 3A4 should be closely monitored for either toxicities or reduced efficacy).
No products indexed under this heading.

Zonisamide (Bortezomib may inhibit 2C19 activity and increase exposure to drugs that are substrates for this enzyme). Products include:
Zonegran Capsules 1089

Food Interactions

Grapefruit (Patients who are concomitantly receiving bortezomib and drugs that are inhibitors or inducers of cytochrome P450 3A4 should be closely monitored for either toxicities or reduced efficacy).

Grapefruit Juice (Patients who are concomitantly receiving bortezomib and drugs that are inhibitors or inducers of cytochrome P450 3A4 should be closely monitored for either toxicities or reduced efficacy).

VENLAFAXINE HYDROCHLORIDE TABLETS

(Venlafaxine Hydrochloride) 2199
May interact with aspirin-acetylsalicylic acid, central nervous system depressants, central nervous system stimulants, cytochrome p450 2d6 inhibitors (selected), cytochrome p450 3a4 inhibitors (selected), diuretics, lithium preparations, monoamine oxidase inhibitors, non-steroidal anti-inflammatory agents, serotoninergic agents, Serotonin and Norepinephrine Reuptake Inhibitors, selective serotonin reuptake inhibitors, triptans, and certain other agents. Compounds in these categories include:

5-hydroxytryptophan (The concomitant use of venlafaxine with tryptophan supplements is not recommended).
No products indexed under this heading.

Acetazolamide (Concomitant use of CYP3A4 inhibitors and venlafaxine may increase levels of venlafaxine and ODV. Therefore, caution is advised if a patient's therapy includes a CYP3A4 inhibitor and venlafaxine concomitantly. The concomitant use of venlafaxine with a drug treatment(s) that potently inhibits both CYP2D6 and CYP3A4, the primary metabolizing enzymes for venlafaxine, has not been studied. Therefore, caution is advised should a patient's therapy include venlafaxine and any agent(s) that produce potent simultaneous inhibition of these two enzyme systems).
No products indexed under this heading.

Alfentanil Hydrochloride (The risk of using venlafaxine in combination with other CNS active drugs has not been systematically evaluated. Consequently, caution is advised if the concomitant administration of venlafaxine and such drugs is required).
No products indexed under this heading.

Almotriptan Malate (Based on the mechanism of action of venlafaxine and the potential for serotonin syndrome, caution is advised when venlafaxine is co-administered with other drugs that may affect the serotonergic neurotransmitter systems, such as triptans. If concomitant treatment of venlafaxine with a triptan is clinically warranted, careful observation of the patient is advised, particularly during treatment initiation and dose increases). Products include:

Axert Tablets 2431

Alprazolam (The risk of using venlafaxine in combination with other CNS active drugs has not been systematically evaluated. Consequently, caution is advised if the concomitant administration of venlafaxine and such drugs is required).

No products indexed under this heading.

Amiloride Hydrochloride (Hyponatremia may occur as a result of treatment with SNRIs, including venlafaxine. In many cases, this hyponatremia appears to be the result of the syndrome of inappropriate antidiuretic hormone secretion (SIADH). Cases with serum sodium lower than 110 mmol/L have been reported. Elderly patients may be at greater risk of developing hyponatremia with SSRIs and SNRIs. Also patients taking diuretics or who are otherwise volume depleted may be at greater risk. Discontinuation of venlafaxine should be considered in patients with symptomatic hyponatremia and appropriate medical intervention should be instituted).

No products indexed under this heading.

Amiodarone Hydrochloride (Concomitant use of CYP3A4 inhibitors and venlafaxine may increase levels of venlafaxine and ODV. Therefore, caution is advised if a patient's therapy includes a CYP3A4 inhibitor and venlafaxine concomitantly. The concomitant use of venlafaxine with a drug treatment(s) that potently inhibits both CYP2D6 and CYP3A4, the primary metabolizing enzymes for venlafaxine, has not been studied. Therefore, caution is advised should a patient's therapy include venlafaxine and any agent(s) that produce potent simultaneous inhibition of these two enzyme systems).

No products indexed under this heading.

Amitriptyline Hydrochloride (Studies indicate that venlafaxine is metabolized to its active metabolite, ODV, by CYP2D6. Thus the potential exists for a drug interaction between drugs that inhibit CYP2D6-mediated metabolism and venlafaxine. However, although imipramine partially inhibited the CYP2D6-mediated metabolism of venlafaxine, resulting in higher plasma concentrations of venlafaxine and lower plasma concentrations of ODV, the total concentration of active compounds (venlafaxine plus ODV) was not affected. Also, in a clinical study involving CYP2D6 poor and extensive metabolizers, the total concentration of active compounds (venlafaxine plus ODV), was similar in both groups. No dosage adjustment is required when venlafaxine is co-administered with a CYP2D6 inhibitor).

No products indexed under this heading.

Amoxapine (Studies indicate that venlafaxine is metabolized to its active metabolite, ODV, by CYP2D6. Thus the potential exists for a drug interaction between drugs that inhibit CYP2D6-mediated metabolism and venlafaxine. However, although imipramine partially inhibited the CYP2D6-mediated metabolism of venlafaxine, resulting in higher plasma concentrations of venlafaxine and lower plasma concentrations of ODV, the total concentration of active compounds (venlafaxine plus ODV) was not affected. Also, in a clinical study involving CYP2D6 poor and extensive metabolizers, the total concentration of active compounds (venlafaxine plus ODV), was similar in both groups. No dosage adjustment is required when venlafaxine is co-administered with a CYP2D6 inhibitor).

No products indexed under this heading.

Amphetamine Resins (The risk of using venlafaxine in combination with other CNS active drugs has not been systematically evaluated. Consequently, caution is advised if the concomitant administration of venlafaxine and such drugs is required).

No products indexed under this heading.

Amprenavir (Concomitant use of CYP3A4 inhibitors and venlafaxine may increase levels of venlafaxine and ODV. Therefore, caution is advised if a patient's therapy includes a CYP3A4 inhibitor and venlafaxine concomitantly. The concomitant use of venlafaxine with a drug treatment(s) that potently inhibits both CYP2D6 and CYP3A4, the primary metabolizing enzymes for venlafaxine, has not been studied. Therefore, caution is advised should a patient's therapy include venlafaxine and any agent(s) that produce potent simultaneous inhibition of these two enzyme systems).

No products indexed under this heading.

Anastrozole (Concomitant use of CYP3A4 inhibitors and venlafaxine may increase levels of venlafaxine and ODV. Therefore, caution is advised if a patient's therapy includes a CYP3A4 inhibitor and venlafaxine concomitantly. The concomitant use of venlafaxine with a drug treatment(s) that potently inhibits both CYP2D6 and CYP3A4, the primary metabolizing enzymes for venlafaxine, has not been studied. Therefore, caution is advised should a patient's therapy include venlafaxine and any agent(s) that produce potent simultaneous inhibition of these two enzyme systems). Products include:

Arimidex Tablets 672

Aprepitant (Concomitant use of CYP3A4 inhibitors and venlafaxine may increase levels of venlafaxine and ODV. Therefore, caution is advised if a patient's therapy includes a CYP3A4 inhibitor and venlafaxine concomitantly. The concomitant use of venlafaxine with a drug treatment(s) that potently inhibits both CYP2D6 and CYP3A4, the primary metabolizing enzymes for venlafaxine, has not been studied. Therefore, caution is advised should a patient's therapy include venlafaxine and any agent(s) that produce potent simultaneous inhibition of these two enzyme systems). Products include:

Emend Capsules 1992

Aprobarbital (The risk of using venlafaxine in combination with other CNS active drugs has not been systematically evaluated. Consequently, caution is advised if the concomitant administration of venlafaxine and such drugs is required).

No products indexed under this heading.

Aspirin (Serotonin release by platelets plays an important role in hemostasis. Epidemiological studies of the case control and cohort design have demonstrated an association between use of psychotropic drugs that interfere with serotonin reuptake and the occurrence of upper gastrointestinal bleeding have also shown that concurrent use of an aspirin may potentiate this risk of bleeding). Products include:

Aggrenox Capsules 819
Bayer Aspirin 750
Percodan Tablets 1130
St. Joseph 81 mg Aspirin Chewable and Enteric Coated Tablets 1903

Aspirin, Enteric Coated (Serotonin release by platelets plays an important role in hemostasis. Epidemiological studies of the case control and cohort design have demonstrated an association between use of psychotropic drugs that interfere with serotonin reuptake and the occurrence of upper gastrointestinal bleeding have also shown that concurrent use of an aspirin may potentiate this risk of bleeding).

No products indexed under this heading.

Aspirin Buffered (Serotonin release by platelets plays an important role in hemostasis. Epidemiological studies of the case control and cohort design have demonstrated an association between use of psychotropic drugs that interfere with serotonin reuptake and the occurrence of upper gastrointestinal bleeding have also shown that concurrent use of an aspirin may potentiate this risk of bleeding).

No products indexed under this heading.

Atazanavir (Concomitant use of CYP3A4 inhibitors and venlafaxine may increase levels of venlafaxine and ODV. Therefore, caution is advised if a patient's therapy includes a CYP3A4 inhibitor and venlafaxine concomitantly. The concomitant use of venlafaxine with a drug treatment(s) that potently inhibits both CYP2D6 and CYP3A4, the primary metabolizing enzymes for venlafaxine, has not been studied. Therefore, caution is advised should a patient's therapy include venlafaxine and any agent(s) that produce potent simultaneous inhibition of these two enzyme systems).

No products indexed under this heading.

Atazanavir Sulfate (Concomitant use of CYP3A4 inhibitors and venlafaxine may increase levels of venlafaxine and ODV. Therefore, caution is advised if a patient's therapy includes a CYP3A4 inhibitor and venlafaxine concomitantly. The concomitant use of venlafaxine with a drug treatment(s) that potently inhibits both CYP2D6 and CYP3A4, the primary metabolizing enzymes for venlafaxine, has not been studied. Therefore, caution is advised should a patient's therapy include venlafaxine and any agent(s) that produce potent simultaneous inhibition of these two enzyme systems). Products include:

Reyataz Capsules 3299

Bendroflumethiazide (Hyponatremia may occur as a result of treatment with SNRIs, including venlafaxine. In many cases, this hyponatremia appears to be the result of the syndrome of inappropriate antidiuretic hormone secretion (SIADH). Cases with serum sodium lower than 110 mmol/L have been reported. Elderly patients may be at greater risk of developing hyponatremia with SSRIs and SNRIs. Also patients taking diuretics or who are otherwise volume depleted may be at greater risk. Discontinuation of venlafaxine should be considered in patients with symptomatic hyponatremia and appropriate medical intervention should be instituted).

No products indexed under this heading.

Bumetanide (Hyponatremia may occur as a result of treatment with SNRIs, including venlafaxine. In many cases, this hyponatremia appears to be the result of the syndrome of inappropriate antidiuretic hormone secretion (SIADH). Cases with serum sodium lower than 110 mmol/L have been reported. Elderly patients may be at greater risk of developing hyponatremia with SSRIs and SNRIs. Also patients taking diuretics or who are otherwise volume depleted may be at greater risk. Discontinuation of venlafaxine should be considered in patients with symptomatic hyponatremia and appropriate medical intervention should be instituted).

No products indexed under this heading.

Buprenorphine Hydrochloride (The risk of using venlafaxine in combination with other CNS active drugs has not been systematically evaluated. Consequently, caution is advised if the concomitant administration of venlafaxine and such drugs is required). Products include:

Suboxone Tablets 2601
Subutex Tablets 2601

Bupropion Hydrochloride (Studies indicate that venlafaxine is metabolized to its active metabolite, ODV, by CYP2D6. Thus the potential exists for a drug interaction between drugs that inhibit CYP2D6-mediated metabolism and venlafaxine. However, although imipramine partially inhibited the CYP2D6-mediated metabolism of venlafaxine, resulting in higher plasma concentrations of venlafaxine and lower plasma concentrations of ODV, the total concentration of active compounds (venlafaxine plus ODV) was not affected. Also, in a clinical study involving CYP2D6 poor and extensive metabolizers, the total concentration of active compounds (venlafaxine plus ODV), was similar in both groups. No dosage adjustment is required when venlafaxine is co-administered with a CYP2D6 inhibitor). Products include:

Wellbutrin Tablets 1648
Wellbutrin SR Sustained-Release Tablets 1653
Wellbutrin XL Extended-Release Tablets 1659
Zyban Sustained-Release Tablets 1692

Buspirone Hydrochloride (The risk of using venlafaxine in combination with other CNS active drugs has not been systematically evaluated. Consequently, caution is advised if the concomitant administration of venlafaxine and such drugs is required).
No products indexed under this heading.

Butabarbital (The risk of using venlafaxine in combination with other CNS active drugs has not been systematically evaluated. Consequently, caution is advised if the concomitant administration of venlafaxine and such drugs is required).
No products indexed under this heading.

Butalbital (The risk of using venlafaxine in combination with other CNS active drugs has not been systematically evaluated. Consequently, caution is advised if the concomitant administration of venlafaxine and such drugs is required).
No products indexed under this heading.

Celecoxib (Serotonin release by platelets plays an important role in hemostasis. Epidemiological studies of the case control and cohort design have demonstrated an association between use of psychotropic drugs that interfere with serotonin reuptake and the occurrence of upper gastrointestinal bleeding have also shown that concurrent use of an NSAID may potentiate this risk of bleeding). Products include:
Celebrex Capsules 2979

Chlordiazepoxide (The risk of using venlafaxine in combination with other CNS active drugs has not been systematically evaluated. Consequently, caution is advised if the concomitant administration of venlafaxine and such drugs is required).
No products indexed under this heading.

Chlordiazepoxide Hydrochloride (The risk of using venlafaxine in combination with other CNS active drugs has not been systematically evaluated. Consequently, caution is advised if the concomitant administration of venlafaxine and such drugs is required).
No products indexed under this heading.

Chloroquine Hydrochloride (Studies indicate that venlafaxine is metabolized to its active metabolite, ODV, by CYP2D6. Thus the potential exists for a drug interaction between drugs that inhibit CYP2D6-mediated metabolism and venlafaxine. However, although imipramine partially inhibited the CYP2D6-mediated metabolism of venlafaxine, resulting in higher plasma concentrations of venlafaxine and lower plasma concentrations of ODV, the total concentration of active compounds (venlafaxine plus ODV) was not affected. Also, in a clinical study involving CYP2D6 poor and extensive metabolizers, the total concentration of active compounds (venlafaxine plus ODV), was similar in both groups. No dosage adjustment is required when venlafaxine is co-administered with a CYP2D6 inhibitor).
No products indexed under this heading.

Chloroquine Phosphate (Studies indicate that venlafaxine is metabolized to its active metabolite, ODV, by CYP2D6. Thus the potential exists for a drug interaction between drugs that inhibit CYP2D6-mediated metabolism and venlafaxine. However, although imipramine partially inhibited the CYP2D6-mediated metabolism of venlafaxine, resulting in higher plasma concentrations of venlafaxine and lower plasma concentrations of ODV, the total concentration of active compounds (venlafaxine plus ODV) was not affected. Also, in a clinical study involving CYP2D6 poor and extensive metabolizers, the total concentration of active compounds (venlafaxine plus ODV), was similar in both groups. No dosage adjustment is required when venlafaxine is co-administered with a CYP2D6 inhibitor).
No products indexed under this heading.

Chlorothiazide (Hyponatremia may occur as a result of treatment with SNRIs, including venlafaxine. In many cases, this hyponatremia appears to be the result of the syndrome of inappropriate antidiuretic hormone secretion (SIADH). Cases with serum sodium lower than 110 mmol/L have been reported. Elderly patients may be at greater risk of developing hyponatremia with SSRIs and SNRIs. Also patients taking diuretics or who are otherwise volume depleted may be at greater risk. Discontinuation of venlafaxine should be considered in patients with symptomatic hyponatremia and appropriate medical intervention should be instituted).
No products indexed under this heading.

Chlorothiazide Sodium (Hyponatremia may occur as a result of treatment with SNRIs, including venlafaxine. In many cases, this hyponatremia appears to be the result of the syndrome of inappropriate antidiuretic hormone secretion (SIADH). Cases with serum sodium lower than 110 mmol/L have been reported. Elderly patients may be at greater risk of developing hyponatremia with SSRIs and SNRIs. Also patients taking diuretics or who are otherwise volume depleted may be at greater risk. Discontinuation of venlafaxine should be considered in patients with symptomatic hyponatremia and appropriate medical intervention should be instituted). Products include:
Intravenous Sodium Diuril 2490

Chlorpheniramine (Studies indicate that venlafaxine is metabolized to its active metabolite, ODV, by CYP2D6. Thus the potential exists for a drug interaction between drugs that inhibit CYP2D6-mediated metabolism and venlafaxine. However, although imipramine partially inhibited the CYP2D6-mediated metabolism of venlafaxine, resulting in higher plasma concentrations of venlafaxine and lower plasma concentrations of ODV, the total concentration of active compounds (venlafaxine plus ODV) was not affected. Also, in a clinical study involving CYP2D6 poor and extensive metabolizers, the total concentration of active compounds (venlafaxine plus ODV), was similar in both groups. No dosage adjustment is required when venlafaxine is co-administered with a CYP2D6 inhibitor).
No products indexed under this heading.

Chlorpheniramine Maleate (Studies indicate that venlafaxine is metabolized to its active metabolite, ODV, by CYP2D6. Thus the potential exists for a drug interaction between drugs that inhibit CYP2D6-mediated metabolism and venlafaxine. However, although imipramine partially inhibited the CYP2D6-mediated metabolism of venlafaxine, resulting in higher plasma concentrations of venlafaxine and lower plasma concentrations of ODV, the total concentration of active compounds (venlafaxine plus ODV) was not affected. Also, in a clinical study involving CYP2D6 poor and extensive metabolizers, the total concentration of active compounds (venlafaxine plus ODV), was similar in both groups. No dosage adjustment is required when venlafaxine is co-administered with a CYP2D6 inhibitor). Products include:
Actifed Cold & Allergy Tablets 1895
Sudafed PE Sinus & Allergy Tablets 1908
Tylenol Allergy Multi-Symptom Caplets with Cool Burst and Rapid Release Gelcaps 1916
Children's Tylenol Plus Cold Suspension Liquid 1912
Children's Tylenol Plus Cough & Runny Nose Suspension Liquid 1912
Children's Tylenol Plus Flu Suspension Liquid 1914
Children's Tylenol Plus Multi-Symptom Cold Suspension Liquid 1912
Tylenol Cold Head Congestion Nighttime Caplets with Cool Burst 1910
Tylenol Cold Multi-Symptom Nighttime Caplets with Cool Burst 1913
Tylenol Sinus Congestion & Pain Nighttime Caplets with Cool Burst 1917

Chlorpheniramine Polistirex (Studies indicate that venlafaxine is metabolized to its active metabolite, ODV, by CYP2D6. Thus the potential exists for a drug interaction between drugs that inhibit CYP2D6-mediated metabolism and venlafaxine. However, although imipramine partially inhibited the CYP2D6-mediated metabolism of venlafaxine, resulting in higher plasma concentrations of venlafaxine and lower plasma concentrations of ODV, the total concentration of active compounds (venlafaxine plus ODV) was not affected. Also, in a clinical study involving CYP2D6 poor and extensive metabolizers, the total concentration of active compounds (venlafaxine plus ODV), was similar in both groups. No dosage adjustment is required when venlafaxine is co-administered with a CYP2D6 inhibitor). Products include:
Tussionex Pennkinetic Extended-Release Suspension 3154

Chlorpheniramine Tannate (Studies indicate that venlafaxine is metabolized to its active metabolite, ODV, by CYP2D6. Thus the potential exists for a drug interaction between drugs that inhibit CYP2D6-mediated metabolism and venlafaxine. However, although imipramine partially inhibited the CYP2D6-mediated metabolism of venlafaxine, resulting in higher plasma concentrations of venlafaxine and lower plasma concentrations of ODV, the total concentration of active compounds (venlafaxine plus ODV) was not affected. Also, in a clinical study involving CYP2D6 poor and extensive metabolizers, the total concentration of active compounds (venlafaxine plus ODV), was similar in both groups. No dosage adjustment is required when venlafaxine is co-administered with a CYP2D6 inhibitor).
No products indexed under this heading.

Chlorpromazine (The risk of using venlafaxine in combination with other CNS active drugs has not been systematically evaluated. Consequently, caution is advised if the concomitant administration of venlafaxine and such drugs is required).
No products indexed under this heading.

Chlorpromazine Hydrochloride (The risk of using venlafaxine in combination with other CNS active drugs has not been systematically evaluated. Consequently, caution is advised if the concomitant administration of venlafaxine and such drugs is required).
No products indexed under this heading.

Chlorprothixene (The risk of using venlafaxine in combination with other CNS active drugs has not been systematically evaluated. Consequently, caution is advised if the concomitant administration of venlafaxine and such drugs is required).
No products indexed under this heading.

Chlorprothixene Hydrochloride (The risk of using venlafaxine in combination with other CNS active drugs has not been systematically evaluated. Consequently, caution is advised if the concomitant administration of venlafaxine and such drugs is required).
No products indexed under this heading.

Chlorprothixene Lactate (The risk of using venlafaxine in combination with other CNS active drugs has not been systematically evaluated. Consequently, caution is advised if the concomitant administration of venlafaxine and such drugs is required).
No products indexed under this heading.

Chlorthalidone (Hyponatremia may occur as a result of treatment with SNRIs, including venlafaxine. In many cases, this hyponatremia appears to be the result of the syndrome of inappropriate antidiuretic hormone secretion (SIADH). Cases with serum sodium lower than 110 mmol/L have been reported. Elderly patients may be at greater risk of developing hyponatremia with SSRIs and SNRIs. Also patients taking diuretics or who are otherwise volume depleted may be at greater risk. Discontinuation of venlafaxine should be considered in patients with symptomatic hyponatremia and appropriate medical intervention should be instituted). Products include:
Clorpres Tablets 2185

Cimetidine (Concomitant administration of cimetidine and venlafaxine resulted in inhibition of first-pass metabolism of venlafaxine. The oral clearance of venlafaxine was reduced by about 43%, and the exposure (AUC) and maximum concentration (Cmax) of the drug were increased by about 60%. However, co-administration of cimetidine had no apparent effect on the pharmacokinetics of O-desmethylvenlafaxine (ODV). The overall pharmacological activity of venlafaxine plus ODV is

expected to increase only slightly, and no dosage adjustment should be necessary for most normal adults. However, in elderly patients, patients with pre-existing hypertension or hepatic dysfunction, the interaction of venlafaxine and cimetidine is not known and potentially could be more pronounced).

No products indexed under this heading.

Cimetidine Hydrochloride (Concomitant administration of cimetidine and venlafaxine resulted in inhibition of first-pass metabolism of venlafaxine. The oral clearance of venlafaxine was reduced by about 43%, and the exposure (AUC) and maximum concentration (Cmax) of the drug were increased by about 60%. However, co-administration of cimetidine had no apparent effect on the pharmacokinetics of O-desmethylvenlafaxine (ODV). The overall pharmacological activity of venlafaxine plus ODV is expected to increase only slightly, and no dosage adjustment should be necessary for most normal adults. However, in elderly patients, patients with pre-existing hypertension or hepatic dysfunction, the interaction of venlafaxine and cimetidine is not known and potentially could be more pronounced).

No products indexed under this heading.

Ciprofloxacin (Concomitant use of CYP3A4 inhibitors and venlafaxine may increase levels of venlafaxine and ODV. Therefore, caution is advised if a patient's therapy includes a CYP3A4 inhibitor and venlafaxine concomitantly. The concomitant use of venlafaxine with a drug treatment(s) that potently inhibits both CYP2D6 and CYP3A4, the primary metabolizing enzymes for venlafaxine, has not been studied. Therefore, caution is advised should a patient's therapy include venlafaxine and any agent(s) that produce potent simultaneous inhibition of these two enzyme systems). Products include:

Cipro I.V. **2817**
Cipro Oral Suspension **2810**
Cipro XR Tablets **2823**
Ciprodex Otic Suspension **541**

Citalopram Hydrobromide (Based on the mechanism of action of venlafaxine and the potential for serotonin syndrome, caution is advised when venlafaxine is co-administered with other drugs that may affect the serotonergic neurotransmitter systems. If concomitant treatment of venlafaxine with these drugs is clinically warranted, careful observation of the patient is advised, particularly during treatment initiation and dose increases). Products include:

Celexa **1160**

Clarithromycin (Concomitant use of CYP3A4 inhibitors and venlafaxine may increase levels of venlafaxine and ODV. Therefore, caution is advised if a patient's therapy includes a CYP3A4 inhibitor and venlafaxine concomitantly. The concomitant use of venlafaxine with a drug treatment(s) that potently inhibits both CYP2D6 and CYP3A4, the primary metabolizing enzymes for venlafaxine, has not been studied. Therefore, caution is advised should a patient's therapy include venlafaxine and any agent(s) that produce potent simultaneous inhibition of these two enzyme systems). Products include:

Biaxin/Biaxin XL **411**

Clomipramine Hydrochloride (Studies indicate that venlafaxine is metabolized to its active metabolite, ODV, by CYP2D6. Thus the potential exists for a drug interaction between drugs that inhibit CYP2D6-mediated metabolism and venlafaxine. However, although imipramine partially inhibited the CYP2D6-mediated metabolism of venlafaxine, resulting in higher plasma concentrations of venlafaxine and lower plasma concentrations of ODV, the total concentration of active compounds (venlafaxine plus ODV) was not affected. Also, in a clinical study involving CYP2D6 poor and extensive metabolizers, the total concentration of active compounds (venlafaxine plus ODV), was similar in both groups. No dosage adjustment is required when venlafaxine is co-administered with a CYP2D6 inhibitor).

No products indexed under this heading.

Clorazepate Dipotassium (The risk of using venlafaxine in combination with other CNS active drugs has not been systematically evaluated. Consequently, caution is advised if the concomitant administration of venlafaxine and such drugs is required).

No products indexed under this heading.

Clotrimazole (Concomitant use of CYP3A4 inhibitors and venlafaxine may increase levels of venlafaxine and ODV. Therefore, caution is advised if a patient's therapy includes a CYP3A4 inhibitor and venlafaxine concomitantly. The concomitant use of venlafaxine with a drug treatment(s) that potently inhibits both CYP2D6 and CYP3A4, the primary metabolizing enzymes for venlafaxine, has not been studied. Therefore, caution is advised should a patient's therapy include venlafaxine and any agent(s) that produce potent simultaneous inhibition of these two enzyme systems). Products include:

Lotrisone **2881**

Clozapine (There have been reports of elevated clozapine levels that were temporally associated with adverse events, including seizures, following the addition of venlafaxine).

No products indexed under this heading.

Cocaine Hydrochloride (Studies indicate that venlafaxine is metabolized to its active metabolite, ODV, by CYP2D6. Thus the potential exists for a drug interaction between drugs that inhibit CYP2D6-mediated metabolism and venlafaxine. However, although imipramine partially inhibited the CYP2D6-mediated metabolism of venlafaxine, resulting in higher plasma concentrations of venlafaxine and lower plasma concentrations of ODV, the total concentration of active compounds (venlafaxine plus ODV) was not affected. Also, in a clinical study involving CYP2D6 poor and extensive metabolizers, the total concentration of active compounds (venlafaxine plus ODV), was similar in both groups. No dosage adjustment is required when venlafaxine is co-administered with a CYP2D6 inhibitor).

No products indexed under this heading.

Codeine Phosphate (The risk of using venlafaxine in combination with other CNS active drugs has not been systematically evaluated. Consequently, caution is advised if the concomitant administration of venlafaxine and such drugs is required). Products include:

Tylenol with Codeine Tablets **2427**

Cyclosporine (Concomitant use of CYP3A4 inhibitors and venlafaxine may increase levels of venlafaxine and ODV. Therefore, caution is advised if a patient's therapy includes a CYP3A4 inhibitor and venlafaxine concomitantly. The concomitant use of venlafaxine with a drug treatment(s) that potently inhibits both CYP2D6 and CYP3A4, the primary metabolizing enzymes for venlafaxine, has not been studied. Therefore, caution is advised should a patient's therapy include venlafaxine and any agent(s) that produce potent simultaneous inhibition of these two enzyme systems). Products include:

Gengraf Capsules **435**
Neoral Oral Solution **2280**
Neoral Soft Gelatin Capsules **2280**
Restasis Ophthalmic Emulsion **557**
Sandimmune **2296**

Dalfopristin (Concomitant use of CYP3A4 inhibitors and venlafaxine may increase levels of venlafaxine and ODV. Therefore, caution is advised if a patient's therapy includes a CYP3A4 inhibitor and venlafaxine concomitantly. The concomitant use of venlafaxine with a drug treatment(s) that potently inhibits both CYP2D6 and CYP3A4, the primary metabolizing enzymes for venlafaxine, has not been studied. Therefore, caution is advised should a patient's therapy include venlafaxine and any agent(s) that produce potent simultaneous inhibition of these two enzyme systems).

No products indexed under this heading.

Danazol (Concomitant use of CYP3A4 inhibitors and venlafaxine may increase levels of venlafaxine and ODV. Therefore, caution is advised if a patient's therapy includes a CYP3A4 inhibitor and venlafaxine concomitantly. The concomitant use of venlafaxine with a drug treatment(s) that potently inhibits both CYP2D6 and CYP3A4, the primary metabolizing enzymes for venlafaxine, has not been studied. Therefore, caution is advised should a patient's therapy include venlafaxine and any agent(s) that produce potent simultaneous inhibition of these two enzyme systems).

No products indexed under this heading.

Delavirdine Mesylate (Concomitant use of CYP3A4 inhibitors and venlafaxine may increase levels of venlafaxine and ODV. Therefore, caution is advised if a patient's therapy includes a CYP3A4 inhibitor and venlafaxine concomitantly. The concomitant use of venlafaxine with a drug treatment(s) that potently inhibits both CYP2D6 and CYP3A4, the primary metabolizing enzymes for venlafaxine, has not been studied. Therefore, caution is advised should a patient's therapy include venlafaxine and any agent(s) that produce potent simultaneous inhibition of these two enzyme systems).

No products indexed under this heading.

Desflurane (The risk of using venlafaxine in combination with other CNS active drugs has not been systematically evaluated. Consequently, caution is advised if the concomitant administration of venlafaxine and such drugs is required).

No products indexed under this heading.

Desipramine Hydrochloride (Studies indicate that venlafaxine is metabolized to its active metabolite, ODV, by CYP2D6. Thus the potential exists for a drug interaction between drugs that inhibit CYP2D6-mediated metabolism and venlafaxine. However, although imipramine partially inhibited the CYP2D6-mediated metabolism of venlafaxine, resulting in higher plasma concentrations of venlafaxine and lower plasma concentrations of ODV, the total concentration of active compounds (venlafaxine plus ODV) was not affected. Also, in a clinical study involving CYP2D6 poor and extensive metabolizers, the total concentration of active compounds (venlafaxine plus ODV), was similar in both groups. No dosage adjustment is required when venlafaxine is co-administered with a CYP2D6 inhibitor).

No products indexed under this heading.

Desvenlafaxine Succinate (Based on the mechanism of action of venlafaxine and the potential for serotonin syndrome, caution is advised when venlafaxine is co-administered with other drugs that may affect the serotonergic neurotransmitter systems, such as other SNRIs. If concomitant treatment of venlafaxine with another SNRI is clinically warranted, careful observation of the patient is advised, particularly during treatment initiation and dose increases). Products include:

Pristiq Extended-Release Tablets **3247**

Dextroamphetamine Sulfate (The risk of using venlafaxine in combination with other CNS active drugs has not been systematically evaluated. Consequently, caution is advised if the concomitant administration of venlafaxine and such drugs is required). Products include:

Adderall XR Capsules **3012**
Dexedrine **1401**

Dezocine (The risk of using venlafaxine in combination with other CNS active drugs has not been systematically evaluated. Consequently, caution is advised if the concomitant administration of venlafaxine and such drugs is required).

No products indexed under this heading.

Diazepam (The risk of using venlafaxine in combination with other CNS active drugs has not been systematically evaluated. Consequently, caution is advised if the concomitant administration of venlafaxine and such drugs is required). Products include:

Valium Tablets **2658**

Diclofenac Epolamine (Serotonin release by platelets plays an important role in hemostasis. Epidemiological studies of the case control and cohort design have demonstrated an association between use of psychotropic drugs that interfere with serotonin reuptake and the occurrence of upper gastrointestinal bleeding have also shown that concurrent use of an NSAID may potentiate this risk of bleeding). Products include:

Flector Patch 561

Diclofenac Potassium (Serotonin release by platelets plays an important role in hemostasis. Epidemiological studies of the case control and cohort design have demonstrated an association between use of psychotropic drugs that interfere with serotonin reuptake and the occurrence of upper gastrointestinal bleeding have also shown that concurrent use of an NSAID may potentiate this risk of bleeding).

No products indexed under this heading.

Diclofenac Sodium (Serotonin release by platelets plays an important role in hemostasis. Epidemiological studies of the case control and cohort design have demonstrated an association between use of psychotropic drugs that interfere with serotonin reuptake and the occurrence of upper gastrointestinal bleeding have also shown that concurrent use of an NSAID may potentiate this risk of bleeding). Products include:

Diclofenac Sodium Ophthalmic Solution................................ ⊙240
Voltaren Ophthalmic Solution 2336
Voltaren Tablets 2334
Voltaren-XR Tablets 2337

Diltiazem Hydrochloride (Concomitant use of CYP3A4 inhibitors and venlafaxine may increase levels of venlafaxine and ODV. Therefore, caution is advised if a patient's therapy includes a CYP3A4 inhibitor and venlafaxine concomitantly. The concomitant use of venlafaxine with a drug treatment(s) that potently inhibits both CYP2D6 and CYP3A4, the primary metabolizing enzymes for venlafaxine, has not been studied. Therefore, caution is advised should a patient's therapy include venlafaxine and any agent(s) that produce potent simultaneous inhibition of these two enzyme systems). Products include:

Cardizem LA Extended Release Tablets....................................... 421

Diltiazem Maleate (Concomitant use of CYP3A4 inhibitors and venlafaxine may increase levels of venlafaxine and ODV. Therefore, caution is advised if a patient's therapy includes a CYP3A4 inhibitor and venlafaxine concomitantly. The concomitant use of venlafaxine with a drug treatment(s) that potently inhibits both CYP2D6 and CYP3A4, the primary metabolizing enzymes for venlafaxine, has not been studied. Therefore, caution is advised should a patient's therapy include venlafaxine and any agent(s) that produce potent simultaneous inhibition of these two enzyme systems).

No products indexed under this heading.

Diphenhydramine (Studies indicate that venlafaxine is metabolized to its active metabolite, ODV, by CYP2D6. Thus the potential exists for a drug interaction between drugs that inhibit CYP2D6-mediated metabolism and venlafaxine. However, although imipramine partially inhibited the CYP2D6-mediated metabolism of venlafaxine, resulting in higher plasma concentrations of venlafaxine and lower plasma concentrations of ODV, the total concentration of active compounds (venlafaxine plus ODV) was not affected. Also, in a clinical study involving CYP2D6 poor and extensive metabolizers, the total concentration of active compounds (venlafaxine plus ODV), was similar in both groups. No dosage adjustment is required when venlafaxine is co-administered with a CYP2D6 inhibitor).

No products indexed under this heading.

Diphenhydramine Hydrochloride (Studies indicate that venlafaxine is metabolized to its active metabolite, ODV, by CYP2D6. Thus the potential exists for a drug interaction between drugs that inhibit CYP2D6-mediated metabolism and venlafaxine. However, although imipramine partially inhibited the CYP2D6-mediated metabolism of venlafaxine, resulting in higher plasma concentrations of venlafaxine and lower plasma concentrations of ODV, the total concentration of active compounds (venlafaxine plus ODV) was not affected. Also, in a clinical study involving CYP2D6 poor and extensive metabolizers, the total concentration of active compounds (venlafaxine plus ODV), was similar in both groups. No dosage adjustment is required when venlafaxine is co-administered with a CYP2D6 inhibitor). Products include:

Benadryl Allergy & Cold Kapgels 1895
Benadryl Allergy & Sinus Headache Kapgels 1895
Benadryl Severe Allergy & Sinus Headache Caplets 1897
Benadryl Dye-Free Allergy Liqui-gels Softgels...................... 1897
Benadryl Allergy Kapgels 1895
Benadryl Allergy Quick Dissolve Strips 1896
Benadryl Allergy Ultratab Tablets 1896
Children's Benadryl Dye-Free Allergy Liquid.............................. 1897
Children's Benadryl Allergy Fastmelts................................... 1897
Children's Benadryl Allergy Liquid 1898
Children's Benadryl Allergy Perfect Measure.......................... 1896
Children's Benadryl-D Allergy & Sinus Liquid................................. 1896
Benadryl-D Allergy & Sinus Tablet 1896
PediaCare Children's Allergy & Cold Liquid................................ 1902
PediaCare Children's Allergy Liquid.. 1902
Simply Sleep Caplets 1905
Sudafed PE Nighttime Cold Caplets.. 1907
Sudafed PE Severe Cold Caplets 1908
Extra Strength Tylenol PM Caplets, Geltabs, Liquid, and Rapid Release Gels..................... 1915
Tylenol Allergy Multi-Symptom Nighttime Caplets with Cool Burst.. 1916
Tylenol Severe Allergy Caplets 1916
Children's Tylenol Plus Cold & Allergy Suspension Liquid............ 1914
Tylenol Sore Throat Nighttime Liquid with Cool Burst.................. 1918

Doxepin Hydrochloride (Studies indicate that venlafaxine is metabolized to its active metabolite, ODV, by CYP2D6. Thus the potential exists for a drug interaction between drugs that inhibit CYP2D6-mediated metabolism and venlafaxine. However, although imipramine partially inhibited the CYP2D6-mediated metabolism of venlafaxine, resulting in higher plasma concentrations of venlafaxine and lower plasma concentrations of ODV, the total concentration of active compounds (venlafaxine plus ODV) was not affected. Also, in a clinical study involving CYP2D6 poor and extensive metabolizers, the total concentration of active compounds (venlafaxine plus ODV), was similar in both groups. No dosage adjustment is required when venlafaxine is co-administered with a CYP2D6 inhibitor).

No products indexed under this heading.

Droperidol (The risk of using venlafaxine in combination with other CNS active drugs has not been systematically evaluated. Consequently, caution is advised if the concomitant administration of venlafaxine and such drugs is required).

No products indexed under this heading.

Duloxetine Hydrochloride (Based on the mechanism of action of venlafaxine and the potential for serotonin syndrome, caution is advised when venlafaxine is co-administered with other drugs that may affect the serotonergic neurotransmitter systems, such as other SNRIs. If concomitant treatment of venlafaxine with another SNRI is clinically warranted, careful observation of the patient is advised, particularly during treatment initiation and dose increases). Products include:

Cymbalta Delayed-Release Capsules.................................. 1801

Efavirenz (Concomitant use of CYP3A4 inhibitors and venlafaxine may increase levels of venlafaxine and ODV. Therefore, caution is advised if a patient's therapy includes a CYP3A4 inhibitor and venlafaxine concomitantly. The concomitant use of venlafaxine with a drug treatment(s) that potently inhibits both CYP2D6 and CYP3A4, the primary metabolizing enzymes for venlafaxine, has not been studied. Therefore, caution is advised should a patient's therapy include venlafaxine and any agent(s) that produce potent simultaneous inhibition of these two enzyme systems). Products include:

Atripla Tablets 938
Sustiva Capsules 930
Sustiva Tablets 930

Eletriptan Hydrobromide (Based on the mechanism of action of venlafaxine and the potential for serotonin syndrome, caution is advised when venlafaxine is co-administered with other drugs that may affect the serotonergic neurotransmitter systems, such as triptans. If concomitant treatment of venlafaxine with a triptan is clinically warranted, careful observation of the patient is advised, particularly during treatment initiation and dose increases).

No products indexed under this heading.

Enflurane (The risk of using venlafaxine in combination with other CNS active drugs has not been systematically evaluated. Consequently, caution is advised if the concomitant administration of venlafaxine and such drugs is required).

No products indexed under this heading.

Erythromycin (Concomitant use of CYP3A4 inhibitors and venlafaxine may increase levels of venlafaxine and ODV. Therefore, caution is advised if a patient's therapy includes a CYP3A4 inhibitor and venlafaxine concomitantly. The concomitant use of venlafaxine with a drug treatment(s) that potently inhibits both CYP2D6 and CYP3A4, the primary metabolizing enzymes for venlafaxine, has not been studied. Therefore, caution is advised should a patient's therapy include venlafaxine and any agent(s) that produce potent simultaneous inhibition of these two enzyme systems).

No products indexed under this heading.

Erythromycin Estolate (Concomitant use of CYP3A4 inhibitors and venlafaxine may increase levels of venlafaxine and ODV. Therefore, caution is advised if a patient's therapy includes a CYP3A4 inhibitor and venlafaxine concomitantly. The concomitant use of venlafaxine with a drug treatment(s) that potently inhibits both CYP2D6 and CYP3A4, the primary metabolizing enzymes for venlafaxine, has not been studied. Therefore, caution is advised should a patient's therapy include venlafaxine and any agent(s) that produce potent simultaneous inhibition of these two enzyme systems).

No products indexed under this heading.

Erythromycin Ethylsuccinate (Concomitant use of CYP3A4 inhibitors and venlafaxine may increase levels of venlafaxine and ODV. Therefore, caution is advised if a patient's therapy includes a CYP3A4 inhibitor and venlafaxine concomitantly. The concomitant use of venlafaxine with a drug treatment(s) that potently inhibits both CYP2D6 and CYP3A4, the primary metabolizing enzymes for venlafaxine, has not been studied. Therefore, caution is advised should a patient's therapy include venlafaxine and any agent(s) that produce potent simultaneous inhibition of these two enzyme systems). Products include:

E.E.S. 433
EryPed 431

Erythromycin Gluceptate (Concomitant use of CYP3A4 inhibitors and venlafaxine may increase levels of venlafaxine and ODV. Therefore, caution is advised if a patient's therapy includes a CYP3A4 inhibitor and venlafaxine concomitantly. The concomitant use of venlafaxine with a drug treatment(s) that potently inhibits both CYP2D6 and CYP3A4, the primary metabolizing enzymes for venlafaxine, has not been studied. Therefore, caution is advised should a patient's therapy include venlafaxine and any agent(s) that produce potent simultaneous inhibition of these two enzyme systems).

No products indexed under this heading.

Erythromycin Lactobionate (Concomitant use of CYP3A4 inhibitors and venlafaxine may increase levels of venlafaxine and ODV. Therefore, caution is advised if a patient's therapy includes a CYP3A4 inhibitor and venlafaxine concomitantly. The concomitant use of venlafaxine with a drug treatment(s) that potently inhibits both CYP2D6 and CYP3A4, the primary metabolizing enzymes for venlafaxine, has not been studied. Therefore, caution is advised should a patient's therapy include venlafaxine and any agent(s) that produce potent simultaneous inhibition of these two enzyme systems).

No products indexed under this heading.

Erythromycin Stearate (Concomitant use of CYP3A4 inhibitors and venlafaxine may increase levels of venlafaxine and ODV. Therefore, caution is advised if a patient's therapy includes a CYP3A4 inhibitor and venlafaxine concomitantly. The concomitant use of venlafaxine with a drug treatment(s) that potently inhibits both CYP2D6 and CYP3A4, the primary metabolizing enzymes for venlafaxine, has not been studied. Therefore, caution is advised should a patient's therapy include venlafaxine and any agent(s) that produce potent simultaneous inhibition of these two enzyme systems).
No products indexed under this heading.

Escitalopram Oxalate (Based on the mechanism of action of venlafaxine and the potential for serotonin syndrome, caution is advised when venlafaxine is co-administered with other drugs that may affect the serotonergic neurotransmitter systems. If concomitant treatment of venlafaxine with these drugs is clinically warranted, careful observation of the patient is advised, particularly during treatment initiation and dose increases). Products include:
Lexapro Oral Suspension 1174
Lexapro Tablets 1174

Esomeprazole Magnesium (Concomitant use of CYP3A4 inhibitors and venlafaxine may increase levels of venlafaxine and ODV. Therefore, caution is advised if a patient's therapy includes a CYP3A4 inhibitor and venlafaxine concomitantly. The concomitant use of venlafaxine with a drug treatment(s) that potently inhibits both CYP2D6 and CYP3A4, the primary metabolizing enzymes for venlafaxine, has not been studied. Therefore, caution is advised should a patient's therapy include venlafaxine and any agent(s) that produce potent simultaneous inhibition of these two enzyme systems). Products include:
Nexium Delayed-Release Capsules 645
Nexium Delayed-Release Oral Suspension 645

Estazolam (The risk of using venlafaxine in combination with other CNS active drugs has not been systematically evaluated. Consequently, caution is advised if the concomitant administration of venlafaxine and such drugs is required).
No products indexed under this heading.

Ethacrynic Acid (Hyponatremia may occur as a result of treatment with SNRIs, including venlafaxine. In many cases, this hyponatremia appears to be the result of the syndrome of inappropriate antidiuretic hormone secretion (SIADH). Cases with serum sodium lower than 110 mmol/L have been reported. Elderly patients may be at greater risk of developing hyponatremia with SSRIs and SNRIs. Also patients taking diuretics or who are otherwise volume depleted may be at greater risk. Discontinuation of venlafaxine should be considered in patients with symptomatic hyponatremia and appropriate medical intervention should be instituted). Products include:
Edecrin Tablets 698

Ethanol (Although venlafaxine has not been shown to increase the impairment of mental and motor skills caused by alcohol, patients should be advised to avoid alcohol while taking venlafaxine).
No products indexed under this heading.

Ethchlorvynol (The risk of using venlafaxine in combination with other CNS active drugs has not been systematically evaluated. Consequently, caution is advised if the concomitant administration of venlafaxine and such drugs is required).
No products indexed under this heading.

Ethinamate (The risk of using venlafaxine in combination with other CNS active drugs has not been systematically evaluated. Consequently, caution is advised if the concomitant administration of venlafaxine and such drugs is required).
No products indexed under this heading.

Ethyl Alcohol (Although venlafaxine has not been shown to increase the impairment of mental and motor skills caused by alcohol, patients should be advised to avoid alcohol while taking venlafaxine).
No products indexed under this heading.

Etodolac (Serotonin release by platelets plays an important role in hemostasis. Epidemiological studies of the case control and cohort design have demonstrated an association between use of psychotropic drugs that interfere with serotonin reuptake and the occurrence of upper gastrointestinal bleeding have also shown that concurrent use of an NSAID may potentiate this risk of bleeding).
No products indexed under this heading.

Fenoprofen Calcium (Serotonin release by platelets plays an important role in hemostasis. Epidemiological studies of the case control and cohort design have demonstrated an association between use of psychotropic drugs that interfere with serotonin reuptake and the occurrence of upper gastrointestinal bleeding have also shown that concurrent use of an NSAID may potentiate this risk of bleeding). Products include:
Nalfon Capsules 2508

Fentanyl (The risk of using venlafaxine in combination with other CNS active drugs has not been systematically evaluated. Consequently, caution is advised if the concomitant administration of venlafaxine and such drugs is required). Products include:
Duragesic Transdermal System 2405
Ionsys Transdermal System 2410

Fentanyl Citrate (The risk of using venlafaxine in combination with other CNS active drugs has not been systematically evaluated. Consequently, caution is advised if the concomitant administration of venlafaxine and such drugs is required). Products include:
Actiq 959
Fentora Tablets 968

Fluconazole (Concomitant use of CYP3A4 inhibitors and venlafaxine may increase levels of venlafaxine and ODV. Therefore, caution is advised if a patient's therapy includes a CYP3A4 inhibitor and venlafaxine concomitantly. The concomitant use of venlafaxine with a drug treatment(s) that potently inhibits both CYP2D6 and CYP3A4, the primary metabolizing enzymes for venlafaxine, has not been studied. Therefore, caution is advised should a patient's therapy include venlafaxine and any agent(s) that produce potent simultaneous inhibition of these two enzyme systems).
No products indexed under this heading.

Fluoxetine (Based on the mechanism of action of venlafaxine and the potential for serotonin syndrome, caution is advised when venlafaxine is co-administered with other drugs that may affect the serotonergic neurotransmitter systems, such as SSRIs. If concomitant treatment of venlafaxine with an SSRI is clinically warranted, careful observation of the patient is advised, particularly during treatment initiation and dose increases).
No products indexed under this heading.

Fluoxetine Hydrochloride (Based on the mechanism of action of venlafaxine and the potential for serotonin syndrome, caution is advised when venlafaxine is co-administered with other drugs that may affect the serotonergic neurotransmitter systems. If concomitant treatment of venlafaxine with these drugs is clinically warranted, careful observation of the patient is advised, particularly during treatment initiation and dose increases). Products include:
Prozac Weekly Capsules 1852
Prozac Pulvules and Liquid 1852
Symbyax Capsules 1871

Fluphenazine Decanoate (The risk of using venlafaxine in combination with other CNS active drugs has not been systematically evaluated. Consequently, caution is advised if the concomitant administration of venlafaxine and such drugs is required).
No products indexed under this heading.

Fluphenazine Enanthate (The risk of using venlafaxine in combination with other CNS active drugs has not been systematically evaluated. Consequently, caution is advised if the concomitant administration of venlafaxine and such drugs is required).
No products indexed under this heading.

Fluphenazine Hydrochloride (The risk of using venlafaxine in combination with other CNS active drugs has not been systematically evaluated. Consequently, caution is advised if the concomitant administration of venlafaxine and such drugs is required).
No products indexed under this heading.

Flurazepam Hydrochloride (The risk of using venlafaxine in combination with other CNS active drugs has not been systematically evaluated. Consequently, caution is advised if the concomitant administration of venlafaxine and such drugs is required).
No products indexed under this heading.

Flurbiprofen (Serotonin release by platelets plays an important role in hemostasis. Epidemiological studies of the case control and cohort design have demonstrated an association between use of psychotropic drugs that interfere with serotonin reuptake and the occurrence of upper gastrointestinal bleeding have also shown that concurrent use of an NSAID may potentiate this risk of bleeding).
No products indexed under this heading.

Fluvoxamine Maleate (Based on the mechanism of action of venlafaxine and the potential for serotonin syndrome, caution is advised when venlafaxine is co-administered with other drugs that may affect the serotonergic neurotransmitter systems. If concomitant treatment of venlafaxine with these drugs is clinically warranted, careful observation of the patient is advised, particularly during treatment initiation and dose increases). Products include:
Luvox CR Extended-Release Capsules 1759

Fosamprenavir Calcium (Concomitant use of CYP3A4 inhibitors and venlafaxine may increase levels of venlafaxine and ODV. Therefore, caution is advised if a patient's therapy includes a CYP3A4 inhibitor and venlafaxine concomitantly. The concomitant use of venlafaxine with a drug treatment(s) that potently inhibits both CYP2D6 and CYP3A4, the primary metabolizing enzymes for venlafaxine, has not been studied. Therefore, caution is advised should a patient's therapy include venlafaxine and any agent(s) that produce potent simultaneous inhibition of these two enzyme systems). Products include:
Lexiva Oral Suspension 1510
Lexiva Tablets 1510

Frovatriptan Succinate (Based on the mechanism of action of venlafaxine and the potential for serotonin syndrome, caution is advised when venlafaxine is co-administered with other drugs that may affect the serotonergic neurotransmitter systems, such as triptans. If concomitant treatment of venlafaxine with a triptan is clinically warranted, careful observation of the patient is advised, particularly during treatment initiation and dose increases). Products include:
Frova Tablets 1111

Furosemide (Hyponatremia may occur as a result of treatment with SNRIs, including venlafaxine. In many cases, this hyponatremia appears to be the result of the syndrome of inappropriate antidiuretic hormone secretion (SIADH). Cases with serum sodium lower than 110 mmol/L have been reported. Elderly patients may be at greater risk of developing hyponatremia with SSRIs and SNRIs. Also patients taking diuretics or who are otherwise volume depleted may be at greater risk. Discontinuation of venlafaxine should be considered in patients with symptomatic hyponatremia and appropriate medical intervention should be instituted). Products include:
Furosemide Tablets 2186

Glutethimide (The risk of using venlafaxine in combination with other CNS active drugs has not been systematically evaluated. Consequently, caution is advised if the concomitant administration of venlafaxine and such drugs is required).
No products indexed under this heading.

Halofantrine Hydrochloride (Studies indicate that venlafaxine is metabolized to its active metabolite, ODV, by CYP2D6. Thus the potential exists for a drug interaction between drugs that inhibit CYP2D6-mediated metabolism and venlafaxine. However, although imipramine partially inhibited the CYP2D6-mediated metabolism of venlafaxine, resulting in higher plasma concentrations of venlafaxine and lower plasma concentrations of ODV, the total concentration of active compounds (venlafaxine plus ODV) was not affected. Also, in a clinical study involving CYP2D6 poor and extensive metabolizers, the total concentration of active compounds (venlafaxine plus ODV), was similar in both groups. No dosage adjustment is required when venlafaxine is co-administered with a CYP2D6 inhibitor).

No products indexed under this heading.

Haloperidol (Venlafaxine administered under steady-state conditions at 150 mg/day in 24 healthy subjects decreased total oral-dose clearance (Cl/F) of a single 2 mg dose of haloperidol by 42%, which resulted in a 70% increase in haloperidol AUC. In addition, the haloperidol Cmax increased 88% when co-administered with venlafaxine, but the haloperidol elimination half-life (t1/2) was unchanged. The mechanism explaining this finding is unknown).

No products indexed under this heading.

Haloperidol Decanoate (Venlafaxine administered under steady-state conditions at 150 mg/day in 24 healthy subjects decreased total oral-dose clearance (Cl/F) of a single 2 mg dose of haloperidol by 42%, which resulted in a 70% increase in haloperidol AUC. In addition, the haloperidol Cmax increased 88% when co-administered with venlafaxine, but the haloperidol elimination half-life (t1/2) was unchanged. The mechanism explaining this finding is unknown).

No products indexed under this heading.

Haloperidol Lactate (Venlafaxine administered under steady-state conditions at 150 mg/day in 24 healthy subjects decreased total oral-dose clearance (Cl/F) of a single 2 mg dose of haloperidol by 42%, which resulted in a 70% increase in haloperidol AUC. In addition, the haloperidol Cmax increased 88% when co-administered with venlafaxine, but the haloperidol elimination half-life (t1/2) was unchanged. The mechanism explaining this finding is unknown).

No products indexed under this heading.

Hydrochlorothiazide (Hyponatremia may occur as a result of treatment with SNRIs, including venlafaxine. In many cases, this hyponatremia appears to be the result of the syndrome of inappropriate antidiuretic hormone secretion (SIADH). Cases with serum sodium lower than 110 mmol/L have been reported. Elderly patients may be at greater risk of developing hyponatremia with SSRIs and SNRIs. Also patients taking diuretics or who are otherwise volume depleted may be at greater risk. Discontinuation of venlafaxine should be considered in patients with symptomatic hyponatremia and appropriate medical intervention should be instituted).

Products include:

Atacand HCT 642
Avalide Tablets 892
Avalide Tablets 2713
Benicar HCT Tablets 1010
Diovan HCT Tablets 2216
Dyazide Capsules 1405
Micardis HCT Tablets 854
Prinzide Tablets 2092
Tekturna HCT Tablets 2324
Teveten HCT Tablets 517

Hydrocodone Bitartrate (The risk of using venlafaxine in combination with other CNS active drugs has not been systematically evaluated. Consequently, caution is advised if the concomitant administration of venlafaxine and such drugs is required).

Products include:

Lortab 5/500 Tablets 3143
Lortab 7.5/500 Tablets 3144
Lortab 10/500 Tablets 3144
Vicodin Tablets 529
Vicodin ES Tablets 530
Vicodin HP Tablets 531
Vicoprofen Tablets 533
Zydone Tablets 1132

Hydrocodone Polistirex (The risk of using venlafaxine in combination with other CNS active drugs has not been systematically evaluated. Consequently, caution is advised if the concomitant administration of venlafaxine and such drugs is required).

Products include:

Tussionex Pennkinetic Extended-Release Suspension 3154

Hydroflumethiazide (Hyponatremia may occur as a result of treatment with SNRIs, including venlafaxine. In many cases, this hyponatremia appears to be the result of the syndrome of inappropriate antidiuretic hormone secretion (SIADH). Cases with serum sodium lower than 110 mmol/L have been reported. Elderly patients may be at greater risk of developing hyponatremia with SSRIs and SNRIs. Also patients taking diuretics or who are otherwise volume depleted may be at greater risk. Discontinuation of venlafaxine should be considered in patients with symptomatic hyponatremia and appropriate medical intervention should be instituted).

No products indexed under this heading.

Hydromorphone Hydrochloride (The risk of using venlafaxine in combination with other CNS active drugs has not been systematically evaluated. Consequently, caution is advised if the concomitant administration of venlafaxine and such drugs is required).

No products indexed under this heading.

Hydroxychloroquine Sulfate (Studies indicate that venlafaxine is metabolized to its active metabolite, ODV, by CYP2D6. Thus the potential exists for a drug interaction between drugs that inhibit CYP2D6-mediated metabolism and venlafaxine. However, although imipramine partially inhibited the CYP2D6-mediated metabolism of venlafaxine, resulting in higher plasma concentrations of venlafaxine and lower plasma concentrations of ODV, the total concentration of active compounds (venlafaxine plus ODV) was not affected. Also, in a clinical study involving CYP2D6 poor and extensive metabolizers, the total concentration of active compounds (venlafaxine plus ODV), was similar in both groups. No dosage adjustment is required when venlafaxine is co-administered with a CYP2D6 inhibitor).

No products indexed under this heading.

Hydroxyzine Hydrochloride (The risk of using venlafaxine in combination with other CNS active drugs has not been systematically evaluated. Consequently, caution is advised if the concomitant administration of venlafaxine and such drugs is required).

No products indexed under this heading.

Hypericum (Based on the mechanism of action of venlafaxine and the potential for serotonin syndrome, caution is advised when venlafaxine is co-administered with other drugs that may affect the serotonergic neurotransmitter systems, such as St. John's Wort. If concomitant treatment of venlafaxine with St. John's Wort is clinically warranted, careful observation of the patient is advised, particularly during treatment initiation and dose increases). Products include:

Satieté Tablets 640

Ibuprofen (Serotonin release by platelets plays an important role in hemostasis. Epidemiological studies of the case control and cohort design have demonstrated an association between use of psychotropic drugs that interfere with serotonin reuptake and the occurrence of upper gastrointestinal bleeding have also shown that concurrent use of an NSAID may potentiate this risk of bleeding). Products include:

Motrin IB Tablets and Caplets 1900
Children's Motrin Oral Suspension ... 1901
Children's Motrin Non-Staining Dye-Free Oral Suspension 1901
Children's Motrin Cold Oral Suspension 1899
Infants' Motrin Concentrated Drops 1901
Infants' Motrin Non-Staining Dye-Free Concentrated Drops 1901
Junior Strength Motrin Caplets and Chewable Tablets 1901
Vicoprofen Tablets 533

Imatinib Mesylate (Studies indicate that venlafaxine is metabolized to its active metabolite, ODV, by CYP2D6. Thus the potential exists for a drug interaction between drugs that inhibit CYP2D6-mediated metabolism and venlafaxine. However, although imipramine partially inhibited the CYP2D6-mediated metabolism of venlafaxine, resulting in higher plasma concentrations of venlafaxine and lower plasma concentrations of ODV, the total concentration of active compounds (venlafaxine plus ODV) was not affected. Also, in a clinical study involving CYP2D6 poor and extensive metabolizers, the total concentration of active compounds (venlafaxine plus ODV), was similar in both groups. No dosage adjustment is required when venlafaxine is co-administered with a CYP2D6 inhibitor). Products include:

Gleevec Tablets 2255

Imipramine Hydrochloride (Venlafaxine did not affect the pharmacokinetics of imipramine and 2-OH-imipramine. However desipramine AUC, Cmax, and Cmin increased by about 35% in the presence of venlafaxine. The 2-OH-desipramine AUCs increased by at least 2.5-fold (with venlafaxine 37.5 mg q 12h) and 4.5-fold (with venlafaxine 75 mg q 12h). Imipramine did not affect the pharmacokinetics of venlafaxine and ODV. The clinical significance of elevated 2-OH-desipramine levels is unknown).

No products indexed under this heading.

Imipramine Pamoate (Venlafaxine did not affect the pharmacokinetics of imipramine and 2-OH-imipramine. However desipramine AUC, Cmax, and Cmin increased by about 35% in the presence of venlafaxine. The 2-OH-desipramine AUCs increased by at least 2.5-fold (with venlafaxine 37.5 mg q 12h) and 4.5-fold (with venlafaxine 75 mg q 12h). Imipramine did not affect the pharmacokinetics of venlafaxine and ODV. The clinical significance of elevated 2-OH-desipramine levels is unknown).

No products indexed under this heading.

Indapamide (Hyponatremia may occur as a result of treatment with SNRIs, including venlafaxine. In many cases, this hyponatremia appears to be the result of the syndrome of inappropriate antidiuretic hormone secretion (SIADH). Cases with serum sodium lower than 110 mmol/L have been reported. Elderly patients may be at greater risk of developing hyponatremia with SSRIs and SNRIs. Also patients taking diuretics or who are otherwise volume depleted may be at greater risk. Discontinuation of venlafaxine should be considered in patients with symptomatic hyponatremia and appropriate medical intervention should be instituted).

Products include:

Indapamide Tablets 2188

Indinavir Sulfate (In a study of nine healthy volunteers, venlafaxine administered under steady-state conditions at 150 mg/day resulted in a 28% decrease in the AUC of a single 800 mg dose of indinavir and a 36% decrease in indinavir Cmax. Indinavir did not affect the pharmacokinetics of venlafaxine and ODV. The clinical significance of this finding is unknown). Products include:

Crixivan Capsules 1979

Indomethacin (Serotonin release by platelets plays an important role in hemostasis. Epidemiological studies of the case control and cohort design have demonstrated an association between use of psychotropic drugs that interfere with serotonin reuptake and the occurrence of upper gastrointestinal bleeding have also shown that concurrent use of an NSAID may potentiate this risk of bleeding). Products include:

Indocin 2024

Indomethacin Sodium Trihydrate (Serotonin release by platelets plays an important role in hemostasis. Epidemiological studies of the case control and cohort design have demonstrated an association between use of psychotropic drugs that interfere with serotonin reuptake and the occurrence of upper gastrointestinal bleeding have also shown that concurrent use of an NSAID may potentiate this risk of bleeding).

Products include:

Indocin I.V. 2489

Isocarboxazid (Adverse reactions, some of which were serious, have been reported in patients who have recently been discontinued from a monoamine oxidase inhibitor (MAOI) and started on venlafaxine, or who have recently had venlafaxine therapy discontinued prior to initiation of an MAOI. Therefore, it is recommended that venlafaxine not be used in combination with an MAOI, or within at least 14 days of discontinuing treatment with an MAOI. Based on the half-life of venlafaxine, at least 7 days should be allowed after stopping venlafaxine before starting an MAOI. The concomitant use of venlafaxine with MAOIs intended to treat depression is contraindicated). Products include:

Marplan Tablets 3177

Isoflurane (The risk of using venlafaxine in combination with other CNS active drugs has not been systematically evaluated. Consequently, caution is advised if the concomitant administration of venlafaxine and such drugs is required).

No products indexed under this heading.

Isoniazid (Concomitant use of CYP3A4 inhibitors and venlafaxine may increase levels of venlafaxine and ODV. Therefore, caution is advised if a patient's therapy includes a CYP3A4 inhibitor and venlafaxine concomitantly. The concomitant use of venlafaxine with a drug treatment(s) that potently inhibits both CYP2D6 and CYP3A4, the primary metabolizing enzymes for venlafaxine, has not been studied. Therefore, caution is advised should a patient's therapy include venlafaxine and any agent(s) that produce potent simultaneous inhibition of these two enzyme systems).

No products indexed under this heading.

Itraconazole (Concomitant use of CYP3A4 inhibitors and venlafaxine may increase levels of venlafaxine and ODV. Therefore, caution is advised if a patient's therapy includes a CYP3A4 inhibitor and venlafaxine concomitantly. The concomitant use of venlafaxine with a drug treatment(s) that potently inhibits both CYP2D6 and CYP3A4, the primary metabolizing enzymes for venlafaxine, has not been studied. Therefore, caution is advised should a patient's therapy include venlafaxine and any agent(s) that produce potent simultaneous inhibition of these two enzyme systems).

No products indexed under this heading.

Ketamine Hydrochloride (The risk of using venlafaxine in combination with other CNS active drugs has not been systematically evaluated. Consequently, caution is advised if the concomitant administration of venlafaxine and such drugs is required).

No products indexed under this heading.

Ketoconazole (A study of ketoconazole 100 mg b.i.d. with a single dose of venlafaxine 50 mg in extensive metabolizers and 25 mg in poor metabolizers of CYP2D6 resulted in higher plasma concentrations of both venlafaxine and O-desvenlafaxine (ODV) in most subjects following administration of ketoconazole. Venlafaxine Cmax increased by 26% in EM subjects and 48% in PM subjects. Cmax values for ODV increased by 14% and 29% in EM and PM subjects, respectively. Venlafaxine AUC increased by 21% in EM subjects and 70% in PM subjects, and AUC values for ODV increased by 23% and 141% in EM and PM subjects, respectively. Combined AUCs of venlafaxine and ODV increased on an average of approximately 23% in EMs and 53% in PMs). Products include:

Extina Foam, 2% 3057
Nizoral A-D Shampoo 1901

Ketoprofen (Serotonin release by platelets plays an important role in hemostasis. Epidemiological studies of the case control and cohort design have demonstrated an association between use of psychotropic drugs that interfere with serotonin reuptake and the occurrence of upper gastrointestinal bleeding have also shown that concurrent use of an NSAID may potentiate this risk of bleeding).

No products indexed under this heading.

Ketorolac Tromethamine (Serotonin release by platelets plays an important role in hemostasis. Epidemiological studies of the case control and cohort design have demonstrated an association between use of psychotropic drugs that interfere with serotonin reuptake and the occurrence of upper gastrointestinal bleeding have also shown that concurrent use of an NSAID may potentiate this risk of bleeding).

No products indexed under this heading.

Levomethadyl Acetate Hydrochloride (The risk of using venlafaxine in combination with other CNS active drugs has not been systematically evaluated. Consequently, caution is advised if the concomitant administration of venlafaxine and such drugs is required).

No products indexed under this heading.

Levorphanol Tartrate (The risk of using venlafaxine in combination with other CNS active drugs has not been systematically evaluated. Consequently, caution is advised if the concomitant administration of venlafaxine and such drugs is required).

No products indexed under this heading.

Linezolid (Based on the mechanism of action of venlafaxine and the potential for serotonin syndrome, caution is advised when venlafaxine is co-administered with other drugs that may affect the serotonergic neurotransmitter systems, such as linezolid (an antibiotic which is a reversible non-selective MAOI). If concomitant treatment of venlafaxine with linezolid is clinically warranted, careful observation of the patient is advised, particularly during treatment initiation and dose increases). Products include:

Zyvox 2552

Lithium (Based on the mechanism of action of venlafaxine and the potential for serotonin syndrome, caution is advised when venlafaxine is co-administered with other drugs that may affect the serotonergic neurotransmitter systems, such as lithium. If concomitant treatment of venlafaxine with lithium is clinically warranted, careful observation of the patient is advised, particularly during treatment initiation and dose increases).

No products indexed under this heading.

Lithium Carbonate (Based on the mechanism of action of venlafaxine and the potential for serotonin syndrome, caution is advised when venlafaxine is co-administered with other drugs that may affect the serotonergic neurotransmitter systems, such as lithium. If concomitant treatment of venlafaxine with lithium is clinically warranted, careful observation of the patient is advised, particularly during treatment initiation and dose increases).

No products indexed under this heading.

Lithium Citrate (Based on the mechanism of action of venlafaxine and the potential for serotonin syndrome, caution is advised when venlafaxine is co-administered with other drugs that may affect the serotonergic neurotransmitter systems, such as lithium. If concomitant treatment of venlafaxine with lithium is clinically warranted, careful observation of the patient is advised, particularly during treatment initiation and dose increases).

No products indexed under this heading.

Lopinavir (Concomitant use of CYP3A4 inhibitors and venlafaxine may increase levels of venlafaxine and ODV. Therefore, caution is advised if a patient's therapy includes a CYP3A4 inhibitor and venlafaxine concomitantly. The concomitant use of venlafaxine with a drug treatment(s) that potently inhibits both CYP2D6 and CYP3A4, the primary metabolizing enzymes for venlafaxine, has not been studied. Therefore, caution is advised should a patient's therapy include venlafaxine and any agent(s) that produce potent simultaneous inhibition of these two enzyme systems). Products include:

Kaletra 452

Loratadine (Concomitant use of CYP3A4 inhibitors and venlafaxine may increase levels of venlafaxine and ODV. Therefore, caution is advised if a patient's therapy includes a CYP3A4 inhibitor and venlafaxine concomitantly. The concomitant use of venlafaxine with a drug treatment(s) that potently inhibits both CYP2D6 and CYP3A4, the primary metabolizing enzymes for venlafaxine, has not been studied. Therefore, caution is advised should a patient's therapy include venlafaxine and any agent(s) that produce potent simultaneous inhibition of these two enzyme systems).

No products indexed under this heading.

Lorazepam (The risk of using venlafaxine in combination with other CNS active drugs has not been systematically evaluated. Consequently, caution is advised if the concomitant administration of venlafaxine and such drugs is required).

No products indexed under this heading.

Loxapine Hydrochloride (The risk of using venlafaxine in combination with other CNS active drugs has not been systematically evaluated. Consequently, caution is advised if the concomitant administration of venlafaxine and such drugs is required).

No products indexed under this heading.

Loxapine Succinate (The risk of using venlafaxine in combination with other CNS active drugs has not been systematically evaluated. Consequently, caution is advised if the concomitant administration of venlafaxine and such drugs is required).

No products indexed under this heading.

Maprotiline Hydrochloride (Studies indicate that venlafaxine is metabolized to its active metabolite, ODV, by CYP2D6. Thus the potential exists for a drug interaction between drugs that inhibit CYP2D6-mediated metabolism and venlafaxine. However, although imipramine partially inhibited the CYP2D6-mediated metabolism of venlafaxine, resulting in higher plasma concentrations of venlafaxine and lower plasma concentrations of ODV, the total concentration of active compounds (venlafaxine plus ODV) was not affected. Also, in a clinical study involving CYP2D6 poor and extensive metabolizers, the total concentration of active compounds (venlafaxine plus ODV), was similar in both groups. No dosage adjustment is required when venlafaxine is co-administered with a CYP2D6 inhibitor).

No products indexed under this heading.

Meclofenamate Sodium (Serotonin release by platelets plays an important role in hemostasis. Epidemiological studies of the case control and cohort design have demonstrated an association between use of psychotropic drugs that interfere with serotonin reuptake and the occurrence of upper gastrointestinal bleeding have also shown that concurrent use of an NSAID may potentiate this risk of bleeding).

No products indexed under this heading.

Mefenamic Acid (Serotonin release by platelets plays an important role in hemostasis. Epidemiological studies of the case control and cohort design have demonstrated an association between use of psychotropic drugs that interfere with serotonin reuptake and the occurrence of upper gastrointestinal bleeding have also shown that concurrent use of an NSAID may potentiate this risk of bleeding).

No products indexed under this heading.

Meloxicam (Serotonin release by platelets plays an important role in hemostasis. Epidemiological studies of the case control and cohort design have demonstrated an association between use of psychotropic drugs that interfere with serotonin reuptake and the occurrence of upper gastrointestinal bleeding have also shown that concurrent use of an NSAID may potentiate this risk of bleeding). Products include:

Mobic Oral Suspension 863
Mobic Tablets 863

Meperidine Hydrochloride (The risk of using venlafaxine in combination with other CNS active drugs has not been systematically evaluated. Consequently, caution is advised if the concomitant administration of venlafaxine and such drugs is required).

No products indexed under this heading.

Mephobarbital (The risk of using venlafaxine in combination with other CNS active drugs has not been systematically evaluated. Consequently, caution is advised if the concomitant administration of venlafaxine and such drugs is required).
No products indexed under this heading.

Meprobamate (The risk of using venlafaxine in combination with other CNS active drugs has not been systematically evaluated. Consequently, caution is advised if the concomitant administration of venlafaxine and such drugs is required).
No products indexed under this heading.

Mesoridazine Besylate (The risk of using venlafaxine in combination with other CNS active drugs has not been systematically evaluated. Consequently, caution is advised if the concomitant administration of venlafaxine and such drugs is required).
No products indexed under this heading.

Methadone Hydrochloride (The risk of using venlafaxine in combination with other CNS active drugs has not been systematically evaluated. Consequently, caution is advised if the concomitant administration of venlafaxine and such drugs is required).
No products indexed under this heading.

Methamphetamine Hydrochloride (The risk of using venlafaxine in combination with other CNS active drugs has not been systematically evaluated. Consequently, caution is advised if the concomitant administration of venlafaxine and such drugs is required).
No products indexed under this heading.

Methohexital Sodium (The risk of using venlafaxine in combination with other CNS active drugs has not been systematically evaluated. Consequently, caution is advised if the concomitant administration of venlafaxine and such drugs is required).
No products indexed under this heading.

Methotrimeprazine (The risk of using venlafaxine in combination with other CNS active drugs has not been systematically evaluated. Consequently, caution is advised if the concomitant administration of venlafaxine and such drugs is required).
No products indexed under this heading.

Methoxyflurane (The risk of using venlafaxine in combination with other CNS active drugs has not been systematically evaluated. Consequently, caution is advised if the concomitant administration of venlafaxine and such drugs is required).
No products indexed under this heading.

Methyclothiazide (Hyponatremia may occur as a result of treatment with SNRIs, including venlafaxine. In many cases, this hyponatremia appears to be the result of the syndrome of inappropriate antidiuretic hormone secretion (SIADH). Cases with serum sodium lower than 110 mmol/L have been reported. Elderly patients may be at greater risk of developing hyponatremia with SSRIs and SNRIs. Also patients taking diuretics or who are otherwise volume depleted may be at greater risk. Discontinuation of venlafaxine should be considered in patients with symptomatic hyponatremia and appropriate medical intervention should be instituted).
No products indexed under this heading.

Methylphenidate (The risk of using venlafaxine in combination with other CNS active drugs has not been systematically evaluated. Consequently, caution is advised if the concomitant administration of venlafaxine and such drugs is required). Products include:
Daytrana Transdermal Patch 3022

Methylphenidate Hydrochloride (The risk of using venlafaxine in combination with other CNS active drugs has not been systematically evaluated. Consequently, caution is advised if the concomitant administration of venlafaxine and such drugs is required). Products include:
Concerta Extended-Release Tablets 1925
Metadate CD Capsules 3146

Metolazone (Hyponatremia may occur as a result of treatment with SNRIs, including venlafaxine. In many cases, this hyponatremia appears to be the result of the syndrome of inappropriate antidiuretic hormone secretion (SIADH). Cases with serum sodium lower than 110 mmol/L have been reported. Elderly patients may be at greater risk of developing hyponatremia with SSRIs and SNRIs. Also patients taking diuretics or who are otherwise volume depleted may be at greater risk. Discontinuation of venlafaxine should be considered in patients with symptomatic hyponatremia and appropriate medical intervention should be instituted).
No products indexed under this heading.

Metoprolol Succinate (Concomitant administration of venlafaxine (50 mg every 8 hours for 5 days) and metoprolol (100 mg every 24 hours for 5 days) to 18 healthy male subjects in a pharmacokinetic interaction study for both drugs resulted in an increase of plasma concentrations of metoprolol by approximately 30% to 40% without altering the plasma concentrations of its active metabolite, alpha-hydroxymetoprolol. Metoprolol did not alter the pharmacokinetic profile of venlafaxine or its active metabolite, O-desmethylvenlafaxine. Venlafaxine appeared to reduce the blood pressure-lowering effect of metoprolol in this study. The clinical relevance of this finding for hypertensive patients is unknown. Caution should be exercised with co-administration of venlafaxine and metoprolol). Products include:
Toprol-XL Tablets 666

Metoprolol Tartrate (Concomitant administration of venlafaxine (50 mg every 8 hours for 5 days) and metoprolol (100 mg every 24 hours for 5 days) to 18 healthy male subjects in a pharmacokinetic interaction study for both drugs resulted in an increase of plasma concentrations of metoprolol by approximately 30% to 40% without altering the plasma concentrations of its active metabolite, alpha-hydroxymetoprolol. Metoprolol did not alter the pharmacokinetic profile of venlafaxine or its active metabolite, O-desmethylvenlafaxine. Venlafaxine appeared to reduce the blood pressure-lowering effect of metoprolol in this study. The clinical relevance of this finding for hypertensive patients is unknown. Caution should be exercised with co-administration of venlafaxine and metoprolol).
No products indexed under this heading.

Metronidazole (Concomitant use of CYP3A4 inhibitors and venlafaxine may increase levels of venlafaxine and ODV. Therefore, caution is advised if a patient's therapy includes a CYP3A4 inhibitor and venlafaxine concomitantly. The concomitant use of venlafaxine with a drug treatment(s) that potently inhibits both CYP2D6 and CYP3A4, the primary metabolizing enzymes for venlafaxine, has not been studied. Therefore, caution is advised should a patient's therapy include venlafaxine and any agent(s) that produce potent simultaneous inhibition of these two enzyme systems). Products include:
Pylera Capsules 714

Metronidazole Benzoate (Concomitant use of CYP3A4 inhibitors and venlafaxine may increase levels of venlafaxine and ODV. Therefore, caution is advised if a patient's therapy includes a CYP3A4 inhibitor and venlafaxine concomitantly. The concomitant use of venlafaxine with a drug treatment(s) that potently inhibits both CYP2D6 and CYP3A4, the primary metabolizing enzymes for venlafaxine, has not been studied. Therefore, caution is advised should a patient's therapy include venlafaxine and any agent(s) that produce potent simultaneous inhibition of these two enzyme systems).
No products indexed under this heading.

Metronidazole Hydrochloride (Concomitant use of CYP3A4 inhibitors and venlafaxine may increase levels of venlafaxine and ODV. Therefore, caution is advised if a patient's therapy includes a CYP3A4 inhibitor and venlafaxine concomitantly. The concomitant use of venlafaxine with a drug treatment(s) that potently inhibits both CYP2D6 and CYP3A4, the primary metabolizing enzymes for venlafaxine, has not been studied. Therefore, caution is advised should a patient's therapy include venlafaxine and any agent(s) that produce potent simultaneous inhibition of these two enzyme systems).
No products indexed under this heading.

Metronidazole Sodium (Concomitant use of CYP3A4 inhibitors and venlafaxine may increase levels of venlafaxine and ODV. Therefore, caution is advised if a patient's therapy includes a CYP3A4 inhibitor and venlafaxine concomitantly. The concomitant use of venlafaxine with a drug treatment(s) that potently inhibits both CYP2D6 and CYP3A4, the primary metabolizing enzymes for venlafaxine, has not been studied. Therefore, caution is advised should a patient's therapy include venlafaxine and any agent(s) that produce potent simultaneous inhibition of these two enzyme systems).
No products indexed under this heading.

Mibefradil Dihydrochloride (Studies indicate that venlafaxine is metabolized to its active metabolite, ODV, by CYP2D6. Thus the potential exists for a drug interaction between drugs that inhibit CYP2D6-mediated metabolism and venlafaxine. However, although imipramine partially inhibited the CYP2D6-mediated metabolism of venlafaxine, resulting in higher plasma concentrations of venlafaxine and lower plasma concentrations of ODV, the total concentration of active compounds (venlafaxine plus ODV) was not affected. Also, in a clinical study involving CYP2D6 poor and extensive metabolizers, the total concentration of active compounds (venlafaxine plus ODV), was similar in both groups. No dosage adjustment is required when venlafaxine is co-administered with a CYP2D6 inhibitor).
No products indexed under this heading.

Miconazole (Concomitant use of CYP3A4 inhibitors and venlafaxine may increase levels of venlafaxine and ODV. Therefore, caution is advised if a patient's therapy includes a CYP3A4 inhibitor and venlafaxine concomitantly. The concomitant use of venlafaxine with a drug treatment(s) that potently inhibits both CYP2D6 and CYP3A4, the primary metabolizing enzymes for venlafaxine, has not been studied. Therefore, caution is advised should a patient's therapy include venlafaxine and any agent(s) that produce potent simultaneous inhibition of these two enzyme systems).
No products indexed under this heading.

Miconazole Nitrate (Concomitant use of CYP3A4 inhibitors and venlafaxine may increase levels of venlafaxine and ODV. Therefore, caution is advised if a patient's therapy includes a CYP3A4 inhibitor and venlafaxine concomitantly. The concomitant use of venlafaxine with a drug treatment(s) that potently inhibits both CYP2D6 and CYP3A4, the primary metabolizing enzymes for venlafaxine, has not been studied. Therefore, caution is advised should a patient's therapy include venlafaxine and any agent(s) that produce potent simultaneous inhibition of these two enzyme systems).
No products indexed under this heading.

Midazolam Hydrochloride (The risk of using venlafaxine in combination with other CNS active drugs has not been systematically evaluated. Consequently, caution is advised if the concomitant administration of venlafaxine and such drugs is required).
No products indexed under this heading.

Moclobemide (Adverse reactions, some of which were serious, have been reported in patients who have recently been discontinued from a monoamine oxidase inhibitor (MAOI) and started on venlafaxine, or who have recently had venlafaxine therapy discontinued prior to initiation of an MAOI. Therefore, it is recommended that venlafaxine not be used in combination with an MAOI, or within at least 14 days of discontinuing treatment with an MAOI. Based on the half-life of venlafaxine, at least 7 days should be allowed after stopping venlafaxine before starting an MAOI. The concomitant use of ven-

lafaxine with MAOIs intended to treat depression is contraindicated).

No products indexed under this heading.

Molindone Hydrochloride (The risk of using venlafaxine in combination with other CNS active drugs has not been systematically evaluated. Consequently, caution is advised if the concomitant administration of venlafaxine and such drugs is required). Products include:

Moban Tablets 1116

Morphine Sulfate (The risk of using venlafaxine in combination with other CNS active drugs has not been systematically evaluated. Consequently, caution is advised if the concomitant administration of venlafaxine and such drugs is required). Products include:

Avinza Capsules 1772
DepoDur Injection 1095
MS Contin Tablets 2585

Nabumetone (Serotonin release by platelets plays an important role in hemostasis. Epidemiological studies of the case control and cohort design have demonstrated an association between use of psychotropic drugs that interfere with serotonin reuptake and the occurrence of upper gastrointestinal bleeding have also shown that concurrent use of an NSAID may potentiate this risk of bleeding).

No products indexed under this heading.

Naproxen (Serotonin release by platelets plays an important role in hemostasis. Epidemiological studies of the case control and cohort design have demonstrated an association between use of psychotropic drugs that interfere with serotonin reuptake and the occurrence of upper gastrointestinal bleeding have also shown that concurrent use of an NSAID may potentiate this risk of bleeding). Products include:

EC-Naprosyn Delayed-Release Tablets 2632
Naprosyn Suspension 2632
Naprosyn Tablets 2632

Naproxen Sodium (Serotonin release by platelets plays an important role in hemostasis. Epidemiological studies of the case control and cohort design have demonstrated an association between use of psychotropic drugs that interfere with serotonin reuptake and the occurrence of upper gastrointestinal bleeding have also shown that concurrent use of an NSAID may potentiate this risk of bleeding). Products include:

Anaprox Tablets 2632
Anaprox DS Tablets 2632
Treximet Tablets 1616

Naratriptan Hydrochloride (Based on the mechanism of action of venlafaxine and the potential for serotonin syndrome, caution is advised when venlafaxine is co-administered with other drugs that may affect the serotonergic neurotransmitter systems, such as triptans. If concomitant treatment of venlafaxine with a triptan is clinically warranted, careful observation of the patient is advised, particularly during treatment initiation and dose increases). Products include:

Amerge Tablets 1301

Nefazodone Hydrochloride (Based on the mechanism of action of venlafaxine and the potential for serotonin syndrome, caution is advised when venlafaxine is co-administered with other drugs that may affect the serotonergic neurotransmitter systems, such as other SNRIs. If concomitant treatment of venlafaxine with another SNRI is clinically warranted, careful observation of the patient is advised, particularly during treatment initiation and dose increases).

No products indexed under this heading.

Nelfinavir Mesylate (Concomitant use of CYP3A4 inhibitors and venlafaxine may increase levels of venlafaxine and ODV. Therefore, caution is advised if a patient's therapy includes a CYP3A4 inhibitor and venlafaxine concomitantly. The concomitant use of venlafaxine with a drug treatment(s) that potently inhibits both CYP2D6 and CYP3A4, the primary metabolizing enzymes for venlafaxine, has not been studied. Therefore, caution is advised should a patient's therapy include venlafaxine and any agent(s) that produce potent simultaneous inhibition of these two enzyme systems).

No products indexed under this heading.

Nevirapine (Concomitant use of CYP3A4 inhibitors and venlafaxine may increase levels of venlafaxine and ODV. Therefore, caution is advised if a patient's therapy includes a CYP3A4 inhibitor and venlafaxine concomitantly. The concomitant use of venlafaxine with a drug treatment(s) that potently inhibits both CYP2D6 and CYP3A4, the primary metabolizing enzymes for venlafaxine, has not been studied. Therefore, caution is advised should a patient's therapy include venlafaxine and any agent(s) that produce potent simultaneous inhibition of these two enzyme systems). Products include:

Viramune Oral Suspension 873
Viramune Tablets 873

Niacinamide (Concomitant use of CYP3A4 inhibitors and venlafaxine may increase levels of venlafaxine and ODV. Therefore, caution is advised if a patient's therapy includes a CYP3A4 inhibitor and venlafaxine concomitantly. The concomitant use of venlafaxine with a drug treatment(s) that potently inhibits both CYP2D6 and CYP3A4, the primary metabolizing enzymes for venlafaxine, has not been studied. Therefore, caution is advised should a patient's therapy include venlafaxine and any agent(s) that produce potent simultaneous inhibition of these two enzyme systems). Products include:

BioLean Free Tablets .... ▣635

Nicotinamide (Concomitant use of CYP3A4 inhibitors and venlafaxine may increase levels of venlafaxine and ODV. Therefore, caution is advised if a patient's therapy includes a CYP3A4 inhibitor and venlafaxine concomitantly. The concomitant use of venlafaxine with a drug treatment(s) that potently inhibits both CYP2D6 and CYP3A4, the primary metabolizing enzymes for venlafaxine, has not been studied. Therefore, caution is advised should a patient's therapy include venlafaxine and any agent(s) that produce potent simultaneous inhibition of these two enzyme systems).

No products indexed under this heading.

Nifedipine (Concomitant use of CYP3A4 inhibitors and venlafaxine may increase levels of venlafaxine and ODV. Therefore, caution is advised if a patient's therapy includes a CYP3A4 inhibitor and venlafaxine concomitantly. The concomitant use of venlafaxine with a drug treatment(s) that potently inhibits both CYP2D6 and CYP3A4, the primary metabolizing enzymes for venlafaxine, has not been studied. Therefore, caution is advised should a patient's therapy include venlafaxine and any agent(s) that produce potent simultaneous inhibition of these two enzyme systems).

No products indexed under this heading.

Norfloxacin (Concomitant use of CYP3A4 inhibitors and venlafaxine may increase levels of venlafaxine and ODV. Therefore, caution is advised if a patient's therapy includes a CYP3A4 inhibitor and venlafaxine concomitantly. The concomitant use of venlafaxine with a drug treatment(s) that potently inhibits both CYP2D6 and CYP3A4, the primary metabolizing enzymes for venlafaxine, has not been studied. Therefore, caution is advised should a patient's therapy include venlafaxine and any agent(s) that produce potent simultaneous inhibition of these two enzyme systems). Products include:

Noroxin Tablets 2069

Nortriptyline Hydrochloride (Studies indicate that venlafaxine is metabolized to its active metabolite, ODV, by CYP2D6. Thus the potential exists for a drug interaction between drugs that inhibit CYP2D6-mediated metabolism and venlafaxine. However, although imipramine partially inhibited the CYP2D6-mediated metabolism of venlafaxine, resulting in higher plasma concentrations of venlafaxine and lower plasma concentrations of ODV, the total concentration of active compounds (venlafaxine plus ODV) was not affected. Also, in a clinical study involving CYP2D6 poor and extensive metabolizers, the total concentration of active compounds (venlafaxine plus ODV), was similar in both groups. No dosage adjustment is required when venlafaxine is co-administered with a CYP2D6 inhibitor).

No products indexed under this heading.

Olanzapine (The risk of using venlafaxine in combination with other CNS active drugs has not been systematically evaluated. Consequently, caution is advised if the concomitant administration of venlafaxine and such drugs is required). Products include:

Symbyax Capsules 1871
Zyprexa Tablets 1883
Zyprexa IntraMuscular 1883
Zyprexa ZYDIS Orally Disintegrating Tablets 1883

Omeprazole (Concomitant use of CYP3A4 inhibitors and venlafaxine may increase levels of venlafaxine and ODV. Therefore, caution is advised if a patient's therapy includes a CYP3A4 inhibitor and venlafaxine concomitantly. The concomitant use of venlafaxine with a drug treatment(s) that potently inhibits both CYP2D6 and CYP3A4, the primary metabolizing enzymes for venlafaxine, has not been studied. Therefore, caution is advised should a patient's therapy include venlafaxine and any agent(s) that produce potent simultaneous inhibition of these two enzyme systems).

No products indexed under this heading.

Oxaprozin (Serotonin release by platelets plays an important role in hemostasis. Epidemiological studies of the case control and cohort design have demonstrated an association between use of psychotropic drugs that interfere with serotonin reuptake and the occurrence of upper gastrointestinal bleeding have also shown that concurrent use of an NSAID may potentiate this risk of bleeding).

No products indexed under this heading.

Oxazepam (The risk of using venlafaxine in combination with other CNS active drugs has not been systematically evaluated. Consequently, caution is advised if the concomitant administration of venlafaxine and such drugs is required).

No products indexed under this heading.

Oxycodone Hydrochloride (The risk of using venlafaxine in combination with other CNS active drugs has not been systematically evaluated. Consequently, caution is advised if the concomitant administration of venlafaxine and such drugs is required). Products include:

OxyContin Tablets 2589
OxyIR Capsules 2593
Percocet Tablets 1127
Percodan Tablets 1130

Pargyline Hydrochloride (Adverse reactions, some of which were serious, have been reported in patients who have recently been discontinued from a monoamine oxidase inhibitor (MAOI) and started on venlafaxine, or who have recently had venlafaxine therapy discontinued prior to initiation of an MAOI. Therefore, it is recommended that venlafaxine not be used in combination with an MAOI, or within at least 14 days of discontinuing treatment with an MAOI. Based on the half-life of venlafaxine, at least 7 days should be allowed after stopping venlafaxine before starting an MAOI. The concomitant use of venlafaxine with MAOIs intended to treat depression is contraindicated).

No products indexed under this heading.

Paroxetine Hydrochloride (Based on the mechanism of action of venlafaxine and the potential for serotonin syndrome, caution is advised when venlafaxine is co-administered with other drugs that may affect the serotonergic neurotransmitter systems. If concomitant treatment of venlafaxine with these drugs is clinically warranted, careful observation of the patient is advised, particularly during treatment initiation and dose increases). Products include:

Paxil 1535
Paxil CR Controlled-Release Tablets 1544

Pemoline (The risk of using venlafaxine in combination with other CNS active drugs has not been systematically evaluated. Consequently, caution is advised if the concomitant administration of venlafaxine and such drugs is required).

No products indexed under this heading.

Pentobarbital Sodium (The risk of using venlafaxine in combination with other CNS active drugs has not been systematically evaluated. Consequently, caution is advised if the concomitant administration of venlafaxine and such drugs is required). Products include:

Nembutal Sodium Solution, USP 2494

Perphenazine (The risk of using venlafaxine in combination with other CNS active drugs has not been systematically evaluated. Consequently, caution is advised if the concomitant administration of venlafaxine and such drugs is required).

No products indexed under this heading.

Phenelzine Sulfate (Adverse reactions, some of which were serious, have been reported in patients who have recently been discontinued from a monoamine oxidase inhibitor (MAOI) and started on venlafaxine, or who have recently had venlafaxine therapy discontinued prior to initiation of an MAOI. Therefore, it is recommended that venlafaxine not be used in combination with an MAOI, or within at least 14 days of discontinuing treatment with an MAOI. Based on the half-life of venlafaxine, at least 7 days should be allowed after stopping venlafaxine before starting an MAOI. The concomitant use of venlafaxine with MAOIs intended to treat depression is contraindicated).

No products indexed under this heading.

Phenobarbital (The risk of using venlafaxine in combination with other CNS active drugs has not been systematically evaluated. Consequently, caution is advised if the concomitant administration of venlafaxine and such drugs is required). Products include:

Donnatal Extentabs 2507

Phentermine Hydrochloride (The safety and efficacy of venlafaxine therapy in combination with weight loss agents, including phentermine, have not been established. Coadministration of venlafaxine and weight loss agents is not recommended). Products include:

Adipex-P 1185

Phenylbutazone (Serotonin release by platelets plays an important role in hemostasis. Epidemiological studies of the case control and cohort design have demonstrated an association between use of psychotropic drugs that interfere with serotonin reuptake and the occurrence of upper gastrointestinal bleeding have also shown that concurrent use of an NSAID may potentiate this risk of bleeding).

No products indexed under this heading.

Piroxicam (Serotonin release by platelets plays an important role in hemostasis. Epidemiological studies of the case control and cohort design have demonstrated an association between use of psychotropic drugs that interfere with serotonin reuptake and the occurrence of upper gastrointestinal bleeding have also shown that concurrent use of an NSAID may potentiate this risk of bleeding).

No products indexed under this heading.

Polythiazide (Hyponatremia may occur as a result of treatment with SNRIs, including venlafaxine. In many cases, this hyponatremia appears to be the result of the syndrome of inappropriate antidiuretic hormone secretion (SIADH). Cases with serum sodium lower than 110 mmol/L have been reported. Elderly patients may be at greater risk of developing hyponatremia with SSRIs and SNRIs. Also patients taking diuretics or who are otherwise volume depleted may be at greater risk. Discontinuation of venlafaxine should be considered in patients with symptomatic hyponatremia and appropriate medical intervention should be instituted).

No products indexed under this heading.

Prazepam (The risk of using venlafaxine in combination with other CNS active drugs has not been systematically evaluated. Consequently, caution is advised if the concomitant administration of venlafaxine and such drugs is required).

No products indexed under this heading.

Procarbazine Hydrochloride (Adverse reactions, some of which were serious, have been reported in patients who have recently been discontinued from a monoamine oxidase inhibitor (MAOI) and started on venlafaxine, or who have recently had venlafaxine therapy discontinued prior to initiation of an MAOI. Therefore, it is recommended that venlafaxine not be used in combination with an MAOI, or within at least 14 days of discontinuing treatment with an MAOI. Based on the half-life of venlafaxine, at least 7 days should be allowed after stopping venlafaxine before starting an MAOI. The concomitant use of venlafaxine with MAOIs intended to treat depression is contraindicated).

No products indexed under this heading.

Prochlorperazine (The risk of using venlafaxine in combination with other CNS active drugs has not been systematically evaluated. Consequently, caution is advised if the concomitant administration of venlafaxine and such drugs is required).

No products indexed under this heading.

Promethazine Hydrochloride (The risk of using venlafaxine in combination with other CNS active drugs has not been systematically evaluated. Consequently, caution is advised if the concomitant administration of venlafaxine and such drugs is required).

No products indexed under this heading.

Propafenone Hydrochloride (Studies indicate that venlafaxine is metabolized to its active metabolite, ODV, by CYP2D6. Thus the potential exists for a drug interaction between drugs that inhibit CYP2D6-mediated metabolism and venlafaxine. However, although imipramine partially inhibited the CYP2D6-mediated metabolism of venlafaxine, resulting in higher plasma concentrations of venlafaxine and lower plasma concentrations of ODV, the total concentration of active compounds (venlafaxine plus ODV) was not affected. Also, in a clinical study involving CYP2D6 poor and extensive metabolizers, the total concentration of active compounds (venlafaxine plus ODV), was similar in both groups. No dosage adjustment is required when venlafaxine is co-administered with a CYP2D6 inhibitor). Products include:

Rythmol Tablets 1586
Rythmol SR Capsules 1590

Propofol (The risk of using venlafaxine in combination with other CNS active drugs has not been systematically evaluated. Consequently, caution is advised if the concomitant administration of venlafaxine and such drugs is required).

No products indexed under this heading.

Propoxyphene Hydrochloride (Concomitant use of CYP3A4 inhibitors and venlafaxine may increase levels of venlafaxine and ODV. Therefore, caution is advised if a patient's therapy includes a CYP3A4 inhibitor and venlafaxine concomitantly. The concomitant use of venlafaxine with a drug treatment(s) that potently inhibits both CYP2D6 and CYP3A4, the primary metabolizing enzymes for venlafaxine, has not been studied. Therefore, caution is advised should a patient's therapy include venlafaxine and any agent(s) that produce potent simultaneous inhibition of these two enzyme systems).

No products indexed under this heading.

Propoxyphene Napsylate (Concomitant use of CYP3A4 inhibitors and venlafaxine may increase levels of venlafaxine and ODV. Therefore, caution is advised if a patient's therapy includes a CYP3A4 inhibitor and venlafaxine concomitantly. The concomitant use of venlafaxine with a drug treatment(s) that potently inhibits both CYP2D6 and CYP3A4, the primary metabolizing enzymes for venlafaxine, has not been studied. Therefore, caution is advised should a patient's therapy include venlafaxine and any agent(s) that produce potent simultaneous inhibition of these two enzyme systems).

No products indexed under this heading.

Protriptyline Hydrochloride (Studies indicate that venlafaxine is metabolized to its active metabolite, ODV, by CYP2D6. Thus the potential exists for a drug interaction between drugs that inhibit CYP2D6-mediated metabolism and venlafaxine. However, although imipramine partially inhibited the CYP2D6-mediated metabolism of venlafaxine, resulting in higher plasma concentrations of venlafaxine and lower plasma concentrations of ODV, the total concentration of active compounds (venlafaxine plus ODV) was not affected. Also, in a clinical study involving CYP2D6 poor and extensive metabolizers, the total concentration of active compounds (venlafaxine plus ODV), was similar in both groups. No dosage adjustment is required when venlafaxine is co-administered with a CYP2D6 inhibitor).

No products indexed under this heading.

Quazepam (The risk of using venlafaxine in combination with other CNS active drugs has not been systematically evaluated. Consequently, caution is advised if the concomitant administration of venlafaxine and such drugs is required).

No products indexed under this heading.

Quetiapine Fumarate (The risk of using venlafaxine in combination with other CNS active drugs has not been systematically evaluated. Consequently, caution is advised if the concomitant administration of venlafaxine and such drugs is required).

No products indexed under this heading.

Quinacrine Hydrochloride (Studies indicate that venlafaxine is metabolized to its active metabolite, ODV, by CYP2D6. Thus the potential exists for a drug interaction between drugs that inhibit CYP2D6-mediated metabolism and venlafaxine. However, although imipramine partially inhibited the CYP2D6-mediated metabolism of venlafaxine, resulting in higher plasma concentrations of venlafaxine and lower plasma concentrations of ODV, the total concentration of active compounds (venlafaxine plus ODV) was not affected. Also, in a clinical study involving CYP2D6 poor and extensive metabolizers, the total concentration of active compounds (venlafaxine plus ODV), was similar in both groups. No dosage adjustment is required when venlafaxine is co-administered with a CYP2D6 inhibitor).

No products indexed under this heading.

Quinidine (Concomitant use of CYP3A4 inhibitors and venlafaxine may increase levels of venlafaxine and ODV. Therefore, caution is advised if a patient's therapy includes a CYP3A4 inhibitor and venlafaxine concomitantly. The concomitant use of venlafaxine with a drug treatment(s) that potently inhibits both CYP2D6 and CYP3A4, the primary metabolizing enzymes for venlafaxine, has not been studied. Therefore, caution is advised should a patient's therapy include venlafaxine and any agent(s) that produce potent simultaneous inhibition of these two enzyme systems).

No products indexed under this heading.

Quinidine Gluconate (Studies indicate that venlafaxine is metabolized to its active metabolite, ODV, by CYP2D6. Thus the potential exists for a drug interaction between drugs that inhibit CYP2D6-mediated metabolism and venlafaxine. However, although imipramine partially inhibited the CYP2D6-mediated metabolism of venlafaxine, resulting in higher plasma concentrations of venlafaxine and lower plasma concentrations of ODV, the total concentration of active compounds (venlafaxine plus ODV) was not affected. Also, in a clinical study involving CYP2D6 poor and extensive metabolizers, the total concentration of active compounds (venlafaxine plus ODV), was similar in both groups. No dosage adjustment is required when venlafaxine is co-administered with a CYP2D6 inhibitor).

No products indexed under this heading.

Quinidine Hydrochloride (Concomitant use of CYP3A4 inhibitors and venlafaxine may increase levels of venlafaxine and ODV. Therefore, caution is advised if a patient's therapy includes a CYP3A4 inhibitor and venlafaxine concomitantly. The concomitant use of venlafaxine with a drug treatment(s) that potently inhibits both CYP2D6 and CYP3A4, the primary metabolizing enzymes for venlafaxine, has not been studied. Therefore, caution is advised should a patient's therapy include venlafaxine and any agent(s) that produce potent simultaneous inhibition of these two enzyme systems).

No products indexed under this heading.

Quinidine Polygalacturonate (Concomitant use of CYP3A4 inhibitors and venlafaxine may increase levels of venlafaxine and ODV. Therefore, caution is advised if a patient's therapy includes a CYP3A4 inhibitor and venlafaxine concomitantly. The concomitant use of venlafaxine with a drug treatment(s) that potently inhibits both CYP2D6 and CYP3A4, the primary metabolizing enzymes for venlafaxine, has not been studied. Therefore, caution is advised should a patient's therapy include venlafaxine and any agent(s) that produce potent simultaneous inhibition of these two enzyme systems).

No products indexed under this heading.

Quinidine Sulfate (Concomitant use of CYP3A4 inhibitors and venlafaxine may increase levels of venlafaxine and ODV. Therefore, caution is advised if a patient's therapy includes a CYP3A4 inhibitor and venlafaxine concomitantly. The concomitant use of venlafaxine with a drug treatment(s) that potently inhibits both CYP2D6 and CYP3A4, the primary metabolizing enzymes for venlafaxine, has not been studied. Therefore, caution is advised should a patient's therapy include venlafaxine and any agent(s) that produce potent simultaneous inhibition of these two enzyme systems).

No products indexed under this heading.

Quinine (Concomitant use of CYP3A4 inhibitors and venlafaxine may increase levels of venlafaxine and ODV. Therefore, caution is advised if a patient's therapy includes a CYP3A4 inhibitor and venlafaxine concomitantly. The concomitant use of venlafaxine with a drug treatment(s) that potently inhibits both CYP2D6 and CYP3A4, the primary metabolizing enzymes for venlafaxine, has not been studied. Therefore, caution is advised should a patient's therapy include venlafaxine and any agent(s) that produce potent simultaneous inhibition of these two enzyme systems).

No products indexed under this heading.

Quinine Sulfate (Concomitant use of CYP3A4 inhibitors and venlafaxine may increase levels of venlafaxine and ODV. Therefore, caution is advised if a patient's therapy includes a CYP3A4 inhibitor and venlafaxine concomitantly. The concomitant use of venlafaxine with a drug treatment(s) that potently inhibits both CYP2D6 and CYP3A4, the primary metabolizing enzymes for venlafaxine, has not been studied. Therefore, caution is advised should a patient's therapy include venlafaxine and any agent(s) that produce potent simultaneous inhibition of these two enzyme systems).

No products indexed under this heading.

Quinupristin (Concomitant use of CYP3A4 inhibitors and venlafaxine may increase levels of venlafaxine and ODV. Therefore, caution is advised if a patient's therapy includes a CYP3A4 inhibitor and venlafaxine concomitantly. The concomitant use of venlafaxine with a drug treatment(s) that potently inhibits both CYP2D6 and CYP3A4, the primary metabolizing enzymes for venlafaxine, has not been studied. Therefore, caution is advised should a patient's therapy include venlafaxine and any agent(s) that produce potent simultaneous inhibition of these two enzyme systems).

No products indexed under this heading.

Ranitidine Bismuth Citrate (Concomitant use of CYP3A4 inhibitors and venlafaxine may increase levels of venlafaxine and ODV. Therefore, caution is advised if a patient's therapy includes a CYP3A4 inhibitor and venlafaxine concomitantly. The concomitant use of venlafaxine with a drug treatment(s) that potently inhibits both CYP2D6 and CYP3A4, the primary metabolizing enzymes for venlafaxine, has not been studied. Therefore, caution is advised should a patient's therapy include venlafaxine and any agent(s) that produce potent simultaneous inhibition of these two enzyme systems).

No products indexed under this heading.

Ranitidine Hydrochloride (Concomitant use of CYP3A4 inhibitors and venlafaxine may increase levels of venlafaxine and ODV. Therefore, caution is advised if a patient's therapy includes a CYP3A4 inhibitor and venlafaxine concomitantly. The concomitant use of venlafaxine with a drug treatment(s) that potently inhibits both CYP2D6 and CYP3A4, the primary metabolizing enzymes for venlafaxine, has not been studied. Therefore, caution is advised should a patient's therapy include venlafaxine and any agent(s) that produce potent simultaneous inhibition of these two enzyme systems).

Products include:

- Zantac 75 Tablets .... ▣603
- Zantac 1670
- Zantac Injection 1666
- Zantac Injection Pharmacy Bulk Package 1668
- Maximum Strength Zantac 150 Tablets .... ▣603
- Maximum Strength Zantac 150 Cool Mint Tablets .... ▣603

Rasagiline Mesylate (Adverse reactions, some of which were serious, have been reported in patients who have recently been discontinued from a monoamine oxidase inhibitor (MAOI) and started on venlafaxine, or who have recently had venlafaxine therapy discontinued prior to initiation of an MAOI. Therefore, it is recommended that venlafaxine not be used in combination with an MAOI, or within at least 14 days of discontinuing treatment with an MAOI. Based on the half-life of venlafaxine, at least 7 days should be allowed after stopping venlafaxine before starting an MAOI. The concomitant use of venlafaxine with MAOIs intended to treat depression is contraindicated).

Products include:

- Azilect Tablets 3106

Remifentanil Hydrochloride (The risk of using venlafaxine in combination with other CNS active drugs has not been systematically evaluated. Consequently, caution is advised if the concomitant administration of venlafaxine and such drugs is required).

No products indexed under this heading.

Risperidone (Venlafaxine administered under steady-state conditions at 150 mg/day slightly inhibited the CYP2D6-mediated metabolism of risperidone (administered as a single 1 mg oral dose) to its active metabolite, 9-hydroxyrisperidone, resulting in an approximately 32% increase in risperidone AUC. However venlafaxine co-administration did not significantly alter the pharmacokinetic profile of the total active moiety (risperidone plus 9-hydroxyrisperidone)). Products include:

- Risperdal Consta Long-Acting Injection 1753

Ritonavir (Concomitant use of CYP3A4 inhibitors and venlafaxine may increase levels of venlafaxine and ODV. Therefore, caution is advised if a patient's therapy includes a CYP3A4 inhibitor and venlafaxine concomitantly. The concomitant use of venlafaxine with a drug treatment(s) that potently inhibits both CYP2D6 and CYP3A4, the primary metabolizing enzymes for venlafaxine, has not been studied. Therefore, caution is advised should a patient's therapy include venlafaxine and any agent(s) that produce potent simultaneous inhibition of these two enzyme systems).

Products include:

- Kaletra 452
- Norvir 489

Rizatriptan Benzoate (Based on the mechanism of action of venlafaxine and the potential for serotonin syndrome, caution is advised when venlafaxine is co-administered with other drugs that may affect the serotonergic neurotransmitter systems, such as triptans. If concomitant treatment of venlafaxine with a triptan is clinically warranted, careful observation of the patient is advised, particularly during treatment initiation and dose increases). Products include:

- Maxalt Tablets 2056
- Maxalt-MLT Orally Disintegrating Tablets 2056

Rofecoxib (Serotonin release by platelets plays an important role in hemostasis. Epidemiological studies of the case control and cohort design have demonstrated an association between use of psychotropic drugs that interfere with serotonin reuptake and the occurrence of upper gastrointestinal bleeding have also shown that concurrent use of an NSAID may potentiate this risk of bleeding).

No products indexed under this heading.

Saquinavir (Concomitant use of CYP3A4 inhibitors and venlafaxine may increase levels of venlafaxine and ODV. Therefore, caution is advised if a patient's therapy includes a CYP3A4 inhibitor and venlafaxine concomitantly. The concomitant use of venlafaxine with a drug treatment(s) that potently inhibits both CYP2D6 and CYP3A4, the primary metabolizing enzymes for venlafaxine, has not been studied. Therefore, caution is advised should a patient's therapy include venlafaxine and any agent(s) that produce potent simultaneous inhibition of these two enzyme systems).

No products indexed under this heading.

Saquinavir Mesylate (Concomitant use of CYP3A4 inhibitors and venlafaxine may increase levels of venlafaxine and ODV. Therefore, caution is advised if a patient's therapy includes a CYP3A4 inhibitor and venlafaxine concomitantly. The concomitant use of venlafaxine with a drug treatment(s) that potently inhibits both CYP2D6 and CYP3A4, the primary metabolizing enzymes for venlafaxine, has not been studied. Therefore, caution is advised should a patient's therapy include venlafaxine and any agent(s) that produce potent simultaneous inhibition of these two enzyme systems).

No products indexed under this heading.

Secobarbital Sodium (The risk of using venlafaxine in combination with other CNS active drugs has not been systematically evaluated. Consequently, caution is advised if the concomitant administration of venlafaxine and such drugs is required).

No products indexed under this heading.

Selegiline (Adverse reactions, some of which were serious, have been reported in patients who have recently been discontinued from a monoamine oxidase inhibitor (MAOI) and started on venlafaxine, or who have recently had venlafaxine therapy discontinued prior to initiation of an MAOI. Therefore, it is recommended that venlafaxine not be used in combination with an MAOI, or within at least 14 days of discontinuing treatment with an MAOI. Based on the half-life of venlafaxine, at least 7 days should be allowed after stopping venlafaxine before starting an MAOI. The concomitant use of venlafaxine with MAOIs intended to treat depression is contraindicated).

Products include:

- Emsam Transdermal System 905

Selegiline Hydrochloride (Adverse reactions, some of which were serious, have been reported in patients who have recently been discontinued from a monoamine oxidase inhibitor (MAOI) and started on venlafaxine, or who have recently had venlafaxine therapy discontinued prior to initiation of an MAOI. Therefore, it is recommended that venlafaxine not be used in combination with an MAOI, or within at least 14 days of discontinuing treatment with an MAOI. Based on the half-life of venlafaxine, at least 7 days should be allowed after stopping venlafaxine before starting an MAOI. The concomitant use of venlafaxine with

MAOIs intended to treat depression is contraindicated). Products include:

Eldepryl Capsules 3052

Sertraline Hydrochloride (Based on the mechanism of action of venlafaxine and the potential for serotonin syndrome, caution is advised when venlafaxine is co-administered with other drugs that may affect the serotonergic neurotransmitter systems. If concomitant treatment of venlafaxine with these drugs is clinically warranted, careful observation of the patient is advised, particularly during treatment initiation and dose increases).

No products indexed under this heading.

Sevoflurane (The risk of using venlafaxine in combination with other CNS active drugs has not been systematically evaluated. Consequently, caution is advised if the concomitant administration of venlafaxine and such drugs is required). Products include:

Ultane Liquid for Inhalation 524

Sildenafil Citrate (Concomitant use of CYP3A4 inhibitors and venlafaxine may increase levels of venlafaxine and ODV. Therefore, caution is advised if a patient's therapy includes a CYP3A4 inhibitor and venlafaxine concomitantly. The concomitant use of venlafaxine with a drug treatment(s) that potently inhibits both CYP2D6 and CYP3A4, the primary metabolizing enzymes for venlafaxine, has not been studied. Therefore, caution is advised should a patient's therapy include venlafaxine and any agent(s) that produce potent simultaneous inhibition of these two enzyme systems).

No products indexed under this heading.

Sodium Oxybate (The risk of using venlafaxine in combination with other CNS active drugs has not been systematically evaluated. Consequently, caution is advised if the concomitant administration of venlafaxine and such drugs is required). Products include:

Xyrem Oral Solution 1766

Spironolactone (Hyponatremia may occur as a result of treatment with SNRIs, including venlafaxine. In many cases, this hyponatremia appears to be the result of the syndrome of inappropriate antidiuretic hormone secretion (SIADH). Cases with serum sodium lower than 110 mmol/L have been reported. Elderly patients may be at greater risk of developing hyponatremia with SSRIs and SNRIs. Also patients taking diuretics or who are otherwise volume depleted may be at greater risk. Discontinuation of venlafaxine should be considered in patients with symptomatic hyponatremia and appropriate medical intervention should be instituted).

No products indexed under this heading.

Sufentanil Citrate (The risk of using venlafaxine in combination with other CNS active drugs has not been systematically evaluated. Consequently, caution is advised if the concomitant administration of venlafaxine and such drugs is required).

No products indexed under this heading.

Sulindac (Serotonin release by platelets plays an important role in hemostasis. Epidemiological studies of the case control and cohort design have demonstrated an association between use of psychotropic drugs that interfere with serotonin reuptake and the occurrence of upper gastrointestinal bleeding have also shown that concurrent use of an NSAID may potentiate this risk of bleeding). Products include:

Clinoril Tablets 1962

Sumatriptan (Based on the mechanism of action of venlafaxine and the potential for serotonin syndrome, caution is advised when venlafaxine is co-administered with other drugs that may affect the serotonergic neurotransmitter systems, such as triptans. If concomitant treatment of venlafaxine with a triptan is clinically warranted, careful observation of the patient is advised, particularly during treatment initiation and dose increases). Products include:

Imitrex Nasal Spray 1470

Sumatriptan Succinate (Based on the mechanism of action of venlafaxine and the potential for serotonin syndrome, caution is advised when venlafaxine is co-administered with other drugs that may affect the serotonergic neurotransmitter systems, such as triptans. If concomitant treatment of venlafaxine with a triptan is clinically warranted, careful observation of the patient is advised, particularly during treatment initiation and dose increases). Products include:

Imitrex Injection 1465
Imitrex Tablets 1474
Treximet Tablets 1616

Telithromycin (Concomitant use of CYP3A4 inhibitors and venlafaxine may increase levels of venlafaxine and ODV. Therefore, caution is advised if a patient's therapy includes a CYP3A4 inhibitor and venlafaxine concomitantly. The concomitant use of venlafaxine with a drug treatment(s) that potently inhibits both CYP2D6 and CYP3A4, the primary metabolizing enzymes for venlafaxine, has not been studied. Therefore, caution is advised should a patient's therapy include venlafaxine and any agent(s) that produce potent simultaneous inhibition of these two enzyme systems). Products include:

Ketek Tablets 2744

Temazepam (The risk of using venlafaxine in combination with other CNS active drugs has not been systematically evaluated. Consequently, caution is advised if the concomitant administration of venlafaxine and such drugs is required).

No products indexed under this heading.

Terbinafine Hydrochloride (Studies indicate that venlafaxine is metabolized to its active metabolite, ODV, by CYP2D6. Thus the potential exists for a drug interaction between drugs that inhibit CYP2D6-mediated metabolism and venlafaxine. However, although imipramine partially inhibited the CYP2D6-mediated metabolism of venlafaxine, resulting in higher plasma concentrations of venlafaxine and lower plasma concentrations of ODV, the total concentration of active compounds (venlafaxine plus ODV) was not affected. Also, in a clinical study involving CYP2D6 poor and extensive metabolizers, the total concentration of active compounds (venlafaxine plus ODV), was similar in both groups. No dosage adjustment is required when venlafaxine is co-administered with a CYP2D6 inhibitor). Products include:

Lamisil Oral Granules 2264
Lamisil Tablets 2266

Thiamylal Sodium (The risk of using venlafaxine in combination with other CNS active drugs has not been systematically evaluated. Consequently, caution is advised if the concomitant administration of venlafaxine and such drugs is required).

No products indexed under this heading.

Thioridazine Hydrochloride (The risk of using venlafaxine in combination with other CNS active drugs has not been systematically evaluated. Consequently, caution is advised if the concomitant administration of venlafaxine and such drugs is required). Products include:

Thioridazine Hydrochloride Tablets 2195

Thiothixene (The risk of using venlafaxine in combination with other CNS active drugs has not been systematically evaluated. Consequently, caution is advised if the concomitant administration of venlafaxine and such drugs is required). Products include:

Thiothixene Capsules 2197

Tolmetin Sodium (Serotonin release by platelets plays an important role in hemostasis. Epidemiological studies of the case control and cohort design have demonstrated an association between use of psychotropic drugs that interfere with serotonin reuptake and the occurrence of upper gastrointestinal bleeding have also shown that concurrent use of an NSAID may potentiate this risk of bleeding).

No products indexed under this heading.

Torsemide (Hyponatremia may occur as a result of treatment with SNRIs, including venlafaxine. In many cases, this hyponatremia appears to be the result of the syndrome of inappropriate antidiuretic hormone secretion (SIADH). Cases with serum sodium lower than 110 mmol/L have been reported. Elderly patients may be at greater risk of developing hyponatremia with SSRIs and SNRIs. Also patients taking diuretics or who are otherwise volume depleted may be at greater risk. Discontinuation of venlafaxine should be considered in patients with symptomatic hyponatremia and appropriate medical intervention should be instituted). Products include:

Demadex Injection 2630
Demadex Tablets 2630

Tramadol Hydrochloride (Based on the mechanism of action of venlafaxine and the potential for serotonin syndrome, caution is advised when venlafaxine is co-administered with other drugs that may affect the serotonergic neurotransmitter systems, such as tramadol. If concomitant treatment of venlafaxine with tramadol is clinically warranted, careful observation of the patient is advised, particularly during treatment initiation and dose increases). Products include:

Ultram ER Extended-Release Tablets 2428

Tranylcypromine Sulfate (Adverse reactions, some of which were serious, have been reported in patients who have recently been discontinued from a monoamine oxidase inhibitor (MAOI) and started on venlafaxine, or who have recently had venlafaxine therapy discontinued prior to initiation of an MAOI. Therefore, it is recommended that venlafaxine not be used in combination with an MAOI, or within at least 14 days of discontinuing treatment with an MAOI. Based on the half-life of venlafaxine, at least 7 days should be allowed after stopping venlafaxine before starting an MAOI. The concomitant use of venlafaxine with MAOIs intended to treat depression is contraindicated). Products include:

Parnate Tablets 1532

Triamterene (Hyponatremia may occur as a result of treatment with SNRIs, including venlafaxine. In many cases, this hyponatremia appears to be the result of the syndrome of inappropriate antidiuretic hormone secretion (SIADH). Cases with serum sodium lower than 110 mmol/L have been reported. Elderly patients may be at greater risk of developing hyponatremia with SSRIs and SNRIs. Also patients taking diuretics or who are otherwise volume depleted may be at greater risk. Discontinuation of venlafaxine should be considered in patients with symptomatic hyponatremia and appropriate medical intervention should be instituted). Products include:

Dyazide Capsules 1405
Dyrenium Capsules 3189

Triazolam (The risk of using venlafaxine in combination with other CNS active drugs has not been systematically evaluated. Consequently, caution is advised if the concomitant administration of venlafaxine and such drugs is required).

No products indexed under this heading.

Trifluoperazine Hydrochloride (The risk of using venlafaxine in combination with other CNS active drugs has not been systematically evaluated. Consequently, caution is advised if the concomitant administration of venlafaxine and such drugs is required).

No products indexed under this heading.

Trimipramine Maleate (Studies indicate that venlafaxine is metabolized to its active metabolite, ODV, by CYP2D6. Thus the potential exists for a drug interaction between drugs that inhibit CYP2D6-mediated metabolism and venlafaxine. However, although imipramine partially inhibited the CYP2D6-mediated metabolism of venlafaxine, resulting in higher plasma concentrations of venlafaxine and lower plasma concentrations of ODV, the total concentration of active compounds (venlafaxine plus ODV) was not affected. Also, in a clinical study involving CYP2D6 poor and extensive metabolizers, the total concentration of active compounds (venlafaxine plus ODV), was similar in both groups. No dosage adjustment is required when venlafaxine is co-administered with a CYP2D6 inhibitor).

No products indexed under this heading.

Troglitazone (Concomitant use of CYP3A4 inhibitors and venlafaxine may increase levels of venlafaxine and ODV. Therefore, caution is advised if a patient's therapy includes a CYP3A4 inhibitor and venlafaxine concomitantly. The concomitant use of venlafaxine with a drug treatment(s) that potently inhibits both CYP2D6 and CYP3A4, the primary metabolizing enzymes for venlafaxine, has not been studied. Therefore, caution is advised should a patient's therapy include venlafaxine and any agent(s) that produce potent simultaneous inhibition of these two enzyme systems).

No products indexed under this heading.

Troleandomycin (Concomitant use of CYP3A4 inhibitors and venlafaxine may increase levels of venlafaxine and ODV. Therefore, caution is advised if a patient's therapy includes a CYP3A4 inhibitor and venlafaxine concomitantly. The concomitant use of venlafaxine with a drug treatment(s) that potently inhibits both CYP2D6 and CYP3A4, the primary metabolizing enzymes for venlafaxine, has not been studied. Therefore, caution is advised should a patient's therapy include venlafaxine and any agent(s) that produce potent simultaneous inhibition of these two enzyme systems).

No products indexed under this heading.

Tryptophan (The concomitant use of venlafaxine with tryptophan supplements is not recommended).

No products indexed under this heading.

L-Tryptophan (The concomitant use of venlafaxine with tryptophan supplements is not recommended).

No products indexed under this heading.

Valdecoxib (Serotonin release by platelets plays an important role in hemostasis. Epidemiological studies of the case control and cohort design have demonstrated an association between use of psychotropic drugs that interfere with serotonin reuptake and the occurrence of upper gastrointestinal bleeding have also shown that concurrent use of an NSAID may potentiate this risk of bleeding).

No products indexed under this heading.

Valproate Sodium (Concomitant use of CYP3A4 inhibitors and venlafaxine may increase levels of venlafaxine and ODV. Therefore, caution is advised if a patient's therapy includes a CYP3A4 inhibitor and venlafaxine concomitantly. The concomitant use of venlafaxine with a drug treatment(s) that potently inhibits both CYP2D6 and CYP3A4, the primary metabolizing enzymes for venlafaxine, has not been studied. Therefore, caution is advised should a patient's therapy include venlafaxine and any agent(s) that produce potent simultaneous inhibition of these two enzyme systems).

No products indexed under this heading.

Vardenafil Hydrochloride (Concomitant use of CYP3A4 inhibitors and venlafaxine may increase levels of venlafaxine and ODV. Therefore, caution is advised if a patient's therapy includes a CYP3A4 inhibitor and venlafaxine concomitantly. The concomitant use of venlafaxine with a drug treatment(s) that potently inhibits both CYP2D6 and CYP3A4, the primary metabolizing enzymes for venlafaxine, has not been studied. Therefore, caution is advised should a patient's therapy include venlafaxine and any agent(s) that produce potent simultaneous inhibition of these two enzyme systems). Products include:

Levitra Tablets 2876

Verapamil Hydrochloride (Concomitant use of CYP3A4 inhibitors and venlafaxine may increase levels of venlafaxine and ODV. Therefore, caution is advised if a patient's therapy includes a CYP3A4 inhibitor and venlafaxine concomitantly. The concomitant use of venlafaxine with a drug treatment(s) that potently inhibits both CYP2D6 and CYP3A4, the primary metabolizing enzymes for venlafaxine, has not been studied. Therefore, caution is advised should a patient's therapy include venlafaxine and any agent(s) that produce potent simultaneous inhibition of these two enzyme systems). Products include:

Tarka Tablets 511

Voriconazole (Concomitant use of CYP3A4 inhibitors and venlafaxine may increase levels of venlafaxine and ODV. Therefore, caution is advised if a patient's therapy includes a CYP3A4 inhibitor and venlafaxine concomitantly. The concomitant use of venlafaxine with a drug treatment(s) that potently inhibits both CYP2D6 and CYP3A4, the primary metabolizing enzymes for venlafaxine, has not been studied. Therefore, caution is advised should a patient's therapy include venlafaxine and any agent(s) that produce potent simultaneous inhibition of these two enzyme systems).

No products indexed under this heading.

Warfarin Sodium (Altered anticoagulant effects, including increased bleeding, have been reported when SNRIs are co-administered with warfarin. Patients receiving warfarin therapy should be carefully monitored when venlafaxine is initiated or discontinued).

No products indexed under this heading.

Zafirlukast (Concomitant use of CYP3A4 inhibitors and venlafaxine may increase levels of venlafaxine and ODV. Therefore, caution is advised if a patient's therapy includes a CYP3A4 inhibitor and venlafaxine concomitantly. The concomitant use of venlafaxine with a drug treatment(s) that potently inhibits both CYP2D6 and CYP3A4, the primary metabolizing enzymes for venlafaxine, has not been studied. Therefore, caution is advised should a patient's therapy include venlafaxine and any agent(s) that produce potent simultaneous inhibition of these two enzyme systems). Products include:

Accolate Tablets 669

Zaleplon (The risk of using venlafaxine in combination with other CNS active drugs has not been systematically evaluated. Consequently, caution is advised if the concomitant administration of venlafaxine and such drugs is required).

No products indexed under this heading.

Zileuton (Concomitant use of CYP3A4 inhibitors and venlafaxine may increase levels of venlafaxine and ODV. Therefore, caution is advised if a patient's therapy includes a CYP3A4 inhibitor and venlafaxine concomitantly. The concomitant use of venlafaxine with a drug treatment(s) that potently inhibits both CYP2D6 and CYP3A4, the primary metabolizing enzymes for venlafaxine, has not been studied. Therefore, caution is advised should a patient's therapy include venlafaxine and any agent(s) that produce potent simultaneous inhibition of these two enzyme systems).

No products indexed under this heading.

Ziprasidone Hydrochloride (The risk of using venlafaxine in combination with other CNS active drugs has not been systematically evaluated. Consequently, caution is advised if the concomitant administration of venlafaxine and such drugs is required). Products include:

Geodon Capsules 2520

Zolmitriptan (Based on the mechanism of action of venlafaxine and the potential for serotonin syndrome, caution is advised when venlafaxine is co-administered with other drugs that may affect the serotonergic neurotransmitter systems, such as triptans. If concomitant treatment of venlafaxine with a triptan is clinically warranted, careful observation of the patient is advised, particularly during treatment initiation and dose increases). Products include:

Zomig Tablets 694
Zomig Nasal Spray 689
Zomig-ZMT Tablets 694

Zolpidem Tartrate (The risk of using venlafaxine in combination with other CNS active drugs has not been systematically evaluated. Consequently, caution is advised if the concomitant administration of venlafaxine and such drugs is required). Products include:

Ambien Tablets 2692
Ambien CR Tablets 2696

Food Interactions

Alcohol (Although venlafaxine has not been shown to increase the impairment of mental and motor skills caused by alcohol, patients should be advised to avoid alcohol while taking venlafaxine).

Grapefruit (Concomitant use of CYP3A4 inhibitors and venlafaxine may increase levels of venlafaxine and ODV. Therefore, caution is advised if a patient's therapy includes a CYP3A4 inhibitor and venlafaxine concomitantly. The concomitant use of venlafaxine with a drug treatment(s) that potently inhibits both CYP2D6 and CYP3A4, the primary metabolizing enzymes for venlafaxine, has not been studied. Therefore, caution is advised should a patient's therapy include venlafaxine and any agent(s) that produce potent simultaneous inhibition of these two enzyme systems).

Grapefruit Juice (Concomitant use of CYP3A4 inhibitors and venlafaxine may increase levels of venlafaxine and ODV. Therefore, caution is advised if a patient's therapy includes a CYP3A4 inhibitor and venlafaxine concomitantly. The concomitant use of venlafaxine with a drug treatment(s) that potently inhibits both CYP2D6 and CYP3A4, the primary metabolizing enzymes for venlafaxine, has not been studied. Therefore, caution is advised should a patient's therapy include venlafaxine and any agent(s) that produce potent simultaneous inhibition of these two enzyme systems).

VENTOLIN HFA INHALATION AEROSOL

(Albuterol Sulfate) 1638

May interact with beta blockers, monoamine oxidase inhibitors, nonpotassium-sparing diuretics, sympathomimetic bronchodilators, sympathomimetics, tricyclic antidepressants, and certain other agents. Compounds in these categories include:

Acebutolol Hydrochloride (Beta-adrenergic receptor blocking agents not only block the pulmonary effect of beta agonists such as albuterol sulfate inhalation aerosol, but may produce severe bronchospasm in patients with asthma. Therefore, patients with asthma should not normally be treated with beta-blockers. However under certain circumstances, eg, as prophylaxis after myocardial infarction, there may be no acceptable alternatives to the use of beta-adrenergic blocking agents in patients with asthma. In this setting, cardioselective beta-blockers should be considered, although they should be administered with caution).

No products indexed under this heading.

Albuterol (Other short-acting sympathomimetic aerosol bronchodilators should not be used concomitantly with albuterol).

No products indexed under this heading.

Amitriptyline Hydrochloride (Albuterol sulfate inhalation aerosol should be administered with extreme caution to patients being treated with tricyclic antidepressants, or within 2 weeks of discontinuation of such agents, because the action of albuterol on the vascular system may be potentiated. Consider alternative therapy in patients taking tricyclic antidepressants).

No products indexed under this heading.

Amoxapine (Albuterol sulfate inhalation aerosol should be administered with extreme caution to patients being treated with tricyclic antidepressants, or within 2 weeks of discontinuation of such agents, because the action of albuterol on the vascular system may be potentiated. Consider alternative therapy in patients taking tricyclic antidepressants).

No products indexed under this heading.

Atenolol (Beta-adrenergic receptor blocking agents not only block the pulmonary effect of beta agonists such as albuterol sulfate inhalation aerosol, but may produce severe bronchospasm in patients with asthma. Therefore, patients with asthma should not normally be treated with beta-blockers. However under certain circumstances, eg, as prophylaxis after myocardial infarction, there may be no acceptable alternatives to the use of beta-adrenergic blocking agents in patients with asthma. In this setting, cardioselective beta-blockers should be considered, although they should be administered with caution).

No products indexed under this heading.

Bendroflumethiazide (The ECG changes and/or hypokalemia that may result from the administration of nonpotassium-sparing diuretics (eg,

loop or thiazide diuretics) can be acutely worsened by beta-agonists, especially when the recommended dose of the beta-agonist is exceeded.Although the clinical relevance of these effects is not known, caution is advised in the co-administration of beta-agonists with nonpotassium-sparing diuretics. Consider monitoring potassium levels).
No products indexed under this heading.

Betaxolol Hydrochloride (Beta-adrenergic receptor blocking agents not only block the pulmonary effect of beta agonists such as albuterol sulfate inhalation aerosol, but may produce severe bronchospasm in patients with asthma. Therefore, patients with asthma should not normally be treated with beta-blockers. However under certain circumstances, eg, as prophylaxis after myocardial infarction, there may be no acceptable alternatives to the use of beta-adrenergic blocking agents in patients with asthma. In this setting, cardioselective beta-blockers should be considered, although they should be administered with caution).
No products indexed under this heading.

Bisoprolol Fumarate (Beta-adrenergic receptor blocking agents not only block the pulmonary effect of beta agonists such as albuterol sulfate inhalation aerosol, but may produce severe bronchospasm in patients with asthma. Therefore, patients with asthma should not normally be treated with beta-blockers. However under certain circumstances, eg, as prophylaxis after myocardial infarction, there may be no acceptable alternatives to the use of beta-adrenergic blocking agents in patients with asthma. In this setting, cardioselective beta-blockers should be considered, although they should be administered with caution).
No products indexed under this heading.

Bitolterol Mesylate (Other short-acting sympathomimetic aerosol bronchodilators should not be used concomitantly with albuterol).
No products indexed under this heading.

Bumetanide (The ECG changes and/or hypokalemia that may result from the administration of nonpotassium-sparing diuretics (eg, loop or thiazide diuretics) can be acutely worsened by beta-agonists, especially when the recommended dose of the beta-agonist is exceeded.Although the clinical relevance of these effects is not known, caution is advised in the co-administration of beta-agonists with nonpotassium-sparing diuretics. Consider monitoring potassium levels).
No products indexed under this heading.

Carteolol Hydrochloride (Beta-adrenergic receptor blocking agents not only block the pulmonary effect of beta agonists such as albuterol sulfate inhalation aerosol, but may produce severe bronchospasm in patients with asthma. Therefore, patients with asthma should not normally be treated with beta-blockers. However under certain circumstances, eg, as prophylaxis after myocardial infarction, there may be no acceptable alternatives to the use of beta-adrenergic blocking agents in patients with asthma. In this setting, cardioselective beta-blockers should be considered, although they should be administered with caution).
No products indexed under this heading.

Chlorothiazide (The ECG changes and/or hypokalemia that may result from the administration of nonpotassium-sparing diuretics (eg, loop or thiazide diuretics) can be acutely worsened by beta-agonists, especially when the recommended dose of the beta-agonist is exceeded.Although the clinical relevance of these effects is not known, caution is advised in the co-administration of beta-agonists with nonpotassium-sparing diuretics. Consider monitoring potassium levels).
No products indexed under this heading.

Chlorothiazide Sodium (The ECG changes and/or hypokalemia that may result from the administration of nonpotassium-sparing diuretics (eg, loop or thiazide diuretics) can be acutely worsened by beta-agonists, especially when the recommended dose of the beta-agonist is exceeded.Although the clinical relevance of these effects is not known, caution is advised in the co-administration of beta-agonists with nonpotassium-sparing diuretics. Consider monitoring potassium levels). Products include:
Intravenous Sodium Diuril 2490

Clomipramine Hydrochloride (Albuterol sulfate inhalation aerosol should be administered with extreme caution to patients being treated with tricyclic antidepressants, or within 2 weeks of discontinuation of such agents, because the action of albuterol on the vascular system may be potentiated. Consider alternative therapy in patients taking tricyclic antidepressants).
No products indexed under this heading.

Desipramine Hydrochloride (Albuterol sulfate inhalation aerosol should be administered with extreme caution to patients being treated with tricyclic antidepressants, or within 2 weeks of discontinuation of such agents, because the action of albuterol on the vascular system may be potentiated. Consider alternative therapy in patients taking tricyclic antidepressants).
No products indexed under this heading.

Digoxin (Mean decreases of 16% to 22% in serum digoxin levels were demonstrated after single dose intravenous and oral administration of albuterol, respectively, to normal volunteers who had received digoxin for 10 days. The clinical relevance of these findings for patients with obstructive airway disease who are receiving inhaled albuterol and digoxin on a chronic basis is unclear. Nevertheless it would be prudent to carefully evaluate the serum digoxin levels in patients who are currently receiving digoxin and albuterol). Products include:
Lanoxin Injection 1498
Lanoxin Injection Pediatric 1502
Lanoxin Tablets 1505

Dobutamine Hydrochloride (If additional adrenergic drugs are to be administered by any route, they should be used with caution to avoid deleterious cardiovascular effects).
No products indexed under this heading.

Dopamine Hydrochloride (If additional adrenergic drugs are to be administered by any route, they should be used with caution to avoid deleterious cardiovascular effects).
No products indexed under this heading.

Doxepin Hydrochloride (Albuterol sulfate inhalation aerosol should be administered with extreme caution to patients being treated with tricyclic antidepressants, or within 2 weeks of discontinuation of such agents, because the action of albuterol on the vascular system may be potentiated. Consider alternative therapy in patients taking tricyclic antidepressants).
No products indexed under this heading.

Ephedrine Hydrochloride (Other short-acting sympathomimetic aerosol bronchodilators should not be used concomitantly with albuterol).
No products indexed under this heading.

Ephedrine Sulfate (Other short-acting sympathomimetic aerosol bronchodilators should not be used concomitantly with albuterol).
No products indexed under this heading.

Ephedrine Tannate (Other short-acting sympathomimetic aerosol bronchodilators should not be used concomitantly with albuterol).
No products indexed under this heading.

Epinephrine (Other short-acting sympathomimetic aerosol bronchodilators should not be used concomitantly with albuterol). Products include:
EpiPen 1024

Epinephrine Bitartrate (If additional adrenergic drugs are to be administered by any route, they should be used with caution to avoid deleterious cardiovascular effects).
No products indexed under this heading.

Epinephrine Hydrochloride (Other short-acting sympathomimetic aerosol bronchodilators should not be used concomitantly with albuterol).
No products indexed under this heading.

Esmolol Hydrochloride (Beta-adrenergic receptor blocking agents not only block the pulmonary effect of beta agonists such as albuterol sulfate inhalation aerosol, but may produce severe bronchospasm in patients with asthma. Therefore, patients with asthma should not normally be treated with beta-blockers. However under certain circumstances, eg, as prophylaxis after myocardial infarction, there may be no acceptable alternatives to the use of beta-adrenergic blocking agents in patients with asthma. In this setting, cardioselective beta-blockers should be considered, although they should be administered with caution).
No products indexed under this heading.

Ethacrynic Acid (The ECG changes and/or hypokalemia that may result from the administration of nonpotassium-sparing diuretics (eg, loop or thiazide diuretics) can be acutely worsened by beta-agonists, especially when the recommended dose of the beta-agonist is exceeded.Although the clinical relevance of these effects is not known, caution is advised in the co-administration of beta-agonists with nonpotassium-sparing diuretics. Consider monitoring potassium levels). Products include:
Edecrin Tablets 698

Furosemide (The ECG changes and/or hypokalemia that may result from the administration of nonpotassium-sparing diuretics (eg, loop or thiazide diuretics) can be acutely worsened by beta-agonists, especially when the recommended dose of the beta-agonist is exceeded.Although the clinical relevance of these effects is not known, caution is advised in the co-administration of beta-agonists with nonpotassium-sparing diuretics. Consider monitoring potassium levels). Products include:
Furosemide Tablets 2186

Hydrochlorothiazide (The ECG changes and/or hypokalemia that may result from the administration of nonpotassium-sparing diuretics (eg, loop or thiazide diuretics) can be acutely worsened by beta-agonists, especially when the recommended dose of the beta-agonist is exceeded.Although the clinical relevance of these effects is not known, caution is advised in the co-administration of beta-agonists with nonpotassium-sparing diuretics. Consider monitoring potassium levels). Products include:
Atacand HCT 642
Avalide Tablets 892
Avalide Tablets 2713
Benicar HCT Tablets 1010
Diovan HCT Tablets 2216
Dyazide Capsules 1405
Micardis HCT Tablets 854
Prinzide Tablets 2092
Tekturna HCT Tablets 2324
Teveten HCT Tablets 517

Hydroflumethiazide (The ECG changes and/or hypokalemia that may result from the administration of nonpotassium-sparing diuretics (eg, loop or thiazide diuretics) can be acutely worsened by beta-agonists, especially when the recommended dose of the beta-agonist is exceeded.Although the clinical relevance of these effects is not known, caution is advised in the co-administration of beta-agonists with nonpotassium-sparing diuretics. Consider monitoring potassium levels).
No products indexed under this heading.

Imipramine Hydrochloride (Albuterol sulfate inhalation aerosol should be administered with extreme caution to patients being treated with tricyclic antidepressants, or within 2 weeks of discontinuation of such agents, because the action of albuterol on the vascular system may be potentiated. Consider alternative therapy in patients taking tricyclic antidepressants).
No products indexed under this heading.

Imipramine Pamoate (Albuterol sulfate inhalation aerosol should be administered with extreme caution to patients being treated with tricyclic antidepressants, or within 2 weeks of discontinuation of such agents, because the action of albuterol on the vascular system may be potentiated. Consider alternative therapy in patients taking tricyclic antidepressants).
No products indexed under this heading.

Isocarboxazid (Albuterol sulfate inhalation aerosol should be administered with extreme caution to patients being treated with monoamine oxidase inhibitors, or within 2 weeks of discontinuation of such agents, because the action of albuterol on the vascular system may be potentiated. Consider alternative therapy in patients taking MAO inhibitors). Products include:
Marplan Tablets 3177

Isoetharine (Other short-acting sympathomimetic aerosol bronchodilators should not be used concomitantly with albuterol).
No products indexed under this heading.

Isoproterenol Hydrochloride (Other short-acting sympathomimetic aerosol bronchodilators should not be used concomitantly with albuterol).
No products indexed under this heading.

Isoproterenol Sulfate (Other short-acting sympathomimetic aerosol bronchodilators should not be used concomitantly with albuterol).
No products indexed under this heading.

Labetalol Hydrochloride (Beta-adrenergic receptor blocking agents not only block the pulmonary effect of beta agonists such as albuterol sulfate inhalation aerosol, but may produce severe bronchospasm in patients with asthma. Therefore, patients with asthma should not normally be treated with beta-blockers. However under certain circumstances, eg, as prophylaxis after myocardial infarction, there may be no acceptable alternatives to the use of beta-adrenergic blocking agents in patients with asthma. In this setting, cardioselective beta-blockers should be considered, although they should be administered with caution).
No products indexed under this heading.

Levalbuterol Hydrochloride (Other short-acting sympathomimetic aerosol bronchodilators should not be used concomitantly with albuterol). Products include:
Xopenex Inhalation Solution 3001
Xopenex Inhalation Solution Concentrate 3005

Levobunolol Hydrochloride (Beta-adrenergic receptor blocking agents not only block the pulmonary effect of beta agonists such as albuterol sulfate inhalation aerosol, but may produce severe bronchospasm in patients with asthma. Therefore, patients with asthma should not normally be treated with beta-blockers. However under certain circumstances, eg, as prophylaxis after myocardial infarction, there may be no acceptable alternatives to the use of beta-adrenergic blocking agents in patients with asthma. In this setting, cardioselective beta-blockers should be considered, although they should be administered with caution).
No products indexed under this heading.

Maprotiline Hydrochloride (Albuterol sulfate inhalation aerosol should be administered with extreme caution to patients being treated with tricyclic antidepressants, or within 2 weeks of discontinuation of such agents, because the action of albuterol on the vascular system may be potentiated. Consider alternative therapy in patients taking tricyclic antidepressants).
No products indexed under this heading.

Metaproterenol Sulfate (Other short-acting sympathomimetic aerosol bronchodilators should not be used concomitantly with albuterol).
No products indexed under this heading.

Metaraminol Bitartrate (If additional adrenergic drugs are to be administered by any route, they should be used with caution to avoid deleterious cardiovascular effects).
No products indexed under this heading.

Methoxamine Hydrochloride (If additional adrenergic drugs are to be administered by any route, they should be used with caution to avoid deleterious cardiovascular effects).
No products indexed under this heading.

Methyclothiazide (The ECG changes and/or hypokalemia that may result from the administration of nonpotassium-sparing diuretics (eg, loop or thiazide diuretics) can be acutely worsened by beta-agonists, especially when the recommended dose of the beta-agonist is exceeded.Although the clinical relevance of these effects is not known, caution is advised in the co-administration of beta-agonists with nonpotassium-sparing diuretics. Consider monitoring potassium levels).
No products indexed under this heading.

Metipranolol Hydrochloride (Beta-adrenergic receptor blocking agents not only block the pulmonary effect of beta agonists such as albuterol sulfate inhalation aerosol, but may produce severe bronchospasm in patients with asthma. Therefore, patients with asthma should not normally be treated with beta-blockers. However under certain circumstances, eg, as prophylaxis after myocardial infarction, there may be no acceptable alternatives to the use of beta-adrenergic blocking agents in patients with asthma. In this setting, cardioselective beta-blockers should be considered, although they should be administered with caution).
No products indexed under this heading.

Metoprolol Succinate (Beta-adrenergic receptor blocking agents not only block the pulmonary effect of beta agonists such as albuterol sulfate inhalation aerosol, but may produce severe bronchospasm in patients with asthma. Therefore, patients with asthma should not normally be treated with beta-blockers. However under certain circumstances, eg, as prophylaxis after myocardial infarction, there may be no acceptable alternatives to the use of beta-adrenergic blocking agents in patients with asthma. In this setting, cardioselective beta-blockers should be considered, although they should be administered with caution). Products include:
Toprol-XL Tablets 666

Metoprolol Tartrate (Beta-adrenergic receptor blocking agents not only block the pulmonary effect of beta agonists such as albuterol sulfate inhalation aerosol, but may produce severe bronchospasm in patients with asthma. Therefore, patients with asthma should not normally be treated with beta-blockers. However under certain circumstances, eg, as prophylaxis after myocardial infarction, there may be no acceptable alternatives to the use of beta-adrenergic blocking agents in patients with asthma. In this setting, cardioselective beta-blockers should be considered, although they should be administered with caution).
No products indexed under this heading.

Moclobemide (Albuterol sulfate inhalation aerosol should be administered with extreme caution to patients being treated with monoamine oxidase inhibitors, or within 2 weeks of discontinuation of such agents, because the action of albuterol on the vascular system may be potentiated. Consider alternative therapy in patients taking MAO inhibitors).
No products indexed under this heading.

Nadolol (Beta-adrenergic receptor blocking agents not only block the pulmonary effect of beta agonists such as albuterol sulfate inhalation aerosol, but may produce severe bronchospasm in patients with asthma. Therefore, patients with asthma should not normally be treated with beta-blockers. However under certain circumstances, eg, as prophylaxis after myocardial infarction, there may be no acceptable alternatives to the use of beta-adrenergic blocking agents in patients with asthma. In this setting, cardioselective beta-blockers should be considered, although they should be administered with caution). Products include:
Nadolol Tablets 2191

Nebivolol (Beta-adrenergic receptor blocking agents not only block the pulmonary effect of beta agonists such as albuterol sulfate inhalation aerosol, but may produce severe bronchospasm in patients with asthma. Therefore, patients with asthma should not normally be treated with beta-blockers. However under certain circumstances, eg, as prophylaxis after myocardial infarction, there may be no acceptable alternatives to the use of beta-adrenergic blocking agents in patients with asthma. In this setting, cardioselective beta-blockers should be considered, although they should be administered with caution). Products include:
Bystolic Tablets 1155

Norepinephrine Bitartrate (If additional adrenergic drugs are to be administered by any route, they should be used with caution to avoid deleterious cardiovascular effects).
No products indexed under this heading.

Nortriptyline Hydrochloride (Albuterol sulfate inhalation aerosol should be administered with extreme caution to patients being treated with tricyclic antidepressants, or within 2 weeks of discontinuation of such agents, because the action of albuterol on the vascular system may be potentiated. Consider alternative therapy in patients taking tricyclic antidepressants).
No products indexed under this heading.

Pargyline Hydrochloride (Albuterol sulfate inhalation aerosol should be administered with extreme caution to patients being treated with monoamine oxidase inhibitors, or within 2 weeks of discontinuation of such agents, because the action of albuterol on the vascular system may be potentiated. Consider alternative therapy in patients taking MAO inhibitors).
No products indexed under this heading.

Penbutolol Sulfate (Beta-adrenergic receptor blocking agents not only block the pulmonary effect of beta agonists such as albuterol sulfate inhalation aerosol, but may produce severe bronchospasm in patients with asthma. Therefore, patients with asthma should not normally be treated with beta-blockers. However under certain circumstances, eg, as prophylaxis after myocardial infarction, there may be no acceptable alternatives to the use of beta-adrenergic blocking agents in patients with asthma. In this setting, cardioselective beta-blockers should be considered, although they should be administered with caution).
No products indexed under this heading.

Phenelzine Sulfate (Albuterol sulfate inhalation aerosol should be administered with extreme caution to patients being treated with monoamine oxidase inhibitors, or within 2 weeks of discontinuation of such agents, because the action of albuterol on the vascular system may be potentiated. Consider alternative therapy in patients taking MAO inhibitors).
No products indexed under this heading.

Phenylephrine Bitartrate (If additional adrenergic drugs are to be administered by any route, they should be used with caution to avoid deleterious cardiovascular effects).
No products indexed under this heading.

Phenylephrine Hydrochloride (If additional adrenergic drugs are to be administered by any route, they should be used with caution to avoid deleterious cardiovascular effects). Products include:
Actifed Cold & Allergy Tablets 1895
Benadryl Allergy & Cold Kapgels 1895
Benadryl Allergy & Sinus Headache Kapgels 1895
Benadryl Severe Allergy & Sinus Headache Caplets 1897
Children's Benadryl-D Allergy & Sinus Liquid................................ 1896
Benadryl-D Allergy & Sinus Tablet 1896
PediaCare Children's Allergy & Cold Liquid 1902
PediaCare Children's Decongestant Liquid.................... 1902
PediaCare Children's Liquid Multi-Symptom Cold..................... 1902
Sinutab Non-Drying Caplets 1905
Sinutab Sinus Caplets 1905

Children's Sudafed PE Cold & Cough Liquid 1907
Children's Sudafed PE Nasal Decongestant Liquid 1906
Sudafed PE Cold & Cough Caplets 1907
Sudafed PE Nasal Decongestant Tablets 1907
Sudafed PE Nighttime Cold Caplets 1907
Sudafed PE Non-Drying Sinus Caplets 1908
Sudafed PE Severe Cold Caplets 1908
Sudafed PE Sinus & Allergy Tablets 1908
Sudafed PE Sinus Headache Caplets 1908
Tylenol Allergy Multi-Symptom Caplets with Cool Burst and Rapid Release Gelcaps 1916
Tylenol Allergy Multi-Symptom Nighttime Caplets with Cool Burst 1916
Children's Tylenol Plus Cold Suspension Liquid 1912
Children's Tylenol Plus Cold & Allergy Suspension Liquid 1914
Children's Tylenol Plus Flu Suspension Liquid 1914
Children's Tylenol Plus Multi-Symptom Cold Suspension Liquid 1912
Tylenol Cold Head Congestion Daytime Caplets with Cool Burst 1910
Tylenol Cold Head Congestion Nighttime Caplets with Cool Burst 1910
Tylenol Cold Head Congestion Severe Daytime Caplets with Cool Burst 1910
Tylenol Cold Multi-Symptom Daytime Caplets with Cool Burst and Rapid Release Gels 1913
Tylenol Cold Multi-Symptom Daytime Liquid with Citrus Burst 1913
Tylenol Cold Multi-Symptom Nighttime Caplets with Cool Burst 1913
Tylenol Cold Multi-Symptom Nighttime Liquid with Cool Burst 1913
Tylenol Cold Multi-Symptom Severe Caplets with Cool Burst 1913
Tylenol Cold Multi-Symptom Severe Daytime Liquid with Citrus Burst 1913
Tylenol Sinus Congestion & Pain Daytime Caplets with Cool Burst and Gelcaps 1917
Tylenol Sinus Congestion & Pain Nighttime Caplets with Cool Burst 1917
Tylenol Sinus Congestion & Pain Severe Caplets with Cool Burst 1917
Vicks DayQuil Cold & Flu Multi-Symptom Relief 616
Vicks DayQuil LiquiCaps 2567
Vicks DayQuil Liquid 2567
Vicks DayQuil Multi-Symptom Cold/Flu Relief 2567

Phenylephrine Tannate (If additional adrenergic drugs are to be administered by any route, they should be used with caution to avoid deleterious cardiovascular effects).
No products indexed under this heading.

Phenylpropanolamine Hydrochloride (If additional adrenergic drugs are to be administered by any route, they should be used with caution to avoid deleterious cardiovascular effects).
No products indexed under this heading.

Pindolol (Beta-adrenergic receptor blocking agents not only block the pulmonary effect of beta agonists such as albuterol sulfate inhalation aerosol, but may produce severe bronchospasm in patients with asthma. Therefore, patients with asthma should not normally be treated with beta-blockers. However under certain circumstances, eg, as prophylaxis after myocardial infarction, there may be no acceptable alternatives to the use of beta-adrenergic blocking agents in patients with asthma. In this setting, cardioselective beta-blockers should be considered, although they should be administered with caution).
No products indexed under this heading.

Pirbuterol Acetate (Other short-acting sympathomimetic aerosol bronchodilators should not be used concomitantly with albuterol). Products include:
Maxair Autohaler 1705

Polythiazide (The ECG changes and/or hypokalemia that may result from the administration of nonpotassium-sparing diuretics (eg, loop or thiazide diuretics) can be acutely worsened by beta-agonists, especially when the recommended dose of the beta-agonist is exceeded.Although the clinical relevance of these effects is not known, caution is advised in the co-administration of beta-agonists with nonpotassium-sparing diuretics. Consider monitoring potassium levels).
No products indexed under this heading.

Procarbazine Hydrochloride (Albuterol sulfate inhalation aerosol should be administered with extreme caution to patients being treated with monoamine oxidase inhibitors, or within 2 weeks of discontinuation of such agents, because the action of albuterol on the vascular system may be potentiated. Consider alternative therapy in patients taking MAO inhibitors).
No products indexed under this heading.

Propranolol Hydrochloride (Beta-adrenergic receptor blocking agents not only block the pulmonary effect of beta agonists such as albuterol sulfate inhalation aerosol, but may produce severe bronchospasm in patients with asthma. Therefore, patients with asthma should not normally be treated with beta-blockers. However under certain circumstances, eg, as prophylaxis after myocardial infarction, there may be no acceptable alternatives to the use of beta-adrenergic blocking agents in patients with asthma. In this setting, cardioselective beta-blockers should be considered, although they should be administered with caution). Products include:
InnoPran XL Extended Release Capsules 1484

Protriptyline Hydrochloride (Albuterol sulfate inhalation aerosol should be administered with extreme caution to patients being treated with tricyclic antidepressants, or within 2 weeks of discontinuation of such agents, because the action of albuterol on the vascular system may be potentiated. Consider alternative therapy in patients taking tricyclic antidepressants).
No products indexed under this heading.

Pseudoephedrine Hydrochloride (If additional adrenergic drugs are to be administered by any route, they should be used with caution to avoid deleterious cardiovascular effects). Products include:
Allegra-D 12 Hour Extended-Release Tablets 2687
Allegra-D 24 Hour Extended-Release Tablets 2690
Children's Motrin Cold Oral Suspension 1899
Sudafed 12 Hour Nasal Decongestant Non-Drowsy Caplets 1909
Sudafed 24 Hour Non-Drowsy Nasal Decongestant Tablets 1906
Children's Sudafed Nasal Decongestant Liquid 1906
Sudafed Nasal Decongestant Tablets 1906
Tylenol Cold Severe Congestion Daytime Caplets with Cool Burst 1912
Tylenol Sinus Severe Congestion Caplets with Cool Burst 1917
Vicks NyQuil LiquiCaps 2567
Vicks NyQuil Liquid 2567
Vicks NyQuil Multi-Symptom Cold/Flu Relief 2567
Zyrtec-D 12 Hour Extended Release Tablets 1923
Zyrtec-D Allergy & Congestion Extended-Release Tablets 1923

Pseudoephedrine Sulfate (If additional adrenergic drugs are to be administered by any route, they should be used with caution to avoid deleterious cardiovascular effects). Products include:
Clarinex-D 12-Hour Extended-Release Tablets 2831
Clarinex-D 24-Hour Extended-Release Tablets 2834

Rasagiline Mesylate (Albuterol sulfate inhalation aerosol should be administered with extreme caution to patients being treated with monoamine oxidase inhibitors, or within 2 weeks of discontinuation of such agents, because the action of albuterol on the vascular system may be potentiated. Consider alternative therapy in patients taking MAO inhibitors). Products include:
Azilect Tablets 3106

Salmeterol Xinafoate (Other short-acting sympathomimetic aerosol bronchodilators should not be used concomitantly with albuterol). Products include:
Advair Diskus 100/50 1276
Advair Diskus 250/50 1276
Advair Diskus 500/50 1276
Advair HFA 45/21 Inhalation Aerosol 1288
Advair HFA 115/21 Inhalation Aerosol 1288
Advair HFA 230/21 Inhalation Aerosol 1288
Serevent Diskus 1594

Selegiline (Albuterol sulfate inhalation aerosol should be administered with extreme caution to patients being treated with monoamine oxidase inhibitors, or within 2 weeks of discontinuation of such agents, because the action of albuterol on the vascular system may be potentiated. Consider alternative therapy in patients taking MAO inhibitors). Products include:
Emsam Transdermal System 905

Selegiline Hydrochloride (Albuterol sulfate inhalation aerosol should be administered with extreme caution to patients being treated with monoamine oxidase inhibitors, or within 2 weeks of discontinuation of such agents, because the action of albuterol on the vascular system may be potentiated. Consider alternative therapy in patients taking MAO inhibitors). Products include:
Eldepryl Capsules 3052

Sotalol Hydrochloride (Beta-adrenergic receptor blocking agents not only block the pulmonary effect of beta agonists such as albuterol sulfate inhalation aerosol, but may produce severe bronchospasm in patients with asthma. Therefore, patients with asthma should not normally be treated with beta-blockers. However under certain circumstances, eg, as prophylaxis after myocardial infarction, there may be no acceptable alternatives to the use of beta-adrenergic blocking agents in patients with asthma. In this setting, cardioselective beta-blockers should be considered, although they should be administered with caution).
No products indexed under this heading.

Terbutaline Sulfate (Other short-acting sympathomimetic aerosol bronchodilators should not be used concomitantly with albuterol).
No products indexed under this heading.

Timolol Hemihydrate (Beta-adrenergic receptor blocking agents not only block the pulmonary effect of beta agonists such as albuterol sulfate inhalation aerosol, but may produce severe bronchospasm in patients with asthma. Therefore, patients with asthma should not normally be treated with beta-blockers. However under certain circumstances, eg, as prophylaxis after myocardial infarction, there may be no acceptable alternatives to the use of beta-adrenergic blocking agents in patients with asthma. In this setting, cardioselective beta-blockers should be considered, although they should be administered with caution). Products include:
Betimol Ophthalmic Solution 3181

Timolol Maleate (Beta-adrenergic receptor blocking agents not only block the pulmonary effect of beta agonists such as albuterol sulfate inhalation aerosol, but may produce severe bronchospasm in patients with asthma. Therefore, patients with asthma should not normally be treated with beta-blockers. However under certain circumstances, eg, as prophylaxis after myocardial infarction, there may be no acceptable alternatives to the use of beta-adrenergic blocking agents in patients with asthma. In this setting, cardioselective beta-blockers should be considered, although they should be administered with caution). Products include:
Combigan Ophthalmic Solution 553
Cosopt Sterile Ophthalmic Solution 1969
Timoptic Sterile Ophthalmic Solution 2121
Timoptic in Ocudose 2124
Timoptic-XE Sterile Ophthalmic Gel Forming Solution 2125

Torsemide (The ECG changes and/or hypokalemia that may result from the administration of nonpotassium-sparing diuretics (eg, loop or thiazide diuretics) can be acutely worsened by beta-agonists, especially when the recommended dose of the beta-agonist is exceeded.Although the clinical relevance of these effects is not known, caution is advised in the co-administration of beta-agonists with nonpotassium-sparing diuretics. Consider monitoring potassium levels). Products include:
Demadex Injection 2630
Demadex Tablets 2630

Tranylcypromine Sulfate (Albuterol sulfate inhalation aerosol should be administered with extreme caution to patients being treated with monoamine oxidase inhibitors, or within 2 weeks of discontinuation of such agents, because the action of albuterol on the vascular system may be potentiated. Consider alternative therapy in patients taking MAO inhibitors). Products include:
Parnate Tablets ... 1532

Trimipramine Maleate (Albuterol sulfate inhalation aerosol should be administered with extreme caution to patients being treated with tricyclic antidepressants, or within 2 weeks of discontinuation of such agents, because the action of albuterol on the vascular system may be potentiated. Consider alternative therapy in patients taking tricyclic antidepressants).
No products indexed under this heading.

VERAMYST NASAL SPRAY

(Fluticasone Furoate) ... 1643
May interact with cytochrome p450 3a4 inhibitors, potent and certain other agents. Compounds in these categories include:

Amprenavir (Use caution with the co-administration of fluticasone furoate nasal spray and ketoconazole or other potent CYP3A4 inhibitors).
No products indexed under this heading.

Atazanavir (Use caution with the co-administration of fluticasone furoate nasal spray and ketoconazole or other potent CYP3A4 inhibitors).
No products indexed under this heading.

Atazanavir Sulfate (Use caution with the co-administration of fluticasone furoate nasal spray and ketoconazole or other potent CYP3A4 inhibitors). Products include:
Reyataz Capsules ... 3299

Clarithromycin (Use caution with the co-administration of fluticasone furoate nasal spray and ketoconazole or other potent CYP3A4 inhibitors). Products include:
Biaxin/Biaxin XL ... 411

Delavirdine Mesylate (Use caution with the co-administration of fluticasone furoate nasal spray and ketoconazole or other potent CYP3A4 inhibitors).
No products indexed under this heading.

Delavirine (Use caution with the co-administration of fluticasone furoate nasal spray and ketoconazole or other potent CYP3A4 inhibitors).
No products indexed under this heading.

Fosamprenavir Calcium (Use caution with the co-administration of fluticasone furoate nasal spray and ketoconazole or other potent CYP3A4 inhibitors). Products include:
Lexiva Oral Suspension ... 1510
Lexiva Tablets ... 1510

Indinavir Sulfate (Use caution with the co-administration of fluticasone furoate nasal spray and ketoconazole or other potent CYP3A4 inhibitors). Products include:
Crixivan Capsules ... 1979

Itraconazole (Use caution with the co-administration of fluticasone furoate nasal spray and ketoconazole or other potent CYP3A4 inhibitors).
No products indexed under this heading.

Ketoconazole (Use caution with the co-administration of fluticasone furoate nasal spray and ketoconazole or other potent CYP3A4 inhibitors). Products include:
Extina Foam, 2% ... 3057
Nizoral A-D Shampoo ... 1901

Lopinavir (Use caution with the co-administration of fluticasone furoate nasal spray and ketoconazole or other potent CYP3A4 inhibitors). Products include:
Kaletra ... 452

Nefazodone Hydrochloride (Use caution with the co-administration of fluticasone furoate nasal spray and ketoconazole or other potent CYP3A4 inhibitors).
No products indexed under this heading.

Nelfinavir Mesylate (Use caution with the co-administration of fluticasone furoate nasal spray and ketoconazole or other potent CYP3A4 inhibitors).
No products indexed under this heading.

Ritonavir (Co-administration with ritonavir is not recommended because of the risk of systemic effects secondary to increased exposure to fluticasone furoate). Products include:
Kaletra ... 452
Norvir ... 489

Saquinavir (Use caution with the co-administration of fluticasone furoate nasal spray and ketoconazole or other potent CYP3A4 inhibitors).
No products indexed under this heading.

Saquinavir Mesylate (Use caution with the co-administration of fluticasone furoate nasal spray and ketoconazole or other potent CYP3A4 inhibitors).
No products indexed under this heading.

Telithromycin (Use caution with the co-administration of fluticasone furoate nasal spray and ketoconazole or other potent CYP3A4 inhibitors). Products include:
Ketek Tablets ... 2744

Troleandomycin (Use caution with the co-administration of fluticasone furoate nasal spray and ketoconazole or other potent CYP3A4 inhibitors).
No products indexed under this heading.

Voriconazole (Use caution with the co-administration of fluticasone furoate nasal spray and ketoconazole or other potent CYP3A4 inhibitors).
No products indexed under this heading.

VERDESO FOAM

(Desonide) ... 3069
None cited in PDR database.

VESANOID CAPSULES

(Tretinoin) ... 2660
May interact with cytochrome p450 3a4 inducers (selected), cytochrome p450 3a4 inhibitors (selected), erythromycin, glucocorticoids, tetracyclines, and certain other agents. Compounds in these categories include:

Acetazolamide (Tretinoin is metaboized by the hepatic P450 system; therefore, there is a potential for alteration of pharmacokinetic parameters in patients administered concomitant medications that are also inducers of this system. To date, there is no data to suggest that co-use with these medications increases or decreases either efficacy or toxicity of tretinoin).
No products indexed under this heading.

Allium sativum (Tretinoin is metaboized by the hepatic P450 system; therefore, there is a potential for alteration of pharmacokinetic parameters in patients administered concomitant medications that are also inducers of this system. To date, there is no data to suggest that co-use with these medications increases or decreases either efficacy or toxicity of tretinoin).
No products indexed under this heading.

Aminocaproic Acid (Cases of fatal thrombotic complications have been reported rarely in patients concomitantly treated with tretinoin and antifibrinolytic agents. Therefore, caution should be exercised when administering tretinoin concomitantly with these agents).
No products indexed under this heading.

Amiodarone Hydrochloride (Tretinoin is metaboized by the hepatic P450 system; therefore, there is a potential for alteration of pharmacokinetic parameters in patients administered concomitant medications that are also inducers of this system. To date, there is no data to suggest that co-use with these medications increases or decreases either efficacy or toxicity of tretinoin).
No products indexed under this heading.

Amprenavir (Tretinoin is metaboized by the hepatic P450 system; therefore, there is a potential for alteration of pharmacokinetic parameters in patients administered concomitant medications that are also inducers of this system. To date, there is no data to suggest that co-use with these medications increases or decreases either efficacy or toxicity of tretinoin).
No products indexed under this heading.

Anastrozole (Tretinoin is metaboized by the hepatic P450 system; therefore, there is a potential for alteration of pharmacokinetic parameters in patients administered concomitant medications that are also inducers of this system. To date, there is no data to suggest that co-use with these medications increases or decreases either efficacy or toxicity of tretinoin). Products include:
Arimidex Tablets ... 672

Aprepitant (Tretinoin is metaboized by the hepatic P450 system; therefore, there is a potential for alteration of pharmacokinetic parameters in patients administered concomitant medications that are also inducers of this system. To date, there is no data to suggest that co-use with these medications increases or decreases either efficacy or toxicity of tretinoin). Products include:
Emend Capsules ... 1992

Aprotinin (Cases of fatal thrombotic complications have been reported rarely in patients concomitantly treated with tretinoin and anti-fibrinolytic agents. Therefore, caution should be exercised when administering tretinoin concomitantly with these agents). Products include:
Trasylol Injection ... 799

Atazanavir (Tretinoin is metaboized by the hepatic P450 system; therefore, there is a potential for alteration of pharmacokinetic parameters in patients administered concomitant medications that are also inducers of this system. To date, there is no data to suggest that co-use with these medications increases or decreases either efficacy or toxicity of tretinoin).
No products indexed under this heading.

Atazanavir Sulfate (Tretinoin is metaboized by the hepatic P450 system; therefore, there is a potential for alteration of pharmacokinetic parameters in patients administered concomitant medications that are also inducers of this system. To date, there is no data to suggest that co-use with these medications increases or decreases either efficacy or toxicity of tretinoin). Products include:
Reyataz Capsules ... 3299

Betamethasone Acetate (Potential for alteration of pharmacokinetic parameters in patients on concomitant drugs that are inducers of hepatic CYP enzymes).
No products indexed under this heading.

Betamethasone Sodium Phosphate (Potential for alteration of pharmacokinetic parameters in patients on concomitant drugs that are inducers of hepatic CYP enzymes).
No products indexed under this heading.

Carbamazepine (Tretinoin is metaboized by the hepatic P450 system; therefore, there is a potential for alteration of pharmacokinetic parameters in patients administered concomitant medications that are also inducers of this system. To date, there is no data to suggest that co-use with these medications increases or decreases either efficacy or toxicity of tretinoin). Products include:
Carbatrol Capsules ... 3019
Equetro Extended-Release Capsules ... 3174

Cimetidine (Potential for alteration of pharmacokinetic parameters in patients on concomitant drugs that inhibit hepatic CYP enzymes).
No products indexed under this heading.

Cimetidine Hydrochloride (Potential for alteration of pharmacokinetic parameters in patients on concomitant drugs that inhibit hepatic CYP enzymes).
No products indexed under this heading.

Ciprofloxacin (Tretinoin is metaboized by the hepatic P450 system; therefore, there is a potential for alteration of pharmacokinetic parameters in patients administered concomitant medications that are also inducers of this system. To date, there is no data to suggest that co-use with these medications increases or decreases either efficacy or toxicity of tretinoin). Products include:

Cipro I.V. **2817**
Cipro Oral Suspension **2810**
Cipro XR Tablets **2823**
Ciprodex Otic Suspension **541**

Ciprofloxacin Hydrochloride (Tretinoin is metaboized by the hepatic P450 system; therefore, there is a potential for alteration of pharmacokinetic parameters in patients administered concomitant medications that are also inducers of this system. To date, there is no data to suggest that co-use with these medications increases or decreases either efficacy or toxicity of tretinoin). Products include:

Cipro Tablets **2810**

Cisplatin (Tretinoin is metaboized by the hepatic P450 system; therefore, there is a potential for alteration of pharmacokinetic parameters in patients administered concomitant medications that are also inducers of this system. To date, there is no data to suggest that co-use with these medications increases or decreases either efficacy or toxicity of tretinoin).

No products indexed under this heading.

Clarithromycin (Tretinoin is metaboized by the hepatic P450 system; therefore, there is a potential for alteration of pharmacokinetic parameters in patients administered concomitant medications that are also inducers of this system. To date, there is no data to suggest that co-use with these medications increases or decreases either efficacy or toxicity of tretinoin). Products include:

Biaxin/Biaxin XL **411**

Clotrimazole (Tretinoin is metaboized by the hepatic P450 system; therefore, there is a potential for alteration of pharmacokinetic parameters in patients administered concomitant medications that are also inducers of this system. To date, there is no data to suggest that co-use with these medications increases or decreases either efficacy or toxicity of tretinoin). Products include:

Lotrisone **2881**

Cortisone Acetate (Potential for alteration of pharmacokinetic parameters in patients on concomitant drugs that are inducers of hepatic CYP enzymes).

No products indexed under this heading.

Cyclosporine (Potential for alteration of pharmacokinetic parameters in patients on concomitant drugs that inhibit hepatic CYP enzymes). Products include:

Gengraf Capsules **435**
Neoral Oral Solution **2280**
Neoral Soft Gelatin Capsules **2280**
Restasis Ophthalmic Emulsion **557**
Sandimmune **2296**

Dalfopristin (Tretinoin is metaboized by the hepatic P450 system; therefore, there is a potential for alteration of pharmacokinetic parameters in patients administered concomitant medications that are also inducers of this system. To date, there is no data to suggest that co-use with these medications increases or decreases either efficacy or toxicity of tretinoin).

No products indexed under this heading.

Danazol (Tretinoin is metaboized by the hepatic P450 system; therefore, there is a potential for alteration of pharmacokinetic parameters in patients administered concomitant medications that are also inducers of this system. To date, there is no data to suggest that co-use with these medications increases or decreases either efficacy or toxicity of tretinoin).

No products indexed under this heading.

Delavirdine Mesylate (Tretinoin is metaboized by the hepatic P450 system; therefore, there is a potential for alteration of pharmacokinetic parameters in patients administered concomitant medications that are also inducers of this system. To date, there is no data to suggest that co-use with these medications increases or decreases either efficacy or toxicity of tretinoin).

No products indexed under this heading.

Demeclocycline Hydrochloride (Tretinoin may cause pseudotumor cerebri/intracranial hypertension. Concomitant administration of tretinoin and agents known to cause pseudotumor cerebri/intracranial hypertension as well might increase the risk of this condition).

No products indexed under this heading.

Dexamethasone (Potential for alteration of pharmacokinetic parameters in patients on concomitant drugs that are inducers of hepatic CYP enzymes). Products include:

Ciprodex Otic Suspension **541**

Dexamethasone Acetate (Potential for alteration of pharmacokinetic parameters in patients on concomitant drugs that are inducers of hepatic CYP enzymes).

No products indexed under this heading.

Dexamethasone Sodium Phosphate (Potential for alteration of pharmacokinetic parameters in patients on concomitant drugs that are inducers of hepatic CYP enzymes).

No products indexed under this heading.

Diltiazem Hydrochloride (Potential for alteration of pharmacokinetic parameters in patients on concomitant drugs that inhibit hepatic CYP enzymes). Products include:

Cardizem LA Extended Release Tablets **421**

Diltiazem Maleate (Tretinoin is metaboized by the hepatic P450 system; therefore, there is a potential for alteration of pharmacokinetic parameters in patients administered concomitant medications that are also inducers of this system. To date, there is no data to suggest that co-use with these medications increases or decreases either efficacy or toxicity of tretinoin).

No products indexed under this heading.

Doxorubicin Hydrochloride (Tretinoin is metaboized by the hepatic P450 system; therefore, there is a potential for alteration of pharmacokinetic parameters in patients administered concomitant medications that are also inducers of this system. To date, there is no data to suggest that co-use with these medications increases or decreases either efficacy or toxicity of tretinoin).

No products indexed under this heading.

Doxycycline Calcium (Tretinoin may cause pseudotumor cerebri/intracranial hypertension. Concomitant administration of tretinoin and agents known to cause pseudotumor cerebri/intracranial hypertension as well might increase the risk of this condition).

No products indexed under this heading.

Doxycycline Hyclate (Tretinoin may cause pseudotumor cerebri/intracranial hypertension. Concomitant administration of tretinoin and agents known to cause pseudotumor cerebri/intracranial hypertension as well might increase the risk of this condition).

No products indexed under this heading.

Doxycycline Monohydrate (Tretinoin may cause pseudotumor cerebri/intracranial hypertension. Concomitant administration of tretinoin and agents known to cause pseudotumor cerebri/intracranial hypertension as well might increase the risk of this condition).

No products indexed under this heading.

Efavirenz (Tretinoin is metaboized by the hepatic P450 system; therefore, there is a potential for alteration of pharmacokinetic parameters in patients administered concomitant medications that are also inducers of this system. To date, there is no data to suggest that co-use with these medications increases or decreases either efficacy or toxicity of tretinoin). Products include:

Atripla Tablets **938**
Sustiva Capsules **930**
Sustiva Tablets **930**

Erythromycin (Potential for alteration of pharmacokinetic parameters in patients on concomitant drugs that inhibit hepatic CYP enzymes).

No products indexed under this heading.

Erythromycin Estolate (Potential for alteration of pharmacokinetic parameters in patients on concomitant drugs that inhibit hepatic CYP enzymes).

No products indexed under this heading.

Erythromycin Ethylsuccinate (Potential for alteration of pharmacokinetic parameters in patients on concomitant drugs that inhibit hepatic CYP enzymes). Products include:

E.E.S. **433**
EryPed **431**

Erythromycin Gluceptate (Potential for alteration of pharmacokinetic parameters in patients on concomitant drugs that inhibit hepatic CYP enzymes).

No products indexed under this heading.

Erythromycin Lactobionate (Potential for alteration of pharmacokinetic parameters in patients on concomitant drugs that inhibit hepatic CYP enzymes).

No products indexed under this heading.

Erythromycin Stearate (Potential for alteration of pharmacokinetic parameters in patients on concomitant drugs that inhibit hepatic CYP enzymes).

No products indexed under this heading.

Esomeprazole Magnesium (Tretinoin is metaboized by the hepatic P450 system; therefore, there is a potential for alteration of pharmacokinetic parameters in patients administered concomitant medications that are also inducers of this system. To date, there is no data to suggest that co-use with these medications increases or decreases either efficacy or toxicity of tretinoin). Products include:

Nexium Delayed-Release Capsules **645**
Nexium Delayed-Release Oral Suspension **645**

Ethosuximide (Tretinoin is metaboized by the hepatic P450 system; therefore, there is a potential for alteration of pharmacokinetic parameters in patients administered concomitant medications that are also inducers of this system. To date, there is no data to suggest that co-use with these medications increases or decreases either efficacy or toxicity of tretinoin).

No products indexed under this heading.

Felbamate (Tretinoin is metaboized by the hepatic P450 system; therefore, there is a potential for alteration of pharmacokinetic parameters in patients administered concomitant medications that are also inducers of this system. To date, there is no data to suggest that co-use with these medications increases or decreases either efficacy or toxicity of tretinoin).

No products indexed under this heading.

Fluconazole (Tretinoin is metaboized by the hepatic P450 system; therefore, there is a potential for alteration of pharmacokinetic parameters in patients administered concomitant medications that are also inducers of this system. To date, there is no data to suggest that co-use with these medications increases or decreases either efficacy or toxicity of tretinoin).

No products indexed under this heading.

Fludrocortisone Acetate (Potential for alteration of pharmacokinetic parameters in patients on concomitant drugs that are inducers of hepatic CYP enzymes).

No products indexed under this heading.

Fluoxetine (Tretinoin is metaboized by the hepatic P450 system; therefore, there is a potential for alteration of pharmacokinetic parameters in patients administered concomitant medications that are also inducers of this system. To date, there is no data to suggest that co-use with these medications increases or decreases either efficacy or toxicity of tretinoin).
No products indexed under this heading.

Fluoxetine Hydrochloride (Tretinoin is metaboized by the hepatic P450 system; therefore, there is a potential for alteration of pharmacokinetic parameters in patients administered concomitant medications that are also inducers of this system. To date, there is no data to suggest that co-use with these medications increases or decreases either efficacy or toxicity of tretinoin). Products include:
Prozac Weekly Capsules 1852
Prozac Pulvules and Liquid 1852
Symbyax Capsules 1871

Fluvoxamine Maleate (Tretinoin is metaboized by the hepatic P450 system; therefore, there is a potential for alteration of pharmacokinetic parameters in patients administered concomitant medications that are also inducers of this system. To date, there is no data to suggest that co-use with these medications increases or decreases either efficacy or toxicity of tretinoin). Products include:
Luvox CR Extended-Release Capsules 1759

Fosamprenavir Calcium (Tretinoin is metaboized by the hepatic P450 system; therefore, there is a potential for alteration of pharmacokinetic parameters in patients administered concomitant medications that are also inducers of this system. To date, there is no data to suggest that co-use with these medications increases or decreases either efficacy or toxicity of tretinoin). Products include:
Lexiva Oral Suspension 1510
Lexiva Tablets 1510

Fosphenytoin Sodium (Tretinoin is metaboized by the hepatic P450 system; therefore, there is a potential for alteration of pharmacokinetic parameters in patients administered concomitant medications that are also inducers of this system. To date, there is no data to suggest that co-use with these medications increases or decreases either efficacy or toxicity of tretinoin).
No products indexed under this heading.

Garlic Extract (Tretinoin is metaboized by the hepatic P450 system; therefore, there is a potential for alteration of pharmacokinetic parameters in patients administered concomitant medications that are also inducers of this system. To date, there is no data to suggest that co-use with these medications increases or decreases either efficacy or toxicity of tretinoin).
No products indexed under this heading.

Garlic Oil (Tretinoin is metaboized by the hepatic P450 system; therefore, there is a potential for alteration of pharmacokinetic parameters in patients administered concomitant medications that are also inducers of this system. To date, there is no data to suggest that co-use with these medications increases or decreases either efficacy or toxicity of tretinoin).
No products indexed under this heading.

Hydrocortisone (Potential for alteration of pharmacokinetic parameters in patients on concomitant drugs that are inducers of hepatic CYP enzymes).
No products indexed under this heading.

Hydrocortisone Acetate (Potential for alteration of pharmacokinetic parameters in patients on concomitant drugs that are inducers of hepatic CYP enzymes). Products include:
Analpram-HC 1140
Pramosone 1141

Hydrocortisone Butyrate (Tretinoin is metaboized by the hepatic P450 system; therefore, there is a potential for alteration of pharmacokinetic parameters in patients administered concomitant medications that are also inducers of this system. To date, there is no data to suggest that co-use with these medications increases or decreases either efficacy or toxicity of tretinoin).
No products indexed under this heading.

Hydrocortisone Cypionate (Tretinoin is metaboized by the hepatic P450 system; therefore, there is a potential for alteration of pharmacokinetic parameters in patients administered concomitant medications that are also inducers of this system. To date, there is no data to suggest that co-use with these medications increases or decreases either efficacy or toxicity of tretinoin).
No products indexed under this heading.

Hydrocortisone Hemisuccinate (Tretinoin is metaboized by the hepatic P450 system; therefore, there is a potential for alteration of pharmacokinetic parameters in patients administered concomitant medications that are also inducers of this system. To date, there is no data to suggest that co-use with these medications increases or decreases either efficacy or toxicity of tretinoin).
No products indexed under this heading.

Hydrocortisone Probutate (Tretinoin is metaboized by the hepatic P450 system; therefore, there is a potential for alteration of pharmacokinetic parameters in patients administered concomitant medications that are also inducers of this system. To date, there is no data to suggest that co-use with these medications increases or decreases either efficacy or toxicity of tretinoin).
No products indexed under this heading.

Hydrocortisone Sodium Phosphate (Potential for alteration of pharmacokinetic parameters in patients on concomitant drugs that are inducers of hepatic CYP enzymes).
No products indexed under this heading.

Hydrocortisone Sodium Succinate (Potential for alteration of pharmacokinetic parameters in patients on concomitant drugs that are inducers of hepatic CYP enzymes).
No products indexed under this heading.

Hydrocortisone Valerate (Tretinoin is metaboized by the hepatic P450 system; therefore, there is a potential for alteration of pharmacokinetic parameters in patients administered concomitant medications that are also inducers of this system. To date, there is no data to suggest that co-use with these medications increases or decreases either efficacy or toxicity of tretinoin).
No products indexed under this heading.

Hypericum (Tretinoin is metaboized by the hepatic P450 system; therefore, there is a potential for alteration of pharmacokinetic parameters in patients administered concomitant medications that are also inducers of this system. To date, there is no data to suggest that co-use with these medications increases or decreases either efficacy or toxicity of tretinoin). Products include:
Satieté Tablets .... ▣ 640

Hypericum Perforatum (Tretinoin is metaboized by the hepatic P450 system; therefore, there is a potential for alteration of pharmacokinetic parameters in patients administered concomitant medications that are also inducers of this system. To date, there is no data to suggest that co-use with these medications increases or decreases either efficacy or toxicity of tretinoin).
No products indexed under this heading.

Indinavir Sulfate (Tretinoin is metaboized by the hepatic P450 system; therefore, there is a potential for alteration of pharmacokinetic parameters in patients administered concomitant medications that are also inducers of this system. To date, there is no data to suggest that co-use with these medications increases or decreases either efficacy or toxicity of tretinoin). Products include:
Crixivan Capsules 1979

Isoniazid (Tretinoin is metaboized by the hepatic P450 system; therefore, there is a potential for alteration of pharmacokinetic parameters in patients administered concomitant medications that are also inducers of this system. To date, there is no data to suggest that co-use with these medications increases or decreases either efficacy or toxicity of tretinoin).
No products indexed under this heading.

Itraconazole (Tretinoin is metaboized by the hepatic P450 system; therefore, there is a potential for alteration of pharmacokinetic parameters in patients administered concomitant medications that are also inducers of this system. To date, there is no data to suggest that co-use with these medications increases or decreases either efficacy or toxicity of tretinoin).
No products indexed under this heading.

Ketoconazole (Potential for alteration of pharmacokinetic parameters in patients on concomitant drugs that inhibit hepatic CYP enzymes). Products include:
Extina Foam, 2% 3057
Nizoral A-D Shampoo 1901

Lopinavir (Tretinoin is metaboized by the hepatic P450 system; therefore, there is a potential for alteration of pharmacokinetic parameters in patients administered concomitant medications that are also inducers of this system. To date, there is no data to suggest that co-use with these medications increases or decreases either efficacy or toxicity of tretinoin). Products include:
Kaletra 452

Loratadine (Tretinoin is metaboized by the hepatic P450 system; therefore, there is a potential for alteration of pharmacokinetic parameters in patients administered concomitant medications that are also inducers of this system. To date, there is no data to suggest that co-use with these medications increases or decreases either efficacy or toxicity of tretinoin).
No products indexed under this heading.

Mephenytoin (Tretinoin is metaboized by the hepatic P450 system; therefore, there is a potential for alteration of pharmacokinetic parameters in patients administered concomitant medications that are also inducers of this system. To date, there is no data to suggest that co-use with these medications increases or decreases either efficacy or toxicity of tretinoin).
No products indexed under this heading.

Methacycline Hydrochloride (Tretinoin may cause pseudotumor cerebri/intracranial hypertension. Concomitant administration of tretinoin and agents known to cause pseudotumor cerebri/intracranial hypertension as well might increase the risk of this condition).
No products indexed under this heading.

Methsuximide (Tretinoin is metaboized by the hepatic P450 system; therefore, there is a potential for alteration of pharmacokinetic parameters in patients administered concomitant medications that are also inducers of this system. To date, there is no data to suggest that co-use with these medications increases or decreases either efficacy or toxicity of tretinoin).
No products indexed under this heading.

Methylprednisolone (Tretinoin is metaboized by the hepatic P450 system; therefore, there is a potential for alteration of pharmacokinetic parameters in patients administered concomitant medications that are also inducers of this system. To date, there is no data to suggest that co-use with these medications increases or decreases either efficacy or toxicity of tretinoin).
No products indexed under this heading.

Methylprednisolone Acetate (Potential for alteration of pharmacokinetic parameters in patients on concomitant drugs that are inducers of hepatic CYP enzymes).
No products indexed under this heading.

Methylprednisolone Sodium Succinate (Potential for alteration of pharmacokinetic parameters in patients on concomitant drugs that are inducers of hepatic CYP enzymes).
No products indexed under this heading.

Metronidazole (Tretinoin is metabolized by the hepatic P450 system; therefore, there is a potential for alteration of pharmacokinetic parameters in patients administered concomitant medications that are also inducers of this system. To date, there is no data to suggest that co-use with these medications increases or decreases either efficacy or toxicity of tretinoin). Products include:
Pylera Capsules 714

Metronidazole Benzoate (Tretinoin is metabolized by the hepatic P450 system; therefore, there is a potential for alteration of pharmacokinetic parameters in patients administered concomitant medications that are also inducers of this system. To date, there is no data to suggest that co-use with these medications increases or decreases either efficacy or toxicity of tretinoin).
No products indexed under this heading.

Metronidazole Hydrochloride (Tretinoin is metabolized by the hepatic P450 system; therefore, there is a potential for alteration of pharmacokinetic parameters in patients administered concomitant medications that are also inducers of this system. To date, there is no data to suggest that co-use with these medications increases or decreases either efficacy or toxicity of tretinoin).
No products indexed under this heading.

Miconazole (Tretinoin is metabolized by the hepatic P450 system; therefore, there is a potential for alteration of pharmacokinetic parameters in patients administered concomitant medications that are also inducers of this system. To date, there is no data to suggest that co-use with these medications increases or decreases either efficacy or toxicity of tretinoin).
No products indexed under this heading.

Miconazole Nitrate (Tretinoin is metabolized by the hepatic P450 system; therefore, there is a potential for alteration of pharmacokinetic parameters in patients administered concomitant medications that are also inducers of this system. To date, there is no data to suggest that co-use with these medications increases or decreases either efficacy or toxicity of tretinoin).
No products indexed under this heading.

Minocycline Hydrochloride (Tretinoin may cause pseudotumor cerebri/intracranial hypertension. Concomitant administration of tretinoin and agents known to cause pseudotumor cerebri/intracranial hypertension as well might increase the risk of this condition). Products include:
Solodyn Extended Release Tablets 1938

Modafinil (Tretinoin is metabolized by the hepatic P450 system; therefore, there is a potential for alteration of pharmacokinetic parameters in patients administered concomitant medications that are also inducers of this system. To date, there is no data to suggest that co-use with these medications increases or decreases either efficacy or toxicity of tretinoin). Products include:
Provigil Tablets 977

Nefazodone Hydrochloride (Tretinoin is metabolized by the hepatic P450 system; therefore, there is a potential for alteration of pharmacokinetic parameters in patients administered concomitant medications that are also inducers of this system. To date, there is no data to suggest that co-use with these medications increases or decreases either efficacy or toxicity of tretinoin).
No products indexed under this heading.

Nelfinavir Mesylate (Tretinoin is metabolized by the hepatic P450 system; therefore, there is a potential for alteration of pharmacokinetic parameters in patients administered concomitant medications that are also inducers of this system. To date, there is no data to suggest that co-use with these medications increases or decreases either efficacy or toxicity of tretinoin).
No products indexed under this heading.

Nevirapine (Tretinoin is metabolized by the hepatic P450 system; therefore, there is a potential for alteration of pharmacokinetic parameters in patients administered concomitant medications that are also inducers of this system. To date, there is no data to suggest that co-use with these medications increases or decreases either efficacy or toxicity of tretinoin). Products include:
Viramune Oral Suspension 873
Viramune Tablets 873

Niacinamide (Tretinoin is metabolized by the hepatic P450 system; therefore, there is a potential for alteration of pharmacokinetic parameters in patients administered concomitant medications that are also inducers of this system. To date, there is no data to suggest that co-use with these medications increases or decreases either efficacy or toxicity of tretinoin). Products include:
BioLean Free Tablets .... ▣ 635

Nicotinamide (Tretinoin is metabolized by the hepatic P450 system; therefore, there is a potential for alteration of pharmacokinetic parameters in patients administered concomitant medications that are also inducers of this system. To date, there is no data to suggest that co-use with these medications increases or decreases either efficacy or toxicity of tretinoin).
No products indexed under this heading.

Nifedipine (Tretinoin is metabolized by the hepatic P450 system; therefore, there is a potential for alteration of pharmacokinetic parameters in patients administered concomitant medications that are also inducers of this system. To date, there is no data to suggest that co-use with these medications increases or decreases either efficacy or toxicity of tretinoin).
No products indexed under this heading.

Norfloxacin (Tretinoin is metabolized by the hepatic P450 system; therefore, there is a potential for alteration of pharmacokinetic parameters in patients administered concomitant medications that are also inducers of this system. To date, there is no data to suggest that co-use with these medications increases or decreases either efficacy or toxicity of tretinoin). Products include:
Noroxin Tablets 2069

Omeprazole (Tretinoin is metabolized by the hepatic P450 system; therefore, there is a potential for alteration of pharmacokinetic parameters in patients administered concomitant medications that are also inducers of this system. To date, there is no data to suggest that co-use with these medications increases or decreases either efficacy or toxicity of tretinoin).
No products indexed under this heading.

Oxcarbazepine (Tretinoin is metabolized by the hepatic P450 system; therefore, there is a potential for alteration of pharmacokinetic parameters in patients administered concomitant medications that are also inducers of this system. To date, there is no data to suggest that co-use with these medications increases or decreases either efficacy or toxicity of tretinoin).
No products indexed under this heading.

Oxytetracycline Hydrochloride (Tretinoin may cause pseudotumor cerebri/intracranial hypertension. Concomitant administration of tretinoin and agents known to cause pseudotumor cerebri/intracranial hypertension as well might increase the risk of this condition).
No products indexed under this heading.

Paroxetine Hydrochloride (Tretinoin is metabolized by the hepatic P450 system; therefore, there is a potential for alteration of pharmacokinetic parameters in patients administered concomitant medications that are also inducers of this system. To date, there is no data to suggest that co-use with these medications increases or decreases either efficacy or toxicity of tretinoin). Products include:
Paxil 1535
Paxil CR Controlled-Release Tablets 1544

Pentobarbital Sodium (Potential for alteration of pharmacokinetic parameters in patients on concomitant drugs that are inducers of hepatic CYP enzymes). Products include:
Nembutal Sodium Solution, USP 2494

Phenobarbital (Potential for alteration of pharmacokinetic parameters in patients on concomitant drugs that are inducers of hepatic CYP enzymes). Products include:
Donnatal Extentabs 2507

Phenobarbital Sodium (Tretinoin is metabolized by the hepatic P450 system; therefore, there is a potential for alteration of pharmacokinetic parameters in patients administered concomitant medications that are also inducers of this system. To date, there is no data to suggest that co-use with these medications increases or decreases either efficacy or toxicity of tretinoin).
No products indexed under this heading.

Phenytoin (Tretinoin is metabolized by the hepatic P450 system; therefore, there is a potential for alteration of pharmacokinetic parameters in patients administered concomitant medications that are also inducers of this system. To date, there is no data to suggest that co-use with these medications increases or decreases either efficacy or toxicity of tretinoin).
No products indexed under this heading.

Phenytoin Sodium (Tretinoin is metabolized by the hepatic P450 system; therefore, there is a potential for alteration of pharmacokinetic parameters in patients administered concomitant medications that are also inducers of this system. To date, there is no data to suggest that co-use with these medications increases or decreases either efficacy or toxicity of tretinoin). Products include:
Phenytek Capsules 2192

Prednisolone Acetate (Potential for alteration of pharmacokinetic parameters in patients on concomitant drugs that are inducers of hepatic CYP enzymes). Products include:
Pred Forte Ophthalmic Suspension .... ⊙ 227
Pred Mild Ophthalmic Suspension .... ⊙ 230
Pred-G Ophthalmic Ointment .... ⊙ 229
Pred-G Ophthalmic Suspension ...... ⊙ 228

Prednisolone Sodium Phosphate (Potential for alteration of pharmacokinetic parameters in patients on concomitant drugs that are inducers of hepatic CYP enzymes).
No products indexed under this heading.

Prednisolone Tebutate (Potential for alteration of pharmacokinetic parameters in patients on concomitant drugs that are inducers of hepatic CYP enzymes).
No products indexed under this heading.

Prednisone (Potential for alteration of pharmacokinetic parameters in patients on concomitant drugs that are inducers of hepatic CYP enzymes).
No products indexed under this heading.

Primidone (Tretinoin is metabolized by the hepatic P450 system; therefore, there is a potential for alteration of pharmacokinetic parameters in patients administered concomitant medications that are also inducers of this system. To date, there is no data to suggest that co-use with these medications increases or decreases either efficacy or toxicity of tretinoin).
No products indexed under this heading.

Propoxyphene Hydrochloride (Tretinoin is metaboized by the hepatic P450 system; therefore, there is a potential for alteration of pharmacokinetic parameters in patients administered concomitant medications that are also inducers of this system. To date, there is no data to suggest that co-use with these medications increases or decreases either efficacy or toxicity of tretinoin).
No products indexed under this heading.

Propoxyphene Napsylate (Tretinoin is metaboized by the hepatic P450 system; therefore, there is a potential for alteration of pharmacokinetic parameters in patients administered concomitant medications that are also inducers of this system. To date, there is no data to suggest that co-use with these medications increases or decreases either efficacy or toxicity of tretinoin).
No products indexed under this heading.

Quinidine (Tretinoin is metaboized by the hepatic P450 system; therefore, there is a potential for alteration of pharmacokinetic parameters in patients administered concomitant medications that are also inducers of this system. To date, there is no data to suggest that co-use with these medications increases or decreases either efficacy or toxicity of tretinoin).
No products indexed under this heading.

Quinidine Hydrochloride (Tretinoin is metaboized by the hepatic P450 system; therefore, there is a potential for alteration of pharmacokinetic parameters in patients administered concomitant medications that are also inducers of this system. To date, there is no data to suggest that co-use with these medications increases or decreases either efficacy or toxicity of tretinoin).
No products indexed under this heading.

Quinidine Polygalacturonate (Tretinoin is metaboized by the hepatic P450 system; therefore, there is a potential for alteration of pharmacokinetic parameters in patients administered concomitant medications that are also inducers of this system. To date, there is no data to suggest that co-use with these medications increases or decreases either efficacy or toxicity of tretinoin).
No products indexed under this heading.

Quinidine Sulfate (Tretinoin is metaboized by the hepatic P450 system; therefore, there is a potential for alteration of pharmacokinetic parameters in patients administered concomitant medications that are also inducers of this system. To date, there is no data to suggest that co-use with these medications increases or decreases either efficacy or toxicity of tretinoin).
No products indexed under this heading.

Quinine (Tretinoin is metaboized by the hepatic P450 system; therefore, there is a potential for alteration of pharmacokinetic parameters in patients administered concomitant medications that are also inducers of this system. To date, there is no data to suggest that co-use with these medications increases or decreases either efficacy or toxicity of tretinoin).
No products indexed under this heading.

Quinine Sulfate (Tretinoin is metaboized by the hepatic P450 system; therefore, there is a potential for alteration of pharmacokinetic parameters in patients administered concomitant medications that are also inducers of this system. To date, there is no data to suggest that co-use with these medications increases or decreases either efficacy or toxicity of tretinoin).
No products indexed under this heading.

Quinupristin (Tretinoin is metaboized by the hepatic P450 system; therefore, there is a potential for alteration of pharmacokinetic parameters in patients administered concomitant medications that are also inducers of this system. To date, there is no data to suggest that co-use with these medications increases or decreases either efficacy or toxicity of tretinoin).
No products indexed under this heading.

Ranitidine Bismuth Citrate (Tretinoin is metaboized by the hepatic P450 system; therefore, there is a potential for alteration of pharmacokinetic parameters in patients administered concomitant medications that are also inducers of this system. To date, there is no data to suggest that co-use with these medications increases or decreases either efficacy or toxicity of tretinoin).
No products indexed under this heading.

Ranitidine Hydrochloride (Tretinoin is metaboized by the hepatic P450 system; therefore, there is a potential for alteration of pharmacokinetic parameters in patients administered concomitant medications that are also inducers of this system. To date, there is no data to suggest that co-use with these medications increases or decreases either efficacy or toxicity of tretinoin). Products include:
Zantac 75 Tablets .... ▣ 603
Zantac 1670
Zantac Injection 1666
Zantac Injection Pharmacy Bulk Package 1668
Maximum Strength Zantac 150 Tablets .... ▣ 603
Maximum Strength Zantac 150 Cool Mint Tablets .... ▣ 603

Rifabutin (Tretinoin is metaboized by the hepatic P450 system; therefore, there is a potential for alteration of pharmacokinetic parameters in patients administered concomitant medications that are also inducers of this system. To date, there is no data to suggest that co-use with these medications increases or decreases either efficacy or toxicity of tretinoin).
No products indexed under this heading.

Rifampicin (Tretinoin is metaboized by the hepatic P450 system; therefore, there is a potential for alteration of pharmacokinetic parameters in patients administered concomitant medications that are also inducers of this system. To date, there is no data to suggest that co-use with these medications increases or decreases either efficacy or toxicity of tretinoin).
No products indexed under this heading.

Rifampin (Potential for alteration of pharmacokinetic parameters in patients on concomitant drugs that are inducers of hepatic CYP enzymes).
No products indexed under this heading.

Rifapentine (Tretinoin is metaboized by the hepatic P450 system; therefore, there is a potential for alteration of pharmacokinetic parameters in patients administered concomitant medications that are also inducers of this system. To date, there is no data to suggest that co-use with these medications increases or decreases either efficacy or toxicity of tretinoin).
No products indexed under this heading.

Ritonavir (Tretinoin is metaboized by the hepatic P450 system; therefore, there is a potential for alteration of pharmacokinetic parameters in patients administered concomitant medications that are also inducers of this system. To date, there is no data to suggest that co-use with these medications increases or decreases either efficacy or toxicity of tretinoin). Products include:
Kaletra 452
Norvir 489

Saquinavir (Tretinoin is metaboized by the hepatic P450 system; therefore, there is a potential for alteration of pharmacokinetic parameters in patients administered concomitant medications that are also inducers of this system. To date, there is no data to suggest that co-use with these medications increases or decreases either efficacy or toxicity of tretinoin).
No products indexed under this heading.

Saquinavir Mesylate (Tretinoin is metaboized by the hepatic P450 system; therefore, there is a potential for alteration of pharmacokinetic parameters in patients administered concomitant medications that are also inducers of this system. To date, there is no data to suggest that co-use with these medications increases or decreases either efficacy or toxicity of tretinoin).
No products indexed under this heading.

Sertraline Hydrochloride (Tretinoin is metaboized by the hepatic P450 system; therefore, there is a potential for alteration of pharmacokinetic parameters in patients administered concomitant medications that are also inducers of this system. To date, there is no data to suggest that co-use with these medications increases or decreases either efficacy or toxicity of tretinoin).
No products indexed under this heading.

Sildenafil Citrate (Tretinoin is metaboized by the hepatic P450 system; therefore, there is a potential for alteration of pharmacokinetic parameters in patients administered concomitant medications that are also inducers of this system. To date, there is no data to suggest that co-use with these medications increases or decreases either efficacy or toxicity of tretinoin).
No products indexed under this heading.

Sulfinpyrazone (Tretinoin is metaboized by the hepatic P450 system; therefore, there is a potential for alteration of pharmacokinetic parameters in patients administered concomitant medications that are also inducers of this system. To date, there is no data to suggest that co-use with these medications increases or decreases either efficacy or toxicity of tretinoin).
No products indexed under this heading.

Telithromycin (Tretinoin is metaboized by the hepatic P450 system; therefore, there is a potential for alteration of pharmacokinetic parameters in patients administered concomitant medications that are also inducers of this system. To date, there is no data to suggest that co-use with these medications increases or decreases either efficacy or toxicity of tretinoin). Products include:
Ketek Tablets 2744

Tetracycline Hydrochloride (Tretinoin may cause pseudotumor cerebri/intracranial hypertension. Concomitant administration of tretinoin and agents known to cause pseudotumor cerebri/intracranial hypertension as well might increase the risk of this condition). Products include:
Pylera Capsules 714

Theophylline (Tretinoin is metaboized by the hepatic P450 system; therefore, there is a potential for alteration of pharmacokinetic parameters in patients administered concomitant medications that are also inducers of this system. To date, there is no data to suggest that co-use with these medications increases or decreases either efficacy or toxicity of tretinoin).
No products indexed under this heading.

Theophylline Anhydrous (Tretinoin is metaboized by the hepatic P450 system; therefore, there is a potential for alteration of pharmacokinetic parameters in patients administered concomitant medications that are also inducers of this system. To date, there is no data to suggest that co-use with these medications increases or decreases either efficacy or toxicity of tretinoin). Products include:
Uniphyl Tablets 2595

Theophylline Calcium Salicylate (Tretinoin is metaboized by the hepatic P450 system; therefore, there is a potential for alteration of pharmacokinetic parameters in patients administered concomitant medications that are also inducers of this system. To date, there is no data to suggest that co-use with these medications increases or decreases either efficacy or toxicity of tretinoin).
No products indexed under this heading.

Theophylline Dihydroxypropyl (Glyceryl) (Tretinoin is metaboized by the hepatic P450 system; therefore, there is a potential for alteration of pharmacokinetic parameters in patients administered concomitant medications that are also inducers of this system. To date, there is no data to suggest that co-use with these medications increases or decreases either efficacy or toxicity of tretinoin).
No products indexed under this heading.

Theophylline Ethylenediamine (Tretinoin is metaboized by the hepatic P450 system; therefore, there is a potential for alteration of pharmacokinetic parameters in patients administered concomitant medications that are also inducers of this system. To date, there is no data to suggest that co-use with these medications increases or decreases either efficacy or toxicity of tretinoin).
No products indexed under this heading.

Tranexamic Acid (Cases of fatal thrombotic complications have been reported rarely in patients concomitantly treated with tretinoin and antifibrinolytic agents. Therefore, caution should be exercised when administering tretinoin concomitantly with these agents).
No products indexed under this heading.

Triamcinolone (Potential for alteration of pharmacokinetic parameters in patients on concomitant drugs that are inducers of hepatic CYP enzymes).
No products indexed under this heading.

Triamcinolone Acetonide (Potential for alteration of pharmacokinetic parameters in patients on concomitant drugs that are inducers of hepatic CYP enzymes). Products include:
Azmacort Inhalation Aerosol 407
Nasacort AQ Nasal Spray 2765
Triesence Injectable Suspension .... ⊙209

Triamcinolone Diacetate (Potential for alteration of pharmacokinetic parameters in patients on concomitant drugs that are inducers of hepatic CYP enzymes).
No products indexed under this heading.

Triamcinolone Hexacetonide (Potential for alteration of pharmacokinetic parameters in patients on concomitant drugs that are inducers of hepatic CYP enzymes).
No products indexed under this heading.

Troglitazone (Tretinoin is metaboized by the hepatic P450 system; therefore, there is a potential for alteration of pharmacokinetic parameters in patients administered concomitant medications that are also inducers of this system. To date, there is no data to suggest that co-use with these medications increases or decreases either efficacy or toxicity of tretinoin).
No products indexed under this heading.

Troleandomycin (Tretinoin is metaboized by the hepatic P450 system; therefore, there is a potential for alteration of pharmacokinetic parameters in patients administered concomitant medications that are also inducers of this system. To date, there is no data to suggest that co-use with these medications increases or decreases either efficacy or toxicity of tretinoin).
No products indexed under this heading.

Valproate Sodium (Tretinoin is metaboized by the hepatic P450 system; therefore, there is a potential for alteration of pharmacokinetic parameters in patients administered concomitant medications that are also inducers of this system. To date, there is no data to suggest that co-use with these medications increases or decreases either efficacy or toxicity of tretinoin).
No products indexed under this heading.

Vardenafil Hydrochloride (Tretinoin is metaboized by the hepatic P450 system; therefore, there is a potential for alteration of pharmacokinetic parameters in patients administered concomitant medications that are also inducers of this system. To date, there is no data to suggest that co-use with these medications increases or decreases either efficacy or toxicity of tretinoin). Products include:
Levitra Tablets 2876

Verapamil Hydrochloride (Potential for alteration of pharmacokinetic parameters in patients on concomitant drugs that inhibit hepatic CYP enzymes). Products include:
Tarka Tablets 511

Vitamin A (Vesanoid must not be administered in combination with vitamin A because of symptoms of hypervitaminosis A could be aggravated). Products include:
Norwegian Cod Liver Oil 949

Voriconazole (Tretinoin is metaboized by the hepatic P450 system; therefore, there is a potential for alteration of pharmacokinetic parameters in patients administered concomitant medications that are also inducers of this system. To date, there is no data to suggest that co-use with these medications increases or decreases either efficacy or toxicity of tretinoin).
No products indexed under this heading.

Zafirlukast (Tretinoin is metaboized by the hepatic P450 system; therefore, there is a potential for alteration of pharmacokinetic parameters in patients administered concomitant medications that are also inducers of this system. To date, there is no data to suggest that co-use with these medications increases or decreases either efficacy or toxicity of tretinoin). Products include:
Accolate Tablets 669

Zileuton (Tretinoin is metaboized by the hepatic P450 system; therefore, there is a potential for alteration of pharmacokinetic parameters in patients administered concomitant medications that are also inducers of this system. To date, there is no data to suggest that co-use with these medications increases or decreases either efficacy or toxicity of tretinoin).
No products indexed under this heading.

Food Interactions

Food, unspecified (The absorption of retinoids as a class has been shown to be enhanced when taken with food).

Grapefruit (Tretinoin is metaboized by the hepatic P450 system; therefore, there is a potential for alteration of pharmacokinetic parameters in patients administered concomitant medications that are also inducers of this system. To date, there is no data to suggest that co-use with these medications increases or decreases either efficacy or toxicity of tretinoin).

Grapefruit Juice (Tretinoin is metaboized by the hepatic P450 system; therefore, there is a potential for alteration of pharmacokinetic parameters in patients administered concomitant medications that are also inducers of this system. To date, there is no data to suggest that co-use with these medications increases or decreases either efficacy or toxicity of tretinoin).

VESICARE TABLETS

(Solifenacin Succinate) 636

May interact with cytochrome p450 3a4 inhibitors, potent and drugs that prolong the QT interval. Compounds in these categories include:

Alprazolam (In a study of the effect of solifenacin on the QT interval in 76 healthy women, the QT prolonging effect appered less with solifenacin 10 mg than with 30 mg (three times the maximum recommended dose), and the effect of solifenacin 30 mg did not appear as large as that of the positive control moxifloxacin at its therapeutic dose. This observation should be considered in clinical decisions to prescribe solifenacin succinate for patients with a known history of QT prolongation or patients who are taking medications known to prolong the QT interval).
No products indexed under this heading.

Amiodarone Hydrochloride (In a study of the effect of solifenacin on the QT interval in 76 healthy women, the QT prolonging effect appered less with solifenacin 10 mg than with 30 mg (three times the maximum recommended dose), and the effect of solifenacin 30 mg did not appear as large as that of the positive control moxifloxacin at its therapeutic dose. This observation should be considered in clinical decisions to prescribe solifenacin succinate for patients with a known history of QT prolongation or patients who are taking medications known to prolong the QT interval).
No products indexed under this heading.

Amitriptyline Hydrochloride (In a study of the effect of solifenacin on the QT interval in 76 healthy women, the QT prolonging effect appered less with solifenacin 10 mg than with 30 mg (three times the maximum recommended dose), and the effect of solifenacin 30 mg did not appear as large as that of the positive control moxifloxacin at its therapeutic dose. This observation should be considered in clinical decisions to prescribe solifenacin succinate for patients with a known history of QT prolongation or patients who are taking medications known to prolong the QT interval).
No products indexed under this heading.

Amoxapine (In a study of the effect of solifenacin on the QT interval in 76 healthy women, the QT prolonging effect appered less with solifenacin 10 mg than with 30 mg (three times the maximum recommended dose), and the effect of solifenacin 30 mg did not appear as large as that of the positive control moxifloxacin at its therapeutic dose. This observation should be considered in clinical decisions to prescribe solifenacin succinate for patients with a known history of QT prolongation or patients who are taking medications known to prolong the QT interval).
No products indexed under this heading.

Amprenavir (Do not exceed a 5 mg daily dose of solifenacin succinate when administered with therapeutic doses of ketoconazole or other potent CYP3A4 inhibitors).
No products indexed under this heading.

Astemizole (In a study of the effect of solifenacin on the QT interval in 76 healthy women, the QT prolonging effect appered less with solifenacin 10 mg than with 30 mg (three times the maximum recommended dose), and the effect of solifenacin 30 mg did not appear as large as that of the positive control moxifloxacin at its therapeutic dose. This observation should be considered in clinical decisions to prescribe solifenacin succinate for patients with a known history of QT prolongation or patients who are taking medications known to prolong the QT interval).
No products indexed under this heading.

Atazanavir (Do not exceed a 5 mg daily dose of solifenacin succinate when administered with therapeutic doses of ketoconazole or other potent CYP3A4 inhibitors).
No products indexed under this heading.

Atazanavir Sulfate (Do not exceed a 5 mg daily dose of solifenacin succinate when administered with therapeutic doses of ketoconazole or other potent CYP3A4 inhibitors). Products include:
Reyataz Capsules 3299

Bretylium Tosylate (In a study of the effect of solifenacin on the QT interval in 76 healthy women, the QT prolonging effect appered less with solifenacin 10 mg than with 30 mg (three times the maximum recommended dose), and the effect of solifenacin 30 mg did not appear as large as that of the positive control moxifloxacin at its therapeutic dose. This observation should be considered in clinical decisions to prescribe solifenacin succinate for patients with a known history of QT prolongation or patients who are taking medications known to prolong the QT interval).
No products indexed under this heading.

Buspirone Hydrochloride (In a study of the effect of solifenacin on the QT interval in 76 healthy women, the QT prolonging effect appered less with solifenacin 10 mg than with 30 mg (three times the maximum recommended dose), and the effect of solifenacin 30 mg did not appear as large as that of the positive control moxifloxacin at its therapeutic dose. This observation should be considered in clinical decisions to

prescribe solifenacin succinate for patients with a known history of QT prolongation or patients who are taking medications known to prolong the QT interval).
No products indexed under this heading.

Chlordiazepoxide (In a study of the effect of solifenacin on the QT interval in 76 healthy women, the QT prolonging effect appered less with solifenacin 10 mg than with 30 mg (three times the maximum recommended dose), and the effect of solifenacin 30 mg did not appear as large as that of the positive control moxifloxacin at its therapeutic dose. This observation should be considered in clinical decisions to prescribe solifenacin succinate for patients with a known history of QT prolongation or patients who are taking medications known to prolong the QT interval).
No products indexed under this heading.

Chlordiazepoxide Hydrochloride (In a study of the effect of solifenacin on the QT interval in 76 healthy women, the QT prolonging effect appered less with solifenacin 10 mg than with 30 mg (three times the maximum recommended dose), and the effect of solifenacin 30 mg did not appear as large as that of the positive control moxifloxacin at its therapeutic dose. This observation should be considered in clinical decisions to prescribe solifenacin succinate for patients with a known history of QT prolongation or patients who are taking medications known to prolong the QT interval).
No products indexed under this heading.

Chlorpromazine (In a study of the effect of solifenacin on the QT interval in 76 healthy women, the QT prolonging effect appered less with solifenacin 10 mg than with 30 mg (three times the maximum recommended dose), and the effect of solifenacin 30 mg did not appear as large as that of the positive control moxifloxacin at its therapeutic dose. This observation should be considered in clinical decisions to prescribe solifenacin succinate for patients with a known history of QT prolongation or patients who are taking medications known to prolong the QT interval).
No products indexed under this heading.

Chlorpromazine Hydrochloride (In a study of the effect of solifenacin on the QT interval in 76 healthy women, the QT prolonging effect appered less with solifenacin 10 mg than with 30 mg (three times the maximum recommended dose), and the effect of solifenacin 30 mg did not appear as large as that of the positive control moxifloxacin at its therapeutic dose. This observation should be considered in clinical decisions to prescribe solifenacin succinate for patients with a known history of QT prolongation or patients who are taking medications known to prolong the QT interval).
No products indexed under this heading.

Chlorprothixene (In a study of the effect of solifenacin on the QT interval in 76 healthy women, the QT prolonging effect appered less with solifenacin 10 mg than with 30 mg (three times the maximum recommended dose), and the effect of solifenacin 30 mg did not appear as large as that of the positive control moxifloxacin at its therapeutic dose. This observation should be considered in clinical decisions to prescribe solifenacin succinate for patients with a known history of QT prolongation or patients who are taking medications known to prolong the QT interval).
No products indexed under this heading.

Chlorprothixene Hydrochloride (In a study of the effect of solifenacin on the QT interval in 76 healthy women, the QT prolonging effect appered less with solifenacin 10 mg than with 30 mg (three times the maximum recommended dose), and the effect of solifenacin 30 mg did not appear as large as that of the positive control moxifloxacin at its therapeutic dose. This observation should be considered in clinical decisions to prescribe solifenacin succinate for patients with a known history of QT prolongation or patients who are taking medications known to prolong the QT interval).
No products indexed under this heading.

Clarithromycin (Do not exceed a 5 mg daily dose of solifenacin succinate when administered with therapeutic doses of ketoconazole or other potent CYP3A4 inhibitors).
Products include:
Biaxin/Biaxin XL 411

Clomipramine Hydrochloride (In a study of the effect of solifenacin on the QT interval in 76 healthy women, the QT prolonging effect appered less with solifenacin 10 mg than with 30 mg (three times the maximum recommended dose), and the effect of solifenacin 30 mg did not appear as large as that of the positive control moxifloxacin at its therapeutic dose. This observation should be considered in clinical decisions to prescribe solifenacin succinate for patients with a known history of QT prolongation or patients who are taking medications known to prolong the QT interval).
No products indexed under this heading.

Clorazepate Dipotassium (In a study of the effect of solifenacin on the QT interval in 76 healthy women, the QT prolonging effect appered less with solifenacin 10 mg than with 30 mg (three times the maximum recommended dose), and the effect of solifenacin 30 mg did not appear as large as that of the positive control moxifloxacin at its therapeutic dose. This observation should be considered in clinical decisions to prescribe solifenacin succinate for patients with a known history of QT prolongation or patients who are taking medications known to prolong the QT interval).
No products indexed under this heading.

Clozapine (In a study of the effect of solifenacin on the QT interval in 76 healthy women, the QT prolonging effect appered less with solifenacin 10 mg than with 30 mg (three times the maximum recommended dose), and the effect of solifenacin 30 mg did not appear as large as that of the positive control moxifloxacin at its therapeutic dose. This observation should be considered in clinical decisions to prescribe solifenacin succinate for patients with a known history of QT prolongation or patients who are taking medications known to prolong the QT interval).
No products indexed under this heading.

Delavirdine Mesylate (Do not exceed a 5 mg daily dose of solifenacin succinate when administered with therapeutic doses of ketoconazole or other potent CYP3A4 inhibitors).
No products indexed under this heading.

Delavirine (Do not exceed a 5 mg daily dose of solifenacin succinate when administered with therapeutic doses of ketoconazole or other potent CYP3A4 inhibitors).
No products indexed under this heading.

Desipramine Hydrochloride (In a study of the effect of solifenacin on the QT interval in 76 healthy women, the QT prolonging effect appered less with solifenacin 10 mg than with 30 mg (three times the maximum recommended dose), and the effect of solifenacin 30 mg did not appear as large as that of the positive control moxifloxacin at its therapeutic dose. This observation should be considered in clinical decisions to prescribe solifenacin succinate for patients with a known history of QT prolongation or patients who are taking medications known to prolong the QT interval).
No products indexed under this heading.

Diazepam (In a study of the effect of solifenacin on the QT interval in 76 healthy women, the QT prolonging effect appered less with solifenacin 10 mg than with 30 mg (three times the maximum recommended dose), and the effect of solifenacin 30 mg did not appear as large as that of the positive control moxifloxacin at its therapeutic dose. This observation should be considered in clinical decisions to prescribe solifenacin succinate for patients with a known history of QT prolongation or patients who are taking medications known to prolong the QT interval).
Products include:
Valium Tablets 2658

Disopyramide Phosphate (In a study of the effect of solifenacin on the QT interval in 76 healthy women, the QT prolonging effect appered less with solifenacin 10 mg than with 30 mg (three times the maximum recommended dose), and the effect of solifenacin 30 mg did not appear as large as that of the positive control moxifloxacin at its therapeutic dose. This observation should be considered in clinical decisions to prescribe solifenacin succinate for patients with a known history of QT prolongation or patients who are taking medications known to prolong the QT interval).
No products indexed under this heading.

Dofetilide (In a study of the effect of solifenacin on the QT interval in 76 healthy women, the QT prolonging effect appered less with solifenacin 10 mg than with 30 mg (three times the maximum recommended dose), and the effect of solifenacin 30 mg did not appear as large as that of the positive control moxifloxacin at its therapeutic dose. This observation should be considered in clinical decisions to prescribe solifenacin succinate for patients with a known history of QT prolongation or patients who are taking medications known to prolong the QT interval).
No products indexed under this heading.

Doxepin Hydrochloride (In a study of the effect of solifenacin on the QT interval in 76 healthy women, the QT prolonging effect appered less with solifenacin 10 mg than with 30 mg (three times the maximum recommended dose), and the effect of solifenacin 30 mg did not appear as large as that of the positive control moxifloxacin at its therapeutic dose. This observation should be considered in clinical decisions to prescribe solifenacin succinate for patients with a known history of QT prolongation or patients who are taking medications known to prolong the QT interval).
No products indexed under this heading.

Droperidol (In a study of the effect of solifenacin on the QT interval in 76 healthy women, the QT prolonging effect appered less with solifenacin 10 mg than with 30 mg (three times the maximum recommended dose), and the effect of solifenacin 30 mg did not appear as large as that of the positive control moxifloxacin at its therapeutic dose. This observation should be considered in clinical decisions to prescribe solifenacin succinate for patients with a known history of QT prolongation or patients who are taking medications known to prolong the QT interval).
No products indexed under this heading.

Erythromycin (In a study of the effect of solifenacin on the QT interval in 76 healthy women, the QT prolonging effect appered less with solifenacin 10 mg than with 30 mg (three times the maximum recommended dose), and the effect of solifenacin 30 mg did not appear as large as that of the positive control moxifloxacin at its therapeutic dose. This observation should be considered in clinical decisions to prescribe solifenacin succinate for patients with a known history of QT prolongation or patients who are taking medications known to prolong the QT interval).
No products indexed under this heading.

Erythromycin Estolate (In a study of the effect of solifenacin on the QT interval in 76 healthy women, the QT prolonging effect appered less with solifenacin 10 mg than with 30 mg (three times the maximum recommended dose), and the effect of solifenacin 30 mg did not appear as large as that of the positive control moxifloxacin at its therapeutic dose. This observation should be considered in clinical decisions to prescribe solifenacin succinate for patients with a known history of QT prolongation or patients who are taking medications known to prolong the QT interval).
No products indexed under this heading.

Erythromycin Ethylsuccinate (In a study of the effect of solifenacin on the QT interval in 76 healthy women, the QT prolonging effect appered less with solifenacin 10 mg than with 30 mg (three times the maximum recommended dose), and the effect of solifenacin 30 mg did not appear as large as that of the positive control moxifloxacin at its therapeutic dose. This observation should be considered in clinical decisions to prescribe solifenacin succinate for patients with a known history of QT prolongation or patients who are taking medications known to prolong the QT interval). Products include:

E.E.S. 433
EryPed 431

Erythromycin Gluceptate (In a study of the effect of solifenacin on the QT interval in 76 healthy women, the QT prolonging effect appered less with solifenacin 10 mg than with 30 mg (three times the maximum recommended dose), and the effect of solifenacin 30 mg did not appear as large as that of the positive control moxifloxacin at its therapeutic dose. This observation should be considered in clinical decisions to prescribe solifenacin succinate for patients with a known history of QT prolongation or patients who are taking medications known to prolong the QT interval).

No products indexed under this heading.

Erythromycin Lactobionate (In a study of the effect of solifenacin on the QT interval in 76 healthy women, the QT prolonging effect appered less with solifenacin 10 mg than with 30 mg (three times the maximum recommended dose), and the effect of solifenacin 30 mg did not appear as large as that of the positive control moxifloxacin at its therapeutic dose. This observation should be considered in clinical decisions to prescribe solifenacin succinate for patients with a known history of QT prolongation or patients who are taking medications known to prolong the QT interval).

No products indexed under this heading.

Erythromycin Stearate (In a study of the effect of solifenacin on the QT interval in 76 healthy women, the QT prolonging effect appered less with solifenacin 10 mg than with 30 mg (three times the maximum recommended dose), and the effect of solifenacin 30 mg did not appear as large as that of the positive control moxifloxacin at its therapeutic dose. This observation should be considered in clinical decisions to prescribe solifenacin succinate for patients with a known history of QT prolongation or patients who are taking medications known to prolong the QT interval).

No products indexed under this heading.

Flecainide Acetate (In a study of the effect of solifenacin on the QT interval in 76 healthy women, the QT prolonging effect appered less with solifenacin 10 mg than with 30 mg (three times the maximum recommended dose), and the effect of solifenacin 30 mg did not appear as large as that of the positive control moxifloxacin at its therapeutic dose. This observation should be considered in clinical decisions to prescribe solifenacin succinate for patients with a known history of QT prolongation or patients who are taking medications known to prolong the QT interval).

No products indexed under this heading.

Fluphenazine Decanoate (In a study of the effect of solifenacin on the QT interval in 76 healthy women, the QT prolonging effect appered less with solifenacin 10 mg than with 30 mg (three times the maximum recommended dose), and the effect of solifenacin 30 mg did not appear as large as that of the positive control moxifloxacin at its therapeutic dose. This observation should be considered in clinical decisions to prescribe solifenacin succinate for patients with a known history of QT prolongation or patients who are taking medications known to prolong the QT interval).

No products indexed under this heading.

Fluphenazine Enanthate (In a study of the effect of solifenacin on the QT interval in 76 healthy women, the QT prolonging effect appered less with solifenacin 10 mg than with 30 mg (three times the maximum recommended dose), and the effect of solifenacin 30 mg did not appear as large as that of the positive control moxifloxacin at its therapeutic dose. This observation should be considered in clinical decisions to prescribe solifenacin succinate for patients with a known history of QT prolongation or patients who are taking medications known to prolong the QT interval).

No products indexed under this heading.

Fluphenazine Hydrochloride (In a study of the effect of solifenacin on the QT interval in 76 healthy women, the QT prolonging effect appered less with solifenacin 10 mg than with 30 mg (three times the maximum recommended dose), and the effect of solifenacin 30 mg did not appear as large as that of the positive control moxifloxacin at its therapeutic dose. This observation should be considered in clinical decisions to prescribe solifenacin succinate for patients with a known history of QT prolongation or patients who are taking medications known to prolong the QT interval).

No products indexed under this heading.

Fosamprenavir Calcium (Do not exceed a 5 mg daily dose of solifenacin succinate when administered with therapeutic doses of ketoconazole or other potent CYP3A4 inhibitors). Products include:

Lexiva Oral Suspension 1510
Lexiva Tablets 1510

Haloperidol (In a study of the effect of solifenacin on the QT interval in 76 healthy women, the QT prolonging effect appered less with solifenacin 10 mg than with 30 mg (three times the maximum recommended dose), and the effect of solifenacin 30 mg did not appear as large as that of the positive control moxifloxacin at its therapeutic dose. This observation should be considered in clinical decisions to prescribe solifenacin succinate for patients with a known history of QT prolongation or patients who are taking medications known to prolong the QT interval).

No products indexed under this heading.

Haloperidol Decanoate (In a study of the effect of solifenacin on the QT interval in 76 healthy women, the QT prolonging effect appered less with solifenacin 10 mg than with 30 mg (three times the maximum recommended dose), and the effect of solifenacin 30 mg did not appear as large as that of the positive control moxifloxacin at its therapeutic dose. This observation should be considered in clinical decisions to prescribe solifenacin succinate for patients with a known history of QT prolongation or patients who are taking medications known to prolong the QT interval).

No products indexed under this heading.

Hydroxyzine Hydrochloride (In a study of the effect of solifenacin on the QT interval in 76 healthy women, the QT prolonging effect appered less with solifenacin 10 mg than with 30 mg (three times the maximum recommended dose), and the effect of solifenacin 30 mg did not appear as large as that of the positive control moxifloxacin at its therapeutic dose. This observation should be considered in clinical decisions to prescribe solifenacin succinate for patients with a known history of QT prolongation or patients who are taking medications known to prolong the QT interval).

No products indexed under this heading.

Imipramine Hydrochloride (In a study of the effect of solifenacin on the QT interval in 76 healthy women, the QT prolonging effect appered less with solifenacin 10 mg than with 30 mg (three times the maximum recommended dose), and the effect of solifenacin 30 mg did not appear as large as that of the positive control moxifloxacin at its therapeutic dose. This observation should be considered in clinical decisions to prescribe solifenacin succinate for patients with a known history of QT prolongation or patients who are taking medications known to prolong the QT interval).

No products indexed under this heading.

Imipramine Pamoate (In a study of the effect of solifenacin on the QT interval in 76 healthy women, the QT prolonging effect appered less with solifenacin 10 mg than with 30 mg (three times the maximum recommended dose), and the effect of solifenacin 30 mg did not appear as large as that of the positive control moxifloxacin at its therapeutic dose. This observation should be considered in clinical decisions to prescribe solifenacin succinate for patients with a known history of QT prolongation or patients who are taking medications known to prolong the QT interval).

No products indexed under this heading.

Indinavir Sulfate (Do not exceed a 5 mg daily dose of solifenacin succinate when administered with therapeutic doses of ketoconazole or other potent CYP3A4 inhibitors). Products include:

Crixivan Capsules 1979

Isocarboxazid (In a study of the effect of solifenacin on the QT interval in 76 healthy women, the QT prolonging effect appered less with solifenacin 10 mg than with 30 mg (three times the maximum recommended dose), and the effect of solifenacin 30 mg did not appear as large as that of the positive control moxifloxacin at its therapeutic dose. This observation should be considered in clinical decisions to prescribe solifenacin succinate for patients with a known history of QT prolongation or patients who are taking medications known to prolong the QT interval). Products include:

Marplan Tablets 3177

Itraconazole (Do not exceed a 5 mg daily dose of solifenacin succinate when administered with therapeutic doses of ketoconazole or other potent CYP3A4 inhibitors).

No products indexed under this heading.

Ketoconazole (Do not exceed a 5 mg daily dose of solifenacin succinate when administered with therapeutic doses of ketoconazole or other potent CYP3A4 inhibitors). Products include:

Extina Foam, 2% 3057
Nizoral A-D Shampoo 1901

Lidocaine Hydrochloride (In a study of the effect of solifenacin on the QT interval in 76 healthy women, the QT prolonging effect appered less with solifenacin 10 mg than with 30 mg (three times the maximum recommended dose), and the effect of solifenacin 30 mg did not appear as large as that of the positive control moxifloxacin at its therapeutic dose. This observation should be considered in clinical decisions to prescribe solifenacin succinate for patients with a known history of QT prolongation or patients who are taking medications known to prolong the QT interval).

No products indexed under this heading.

Lithium Carbonate (In a study of the effect of solifenacin on the QT interval in 76 healthy women, the QT prolonging effect appered less with solifenacin 10 mg than with 30 mg (three times the maximum recommended dose), and the effect of solifenacin 30 mg did not appear as large as that of the positive control moxifloxacin at its therapeutic dose. This observation should be considered in clinical decisions to prescribe solifenacin succinate for patients with a known history of QT prolongation or patients who are taking medications known to prolong the QT interval).

No products indexed under this heading.

Lithium Citrate (In a study of the effect of solifenacin on the QT interval in 76 healthy women, the QT prolonging effect appered less with solifenacin 10 mg than with 30 mg (three times the maximum recommended dose), and the effect of solifenacin 30 mg did not appear as large as that of the positive control moxifloxacin at its therapeutic dose. This observation should be considered in clinical decisions to prescribe solifenacin succinate for patients with a known history of QT prolongation or patients who are taking medications known to prolong the QT interval).

No products indexed under this heading.

Lopinavir (Do not exceed a 5 mg daily dose of solifenacin succinate when administered with therapeutic doses of ketoconazole or other potent CYP3A4 inhibitors). Products include:

Kaletra ... 452

Lorazepam (In a study of the effect of solifenacin on the QT interval in 76 healthy women, the QT prolonging effect appered less with solifenacin 10 mg than with 30 mg (three times the maximum recommended dose), and the effect of solifenacin 30 mg did not appear as large as that of the positive control moxifloxacin at its therapeutic dose. This observation should be considered in clinical decisions to prescribe solifenacin succinate for patients with a known history of QT prolongation or patients who are taking medications known to prolong the QT interval).

No products indexed under this heading.

Loxapine Hydrochloride (In a study of the effect of solifenacin on the QT interval in 76 healthy women, the QT prolonging effect appered less with solifenacin 10 mg than with 30 mg (three times the maximum recommended dose), and the effect of solifenacin 30 mg did not appear as large as that of the positive control moxifloxacin at its therapeutic dose. This observation should be considered in clinical decisions to prescribe solifenacin succinate for patients with a known history of QT prolongation or patients who are taking medications known to prolong the QT interval).

No products indexed under this heading.

Loxapine Succinate (In a study of the effect of solifenacin on the QT interval in 76 healthy women, the QT prolonging effect appered less with solifenacin 10 mg than with 30 mg (three times the maximum recommended dose), and the effect of solifenacin 30 mg did not appear as large as that of the positive control moxifloxacin at its therapeutic dose. This observation should be considered in clinical decisions to prescribe solifenacin succinate for patients with a known history of QT prolongation or patients who are taking medications known to prolong the QT interval).

No products indexed under this heading.

Maprotiline Hydrochloride (In a study of the effect of solifenacin on the QT interval in 76 healthy women, the QT prolonging effect appered less with solifenacin 10 mg than with 30 mg (three times the maximum recommended dose), and the effect of solifenacin 30 mg did not appear as large as that of the positive control moxifloxacin at its therapeutic dose. This observation should be considered in clinical decisions to prescribe solifenacin succinate for patients with a known history of QT prolongation or patients who are taking medications known to prolong the QT interval).

No products indexed under this heading.

Meprobamate (In a study of the effect of solifenacin on the QT interval in 76 healthy women, the QT prolonging effect appered less with solifenacin 10 mg than with 30 mg (three times the maximum recommended dose), and the effect of solifenacin 30 mg did not appear as large as that of the positive control moxifloxacin at its therapeutic dose. This observation should be considered in clinical decisions to prescribe solifenacin succinate for patients with a known history of QT prolongation or patients who are taking medications known to prolong the QT interval).

No products indexed under this heading.

Mesoridazine Besylate (In a study of the effect of solifenacin on the QT interval in 76 healthy women, the QT prolonging effect appered less with solifenacin 10 mg than with 30 mg (three times the maximum recommended dose), and the effect of solifenacin 30 mg did not appear as large as that of the positive control moxifloxacin at its therapeutic dose. This observation should be considered in clinical decisions to prescribe solifenacin succinate for patients with a known history of QT prolongation or patients who are taking medications known to prolong the QT interval).

No products indexed under this heading.

Mexiletine Hydrochloride (In a study of the effect of solifenacin on the QT interval in 76 healthy women, the QT prolonging effect appered less with solifenacin 10 mg than with 30 mg (three times the maximum recommended dose), and the effect of solifenacin 30 mg did not appear as large as that of the positive control moxifloxacin at its therapeutic dose. This observation should be considered in clinical decisions to prescribe solifenacin succinate for patients with a known history of QT prolongation or patients who are taking medications known to prolong the QT interval).

No products indexed under this heading.

Midazolam Hydrochloride (In a study of the effect of solifenacin on the QT interval in 76 healthy women, the QT prolonging effect appered less with solifenacin 10 mg than with 30 mg (three times the maximum recommended dose), and the effect of solifenacin 30 mg did not appear as large as that of the positive control moxifloxacin at its therapeutic dose. This observation should be considered in clinical decisions to prescribe solifenacin succinate for patients with a known history of QT prolongation or patients who are taking medications known to prolong the QT interval).

No products indexed under this heading.

Molindone Hydrochloride (In a study of the effect of solifenacin on the QT interval in 76 healthy women, the QT prolonging effect appered less with solifenacin 10 mg than with 30 mg (three times the maximum recommended dose), and the effect of solifenacin 30 mg did not appear as large as that of the positive control moxifloxacin at its therapeutic dose. This observation should be considered in clinical decisions to prescribe solifenacin succinate for patients with a known history of QT prolongation or patients who are taking medications known to prolong the QT interval). Products include:

Moban Tablets ... 1116

Nefazodone Hydrochloride (Do not exceed a 5 mg daily dose of solifenacin succinate when administered with therapeutic doses of ketoconazole or other potent CYP3A4 inhibitors).

No products indexed under this heading.

Nelfinavir Mesylate (Do not exceed a 5 mg daily dose of solifenacin succinate when administered with therapeutic doses of ketoconazole or other potent CYP3A4 inhibitors).

No products indexed under this heading.

Nortriptyline Hydrochloride (In a study of the effect of solifenacin on the QT interval in 76 healthy women, the QT prolonging effect appered less with solifenacin 10 mg than with 30 mg (three times the maximum recommended dose), and the effect of solifenacin 30 mg did not appear as large as that of the positive control moxifloxacin at its therapeutic dose. This observation should be considered in clinical decisions to prescribe solifenacin succinate for patients with a known history of QT prolongation or patients who are taking medications known to prolong the QT interval).

No products indexed under this heading.

Olanzapine (In a study of the effect of solifenacin on the QT interval in 76 healthy women, the QT prolonging effect appered less with solifenacin 10 mg than with 30 mg (three times the maximum recommended dose), and the effect of solifenacin 30 mg did not appear as large as that of the positive control moxifloxacin at its therapeutic dose. This observation should be considered in clinical decisions to prescribe solifenacin succinate for patients with a known history of QT prolongation or patients who are taking medications known to prolong the QT interval). Products include:

Symbyax Capsules ... 1871
Zyprexa Tablets ... 1883
Zyprexa IntraMuscular ... 1883
Zyprexa ZYDIS Orally Disintegrating Tablets ... 1883

Oxazepam (In a study of the effect of solifenacin on the QT interval in 76 healthy women, the QT prolonging effect appered less with solifenacin 10 mg than with 30 mg (three times the maximum recommended dose), and the effect of solifenacin 30 mg did not appear as large as that of the positive control moxifloxacin at its therapeutic dose. This observation should be considered in clinical decisions to prescribe solifenacin succinate for patients with a known history of QT prolongation or patients who are taking medications known to prolong the QT interval).

No products indexed under this heading.

Perphenazine (In a study of the effect of solifenacin on the QT interval in 76 healthy women, the QT prolonging effect appered less with solifenacin 10 mg than with 30 mg (three times the maximum recommended dose), and the effect of solifenacin 30 mg did not appear as large as that of the positive control moxifloxacin at its therapeutic dose. This observation should be considered in clinical decisions to prescribe solifenacin succinate for patients with a known history of QT prolongation or patients who are taking medications known to prolong the QT interval).

No products indexed under this heading.

Phenelzine Sulfate (In a study of the effect of solifenacin on the QT interval in 76 healthy women, the QT prolonging effect appered less with solifenacin 10 mg than with 30 mg (three times the maximum recommended dose), and the effect of solifenacin 30 mg did not appear as large as that of the positive control moxifloxacin at its therapeutic dose. This observation should be considered in clinical decisions to prescribe solifenacin succinate for patients with a known history of QT prolongation or patients who are taking medications known to prolong the QT interval).

No products indexed under this heading.

Prazepam (In a study of the effect of solifenacin on the QT interval in 76 healthy women, the QT prolonging effect appered less with solifenacin 10 mg than with 30 mg (three times the maximum recommended dose), and the effect of solifenacin 30 mg did not appear as large as that of the positive control moxifloxacin at its therapeutic dose. This observation should be considered in clinical decisions to prescribe solifenacin succinate for patients with a known history of QT prolongation or patients who are taking medications known to prolong the QT interval).

No products indexed under this heading.

Procainamide Hydrochloride (In a study of the effect of solifenacin on the QT interval in 76 healthy women, the QT prolonging effect appered less with solifenacin 10 mg than with 30 mg (three times the maximum recommended dose), and the effect of solifenacin 30 mg did not appear as large as that of the positive control moxifloxacin at its therapeutic dose. This observation should be considered in clinical decisions to prescribe solifenacin succinate for patients with a known history of QT prolongation or patients who are taking medications known to prolong the QT interval).

No products indexed under this heading.

Prochlorperazine (In a study of the effect of solifenacin on the QT interval in 76 healthy women, the QT prolonging effect appered less with solifenacin 10 mg than with 30 mg (three times the maximum recommended dose), and the effect of solifenacin 30 mg did not appear as large as that of the positive control moxifloxacin at its therapeutic dose. This observation should be considered in clinical decisions to prescribe solifenacin succinate for patients with a known history of QT prolongation or patients who are taking medications known to prolong the QT interval).

No products indexed under this heading.

Promethazine Hydrochloride (In a study of the effect of solifenacin on the QT interval in 76 healthy women, the QT prolonging effect appered less with solifenacin 10 mg than with 30 mg (three times the maximum recommended dose), and the effect

of solifenacin 30 mg did not appear as large as that of the positive control moxifloxacin at its therapeutic dose. This observation should be considered in clinical decisions to prescribe solifenacin succinate for patients with a known history of QT prolongation or patients who are taking medications known to prolong the QT interval).
No products indexed under this heading.

Propafenone Hydrochloride (In a study of the effect of solifenacin on the QT interval in 76 healthy women, the QT prolonging effect appered less with solifenacin 10 mg than with 30 mg (three times the maximum recommended dose), and the effect of solifenacin 30 mg did not appear as large as that of the positive control moxifloxacin at its therapeutic dose. This observation should be considered in clinical decisions to prescribe solifenacin succinate for patients with a known history of QT prolongation or patients who are taking medications known to prolong the QT interval). Products include:
Rythmol Tablets 1586
Rythmol SR Capsules 1590

Protriptyline Hydrochloride (In a study of the effect of solifenacin on the QT interval in 76 healthy women, the QT prolonging effect appered less with solifenacin 10 mg than with 30 mg (three times the maximum recommended dose), and the effect of solifenacin 30 mg did not appear as large as that of the positive control moxifloxacin at its therapeutic dose. This observation should be considered in clinical decisions to prescribe solifenacin succinate for patients with a known history of QT prolongation or patients who are taking medications known to prolong the QT interval).
No products indexed under this heading.

Quetiapine Fumarate (In a study of the effect of solifenacin on the QT interval in 76 healthy women, the QT prolonging effect appered less with solifenacin 10 mg than with 30 mg (three times the maximum recommended dose), and the effect of solifenacin 30 mg did not appear as large as that of the positive control moxifloxacin at its therapeutic dose. This observation should be considered in clinical decisions to prescribe solifenacin succinate for patients with a known history of QT prolongation or patients who are taking medications known to prolong the QT interval).
No products indexed under this heading.

Quinidine Gluconate (In a study of the effect of solifenacin on the QT interval in 76 healthy women, the QT prolonging effect appered less with solifenacin 10 mg than with 30 mg (three times the maximum recommended dose), and the effect of solifenacin 30 mg did not appear as large as that of the positive control moxifloxacin at its therapeutic dose. This observation should be considered in clinical decisions to prescribe solifenacin succinate for patients with a known history of QT prolongation or patients who are taking medications known to prolong the QT interval).
No products indexed under this heading.

Quinidine Polygalacturonate (In a study of the effect of solifenacin on the QT interval in 76 healthy women, the QT prolonging effect appered less with solifenacin 10 mg than with 30 mg (three times the maximum recommended dose), and the effect of solifenacin 30 mg did not appear as large as that of the positive control moxifloxacin at its therapeutic dose. This observation should be considered in clinical decisions to prescribe solifenacin succinate for patients with a known history of QT prolongation or patients who are taking medications known to prolong the QT interval).
No products indexed under this heading.

Quinidine Sulfate (In a study of the effect of solifenacin on the QT interval in 76 healthy women, the QT prolonging effect appered less with solifenacin 10 mg than with 30 mg (three times the maximum recommended dose), and the effect of solifenacin 30 mg did not appear as large as that of the positive control moxifloxacin at its therapeutic dose. This observation should be considered in clinical decisions to prescribe solifenacin succinate for patients with a known history of QT prolongation or patients who are taking medications known to prolong the QT interval).
No products indexed under this heading.

Risperidone (In a study of the effect of solifenacin on the QT interval in 76 healthy women, the QT prolonging effect appered less with solifenacin 10 mg than with 30 mg (three times the maximum recommended dose), and the effect of solifenacin 30 mg did not appear as large as that of the positive control moxifloxacin at its therapeutic dose. This observation should be considered in clinical decisions to prescribe solifenacin succinate for patients with a known history of QT prolongation or patients who are taking medications known to prolong the QT interval). Products include:
Risperdal Consta Long-Acting Injection 1753

Ritonavir (Do not exceed a 5 mg daily dose of solifenacin succinate when administered with therapeutic doses of ketoconazole or other potent CYP3A4 inhibitors). Products include:
Kaletra 452
Norvir 489

Saquinavir (Do not exceed a 5 mg daily dose of solifenacin succinate when administered with therapeutic doses of ketoconazole or other potent CYP3A4 inhibitors).
No products indexed under this heading.

Saquinavir Mesylate (Do not exceed a 5 mg daily dose of solifenacin succinate when administered with therapeutic doses of ketoconazole or other potent CYP3A4 inhibitors).
No products indexed under this heading.

Telithromycin (Do not exceed a 5 mg daily dose of solifenacin succinate when administered with therapeutic doses of ketoconazole or other potent CYP3A4 inhibitors). Products include:
Ketek Tablets 2744

Thioridazine Hydrochloride (In a study of the effect of solifenacin on the QT interval in 76 healthy women, the QT prolonging effect appered less with solifenacin 10 mg than with 30 mg (three times the maximum recommended dose), and the effect of solifenacin 30 mg did not appear as large as that of the positive control moxifloxacin at its therapeutic dose. This observation should be considered in clinical decisions to prescribe solifenacin succinate for patients with a known history of QT prolongation or patients who are taking medications known to prolong the QT interval). Products include:
Thioridazine Hydrochloride Tablets 2195

Thiothixene (In a study of the effect of solifenacin on the QT interval in 76 healthy women, the QT prolonging effect appered less with solifenacin 10 mg than with 30 mg (three times the maximum recommended dose), and the effect of solifenacin 30 mg did not appear as large as that of the positive control moxifloxacin at its therapeutic dose. This observation should be considered in clinical decisions to prescribe solifenacin succinate for patients with a known history of QT prolongation or patients who are taking medications known to prolong the QT interval). Products include:
Thiothixene Capsules 2197

Tocainide Hydrochloride (In a study of the effect of solifenacin on the QT interval in 76 healthy women, the QT prolonging effect appered less with solifenacin 10 mg than with 30 mg (three times the maximum recommended dose), and the effect of solifenacin 30 mg did not appear as large as that of the positive control moxifloxacin at its therapeutic dose. This observation should be considered in clinical decisions to prescribe solifenacin succinate for patients with a known history of QT prolongation or patients who are taking medications known to prolong the QT interval).
No products indexed under this heading.

Tranylcypromine Sulfate (In a study of the effect of solifenacin on the QT interval in 76 healthy women, the QT prolonging effect appered less with solifenacin 10 mg than with 30 mg (three times the maximum recommended dose), and the effect of solifenacin 30 mg did not appear as large as that of the positive control moxifloxacin at its therapeutic dose. This observation should be considered in clinical decisions to prescribe solifenacin succinate for patients with a known history of QT prolongation or patients who are taking medications known to prolong the QT interval). Products include:
Parnate Tablets 1532

Trifluoperazine Hydrochloride (In a study of the effect of solifenacin on the QT interval in 76 healthy women, the QT prolonging effect appered less with solifenacin 10 mg than with 30 mg (three times the maximum recommended dose), and the effect of solifenacin 30 mg did not appear as large as that of the positive control moxifloxacin at its therapeutic dose. This observation should be considered in clinical decisions to prescribe solifenacin succinate for patients with a known history of QT prolongation or patients who are taking medications known to prolong the QT interval).
No products indexed under this heading.

Trimipramine Maleate (In a study of the effect of solifenacin on the QT interval in 76 healthy women, the QT prolonging effect appered less with solifenacin 10 mg than with 30 mg (three times the maximum recommended dose), and the effect of solifenacin 30 mg did not appear as large as that of the positive control moxifloxacin at its therapeutic dose. This observation should be considered in clinical decisions to prescribe solifenacin succinate for patients with a known history of QT prolongation or patients who are taking medications known to prolong the QT interval).
No products indexed under this heading.

Troleandomycin (Do not exceed a 5 mg daily dose of solifenacin succinate when administered with therapeutic doses of ketoconazole or other potent CYP3A4 inhibitors).
No products indexed under this heading.

Voriconazole (Do not exceed a 5 mg daily dose of solifenacin succinate when administered with therapeutic doses of ketoconazole or other potent CYP3A4 inhibitors).
No products indexed under this heading.

Ziprasidone Hydrochloride (In a study of the effect of solifenacin on the QT interval in 76 healthy women, the QT prolonging effect appered less with solifenacin 10 mg than with 30 mg (three times the maximum recommended dose), and the effect of solifenacin 30 mg did not appear as large as that of the positive control moxifloxacin at its therapeutic dose. This observation should be considered in clinical decisions to prescribe solifenacin succinate for patients with a known history of QT prolongation or patients who are taking medications known to prolong the QT interval). Products include:
Geodon Capsules 2520

VIADUR IMPLANT

(Leuprolide Acetate) 802
None cited in PDR database.

VIBE LIQUID MULTI-NUTRIENT SUPPLEMENT

(Aloe vera, Amino Acid Preparations, Antioxidants, Bioflavonoids, Calcium, Dietary Supplement, Folic Acid, Green Tea Extract, Herbals, Multiple, Herbals with Minerals, Herbals with Vitamins, Herbals with Vitamins & Minerals, Magnesium, Minerals, Minerals, Multiple, Phytonutrients, Potassium, Vitamin B_6, Vitamin C, Vitamin E, Vitamins, Multiple, Vitamins with Minerals, Zinc) 626
None cited in PDR database.

VICKS DAYQUIL COLD & FLU MULTI-SYMPTOM RELIEF

(Acetaminophen, Dextromethorphan Hydrobromide, Phenylephrine Hydrochloride)............ 616

See Vicks DayQuil LiquiCaps

IMPORTANT NOTE: Always consult each drug listing in the patient's regimen for possible interactions.

VICKS DAYQUIL LIQUICAPS
(Acetaminophen, Dextromethorphan Hydrobromide, Phenylephrine Hydrochloride) 2567
May interact with monoamine oxidase inhibitors and certain other agents. Compounds in these categories include:

Isocarboxazid (Concurrent and/or sequential use with MAO inhibitors is not recommended). Products include:
Marplan Tablets 3177

Moclobemide (Concurrent and/or sequential use with MAO inhibitors is not recommended).
No products indexed under this heading.

Pargyline Hydrochloride (Concurrent and/or sequential use with MAO inhibitors is not recommended).
No products indexed under this heading.

Phenelzine Sulfate (Concurrent and/or sequential use with MAO inhibitors is not recommended).
No products indexed under this heading.

Procarbazine Hydrochloride (Concurrent and/or sequential use with MAO inhibitors is not recommended).
No products indexed under this heading.

Rasagiline Mesylate (Concurrent and/or sequential use with MAO inhibitors is not recommended). Products include:
Azilect Tablets 3106

Selegiline (Concurrent and/or sequential use with MAO inhibitors is not recommended). Products include:
Emsam Transdermal System 905

Selegiline Hydrochloride (Concurrent and/or sequential use with MAO inhibitors is not recommended). Products include:
Eldepryl Capsules 3052

Tranylcypromine Sulfate (Concurrent and/or sequential use with MAO inhibitors is not recommended). Products include:
Parnate Tablets 1532

Food Interactions

Alcohol (Consuming 3 or more alcoholic drinks every day while using this product may cause severe liver damage).

VICKS DAYQUIL LIQUID
(Acetaminophen, Dextromethorphan Hydrobromide, Phenylephrine Hydrochloride) 2567
See Vicks DayQuil LiquiCaps

VICKS DAYQUIL MULTI-SYMPTOM COLD/FLU RELIEF
(Acetaminophen, Dextromethorphan Hydrobromide, Phenylephrine Hydrochloride) 2567
See Vicks DayQuil LiquiCaps

VICKS NYQUIL COLD & FLU MULTI-SYMPTOM RELIEF
(Acetaminophen, Dextromethorphan Hydrobromide, Doxylamine Succinate) .... ▣617
See Vicks NyQuil LiquiCaps

VICKS NYQUIL LIQUICAPS
(Acetaminophen, Dextromethorphan Hydrobromide, Doxylamine Succinate, Pseudoephedrine Hydrochloride) 2567
May interact with hypnotics and sedatives, monoamine oxidase inhibitors, tranquilizers, and certain other agents. Compounds in these categories include:

Alprazolam (May increase drowsiness effect).
No products indexed under this heading.

Buspirone Hydrochloride (May increase drowsiness effect).
No products indexed under this heading.

Butabarbital (May increase drowsiness effect).
No products indexed under this heading.

Butabarbital Sodium (May increase drowsiness effect).
No products indexed under this heading.

Chloral Hydrate (May increase drowsiness effect).
No products indexed under this heading.

Chlordiazepoxide (May increase drowsiness effect).
No products indexed under this heading.

Chlordiazepoxide Hydrochloride (May increase drowsiness effect).
No products indexed under this heading.

Chlorpromazine (May increase drowsiness effect).
No products indexed under this heading.

Chlorpromazine Hydrochloride (May increase drowsiness effect).
No products indexed under this heading.

Chlorprothixene (May increase drowsiness effect).
No products indexed under this heading.

Chlorprothixene Hydrochloride (May increase drowsiness effect).
No products indexed under this heading.

Clorazepate Dipotassium (May increase drowsiness effect).
No products indexed under this heading.

Diazepam (May increase drowsiness effect). Products include:
Valium Tablets 2658

Droperidol (May increase drowsiness effect).
No products indexed under this heading.

Estazolam (May increase drowsiness effect).
No products indexed under this heading.

Ethchlorvynol (May increase drowsiness effect).
No products indexed under this heading.

Ethinamate (May increase drowsiness effect).
No products indexed under this heading.

Fluphenazine Decanoate (May increase drowsiness effect).
No products indexed under this heading.

Fluphenazine Enanthate (May increase drowsiness effect).
No products indexed under this heading.

Fluphenazine Hydrochloride (May increase drowsiness effect).
No products indexed under this heading.

Flurazepam Hydrochloride (May increase drowsiness effect).
No products indexed under this heading.

Glutethimide (May increase drowsiness effect).
No products indexed under this heading.

Haloperidol (May increase drowsiness effect).
No products indexed under this heading.

Haloperidol Decanoate (May increase drowsiness effect).
No products indexed under this heading.

Hydroxyzine Hydrochloride (May increase drowsiness effect).
No products indexed under this heading.

Isocarboxazid (Concurrent and/or sequential use with MAO inhibitors is not recommended). Products include:
Marplan Tablets 3177

Lorazepam (May increase drowsiness effect).
No products indexed under this heading.

Loxapine Hydrochloride (May increase drowsiness effect).
No products indexed under this heading.

Loxapine Succinate (May increase drowsiness effect).
No products indexed under this heading.

Meprobamate (May increase drowsiness effect).
No products indexed under this heading.

Mesoridazine Besylate (May increase drowsiness effect).
No products indexed under this heading.

Midazolam Hydrochloride (May increase drowsiness effect).
No products indexed under this heading.

Moclobemide (Concurrent and/or sequential use with MAO inhibitors is not recommended).
No products indexed under this heading.

Molindone Hydrochloride (May increase drowsiness effect). Products include:
Moban Tablets 1116

Oxazepam (May increase drowsiness effect).
No products indexed under this heading.

Pargyline Hydrochloride (Concurrent and/or sequential use with MAO inhibitors is not recommended).
No products indexed under this heading.

Perphenazine (May increase drowsiness effect).
No products indexed under this heading.

Phenelzine Sulfate (Concurrent and/or sequential use with MAO inhibitors is not recommended).
No products indexed under this heading.

Prazepam (May increase drowsiness effect).
No products indexed under this heading.

Procarbazine Hydrochloride (Concurrent and/or sequential use with MAO inhibitors is not recommended).
No products indexed under this heading.

Prochlorperazine (May increase drowsiness effect).
No products indexed under this heading.

Promethazine Hydrochloride (May increase drowsiness effect).
No products indexed under this heading.

Propofol (May increase drowsiness effect).
No products indexed under this heading.

Quazepam (May increase drowsiness effect).
No products indexed under this heading.

Ramelteon (May increase drowsiness effect). Products include:
Rozerem Tablets 3091

Rasagiline Mesylate (Concurrent and/or sequential use with MAO inhibitors is not recommended). Products include:
Azilect Tablets 3106

Secobarbital Sodium (May increase drowsiness effect).
No products indexed under this heading.

Selegiline (Concurrent and/or sequential use with MAO inhibitors is not recommended). Products include:
Emsam Transdermal System 905

Selegiline Hydrochloride (Concurrent and/or sequential use with MAO inhibitors is not recommended). Products include:
Eldepryl Capsules 3052

Sodium Butabarbital (May increase drowsiness effect).
No products indexed under this heading.

Temazepam (May increase drowsiness effect).
No products indexed under this heading.

Thioridazine Hydrochloride (May increase drowsiness effect). Products include:
Thioridazine Hydrochloride Tablets 2195

Thiothixene (May increase drowsiness effect). Products include:
Thiothixene Capsules 2197

Tranylcypromine Sulfate (Concurrent and/or sequential use with MAO inhibitors is not recommended). Products include:
Parnate Tablets 1532

Triazolam (May increase drowsiness effect).
No products indexed under this heading.

Trifluoperazine Hydrochloride (May increase drowsiness effect).
No products indexed under this heading.

Zaleplon (May increase drowsiness effect).
No products indexed under this heading.

Zolpidem Tartrate (May increase drowsiness effect). Products include:
Ambien Tablets 2692
Ambien CR Tablets 2696

Food Interactions

Alcohol (May increase drowsiness effect; patients consuming 3 or more alcoholic drinks per day should consult their physician for advice on when and how they should take this medication).

VICKS NYQUIL LIQUID
(Acetaminophen, Dextromethorphan Hydrobromide, Doxylamine Succinate, Pseudoephedrine Hydrochloride)........ 2567
See Vicks NyQuil LiquiCaps

VICKS NYQUIL MULTI-SYMPTOM COLD/FLU RELIEF
(Acetaminophen, Dextromethorphan Hydrobromide, Doxylamine Succinate, Pseudoephedrine Hydrochloride)........ 2567
See Vicks NyQuil LiquiCaps

VICODIN TABLETS
(Acetaminophen, Hydrocodone Bitartrate)........ 529
May interact with antihistamines, central nervous system depressants, monoamine oxidase inhibitors, narcotic analgesics, antipsychotic agents, tricyclic antidepressants, and certain other agents. Compounds in these categories include:

Acrivastine (May exhibit an additive CNS depression).
No products indexed under this heading.

Alfentanil Hydrochloride (May exhibit an additive CNS depression).
No products indexed under this heading.

Alprazolam (May exhibit an additive CNS depression).
No products indexed under this heading.

Amitriptyline Hydrochloride (Co-administration may increase the effect of either antidepressant or hydrocodone).
No products indexed under this heading.

Amoxapine (Co-administration may increase the effect of either antidepressant or hydrocodone).
No products indexed under this heading.

Aprobarbital (May exhibit an additive CNS depression).
No products indexed under this heading.

Aripiprazole (May exhibit an additive CNS depression). Products include:
- Abilify Injection........ 881
- Abilify Injection........ 2466
- Abilify Oral Solution........ 881
- Abilify Oral Solution........ 2466
- Abilify Discmelt Orally Disintegrating Tablets........ 881
- Abilify Discmelt Orally Disintegrating Tablets........ 2466
- Abilify Tablets........ 881
- Abilify Tablets........ 2466

Astemizole (May exhibit an additive CNS depression).
No products indexed under this heading.

Azatadine Maleate (May exhibit an additive CNS depression).
No products indexed under this heading.

Bromodiphenhydramine Hydrochloride (May exhibit an additive CNS depression).
No products indexed under this heading.

Brompheniramine Maleate (May exhibit an additive CNS depression).
No products indexed under this heading.

Buprenorphine Hydrochloride (May exhibit an additive CNS depression). Products include:
- Suboxone Tablets........ 2601
- Subutex Tablets........ 2601

Buspirone Hydrochloride (May exhibit an additive CNS depression).
No products indexed under this heading.

Butabarbital (May exhibit an additive CNS depression).
No products indexed under this heading.

Butalbital (May exhibit an additive CNS depression).
No products indexed under this heading.

Cetirizine Hydrochloride (May exhibit an additive CNS depression). Products include:
- Zyrtec Allergy Tablets........ 1919
- Zyrtec Chewable Tablets........ 1920
- Children's Zyrtec Allergy Chewable Tablets........ 1922
- Children's Zyrtec Allergy Syrup........ 1920
- Children's Zyrtec Hives Relief Syrup........ 1920
- Zyrtec Syrup........ 1920
- Zyrtec Tablets........ 1920
- Zyrtec-D 12 Hour Extended Release Tablets........ 1923
- Zyrtec-D Allergy & Congestion Extended-Release Tablets........ 1923

Chlordiazepoxide (May exhibit an additive CNS depression).
No products indexed under this heading.

Chlordiazepoxide Hydrochloride (May exhibit an additive CNS depression).
No products indexed under this heading.

Chlorpheniramine Maleate (May exhibit an additive CNS depression). Products include:
- Actifed Cold & Allergy Tablets........ 1895
- Sudafed PE Sinus & Allergy Tablets........ 1908
- Tylenol Allergy Multi-Symptom Caplets with Cool Burst and Rapid Release Gelcaps........ 1916
- Children's Tylenol Plus Cold Suspension Liquid........ 1912
- Children's Tylenol Plus Cough & Runny Nose Suspension Liquid........ 1912
- Children's Tylenol Plus Flu Suspension Liquid........ 1914
- Children's Tylenol Plus Multi-Symptom Cold Suspension Liquid........ 1912
- Tylenol Cold Head Congestion Nighttime Caplets with Cool Burst........ 1910
- Tylenol Cold Multi-Symptom Nighttime Caplets with Cool Burst........ 1913
- Tylenol Sinus Congestion & Pain Nighttime Caplets with Cool Burst........ 1917

Chlorpheniramine Polistirex (May exhibit an additive CNS depression). Products include:
- Tussionex Pennkinetic Extended-Release Suspension........ 3154

Chlorpheniramine Tannate (May exhibit an additive CNS depression).
No products indexed under this heading.

Chlorpromazine (May exhibit an additive CNS depression).
No products indexed under this heading.

Chlorpromazine Hydrochloride (May exhibit an additive CNS depression).
No products indexed under this heading.

Chlorprothixene (May exhibit an additive CNS depression).
No products indexed under this heading.

Chlorprothixene Hydrochloride (May exhibit an additive CNS depression).
No products indexed under this heading.

Chlorprothixene Lactate (May exhibit an additive CNS depression).
No products indexed under this heading.

Clemastine Fumarate (May exhibit an additive CNS depression).
No products indexed under this heading.

Clomipramine Hydrochloride (Co-administration may increase the effect of either antidepressant or hydrocodone).
No products indexed under this heading.

Clorazepate Dipotassium (May exhibit an additive CNS depression).
No products indexed under this heading.

Clozapine (May exhibit an additive CNS depression).
No products indexed under this heading.

Codeine Phosphate (May exhibit an additive CNS depression). Products include:
- Tylenol with Codeine Tablets........ 2427

Cyproheptadine Hydrochloride (May exhibit an additive CNS depression).
No products indexed under this heading.

Desflurane (May exhibit an additive CNS depression).
No products indexed under this heading.

Desipramine Hydrochloride (Co-administration may increase the effect of either antidepressant or hydrocodone).
No products indexed under this heading.

Dexchlorpheniramine Maleate (May exhibit an additive CNS depression).
No products indexed under this heading.

Dezocine (May exhibit an additive CNS depression).
No products indexed under this heading.

Diazepam (May exhibit an additive CNS depression). Products include:
- Valium Tablets........ 2658

Diphenhydramine Citrate (May exhibit an additive CNS depression).
No products indexed under this heading.

Diphenhydramine Hydrochloride (May exhibit an additive CNS depression). Products include:
- Benadryl Allergy & Cold Kapgels........ 1895
- Benadryl Allergy & Sinus Headache Kapgels........ 1895
- Benadryl Severe Allergy & Sinus Headache Caplets........ 1897
- Benadryl Dye-Free Allergy Liqui-gels Softgels........ 1897
- Benadryl Allergy Kapgels........ 1895
- Benadryl Allergy Quick Dissolve Strips........ 1896
- Benadryl Allergy Ultratab Tablets........ 1896
- Children's Benadryl Dye-Free Allergy Liquid........ 1897
- Children's Benadryl Allergy Fastmelts........ 1897
- Children's Benadryl Allergy Liquid........ 1898
- Children's Benadryl Allergy Perfect Measure........ 1896
- Children's Benadryl-D Allergy & Sinus Liquid........ 1896
- Benadryl-D Allergy & Sinus Tablet........ 1896
- PediaCare Children's Allergy & Cold Liquid........ 1902
- PediaCare Children's Allergy Liquid........ 1902
- Simply Sleep Caplets........ 1905
- Sudafed PE Nighttime Cold Caplets........ 1907
- Sudafed PE Severe Cold Caplets........ 1908
- Extra Strength Tylenol PM Caplets, Geltabs, Liquid, and Rapid Release Gels........ 1915
- Tylenol Allergy Multi-Symptom Nighttime Caplets with Cool Burst........ 1916
- Tylenol Severe Allergy Caplets........ 1916
- Children's Tylenol Plus Cold & Allergy Suspension Liquid........ 1914
- Tylenol Sore Throat Nighttime Liquid with Cool Burst........ 1918

Diphenylpyraline Hydrochloride (May exhibit an additive CNS depression).
No products indexed under this heading.

Doxepin Hydrochloride (Co-administration may increase the effect of either antidepressant or hydrocodone).
No products indexed under this heading.

Droperidol (May exhibit an additive CNS depression).
No products indexed under this heading.

Enflurane (May exhibit an additive CNS depression).
No products indexed under this heading.

Estazolam (May exhibit an additive CNS depression).
No products indexed under this heading.

Ethanol (May exhibit an additive CNS depression).
No products indexed under this heading.

Ethchlorvynol (May exhibit an additive CNS depression).
No products indexed under this heading.

Ethinamate (May exhibit an additive CNS depression).
No products indexed under this heading.

Ethyl Alcohol (May exhibit an additive CNS depression).
No products indexed under this heading.

Fentanyl (May exhibit an additive CNS depression). Products include:
- Duragesic Transdermal System........ 2405
- Ionsys Transdermal System........ 2410

Fentanyl Citrate (May exhibit an additive CNS depression). Products include:
- Actiq........ 959
- Fentora Tablets........ 968

Fexofenadine Hydrochloride (May exhibit an additive CNS depression). Products include:
- Allegra Oral Solution........ 2684
- Allegra Tablets........ 2684
- Allegra-D 12 Hour Extended-Release Tablets........ 2687
- Allegra-D 24 Hour Extended-Release Tablets........ 2690

Fluphenazine Decanoate (May exhibit an additive CNS depression).
No products indexed under this heading.

Fluphenazine Enanthate (May exhibit an additive CNS depression).
No products indexed under this heading.

Fluphenazine Hydrochloride (May exhibit an additive CNS depression).
No products indexed under this heading.

Flurazepam Hydrochloride (May exhibit an additive CNS depression).
No products indexed under this heading.

Glutethimide (May exhibit an additive CNS depression).
No products indexed under this heading.

Haloperidol (May exhibit an additive CNS depression).
No products indexed under this heading.

Haloperidol Decanoate (May exhibit an additive CNS depression).
No products indexed under this heading.

Hydrocodone Polistirex (May exhibit an additive CNS depression). Products include:
Tussionex Pennkinetic Extended-Release Suspension 3154

Hydromorphone Hydrochloride (May exhibit an additive CNS depression).
No products indexed under this heading.

Hydroxyzine Hydrochloride (May exhibit an additive CNS depression).
No products indexed under this heading.

Imipramine Hydrochloride (Co-administration may increase the effect of either antidepressant or hydrocodone).
No products indexed under this heading.

Imipramine Pamoate (Co-administration may increase the effect of either antidepressant or hydrocodone).
No products indexed under this heading.

Isocarboxazid (Co-administration may increase the effect of either the MAO inhibitor or hydrocodone). Products include:
Marplan Tablets 3177

Isoflurane (May exhibit an additive CNS depression).
No products indexed under this heading.

Ketamine Hydrochloride (May exhibit an additive CNS depression).
No products indexed under this heading.

Levomethadyl Acetate Hydrochloride (May exhibit an additive CNS depression).
No products indexed under this heading.

Levorphanol Tartrate (May exhibit an additive CNS depression).
No products indexed under this heading.

Lithium Carbonate (May exhibit an additive CNS depression).
No products indexed under this heading.

Lithium Citrate (May exhibit an additive CNS depression).
No products indexed under this heading.

Loratadine (May exhibit an additive CNS depression).
No products indexed under this heading.

Lorazepam (May exhibit an additive CNS depression).
No products indexed under this heading.

Loxapine Hydrochloride (May exhibit an additive CNS depression).
No products indexed under this heading.

Loxapine Succinate (May exhibit an additive CNS depression).
No products indexed under this heading.

Maprotiline Hydrochloride (Co-administration may increase the effect of either antidepressant or hydrocodone).
No products indexed under this heading.

Meperidine Hydrochloride (May exhibit an additive CNS depression).
No products indexed under this heading.

Mephobarbital (May exhibit an additive CNS depression).
No products indexed under this heading.

Meprobamate (May exhibit an additive CNS depression).
No products indexed under this heading.

Mesoridazine Besylate (May exhibit an additive CNS depression).
No products indexed under this heading.

Methadone Hydrochloride (May exhibit an additive CNS depression).
No products indexed under this heading.

Methdilazine Hydrochloride (May exhibit an additive CNS depression).
No products indexed under this heading.

Methohexital Sodium (May exhibit an additive CNS depression).
No products indexed under this heading.

Methotrimeprazine (May exhibit an additive CNS depression).
No products indexed under this heading.

Methoxyflurane (May exhibit an additive CNS depression).
No products indexed under this heading.

Midazolam Hydrochloride (May exhibit an additive CNS depression).
No products indexed under this heading.

Moclobemide (Co-administration may increase the effect of either the MAO inhibitor or hydrocodone).
No products indexed under this heading.

Molindone Hydrochloride (May exhibit an additive CNS depression). Products include:
Moban Tablets 1116

Morphine Sulfate (May exhibit an additive CNS depression). Products include:
Avinza Capsules 1772
DepoDur Injection 1095
MS Contin Tablets 2585

Nortriptyline Hydrochloride (Co-administration may increase the effect of either antidepressant or hydrocodone).
No products indexed under this heading.

Olanzapine (May exhibit an additive CNS depression). Products include:
Symbyax Capsules 1871
Zyprexa Tablets 1883
Zyprexa IntraMuscular 1883
Zyprexa ZYDIS Orally Disintegrating Tablets 1883

Oxazepam (May exhibit an additive CNS depression).
No products indexed under this heading.

Oxycodone Hydrochloride (May exhibit an additive CNS depression). Products include:
OxyContin Tablets 2589
OxyIR Capsules 2593
Percocet Tablets 1127
Percodan Tablets 1130

Paliperidone (May exhibit an additive CNS depression). Products include:
Invega Extended-Release Tablets 1748

Pargyline Hydrochloride (Co-administration may increase the effect of either the MAO inhibitor or hydrocodone).
No products indexed under this heading.

Pentobarbital Sodium (May exhibit an additive CNS depression). Products include:
Nembutal Sodium Solution, USP 2494

Perphenazine (May exhibit an additive CNS depression).
No products indexed under this heading.

Phenelzine Sulfate (Co-administration may increase the effect of either the MAO inhibitor or hydrocodone).
No products indexed under this heading.

Phenobarbital (May exhibit an additive CNS depression). Products include:
Donnatal Extentabs 2507

Pimozide (May exhibit an additive CNS depression).
No products indexed under this heading.

Prazepam (May exhibit an additive CNS depression).
No products indexed under this heading.

Procarbazine Hydrochloride (Co-administration may increase the effect of either the MAO inhibitor or hydrocodone).
No products indexed under this heading.

Prochlorperazine (May exhibit an additive CNS depression).
No products indexed under this heading.

Promethazine Hydrochloride (May exhibit an additive CNS depression).
No products indexed under this heading.

Propofol (May exhibit an additive CNS depression).
No products indexed under this heading.

Propoxyphene Hydrochloride (May exhibit an additive CNS depression).
No products indexed under this heading.

Propoxyphene Napsylate (May exhibit an additive CNS depression).
No products indexed under this heading.

Protriptyline Hydrochloride (Co-administration may increase the effect of either antidepressant or hydrocodone).
No products indexed under this heading.

Pyrilamine Maleate (May exhibit an additive CNS depression).
No products indexed under this heading.

Pyrilamine Tannate (May exhibit an additive CNS depression).
No products indexed under this heading.

Quazepam (May exhibit an additive CNS depression).
No products indexed under this heading.

Quetiapine Fumarate (May exhibit an additive CNS depression).
No products indexed under this heading.

Rasagiline Mesylate (Co-administration may increase the effect of either the MAO inhibitor or hydrocodone). Products include:
Azilect Tablets 3106

Remifentanil Hydrochloride (May exhibit an additive CNS depression).
No products indexed under this heading.

Risperidone (May exhibit an additive CNS depression). Products include:
Risperdal Consta Long-Acting Injection 1753

Secobarbital Sodium (May exhibit an additive CNS depression).
No products indexed under this heading.

Selegiline (Co-administration may increase the effect of either the MAO inhibitor or hydrocodone). Products include:
Emsam Transdermal System 905

Selegiline Hydrochloride (Co-administration may increase the effect of either the MAO inhibitor or hydrocodone). Products include:
Eldepryl Capsules 3052

Sevoflurane (May exhibit an additive CNS depression). Products include:
Ultane Liquid for Inhalation 524

Sodium Oxybate (May exhibit an additive CNS depression). Products include:
Xyrem Oral Solution 1766

Sufentanil Citrate (May exhibit an additive CNS depression).
No products indexed under this heading.

Temazepam (May exhibit an additive CNS depression).
No products indexed under this heading.

Terfenadine (May exhibit an additive CNS depression).
No products indexed under this heading.

Thiamylal Sodium (May exhibit an additive CNS depression).
No products indexed under this heading.

Thioridazine Hydrochloride (May exhibit an additive CNS depression). Products include:
Thioridazine Hydrochloride Tablets 2195

Thiothixene (May exhibit an additive CNS depression). Products include:
Thiothixene Capsules 2197

Tranylcypromine Sulfate (Co-administration may increase the effect of either the MAO inhibitor or hydrocodone). Products include:
Parnate Tablets 1532

Triazolam (May exhibit an additive CNS depression).
No products indexed under this heading.

Trifluoperazine Hydrochloride (May exhibit an additive CNS depression).
No products indexed under this heading.

Trimeprazine Tartrate (May exhibit an additive CNS depression).
No products indexed under this heading.

Trimipramine Maleate (Co-administration may increase the effect of either antidepressant or hydrocodone).
No products indexed under this heading.

Tripelennamine Hydrochloride (May exhibit an additive CNS depression).
No products indexed under this heading.

Triprolidine Hydrochloride (May exhibit an additive CNS depression).
No products indexed under this heading.

Zaleplon (May exhibit an additive CNS depression).
No products indexed under this heading.

Ziprasidone Hydrochloride (May exhibit an additive CNS depression). Products include:
Geodon Capsules 2520

Zolpidem Tartrate (May exhibit an additive CNS depression). Products include:
Ambien Tablets 2692
Ambien CR Tablets 2696

Food Interactions

Alcohol (May exhibit an additive CNS depression).

VICODIN ES TABLETS

(Acetaminophen, Hydrocodone Bitartrate) 530

May interact with anticholinergics, central nervous system depressants, narcotic analgesics, psychotropics, tranquilizers, tricyclic antidepressants, and certain other agents. Compounds in these categories include:

Alfentanil Hydrochloride (Additive CNS depression; the dose of one or both agents should be reduced).
No products indexed under this heading.

Alprazolam (Additive CNS depression; the dose of one or both agents should be reduced).
No products indexed under this heading.

Amitriptyline Hydrochloride (Concurrent use of tricyclic antidepressants and hydrocodone preparations may increase the effect of either the antidepressant or hydrocodone).
No products indexed under this heading.

Amoxapine (Concurrent use of tricyclic antidepressants and hydrocodone preparations may increase the effect of either the antidepressant or hydrocodone).
No products indexed under this heading.

Aprobarbital (Additive CNS depression; the dose of one or both agents should be reduced).
No products indexed under this heading.

Atropine Sulfate (May produce paralytic ileus). Products include:
Donnatal Extentabs 2507

Belladonna Alkaloids (May produce paralytic ileus). Products include:
Hyland's Teething Tablets 621

Benztropine Mesylate (May produce paralytic ileus).
No products indexed under this heading.

Biperiden Hydrochloride (May produce paralytic ileus).
No products indexed under this heading.

Buprenorphine Hydrochloride (Additive CNS depression; the dose of one or both agents should be reduced). Products include:
Suboxone Tablets 2601
Subutex Tablets 2601

Buspirone Hydrochloride (Additive CNS depression; the dose of one or both agents should be reduced).
No products indexed under this heading.

Butabarbital (Additive CNS depression; the dose of one or both agents should be reduced).
No products indexed under this heading.

Butalbital (Additive CNS depression; the dose of one or both agents should be reduced).
No products indexed under this heading.

Chlordiazepoxide (Additive CNS depression; the dose of one or both agents should be reduced).
No products indexed under this heading.

Chlordiazepoxide Hydrochloride (Additive CNS depression; the dose of one or both agents should be reduced).
No products indexed under this heading.

Chlorpromazine (Additive CNS depression; the dose of one or both agents should be reduced).
No products indexed under this heading.

Chlorpromazine Hydrochloride (Additive CNS depression; the dose of one or both agents should be reduced).
No products indexed under this heading.

Chlorprothixene (Additive CNS depression; the dose of one or both agents should be reduced).
No products indexed under this heading.

Chlorprothixene Hydrochloride (Additive CNS depression; the dose of one or both agents should be reduced).
No products indexed under this heading.

Chlorprothixene Lactate (Additive CNS depression; the dose of one or both agents should be reduced).
No products indexed under this heading.

Clidinium Bromide (May produce paralytic ileus).
No products indexed under this heading.

Clomipramine Hydrochloride (Concurrent use of tricyclic antidepressants and hydrocodone preparations may increase the effect of either the antidepressant or hydrocodone).
No products indexed under this heading.

Clorazepate Dipotassium (Additive CNS depression; the dose of one or both agents should be reduced).
No products indexed under this heading.

Clozapine (Additive CNS depression; the dose of one or both agents should be reduced).
No products indexed under this heading.

Codeine Phosphate (Additive CNS depression; the dose of one or both agents should be reduced). Products include:
Tylenol with Codeine Tablets 2427

Desflurane (Additive CNS depression; the dose of one or both agents should be reduced).
No products indexed under this heading.

Desipramine Hydrochloride (Concurrent use of tricyclic antidepressants and hydrocodone preparations may increase the effect of either the antidepressant or hydrocodone).
No products indexed under this heading.

Dezocine (Additive CNS depression; the dose of one or both agents should be reduced).
No products indexed under this heading.

Diazepam (Additive CNS depression; the dose of one or both agents should be reduced). Products include:
Valium Tablets 2658

Dicyclomine Hydrochloride (May produce paralytic ileus). Products include:
Bentyl Capsules 703
Bentyl Injection 703
Bentyl Syrup 703
Bentyl Tablets 703

Doxepin Hydrochloride (Concurrent use of tricyclic antidepressants and hydrocodone preparations may increase the effect of either the antidepressant or hydrocodone).
No products indexed under this heading.

Droperidol (Additive CNS depression; the dose of one or both agents should be reduced).
No products indexed under this heading.

Enflurane (Additive CNS depression; the dose of one or both agents should be reduced).
No products indexed under this heading.

Estazolam (Additive CNS depression; the dose of one or both agents should be reduced).
No products indexed under this heading.

Ethanol (Additive CNS depression; the dose of one or both agents should be reduced).
No products indexed under this heading.

Ethchlorvynol (Additive CNS depression; the dose of one or both agents should be reduced).
No products indexed under this heading.

Ethinamate (Additive CNS depression; the dose of one or both agents should be reduced).
No products indexed under this heading.

Ethyl Alcohol (Additive CNS depression; the dose of one or both agents should be reduced).
No products indexed under this heading.

Fentanyl (Additive CNS depression; the dose of one or both agents should be reduced). Products include:
Duragesic Transdermal System 2405
Ionsys Transdermal System 2410

Fentanyl Citrate (Additive CNS depression; the dose of one or both agents should be reduced). Products include:
Actiq 959
Fentora Tablets 968

Fluphenazine Decanoate (Additive CNS depression; the dose of one or both agents should be reduced).
No products indexed under this heading.

Fluphenazine Enanthate (Additive CNS depression; the dose of one or both agents should be reduced).
No products indexed under this heading.

Fluphenazine Hydrochloride (Additive CNS depression; the dose of one or both agents should be reduced).
No products indexed under this heading.

Flurazepam Hydrochloride (Additive CNS depression; the dose of one or both agents should be reduced).
No products indexed under this heading.

Glutethimide (Additive CNS depression; the dose of one or both agents should be reduced).
No products indexed under this heading.

Glycopyrrolate (May produce paralytic ileus).
No products indexed under this heading.

Haloperidol (Additive CNS depression; the dose of one or both agents should be reduced).
No products indexed under this heading.

Haloperidol Decanoate (Additive CNS depression; the dose of one or both agents should be reduced).
No products indexed under this heading.

Hydrocodone Polistirex (Additive CNS depression; the dose of one or both agents should be reduced). Products include:
Tussionex Pennkinetic Extended-Release Suspension 3154

Hydromorphone Hydrochloride (Additive CNS depression; the dose of one or both agents should be reduced).
No products indexed under this heading.

Hydroxyzine Hydrochloride (Additive CNS depression; the dose of one or both agents should be reduced).
No products indexed under this heading.

Hyoscyamine (May produce paralytic ileus).
No products indexed under this heading.

Hyoscyamine Sulfate (May produce paralytic ileus). Products include:
Donnatal Extentabs 2507

Imipramine Hydrochloride (Concurrent use of tricyclic antidepressants and hydrocodone preparations may increase the effect of either the antidepressant or hydrocodone).
No products indexed under this heading.

Imipramine Pamoate (Concurrent use of tricyclic antidepressants and hydrocodone preparations may increase the effect of either the antidepressant or hydrocodone).
No products indexed under this heading.

Ipratropium Bromide (May produce paralytic ileus). Products include:
Atrovent HFA Inhalation Aerosol 839
Atrovent Nasal Spray 0.03% 834
Atrovent Nasal Spray 0.06% 836
Combivent Inhalation Aerosol 845

Isocarboxazid (Concurrent use of MAO inhibitor and hydrocodone preparations may increase the effect of either the MAO inhibitor or hydrocodone). Products include:
Marplan Tablets 3177

Isoflurane (Additive CNS depression; the dose of one or both agents should be reduced).
No products indexed under this heading.

Ketamine Hydrochloride (Additive CNS depression; the dose of one or both agents should be reduced).
No products indexed under this heading.

Levomethadyl Acetate Hydrochloride (Additive CNS depression; the dose of one or both agents should be reduced).
No products indexed under this heading.

Levorphanol Tartrate (Additive CNS depression; the dose of one or both agents should be reduced).
No products indexed under this heading.

Lithium Carbonate (Additive CNS depression; the dose of one or both agents should be reduced).
No products indexed under this heading.

Lithium Citrate (Additive CNS depression; the dose of one or both agents should be reduced).
No products indexed under this heading.

Lorazepam (Additive CNS depression; the dose of one or both agents should be reduced).
No products indexed under this heading.

Loxapine Hydrochloride (Additive CNS depression; the dose of one or both agents should be reduced).
No products indexed under this heading.

Loxapine Succinate (Additive CNS depression; the dose of one or both agents should be reduced).
No products indexed under this heading.

Maprotiline Hydrochloride (Concurrent use of tricyclic antidepressants and hydrocodone preparations may increase the effect of either the antidepressant or hydrocodone).
No products indexed under this heading.

Mepenzolate Bromide (May produce paralytic ileus).
No products indexed under this heading.

Meperidine Hydrochloride (Additive CNS depression; the dose of one or both agents should be reduced).
No products indexed under this heading.

Mephobarbital (Additive CNS depression; the dose of one or both agents should be reduced).
No products indexed under this heading.

Meprobamate (Additive CNS depression; the dose of one or both agents should be reduced).
No products indexed under this heading.

Mesoridazine Besylate (Additive CNS depression; the dose of one or both agents should be reduced).
No products indexed under this heading.

Methadone Hydrochloride (Additive CNS depression; the dose of one or both agents should be reduced).
No products indexed under this heading.

Methohexital Sodium (Additive CNS depression; the dose of one or both agents should be reduced).
No products indexed under this heading.

Methotrimeprazine (Additive CNS depression; the dose of one or both agents should be reduced).
No products indexed under this heading.

Methoxyflurane (Additive CNS depression; the dose of one or both agents should be reduced).
No products indexed under this heading.

Midazolam Hydrochloride (Additive CNS depression; the dose of one or both agents should be reduced).
No products indexed under this heading.

Molindone Hydrochloride (Additive CNS depression; the dose of one or both agents should be reduced). Products include:
Moban Tablets 1116

Morphine Sulfate (Additive CNS depression; the dose of one or both agents should be reduced). Products include:
Avinza Capsules 1772
DepoDur Injection 1095
MS Contin Tablets 2585

Nortriptyline Hydrochloride (Concurrent use of tricyclic antidepressants and hydrocodone preparations may increase the effect of either the antidepressant or hydrocodone).
No products indexed under this heading.

Olanzapine (Additive CNS depression; the dose of one or both agents should be reduced). Products include:
Symbyax Capsules 1871
Zyprexa Tablets 1883
Zyprexa IntraMuscular 1883
Zyprexa ZYDIS Orally Disintegrating Tablets 1883

Oxazepam (Additive CNS depression; the dose of one or both agents should be reduced).
No products indexed under this heading.

Oxybutynin Chloride (May produce paralytic ileus).
No products indexed under this heading.

Oxycodone Hydrochloride (Additive CNS depression; the dose of one or both agents should be reduced). Products include:
OxyContin Tablets 2589
OxyIR Capsules 2593
Percocet Tablets 1127
Percodan Tablets 1130

Paliperidone (Additive CNS depression; the dose of one or both agents should be reduced). Products include:
Invega Extended-Release Tablets 1748

Pentobarbital Sodium (Additive CNS depression; the dose of one or both agents should be reduced). Products include:
Nembutal Sodium Solution, USP 2494

Perphenazine (Additive CNS depression; the dose of one or both agents should be reduced).
No products indexed under this heading.

Phenelzine Sulfate (Concurrent use of MAO inhibitor and hydrocodone preparations may increase the effect of either the MAO inhibitor or hydrocodone).
No products indexed under this heading.

Phenobarbital (Additive CNS depression; the dose of one or both agents should be reduced). Products include:
Donnatal Extentabs 2507

Prazepam (Additive CNS depression; the dose of one or both agents should be reduced).
No products indexed under this heading.

Prochlorperazine (Additive CNS depression; the dose of one or both agents should be reduced).
No products indexed under this heading.

Procyclidine Hydrochloride (May produce paralytic ileus).
No products indexed under this heading.

Promethazine Hydrochloride (Additive CNS depression; the dose of one or both agents should be reduced).
No products indexed under this heading.

Propantheline Bromide (May produce paralytic ileus).
No products indexed under this heading.

Propofol (Additive CNS depression; the dose of one or both agents should be reduced).
No products indexed under this heading.

Propoxyphene Hydrochloride (Additive CNS depression; the dose of one or both agents should be reduced).
No products indexed under this heading.

Propoxyphene Napsylate (Additive CNS depression; the dose of one or both agents should be reduced).
No products indexed under this heading.

Protriptyline Hydrochloride (Concurrent use of tricyclic antidepressants and hydrocodone preparations may increase the effect of either the antidepressant or hydrocodone).
No products indexed under this heading.

Quazepam (Additive CNS depression; the dose of one or both agents should be reduced).
No products indexed under this heading.

Quetiapine Fumarate (Additive CNS depression; the dose of one or both agents should be reduced).
No products indexed under this heading.

Remifentanil Hydrochloride (Additive CNS depression; the dose of one or both agents should be reduced).
No products indexed under this heading.

Risperidone (Additive CNS depression; the dose of one or both agents should be reduced). Products include:
Risperdal Consta Long-Acting Injection 1753

Scopolamine (May produce paralytic ileus). Products include:
Transderm Scōp Transdermal Therapeutic System 2206

Scopolamine Hydrobromide (May produce paralytic ileus). Products include:
Donnatal Extentabs 2507

Secobarbital Sodium (Additive CNS depression; the dose of one or both agents should be reduced).
No products indexed under this heading.

Selegiline Hydrochloride (Concurrent use of MAO inhibitor and hydrocodone preparations may increase the effect of either the MAO inhibitor or hydrocodone). Products include:
Eldepryl Capsules 3052

Sevoflurane (Additive CNS depression; the dose of one or both agents should be reduced). Products include:
Ultane Liquid for Inhalation 524

Sufentanil Citrate (Additive CNS depression; the dose of one or both agents should be reduced).
No products indexed under this heading.

Temazepam (Additive CNS depression; the dose of one or both agents should be reduced).
No products indexed under this heading.

Thiamylal Sodium (Additive CNS depression; the dose of one or both agents should be reduced).
No products indexed under this heading.

Thioridazine Hydrochloride (Additive CNS depression; the dose of one or both agents should be reduced). Products include:
Thioridazine Hydrochloride Tablets 2195

Thiothixene (Additive CNS depression; the dose of one or both agents should be reduced). Products include:
Thiothixene Capsules 2197

Tolterodine Tartrate (May produce paralytic ileus).
No products indexed under this heading.

Tranylcypromine Sulfate (Concurrent use of MAO inhibitor and hydrocodone preparations may increase the effect of either the MAO inhibitor or hydrocodone). Products include:
Parnate Tablets 1532

Triazolam (Additive CNS depression; the dose of one or both agents should be reduced).
No products indexed under this heading.

Tridihexethyl Chloride (May produce paralytic ileus).
No products indexed under this heading.

Trifluoperazine Hydrochloride (Additive CNS depression; the dose of one or both agents should be reduced).
No products indexed under this heading.

Trihexyphenidyl Hydrochloride (May produce paralytic ileus).
No products indexed under this heading.

Trimipramine Maleate (Concurrent use of tricyclic antidepressants and hydrocodone preparations may increase the effect of either the antidepressant or hydrocodone).
No products indexed under this heading.

Zaleplon (Additive CNS depression; the dose of one or both agents should be reduced).
No products indexed under this heading.

Ziprasidone Hydrochloride (Additive CNS depression; the dose of one or both agents should be reduced). Products include:
Geodon Capsules 2520

Zolpidem Tartrate (Additive CNS depression; the dose of one or both agents should be reduced). Products include:
Ambien Tablets 2692
Ambien CR Tablets 2696

Food Interactions

Alcohol (Additive CNS depression).

VICODIN HP TABLETS

(Acetaminophen, Hydrocodone Bitartrate) 531

May interact with antihistamines, central nervous system depressants, monoamine oxidase inhibitors, narcotic analgesics, tranquilizers, tricyclic antidepressants, and certain other agents. Compounds in these categories include:

Acrivastine (Co-administration may result in an additive CNS depression).
No products indexed under this heading.

Alfentanil Hydrochloride (Co-administration may result in an additive CNS depression).
No products indexed under this heading.

Alprazolam (Co-administration may result in an additive CNS depression).
No products indexed under this heading.

Amitriptyline Hydrochloride (Co-administration with tricyclic antidepressants may increase the effect of either hydrocodone or the tricyclic antidepressant).
No products indexed under this heading.

Amoxapine (Co-administration with tricyclic antidepressants may increase the effect of either hydrocodone or the tricyclic antidepressant).
No products indexed under this heading.

Aprobarbital (Co-administration may result in an additive CNS depression).
No products indexed under this heading.

Astemizole (Co-administration may result in an additive CNS depression).
No products indexed under this heading.

Azatadine Maleate (Co-administration may result in an additive CNS depression).
No products indexed under this heading.

Bromodiphenhydramine Hydrochloride (Co-administration may result in an additive CNS depression).
No products indexed under this heading.

Brompheniramine Maleate (Co-administration may result in an additive CNS depression).
No products indexed under this heading.

Buprenorphine Hydrochloride (Co-administration may result in an additive CNS depression). Products include:
Suboxone Tablets 2601
Subutex Tablets 2601

Buspirone Hydrochloride (Co-administration may result in an additive CNS depression).
No products indexed under this heading.

Butabarbital (Co-administration may result in an additive CNS depression).
No products indexed under this heading.

Butalbital (Co-administration may result in an additive CNS depression).
No products indexed under this heading.

Cetirizine Hydrochloride (Co-administration may result in an additive CNS depression). Products include:
Zyrtec Allergy Tablets 1919
Zyrtec Chewable Tablets 1920
Children's Zyrtec Allergy Chewable Tablets 1922
Children's Zyrtec Allergy Syrup 1920
Children's Zyrtec Hives Relief Syrup 1920
Zyrtec Syrup 1920
Zyrtec Tablets 1920
Zyrtec-D 12 Hour Extended Release Tablets 1923
Zyrtec-D Allergy & Congestion Extended-Release Tablets 1923

Chlordiazepoxide (Co-administration may result in an additive CNS depression).
No products indexed under this heading.

Chlordiazepoxide Hydrochloride (Co-administration may result in an additive CNS depression).
No products indexed under this heading.

Chlorpheniramine Maleate (Co-administration may result in an additive CNS depression). Products include:
Actifed Cold & Allergy Tablets 1895
Sudafed PE Sinus & Allergy Tablets 1908
Tylenol Allergy Multi-Symptom Caplets with Cool Burst and Rapid Release Gelcaps 1916
Children's Tylenol Plus Cold Suspension Liquid 1912
Children's Tylenol Plus Cough & Runny Nose Suspension Liquid 1912
Children's Tylenol Plus Flu Suspension Liquid 1914
Children's Tylenol Plus Multi-Symptom Cold Suspension Liquid 1912
Tylenol Cold Head Congestion Nighttime Caplets with Cool Burst 1910
Tylenol Cold Multi-Symptom Nighttime Caplets with Cool Burst 1913
Tylenol Sinus Congestion & Pain Nighttime Caplets with Cool Burst 1917

Chlorpheniramine Polistirex (Co-administration may result in an additive CNS depression). Products include:
Tussionex Pennkinetic Extended-Release Suspension 3154

Chlorpheniramine Tannate (Co-administration may result in an additive CNS depression).
No products indexed under this heading.

Chlorpromazine (Co-administration may result in an additive CNS depression).
No products indexed under this heading.

Chlorpromazine Hydrochloride (Co-administration may result in an additive CNS depression).
No products indexed under this heading.

Chlorprothixene (Co-administration may result in an additive CNS depression).
No products indexed under this heading.

Chlorprothixene Hydrochloride (Co-administration may result in an additive CNS depression).
No products indexed under this heading.

Chlorprothixene Lactate (Co-administration may result in an additive CNS depression).
No products indexed under this heading.

Clemastine Fumarate (Co-administration may result in an additive CNS depression).
No products indexed under this heading.

Clomipramine Hydrochloride (Co-administration with tricyclic antidepressants may increase the effect of either hydrocodone or the tricyclic antidepressant).
No products indexed under this heading.

Clorazepate Dipotassium (Co-administration may result in an additive CNS depression).
No products indexed under this heading.

Clozapine (Co-administration may result in an additive CNS depression).
No products indexed under this heading.

Codeine Phosphate (Co-administration may result in an additive CNS depression). Products include:
Tylenol with Codeine Tablets 2427

Cyproheptadine Hydrochloride (Co-administration may result in an additive CNS depression).
No products indexed under this heading.

Desflurane (Co-administration may result in an additive CNS depression).
No products indexed under this heading.

Desipramine Hydrochloride (Co-administration with tricyclic antidepressants may increase the effect of either hydrocodone or the tricyclic antidepressant).
No products indexed under this heading.

Dexchlorpheniramine Maleate (Co-administration may result in an additive CNS depression).
No products indexed under this heading.

Dezocine (Co-administration may result in an additive CNS depression).
No products indexed under this heading.

Diazepam (Co-administration may result in an additive CNS depression). Products include:
Valium Tablets 2658

Diphenhydramine Citrate (Co-administration may result in an additive CNS depression).
No products indexed under this heading.

Diphenhydramine Hydrochloride (Co-administration may result in an additive CNS depression). Products include:
Benadryl Allergy & Cold Kapgels 1895
Benadryl Allergy & Sinus Headache Kapgels 1895
Benadryl Severe Allergy & Sinus Headache Caplets 1897
Benadryl Dye-Free Allergy Liqui-gels Softgels 1897
Benadryl Allergy Kapgels 1895
Benadryl Allergy Quick Dissolve Strips 1896
Benadryl Allergy Ultratab Tablets 1896
Children's Benadryl Dye-Free Allergy Liquid 1897
Children's Benadryl Allergy Fastmelts 1897
Children's Benadryl Allergy Liquid 1898
Children's Benadryl Allergy Perfect Measure 1896
Children's Benadryl-D Allergy & Sinus Liquid 1896
Benadryl-D Allergy & Sinus Tablet 1896
PediaCare Children's Allergy & Cold Liquid 1902
PediaCare Children's Allergy Liquid 1902
Simply Sleep Caplets 1905
Sudafed PE Nighttime Cold Caplets 1907
Sudafed PE Severe Cold Caplets 1908
Extra Strength Tylenol PM Caplets, Geltabs, Liquid, and Rapid Release Gels 1915
Tylenol Allergy Multi-Symptom Nighttime Caplets with Cool Burst 1916
Tylenol Severe Allergy Caplets 1916
Children's Tylenol Plus Cold & Allergy Suspension Liquid 1914
Tylenol Sore Throat Nighttime Liquid with Cool Burst 1918

Diphenylpyraline Hydrochloride (Co-administration may result in an additive CNS depression).
No products indexed under this heading.

Doxepin Hydrochloride (Co-administration with tricyclic antidepressants may increase the effect of either hydrocodone or the tricyclic antidepressant).
No products indexed under this heading.

Droperidol (Co-administration may result in an additive CNS depression).
No products indexed under this heading.

Enflurane (Co-administration may result in an additive CNS depression).
No products indexed under this heading.

Estazolam (Co-administration may result in an additive CNS depression).
No products indexed under this heading.

Ethanol (Co-administration may result in an additive CNS depression).
No products indexed under this heading.

Ethchlorvynol (Co-administration may result in an additive CNS depression).
No products indexed under this heading.

Ethinamate (Co-administration may result in an additive CNS depression).
No products indexed under this heading.

Ethyl Alcohol (Co-administration may result in an additive CNS depression).
No products indexed under this heading.

Fentanyl (Co-administration may result in an additive CNS depression). Products include:
Duragesic Transdermal System 2405
Ionsys Transdermal System 2410

Fentanyl Citrate (Co-administration may result in an additive CNS depression). Products include:
Actiq 959
Fentora Tablets 968

Fexofenadine Hydrochloride (Co-administration may result in an additive CNS depression). Products include:
Allegra Oral Solution 2684
Allegra Tablets 2684
Allegra-D 12 Hour Extended-Release Tablets 2687
Allegra-D 24 Hour Extended-Release Tablets 2690

Fluphenazine Decanoate (Co-administration may result in an additive CNS depression).
No products indexed under this heading.

Fluphenazine Enanthate (Co-administration may result in an additive CNS depression).
No products indexed under this heading.

Fluphenazine Hydrochloride (Co-administration may result in an additive CNS depression).
No products indexed under this heading.

Flurazepam Hydrochloride (Co-administration may result in an additive CNS depression).
No products indexed under this heading.

Glutethimide (Co-administration may result in an additive CNS depression).
No products indexed under this heading.

Haloperidol (Co-administration may result in an additive CNS depression).
No products indexed under this heading.

Haloperidol Decanoate (Co-administration may result in an additive CNS depression).
No products indexed under this heading.

Hydrocodone Polistirex (Co-administration may result in an additive CNS depression). Products include:
Tussionex Pennkinetic Extended-Release Suspension 3154

Hydromorphone Hydrochloride (Co-administration may result in an additive CNS depression).
No products indexed under this heading.

Hydroxyzine Hydrochloride (Co-administration may result in an additive CNS depression).
No products indexed under this heading.

Imipramine Hydrochloride (Co-administration with tricyclic antidepressants may increase the effect of either hydrocodone or the tricyclic antidepressant).
No products indexed under this heading.

Imipramine Pamoate (Co-administration with tricyclic antidepressants may increase the effect of either hydrocodone or the tricyclic antidepressant).
No products indexed under this heading.

Isocarboxazid (Co-administration with an MAO inhibitor may increase the effect of either hydrocodone or the MAO inhibitor). Products include:
Marplan Tablets 3177

Isoflurane (Co-administration may result in an additive CNS depression).
No products indexed under this heading.

Ketamine Hydrochloride (Co-administration may result in an additive CNS depression).
No products indexed under this heading.

Levomethadyl Acetate Hydrochloride (Co-administration may result in an additive CNS depression).
No products indexed under this heading.

Levorphanol Tartrate (Co-administration may result in an additive CNS depression).
No products indexed under this heading.

Loratadine (Co-administration may result in an additive CNS depression).
No products indexed under this heading.

Lorazepam (Co-administration may result in an additive CNS depression).
No products indexed under this heading.

Loxapine Hydrochloride (Co-administration may result in an additive CNS depression).
No products indexed under this heading.

Loxapine Succinate (Co-administration may result in an additive CNS depression).
No products indexed under this heading.

Maprotiline Hydrochloride (Co-administration with tricyclic antidepressants may increase the effect of either hydrocodone or the tricyclic antidepressant).
No products indexed under this heading.

Meperidine Hydrochloride (Co-administration may result in an additive CNS depression).
No products indexed under this heading.

Mephobarbital (Co-administration may result in an additive CNS depression).
No products indexed under this heading.

Meprobamate (Co-administration may result in an additive CNS depression).
No products indexed under this heading.

Mesoridazine Besylate (Co-administration may result in an additive CNS depression).
No products indexed under this heading.

Methadone Hydrochloride (Co-administration may result in an additive CNS depression).
No products indexed under this heading.

Methdilazine Hydrochloride (Co-administration may result in an additive CNS depression).
No products indexed under this heading.

Methohexital Sodium (Co-administration may result in an additive CNS depression).
No products indexed under this heading.

Methotrimeprazine (Co-administration may result in an additive CNS depression).
No products indexed under this heading.

Methoxyflurane (Co-administration may result in an additive CNS depression).
No products indexed under this heading.

Midazolam Hydrochloride (Co-administration may result in an additive CNS depression).
No products indexed under this heading.

Moclobemide (Co-administration with an MAO inhibitor may increase the effect of either hydrocodone or the MAO inhibitor).
No products indexed under this heading.

Molindone Hydrochloride (Co-administration may result in an additive CNS depression). Products include:
Moban Tablets 1116

Morphine Sulfate (Co-administration may result in an additive CNS depression). Products include:
Avinza Capsules 1772
DepoDur Injection 1095
MS Contin Tablets 2585

Nortriptyline Hydrochloride (Co-administration with tricyclic antidepressants may increase the effect of either hydrocodone or the tricyclic antidepressant).
No products indexed under this heading.

Olanzapine (Co-administration may result in an additive CNS depression). Products include:
Symbyax Capsules 1871
Zyprexa Tablets 1883
Zyprexa IntraMuscular 1883
Zyprexa ZYDIS Orally Disintegrating Tablets 1883

Oxazepam (Co-administration may result in an additive CNS depression).
No products indexed under this heading.

Oxycodone Hydrochloride (Co-administration may result in an additive CNS depression). Products include:
OxyContin Tablets 2589
OxyIR Capsules 2593
Percocet Tablets 1127
Percodan Tablets 1130

Pargyline Hydrochloride (Co-administration with an MAO inhibitor may increase the effect of either hydrocodone or the MAO inhibitor).
No products indexed under this heading.

Pentobarbital Sodium (Co-administration may result in an additive CNS depression). Products include:
Nembutal Sodium Solution, USP 2494

Perphenazine (Co-administration may result in an additive CNS depression).
No products indexed under this heading.

Phenelzine Sulfate (Co-administration with an MAO inhibitor may increase the effect of either hydrocodone or the MAO inhibitor).
No products indexed under this heading.

Phenobarbital (Co-administration may result in an additive CNS depression). Products include:
Donnatal Extentabs 2507

Prazepam (Co-administration may result in an additive CNS depression).
No products indexed under this heading.

Procarbazine Hydrochloride (Co-administration with an MAO inhibitor may increase the effect of either hydrocodone or the MAO inhibitor).
No products indexed under this heading.

Prochlorperazine (Co-administration may result in an additive CNS depression).
No products indexed under this heading.

Promethazine Hydrochloride (Co-administration may result in an additive CNS depression).
No products indexed under this heading.

Propofol (Co-administration may result in an additive CNS depression).
No products indexed under this heading.

Propoxyphene Hydrochloride (Co-administration may result in an additive CNS depression).
No products indexed under this heading.

Propoxyphene Napsylate (Co-administration may result in an additive CNS depression).
No products indexed under this heading.

Protriptyline Hydrochloride (Co-administration with tricyclic antidepressants may increase the effect of either hydrocodone or the tricyclic antidepressant).
No products indexed under this heading.

Pyrilamine Maleate (Co-administration may result in an additive CNS depression).
No products indexed under this heading.

Pyrilamine Tannate (Co-administration may result in an additive CNS depression).
No products indexed under this heading.

Quazepam (Co-administration may result in an additive CNS depression).
No products indexed under this heading.

Quetiapine Fumarate (Co-administration may result in an additive CNS depression).
No products indexed under this heading.

Rasagiline Mesylate (Co-administration with an MAO inhibitor may increase the effect of either hydrocodone or the MAO inhibitor). Products include:
Azilect Tablets 3106

Remifentanil Hydrochloride (Co-administration may result in an additive CNS depression).
No products indexed under this heading.

Risperidone (Co-administration may result in an additive CNS depression). Products include:
Risperdal Consta Long-Acting Injection 1753

Secobarbital Sodium (Co-administration may result in an additive CNS depression).
No products indexed under this heading.

Selegiline (Co-administration with an MAO inhibitor may increase the effect of either hydrocodone or the MAO inhibitor). Products include:
Emsam Transdermal System 905

Selegiline Hydrochloride (Co-administration with an MAO inhibitor may increase the effect of either hydrocodone or the MAO inhibitor). Products include:
Eldepryl Capsules 3052

Sevoflurane (Co-administration may result in an additive CNS depression). Products include:
Ultane Liquid for Inhalation 524

Sufentanil Citrate (Co-administration may result in an additive CNS depression).
No products indexed under this heading.

Temazepam (Co-administration may result in an additive CNS depression).
No products indexed under this heading.

Terfenadine (Co-administration may result in an additive CNS depression).
No products indexed under this heading.

Thiamylal Sodium (Co-administration may result in an additive CNS depression).
No products indexed under this heading.

Thioridazine Hydrochloride (Co-administration may result in an additive CNS depression). Products include:
Thioridazine Hydrochloride Tablets 2195

Thiothixene (Co-administration may result in an additive CNS depression). Products include:
Thiothixene Capsules 2197

Tranylcypromine Sulfate (Co-administration with an MAO inhibitor may increase the effect of either hydrocodone or the MAO inhibitor). Products include:
Parnate Tablets 1532

Triazolam (Co-administration may result in an additive CNS depression).
No products indexed under this heading.

Trifluoperazine Hydrochloride (Co-administration may result in an additive CNS depression).
No products indexed under this heading.

Trimeprazine Tartrate (Co-administration may result in an additive CNS depression).
No products indexed under this heading.

Trimipramine Maleate (Co-administration with tricyclic antidepressants may increase the effect of either hydrocodone or the tricyclic antidepressant).
No products indexed under this heading.

Tripelennamine Hydrochloride (Co-administration may result in an additive CNS depression).
No products indexed under this heading.

Triprolidine Hydrochloride (Co-administration may result in an additive CNS depression).
No products indexed under this heading.

Zaleplon (Co-administration may result in an additive CNS depression).
No products indexed under this heading.

Ziprasidone Hydrochloride (Co-administration may result in an additive CNS depression). Products include:
Geodon Capsules 2520

Zolpidem Tartrate (Co-administration may result in an additive CNS depression). Products include:
Ambien Tablets 2692
Ambien CR Tablets 2696

Food Interactions

Alcohol (Concurrent use results in an additive CNS depression).

VICOPROFEN TABLETS

(Hydrocodone Bitartrate, Ibuprofen).......... 533

May interact with ACE inhibitors, anticholinergics, aspirin-acetylsalicylic acid, central nervous system depressants, diuretics, lithium preparations, monoamine oxidase inhibitors, neuromuscular blocking agents, thiazides, tricyclic antidepressants, and certain other agents. Compounds in these categories include:

Alfentanil Hydrochloride (May exhibit additive CNS depression).
No products indexed under this heading.

Alprazolam (May exhibit additive CNS depression).
No products indexed under this heading.

Amiloride Hydrochloride (Ibuprofen has been shown to reduce the natriuretic effect of furosemide and thiazides in some patients. This response has been attributed to inhibition of renal prostaglandin synthesis. During concomitant therapy with Vicoprofen the patient should be observed closely for signs of renal failure).
No products indexed under this heading.

Amitriptyline Hydrochloride (Co-administration of tricyclic antidepressants with hydrocodone preparations may increase the effect of either the antidepressant or hydrocodone).
No products indexed under this heading.

Amoxapine (Co-administration of tricyclic antidepressants with hydrocodone preparations may increase the effect of either the antidepressant or hydrocodone).
No products indexed under this heading.

Aprobarbital (May exhibit additive CNS depression).
No products indexed under this heading.

Aspirin (Co-administration of Vicoprofen and aspirin may increase the risk of adverse effects; concurrent use should be avoided). Products include:
Aggrenox Capsules 819
Bayer Aspirin 750
Percodan Tablets 1130
St. Joseph 81 mg Aspirin Chewable and Enteric Coated Tablets 1903

Aspirin, Enteric Coated (Co-administration of Vicoprofen and aspirin may increase the risk of adverse effects; concurrent use should be avoided).
No products indexed under this heading.

Aspirin Buffered (Co-administration of Vicoprofen and aspirin may increase the risk of adverse effects; concurrent use should be avoided).
No products indexed under this heading.

Atracurium Besylate (Hydrocodone as well as other opioid analgesics may enhance the neuromuscular blocking action of skeletal muscle relaxants and produce an increased degree of respiratory depression).
No products indexed under this heading.

Atropine Sulfate (Concurrent use of anticholinergics with hydrocodone preparations may produce paralytic ileus). Products include:
Donnatal Extentabs 2507

Belladonna Alkaloids (Concurrent use of anticholinergics with hydrocodone preparations may produce paralytic ileus). Products include:
Hyland's Teething Tablets 621

Benazepril Hydrochloride (NSAIDs may diminish the antihypertensive effect of ACE inhibitors).
No products indexed under this heading.

Bendroflumethiazide (Ibuprofen has been shown to reduce the natriuretic effect of thiazides in some patients).
No products indexed under this heading.

Benztropine Mesylate (Concurrent use of anticholinergics with hydrocodone preparations may produce paralytic ileus).
No products indexed under this heading.

Biperiden Hydrochloride (Concurrent use of anticholinergics with hydrocodone preparations may produce paralytic ileus).
No products indexed under this heading.

Bumetanide (Ibuprofen has been shown to reduce the natriuretic effect of furosemide and thiazides in some patients. This response has been attributed to inhibition of renal prostaglandin synthesis. During concomitant therapy with Vicoprofen the patient should be observed closely for signs of renal failure).
No products indexed under this heading.

Buprenorphine Hydrochloride (May exhibit additive CNS depression). Products include:
Suboxone Tablets 2601
Subutex Tablets 2601

Buspirone Hydrochloride (May exhibit additive CNS depression).
No products indexed under this heading.

Butabarbital (May exhibit additive CNS depression).
No products indexed under this heading.

Butalbital (May exhibit additive CNS depression).
No products indexed under this heading.

Captopril (NSAIDs may diminish the antihypertensive effect of ACE inhibitors). Products include:
Captopril Tablets 2182

Chlordiazepoxide (May exhibit additive CNS depression).
No products indexed under this heading.

Chlordiazepoxide Hydrochloride (May exhibit additive CNS depression).
No products indexed under this heading.

Chlorothiazide (Ibuprofen has been shown to reduce the natriuretic effect of thiazides in some patients).
No products indexed under this heading.

Chlorothiazide Sodium (Ibuprofen has been shown to reduce the natriuretic effect of thiazides in some patients). Products include:
Intravenous Sodium Diuril 2490

Chlorpromazine (May exhibit additive CNS depression).
No products indexed under this heading.

Chlorpromazine Hydrochloride (May exhibit additive CNS depression).
No products indexed under this heading.

Chlorprothixene (May exhibit additive CNS depression).
No products indexed under this heading.

Chlorprothixene Hydrochloride (May exhibit additive CNS depression).
No products indexed under this heading.

Chlorprothixene Lactate (May exhibit additive CNS depression).
No products indexed under this heading.

Chlorthalidone (Ibuprofen has been shown to reduce the natriuretic effect of furosemide and thiazides in some patients. This response has been attributed to inhibition of renal prostaglandin synthesis. During concomitant therapy with Vicoprofen the patient should be observed closely for signs of renal failure). Products include:
Clorpres Tablets 2185

Cisatracurium Besylate (Hydrocodone as well as other opioid analgesics may enhance the neuromuscular blocking action of skeletal muscle relaxants and produce an increased degree of respiratory depression). Products include:

Nimbex Injection 484

Clidinium Bromide (Concurrent use of anticholinergics with hydrocodone preparations may produce paralytic ileus).

No products indexed under this heading.

Clomipramine Hydrochloride (Co-administration of tricyclic antidepressants with hydrocodone preparations may increase the effect of either the antidepressant or hydrocodone).

No products indexed under this heading.

Clorazepate Dipotassium (May exhibit additive CNS depression).

No products indexed under this heading.

Clozapine (May exhibit additive CNS depression).

No products indexed under this heading.

Codeine Phosphate (May exhibit additive CNS depression). Products include:

Tylenol with Codeine Tablets 2427

Desflurane (May exhibit additive CNS depression).

No products indexed under this heading.

Desipramine Hydrochloride (Co-administration of tricyclic antidepressants with hydrocodone preparations may increase the effect of either the antidepressant or hydrocodone).

No products indexed under this heading.

Dezocine (May exhibit additive CNS depression).

No products indexed under this heading.

Diazepam (May exhibit additive CNS depression). Products include:

Valium Tablets 2658

Dicyclomine Hydrochloride (Concurrent use of anticholinergics with hydrocodone preparations may produce paralytic ileus). Products include:

Bentyl Capsules 703
Bentyl Injection 703
Bentyl Syrup 703
Bentyl Tablets 703

Doxacurium Chloride (Hydrocodone as well as other opioid analgesics may enhance the neuromuscular blocking action of skeletal muscle relaxants and produce an increased degree of respiratory depression).

No products indexed under this heading.

Doxepin Hydrochloride (Co-administration of tricyclic antidepressants with hydrocodone preparations may increase the effect of either the antidepressant or hydrocodone).

No products indexed under this heading.

Droperidol (May exhibit additive CNS depression).

No products indexed under this heading.

Enalapril Maleate (NSAIDs may diminish the antihypertensive effect of ACE inhibitors).

No products indexed under this heading.

Enalaprilat (NSAIDs may diminish the antihypertensive effect of ACE inhibitors).

No products indexed under this heading.

Enflurane (May exhibit additive CNS depression).

No products indexed under this heading.

Estazolam (May exhibit additive CNS depression).

No products indexed under this heading.

Ethacrynic Acid (Ibuprofen has been shown to reduce the natriuretic effect of furosemide and thiazides in some patients. This response has been attributed to inhibition of renal prostaglandin synthesis. During concomitant therapy with Vicoprofen the patient should be observed closely for signs of renal failure). Products include:

Edecrin Tablets 698

Ethanol (May exhibit additive CNS depression).

No products indexed under this heading.

Ethchlorvynol (May exhibit additive CNS depression).

No products indexed under this heading.

Ethinamate (May exhibit additive CNS depression).

No products indexed under this heading.

Ethyl Alcohol (May exhibit additive CNS depression).

No products indexed under this heading.

Fentanyl (May exhibit additive CNS depression). Products include:

Duragesic Transdermal System 2405
Ionsys Transdermal System 2410

Fentanyl Citrate (May exhibit additive CNS depression). Products include:

Actiq 959
Fentora Tablets 968

Fluphenazine Decanoate (May exhibit additive CNS depression).

No products indexed under this heading.

Fluphenazine Enanthate (May exhibit additive CNS depression).

No products indexed under this heading.

Fluphenazine Hydrochloride (May exhibit additive CNS depression).

No products indexed under this heading.

Flurazepam Hydrochloride (May exhibit additive CNS depression).

No products indexed under this heading.

Fosinopril Sodium (NSAIDs may diminish the antihypertensive effect of ACE inhibitors).

No products indexed under this heading.

Furosemide (Ibuprofen has been shown to reduce the natriuretic effect of furosemide). Products include:

Furosemide Tablets 2186

Glutethimide (May exhibit additive CNS depression).

No products indexed under this heading.

Glycopyrrolate (Concurrent use of anticholinergics with hydrocodone preparations may produce paralytic ileus).

No products indexed under this heading.

Haloperidol (May exhibit additive CNS depression).

No products indexed under this heading.

Haloperidol Decanoate (May exhibit additive CNS depression).

No products indexed under this heading.

Hydrochlorothiazide (Ibuprofen has been shown to reduce the natriuretic effect of thiazides in some patients). Products include:

Atacand HCT 642
Avalide Tablets 892
Avalide Tablets 2713
Benicar HCT Tablets 1010
Diovan HCT Tablets 2216
Dyazide Capsules 1405
Micardis HCT Tablets 854
Prinzide Tablets 2092
Tekturna HCT Tablets 2324
Teveten HCT Tablets 517

Hydrocodone Polistirex (May exhibit additive CNS depression). Products include:

Tussionex Pennkinetic Extended-Release Suspension 3154

Hydroflumethiazide (Ibuprofen has been shown to reduce the natriuretic effect of thiazides in some patients).

No products indexed under this heading.

Hydromorphone Hydrochloride (May exhibit additive CNS depression).

No products indexed under this heading.

Hydroxyzine Hydrochloride (May exhibit additive CNS depression).

No products indexed under this heading.

Hyoscyamine (Concurrent use of anticholinergics with hydrocodone preparations may produce paralytic ileus).

No products indexed under this heading.

Hyoscyamine Sulfate (Concurrent use of anticholinergics with hydrocodone preparations may produce paralytic ileus). Products include:

Donnatal Extentabs 2507

Imipramine Hydrochloride (Co-administration of tricyclic antidepressants with hydrocodone preparations may increase the effect of either the antidepressant or hydrocodone).

No products indexed under this heading.

Imipramine Pamoate (Co-administration of tricyclic antidepressants with hydrocodone preparations may increase the effect of either the antidepressant or hydrocodone).

No products indexed under this heading.

Indapamide (Ibuprofen has been shown to reduce the natriuretic effect of furosemide and thiazides in some patients. This response has been attributed to inhibition of renal prostaglandin synthesis. During concomitant therapy with Vicoprofen the patient should be observed closely for signs of renal failure). Products include:

Indapamide Tablets 2188

Ipratropium Bromide (Concurrent use of anticholinergics with hydrocodone preparations may produce paralytic ileus). Products include:

Atrovent HFA Inhalation Aerosol 839
Atrovent Nasal Spray 0.03% 834
Atrovent Nasal Spray 0.06% 836
Combivent Inhalation Aerosol 845

Isocarboxazid (Co-administration of MAO inhibitors with hydrocodone preparations may increase the effect of either the MAO inhibitors or hydrocodone. The use of hydrocodone is not recommended for patients taking MAOIs or within 14 days of stopping such treatment). Products include:

Marplan Tablets 3177

Isoflurane (May exhibit additive CNS depression).

No products indexed under this heading.

Ketamine Hydrochloride (May exhibit additive CNS depression).

No products indexed under this heading.

Levomethadyl Acetate Hydrochloride (May exhibit additive CNS depression).

No products indexed under this heading.

Levorphanol Tartrate (May exhibit additive CNS depression).

No products indexed under this heading.

Lisinopril (NSAIDs may diminish the antihypertensive effect of ACE inhibitors). Products include:

Prinivil Tablets 2087
Prinzide Tablets 2092

Lithium (Ibuprofen has been shown to elevate plasma lithium concentration and reduce renal clearance. The mean minimum lithium concentration is increased 15% and the renal clearance is decreased by approximately 20%. Patients should be observed for signs of lithium toxicity when Vicoprofen and lithium are administered concurrently).

No products indexed under this heading.

Lithium Carbonate (Ibuprofen has been shown to elevate plasma lithium concentration and reduce renal clearance. The mean minimum lithium concentration is increased 15% and the renal clearance is decreased by approximately 20%. Patients should be observed for signs of lithium toxicity when Vicoprofen and lithium are administered concurrently).

No products indexed under this heading.

Lithium Citrate (Ibuprofen has been shown to elevate plasma lithium concentration and reduce renal clearance. The mean minimum lithium concentration is increased 15% and the renal clearance is decreased by approximately 20%. Patients should be observed for signs of lithium toxicity when Vicoprofen and lithium are administered concurrently).

No products indexed under this heading.

Lorazepam (May exhibit additive CNS depression).

No products indexed under this heading.

Loxapine Hydrochloride (May exhibit additive CNS depression).

No products indexed under this heading.

Loxapine Succinate (May exhibit additive CNS depression).

No products indexed under this heading.

Maprotiline Hydrochloride (Co-administration of tricyclic antidepressants with hydrocodone preparations may increase the effect of either the antidepressant or hydrocodone).
No products indexed under this heading.

Mepenzolate Bromide (Concurrent use of anticholinergics with hydrocodone preparations may produce paralytic ileus).
No products indexed under this heading.

Meperidine Hydrochloride (May exhibit additive CNS depression).
No products indexed under this heading.

Mephobarbital (May exhibit additive CNS depression).
No products indexed under this heading.

Meprobamate (May exhibit additive CNS depression).
No products indexed under this heading.

Mesoridazine Besylate (May exhibit additive CNS depression).
No products indexed under this heading.

Methadone Hydrochloride (May exhibit additive CNS depression).
No products indexed under this heading.

Methohexital Sodium (May exhibit additive CNS depression).
No products indexed under this heading.

Methotrexate Sodium (Ibuprofen, in animal studies, has been reported to competitively inhibit methotrexate accumulation; this could lead to enhanced toxicity of methotrexate).
No products indexed under this heading.

Methotrimeprazine (May exhibit additive CNS depression).
No products indexed under this heading.

Methoxyflurane (May exhibit additive CNS depression).
No products indexed under this heading.

Methyclothiazide (Ibuprofen has been shown to reduce the natriuretic effect of thiazides in some patients).
No products indexed under this heading.

Metocurine Iodide (Hydrocodone as well as other opioid analgesics may enhance the neuromuscular blocking action of skeletal muscle relaxants and produce an increased degree of respiratory depression).
No products indexed under this heading.

Metolazone (Ibuprofen has been shown to reduce the natriuretic effect of furosemide and thiazides in some patients. This response has been attributed to inhibition of renal prostaglandin synthesis. During concomitant therapy with Vicoprofen the patient should be observed closely for signs of renal failure).
No products indexed under this heading.

Midazolam Hydrochloride (May exhibit additive CNS depression).
No products indexed under this heading.

Mivacurium Chloride (Hydrocodone as well as other opioid analgesics may enhance the neuromuscular blocking action of skeletal muscle relaxants and produce an increased degree of respiratory depression).
No products indexed under this heading.

Moclobemide (Co-administration of MAO inhibitors with hydrocodone preparations may increase the effect of either the MAO inhibitors or hydrocodone. The use of hydrocodone is not recommended for patients taking MAOIs or within 14 days of stopping such treatment).
No products indexed under this heading.

Moexipril Hydrochloride (NSAIDs may diminish the antihypertensive effect of ACE inhibitors).
No products indexed under this heading.

Molindone Hydrochloride (May exhibit additive CNS depression). Products include:
Moban Tablets ... **1116**

Morphine Sulfate (May exhibit additive CNS depression). Products include:
Avinza Capsules ... **1772**
DepoDur Injection ... **1095**
MS Contin Tablets ... **2585**

Nortriptyline Hydrochloride (Co-administration of tricyclic antidepressants with hydrocodone preparations may increase the effect of either the antidepressant or hydrocodone).
No products indexed under this heading.

Olanzapine (May exhibit additive CNS depression). Products include:
Symbyax Capsules ... **1871**
Zyprexa Tablets ... **1883**
Zyprexa IntraMuscular ... **1883**
Zyprexa ZYDIS Orally Disintegrating Tablets ... **1883**

Oxazepam (May exhibit additive CNS depression).
No products indexed under this heading.

Oxybutynin Chloride (Concurrent use of anticholinergics with hydrocodone preparations may produce paralytic ileus).
No products indexed under this heading.

Oxycodone Hydrochloride (May exhibit additive CNS depression). Products include:
OxyContin Tablets ... **2589**
OxyIR Capsules ... **2593**
Percocet Tablets ... **1127**
Percodan Tablets ... **1130**

Pancuronium Bromide (Hydrocodone as well as other opioid analgesics may enhance the neuromuscular blocking action of skeletal muscle relaxants and produce an increased degree of respiratory depression).
No products indexed under this heading.

Pargyline Hydrochloride (Co-administration of MAO inhibitors with hydrocodone preparations may increase the effect of either the MAO inhibitors or hydrocodone. The use of hydrocodone is not recommended for patients taking MAOIs or within 14 days of stopping such treatment).
No products indexed under this heading.

Pentobarbital Sodium (May exhibit additive CNS depression). Products include:
Nembutal Sodium Solution, USP ... **2494**

Perindopril Erbumine (NSAIDs may diminish the antihypertensive effect of ACE inhibitors). Products include:
Aceon Tablets (2 mg, 4 mg, 8 mg) ... **3038**

Perphenazine (May exhibit additive CNS depression).
No products indexed under this heading.

Phenelzine Sulfate (Co-administration of MAO inhibitors with hydrocodone preparations may increase the effect of either the MAO inhibitors or hydrocodone. The use of hydrocodone is not recommended for patients taking MAOIs or within 14 days of stopping such treatment).
No products indexed under this heading.

Phenobarbital (May exhibit additive CNS depression). Products include:
Donnatal Extentabs ... **2507**

Polythiazide (Ibuprofen has been shown to reduce the natriuretic effect of thiazides in some patients).
No products indexed under this heading.

Prazepam (May exhibit additive CNS depression).
No products indexed under this heading.

Procarbazine Hydrochloride (Co-administration of MAO inhibitors with hydrocodone preparations may increase the effect of either the MAO inhibitors or hydrocodone. The use of hydrocodone is not recommended for patients taking MAOIs or within 14 days of stopping such treatment).
No products indexed under this heading.

Prochlorperazine (May exhibit additive CNS depression).
No products indexed under this heading.

Procyclidine Hydrochloride (Concurrent use of anticholinergics with hydrocodone preparations may produce paralytic ileus).
No products indexed under this heading.

Promethazine Hydrochloride (May exhibit additive CNS depression).
No products indexed under this heading.

Propantheline Bromide (Concurrent use of anticholinergics with hydrocodone preparations may produce paralytic ileus).
No products indexed under this heading.

Propofol (May exhibit additive CNS depression).
No products indexed under this heading.

Propoxyphene Hydrochloride (May exhibit additive CNS depression).
No products indexed under this heading.

Propoxyphene Napsylate (May exhibit additive CNS depression).
No products indexed under this heading.

Protriptyline Hydrochloride (Co-administration of tricyclic antidepressants with hydrocodone preparations may increase the effect of either the antidepressant or hydrocodone).
No products indexed under this heading.

Quazepam (May exhibit additive CNS depression).
No products indexed under this heading.

Quetiapine Fumarate (May exhibit additive CNS depression).
No products indexed under this heading.

Quinapril Hydrochloride (NSAIDs may diminish the antihypertensive effect of ACE inhibitors).
No products indexed under this heading.

Ramipril (NSAIDs may diminish the antihypertensive effect of ACE inhibitors).
No products indexed under this heading.

Rapacuronium Bromide (Hydrocodone as well as other opioid analgesics may enhance the neuromuscular blocking action of skeletal muscle relaxants and produce an increased degree of respiratory depression).
No products indexed under this heading.

Rasagiline Mesylate (Co-administration of MAO inhibitors with hydrocodone preparations may increase the effect of either the MAO inhibitors or hydrocodone. The use of hydrocodone is not recommended for patients taking MAOIs or within 14 days of stopping such treatment). Products include:
Azilect Tablets ... **3106**

Remifentanil Hydrochloride (May exhibit additive CNS depression).
No products indexed under this heading.

Risperidone (May exhibit additive CNS depression). Products include:
Risperdal Consta Long-Acting Injection ... **1753**

Rocuronium Bromide (Hydrocodone as well as other opioid analgesics may enhance the neuromuscular blocking action of skeletal muscle relaxants and produce an increased degree of respiratory depression). Products include:
Zemuron Injection ... **2947**

Scopolamine (Concurrent use of anticholinergics with hydrocodone preparations may produce paralytic ileus). Products include:
Transderm Scōp Transdermal Therapeutic System ... **2206**

Scopolamine Hydrobromide (Concurrent use of anticholinergics with hydrocodone preparations may produce paralytic ileus). Products include:
Donnatal Extentabs ... **2507**

Secobarbital Sodium (May exhibit additive CNS depression).
No products indexed under this heading.

Selegiline (Co-administration of MAO inhibitors with hydrocodone preparations may increase the effect of either the MAO inhibitors or hydrocodone. The use of hydrocodone is not recommended for patients taking MAOIs or within 14 days of stopping such treatment). Products include:
Emsam Transdermal System ... **905**

Selegiline Hydrochloride (Co-administration of MAO inhibitors with hydrocodone preparations may increase the effect of either the MAO inhibitors or hydrocodone. The use of hydrocodone is not recommended

for patients taking MAOIs or within 14 days of stopping such treatment). Products include:
Eldepryl Capsules 3052

Sevoflurane (May exhibit additive CNS depression). Products include:
Ultane Liquid for Inhalation 524

Sodium Oxybate (May exhibit additive CNS depression). Products include:
Xyrem Oral Solution 1766

Spirapril Hydrochloride (NSAIDs may diminish the antihypertensive effect of ACE inhibitors).
No products indexed under this heading.

Spironolactone (Ibuprofen has been shown to reduce the natriuretic effect of furosemide and thiazides in some patients. This response has been attributed to inhibition of renal prostaglandin synthesis. During concomitant therapy with Vicoprofen the patient should be observed closely for signs of renal failure).
No products indexed under this heading.

Succinylcholine Chloride (Hydrocodone as well as other opioid analgesics may enhance the neuromuscular blocking action of skeletal muscle relaxants and produce an increased degree of respiratory depression).
No products indexed under this heading.

Sufentanil Citrate (May exhibit additive CNS depression).
No products indexed under this heading.

Temazepam (May exhibit additive CNS depression).
No products indexed under this heading.

Thiamylal Sodium (May exhibit additive CNS depression).
No products indexed under this heading.

Thioridazine Hydrochloride (May exhibit additive CNS depression). Products include:
Thioridazine Hydrochloride Tablets 2195

Thiothixene (May exhibit additive CNS depression). Products include:
Thiothixene Capsules 2197

Tolterodine Tartrate (Concurrent use of anticholinergics with hydrocodone preparations may produce paralytic ileus).
No products indexed under this heading.

Torsemide (Ibuprofen has been shown to reduce the natriuretic effect of furosemide and thiazides in some patients. This response has been attributed to inhibition of renal prostaglandin synthesis. During concomitant therapy with Vicoprofen the patient should be observed closely for signs of renal failure). Products include:
Demadex Injection 2630
Demadex Tablets 2630

Trandolapril (NSAIDs may diminish the antihypertensive effect of ACE inhibitors). Products include:
Mavik Tablets 472
Tarka Tablets 511

Tranylcypromine Sulfate (Coadministration of MAO inhibitors with hydrocodone preparations may increase the effect of either the MAO inhibitors or hydrocodone. The use of hydrocodone is not recommended for patients taking MAOIs or within 14 days of stopping such treatment). Products include:
Parnate Tablets 1532

Triamterene (Ibuprofen has been shown to reduce the natriuretic effect of furosemide and thiazides in some patients. This response has been attributed to inhibition of renal prostaglandin synthesis. During concomitant therapy with Vicoprofen the patient should be observed closely for signs of renal failure). Products include:
Dyazide Capsules 1405
Dyrenium Capsules 3189

Triazolam (May exhibit additive CNS depression).
No products indexed under this heading.

Tridihexethyl Chloride (Concurrent use of anticholinergics with hydrocodone preparations may produce paralytic ileus).
No products indexed under this heading.

Trifluoperazine Hydrochloride (May exhibit additive CNS depression).
No products indexed under this heading.

Trihexyphenidyl Hydrochloride (Concurrent use of anticholinergics with hydrocodone preparations may produce paralytic ileus).
No products indexed under this heading.

Trimipramine Maleate (Coadministration of tricyclic antidepressants with hydrocodone preparations may increase the effect of either the antidepressant or hydrocodone).
No products indexed under this heading.

Vecuronium Bromide (Hydrocodone as well as other opioid analgesics may enhance the neuromuscular blocking action of skeletal muscle relaxants and produce an increased degree of respiratory depression).
No products indexed under this heading.

Warfarin Sodium (The effects of warfarin and NSAIDs on GI bleeding are synergistic).
No products indexed under this heading.

Zaleplon (May exhibit additive CNS depression).
No products indexed under this heading.

Ziprasidone Hydrochloride (May exhibit additive CNS depression). Products include:
Geodon Capsules 2520

Zolpidem Tartrate (May exhibit additive CNS depression). Products include:
Ambien Tablets 2692
Ambien CR Tablets 2696

Food Interactions

Alcohol (May exhibit additive CNS depression).

VIGAMOX OPHTHALMIC SOLUTION

(Moxifloxacin Hydrochloride) 548
None cited in PDR database.

VIOKASE POWDER

(Pancrelipase) 721
None cited in PDR database.

VIOKASE TABLETS

(Pancrelipase) 721
None cited in PDR database.

VIRAMUNE ORAL SUSPENSION

(Nevirapine) 873
See Viramune Tablets

VIRAMUNE TABLETS

(Nevirapine) 873
May interact with antiarrhythmics, azole antifungals, calcium channel blockers, antineoplastics, anticoagulants, cytochrome p450 3a substrates (selected), anticonvulsants, ergot-containing drugs, drugs affecting gastrointestinal motility, immunosuppressive agents, narcotic analgesics, oral contraceptives, and certain other agents. Compounds in these categories include:

Acebutolol Hydrochloride (Plasma concentrations of antiarrhythmics may be decreased with concomitant use of nevirapine).
No products indexed under this heading.

Adenosine (Plasma concentrations of antiarrhythmics may be decreased with concomitant use of nevirapine). Products include:
Adenocard IV Injection 603
Adenoscan 605

Albuterol (Plasma concentrations of motility agents may be decreased with concomitant use of nevirapine).
No products indexed under this heading.

Albuterol Sulfate (Plasma concentrations of motility agents may be decreased with concomitant use of nevirapine). Products include:
Combivent Inhalation Aerosol 845
ProAir HFA Inhalation Aerosol 3113
Proventil HFA Inhalation Aerosol 2914
Ventolin HFA Inhalation Aerosol 1638

Alfentanil Hydrochloride (Plasma concentrations of motility agents may be decreased with concomitant use of nevirapine).
No products indexed under this heading.

Alprazolam (Nevirapine is principally metabolized by the liver via cytochrome P450 isoenzymes 3A and 2B6. Nevirapine is known to be an inducer of these enzymes. As a result, drugs that are metabolized by these enzyme systems may have lower than expected plasma levels when co-administered with nevirapine).
No products indexed under this heading.

Altretamine (Plasma concentrations of cancer chemotherapeutic agents may be decreased with concomitant use of nevirapine). Products include:
Hexalen Capsules 1078

Aminophylline (Nevirapine is principally metabolized by the liver via cytochrome P450 isoenzymes 3A and 2B6. Nevirapine is known to be an inducer of these enzymes. As a result, drugs that are metabolized by these enzyme systems may have lower than expected plasma levels when co-administered with nevirapine).
No products indexed under this heading.

Amiodarone Hydrochloride (Plasma concentrations of antiarrhythmics may be decreased with concomitant use of nevirapine).
No products indexed under this heading.

Amitriptyline Hydrochloride (Plasma concentrations of motility agents may be decreased with concomitant use of nevirapine).
No products indexed under this heading.

Amlodipine Besylate (Plasma concentrations of calcium channel blockers may be decreased with concomitant use of nevirapine). Products include:
Azor Tablets 1005
Exforge Tablets 2238

Amoxapine (Plasma concentrations of motility agents may be decreased with concomitant use of nevirapine).
No products indexed under this heading.

Anastrozole (Plasma concentrations of cancer chemotherapeutic agents may be decreased with concomitant use of nevirapine). Products include:
Arimidex Tablets 672

Anisindione (Plasma concentrations of antithrombotics may be increased with concomitant use of nevirapine. This may have a potential effect on anticoagulation. Monitoring of anticoagulation levels is recommended).
No products indexed under this heading.

Aprepitant (Nevirapine is principally metabolized by the liver via cytochrome P450 isoenzymes 3A and 2B6. Nevirapine is known to be an inducer of these enzymes. As a result, drugs that are metabolized by these enzyme systems may have lower than expected plasma levels when co-administered with nevirapine). Products include:
Emend Capsules 1992

Ardeparin Sodium (Plasma concentrations of antithrombotics may be increased with concomitant use of nevirapine. This may have a potential effect on anticoagulation. Monitoring of anticoagulation levels is recommended).
No products indexed under this heading.

Asparaginase (Plasma concentrations of cancer chemotherapeutic agents may be decreased with concomitant use of nevirapine). Products include:
Elspar for Injection 1990
Elspar for Injection 2488

Astemizole (Plasma concentrations of motility agents may be decreased with concomitant use of nevirapine).
No products indexed under this heading.

Atorvastatin Calcium (Nevirapine is principally metabolized by the liver via cytochrome P450 isoenzymes 3A and 2B6. Nevirapine is known to be an inducer of these enzymes. As a result, drugs that are metabolized by these enzyme systems may have lower than expected plasma levels when co-administered with nevirapine). Products include:
Lipitor Tablets 2501

Atropine Sulfate (Plasma concentrations of motility agents may be decreased with concomitant use of nevirapine). Products include:
Donnatal Extentabs 2507

Azatadine Maleate (Plasma concentrations of motility agents may be decreased with concomitant use of nevirapine).
No products indexed under this heading.

Azathioprine (Plasma concentrations of cancer immunosuppressants agents may be decreased with concomitant use of nevirapine).
No products indexed under this heading.

Basiliximab (Plasma concentrations of cancer immunosuppressants agents may be decreased with concomitant use of nevirapine). Products include:
Simulect for Injection 2306

Belladonna Alkaloids (Plasma concentrations of motility agents may be decreased with concomitant use of nevirapine). Products include:
Hyland's Teething Tablets 621

Benztropine Mesylate (Plasma concentrations of motility agents may be decreased with concomitant use of nevirapine).
No products indexed under this heading.

Bepridil Hydrochloride (Plasma concentrations of calcium channel blockers may be decreased with concomitant use of nevirapine).
No products indexed under this heading.

Bethanechol Chloride (Plasma concentrations of motility agents may be decreased with concomitant use of nevirapine).
No products indexed under this heading.

Bicalutamide (Plasma concentrations of cancer chemotherapeutic agents may be decreased with concomitant use of nevirapine). Products include:
No products indexed under this heading.

Biperiden Hydrochloride (Plasma concentrations of motility agents may be decreased with concomitant use of nevirapine).
No products indexed under this heading.

Bitolterol Mesylate (Plasma concentrations of motility agents may be decreased with concomitant use of nevirapine).
No products indexed under this heading.

Bleomycin Sulfate (Plasma concentrations of cancer chemotherapeutic agents may be decreased with concomitant use of nevirapine).
No products indexed under this heading.

Bretylium Tosylate (Plasma concentrations of antiarrhythmics may be decreased with concomitant use of nevirapine).
No products indexed under this heading.

Bromocriptine Mesylate (Plasma concentrations of motility agents may be decreased with concomitant use of nevirapine).
No products indexed under this heading.

Bromodiphenhydramine Hydrochloride (Plasma concentrations of motility agents may be decreased with concomitant use of nevirapine).
No products indexed under this heading.

Brompheniramine Maleate (Plasma concentrations of motility agents may be decreased with concomitant use of nevirapine).
No products indexed under this heading.

Buprenorphine Hydrochloride (Plasma concentrations of motility agents may be decreased with concomitant use of nevirapine). Products include:
Suboxone Tablets 2601
Subutex Tablets 2601

Buspirone Hydrochloride (Nevirapine is principally metabolized by the liver via cytochrome P450 isoenzymes 3A and 2B6. Nevirapine is known to be an inducer of these enzymes. As a result, drugs that are metabolized by these enzyme systems may have lower than expected plasma levels when co-administered with nevirapine).
No products indexed under this heading.

Busulfan (Plasma concentrations of cancer chemotherapeutic agents may be decreased with concomitant use of nevirapine). Products include:
Busulfex Injection 2477
Myleran Tablets 1530

Carbamazepine (Plasma concentrations of anticonvulsants may be decreased with concomitant use of nevirapine). Products include:
Carbatrol Capsules 3019
Equetro Extended-Release Capsules 3174

Carboplatin (Plasma concentrations of cancer chemotherapeutic agents may be decreased with concomitant use of nevirapine).
No products indexed under this heading.

Carmustine (BCNU) (Plasma concentrations of cancer chemotherapeutic agents may be decreased with concomitant use of nevirapine).
No products indexed under this heading.

Cerivastatin Sodium (Nevirapine is principally metabolized by the liver via cytochrome P450 isoenzymes 3A and 2B6. Nevirapine is known to be an inducer of these enzymes. As a result, drugs that are metabolized by these enzyme systems may have lower than expected plasma levels when co-administered with nevirapine).
No products indexed under this heading.

Cevimeline Hydrochloride (Plasma concentrations of motility agents may be decreased with concomitant use of nevirapine). Products include:
Evoxac Capsules 1013

Chlorambucil (Plasma concentrations of cancer chemotherapeutic agents may be decreased with concomitant use of nevirapine). Products include:
Leukeran Tablets 1508

Chlorpheniramine (Nevirapine is principally metabolized by the liver via cytochrome P450 isoenzymes 3A and 2B6. Nevirapine is known to be an inducer of these enzymes. As a result, drugs that are metabolized by these enzyme systems may have lower than expected plasma levels when co-administered with nevirapine).
No products indexed under this heading.

Chlorpheniramine Maleate (Plasma concentrations of motility agents may be decreased with concomitant use of nevirapine). Products include:
Actifed Cold & Allergy Tablets 1895
Sudafed PE Sinus & Allergy Tablets 1908
Tylenol Allergy Multi-Symptom Caplets with Cool Burst and Rapid Release Gelcaps 1916
Children's Tylenol Plus Cold Suspension Liquid 1912
Children's Tylenol Plus Cough & Runny Nose Suspension Liquid 1912
Children's Tylenol Plus Flu Suspension Liquid 1914
Children's Tylenol Plus Multi-Symptom Cold Suspension Liquid 1912
Tylenol Cold Head Congestion Nighttime Caplets with Cool Burst 1910
Tylenol Cold Multi-Symptom Nighttime Caplets with Cool Burst 1913
Tylenol Sinus Congestion & Pain Nighttime Caplets with Cool Burst 1917

Chlorpheniramine Polistirex (Plasma concentrations of motility agents may be decreased with concomitant use of nevirapine). Products include:
Tussionex Pennkinetic Extended-Release Suspension 3154

Chlorpheniramine Tannate (Plasma concentrations of motility agents may be decreased with concomitant use of nevirapine).
No products indexed under this heading.

Cisapride (Plasma concentrations of motility agents may be decreased with concomitant use of nevirapine).
No products indexed under this heading.

Cisplatin (Plasma concentrations of cancer chemotherapeutic agents may be decreased with concomitant use of nevirapine).
No products indexed under this heading.

Clarithromycin (Clarithromycin exposure was significantly decreased by nevirapine; however, 14-OH metabolite concentrations were increased. Because clarithromycin active metabolite has reduced activity against mycobacterium avium-intracellulare complex, overall activity against this pathogen may be altered. Alternatives to clarithromycin, such as azithromycin, should be considered). Products include:
Biaxin/Biaxin XL 411

Clemastine Fumarate (Plasma concentrations of motility agents may be decreased with concomitant use of nevirapine).
No products indexed under this heading.

Clidinium Bromide (Plasma concentrations of motility agents may be decreased with concomitant use of nevirapine).
No products indexed under this heading.

Clomipramine Hydrochloride (Plasma concentrations of motility agents may be decreased with concomitant use of nevirapine).
No products indexed under this heading.

Clotrimazole (Plasma concentrations of antifungals may be decreased with concomitant use of nevirapine). Products include:
Lotrisone 2881

Codeine Phosphate (Plasma concentrations of motility agents may be decreased with concomitant use of nevirapine). Products include:
Tylenol with Codeine Tablets 2427

Cyclophosphamide (Plasma concentrations of cancer chemotherapeutic agents may be decreased with concomitant use of nevirapine).
No products indexed under this heading.

Cyclosporine (Plasma concentrations of cancer immunosuppressants agents may be decreased with concomitant use of nevirapine). Products include:
Gengraf Capsules 435
Neoral Oral Solution 2280
Neoral Soft Gelatin Capsules 2280
Restasis Ophthalmic Emulsion 557
Sandimmune 2296

Cyproheptadine Hydrochloride (Plasma concentrations of motility agents may be decreased with concomitant use of nevirapine).
No products indexed under this heading.

Dacarbazine (Plasma concentrations of cancer chemotherapeutic agents may be decreased with concomitant use of nevirapine).
No products indexed under this heading.

Dalteparin Sodium (Plasma concentrations of antithrombotics may be increased with concomitant use of nevirapine. This may have a potential effect on anticoagulation. Monitoring of anticoagulation levels is recommended). Products include:
Fragmin Injection 1070

Danaparoid Sodium (Plasma concentrations of antithrombotics may be increased with concomitant use of nevirapine. This may have a potential effect on anticoagulation. Monitoring of anticoagulation levels is recommended).
No products indexed under this heading.

Daunorubicin Citrate (Plasma concentrations of cancer chemotherapeutic agents may be decreased with concomitant use of nevirapine).
No products indexed under this heading.

Daunorubicin Hydrochloride (Plasma concentrations of cancer chemotherapeutic agents may be decreased with concomitant use of nevirapine).
No products indexed under this heading.

Denileukin Diftitox (Plasma concentrations of cancer chemotherapeutic agents may be decreased with concomitant use of nevirapine). Products include:
Ontak Vials 1079

Desipramine Hydrochloride (Plasma concentrations of motility agents may be decreased with concomitant use of nevirapine).
No products indexed under this heading.

Desogestrel (Oral contraceptives and other hormonal methods of birth control should not be used as the sole method of contraception in women taking nevirapine, since nevirapine may lower the plasma levels of these medications. An alternative or additional method of contraception is recommended). Products include:
Mircette Tablets 1034

Dexamethasone (Nevirapine is principally metabolized by the liver via cytochrome P450 isoenzymes 3A and 2B6. Nevirapine is known to be an inducer of these enzymes. As a result, drugs that are metabolized by these enzyme systems may have lower than expected plasma levels when co-administered with nevirapine). Products include:
Ciprodex Otic Suspension 541

IMPORTANT NOTE: Always consult each drug listing in the patient's regimen for possible interactions.

Dexamethasone Acetate (Nevirapine is principally metabolized by the liver via cytochrome P450 isoenzymes 3A and 2B6. Nevirapine is known to be an inducer of these enzymes. As a result, drugs that are metabolized by these enzyme systems may have lower than expected plasma levels when co-administered with nevirapine).

No products indexed under this heading.

Dexamethasone Phosphate (Nevirapine is principally metabolized by the liver via cytochrome P450 isoenzymes 3A and 2B6. Nevirapine is known to be an inducer of these enzymes. As a result, drugs that are metabolized by these enzyme systems may have lower than expected plasma levels when co-administered with nevirapine).

No products indexed under this heading.

Dexamethasone Sodium (Nevirapine is principally metabolized by the liver via cytochrome P450 isoenzymes 3A and 2B6. Nevirapine is known to be an inducer of these enzymes. As a result, drugs that are metabolized by these enzyme systems may have lower than expected plasma levels when co-administered with nevirapine).

No products indexed under this heading.

Dexamethasone Sodium Phosphate (Nevirapine is principally metabolized by the liver via cytochrome P450 isoenzymes 3A and 2B6. Nevirapine is known to be an inducer of these enzymes. As a result, drugs that are metabolized by these enzyme systems may have lower than expected plasma levels when co-administered with nevirapine).

No products indexed under this heading.

Dexchlorpheniramine Maleate (Plasma concentrations of motility agents may be decreased with concomitant use of nevirapine).

No products indexed under this heading.

Dezocine (Plasma concentrations of motility agents may be decreased with concomitant use of nevirapine).

No products indexed under this heading.

Diazepam (Nevirapine is principally metabolized by the liver via cytochrome P450 isoenzymes 3A and 2B6. Nevirapine is known to be an inducer of these enzymes. As a result, drugs that are metabolized by these enzyme systems may have lower than expected plasma levels when co-administered with nevirapine). Products include:

Valium Tablets 2658

Dicumarol (Plasma concentrations of antithrombotics may be increased with concomitant use of nevirapine. This may have a potential effect on anticoagulation. Monitoring of anticoagulation levels is recommended).

No products indexed under this heading.

Dicyclomine Hydrochloride (Plasma concentrations of motility agents may be decreased with concomitant use of nevirapine). Products include:

Bentyl Capsules 703
Bentyl Injection 703
Bentyl Syrup 703
Bentyl Tablets 703

Dihydroergotamine Mesylate (Plasma concentrations of ergot alkaloids may be decreased with concomitant use of nevirapine).

No products indexed under this heading.

Diltiazem Hydrochloride (Plasma concentrations of calcium channel blockers may be decreased with concomitant use of nevirapine). Products include:

Cardizem LA Extended Release Tablets 421

Diltiazem Maleate (Nevirapine is principally metabolized by the liver via cytochrome P450 isoenzymes 3A and 2B6. Nevirapine is known to be an inducer of these enzymes. As a result, drugs that are metabolized by these enzyme systems may have lower than expected plasma levels when co-administered with nevirapine).

No products indexed under this heading.

Diphenhydramine Citrate (Plasma concentrations of motility agents may be decreased with concomitant use of nevirapine).

No products indexed under this heading.

Diphenhydramine Hydrochloride (Plasma concentrations of motility agents may be decreased with concomitant use of nevirapine). Products include:

Benadryl Allergy & Cold Kapgels 1895
Benadryl Allergy & Sinus Headache Kapgels 1895
Benadryl Severe Allergy & Sinus Headache Caplets 1897
Benadryl Dye-Free Allergy Liqui-gels Softgels 1897
Benadryl Allergy Kapgels 1895
Benadryl Allergy Quick Dissolve Strips 1896
Benadryl Allergy Ultratab Tablets 1896
Children's Benadryl Dye-Free Allergy Liquid 1897
Children's Benadryl Allergy Fastmelts 1897
Children's Benadryl Allergy Liquid 1898
Children's Benadryl Allergy Perfect Measure 1896
Children's Benadryl-D Allergy & Sinus Liquid 1896
Benadryl-D Allergy & Sinus Tablet 1896
PediaCare Children's Allergy & Cold Liquid 1902
PediaCare Children's Allergy Liquid 1902
Simply Sleep Caplets 1905
Sudafed PE Nighttime Cold Caplets 1907
Sudafed PE Severe Cold Caplets 1908
Extra Strength Tylenol PM Caplets, Geltabs, Liquid, and Rapid Release Gels 1915
Tylenol Allergy Multi-Symptom Nighttime Caplets with Cool Burst 1916
Tylenol Severe Allergy Caplets 1916
Children's Tylenol Plus Cold & Allergy Suspension Liquid 1914
Tylenol Sore Throat Nighttime Liquid with Cool Burst 1918

Diphenylpyraline Hydrochloride (Plasma concentrations of motility agents may be decreased with concomitant use of nevirapine).

No products indexed under this heading.

Disopyramide Phosphate (Plasma concentrations of antiarrhythmics may be decreased with concomitant use of nevirapine).

No products indexed under this heading.

Divalproex Sodium (Plasma concentrations of anticonvulsants may be decreased with concomitant use of nevirapine). Products include:

Depakote ER Tablets 423

Dobutamine (Plasma concentrations of motility agents may be decreased with concomitant use of nevirapine).

No products indexed under this heading.

Dobutamine Hydrochloride (Plasma concentrations of motility agents may be decreased with concomitant use of nevirapine).

No products indexed under this heading.

Docetaxel (Plasma concentrations of cancer chemotherapeutic agents may be decreased with concomitant use of nevirapine). Products include:

Taxotere Injection Concentrate 2773

Dofetilide (Plasma concentrations of antiarrhythmics may be decreased with concomitant use of nevirapine).

No products indexed under this heading.

Domperidone (Plasma concentrations of motility agents may be decreased with concomitant use of nevirapine).

No products indexed under this heading.

Donepezil Hydrochloride (Plasma concentrations of motility agents may be decreased with concomitant use of nevirapine). Products include:

Aricept Tablets 1062
Aricept ODT Tablets 1062

Dopamine Hydrochloride (Plasma concentrations of motility agents may be decreased with concomitant use of nevirapine).

No products indexed under this heading.

Doxepin Hydrochloride (Plasma concentrations of motility agents may be decreased with concomitant use of nevirapine).

No products indexed under this heading.

Doxorubicin Hydrochloride (Plasma concentrations of cancer chemotherapeutic agents may be decreased with concomitant use of nevirapine).

No products indexed under this heading.

Dronabinol (Nevirapine is principally metabolized by the liver via cytochrome P450 isoenzymes 3A and 2B6. Nevirapine is known to be an inducer of these enzymes. As a result, drugs that are metabolized by these enzyme systems may have lower than expected plasma levels when co-administered with nevirapine). Products include:

Marinol Capsules 3163

Dyphylline (Nevirapine is principally metabolized by the liver via cytochrome P450 isoenzymes 3A and 2B6. Nevirapine is known to be an inducer of these enzymes. As a result, drugs that are metabolized by these enzyme systems may have lower than expected plasma levels when co-administered with nevirapine).

No products indexed under this heading.

Edrophonium Chloride (Plasma concentrations of motility agents may be decreased with concomitant use of nevirapine).

No products indexed under this heading.

Efavirenz (Efavirenz concentrations are decreased when used concomitantly with nevirapine. Appropriate doses for this combination are not established). Products include:

Atripla Tablets 938
Sustiva Capsules 930
Sustiva Tablets 930

Enoxaparin Sodium (Plasma concentrations of antithrombotics may be increased with concomitant use of nevirapine. This may have a potential effect on anticoagulation. Monitoring of anticoagulation levels is recommended). Products include:

Lovenox Injection 2756

Ephedrine Hydrochloride (Plasma concentrations of motility agents may be decreased with concomitant use of nevirapine).

No products indexed under this heading.

Ephedrine Sulfate (Plasma concentrations of motility agents may be decreased with concomitant use of nevirapine).

No products indexed under this heading.

Ephedrine Tannate (Plasma concentrations of motility agents may be decreased with concomitant use of nevirapine).

No products indexed under this heading.

Epinephrine (Plasma concentrations of motility agents may be decreased with concomitant use of nevirapine). Products include:

EpiPen 1024

Epinephrine Hydrochloride (Plasma concentrations of motility agents may be decreased with concomitant use of nevirapine).

No products indexed under this heading.

Epirubicin Hydrochloride (Plasma concentrations of cancer chemotherapeutic agents may be decreased with concomitant use of nevirapine).

No products indexed under this heading.

Ergonovine Maleate (Plasma concentrations of ergot alkaloids may be decreased with concomitant use of nevirapine).

No products indexed under this heading.

Ergotamine Tartrate (Plasma concentrations of ergot alkaloids may be decreased with concomitant use of nevirapine).

No products indexed under this heading.

Erythromycin (Plasma concentrations of motility agents may be decreased with concomitant use of nevirapine).

No products indexed under this heading.

Erythromycin Estolate (Plasma concentrations of motility agents may be decreased with concomitant use of nevirapine).

No products indexed under this heading.

Erythromycin Ethylsuccinate (Plasma concentrations of motility agents may be decreased with concomitant use of nevirapine). Products include:

E.E.S. 433
EryPed 431

Erythromycin Gluceptate (Plasma concentrations of motility agents may be decreased with concomitant use of nevirapine).
No products indexed under this heading.

Erythromycin Lactobionate (Nevirapine is principally metabolized by the liver via cytochrome P450 isoenzymes 3A and 2B6. Nevirapine is known to be an inducer of these enzymes. As a result, drugs that are metabolized by these enzyme systems may have lower than expected plasma levels when co-administered with nevirapine).
No products indexed under this heading.

Erythromycin Stearate (Plasma concentrations of motility agents may be decreased with concomitant use of nevirapine).
No products indexed under this heading.

Estramustine Phosphate Sodium (Plasma concentrations of cancer chemotherapeutic agents may be decreased with concomitant use of nevirapine).
No products indexed under this heading.

Estrogen (Nevirapine is principally metabolized by the liver via cytochrome P450 isoenzymes 3A and 2B6. Nevirapine is known to be an inducer of these enzymes. As a result, drugs that are metabolized by these enzyme systems may have lower than expected plasma levels when co-administered with nevirapine).
No products indexed under this heading.

Estrogens, Conjugated (Nevirapine is principally metabolized by the liver via cytochrome P450 isoenzymes 3A and 2B6. Nevirapine is known to be an inducer of these enzymes. As a result, drugs that are metabolized by these enzyme systems may have lower than expected plasma levels when co-administered with nevirapine). Products include:
Premarin Intravenous 3217
Premarin Tablets 3221
Premarin Vaginal Cream 3228
Premphase Tablets 3232
Prempro Tablets 3232

Estrogens, Conjugated, Synthetic A (Nevirapine is principally metabolized by the liver via cytochrome P450 isoenzymes 3A and 2B6. Nevirapine is known to be an inducer of these enzymes. As a result, drugs that are metabolized by these enzyme systems may have lower than expected plasma levels when co-administered with nevirapine).
No products indexed under this heading.

Estrogens, Esterified (Nevirapine is principally metabolized by the liver via cytochrome P450 isoenzymes 3A and 2B6. Nevirapine is known to be an inducer of these enzymes. As a result, drugs that are metabolized by these enzyme systems may have lower than expected plasma levels when co-administered with nevirapine). Products include:
Estratest Tablets 3043
Estratest H.S. Tablets 3043

Ethinyl Estradiol (Oral contraceptives and other hormonal methods of birth control should not be used as the sole method of contraception in women taking nevirapine, since nevirapine may lower the plasma levels of these medications. An alternative or additional method of contraception is recommended). Products include:
Lybrel Tablets 3204
Mircette Tablets 1034
NuvaRing 2897
Ortho-Cyclen/Ortho Tri-Cyclen 2449
Ortho Evra Transdermal System 2437
Ortho Tri-Cyclen Lo Tablets 2458
Seasonique Tablets 1046
Yaz Tablets 805

Ethosuximide (Plasma concentrations of anticonvulsants may be decreased with concomitant use of nevirapine).
No products indexed under this heading.

Ethotoin (Plasma concentrations of anticonvulsants may be decreased with concomitant use of nevirapine).
No products indexed under this heading.

Ethynodiol Diacetate (Oral contraceptives and other hormonal methods of birth control should not be used as the sole method of contraception in women taking nevirapine, since nevirapine may lower the plasma levels of these medications. An alternative or additional method of contraception is recommended).
No products indexed under this heading.

Etoposide (Plasma concentrations of cancer chemotherapeutic agents may be decreased with concomitant use of nevirapine).
No products indexed under this heading.

Etoposide Phosphate (Nevirapine is principally metabolized by the liver via cytochrome P450 isoenzymes 3A and 2B6. Nevirapine is known to be an inducer of these enzymes. As a result, drugs that are metabolized by these enzyme systems may have lower than expected plasma levels when co-administered with nevirapine).
No products indexed under this heading.

Exemestane (Plasma concentrations of cancer chemotherapeutic agents may be decreased with concomitant use of nevirapine).
No products indexed under this heading.

Felbamate (Plasma concentrations of anticonvulsants may be decreased with concomitant use of nevirapine).
No products indexed under this heading.

Felodipine (Plasma concentrations of calcium channel blockers may be decreased with concomitant use of nevirapine).
No products indexed under this heading.

Fentanyl (Plasma concentrations of motility agents may be decreased with concomitant use of nevirapine). Products include:
Duragesic Transdermal System 2405
Ionsys Transdermal System 2410

Fentanyl Citrate (Plasma concentrations of motility agents may be decreased with concomitant use of nevirapine). Products include:
Actiq 959
Fentora Tablets 968

Flecainide Acetate (Plasma concentrations of antiarrhythmics may be decreased with concomitant use of nevirapine).
No products indexed under this heading.

Floxuridine (Plasma concentrations of cancer chemotherapeutic agents may be decreased with concomitant use of nevirapine).
No products indexed under this heading.

Fluconazole (Nevirapine concentrations are increased when used concomitantly with fluconazole. Because of the risk of increased exposure to nevirapine, caution should be used in concomitant administration and patients should be monitored closely for nevirapine-associated adverse events).
No products indexed under this heading.

Fluorouracil (Plasma concentrations of cancer chemotherapeutic agents may be decreased with concomitant use of nevirapine). Products include:
Carac Cream 0.5% 2722

Flutamide (Plasma concentrations of cancer chemotherapeutic agents may be decreased with concomitant use of nevirapine).
No products indexed under this heading.

Fondaparinux Sodium (Plasma concentrations of antithrombotics may be increased with concomitant use of nevirapine. This may have a potential effect on anticoagulation. Monitoring of anticoagulation levels is recommended). Products include:
Arixtra Injection 1313

Fosphenytoin (Plasma concentrations of anticonvulsants may be decreased with concomitant use of nevirapine).
No products indexed under this heading.

Fosphenytoin Sodium (Plasma concentrations of anticonvulsants may be decreased with concomitant use of nevirapine).
No products indexed under this heading.

Gabapentin (Plasma concentrations of anticonvulsants may be decreased with concomitant use of nevirapine).
No products indexed under this heading.

Galantamine Hydrobromide (Plasma concentrations of motility agents may be decreased with concomitant use of nevirapine).
No products indexed under this heading.

Gemcitabine Hydrochloride (Plasma concentrations of cancer chemotherapeutic agents may be decreased with concomitant use of nevirapine). Products include:
Gemzar for Injection 1820

Glyburide (Nevirapine is principally metabolized by the liver via cytochrome P450 isoenzymes 3A and 2B6. Nevirapine is known to be an inducer of these enzymes. As a result, drugs that are metabolized by these enzyme systems may have lower than expected plasma levels when co-administered with nevirapine).
No products indexed under this heading.

Glycopyrrolate (Plasma concentrations of motility agents may be decreased with concomitant use of nevirapine).
No products indexed under this heading.

Haloperidol (Nevirapine is principally metabolized by the liver via cytochrome P450 isoenzymes 3A and 2B6. Nevirapine is known to be an inducer of these enzymes. As a result, drugs that are metabolized by these enzyme systems may have lower than expected plasma levels when co-administered with nevirapine).
No products indexed under this heading.

Haloperidol Decanoate (Nevirapine is principally metabolized by the liver via cytochrome P450 isoenzymes 3A and 2B6. Nevirapine is known to be an inducer of these enzymes. As a result, drugs that are metabolized by these enzyme systems may have lower than expected plasma levels when co-administered with nevirapine).
No products indexed under this heading.

Heparin Calcium (Plasma concentrations of antithrombotics may be increased with concomitant use of nevirapine. This may have a potential effect on anticoagulation. Monitoring of anticoagulation levels is recommended).
No products indexed under this heading.

Heparin Sodium (Plasma concentrations of antithrombotics may be increased with concomitant use of nevirapine. This may have a potential effect on anticoagulation. Monitoring of anticoagulation levels is recommended).
No products indexed under this heading.

Hydrocodone Bitartrate (Plasma concentrations of motility agents may be decreased with concomitant use of nevirapine). Products include:
Lortab 5/500 Tablets 3143
Lortab 7.5/500 Tablets 3144
Lortab 10/500 Tablets 3144
Vicodin Tablets 529
Vicodin ES Tablets 530
Vicodin HP Tablets 531
Vicoprofen Tablets 533
Zydone Tablets 1132

Hydrocodone Polistirex (Plasma concentrations of motility agents may be decreased with concomitant use of nevirapine). Products include:
Tussionex Pennkinetic Extended-Release Suspension 3154

Hydromorphone Hydrochloride (Plasma concentrations of motility agents may be decreased with concomitant use of nevirapine).
No products indexed under this heading.

Hydroxyurea (Plasma concentrations of cancer chemotherapeutic agents may be decreased with concomitant use of nevirapine).
No products indexed under this heading.

Hyoscyamine (Plasma concentrations of motility agents may be decreased with concomitant use of nevirapine).
No products indexed under this heading.

Hyoscyamine Sulfate (Plasma concentrations of motility agents may be decreased with concomitant use of nevirapine). Products include:

Donnatal Extentabs ... 2507

Hypericum (Concomitant use of St. John's wort or St. John's wort-containing products and nevirapine is not recommended. Co-administration of St. John's wort with non-nucleoside reverse transcriptase inhibitors (NNRTIs), including nevirapine, is expected to substantially decrease NNRTI concentrations and may result in sub-optimal levels of nevirapine and lead to loss of virologic response and possibly resistance to nevirapine or to the class of NNRTIs). Products include:

Satieté Tablets ... ▣640

Idarubicin Hydrochloride (Plasma concentrations of cancer chemotherapeutic agents may be decreased with concomitant use of nevirapine).

No products indexed under this heading.

Ifosfamide (Plasma concentrations of cancer chemotherapeutic agents may be decreased with concomitant use of nevirapine).

No products indexed under this heading.

Imipramine Hydrochloride (Plasma concentrations of motility agents may be decreased with concomitant use of nevirapine).

No products indexed under this heading.

Imipramine Pamoate (Plasma concentrations of motility agents may be decreased with concomitant use of nevirapine).

No products indexed under this heading.

Indinavir Sulfate (Indinavir concentrations are decreased when used concomitantly with nevirapine. Appropriate doses for this combination are not established, but an increase in the dosage of indinavir may be required). Products include:

Crixivan Capsules ... 1979

Interferon alfa-2a, Recombinant (Plasma concentrations of cancer chemotherapeutic agents may be decreased with concomitant use of nevirapine).

No products indexed under this heading.

Interferon alfa-2b, Recombinant (Plasma concentrations of cancer chemotherapeutic agents may be decreased with concomitant use of nevirapine). Products include:

Intron A for Injection ... 2859

Ipratropium Bromide (Plasma concentrations of motility agents may be decreased with concomitant use of nevirapine). Products include:

Atrovent HFA Inhalation Aerosol ... 839
Atrovent Nasal Spray 0.03% ... 834
Atrovent Nasal Spray 0.06% ... 836
Combivent Inhalation Aerosol ... 845

Irinotecan Hydrochloride (Plasma concentrations of cancer chemotherapeutic agents may be decreased with concomitant use of nevirapine).

No products indexed under this heading.

Isoetharine (Plasma concentrations of motility agents may be decreased with concomitant use of nevirapine).

No products indexed under this heading.

Isoproterenol Hydrochloride (Plasma concentrations of motility agents may be decreased with concomitant use of nevirapine).

No products indexed under this heading.

Isoproterenol Sulfate (Plasma concentrations of motility agents may be decreased with concomitant use of nevirapine).

No products indexed under this heading.

Isradipine (Plasma concentrations of calcium channel blockers may be decreased with concomitant use of nevirapine). Products include:

DynaCirc CR Controlled Release Tablets ... 1407

Itraconazole (Plasma concentrations of antifungals may be decreased with concomitant use of nevirapine).

No products indexed under this heading.

Ketoconazole (Nevirapine and ketoconazole should not be administered concomitantly because decreases in ketoconazole plasma concentrations may reduce the efficacy of the drug). Products include:

Extina Foam, 2% ... 3057
Nizoral A-D Shampoo ... 1901

Lamotrigine (Plasma concentrations of anticonvulsants may be decreased with concomitant use of nevirapine). Products include:

Lamictal ... 1488

Levalbuterol Hydrochloride (Plasma concentrations of motility agents may be decreased with concomitant use of nevirapine). Products include:

Xopenex Inhalation Solution ... 3001
Xopenex Inhalation Solution Concentrate ... 3005

Levamisole Hydrochloride (Plasma concentrations of cancer chemotherapeutic agents may be decreased with concomitant use of nevirapine).

No products indexed under this heading.

Levetiracetam (Plasma concentrations of anticonvulsants may be decreased with concomitant use of nevirapine). Products include:

Keppra Injection ... 3137
Keppra Oral Solution ... 3131
Keppra Tablets ... 3131

Levonorgestrel (Oral contraceptives and other hormonal methods of birth control should not be used as the sole method of contraception in women taking nevirapine, since nevirapine may lower the plasma levels of these medications. An alternative or additional method of contraception is recommended). Products include:

Climara Pro Transdermal System ... 768
Lybrel Tablets ... 3204
Mirena Intrauterine System ... 779
Plan B Tablets ... 1044
Seasonique Tablets ... 1046

Levorphanol Tartrate (Plasma concentrations of motility agents may be decreased with concomitant use of nevirapine).

No products indexed under this heading.

Lidocaine (Nevirapine is principally metabolized by the liver via cytochrome P450 isoenzymes 3A and 2B6. Nevirapine is known to be an inducer of these enzymes. As a result, drugs that are metabolized by these enzyme systems may have lower than expected plasma levels when co-administered with nevirapine). Products include:

Lidoderm Patch ... 1114

Lidocaine Hydrochloride (Plasma concentrations of antiarrhythmics may be decreased with concomitant use of nevirapine).

No products indexed under this heading.

Lomustine (CCNU) (Plasma concentrations of cancer chemotherapeutic agents may be decreased with concomitant use of nevirapine).

No products indexed under this heading.

Lopinavir (A dose increase of lopinavir/ritonavir tablets to 100/150 mg b.i.d. may be considered when used in combination with nevirapine in treatment experienced patients where decreased susceptibility to lopinavir is suspected. A dose increase of lopinavir/ritonavir oral solution to 533/133 mg b.i.d. with food is recommended in combination with nevirapine. In children 6 months to 12 years of age, consideration should be given to increasing the dose of lopinavir/ritonavir to 12/3.25 mg/kg for those 7 to less than 15 kg; 11/2.75 mg/kg for those 15 to 45 kg; and a maximum dose of 533/133 mg for those greater than 45 kg b.i.d. when used in combination with nevirapine, particularly for patients in who reduced susceptibility to lopinavir/ritonavir is suspected). Products include:

Kaletra ... 452

Lovastatin (Nevirapine is principally metabolized by the liver via cytochrome P450 isoenzymes 3A and 2B6. Nevirapine is known to be an inducer of these enzymes. As a result, drugs that are metabolized by these enzyme systems may have lower than expected plasma levels when co-administered with nevirapine). Products include:

Advicor Tablets ... 402
Mevacor Tablets ... 2063

Low Molecular Weight Heparins (Plasma concentrations of antithrombotics may be increased with concomitant use of nevirapine. This may have a potential effect on anticoagulation. Monitoring of anticoagulation levels is recommended).

No products indexed under this heading.

Maprotiline Hydrochloride (Plasma concentrations of motility agents may be decreased with concomitant use of nevirapine).

No products indexed under this heading.

Mechlorethamine Hydrochloride (Plasma concentrations of cancer chemotherapeutic agents may be decreased with concomitant use of nevirapine). Products include:

Mustargen for Injection ... 2492

Megestrol Acetate (Plasma concentrations of cancer chemotherapeutic agents may be decreased with concomitant use of nevirapine). Products include:

Megace ES Oral Suspension ... 2499

Melphalan (Plasma concentrations of cancer chemotherapeutic agents may be decreased with concomitant use of nevirapine).

No products indexed under this heading.

Mepenzolate Bromide (Plasma concentrations of motility agents may be decreased with concomitant use of nevirapine).

No products indexed under this heading.

Meperidine Hydrochloride (Plasma concentrations of motility agents may be decreased with concomitant use of nevirapine).

No products indexed under this heading.

Mephenytoin (Plasma concentrations of anticonvulsants may be decreased with concomitant use of nevirapine).

No products indexed under this heading.

Mercaptopurine (Plasma concentrations of cancer chemotherapeutic agents may be decreased with concomitant use of nevirapine).

No products indexed under this heading.

Mestranol (Oral contraceptives and other hormonal methods of birth control should not be used as the sole method of contraception in women taking nevirapine, since nevirapine may lower the plasma levels of these medications. An alternative or additional method of contraception is recommended).

No products indexed under this heading.

Metaproterenol Sulfate (Plasma concentrations of motility agents may be decreased with concomitant use of nevirapine).

No products indexed under this heading.

Methadone Hydrochloride (Methadone levels were decreased; increased dosages may be required to prevent symptoms of opiate withdrawal. Methadone maintained patients beginning nevirapine therapy should be monitored for evidence of withdrawal and methadone dose should be adjusted accordingly).

No products indexed under this heading.

Methdilazine Hydrochloride (Plasma concentrations of motility agents may be decreased with concomitant use of nevirapine).

No products indexed under this heading.

Methotrexate Sodium (Plasma concentrations of cancer chemotherapeutic agents may be decreased with concomitant use of nevirapine).

No products indexed under this heading.

Methsuximide (Plasma concentrations of anticonvulsants may be decreased with concomitant use of nevirapine).

No products indexed under this heading.

Methylergonovine Maleate (Plasma concentrations of ergot alkaloids may be decreased with concomitant use of nevirapine).

No products indexed under this heading.

Methysergide Maleate (Plasma concentrations of ergot alkaloids may be decreased with concomitant use of nevirapine).

No products indexed under this heading.

Metoclopramide Hydrochloride (Plasma concentrations of motility agents may be decreased with concomitant use of nevirapine).

No products indexed under this heading.

Mexiletine Hydrochloride (Plasma concentrations of antiarrhythmics may be decreased with concomitant use of nevirapine).
No products indexed under this heading.

Mibefradil Dihydrochloride (Plasma concentrations of calcium channel blockers may be decreased with concomitant use of nevirapine).
No products indexed under this heading.

Miconazole (Plasma concentrations of antifungals may be decreased with concomitant use of nevirapine).
No products indexed under this heading.

Midazolam Hydrochloride (Nevirapine is principally metabolized by the liver via cytochrome P450 isoenzymes 3A and 2B6. Nevirapine is known to be an inducer of these enzymes. As a result, drugs that are metabolized by these enzyme systems may have lower than expected plasma levels when co-administered with nevirapine).
No products indexed under this heading.

Mitomycin (Mitomycin-C) (Plasma concentrations of cancer chemotherapeutic agents may be decreased with concomitant use of nevirapine).
No products indexed under this heading.

Mitotane (Plasma concentrations of cancer chemotherapeutic agents may be decreased with concomitant use of nevirapine).
No products indexed under this heading.

Mitoxantrone Hydrochloride (Plasma concentrations of cancer chemotherapeutic agents may be decreased with concomitant use of nevirapine). Products include:
Novantrone for Injection Concentrate ... **1100**

Moricizine Hydrochloride (Plasma concentrations of antiarrhythmics may be decreased with concomitant use of nevirapine).
No products indexed under this heading.

Morphine Sulfate (Plasma concentrations of motility agents may be decreased with concomitant use of nevirapine). Products include:
Avinza Capsules ... **1772**
DepoDur Injection ... **1095**
MS Contin Tablets ... **2585**

Muromonab-CD3 (Plasma concentrations of cancer immunosuppressants agents may be decreased with concomitant use of nevirapine). Products include:
Orthoclone OKT3 Sterile Solution ... **2387**

Mycophenolate Mofetil (Plasma concentrations of cancer immunosuppressants agents may be decreased with concomitant use of nevirapine). Products include:
CellCept Capsules ... **2622**
CellCept Oral Suspension ... **2622**
CellCept Tablets ... **2622**

Nefazodone Hydrochloride (Nevirapine is principally metabolized by the liver via cytochrome P450 isoenzymes 3A and 2B6. Nevirapine is known to be an inducer of these enzymes. As a result, drugs that are metabolized by these enzyme systems may have lower than expected plasma levels when co-administered with nevirapine).
No products indexed under this heading.

Nelfinavir Mesylate (Concomitant use with nevirapine has shown a decrease in nelfinavir M8 metabolite concentrations and a decrease in nevirapine Cmin. The appropriate dose for nelfinavir in combination with nevirapine, with respect to safety and efficacy, has not been established).
No products indexed under this heading.

Neostigmine Bromide (Plasma concentrations of motility agents may be decreased with concomitant use of nevirapine).
No products indexed under this heading.

Neostigmine Methylsulfate (Plasma concentrations of motility agents may be decreased with concomitant use of nevirapine).
No products indexed under this heading.

Nicardipine (Nevirapine is principally metabolized by the liver via cytochrome P450 isoenzymes 3A and 2B6. Nevirapine is known to be an inducer of these enzymes. As a result, drugs that are metabolized by these enzyme systems may have lower than expected plasma levels when co-administered with nevirapine).
No products indexed under this heading.

Nicardipine Hydrochloride (Plasma concentrations of calcium channel blockers may be decreased with concomitant use of nevirapine). Products include:
Cardene I.V. ... **1093**

Nifedipine (Plasma concentrations of calcium channel blockers may be decreased with concomitant use of nevirapine).
No products indexed under this heading.

Nimodipine (Plasma concentrations of calcium channel blockers may be decreased with concomitant use of nevirapine). Products include:
Nimotop Capsules ... **790**

Nisoldipine (Plasma concentrations of calcium channel blockers may be decreased with concomitant use of nevirapine). Products include:
Sular Extended Release Tablets ... **2975**

Norethindrone (Oral contraceptives and other hormonal methods of birth control should not be used as the sole method of contraception in women taking nevirapine, since nevirapine may lower the plasma levels of these medications. An alternative or additional method of contraception is recommended). Products include:
Ortho Micronor Tablets ... **2446**

Norethindrone Acetate (Oral contraceptives and other hormonal methods of birth control should not be used as the sole method of contraception in women taking nevirapine, since nevirapine may lower the plasma levels of these medications. An alternative or additional method of contraception is recommended). Products include:
Activella Tablets ... **2347**

Norethynodrel (Oral contraceptives and other hormonal methods of birth control should not be used as the sole method of contraception in women taking nevirapine, since nevirapine may lower the plasma levels of these medications. An alternative or additional method of contraception is recommended).
No products indexed under this heading.

Norgestimate (Oral contraceptives and other hormonal methods of birth control should not be used as the sole method of contraception in women taking nevirapine, since nevirapine may lower the plasma levels of these medications. An alternative or additional method of contraception is recommended). Products include:
Ortho-Cyclen/Ortho Tri-Cyclen ... **2449**
Ortho Tri-Cyclen Lo Tablets ... **2458**

Norgestrel (Oral contraceptives and other hormonal methods of birth control should not be used as the sole method of contraception in women taking nevirapine, since nevirapine may lower the plasma levels of these medications. An alternative or additional method of contraception is recommended).
No products indexed under this heading.

Nortriptyline Hydrochloride (Plasma concentrations of motility agents may be decreased with concomitant use of nevirapine).
No products indexed under this heading.

Octreotide Acetate (Plasma concentrations of motility agents may be decreased with concomitant use of nevirapine). Products include:
Sandostatin Injection ... **2300**
Sandostatin LAR Depot ... **2302**

Ondansetron Hydrochloride (Nevirapine is principally metabolized by the liver via cytochrome P450 isoenzymes 3A and 2B6. Nevirapine is known to be an inducer of these enzymes. As a result, drugs that are metabolized by these enzyme systems may have lower than expected plasma levels when co-administered with nevirapine). Products include:
Zofran Injection ... **1682**
Zofran ... **1687**

Oxaliplatin (Plasma concentrations of cancer chemotherapeutic agents may be decreased with concomitant use of nevirapine). Products include:
Eloxatin for Injection ... **2731**

Oxcarbazepine (Plasma concentrations of anticonvulsants may be decreased with concomitant use of nevirapine).
No products indexed under this heading.

Oxiconazole Nitrate (Plasma concentrations of antifungals may be decreased with concomitant use of nevirapine).
No products indexed under this heading.

Oxybutynin Chloride (Plasma concentrations of motility agents may be decreased with concomitant use of nevirapine).
No products indexed under this heading.

Oxycodone Hydrochloride (Plasma concentrations of motility agents may be decreased with concomitant use of nevirapine). Products include:
OxyContin Tablets ... **2589**
OxyIR Capsules ... **2593**
Percocet Tablets ... **1127**
Percodan Tablets ... **1130**

Oxyphenonium Bromide (Plasma concentrations of motility agents may be decreased with concomitant use of nevirapine).
No products indexed under this heading.

Paclitaxel (Plasma concentrations of cancer chemotherapeutic agents may be decreased with concomitant use of nevirapine).
No products indexed under this heading.

Paramethadione (Plasma concentrations of anticonvulsants may be decreased with concomitant use of nevirapine).
No products indexed under this heading.

Pergolide Mesylate (Plasma concentrations of motility agents may be decreased with concomitant use of nevirapine).
No products indexed under this heading.

Phenacemide (Plasma concentrations of anticonvulsants may be decreased with concomitant use of nevirapine).
No products indexed under this heading.

Phenobarbital (Plasma concentrations of anticonvulsants may be decreased with concomitant use of nevirapine). Products include:
Donnatal Extentabs ... **2507**

Phensuximide (Plasma concentrations of anticonvulsants may be decreased with concomitant use of nevirapine).
No products indexed under this heading.

Phenytoin (Plasma concentrations of anticonvulsants may be decreased with concomitant use of nevirapine).
No products indexed under this heading.

Phenytoin Sodium (Plasma concentrations of anticonvulsants may be decreased with concomitant use of nevirapine). Products include:
Phenytek Capsules ... **2192**

Pimozide (Nevirapine is principally metabolized by the liver via cytochrome P450 isoenzymes 3A and 2B6. Nevirapine is known to be an inducer of these enzymes. As a result, drugs that are metabolized by these enzyme systems may have lower than expected plasma levels when co-administered with nevirapine).
No products indexed under this heading.

Pirbuterol Acetate (Plasma concentrations of motility agents may be decreased with concomitant use of nevirapine). Products include:
Maxair Autohaler ... **1705**

Posaconazole (Plasma concentrations of antifungals may be decreased with concomitant use of nevirapine). Products include:
Noxafil Oral Suspension ... **2889**

Pramipexole Dihydrochloride (Plasma concentrations of motility agents may be decreased with concomitant use of nevirapine). Products include:
Mirapex Tablets ... **857**

Primidone (Plasma concentrations of anticonvulsants may be decreased with concomitant use of nevirapine).

No products indexed under this heading.

Procainamide Hydrochloride (Plasma concentrations of antiarrhythmics may be decreased with concomitant use of nevirapine).

No products indexed under this heading.

Procarbazine Hydrochloride (Plasma concentrations of cancer chemotherapeutic agents may be decreased with concomitant use of nevirapine).

No products indexed under this heading.

Procyclidine Hydrochloride (Plasma concentrations of motility agents may be decreased with concomitant use of nevirapine).

No products indexed under this heading.

Promethazine Hydrochloride (Plasma concentrations of motility agents may be decreased with concomitant use of nevirapine).

No products indexed under this heading.

Propafenone Hydrochloride (Plasma concentrations of antiarrhythmics may be decreased with concomitant use of nevirapine). Products include:

Rythmol Tablets **1586**
Rythmol SR Capsules **1590**

Propantheline Bromide (Plasma concentrations of motility agents may be decreased with concomitant use of nevirapine).

No products indexed under this heading.

Propoxyphene Hydrochloride (Plasma concentrations of motility agents may be decreased with concomitant use of nevirapine).

No products indexed under this heading.

Propoxyphene Napsylate (Plasma concentrations of motility agents may be decreased with concomitant use of nevirapine).

No products indexed under this heading.

Propranolol Hydrochloride (Plasma concentrations of antiarrhythmics may be decreased with concomitant use of nevirapine). Products include:

InnoPran XL Extended Release Capsules **1484**

Protriptyline Hydrochloride (Plasma concentrations of motility agents may be decreased with concomitant use of nevirapine).

No products indexed under this heading.

Pyridostigmine Bromide (Plasma concentrations of motility agents may be decreased with concomitant use of nevirapine).

No products indexed under this heading.

Pyrilamine Maleate (Plasma concentrations of motility agents may be decreased with concomitant use of nevirapine).

No products indexed under this heading.

Pyrilamine Tannate (Plasma concentrations of motility agents may be decreased with concomitant use of nevirapine).

No products indexed under this heading.

Quinidine Gluconate (Plasma concentrations of antiarrhythmics may be decreased with concomitant use of nevirapine).

No products indexed under this heading.

Quinidine Polygalacturonate (Plasma concentrations of antiarrhythmics may be decreased with concomitant use of nevirapine).

No products indexed under this heading.

Quinidine Sulfate (Plasma concentrations of antiarrhythmics may be decreased with concomitant use of nevirapine).

No products indexed under this heading.

Quinine (Nevirapine is principally metabolized by the liver via cytochrome P450 isoenzymes 3A and 2B6. Nevirapine is known to be an inducer of these enzymes. As a result, drugs that are metabolized by these enzyme systems may have lower than expected plasma levels when co-administered with nevirapine).

No products indexed under this heading.

Quinine Sulfate (Nevirapine is principally metabolized by the liver via cytochrome P450 isoenzymes 3A and 2B6. Nevirapine is known to be an inducer of these enzymes. As a result, drugs that are metabolized by these enzyme systems may have lower than expected plasma levels when co-administered with nevirapine).

No products indexed under this heading.

Remifentanil Hydrochloride (Plasma concentrations of motility agents may be decreased with concomitant use of nevirapine).

No products indexed under this heading.

Rifabutin (Rifabutin and its metabolite concentrations were moderately increased. Due to high inter-subject variability; however, some patients may experience large increases in rifabutin exposure and may be at higher risk for rifabutin toxicity. Therefore, caution should be used in concomitant administration).

No products indexed under this heading.

Rifampin (Nevirapine and rifampin should not be administered concomitantly because decreases in nevirapine plasma concentrations may reduce the efficacy of the drug. Physicians needing to treat patients co-infected with tuberculosis and using a nevirapine-containing regimen may use rifabutin instead).

No products indexed under this heading.

Ritonavir (A dose increase of lopinavir/ritonavir tablets to 100/150 mg b.i.d. may be considered when used in combination with nevirapine in treatment experienced patients where decreased susceptibility to lopinavir is suspected. A dose increase of lopinavir/ritonavir oral solution to 533/133 mg b.i.d. with food is recommended in combination with nevirapine. In children 6 months to 12 years of age, consideration should be given to increasing the dose of lopinavir/ritonavir to 12/3.25 mg/kg for those 7 to less than 15 kg; 11/2.75 mg/kg for those 15 to 45 kg; and a maximum dose of 533/133 mg for those greater than 45 kg b.i.d. when used in combination with nevirapine, particularly for patients in who reduced susceptibility to lopinavir/ritonavir is suspected). Products include:

Kaletra **452**
Norvir **489**

Rivastigmine Tartrate (Plasma concentrations of motility agents may be decreased with concomitant use of nevirapine). Products include:

Exelon Capsules **2229**
Exelon Oral Solution **2229**
Exelon Patch **2233**

Ropinirole Hydrochloride (Plasma concentrations of motility agents may be decreased with concomitant use of nevirapine). Products include:

Requip Tablets **1561**
Requip XL Tablets **1568**

Salmeterol Xinafoate (Plasma concentrations of motility agents may be decreased with concomitant use of nevirapine). Products include:

Advair Diskus 100/50 .... **1276**
Advair Diskus 250/50 .... **1276**
Advair Diskus 500/50 .... **1276**
Advair HFA 45/21 Inhalation Aerosol **1288**
Advair HFA 115/21 Inhalation Aerosol **1288**
Advair HFA 230/21 Inhalation Aerosol **1288**
Serevent Diskus **1594**

Saquinavir (Concomitant use with nevirapine may decrease the concentrations of saquinavir. Appropriate doses for this combination are not established, but an increase in the dosage of saquinavir may be required).

No products indexed under this heading.

Saquinavir Mesylate (Concomitant use with nevirapine may decrease the concentrations of saquinavir. Appropriate doses for this combination are not established, but an increase in the dosage of saquinavir may be required).

No products indexed under this heading.

Scopolamine (Plasma concentrations of motility agents may be decreased with concomitant use of nevirapine). Products include:

Transderm Scōp Transdermal Therapeutic System **2206**

Scopolamine Hydrobromide (Plasma concentrations of motility agents may be decreased with concomitant use of nevirapine). Products include:

Donnatal Extentabs **2507**

Sertraline Hydrochloride (Nevirapine is principally metabolized by the liver via cytochrome P450 isoenzymes 3A and 2B6. Nevirapine is known to be an inducer of these enzymes. As a result, drugs that are metabolized by these enzyme systems may have lower than expected plasma levels when co-administered with nevirapine).

No products indexed under this heading.

Sildenafil Citrate (Nevirapine is principally metabolized by the liver via cytochrome P450 isoenzymes 3A and 2B6. Nevirapine is known to be an inducer of these enzymes. As a result, drugs that are metabolized by these enzyme systems may have lower than expected plasma levels when co-administered with nevirapine).

No products indexed under this heading.

Simvastatin (Nevirapine is principally metabolized by the liver via cytochrome P450 isoenzymes 3A and 2B6. Nevirapine is known to be an inducer of these enzymes. As a result, drugs that are metabolized by these enzyme systems may have lower than expected plasma levels when co-administered with nevirapine). Products include:

Simcor Tablets **502**
Vytorin 10/10 Tablets **2149**
Vytorin 10/10 Tablets **2939**
Vytorin 10/20 Tablets **2149**
Vytorin 10/20 Tablets **2939**
Vytorin 10/40 Tablets **2149**
Vytorin 10/40 Tablets **2939**
Vytorin 10/80 Tablets **2149**
Vytorin 10/80 Tablets **2939**
Zocor Tablets **2136**

Sirolimus (Plasma concentrations of cancer immunosuppressants agents may be decreased with concomitant use of nevirapine). Products include:

Rapamune **3260**

Sotalol Hydrochloride (Plasma concentrations of antiarrhythmics may be decreased with concomitant use of nevirapine).

No products indexed under this heading.

Streptozocin (Plasma concentrations of cancer chemotherapeutic agents may be decreased with concomitant use of nevirapine).

No products indexed under this heading.

Sucralfate (Plasma concentrations of motility agents may be decreased with concomitant use of nevirapine). Products include:

Carafate Suspension **706**
Carafate Tablets **707**

Sufentanil Citrate (Plasma concentrations of motility agents may be decreased with concomitant use of nevirapine).

No products indexed under this heading.

Tacrine Hydrochloride (Plasma concentrations of motility agents may be decreased with concomitant use of nevirapine).

No products indexed under this heading.

Tacrolimus (Plasma concentrations of cancer immunosuppressants agents may be decreased with concomitant use of nevirapine). Products include:

Prograf Capsules and Injection **622**
Protopic Ointment **628**

Tamoxifen Citrate (Plasma concentrations of cancer chemotherapeutic agents may be decreased with concomitant use of nevirapine).

No products indexed under this heading.

Teniposide (Plasma concentrations of cancer chemotherapeutic agents may be decreased with concomitant use of nevirapine).

No products indexed under this heading.

Terbutaline Sulfate (Plasma concentrations of motility agents may be decreased with concomitant use of nevirapine).

No products indexed under this heading.

Terconazole (Plasma concentrations of antifungals may be decreased with concomitant use of nevirapine).

No products indexed under this heading.

Terfenadine (Nevirapine is principally metabolized by the liver via cytochrome P450 isoenzymes 3A and 2B6. Nevirapine is known to be an inducer of these enzymes. As a result, drugs that are metabolized by these enzyme systems may have lower than expected plasma levels when co-administered with nevirapine).
No products indexed under this heading.

Testosterone (Nevirapine is principally metabolized by the liver via cytochrome P450 isoenzymes 3A and 2B6. Nevirapine is known to be an inducer of these enzymes. As a result, drugs that are metabolized by these enzyme systems may have lower than expected plasma levels when co-administered with nevirapine). Products include:
AndroGel 3159
Testim 1% Gel 701

Testosterone Cypionate (Nevirapine is principally metabolized by the liver via cytochrome P450 isoenzymes 3A and 2B6. Nevirapine is known to be an inducer of these enzymes. As a result, drugs that are metabolized by these enzyme systems may have lower than expected plasma levels when co-administered with nevirapine).
No products indexed under this heading.

Testosterone Enanthate (Nevirapine is principally metabolized by the liver via cytochrome P450 isoenzymes 3A and 2B6. Nevirapine is known to be an inducer of these enzymes. As a result, drugs that are metabolized by these enzyme systems may have lower than expected plasma levels when co-administered with nevirapine). Products include:
Delatestryl Injection 1730

Testosterone Propionate (Nevirapine is principally metabolized by the liver via cytochrome P450 isoenzymes 3A and 2B6. Nevirapine is known to be an inducer of these enzymes. As a result, drugs that are metabolized by these enzyme systems may have lower than expected plasma levels when co-administered with nevirapine).
No products indexed under this heading.

Theophylline (Nevirapine is principally metabolized by the liver via cytochrome P450 isoenzymes 3A and 2B6. Nevirapine is known to be an inducer of these enzymes. As a result, drugs that are metabolized by these enzyme systems may have lower than expected plasma levels when co-administered with nevirapine).
No products indexed under this heading.

Theophylline Anhydrous (Nevirapine is principally metabolized by the liver via cytochrome P450 isoenzymes 3A and 2B6. Nevirapine is known to be an inducer of these enzymes. As a result, drugs that are metabolized by these enzyme systems may have lower than expected plasma levels when co-administered with nevirapine). Products include:
Uniphyl Tablets 2595

Theophylline Calcium Salicylate (Nevirapine is principally metabolized by the liver via cytochrome P450 isoenzymes 3A and 2B6. Nevirapine is known to be an inducer of these enzymes. As a result, drugs that are metabolized by these enzyme systems may have lower than expected plasma levels when co-administered with nevirapine).
No products indexed under this heading.

Theophylline Sodium Glycinate (Nevirapine is principally metabolized by the liver via cytochrome P450 isoenzymes 3A and 2B6. Nevirapine is known to be an inducer of these enzymes. As a result, drugs that are metabolized by these enzyme systems may have lower than expected plasma levels when co-administered with nevirapine).
No products indexed under this heading.

Thioguanine (Plasma concentrations of cancer chemotherapeutic agents may be decreased with concomitant use of nevirapine). Products include:
Tabloid Tablets 1601

Thiotepa (Plasma concentrations of cancer chemotherapeutic agents may be decreased with concomitant use of nevirapine).
No products indexed under this heading.

Tiagabine Hydrochloride (Plasma concentrations of anticonvulsants may be decreased with concomitant use of nevirapine). Products include:
Gabitril Tablets 973

Tinzaparin Sodium (Plasma concentrations of antithrombotics may be increased with concomitant use of nevirapine. This may have a potential effect on anticoagulation. Monitoring of anticoagulation levels is recommended).
No products indexed under this heading.

Tocainide Hydrochloride (Plasma concentrations of antiarrhythmics may be decreased with concomitant use of nevirapine).
No products indexed under this heading.

Tolterodine Tartrate (Plasma concentrations of motility agents may be decreased with concomitant use of nevirapine).
No products indexed under this heading.

Topiramate (Plasma concentrations of anticonvulsants may be decreased with concomitant use of nevirapine).
No products indexed under this heading.

Topotecan Hydrochloride (Plasma concentrations of cancer chemotherapeutic agents may be decreased with concomitant use of nevirapine). Products include:
Hycamtin for Injection 1459
Hycamtin Capsules 1456

Toremifene Citrate (Plasma concentrations of cancer chemotherapeutic agents may be decreased with concomitant use of nevirapine).
No products indexed under this heading.

Trazodone Hydrochloride (Nevirapine is principally metabolized by the liver via cytochrome P450 isoenzymes 3A and 2B6. Nevirapine is known to be an inducer of these enzymes. As a result, drugs that are metabolized by these enzyme systems may have lower than expected plasma levels when co-administered with nevirapine).
No products indexed under this heading.

Triazolam (Nevirapine is principally metabolized by the liver via cytochrome P450 isoenzymes 3A and 2B6. Nevirapine is known to be an inducer of these enzymes. As a result, drugs that are metabolized by these enzyme systems may have lower than expected plasma levels when co-administered with nevirapine).
No products indexed under this heading.

Tridihexethyl Chloride (Plasma concentrations of motility agents may be decreased with concomitant use of nevirapine).
No products indexed under this heading.

Trihexyphenidyl Hydrochloride (Plasma concentrations of motility agents may be decreased with concomitant use of nevirapine).
No products indexed under this heading.

Trimeprazine Tartrate (Plasma concentrations of motility agents may be decreased with concomitant use of nevirapine).
No products indexed under this heading.

Trimethadione (Plasma concentrations of anticonvulsants may be decreased with concomitant use of nevirapine).
No products indexed under this heading.

Trimipramine Maleate (Plasma concentrations of motility agents may be decreased with concomitant use of nevirapine).
No products indexed under this heading.

Tripelennamine Hydrochloride (Plasma concentrations of motility agents may be decreased with concomitant use of nevirapine).
No products indexed under this heading.

Triprolidine Hydrochloride (Plasma concentrations of motility agents may be decreased with concomitant use of nevirapine).
No products indexed under this heading.

Valproate Sodium (Plasma concentrations of anticonvulsants may be decreased with concomitant use of nevirapine).
No products indexed under this heading.

Valproic Acid (Plasma concentrations of anticonvulsants may be decreased with concomitant use of nevirapine).
No products indexed under this heading.

Valrubicin (Plasma concentrations of cancer chemotherapeutic agents may be decreased with concomitant use of nevirapine). Products include:
Valstar Sterile Solution for Intravesical Instillation 1735

Venlafaxine Hydrochloride (Nevirapine is principally metabolized by the liver via cytochrome P450 isoenzymes 3A and 2B6. Nevirapine is known to be an inducer of these enzymes. As a result, drugs that are metabolized by these enzyme systems may have lower than expected plasma levels when co-administered with nevirapine). Products include:
Effexor XR Extended-Release Capsules 3195
Venlafaxine Hydrochloride Tablets ... 2199

Verapamil Hydrochloride (Plasma concentrations of antiarrhythmics may be decreased with concomitant use of nevirapine). Products include:
Tarka Tablets 511

Vinblastine Sulfate (Nevirapine is principally metabolized by the liver via cytochrome P450 isoenzymes 3A and 2B6. Nevirapine is known to be an inducer of these enzymes. As a result, drugs that are metabolized by these enzyme systems may have lower than expected plasma levels when co-administered with nevirapine).
No products indexed under this heading.

Vincristine Sulfate (Plasma concentrations of cancer chemotherapeutic agents may be decreased with concomitant use of nevirapine).
No products indexed under this heading.

Vinorelbine Tartrate (Plasma concentrations of cancer chemotherapeutic agents may be decreased with concomitant use of nevirapine).
No products indexed under this heading.

Voriconazole (Plasma concentrations of antifungals may be decreased with concomitant use of nevirapine).
No products indexed under this heading.

Warfarin Sodium (The interaction between nevirapine and the antithrombotic agent warfarin is complex. As a result, when giving these drugs concomitantly, plasma warfarin levels may change with the potential for increases in coagulation time. When warfarin is co-administered with nevirapine, anticoagulation levels should be monitored frequently).
No products indexed under this heading.

Zidovudine (When zidovudine was co-administered with nevirapine, the AUC and Cmax of zidovudine were decreased by 28% and 30%, respectively). Products include:
Combivir Tablets 1384
Retrovir 1574
Retrovir IV Infusion 1579
Trizivir Tablets 1622

Zonisamide (Plasma concentrations of anticonvulsants may be decreased with concomitant use of nevirapine). Products include:
Zonegran Capsules 1089

VIREAD TABLETS

(Tenofovir Disoproxil Fumarate) 1268
May interact with nephrotoxic agents, inhibitors of renal tubular secretion or resorption, and certain other agents. Compounds in these categories include:

Abacavir Sulfate (Drugs that decrease renal function may increase serum concentrations of tenofovir. Tenofovir should be avoided with concomitant or recent use of a nephrotoxic agent). Products include:
Epzicom Tablets 1422

IMPORTANT NOTE: Always consult each drug listing in the patient's regimen for possible interactions.

Trizivir Tablets 1622
Ziagen 1673

Acyclovir (Co-administration with drugs that reduce renal function or compete for active tubular secretion may increase serum concentrations of tenofovir and/or increase the concentrations of other renally eliminated drugs, such as acyclovir).
Products include:
Zovirax 1690
Zovirax Cream 817
Zovirax Ointment 819

Acyclovir Sodium (Co-administration with drugs that reduce renal function or compete for active tubular secretion may increase serum concentrations of tenofovir and/or increase the concentrations of other renally eliminated drugs, such as acyclovir).
No products indexed under this heading.

Alatrofloxacin Mesylate (Drugs that decrease renal function may increase serum concentrations of tenofovir. Tenofovir should be avoided with concomittant or recent use of a nephrotoxic agent).
No products indexed under this heading.

Aldesleukin (Drugs that decrease renal function may increase serum concentrations of tenofovir. Tenofovir should be avoided with concomittant or recent use of a nephrotoxic agent). Products include:
Proleukin for Injection 2287

Amikacin Sulfate (Drugs that decrease renal function may increase serum concentrations of tenofovir. Tenofovir should be avoided with concomittant or recent use of a nephrotoxic agent).
No products indexed under this heading.

Amoxicillin (Drugs that decrease renal function may increase serum concentrations of tenofovir. Tenofovir should be avoided with concomittant or recent use of a nephrotoxic agent). Products include:
Amoxil Capsules 1305
Amoxil Chewable Tablets 1305
Amoxil Pediatric Drops for Oral Suspension 1305
Amoxil Powder for Oral Suspension 1305
Amoxil Tablets 1305
Augmentin 1323
Augmentin Tablets 1327
Augmentin XR Extended Release Tablets 1333
Augmentin ES-600 Powder for Oral Suspension 1329
Moxatag Tablets 2165

Amoxicillin Trihydrate (Drugs that decrease renal function may increase serum concentrations of tenofovir. Tenofovir should be avoided with concomittant or recent use of a nephrotoxic agent).
No products indexed under this heading.

Amphotericin B (Drugs that decrease renal function may increase serum concentrations of tenofovir. Tenofovir should be avoided with concomittant or recent use of a nephrotoxic agent).
No products indexed under this heading.

Amphotericin B, liposomal (Drugs that decrease renal function may increase serum concentrations of tenofovir. Tenofovir should be avoided with concomittant or recent use of a nephrotoxic agent).
Products include:
AmBisome for Injection 606

Amphotericin B Cholesteryl Sulfate (Drugs that decrease renal function may increase serum concentrations of tenofovir. Tenofovir should be avoided with concomittant or recent use of a nephrotoxic agent).
No products indexed under this heading.

Amphotericin B Lipid Complex (Drugs that decrease renal function may increase serum concentrations of tenofovir. Tenofovir should be avoided with concomittant or recent use of a nephrotoxic agent).
Products include:
Abelcet Injection 1134

Ampicillin (Drugs that decrease renal function may increase serum concentrations of tenofovir. Tenofovir should be avoided with concomittant or recent use of a nephrotoxic agent).
No products indexed under this heading.

Ampicillin Sodium (Drugs that decrease renal function may increase serum concentrations of tenofovir. Tenofovir should be avoided with concomittant or recent use of a nephrotoxic agent).
No products indexed under this heading.

Ampicillin Trihydrate (Drugs that decrease renal function may increase serum concentrations of tenofovir. Tenofovir should be avoided with concomittant or recent use of a nephrotoxic agent).
No products indexed under this heading.

Amprenavir (Drugs that decrease renal function may increase serum concentrations of tenofovir. Tenofovir should be avoided with concomittant or recent use of a nephrotoxic agent).
No products indexed under this heading.

Aspirin (Drugs that decrease renal function may increase serum concentrations of tenofovir. Tenofovir should be avoided with concomittant or recent use of a nephrotoxic agent). Products include:
Aggrenox Capsules 819
Bayer Aspirin 750
Percodan Tablets 1130
St. Joseph 81 mg Aspirin Chewable and Enteric Coated Tablets 1903

Atazanavir (Tenofovir decreases the AUC and Cmin of atazanavir. When co-administered with tenofovir, it is recommended that atazanavir 300mg is given with ritonavir 100mg. Atazanavir without ritonavir should not be co-administered with tenofovir. Atazanavir may increase the Cmax, AUC and Cmin of tenofovir).
No products indexed under this heading.

Atazanavir Sulfate (Tenofovir decreases the AUC and Cmin of atazanavir. When co-administered with tenofovir, it is recommended that atazanavir 300mg is given with ritonavir 100mg. Atazanavir without ritonavir should not be co-administered with tenofovir. Atazanavir may increase the Cmax, AUC and Cmin of tenofovir). Products include:
Reyataz Capsules 3299

Atorvastatin Calcium (Drugs that decrease renal function may increase serum concentrations of tenofovir. Tenofovir should be avoided with concomittant or recent use of a nephrotoxic agent).
Products include:
Lipitor Tablets 2501

Azithromycin Dihydrate (Drugs that decrease renal function may increase serum concentrations of tenofovir. Tenofovir should be avoided with concomittant or recent use of a nephrotoxic agent).
No products indexed under this heading.

Azlocillin Sodium (Drugs that decrease renal function may increase serum concentrations of tenofovir. Tenofovir should be avoided with concomittant or recent use of a nephrotoxic agent).
No products indexed under this heading.

Aztreonam (Drugs that decrease renal function may increase serum concentrations of tenofovir. Tenofovir should be avoided with concomittant or recent use of a nephrotoxic agent).
No products indexed under this heading.

Bacampicillin Hydrochloride (Drugs that decrease renal function may increase serum concentrations of tenofovir. Tenofovir should be avoided with concomittant or recent use of a nephrotoxic agent).
No products indexed under this heading.

Balsalazide Disodium (Drugs that decrease renal function may increase serum concentrations of tenofovir. Tenofovir should be avoided with concomittant or recent use of a nephrotoxic agent).
No products indexed under this heading.

Benazepril Hydrochloride (Drugs that decrease renal function may increase serum concentrations of tenofovir. Tenofovir should be avoided with concomittant or recent use of a nephrotoxic agent).
No products indexed under this heading.

Bendroflumethiazide (Drugs that decrease renal function may increase serum concentrations of tenofovir. Tenofovir should be avoided with concomittant or recent use of a nephrotoxic agent).
No products indexed under this heading.

Caffeine (Drugs that decrease renal function may increase serum concentrations of tenofovir. Tenofovir should be avoided with concomittant or recent use of a nephrotoxic agent). Products include:
BioLean Free Tablets .... ▣635
BioLean II Tablets .... ▣635
Winrgy Dietary Supplement .... ▣642

Captopril (Drugs that decrease renal function may increase serum concentrations of tenofovir. Tenofovir should be avoided with concomittant or recent use of a nephrotoxic agent). Products include:
Captopril Tablets 2182

Carbenicillin Disodium (Drugs that decrease renal function may increase serum concentrations of tenofovir. Tenofovir should be avoided with concomittant or recent use of a nephrotoxic agent).
No products indexed under this heading.

Carbenicillin Indanyl Sodium (Drugs that decrease renal function may increase serum concentrations of tenofovir. Tenofovir should be avoided with concomittant or recent use of a nephrotoxic agent).
No products indexed under this heading.

Carboplatin (Drugs that decrease renal function may increase serum concentrations of tenofovir. Tenofovir should be avoided with concomittant or recent use of a nephrotoxic agent).
No products indexed under this heading.

Carmustine (BCNU) (Drugs that decrease renal function may increase serum concentrations of tenofovir. Tenofovir should be avoided with concomittant or recent use of a nephrotoxic agent).
No products indexed under this heading.

Cefaclor (Drugs that decrease renal function may increase serum concentrations of tenofovir. Tenofovir should be avoided with concomittant or recent use of a nephrotoxic agent).
No products indexed under this heading.

Cefadroxil (Drugs that decrease renal function may increase serum concentrations of tenofovir. Tenofovir should be avoided with concomittant or recent use of a nephrotoxic agent).
No products indexed under this heading.

Cefamandole Nafate (Drugs that decrease renal function may increase serum concentrations of tenofovir. Tenofovir should be avoided with concomittant or recent use of a nephrotoxic agent).
No products indexed under this heading.

Cefazolin Sodium (Drugs that decrease renal function may increase serum concentrations of tenofovir. Tenofovir should be avoided with concomittant or recent use of a nephrotoxic agent).
No products indexed under this heading.

Cefdinir (Drugs that decrease renal function may increase serum concentrations of tenofovir. Tenofovir should be avoided with concomittant or recent use of a nephrotoxic agent). Products include:
Omnicef Capsules 497
Omnicef for Oral Suspension 497

Cefepime Hydrochloride (Drugs that decrease renal function may increase serum concentrations of tenofovir. Tenofovir should be avoided with concomittant or recent use of a nephrotoxic agent).
No products indexed under this heading.

Cefixime (Drugs that decrease renal function may increase serum concentrations of tenofovir. Tenofovir should be avoided with concomittant or recent use of a nephrotoxic agent). Products include:

Suprax for Oral Suspension 1891
Suprax Tablets 1891

Cefmetazole Sodium (Drugs that decrease renal function may increase serum concentrations of tenofovir. Tenofovir should be avoided with concomittant or recent use of a nephrotoxic agent).
No products indexed under this heading.

Cefonicid Sodium (Drugs that decrease renal function may increase serum concentrations of tenofovir. Tenofovir should be avoided with concomittant or recent use of a nephrotoxic agent).
No products indexed under this heading.

Cefoperazone Sodium (Drugs that decrease renal function may increase serum concentrations of tenofovir. Tenofovir should be avoided with concomittant or recent use of a nephrotoxic agent).
No products indexed under this heading.

Ceforanide (Drugs that decrease renal function may increase serum concentrations of tenofovir. Tenofovir should be avoided with concomittant or recent use of a nephrotoxic agent).
No products indexed under this heading.

Cefotaxime Sodium (Drugs that decrease renal function may increase serum concentrations of tenofovir. Tenofovir should be avoided with concomittant or recent use of a nephrotoxic agent).
No products indexed under this heading.

Cefotetan (Drugs that decrease renal function may increase serum concentrations of tenofovir. Tenofovir should be avoided with concomittant or recent use of a nephrotoxic agent).
No products indexed under this heading.

Cefoxitin Sodium (Drugs that decrease renal function may increase serum concentrations of tenofovir. Tenofovir should be avoided with concomittant or recent use of a nephrotoxic agent).
No products indexed under this heading.

Cefpodoxime Proxetil (Drugs that decrease renal function may increase serum concentrations of tenofovir. Tenofovir should be avoided with concomittant or recent use of a nephrotoxic agent).
No products indexed under this heading.

Cefprozil (Drugs that decrease renal function may increase serum concentrations of tenofovir. Tenofovir should be avoided with concomittant or recent use of a nephrotoxic agent).
No products indexed under this heading.

Ceftazidime (Drugs that decrease renal function may increase serum concentrations of tenofovir. Tenofovir should be avoided with concomittant or recent use of a nephrotoxic agent). Products include:
Fortaz 1450

Ceftizoxime Sodium (Drugs that decrease renal function may increase serum concentrations of tenofovir. Tenofovir should be avoided with concomittant or recent use of a nephrotoxic agent).
No products indexed under this heading.

Ceftriaxone Sodium (Drugs that decrease renal function may increase serum concentrations of tenofovir. Tenofovir should be avoided with concomittant or recent use of a nephrotoxic agent).
Products include:
Rocephin Injectable Vials, ADD-Vantage, Galaxy, Bulk 2642

Cefuroxime Axetil (Drugs that decrease renal function may increase serum concentrations of tenofovir. Tenofovir should be avoided with concomittant or recent use of a nephrotoxic agent).
Products include:
Ceftin 1380

Cefuroxime Sodium (Drugs that decrease renal function may increase serum concentrations of tenofovir. Tenofovir should be avoided with concomittant or recent use of a nephrotoxic agent).
No products indexed under this heading.

Celecoxib (Drugs that decrease renal function may increase serum concentrations of tenofovir. Tenofovir should be avoided with concomittant or recent use of a nephrotoxic agent). Products include:
Celebrex Capsules 2979

Cephalexin (Drugs that decrease renal function may increase serum concentrations of tenofovir. Tenofovir should be avoided with concomittant or recent use of a nephrotoxic agent).
No products indexed under this heading.

Cephalothin Sodium (Drugs that decrease renal function may increase serum concentrations of tenofovir. Tenofovir should be avoided with concomittant or recent use of a nephrotoxic agent).
No products indexed under this heading.

Cephapirin Sodium (Drugs that decrease renal function may increase serum concentrations of tenofovir. Tenofovir should be avoided with concomittant or recent use of a nephrotoxic agent).
No products indexed under this heading.

Cephradine (Drugs that decrease renal function may increase serum concentrations of tenofovir. Tenofovir should be avoided with concomittant or recent use of a nephrotoxic agent).
No products indexed under this heading.

Cerivastatin Sodium (Drugs that decrease renal function may increase serum concentrations of tenofovir. Tenofovir should be avoided with concomittant or recent use of a nephrotoxic agent).
No products indexed under this heading.

Chlorothiazide (Drugs that decrease renal function may increase serum concentrations of tenofovir. Tenofovir should be avoided with concomittant or recent use of a nephrotoxic agent).
No products indexed under this heading.

Chlorothiazide Sodium (Drugs that decrease renal function may increase serum concentrations of tenofovir. Tenofovir should be avoided with concomittant or recent use of a nephrotoxic agent).
Products include:
Intravenous Sodium Diuril 2490

Chlorpropamide (Drugs that decrease renal function may increase serum concentrations of tenofovir. Tenofovir should be avoided with concomittant or recent use of a nephrotoxic agent).
No products indexed under this heading.

Cidofovir (Co-administration with drugs that reduce renal function or compete for active tubular secretion may increase serum concentrations of tenofovir and/or increase the concentrations of other renally eliminated drugs, such as cidofovir).
No products indexed under this heading.

Cilastatin Sodium (Drugs that decrease renal function may increase serum concentrations of tenofovir. Tenofovir should be avoided with concomittant or recent use of a nephrotoxic agent).
Products include:
Primaxin I.M. 2080
Primaxin I.V. 2083

Cimetidine (Drugs that decrease renal function may increase serum concentrations of tenofovir. Tenofovir should be avoided with concomittant or recent use of a nephrotoxic agent).
No products indexed under this heading.

Cimetidine Hydrochloride (Drugs that decrease renal function may increase serum concentrations of tenofovir. Tenofovir should be avoided with concomittant or recent use of a nephrotoxic agent).
No products indexed under this heading.

Cisplatin (Drugs that decrease renal function may increase serum concentrations of tenofovir. Tenofovir should be avoided with concomittant or recent use of a nephrotoxic agent).
No products indexed under this heading.

Cladribine (Drugs that decrease renal function may increase serum concentrations of tenofovir. Tenofovir should be avoided with concomittant or recent use of a nephrotoxic agent). Products include:
Leustatin Injection 2384

Clozapine (Drugs that decrease renal function may increase serum concentrations of tenofovir. Tenofovir should be avoided with concomittant or recent use of a nephrotoxic agent).
No products indexed under this heading.

Colistimethate Sodium (Drugs that decrease renal function may increase serum concentrations of tenofovir. Tenofovir should be avoided with concomittant or recent use of a nephrotoxic agent).
No products indexed under this heading.

Colistin Sulfate (Drugs that decrease renal function may increase serum concentrations of tenofovir. Tenofovir should be avoided with concomittant or recent use of a nephrotoxic agent).
No products indexed under this heading.

Cyclophosphamide (Drugs that decrease renal function may increase serum concentrations of tenofovir. Tenofovir should be avoided with concomittant or recent use of a nephrotoxic agent).
No products indexed under this heading.

Cyclosporine (Drugs that decrease renal function may increase serum concentrations of tenofovir. Tenofovir should be avoided with concomittant or recent use of a nephrotoxic agent). Products include:
Gengraf Capsules 435
Neoral Oral Solution 2280
Neoral Soft Gelatin Capsules 2280
Restasis Ophthalmic Emulsion 557
Sandimmune 2296

Cytarabine (Drugs that decrease renal function may increase serum concentrations of tenofovir. Tenofovir should be avoided with concomittant or recent use of a nephrotoxic agent).
No products indexed under this heading.

Cytarabine Liposome (Drugs that decrease renal function may increase serum concentrations of tenofovir. Tenofovir should be avoided with concomittant or recent use of a nephrotoxic agent).
Products include:
DepoCyt Injection 1136

Delavirdine Mesylate (Drugs that decrease renal function may increase serum concentrations of tenofovir. Tenofovir should be avoided with concomittant or recent use of a nephrotoxic agent).
No products indexed under this heading.

Diatrizoate Meglumine (Drugs that decrease renal function may increase serum concentrations of tenofovir. Tenofovir should be avoided with concomittant or recent use of a nephrotoxic agent).
No products indexed under this heading.

Diatrizoate Sodium (Drugs that decrease renal function may increase serum concentrations of tenofovir. Tenofovir should be avoided with concomittant or recent use of a nephrotoxic agent).
No products indexed under this heading.

Diclofenac Potassium (Drugs that decrease renal function may increase serum concentrations of tenofovir. Tenofovir should be avoided with concomittant or recent use of a nephrotoxic agent).
No products indexed under this heading.

Diclofenac Sodium (Drugs that decrease renal function may increase serum concentrations of tenofovir. Tenofovir should be

avoided with concomittant or recent use of a nephrotoxic agent).
Products include:
Diclofenac Sodium Ophthalmic Solution .... ⊙ 240
Voltaren Ophthalmic Solution 2336
Voltaren Tablets 2334
Voltaren-XR Tablets 2337

Dicloxacillin Sodium (Drugs that decrease renal function may increase serum concentrations of tenofovir. Tenofovir should be avoided with concomittant or recent use of a nephrotoxic agent).
No products indexed under this heading.

Didanosine (Co-administration results in increased AUC and Cmax of didanosine and could potentiate didanosine-associated adverse events. Discontinue didanosine if didanosine-associated adverse events develop).
No products indexed under this heading.

Efavirenz (Drugs that decrease renal function may increase serum concentrations of tenofovir. Tenofovir should be avoided with concomittant or recent use of a nephrotoxic agent). Products include:
Atripla Tablets 938
Sustiva Capsules 930
Sustiva Tablets 930

Emtricitabine (Drugs that decrease renal function may increase serum concentrations of tenofovir. Tenofovir should be avoided with concomittant or recent use of a nephrotoxic agent). Products include:
Atripla Tablets 938
Emtriva Capsules 1246
Emtriva Oral Solution 1246
Truvada Tablets 1262

Enalapril Maleate (Drugs that decrease renal function may increase serum concentrations of tenofovir. Tenofovir should be avoided with concomittant or recent use of a nephrotoxic agent).
No products indexed under this heading.

Enalaprilat (Drugs that decrease renal function may increase serum concentrations of tenofovir. Tenofovir should be avoided with concomittant or recent use of a nephrotoxic agent).
No products indexed under this heading.

Enfuvirtide (Drugs that decrease renal function may increase serum concentrations of tenofovir. Tenofovir should be avoided with concomittant or recent use of a nephrotoxic agent).
No products indexed under this heading.

Ethiodized Oil (Drugs that decrease renal function may increase serum concentrations of tenofovir. Tenofovir should be avoided with concomittant or recent use of a nephrotoxic agent).
No products indexed under this heading.

Etodolac (Drugs that decrease renal function may increase serum concentrations of tenofovir. Tenofovir should be avoided with concomittant or recent use of a nephrotoxic agent).
No products indexed under this heading.

Fenoprofen Calcium (Drugs that decrease renal function may increase serum concentrations of tenofovir. Tenofovir should be avoided with concomittant or recent use of a nephrotoxic agent).
Products include:
Nalfon Capsules 2508

Filgrastim (Drugs that decrease renal function may increase serum concentrations of tenofovir. Tenofovir should be avoided with concomittant or recent use of a nephrotoxic agent). Products include:
Neupogen for Injection 589

Fluorouracil (Drugs that decrease renal function may increase serum concentrations of tenofovir. Tenofovir should be avoided with concomittant or recent use of a nephrotoxic agent). Products include:
Carac Cream 0.5% 2722

Flurbiprofen (Drugs that decrease renal function may increase serum concentrations of tenofovir. Tenofovir should be avoided with concomittant or recent use of a nephrotoxic agent).
No products indexed under this heading.

Fluvastatin Sodium (Drugs that decrease renal function may increase serum concentrations of tenofovir. Tenofovir should be avoided with concomittant or recent use of a nephrotoxic agent).
Products include:
Lescol Capsules 2268
Lescol XL Tablets 2268

Foscarnet Sodium (Drugs that decrease renal function may increase serum concentrations of tenofovir. Tenofovir should be avoided with concomittant or recent use of a nephrotoxic agent).
No products indexed under this heading.

Fosinopril Sodium (Drugs that decrease renal function may increase serum concentrations of tenofovir. Tenofovir should be avoided with concomittant or recent use of a nephrotoxic agent).
No products indexed under this heading.

Furosemide (Drugs that decrease renal function may increase serum concentrations of tenofovir. Tenofovir should be avoided with concomittant or recent use of a nephrotoxic agent). Products include:
Furosemide Tablets 2186

Gadopentetate Dimeglumine (Drugs that decrease renal function may increase serum concentrations of tenofovir. Tenofovir should be avoided with concomittant or recent use of a nephrotoxic agent).
No products indexed under this heading.

Ganciclovir (Co-administration with drugs that reduce renal function or compete for active tubular secretion may increase serum concentrations of tenofovir and/or increase the concentrations of other renally eliminated drugs, such as ganciclovir).
No products indexed under this heading.

Gentamicin (Drugs that decrease renal function may increase serum concentrations of tenofovir. Tenofovir should be avoided with concomittant or recent use of a nephrotoxic agent).
No products indexed under this heading.

Gentamicin Sulfate (Drugs that decrease renal function may increase serum concentrations of tenofovir. Tenofovir should be avoided with concomittant or recent use of a nephrotoxic agent).
Products include:
Pred-G Ophthalmic Ointment .... ⊙ 229
Pred-G Ophthalmic Suspension .... ⊙ 228

Glipizide (Drugs that decrease renal function may increase serum concentrations of tenofovir. Tenofovir should be avoided with concomittant or recent use of a nephrotoxic agent).
No products indexed under this heading.

Globulin, Immune (Human) (Drugs that decrease renal function may increase serum concentrations of tenofovir. Tenofovir should be avoided with concomittant or recent use of a nephrotoxic agent).
Products include:
Flebogamma 5% 1715

Glyburide (Drugs that decrease renal function may increase serum concentrations of tenofovir. Tenofovir should be avoided with concomittant or recent use of a nephrotoxic agent).
No products indexed under this heading.

Gold Therapy (Drugs that decrease renal function may increase serum concentrations of tenofovir. Tenofovir should be avoided with concomittant or recent use of a nephrotoxic agent).
No products indexed under this heading.

HMG-CoA Reductase Inhibitors (Drugs that decrease renal function may increase serum concentrations of tenofovir. Tenofovir should be avoided with concomittant or recent use of a nephrotoxic agent).
No products indexed under this heading.

Hydrochlorothiazide (Drugs that decrease renal function may increase serum concentrations of tenofovir. Tenofovir should be avoided with concomittant or recent use of a nephrotoxic agent).
Products include:
Atacand HCT 642
Avalide Tablets 892
Avalide Tablets 2713
Benicar HCT Tablets 1010
Diovan HCT Tablets 2216
Dyazide Capsules 1405
Micardis HCT Tablets 854
Prinzide Tablets 2092
Tekturna HCT Tablets 2324
Teveten HCT Tablets 517

Hydroflumethiazide (Drugs that decrease renal function may increase serum concentrations of tenofovir. Tenofovir should be avoided with concomittant or recent use of a nephrotoxic agent).
No products indexed under this heading.

Ibuprofen (Drugs that decrease renal function may increase serum concentrations of tenofovir. Tenofovir should be avoided with concomittant or recent use of a nephrotoxic agent). Products include:
Motrin IB Tablets and Caplets 1900
Children's Motrin Oral Suspension 1901
Children's Motrin Non-Staining Dye-Free Oral Suspension 1901
Children's Motrin Cold Oral Suspension 1899
Infants' Motrin Concentrated Drops 1901
Infants' Motrin Non-Staining Dye-Free Concentrated Drops 1901
Junior Strength Motrin Caplets and Chewable Tablets 1901
Vicoprofen Tablets 533

Idarubicin Hydrochloride (Drugs that decrease renal function may increase serum concentrations of tenofovir. Tenofovir should be avoided with concomittant or recent use of a nephrotoxic agent).
No products indexed under this heading.

Ifosfamide (Drugs that decrease renal function may increase serum concentrations of tenofovir. Tenofovir should be avoided with concomittant or recent use of a nephrotoxic agent).
No products indexed under this heading.

Imipenem (Drugs that decrease renal function may increase serum concentrations of tenofovir. Tenofovir should be avoided with concomittant or recent use of a nephrotoxic agent). Products include:
Primaxin I.M. 2080
Primaxin I.V. 2083

Immune Globulin Intravenous (Human) (Drugs that decrease renal function may increase serum concentrations of tenofovir. Tenofovir should be avoided with concomittant or recent use of a nephrotoxic agent). Products include:
Flebogamma 5% DIF 1718
Gammagard Liquid 730
Gammagard S/D 734
Gamunex 3094

Indinavir Sulfate (Co-administration of tenofovir with indinavir has resulted in increased Cmax tenofovir and decreased Cmax for indinavir). Products include:
Crixivan Capsules 1979

Indomethacin (Drugs that decrease renal function may increase serum concentrations of tenofovir. Tenofovir should be avoided with concomittant or recent use of a nephrotoxic agent).
Products include:
Indocin 2024

Indomethacin Sodium Trihydrate (Drugs that decrease renal function may increase serum concentrations of tenofovir. Tenofovir should be avoided with concomittant or recent use of a nephrotoxic agent). Products include:
Indocin I.V. 2489

Interferon Beta-1b (Drugs that decrease renal function may increase serum concentrations of tenofovir. Tenofovir should be avoided with concomittant or recent use of a nephrotoxic agent).
Products include:
Betaseron for SC Injection 756

Interleukin-2 (Drugs that decrease renal function may increase serum concentrations of tenofovir. Tenofovir should be avoided with concomittant or recent use of a nephrotoxic agent).
No products indexed under this heading.

Iodamide Meglumine (Drugs that decrease renal function may increase serum concentrations of tenofovir. Tenofovir should be avoided with concomittant or recent use of a nephrotoxic agent).
No products indexed under this heading.

Iohexol (Drugs that decrease renal function may increase serum concentrations of tenofovir. Tenofovir should be avoided with concomittant or recent use of a nephrotoxic agent).
No products indexed under this heading.

Iopamidol (Drugs that decrease renal function may increase serum concentrations of tenofovir. Tenofovir should be avoided with concomittant or recent use of a nephrotoxic agent).
No products indexed under this heading.

Iopanoic Acid (Drugs that decrease renal function may increase serum concentrations of tenofovir. Tenofovir should be avoided with concomittant or recent use of a nephrotoxic agent).
No products indexed under this heading.

Iothalamate Meglumine (Drugs that decrease renal function may increase serum concentrations of tenofovir. Tenofovir should be avoided with concomittant or recent use of a nephrotoxic agent).
No products indexed under this heading.

Ioxaglate Meglumine (Drugs that decrease renal function may increase serum concentrations of tenofovir. Tenofovir should be avoided with concomittant or recent use of a nephrotoxic agent).
No products indexed under this heading.

Ioxaglate Sodium (Drugs that decrease renal function may increase serum concentrations of tenofovir. Tenofovir should be avoided with concomittant or recent use of a nephrotoxic agent).
No products indexed under this heading.

Kanamycin Sulfate (Drugs that decrease renal function may increase serum concentrations of tenofovir. Tenofovir should be avoided with concomittant or recent use of a nephrotoxic agent).
No products indexed under this heading.

Ketoprofen (Drugs that decrease renal function may increase serum concentrations of tenofovir. Tenofovir should be avoided with concomittant or recent use of a nephrotoxic agent).
No products indexed under this heading.

Ketorolac Tromethamine (Drugs that decrease renal function may increase serum concentrations of tenofovir. Tenofovir should be avoided with concomittant or recent use of a nephrotoxic agent).
No products indexed under this heading.

Lamium album (Drugs that decrease renal function may increase serum concentrations of tenofovir. Tenofovir should be avoided with concomittant or recent use of a nephrotoxic agent).
No products indexed under this heading.

Lamivudine (Co-administration of tenofovir with lamivudine has resulted in decreased Cmax for lamivudine). Products include:
Combivir Tablets **1384**
Epivir **1412**
Epivir-HBV **1417**
Epzicom Tablets **1422**
Trizivir Tablets **1622**

Lisinopril (Drugs that decrease renal function may increase serum concentrations of tenofovir. Tenofovir should be avoided with concomittant or recent use of a nephrotoxic agent). Products include:
Prinivil Tablets **2087**
Prinzide Tablets **2092**

Lithium (Drugs that decrease renal function may increase serum concentrations of tenofovir. Tenofovir should be avoided with concomittant or recent use of a nephrotoxic agent).
No products indexed under this heading.

Lithium Carbonate (Drugs that decrease renal function may increase serum concentrations of tenofovir. Tenofovir should be avoided with concomittant or recent use of a nephrotoxic agent).
No products indexed under this heading.

Lithium Citrate (Drugs that decrease renal function may increase serum concentrations of tenofovir. Tenofovir should be avoided with concomittant or recent use of a nephrotoxic agent).
No products indexed under this heading.

Lopinavir (Co-administration of tenofovir with lopinavir has resulted in increased Cmax, AUC, and Cmin for tenofovir and decreased AUC, Cmax, and Cmin for lopinavir). Products include:
Kaletra **452**

Loracarbef (Drugs that decrease renal function may increase serum concentrations of tenofovir. Tenofovir should be avoided with concomittant or recent use of a nephrotoxic agent).
No products indexed under this heading.

Lovastatin (Drugs that decrease renal function may increase serum concentrations of tenofovir. Tenofovir should be avoided with concomittant or recent use of a nephrotoxic agent). Products include:
Advicor Tablets **402**
Mevacor Tablets **2063**

Meclofenamate Sodium (Drugs that decrease renal function may increase serum concentrations of tenofovir. Tenofovir should be avoided with concomittant or recent use of a nephrotoxic agent).
No products indexed under this heading.

Mefenamic Acid (Drugs that decrease renal function may increase serum concentrations of tenofovir. Tenofovir should be avoided with concomittant or recent use of a nephrotoxic agent).
No products indexed under this heading.

Meloxicam (Drugs that decrease renal function may increase serum concentrations of tenofovir. Tenofovir should be avoided with concomittant or recent use of a nephrotoxic agent). Products include:
Mobic Oral Suspension **863**
Mobic Tablets **863**

Melphalan Hydrochloride (Drugs that decrease renal function may increase serum concentrations of tenofovir. Tenofovir should be avoided with concomittant or recent use of a nephrotoxic agent).
No products indexed under this heading.

Mesalamine (Drugs that decrease renal function may increase serum concentrations of tenofovir. Tenofovir should be avoided with concomittant or recent use of a nephrotoxic agent). Products include:
Asacol Delayed-Release Tablets **2579**
Canasa Rectal Suppositories **705**
Lialda Tablets **3029**
Pentasa Capsules **3030**

Methimazole (Drugs that decrease renal function may increase serum concentrations of tenofovir. Tenofovir should be avoided with concomittant or recent use of a nephrotoxic agent).
No products indexed under this heading.

Methotrexate (Drugs that decrease renal function may increase serum concentrations of tenofovir. Tenofovir should be avoided with concomittant or recent use of a nephrotoxic agent).
No products indexed under this heading.

Methotrexate Sodium (Drugs that decrease renal function may increase serum concentrations of tenofovir. Tenofovir should be avoided with concomittant or recent use of a nephrotoxic agent).
No products indexed under this heading.

Methyclothiazide (Drugs that decrease renal function may increase serum concentrations of tenofovir. Tenofovir should be avoided with concomittant or recent use of a nephrotoxic agent).
No products indexed under this heading.

Mezlocillin Sodium (Drugs that decrease renal function may increase serum concentrations of tenofovir. Tenofovir should be avoided with concomittant or recent use of a nephrotoxic agent).
No products indexed under this heading.

Minocycline Hydrochloride (Drugs that decrease renal function may increase serum concentrations of tenofovir. Tenofovir should be avoided with concomittant or recent use of a nephrotoxic agent). Products include:
Solodyn Extended Release Tablets **1938**

Mitomycin (Mitomycin-C) (Drugs that decrease renal function may increase serum concentrations of tenofovir. Tenofovir should be avoided with concomittant or recent use of a nephrotoxic agent).
No products indexed under this heading.

Moexipril Hydrochloride (Drugs that decrease renal function may increase serum concentrations of tenofovir. Tenofovir should be avoided with concomittant or recent use of a nephrotoxic agent).
No products indexed under this heading.

Muromonab-CD3 (Drugs that decrease renal function may increase serum concentrations of tenofovir. Tenofovir should be avoided with concomittant or recent use of a nephrotoxic agent). Products include:
Orthoclone OKT3 Sterile Solution **2387**

Nabumetone (Drugs that decrease renal function may increase serum concentrations of tenofovir. Tenofovir should be avoided with concomittant or recent use of a nephrotoxic agent).
No products indexed under this heading.

Nafcillin Sodium (Drugs that decrease renal function may increase serum concentrations of tenofovir. Tenofovir should be avoided with concomittant or recent use of a nephrotoxic agent).
No products indexed under this heading.

Naproxen (Drugs that decrease renal function may increase serum concentrations of tenofovir. Tenofovir should be avoided with concomittant or recent use of a nephrotoxic agent). Products include:
EC-Naprosyn Delayed-Release Tablets **2632**
Naprosyn Suspension **2632**
Naprosyn Tablets **2632**

Naproxen Sodium (Drugs that decrease renal function may increase serum concentrations of tenofovir. Tenofovir should be avoided with concomittant or recent use of a nephrotoxic agent). Products include:
Anaprox Tablets **2632**
Anaprox DS Tablets **2632**
Treximet Tablets **1616**

Nelfinavir Mesylate (Drugs that decrease renal function may increase serum concentrations of tenofovir. Tenofovir should be avoided with concomittant or recent use of a nephrotoxic agent).
No products indexed under this heading.

Neomycin (Drugs that decrease renal function may increase serum concentrations of tenofovir. Tenofovir should be avoided with concomittant or recent use of a nephrotoxic agent).
No products indexed under this heading.

Neomycin, oral (Drugs that decrease renal function may increase serum concentrations of tenofovir. Tenofovir should be avoided with concomittant or recent use of a nephrotoxic agent).
No products indexed under this heading.

Neomycin Sulfate (Drugs that decrease renal function may increase serum concentrations of tenofovir. Tenofovir should be avoided with concomittant or recent use of a nephrotoxic agent). Products include:
Neosporin Ophthalmic Solution Sterile .... ⊙ **252**

Nevirapine (Drugs that decrease renal function may increase serum concentrations of tenofovir. Tenofovir should be avoided with concomittant or recent use of a nephrotoxic agent). Products include:
Viramune Oral Suspension **873**
Viramune Tablets **873**

Norfloxacin (Drugs that decrease renal function may increase serum concentrations of tenofovir. Tenofovir should be avoided with concomittant or recent use of a nephrotoxic agent). Products include:

Noroxin Tablets 2069

Olsalazine Sodium (Drugs that decrease renal function may increase serum concentrations of tenofovir. Tenofovir should be avoided with concomittant or recent use of a nephrotoxic agent).
No products indexed under this heading.

Omeprazole (Drugs that decrease renal function may increase serum concentrations of tenofovir. Tenofovir should be avoided with concomittant or recent use of a nephrotoxic agent).
No products indexed under this heading.

Oxaprozin (Drugs that decrease renal function may increase serum concentrations of tenofovir. Tenofovir should be avoided with concomittant or recent use of a nephrotoxic agent).
No products indexed under this heading.

Pamidronate Disodium (Drugs that decrease renal function may increase serum concentrations of tenofovir. Tenofovir should be avoided with concomittant or recent use of a nephrotoxic agent).
No products indexed under this heading.

Paroxetine Hydrochloride (Drugs that decrease renal function may increase serum concentrations of tenofovir. Tenofovir should be avoided with concomittant or recent use of a nephrotoxic agent).
Products include:
Paxil 1535
Paxil CR Controlled-Release Tablets 1544

Penicillamine (Drugs that decrease renal function may increase serum concentrations of tenofovir. Tenofovir should be avoided with concomittant or recent use of a nephrotoxic agent).
Products include:
Cuprimine Capsules 1986

Penicillin G Benzathine (Drugs that decrease renal function may increase serum concentrations of tenofovir. Tenofovir should be avoided with concomittant or recent use of a nephrotoxic agent).
Products include:
Bicillin C-R Injectable Suspension 1775
Bicillin L-A Injection 1777

Penicillin G Potassium (Drugs that decrease renal function may increase serum concentrations of tenofovir. Tenofovir should be avoided with concomittant or recent use of a nephrotoxic agent).
No products indexed under this heading.

Penicillin G Procaine (Drugs that decrease renal function may increase serum concentrations of tenofovir. Tenofovir should be avoided with concomittant or recent use of a nephrotoxic agent).
Products include:
Bicillin C-R Injectable Suspension 1775
Bicillin L-A Injection 1777

Penicillin G Sodium (Drugs that decrease renal function may increase serum concentrations of tenofovir. Tenofovir should be avoided with concomittant or recent use of a nephrotoxic agent).
No products indexed under this heading.

Penicillin V Potassium (Drugs that decrease renal function may increase serum concentrations of tenofovir. Tenofovir should be avoided with concomittant or recent use of a nephrotoxic agent).
No products indexed under this heading.

Pentamidine Isethionate (Drugs that decrease renal function may increase serum concentrations of tenofovir. Tenofovir should be avoided with concomittant or recent use of a nephrotoxic agent).
No products indexed under this heading.

Perindopril Erbumine (Drugs that decrease renal function may increase serum concentrations of tenofovir. Tenofovir should be avoided with concomittant or recent use of a nephrotoxic agent).
Products include:
Aceon Tablets (2 mg, 4 mg, 8 mg) 3038

Phenylbutazone (Drugs that decrease renal function may increase serum concentrations of tenofovir. Tenofovir should be avoided with concomittant or recent use of a nephrotoxic agent).
No products indexed under this heading.

Piroxicam (Drugs that decrease renal function may increase serum concentrations of tenofovir. Tenofovir should be avoided with concomittant or recent use of a nephrotoxic agent).
No products indexed under this heading.

Plicamycin (Drugs that decrease renal function may increase serum concentrations of tenofovir. Tenofovir should be avoided with concomittant or recent use of a nephrotoxic agent).
No products indexed under this heading.

Polymyxin (Drugs that decrease renal function may increase serum concentrations of tenofovir. Tenofovir should be avoided with concomittant or recent use of a nephrotoxic agent).
No products indexed under this heading.

Polymyxin B Sulfate (Drugs that decrease renal function may increase serum concentrations of tenofovir. Tenofovir should be avoided with concomittant or recent use of a nephrotoxic agent).
Products include:
Neosporin Ophthalmic Solution Sterile .... ⊙252

Polythiazide (Drugs that decrease renal function may increase serum concentrations of tenofovir. Tenofovir should be avoided with concomittant or recent use of a nephrotoxic agent).
No products indexed under this heading.

Pravastatin Sodium (Drugs that decrease renal function may increase serum concentrations of tenofovir. Tenofovir should be avoided with concomittant or recent use of a nephrotoxic agent).
No products indexed under this heading.

Probenecid (Co-administration of tenofovir with drugs that are eliminated by active tubular secretion may increase serum concentrations of either tenofovir or the co-administered drug).
No products indexed under this heading.

Quinapril Hydrochloride (Drugs that decrease renal function may increase serum concentrations of tenofovir. Tenofovir should be avoided with concomittant or recent use of a nephrotoxic agent).
No products indexed under this heading.

Rabeprazole Sodium (Drugs that decrease renal function may increase serum concentrations of tenofovir. Tenofovir should be avoided with concomittant or recent use of a nephrotoxic agent).
Products include:
Aciphex Tablets 1053

Ramipril (Drugs that decrease renal function may increase serum concentrations of tenofovir. Tenofovir should be avoided with concomittant or recent use of a nephrotoxic agent).
No products indexed under this heading.

Rifampin (Drugs that decrease renal function may increase serum concentrations of tenofovir. Tenofovir should be avoided with concomittant or recent use of a nephrotoxic agent).
No products indexed under this heading.

Riluzole (Drugs that decrease renal function may increase serum concentrations of tenofovir. Tenofovir should be avoided with concomittant or recent use of a nephrotoxic agent). Products include:
Rilutek Tablets 2771

Ritonavir (Co-administration of tenofovir and ritonavir resulted in a 23% increase in Cmin). Products include:
Kaletra 452
Norvir 489

Rofecoxib (Drugs that decrease renal function may increase serum concentrations of tenofovir. Tenofovir should be avoided with concomittant or recent use of a nephrotoxic agent).
No products indexed under this heading.

Saquinavir (Co-administration of tenofovir and saquinavir resulted in a 22% increase in Cmax).
No products indexed under this heading.

Sibutramine Hydrochloride Monohydrate (Drugs that decrease renal function may increase serum concentrations of tenofovir. Tenofovir should be avoided with concomittant or recent use of a nephrotoxic agent). Products include:
Meridia Capsules 475

Simvastatin (Drugs that decrease renal function may increase serum concentrations of tenofovir. Tenofovir should be avoided with concomittant or recent use of a nephrotoxic agent). Products include:
Simcor Tablets 502
Vytorin 10/10 Tablets 2149
Vytorin 10/10 Tablets 2939
Vytorin 10/20 Tablets 2149
Vytorin 10/20 Tablets 2939
Vytorin 10/40 Tablets 2149
Vytorin 10/40 Tablets 2939
Vytorin 10/80 Tablets 2149
Vytorin 10/80 Tablets 2939
Zocor Tablets 2136

Spirapril Hydrochloride (Drugs that decrease renal function may increase serum concentrations of tenofovir. Tenofovir should be avoided with concomittant or recent use of a nephrotoxic agent).
No products indexed under this heading.

Stavudine (Drugs that decrease renal function may increase serum concentrations of tenofovir. Tenofovir should be avoided with concomittant or recent use of a nephrotoxic agent).
No products indexed under this heading.

Streptomycin Sulfate (Drugs that decrease renal function may increase serum concentrations of tenofovir. Tenofovir should be avoided with concomittant or recent use of a nephrotoxic agent).
No products indexed under this heading.

Streptozocin (Drugs that decrease renal function may increase serum concentrations of tenofovir. Tenofovir should be avoided with concomittant or recent use of a nephrotoxic agent).
No products indexed under this heading.

Sulfacytine (Drugs that decrease renal function may increase serum concentrations of tenofovir. Tenofovir should be avoided with concomittant or recent use of a nephrotoxic agent).
No products indexed under this heading.

Sulfamethizole (Drugs that decrease renal function may increase serum concentrations of tenofovir. Tenofovir should be avoided with concomittant or recent use of a nephrotoxic agent).
No products indexed under this heading.

Sulfamethoxazole (Drugs that decrease renal function may increase serum concentrations of tenofovir. Tenofovir should be avoided with concomittant or recent use of a nephrotoxic agent).
No products indexed under this heading.

Sulfasalazine (Drugs that decrease renal function may increase serum concentrations of tenofovir. Tenofovir should be avoided with concomittant or recent use of a nephrotoxic agent).
No products indexed under this heading.

Sulfinpyrazone (Co-administration of tenofovir with drugs that are eliminated by active tubular secretion may increase serum concentrations of either tenofovir or the co-administered drug).
No products indexed under this heading.

Sulfisoxazole Acetyl (Drugs that decrease renal function may increase serum concentrations of tenofovir. Tenofovir should be avoided with concomittant or recent use of a nephrotoxic agent).
No products indexed under this heading.

Sulfisoxazole Diolamine (Drugs that decrease renal function may increase serum concentrations of tenofovir. Tenofovir should be avoided with concomittant or recent use of a nephrotoxic agent).
No products indexed under this heading.

Sulindac (Drugs that decrease renal function may increase serum concentrations of tenofovir. Tenofovir should be avoided with concomittant or recent use of a nephrotoxic agent). Products include:
Clinoril Tablets 1962

Tacrolimus (Drugs that decrease renal function may increase serum concentrations of tenofovir. Tenofovir should be avoided with concomittant or recent use of a nephrotoxic agent). Products include:
Prograf Capsules and Injection 622
Protopic Ointment 628

Thioguanine (Drugs that decrease renal function may increase serum concentrations of tenofovir. Tenofovir should be avoided with concomittant or recent use of a nephrotoxic agent). Products include:
Tabloid Tablets 1601

Ticarcillin Disodium (Drugs that decrease renal function may increase serum concentrations of tenofovir. Tenofovir should be avoided with concomittant or recent use of a nephrotoxic agent).
Products include:
Timentin ADD-Vantage 1606
Timentin Injection Galaxy Container 1609
Timentin IV Infusion 1603
Timentin Pharmacy Bulk Package 1613

Tobramycin (Drugs that decrease renal function may increase serum concentrations of tenofovir. Tenofovir should be avoided with concomittant or recent use of a nephrotoxic agent). Products include:
Zylet Ophthalmic Suspension .... ⊙247

Tobramycin Sulfate (Drugs that decrease renal function may increase serum concentrations of tenofovir. Tenofovir should be avoided with concomittant or recent use of a nephrotoxic agent).
No products indexed under this heading.

Tolazamide (Drugs that decrease renal function may increase serum concentrations of tenofovir. Tenofovir should be avoided with concomittant or recent use of a nephrotoxic agent).
No products indexed under this heading.

Tolbutamide (Drugs that decrease renal function may increase serum concentrations of tenofovir. Tenofovir should be avoided with concomittant or recent use of a nephrotoxic agent).
No products indexed under this heading.

Tolmetin Sodium (Drugs that decrease renal function may increase serum concentrations of tenofovir. Tenofovir should be avoided with concomittant or recent use of a nephrotoxic agent).
No products indexed under this heading.

Trandolapril (Drugs that decrease renal function may increase serum concentrations of tenofovir. Tenofovir should be avoided with concomittant or recent use of a nephrotoxic agent). Products include:
Mavik Tablets 472
Tarka Tablets 511

Triamterene (Drugs that decrease renal function may increase serum concentrations of tenofovir. Tenofovir should be avoided with concomittant or recent use of a nephrotoxic agent). Products include:
Dyazide Capsules 1405
Dyrenium Capsules 3189

Trimethadione (Drugs that decrease renal function may increase serum concentrations of tenofovir. Tenofovir should be avoided with concomittant or recent use of a nephrotoxic agent).
No products indexed under this heading.

Trovafloxacin Mesylate (Drugs that decrease renal function may increase serum concentrations of tenofovir. Tenofovir should be avoided with concomittant or recent use of a nephrotoxic agent).
No products indexed under this heading.

Tyropanoate Sodium (Drugs that decrease renal function may increase serum concentrations of tenofovir. Tenofovir should be avoided with concomittant or recent use of a nephrotoxic agent).
No products indexed under this heading.

Valacyclovir Hydrochloride (Co-administration with drugs that reduce renal function or compete for active tubular secretion may increase serum concentrations of tenofovir and/or increase the concentrations of other renally eliminated drugs, such as valacyclovir).
Products include:
Valtrex Caplets 1635

Valdecoxib (Drugs that decrease renal function may increase serum concentrations of tenofovir. Tenofovir should be avoided with concomittant or recent use of a nephrotoxic agent).
No products indexed under this heading.

Valganciclovir Hydrochloride (Co-administration with drugs that reduce renal function or compete for active tubular secretion may increase serum concentrations of tenofovir and/or increase the concentrations of other renally eliminated drugs, such as valganciclovir).
Products include:
Valcyte Tablets 2654

Vancomycin Hydrochloride (Drugs that decrease renal function may increase serum concentrations of tenofovir. Tenofovir should be avoided with concomittant or recent use of a nephrotoxic agent).
No products indexed under this heading.

Voriconazole (Drugs that decrease renal function may increase serum concentrations of tenofovir. Tenofovir should be avoided with concomittant or recent use of a nephrotoxic agent).
No products indexed under this heading.

Zalcitabine (Drugs that decrease renal function may increase serum concentrations of tenofovir. Tenofovir should be avoided with concomittant or recent use of a nephrotoxic agent).
No products indexed under this heading.

Zidovudine (Drugs that decrease renal function may increase serum concentrations of tenofovir. Tenofovir should be avoided with concomittant or recent use of a nephrotoxic agent). Products include:
Combivir Tablets 1384
Retrovir 1574
Retrovir IV Infusion 1579
Trizivir Tablets 1622

Zoledronic acid (Drugs that decrease renal function may increase serum concentrations of tenofovir. Tenofovir should be avoided with concomittant or recent use of a nephrotoxic agent).
Products include:
Reclast Injection 2291
Zometa for Intravenous Infusion 2341

Food Interactions

Food, unspecified (Increases the bioavailability and delays the time to tenofovir Cmax; Viread should be taken with a meal).

VIROPTIC OPHTHALMIC SOLUTION

(Trifluridine) .... ⊙253
None cited in PDR database.

VISINE PURE TEARS DRY EYE RELIEF LUBRICANT EYE DROPS

(Glycerin, Hypromellose, Polyethylene Glycol) .... ⊙251
None cited in PDR database.

VISUDYNE FOR INJECTION

(Verteporfin) 2332
May interact with calcium channel blockers, anticoagulants, phenothiazines, sulfonamides, sulfonylureas, tetracyclines, thiazides, and certain other agents. Compounds in these categories include:

Amlodipine Besylate (Co-administration with calcium channel blockers could enhance the rate of verteporfin's uptake by the vascular endothelium). Products include:
Azor Tablets 1005
Exforge Tablets 2238

Anisindione (Co-administration with drugs that decrease clotting would be expected to decrease verteporfin activity).
No products indexed under this heading.

Ardeparin Sodium (Co-administration with drugs that decrease clotting would be expected to decrease verteporfin activity).
No products indexed under this heading.

Aspirin (Co-administration with drugs that decrease platelet aggregation would be expected to decrease verteporfin activity).
Products include:
Aggrenox Capsules 819
Bayer Aspirin 750
Percodan Tablets 1130
St. Joseph 81 mg Aspirin Chewable and Enteric Coated Tablets 1903

Bendroflumethiazide (Co-administration with other photosensitizing agents, such as thiazide diuretics, could increase the potential for skin photosensitivity reactions).
No products indexed under this heading.

Bepridil Hydrochloride (Co-administration with calcium channel blockers could enhance the rate of verteporfin's uptake by the vascular endothelium).
No products indexed under this heading.

Chlorothiazide (Co-administration with other photosensitizing agents, such as thiazide diuretics, could increase the potential for skin photosensitivity reactions).
No products indexed under this heading.

Chlorothiazide Sodium (Co-administration with other photosensitizing agents, such as thiazide diuretics, could increase the potential for skin photosensitivity reactions).
Products include:
Intravenous Sodium Diuril 2490

Chlorpromazine (Co-administration with other photosensitizing agents, such as phenothiazines, could increase the potential for skin photosensitivity reactions).
No products indexed under this heading.

Chlorpromazine Hydrochloride (Co-administration with other photosensitizing agents, such as phenothiazines, could increase the potential for skin photosensitivity reactions).
No products indexed under this heading.

Chlorpropamide (Co-administration with other photosensitizing agents, such as sulfonylurea hypoglycemic agents, could increase the potential for skin photosensitivity reactions).
No products indexed under this heading.

Clopidogrel Bisulfate (Co-administration with drugs that decrease platelet aggregation would be expected to decrease verteporfin activity). Products include:
Plavix Tablets 926
Plavix Tablets 2767

Dalteparin Sodium (Co-administration with drugs that decrease clotting would be expected to decrease verteporfin activity).
Products include:
Fragmin Injection 1070

Danaparoid Sodium (Co-administration with drugs that decrease clotting would be expected to decrease verteporfin activity).
No products indexed under this heading.

Demeclocycline Hydrochloride (Co-administration with other photosensitizing agents, such as tetracyclines, could increase the potential for skin photosensitivity reactions).
No products indexed under this heading.

Dicumarol (Co-administration with drugs that decrease clotting would be expected to decrease verteporfin activity).
No products indexed under this heading.

Diltiazem Hydrochloride (Co-administration with calcium channel blockers could enhance the rate of verteporfin's uptake by the vascular endothelium). Products include:
Cardizem LA Extended Release Tablets 421

Dimethyl Sulfoxide (Co-administration with compounds that quench active oxygen species or scavenge radicals, such as dimethyl sulfoxide, would be expected to decrease verteporfin activity).
No products indexed under this heading.

Dipyridamole (Co-administration with drugs that decrease platelet aggregation would be expected to decrease verteporfin activity).
Products include:
Aggrenox Capsules 819
Persantine Tablets 869

Doxycycline Calcium (Co-administration with other photosensitizing agents, such as tetracyclines, could increase the potential for skin photosensitivity reactions).
No products indexed under this heading.

Doxycycline Hyclate (Co-administration with other photosensitizing agents, such as tetracyclines, could increase the potential for skin photosensitivity reactions).
No products indexed under this heading.

Doxycycline Monohydrate (Co-administration with other photosensitizing agents, such as tetracyclines, could increase the potential for skin photosensitivity reactions).
No products indexed under this heading.

Enoxaparin Sodium (Co-administration with drugs that decrease clotting would be expected to decrease verteporfin activity).
Products include:
Lovenox Injection 2756

Felodipine (Co-administration with calcium channel blockers could enhance the rate of verteporfin's uptake by the vascular endothelium).
No products indexed under this heading.

Fluphenazine Decanoate (Co-administration with other photosensitizing agents, such as phenothiazines, could increase the potential for skin photosensitivity reactions).
No products indexed under this heading.

Fluphenazine Enanthate (Co-administration with other photosensitizing agents, such as phenothiazines, could increase the potential for skin photosensitivity reactions).
No products indexed under this heading.

Fluphenazine Hydrochloride (Co-administration with other photosensitizing agents, such as phenothiazines, could increase the potential for skin photosensitivity reactions).
No products indexed under this heading.

Fondaparinux Sodium (Co-administration with drugs that decrease clotting would be expected to decrease verteporfin activity).
Products include:
Arixtra Injection 1313

Glimepiride (Co-administration with other photosensitizing agents, such as sulfonylurea hypoglycemic agents, could increase the potential for skin photosensitivity reactions).
Products include:
Avandaryl Tablets 1344
Duetact Tablets 3085

Glipizide (Co-administration with other photosensitizing agents, such as sulfonylurea hypoglycemic agents, could increase the potential for skin photosensitivity reactions).
No products indexed under this heading.

Glyburide (Co-administration with other photosensitizing agents, such as sulfonylurea hypoglycemic agents, could increase the potential for skin photosensitivity reactions).
No products indexed under this heading.

Griseofulvin (Co-administration with other photosensitizing agents, such as griseofulvin, could increase the potential for skin photosensitivity reactions). Products include:
Gris-PEG Tablets 2507

Heparin Calcium (Co-administration with drugs that decrease clotting would be expected to decrease verteporfin activity).
No products indexed under this heading.

Heparin Sodium (Co-administration with drugs that decrease clotting would be expected to decrease verteporfin activity).
No products indexed under this heading.

Hydrochlorothiazide (Co-administration with other photosensitizing agents, such as thiazide diuretics, could increase the potential for skin photosensitivity reactions).
Products include:
Atacand HCT 642
Avalide Tablets 892
Avalide Tablets 2713
Benicar HCT Tablets 1010
Diovan HCT Tablets 2216
Dyazide Capsules 1405
Micardis HCT Tablets 854
Prinzide Tablets 2092
Tekturna HCT Tablets 2324
Teveten HCT Tablets 517

Hydroflumethiazide (Co-administration with other photosensitizing agents, such as thiazide diuretics, could increase the potential for skin photosensitivity reactions).
No products indexed under this heading.

Isradipine (Co-administration with calcium channel blockers could enhance the rate of verteporfin's uptake by the vascular endothelium).
Products include:
DynaCirc CR Controlled Release Tablets 1407

Low Molecular Weight Heparins (Co-administration with drugs that decrease clotting would be expected to decrease verteporfin activity).
No products indexed under this heading.

Mannitol (Co-administration with compounds that quench active oxygen species or scavenge radicals, such as mannitol, would be expected to decrease verteporfin activity).
No products indexed under this heading.

Mesoridazine Besylate (Co-administration with other photosensitizing agents, such as phenothiazines, could increase the potential for skin photosensitivity reactions).
No products indexed under this heading.

Methacycline Hydrochloride (Co-administration with other photosensitizing agents, such as tetracyclines, could increase the potential for skin photosensitivity reactions).
No products indexed under this heading.

Methotrimeprazine (Co-administration with other photosensitizing agents, such as phenothiazines, could increase the potential for skin photosensitivity reactions).
No products indexed under this heading.

Methyclothiazide (Co-administration with other photosensitizing agents, such as thiazide diuretics, could increase the potential for skin photosensitivity reactions).
No products indexed under this heading.

Mibefradil Dihydrochloride (Co-administration with calcium channel blockers could enhance the rate of verteporfin's uptake by the vascular endothelium).
No products indexed under this heading.

Minocycline Hydrochloride (Co-administration with other photosensitizing agents, such as tetracyclines, could increase the potential for skin photosensitivity reactions). Products include:
Solodyn Extended Release Tablets 1938

Nicardipine Hydrochloride (Co-administration with calcium channel blockers could enhance the rate of verteporfin's uptake by the vascular endothelium). Products include:
Cardene I.V. 1093

Nifedipine (Co-administration with calcium channel blockers could enhance the rate of verteporfin's uptake by the vascular endothelium).
No products indexed under this heading.

Nimodipine (Co-administration with calcium channel blockers could enhance the rate of verteporfin's uptake by the vascular endothelium).
Products include:
Nimotop Capsules 790

Nisoldipine (Co-administration with calcium channel blockers could enhance the rate of verteporfin's uptake by the vascular endothelium).
Products include:
Sular Extended Release Tablets 2975

Oxytetracycline Hydrochloride (Co-administration with other photosensitizing agents, such as tetracyclines, could increase the potential for skin photosensitivity reactions).
No products indexed under this heading.

Perphenazine (Co-administration with other photosensitizing agents, such as phenothiazines, could increase the potential for skin photosensitivity reactions).
No products indexed under this heading.

Polymyxin B Sulfate (Co-administration with polymyxin B could enhance the rate of verteporfin's uptake by the vascular endothelium). Products include:
Neosporin Ophthalmic Solution Sterile .... ⊙252

Polythiazide (Co-administration with other photosensitizing agents, such as thiazide diuretics, could increase the potential for skin photosensitivity reactions).
No products indexed under this heading.

Prochlorperazine (Co-administration with other photosensitizing agents, such as phenothiazines, could increase the potential for skin photosensitivity reactions).
No products indexed under this heading.

Promethazine Hydrochloride (Co-administration with other photosensitizing agents, such as phenothiazines, could increase the potential for skin photosensitivity reactions).
No products indexed under this heading.

Sulfacytine (Co-administration with other photosensitizing agents, such as sulfonamides, could increase the potential for skin photosensitivity reactions).
No products indexed under this heading.

Sulfamethizole (Co-administration with other photosensitizing agents, such as sulfonamides, could increase the potential for skin photosensitivity reactions).
No products indexed under this heading.

Sulfamethoxazole (Co-administration with other photosensitizing agents, such as sulfonamides, could increase the potential for skin photosensitivity reactions).
No products indexed under this heading.

Sulfasalazine (Co-administration with other photosensitizing agents, such as sulfonamides, could increase the potential for skin photosensitivity reactions).
No products indexed under this heading.

Sulfinpyrazone (Co-administration with other photosensitizing agents, such as sulfonamides, could increase the potential for skin photosensitivity reactions).
No products indexed under this heading.

Sulfisoxazole Acetyl (Co-administration with other photosensitizing agents, such as sulfonamides, could increase the potential for skin photosensitivity reactions).
No products indexed under this heading.

Sulfisoxazole Diolamine (Co-administration with other photosensitizing agents, such as sulfonamides, could increase the potential for skin photosensitivity reactions).
No products indexed under this heading.

Tetracycline Hydrochloride (Co-administration with other photosensitizing agents, such as tetracyclines, could increase the potential for skin photosensitivity reactions). Products include:
Pylera Capsules 714

Thioridazine Hydrochloride (Co-administration with other photosensitizing agents, such as phenothiazines, could increase the potential for skin photosensitivity reactions).
Products include:
Thioridazine Hydrochloride Tablets 2195

Tinzaparin Sodium (Co-administration with drugs that decrease clotting would be expected to decrease verteporfin activity).
No products indexed under this heading.

Tolazamide (Co-administration with other photosensitizing agents, such as sulfonylurea hypoglycemic agents, could increase the potential for skin photosensitivity reactions).
No products indexed under this heading.

Tolbutamide (Co-administration with other photosensitizing agents, such as sulfonylurea hypoglycemic agents, could increase the potential for skin photosensitivity reactions).
No products indexed under this heading.

Trifluoperazine Hydrochloride (Co-administration with other photosensitizing agents, such as phenothiazines, could increase the potential for skin photosensitivity reactions).
No products indexed under this heading.

Verapamil Hydrochloride (Co-administration with calcium channel blockers could enhance the rate of verteporfin's uptake by the vascular endothelium). Products include:
Tarka Tablets **511**

Warfarin Sodium (Co-administration with drugs that decrease clotting would be expected to decrease verteporfin activity).
No products indexed under this heading.

Food Interactions

Alcohol (Co-administration with compounds that quench active oxygen species or scavenge radicals, such as ethanol, would be expected to decrease verteporfin activity).

VISUTEIN CAPSULES

(Acetylcysteine, Carotenoids, Lutein, Vitamin B_2, Zinc) **3159**
None cited in PDR database.

VIVITROL

(Naltrexone) **988**
May interact with narcotic analgesics and certain other agents. Compounds in these categories include:

Alfentanil Hydrochloride (Naltrexone is contraindicated in patients receiving opioid analgesics).
No products indexed under this heading.

Buprenorphine Hydrochloride (Naltrexone is contraindicated in patients receiving opioid analgesics). Products include:
Suboxone Tablets **2601**
Subutex Tablets **2601**

Codeine Phosphate (Naltrexone is contraindicated in patients receiving opioid analgesics). Products include:
Tylenol with Codeine Tablets **2427**

Dezocine (Naltrexone is contraindicated in patients receiving opioid analgesics).
No products indexed under this heading.

Fentanyl (Naltrexone is contraindicated in patients receiving opioid analgesics). Products include:
Duragesic Transdermal System **2405**
Ionsys Transdermal System **2410**

Fentanyl Citrate (Naltrexone is contraindicated in patients receiving opioid analgesics). Products include:
Actiq **959**
Fentora Tablets **968**

Hydrocodone Bitartrate (Naltrexone is contraindicated in patients receiving opioid analgesics). Products include:
Lortab 5/500 Tablets **3143**
Lortab 7.5/500 Tablets **3144**
Lortab 10/500 Tablets **3144**
Vicodin Tablets **529**
Vicodin ES Tablets **530**
Vicodin HP Tablets **531**
Vicoprofen Tablets **533**
Zydone Tablets **1132**

Hydrocodone Polistirex (Naltrexone is contraindicated in patients receiving opioid analgesics). Products include:
Tussionex Pennkinetic Extended-Release Suspension **3154**

Hydromorphone Hydrochloride (Naltrexone is contraindicated in patients receiving opioid analgesics).
No products indexed under this heading.

Levorphanol Tartrate (Naltrexone is contraindicated in patients receiving opioid analgesics).
No products indexed under this heading.

Meperidine Hydrochloride (Naltrexone is contraindicated in patients receiving opioid analgesics).
No products indexed under this heading.

Methadone Hydrochloride (Naltrexone is contraindicated in patients receiving opioid analgesics).
No products indexed under this heading.

Morphine Sulfate (Naltrexone is contraindicated in patients receiving opioid analgesics). Products include:
Avinza Capsules **1772**
DepoDur Injection **1095**
MS Contin Tablets **2585**

Opioid Analgesics (Naltrexone is contraindicated in patients receiving opioid analgesics).
No products indexed under this heading.

Opium Preparations (Naltrexone antagonizes the effects of opioid containing medicines, such as cough and cold remedies, antidiarrheal preparations and opioid analgesics).
No products indexed under this heading.

Oxycodone Hydrochloride (Naltrexone is contraindicated in patients receiving opioid analgesics). Products include:
OxyContin Tablets **2589**
OxyIR Capsules **2593**
Percocet Tablets **1127**
Percodan Tablets **1130**

Propoxyphene Hydrochloride (Naltrexone is contraindicated in patients receiving opioid analgesics).
No products indexed under this heading.

Propoxyphene Napsylate (Naltrexone is contraindicated in patients receiving opioid analgesics).
No products indexed under this heading.

Remifentanil Hydrochloride (Naltrexone is contraindicated in patients receiving opioid analgesics).
No products indexed under this heading.

Sufentanil Citrate (Naltrexone is contraindicated in patients receiving opioid analgesics).
No products indexed under this heading.

VOLTAREN OPHTHALMIC SOLUTION

(Diclofenac Sodium) **2336**
May interact with anticoagulants and corticosteroids. Compounds in these categories include:

Anisindione (It is recommended that diclofenac ophthalmic suspension be used with caution in patients who are receiving other medications which may prolong bleeding time).
No products indexed under this heading.

Ardeparin Sodium (It is recommended that diclofenac ophthalmic suspension be used with caution in patients who are receiving other medications which may prolong bleeding time).
No products indexed under this heading.

Betamethasone Acetate (All topical nonsteroidal anti-inflammatory drugs (NSAIDs) may slow or delay healing. Topical corticosteroids are also known to slow or delay healing. Concomitant use of topical NSAIDs and topical steroids may increase the potential for healing problems).
No products indexed under this heading.

Betamethasone Sodium Phosphate (All topical nonsteroidal anti-inflammatory drugs (NSAIDs) may slow or delay healing. Topical corticosteroids are also known to slow or delay healing. Concomitant use of topical NSAIDs and topical steroids may increase the potential for healing problems).
No products indexed under this heading.

Budesonide (All topical nonsteroidal anti-inflammatory drugs (NSAIDs) may slow or delay healing. Topical corticosteroids are also known to slow or delay healing. Concomitant use of topical NSAIDs and topical steroids may increase the potential for healing problems). Products include:
Pulmicort Flexhaler **654**
Symbicort 80/4.5 Inhalation Aerosol **659**
Symbicort 160/4.5 Inhalation Aerosol **659**

Ciclesonide (All topical nonsteroidal anti-inflammatory drugs (NSAIDs) may slow or delay healing. Topical corticosteroids are also known to slow or delay healing. Concomitant use of topical NSAIDs and topical steroids may increase the potential for healing problems). Products include:
Alvesco Inhalation Aerosol **2985**
Omnaris Nasal Spray **2998**

Cortisone Acetate (All topical nonsteroidal anti-inflammatory drugs (NSAIDs) may slow or delay healing. Topical corticosteroids are also known to slow or delay healing. Concomitant use of topical NSAIDs and topical steroids may increase the potential for healing problems).
No products indexed under this heading.

Dalteparin Sodium (It is recommended that diclofenac ophthalmic suspension be used with caution in patients who are receiving other medications which may prolong bleeding time). Products include:
Fragmin Injection **1070**

Danaparoid Sodium (It is recommended that diclofenac ophthalmic suspension be used with caution in patients who are receiving other medications which may prolong bleeding time).
No products indexed under this heading.

Dexamethasone (All topical nonsteroidal anti-inflammatory drugs (NSAIDs) may slow or delay healing. Topical corticosteroids are also known to slow or delay healing. Concomitant use of topical NSAIDs and topical steroids may increase the potential for healing problems). Products include:
Ciprodex Otic Suspension **541**

Dexamethasone Acetate (All topical nonsteroidal anti-inflammatory drugs (NSAIDs) may slow or delay healing. Topical corticosteroids are also known to slow or delay healing. Concomitant use of topical NSAIDs and topical steroids may increase the potential for healing problems).
No products indexed under this heading.

Dexamethasone Sodium Phosphate (All topical nonsteroidal anti-inflammatory drugs (NSAIDs) may slow or delay healing. Topical corticosteroids are also known to slow or delay healing. Concomitant use of topical NSAIDs and topical steroids may increase the potential for healing problems).
No products indexed under this heading.

Dicumarol (It is recommended that diclofenac ophthalmic suspension be used with caution in patients who are receiving other medications which may prolong bleeding time).
No products indexed under this heading.

Enoxaparin Sodium (It is recommended that diclofenac ophthalmic suspension be used with caution in patients who are receiving other medications which may prolong bleeding time). Products include:
Lovenox Injection **2756**

Fludrocortisone Acetate (All topical nonsteroidal anti-inflammatory drugs (NSAIDs) may slow or delay healing. Topical corticosteroids are also known to slow or delay healing. Concomitant use of topical NSAIDs and topical steroids may increase the potential for healing problems).
No products indexed under this heading.

Flunisolide (All topical nonsteroidal anti-inflammatory drugs (NSAIDs) may slow or delay healing. Topical corticosteroids are also known to slow or delay healing. Concomitant use of topical NSAIDs and topical steroids may increase the potential for healing problems). Products include:
Aerobid/Aerobid-M **1153**

Fluticasone Propionate (All topical nonsteroidal anti-inflammatory drugs (NSAIDs) may slow or delay healing. Topical corticosteroids are also known to slow or delay healing. Concomitant use of topical NSAIDs and topical steroids may increase the potential for healing problems). Products include:
Advair Diskus 100/50 ..... **1276**
Advair Diskus 250/50 ..... **1276**
Advair Diskus 500/50 ..... **1276**
Advair HFA 45/21 Inhalation Aerosol **1288**

Advair HFA 115/21 Inhalation Aerosol 1288
Advair HFA 230/21 Inhalation Aerosol 1288
Flonase Nasal Spray 1431
Flovent Diskus 50 mcg 1435

Fluticasone Propionate HFA (All topical nonsteroidal anti-inflammatory drugs (NSAIDs) may slow or delay healing. Topical corticosteroids are also known to slow or delay healing. Concomitant use of topical NSAIDs and topical steroids may increase the potential for healing problems). Products include:
Flovent HFA 1440

Fondaparinux Sodium (It is recommended that diclofenac ophthalmic suspension be used with caution in patients who are receiving other medications which may prolong bleeding time). Products include:
Arixtra Injection 1313

Heparin Calcium (It is recommended that diclofenac ophthalmic suspension be used with caution in patients who are receiving other medications which may prolong bleeding time).
No products indexed under this heading.

Heparin Sodium (It is recommended that diclofenac ophthalmic suspension be used with caution in patients who are receiving other medications which may prolong bleeding time).
No products indexed under this heading.

Hydrocortisone (All topical nonsteroidal anti-inflammatory drugs (NSAIDs) may slow or delay healing. Topical corticosteroids are also known to slow or delay healing. Concomitant use of topical NSAIDs and topical steroids may increase the potential for healing problems).
No products indexed under this heading.

Hydrocortisone Acetate (All topical nonsteroidal anti-inflammatory drugs (NSAIDs) may slow or delay healing. Topical corticosteroids are also known to slow or delay healing. Concomitant use of topical NSAIDs and topical steroids may increase the potential for healing problems). Products include:
Analpram-HC 1140
Pramosone 1141

Hydrocortisone Sodium Phosphate (All topical nonsteroidal anti-inflammatory drugs (NSAIDs) may slow or delay healing. Topical corticosteroids are also known to slow or delay healing. Concomitant use of topical NSAIDs and topical steroids may increase the potential for healing problems).
No products indexed under this heading.

Hydrocortisone Sodium Succinate (All topical nonsteroidal anti-inflammatory drugs (NSAIDs) may slow or delay healing. Topical corticosteroids are also known to slow or delay healing. Concomitant use of topical NSAIDs and topical steroids may increase the potential for healing problems).
No products indexed under this heading.

Low Molecular Weight Heparins (It is recommended that diclofenac ophthalmic suspension be used with caution in patients who are receiving other medications which may prolong bleeding time).
No products indexed under this heading.

Methylprednisolone Acetate (All topical nonsteroidal anti-inflammatory drugs (NSAIDs) may slow or delay healing. Topical corticosteroids are also known to slow or delay healing. Concomitant use of topical NSAIDs and topical steroids may increase the potential for healing problems).
No products indexed under this heading.

Methylprednisolone Sodium Succinate (All topical nonsteroidal anti-inflammatory drugs (NSAIDs) may slow or delay healing. Topical corticosteroids are also known to slow or delay healing. Concomitant use of topical NSAIDs and topical steroids may increase the potential for healing problems).
No products indexed under this heading.

Mometasone Furoate (All topical nonsteroidal anti-inflammatory drugs (NSAIDs) may slow or delay healing. Topical corticosteroids are also known to slow or delay healing. Concomitant use of topical NSAIDs and topical steroids may increase the potential for healing problems). Products include:
Asmanex Twisthaler 2797
Elocon Cream 0.1% 2840
Elocon Lotion 0.1% 2841
Elocon Ointment 0.1% 2842

Mometasone Furoate Monohydrate (All topical nonsteroidal anti-inflammatory drugs (NSAIDs) may slow or delay healing. Topical corticosteroids are also known to slow or delay healing. Concomitant use of topical NSAIDs and topical steroids may increase the potential for healing problems). Products include:
Nasonex Nasal Spray 2883

Prednisolone Acetate (All topical nonsteroidal anti-inflammatory drugs (NSAIDs) may slow or delay healing. Topical corticosteroids are also known to slow or delay healing. Concomitant use of topical NSAIDs and topical steroids may increase the potential for healing problems). Products include:
Pred Forte Ophthalmic Suspension .... ⊙ 227
Pred Mild Ophthalmic Suspension .... ⊙ 230
Pred-G Ophthalmic Ointment .... ⊙ 229
Pred-G Ophthalmic Suspension .... ⊙ 228

Prednisolone Sodium Phosphate (All topical nonsteroidal anti-inflammatory drugs (NSAIDs) may slow or delay healing. Topical corticosteroids are also known to slow or delay healing. Concomitant use of topical NSAIDs and topical steroids may increase the potential for healing problems).
No products indexed under this heading.

Prednisolone Tebutate (All topical nonsteroidal anti-inflammatory drugs (NSAIDs) may slow or delay healing. Topical corticosteroids are also known to slow or delay healing. Concomitant use of topical NSAIDs and topical steroids may increase the potential for healing problems).
No products indexed under this heading.

Prednisone (All topical nonsteroidal anti-inflammatory drugs (NSAIDs) may slow or delay healing. Topical corticosteroids are also known to slow or delay healing. Concomitant use of topical NSAIDs and topical steroids may increase the potential for healing problems).
No products indexed under this heading.

Tinzaparin Sodium (It is recommended that diclofenac ophthalmic suspension be used with caution in patients who are receiving other medications which may prolong bleeding time).
No products indexed under this heading.

Triamcinolone (All topical nonsteroidal anti-inflammatory drugs (NSAIDs) may slow or delay healing. Topical corticosteroids are also known to slow or delay healing. Concomitant use of topical NSAIDs and topical steroids may increase the potential for healing problems).
No products indexed under this heading.

Triamcinolone Acetonide (All topical nonsteroidal anti-inflammatory drugs (NSAIDs) may slow or delay healing. Topical corticosteroids are also known to slow or delay healing. Concomitant use of topical NSAIDs and topical steroids may increase the potential for healing problems). Products include:
Azmacort Inhalation Aerosol 407
Nasacort AQ Nasal Spray 2765
Triesence Injectable Suspension .... ⊙ 209

Triamcinolone Diacetate (All topical nonsteroidal anti-inflammatory drugs (NSAIDs) may slow or delay healing. Topical corticosteroids are also known to slow or delay healing. Concomitant use of topical NSAIDs and topical steroids may increase the potential for healing problems).
No products indexed under this heading.

Triamcinolone Hexacetonide (All topical nonsteroidal anti-inflammatory drugs (NSAIDs) may slow or delay healing. Topical corticosteroids are also known to slow or delay healing. Concomitant use of topical NSAIDs and topical steroids may increase the potential for healing problems).
No products indexed under this heading.

Warfarin Sodium (It is recommended that diclofenac ophthalmic suspension be used with caution in patients who are receiving other medications which may prolong bleeding time).
No products indexed under this heading.

VOLTAREN TABLETS

(Diclofenac Sodium) 2334
May interact with ACE inhibitors, lithium preparations, thiazides, and certain other agents. Compounds in these categories include:

Aspirin (When diclofenac is administered with aspirin, its protein binding is reduced; the clinical significance of this interaction is not known). Products include:
Aggrenox Capsules 819
Bayer Aspirin 750
Percodan Tablets 1130
St. Joseph 81 mg Aspirin Chewable and Enteric Coated Tablets 1903

Benazepril Hydrochloride (Reports suggest that NSAIDs may diminish the antihypertensive effect of ACE inhibitors; this interaction should be given consideration in patients taking NSAIDs concomitantly with ACE inhibitors).
No products indexed under this heading.

Bendroflumethiazide (Studies have shown that diclofenac can reduce the natriuretic effect of furosemide and thiazides in some patients; during concomitant therapy with NSAIDs, the patient should be observed closely for signs of renal failure, as well as to assure diuretic efficacy).
No products indexed under this heading.

Captopril (Reports suggest that NSAIDs may diminish the antihypertensive effect of ACE inhibitors; this interaction should be given consideration in patients taking NSAIDs concomitantly with ACE inhibitors). Products include:
Captopril Tablets 2182

Chlorothiazide (Studies have shown that diclofenac can reduce the natriuretic effect of furosemide and thiazides in some patients; during concomitant therapy with NSAIDs, the patient should be observed closely for signs of renal failure, as well as to assure diuretic efficacy).
No products indexed under this heading.

Chlorothiazide Sodium (Studies have shown that diclofenac can reduce the natriuretic effect of furosemide and thiazides in some patients; during concomitant therapy with NSAIDs, the patient should be observed closely for signs of renal failure, as well as to assure diuretic efficacy). Products include:
Intravenous Sodium Diuril 2490

Cyclosporine (Diclofenac may affect renal prostaglandins and increase the toxicity of certain drugs; concomitant therapy with diclofenac may increase cyclosporine's nephrotoxicity; caution should be used when administered concomitantly with cyclosporine). Products include:
Gengraf Capsules 435
Neoral Oral Solution 2280
Neoral Soft Gelatin Capsules 2280
Restasis Ophthalmic Emulsion 557
Sandimmune 2296

Enalapril Maleate (Reports suggest that NSAIDs may diminish the antihypertensive effect of ACE inhibitors; this interaction should be given consideration in patients taking NSAIDs concomitantly with ACE inhibitors).
No products indexed under this heading.

Enalaprilat (Reports suggest that NSAIDs may diminish the antihypertensive effect of ACE inhibitors; this interaction should be given consideration in patients taking NSAIDs concomitantly with ACE inhibitors).
No products indexed under this heading.

Fosinopril Sodium (Reports suggest that NSAIDs may diminish the antihypertensive effect of ACE inhibitors; this interaction should be given consideration in patients taking NSAIDs concomitantly with ACE inhibitors).
No products indexed under this heading.

Furosemide (Studies have shown that diclofenac can reduce the natriuretic effect of furosemide and thiazides in some patients; during concomitant therapy with NSAIDs, the patient should be observed closely for signs of renal failure, as well as to assure diuretic efficacy). Products include:
Furosemide Tablets 2186

Hydrochlorothiazide (Studies have shown that diclofenac can reduce the natriuretic effect of furosemide and thiazides in some patients; during concomitant therapy with NSAIDs, the patient should be observed closely for signs of renal failure, as well as to assure diuretic efficacy). Products include:
Atacand HCT 642
Avalide Tablets 892
Avalide Tablets 2713
Benicar HCT Tablets 1010
Diovan HCT Tablets 2216
Dyazide Capsules 1405
Micardis HCT Tablets 854
Prinzide Tablets 2092
Tekturna HCT Tablets 2324
Teveten HCT Tablets 517

Hydroflumethiazide (Studies have shown that diclofenac can reduce the natriuretic effect of furosemide and thiazides in some patients; during concomitant therapy with NSAIDs, the patient should be observed closely for signs of renal failure, as well as to assure diuretic efficacy).
No products indexed under this heading.

Lisinopril (Reports suggest that NSAIDs may diminish the antihypertensive effect of ACE inhibitors; this interaction should be given consideration in patients taking NSAIDs concomitantly with ACE inhibitors).
Products include:
Prinivil Tablets 2087
Prinzide Tablets 2092

Lithium (NSAIDs have produced an elevation of plasma lithium levels and a reduction in renal lithium clearance; these effects have been attributed to inhibition of renal prostaglandin synthesis by the NSAID; monitor for signs of lithium toxicity).
No products indexed under this heading.

Lithium Carbonate (NSAIDs have produced an elevation of plasma lithium levels and a reduction in renal lithium clearance; these effects have been attributed to inhibition of renal prostaglandin synthesis by the NSAID; monitor for signs of lithium toxicity).
No products indexed under this heading.

Lithium Citrate (NSAIDs have produced an elevation of plasma lithium levels and a reduction in renal lithium clearance; these effects have been attributed to inhibition of renal prostaglandin synthesis by the NSAID; monitor for signs of lithium toxicity).
No products indexed under this heading.

Methotrexate Sodium (NSAIDs have been reported to competitively inhibit methotrexate accumulation in animal studies; this may indicate that they could enhance the toxicity of methotrexate; caution should be given when NSAIDs are administered concomitantly with methotrexate).
No products indexed under this heading.

Methyclothiazide (Studies have shown that diclofenac can reduce the natriuretic effect of furosemide and thiazides in some patients; during concomitant therapy with NSAIDs, the patient should be observed closely for signs of renal failure, as well as to assure diuretic efficacy).
No products indexed under this heading.

Moexipril Hydrochloride (Reports suggest that NSAIDs may diminish the antihypertensive effect of ACE inhibitors; this interaction should be given consideration in patients taking NSAIDs concomitantly with ACE inhibitors).
No products indexed under this heading.

Perindopril Erbumine (Reports suggest that NSAIDs may diminish the antihypertensive effect of ACE inhibitors; this interaction should be given consideration in patients taking NSAIDs concomitantly with ACE inhibitors). Products include:
Aceon Tablets (2 mg, 4 mg, 8 mg) 3038

Polythiazide (Studies have shown that diclofenac can reduce the natriuretic effect of furosemide and thiazides in some patients; during concomitant therapy with NSAIDs, the patient should be observed closely for signs of renal failure, as well as to assure diuretic efficacy).
No products indexed under this heading.

Quinapril Hydrochloride (Reports suggest that NSAIDs may diminish the antihypertensive effect of ACE inhibitors; this interaction should be given consideration in patients taking NSAIDs concomitantly with ACE inhibitors).
No products indexed under this heading.

Ramipril (Reports suggest that NSAIDs may diminish the antihypertensive effect of ACE inhibitors; this interaction should be given consideration in patients taking NSAIDs concomitantly with ACE inhibitors).
No products indexed under this heading.

Spirapril Hydrochloride (Reports suggest that NSAIDs may diminish the antihypertensive effect of ACE inhibitors; this interaction should be given consideration in patients taking NSAIDs concomitantly with ACE inhibitors).
No products indexed under this heading.

Trandolapril (Reports suggest that NSAIDs may diminish the antihypertensive effect of ACE inhibitors; this interaction should be given consideration in patients taking NSAIDs concomitantly with ACE inhibitors).
Products include:
Mavik Tablets 472
Tarka Tablets 511

Warfarin Sodium (The effects of warfarin and NSAIDs on GI bleeding are synergistic, such that users of both drugs together have a risk of serious GI bleeding higher than users of either drug alone).
No products indexed under this heading.

VOLTAREN-XR TABLETS
(Diclofenac Sodium) 2337
See Voltaren Tablets

VYTORIN 10/10 TABLETS
(Ezetimibe, Simvastatin) 2149
May interact with bile acid sequestering agents, oral anticoagulants, cytochrome p450 3a4 inhibitors, potent, erythromycin, fibrates, protease inhibitors, and certain other agents. Compounds in these categories include:

Amiodarone Hydrochloride (The risk of myopathy/rhabdomyolysis is increased by concomitant administration of amiodarone with higher doses of Vytorin. In patients taking amiodarone concomitantly with Vytorin, the dose of Vytorin should not exceed 10/20 mg/day).
No products indexed under this heading.

Amprenavir (Simvastatin is metabolized by the cytochrome P450 isoform 3A4. Certain drugs that inhibit this metabolic pathway can raise plasma levels of simvastatin and may increase the risk of myopathy. This includes HIV protease inhibitors. The use of Vytorin concomitantly with these CYP3A4 inhibitors should be avoided).
No products indexed under this heading.

Anisindione (Simvastatin 20-40 mg/day modestly potentiated the effect of coumarin anticoagulants: the prothrombin time, reported as International Normalized Ratio (INR), increased from a baseline of 1.7 to 1.8 and from 2.6 to 3.4 in a normal volunteer study and in a hypercholesterolemic patient study, respectively. Prothrombin time should be determined before starting Vytorin and frequently enough during early therapy to ensure that no significant alteration of prothrombin time occurs. Once a stable prothrombin time has been documented, prothrombin times can be monitored at the intervals usually recommended for patients on coumarin anticoagulants. If the dose of Vytorin is changed or discontinued, the same procedure should be repeated).
No products indexed under this heading.

Atazanavir (Simvastatin is metabolized by the cytochrome P450 isoform 3A4. Certain drugs that inhibit this metabolic pathway can raise plasma levels of simvastatin and may increase the risk of myopathy. Concomitant use of any medication labeled as having a strong inhibitory effect on CYP3A4 should be avoided unless the benefits of combined therapy outweigh the increased risk).
No products indexed under this heading.

Atazanavir Sulfate (Simvastatin is metabolized by the cytochrome P450 isoform 3A4. Certain drugs that inhibit this metabolic pathway can raise plasma levels of simvastatin and may increase the risk of myopathy. Concomitant use of any medication labeled as having a strong inhibitory effect on CYP3A4 should be avoided unless the benefits of combined therapy outweigh the increased risk). Products include:
Reyataz Capsules 3299

Cholestyramine (Concomitant cholestyramine administration decreased the mean AUC of total ezetimibe approximately 55%. The incremental LDL-C reduction due to adding Vytorin to cholestyramine may be reduced by this interaction. Dosing of Vytorin should occur either greater than or equal to 2 hours before or greater than or equal to 4 hours after administration of a bile acid sequestrant).
No products indexed under this heading.

Clarithromycin (Simvastatin is metabolized by the cytochrome P450 isoform 3A4. Certain drugs that inhibit this metabolic pathway can raise plasma levels of simvastatin and may increase the risk of myopathy. This includes the macrolide antibiotic clarithromycin. The use of Vytorin concomitantly with this CYP3A4 inhibitor should be avoided. If treatment with clarithromycin is unavoidable, therapy with Vytorin should be suspended during the course of treatment). Products include:
Biaxin/Biaxin XL 411

Clofibrate (The safety and effectiveness of Vytorin administered with fibrates have not been established. Therefore the combination of Vytorin and fibrates should be avoided. There is an increased risk of myopathy when simvastatin is used concomitantly with fibrates).
No products indexed under this heading.

Colesevelam Hydrochloride (Dosing of Vytorin should occur either greater than or equal to 2 hours before or greater than or equal to 4 hours after administration of a bile acid sequestrant). Products include:
WelChol Tablets 1015

Colestipol Hydrochloride (Dosing of Vytorin should occur either greater than or equal to 2 hours before or greater than or equal to 4 hours after administration of a bile acid sequestrant).
No products indexed under this heading.

Cyclosporine (Caution should be exercised when using Vytorin and cyclosporine concurrently due to increased exposure to both ezetimibe and cyclosporine. The risk of myopathy/rhabdomyolysis is increased by concomitant administration of cyclosporine with Vytorin. Cyclosporine concentrations should be monitored if using Vytorin concomitantly. In patients treated with cyclosporine, the potential effects of the increased exposure to ezetimibe from concomitant use should be carefully weighed against the benefits of alterations in lipid levels provided by ezetimibe. In patients taking cyclosporine, Vytorin should not be started unless the patient has already tolerated treatment with simvastatin at a dose of 5 mg or higher. The dose of Vytorin should not exceed 10/10 mg/day). Products include:

Gengraf Capsules 435
Neoral Oral Solution 2280
Neoral Soft Gelatin Capsules 2280
Restasis Ophthalmic Emulsion 557
Sandimmune 2296

Danazol (The risk of myopathy/ rhabdomyolysis is increased by concomitant administration of danazol particularly with higher doses of Vytorin. In patients taking danazol, Vytorin should not be started unless the patient has already tolerated treatment with simvastatin at a dose of 5 mg or higher. The dose of Vytorin should not exceed 10/10 mg/day).

No products indexed under this heading.

Darunavir (Simvastatin is metabolized by the cytochrome P450 isoform 3A4. Certain drugs that inhibit this metabolic pathway can raise plasma levels of simvastatin and may increase the risk of myopathy. This includes HIV protease inhibitors. The use of Vytorin concomitantly with these CYP3A4 inhibitors should be avoided).

No products indexed under this heading.

Delavirdine Mesylate (Simvastatin is metabolized by the cytochrome P450 isoform 3A4. Certain drugs that inhibit this metabolic pathway can raise plasma levels of simvastatin and may increase the risk of myopathy. Concomitant use of any medication labeled as having a strong inhibitory effect on CYP3A4 should be avoided unless the benefits of combined therapy outweigh the increased risk).

No products indexed under this heading.

Delavirine (Simvastatin is metabolized by the cytochrome P450 isoform 3A4. Certain drugs that inhibit this metabolic pathway can raise plasma levels of simvastatin and may increase the risk of myopathy. Concomitant use of any medication labeled as having a strong inhibitory effect on CYP3A4 should be avoided unless the benefits of combined therapy outweigh the increased risk).

No products indexed under this heading.

Dicumarol (Simvastatin 20-40 mg/ day modestly potentiated the effect of coumarin anticoagulants: the prothrombin time, reported as International Normalized Ratio (INR), increased from a baseline of 1.7 to 1.8 and from 2.6 to 3.4 in a normal volunteer study and in a hypercholesterolemic patient study, respectively. Prothrombin time should be determined before starting Vytorin and frequently enough during early therapy to ensure that no significant alteration of prothrombin time occurs. Once a stable prothrombin time has been documented, prothrombin times can be monitored at the intervals usually recommended for patients on coumarin anticoagulants. If the dose of Vytorin is changed or discontinued, the same procedure should be repeated).

No products indexed under this heading.

Digoxin (In one study, concomitant administration of digoxin with simvastatin resulted in a slight elevation of plasma digoxin concentrations. Patients taking digoxin should be monitored appropriately when Vytorin is initiated). Products include:

Lanoxin Injection 1498
Lanoxin Injection Pediatric 1502
Lanoxin Tablets 1505

Erythromycin (Simvastatin is metabolized by the cytochrome P450 isoform 3A4. Certain drugs that inhibit this metabolic pathway can raise plasma levels of simvastatin and may increase the risk of myopathy. This includes the macrolide antibiotic erythromycin. The use of Vytorin concomitantly with this CYP3A4 inhibitor should be avoided. If treatment with erythromycin is unavoidable, therapy with Vytorin should be suspended during the course of treatment).

No products indexed under this heading.

Erythromycin Estolate (Simvastatin is metabolized by the cytochrome P450 isoform 3A4. Certain drugs that inhibit this metabolic pathway can raise plasma levels of simvastatin and may increase the risk of myopathy. This includes the macrolide antibiotic erythromycin. The use of Vytorin concomitantly with this CYP3A4 inhibitor should be avoided. If treatment with erythromycin is unavoidable, therapy with Vytorin should be suspended during the course of treatment).

No products indexed under this heading.

Erythromycin Ethylsuccinate (Simvastatin is metabolized by the cytochrome P450 isoform 3A4. Certain drugs that inhibit this metabolic pathway can raise plasma levels of simvastatin and may increase the risk of myopathy. This includes the macrolide antibiotic erythromycin. The use of Vytorin concomitantly with this CYP3A4 inhibitor should be avoided. If treatment with erythromycin is unavoidable, therapy with Vytorin should be suspended during the course of treatment). Products include:

E.E.S. 433
EryPed 431

Erythromycin Gluceptate (Simvastatin is metabolized by the cytochrome P450 isoform 3A4. Certain drugs that inhibit this metabolic pathway can raise plasma levels of simvastatin and may increase the risk of myopathy. This includes the macrolide antibiotic erythromycin. The use of Vytorin concomitantly with this CYP3A4 inhibitor should be avoided. If treatment with erythromycin is unavoidable, therapy with Vytorin should be suspended during the course of treatment).

No products indexed under this heading.

Erythromycin Lactobionate (Simvastatin is metabolized by the cytochrome P450 isoform 3A4. Certain drugs that inhibit this metabolic pathway can raise plasma levels of simvastatin and may increase the risk of myopathy. This includes the macrolide antibiotic erythromycin. The use of Vytorin concomitantly with this CYP3A4 inhibitor should be avoided. If treatment with erythromycin is unavoidable, therapy with Vytorin should be suspended during the course of treatment).

No products indexed under this heading.

Erythromycin Stearate (Simvastatin is metabolized by the cytochrome P450 isoform 3A4. Certain drugs that inhibit this metabolic pathway can raise plasma levels of simvastatin and may increase the risk of myopathy. This includes the macrolide antibiotic erythromycin. The use of Vytorin concomitantly with this CYP3A4 inhibitor should be avoided. If treatment with erythromycin is unavoidable, therapy with Vytorin should be suspended during the course of treatment).

No products indexed under this heading.

Fenofibrate (The safety and effectiveness of Vytorin administered with fibrates have not been established. Therefore the combination of Vytorin and fibrates should be avoided. There is an increased risk of myopathy when simvastatin is used concomitantly with fibrates). Products include:

Fenoglide Tablets 2960
Tricor Tablets 520

Fosamprenavir Calcium (Simvastatin is metabolized by the cytochrome P450 isoform 3A4. Certain drugs that inhibit this metabolic pathway can raise plasma levels of simvastatin and may increase the risk of myopathy. This includes HIV protease inhibitors. The use of Vytorin concomitantly with these CYP3A4 inhibitors should be avoided). Products include:

Lexiva Oral Suspension 1510
Lexiva Tablets 1510

Gemfibrozil (The safety and effectiveness of Vytorin administered with fibrates have not been established. Therefore the combination of Vytorin and fibrates should be avoided. There is an increased risk of myopathy when simvastatin is used concomitantly with fibrates (especially gemfibrozil). Combination therapy with gemfibrozil should be avoided because of an increase in simvastatin exposure with concomitant use).

No products indexed under this heading.

Indinavir Sulfate (Simvastatin is metabolized by the cytochrome P450 isoform 3A4. Certain drugs that inhibit this metabolic pathway can raise plasma levels of simvastatin and may increase the risk of myopathy. This includes HIV protease inhibitors. The use of Vytorin concomitantly with these CYP3A4 inhibitors should be avoided). Products include:

Crixivan Capsules 1979

Itraconazole (Simvastatin is metabolized by the cytochrome P450 isoform 3A4. Certain drugs that inhibit this metabolic pathway can raise plasma levels of simvastatin and may increase the risk of myopathy. This includes itraconazole. The use of Vytorin concomitantly with this CYP3A4 inhibitor should be avoided. If treatment with itraconazole is unavoidable, therapy with Vytorin should be suspended during the course of treatment).

No products indexed under this heading.

Ketoconazole (Simvastatin is metabolized by the cytochrome P450 isoform 3A4. Certain drugs that inhibit this metabolic pathway can raise plasma levels of simvastatin and may increase the risk of myopathy. This includes ketoconazole. The use of Vytorin concomitantly with this CYP3A4 inhibitor should be avoided. If treatment with ketoconazole is unavoidable, therapy with Vytorin should be suspended during the course of treatment). Products include:

Extina Foam, 2% 3057
Nizoral A-D Shampoo 1901

Lopinavir (Simvastatin is metabolized by the cytochrome P450 isoform 3A4. Certain drugs that inhibit this metabolic pathway can raise plasma levels of simvastatin and may increase the risk of myopathy. This includes HIV protease inhibitors. The use of Vytorin concomitantly with these CYP3A4 inhibitors should be avoided). Products include:

Kaletra 452

Nefazodone Hydrochloride (Simvastatin is metabolized by the cytochrome P450 isoform 3A4. Certain drugs that inhibit this metabolic pathway can raise plasma levels of simvastatin and may increase the risk of myopathy. This includes the antidepressant nefazodone. The use of Vytorin concomitantly with this CYP3A4 inhibitor should be avoided).

No products indexed under this heading.

Nelfinavir Mesylate (Simvastatin is metabolized by the cytochrome P450 isoform 3A4. Certain drugs that inhibit this metabolic pathway can raise plasma levels of simvastatin and may increase the risk of myopathy. This includes HIV protease inhibitors. The use of Vytorin concomitantly with these CYP3A4 inhibitors should be avoided).

No products indexed under this heading.

Niacin (Caution should be used when prescribing lipid-lowering doses (greater than or equal to 1 g/day) of niacin with Vytorin, as this agent can cause myopathy when given alone. The benefits of the combined use of Vytorin and other lipid lowering drugs (greater than or equal to 1 g/day of niacin) should be carefully weighed against the potential risks of this combination). Products include:

Advicor Tablets 402
Bausch & Lomb Ocuvite DF Vitamin Supplement.................... ⊙238
Dismutax Dietary Supplement 995
Niaspan Extended-Release Tablets.. 480
NT-Kinase Dietary Supplement 995
Simcor Tablets 502

Niacinamide (Caution should be used when prescribing lipid-lowering doses (greater than or equal to 1 g/day) of niacin with Vytorin, as this agent can cause myopathy when given alone. The benefits of the combined use of Vytorin and other lipid lowering drugs (greater than or equal to 1 g/day of niacin) should be carefully weighed against the potential risks of this combination). Products include:

BioLean Free Tablets .... ▣635

Niacinamide Hydroiodide (Caution should be used when prescribing lipid-lowering doses (greater than or equal to 1 g/day) of niacin with Vytorin, as this agent can cause myopathy when given alone. The benefits of the combined use of Vytorin and other lipid lowering drugs (greater than or equal to 1 g/day of niacin) should be carefully weighed against the potential risks of this combination).

No products indexed under this heading.

Ritonavir (Simvastatin is metabolized by the cytochrome P450 isoform 3A4. Certain drugs that inhibit this metabolic pathway can raise plasma levels of simvastatin and may increase the risk of myopathy. This includes HIV protease inhibitors. The use of Vytorin concomitantly with these CYP3A4 inhibitors should be avoided). Products include:
Kaletra 452
Norvir 489

Saquinavir (Simvastatin is metabolized by the cytochrome P450 isoform 3A4. Certain drugs that inhibit this metabolic pathway can raise plasma levels of simvastatin and may increase the risk of myopathy. This includes HIV protease inhibitors. The use of Vytorin concomitantly with these CYP3A4 inhibitors should be avoided).
No products indexed under this heading.

Saquinavir Mesylate (Simvastatin is metabolized by the cytochrome P450 isoform 3A4. Certain drugs that inhibit this metabolic pathway can raise plasma levels of simvastatin and may increase the risk of myopathy. This includes HIV protease inhibitors. The use of Vytorin concomitantly with these CYP3A4 inhibitors should be avoided).
No products indexed under this heading.

Telithromycin (Simvastatin is metabolized by the cytochrome P450 isoform 3A4. Certain drugs that inhibit this metabolic pathway can raise plasma levels of simvastatin and may increase the risk of myopathy. This includes the ketolide antibiotic telithromycin. The use of Vytorin concomitantly with this CYP3A4 inhibitor should be avoided. If treatment with telithromycin is unavoidable, therapy with Vytorin should be suspended during the course of treatment). Products include:
Ketek Tablets 2744

Tipranavir (Simvastatin is metabolized by the cytochrome P450 isoform 3A4. Certain drugs that inhibit this metabolic pathway can raise plasma levels of simvastatin and may increase the risk of myopathy. This includes HIV protease inhibitors. The use of Vytorin concomitantly with these CYP3A4 inhibitors should be avoided). Products include:
Aptivus Capsules 823
Aptivus Oral Solution 823

Troleandomycin (Simvastatin is metabolized by the cytochrome P450 isoform 3A4. Certain drugs that inhibit this metabolic pathway can raise plasma levels of simvastatin and may increase the risk of myopathy. Concomitant use of any medication labeled as having a strong inhibitory effect on CYP3A4 should be avoided unless the benefits of combined therapy outweigh the increased risk).
No products indexed under this heading.

Verapamil Hydrochloride (The risk of myopathy/rhabdomyolysis is increased by concomitant administration of verapamil with higher doses of Vytorin. In patients taking verapamil concomitantly with Vytorin, the dose of Vytorin should not exceed 10/20 mg/day). Products include:
Tarka Tablets 511

Voriconazole (Simvastatin is metabolized by the cytochrome P450 isoform 3A4. Certain drugs that inhibit this metabolic pathway can raise plasma levels of simvastatin and may increase the risk of myopathy. Concomitant use of any medication labeled as having a strong inhibitory effect on CYP3A4 should be avoided unless the benefits of combined therapy outweigh the increased risk).
No products indexed under this heading.

Warfarin Sodium (Simvastatin 20-40 mg/day modestly potentiated the effect of coumarin anticoagulants: the prothrombin time, reported as International Normalized Ratio (INR), increased from a baseline of 1.7 to 1.8 and from 2.6 to 3.4 in a normal volunteer study and in a hypercholesterolemic patient study, respectively. Prothrombin time should be determined before starting Vytorin and frequently enough during early therapy to ensure that no significant alteration of prothrombin time occurs. Once a stable prothrombin time has been documented, prothrombin times can be monitored at the intervals usually recommended for patients on coumarin anticoagulants. If the dose of Vytorin is changed or discontinued, the same procedure should be repeated).
No products indexed under this heading.

Food Interactions

Grapefruit (Simvastatin is metabolized by the cytochrome P450 isoform 3A4. Certain drugs that inhibit this metabolic pathway can raise plasma levels of simvastatin and may increase the risk of myopathy. This includes large quantities of grapefruit juice (greater than 1 quart daily). The use of Vytorin concomitantly with this CYP3A4 inhibitor should be avoided).

Grapefruit Juice (Simvastatin is metabolized by the cytochrome P450 isoform 3A4. Certain drugs that inhibit this metabolic pathway can raise plasma levels of simvastatin and may increase the risk of myopathy. This includes large quantities of grapefruit juice (greater than 1 quart daily). The use of Vytorin concomitantly with this CYP3A4 inhibitor should be avoided).

VYTORIN 10/10 TABLETS

(Ezetimibe, Simvastatin) 2939
May interact with azole antifungals, oral anticoagulants, erythromycin, fibrates, macrolide antibiotics, protease inhibitors, and certain other agents. Compounds in these categories include:

Amiodarone Hydrochloride (The risk of myopathy/rhabdomyolysis is increased by concomitant administration of amiodarone of verapamil with higher doses of Vytorin. The combined use of Vytorin at doses higher than 10/20 mg daily with amiodarone or verapamil should be avoided unless the clinical benefit is likely to outweigh the increased risk of myopathy).
No products indexed under this heading.

Amprenavir (The risk of myopathy and rhabdomyolysis is increased by high levels of statin activity in plasma. Simvastatin is metabolized by the cytochrome P450 isoform 3A4. Certain drugs that inhibit this metabolic pathway can raise the plasma levels of simvastatin and may increase the risk of myopathy. These include HIV protease inhibitors. The use of Vytorin concomitantly with these CYP3A4 inhibitors should be avoided. If treatment is unavoidable, therapy with Vytorin should be suspended during the course of treatment).
No products indexed under this heading.

Anisindione (Simvastatin may prolong INR. Achieve stable INR prior to starting Vytorin. Monitor INR frequently until stable upon initiation or alteration of Vytorin therapy).
No products indexed under this heading.

Azithromycin Dihydrate (The risk of myopathy and rhabdomyolysis is increased by high levels of statin activity in plasma. Simvastatin is metabolized by the cytochrome P450 isoform 3A4. Certain drugs that inhibit this metabolic pathway can raise the plasma levels of simvastatin and may increase the risk of myopathy. These include the macrolide antibiotics erythromycin and clarithromycin, and the keolide antibiotic telithromycin. The use of Vytorin concomitantly with these CYP3A4 inhibitors should be avoided. If treatment with erythromycin, clarithromycin or telithromycin is unavoidable, therapy with Vytorin should be suspended during the course of treatment).
No products indexed under this heading.

Cholestyramine (Concomitant cholestyramine administration decreased the mean AUC of total ezetimibe approximately 55%. The incremental LDL-C reduction due to adding Vytorin to cholestyramine may be reduced by this interaction).
No products indexed under this heading.

Clarithromycin (The risk of myopathy and rhabdomyolysis is increased by high levels of statin activity in plasma. Simvastatin is metabolized by the cytochrome P450 isoform 3A4. Certain drugs that inhibit this metabolic pathway can raise the plasma levels of simvastatin and may increase the risk of myopathy. These include the macrolide antibiotics erythromycin and clarithromycin, and the keolide antibiotic telithromycin. The use of Vytorin concomitantly with these CYP3A4 inhibitors should be avoided. If treatment with erythromycin, clarithromycin or telithromycin is unavoidable, therapy with Vytorin should be suspended during the course of treatment). Products include:
Biaxin/Biaxin XL 411

Clofibrate (Combination therapy with fibrates should be avoided. However, although not recommended, if Vytorin is used in combination with gemfibrozil, the dose should not exceed 10/10 mg daily. Caution should be used when prescribing other fibrates or lipid-lowering doses (greater than or equal to 1 gram per day) of niacin with Vytorin, as these agents can cause myopathy when given alone).
No products indexed under this heading.

Clotrimazole (The risk of myopathy and rhabdomyolysis is increased by high levels of statin activity in plasma. Simvastatin is metabolized by the cytochrome P450 isoform 3A4. Certain drugs that inhibit this metabolic pathway can raise the plasma levels of simvastatin and may increase the risk of mypathy. These include itraconazole, ketoconazole, and other antifungal azoles. The use of Vytorin concomitantly with these CYP3A4 inhibitors should be avoided. If treatment with itraconazole or ketoconazole is unavoidable, therapy with Vytorin should be suspended during course of treatment). Products include:
Lotrisone 2881

Cyclosporine (The risk of myopathy/rhabdomyolysis is increased by concomitant administration of cyclosporine particularly with higher doses of Vytorin. Caution should be exercised when using Vytorin and cyclosporine concomitantly due to increased exposure to both ezetimibe and cyclosporine. Cyclosporine concentrations should be monitored in patients receiving Vytorin and cyclopsporine. Do not exceed 10/10 mg Vytorin daily). Products include:
Gengraf Capsules 435
Neoral Oral Solution 2280
Neoral Soft Gelatin Capsules 2280
Restasis Ophthalmic Emulsion 557
Sandimmune 2296

Danazol (The risk of myopathy/rhabdomyolysis is increased by concomitant administration of danazol, particularly with higher doses of Vytorin. Do no exceed 10/10 mg Vytorin dialy).
No products indexed under this heading.

Darunavir (The risk of myopathy and rhabdomyolysis is increased by high levels of statin activity in plasma. Simvastatin is metabolized by the cytochrome P450 isoform 3A4. Certain drugs that inhibit this metabolic pathway can raise the plasma levels of simvastatin and may increase the risk of myopathy. These include HIV protease inhibitors. The use of Vytorin concomitantly with these CYP3A4 inhibitors should be avoided. If treatment is unavoidable, therapy with Vytorin should be suspended during the course of treatment).
No products indexed under this heading.

Dicumarol (Simvastatin may prolong INR. Achieve stable INR prior to starting Vytorin. Monitor INR frequently until stable upon initiation or alteration of Vytorin therapy).
No products indexed under this heading.

Digoxin (In one study, concomitant administration of digoxin with simvastatin resulted in a slight elevation in plasma digoxin concentrations. Patients taking digoxin should be monitored appropriately when Vytorin is initiated). Products include:
Lanoxin Injection 1498
Lanoxin Injection Pediatric 1502
Lanoxin Tablets 1505

Dirithromycin (The risk of myopathy and rhabdomyolysis is increased by high levels of statin activity in plasma. Simvastatin is metabolized by the cytochrome P450 isoform 3A4. Certain drugs that inhibit this metabolic pathway can raise the

plasma levels of simvastatin and may increase the risk of myopathy. These include the macrolide antibiotics erythromycin and clarithromycin, and the keolide antibiotic telithromycin. The use of Vytorin concomitantly with these CYP3A4 inhibitors should be avoided. If treatment with erythromycin, clarithromycin or telithromycin is unavoidable, therapy with Vytorin should be suspended during the course of treatment).

No products indexed under this heading.

Erythromycin (The risk of myopathy and rhabdomyolysis is increased by high levels of statin activity in plasma. Simvastatin is metabolized by the cytochrome P450 isoform 3A4. Certain drugs that inhibit this metabolic pathway can raise the plasma levels of simvastatin and may increase the risk of myopathy. These include the macrolide antibiotics erythromycin and clarithromycin, and the keolide antibiotic telithromycin. The use of Vytorin concomitantly with these CYP3A4 inhibitors should be avoided. If treatment with erythromycin, clarithromycin or telithromycin is unavoidable, therapy with Vytorin should be suspended during the course of treatment).

No products indexed under this heading.

Erythromycin Estolate (The risk of myopathy and rhabdomyolysis is increased by high levels of statin activity in plasma. Simvastatin is metabolized by the cytochrome P450 isoform 3A4. Certain drugs that inhibit this metabolic pathway can raise the plasma levels of simvastatin and may increase the risk of myopathy. These include the macrolide antibiotics erythromycin and clarithromycin, and the keolide antibiotic telithromycin. The use of Vytorin concomitantly with these CYP3A4 inhibitors should be avoided. If treatment with erythromycin, clarithromycin or telithromycin is unavoidable, therapy with Vytorin should be suspended during the course of treatment).

No products indexed under this heading.

Erythromycin Ethylsuccinate (The risk of myopathy and rhabdomyolysis is increased by high levels of statin activity in plasma. Simvastatin is metabolized by the cytochrome P450 isoform 3A4. Certain drugs that inhibit this metabolic pathway can raise the plasma levels of simvastatin and may increase the risk of myopathy. These include the macrolide antibiotics erythromycin and clarithromycin, and the keolide antibiotic telithromycin. The use of Vytorin concomitantly with these CYP3A4 inhibitors should be avoided. If treatment with erythromycin, clarithromycin or telithromycin is unavoidable, therapy with Vytorin should be suspended during the course of treatment). Products include:

E.E.S. 433
EryPed 431

Erythromycin Gluceptate (The risk of myopathy and rhabdomyolysis is increased by high levels of statin activity in plasma. Simvastatin is metabolized by the cytochrome P450 isoform 3A4. Certain drugs that inhibit this metabolic pathway can raise the plasma levels of simvastatin and may increase the risk of myopathy. These include the macrolide antibiotics erythromycin and clarithromycin, and the keolide antibiotic telithromycin. The use of Vytorin concomitantly with these CYP3A4 inhibitors should be avoided. If treatment with erythromycin, clarithromycin or telithromycin is unavoidable, therapy with Vytorin should be suspended during the course of treatment).

No products indexed under this heading.

Erythromycin Lactobionate (The risk of myopathy and rhabdomyolysis is increased by high levels of statin activity in plasma. Simvastatin is metabolized by the cytochrome P450 isoform 3A4. Certain drugs that inhibit this metabolic pathway can raise the plasma levels of simvastatin and may increase the risk of myopathy. These include the macrolide antibiotics erythromycin, and clarithromycin, and the ketolide antiobiotic telithromycin. The use of Vytorin concomitantly with these CYP3A4 inhibitors should be avoided. If treatment with erythromycin, clarithromycin or telithromycin is unavoidable, therapy with Vytorin should be suspended during the course of treatment).

No products indexed under this heading.

Erythromycin Stearate (The risk of myopathy and rhabdomyolysis is increased by high levels of statin activity in plasma. Simvastatin is metabolized by the cytochrome P450 isoform 3A4. Certain drugs that inhibit this metabolic pathway can raise the plasma levels of simvastatin and may increase the risk of myopathy. These include the macrolide antibiotics erythromycin and clarithromycin, and the keolide antibiotic telithromycin. The use of Vytorin concomitantly with these CYP3A4 inhibitors should be avoided. If treatment with erythromycin, clarithromycin or telithromycin is unavoidable, therapy with Vytorin should be suspended during the course of treatment).

No products indexed under this heading.

Fenofibrate (Combination therapy with fibrates should be avoided. However, although not recommended, if Vytorin is used in combination with gemfibrozil, the dose should not exceed 10/10 mg daily. Caution should be used when prescribing other fibrates or lipid-lowering doses (greater than or equal to 1 gram per day) of niacin with Vytorin, as these agents can cause myopathy when given alone). Products include:

Fenoglide Tablets 2960
Tricor Tablets 520

Fluconazole (The risk of myopathy and rhabdomyolysis is increased by high levels of statin activity in plasma. Simvastatin is metabolized by the cytochrome P450 isoform 3A4. Certain drugs that inhibit this metabolic pathway can raise the plasma levels of simvastatin and may increase the risk of mypathy. These include itraconazole, ketoconazole, and other antifungal azoles. The use of Vytorin concomitantly with these CYP3A4 inhibitors should be avoided. If treatment with itraconazole or ketoconazole is unavoidable, therapy with Vytorin should be suspended during course of treatment).

No products indexed under this heading.

Fosamprenavir Calcium (The risk of myopathy and rhabdomyolysis is increased by high levels of statin activity in plasma. Simvastatin is metabolized by the cytochrome P450 isoform 3A4. Certain drugs that inhibit this metabolic pathway can raise the plasma levels of simvastatin and may increase the risk of myopathy. These include HIV protease inhibitors. The use of Vytorin concomitantly with these CYP3A4 inhibitors should be avoided. If treatment is unavoidable, therapy with Vytorin should be suspended during the course of treatment). Products include:

Lexiva Oral Suspension 1510
Lexiva Tablets 1510

Gemfibrozil (Combination therapy with fibrates should be avoided. However, although not recommended, if Vytorin is used in combination with gemfibrozil, the dose should not exceed 10/10 mg daily. Caution should be used when prescribing other fibrates or lipid-lowering doses (greater than or equal to 1 gram per day) of niacin with Vytorin, as these agents can cause myopathy when given alone).

No products indexed under this heading.

Indinavir Sulfate (The risk of myopathy and rhabdomyolysis is increased by high levels of statin activity in plasma. Simvastatin is metabolized by the cytochrome P450 isoform 3A4. Certain drugs that inhibit this metabolic pathway can raise the plasma levels of simvastatin and may increase the risk of myopathy. These include HIV protease inhibitors. The use of Vytorin concomitantly with these CYP3A4 inhibitors should be avoided. If treatment is unavoidable, therapy with Vytorin should be suspended during the course of treatment). Products include:

Crixivan Capsules 1979

Itraconazole (The risk of myopathy and rhabdomyolysis is increased by high levels of statin activity in plasma. Simvastatin is metabolized by the cytochrome P450 isoform 3A4. Certain drugs that inhibit this metabolic pathway can raise the plasma levels of simvastatin and may increase the risk of mypathy. These include itraconazole, ketoconazole, and other antifungal azoles. The use of Vytorin concomitantly with these CYP3A4 inhibitors should be avoided. If treatment with itraconazole or ketoconazole is unavoidable, therapy with Vytorin should be suspended during course of treatment).

No products indexed under this heading.

Ketoconazole (The risk of myopathy and rhabdomyolysis is increased by high levels of statin activity in plasma. Simvastatin is metabolized by the cytochrome P450 isoform 3A4. Certain drugs that inhibit this metabolic pathway can raise the plasma levels of simvastatin and may increase the risk of mypathy. These include itraconazole, ketoconazole, and other antifungal azoles. The use of Vytorin concomitantly with these CYP3A4 inhibitors should be avoided. If treatment with itraconazole or ketoconazole is unavoidable, therapy with Vytorin should be suspended during course of treatment). Products include:

Extina Foam, 2% 3057
Nizoral A-D Shampoo 1901

Lopinavir (The risk of myopathy and rhabdomyolysis is increased by high levels of statin activity in plasma. Simvastatin is metabolized by the cytochrome P450 isoform 3A4. Certain drugs that inhibit this metabolic pathway can raise the plasma levels of simvastatin and may increase the risk of myopathy. These include HIV protease inhibitors. The use of Vytorin concomitantly with these CYP3A4 inhibitors should be avoided. If treatment is unavoidable, therapy with Vytorin should be suspended during the course of treatment). Products include:

Kaletra 452

Miconazole (The risk of myopathy and rhabdomyolysis is increased by high levels of statin activity in plasma. Simvastatin is metabolized by the cytochrome P450 isoform 3A4. Certain drugs that inhibit this metabolic pathway can raise the plasma levels of simvastatin and may increase the risk of mypathy. These include itraconazole, ketoconazole, and other antifungal azoles. The use of Vytorin concomitantly with these CYP3A4 inhibitors should be avoided. If treatment with itraconazole or ketoconazole is unavoidable, therapy with Vytorin should be suspended during course of treatment).

No products indexed under this heading.

Nefazodone Hydrochloride (The risk of myopathy and rhabdomyolysis is increased by high levels of statin activity in plasma. Simvastatin is metabolized by cytochrome P450 isoform 3A4. Certain drugs that inhibit this metabolic pathway can raise the plasma levels of simvastatin and may increase the risk of myopathy. These include the antidepressant nefazodone. The use of Vytorin concomitantly with these CYP3A4 inhibitors should be avoided. If treatment is unavoidable, therapy with Vytorin should be suspended during the course of treatment).

No products indexed under this heading.

Nelfinavir Mesylate (The risk of myopathy and rhabdomyolysis is increased by high levels of statin activity in plasma. Simvastatin is metabolized by the cytochrome P450 isoform 3A4. Certain drugs that inhibit this metabolic pathway can raise the plasma levels of simvastatin and may increase the risk of myopathy. These include HIV protease inhibitors. The use of Vytorin concomitantly with these CYP3A4 inhibitors should be avoided. If treatment is unavoidable, therapy with Vytorin should be suspended during the course of treatment).

No products indexed under this heading.

Niacin (The risk of myopathy is increased by gemfibrozil and to a lesser extent by other fibrates and niacin (nicotinic acid) (greater than or equal to 1 gram per day). Caution should be used when prescribing other fibrates or lipid-lowering doses (greater than or equal to 1 gram per

day) of niacin with Vytorin, as these agents can cause myopathy when given alone). Products include:

Advicor Tablets 402
Bausch & Lomb Ocuvite DF Vitamin Supplement.................... ⊙ 238
Dismutax Dietary Supplement 995
Niaspan Extended-Release Tablets.. 480
NT-Kinase Dietary Supplement 995
Simcor Tablets 502

Niacinamide (The risk of myopathy is increased by gemfibrozil and to a lesser extent by other fibrates and niacin (nicotinic acid) (greater than or equal to 1 gram per day). Caution should be used when prescribing other fibrates or lipid-lowering doses (greater than or equal to 1 gram per day) of niacin with Vytorin, as these agents can cause myopathy when given alone). Products include:

BioLean Free Tablets 635

Oxiconazole Nitrate (The risk of myopathy and rhabdomyolysis is increased by high levels of statin activity in plasma. Simvastatin is metabolized by the cytochrome P450 isoform 3A4. Certain drugs that inhibit this metabolic pathway can raise the plasma levels of simvastatin and may increase the risk of mypathy. These include itraconazole, ketoconazole, and other antifungal azoles. The use of Vytorin concomitantly with these CYP3A4 inhibitors should be avoided. If treatment with itraconazole or ketoconazole is unavoidable, therapy with Vytorin should be suspended during course of treatment).

No products indexed under this heading.

Posaconazole (The risk of myopathy and rhabdomyolysis is increased by high levels of statin activity in plasma. Simvastatin is metabolized by the cytochrome P450 isoform 3A4. Certain drugs that inhibit this metabolic pathway can raise the plasma levels of simvastatin and may increase the risk of mypathy. These include itraconazole, ketoconazole, and other antifungal azoles. The use of Vytorin concomitantly with these CYP3A4 inhibitors should be avoided. If treatment with itraconazole or ketoconazole is unavoidable, therapy with Vytorin should be suspended during course of treatment). Products include:

Noxafil Oral Suspension 2889

Ritonavir (The risk of myopathy and rhabdomyolysis is increased by high levels of statin activity in plasma. Simvastatin is metabolized by the cytochrome P450 isoform 3A4. Certain drugs that inhibit this metabolic pathway can raise the plasma levels of simvastatin and may increase the risk of myopathy. These include HIV protease inhibitors. The use of Vytorin concomitantly with these CYP3A4 inhibitors should be avoided. If treatment is unavoidable, therapy with Vytorin should be suspended during the course of treatment). Products include:

Kaletra 452
Norvir 489

Saquinavir (The risk of myopathy and rhabdomyolysis is increased by high levels of statin activity in plasma. Simvastatin is metabolized by the cytochrome P450 isoform 3A4. Certain drugs that inhibit this metabolic pathway can raise the plasma levels of simvastatin and may increase the risk of myopathy. These include HIV protease inhibitors. The use of Vytorin concomitantly with these CYP3A4 inhibitors should be avoided. If treatment is unavoidable, therapy with Vytorin should be suspended during the course of treatment).

No products indexed under this heading.

Saquinavir Mesylate (The risk of myopathy and rhabdomyolysis is increased by high levels of statin activity in plasma. Simvastatin is metabolized by the cytochrome P450 isoform 3A4. Certain drugs that inhibit this metabolic pathway can raise the plasma levels of simvastatin and may increase the risk of myopathy. These include HIV protease inhibitors. The use of Vytorin concomitantly with these CYP3A4 inhibitors should be avoided. If treatment is unavoidable, therapy with Vytorin should be suspended during the course of treatment).

No products indexed under this heading.

Telithromycin (The risk of myopathy and rhabdomyolysis is increased by high levels of statin activity in plasma. Simvastatin is metabolized by the cytochrome P450 3A4. Certain drugs that inhibit metabolic pathway can raise the plasma levels of simvastatin and may increase the risk of myopathy. These include the macrolide antibiotics erythromycin and clarithromycin, and the ketolide antibiotic telithromycin. The use of Vytorin concomitantly with these CYP3A4 inhibitors should be avoided. If treatment with erythromycin, clarithromycin or telithromycin is unavoidable, therapy with Vytorin should be suspended during course of treatment). Products include:

Ketek Tablets 2744

Terconazole (The risk of myopathy and rhabdomyolysis is increased by high levels of statin activity in plasma. Simvastatin is metabolized by the cytochrome P450 isoform 3A4. Certain drugs that inhibit this metabolic pathway can raise the plasma levels of simvastatin and may increase the risk of mypathy. These include itraconazole, ketoconazole, and other antifungal azoles. The use of Vytorin concomitantly with these CYP3A4 inhibitors should be avoided. If treatment with itraconazole or ketoconazole is unavoidable, therapy with Vytorin should be suspended during course of treatment).

No products indexed under this heading.

Tipranavir (The risk of myopathy and rhabdomyolysis is increased by high levels of statin activity in plasma. Simvastatin is metabolized by the cytochrome P450 isoform 3A4. Certain drugs that inhibit this metabolic pathway can raise the plasma levels of simvastatin and may increase the risk of myopathy. These include HIV protease inhibitors. The use of Vytorin concomitantly with these CYP3A4 inhibitors should be avoided. If treatment is unavoidable, therapy with Vytorin should be suspended during the course of treatment). Products include:

Aptivus Capsules 823
Aptivus Oral Solution 823

Troleandomycin (The risk of myopathy and rhabdomyolysis is increased by high levels of statin activity in plasma. Simvastatin is metabolized by the cytochrome P450 isoform 3A4. Certain drugs that inhibit this metabolic pathway can raise the plasma levels of simvastatin and may increase the risk of myopathy. These include the macrolide antibiotics erythromycin and clarithromycin, and the keolide antibiotic telithromycin. The use of Vytorin concomitantly with these CYP3A4 inhibitors should be avoided. If treatment with erythromycin, clarithromycin or telithromycin is unavoidable, therapy with Vytorin should be suspended during the course of treatment).

No products indexed under this heading.

Verapamil Hydrochloride (The risk of myopathy/rhabdomyolysis is increased by concomitant administration of amiodarone or verapamil with higher doses of Vytorin. The combined use of Vytorin at doses higher than 10/20 mg daily with amiodarone or verapamil should be avoided unless the clinical benefit is likely to outweigh the increased risk of myopathy). Products include:

Tarka Tablets 511

Voriconazole (The risk of myopathy and rhabdomyolysis is increased by high levels of statin activity in plasma. Simvastatin is metabolized by the cytochrome P450 isoform 3A4. Certain drugs that inhibit this metabolic pathway can raise the plasma levels of simvastatin and may increase the risk of mypathy. These include itraconazole, ketoconazole, and other antifungal azoles. The use of Vytorin concomitantly with these CYP3A4 inhibitors should be avoided. If treatment with itraconazole or ketoconazole is unavoidable, therapy with Vytorin should be suspended during course of treatment).

No products indexed under this heading.

Warfarin Sodium (Simvastatin may prolong INR. Achieve stable INR prior to starting Vytorin. Monitor INR frequently until stable upon initiation or alteration of Vytorin therapy).

No products indexed under this heading.

Food Interactions

Grapefruit (The risk of myopathy and rhabdomyolysis is increased by high levels of statin activity in plasma. Simvastatin is metabolized by the cytochrome P450 3A4. Certain drugs that inhibit this metabolic pathway can raise the plasma levels of simvastatin and may increase the risk of myopathy. These include large quantities of grapefruit juice (greater than 1 quart daily); concurrent use should be avoided).

Grapefruit Juice (The risk of myopathy and rhabdomyolysis is increased by high levels of statin activity in plasma. Simvastatin is metabolized by the cytochrome P450 3A4. Certain drugs that inhibit this metabolic pathway can raise the plasma levels of simvastatin and may increase the risk of myopathy. These include large quantities of grapefruit juice (greater than 1 quart daily); concurrent use should be avoided).

VYTORIN 10/20 TABLETS

(Ezetimibe, Simvastatin) 2149
See Vytorin 10/10 Tablets

VYTORIN 10/20 TABLETS

(Ezetimibe, Simvastatin) 2939
See Vytorin 10/10 Tablets

VYTORIN 10/40 TABLETS

(Ezetimibe, Simvastatin) 2149
See Vytorin 10/10 Tablets

VYTORIN 10/40 TABLETS

(Ezetimibe, Simvastatin) 2939
See Vytorin 10/10 Tablets

VYTORIN 10/80 TABLETS

(Ezetimibe, Simvastatin) 2149
See Vytorin 10/10 Tablets

VYTORIN 10/80 TABLETS

(Ezetimibe, Simvastatin) 2939
See Vytorin 10/10 Tablets

VYVANSE CAPSULES

(Lisdexamfetamine Dimesylate) 3033
May interact with alpha adrenergic blockers, antihistamines, antihypertensives, beta blockers, monoamine oxidase inhibitors, phenytoin, sympathomimetics, thiazides, tricyclic antidepressants, urinary alkalinizing agents, veratrum alkaloids, and certain other agents. Compounds in these categories include:

Acebutolol Hydrochloride (Adrenergic blockers are inhibited by amphetamines).

No products indexed under this heading.

Acetazolamide (Urinary alkalinizing agents such as acetazolamide increase the concentration of the non-ionized species of the amphetamine molecule, thereby decreasing urinary excretion).

No products indexed under this heading.

Acrivastine (Amphetamines may counteract the sedative effect of antihistamines).

No products indexed under this heading.

Albuterol (Amphetamines may enhance the activity of sympathomimetic agents).

No products indexed under this heading.

Albuterol Sulfate (Amphetamines may enhance the activity of sympathomimetic agents). Products include:

Combivent Inhalation Aerosol 845
ProAir HFA Inhalation Aerosol 3113
Proventil HFA Inhalation Aerosol 2914
Ventolin HFA Inhalation Aerosol 1638

Aliskiren (Amphetamines may antagonize the hypotensive effects of antihypertensives). Products include:

Tekturna Tablets 2321
Tekturna HCT Tablets 2324

Amitriptyline Hydrochloride (Amphetamines may enhance the activity of tricyclic antidepressants; d-amphetamine with desipramine or protriptyline and possibly other tricyclics cause striking and sustained increases in the concentration of d-amphetamine in the brain; cardiovascular effects can be potentiated).

No products indexed under this heading.

Amlodipine Besylate (Amphetamines may antagonize the hypotensive effects of antihypertensives). Products include:

Azor Tablets 1005
Exforge Tablets 2238

Ammonium Chloride (Urinary acidifying agents such as ammonium chloride increase the concentration of the ionized species of the amphetamine molecule, thereby increasing urinary excretion).
No products indexed under this heading.

Amoxapine (Amphetamines may enhance the activity of tricyclic antidepressants; d-amphetamine with desipramine or protriptyline and possibly other tricyclics cause striking and sustained increases in the concentration of d-amphetamine in the brain; cardiovascular effects can be potentiated).
No products indexed under this heading.

Astemizole (Amphetamines may counteract the sedative effect of antihistamines).
No products indexed under this heading.

Atenolol (Adrenergic blockers are inhibited by amphetamines).
No products indexed under this heading.

Azatadine Maleate (Amphetamines may counteract the sedative effect of antihistamines).
No products indexed under this heading.

Benazepril Hydrochloride (Amphetamines may antagonize the hypotensive effects of antihypertensives).
No products indexed under this heading.

Bendroflumethiazide (Urinary alkalinizing agents including some thiazides, increase the concentration of the non-ionized species of the amphetamine molecule, thereby decreasing urinary excretion).
No products indexed under this heading.

Betaxolol Hydrochloride (Adrenergic blockers are inhibited by amphetamines).
No products indexed under this heading.

Bisoprolol Fumarate (Adrenergic blockers are inhibited by amphetamines).
No products indexed under this heading.

Bromodiphenhydramine Hydrochloride (Amphetamines may counteract the sedative effect of antihistamines).
No products indexed under this heading.

Brompheniramine Maleate (Amphetamines may counteract the sedative effect of antihistamines).
No products indexed under this heading.

Candesartan Cilexetil (Amphetamines may antagonize the hypotensive effects of antihypertensives).
Products include:
Atacand Tablets 639
Atacand HCT 642

Captopril (Amphetamines may antagonize the hypotensive effects of antihypertensives). Products include:
Captopril Tablets 2182

Carteolol Hydrochloride (Adrenergic blockers are inhibited by amphetamines).
No products indexed under this heading.

Cetirizine Hydrochloride (Amphetamines may counteract the sedative effect of antihistamines).
Products include:
Zyrtec Allergy Tablets 1919
Zyrtec Chewable Tablets 1920
Children's Zyrtec Allergy Chewable Tablets 1922
Children's Zyrtec Allergy Syrup 1920
Children's Zyrtec Hives Relief Syrup 1920
Zyrtec Syrup 1920
Zyrtec Tablets 1920
Zyrtec-D 12 Hour Extended Release Tablets 1923
Zyrtec-D Allergy & Congestion Extended-Release Tablets 1923

Chlorothiazide (Urinary alkalinizing agents including some thiazides, increase the concentration of the non-ionized species of the amphetamine molecule, thereby decreasing urinary excretion).
No products indexed under this heading.

Chlorothiazide Sodium (Urinary alkalinizing agents including some thiazides, increase the concentration of the non-ionized species of the amphetamine molecule, thereby decreasing urinary excretion).
Products include:
Intravenous Sodium Diuril 2490

Chlorpheniramine Maleate (Amphetamines may counteract the sedative effect of antihistamines).
Products include:
Actifed Cold & Allergy Tablets 1895
Sudafed PE Sinus & Allergy Tablets 1908
Tylenol Allergy Multi-Symptom Caplets with Cool Burst and Rapid Release Gelcaps 1916
Children's Tylenol Plus Cold Suspension Liquid 1912
Children's Tylenol Plus Cough & Runny Nose Suspension Liquid 1912
Children's Tylenol Plus Flu Suspension Liquid 1914
Children's Tylenol Plus Multi-Symptom Cold Suspension Liquid 1912
Tylenol Cold Head Congestion Nighttime Caplets with Cool Burst 1910
Tylenol Cold Multi-Symptom Nighttime Caplets with Cool Burst 1913
Tylenol Sinus Congestion & Pain Nighttime Caplets with Cool Burst 1917

Chlorpheniramine Polistirex (Amphetamines may counteract the sedative effect of antihistamines).
Products include:
Tussionex Pennkinetic Extended-Release Suspension 3154

Chlorpheniramine Tannate (Amphetamines may counteract the sedative effect of antihistamines).
No products indexed under this heading.

Chlorpromazine (Chlorpromazine blocks dopamine and norepinephrine receptors, thus inhibiting the central stimulant effects of amphetamines, and can be used to treat amphetamine poisoning).
No products indexed under this heading.

Chlorpromazine Hydrochloride (Chlorpromazine blocks dopamine and norepinephrine receptors, thus inhibiting the central stimulant effects of amphetamines, and can be used to treat amphetamine poisoning).
No products indexed under this heading.

Chlorthalidone (Amphetamines may antagonize the hypotensive effects of antihypertensives).
Products include:
Clorpres Tablets 2185

Clemastine Fumarate (Amphetamines may counteract the sedative effect of antihistamines).
No products indexed under this heading.

Clomipramine Hydrochloride (Amphetamines may enhance the activity of tricyclic antidepressants; d-amphetamine with desipramine or protriptyline and possibly other tricyclics cause striking and sustained increases in the concentration of d-amphetamine in the brain; cardiovascular effects can be potentiated).
No products indexed under this heading.

Clonidine (Amphetamines may antagonize the hypotensive effects of antihypertensives). Products include:
Catapres-TTS 842

Clonidine Hydrochloride (Amphetamines may antagonize the hypotensive effects of antihypertensives).
Products include:
Catapres Tablets 841
Clorpres Tablets 2185

Cryptenamine Preparations (Amphetamines may inhibit the hypotensive effects of veratrum alkaloids).
No products indexed under this heading.

Cyproheptadine Hydrochloride (Amphetamines may counteract the sedative effect of antihistamines).
No products indexed under this heading.

Deserpidine (Amphetamines may antagonize the hypotensive effects of antihypertensives).
No products indexed under this heading.

Desipramine Hydrochloride (Amphetamines may enhance the activity of tricyclic antidepressants; d-amphetamine with desipramine or protriptyline and possibly other tricyclics cause striking and sustained increases in the concentration of d-amphetamine in the brain; cardiovascular effects can be potentiated).
No products indexed under this heading.

Dexchlorpheniramine Maleate (Amphetamines may counteract the sedative effect of antihistamines).
No products indexed under this heading.

Diazoxide (Amphetamines may antagonize the hypotensive effects of antihypertensives). Products include:
Proglycem Capsules 1185
Proglycem Suspension 1185

Diltiazem Hydrochloride (Amphetamines may antagonize the hypotensive effects of antihypertensives).
Products include:
Cardizem LA Extended Release Tablets 421

Diphenhydramine Citrate (Amphetamines may counteract the sedative effect of antihistamines).
No products indexed under this heading.

Diphenhydramine Hydrochloride (Amphetamines may counteract the sedative effect of antihistamines).
Products include:
Benadryl Allergy & Cold Kapgels 1895
Benadryl Allergy & Sinus Headache Kapgels 1895
Benadryl Severe Allergy & Sinus Headache Caplets 1897
Benadryl Dye-Free Allergy Liqui-gels Softgels 1897
Benadryl Allergy Kapgels 1895
Benadryl Allergy Quick Dissolve Strips 1896
Benadryl Allergy Ultratab Tablets 1896
Children's Benadryl Dye-Free Allergy Liquid 1897
Children's Benadryl Allergy Fastmelts 1897
Children's Benadryl Allergy Liquid 1898
Children's Benadryl Allergy Perfect Measure 1896
Children's Benadryl-D Allergy & Sinus Liquid 1896
Benadryl-D Allergy & Sinus Tablet 1896
PediaCare Children's Allergy & Cold Liquid 1902
PediaCare Children's Allergy Liquid 1902
Simply Sleep Caplets 1905
Sudafed PE Nighttime Cold Caplets 1907
Sudafed PE Severe Cold Caplets 1908
Extra Strength Tylenol PM Caplets, Geltabs, Liquid, and Rapid Release Gels 1915
Tylenol Allergy Multi-Symptom Nighttime Caplets with Cool Burst 1916
Tylenol Severe Allergy Caplets 1916
Children's Tylenol Plus Cold & Allergy Suspension Liquid 1914
Tylenol Sore Throat Nighttime Liquid with Cool Burst 1918

Diphenylpyraline Hydrochloride (Amphetamines may counteract the sedative effect of antihistamines).
No products indexed under this heading.

Dobutamine Hydrochloride (Amphetamines may enhance the activity of sympathomimetic agents).
No products indexed under this heading.

Dopamine Hydrochloride (Amphetamines may enhance the activity of sympathomimetic agents).
No products indexed under this heading.

Doxazosin Mesylate (Adrenergic blockers are inhibited by amphetamines).
No products indexed under this heading.

Doxepin Hydrochloride (Amphetamines may enhance the activity of tricyclic antidepressants; d-amphetamine with desipramine or protriptyline and possibly other tricyclics cause striking and sustained increases in the concentration of d-amphetamine in the brain; cardiovascular effects can be potentiated).
No products indexed under this heading.

Enalapril Maleate (Amphetamines may antagonize the hypotensive effects of antihypertensives).
No products indexed under this heading.

Enalaprilat (Amphetamines may antagonize the hypotensive effects of antihypertensives).
No products indexed under this heading.

Ephedrine Hydrochloride (Amphetamines may enhance the activity of sympathomimetic agents).
No products indexed under this heading.

Ephedrine Sulfate (Amphetamines may enhance the activity of sympathomimetic agents).
No products indexed under this heading.

Ephedrine Tannate (Amphetamines may enhance the activity of sympathomimetic agents).
No products indexed under this heading.

Epinephrine (Amphetamines may enhance the activity of sympathomimetic agents). Products include:
EpiPen 1024

Epinephrine Bitartrate (Amphetamines may enhance the activity of sympathomimetic agents).
No products indexed under this heading.

Epinephrine Hydrochloride (Amphetamines may enhance the activity of sympathomimetic agents).
No products indexed under this heading.

Eprosartan Mesylate (Amphetamines may antagonize the hypotensive effects of antihypertensives).
Products include:
Teveten Tablets 515
Teveten HCT Tablets 517

Esmolol Hydrochloride (Adrenergic blockers are inhibited by amphetamines).
No products indexed under this heading.

Ethosuximide (Amphetamines may delay intestinal absorption of ethosuximide).
No products indexed under this heading.

Felodipine (Amphetamines may antagonize the hypotensive effects of antihypertensives).
No products indexed under this heading.

Fexofenadine Hydrochloride (Amphetamines may counteract the sedative effect of antihistamines).
Products include:
Allegra Oral Solution 2684
Allegra Tablets 2684
Allegra-D 12 Hour Extended-Release Tablets 2687
Allegra-D 24 Hour Extended-Release Tablets 2690

Fosinopril Sodium (Amphetamines may antagonize the hypotensive effects of antihypertensives).
No products indexed under this heading.

Fosphenytoin Sodium (Amphetamines may delay intestinal absorption of phenytoin; co-administration of phenytoin may produce a synergistic anticonvulsant action).
No products indexed under this heading.

Furazolidone (A metabolite of furazolidone slows amphetamine metabolism).
No products indexed under this heading.

Furosemide (Amphetamines may antagonize the hypotensive effects of antihypertensives). Products include:
Furosemide Tablets 2186

Guanabenz Acetate (Amphetamines may antagonize the hypotensive effects of antihypertensives).
No products indexed under this heading.

Guanethidine Monosulfate (Amphetamines may antagonize the hypotensive effects of antihypertensives).
No products indexed under this heading.

Haloperidol (Haloperidol blocks dopamine receptors, thus inhibiting the central stimulant effects of amphetamines).
No products indexed under this heading.

Haloperidol Decanoate (Haloperidol blocks dopamine receptors, thus inhibiting the central stimulant effects of amphetamines).
No products indexed under this heading.

Haloperidol Lactate (Haloperidol blocks dopamine receptors, thus inhibiting the central stimulant effects of amphetamines).
No products indexed under this heading.

Hydralazine Hydrochloride (Amphetamines may antagonize the hypotensive effects of antihypertensives).
No products indexed under this heading.

Hydrochlorothiazide (Urinary alkalinizing agents including some thiazides, increase the concentration of the non-ionized species of the amphetamine molecule, thereby decreasing urinary excretion).
Products include:
Atacand HCT 642
Avalide Tablets 892
Avalide Tablets 2713
Benicar HCT Tablets 1010
Diovan HCT Tablets 2216
Dyazide Capsules 1405
Micardis HCT Tablets 854
Prinzide Tablets 2092
Tekturna HCT Tablets 2324
Teveten HCT Tablets 517

Hydroflumethiazide (Urinary alkalinizing agents including some thiazides, increase the concentration of the non-ionized species of the amphetamine molecule, thereby decreasing urinary excretion).
No products indexed under this heading.

Imipramine Hydrochloride (Amphetamines may enhance the activity of tricyclic antidepressants; d-amphetamine with desipramine or protriptyline and possibly other tricyclics cause striking and sustained increases in the concentration of d-amphetamine in the brain; cardiovascular effects can be potentiated).
No products indexed under this heading.

Imipramine Pamoate (Amphetamines may enhance the activity of tricyclic antidepressants; d-amphetamine with desipramine or protriptyline and possibly other tricyclics cause striking and sustained increases in the concentration of d-amphetamine in the brain; cardiovascular effects can be potentiated).
No products indexed under this heading.

Indapamide (Amphetamines may antagonize the hypotensive effects of antihypertensives). Products include:
Indapamide Tablets 2188

Irbesartan (Amphetamines may antagonize the hypotensive effects of antihypertensives). Products include:
Avalide Tablets 892
Avalide Tablets 2713
Avapro Tablets 897
Avapro Tablets 2718

Isocarboxazid (Monoamine oxidase inhibitors (MAIO) antidepressants slow amphetamine metabolism. This slowing potentiates amphetamines, increasing their effect on the release of norepinephrine and other monoamines from adrenergic nerve endings; this can cause headaches and other signs of hypertensive crisis. A variety of toxic neurological effects and malignant hyperpyrexia can occur, sometimes with fatal results. Use of lisdexamfetamine is contraindicated during or within the 14 days following the administration of MAOIs). Products include:
Marplan Tablets 3177

Isoproterenol Hydrochloride (Amphetamines may enhance the activity of sympathomimetic agents).
No products indexed under this heading.

Isoproterenol Sulfate (Amphetamines may enhance the activity of sympathomimetic agents).
No products indexed under this heading.

Isradipine (Amphetamines may antagonize the hypotensive effects of antihypertensives). Products include:
DynaCirc CR Controlled Release Tablets 1407

Labetalol Hydrochloride (Adrenergic blockers are inhibited by amphetamines).
No products indexed under this heading.

Levalbuterol Hydrochloride (Amphetamines may enhance the activity of sympathomimetic agents).
Products include:
Xopenex Inhalation Solution 3001
Xopenex Inhalation Solution Concentrate 3005

Levobunolol Hydrochloride (Adrenergic blockers are inhibited by amphetamines).
No products indexed under this heading.

Lisinopril (Amphetamines may antagonize the hypotensive effects of antihypertensives). Products include:
Prinivil Tablets 2087
Prinzide Tablets 2092

Lithium Carbonate (The anorectic and stimulatory effects of amphetamines may be inhibited by lithium carbonate).
No products indexed under this heading.

Loratadine (Amphetamines may counteract the sedative effect of antihistamines).
No products indexed under this heading.

Losartan Potassium (Amphetamines may antagonize the hypotensive effects of antihypertensives).
Products include:
Cozaar Tablets 1973

Maprotiline Hydrochloride (Amphetamines may enhance the activity of tricyclic antidepressants; d-amphetamine with desipramine or protriptyline and possibly other tricyclics cause striking and sustained increases in the concentration of d-amphetamine in the brain; cardiovascular effects can be potentiated).
No products indexed under this heading.

Mecamylamine Hydrochloride (Amphetamines may antagonize the hypotensive effects of antihypertensives).
No products indexed under this heading.

Meperidine Hydrochloride (Amphetamines potentiate the analgesic effect of meperidine).
No products indexed under this heading.

Metaproterenol Sulfate (Amphetamines may enhance the activity of sympathomimetic agents).
No products indexed under this heading.

Metaraminol Bitartrate (Amphetamines may enhance the activity of sympathomimetic agents).
No products indexed under this heading.

Methdilazine Hydrochloride (Amphetamines may counteract the sedative effect of antihistamines).
No products indexed under this heading.

Methenamine (Urinary excretion of amphetamines is increased and efficacy is reduced by acidifying agents used in methenamine therapy).
No products indexed under this heading.

Methenamine Hippurate (Urinary excretion of amphetamines is increased and efficacy is reduced by acidifying agents used in methenamine therapy).
No products indexed under this heading.

Methenamine Mandelate (Urinary excretion of amphetamines is increased and efficacy is reduced by acidifying agents used in methenamine therapy). Products include:
Uroqid-Acid No. 2 Tablets 814

Methoxamine Hydrochloride (Amphetamines may enhance the activity of sympathomimetic agents).
No products indexed under this heading.

Methyclothiazide (Urinary alkalinizing agents including some thiazides, increase the concentration of the non-ionized species of the amphetamine molecule, thereby decreasing urinary excretion).
No products indexed under this heading.

Methyldopa (Amphetamines may antagonize the hypotensive effects of antihypertensives).
No products indexed under this heading.

Methyldopate Hydrochloride (Amphetamines may antagonize the hypotensive effects of antihypertensives).
No products indexed under this heading.

Metipranolol Hydrochloride (Adrenergic blockers are inhibited by amphetamines).
No products indexed under this heading.

Metolazone (Amphetamines may antagonize the hypotensive effects of antihypertensives).
No products indexed under this heading.

Metoprolol Succinate (Adrenergic blockers are inhibited by amphetamines). Products include:
Toprol-XL Tablets 666

Metoprolol Tartrate (Adrenergic blockers are inhibited by amphetamines).
No products indexed under this heading.

Metyrosine (Amphetamines may antagonize the hypotensive effects of antihypertensives). Products include:

Demser Capsules 1989

Mibefradil Dihydrochloride (Amphetamines may antagonize the hypotensive effects of antihypertensives).
No products indexed under this heading.

Minoxidil (Amphetamines may antagonize the hypotensive effects of antihypertensives).
No products indexed under this heading.

Moclobemide (Monoamine oxidase inhibitors (MAIO) antidepressants slow amphetamine metabolism. This slowing potentiates amphetamines, increasing their effect on the release of norepinephrine and other monoamines from adrenergic nerve endings; this can cause headaches and other signs of hypertensive crisis. A variety of toxic neurological effects and malignant hyperpyrexia can occur, sometimes with fatal results. Use of lisdexamfetamine is contraindicated during or within the 14 days following the administration of MAOIs).
No products indexed under this heading.

Moexipril Hydrochloride (Amphetamines may antagonize the hypotensive effects of antihypertensives).
No products indexed under this heading.

Nadolol (Adrenergic blockers are inhibited by amphetamines).
Products include:
Nadolol Tablets 2191

Nebivolol (Adrenergic blockers are inhibited by amphetamines).
Products include:
Bystolic Tablets 1155

Nicardipine Hydrochloride (Amphetamines may antagonize the hypotensive effects of antihypertensives). Products include:
Cardene I.V. 1093

Nifedipine (Amphetamines may antagonize the hypotensive effects of antihypertensives).
No products indexed under this heading.

Nisoldipine (Amphetamines may antagonize the hypotensive effects of antihypertensives). Products include:
Sular Extended Release Tablets 2975

Nitroglycerin (Amphetamines may antagonize the hypotensive effects of antihypertensives). Products include:
Nitro-Dur Transdermal Infusion System 2887
Nitrolingual Pumpspray 2965

Norepinephrine Bitartrate (Amphetamines enhance the adrenergic effect of norepinephrine).
No products indexed under this heading.

Norepinephrine Hydrochloride (Amphetamines enhance the adrenergic effect of norepinephrine).
No products indexed under this heading.

Nortriptyline Hydrochloride (Amphetamines may enhance the activity of tricyclic antidepressants; d-amphetamine with desipramine or protriptyline and possibly other tricyclics cause striking and sustained increases in the concentration of d-amphetamine in the brain; cardiovascular effects can be potentiated).
No products indexed under this heading.

Pargyline Hydrochloride (Monoamine oxidase inhibitors (MAIO) antidepressants slow amphetamine metabolism. This slowing potentiates amphetamines, increasing their effect on the release of norepinephrine and other monoamines from adrenergic nerve endings; this can cause headaches and other signs of hypertensive crisis. A variety of toxic neurological effects and malignant hyperpyrexia can occur, sometimes with fatal results. Use of lisdexamfetamine is contraindicated during or within the 14 days following the administration of MAOIs).
No products indexed under this heading.

Penbutolol Sulfate (Adrenergic blockers are inhibited by amphetamines).
No products indexed under this heading.

Perindopril Erbumine (Amphetamines may antagonize the hypotensive effects of antihypertensives).
Products include:
Aceon Tablets (2 mg, 4 mg, 8 mg) 3038

Phenelzine Sulfate (Monoamine oxidase inhibitors (MAIO) antidepressants slow amphetamine metabolism. This slowing potentiates amphetamines, increasing their effect on the release of norepinephrine and other monoamines from adrenergic nerve endings; this can cause headaches and other signs of hypertensive crisis. A variety of toxic neurological effects and malignant hyperpyrexia can occur, sometimes with fatal results. Use of lisdexamfetamine is contraindicated during or within the 14 days following the administration of MAOIs).
No products indexed under this heading.

Phenobarbital (Amphetamines may delay intestinal absorption of phenobarbital; co-administration of phenobarbital may produce a synergistic anticonvulsant action). Products include:
Donnatal Extentabs 2507

Phenobarbital Sodium (Amphetamines may delay intestinal absorption of phenobarbital; co-administration of phenobarbital may produce a synergistic anticonvulsant action).
No products indexed under this heading.

Phenoxybenzamine Hydrochloride (Amphetamines may antagonize the hypotensive effects of antihypertensives). Products include:
Dibenzyline Capsules 3188

Phentolamine Mesylate (Amphetamines may antagonize the hypotensive effects of antihypertensives).
No products indexed under this heading.

Phenylephrine Bitartrate (Amphetamines may enhance the activity of sympathomimetic agents).
No products indexed under this heading.

Phenylephrine Hydrochloride (Amphetamines may enhance the activity of sympathomimetic agents).
Products include:
Actifed Cold & Allergy Tablets 1895
Benadryl Allergy & Cold Kapgels 1895
Benadryl Allergy & Sinus Headache Kapgels 1895
Benadryl Severe Allergy & Sinus Headache Caplets 1897
Children's Benadryl-D Allergy & Sinus Liquid 1896
Benadryl-D Allergy & Sinus Tablet 1896
PediaCare Children's Allergy & Cold Liquid 1902
PediaCare Children's Decongestant Liquid 1902
PediaCare Children's Liquid Multi-Symptom Cold 1902
Sinutab Non-Drying Caplets 1905
Sinutab Sinus Caplets 1905
Children's Sudafed PE Cold & Cough Liquid 1907
Children's Sudafed PE Nasal Decongestant Liquid 1906
Sudafed PE Cold & Cough Caplets 1907
Sudafed PE Nasal Decongestant Tablets 1907
Sudafed PE Nighttime Cold Caplets 1907
Sudafed PE Non-Drying Sinus Caplets 1908
Sudafed PE Severe Cold Caplets 1908
Sudafed PE Sinus & Allergy Tablets 1908
Sudafed PE Sinus Headache Caplets 1908
Tylenol Allergy Multi-Symptom Caplets with Cool Burst and Rapid Release Gelcaps 1916
Tylenol Allergy Multi-Symptom Nighttime Caplets with Cool Burst 1916
Children's Tylenol Plus Cold Suspension Liquid 1912
Children's Tylenol Plus Cold & Allergy Suspension Liquid 1914
Children's Tylenol Plus Flu Suspension Liquid 1914
Children's Tylenol Plus Multi-Symptom Cold Suspension Liquid 1912
Tylenol Cold Head Congestion Daytime Caplets with Cool Burst 1910
Tylenol Cold Head Congestion Nighttime Caplets with Cool Burst 1910
Tylenol Cold Head Congestion Severe Daytime Caplets with Cool Burst 1910
Tylenol Cold Multi-Symptom Daytime Caplets with Cool Burst and Rapid Release Gels 1913
Tylenol Cold Multi-Symptom Daytime Liquid with Citrus Burst 1913
Tylenol Cold Multi-Symptom Nighttime Caplets with Cool Burst 1913
Tylenol Cold Multi-Symptom Nighttime Liquid with Cool Burst 1913
Tylenol Cold Multi-Symptom Severe Caplets with Cool Burst 1913
Tylenol Cold Multi-Symptom Severe Daytime Liquid with Citrus Burst 1913
Tylenol Sinus Congestion & Pain Daytime Caplets with Cool Burst and Gelcaps 1917
Tylenol Sinus Congestion & Pain Nighttime Caplets with Cool Burst 1917
Tylenol Sinus Congestion & Pain Severe Caplets with Cool Burst 1917
Vicks DayQuil Cold & Flu Multi-Symptom Relief .... ▣616
Vicks DayQuil LiquiCaps 2567
Vicks DayQuil Liquid 2567
Vicks DayQuil Multi-Symptom Cold/Flu Relief 2567

Phenylephrine Tannate (Amphetamines may enhance the activity of sympathomimetic agents).
No products indexed under this heading.

Phenylpropanolamine Hydrochloride (Amphetamines may enhance the activity of sympathomimetic agents).
No products indexed under this heading.

Phenytoin (Amphetamines may delay intestinal absorption of phenytoin; co-administration of phenytoin may produce a synergistic anticonvulsant action).
No products indexed under this heading.

Phenytoin Sodium (Amphetamines may delay intestinal absorption of phenytoin; co-administration of phenytoin may produce a synergistic anticonvulsant action). Products include:
Phenytek Capsules 2192

Pindolol (Adrenergic blockers are inhibited by amphetamines).
No products indexed under this heading.

Pirbuterol Acetate (Amphetamines may enhance the activity of sympathomimetic agents). Products include:
Maxair Autohaler 1705

Polythiazide (Urinary alkalinizing agents including some thiazides, increase the concentration of the non-ionized species of the amphetamine molecule, thereby decreasing urinary excretion).
No products indexed under this heading.

Potassium Citrate (Urinary alkalinizing agents increase the concentration of the non-ionized species of the amphetamine molecule, thereby decreasing urinary excretion).
Products include:
BioLean Free Tablets .... ▣635
Urocit-K Tablets 2176

Prazosin Hydrochloride (Adrenergic blockers are inhibited by amphetamines).
No products indexed under this heading.

Procarbazine Hydrochloride (Monoamine oxidase inhibitors (MAIO) antidepressants slow amphetamine metabolism. This slowing potentiates amphetamines, increasing their effect on the release of norepinephrine and other monoamines from adrenergic nerve endings; this can cause headaches and other signs of hypertensive crisis. A variety of toxic neurological effects and malignant hyperpyrexia can occur, sometimes with fatal results. Use of lisdexamfetamine is contraindicated during or within the 14 days following the administration of MAOIs).
No products indexed under this heading.

Promethazine Hydrochloride (Amphetamines may counteract the sedative effect of antihistamines).
No products indexed under this heading.

Propoxyphene Hydrochloride (In cases of propoxyphene overdosage, amphetamine CNS stimulation is potentiated and fatal convulsions can occur).
No products indexed under this heading.

Propoxyphene Napsylate (In cases of propoxyphene overdosage, amphetamine CNS stimulation is potentiated and fatal convulsions can occur).
No products indexed under this heading.

Propranolol Hydrochloride (Adrenergic blockers are inhibited by amphetamines). Products include:
InnoPran XL Extended Release Capsules 1484

Protriptyline Hydrochloride (Amphetamines may enhance the activity of tricyclic antidepressants; d-amphetamine with desipramine or protriptyline and possibly other tricyclics cause striking and sustained increases in the concentration of d-amphetamine in the brain; cardiovascular effects can be potentiated).
No products indexed under this heading.

Pseudoephedrine Hydrochloride (Amphetamines may enhance the activity of sympathomimetic agents). Products include:
Allegra-D 12 Hour Extended-Release Tablets 2687
Allegra-D 24 Hour Extended-Release Tablets 2690
Children's Motrin Cold Oral Suspension 1899
Sudafed 12 Hour Nasal Decongestant Non-Drowsy Caplets 1909
Sudafed 24 Hour Non-Drowsy Nasal Decongestant Tablets 1906
Children's Sudafed Nasal Decongestant Liquid 1906
Sudafed Nasal Decongestant Tablets 1906
Tylenol Cold Severe Congestion Daytime Caplets with Cool Burst 1912
Tylenol Sinus Severe Congestion Caplets with Cool Burst 1917
Vicks NyQuil LiquiCaps 2567
Vicks NyQuil Liquid 2567
Vicks NyQuil Multi-Symptom Cold/Flu Relief 2567
Zyrtec-D 12 Hour Extended Release Tablets 1923
Zyrtec-D Allergy & Congestion Extended-Release Tablets 1923

Pseudoephedrine Sulfate (Amphetamines may enhance the activity of sympathomimetic agents). Products include:
Clarinex-D 12-Hour Extended-Release Tablets 2831
Clarinex-D 24-Hour Extended-Release Tablets 2834

Pyrilamine Maleate (Amphetamines may counteract the sedative effect of antihistamines).
No products indexed under this heading.

Pyrilamine Tannate (Amphetamines may counteract the sedative effect of antihistamines).
No products indexed under this heading.

Quinapril Hydrochloride (Amphetamines may antagonize the hypotensive effects of antihypertensives).
No products indexed under this heading.

Ramipril (Amphetamines may antagonize the hypotensive effects of antihypertensives).
No products indexed under this heading.

Rasagiline Mesylate (Monoamine oxidase inhibitors (MAIO) antidepressants slow amphetamine metabolism. This slowing potentiates amphetamines, increasing their effect on the release of norepinephrine and other monoamines from adrenergic nerve endings; this can cause headaches and other signs of hypertensive crisis. A variety of toxic neurological effects and malignant hyperpyrexia can occur, sometimes with fatal results. Use of lisdexamfetamine is contraindicated during or within the 14 days following the administration of MAOIs). Products include:
Azilect Tablets 3106

Rauwolfia Serpentina (Amphetamines may antagonize the hypotensive effects of antihypertensives).
No products indexed under this heading.

Rescinnamine (Amphetamines may antagonize the hypotensive effects of antihypertensives).
No products indexed under this heading.

Reserpine (Amphetamines may antagonize the hypotensive effects of antihypertensives).
No products indexed under this heading.

Salmeterol Xinafoate (Amphetamines may enhance the activity of sympathomimetic agents). Products include:
Advair Diskus 100/50 1276
Advair Diskus 250/50 1276
Advair Diskus 500/50 1276
Advair HFA 45/21 Inhalation Aerosol 1288
Advair HFA 115/21 Inhalation Aerosol 1288
Advair HFA 230/21 Inhalation Aerosol 1288
Serevent Diskus 1594

Selegiline (Monoamine oxidase inhibitors (MAIO) antidepressants slow amphetamine metabolism. This slowing potentiates amphetamines, increasing their effect on the release of norepinephrine and other monoamines from adrenergic nerve endings; this can cause headaches and other signs of hypertensive crisis. A variety of toxic neurological effects and malignant hyperpyrexia can occur, sometimes with fatal results. Use of lisdexamfetamine is contraindicated during or within the 14 days following the administration of MAOIs). Products include:
Emsam Transdermal System 905

Selegiline Hydrochloride (Monoamine oxidase inhibitors (MAIO) antidepressants slow amphetamine metabolism. This slowing potentiates amphetamines, increasing their effect on the release of norepinephrine and other monoamines from adrenergic nerve endings; this can cause headaches and other signs of hypertensive crisis. A variety of toxic neurological effects and malignant hyperpyrexia can occur, sometimes with fatal results. Use of lisdexamfetamine is contraindicated during or within the 14 days following the administration of MAOIs). Products include:
Eldepryl Capsules 3052

Sodium Acid Phosphate (Amphetamines inhibit the hypotensive effect of veratrum alkaloids). Products include:
Uroqid-Acid No. 2 Tablets 814

Sodium Bicarbonate (Urinary alkalinizing agents increase the concentration of the non-ionized species of the amphetamine molecule, thereby decreasing urinary excretion). Products include:
Ceo-Two Laxative Suppository 815

Sodium Citrate (Urinary alkalinizing agents increase the concentration of the non-ionized species of the amphetamine molecule, thereby decreasing urinary excretion).
No products indexed under this heading.

Sodium Nitroprusside (Amphetamines may antagonize the hypotensive effects of antihypertensives).
No products indexed under this heading.

Sotalol Hydrochloride (Adrenergic blockers are inhibited by amphetamines).
No products indexed under this heading.

Spirapril Hydrochloride (Amphetamines may antagonize the hypotensive effects of antihypertensives).
No products indexed under this heading.

Tamsulosin Hydrochloride (Adrenergic blockers are inhibited by amphetamines). Products include:
Flomax Capsules 848

Telmisartan (Amphetamines may antagonize the hypotensive effects of antihypertensives). Products include:
Micardis Tablets 852
Micardis HCT Tablets 854

Terazosin Hydrochloride (Adrenergic blockers are inhibited by amphetamines).
No products indexed under this heading.

Terbutaline Sulfate (Amphetamines may enhance the activity of sympathomimetic agents).
No products indexed under this heading.

Terfenadine (Amphetamines may counteract the sedative effect of antihistamines).
No products indexed under this heading.

Timolol Hemihydrate (Adrenergic blockers are inhibited by amphetamines). Products include:
Betimol Ophthalmic Solution 3181

Timolol Maleate (Adrenergic blockers are inhibited by amphetamines). Products include:
Combigan Ophthalmic Solution 553
Cosopt Sterile Ophthalmic Solution 1969
Timoptic Sterile Ophthalmic Solution 2121
Timoptic in Ocudose 2124
Timoptic-XE Sterile Ophthalmic Gel Forming Solution 2125

Torsemide (Amphetamines may antagonize the hypotensive effects of antihypertensives). Products include:
Demadex Injection 2630
Demadex Tablets 2630

Trandolapril (Amphetamines may antagonize the hypotensive effects of antihypertensives). Products include:
Mavik Tablets 472
Tarka Tablets 511

Tranylcypromine Sulfate (Monoamine oxidase inhibitors (MAIO) antidepressants slow amphetamine metabolism. This slowing potentiates amphetamines, increasing their effect on the release of norepinephrine and other monoamines from adrenergic nerve endings; this can cause headaches and other signs of hypertensive crisis. A variety of toxic neurological effects and malignant hyperpyrexia can occur, sometimes with fatal results. Use of lisdexamfetamine is contraindicated during or within the 14 days following the administration of MAOIs). Products include:
Parnate Tablets 1532

Trimeprazine Tartrate (Amphetamines may counteract the sedative effect of antihistamines).
No products indexed under this heading.

Trimethaphan Camsylate (Amphetamines may antagonize the hypotensive effects of antihypertensives).
No products indexed under this heading.

Trimipramine Maleate (Amphetamines may enhance the activity of tricyclic antidepressants; d-amphetamine with desipramine or protriptyline and possibly other tricyclics cause striking and sustained increases in the concentration of d-amphetamine in the brain; cardiovascular effects can be potentiated).
No products indexed under this heading.

Tripelennamine Hydrochloride (Amphetamines may counteract the sedative effect of antihistamines).
No products indexed under this heading.

Triprolidine Hydrochloride (Amphetamines may counteract the sedative effect of antihistamines).
No products indexed under this heading.

Valsartan (Amphetamines may antagonize the hypotensive effects of antihypertensives). Products include:
Diovan Tablets 2212
Diovan HCT Tablets 2216
Exforge Tablets 2238

Verapamil Hydrochloride (Amphetamines may antagonize the hypotensive effects of antihypertensives). Products include:
Tarka Tablets 511

WELCHOL TABLETS

(Colesevelam Hydrochloride) 1015
May interact with oral contraceptives, phenytoin, and certain other agents. Compounds in these categories include:

Desogestrel (In drug interaction studies, colesevelam hydrochloride reduced levels of oral contraceptives containing ethinyl estradiol and norethindrone). Products include:
Mircette Tablets 1034

Drugs, unspecified (When administering a drug with a narrow therapeutic index or margin of safety that has not been evaluated in formal drug-drug interaction studies, the drug should be administered at least 1 hr before or 4 hrs after colesevelam hydrochloride).
No products indexed under this heading.

Ethinyl Estradiol (In drug interaction studies, colesevelam hydrochloride reduced levels of oral contraceptives containing ethinyl estradiol and norethindrone). Products include:
Lybrel Tablets 3204
Mircette Tablets 1034
NuvaRing 2897
Ortho-Cyclen/Ortho Tri-Cyclen 2449
Ortho Evra Transdermal System 2437
Ortho Tri-Cyclen Lo Tablets 2458
Seasonique Tablets 1046
Yaz Tablets 805

Ethynodiol Diacetate (In drug interaction studies, colesevelam hydrochloride reduced levels of oral contraceptives containing ethinyl estradiol and norethindrone).
No products indexed under this heading.

Fosphenytoin Sodium (There have been postmarketing reports of decreases in phenytoin levels in patients receiving phenytoin concomitantly with colesevelam hydrochloride).
No products indexed under this heading.

Glyburide (In drug interaction studies, colesevelam reduced levels of glyburide).
No products indexed under this heading.

Levonorgestrel (In drug interaction studies, colesevelam hydrochloride reduced levels of oral contraceptives containing ethinyl estradiol and norethindrone). Products include:
Climara Pro Transdermal System 768
Lybrel Tablets 3204
Mirena Intrauterine System 779
Plan B Tablets 1044
Seasonique Tablets 1046

Levothyroxine (In drug interaction studies, colesevelam reduced levels of levothyroxine). Products include:
Naturethroid Tablets 2605

Levothyroxine Sodium (In drug interaction studies, colesevelam reduced levels of levothyroxine). Products include:
Levothroid Tablets 1170
Levoxyl Tablets 1780
Synthroid Tablets 507

Mestranol (In drug interaction studies, colesevelam hydrochloride reduced levels of oral contraceptives containing ethinyl estradiol and norethindrone).
No products indexed under this heading.

Norethindrone (In drug interaction studies, colesevelam hydrochloride reduced levels of oral contraceptives containing ethinyl estradiol and norethindrone). Products include:
Ortho Micronor Tablets 2446

Norethynodrel (In drug interaction studies, colesevelam hydrochloride reduced levels of oral contraceptives containing ethinyl estradiol and norethindrone).
No products indexed under this heading.

Norgestimate (In drug interaction studies, colesevelam hydrochloride reduced levels of oral contraceptives containing ethinyl estradiol and norethindrone). Products include:
Ortho-Cyclen/Ortho Tri-Cyclen 2449
Ortho Tri-Cyclen Lo Tablets 2458

Norgestrel (In drug interaction studies, colesevelam hydrochloride reduced levels of oral contraceptives containing ethinyl estradiol and norethindrone).
No products indexed under this heading.

Phenytoin (There have been postmarketing reports of decreases in phenytoin levels in patients receiving phenytoin concomitantly with colesevelam hydrochloride).
No products indexed under this heading.

Phenytoin Sodium (There have been postmarketing reports of decreases in phenytoin levels in patients receiving phenytoin concomitantly with colesevelam hydrochloride). Products include:
Phenytek Capsules 2192

Warfarin Sodium (There have been postmarketing reports of decreases in INR in patients receiving warfarin concomitantly with colesevelam hydrochloride).
No products indexed under this heading.

WELLBUTRIN TABLETS
(Bupropion Hydrochloride) 1648
See Wellbutrin SR Sustained-Release Tablets

WELLBUTRIN SR SUSTAINED-RELEASE TABLETS
(Bupropion Hydrochloride) 1653
May interact with benzodiazepines, corticosteroids, cytochrome p450 2d6 substrates (selected), antidepressant drugs, monoamine oxidase inhibitors, antipsychotic agents, phenytoin, drugs which lower seizure threshold, xanthines, and certain other agents. Compounds in these categories include:

Alprazolam (Bupropion is associated with a dose-related risk of seizures; excessive use of benzodiazepine sedatives is associated with increased risk of seizures; bupropion is contraindicated in patients undergoing abrupt discontinuation of benzodiazepine sedatives).
No products indexed under this heading.

Amantadine Hydrochloride (Limited clinical data suggest higher incidence of adverse experiences with co-administration; use small initial dose and gradually increase doses).
No products indexed under this heading.

Aminophylline (Bupropion is associated with a dose-related risk of seizures; co-administration with drugs that lower seizure threshold may increase the risk of seizures with bupropion; concurrent use should be undertaken with extreme caution).
No products indexed under this heading.

Amitriptyline Hydrochloride (Bupropion is associated with a dose-related risk of seizures; co-administration with drugs that lower seizure threshold may increase the risk of seizure with bupropion; concurrent use should be undertaken with extreme caution).
No products indexed under this heading.

Amoxapine (Bupropion is associated with a dose-related risk of seizures; co-administration with drugs that lower seizure threshold may increase the risk of seizure with bupropion; concurrent use should be undertaken with extreme caution).
No products indexed under this heading.

Amphetamine Aspartate (Co-administration of bupropion with drugs that are metabolized by the CYP2D6 isoenzyme should be approached with caution and should be initiated at the lower end of the dose range of the concomitant medication. If bupropion is added to the treatment regimen of a patient already receiving a drug metabolized by CYP2D6, the need to decrease the dose of the original medication should be considered, particularly for those concomitant medications with a narrow therapeutic index). Products include:
Adderall XR Capsules 3012

Amphetamine Aspartate Monohydrate (Co-administration of bupropion with drugs that are metabolized by the CYP2D6 isoenzyme should be approached with caution and should be initiated at the lower end of the dose range of the concomitant medication. If bupropion is added to the treatment regimen of a patient already receiving a drug metabolized by CYP2D6, the need to decrease the dose of the original medication should be considered, particularly for those concomitant medications with a narrow therapeutic index).
No products indexed under this heading.

Amphetamine Sulfate (Co-administration of bupropion with drugs that are metabolized by the CYP2D6 isoenzyme should be approached with caution and should be initiated at the lower end of the dose range of the concomitant medication. If bupropion is added to the treatment regimen of a patient already receiving a drug metabolized by CYP2D6, the need to decrease the dose of the original medication should be considered, particularly for those concomitant medications with a narrow therapeutic index). Products include:
Adderall XR Capsules 3012

Aripiprazole (Concurrent administration of bupropion and agents that lower seizure threshold (e.g., antipsychotics) should be undertaken only with extreme caution. Low initial dosing and gradual dose increases should be employed). Products include:
Abilify Injection 881
Abilify Injection 2466
Abilify Oral Solution 881
Abilify Oral Solution 2466
Abilify Discmelt Orally Disintegrating Tablets 881
Abilify Discmelt Orally Disintegrating Tablets 2466
Abilify Tablets 881
Abilify Tablets 2466

Atomoxetine Hydrochloride (Co-administration of bupropion with drugs that are metabolized by the CYP2D6 isoenzyme should be approached with caution and should be initiated at the lower end of the dose range of the concomitant medication. If bupropion is added to the treatment regimen of a patient already receiving a drug metabolized by CYP2D6, the need to decrease the dose of the original medication should be considered, particularly for those concomitant medications with a narrow therapeutic index). Products include:
Strattera Capsules 1864

Betamethasone Acetate (Bupropion is associated with a dose-related risk of seizures; co-administration with drugs that lower seizure threshold, such as systemic steroids, may increase the risk of seizure with bupropion).
No products indexed under this heading.

Betamethasone Sodium Phosphate (Bupropion is associated with a dose-related risk of seizures; co-administration with drugs that lower seizure threshold, such as systemic steroids, may increase the risk of seizure with bupropion).
No products indexed under this heading.

Bisoprolol Fumarate (Co-administration of bupropion with drugs that are metabolized by the CYP2D6 isoenzyme should be approached with caution and should be initiated at the lower end of the dose range of the concomitant medication. If bupropion is added to the treatment regimen of a patient already receiving a drug metabolized by CYP2D6, the need to decrease the dose of the original medication should be considered, particularly for those concomitant medications with a narrow therapeutic index).
No products indexed under this heading.

Budesonide (Bupropion is associated with a dose-related risk of seizures; co-administration with drugs that lower seizure threshold, such as systemic steroids, may increase the risk of seizure with bupropion). Products include:
Pulmicort Flexhaler 654
Symbicort 80/4.5 Inhalation Aerosol 659
Symbicort 160/4.5 Inhalation Aerosol 659

Bupropion (Patients should be made aware that both formulations of Wellbutrin contain the same active moiety found in Zyban, an aid to smoking cessation; combination is contraindicated).
No products indexed under this heading.

Captopril (Co-administration of bupropion with drugs that are metabolized by the CYP2D6 isoenzyme should be approached with caution and should be initiated at the lower end of the dose range of the concomitant medication. If bupropion is added to the treatment regimen of a patient already receiving a drug metabolized by CYP2D6, the need to decrease the dose of the original medication should be considered, particularly for those concomitant medications with a narrow therapeutic index). Products include:
Captopril Tablets 2182

Carbamazepine (May induce the metabolism of bupropion). Products include:
Carbatrol Capsules 3019
Equetro Extended-Release Capsules 3174

Carvedilol (Co-administration of bupropion with drugs that are metabolized by the CYP2D6 isoenzyme should be approached with caution and should be initiated at the lower end of the dose range of the concomitant medication. If bupropion is added to the treatment regimen of a patient already receiving a drug metabolized by CYP2D6, the need to decrease the dose of the original medication should be considered, particularly for those concomitant medications with a narrow therapeutic index). Products include:
Coreg Tablets 1387

Cevimeline Hydrochloride (Co-administration of bupropion with drugs that are metabolized by the CYP2D6 isoenzyme should be approached with caution and should be initiated at the lower end of the dose range of the concomitant medication. If bupropion is added to the treatment regimen of a patient already receiving a drug metabolized by CYP2D6, the need to decrease the dose of the original medication should be considered, particularly

for those concomitant medications with a narrow therapeutic index).
Products include:
Evoxac Capsules 1013

Chlordiazepoxide (Bupropion is associated with a dose-related risk of seizures; excessive use of benzodiazepine sedatives is associated with increased risk of seizures; bupropion is contraindicated in patients undergoing abrupt discontinuation of benzodiazepine sedatives).
No products indexed under this heading.

Chlordiazepoxide Hydrochloride (Bupropion is associated with a dose-related risk of seizures; excessive use of benzodiazepine sedatives is associated with increased risk of seizures; bupropion is contraindicated in patients undergoing abrupt discontinuation of benzodiazepine sedatives).
No products indexed under this heading.

Chlorpromazine (Bupropion is associated with a dose-related risk of seizures; co-administration with drugs that lower seizure threshold may increase the risk of seizure with bupropion; concurrent use should be undertaken with extreme caution).
No products indexed under this heading.

Chlorpromazine Hydrochloride (Bupropion is associated with a dose-related risk of seizures; co-administration with drugs that lower seizure threshold may increase the risk of seizure with bupropion; concurrent use should be undertaken with extreme caution).
No products indexed under this heading.

Chlorpropamide (Co-administration of bupropion with drugs that are metabolized by the CYP2D6 isoenzyme should be approached with caution and should be initiated at the lower end of the dose range of the concomitant medication. If bupropion is added to the treatment regimen of a patient already receiving a drug metabolized by CYP2D6, the need to decrease the dose of the original medication should be considered, particularly for those concomitant medications with a narrow therapeutic index).
No products indexed under this heading.

Chlorprothixene (Concurrent administration of bupropion and agents that lower seizure threshold (e.g., antipsychotics) should be undertaken only with extreme caution. Low initial dosing and gradual dose increases should be employed).
No products indexed under this heading.

Chlorprothixene Hydrochloride (Concurrent administration of bupropion and agents that lower seizure threshold (e.g., antipsychotics) should be undertaken only with extreme caution. Low initial dosing and gradual dose increases should be employed).
No products indexed under this heading.

Ciclesonide (Bupropion is associated with a dose-related risk of seizures; co-administration with drugs that lower seizure threshold, such as systemic steroids, may increase the risk of seizure with bupropion).
Products include:
Alvesco Inhalation Aerosol 2985
Omnaris Nasal Spray 2998

Cimetidine (May inhibit the metabolism of bupropion).
No products indexed under this heading.

Cimetidine Hydrochloride (May induce the metabolism of bupropion).
No products indexed under this heading.

Citalopram Hydrobromide (Concurrent administration of bupropion and agents that lower seizure threshold (e.g., other antidepressants) should be undertaken only with extreme caution. Low initial dosing and gradual dose increases should be employed). Products include:
Celexa 1160

Clomipramine Hydrochloride (Co-administration of bupropion with drugs that are metabolized by the CYP2D6 isoenzyme should be approached with caution and should be initiated at the lower end of the dose range of the concomitant medication. If bupropion is added to the treatment regimen of a patient already receiving a drug metabolized by CYP2D6, the need to decrease the dose of the original medication should be considered, particularly for those concomitant medications with a narrow therapeutic index).
No products indexed under this heading.

Clorazepate Dipotassium (Bupropion is associated with a dose-related risk of seizures; excessive use of benzodiazepine sedatives is associated with increased risk of seizures; bupropion is contraindicated in patients undergoing abrupt discontinuation of benzodiazepine sedatives).
No products indexed under this heading.

Clozapine (Co-administration of bupropion with drugs that are metabolized by the CYP2D6 isoenzyme should be approached with caution and should be initiated at the lower end of the dose range of the concomitant medication. If bupropion is added to the treatment regimen of a patient already receiving a drug metabolized by CYP2D6, the need to decrease the dose of the original medication should be considered, particularly for those concomitant medications with a narrow therapeutic index).
No products indexed under this heading.

Codeine Phosphate (Co-administration of bupropion with drugs that are metabolized by the CYP2D6 isoenzyme should be approached with caution and should be initiated at the lower end of the dose range of the concomitant medication. If bupropion is added to the treatment regimen of a patient already receiving a drug metabolized by CYP2D6, the need to decrease the dose of the original medication should be considered, particularly for those concomitant medications with a narrow therapeutic index).
Products include:
Tylenol with Codeine Tablets 2427

Codeine Sulfate (Co-administration of bupropion with drugs that are metabolized by the CYP2D6 isoenzyme should be approached with caution and should be initiated at the lower end of the dose range of the concomitant medication. If bupropion is added to the treatment regimen of a patient already receiving a drug metabolized by CYP2D6, the need to decrease the dose of the original medication should be considered, particularly for those concomitant medications with a narrow therapeutic index).
No products indexed under this heading.

Cortisone Acetate (Bupropion is associated with a dose-related risk of seizures; co-administration with drugs that lower seizure threshold, such as systemic steroids, may increase the risk of seizure with bupropion).
No products indexed under this heading.

Cyclobenzaprine Hydrochloride (Co-administration of bupropion with drugs that are metabolized by the CYP2D6 isoenzyme should be approached with caution and should be initiated at the lower end of the dose range of the concomitant medication. If bupropion is added to the treatment regimen of a patient already receiving a drug metabolized by CYP2D6, the need to decrease the dose of the original medication should be considered, particularly for those concomitant medications with a narrow therapeutic index).
Products include:
Amrix Capsules 966

Cyclophosphamide (Bupropion is primarily metabolized, based on *in vitro* studies, to the morpholinol metabolite by cytochrome P450IIB6 isoenzyme; therefore, the potential exists for a drug interaction with agents that affect the cytochrome P450IIB6 metabolism, such as cyclophosphamide).
No products indexed under this heading.

Desipramine Hydrochloride (Co-administration of bupropion with drugs that are metabolized by the CYP2D6 isoenzyme, including desipramine, should be approached with caution and should be initiated at the lower end of the dose range of the concomitant medication. If bupropion is added to the treatment regimen of a patient already receiving a drug metabolized by CYP2D6, the need to decrease the dose of the original medication should be considered, particularly for those concomitant medications with a narrow therapeutic index).
No products indexed under this heading.

Dexamethasone (Bupropion is associated with a dose-related risk of seizures; co-administration with drugs that lower seizure threshold, such as systemic steroids, may increase the risk of seizure with bupropion). Products include:
Ciprodex Otic Suspension 541

Dexamethasone Acetate (Bupropion is associated with a dose-related risk of seizures; co-administration with drugs that lower seizure threshold, such as systemic steroids, may increase the risk of seizure with bupropion).
No products indexed under this heading.

Dexamethasone Sodium Phosphate (Bupropion is associated with a dose-related risk of seizures; co-administration with drugs that lower seizure threshold, such as systemic steroids, may increase the risk of seizure with bupropion).
No products indexed under this heading.

Dexfenfluramine Hydrochloride (Co-administration of bupropion with drugs that are metabolized by the CYP2D6 isoenzyme should be approached with caution and should be initiated at the lower end of the dose range of the concomitant medication. If bupropion is added to the treatment regimen of a patient already receiving a drug metabolized by CYP2D6, the need to decrease the dose of the original medication should be considered, particularly for those concomitant medications with a narrow therapeutic index).
No products indexed under this heading.

Dextromethorphan Hydrobromide (Co-administration of bupropion with drugs that are metabolized by the CYP2D6 isoenzyme should be approached with caution and should be initiated at the lower end of the dose range of the concomitant medication. If bupropion is added to the treatment regimen of a patient already receiving a drug metabolized by CYP2D6, the need to decrease the dose of the original medication should be considered, particularly for those concomitant medications with a narrow therapeutic index).
Products include:
PediaCare Children's Liquid Multi-Symptom Cold........................ 1902
PediaCare Children's Long-Acting Cough.. 1902
Children's Sudafed PE Cold & Cough Liquid 1907
Sudafed PE Cold & Cough Caplets... 1907
Children's Tylenol Plus Cough & Runny Nose Suspension Liquid..... 1912
Children's Tylenol Plus Cough & Sore Throat Suspension Liquid..... 1912
Children's Tylenol Plus Flu Suspension Liquid 1914
Children's Tylenol Plus Multi-Symptom Cold Suspension Liquid 1912
Tylenol Cold Severe Congestion Daytime Caplets with Cool Burst.. 1912
Tylenol Cold Head Congestion Daytime Caplets with Cool Burst.. 1910
Tylenol Cold Head Congestion Nighttime Caplets with Cool Burst.. 1910
Tylenol Cold Head Congestion Severe Daytime Caplets with Cool Burst.. 1910
Tylenol Cold Multi-Symptom Daytime Caplets with Cool Burst and Rapid Release Gels....... 1913
Tylenol Cold Multi-Symptom Daytime Liquid with Citrus Burst... 1913
Tylenol Cold Multi-Symptom Nighttime Caplets with Cool Burst.. 1913
Tylenol Cold Multi-Symptom Nighttime Liquid with Cool Burst... 1913
Tylenol Cold Multi-Symptom Severe Caplets with Cool Burst..... 1913
Tylenol Cold Multi-Symptom Severe Daytime Liquid with Citrus Burst.. 1913
Tylenol Cough & Sore Throat Daytime Liquid with Cool Burst...... 1918
Tylenol Cough & Sore Throat Nighttime Liquid with Cool Burst... 1918
Vicks DayQuil Cold & Flu Multi-Symptom Relief 616
Vicks DayQuil LiquiCaps 2567

IMPORTANT NOTE: Always consult each drug listing in the patient's regimen for possible interactions.

Vicks DayQuil Liquid 2567
Vicks DayQuil Multi-Symptom Cold/Flu Relief 2567
Vicks NyQuil Cold & Flu Multi-Symptom Relief .... ▣617
Vicks NyQuil LiquiCaps 2567
Vicks NyQuil Liquid 2567
Vicks NyQuil Multi-Symptom Cold/Flu Relief 2567

Dextromethorphan Polistirex (Co-administration of bupropion with drugs that are metabolized by the CYP2D6 isoenzyme should be approached with caution and should be initiated at the lower end of the dose range of the concomitant medication. If bupropion is added to the treatment regimen of a patient already receiving a drug metabolized by CYP2D6, the need to decrease the dose of the original medication should be considered, particularly for those concomitant medications with a narrow therapeutic index).
No products indexed under this heading.

Diazepam (Bupropion is associated with a dose-related risk of seizures; excessive use of benzodiazepine sedatives is associated with increased risk of seizures; bupropion is contraindicated in patients undergoing abrupt discontinuation of benzodiazepine sedatives). Products include:
Valium Tablets 2658

Dolasetron Mesylate (Co-administration of bupropion with drugs that are metabolized by the CYP2D6 isoenzyme should be approached with caution and should be initiated at the lower end of the dose range of the concomitant medication. If bupropion is added to the treatment regimen of a patient already receiving a drug metabolized by CYP2D6, the need to decrease the dose of the original medication should be considered, particularly for those concomitant medications with a narrow therapeutic index). Products include:
Anzemet Injection 2701
Anzemet Tablets 2704

Donepezil Hydrochloride (Co-administration of bupropion with drugs that are metabolized by the CYP2D6 isoenzyme should be approached with caution and should be initiated at the lower end of the dose range of the concomitant medication. If bupropion is added to the treatment regimen of a patient already receiving a drug metabolized by CYP2D6, the need to decrease the dose of the original medication should be considered, particularly for those concomitant medications with a narrow therapeutic index). Products include:
Aricept Tablets 1062
Aricept ODT Tablets 1062

Doxepin Hydrochloride (Bupropion is associated with a dose-related risk of seizures; co-administration with drugs that lower seizure threshold may increase the risk of seizure with bupropion; concurrent use should be undertaken with extreme caution).
No products indexed under this heading.

Dyphylline (Bupropion is associated with a dose-related risk of seizures; co-administration with drugs that lower seizure threshold may increase the risk of seizures with bupropion; concurrent use should be undertaken with extreme caution).
No products indexed under this heading.

Encainide Hydrochloride (Co-administration of bupropion with drugs that are metabolized by the CYP2D6 isoenzyme should be approached with caution and should be initiated at the lower end of the dose range of the concomitant medication. If bupropion is added to the treatment regimen of a patient already receiving a drug metabolized by CYP2D6, the need to decrease the dose of the original medication should be considered, particularly for those concomitant medications with a narrow therapeutic index).
No products indexed under this heading.

Escitalopram Oxalate (Concurrent administration of bupropion and agents that lower seizure threshold (e.g., other antidepressants) should be undertaken only with extreme caution. Low initial dosing and gradual dose increases should be employed). Products include:
Lexapro Oral Suspension 1174
Lexapro Tablets 1174

Estazolam (Bupropion is associated with a dose-related risk of seizures; excessive use of benzodiazepine sedatives is associated with increased risk of seizures; bupropion is contraindicated in patients undergoing abrupt discontinuation of benzodiazepine sedatives).
No products indexed under this heading.

Fentanyl (Co-administration of bupropion with drugs that are metabolized by the CYP2D6 isoenzyme should be approached with caution and should be initiated at the lower end of the dose range of the concomitant medication. If bupropion is added to the treatment regimen of a patient already receiving a drug metabolized by CYP2D6, the need to decrease the dose of the original medication should be considered, particularly for those concomitant medications with a narrow therapeutic index). Products include:
Duragesic Transdermal System 2405
Ionsys Transdermal System 2410

Fentanyl Citrate (Co-administration of bupropion with drugs that are metabolized by the CYP2D6 isoenzyme should be approached with caution and should be initiated at the lower end of the dose range of the concomitant medication. If bupropion is added to the treatment regimen of a patient already receiving a drug metabolized by CYP2D6, the need to decrease the dose of the original medication should be considered, particularly for those concomitant medications with a narrow therapeutic index). Products include:
Actiq 959
Fentora Tablets 968

Flecainide Acetate (Co-administration of bupropion with drugs that are metabolized by the CYP2D6 isoenzyme, including flecainide, should be approached with caution and should be initiated at the lower end of the dose range of the concomitant medication. If bupropion is added to the treatment regimen of a patient already receiving a drug metabolized by CYP2D6, the need to decrease the dose of the original medication should be considered, particularly for those concomitant medications with a narrow therapeutic index).
No products indexed under this heading.

Fludrocortisone Acetate (Bupropion is associated with a dose-related risk of seizures; co-administration with drugs that lower seizure threshold, such as systemic steroids, may increase the risk of seizure with bupropion).
No products indexed under this heading.

Flunisolide (Bupropion is associated with a dose-related risk of seizures; co-administration with drugs that lower seizure threshold, such as systemic steroids, may increase the risk of seizure with bupropion). Products include:
Aerobid/Aerobid-M 1153

Fluoxetine (Co-administration of bupropion with drugs that are metabolized by the CYP2D6 isoenzyme, including fluoxetine, should be approached with caution and should be initiated at the lower end of the dose range of the concomitant medication. If bupropion is added to the treatment regimen of a patient already receiving a drug metabolized by CYP2D6, the need to decrease the dose of the original medication should be considered, particularly for those concomitant medications with a narrow therapeutic index).
No products indexed under this heading.

Fluoxetine Hydrochloride (Co-administration of bupropion with drugs that are metabolized by the CYP2D6 isoenzyme, including fluoxetine, should be approached with caution and should be initiated at the lower end of the dose range of the concomitant medication. If bupropion is added to the treatment regimen of a patient already receiving a drug metabolized by CYP2D6, the need to decrease the dose of the original medication should be considered, particularly for those concomitant medications with a narrow therapeutic index). Products include:
Prozac Weekly Capsules 1852
Prozac Pulvules and Liquid 1852
Symbyax Capsules 1871

Fluphenazine Decanoate (Bupropion is associated with a dose-related risk of seizures; co-administration with drugs that lower seizure threshold may increase the risk of seizure with bupropion; concurrent use should be undertaken with extreme caution).
No products indexed under this heading.

Fluphenazine Enanthate (Bupropion is associated with a dose-related risk of seizures; co-administration with drugs that lower seizure threshold may increase the risk of seizure with bupropion; concurrent use should be undertaken with extreme caution).
No products indexed under this heading.

Fluphenazine Hydrochloride (Bupropion is associated with a dose-related risk of seizures; co-administration with drugs that lower seizure threshold may increase the risk of seizure with bupropion; concurrent use should be undertaken with extreme caution).
No products indexed under this heading.

Flurazepam Hydrochloride (Bupropion is associated with a dose-related risk of seizures; excessive use of benzodiazepine sedatives is associated with increased risk of seizures; bupropion is contraindicated in patients undergoing abrupt discontinuation of benzodiazepine sedatives).
No products indexed under this heading.

Fluticasone Propionate (Bupropion is associated with a dose-related risk of seizures; co-administration with drugs that lower seizure threshold, such as systemic steroids, may increase the risk of seizure with bupropion). Products include:
Advair Diskus 100/50 1276
Advair Diskus 250/50 1276
Advair Diskus 500/50 1276
Advair HFA 45/21 Inhalation Aerosol 1288
Advair HFA 115/21 Inhalation Aerosol 1288
Advair HFA 230/21 Inhalation Aerosol 1288
Flonase Nasal Spray 1431
Flovent Diskus 50 mcg 1435

Fluticasone Propionate HFA (Bupropion is associated with a dose-related risk of seizures; co-administration with drugs that lower seizure threshold, such as systemic steroids, may increase the risk of seizure with bupropion). Products include:
Flovent HFA 1440

Fluvoxamine Maleate (Co-administration of bupropion with drugs that are metabolized by the CYP2D6 isoenzyme should be approached with caution and should be initiated at the lower end of the dose range of the concomitant medication. If bupropion is added to the treatment regimen of a patient already receiving a drug metabolized by CYP2D6, the need to decrease the dose of the original medication should be considered, particularly for those concomitant medications with a narrow therapeutic index). Products include:
Luvox CR Extended-Release Capsules 1759

Formoterol Fumarate (Co-administration of bupropion with drugs that are metabolized by the CYP2D6 isoenzyme should be approached with caution and should be initiated at the lower end of the dose range of the concomitant medication. If bupropion is added to the treatment regimen of a patient already receiving a drug metabolized by CYP2D6, the need to decrease the dose of the original medication should be considered, particularly for those concomitant medications with a narrow therapeutic index). Products include:
Foradil Aerolizer 2849
Perforomist Inhalation Solution 1025

Fosphenytoin Sodium (May induce the metabolism of bupropion).
No products indexed under this heading.

Galantamine Hydrobromide (Co-administration of bupropion with drugs that are metabolized by the CYP2D6 isoenzyme should be approached with caution and should be initiated at the lower end of the dose range of the concomitant medication. If bupropion is added to the treatment regimen of a patient already receiving a drug metabolized by CYP2D6, the need to decrease the dose of the original medication should be considered, particularly for those concomitant medications with a narrow therapeutic index).
No products indexed under this heading.

Halazepam (Bupropion is associated with a dose-related risk of seizures; excessive use of benzodiazepine sedatives is associated with increased risk of seizures; bupropion is contraindicated in patients undergoing abrupt discontinuation of benzodiazepine sedatives).
No products indexed under this heading.

Haloperidol (Co-administration of bupropion with drugs that are metabolized by the CYP2D6 isoenzyme, including haloperidol, should be approached with caution and should be initiated at the lower end of the dose range of the concomitant medication. If bupropion is added to the treatment regimen of a patient already receiving a drug metabolized by CYP2D6, the need to decrease the dose of the original medication should be considered, particularly for those concomitant medications with a narrow therapeutic index).
No products indexed under this heading.

Haloperidol Decanoate (Co-administration of bupropion with drugs that are metabolized by the CYP2D6 isoenzyme, including haloperidol, should be approached with caution and should be initiated at the lower end of the dose range of the concomitant medication. If bupropion is added to the treatment regimen of a patient already receiving a drug metabolized by CYP2D6, the need to decrease the dose of the original medication should be considered, particularly for those concomitant medications with a narrow therapeutic index).
No products indexed under this heading.

Haloperidol Lactate (Co-administration of bupropion with drugs that are metabolized by the CYP2D6 isoenzyme, including haloperidol, should be approached with caution and should be initiated at the lower end of the dose range of the concomitant medication. If bupropion is added to the treatment regimen of a patient already receiving a drug metabolized by CYP2D6, the need to decrease the dose of the original medication should be considered, particularly for those concomitant medications with a narrow therapeutic index).
No products indexed under this heading.

Hydrocodone Bitartrate (Co-administration of bupropion with drugs that are metabolized by the CYP2D6 isoenzyme should be approached with caution and should be initiated at the lower end of the dose range of the concomitant medication. If bupropion is added to the treatment regimen of a patient already receiving a drug metabolized by CYP2D6, the need to decrease the dose of the original medication should be considered, particularly for those concomitant medications with a narrow therapeutic index). Products include:
Lortab 5/500 Tablets **3143**
Lortab 7.5/500 Tablets **3144**
Lortab 10/500 Tablets **3144**
Vicodin Tablets **529**
Vicodin ES Tablets **530**
Vicodin HP Tablets **531**
Vicoprofen Tablets **533**
Zydone Tablets **1132**

Hydrocortisone (Bupropion is associated with a dose-related risk of seizures; co-administration with drugs that lower seizure threshold, such as systemic steroids, may increase the risk of seizure with bupropion).
No products indexed under this heading.

Hydrocortisone Acetate (Bupropion is associated with a dose-related risk of seizures; co-administration with drugs that lower seizure threshold, such as systemic steroids, may increase the risk of seizure with bupropion). Products include:
Analpram-HC **1140**
Pramosone **1141**

Hydrocortisone Sodium Phosphate (Bupropion is associated with a dose-related risk of seizures; co-administration with drugs that lower seizure threshold, such as systemic steroids, may increase the risk of seizure with bupropion).
No products indexed under this heading.

Hydrocortisone Sodium Succinate (Bupropion is associated with a dose-related risk of seizures; co-administration with drugs that lower seizure threshold, such as systemic steroids, may increase the risk of seizure with bupropion).
No products indexed under this heading.

Imipramine Hydrochloride (Co-administration of bupropion with drugs that are metabolized by the CYP2D6 isoenzyme, including imipramine, should be approached with caution and should be initiated at the lower end of the dose range of the concomitant medication. If bupropion is added to the treatment regimen of a patient already receiving a drug metabolized by CYP2D6, the need to decrease the dose of the original medication should be considered, particularly for those concomitant medications with a narrow therapeutic index).
No products indexed under this heading.

Imipramine Pamoate (Co-administration of bupropion with drugs that are metabolized by the CYP2D6 isoenzyme, including imipramine, should be approached with caution and should be initiated at the lower end of the dose range of the concomitant medication. If bupropion is added to the treatment regimen of a patient already receiving a drug metabolized by CYP2D6, the need to decrease the dose of the original medication should be considered, particularly for those concomitant medications with a narrow therapeutic index).
No products indexed under this heading.

Indoramin Hydrochloride (Co-administration of bupropion with drugs that are metabolized by the CYP2D6 isoenzyme should be approached with caution and should be initiated at the lower end of the dose range of the concomitant medication. If bupropion is added to the treatment regimen of a patient already receiving a drug metabolized by CYP2D6, the need to decrease the dose of the original medication should be considered, particularly for those concomitant medications with a narrow therapeutic index).
No products indexed under this heading.

Isocarboxazid (Concurrent and/or sequential use with MAO inhibitors is contraindicated). Products include:
Marplan Tablets **3177**

Labetalol Hydrochloride (Co-administration of bupropion with drugs that are metabolized by the CYP2D6 isoenzyme should be approached with caution and should be initiated at the lower end of the dose range of the concomitant medication. If bupropion is added to the treatment regimen of a patient already receiving a drug metabolized by CYP2D6, the need to decrease the dose of the original medication should be considered, particularly for those concomitant medications with a narrow therapeutic index).
No products indexed under this heading.

Levodopa (Limited clinical data suggest higher incidence of adverse experiences with co-administration; use small initial dose and gradually increase doses). Products include:
Stalevo Tablets **2309**

Lidocaine (Co-administration of bupropion with drugs that are metabolized by the CYP2D6 isoenzyme should be approached with caution and should be initiated at the lower end of the dose range of the concomitant medication. If bupropion is added to the treatment regimen of a patient already receiving a drug metabolized by CYP2D6, the need to decrease the dose of the original medication should be considered, particularly for those concomitant medications with a narrow therapeutic index). Products include:
Lidoderm Patch **1114**

Lidocaine Hydrochloride (Co-administration of bupropion with drugs that are metabolized by the CYP2D6 isoenzyme should be approached with caution and should be initiated at the lower end of the dose range of the concomitant medication. If bupropion is added to the treatment regimen of a patient already receiving a drug metabolized by CYP2D6, the need to decrease the dose of the original medication should be considered, particularly for those concomitant medications with a narrow therapeutic index).
No products indexed under this heading.

Lithium Carbonate (Concurrent administration of bupropion and agents that lower seizure threshold (e.g., antipsychotics) should be undertaken only with extreme caution. Low initial dosing and gradual dose increases should be employed).
No products indexed under this heading.

Lithium Citrate (Concurrent administration of bupropion and agents that lower seizure threshold (e.g., antipsychotics) should be undertaken only with extreme caution. Low initial dosing and gradual dose increases should be employed).
No products indexed under this heading.

Lorazepam (Bupropion is associated with a dose-related risk of seizures; excessive use of benzodiazepine sedatives is associated with increased risk of seizures; bupropion is contraindicated in patients undergoing abrupt discontinuation of benzodiazepine sedatives).
No products indexed under this heading.

Loxapine Hydrochloride (Concurrent administration of bupropion and agents that lower seizure threshold (e.g., antipsychotics) should be undertaken only with extreme caution. Low initial dosing and gradual dose increases should be employed).
No products indexed under this heading.

Loxapine Succinate (Concurrent administration of bupropion and agents that lower seizure threshold (e.g., antipsychotics) should be undertaken only with extreme caution. Low initial dosing and gradual dose increases should be employed).
No products indexed under this heading.

Maprotiline Hydrochloride (Bupropion is associated with a dose-related risk of seizures; co-administration with drugs that lower seizure threshold may increase the risk of seizure with bupropion; concurrent use should be undertaken with extreme caution).
No products indexed under this heading.

Meperidine Hydrochloride (Co-administration of bupropion with drugs that are metabolized by the CYP2D6 isoenzyme should be approached with caution and should be initiated at the lower end of the dose range of the concomitant medication. If bupropion is added to the treatment regimen of a patient already receiving a drug metabolized by CYP2D6, the need to decrease the dose of the original medication should be considered, particularly for those concomitant medications with a narrow therapeutic index).
No products indexed under this heading.

Mesoridazine Besylate (Bupropion is associated with a dose-related risk of seizures; co-administration with drugs that lower seizure threshold may increase the risk of seizure with bupropion; concurrent use should be undertaken with extreme caution).
No products indexed under this heading.

Methadone Hydrochloride (Co-administration of bupropion with

drugs that are metabolized by the CYP2D6 isoenzyme should be approached with caution and should be initiated at the lower end of the dose range of the concomitant medication. If bupropion is added to the treatment regimen of a patient already receiving a drug metabolized by CYP2D6, the need to decrease the dose of the original medication should be considered, particularly for those concomitant medications with a narrow therapeutic index).
No products indexed under this heading.

Methamphetamine Hydrochloride (Co-administration of bupropion with drugs that are metabolized by the CYP2D6 isoenzyme should be approached with caution and should be initiated at the lower end of the dose range of the concomitant medication. If bupropion is added to the treatment regimen of a patient already receiving a drug metabolized by CYP2D6, the need to decrease the dose of the original medication should be considered, particularly for those concomitant medications with a narrow therapeutic index).
No products indexed under this heading.

Methotrimeprazine (Concurrent administration of bupropion and agents that lower seizure threshold (e.g., antipsychotics) should be undertaken only with extreme caution. Low initial dosing and gradual dose increases should be employed).
No products indexed under this heading.

Methylprednisolone Acetate (Bupropion is associated with a dose-related risk of seizures; co-administration with drugs that lower seizure threshold, such as systemic steroids, may increase the risk of seizure with bupropion).
No products indexed under this heading.

Methylprednisolone Sodium Succinate (Bupropion is associated with a dose-related risk of seizures; co-administration with drugs that lower seizure threshold, such as systemic steroids, may increase the risk of seizure with bupropion).
No products indexed under this heading.

Metoprolol Succinate (Co-administration of bupropion with drugs that are metabolized by the CYP2D6 isoenzyme, including metoprolol, should be approached with caution and should be initiated at the lower end of the dose range of the concomitant medication. If bupropion is added to the treatment regimen of a patient already receiving a drug metabolized by CYP2D6, the need to decrease the dose of the original medication should be considered, particularly for those concomitant medications with a narrow therapeutic index). Products include:
Toprol-XL Tablets 666

Metoprolol Tartrate (Co-administration of bupropion with drugs that are metabolized by the CYP2D6 isoenzyme, including metoprolol, should be approached with caution and should be initiated at the lower end of the dose range of the concomitant medication. If bupropion is added to the treatment regimen of a patient already receiving a drug metabolized by CYP2D6, the need to decrease the dose of the original medication should be considered, particularly for those concomitant medications with a narrow therapeutic index).
No products indexed under this heading.

Mexiletine Hydrochloride (Co-administration of bupropion with drugs that are metabolized by the CYP2D6 isoenzyme should be approached with caution and should be initiated at the lower end of the dose range of the concomitant medication. If bupropion is added to the treatment regimen of a patient already receiving a drug metabolized by CYP2D6, the need to decrease the dose of the original medication should be considered, particularly for those concomitant medications with a narrow therapeutic index).
No products indexed under this heading.

Midazolam Hydrochloride (Bupropion is associated with a dose-related risk of seizures; excessive use of benzodiazepine sedatives is associated with increased risk of seizures; bupropion is contraindicated in patients undergoing abrupt discontinuation of benzodiazepine sedatives).
No products indexed under this heading.

Mirtazapine (Co-administration of bupropion with drugs that are metabolized by the CYP2D6 isoenzyme should be approached with caution and should be initiated at the lower end of the dose range of the concomitant medication. If bupropion is added to the treatment regimen of a patient already receiving a drug metabolized by CYP2D6, the need to decrease the dose of the original medication should be considered, particularly for those concomitant medications with a narrow therapeutic index). Products include:
Remeron Tablets 2924
RemeronSolTab Tablets 2927

Moclobemide (Concurrent and/or sequential use with MAO inhibitors is contraindicated).
No products indexed under this heading.

Molindone Hydrochloride (Concurrent administration of bupropion and agents that lower seizure threshold (e.g., antipsychotics) should be undertaken only with extreme caution. Low initial dosing and gradual dose increases should be employed). Products include:
Moban Tablets 1116

Mometasone Furoate (Bupropion is associated with a dose-related risk of seizures; co-administration with drugs that lower seizure threshold, such as systemic steroids, may increase the risk of seizure with bupropion). Products include:
Asmanex Twisthaler 2797
Elocon Cream 0.1% 2840
Elocon Lotion 0.1% 2841
Elocon Ointment 0.1% 2842

Mometasone Furoate Monohydrate (Bupropion is associated with a dose-related risk of seizures; co-administration with drugs that lower seizure threshold, such as systemic steroids, may increase the risk of seizure with bupropion). Products include:
Nasonex Nasal Spray 2883

Morphine Sulfate (Co-administration of bupropion with drugs that are metabolized by the CYP2D6 isoenzyme should be approached with caution and should be initiated at the lower end of the dose range of the concomitant medication. If bupropion is added to the treatment regimen of a patient already receiving a drug metabolized by CYP2D6, the need to decrease the dose of the original medication should be considered, particularly for those concomitant medications with a narrow therapeutic index). Products include:
Avinza Capsules 1772
DepoDur Injection 1095
MS Contin Tablets 2585

Nefazodone Hydrochloride (Concurrent administration of bupropion and agents that lower seizure threshold (e.g., other antidepressants) should be undertaken only with extreme caution. Low initial dosing and gradual dose increases should be employed).
No products indexed under this heading.

Nelfinavir Mesylate (Co-administration of bupropion with drugs that are metabolized by the CYP2D6 isoenzyme should be approached with caution and should be initiated at the lower end of the dose range of the concomitant medication. If bupropion is added to the treatment regimen of a patient already receiving a drug metabolized by CYP2D6, the need to decrease the dose of the original medication should be considered, particularly for those concomitant medications with a narrow therapeutic index).
No products indexed under this heading.

Nicotine (Co-administration has resulted in a higher incidence of treatment-emergent hypertension).
No products indexed under this heading.

Nortriptyline Hydrochloride (Co-administration of bupropion with drugs that are metabolized by the CYP2D6 isoenzyme, including nortriptyline, should be approached with caution and should be initiated at the lower end of the dose range of the concomitant medication. If bupropion is added to the treatment regimen of a patient already receiving a drug metabolized by CYP2D6, the need to decrease the dose of the original medication should be considered, particularly for those concomitant medications with a narrow therapeutic index).
No products indexed under this heading.

Olanzapine (Co-administration of bupropion with drugs that are metabolized by the CYP2D6 isoenzyme should be approached with caution and should be initiated at the lower end of the dose range of the concomitant medication. If bupropion is added to the treatment regimen of a patient already receiving a drug metabolized by CYP2D6, the need to decrease the dose of the original medication should be considered, particularly for those concomitant medications with a narrow therapeutic index). Products include:
Symbyax Capsules 1871
Zyprexa Tablets 1883
Zyprexa IntraMuscular 1883
Zyprexa ZYDIS Orally Disintegrating Tablets 1883

Omeprazole (Co-administration of bupropion with drugs that are metabolized by the CYP2D6 isoenzyme should be approached with caution and should be initiated at the lower end of the dose range of the concomitant medication. If bupropion is added to the treatment regimen of a patient already receiving a drug metabolized by CYP2D6, the need to decrease the dose of the original medication should be considered, particularly for those concomitant medications with a narrow therapeutic index).
No products indexed under this heading.

Ondansetron (Co-administration of bupropion with drugs that are metabolized by the CYP2D6 isoenzyme should be approached with caution and should be initiated at the lower end of the dose range of the concomitant medication. If bupropion is added to the treatment regimen of a patient already receiving a drug metabolized by CYP2D6, the need to decrease the dose of the original medication should be considered, particularly for those concomitant medications with a narrow therapeutic index). Products include:
Zofran ODT Orally Disintegrating Tablets 1687

Ondansetron Hydrochloride (Co-administration of bupropion with drugs that are metabolized by the CYP2D6 isoenzyme should be approached with caution and should be initiated at the lower end of the dose range of the concomitant medication. If bupropion is added to the treatment regimen of a patient already receiving a drug metabolized by CYP2D6, the need to decrease the dose of the original medication should be considered, particularly for those concomitant medications with a narrow therapeutic index). Products include:
Zofran Injection 1682
Zofran 1687

Orphenadrine Citrate (Bupropion is primarily metabolized, based on *in vitro* studies, to hydroxybupropion by cytochrome P450IIB6 isoenzyme; therefore, the potential exists for a drug interaction with agents that affect the cytochrome P450IIB6 metabolism, such as orphenadrine).
No products indexed under this heading.

Oxazepam (Bupropion is associated with a dose-related risk of seizures; excessive use of benzodiazepine sedatives is associated with increased risk of seizures; bupropion is contraindicated in patients undergoing abrupt discontinuation of benzodiazepine sedatives).
No products indexed under this heading.

Oxycodone Hydrochloride (Co-administration of bupropion with drugs that are metabolized by the CYP2D6 isoenzyme should be approached with caution and should be initiated at the lower end of the dose range of the concomitant medication. If bupropion is added to the treatment regimen of a patient already receiving a drug metabolized by CYP2D6, the need to decrease the dose of the original medication should be considered, particularly

for those concomitant medications with a narrow therapeutic index). Products include:

- OxyContin Tablets 2589
- OxyIR Capsules 2593
- Percocet Tablets 1127
- Percodan Tablets 1130

Paclitaxel (Co-administration of bupropion with drugs that are metabolized by the CYP2D6 isoenzyme should be approached with caution and should be initiated at the lower end of the dose range of the concomitant medication. If bupropion is added to the treatment regimen of a patient already receiving a drug metabolized by CYP2D6, the need to decrease the dose of the original medication should be considered, particularly for those concomitant medications with a narrow therapeutic index).
No products indexed under this heading.

Paliperidone (Concurrent administration of bupropion and agents that lower seizure threshold (e.g., antipsychotics) should be undertaken only with extreme caution. Low initial dosing and gradual dose increases should be employed). Products include:

- Invega Extended-Release Tablets 1748

Pargyline Hydrochloride (Concurrent and/or sequential use with MAO inhibitors is contraindicated).
No products indexed under this heading.

Paroxetine Hydrochloride (Co-administration of bupropion with drugs that are metabolized by the CYP2D6 isoenzyme, including paroxetine, should be approached with caution and should be initiated at the lower end of the dose range of the concomitant medication. If bupropion is added to the treatment regimen of a patient already receiving a drug metabolized by CYP2D6, the need to decrease the dose of the original medication should be considered, particularly for those concomitant medications with a narrow therapeutic index). Products include:

- Paxil 1535
- Paxil CR Controlled-Release Tablets 1544

Perphenazine (Bupropion is associated with a dose-related risk of seizures; co-administration with drugs that lower seizure threshold may increase the risk of seizure with bupropion; concurrent use should be undertaken with extreme caution).
No products indexed under this heading.

Phenelzine Sulfate (Concurrent and/or sequential use with MAO inhibitors is contraindicated; acute toxicity of bupropion is enhanced by phenelzine in animal models).
No products indexed under this heading.

Phenobarbital (May induce the metabolism of bupropion). Products include:

- Donnatal Extentabs 2507

Phenytoin (May induce the metabolism of bupropion).
No products indexed under this heading.

Phenytoin Sodium (May induce the metabolism of bupropion). Products include:

- Phenytek Capsules 2192

Pimozide (Concurrent administration of bupropion and agents that lower seizure threshold (e.g., antipsychotics) should be undertaken only with extreme caution. Low initial dosing and gradual dose increases should be employed).
No products indexed under this heading.

Pindolol (Co-administration of bupropion with drugs that are metabolized by the CYP2D6 isoenzyme should be approached with caution and should be initiated at the lower end of the dose range of the concomitant medication. If bupropion is added to the treatment regimen of a patient already receiving a drug metabolized by CYP2D6, the need to decrease the dose of the original medication should be considered, particularly for those concomitant medications with a narrow therapeutic index).
No products indexed under this heading.

Prazepam (Bupropion is associated with a dose-related risk of seizures; excessive use of benzodiazepine sedatives is associated with increased risk of seizures; bupropion is contraindicated in patients undergoing abrupt discontinuation of benzodiazepine sedatives).
No products indexed under this heading.

Prednisolone Acetate (Bupropion is associated with a dose-related risk of seizures; co-administration with drugs that lower seizure threshold, such as systemic steroids, may increase the risk of seizure with bupropion). Products include:

- Pred Forte Ophthalmic Suspension .... ⊙ 227
- Pred Mild Ophthalmic Suspension .... ⊙ 230
- Pred-G Ophthalmic Ointment .... ⊙ 229
- Pred-G Ophthalmic Suspension .... ⊙ 228

Prednisolone Sodium Phosphate (Bupropion is associated with a dose-related risk of seizures; co-administration with drugs that lower seizure threshold, such as systemic steroids, may increase the risk of seizure with bupropion).
No products indexed under this heading.

Prednisolone Tebutate (Bupropion is associated with a dose-related risk of seizures; co-administration with drugs that lower seizure threshold, such as systemic steroids, may increase the risk of seizure with bupropion).
No products indexed under this heading.

Prednisone (Bupropion is associated with a dose-related risk of seizures; co-administration with drugs that lower seizure threshold, such as systemic steroids, may increase the risk of seizure with bupropion).
No products indexed under this heading.

Procarbazine Hydrochloride (Concurrent and/or sequential use with MAO inhibitors is contraindicated).
No products indexed under this heading.

Prochlorperazine (Bupropion is associated with a dose-related risk of seizures; co-administration with drugs that lower seizure threshold may increase the risk of seizure with bupropion; concurrent use should be undertaken with extreme caution).
No products indexed under this heading.

Promethazine Hydrochloride (Bupropion is associated with a dose-related risk of seizures; co-administration with drugs that lower seizure threshold may increase the risk of seizure with bupropion; concurrent use should be undertaken with extreme caution).
No products indexed under this heading.

Propafenone Hydrochloride (Co-administration of bupropion with drugs that are metabolized by the CYP2D6 isoenzyme, including propafenone, should be approached with caution and should be initiated at the lower end of the dose range of the concomitant medication. If bupropion is added to the treatment regimen of a patient already receiving a drug metabolized by CYP2D6, the need to decrease the dose of the original medication should be considered, particularly for those concomitant medications with a narrow therapeutic index). Products include:

- Rythmol Tablets 1586
- Rythmol SR Capsules 1590

Propoxyphene Hydrochloride (Co-administration of bupropion with drugs that are metabolized by the CYP2D6 isoenzyme should be approached with caution and should be initiated at the lower end of the dose range of the concomitant medication. If bupropion is added to the treatment regimen of a patient already receiving a drug metabolized by CYP2D6, the need to decrease the dose of the original medication should be considered, particularly for those concomitant medications with a narrow therapeutic index).
No products indexed under this heading.

Propoxyphene Napsylate (Co-administration of bupropion with drugs that are metabolized by the CYP2D6 isoenzyme should be approached with caution and should be initiated at the lower end of the dose range of the concomitant medication. If bupropion is added to the treatment regimen of a patient already receiving a drug metabolized by CYP2D6, the need to decrease the dose of the original medication should be considered, particularly for those concomitant medications with a narrow therapeutic index).
No products indexed under this heading.

Propranolol Hydrochloride (Co-administration of bupropion with drugs that are metabolized by the CYP2D6 isoenzyme should be approached with caution and should be initiated at the lower end of the dose range of the concomitant medication. If bupropion is added to the treatment regimen of a patient already receiving a drug metabolized by CYP2D6, the need to decrease the dose of the original medication should be considered, particularly for those concomitant medications with a narrow therapeutic index). Products include:

- InnoPran XL Extended Release Capsules 1484

Protriptyline Hydrochloride (Bupropion is associated with a dose-related risk of seizures; co-administration with drugs that lower seizure threshold may increase the risk of seizure with bupropion; concurrent use should be undertaken with extreme caution).
No products indexed under this heading.

Quazepam (Bupropion is associated with a dose-related risk of seizures; excessive use of benzodiazepine sedatives is associated with increased risk of seizures; bupropion is contraindicated in patients undergoing abrupt discontinuation of benzodiazepine sedatives).
No products indexed under this heading.

Quetiapine Fumarate (Co-administration of bupropion with drugs that are metabolized by the CYP2D6 isoenzyme should be approached with caution and should be initiated at the lower end of the dose range of the concomitant medication. If bupropion is added to the treatment regimen of a patient already receiving a drug metabolized by CYP2D6, the need to decrease the dose of the original medication should be considered, particularly for those concomitant medications with a narrow therapeutic index).
No products indexed under this heading.

Quinidine Gluconate (Co-administration of bupropion with drugs that are metabolized by the CYP2D6 isoenzyme should be approached with caution and should be initiated at the lower end of the dose range of the concomitant medication. If bupropion is added to the treatment regimen of a patient already receiving a drug metabolized by CYP2D6, the need to decrease the dose of the original medication should be considered, particularly for those concomitant medications with a narrow therapeutic index).
No products indexed under this heading.

Quinidine Hydrochloride (Co-administration of bupropion with drugs that are metabolized by the CYP2D6 isoenzyme should be approached with caution and should be initiated at the lower end of the dose range of the concomitant medication. If bupropion is added to the treatment regimen of a patient already receiving a drug metabolized by CYP2D6, the need to decrease the dose of the original medication should be considered, particularly for those concomitant medications with a narrow therapeutic index).
No products indexed under this heading.

Quinidine Polygalacturonate (Co-administration of bupropion with drugs that are metabolized by the CYP2D6 isoenzyme should be approached with caution and should be initiated at the lower end of the dose range of the concomitant medication. If bupropion is added to the treatment regimen of a patient already receiving a drug metabolized by CYP2D6, the need to decrease the dose of the original medication should be considered, particularly for those concomitant medications

with a narrow therapeutic index).
No products indexed under this heading.

Quinidine Sulfate (Co-administration of bupropion with drugs that are metabolized by the CYP2D6 isoenzyme should be approached with caution and should be initiated at the lower end of the dose range of the concomitant medication. If bupropion is added to the treatment regimen of a patient already receiving a drug metabolized by CYP2D6, the need to decrease the dose of the original medication should be considered, particularly for those concomitant medications with a narrow therapeutic index).
No products indexed under this heading.

Rasagiline Mesylate (Concurrent and/or sequential use with MAO inhibitors is contraindicated). Products include:
Azilect Tablets 3106

Risperidone (Co-administration of bupropion with drugs that are metabolized by the CYP2D6 isoenzyme, including risperidone, should be approached with caution and should be initiated at the lower end of the dose range of the concomitant medication. If bupropion is added to the treatment regimen of a patient already receiving a drug metabolized by CYP2D6, the need to decrease the dose of the original medication should be considered, particularly for those concomitant medications with a narrow therapeutic index). Products include:
Risperdal Consta Long-Acting Injection 1753

Ritonavir (Co-administration of bupropion with drugs that are metabolized by the CYP2D6 isoenzyme should be approached with caution and should be initiated at the lower end of the dose range of the concomitant medication. If bupropion is added to the treatment regimen of a patient already receiving a drug metabolized by CYP2D6, the need to decrease the dose of the original medication should be considered, particularly for those concomitant medications with a narrow therapeutic index). Products include:
Kaletra 452
Norvir 489

Selegiline (Concurrent and/or sequential use with MAO inhibitors is contraindicated). Products include:
Emsam Transdermal System 905

Selegiline Hydrochloride (Concurrent and/or sequential use with MAO inhibitors is contraindicated). Products include:
Eldepryl Capsules 3052

Sertraline Hydrochloride (Co-administration of bupropion with drugs that are metabolized by the CYP2D6 isoenzyme, including sertraline, should be approached with caution and should be initiated at the lower end of the dose range of the concomitant medication. If bupropion is added to the treatment regimen of a patient already receiving a drug metabolized by CYP2D6, the need to decrease the dose of the original medication should be considered, particularly for those concomitant medications with a narrow therapeutic index).
No products indexed under this heading.

Tamoxifen Citrate (Co-administration of bupropion with drugs that are metabolized by the CYP2D6 isoenzyme should be approached with caution and should be initiated at the lower end of the dose range of the concomitant medication. If bupropion is added to the treatment regimen of a patient already receiving a drug metabolized by CYP2D6, the need to decrease the dose of the original medication should be considered, particularly for those concomitant medications with a narrow therapeutic index).
No products indexed under this heading.

Temazepam (Bupropion is associated with a dose-related risk of seizures; excessive use of benzodiazepine sedatives is associated with increased risk of seizures; bupropion is contraindicated in patients undergoing abrupt discontinuation of benzodiazepine sedatives).
No products indexed under this heading.

Teniposide (Co-administration of bupropion with drugs that are metabolized by the CYP2D6 isoenzyme should be approached with caution and should be initiated at the lower end of the dose range of the concomitant medication. If bupropion is added to the treatment regimen of a patient already receiving a drug metabolized by CYP2D6, the need to decrease the dose of the original medication should be considered, particularly for those concomitant medications with a narrow therapeutic index).
No products indexed under this heading.

Testosterone (Co-administration of bupropion with drugs that are metabolized by the CYP2D6 isoenzyme should be approached with caution and should be initiated at the lower end of the dose range of the concomitant medication. If bupropion is added to the treatment regimen of a patient already receiving a drug metabolized by CYP2D6, the need to decrease the dose of the original medication should be considered, particularly for those concomitant medications with a narrow therapeutic index). Products include:
AndroGel 3159
Testim 1% Gel 701

Testosterone Cypionate (Co-administration of bupropion with drugs that are metabolized by the CYP2D6 isoenzyme should be approached with caution and should be initiated at the lower end of the dose range of the concomitant medication. If bupropion is added to the treatment regimen of a patient already receiving a drug metabolized by CYP2D6, the need to decrease the dose of the original medication should be considered, particularly for those concomitant medications with a narrow therapeutic index).
No products indexed under this heading.

Testosterone Enanthate (Co-administration of bupropion with drugs that are metabolized by the CYP2D6 isoenzyme should be approached with caution and should be initiated at the lower end of the dose range of the concomitant medication. If bupropion is added to the treatment regimen of a patient already receiving a drug metabolized by CYP2D6, the need to decrease the dose of the original medication should be considered, particularly for those concomitant medications with a narrow therapeutic index). Products include:
Delatestryl Injection 1730

Testosterone Propionate (Co-administration of bupropion with drugs that are metabolized by the CYP2D6 isoenzyme should be approached with caution and should be initiated at the lower end of the dose range of the concomitant medication. If bupropion is added to the treatment regimen of a patient already receiving a drug metabolized by CYP2D6, the need to decrease the dose of the original medication should be considered, particularly for those concomitant medications with a narrow therapeutic index).
No products indexed under this heading.

Theophylline (Bupropion is associated with a dose-related risk of seizures; co-administration with drugs that lower seizure threshold may increase the risk of seizures with bupropion; concurrent use should be undertaken with extreme caution).
No products indexed under this heading.

Theophylline Anhydrous (Bupropion is associated with a dose-related risk of seizures; co-administration with drugs that lower seizure threshold may increase the risk of seizures with bupropion; concurrent use should be undertaken with extreme caution). Products include:
Uniphyl Tablets 2595

Theophylline Calcium Salicylate (Bupropion is associated with a dose-related risk of seizures; co-administration with drugs that lower seizure threshold may increase the risk of seizures with bupropion; concurrent use should be undertaken with extreme caution).
No products indexed under this heading.

Theophylline Dihydroxypropyl (Glyceryl) (Bupropion is associated with a dose-related risk of seizures; co-administration with drugs that lower seizure threshold may increase the risk of seizures with bupropion; concurrent use should be undertaken with extreme caution).
No products indexed under this heading.

Theophylline Ethylenediamine (Bupropion is associated with a dose-related risk of seizures; co-administration with drugs that lower seizure threshold may increase the risk of seizures with bupropion; concurrent use should be undertaken with extreme caution).
No products indexed under this heading.

Theophylline Sodium Glycinate (Bupropion is associated with a dose-related risk of seizures; co-administration with drugs that lower seizure threshold may increase the risk of seizures with bupropion; concurrent use should be undertaken with extreme caution).
No products indexed under this heading.

Thioridazine (Co-administration of bupropion with drugs that are metabolized by the CYP2D6 isoenzyme, including thioridazine, should be approached with caution and should be initiated at the lower end of the dose range of the concomitant medication. If bupropion is added to the treatment regimen of a patient already receiving a drug metabolized by CYP2D6, the need to decrease the dose of the original medication should be considered, particularly for those concomitant medications with a narrow therapeutic index).
No products indexed under this heading.

Thioridazine Hydrochloride (Co-administration of bupropion with drugs that are metabolized by the CYP2D6 isoenzyme, including thioridazine, should be approached with caution and should be initiated at the lower end of the dose range of the concomitant medication. If bupropion is added to the treatment regimen of a patient already receiving a drug metabolized by CYP2D6, the need to decrease the dose of the original medication should be considered, particularly for those concomitant medications with a narrow therapeutic index). Products include:
Thioridazine Hydrochloride Tablets 2195

Thiotepa (Bupropion is primarily metabolized, based on in vitro studies, to hydroxybupropion by cytochrome P450IIB6 isoenzyme; therefore, the potential exists for a drug interaction with agents that affect the cytochrome P450IIB6 metabolism, such as thiotepa).
No products indexed under this heading.

Thiothixene (Concurrent administration of bupropion and agents that lower seizure threshold (e.g., antipsychotics) should be undertaken only with extreme caution. Low initial dosing and gradual dose increases should be employed). Products include:
Thiothixene Capsules 2197

Timolol Maleate (Co-administration of bupropion with drugs that are metabolized by the CYP2D6 isoenzyme should be approached with caution and should be initiated at the lower end of the dose range of the concomitant medication. If bupropion is added to the treatment regimen of a patient already receiving a drug metabolized by CYP2D6, the need to decrease the dose of the original medication should be considered, particularly for those concomitant medications with a narrow therapeutic index). Products include:
Combigan Ophthalmic Solution 553
Cosopt Sterile Ophthalmic Solution 1969
Timoptic Sterile Ophthalmic Solution 2121
Timoptic in Ocudose 2124
Timoptic-XE Sterile Ophthalmic Gel Forming Solution 2125

Tolterodine Tartrate (Co-administration of bupropion with drugs that are metabolized by the CYP2D6 isoenzyme should be approached with caution and should be initiated at the lower end of the dose range of the concomitant medication. If bupropion is added to the treatment regimen of a patient already receiving a drug metabolized by CYP2D6, the need to decrease the dose of the original medication should be considered, particularly for those concomitant medications

with a narrow therapeutic index).
No products indexed under this heading.

Tramadol Hydrochloride (Co-administration of bupropion with drugs that are metabolized by the CYP2D6 isoenzyme should be approached with caution and should be initiated at the lower end of the dose range of the concomitant medication. If bupropion is added to the treatment regimen of a patient already receiving a drug metabolized by CYP2D6, the need to decrease the dose of the original medication should be considered, particularly for those concomitant medications with a narrow therapeutic index).
Products include:
Ultram ER Extended-Release Tablets 2428

Tranylcypromine Sulfate (Concurrent and/or sequential use with MAO inhibitors is contraindicated).
Products include:
Parnate Tablets 1532

Trazodone Hydrochloride (Bupropion is associated with a dose-related risk of seizures; co-administration with drugs that lower seizure threshold may increase the risk of seizure with bupropion; concurrent use should be undertaken with extreme caution).
No products indexed under this heading.

Triamcinolone (Bupropion is associated with a dose-related risk of seizures; co-administration with drugs that lower seizure threshold, such as systemic steroids, may increase the risk of seizure with bupropion).
No products indexed under this heading.

Triamcinolone Acetonide (Bupropion is associated with a dose-related risk of seizures; co-administration with drugs that lower seizure threshold, such as systemic steroids, may increase the risk of seizure with bupropion). Products include:
Azmacort Inhalation Aerosol 407
Nasacort AQ Nasal Spray 2765
Triesence Injectable Suspension .... ⊙209

Triamcinolone Diacetate (Bupropion is associated with a dose-related risk of seizures; co-administration with drugs that lower seizure threshold, such as systemic steroids, may increase the risk of seizure with bupropion).
No products indexed under this heading.

Triamcinolone Hexacetonide (Bupropion is associated with a dose-related risk of seizures; co-administration with drugs that lower seizure threshold, such as systemic steroids, may increase the risk of seizure with bupropion).
No products indexed under this heading.

Triazolam (Bupropion is associated with a dose-related risk of seizures; excessive use of benzodiazepine sedatives is associated with increased risk of seizures; bupropion is contraindicated in patients undergoing abrupt discontinuation of benzodiazepine sedatives).
No products indexed under this heading.

Trifluoperazine Hydrochloride (Bupropion is associated with a dose-related risk of seizures; co-administration with drugs that lower seizure threshold may increase the risk of seizure with bupropion; concurrent use should be undertaken with extreme caution).
No products indexed under this heading.

Trimipramine Maleate (Bupropion is associated with a dose-related risk of seizures; co-administration with drugs that lower seizure threshold may increase the risk of seizure with bupropion; concurrent use should be undertaken with extreme caution).
No products indexed under this heading.

Venlafaxine Hydrochloride (Co-administration of bupropion with drugs that are metabolized by the CYP2D6 isoenzyme should be approached with caution and should be initiated at the lower end of the dose range of the concomitant medication. If bupropion is added to the treatment regimen of a patient already receiving a drug metabolized by CYP2D6, the need to decrease the dose of the original medication should be considered, particularly for those concomitant medications with a narrow therapeutic index).
Products include:
Effexor XR Extended-Release Capsules 3195
Venlafaxine Hydrochloride Tablets ... 2199

Vinblastine Sulfate (Co-administration of bupropion with drugs that are metabolized by the CYP2D6 isoenzyme should be approached with caution and should be initiated at the lower end of the dose range of the concomitant medication. If bupropion is added to the treatment regimen of a patient already receiving a drug metabolized by CYP2D6, the need to decrease the dose of the original medication should be considered, particularly for those concomitant medications with a narrow therapeutic index).
No products indexed under this heading.

Warfarin Sodium (Altered PT and/or INR, infrequently associated with hemorrhagic or thrombotic complications, were observed when bupropion was co-administered with warfarin).
No products indexed under this heading.

Ziprasidone Hydrochloride (Concurrent administration of bupropion and agents that lower seizure threshold (e.g., antipsychotics) should be undertaken only with extreme caution. Low initial dosing and gradual dose increases should be employed). Products include:
Geodon Capsules 2520

Zonisamide (Co-administration of bupropion with drugs that are metabolized by the CYP2D6 isoenzyme should be approached with caution and should be initiated at the lower end of the dose range of the concomitant medication. If bupropion is added to the treatment regimen of a patient already receiving a drug metabolized by CYP2D6, the need to decrease the dose of the original medication should be considered, particularly for those concomitant medications with a narrow therapeutic index). Products include:
Zonegran Capsules 1089

Food Interactions

Alcohol (Bupropion hydrochloride is contraindicated in patients undergoing abrupt discontinuation of alcohol. The consumption of alcohol during treatment with bupropion hydrochloride should be minimized or avoided).

Food, unspecified (Food increases Cmax and AUC of bupropion by 11% and 17%, respectively; no clinically significant food effect).

WELLBUTRIN XL EXTENDED-RELEASE TABLETS
(Bupropion Hydrochloride) 1659
See Wellbutrin SR Sustained-Release Tablets

WIN COQ10 GELCAPS
(Coenzyme Q-10) .... ▣641
None cited in PDR database.

WINOMEG3COMPLEX GELCAPS
(Docosahexaenoic Acid (DHA), Eicosapentaenoic Acid (EPA), Omega-3-acid ethyl esters, Omega-3 Acids, Omega-6 Polyunsaturates) .... ▣642
None cited in PDR database.

WINRGY DIETARY SUPPLEMENT
(Amino Acid Preparations, Caffeine, Vitamins with Minerals)........ ▣642
May interact with:

Aluminum Carbonate (Concomitant use with aluminum-containing antacids should be avoided).
No products indexed under this heading.

Aluminum Hydroxide (Concomitant use with aluminum-containing antacids should be avoided).
No products indexed under this heading.

WINRHO SDF
(Rh_o (D) Immune Globulin (Human)) 741
May interact with vaccines, live. Compounds in these categories include:

BCG Vaccine (Other antibodies contained in WinRho SDF may interfere with the response to live virus vaccines such as measles, mumps, polio or rubella. Therefore, immunization with live vaccines should not be given within 3 months after WinRho SDF administration).
No products indexed under this heading.

Influenza Vaccine, Live Attenuated (Other antibodies contained in WinRho SDF may interfere with the response to live virus vaccines such as measles, mumps, polio or rubella. Therefore, immunization with live vaccines should not be given within 3 months after WinRho SDF administration).
No products indexed under this heading.

Influenza Virus Vaccine Live, Intranasal (Other antibodies contained in WinRho SDF may interfere with the response to live virus vaccines such as measles, mumps, polio or rubella. Therefore, immunization with live vaccines should not be given within 3 months after WinRho SDF administration). Products include:
FluMist Vaccine 1945

Measles, Mumps, Rubella and Varicella Virus Vaccine Live (Other antibodies contained in WinRho SDF may interfere with the response to live virus vaccines such as measles, mumps, polio or rubella. Therefore, immunization with live vaccines should not be given within 3 months after WinRho SDF administration).
Products include:
ProQuad 2099

Measles, Mumps & Rubella Virus Vaccine, Live (Other antibodies contained in WinRho SDF may interfere with the response to live virus vaccines such as measles, mumps, polio or rubella. Therefore, immunization with live vaccines should not be given within 3 months after WinRho SDF administration).
Products include:
M-M-R II 2054

Measles & Rubella Virus Vaccine Live (Other antibodies contained in WinRho SDF may interfere with the response to live virus vaccines such as measles, mumps, polio or rubella. Therefore, immunization with live vaccines should not be given within 3 months after WinRho SDF administration).
No products indexed under this heading.

Measles Virus Vaccine Live (Other antibodies contained in WinRho SDF may interfere with the response to live virus vaccines such as measles, mumps, polio or rubella. Therefore, immunization with live vaccines should not be given within 3 months after WinRho SDF administration).
Products include:
Attenuvax 1951

Mumps Virus Vaccine, Live (Other antibodies contained in WinRho SDF may interfere with the response to live virus vaccines such as measles, mumps, polio or rubella. Therefore, immunization with live vaccines should not be given within 3 months after WinRho SDF administration).
Products include:
Mumpsvax 2068

Poliovirus Vaccine, Live, Oral, Trivalent, Types 1,2,3 (Sabin) (Other antibodies contained in WinRho SDF may interfere with the response to live virus vaccines such as measles, mumps, polio or rubella. Therefore, immunization with live vaccines should not be given within 3 months after WinRho SDF administration).
No products indexed under this heading.

Rotavirus Vaccine, Live, Oral, Tetravalent (Other antibodies contained in WinRho SDF may interfere with the response to live virus vaccines such as measles, mumps, polio or rubella. Therefore, immunization with live vaccines should not be given within 3 months after WinRho SDF administration).
No products indexed under this heading.

Rubella & Mumps Virus Vaccine Live (Other antibodies contained in WinRho SDF may interfere with the response to live virus vaccines such as measles, mumps, polio or rubella. Therefore, immunization with live vaccines should not be given within 3 months after WinRho SDF administration).
No products indexed under this heading.

Rubella Virus Vaccine Live (Other antibodies contained in WinRho SDF may interfere with the response to live virus vaccines such as measles, mumps, polio or rubella. Therefore, immunization with live vaccines should not be given within 3 months after WinRho SDF administration). Products include:

Meruvax II 2061

Smallpox Vaccine (Other antibodies contained in WinRho SDF may interfere with the response to live virus vaccines such as measles, mumps, polio or rubella. Therefore, immunization with live vaccines should not be given within 3 months after WinRho SDF administration).

No products indexed under this heading.

Typhoid Vaccine (Other antibodies contained in WinRho SDF may interfere with the response to live virus vaccines such as measles, mumps, polio or rubella. Therefore, immunization with live vaccines should not be given within 3 months after WinRho SDF administration).

No products indexed under this heading.

Varicella Virus Vaccine Live (Other antibodies contained in WinRho SDF may interfere with the response to live virus vaccines such as measles, mumps, polio or rubella. Therefore, immunization with live vaccines should not be given within 3 months after WinRho SDF administration). Products include:

Varivax 2133

Yellow Fever Vaccine (Other antibodies contained in WinRho SDF may interfere with the response to live virus vaccines such as measles, mumps, polio or rubella. Therefore, immunization with live vaccines should not be given within 3 months after WinRho SDF administration).

No products indexed under this heading.

Zoster Vaccine Live (Other antibodies contained in WinRho SDF may interfere with the response to live virus vaccines such as measles, mumps, polio or rubella. Therefore, immunization with live vaccines should not be given within 3 months after WinRho SDF administration). Products include:

Zostavax Injection 2145

XALATAN OPHTHALMIC SOLUTION

(Latanoprost) .... ⊙273

None cited in PDR database.

XELODA TABLETS

(Capecitabine) 2662

May interact with oral anticoagulants, phenytoin, and certain other agents. Compounds in these categories include:

Aluminum Hydroxide (Co-administration of capecitabine with aluminum hydroxide- and magnesium hydroxide-containing antacids has resulted in a small increase in plasma concentrations of capecitabine and one metabolite (5'DFCR)).

No products indexed under this heading.

Anisindione (Co-administration has resulted in altered coagulation parameters and/or bleeding).

No products indexed under this heading.

Dicumarol (Co-administration has resulted in altered coagulation parameters and/or bleeding).

No products indexed under this heading.

Fosphenytoin Sodium (Co-administration has resulted in toxicity associated with elevated phenytoin levels).

No products indexed under this heading.

Leucovorin Calcium (The concentrations of 5-fluorouracil, capecitabine is a prodrug and it is converted to 5-FU, is increased and its toxicity may be enhanced by leucovorin; deaths from severe enterocolitis, diarrhea, and dehydration have been reported in elderly patients receiving fluorouracil and leucovorin).

No products indexed under this heading.

Magnesium Hydroxide (Co-administration of capecitabine with aluminum hydroxide- and magnesium hydroxide-containing antacids has resulted in a small increase in plasma concentrations of capecitabine and one metabolite (5'DFCR)). Products include:

Fleet Pedia-Lax Chewable Tablets 1145
Pepcid Complete Chewable Tablets 1771
Extra Strength Rolaids Freshmint Tablets 1903
Rolaids Multi-Symptom Berry Tablets 1903
Rolaids Original Peppermint Tablets 1903

Phenytoin (Co-administration has resulted in toxicity associated with elevated phenytoin levels).

No products indexed under this heading.

Phenytoin Sodium (Co-administration has resulted in toxicity associated with elevated phenytoin levels). Products include:

Phenytek Capsules 2192

Warfarin Sodium (Co-administration has resulted in altered coagulation parameters and/or bleeding).

No products indexed under this heading.

Food Interactions

Food, unspecified (Reduces both rate and extent of absorption of capecitabine and delays Tmax of both parent and 5-FU).

XENADERM OINTMENT

(Balsam Peru, Castor Oil, Trypsin) 1725

None cited in PDR database.

XENICAL CAPSULES

(Orlistat) 2672

May interact with:

Beta-Carotene (Orlistat has been shown to reduce the absorption of some fat soluble vitamins; the vitamin supplement should be taken once a day at least 2 hours before or after the administration of orlistat).

No products indexed under this heading.

Cyclosporine (Co-administration has resulted in reduction in cyclosporine plasma levels; concurrent use is not recommended; if used concurrently, cyclosporine should be taken at least 2 hours before or after Xenical). Products include:

Gengraf Capsules 435
Neoral Oral Solution 2280
Neoral Soft Gelatin Capsules 2280
Restasis Ophthalmic Emulsion 557
Sandimmune 2296

Levothyroxine (Hypothyroidism has been reported in patients treated concomitantly with orlistat and levothyroxine post-marketing. Patients treated concomitantly with orlistat and levothyroxine should be monitored for changes in thyroid function. Administer levothyroxine and orlistat at least 4 hours apart). Products include:

Naturethroid Tablets 2605

Pravastatin Sodium (Co-administration results in additive lipid lowering effect of pravastatin; modest increases in pravastatin plasma concentrations were observed during co-administration).

No products indexed under this heading.

Vitamin A (Orlistat has been shown to reduce the absorption of some fat soluble vitamins; the vitamin supplement should be taken once a day at least 2 hours before or after the administration of orlistat). Products include:

Norwegian Cod Liver Oil 949

Vitamin D (Orlistat has been shown to reduce the absorption of some fat soluble vitamins; the vitamin supplement should be taken once a day at least 2 hours before or after the administration of orlistat). Products include:

Active Calcium Tablets 3173
D-Cal Chewable Caplets .... ▣624
Norwegian Cod Liver Oil 949

Vitamin E (Orlistat has been shown to reduce the absorption of some fat soluble vitamins; the vitamin supplement should be taken once a day at least 2 hours before or after the administration of orlistat). Products include:

Bausch & Lomb Ocuvite Adult 50+ Vitamin and Mineral Supplement .... ⊙237
Comax Dietary Supplement 995
Glaucofit Dietary Supplement 995
Glauma Dietary Supplement 995
MarineOmega Softgel Capsules 2560
Norwegian Cod Liver Oil 949
Tonox Dietary Supplement 995
Vibe Liquid Multi-Nutrient Supplement .... ▣626

Vitamin K_1 (Absorption of vitamin K may be decreased). Products include:

Mephyton Tablets 700

Warfarin Sodium (Vitamin K absorption may be decreased with orlistat; patients on chronic stable doses of warfarin who are prescribed orlistat should be monitored closely for changes in coagulation parameters).

No products indexed under this heading.

Food Interactions

Food, unspecified (Gastrointestinal events may increase when orlistat is taken with a diet high in fat).

XIFAXAN TABLETS

(Rifaximin) 2682

None cited in PDR database.

XIGRIS POWDER FOR INTRAVENOUS INFUSION

(Drotrecogin alfa (activated)) 1880

May interact with oral anticoagulants, glycoprotein (GP) IIb/IIIa inhibitors, platelet inhibitors, thrombolytics, and certain other agents. Compounds in these categories include:

Abciximab (Bleeding is the most common serious adverse effect associated with drotrecogin alfa therapy; recent administration (within 7 days) of glycoprotein IIb/IIIa therapy increases the risk of bleeding). Products include:

ReoPro Vials 1860

Alteplase (Bleeding is the most common serious adverse effect associated with drotrecogin alfa therapy; recent administration (within 3 days) of thrombolytic therapy increases the risk of bleeding). Products include:

Activase I.V. 1188
Cathflo Activase 1198

Anisindione (Bleeding is the most common serious adverse effect associated with drotrecogin alfa therapy; recent administration (within 7 days) of oral anticoagulant therapy increases the risk of bleeding).

No products indexed under this heading.

Anistreplase (Bleeding is the most common serious adverse effect associated with drotrecogin alfa therapy; recent administration (within 3 days) of thrombolytic therapy increases the risk of bleeding).

No products indexed under this heading.

Aspirin (Bleeding is the most common serious adverse effect associated with drotrecogin alfa therapy; recent administration (within 7 days) of more than 650mg per day of aspirin or other platelet inhibitors increases the risk of bleeding). Products include:

Aggrenox Capsules 819
Bayer Aspirin 750
Percodan Tablets 1130
St. Joseph 81 mg Aspirin Chewable and Enteric Coated Tablets 1903

Aspirin, Enteric Coated (Bleeding is the most common serious adverse effect associated with drotrecogin alfa therapy; recent administration (within 7 days) of more than 650mg per day of aspirin or other platelet inhibitors increases the risk of bleeding).

No products indexed under this heading.

Aspirin Buffered (Bleeding is the most common serious adverse effect associated with drotrecogin alfa therapy; recent administration (within 7 days) of more than 650mg per day of aspirin or other platelet inhibitors increases the risk of bleeding).

No products indexed under this heading.

Azlocillin Sodium (Bleeding is the most common serious adverse effect associated with drotrecogin alfa therapy; recent administration (within 7 days) of more than 650mg per day of aspirin or other platelet inhibitors increases the risk of bleeding).

No products indexed under this heading.

Bivalirudin (Bleeding is the most common serious adverse effect associated with drotrecogin alfa therapy; recent administration (within 3 days) of thrombolytic therapy increases the risk of bleeding). Products include:

Angiomax for Injection 1933

Carbenicillin Indanyl Sodium (Bleeding is the most common serious adverse effect associated with drotrecogin alfa therapy; recent administration (within 7 days) of more than 650mg per day of aspirin or other platelet inhibitors increases the risk of bleeding).

No products indexed under this heading.

Choline Magnesium Trisalicylate (Bleeding is the most common serious adverse effect associated with drotrecogin alfa therapy; recent administration (within 7 days) of more than 650mg per day of aspirin or other platelet inhibitors increases the risk of bleeding).

No products indexed under this heading.

Clopidogrel Bisulfate (Bleeding is the most common serious adverse effect associated with drotrecogin alfa therapy; recent administration (within 7 days) of more than 650mg per day of aspirin or other platelet inhibitors increases the risk of bleeding). Products include:

Plavix Tablets 926
Plavix Tablets 2767

Diclofenac Potassium (Bleeding is the most common serious adverse effect associated with drotrecogin alfa therapy; recent administration (within 7 days) of more than 650mg per day of aspirin or other platelet inhibitors increases the risk of bleeding).

No products indexed under this heading.

Diclofenac Sodium (Bleeding is the most common serious adverse effect associated with drotrecogin alfa therapy; recent administration (within 7 days) of more than 650mg per day of aspirin or other platelet inhibitors increases the risk of bleeding). Products include:

Diclofenac Sodium Ophthalmic Solution .... ⊙240
Voltaren Ophthalmic Solution 2336
Voltaren Tablets 2334
Voltaren-XR Tablets 2337

Dicumarol (Bleeding is the most common serious adverse effect associated with drotrecogin alfa therapy; recent administration (within 7 days) of oral anticoagulant therapy increases the risk of bleeding).

No products indexed under this heading.

Diflunisal (Bleeding is the most common serious adverse effect associated with drotrecogin alfa therapy; recent administration (within 7 days) of more than 650mg per day of aspirin or other platelet inhibitors increases the risk of bleeding).

No products indexed under this heading.

Dipyridamole (Bleeding is the most common serious adverse effect associated with drotrecogin alfa therapy; recent administration (within 7 days) of more than 650mg per day of aspirin or other platelet inhibitors increases the risk of bleeding). Products include:

Aggrenox Capsules 819
Persantine Tablets 869

Eptifibatide (Bleeding is the most common serious adverse effect associated with drotrecogin alfa therapy; recent administration (within 7 days) of glycoprotein IIb/IIIa therapy increases the risk of bleeding). Products include:

Integrilin Injection 2855

Fenoprofen Calcium (Bleeding is the most common serious adverse effect associated with drotrecogin alfa therapy; recent administration (within 7 days) of more than 650mg per day of aspirin or other platelet inhibitors increases the risk of bleeding). Products include:

Nalfon Capsules 2508

Flurbiprofen (Bleeding is the most common serious adverse effect associated with drotrecogin alfa therapy; recent administration (within 7 days) of more than 650mg per day of aspirin or other platelet inhibitors increases the risk of bleeding).

No products indexed under this heading.

Heparin Sodium (Bleeding is the most common serious adverse effect associated with drotrecogin alfa therapy; concurrent therapeutic dosing of heparin used to treat an active thrombotic or embolic event increases the risk of bleeding; low dose heparin does not appear to affect safety).

No products indexed under this heading.

Ibuprofen (Bleeding is the most common serious adverse effect associated with drotrecogin alfa therapy; recent administration (within 7 days) of more than 650mg per day of aspirin or other platelet inhibitors increases the risk of bleeding). Products include:

Motrin IB Tablets and Caplets 1900
Children's Motrin Oral Suspension ... 1901
Children's Motrin Non-Staining Dye-Free Oral Suspension............ 1901
Children's Motrin Cold Oral Suspension 1899
Infants' Motrin Concentrated Drops.. 1901
Infants' Motrin Non-Staining Dye-Free Concentrated Drops....... 1901
Junior Strength Motrin Caplets and Chewable Tablets.................. 1901
Vicoprofen Tablets 533

Indomethacin (Bleeding is the most common serious adverse effect associated with drotrecogin alfa therapy; recent administration (within 7 days) of more than 650mg per day of aspirin or other platelet inhibitors increases the risk of bleeding). Products include:

Indocin 2024

Indomethacin Sodium Trihydrate (Bleeding is the most common serious adverse effect associated with drotrecogin alfa therapy; recent administration (within 7 days) of more than 650mg per day of aspirin or other platelet inhibitors increases the risk of bleeding). Products include:

Indocin I.V. 2489

Ketoprofen (Bleeding is the most common serious adverse effect associated with drotrecogin alfa therapy; recent administration (within 7 days) of more than 650mg per day of aspirin or other platelet inhibitors increases the risk of bleeding).

No products indexed under this heading.

Magnesium Salicylate (Bleeding is the most common serious adverse effect associated with drotrecogin alfa therapy; recent administration (within 7 days) of more than 650mg per day of aspirin or other platelet inhibitors increases the risk of bleeding).

No products indexed under this heading.

Meclofenamate Sodium (Bleeding is the most common serious adverse effect associated with drotrecogin alfa therapy; recent administration (within 7 days) of more than 650mg per day of aspirin or other platelet inhibitors increases the risk of bleeding).

No products indexed under this heading.

Mefenamic Acid (Bleeding is the most common serious adverse effect associated with drotrecogin alfa therapy; recent administration (within 7 days) of more than 650mg per day of aspirin or other platelet inhibitors increases the risk of bleeding).

No products indexed under this heading.

Mezlocillin Sodium (Bleeding is the most common serious adverse effect associated with drotrecogin alfa therapy; recent administration (within 7 days) of more than 650mg per day of aspirin or other platelet inhibitors increases the risk of bleeding).

No products indexed under this heading.

Nafcillin Sodium (Bleeding is the most common serious adverse effect associated with drotrecogin alfa therapy; recent administration (within 7 days) of more than 650mg per day of aspirin or other platelet inhibitors increases the risk of bleeding).

No products indexed under this heading.

Naproxen (Bleeding is the most common serious adverse effect associated with drotrecogin alfa therapy; recent administration (within 7 days) of more than 650mg per day of aspirin or other platelet inhibitors increases the risk of bleeding). Products include:

EC-Naprosyn Delayed-Release Tablets 2632
Naprosyn Suspension 2632
Naprosyn Tablets 2632

Naproxen Sodium (Bleeding is the most common serious adverse effect associated with drotrecogin alfa therapy; recent administration (within 7 days) of more than 650mg per day of aspirin or other platelet inhibitors increases the risk of bleeding). Products include:

Anaprox Tablets 2632
Anaprox DS Tablets 2632
Treximet Tablets 1616

Penicillin G Benzathine (Bleeding is the most common serious adverse effect associated with drotrecogin alfa therapy; recent administration (within 7 days) of more than 650mg per day of aspirin or other platelet inhibitors increases the risk of bleeding). Products include:

Bicillin C-R Injectable Suspension 1775
Bicillin L-A Injection 1777

Penicillin G Procaine (Bleeding is the most common serious adverse effect associated with drotrecogin alfa therapy; recent administration (within 7 days) of more than 650mg per day of aspirin or other platelet inhibitors increases the risk of bleeding). Products include:

Bicillin C-R Injectable Suspension 1775
Bicillin L-A Injection 1777

Phenylbutazone (Bleeding is the most common serious adverse effect associated with drotrecogin alfa therapy; recent administration (within 7 days) of more than 650mg per day of aspirin or other platelet inhibitors increases the risk of bleeding).

No products indexed under this heading.

Piroxicam (Bleeding is the most common serious adverse effect associated with drotrecogin alfa therapy; recent administration (within 7 days) of more than 650mg per day of aspirin or other platelet inhibitors increases the risk of bleeding).

No products indexed under this heading.

Reteplase (Bleeding is the most common serious adverse effect associated with drotrecogin alfa therapy; recent administration (within 3 days) of thrombolytic therapy increases the risk of bleeding).

No products indexed under this heading.

Salsalate (Bleeding is the most common serious adverse effect associated with drotrecogin alfa therapy; recent administration (within 7 days) of more than 650mg per day of aspirin or other platelet inhibitors increases the risk of bleeding).

No products indexed under this heading.

Streptokinase (Bleeding is the most common serious adverse effect associated with drotrecogin alfa therapy; recent administration (within 3 days) of thrombolytic therapy increases the risk of bleeding).

No products indexed under this heading.

Sulindac (Bleeding is the most common serious adverse effect associated with drotrecogin alfa therapy; recent administration (within 7 days) of more than 650mg per day of aspirin or other platelet inhibitors increases the risk of bleeding). Products include:

Clinoril Tablets 1962

Ticarcillin Disodium (Bleeding is the most common serious adverse effect associated with drotrecogin alfa therapy; recent administration (within 7 days) of more than 650mg per day of aspirin or other platelet inhibitors increases the risk of bleeding). Products include:

Timentin ADD-Vantage 1606
Timentin Injection Galaxy Container 1609
Timentin IV Infusion 1603
Timentin Pharmacy Bulk Package 1613

Ticlopidine Hydrochloride (Bleeding is the most common serious adverse effect associated with drotrecogin alfa therapy; recent administration (within 7 days) of more than 650mg per day of aspirin or other platelet inhibitors increases the risk of bleeding).

No products indexed under this heading.

IMPORTANT NOTE: Always consult each drug listing in the patient's regimen for possible interactions.

Tirofiban Hydrochloride (Bleeding is the most common serious adverse effect associated with drotrecogin alfa therapy; recent administration (within 7 days) of glycoprotein IIb/IIIa therapy increases the risk of bleeding).
No products indexed under this heading.

Tolmetin Sodium (Bleeding is the most common serious adverse effect associated with drotrecogin alfa therapy; recent administration (within 7 days) of more than 650mg per day of aspirin or other platelet inhibitors increases the risk of bleeding).
No products indexed under this heading.

Urokinase (Bleeding is the most common serious adverse effect associated with drotrecogin alfa therapy; recent administration (within 3 days) of thrombolytic therapy increases the risk of bleeding).
No products indexed under this heading.

Warfarin Sodium (Bleeding is the most common serious adverse effect associated with drotrecogin alfa therapy; recent administration (within 7 days) of oral anticoagulant therapy increases the risk of bleeding).
No products indexed under this heading.

XOLAIR

(Omalizumab) 2339
None cited in PDR database.

XOLAIR

(Omalizumab) 1235
None cited in PDR database.

XOPENEX INHALATION SOLUTION

(Levalbuterol Hydrochloride) 3001
May interact with beta blockers, monoamine oxidase inhibitors, potassium-depleting diuretics, sympathomimetic aerosol bronchodilators, tricyclic antidepressants, and certain other agents. Compounds in these categories include:

Acebutolol Hydrochloride (Beta-adrenergic receptor blocking agents block the pulmonary effect of beta agonist and may produce severe bronchospasm in asthmatic patients).
No products indexed under this heading.

Albuterol (Potential for deleterious cardiovascular effects with concomitant use).
No products indexed under this heading.

Amitriptyline Hydrochloride (Action of levalbuterol on the vascular system may be potentiated).
No products indexed under this heading.

Amoxapine (Action of levalbuterol on the vascular system may be potentiated).
No products indexed under this heading.

Atenolol (Beta-adrenergic receptor blocking agents block the pulmonary effect of beta agonist and may produce severe bronchospasm in asthmatic patients).
No products indexed under this heading.

Bendroflumethiazide (The ECG changes and/or hypokalemia that may result from the administration of non-potassium sparing diuretics can be acutely worsened by beta-agonists).
No products indexed under this heading.

Betaxolol Hydrochloride (Beta-adrenergic receptor blocking agents block the pulmonary effect of beta agonist and may produce severe bronchospasm in asthmatic patients).
No products indexed under this heading.

Bisoprolol Fumarate (Beta-adrenergic receptor blocking agents block the pulmonary effect of beta agonist and may produce severe bronchospasm in asthmatic patients).
No products indexed under this heading.

Bitolterol Mesylate (Potential for deleterious cardiovascular effects with concomitant use).
No products indexed under this heading.

Bumetanide (The ECG changes and/or hypokalemia that may result from the administration of non-potassium sparing diuretics can be acutely worsened by beta-agonists).
No products indexed under this heading.

Carteolol Hydrochloride (Beta-adrenergic receptor blocking agents block the pulmonary effect of beta agonist and may produce severe bronchospasm in asthmatic patients).
No products indexed under this heading.

Chlorothiazide (The ECG changes and/or hypokalemia that may result from the administration of non-potassium sparing diuretics can be acutely worsened by beta-agonists).
No products indexed under this heading.

Chlorothiazide Sodium (The ECG changes and/or hypokalemia that may result from the administration of non-potassium sparing diuretics can be acutely worsened by beta-agonists). Products include:
Intravenous Sodium Diuril 2490

Clomipramine Hydrochloride (Action of levalbuterol on the vascular system may be potentiated).
No products indexed under this heading.

Desipramine Hydrochloride (Action of levalbuterol on the vascular system may be potentiated).
No products indexed under this heading.

Digoxin (Mean decreases of 16% and 22% in serum digoxin levels were demonstrated after the single-dose intravenous and oral administration of racemic albuterol, respectively; clinical significance of this finding is unclear). Products include:
Lanoxin Injection 1498
Lanoxin Injection Pediatric 1502
Lanoxin Tablets 1505

Doxepin Hydrochloride (Action of levalbuterol on the vascular system may be potentiated).
No products indexed under this heading.

Esmolol Hydrochloride (Beta-adrenergic receptor blocking agents block the pulmonary effect of beta agonist and may produce severe bronchospasm in asthmatic patients).
No products indexed under this heading.

Ethacrynic Acid (The ECG changes and/or hypokalemia that may result from the administration of non-potassium sparing diuretics can be acutely worsened by beta-agonists). Products include:
Edecrin Tablets 698

Furosemide (The ECG changes and/or hypokalemia that may result from the administration of non-potassium sparing diuretics can be acutely worsened by beta-agonists). Products include:
Furosemide Tablets 2186

Hydrochlorothiazide (The ECG changes and/or hypokalemia that may result from the administration of non-potassium sparing diuretics can be acutely worsened by beta-agonists). Products include:
Atacand HCT 642
Avalide Tablets 892
Avalide Tablets 2713
Benicar HCT Tablets 1010
Diovan HCT Tablets 2216
Dyazide Capsules 1405
Micardis HCT Tablets 854
Prinzide Tablets 2092
Tekturna HCT Tablets 2324
Teveten HCT Tablets 517

Hydroflumethiazide (The ECG changes and/or hypokalemia that may result from the administration of non-potassium sparing diuretics can be acutely worsened by beta-agonists).
No products indexed under this heading.

Imipramine Hydrochloride (Action of levalbuterol on the vascular system may be potentiated).
No products indexed under this heading.

Imipramine Pamoate (Action of levalbuterol on the vascular system may be potentiated).
No products indexed under this heading.

Isocarboxazid (Action of levalbuterol on the vascular system may be potentiated). Products include:
Marplan Tablets 3177

Isoetharine (Potential for deleterious cardiovascular effects with concomitant use).
No products indexed under this heading.

Isoproterenol Hydrochloride (Potential for deleterious cardiovascular effects with concomitant use).
No products indexed under this heading.

Labetalol Hydrochloride (Beta-adrenergic receptor blocking agents block the pulmonary effect of beta agonist and may produce severe bronchospasm in asthmatic patients).
No products indexed under this heading.

Levobunolol Hydrochloride (Beta-adrenergic receptor blocking agents block the pulmonary effect of beta agonist and may produce severe bronchospasm in asthmatic patients).
No products indexed under this heading.

Maprotiline Hydrochloride (Action of levalbuterol on the vascular system may be potentiated).
No products indexed under this heading.

Metaproterenol Sulfate (Potential for deleterious cardiovascular effects with concomitant use).
No products indexed under this heading.

Methyclothiazide (The ECG changes and/or hypokalemia that may result from the administration of non-potassium sparing diuretics can be acutely worsened by beta-agonists).
No products indexed under this heading.

Metipranolol Hydrochloride (Beta-adrenergic receptor blocking agents block the pulmonary effect of beta agonist and may produce severe bronchospasm in asthmatic patients).
No products indexed under this heading.

Metoprolol Succinate (Beta-adrenergic receptor blocking agents block the pulmonary effect of beta agonist and may produce severe bronchospasm in asthmatic patients). Products include:
Toprol-XL Tablets 666

Metoprolol Tartrate (Beta-adrenergic receptor blocking agents block the pulmonary effect of beta agonist and may produce severe bronchospasm in asthmatic patients).
No products indexed under this heading.

Moclobemide (Action of levalbuterol on the vascular system may be potentiated).
No products indexed under this heading.

Nadolol (Beta-adrenergic receptor blocking agents block the pulmonary effect of beta agonist and may produce severe bronchospasm in asthmatic patients). Products include:
Nadolol Tablets 2191

Nebivolol (Beta-adrenergic receptor blocking agents block the pulmonary effect of beta agonist and may produce severe bronchospasm in asthmatic patients). Products include:
Bystolic Tablets 1155

Nortriptyline Hydrochloride (Action of levalbuterol on the vascular system may be potentiated).
No products indexed under this heading.

Pargyline Hydrochloride (Action of levalbuterol on the vascular system may be potentiated).
No products indexed under this heading.

Penbutolol Sulfate (Beta-adrenergic receptor blocking agents block the pulmonary effect of beta agonist and may produce severe bronchospasm in asthmatic patients).
No products indexed under this heading.

Phenelzine Sulfate (Action of levalbuterol on the vascular system may be potentiated).
No products indexed under this heading.

Pindolol (Beta-adrenergic receptor blocking agents block the pulmonary effect of beta agonist and may produce severe bronchospasm in asthmatic patients).
No products indexed under this heading.

Pirbuterol Acetate (Potential for deleterious cardiovascular effects with concomitant use). Products include:
Maxair Autohaler 1705

Polythiazide (The ECG changes and/or hypokalemia that may result from the administration of non-potassium sparing diuretics can be acutely worsened by beta-agonists).
No products indexed under this heading.

Procarbazine Hydrochloride (Action of levalbuterol on the vascular system may be potentiated).
No products indexed under this heading.

Propranolol Hydrochloride (Beta-adrenergic receptor blocking agents block the pulmonary effect of beta agonist and may produce severe bronchospasm in asthmatic patients). Products include:
InnoPran XL Extended Release Capsules 1484

Protriptyline Hydrochloride (Action of levalbuterol on the vascular system may be potentiated).
No products indexed under this heading.

Rasagiline Mesylate (Action of levalbuterol on the vascular system may be potentiated). Products include:
Azilect Tablets 3106

Salmeterol Xinafoate (Potential for deleterious cardiovascular effects with concomitant use). Products include:
Advair Diskus 100/50 1276
Advair Diskus 250/50 1276
Advair Diskus 500/50 1276
Advair HFA 45/21 Inhalation Aerosol 1288
Advair HFA 115/21 Inhalation Aerosol 1288
Advair HFA 230/21 Inhalation Aerosol 1288
Serevent Diskus 1594

Selegiline (Action of levalbuterol on the vascular system may be potentiated). Products include:
Emsam Transdermal System 905

Selegiline Hydrochloride (Action of levalbuterol on the vascular system may be potentiated). Products include:
Eldepryl Capsules 3052

Sotalol Hydrochloride (Beta-adrenergic receptor blocking agents block the pulmonary effect of beta agonist and may produce severe bronchospasm in asthmatic patients).
No products indexed under this heading.

Terbutaline Sulfate (Potential for deleterious cardiovascular effects with concomitant use).
No products indexed under this heading.

Timolol Hemihydrate (Beta-adrenergic receptor blocking agents block the pulmonary effect of beta agonist and may produce severe bronchospasm in asthmatic patients). Products include:
Betimol Ophthalmic Solution 3181

Timolol Maleate (Beta-adrenergic receptor blocking agents block the pulmonary effect of beta agonist and may produce severe bronchospasm in asthmatic patients). Products include:
Combigan Ophthalmic Solution 553
Cosopt Sterile Ophthalmic Solution 1969
Timoptic Sterile Ophthalmic Solution 2121
Timoptic in Ocudose 2124
Timoptic-XE Sterile Ophthalmic Gel Forming Solution 2125

Torsemide (The ECG changes and/or hypokalemia that may result from the administration of non-potassium sparing diuretics can be acutely worsened by beta-agonists). Products include:
Demadex Injection 2630
Demadex Tablets 2630

Tranylcypromine Sulfate (Action of levalbuterol on the vascular system may be potentiated). Products include:
Parnate Tablets 1532

Trimipramine Maleate (Action of levalbuterol on the vascular system may be potentiated).
No products indexed under this heading.

XOPENEX INHALATION SOLUTION CONCENTRATE

(Levalbuterol Hydrochloride) 3005
See Xopenex Inhalation Solution

XOPENEX HFA INHALATION AEROSOL

(Levalbuterol Tartrate) 3009
See Xopenex Inhalation Solution

XYNTHA VIALS

(Antihemophilic Factor (Recombinant), Plasma/Albumin-Free)............................ 3280
None cited in PDR database.

XYREM ORAL SOLUTION

(Sodium Oxybate) 1766
May interact with central nervous system depressants, hypnotics and sedatives, and certain other agents. Compounds in these categories include:

Alfentanil Hydrochloride (Sodium oxybate should not be used in combination with other CNS depressants).
No products indexed under this heading.

Alprazolam (Sodium oxybate should not be used in combination with other CNS depressants).
No products indexed under this heading.

Aprobarbital (Sodium oxybate should not be used in combination with other CNS depressants).
No products indexed under this heading.

Buprenorphine Hydrochloride (Sodium oxybate should not be used in combination with other CNS depressants). Products include:
Suboxone Tablets 2601
Subutex Tablets 2601

Buspirone Hydrochloride (Sodium oxybate should not be used in combination with other CNS depressants).
No products indexed under this heading.

Butabarbital (Sodium oxybate is contraindicated in patients being treated with sedative hypnotic agents).
No products indexed under this heading.

Butabarbital Sodium (Sodium oxybate is contraindicated in patients being treated with sedative hypnotic agents).
No products indexed under this heading.

Butalbital (Sodium oxybate should not be used in combination with other CNS depressants).
No products indexed under this heading.

Chloral Hydrate (Sodium oxybate is contraindicated in patients being treated with sedative hypnotic agents).
No products indexed under this heading.

Chlordiazepoxide (Sodium oxybate should not be used in combination with other CNS depressants).
No products indexed under this heading.

Chlordiazepoxide Hydrochloride (Sodium oxybate should not be used in combination with other CNS depressants).
No products indexed under this heading.

Chlorpromazine (Sodium oxybate should not be used in combination with other CNS depressants).
No products indexed under this heading.

Chlorpromazine Hydrochloride (Sodium oxybate should not be used in combination with other CNS depressants).
No products indexed under this heading.

Chlorprothixene (Sodium oxybate should not be used in combination with other CNS depressants).
No products indexed under this heading.

Chlorprothixene Hydrochloride (Sodium oxybate should not be used in combination with other CNS depressants).
No products indexed under this heading.

Chlorprothixene Lactate (Sodium oxybate should not be used in combination with other CNS depressants).
No products indexed under this heading.

Clorazepate Dipotassium (Sodium oxybate should not be used in combination with other CNS depressants).
No products indexed under this heading.

Clozapine (Sodium oxybate should not be used in combination with other CNS depressants).
No products indexed under this heading.

Codeine Phosphate (Sodium oxybate should not be used in combination with other CNS depressants). Products include:
Tylenol with Codeine Tablets 2427

Desflurane (Sodium oxybate should not be used in combination with other CNS depressants).
No products indexed under this heading.

Dezocine (Sodium oxybate should not be used in combination with other CNS depressants).
No products indexed under this heading.

Diazepam (Sodium oxybate should not be used in combination with other CNS depressants). Products include:
Valium Tablets 2658

Droperidol (Sodium oxybate should not be used in combination with other CNS depressants).
No products indexed under this heading.

Enflurane (Sodium oxybate should not be used in combination with other CNS depressants).
No products indexed under this heading.

Estazolam (Sodium oxybate is contraindicated in patients being treated with sedative hypnotic agents).
No products indexed under this heading.

Ethanol (Sodium oxybate should not be used in combination with other CNS depressants).
No products indexed under this heading.

Ethchlorvynol (Sodium oxybate is contraindicated in patients being treated with sedative hypnotic agents).
No products indexed under this heading.

Ethinamate (Sodium oxybate is contraindicated in patients being treated with sedative hypnotic agents).
No products indexed under this heading.

Ethyl Alcohol (Sodium oxybate should not be used in combination with other CNS depressants).
No products indexed under this heading.

Fentanyl (Sodium oxybate should not be used in combination with other CNS depressants). Products include:
Duragesic Transdermal System 2405
Ionsys Transdermal System 2410

Fentanyl Citrate (Sodium oxybate should not be used in combination with other CNS depressants). Products include:
Actiq 959
Fentora Tablets 968

Fluphenazine Decanoate (Sodium oxybate should not be used in combination with other CNS depressants).
No products indexed under this heading.

Fluphenazine Enanthate (Sodium oxybate should not be used in combination with other CNS depressants).
No products indexed under this heading.

Fluphenazine Hydrochloride (Sodium oxybate should not be used in combination with other CNS depressants).
No products indexed under this heading.

Flurazepam Hydrochloride (Sodium oxybate is contraindicated in patients being treated with sedative hypnotic agents).
No products indexed under this heading.

Glutethimide (Sodium oxybate is contraindicated in patients being treated with sedative hypnotic agents).
No products indexed under this heading.

Haloperidol (Sodium oxybate should not be used in combination with other CNS depressants).
No products indexed under this heading.

Haloperidol Decanoate (Sodium oxybate should not be used in combination with other CNS depressants).
No products indexed under this heading.

Hydrocodone Bitartrate (Sodium oxybate should not be used in combination with other CNS depressants). Products include:
Lortab 5/500 Tablets 3143
Lortab 7.5/500 Tablets 3144
Lortab 10/500 Tablets 3144
Vicodin Tablets 529
Vicodin ES Tablets 530
Vicodin HP Tablets 531
Vicoprofen Tablets 533
Zydone Tablets 1132

Hydrocodone Polistirex (Sodium oxybate should not be used in combination with other CNS depressants). Products include:
Tussionex Pennkinetic Extended-Release Suspension 3154

Hydromorphone Hydrochloride (Sodium oxybate should not be used in combination with other CNS depressants).
No products indexed under this heading.

Hydroxyzine Hydrochloride (Sodium oxybate should not be used in combination with other CNS depressants).
No products indexed under this heading.

Isoflurane (Sodium oxybate should not be used in combination with other CNS depressants).
No products indexed under this heading.

Ketamine Hydrochloride (Sodium oxybate should not be used in combination with other CNS depressants).
No products indexed under this heading.

Levomethadyl Acetate Hydrochloride (Sodium oxybate should not be used in combination with other CNS depressants).
No products indexed under this heading.

Levorphanol Tartrate (Sodium oxybate should not be used in combination with other CNS depressants).
No products indexed under this heading.

Lorazepam (Sodium oxybate is contraindicated in patients being treated with sedative hypnotic agents).
No products indexed under this heading.

Loxapine Hydrochloride (Sodium oxybate should not be used in combination with other CNS depressants).
No products indexed under this heading.

Loxapine Succinate (Sodium oxybate should not be used in combination with other CNS depressants).
No products indexed under this heading.

Meperidine Hydrochloride (Sodium oxybate should not be used in combination with other CNS depressants).
No products indexed under this heading.

Mephobarbital (Sodium oxybate should not be used in combination with other CNS depressants).
No products indexed under this heading.

Meprobamate (Sodium oxybate should not be used in combination with other CNS depressants).
No products indexed under this heading.

Mesoridazine Besylate (Sodium oxybate should not be used in combination with other CNS depressants).
No products indexed under this heading.

Methadone Hydrochloride (Sodium oxybate should not be used in combination with other CNS depressants).
No products indexed under this heading.

Methohexital Sodium (Sodium oxybate should not be used in combination with other CNS depressants).
No products indexed under this heading.

Methotrimeprazine (Sodium oxybate should not be used in combination with other CNS depressants).
No products indexed under this heading.

Methoxyflurane (Sodium oxybate should not be used in combination with other CNS depressants).
No products indexed under this heading.

Midazolam Hydrochloride (Sodium oxybate is contraindicated in patients being treated with sedative hypnotic agents).
No products indexed under this heading.

Molindone Hydrochloride (Sodium oxybate should not be used in combination with other CNS depressants). Products include:
Moban Tablets 1116

Morphine Sulfate (Sodium oxybate should not be used in combination with other CNS depressants). Products include:
Avinza Capsules 1772
DepoDur Injection 1095
MS Contin Tablets 2585

Olanzapine (Sodium oxybate should not be used in combination with other CNS depressants). Products include:
Symbyax Capsules 1871
Zyprexa Tablets 1883
Zyprexa IntraMuscular 1883
Zyprexa ZYDIS Orally Disintegrating Tablets 1883

Oxazepam (Sodium oxybate should not be used in combination with other CNS depressants).
No products indexed under this heading.

Oxycodone Hydrochloride (Sodium oxybate should not be used in combination with other CNS depressants). Products include:
OxyContin Tablets 2589
OxyIR Capsules 2593
Percocet Tablets 1127
Percodan Tablets 1130

Pentobarbital Sodium (Sodium oxybate should not be used in combination with other CNS depressants). Products include:
Nembutal Sodium Solution, USP 2494

Perphenazine (Sodium oxybate should not be used in combination with other CNS depressants).
No products indexed under this heading.

Phenobarbital (Sodium oxybate should not be used in combination with other CNS depressants). Products include:
Donnatal Extentabs 2507

Prazepam (Sodium oxybate should not be used in combination with other CNS depressants).
No products indexed under this heading.

Prochlorperazine (Sodium oxybate should not be used in combination with other CNS depressants).
No products indexed under this heading.

Promethazine Hydrochloride (Sodium oxybate should not be used in combination with other CNS depressants).
No products indexed under this heading.

Propofol (Sodium oxybate is contraindicated in patients being treated with sedative hypnotic agents).
No products indexed under this heading.

Propoxyphene Hydrochloride (Sodium oxybate should not be used in combination with other CNS depressants).
No products indexed under this heading.

Propoxyphene Napsylate (Sodium oxybate should not be used in combination with other CNS depressants).
No products indexed under this heading.

Quazepam (Sodium oxybate is contraindicated in patients being treated with sedative hypnotic agents).
No products indexed under this heading.

Quetiapine Fumarate (Sodium oxybate should not be used in combination with other CNS depressants).
No products indexed under this heading.

Ramelteon (Sodium oxybate is contraindicated in patients being treated with sedative hypnotic agents). Products include:
Rozerem Tablets 3091

Remifentanil Hydrochloride (Sodium oxybate should not be used in combination with other CNS depressants).
No products indexed under this heading.

Risperidone (Sodium oxybate should not be used in combination with other CNS depressants). Products include:
Risperdal Consta Long-Acting Injection 1753

Secobarbital Sodium (Sodium oxybate is contraindicated in patients being treated with sedative hypnotic agents).
No products indexed under this heading.

Sevoflurane (Sodium oxybate should not be used in combination with other CNS depressants). Products include:
Ultane Liquid for Inhalation 524

Sodium Butabarbital (Sodium oxybate is contraindicated in patients being treated with sedative hypnotic agents).
No products indexed under this heading.

Sufentanil Citrate (Sodium oxybate should not be used in combination with other CNS depressants).
No products indexed under this heading.

Temazepam (Sodium oxybate is contraindicated in patients being treated with sedative hypnotic agents).
No products indexed under this heading.

Thiamylal Sodium (Sodium oxybate should not be used in combination with other CNS depressants).
No products indexed under this heading.

Thioridazine Hydrochloride (Sodium oxybate should not be used in combination with other CNS depressants). Products include:
Thioridazine Hydrochloride Tablets 2195

Thiothixene (Sodium oxybate should not be used in combination with other CNS depressants). Products include:
Thiothixene Capsules 2197

Triazolam (Sodium oxybate is contraindicated in patients being treated with sedative hypnotic agents).
No products indexed under this heading.

Trifluoperazine Hydrochloride (Sodium oxybate should not be used in combination with other CNS depressants).
No products indexed under this heading.

Zaleplon (Sodium oxybate is contraindicated in patients being treated with sedative hypnotic agents).
No products indexed under this heading.

Ziprasidone Hydrochloride (Sodium oxybate should not be used in combination with other CNS depressants). Products include:
Geodon Capsules 2520

Zolpidem Tartrate (Sodium oxybate is contraindicated in patients being treated with sedative hypnotic agents). Products include:
Ambien Tablets 2692
Ambien CR Tablets 2696

Food Interactions

Alcohol (The combined use of alcohol with sodium oxybate may result in potentiation of the central nervous system-depressant effects of sodium oxybate and alcohol).

XYZAL ORAL SOLUTION

(Levocetirizine Dihydrochloride) 3155
May interact with central nervous system depressants, theophyllines, and certain other agents. Compounds in these categories include:

Alfentanil Hydrochloride (Concurrent use of levocetirizine dihydrochloride with other central nervous system depressants should be avoided because additional reductions in alertness and additional impairment of central nervous system performance may occur).
No products indexed under this heading.

Alprazolam (Concurrent use of levocetirizine dihydrochloride with other central nervous system depressants should be avoided because additional reductions in alertness and additional impairment of central nervous system performance may occur).
No products indexed under this heading.

Aprobarbital (Concurrent use of levocetirizine dihydrochloride with other central nervous system depressants should be avoided because additional reductions in alertness and additional impairment of central nervous system performance may occur).
No products indexed under this heading.

Buprenorphine Hydrochloride (Concurrent use of levocetirizine dihydrochloride with other central nervous system depressants should be avoided because additional reductions in alertness and additional impairment of central nervous system performance may occur). Products include:
Suboxone Tablets ... **2601**
Subutex Tablets ... **2601**

Buspirone Hydrochloride (Concurrent use of levocetirizine dihydrochloride with other central nervous system depressants should be avoided because additional reductions in alertness and additional impairment of central nervous system performance may occur).
No products indexed under this heading.

Butabarbital (Concurrent use of levocetirizine dihydrochloride with other central nervous system depressants should be avoided because additional reductions in alertness and additional impairment of central nervous system performance may occur).
No products indexed under this heading.

Butalbital (Concurrent use of levocetirizine dihydrochloride with other central nervous system depressants should be avoided because additional reductions in alertness and additional impairment of central nervous system performance may occur).
No products indexed under this heading.

Chlordiazepoxide (Concurrent use of levocetirizine dihydrochloride with other central nervous system depressants should be avoided because additional reductions in alertness and additional impairment of central nervous system performance may occur).
No products indexed under this heading.

Chlordiazepoxide Hydrochloride (Concurrent use of levocetirizine dihydrochloride with other central nervous system depressants should be avoided because additional reductions in alertness and additional impairment of central nervous system performance may occur).
No products indexed under this heading.

Chlorpromazine (Concurrent use of levocetirizine dihydrochloride with other central nervous system depressants should be avoided because additional reductions in alertness and additional impairment of central nervous system performance may occur).
No products indexed under this heading.

Chlorpromazine Hydrochloride (Concurrent use of levocetirizine dihydrochloride with other central nervous system depressants should be avoided because additional reductions in alertness and additional impairment of central nervous system performance may occur).
No products indexed under this heading.

Chlorprothixene (Concurrent use of levocetirizine dihydrochloride with other central nervous system depressants should be avoided because additional reductions in alertness and additional impairment of central nervous system performance may occur).
No products indexed under this heading.

Chlorprothixene Hydrochloride (Concurrent use of levocetirizine dihydrochloride with other central nervous system depressants should be avoided because additional reductions in alertness and additional impairment of central nervous system performance may occur).
No products indexed under this heading.

Chlorprothixene Lactate (Concurrent use of levocetirizine dihydrochloride with other central nervous system depressants should be avoided because additional reductions in alertness and additional impairment of central nervous system performance may occur).
No products indexed under this heading.

Clorazepate Dipotassium (Concurrent use of levocetirizine dihydrochloride with other central nervous system depressants should be avoided because additional reductions in alertness and additional impairment of central nervous system performance may occur).
No products indexed under this heading.

Clozapine (Concurrent use of levocetirizine dihydrochloride with other central nervous system depressants should be avoided because additional reductions in alertness and additional impairment of central nervous system performance may occur).
No products indexed under this heading.

Codeine Phosphate (Concurrent use of levocetirizine dihydrochloride with other central nervous system depressants should be avoided because additional reductions in alertness and additional impairment of central nervous system performance may occur). Products include:
Tylenol with Codeine Tablets ... **2427**

Desflurane (Concurrent use of levocetirizine dihydrochloride with other central nervous system depressants should be avoided because additional reductions in alertness and additional impairment of central nervous system performance may occur).
No products indexed under this heading.

Dezocine (Concurrent use of levocetirizine dihydrochloride with other central nervous system depressants should be avoided because additional reductions in alertness and additional impairment of central nervous system performance may occur).
No products indexed under this heading.

Diazepam (Concurrent use of levocetirizine dihydrochloride with other central nervous system depressants should be avoided because additional reductions in alertness and additional impairment of central nervous system performance may occur). Products include:
Valium Tablets ... **2658**

Droperidol (Concurrent use of levocetirizine dihydrochloride with other central nervous system depressants should be avoided because additional reductions in alertness and additional impairment of central nervous system performance may occur).
No products indexed under this heading.

Enflurane (Concurrent use of levocetirizine dihydrochloride with other central nervous system depressants should be avoided because additional reductions in alertness and additional impairment of central nervous system performance may occur).
No products indexed under this heading.

Estazolam (Concurrent use of levocetirizine dihydrochloride with other central nervous system depressants should be avoided because additional reductions in alertness and additional impairment of central nervous system performance may occur).
No products indexed under this heading.

Ethanol (Concurrent use of levocetirizine dihydrochloride with alcohol should be avoided because additional reductions in alertness and additional impairment of central nervous system performance may occur).
No products indexed under this heading.

Ethchlorvynol (Concurrent use of levocetirizine dihydrochloride with other central nervous system depressants should be avoided because additional reductions in alertness and additional impairment of central nervous system performance may occur).
No products indexed under this heading.

Ethinamate (Concurrent use of levocetirizine dihydrochloride with other central nervous system depressants should be avoided because additional reductions in alertness and additional impairment of central nervous system performance may occur).
No products indexed under this heading.

Ethyl Alcohol (Concurrent use of levocetirizine dihydrochloride with alcohol should be avoided because additional reductions in alertness and additional impairment of central nervous system performance may occur).
No products indexed under this heading.

Fentanyl (Concurrent use of levocetirizine dihydrochloride with other central nervous system depressants should be avoided because additional reductions in alertness and additional impairment of central nervous system performance may occur). Products include:
Duragesic Transdermal System ... **2405**
Ionsys Transdermal System ... **2410**

Fentanyl Citrate (Concurrent use of levocetirizine dihydrochloride with other central nervous system depressants should be avoided because additional reductions in alertness and additional impairment of central nervous system performance may occur). Products include:
Actiq ... **959**
Fentora Tablets ... **968**

Fluphenazine Decanoate (Concurrent use of levocetirizine dihydrochloride with other central nervous system depressants should be avoided because additional reductions in alertness and additional impairment of central nervous system performance may occur).
No products indexed under this heading.

Fluphenazine Enanthate (Concurrent use of levocetirizine dihydrochloride with other central nervous system depressants should be avoided because additional reductions in alertness and additional impairment of central nervous system performance may occur).
No products indexed under this heading.

Fluphenazine Hydrochloride (Concurrent use of levocetirizine dihydrochloride with other central nervous system depressants should be avoided because additional reductions in alertness and additional impairment of central nervous system performance may occur).
No products indexed under this heading.

Flurazepam Hydrochloride (Concurrent use of levocetirizine dihydrochloride with other central nervous system depressants should be avoided because additional reductions in alertness and additional impairment of central nervous system performance may occur).
No products indexed under this heading.

Glutethimide (Concurrent use of levocetirizine dihydrochloride with other central nervous system depressants should be avoided because additional reductions in alertness and additional impairment of central nervous system performance may occur).
No products indexed under this heading.

Haloperidol (Concurrent use of levocetirizine dihydrochloride with other central nervous system depressants should be avoided because additional reductions in alertness and additional impairment of central nervous system performance may occur).
No products indexed under this heading.

Haloperidol Decanoate (Concurrent use of levocetirizine dihydrochloride with other central nervous system depressants should be avoided because additional reductions in alertness and additional impairment of central nervous system performance may occur).
No products indexed under this heading.

Hydrocodone Bitartrate (Concurrent use of levocetirizine dihydrochloride with other central nervous system depressants should be avoided because additional reductions in alertness and additional impairment of central nervous system performance may occur). Products include:
Lortab 5/500 Tablets ... **3143**

Lortab 7.5/500 Tablets 3144
Lortab 10/500 Tablets 3144
Vicodin Tablets 529
Vicodin ES Tablets 530
Vicodin HP Tablets 531
Vicoprofen Tablets 533
Zydone Tablets 1132

Hydrocodone Polistirex (Concurrent use of levocetirizine dihydrochloride with other central nervous system depressants should be avoided because additional reductions in alertness and additional impairment of central nervous system performance may occur).
Products include:
Tussionex Pennkinetic Extended-Release Suspension 3154

Hydromorphone Hydrochloride (Concurrent use of levocetirizine dihydrochloride with other central nervous system depressants should be avoided because additional reductions in alertness and additional impairment of central nervous system performance may occur).
No products indexed under this heading.

Hydroxyzine Hydrochloride (Concurrent use of levocetirizine dihydrochloride with other central nervous system depressants should be avoided because additional reductions in alertness and additional impairment of central nervous system performance may occur).
No products indexed under this heading.

Isoflurane (Concurrent use of levocetirizine dihydrochloride with other central nervous system depressants should be avoided because additional reductions in alertness and additional impairment of central nervous system performance may occur).
No products indexed under this heading.

Ketamine Hydrochloride (Concurrent use of levocetirizine dihydrochloride with other central nervous system depressants should be avoided because additional reductions in alertness and additional impairment of central nervous system performance may occur).
No products indexed under this heading.

Levomethadyl Acetate Hydrochloride (Concurrent use of levocetirizine dihydrochloride with other central nervous system depressants should be avoided because additional reductions in alertness and additional impairment of central nervous system performance may occur).
No products indexed under this heading.

Levorphanol Tartrate (Concurrent use of levocetirizine dihydrochloride with other central nervous system depressants should be avoided because additional reductions in alertness and additional impairment of central nervous system performance may occur).
No products indexed under this heading.

Lorazepam (Concurrent use of levocetirizine dihydrochloride with other central nervous system depressants should be avoided because additional reductions in alertness and additional impairment of central nervous system performance may occur).
No products indexed under this heading.

Loxapine Hydrochloride (Concurrent use of levocetirizine dihydrochloride with other central nervous system depressants should be avoided because additional reductions in alertness and additional impairment of central nervous system performance may occur).
No products indexed under this heading.

Loxapine Succinate (Concurrent use of levocetirizine dihydrochloride with other central nervous system depressants should be avoided because additional reductions in alertness and additional impairment of central nervous system performance may occur).
No products indexed under this heading.

Meperidine Hydrochloride (Concurrent use of levocetirizine dihydrochloride with other central nervous system depressants should be avoided because additional reductions in alertness and additional impairment of central nervous system performance may occur).
No products indexed under this heading.

Mephobarbital (Concurrent use of levocetirizine dihydrochloride with other central nervous system depressants should be avoided because additional reductions in alertness and additional impairment of central nervous system performance may occur).
No products indexed under this heading.

Meprobamate (Concurrent use of levocetirizine dihydrochloride with other central nervous system depressants should be avoided because additional reductions in alertness and additional impairment of central nervous system performance may occur).
No products indexed under this heading.

Mesoridazine Besylate (Concurrent use of levocetirizine dihydrochloride with other central nervous system depressants should be avoided because additional reductions in alertness and additional impairment of central nervous system performance may occur).
No products indexed under this heading.

Methadone Hydrochloride (Concurrent use of levocetirizine dihydrochloride with other central nervous system depressants should be avoided because additional reductions in alertness and additional impairment of central nervous system performance may occur).
No products indexed under this heading.

Methohexital Sodium (Concurrent use of levocetirizine dihydrochloride with other central nervous system depressants should be avoided because additional reductions in alertness and additional impairment of central nervous system performance may occur).
No products indexed under this heading.

Methotrimeprazine (Concurrent use of levocetirizine dihydrochloride with other central nervous system depressants should be avoided because additional reductions in alertness and additional impairment of central nervous system performance may occur).
No products indexed under this heading.

Methoxyflurane (Concurrent use of levocetirizine dihydrochloride with other central nervous system depressants should be avoided because additional reductions in alertness and additional impairment of central nervous system performance may occur).
No products indexed under this heading.

Midazolam Hydrochloride (Concurrent use of levocetirizine dihydrochloride with other central nervous system depressants should be avoided because additional reductions in alertness and additional impairment of central nervous system performance may occur).
No products indexed under this heading.

Molindone Hydrochloride (Concurrent use of levocetirizine dihydrochloride with other central nervous system depressants should be avoided because additional reductions in alertness and additional impairment of central nervous system performance may occur).
Products include:
Moban Tablets 1116

Morphine Sulfate (Concurrent use of levocetirizine dihydrochloride with other central nervous system depressants should be avoided because additional reductions in alertness and additional impairment of central nervous system performance may occur). Products include:
Avinza Capsules 1772
DepoDur Injection 1095
MS Contin Tablets 2585

Olanzapine (Concurrent use of levocetirizine dihydrochloride with other central nervous system depressants should be avoided because additional reductions in alertness and additional impairment of central nervous system performance may occur). Products include:
Symbyax Capsules 1871
Zyprexa Tablets 1883
Zyprexa IntraMuscular 1883
Zyprexa ZYDIS Orally Disintegrating Tablets 1883

Oxazepam (Concurrent use of levocetirizine dihydrochloride with other central nervous system depressants should be avoided because additional reductions in alertness and additional impairment of central nervous system performance may occur).
No products indexed under this heading.

Oxycodone Hydrochloride (Concurrent use of levocetirizine dihydrochloride with other central nervous system depressants should be avoided because additional reductions in alertness and additional impairment of central nervous system performance may occur).
Products include:
OxyContin Tablets 2589
OxyIR Capsules 2593
Percocet Tablets 1127
Percodan Tablets 1130

Pentobarbital Sodium (Concurrent use of levocetirizine dihydrochloride with other central nervous system depressants should be avoided because additional reductions in alertness and additional impairment of central nervous system performance may occur).
Products include:
Nembutal Sodium Solution, USP 2494

Perphenazine (Concurrent use of levocetirizine dihydrochloride with other central nervous system depressants should be avoided because additional reductions in alertness and additional impairment of central nervous system performance may occur).
No products indexed under this heading.

Phenobarbital (Concurrent use of levocetirizine dihydrochloride with other central nervous system depressants should be avoided because additional reductions in alertness and additional impairment of central nervous system performance may occur). Products include:
Donnatal Extentabs 2507

Prazepam (Concurrent use of levocetirizine dihydrochloride with other central nervous system depressants should be avoided because additional reductions in alertness and additional impairment of central nervous system performance may occur).
No products indexed under this heading.

Prochlorperazine (Concurrent use of levocetirizine dihydrochloride with other central nervous system depressants should be avoided because additional reductions in alertness and additional impairment of central nervous system performance may occur).
No products indexed under this heading.

Promethazine Hydrochloride (Concurrent use of levocetirizine dihydrochloride with other central nervous system depressants should be avoided because additional reductions in alertness and additional impairment of central nervous system performance may occur).
No products indexed under this heading.

Propofol (Concurrent use of levocetirizine dihydrochloride with other central nervous system depressants should be avoided because additional reductions in alertness and additional impairment of central nervous system performance may occur).
No products indexed under this heading.

Propoxyphene Hydrochloride (Concurrent use of levocetirizine dihydrochloride with other central nervous system depressants should be avoided because additional reductions in alertness and additional impairment of central nervous system performance may occur).
No products indexed under this heading.

Food Interactions

XYZAL ORAL SOLUTION

Chlordiazepoxide (Concurrent use of levocetirizine dihydrochloride with other central nervous system depressants should be avoided because additional reductions in alertness and additional impairment of central nervous system performance may occur).
No products indexed under this heading.

Chlordiazepoxide Hydrochloride (Concurrent use of levocetirizine dihydrochloride with other central nervous system depressants should be avoided because additional reductions in alertness and additional impairment of central nervous system performance may occur).
No products indexed under this heading.

Chlorpromazine (Concurrent use of levocetirizine dihydrochloride with other central nervous system depressants should be avoided because additional reductions in alertness and additional impairment of central nervous system performance may occur).
No products indexed under this heading.

Chlorpromazine Hydrochloride (Concurrent use of levocetirizine dihydrochloride with other central nervous system depressants should be avoided because additional reductions in alertness and additional impairment of central nervous system performance may occur).
No products indexed under this heading.

Chlorprothixene (Concurrent use of levocetirizine dihydrochloride with other central nervous system depressants should be avoided because additional reductions in alertness and additional impairment of central nervous system performance may occur).
No products indexed under this heading.

Chlorprothixene Hydrochloride (Concurrent use of levocetirizine dihydrochloride with other central nervous system depressants should be avoided because additional reductions in alertness and additional impairment of central nervous system performance may occur).
No products indexed under this heading.

Chlorprothixene Lactate (Concurrent use of levocetirizine dihydrochloride with other central nervous system depressants should be avoided because additional reductions in alertness and additional impairment of central nervous system performance may occur).
No products indexed under this heading.

Clorazepate Dipotassium (Concurrent use of levocetirizine dihydrochloride with other central nervous system depressants should be avoided because additional reductions in alertness and additional impairment of central nervous system performance may occur).
No products indexed under this heading.

Clozapine (Concurrent use of levocetirizine dihydrochloride with other central nervous system depressants should be avoided because additional reductions in alertness and additional impairment of central nervous system performance may occur).
No products indexed under this heading.

Codeine Phosphate (Concurrent use of levocetirizine dihydrochloride with other central nervous system depressants should be avoided because additional reductions in alertness and additional impairment of central nervous system performance may occur). Products include:
Tylenol with Codeine Tablets **2427**

Desflurane (Concurrent use of levocetirizine dihydrochloride with other central nervous system depressants should be avoided because additional reductions in alertness and additional impairment of central nervous system performance may occur).
No products indexed under this heading.

Dezocine (Concurrent use of levocetirizine dihydrochloride with other central nervous system depressants should be avoided because additional reductions in alertness and additional impairment of central nervous system performance may occur).
No products indexed under this heading.

Diazepam (Concurrent use of levocetirizine dihydrochloride with other central nervous system depressants should be avoided because additional reductions in alertness and additional impairment of central nervous system performance may occur). Products include:
Valium Tablets **2658**

Droperidol (Concurrent use of levocetirizine dihydrochloride with other central nervous system depressants should be avoided because additional reductions in alertness and additional impairment of central nervous system performance may occur).
No products indexed under this heading.

Enflurane (Concurrent use of levocetirizine dihydrochloride with other central nervous system depressants should be avoided because additional reductions in alertness and additional impairment of central nervous system performance may occur).
No products indexed under this heading.

Estazolam (Concurrent use of levocetirizine dihydrochloride with other central nervous system depressants should be avoided because additional reductions in alertness and additional impairment of central nervous system performance may occur).
No products indexed under this heading.

Ethanol (Concurrent use of levocetirizine dihydrochloride with alcohol because additional reductions in alertness and additional impairment of central nervous system performance may occur).
No products indexed under this heading.

Ethchlorvynol (Concurrent use of levocetirizine dihydrochloride with other central nervous system depressants should be avoided because additional reductions in alertness and additional impairment of central nervous system performance may occur).
No products indexed under this heading.

Ethinamate (Concurrent use of levocetirizine dihydrochloride with other central nervous system depressants should be avoided because additional reductions in alertness and additional impairment of central nervous system performance may occur).
No products indexed under this heading.

Ethyl Alcohol (Concurrent use of levocetirizine dihydrochloride with alcohol because additional reductions in alertness and additional impairment of central nervous system performance may occur).
No products indexed under this heading.

Fentanyl (Concurrent use of levocetirizine dihydrochloride with other central nervous system depressants should be avoided because additional reductions in alertness and additional impairment of central nervous system performance may occur). Products include:
Duragesic Transdermal System **2405**
Ionsys Transdermal System **2410**

Fentanyl Citrate (Concurrent use of levocetirizine dihydrochloride with other central nervous system depressants should be avoided because additional reductions in alertness and additional impairment of central nervous system performance may occur). Products include:
Actiq **959**
Fentora Tablets **968**

Fluphenazine Decanoate (Concurrent use of levocetirizine dihydrochloride with other central nervous system depressants should be avoided because additional reductions in alertness and additional impairment of central nervous system performance may occur).
No products indexed under this heading.

Fluphenazine Enanthate (Concurrent use of levocetirizine dihydrochloride with other central nervous system depressants should be avoided because additional reductions in alertness and additional impairment of central nervous system performance may occur).
No products indexed under this heading.

Fluphenazine Hydrochloride (Concurrent use of levocetirizine dihydrochloride with other central nervous system depressants should be avoided because additional reductions in alertness and additional impairment of central nervous system performance may occur).
No products indexed under this heading.

Flurazepam Hydrochloride (Concurrent use of levocetirizine dihydrochloride with other central nervous system depressants should be avoided because additional reductions in alertness and additional impairment of central nervous system performance may occur).
No products indexed under this heading.

Glutethimide (Concurrent use of levocetirizine dihydrochloride with other central nervous system depressants should be avoided because additional reductions in alertness and additional impairment of central nervous system performance may occur).
No products indexed under this heading.

Haloperidol (Concurrent use of levocetirizine dihydrochloride with other central nervous system depressants should be avoided because additional reductions in alertness and additional impairment of central nervous system performance may occur).
No products indexed under this heading.

Haloperidol Decanoate (Concurrent use of levocetirizine dihydrochloride with other central nervous system depressants should be avoided because additional reductions in alertness and additional impairment of central nervous system performance may occur).
No products indexed under this heading.

Hydrocodone Bitartrate (Concurrent use of levocetirizine dihydrochloride with other central nervous system depressants should be avoided because additional reductions in alertness and additional impairment of central nervous system performance may occur).
Products include:
Lortab 5/500 Tablets **3143**
Lortab 7.5/500 Tablets **3144**
Lortab 10/500 Tablets **3144**
Vicodin Tablets **529**
Vicodin ES Tablets **530**
Vicodin HP Tablets **531**
Vicoprofen Tablets **533**
Zydone Tablets **1132**

Hydrocodone Polistirex (Concurrent use of levocetirizine dihydrochloride with other central nervous system depressants should be avoided because additional reductions in alertness and additional impairment of central nervous system performance may occur).
Products include:
Tussionex Pennkinetic
Extended-Release Suspension **3154**

Hydromorphone Hydrochloride (Concurrent use of levocetirizine dihydrochloride with other central nervous system depressants should be avoided because additional reductions in alertness and additional impairment of central nervous system performance may occur).
No products indexed under this heading.

Hydroxyzine Hydrochloride (Concurrent use of levocetirizine dihydrochloride with other central nervous system depressants should be avoided because additional reductions in alertness and additional impairment of central nervous system performance may occur).
No products indexed under this heading.

Isoflurane (Concurrent use of levocetirizine dihydrochloride with other central nervous system depressants should be avoided because additional reductions in alertness and additional impairment of central nervous system performance may occur).
No products indexed under this heading.

Ketamine Hydrochloride (Concurrent use of levocetirizine dihydrochloride with other central nervous system depressants should be avoided because additional reductions in alertness and additional impairment of central nervous system performance may occur).
No products indexed under this heading.

Levomethadyl Acetate Hydrochloride (Concurrent use of levocetirizine dihydrochloride with other central nervous system depressants should be avoided because additional reductions in alertness and additional impairment of central nervous system performance may occur).
No products indexed under this heading.

Levorphanol Tartrate (Concurrent use of levocetirizine dihydrochloride with other central nervous system depressants should be avoided because additional reductions in alertness and additional impairment of central nervous system performance may occur).
No products indexed under this heading.

Lorazepam (Concurrent use of levocetirizine dihydrochloride with other central nervous system depressants should be avoided because additional reductions in alertness and additional impairment of central nervous system performance may occur).
No products indexed under this heading.

Loxapine Hydrochloride (Concurrent use of levocetirizine dihydrochloride with other central nervous system depressants should be avoided because additional reductions in alertness and additional impairment of central nervous system performance may occur).
No products indexed under this heading.

Loxapine Succinate (Concurrent use of levocetirizine dihydrochloride with other central nervous system depressants should be avoided because additional reductions in alertness and additional impairment of central nervous system performance may occur).
No products indexed under this heading.

Meperidine Hydrochloride (Concurrent use of levocetirizine dihydrochloride with other central nervous system depressants should be avoided because additional reductions in alertness and additional impairment of central nervous system performance may occur).
No products indexed under this heading.

Mephobarbital (Concurrent use of levocetirizine dihydrochloride with other central nervous system depressants should be avoided because additional reductions in alertness and additional impairment of central nervous system performance may occur).
No products indexed under this heading.

Meprobamate (Concurrent use of levocetirizine dihydrochloride with other central nervous system depressants should be avoided because additional reductions in alertness and additional impairment of central nervous system performance may occur).
No products indexed under this heading.

Mesoridazine Besylate (Concurrent use of levocetirizine dihydrochloride with other central nervous system depressants should be avoided because additional reductions in alertness and additional impairment of central nervous system performance may occur).
No products indexed under this heading.

Methadone Hydrochloride (Concurrent use of levocetirizine dihydrochloride with other central nervous system depressants should be avoided because additional reductions in alertness and additional impairment of central nervous system performance may occur).
No products indexed under this heading.

Methohexital Sodium (Concurrent use of levocetirizine dihydrochloride with other central nervous system depressants should be avoided because additional reductions in alertness and additional impairment of central nervous system performance may occur).
No products indexed under this heading.

Methotrimeprazine (Concurrent use of levocetirizine dihydrochloride with other central nervous system depressants should be avoided because additional reductions in alertness and additional impairment of central nervous system performance may occur).
No products indexed under this heading.

Methoxyflurane (Concurrent use of levocetirizine dihydrochloride with other central nervous system depressants should be avoided because additional reductions in alertness and additional impairment of central nervous system performance may occur).
No products indexed under this heading.

Midazolam Hydrochloride (Concurrent use of levocetirizine dihydrochloride with other central nervous system depressants should be avoided because additional reductions in alertness and additional impairment of central nervous system performance may occur).
No products indexed under this heading.

Molindone Hydrochloride (Concurrent use of levocetirizine dihydrochloride with other central nervous system depressants should be avoided because additional reductions in alertness and additional impairment of central nervous system performance may occur).
Products include:
Moban Tablets 1116

Morphine Sulfate (Concurrent use of levocetirizine dihydrochloride with other central nervous system depressants should be avoided because additional reductions in alertness and additional impairment of central nervous system performance may occur). Products include:
Avinza Capsules 1772
DepoDur Injection 1095
MS Contin Tablets 2585

Olanzapine (Concurrent use of levocetirizine dihydrochloride with other central nervous system depressants should be avoided because additional reductions in alertness and additional impairment of central nervous system performance may occur). Products include:
Symbyax Capsules 1871
Zyprexa Tablets 1883
Zyprexa IntraMuscular 1883
Zyprexa ZYDIS Orally Disintegrating Tablets 1883

Oxazepam (Concurrent use of levocetirizine dihydrochloride with other central nervous system depressants should be avoided because additional reductions in alertness and additional impairment of central nervous system performance may occur).
No products indexed under this heading.

Oxycodone Hydrochloride (Concurrent use of levocetirizine dihydrochloride with other central nervous system depressants should be avoided because additional reductions in alertness and additional impairment of central nervous system performance may occur).
Products include:
OxyContin Tablets 2589
OxyIR Capsules 2593
Percocet Tablets 1127
Percodan Tablets 1130

Pentobarbital Sodium (Concurrent use of levocetirizine dihydrochloride with other central nervous system depressants should be avoided because additional reductions in alertness and additional impairment of central nervous system performance may occur).
Products include:
Nembutal Sodium Solution, USP 2494

Perphenazine (Concurrent use of levocetirizine dihydrochloride with other central nervous system depressants should be avoided because additional reductions in alertness and additional impairment of central nervous system performance may occur).
No products indexed under this heading.

Phenobarbital (Concurrent use of levocetirizine dihydrochloride with other central nervous system depressants should be avoided because additional reductions in alertness and additional impairment of central nervous system performance may occur). Products include:
Donnatal Extentabs 2507

Prazepam (Concurrent use of levocetirizine dihydrochloride with other central nervous system depressants should be avoided because additional reductions in alertness and additional impairment of central nervous system performance may occur).
No products indexed under this heading.

Prochlorperazine (Concurrent use of levocetirizine dihydrochloride with other central nervous system depressants should be avoided because additional reductions in alertness and additional impairment of central nervous system performance may occur).
No products indexed under this heading.

Promethazine Hydrochloride (Concurrent use of levocetirizine dihydrochloride with other central nervous system depressants should be avoided because additional reductions in alertness and additional impairment of central nervous system performance may occur).
No products indexed under this heading.

Propofol (Concurrent use of levocetirizine dihydrochloride with other central nervous system depressants should be avoided because additional reductions in alertness and additional impairment of central nervous system performance may occur).
No products indexed under this heading.

Propoxyphene Hydrochloride (Concurrent use of levocetirizine dihydrochloride with other central nervous system depressants should be avoided because additional reductions in alertness and additional impairment of central nervous system performance may occur).
No products indexed under this heading.

Propoxyphene Napsylate (Concurrent use of levocetirizine dihydrochloride with other central nervous system depressants should be avoided because additional reductions in alertness and additional impairment of central nervous system performance may occur).
No products indexed under this heading.

Quazepam (Concurrent use of levocetirizine dihydrochloride with other central nervous system depressants should be avoided because additional reductions in alertness and additional impairment of central nervous system performance may occur).
No products indexed under this heading.

Quetiapine Fumarate (Concurrent use of levocetirizine dihydrochloride with other central nervous system depressants should be avoided because additional reductions in alertness and additional impairment of central nervous system performance may occur).
No products indexed under this heading.

Remifentanil Hydrochloride (Concurrent use of levocetirizine dihydrochloride with other central nervous system depressants should be avoided because additional reductions in alertness and additional impairment of central nervous system performance may occur).
No products indexed under this heading.

Risperidone (Concurrent use of levocetirizine dihydrochloride with other central nervous system depressants should be avoided because additional reductions in alertness and additional impairment of central nervous system performance may occur). Products include:
Risperdal Consta Long-Acting Injection 1753

Ritonavir (Ritonavir increased the plasma AUC of cetirizine by about 42% accompanied by an increase in half-life (53%) and a decrease in clearance (29%) of cetirizine. The disposition of ritonavir was not altered by concomitant cetirizine administration). Products include:

Kaletra 452
Norvir 489

Secobarbital Sodium (Concurrent use of levocetirizine dihydrochloride with other central nervous system depressants should be avoided because additional reductions in alertness and additional impairment of central nervous system performance may occur).
No products indexed under this heading.

Sevoflurane (Concurrent use of levocetirizine dihydrochloride with other central nervous system depressants should be avoided because additional reductions in alertness and additional impairment of central nervous system performance may occur). Products include:
Ultane Liquid for Inhalation 524

Sodium Oxybate (Concurrent use of levocetirizine dihydrochloride with other central nervous system depressants should be avoided because additional reductions in alertness and additional impairment of central nervous system performance may occur). Products include:
Xyrem Oral Solution 1766

Sufentanil Citrate (Concurrent use of levocetirizine dihydrochloride with other central nervous system depressants should be avoided because additional reductions in alertness and additional impairment of central nervous system performance may occur).
No products indexed under this heading.

Temazepam (Concurrent use of levocetirizine dihydrochloride with other central nervous system depressants should be avoided because additional reductions in alertness and additional impairment of central nervous system performance may occur).
No products indexed under this heading.

Theophylline (There was a small decrease (approximately 16%) in the clearance of cetirizine caused by a 400 mg dose of theophylline. It is possible that higher theophylline doses could have greater effect).
No products indexed under this heading.

Theophylline Anhydrous (There was a small decrease (approximately 16%) in the clearance of cetirizine caused by a 400 mg dose of theophylline. It is possible that higher theophylline doses could have greater effect). Products include:
Uniphyl Tablets 2595

Theophylline Calcium Salicylate (There was a small decrease (approximately 16%) in the clearance of cetirizine caused by a 400 mg dose of theophylline. It is possible that higher theophylline doses could have greater effect).
No products indexed under this heading.

Theophylline Dihydroxypropyl (Glyceryl) (There was a small decrease (approximately 16%) in the clearance of cetirizine caused by a 400 mg dose of theophylline. It is possible that higher theophylline doses could have greater effect).
No products indexed under this heading.

Theophylline Ethylenediamine (There was a small decrease (approximately 16%) in the clearance of cetirizine caused by a 400 mg dose of theophylline. It is possible that higher theophylline doses could have greater effect).
No products indexed under this heading.

Theophylline Sodium Glycinate (There was a small decrease (approximately 16%) in the clearance of cetirizine caused by a 400 mg dose of theophylline. It is possible that higher theophylline doses could have greater effect).
No products indexed under this heading.

Thiamylal Sodium (Concurrent use of levocetirizine dihydrochloride with other central nervous system depressants should be avoided because additional reductions in alertness and additional impairment of central nervous system performance may occur).
No products indexed under this heading.

Thioridazine Hydrochloride (Concurrent use of levocetirizine dihydrochloride with other central nervous system depressants should be avoided because additional reductions in alertness and additional impairment of central nervous system performance may occur). Products include:
Thioridazine Hydrochloride Tablets 2195

Thiothixene (Concurrent use of levocetirizine dihydrochloride with other central nervous system depressants should be avoided because additional reductions in alertness and additional impairment of central nervous system performance may occur). Products include:
Thiothixene Capsules 2197

Triazolam (Concurrent use of levocetirizine dihydrochloride with other central nervous system depressants should be avoided because additional reductions in alertness and additional impairment of central nervous system performance may occur).
No products indexed under this heading.

Trifluoperazine Hydrochloride (Concurrent use of levocetirizine dihydrochloride with other central nervous system depressants should be avoided because additional reductions in alertness and additional impairment of central nervous system performance may occur).
No products indexed under this heading.

Zaleplon (Concurrent use of levocetirizine dihydrochloride with other central nervous system depressants should be avoided because additional reductions in alertness and additional impairment of central nervous system performance may occur).
No products indexed under this heading.

Ziprasidone Hydrochloride (Concurrent use of levocetirizine dihydrochloride with other central nervous system depressants should be avoided because additional reductions in alertness and additional impairment of central nervous system performance may occur). Products include:
Geodon Capsules 2520

Zolpidem Tartrate (Concurrent use of levocetirizine dihydrochloride with other central nervous system depressants should be avoided because additional reductions in alertness and additional impairment of central nervous system performance may occur). Products include:
Ambien Tablets 2692
Ambien CR Tablets 2696

Food Interactions

Alcohol (Concurrent use of levocetirizine dihydrochloride with alcohol because additional reductions in alertness and additional impairment of central nervous system performance may occur).

XYZAL TABLETS

(Levocetirizine Dihydrochloride) 3155
May interact with:

Ritonavir (Ritonavir increased the plasma AUC of cetirizine by about 42% accompanied by an increase in half-life (53%) and a decrease in clearance (29%) of cetirizine. The disposition of ritonavir was not altered by concomitant cetirizine administration). Products include:
Kaletra 452
Norvir 489

XYZAL TABLETS

(Levocetirizine Dihydrochloride) 2789
May interact with:

Ritonavir (Ritonavir increased the plasma AUC of cetirizine by about 42% accompanied by an increase in half-life (53%) and a decrease in clearance (29%) of cetirizine. The disposition of ritonavir was not altered by concomitant cetirizine administration). Products include:
Kaletra 452
Norvir 489

YAZ TABLETS

(Drospirenone, Ethinyl Estradiol) 805
May interact with ACE inhibitors, aldosterone-inhibiting diuretic agents, angiotensin-II receptor antagonists, anticonvulsants, non-steroidal anti-inflammatory agents, potassium preparations, prednisolone, potassium sparing diuretics, tetracyclines, theophyllines, and certain other agents. Compounds in these categories include:

Acetaminophen (Ascorbic acid and acetaminophen may increase plasma concentrations of some synthetic estrogents, possibly by inhibition of conjugation. Decreased plasma concentrations of acetaminophen have been noted when administered with oral contraceptives). Products include:
Benadryl Allergy & Cold Kapgels 1895
Benadryl Allergy & Sinus Headache Kapgels 1895
Benadryl Severe Allergy & Sinus Headache Caplets 1897
Lortab 5/500 Tablets 3143
Lortab 7.5/500 Tablets 3144
Lortab 10/500 Tablets 3144
Percocet Tablets 1127
Sinutab Sinus Caplets 1905
Sudafed PE Cold & Cough Caplets 1907
Sudafed PE Nighttime Cold Caplets 1907
Sudafed PE Severe Cold Caplets 1908
Sudafed PE Sinus Headache Caplets 1908
Regular Strength Tylenol Tablets 1915
Tylenol 8 Hour Extended Release Caplets 1915
Extra Strength Tylenol Caplets, Cool Caplets, and EZ Tabs 1915
Extra Strength Tylenol Adult Rapid Blast Liquid 1915
Extra Strength Tylenol PM Caplets, Geltabs, Liquid, and Rapid Release Gels 1915
Extra Strength Tylenol Rapid Release Gels 1915
Tylenol with Codeine Tablets 2427
Tylenol Allergy Multi-Symptom Caplets with Cool Burst and Rapid Release Gelcaps 1916
Tylenol Allergy Multi-Symptom Nighttime Caplets with Cool Burst 1916
Tylenol Severe Allergy Caplets 1916
Tylenol Arthritis Pain Extended Release Geltabs/Caplets 1915
Tylenol Chest Congestion Caplets with Cool Burst 1910
Tylenol Chest Congestion Liquid with Cool Burst 1910
Children's Tylenol Plus Cold Suspension Liquid 1912
Children's Tylenol Plus Cold & Allergy Suspension Liquid 1914
Children's Tylenol Plus Cough & Runny Nose Suspension Liquid 1912
Children's Tylenol Plus Cough & Sore Throat Suspension Liquid 1912
Children's Tylenol Plus Flu Suspension Liquid 1914
Children's Tylenol Suspension Liquid 1909
Children's Tylenol Meltaways 1909
Children's Tylenol Plus Multi-Symptom Cold Suspension Liquid 1912
Tylenol Cold Severe Congestion Daytime Caplets with Cool Burst 1912
Tylenol Cold Head Congestion Daytime Caplets with Cool Burst 1910
Tylenol Cold Head Congestion Nighttime Caplets with Cool Burst 1910
Tylenol Cold Head Congestion Severe Daytime Caplets with Cool Burst 1910
Tylenol Cold Multi-Symptom Daytime Caplets with Cool Burst and Rapid Release Gels 1913
Tylenol Cold Multi-Symptom Daytime Liquid with Citrus Burst 1913
Tylenol Cold Multi-Symptom Nighttime Caplets with Cool Burst 1913
Tylenol Cold Multi-Symptom Nighttime Liquid with Cool Burst 1913
Tylenol Cold Multi-Symptom Severe Caplets with Cool Burst 1913
Tylenol Cold Multi-Symptom Severe Daytime Liquid with Citrus Burst 1913
Tylenol Cough & Sore Throat Daytime Liquid with Cool Burst 1918
Tylenol Cough & Sore Throat Nighttime Liquid with Cool Burst 1918
Concentrated Tylenol Infants' Drops 1909
Jr. Tylenol Meltaways 1909
Tylenol Sinus Congestion & Pain Daytime Caplets with Cool Burst and Gelcaps 1917
Tylenol Sinus Congestion & Pain Nighttime Caplets with Cool Burst 1917
Tylenol Sinus Congestion & Pain Severe Caplets with Cool Burst 1917
Tylenol Sinus Severe Congestion Caplets with Cool Burst 1917
Tylenol Sore Throat Daytime Liquid with Cool Burst 1918
Tylenol Sore Throat Nighttime Liquid with Cool Burst 1918
Women's Tylenol Menstrual Relief Caplets 1919
Vicks DayQuil Cold & Flu Multi-Symptom Relief .... ▣616
Vicks DayQuil LiquiCaps 2567
Vicks DayQuil Liquid 2567
Vicks DayQuil Multi-Symptom Cold/Flu Relief 2567
Vicks NyQuil Cold & Flu Multi-Symptom Relief .... ▣617
Vicks NyQuil LiquiCaps 2567

Vicks NyQuil Liquid 2567
Vicks NyQuil Multi-Symptom Cold/Flu Relief 2567
Vicodin Tablets 529
Vicodin ES Tablets 530
Vicodin HP Tablets 531
Zydone Tablets 1132

Amiloride Hydrochloride (YAZ has the potential to cause hyperkalemia in high-risk patients; co-administration with other drugs that have the potential to increase serum potassium, such as potassium-sparing diuretics, may increase the risk further).
No products indexed under this heading.

Ampicillin (Pregnancy while taking combined hormonal contraceptives has been reported when the combined hormonal contraceptives were administered with antimicrobials such as ampicillin).
No products indexed under this heading.

Ampicillin Sodium (Pregnancy while taking combined hormonal contraceptives has been reported when the combined hormonal contraceptives were administered with antimicrobials such as ampicillin).
No products indexed under this heading.

Ampicillin Trihydrate (Pregnancy while taking combined hormonal contraceptives has been reported when the combined hormonal contraceptives were administered with antimicrobials such as ampicillin).
No products indexed under this heading.

Ascorbic Acid (Ascorbic acid and acetaminophen may increase plasma concentrations of some synthetic estrogens, possibly by inhibition of conjugation).
No products indexed under this heading.

Atorvastatin Calcium (Co-administration of atorvastatin and an oral contraceptive increased AUC values for norethindrone and ethinyl estradiol by approximately 30% and 20%, respectively). Products include:
Lipitor Tablets 2501

Benazepril Hydrochloride (YAZ has the potential to cause hyperkalemia in high-risk patients; co-administration with other drugs that have the potential to increase serum potassium, such as ACE inhibitors, may increase the risk further).
No products indexed under this heading.

Candesartan Cilexetil (YAZ has the potential to cause hyperkalemia in high-risk patients; co-administration with other drugs that have the potential to increase serum potassium, such as angiotensin-II receptor antagonists, may increase the risk further). Products include:
Atacand Tablets 639
Atacand HCT 642

Captopril (YAZ has the potential to cause hyperkalemia in high-risk patients; co-administration with other drugs that have the potential to increase serum potassium, such as ACE inhibitors, may increase the risk further). Products include:
Captopril Tablets 2182

Carbamazepine (Co-administration results in increased metabolism of ethinyl estradiol and/or some progestins which could result in a reduction of contraceptive effectiveness). Products include:
Carbatrol Capsules 3019
Equetro Extended-Release Capsules 3174

Celecoxib (YAZ has the potential to cause hyperkalemia in high-risk patients; co-administration with other drugs that have the potential to increase serum potassium, such as NSAIDs, may increase the risk further). Products include:
Celebrex Capsules 2979

Clofibrate (Co-administration of products containing ethinyl estradiol may increase clearance of clofibric acid).
No products indexed under this heading.

Clofibric Acid (Increased clearance of clofibric acid has been noted when administered with oral contraceptives).
No products indexed under this heading.

Cyclosporine (Increased plasma concentrations of cyclosporine have been reported with concomitant administration of oral contraceptives). Products include:
Gengraf Capsules 435
Neoral Oral Solution 2280
Neoral Soft Gelatin Capsules 2280
Restasis Ophthalmic Emulsion 557
Sandimmune 2296

Demeclocycline Hydrochloride (Pregnancy while taking combined hormonal contraceptives has been reported when the combined hormonal contraceptives were administered with antimicrobials such as tetracycline).
No products indexed under this heading.

Diclofenac Epolamine (YAZ has the potential to cause hyperkalemia in high-risk patients; co-administration with other drugs that have the potential to increase serum potassium, such as NSAIDs, may increase the risk further). Products include:
Flector Patch 561

Diclofenac Potassium (YAZ has the potential to cause hyperkalemia in high-risk patients; co-administration with other drugs that have the potential to increase serum potassium, such as NSAIDs, may increase the risk further).
No products indexed under this heading.

Diclofenac Sodium (YAZ has the potential to cause hyperkalemia in high-risk patients; co-administration with other drugs that have the potential to increase serum potassium, such as NSAIDs, may increase the risk further). Products include:
Diclofenac Sodium Ophthalmic Solution .... ⊙240
Voltaren Ophthalmic Solution 2336
Voltaren Tablets 2334
Voltaren-XR Tablets 2337

Divalproex Sodium (Anticonvulsants have been shown to increase the metabolism of ethinyl estradiol and/or some progestins, which could result in a reduction of contraceptive effectiveness). Products include:
Depakote ER Tablets 423

Doxycycline Calcium (Pregnancy while taking combined hormonal contraceptives has been reported when the combined hormonal contraceptives were administered with antimicrobials such as tetracycline).
No products indexed under this heading.

Doxycycline Hyclate (Pregnancy while taking combined hormonal contraceptives has been reported when the combined hormonal contraceptives were administered with antimicrobials such as tetracycline).
No products indexed under this heading.

Doxycycline Monohydrate (Pregnancy while taking combined hormonal contraceptives has been reported when the combined hormonal contraceptives were administered with antimicrobials such as tetracycline).
No products indexed under this heading.

Enalapril Maleate (YAZ has the potential to cause hyperkalemia in high-risk patients; co-administration with other drugs that have the potential to increase serum potassium, such as ACE inhibitors, may increase the risk further).
No products indexed under this heading.

Enalaprilat (YAZ has the potential to cause hyperkalemia in high-risk patients; co-administration with other drugs that have the potential to increase serum potassium, such as ACE inhibitors, may increase the risk further).
No products indexed under this heading.

Eprosartan Mesylate (YAZ has the potential to cause hyperkalemia in high-risk patients; co-administration with other drugs that have the potential to increase serum potassium, such as angiotensin-II receptor antagonists, may increase the risk further). Products include:
Teveten Tablets 515
Teveten HCT Tablets 517

Ethosuximide (Anticonvulsants have been shown to increase the metabolism of ethinyl estradiol and/or some progestins, which could result in a reduction of contraceptive effectiveness).
No products indexed under this heading.

Ethotoin (Anticonvulsants have been shown to increase the metabolism of ethinyl estradiol and/or some progestins, which could result in a reduction of contraceptive effectiveness).
No products indexed under this heading.

Etodolac (YAZ has the potential to cause hyperkalemia in high-risk patients; co-administration with other drugs that have the potential to increase serum potassium, such as NSAIDs, may increase the risk further).
No products indexed under this heading.

Felbamate (Anticonvulsants have been shown to increase the metabolism of ethinyl estradiol and/or some progestins, which could result in a reduction of contraceptive effectiveness).
No products indexed under this heading.

Fenoprofen Calcium (YAZ has the potential to cause hyperkalemia in high-risk patients; co-administration with other drugs that have the potential to increase serum potassium, such as NSAIDs, may increase the risk further). Products include:
Nalfon Capsules 2508

Flurbiprofen (YAZ has the potential to cause hyperkalemia in high-risk patients; co-administration with other drugs that have the potential to increase serum potassium, such as NSAIDs, may increase the risk further).
No products indexed under this heading.

Fosinopril Sodium (YAZ has the potential to cause hyperkalemia in high-risk patients; co-administration with other drugs that have the potential to increase serum potassium, such as ACE inhibitors, may increase the risk further).
No products indexed under this heading.

Fosphenytoin (Anticonvulsants have been shown to increase the metabolism of ethinyl estradiol and/or some progestins, which could result in a reduction of contraceptive effectiveness).
No products indexed under this heading.

Gabapentin (Anticonvulsants have been shown to increase the metabolism of ethinyl estradiol and/or some progestins, which could result in a reduction of contraceptive effectiveness).
No products indexed under this heading.

Griseofulvin (Pregnancy while taking combined hormonal contraceptives has been reported when the combined hormonal contraceptives were administered with antimicrobials such as griseofulvin). Products include:
Gris-PEG Tablets 2507

Heparin Calcium (YAZ has the potential to cause hyperkalemia in high-risk patients; co-administration with other drugs that have the potential to increase serum potassium, such as heparin, may increase the risk further).
No products indexed under this heading.

Heparin Sodium (YAZ has the potential to cause hyperkalemia in high-risk patients; co-administration with other drugs that have the potential to increase serum potassium, such as heparin, may increase the risk further).
No products indexed under this heading.

Hypericum (Herbal products containing St. John's Wort may induce hepatic enzyme and p-glycoprotein transporter and may reduce the effectiveness of oral contraceptives and emergency contraceptive pills. This may also result in breakthrough bleeding). Products include:
Satieté Tablets .... ▣640

Hypericum Perforatum (Herbal products containing St. John's Wort may induce hepatic enzyme and p-glycoprotein transporter and may reduce the effectiveness of oral contraceptives and emergency contraceptive pills. This may also result in breakthrough bleeding).
No products indexed under this heading.

Ibuprofen (YAZ has the potential to cause hyperkalemia in high-risk patients; co-administration with other drugs that have the potential to increase serum potassium, such as NSAIDs, may increase the risk further). Products include:

Motrin IB Tablets and Caplets 1900
Children's Motrin Oral Suspension ... 1901
Children's Motrin Non-Staining Dye-Free Oral Suspension............ 1901
Children's Motrin Cold Oral Suspension 1899
Infants' Motrin Concentrated Drops.................................... 1901
Infants' Motrin Non-Staining Dye-Free Concentrated Drops....... 1901
Junior Strength Motrin Caplets and Chewable Tablets.................. 1901
Vicoprofen Tablets 533

Indomethacin (YAZ has the potential to cause hyperkalemia in high-risk patients; co-administration with other drugs that have the potential to increase serum potassium, such as NSAIDs, may increase the risk further). Products include:

Indocin 2024

Indomethacin Sodium Trihydrate (YAZ has the potential to cause hyperkalemia in high-risk patients; co-administration with other drugs that have the potential to increase serum potassium, such as NSAIDs, may increase the risk further). Products include:

Indocin I.V. 2489

Irbesartan (YAZ has the potential to cause hyperkalemia in high-risk patients; co-administration with other drugs that have the potential to increase serum potassium, such as angiotensin-II receptor antagonists, may increase the risk further). Products include:

Avalide Tablets 892
Avalide Tablets 2713
Avapro Tablets 897
Avapro Tablets 2718

Ketoprofen (YAZ has the potential to cause hyperkalemia in high-risk patients; co-administration with other drugs that have the potential to increase serum potassium, such as NSAIDs, may increase the risk further).

No products indexed under this heading.

Ketorolac Tromethamine (YAZ has the potential to cause hyperkalemia in high-risk patients; co-administration with other drugs that have the potential to increase serum potassium, such as NSAIDs, may increase the risk further).

No products indexed under this heading.

Lamotrigine (Anticonvulsants have been shown to increase the metabolism of ethinyl estradiol and/or some progestins, which could result in a reduction of contraceptive effectiveness). Products include:

Lamictal 1488

Levetiracetam (Anticonvulsants have been shown to increase the metabolism of ethinyl estradiol and/or some progestins, which could result in a reduction of contraceptive effectiveness). Products include:

Keppra Injection 3137
Keppra Oral Solution 3131
Keppra Tablets 3131

Lisinopril (YAZ has the potential to cause hyperkalemia in high-risk patients; co-administration with other drugs that have the potential to increase serum potassium, such as ACE inhibitors, may increase the risk further). Products include:

Prinivil Tablets 2087
Prinzide Tablets 2092

Losartan Potassium (YAZ has the potential to cause hyperkalemia in high-risk patients; co-administration with other drugs that have the potential to increase serum potassium, such as angiotensin-II receptor antagonists, may increase the risk further). Products include:

Cozaar Tablets 1973

Low Molecular Weight Heparins (YAZ has the potential to cause hyperkalemia in high-risk patients; co-administration with other drugs that have the potential to increase serum potassium, such as heparin, may increase the risk further).

No products indexed under this heading.

Meclofenamate Sodium (YAZ has the potential to cause hyperkalemia in high-risk patients; co-administration with other drugs that have the potential to increase serum potassium, such as NSAIDs, may increase the risk further).

No products indexed under this heading.

Mefenamic Acid (YAZ has the potential to cause hyperkalemia in high-risk patients; co-administration with other drugs that have the potential to increase serum potassium, such as NSAIDs, may increase the risk further).

No products indexed under this heading.

Meloxicam (YAZ has the potential to cause hyperkalemia in high-risk patients; co-administration with other drugs that have the potential to increase serum potassium, such as NSAIDs, may increase the risk further). Products include:

Mobic Oral Suspension 863
Mobic Tablets 863

Mephenytoin (Anticonvulsants have been shown to increase the metabolism of ethinyl estradiol and/or some progestins, which could result in a reduction of contraceptive effectiveness).

No products indexed under this heading.

Methacycline Hydrochloride (Pregnancy while taking combined hormonal contraceptives has been reported when the combined hormonal contraceptives were administered with antimicrobials such as tetracycline).

No products indexed under this heading.

Methsuximide (Anticonvulsants have been shown to increase the metabolism of ethinyl estradiol and/or some progestins, which could result in a reduction of contraceptive effectiveness).

No products indexed under this heading.

Minocycline Hydrochloride (Minocycline-related changes in estradiol, progesterone, FSH, and LH plasma levels, breakthrough bleeding, or contraceptive failure cannot be ruled out). Products include:

Solodyn Extended Release Tablets.. 1938

Moexipril Hydrochloride (YAZ has the potential to cause hyperkalemia in high-risk patients; co-administration with other drugs that have the potential to increase serum potassium, such as ACE inhibitors, may increase the risk further).

No products indexed under this heading.

Morphine Sulfate (Increased clearance of morphine has been noted when administered with oral contraceptives). Products include:

Avinza Capsules 1772
DepoDur Injection 1095
MS Contin Tablets 2585

Morphine sulfate, liposomal (Increased clearance of morphine has been noted when administered with oral contraceptives).

No products indexed under this heading.

Nabumetone (YAZ has the potential to cause hyperkalemia in high-risk patients; co-administration with other drugs that have the potential to increase serum potassium, such as NSAIDs, may increase the risk further).

No products indexed under this heading.

Naproxen (YAZ has the potential to cause hyperkalemia in high-risk patients; co-administration with other drugs that have the potential to increase serum potassium, such as NSAIDs, may increase the risk further). Products include:

EC-Naprosyn Delayed-Release Tablets... 2632
Naprosyn Suspension 2632
Naprosyn Tablets 2632

Naproxen Sodium (YAZ has the potential to cause hyperkalemia in high-risk patients; co-administration with other drugs that have the potential to increase serum potassium, such as NSAIDs, may increase the risk further). Products include:

Anaprox Tablets 2632
Anaprox DS Tablets 2632
Treximet Tablets 1616

Oxaprozin (YAZ has the potential to cause hyperkalemia in high-risk patients; co-administration with other drugs that have the potential to increase serum potassium, such as NSAIDs, may increase the risk further).

No products indexed under this heading.

Oxcarbazepine (Anticonvulsants have been shown to increase the metabolism of ethinyl estradiol and/or some progestins, which could result in a reduction of contraceptive effectiveness).

No products indexed under this heading.

Oxytetracycline Hydrochloride (Pregnancy while taking combined hormonal contraceptives has been reported when the combined hormonal contraceptives were administered with antimicrobials such as tetracycline).

No products indexed under this heading.

Paramethadione (Anticonvulsants have been shown to increase the metabolism of ethinyl estradiol and/or some progestins, which could result in a reduction of contraceptive effectiveness).

No products indexed under this heading.

Perindopril Erbumine (YAZ has the potential to cause hyperkalemia in high-risk patients; co-administration with other drugs that have the potential to increase serum potassium, such as ACE inhibitors, may increase the risk further). Products include:

Aceon Tablets (2 mg, 4 mg, 8 mg)... 3038

Phenacemide (Anticonvulsants have been shown to increase the metabolism of ethinyl estradiol and/or some progestins, which could result in a reduction of contraceptive effectiveness).

No products indexed under this heading.

Phenobarbital (Co-administration results in increased metabolism of ethinyl estradiol and/or some progestins which could result in a reduction of contraceptive effectiveness). Products include:

Donnatal Extentabs 2507

Phensuximide (Anticonvulsants have been shown to increase the metabolism of ethinyl estradiol and/or some progestins, which could result in a reduction of contraceptive effectiveness).

No products indexed under this heading.

Phenylbutazone (A reduction in contraceptive effectiveness and an increased incidence of menstrual irregularities has been suggested with phenylbutazone).

No products indexed under this heading.

Piroxicam (YAZ has the potential to cause hyperkalemia in high-risk patients; co-administration with other drugs that have the potential to increase serum potassium, such as NSAIDs, may increase the risk further).

No products indexed under this heading.

Potassium Acid Phosphate (YAZ has the potential to cause hyperkalemia in high-risk patients; co-administration with other drugs that have the potential to increase serum potassium, such as potassium supplementation, may increase the risk further). Products include:

K-Phos Original (Sodium Free) Tablets... 814

Potassium Bicarbonate (YAZ has the potential to cause hyperkalemia in high-risk patients; co-administration with other drugs that have the potential to increase serum potassium, such as potassium supplementation, may increase the risk further).

No products indexed under this heading.

Potassium Chloride (YAZ has the potential to cause hyperkalemia in high-risk patients; co-administration with other drugs that have the potential to increase serum potassium, such as potassium supplementation, may increase the risk further). Products include:

MoviPrep Oral Solution 2679

Potassium Citrate (YAZ has the potential to cause hyperkalemia in high-risk patients; co-administration with other drugs that have the potential to increase serum potassium, such as potassium supplementation, may increase the risk further). Products include:

BioLean Free Tablets 635
Urocit-K Tablets 2176

Potassium Gluconate (YAZ has the potential to cause hyperkalemia in high-risk patients; co-administration with other drugs that have the potential to increase serum potassium, such as potassium supplementation, may increase the risk further).
No products indexed under this heading.

Potassium Phosphate (YAZ has the potential to cause hyperkalemia in high-risk patients; co-administration with other drugs that have the potential to increase serum potassium, such as potassium supplementation, may increase the risk further). Products include:
K-Phos Neutral Tablets 813

Prednisolone (Increased plasma concentrations of prednisolone have been reported with concomitant administration of oral contraceptives).
No products indexed under this heading.

Prednisolone Acetate (Increased plasma concentrations of prednisolone have been reported with concomitant administration of oral contraceptives). Products include:
Pred Forte Ophthalmic Suspension .... ⊙ 227
Pred Mild Ophthalmic Suspension .... ⊙ 230
Pred-G Ophthalmic Ointment .... ⊙ 229
Pred-G Ophthalmic Suspension ...... ⊙ 228

Prednisolone Sodium Phosphate (Increased plasma concentrations of prednisolone have been reported with concomitant administration of oral contraceptives).
No products indexed under this heading.

Prednisolone Tebutate (Increased plasma concentrations of prednisolone have been reported with concomitant administration of oral contraceptives).
No products indexed under this heading.

Primidone (Anticonvulsants have been shown to increase the metabolism of ethinyl estradiol and/or some progestins, which could result in a reduction of contraceptive effectiveness).
No products indexed under this heading.

Quinapril Hydrochloride (YAZ has the potential to cause hyperkalemia in high-risk patients; co-administration with other drugs that have the potential to increase serum potassium, such as ACE inhibitors, may increase the risk further).
No products indexed under this heading.

Ramipril (YAZ has the potential to cause hyperkalemia in high-risk patients; co-administration with other drugs that have the potential to increase serum potassium, such as ACE inhibitors, may increase the risk further).
No products indexed under this heading.

Rifampin (Co-administration results in increased metabolism of ethinyl estradiol precipitating a reduction in contraceptive effectiveness and an increase in menstrual irregularities).
No products indexed under this heading.

Rofecoxib (YAZ has the potential to cause hyperkalemia in high-risk patients; co-administration with other drugs that have the potential to increase serum potassium, such as NSAIDs, may increase the risk further).
No products indexed under this heading.

Salicylic Acid (Increased clearance of salicylic acid has been noted when administered with oral contraceptives).
No products indexed under this heading.

Spirapril Hydrochloride (YAZ has the potential to cause hyperkalemia in high-risk patients; co-administration with other drugs that have the potential to increase serum potassium, such as ACE inhibitors, may increase the risk further).
No products indexed under this heading.

Spironolactone (YAZ has the potential to cause hyperkalemia in high-risk patients; co-administration with other drugs that have the potential to increase serum potassium, such as aldosterone antagonists, may increase the risk further).
No products indexed under this heading.

Sulindac (YAZ has the potential to cause hyperkalemia in high-risk patients; co-administration with other drugs that have the potential to increase serum potassium, such as NSAIDs, may increase the risk further). Products include:
Clinoril Tablets 1962

Telmisartan (YAZ has the potential to cause hyperkalemia in high-risk patients; co-administration with other drugs that have the potential to increase serum potassium, such as angiotensin-II receptor antagonists, may increase the risk further). Products include:
Micardis Tablets 852
Micardis HCT Tablets 854

Temazepam (Increased clearance of temazepam has been noted when administered with oral contraceptives).
No products indexed under this heading.

Tetracycline Hydrochloride (Pregnancy while taking combined hormonal contraceptives has been reported when the combined hormonal contraceptives were administered with antimicrobials such as tetracycline). Products include:
Pylera Capsules 714

Theophylline (Increased plasma concentrations of theophylline have been reported with concomitant administration of oral contraceptives).
No products indexed under this heading.

Theophylline Anhydrous (Increased plasma concentrations of theophylline have been reported with concomitant administration of oral contraceptives). Products include:
Uniphyl Tablets 2595

Theophylline Calcium Salicylate (Increased plasma concentrations of theophylline have been reported with concomitant administration of oral contraceptives).
No products indexed under this heading.

Theophylline Dihydroxypropyl (Glyceryl) (Increased plasma concentrations of theophylline have been reported with concomitant administration of oral contraceptives).
No products indexed under this heading.

Theophylline Ethylenediamine (Increased plasma concentrations of theophylline have been reported with concomitant administration of oral contraceptives).
No products indexed under this heading.

Theophylline Sodium Glycinate (Increased plasma concentrations of theophylline have been reported with concomitant administration of oral contraceptives).
No products indexed under this heading.

Tiagabine Hydrochloride (Anticonvulsants have been shown to increase the metabolism of ethinyl estradiol and/or some progestins, which could result in a reduction of contraceptive effectiveness). Products include:
Gabitril Tablets 973

Tolmetin Sodium (YAZ has the potential to cause hyperkalemia in high-risk patients; co-administration with other drugs that have the potential to increase serum potassium, such as NSAIDs, may increase the risk further).
No products indexed under this heading.

Topiramate (Anticonvulsants have been shown to increase the metabolism of ethinyl estradiol and/or some progestins, which could result in a reduction of contraceptive effectiveness).
No products indexed under this heading.

Trandolapril (YAZ has the potential to cause hyperkalemia in high-risk patients; co-administration with other drugs that have the potential to increase serum potassium, such as ACE inhibitors, may increase the risk further). Products include:
Mavik Tablets 472
Tarka Tablets 511

Triamterene (YAZ has the potential to cause hyperkalemia in high-risk patients; co-administration with other drugs that have the potential to increase serum potassium, such as potassium-sparing diuretics, may increase the risk further). Products include:
Dyazide Capsules 1405
Dyrenium Capsules 3189

Trimethadione (Anticonvulsants have been shown to increase the metabolism of ethinyl estradiol and/or some progestins, which could result in a reduction of contraceptive effectiveness).
No products indexed under this heading.

Valdecoxib (YAZ has the potential to cause hyperkalemia in high-risk patients; co-administration with other drugs that have the potential to increase serum potassium, such as NSAIDs, may increase the risk further).
No products indexed under this heading.

Valproate Sodium (Anticonvulsants have been shown to increase the metabolism of ethinyl estradiol and/or some progestins, which could result in a reduction of contraceptive effectiveness).
No products indexed under this heading.

Valproic Acid (Anticonvulsants have been shown to increase the metabolism of ethinyl estradiol and/or some progestins, which could result in a reduction of contraceptive effectiveness).
No products indexed under this heading.

Valsartan (YAZ has the potential to cause hyperkalemia in high-risk patients; co-administration with other drugs that have the potential to increase serum potassium, such as angiotensin-II receptor antagonists, may increase the risk further). Products include:
Diovan Tablets 2212
Diovan HCT Tablets 2216
Exforge Tablets 2238

Vitamin C (May increase plasma levels of ethinyl estradiol possibly by inhibition of conjugation). Products include:
Bausch & Lomb Ocuvite Adult 50+ Vitamin and Mineral Supplement................................ ⊙ 237
Comax Dietary Supplement 995
Ferralet 90 Tablets 2175
Glaucofit Dietary Supplement 995
Glauma Dietary Supplement 995
MoviPrep Oral Solution 2679
Procosa II Tablets 3174
Proflavanol 90 Tablets 3174
Tonox Dietary Supplement 995
Vibe Liquid Multi-Nutrient Supplement 626

Zonisamide (Anticonvulsants have been shown to increase the metabolism of ethinyl estradiol and/or some progestins, which could result in a reduction of contraceptive effectiveness). Products include:
Zonegran Capsules 1089

YOUTHGENES SPRAY
(Placenta factor) 564
None cited in PDR database.

ZANTAC 75 TABLETS
(Ranitidine Hydrochloride) 603
None cited in PDR database.

ZANTAC 25 EFFERDOSE TABLETS
(Ranitidine Hydrochloride) 1670
See Zantac 150 Tablets

ZANTAC INJECTION
(Ranitidine Hydrochloride) 1666
See Zantac 150 Tablets

ZANTAC INJECTION PHARMACY BULK PACKAGE
(Ranitidine Hydrochloride) 1668
May interact with:

Atazanavir Sulfate (The bioavailability of certain drugs may be affected by the alteration of gastric pH. This can result in a decrease in atazanavir absorption). Products include:
Reyataz Capsules 3299

Delaviridine (The bioavailability of certain drugs may be affected by the alteration of gastric pH. This can result in a decrease in delavirdine absorption).
No products indexed under this heading.

Gefitinib (The bioavailability of certain drugs may be affected by the alteration of gastric pH. This can result in a decrease in gefitnib absorption).
No products indexed under this heading.

Glipizide (The bioavailability of certain drugs may be affected by the alteration of gastric pH. This can result in an increase in glipizide absorption).
No products indexed under this heading.

Ketoconazole (The bioavailability of certain drugs may be affected by the alteration of gastric pH. This can result in a decrease in ketoconazole absorption). Products include:
Extina Foam, 2% 3057
Nizoral A-D Shampoo 1901

Midazolam Hydrochloride (The bioavailability of certain drugs may be affected by the alteration of gastric pH. This can result in an increase in midazolam absorption).
No products indexed under this heading.

Procainamide Hydrochloride (Ranitidine may affect the clearance of other drugs eliminated by cationic system. High doses of ranitidine (eg, such as those used in the treatment of Zollinger-Ellison syndrome) may reduce the excretion of procainamide and N-acetylprocainamide resulting in increased plasma levels of these drugs).
No products indexed under this heading.

Triazolam (The bioavailability of certain drugs may be affected by the alteration of gastric pH. This can result in an increase in triazolam absorption).
No products indexed under this heading.

Warfarin Sodium (Potential for increased or decreased prothrombin time. Due to the narrow therapeutic index, close monitoring of increased or decreased prothrombin time is recommended during concurrent treatment with ranitidine).
No products indexed under this heading.

ZANTAC INJECTION PREMIXED
(Ranitidine Hydrochloride) 1666
See Zantac 150 Tablets

MAXIMUM STRENGTH ZANTAC 150 TABLETS
(Ranitidine Hydrochloride) .... ▣603
None cited in PDR database.

MAXIMUM STRENGTH ZANTAC 150 COOL MINT TABLETS
(Ranitidine Hydrochloride) .... ▣603
None cited in PDR database.

ZANTAC SYRUP
(Ranitidine Hydrochloride) 1670
See Zantac 150 Tablets

ZANTAC 150 TABLETS
(Ranitidine Hydrochloride) 1670
May interact with:

Atazanavir Sulfate (The bioavailability of certain drugs may be affected by the alteration of gastric pH. This can result in an increase in atazanavir absorption). Products include:
Reyataz Capsules 3299

Delaviridine (The bioavailability of certain drugs may be affected by the alteration of gastric pH. This can result in an increase in delaviridine absorption).
No products indexed under this heading.

Gefitinib (The bioavailability of certain drugs may be affected by the alteration of gastric pH. This can result in an increase in gefitnib absorption).
No products indexed under this heading.

Glipizide (The bioavailability of certain drugs may be affected by the alteration of gastric pH. This can result in an increase in glipizide absorption).
No products indexed under this heading.

Ketoconazole (The bioavailability of certain drugs may be affected by the alteration of gastric pH. This can result in an increase in ketoconazole absorption). Products include:
Extina Foam, 2% 3057
Nizoral A-D Shampoo 1901

Midazolam Hydrochloride (The bioavailability of certain drugs may be affected by the alteration of gastric pH. This can result in an increase in midazolam absorption).
No products indexed under this heading.

Procainamide Hydrochloride (Ranitidine may affect the clearance of other drugs eliminated by cationic system. High doses of ranitidine (eg, such as those used in the treatment of Zollinger-Ellison syndrome) may reduce the excretion of procainamide and N-acetylprocainamide resulting in increased plasma levels of these drugs).
No products indexed under this heading.

Triazolam (The bioavailability of certain drugs may be affected by the alteration of gastric pH. This can result in an increase in triazolam absorption).
No products indexed under this heading.

Warfarin Sodium (There have been reports of altered prothrombin time with coumarin anticoagulants (eg, warfarin). Due to the narrow therapeutic index, close monitoring of altered prothrombin time is recommended during concurrent treatment with ranitidine).
No products indexed under this heading.

ZANTAC 300 TABLETS
(Ranitidine Hydrochloride) 1670
See Zantac 150 Tablets

ZEEL INJECTION SOLUTION
(Homeopathic Formulations) 1726
None cited in PDR database.

ZEMPLAR CAPSULES
(Paricalcitol) 536
May interact with cytochrome p450 3a4 inhibitors, potent and certain other agents. Compounds in these categories include:

Amprenavir (A study has demonstrated that ketoconazole approximately doubled paricalcitol AUC. Since paricalcitol is partially metabolized by CYP3A and ketoconazole is known to be a strong inhibitor of cytochrome P450 3A enzyme, care should be taken while dosing paricalcitol with ketoconazole and other strong P450 3A inhibitors. Dose adjustment of paricalcitol capsules may be required and iPTH and serum calcium concentrations should be closely monitored if a patient initiates or discontinues therapy with a strong CYP3A4 inhibitor, such as ketoconazole).
No products indexed under this heading.

Atazanavir (A study has demonstrated that ketoconazole approximately doubled paricalcitol AUC. Since paricalcitol is partially metabolized by CYP3A and ketoconazole is known to be a strong inhibitor of cytochrome P450 3A enzyme, care should be taken while dosing paricalcitol with ketoconazole and other strong P450 3A inhibitors. Dose adjustment of paricalcitol capsules may be required and iPTH and serum calcium concentrations should be closely monitored if a patient initiates or discontinues therapy with a strong CYP3A4 inhibitor, such as ketoconazole).
No products indexed under this heading.

Atazanavir Sulfate (A study has demonstrated that ketoconazole approximately doubled paricalcitol AUC. Since paricalcitol is partially metabolized by CYP3A and ketoconazole is known to be a strong inhibitor of cytochrome P450 3A enzyme, care should be taken while dosing paricalcitol with ketoconazole and other strong P450 3A inhibitors. Dose adjustment of paricalcitol capsules may be required and iPTH and serum calcium concentrations should be closely monitored if a patient initiates or discontinues therapy with a strong CYP3A4 inhibitor, such as ketoconazole). Products include:
Reyataz Capsules 3299

Cholestyramine (Drugs that impair intestinal absorption of fat-soluble vitamins, such as cholestyramine, may interfere with the absorption of paricalcitol).
No products indexed under this heading.

Clarithromycin (A study has demonstrated that ketoconazole approximately doubled paricalcitol AUC. Since paricalcitol is partially metabolized by CYP3A and ketoconazole is known to be a strong inhibitor of cytochrome P450 3A enzyme, care should be taken while dosing paricalcitol with ketoconazole and other strong P450 3A inhibitors. Dose adjustment of paricalcitol capsules may be required and iPTH and serum calcium concentrations should be closely monitored if a patient initiates or discontinues therapy with a strong CYP3A4 inhibitor, such as ketoconazole). Products include:
Biaxin/Biaxin XL 411

Delavirdine Mesylate (A study has demonstrated that ketoconazole approximately doubled paricalcitol AUC. Since paricalcitol is partially metabolized by CYP3A and ketoconazole is known to be a strong inhibitor of cytochrome P450 3A enzyme, care should be taken while dosing paricalcitol with ketoconazole and other strong P450 3A inhibitors. Dose adjustment of paricalcitol capsules may be required and iPTH and serum calcium concentrations should be closely monitored if a patient initiates or discontinues therapy with a strong CYP3A4 inhibitor, such as ketoconazole).
No products indexed under this heading.

Delavirine (A study has demonstrated that ketoconazole approximately doubled paricalcitol AUC. Since paricalcitol is partially metabolized by CYP3A and ketoconazole is known to be a strong inhibitor of cytochrome P450 3A enzyme, care should be taken while dosing paricalcitol with ketoconazole and other strong P450 3A inhibitors. Dose adjustment of paricalcitol capsules may be required and iPTH and serum calcium concentrations should be closely monitored if a patient initiates or discontinues therapy with a strong CYP3A4 inhibitor, such as ketoconazole).
No products indexed under this heading.

Fosamprenavir Calcium (A study has demonstrated that ketoconazole approximately doubled paricalcitol AUC. Since paricalcitol is partially metabolized by CYP3A and ketoconazole is known to be a strong inhibitor of cytochrome P450 3A enzyme, care should be taken while dosing paricalcitol with ketoconazole and other strong P450 3A inhibitors. Dose adjustment of paricalcitol capsules may be required and iPTH and serum calcium concentrations should be closely monitored if a patient initiates or discontinues therapy with a strong CYP3A4 inhibitor, such as ketoconazole). Products include:
Lexiva Oral Suspension 1510
Lexiva Tablets 1510

Indinavir Sulfate (A study has demonstrated that ketoconazole approximately doubled paricalcitol AUC. Since paricalcitol is partially metabolized by CYP3A and ketoconazole is known to be a strong inhibitor of cytochrome P450 3A enzyme, care should be taken while dosing paricalcitol with ketoconazole and other strong P450 3A inhibitors. Dose adjustment of paricalcitol capsules may be required and iPTH and serum calcium concentrations should be closely monitored if a patient initiates or discontinues therapy with a strong CYP3A4 inhibitor, such as ketoconazole). Products include:
Crixivan Capsules 1979

Itraconazole (A study has demonstrated that ketoconazole approximately doubled paricalcitol AUC. Since paricalcitol is partially metabolized by CYP3A and ketoconazole is known to be a strong inhibitor of cytochrome P450 3A enzyme, care should be taken while dosing paricalcitol with ketoconazole and other strong P450 3A inhibitors. Dose adjustment of paricalcitol capsules may be required and iPTH and serum calcium concentrations should be closely monitored if a patient initiates or discontinues therapy with a strong CYP3A4 inhibitor, such as ketoconazole).
No products indexed under this heading.

Ketoconazole (A study has demonstrated that ketoconazole approximately doubled paricalcitol AUC. Since paricalcitol is partially metabolized by CYP3A and ketoconazole is known to be a strong inhibitor of cytochrome P450 3A enzyme, care should be taken while dosing paricalcitol with ketoconazole and other strong P450 3A inhibitors. Dose adjustment of paricalcitol capsules may be required and iPTH and serum calcium concentrations should be closely monitored if a patient initiates or discontinues therapy with a strong CYP3A4 inhibitor, such as ketoconazole). Products include:

Extina Foam, 2% 3057
Nizoral A-D Shampoo 1901

Lopinavir (A study has demonstrated that ketoconazole approximately doubled paricalcitol AUC. Since paricalcitol is partially metabolized by CYP3A and ketoconazole is known to be a strong inhibitor of cytochrome P450 3A enzyme, care should be taken while dosing paricalcitol with ketoconazole and other strong P450 3A inhibitors. Dose adjustment of paricalcitol capsules may be required and iPTH and serum calcium concentrations should be closely monitored if a patient initiates or discontinues therapy with a strong CYP3A4 inhibitor, such as ketoconazole). Products include:

Kaletra 452

Nefazodone Hydrochloride (A study has demonstrated that ketoconazole approximately doubled paricalcitol AUC. Since paricalcitol is partially metabolized by CYP3A and ketoconazole is known to be a strong inhibitor of cytochrome P450 3A enzyme, care should be taken while dosing paricalcitol with ketoconazole and other strong P450 3A inhibitors. Dose adjustment of paricalcitol capsules may be required and iPTH and serum calcium concentrations should be closely monitored if a patient initiates or discontinues therapy with a strong CYP3A4 inhibitor, such as ketoconazole).

No products indexed under this heading.

Nelfinavir Mesylate (A study has demonstrated that ketoconazole approximately doubled paricalcitol AUC. Since paricalcitol is partially metabolized by CYP3A and ketoconazole is known to be a strong inhibitor of cytochrome P450 3A enzyme, care should be taken while dosing paricalcitol with ketoconazole and other strong P450 3A inhibitors. Dose adjustment of paricalcitol capsules may be required and iPTH and serum calcium concentrations should be closely monitored if a patient initiates or discontinues therapy with a strong CYP3A4 inhibitor, such as ketoconazole).

No products indexed under this heading.

Ritonavir (A study has demonstrated that ketoconazole approximately doubled paricalcitol AUC. Since paricalcitol is partially metabolized by CYP3A and ketoconazole is known to be a strong inhibitor of cytochrome P450 3A enzyme, care should be taken while dosing paricalcitol with ketoconazole and other strong P450 3A inhibitors. Dose adjustment of paricalcitol capsules may be required and iPTH and serum calcium concentrations should be closely monitored if a patient initiates or discontinues therapy with a strong CYP3A4 inhibitor, such as ketoconazole). Products include:

Kaletra 452
Norvir 489

Saquinavir (A study has demonstrated that ketoconazole approximately doubled paricalcitol AUC. Since paricalcitol is partially metabolized by CYP3A and ketoconazole is known to be a strong inhibitor of cytochrome P450 3A enzyme, care should be taken while dosing paricalcitol with ketoconazole and other strong P450 3A inhibitors. Dose adjustment of paricalcitol capsules may be required and iPTH and serum calcium concentrations should be closely monitored if a patient initiates or discontinues therapy with a strong CYP3A4 inhibitor, such as ketoconazole).

No products indexed under this heading.

Saquinavir Mesylate (A study has demonstrated that ketoconazole approximately doubled paricalcitol AUC. Since paricalcitol is partially metabolized by CYP3A and ketoconazole is known to be a strong inhibitor of cytochrome P450 3A enzyme, care should be taken while dosing paricalcitol with ketoconazole and other strong P450 3A inhibitors. Dose adjustment of paricalcitol capsules may be required and iPTH and serum calcium concentrations should be closely monitored if a patient initiates or discontinues therapy with a strong CYP3A4 inhibitor, such as ketoconazole).

No products indexed under this heading.

Telithromycin (A study has demonstrated that ketoconazole approximately doubled paricalcitol AUC. Since paricalcitol is partially metabolized by CYP3A and ketoconazole is known to be a strong inhibitor of cytochrome P450 3A enzyme, care should be taken while dosing paricalcitol with ketoconazole and other strong P450 3A inhibitors. Dose adjustment of paricalcitol capsules may be required and iPTH and serum calcium concentrations should be closely monitored if a patient initiates or discontinues therapy with a strong CYP3A4 inhibitor, such as ketoconazole). Products include:

Ketek Tablets 2744

Troleandomycin (A study has demonstrated that ketoconazole approximately doubled paricalcitol AUC. Since paricalcitol is partially metabolized by CYP3A and ketoconazole is known to be a strong inhibitor of cytochrome P450 3A enzyme, care should be taken while dosing paricalcitol with ketoconazole and other strong P450 3A inhibitors. Dose adjustment of paricalcitol capsules may be required and iPTH and serum calcium concentrations should be closely monitored if a patient initiates or discontinues therapy with a strong CYP3A4 inhibitor, such as ketoconazole).

No products indexed under this heading.

Voriconazole (A study has demonstrated that ketoconazole approximately doubled paricalcitol AUC. Since paricalcitol is partially metabolized by CYP3A and ketoconazole is known to be a strong inhibitor of cytochrome P450 3A enzyme, care should be taken while dosing paricalcitol with ketoconazole and other strong P450 3A inhibitors. Dose adjustment of paricalcitol capsules may be required and iPTH and serum calcium concentrations should be closely monitored if a patient initiates or discontinues therapy with a strong CYP3A4 inhibitor, such as ketoconazole).

No products indexed under this heading.

ZEMPLAR INJECTION

(Paricalcitol) 538

May interact with cardiac glycosides and certain other agents. Compounds in these categories include:

Atazanavir (Care should be taken while dosing paricalcitol with ketoconazole and other strong P450 3A inhibitiors including atazanavir, clarithromycin, indinavir, itraconazole, nefazodone, nelfinavir, ritonavir, saquinavir, telithromycin, or voriconazole due to a doubling of paricalcitol AUC and an increased mean half life when co-administered with these agents).

No products indexed under this heading.

Atazanavir Sulfate (Care should be taken while dosing paricalcitol with ketoconazole and other strong P450 3A inhibitiors including atazanavir, clarithromycin, indinavir, itraconazole, nefazodone, nelfinavir, ritonavir, saquinavir, telithromycin, or voriconazole due to a doubling of paricalcitol AUC and an increased mean half life when co-administered with these agents). Products include:

Reyataz Capsules 3299

Calcitriol (Vitamin D-related compounds should not be taken concomitantly with paricalcitol). Products include:

Calcijex Injection 419
Rocaltrol Capsules 1150
Rocaltrol Oral Solution 1150

Clarithromycin (Care should be taken while dosing paricalcitol with ketoconazole and other strong P450 3A inhibitiors including atazanavir, clarithromycin, indinavir, itraconazole, nefazodone, nelfinavir, ritonavir, saquinavir, telithromycin, or voriconazole due to a doubling of paricalcitol AUC and an increased mean half life when co-administered with these agents). Products include:

Biaxin/Biaxin XL 411

Deslanoside (Digitalis toxicity is potentiated by hypercalcemia of any cause, so caution should be applied when digitalis compounds are prescribed concomitantly with paricalcitol).

No products indexed under this heading.

Digitalis Glycoside Preparations (Digitalis toxicity is potentiated by hypercalcemia of any cause, so caution should be applied when digitalis compounds are prescribed concomitantly with paricalcitol).

No products indexed under this heading.

Digitoxin (Digitalis toxicity is potentiated by hypercalcemia of any cause, so caution should be applied when digitalis compounds are prescribed concomitantly with paricalcitol).

No products indexed under this heading.

Digoxin (Digitalis toxicity is potentiated by hypercalcemia of any cause, so caution should be applied when digitalis compounds are prescribed concomitantly with paricalcitol). Products include:

Lanoxin Injection 1498
Lanoxin Injection Pediatric 1502
Lanoxin Tablets 1505

Indinavir Sulfate (Care should be taken while dosing paricalcitol with ketoconazole and other strong P450 3A inhibitiors including atazanavir, clarithromycin, indinavir, itraconazole, nefazodone, nelfinavir, ritonavir, saquinavir, telithromycin, or voriconazole due to a doubling of paricalcitol AUC and an increased mean half life when co-administered with these agents). Products include:

Crixivan Capsules 1979

Itraconazole (Care should be taken while dosing paricalcitol with ketoconazole and other strong P450 3A inhibitiors including atazanavir, clarithromycin, indinavir, itraconazole, nefazodone, nelfinavir, ritonavir, saquinavir, telithromycin, or voriconazole due to a doubling of paricalcitol AUC and an increased mean half life when co-administered with these agents).

No products indexed under this heading.

Ketoconazole (Care should be taken while dosing paricalcitol with ketoconazole and other strong P450 3A inhibitiors including atazanavir, clarithromycin, indinavir, itraconazole, nefazodone, nelfinavir, ritonavir, saquinavir, telithromycin, or voriconazole due to a doubling of paricalcitol AUC and an increased mean half life when co-administered with these agents). Products include:

Extina Foam, 2% 3057
Nizoral A-D Shampoo 1901

Nefazodone Hydrochloride (Care should be taken while dosing paricalcitol with ketoconazole and other strong P450 3A inhibitiors including atazanavir, clarithromycin, indinavir, itraconazole, nefazodone, nelfinavir, ritonavir, saquinavir, telithromycin, or voriconazole due to a doubling of paricalcitol AUC and an increased mean half life when co-administered with these agents).

No products indexed under this heading.

Nelfinavir Mesylate (Care should be taken while dosing paricalcitol with ketoconazole and other strong P450 3A inhibitiors including atazanavir, clarithromycin, indinavir, itraconazole, nefazodone, nelfinavir, ritonavir, saquinavir, telithromycin, or voriconazole due to a doubling of paricalcitol AUC and an increased mean half life when co-administered with these agents).

No products indexed under this heading.

Potassium Acid Phosphate (Phosphate compounds should not be taken concomitantly with paricalcitol). Products include:

K-Phos Original (Sodium Free) Tablets 814

Potassium Phosphate (Phosphate compounds should not be taken concomitantly with paricalcitol). Products include:

K-Phos Neutral Tablets 813

Ritonavir (Care should be taken while dosing paricalcitol with ketoconazole and other strong P450 3A inhibitions including atazanavir, clarithromycin, indinavir, itraconazole, nefazodone, nelfinavir, ritonavir, saquinavir, telithromycin, or voriconazole due to a doubling of paricalcitol AUC and an increased

mean half life when co-administered with these agents). Products include:

Kaletra 452
Norvir 489

Saquinavir (Care should be taken while dosing paricalcitol with ketoconazole and other strong P450 3A inhibitiors including atazanavir, clarithromycin, indinavir, itraconazole, nefazodone, nelfinavir, ritonavir, saquinavir, telithromycin, or voriconazole due to a doubling of paricalcitol AUC and an increased mean half life when co-administered with these agents).

No products indexed under this heading.

Saquinavir Mesylate (Care should be taken while dosing paricalcitol with ketoconazole and other strong P450 3A inhibitors including atazanavir, clarithromycin, indinavir, itraconazole, nefazodone, nelfinavir, ritonavir, saquinavir, telithromycin, or voriconazole due to a doubling of paricalcitol AUC and an increased mean half life when co-administered with these agents).

No products indexed under this heading.

Telithromycin (Care should be taken while dosing paricalcitol with ketoconazole and other strong P450 3A inhibitiors including atazanavir, clarithromycin, indinavir, itraconazole, nefazodone, nelfinavir, ritonavir, saquinavir, telithromycin, or voriconazole due to a doubling of paricalcitol AUC and an increased mean half life when co-administered with these agents). Products include:

Ketek Tablets 2744

Voriconazole (Care should be taken while dosing paricalcitol with ketoconazole and other strong P450 3A inhibitiors including atazanavir, clarithromycin, indinavir, itraconazole, nefazodone, nelfinavir, ritonavir, saquinavir, telithromycin, or voriconazole due to a doubling of paricalcitol AUC and an increased mean half life when co-administered with these agents).

No products indexed under this heading.

ZEMURON INJECTION

(Rocuronium Bromide) 2947

May interact with aminoglycosides, barbiturates, anticonvulsants, inhalant anesthetics, lithium preparations, local anesthetics, nondepolarizing neuromuscular blocking agents, quinidine, tetracyclines, and certain other agents. Compounds in these categories include:

Alkaline Drugs (Rocuronium, which has an acid pH, should not be mixed with alkaline solutions (e.g., barbiturate solutions) in the same syringe or administered simultaneously during intravenous infusion through the same needle).

No products indexed under this heading.

Amikacin Sulfate (Drugs which may enhance the neuromuscular blocking action of rocuronium include certain antibiotics, such as aminoglyosides. If aminoglycosides are used in conjunction with rocuronium, prolongation of neuromuscular block should be considered a possibility. In patients in whom potentiation of neuromuscular block may be anticipated, a decrease from the recommended initial dose should be considered).

No products indexed under this heading.

Aprobarbital (Rocuronium, which has an acid pH, should not be mixed with alkaline solutions (eg, barbiturate solutions) in the same syringe or administered simultaneously during intravenous infusion through the same needle).

No products indexed under this heading.

Atracurium Besylate (There are no controlled studies documenting the use of rocuronium before or after other nondepolarizing muscle relaxants. Interactions have been observed when other nondepolarizing muscle relaxants have been administered in succession).

No products indexed under this heading.

Bacitracin (Drugs which may enhance the neuromuscular blocking action of rocuronium include certain antibiotics, such as bacitracin. If bacitracin is used in conjunction with rocuronium, prolongation of neuromuscular block should be considered a possibility. In patients in whom potentiation of neuromuscular block may be anticipated, a decrease from the recommended initial dose should be considered).

No products indexed under this heading.

Bupivacaine Hydrochloride (Local anesthetics have been shown to increase the duration of neuromuscular block and decrease infusion requirements of other neuromuscular blocking agents. In patients in whom potentiation of neuromuscular block may be anticipated, a decrease from the recommended initial dose should be considered).

No products indexed under this heading.

Butabarbital (Rocuronium, which has an acid pH, should not be mixed with alkaline solutions (eg, barbiturate solutions) in the same syringe or administered simultaneously during intravenous infusion through the same needle).

No products indexed under this heading.

Butalbital (Rocuronium, which has an acid pH, should not be mixed with alkaline solutions (eg, barbiturate solutions) in the same syringe or administered simultaneously during intravenous infusion through the same needle).

No products indexed under this heading.

Carbamazepine (In two out of four patients receiving chronic anticonvulsant therapy, apparent resistance to the effects of rocuronium was observed in the form of diminshed magnitude of neuromuscular block, or shortened clinical duration. As with other nondepolarizing neuromuscular blocking drugs, if rouronium is administered to patients chronically receiving anticonvulsant agents, such as carbamazepine or phenytoin, shorter durations of neuromuscular block may occur and infusion rates may be higher due to the development of resistance to non-depolarizing muscle relaxants. While the mechanism for development of this resistance is not known, receptor upregulation may be a contributing factor). Products include:

Carbatrol Capsules 3019
Equetro Extended-Release Capsules 3174

Chloroprocaine Hydrochloride (Local anesthetics have been shown to increase the duration of neuromuscular block and decrease infusion requirements of other neuromuscular blocking agents. In patients in whom potentiation of neuromuscular block may be anticipated, a decrease from the recommended initial dose should be considered).

No products indexed under this heading.

Cisatracurium Besylate (There are no controlled studies documenting the use of rocuronium before or after other nondepolarizing muscle relaxants. Interactions have been observed when other nondepolarizing muscle relaxants have been administered in succession). Products include:

Nimbex Injection 484

Colistimethate Sodium (Drugs which may enhance the neuromuscular blocking action of rocuronium include certain antibiotics, such as colistimethate sodium. If colistimethate sodium is used in conjunction with rocuronium, prolongation of neuromuscular block should be considereda possibility. In patients in whom potentiation of neuromuscular block may be anticipated, a decrease from the recommended initial dose should be considered).

No products indexed under this heading.

Colistin Sulfate (Drugs which may enhance the neuromuscular blocking action of rocuronium include certain antibiotics, such as colistin. If colistin is used in conjunction with rocuronium, prolongation of neuromuscular block should be considered a possibility. In patients in whom potentiation of neuromuscular block may be anticipated, a decrease from the recommended initial dose should be considered).

No products indexed under this heading.

Demeclocycline Hydrochloride (Drugs which may enhance the neuromuscular blocking action of rocuronium include certain antibiotics, such as tetracyclines. If tetracyclines are used in conjunction with rocuronium, prolongation of neuromuscular block should be considered a possibility. In patients in whom potentiation of neuromuscular block may be anticipated, a decrease from the recommended initial dose should be considered).

No products indexed under this heading.

Desflurane (Use of inhalation anesthetics as been shown to enhance the activity of other neuromuscular blocking agents).

No products indexed under this heading.

Divalproex Sodium (In two out of four patients receiving chronic anticonvulsant therapy, apparent resistance to the effects of rocuronium was observed in the form of diminshed magnitude of neuromuscular block, or shortened clinical duration. As with other nondepolarizing neuromuscular blocking drugs, if rouronium is administered to patients chronically receiving anticonvulsant agents, such as carbamazepine or phenytoin, shorter durations of neuromuscular block may occur and infusion rates may be higher due to the development of resistance to non-depolarizing muscle relaxants. While the mechanism for development of this resistance is not known, receptor upregulation may be a contributing factor). Products include:

Depakote ER Tablets 423

Doxycycline Calcium (Drugs which may enhance the neuromuscular blocking action of rocuronium include certain antibiotics, such as tetracyclines. If tetracyclines are used in conjunction with rocuronium, prolongation of neuromuscular block should be considered a possibility. In patients in whom potentiation of neuromuscular block may be anticipated, a decrease from the recommended initial dose should be considered).

No products indexed under this heading.

Doxycycline Hyclate (Drugs which may enhance the neuromuscular blocking action of rocuronium include certain antibiotics, such as tetracyclines. If tetracyclines are used in conjunction with rocuronium, prolongation of neuromuscular block should be considered a possibility. In patients in whom potentiation of neuromuscular block may be anticipated, a decrease from the recommended initial dose should be considered).

No products indexed under this heading.

Doxycycline Monohydrate (Drugs which may enhance the neuromuscular blocking action of rocuronium include certain antibiotics, such as tetracyclines. If tetracyclines are used in conjunction with rocuronium, prolongation of neuromuscular block should be considered a possibility. In patients in whom potentiation of neuromuscular block may be anticipated, a decrease from the recommended initial dose should be considered).

No products indexed under this heading.

Enflurane (Enflurane potentiates neuromuscular blocking actions. Enflurane may prolong the duration of action of initial and maintenance doses of rocuronium and decrease the average infusion requirement of rocuronium by 40% compared to opioid/nitrous oxide/oxygen anesthesia. The clinical duration of initial doses of rocuronium of 0.57 to 0.85 mg/kg under enflurane anesthesia was increased by 11%. The duration of maintenance doses was increased by 30% to 50% under enflurane. Potentiation by enflurane is also seen with the infusion rates of rocuronium required to maintain 95% neuromuscular block. Infusion rates are decreased by 40% compared to opioid/nitrous oxide/oxygen anesthesia. The median spontaneous recovery time is prolonged by enflurane (15% longer)).

No products indexed under this heading.

Ethosuximide (In two out of four patients receiving chronic anticonvulsant therapy, apparent resistance to the effects of rocuronium was observed in the form of diminshed magnitude of neuromuscular block, or shortened clinical duration. As with other nondepolarizing neuro-

muscular blocking drugs, if rouronium is administered to patients chronically receiving anticonvulsant agents, such as carbamazepine or phenytoin, shorter durations of neuromuscular block may occur and infusion rates may be higher due to the development of resistance to non-depolarizing muscle relaxants. While the mechanism for development of this resistance is not known, receptor upregulation may be a contributing factor).
No products indexed under this heading.

Ethotoin (In two out of four patients receiving chronic anticonvulsant therapy, apparent resistance to the effects of rocuronium was observed in the form of diminshed magnitude of neuromuscular block, or shortened clinical duration. As with other nondepolarizing neuromuscular blocking drugs, if rouronium is administered to patients chronically receiving anticonvulsant agents, such as carbamazepine or phenytoin, shorter durations of neuromuscular block may occur and infusion rates may be higher due to the development of resistance to non-depolarizing muscle relaxants. While the mechanism for development of this resistance is not known, receptor upregulation may be a contributing factor).
No products indexed under this heading.

Etidocaine Hydrochloride (Local anesthetics have been shown to increase the duration of neuromuscular block and decrease infusion requirements of other neuromuscular blocking agents. In patients in whom potentiation of neuromuscular block may be anticipated, a decrease from the recommended initial dose should be considered).
No products indexed under this heading.

Felbamate (In two out of four patients receiving chronic anticonvulsant therapy, apparent resistance to the effects of rocuronium was observed in the form of diminshed magnitude of neuromuscular block, or shortened clinical duration. As with other nondepolarizing neuromuscular blocking drugs, if rouronium is administered to patients chronically receiving anticonvulsant agents, such as carbamazepine or phenytoin, shorter durations of neuromuscular block may occur and infusion rates may be higher due to the development of resistance to non-depolarizing muscle relaxants. While the mechanism for development of this resistance is not known, receptor upregulation may be a contributing factor).
No products indexed under this heading.

Fosphenytoin (In two out of four patients receiving chronic anticonvulsant therapy, apparent resistance to the effects of rocuronium was observed in the form of diminshed magnitude of neuromuscular block, or shortened clinical duration. As with other nondepolarizing neuromuscular blocking drugs, if rouronium is administered to patients chronically receiving anticonvulsant agents, such as carbamazepine or phenytoin, shorter durations of neuromuscular block may occur and infusion rates may be higher due to the development of resistance to non-depolarizing muscle relaxants. While the mechanism for development of this resistance is not known, receptor upregulation may be a contributing factor).
No products indexed under this heading.

Fosphenytoin Sodium (In two out of four patients receiving chronic anticonvulsant therapy, apparent resistance to the effects of rocuronium was observed in the form of diminshed magnitude of neuromuscular block, or shortened clinical duration. As with other nondepolarizing neuromuscular blocking drugs, if rouronium is administered to patients chronically receiving anticonvulsant agents, such as carbamazepine or phenytoin, shorter durations of neuromuscular block may occur and infusion rates may be higher due to the development of resistance to non-depolarizing muscle relaxants. While the mechanism for development of this resistance is not known, receptor upregulation may be a contributing factor).
No products indexed under this heading.

Gabapentin (In two out of four patients receiving chronic anticonvulsant therapy, apparent resistance to the effects of rocuronium was observed in the form of diminshed magnitude of neuromuscular block, or shortened clinical duration. As with other nondepolarizing neuromuscular blocking drugs, if rouronium is administered to patients chronically receiving anticonvulsant agents, such as carbamazepine or phenytoin, shorter durations of neuromuscular block may occur and infusion rates may be higher due to the development of resistance to non-depolarizing muscle relaxants. While the mechanism for development of this resistance is not known, receptor upregulation may be a contributing factor).
No products indexed under this heading.

Gentamicin Sulfate (Drugs which may enhance the neuromuscular blocking action of rocuronium include certain antibiotics, such as aminoglyosides. If aminoglycosides are used in conjunction with rocuronium, prolongation of neuromuscular block should be considered a possibility. In patients in whom potentiation of neuromuscular block may be anticipated, a decrease from the recommended initial dose should be considered). Products include:

Pred-G Ophthalmic Ointment .... ⊙229
Pred-G Ophthalmic Suspension ...... ⊙228

Halothane (Use of inhalation anesthetics has been shown to enhance the activity of other neuromuscular blocking agents. However, there has been no definite interaction demonstrated between rocuronium and halothane).
No products indexed under this heading.

Isoflurane (Isoflurane potentiates neuromuscular blocking actions. Isoflurane may prolong the duration of action of initial and maintenance doses of rocuronium and decrease the average infusion requirement of rocuronium by 40% compared to opioid/nitrous oxide/oxygenanesthesia. The clinical duration of initial doses of rocuronium of 0.57 to 0.85 mg/kg under isoflurane anesthesia was increased by 23%. The duration of maintenance doses was increased by 30% to 50% under isoflurane. Potentiation by isoflurane is alsoseen with the infusion rates of rocuronium required to maintain 95% neuromuscular block. Infusion rates are decreased by 40% compared to opioid/nitrous oxide/ oxygen anesthesia. The median spontaneous recovery time is prolonged by isoflurane (62% longer)).
No products indexed under this heading.

Kanamycin Sulfate (Drugs which may enhance the neuromuscular blocking action of rocuronium include certain antibiotics, such as aminoglyosides. If aminoglycosides are used in conjunction with rocuronium, prolongation of neuromuscular block should be considered a possibility. In patients in whom potentiation of neuromuscular block may be anticipated, a decrease from the recommended initial dose should be considered).
No products indexed under this heading.

Lamotrigine (In two out of four patients receiving chronic anticonvulsant therapy, apparent resistance to the effects of rocuronium was observed in the form of diminshed magnitude of neuromuscular block, or shortened clinical duration. As with other nondepolarizing neuromuscular blocking drugs, if rouronium is administered to patients chronically receiving anticonvulsant agents, such as carbamazepine or phenytoin, shorter durations of neuromuscular block may occur and infusion rates may be higher due to the development of resistance to non-depolarizing muscle relaxants. While the mechanism for development of this resistance is not known, receptor upregulation may be a contributing factor). Products include:

Lamictal 1488

Levetiracetam (In two out of four patients receiving chronic anticonvulsant therapy, apparent resistance to the effects of rocuronium was observed in the form of diminshed magnitude of neuromuscular block, or shortened clinical duration. As with other nondepolarizing neuromuscular blocking drugs, if rouronium is administered to patients chronically receiving anticonvulsant agents, such as carbamazepine or phenytoin, shorter durations of neuromuscular block may occur and infusion rates may be higher due to the development of resistance to non-depolarizing muscle relaxants. While the mechanism for development of this resistance is not known, receptor upregulation may be a contributing factor). Products include:

Keppra Injection 3137
Keppra Oral Solution 3131
Keppra Tablets 3131

Levobupivacaine Hydrochloride (Local anesthetics have been shown to increase the duration of neuromuscular block and decrease infusion requirements of other neuromuscular blocking agents. In patients in whom potentiation of neuromuscular block may be anticipated, a decrease from the recommended initial dose should be considered).
No products indexed under this heading.

Lidocaine Hydrochloride (Local anesthetics have been shown to increase the duration of neuromuscular block and decrease infusion requirements of other neuromuscular blocking agents. In patients in whom potentiation of neuromuscular block may be anticipated, a decrease from the recommended initial dose should be considered).
No products indexed under this heading.

Lithium (Lithium has been shown to increase the duration of neuromuscular block and decrease infusion requirements of other neuromuscular blocking agents. In patients in whom potentiation of neuromuscular block may be anticipated, a decrease from the recommended initial dose should be considered).
No products indexed under this heading.

Lithium Carbonate (Lithium has been shown to increase the duration of neuromuscular block and decrease infusion requirements of other neuromuscular blocking agents. In patients in whom potentiation of neuromuscular block may be anticipated, a decrease from the recommended initial dose should be considered).
No products indexed under this heading.

Lithium Citrate (Lithium has been shown to increase the duration of neuromuscular block and decrease infusion requirements of other neuromuscular blocking agents. In patients in whom potentiation of neuromuscular block may be anticipated, a decrease from the recommended initial dose should be considered).
No products indexed under this heading.

Magnesium Salts (Magnesium salts have been shown to increase the duration of neuromuscular block and decrease infusion requirements of other neuromuscular blocking agents. In patients in whom potentiation of neuromuscular block may be anticipated, a decrease from the recommended initial dose should be considered).
No products indexed under this heading.

Mephenytoin (In two out of four patients receiving chronic anticonvulsant therapy, apparent resistance to the effects of rocuronium was observed in the form of diminshed magnitude of neuromuscular block, or shortened clinical duration. As with other nondepolarizing neuromuscular blocking drugs, if rouronium is administered to patients chronically receiving anticonvulsant agents, such as carbamazepine or phenytoin, shorter durations of neuromuscular block may occur and infusion rates may be higher due to the development of resistance to non-depolarizing muscle relaxants. While the mechanism for development of this resistance is not known, receptor upregulation may be a contributing factor).
No products indexed under this heading.

Mephobarbital (Rocuronium, which has an acid pH, should not be mixed with alkaline solutions (eg, barbiturate solutions) in the same syringe or administered simultaneously during intravenous infusion through the same needle).
No products indexed under this heading.

Mepivacaine Hydrochloride (Local anesthetics have been shown to increase the duration of neuromuscular block and decrease infusion requirements of other neuromuscular blocking agents. In patients in whom potentiation of neuromuscular block may be anticipated, a decrease from the recommended initial dose should be considered).
No products indexed under this heading.

Methacycline Hydrochloride (Drugs which may enhance the neuromuscular blocking action of rocuronium include certain antibiotics, such as tetracyclines. If tetracyclines are used in conjunction with rocuronium, prolongation of neuromuscular block should be considered a possibility. In patients in whom potentiation of neuromuscular block may be anticipated, a decrease from the recommended initial dose should be considered).
No products indexed under this heading.

Methoxyflurane (Use of inhalation anesthetics as been shown to enhance the activity of other neuromuscular blocking agents).
No products indexed under this heading.

Methsuximide (In two out of four patients receiving chronic anticonvulsant therapy, apparent resistance to the effects of rocuronium was observed in the form of diminshed magnitude of neuromuscular block, or shortened clinical duration. As with other nondepolarizing neuromuscular blocking drugs, if rouronium is administered to patients chronically receiving anticonvulsant agents, such as carbamazepine or phenytoin, shorter durations of neuromuscular block may occur and infusion rates may be higher due to the development of resistance to non-depolarizing muscle relaxants. While the mechanism for development of this resistance is not known, receptor upregulation may be a contributing factor).
No products indexed under this heading.

Metocurine Iodide (There are no controlled studies documenting the use of rocuronium before or after other nondepolarizing muscle relaxants. Interactions have been observed when other nondepolarizing muscle relaxants have been administered in succession).
No products indexed under this heading.

Minocycline Hydrochloride (Drugs which may enhance the neuromuscular blocking action of rocuronium include certain antibiotics, such as tetracyclines. If tetracyclines are used in conjunction with rocuronium, prolongation of neuromuscular block should be considered a possibility. In patients in whom potentiation of neuromuscular block may be anticipated, a decrease from the recommended initial dose should be considered). Products include:
Solodyn Extended Release Tablets **1938**

Mivacurium Chloride (There are no controlled studies documenting the use of rocuronium before or after other nondepolarizing muscle relaxants. Interactions have been observed when other nondepolarizing muscle relaxants have been administered in succession).
No products indexed under this heading.

Oxcarbazepine (In two out of four patients receiving chronic anticonvulsant therapy, apparent resistance to the effects of rocuronium was observed in the form of diminshed magnitude of neuromuscular block, or shortened clinical duration. As with other nondepolarizing neuromuscular blocking drugs, if rouronium is administered to patients chronically receiving anticonvulsant agents, such as carbamazepine or phenytoin, shorter durations of neuromuscular block may occur and infusion rates may be higher due to the development of resistance to non-depolarizing muscle relaxants. While the mechanism for development of this resistance is not known, receptor upregulation may be a contributing factor).
No products indexed under this heading.

Oxytetracycline Hydrochloride (Drugs which may enhance the neuromuscular blocking action of rocuronium include certain antibiotics, such as tetracyclines. If tetracyclines are used in conjunction with rocuronium, prolongation of neuromuscular block should be considered a possibility. In patients in whom potentiation of neuromuscular block may be anticipated, a decrease from the recommended initial dose should be considered).
No products indexed under this heading.

Pancuronium Bromide (There are no controlled studies documenting the use of rocuronium before or after other nondepolarizing muscle relaxants. Interactions have been observed when other nondepolarizing muscle relaxants have been administered in succession).
No products indexed under this heading.

Paramethadione (In two out of four patients receiving chronic anticonvulsant therapy, apparent resistance to the effects of rocuronium was observed in the form of diminshed magnitude of neuromuscular block, or shortened clinical duration. As with other nondepolarizing neuromuscular blocking drugs, if rouronium is administered to patients chronically receiving anticonvulsant agents, such as carbamazepine or phenytoin, shorter durations of neuromuscular block may occur and infusion rates may be higher due to the development of resistance to non-depolarizing muscle relaxants. While the mechanism for development of this resistance is not known, receptor upregulation may be a contributing factor).
No products indexed under this heading.

Pentobarbital Sodium (Rocuronium, which has an acid pH, should not be mixed with alkaline solutions (eg, barbiturate solutions) in the same syringe or administered simultaneously during intravenous infusion through the same needle). Products include:
Nembutal Sodium Solution, USP **2494**

Phenacemide (In two out of four patients receiving chronic anticonvulsant therapy, apparent resistance to the effects of rocuronium was observed in the form of diminshed magnitude of neuromuscular block, or shortened clinical duration. As with other nondepolarizing neuromuscular blocking drugs, if rouronium is administered to patients chronically receiving anticonvulsant agents, such as carbamazepine or phenytoin, shorter durations of neuromuscular block may occur and infusion rates may be higher due to the development of resistance to non-depolarizing muscle relaxants. While the mechanism for development of this resistance is not known, receptor upregulation may be a contributing factor).
No products indexed under this heading.

Phenobarbital (In two out of four patients receiving chronic anticonvulsant therapy, apparent resistance to the effects of rocuronium was observed in the form of diminshed magnitude of neuromuscular block, or shortened clinical duration. As with other nondepolarizing neuromuscular blocking drugs, if rouronium is administered to patients chronically receiving anticonvulsant agents, such as carbamazepine or phenytoin, shorter durations of neuromuscular block may occur and infusion rates may be higher due to the development of resistance to non-depolarizing muscle relaxants. While the mechanism for development of this resistance is not known, receptor upregulation may be a contributing factor). Products include:
Donnatal Extentabs **2507**

Phensuximide (In two out of four patients receiving chronic anticonvulsant therapy, apparent resistance to the effects of rocuronium was observed in the form of diminshed magnitude of neuromuscular block, or shortened clinical duration. As with other nondepolarizing neuromuscular blocking drugs, if rouronium is administered to patients chronically receiving anticonvulsant agents, such as carbamazepine or phenytoin, shorter durations of neuromuscular block may occur and infusion rates may be higher due to the development of resistance to non-depolarizing muscle relaxants. While the mechanism for development of this resistance is not known, receptor upregulation may be a contributing factor).
No products indexed under this heading.

Phenytoin (In two out of four patients receiving chronic anticonvulsant therapy, apparent resistance to the effects of rocuronium was observed in the form of diminshed magnitude of neuromuscular block, or shortened clinical duration. As with other nondepolarizing neuromuscular blocking drugs, if rouronium is administered to patients chronically receiving anticonvulsant agents, such as carbamazepine or phenytoin, shorter durations of neuromuscular block may occur and infusion rates may be higher due to the development of resistance to non-depolarizing muscle relaxants. While the mechanism for development of this resistance is not known, receptor upregulation may be a contributing factor).
No products indexed under this heading.

Phenytoin Sodium (In two out of four patients receiving chronic anticonvulsant therapy, apparent resistance to the effects of rocuronium was observed in the form of diminshed magnitude of neuromuscular block, or shortened clinical duration. As with other nondepolarizing neuromuscular blocking drugs, if rouronium is administered to patients chronically receiving anticonvulsant agents, such as carbamazepine or phenytoin, shorter durations of neuromuscular block may occur and infusion rates may be higher due to the development of resistance to non-depolarizing muscle relaxants. While the mechanism for development of this resistance is not known, receptor upregulation may be a contributing factor). Products include:
Phenytek Capsules **2192**

Polymyxin (Drugs which may enhance the neuromuscular blocking action of rocuronium include certain antibiotics, such as polymyxin. If polymyxin is used in conjunction with rocuronium, prolongation of neuromuscular block should be considered a possibility. In patients in whom potentiation of neuromuscular block may be anticipated, a decrease from the recommended initial dose should be considered).
No products indexed under this heading.

Polymyxin B Sulfate (Drugs which may enhance the neuromuscular blocking action of rocuronium include certain antibiotics, such as polymyxin. If polymyxin is used in conjunction with rocuronium, prolongation of neuromuscular block should be considered a possibility. In patients in whom potentiation of neuromuscular block may be anticipated, a decrease from the recommended initial dose should be considered). Products include:
Neosporin Ophthalmic Solution Sterile .... ⊙**252**

Polymyxin Preparations (Drugs which may enhance the neuromuscular blocking action of rocuronium include certain antibiotics, such as polymyxin. If polymyxin is used in conjunction with rocuronium, prolongation of neuromuscular block should be considered a possibility. In patients in whom potentiation of neuromuscular block may be anticipated, a decrease from the recommended initial dose should be considered).
No products indexed under this heading.

Primidone (In two out of four patients receiving chronic anticonvulsant therapy, apparent resistance to the effects of rocuronium was observed in the form of diminshed magnitude of neuromuscular block, or shortened clinical duration. As with other nondepolarizing neuromuscular blocking drugs, if rouronium is administered to patients chronically receiving anticonvulsant agents, such as carbamazepine or

phenytoin, shorter durations of neuromuscular block may occur and infusion rates may be higher due to the development of resistance to non-depolarizing muscle relaxants. While the mechanism for development of this resistance is not known, receptor upregulation may be a contributing factor).

No products indexed under this heading.

Procainamide (Procainamide has been shown to increase the duration of neuromuscular block and decrease infusion requirements of other neuromuscular blocking agents. In patients in whom potentiation of neuromuscular block may be anticipated, a decrease from the recommended initial dose should be considered).

No products indexed under this heading.

Procainamide Hydrochloride (Procainamide has been shown to increase the duration of neuromuscular block and decrease infusion requirements of other neuromuscular blocking agents. In patients in whom potentiation of neuromuscular block may be anticipated, a decrease from the recommended initial dose should be considered).

No products indexed under this heading.

Procaine Hydrochloride (Local anesthetics have been shown to increase the duration of neuromuscular block and decrease infusion requirements of other neuromuscular blocking agents. In patients in whom potentiation of neuromuscular block may be anticipated, a decrease from the recommended initial dose should be considered).

No products indexed under this heading.

Quinidine (Quinidine has been shown to increase the duration of neuromuscular block and decrease infusion requirements of other neuromuscular blocking agents. In patients in whom potentiation of neuromuscular block may be anticipated, a decrease from the recommended initial dose should be considered. Also, experience concerning injection of quinidine during recovery from use of other muscle relaxants suggests that recurrent paralysis may occur. This possibility must also be considered for rocuronium).

No products indexed under this heading.

Quinidine Gluconate (Quinidine has been shown to increase the duration of neuromuscular block and decrease infusion requirements of other neuromuscular blocking agents. In patients in whom potentiation of neuromuscular block may be anticipated, a decrease from the recommended initial dose should be considered. Also, experience concerning injection of quinidine during recovery from use of other muscle relaxants suggests that recurrent paralysis may occur. This possibility must also be considered for rocuronium).

No products indexed under this heading.

Quinidine Hydrochloride (Quinidine has been shown to increase the duration of neuromuscular block and decrease infusion requirements of other neuromuscular blocking agents. In patients in whom potentiation of neuromuscular block may be anticipated, a decrease from the recommended initial dose should be considered. Also, experience concerning injection of quinidine during recovery from use of other muscle relaxants suggests that recurrent paralysis may occur. This possibility must also be considered for rocuronium).

No products indexed under this heading.

Quinidine Polygalacturonate (Quinidine has been shown to increase the duration of neuromuscular block and decrease infusion requirements of other neuromuscular blocking agents. In patients in whom potentiation of neuromuscular block may be anticipated, a decrease from the recommended initial dose should be considered. Also, experience concerning injection of quinidine during recovery from use of other muscle relaxants suggests that recurrent paralysis may occur. This possibility must also be considered for rocuronium).

No products indexed under this heading.

Quinidine Sulfate (Quinidine has been shown to increase the duration of neuromuscular block and decrease infusion requirements of other neuromuscular blocking agents. In patients in whom potentiation of neuromuscular block may be anticipated, a decrease from the recommended initial dose should be considered. Also, experience concerning injection of quinidine during recovery from use of other muscle relaxants suggests that recurrent paralysis may occur. This possibility must also be considered for rocuronium).

No products indexed under this heading.

Rapacuronium Bromide (There are no controlled studies documenting the use of rocuronium before or after other nondepolarizing muscle relaxants. Interactions have been observed when other nondepolarizing muscle relaxants have been administered in succession).

No products indexed under this heading.

Secobarbital Sodium (Rocuronium, which has an acid pH, should not be mixed with alkaline solutions (eg, barbiturate solutions) in the same syringe or administered simultaneously during intravenous infusion through the same needle).

No products indexed under this heading.

Streptomycin Sulfate (Drugs which may enhance the neuromuscular blocking action of rocuronium include certain antibiotics, such as aminoglyosides. If aminoglycosides are used in conjunction with rocuronium, prolongation of neuromuscular block should be considered a possibility. In patients in whom potentiation of neuromuscular block may be anticipated, a decrease from the recommended initial dose should be considered).

No products indexed under this heading.

Succinylcholine Chloride (The use of rocuronium before succinylcholine, for the purpose of attenuating some of the side effects of succinylcholine, has not been studied. If rocuronium is administered following administration of succinylcholine, it should not be given until recovery from succinylcholine has been observed. The median duration of action of rocuronium 0.6 mg/kg administered after a 1 mg/kg dose of succinylcholine when T returned to 75% of control was 36 minutes (range 14 to 57, n equals 12) versus 28 minutes (17 to 51, n equals 12) without succinylcholine).

No products indexed under this heading.

Tetracaine Hydrochloride (Local anesthetics have been shown to increase the duration of neuromuscular block and decrease infusion requirements of other neuromuscular blocking agents. In patients in whom potentiation of neuromuscular block may be anticipated, a decrease from the recommended initial dose should be considered).

No products indexed under this heading.

Tetracycline Hydrochloride (Drugs which may enhance the neuromuscular blocking action of rocuronium include certain antibiotics, such as tetracyclines. If tetracyclines are used in conjunction with rocuronium, prolongation of neuromuscular block should be considered a possibility. In patients in whom potentiation of neuromuscular block may be anticipated, a decrease from the recommended initial dose should be considered). Products include:

Pylera Capsules **714**

Thiamylal Sodium (Rocuronium, which has an acid pH, should not be mixed with alkaline solutions (eg, barbiturate solutions) in the same syringe or administered simultaneously during intravenous infusion through the same needle).

No products indexed under this heading.

Tiagabine Hydrochloride (In two out of four patients receiving chronic anticonvulsant therapy, apparent resistance to the effects of rocuronium was observed in the form of diminshed magnitude of neuromuscular block, or shortened clinical duration. As with other nondepolarizing neuromuscular blocking drugs, if rouronium is administered to patients chronically receiving anticonvulsant agents, such as carbamazepine or phenytoin, shorter durations of neuromuscular block may occur and infusion rates may be higher due to the development of resistance to non-depolarizing muscle relaxants. While the mechanism for development of this resistance is not known, receptor upregulation may be a contributing factor). Products include:

Gabitril Tablets **973**

Tobramycin (Drugs which may enhance the neuromuscular blocking action of rocuronium include certain antibiotics, such as aminoglyosides. If aminoglycosides are used in conjunction with rocuronium, prolongation of neuromuscular block should be considered a possibility. In patients in whom potentiation of neuromuscular block may be anticipated, a decrease from the recommended initial dose should be considered). Products include:

Zylet Ophthalmic Suspension .... ⊙**247**

Tobramycin Sulfate (Drugs which may enhance the neuromuscular blocking action of rocuronium include certain antibiotics, such as aminoglyosides. If aminoglycosides are used in conjunction with rocuronium, prolongation of neuromuscular block should be considered a possibility. In patients in whom potentiation of neuromuscular block may be anticipated, a decrease from the recommended initial dose should be considered).

No products indexed under this heading.

Topiramate (In two out of four patients receiving chronic anticonvulsant therapy, apparent resistance to the effects of rocuronium was observed in the form of diminshed magnitude of neuromuscular block, or shortened clinical duration. As with other nondepolarizing neuromuscular blocking drugs, if rouronium is administered to patients chronically receiving anticonvulsant agents, such as carbamazepine or phenytoin, shorter durations of neuromuscular block may occur and infusion rates may be higher due to the development of resistance to non-depolarizing muscle relaxants. While the mechanism for development of this resistance is not known, receptor upregulation may be a contributing factor).

No products indexed under this heading.

Trimethadione (In two out of four patients receiving chronic anticonvulsant therapy, apparent resistance to the effects of rocuronium was observed in the form of diminshed magnitude of neuromuscular block, or shortened clinical duration. As with other nondepolarizing neuromuscular blocking drugs, if rouronium is administered to patients chronically receiving anticonvulsant agents, such as carbamazepine or phenytoin, shorter durations of neuromuscular block may occur and infusion rates may be higher due to the development of resistance to non-depolarizing muscle relaxants. While the mechanism for development of this resistance is not known, receptor upregulation may be a contributing factor).

No products indexed under this heading.

Valproate Sodium (In two out of four patients receiving chronic anticonvulsant therapy, apparent resistance to the effects of rocuronium was observed in the form of diminshed magnitude of neuromuscular block, or shortened clinical duration. As with other nondepolarizing neuromuscular blocking drugs, if rouronium is administered to patients chronically receiving anticonvulsant agents, such as carbamazepine or phenytoin, shorter durations of neuromuscular block may occur and infusion rates may be higher due to the development of resistance to non-depolarizing muscle relaxants. While the mechanism for development of this resistance is not known, receptor upregulation may be a contributing factor).

No products indexed under this heading.

Valproic Acid (In two out of four patients receiving chronic anticonvulsant therapy, apparent resistance to the effects of rocuronium was

observed in the form of diminshed magnitude of neuromuscular block, or shortened clinical duration. As with other nondepolarizing neuromuscular blocking drugs, if rocuronium is administered to patients chronically receiving anticonvulsant agents, such as carbamazepine or phenytoin, shorter durations of neuromuscular block may occur and infusion rates may be higher due to the development of resistance to non-depolarizing muscle relaxants. While the mechanism for development of this resistance is not known, receptor upregulation may be a contributing factor).
No products indexed under this heading.

Vancomycin Hydrochloride (Drugs which may enhance the neuromuscular blocking action of rocuronium include certain antibiotics, such as vancomycin. If vancomycin is used in conjunction with rocuronium, prolongation of neuromuscular block should be considered a possibility. In patients in whom potentiation of neuromuscular block my be anticipated, a decrease from the recommended initial dose should be considered).
No products indexed under this heading.

Vecuronium Bromide (There are no controlled studies documenting the use of rocuronium before or after other nondepolarizing muscle relaxants. Interactions have been observed when other nondepolarizing muscle relaxants have been administered in succession).
No products indexed under this heading.

Zonisamide (In two out of four patients receiving chronic anticonvulsant therapy, apparent resistance to the effects of rocuronium was observed in the form of diminshed magnitude of neuromuscular block, or shortened clinical duration. As with other nondepolarizing neuromuscular blocking drugs, if rocuronium is administered to patients chronically receiving anticonvulsant agents, such as carbamazepine or phenytoin, shorter durations of neuromuscular block may occur and infusion rates may be higher due to the development of resistance to non-depolarizing muscle relaxants. While the mechanism for development of this resistance is not known, receptor upregulation may be a contributing factor). Products include:
Zonegran Capsules ... 1089

ZETIA TABLETS

(Ezetimibe) ... 2157
May interact with antacids, fibrates, and certain other agents. Compounds in these categories include:

Aluminum Carbonate (Co-administration with aluminum and magnesium hydroxide combination antacid may decrease exposure to ezetimibe).
No products indexed under this heading.

Aluminum Hydroxide (Co-administration with aluminum and magnesium hydroxide combination antacid may decrease exposure to ezetimibe).
No products indexed under this heading.

Cholestyramine (Concomitant cholestyramine administration decreased the mean AUC of total ezetimibe approximately 55%. The incremental LDL-C reduction to adding ezetimibe to cholestyramine may be reduced by this interaction).
No products indexed under this heading.

Clofibrate (The efficacy and safety of co-administration of ezetimibe with fibrates other than fenofibrate have not been studied. Fibrates may increase cholesterol excretion into the bile, leading to cholelithiasis. In a preclinical study in dogs, ezetimibe increased cholesterol in the gallbladder bile. Co-administration of ezetimibe with fibrates other than fenofibrate is not recommended until use in patients is adequately studied).
No products indexed under this heading.

Cyclosporine (Caution should be exercised when using ezetimibe and cyclosporine concomitantly due to increased exposure to both ezetimibe and cyclosporine. Cyclosporine concentrations should be monitored in patients receiving ezetimibe and cyclosporine. The degree of increase in ezetimibe exposure may be greater in patients with severe renal insufficiency. In patients treated with cyclosporine, the potential effects of the increased exposure to ezetimibe from concomitant use should be carefully weighed against the benefits of alterations in lipid levels provided by ezetimibe). Products include:
Gengraf Capsules ... 435
Neoral Oral Solution ... 2280
Neoral Soft Gelatin Capsules ... 2280
Restasis Ophthalmic Emulsion ... 557
Sandimmune ... 2296

Fenofibrate (If cholelithiasis is suspected in a patient receiving ezetimibe and fenofibrate, gallbladder studies are indicated and alternative lipid-lowering therapy should be considered). Products include:
Fenoglide Tablets ... 2960
Tricor Tablets ... 520

Gemfibrozil (The efficacy and safety of co-administration of ezetimibe with fibrates other than fenofibrate have not been studied. Fibrates may increase cholesterol excretion into the bile, leading to cholelithiasis. In a preclinical study in dogs, ezetimibe increased cholesterol in the gallbladder bile. Co-administration of ezetimibe with fibrates other than fenofibrate is not recommended until use in patients is adequately studied).
No products indexed under this heading.

Magaldrate (Co-administration with aluminum and magnesium hydroxide combination antacid may decrease exposure to ezetimibe).
No products indexed under this heading.

Magnesium Hydroxide (Co-administration with aluminum and magnesium hydroxide combination antacid may decrease exposure to ezetimibe). Products include:
Fleet Pedia-Lax Chewable Tablets ... 1145
Pepcid Complete Chewable Tablets ... 1771
Extra Strength Rolaids Freshmint Tablets ... 1903
Rolaids Multi-Symptom Berry Tablets ... 1903
Rolaids Original Peppermint Tablets ... 1903

Magnesium Oxide (Co-administration with aluminum and magnesium hydroxide combination antacid may decrease exposure to ezetimibe). Products include:
Beelith Tablets ... 813

Sodium Bicarbonate (Co-administration with aluminum and magnesium hydroxide combination antacid may decrease exposure to ezetimibe). Products include:
Ceo-Two Laxative Suppository ... 815

Warfarin Sodium (If ezetimibe is added to warfarn, a coumarin anticoagulant, the International Normalized Ratio (INR) should be appropriately monitored).
No products indexed under this heading.

ZETIA TABLETS

(Ezetimibe) ... 2951
May interact with bile acid sequestering agents, fibrates, HMG-CoA reductase inhibitors, and certain other agents. Compounds in these categories include:

Aluminum Carbonate (Co-administration may decrease AUC and Cmax of ezetimibe).
No products indexed under this heading.

Aluminum Hydroxide (Co-administration may decrease AUC and Cmax of ezetimibe).
No products indexed under this heading.

Atorvastatin Calcium (In 28 double-blind, controlled clinical trials, 11,308 patients with primary hyperlipidemia and elevated LDL-C were treated with ezetimibe 10 mg/day concurrently with or added to on-going statin therapy for a median treatment duration of 8 weeks. The incidence of consecutive increased transaminases (greater than or equal to 3x ULN) was higher in patients receiving ezetimibe administered with statins (1.3%) than in patients treated with statins alone (0.4%). The combination of ezetimibe with a statin is contraindicated in patients with active liver disease or unexplained persistent elevations in hepatic transaminase levels. The use of a statin is also contraindicated in women who are pregnant or whom may become pregnant and in women who are nursing). Products include:
Lipitor Tablets ... 2501

Cerivastatin Sodium (In 28 double-blind, controlled clinical trials, 11,308 patients with primary hyperlipidemia and elevated LDL-C were treated with ezetimibe 10 mg/day concurrently with or added to on-going statin therapy for a median treatment duration of 8 weeks. The incidence of consecutive increased transaminases (greater than or equal to 3x ULN) was higher in patients receiving ezetimibe administered with statins (1.3%) than in patients treated with statins alone (0.4%). The combination of ezetimibe with a statin is contraindicated in patients with active liver disease or unexplained persistent elevations in hepatic transaminase levels. The use of a statin is also contraindicated in women who are pregnant or whom may become pregnant and in women who are nursing).
No products indexed under this heading.

Cholestyramine (Concomitant cholestyramine administration decreased the mean area under the curve (AUC) of total ezetimibe approximately 55%. The incremental LDL-C reduction to adding ezetimibe to cholestyramine may be reduced by this interaction. Dosing of ezetimibe should occur either greater or equal to 2 hours before or greater or equal to 4 hours after administration of a bile acid sequestrant).
No products indexed under this heading.

Clofibrate (The efficacy and safety of co-administration of ezetimibe with fibrates other than fenofibrate have not been studied. Fibrates may increase cholesterol excretion into the bile, leading to cholelithiasis. Co-administration of ezetimibe with fibrates other than fenofibrate is not recommended until use in patients is adequately studied).
No products indexed under this heading.

Colesevelam Hydrochloride (Dosing of ezetimibe should occur either greater or equal to 2 hours before or greater or equal to 4 hours after administration of a bile acid sequestrant). Products include:
WelChol Tablets ... 1015

Colestipol Hydrochloride (Dosing of ezetimibe should occur either greater or equal to 2 hours before or greater or equal to 4 hours after administration of a bile acid sequestrant).
No products indexed under this heading.

Cyclosporine (Caution should be exercised when using ezetimibe and cyclosporine concomitantly due to increased exposure to both ezetimibe and cyclosporine. Cyclosporine concentrations should be monitored in patients receiving ezetimibe and cyclosporine. The degree of increase in ezetimibe exposure may be greater in patients with severe renal insufficiency. In patients treated with cyclosporine, the potential effects of the increased exposure to ezetimibe from concomitant use should be carefully weighed against the benefits of alterations in lipid levels provided by ezetimibe). Products include:
Gengraf Capsules ... 435
Neoral Oral Solution ... 2280
Neoral Soft Gelatin Capsules ... 2280
Restasis Ophthalmic Emulsion ... 557
Sandimmune ... 2296

Fenofibrate (Concomitant use increases exposure of ezetimibe. If cholelithiasis is suspected in a patient receiving ezetimibe and fenofibrate, gallbladder studies are indicated and alternative lipid-lowering therapy should be considered). Products include:
Fenoglide Tablets ... 2960
Tricor Tablets ... 520

Fluvastatin Sodium (In 28 double-blind, controlled clinical trials, 11,308 patients with primary hyperlipidemia and elevated LDL-C were treated with ezetimibe 10 mg/day concurrently with or added to on-going statin therapy for a median treatment duration of 8 weeks. The incidence of consecutive increased transaminases (greater than or equal to 3x ULN) was higher in patients receiving ezetimibe administered with statins (1.3%) than in patients

treated with statins alone (0.4%). The combination of ezetimibe with a statin is contraindicated in patients with active liver disease or unexplained persistent elevations in hepatic transaminase levels. The use of a statin is also contraindicated in women who are pregnant or whom may become pregnant and in women who are nursing). Products include:

Lescol Capsules 2268
Lescol XL Tablets 2268

Gemfibrozil (Co-administration increased total ezetimibe concentrations by approximately 1.7-fold).

No products indexed under this heading.

Lovastatin (In 28 double-blind, controlled clinical trials, 11,308 patients with primary hyperlipidemia and elevated LDL-C were treated with ezetimibe 10 mg/day concurrently with or added to on-going statin therapy for a median treatment duration of 8 weeks. The incidence of consecutive increased transaminases (greater than or equal to 3x ULN) was higher in patients receiving ezetimibe administered with statins (1.3%) than in patients treated with statins alone (0.4%). The combination of ezetimibe with a statin is contraindicated in patients with active liver disease or unexplained persistent elevations in hepatic transaminase levels. The use of a statin is also contraindicated in women who are pregnant or whom may become pregnant and in women who are nursing). Products include:

Advicor Tablets 402
Mevacor Tablets 2063

Magnesium Hydroxide (Co-administration may decrease AUC and Cmax of ezetimibe). Products include:

Fleet Pedia-Lax Chewable Tablets 1145
Pepcid Complete Chewable Tablets 1771
Extra Strength Rolaids Freshmint Tablets 1903
Rolaids Multi-Symptom Berry Tablets 1903
Rolaids Original Peppermint Tablets 1903

Pravastatin Sodium (In 28 double-blind, controlled clinical trials, 11,308 patients with primary hyperlipidemia and elevated LDL-C were treated with ezetimibe 10 mg/day concurrently with or added to on-going statin therapy for a median treatment duration of 8 weeks. The incidence of consecutive increased transaminases (greater than or equal to 3x ULN) was higher in patients receiving ezetimibe administered with statins (1.3%) than in patients treated with statins alone (0.4%). The combination of ezetimibe with a statin is contraindicated in patients with active liver disease or unexplained persistent elevations in hepatic transaminase levels. The use of a statin is also contraindicated in women who are pregnant or whom may become pregnant and in women who are nursing).

No products indexed under this heading.

Rosuvastatin Calcium (In 28 double-blind, controlled clinical trials, 11,308 patients with primary hyperlipidemia and elevated LDL-C were treated with ezetimibe 10 mg/day concurrently with or added to on-going statin therapy for a median treatment duration of 8 weeks. The incidence of consecutive increased transaminases (greater than or equal to 3x ULN) was higher in patients receiving ezetimibe administered with statins (1.3%) than in patients treated with statins alone (0.4%). The combination of ezetimibe with a statin is contraindicated in patients with active liver disease or unexplained persistent elevations in hepatic transaminase levels. The use of a statin is also contraindicated in women who are pregnant or whom may become pregnant and in women who are nursing). Products include:

Crestor Tablets 677

Simvastatin (In 28 double-blind, controlled clinical trials, 11,308 patients with primary hyperlipidemia and elevated LDL-C were treated with ezetimibe 10 mg/day concurrently with or added to on-going statin therapy for a median treatment duration of 8 weeks. The incidence of consecutive increased transaminases (greater than or equal to 3x ULN) was higher in patients receiving ezetimibe administered with statins (1.3%) than in patients treated with statins alone (0.4%). The combination of ezetimibe with a statin is contraindicated in patients with active liver disease or unexplained persistent elevations in hepatic transaminase levels. The use of a statin is also contraindicated in women who are pregnant or whom may become pregnant and in women who are nursing). Products include:

Simcor Tablets 502
Vytorin 10/10 Tablets 2149
Vytorin 10/10 Tablets 2939
Vytorin 10/20 Tablets 2149
Vytorin 10/20 Tablets 2939
Vytorin 10/40 Tablets 2149
Vytorin 10/40 Tablets 2939
Vytorin 10/80 Tablets 2149
Vytorin 10/80 Tablets 2939
Zocor Tablets 2136

Warfarin Sodium (If ezetimibe is added to warfarin, a coumarin anticoagulatn, the International Normalized Ratio (INR) should be appropriately monitored).

No products indexed under this heading.

ZIAGEN ORAL SOLUTION

(Abacavir Sulfate) 1673

See Ziagen Tablets

ZIAGEN TABLETS

(Abacavir Sulfate) 1673

May interact with:

Lamivudine (Ziagen should not be co-administered with Epzicom or Trizivir). Products include:

Combivir Tablets 1384
Epivir 1412
Epivir-HBV 1417
Epzicom Tablets 1422
Trizivir Tablets 1622

Methadone Hydrochloride (Co-administration in patients on methadone-maintenance therapy has resulted in increased methadone clearance by 22%. This alteration will not result in a methadone dose modification in the majority of patients; however, an increased methadone dose may be required in a small number of patients).

No products indexed under this heading.

Food Interactions

Alcohol (Decreases the elimination of abacavir causing an increase in overall exposure).

ZIANA GEL

(Clindamycin Phosphate, Tretinoin) 1942

May interact with erythromycin, neuromuscular blocking agents, and certain other agents. Compounds in these categories include:

Atracurium Besylate (Clindamycin has been shown to have neuromuscular blocking properties that may enhance the action of other neuromuscular blocking agents. Therefore, ZIANA Gel should be used with caution in patients receiving such agents).

No products indexed under this heading.

Cisatracurium Besylate (Clindamycin has been shown to have neuromuscular blocking properties that may enhance the action of other neuromuscular blocking agents. Therefore, ZIANA Gel should be used with caution in patients receiving such agents). Products include:

Nimbex Injection 484

Doxacurium Chloride (Clindamycin has been shown to have neuromuscular blocking properties that may enhance the action of other neuromuscular blocking agents. Therefore, ZIANA Gel should be used with caution in patients receiving such agents).

No products indexed under this heading.

Erythromycin (ZIANA Gel should not be used in combination with erythromycin-containing products due to its clindamycin component).

No products indexed under this heading.

Erythromycin Estolate (ZIANA Gel should not be used in combination with erythromycin-containing products due to its clindamycin component).

No products indexed under this heading.

Erythromycin Ethylsuccinate (ZIANA Gel should not be used in combination with erythromycin-containing products due to its clindamycin component). Products include:

E.E.S. 433
EryPed 431

Erythromycin Gluceptate (ZIANA Gel should not be used in combination with erythromycin-containing products due to its clindamycin component).

No products indexed under this heading.

Erythromycin Lactobionate (ZIANA Gel should not be used in combination with erythromycin-containing products due to its clindamycin component).

No products indexed under this heading.

Erythromycin Stearate (ZIANA Gel should not be used in combination with erythromycin-containing products due to its clindamycin component).

No products indexed under this heading.

Metocurine Iodide (Clindamycin has been shown to have neuromuscular blocking properties that may enhance the action of other neuromuscular blocking agents. Therefore, ZIANA Gel should be used with caution in patients receiving such agents).

No products indexed under this heading.

Mivacurium Chloride (Clindamycin has been shown to have neuromuscular blocking properties that may enhance the action of other neuromuscular blocking agents. Therefore, ZIANA Gel should be used with caution in patients receiving such agents).

No products indexed under this heading.

Pancuronium Bromide (Clindamycin has been shown to have neuromuscular blocking properties that may enhance the action of other neuromuscular blocking agents. Therefore, ZIANA Gel should be used with caution in patients receiving such agents).

No products indexed under this heading.

Rapacuronium Bromide (Clindamycin has been shown to have neuromuscular blocking properties that may enhance the action of other neuromuscular blocking agents. Therefore, ZIANA Gel should be used with caution in patients receiving such agents).

No products indexed under this heading.

Rocuronium Bromide (Clindamycin has been shown to have neuromuscular blocking properties that may enhance the action of other neuromuscular blocking agents. Therefore, ZIANA Gel should be used with caution in patients receiving such agents). Products include:

Zemuron Injection 2947

Succinylcholine Chloride (Clindamycin has been shown to have neuromuscular blocking properties that may enhance the action of other neuromuscular blocking agents. Therefore, ZIANA Gel should be used with caution in patients receiving such agents).

No products indexed under this heading.

Topical Medications (Concomitant topical medication, medicated or abrasive soaps and cleansers, soaps and cosmetics that have a strong drying effect, and products with high concentrations of alcohol, astringents, spices or lime should be used with caution. When used with ZIANA Gel, there may be increased skin irritation).

No products indexed under this heading.

Vecuronium Bromide (Clindamycin has been shown to have neuromuscular blocking properties that may enhance the action of other neuromuscular blocking agents. Therefore, ZIANA Gel should be used with caution in patients receiving such agents).

No products indexed under this heading.

ZINACEF FOR INJECTION

(Cefuroxime) 1678

See Zinacef Injection

ZINACEF INJECTION

(Cefuroxime) 1678

May interact with aminoglycosides, oral anticoagulants, and certain other agents. Compounds in these categories include:

Amikacin Sulfate (Concomitant administration may produce nephrotoxicity).

No products indexed under this heading.

Anisindione (Cephalosporins may be associated with a fall in prothrombin activity; those at risk include patients stabilized on anticoagulants).
No products indexed under this heading.

Dicumarol (Cephalosporins may be associated with a fall in prothrombin activity; those at risk include patients stabilized on anticoagulants).
No products indexed under this heading.

Gentamicin Sulfate (Concomitant administration may produce nephrotoxicity). Products include:
Pred-G Ophthalmic Ointment .... ⊙ **229**
Pred-G Ophthalmic Suspension ...... ⊙ **228**

Kanamycin Sulfate (Concomitant administration may produce nephrotoxicity).
No products indexed under this heading.

Probenecid (Concurrent administration of probenecid decreases renal clearance and increases peak serum levels of cefuroxime).
No products indexed under this heading.

Streptomycin Sulfate (Concomitant administration may produce nephrotoxicity).
No products indexed under this heading.

Tobramycin (Concomitant administration may produce nephrotoxicity). Products include:
Zylet Ophthalmic Suspension .... ⊙ **247**

Tobramycin Sulfate (Concomitant administration may produce nephrotoxicity).
No products indexed under this heading.

Warfarin Sodium (Cephalosporins may be associated with a fall in prothrombin activity; those at risk include patients stabilized on anticoagulants).
No products indexed under this heading.

ZINC-220 CAPSULES

(Zinc Sulfate) **564**
None cited in PDR database.

ZOCOR TABLETS

(Simvastatin) **2136**
May interact with azole antifungals, oral anticoagulants, cytochrome p450 3a4 inhibitors (selected), cytochrome p450 3a4 inhibitors, potent, fibrates, macrolide antibiotics, protease inhibitors, and certain other agents. Compounds in these categories include:

Acetazolamide (The risk of myopathy is increased by reducing the elimination of simvastatin. Hence when simvastatin is used with an inhibitor of CYP3A4, elevated plasma levels of HMG-CoA reductase inhibitory activity can increase the risk of myopathy and rhabdomyolysis, particularly with higher doses of simvastatin).
No products indexed under this heading.

Amiodarone Hydrochloride (The risk of myopathy/rhabdomyolysis is increased by concomitant administration of amiodarone hydrochloride with higher doses of simvastatin. The combined use of simvastatin at doses higher than 20 mg with amiodarone should be avoided unless the clinical benefit is likely to outweigh the increased risk of myopathy).
No products indexed under this heading.

Amprenavir (The risk of myopathy and rhabdomyolysis is increased by high levels of statin activity in plasma. Simvastatin is metabolized by the cytochrome P450 isoform 3A4. Certain drugs, including the HIV protease inhibitors, which inhibit this metabolic pathway can raise the plasma levels of simvastatin and may increase the risk of myopathy. The use of simvastatin concomitantly with these CYP3A4 inhibitors should be avoided).
No products indexed under this heading.

Anastrozole (The risk of myopathy is increased by reducing the elimination of simvastatin. Hence when simvastatin is used with an inhibitor of CYP3A4, elevated plasma levels of HMG-CoA reductase inhibitory activity can increase the risk of myopathy and rhabdomyolysis, particularly with higher doses of simvastatin). Products include:
Arimidex Tablets **672**

Anisindione (Concomitant use with simvastatin may prolong INR. Achieve stable INR prior to initiation of simvastatin. Monitor INR frequently until stable upon initiation or alteration of simvastatin therapy).
No products indexed under this heading.

Aprepitant (The risk of myopathy is increased by reducing the elimination of simvastatin. Hence when simvastatin is used with an inhibitor of CYP3A4, elevated plasma levels of HMG-CoA reductase inhibitory activity can increase the risk of myopathy and rhabdomyolysis, particularly with higher doses of simvastatin). Products include:
Emend Capsules **1992**

Atazanavir (The risk of myopathy is increased by reducing the elimination of simvastatin. Hence when simvastatin is used with an inhibitor of CYP3A4, elevated plasma levels of HMG-CoA reductase inhibitory activity can increase the risk of myopathy and rhabdomyolysis, particularly with higher doses of simvastatin. Concomitant use should be avoided unless the benefits of combined therapy outweigh the risk. If treatment with itraconazole, ketoconazole, erythromycin, clarithromycin, or telithromycin is unavoidable, therapy with simvastatin should be suspended during the course of treatment).
No products indexed under this heading.

Atazanavir Sulfate (The risk of myopathy is increased by reducing the elimination of simvastatin. Hence when simvastatin is used with an inhibitor of CYP3A4, elevated plasma levels of HMG-CoA reductase inhibitory activity can increase the risk of myopathy and rhabdomyolysis, particularly with higher doses of simvastatin. Concomitant use should be avoided unless the benefits of combined therapy outweigh the risk. If treatment with itraconazole, ketoconazole, erythromycin, clarithromycin, or telithromycin is unavoidable, therapy with simvastatin should be suspended during the course of treatment). Products include:
Reyataz Capsules **3299**

Azithromycin Dihydrate (The risk of myopathy and rhabdomyolysis is increased by high levels of statin activity in plasma. Simvastatin is metabolized by the cytochrome P450 isoform 3A4. Certain drugs, including the macrolide antibiotics erythromycin and clarithromycin, which inhibit this metabolic pathway can raise the plasma levels of simvastatin and may increase the risk of myopathy. The use of simvastatin concomitantly with these CYP3A4 inhibitors should be avoided. If treatment with erythromycin or clarithromycin is unavoidable, therapy with simvastatin should be suspended during the course of treatment).
No products indexed under this heading.

Cimetidine (The risk of myopathy is increased by reducing the elimination of simvastatin. Hence when simvastatin is used with an inhibitor of CYP3A4, elevated plasma levels of HMG-CoA reductase inhibitory activity can increase the risk of myopathy and rhabdomyolysis, particularly with higher doses of simvastatin).
No products indexed under this heading.

Cimetidine Hydrochloride (The risk of myopathy is increased by reducing the elimination of simvastatin. Hence when simvastatin is used with an inhibitor of CYP3A4, elevated plasma levels of HMG-CoA reductase inhibitory activity can increase the risk of myopathy and rhabdomyolysis, particularly with higher doses of simvastatin).
No products indexed under this heading.

Ciprofloxacin (The risk of myopathy is increased by reducing the elimination of simvastatin. Hence when simvastatin is used with an inhibitor of CYP3A4, elevated plasma levels of HMG-CoA reductase inhibitory activity can increase the risk of myopathy and rhabdomyolysis, particularly with higher doses of simvastatin). Products include:
Cipro I.V. **2817**
Cipro Oral Suspension **2810**
Cipro XR Tablets **2823**
Ciprodex Otic Suspension **541**

Clarithromycin (Simvastatin is metabolized by CYP3A4; coadministration with potent inhibitors of CYP3A4, such as clarithromycin increases the risk of myopathy by reducing the elimination of simvastatin; concurrent use should be avoided). Products include:
Biaxin/Biaxin XL **411**

Clofibrate (The risk of myopathy is increased by gemfibrozil and to a lesser extent by other fibrates. The combined use of simvastatin with gemfibrozil should be avoided, unless benefits are likely to outweight the increased risks. If concurrent use is deemed necessary, the dose of simvastatin should not exceed 10 mg daily. Caution should be used when prescribing other fibrates with simvastatin).
No products indexed under this heading.

Clotrimazole (The risk of myopathy and rhabdomyolysis is increased by high levels of statin activity in plasma. Simvastatin is metabolized by the cytochrome P450 isoform 3A4. Certain drugs, including itraconazole, ketoconazole, and other antifungal azoles, which inhibit this metabolic pathway can raise the plasma levels of simvastatin and may increase the risk of myopathy. The use of simvastatin concomitantly with these CYP3A4 inhibitors should be avoided. If treatment with itraconazole or ketoconazole is unavoidable, therapy with simvastatin should be suspended during the course of treatment). Products include:
Lotrisone **2881**

Cyclosporine (The risk of myopathy/rhabdomyolysis is increased by concomitant administration of cyclosporine particularly with higher doses of simvastatin. The benefits of the use of simvastatin in patients receiving cyclosporine should be carefully weighed against the risks. If concurrent use is deemed necessary, the dose of simvastatin should not exceed 10 mg daily). Products include:
Gengraf Capsules **435**
Neoral Oral Solution **2280**
Neoral Soft Gelatin Capsules **2280**
Restasis Ophthalmic Emulsion **557**
Sandimmune **2296**

Dalfopristin (The risk of myopathy is increased by reducing the elimination of simvastatin. Hence when simvastatin is used with an inhibitor of CYP3A4, elevated plasma levels of HMG-CoA reductase inhibitory activity can increase the risk of myopathy and rhabdomyolysis, particularly with higher doses of simvastatin).
No products indexed under this heading.

Danazol (The risk of myopathy/rhabdomyolysis is increased by concomitant administration of danazol particularly with higher doses of simvastatin. The benefits of the use of simvastatin in patients receiving danazol should be carefully weighed against the risks. If concurrent use is deemed necessary, the dose of simvastatin should not exceed 10 mg daily).
No products indexed under this heading.

Darunavir (The risk of myopathy and rhabdomyolysis is increased by high levels of statin activity in plasma. Simvastatin is metabolized by the cytochrome P450 isoform 3A4. Certain drugs, including the HIV protease inhibitors, which inhibit this metabolic pathway can raise the plasma levels of simvastatin and may increase the risk of myopathy. The use of simvastatin concomitantly with these CYP3A4 inhibitors should be avoided).
No products indexed under this heading.

Delavirdine Mesylate (The risk of myopathy is increased by reducing the elimination of simvastatin. Hence when simvastatin is used with an inhibitor of CYP3A4, elevated plasma levels of HMG-CoA reductase inhibitory activity can increase the risk of myopathy and rhabdomyolysis, particularly with higher doses of simvastatin. Concomitant use should be avoided unless the benefits of combined therapy outweigh the risk. If treatment with itraconazole, keto-

conazole, erythromycin, clarithromycin, or telithromycin is unavoidable, therapy with simvastatin should be suspended during the course of treatment).
No products indexed under this heading.

Delavirine (The risk of myopathy is increased by reducing the elimination of simvastatin. Hence when simvastatin is used with an inhibitor of CYP3A4, elevated plasma levels of HMG-CoA reductase inhibitory activity can increase the risk of myopathy and rhabdomyolysis, particularly with higher doses of simvastatin. Concomitant use should be avoided unless the benefits of combined therapy outweigh the risk. If treatment with itraconazole, ketoconazole, erythromycin, clarithromycin, or telithromycin is unavoidable, therapy with simvastatin should be suspended during the course of treatment).
No products indexed under this heading.

Dicumarol (Concomitant use with simvastatin may prolong INR. Achieve stable INR prior to initiation of simvastatin. Monitor INR frequently until stable upon initiation or alteration of simvastatin therapy).
No products indexed under this heading.

Digoxin (In one study, concomitant administration of digoxin with simvastatin resulted in a slight elevation of digoxin concentrations in plasma. Patients taking digoxin should be monitored appropriately when simvastatin is initiated). Products include:
Lanoxin Injection **1498**
Lanoxin Injection Pediatric **1502**
Lanoxin Tablets **1505**

Diltiazem Hydrochloride (The risk of myopathy is increased by reducing the elimination of simvastatin. Hence when simvastatin is used with an inhibitor of CYP3A4, elevated plasma levels of HMG-CoA reductase inhibitory activity can increase the risk of myopathy and rhabdomyolysis, particularly with higher doses of simvastatin). Products include:
Cardizem LA Extended Release Tablets **421**

Diltiazem Maleate (The risk of myopathy is increased by reducing the elimination of simvastatin. Hence when simvastatin is used with an inhibitor of CYP3A4, elevated plasma levels of HMG-CoA reductase inhibitory activity can increase the risk of myopathy and rhabdomyolysis, particularly with higher doses of simvastatin).
No products indexed under this heading.

Dirithromycin (The risk of myopathy and rhabdomyolysis is increased by high levels of statin activity in plasma. Simvastatin is metabolized by the cytochrome P450 isoform 3A4. Certain drugs, including the macrolide antibiotics erythromycin and clarithromycin, which inhibit this metabolic pathway can raise the plasma levels of simvastatin and may increase the risk of myopathy. The use of simvastatin concomitantly with these CYP3A4 inhibitors should be avoided. If treatment with erythromycin or clarithromycin is unavoidable, therapy with simvastatin should be suspended during the course of treatment).
No products indexed under this heading.

Efavirenz (The risk of myopathy is increased by reducing the elimination of simvastatin. Hence when simvastatin is used with an inhibitor of CYP3A4, elevated plasma levels of HMG-CoA reductase inhibitory activity can increase the risk of myopathy and rhabdomyolysis, particularly with higher doses of simvastatin).
Products include:
Atripla Tablets **938**
Sustiva Capsules **930**
Sustiva Tablets **930**

Erythromycin (The risk of myopathy and rhabdomyolysis is increased by high levels of statin activity in plasma. Simvastatin is metabolized by the cytochrome P450 isoform 3A4. Certain drugs, including the macrolide antibiotics erythromycin and clarithromycin, which inhibit this metabolic pathway can raise the plasma levels of simvastatin and may increase the risk of myopathy. The use of simvastatin concomitantly with these CYP3A4 inhibitors should be avoided. If treatment with erythromycin or clarithromycin is unavoidable, therapy with simvastatin should be suspended during the course of treatment).
No products indexed under this heading.

Erythromycin Estolate (The risk of myopathy and rhabdomyolysis is increased by high levels of statin activity in plasma. Simvastatin is metabolized by the cytochrome P450 isoform 3A4. Certain drugs, including the macrolide antibiotics erythromycin and clarithromycin, which inhibit this metabolic pathway can raise the plasma levels of simvastatin and may increase the risk of myopathy. The use of simvastatin concomitantly with these CYP3A4 inhibitors should be avoided. If treatment with erythromycin or clarithromycin is unavoidable, therapy with simvastatin should be suspended during the course of treatment).
No products indexed under this heading.

Erythromycin Ethylsuccinate (The risk of myopathy and rhabdomyolysis is increased by high levels of statin activity in plasma. Simvastatin is metabolized by the cytochrome P450 isoform 3A4. Certain drugs, including the macrolide antibiotics erythromycin and clarithromycin, which inhibit this metabolic pathway can raise the plasma levels of simvastatin and may increase the risk of myopathy. The use of simvastatin concomitantly with these CYP3A4 inhibitors should be avoided. If treatment with erythromycin or clarithromycin is unavoidable, therapy with simvastatin should be suspended during the course of treatment).
Products include:
E.E.S. **433**
EryPed **431**

Erythromycin Gluceptate (The risk of myopathy and rhabdomyolysis is increased by high levels of statin activity in plasma. Simvastatin is metabolized by the cytochrome P450 isoform 3A4. Certain drugs, including the macrolide antibiotics erythromycin and clarithromycin, which inhibit this metabolic pathway can raise the plasma levels of simvastatin and may increase the risk of myopathy. The use of simvastatin concomitantly with these CYP3A4 inhibitors should be avoided. If treatment with erythromycin or clarithromycin is unavoidable, therapy with simvastatin should be suspended during the course of treatment).
No products indexed under this heading.

Erythromycin Lactobionate (The risk of myopathy is increased by reducing the elimination of simvastatin. Hence when simvastatin is used with an inhibitor of CYP3A4, elevated plasma levels of HMG-CoA reductase inhibitory activity can increase the risk of myopathy and rhabdomyolysis, particularly with higher doses of simvastatin).
No products indexed under this heading.

Erythromycin Stearate (The risk of myopathy and rhabdomyolysis is increased by high levels of statin activity in plasma. Simvastatin is metabolized by the cytochrome P450 isoform 3A4. Certain drugs, including the macrolide antibiotics erythromycin and clarithromycin, which inhibit this metabolic pathway can raise the plasma levels of simvastatin and may increase the risk of myopathy. The use of simvastatin concomitantly with these CYP3A4 inhibitors should be avoided. If treatment with erythromycin or clarithromycin is unavoidable, therapy with simvastatin should be suspended during the course of treatment).
No products indexed under this heading.

Esomeprazole Magnesium (The risk of myopathy is increased by reducing the elimination of simvastatin. Hence when simvastatin is used with an inhibitor of CYP3A4, elevated plasma levels of HMG-CoA reductase inhibitory activity can increase the risk of myopathy and rhabdomyolysis, particularly with higher doses of simvastatin). Products include:
Nexium Delayed-Release Capsules **645**
Nexium Delayed-Release Oral Suspension **645**

Ethanol (Simvastatin should be used with caution in patients who consume substantial quantities of alcohol).
No products indexed under this heading.

Ethyl Alcohol (Simvastatin should be used with caution in patients who consume substantial quantities of alcohol).
No products indexed under this heading.

Fenofibrate (The risk of myopathy is increased by gemfibrozil and to a lesser extent by other fibrates. The combined use of simvastatin with gemfibrozil should be avoided, unless benefits are likely to outweigh the increased risks. If concurrent use is deemed necessary, the dose of simvastatin should not exceed 10 mg daily. Caution should be used when prescribing other fibrates with simvastatin). Products include:
Fenoglide Tablets **2960**
Tricor Tablets **520**

Fluconazole (The risk of myopathy and rhabdomyolysis is increased by high levels of statin activity in plasma. Simvastatin is metabolized by the cytochrome P450 isoform 3A4. Certain drugs, including itraconazole, ketoconazole, and other antifungal azoles, which inhibit this metabolic pathway can raise the plasma levels of simvastatin and may increase the risk of myopathy. The use of simvastatin concomitantly with these CYP3A4 inhibitors should be avoided. If treatment with itraconazole or ketoconazole is unavoidable, therapy with simvastatin should be suspended during the course of treatment).
No products indexed under this heading.

Fluoxetine (The risk of myopathy is increased by reducing the elimination of simvastatin. Hence when simvastatin is used with an inhibitor of CYP3A4, elevated plasma levels of HMG-CoA reductase inhibitory activity can increase the risk of myopathy and rhabdomyolysis, particularly with higher doses of simvastatin).
No products indexed under this heading.

Fluoxetine Hydrochloride (The risk of myopathy is increased by reducing the elimination of simvastatin. Hence when simvastatin is used with an inhibitor of CYP3A4, elevated plasma levels of HMG-CoA reductase inhibitory activity can increase the risk of myopathy and rhabdomyolysis, particularly with higher doses of simvastatin). Products include:
Prozac Weekly Capsules **1852**
Prozac Pulvules and Liquid **1852**
Symbyax Capsules **1871**

Fluvoxamine Maleate (The risk of myopathy is increased by reducing the elimination of simvastatin. Hence when simvastatin is used with an inhibitor of CYP3A4, elevated plasma levels of HMG-CoA reductase inhibitory activity can increase the risk of myopathy and rhabdomyolysis, particularly with higher doses of simvastatin). Products include:
Luvox CR Extended-Release Capsules **1759**

Fosamprenavir Calcium (The risk of myopathy and rhabdomyolysis is increased by high levels of statin activity in plasma. Simvastatin is metabolized by the cytochrome P450 isoform 3A4. Certain drugs, including the HIV protease inhibitors, which inhibit this metabolic pathway can raise the plasma levels of simvastatin and may increase the risk of myopathy. The use of simvastatin concomitantly with these CYP3A4 inhibitors should be avoided).
Products include:
Lexiva Oral Suspension **1510**
Lexiva Tablets **1510**

Gemfibrozil (The risk of myopathy is increased by gemfibrozil and to a lesser extent by other fibrates. The combined use of simvastatin with gemfibrozil should be avoided, unless benefits are likely to outweigh the increased risks. If concurrent use is deemed necessary, the dose of simvastatin should not exceed 10 mg daily. Caution should be used when prescribing other fibrates with simvastatin).
No products indexed under this heading.

Indinavir Sulfate (The risk of myopathy and rhabdomyolysis is increased by high levels of statin activity in plasma. Simvastatin is metabolized by the cytochrome P450 isoform 3A4. Certain drugs, including the HIV protease inhibitors, which inhibit this metabolic pathway can raise the plasma levels of simvastatin and may increase the risk of myopathy. The use of simvastatin

concomitantly with these CYP3A4 inhibitors should be avoided). Products include:

Crixivan Capsules 1979

Isoniazid (The risk of myopathy is increased by reducing the elimination of simvastatin. Hence when simvastatin is used with an inhibitor of CYP3A4, elevated plasma levels of HMG-CoA reductase inhibitory activity can increase the risk of myopathy and rhabdomyolysis, particularly with higher doses of simvastatin).

No products indexed under this heading.

Itraconazole (Simvastatin is metabolized by CYP3A4; co-administration with potent inhibitors of CYP3A4, such as itraconazole, increases the risk of myopathy by reducing the elimination of simvastatin; concurrent use should be avoided).

No products indexed under this heading.

Ketoconazole (Simvastatin is metabolized by CYP3A4; co-administration with potent inhibitors of CYP3A4, such as ketoconazole, increases the risk of myopathy by reducing the elimination of simvastatin; concurrent use should be avoided). Products include:

Extina Foam, 2% 3057
Nizoral A-D Shampoo 1901

Lopinavir (The risk of myopathy and rhabdomyolysis is increased by high levels of statin activity in plasma. Simvastatin is metabolized by the cytochrome P450 isoform 3A4. Certain drugs, including the HIV protease inhibitors, which inhibit this metabolic pathway can raise the plasma levels of simvastatin and may increase the risk of myopathy. The use of simvastatin concomitantly with these CYP3A4 inhibitors should be avoided). Products include:

Kaletra 452

Loratadine (The risk of myopathy is increased by reducing the elimination of simvastatin. Hence when simvastatin is used with an inhibitor of CYP3A4, elevated plasma levels of HMG-CoA reductase inhibitory activity can increase the risk of myopathy and rhabdomyolysis, particularly with higher doses of simvastatin).

No products indexed under this heading.

Metronidazole (The risk of myopathy is increased by reducing the elimination of simvastatin. Hence when simvastatin is used with an inhibitor of CYP3A4, elevated plasma levels of HMG-CoA reductase inhibitory activity can increase the risk of myopathy and rhabdomyolysis, particularly with higher doses of simvastatin). Products include:

Pylera Capsules 714

Metronidazole Benzoate (The risk of myopathy is increased by reducing the elimination of simvastatin. Hence when simvastatin is used with an inhibitor of CYP3A4, elevated plasma levels of HMG-CoA reductase inhibitory activity can increase the risk of myopathy and rhabdomyolysis, particularly with higher doses of simvastatin).

No products indexed under this heading.

Metronidazole Hydrochloride (The risk of myopathy is increased by reducing the elimination of simvastatin. Hence when simvastatin is used with an inhibitor of CYP3A4, elevated plasma levels of HMG-CoA reductase inhibitory activity can increase the risk of myopathy and rhabdomyolysis, particularly with higher doses of simvastatin).

No products indexed under this heading.

Metronidazole Sodium (The risk of myopathy is increased by reducing the elimination of simvastatin. Hence when simvastatin is used with an inhibitor of CYP3A4, elevated plasma levels of HMG-CoA reductase inhibitory activity can increase the risk of myopathy and rhabdomyolysis, particularly with higher doses of simvastatin).

No products indexed under this heading.

Miconazole (The risk of myopathy and rhabdomyolysis is increased by high levels of statin activity in plasma. Simvastatin is metabolized by the cytochrome P450 isoform 3A4. Certain drugs, including itraconazole, ketoconazole, and other antifungal azoles, which inhibit this metabolic pathway can raise the plasma levels of simvastatin and may increase the risk of myopathy. The use of simvastatin concomitantly with these CYP3A4 inhibitors should be avoided. If treatment with itraconazole or ketoconazole is unavoidable, therapy with simvastatin should be suspended during the course of treatment).

No products indexed under this heading.

Miconazole Nitrate (The risk of myopathy is increased by reducing the elimination of simvastatin. Hence when simvastatin is used with an inhibitor of CYP3A4, elevated plasma levels of HMG-CoA reductase inhibitory activity can increase the risk of myopathy and rhabdomyolysis, particularly with higher doses of simvastatin).

No products indexed under this heading.

Nefazodone Hydrochloride (The risk of myopathy and rhabdomyolysis is increased by high level of statin activity in plasma. Simvastatin is metabolized by the cytochrome P450 isoform 3A4. Certain drugs, including the antidepressant nefazodone, which inhibit this metabolic pathwaycan raise the plasma levels of simvastatin and may increase the risk of myopathy. The use of simvastatin concomitantly with this CYP3A4 inhibitor should be avoided).

No products indexed under this heading.

Nelfinavir Mesylate (The risk of myopathy and rhabdomyolysis is increased by high levels of statin activity in plasma. Simvastatin is metabolized by the cytochrome P450 isoform 3A4. Certain drugs, including the HIV protease inhibitors, which inhibit this metabolic pathway can raise the plasma levels of simvastatin and may increase the risk of myopathy. The use of simvastatin concomitantly with these CYP3A4 inhibitors should be avoided).

No products indexed under this heading.

Nevirapine (The risk of myopathy is increased by reducing the elimination of simvastatin. Hence when simvastatin is used with an inhibitor of CYP3A4, elevated plasma levels of HMG-CoA reductase inhibitory activity can increase the risk of myopathy and rhabdomyolysis, particularly with higher doses of simvastatin). Products include:

Viramune Oral Suspension 873
Viramune Tablets 873

Niacin (The risk of myopathy is increased by niacin (nicotinic acid) (greater or equal to 1 gm/day). Caution should be used when prescribing lipid-lowering doses (greater or equal to 1 gm/day) of niacin with simvastatin). Products include:

Advicor Tablets 402
Bausch & Lomb Ocuvite DF Vitamin Supplement.................. ⊙238
Dismutax Dietary Supplement 995
Niaspan Extended-Release Tablets 480
NT-Kinase Dietary Supplement 995
Simcor Tablets 502

Niacinamide (The risk of myopathy is increased by niacin (nicotinic acid) (greater or equal to 1 gm/day). Caution should be used when prescribing lipid-lowering doses (greater or equal to 1 gm/day) of niacin with simvastatin). Products include:

BioLean Free Tablets .... ■□635

Nicotinamide (The risk of myopathy is increased by reducing the elimination of simvastatin. Hence when simvastatin is used with an inhibitor of CYP3A4, elevated plasma levels of HMG-CoA reductase inhibitory activity can increase the risk of myopathy and rhabdomyolysis, particularly with higher doses of simvastatin).

No products indexed under this heading.

Nifedipine (The risk of myopathy is increased by reducing the elimination of simvastatin. Hence when simvastatin is used with an inhibitor of CYP3A4, elevated plasma levels of HMG-CoA reductase inhibitory activity can increase the risk of myopathy and rhabdomyolysis, particularly with higher doses of simvastatin).

No products indexed under this heading.

Norfloxacin (The risk of myopathy is increased by reducing the elimination of simvastatin. Hence when simvastatin is used with an inhibitor of CYP3A4, elevated plasma levels of HMG-CoA reductase inhibitory activity can increase the risk of myopathy and rhabdomyolysis, particularly with higher doses of simvastatin). Products include:

Noroxin Tablets 2069

Omeprazole (The risk of myopathy is increased by reducing the elimination of simvastatin. Hence when simvastatin is used with an inhibitor of CYP3A4, elevated plasma levels of HMG-CoA reductase inhibitory activity can increase the risk of myopathy and rhabdomyolysis, particularly with higher doses of simvastatin).

No products indexed under this heading.

Oxiconazole Nitrate (The risk of myopathy and rhabdomyolysis is increased by high levels of statin activity in plasma. Simvastatin is metabolized by the cytochrome P450 isoform 3A4. Certain drugs, including itraconazole, ketoconazole, and other antifungal azoles, which inhibit this metabolic pathway can raise the plasma levels of simvastatin and may increase the risk of myopathy. The use of simvastatin concomitantly with these CYP3A4 inhibitors should be avoided. If treatment with itraconazole or ketoconazole is unavoidable, therapy with simvastatin should be suspended during the course of treatment).

No products indexed under this heading.

Paroxetine Hydrochloride (The risk of myopathy is increased by reducing the elimination of simvastatin. Hence when simvastatin is used with an inhibitor of CYP3A4, elevated plasma levels of HMG-CoA reductase inhibitory activity can increase the risk of myopathy and rhabdomyolysis, particularly with higher doses of simvastatin). Products include:

Paxil 1535
Paxil CR Controlled-Release Tablets 1544

Posaconazole (The risk of myopathy and rhabdomyolysis is increased by high levels of statin activity in plasma. Simvastatin is metabolized by the cytochrome P450 isoform 3A4. Certain drugs, including itraconazole, ketoconazole, and other antifungal azoles, which inhibit this metabolic pathway can raise the plasma levels of simvastatin and may increase the risk of myopathy. The use of simvastatin concomitantly with these CYP3A4 inhibitors should be avoided. If treatment with itraconazole or ketoconazole is unavoidable, therapy with simvastatin should be suspended during the course of treatment). Products include:

Noxafil Oral Suspension 2889

Propoxyphene Hydrochloride (The risk of myopathy is increased by reducing the elimination of simvastatin. Hence when simvastatin is used with an inhibitor of CYP3A4, elevated plasma levels of HMG-CoA reductase inhibitory activity can increase the risk of myopathy and rhabdomyolysis, particularly with higher doses of simvastatin).

No products indexed under this heading.

Propoxyphene Napsylate (The risk of myopathy is increased by reducing the elimination of simvastatin. Hence when simvastatin is used with an inhibitor of CYP3A4, elevated plasma levels of HMG-CoA reductase inhibitory activity can increase the risk of myopathy and rhabdomyolysis, particularly with higher doses of simvastatin).

No products indexed under this heading.

Propranolol Hydrochloride (Significant decreases in mean Cmax, but no change in AUC). Products include:

InnoPran XL Extended Release Capsules.................................. 1484

Quinidine (The risk of myopathy is increased by reducing the elimination of simvastatin. Hence when simvastatin is used with an inhibitor of CYP3A4, elevated plasma levels of HMG-CoA reductase inhibitory activity can increase the risk of myopathy and rhabdomyolysis, particularly with higher doses of simvastatin).

No products indexed under this heading.

Quinidine Hydrochloride (The risk of myopathy is increased by reducing the elimination of simvastatin. Hence when simvastatin is used with an inhibitor of CYP3A4, elevated plasma levels of HMG-CoA reductase inhibitory activity can increase the risk of myopathy and rhabdomyolysis, particularly with higher doses of simvastatin).
No products indexed under this heading.

Quinidine Polygalacturonate (The risk of myopathy is increased by reducing the elimination of simvastatin. Hence when simvastatin is used with an inhibitor of CYP3A4, elevated plasma levels of HMG-CoA reductase inhibitory activity can increase the risk of myopathy and rhabdomyolysis, particularly with higher doses of simvastatin).
No products indexed under this heading.

Quinidine Sulfate (The risk of myopathy is increased by reducing the elimination of simvastatin. Hence when simvastatin is used with an inhibitor of CYP3A4, elevated plasma levels of HMG-CoA reductase inhibitory activity can increase the risk of myopathy and rhabdomyolysis, particularly with higher doses of simvastatin).
No products indexed under this heading.

Quinine (The risk of myopathy is increased by reducing the elimination of simvastatin. Hence when simvastatin is used with an inhibitor of CYP3A4, elevated plasma levels of HMG-CoA reductase inhibitory activity can increase the risk of myopathy and rhabdomyolysis, particularly with higher doses of simvastatin).
No products indexed under this heading.

Quinine Sulfate (The risk of myopathy is increased by reducing the elimination of simvastatin. Hence when simvastatin is used with an inhibitor of CYP3A4, elevated plasma levels of HMG-CoA reductase inhibitory activity can increase the risk of myopathy and rhabdomyolysis, particularly with higher doses of simvastatin).
No products indexed under this heading.

Quinupristin (The risk of myopathy is increased by reducing the elimination of simvastatin. Hence when simvastatin is used with an inhibitor of CYP3A4, elevated plasma levels of HMG-CoA reductase inhibitory activity can increase the risk of myopathy and rhabdomyolysis, particularly with higher doses of simvastatin).
No products indexed under this heading.

Ranitidine Bismuth Citrate (The risk of myopathy is increased by reducing the elimination of simvastatin. Hence when simvastatin is used with an inhibitor of CYP3A4, elevated plasma levels of HMG-CoA reductase inhibitory activity can increase the risk of myopathy and rhabdomyolysis, particularly with higher doses of simvastatin).
No products indexed under this heading.

Ranitidine Hydrochloride (The risk of myopathy is increased by reducing the elimination of simvastatin. Hence when simvastatin is used with an inhibitor of CYP3A4, elevated plasma levels of HMG-CoA reductase inhibitory activity can increase the risk of myopathy and rhabdomyolysis, particularly with higher doses of simvastatin). Products include:
Zantac 75 Tablets 603
Zantac 1670
Zantac Injection 1666
Zantac Injection Pharmacy Bulk Package 1668
Maximum Strength Zantac 150 Tablets 603
Maximum Strength Zantac 150 Cool Mint Tablets 603

Ritonavir (The risk of myopathy and rhabdomyolysis is increased by high levels of statin activity in plasma. Simvastatin is metabolized by the cytochrome P450 isoform 3A4. Certain drugs, including the HIV protease inhibitors, which inhibit this metabolic pathway can raise the plasma levels of simvastatin and may increase the risk of myopathy. The use of simvastatin concomitantly with these CYP3A4 inhibitors should be avoided). Products include:
Kaletra 452
Norvir 489

Saquinavir (The risk of myopathy and rhabdomyolysis is increased by high levels of statin activity in plasma. Simvastatin is metabolized by the cytochrome P450 isoform 3A4. Certain drugs, including the HIV protease inhibitors, which inhibit this metabolic pathway can raise the plasma levels of simvastatin and may increase the risk of myopathy. The use of simvastatin concomitantly with these CYP3A4 inhibitors should be avoided).
No products indexed under this heading.

Saquinavir Mesylate (The risk of myopathy and rhabdomyolysis is increased by high levels of statin activity in plasma. Simvastatin is metabolized by the cytochrome P450 isoform 3A4. Certain drugs, including the HIV protease inhibitors, which inhibit this metabolic pathway can raise the plasma levels of simvastatin and may increase the risk of myopathy. The use of simvastatin concomitantly with these CYP3A4 inhibitors should be avoided).
No products indexed under this heading.

Sertraline Hydrochloride (The risk of myopathy is increased by reducing the elimination of simvastatin. Hence when simvastatin is used with an inhibitor of CYP3A4, elevated plasma levels of HMG-CoA reductase inhibitory activity can increase the risk of myopathy and rhabdomyolysis, particularly with higher doses of simvastatin).
No products indexed under this heading.

Sildenafil Citrate (The risk of myopathy is increased by reducing the elimination of simvastatin. Hence when simvastatin is used with an inhibitor of CYP3A4, elevated plasma levels of HMG-CoA reductase inhibitory activity can increase the risk of myopathy and rhabdomyolysis, particularly with higher doses of simvastatin).
No products indexed under this heading.

Telithromycin (The risk of myopathy and rhabdomyolysis is increased by high level of statin activity in plasma. Simvastatin is metabolized by the cytochrome P450 isoform 3A4. Certain drugs, including telithromycin, which inhibit this metabolic pathway can raise the plasma levels of simvastatin and may increase the risk of myopathy. The use of simvastatin concomitantly with this CYP3A4 inhibitor should be avoided). Products include:
Ketek Tablets 2744

Terconazole (The risk of myopathy and rhabdomyolysis is increased by high levels of statin activity in plasma. Simvastatin is metabolized by the cytochrome P450 isoform 3A4. Certain drugs, including itraconazole, ketoconazole, and other antifungal azoles, which inhibit this metabolic pathway can raise the plasma levels of simvastatin and may increase the risk of myopathy. The use of simvastatin concomitantly with these CYP3A4 inhibitors should be avoided. If treatment with itraconazole or ketoconazole is unavoidable, therapy with simvastatin should be suspended during the course of treatment).
No products indexed under this heading.

Tipranavir (The risk of myopathy and rhabdomyolysis is increased by high levels of statin activity in plasma. Simvastatin is metabolized by the cytochrome P450 isoform 3A4. Certain drugs, including the HIV protease inhibitors, which inhibit this metabolic pathway can raise the plasma levels of simvastatin and may increase the risk of myopathy. The use of simvastatin concomitantly with these CYP3A4 inhibitors should be avoided). Products include:
Aptivus Capsules 823
Aptivus Oral Solution 823

Troglitazone (The risk of myopathy is increased by reducing the elimination of simvastatin. Hence when simvastatin is used with an inhibitor of CYP3A4, elevated plasma levels of HMG-CoA reductase inhibitory activity can increase the risk of myopathy and rhabdomyolysis, particularly with higher doses of simvastatin).
No products indexed under this heading.

Troleandomycin (The risk of myopathy and rhabdomyolysis is increased by high levels of statin activity in plasma. Simvastatin is metabolized by the cytochrome P450 isoform 3A4. Certain drugs, including the macrolide antibiotics erythromycin and clarithromycin, which inhibit this metabolic pathway can raise the plasma levels of simvastatin and may increase the risk of myopathy. The use of simvastatin concomitantly with these CYP3A4 inhibitors should be avoided. If treatment with erythromycin or clarithromycin is unavoidable, therapy with simvastatin should be suspended during the course of treatment).
No products indexed under this heading.

Valproate Sodium (The risk of myopathy is increased by reducing the elimination of simvastatin. Hence when simvastatin is used with an inhibitor of CYP3A4, elevated plasma levels of HMG-CoA reductase inhibitory activity can increase the risk of myopathy and rhabdomyolysis, particularly with higher doses of simvastatin).
No products indexed under this heading.

Vardenafil Hydrochloride (The risk of myopathy is increased by reducing the elimination of simvastatin. Hence when simvastatin is used with an inhibitor of CYP3A4, elevated plasma levels of HMG-CoA reductase inhibitory activity can increase the risk of myopathy and rhabdomyolysis, particularly with higher doses of simvastatin). Products include:
Levitra Tablets 2876

Verapamil Hydrochloride (The risk of myopathy/rhabdomyolysis is increased by concomitant administration of verapamil with higher doses of simvastatin. The combined use of simvastatin at doses higher than 20 mg with verapamil should be avoided unless the clinical benefit is likely to outweigh the increased risk of myopathy). Products include:
Tarka Tablets 511

Voriconazole (The risk of myopathy and rhabdomyolysis is increased by high levels of statin activity in plasma. Simvastatin is metabolized by the cytochrome P450 isoform 3A4. Certain drugs, including itraconazole, ketoconazole, and other antifungal azoles, which inhibit this metabolic pathway can raise the plasma levels of simvastatin and may increase the risk of myopathy. The use of simvastatin concomitantly with these CYP3A4 inhibitors should be avoided. If treatment with itraconazole or ketoconazole is unavoidable, therapy with simvastatin should be suspended during the course of treatment).
No products indexed under this heading.

Warfarin Sodium (Concomitant use with simvastatin may prolong INR. Achieve stable INR prior to initiation of simvastatin. Monitor INR frequently until stable upon initiation or alteration of simvastatin therapy).
No products indexed under this heading.

Zafirlukast (The risk of myopathy is increased by reducing the elimination of simvastatin. Hence when simvastatin is used with an inhibitor of CYP3A4, elevated plasma levels of HMG-CoA reductase inhibitory activity can increase the risk of myopathy and rhabdomyolysis, particularly with higher doses of simvastatin). Products include:
Accolate Tablets 669

Zileuton (The risk of myopathy is increased by reducing the elimination of simvastatin. Hence when simvastatin is used with an inhibitor of CYP3A4, elevated plasma levels of HMG-CoA reductase inhibitory activity can increase the risk of myopathy and rhabdomyolysis, particularly with higher doses of simvastatin).
No products indexed under this heading.

Food Interactions

Alcohol (Simvastatin should be used with caution in patients who consume substantial quantities of alcohol).

Grapefruit (The risk of myopathy and rhabdomyolysis is increased by high level of statin activity in plasma. Simvastatin is metabolized by the cytochrome P450 isoform 3A4. Certain drugs, including the large quantities of grapefruit juice (greater than 1 quart daily), which inhibit this metabolic pathway can raise the plasma levels of simvastatin and may increase the risk of myopathy. The use of simvastatin concomitantly with this CYP3A4 inhibitor should be avoided).

Grapefruit Juice (The risk of myopathy and rhabdomyolysis is increased by high level of statin activity in plasma. Simvastatin is metabolized by the cytochrome P450 isoform 3A4. Certain drugs, including the large quantities of grapefruit juice (greater than 1 quart daily), which inhibit this metabolic pathway can raise the plasma levels of simvastatin and may increase the risk of myopathy. The use of simvastatin concomitantly with this CYP3A4 inhibitor should be avoided).

ZOFRAN INJECTION

(Ondansetron Hydrochloride) 1682
See Zofran Tablets

ZOFRAN INJECTION PREMIXED

(Ondansetron Hydrochloride) 1682
See Zofran Tablets

ZOFRAN ORAL SOLUTION

(Ondansetron Hydrochloride) 1687
See Zofran Tablets

ZOFRAN TABLETS

(Ondansetron Hydrochloride) 1687
May interact with phenytoin and certain other agents. Compounds in these categories include:

Carbamazepine (Co-administration with potent inducers of CYP3A4, such as carbamazepine, may increase the clearance and decrease ondansetron blood concentrations; based on available data, no dosage adjustment is recommended). Products include:
- Carbatrol Capsules 3019
- Equetro Extended-Release Capsules 3174

Fosphenytoin Sodium (Co-administration with potent inducers of CYP3A4, such as phenytoin, may increase the clearance and decrease ondansetron blood concentrations; based on the available data, no dosage adjustment is recommended).
No products indexed under this heading.

Phenytoin (Co-administration with potent inducers of CYP3A4, such as phenytoin, may increase the clearance and decrease ondansetron blood concentrations; based on the available data, no dosage adjustment is recommended).
No products indexed under this heading.

Phenytoin Sodium (Co-administration with potent inducers of CYP3A4, such as phenytoin, may increase the clearance and decrease ondansetron blood concentrations; based on the available data, no dosage adjustment is recommended). Products include:
- Phenytek Capsules 2192

Rifampin (Co-administration with potent inducers of CYP3A4, such as rifampin, may increase the clearance and decrease ondansetron blood concentrations; based on available data, no dosage adjustment is recommended).
No products indexed under this heading.

Tramadol Hydrochloride (Ondansetron may be associated with an increase in patient-controlled administration of tramadol). Products include:
- Ultram ER Extended-Release Tablets 2428

Food Interactions

Food, unspecified (Bioavailability slightly enhanced by food).

ZOFRAN ODT ORALLY DISINTEGRATING TABLETS

(Ondansetron) 1687
See Zofran Tablets

ZOLINZA CAPSULES

(Vorinostat) 2142
May interact with oral anticoagulants and valproate. Compounds in these categories include:

Anisindione (Prolongation of PT and INR were observed in patients receiving vorinostat concomitantly with coumarin-derivative anticoagulants; carefully monitor PT and INR in patients concurrently administered vorinostat and coumarin derivatives).
No products indexed under this heading.

Dicumarol (Prolongation of PT and INR were observed in patients receiving vorinostat concomitantly with coumarin-derivative anticoagulants; carefully monitor PT and INR in patients concurrently administered vorinostat and coumarin derivatives).
No products indexed under this heading.

Divalproex Sodium (Severe thrombocytopenia and GI bleeding have been reported with concomitant use of vorinostat and other histone deacetylase inhibitors (eg, valproic acid). Monitor platelet count every two weeks for the first two months). Products include:
- Depakote ER Tablets 423

Valproate Sodium (Severe thrombocytopenia and GI bleeding have been reported with concomitant use of vorinostat and other histone deacetylase inhibitors (eg, valproic acid). Monitor platelet count every two weeks for the first two months).
No products indexed under this heading.

Valproic Acid (Severe thrombocytopenia and GI bleeding have been reported with concomitant use of vorinostat and other histone deacetylase inhibitors (eg, valproic acid). Monitor platelet count every two weeks for the first two months).
No products indexed under this heading.

Warfarin Sodium (Prolongation of PT and INR were observed in patients receiving vorinostat concomitantly with coumarin-derivative anticoagulants; carefully monitor PT and INR in patients concurrently administered vorinostat and coumarin derivatives).
No products indexed under this heading.

ZOMETA FOR INTRAVENOUS INFUSION

(Zoledronic acid) 2341
May interact with aminoglycosides, loop diuretics, nephrotoxic agents, and certain other agents. Compounds in these categories include:

Abacavir Sulfate (Caution is indicated when zoledronic acid is used with other potentially nephrotoxic drugs). Products include:
- Epzicom Tablets 1422
- Trizivir Tablets 1622
- Ziagen 1673

Acyclovir (Caution is indicated when zoledronic acid is used with other potentially nephrotoxic drugs). Products include:
- Zovirax 1690
- Zovirax Cream 817
- Zovirax Ointment 819

Acyclovir Sodium (Caution is indicated when zoledronic acid is used with other potentially nephrotoxic drugs).
No products indexed under this heading.

Alatrofloxacin Mesylate (Caution is indicated when zoledronic acid is used with other potentially nephrotoxic drugs).
No products indexed under this heading.

Aldesleukin (Caution is indicated when zoledronic acid is used with other potentially nephrotoxic drugs). Products include:
- Proleukin for Injection 2287

Amikacin Sulfate (Co-administration with aminoglycosides may have an additive effect to lower serum calcium for prolonged periods).
No products indexed under this heading.

Amoxicillin (Caution is indicated when zoledronic acid is used with other potentially nephrotoxic drugs). Products include:
- Amoxil Capsules 1305
- Amoxil Chewable Tablets 1305
- Amoxil Pediatric Drops for Oral Suspension 1305
- Amoxil Powder for Oral Suspension 1305
- Amoxil Tablets 1305
- Augmentin 1323
- Augmentin Tablets 1327
- Augmentin XR Extended Release Tablets 1333
- Augmentin ES-600 Powder for Oral Suspension 1329
- Moxatag Tablets 2165

Amoxicillin Trihydrate (Caution is indicated when zoledronic acid is used with other potentially nephrotoxic drugs).
No products indexed under this heading.

Amphotericin B (Caution is indicated when zoledronic acid is used with other potentially nephrotoxic drugs).
No products indexed under this heading.

Amphotericin B, liposomal (Caution is indicated when zoledronic acid is used with other potentially nephrotoxic drugs). Products include:
- AmBisome for Injection 606

Amphotericin B Cholesteryl Sulfate (Caution is indicated when zoledronic acid is used with other potentially nephrotoxic drugs).
No products indexed under this heading.

Amphotericin B Lipid Complex (Caution is indicated when zoledronic acid is used with other potentially nephrotoxic drugs). Products include:
- Abelcet Injection 1134

Ampicillin (Caution is indicated when zoledronic acid is used with other potentially nephrotoxic drugs).
No products indexed under this heading.

Ampicillin Sodium (Caution is indicated when zoledronic acid is used with other potentially nephrotoxic drugs).
No products indexed under this heading.

Ampicillin Trihydrate (Caution is indicated when zoledronic acid is used with other potentially nephrotoxic drugs).
No products indexed under this heading.

Amprenavir (Caution is indicated when zoledronic acid is used with other potentially nephrotoxic drugs).
No products indexed under this heading.

Aspirin (Caution is indicated when zoledronic acid is used with other potentially nephrotoxic drugs). Products include:
- Aggrenox Capsules 819
- Bayer Aspirin 750
- Percodan Tablets 1130
- St. Joseph 81 mg Aspirin Chewable and Enteric Coated Tablets 1903

Atazanavir (Caution is indicated when zoledronic acid is used with other potentially nephrotoxic drugs).
No products indexed under this heading.

Atorvastatin Calcium (Caution is indicated when zoledronic acid is used with other potentially nephrotoxic drugs). Products include:
- Lipitor Tablets 2501

Azithromycin Dihydrate (Caution is indicated when zoledronic acid is used with other potentially nephrotoxic drugs).
No products indexed under this heading.

Azlocillin Sodium (Caution is indicated when zoledronic acid is used with other potentially nephrotoxic drugs).
No products indexed under this heading.

Aztreonam (Caution is indicated when zoledronic acid is used with other potentially nephrotoxic drugs).
No products indexed under this heading.

Bacampicillin Hydrochloride (Caution is indicated when zoledronic acid is used with other potentially nephrotoxic drugs).
No products indexed under this heading.

Balsalazide Disodium (Caution is indicated when zoledronic acid is used with other potentially nephrotoxic drugs).
No products indexed under this heading.

Benazepril Hydrochloride (Caution is indicated when zoledronic acid is used with other potentially nephrotoxic drugs).
No products indexed under this heading.

Bendroflumethiazide (Caution is indicated when zoledronic acid is used with other potentially nephrotoxic drugs).
No products indexed under this heading.

Bumetanide (Concomitant use may increase risk of hypocalcemia).
No products indexed under this heading.

Caffeine (Caution is indicated when zoledronic acid is used with other potentially nephrotoxic drugs). Products include:

BioLean Free Tablets 635
BioLean II Tablets 635
Winrgy Dietary Supplement 642

Captopril (Caution is indicated when zoledronic acid is used with other potentially nephrotoxic drugs). Products include:
Captopril Tablets 2182

Carbenicillin Disodium (Caution is indicated when zoledronic acid is used with other potentially nephrotoxic drugs).
No products indexed under this heading.

Carbenicillin Indanyl Sodium (Caution is indicated when zoledronic acid is used with other potentially nephrotoxic drugs).
No products indexed under this heading.

Carboplatin (Caution is indicated when zoledronic acid is used with other potentially nephrotoxic drugs).
No products indexed under this heading.

Carmustine (BCNU) (Caution is indicated when zoledronic acid is used with other potentially nephrotoxic drugs).
No products indexed under this heading.

Cefaclor (Caution is indicated when zoledronic acid is used with other potentially nephrotoxic drugs).
No products indexed under this heading.

Cefadroxil (Caution is indicated when zoledronic acid is used with other potentially nephrotoxic drugs).
No products indexed under this heading.

Cefamandole Nafate (Caution is indicated when zoledronic acid is used with other potentially nephrotoxic drugs).
No products indexed under this heading.

Cefazolin Sodium (Caution is indicated when zoledronic acid is used with other potentially nephrotoxic drugs).
No products indexed under this heading.

Cefdinir (Caution is indicated when zoledronic acid is used with other potentially nephrotoxic drugs). Products include:
Omnicef Capsules 497
Omnicef for Oral Suspension 497

Cefepime Hydrochloride (Caution is indicated when zoledronic acid is used with other potentially nephrotoxic drugs).
No products indexed under this heading.

Cefixime (Caution is indicated when zoledronic acid is used with other potentially nephrotoxic drugs). Products include:
Suprax for Oral Suspension 1891
Suprax Tablets 1891

Cefmetazole Sodium (Caution is indicated when zoledronic acid is used with other potentially nephrotoxic drugs).
No products indexed under this heading.

Cefonicid Sodium (Caution is indicated when zoledronic acid is used with other potentially nephrotoxic drugs).
No products indexed under this heading.

Cefoperazone Sodium (Caution is indicated when zoledronic acid is used with other potentially nephrotoxic drugs).
No products indexed under this heading.

Ceforanide (Caution is indicated when zoledronic acid is used with other potentially nephrotoxic drugs).
No products indexed under this heading.

Cefotaxime Sodium (Caution is indicated when zoledronic acid is used with other potentially nephrotoxic drugs).
No products indexed under this heading.

Cefotetan (Caution is indicated when zoledronic acid is used with other potentially nephrotoxic drugs).
No products indexed under this heading.

Cefoxitin Sodium (Caution is indicated when zoledronic acid is used with other potentially nephrotoxic drugs).
No products indexed under this heading.

Cefpodoxime Proxetil (Caution is indicated when zoledronic acid is used with other potentially nephrotoxic drugs).
No products indexed under this heading.

Cefprozil (Caution is indicated when zoledronic acid is used with other potentially nephrotoxic drugs).
No products indexed under this heading.

Ceftazidime (Caution is indicated when zoledronic acid is used with other potentially nephrotoxic drugs). Products include:
Fortaz 1450

Ceftizoxime Sodium (Caution is indicated when zoledronic acid is used with other potentially nephrotoxic drugs).
No products indexed under this heading.

Ceftriaxone Sodium (Caution is indicated when zoledronic acid is used with other potentially nephrotoxic drugs). Products include:
Rocephin Injectable Vials, ADD-Vantage, Galaxy, Bulk 2642

Cefuroxime Axetil (Caution is indicated when zoledronic acid is used with other potentially nephrotoxic drugs). Products include:
Ceftin 1380

Cefuroxime Sodium (Caution is indicated when zoledronic acid is used with other potentially nephrotoxic drugs).
No products indexed under this heading.

Celecoxib (Caution is indicated when zoledronic acid is used with other potentially nephrotoxic drugs). Products include:
Celebrex Capsules 2979

Cephalexin (Caution is indicated when zoledronic acid is used with other potentially nephrotoxic drugs).
No products indexed under this heading.

Cephalothin Sodium (Caution is indicated when zoledronic acid is used with other potentially nephrotoxic drugs).
No products indexed under this heading.

Cephapirin Sodium (Caution is indicated when zoledronic acid is used with other potentially nephrotoxic drugs).
No products indexed under this heading.

Cephradine (Caution is indicated when zoledronic acid is used with other potentially nephrotoxic drugs).
No products indexed under this heading.

Cerivastatin Sodium (Caution is indicated when zoledronic acid is used with other potentially nephrotoxic drugs).
No products indexed under this heading.

Chlorothiazide (Caution is indicated when zoledronic acid is used with other potentially nephrotoxic drugs).
No products indexed under this heading.

Chlorothiazide Sodium (Caution is indicated when zoledronic acid is used with other potentially nephrotoxic drugs). Products include:
Intravenous Sodium Diuril 2490

Chlorpropamide (Caution is indicated when zoledronic acid is used with other potentially nephrotoxic drugs).
No products indexed under this heading.

Cidofovir (Caution is indicated when zoledronic acid is used with other potentially nephrotoxic drugs).
No products indexed under this heading.

Cilastatin Sodium (Caution is indicated when zoledronic acid is used with other potentially nephrotoxic drugs). Products include:
Primaxin I.M. 2080
Primaxin I.V. 2083

Cimetidine (Caution is indicated when zoledronic acid is used with other potentially nephrotoxic drugs).
No products indexed under this heading.

Cimetidine Hydrochloride (Caution is indicated when zoledronic acid is used with other potentially nephrotoxic drugs).
No products indexed under this heading.

Cisplatin (Caution is indicated when zoledronic acid is used with other potentially nephrotoxic drugs).
No products indexed under this heading.

Cladribine (Caution is indicated when zoledronic acid is used with other potentially nephrotoxic drugs). Products include:
Leustatin Injection 2384

Clozapine (Caution is indicated when zoledronic acid is used with other potentially nephrotoxic drugs).
No products indexed under this heading.

Colistimethate Sodium (Caution is indicated when zoledronic acid is used with other potentially nephrotoxic drugs).
No products indexed under this heading.

Colistin Sulfate (Caution is indicated when zoledronic acid is used with other potentially nephrotoxic drugs).
No products indexed under this heading.

Cyclophosphamide (Caution is indicated when zoledronic acid is used with other potentially nephrotoxic drugs).
No products indexed under this heading.

Cyclosporine (Caution is indicated when zoledronic acid is used with other potentially nephrotoxic drugs). Products include:
Gengraf Capsules 435
Neoral Oral Solution 2280
Neoral Soft Gelatin Capsules 2280
Restasis Ophthalmic Emulsion 557
Sandimmune 2296

Cytarabine (Caution is indicated when zoledronic acid is used with other potentially nephrotoxic drugs).
No products indexed under this heading.

Cytarabine Liposome (Caution is indicated when zoledronic acid is used with other potentially nephrotoxic drugs). Products include:
DepoCyt Injection 1136

Delavirdine Mesylate (Caution is indicated when zoledronic acid is used with other potentially nephrotoxic drugs).
No products indexed under this heading.

Diatrizoate Meglumine (Caution is indicated when zoledronic acid is used with other potentially nephrotoxic drugs).
No products indexed under this heading.

Diatrizoate Sodium (Caution is indicated when zoledronic acid is used with other potentially nephrotoxic drugs).
No products indexed under this heading.

Diclofenac Potassium (Caution is indicated when zoledronic acid is used with other potentially nephrotoxic drugs).
No products indexed under this heading.

Diclofenac Sodium (Caution is indicated when zoledronic acid is used with other potentially nephrotoxic drugs). Products include:
Diclofenac Sodium Ophthalmic Solution .... ⊙240
Voltaren Ophthalmic Solution 2336
Voltaren Tablets 2334
Voltaren-XR Tablets 2337

Dicloxacillin Sodium (Caution is indicated when zoledronic acid is used with other potentially nephrotoxic drugs).
No products indexed under this heading.

Didanosine (Caution is indicated when zoledronic acid is used with other potentially nephrotoxic drugs).
No products indexed under this heading.

Efavirenz (Caution is indicated when zoledronic acid is used with other potentially nephrotoxic drugs). Products include:
Atripla Tablets 938
Sustiva Capsules 930
Sustiva Tablets 930

Emtricitabine (Caution is indicated when zoledronic acid is used with other potentially nephrotoxic drugs). Products include:
Atripla Tablets 938
Emtriva Capsules 1246
Emtriva Oral Solution 1246
Truvada Tablets 1262

Enalapril Maleate (Caution is indicated when zoledronic acid is used with other potentially nephrotoxic drugs).
No products indexed under this heading.

Enalaprilat (Caution is indicated when zoledronic acid is used with other potentially nephrotoxic drugs).
No products indexed under this heading.

Enfuvirtide (Caution is indicated when zoledronic acid is used with other potentially nephrotoxic drugs).
No products indexed under this heading.

Ethacrynic Acid (Concomitant use may increase risk of hypocalcemia). Products include:
Edecrin Tablets 698

Ethiodized Oil (Caution is indicated when zoledronic acid is used with other potentially nephrotoxic drugs).
No products indexed under this heading.

Etodolac (Caution is indicated when zoledronic acid is used with other potentially nephrotoxic drugs).
No products indexed under this heading.

Fenoprofen Calcium (Caution is indicated when zoledronic acid is used with other potentially nephrotoxic drugs). Products include:
Nalfon Capsules 2508

Filgrastim (Caution is indicated when zoledronic acid is used with other potentially nephrotoxic drugs). Products include:
Neupogen for Injection 589

Fluorouracil (Caution is indicated when zoledronic acid is used with other potentially nephrotoxic drugs). Products include:
Carac Cream 0.5% 2722

Flurbiprofen (Caution is indicated when zoledronic acid is used with other potentially nephrotoxic drugs).
No products indexed under this heading.

Fluvastatin Sodium (Caution is indicated when zoledronic acid is used with other potentially nephrotoxic drugs). Products include:
Lescol Capsules 2268
Lescol XL Tablets 2268

Foscarnet Sodium (Caution is indicated when zoledronic acid is used with other potentially nephrotoxic drugs).
No products indexed under this heading.

Fosinopril Sodium (Caution is indicated when zoledronic acid is used with other potentially nephrotoxic drugs).
No products indexed under this heading.

Furosemide (Concomitant use may increase risk of hypocalcemia). Products include:
Furosemide Tablets 2186

Gadopentetate Dimeglumine (Caution is indicated when zoledronic acid is used with other potentially nephrotoxic drugs).
No products indexed under this heading.

Gentamicin (Caution is indicated when zoledronic acid is used with other potentially nephrotoxic drugs).
No products indexed under this heading.

Gentamicin Sulfate (Co-administration with aminoglycosides may have an additive effect to lower serum calcium for prolonged periods). Products include:
Pred-G Ophthalmic Ointment .... ⊙229
Pred-G Ophthalmic Suspension .... ⊙228

Glipizide (Caution is indicated when zoledronic acid is used with other potentially nephrotoxic drugs).
No products indexed under this heading.

Globulin, Immune (Human) (Caution is indicated when zoledronic acid is used with other potentially nephrotoxic drugs). Products include:
Flebogamma 5% 1715

Glyburide (Caution is indicated when zoledronic acid is used with other potentially nephrotoxic drugs).
No products indexed under this heading.

Gold Therapy (Caution is indicated when zoledronic acid is used with other potentially nephrotoxic drugs).
No products indexed under this heading.

HMG-CoA Reductase Inhibitors (Caution is indicated when zoledronic acid is used with other potentially nephrotoxic drugs).
No products indexed under this heading.

Hydrochlorothiazide (Caution is indicated when zoledronic acid is used with other potentially nephrotoxic drugs). Products include:
Atacand HCT 642
Avalide Tablets 892
Avalide Tablets 2713
Benicar HCT Tablets 1010
Diovan HCT Tablets 2216
Dyazide Capsules 1405
Micardis HCT Tablets 854
Prinzide Tablets 2092
Tekturna HCT Tablets 2324
Teveten HCT Tablets 517

Hydroflumethiazide (Caution is indicated when zoledronic acid is used with other potentially nephrotoxic drugs).
No products indexed under this heading.

Ibuprofen (Caution is indicated when zoledronic acid is used with other potentially nephrotoxic drugs). Products include:
Motrin IB Tablets and Caplets 1900
Children's Motrin Oral Suspension 1901
Children's Motrin Non-Staining Dye-Free Oral Suspension 1901
Children's Motrin Cold Oral Suspension 1899
Infants' Motrin Concentrated Drops 1901
Infants' Motrin Non-Staining Dye-Free Concentrated Drops 1901
Junior Strength Motrin Caplets and Chewable Tablets 1901
Vicoprofen Tablets 533

Idarubicin Hydrochloride (Caution is indicated when zoledronic acid is used with other potentially nephrotoxic drugs).
No products indexed under this heading.

Ifosfamide (Caution is indicated when zoledronic acid is used with other potentially nephrotoxic drugs).
No products indexed under this heading.

Imipenem (Caution is indicated when zoledronic acid is used with other potentially nephrotoxic drugs). Products include:
Primaxin I.M. 2080
Primaxin I.V. 2083

Immune Globulin Intravenous (Human) (Caution is indicated when zoledronic acid is used with other potentially nephrotoxic drugs). Products include:
Flebogamma 5% DIF 1718
Gammagard Liquid 730
Gammagard S/D 734
Gamunex 3094

Indinavir Sulfate (Caution is indicated when zoledronic acid is used with other potentially nephrotoxic drugs). Products include:
Crixivan Capsules 1979

Indomethacin (Caution is indicated when zoledronic acid is used with other potentially nephrotoxic drugs). Products include:
Indocin 2024

Indomethacin Sodium Trihydrate (Caution is indicated when zoledronic acid is used with other potentially nephrotoxic drugs). Products include:
Indocin I.V. 2489

Interferon Beta-1b (Caution is indicated when zoledronic acid is used with other potentially nephrotoxic drugs). Products include:
Betaseron for SC Injection 756

Interleukin-2 (Caution is indicated when zoledronic acid is used with other potentially nephrotoxic drugs).
No products indexed under this heading.

Iodamide Meglumine (Caution is indicated when zoledronic acid is used with other potentially nephrotoxic drugs).
No products indexed under this heading.

Iohexol (Caution is indicated when zoledronic acid is used with other potentially nephrotoxic drugs).
No products indexed under this heading.

Iopamidol (Caution is indicated when zoledronic acid is used with other potentially nephrotoxic drugs).
No products indexed under this heading.

Iopanoic Acid (Caution is indicated when zoledronic acid is used with other potentially nephrotoxic drugs).
No products indexed under this heading.

Iothalamate Meglumine (Caution is indicated when zoledronic acid is used with other potentially nephrotoxic drugs).
No products indexed under this heading.

Ioxaglate Meglumine (Caution is indicated when zoledronic acid is used with other potentially nephrotoxic drugs).
No products indexed under this heading.

Ioxaglate Sodium (Caution is indicated when zoledronic acid is used with other potentially nephrotoxic drugs).
No products indexed under this heading.

Kanamycin Sulfate (Co-administration with aminoglycosides may have an additive effect to lower serum calcium for prolonged periods).
No products indexed under this heading.

Ketoprofen (Caution is indicated when zoledronic acid is used with other potentially nephrotoxic drugs).
No products indexed under this heading.

Ketorolac Tromethamine (Caution is indicated when zoledronic acid is used with other potentially nephrotoxic drugs).
No products indexed under this heading.

Lamium album (Caution is indicated when zoledronic acid is used with other potentially nephrotoxic drugs).
No products indexed under this heading.

Lisinopril (Caution is indicated when zoledronic acid is used with other potentially nephrotoxic drugs). Products include:
Prinivil Tablets 2087
Prinzide Tablets 2092

Lithium (Caution is indicated when zoledronic acid is used with other potentially nephrotoxic drugs).
No products indexed under this heading.

Lithium Carbonate (Caution is indicated when zoledronic acid is used with other potentially nephrotoxic drugs).
No products indexed under this heading.

Lithium Citrate (Caution is indicated when zoledronic acid is used with other potentially nephrotoxic drugs).
No products indexed under this heading.

Lopinavir (Caution is indicated when zoledronic acid is used with other potentially nephrotoxic drugs). Products include:
Kaletra 452

Loracarbef (Caution is indicated when zoledronic acid is used with other potentially nephrotoxic drugs).
No products indexed under this heading.

Lovastatin (Caution is indicated when zoledronic acid is used with other potentially nephrotoxic drugs). Products include:
Advicor Tablets 402
Mevacor Tablets 2063

Meclofenamate Sodium (Caution is indicated when zoledronic acid is used with other potentially nephrotoxic drugs).
No products indexed under this heading.

Mefenamic Acid (Caution is indicated when zoledronic acid is used with other potentially nephrotoxic drugs).
No products indexed under this heading.

Meloxicam (Caution is indicated when zoledronic acid is used with other potentially nephrotoxic drugs). Products include:
Mobic Oral Suspension 863
Mobic Tablets 863

Melphalan Hydrochloride (Caution is indicated when zoledronic acid is used with other potentially nephrotoxic drugs).
No products indexed under this heading.

Mesalamine (Caution is indicated when zoledronic acid is used with other potentially nephrotoxic drugs). Products include:
Asacol Delayed-Release Tablets 2579
Canasa Rectal Suppositories 705
Lialda Tablets 3029
Pentasa Capsules 3030

Methimazole (Caution is indicated when zoledronic acid is used with other potentially nephrotoxic drugs).
No products indexed under this heading.

Methotrexate (Caution is indicated when zoledronic acid is used with other potentially nephrotoxic drugs).
No products indexed under this heading.

Methotrexate Sodium (Caution is indicated when zoledronic acid is used with other potentially nephrotoxic drugs).
No products indexed under this heading.

Methyclothiazide (Caution is indicated when zoledronic acid is used with other potentially nephrotoxic drugs).
No products indexed under this heading.

Mezlocillin Sodium (Caution is indicated when zoledronic acid is used with other potentially nephrotoxic drugs).
No products indexed under this heading.

Minocycline Hydrochloride (Caution is indicated when zoledronic acid is used with other potentially nephrotoxic drugs). Products include:
Solodyn Extended Release Tablets 1938

Mitomycin (Mitomycin-C) (Caution is indicated when zoledronic acid is used with other potentially nephrotoxic drugs).
No products indexed under this heading.

Moexipril Hydrochloride (Caution is indicated when zoledronic acid is used with other potentially nephrotoxic drugs).
No products indexed under this heading.

Muromonab-CD3 (Caution is indicated when zoledronic acid is used with other potentially nephrotoxic drugs). Products include:
Orthoclone OKT3 Sterile Solution 2387

Nabumetone (Caution is indicated when zoledronic acid is used with other potentially nephrotoxic drugs).
No products indexed under this heading.

Nafcillin Sodium (Caution is indicated when zoledronic acid is used with other potentially nephrotoxic drugs).
No products indexed under this heading.

Naproxen (Caution is indicated when zoledronic acid is used with other potentially nephrotoxic drugs). Products include:
EC-Naprosyn Delayed-Release Tablets 2632
Naprosyn Suspension 2632
Naprosyn Tablets 2632

Naproxen Sodium (Caution is indicated when zoledronic acid is used with other potentially nephrotoxic drugs). Products include:
Anaprox Tablets 2632
Anaprox DS Tablets 2632
Treximet Tablets 1616

Nelfinavir Mesylate (Caution is indicated when zoledronic acid is used with other potentially nephrotoxic drugs).
No products indexed under this heading.

Neomycin (Caution is indicated when zoledronic acid is used with other potentially nephrotoxic drugs).
No products indexed under this heading.

Neomycin, oral (Caution is indicated when zoledronic acid is used with other potentially nephrotoxic drugs).
No products indexed under this heading.

Neomycin Sulfate (Caution is indicated when zoledronic acid is used with other potentially nephrotoxic drugs). Products include:
Neosporin Ophthalmic Solution Sterile .... ⊙252

Nevirapine (Caution is indicated when zoledronic acid is used with other potentially nephrotoxic drugs). Products include:
Viramune Oral Suspension 873
Viramune Tablets 873

Norfloxacin (Caution is indicated when zoledronic acid is used with other potentially nephrotoxic drugs). Products include:
Noroxin Tablets 2069

Olsalazine Sodium (Caution is indicated when zoledronic acid is used with other potentially nephrotoxic drugs).
No products indexed under this heading.

Omeprazole (Caution is indicated when zoledronic acid is used with other potentially nephrotoxic drugs).
No products indexed under this heading.

Oxaprozin (Caution is indicated when zoledronic acid is used with other potentially nephrotoxic drugs).
No products indexed under this heading.

Pamidronate Disodium (Caution is indicated when zoledronic acid is used with other potentially nephrotoxic drugs).
No products indexed under this heading.

Paroxetine Hydrochloride (Caution is indicated when zoledronic acid is used with other potentially nephrotoxic drugs). Products include:
Paxil 1535
Paxil CR Controlled-Release Tablets 1544

Penicillamine (Caution is indicated when zoledronic acid is used with other potentially nephrotoxic drugs). Products include:
Cuprimine Capsules 1986

Penicillin G Benzathine (Caution is indicated when zoledronic acid is used with other potentially nephrotoxic drugs). Products include:
Bicillin C-R Injectable Suspension 1775
Bicillin L-A Injection 1777

Penicillin G Potassium (Caution is indicated when zoledronic acid is used with other potentially nephrotoxic drugs).
No products indexed under this heading.

Penicillin G Procaine (Caution is indicated when zoledronic acid is used with other potentially nephrotoxic drugs). Products include:
Bicillin C-R Injectable Suspension 1775
Bicillin L-A Injection 1777

Penicillin G Sodium (Caution is indicated when zoledronic acid is used with other potentially nephrotoxic drugs).
No products indexed under this heading.

Penicillin V Potassium (Caution is indicated when zoledronic acid is used with other potentially nephrotoxic drugs).
No products indexed under this heading.

Pentamidine Isethionate (Caution is indicated when zoledronic acid is used with other potentially nephrotoxic drugs).
No products indexed under this heading.

Perindopril Erbumine (Caution is indicated when zoledronic acid is used with other potentially nephrotoxic drugs). Products include:
Aceon Tablets (2 mg, 4 mg, 8 mg) 3038

Phenylbutazone (Caution is indicated when zoledronic acid is used with other potentially nephrotoxic drugs).
No products indexed under this heading.

Piroxicam (Caution is indicated when zoledronic acid is used with other potentially nephrotoxic drugs).
No products indexed under this heading.

Plicamycin (Caution is indicated when zoledronic acid is used with other potentially nephrotoxic drugs).
No products indexed under this heading.

Polymyxin (Caution is indicated when zoledronic acid is used with other potentially nephrotoxic drugs).
No products indexed under this heading.

Polymyxin B Sulfate (Caution is indicated when zoledronic acid is used with other potentially nephrotoxic drugs). Products include:
Neosporin Ophthalmic Solution Sterile .... ⊙252

Polythiazide (Caution is indicated when zoledronic acid is used with other potentially nephrotoxic drugs).
No products indexed under this heading.

Pravastatin Sodium (Caution is indicated when zoledronic acid is used with other potentially nephrotoxic drugs).
No products indexed under this heading.

Probenecid (Caution is indicated when zoledronic acid is used with other potentially nephrotoxic drugs).
No products indexed under this heading.

Quinapril Hydrochloride (Caution is indicated when zoledronic acid is used with other potentially nephrotoxic drugs).
No products indexed under this heading.

Rabeprazole Sodium (Caution is indicated when zoledronic acid is used with other potentially nephrotoxic drugs). Products include:
Aciphex Tablets 1053

Ramipril (Caution is indicated when zoledronic acid is used with other potentially nephrotoxic drugs).
No products indexed under this heading.

Rifampin (Caution is indicated when zoledronic acid is used with other potentially nephrotoxic drugs).
No products indexed under this heading.

Riluzole (Caution is indicated when zoledronic acid is used with other potentially nephrotoxic drugs). Products include:
Rilutek Tablets 2771

Ritonavir (Caution is indicated when zoledronic acid is used with other potentially nephrotoxic drugs). Products include:
Kaletra 452
Norvir 489

Rofecoxib (Caution is indicated when zoledronic acid is used with other potentially nephrotoxic drugs).
No products indexed under this heading.

Saquinavir (Caution is indicated when zoledronic acid is used with other potentially nephrotoxic drugs).
No products indexed under this heading.

Sibutramine Hydrochloride Monohydrate (Caution is indicated when zoledronic acid is used with other potentially nephrotoxic drugs). Products include:
Meridia Capsules 475

Simvastatin (Caution is indicated when zoledronic acid is used with other potentially nephrotoxic drugs). Products include:
Simcor Tablets 502
Vytorin 10/10 Tablets 2149
Vytorin 10/10 Tablets 2939
Vytorin 10/20 Tablets 2149
Vytorin 10/20 Tablets 2939
Vytorin 10/40 Tablets 2149
Vytorin 10/40 Tablets 2939
Vytorin 10/80 Tablets 2149
Vytorin 10/80 Tablets 2939
Zocor Tablets 2136

Spirapril Hydrochloride (Caution is indicated when zoledronic acid is used with other potentially nephrotoxic drugs).
No products indexed under this heading.

Stavudine (Caution is indicated when zoledronic acid is used with other potentially nephrotoxic drugs).
No products indexed under this heading.

Streptomycin Sulfate (Coadministration with aminoglycosides may have an additive effect to lower serum calcium for prolonged periods).
No products indexed under this heading.

Streptozocin (Caution is indicated when zoledronic acid is used with other potentially nephrotoxic drugs).
No products indexed under this heading.

Sulfacytine (Caution is indicated when zoledronic acid is used with other potentially nephrotoxic drugs).
No products indexed under this heading.

Sulfamethizole (Caution is indicated when zoledronic acid is used with other potentially nephrotoxic drugs).
No products indexed under this heading.

Sulfamethoxazole (Caution is indicated when zoledronic acid is used with other potentially nephrotoxic drugs).
No products indexed under this heading.

Sulfasalazine (Caution is indicated when zoledronic acid is used with other potentially nephrotoxic drugs).
No products indexed under this heading.

Sulfinpyrazone (Caution is indicated when zoledronic acid is used with other potentially nephrotoxic drugs).
No products indexed under this heading.

Sulfisoxazole Acetyl (Caution is indicated when zoledronic acid is used with other potentially nephrotoxic drugs).
No products indexed under this heading.

Sulfisoxazole Diolamine (Caution is indicated when zoledronic acid is used with other potentially nephrotoxic drugs).
No products indexed under this heading.

Sulindac (Caution is indicated when zoledronic acid is used with other potentially nephrotoxic drugs).
Products include:
Clinoril Tablets ... 1962

Tacrolimus (Caution is indicated when zoledronic acid is used with other potentially nephrotoxic drugs).
Products include:
Prograf Capsules and Injection ... 622
Protopic Ointment ... 628

Tenofovir Disoproxil Fumarate (Caution is indicated when zoledronic acid is used with other potentially nephrotoxic drugs). Products include:
Atripla Tablets ... 938
Truvada Tablets ... 1262
Viread Tablets ... 1268

Thalidomide (In multiple myeloma patients, the risk of renal dysfunction may be increased with zoledronic acid is used in combination with thalidomide).
No products indexed under this heading.

Thioguanine (Caution is indicated when zoledronic acid is used with other potentially nephrotoxic drugs).
Products include:
Tabloid Tablets ... 1601

Ticarcillin Disodium (Caution is indicated when zoledronic acid is used with other potentially nephrotoxic drugs). Products include:
Timentin ADD-Vantage ... 1606
Timentin Injection Galaxy Container ... 1609
Timentin IV Infusion ... 1603
Timentin Pharmacy Bulk Package ... 1613

Tobramycin (Co-administration with aminoglycosides may have an additive effect to lower serum calcium for prolonged periods). Products include:
Zylet Ophthalmic Suspension ... ⊙247

Tobramycin Sulfate (Co-administration with aminoglycosides may have an additive effect to lower serum calcium for prolonged periods).
No products indexed under this heading.

Tolazamide (Caution is indicated when zoledronic acid is used with other potentially nephrotoxic drugs).
No products indexed under this heading.

Tolbutamide (Caution is indicated when zoledronic acid is used with other potentially nephrotoxic drugs).
No products indexed under this heading.

Tolmetin Sodium (Caution is indicated when zoledronic acid is used with other potentially nephrotoxic drugs).
No products indexed under this heading.

Torsemide (Concomitant use may increase risk of hypocalcemia).
Products include:
Demadex Injection ... 2630
Demadex Tablets ... 2630

Trandolapril (Caution is indicated when zoledronic acid is used with other potentially nephrotoxic drugs).
Products include:
Mavik Tablets ... 472
Tarka Tablets ... 511

Triamterene (Caution is indicated when zoledronic acid is used with other potentially nephrotoxic drugs).
Products include:
Dyazide Capsules ... 1405
Dyrenium Capsules ... 3189

Trimethadione (Caution is indicated when zoledronic acid is used with other potentially nephrotoxic drugs).
No products indexed under this heading.

Trovafloxacin Mesylate (Caution is indicated when zoledronic acid is used with other potentially nephrotoxic drugs).
No products indexed under this heading.

Tyropanoate Sodium (Caution is indicated when zoledronic acid is used with other potentially nephrotoxic drugs).
No products indexed under this heading.

Valacyclovir Hydrochloride (Caution is indicated when zoledronic acid is used with other potentially nephrotoxic drugs). Products include:
Valtrex Caplets ... 1635

Valdecoxib (Caution is indicated when zoledronic acid is used with other potentially nephrotoxic drugs).
No products indexed under this heading.

Vancomycin Hydrochloride (Caution is indicated when zoledronic acid is used with other potentially nephrotoxic drugs).
No products indexed under this heading.

Voriconazole (Caution is indicated when zoledronic acid is used with other potentially nephrotoxic drugs).
No products indexed under this heading.

Zalcitabine (Caution is indicated when zoledronic acid is used with other potentially nephrotoxic drugs).
No products indexed under this heading.

Zidovudine (Caution is indicated when zoledronic acid is used with other potentially nephrotoxic drugs).
Products include:
Combivir Tablets ... 1384
Retrovir ... 1574
Retrovir IV Infusion ... 1579
Trizivir Tablets ... 1622

ZOMIG TABLETS

(Zolmitriptan) ... 694
See Zomig Nasal Spray

ZOMIG NASAL SPRAY

(Zolmitriptan) ... 689
May interact with 5HT1-receptor agonists, ergot-containing drugs, monoamine oxidase inhibitors, oral contraceptives, Serotonin and Norepinephrine Reuptake Inhibitors, selective serotonin reuptake inhibitors, and certain other agents. Compounds in these categories include:

Acetaminophen (Zolmitriptan delayed the Tmax of acetaminophen by one hour in a single dose study).
Products include:
Benadryl Allergy & Cold Kapgels ... 1895
Benadryl Allergy & Sinus Headache Kapgels ... 1895
Benadryl Severe Allergy & Sinus Headache Caplets ... 1897
Lortab 5/500 Tablets ... 3143
Lortab 7.5/500 Tablets ... 3144
Lortab 10/500 Tablets ... 3144
Percocet Tablets ... 1127
Sinutab Sinus Caplets ... 1905
Sudafed PE Cold & Cough Caplets ... 1907
Sudafed PE Nighttime Cold Caplets ... 1907
Sudafed PE Severe Cold Caplets ... 1908
Sudafed PE Sinus Headache Caplets ... 1908
Regular Strength Tylenol Tablets ... 1915
Tylenol 8 Hour Extended Release Caplets ... 1915
Extra Strength Tylenol Caplets, Cool Caplets, and EZ Tabs ... 1915
Extra Strength Tylenol Adult Rapid Blast Liquid ... 1915
Extra Strength Tylenol PM Caplets, Geltabs, Liquid, and Rapid Release Gels ... 1915
Extra Strength Tylenol Rapid Release Gels ... 1915
Tylenol with Codeine Tablets ... 2427
Tylenol Allergy Multi-Symptom Caplets with Cool Burst and Rapid Release Gelcaps ... 1916
Tylenol Allergy Multi-Symptom Nighttime Caplets with Cool Burst ... 1916
Tylenol Severe Allergy Caplets ... 1916
Tylenol Arthritis Pain Extended Release Geltabs/Caplets ... 1915
Tylenol Chest Congestion Caplets with Cool Burst ... 1910
Tylenol Chest Congestion Liquid with Cool Burst ... 1910
Children's Tylenol Plus Cold Suspension Liquid ... 1912
Children's Tylenol Plus Cold & Allergy Suspension Liquid ... 1914
Children's Tylenol Plus Cough & Runny Nose Suspension Liquid ... 1912
Children's Tylenol Plus Cough & Sore Throat Suspension Liquid ... 1912
Children's Tylenol Plus Flu Suspension Liquid ... 1914
Children's Tylenol Suspension Liquid ... 1909
Children's Tylenol Meltaways ... 1909
Children's Tylenol Plus Multi-Symptom Cold Suspension Liquid ... 1912
Tylenol Cold Severe Congestion Daytime Caplets with Cool Burst ... 1912
Tylenol Cold Head Congestion Daytime Caplets with Cool Burst ... 1910
Tylenol Cold Head Congestion Nighttime Caplets with Cool Burst ... 1910
Tylenol Cold Head Congestion Severe Daytime Caplets with Cool Burst ... 1910
Tylenol Cold Multi-Symptom Daytime Caplets with Cool Burst and Rapid Release Gels ... 1913
Tylenol Cold Multi-Symptom Daytime Liquid with Citrus Burst ... 1913
Tylenol Cold Multi-Symptom Nighttime Caplets with Cool Burst ... 1913
Tylenol Cold Multi-Symptom Nighttime Liquid with Cool Burst ... 1913
Tylenol Cold Multi-Symptom Severe Caplets with Cool Burst ... 1913
Tylenol Cold Multi-Symptom Severe Daytime Liquid with Citrus Burst ... 1913
Tylenol Cough & Sore Throat Daytime Liquid with Cool Burst ... 1918
Tylenol Cough & Sore Throat Nighttime Liquid with Cool Burst ... 1918
Concentrated Tylenol Infants' Drops ... 1909
Jr. Tylenol Meltaways ... 1909
Tylenol Sinus Congestion & Pain Daytime Caplets with Cool Burst and Gelcaps ... 1917
Tylenol Sinus Congestion & Pain Nighttime Caplets with Cool Burst ... 1917
Tylenol Sinus Congestion & Pain Severe Caplets with Cool Burst ... 1917
Tylenol Sinus Severe Congestion Caplets with Cool Burst ... 1917
Tylenol Sore Throat Daytime Liquid with Cool Burst ... 1918
Tylenol Sore Throat Nighttime Liquid with Cool Burst ... 1918
Women's Tylenol Menstrual Relief Caplets ... 1919
Vicks DayQuil Cold & Flu Multi-Symptom Relief ... ▣616
Vicks DayQuil LiquiCaps ... 2567
Vicks DayQuil Liquid ... 2567
Vicks DayQuil Multi-Symptom Cold/Flu Relief ... 2567
Vicks NyQuil Cold & Flu Multi-Symptom Relief ... ▣617
Vicks NyQuil LiquiCaps ... 2567
Vicks NyQuil Liquid ... 2567
Vicks NyQuil Multi-Symptom Cold/Flu Relief ... 2567
Vicodin Tablets ... 529
Vicodin ES Tablets ... 530
Vicodin HP Tablets ... 531
Zydone Tablets ... 1132

Almotriptan Malate (Co-administration with other 5-HT1 agonists within 24 hours of each other is contraindicated). Products include:
Axert Tablets ... 2431

Cimetidine (Following administration of cimetidine, the half-life and AUC of zolmitriptan and its active metabolites were approximately doubled).
No products indexed under this heading.

Cimetidine Hydrochloride (Following administration of cimetidine, the half-life and AUC of zolmitriptan and its active metabolites were approximately doubled).
No products indexed under this heading.

Citalopram Hydrobromide (Cases of life-threatening serotonin syndrome, including mental status changes, autonomic instability, neuromuscular aberrations, and/or GI symptoms, have been reported during combination use of selective serotonin reuptake inhibitors and triptans. If concomitant treatment with zolmitriptan and an SSRI is clinically warranted, careful observation of the patient is advised, particularly during treatment initiation and dose increases). Products include:
Celexa ... 1160

Desogestrel (Retrospective analysis of pharmacokinetic data indicates the mean plasma concentrations, Cmax and AUC, of zolmitriptan were generally higher in females taking oral contraceptives, Tmax was delayed by one-half hour in these females). Products include:
Mircette Tablets ... 1034

Desvenlafaxine Succinate (Cases of life-threatening serotonin syndrome, including mental status changes, autonomic instability, neuromuscular aberrations, and/or GI

symptoms, have been reported during combination use of serotonin/norepinephrine reuptake inhibitors and triptans. If concomitant treatment with zolmitriptan and an SNRI is clinically warranted, careful observation of the patient is advised, particularly during treatment initiation and dose increases). Products include:

Pristiq Extended-Release Tablets 3247

Dihydroergotamine Mesylate (Ergot-containing drugs have been reported to cause prolonged vasospastic reactions; because there is a theoretical basis that these effects may be additive, use of ergot-type agents and zolmitriptan within 24 hours is contraindicated).

No products indexed under this heading.

Duloxetine Hydrochloride (Cases of life-threatening serotonin syndrome, including mental status changes, autonomic instability, neuromuscular aberrations, and/or GI symptoms, have been reported during combination use of serotonin and norepinephrine reuptake inhibitors and triptans. If concomitant treatment with zolmitriptan and an SNRI is clinically warranted, careful observation of the patient is advised, particularly during treatment initiation and dose increases). Products include:

Cymbalta Delayed-Release Capsules 1801

Eletriptan Hydrobromide (Co-administration with other 5-HT1 agonists within 24 hours of each other is contraindicated).

No products indexed under this heading.

Ergonovine Maleate (Ergot-containing drugs have been reported to cause prolonged vasospastic reactions; because there is a theoretical basis that these effects may be additive, use of ergot-type agents and zolmitriptan within 24 hours is contraindicated).

No products indexed under this heading.

Ergotamine Tartrate (Ergot-containing drugs have been reported to cause prolonged vasospastic reactions; because there is a theoretical basis that these effects may be additive, use of ergot-type agents and zolmitriptan within 24 hours is contraindicated).

No products indexed under this heading.

Escitalopram Oxalate (Cases of life-threatening serotonin syndrome, including mental status changes, autonomic instability, neuromuscular aberrations, and/or GI symptoms, have been reported during combination use of selective serotonin reuptake inhibitors and triptans. If concomitant treatment with zolmitriptan and an SSRI is clinically warranted, careful observation of the patient is advised, particularly during treatment initiation and dose increases). Products include:

Lexapro Oral Suspension 1174
Lexapro Tablets 1174

Ethinyl Estradiol (Retrospective analysis of pharmacokinetic data indicates the mean plasma concentrations, Cmax and AUC, of zolmitriptan were generally higher in females taking oral contraceptives, Tmax was delayed by one-half hour in these females). Products include:

Lybrel Tablets 3204
Mircette Tablets 1034
NuvaRing 2897
Ortho-Cyclen/Ortho Tri-Cyclen 2449
Ortho Evra Transdermal System 2437
Ortho Tri-Cyclen Lo Tablets 2458
Seasonique Tablets 1046
Yaz Tablets 805

Ethynodiol Diacetate (Retrospective analysis of pharmacokinetic data indicates the mean plasma concentrations, Cmax and AUC, of zolmitriptan were generally higher in females taking oral contraceptives, Tmax was delayed by one-half hour in these females).

No products indexed under this heading.

Fluoxetine (Cases of life-threatening serotonin syndrome, including mental status changes, autonomic instability, neuromuscular aberrations, and/or GI symptoms, have been reported during combination use of selective serotonin reuptake inhibitors and triptans. If concomitant treatment with zolmitriptan and an SSRI is clinically warranted, careful observation of the patient is advised, particularly during treatment initiation and dose increases).

No products indexed under this heading.

Fluoxetine Hydrochloride (Cases of life-threatening serotonin syndrome, including mental status changes, autonomic instability, neuromuscular aberrations, and/or GI symptoms, have been reported during combination use of selective serotonin reuptake inhibitors and triptans. If concomitant treatment with zolmitriptan and an SSRI is clinically warranted, careful observation of the patient is advised, particularly during treatment initiation and dose increases). Products include:

Prozac Weekly Capsules 1852
Prozac Pulvules and Liquid 1852
Symbyax Capsules 1871

Fluvoxamine Maleate (Cases of life-threatening serotonin syndrome, including mental status changes, autonomic instability, neuromuscular aberrations, and/or GI symptoms, have been reported during combination use of selective serotonin reuptake inhibitors and triptans. If concomitant treatment with zolmitriptan and an SSRI is clinically warranted, careful observation of the patient is advised, particularly during treatment initiation and dose increases). Products include:

Luvox CR Extended-Release Capsules 1759

Frovatriptan Succinate (Co-administration with other 5-HT1 agonists within 24 hours of each other is contraindicated). Products include:

Frova Tablets 1111

Isocarboxazid (MAO-A inhibitors increase the systemic exposure of zolmitriptan; concurrent and/or sequential use is contraindicated). Products include:

Marplan Tablets 3177

Levonorgestrel (Retrospective analysis of pharmacokinetic data indicates the mean plasma concentrations, Cmax and AUC, of zolmitriptan were generally higher in females taking oral contraceptives, Tmax was delayed by one-half hour in these females). Products include:

Climara Pro Transdermal System 768
Lybrel Tablets 3204
Mirena Intrauterine System 779
Plan B Tablets 1044
Seasonique Tablets 1046

Mestranol (Retrospective analysis of pharmacokinetic data indicates the mean plasma concentrations, Cmax and AUC, of zolmitriptan were generally higher in females taking oral contraceptives, Tmax was delayed by one-half hour in these females).

No products indexed under this heading.

Methylergonovine Maleate (Ergot-containing drugs have been reported to cause prolonged vasospastic reactions; because there is a theoretical basis that these effects may be additive, use of ergot-type agents and zolmitriptan within 24 hours is contraindicated).

No products indexed under this heading.

Methysergide Maleate (Ergot-containing drugs have been reported to cause prolonged vasospastic reactions; because there is a theoretical basis that these effects may be additive, use of ergot-type agents and zolmitriptan within 24 hours is contraindicated).

No products indexed under this heading.

Moclobemide (MAO-A inhibitors increase the systemic exposure of zolmitriptan; concurrent and/or sequential use is contraindicated).

No products indexed under this heading.

Naratriptan Hydrochloride (Co-administration with other 5-HT1 agonists within 24 hours of each other is contraindicated). Products include:

Amerge Tablets 1301

Nefazodone Hydrochloride (Cases of life-threatening serotonin syndrome, including mental status changes, autonomic instability, neuromuscular aberrations, and/or GI symptoms, have been reported during combination use of serotonin/norepinephrine reuptake inhibitors and triptans. If concomitant treatment with zolmitriptan and an SNRI is clinically warranted, careful observation of the patient is advised, particularly during treatment initiation and dose increases).

No products indexed under this heading.

Norethindrone (Retrospective analysis of pharmacokinetic data indicates the mean plasma concentrations, Cmax and AUC, of zolmitriptan were generally higher in females taking oral contraceptives, Tmax was delayed by one-half hour in these females). Products include:

Ortho Micronor Tablets 2446

Norethynodrel (Retrospective analysis of pharmacokinetic data indicates the mean plasma concentrations, Cmax and AUC, of zolmitriptan were generally higher in females taking oral contraceptives, Tmax was delayed by one-half hour in these females).

No products indexed under this heading.

Norgestimate (Retrospective analysis of pharmacokinetic data indicates the mean plasma concentrations, Cmax and AUC, of zolmitriptan were generally higher in females taking oral contraceptives, Tmax was delayed by one-half hour in these females). Products include:

Ortho-Cyclen/Ortho Tri-Cyclen 2449
Ortho Tri-Cyclen Lo Tablets 2458

Norgestrel (Retrospective analysis of pharmacokinetic data indicates the mean plasma concentrations, Cmax and AUC, of zolmitriptan were generally higher in females taking oral contraceptives, Tmax was delayed by one-half hour in these females).

No products indexed under this heading.

Pargyline Hydrochloride (MAO-A inhibitors increase the systemic exposure of zolmitriptan; concurrent and/or sequential use is contraindicated).

No products indexed under this heading.

Paroxetine Hydrochloride (Cases of life-threatening serotonin syndrome, including mental status changes, autonomic instability, neuromuscular aberrations, and/or GI symptoms, have been reported during combination use of selective serotonin reuptake inhibitors and triptans. If concomitant treatment with zolmitriptan and an SSRI is clinically warranted, careful observation of the patient is advised, particularly during treatment initiation and dose increases). Products include:

Paxil 1535
Paxil CR Controlled-Release Tablets 1544

Phenelzine Sulfate (MAO-A inhibitors increase the systemic exposure of zolmitriptan; concurrent and/or sequential use is contraindicated).

No products indexed under this heading.

Procarbazine Hydrochloride (MAO-A inhibitors increase the systemic exposure of zolmitriptan; concurrent and/or sequential use is contraindicated).

No products indexed under this heading.

Propranolol (Cmax and AUC of zolmitriptan increased after one week of dosing with propanolol; Cmax and AUC of N-desmethyl metabolite was reduced).

No products indexed under this heading.

Rasagiline Mesylate (MAO-A inhibitors increase the systemic exposure of zolmitriptan; concurrent and/or sequential use is contraindicated). Products include:

Azilect Tablets 3106

Rizatriptan Benzoate (Co-administration with other 5-HT1 agonists within 24 hours of each other is contraindicated). Products include:

Maxalt Tablets 2056
Maxalt-MLT Orally Disintegrating Tablets 2056

Selegiline (MAO-A inhibitors increase the systemic exposure of zolmitriptan; concurrent and/or sequential use is contraindicated). Products include:

Emsam Transdermal System 905

Selegiline Hydrochloride (MAO-A inhibitors increase the systemic exposure of zolmitriptan; concurrent and/or sequential use is contraindicated). Products include:

Eldepryl Capsules 3052

Sertraline Hydrochloride (Cases of life-threatening serotonin syndrome, including mental status changes, autonomic instability, neuromuscular aberrations, and/or GI symptoms, have been reported dur-

ing combination use of selective serotonin reuptake inhibitors and triptans. If concomitant treatment with zolmitriptan and an SSRI is clinically warranted, careful observation of the patient is advised, particularly during treatment initiation and dose increases).
No products indexed under this heading.

Sumatriptan (Co-administration with other 5-HT1 agonists within 24 hours of each other is contraindicated). Products include:
Imitrex Nasal Spray 1470

Sumatriptan Succinate (Co-administration with other 5-HT1 agonists within 24 hours of each other is contraindicated). Products include:
Imitrex Injection 1465
Imitrex Tablets 1474
Treximet Tablets 1616

Tranylcypromine Sulfate (MAO-A inhibitors increase the systemic exposure of zolmitriptan; concurrent and/or sequential use is contraindicated). Products include:
Parnate Tablets 1532

Venlafaxine Hydrochloride (Cases of life-threatening serotonin syndrome, including mental status changes, autonomic instability, neuromuscular aberrations, and/or GI symptoms, have been reported during combination use of serotonin and norepinephrine reuptake inhibitors and triptans. If concomitant treatment with zolmitriptan and an SNRI is clinically warranted, careful observation of the patient is advised, particularly during treatment initiation and dose increases). Products include:
Effexor XR Extended-Release Capsules 3195
Venlafaxine Hydrochloride Tablets ... 2199

ZOMIG-ZMT TABLETS

(Zolmitriptan) 694
See Zomig Nasal Spray

ZONEGRAN CAPSULES

(Zonisamide) 1089
May interact with phenytoin, valproate, and certain other agents. Compounds in these categories include:

Carbamazepine (Co-administration with drugs that induce liver enzymes increases the metabolism and clearance of zonisamide and decreases the half-life to 38 hours). Products include:
Carbatrol Capsules 3019
Equetro Extended-Release Capsules 3174

Divalproex Sodium (The half-life of zonisamide in patients concurrently on the non-enzyme inducing AED, valproate, was 46 hours). Products include:
Depakote ER Tablets 423

Fosphenytoin Sodium (Co-administration with drugs that induce liver enzymes increases the metabolism and clearance of zonisamide and decreases the half-life to 27 hours).
No products indexed under this heading.

Phenobarbital (Co-administration with drugs that induce liver enzymes increases the metabolism and clearance of zonisamide and decreases the half-life to 38 hours). Products include:
Donnatal Extentabs 2507

Phenytoin (Co-administration with drugs that induce liver enzymes increases the metabolism and clearance of zonisamide and decreases the half-life to 27 hours).
No products indexed under this heading.

Phenytoin Sodium (Co-administration with drugs that induce liver enzymes increases the metabolism and clearance of zonisamide and decreases the half-life to 27 hours). Products include:
Phenytek Capsules 2192

Valproate Sodium (The half-life of zonisamide in patients concurrently on the non-enzyme inducing AED, valproate, was 46 hours).
No products indexed under this heading.

Valproic Acid (The half-life of zonisamide in patients concurrently on the non-enzyme inducing AED, valproate, was 46 hours).
No products indexed under this heading.

ZOSTAVAX INJECTION

(Zoster Vaccine Live) 2145
None cited in PDR database.

ZOSYN FOR INJECTION

(Piperacillin Sodium, Tazobactam Sodium)... 3284
May interact with aminoglycosides, anticoagulants, nondepolarizing neuromuscular blocking agents, and certain other agents. Compounds in these categories include:

Amikacin Sulfate (The mixing of beta-lactam antibiotics with aminoglycosides in-vitro can result in substantial inactivation of the aminoglycoside. However, amikacin and gentamicin have been shown to be compatible *in vitro* with reformulated Zosyn containing EDTA supplied in vials or bulk pharmacy containers in certain diluents at specific concentrations for a simultaneous Y-site infusion. Reformulated Zosyn containing EDTA is not compatible with tobramycin for simultaneous administration via Y-site infusion).
No products indexed under this heading.

Anisindione (Coagulation parameters should be tested more frequently and monitored regularly during simultaneous administration; effect of concurrent use is not specified).
No products indexed under this heading.

Ardeparin Sodium (Coagulation parameters should be tested more frequently and monitored regularly during simultaneous administration; effect of concurrent use is not specified).
No products indexed under this heading.

Atracurium Besylate (Due to similar mechanism of action as vecuronium, it is expected that the neuromuscular blockade produced by other non-depolarizing muscle relaxants could be prolonged in the presence of piperacillin).
No products indexed under this heading.

Cisatracurium Besylate (Due to similar mechanism of action as vecuronium, it is expected that the neuromuscular blockade produced by other non-depolarizing muscle relaxants could be prolonged in the presence of piperacillin). Products include:
Nimbex Injection 484

Dalteparin Sodium (Coagulation parameters should be tested more frequently and monitored regularly during simultaneous administration; effect of concurrent use is not specified). Products include:
Fragmin Injection 1070

Danaparoid Sodium (Coagulation parameters should be tested more frequently and monitored regularly during simultaneous administration; effect of concurrent use is not specified).
No products indexed under this heading.

Dicumarol (Coagulation parameters should be tested more frequently and monitored regularly during simultaneous administration; effect of concurrent use is not specified).
No products indexed under this heading.

Enoxaparin Sodium (Coagulation parameters should be tested more frequently and monitored regularly during simultaneous administration; effect of concurrent use is not specified). Products include:
Lovenox Injection 2756

Fondaparinux Sodium (Coagulation parameters should be tested more frequently and monitored regularly during simultaneous administration; effect of concurrent use is not specified). Products include:
Arixtra Injection 1313

Gentamicin Sulfate (The mixing of beta-lactam antibiotics with aminoglycosides in-vitro can result in substantial inactivation of the aminoglycoside. However, amikacin and gentamicin have been shown to be compatible *in vitro* with reformulated Zosyn containing EDTA supplied in vials or bulk pharmacy containers in certain diluents at specific concentrations for a simultaneous Y-site infusion. Reformulated Zosyn containing EDTA is not compatible with tobramycin for simultaneous administration via Y-site infusion). Products include:
Pred-G Ophthalmic Ointment .... ⊙229
Pred-G Ophthalmic Suspension ...... ⊙228

Heparin Calcium (Coagulation parameters should be tested more frequently and monitored regularly during simultaneous administration; effect of concurrent use is not specified).
No products indexed under this heading.

Heparin Sodium (Coagulation parameters should be tested more frequently and monitored regularly during simultaneous administration; effect of concurrent use is not specified).
No products indexed under this heading.

Kanamycin Sulfate (The mixing of beta-lactam antibiotics with aminoglycosides *in-vitro* can result in substantial inactivation of the aminoglycoside. However, amikacin and gentamicin have been shown to be compatible *in vitro* with reformulated Zosyn containing EDTA supplied in vials or bulk pharmacy containers in certain diluents at specific concentrations for a simultaneous Y-site infusion. Reformulated Zosyn containing EDTA is not compatible with tobramycin for simultaneous administration via Y-site infusion).
No products indexed under this heading.

Low Molecular Weight Heparins (Coagulation parameters should be tested more frequently and monitored regularly during simultaneous administration; effect of concurrent use is not specified).
No products indexed under this heading.

Methotrexate (Limited data suggests that co-administration of methotrexate and piperacillin may reduce the clearance of methotrexate due to competition for renal excretion).
No products indexed under this heading.

Metocurine Iodide (Due to similar mechanism of action as vecuronium, it is expected that the neuromuscular blockade produced by other non-depolarizing muscle relaxants could be prolonged in the presence of piperacillin).
No products indexed under this heading.

Mivacurium Chloride (Due to similar mechanism of action as vecuronium, it is expected that the neuromuscular blockade produced by other non-depolarizing muscle relaxants could be prolonged in the presence of piperacillin).
No products indexed under this heading.

Pancuronium Bromide (Due to similar mechanism of action as vecuronium, it is expected that the neuromuscular blockade produced by other non-depolarizing muscle relaxants could be prolonged in the presence of piperacillin).
No products indexed under this heading.

Probenecid (Concomitant administration prolongs half-life of piperacillin by 21% and of tazobactam by 71%).
No products indexed under this heading.

Rapacuronium Bromide (Due to similar mechanism of action as vecuronium, it is expected that the neuromuscular blockade produced by other non-depolarizing muscle relaxants could be prolonged in the presence of piperacillin).
No products indexed under this heading.

Rocuronium Bromide (Due to similar mechanism of action as vecuronium, it is expected that the neuromuscular blockade produced by other non-depolarizing muscle relaxants could be prolonged in the presence of piperacillin). Products include:
Zemuron Injection 2947

Streptomycin Sulfate (The mixing of beta-lactam antibiotics with aminoglycosides in-vitro can result in substantial inactivation of the aminoglycoside. However, amikacin and gentamicin have been shown to be compatible *in vitro* with reformulated Zosyn containing EDTA supplied in vials or bulk pharmacy containers in certain diluents at specific concentrations for a simultaneous Y-site infusion. Reformulated Zosyn containing EDTA is not compatible with tobramycin for simultaneous administration via Y-site infusion).
No products indexed under this heading.

Tinzaparin Sodium (Coagulation parameters should be tested more frequently and monitored regularly during simultaneous administration; effect of concurrent use is not specified).
No products indexed under this heading.

Tobramycin (The mixing of beta-lactam antibiotics with aminoglycosides *in-vitro* can result in substantial inactivation of the aminoglycoside. However, amikacin and gentamicin have been shown to be compatible *in vitro* with reformulated Zosyn containing EDTA supplied in vials or bulk pharmacy containers in certain diluents at specific concentrations for a simultaneous Y-site infusion. Reformulated Zosyn containing EDTA is not compatible with tobramycin for simultaneous administration via Y-site infusion). Products include:
Zylet Ophthalmic Suspension .... ⊙247

Tobramycin Sulfate (Coadministration has resulted in the alteration of tobramycin pharmacokinetics which may be due to *in vitro* and in vivo inactivation of tobramycin).
No products indexed under this heading.

Vecuronium Bromide (Coadministration of piperacillin and vecuronium has been implicated in the prolongation of the neuromuscular blockade).
No products indexed under this heading.

Warfarin Sodium (Coagulation parameters should be tested more frequently and monitored regularly during simultaneous administration; effect of concurrent use is not specified).
No products indexed under this heading.

ZOVIRAX CAPSULES

(Acyclovir) **1690**

May interact with nephrotoxic agents and certain other agents. Compounds in these categories include:

Abacavir Sulfate (Caution should be exercised when administering acyclovir to patients receiving potentially nephrotoxic agents since this may increase the risk of renal dysfunction and/or the risk of reversible CNS symptoms such as those that have been reported in patients treated with intravenous acyclovir. Adequate hydration should be maintained). Products include:
Epzicom Tablets **1422**
Trizivir Tablets **1622**
Ziagen **1673**

Acyclovir Sodium (Caution should be exercised when administering acyclovir to patients receiving potentially nephrotoxic agents since this may increase the risk of renal dysfunction and/or the risk of reversible CNS symptoms such as those that have been reported in patients treated with intravenous acyclovir. Adequate hydration should be maintained).
No products indexed under this heading.

Alatrofloxacin Mesylate (Caution should be exercised when administering acyclovir to patients receiving potentially nephrotoxic agents since this may increase the risk of renal dysfunction and/or the risk of reversible CNS symptoms such as those that have been reported in patients treated with intravenous acyclovir. Adequate hydration should be maintained).
No products indexed under this heading.

Aldesleukin (Caution should be exercised when administering acyclovir to patients receiving potentially nephrotoxic agents since this may increase the risk of renal dysfunction and/or the risk of reversible CNS symptoms such as those that have been reported in patients treated with intravenous acyclovir. Adequate hydration should be maintained). Products include:
Proleukin for Injection **2287**

Amikacin Sulfate (Caution should be exercised when administering acyclovir to patients receiving potentially nephrotoxic agents since this may increase the risk of renal dysfunction and/or the risk of reversible CNS symptoms such as those that have been reported in patients treated with intravenous acyclovir. Adequate hydration should be maintained).
No products indexed under this heading.

Amoxicillin (Caution should be exercised when administering acyclovir to patients receiving potentially nephrotoxic agents since this may increase the risk of renal dysfunction and/or the risk of reversible CNS symptoms such as those that have been reported in patients treated with intravenous acyclovir. Adequate hydration should be maintained). Products include:
Amoxil Capsules **1305**
Amoxil Chewable Tablets **1305**
Amoxil Pediatric Drops for Oral Suspension **1305**
Amoxil Powder for Oral Suspension **1305**
Amoxil Tablets **1305**
Augmentin **1323**
Augmentin Tablets **1327**
Augmentin XR Extended Release Tablets **1333**
Augmentin ES-600 Powder for Oral Suspension **1329**
Moxatag Tablets **2165**

Amoxicillin Trihydrate (Caution should be exercised when administering acyclovir to patients receiving potentially nephrotoxic agents since this may increase the risk of renal dysfunction and/or the risk of reversible CNS symptoms such as those that have been reported in patients treated with intravenous acyclovir. Adequate hydration should be maintained).
No products indexed under this heading.

Amphotericin B (Caution should be exercised when administering acyclovir to patients receiving potentially nephrotoxic agents since this may increase the risk of renal dysfunction and/or the risk of reversible CNS symptoms such as those that have been reported in patients treated with intravenous acyclovir. Adequate hydration should be maintained).
No products indexed under this heading.

Amphotericin B, liposomal (Caution should be exercised when administering acyclovir to patients receiving potentially nephrotoxic agents since this may increase the risk of renal dysfunction and/or the risk of reversible CNS symptoms such as those that have been reported in patients treated with intravenous acyclovir. Adequate hydration should be maintained). Products include:
AmBisome for Injection **606**

Amphotericin B Cholesteryl Sulfate (Caution should be exercised when administering acyclovir to patients receiving potentially nephrotoxic agents since this may increase the risk of renal dysfunction and/or the risk of reversible CNS symptoms such as those that have been reported in patients treated with intravenous acyclovir. Adequate hydration should be maintained).
No products indexed under this heading.

Amphotericin B Lipid Complex (Caution should be exercised when administering acyclovir to patients receiving potentially nephrotoxic agents since this may increase the risk of renal dysfunction and/or the risk of reversible CNS symptoms such as those that have been reported in patients treated with intravenous acyclovir. Adequate hydration should be maintained). Products include:
Abelcet Injection **1134**

Ampicillin (Caution should be exercised when administering acyclovir to patients receiving potentially nephrotoxic agents since this may increase the risk of renal dysfunction and/or the risk of reversible CNS symptoms such as those that have been reported in patients treated with intravenous acyclovir. Adequate hydration should be maintained).
No products indexed under this heading.

Ampicillin Sodium (Caution should be exercised when administering acyclovir to patients receiving potentially nephrotoxic agents since this may increase the risk of renal dysfunction and/or the risk of reversible CNS symptoms such as those that have been reported in patients treated with intravenous acyclovir. Adequate hydration should be maintained).
No products indexed under this heading.

Ampicillin Trihydrate (Caution should be exercised when administering acyclovir to patients receiving potentially nephrotoxic agents since this may increase the risk of renal dysfunction and/or the risk of reversible CNS symptoms such as those that have been reported in patients treated with intravenous acyclovir. Adequate hydration should be maintained).
No products indexed under this heading.

Amprenavir (Caution should be exercised when administering acyclovir to patients receiving potentially nephrotoxic agents since this may increase the risk of renal dysfunction and/or the risk of reversible CNS symptoms such as those that have been reported in patients treated with intravenous acyclovir. Adequate hydration should be maintained).
No products indexed under this heading.

Aspirin (Caution should be exercised when administering acyclovir to patients receiving potentially nephrotoxic agents since this may increase the risk of renal dysfunction and/or the risk of reversible CNS symptoms such as those that have been reported in patients treated with intravenous acyclovir. Adequate hydration should be maintained). Products include:
Aggrenox Capsules **819**
Bayer Aspirin **750**
Percodan Tablets **1130**
St. Joseph 81 mg Aspirin Chewable and Enteric Coated Tablets **1903**

Atazanavir (Caution should be exercised when administering acyclovir to patients receiving potentially nephrotoxic agents since this may increase the risk of renal dysfunction and/or the risk of reversible CNS symptoms such as those that have been reported in patients treated with intravenous acyclovir. Adequate hydration should be maintained).
No products indexed under this heading.

Atorvastatin Calcium (Caution should be exercised when administering acyclovir to patients receiving potentially nephrotoxic agents since this may increase the risk of renal dysfunction and/or the risk of reversible CNS symptoms such as those that have been reported in patients treated with intravenous acyclovir. Adequate hydration should be maintained). Products include:
Lipitor Tablets **2501**

Azithromycin Dihydrate (Caution should be exercised when administering acyclovir to patients receiving potentially nephrotoxic agents since this may increase the risk of renal dysfunction and/or the risk of reversible CNS symptoms such as those that have been reported in patients treated with intravenous acyclovir. Adequate hydration should be maintained).
No products indexed under this heading.

Azlocillin Sodium (Caution should be exercised when administering acyclovir to patients receiving potentially nephrotoxic agents since this may increase the risk of renal dysfunction and/or the risk of reversible CNS symptoms such as those that have been reported in patients treated with intravenous acyclovir. Adequate hydration should be maintained).
No products indexed under this heading.

Aztreonam (Caution should be exercised when administering acyclovir to patients receiving potentially nephrotoxic agents since this may increase the risk of renal dysfunction and/or the risk of reversible CNS symptoms such as those that have been reported in patients treated with intravenous acyclovir. Adequate hydration should be maintained).
No products indexed under this heading.

Bacampicillin Hydrochloride (Caution should be exercised when administering acyclovir to patients receiving potentially nephrotoxic agents since this may increase the risk of renal dysfunction and/or the risk of reversible CNS symptoms such as those that have been reported in patients treated with intravenous acyclovir. Adequate hydration should be maintained).
No products indexed under this heading.

Balsalazide Disodium (Caution should be exercised when administering acyclovir to patients receiving potentially nephrotoxic agents since this may increase the risk of renal dysfunction and/or the risk of reversible CNS symptoms such as those that have been reported in patients treated with intravenous acyclovir. Adequate hydration should be maintained).
No products indexed under this heading.

Benazepril Hydrochloride (Caution should be exercised when administering acyclovir to patients receiving potentially nephrotoxic agents since this may increase the risk of renal dysfunction and/or the risk of reversible CNS symptoms such as those that have been reported in patients treated with intravenous acyclovir. Adequate hydration should be maintained).
No products indexed under this heading.

Bendroflumethiazide (Caution should be exercised when administering acyclovir to patients receiving potentially nephrotoxic agents since this may increase the risk of renal dysfunction and/or the risk of reversible CNS symptoms such as those that have been reported in patients treated with intravenous acyclovir. Adequate hydration should be maintained).
No products indexed under this heading.

Caffeine (Caution should be exercised when administering acyclovir to patients receiving potentially nephrotoxic agents since this may increase the risk of renal dysfunction and/or the risk of reversible CNS symptoms such as those that have been reported in patients treated with intravenous acyclovir. Adequate hydration should be maintained).
Products include:
BioLean Free Tablets .... ▣635
BioLean II Tablets .... ▣635
Winrgy Dietary Supplement .... ▣642

Captopril (Caution should be exercised when administering acyclovir to patients receiving potentially nephrotoxic agents since this may increase the risk of renal dysfunction and/or the risk of reversible CNS symptoms such as those that have been reported in patients treated with intravenous acyclovir. Adequate hydration should be maintained).
Products include:
Captopril Tablets 2182

Carbenicillin Disodium (Caution should be exercised when administering acyclovir to patients receiving potentially nephrotoxic agents since this may increase the risk of renal dysfunction and/or the risk of reversible CNS symptoms such as those that have been reported in patients treated with intravenous acyclovir. Adequate hydration should be maintained).
No products indexed under this heading.

Carbenicillin Indanyl Sodium (Caution should be exercised when administering acyclovir to patients receiving potentially nephrotoxic agents since this may increase the risk of renal dysfunction and/or the risk of reversible CNS symptoms such as those that have been reported in patients treated with intravenous acyclovir. Adequate hydration should be maintained).
No products indexed under this heading.

Carboplatin (Caution should be exercised when administering acyclovir to patients receiving potentially nephrotoxic agents since this may increase the risk of renal dysfunction and/or the risk of reversible CNS symptoms such as those that have been reported in patients treated with intravenous acyclovir. Adequate hydration should be maintained).
No products indexed under this heading.

Carmustine (BCNU) (Caution should be exercised when administering acyclovir to patients receiving potentially nephrotoxic agents since this may increase the risk of renal dysfunction and/or the risk of reversible CNS symptoms such as those that have been reported in patients treated with intravenous acyclovir. Adequate hydration should be maintained).
No products indexed under this heading.

Cefaclor (Caution should be exercised when administering acyclovir to patients receiving potentially nephrotoxic agents since this may increase the risk of renal dysfunction and/or the risk of reversible CNS symptoms such as those that have been reported in patients treated with intravenous acyclovir. Adequate hydration should be maintained).
No products indexed under this heading.

Cefadroxil (Caution should be exercised when administering acyclovir to patients receiving potentially nephrotoxic agents since this may increase the risk of renal dysfunction and/or the risk of reversible CNS symptoms such as those that have been reported in patients treated with intravenous acyclovir. Adequate hydration should be maintained).
No products indexed under this heading.

Cefamandole Nafate (Caution should be exercised when administering acyclovir to patients receiving potentially nephrotoxic agents since this may increase the risk of renal dysfunction and/or the risk of reversible CNS symptoms such as those that have been reported in patients treated with intravenous acyclovir. Adequate hydration should be maintained).
No products indexed under this heading.

Cefazolin Sodium (Caution should be exercised when administering acyclovir to patients receiving potentially nephrotoxic agents since this may increase the risk of renal dysfunction and/or the risk of reversible CNS symptoms such as those that have been reported in patients treated with intravenous acyclovir. Adequate hydration should be maintained).
No products indexed under this heading.

Cefdinir (Caution should be exercised when administering acyclovir to patients receiving potentially nephrotoxic agents since this may increase the risk of renal dysfunction and/or the risk of reversible CNS symptoms such as those that have been reported in patients treated with intravenous acyclovir. Adequate hydration should be maintained).
Products include:
Omnicef Capsules 497
Omnicef for Oral Suspension 497

Cefepime Hydrochloride (Caution should be exercised when administering acyclovir to patients receiving potentially nephrotoxic agents since this may increase the risk of renal dysfunction and/or the risk of reversible CNS symptoms such as those that have been reported in patients treated with intravenous acyclovir. Adequate hydration should be maintained).
No products indexed under this heading.

Cefixime (Caution should be exercised when administering acyclovir to patients receiving potentially nephrotoxic agents since this may increase the risk of renal dysfunction and/or the risk of reversible CNS symptoms such as those that have been reported in patients treated with intravenous acyclovir. Adequate hydration should be maintained).
Products include:
Suprax for Oral Suspension 1891
Suprax Tablets 1891

Cefmetazole Sodium (Caution should be exercised when administering acyclovir to patients receiving potentially nephrotoxic agents since this may increase the risk of renal dysfunction and/or the risk of reversible CNS symptoms such as those that have been reported in patients treated with intravenous acyclovir. Adequate hydration should be maintained).
No products indexed under this heading.

Cefonicid Sodium (Caution should be exercised when administering acyclovir to patients receiving potentially nephrotoxic agents since this may increase the risk of renal dysfunction and/or the risk of reversible CNS symptoms such as those that have been reported in patients treated with intravenous acyclovir. Adequate hydration should be maintained).
No products indexed under this heading.

Cefoperazone Sodium (Caution should be exercised when administering acyclovir to patients receiving potentially nephrotoxic agents since this may increase the risk of renal dysfunction and/or the risk of reversible CNS symptoms such as those that have been reported in patients treated with intravenous acyclovir. Adequate hydration should be maintained).
No products indexed under this heading.

Ceforanide (Caution should be exercised when administering acyclovir to patients receiving potentially nephrotoxic agents since this may increase the risk of renal dysfunction and/or the risk of reversible CNS symptoms such as those that have been reported in patients treated with intravenous acyclovir. Adequate hydration should be maintained).
No products indexed under this heading.

Cefotaxime Sodium (Caution should be exercised when administering acyclovir to patients receiving potentially nephrotoxic agents since this may increase the risk of renal dysfunction and/or the risk of reversible CNS symptoms such as those that have been reported in patients treated with intravenous acyclovir. Adequate hydration should be maintained).
No products indexed under this heading.

Cefotetan (Caution should be exercised when administering acyclovir to patients receiving potentially nephrotoxic agents since this may increase the risk of renal dysfunction and/or the risk of reversible CNS symptoms such as those that have been reported in patients treated with intravenous acyclovir. Adequate hydration should be maintained).
No products indexed under this heading.

Cefoxitin Sodium (Caution should be exercised when administering acyclovir to patients receiving potentially nephrotoxic agents since this may increase the risk of renal dysfunction and/or the risk of reversible CNS symptoms such as those that have been reported in patients treated with intravenous acyclovir. Adequate hydration should be maintained).
No products indexed under this heading.

Cefpodoxime Proxetil (Caution should be exercised when administering acyclovir to patients receiving potentially nephrotoxic agents since this may increase the risk of renal dysfunction and/or the risk of reversible CNS symptoms such as those that have been reported in patients treated with intravenous acyclovir. Adequate hydration should be maintained).
No products indexed under this heading.

Cefprozil (Caution should be exercised when administering acyclovir to patients receiving potentially nephrotoxic agents since this may increase the risk of renal dysfunction and/or the risk of reversible CNS symptoms such as those that have been reported in patients treated with intravenous acyclovir. Adequate hydration should be maintained).
No products indexed under this heading.

Ceftazidime (Caution should be exercised when administering acyclovir to patients receiving potentially nephrotoxic agents since this may increase the risk of renal dysfunction and/or the risk of reversible CNS symptoms such as those that have been reported in patients treated with intravenous acyclovir. Adequate hydration should be maintained). Products include:

Fortaz ... 1450

Ceftizoxime Sodium (Caution should be exercised when administering acyclovir to patients receiving potentially nephrotoxic agents since this may increase the risk of renal dysfunction and/or the risk of reversible CNS symptoms such as those that have been reported in patients treated with intravenous acyclovir. Adequate hydration should be maintained).

No products indexed under this heading.

Ceftriaxone Sodium (Caution should be exercised when administering acyclovir to patients receiving potentially nephrotoxic agents since this may increase the risk of renal dysfunction and/or the risk of reversible CNS symptoms such as those that have been reported in patients treated with intravenous acyclovir. Adequate hydration should be maintained). Products include:

Rocephin Injectable Vials, ADD-Vantage, Galaxy, Bulk ... 2642

Cefuroxime Axetil (Caution should be exercised when administering acyclovir to patients receiving potentially nephrotoxic agents since this may increase the risk of renal dysfunction and/or the risk of reversible CNS symptoms such as those that have been reported in patients treated with intravenous acyclovir. Adequate hydration should be maintained). Products include:

Ceftin ... 1380

Cefuroxime Sodium (Caution should be exercised when administering acyclovir to patients receiving potentially nephrotoxic agents since this may increase the risk of renal dysfunction and/or the risk of reversible CNS symptoms such as those that have been reported in patients treated with intravenous acyclovir. Adequate hydration should be maintained).

No products indexed under this heading.

Celecoxib (Caution should be exercised when administering acyclovir to patients receiving potentially nephrotoxic agents since this may increase the risk of renal dysfunction and/or the risk of reversible CNS symptoms such as those that have been reported in patients treated with intravenous acyclovir. Adequate hydration should be maintained). Products include:

Celebrex Capsules ... 2979

Cephalexin (Caution should be exercised when administering acyclovir to patients receiving potentially nephrotoxic agents since this may increase the risk of renal dysfunction and/or the risk of reversible CNS symptoms such as those that have been reported in patients treated with intravenous acyclovir. Adequate hydration should be maintained).

No products indexed under this heading.

Cephalothin Sodium (Caution should be exercised when administering acyclovir to patients receiving potentially nephrotoxic agents since this may increase the risk of renal dysfunction and/or the risk of reversible CNS symptoms such as those that have been reported in patients treated with intravenous acyclovir. Adequate hydration should be maintained).

No products indexed under this heading.

Cephapirin Sodium (Caution should be exercised when administering acyclovir to patients receiving potentially nephrotoxic agents since this may increase the risk of renal dysfunction and/or the risk of reversible CNS symptoms such as those that have been reported in patients treated with intravenous acyclovir. Adequate hydration should be maintained).

No products indexed under this heading.

Cephradine (Caution should be exercised when administering acyclovir to patients receiving potentially nephrotoxic agents since this may increase the risk of renal dysfunction and/or the risk of reversible CNS symptoms such as those that have been reported in patients treated with intravenous acyclovir. Adequate hydration should be maintained).

No products indexed under this heading.

Cerivastatin Sodium (Caution should be exercised when administering acyclovir to patients receiving potentially nephrotoxic agents since this may increase the risk of renal dysfunction and/or the risk of reversible CNS symptoms such as those that have been reported in patients treated with intravenous acyclovir. Adequate hydration should be maintained).

No products indexed under this heading.

Chlorothiazide (Caution should be exercised when administering acyclovir to patients receiving potentially nephrotoxic agents since this may increase the risk of renal dysfunction and/or the risk of reversible CNS symptoms such as those that have been reported in patients treated with intravenous acyclovir. Adequate hydration should be maintained).

No products indexed under this heading.

Chlorothiazide Sodium (Caution should be exercised when administering acyclovir to patients receiving potentially nephrotoxic agents since this may increase the risk of renal dysfunction and/or the risk of reversible CNS symptoms such as those that have been reported in patients treated with intravenous acyclovir. Adequate hydration should be maintained). Products include:

Intravenous Sodium Diuril ... 2490

Chlorpropamide (Caution should be exercised when administering acyclovir to patients receiving potentially nephrotoxic agents since this may increase the risk of renal dysfunction and/or the risk of reversible CNS symptoms such as those that have been reported in patients treated with intravenous acyclovir. Adequate hydration should be maintained).

No products indexed under this heading.

Cidofovir (Caution should be exercised when administering acyclovir to patients receiving potentially nephrotoxic agents since this may increase the risk of renal dysfunction and/or the risk of reversible CNS symptoms such as those that have been reported in patients treated with intravenous acyclovir. Adequate hydration should be maintained).

No products indexed under this heading.

Cilastatin Sodium (Caution should be exercised when administering acyclovir to patients receiving potentially nephrotoxic agents since this may increase the risk of renal dysfunction and/or the risk of reversible CNS symptoms such as those that have been reported in patients treated with intravenous acyclovir. Adequate hydration should be maintained). Products include:

Primaxin I.M. ... 2080
Primaxin I.V. ... 2083

Cimetidine (Caution should be exercised when administering acyclovir to patients receiving potentially nephrotoxic agents since this may increase the risk of renal dysfunction and/or the risk of reversible CNS symptoms such as those that have been reported in patients treated with intravenous acyclovir. Adequate hydration should be maintained).

No products indexed under this heading.

Cimetidine Hydrochloride (Caution should be exercised when administering acyclovir to patients receiving potentially nephrotoxic agents since this may increase the risk of renal dysfunction and/or the risk of reversible CNS symptoms such as those that have been reported in patients treated with intravenous acyclovir. Adequate hydration should be maintained).

No products indexed under this heading.

Cisplatin (Caution should be exercised when administering acyclovir to patients receiving potentially nephrotoxic agents since this may increase the risk of renal dysfunction and/or the risk of reversible CNS symptoms such as those that have been reported in patients treated with intravenous acyclovir. Adequate hydration should be maintained).

No products indexed under this heading.

Cladribine (Caution should be exercised when administering acyclovir to patients receiving potentially nephrotoxic agents since this may increase the risk of renal dysfunction and/or the risk of reversible CNS symptoms such as those that have been reported in patients treated with intravenous acyclovir. Adequate hydration should be maintained). Products include:

Leustatin Injection ... 2384

Clozapine (Caution should be exercised when administering acyclovir to patients receiving potentially nephrotoxic agents since this may increase the risk of renal dysfunction and/or the risk of reversible CNS symptoms such as those that have been reported in patients treated with intravenous acyclovir. Adequate hydration should be maintained).

No products indexed under this heading.

Colistimethate Sodium (Caution should be exercised when administering acyclovir to patients receiving potentially nephrotoxic agents since this may increase the risk of renal dysfunction and/or the risk of reversible CNS symptoms such as those that have been reported in patients treated with intravenous acyclovir. Adequate hydration should be maintained).

No products indexed under this heading.

Colistin Sulfate (Caution should be exercised when administering acyclovir to patients receiving potentially nephrotoxic agents since this may increase the risk of renal dysfunction and/or the risk of reversible CNS symptoms such as those that have been reported in patients treated with intravenous acyclovir. Adequate hydration should be maintained).

No products indexed under this heading.

Cyclophosphamide (Caution should be exercised when administering acyclovir to patients receiving potentially nephrotoxic agents since this may increase the risk of renal dysfunction and/or the risk of reversible CNS symptoms such as those that have been reported in patients treated with intravenous acyclovir. Adequate hydration should be maintained).

No products indexed under this heading.

Cyclosporine (Caution should be exercised when administering acyclovir to patients receiving potentially nephrotoxic agents since this may increase the risk of renal dysfunction and/or the risk of reversible CNS symptoms such as those that have been reported in patients treated with intravenous acyclovir. Adequate hydration should be maintained). Products include:

Gengraf Capsules ... 435
Neoral Oral Solution ... 2280
Neoral Soft Gelatin Capsules ... 2280
Restasis Ophthalmic Emulsion ... 557
Sandimmune ... 2296

Cytarabine (Caution should be exercised when administering acyclovir to patients receiving potentially nephrotoxic agents since this may increase the risk of renal dysfunction and/or the risk of reversible CNS symptoms such as those that have been reported in patients treated with intravenous acyclovir. Adequate hydration should be maintained).

No products indexed under this heading.

Cytarabine Liposome (Caution should be exercised when administering acyclovir to patients receiving potentially nephrotoxic agents since this may increase the risk of renal dysfunction and/or the risk of reversible CNS symptoms such as those that have been reported in patients treated with intravenous acyclovir. Adequate hydration should be maintained). Products include:

DepoCyt Injection ... 1136

Delavirdine Mesylate (Caution should be exercised when administering acyclovir to patients receiving potentially nephrotoxic agents since this may increase the risk of renal dysfunction and/or the risk of reversible CNS symptoms such as those that have been reported in patients treated with intravenous acyclovir. Adequate hydration should be maintained).
No products indexed under this heading.

Diatrizoate Meglumine (Caution should be exercised when administering acyclovir to patients receiving potentially nephrotoxic agents since this may increase the risk of renal dysfunction and/or the risk of reversible CNS symptoms such as those that have been reported in patients treated with intravenous acyclovir. Adequate hydration should be maintained).
No products indexed under this heading.

Diatrizoate Sodium (Caution should be exercised when administering acyclovir to patients receiving potentially nephrotoxic agents since this may increase the risk of renal dysfunction and/or the risk of reversible CNS symptoms such as those that have been reported in patients treated with intravenous acyclovir. Adequate hydration should be maintained).
No products indexed under this heading.

Diclofenac Potassium (Caution should be exercised when administering acyclovir to patients receiving potentially nephrotoxic agents since this may increase the risk of renal dysfunction and/or the risk of reversible CNS symptoms such as those that have been reported in patients treated with intravenous acyclovir. Adequate hydration should be maintained).
No products indexed under this heading.

Diclofenac Sodium (Caution should be exercised when administering acyclovir to patients receiving potentially nephrotoxic agents since this may increase the risk of renal dysfunction and/or the risk of reversible CNS symptoms such as those that have been reported in patients treated with intravenous acyclovir. Adequate hydration should be maintained). Products include:
Diclofenac Sodium Ophthalmic Solution .... ⊙ 240
Voltaren Ophthalmic Solution 2336
Voltaren Tablets 2334
Voltaren-XR Tablets 2337

Dicloxacillin Sodium (Caution should be exercised when administering acyclovir to patients receiving potentially nephrotoxic agents since this may increase the risk of renal dysfunction and/or the risk of reversible CNS symptoms such as those that have been reported in patients treated with intravenous acyclovir. Adequate hydration should be maintained).
No products indexed under this heading.

Didanosine (Caution should be exercised when administering acyclovir to patients receiving potentially nephrotoxic agents since this may increase the risk of renal dysfunction and/or the risk of reversible CNS symptoms such as those that have been reported in patients treated with intravenous acyclovir. Adequate hydration should be maintained).
No products indexed under this heading.

Efavirenz (Caution should be exercised when administering acyclovir to patients receiving potentially nephrotoxic agents since this may increase the risk of renal dysfunction and/or the risk of reversible CNS symptoms such as those that have been reported in patients treated with intravenous acyclovir. Adequate hydration should be maintained). Products include:
Atripla Tablets 938
Sustiva Capsules 930
Sustiva Tablets 930

Emtricitabine (Caution should be exercised when administering acyclovir to patients receiving potentially nephrotoxic agents since this may increase the risk of renal dysfunction and/or the risk of reversible CNS symptoms such as those that have been reported in patients treated with intravenous acyclovir. Adequate hydration should be maintained). Products include:
Atripla Tablets 938
Emtriva Capsules 1246
Emtriva Oral Solution 1246
Truvada Tablets 1262

Enalapril Maleate (Caution should be exercised when administering acyclovir to patients receiving potentially nephrotoxic agents since this may increase the risk of renal dysfunction and/or the risk of reversible CNS symptoms such as those that have been reported in patients treated with intravenous acyclovir. Adequate hydration should be maintained).
No products indexed under this heading.

Enalaprilat (Caution should be exercised when administering acyclovir to patients receiving potentially nephrotoxic agents since this may increase the risk of renal dysfunction and/or the risk of reversible CNS symptoms such as those that have been reported in patients treated with intravenous acyclovir. Adequate hydration should be maintained).
No products indexed under this heading.

Enfuvirtide (Caution should be exercised when administering acyclovir to patients receiving potentially nephrotoxic agents since this may increase the risk of renal dysfunction and/or the risk of reversible CNS symptoms such as those that have been reported in patients treated with intravenous acyclovir. Adequate hydration should be maintained).
No products indexed under this heading.

Ethiodized Oil (Caution should be exercised when administering acyclovir to patients receiving potentially nephrotoxic agents since this may increase the risk of renal dysfunction and/or the risk of reversible CNS symptoms such as those that have been reported in patients treated with intravenous acyclovir. Adequate hydration should be maintained).
No products indexed under this heading.

Etodolac (Caution should be exercised when administering acyclovir to patients receiving potentially nephrotoxic agents since this may increase the risk of renal dysfunction and/or the risk of reversible CNS symptoms such as those that have been reported in patients treated with intravenous acyclovir. Adequate hydration should be maintained).
No products indexed under this heading.

Fenoprofen Calcium (Caution should be exercised when administering acyclovir to patients receiving potentially nephrotoxic agents since this may increase the risk of renal dysfunction and/or the risk of reversible CNS symptoms such as those that have been reported in patients treated with intravenous acyclovir. Adequate hydration should be maintained). Products include:
Nalfon Capsules 2508

Filgrastim (Caution should be exercised when administering acyclovir to patients receiving potentially nephrotoxic agents since this may increase the risk of renal dysfunction and/or the risk of reversible CNS symptoms such as those that have been reported in patients treated with intravenous acyclovir. Adequate hydration should be maintained). Products include:
Neupogen for Injection 589

Fluorouracil (Caution should be exercised when administering acyclovir to patients receiving potentially nephrotoxic agents since this may increase the risk of renal dysfunction and/or the risk of reversible CNS symptoms such as those that have been reported in patients treated with intravenous acyclovir. Adequate hydration should be maintained). Products include:
Carac Cream 0.5% 2722

Flurbiprofen (Caution should be exercised when administering acyclovir to patients receiving potentially nephrotoxic agents since this may increase the risk of renal dysfunction and/or the risk of reversible CNS symptoms such as those that have been reported in patients treated with intravenous acyclovir. Adequate hydration should be maintained).
No products indexed under this heading.

Fluvastatin Sodium (Caution should be exercised when administering acyclovir to patients receiving potentially nephrotoxic agents since this may increase the risk of renal dysfunction and/or the risk of reversible CNS symptoms such as those that have been reported in patients treated with intravenous acyclovir. Adequate hydration should be maintained). Products include:
Lescol Capsules 2268
Lescol XL Tablets 2268

Foscarnet Sodium (Caution should be exercised when administering acyclovir to patients receiving potentially nephrotoxic agents since this may increase the risk of renal dysfunction and/or the risk of reversible CNS symptoms such as those that have been reported in patients treated with intravenous acyclovir. Adequate hydration should be maintained).
No products indexed under this heading.

Fosinopril Sodium (Caution should be exercised when administering acyclovir to patients receiving potentially nephrotoxic agents since this may increase the risk of renal dysfunction and/or the risk of reversible CNS symptoms such as those that have been reported in patients treated with intravenous acyclovir. Adequate hydration should be maintained).
No products indexed under this heading.

Furosemide (Caution should be exercised when administering acyclovir to patients receiving potentially nephrotoxic agents since this may increase the risk of renal dysfunction and/or the risk of reversible CNS symptoms such as those that have been reported in patients treated with intravenous acyclovir. Adequate hydration should be maintained). Products include:
Furosemide Tablets 2186

Gadopentetate Dimeglumine (Caution should be exercised when administering acyclovir to patients receiving potentially nephrotoxic agents since this may increase the risk of renal dysfunction and/or the risk of reversible CNS symptoms such as those that have been reported in patients treated with intravenous acyclovir. Adequate hydration should be maintained).
No products indexed under this heading.

Gentamicin (Caution should be exercised when administering acyclovir to patients receiving potentially nephrotoxic agents since this may increase the risk of renal dysfunction and/or the risk of reversible CNS symptoms such as those that have been reported in patients treated with intravenous acyclovir. Adequate hydration should be maintained).
No products indexed under this heading.

Gentamicin Sulfate (Caution should be exercised when administering acyclovir to patients receiving potentially nephrotoxic agents since this may increase the risk of renal dysfunction and/or the risk of reversible CNS symptoms such as those that have been reported in patients treated with intravenous acyclovir. Adequate hydration should be maintained). Products include:
Pred-G Ophthalmic Ointment .... ⊙ 229
Pred-G Ophthalmic Suspension .... ⊙ 228

Glipizide (Caution should be exercised when administering acyclovir to patients receiving potentially nephrotoxic agents since this may increase the risk of renal dysfunction and/or the risk of reversible CNS symptoms such as those that have been reported in patients treated with intravenous acyclovir. Adequate hydration should be maintained).
No products indexed under this heading.

Globulin, Immune (Human) (Caution should be exercised when administering acyclovir to patients receiving potentially nephrotoxic agents since this may increase the risk of renal dysfunction and/or the risk of reversible CNS symptoms such as those that have been reported in patients treated with intravenous acyclovir. Adequate hydration should be maintained). Products include:

Flebogamma 5% ... **1715**

Glyburide (Caution should be exercised when administering acyclovir to patients receiving potentially nephrotoxic agents since this may increase the risk of renal dysfunction and/or the risk of reversible CNS symptoms such as those that have been reported in patients treated with intravenous acyclovir. Adequate hydration should be maintained).

No products indexed under this heading.

Gold Therapy (Caution should be exercised when administering acyclovir to patients receiving potentially nephrotoxic agents since this may increase the risk of renal dysfunction and/or the risk of reversible CNS symptoms such as those that have been reported in patients treated with intravenous acyclovir. Adequate hydration should be maintained).

No products indexed under this heading.

HMG-CoA Reductase Inhibitors (Caution should be exercised when administering acyclovir to patients receiving potentially nephrotoxic agents since this may increase the risk of renal dysfunction and/or the risk of reversible CNS symptoms such as those that have been reported in patients treated with intravenous acyclovir. Adequate hydration should be maintained).

No products indexed under this heading.

Hydrochlorothiazide (Caution should be exercised when administering acyclovir to patients receiving potentially nephrotoxic agents since this may increase the risk of renal dysfunction and/or the risk of reversible CNS symptoms such as those that have been reported in patients treated with intravenous acyclovir. Adequate hydration should be maintained). Products include:

Atacand HCT ... **642**
Avalide Tablets ... **892**
Avalide Tablets ... **2713**
Benicar HCT Tablets ... **1010**
Diovan HCT Tablets ... **2216**
Dyazide Capsules ... **1405**
Micardis HCT Tablets ... **854**
Prinzide Tablets ... **2092**
Tekturna HCT Tablets ... **2324**
Teveten HCT Tablets ... **517**

Hydroflumethiazide (Caution should be exercised when administering acyclovir to patients receiving potentially nephrotoxic agents since this may increase the risk of renal dysfunction and/or the risk of reversible CNS symptoms such as those that have been reported in patients treated with intravenous acyclovir. Adequate hydration should be maintained).

No products indexed under this heading.

Ibuprofen (Caution should be exercised when administering acyclovir to patients receiving potentially nephrotoxic agents since this may increase the risk of renal dysfunction and/or the risk of reversible CNS symptoms such as those that have been reported in patients treated with intravenous acyclovir. Adequate hydration should be maintained). Products include:

Motrin IB Tablets and Caplets ... **1900**
Children's Motrin Oral Suspension ... **1901**
Children's Motrin Non-Staining Dye-Free Oral Suspension ... **1901**
Children's Motrin Cold Oral Suspension ... **1899**
Infants' Motrin Concentrated Drops ... **1901**
Infants' Motrin Non-Staining Dye-Free Concentrated Drops ... **1901**
Junior Strength Motrin Caplets and Chewable Tablets ... **1901**
Vicoprofen Tablets ... **533**

Idarubicin Hydrochloride (Caution should be exercised when administering acyclovir to patients receiving potentially nephrotoxic agents since this may increase the risk of renal dysfunction and/or the risk of reversible CNS symptoms such as those that have been reported in patients treated with intravenous acyclovir. Adequate hydration should be maintained).

No products indexed under this heading.

Ifosfamide (Caution should be exercised when administering acyclovir to patients receiving potentially nephrotoxic agents since this may increase the risk of renal dysfunction and/or the risk of reversible CNS symptoms such as those that have been reported in patients treated with intravenous acyclovir. Adequate hydration should be maintained).

No products indexed under this heading.

Imipenem (Caution should be exercised when administering acyclovir to patients receiving potentially nephrotoxic agents since this may increase the risk of renal dysfunction and/or the risk of reversible CNS symptoms such as those that have been reported in patients treated with intravenous acyclovir. Adequate hydration should be maintained). Products include:

Primaxin I.M. ... **2080**
Primaxin I.V. ... **2083**

Immune Globulin Intravenous (Human) (Caution should be exercised when administering acyclovir to patients receiving potentially nephrotoxic agents since this may increase the risk of renal dysfunction and/or the risk of reversible CNS symptoms such as those that have been reported in patients treated with intravenous acyclovir. Adequate hydration should be maintained). Products include:

Flebogamma 5% DIF ... **1718**
Gammagard Liquid ... **730**
Gammagard S/D ... **734**
Gamunex ... **3094**

Indinavir Sulfate (Caution should be exercised when administering acyclovir to patients receiving potentially nephrotoxic agents since this may increase the risk of renal dysfunction and/or the risk of reversible CNS symptoms such as those that have been reported in patients treated with intravenous acyclovir. Adequate hydration should be maintained). Products include:

Crixivan Capsules ... **1979**

Indomethacin (Caution should be exercised when administering acyclovir to patients receiving potentially nephrotoxic agents since this may increase the risk of renal dysfunction and/or the risk of reversible CNS symptoms such as those that have been reported in patients treated with intravenous acyclovir. Adequate hydration should be maintained). Products include:

Indocin ... **2024**

Indomethacin Sodium Trihydrate (Caution should be exercised when administering acyclovir to patients receiving potentially nephrotoxic agents since this may increase the risk of renal dysfunction and/or the risk of reversible CNS symptoms such as those that have been reported in patients treated with intravenous acyclovir. Adequate hydration should be maintained). Products include:

Indocin I.V. ... **2489**

Interferon Beta-1b (Caution should be exercised when administering acyclovir to patients receiving potentially nephrotoxic agents since this may increase the risk of renal dysfunction and/or the risk of reversible CNS symptoms such as those that have been reported in patients treated with intravenous acyclovir. Adequate hydration should be maintained). Products include:

Betaseron for SC Injection ... **756**

Interleukin-2 (Caution should be exercised when administering acyclovir to patients receiving potentially nephrotoxic agents since this may increase the risk of renal dysfunction and/or the risk of reversible CNS symptoms such as those that have been reported in patients treated with intravenous acyclovir. Adequate hydration should be maintained).

No products indexed under this heading.

Iodamide Meglumine (Caution should be exercised when administering acyclovir to patients receiving potentially nephrotoxic agents since this may increase the risk of renal dysfunction and/or the risk of reversible CNS symptoms such as those that have been reported in patients treated with intravenous acyclovir. Adequate hydration should be maintained).

No products indexed under this heading.

Iohexol (Caution should be exercised when administering acyclovir to patients receiving potentially nephrotoxic agents since this may increase the risk of renal dysfunction and/or the risk of reversible CNS symptoms such as those that have been reported in patients treated with intravenous acyclovir. Adequate hydration should be maintained).

No products indexed under this heading.

Iopamidol (Caution should be exercised when administering acyclovir to patients receiving potentially nephrotoxic agents since this may increase the risk of renal dysfunction and/or the risk of reversible CNS symptoms such as those that have been reported in patients treated with intravenous acyclovir. Adequate hydration should be maintained).

No products indexed under this heading.

Iopanoic Acid (Caution should be exercised when administering acyclovir to patients receiving potentially nephrotoxic agents since this may increase the risk of renal dysfunction and/or the risk of reversible CNS symptoms such as those that have been reported in patients treated with intravenous acyclovir. Adequate hydration should be maintained).

No products indexed under this heading.

Iothalamate Meglumine (Caution should be exercised when administering acyclovir to patients receiving potentially nephrotoxic agents since this may increase the risk of renal dysfunction and/or the risk of reversible CNS symptoms such as those that have been reported in patients treated with intravenous acyclovir. Adequate hydration should be maintained).

No products indexed under this heading.

Ioxaglate Meglumine (Caution should be exercised when administering acyclovir to patients receiving potentially nephrotoxic agents since this may increase the risk of renal dysfunction and/or the risk of reversible CNS symptoms such as those that have been reported in patients treated with intravenous acyclovir. Adequate hydration should be maintained).

No products indexed under this heading.

Ioxaglate Sodium (Caution should be exercised when administering acyclovir to patients receiving potentially nephrotoxic agents since this may increase the risk of renal dysfunction and/or the risk of reversible CNS symptoms such as those that have been reported in patients treated with intravenous acyclovir. Adequate hydration should be maintained).

No products indexed under this heading.

Kanamycin Sulfate (Caution should be exercised when administering acyclovir to patients receiving potentially nephrotoxic agents since this may increase the risk of renal dysfunction and/or the risk of reversible CNS symptoms such as those that have been reported in patients treated with intravenous acyclovir. Adequate hydration should be maintained).

No products indexed under this heading.

Ketoprofen (Caution should be exercised when administering acyclovir to patients receiving potentially nephrotoxic agents since this may increase the risk of renal dysfunction and/or the risk of reversible CNS symptoms such as those that have been reported in patients treated with intravenous acyclovir. Adequate hydration should be maintained).

No products indexed under this heading.

Ketorolac Tromethamine (Caution should be exercised when administering acyclovir to patients receiving potentially nephrotoxic agents since this may increase the risk of renal dysfunction and/or the risk of reversible CNS symptoms such as those that have been reported in patients treated with intravenous acyclovir. Adequate hydration should be maintained).

No products indexed under this heading.

Lamium album (Caution should be exercised when administering acyclovir to patients receiving potentially nephrotoxic agents since this may increase the risk of renal dysfunction and/or the risk of reversible CNS symptoms such as those that have been reported in patients treated with intravenous acyclovir. Adequate hydration should be maintained).
No products indexed under this heading.

Lisinopril (Caution should be exercised when administering acyclovir to patients receiving potentially nephrotoxic agents since this may increase the risk of renal dysfunction and/or the risk of reversible CNS symptoms such as those that have been reported in patients treated with intravenous acyclovir. Adequate hydration should be maintained).
Products include:
Prinivil Tablets 2087
Prinzide Tablets 2092

Lithium (Caution should be exercised when administering acyclovir to patients receiving potentially nephrotoxic agents since this may increase the risk of renal dysfunction and/or the risk of reversible CNS symptoms such as those that have been reported in patients treated with intravenous acyclovir. Adequate hydration should be maintained).
No products indexed under this heading.

Lithium Carbonate (Caution should be exercised when administering acyclovir to patients receiving potentially nephrotoxic agents since this may increase the risk of renal dysfunction and/or the risk of reversible CNS symptoms such as those that have been reported in patients treated with intravenous acyclovir. Adequate hydration should be maintained).
No products indexed under this heading.

Lithium Citrate (Caution should be exercised when administering acyclovir to patients receiving potentially nephrotoxic agents since this may increase the risk of renal dysfunction and/or the risk of reversible CNS symptoms such as those that have been reported in patients treated with intravenous acyclovir. Adequate hydration should be maintained).
No products indexed under this heading.

Lopinavir (Caution should be exercised when administering acyclovir to patients receiving potentially nephrotoxic agents since this may increase the risk of renal dysfunction and/or the risk of reversible CNS symptoms such as those that have been reported in patients treated with intravenous acyclovir. Adequate hydration should be maintained).
Products include:
Kaletra 452

Loracarbef (Caution should be exercised when administering acyclovir to patients receiving potentially nephrotoxic agents since this may increase the risk of renal dysfunction and/or the risk of reversible CNS symptoms such as those that have been reported in patients treated with intravenous acyclovir. Adequate hydration should be maintained).
No products indexed under this heading.

Lovastatin (Caution should be exercised when administering acyclovir to patients receiving potentially nephrotoxic agents since this may increase the risk of renal dysfunction and/or the risk of reversible CNS symptoms such as those that have been reported in patients treated with intravenous acyclovir. Adequate hydration should be maintained).
Products include:
Advicor Tablets 402
Mevacor Tablets 2063

Meclofenamate Sodium (Caution should be exercised when administering acyclovir to patients receiving potentially nephrotoxic agents since this may increase the risk of renal dysfunction and/or the risk of reversible CNS symptoms such as those that have been reported in patients treated with intravenous acyclovir. Adequate hydration should be maintained).
No products indexed under this heading.

Mefenamic Acid (Caution should be exercised when administering acyclovir to patients receiving potentially nephrotoxic agents since this may increase the risk of renal dysfunction and/or the risk of reversible CNS symptoms such as those that have been reported in patients treated with intravenous acyclovir. Adequate hydration should be maintained).
No products indexed under this heading.

Meloxicam (Caution should be exercised when administering acyclovir to patients receiving potentially nephrotoxic agents since this may increase the risk of renal dysfunction and/or the risk of reversible CNS symptoms such as those that have been reported in patients treated with intravenous acyclovir. Adequate hydration should be maintained).
Products include:
Mobic Oral Suspension 863
Mobic Tablets 863

Melphalan Hydrochloride (Caution should be exercised when administering acyclovir to patients receiving potentially nephrotoxic agents since this may increase the risk of renal dysfunction and/or the risk of reversible CNS symptoms such as those that have been reported in patients treated with intravenous acyclovir. Adequate hydration should be maintained).
No products indexed under this heading.

Mesalamine (Caution should be exercised when administering acyclovir to patients receiving potentially nephrotoxic agents since this may increase the risk of renal dysfunction and/or the risk of reversible CNS symptoms such as those that have been reported in patients treated with intravenous acyclovir. Adequate hydration should be maintained).
Products include:
Asacol Delayed-Release Tablets 2579
Canasa Rectal Suppositories 705
Lialda Tablets 3029
Pentasa Capsules 3030

Methimazole (Caution should be exercised when administering acyclovir to patients receiving potentially nephrotoxic agents since this may increase the risk of renal dysfunction and/or the risk of reversible CNS symptoms such as those that have been reported in patients treated with intravenous acyclovir. Adequate hydration should be maintained).
No products indexed under this heading.

Methotrexate (Caution should be exercised when administering acyclovir to patients receiving potentially nephrotoxic agents since this may increase the risk of renal dysfunction and/or the risk of reversible CNS symptoms such as those that have been reported in patients treated with intravenous acyclovir. Adequate hydration should be maintained).
No products indexed under this heading.

Methotrexate Sodium (Caution should be exercised when administering acyclovir to patients receiving potentially nephrotoxic agents since this may increase the risk of renal dysfunction and/or the risk of reversible CNS symptoms such as those that have been reported in patients treated with intravenous acyclovir. Adequate hydration should be maintained).
No products indexed under this heading.

Methyclothiazide (Caution should be exercised when administering acyclovir to patients receiving potentially nephrotoxic agents since this may increase the risk of renal dysfunction and/or the risk of reversible CNS symptoms such as those that have been reported in patients treated with intravenous acyclovir. Adequate hydration should be maintained).
No products indexed under this heading.

Mezlocillin Sodium (Caution should be exercised when administering acyclovir to patients receiving potentially nephrotoxic agents since this may increase the risk of renal dysfunction and/or the risk of reversible CNS symptoms such as those that have been reported in patients treated with intravenous acyclovir. Adequate hydration should be maintained).
No products indexed under this heading.

Minocycline Hydrochloride (Caution should be exercised when administering acyclovir to patients receiving potentially nephrotoxic agents since this may increase the risk of renal dysfunction and/or the risk of reversible CNS symptoms such as those that have been reported in patients treated with intravenous acyclovir. Adequate hydration should be maintained). Products include:
Solodyn Extended Release Tablets 1938

Mitomycin (Mitomycin-C) (Caution should be exercised when administering acyclovir to patients receiving potentially nephrotoxic agents since this may increase the risk of renal dysfunction and/or the risk of reversible CNS symptoms such as those that have been reported in patients treated with intravenous acyclovir. Adequate hydration should be maintained).
No products indexed under this heading.

Moexipril Hydrochloride (Caution should be exercised when administering acyclovir to patients receiving potentially nephrotoxic agents since this may increase the risk of renal dysfunction and/or the risk of reversible CNS symptoms such as those that have been reported in patients treated with intravenous acyclovir. Adequate hydration should be maintained).
No products indexed under this heading.

Muromonab-CD3 (Caution should be exercised when administering acyclovir to patients receiving potentially nephrotoxic agents since this may increase the risk of renal dysfunction and/or the risk of reversible CNS symptoms such as those that have been reported in patients treated with intravenous acyclovir. Adequate hydration should be maintained). Products include:
Orthoclone OKT3 Sterile Solution 2387

Nabumetone (Caution should be exercised when administering acyclovir to patients receiving potentially nephrotoxic agents since this may increase the risk of renal dysfunction and/or the risk of reversible CNS symptoms such as those that have been reported in patients treated with intravenous acyclovir. Adequate hydration should be maintained).
No products indexed under this heading.

Nafcillin Sodium (Caution should be exercised when administering acyclovir to patients receiving potentially nephrotoxic agents since this may increase the risk of renal dysfunction and/or the risk of reversible CNS symptoms such as those that have been reported in patients treated with intravenous acyclovir. Adequate hydration should be maintained).
No products indexed under this heading.

Naproxen (Caution should be exercised when administering acyclovir to patients receiving potentially nephrotoxic agents since this may increase the risk of renal dysfunction and/or the risk of reversible CNS symptoms such as those that have been reported in patients treated with intravenous acyclovir. Adequate hydration should be maintained).
Products include:
EC-Naprosyn Delayed-Release Tablets 2632
Naprosyn Suspension 2632
Naprosyn Tablets 2632

Naproxen Sodium (Caution should be exercised when administering acyclovir to patients receiving potentially nephrotoxic agents since this may increase the risk of renal dysfunction and/or the risk of reversible CNS symptoms such as those that have been reported in patients treated with intravenous acyclovir. Adequate hydration should be maintained). Products include:
Anaprox Tablets 2632
Anaprox DS Tablets 2632
Treximet Tablets 1616

Nelfinavir Mesylate (Caution should be exercised when administering acyclovir to patients receiving potentially nephrotoxic agents since this may increase the risk of renal dysfunction and/or the risk of reversible CNS symptoms such as those that have been reported in patients treated with intravenous acyclovir. Adequate hydration should be maintained).
No products indexed under this heading.

Neomycin (Caution should be exercised when administering acyclovir to patients receiving potentially nephrotoxic agents since this may increase the risk of renal dysfunction and/or the risk of reversible CNS symptoms such as those that have been reported in patients treated with intravenous acyclovir. Adequate hydration should be maintained).
No products indexed under this heading.

Neomycin, oral (Caution should be exercised when administering acyclovir to patients receiving potentially nephrotoxic agents since this may increase the risk of renal dysfunction and/or the risk of reversible CNS symptoms such as those that have been reported in patients treated with intravenous acyclovir. Adequate hydration should be maintained).
No products indexed under this heading.

Neomycin Sulfate (Caution should be exercised when administering acyclovir to patients receiving potentially nephrotoxic agents since this may increase the risk of renal dysfunction and/or the risk of reversible CNS symptoms such as those that have been reported in patients treated with intravenous acyclovir. Adequate hydration should be maintained). Products include:
Neosporin Ophthalmic Solution Sterile .... ⊙ 252

Nephrotoxic Drugs (Caution should be exercised when administering acyclovir to patients receiving potentially nephrotoxic agents since this may increase the risk of renal dysfunction and/or the risk of reversible CNS symptoms such as those that have been reported in patients treated with intravenous acyclovir. Adequate hydration should be maintained).
No products indexed under this heading.

Nevirapine (Caution should be exercised when administering acyclovir to patients receiving potentially nephrotoxic agents since this may increase the risk of renal dysfunction and/or the risk of reversible CNS symptoms such as those that have been reported in patients treated with intravenous acyclovir. Adequate hydration should be maintained). Products include:
Viramune Oral Suspension 873
Viramune Tablets 873

Norfloxacin (Caution should be exercised when administering acyclovir to patients receiving potentially nephrotoxic agents since this may increase the risk of renal dysfunction and/or the risk of reversible CNS symptoms such as those that have been reported in patients treated with intravenous acyclovir. Adequate hydration should be maintained). Products include:
Noroxin Tablets 2069

Olsalazine Sodium (Caution should be exercised when administering acyclovir to patients receiving potentially nephrotoxic agents since this may increase the risk of renal dysfunction and/or the risk of reversible CNS symptoms such as those that have been reported in patients treated with intravenous acyclovir. Adequate hydration should be maintained).
No products indexed under this heading.

Omeprazole (Caution should be exercised when administering acyclovir to patients receiving potentially nephrotoxic agents since this may increase the risk of renal dysfunction and/or the risk of reversible CNS symptoms such as those that have been reported in patients treated with intravenous acyclovir. Adequate hydration should be maintained).
No products indexed under this heading.

Oxaprozin (Caution should be exercised when administering acyclovir to patients receiving potentially nephrotoxic agents since this may increase the risk of renal dysfunction and/or the risk of reversible CNS symptoms such as those that have been reported in patients treated with intravenous acyclovir. Adequate hydration should be maintained).
No products indexed under this heading.

Pamidronate Disodium (Caution should be exercised when administering acyclovir to patients receiving potentially nephrotoxic agents since this may increase the risk of renal dysfunction and/or the risk of reversible CNS symptoms such as those that have been reported in patients treated with intravenous acyclovir. Adequate hydration should be maintained).
No products indexed under this heading.

Paroxetine Hydrochloride (Caution should be exercised when administering acyclovir to patients receiving potentially nephrotoxic agents since this may increase the risk of renal dysfunction and/or the risk of reversible CNS symptoms such as those that have been reported in patients treated with intravenous acyclovir. Adequate hydration should be maintained). Products include:
Paxil 1535
Paxil CR Controlled-Release Tablets 1544

Penicillamine (Caution should be exercised when administering acyclovir to patients receiving potentially nephrotoxic agents since this may increase the risk of renal dysfunction and/or the risk of reversible CNS symptoms such as those that have been reported in patients treated with intravenous acyclovir. Adequate hydration should be maintained). Products include:
Cuprimine Capsules 1986

Penicillin G Benzathine (Caution should be exercised when administering acyclovir to patients receiving potentially nephrotoxic agents since this may increase the risk of renal dysfunction and/or the risk of reversible CNS symptoms such as those that have been reported in patients treated with intravenous acyclovir. Adequate hydration should be maintained). Products include:
Bicillin C-R Injectable Suspension 1775
Bicillin L-A Injection 1777

Penicillin G Potassium (Caution should be exercised when administering acyclovir to patients receiving potentially nephrotoxic agents since this may increase the risk of renal dysfunction and/or the risk of reversible CNS symptoms such as those that have been reported in patients treated with intravenous acyclovir. Adequate hydration should be maintained).
No products indexed under this heading.

Penicillin G Procaine (Caution should be exercised when administering acyclovir to patients receiving potentially nephrotoxic agents since this may increase the risk of renal dysfunction and/or the risk of reversible CNS symptoms such as those that have been reported in patients treated with intravenous acyclovir. Adequate hydration should be maintained). Products include:
Bicillin C-R Injectable Suspension 1775
Bicillin L-A Injection 1777

Penicillin G Sodium (Caution should be exercised when administering acyclovir to patients receiving potentially nephrotoxic agents since this may increase the risk of renal dysfunction and/or the risk of reversible CNS symptoms such as those that have been reported in patients treated with intravenous acyclovir. Adequate hydration should be maintained).
No products indexed under this heading.

Penicillin V Potassium (Caution should be exercised when administering acyclovir to patients receiving potentially nephrotoxic agents since this may increase the risk of renal dysfunction and/or the risk of reversible CNS symptoms such as those that have been reported in patients treated with intravenous acyclovir. Adequate hydration should be maintained).
No products indexed under this heading.

Pentamidine Isethionate (Caution should be exercised when administering acyclovir to patients receiving potentially nephrotoxic agents since this may increase the risk of renal dysfunction and/or the risk of reversible CNS symptoms such as those that have been reported in patients treated with intravenous acyclovir. Adequate hydration should be maintained).
No products indexed under this heading.

Perindopril Erbumine (Caution should be exercised when administering acyclovir to patients receiving potentially nephrotoxic agents since this may increase the risk of renal dysfunction and/or the risk of reversible CNS symptoms such as those that have been reported in patients treated with intravenous acyclovir. Adequate hydration should be maintained). Products include:
Aceon Tablets (2 mg, 4 mg, 8 mg) 3038

Phenylbutazone (Caution should be exercised when administering acyclovir to patients receiving potentially nephrotoxic agents since this may increase the risk of renal dysfunction and/or the risk of reversible CNS symptoms such as those that have been reported in patients treated with intravenous acyclovir. Adequate hydration should be maintained).
No products indexed under this heading.

Piroxicam (Caution should be exercised when administering acyclovir to patients receiving potentially nephrotoxic agents since this may increase the risk of renal dysfunction and/or the risk of reversible CNS symptoms such as those that have been reported in patients treated with intravenous acyclovir. Adequate hydration should be maintained).
No products indexed under this heading.

Plicamycin (Caution should be exercised when administering acyclovir to patients receiving potentially nephrotoxic agents since this may increase the risk of renal dysfunction and/or the risk of reversible CNS symptoms such as those that have been reported in patients treated with intravenous acyclovir. Adequate hydration should be maintained).
No products indexed under this heading.

Polymyxin (Caution should be exercised when administering acyclovir to patients receiving potentially nephrotoxic agents since this may increase the risk of renal dysfunction and/or the risk of reversible CNS symptoms such as those that have been reported in patients treated with intravenous acyclovir. Adequate hydration should be maintained).
No products indexed under this heading.

Polymyxin B Sulfate (Caution should be exercised when administering acyclovir to patients receiving potentially nephrotoxic agents since this may increase the risk of renal dysfunction and/or the risk of reversible CNS symptoms such as those that have been reported in patients treated with intravenous acyclovir. Adequate hydration should be maintained). Products include:
Neosporin Ophthalmic Solution Sterile .... ⊙ 252

Polythiazide (Caution should be exercised when administering acyclovir to patients receiving potentially nephrotoxic agents since this may increase the risk of renal dysfunction and/or the risk of reversible CNS symptoms such as those that have been reported in patients treated with intravenous acyclovir. Adequate hydration should be maintained).
No products indexed under this heading.

Pravastatin Sodium (Caution should be exercised when administering acyclovir to patients receiving potentially nephrotoxic agents since this may increase the risk of renal dysfunction and/or the risk of reversible CNS symptoms such as those that have been reported in patients treated with intravenous acyclovir. Adequate hydration should be maintained).
No products indexed under this heading.

Probenecid (Co-administration of probenecid with intravenous acyclovir has been shown to increase acyclovir half-life and systemic exposure; urinary excretion and renal clearance were correspondingly reduced).
No products indexed under this heading.

Quinapril Hydrochloride (Caution should be exercised when administering acyclovir to patients receiving potentially nephrotoxic agents since this may increase the risk of renal dysfunction and/or the risk of reversible CNS symptoms such as those that have been reported in patients treated with intravenous acyclovir. Adequate hydration should be maintained).
No products indexed under this heading.

Rabeprazole Sodium (Caution should be exercised when administering acyclovir to patients receiving potentially nephrotoxic agents since this may increase the risk of renal dysfunction and/or the risk of reversible CNS symptoms such as those that have been reported in patients treated with intravenous acyclovir. Adequate hydration should be maintained). Products include:
Aciphex Tablets 1053

Ramipril (Caution should be exercised when administering acyclovir to patients receiving potentially nephrotoxic agents since this may increase the risk of renal dysfunction and/or the risk of reversible CNS symptoms such as those that have been reported in patients treated with intravenous acyclovir. Adequate hydration should be maintained).
No products indexed under this heading.

Rifampin (Caution should be exercised when administering acyclovir to patients receiving potentially nephrotoxic agents since this may increase the risk of renal dysfunction and/or the risk of reversible CNS symptoms such as those that have been reported in patients treated with intravenous acyclovir. Adequate hydration should be maintained).
No products indexed under this heading.

Riluzole (Caution should be exercised when administering acyclovir to patients receiving potentially nephrotoxic agents since this may increase the risk of renal dysfunction and/or the risk of reversible CNS symptoms such as those that have been reported in patients treated with intravenous acyclovir. Adequate hydration should be maintained). Products include:
Rilutek Tablets 2771

Ritonavir (Caution should be exercised when administering acyclovir to patients receiving potentially nephrotoxic agents since this may increase the risk of renal dysfunction and/or the risk of reversible CNS symptoms such as those that have been reported in patients treated with intravenous acyclovir. Adequate hydration should be maintained). Products include:
Kaletra 452
Norvir 489

Rofecoxib (Caution should be exercised when administering acyclovir to patients receiving potentially nephrotoxic agents since this may increase the risk of renal dysfunction and/or the risk of reversible CNS symptoms such as those that have been reported in patients treated with intravenous acyclovir. Adequate hydration should be maintained).
No products indexed under this heading.

Saquinavir (Caution should be exercised when administering acyclovir to patients receiving potentially nephrotoxic agents since this may increase the risk of renal dysfunction and/or the risk of reversible CNS symptoms such as those that have been reported in patients treated with intravenous acyclovir. Adequate hydration should be maintained).
No products indexed under this heading.

Sibutramine Hydrochloride Monohydrate (Caution should be exercised when administering acyclovir to patients receiving potentially nephrotoxic agents since this may increase the risk of renal dysfunction and/or the risk of reversible CNS symptoms such as those that have been reported in patients treated with intravenous acyclovir. Adequate hydration should be maintained). Products include:
Meridia Capsules 475

Simvastatin (Caution should be exercised when administering acyclovir to patients receiving potentially nephrotoxic agents since this may increase the risk of renal dysfunction and/or the risk of reversible CNS symptoms such as those that have been reported in patients treated with intravenous acyclovir. Adequate hydration should be maintained). Products include:
Simcor Tablets 502
Vytorin 10/10 Tablets 2149
Vytorin 10/10 Tablets 2939
Vytorin 10/20 Tablets 2149
Vytorin 10/20 Tablets 2939
Vytorin 10/40 Tablets 2149
Vytorin 10/40 Tablets 2939
Vytorin 10/80 Tablets 2149
Vytorin 10/80 Tablets 2939
Zocor Tablets 2136

Spirapril Hydrochloride (Caution should be exercised when administering acyclovir to patients receiving potentially nephrotoxic agents since this may increase the risk of renal dysfunction and/or the risk of reversible CNS symptoms such as those that have been reported in patients treated with intravenous acyclovir. Adequate hydration should be maintained).
No products indexed under this heading.

Stavudine (Caution should be exercised when administering acyclovir to patients receiving potentially nephrotoxic agents since this may increase the risk of renal dysfunction and/or the risk of reversible CNS symptoms such as those that have been reported in patients treated with intravenous acyclovir. Adequate hydration should be maintained).
No products indexed under this heading.

Streptomycin Sulfate (Caution should be exercised when administering acyclovir to patients receiving potentially nephrotoxic agents since this may increase the risk of renal dysfunction and/or the risk of reversible CNS symptoms such as those that have been reported in patients treated with intravenous acyclovir. Adequate hydration should be maintained).
No products indexed under this heading.

Streptozocin (Caution should be exercised when administering acyclovir to patients receiving potentially nephrotoxic agents since this may increase the risk of renal dysfunction and/or the risk of reversible CNS symptoms such as those that have been reported in patients treated with intravenous acyclovir. Adequate hydration should be maintained).
No products indexed under this heading.

Sulfacytine (Caution should be exercised when administering acyclovir to patients receiving potentially nephrotoxic agents since this may increase the risk of renal dysfunction and/or the risk of reversible CNS symptoms such as those that have been reported in patients treated with intravenous acyclovir. Adequate hydration should be maintained).
No products indexed under this heading.

Sulfamethizole (Caution should be exercised when administering acyclovir to patients receiving potentially nephrotoxic agents since this may increase the risk of renal dysfunction and/or the risk of reversible CNS symptoms such as those that have been reported in patients treated with intravenous acyclovir. Adequate hydration should be maintained).
No products indexed under this heading.

Sulfamethoxazole (Caution should be exercised when administering acyclovir to patients receiving potentially nephrotoxic agents since this may increase the risk of renal dysfunction and/or the risk of reversible CNS symptoms such as those that have been reported in patients treated with intravenous acyclovir. Adequate hydration should be maintained).
No products indexed under this heading.

Sulfasalazine (Caution should be exercised when administering acyclovir to patients receiving potentially nephrotoxic agents since this may increase the risk of renal dysfunction and/or the risk of reversible CNS symptoms such as those that have been reported in patients treated with intravenous acyclovir. Adequate hydration should be maintained).
No products indexed under this heading.

Sulfinpyrazone (Caution should be exercised when administering acyclovir to patients receiving potentially nephrotoxic agents since this may increase the risk of renal dysfunction and/or the risk of reversible CNS symptoms such as those that have been reported in patients treated with intravenous acyclovir. Adequate hydration should be maintained).
No products indexed under this heading.

Sulfisoxazole Acetyl (Caution should be exercised when administering acyclovir to patients receiving potentially nephrotoxic agents since this may increase the risk of renal dysfunction and/or the risk of reversible CNS symptoms such as those that have been reported in patients treated with intravenous acyclovir. Adequate hydration should be maintained).
No products indexed under this heading.

Sulfisoxazole Diolamine (Caution should be exercised when administering acyclovir to patients receiving potentially nephrotoxic agents since this may increase the risk of renal dysfunction and/or the risk of reversible CNS symptoms such as those that have been reported in patients treated with intravenous acyclovir. Adequate hydration should be maintained).
No products indexed under this heading.

Sulindac (Caution should be exercised when administering acyclovir to patients receiving potentially nephrotoxic agents since this may increase the risk of renal dysfunction and/or the risk of reversible CNS symptoms such as those that have been reported in patients treated with intravenous acyclovir. Adequate hydration should be maintained). Products include:
Clinoril Tablets 1962

Tacrolimus (Caution should be exercised when administering acyclovir to patients receiving potentially nephrotoxic agents since this may increase the risk of renal dysfunction and/or the risk of reversible CNS symptoms such as those that have been reported in patients treated with intravenous acyclovir. Adequate hydration should be maintained). Products include:
Prograf Capsules and Injection 622
Protopic Ointment 628

Tenofovir Disoproxil Fumarate (Caution should be exercised when administering acyclovir to patients receiving potentially nephrotoxic agents since this may increase the risk of renal dysfunction and/or the risk of reversible CNS symptoms such as those that have been reported in patients treated with intravenous acyclovir. Adequate hydration should be maintained). Products include:
Atripla Tablets 938
Truvada Tablets 1262
Viread Tablets 1268

Thioguanine (Caution should be exercised when administering acyclovir to patients receiving potentially nephrotoxic agents since this may increase the risk of renal dysfunction and/or the risk of reversible CNS symptoms such as those that have been reported in patients treated with intravenous acyclovir. Adequate hydration should be maintained). Products include:
Tabloid Tablets 1601

Ticarcillin Disodium (Caution should be exercised when administering acyclovir to patients receiving potentially nephrotoxic agents since this may increase the risk of renal dysfunction and/or the risk of reversible CNS symptoms such as those that have been reported in patients treated with intravenous acyclovir. Adequate hydration should be maintained). Products include:

Timentin ADD-Vantage 1606
Timentin Injection Galaxy Container 1609
Timentin IV Infusion 1603
Timentin Pharmacy Bulk Package 1613

Tobramycin (Caution should be exercised when administering acyclovir to patients receiving potentially nephrotoxic agents since this may increase the risk of renal dysfunction and/or the risk of reversible CNS symptoms such as those that have been reported in patients treated with intravenous acyclovir. Adequate hydration should be maintained). Products include:

Zylet Ophthalmic Suspension .... ⊙ 247

Tobramycin Sulfate (Caution should be exercised when administering acyclovir to patients receiving potentially nephrotoxic agents since this may increase the risk of renal dysfunction and/or the risk of reversible CNS symptoms such as those that have been reported in patients treated with intravenous acyclovir. Adequate hydration should be maintained).
No products indexed under this heading.

Tolazamide (Caution should be exercised when administering acyclovir to patients receiving potentially nephrotoxic agents since this may increase the risk of renal dysfunction and/or the risk of reversible CNS symptoms such as those that have been reported in patients treated with intravenous acyclovir. Adequate hydration should be maintained).
No products indexed under this heading.

Tolbutamide (Caution should be exercised when administering acyclovir to patients receiving potentially nephrotoxic agents since this may increase the risk of renal dysfunction and/or the risk of reversible CNS symptoms such as those that have been reported in patients treated with intravenous acyclovir. Adequate hydration should be maintained).
No products indexed under this heading.

Tolmetin Sodium (Caution should be exercised when administering acyclovir to patients receiving potentially nephrotoxic agents since this may increase the risk of renal dysfunction and/or the risk of reversible CNS symptoms such as those that have been reported in patients treated with intravenous acyclovir. Adequate hydration should be maintained).
No products indexed under this heading.

Trandolapril (Caution should be exercised when administering acyclovir to patients receiving potentially nephrotoxic agents since this may increase the risk of renal dysfunction and/or the risk of reversible CNS symptoms such as those that have been reported in patients treated with intravenous acyclovir. Adequate hydration should be maintained). Products include:

Mavik Tablets 472
Tarka Tablets 511

Triamterene (Caution should be exercised when administering acyclovir to patients receiving potentially nephrotoxic agents since this may increase the risk of renal dysfunction and/or the risk of reversible CNS symptoms such as those that have been reported in patients treated with intravenous acyclovir. Adequate hydration should be maintained). Products include:

Dyazide Capsules 1405
Dyrenium Capsules 3189

Trimethadione (Caution should be exercised when administering acyclovir to patients receiving potentially nephrotoxic agents since this may increase the risk of renal dysfunction and/or the risk of reversible CNS symptoms such as those that have been reported in patients treated with intravenous acyclovir. Adequate hydration should be maintained).
No products indexed under this heading.

Trovafloxacin Mesylate (Caution should be exercised when administering acyclovir to patients receiving potentially nephrotoxic agents since this may increase the risk of renal dysfunction and/or the risk of reversible CNS symptoms such as those that have been reported in patients treated with intravenous acyclovir. Adequate hydration should be maintained).
No products indexed under this heading.

Tyropanoate Sodium (Caution should be exercised when administering acyclovir to patients receiving potentially nephrotoxic agents since this may increase the risk of renal dysfunction and/or the risk of reversible CNS symptoms such as those that have been reported in patients treated with intravenous acyclovir. Adequate hydration should be maintained).
No products indexed under this heading.

Valacyclovir Hydrochloride (Caution should be exercised when administering acyclovir to patients receiving potentially nephrotoxic agents since this may increase the risk of renal dysfunction and/or the risk of reversible CNS symptoms such as those that have been reported in patients treated with intravenous acyclovir. Adequate hydration should be maintained). Products include:

Valtrex Caplets 1635

Valdecoxib (Caution should be exercised when administering acyclovir to patients receiving potentially nephrotoxic agents since this may increase the risk of renal dysfunction and/or the risk of reversible CNS symptoms such as those that have been reported in patients treated with intravenous acyclovir. Adequate hydration should be maintained).
No products indexed under this heading.

Vancomycin Hydrochloride (Caution should be exercised when administering acyclovir to patients receiving potentially nephrotoxic agents since this may increase the risk of renal dysfunction and/or the risk of reversible CNS symptoms such as those that have been reported in patients treated with intravenous acyclovir. Adequate hydration should be maintained).
No products indexed under this heading.

Voriconazole (Caution should be exercised when administering acyclovir to patients receiving potentially nephrotoxic agents since this may increase the risk of renal dysfunction and/or the risk of reversible CNS symptoms such as those that have been reported in patients treated with intravenous acyclovir. Adequate hydration should be maintained).
No products indexed under this heading.

Zalcitabine (Caution should be exercised when administering acyclovir to patients receiving potentially nephrotoxic agents since this may increase the risk of renal dysfunction and/or the risk of reversible CNS symptoms such as those that have been reported in patients treated with intravenous acyclovir. Adequate hydration should be maintained).
No products indexed under this heading.

Zidovudine (Caution should be exercised when administering acyclovir to patients receiving potentially nephrotoxic agents since this may increase the risk of renal dysfunction and/or the risk of reversible CNS symptoms such as those that have been reported in patients treated with intravenous acyclovir. Adequate hydration should be maintained). Products include:

Combivir Tablets 1384
Retrovir 1574
Retrovir IV Infusion 1579
Trizivir Tablets 1622

Zoledronic acid (Caution should be exercised when administering acyclovir to patients receiving potentially nephrotoxic agents since this may increase the risk of renal dysfunction and/or the risk of reversible CNS symptoms such as those that have been reported in patients treated with intravenous acyclovir. Adequate hydration should be maintained). Products include:

Reclast Injection 2291
Zometa for Intravenous Infusion 2341

ZOVIRAX CREAM

(Acyclovir) 817
None cited in PDR database.

ZOVIRAX OINTMENT

(Acyclovir) 819
None cited in PDR database.

ZOVIRAX SUSPENSION

(Acyclovir) 1690
See Zovirax Capsules

ZOVIRAX TABLETS

(Acyclovir) 1690
See Zovirax Capsules

ZYBAN SUSTAINED-RELEASE TABLETS

(Bupropion Hydrochloride) 1692

May interact with benzodiazepines, corticosteroids, antidepressant drugs, hypnotics and sedatives, monoamine oxidase inhibitors, antipsychotic agents, phenytoin, drugs which lower seizure threshold, xanthines, and certain other agents. Compounds in these categories include:

Alprazolam (Bupropion is associated with a dose-related risk of seizures; excessive use of benzodiazepine sedatives is associated with increased risk of seizures; bupropion is contraindicated in patients undergoing abrupt discontinuation of benzodiazepine sedatives).
No products indexed under this heading.

Amantadine Hydrochloride (Limited clinical data suggests higher incidence of adverse experiences with co-administration; use small initial dose and gradually increase doses).
No products indexed under this heading.

Aminophylline (Bupropion is associated with a dose-related risk of seizures; co-administration with drugs that lower seizure threshold may increase the risk of seizures with bupropion; concurrent use should be undertaken with extreme caution).
No products indexed under this heading.

Amitriptyline Hydrochloride (Bupropion is associated with dose-dependent risk of seizures; co-administration with drugs that lower seizure threshold may increase the risk of seizure with bupropion).
No products indexed under this heading.

Amoxapine (Bupropion is associated with dose-dependent risk of seizures; co-administration with drugs that lower seizure threshold may increase the risk of seizure with bupropion).
No products indexed under this heading.

Aripiprazole (Bupropion is associated with dose-dependent risk of seizures; co-administration with drugs that lower seizure threshold, such as antipsychotics, may increase the risk of seizure with bupropion). Products include:

Abilify Injection 881
Abilify Injection 2466
Abilify Oral Solution 881
Abilify Oral Solution 2466
Abilify Discmelt Orally Disintegrating Tablets 881
Abilify Discmelt Orally Disintegrating Tablets 2466
Abilify Tablets 881
Abilify Tablets 2466

Atazanavir (Co-administration with fosamprenavir/ritonavir combination may lead to decreased levels of atazanavir).
No products indexed under this heading.

Atazanavir Sulfate (Co-administration with fosamprenavir/ritonavir combination may lead to decreased levels of atazanavir). Products include:

Reyataz Capsules 3299

Betamethasone Acetate (Concurrent administration of bupropion hydrochloride and agents that lower seizure threshold, such as systemic steroids, should be undertaken only with extreme caution).
No products indexed under this heading.

Betamethasone Sodium Phosphate (Concurrent administration of bupropion hydrochloride and agents that lower seizure threshold, such as systemic steroids, should be undertaken only with extreme caution).
No products indexed under this heading.

IMPORTANT NOTE: Always consult each drug listing in the patient's regimen for possible interactions.

Budesonide (Concurrent administration of bupropion hydrochloride and agents that lower seizure threshold, such as systemic steroids, should be undertaken only with extreme caution). Products include:
Pulmicort Flexhaler 654
Symbicort 80/4.5 Inhalation Aerosol 659
Symbicort 160/4.5 Inhalation Aerosol 659

Bupropion (Zyban should not be used in combination with any other medications containing bupropion, such as Wellbutrin or Wellbutrin SR).
No products indexed under this heading.

Butabarbital (Bupropion hydrochloride is contraindicated in patients undergoing abrupt discontinuation of sedatives).
No products indexed under this heading.

Butabarbital Sodium (Bupropion hydrochloride is contraindicated in patients undergoing abrupt discontinuation of sedatives).
No products indexed under this heading.

Carbamazepine (May induce the metabolism of bupropion). Products include:
Carbatrol Capsules 3019
Equetro Extended-Release Capsules 3174

Chloral Hydrate (Bupropion hydrochloride is contraindicated in patients undergoing abrupt discontinuation of sedatives).
No products indexed under this heading.

Chlordiazepoxide (Bupropion is associated with a dose-related risk of seizures; excessive use of benzodiazepine sedatives is associated with increased risk of seizures; bupropion is contraindicated in patients undergoing abrupt discontinuation of benzodiazepine sedatives).
No products indexed under this heading.

Chlordiazepoxide Hydrochloride (Bupropion is associated with a dose-related risk of seizures; excessive use of benzodiazepine sedatives is associated with increased risk of seizures; bupropion is contraindicated in patients undergoing abrupt discontinuation of benzodiazepine sedatives).
No products indexed under this heading.

Chlorpromazine (Bupropion is associated with dose-dependent risk of seizures; co-administration with drugs that lower seizure threshold, such as antipsychotics, may increase the risk of seizure with bupropion).
No products indexed under this heading.

Chlorpromazine Hydrochloride (Bupropion is associated with dose-dependent risk of seizures; co-administration with drugs that lower seizure threshold, such as antipsychotics, may increase the risk of seizure with bupropion).
No products indexed under this heading.

Chlorprothixene (Bupropion is associated with dose-dependent risk of seizures; co-administration with drugs that lower seizure threshold, such as antipsychotics, may increase the risk of seizure with bupropion).
No products indexed under this heading.

Chlorprothixene Hydrochloride (Bupropion is associated with dose-dependent risk of seizures; co-administration with drugs that lower seizure threshold, such as antipsychotics, may increase the risk of seizure with bupropion).
No products indexed under this heading.

Ciclesonide (Concurrent administration of bupropion hydrochloride and agents that lower seizure threshold, such as systemic steroids, should be undertaken only with extreme caution). Products include:
Alvesco Inhalation Aerosol 2985
Omnaris Nasal Spray 2998

Cimetidine (May inhibit the metabolism of bupropion).
No products indexed under this heading.

Cimetidine Hydrochloride (May inhibit the metabolism of bupropion).
No products indexed under this heading.

Citalopram Hydrobromide (Bupropion is associated with dose-dependent risk of seizures; co-administration with drugs that lower seizure threshold, such as antidepressants, may increase the risk of seizure with bupropion). Products include:
Celexa 1160

Clorazepate Dipotassium (Bupropion is associated with a dose-related risk of seizures; excessive use of benzodiazepine sedatives is associated with increased risk of seizures; bupropion is contraindicated in patients undergoing abrupt discontinuation of benzodiazepine sedatives).
No products indexed under this heading.

Clozapine (Bupropion is associated with dose-dependent risk of seizures; co-administration with drugs that lower seizure threshold, such as antipsychotics, may increase the risk of seizure with bupropion).
No products indexed under this heading.

Cortisone Acetate (Concurrent administration of bupropion hydrochloride and agents that lower seizure threshold, such as systemic steroids, should be undertaken only with extreme caution).
No products indexed under this heading.

Cyclophosphamide (Bupropion is primarily metabolized, based on in vitro studies, to hydroxybupropion by the CYP2B6 isoenzyme, therefore the potential exists for a drug interaction with agents that affect the CYP2B6 isoenzyme metabolism, such as cyclophosphamide).
No products indexed under this heading.

Desipramine Hydrochloride (Co-administration in male subjects who were extensive metabolizers of the CYP2D6 isoenzyme with daily doses of bupropion followed by a single dose of desipramine increased the Cmax, AUC and t1/2 of desipramine by an average of approximately two-, five-, and two-fold respectively; co-administration should be initiated at the lower end of the dose range of desipramine; potential for increased risk of seizures).
No products indexed under this heading.

Dexamethasone (Concurrent administration of bupropion hydrochloride and agents that lower seizure threshold, such as systemic steroids, should be undertaken only with extreme caution). Products include:
Ciprodex Otic Suspension 541

Dexamethasone Acetate (Concurrent administration of bupropion hydrochloride and agents that lower seizure threshold, such as systemic steroids, should be undertaken only with extreme caution).
No products indexed under this heading.

Dexamethasone Sodium Phosphate (Concurrent administration of bupropion hydrochloride and agents that lower seizure threshold, such as systemic steroids, should be undertaken only with extreme caution).
No products indexed under this heading.

Diazepam (Bupropion is associated with a dose-related risk of seizures; excessive use of benzodiazepine sedatives is associated with increased risk of seizures; bupropion is contraindicated in patients undergoing abrupt discontinuation of benzodiazepine sedatives). Products include:
Valium Tablets 2658

Doxepin Hydrochloride (Bupropion is associated with dose-dependent risk of seizures; co-administration with drugs that lower seizure threshold may increase the risk of seizure with bupropion).
No products indexed under this heading.

Dyphylline (Bupropion is associated with a dose-related risk of seizures; co-administration with drugs that lower seizure threshold may increase the risk of seizures with bupropion; concurrent use should be undertaken with extreme caution).
No products indexed under this heading.

Escitalopram Oxalate (Bupropion is associated with dose-dependent risk of seizures; co-administration with drugs that lower seizure threshold, such as antidepressants, may increase the risk of seizure with bupropion). Products include:
Lexapro Oral Suspension 1174
Lexapro Tablets 1174

Estazolam (Bupropion is associated with a dose-related risk of seizures; excessive use of benzodiazepine sedatives is associated with increased risk of seizures; bupropion is contraindicated in patients undergoing abrupt discontinuation of benzodiazepine sedatives).
No products indexed under this heading.

Ethchlorvynol (Bupropion hydrochloride is contraindicated in patients undergoing abrupt discontinuation of sedatives).
No products indexed under this heading.

Ethinamate (Bupropion hydrochloride is contraindicated in patients undergoing abrupt discontinuation of sedatives).
No products indexed under this heading.

Flecainide Acetate (Co-administration of bupropion with drugs that are metabolized by CYP2D6 isoenzyme, such as flecainide, may result in, based on data with desipramine, increased Cmax, AUC and t1/2; co-administration should be initiated at the lower end of the dose range of flecainide).
No products indexed under this heading.

Fludrocortisone Acetate (Concurrent administration of bupropion hydrochloride and agents that lower seizure threshold, such as systemic steroids, should be undertaken only with extreme caution).
No products indexed under this heading.

Flunisolide (Concurrent administration of bupropion hydrochloride and agents that lower seizure threshold, such as systemic steroids, should be undertaken only with extreme caution). Products include:
Aerobid/Aerobid-M 1153

Fluoxetine Hydrochloride (Co-administration of bupropion with drugs that are metabolized by CYP2D6 isoenzyme, such as fluoxetine, may result in, based on data with desipramine, increased Cmax, AUC and t1/2; co-administration should be initiated at the lower end of the dose range of fluoxetine). Products include:
Prozac Weekly Capsules 1852
Prozac Pulvules and Liquid 1852
Symbyax Capsules 1871

Fluphenazine Decanoate (Bupropion is associated with dose-dependent risk of seizures; co-administration with drugs that lower seizure threshold, such as antipsychotics, may increase the risk of seizure with bupropion).
No products indexed under this heading.

Fluphenazine Enanthate (Bupropion is associated with dose-dependent risk of seizures; co-administration with drugs that lower seizure threshold, such as antipsychotics, may increase the risk of seizure with bupropion).
No products indexed under this heading.

Fluphenazine Hydrochloride (Bupropion is associated with dose-dependent risk of seizures; co-administration with drugs that lower seizure threshold, such as antipsychotics, may increase the risk of seizure with bupropion).
No products indexed under this heading.

Flurazepam Hydrochloride (Bupropion is associated with a dose-related risk of seizures; excessive use of benzodiazepine sedatives is associated with increased risk of seizures; bupropion is contraindicated in patients undergoing abrupt discontinuation of benzodiazepine sedatives).
No products indexed under this heading.

Fluticasone Propionate (Concurrent administration of bupropion hydrochloride and agents that lower seizure threshold, such as systemic

steroids, should be undertaken only with extreme caution). Products include:
Advair Diskus 100/50 1276
Advair Diskus 250/50 1276
Advair Diskus 500/50 1276
Advair HFA 45/21 Inhalation Aerosol.................................... 1288
Advair HFA 115/21 Inhalation Aerosol.................................... 1288
Advair HFA 230/21 Inhalation Aerosol.................................... 1288
Flonase Nasal Spray 1431
Flovent Diskus 50 mcg 1435

Fluticasone Propionate HFA (Concurrent administration of bupropion hydrochloride and agents that lower seizure threshold, such as systemic steroids, should be undertaken only with extreme caution). Products include:
Flovent HFA 1440

Fosphenytoin Sodium (May induce the metabolism of bupropion).
No products indexed under this heading.

Glutethimide (Bupropion hydrochloride is contraindicated in patients undergoing abrupt discontinuation of sedatives).
No products indexed under this heading.

Halazepam (Bupropion is associated with a dose-related risk of seizures; excessive use of benzodiazepine sedatives is associated with increased risk of seizures; bupropion is contraindicated in patients undergoing abrupt discontinuation of benzodiazepine sedatives).
No products indexed under this heading.

Haloperidol (Co-administration of bupropion with drugs that are metabolized by CYP2D6 isoenzyme, such as haloperidol, may result in, based on data with desipramine, increased Cmax, AUC and t1/2; co-administration should be initiated at the lower end of the dose range of haloperidol; potential for increased risk of seizures).
No products indexed under this heading.

Haloperidol Decanoate (Co-administration of bupropion with drugs that are metabolized by CYP2D6 isoenzyme, such as haloperidol, may result in, based on data with desipramine, increased Cmax, AUC and t1/2; co-administration should be initiated at the lower end of the dose range of haloperidol; potential for increased risk of seizures).
No products indexed under this heading.

Hydrocortisone (Concurrent administration of bupropion hydrochloride and agents that lower seizure threshold, such as systemic steroids, should be undertaken only with extreme caution).
No products indexed under this heading.

Hydrocortisone Acetate (Concurrent administration of bupropion hydrochloride and agents that lower seizure threshold, such as systemic steroids, should be undertaken only with extreme caution). Products include:
Analpram-HC 1140
Pramosone 1141

Hydrocortisone Sodium Phosphate (Concurrent administration of bupropion hydrochloride and agents that lower seizure threshold, such as systemic steroids, should be undertaken only with extreme caution).
No products indexed under this heading.

Hydrocortisone Sodium Succinate (Concurrent administration of bupropion hydrochloride and agents that lower seizure threshold, such as systemic steroids, should be undertaken only with extreme caution).
No products indexed under this heading.

Imipramine Hydrochloride (Co-administration of bupropion with drugs that are metabolized by CYP2D6 isoenzyme, such as imipramine, may result in, based on data with desipramine, increased Cmax, AUC and t1/2; co-administration should be initiated at the lower end of the dose range of imipramine; potential for increased risk of seizures).
No products indexed under this heading.

Imipramine Pamoate (Co-administration of bupropion with drugs that are metabolized by CYP2D6 isoenzyme, such as imipramine, may result in, based on data with desipramine, increased Cmax, AUC and t1/2; co-administration should be initiated at the lower end of the dose range of imipramine; potential for increased risk of seizures).
No products indexed under this heading.

Isocarboxazid (Concurrent and/or sequential use with MAO inhibitors is contraindicated). Products include:
Marplan Tablets 3177

Levodopa (Limited clinical data suggests higher incidence of adverse experiences with co-administration; use small initial dose and gradually increase doses). Products include:
Stalevo Tablets 2309

Lithium Carbonate (Bupropion is associated with dose-dependent risk of seizures; co-administration with drugs that lower seizure threshold, such as antipsychotics, may increase the risk of seizure with bupropion).
No products indexed under this heading.

Lithium Citrate (Bupropion is associated with dose-dependent risk of seizures; co-administration with drugs that lower seizure threshold, such as antipsychotics, may increase the risk of seizure with bupropion).
No products indexed under this heading.

Lorazepam (Bupropion is associated with a dose-related risk of seizures; excessive use of benzodiazepine sedatives is associated with increased risk of seizures; bupropion is contraindicated in patients undergoing abrupt discontinuation of benzodiazepine sedatives).
No products indexed under this heading.

Loxapine Hydrochloride (Bupropion is associated with dose-dependent risk of seizures; co-administration with drugs that lower seizure threshold, such as antipsychotics, may increase the risk of seizure with bupropion).
No products indexed under this heading.

Loxapine Succinate (Bupropion is associated with dose-dependent risk of seizures; co-administration with drugs that lower seizure threshold, such as antipsychotics, may increase the risk of seizure with bupropion).
No products indexed under this heading.

Maprotiline Hydrochloride (Bupropion is associated with dose-dependent risk of seizures; co-administration with drugs that lower seizure threshold may increase the risk of seizure with bupropion).
No products indexed under this heading.

Mesoridazine Besylate (Bupropion is associated with dose-dependent risk of seizures; co-administration with drugs that lower seizure threshold, such as antipsychotics, may increase the risk of seizure with bupropion).
No products indexed under this heading.

Methotrimeprazine (Bupropion is associated with dose-dependent risk of seizures; co-administration with drugs that lower seizure threshold, such as antipsychotics, may increase the risk of seizure with bupropion).
No products indexed under this heading.

Methylprednisolone Acetate (Concurrent administration of bupropion hydrochloride and agents that lower seizure threshold, such as systemic steroids, should be undertaken only with extreme caution).
No products indexed under this heading.

Methylprednisolone Sodium Succinate (Concurrent administration of bupropion hydrochloride and agents that lower seizure threshold, such as systemic steroids, should be undertaken only with extreme caution).
No products indexed under this heading.

Metoprolol Succinate (Co-administration of bupropion with drugs that are metabolized by CYP2D6 isoenzyme, such as metoprolol, may result in, based on data with desipramine, increased Cmax, AUC and t1/2; co-administration should be initiated at the lower end of the dose range of metoprolol). Products include:
Toprol-XL Tablets 666

Metoprolol Tartrate (Co-administration of bupropion with drugs that are metabolized by CYP2D6 isoenzyme, such as metoprolol, may result in, based on data with desipramine, increased Cmax, AUC and t1/2; co-administration should be initiated at the lower end of the dose range of metoprolol).
No products indexed under this heading.

Midazolam Hydrochloride (Bupropion is associated with a dose-related risk of seizures; excessive use of benzodiazepine sedatives is associated with increased risk of seizures; bupropion is contraindicated in patients undergoing abrupt discontinuation of benzodiazepine sedatives).
No products indexed under this heading.

Mirtazapine (Bupropion is associated with dose-dependent risk of seizures; co-administration with drugs that lower seizure threshold, such as antidepressants, may increase the risk of seizure with bupropion). Products include:
Remeron Tablets 2924
RemeronSolTab Tablets 2927

Moclobemide (Concurrent and/or sequential use with MAO inhibitors is contraindicated).
No products indexed under this heading.

Molindone Hydrochloride (Bupropion is associated with dose-dependent risk of seizures; co-administration with drugs that lower seizure threshold, such as antipsychotics, may increase the risk of seizure with bupropion). Products include:
Moban Tablets 1116

Mometasone Furoate (Concurrent administration of bupropion hydrochloride and agents that lower seizure threshold, such as systemic steroids, should be undertaken only with extreme caution). Products include:
Asmanex Twisthaler 2797
Elocon Cream 0.1% 2840
Elocon Lotion 0.1% 2841
Elocon Ointment 0.1% 2842

Mometasone Furoate Monohydrate (Concurrent administration of bupropion hydrochloride and agents that lower seizure threshold, such as systemic steroids, should be undertaken only with extreme caution). Products include:
Nasonex Nasal Spray 2883

Nefazodone Hydrochloride (Bupropion is associated with dose-dependent risk of seizures; co-administration with drugs that lower seizure threshold, such as antidepressants, may increase the risk of seizure with bupropion).
No products indexed under this heading.

Nicotine (Co-administration of bupropion and nicotine transdermal system has resulted in a higher incidence of treatment-emergent hypertension).
No products indexed under this heading.

Nortriptyline Hydrochloride (Co-administration of bupropion with drugs that are metabolized by CYP2D6 isoenzyme, such as nortriptyline, may result in, based on data with desipramine, increased Cmax, AUC and t1/2; co-administration should be initiated at the lower end of the dose range of nortriptyline; potential for increased risk of seizures).
No products indexed under this heading.

Olanzapine (Bupropion is associated with dose-dependent risk of seizures; co-administration with drugs that lower seizure threshold, such as

antipsychotics, may increase the risk of seizure with bupropion). Products include:
Symbyax Capsules 1871
Zyprexa Tablets 1883
Zyprexa IntraMuscular 1883
Zyprexa ZYDIS Orally Disintegrating Tablets 1883

Orphenadrine Citrate (Bupropion is primarily metabolized, based on in vitro studies, to hydroxybupropion by the CYP2B6 isoenzyme; therefore the potential exists for a drug interaction with agents that affect the CYP2B6 isoenzyme metabolism, such as orphenadrine).
No products indexed under this heading.

Oxazepam (Bupropion is associated with a dose-related risk of seizures; excessive use of benzodiazepine sedatives is associated with increased risk of seizures; bupropion is contraindicated in patients undergoing abrupt discontinuation of benzodiazepine sedatives).
No products indexed under this heading.

Paliperidone (Bupropion is associated with dose-dependent risk of seizures; co-administration with drugs that lower seizure threshold, such as antipsychotics, may increase the risk of seizure with bupropion). Products include:
Invega Extended-Release Tablets 1748

Pargyline Hydrochloride (Concurrent and/or sequential use with MAO inhibitors is contraindicated).
No products indexed under this heading.

Paroxetine Hydrochloride (Co-administration of bupropion with drugs that are metabolized by CYP2D6 isoenzyme, such as paroxetine, may result in, based on data with desipramine, increased Cmax, AUC and t1/2; co-administration should be initiated at the lower end of the dose range of paroxetine). Products include:
Paxil 1535
Paxil CR Controlled-Release Tablets 1544

Perphenazine (Bupropion is associated with dose-dependent risk of seizures; co-administration with drugs that lower seizure threshold, such as antipsychotics, may increase the risk of seizure with bupropion).
No products indexed under this heading.

Phenelzine Sulfate (Concurrent and/or sequential use with MAO inhibitors is contraindicated; acute toxicity of bupropion is enhanced by phenelzine in animal models).
No products indexed under this heading.

Phenobarbital (May induce the metabolism of bupropion). Products include:
Donnatal Extentabs 2507

Phenytoin (May induce the metabolism of bupropion).
No products indexed under this heading.

Phenytoin Sodium (May induce the metabolism of bupropion). Products include:
Phenytek Capsules 2192

Pimozide (Bupropion is associated with dose-dependent risk of seizures; co-administration with drugs that lower seizure threshold, such as antipsychotics, may increase the risk of seizure with bupropion).
No products indexed under this heading.

Prazepam (Bupropion is associated with a dose-related risk of seizures; excessive use of benzodiazepine sedatives is associated with increased risk of seizures; bupropion is contraindicated in patients undergoing abrupt discontinuation of benzodiazepine sedatives).
No products indexed under this heading.

Prednisolone Acetate (Concurrent administration of bupropion hydrochloride and agents that lower seizure threshold, such as systemic steroids, should be undertaken only with extreme caution). Products include:
Pred Forte Ophthalmic Suspension .... ⊙ 227
Pred Mild Ophthalmic Suspension .... ⊙ 230
Pred-G Ophthalmic Ointment .... ⊙ 229
Pred-G Ophthalmic Suspension .... ⊙ 228

Prednisolone Sodium Phosphate (Concurrent administration of bupropion hydrochloride and agents that lower seizure threshold, such as systemic steroids, should be undertaken only with extreme caution).
No products indexed under this heading.

Prednisolone Tebutate (Concurrent administration of bupropion hydrochloride and agents that lower seizure threshold, such as systemic steroids, should be undertaken only with extreme caution).
No products indexed under this heading.

Prednisone (Concurrent administration of bupropion hydrochloride and agents that lower seizure threshold, such as systemic steroids, should be undertaken only with extreme caution).
No products indexed under this heading.

Procarbazine Hydrochloride (Concurrent and/or sequential use with MAO inhibitors is contraindicated).
No products indexed under this heading.

Prochlorperazine (Bupropion is associated with dose-dependent risk of seizures; co-administration with drugs that lower seizure threshold, such as antipsychotics, may increase the risk of seizure with bupropion).
No products indexed under this heading.

Promethazine Hydrochloride (Bupropion is associated with dose-dependent risk of seizures; co-administration with drugs that lower seizure threshold, such as antipsychotics, may increase the risk of seizure with bupropion).
No products indexed under this heading.

Propafenone Hydrochloride (Co-administration of bupropion with drugs that are metabolized by CYP2D6 isoenzyme, such as propafenone, may result in, based on data with desipramine, increased Cmax, AUC and t1/2; co-administration should be initiated at the lower end of the dose range of propafenone). Products include:
Rythmol Tablets 1586
Rythmol SR Capsules 1590

Propofol (Bupropion hydrochloride is contraindicated in patients undergoing abrupt discontinuation of sedatives).
No products indexed under this heading.

Protriptyline Hydrochloride (Bupropion is associated with dose-dependent risk of seizures; co-administration with drugs that lower seizure threshold may increase the risk of seizure with bupropion).
No products indexed under this heading.

Quazepam (Bupropion is associated with a dose-related risk of seizures; excessive use of benzodiazepine sedatives is associated with increased risk of seizures; bupropion is contraindicated in patients undergoing abrupt discontinuation of benzodiazepine sedatives).
No products indexed under this heading.

Quetiapine Fumarate (Bupropion is associated with dose-dependent risk of seizures; co-administration with drugs that lower seizure threshold, such as antipsychotics, may increase the risk of seizure with bupropion).
No products indexed under this heading.

Ramelteon (Bupropion hydrochloride is contraindicated in patients undergoing abrupt discontinuation of sedatives). Products include:
Rozerem Tablets 3091

Rasagiline Mesylate (Concurrent and/or sequential use with MAO inhibitors is contraindicated). Products include:
Azilect Tablets 3106

Risperidone (Co-administration of bupropion with drugs that are metabolized by CYP2D6 isoenzyme, such as risperidone, may result in, based on data with desipramine, increased Cmax, AUC and t1/2; co-administration should be initiated at the lower end of the dose range of risperidone; potential for increased risk of seizures). Products include:
Risperdal Consta Long-Acting Injection 1753

Secobarbital Sodium (Bupropion hydrochloride is contraindicated in patients undergoing abrupt discontinuation of sedatives).
No products indexed under this heading.

Selegiline (Concurrent and/or sequential use with MAO inhibitors is contraindicated). Products include:
Emsam Transdermal System 905

Selegiline Hydrochloride (Concurrent and/or sequential use with MAO inhibitors is contraindicated). Products include:
Eldepryl Capsules 3052

Sertraline Hydrochloride (Co-administration of bupropion with drugs that are metabolized by CYP2D6 isoenzyme, such as sertraline, may result in, based on data with desipramine, increased Cmax, AUC and t1/2; co-administration should be initiated at the lower end of the dose range of sertraline).
No products indexed under this heading.

Sodium Butabarbital (Bupropion hydrochloride is contraindicated in patients undergoing abrupt discontinuation of sedatives).
No products indexed under this heading.

Temazepam (Bupropion is associated with a dose-related risk of seizures; excessive use of benzodiazepine sedatives is associated with increased risk of seizures; bupropion is contraindicated in patients undergoing abrupt discontinuation of benzodiazepine sedatives).
No products indexed under this heading.

Theophylline (Bupropion is associated with a dose-related risk of seizures; co-administration with drugs that lower seizure threshold may increase the risk of seizures with bupropion; concurrent use should be undertaken with extreme caution).
No products indexed under this heading.

Theophylline Anhydrous (Bupropion is associated with a dose-related risk of seizures; co-administration with drugs that lower seizure threshold may increase the risk of seizures with bupropion; concurrent use should be undertaken with extreme caution). Products include:
Uniphyl Tablets 2595

Theophylline Calcium Salicylate (Bupropion is associated with a dose-related risk of seizures; co-administration with drugs that lower seizure threshold may increase the risk of seizures with bupropion; concurrent use should be undertaken with extreme caution).
No products indexed under this heading.

Theophylline Dihydroxypropyl (Glyceryl) (Bupropion is associated with a dose-related risk of seizures; co-administration with drugs that lower seizure threshold may increase the risk of seizures with bupropion; concurrent use should be undertaken with extreme caution).
No products indexed under this heading.

Theophylline Ethylenediamine (Bupropion is associated with a dose-related risk of seizures; co-administration with drugs that lower seizure threshold may increase the risk of seizures with bupropion; concurrent use should be undertaken with extreme caution).
No products indexed under this heading.

Theophylline Sodium Glycinate (Bupropion is associated with a dose-related risk of seizures; co-administration with drugs that lower seizure threshold may increase the risk of seizures with bupropion; concurrent use should be undertaken with extreme caution).
No products indexed under this heading.

Thioridazine Hydrochloride (Co-administration of bupropion with drugs that are metabolized by CYP2D6 isoenzyme, such as thioridazine, may result in, based on data with desipramine, increased Cmax, AUC and t1/2; co-administration should be initiated at the lower end of the dose range of thioridazine; potential for increased risk of seizures). Products include:

Thioridazine Hydrochloride Tablets 2195

Thiotepa (Bupropion is primarily metabolized, based on in vitro studies, to hydroxybupropion by the CYP2B6 isoenzyme; therefore the potential exists for a drug interaction with agents that affect the CYP2B6 isoenzyme metabolism, such as thiotepa).
No products indexed under this heading.

Thiothixene (Bupropion is associated with dose-dependent risk of seizures; co-administration with drugs that lower seizure threshold, such as antipsychotics, may increase the risk of seizure with bupropion). Products include:
Thiothixene Capsules 2197

Tranylcypromine Sulfate (Concurrent and/or sequential use with MAO inhibitors is contraindicated). Products include:
Parnate Tablets 1532

Trazodone Hydrochloride (Bupropion is associated with dose-dependent risk of seizures; co-administration with drugs that lower seizure threshold may increase the risk of seizure with bupropion).
No products indexed under this heading.

Triamcinolone (Concurrent administration of bupropion hydrochloride and agents that lower seizure threshold, such as systemic steroids, should be undertaken only with extreme caution).
No products indexed under this heading.

Triamcinolone Acetonide (Concurrent administration of bupropion hydrochloride and agents that lower seizure threshold, such as systemic steroids, should be undertaken only with extreme caution). Products include:
Azmacort Inhalation Aerosol 407
Nasacort AQ Nasal Spray 2765
Triesence Injectable Suspension .... ⊙209

Triamcinolone Diacetate (Concurrent administration of bupropion hydrochloride and agents that lower seizure threshold, such as systemic steroids, should be undertaken only with extreme caution).
No products indexed under this heading.

Triamcinolone Hexacetonide (Concurrent administration of bupropion hydrochloride and agents that lower seizure threshold, such as systemic steroids, should be undertaken only with extreme caution).
No products indexed under this heading.

Triazolam (Bupropion is associated with a dose-related risk of seizures; excessive use of benzodiazepine sedatives is associated with increased risk of seizures; bupropion is contraindicated in patients undergoing abrupt discontinuation of benzodiazepine sedatives).
No products indexed under this heading.

Trifluoperazine Hydrochloride (Bupropion is associated with dose-dependent risk of seizures; co-administration with drugs that lower seizure threshold, such as antipsychotics, may increase the risk of seizure with bupropion).
No products indexed under this heading.

Trimipramine Maleate (Bupropion is associated with dose-dependent risk of seizures; co-administration with drugs that lower seizure threshold may increase the risk of seizure with bupropion).
No products indexed under this heading.

Venlafaxine Hydrochloride (Bupropion is associated with dose-dependent risk of seizures; co-administration with drugs that lower seizure threshold, such as antidepressants, may increase the risk of seizure with bupropion). Products include:
Effexor XR Extended-Release Capsules 3195
Venlafaxine Hydrochloride Tablets ... 2199

Warfarin Sodium (Altered PT and/or INR infrequently associated with hemorrhagic or thrombotic complications were observed when bupropion was co-administered with warfarin).
No products indexed under this heading.

Zaleplon (Bupropion hydrochloride is contraindicated in patients undergoing abrupt discontinuation of sedatives).
No products indexed under this heading.

Ziprasidone Hydrochloride (Bupropion is associated with dose-dependent risk of seizures; co-administration with drugs that lower seizure threshold, such as antipsychotics, may increase the risk of seizure with bupropion). Products include:
Geodon Capsules 2520

Zolpidem Tartrate (Bupropion hydrochloride is contraindicated in patients undergoing abrupt discontinuation of sedatives). Products include:
Ambien Tablets 2692
Ambien CR Tablets 2696

Food Interactions

Alcohol (Bupropion hydrochloride is contraindicated in patients undergoing abrupt discontinuation of alcohol. The consumption of alcohol during treatment with bupropion hydrochloride should be minimized or avoided).

Food, unspecified (Food increases Cmax and AUC of bupropion by 11% and 17% respectively. The mean time to peak concentration Tmax was prolonged by 1 hour; this effect was of no clinical significance).

ZYDONE TABLETS

(Acetaminophen, Hydrocodone Bitartrate)........ 1132

May interact with anticholinergics, central nervous system depressants, monoamine oxidase inhibitors, narcotic analgesics, tricyclic antidepressants, and certain other agents. Compounds in these categories include:

Alfentanil Hydrochloride (Co-administration may exhibit additive CNS depression).
No products indexed under this heading.

Alprazolam (Co-administration may exhibit additive CNS depression).
No products indexed under this heading.

Amitriptyline Hydrochloride (Co-administration of tricyclic antidepressants with hydrocodone may increase the effect of either hydrocodone or antidepressant).
No products indexed under this heading.

Amoxapine (Co-administration of tricyclic antidepressants with hydrocodone may increase the effect of either hydrocodone or antidepressant).
No products indexed under this heading.

Aprobarbital (Co-administration may exhibit additive CNS depression).
No products indexed under this heading.

Atropine Sulfate (Co-administration may produce paralytic ileus). Products include:
Donnatal Extentabs 2507

Belladonna Alkaloids (Co-administration may produce paralytic ileus). Products include:
Hyland's Teething Tablets 621

Benztropine Mesylate (Co-administration may produce paralytic ileus).
No products indexed under this heading.

Biperiden Hydrochloride (Co-administration may produce paralytic ileus).
No products indexed under this heading.

Buprenorphine Hydrochloride (Co-administration may exhibit additive CNS depression). Products include:
Suboxone Tablets 2601
Subutex Tablets 2601

Buspirone Hydrochloride (Co-administration may exhibit additive CNS depression).
No products indexed under this heading.

Butabarbital (Co-administration may exhibit additive CNS depression).
No products indexed under this heading.

Butalbital (Co-administration may exhibit additive CNS depression).
No products indexed under this heading.

Chlordiazepoxide (Co-administration may exhibit additive CNS depression).
No products indexed under this heading.

Chlordiazepoxide Hydrochloride (Co-administration may exhibit additive CNS depression).
No products indexed under this heading.

Chlorpromazine (Co-administration may exhibit additive CNS depression).
No products indexed under this heading.

Chlorpromazine Hydrochloride (Co-administration may exhibit additive CNS depression).
No products indexed under this heading.

Chlorprothixene (Co-administration may exhibit additive CNS depression).
No products indexed under this heading.

Chlorprothixene Hydrochloride (Co-administration may exhibit additive CNS depression).
No products indexed under this heading.

Chlorprothixene Lactate (Co-administration may exhibit additive CNS depression).
No products indexed under this heading.

Clidinium Bromide (Co-administration may produce paralytic ileus).
No products indexed under this heading.

Clomipramine Hydrochloride (Co-administration of tricyclic antidepressants with hydrocodone may increase the effect of either hydrocodone or antidepressant).
No products indexed under this heading.

Clorazepate Dipotassium (Co-administration may exhibit additive CNS depression).
No products indexed under this heading.

Clozapine (Co-administration may exhibit additive CNS depression).
No products indexed under this heading.

Codeine Phosphate (Co-administration may exhibit additive CNS depression). Products include:
Tylenol with Codeine Tablets 2427

Desflurane (Co-administration may exhibit additive CNS depression).
No products indexed under this heading.

Desipramine Hydrochloride (Co-administration of tricyclic antidepressants with hydrocodone may increase the effect of either hydrocodone or antidepressant).
No products indexed under this heading.

Dezocine (Co-administration may exhibit additive CNS depression).
No products indexed under this heading.

Diazepam (Co-administration may exhibit additive CNS depression). Products include:
Valium Tablets 2658

Dicyclomine Hydrochloride (Co-administration may produce paralytic ileus). Products include:
Bentyl Capsules 703
Bentyl Injection 703
Bentyl Syrup 703
Bentyl Tablets 703

Doxepin Hydrochloride (Co-administration of tricyclic antidepressants with hydrocodone may increase the effect of either hydrocodone or antidepressant).
No products indexed under this heading.

Droperidol (Co-administration may exhibit additive CNS depression).
No products indexed under this heading.

Enflurane (Co-administration may exhibit additive CNS depression).
No products indexed under this heading.

Estazolam (Co-administration may exhibit additive CNS depression).
No products indexed under this heading.

Ethanol (Co-administration may exhibit additive CNS depression).
No products indexed under this heading.

Ethchlorvynol (Co-administration may exhibit additive CNS depression).
No products indexed under this heading.

Ethinamate (Co-administration may exhibit additive CNS depression).
No products indexed under this heading.

Ethyl Alcohol (Co-administration may exhibit additive CNS depression).
No products indexed under this heading.

Fentanyl (Co-administration may exhibit additive CNS depression). Products include:
Duragesic Transdermal System 2405
Ionsys Transdermal System 2410

Fentanyl Citrate (Co-administration may exhibit additive CNS depression). Products include:
Actiq 959
Fentora Tablets 968

Fluphenazine Decanoate (Co-administration may exhibit additive CNS depression).
No products indexed under this heading.

Fluphenazine Enanthate (Co-administration may exhibit additive CNS depression).
No products indexed under this heading.

Fluphenazine Hydrochloride (Co-administration may exhibit additive CNS depression).
No products indexed under this heading.

Flurazepam Hydrochloride (Co-administration may exhibit additive CNS depression).
No products indexed under this heading.

Glutethimide (Co-administration may exhibit additive CNS depression).
No products indexed under this heading.

Glycopyrrolate (Co-administration may produce paralytic ileus).
No products indexed under this heading.

Haloperidol (Co-administration may exhibit additive CNS depression).
No products indexed under this heading.

Haloperidol Decanoate (Co-administration may exhibit additive CNS depression).
No products indexed under this heading.

Hydrocodone Polistirex (Co-administration may exhibit additive CNS depression). Products include:
Tussionex Pennkinetic Extended-Release Suspension 3154

Hydromorphone Hydrochloride (Co-administration may exhibit additive CNS depression).
No products indexed under this heading.

Hydroxyzine Hydrochloride (Co-administration may exhibit additive CNS depression).
No products indexed under this heading.

Hyoscyamine (Co-administration may produce paralytic ileus).
No products indexed under this heading.

Hyoscyamine Sulfate (Co-administration may produce paralytic ileus). Products include:
Donnatal Extentabs 2507

Imipramine Hydrochloride (Co-administration of tricyclic antidepressants with hydrocodone may increase the effect of either hydrocodone or antidepressant).
No products indexed under this heading.

Imipramine Pamoate (Co-administration of tricyclic antidepressants with hydrocodone may increase the effect of either hydrocodone or antidepressant).
No products indexed under this heading.

Ipratropium Bromide (Co-administration may produce paralytic ileus). Products include:
Atrovent HFA Inhalation Aerosol 839
Atrovent Nasal Spray 0.03% 834
Atrovent Nasal Spray 0.06% 836
Combivent Inhalation Aerosol 845

Isocarboxazid (Co-administration of MAO inhibitors with hydrocodone may increase the effect of either hydrocodone or MAO inhibitor). Products include:
Marplan Tablets 3177

Isoflurane (Co-administration may exhibit additive CNS depression).
No products indexed under this heading.

Ketamine Hydrochloride (Co-administration may exhibit additive CNS depression).
No products indexed under this heading.

Levomethadyl Acetate Hydrochloride (Co-administration may exhibit additive CNS depression).
No products indexed under this heading.

Levorphanol Tartrate (Co-administration may exhibit additive CNS depression).
No products indexed under this heading.

Lorazepam (Co-administration may exhibit additive CNS depression).
No products indexed under this heading.

Loxapine Hydrochloride (Co-administration may exhibit additive CNS depression).
No products indexed under this heading.

Loxapine Succinate (Co-administration may exhibit additive CNS depression).
No products indexed under this heading.

Maprotiline Hydrochloride (Co-administration of tricyclic antidepressants with hydrocodone may increase the effect of either hydrocodone or antidepressant).
No products indexed under this heading.

Mepenzolate Bromide (Co-administration may produce paralytic ileus).
No products indexed under this heading.

Meperidine Hydrochloride (Co-administration may exhibit additive CNS depression).
No products indexed under this heading.

Mephobarbital (Co-administration may exhibit additive CNS depression).
No products indexed under this heading.

Meprobamate (Co-administration may exhibit additive CNS depression).
No products indexed under this heading.

Mesoridazine Besylate (Co-administration may exhibit additive CNS depression).
No products indexed under this heading.

Methadone Hydrochloride (Co-administration may exhibit additive CNS depression).
No products indexed under this heading.

Methohexital Sodium (Co-administration may exhibit additive CNS depression).
No products indexed under this heading.

Methotrimeprazine (Co-administration may exhibit additive CNS depression).
No products indexed under this heading.

Methoxyflurane (Co-administration may exhibit additive CNS depression).
No products indexed under this heading.

Midazolam Hydrochloride (Co-administration may exhibit additive CNS depression).
No products indexed under this heading.

Moclobemide (Co-administration of MAO inhibitors with hydrocodone may increase the effect of either hydrocodone or MAO inhibitor).
No products indexed under this heading.

Molindone Hydrochloride (Co-administration may exhibit additive CNS depression). Products include:
Moban Tablets 1116

Morphine Sulfate (Co-administration may exhibit additive CNS depression). Products include:
Avinza Capsules 1772
DepoDur Injection 1095
MS Contin Tablets 2585

Nortriptyline Hydrochloride (Co-administration of tricyclic antidepressants with hydrocodone may increase the effect of either hydrocodone or antidepressant).
No products indexed under this heading.

Olanzapine (Co-administration may exhibit additive CNS depression). Products include:
Symbyax Capsules 1871
Zyprexa Tablets 1883
Zyprexa IntraMuscular 1883
Zyprexa ZYDIS Orally Disintegrating Tablets 1883

Oxazepam (Co-administration may exhibit additive CNS depression).
No products indexed under this heading.

Oxybutynin Chloride (Co-administration may produce paralytic ileus).
No products indexed under this heading.

Oxycodone Hydrochloride (Co-administration may exhibit additive CNS depression). Products include:
OxyContin Tablets 2589
OxyIR Capsules 2593
Percocet Tablets 1127
Percodan Tablets 1130

Pargyline Hydrochloride (Co-administration of MAO inhibitors with hydrocodone may increase the effect of either hydrocodone or MAO inhibitor).
No products indexed under this heading.

Pentobarbital Sodium (Co-administration may exhibit additive CNS depression). Products include:
Nembutal Sodium Solution, USP 2494

Perphenazine (Co-administration may exhibit additive CNS depression).
No products indexed under this heading.

Phenelzine Sulfate (Co-administration of MAO inhibitors with hydrocodone may increase the effect of either hydrocodone or MAO inhibitor).
No products indexed under this heading.

Phenobarbital (Co-administration may exhibit additive CNS depression). Products include:
Donnatal Extentabs 2507

Prazepam (Co-administration may exhibit additive CNS depression).
No products indexed under this heading.

Procarbazine Hydrochloride (Co-administration of MAO inhibitors with hydrocodone may increase the effect of either hydrocodone or MAO inhibitor).
No products indexed under this heading.

Prochlorperazine (Co-administration may exhibit additive CNS depression).
No products indexed under this heading.

Procyclidine Hydrochloride (Co-administration may produce paralytic ileus).
No products indexed under this heading.

Promethazine Hydrochloride (Co-administration may exhibit additive CNS depression).
No products indexed under this heading.

Propantheline Bromide (Co-administration may produce paralytic ileus).
No products indexed under this heading.

Propofol (Co-administration may exhibit additive CNS depression).
No products indexed under this heading.

Propoxyphene Hydrochloride (Co-administration may exhibit additive CNS depression).
No products indexed under this heading.

Propoxyphene Napsylate (Co-administration may exhibit additive CNS depression).
No products indexed under this heading.

Protriptyline Hydrochloride (Co-administration of tricyclic antidepressants with hydrocodone may increase the effect of either hydrocodone or antidepressant).
No products indexed under this heading.

Quazepam (Co-administration may exhibit additive CNS depression).
No products indexed under this heading.

Quetiapine Fumarate (Co-administration may exhibit additive CNS depression).
No products indexed under this heading.

Rasagiline Mesylate (Co-administration of MAO inhibitors with hydrocodone may increase the effect of either hydrocodone or MAO inhibitor). Products include:

Azilect Tablets 3106

Remifentanil Hydrochloride (Co-administration may exhibit additive CNS depression).
No products indexed under this heading.

Risperidone (Co-administration may exhibit additive CNS depression). Products include:
Risperdal Consta Long-Acting Injection 1753

Scopolamine (Co-administration may produce paralytic ileus). Products include:
Transderm Scōp Transdermal Therapeutic System 2206

Scopolamine Hydrobromide (Co-administration may produce paralytic ileus). Products include:
Donnatal Extentabs 2507

Secobarbital Sodium (Co-administration may exhibit additive CNS depression).
No products indexed under this heading.

Selegiline (Co-administration of MAO inhibitors with hydrocodone may increase the effect of either hydrocodone or MAO inhibitor). Products include:
Emsam Transdermal System 905

Selegiline Hydrochloride (Co-administration of MAO inhibitors with hydrocodone may increase the effect of either hydrocodone or MAO inhibitor). Products include:
Eldepryl Capsules 3052

Sevoflurane (Co-administration may exhibit additive CNS depression). Products include:
Ultane Liquid for Inhalation 524

Sodium Oxybate (Co-administration may exhibit additive CNS depression). Products include:
Xyrem Oral Solution 1766

Sufentanil Citrate (Co-administration may exhibit additive CNS depression).
No products indexed under this heading.

Temazepam (Co-administration may exhibit additive CNS depression).
No products indexed under this heading.

Thiamylal Sodium (Co-administration may exhibit additive CNS depression).
No products indexed under this heading.

Thioridazine Hydrochloride (Co-administration may exhibit additive CNS depression). Products include:
Thioridazine Hydrochloride Tablets 2195

Thiothixene (Co-administration may exhibit additive CNS depression). Products include:
Thiothixene Capsules 2197

Tolterodine Tartrate (Co-administration may produce paralytic ileus).
No products indexed under this heading.

Tranylcypromine Sulfate (Co administration of MAO inhibitors with hydrocodone may increase the effect of either hydrocodone or MAO inhibitor). Products include:
Parnate Tablets 1532

Triazolam (Co-administration may exhibit additive CNS depression).
No products indexed under this heading.

Tridihexethyl Chloride (Co-administration may produce paralytic ileus).
No products indexed under this heading.

Trifluoperazine Hydrochloride (Co-administration may exhibit additive CNS depression).
No products indexed under this heading.

Trihexyphenidyl Hydrochloride (Co-administration may produce paralytic ileus).
No products indexed under this heading.

Trimipramine Maleate (Co-administration of tricyclic antidepressants with hydrocodone may increase the effect of either hydrocodone or antidepressant).
No products indexed under this heading.

Zaleplon (Co-administration may exhibit additive CNS depression).
No products indexed under this heading.

Ziprasidone Hydrochloride (Co-administration may exhibit additive CNS depression). Products include:
Geodon Capsules 2520

Zolpidem Tartrate (Co-administration may exhibit additive CNS depression). Products include:
Ambien Tablets 2692
Ambien CR Tablets 2696

Food Interactions

Alcohol (Co-administration may exhibit additive CNS depression).

ZYLET OPHTHALMIC SUSPENSION

(Loteprednol Etabonate, Tobramycin) .... ⊙247
None cited in PDR database.

ZYPREXA TABLETS

(Olanzapine) 1883
May interact with antihypertensives, central nervous system depressants, cytochrome p450 1a2 inducers (selected), cytochrome p450 1a2 inhibitors (selected), dopamine agonists, drugs that elevate levels of glucuronosyl transferase, and certain other agents. Compounds in these categories include:

Acebutolol Hydrochloride (Olanzapine, because of its potential for inducing hypotension, may enhance the effects of certain antihypertensive agents).
No products indexed under this heading.

Alatrofloxacin Mesylate (Can potentially inhibit olanzapine clearance; therefore, a dosage decrease might be considered).
No products indexed under this heading.

Alfentanil Hydrochloride (Given the primary CNS effects of olanzapine, caution should be used when olanzapine is taken in combination with other centrally-acting drugs).
No products indexed under this heading.

Aliskiren (Olanzapine, because of its potential for inducing hypotension, may enhance the effects of certain antihypertensive agents). Products include:
Tekturna Tablets 2321
Tekturna HCT Tablets 2324

Alprazolam (Given the primary CNS effects of olanzapine, caution should be used when olanzapine is taken in combination with other centrally-acting drugs).
No products indexed under this heading.

Amiodarone Hydrochloride (Can potentially inhibit olanzapine clearance; therefore, a dosage decrease might be considered).
No products indexed under this heading.

Amlodipine Besylate (Olanzapine, because of its potential for inducing hypotension, may enhance the effects of certain antihypertensive agents). Products include:
Azor Tablets 1005
Exforge Tablets 2238

Anastrozole (Can potentially inhibit olanzapine clearance; therefore, a dosage decrease might be considered). Products include:
Arimidex Tablets 672

Aprobarbital (Given the primary CNS effects of olanzapine, caution should be used when olanzapine is taken in combination with other centrally-acting drugs).
No products indexed under this heading.

Atenolol (Olanzapine, because of its potential for inducing hypotension, may enhance the effects of certain antihypertensive agents).
No products indexed under this heading.

Benazepril Hydrochloride (Olanzapine, because of its potential for inducing hypotension, may enhance the effects of certain antihypertensive agents).
No products indexed under this heading.

Bendroflumethiazide (Olanzapine, because of its potential for inducing hypotension, may enhance the effects of certain antihypertensive agents).
No products indexed under this heading.

Betaxolol Hydrochloride (Olanzapine, because of its potential for inducing hypotension, may enhance the effects of certain antihypertensive agents).
No products indexed under this heading.

Bisoprolol Fumarate (Olanzapine, because of its potential for inducing hypotension, may enhance the effects of certain antihypertensive agents).
No products indexed under this heading.

Bromocriptine Mesylate (Olanzapine may antagonize the effects of dopamine agonists).
No products indexed under this heading.

Buprenorphine Hydrochloride (Given the primary CNS effects of olanzapine, caution should be used when olanzapine is taken in combination with other centrally-acting drugs). Products include:
Suboxone Tablets 2601
Subutex Tablets 2601

Buspirone Hydrochloride (Given the primary CNS effects of olanzapine, caution should be used when olanzapine is taken in combination with other centrally-acting drugs).
No products indexed under this heading.

Butabarbital (Given the primary CNS effects of olanzapine, caution should be used when olanzapine is taken in combination with other centrally-acting drugs).
No products indexed under this heading.

Butalbital (Given the primary CNS effects of olanzapine, caution should be used when olanzapine is taken in combination with other centrally-acting drugs).
No products indexed under this heading.

Candesartan Cilexetil (Olanzapine, because of its potential for inducing hypotension, may enhance the effects of certain antihypertensive agents). Products include:
Atacand Tablets 639
Atacand HCT 642

Captopril (Olanzapine, because of its potential for inducing hypotension, may enhance the effects of certain antihypertensive agents). Products include:
Captopril Tablets 2182

Carbamazepine (Causes an approximately 50% increase in the clearance of olanzapine at 400 mg daily; higher daily doses of carbamazepine may cause an even greater increase in olanzapine clearance). Products include:
Carbatrol Capsules 3019
Equetro Extended-Release Capsules 3174

Carteolol Hydrochloride (Olanzapine, because of its potential for inducing hypotension, may enhance the effects of certain antihypertensive agents).
No products indexed under this heading.

Charcoal, Activated (Co-administration with activated charcoal reduces the Cmax and AUC of olanzapine by about 60%).
No products indexed under this heading.

Chlordiazepoxide (Given the primary CNS effects of olanzapine, caution should be used when olanzapine is taken in combination with other centrally-acting drugs).
No products indexed under this heading.

Chlordiazepoxide Hydrochloride (Given the primary CNS effects of olanzapine, caution should be used when olanzapine is taken in combination with other centrally-acting drugs).
No products indexed under this heading.

Chlorothiazide (Olanzapine, because of its potential for inducing hypotension, may enhance the effects of certain antihypertensive agents).
No products indexed under this heading.

Chlorothiazide Sodium (Olanzapine, because of its potential for inducing hypotension, may enhance the effects of certain antihypertensive agents). Products include:
Intravenous Sodium Diuril 2490

Chlorpromazine (Given the primary CNS effects of olanzapine, caution should be used when olanzapine is taken in combination with other centrally-acting drugs).
No products indexed under this heading.

Chlorpromazine Hydrochloride (Given the primary CNS effects of olanzapine, caution should be used when olanzapine is taken in combination with other centrally-acting drugs).
No products indexed under this heading.

Chlorprothixene (Given the primary CNS effects of olanzapine, caution should be used when olanzapine is taken in combination with other centrally-acting drugs).
No products indexed under this heading.

Chlorprothixene Hydrochloride (Given the primary CNS effects of olanzapine, caution should be used when olanzapine is taken in combination with other centrally-acting drugs).
No products indexed under this heading.

Chlorprothixene Lactate (Given the primary CNS effects of olanzapine, caution should be used when olanzapine is taken in combination with other centrally-acting drugs).
No products indexed under this heading.

Chlorthalidone (Olanzapine, because of its potential for inducing hypotension, may enhance the effects of certain antihypertensive agents). Products include:
Clorpres Tablets **2185**

Cimetidine (Can potentially inhibit olanzapine clearance; therefore, a dosage decrease might be considered).
No products indexed under this heading.

Cimetidine Hydrochloride (Can potentially inhibit olanzapine clearance; therefore, a dosage decrease might be considered).
No products indexed under this heading.

Ciprofloxacin (Can potentially inhibit olanzapine clearance; therefore, a dosage decrease might be considered). Products include:
Cipro I.V. **2817**
Cipro Oral Suspension **2810**
Cipro XR Tablets **2823**
Ciprodex Otic Suspension **541**

Ciprofloxacin Hydrochloride (Can potentially inhibit olanzapine clearance; therefore, a dosage decrease might be considered). Products include:
Cipro Tablets **2810**

Citalopram Hydrobromide (May cause an increase in olanzapine clearance; therefore, a dosage increase might be considered). Products include:
Celexa **1160**

Clarithromycin (Can potentially inhibit olanzapine clearance; therefore, a dosage decrease might be considered). Products include:
Biaxin/Biaxin XL **411**

Clonidine (Olanzapine, because of its potential for inducing hypotension, may enhance the effects of certain antihypertensive agents). Products include:
Catapres-TTS **842**

Clonidine Hydrochloride (Olanzapine, because of its potential for inducing hypotension, may enhance the effects of certain antihypertensive agents). Products include:
Catapres Tablets **841**
Clorpres Tablets **2185**

Clorazepate Dipotassium (Given the primary CNS effects of olanzapine, caution should be used when olanzapine is taken in combination with other centrally-acting drugs).
No products indexed under this heading.

Clozapine (Given the primary CNS effects of olanzapine, caution should be used when olanzapine is taken in combination with other centrally-acting drugs).
No products indexed under this heading.

Codeine Phosphate (Given the primary CNS effects of olanzapine, caution should be used when olanzapine is taken in combination with other centrally-acting drugs). Products include:
Tylenol with Codeine Tablets **2427**

Deserpidine (Olanzapine, because of its potential for inducing hypotension, may enhance the effects of certain antihypertensive agents).
No products indexed under this heading.

Desflurane (Given the primary CNS effects of olanzapine, caution should be used when olanzapine is taken in combination with other centrally-acting drugs).
No products indexed under this heading.

Desogestrel (Can potentially inhibit olanzapine clearance; therefore, a dosage decrease might be considered). Products include:
Mircette Tablets **1034**

Dezocine (Given the primary CNS effects of olanzapine, caution should be used when olanzapine is taken in combination with other centrally-acting drugs).
No products indexed under this heading.

Diazepam (Co-administration of diazepam with olanzapine may potentiate orthostatic hypotension). Products include:
Valium Tablets **2658**

Diazoxide (Olanzapine, because of its potential for inducing hypotension, may enhance the effects of certain antihypertensive agents). Products include:
Proglycem Capsules **1185**
Proglycem Suspension **1185**

Diltiazem Hydrochloride (Olanzapine, because of its potential for inducing hypotension, may enhance the effects of certain antihypertensive agents). Products include:
Cardizem LA Extended Release Tablets **421**

Diltiazem Maleate (May cause an increase in olanzapine clearance; therefore, a dosage increase might be considered).
No products indexed under this heading.

Dopamine Hydrochloride (Olanzapine may antagonize the effects of dopamine agonists).
No products indexed under this heading.

Doxazosin Mesylate (Olanzapine, because of its potential for inducing hypotension, may enhance the effects of certain antihypertensive agents).
No products indexed under this heading.

Droperidol (Given the primary CNS effects of olanzapine, caution should be used when olanzapine is taken in combination with other centrally-acting drugs).
No products indexed under this heading.

Enalapril Maleate (Olanzapine, because of its potential for inducing hypotension, may enhance the effects of certain antihypertensive agents).
No products indexed under this heading.

Enalaprilat (Olanzapine, because of its potential for inducing hypotension, may enhance the effects of certain antihypertensive agents).
No products indexed under this heading.

Enflurane (Given the primary CNS effects of olanzapine, caution should be used when olanzapine is taken in combination with other centrally-acting drugs).
No products indexed under this heading.

Enoxacin (Can potentially inhibit olanzapine clearance; therefore, a dosage decrease might be considered).
No products indexed under this heading.

Eprosartan Mesylate (Olanzapine, because of its potential for inducing hypotension, may enhance the effects of certain antihypertensive agents). Products include:
Teveten Tablets **515**
Teveten HCT Tablets **517**

Erythromycin (May cause an increase in olanzapine clearance; therefore, a dosage increase might be considered).
No products indexed under this heading.

Erythromycin Estolate (May cause an increase in olanzapine clearance; therefore, a dosage increase might be considered).
No products indexed under this heading.

Erythromycin Ethylsuccinate (May cause an increase in olanzapine clearance; therefore, a dosage increase might be considered). Products include:
E.E.S. **433**
EryPed **431**

Erythromycin Gluceptate (May cause an increase in olanzapine clearance; therefore, a dosage increase might be considered).
No products indexed under this heading.

Erythromycin Lactobionate (May cause an increase in olanzapine clearance; therefore, a dosage increase might be considered).
No products indexed under this heading.

Erythromycin Stearate (May cause an increase in olanzapine clearance; therefore, a dosage increase might be considered).
No products indexed under this heading.

Esmolol Hydrochloride (Olanzapine, because of its potential for inducing hypotension, may enhance the effects of certain antihypertensive agents).
No products indexed under this heading.

Estazolam (Given the primary CNS effects of olanzapine, caution should be used when olanzapine is taken in combination with other centrally-acting drugs).
No products indexed under this heading.

Ethanol (Given the primary CNS effects of olanzapine, caution should be used when olanzapine is taken in combination with other centrally-acting drugs).
No products indexed under this heading.

Ethchlorvynol (Given the primary CNS effects of olanzapine, caution should be used when olanzapine is taken in combination with other centrally-acting drugs).
No products indexed under this heading.

Ethinamate (Given the primary CNS effects of olanzapine, caution should be used when olanzapine is taken in combination with other centrally-acting drugs).
No products indexed under this heading.

Ethinyl Estradiol (Can potentially inhibit olanzapine clearance; therefore, a dosage decrease might be considered). Products include:
Lybrel Tablets **3204**
Mircette Tablets **1034**
NuvaRing **2897**
Ortho-Cyclen/Ortho Tri-Cyclen **2449**
Ortho Evra Transdermal System **2437**
Ortho Tri-Cyclen Lo Tablets **2458**
Seasonique Tablets **1046**
Yaz Tablets **805**

Ethyl Alcohol (Given the primary CNS effects of olanzapine, caution should be used when olanzapine is taken in combination with other centrally-acting drugs).
No products indexed under this heading.

Felodipine (Olanzapine, because of its potential for inducing hypotension, may enhance the effects of certain antihypertensive agents).
No products indexed under this heading.

Fentanyl (Given the primary CNS effects of olanzapine, caution should be used when olanzapine is taken in combination with other centrally-acting drugs). Products include:
Duragesic Transdermal System **2405**
Ionsys Transdermal System **2410**

Fentanyl Citrate (Given the primary CNS effects of olanzapine, caution should be used when olanzapine is taken in combination with other centrally-acting drugs). Products include:
Actiq **959**
Fentora Tablets **968**

Fluoxetine Hydrochloride (Co-administration causes a small increase in the maximum concentration of olanzapine and a small decrease in olanzapine clearance; the magnitude of the impact of this factor is small in comparison to the overall variability between individuals and; therefore, dose modification is not routinely recommended). Products include:
Prozac Weekly Capsules **1852**
Prozac Pulvules and Liquid **1852**
Symbyax Capsules **1871**

Fluphenazine Decanoate (Given the primary CNS effects of olanzapine, caution should be used when olanzapine is taken in combination with other centrally-acting drugs).
No products indexed under this heading.

Fluphenazine Enanthate (Given the primary CNS effects of olanzapine, caution should be used when olanzapine is taken in combination with other centrally-acting drugs).
No products indexed under this heading.

Fluphenazine Hydrochloride (Given the primary CNS effects of olanzapine, caution should be used when olanzapine is taken in combination with other centrally-acting drugs).
No products indexed under this heading.

Flurazepam Hydrochloride (Given the primary CNS effects of olanzapine, caution should be used when olanzapine is taken in combination with other centrally-acting drugs).
No products indexed under this heading.

Fluvoxamine (Can potentially inhibit olanzapine clearance; therefore, a dosage decrease might be considered).
No products indexed under this heading.

Fluvoxamine Maleate (Decreases the clearance of olanzapine leading to a mean increase in olanzapine Cmax and AUC; lower doses of olanzapine should be considered or co-administered). Products include:
Luvox CR Extended-Release Capsules **1759**

Fosinopril Sodium (Olanzapine, because of its potential for inducing hypotension, may enhance the effects of certain antihypertensive agents).
No products indexed under this heading.

Furosemide (Olanzapine, because of its potential for inducing hypotension, may enhance the effects of certain antihypertensive agents). Products include:
Furosemide Tablets **2186**

Gatifloxacin (Can potentially inhibit olanzapine clearance; therefore, a dosage decrease might be considered).
No products indexed under this heading.

Gemifloxacin Mesylate (Can potentially inhibit olanzapine clearance; therefore, a dosage decrease might be considered).
No products indexed under this heading.

Glutethimide (Given the primary CNS effects of olanzapine, caution should be used when olanzapine is taken in combination with other centrally-acting drugs).
No products indexed under this heading.

Grepafloxacin Hydrochloride (Can potentially inhibit olanzapine clearance; therefore, a dosage decrease might be considered).
No products indexed under this heading.

Guanabenz Acetate (Olanzapine, because of its potential for inducing hypotension, may enhance the effects of certain antihypertensive agents).
No products indexed under this heading.

Guanethidine Monosulfate (Olanzapine, because of its potential for inducing hypotension, may enhance the effects of certain antihypertensive agents).
No products indexed under this heading.

Haloperidol (Given the primary CNS effects of olanzapine, caution should be used when olanzapine is taken in combination with other centrally-acting drugs).
No products indexed under this heading.

Haloperidol Decanoate (Given the primary CNS effects of olanzapine, caution should be used when olanzapine is taken in combination with other centrally-acting drugs).
No products indexed under this heading.

Hydralazine Hydrochloride (Olanzapine, because of its potential for inducing hypotension, may enhance the effects of certain antihypertensive agents).
No products indexed under this heading.

Hydrochlorothiazide (Olanzapine, because of its potential for inducing hypotension, may enhance the effects of certain antihypertensive agents). Products include:
Atacand HCT **642**
Avalide Tablets **892**
Avalide Tablets **2713**
Benicar HCT Tablets **1010**
Diovan HCT Tablets **2216**
Dyazide Capsules **1405**
Micardis HCT Tablets **854**
Prinzide Tablets **2092**
Tekturna HCT Tablets **2324**
Teveten HCT Tablets **517**

Hydrocodone Bitartrate (Given the primary CNS effects of olanzapine, caution should be used when olanzapine is taken in combination with other centrally-acting drugs). Products include:
Lortab 5/500 Tablets **3143**
Lortab 7.5/500 Tablets **3144**
Lortab 10/500 Tablets **3144**
Vicodin Tablets **529**
Vicodin ES Tablets **530**
Vicodin HP Tablets **531**
Vicoprofen Tablets **533**
Zydone Tablets **1132**

Hydrocodone Polistirex (Given the primary CNS effects of olanzapine, caution should be used when olanzapine is taken in combination with other centrally-acting drugs). Products include:
Tussionex Pennkinetic Extended-Release Suspension **3154**

Hydroflumethiazide (Olanzapine, because of its potential for inducing hypotension, may enhance the effects of certain antihypertensive agents).
No products indexed under this heading.

Hydromorphone Hydrochloride (Given the primary CNS effects of olanzapine, caution should be used when olanzapine is taken in combination with other centrally-acting drugs).
No products indexed under this heading.

Hydroxyzine Hydrochloride (Given the primary CNS effects of olanzapine, caution should be used when olanzapine is taken in combination with other centrally-acting drugs).
No products indexed under this heading.

Hypericum (May cause an increase in olanzapine clearance; therefore, a dosage increase might be considered). Products include:
Satieté Tablets **640**

Indapamide (Olanzapine, because of its potential for inducing hypotension, may enhance the effects of certain antihypertensive agents). Products include:
Indapamide Tablets **2188**

Insulin (May cause an increase in olanzapine clearance; therefore, a dosage increase might be considered).
No products indexed under this heading.

Irbesartan (Olanzapine, because of its potential for inducing hypotension, may enhance the effects of certain antihypertensive agents). Products include:
Avalide Tablets **892**
Avalide Tablets **2713**
Avapro Tablets **897**
Avapro Tablets **2718**

Isoflurane (Given the primary CNS effects of olanzapine, caution should be used when olanzapine is taken in combination with other centrally-acting drugs).
No products indexed under this heading.

Isoniazid (Can potentially inhibit olanzapine clearance; therefore, a dosage decrease might be considered).
No products indexed under this heading.

Isradipine (Olanzapine, because of its potential for inducing hypotension, may enhance the effects of certain antihypertensive agents). Products include:
DynaCirc CR Controlled Release Tablets **1407**

Ketamine Hydrochloride (Given the primary CNS effects of olanzapine, caution should be used when olanzapine is taken in combination with other centrally-acting drugs).
No products indexed under this heading.

Ketoconazole (Can potentially inhibit olanzapine clearance; therefore, a dosage decrease might be considered). Products include:
Extina Foam, 2% **3057**
Nizoral A-D Shampoo **1901**

Labetalol Hydrochloride (Olanzapine, because of its potential for inducing hypotension, may enhance the effects of certain antihypertensive agents).
No products indexed under this heading.

Lansoprazole (May cause an increase in olanzapine clearance; therefore, a dosage increase might be considered).
No products indexed under this heading.

Levodopa (Olanzapine may antagonize the effects of levodopa). Products include:
Stalevo Tablets **2309**

Levofloxacin (Can potentially inhibit olanzapine clearance; therefore, a dosage decrease might be considered). Products include:
Iquix Ophthalmic Solution **3183**
Levaquin **2416**
Levaquin in 5% Dextrose Injection **2416**
Quixin Ophthalmic Solution **3184**

Levomethadyl Acetate Hydrochloride (Given the primary CNS effects of olanzapine, caution should be used when olanzapine is taken in combination with other centrally-acting drugs).
No products indexed under this heading.

Levonorgestrel (Can potentially inhibit olanzapine clearance; therefore, a dosage decrease might be considered). Products include:
Climara Pro Transdermal System **768**
Lybrel Tablets **3204**
Mirena Intrauterine System **779**
Plan B Tablets **1044**
Seasonique Tablets **1046**

Levorphanol Tartrate (Given the primary CNS effects of olanzapine, caution should be used when olanzapine is taken in combination with other centrally-acting drugs).
No products indexed under this heading.

Lisinopril (Olanzapine, because of its potential for inducing hypotension, may enhance the effects of certain antihypertensive agents). Products include:
Prinivil Tablets **2087**
Prinzide Tablets **2092**

Lomefloxacin Hydrochloride (Can potentially inhibit olanzapine clearance; therefore, a dosage decrease might be considered).
No products indexed under this heading.

Lorazepam (Given the primary CNS effects of olanzapine, caution should be used when olanzapine is taken in combination with other centrally-acting drugs).
No products indexed under this heading.

Losartan Potassium (Olanzapine, because of its potential for inducing hypotension, may enhance the effects of certain antihypertensive agents). Products include:
Cozaar Tablets **1973**

Loxapine Hydrochloride (Given the primary CNS effects of olanzapine, caution should be used when olanzapine is taken in combination with other centrally-acting drugs).
No products indexed under this heading.

Loxapine Succinate (Given the primary CNS effects of olanzapine, caution should be used when olanzapine is taken in combination with other centrally-acting drugs).
No products indexed under this heading.

Mecamylamine Hydrochloride (Olanzapine, because of its potential for inducing hypotension, may enhance the effects of certain antihypertensive agents).
No products indexed under this heading.

Meperidine Hydrochloride (Given the primary CNS effects of olanzapine, caution should be used when olanzapine is taken in combination with other centrally-acting drugs).
No products indexed under this heading.

Mephobarbital (Given the primary CNS effects of olanzapine, caution should be used when olanzapine is taken in combination with other centrally-acting drugs).
No products indexed under this heading.

Trifluoperazine Hydrochloride (Given the primary CNS effects of olanzapine, caution should be used when olanzapine is taken in combination with other centrally-acting drugs).
No products indexed under this heading.

Trimethaphan Camsylate (Olanzapine, because of its potential for inducing hypotension, may enhance the effects of certain antihypertensive agents).
No products indexed under this heading.

Troleandomycin (Can potentially inhibit olanzapine clearance; therefore, a dosage decrease might be considered).
No products indexed under this heading.

Trovafloxacin Mesylate (Can potentially inhibit olanzapine clearance; therefore, a dosage decrease might be considered).
No products indexed under this heading.

Valsartan (Olanzapine, because of its potential for inducing hypotension, may enhance the effects of certain antihypertensive agents).
Products include:
Diovan Tablets ... 2212
Diovan HCT Tablets ... 2216
Exforge Tablets ... 2238

Vardenafil Hydrochloride (Can potentially inhibit olanzapine clearance; therefore, a dosage decrease might be considered). Products include:
Levitra Tablets ... 2876

Verapamil Hydrochloride (Olanzapine, because of its potential for inducing hypotension, may enhance the effects of certain antihypertensive agents). Products include:
Tarka Tablets ... 511

Zaleplon (Given the primary CNS effects of olanzapine, caution should be used when olanzapine is taken in combination with other centrally-acting drugs).
No products indexed under this heading.

Zileuton (Can potentially inhibit olanzapine clearance; therefore, a dosage decrease might be considered).
No products indexed under this heading.

Ziprasidone Hydrochloride (Given the primary CNS effects of olanzapine, caution should be used when olanzapine is taken in combination with other centrally-acting drugs).
Products include:
Geodon Capsules ... 2520

Zolpidem Tartrate (Given the primary CNS effects of olanzapine, caution should be used when olanzapine is taken in combination with other centrally-acting drugs).
Products include:
Ambien Tablets ... 2692
Ambien CR Tablets ... 2696

Food Interactions

Alcohol (Co-administration of alcohol with olanzapine potentiates orthostatic hypotension; concurrent use should be avoided).

Broccoli (May cause an increase in olanzapine clearance; therefore, a dosage increase might be considered).

Brussel Sprouts (May cause an increase in olanzapine clearance; therefore, a dosage increase might be considered).

Charbroiled Food (May cause an increase in olanzapine clearance; therefore, a dosage increase might be considered).

Grapefruit Juice (Can potentially inhibit olanzapine clearance; therefore, a dosage decrease might be considered).

ZYPREXA INTRAMUSCULAR

(Olanzapine) ... 1883
May interact with antihypertensives, benzodiazepines, central nervous system depressants, cytochrome p450 1a2 inducers (selected), cytochrome p450 1a2 inhibitors (selected), dopamine agonists, drugs that elevate levels of glucuronosyl transferase, and certain other agents. Compounds in these categories include:

Acebutolol Hydrochloride (Olanzapine, because of its potential for inducing hypotension, may enhance the effects of certain antihypertensive agents).
No products indexed under this heading.

Alatrofloxacin Mesylate (Can potentially inhibit olanzapine clearance; therefore, a dosage decrease might be considered).
No products indexed under this heading.

Alfentanil Hydrochloride (Given the primary CNS effects of olanzapine, caution should be used when olanzapine is taken in combination with other centrally-acting drugs).
No products indexed under this heading.

Aliskiren (Olanzapine, because of its potential for inducing hypotension, may enhance the effects of certain antihypertensive agents).
Products include:
Tekturna Tablets ... 2321
Tekturna HCT Tablets ... 2324

Alprazolam (Given the primary CNS effects of olanzapine, caution should be used when olanzapine is taken in combination with other centrally-acting drugs).
No products indexed under this heading.

Amiodarone Hydrochloride (Can potentially inhibit olanzapine clearance; therefore, a dosage decrease might be considered).
No products indexed under this heading.

Amlodipine Besylate (Olanzapine, because of its potential for inducing hypotension, may enhance the effects of certain antihypertensive agents). Products include:
Azor Tablets ... 1005
Exforge Tablets ... 2238

Anastrozole (Can potentially inhibit olanzapine clearance; therefore, a dosage decrease might be considered). Products include:
Arimidex Tablets ... 672

Aprobarbital (Given the primary CNS effects of olanzapine, caution should be used when olanzapine is taken in combination with other centrally-acting drugs).
No products indexed under this heading.

Atenolol (Olanzapine, because of its potential for inducing hypotension, may enhance the effects of certain antihypertensive agents).
No products indexed under this heading.

Benazepril Hydrochloride (Olanzapine, because of its potential for inducing hypotension, may enhance the effects of certain antihypertensive agents).
No products indexed under this heading.

Bendroflumethiazide (Olanzapine, because of its potential for inducing hypotension, may enhance the effects of certain antihypertensive agents).
No products indexed under this heading.

Betaxolol Hydrochloride (Olanzapine, because of its potential for inducing hypotension, may enhance the effects of certain antihypertensive agents).
No products indexed under this heading.

Bisoprolol Fumarate (Olanzapine, because of its potential for inducing hypotension, may enhance the effects of certain antihypertensive agents).
No products indexed under this heading.

Bromocriptine Mesylate (Olanzapine may antagonize the effects of dopamine agonists).
No products indexed under this heading.

Buprenorphine Hydrochloride (Given the primary CNS effects of olanzapine, caution should be used when olanzapine is taken in combination with other centrally-acting drugs). Products include:
Suboxone Tablets ... 2601
Subutex Tablets ... 2601

Buspirone Hydrochloride (Given the primary CNS effects of olanzapine, caution should be used when olanzapine is taken in combination with other centrally-acting drugs).
No products indexed under this heading.

Butabarbital (Given the primary CNS effects of olanzapine, caution should be used when olanzapine is taken in combination with other centrally-acting drugs).
No products indexed under this heading.

Butalbital (Given the primary CNS effects of olanzapine, caution should be used when olanzapine is taken in combination with other centrally-acting drugs).
No products indexed under this heading.

Candesartan Cilexetil (Olanzapine, because of its potential for inducing hypotension, may enhance the effects of certain antihypertensive agents). Products include:
Atacand Tablets ... 639
Atacand HCT ... 642

Captopril (Olanzapine, because of its potential for inducing hypotension, may enhance the effects of certain antihypertensive agents).
Products include:
Captopril Tablets ... 2182

Carbamazepine (Causes an approximately 50% increase in the clearance of olanzapine at 400 mg daily; higher daily doses of carbamazepine may cause an even greater increase in olanzapine clearance).
Products include:
Carbatrol Capsules ... 3019
Equetro Extended-Release Capsules ... 3174

Carteolol Hydrochloride (Olanzapine, because of its potential for inducing hypotension, may enhance the effects of certain antihypertensive agents).
No products indexed under this heading.

Chlordiazepoxide (Given the primary CNS effects of olanzapine, caution should be used when olanzapine is taken in combination with other centrally-acting drugs).
No products indexed under this heading.

Chlordiazepoxide Hydrochloride (Given the primary CNS effects of olanzapine, caution should be used when olanzapine is taken in combination with other centrally-acting drugs).
No products indexed under this heading.

Chlorothiazide (Olanzapine, because of its potential for inducing hypotension, may enhance the effects of certain antihypertensive agents).
No products indexed under this heading.

Chlorothiazide Sodium (Olanzapine, because of its potential for inducing hypotension, may enhance the effects of certain antihypertensive agents). Products include:
Intravenous Sodium Diuril ... 2490

Chlorpromazine (Given the primary CNS effects of olanzapine, caution should be used when olanzapine is taken in combination with other centrally-acting drugs).
No products indexed under this heading.

Chlorpromazine Hydrochloride (Given the primary CNS effects of olanzapine, caution should be used when olanzapine is taken in combination with other centrally-acting drugs).
No products indexed under this heading.

Chlorprothixene (Given the primary CNS effects of olanzapine, caution should be used when olanzapine is taken in combination with other centrally-acting drugs).
No products indexed under this heading.

Chlorprothixene Hydrochloride (Given the primary CNS effects of olanzapine, caution should be used when olanzapine is taken in combination with other centrally-acting drugs).
No products indexed under this heading.

Chlorprothixene Lactate (Given the primary CNS effects of olanzapine, caution should be used when olanzapine is taken in combination with other centrally-acting drugs).
No products indexed under this heading.

Chlorthalidone (Olanzapine, because of its potential for inducing hypotension, may enhance the effects of certain antihypertensive agents). Products include:
Clorpres Tablets ... 2185

Cimetidine (Can potentially inhibit olanzapine clearance; therefore, a dosage decrease might be considered).
No products indexed under this heading.

Cimetidine Hydrochloride (Can potentially inhibit olanzapine clearance; therefore, a dosage decrease might be considered).
No products indexed under this heading.

Ciprofloxacin (Can potentially inhibit olanzapine clearance; therefore, a dosage decrease might be considered). Products include:
Cipro I.V. 2817
Cipro Oral Suspension 2810
Cipro XR Tablets 2823
Ciprodex Otic Suspension 541

Ciprofloxacin Hydrochloride (Can potentially inhibit olanzapine clearance; therefore, a dosage decrease might be considered). Products include:
Cipro Tablets 2810

Citalopram Hydrobromide (May cause an increase in olanzapine clearance; therefore, a dosage increase might be considered). Products include:
Celexa 1160

Clarithromycin (Can potentially inhibit olanzapine clearance; therefore, a dosage decrease might be considered). Products include:
Biaxin/Biaxin XL 411

Clonidine (Olanzapine, because of its potential for inducing hypotension, may enhance the effects of certain antihypertensive agents). Products include:
Catapres-TTS 842

Clonidine Hydrochloride (Olanzapine, because of its potential for inducing hypotension, may enhance the effects of certain antihypertensive agents). Products include:
Catapres Tablets 841
Clorpres Tablets 2185

Clorazepate Dipotassium (Given the primary CNS effects of olanzapine, caution should be used when olanzapine is taken in combination with other centrally-acting drugs).
No products indexed under this heading.

Clozapine (Given the primary CNS effects of olanzapine, caution should be used when olanzapine is taken in combination with other centrally-acting drugs).
No products indexed under this heading.

Codeine Phosphate (Given the primary CNS effects of olanzapine, caution should be used when olanzapine is taken in combination with other centrally-acting drugs). Products include:
Tylenol with Codeine Tablets 2427

Deserpidine (Olanzapine, because of its potential for inducing hypotension, may enhance the effects of certain antihypertensive agents).
No products indexed under this heading.

Desflurane (Given the primary CNS effects of olanzapine, caution should be used when olanzapine is taken in combination with other centrally-acting drugs).
No products indexed under this heading.

Desogestrel (Can potentially inhibit olanzapine clearance; therefore, a dosage decrease might be considered). Products include:
Mircette Tablets 1034

Dezocine (Given the primary CNS effects of olanzapine, caution should be used when olanzapine is taken in combination with other centrally-acting drugs).
No products indexed under this heading.

Diazepam (Co-administration of diazepam with olanzapine may potentiate orthostatic hypotension. Concomitant administration of intramuscular olanzapine and parenteral benzodiazepine has not been studied and is therefore not recommended. If use of intramuscular olanzapine in combination with parenteral benzodiazepines is considered, careful evaluation of clinical status for excessive sedation and cardiorespiratory depression is recommended). Products include:
Valium Tablets 2658

Diazoxide (Olanzapine, because of its potential for inducing hypotension, may enhance the effects of certain antihypertensive agents). Products include:
Proglycem Capsules 1185
Proglycem Suspension 1185

Diltiazem Hydrochloride (Olanzapine, because of its potential for inducing hypotension, may enhance the effects of certain antihypertensive agents). Products include:
Cardizem LA Extended Release Tablets 421

Diltiazem Maleate (May cause an increase in olanzapine clearance; therefore, a dosage increase might be considered).
No products indexed under this heading.

Dopamine Hydrochloride (Olanzapine may antagonize the effects of dopamine agonists).
No products indexed under this heading.

Doxazosin Mesylate (Olanzapine, because of its potential for inducing hypotension, may enhance the effects of certain antihypertensive agents).
No products indexed under this heading.

Droperidol (Given the primary CNS effects of olanzapine, caution should be used when olanzapine is taken in combination with other centrally-acting drugs).
No products indexed under this heading.

Enalapril Maleate (Olanzapine, because of its potential for inducing hypotension, may enhance the effects of certain antihypertensive agents).
No products indexed under this heading.

Enalaprilat (Olanzapine, because of its potential for inducing hypotension, may enhance the effects of certain antihypertensive agents).
No products indexed under this heading.

Enflurane (Given the primary CNS effects of olanzapine, caution should be used when olanzapine is taken in combination with other centrally-acting drugs).
No products indexed under this heading.

Enoxacin (Can potentially inhibit olanzapine clearance; therefore, a dosage decrease might be considered).
No products indexed under this heading.

Eprosartan Mesylate (Olanzapine, because of its potential for inducing hypotension, may enhance the effects of certain antihypertensive agents). Products include:
Teveten Tablets 515
Teveten HCT Tablets 517

Erythromycin (May cause an increase in olanzapine clearance; therefore, a dosage increase might be considered).
No products indexed under this heading.

Erythromycin Estolate (May cause an increase in olanzapine clearance; therefore, a dosage increase might be considered).
No products indexed under this heading.

Erythromycin Ethylsuccinate (May cause an increase in olanzapine clearance; therefore, a dosage increase might be considered). Products include:
E.E.S. 433
EryPed 431

Erythromycin Gluceptate (May cause an increase in olanzapine clearance; therefore, a dosage increase might be considered).
No products indexed under this heading.

Erythromycin Lactobionate (May cause an increase in olanzapine clearance; therefore, a dosage increase might be considered).
No products indexed under this heading.

Erythromycin Stearate (May cause an increase in olanzapine clearance; therefore, a dosage increase might be considered).
No products indexed under this heading.

Esmolol Hydrochloride (Olanzapine, because of its potential for inducing hypotension, may enhance the effects of certain antihypertensive agents).
No products indexed under this heading.

Estazolam (Given the primary CNS effects of olanzapine, caution should be used when olanzapine is taken in combination with other centrally-acting drugs).
No products indexed under this heading.

Ethanol (Given the primary CNS effects of olanzapine, caution should be used when olanzapine is taken in combination with other centrally-acting drugs).
No products indexed under this heading.

Ethchlorvynol (Given the primary CNS effects of olanzapine, caution should be used when olanzapine is taken in combination with other centrally-acting drugs).
No products indexed under this heading.

Ethinamate (Given the primary CNS effects of olanzapine, caution should be used when olanzapine is taken in combination with other centrally-acting drugs).
No products indexed under this heading.

Ethinyl Estradiol (Can potentially inhibit olanzapine clearance; therefore, a dosage decrease might be considered). Products include:
Lybrel Tablets 3204
Mircette Tablets 1034
NuvaRing 2897
Ortho-Cyclen/Ortho Tri-Cyclen 2449
Ortho Evra Transdermal System 2437
Ortho Tri-Cyclen Lo Tablets 2458
Seasonique Tablets 1046
Yaz Tablets 805

Ethyl Alcohol (Given the primary CNS effects of olanzapine, caution should be used when olanzapine is taken in combination with other centrally-acting drugs).
No products indexed under this heading.

Felodipine (Olanzapine, because of its potential for inducing hypotension, may enhance the effects of certain antihypertensive agents).
No products indexed under this heading.

Fentanyl (Given the primary CNS effects of olanzapine, caution should be used when olanzapine is taken in combination with other centrally-acting drugs). Products include:
Duragesic Transdermal System 2405
Ionsys Transdermal System 2410

Fentanyl Citrate (Given the primary CNS effects of olanzapine, caution should be used when olanzapine is taken in combination with other centrally-acting drugs). Products include:
Actiq 959
Fentora Tablets 968

Fluoxetine Hydrochloride (Co-administration causes a small increase in the maximum concentration of olanzapine and a small decrease in olanzapine clearance; the magnitude of the impact of this factor is small in comparison to the overall variability between individuals and, therefore, dose modification is not routinely recommended). Products include:
Prozac Weekly Capsules 1852
Prozac Pulvules and Liquid 1852
Symbyax Capsules 1871

Fluphenazine Decanoate (Given the primary CNS effects of olanzapine, caution should be used when olanzapine is taken in combination with other centrally-acting drugs).
No products indexed under this heading.

Fluphenazine Enanthate (Given the primary CNS effects of olanzapine, caution should be used when olanzapine is taken in combination with other centrally-acting drugs).
No products indexed under this heading.

Fluphenazine Hydrochloride (Given the primary CNS effects of olanzapine, caution should be used when olanzapine is taken in combination with other centrally-acting drugs).
No products indexed under this heading.

Flurazepam Hydrochloride (Given the primary CNS effects of olanzapine, caution should be used when olanzapine is taken in combination with other centrally-acting drugs).
No products indexed under this heading.

Fluvoxamine (Can potentially inhibit olanzapine clearance; therefore, a dosage decrease might be considered).
No products indexed under this heading.

Fluvoxamine Maleate (Decreases the clearance of olanzapine leading to a mean increase in olanzapine Cmax and AUC; lower doses of olanzapine should be considered or co-administered). Products include:

Methohexital Sodium (Given the primary CNS effects of olanzapine, caution should be used when olanzapine is taken in combination with other centrally-acting drugs).
No products indexed under this heading.

Methotrimeprazine (Given the primary CNS effects of olanzapine, caution should be used when olanzapine is taken in combination with other centrally-acting drugs).
No products indexed under this heading.

Methoxsalen (Can potentially inhibit olanzapine clearance; therefore, a dosage decrease might be considered).
No products indexed under this heading.

Methoxyflurane (Given the primary CNS effects of olanzapine, caution should be used when olanzapine is taken in combination with other centrally-acting drugs).
No products indexed under this heading.

Methyclothiazide (Olanzapine, because of its potential for inducing hypotension, may enhance the effects of certain antihypertensive agents).
No products indexed under this heading.

Methyldopa (Olanzapine, because of its potential for inducing hypotension, may enhance the effects of certain antihypertensive agents).
No products indexed under this heading.

Methyldopate Hydrochloride (Olanzapine, because of its potential for inducing hypotension, may enhance the effects of certain antihypertensive agents).
No products indexed under this heading.

Metolazone (Olanzapine, because of its potential for inducing hypotension, may enhance the effects of certain antihypertensive agents).
No products indexed under this heading.

Metoprolol Succinate (Olanzapine, because of its potential for inducing hypotension, may enhance the effects of certain antihypertensive agents). Products include:
Toprol-XL Tablets 666

Metoprolol Tartrate (Olanzapine, because of its potential for inducing hypotension, may enhance the effects of certain antihypertensive agents).
No products indexed under this heading.

Metyrosine (Olanzapine, because of its potential for inducing hypotension, may enhance the effects of certain antihypertensive agents). Products include:
Demser Capsules 1989

Mexiletine Hydrochloride (Can potentially inhibit olanzapine clearance; therefore, a dosage decrease might be considered).
No products indexed under this heading.

Mibefradil Dihydrochloride (Olanzapine, because of its potential for inducing hypotension, may enhance the effects of certain antihypertensive agents).
No products indexed under this heading.

Midazolam Hydrochloride (Given the primary CNS effects of olanzapine, caution should be used when olanzapine is taken in combination with other centrally-acting drugs).
No products indexed under this heading.

Minoxidil (Olanzapine, because of its potential for inducing hypotension, may enhance the effects of certain antihypertensive agents).
No products indexed under this heading.

Moexipril Hydrochloride (Olanzapine, because of its potential for inducing hypotension, may enhance the effects of certain antihypertensive agents).
No products indexed under this heading.

Molindone Hydrochloride (Given the primary CNS effects of olanzapine, caution should be used when olanzapine is taken in combination with other centrally-acting drugs). Products include:
Moban Tablets 1116

Morphine Sulfate (Given the primary CNS effects of olanzapine, caution should be used when olanzapine is taken in combination with other centrally-acting drugs). Products include:
Avinza Capsules 1772
DepoDur Injection 1095
MS Contin Tablets 2585

Moxifloxacin Hydrochloride (Can potentially inhibit olanzapine clearance; therefore, a dosage decrease might be considered). Products include:
Avelox 2803
Vigamox Ophthalmic Solution 548

Nadolol (Olanzapine, because of its potential for inducing hypotension, may enhance the effects of certain antihypertensive agents). Products include:
Nadolol Tablets 2191

Nafcillin Sodium (May cause an increase in olanzapine clearance; therefore, a dosage increase might be considered).
No products indexed under this heading.

Nalidixic Acid (Can potentially inhibit olanzapine clearance; therefore, a dosage decrease might be considered).
No products indexed under this heading.

Nebivolol (Olanzapine, because of its potential for inducing hypotension, may enhance the effects of certain antihypertensive agents). Products include:
Bystolic Tablets 1155

Nicardipine Hydrochloride (Olanzapine, because of its potential for inducing hypotension, may enhance the effects of certain antihypertensive agents). Products include:
Cardene I.V. 1093

Nicotine (May cause an increase in olanzapine clearance; therefore, a dosage increase might be considered).
No products indexed under this heading.

Nicotine Polacrilex (May cause an increase in olanzapine clearance; therefore, a dosage increase might be considered).
No products indexed under this heading.

Nicotine Salicylate (May cause an increase in olanzapine clearance; therefore, a dosage increase might be considered).
No products indexed under this heading.

Nicotine Sulfate (May cause an increase in olanzapine clearance; therefore, a dosage increase might be considered).
No products indexed under this heading.

Nifedipine (Olanzapine, because of its potential for inducing hypotension, may enhance the effects of certain antihypertensive agents).
No products indexed under this heading.

Nisoldipine (Olanzapine, because of its potential for inducing hypotension, may enhance the effects of certain antihypertensive agents). Products include:
Sular Extended Release Tablets 2975

Nitroglycerin (Olanzapine, because of its potential for inducing hypotension, may enhance the effects of certain antihypertensive agents). Products include:
Nitro-Dur Transdermal Infusion System 2887
Nitrolingual Pumpspray 2965

Norethindrone (Can potentially inhibit olanzapine clearance; therefore, a dosage decrease might be considered). Products include:
Ortho Micronor Tablets 2446

Norfloxacin (Can potentially inhibit olanzapine clearance; therefore, a dosage decrease might be considered). Products include:
Noroxin Tablets 2069

Norgestrel (Can potentially inhibit olanzapine clearance; therefore, a dosage decrease might be considered).
No products indexed under this heading.

Ofloxacin (Can potentially inhibit olanzapine clearance; therefore, a dosage decrease might be considered). Products include:
Ofloxacin Ophthalmic Solution 0.3% ..... ⊙243

Omeprazole (May cause an increase in olanzapine clearance by inducing CYP1A2 or glucuronyl transferase clearance).
No products indexed under this heading.

Oxazepam (Given the primary CNS effects of olanzapine, caution should be used when olanzapine is taken in combination with other centrally-acting drugs).
No products indexed under this heading.

Oxycodone Hydrochloride (Given the primary CNS effects of olanzapine, caution should be used when olanzapine is taken in combination with other centrally-acting drugs). Products include:
OxyContin Tablets 2589
OxyIR Capsules 2593
Percocet Tablets 1127
Percodan Tablets 1130

Paroxetine Hydrochloride (Can potentially inhibit olanzapine clearance; therefore, a dosage decrease might be considered). Products include:
Paxil 1535
Paxil CR Controlled-Release Tablets 1544

Penbutolol Sulfate (Olanzapine, because of its potential for inducing hypotension, may enhance the effects of certain antihypertensive agents).
No products indexed under this heading.

Pentobarbital Sodium (Given the primary CNS effects of olanzapine, caution should be used when olanzapine is taken in combination with other centrally-acting drugs). Products include:
Nembutal Sodium Solution, USP 2494

Pergolide Mesylate (Olanzapine may antagonize the effects of dopamine agonists).
No products indexed under this heading.

Perindopril Erbumine (Olanzapine, because of its potential for inducing hypotension, may enhance the effects of certain antihypertensive agents). Products include:
Aceon Tablets (2 mg, 4 mg, 8 mg) 3038

Perphenazine (Given the primary CNS effects of olanzapine, caution should be used when olanzapine is taken in combination with other centrally-acting drugs).
No products indexed under this heading.

Phenobarbital (Given the primary CNS effects of olanzapine, caution should be used when olanzapine is taken in combination with other centrally-acting drugs). Products include:
Donnatal Extentabs 2507

Phenoxybenzamine Hydrochloride (Olanzapine, because of its potential for inducing hypotension, may enhance the effects of certain antihypertensive agents). Products include:
Dibenzyline Capsules 3188

Phentolamine Mesylate (Olanzapine, because of its potential for inducing hypotension, may enhance the effects of certain antihypertensive agents).
No products indexed under this heading.

Phenytoin (May cause an increase in olanzapine clearance; therefore, a dosage increase might be considered).
No products indexed under this heading.

Phenytoin Sodium (May cause an increase in olanzapine clearance; therefore, a dosage increase might be considered). Products include:
Phenytek Capsules 2192

Pindolol (Olanzapine, because of its potential for inducing hypotension, may enhance the effects of certain antihypertensive agents).
No products indexed under this heading.

Polythiazide (Olanzapine, because of its potential for inducing hypotension, may enhance the effects of certain antihypertensive agents).
No products indexed under this heading.

Pramipexole Dihydrochloride (Olanzapine may antagonize the effects of dopamine agonists). Products include:
Mirapex Tablets 857

Prazepam (Given the primary CNS effects of olanzapine, caution should be used when olanzapine is taken in combination with other centrally-acting drugs).
No products indexed under this heading.

Prazosin Hydrochloride (Olanzapine, because of its potential for inducing hypotension, may enhance the effects of certain antihypertensive agents).
No products indexed under this heading.

Primidone (May cause an increase in olanzapine clearance; therefore, a dosage increase might be considered).
No products indexed under this heading.

Prochlorperazine (Given the primary CNS effects of olanzapine, caution should be used when olanzapine is taken in combination with other centrally-acting drugs).
No products indexed under this heading.

Promethazine Hydrochloride (Given the primary CNS effects of olanzapine, caution should be used when olanzapine is taken in combination with other centrally-acting drugs).
No products indexed under this heading.

Propofol (Given the primary CNS effects of olanzapine, caution should be used when olanzapine is taken in combination with other centrally-acting drugs).
No products indexed under this heading.

Propoxyphene Hydrochloride (Given the primary CNS effects of olanzapine, caution should be used when olanzapine is taken in combination with other centrally-acting drugs).
No products indexed under this heading.

Propoxyphene Napsylate (Given the primary CNS effects of olanzapine, caution should be used when olanzapine is taken in combination with other centrally-acting drugs).
No products indexed under this heading.

Propranolol Hydrochloride (Olanzapine, because of its potential for inducing hypotension, may enhance the effects of certain antihypertensive agents). Products include:
InnoPran XL Extended Release Capsules 1484

Quazepam (Given the primary CNS effects of olanzapine, caution should be used when olanzapine is taken in combination with other centrally-acting drugs).
No products indexed under this heading.

Quetiapine Fumarate (Given the primary CNS effects of olanzapine, caution should be used when olanzapine is taken in combination with other centrally-acting drugs).
No products indexed under this heading.

Quinapril Hydrochloride (Olanzapine, because of its potential for inducing hypotension, may enhance the effects of certain antihypertensive agents).
No products indexed under this heading.

Ramipril (Olanzapine, because of its potential for inducing hypotension, may enhance the effects of certain antihypertensive agents).
No products indexed under this heading.

Ranitidine Hydrochloride (Can potentially inhibit olanzapine clearance; therefore, a dosage decrease might be considered). Products include:
Zantac 75 Tablets .... ◘ 603
Zantac 1670
Zantac Injection 1666
Zantac Injection Pharmacy Bulk Package 1668
Maximum Strength Zantac 150 Tablets .... ◘ 603
Maximum Strength Zantac 150 Cool Mint Tablets .... ◘ 603

Rauwolfia Serpentina (Olanzapine, because of its potential for inducing hypotension, may enhance the effects of certain antihypertensive agents).
No products indexed under this heading.

Remifentanil Hydrochloride (Given the primary CNS effects of olanzapine, caution should be used when olanzapine is taken in combination with other centrally-acting drugs).
No products indexed under this heading.

Rescinnamine (Olanzapine, because of its potential for inducing hypotension, may enhance the effects of certain antihypertensive agents).
No products indexed under this heading.

Reserpine (Olanzapine, because of its potential for inducing hypotension, may enhance the effects of certain antihypertensive agents).
No products indexed under this heading.

Rifampicin (May cause an increase in olanzapine clearance; therefore, a dosage increase might be considered).
No products indexed under this heading.

Rifampin (May cause an increase in olanzapine clearance by inducing CYP1A2 or glucuronyl tranferase clearance).
No products indexed under this heading.

Risperidone (Given the primary CNS effects of olanzapine, caution should be used when olanzapine is taken in combination with other centrally-acting drugs). Products include:
Risperdal Consta Long-Acting Injection 1753

Ritonavir (May cause an increase in olanzapine clearance; therefore, a dosage increase might be considered). Products include:
Kaletra 452
Norvir 489

Ropinirole Hydrochloride (Olanzapine may antagonize the effects of dopamine agonists). Products include:
Requip Tablets 1561
Requip XL Tablets 1568

Secobarbital Sodium (Given the primary CNS effects of olanzapine, caution should be used when olanzapine is taken in combination with other centrally-acting drugs).
No products indexed under this heading.

Sevoflurane (Given the primary CNS effects of olanzapine, caution should be used when olanzapine is taken in combination with other centrally-acting drugs). Products include:
Ultane Liquid for Inhalation 524

Sildenafil Citrate (Can potentially inhibit olanzapine clearance; therefore, a dosage decrease might be considered).
No products indexed under this heading.

Sodium Nitroprusside (Olanzapine, because of its potential for inducing hypotension, may enhance the effects of certain antihypertensive agents).
No products indexed under this heading.

Sodium Oxybate (Given the primary CNS effects of olanzapine, caution should be used when olanzapine is taken in combination with other centrally-acting drugs). Products include:
Xyrem Oral Solution 1766

Sotalol Hydrochloride (Olanzapine, because of its potential for inducing hypotension, may enhance the effects of certain antihypertensive agents).
No products indexed under this heading.

Sparfloxacin (Can potentially inhibit olanzapine clearance; therefore, a dosage decrease might be considered).
No products indexed under this heading.

Spirapril Hydrochloride (Olanzapine, because of its potential for inducing hypotension, may enhance the effects of certain antihypertensive agents).
No products indexed under this heading.

Sufentanil Citrate (Given the primary CNS effects of olanzapine, caution should be used when olanzapine is taken in combination with other centrally-acting drugs).
No products indexed under this heading.

Tacrine Hydrochloride (Can potentially inhibit olanzapine clearance; therefore, a dosage decrease might be considered).
No products indexed under this heading.

Telmisartan (Olanzapine, because of its potential for inducing hypotension, may enhance the effects of certain antihypertensive agents). Products include:
Micardis Tablets 852
Micardis HCT Tablets 854

Temazepam (Given the primary CNS effects of olanzapine, caution should be used when olanzapine is taken in combination with other centrally-acting drugs).
No products indexed under this heading.

Terazosin Hydrochloride (Olanzapine, because of its potential for inducing hypotension, may enhance the effects of certain antihypertensive agents).
No products indexed under this heading.

Thiamylal Sodium (Given the primary CNS effects of olanzapine, caution should be used when olanzapine is taken in combination with other centrally-acting drugs).
No products indexed under this heading.

Thioridazine Hydrochloride (Given the primary CNS effects of olanzapine, caution should be used when olanzapine is taken in combination with other centrally-acting drugs). Products include:
Thioridazine Hydrochloride Tablets 2195

Thiothixene (Given the primary CNS effects of olanzapine, caution should be used when olanzapine is taken in combination with other centrally-acting drugs). Products include:
Thiothixene Capsules 2197

Ticlopidine Hydrochloride (Can potentially inhibit olanzapine clearance; therefore, a dosage decrease might be considered).
No products indexed under this heading.

Timolol Maleate (Olanzapine, because of its potential for inducing hypotension, may enhance the effects of certain antihypertensive agents). Products include:
Combigan Ophthalmic Solution 553
Cosopt Sterile Ophthalmic Solution 1969
Timoptic Sterile Ophthalmic Solution 2121
Timoptic in Ocudose 2124
Timoptic-XE Sterile Ophthalmic Gel Forming Solution 2125

Tobacco (May cause an increase in olanzapine clearance; therefore, a dosage increase might be considered).
No products indexed under this heading.

Torsemide (Olanzapine, because of its potential for inducing hypotension, may enhance the effects of certain antihypertensive agents). Products include:
Demadex Injection 2630
Demadex Tablets 2630

Trandolapril (Olanzapine, because of its potential for inducing hypotension, may enhance the effects of certain antihypertensive agents). Products include:
Mavik Tablets 472
Tarka Tablets 511

Triazolam (Given the primary CNS effects of olanzapine, caution should be used when olanzapine is taken in combination with other centrally-acting drugs).
No products indexed under this heading.

Trifluoperazine Hydrochloride (Given the primary CNS effects of olanzapine, caution should be used when olanzapine is taken in combination with other centrally-acting drugs).
No products indexed under this heading.

Trimethaphan Camsylate (Olanzapine, because of its potential for inducing hypotension, may enhance the effects of certain antihypertensive agents).
No products indexed under this heading.

Troleandomycin (Can potentially inhibit olanzapine clearance; therefore, a dosage decrease might be considered).
No products indexed under this heading.

Trovafloxacin Mesylate (Can potentially inhibit olanzapine clearance; therefore, a dosage decrease might be considered).
No products indexed under this heading.

Valsartan (Olanzapine, because of its potential for inducing hypotension, may enhance the effects of certain antihypertensive agents). Products include:
- Diovan Tablets 2212
- Diovan HCT Tablets 2216
- Exforge Tablets 2238

Vardenafil Hydrochloride (Can potentially inhibit olanzapine clearance; therefore, a dosage decrease might be considered). Products include:
- Levitra Tablets 2876

Verapamil Hydrochloride (Olanzapine, because of its potential for inducing hypotension, may enhance the effects of certain antihypertensive agents). Products include:
- Tarka Tablets 511

Zaleplon (Given the primary CNS effects of olanzapine, caution should be used when olanzapine is taken in combination with other centrally-acting drugs).
No products indexed under this heading.

Zileuton (Can potentially inhibit olanzapine clearance; therefore, a dosage decrease might be considered).
No products indexed under this heading.

Ziprasidone Hydrochloride (Given the primary CNS effects of olanzapine, caution should be used when olanzapine is taken in combination with other centrally-acting drugs). Products include:
- Geodon Capsules 2520

Zolpidem Tartrate (Given the primary CNS effects of olanzapine, caution should be used when olanzapine is taken in combination with other centrally-acting drugs). Products include:
- Ambien Tablets 2692
- Ambien CR Tablets 2696

Food Interactions

Alcohol (Co-administration of alcohol with olanzapine potentiates orthostatic hypotension; concurrent use should be avoided).

Broccoli (May cause an increase in olanzapine clearance; therefore, a dosage increase might be considered).

Brussel Sprouts (May cause an increase in olanzapine clearance; therefore, a dosage increase might be considered).

Charbroiled Food (May cause an increase in olanzapine clearance; therefore, a dosage increase might be considered).

Grapefruit Juice (Can potentially inhibit olanzapine clearance; therefore, a dosage decrease might be considered).

ZYPREXA ZYDIS ORALLY DISINTEGRATING TABLETS

(Olanzapine) 1883
See Zyprexa Tablets

ZYRTEC ALLERGY TABLETS

(Cetirizine Hydrochloride) 1919
May interact with hypnotics and sedatives, tranquilizers, and certain other agents. Compounds in these categories include:

Alprazolam (Concomitant use may increase drowsiness).
No products indexed under this heading.

Buspirone Hydrochloride (Concomitant use may increase drowsiness).
No products indexed under this heading.

Butabarbital (Concomitant use may increase drowsiness).
No products indexed under this heading.

Butabarbital Sodium (Concomitant use may increase drowsiness).
No products indexed under this heading.

Chloral Hydrate (Concomitant use may increase drowsiness).
No products indexed under this heading.

Chlordiazepoxide (Concomitant use may increase drowsiness).
No products indexed under this heading.

Chlordiazepoxide Hydrochloride (Concomitant use may increase drowsiness).
No products indexed under this heading.

Chlorpromazine (Concomitant use may increase drowsiness).
No products indexed under this heading.

Chlorpromazine Hydrochloride (Concomitant use may increase drowsiness).
No products indexed under this heading.

Chlorprothixene (Concomitant use may increase drowsiness).
No products indexed under this heading.

Chlorprothixene Hydrochloride (Concomitant use may increase drowsiness).
No products indexed under this heading.

Clorazepate Dipotassium (Concomitant use may increase drowsiness).
No products indexed under this heading.

Diazepam (Concomitant use may increase drowsiness). Products include:
- Valium Tablets 2658

Droperidol (Concomitant use may increase drowsiness).
No products indexed under this heading.

Estazolam (Concomitant use may increase drowsiness).
No products indexed under this heading.

Ethanol (Alcohol may increase drowsiness. Avoid alcoholic drinks).
No products indexed under this heading.

Ethchlorvynol (Concomitant use may increase drowsiness).
No products indexed under this heading.

Ethinamate (Concomitant use may increase drowsiness).
No products indexed under this heading.

Ethyl Alcohol (Alcohol may increase drowsiness. Avoid alcoholic drinks).
No products indexed under this heading.

Fluphenazine Decanoate (Concomitant use may increase drowsiness).
No products indexed under this heading.

Fluphenazine Enanthate (Concomitant use may increase drowsiness).
No products indexed under this heading.

Fluphenazine Hydrochloride (Concomitant use may increase drowsiness).
No products indexed under this heading.

Flurazepam Hydrochloride (Concomitant use may increase drowsiness).
No products indexed under this heading.

Glutethimide (Concomitant use may increase drowsiness).
No products indexed under this heading.

Haloperidol (Concomitant use may increase drowsiness).
No products indexed under this heading.

Haloperidol Decanoate (Concomitant use may increase drowsiness).
No products indexed under this heading.

Hydroxyzine Hydrochloride (Concomitant use may increase drowsiness).
No products indexed under this heading.

Lorazepam (Concomitant use may increase drowsiness).
No products indexed under this heading.

Loxapine Hydrochloride (Concomitant use may increase drowsiness).
No products indexed under this heading.

Loxapine Succinate (Concomitant use may increase drowsiness).
No products indexed under this heading.

Meprobamate (Concomitant use may increase drowsiness).
No products indexed under this heading.

Mesoridazine Besylate (Concomitant use may increase drowsiness).
No products indexed under this heading.

Midazolam Hydrochloride (Concomitant use may increase drowsiness).
No products indexed under this heading.

Molindone Hydrochloride (Concomitant use may increase drowsiness). Products include:
- Moban Tablets 1116

Oxazepam (Concomitant use may increase drowsiness).
No products indexed under this heading.

Perphenazine (Concomitant use may increase drowsiness).
No products indexed under this heading.

Prazepam (Concomitant use may increase drowsiness).
No products indexed under this heading.

Prochlorperazine (Concomitant use may increase drowsiness).
No products indexed under this heading.

Promethazine Hydrochloride (Concomitant use may increase drowsiness).
No products indexed under this heading.

Propofol (Concomitant use may increase drowsiness).
No products indexed under this heading.

Quazepam (Concomitant use may increase drowsiness).
No products indexed under this heading.

Ramelteon (Concomitant use may increase drowsiness). Products include:
- Rozerem Tablets 3091

Secobarbital Sodium (Concomitant use may increase drowsiness).
No products indexed under this heading.

Sodium Butabarbital (Concomitant use may increase drowsiness).
No products indexed under this heading.

Temazepam (Concomitant use may increase drowsiness).
No products indexed under this heading.

Thioridazine Hydrochloride (Concomitant use may increase drowsiness). Products include:
- Thioridazine Hydrochloride Tablets 2195

Thiothixene (Concomitant use may increase drowsiness). Products include:
- Thiothixene Capsules 2197

Triazolam (Concomitant use may increase drowsiness).
No products indexed under this heading.

Trifluoperazine Hydrochloride (Concomitant use may increase drowsiness).
No products indexed under this heading.

Zaleplon (Concomitant use may increase drowsiness).
No products indexed under this heading.

Zolpidem Tartrate (Concomitant use may increase drowsiness). Products include:
- Ambien Tablets 2692
- Ambien CR Tablets 2696

Food Interactions

Alcohol (Alcohol may increase drowsiness. Avoid alcoholic drinks).

ZYRTEC CHEWABLE TABLETS

(Cetirizine Hydrochloride) 1920
See Zyrtec Tablets

CHILDREN'S ZYRTEC ALLERGY SYRUP

(Cetirizine Hydrochloride) 1920
May interact with hypnotics and sedatives, tranquilizers, and certain other agents. Compounds in these categories include:

Alprazolam (Concomitant use may increase drowsiness).
No products indexed under this heading.

Buspirone Hydrochloride (Concomitant use may increase drowsiness).
No products indexed under this heading.

Butabarbital (Concomitant use may increase drowsiness).
No products indexed under this heading.

Butabarbital Sodium (Concomitant use may increase drowsiness).
No products indexed under this heading.

Chloral Hydrate (Concomitant use may increase drowsiness).
No products indexed under this heading.

Chlordiazepoxide (Concomitant use may increase drowsiness).
No products indexed under this heading.

Chlordiazepoxide Hydrochloride (Concomitant use may increase drowsiness).
No products indexed under this heading.

Chlorpromazine (Concomitant use may increase drowsiness).
No products indexed under this heading.

Chlorpromazine Hydrochloride (Concomitant use may increase drowsiness).
No products indexed under this heading.

Chlorprothixene (Concomitant use may increase drowsiness).
No products indexed under this heading.

Chlorprothixene Hydrochloride (Concomitant use may increase drowsiness).
No products indexed under this heading.

Clorazepate Dipotassium (Concomitant use may increase drowsiness).
No products indexed under this heading.

Diazepam (Concomitant use may increase drowsiness). Products include:
Valium Tablets 2658

Droperidol (Concomitant use may increase drowsiness).
No products indexed under this heading.

Estazolam (Concomitant use may increase drowsiness).
No products indexed under this heading.

Ethanol (Concomitant use may increase drowsiness).
No products indexed under this heading.

Ethchlorvynol (Concomitant use may increase drowsiness).
No products indexed under this heading.

Ethinamate (Concomitant use may increase drowsiness).
No products indexed under this heading.

Ethyl Alcohol (Concomitant use may increase drowsiness).
No products indexed under this heading.

Fluphenazine Decanoate (Concomitant use may increase drowsiness).
No products indexed under this heading.

Fluphenazine Enanthate (Concomitant use may increase drowsiness).
No products indexed under this heading.

Fluphenazine Hydrochloride (Concomitant use may increase drowsiness).
No products indexed under this heading.

Flurazepam Hydrochloride (Concomitant use may increase drowsiness).
No products indexed under this heading.

Glutethimide (Concomitant use may increase drowsiness).
No products indexed under this heading.

Haloperidol (Concomitant use may increase drowsiness).
No products indexed under this heading.

Haloperidol Decanoate (Concomitant use may increase drowsiness).
No products indexed under this heading.

Hydroxyzine Hydrochloride (Concomitant use may increase drowsiness).
No products indexed under this heading.

Lorazepam (Concomitant use may increase drowsiness).
No products indexed under this heading.

Midazolam Hydrochloride (Concomitant use may increase drowsiness).
No products indexed under this heading.

Propofol (Concomitant use may increase drowsiness).
No products indexed under this heading.

Quazepam (Concomitant use may increase drowsiness).
No products indexed under this heading.

Ramelteon (Concomitant use may increase drowsiness). Products include:
Rozerem Tablets 3091

Secobarbital Sodium (Concomitant use may increase drowsiness).
No products indexed under this heading.

Sodium Butabarbital (Concomitant use may increase drowsiness).
No products indexed under this heading.

Temazepam (Concomitant use may increase drowsiness).
No products indexed under this heading.

Triazolam (Concomitant use may increase drowsiness).
No products indexed under this heading.

Zaleplon (Concomitant use may increase drowsiness).
No products indexed under this heading.

Zolpidem Tartrate (Concomitant use may increase drowsiness). Products include:
Ambien Tablets 2692
Ambien CR Tablets 2696

Food Interactions

Alcohol (Concomitant use may increase drowsiness).

CHILDREN'S ZYRTEC ALLERGY CHEWABLE TABLETS

(Cetirizine Hydrochloride) 1922

May interact with hypnotics and sedatives, tranquilizers, and certain other agents. Compounds in these categories include:

Alprazolam (Concomitant use may increase drowsiness).
No products indexed under this heading.

Buspirone Hydrochloride (Concomitant use may increase drowsiness).
No products indexed under this heading.

Butabarbital (Concomitant use may increase drowsiness).
No products indexed under this heading.

Butabarbital Sodium (Concomitant use may increase drowsiness).
No products indexed under this heading.

Chloral Hydrate (Concomitant use may increase drowsiness).
No products indexed under this heading.

Chlordiazepoxide (Concomitant use may increase drowsiness).
No products indexed under this heading.

Chlordiazepoxide Hydrochloride (Concomitant use may increase drowsiness).
No products indexed under this heading.

Chlorpromazine (Concomitant use may increase drowsiness).
No products indexed under this heading.

Chlorpromazine Hydrochloride (Concomitant use may increase drowsiness).
No products indexed under this heading.

Chlorprothixene (Concomitant use may increase drowsiness).
No products indexed under this heading.

Chlorprothixene Hydrochloride (Concomitant use may increase drowsiness).
No products indexed under this heading.

Clorazepate Dipotassium (Concomitant use may increase drowsiness).
No products indexed under this heading.

Diazepam (Concomitant use may increase drowsiness). Products include:
Valium Tablets 2658

Droperidol (Concomitant use may increase drowsiness).
No products indexed under this heading.

Estazolam (Concomitant use may increase drowsiness).
No products indexed under this heading.

Ethanol (Alcohol may increase drowsiness. Avoid alcoholic drinks).
No products indexed under this heading.

Ethchlorvynol (Concomitant use may increase drowsiness).
No products indexed under this heading.

Ethinamate (Concomitant use may increase drowsiness).
No products indexed under this heading.

Ethyl Alcohol (Alcohol may increase drowsiness. Avoid alcoholic drinks).
No products indexed under this heading.

Fluphenazine Decanoate (Concomitant use may increase drowsiness).
No products indexed under this heading.

Fluphenazine Enanthate (Concomitant use may increase drowsiness).
No products indexed under this heading.

Fluphenazine Hydrochloride (Concomitant use may increase drowsiness).
No products indexed under this heading.

Flurazepam Hydrochloride (Concomitant use may increase drowsiness).
No products indexed under this heading.

Glutethimide (Concomitant use may increase drowsiness).
No products indexed under this heading.

Haloperidol (Concomitant use may increase drowsiness).
No products indexed under this heading.

Haloperidol Decanoate (Concomitant use may increase drowsiness).
No products indexed under this heading.

Hydroxyzine Hydrochloride (Concomitant use may increase drowsiness).
No products indexed under this heading.

Lorazepam (Concomitant use may increase drowsiness).
No products indexed under this heading.

Loxapine Hydrochloride (Concomitant use may increase drowsiness).
No products indexed under this heading.

Loxapine Succinate (Concomitant use may increase drowsiness).
No products indexed under this heading.

Meprobamate (Concomitant use may increase drowsiness).
No products indexed under this heading.

Mesoridazine Besylate (Concomitant use may increase drowsiness).
No products indexed under this heading.

Midazolam Hydrochloride (Concomitant use may increase drowsiness).
No products indexed under this heading.

Molindone Hydrochloride (Concomitant use may increase drowsiness). Products include:
Moban Tablets 1116

Oxazepam (Concomitant use may increase drowsiness).
No products indexed under this heading.

Perphenazine (Concomitant use may increase drowsiness).
No products indexed under this heading.

Prazepam (Concomitant use may increase drowsiness).
No products indexed under this heading.

Prochlorperazine (Concomitant use may increase drowsiness).
No products indexed under this heading.

Promethazine Hydrochloride (Concomitant use may increase drowsiness).
No products indexed under this heading.

Propofol (Concomitant use may increase drowsiness).
No products indexed under this heading.

Quazepam (Concomitant use may increase drowsiness).
No products indexed under this heading.

Ramelteon (Concomitant use may increase drowsiness). Products include:
Rozerem Tablets 3091

Secobarbital Sodium (Concomitant use may increase drowsiness).
No products indexed under this heading.

Sodium Butabarbital (Concomitant use may increase drowsiness).
No products indexed under this heading.

Temazepam (Concomitant use may increase drowsiness).
No products indexed under this heading.

Thioridazine Hydrochloride (Concomitant use may increase drowsiness). Products include:
Thioridazine Hydrochloride Tablets 2195

Thiothixene (Concomitant use may increase drowsiness). Products include:
Thiothixene Capsules 2197

Triazolam (Concomitant use may increase drowsiness).
No products indexed under this heading.

Trifluoperazine Hydrochloride (Concomitant use may increase drowsiness).
No products indexed under this heading.

Zaleplon (Concomitant use may increase drowsiness).
No products indexed under this heading.

Zolpidem Tartrate (Concomitant use may increase drowsiness). Products include:
Ambien Tablets 2692
Ambien CR Tablets 2696

Food Interactions

Alcohol (Alcohol may increase drowsiness. Avoid alcoholic drinks).

CHILDREN'S ZYRTEC HIVES RELIEF SYRUP
(Cetirizine Hydrochloride) 1920
May interact with hypnotics and sedatives, tranquilizers, and certain other agents. Compounds in these categories include:

Alprazolam (Concomitant use may increase drowsiness).
No products indexed under this heading.

Buspirone Hydrochloride (Concomitant use may increase drowsiness).
No products indexed under this heading.

Butabarbital (Concomitant use may increase drowsiness).
No products indexed under this heading.

Butabarbital Sodium (Concomitant use may increase drowsiness).
No products indexed under this heading.

Chloral Hydrate (Concomitant use may increase drowsiness).
No products indexed under this heading.

Chlordiazepoxide (Concomitant use may increase drowsiness).
No products indexed under this heading.

Chlordiazepoxide Hydrochloride (Concomitant use may increase drowsiness).
No products indexed under this heading.

Chlorpromazine (Concomitant use may increase drowsiness).
No products indexed under this heading.

Chlorpromazine Hydrochloride (Concomitant use may increase drowsiness).
No products indexed under this heading.

Chlorprothixene (Concomitant use may increase drowsiness).
No products indexed under this heading.

Chlorprothixene Hydrochloride (Concomitant use may increase drowsiness).
No products indexed under this heading.

Clorazepate Dipotassium (Concomitant use may increase drowsiness).
No products indexed under this heading.

Diazepam (Concomitant use may increase drowsiness). Products include:
Valium Tablets 2658

Droperidol (Concomitant use may increase drowsiness).
No products indexed under this heading.

Estazolam (Concomitant use may increase drowsiness).
No products indexed under this heading.

Ethanol (Concomitant use may increase drowsiness).
No products indexed under this heading.

Ethchlorvynol (Concomitant use may increase drowsiness).
No products indexed under this heading.

Ethinamate (Concomitant use may increase drowsiness).
No products indexed under this heading.

Ethyl Alcohol (Concomitant use may increase drowsiness).
No products indexed under this heading.

Fluphenazine Decanoate (Concomitant use may increase drowsiness).
No products indexed under this heading.

Fluphenazine Enanthate (Concomitant use may increase drowsiness).
No products indexed under this heading.

Fluphenazine Hydrochloride (Concomitant use may increase drowsiness).
No products indexed under this heading.

Flurazepam Hydrochloride (Concomitant use may increase drowsiness).
No products indexed under this heading.

Glutethimide (Concomitant use may increase drowsiness).
No products indexed under this heading.

Haloperidol (Concomitant use may increase drowsiness).
No products indexed under this heading.

Haloperidol Decanoate (Concomitant use may increase drowsiness).
No products indexed under this heading.

Hydroxyzine Hydrochloride (Concomitant use may increase drowsiness).
No products indexed under this heading.

Lorazepam (Concomitant use may increase drowsiness).
No products indexed under this heading.

Loxapine Hydrochloride (Concomitant use may increase drowsiness).
No products indexed under this heading.

Loxapine Succinate (Concomitant use may increase drowsiness).
No products indexed under this heading.

Meprobamate (Concomitant use may increase drowsiness).
No products indexed under this heading.

Mesoridazine Besylate (Concomitant use may increase drowsiness).
No products indexed under this heading.

Midazolam Hydrochloride (Concomitant use may increase drowsiness).
No products indexed under this heading.

Molindone Hydrochloride (Concomitant use may increase drowsiness). Products include:
Moban Tablets 1116

Oxazepam (Concomitant use may increase drowsiness).
No products indexed under this heading.

Perphenazine (Concomitant use may increase drowsiness).
No products indexed under this heading.

Prazepam (Concomitant use may increase drowsiness).
No products indexed under this heading.

Prochlorperazine (Concomitant use may increase drowsiness).
No products indexed under this heading.

Promethazine Hydrochloride (Concomitant use may increase drowsiness).
No products indexed under this heading.

Propofol (Concomitant use may increase drowsiness).
No products indexed under this heading.

Quazepam (Concomitant use may increase drowsiness).
No products indexed under this heading.

Ramelteon (Concomitant use may increase drowsiness). Products include:
Rozerem Tablets 3091

Secobarbital Sodium (Concomitant use may increase drowsiness).
No products indexed under this heading.

Sodium Butabarbital (Concomitant use may increase drowsiness).
No products indexed under this heading.

Temazepam (Concomitant use may increase drowsiness).
No products indexed under this heading.

Thioridazine Hydrochloride (Concomitant use may increase drowsiness). Products include:
Thioridazine Hydrochloride Tablets 2195

Thiothixene (Concomitant use may increase drowsiness). Products include:
Thiothixene Capsules 2197

Triazolam (Concomitant use may increase drowsiness).
No products indexed under this heading.

Trifluoperazine Hydrochloride (Concomitant use may increase drowsiness).
No products indexed under this heading.

Zaleplon (Concomitant use may increase drowsiness).
No products indexed under this heading.

Zolpidem Tartrate (Concomitant use may increase drowsiness). Products include:
Ambien Tablets 2692
Ambien CR Tablets 2696

Food Interactions

Alcohol (Concomitant use may increase drowsiness).

ZYRTEC SYRUP
(Cetirizine Hydrochloride) 1920
See Zyrtec Tablets

ZYRTEC TABLETS
(Cetirizine Hydrochloride) 1920
May interact with central nervous system depressants, theophyllines, and certain other agents. Compounds in these categories include:

Alfentanil Hydrochloride (Concurrent use of cetirizine with CNS depressants should be avoided because additional reductions in alertness and additional impairment of CNS performance may occur).
No products indexed under this heading.

Alprazolam (Concurrent use of cetirizine with CNS depressants should be avoided because additional reductions in alertness and additional impairment of CNS performance may occur).
No products indexed under this heading.

Aprobarbital (Concurrent use of cetirizine with CNS depressants should be avoided because additional reductions in alertness and additional impairment of CNS performance may occur).
No products indexed under this heading.

Buprenorphine Hydrochloride (Concurrent use of cetirizine with CNS depressants should be avoided because additional reductions in alertness and additional impairment of CNS performance may occur). Products include:
Suboxone Tablets 2601
Subutex Tablets 2601

Buspirone Hydrochloride (Concurrent use of cetirizine with CNS depressants should be avoided because additional reductions in alertness and additional impairment of CNS performance may occur).
No products indexed under this heading.

Butabarbital (Concurrent use of cetirizine with CNS depressants should be avoided because additional reductions in alertness and additional impairment of CNS performance may occur).
No products indexed under this heading.

Butalbital (Concurrent use of cetirizine with CNS depressants should be avoided because additional reductions in alertness and additional impairment of CNS performance may occur).
No products indexed under this heading.

Chlordiazepoxide (Concurrent use of cetirizine with CNS depressants should be avoided because additional reductions in alertness and additional impairment of CNS performance may occur).
No products indexed under this heading.

Chlordiazepoxide Hydrochloride (Concurrent use of cetirizine with CNS depressants should be avoided because additional reductions in alertness and additional impairment of CNS performance may occur).
No products indexed under this heading.

Chlorpromazine (Concurrent use of cetirizine with CNS depressants should be avoided because additional reductions in alertness and additional impairment of CNS performance may occur).
No products indexed under this heading.

Chlorpromazine Hydrochloride (Concurrent use of cetirizine with CNS depressants should be avoided because additional reductions in alertness and additional impairment of CNS performance may occur).
No products indexed under this heading.

Chlorprothixene (Concurrent use of cetirizine with CNS depressants should be avoided because additional reductions in alertness and additional impairment of CNS performance may occur).
No products indexed under this heading.

Chlorprothixene Hydrochloride (Concurrent use of cetirizine with CNS depressants should be avoided because additional reductions in alertness and additional impairment of CNS performance may occur).
No products indexed under this heading.

Chlorprothixene Lactate (Concurrent use of cetirizine with CNS depressants should be avoided because additional reductions in alertness and additional impairment of CNS performance may occur).
No products indexed under this heading.

Clorazepate Dipotassium (Concurrent use of cetirizine with CNS depressants should be avoided because additional reductions in alertness and additional impairment of CNS performance may occur).
No products indexed under this heading.

Clozapine (Concurrent use of cetirizine with CNS depressants should be avoided because additional reductions in alertness and additional impairment of CNS performance may occur).
No products indexed under this heading.

Codeine Phosphate (Concurrent use of cetirizine with CNS depressants should be avoided because additional reductions in alertness and additional impairment of CNS performance may occur). Products include:
Tylenol with Codeine Tablets 2427

Desflurane (Concurrent use of cetirizine with CNS depressants should be avoided because additional reductions in alertness and additional impairment of CNS performance may occur).
No products indexed under this heading.

Dezocine (Concurrent use of cetirizine with CNS depressants should be avoided because additional reductions in alertness and additional impairment of CNS performance may occur).
No products indexed under this heading.

Diazepam (Concurrent use of cetirizine with CNS depressants should be avoided because additional reductions in alertness and additional impairment of CNS performance may occur). Products include:
Valium Tablets 2658

Droperidol (Concurrent use of cetirizine with CNS depressants should be avoided because additional reductions in alertness and additional impairment of CNS performance may occur).
No products indexed under this heading.

Enflurane (Concurrent use of cetirizine with CNS depressants should be avoided because additional reductions in alertness and additional impairment of CNS performance may occur).
No products indexed under this heading.

Estazolam (Concurrent use of cetirizine with CNS depressants should be avoided because additional reductions in alertness and additional impairment of CNS performance may occur).
No products indexed under this heading.

Ethanol (Concurrent use of cetirizine with alcohol should be avoided because additional reductions in alertness and additional impairment of CNS performance may occur).
No products indexed under this heading.

Ethchlorvynol (Concurrent use of cetirizine with CNS depressants should be avoided because additional reductions in alertness and additional impairment of CNS performance may occur).
No products indexed under this heading.

Ethinamate (Concurrent use of cetirizine with CNS depressants should be avoided because additional reductions in alertness and additional impairment of CNS performance may occur).
No products indexed under this heading.

Ethyl Alcohol (Concurrent use of cetirizine with alcohol should be avoided because additional reductions in alertness and additional impairment of CNS performance may occur).
No products indexed under this heading.

Fentanyl (Concurrent use of cetirizine with CNS depressants should be avoided because additional reductions in alertness and additional impairment of CNS performance may occur). Products include:
Duragesic Transdermal System 2405
Ionsys Transdermal System 2410

Fentanyl Citrate (Concurrent use of cetirizine with CNS depressants should be avoided because additional reductions in alertness and additional impairment of CNS performance may occur). Products include:
Actiq 959
Fentora Tablets 968

Fluphenazine Decanoate (Concurrent use of cetirizine with CNS depressants should be avoided because additional reductions in alertness and additional impairment of CNS performance may occur).
No products indexed under this heading.

Fluphenazine Enanthate (Concurrent use of cetirizine with CNS depressants should be avoided because additional reductions in alertness and additional impairment of CNS performance may occur).
No products indexed under this heading.

Fluphenazine Hydrochloride (Concurrent use of cetirizine with CNS depressants should be avoided because additional reductions in alertness and additional impairment of CNS performance may occur).
No products indexed under this heading.

Flurazepam Hydrochloride (Concurrent use of cetirizine with CNS depressants should be avoided because additional reductions in alertness and additional impairment of CNS performance may occur).
No products indexed under this heading.

Glutethimide (Concurrent use of cetirizine with CNS depressants should be avoided because additional reductions in alertness and additional impairment of CNS performance may occur).
No products indexed under this heading.

Haloperidol (Concurrent use of cetirizine with CNS depressants should be avoided because additional reductions in alertness and additional impairment of CNS performance may occur).
No products indexed under this heading.

Haloperidol Decanoate (Concurrent use of cetirizine with CNS depressants should be avoided because additional reductions in alertness and additional impairment of CNS performance may occur).
No products indexed under this heading.

Hydrocodone Bitartrate (Concurrent use of cetirizine with CNS depressants should be avoided because additional reductions in alertness and additional impairment of CNS performance may occur). Products include:
Lortab 5/500 Tablets 3143
Lortab 7.5/500 Tablets 3144
Lortab 10/500 Tablets 3144
Vicodin Tablets 529
Vicodin ES Tablets 530
Vicodin HP Tablets 531
Vicoprofen Tablets 533
Zydone Tablets 1132

Hydrocodone Polistirex (Concurrent use of cetirizine with CNS depressants should be avoided because additional reductions in alertness and additional impairment of CNS performance may occur). Products include:
Tussionex Pennkinetic Extended-Release Suspension...... 3154

Hydromorphone Hydrochloride (Concurrent use of cetirizine with CNS depressants should be avoided because additional reductions in alertness and additional impairment of CNS performance may occur).
No products indexed under this heading.

Hydroxyzine Hydrochloride (Concurrent use of cetirizine with CNS depressants should be avoided because additional reductions in alertness and additional impairment of CNS performance may occur).
No products indexed under this heading.

Isoflurane (Concurrent use of cetirizine with CNS depressants should be avoided because additional reductions in alertness and additional impairment of CNS performance may occur).
No products indexed under this heading.

Ketamine Hydrochloride (Concurrent use of cetirizine with CNS depressants should be avoided because additional reductions in alertness and additional impairment of CNS performance may occur).
No products indexed under this heading.

Levomethadyl Acetate Hydrochloride (Concurrent use of cetirizine with CNS depressants should be avoided because additional reductions in alertness and additional impairment of CNS performance may occur).
No products indexed under this heading.

Levorphanol Tartrate (Concurrent use of cetirizine with CNS depressants should be avoided because additional reductions in alertness and additional impairment of CNS performance may occur).
No products indexed under this heading.

Lorazepam (Concurrent use of cetirizine with CNS depressants should be avoided because additional reductions in alertness and additional impairment of CNS performance may occur).
No products indexed under this heading.

Loxapine Hydrochloride (Concurrent use of cetirizine with CNS depressants should be avoided because additional reductions in alertness and additional impairment of CNS performance may occur).
No products indexed under this heading.

Loxapine Succinate (Concurrent use of cetirizine with CNS depressants should be avoided because additional reductions in alertness and additional impairment of CNS performance may occur).
No products indexed under this heading.

Meperidine Hydrochloride (Concurrent use of cetirizine with CNS depressants should be avoided because additional reductions in alertness and additional impairment of CNS performance may occur).
No products indexed under this heading.

Mephobarbital (Concurrent use of cetirizine with CNS depressants should be avoided because additional reductions in alertness and additional impairment of CNS performance may occur).
No products indexed under this heading.

Meprobamate (Concurrent use of cetirizine with CNS depressants should be avoided because additional reductions in alertness and additional impairment of CNS performance may occur).
No products indexed under this heading.

Mesoridazine Besylate (Concurrent use of cetirizine with CNS depressants should be avoided because additional reductions in alertness and additional impairment of CNS performance may occur).
No products indexed under this heading.

Methadone Hydrochloride (Concurrent use of cetirizine with CNS depressants should be avoided because additional reductions in alertness and additional impairment of CNS performance may occur).
No products indexed under this heading.

Methohexital Sodium (Concurrent use of cetirizine with CNS depressants should be avoided because additional reductions in alertness and additional impairment of CNS performance may occur).
No products indexed under this heading.

Methotrimeprazine (Concurrent use of cetirizine with CNS depressants should be avoided because additional reductions in alertness and additional impairment of CNS performance may occur).
No products indexed under this heading.

Methoxyflurane (Concurrent use of cetirizine with CNS depressants should be avoided because additional reductions in alertness and additional impairment of CNS performance may occur).
No products indexed under this heading.

Midazolam Hydrochloride (Concurrent use of cetirizine with CNS depressants should be avoided because additional reductions in alertness and additional impairment of CNS performance may occur).
No products indexed under this heading.

Molindone Hydrochloride (Concurrent use of cetirizine with CNS depressants should be avoided because additional reductions in alertness and additional impairment of CNS performance may occur). Products include:
Moban Tablets ... **1116**

Morphine Sulfate (Concurrent use of cetirizine with CNS depressants should be avoided because additional reductions in alertness and additional impairment of CNS performance may occur). Products include:
Avinza Capsules ... **1772**
DepoDur Injection ... **1095**
MS Contin Tablets ... **2585**

Olanzapine (Concurrent use of cetirizine with CNS depressants should be avoided because additional reductions in alertness and additional impairment of CNS performance may occur). Products include:
Symbyax Capsules ... **1871**
Zyprexa Tablets ... **1883**
Zyprexa IntraMuscular ... **1883**
Zyprexa ZYDIS Orally Disintegrating Tablets ... **1883**

Oxazepam (Concurrent use of cetirizine with CNS depressants should be avoided because additional reductions in alertness and additional impairment of CNS performance may occur).
No products indexed under this heading.

Oxycodone Hydrochloride (Concurrent use of cetirizine with CNS depressants should be avoided because additional reductions in alertness and additional impairment of CNS performance may occur). Products include:
OxyContin Tablets ... **2589**
OxyIR Capsules ... **2593**
Percocet Tablets ... **1127**
Percodan Tablets ... **1130**

Pentobarbital Sodium (Concurrent use of cetirizine with CNS depressants should be avoided because additional reductions in alertness and additional impairment of CNS performance may occur). Products include:
Nembutal Sodium Solution, USP ... **2494**

Perphenazine (Concurrent use of cetirizine with CNS depressants should be avoided because additional reductions in alertness and additional impairment of CNS performance may occur).
No products indexed under this heading.

Phenobarbital (Concurrent use of cetirizine with CNS depressants should be avoided because additional reductions in alertness and additional impairment of CNS performance may occur). Products include:
Donnatal Extentabs ... **2507**

Prazepam (Concurrent use of cetirizine with CNS depressants should be avoided because additional reductions in alertness and additional impairment of CNS performance may occur).
No products indexed under this heading.

Prochlorperazine (Concurrent use of cetirizine with CNS depressants should be avoided because additional reductions in alertness and additional impairment of CNS performance may occur).
No products indexed under this heading.

Promethazine Hydrochloride (Concurrent use of cetirizine with CNS depressants should be avoided because additional reductions in alertness and additional impairment of CNS performance may occur).
No products indexed under this heading.

Propofol (Concurrent use of cetirizine with CNS depressants should be avoided because additional reductions in alertness and additional impairment of CNS performance may occur).
No products indexed under this heading.

Propoxyphene Hydrochloride (Concurrent use of cetirizine with CNS depressants should be avoided because additional reductions in alertness and additional impairment of CNS performance may occur).
No products indexed under this heading.

Propoxyphene Napsylate (Concurrent use of cetirizine with CNS depressants should be avoided because additional reductions in alertness and additional impairment of CNS performance may occur).
No products indexed under this heading.

Quazepam (Concurrent use of cetirizine with CNS depressants should be avoided because additional reductions in alertness and additional impairment of CNS performance may occur).
No products indexed under this heading.

Quetiapine Fumarate (Concurrent use of cetirizine with CNS depressants should be avoided because additional reductions in alertness and additional impairment of CNS performance may occur).
No products indexed under this heading.

Remifentanil Hydrochloride (Concurrent use of cetirizine with CNS depressants should be avoided because additional reductions in alertness and additional impairment of CNS performance may occur).
No products indexed under this heading.

Risperidone (Concurrent use of cetirizine with CNS depressants should be avoided because additional reductions in alertness and additional impairment of CNS performance may occur). Products include:
Risperdal Consta Long-Acting Injection ... **1753**

Secobarbital Sodium (Concurrent use of cetirizine with CNS depressants should be avoided because additional reductions in alertness and additional impairment of CNS performance may occur).
No products indexed under this heading.

Sevoflurane (Concurrent use of cetirizine with CNS depressants should be avoided because additional reductions in alertness and additional impairment of CNS performance may occur). Products include:
Ultane Liquid for Inhalation ... **524**

Sodium Oxybate (Concurrent use of cetirizine with CNS depressants should be avoided because additional reductions in alertness and additional impairment of CNS performance may occur). Products include:
Xyrem Oral Solution ... **1766**

Sufentanil Citrate (Concurrent use of cetirizine with CNS depressants should be avoided because additional reductions in alertness and additional impairment of CNS performance may occur).
No products indexed under this heading.

Temazepam (Concurrent use of cetirizine with CNS depressants should be avoided because additional reductions in alertness and additional impairment of CNS performance may occur).
No products indexed under this heading.

Theophylline (There was a small decrease in the clearance of cetirizine caused by a 400 mg dose of theophylline; it is possible that larger theophylline doses could have a greater effect).
No products indexed under this heading.

Theophylline Anhydrous (There was a small decrease in the clearance of cetirizine caused by a 400 mg dose of theophylline; it is possible that larger theophylline doses could have a greater effect). Products include:
Uniphyl Tablets ... **2595**

Theophylline Calcium Salicylate (There was a small decrease in the clearance of cetirizine caused by a 400 mg dose of theophylline; it is possible that larger theophylline doses could have a greater effect).
No products indexed under this heading.

Theophylline Dihydroxypropyl (Glyceryl) (There was a small decrease in the clearance of cetirizine caused by a 400 mg dose of theophylline; it is possible that larger theophylline doses could have a greater effect).
No products indexed under this heading.

Theophylline Ethylenediamine (There was a small decrease in the clearance of cetirizine caused by a 400 mg dose of theophylline; it is possible that larger theophylline doses could have a greater effect).
No products indexed under this heading.

Theophylline Sodium Glycinate (There was a small decrease in the clearance of cetirizine caused by a 400 mg dose of theophylline; it is possible that larger theophylline doses could have a greater effect).
No products indexed under this heading.

Thiamylal Sodium (Concurrent use of cetirizine with CNS depressants should be avoided because additional reductions in alertness and additional impairment of CNS performance may occur).
No products indexed under this heading.

Thioridazine Hydrochloride (Concurrent use of cetirizine with CNS depressants should be avoided because additional reductions in alertness and additional impairment of CNS performance may occur). Products include:
Thioridazine Hydrochloride Tablets ... **2195**

Thiothixene (Concurrent use of cetirizine with CNS depressants should be avoided because additional reductions in alertness and additional impairment of CNS performance may occur). Products include:
Thiothixene Capsules 2197

Triazolam (Concurrent use of cetirizine with CNS depressants should be avoided because additional reductions in alertness and additional impairment of CNS performance may occur).
No products indexed under this heading.

Trifluoperazine Hydrochloride (Concurrent use of cetirizine with CNS depressants should be avoided because additional reductions in alertness and additional impairment of CNS performance may occur).
No products indexed under this heading.

Zaleplon (Concurrent use of cetirizine with CNS depressants should be avoided because additional reductions in alertness and additional impairment of CNS performance may occur).
No products indexed under this heading.

Ziprasidone Hydrochloride (Concurrent use of cetirizine with CNS depressants should be avoided because additional reductions in alertness and additional impairment of CNS performance may occur). Products include:
Geodon Capsules 2520

Zolpidem Tartrate (Concurrent use of cetirizine with CNS depressants should be avoided because additional reductions in alertness and additional impairment of CNS performance may occur). Products include:
Ambien Tablets 2692
Ambien CR Tablets 2696

Food Interactions

Alcohol (Concurrent use of cetirizine with alcohol should be avoided because additional reductions in alertness and additional impairment of CNS performance may occur).

ZYRTEC-D 12 HOUR EXTENDED RELEASE TABLETS

(Cetirizine Hydrochloride, Pseudoephedrine Hydrochloride)........ 1923
May interact with central nervous system depressants, monoamine oxidase inhibitors, sympathomimetics, theophyllines, and certain other agents. Compounds in these categories include:

Albuterol (Care should be taken in the administration of Zyrtec-D 12 Hour extended release tablets concomitantly with other sympathomimetic amines because combined effects on the cardiovascular system may be harmful to the patient).
No products indexed under this heading.

Albuterol Sulfate (Care should be taken in the administration of Zyrtec-D 12 Hour extended release tablets concomitantly with other sympathomimetic amines because combined effects on the cardiovascular system may be harmful to the patient). Products include:
Combivent Inhalation Aerosol 845
ProAir HFA Inhalation Aerosol 3113
Proventil HFA Inhalation Aerosol 2914
Ventolin HFA Inhalation Aerosol 1638

Alfentanil Hydrochloride (Concurrent use of Zyrtec-D 12 Hour extended release tablets with other CNS depressants should be avoided because additional reductions in alertness and additional impairment of CNS performance may occur).
No products indexed under this heading.

Alprazolam (Concurrent use of Zyrtec-D 12 Hour extended release tablets with other CNS depressants should be avoided because additional reductions in alertness and additional impairment of CNS performance may occur).
No products indexed under this heading.

Aprobarbital (Concurrent use of Zyrtec-D 12 Hour extended release tablets with other CNS depressants should be avoided because additional reductions in alertness and additional impairment of CNS performance may occur).
No products indexed under this heading.

Buprenorphine Hydrochloride (Concurrent use of Zyrtec-D 12 Hour extended release tablets with other CNS depressants should be avoided because additional reductions in alertness and additional impairment of CNS performance may occur). Products include:
Suboxone Tablets 2601
Subutex Tablets 2601

Buspirone Hydrochloride (Concurrent use of Zyrtec-D 12 Hour extended release tablets with other CNS depressants should be avoided because additional reductions in alertness and additional impairment of CNS performance may occur).
No products indexed under this heading.

Butabarbital (Concurrent use of Zyrtec-D 12 Hour extended release tablets with other CNS depressants should be avoided because additional reductions in alertness and additional impairment of CNS performance may occur).
No products indexed under this heading.

Butalbital (Concurrent use of Zyrtec-D 12 Hour extended release tablets with other CNS depressants should be avoided because additional reductions in alertness and additional impairment of CNS performance may occur).
No products indexed under this heading.

Chlordiazepoxide (Concurrent use of Zyrtec-D 12 Hour extended release tablets with other CNS depressants should be avoided because additional reductions in alertness and additional impairment of CNS performance may occur).
No products indexed under this heading.

Chlordiazepoxide Hydrochloride (Concurrent use of Zyrtec-D 12 Hour extended release tablets with other CNS depressants should be avoided because additional reductions in alertness and additional impairment of CNS performance may occur).
No products indexed under this heading.

Chlorpromazine (Concurrent use of Zyrtec-D 12 Hour extended release tablets with other CNS depressants should be avoided because additional reductions in alertness and additional impairment of CNS performance may occur).
No products indexed under this heading.

Chlorpromazine Hydrochloride (Concurrent use of Zyrtec-D 12 Hour extended release tablets with other CNS depressants should be avoided because additional reductions in alertness and additional impairment of CNS performance may occur).
No products indexed under this heading.

Chlorprothixene (Concurrent use of Zyrtec-D 12 Hour extended release tablets with other CNS depressants should be avoided because additional reductions in alertness and additional impairment of CNS performance may occur).
No products indexed under this heading.

Chlorprothixene Hydrochloride (Concurrent use of Zyrtec-D 12 Hour extended release tablets with other CNS depressants should be avoided because additional reductions in alertness and additional impairment of CNS performance may occur).
No products indexed under this heading.

Chlorprothixene Lactate (Concurrent use of Zyrtec-D 12 Hour extended release tablets with other CNS depressants should be avoided because additional reductions in alertness and additional impairment of CNS performance may occur).
No products indexed under this heading.

Clorazepate Dipotassium (Concurrent use of Zyrtec-D 12 Hour extended release tablets with other CNS depressants should be avoided because additional reductions in alertness and additional impairment of CNS performance may occur).
No products indexed under this heading.

Clozapine (Concurrent use of Zyrtec-D 12 Hour extended release tablets with other CNS depressants should be avoided because additional reductions in alertness and additional impairment of CNS performance may occur).
No products indexed under this heading.

Codeine Phosphate (Concurrent use of Zyrtec-D 12 Hour extended release tablets with other CNS depressants should be avoided because additional reductions in alertness and additional impairment of CNS performance may occur). Products include:
Tylenol with Codeine Tablets 2427

Desflurane (Concurrent use of Zyrtec-D 12 Hour extended release tablets with other CNS depressants should be avoided because additional reductions in alertness and additional impairment of CNS performance may occur).
No products indexed under this heading.

Dezocine (Concurrent use of Zyrtec-D 12 Hour extended release tablets with other CNS depressants should be avoided because additional reductions in alertness and additional impairment of CNS performance may occur).
No products indexed under this heading.

Diazepam (Concurrent use of Zyrtec-D 12 Hour extended release tablets with other CNS depressants should be avoided because additional reductions in alertness and additional impairment of CNS performance may occur). Products include:
Valium Tablets 2658

Digoxin (Increased ectopic pacemaker activity can occur when pseudoephedrine is used concomitantly with digitalis). Products include:
Lanoxin Injection 1498
Lanoxin Injection Pediatric 1502
Lanoxin Tablets 1505

Dobutamine Hydrochloride (Care should be taken in the administration of Zyrtec-D 12 Hour extended release tablets concomitantly with other sympathomimetic amines because combined effects on the cardiovascular system may be harmful to the patient).
No products indexed under this heading.

Dopamine Hydrochloride (Care should be taken in the administration of Zyrtec-D 12 Hour extended release tablets concomitantly with other sympathomimetic amines because combined effects on the cardiovascular system may be harmful to the patient).
No products indexed under this heading.

Droperidol (Concurrent use of Zyrtec-D 12 Hour extended release tablets with other CNS depressants should be avoided because additional reductions in alertness and additional impairment of CNS performance may occur).
No products indexed under this heading.

Enflurane (Concurrent use of Zyrtec-D 12 Hour extended release tablets with other CNS depressants should be avoided because additional reductions in alertness and additional impairment of CNS performance may occur).
No products indexed under this heading.

Ephedrine Hydrochloride (Care should be taken in the administration of Zyrtec-D 12 Hour extended release tablets concomitantly with other sympathomimetic amines because combined effects on the cardiovascular system may be harmful to the patient).
No products indexed under this heading.

Ephedrine Sulfate (Care should be taken in the administration of Zyrtec-D 12 Hour extended release tablets concomitantly with other sympathomimetic amines because combined effects on the cardiovascular system may be harmful to the patient).
No products indexed under this heading.

Ephedrine Tannate (Care should be taken in the administration of Zyrtec-D 12 Hour extended release tablets concomitantly with other sympathomimetic amines because combined effects on the cardiovascular system may be harmful to the patient).
No products indexed under this heading.

Epinephrine (Care should be taken in the administration of Zyrtec-D 12 Hour extended release tablets concomitantly with other sympathomimetic amines because combined effects on the cardiovascular system may be harmful to the patient). Products include:
EpiPen ... 1024

Epinephrine Bitartrate (Care should be taken in the administration of Zyrtec-D 12 Hour extended release tablets concomitantly with other sympathomimetic amines because combined effects on the cardiovascular system may be harmful to the patient).
No products indexed under this heading.

Epinephrine Hydrochloride (Care should be taken in the administration of Zyrtec-D 12 Hour extended release tablets concomitantly with other sympathomimetic amines because combined effects on the cardiovascular system may be harmful to the patient).
No products indexed under this heading.

Estazolam (Concurrent use of Zyrtec-D 12 Hour extended release tablets with other CNS depressants should be avoided because additional reductions in alertness and additional impairment of CNS performance may occur).
No products indexed under this heading.

Ethanol (Concurrent use of Zyrtec-D 12 Hour extended release tablets with alcohol should be avoided because additional reductions in alertness and additional impairment of CNS performance may occur).
No products indexed under this heading.

Ethchlorvynol (Concurrent use of Zyrtec-D 12 Hour extended release tablets with other CNS depressants should be avoided because additional reductions in alertness and additional impairment of CNS performance may occur).
No products indexed under this heading.

Ethinamate (Concurrent use of Zyrtec-D 12 Hour extended release tablets with other CNS depressants should be avoided because additional reductions in alertness and additional impairment of CNS performance may occur).
No products indexed under this heading.

Ethyl Alcohol (Concurrent use of Zyrtec-D 12 Hour extended release tablets with alcohol should be avoided because additional reductions in alertness and additional impairment of CNS performance may occur).
No products indexed under this heading.

Fentanyl (Concurrent use of Zyrtec-D 12 Hour extended release tablets with other CNS depressants should be avoided because additional reductions in alertness and additional impairment of CNS performance may occur). Products include:
Duragesic Transdermal System ... 2405
Ionsys Transdermal System ... 2410

Fentanyl Citrate (Concurrent use of Zyrtec-D 12 Hour extended release tablets with other CNS depressants should be avoided because additional reductions in alertness and additional impairment of CNS performance may occur). Products include:
Actiq ... 959
Fentora Tablets ... 968

Fluphenazine Decanoate (Concurrent use of Zyrtec-D 12 Hour extended release tablets with other CNS depressants should be avoided because additional reductions in alertness and additional impairment of CNS performance may occur).
No products indexed under this heading.

Fluphenazine Enanthate (Concurrent use of Zyrtec-D 12 Hour extended release tablets with other CNS depressants should be avoided because additional reductions in alertness and additional impairment of CNS performance may occur).
No products indexed under this heading.

Fluphenazine Hydrochloride (Concurrent use of Zyrtec-D 12 Hour extended release tablets with other CNS depressants should be avoided because additional reductions in alertness and additional impairment of CNS performance may occur).
No products indexed under this heading.

Flurazepam Hydrochloride (Concurrent use of Zyrtec-D 12 Hour extended release tablets with other CNS depressants should be avoided because additional reductions in alertness and additional impairment of CNS performance may occur).
No products indexed under this heading.

Glutethimide (Concurrent use of Zyrtec-D 12 Hour extended release tablets with other CNS depressants should be avoided because additional reductions in alertness and additional impairment of CNS performance may occur).
No products indexed under this heading.

Haloperidol (Concurrent use of Zyrtec-D 12 Hour extended release tablets with other CNS depressants should be avoided because additional reductions in alertness and additional impairment of CNS performance may occur).
No products indexed under this heading.

Haloperidol Decanoate (Concurrent use of Zyrtec-D 12 Hour extended release tablets with other CNS depressants should be avoided because additional reductions in alertness and additional impairment of CNS performance may occur).
No products indexed under this heading.

Hydrocodone Bitartrate (Concurrent use of Zyrtec-D 12 Hour extended release tablets with other CNS depressants should be avoided because additional reductions in alertness and additional impairment of CNS performance may occur). Products include:
Lortab 5/500 Tablets ... 3143
Lortab 7.5/500 Tablets ... 3144
Lortab 10/500 Tablets ... 3144
Vicodin Tablets ... 529
Vicodin ES Tablets ... 530
Vicodin HP Tablets ... 531
Vicoprofen Tablets ... 533
Zydone Tablets ... 1132

Hydrocodone Polistirex (Concurrent use of Zyrtec-D 12 Hour extended release tablets with other CNS depressants should be avoided because additional reductions in alertness and additional impairment of CNS performance may occur). Products include:
Tussionex Pennkinetic Extended-Release Suspension ... 3154

Hydromorphone Hydrochloride (Concurrent use of Zyrtec-D 12 Hour extended release tablets with other CNS depressants should be avoided because additional reductions in alertness and additional impairment of CNS performance may occur).
No products indexed under this heading.

Hydroxyzine Hydrochloride (Concurrent use of Zyrtec-D 12 Hour extended release tablets with other CNS depressants should be avoided because additional reductions in alertness and additional impairment of CNS performance may occur).
No products indexed under this heading.

Isocarboxazid (Due to the pseudoephedrine component, Zyrtec-D 12 Hour extended release tablets are contraindicated in patients taking monoamine oxidase (MAO) inhibitors and for 14 days after stopping use of an MAO inhibitor). Products include:
Marplan Tablets ... 3177

Isoflurane (Concurrent use of Zyrtec-D 12 Hour extended release tablets with other CNS depressants should be avoided because additional reductions in alertness and additional impairment of CNS performance may occur).
No products indexed under this heading.

Isoproterenol Hydrochloride (Care should be taken in the administration of Zyrtec-D 12 Hour extended release tablets concomitantly with other sympathomimetic amines because combined effects on the cardiovascular system may be harmful to the patient).
No products indexed under this heading.

Isoproterenol Sulfate (Care should be taken in the administration of Zyrtec-D 12 Hour extended release tablets concomitantly with other sympathomimetic amines because combined effects on the cardiovascular system may be harmful to the patient).
No products indexed under this heading.

Ketamine Hydrochloride (Concurrent use of Zyrtec-D 12 Hour extended release tablets with other CNS depressants should be avoided because additional reductions in alertness and additional impairment of CNS performance may occur).
No products indexed under this heading.

Levalbuterol Hydrochloride (Care should be taken in the administration of Zyrtec-D 12 Hour extended release tablets concomitantly with other sympathomimetic amines because combined effects on the cardiovascular system may be harmful to the patient). Products include:
Xopenex Inhalation Solution ... 3001
Xopenex Inhalation Solution Concentrate ... 3005

Levomethadyl Acetate Hydrochloride (Concurrent use of Zyrtec-D 12 Hour extended release tablets with other CNS depressants should be avoided because additional reductions in alertness and additional impairment of CNS performance may occur).
No products indexed under this heading.

Levorphanol Tartrate (Concurrent use of Zyrtec-D 12 Hour extended release tablets with other CNS depressants should be avoided because additional reductions in alertness and additional impairment of CNS performance may occur).
No products indexed under this heading.

Lorazepam (Concurrent use of Zyrtec-D 12 Hour extended release tablets with other CNS depressants should be avoided because additional reductions in alertness and additional impairment of CNS performance may occur).
No products indexed under this heading.

Loxapine Hydrochloride (Concurrent use of Zyrtec-D 12 Hour extended release tablets with other CNS depressants should be avoided because additional reductions in alertness and additional impairment of CNS performance may occur).
No products indexed under this heading.

Loxapine Succinate (Concurrent use of Zyrtec-D 12 Hour extended release tablets with other CNS depressants should be avoided because additional reductions in alertness and additional impairment of CNS performance may occur).
No products indexed under this heading.

Mecamylamine Hydrochloride (Concomitant use with antihypertensive drugs that interfere with sympathetic activity (eg, mecamylamine), may reduce the antihypertensive effects of mecamylamine).
No products indexed under this heading.

Meperidine Hydrochloride (Concurrent use of Zyrtec-D 12 Hour extended release tablets with other CNS depressants should be avoided because additional reductions in alertness and additional impairment of CNS performance may occur).
No products indexed under this heading.

Mephobarbital (Concurrent use of Zyrtec-D 12 Hour extended release tablets with other CNS depressants should be avoided because additional reductions in alertness and additional impairment of CNS performance may occur).
No products indexed under this heading.

Meprobamate (Concurrent use of Zyrtec-D 12 Hour extended release tablets with other CNS depressants should be avoided because additional reductions in alertness and additional impairment of CNS performance may occur).
No products indexed under this heading.

Mesoridazine Besylate (Concurrent use of Zyrtec-D 12 Hour extended release tablets with other CNS depressants should be avoided because additional reductions in alertness and additional impairment of CNS performance may occur).
No products indexed under this heading.

Metaproterenol Sulfate (Care should be taken in the administration of Zyrtec-D 12 Hour extended release tablets concomitantly with other sympathomimetic amines because combined effects on the cardiovascular system may be harmful to the patient).
No products indexed under this heading.

Metaraminol Bitartrate (Care should be taken in the administration of Zyrtec-D 12 Hour extended release tablets concomitantly with other sympathomimetic amines because combined effects on the cardiovascular system may be harmful to the patient).
No products indexed under this heading.

Methadone Hydrochloride (Concurrent use of Zyrtec-D 12 Hour extended release tablets with other CNS depressants should be avoided because additional reductions in alertness and additional impairment of CNS performance may occur).
No products indexed under this heading.

Methohexital Sodium (Concurrent use of Zyrtec-D 12 Hour extended release tablets with other CNS depressants should be avoided because additional reductions in alertness and additional impairment of CNS performance may occur).
No products indexed under this heading.

Methotrimeprazine (Concurrent use of Zyrtec-D 12 Hour extended release tablets with other CNS depressants should be avoided because additional reductions in alertness and additional impairment of CNS performance may occur).
No products indexed under this heading.

Methoxamine Hydrochloride (Care should be taken in the administration of Zyrtec-D 12 Hour extended release tablets concomitantly with other sympathomimetic amines because combined effects on the cardiovascular system may be harmful to the patient).
No products indexed under this heading.

Methoxyflurane (Concurrent use of Zyrtec-D 12 Hour extended release tablets with other CNS depressants should be avoided because additional reductions in alertness and additional impairment of CNS performance may occur).
No products indexed under this heading.

Methyldopa (Concomitant use with antihypertensive drugs that interfere with sympathetic activity (eg, methyldopa), may reduce the antihypertensive effects of methyldopa).
No products indexed under this heading.

Midazolam Hydrochloride (Concurrent use of Zyrtec-D 12 Hour extended release tablets with other CNS depressants should be avoided because additional reductions in alertness and additional impairment of CNS performance may occur).
No products indexed under this heading.

Moclobemide (Due to the pseudoephedrine component, Zyrtec-D 12 Hour extended release tablets are contraindicated in patients taking monoamine oxidase (MAO) inhibitors and for 14 days after stopping use of an MAO inhibitor).
No products indexed under this heading.

Molindone Hydrochloride (Concurrent use of Zyrtec-D 12 Hour extended release tablets with other CNS depressants should be avoided because additional reductions in alertness and additional impairment of CNS performance may occur).
Products include:
Moban Tablets 1116

Morphine Sulfate (Concurrent use of Zyrtec-D 12 Hour extended release tablets with other CNS depressants should be avoided because additional reductions in alertness and additional impairment of CNS performance may occur).
Products include:
Avinza Capsules 1772
DepoDur Injection 1095
MS Contin Tablets 2585

Norepinephrine Bitartrate (Care should be taken in the administration of Zyrtec-D 12 Hour extended release tablets concomitantly with other sympathomimetic amines because combined effects on the cardiovascular system may be harmful to the patient).
No products indexed under this heading.

Olanzapine (Concurrent use of Zyrtec-D 12 Hour extended release tablets with other CNS depressants should be avoided because additional reductions in alertness and additional impairment of CNS performance may occur). Products include:
Symbyax Capsules 1871
Zyprexa Tablets 1883
Zyprexa IntraMuscular 1883
Zyprexa ZYDIS Orally Disintegrating Tablets 1883

Oxazepam (Concurrent use of Zyrtec-D 12 Hour extended release tablets with other CNS depressants should be avoided because additional reductions in alertness and additional impairment of CNS performance may occur).
No products indexed under this heading.

Oxycodone Hydrochloride (Concurrent use of Zyrtec-D 12 Hour extended release tablets with other CNS depressants should be avoided because additional reductions in alertness and additional impairment of CNS performance may occur).
Products include:
OxyContin Tablets 2589
OxyIR Capsules 2593
Percocet Tablets 1127
Percodan Tablets 1130

Pargyline Hydrochloride (Due to the pseudoephedrine component, Zyrtec-D 12 Hour extended release tablets are contraindicated in patients taking monoamine oxidase (MAO) inhibitors and for 14 days after stopping use of an MAO inhibitor).
No products indexed under this heading.

Pentobarbital Sodium (Concurrent use of Zyrtec-D 12 Hour extended release tablets with other CNS depressants should be avoided because additional reductions in alertness and additional impairment of CNS performance may occur).
Products include:
Nembutal Sodium Solution, USP 2494

Perphenazine (Concurrent use of Zyrtec-D 12 Hour extended release tablets with other CNS depressants should be avoided because additional reductions in alertness and additional impairment of CNS performance may occur).
No products indexed under this heading.

Phenelzine Sulfate (Due to the pseudoephedrine component, Zyrtec-D 12 Hour extended release tablets are contraindicated in patients taking monoamine oxidase (MAO) inhibitors and for 14 days after stopping use of an MAO inhibitor).
No products indexed under this heading.

Phenobarbital (Concurrent use of Zyrtec-D 12 Hour extended release tablets with other CNS depressants should be avoided because additional reductions in alertness and additional impairment of CNS performance may occur). Products include:
Donnatal Extentabs 2507

Phenylephrine Bitartrate (Care should be taken in the administration of Zyrtec-D 12 Hour extended release tablets concomitantly with other sympathomimetic amines because combined effects on the cardiovascular system may be harmful to the patient).
No products indexed under this heading.

Phenylephrine Hydrochloride (Care should be taken in the administration of Zyrtec-D 12 Hour extended release tablets concomitantly with other sympathomimetic amines because combined effects on the cardiovascular system may be harmful to the patient). Products include:
Actifed Cold & Allergy Tablets 1895
Benadryl Allergy & Cold Kapgels 1895
Benadryl Allergy & Sinus Headache Kapgels 1895
Benadryl Severe Allergy & Sinus Headache Caplets 1897
Children's Benadryl-D Allergy & Sinus Liquid 1896
Benadryl-D Allergy & Sinus Tablet 1896
PediaCare Children's Allergy & Cold Liquid 1902
PediaCare Children's Decongestant Liquid 1902
PediaCare Children's Liquid Multi-Symptom Cold 1902
Sinutab Non-Drying Caplets 1905
Sinutab Sinus Caplets 1905
Children's Sudafed PE Cold & Cough Liquid 1907
Children's Sudafed PE Nasal Decongestant Liquid 1906
Sudafed PE Cold & Cough Caplets 1907
Sudafed PE Nasal Decongestant Tablets 1907
Sudafed PE Nighttime Cold Caplets 1907
Sudafed PE Non-Drying Sinus Caplets 1908
Sudafed PE Severe Cold Caplets 1908
Sudafed PE Sinus & Allergy Tablets 1908
Sudafed PE Sinus Headache Caplets 1908
Tylenol Allergy Multi-Symptom Caplets with Cool Burst and Rapid Release Gelcaps 1916
Tylenol Allergy Multi-Symptom Nighttime Caplets with Cool Burst 1916
Children's Tylenol Plus Cold Suspension Liquid 1912
Children's Tylenol Plus Cold & Allergy Suspension Liquid 1914
Children's Tylenol Plus Flu Suspension Liquid 1914
Children's Tylenol Plus Multi-Symptom Cold Suspension Liquid 1912
Tylenol Cold Head Congestion Daytime Caplets with Cool Burst 1910
Tylenol Cold Head Congestion Nighttime Caplets with Cool Burst 1910
Tylenol Cold Head Congestion Severe Daytime Caplets with Cool Burst 1910
Tylenol Cold Multi-Symptom Daytime Caplets with Cool Burst and Rapid Release Gels 1913
Tylenol Cold Multi-Symptom Daytime Liquid with Citrus Burst 1913
Tylenol Cold Multi-Symptom Nighttime Caplets with Cool Burst 1913
Tylenol Cold Multi-Symptom Nighttime Liquid with Cool Burst 1913
Tylenol Cold Multi-Symptom Severe Caplets with Cool Burst 1913
Tylenol Cold Multi-Symptom Severe Daytime Liquid with Citrus Burst 1913
Tylenol Sinus Congestion & Pain Daytime Caplets with Cool Burst and Gelcaps 1917
Tylenol Sinus Congestion & Pain Nighttime Caplets with Cool Burst 1917
Tylenol Sinus Congestion & Pain Severe Caplets with Cool Burst 1917
Vicks DayQuil Cold & Flu Multi-Symptom Relief .... ▣616
Vicks DayQuil LiquiCaps 2567
Vicks DayQuil Liquid 2567
Vicks DayQuil Multi-Symptom Cold/Flu Relief 2567

Phenylephrine Tannate (Care should be taken in the administration of Zyrtec-D 12 Hour extended release tablets concomitantly with other sympathomimetic amines because combined effects on the cardiovascular system may be harmful to the patient).
No products indexed under this heading.

Phenylpropanolamine Hydrochloride (Care should be taken in the administration of Zyrtec-D 12 Hour extended release tablets concomitantly with other sympathomimetic amines because combined effects on the cardiovascular system may be harmful to the patient).
No products indexed under this heading.

Pirbuterol Acetate (Care should be taken in the administration of Zyrtec-D 12 Hour extended release tablets concomitantly with other sympathomimetic amines because combined effects on the cardiovascular system may be harmful to the patient). Products include:
Maxair Autohaler 1705

Prazepam (Concurrent use of Zyrtec-D 12 Hour extended release tablets with other CNS depressants should be avoided because additional reductions in alertness and additional impairment of CNS performance may occur).
No products indexed under this heading.

Procarbazine Hydrochloride (Due to the pseudoephedrine component, Zyrtec-D 12 Hour extended release tablets are contraindicated in patients taking monoamine oxidase (MAO) inhibitors and for 14 days after stopping use of an MAO inhibitor).
No products indexed under this heading.

Prochlorperazine (Concurrent use of Zyrtec-D 12 Hour extended release tablets with other CNS depressants should be avoided because additional reductions in alertness and additional impairment of CNS performance may occur).
No products indexed under this heading.

Promethazine Hydrochloride (Concurrent use of Zyrtec-D 12 Hour extended release tablets with other CNS depressants should be avoided because additional reductions in alertness and additional impairment of CNS performance may occur).
No products indexed under this heading.

Propofol (Concurrent use of Zyrtec-D 12 Hour extended release tablets with other CNS depressants should be avoided because additional reductions in alertness and additional impairment of CNS performance may occur).
No products indexed under this heading.

Propoxyphene Hydrochloride (Concurrent use of Zyrtec-D 12 Hour extended release tablets with other CNS depressants should be avoided because additional reductions in alertness and additional impairment of CNS performance may occur).
No products indexed under this heading.

Propoxyphene Napsylate (Concurrent use of Zyrtec-D 12 Hour extended release tablets with other CNS depressants should be avoided because additional reductions in alertness and additional impairment of CNS performance may occur).
No products indexed under this heading.

Pseudoephedrine Sulfate (Care should be taken in the administration of Zyrtec-D 12 Hour extended release tablets concomitantly with other sympathomimetic amines because combined effects on the cardiovascular system may be harmful to the patient). Products include:
Clarinex-D 12-Hour Extended-Release Tablets 2831
Clarinex-D 24-Hour Extended-Release Tablets 2834

Quazepam (Concurrent use of Zyrtec-D 12 Hour extended release tablets with other CNS depressants should be avoided because additional reductions in alertness and additional impairment of CNS performance may occur).
No products indexed under this heading.

Quetiapine Fumarate (Concurrent use of Zyrtec-D 12 Hour extended release tablets with other CNS depressants should be avoided because additional reductions in alertness and additional impairment of CNS performance may occur).
No products indexed under this heading.

Rasagiline Mesylate (Due to the pseudoephedrine component, Zyrtec-D 12 Hour extended release tablets are contraindicated in patients taking monoamine oxidase (MAO) inhibitors and for 14 days after stopping use of an MAO inhibitor). Products include:
Azilect Tablets 3106

Remifentanil Hydrochloride (Concurrent use of Zyrtec-D 12 Hour extended release tablets with other CNS depressants should be avoided because additional reductions in alertness and additional impairment of CNS performance may occur).
No products indexed under this heading.

Reserpine (Concomitant use with antihypertensive drugs that interfere with sympathetic activity (eg, reserpine), may reduce the antihypertensive effects of reserpine).
No products indexed under this heading.

Risperidone (Concurrent use of Zyrtec-D 12 Hour extended release tablets with other CNS depressants should be avoided because additional reductions in alertness and additional impairment of CNS performance may occur). Products include:
Risperdal Consta Long-Acting Injection 1753

Salmeterol Xinafoate (Care should be taken in the administration of Zyrtec-D 12 Hour extended release tablets concomitantly with other sympathomimetic amines because combined effects on the cardiovascular system may be harmful to the patient). Products include:
Advair Diskus 100/50 1276
Advair Diskus 250/50 1276
Advair Diskus 500/50 1276
Advair HFA 45/21 Inhalation Aerosol 1288
Advair HFA 115/21 Inhalation Aerosol 1288
Advair HFA 230/21 Inhalation Aerosol 1288
Serevent Diskus 1594

Secobarbital Sodium (Concurrent use of Zyrtec-D 12 Hour extended release tablets with other CNS depressants should be avoided because additional reductions in alertness and additional impairment of CNS performance may occur).
No products indexed under this heading.

Selegiline (Due to the pseudoephedrine component, Zyrtec-D 12 Hour extended release tablets are contraindicated in patients taking monoamine oxidase (MAO) inhibitors and for 14 days after stopping use of an MAO inhibitor). Products include:
Emsam Transdermal System 905

Selegiline Hydrochloride (Due to the pseudoephedrine component, Zyrtec-D 12 Hour extended release tablets are contraindicated in patients taking monoamine oxidase (MAO) inhibitors and for 14 days after stopping use of an MAO inhibitor). Products include:
Eldepryl Capsules 3052

Sevoflurane (Concurrent use of Zyrtec-D 12 Hour extended release tablets with other CNS depressants should be avoided because additional reductions in alertness and additional impairment of CNS performance may occur). Products include:
Ultane Liquid for Inhalation 524

Sodium Oxybate (Concurrent use of Zyrtec-D 12 Hour extended release tablets with other CNS depressants should be avoided because additional reductions in alertness and additional impairment of CNS performance may occur). Products include:
Xyrem Oral Solution 1766

Sufentanil Citrate (Concurrent use of Zyrtec-D 12 Hour extended release tablets with other CNS depressants should be avoided because additional reductions in alertness and additional impairment of CNS performance may occur).
No products indexed under this heading.

Temazepam (Concurrent use of Zyrtec-D 12 Hour extended release tablets with other CNS depressants should be avoided because additional reductions in alertness and additional impairment of CNS performance may occur).
No products indexed under this heading.

Terbutaline Sulfate (Care should be taken in the administration of Zyrtec-D 12 Hour extended release tablets concomitantly with other sympathomimetic amines because combined effects on the cardiovascular system may be harmful to the patient).
No products indexed under this heading.

Theophylline (There was a small decrease in the clearance of cetirizine caused by a 400 mg dose of theophylline; it is possible that larger theophylline doses could have a greater effect).
No products indexed under this heading.

Theophylline Anhydrous (There was a small decrease in the clearance of cetirizine caused by a 400 mg dose of theophylline; it is possible that larger theophylline doses could have a greater effect). Products include:
Uniphyl Tablets 2595

Theophylline Calcium Salicylate (There was a small decrease in the clearance of cetirizine caused by a 400 mg dose of theophylline; it is possible that larger theophylline doses could have a greater effect).
No products indexed under this heading.

Theophylline Dihydroxypropyl (Glyceryl) (There was a small decrease in the clearance of cetirizine caused by a 400 mg dose of theophylline; it is possible that larger theophylline doses could have a greater effect).
No products indexed under this heading.

Theophylline Ethylenediamine (There was a small decrease in the clearance of cetirizine caused by a 400 mg dose of theophylline; it is possible that larger theophylline doses could have a greater effect).
No products indexed under this heading.

Theophylline Sodium Glycinate (There was a small decrease in the clearance of cetirizine caused by a 400 mg dose of theophylline; it is possible that larger theophylline doses could have a greater effect).
No products indexed under this heading.

Thiamylal Sodium (Concurrent use of Zyrtec-D 12 Hour extended release tablets with other CNS depressants should be avoided because additional reductions in alertness and additional impairment of CNS performance may occur).
No products indexed under this heading.

Thioridazine Hydrochloride (Concurrent use of Zyrtec-D 12 Hour extended release tablets with other CNS depressants should be avoided because additional reductions in alertness and additional impairment of CNS performance may occur). Products include:
Thioridazine Hydrochloride Tablets 2195

Thiothixene (Concurrent use of Zyrtec-D 12 Hour extended release tablets with other CNS depressants should be avoided because additional reductions in alertness and additional impairment of CNS performance may occur). Products include:
Thiothixene Capsules 2197

Tranylcypromine Sulfate (Due to the pseudoephedrine component, Zyrtec-D 12 Hour extended release tablets are contraindicated in patients taking monoamine oxidase (MAO) inhibitors and for 14 days after stopping use of an MAO inhibitor). Products include:
Parnate Tablets 1532

Triazolam (Concurrent use of Zyrtec-D 12 Hour extended release tablets with other CNS depressants should be avoided because additional reductions in alertness and additional impairment of CNS performance may occur).
No products indexed under this heading.

Trifluoperazine Hydrochloride (Concurrent use of Zyrtec-D 12 Hour extended release tablets with other CNS depressants should be avoided because additional reductions in alertness and additional impairment of CNS performance may occur).
No products indexed under this heading.

Zaleplon (Concurrent use of Zyrtec-D 12 Hour extended release tablets with other CNS depressants should be avoided because additional reductions in alertness and additional impairment of CNS performance may occur).
No products indexed under this heading.

Ziprasidone Hydrochloride (Concurrent use of Zyrtec-D 12 Hour extended release tablets with other CNS depressants should be avoided because additional reductions in

alertness and additional impairment of CNS performance may occur). Products include:
Geodon Capsules 2520

Zolpidem Tartrate (Concurrent use of Zyrtec-D 12 Hour extended release tablets with other CNS depressants should be avoided because additional reductions in alertness and additional impairment of CNS performance may occur). Products include:
Ambien Tablets 2692
Ambien CR Tablets 2696

Food Interactions

Alcohol (Concurrent use of Zyrtec-D 12 Hour extended release tablets with alcohol should be avoided because additional reductions in alertness and additional impairment of CNS performance may occur).

ZYRTEC-D ALLERGY & CONGESTION EXTENDED-RELEASE TABLETS

(Cetirizine Hydrochloride, Pseudoephedrine Hydrochloride)........ 1923

May interact with hypnotics and sedatives, monoamine oxidase inhibitors, tranquilizers, and certain other agents. Compounds in these categories include:

Alprazolam (Concurrent use with tranquilizers may increase drowsiness).
No products indexed under this heading.

Buspirone Hydrochloride (Concurrent use with tranquilizers may increase drowsiness).
No products indexed under this heading.

Butabarbital (Concurrent use with sedatives may increase drowsiness).
No products indexed under this heading.

Butabarbital Sodium (Concurrent use with sedatives may increase drowsiness).
No products indexed under this heading.

Chloral Hydrate (Concurrent use with sedatives may increase drowsiness).
No products indexed under this heading.

Chlordiazepoxide (Concurrent use with tranquilizers may increase drowsiness).
No products indexed under this heading.

Chlordiazepoxide Hydrochloride (Concurrent use with tranquilizers may increase drowsiness).
No products indexed under this heading.

Chlorpromazine (Concurrent use with tranquilizers may increase drowsiness).
No products indexed under this heading.

Chlorpromazine Hydrochloride (Concurrent use with tranquilizers may increase drowsiness).
No products indexed under this heading.

Chlorprothixene (Concurrent use with tranquilizers may increase drowsiness).
No products indexed under this heading.

Chlorprothixene Hydrochloride (Concurrent use with tranquilizers may increase drowsiness).
No products indexed under this heading.

Clorazepate Dipotassium (Concurrent use with tranquilizers may increase drowsiness).
No products indexed under this heading.

Diazepam (Concurrent use with tranquilizers may increase drowsiness). Products include:
Valium Tablets 2658

Droperidol (Concurrent use with tranquilizers may increase drowsiness).
No products indexed under this heading.

Estazolam (Concurrent use with sedatives may increase drowsiness).
No products indexed under this heading.

Ethanol (Concurrent use with alcohol may increase drowsiness; avoid alcohol).
No products indexed under this heading.

Ethchlorvynol (Concurrent use with sedatives may increase drowsiness).
No products indexed under this heading.

Ethinamate (Concurrent use with sedatives may increase drowsiness).
No products indexed under this heading.

Ethyl Alcohol (Concurrent use with alcohol may increase drowsiness; avoid alcohol).
No products indexed under this heading.

Fluphenazine Decanoate (Concurrent use with tranquilizers may increase drowsiness).
No products indexed under this heading.

Fluphenazine Enanthate (Concurrent use with tranquilizers may increase drowsiness).
No products indexed under this heading.

Fluphenazine Hydrochloride (Concurrent use with tranquilizers may increase drowsiness).
No products indexed under this heading.

Flurazepam Hydrochloride (Concurrent use with sedatives may increase drowsiness).
No products indexed under this heading.

Glutethimide (Concurrent use with sedatives may increase drowsiness).
No products indexed under this heading.

Haloperidol (Concurrent use with tranquilizers may increase drowsiness).
No products indexed under this heading.

Haloperidol Decanoate (Concurrent use with tranquilizers may increase drowsiness).
No products indexed under this heading.

Hydroxyzine Hydrochloride (Concurrent use with tranquilizers may increase drowsiness).
No products indexed under this heading.

Isocarboxazid (Avoid concurrent use with MAO inhibitors. Also, Zyrtec-D should not be used for two weeks after stopping an MAO inhibitor). Products include:
Marplan Tablets 3177

Lorazepam (Concurrent use with sedatives may increase drowsiness).
No products indexed under this heading.

Loxapine Hydrochloride (Concurrent use with tranquilizers may increase drowsiness).
No products indexed under this heading.

Loxapine Succinate (Concurrent use with tranquilizers may increase drowsiness).
No products indexed under this heading.

Meprobamate (Concurrent use with tranquilizers may increase drowsiness).
No products indexed under this heading.

Mesoridazine Besylate (Concurrent use with tranquilizers may increase drowsiness).
No products indexed under this heading.

Midazolam Hydrochloride (Concurrent use with sedatives may increase drowsiness).
No products indexed under this heading.

Moclobemide (Avoid concurrent use with MAO inhibitors. Also, Zyrtec-D should not be used for two weeks after stopping an MAO inhibitor).
No products indexed under this heading.

Molindone Hydrochloride (Concurrent use with tranquilizers may increase drowsiness). Products include:
Moban Tablets 1116

Oxazepam (Concurrent use with tranquilizers may increase drowsiness).
No products indexed under this heading.

Pargyline Hydrochloride (Avoid concurrent use with MAO inhibitors. Also, Zyrtec-D should not be used for two weeks after stopping an MAO inhibitor).
No products indexed under this heading.

Perphenazine (Concurrent use with tranquilizers may increase drowsiness).
No products indexed under this heading.

Phenelzine Sulfate (Avoid concurrent use with MAO inhibitors. Also, Zyrtec-D should not be used for two weeks after stopping an MAO inhibitor).
No products indexed under this heading.

Prazepam (Concurrent use with tranquilizers may increase drowsiness).
No products indexed under this heading.

Procarbazine Hydrochloride (Avoid concurrent use with MAO inhibitors. Also, Zyrtec-D should not be used for two weeks after stopping an MAO inhibitor).
No products indexed under this heading.

Prochlorperazine (Concurrent use with tranquilizers may increase drowsiness).
No products indexed under this heading.

Promethazine Hydrochloride (Concurrent use with tranquilizers may increase drowsiness).
No products indexed under this heading.

Propofol (Concurrent use with sedatives may increase drowsiness).
No products indexed under this heading.

Quazepam (Concurrent use with sedatives may increase drowsiness).
No products indexed under this heading.

Ramelteon (Concurrent use with sedatives may increase drowsiness). Products include:
Rozerem Tablets 3091

Rasagiline Mesylate (Avoid concurrent use with MAO inhibitors. Also, Zyrtec-D should not be used for two weeks after stopping an MAO inhibitor). Products include:
Azilect Tablets 3106

Secobarbital Sodium (Concurrent use with sedatives may increase drowsiness).
No products indexed under this heading.

Selegiline (Avoid concurrent use with MAO inhibitors. Also, Zyrtec-D should not be used for two weeks after stopping an MAO inhibitor). Products include:
Emsam Transdermal System 905

Selegiline Hydrochloride (Avoid concurrent use with MAO inhibitors. Also, Zyrtec-D should not be used for two weeks after stopping an MAO inhibitor). Products include:
Eldepryl Capsules 3052

Sodium Butabarbital (Concurrent use with sedatives may increase drowsiness).
No products indexed under this heading.

Temazepam (Concurrent use with sedatives may increase drowsiness).
No products indexed under this heading.

Thioridazine Hydrochloride (Concurrent use with tranquilizers may increase drowsiness). Products include:
Thioridazine Hydrochloride Tablets 2195

Thiothixene (Concurrent use with tranquilizers may increase drowsiness). Products include:
Thiothixene Capsules 2197

Tranylcypromine Sulfate (Avoid concurrent use with MAO inhibitors. Also, Zyrtec-D should not be used for two weeks after stopping an MAO inhibitor). Products include:
Parnate Tablets 1532

Triazolam (Concurrent use with sedatives may increase drowsiness).
No products indexed under this heading.

Trifluoperazine Hydrochloride (Concurrent use with tranquilizers may increase drowsiness).
No products indexed under this heading.

Zaleplon (Concurrent use with sedatives may increase drowsiness).
No products indexed under this heading.

Zolpidem Tartrate (Concurrent use with sedatives may increase drowsiness). Products include:
Ambien Tablets 2692
Ambien CR Tablets 2696

Food Interactions

Alcohol (Concurrent use with alcohol may increase drowsiness; avoid alcohol).

ZYVOX FOR ORAL SUSPENSION
(Linezolid) 2552
See Zyvox Tablets

ZYVOX INJECTION
(Linezolid) 2552
See Zyvox Tablets

ZYVOX TABLETS
(Linezolid) 2552
May interact with 5HT1-receptor agonists, dopamine agonists, monoamine oxidase inhibitors, serotoninergic agents, selective serotonin reuptake inhibitors, sympathomimetics, tricyclic antidepressants, vasopressors, and certain other agents. Compounds in these categories include:

Albuterol (Unless patients are monitored for potential increases in BP, linezolid should not be administered to patients taking directly and indirectly acting sympathomimetic agents (eg, pseudoephedrine)).
No products indexed under this heading.

Albuterol Sulfate (Unless patients are monitored for potential increases in BP, linezolid should not be administered to patients taking directly and indirectly acting sympathomimetic agents (eg, pseudoephedrine)). Products include:
Combivent Inhalation Aerosol 845
ProAir HFA Inhalation Aerosol 3113
Proventil HFA Inhalation Aerosol 2914
Ventolin HFA Inhalation Aerosol 1638

Almotriptan Malate (Unless patients are carefully observed for signs and/or symptoms of serotonin syndrome, linezolid should not be administered to patients taking 5-HT1 receptor agonists (triptans)). Products include:
Axert Tablets 2431

Amitriptyline Hydrochloride (Unless patients are carefully observed for signs and/or symptoms of serotonin syndrome, linezolid should not be administered to patients taking tricyclic antidepressants).
No products indexed under this heading.

Amoxapine (Unless patients are carefully observed for signs and/or symptoms of serotonin syndrome, linezolid should not be administered to patients taking tricyclic antidepressants).
No products indexed under this heading.

Bromocriptine Mesylate (Unless patients are monitored for potential increases in BP, linezolid should not be administered to patients taking dopaminergic agents (eg, dopamine, dobutamine)).
No products indexed under this heading.

Buspirone Hydrochloride (Unless patients are carefully observed for signs and/or symptoms of serotonin syndrome, linezolid should not be administered to patients taking buspirone).
No products indexed under this heading.

Citalopram Hydrobromide (Spontaneous reports of serotonin syndrome associated with the co-administration of linezolid and serotonergic agents, including antidepressants such as selective serotonin reuptake inhibitors (SSRIs), have been reported. Unless patients are carefully observed for signs and/or symptoms of serotonin syndrome, linezolid should not be administered to patients taking serotonin re-uptake inhibitors. Where administration of linezolid and concomitant serotonergic agents is clinically appropriate, patients should be closely observed for signs/symptoms of serotonin syndrome. If signs/symptoms occur, discontinuation of either one or both agents should be considered. If the concomitant serotonergic agent is withdrawn, discontinuation symptoms can be observed). Products include:
Celexa 1160

Clomipramine Hydrochloride (Unless patients are carefully observed for signs and/or symptoms of serotonin syndrome, linezolid should not be administered to patients taking tricyclic antidepressants).
No products indexed under this heading.

Desipramine Hydrochloride (Unless patients are carefully observed for signs and/or symptoms of serotonin syndrome, linezolid should not be administered to patients taking tricyclic antidepressants).
No products indexed under this heading.

Dobutamine (Unless patients are monitored for potential increases in BP, linezolid should not be administered to patients taking dopaminergic agents (eg, dopamine, dobutamine)).
No products indexed under this heading.

Dobutamine Hydrochloride (Unless patients are monitored for potential increases in BP, linezolid should not be administered to patients taking dopaminergic agents (eg, dopamine, dobutamine)).
No products indexed under this heading.

Dopamine Hydrochloride (Unless patients are monitored for potential increases in BP, linezolid should not be administered to patients taking directly and indirectly acting sympathomimetic agents (eg, pseudoephedrine)).
No products indexed under this heading.

Doxepin Hydrochloride (Unless patients are carefully observed for signs and/or symptoms of serotonin syndrome, linezolid should not be administered to patients taking tricyclic antidepressants).
No products indexed under this heading.

Eletriptan Hydrobromide (Unless patients are carefully observed for signs and/or symptoms of serotonin syndrome, linezolid should not be administered to patients taking 5-HT1 receptor agonists (triptans)).
No products indexed under this heading.

Ephedrine Hydrochloride (Unless patients are monitored for potential increases in BP, linezolid should not be administered to patients taking directly and indirectly acting sympathomimetic agents (eg, pseudoephedrine)).
No products indexed under this heading.

Ephedrine Sulfate (Unless patients are monitored for potential increases in BP, linezolid should not be administered to patients taking directly and indirectly acting sympathomimetic agents (eg, pseudoephedrine)).
No products indexed under this heading.

Ephedrine Tannate (Unless patients are monitored for potential increases in BP, linezolid should not be administered to patients taking directly and indirectly acting sympathomimetic agents (eg, pseudoephedrine)).
No products indexed under this heading.

Epinephrine (Unless patients are monitored for potential increases in BP, linezolid should not be administered to patients taking directly and indirectly acting sympathomimetic agents (eg, pseudoephedrine)). Products include:
EpiPen 1024

Epinephrine Bitartrate (Unless patients are monitored for potential increases in BP, linezolid should not be administered to patients taking directly and indirectly acting sympathomimetic agents (eg, pseudoephedrine)).
No products indexed under this heading.

Epinephrine Hydrochloride (Unless patients are monitored for potential increases in BP, linezolid should not be administered to patients taking directly and indirectly acting sympathomimetic agents (eg, pseudoephedrine)).
No products indexed under this heading.

Escitalopram Oxalate (Spontaneous reports of serotonin syndrome associated with the co-administration of linezolid and serotonergic agents, including antidepressants such as selective serotonin reuptake inhibitors (SSRIs), have been reported. Unless patients are carefully observed for signs and/or symptoms of serotonin syndrome, linezolid should not be administered to patients taking serotonin re-uptake inhibitors. Where administration of linezolid and concomitant serotonergic agents is clinically appropriate, patients should be closely observed for signs/symptoms of serotonin syndrome. If signs/symptoms occur, discontinuation of either one or both agents should be considered. If the concomitant serotonergic agent is withdrawn, discontinuation symptoms can be observed). Products include:
Lexapro Oral Suspension 1174
Lexapro Tablets 1174

Fluoxetine (Spontaneous reports of serotonin syndrome associated with the co-administration of linezolid and serotonergic agents, including antidepressants such as selective serotonin reuptake inhibitors (SSRIs), have been reported. Unless patients are carefully observed for signs and/or symptoms of serotonin syndrome, linezolid should not be administered to patients taking serotonin re-uptake inhibitors. Where administration of linezolid and concomitant serotonergic agents is clinically appropriate, patients should be closely observed for signs/symptoms of serotonin syndrome. If signs/symptoms occur, discontinuation of either one or both agents should be considered. If the concomitant serotonergic agent is withdrawn, discontinuation symptoms can be observed).
No products indexed under this heading.

Fluoxetine Hydrochloride (Spontaneous reports of serotonin syndrome associated with the co-administration of linezolid and serotonergic agents, including antidepressants such as selective serotonin reuptake inhibitors (SSRIs), have been reported. Unless patients are carefully observed for signs and/or symptoms of serotonin syndrome, linezolid should not be administered to patients taking serotonin re-uptake inhibitors. Where administration of linezolid and concomitant serotonergic agents is clinically appropriate, patients should be closely observed for signs/symptoms of serotonin syndrome. If signs/symptoms occur, discontinuation of either one or both agents should be considered. If the concomitant serotonergic agent is withdrawn, discontinuation symptoms can be observed). Products include:
Prozac Weekly Capsules 1852
Prozac Pulvules and Liquid 1852
Symbyax Capsules 1871

Fluvoxamine Maleate (Spontaneous reports of serotonin syndrome associated with the co-administration of linezolid and serotonergic agents, including antidepressants such as selective serotonin reuptake inhibitors (SSRIs), have been reported. Unless patients are carefully observed for signs and/or symptoms of serotonin syndrome, linezolid should not be administered to patients taking serotonin re-uptake inhibitors. Where administration of linezolid and concomitant serotonergic agents is clinically appropriate, patients should be closely observed for signs/symptoms of serotonin syndrome. If signs/symptoms occur, discontinuation of either one or both agents should be considered. If the concomitant serotonergic agent is withdrawn, discontinuation symptoms can be observed). Products include:
Luvox CR Extended-Release Capsules 1759

Frovatriptan Succinate (Unless patients are carefully observed for signs and/or symptoms of serotonin syndrome, linezolid should not be administered to patients taking 5-HT1 receptor agonists (triptans)). Products include:
Frova Tablets 1111

Imipramine Hydrochloride (Unless patients are carefully observed for signs and/or symptoms of serotonin syndrome, linezolid should not be administered to patients taking tricyclic antidepressants).
No products indexed under this heading.

Imipramine Pamoate (Unless patients are carefully observed for signs and/or symptoms of serotonin syndrome, linezolid should not be administered to patients taking tricyclic antidepressants).
No products indexed under this heading.

Isocarboxazid (Linezolid should not be used in patients taking any medicinal product which inhibits monoamine oxidases A or B (eg, phenelzine, isocarboxazid) or within 2 weeks of taking such medicinal product). Products include:
Marplan Tablets 3177

Isoproterenol Hydrochloride (Unless patients are monitored for potential increases in BP, linezolid should not be administered to patients taking directly and indirectly acting sympathomimetic agents (eg, pseudoephedrine)).
No products indexed under this heading.

Isoproterenol Sulfate (Unless patients are monitored for potential increases in BP, linezolid should not be administered to patients taking directly and indirectly acting sympathomimetic agents (eg, pseudoephedrine)).
No products indexed under this heading.

Levalbuterol Hydrochloride (Unless patients are monitored for potential increases in BP, linezolid should not be administered to patients taking directly and indirectly acting sympathomimetic agents (eg, pseudoephedrine)). Products include:
Xopenex Inhalation Solution 3001
Xopenex Inhalation Solution Concentrate 3005

Levodopa (Unless patients are monitored for potential increases in BP, linezolid should not be administered to patients taking dopaminergic agents (eg, dopamine, dobutamine)). Products include:
Stalevo Tablets 2309

Maprotiline Hydrochloride (Unless patients are carefully observed for signs and/or symptoms of serotonin syndrome, linezolid should not be administered to patients taking tricyclic antidepressants).
No products indexed under this heading.

Meperidine Hydrochloride (Unless patients are carefully observed for signs and/or symptoms of serotonin syndrome, linezolid should not be administered to patients taking meperidine).
No products indexed under this heading.

Mephentermine Sulfate (Unless patients are monitored for potential increases in BP, linezolid should not be administered to patients taking vasopressive agents (eg, epinephrine, norepinephrine)).
No products indexed under this heading.

Metaproterenol Sulfate (Unless patients are monitored for potential increases in BP, linezolid should not be administered to patients taking directly and indirectly acting sympathomimetic agents (eg, pseudoephedrine)).
No products indexed under this heading.

Metaraminol Bitartrate (Unless patients are monitored for potential increases in BP, linezolid should not be administered to patients taking directly and indirectly acting sympathomimetic agents (eg, pseudoephedrine)).
No products indexed under this heading.

Methoxamine Hydrochloride (Unless patients are monitored for potential increases in BP, linezolid should not be administered to patients taking directly and indirectly acting sympathomimetic agents (eg, pseudoephedrine)).
No products indexed under this heading.

Moclobemide (Linezolid should not be used in patients taking any medicinal product which inhibits monoamine oxidases A or B (eg, phenelzine, isocarboxazid) or within 2 weeks of taking such medicinal product).
No products indexed under this heading.

Naratriptan Hydrochloride (Unless patients are carefully observed for signs and/or symptoms of serotonin syndrome, linezolid should not be administered to patients taking 5-HT1 receptor agonists (triptans)). Products include:
Amerge Tablets 1301

Norepinephrine Bitartrate (Unless patients are monitored for potential increases in BP, linezolid should not be administered to patients taking directly and indirectly acting sympathomimetic agents (eg, pseudoephedrine)).
No products indexed under this heading.

Nortriptyline Hydrochloride (Unless patients are carefully observed for signs and/or symptoms of serotonin syndrome, linezolid should not be administered to patients taking tricyclic antidepressants).
No products indexed under this heading.

Pargyline Hydrochloride (Linezolid should not be used in patients taking any medicinal product which inhibits monoamine oxidases A or B (eg, phenelzine, isocarboxazid) or within 2 weeks of taking such medicinal product).
No products indexed under this heading.

Paroxetine Hydrochloride (Spontaneous reports of serotonin syndrome associated with the co-administration of linezolid and serotonergic agents, including antidepressants such as selective serotonin reuptake inhibitors (SSRIs), have been reported. Unless patients are carefully observed for signs and/or symptoms of serotonin syndrome, linezolid should not be administered to patients taking serotonin re-uptake inhibitors. Where administration of linezolid and concomitant serotonergic agents is clinically appropriate, patients should be closely observed for signs/symptoms of serotonin syndrome. If signs/symptoms occur, discontinuation of either one or both agents should be considered. If the concomitant serotonergic agent is withdrawn, discontinuation symptoms can be observed). Products include:
Paxil 1535
Paxil CR Controlled-Release Tablets 1544

Pergolide Mesylate (Unless patients are monitored for potential increases in BP, linezolid should not be administered to patients taking dopaminergic agents (eg, dopamine, dobutamine)).
No products indexed under this heading.

Phenelzine Sulfate (Linezolid should not be used in patients taking any medicinal product which inhibits monoamine oxidases A or B (eg, phenelzine, isocarboxazid) or within 2 weeks of taking such medicinal product).
No products indexed under this heading.

Phenylephrine Bitartrate (Unless patients are monitored for potential increases in BP, linezolid should not be administered to patients taking directly and indirectly acting sympathomimetic agents (eg, pseudoephedrine)).
No products indexed under this heading.

Phenylephrine Hydrochloride (Unless patients are monitored for potential increases in BP, linezolid should not be administered to patients taking directly and indirectly acting sympathomimetic agents (eg, pseudoephedrine)). Products include:
Actifed Cold & Allergy Tablets 1895
Benadryl Allergy & Cold Kapgels 1895
Benadryl Allergy & Sinus Headache Kapgels 1895
Benadryl Severe Allergy & Sinus Headache Caplets 1897
Children's Benadryl-D Allergy & Sinus Liquid 1896
Benadryl-D Allergy & Sinus Tablet 1896
PediaCare Children's Allergy & Cold Liquid 1902
PediaCare Children's Decongestant Liquid.................... 1902
PediaCare Children's Liquid Multi-Symptom Cold..................... 1902
Sinutab Non-Drying Caplets 1905
Sinutab Sinus Caplets 1905
Children's Sudafed PE Cold & Cough Liquid 1907
Children's Sudafed PE Nasal Decongestant Liquid.................... 1906
Sudafed PE Cold & Cough Caplets.. 1907
Sudafed PE Nasal Decongestant Tablets 1907
Sudafed PE Nighttime Cold Caplets.. 1907
Sudafed PE Non-Drying Sinus Caplets.. 1908
Sudafed PE Severe Cold Caplets 1908
Sudafed PE Sinus & Allergy Tablets 1908
Sudafed PE Sinus Headache Caplets.. 1908
Tylenol Allergy Multi-Symptom Caplets with Cool Burst and Rapid Release Gelcaps................ 1916
Tylenol Allergy Multi-Symptom Nighttime Caplets with Cool Burst.. 1916
Children's Tylenol Plus Cold Suspension Liquid 1912
Children's Tylenol Plus Cold & Allergy Suspension Liquid............ 1914
Children's Tylenol Plus Flu Suspension Liquid 1914
Children's Tylenol Plus Multi-Symptom Cold Suspension Liquid 1912
Tylenol Cold Head Congestion Daytime Caplets with Cool Burst.. 1910
Tylenol Cold Head Congestion Nighttime Caplets with Cool Burst.. 1910
Tylenol Cold Head Congestion Severe Daytime Caplets with Cool Burst.................................. 1910
Tylenol Cold Multi-Symptom Daytime Caplets with Cool Burst and Rapid Release Gels....... 1913
Tylenol Cold Multi-Symptom Daytime Liquid with Citrus Burst... 1913
Tylenol Cold Multi-Symptom Nighttime Caplets with Cool Burst.. 1913
Tylenol Cold Multi-Symptom Nighttime Liquid with Cool Burst... 1913
Tylenol Cold Multi-Symptom Severe Caplets with Cool Burst..... 1913
Tylenol Cold Multi-Symptom Severe Daytime Liquid with Citrus Burst................................ 1913
Tylenol Sinus Congestion & Pain Daytime Caplets with Cool Burst and Gelcaps...................... 1917
Tylenol Sinus Congestion & Pain Nighttime Caplets with Cool Burst.. 1917
Tylenol Sinus Congestion & Pain Severe Caplets with Cool Burst..... 1917
Vicks DayQuil Cold & Flu Multi-Symptom Relief .... ▣616
Vicks DayQuil LiquiCaps 2567
Vicks DayQuil Liquid 2567
Vicks DayQuil Multi-Symptom Cold/Flu Relief............................ 2567

Phenylephrine Tannate (Unless patients are monitored for potential increases in BP, linezolid should not be administered to patients taking directly and indirectly acting sympathomimetic agents (eg, pseudoephedrine)).
No products indexed under this heading.

Phenylpropanolamine Hydrochloride (Unless patients are monitored for potential increases in BP, linezolid should not be administered to patients taking directly and indirectly acting sympathomimetic agents (eg, pseudoephedrine)).
No products indexed under this heading.

Pirbuterol Acetate (Unless patients are monitored for potential increases in BP, linezolid should not be administered to patients taking directly and indirectly acting sympathomimetic agents (eg, pseudoephedrine)). Products include:
Maxair Autohaler 1705

Pramipexole Dihydrochloride (Unless patients are monitored for potential increases in BP, linezolid should not be administered to patients taking dopaminergic agents (eg, dopamine, dobutamine)). Products include:
Mirapex Tablets 857

Procarbazine Hydrochloride (Linezolid should not be used in patients taking any medicinal product which inhibits monoamine oxidases A or B (eg, phenelzine, isocarboxazid) or within 2 weeks of taking such medicinal product).
No products indexed under this heading.

Protriptyline Hydrochloride (Unless patients are carefully observed for signs and/or symptoms of serotonin syndrome, linezolid should not be administered to patients taking tricyclic antidepressants).
No products indexed under this heading.

Pseudoephedrine Hydrochloride (Unless patients are monitored for potential increases in BP, linezolid should not be administered to patients taking directly and indirectly

acting sympathomimetic agents (eg, pseudoephedrine)). Products include:
Allegra-D 12 Hour Extended-Release Tablets 2687
Allegra-D 24 Hour Extended-Release Tablets 2690
Children's Motrin Cold Oral Suspension 1899
Sudafed 12 Hour Nasal Decongestant Non-Drowsy Caplets 1909
Sudafed 24 Hour Non-Drowsy Nasal Decongestant Tablets 1906
Children's Sudafed Nasal Decongestant Liquid 1906
Sudafed Nasal Decongestant Tablets 1906
Tylenol Cold Severe Congestion Daytime Caplets with Cool Burst 1912
Tylenol Sinus Severe Congestion Caplets with Cool Burst 1917
Vicks NyQuil LiquiCaps 2567
Vicks NyQuil Liquid 2567
Vicks NyQuil Multi-Symptom Cold/Flu Relief 2567
Zyrtec-D 12 Hour Extended Release Tablets 1923
Zyrtec-D Allergy & Congestion Extended-Release Tablets 1923

Pseudoephedrine Sulfate (Unless patients are monitored for potential increases in BP, linezolid should not be administered to patients taking directly and indirectly acting sympathomimetic agents (eg, pseudoephedrine)). Products include:
Clarinex-D 12-Hour Extended-Release Tablets 2831
Clarinex-D 24-Hour Extended-Release Tablets 2834

Rasagiline Mesylate (Linezolid should not be used in patients taking any medicinal product which inhibits monoamine oxidases A or B (eg, phenelzine, isocarboxazid) or within 2 weeks of taking such medicinal product). Products include:
Azilect Tablets 3106

Rifampin (In health volunteers, co-administration of rifampin with linezolid resulted in a 21% decrease in linezolid Cmax and a 32% decrease in linezolid AUC. The clinical significance of this interaction is unknown).
No products indexed under this heading.

Rizatriptan Benzoate (Unless patients are carefully observed for signs and/or symptoms of serotonin syndrome, linezolid should not be administered to patients taking 5-HT1 receptor agonists (triptans)). Products include:
Maxalt Tablets 2056
Maxalt-MLT Orally Disintegrating Tablets 2056

Ropinirole Hydrochloride (Unless patients are monitored for potential increases in BP, linezolid should not be administered to patients taking dopaminergic agents (eg, dopamine, dobutamine)). Products include:
Requip Tablets 1561
Requip XL Tablets 1568

Salmeterol Xinafoate (Unless patients are monitored for potential increases in BP, linezolid should not be administered to patients taking directly and indirectly acting sympathomimetic agents (eg, pseudoephedrine)). Products include:
Advair Diskus 100/50 1276
Advair Diskus 250/50 1276
Advair Diskus 500/50 1276
Advair HFA 45/21 Inhalation Aerosol 1288
Advair HFA 115/21 Inhalation Aerosol 1288
Advair HFA 230/21 Inhalation Aerosol 1288
Serevent Diskus 1594

Selegiline (Linezolid should not be used in patients taking any medicinal product which inhibits monoamine oxidases A or B (eg, phenelzine, isocarboxazid) or within 2 weeks of taking such medicinal product). Products include:
Emsam Transdermal System 905

Selegiline Hydrochloride (Linezolid should not be used in patients taking any medicinal product which inhibits monoamine oxidases A or B (eg, phenelzine, isocarboxazid) or within 2 weeks of taking such medicinal product). Products include:
Eldepryl Capsules 3052

Sertraline Hydrochloride (Spontaneous reports of serotonin syndrome associated with the co-administration of linezolid and serotonergic agents, including antidepressants such as selective serotonin reuptake inhibitors (SSRIs), have been reported. Unless patients are carefully observed for signs and/or symptoms of serotonin syndrome, linezolid should not be administered to patients taking serotonin re-uptake inhibitors. Where administration of linezolid and concomitant serotonergic agents is clinically appropriate, patients should be closely observed for signs/symptoms of serotonin syndrome. If signs/symptoms occur, discontinuation of either one or both agents should be considered. If the concomitant serotonergic agent is withdrawn, discontinuation symptoms can be observed).
No products indexed under this heading.

Sumatriptan (Unless patients are carefully observed for signs and/or symptoms of serotonin syndrome, linezolid should not be administered to patients taking 5-HT1 receptor agonists (triptans)). Products include:
Imitrex Nasal Spray 1470

Sumatriptan Succinate (Unless patients are carefully observed for signs and/or symptoms of serotonin syndrome, linezolid should not be administered to patients taking 5-HT1 receptor agonists (triptans)). Products include:
Imitrex Injection 1465
Imitrex Tablets 1474
Treximet Tablets 1616

Terbutaline Sulfate (Unless patients are monitored for potential increases in BP, linezolid should not be administered to patients taking directly and indirectly acting sympathomimetic agents (eg, pseudoephedrine)).
No products indexed under this heading.

Tranylcypromine Sulfate (Linezolid should not be used in patients taking any medicinal product which inhibits monoamine oxidases A or B (eg, phenelzine, isocarboxazid) or within 2 weeks of taking such medicinal product). Products include:
Parnate Tablets 1532

Trimipramine Maleate (Unless patients are carefully observed for signs and/or symptoms of serotonin syndrome, linezolid should not be administered to patients taking tricyclic antidepressants).
No products indexed under this heading.

Tyramine (A significant pressor response has been observed in normal adult subjects receiving linezolid and tyramine doses of more than 100 mg. Therefore, patients receiving linezolid need to avoid consuming large amounts of foods or beverages with high tyramine content).
No products indexed under this heading.

Venlafaxine Hydrochloride (Spontaneous reports of serotonin syndrome associated with the co-administration of linezolid and serotonergic agents, including antidepressants such as selective serotonin reuptake inhibitors (SSRIs), have been reported. Where administration of linezolid and concomitant serotonergic agents is clinically appropriate, patients should be closely observed for signs/symptoms of serotonin syndrome. If signs/symptoms occur, discontinuation of either one or both agents. If the concomitant serotonergic agent is withdrawn, discontinuation symptoms can be observed). Products include:
Effexor XR Extended-Release Capsules 3195
Venlafaxine Hydrochloride Tablets ... 2199

Zolmitriptan (Unless patients are carefully observed for signs and/or symptoms of serotonin syndrome, linezolid should not be administered to patients taking 5-HT1 receptor agonists (triptans)). Products include:
Zomig Tablets 694
Zomig Nasal Spray 689
Zomig-ZMT Tablets 694

Food Interactions

Food, unspecified (Linezolid may be administered without regard to the timing of meals. The time to reach maximum concentration is delayed from 1.5 hours to 2.2 hours and Cmax is decreased by about 17% when high fat food is given with linezolid. However, the total exposure measured as AUC values is similar under both conditions).

Food high in tyramine (A significant pressor response has been observed in normal adult subjects receiving linezolid and tyramine doses of more than 100 mg. Therefore, patients receiving linezolid need to avoid consuming large amounts of foods or beverages with high tyramine content).

SECTION 2

FOOD INTERACTIONS CROSS-REFERENCE

In this section, drug/food and drug/alcohol interactions listed in the preceding index are cross-referenced by dietary item. Under each entry is an alphabetical list, by brand name, of drugs said to interact with the item. A brief description of the interaction follows each brand, along with the page number of the underlying text. Page numbers refer to the 2009 editions of *PDR®*, *PDR® For Ophthalmic Medicines* and *PDR® For Nonprescription Drugs, Dietary Supplements and Herbs*. A key to the symbols denoting the companion volumes appears in the bottom margin.

Entries in this section are limited to drug/food and drug/alcohol interactions listed in official prescribing information as published by *PDR®*.

Alcohol

Abilify Tablets (Given the primary CNS effects of aripiprazole, caution should be used when co-administered with alcohol; patients should be advised to avoid alcohol while taking aripiprazole) ... 881

Abilify Tablets (Given the primary CNS effects of aripiprazole, caution should be used when co-administered with alcohol; patients should be advised to avoid alcohol while taking aripiprazole) ... 2466

Actifed Cold & Allergy Tablets (Concomitant use may cause increased drowsiness) ... 1895

Actiq (Concurrent use with alcoholic beverages may result in increased depressant effects; hypoventilation, hypotension, and profound sedation may occur) ... 959

ActoPlus Met Tablets (Alcohol is known to potentiate the effect of metformin on lactate metabolism. Patients, therefore, should be warned against excessive alcohol intake, acute or chronic, while receiving Actoplus Met) ... 3071

Adipex-P Tablets (May result in adverse drug interaction) ... 1185

Advicor Tablets (Concomitant alcohol may increase the flushing and its use should be avoided around the time of Advicor administration) ... 402

Aggrenox Capsules (Patients who consume three or more alcoholic drinks every day should be counseled about the bleeding risks involved with chronic, heavy alcohol use while taking aspirin) ... 819

Alphagan P Ophthalmic Solution (Possible additive or potentiating effect with CNS depressants) ... 549

Ambien Tablets (An additive effect on psychomotor performance between alcohol and zolpidem was demonstrated. Zolpidem should not be taken with alcohol) ... 2692

Ambien CR Tablets (Zolpidem tartrate has shown additive effects when combined with alcohol and should not be taken with alcohol) ... 2696

Amrix Capsules (Concomitant use with cyclobenzaprine HCl may enhance the effects of alcohol) ... 966

Apidra Injection (Alcohol may either potentiate or weaken the blood glucose-lowering effect of insulin) ... 2706

Atacand HCT 16-12.5 Tablets (May aggravate orthostatic hypotension produced by hydrochlorothiazide) ... 642

Avalide Tablets (Potentiation of orthostatic hypotension may occur) ... 892

Avalide Tablets (Potentiation of orthostatic hypertension may occur) ... 2713

Avandamet Tablets (Alcohol potentiates the effect of metformin on lactate metabolism; patients should be warned against excessive alcohol intake, acute or chronic) ... 1336

Avinza Capsules (Patients must not consume alcoholic beverages, prescription or non-prescription medications containing alcohol while on morphine sulfate therapy. Consumption of alcohol while taking morphine sulfate may result in the rapid release and absoption of a potentially fatal dose of morphine) ... 1772

Benadryl Allergy & Cold Kapgels (Concurrent use may increase drowsiness) ... 1895

Benadryl Allergy & Sinus Headache Kapgels (Increases drowsiness effect; avoid concomitant use) ... 1895

Benadryl Severe Allergy & Sinus Headache Caplets (Increases drowsiness effect; avoid concomitant use) ... 1897

Benadryl Dye-Free Allergy Liqui-gels Softgels (Increases drowsiness effect; avoid concomitant use) ... 1897

Benadryl Allergy Kapgels (Increases drowsiness effect; avoid concomittant use) ... 1895

Benadryl Allergy Quick Dissolve Strips (Increases drowsiness effect; avoid concomitant use) ... 1896

Benadryl Allergy Ultratab Tablets (Increases drowsiness effect; avoid concomitant use) ... 1896

Children's Benadryl Allergy Fastmelts (Increases drowsiness effect; avoid concurrent use) ... 1897

Children's Benadryl Allergy Perfect Measure (Concurrent use may increase drowsiness) ... 1896

Children's Benadryl-D Allergy & Sinus Liquid (Concurrent use may increase drowsiness) ... 1896

Benadryl-D Allergy & Sinus Tablet (Increases drowsiness effect; avoid concomitant use) ... 1896

Benicar HCT Tablets (Concurrent administration could cause potentiation of orthostatic hypotension) ... 1010

Captopril Tablets (Drugs having vasodilator activity should, if possible, be discontinued before starting captopril) ... 2182

Catapres Tablets (Clonidine may potentiate the CNS-depressive effects) ... 841

Catapres-TTS (Clonidine may potentiate the CNS-depressive effects) ... 842

Celexa Tablets (Although citalopram did not potentiate cognitive and motor effects of alcohol, concurrent use is not recommended) ... 1160

Cialis Tablets (Both tadalafil and alcohol act as mild vasodilators. When mild vasodilators are taken in combination, blood-pressure lowering effects of each individual compound may be increased. Substantial consumption of alcohol in combination with tadalafil may increase the potential for orthostatic signs and symptoms, including increase in heart rate, decrease in standing, blood pressure, dizziness, and headache) ... 1792

Clorpres Tablets (Clonidine may enhance the CNS-depressive effects of alcohol; orthostatic hypotension may be aggravated by alcohol) ... 2185

Combigan Ophthalmic Solution (Although specific drug interaction studies have not been conducted with Combigan, the possibility of an additive or potentiating effect with CNS depressants (alcohol, barbiturates, opiates, sedatives or anesthetics) should be considered) 553
Comtan Tablets (Possible additive sedative effects) 2208
Coreg CR Extended-Release Capsules (Concomitant administration of Coreg CR with alcohol may affect the modified release properties of Coreg CR, potentially resulting in a faster rate of release and higher than expected peak and lower than expected trough plasma concentrations of carvedilol phosphate. To avoid the potential for this interaction, the administration of Coreg CR with alcohol (including prescription and OTC medications that contain ethanol) should be separated by at least two hours) 1393
Cymbalta Delayed-Release Capsules (Use of duloxetine concomitantly with heavy alcohol intake may be associated with severe liver injury; for this reason, duloxetine should ordinarily not be prescribed for patients with substantial alcohol use) 1801
Dantrium Capsules (Co-administration may result in increased drowsiness; caution should be exercised) 2580
Demser Capsules (Concurrent use of metyrosine with alcohol or other CNS depressants can increase their sedative effects) 1989
Depakote ER Tablets (Valproate produces CNS depression, especially when combined with another CNS depressant, such as alcohol) 423
DepoDur Injection (The concurrent use of other central nervous system (CNS) depressants increase the risk of respiratory depression, hypotension, profound sedation, or coma. Use with caution and with vigilant monitoring in patients taking these agents) 1095
Diovan HCT Tablets (Co-administration of thiazide diuretics and alcohol may result in potentiation of orthostatic hypotension) 2216
Dramamine Original Tablets (May increase drowsiness effect) 1898
Duragesic Transdermal System (The concomitant use of fentanyl with other CNS depressants, including alcohol, may cause respiratory depression, hypotension, and profound sedation or potentially result in coma. When such combined therapy is contemplated, the dose of one or both agents should be significantly reduced) 2405
Effexor XR Extended-Release Capsules (Co-administration of venlafaxine as a stable regimen did not exaggerate the psychomotor and psychometric effects of alcohol; however, patiénts should be advised to avoid alcohol while taking venlafaxine) 3195
Emsam Transdermal System (The use of alcohol is not recommended while using selegiline transdermal system.) 905
Equetro Extended-Release Capsules (Because of its primary CNS effect, caution should be used when carbamazepine is taken with alcohol) 3174
Exubera Inhalation Powder (Alcohol may either increase or reduce the blood glucose-lowering effect of insulin. Co-administration may require insulin dose adjustment and particularly close monitoring) 2515
Fentora Tablets (The concomitant use of other CNS depressants, including alcoholic beverages, may produce increased depressant effects. Hypoventilation, hypotension, and profound sedation may occur) 968
Flolan for Injection (Additional reductions in blood pressure may occur) 1426
Furosemide Tablets (Aggravates orthostatic hypotension) 2186
Gabitril Tablets (Possible additive depressive effects) 973
Geodon Capsules (Somnolence was a commonly reported adverse event in patients treated with ziprasidone; concurrent use with alcohol or other CNS active drugs, such as depressants, should be undertaken with caution) 2520
Gris-PEG Tablets (The effects of alcohol may be potentiated by griseofulvin, producing such effects as tachycardia and flushing) 2507
Humalog-Pen and KwikPen (Co-administration with drugs with hypoglycemic activity may result in decreased insulin requirements) 1829
Humalog Mix 50/50-Pen and KwikPen (Insulin requirements may be decreased in the presence of drugs with hypoglycemic activity, such as alcohol) 1833
Humulin N Vial (Insulin requirements may be reduced in the presence of drugs that lower blood glucose or affect how the body responds to insulin) 1846
Humulin R (U-500) (Insulin requirements may be decreased in the presence of drugs that increase insulin sensitivity or have hypoglycemic activity, such as alcohol) 1850
Indapamide Tablets (Aggravates orthostatic hypotension) 2188
Intravenous Sodium Diuril (Potentiation of orthostatic hypotension may occur) 2490
Invega Extended-Release Tablets (Given the primary CNS effects of paliperidone, caution should be used if taken with other centrally-acting drugs) 1748
Ionsys Transdermal System (The concomitant use of other central nervous system depressants, such as alcoholic beverages, may produce additive depressant effects. Hypoventilation, hypotension, profound sedation, and coma may occur. Therefore, use of concomitant CNS depressants requires individual adjustment of dosage of the concomitant medication and observation of a given patient) 2410
Klonopin Tablets (Potentiates CNS-depressant action) 2639
Lantus Injection (May either potentiate or weaken the blood-glucose-lowering effect of insulin) 2749
Levemir Injection (Co-administration may either potentiate or weaken the blood-glucose lowering effect of insulin) 2352
Lexapro Tablets (Although escitalopram did not potentiate the cognitive and motor effects of alcohol in a clinical trial, as with other psychotropic medications, the use of alcohol by patients taking escitalopram is not recommended) 1174
Lortab 5/500 Tablets (Concomitant use may cause additive CBS depression. When combined therapy is contemplated, the dose of one or both agents should be reduced) 3143
Lortab 7.5/500 Tablets (Co-administration may exhibit additive CNS-depression; concurrent use should be avoided) 3144
Lunesta Tablets (An additive effect on psychomotor performance was seen with co-administration of eszopiclone and alcohol 0.70 g/kg for up to 4 hours after alcohol consumption) 2994
Luvox CR Extended-Release Capsules (Patients should be advised to avoid taking alcohol while taking Luvox CR capsules) 1759
Lyrica Capsules (Alcohol consumption should be avoided while taking pregabalin, as pregabalin may potentiate the impairment of motor skills and sedation of alcohol) 2527
Marinol Capsules (Co-administration results in additive drowsiness and CNS depression) 3163
Marplan Tablets (Isocarboxazid should not be administered in combination with some central nervous systems depressants including alcohol) 3177
Meridia Capsules (Concurrent use has not resulted in psychomotor reactions of clinical significance, however, concomitant use with excessive alcohol is not recommended) 475
Mevacor Tablets (Lovastatin should be used with caution in patients who have consumed substantial quantity of alcohol and have a past history of liver disease; active liver disease and unexplained elevation in transaminase are contraindications to the use of lovastatin) 2063
Micardis HCT Tablets (Potentiation of orthostatic hypotension) 854
MS Contin Tablets (Respiratory depression, hypotension and profound sedation or coma may result) 2585
Nembutal Sodium Solution, USP (Concomitant use of other CNS depressants may produce additive depressant effects. Alcohol should not be consumed while taking barbiturates) 2494
Niaspan Extended-Release Tablets (Concomitant alcohol may increase the side effects of flushing and pruritus and should be avoided around the time of Niaspan ingestion) 480
Nitro-Dur Transdermal Infusion System (Enhances sensitivity to the hypotensive effects) 2887
Nitrolingual Pumpspray (Enhanced sensitivity to hypotensive effects) 2965
NovoLog Injection (May either potentiate or weaken the blood-glucose-lowering effect of insulin) 2359
Opana Tablets (The concomitant use of other CNS depressants including sedatives, hypnotics, tranquilizers, general anesthetics, phenothiazines, other opioids, and alcohol may produce additive CNS depressant effects. Additive effects resulting in respiratory depression, hypotension, profound sedation or coma may result if these drugs are taken in combination with the usual doses of oxymorphone hydrochloride) 1117
OxyContin Tablets (Concurrent use with the usual dose of OxyContin may result in respiratory depression, profound sedation or coma) 2589
OxyIR Capsules (Concomitant use may exhibit an additive CNS depression) 2593
Parnate Tablets (Concurrent use is contraindicated; a marked potentiating effect on alcohol has been reported) 1532
Patanase Nasal Spray (Concurrent use of olopatadine nasal spray with alcohol should be avoided because additional reductions in alertness and additional impairment of central nervous system performance may occur) 544
Paxil Tablets (Concurrent use should be avoided) 1535
Percocet Tablets (Additive CNS depression) 1127
Percodan Tablets (Additive CNS depression) 1130
Phenytek Capsules (Acute alcohol intake may increase phenytoin serum levels; chronic alcohol abuse may decrease phenytoin serum levels) 2192
Photofrin for Injection (Compounds that quench active oxygen species or scavenge radicals, such as ethanol, would be expected to decrease photodynamic therapy; no human data available to support or rebut this possibility) 708
PrandiMet Tablets (Alcohol potentiates the effect of metformin on lactate metabolism. Patients should be warned against excessive alcohol intake while receiving PrandiMet) 2967
Prinzide Tablets (Co-administration of thiazide and alcohol may potentiate orthostatic hypotension) 2092
Pristiq Extended-Release Tablets (Caution is advised when desvenlafaxine is taken in combination with other CNS-active drugs) 3247
Provigil Tablets (The use of modafinil in combination with alcohol has not been studied. It is advisable to avoid alcohol while taking modafinil) 977
Prozac Weekly Capsules (The risk of using fluoxetine in combination with other CNS active drugs has not been systematically evaluated. Nonetheless, caution is advised if the concomitant administration of fluoxetine and such drugs is required. In evaluating individual cases, consideration should be given to using lower initial doses of the concomitantly administered drugs, using conservative titration schedules, and monitoring of clinical status) 1852
Prozac Pulvules and Liquid (Concurrent use with CNS active agents, such as alcohol, requires caution) 1852

Pylera Capsules (Alcoholic beverages should not be consumed during Pylera therapy and for at least 1 day afterward. Psychotic reactions have been reported in alcoholic patients who are using Pylera and disulfiram concurrently. Pylera should not be given to patients who have taken disulfiram within the last 2 weeks) ... 714

Remeron Tablets (Co-administration has shown to result in an additive impairment of motor skills) ... 2924

Requip Tablets (Sedating medications (such as alcohol or CNS depressants), the presence of sleeping disorders, or other medications that increase plasma levels of ropinirole, may increase the risk of somnolence or falling asleep while engaged in activities of daily living. Because of possible additive effects, caution should be advised when patients are taking other sedating medications, alcohol, or other CNS depressants (e.g., benzodiazepines, antipsychotics, antidepressants) in combination with ropinirole) ... 1561

Requip XL Tablets (Sedating medications (such as alcohol or CNS depressants), the presence of sleeping disorders, or other medications that increase plasma levels of ropinirole, may increase the risk of somnolence or falling asleep while engaged in activities of daily living. Because of possible additive effects, caution should be advised when patients are taking other sedating medications, alcohol, or other CNS depressants (e.g., benzodiazepines, antipsychotics, antidepressants) in combination with ropinirole) ... 1568

Rilutek Tablets (Alcohol may increase the risk of hepatotoxicity; patients on riluzole should be discouraged from drinking excessive amounts of alcohol) ... 2771

Risperdal Consta Long-Acting Injection (Caution should be used when risperidone is taken in combination with alcohol) ... 1753

Rozerem Tablets (With single-dose, daytime co-administration of ramelteon 32 mg and alcohol (0.6 g/kg), there were no clinically meaningful or statistically significant effects on peak or total exposure to ramelteon. However, an additive effect was seen on some measures of psychomotor performance (ie. the Digit Symbol Substitution Test, the Psychomotor Vigilance Task Test, and a Visual Analog Scale of sedation) at some post-dose time points. No additive effect was seen on the Delayed Word Recognition Test. Because alcohol by itself impairs performance, and the intended effect of ramelteon is to promote sleep, patients should be cautioned not to consume alcohol when using ramelteon) ... 3091

St. Joseph 81 mg Aspirin Chewable and Enteric Coated Tablets (Chronic heavy alcohol users, 3 or more drinks per day, in combination with analgesic/antipyretic drug products containing aspirin increases the risk of adverse GI events, including stomach bleeding) ... 1903

Salonpas Arthritis Pain Patches (Having 3 or more alcoholic drinks every day while using this product increases the chance of stomach bleeding) ... ▣ 608

Seromycin Capsules (Concurrent use increases the possibility and risk of epileptic episodes) ... 1864

Simply Sleep Caplets (Diphenhydramine is an antihistamine with sedative properties; concurrent use with alcoholic beverages should be avoided) ... 1905

Sinutab Non-Drying Caplets (Patients consuming 3 or more alcohol-containing drinks per day should consult physician for advice on when and how they should take this product) ... 1905

Sinutab Sinus Caplets (Patients consuming 3 or more alcohol-containing drinks per day should consult physician for advice on when and how they should take this product) ... 1905

Skelaxin Tablets (Skelaxin may enhance the effects of alcohol, barbiturates and other CNS depressants) ... 1784

Sleep-Tite Caplets (Concurrent use is not recommended) ... ▣ 640

Soma Tablets (The sedative effects of carisoprodol and other CNS depressants (eg, alcohol) may be additive. Therefore, caution should be exercised with patients who take more than one CNS depressant simultaneously) ... 1931

Soriatane Capsules (Clinical evidence has shown that etretinate can be formed with concurrent ingestion of acitretin and ethanol) ... 3062

Sudafed PE Severe Cold Caplets (Chronic heavy alcohol abusers, 3 or more drinks per day, should consult their physicians for advice on when and how they should take pain relievers/fever reducers including acetaminophen. Acetaminophen may cause liver damage) ... 1908

Sudafed PE Sinus & Allergy Tablets (Concomitant use may cause increased drowsiness) ... 1908

Sudafed PE Sinus Headache Caplets (Chronic heavy alcohol abusers, 3 or more drinks per day, should consult their physicians for advice on when and how they should take pain relievers/fever reducers including acetaminophen. Acetaminophen may cause liver damage) ... 1908

Sustiva Capsules (Potential for additive central nervous system effects when Sustiva is used concomitantly with alcohol) ... 930

Symbyax Capsules (Alcohol may potentiate the orthostatic effect of olanzapine, increasing the risk of orthostatic hypotension. Therefore, patients should be advised to avoid alcohol while taking Symbyax) ... 1871

Tekturna HCT Tablets (Potentiation of orthostatic hypotension may occur with concurrent use) ... 2324

Teveten HCT Tablets (May potentiate orthostatic hypotension) ... 517

Thioridazine Hydrochloride Tablets (Thioridazine is capable of potentiating CNS depressants) ... 2195

Thiothixene Capsules (As with the case of other CNS-acting drugs, patients receiving thiothixene should be cautioned about the possible additive effects (which may include hypotension) with alcohol) ... 2197

Transderm Scōp Transdermal Therapeutic System (Scopolamine is an anticholinergic agent and causes certain CNS effects, such as drowsiness and dizziness, and hence it should be used with care in patients on concomitant therapy) ... 2206

Trizivir Tablets (Concurrent use decreases the elimination of abacavir causing an increase in overall exposure) ... 1622

Tussionex Pennkinetic Extended-Release Suspension (Combined use may result in additive CNS depression) ... 3154

Regular Strength Tylenol Tablets (Chronic heavy alcohol users, 3 or more drinks per day, should consult their physicians for advice on when and how they should take pain relievers including acetaminophen) ... 1915

Extra Strength Tylenol PM Caplets, Geltabs, Liquid, and Rapid Release Gels (Concurrent use may increase drowsiness effect; chronic heavy alcohol abusers, 3 or more drinks per day, may be at increased risk of liver toxicity from excessive acetaminophen use) ... 1915

Tylenol with Codeine Tablets (Concomitant use with alcohol may produce an additive CNS depression and should be avoided) ... 2427

Tylenol Severe Allergy Caplets (Concurrent use may increase drowsiness effect; chronic heavy alcohol abusers, 3 or more drinks per day, may be at increased risk of liver toxicity from excessive acetaminophen use) ... 1916

Tylenol Chest Congestion Caplets with Cool Burst (Concurrent use may increase drowsiness effect; chronic heavy alcohol abusers, 3 or more drinks per day, may be at increased risk of liver toxicity from excessive acetaminophen use) ... 1910

Tylenol Cold Severe Congestion Daytime Caplets with Cool Burst (Chronic heavy alcohol abusers, 3 or more drinks per day, may be at increased risk of liver toxicity from acetaminophen use) ... 1912

Tylenol Cold Head Congestion Daytime Caplets with Cool Burst (Concurrent use may increase drowsiness effect; chronic heavy alcohol abusers, 3 or more drinks per day, may be at increased risk of liver toxicity from excessive acetaminophen use) ... 1910

Tylenol Cold Head Congestion Nighttime Caplets with Cool Burst (Concurrent use may increase drowsiness effect; chronic heavy alcohol abusers, 3 or more drinks per day, may be at increased risk of liver toxicity from excessive acetaminophen use) ... 1910

Tylenol Cold Multi-Symptom Daytime Caplets with Cool Burst and Rapid Release Gels (Consumption of 3 or more alcoholic drinks every day, need to ask your doctor whether you should take acetaminophen; may be at increased risk of liver toxicity from acetaminophen use) ... 1913

Tylenol Cough & Sore Throat Nighttime Liquid with Cool Burst (Concurrent use with alcohol may increase drowsiness. Avoid alcoholic drinks) ... 1918

Tylenol Sinus Congestion & Pain Nighttime Caplets with Cool Burst (May increase drowsiness effect) ... 1917

Tylenol Sinus Congestion & Pain Severe Caplets with Cool Burst (Avoid concurrent use; chronic heavy alcohol abusers, 3 or more drinks per day, may be at increased risk of liver toxicity from acetaminophen use) ... 1917

Tylenol Sinus Severe Congestion Caplets with Cool Burst (Concurrent use may increase drowsiness effect; chronic heavy alcohol abusers, 3 or more drinks per day, may be at increased risk of liver toxicity from excessive acetaminophen use) ... 1917

Tylenol Sore Throat Nighttime Liquid with Cool Burst (Concomitant use may increase drowsiness. Avoid alcoholic drinks) ... 1918

Women's Tylenol Menstrual Relief Caplets (Chronic heavy alcohol users, 3 or more drinks per day, should consult their physicians for advice on when and how they should take pain relievers, including acetaminophen. Acetaminophen may cause liver damage) ... 1919

Ultram ER Extended-Release Tablets (Tramadol hydrochloride is contraindicated in acute intoxication with alcohol. Tramadol hydrochloride should be used with caution and in reduced dosages when administered to patients receiving CNS depressants, such as alcohol. Tramadol may be expected to have additive effects when used in conjunction with alcohol) ... 2428

Uniphyl Tablets (Concurrent use with a single dose of alcohol (3mL/kg of whiskey) decreases theophylline clearance for up to 24 hours) ... 2595

Valium Tablets (Concomitant use with alcohol is not recommended due to enhancement of the sedative effect) ... 2658

Venlafaxine Hydrochloride Tablets (Although venlafaxine has not been shown to increase the impairment of mental and motor skills caused by alcohol, patients should be advised to avoid alcohol while taking venlafaxine) ... 2199

Vicks DayQuil LiquiCaps (Consuming 3 or more alcoholic drinks every day while using this product may cause severe liver damage) ... 2567

Vicks NyQuil LiquiCaps (May increase drowsiness effect; patients consuming 3 or more alcoholic drinks per day should consult their physician for advice on when and how they should take this medication) ... 2567

Vicodin Tablets (May exhibit an additive CNS depression) ... 529

Vicodin ES Tablets (Additive CNS depression) ... 530

Vicodin HP Tablets (Concurrent use results in an additive CNS depression) ... 531

Vicoprofen Tablets (May exhibit additive CNS depression) ... 533

Visudyne for Injection (Co-administration with compounds that quench active oxygen species or scavenge radicals, such as ethanol, would be expected to decrease verteporfin activity) ... 2332

Wellbutrin SR Sustained-Release Tablets (Bupropion hydrochloride is contraindicated in patients undergoing abrupt discontinuation of alcohol. The consumption of alcohol during treatment with bupropion hydrochloride should be minimized or avoided) 1653

Xyrem Oral Solution (The combined use of alcohol with sodium oxybate may result in potentiation of the central nervous system-depressant effects of sodium oxybate and alcohol) 1766

Xyzal Oral Solution (Concurrent use of levocetirizine dihydrochloride with alcohol because additional reductions in alertness and additional impairment of central nervous system performance may occur) 2789

Xyzal Oral Solution (Concurrent use of levocetirizine dihydrochloride with alcohol should be avoided because additional reductions in alertness and additional impairment of central nervous system performance may occur) 3155

Ziagen Tablets (Decreases the elimination of abacavir causing an increase in overall exposure) 1673

Zocor Tablets (Simvastatin should be used with caution in patients who consume substantial quantities of alcohol) 2136

Zyban Sustained-Release Tablets (Bupropion hydrochloride is contraindicated in patients undergoing abrupt discontinuation of alcohol. The consumption of alcohol during treatment with bupropion hydrochloride should be minimized or avoided) 1692

Zydone Tablets (Co-administration may exhibit additive CNS depression) 1132

Zyprexa Tablets (Co-administration of alcohol with olanzapine potentiates orthostatic hypotension; concurrent use should be avoided) 1883

Zyprexa IntraMuscular (Co-administration of alcohol with olanzapine potentiates orthostatic hypotension; concurrent use should be avoided) 1883

Zyrtec Allergy Tablets (Alcohol may increase drowsiness. Avoid alcoholic drinks) 1919

Children's Zyrtec Allergy Syrup (Concomitant use may increase drowsiness) 1920

Children's Zyrtec Allergy Chewable Tablets (Alcohol may increase drowsiness. Avoid alcoholic drinks) 1922

Children's Zyrtec Hives Relief Syrup (Concomitant use may increase drowsiness) 1920

Zyrtec Tablets (Concurrent use of cetirizine with alcohol should be avoided because additional reductions in alertness and additional impairment of CNS performance may occur) 1920

Zyrtec-D 12 Hour Extended Release Tablets (Concurrent use of Zyrtec-D 12 Hour extended release tablets with alcohol should be avoided because additional reductions in alertness and additional impairment of CNS performance may occur) 1923

Zyrtec-D Allergy & Congestion Extended-Release Tablets (Concurrent use with alcohol may increase drowsiness; avoid alcohol) 1923

Anchovies

Parnate Tablets (Potential for hypertensive crisis; concurrent use is contraindicated) 1532

Apple Juice

Allegra-D 12 Hour Extended-Release Tablets (Co-administration with grapefruit, orange or apple juice will reduce the bioavailability and exposure or fexofenadine) 2687

Avocados

Parnate Tablets (Potential for hypertensive crisis; concurrent use is contraindicated) 1532

Bananas

Parnate Tablets (Potential for hypertensive crisis; concurrent use is contraindicated) 1532

Beans, broad

Parnate Tablets (Potential for hypertensive crisis; concurrent use is contraindicated) 1532

Beans, Fava

Parnate Tablets (Potential for hypertensive crisis; concurrent use is contraindicated) 1532

Beer, alcohol-free

Parnate Tablets (Potential for hypertensive crisis; concurrent use is contraindicated) 1532

Beer, unspecified

Parnate Tablets (Potential for hypertensive crisis; concurrent use is contraindicated) 1532

Beverages, caffeine-containing

Fosamax Tablets (Concomitant administration of alendronate with coffee reduces bioavailability by approximately 60%) 2005

Fosamax Plus D Tablets (Concomitant administration of alendronate with coffee reduces bioavailability by approximately 60%) 2013

Iquix Ophthalmic Solution (Systemic administration of some quinolones has been shown to interfere with the metabolism of caffeine) 3183

Parnate Tablets (Potential for hypertensive crisis; concurrent use is contraindicated) 1532

Beverages with high tyramine

Azilect Tablets (Severe hypertensive reactions have followed the administration of tyramine rich beverages and non-selective MAO inhibitors) 3106

Emsam Transdermal System (As a class, MAO inhibitors have been associated with hypertensive crises caused by the ingestion of foods with a high concentration of tyramine) 905

Broccoli

Letairis Tablets (Use caution when ambrisentan is co-administered with inducers of CYP) 1258

Requip Tablets (In vitro metabolism studies showed that CYP1A2 is the major enzyme responsible for the metabolism of ropinirole. There is thus the potential for inducers or inhibitors of this enzyme to alter the clearance of ropinirole. Therefore, if therapy with a drug known to be a potent inducer or inhibitor of CYP1A2 is stopped or started during treatment with ropinirole, adjustment of the dose of ropinirole may be required) 1561

Requip XL Tablets (In vitro metabolism studies showed that CYP1A2 is the major enzyme responsible for the metabolism of ropinirole. There is thus the potential for inducers or inhibitors of this enzyme to alter the clearance of ropinirole. Therefore, if therapy with a drug known to be a potent inducer or inhibitor of CYP1A2 is stopped or started during treatment with ropinirole, adjustment of the dose of ropinirole may be required) 1568

Rozerem Tablets (Efficacy may be reduced when ramelteon is used in combination with strong CYP enzyme inducers such as rifampin) 3091

Symbyax Capsules (Agents that induce CYP1A2 or glucuronyl transferase enzymes may cause an increase in olanzapine concentration) 1871

Treanda for Injection (Inducers of CYP1A2 (e.g., omeprazole, smoking) have potential to decrease plasma concentrations of bendamustine and increase plasma concentrations of its active metabolites. Caution should be used, or alternative treatments considered if concomitant treatment with CYP1A2 inducers is needed) 983

Zyprexa Tablets (May cause an increase in olanzapine clearance; therefore, a dosage increase might be considered) 1883

Zyprexa IntraMuscular (May cause an increase in olanzapine clearance; therefore, a dosage increase might be considered) 1883

Brussel Sprouts

Letairis Tablets (Use caution when ambrisentan is co-administered with inducers of CYP) 1258

Requip Tablets (In vitro metabolism studies showed that CYP1A2 is the major enzyme responsible for the metabolism of ropinirole. There is thus the potential for inducers or inhibitors of this enzyme to alter the clearance of ropinirole. Therefore, if therapy with a drug known to be a potent inducer or inhibitor of CYP1A2 is stopped or started during treatment with ropinirole, adjustment of the dose of ropinirole may be required) 1561

Requip XL Tablets (In vitro metabolism studies showed that CYP1A2 is the major enzyme responsible for the metabolism of ropinirole. There is thus the potential for inducers or inhibitors of this enzyme to alter the clearance of ropinirole. Therefore, if therapy with a drug known to be a potent inducer or inhibitor of CYP1A2 is stopped or started during treatment with ropinirole, adjustment of the dose of ropinirole may be required) 1568

Rozerem Tablets (Efficacy may be reduced when ramelteon is used in combination with strong CYP enzyme inducers such as rifampin) 3091

Symbyax Capsules (Agents that induce CYP1A2 or glucuronyl transferase enzymes may cause an increase in olanzapine concentration) 1871

Zyprexa Tablets (May cause an increase in olanzapine clearance; therefore, a dosage increase might be considered) 1883

Zyprexa IntraMuscular (May cause an increase in olanzapine clearance; therefore, a dosage increase might be considered) 1883

Caviar

Parnate Tablets (Potential for hypertensive crisis; concurrent use is contraindicated) 1532

Charbroiled Food

Letairis Tablets (Use caution when ambrisentan is co-administered with inducers of CYP) 1258

Requip Tablets (In vitro metabolism studies showed that CYP1A2 is the major enzyme responsible for the metabolism of ropinirole. There is thus the potential for inducers or inhibitors of this enzyme to alter the clearance of ropinirole. Therefore, if therapy with a drug known to be a potent inducer or inhibitor of CYP1A2 is stopped or started during treatment with ropinirole, adjustment of the dose of ropinirole may be required) 1561

Requip XL Tablets (In vitro metabolism studies showed that CYP1A2 is the major enzyme responsible for the metabolism of ropinirole. There is thus the potential for inducers or inhibitors of this enzyme to alter the clearance of ropinirole. Therefore, if therapy with a drug known to be a potent inducer or inhibitor of CYP1A2 is stopped or started during treatment with ropinirole, adjustment of the dose of ropinirole may be required) 1568

Rozerem Tablets (Efficacy may be reduced when ramelteon is used in combination with strong CYP enzyme inducers such as rifampin) 3091

Symbyax Capsules (Agents that induce CYP1A2 or glucuronyl transferase enzymes may cause an increase in olanzapine concentration) 1871

Zyprexa Tablets (May cause an increase in olanzapine clearance; therefore, a dosage increase might be considered) 1883

Zyprexa IntraMuscular (May cause an increase in olanzapine clearance; therefore, a dosage increase might be considered) 1883

Cheese, aged

Parnate Tablets (Potential for hypertensive crisis; concurrent use is contraindicated) 1532

Cheese, strong, unpasteurized

Parnate Tablets (Potential for hypertensive crisis; concurrent use is contraindicated) 1532

Cheese, unspecified

Parnate Tablets (Potential for hypertensive crisis; concurrent use is contraindicated) 1532

Chocolate

Parnate Tablets (Potential for hypertensive crisis; concurrent use is contraindicated) 1532

Cotton seed meal

Levoxyl Tablets (Concurrent use of cotton seed meal may bind and decrease the absorption of levothyroxine sodium from GI tract) 1780

Cream, sour

Parnate Tablets (Potential for hypertensive crisis; concurrent use is contraindicated) 1532

Dairy products

Cipro I.V. (Oral ciprofloxacin should not be taken concurrently with milk or yogurt alone, since absorption of ciprofloxacin may be significantly reduced; dietary calcium as part of a meal; however, does not significantly affect ciprofloxacin absorption) 2817

Cipro Tablets (Ciprofloxacin should not be taken with dairy products (like milk or yogurt) alone since absorption of ciprofloxacin may be significantly reduced; however, ciprofloxacin may be taken with a meal that contains these products) ... 2810
Cipro XR Tablets (Although ciprofloxacin extended release tablets may be taken with meals that include milk, concomitant administration with dairy products should be avoided, since decreased absorption is possible) ... 2823
Dulcolax Tablets (Dulcolax should not be taken within one hour of taking milk) ... ▣ 602
Fleet Prep Kits (Concurrent use within one hour should be avoided) ... 1149
Noroxin Tablets (Avoid simultaneous ingestion; administer norfloxacin at least one hour before or two hours after ingestion of milk and/or other dairy products) ... 2069
Pylera Capsules (Absorption of Pylera is impaired by milk or dairy products) ... 714

Diet, high-lipid

Albenza Tablets (Oral bioavailability appears to be enhanced when albendazole is co-administered with a fatty meal) ... 1297
Allegra-D 12 Hour Extended-Release Tablets (Co-administration with a high-fat meal decreased fexofenadine plasma concentrations Cmax and AUC, and Tmax was delayed by 50%; the rate of extent of pseudoephedrine absorption was not affected by food; administration of Allegra-D with food should be avoided) ... 2687
Gengraf Capsules (A high fat meal within one-half hour before cyclosporine administration decreases the AUC by 13% and Cmax by 33%) ... 435
Neoral Soft Gelatin Capsules (A high-fat meal consumed within one-half hour before Neoral administration decreased the AUC by 13% and Cmax by 33%) ... 2280
Rilutek Tablets (Co-administration with high-fat meal decreases absorption, reduces AUC by about 20% and peak blood levels by about 45%) ... 2771
Sular Extended Release Tablets (Food with a high fat content has a pronounced effect on the release of nisoldipine resulting in a significant increase in peak concentration (Cmax) by up to 300%; concomitant intake of high-fat meal should be avoided) ... 2975
Uniphyl Tablets (Co-administration with a standardized high-fat meal results in increased peak plasma concentration and bioavailability; however, a precipitous increase in the rate and extent of absorption was not evident; the dosing should be ideally administered consistently either with or without food) ... 2595

Dietary Fiber

Levoxyl Tablets (Concurrent use of dietary fiber may bind and decrease the absorption of levothyroxine sodium from GI tract) ... 1780

Drinks, hot, unspecified

Advicor Tablets (Concomitant hot drinks may increase the flushing and its use should be avoided around the time of Advicor administration) ... 402
Niaspan Extended-Release Tablets (Concomitant hot drinks may increase the side effects of flushing and pruritus and should be avoided around the time of Niaspan ingestion) ... 480

Egg Product

FluMist Vaccine (FluMist is contraindicated in individuals with history of hypersensitivity, especially anaphylactic reactions, to eggs and egg proteins) ... 1945

Eggs

FluMist Vaccine (FluMist is contraindicated in individuals with history of hypersensitivity, especially anaphylactic reactions, to eggs and egg proteins) ... 1945

Figs, canned

Parnate Tablets (Potential for hypertensive crisis; concurrent use is contraindicated) ... 1532

Food, caffeine-containing

Iquix Ophthalmic Solution (Systemic administration of some quinolones has been shown to interfere with the metabolism of caffeine) ... 3183

Food, calcium-rich

Cipro XR Tablets (Although ciprofloxacin extended release tablets may be taken with meals that include milk, concomitant administration with dairy products or with calcium-fortified juices alone should be avoided, since decreased absorption is possible) ... 2823

Food, charcoal-broiled

Rilutek Tablets (Potential inducers of CYP1A2, such as charcoal-broiled food, could increase the rate of riluzole elimination) ... 2771

Food, unspecified

Accolate Tablets (The bioavailability of zafirlukast may be decreased when taken with food. Patients should be instructed to take zafirlukast at least 1 hour before or 2 hours after meals) ... 669
Aceon Tablets (2 mg, 4 mg, 8 mg) (The presence of food in the GI tract does not affect the rate or extent of absorption of perindopril but reduces bioavailability of perindoprilat by about 35%; in clinical trials, perindopril was generally administered in a non-fasting state) ... 3038
Actonel Tablets (Mean oral bioavailability is decreased when risedronate is administered with food; risedronate sodium is effective when administered at least 30 minutes before breakfast) ... 2568
Actonel with Calcium Tablets (Mean oral bioavailability is decreased when risedronate is administered with food; risedronate sodium is effective when administered at least 30 minutes before breakfast) ... 2574
Adderall XR Capsules (Concurrent use with food prolongs T_{max} by 2.5 hours, however, food does not affect the extent of absorption) ... 3012
Avandamet Tablets (Food decreases the extent and slightly delays the absorption of metformin) ... 1336
Biaxin Filmtab Tablets (Food slightly delays both the onset of absorption and the formation of the active metabolite, but does not affect the extent of bioavailability; Biaxin may be administered without regard to food) ... 411
Captopril Tablets (Reduces absorption by about 30% to 40%; should be given one hour before meals) ... 2182
Carbatrol Capsules (A high fat meal increased the rat of absorption of a single 400 mg dose but not the AUC; elimination half-life remains unchanged between fasting and fed states) ... 3019
Ceftin Tablets (Absorption is greater when taken after food) ... 1380
Celebrex Capsules (Co-administration with a high-fat meal delayed peak plasma levels for about 1 to 2 hours with an increase in total absorption (AUC) of 10% to 20%; Celebrex can be administered without regard to the timing of meals) ... 2979
Cipro I.V. (Delays the oral absorption of the drug resulting in peak concentrations that are closer to two hours after dosing) ... 2817
Cipro Tablets (When ciprofloxacin tablets are given concomitantly with food, there is a delay in the absorption of the drug, resulting in peak concentrations that occur closer to 2 hours after dosing rather than 1 hour, whereas there is no delay observed when ciprofloxacin suspension is given with food. The overall absorption of ciprofloxacin tablets or ciprofloxacin suspension, however, is not substantially affected. The pharmacokinetics of ciprofloxacin given as the suspension are also not affected by food) ... 2810
Clinoril Tablets (The peak plasma concentrations of biologically active sulfide metabolite is delayed slightly in the presence of food) ... 1962
Coreg Tablets (When carvedilol is administered with food, the rate of absorption is slowed, as evidenced by a delay in the time to reach peak plasma levels, with no significant difference in extent of bioavailability; patients should be instructed to take Coreg with food in order to minimize the risk of hypotension) ... 1387
Coreg CR Extended-Release Capsules (Administration of Coreg CR with a high-fat meal resulted in increases in AUC (~20%) and Cmax compared to Coreg CR administered with a standard meal. Decreases in AUC (27%) and Cmax (43%) were observed when Coreg CR was administered in the fasting state compared to administration after a standard meal. Coreg CR should be taken with food) ... 1393
Crixivan Capsules (Co-administration with a meal high in calories, fat, and protein has resulted in a 77% ± 8% reduction in AUC and an 84% ± 7% reduction in Cmax; administer without food 1 hour before or 2 hours after a meal) ... 1979
Demadex Tablets (Simultaneous food intake delays the time to Cmax by about 30 minutes, but overall bioavailability (AUC) and diuretic activity are unchanged) ... 2630
Diovan Tablets (Decreases the exposure (as measured by AUC) to valsartan about 40% and peak plasma concentration by about 50%) ... 2212
EC-Naprosyn Delayed-Release Tablets (The presence of food prolonged the time the EC-Naprosyn remained in the stomach, time to first detectable serum naproxen levels, and time to maximal naproxen levels (Tmax), but did not affect peak naproxen levels (Cmax)) ... 2632
Eldepryl Capsules (The bioavailability of selegiline is increased 3 to 4 fold when it is taken with food) ... 3052
Epivir Tablets (Absorption of lamivudine was slower in the fed state compared with fasted state; there was no significant difference in systemic exposure in the fed state and fasted states; Epivir may be given with or without food) ... 1412
Evista Tablets (Administration of raloxifene with a standardized, high fat meal increases the absorption of raloxifene, but does not lead to clinically meaningful changes in systemic exposure; Evista can be administered without regard to meals) ... 1810
Evoxac Capsules (Co-administration with food decreases the rate of absorption, with a fasting Tmax of 1.53 hours and a Tmax of 2.86 hours after a meal; the peak concentration is reduced by 17.3%) ... 1013
Exelon Capsules (Co-administration with food delays absorption (Tmax) by 90 minutes, lowers Cmax by approximately 30% and increases AUC by approximately 30%) ... 2229
Flomax Capsules (Tmax is reached by 4 to 5 hours under fasting conditions and by 6 to 7 hours when tamsulosin is administered with food; taking tamsulosin under fasted conditions results in a 30% increase in AUC and 40% to 70% increase in Cmax compared to fed conditions; Flomax should be taken approximately 30 minutes following the meal) ... 848
Gabitril Tablets (A high fat meal decreases the rate (mean Tmax was prolonged to 2.5 hours, and Cmax was reduced by about 40%) but not the extent (AUC) of tiagabine) ... 973
Gengraf Capsules (The administration of food with Gengraf decreases the cyclosporine AUC and Cmax) ... 435
Imitrex Tablets (Delays the Tmax slightly by about 0.5 hour with no significant effect on the bioavailability) ... 1474
Kaletra Tablets (Co-administration with moderate fat meal was associated with a mean increase in AUC and Cmax; to enhance bioavailability Kaletra should be taken with food) ... 452
Keppra Tablets (Food does not affect the extent of absorption of levetiracetam but it decreases Cmax by 20% and delays Tmax by 1.5 hours) ... 3131
Lamisil Tablets (Co-administration has resulted in an increase in the AUC of terbinafine of less than 20%) ... 2266
Lescol Capsules (Administration of regular formulation of fluvastatin with food reduces the rate but not the extent of absorption; administration with evening meal results in a two-fold decrease in Cmax and more than a two-fold increase in tmax as compared to administration 4 hours after the evening meal; administration of Lescol XL with a high fat meal delayed the absorption and increased the bioavailability by 50%) ... 2268
Levaquin Injection (Co-administration slightly prolongs the time to peak concentration by approximately 1 hour and slightly decreases the peak concentration by approximately 14%; levofloxacin can be administered without regard to food) ... 2416

Levaquin Tablets (Co-administration slightly prolongs the time to peak concentration by approximately 1 hour and slightly decreases the peak concentration by approximately 14%; levofloxacin can be administered without regard to food) 2416

Malarone Tablets (Dietary fat intake with atovaquone increases the rate and extent of absorption; Malarone should be taken with food or milky drink) 1521

Mavik Tablets (Slows absorption of trandolapril but does not affect AUC or Cmax) 472

Maxalt Tablets (Delays the time to reach peak concentration by an hour; no significant effect on the bioavailability) 2056

Mepron Suspension (Food enhances absorption by approximately two-fold) 1526

Meridia Capsules (Co-administration with a standard breakfast has resulted in reduced peak M1 and M2 amine concentrations and delayed the time to peak by approximately three hours; the AUCs of M1 and M2 were not significantly altered) 475

Micardis Tablets (Slightly reduces the bioavailability of telmisartan; Micardis tablets may be administered with or without food) 852

Micardis HCT Tablets (Slightly reduces the bioavailability of telmisartan with reduction in AUC of about 6%) 854

Mirapex Tablets (Food does not affect the extent of pramipexole absorption, although the time of maximum plasma concentration is increased by about 1 hour when the drug is taken with a meal) 857

Mobic Tablets (Co-administration with a high-fat breakfast did not affect extent of absorption of meloxicam capsules but led to 22% higher Cmax values; mean Cmax values were achieved between 5 to 6 hours; Mobic tablets can be administered without regard to timing of meals) 863

Neoral Soft Gelatin Capsules (Administration of food with Neoral decreases the AUC and Cmax) 2280

Noroxin Tablets (Co-administration may decrease the absorption of norfloxacin; administer at least one hour before or two hours after a meal) 2069

Omnicef Capsules (Although Cmax and AUC of cefdinir absorption from capsules are reduced by 44% and 33%, respectively, when given with a high-fat meal, the magnitude of these reductions is not likely to be clinically significant; therefore, cefdinir may be taken without regard to food) 497

Paxil Tablets (Co-administration with food resulted in a slight increase (6%) in AUC, but Cmax was 29% greater; time to reach peak plasma concentration decreased from 6.4 hours post-dosing to 4.9 hours) 1535

Pepcid Tablets (Bioavailability may be slightly increased by antacids) 2075

Pletal Tablets (Co-administration with a high-fat meal increases absorption, with an approximately 90% increase in Cmax and a 25% increase in AUC; patients should be advised to take Pletal at least one hour before or two hours after breakfast and dinner) 2481

Premphase Tablets (Administration with a high fat breakfast decreased total estrone Cmax and increased total equilin Cmax compared to fasting state, no other effect on rate or extent of absorption; administration with food doubles MPA Cmax and increases MPA AUC) 3232

Prempro Tablets (Administration with food decreased Cmax of total estrone compared to fasting state, no other effect on rate or extent of absorption; administration with food doubles MPA Cmax and increases MPA AUC) 3232

Prograf Capsules and Injection (The presence and composition of food has decreased both the rate and extent of tacrolimus absorption; this effect was most pronounced with a high-fat meal; the rate and extent of tacrolimus absorption were greatest under fasted conditions) 622

Prometrium Capsules (100 mg, 200 mg) (Concomitant food ingestion increases the bioavailability of Prometrium Capsules relative to the fasting state) 3047

Provigil Tablets (Delays the absorption (tmax) by approximately one hour; no effect on overall bioavailability) 977

Prozac Pulvules and Liquid (May delay absorption of fluoxetine inconsequentially; Prozac may be administered with or without food) 1852

Rapamune Tablets (In healthy subjects, a high-fat meal (861.8 kcal, 54.9% kcal from fat) increased the mean total exposure (AUC) of sirolimus by 23% to 35% compared with fasting. The effect of food on the mean sirolimus Cmax was inconsistent depending on the sirolimus dosage form evaluated) 3260

Remeron Tablets (The presence of food in the stomach has a minimal effect on both the rate and extent of absorption and does not require a dosage adjustment) 2924

Requip Tablets (Food does not affect the extent of absorption of ropinirole, although its Tmax is increased by two and a half hours and its Cmax is decreased by approximately 25% when the drug is taken with a high-fat meal) 1561

Requip XL Tablets (In a single-dose study, administration of ropinirole to healthy volunteers with food (eg, high-fat meal) increased AUC by approximately 30% and Cmax by approximately 44%, compared with dosing under fasted conditions. In a repeat-dose study in patients with Parkinson's disease, food (eg, high-fat meal) increased AUC by approximately 20% and Cmax by approximately 44%; Tmax was prolonged by 3 hours (median prolongation) compared with dosing under fasted conditions) 1568

Romazicon Injection (Ingestion of food during an IV infusion results in a 50% increase in clearance) 2646

Rythmol SR Capsules (Increased peak blood level and bioavailability in a single dose study) 1590

Sanctura XR Capsules (Administration of trospium immediately after a high fat-content meal reduced the oral bioavailability of trospium chloride by 35% for AUC and by 60% for Cmax. It is recommended that trospium be taken on an empty stomach at least one hour before a meal) 557

Skelaxin Tablets (Taking metaxalone with food may enhance general CNS depression, especially in the elderly) 1784

Starlix Tablets (The pharmacokinetics of nateglinide were not affected by the composition of a meal (high protein, fat, or carbohydrate). However, peak plasma levels were significantly reduced when nateglinide was administered 10 minutes prior to a liquid meal) 2314

Sular Extended Release Tablets (A pronounced food-effect is observed when nisldipine is administered with a high-fat meal resulting in an increased peak concentration (Cmax) of up to 245%. Total exposure (AUC) is decreased by 22%. As a result, nisldipine should be taken on an empty stomach (1 hour before or 2 hours after a meal)) 2975

Suprax for Oral Suspension (Cefixime, given orally, is about 40% to 50% absorbed whether administered with or without food; however, time to maximal absorption is increased approximately 0.8 hours when administered with food) 1891

Sustiva Capsules (High fat meal may increase the absorption of Sustiva and should be avoided; it can be taken with or without meals of normal composition) 930

Targretin Capsules (Co-administration with a fat-containing meal has resulted in higher plasma bexarotene AUC and Cmax values; because safety and efficacy data are based upon administration with food, it is recommended that Targretin capsules be administered with or immediately following a meal) 1084

Tarka Tablets (Co-administration with food decreases verapamil bioavailability and the time to peak plasma concentration is delayed; bioavailability of trandolapril is not altered; Tarka should be administered with food) 511

Tasigna Capsules (The bioavailability of nilotinib is increased with food. Nilotinib should not be taken with food. No food should be taken at least 2 hours before and at least one hour after the dose is taken) 2316

Teveten Tablets (Co-administration with food delays absorption and causes variable changes in Cmax and AUC values which do not appear clinically important) 515

Tricor Tablets (The absorption of fenofibrate is increased when administered with food; Tricor should be given with meals) 520

Valcyte Tablets (Co-administration with high fat meals has resulted in increased steady-state ganciclovir AUC and Cmax without any prolongation in time to peak plasma concentrations; Valcyte should be administered with food) 2654

Vesanoid Capsules (The absorption of retinoids as a class has been shown to be enhanced when taken with food) 2660

Viread Tablets (Increases the bioavailability and delays the time to tenofovir Cmax; Viread should be taken with a meal) 1268

Wellbutrin SR Sustained-Release Tablets (Food increases Cmax and AUC of bupropion by 11% and 17%, respectively; no clinically significant food effect) 1653

Xeloda Tablets (Reduces both rate and extent of absorption of capecitabine and delays Tmax of both parent and 5-FU) 2662

Xenical Capsules (Gastrointestinal events may increase when orlistat is taken with a diet high in fat) 2672

Zofran Tablets (Bioavailability slightly enhanced by food) 1687

Zyban Sustained-Release Tablets (Food increases Cmax and AUC of bupropion by 11% and 17% respectively. The mean time to peak concentration Tmax was prolonged by 1 hour; this effect was of no clinical significance) 1692

Zyvox Tablets (Linezolid may be administered without regard to the timing of meals. The time to reach maximum concentration is delayed from 1.5 hours to 2.2 hours and Cmax is decreased by about 17% when high fat food is given with linezolid. However, the total exposure measured as AUC values is similar under both conditions) 2552

Food having a pH greater than 5.5

Creon 5 Capsules (Can dissolve the protective coating resulting in early release of enzymes, irritation of oral mucosa, and/or loss of enzyme activity) 3041

Ultrase Capsules (Can dissolve the protective coating resulting in early release of enzymes, irritation of oral mucosa, and/or loss of enzyme activity) 718

Ultrase MT Capsules (Can dissolve the protective enteric shell) 719

Food high in tyramine

Azilect Tablets (Severe hypertensive reactions have followed the administration of tyramine rich foods and non-selective MAO inhibitors) 3106

Emsam Transdermal System (As a class, MAO inhibitors have been associated with hypertensive crises caused by the ingestion of foods with a high concentration of tyramine) 905

Marplan Tablets (Isocarboxazid should not be administered in combination with cheese or other foods with a high tyramine content. Hypertensive crises have sometimes occurred during isocarboxazid therapy after ingestion of foods with a high tyramine content. In general, patients should avoid protein foods in which aging or protein breakdown is used to increase flavor. In particular, patients should be instructed not to take foods such as cheese, sour cream, Chianti wine, sherry, beer (including non-alcoholic beer), liqueurs, pickled herring, anchovies, caviar, liver, canned figs, raisins, bananas or avocados, chocolate, soy sauce, sauerkraut, the pods of broad beans (fava beans), yeast extracts, yogurt, meat extracts, meat prepared with tenderizers, or dry sausage) 3177

Zyvox Tablets (A significant pressor response has been observed in normal adult subjects receiving linezolid and tyramine doses of more than 100 mg. Therefore, patients receiving linezolid need to avoid consuming large amounts of foods or beverages with high tyramine content) 2552

Food with high concentration of tyramine

Emsam Transdermal System (As a class, MAO inhibitors have been associated with hypertensive crises caused by the ingestion of foods with a high concentration of tyramine) 905

Parnate Tablets (Potential for hypertensive crisis; concurrent use is contraindicated)..................1532

Fruit juices, unspecified

Allegra Tablets (Grapefruit, orange and apple may reduce the bioavailability and exposure of fexofenadine; it is recommended that fexofenadine should be taken with water)....................................2684

Cipro Tablets (Ciprofloxacin should not be taken with calcium-fortified juices alone since absorption of ciprofloxacin may be significantly reduced; however, ciprofloxacin may be taken with a meal that contains these products)....................................2810

Dexedrine Spansule Sustained-Release Capsules (Lowers absorption of amphetamines) 1401

Fruits, dried

Parnate Tablets (Potential for hypertensive crisis; concurrent use is contraindicated)..................1532

Fruits, overripe

Parnate Tablets (Potential for hypertensive crisis; concurrent use is contraindicated)..................1532

Grapefruit

Abilify Tablets (Inhibitors of CYP3A4 can inhibit aripiprazole elimination and cause increased blood levels) 881

Abilify Tablets (Inhibitors of CYP3A4 can inhibit aripiprazole elimination and cause increased blood levels) 2466

Actiq (Grapefruit and grapefruit juice decrease CYP3A4 activity, increasing blood concentrations of fentanyl; concurrent use should be avoided)........................ 959

Advair Diskus 100/50 (Fluticasone propionate and salmeterol, the individual components of Advair Diskus, are substrates of CYP3A4. The use of strong CYP3A4 inhibitors (e.g., ritonavir, atazanavir, clarithromycin, indinavir, itraconazole, nefazodone, nelfinavir, saquinavir, ketoconazole, telithromycin) with Advair Diskus is not recommended because increased corticosteroid and increased cardiovascular adverse effects may occur) 1276

Advair HFA 45/21 Inhalation Aerosol (Concomitant administration of erythromycin (a moderate CYP3A4 inhibitor) and salmeterol inhalation aerosol resulted in a 40% increase in salmeterol Cmax at steady state, a 3.6-beat/min. increase in heart rate, a 5.8-msec increase in QTc interval, and no change in plasma potassium. Due to the potential increased risk of cardiovascular events, the concomitant use of salmeterol with strong CYP3A4 inhibitors (e.g., ketoconazole, ritonavir, atazanavir, clarithromycin, indinavir, itraconazone, nefazodone, nelfinavir, saquinavir, telithromycin) is not recommended) 1288

Advicor Tablets (The risk of myopathy appears to be increased by high levels of HMG-CoA reductase inhibitory activity in plasma. Lovastatin is metabolized by the cytochrome P450 isoform 3A4. Certain drugs which share this metabolic pathway can raise the plasma levels of lovastatin and may increase the risk of myopathy)................................. 402

Ambien Tablets (Some compounds known to inhibit CYP3A may increase exposure to zolpidem).................................2692

Ambien CR Tablets (Some compounds known to inhibit CYP3A4 may increase exposure to zolpidem tartrate) 2696

Angeliq Tablets (Inhibitors of CYP3A4 such as erythromycin, clarithromycin, ketoconazole, itraconazole, ritonavir and grapefruit juice may increase plasma concentrations of estrogens and may result in side effects) 751

Avodart Soft Gelatin Capsules (Blood concentrations of dutasteride may increase in the presence of CYP3A4 inhibitors) 1359

Carbatrol Capsules (Carbamazepine is metabolized mainly by cytochrome P450 (CYP) 3A4 to the active carbamazepine 10,11 -epoxide, which is further metabolized to the trans-diol by epoxide hydrolase. Therefore, the potential exists for interaction between carbamazepine and any agent that inhibits CYP3A4 and/or epoxide hydrolase) 3019

Cardizem LA Extended Release Tablets (Diltiazem is both a substrate and an inhibitor of the CYP3A4 enzyme system. Other drugs that are specific substrates, inhibitors, or inducers of this enzyme system may have a significant impact on the efficacy and side effect profile of diltiazem) 421

Celexa Tablets (In vitro studies indicated that CYP3A4 and CYP2C19 are the primary enzymes involved in the metabolism of citalopram. However, co-administration of citalopram (40 mg) and ketoconazole (200 mg), a potent inhibitor of CYP3A4, did not significantly affect the pharmacokinetics of citalopram. Because citalopram is metabolized by multiple enzyme systems, inhibition of a single enzyme may not appreciably decrease citalopram clearance)......1160

Cialis Tablets (Tadalafil is a substrate of and predominantly metabolized by CYP3A4. Studies have shown that drugs that inhibit CYP3A4 can increase tadalafil exposure. When tadalafil is used on an as-needed basis, patients taking concomitant potent inhibitors of CYP3A4, such as ketoconazole or ritonavir, the maximum recommended dose of tadalafil is 10 mg, not to exceed once every 72 hours. When tadalafil is used in a once-daily regimen, patients taking concomitant potent inhibitors of CYP3A4, such as ketoconazole or ritonavir, the dose should not exceed 2.5 mg).....1792

Climara Transdermal System (Inhibitors of CYP3A4 such as erythromycin, clarithromycin, ketoconazole, itraconazole, ritonavir and grapefruit juice may increase plasma concentrations of estrogens and may result in side effects) 763

Climara Pro Transdermal System (Inhibitors of CYP3A4 such as erythromycin, clarithromycin, ketoconazole, itraconazole, ritonavir and grapefruit juice may increase plasma concentrations of estrogens and may result in side effects) 768

Crixivan Capsules (Co-administration of indinavir and other drugs that inhibit CYP3A4 may decrease the clearance of indinavir and may result in increased plasma concentrations of indinavir) 1979

Divigel (Inhibitors of CYP3A4, such as erythromycin, clarithromycin, ketoconazole, itraconazole, ritonavir, and grapefruit juice, may increase plasma concentrations of estrogens and result in side effects) 3167

Duragesic Transdermal System (The concomitant use of fentanyl with all CYP3A4 inhibitors (such as ritonavir, ketoconazole, itraconazole, troleandomycin, clarithromycin, nelfinavir, nefazodone, amiodarone, amprenavir, aprepitant, diltiazem, erythromycin, fluconazole, fosamprenavir, grapefruit juice, and verapamil) may result in an increase in fentanyl plasma concentrations, which could increase or prolong adverse drug effects and may cause potentially fatal respiratory depression. Patients receiving fentanyl and any CYP3A4 inhibitor should be monitored for an extended period of time and dosage adjustments should be made if warranted) 2405

Effexor XR Extended-Release Capsules (Concomitant use of CYP3A4 inhibitors and venlafaxine may increase levels of venlafaxine and O-desmethylvenlafaxine (ODV). Therefore, caution is advised if venlafaxine is used concomitantly with CYP3A4 inhibitors).......................................3195

Elidel Cream 1% (The concomitant administration of known CYP3A family of inhibitors in patients with widespread and/or erythrodermic disease should be done with caution).....................2221

Emend Capsules (Aprepitant is a substrate for CYP3A4; therefore, co-administration of fosaprepitant or aprepitant with drugs that inhibit CYP3A4 activity may result in increased plasma concentrations of aprepitant. Consequently, concomitant administration of fosaprepitant or aprepitant with strong CYP3A4 inhibitors (e.g., ketoconazole, itraconazole, nefazodone, troleandomycin, clarithromycin, ritonavir, nelfinavir) should be approached with caution. Because moderate CYP3A4 inhibitors (e.g., diltiazem) result in a 2-fold increase in plasma concentrations of aprepitant, concomitant administration should also be approached with caution).......................................1992

Enjuvia Tablets (Inhibitors of CYP3A4 such as erythromycin, clarithromycin, ketoconazole, itraconazole, ritonavir and grapefruit juice may increase plasma concentrations of estrogens and may result in side effects) 1029

Equetro Extended-Release Capsules (Carbamazepine is metabolized mainly by CYP3A4 the active carbamazepine 10,11-epoxide, which is futher metabolized to the trans-diol by epoxide hydrolase. Therefore, the potential exists for interaction between carbamazepine and any agent that inhibits CYP3A4 and/or epoxide hydrolase. Agents that are CYP3A4 inhibitors may increase the plasma levels of carbamazepine. Thus, if a patient has been titrated to a stable dosage of carbamazepine, and then begins a course of treatment with a CYP3A4 or epoxide hydrolase inhibitor, it is reasonable to expect that a dose reduction for carbamazepine may be necessary) 3174

Estratest H.S. Tablets (Co-administration with inhibitors of CYP3A4 may increase plasma concentrations of estrogens and may result in side effects) 3043

Evoxac Capsules (Drugs which inhibit CYP3A3/4 also inhibit the metabolism of cevimeline)........1013

Fentora Tablets (The concomitant use of moderate CYP3A4 inhibitors such as amprenavir, aprepitant, diltiazem, erythromycin, fluconazole, fosamprenavir, grapefruit juice, and verapamil with fentanyl citrate may result in an increase in fentanyl plasma concentrations, which could increase or prolong adverse drug effects and may cause potentially fatal respiratory depression. Patients receiving fentanyl citrate and moderate CYP3A4 inhibitors should be carefully monitored for an extended period of time and dosage increase should be done conservatively) 968

Flomax Capsules (Concomitant administration of tamsulosin HCl and an inhibitor of CYP3A4 may lead to increased tamsulosin HCl plasma exposure. Tamsulosin HCl capsules should be used with caution in combination with moderate or strong inhibitors of CYP3A4 (e.g., ketoconazole), particularly at doses higher than 0.4mg)................................ 848

Flonase Nasal Spray (Caution should be exercised when potent cytochrome P450 3A4 inhibitors are co-administered with fluticasone propionate) 1431

Gengraf Capsules (Affects the metabolism of cyclosporine increasing blood concentration of cyclosporine; concurrent use should be avoided)........................ 435

Gleevec Tablets (There was a significant increase in exposure to imatinib (mean Cmax and AUC increased by 26% and 40% respectively) in healthy subjects when imatinib mesylate was co-administered with a single dose of ketoconazole (a CYP3A4 inhibitor). Caution is recommended when administering imatinib mesylate with strong CYP3A4 inhibitors (eg, ketoconazole, itraconazole, clarithromycin, atazanavir, indinavir, nefazodone, nelfinavir, ritonavir, saquinavir, telithromycin, and voriconazole). Grapefruit juice may also increase plasma concentrations of imatinib and should be avoided. Substances that inhibit the cytochrome P450 isoenzyme (CPY3A4) activity may decrease metabolism and increase imatinib concentrations)................2255

Intelence Tablets (Etravirine is a substrate of CYP3A4, CYP2C9, and CYP2C19. Therefore, co-administration of etravirine with drugs that induce or inhibit CYP3A4, CYP2C9, and CYP2C19 may alter the therapeutic effect or adverse reaction profile of etravirine)..........**3119**

Ionsys Transdermal System (The concomitant use of fentanyl with CYP3A4 inhibitors may result in a decrease in fentanyl clearance, which could increase or prolong adverse drug effects including serious respiratory depression. In this situation, special patient care and observation is appropriate) **2410**

Ixempra Kit for Injection (Grapefruit juice may increase plasma concentrations of ixabepilone and should be avoided) **915**

Lamisil Oral Granules (It is likely that inhibitors of both CYP2C9 and CYP3A4 may lead to substantial increase in the systemic exposure (Cmax and AUC) of terbinafine).......................**2264**

Letairis Tablets (Use caution when ambrisentan is co-administered with strong CYP3A inhibitors)..........**1258**

Levitra Tablets (Although specific interactions have not been studied, other CYP3A4 inhibitors, including grapefruit juice, would likely increase vardenafil exposure).......................**2876**

Lexapro Tablets (In vitro studies indicated that CYP3A4 and -2C19 are the primary enzymes involved in the metabolism of escitalopram. However, co-administration of escitalopram oxalate (20 mg) and ritonavir (600 mg), a potent inhibitor of CYP3A4, did not significantly affect the pharmacokinetics of escitalopram oxalate. Because escitalopram oxalate is metabolized by multiple enzyme systems, inhibition of a single enzyme may not appreciably decrease escitalopram clearance) **1174**

Lexiva Tablets (Amprenavir is metabolized by CYP 3A4. Co-administration of fosamprenavir calcium and drugs that inhibit CYP3A4 may increase amprenavir concentrations and increase the incidence of adverse effects) **1510**

Lipitor Tablets (Contains one or more components that inhibit CYP 3A4 and can increase plasma concentrations of atorvastatin, especially with excessive grapefruit consumption (greater than 1.2 liters per day))...............................**2501**

Luvox CR Extended-Release Capsules (Fluvoxamine is a known potent inhibitor of CYP1A2 and also inhibits CYP3A4, CYP2C9, and CYP2C19)....................................**1759**

Lybrel Tablets (CYP 3A4 inhibitors such as indinavir, itraconazole, ketoconazole, fluconazole, and troleandomycin may increase plasma hormone levels. Troleandomycin may also increase the risk of intrahepatic cholestasis during coadministration with combination oral contraceptives).............................**3204**

Mevacor Tablets (The risk of myopathy/rhabdomyolysis is increased by concomitant use of lovastatin with potent inhibitors of CYP3A4, particularly with higher doses of lovastatin; concomitant use should be avoided unless the benefits of combined therapy outweigh the increased risk)...........**2063**

Neoral Soft Gelatin Capsules (Affects the metabolism of cyclosporine and should be avoided) **2280**

Nimotop Capsules (Grapefruit juice inhibits the cytochrome P450 3A4 system. Administration of dihydropyridine calcium antagonists together with grapefruit juice thus results in elevated concentrations and prolonged action of nimodipine due to a decreased first pass metabolism or reduced clearance. As a consequence, the blood pressure lowering effect may be increased. After intake of grapefruit juice this effect may last for at least 4 days after the last ingestion of grapefruit juice. Ingestion of grapefruit/grapefruit juice is therefore to be avoided while taking nimodipine) **790**

NuvaRing (CYP3A4 inhibitors may increase plasma hormone levels) **2897**

Ortho-Cyclen Tablets (CYP3A4 inhibitors such as itraconazole or ketoconazole may increase plasma hormone levels)................**2449**

Pletal Tablets (A reduced dose of cilostazol should be considered when taken concomitantly with CYP3A4 inhibitors)...............................**2481**

PrandiMet Tablets (Repaglinide is metabolized by CYP2C8 and to a lesser extent by CYP3A4. Drugs that inhibit 3A4 may alter the pharmacokinetics and pharmacodynamics of repaglinide)......................................**2967**

Prandin Tablets (Repaglinide is metabolized by the cytochrome P4502C8 and 3A4 enzymes. Consequently, repaglinide metabolism may be altered by drugs that are CYP3A4 inhibitors. Caution should be used in patients concomitantly using repaglinide and a CYP3A4 inhibitor. The effect may be very significant if both CYP3A4 and CYP2C8 are inhibited at the same time) **2971**

Premarin Tablets (Co-administration of inhibitors of CYP3A4 with estrogens may affect estrogen drug metabolism. Inhibitors of CYP3A4 may increase plasma concentrations of estrogens and may result in side effects) **3221**

Premphase Tablets (Co-administration of estrogens with inhibitors of CYP3A4 may increase plasma concentrations of estrogens and may result in side effects) **3232**

Prempro Tablets (Co-administration of estrogens with inhibitors of CYP3A4 may increase plasma concentrations of estrogens and may result in side effects) **3232**

Pristiq Extended-Release Tablets (CYP3A4 is a minor pathway for the metabolism of desvenlafaxine. In a clinical study, ketoconazole (200 mg b.i.d.) increased the area under the concentration vs. time curve AUC of desvenlafaxine (400 mg single dose) by about 43% and Cmax by about 8%. Concomitant use of desvenlafaxine with potent inhibitors of CYP3A4 may result in higher concentrations of desvenlafaxine) **3247**

Prograf Capsules and Injection (Since tacrolimus is metabolized mainly by the CYP3A enzyme systems, substances known to inhibit these enzymes may decrease the metabolism or increase bioavailability of tacrolimus as indicated by increased whole blood or plasma concentrations. Monitoring of blood concentrations and appropriate dosage adjustments are essential when such drugs are used concomitantly) **622**

Provigil Tablets (Co-administration of potent inhibitors of CYP3A4 could alter the plasma levels of modafinil) **977**

Reyataz Capsules (Co-administration of atazanavir sulfate and other drugs that inhibit CYP3A may increase atazanavir sulfate plasma concentrations)...........................**3299**

Rozerem Tablets (Ramelteon should be administered with caution in subjects taking strong CYP2C9 inhibitors such as fluconazole)...............................**3091**

Rythmol Tablets (Propafenone is metabolized by CYP3A4. Drugs that inhibit CYP3A4 can be expected to cause increased plasma levels of propafenone. Appropriate monitoring is recommended when propafenone is used together with such drugs) **1586**

Rythmol SR Capsules (Drugs that inhibit CYP3A4 might lead to increased plasma levels of propafenone; patients should be closely monitored and the propafenone dose adjusted accordingly) **1590**

Sandimmune I.V. Ampuls for Infusion (Co-administration results in increased blood concentrations of cyclosporine; concurrent use should be avoided) **2296**

Seasonique Tablets (CYP3A4 inhibitors may increase plasma ethinyl estradiol levels) **1046**

Sensipar Tablets (Since cinacalcet hydrochloride is metabolized in part by CYP3A4, dose adjustment of cinacalcet hydrochloride may be required and PTH and serum calcium concentrations closely monitored if a patient initiates or discontinues therapy with a strong CYP3A4 inhibitor) **594**

Serevent Diskus (Coadministration of salmeterol and a strong CYP3A4 inhibitor ketoconazole resulted in a significant increase in plasma salmeterol exposure as determined by a 16-fold increase in AUC mainly due to increased bioavailability of swallowed portion of the dose. Although there was no statistical effect on the mean QTc, coadministration of salmeterol and ketoconazole was associated with more frequent increases in QTc duration compared with salmeterol and placebo administration. Due to the potential increased risk of cardiovascular adverse events, the concomitant use of salmeterol with strong CYP3A4 inhibitors, (eg, ketoconazole, ritonavir, atazanavir, clarithromycin, indinavir, itraconazole, nefazodone, nelfinavir, saquinavir, telithromycin) is not recommended) **1594**

Simcor Tablets (Potent inhibitors of CYP3A4 increase the risk of myopathy by reducing the elimination of simvastatin. Hence when simvastatin is used with a potent inhibitor of CYP3A4, elevated plasma levels of HMG-CoA reductase inhibitory activity can increase the riskof myopathy and rhabdomyolysis, particularly with higher doses of simvastatin. Concomitant use of drugs labeled as potent inhibitors of CYP3A4 should be avoided unless the benefits of combined therapy outweigh the increased risk. If treatment with itraconazole, ketoconazole, erythromycin, clarithromycin or telithromycin is unavoidable, therapy with Simcor should be suspended during the course of treatment) **502**

Suboxone Tablets (Buprenorphine is metabolized to norbuprenorphine by cytochrome CYP3A4. Because CYP3A4 inhibitors may increase plasma concentrations of buprenorphine, patients already on CYP3A4 inhibitors should have their dose of Subutex or Suboxone adjusted.) **2601**

Subutex Tablets (Buprenorphine is metabolized to norbuprenorphine by cytochrome CYP3A4. Because CYP3A4 inhibitors may increase plasma concentrations of buprenorphine, patients already on CYP3A4 inhibitors should have their dose of Subutex or Suboxone adjusted.) **2601**

Sutent Capsules (Grapefruit may increase plasma concentrations of sunitinib maleate) **2540**

Symbicort 80/4.5 Inhalation Aerosol (Concomitant administration of CYP3A4 inhibitors (e.g., itraconazole, clarithromycin, erythromycin, etc.) may inhibit the metabolism of, and increase the systemic exposure to, budesonide. Caution should be exercised with co-administration of Symbicort with potent CYP3A4 inhibitors) **659**

Tarceva Tablets (Caution when administering or taking erlotinib with strong CYP3A4 inhibitors such as atazanavir, clarithromycin, indinavir, itraconazole, nefazodone, nelfinavir, ritonavir, saquinavir, telithromycin, troleandomycin, and voriconazole)..........................**1228**

Targretin Gel 1% (Bexarotene is metabolized by CYP4503A4; co-administration with inhibitors of CYP4503A4, such as grapefruit juice, could lead to an increase in plasma bexarotene concentrations)...............................**1088**

Tasigna Capsules (Grapefruit products may increase serum concentrations of nilotinib and should be avoided)...........................**2316**

Taxotere Injection Concentrate (The metabolism of docetaxel may be modified by the concomitant administration of compounds that inhibit cytochrome P450 3A4. Caution should be exercised with these drugs when treating patients receiving docetaxel as there is a potential for a significant reaction).......................................**2773**

Tracleer Tablets (Co-administration of both a CYP2C9 inhibitor and a CYP3A4 inhibitor with bosentan will likely lead to large increases in plasma concentrations of bosentan and is not recommended) **3289**

Triesence Injectable Suspension (Ketoconazole has been reported to decrease the metabolism of certain corticosteroids by up to 60% leading to an increased risk of corticosteroid side effects)..........⊙ **209**

Tykerb Tablets (Grapefruit may also increase plasma concentrations of lapatinib and should be avoided).........................**1631**

Ultram ER Extended-Release Tablets (Administration of CYP3A4 inhibitors, such as ketoconazole and erythromycin, with tramadol hydrochloride may effect the metabolism of tramadol leading to altered tramadol exposure)........................**2428**

Valium Tablets (There is a potentially relevant interaction between diazepam and certain hepatic enzyme inhibitors such as CYP450 3A4. It has been shown that these compounds influence the pharmacokinetics of diazepam and may lead to increased and prolonged sedation)......................................**2058**

Vaprisol (Conivaptan is a substrate of CYP3A4. Co-administration of conivaptan with CYP3A4 inhibitors could lead to an increase in conivaptan concentrations. Concomitant use of conivaptan with potent CYP3A4 inhibitors is contraindicated) 632

Velcade for Injection (Patients who are concomitantly receiving bortezomib and drugs that are inhibitors or inducers of cytochrome P450 3A4 should be closely monitored for either toxicities or reduced efficacy) 2168

Venlafaxine Hydrochloride Tablets (Concomitant use of CYP3A4 inhibitors and venlafaxine may increase levels of venlafaxine and ODV. Therefore, caution is advised if a patient's therapy includes a CYP3A4 inhibitor and venlafaxine concomitantly. The concomitant use of venlafaxine with a drug treatment(s) that potently inhibits both CYP2D6 and CYP3A4, the primary metabolizing enzymes for venlafaxine, has not been studied. Therefore, caution is advised should a patient's therapy include venlafaxine and any agent(s) that produce potent simultaneous inhibition of these two enzyme systems) 2199

Vesanoid Capsules (Tretinoin is metaboized by the hepatic P450 system; therefore, there is a potential for alteration of pharmacokinetic parameters in patients administered concomitant medications that are also inducers of this system. To date, there is no data to suggest that co-use with these medications increases or decreases either efficacy or toxicity of tretinoin) 2660

Vytorin 10/10 Tablets (Simvastatin is metabolized by the cytochrome P450 isoform 3A4. Certain drugs that inhibit this metabolic pathway can raise plasma levels of simvastatin and may increase the risk of myopathy. This includes large quantities of grapefruit juice (greater than 1 quart daily). The use of Vytorin concomitantly with this CYP3A4 inhibitor should be avoided) 2149

Vytorin 10/10 Tablets (The risk of myopathy and rhabdomyolysis is increased by high levels of statin activity in plasma. Simvastatin is metabolized by the cytochrome P450 3A4. Certain drugs that inhibit this metabolic pathway can raise the plasma levels of simvastatin and may increase the risk of myopathy. These include large quantities of grapefruit juice (greater than 1 quart daily); concurrent use should be avoided) 2939

Zocor Tablets (The risk of myopathy and rhabdomyolysis is increased by high level of statin activity in plasma. Simvastatin is metabolized by the cytochrome P450 isoform 3A4. Certain drugs, including the large quantities of grapefruit juice (greater than 1 quart daily), which inhibit this metabolic pathway can raise the plasma levels of simvastatin and may increase the risk of myopathy. The use of simvastatin concomitantly with this CYP3A4 inhibitor should be avoided) 2136

Grapefruit Juice

Abilify Tablets (Inhibitors of CYP3A4 can inhibit aripiprazole elimination and cause increased blood levels) 881

Abilify Tablets (Inhibitors of CYP3A4 can inhibit aripiprazole elimination and cause increased blood levels) 2466

Actiq (Grapefruit and grapefruit juice decrease CYP3A4 activity, increasing blood concentrations of fentanyl; concurrent use should be avoided) 959

Advair Diskus 100/50 (Fluticasone propionate and salmeterol, the individual components of Advair Diskus, are substrates of CYP3A4. The use of strong CYP3A4 inhibitors (e.g., ritonavir, atazanavir, clarithromycin, indinavir, itraconazole, nefazodone, nelfinavir, saquinavir, ketoconazole, telithromycin) with Advair Diskus is not recommended because increased corticosteroid and increased cardiovascular adverse effects may occur) 1276

Advair HFA 45/21 Inhalation Aerosol (Concomitant administration of erythromycin (a moderate CYP3A4 inhibitor) and salmeterol inhalation aerosol resulted in a 40% increase in salmeterol Cmax at steady state, a 3.6-beat/min. increase in heart rate, a 5.8-msec increase in QTc interval, and no change in plasma potassium. Due to the potential increased risk of cardiovascular events, the concomitant use of salmeterol with strong CYP3A4 inhibitors (e.g., ketoconazole, ritonavir, atazanavir, clarithromycin, indinavir, itraconazone, nefazodone, nelfinavir, saquinavir, telithromycin) is not recommended) 1288

Advicor Tablets (Inhibits CYP3A4 and can increase the plasma concentration of lovastatin; concurrent use should be avoided) 402

Agrylin Capsules (Anagrelide is metabolized at least in part by CYP1A2. Therefore, CYP1A2 inhibitors could theoretically adversely influence the clearance of anagrelide) 3017

Allegra-D 12 Hour Extended-Release Tablets (Co-administration with grapefruit, orange or apple juice will reduce the bioavailability and exposure or fexofenadine) 2687

Angeliq Tablets (Inhibitors of CYP3A4 such as erythromycin, clarithromycin, ketoconazole, itraconazole, ritonavir and grapefruit juice may increase plasma concentrations of estrogens and may result in side effects) 751

Avodart Soft Gelatin Capsules (Blood concentrations of dutasteride may increase in the presence of CYP3A4 inhibitors) 1359

Azilect Tablets (Rasagiline plasma concentrations may increase up to 2 fold in patients using concomitant CYP1A2 inhibitors) 3106

Carbatrol Capsules (Carbamazepine is metabolized mainly by cytochrome P450 (CYP) 3A4 to the active carbamazepine 10,11 -epoxide, which is further metabolized to the trans-diol by epoxide hydrolase. Therefore, the potential exists for interaction between carbamazepine and any agent that inhibits CYP3A4 and/or epoxide hydrolase) 3019

Cardizem LA Extended Release Tablets (Diltiazem is both a substrate and an inhibitor of the CYP3A4 enzyme system. Other drugs that are specific substrates, inhibitors, or inducers of this enzyme system may have a significant impact on the efficacy and side effect profile of diltiazem) 421

Celexa Tablets (In vitro studies indicated that CYP3A4 and CYP2C19 are the primary enzymes involved in the metabolism of citalopram. However, co-administration of citalopram (40 mg) and ketoconazole (200 mg), a potent inhibitor of CYP3A4, did not significantly affect the pharmacokinetics of citalopram. Because citalopram is metabolized by multiple enzyme systems, inhibition of a single enzyme may not appreciably decrease citalopram clearance) 1160

Cialis Tablets (CYP3A4 inhibitors such as grapefruit juice may likely increase tadalafil exposure) 1792

Climara Transdermal System (Inducers of CYP3A4, such as grapefruit juice, may increase plasma concentrations of estrogens and may result in side effects) 763

Climara Pro Transdermal System (Inhibitors of CYP3A4 such as erythromycin, clarithromycin, ketoconazole, itraconazole, ritonavir and grapefruit juice may increase plasma concentrations of estrogens and may result in side effects) 768

Crixivan Capsules (Potential for decrease in indinavir AUC) 1979

Cymbalta Delayed-Release Capsules (Concomitant use of duloxetine with fluvoxamine, an inhibitor of CYP1A2, results in a 6-fold increase in AUC, about 2.5-fold increase in Cmax, and an approximately 3-fold increase in t1/2 of duloxetine. Since duloxetine is metabolized in part by CYP1A2, concomitant use of duloxetine with other inhibitors of CYP1A2, would be expected to have the same effects; these combinations should be avoided) 1801

Divigel (Inhibitors of CYP3A4, such as erythromycin, clarithromycin, ketoconazole, itraconazole, ritonavir, and grapefruit juice, may increase plasma concentrations of estrogens and result in side effects) 3167

Duragesic Transdermal System (The concomitant use of fentanyl with all CYP3A4 inhibitors (such as ritonavir, ketoconazole, itraconazole, troleandomycin, clarithromycin, nelfinavir, nefazodone, amiodarone, amprenavir, aprepitant, diltiazem, erythromycin, fluconazole, fosamprenavir, grapefruit juice, and verapamil) may result in an increase in fentanyl plasma concentrations, which could increase or prolong adverse drug effects and may cause potentially fatal respiratory depression. Patients receiving fentanyl and any CYP3A4 inhibitor should be monitored for an extended period of time and dosage adjustments should be made if warranted) 2405

Effexor XR Extended-Release Capsules (Concomitant use of CYP3A4 inhibitors and venlafaxine may increase levels of venlafaxine and O-desmethylvenlafaxine (ODV). Therefore, caution is advised if venlafaxine is used concomitantly with CYP3A4 inhibitors) 3195

Emend Capsules (Aprepitant is a substrate for CYP3A4; therefore, co-administration of fosaprepitant or aprepitant with drugs that inhibit CYP3A4 activity may result in increased plasma concentrations of aprepitant. Consequently, concomitant administration of fosaprepitant or aprepitant with strong CYP3A4 inhibitors (e.g., ketoconazole, itraconazole, nefazodone, troleandomycin, clarithromycin, ritonavir, nelfinavir) should be approached with caution. Because moderate CYP3A4 inhibitors (e.g., diltiazem) result in a 2-fold increase in plasma concentrations of aprepitant, concomitant administration should also be approached with caution) 1992

Enjuvia Tablets (Inhibitors of CYP3A4 such as erythromycin, clarithromycin, ketoconazole, itraconazole, ritonavir and grapefruit juice may increase plasma concentrations of estrogens and may result in side effects) 1029

Equetro Extended-Release Capsules (Carbamazepine is metabolized mainly by CYP3A4 the active carbamazepine 10,11-epoxide, which is futher metabolized to the trans-diol by epoxide hydrolase. Therefore, the potential exists for interaction between carbamazepine and any agent that inhibits CYP3A4 and/or epoxide hydrolase. Agents that are CYP3A4 inhibitors may increase the plasma levels of carbamazepine. Thus, if a patient has been titrated to a stable dosage of carbamazepine, and then begins a course of treatment with a CYP3A4 or epoxide hydrolase inhibitor, it is reasonable to expect that a dose reduction for carbamazepine may be necessary) 3174

Estratest H.S. Tablets (Co-administration with inhibitors of CYP3A4 may increase plasma concentrations of estrogens and may result in side effects) 3043

Evoxac Capsules (Co-administration with drugs which inhibit CYP3A3/4, such as grapefruit juice, may inhibit the metabolism of cevimeline resulting in a higher risk of adverse events) 1013

Fentora Tablets (The concomitant use of moderate CYP3A4 inhibitors such as amprenavir, aprepitant, diltiazem, erythromycin, fluconazole, fosamprenavir, grapefruit juice, and verapamil with fentanyl citrate may result in an increase in fentanyl plasma concentrations, which could increase or prolong adverse drug effects and may cause potentially fatal respiratory depression. Patients receiving fentanyl citrate and moderate CYP3A4 inhibitors should be carefully monitored for an extended period of time and dosage increase should be done conservatively) 968

Flomax Capsules (Concomitant administration of tamsulosin HCl and an inhibitor of CYP3A4 may lead to increased tamsulosin HCl plasma exposure. Tamsulosin HCl capsules should be used with caution in combination with moderate or strong inhibitors of CYP3A4 (e.g., ketoconazole), particularly at doses higher than 0.4mg) 848

Flonase Nasal Spray (Caution should be exercised when potent cytochrome P450 3A4 inhibitors are co-administered with fluticasone propionate) 1431

Gengraf Capsules (Affects the metabolism of cyclosporine increasing blood concentration of cyclosporine; concurrent use should be avoided)........ 435

Gleevec Tablets (There was a significant increase in exposure to imatinib (mean Cmax and AUC increased by 26% and 40% respectively) in healthy subjects when imatinib mesylate was co-administered with a single dose of ketoconazole (a CYP3A4 inhibitor). Caution is recommended when administering imatinib mesylate with strong CYP3A4 inhibitors (eg, ketoconazole, itraconazole, clarithromycin, atazanavir, indinavir, nefazodone, nelfinavir, ritonavir, saquinavir, telithromycin, and voriconazole). Grapefruit juice may also increase plasma concentrations of imatinib and should be avoided. Substances that inhibit the cytochrome P450 isoenzyme (CPY3A4) activity may decrease metabolism and increase imatinib concentrations)........ 2255

InnoPran XL Extended Release Capsules (Blood levels and/or toxicity of propranolol may be increased by administration of propranolol hydrochloride extended-release capsules with inhibitors of CYP1A2)........ 1484

Intelence Tablets (Etravirine is a substrate of CYP3A4, CYP2C9, and CYP2C19. Therefore, co-administration of etravirine with drugs that induce or inhibit CYP3A4, CYP2C9, and CYP2C19 may alter the therapeutic effect or adverse reaction profile of etravirine)........ 3119

Ionsys Transdermal System (The concomitant use of fentanyl with CYP3A4 inhibitors may result in a decrease in fentanyl clearance, which could increase or prolong adverse drug effects including serious respiratory depression. In this situation, special patient care and observation is appropriate)........ 2410

Ixempra Kit for Injection (Grapefruit juice may increase plasma concentrations of ixabepilone and should be avoided)........ 915

Lamisil Oral Granules (It is likely that inhibitors of both CYP2C9 and CYP3A4 may lead to substantial increase in the systemic exposure (Cmax and AUC) of terbinafine)........ 2264

Levitra Tablets (Although specific interactions have not been studied, other CYP3A4 inhibitors, including grapefruit juice, would likely increase vardenafil exposure)........ 2876

Lexapro Tablets (In vitro studies indicated that CYP3A4 and -2C19 are the primary enzymes involved in the metabolism of escitalopram. However, co-administration of escitalopram oxalate (20 mg) and ritonavir (600 mg), a potent inhibitor of CYP3A4, did not significantly affect the pharmacokinetics of escitalopram oxalate. Because escitalopram oxalate is metabolized by multiple enzyme systems, inhibition of a single enzyme may not appreciably decrease escitalopram clearance)........ 1174

Lexiva Tablets (Amprenavir is metabolized by CYP 3A4. Co-administration of fosamprenavir calcium and drugs that inhibit CYP3A4 may increase amprenavir concentrations and increase the incidence of adverse effects)........ 1510

Lipitor Tablets (Contains one or more components that inhibit CYP 3A4 and can increase plasma concentrations of atorvastatin, especially with excessive grapefruit consumption (greater than 1.2 liters per day))........ 2501

Luvox CR Extended-Release Capsules (Fluvoxamine is a known potent inhibitor of CYP1A2 and also inhibits CYP3A4, CYP2C9, and CYP2C19)........ 1759

Lybrel Tablets (CYP 3A4 inhibitors such as indinavir, itraconazole, ketoconazole, fluconazole, and troleandomycin may increase plasma hormone levels. Troleandomycin may also increase the risk of intrahepatic cholestasis during coadministration with combination oral contraceptives)........ 3204

Mevacor Tablets (The risk of myopathy/rhabdomyolysis is increased by concomitant use of lovastatin with potent inhibitors of CYP3A4, particularly with higher doses of lovastatin; concomitant use should be avoided unless the benefits of combined therapy outweigh the increased risk)........ 2063

Neoral Soft Gelatin Capsules (Affects the metabolism of cyclosporine and should be avoided)........ 2280

Nimotop Capsules (Grapefruit juice inhibits the cytochrome P450 3A4 system. Administration of dihydropyridine calcium antagonists together with grapefruit juice thus results in elevated concentrations and prolonged action of nimodipine due to a decreased first pass metabolism or reduced clearance. As a consequence, the blood pressure lowering effect may be increased. After intake of grapefruit juice this effect may last for at least 4 days after the last ingestion of grapefruit juice. Ingestion of grapefruit/grapefruit juice is therefore to be avoided while taking nimodipine)........ 790

NuvaRing (CYP3A4 inhibitors may increase plasma hormone levels)........ 2897

Ortho-Cyclen Tablets (CYP3A4 inhibitors such as itraconazole or ketoconazole may increase plasma hormone levels)........ 2449

Pletal Tablets (Co-administration of cilostazol with inhibitors of CYP3A4, such as grapefruit juice, increase cilostazol plasma concentration by 50%; concurrent consumption of grapefruit juice should be avoided)........ 2481

PrandiMet Tablets (Repaglinide is metabolized by CYP2C8 and to a lesser extent by CYP3A4. Drugs that inhibit 3A4 may alter the pharmacokinetics and pharmacodynamics of repaglinide)........ 2967

Prandin Tablets (Repaglinide is metabolized by the cytochrome P4502C8 and 3A4 enzymes. Consequently, repaglinide metabolism may be altered by drugs that are CYP3A4 inhibitors. Caution should be used in patients concomitantly using repaglinide and a CYP3A4 inhibitor. The effect may be very significant if both CYP3A4 and CYP2C8 are inhibited at the same time)........ 2971

Premarin Tablets (Co-administration of grapefruit juice with estrogens may increase plasma concentrations of estrogens and may result in side effects)........ 3221

Premphase Tablets (Co-administration of estrogens with inhibitors of CYP3A4, such as grapefruit juice, may increase plasma concentrations of estrogens and may result in side effects)........ 3232

Prempro Tablets (Co-administration of estrogens with inhibitors of CYP3A4, such as grapefruit juice, may increase plasma concentrations of estrogens and may result in side effects)........ 3232

Pristiq Extended-Release Tablets (CYP3A4 is a minor pathway for the metabolism of desvenlafaxine. In a clinical study, ketoconazole (200 mg b.i.d.) increased the area under the concentration vs. time curve AUC of desvenlafaxine (400 mg single dose) by about 43% and Cmax by about 8%. Concomitant use of desvenlafaxine with potent inhibitors of CYP3A4 may result in higher concentrations of desvenlafaxine)........ 3247

Prograf Capsules and Injection (Co-administered grapefruit juice has been reported to increase tacrolimus blood trough concentrations in liver transplant patients; grapefruit juice should be avoided)........ 622

Provigil Tablets (Co-administration of potent inhibitors of CYP3A4 could alter the plasma levels of modafinil)........ 977

Rapamune Tablets (Because grapefruit juice inhibits the CYP3A4-mediated metabolism of sirolimus, it must not be taken with or be used for dilution of sirolimus)........ 3260

Requip Tablets (In vitro metabolism studies showed that CYP1A2 is the major enzyme responsible for the metabolism of ropinirole. There is thus the potential for inducers or inhibitors of this enzyme to alter the clearance of ropinirole. Therefore, if therapy with a drug known to be a potent inducer or inhibitor of CYP1A2 is stopped or started during treatment with ropinirole, adjustment of the dose of ropinirole may be required)........ 1561

Requip XL Tablets (In vitro metabolism studies showed that CYP1A2 is the major enzyme responsible for the metabolism of ropinirole. There is thus the potential for inducers or inhibitors of this enzyme to alter the clearance of ropinirole. Therefore, if therapy with a drug known to be a potent inducer or inhibitor of CYP1A2 is stopped or started during treatment with ropinirole, adjustment of the dose of ropinirole may be required)........ 1568

Rozerem Tablets (Ramelteon should be administered with caution in subjects taking strong CYP2C9 inhibitors such as fluconazole)........ 3091

Rythmol Tablets (Propafenone is metabolized by CYP3A4. Agents that inhibit CYP3A4 (such as grapefruit juice), can be expected to cause increased plasma levels of propafenone. Appropriate monitoring is recommended when propafenone is used together with such agents)........ 1586

Rythmol SR Capsules (Drugs that inhibit CYP1A2 might lead to increased plasma levels of propafenone; patients should be closely monitored and the propafenone dose adjusted accordingly)........ 1590

Sandimmune I.V. Ampuls for Infusion (Co-administration results in increased blood concentrations of cyclosporine; concurrent use should be avoided)........ 2296

Seasonique Tablets (CYP3A4 inhibitors may increase plasma ethinyl estradiol levels)........ 1046

Serevent Diskus (Coadministration of salmeterol and a strong CYP3A4 inhibitor ketoconazole resulted in a significant increase in plasma salmeterol exposure as determined by a 16-fold increase in AUC mainly due to increased bioavailability of swallowed portion of the dose. Although there was no statistical effect on the mean QTc, coadministration of salmeterol and ketoconazole was associated with more frequent increases in QTc duration compared with salmeterol and placebo administration. Due to the potential increased risk of cardiovascular adverse events, the concomitant use of salmeterol with strong CYP3A4 inhibitors, (eg, ketoconazole, ritonavir, atazanavir, clarithromycin, indinavir, itraconazole, nefazodone, nelfinavir, saquinavir, telithromycin) is not recommended)........ 1594

Simcor Tablets (Potent inhibitors of CYP3A4 increase the risk of myopathy by reducing the elimination of simvastatin. Hence when simvastatin is used with a potent inhibitor of CYP3A4, elevated plasma levels of HMG-CoA reductase inhibitory activity can increase the riskof myopathy and rhabdomyolysis, particularly with higher doses of simvastatin. Concomitant use of drugs labeled as potent inhibitors of CYP3A4 should be avoided unless the benefits of combined therapy outweigh the increased risk. If treatment with itraconazole, ketoconazole, erythromycin, clarithromycin or telithromycin is unavoidable, therapy with Simcor should be suspended during the course of treatment)........ 502

Suboxone Tablets (Buprenorphine is metabolized to norbuprenorphine by cytochrome CYP3A4. Because CYP3A4 inhibitors may increase plasma concentrations of buprenorphine, patients already on CYP3A4 inhibitors should have their dose of Subutex or Subuxone adjusted.)........ 2601

Subutex Tablets (Buprenorphine is metabolized to norbuprenorphine by cytochrome CYP3A4. Because CYP3A4 inhibitors may increase plasma concentrations of buprenorphine, patients already on CYP3A4 inhibitors should have their dose of Subutex or Subuxone adjusted.)........ 2601

Sutent Capsules (Grapefruit may increase plasma concentrations of sunitinib maleate)........ 2540

Symbicort 80/4.5 Inhalation Aerosol (Concomitant administration of CYP3A4 inhibitors (e.g., itraconazole, clarithromycin, erythromycin, etc.) may inhibit the metabolism of, and increase the systemic exposure to, budesonide. Caution should be exercised with co-administration of Symbicort with potent CYP3A4 inhibitors)........ 659

Tarceva Tablets (Caution when administering or taking erlotinib with strong CYP3A4 inhibitors such as atazanavir, clarithromycin, indinavir, itraconazole, nefazodone, nelfinavir, ritonavir, saquinavir, telithromycin, troleandomycin, and voriconazole) **1228**

Targretin Capsules (Bexarotene is metabolized by CYP403A4; co-administration with inhibitors of CYP4503A4, such as grapefruit juice, would be expected to lead to an increase in plasma bexarotene concentrations) **1084**

Targretin Gel 1% (Bexarotene is metabolized by CYP4503A4; co-administration with inhibitors of CYP4503A4, such as grapefruit juice, could lead to an increase in plasma bexarotene concentrations) **1088**

Tasigna Capsules (Grapefruit products may increase serum concentrations of nilotinib and should be avoided) **2316**

Taxotere Injection Concentrate (The metabolism of docetaxel may be modified by the concomitant administration of compounds that inhibit cytochrome P450 3A4. Caution should be exercised with these drugs when treating patients receiving docetaxel as there is a potential for a significant reaction) **2773**

Torisel Injection (May increase plasma concentrations of sirolimus (a major metabolite of temsirolimus) and should be avoided) **3272**

Tracleer Tablets (Co-administration of both a CYP2C9 inhibitor and a CYP3A4 inhibitor with bosentan will likely lead to large increases in plasma concentrations of bosentan and is not recommended) **3289**

Treanda for Injection (Inhibitors of CYP1A2 (e.g., fluvoxamine, ciprofloxacin) have potential to increase plasma concentrations of bendamustine and decrease plasma concentrations of active metabolites. Caution should be used, or alternative treatments considered if concomitant treatment with CYP1A2 inhibitors is needed) **983**

Triesence Injectable Suspension (Ketoconazole has been reported to decrease the metabolism of certain corticosteroids by up to 60% leading to an increased risk of corticosteroid side effects) .... ⊙ **209**

Tykerb Tablets (Grapefruit may also increase plasma concentrations of lapatinib and should be avoided) **1631**

Ultram ER Extended-Release Tablets (Administration of CYP3A4 inhibitors, such as ketoconazole and erythromycin, with tramadol hydrochloride may effect the metabolism of tramadol leading to altered tramadol exposure) **2428**

Valium Tablets (There is a potentially relevant interaction between diazepam and certain hepatic enzyme inhibitors such as CYP450 3A4. It has been shown that these compounds influence the pharmacokinetics of diazepam and may lead to increased and prolonged sedation) **2658**

Vaprisol (Conivaptan is a substrate of CYP3A4. Co-administration of conivaptan with CYP3A4 inhibitors could lead to an increase in conivaptan concentrations. Concomitant use of conivaptan with potent CYP3A4 inhibitors is contraindicated) **632**

Velcade for Injection (Patients who are concomitantly receiving bortezomib and drugs that are inhibitors or inducers of cytochrome P450 3A4 should be closely monitored for either toxicities or reduced efficacy) **2168**

Venlafaxine Hydrochloride Tablets (Concomitant use of CYP3A4 inhibitors and venlafaxine may increase levels of venlafaxine and ODV. Therefore, caution is advised if a patient's therapy includes a CYP3A4 inhibitor and venlafaxine concomitantly. The concomitant use of venlafaxine with a drug treatment(s) that potently inhibits both CYP2D6 and CYP3A4, the primary metabolizing enzymes for venlafaxine, has not been studied. Therefore, caution is advised should a patient's therapy include venlafaxine and any agent(s) that produce potent simultaneous inhibition of these two enzyme systems) **2199**

Vesanoid Capsules (Tretinoin is metaboized by the hepatic P450 system; therefore, there is a potential for alteration of pharmacokinetic parameters in patients administered concomitant medications that are also inducers of this system. To date, there is no data to suggest that co-use with these medications increases or decreases either efficacy or toxicity of tretinoin) **2660**

Vytorin 10/10 Tablets (Simvastatin is metabolized by the cytochrome P450 isoform 3A4. Certain drugs that inhibit this metabolic pathway can raise plasma levels of simvastatin and may increase the risk of myopathy. This includes large quantities of grapefruit juice (greater than 1 quart daily). The use of Vytorin concomitantly with this CYP3A4 inhibitor should be avoided) **2149**

Vytorin 10/10 Tablets (The risk of myopathy and rhabdomyolysis is increased by high levels of statin activity in plasma. Simvastatin is metabolized by the cytochrome P450 3A4. Certain drugs that inhibit this metabolic pathway can raise the plasma levels of simvastatin and may increase the risk of myopathy. These include large quantities of grapefruit juice (greater than 1 quart daily); concurrent use should be avoided) **2939**

Zocor Tablets (The risk of myopathy and rhabdomyolysis is increased by high level of statin activity in plasma. Simvastatin is metabolized by the cytochrome P450 isoform 3A4. Certain drugs, including the large quantities of grapefruit juice (greater than 1 quart daily), which inhibit this metabolic pathway can raise the plasma levels of simvastatin and may increase the risk of myopathy. The use of simvastatin concomitantly with this CYP3A4 inhibitor should be avoided) **2136**

Zyprexa Tablets (Can potentially inhibit olanzapine clearance; therefore, a dosage decrease might be considered) **1883**

Zyprexa IntraMuscular (Can potentially inhibit olanzapine clearance; therefore, a dosage decrease might be considered) **1883**

Herring, pickled

Parnate Tablets (Potential for hypertensive crisis; concurrent use is contraindicated) **1532**

Liqueurs

Parnate Tablets (Potential for hypertensive crisis; concurrent use is contraindicated) **1532**

Liver

Parnate Tablets (Potential for hypertensive crisis; concurrent use is contraindicated) **1532**

Meal, high in bran fiber

Lanoxin Tablets (The amount of digoxin from an oral dose may be reduced) **1505**

Meal, unspecified

Ambien Tablets (The effect of zolpidem may be slowed by ingestion with or immediately after a meal) **2692**

Avandaryl Tablets (When glimepiride is given with meals the mean Tmax is slightly increased (12%) and mean Cmax and AUC are slightly decreased) **1344**

Cozaar Tablets (A meal slows absorption and decreases Cmax, but has minor effects on losartan AUC or on the AUC of the metabolite) **1973**

Fosamax Tablets (Standardized breakfast decreases bioavailability by approximately 40% when alendronate is administered either one-half or 1 hour before breakfast) **2005**

Fosamax Plus D Tablets (Bioavailability was decreased (by approximately 40%) when 10 mg alendronate was administered either 0.5 or 1 hour before a standardized breakfast, when compared to dosing 2 hours before eating) **2013**

Lanoxin Tablets (Slows the rate of absorption) **1505**

Mevacor Tablets (When lovastatin was given under fasting conditions, plasma concentrations of total inhibitors were on average about two-thirds those found when lovastatin was administered immediately after a standard meal) **2063**

Nimotop Capsules (In a study of 24 healthy volunteers, administration of nimodipine capsules following a standard breakfast resulted in a 68% lower peak plasma concentrations and 38% lower bioavailability relative to dosing under fasted conditions. In general, nimodipine capsules should be swallowed whole with little liquid, preferably not less than one hour before or two hours after meals) **790**

Norvir Soft Gelatin Capsules (Relative to fasting conditions, the extent of absorption of ritonavir from capsule formulation was 15% higher when administered with a meal; decreased peak ritonavir concentrations when oral solution was given under non-fasting condition) **489**

Meat extracts

Parnate Tablets (Potential for hypertensive crisis; concurrent use is contraindicated) **1532**

Meat prepared with tenderizers

Parnate Tablets (Potential for hypertensive crisis; concurrent use is contraindicated) **1532**

Milk, low fat

Dyazide Capsules (Concurrent use of low-salt milk with triamterene may result in hyperkalemia, especially in patients with renal insufficiency) **1405**

Milk, low salt

Dyrenium Capsules (Co-administration may promote serum potassium accumulation and possibly result in hyperkalemia) **3189**

Orange Juice

Allegra-D 12 Hour Extended-Release Tablets (Co-administration with grapefruit, orange or apple juice will reduce the bioavailability and exposure or fexofenadine) **2687**

Fosamax Tablets (Concomitant administration of alendronate with orange juice reduces bioavailability by approximately 60%) **2005**

Fosamax Plus D Tablets (Concomitant administration of alendronate with orange juice reduces bioavailability by approximately 60%) **2013**

Prunes

Parnate Tablets (Potential for hypertensive crisis; concurrent use is contraindicated) **1532**

Raisins

Parnate Tablets (Potential for hypertensive crisis; concurrent use is contraindicated) **1532**

Raspberries

Parnate Tablets (Potential for hypertensive crisis; concurrent use is contraindicated) **1532**

Salt Substitutes, Potassium-Containing

Prinivil Tablets (Use of lisinopril with potassium-sparing diuretics (such as spironolactone, triamterene or amiloride), potassium supplements or potassium-containing salt substitutes may lead to significant increases in serum potassium. Therefore, if concomitant use of these agents is indicated because of demonstrated hypokalemia, they should be used with caution and with frequent monitoring of serum potassium. Potassium-sparing agents should generally not be used in patients with heart failure who are receiving lisinopril) **2087**

Prinzide Tablets (Risk factors for the development of hyperkalemia include the concomitant use of potassium-sparing diuretics, potassium supplements and/or potassium-containing salt substitutes. Hyperkalemia can cause serious, sometimes, fatal, arrhythmias. Prinzide should be used cautiously, if at all, with these agents and with frequent monitoring of serum potassium) **2092**

Sauerkraut

Parnate Tablets (Potential for hypertensive crisis; concurrent use is contraindicated) **1532**

Sherry
Parnate Tablets (Potential for hypertensive crisis; concurrent use is contraindicated)....1532

Soy Sauce
Parnate Tablets (Potential for hypertensive crisis; concurrent use is contraindicated)....1532

Soybean Formula, Children's
Levoxyl Tablets (Concurrent use of soybean flour may bind and decrease the absorption of levothyroxine sodium from GI tract)....1780
Synthroid Tablets (Binds and decreases absorption of levothyroxine sodium from the gastrointestinal tract).... 507

Walnuts
Levoxyl Tablets (Concurrent use of walnuts may bind and decrease the absorption of levothyroxine sodium from GI tract)....1780

Wine, Chianti
Parnate Tablets (Potential for hypertensive crisis; concurrent use is contraindicated)....1532

Yeast Extract
Parnate Tablets (Potential for hypertensive crisis; concurrent use is contraindicated)....1532

Yogurt
Parnate Tablets (Potential for hypertensive crisis; concurrent use is contraindicated)....1532

SECTION 3

SIDE EFFECTS INDEX

Presented in this section is an alphabetical list of every side effect reported in the "Adverse Reactions" section of the product descriptions in *PDR*® and its companion volumes. Under each side effect is an alphabetical list of brands associated with the reaction.

If noted in the underlying text, incidence is shown in parentheses immediately after the brand name. Products reporting an incidence rate of 3% or more are marked with a ▲ symbol at their left. Because incidence data are sometimes drawn from controlled clinical trials, the rates seen in actual clinical practice may vary from those found in the published reports.

This index lists only side effects noted in official prescribing information as published by *PDR*®. To alert you to the full range of possibilities, the entries include adverse effects shared by an entire class of drugs, but not necessarily reported for the specific drug in question. The index is restricted to reactions that may be expected to occur at recommended dosages in the general patient population. Precautions to be taken under special circumstances are not listed, nor are the effects of overdosage.

The page numbers shown for the products refer to the 2009 editions of *PDR*®, *PDR*® *For Ophthalmic Medicines,* and *PDR*® *For Nonprescription Drugs, Dietary Supplements and Herbs.* A key to the symbols denoting the companion volumes appears in the bottom margin.

A

Abdomen, enlarged

▲ Angeliq Tablets (7%) 751
▲ Busulfex Injection (23%) 2477
Campral Tablets (Rare) 1158
▲ CellCept Capsules (3% to less than 20%) 2622
▲ CellCept Intravenous (3% to less than 20%) 2622
▲ CellCept Oral Suspension (3% to less than 20%) 2622
▲ CellCept Tablets (3% to less than 20%) 2622
▲ Eloxatin for Injection (2% to less than 5%) 2731
▲ Follistim AQ Cartridge (8%) 2844
Ionsys Transdermal System (.1% to less than 1%) 2410
Lovaza Capsules 1520
▲ Proleukin for Injection (10%) 2287
Sandostatin LAR Depot 2302
Yaz Tablets 805
Zyrtec Chewable Tablets (Less than 2%) 1920
Zyrtec Syrup (Less than 2%) 1920
Zyrtec Tablets (Less than 2%) 1920
Zyrtec-D 12 Hour Extended Release Tablets (Less than 2%) 1923

Abdomen, redistribution/accumulation of body fat

Atripla Tablets 938
Kaletra 452
Lexiva Oral Suspension 1510
Lexiva Tablets 1510
Retrovir 1574

Abdominal adhesion

Requip Tablets (Infrequent) 1561

Abdominal bloating

Activella Tablets 2347
Actonel with Calcium Tablets 2574
Aerobid/Aerobid-M (Less than 1%) 1153
Angeliq Tablets 751
Aralast (Greater than or equal to 0.2%) 726
Aricept Tablets (Frequent) 1062
Aricept ODT Tablets (Frequent) 1062
Asacol Delayed-Release Tablets (2% or greater) 2579
Bentyl Capsules 703
Bentyl Injection 703
Bentyl Syrup 703
Bentyl Tablets 703
Climara Transdermal System 763
Climara Pro Transdermal System 768
Creon 5 Capsules (Among most frequent) 3041
Creon 10 Capsules (Among most frequent) 3042
Creon 20 Capsules (Among most frequent) 3042
▲ Crinone 4% Gel (13%) 992
▲ Crinone 8% Gel (7% to 12%) 992
Divigel 3167
Donnatal Extentabs 2507
Enjuvia Tablets 1029
Estratest Tablets 3043
Estratest H.S. Tablets 3043
Fansidar Tablets 2636
Fleet Phospho-soda 1145
Fleet Phospho-soda EZ-PREP 1147
Imitrex Nasal Spray 1470
Indocin Capsules (Less than 1%) 2024
Indocin I.V. (Less than 1%) 2489
Indocin (Less than 1%) 2024
Lexapro Oral Suspension (Infrequent) 1174
Lexapro Tablets (Infrequent) 1174
Lybrel Tablets 3204
Mircette Tablets 1034
Nadolol Tablets (1 to 5 of 1000 patients) 2191
Noroxin Tablets (Less frequent) 2069
Norvir (Less than 2%) 489
Ortho-Cyclen Tablets 2449
Ortho Evra Transdermal System 2437
Ortho Tri-Cyclen Tablets 2449
Ortho Tri-Cyclen Lo Tablets 2458
▲ OsmoPrep Tablets (31% to 39%) 2680
Premarin Intravenous 3217
Premarin Tablets 3221
Premarin Vaginal Cream 3228
Premphase Tablets 3232
Prempro Tablets 3232
▲ Prometrium Capsules (100 mg, 200 mg) (12%) 3047
ProNutra Protein Supplement 1730
Seasonique Tablets 1046
Yaz Tablets 805

Abdominal discomfort
(*see also under* Distress, abdominal; Distress, gastrointestinal)

▲ Abilify Injection (3%) 2466
▲ Abilify Oral Solution (3%) 2466
▲ Abilify Discmelt Orally Disintegrating Tablets (3%) 2466
▲ Abilify Tablets (3%) 2466
Ambien CR Tablets (1%) 2696
▲ Amitiza Capsules (2% to 3%) 3082
Biaxin/Biaxin XL (2%) 411
Carafate Tablets (Less than 0.5%) 707
▲ Chantix Tablets (5% to 7%) 2511
Cipro I.V. (1.7%) 2817
Cipro (Less than 1%) 2810
Concerta Extended-Release Tablets 1925
Cyanokit 5g Antidote 1021
▲ Cymbalta Delayed-Release Capsules (4%) 1801
Dulcolax Suppositories ■ 602
Dulcolax Tablets ■ 602
▲ DynaCirc CR Controlled Release Tablets (1.3% to 5.1%) 1407
▲ Epivir-HBV (16%) 1417
Exforge Tablets (Greater than or equal to 0.2%) 2238
▲ Fabrazyme for Intravenous Infusion (6%) 1241
Fleet Bisacodyl Laxatives 1143
▲ Flovent Diskus 50 mcg (3%) 1435
▲ Gengraf Capsules (Up to 7%) 435
Imitrex Nasal Spray (Infrequent) 1470
Imitrex Tablets 1474
▲ Janumet Tablets (Greater than 5%) 2041
Klonopin (Infrequent) 2639
Lexapro Oral Suspension (Infrequent) 1174
Lexapro Tablets (Infrequent) 1174
▲ Lexiscan Injection (5%) 614
Children's Motrin Oral Suspension 1901
Children's Motrin Non-Staining Dye-Free Oral Suspension 1901
Infants' Motrin Concentrated Drops 1901
Infants' Motrin Non-Staining Dye-Free Concentrated Drops 1901
Junior Strength Motrin Caplets and Chewable Tablets 1901
Nadolol Tablets (1 to 5 of 1000 patients) 2191
▲ Neoral Oral Solution (Up to 7%) 2280
▲ Neoral Soft Gelatin Capsules (Up to 7%) 2280
Pepcid Tablets (Infrequent) 2075
Requip Tablets (Infrequent) 1561
▲ Sandimmune (Less than 1% to 7%) 2296
▲ Sandostatin Injection (34% to 61%) 2300
▲ Sandostatin LAR Depot (29.1%) 2302
Symbicort 80/4.5 Inhalation Aerosol (1.1%) 659
▲ Symbicort 160/4.5 Inhalation Aerosol (6.5%) 659
▲ Tasigna Capsules (1% to 10%) 2316
▲ Trisenox Injection (8%) 986
Tyzeka Tablets (Less than 1%) 2328
Urocit-K Tablets (Some patients) 2176
Vantas (Less than 2%) 1737
▲ Xenical Capsules (25.5%) 2672

Abdominal distention

Actiq (1% or greater) 959
AmBisome for Injection (Less common) 606
▲ Amitiza Capsules (0% to 6%) 3082
Aptivus Capsules (Less than 2%) 823

Aptivus Oral Solution (Less than 2%) 823
▲ Arranon Injection (0% to 6%) 1319
Avalide Tablets 892
Avalide Tablets 2713
Avapro Tablets (Less than 1%) 897
Avapro Tablets (Less than 1%) 2718
Byetta Injection 600
Cancidas for Injection 1953
▲ Chantix Tablets (5% to 7%) 2511
Crixivan Capsules 1979
Cubicin for Injection (Less than 1%) 995
▲ Dacogen Injection (5%) 1066
▲ DepoDur Injection (2% to 5%) 1095
▲ Doxil Injection (1% to 10%) 2378
Duragesic Transdermal System (Less than 1%) 2405
DynaCirc CR Controlled Release Tablets (1.2%) 1407
Evoxac Capsules 1013
Exforge Tablets (Greater than or equal to 0.2%) 2238
Fentora Tablets (Greater than 1%) 968
▲ Flolan for Injection (4%) 1426
Follistim AQ Cartridge 2844
Fosamax (Up to 1.4%) 2005
Fosamax Plus D Tablets (0% to 1.4%) 2013
Gengraf Capsules (1% to less than 3%) 435
Gleevec Tablets (Less common) 2255
Imitrex Nasal Spray 1470
▲ Indocin I.V. (1% to 3%) 2489
Intelence Tablets (Less than 2%) 3119
▲ Intron A for Injection (Less than 5%) 2859
Invanz for Injection (Greater than 0.1%) 2029
Ketek Tablets (Greater than or equal to 0.2% to less than 2%) 2744
Lamictal (Rare) 1488
▲ Leukine (4%) 774
Lialda Tablets (Infrequent) 3029
Lyrica Capsules 2527
Mavik Tablets (0.3% to 1%) 472
Merrem I.V. (Greater than 0.1% to 1%) 684
▲ MoviPrep Oral Solution (59.8%) 2679
▲ Myfortic Tablets (3% to less than 20%) 2276
NeoProfen Injection 2496
Neoral Oral Solution (1% to less than 3%) 2280
Neoral Soft Gelatin Capsules (1% to less than 3%) 2280
Nexium I.V. (Less than 1%) 652
▲ Opana Tablets (1% to less than 10%) 1117
▲ Opana ER Tablets (1% to less than 10%) 1121
Pentasa Capsules (Less than 1%) 3030
Percocet Tablets 1127
▲ Prograf Capsules and Injection (3% to 15%) 622
▲ Prometrium Capsules (100 mg, 200 mg) (6% to 8%) 3047
Reclast Injection (2%) 2291
ReoPro Vials (0.1%) 1860
Requip Tablets (Infrequent) 1561
Rilutek Tablets (Infrequent) 2771
Rythmol SR Capsules 1590
Sanctura XR Capsules (1% to less than 2%) 557
▲ Sandostatin Injection (Less than 10% to 35%) 2300
Sandostatin LAR Depot 2302
▲ Simulect for Injection (3% to 10%) 2306
Tasigna Capsules (0.1% to 1%) 2316
Treximet Tablets (Infrequent) 1616
▲ Trisenox Injection (8%) 986
▲ Valcyte Tablets (Less than 5%) 2654
▲ Vesanoid Capsules (11%) 2660
▲ Xeloda Tablets (Less than 5%) 2662
Xifaxan Tablets (Less than 2%) 2682
Xyrem Oral Solution (Infrequent) 1766
Zyprexa Tablets (Infrequent) 1883
Zyprexa ZYDIS Orally Disintegrating Tablets (Infrequent) 1883

Abdominal guarding
Sandostatin Injection (Rare) 2300
Sandostatin LAR Depot 2302

Abdominal mass
Estratest Tablets 3043
Estratest H.S. Tablets 3043

Abdominal pain, gynecological
▲ Follistim AQ Cartridge (25%) 2844

Abdominal pain, lower
▲ Cymbalta Delayed-Release Capsules (4%) 1801
Requip Tablets (Infrequent) 1561

Abdominal pain, upper
Actonel Tablets (1.4% to 2.5%) 2568
Aptivus Capsules (1.5%) 823
Aptivus Oral Solution (1.5%) 823
Cancidas for Injection 1953
▲ Celebrex Capsules (6% to 8%) 2979
Cialis Tablets (Less than 2%) 1792
▲ Concerta Extended-Release Tablets (5.9%) 1925
▲ Cymbalta Delayed-Release Capsules (4%) 1801
▲ Dacogen Injection (5%) 1066
▲ Elidel Cream 1% (0.3% to 5.5%) 2221
▲ Exelon Patch (1% to 3%) 2233
Exforge Tablets (Greater than or equal to 0.2%) 2238
▲ Exjade Tablets (7.8%) 2244
▲ Invega Extended-Release Tablets (1% to 3%) 1748
▲ Lamisil Oral Granules (4%) 2264
▲ MoviPrep Oral Solution (5.8%) 2679
Mycamine for Injection 616
▲ Reclast Injection (0.9% to 4.6%) 2291
▲ Sandostatin LAR Depot (10.5%) 2302
Strattera Capsules (0.2%) 1864
▲ Ultram ER Extended-Release Tablets (1% to less than 5%) 2428
▲ Velcade for Injection (12%) 2168
▲ Vivitrol (11% to 16%) 988

Abdominal pain/cramps
▲ Abelcet Injection (4%) 1134
▲ Abilify Oral Solution (3%) 881
▲ Abilify Discmelt Orally Disintegrating Tablets (3%) 881
▲ Abilify Tablets (3%) 881
Accolate Tablets (1.8% to 2.8%) 669
Aceon Tablets (2 mg, 4 mg, 8 mg) (2.7%) 3038
▲ Aciphex Tablets (3.6%) 1053
▲ Actimmune (8%) 1743
Actiq (1% or greater) 959
Activella Tablets 2347
▲ Actonel Tablets (7.3% to 12.2%) 2568
▲ Actonel with Calcium Tablets (7.3% to 11.6%) 2574
Aczone Gel 5% 3296
▲ Adderall XR Capsules (11% to 14%) 3012
Advair Diskus 100/50 1276
Advair Diskus 250/50 1276
Advair Diskus 500/50 1276
▲ Advair HFA 45/21 Inhalation Aerosol (1% to 3%) 1288
▲ Advair HFA 115/21 Inhalation Aerosol (1% to 3%) 1288
▲ Advair HFA 230/21 Inhalation Aerosol (1% to 3%) 1288
Advate (0.6%) 721
▲ Advicor Tablets (4%) 402
▲ Aerobid/Aerobid-M (3% to 9%) 1153
▲ Aggrenox Capsules (17.5%) 819
▲ Agrylin Capsules (16.4%) 3017
▲ Albenza Tablets (Up to 6%) 1297
▲ Alinia for Oral Suspension (7.8%) 2677
▲ Alinia Tablets (7.8%) 2677
Allegra-D 12 Hour Extended-Release Tablets (1.4%) 2687
Allegra-D 24 Hour Extended-Release Tablets (1.4%) 2690
Aloxi Injection (Less than 1%) 1059
Ambien Tablets (2%) 2692
▲ AmBisome for Injection (9.9% to 19.8%) 606
Amerge Tablets (Infrequent) 1301
Aminohippurate Sodium "PAH" Injection 1950
▲ Amitiza Capsules (3% to 8%) 3082
▲ Anaprox Tablets (3% to 9%) 2632
▲ Anaprox DS Tablets (3% to 9%) 2632
▲ Angeliq Tablets (11%) 751
▲ Angiomax for Injection (5%) 1933
▲ Anzemet Injection (3.2%) 2701
Anzemet Tablets 2704
▲ Aptivus Capsules (4.4%) 823
▲ Aptivus Oral Solution (4.4%) 823
▲ Aranesp for Injection (10%) 564
▲ Argatroban Injection (2.6% to 3.6%) 1308
Aricept Tablets (Frequent) 1062
Aricept ODT Tablets (Frequent) 1062
▲ Arimidex Tablets (6% to 9%) 672
Arixtra Injection (1.4%) 1313
▲ Arranon Injection (0% to 9%) 1319
▲ Asacol Delayed-Release Tablets (18%) 2579
▲ Asmanex Twisthaler (2% to 6%) 2797
Atacand Tablets (More than 1%) 639
Atacand HCT (0.5% or greater) 642
▲ Atripla Tablets (Greater than or equal to 2%) 938
Augmentin Tablets 1327
Augmentin XR Extended Release Tablets (1.6%) 1333
Augmentin ES-600 Powder for Oral Suspension 1329
Avalide Tablets (2%) 892
Avalide Tablets (2%) 2713
▲ Avandamet Tablets (5%) 1336
Avandaryl Tablets (Less than 1%) 1344
▲ Avandia Tablets (3%) 1351
Avapro Tablets (1% or greater) 897
Avapro Tablets (1% or greater) 2718
▲ Avastin IV (8% to 61%) 1192
Avelox (Greater than or equal to 0.1% to less than 2%) 2803
▲ Avinza Capsules (5% to 10%) 1772
Axert Tablets (Infrequent) 2431
▲ Axid Capsules (7.5%) 1364
▲ Azilect Tablets (5%) 3106
▲ Azmacort Inhalation Aerosol (1% to 3%) 407
Bactroban Cream (Less than 1%) 1366
Benicar Tablets (Greater than 0.5%) 1009
Benicar HCT Tablets (Greater than 1%) 1010
Bentyl Capsules 703
Bentyl Injection 703
Bentyl Syrup 703
Bentyl Tablets 703
▲ Betaseron for SC Injection (18%) 756
▲ Bexxar (3% to 15%) 1371
▲ Biaxin/Biaxin XL (2% to 3%) 411
Bicillin C-R Injectable Suspension 1775
▲ Boniva Injection (5.3% to 7.8%) 2614
▲ Boniva Tablets (5.3% to 7.8%) 2618
▲ Boostrix (3% to 26%) 1377
▲ Busulfex Injection (3% to 72%) 2477
Byetta Injection 600
Bystolic Tablets (Greater than or equal to 1%) 1155
Campath Ampules 761
Campral Tablets (Frequent) 1158
▲ Canasa Rectal Suppositories (5.2%) 705
▲ Cancidas for Injection (6.2% to 8.5%) 1953
Captopril Tablets (About 0.5% to 2%) 2182
Carbatrol Capsules 3019
Cardene I.V. (0.7%) 1093
Catapres Tablets (Rare) 841
Ceftin (0.1% to 1%) 1380
▲ Celebrex Capsules (4% to 7%) 2979
▲ Celexa (3%) 1160
▲ CellCept Capsules (24.7% to 62.5%) 2622
▲ CellCept Intravenous (24.7% to 62.5%) 2622
▲ CellCept Oral Suspension (24.7% to 62.5%) 2622
▲ CellCept Tablets (24.7% to 62.5%) 2622
▲ Cerezyme for Injection (Approximately 6.5%) 1238
Cervidil Vaginal Insert (Less than 1%) 1165
▲ Chantix Tablets (5% to 7%) 2511
▲ Chemet Capsules (5.2% to 15.7%) 2484
Cialis Tablets (1% to 2%) 1792
Cimzia 3127
▲ Cipro I.V. (1% or less to 3.3%) 2817
▲ Cipro (Less than 1% to 3.3%) 2810
Cipro XR Tablets (Less than 1%) 2823
▲ Climara Transdermal System (11% to 16%) 763
▲ Climara Pro Transdermal System (4.2%) 768
▲ Clinoril Tablets (10%) 1962
▲ Clolar for Intravenous Infusion (36%) 1239
▲ Combivir Tablets (6% to 9%) 1384
▲ Comtan Tablets (8%) 2208
▲ Concerta Extended-Release Tablets (Greater than 5%) 1925
Copaxone for Injection (At least 2%) 3110
Cosmegen for Injection 2485
▲ Cosopt Sterile Ophthalmic Solution (1% to 5%) 1969
Cozaar Tablets (1% or greater) 1973
Creon 5 Capsules (Among most frequent) 3041
Creon 10 Capsules (Among most frequent) 3042
Creon 20 Capsules (Among most frequent) 3042
Crestor Tablets (2.4%) 677
▲ Crinone 4% Gel (5%) 992
▲ Crinone 8% Gel (9% to 12%) 992
▲ Crixivan Capsules (16.6%) 1979
▲ Cubicin for Injection (1% to 5.8%) 995
▲ Cymbalta Delayed-Release Capsules (4%) 1801
▲ Dacogen Injection (14%) 1066
Dantrium Capsules (Less frequent) 2580
Dapsone Tablets USP 1746
Daytrana Transdermal Patch 3022
Demser Capsules (Infrequent) 1989
▲ Depakote ER Tablets (7% to 23%) 423
▲ DepoCyt Injection (9% to 15%) 1136
▲ Diclofenac Sodium Ophthalmic Solution (Less than or equal to 3%) ⊙ 240
Diovan Tablets (2%) 2212
Diovan HCT Tablets (Greater than 0.2%) 2216
Divigel 3167
▲ Doxil Injection (1% to 33.5%) 2378
Duac Topical Gel 3054
▲ Duragesic Transdermal System (3% to 10%) 2405
Dyazide Capsules 1405
▲ EC-Naprosyn Delayed-Release Tablets (3% to 9%) 2632
Edecrin 698
E.E.S. (Among most frequent) 433
▲ Effexor XR Extended-Release Capsules (6%) 3195
▲ Eldepryl Capsules (4 of 49 patients) 3052
▲ Elidel Cream 1% (0.3% to 4.4%) 2221
▲ Elitek (20%) 2729
Elmiron Capsules (2%) 2435
▲ Eloxatin for Injection (1% to 39%) 2731
Elspar for Injection 1990
▲ Emend Capsules (4.6%) 1992
▲ Emend for Injection (4.6%) 1999
Emsam Transdermal System 905
▲ Emtriva Capsules (Greater than or equal to 10%) 1246
▲ Emtriva Oral Solution (Greater than or equal to 10%) 1246
▲ Enablex Extended-Release Tablets (2.4% to 3.9%) 2225
▲ Enbrel for Injection (5% to 19%) 569
Engerix-B Vaccine (Less than 1%) 1409
▲ Enjuvia Tablets (4% to 15%) 1029
▲ Epivir (6% to 9%) 1412
▲ Epivir-HBV (16%) 1417
Epogen for Injection 576
▲ Epzicom Tablets (4% to 5%) 1422
Equetro Extended-Release Capsules 3174
▲ Erbitux (14% to 59%) 912
EryPed (Among most frequent) 431
Estratest Tablets 3043
Estratest H.S. Tablets 3043
▲ Evista Tablets (6.6%) 1810
Evoclin Foam, 1% 3056
▲ Evoxac Capsules (7.6%) 1013
▲ Exelon Capsules (4% to 13%) 2229
▲ Exelon Oral Solution (4% to 13%) 2229
▲ Exelon Patch (2% to 4%) 2233
Exforge Tablets (Greater than or equal to 0.2%) 2238
▲ Exjade Tablets (13.9%) 2244
▲ Fabrazyme for Intravenous Infusion (Greater than or equal to 5%) 1241
Fansidar Tablets 2636
▲ Faslodex Injection (11.8%) 682
▲ Femara Tablets (4% to 6%) 2246
▲ Fenoglide Tablets (4.6%) 2960
▲ Fentora Tablets (1% to 11%) 968
Flebogamma 5% 1715
Flebogamma 5% DIF 1718
▲ Flector Patch (3%) 561
Fleet Phospho-soda EZ-PREP 1147
Fleet Prep Kits 1149
▲ Flolan for Injection (5% to 27%) 1426
▲ Flonase Nasal Spray (1% to 3%) 1431
▲ Flovent Diskus 50 mcg (3%) 1435
Fluarix Vaccine 1446
Flumadine (1.4%) 1167
▲ FluMist Vaccine (2% to 12%) 1945
Focalin XR Capsules 2251
▲ Follistim AQ Cartridge (5% to 28%) 2844
Fortaz (1 in 416) 1450
▲ Fosamax (0.9% to 6.6%) 2005
▲ Fosamax Plus D Tablets (0.9% to 6.6%) 2013
▲ Fosrenol Chewable Tablets (5% to 17%) 3027
Fosteum Capsules (1.3% to 2.2%) 2963
Frova Tablets (Frequent) 1111
Furosemide Tablets 2186
▲ Gabitril Tablets (5% to 7%) 973
Gammagard Liquid 730
Gammagard S/D 734
▲ Gamunex (4%) 3094
Gantrisin Pediatric Suspension 2638
▲ Gengraf Capsules (2.7% to 15%) 435
Geodon (Frequent) 2520
▲ Gleevec Tablets (36.5% to 40%) 2255
▲ Gliadel Wafer (8%) 1076
Havrix Injection Vaccine (Less than 1%) 1454
▲ Hepsera Tablets (9%) 1253
▲ Herceptin I.V. (22%) 1199
▲ Humira Injection (7%) 442

▲ Hycamtin for Injection (Less than 1% to 33%) 1459
Imitrex Injection 1465
Imitrex Nasal Spray 1470
Imitrex Tablets 1474
▲ Indapamide Tablets (Less than 5%) 2188
Indocin (Greater than 1%) 2024
InnoPran XL Extended Release Capsules 1484
▲ Intelence Tablets (3%) 3119
Intravenous Sodium Diuril 2490
▲ Intron A for Injection (1% to 21%) 2859
▲ Invanz for Injection (1% to 4.7%) 2029
Invega Extended-Release Tablets 1748
▲ Ionsys Transdermal System (1% to less than 10%) 2410
Isentress Tablets (1% to less than 2%) 2036
▲ Ixempra Kit for Injection (13% to greater than or equal to 20%) 915
Janumet Tablets (2.2%) 2041
Januvia Tablets (2.3%) 2048
▲ Kaletra (3% to 11%) 452
Keppra Oral Solution (1% to greater than or equal to 2%) 3131
Keppra Tablets (1% to greater than or equal to 2%) 3131
Ketek Tablets (Greater than or equal to 0.2% to less than 2%) 2744
▲ Kineret Injection (5%) 585
Klonopin (1%) 2639
Kristalose for Oral Solution 1004
▲ Lamictal (6% to 10%) 1488
Lamisil Oral Granules (2%) 2264
Lamisil Tablets (2.4%) 2266
Lanoxin Injection (Rare) 1498
Lanoxin Injection Pediatric (Rare) 1502
Lanoxin Tablets (Rare) 1505
▲ Lescol Capsules (4.9%) 2268
▲ Lescol XL Tablets (3.7%) 2268
▲ Letairis Tablets (3%) 1258
▲ Leukine (38%) 774
▲ Leustatin Injection (6%) 2384
Levaquin (2%) 2416
Levaquin in 5% Dextrose Injection (2%) 2416
Levitra Tablets (Less than 2%) 2876
Levothroid Tablets 1170
Levoxyl Tablets 1780
Lexapro Oral Suspension (2%) 1174
Lexapro Tablets (2%) 1174
Lexiva Oral Suspension (Less than 1% to 2%) 1510
Lexiva Tablets (Less than 1% to 2%) 1510
▲ Lipitor Tablets (Up to 3.8%) 2501
Lunesta Tablets 2994
▲ Luvox CR Extended-Release Capsules (1% to 5%) 1759
Lybrel Tablets 3204
Lyrica Capsules (Greater than or equal to 1%) 2527
▲ Malarone Pediatric Tablets (2% to 31%) 1521
▲ Malarone Tablets (2% to 31%) 1521
▲ Marinol Capsules (3% to 10%) 3163
Mavik Tablets (0.3% to 1%) 472
Maxair Autohaler 1705
▲ Megace ES Oral Suspension (1% to 3%) 2499
▲ Mepron Suspension (4% to 21%) 1526
▲ Meridia Capsules (4.5%) 475
Merrem I.V. (Greater than 0.1% to 1%) 684
▲ Metadate CD Capsules (7%) 3146
▲ Mevacor Tablets (2% to 5.7%) 2063
Miacalcin Injection 2273
▲ Miacalcin Nasal Spray (1% to 3%) 2274
Micardis Tablets (1%) 852
Micardis HCT Tablets (Less than 2%) 854
Mirapex Tablets (1% or more) 857
Mircette Tablets 1034
▲ Mirena Intrauterine System (5% or more) 779
▲ Mobic Oral Suspension (1.9% to 4.7%) 863
▲ Mobic Tablets (1.9% to 4.7%) 863
▲ MoviPrep Oral Solution (13.3%) 2679
Moxatag Tablets (0.3%) 2165
MS Contin Tablets (Less frequent) 2585
▲ Mycamine for Injection (2% to 27.1%) 616
▲ Myfortic Tablets (3% to less than 20%) 2276
▲ Mylotarg for Injection (26% to 39%) 3212
Nabi-HB 815
Nalfon Capsules (2%) 2508
▲ Naprosyn Suspension (3% to 9%) 2632
▲ Naprosyn Tablets (3% to 9%) 2632
▲ Natrecor for Injection (1% to 3%) 2977
▲ Neoral Oral Solution (2.7% to 15%) 2280
▲ Neoral Soft Gelatin Capsules (2.7% to 15%) 2280
▲ Neulasta Injection (15% to 72%) 587
Neupogen for Injection (Infrequent) 589
Neupro Transdermal System (Greater than or equal to 2%) 3149
▲ Nexavar Tablets (11%) 784
▲ Nexium Delayed-Release Capsules (Greater than or equal to 1% to 3.8%) 645
▲ Nexium I.V. (Greater than or equal to 1% to 3.8%) 652
▲ Nexium Delayed-Release Oral Suspension (Greater than or equal to 1% to 3.8%) 645
▲ Niaspan Extended-Release Tablets (2% to 5%) 480
Noroxin Tablets (0.3% to 1.6%) 2069
▲ Norvir (6% to 8.3%) 489
▲ Novantrone for Injection Concentrate (9% to 15%) 1100
▲ NovoLog Injection (5%) 2359
▲ Noxafil Oral Suspension (1% to 27%) 2889
NuvaRing 2897
Omnicef Capsules (1%) 497
Omnicef for Oral Suspension (0.8%) 497
Opana Tablets (Less than 1%) 1117
Opana ER Tablets (2.5%) 1121
Ortho-Cyclen Tablets 2449
▲ Ortho Evra Transdermal System (9% to 22%) 2437
Ortho Tri-Cyclen Tablets 2449
Ortho Tri-Cyclen Lo Tablets 2458
Orthoclone OKT3 Sterile Solution 2387
▲ OsmoPrep Tablets (23% to 24%) 2680
▲ OxyContin Tablets (Between 1% and 5%) 2589
Parnate Tablets 1532
Paser Granules (Among most common) 1747
Patanase Nasal Spray 544
▲ Paxil (4%) 1535
▲ Paxil CR Controlled-Release Tablets (4%) 1544
Pediarix Vaccine 1552
▲ PegIntron Powder for Injection (15%) 2903
Pentasa Capsules (1.1% to 1.7%) 3030
Percocet Tablets 1127
Percodan Tablets 1130
▲ Photofrin for Injection (12% to 20%) 708
▲ Plan B Tablets (17.6%) 1044
▲ Plavix Tablets (5.6%) 926
▲ Plavix Tablets (5.6%) 2767
▲ Pletal Tablets (4% to 5%) 2481
▲ Precose Tablets (19%) 792
Premarin Intravenous 3217
▲ Premarin Tablets (15% to 17%) 3221
Premarin Vaginal Cream 3228
▲ Premphase Tablets (13% to 23%) 3232
▲ Prempro Tablets (13% to 23%) 3232
Primaxin I.M. 2080
Primaxin I.V. (Less than 0.2%) 2083
▲ Prinivil Tablets (0.3% to 4%) 2087
Prinzide Tablets (0.3% to 1%) 2092
Proglycem Capsules (Frequent) 1185
Proglycem Suspension (Frequent) 1185
▲ Prograf Capsules and Injection (29% to 59%) 622
▲ Proleukin for Injection (11%) 2287
▲ Prometrium Capsules (100 mg, 200 mg) (10% to 20%) 3047
ProNutra Protein Supplement 1730
ProQuad 2099
▲ Protonix for Delayed-Release Oral Suspension (1% to 4%) 3254
▲ Protonix Delayed-Release Tablets (1% to 4%) 3254
▲ Protonix I.V. (12%) 3257
▲ Protopic Ointment (1% to 5%) 628
Provigil Tablets (At least 1%) 977
Prozac Pulvules and Liquid 1852
▲ Pulmicort Flexhaler (Greater than or equal to 1% to 3%) 654
Pulmozyme Inhalation Solution 1217
▲ Rapamune (29% to 36%) 3260
▲ Rebetol (13%) 2917
▲ Rebif Prefilled Syringe for Injection (20% to 22%) 1107
Reclast Injection (2%) 2291
Recombivax HB (Less than 1%) 2107
ReFacto Vials 3269
Relenza Inhalation Powder (Less than 1.5%) 1556
▲ Relistor Injection (28.5%) 3310
Remeron Tablets (Frequent) 2924
RemeronSolTab Tablets (Frequent) 2927
▲ Remicade for IV Injection (12%) 950
▲ Requip Tablets (3% to 9%) 1561
▲ Requip XL Tablets (Greater than or equal to 5%) 1568
▲ Retrovir Capsules (3.2%) 1574
▲ Retrovir IV Infusion (4%) 1579
▲ Retrovir (3.2%) 1574
▲ Reyataz Capsules (4%) 3299
▲ Rilutek Tablets (6.8% to 7.8%) 2771
Risperdal Consta Long-Acting Injection (Frequent) 1753
▲ Rituxan I.V. (1% to 14%) 1223
Rocaltrol Capsules 1150
Rocaltrol Oral Solution 1150
Rocephin Injectable Vials, ADD-Vantage, Galaxy, Bulk (Less than 0.1%) 2642
Rythmol Tablets (2%) 1586
Rythmol SR Capsules 1590
▲ Salagen Tablets (3% to 4%) 1082
Sanctura XR Capsules (1.4% to less than 2%) 557
▲ Sandostatin LAR Depot (10% to 38%) 2302
Seasonique Tablets 1046
Selzentry Tablets 2534
▲ Simcor Tablets (3.5%) 502
▲ Simulect for Injection (Greater than or equal to 10%) 2306
Singulair (Greater than or equal to 2% to 2.9%) 2114
▲ Somatuline Depot Injection (Greater than 5% to 20%) 3102
▲ Soriatane Capsules (1% to 10%) 3062
▲ Spiriva HandiHaler (5% to 6%) 870
▲ Stalevo Tablets (5% to 8%) 2309
▲ Strattera Capsules (0.1% to 18%) 1864
Stromectol Tablets (0.9%) 2120
▲ Suboxone Tablets (11.2%) 2601
▲ Subutex Tablets (11.7%) 2601
▲ Suprax for Oral Suspension (Less than 2% to 3%) 1891
▲ Suprax Tablets (Less than 2% to 3%) 1891
▲ Sustiva Capsules (1% to 3%) 930
▲ Sustiva Tablets (1% to 3%) 930
▲ Sutent Capsules (3% to 33%) 2540
▲ Tamiflu Capsules (2% to 5%) 2649
▲ Tamiflu Oral Suspension (2% to 5%) 2649
▲ Tarceva Tablets (Less than 1% to 46%) 1228
▲ Targretin Capsules (3.8% to 10.7%) 1084
▲ Tasigna Capsules (11% to 13%) 2316
▲ Taxotere Injection Concentrate (0.7% to 10.9%) 2773
Tekturna Tablets 2321
Tekturna HCT Tablets 2324
▲ Temodar Capsules (4% to 9%) 2931
Teveten Tablets (2%) 515
Teveten HCT Tablets (Less than 1%) 517
Tice BCG (2%) 2936
Toprol-XL Tablets (Greater than 1%) 666
▲ Torisel Injection (4% to 21%) 3272
Tracleer Tablets 3289
Treximet Tablets (Frequent) 1616
▲ Tricor Tablets (4.6%) 520
▲ Trisenox Injection (58%) 986
▲ Trizivir Tablets (6% to 9%) 1622
▲ Truvada Tablets (Greater than or equal to 5%) 1262
Twinrix Vaccine (Less than 1%) 1628
▲ Tygacil for Injection (6.8%) 3276
Tylenol with Codeine Tablets 2427
▲ Tyzeka Tablets (Less than 1% to 12%) 2328
▲ Ultram ER Extended-Release Tablets (1% to less than 5%) 2428
Ultrase Capsules 718
▲ Ultrase MT Capsules (5.7%) 719
Uroxatral Tablets (1% to 2%) 2786
▲ Vagifem Tablets (7%) 2375
▲ Valcyte Tablets (15%) 2654
▲ Valstar Sterile Solution for Intravesical Instillation (5%) 1735
▲ Valtrex Caplets (1% to 11%) 1635
Vaqta (1.1% to 1.6%) 2130
Varivax (Greater than or equal to 1%) 2133
▲ Vectibix (1% to 25%) 597
▲ Velcade for Injection (14% to 16%) 2168
▲ Venlafaxine Hydrochloride Tablets (2.2% to 8%) 2199
▲ Vesanoid Capsules (31%) 2660
VESIcare Tablets (1.2% to 1.9%) 636
Viadur Implant (Less than 2%) 802
▲ Vicoprofen Tablets (3% to 9%) 533
Viramune Oral Suspension (0.1% to 2%) 873
Viramune Tablets (0.1% to 2%) 873
▲ Viread Tablets (4% to 7%) 1268
▲ Vivitrol (11% to 16%) 988
▲ Voltaren Ophthalmic Solution (Less than or equal to 3%) 2336
▲ Voltaren Tablets (1% to 10%) 2334
▲ Voltaren-XR Tablets (1% to 10%) 2337
Vytorin 10/10 Tablets 2149
Vytorin 10/10 Tablets 2939
Vytorin 10/20 Tablets 2149
Vytorin 10/20 Tablets 2939
Vytorin 10/40 Tablets 2149
Vytorin 10/40 Tablets 2939
Vytorin 10/80 Tablets 2149
Vytorin 10/80 Tablets 2939
▲ Vyvanse Capsules (12%) 3033
▲ WelChol Tablets (6.7%) 1015
▲ Wellbutrin SR Sustained-Release Tablets (3% to 9%) 1653
▲ Wellbutrin XL Extended-Release Tablets (3% to 9%) 1659
WinRho SDF 741
▲ Xeloda Tablets (9% to 35%) 2662
▲ Xenical Capsules (25.5%) 2672
▲ Xifaxan Tablets (7.2%) 2682
Xopenex Inhalation Solution (1.5%) 3001
Xopenex Inhalation Solution Concentrate (1.5%) 3005
Xopenex HFA Inhalation Aerosol (1.5%) 3009
▲ Xyrem Oral Solution (3% to 11.4%) 1766
Yaz Tablets (Greater than 1%) 805
Zantac 25 EFFERdose Tablets 1670
Zantac Injection 1666
Zantac Injection Pharmacy Bulk Package (Frequent) 1668
Zantac Injection Premixed 1666
Zantac 1670
▲ Ziagen (6%) 1673
Zinacef for Injection 1678
Zinacef Injection 1678
▲ Zocor Tablets (5.9% to 7.3%) 2136
Zofran Injection (2%) 1682
▲ Zofran (1% to 3%) 1687
▲ Zofran ODT Orally Disintegrating Tablets (1% to 3%) 1687
▲ Zometa for Intravenous Infusion (14% to 16%) 2341
Zomig Tablets (Rare) 694
Zomig Nasal Spray (Very rare to less than 2%) 689
Zomig-ZMT Tablets (Rare) 694
▲ Zonegran Capsules (6%) 1089
Zosyn for Injection (1.8%) 3284
▲ Zyban Sustained-Release Tablets (3%) 1692
▲ Zyprexa Tablets (4%) 1883
Zyprexa IntraMuscular (Infrequent) 1883
▲ Zyprexa ZYDIS Orally Disintegrating Tablets (4%) 1883
▲ Zyrtec Chewable Tablets (4.4% to 5.6%) 1920
▲ Zyrtec Syrup (4.4% to 5.6%) 1920
▲ Zyrtec Tablets (4.4% to 5.6%) 1920
Zyvox (0% to 2.4%) 2552

Abdominal symptom complex, acute

Prozac Weekly Capsules (Rare) 1852
Prozac Pulvules and Liquid (Rare) 1852
Remeron Tablets (Frequent) 2924
RemeronSolTab Tablets (Frequent) 2927

Abdominal tenderness

Ambien CR Tablets (1%) 2696
▲ Chantix Tablets (5% to 7%) 2511
▲ Cymbalta Delayed-Release Capsules (4%) 1801
Sandostatin Injection (Rare) 2300
Sandostatin LAR Depot 2302

Abortion

Copaxone for Injection (Infrequent) 3110
Effexor XR Extended-Release Capsules (Rare) 3195
Gabitril Tablets (Infrequent) 973
Imitrex Injection 1465
Imitrex Nasal Spray 1470
Imitrex Tablets (Rare) 1474
Paxil (Infrequent) 1535
Paxil CR Controlled-Release Tablets (Infrequent) 1544
Prozac Weekly Capsules (Infrequent) 1852
Prozac Pulvules and Liquid (Infrequent) 1852
Venlafaxine Hydrochloride Tablets (Rare) 2199

Abortion, septic

ParaGard T 380A Intrauterine Copper Contraceptive 1041

Abortion, spontaneous

Celexa 1160
Lexapro Oral Suspension 1174
Lexapro Tablets 1174
Lupron Depot-PED 7.5 mg, 11.25 mg and 15 mg (Possible) 471
Rebif Prefilled Syringe for Injection 1107

Abrasion

▲ Dacogen Injection (5%) 1066

Abscess
Actiq (Less than 1%) 959
Ambien Tablets (Rare) 2692
▲ Aranesp for Injection (27%) 564
Aricept Tablets (Infrequent) 1062
Aricept ODT Tablets (Infrequent) 1062
Campral Tablets (Infrequent) 1158
Capastat Sulfate for Injection 1791
▲ CellCept Capsules (3% to less than 20%) 2622
▲ CellCept Intravenous (3% to less than 20%) 2622
▲ CellCept Oral Suspension (3% to less than 20%) 2622
▲ CellCept Tablets (3% to less than 20%) 2622
Doxil Injection (Less than 1%) 2378
Enbrel for Injection 569
▲ Evoxac Capsules (1% to 3%) 1013
Gabitril Tablets (Infrequent) 973
▲ Gengraf Capsules (4.4%) 435
▲ Gliadel Wafer (5%) 1076
▲ Intron A for Injection (Less than 5%) 2859
Ionsys Transdermal System (.1% to less than 1%) 2410
Lamictal (Rare) 1488
▲ Lupron Depot-PED 7.5 mg, 11.25 mg and 15 mg (5%) 471
Lyrica Capsules (0.1% to 1%) 2527
Micardis Tablets (More than 0.3%) 852
Micardis HCT Tablets 854
Mirapex Tablets 857
▲ Neoral Soft Gelatin Capsules (1% to 4.4%) 2280
Paxil (Rare) 1535
Paxil CR Controlled-Release Tablets (Rare) 1544
PegIntron Powder for Injection (Less than or equal to 1%) 2903
▲ Prograf Capsules and Injection (3% to 15%) 622
▲ Prometrium Capsules (100 mg, 200 mg) (Less than 5%) 3047
Protonix for Delayed-Release Oral Suspension (Less than 1%) 3254
Protonix Delayed-Release Tablets (Less than 1%) 3254
Protonix I.V. (Less than 1%) 3257
Protopic Ointment (0.2% to less than 1%) 628
Raptiva for Injection 1218
▲ Remicade for IV Injection (15%) 950
ReoPro Vials (0.2%) 1860
Requip Tablets (Infrequent) 1561
Rilutek Tablets (Infrequent) 2771
Risperdal Consta Long-Acting Injection (Infrequent) 1753
▲ Sandimmune (4.4% to 5.3%) 2296
Suboxone Tablets (2%) 2601
Subutex Tablets (2%) 2601
Tice BCG (2%) 2936
▲ Tygacil for Injection (3.2%) 3276
Vectibix 597
Zosyn for Injection (2.2%) 3284

Abscess, abdominal
Avastin IV 1192
Enbrel for Injection 569
Invanz for Injection (1%) 2029

Abscess, dental
Fentora Tablets (Greater than 1%) 968
Mirapex Tablets 857
Requip Tablets (Frequent) 1561
Vivitrol 988
Xyrem Oral Solution (Infrequent) 1766

Abscess, foot
Enbrel for Injection 569

Abscess, peridiverticular
Dacogen Injection 1066

Abscess, periodontal
Actiq (1% or greater) 959
Aricept Tablets (Infrequent) 1062
Aricept ODT Tablets (Infrequent) 1062
Brovana Inhalation Solution (Less than 2%) 2990
Copaxone for Injection (At least 2%) 3110
▲ Depakote ER Tablets (Greater than 1% to less than 5%) 423
Doxil Injection (Less than 1%) 2378
Emsam Transdermal System (Infrequent) 905
Gabitril Tablets (Infrequent) 973
Lyrica Capsules (Rare) 2527
Norvir (Less than 2%) 489
Pletal Tablets (Less than 2%) 2481
Protonix for Delayed-Release Oral Suspension (Less than 1%) 3254
Protonix Delayed-Release Tablets (Less than 1%) 3254
Protonix I.V. (Less than 1%) 3257
▲ Protopic Ointment (Up to 3%) 628
Provigil Tablets (Greater than or equal to 1%) 977
Symbyax Capsules (Infrequent) 1871
Zyprexa Tablets (Infrequent) 1883
Zyprexa ZYDIS Orally Disintegrating Tablets (Infrequent) 1883

Abscess, peritonsillar
Amevive 611
Tamiflu Capsules (Less than 1%) 2649
Tamiflu Oral Suspension (Less than 1%) 2649

Abscess, renal
Gengraf Capsules (1% to less than 3%) 435
Neoral Oral Solution (1% to less than 3%) 2280

Abscess, ruptured
▲ NovoSeven RT (4.7%) 2370

Abscess at injection site
Bicillin C-R Injectable Suspension 1775
Bicillin L-A Injection 1777
Cerezyme for Injection (Less than 1%) 1238
Copaxone for Injection (Frequent) 3110
Fluarix Vaccine 1446
Lupron Depot 3.75 mg 462
Lupron Depot 7.5 mg 469
Lupron Depot–3 Month 11.25 mg 462
Liquid PedvaxHIB 2073
Pentacel 2792
Rebif Prefilled Syringe for Injection 1107
Vivitrol 988

Absorption, impaired, dietary fats
Sandostatin LAR Depot 2302

Absorption, nutrients, alterations in
Sandostatin LAR Depot 2302

Abuse
Ambien Tablets (Rare) 2692
Prozac Pulvules and Liquid 1852

Acanthosis nigricans
Advicor Tablets 402
Niaspan Extended-Release Tablets 480

Accident, road traffic
Xyrem Oral Solution (Infrequent) 1766

Accommodation, changes in
Avandaryl Tablets 1344

Accommodation, impaired
Ambien Tablets (Rare) 2692
Celexa (Frequent) 1160
Concerta Extended-Release Tablets 1925
Daytrana Transdermal Patch 3022
Effexor XR Extended-Release Capsules (Frequent) 3195
Exforge Tablets (Less than or equal to 0.%) 2238
FML Ophthalmic Ointment (Occasional) ⊙ 223
FML Ophthalmic Suspension (Occasional) ⊙ 224
FML Forte Ophthalmic Suspension (Occasional) ⊙ 222
Imitrex Nasal Spray 1470
Lamictal (Infrequent) 1488
Lyrica Capsules (0.1% to 1%) 2527
Metadate CD Capsules 3146
Paxil (Infrequent) 1535
Paxil CR Controlled-Release Tablets (Infrequent) 1544
Pred Forte Ophthalmic Suspension (Occasional) ⊙ 227
Pred Mild Ophthalmic Suspension (Occasional) ⊙ 230
Remeron Tablets (Infrequent) 2924
RemeronSolTab Tablets (Infrequent) 2927
Requip Tablets (Infrequent) 1561
Risperdal Consta Long-Acting Injection (Infrequent) 1753
Symbyax Capsules (Infrequent) 1871
Transderm Scōp Transdermal Therapeutic System 2206
▲ Venlafaxine Hydrochloride Tablets (Frequent to 9.1%) 2199
Wellbutrin SR Sustained-Release Tablets (Infrequent) 1653
Wellbutrin XL Extended-Release Tablets (Infrequent) 1659
Zantac 25 EFFERdose Tablets (Rare) 1670
Zantac Injection (Rare) 1666
Zantac (Rare) 1670
Zofran Injection 1682
Zyban Sustained-Release Tablets (Infrequent) 1692
Zyprexa Tablets (Rare) 1883
Zyprexa ZYDIS Orally Disintegrating Tablets (Rare) 1883
Zyrtec-D 12 Hour Extended Release Tablets (Less than 2%) 1923

Accomodation, loss of
Zyrtec Chewable Tablets (Less than 2%) 1920
Zyrtec Syrup (Less than 2%) 1920
Zyrtec Tablets (Less than 2%) 1920

Aches
Asacol Delayed-Release Tablets 2579
Cipro I.V. (1% or less) 2817
Cipro (Less than 1%) 2810
Cipro XR Tablets 2823
Cosopt Sterile Ophthalmic Solution 1969
Eldepryl Capsules (1 of 49 patients) 3052
▲ Flonase Nasal Spray (1% to 3%) 1431
InnoPran XL Extended Release Capsules 1484
▲ Nabi-HB (3%) 815
Nadolol Tablets 2191
Orthoclone OKT3 Sterile Solution 2387
Recombivax HB (Less than 1%) 2107
▲ Serevent Diskus (1% to 3%) 1594
Tamiflu Capsules (Less than 1%) 2649
Tamiflu Oral Suspension (Less than 1%) 2649
Timoptic Sterile Ophthalmic Solution 2121
Timoptic in Ocudose 2124
Timoptic-XE Sterile Ophthalmic Gel Forming Solution 2125
Toprol-XL Tablets 666

Aches, joints
(*see under* Arthralgia)

Acid-base disturbances
Demadex Injection 2630
Demadex Tablets 2630

Acidosis
▲ Abelcet Injection (3%) 1134
Actiq (Less than 1%) 959
AmBisome for Injection (Less common) 606
▲ CellCept Capsules (3% to less than 20%) 2622
▲ CellCept Intravenous (3% to less than 20%) 2622
▲ CellCept Oral Suspension (3% to less than 20%) 2622
▲ CellCept Tablets (3% to less than 20%) 2622
Cipro I.V. (1% or less) 2817
Cipro (Less than 1%) 2810
Cipro XR Tablets 2823
Dyazide Capsules 1405
Fleet Phospho-soda 1145
Fleet Phospho-soda EZ-PREP 1147
Fleet Prep Kits 1149
Indocin I.V. (Less than 3%) 2489
Mycamine for Injection 616
Percocet Tablets 1127
Percodan Tablets 1130
Perforomist Inhalation Solution 1025
▲ Prograf Capsules and Injection (3% to 15%) 622
▲ Proleukin for Injection (1% to 12%) 2287
Requip Tablets (Infrequent) 1561
▲ Simulect for Injection (3% to 10%) 2306
Symbyax Capsules (Rare) 1871
Trasylol Injection (1% to 2%) 799
▲ Trisenox Injection (5%) 986
Tygacil for Injection 3276
Ultane Liquid for Inhalation (Less than 1%) 524
▲ Vesanoid Capsules (3%) 2660
Zyprexa Tablets (Frequent) 1883
Zyprexa ZYDIS Orally Disintegrating Tablets (Frequent) 1883

Acidosis, hypochloremic metabolic
Gengraf Capsules 435
Sandimmune (Occasional) 2296

Acidosis, metabolic
Aggrenox Capsules 819
Aloxi Injection (Less than 1%) 1059
Bayer Aspirin 750
Brovana Inhalation Solution (Less than 2%) 2990
Eloxatin for Injection 2731
Fleet Enema 1143
Fleet Enema Extra 1143
Fleet Enema for Children 1143
Fleet Pedia-Lax Enema 1143
Fleet Phospho-soda 1145
Fleet Phospho-soda EZ-PREP 1147
Foradil Aerolizer 2849
Ixempra Kit for Injection 915
Percocet Tablets 1127
Percodan Tablets 1130
St. Joseph 81 mg Aspirin Chewable and Enteric Coated Tablets 1903
Sulfamylon Cream 2194
Sulfamylon for 5% Topical Solution 2194
Torisel Injection 3272

Acidosis, renal tubular
Abelcet Injection 1134

Acidosis, respiratory
▲ CellCept Capsules (3% to less than 20%) 2622
▲ CellCept Intravenous (3% to less than 20%) 2622
▲ CellCept Oral Suspension (3% to less than 20%) 2622
▲ CellCept Tablets (3% to less than 20%) 2622
Proleukin for Injection (Less than 1%) 2287
Rilutek Tablets (Infrequent) 2771

Acne
(*see under* Acneiform eruptions)

Acne, cystic, flare-up
Parnate Tablets 1532

Acne fulminaris
Accutane Capsules 2607

Acne vulgaris
Ambien CR Tablets (Rare) 2696
Lialda Tablets (Infrequent) 3029
▲ Nexavar Tablets (1% to less than 10%) 784

Acneiform eruptions
▲ Aerobid/Aerobid-M (1% to 3%) 1153
Ambien Tablets (Rare) 2692
Amerge Tablets (Rare) 1301
Amrix Capsules 966
Analpram-HC 1140
▲ AndroGel (1% to 8%) 3159
Asacol Delayed-Release Tablets (1% to 2%) 2579
Campral Tablets (Infrequent) 1158
Canasa Rectal Suppositories (1.2%) 705
Celexa (Infrequent) 1160
▲ CellCept Capsules (3% to less than 20%) 2622
▲ CellCept Intravenous (3% to less than 20%) 2622
▲ CellCept Oral Suspension (3% to less than 20%) 2622
▲ CellCept Tablets (3% to less than 20%) 2622
Chantix Tablets (Infrequent) 2511
Copaxone for Injection (At least 2%) 3110
Cosmegen for Injection 2485
Crinone 4% Gel 992
Crinone 8% Gel 992
Dantrium Capsules (Less frequent) 2580
Delatestryl Injection 1730
Diprolene Lotion 0.05% (1%) 2838
Diprolene Ointment 0.05% 2839
Diprolene AF Cream 0.05% (Infrequent) 2837
▲ Doxil Injection (1% to 10%) 2378
Effexor XR Extended-Release Capsules (Infrequent) 3195
Elidel Cream 1% (0% to 1.8%) 2221
Elocon Cream 0.1% (Infrequent) 2840
Elocon Lotion 0.1% (Infrequent) 2841
Elocon Ointment 0.1% (Infrequent) 2842
Emend Capsules (Greater than 0.5%) 1992
Emend for Injection (Greater than 0.5%) 1999
Emsam Transdermal System (Frequent) 905
Estratest Tablets 3043
Estratest H.S. Tablets 3043
Evoxac Capsules (Less than 1%) 1013
Finacea Gel (1% or less) 1742
▲ Flovent Diskus 50 mcg (1% to 3%) 1435

Gabitril Tablets (1% or more) 973
▲ Gengraf Capsules (1% to 6%) 435
Herceptin I.V. (2%) 1199
▲ Humatrope Vials and Cartridges (Up to 5.8%) 1838
▲ Intron A for Injection (Less than 5%) 2859
Kaletra 452
Lamictal (Infrequent) 1488
Lexapro Oral Suspension (Infrequent) 1174
Lexapro Tablets (Infrequent) 1174
Lipitor Tablets (Less than 2%) 2501
Lotrisone 2881
Lunesta Tablets (Infrequent) 2994
▲ Lupron Depot–3 Month 11.25 mg (Up to 10%) 462
Lupron Depot-PED 7.5 mg, 11.25 mg and 15 mg (2%) 471
Luvox CR Extended-Release Capsules (2%) 1759
Luxíq Foam (One patient) 3058
Lybrel Tablets 3204
Maxalt Tablets (Rare) 2056
Maxalt-MLT Orally Disintegrating Tablets (Rare) 2056
Meridia Capsules (1%) 475
Mirapex Tablets 857
Mircette Tablets 1034
▲ Mirena Intrauterine System (5% or more) 779
▲ Myfortic Tablets (3% to less than 20%) 2276
Namenda (More than one patient) 1180
▲ Neoral Oral Solution (1% to 6%) 2280
▲ Neoral Soft Gelatin Capsules (1% to 6%) 2280
Nexium Delayed-Release Capsules (Less than 1%) 645
Nexium I.V. (Less than 1%) 652
Nexium Delayed-Release Oral Suspension (Less than 1%) 645
Nimotop Capsules (Up to 1.4%) 790
Norvir (Less than 2%) 489
NuvaRing 2897
Olux Foam 3061
Olux-E Foam 3059
Omnaris Nasal Spray (Very rare) 2998
Ortho-Cyclen Tablets 2449
Ortho Evra Transdermal System 2437
Ortho Micronor Tablets (Rare) 2446
Ortho Tri-Cyclen Tablets 2449
Ortho Tri-Cyclen Lo Tablets 2458
Paxil (Infrequent) 1535
Paxil CR Controlled-Release Tablets (Infrequent) 1544
Pentasa Capsules (0.2%) 3030
Pepcid Tablets (Infrequent) 2075
Pramosone 1141
Premphase Tablets 3232
Prempro Tablets 3232
▲ Prograf Capsules and Injection (3% to 15%) 622
▲ Prometrium Capsules (100 mg, 200 mg) (Less than 5%) 3047
Protonix for Delayed-Release Oral Suspension (Less than 1%) 3254
Protonix Delayed-Release Tablets (Less than 1%) 3254
Protonix I.V. (Less than 1%) 3257
▲ Protopic Ointment (2% to 7%) 628
Prozac Weekly Capsules (Infrequent) 1852
Prozac Pulvules and Liquid (Infrequent) 1852
▲ Rapamune Oral Solution (22%) 3260
▲ Raptiva for Injection (4%) 1218
ReFacto Vials 3269
Requip Tablets (Infrequent) 1561
Retrovir Capsules 1574
Retrovir IV Infusion 1579
Retrovir 1574
Risperdal Consta Long-Acting Injection (2%) 1753
▲ Sandimmune (1% to 6%) 2296
Seasonique Tablets 1046
▲ Simulect for Injection (Greater than or equal to 10%) 2306
Soriatane Capsules (Less than 1%) 3062
Sular Extended Release Tablets (Less than or equal to 1%) 2975
Symbyax Capsules (Infrequent) 1871
Targretin Capsules 1084
Testim 1% Gel (Less than 1%) 701
▲ Torisel Injection (0% to 10%) 3272
Tricor Tablets 520
▲ Valcyte Tablets (Less than 5%) 2654
Vanos Cream 1941
▲ Vectibix (1% to 13%) 597
Venlafaxine Hydrochloride Tablets (Infrequent) 2199
Verdeso Foam 3069
Wellbutrin Tablets (Rare) 1648
Wellbutrin SR Sustained-Release Tablets (At least 1%) 1653
Wellbutrin XL Extended-Release Tablets (At least 1%) 1659
Xyrem Oral Solution (Infrequent) 1766
Yaz Tablets (Greater than 1%) 805
Zonegran Capsules (Infrequent) 1089
Zyban Sustained-Release Tablets (Infrequent) 1692
Zyprexa Tablets (2%) 1883
Zyprexa ZYDIS Orally Disintegrating Tablets (2%) 1883
Zyrtec Chewable Tablets (Less than 2%) 1920
Zyrtec Syrup (Less than 2%) 1920
Zyrtec Tablets (Less than 2%) 1920
Zyrtec-D 12 Hour Extended Release Tablets (Less than 2%) 1923

Acneiform reactions
▲ Busulfex Injection (7%) 2477
Elocon Lotion 0.1% (2 in 209 patients) 2841
▲ Erbitux (14% to 88%) 912

Actinic keratosis
Requip Tablets (Infrequent) 1561

Acute abdomen
Torisel Injection 3272

Adams-Stokes syndrome
Exelon Capsules (Infrequent) 2229
Exelon Oral Solution (Infrequent) 2229

Addiction
Lyrica Capsules (Rare) 2527

Adenitis
Clinoril Tablets 1962

Adenocarcinoma
Mirapex Tablets 857

Adenoma, prostatic
Exelon Capsules (Infrequent) 2229
Exelon Oral Solution (Infrequent) 2229
Mirapex Tablets 857

Adenoma, unspecified
▲ Humira Injection (Less than 5%) 442

Adenomas, benign
Mirapex Tablets 857

Adenomas, benign pituitary
Lupron Depot 3.75 mg 462
Risperdal Consta Long-Acting Injection 1753

Adenopathy
Carbatrol Capsules 3019
Enbrel for Injection 569
Equetro Extended-Release Capsules 3174
Kogenate FS 746
Kogenate FS with Bio-Set 748

ADH syndrome, inappropriate
Avandaryl Tablets 1344
Carbatrol Capsules 3019
Celexa (Several cases) 1160
Depakote ER Tablets 423
Duetact Tablets 3085
Effexor XR Extended-Release Capsules 3195
Equetro Extended-Release Capsules 3174
Lexapro Oral Suspension 1174
Lexapro Tablets 1174
OxyContin Tablets (Less than 1%) 2589
Parnate Tablets 1532
Paxil 1535
Paxil CR Controlled-Release Tablets 1544
Prinivil Tablets 2087
Prinzide Tablets 2092
Requip Tablets (Rare) 1561
Risperdal Consta Long-Acting Injection 1753
Rythmol Tablets (Less than 1%) 1586
Venlafaxine Hydrochloride Tablets 2199
Wellbutrin Tablets 1648
Wellbutrin SR Sustained-Release Tablets 1653
Wellbutrin XL Extended-Release Tablets 1659
Zyban Sustained-Release Tablets 1692

Adnexal torsion, ovarian
Follistim AQ Cartridge 2844

Adrenal hypercorticism
▲ Temodar Capsules (8%) 2931

Adrenal insufficiency
Azmacort Inhalation Aerosol 407
Beconase AQ Nasal Spray 1369
▲ NeoProfen Injection (7%) 2496
Noxafil Oral Suspension (Rare) 2889
Verdeso Foam 3069

Adrenal suppression
(*see also under* HPA axis suppression)
Advair Diskus 100/50 1276
Advair Diskus 250/50 1276
Advair Diskus 500/50 1276
Qvar Inhalation Aerosol 3116
Veramyst Nasal Spray 1643

Adrenergic syndrome, unspecified
Paxil (Rare) 1535
Paxil CR Controlled-Release Tablets (Rare) 1544

Affect lability
Concerta Extended-Release Tablets (1.4%) 1925
▲ Daytrana Transdermal Patch (6%) 3022
Mirapex Tablets 857
▲ Vyvanse Capsules (3%) 3033
Xyrem Oral Solution (Infrequent) 1766

Afibrinogenemia
Depakote ER Tablets 423

Ageusia
▲ Aerobid/Aerobid-M (3% to 9%) 1153
Aggrenox Capsules (Less than 1%) 819
Avelox (Less than 0.1%) 2803
Beconase AQ Nasal Spray (Rare) 1369
Bentyl Capsules 703
Bentyl Injection 703
Bentyl Syrup 703
Bentyl Tablets 703
Captopril Tablets (Approximately 2 to 4 of 100 patients) 2182
Celexa (Rare) 1160
Cipro I.V. 2817
Cipro 2810
Cipro XR Tablets 2823
Clinoril Tablets (Less than 1 in 100) 1962
Copaxone for Injection (Infrequent) 3110
▲ Cuprimine Capsules (12%) 1986
Donnatal Extentabs 2507
Doxil Injection (Less than 1%) 2378
Effexor XR Extended-Release Capsules (Infrequent) 3195
Exelon Capsules (Infrequent) 2229
Exelon Oral Solution (Infrequent) 2229
Flonase Nasal Spray 1431
Flumadine (Less than 0.3%) 1167
Gabitril Tablets (Infrequent) 973
▲ Intron A for Injection (Less than 5%) 2859
Klonopin (Infrequent) 2639
Lamictal (Rare) 1488
Lamisil Oral Granules 2264
Lamisil Tablets (Uncommon) 2266
Levaquin 2416
Levaquin in 5% Dextrose Injection 2416
Lipitor Tablets (Less than 2%) 2501
Lyrica Capsules (0.1% to 1%) 2527
Mirapex Tablets 857
Nexium Delayed-Release Capsules (Less than 1%) 645
Nexium I.V. (Less than 1%) 652
Nexium Delayed-Release Oral Suspension (Less than 1%) 645
Norvir (Less than 2%) 489
Paxil (Infrequent) 1535
Paxil CR Controlled-Release Tablets (Infrequent) 1544
Prozac Weekly Capsules (Rare) 1852
Prozac Pulvules and Liquid (Rare) 1852
Rilutek Tablets (Rare) 2771
Salagen Tablets (Less than 1%) 1082
Soriatane Capsules (Less than 1%) 3062
▲ Sutent Capsules (Less than 1% to 44%) 2540
Venlafaxine Hydrochloride Tablets (Infrequent) 2199
▲ Xeloda Tablets (Less than 5%) 2662
Xifaxan Tablets (Less than 2%) 2682
Zyrtec Chewable Tablets (Less than 2%) 1920
Zyrtec Syrup (Less than 2%) 1920
Zyrtec Tablets (Less than 2%) 1920
Zyrtec-D 12 Hour Extended Release Tablets (Less than 2%) 1923

Aggression
Abilify Injection (Greater than or equal to 1 in 1000 patients and less than 1 in 100 patients) 2466
Abilify Oral Solution (Greater than or equal to 1 in 1000 patients and less than 1 in 100 patients) 881
Abilify Oral Solution (Greater than or equal to 1 in 1000 patients and less than 1 in 100 patients) 2466
Abilify Discmelt Orally Disintegrating Tablets (Greater than or equal to 1 in 1000 patients and less than 1 in 100 patients) 881
Abilify Discmelt Orally Disintegrating Tablets (Greater than or equal to 1 in 1000 patients and less than 1 in 100 patients) 2466
Abilify Tablets (Greater than or equal to 1 in 1000 patients and less than 1 in 100 patients) 881
Abilify Tablets (Greater than or equal to 1 in 1000 patients and less than 1 in 100 patients) 2466
Accutane Capsules 2607
Adderall XR Capsules 3012
Advair Diskus 100/50 1276
Advair Diskus 250/50 1276
Advair Diskus 500/50 1276
Advair HFA 45/21 Inhalation Aerosol 1288
Advair HFA 115/21 Inhalation Aerosol 1288
Advair HFA 230/21 Inhalation Aerosol 1288
Ambien Tablets 2692
Amerge Tablets (Rare) 1301
Aricept Tablets (Frequent) 1062
Aricept ODT Tablets (Frequent) 1062
Celexa (Infrequent) 1160
Chantix Tablets (Infrequent) 2511
Concerta Extended-Release Tablets (1.7%) 1925
Cymbalta Delayed-Release Capsules 1801
Depakote ER Tablets 423
Effexor XR Extended-Release Capsules 3195
Evoxac Capsules 1013
▲ Exelon Capsules (3%) 2229
▲ Exelon Oral Solution (3%) 2229
Flovent Diskus 50 mcg 1435
Flovent HFA 1440
Imitrex Injection 1465
Imitrex Tablets (Rare) 1474
▲ Intron A for Injection (Less than 5%) 2859
▲ Keppra Injection (5% to 13.3%) 3137
Keppra Oral Solution 3131
Keppra Tablets 3131
Klonopin (Infrequent) 2639
Lexapro Oral Suspension (Infrequent) 1174
Lexapro Tablets (Infrequent) 1174
Luvox CR Extended-Release Capsules 1759
Mirapex Tablets 857
Nexium Delayed-Release Capsules 645
Nexium I.V. 652
Nexium Delayed-Release Oral Suspension 645
Parnate Tablets 1532
Paxil 1535
Paxil CR Controlled-Release Tablets 1544
PegIntron Powder for Injection (Less than or equal to 1%) 2903
Provigil Tablets 977
Prozac Pulvules and Liquid 1852
Requip Tablets (Infrequent) 1561
Seromycin Capsules 1864
Singulair 2114
Soriatane Capsules 3062
Strattera Capsules (0.2%) 1864
Sustiva Capsules (0.4%) 930
Sustiva Tablets (0.4%) 930
Symbyax Capsules 1871
Vyvanse Capsules 3033
Wellbutrin Tablets 1648
Wellbutrin SR Sustained-Release Tablets 1653
Wellbutrin XL Extended-Release Tablets 1659
Xyzal Oral Solution 2789
Xyzal Oral Solution 3155
Zyban Sustained-Release Tablets 1692

Aggressive reaction
Ambien Tablets (Rare) 2692
Ambien CR Tablets (Rare) 2696
Atripla Tablets 938
Crinone 4% Gel 992
Crinone 8% Gel 992
Genotropin Lyophilized Powder 2547

Namenda (Frequent) 1180
Pulmicort Flexhaler 654
Remeron Tablets 2924
RemeronSolTab Tablets 2927
Valium Tablets 2658
Zyrtec Chewable Tablets (Rare) 1920
Zyrtec Syrup (Rare) 1920
Zyrtec Tablets (Rare) 1920
Zyrtec-D 12 Hour Extended Release Tablets (Rare) 1923

Agitation

Abilify Injection 881
▲ Abilify Injection (19%) 2466
▲ Abilify Oral Solution (19%) 881
▲ Abilify Oral Solution (19%) 2466
▲ Abilify Discmelt Orally Disintegrating Tablets (19%) 881
▲ Abilify Discmelt Orally Disintegrating Tablets (19%) 2466
▲ Abilify Tablets (19%) 881
▲ Abilify Tablets (19%) 2466
Actiq (Less than 1%) 959
▲ Adderall XR Capsules (8%) 3012
Advair Diskus 100/50 1276
Advair Diskus 250/50 1276
Advair Diskus 500/50 1276
Advair HFA 45/21 Inhalation Aerosol 1288
Advair HFA 115/21 Inhalation Aerosol 1288
Advair HFA 230/21 Inhalation Aerosol 1288
Aggrenox Capsules (Less than 1%) 819
Aldara Cream, 5% 1699
Allegra-D 12 Hour Extended-Release Tablets (1.9%) 2687
Allegra-D 24 Hour Extended-Release Tablets (1.9%) 2690
Ambien Tablets (Infrequent) 2692
Ambien CR Tablets (Infrequent) 2696
AmBisome for Injection (Less common) 606
Amerge Tablets (Rare) 1301
Amoxil Capsules (Rare) 1305
Amoxil Chewable Tablets (Rare) 1305
Amoxil Pediatric Drops for Oral Suspension (Rare) 1305
Amoxil Powder for Oral Suspension (Rare) 1305
Amoxil Tablets (Rare) 1305
Anzemet Injection (Infrequently) 2701
Anzemet Tablets 2704
Aricept Tablets (Frequent) 1062
Aricept ODT Tablets (Frequent) 1062
Atripla Tablets 938
Augmentin (Rare) 1323
Augmentin Tablets (Rare) 1327
Augmentin XR Extended Release Tablets (Rare) 1333
Augmentin ES-600 Powder for Oral Suspension (Rare) 1329
Avelox (Less than 0.1%) 2803
▲ Avinza Capsules (Less than 5%) 1772
Azilect Tablets (Infrequent) 3106
Bayer Aspirin 750
Bicillin C-R Injectable Suspension 1775
Bicillin L-A Injection 1777
Brovana Inhalation Solution (Less than 2%) 2990
Busulfex Injection (2%) 2477
Campral Tablets (Infrequent) 1158
Carbatrol Capsules 3019
Catapres Tablets (About 3 in 100 patients) 841
Catapres-TTS (0.5% or less) 842
▲ Celexa (1% to 3%) 1160
▲ CellCept Capsules (3% to less than 20%) 2622
▲ CellCept Intravenous (3% to less than 20%) 2622
▲ CellCept Oral Suspension (3% to less than 20%) 2622
▲ CellCept Tablets (3% to less than 20%) 2622
Chantix Tablets (Infrequent) 2511
Cipro I.V. 2817
Cipro 2810
Cipro XR Tablets 2823
▲ Clorpres Tablets (About 3%) 2185
Comtan Tablets (1%) 2208
Comvax 1966
Concerta Extended-Release Tablets (2.2%) 1925
▲ Copaxone for Injection (4%) 3110
Cuprimine Capsules 1986
▲ Cymbalta Delayed-Release Capsules (5% to 6%) 1801
Depakote ER Tablets (Greater than 1%) 423
▲ DepoCyt Injection (10% to 15%) 1136
Dexedrine 1401
Donnatal Extentabs 2507
▲ Doxil Injection (1% to 10%) 2378
Duragesic Transdermal System (1% or greater) 2405
▲ Effexor XR Extended-Release Capsules (3%) 3195
Eldepryl Capsules 3052
Elspar for Injection 1990
Emsam Transdermal System (Frequent) 905
Engerix-B Vaccine (Less than 1%) 1409
Equetro Extended-Release Capsules 3174
Evoxac Capsules (Less than 1%) 1013
Exelon Capsules (2% or more) 2229
Exelon Oral Solution (2% or more) 2229
Exforge Tablets (Less than or equal to 0.1%) 2238
▲ Flolan for Injection (11%) 1426
Flovent Diskus 50 mcg 1435
Flovent HFA 1440
Flumadine (0.3% to 1%) 1167
Frova Tablets (Infrequent) 1111
Gabitril Tablets (1%) 973
Geodon Capsules (Frequent) 2520
Imitrex Injection (Infrequent) 1465
Imitrex Nasal Spray (Infrequent) 1470
Imitrex Tablets (Up to 2%) 1474
▲ Indapamide Tablets (Greater than or equal to 5%) 2188
▲ Intron A for Injection (Less than 5%) 2859
▲ Invanz for Injection (3.3% to 5.1%) 2029
Ionsys Transdermal System (.1% to less than 1%) 2410
Kaletra (Less than 2%) 452
▲ Keppra Injection (13.3%) 3137
▲ Keppra Oral Solution (6%) 3131
▲ Keppra Tablets (6%) 3131
Klonopin 2639
▲ Lamictal (Greater than 1% to less than 5%) 1488
Leukeran Tablets (Rare) 1508
Levaquin (0.1% to 1%) 2416
Levaquin in 5% Dextrose Injection (0.1% to 1%) 2416
Lexapro Oral Suspension (Infrequent) 1174
Lexapro Tablets (Infrequent) 1174
Lunesta Tablets (Infrequent) 2994
▲ Lupron Depot 7.5 mg (Less than 5%) 469
Lupron Depot–3 Month 11.25 mg 462
▲ Luvox CR Extended-Release Capsules (1% to 3%) 1759
Lyrica Capsules (0.1% to 1%) 2527
Maxalt Tablets (Infrequent) 2056
Maxalt-MLT Orally Disintegrating Tablets (Infrequent) 2056
Meridia Capsules (Greater than or equal to 1%) 475
Merrem I.V. (Greater than 0.1% to 1%) 684
Miacalcin Nasal Spray (Less than 1%) 2274
Mirapex Tablets (Less than 1%) 857
Moxatag Tablets 2165
MS Contin Tablets (Less frequent) 2585
Namenda (Greater than or equal to 2%) 1180
Nembutal Sodium Solution, USP (Less than 1%) 2494
Nexium Delayed-Release Capsules 645
Nexium I.V. 652
Nexium Delayed-Release Oral Suspension 645
Norvir (Less than 2%) 489
Opana Tablets (Less than 1%) 1117
Opana ER Tablets (Less than 1%) 1121
Orthoclone OKT3 Sterile Solution 2387
OxyContin Tablets (Less than 1%) 2589
Parnate Tablets 1532
▲ Paxil (1.1% to 5%) 1535
▲ Paxil CR Controlled-Release Tablets (1.1% to 5%) 1544
PegIntron Powder for Injection (2%) 2903
Pepcid Tablets (Infrequent) 2075
Percocet Tablets 1127
Percodan Tablets 1130
Pristiq Extended-Release Tablets 3247
▲ Prograf Capsules and Injection (3% to 15%) 622
Proleukin for Injection (Less than 1%) 2287
ProQuad 2099
Provigil Tablets (1%) 977
Prozac Weekly Capsules (Rare to greater than or equal to 2%) 1852
Prozac Pulvules and Liquid (At least 2%) 1852
▲ Rebetol (5% to 8%) 2917
Recombivax HB 2107
Relenza Inhalation Powder 1556
Remeron Tablets (Frequent) 2924
RemeronSolTab Tablets (Frequent) 2927
ReoPro Vials (0.7%) 1860
Requip Tablets (Infrequent) 1561
Rilutek Tablets (Frequent) 2771
Risperdal Consta Long-Acting Injection (Frequent) 1753
▲ Romazicon Injection (3% to 9%) 2646
St. Joseph 81 mg Aspirin Chewable and Enteric Coated Tablets 1903
▲ Simulect for Injection (3% to 10%) 2306
Singulair 2114
Soma Tablets 1931
Stalevo Tablets (1%) 2309
Sustiva Capsules (Less than 2%) 930
Sustiva Tablets (Less than 2%) 930
Symbyax Capsules 1871
Tamiflu Capsules 2649
Tamiflu Oral Suspension 2649
Targretin Capsules 1084
Thioridazine Hydrochloride Tablets 2195
Thiothixene Capsules 2197
Trasylol Injection (1% to 2%) 799
Treximet Tablets 1616
▲ Trisenox Injection (5%) 986
Twinrix Vaccine (Less than 1%) 1628
▲ Ultane Liquid for Inhalation (7% to 15%) 524
Ultram ER Extended-Release Tablets (0.5% to less than 1%) 2428
▲ Valcyte Tablets (Less than 5%) 2654
Valtrex Caplets 1635
Velcade for Injection 2168
▲ Venlafaxine Hydrochloride Tablets (1.1% to 4.5%) 2199
▲ Vesanoid Capsules (9%) 2660
Vicoprofen Tablets (Less than 1%) 533
▲ Vivitrol (8% to 12%) 988
▲ Vyvanse Capsules (3%) 3033
▲ Wellbutrin Tablets (31.9%) 1648
▲ Wellbutrin SR Sustained-Release Tablets (3% to 9%) 1653
▲ Wellbutrin XL Extended-Release Tablets (2% to 9%) 1659
Xyzal Oral Solution 2789
Xyzal Oral Solution 3155
Zantac 25 EFFERdose Tablets (Rare) 1670
Zantac Injection 1666
Zantac Injection Pharmacy Bulk Package (Rare) 1668
Zantac Injection Premixed 1666
Zantac (Rare) 1670
▲ Zofran Injection (2% to 6%) 1682
▲ Zofran (6%) 1687
▲ Zofran ODT Orally Disintegrating Tablets (6%) 1687
▲ Zometa for Intravenous Infusion (13%) 2341
Zomig Tablets (Infrequent) 694
Zomig Nasal Spray (Infrequent to less than 2%) 689
Zomig-ZMT Tablets (Infrequent) 694
▲ Zonegran Capsules (9%) 1089
▲ Zosyn for Injection (2.1% to 7.1%) 3284
Zovirax 1690
Zyban Sustained-Release Tablets (Frequent) 1692
▲ Zyprexa Tablets (23%) 1883
Zyprexa IntraMuscular 1883
▲ Zyprexa ZYDIS Orally Disintegrating Tablets (23%) 1883
Zyrtec Chewable Tablets (Less than 2%) 1920
Zyrtec Syrup (Less than 2%) 1920
Zyrtec Tablets (Less than 2%) 1920
Zyrtec-D 12 Hour Extended Release Tablets (Less than 2%) 1923

Agnosia

▲ Vesanoid Capsules (3%) 2660

Agoraphobia

Luvox CR Extended-Release Capsules (Infrequent) 1759

Agranulocytosis

Abilify Injection (Less than 1 in 1000 patients) 2466
Abilify Oral Solution (Less than 1 in 1000 patients) 2466
Abilify Discmelt Orally Disintegrating Tablets (Less than 1 in 1000 patients) 2466
Abilify Tablets (Less than 1 in 1000 patients) 2466
Accolate Tablets 669
Accutane Capsules 2607
Aceon Tablets (2 mg, 4 mg, 8 mg) 3038
Aciphex Tablets 1053
Albenza Tablets (Rare) 1297
AmBisome for Injection (Infrequent) 606
Amoxil Capsules 1305
Amoxil Chewable Tablets 1305
Amoxil Pediatric Drops for Oral Suspension 1305
Amoxil Powder for Oral Suspension 1305
Amoxil Tablets 1305
Anaprox Tablets (Less than 1%) 2632
Anaprox DS Tablets (Less than 1%) 2632
Asacol Delayed-Release Tablets (Rare) 2579
Atacand Tablets (Very rare) 639
Atacand HCT 642
Augmentin 1323
Augmentin Tablets 1327
Augmentin XR Extended Release Tablets 1333
Augmentin ES-600 Powder for Oral Suspension 1329
Avalide Tablets 892
Avalide Tablets 2713
Avandaryl Tablets 1344
Avelox 2803
Captopril Tablets 2182
Carbatrol Capsules 3019
Ceftin 1380
Cipro I.V. (1% or less) 2817
Cipro 2810
Cipro XR Tablets 2823
Clinoril Tablets (Less than 1%) 1962
Clorpres Tablets 2185
Combigan Ophthalmic Solution 553
Cosmegen for Injection 2485
Cosopt Sterile Ophthalmic Solution 1969
Cuprimine Capsules 1986
Dapsone Tablets USP 1746
Didronel Tablets (Rare) 2583
Diovan HCT Tablets 2216
Duetact Tablets 3085
Dyazide Capsules 1405
EC-Naprosyn Delayed-Release Tablets (Less than 1%) 2632
Edecrin 698
Effexor XR Extended-Release Capsules 3195
Equetro Extended-Release Capsules 3174
Exjade Tablets 2244
Fansidar Tablets 2636
Fortaz (Very rare) 1450
Furosemide Tablets 2186
Gantrisin Pediatric Suspension 2638
▲ Humira Injection (Less than 5%) 442
Indapamide Tablets 2188
Indocin Capsules (Less than 1%) 2024
Indocin I.V. (Less than 1%) 2489
Indocin (Less than 1%) 2024
InnoPran XL Extended Release Capsules 1484
Intravenous Sodium Diuril 2490
Lamictal 1488
Lamisil Oral Granules 2264
Lamisil Tablets (Rare) 2266
▲ Leukine (6%) 774
Levaquin 2416
Levaquin in 5% Dextrose Injection 2416
Lortab 5/500 Tablets 3143
Lortab 7.5/500 Tablets 3144
Lortab 10/500 Tablets 3144
Luvox CR Extended-Release Capsules 1759
Mavik Tablets (Rare) 472
Merrem I.V. 684
Micardis HCT Tablets 854
Mobic Oral Suspension (Less than 0.1%) 863
Mobic Tablets (Less than 0.1%) 863
Moxatag Tablets 2165
Mustargen for Injection (Relatively infrequent) 2492
Nadolol Tablets 2191
Nalfon Capsules (Less than 1%) 2508
Naprosyn Suspension (Less than 1%) 2632
Naprosyn Tablets (Less than 1%) 2632
Nexium Delayed-Release Capsules 645
Nexium I.V. (Rare) 652
Nexium Delayed-Release Oral Suspension 645
Noroxin Tablets 2069
Omnicef Capsules 497
Omnicef for Oral Suspension 497
Parnate Tablets 1532
Paser Granules 1747
Paxil 1535
Paxil CR Controlled-Release Tablets 1544
Pentasa Capsules 3030
Pepcid Tablets (Rare) 2075
Percocet Tablets 1127
Phenytek Capsules (Occasional) 2192

Plavix Tablets (Less than 1%) 926
Plavix Tablets (Less than 1%) 2767
Pletal Tablets 2481
Primaxin I.M. 2080
Primaxin I.V. 2083
Prinivil Tablets (Rare to frequent) 2087
Prinzide Tablets (Rare) 2092
Provigil Tablets 977
Remeron Tablets 2924
RemeronSolTab Tablets 2927
Risperdal Consta Long-Acting Injection 1753
Rocephin Injectable Vials, ADD-Vantage, Galaxy, Bulk (Less than 0.1%) 2642
Rythmol Tablets (Less than 1%) 1586
Stalevo Tablets 2309
Suprax for Oral Suspension 1891
Suprax Tablets 1891
Tekturna HCT Tablets 2324
Teveten HCT Tablets 517
Thioridazine Hydrochloride Tablets (Infrequent) 2195
Thiothixene Capsules 2197
Timoptic Sterile Ophthalmic Solution 2121
Timoptic in Ocudose 2124
Timoptic-XE Sterile Ophthalmic Gel Forming Solution 2125
Toprol-XL Tablets (Rare) 666
Tricor Tablets (Rare) 520
Trusopt Sterile Ophthalmic Solution (Rare) 2128
Tylenol with Codeine Tablets 2427
Venlafaxine Hydrochloride Tablets 2199
Vicodin Tablets 529
Vicodin ES Tablets 530
Vicodin HP Tablets 531
Voltaren Tablets (Rarely) 2334
Voltaren-XR Tablets (Rarely) 2337
▲ Xeloda Tablets (Less than 5%) 2662
Zantac 25 EFFERdose Tablets (Rare) 1670
Zantac Injection (Rare) 1666
Zantac Injection Pharmacy Bulk Package (Rare) 1668
Zantac Injection Premixed (Rare) 1666
Zantac (Rare) 1670
Zinacef for Injection 1678
Zinacef Injection 1678
Zonegran Capsules (Rare) 1089
Zosyn for Injection (1% or less) 3284

Airway constriction
Amerge Tablets (Rare) 1301

Airway obstruction
Amerge Tablets (Rare) 1301
Captopril Tablets 2182
Erbitux 912
▲ Infasurf Intratracheal Suspension (39%) 1168
Levaquin 2416
Levaquin in 5% Dextrose Injection 2416
Orthoclone OKT3 Sterile Solution 2387
Prinivil Tablets 2087
Prinzide Tablets 2092
▲ Ultane Liquid for Inhalation (8%) 524

Airway resistance
Salagen Tablets 1082

Akathisia
▲ Abilify Injection (2% to 25%) 881
▲ Abilify Injection (2% to 25%) 2466
▲ Abilify Oral Solution (5% to 25%) 881
▲ Abilify Oral Solution (2% to 25%) 2466
▲ Abilify Discmelt Orally Disintegrating Tablets (5% to 25%) 881
▲ Abilify Discmelt Orally Disintegrating Tablets (2% to 25%) 2466
▲ Abilify Tablets (2% to 25%) 881
▲ Abilify Tablets (2% to 25%) 2466
Celexa 1160
Effexor XR Extended-Release Capsules (Infrequent) 3195
▲ Geodon (8% to 10%) 2520
▲ Invega Extended-Release Tablets (Greater than 2% to 10%) 1748
Lamictal (Infrequent) 1488
Lexapro Oral Suspension 1174
Lexapro Tablets 1174
Luvox CR Extended-Release Capsules (Infrequent) 1759
Marplan Tablets 3177
▲ Mirapex Tablets (2% to 3%) 857
Moban Tablets 1116
Parnate Tablets 1532
Paxil 1535
Paxil CR Controlled-Release Tablets 1544
Pristiq Extended-Release Tablets 3247
Prozac Weekly Capsules (Infrequent) 1852
Prozac Pulvules and Liquid (Infrequent) 1852
Remeron Tablets (Rare) 2924
RemeronSolTab Tablets (Rare) 2927
▲ Risperdal Consta Long-Acting Injection (5% to 9%) 1753
Symbyax Capsules 1871
Thioridazine Hydrochloride Tablets 2195
Thiothixene Capsules 2197
Venlafaxine Hydrochloride Tablets (Infrequent) 2199
Wellbutrin Tablets (1.5%) 1648
Wellbutrin XL Extended-Release Tablets (2%) 1659
Zomig Tablets (Rare) 694
Zomig-ZMT Tablets (Rare) 694
▲ Zyprexa Tablets (3% to 27%) 1883
▲ Zyprexa IntraMuscular (2% to 5%) 1883
▲ Zyprexa ZYDIS Orally Disintegrating Tablets (3% to 27%) 1883

Akinesia
Abilify Injection (Greater than or equal to 1 in 1000 patients and less than 1 in 100 patients) 881
Abilify Injection (Greater than or equal to 1 in 1000 patients and less than 1 in 100 patients) 2466
Abilify Oral Solution (Greater than or equal to 1 in 1000 patients and less than 1 in 100 patients) 881
Abilify Oral Solution (Greater than or equal to 1 in 1000 patients and less than 1 in 100 patients) 2466
Abilify Discmelt Orally Disintegrating Tablets (Greater than or equal to 1 in 1000 patients and less than 1 in 100 patients) 881
Abilify Discmelt Orally Disintegrating Tablets (Greater than or equal to 1 in 1000 patients and less than 1 in 100 patients) 2466
Abilify Tablets (Greater than or equal to 1 in 1000 patients and less than 1 in 100 patients) 881
Abilify Tablets (Greater than or equal to 1 in 1000 patients and less than 1 in 100 patients) 2466
Effexor XR Extended-Release Capsules (Rare) 3195
Geodon Capsules (Frequent) 2520
Luvox CR Extended-Release Capsules (Rare) 1759
Maxalt Tablets (Rare) 2056
Maxalt-MLT Orally Disintegrating Tablets (Rare) 2056
Mirapex Tablets 857
Moban Tablets 1116
Parnate Tablets 1532
Paxil (Infrequent) 1535
Paxil CR Controlled-Release Tablets (Infrequent) 1544
Thioridazine Hydrochloride Tablets 2195
Venlafaxine Hydrochloride Tablets (Rare) 2199
▲ Wellbutrin Tablets (8%) 1648
Wellbutrin SR Sustained-Release Tablets 1653
Wellbutrin XL Extended-Release Tablets 1659
Zyban Sustained-Release Tablets 1692
▲ Zyprexa Tablets (8% to 20%) 1883
▲ Zyprexa IntraMuscular (2% to 4%) 1883
▲ Zyprexa ZYDIS Orally Disintegrating Tablets (8% to 20%) 1883

Alanine aminotransferase levels, changes in
▲ Eloxatin for Injection (0% to 36%) 2731
Prozac Pulvules and Liquid (Infrequent) 1852
Selzentry Tablets (Greater than or equal to 2%) 2534
▲ Sutent Capsules (2% to 39%) 2540
▲ Tykerb Tablets (0% to 37%) 1631
▲ Zyvox (0% to 10.1%) 2552

Alanine aminotransferase levels, elevation of
Abelcet Injection 1134
Accolate Tablets (1.5%) 669
Accutane Capsules 2607
Aceon Tablets (2 mg, 4 mg, 8 mg) (1.6% to 1.7%) 3038
Actos Tablets (0.3%) 3077
▲ Alimta for Injection (1% to 10%) 1786
Alinia for Oral Suspension (Less than 1.1%) 2677
Alinia Tablets (Less than 1.1%) 2677
Aloxi Injection (Less than 1%) 1059
Ambien Tablets (Rare) 2692
Ambien CR Tablets (Infrequent) 2696
▲ AmBisome for Injection (14.6%) 606
Amevive (1.7%) 611
Amitiza Capsules (Less than 1%) 3082
Amoxil Capsules 1305
Amoxil Chewable Tablets 1305
Amoxil Pediatric Drops for Oral Suspension 1305
Amoxil Powder for Oral Suspension 1305
Amoxil Tablets 1305
Anaprox Tablets (1%) 2632
Anaprox DS Tablets (1%) 2632
AndroGel 3159
Anzemet Injection 2701
Anzemet Tablets (Less than 1%) 2704
▲ Aptivus Capsules (2% to 26%) 823
▲ Aptivus Oral Solution (2% to 26%) 823
▲ Aralast (11.1%) 726
Aricept Tablets (Infrequent) 1062
Aricept ODT Tablets (Infrequent) 1062
▲ Arimidex Tablets (Greater than or equal to 1% to less than 10%) 672
Arixtra Injection (0.3% to 2.6%) 1313
Asacol Delayed-Release Tablets 2579
Atripla Tablets (2%) 938
Augmentin (Infrequent) 1323
Augmentin Tablets (Infrequent) 1327
Augmentin XR Extended Release Tablets (Infrequent) 1333
Augmentin ES-600 Powder for Oral Suspension 1329
Avandamet Tablets (0.2%) 1336
Avandia Tablets (0.2%) 1351
Axid Capsules 1364
▲ Baraclude (2% to 12%) 900
BeneFIX Vials (1.6%) 3191
Benicar HCT Tablets (Greater than 1%) 1010
▲ Betaseron for SC Injection (12%) 756
Biaxin/Biaxin XL 411
▲ Busulfex Injection (7% to 31%) 2477
Bystolic Tablets 1155
Calcijex Injection 419
Campral Tablets (Infrequent) 1158
▲ Cancidas for Injection (5.4% to 18.1%) 1953
Cardizem LA Extended Release Tablets (Less than 2%) 421
Ceftin (0.1% to 1%) 1380
Celebrex Capsules (0.1% to 1.9%) 2979
▲ CellCept Capsules (3% to less than 20%) 2622
▲ CellCept Intravenous (3% to less than 20%) 2622
▲ CellCept Oral Suspension (3% to less than 20%) 2622
▲ CellCept Tablets (3% to less than 20%) 2622
▲ Chemet Capsules (4.2% to 10.4%) 2484
Cipro I.V. (Among most frequent) 2817
Cipro (1.9%) 2810
Cipro XR Tablets 2823
▲ Clolar for Intravenous Infusion (44%) 1239
Combivir Tablets 1384
▲ Coreg Tablets (Greater than 1% to 3%) 1387
▲ Coreg CR Extended-Release Capsules (Greater than 1% to less than or equal to 3%) 1393
Crestor Tablets (2.2%) 677
▲ Crixivan Capsules (4.9%) 1979
Cubicin for Injection (Less than 1%) 995
Cymbalta Delayed-Release Capsules 1801
Doribax Injection (1% to 2%) 2400
▲ Doxil Injection (1% to 5%) 2378
EC-Naprosyn Delayed-Release Tablets (1%) 2632
Effexor XR Extended-Release Capsules (Rare) 3195
Elspar for Injection 1990
▲ Emend Capsules (6%) 1992
▲ Emend for Injection (6%) 1999
Emsam Transdermal System (Infrequent) 905
▲ Emtriva Capsules (2% to 5%) 1246
▲ Emtriva Oral Solution (2% to 5%) 1246
▲ Epivir (1% to 3.8%) 1412
▲ Epivir-HBV (11%) 1417
Evoxac Capsules (Less than 1%) 1013
▲ Exjade Tablets (5.7% to 8.4%) 2244
Femara Tablets 2246
▲ Fenoglide Tablets (3%) 2960
Flebogamma 5% DIF (2.2%) 1718
Flector Patch (1%) 561
▲ Fortaz (1 in 15) 1450
▲ Gamunex (7% to 18%) 3094
▲ Gemzar for Injection (38% to 72%) 1820
▲ Gleevec Tablets (0% to 7%) 2255
▲ Hepsera Tablets (Less than or equal to 25%) 1253
▲ Humatrope Vials and Cartridges (6.25% to 6.67%) 1838
Humira Injection 442
▲ Hycamtin for Injection (Less than 1% to 5%) 1459
Increlex Injection 3100
▲ Intron A for Injection (Up to 15% of patients) 2859
▲ Invanz for Injection (3.8% to 8.8%) 2029
▲ Isentress Tablets (0.6% to 6.9%) 2036
▲ Kaletra (4% to 10%) 452
▲ Leukine (13%) 774
▲ Lexiva Oral Suspension (Less than or equal to 1% to 8%) 1510
▲ Lexiva Tablets (Less than or equal to 1% to 8%) 1510
Lialda Tablets (0.6% to 1.1%) 3029
Lovaza Capsules 1520
▲ Lovenox Injection (Up to 5.5%) 2756
Malarone Pediatric Tablets 1521
Malarone Tablets 1521
Marinol Capsules (Less than 1%) 3163
Mavik Tablets (0.3% to 1%) 472
▲ Mepron Suspension (6%) 1526
Meridia Capsules (1.6%) 475
Merrem I.V. (Greater than 0.2%) 684
Mevacor Tablets 2063
Mobic Oral Suspension (Less than 2%) 863
Mobic Tablets (Less than 2%) 863
Moxatag Tablets 2165
▲ Mycamine for Injection (5.4%) 616
▲ Mylotarg for Injection (9%) 3212
Namenda 1180
Naprosyn Suspension (1%) 2632
Naprosyn Tablets (1%) 2632
Nexium Delayed-Release Capsules (Less than 1%) 645
Nexium I.V. (Less than 1%) 652
Nexium Delayed-Release Oral Suspension (Less than 1%) 645
Niaspan Extended-Release Tablets 480
Nimotop Capsules (0.2%; rare) 790
Noroxin Tablets (1.4%) 2069
▲ Norvir (7.8% to 8.5%) 489
▲ Novantrone for Injection Concentrate (5% to 15%) 1100
▲ Noxafil Oral Suspension (1% to 17%) 2889
Omnicef Capsules (0.7%) 497
Omnicef for Oral Suspension (0.4%) 497
▲ Oncaspar Injection (Greater than or equal to 2% to 11%) 1138
Orthoclone OKT3 Sterile Solution 2387
Paxil (Infrequent) 1535
Paxil CR Controlled-Release Tablets (Infrequent) 1544
▲ PegIntron Powder for Injection (10%) 2903
Pentasa Capsules (Less than 1%) 3030
Precose Tablets 792
Primaxin I.M. 2080
Primaxin I.V. 2083
▲ Prograf Capsules and Injection (3% to 15%) 622
Protonix for Delayed-Release Oral Suspension (Greater than or equal to 1%) 3254
Protonix Delayed-Release Tablets (Greater than or equal to 1%) 3254
Protonix I.V. (Greater than or equal to 1%) 3257
Protopic Ointment (Greater than or equal to 1%) 628
Prozac Weekly Capsules (Rare) 1852
Prozac Pulvules and Liquid (Rare) 1852
Rapamune 3260
▲ Rebif Prefilled Syringe for Injection (20% to 27%) 1107
Remeron Tablets (Rare; 2.0%) 2924
RemeronSolTab Tablets (Rare; 2.0%) 2927
▲ Remicade for IV Injection (Less than 1% to 51%) 950
Risperdal Consta Long-Acting Injection (Infrequent) 1753
Rocaltrol Capsules 1150
Rocaltrol Oral Solution 1150
▲ Rocephin Injectable Vials, ADD-Vantage, Galaxy, Bulk (3.3%) 2642
Rythmol SR Capsules 1590
Singulair (1% to 2.1%) 2114
▲ Soriatane Capsules (Approximately 1 in 3 patients) 3062
Stromectol Tablets (2%) 2120

Suprax for Oral Suspension (Less than 2%) ... 1891
Suprax Tablets (Less than 2%) ... 1891
Sustiva Capsules (2%) ... 930
Sustiva Tablets (2%) ... 930
▲ Symbyax Capsules (6.3%) ... 1871
Synagis Intramuscular Solution (More than 1%) ... 1948
Tarceva Tablets ... 1228
Targretin Capsules ... 1084
Tarka Tablets ... 511
▲ Tasigna Capsules (1% to 10%) ... 2316
▲ Taxotere Injection Concentrate (4.3% to 18.9) ... 2773
Tekturna HCT Tablets (1.2%) ... 2324
Teveten Tablets (Less than 1%) ... 515
Teveten HCT Tablets (Less than 1%) ... 517
Timentin ADD-Vantage ... 1606
Timentin Injection Galaxy Container ... 1609
Timentin IV Infusion ... 1603
Timentin Pharmacy Bulk Package ... 1613
▲ Tracleer Tablets (11%) ... 3289
Trasylol Injection ... 799
Treximet Tablets (1%) ... 1616
▲ Tricor Tablets (3%) ... 520
▲ Trisenox Injection (20%) ... 986
▲ Trizivir Tablets (3.7%) ... 1622
Truvada Tablets (2%) ... 1262
▲ Tygacil for Injection (5.6%) ... 3276
▲ Tyzeka Tablets (3% to 4%) ... 2328
Ultane Liquid for Inhalation (Less than 1%) ... 524
Ultram ER Extended-Release Tablets (0.5% to less than 1%) ... 2428
▲ Valtrex Caplets (14%) ... 1635
Venlafaxine Hydrochloride Tablets (Infrequent) ... 2199
Vicoprofen Tablets (1%) ... 533
▲ Viramune Oral Suspension (5.3% to 14%) ... 873
▲ Viramune Tablets (5.3% to 14%) ... 873
▲ Viread Tablets (3% to 5%) ... 1268
Vivitrol ... 988
Vytorin 10/10 Tablets (3.7%) ... 2149
▲ Vytorin 10/10 Tablets (0.4% to 3.7%) ... 2939
Vytorin 10/20 Tablets (3.7%) ... 2149
▲ Vytorin 10/20 Tablets (0.4% to 3.7%) ... 2939
Vytorin 10/40 Tablets (3.7%) ... 2149
▲ Vytorin 10/40 Tablets (0.4% to 3.7%) ... 2939
Vytorin 10/80 Tablets (3.7%) ... 2149
▲ Vytorin 10/80 Tablets (0.4% to 3.7%) ... 2939
Xeloda Tablets (1.6%) ... 2662
Xyrem Oral Solution (Infrequent) ... 1766
Zantac 25 EFFERdose Tablets ... 1670
Zantac Injection ... 1666
Zantac ... 1670
▲ Ziagen (6%) ... 1673
Zinacef for Injection (1 in 25 patients) ... 1678
Zinacef Injection (1 in 25 patients) ... 1678
Zocor Tablets ... 2136
▲ Zofran Injection (Approximately 5% of patients) ... 1682
Zofran (Approximately 1% to 2%) ... 1687
Zofran ODT Orally Disintegrating Tablets (Approximately 1% to 2%) ... 1687
Zonegran Capsules (Rare) ... 1089
Zosyn for Injection ... 3284
Zyprexa Tablets (2%) ... 1883
Zyprexa IntraMuscular ... 1883
Zyprexa ZYDIS Orally Disintegrating Tablets (2%) ... 1883

Alanine transaminase, increase

Lamictal (Infrequent) ... 1488

Albuminuria

Aricept Tablets (Infrequent) ... 1062
Aricept ODT Tablets (Infrequent) ... 1062
Atacand Tablets (More than 1%) ... 639
Atacand HCT ... 642
Azilect Tablets (Greater than 1%) ... 3106
Calcijex Injection ... 419
Carbatrol Capsules ... 3019
Cardizem LA Extended Release Tablets (Less than 2%) ... 421
Celebrex Capsules (0.1% to 1.9%) ... 2979
▲ CellCept Capsules (3% to less than 20%) ... 2622
▲ CellCept Intravenous (3% to less than 20%) ... 2622
▲ CellCept Oral Suspension (3% to less than 20%) ... 2622
▲ CellCept Tablets (3% to less than 20%) ... 2622
Cipro I.V. ... 2817
Cipro ... 2810
Cipro XR Tablets ... 2823
▲ Coreg Tablets (Greater than 1% to 3%) ... 1387
▲ Coreg CR Extended-Release Capsules (Greater than 1% to less than or equal to 3%) ... 1393
▲ Dacogen Injection (7%) ... 1066
Dapsone Tablets USP ... 1746
▲ Doxil Injection (1% to 5%) ... 2378
Effexor XR Extended-Release Capsules (Frequent) ... 3195
Equetro Extended-Release Capsules ... 3174
Evoxac Capsules (Less than 1%) ... 1013
Exelon Capsules (Infrequent) ... 2229
Exelon Oral Solution (Infrequent) ... 2229
Geodon Capsules (Infrequent) ... 2520
▲ Intron A for Injection (Less than 5%) ... 2859
▲ Keppra Oral Solution (4%) ... 3131
▲ Keppra Tablets (4%) ... 3131
Lipitor Tablets (Less than 2%) ... 2501
Lyrica Capsules (0.1% to 1%) ... 2527
▲ Megace ES Oral Suspension (1% to 3%) ... 2499
Mobic Oral Suspension (Less than 2%) ... 863
Mobic Tablets (Less than 2%) ... 863
Nexium Delayed-Release Capsules (Less than 1%) ... 645
Nexium I.V. (Less than 1%) ... 652
Nexium Delayed-Release Oral Suspension (Less than 1%) ... 645
Noroxin Tablets ... 2069
▲ Ontak Vials (10%) ... 1079
Pentasa Capsules (Less than 1%) ... 3030
Pletal Tablets (Less than 2%) ... 2481
Proglycem Capsules (Infrequent) ... 1185
Proglycem Suspension (Infrequent) ... 1185
▲ Prograf Capsules and Injection (3% to 15%) ... 622
Protonix for Delayed-Release Oral Suspension (Less than 1%) ... 3254
Protonix Delayed-Release Tablets (Less than 1%) ... 3254
Protonix I.V. (Less than 1%) ... 3257
Provigil Tablets (1%) ... 977
Prozac Weekly Capsules (Infrequent) ... 1852
Prozac Pulvules and Liquid (Infrequent) ... 1852
Requip Tablets (Infrequent) ... 1561
Rocaltrol Capsules ... 1150
Rocaltrol Oral Solution ... 1150
▲ Simulect for Injection (3% to 10%) ... 2306
Targretin Capsules ... 1084
Teveten Tablets (Less than 1%) ... 515
Teveten HCT Tablets (Less than 1%) ... 517
Ultane Liquid for Inhalation (Less than 1%) ... 524
Uroqid-Acid No. 2 Tablets ... 814
Venlafaxine Hydrochloride Tablets (Infrequent) ... 2199
▲ Visudyne for Injection (1% to 10%) ... 2332
Zonegran Capsules (Rare) ... 1089
Zyprexa Tablets (Rare) ... 1883
Zyprexa ZYDIS Orally Disintegrating Tablets (Rare) ... 1883

Alcohol, increased sensitivity to

Catapres Tablets ... 841
Celexa (Infrequent) ... 1160
Clorpres Tablets ... 2185
Copaxone for Injection (Infrequent) ... 3110
Effexor XR Extended-Release Capsules (Rare) ... 3195
Emsam Transdermal System (Infrequent) ... 905
Lamictal (Rare) ... 1488
▲ Protopic Ointment (Up to 7%) ... 628
Prozac Weekly Capsules (Rare) ... 1852
Prozac Pulvules and Liquid (Rare) ... 1852
Soriatane Capsules (Less than 1%) ... 3062
Symbyax Capsules (Infrequent) ... 1871
Teveten Tablets (Less than 1%) ... 515
Teveten HCT Tablets (Less than 1%) ... 517
Venlafaxine Hydrochloride Tablets (Rare) ... 2199

Alcohol abuse

Effexor XR Extended-Release Capsules (Rare) ... 3195
Paxil (Infrequent) ... 1535
Paxil CR Controlled-Release Tablets (Infrequent) ... 1544
Venlafaxine Hydrochloride Tablets (Rare) ... 2199
Zyprexa Tablets (Infrequent) ... 1883
Zyprexa ZYDIS Orally Disintegrating Tablets (Infrequent) ... 1883

Alcohol craving

Campral Tablets (Rare) ... 1158

Alkalosis

▲ CellCept Capsules (3% to less than 20%) ... 2622
▲ CellCept Intravenous (3% to less than 20%) ... 2622
▲ CellCept Oral Suspension (3% to less than 20%) ... 2622
▲ CellCept Tablets (3% to less than 20%) ... 2622
Percocet Tablets ... 1127
Percodan Tablets ... 1130
▲ Prograf Capsules and Injection (3% to 15%) ... 622

Alkalosis, metabolic

Indocin I.V. (Less than 3%) ... 2489
Mirapex Tablets ... 857

Alkalosis, respiratory

Adenocard IV Injection ... 603
Bayer Aspirin ... 750
Coreg CR Extended-Release Capsules (Less than or equal to 0.1%) ... 1393
Percocet Tablets ... 1127
Percodan Tablets ... 1130

Allergic interstitial nephritis

Proleukin for Injection ... 2287

Allergic reactions

Abelcet Injection ... 1134
Abilify Injection ... 881
Abilify Injection (Rare) ... 2466
Abilify Oral Solution ... 881
Abilify Oral Solution (Rare) ... 2466
Abilify Discmelt Orally Disintegrating Tablets ... 881
Abilify Discmelt Orally Disintegrating Tablets (Rare) ... 2466
Abilify Tablets ... 881
Abilify Tablets (Rare) ... 2466
Accutane Capsules ... 2607
Aceon Tablets (2 mg, 4 mg, 8 mg) (2%) ... 3038
Actiq (Less than 1%) ... 959
Activase I.V. (Very rare) ... 1188
▲ Actonel Tablets (3.8%) ... 2568
Actonel with Calcium Tablets (1.9% to 2.5%) ... 2574
Adipex-P ... 1185
▲ Advair HFA 45/21 Inhalation Aerosol (1% to 3%) ... 1288
▲ Advair HFA 115/21 Inhalation Aerosol (1% to 3%) ... 1288
▲ Advair HFA 230/21 Inhalation Aerosol (1% to 3%) ... 1288
Aggrenox Capsules (Less than 1%) ... 819
▲ Alamast Ophthalmic Solution (Less than 5%) ... 3181
Albenza Tablets (Rare) ... 1297
Albutein 5% ... 1707
Albutein 25% ... 1708
▲ Alimta for Injection (Up to 8%) ... 1786
Alinia for Oral Suspension (Less than 1%) ... 2677
Alinia Tablets (Less than 1%) ... 2677
▲ Alphagan P Ophthalmic Solution (1% to 4%) ... 549
Alphanate ... 1709
AlphaNine SD ... 1713
▲ Ambien Tablets (Rare to 4%) ... 2692
Ambien CR Tablets (Rare) ... 2696
AmBisome for Injection (Less common) ... 606
Amerge Tablets (Rare) ... 1301
Amoxil Capsules ... 1305
Amoxil Chewable Tablets ... 1305
Amoxil Pediatric Drops for Oral Suspension ... 1305
Amoxil Powder for Oral Suspension ... 1305
Amoxil Tablets ... 1305
Angiomax for Injection ... 1933
Apidra Injection ... 2706
Aranesp for Injection (Rare) ... 564
Argatroban Injection ... 1308
Aricept Tablets (Infrequent) ... 1062
Aricept ODT Tablets (Infrequent) ... 1062
Arimidex Tablets (Very rare) ... 672
▲ Atripla Tablets (Greater than or equal to 5%) ... 938
Atrovent HFA Inhalation Aerosol ... 839
Atrovent Nasal Spray 0.03% ... 834
Attenuvax (Rare) ... 1951
Augmentin ... 1323
Augmentin Tablets ... 1327
Avalide Tablets (1%) ... 2713
Avelox (Greater than or equal to 0.1% to less than 2%) ... 2803
Azilect Tablets (Greater than 1%) ... 3106
Azopt Ophthalmic Suspension (Less than 1%) ... 540
BeneFIX Vials (1.5%) ... 3191
Bentyl Capsules ... 703
Bentyl Injection ... 703
Bentyl Syrup ... 703
Bentyl Tablets ... 703
▲ Betimol Ophthalmic Solution (1% to 5%) ... 3181
Bexxar ... 1371
Biaxin/Biaxin XL ... 411
Bicillin C-R Injectable Suspension ... 1775
Bicillin L-A Injection ... 1777
Boniva Injection (2.5%) ... 2614
Boniva Tablets (2.5%) ... 2618
Brovana Inhalation Solution ... 2990
▲ Busulfex Injection (2% to 26%) ... 2477
Campral Tablets (Infrequent) ... 1158
Carac Cream 0.5% (1.2%) ... 2722
Cardizem LA Extended Release Tablets (Less than 2%) ... 421
Catapres Tablets ... 841
Ceftin ... 1380
Celebrex Capsules (0.1% to 1.9%) ... 2979
Celexa ... 1160
Cipro I.V. (1% or less) ... 2817
Cipro (Less than 1%) ... 2810
Cipro XR Tablets ... 2823
Combigan Ophthalmic Solution (0.1% to 0.2%) ... 553
Combivent Inhalation Aerosol ... 845
Copaxone for Injection (Rare) ... 3110
▲ Coreg Tablets (Greater than 1% to 3%) ... 1387
▲ Coreg CR Extended-Release Capsules (Greater than 1% to less than or equal to 3%) ... 1393
Cosopt Sterile Ophthalmic Solution ... 1969
Creon 5 Capsules (Less frequent) ... 3041
Creon 10 Capsules (Less frequent) ... 3042
Creon 20 Capsules (Less frequent) ... 3042
Crinone 4% Gel ... 992
Crinone 8% Gel ... 992
Cyanokit 5g Antidote ... 1021
Cytomel Tablets (Rare) ... 1778
Depakote ER Tablets ... 423
Digibind for Injection (Rare) ... 1403
Diovan Tablets (Greater than 0.2%) ... 2212
Diovan HCT Tablets ... 2216
▲ Doxil Injection (1% to 5%) ... 2378
Duac Topical Gel ... 3054
Duragesic Transdermal System (1% or greater) ... 2405
E.E.S. ... 433
Effexor XR Extended-Release Capsules (Infrequent) ... 3195
Elitek ... 2729
Elmiron Capsules (Less than or equal to 1%) ... 2435
▲ Eloxatin for Injection (3% to 15%) ... 2731
Elspar for Injection ... 1990
Elspar for Injection ... 2488
▲ Emtriva Capsules (17% to 30%) ... 1246
▲ Emtriva Oral Solution (17% to 30%) ... 1246
Enbrel for Injection (Less than 0.5%) ... 569
Epogen for Injection (Rare) ... 576
▲ Equetro Extended-Release Capsules (Less than 5%) ... 3174
Erbitux ... 912
EryPed ... 431
▲ Evoxac Capsules (1% to 3%) ... 1013
Exelon Capsules (Frequent) ... 2229
Exelon Oral Solution (Frequent) ... 2229
Exforge Tablets (Greater than 0.1% to less than 1%) ... 2238
Feiba VH ... 728
Flomax Capsules ... 848
FML Ophthalmic Suspension ... ⊙ 224
Fortaz (Among most common) ... 1450
Forteo for Injection (Less than 1/1000 patients) ... 1816
Fragmin Injection (Rare) ... 1070
Gabitril Tablets (Frequent) ... 973
Gantrisin Pediatric Suspension ... 2638
Gengraf Capsules (1% to less than 3%) ... 435
Geodon (Rare) ... 2520
Gliadel Wafer (1% to 2%) ... 1076
Glucagon for Injection Vials and Emergency Kit ... 1827
Hemofil M (Extremely rare) ... 737
▲ Herceptin I.V. (3%) ... 1199
Humalog-Pen and KwikPen (Less common) ... 1829
Humalog Mix 50/50-Pen and KwikPen ... 1833

Humalog Mix 75/25-Pen and KwikPen 1835
Humira Injection 442
Humulin 50/50, 100 Units (Less common to occasional) 1843
Humulin 70/30 Vial 1844
Humulin N Vial 1846
Humulin R 1849
Humulin R (U-500) 1850
Hyalgan Solution (Three cases) 2742
▲ Hycamtin for Injection (Infrequent to 6%) 1459
Increlex Injection 3100
Infanrix Vaccine 1479
Integrilin Injection 2855
Janumet Tablets 2041
Januvia Tablets 2048
Kaletra (Less than 2%) 452
Keppra Oral Solution (Greater than or equal to 2%) 3131
Keppra Tablets (Greater than or equal to 2%) 3131
Ketek Tablets (Rare) 2744
Kinrix Injection Vaccine 1486
Klonopin (2%) 2639
Kogenate FS 746
Lamictal (Infrequent) 1488
Lamisil Oral Granules 2264
Lamisil Tablets (Rare) 2266
Lantus Injection 2749
Lescol Capsules (2.3%) 2268
Lescol XL Tablets (1%) 2268
Leukeran Tablets 1508
▲ Leukine (12%) 774
Levaquin (0.1% to 1%) 2416
Levaquin in 5% Dextrose Injection (0.1% to 1%) 2416
Levemir Injection 2352
Lexapro Oral Suspension (Frequent) 1174
Lexapro Tablets (Frequent) 1174
Lipitor Tablets (Up to 2.8%) 2501
Lortab 5/500 Tablets 3143
Lortab 7.5/500 Tablets 3144
Lortab 10/500 Tablets 3144
Lovenox Injection 2756
Lunesta Tablets (Infrequent) 2994
Luvox CR Extended-Release Capsules (Infrequent) 1759
Lyrica Capsules (Greater than or equal to 1%) 2527
Mepron Suspension (0.8% to 1.1%) 1526
Meridia Capsules (1.5%) 475
Merrem I.V. 684
Metamucil 2563
Miacalcin Injection (A few cases) 2273
Miacalcin Nasal Spray (Less than 1%) 2274
Micardis Tablets (More than 0.3%) 852
Micardis HCT Tablets 854
Mirapex Tablets (1% or more) 857
Mobic Oral Suspension (Less than 2%) 863
Mobic Tablets (Less than 2%) 863
Motrin IB Tablets and Caplets 1900
Children's Motrin Oral Suspension 1901
Children's Motrin Non-Staining Dye-Free Oral Suspension 1901
Children's Motrin Cold Oral Suspension 1899
Infants' Motrin Concentrated Drops 1901
Infants' Motrin Non-Staining Dye-Free Concentrated Drops 1901
Junior Strength Motrin Caplets and Chewable Tablets 1901
Mumpsvax (Extremely rare) 2068
Namenda (Infrequent) 1180
Natacyn Antifungal Ophthalmic Suspension (One case) ..... ⊙204
Neoral Oral Solution (1% to less than 3%) 2280
Neoral Soft Gelatin Capsules (1% to less than 3%) 2280
Neulasta Injection 587
Neupogen for Injection (Less than 1 in 4000) 589
Neupro Transdermal System 3149
Nexium Delayed-Release Capsules (Less than 1%) 645
Nexium I.V. (Less than 1%) 652
Nexium Delayed-Release Oral Suspension (Less than 1%) 645
Nitro-Dur Transdermal Infusion System (Uncommon) 2887
Noroxin Tablets (Less frequent) 2069
Norvir (Less than 2%) 489
NoSmo[King] Stop Smoking Aid ..... ▣630
NovoLog Mix 70/30 2364
NovoLog Injection 2359
NovoSeven (1%) 2367
NovoSeven RT (1%) 2370
Noxafil Oral Suspension (Rare) 2889
Nutropin for Injection 1208
Nutropin AQ Injection 1212
Nutropin AQ NuSpin Injection 1212
Nutropin AQ Pen 1212
Nutropin AQ Pen Cartridge 1212
Omnicef Capsules 497
Omnicef for Oral Suspension 497
Oncaspar Injection (1% to greater than or equal to 2%) 1138
Opana Tablets (Less than 1%) 1117
Opana ER Tablets (Less than 1%) 1121
OptiPranolol Metipranolol Ophthalmic Solution 0.3% (A small number of patients) ..... ⊙245
Ortho-Cyclen Tablets 2449
Ortho Evra Transdermal System 2437
Ortho Tri-Cyclen Tablets 2449
Paxil (Infrequent) 1535
Paxil CR Controlled-Release Tablets (Infrequent) 1544
Pentasa Capsules 3030
Percocet Tablets 1127
PhosLo GelCaps 1184
Plavix Tablets (Less than 1%) 926
Plavix Tablets (Less than 1%) 2767
Prandin Tablets (1% to 2%) 2971
Pred Forte Ophthalmic Suspension ..... ⊙227
Pred Mild Ophthalmic Suspension ..... ⊙230
Primaxin I.M. 2080
Procrit for Injection (Rare) 2391
▲ Prograf Capsules and Injection (3% to 15%) 622
Prolastin (Occasional) 3099
Protonix for Delayed-Release Oral Suspension (Less than 1%) 3254
Protonix Delayed-Release Tablets (Less than 1%) 3254
Protonix I.V. (Less than 1%) 3257
▲ Protopic Ointment (6% to 22%) 628
▲ Proventil HFA Inhalation Aerosol (6%) 2914
Provigil Tablets (At least 1%) 977
Quixin Ophthalmic Solution (Less than 1%) 3184
Recombinate (Extremely rare) 738
ReFacto Vials 3269
▲ Refludan for Injection (3.5%) 795
Relenza Inhalation Powder 1556
Remicade for IV Injection (Greater than or equal to 0.2%) 950
ReoPro Vials 1860
Rocaltrol Capsules (One case) 1150
Rocaltrol Oral Solution (One case) 1150
Rocephin Injectable Vials, ADD-Vantage, Galaxy, Bulk 2642
St. Joseph 81 mg Aspirin Chewable and Enteric Coated Tablets 1903
Salagen Tablets (1% to 2%) 1082
Sandimmune (2% or less) 2296
Sandostatin Injection (Less than 1%) 2300
Seromycin Capsules 1864
▲ Spiriva HandiHaler (1% to 3%) 870
Suprax for Oral Suspension 1891
Suprax Tablets 1891
Sustiva Capsules 930
Sustiva Tablets 930
Tamiflu Capsules 2649
▲ Taxotere Injection Concentrate (1.8% to 10.4%) 2773
▲ Temodar Capsules (3% to 5%) 2931
Thiothixene Capsules 2197
Tice BCG (2%) 2936
Timoptic Sterile Ophthalmic Solution 2121
Timoptic in Ocudose 2124
Timoptic-XE Sterile Ophthalmic Gel Forming Solution 2125
TNKase (Less than 1%) 1233
Trasylol Injection (0.3%) 799
Traumeel Injection Solution (Rare) 1725
▲ Travatan Z Ophthalmic Solution (1% to 5%) 547
Tricor Tablets 520
Trusopt Sterile Ophthalmic Solution 2128
Truvada Tablets 1262
Twinrix Vaccine 1628
Tygacil for Injection (0.2% to less than 2%) 3276
Tylenol with Codeine Tablets 2427
Ultane Liquid for Inhalation (Less than 1%) 524
Ultrase Capsules (Less frequent) 718
Ultrase MT Capsules (Less frequent) 719
▲ Vagifem Tablets (3% to 5%) 2375
Varivax (Greater than or equal to 1%) 2133
Vectibix 597
Vicodin Tablets 529
Vicodin ES Tablets 530
Vicodin HP Tablets 531
Vicoprofen Tablets (Less than 1%) 533
Viramune Oral Suspension 873
Viramune Tablets 873
Vivitrol 988
Wellbutrin Tablets 1648
Wellbutrin SR Sustained-Release Tablets 1653
Wellbutrin XL Extended-Release Tablets 1659
Yaz Tablets (Greater than 1%) 805
Zeel Injection Solution 1726
Zemplar Capsules (Rare) 536
Zemplar Injection (Rare) 538
Zemuron Injection 2947
Zinacef for Injection 1678
Zinacef Injection 1678
Zometa for Intravenous Infusion (Rare) 2341
Zomig Tablets (Infrequent) 694
Zomig Nasal Spray (Infrequent) 689
Zomig-ZMT Tablets (Infrequent) 694
Zonegran Capsules (Infrequent) 1089
Zostavax Injection 2145
Zosyn for Injection 3284
Zyban Sustained-Release Tablets (1%) 1692
Zyrtec Allergy Tablets 1919
Children's Zyrtec Allergy Chewable Tablets 1922
Zyrtec-D Allergy & Congestion Extended-Release Tablets 1923

Allergic reactions, ocular

Combigan Ophthalmic Solution (0.1% to 0.2%) 553

Allergic sensitization

▲ Alferon N Injection (1% to 18%) 1726
Animi-3 Capsules 2506
▲ Catapres-TTS (5 of 101 patients) 842
CitraNatal DHA Capsules 2175
CitraNatal DHA Tablets 2175
CitraNatal 90 DHA Capsules 2175
CitraNatal 90 DHA Tablets 2175
Ferralet 90 Tablets 2175
Metamucil Capsules 2563
Pred-G Ophthalmic Ointment ..... ⊙229
Pred-G Ophthalmic Suspension (Most often) ..... ⊙228

Allergy

(*see under* Allergic reactions)

Allergy, seasonal

▲ Cymbalta Delayed-Release Capsules (3%) 1801
Exforge Tablets (Greater than or equal to 0.2%) 2238

Allergy aggravated

Ambien Tablets (Rare) 2692

Alopecia

Abilify Injection (Greater than or equal to 1 in 1000 patients and less than 1 in 100 patients) 2466
Abilify Oral Solution (Greater than or equal to 1 in 1000 patients and less than 1 in 100 patients) 881
Abilify Oral Solution (Greater than or equal to 1 in 1000 patients and less than 1 in 100 patients) 2466
Abilify Discmelt Orally Disintegrating Tablets (Greater than or equal to 1 in 1000 patients and less than 1 in 100 patients) 881
Abilify Discmelt Orally Disintegrating Tablets (Greater than or equal to 1 in 1000 patients and less than 1 in 100 patients) 2466
Abilify Tablets (Greater than or equal to 1 in 1000 patients and less than 1 in 100 patients) 881
Abilify Tablets (Greater than or equal to 1 in 1000 patients and less than 1 in 100 patients) 2466
Accutane Capsules 2607
Actiq (Less than 1%) 959
Advicor Tablets 402
Aggrenox Capsules 819
▲ Agrylin Capsules (1% to less than 5%) 3017
Albenza Tablets (Less than 1% to 1.6%) 1297
Aldara Cream, 5% (1%) 1699
▲ Alimta for Injection (11%) 1786
AmBisome for Injection (Less common) 606
Amerge Tablets (Rare) 1301
Anaprox Tablets (Less than 1%) 2632
Anaprox DS Tablets (Less than 1%) 2632
AndroGel (0% to 1%) 3159
Aricept Tablets (Infrequent) 1062
Aricept ODT Tablets (Infrequent) 1062
Asacol Delayed-Release Tablets 2579
Atacand HCT 642
▲ Avastin IV (6% to 32%) 1192
Azilect Tablets (Greater than 1%) 3106
Azopt Ophthalmic Suspension (Less than 1%) 540
Azor Tablets 1005
Benicar Tablets 1009
Benicar HCT Tablets (Rare) 1010
▲ Betaseron for SC Injection (4%) 756
▲ Betimol Ophthalmic Solution (More than 5%) 3181
▲ Busulfex Injection (2% to 15%) 2477
Campral Tablets (Infrequent) 1158
Canasa Rectal Suppositories 705
Captopril Tablets (About 0.5% to 2%) 2182
Carbatrol Capsules 3019
Cardizem LA Extended Release Tablets (Infrequent) 421
Catapres Tablets 841
Catapres-TTS 842
Celebrex Capsules (0.1% to 1.9%) 2979
Celexa (Infrequent) 1160
▲ CellCept Capsules (3% to less than 20%) 2622
▲ CellCept Intravenous (3% to less than 20%) 2622
▲ CellCept Oral Suspension (3% to less than 20%) 2622
▲ CellCept Tablets (3% to less than 20%) 2622
Cimzia 3127
Climara Transdermal System 763
Climara Pro Transdermal System 768
Clinoril Tablets (Less than 1%) 1962
Clorpres Tablets (About 2 in 1,000) 2185
Combigan Ophthalmic Solution 553
Combivent Inhalation Aerosol 845
Combivir Tablets 1384
Comvax 1966
Concerta Extended-Release Tablets 1925
Copaxone for Injection (At least 2%) 3110
Coreg Tablets (Less than or equal to 0.1%) 1387
Coreg CR Extended-Release Capsules (Less than or equal to 0.1%) 1393
Cosmegen for Injection 2485
Cosopt Sterile Ophthalmic Solution 1969
Cozaar Tablets (Less than 1%) 1973
Crixivan Capsules 1979
Cuprimine Capsules (Rare) 1986
▲ Dacogen Injection (8%) 1066
Daytrana Transdermal Patch 3022
▲ Depakote ER Tablets (6% to 24%) 423
Didronel Tablets 2583
Diovan Tablets 2212
Diovan HCT Tablets 2216
▲ Doxil Injection (8.9% to 19.2%) 2378
EC-Naprosyn Delayed-Release Tablets (Less than 1%) 2632
Effexor XR Extended-Release Capsules (Infrequent) 3195
Eldepryl Capsules 3052
Eligard 7.5 mg (Less than 2%) 2724
Eligard 22.5 mg (Less than 2%) 2724
Eligard 30 mg (Less than 2% to 2.2%) 2724
Eligard 45 mg (Less than 2%) 2724
▲ Elmiron Capsules (4%) 2435
▲ Eloxatin for Injection (3% to 67%) 2731
▲ Emend Capsules (24%) 1992
▲ Emend for Injection (24%) 1999
Emsam Transdermal System (Infrequent) 905
▲ Enbrel for Injection (1% to 6%) 569
Engerix-B Vaccine 1409
Enjuvia Tablets 1029
Epivir 1412
Epivir-HBV 1417
Epzicom Tablets 1422
▲ Equetro Extended-Release Capsules (Less than 5%) 3174
Estratest Tablets 3043
Estratest H.S. Tablets 3043
Evoxac Capsules (Less than 1%) 1013
Exelon Capsules (Infrequent) 2229
Exelon Oral Solution (Infrequent) 2229

Exforge Tablets (Less than or equal to 0.1%) 2238
▲ Femara Tablets (5%) 2246
Focalin XR Capsules 2251
Follistim AQ Cartridge 2844
Fosamax 2005
Fosamax Plus D Tablets 2013
Gabitril Tablets (Frequent) 973
▲ Gemzar for Injection (15% to 49%) 1820
▲ Gengraf Capsules (4%) 435
Genotropin Lyophilized Powder 2547
Geodon Capsules (Infrequent) 2520
Gleevec Tablets (Less common) 2255
▲ Gliadel Wafer (10%) 1076
Hexalen Capsules 1078
▲ Hycamtin Capsules (10% to 20%) 1456
▲ Hycamtin for Injection (31% to 62%) 1459
Indocin Capsules (Less than 1%) 2024
Indocin I.V. (Less than 1%) 2489
Indocin (Less than 1%) 2024
InnoPran XL Extended Release Capsules 1484
Intravenous Sodium Diuril 2490
▲ Intron A for Injection (Up to 38%) 2859
▲ Ixempra Kit for Injection (48%) 915
Kaletra (Less than 2%) 452
Keppra Injection 3137
Keppra Oral Solution 3131
Keppra Tablets 3131
Klonopin (Infrequent) 2639
Lamictal (Infrequent) 1488
Lamisil Oral Granules 2264
Lamisil Tablets 2266
Lescol Capsules 2268
Lescol XL Tablets 2268
▲ Leukine (37% to 73%) 774
Levothroid Tablets 1170
Levoxyl Tablets 1780
Lexapro Oral Suspension (Infrequent) 1174
Lexapro Tablets (Infrequent) 1174
Lialda Tablets (0% to 1.1%) 3029
Lipitor Tablets (Less than 2%) 2501
Lovaza Capsules 1520
Lunesta Tablets (Infrequent) 2994
Lupron Depot 3.75 mg (Among most frequent) 462
▲ Lupron Depot–3 Month 11.25 mg (Less than 5%) 462
Lupron Depot-PED 7.5 mg, 11.25 mg and 15 mg (Less than 2%) 471
Luvox CR Extended-Release Capsules (Infrequent) 1759
Luxíq Foam (One patient) 3058
Lyrica Capsules (0.1% to 1%) 2527
Maxair Autohaler 1705
▲ Megace ES Oral Suspension (1% to 3%) 2499
Meridia Capsules 475
Metadate CD Capsules 3146
Mevacor Tablets (0.5% to 1%) 2063
Miacalcin Nasal Spray (Less than 1%) 2274
Mirapex Tablets 857
Mobic Oral Suspension (Less than 2%) 863
Mobic Tablets (Less than 2%) 863
Mustargen for Injection (Infrequent) 2492
Myleran Tablets (Rare) 1530
Nadolol Tablets (Infrequent) 2191
Nalfon Capsules (Less than 1%) 2508
Namenda (Infrequent) 1180
Naprosyn Suspension (Less than 1%) 2632
Naprosyn Tablets (Less than 1%) 2632
▲ Neoral Oral Solution (4%) 2280
▲ Neoral Soft Gelatin Capsules (4%) 2280
▲ Neulasta Injection (15% to 72%) 587
▲ Neupogen for Injection (18%) 589
▲ Nexavar Tablets (14% to 27%) 784
Nexium Delayed-Release Capsules 645
Nexium I.V. (Rare) 652
Nexium Delayed-Release Oral Suspension 645
▲ Novantrone for Injection Concentrate (20% to 61%) 1100
Ortho-Cyclen Tablets 2449
Ortho Evra Transdermal System 2437
Ortho Tri-Cyclen Tablets 2449
Ortho Tri-Cyclen Lo Tablets 2458
Parnate Tablets 1532
Paxil (Infrequent) 1535
Paxil CR Controlled-Release Tablets (Infrequent) 1544
Pediarix Vaccine 1552
▲ PegIntron Powder for Injection (22%) 2903
Pentasa Capsules (Less than 1%) 3030
Pepcid Tablets (Infrequent) 2075
Persantine Tablets (Rare) 869
PrandiMet Tablets 2967
Prandin Tablets (Rare) 2971
Premarin Intravenous 3217
Premarin Tablets 3221
Premarin Vaginal Cream 3228
Premphase Tablets 3232
Prempro Tablets 3232
Prinivil Tablets (0.3% to 1%) 2087
Prinzide Tablets 2092
▲ Prograf Capsules and Injection (3% to 15%) 622
Protonix for Delayed-Release Oral Suspension (Less than 1%) 3254
Protonix Delayed-Release Tablets (Less than 1%) 3254
Protonix I.V. (Less than 1%) 3257
Protopic Ointment (1%) 628
Prozac Weekly Capsules (Infrequent) 1852
Prozac Pulvules and Liquid (Infrequent) 1852
▲ Rebetol (23% to 36%) 2917
Remeron Tablets (Infrequent) 2924
RemeronSolTab Tablets (Infrequent) 2927
Requip Tablets (Infrequent) 1561
Reyataz Capsules 3299
Rilutek Tablets (Up to 1.2%) 2771
Risperdal Consta Long-Acting Injection (Infrequent) 1753
Rythmol Tablets (Less than 1%) 1586
Rythmol SR Capsules 1590
Salagen Tablets (Less than 1%) 1082
▲ Sandostatin Injection (1% to 4%) 2300
▲ Sandostatin LAR Depot (13.2%) 2302
▲ Soriatane Capsules (50% to 75%) 3062
Stalevo Tablets 2309
Sular Extended Release Tablets (Less than or equal to 1%) 2975
Sustiva Capsules (Less than 2%) 930
Sustiva Tablets (Less than 2%) 930
▲ Sutent Capsules (0% to 12%) 2540
Symbyax Capsules (Infrequent) 1871
Synthroid Tablets 507
▲ Tarceva Tablets (0% to 14%) 1228
▲ Targretin Capsules (3.6% to 11.3%) 1084
Tarka Tablets 511
▲ Tasigna Capsules (1% to 10%) 2316
▲ Taxotere Injection Concentrate (Less than 1% to 97.8%) 2773
▲ Temodar Capsules (69%) 2931
Teveten HCT Tablets 517
Timoptic Sterile Ophthalmic Solution (Less frequent) 2121
Timoptic in Ocudose (Less frequent) 2124
Timoptic-XE Sterile Ophthalmic Gel Forming Solution 2125
Toprol-XL Tablets (Rare) 666
Tricor Tablets 520
Trizivir Tablets 1622
Twinrix Vaccine 1628
Valtrex Caplets 1635
Venlafaxine Hydrochloride Tablets (Infrequent) 2199
▲ Vesanoid Capsules (14%) 2660
Viadur Implant (2.3%) 802
Voltaren Tablets (Occasionally) 2334
Voltaren-XR Tablets (Occasionally) 2337
Vytorin 10/10 Tablets 2149
Vytorin 10/10 Tablets 2939
Vytorin 10/20 Tablets 2149
Vytorin 10/20 Tablets 2939
Vytorin 10/40 Tablets 2149
Vytorin 10/40 Tablets 2939
Vytorin 10/80 Tablets 2149
Vytorin 10/80 Tablets 2939
Wellbutrin Tablets (Infrequent) 1648
Wellbutrin SR Sustained-Release Tablets 1653
Wellbutrin XL Extended-Release Tablets 1659
Xolair 1235
Xolair 2339
Xyrem Oral Solution (Infrequent) 1766
Zantac 25 EFFERdose Tablets (Rare) 1670
Zantac Injection (Rare) 1666
Zantac Injection Pharmacy Bulk Package (Rare) 1668
Zantac Injection Premixed (Rare) 1666
Zantac (Rare) 1670
Zocor Tablets 2136
▲ Zolinza Capsules (16% to 18.6%) 2142
▲ Zometa for Intravenous Infusion (12%) 2341
Zonegran Capsules (Infrequent) 1089
Zovirax 1690
Zyprexa Tablets (Infrequent) 1883
Zyprexa ZYDIS Orally Disintegrating Tablets (Infrequent) 1883
Zyrtec Chewable Tablets (Less than 2%) 1920
Zyrtec Syrup (Less than 2%) 1920
Zyrtec Tablets (Less than 2%) 1920
Zyrtec-D 12 Hour Extended Release Tablets (Less than 2%) 1923

Alopecia hereditaria
Delatestryl Injection 1730
Estratest Tablets 3043
Estratest H.S. Tablets 3043

Alpha-glutamyl transferase, elevation
▲ Eloxatin for Injection (Less than 1% to 42%) 2731

ALT elevation
(*see under* Alanine aminotransferase levels, elevation of)

Altered saliva
Ambien Tablets (Rare) 2692
Ambien CR Tablets (Rare) 2696

Alveolar proteinosis
Rapamune 3260

Alveolitis, allergic
Agrylin Capsules 3017
Cuprimine Capsules (Rare) 1986
Fansidar Tablets 2636
Paxil 1535
Paxil CR Controlled-Release Tablets 1544
Tricor Tablets 520

Alveolitis, fibrosing
Canasa Rectal Suppositories 705

Amaurosis
Zofran Injection (One patient) 1682

Amaurosis fugax
Mirapex Tablets 857

Amblyopia
Advicor Tablets 402
▲ Agrylin Capsules (1% to less than 5%) 3017
Aloxi Injection (Less than 1%) 1059
Avelox (Less then 0.1%) 2803
▲ Avinza Capsules (Less than 5%) 1772
Axid Capsules (1%) 1364
Campral Tablets (Infrequent) 1158
Cardizem LA Extended Release Tablets (Less than 2%) 421
▲ CellCept Capsules (3% to less than 20%) 2622
▲ CellCept Intravenous (3% to less than 20%) 2622
▲ CellCept Oral Suspension (3% to less than 20%) 2622
▲ CellCept Tablets (3% to less than 20%) 2622
Copaxone for Injection (At least 2%) 3110
▲ Depakote ER Tablets (4% to 12%) 423
Doxil Injection (Less than 1%) 2378
Duragesic Transdermal System (Less than 1%) 2405
Elmiron Capsules (Less than or equal to 1%) 2435
▲ Equetro Extended-Release Capsules (6%) 3174
▲ Flolan for Injection (8%) 1426
Flomax Capsules (0.2% to 2%) 848
▲ Gabitril Tablets (1% to 9%) 973
Keppra Oral Solution (1% or 2%) 3131
Keppra Tablets (1% or 2%) 3131
Lamictal (Frequent) 1488
Lipitor Tablets (Less than 2%) 2501
Luvox CR Extended-Release Capsules (2%) 1759
▲ Megace ES Oral Suspension (1% to 3%) 2499
Meridia Capsules (Greater than or equal to 1%) 475
Natrecor for Injection (Greater than or equal to 1%) 2977
Niaspan Extended-Release Tablets 480
Norvir (Less than 2%) 489
Paxil (Rare) 1535
Paxil CR Controlled-Release Tablets (Rare) 1544
Pletal Tablets (Less than 2%) 2481
▲ Prograf Capsules and Injection (3% to 15%) 622
Protonix for Delayed-Release Oral Suspension (Less than 1%) 3254
Protonix Delayed-Release Tablets (Less than 1%) 3254
Protonix I.V. (Less than 1%) 3257
Provigil Tablets (1%) 977
Retrovir Capsules 1574
Retrovir IV Infusion 1579
Retrovir 1574
Rilutek Tablets (Infrequent) 2771
▲ Salagen Tablets (4%) 1082
Sular Extended Release Tablets (Less than or equal to 1%) 2975
▲ Symbyax Capsules (4% to 5%) 1871
Tricor Tablets 520
Ultane Liquid for Inhalation (Less than 1%) 524
▲ Wellbutrin XL Extended-Release Tablets (2% to 3%) 1659
Zomig Tablets (Infrequent) 694
Zomig Nasal Spray (Infrequent) 689
Zomig-ZMT Tablets (Infrequent) 694
Zonegran Capsules (Frequent) 1089
Zyban Sustained-Release Tablets (Frequent) 1692
▲ Zyprexa Tablets (3% to 9%) 1883
▲ Zyprexa ZYDIS Orally Disintegrating Tablets (3% to 9%) 1883

Amblyopia, toxic
Marplan Tablets 3177

Amenorrhea
Abilify Injection (Greater than or equal to 1 in 1000 patients and less than 1 in 100 patients) 2466
Abilify Oral Solution (Greater than or equal to 1 in 1000 patients and less than 1 in 100 patients) 881
Abilify Oral Solution (Greater than or equal to 1 in 1000 patients and less than 1 in 100 patients) 2466
Abilify Discmelt Orally Disintegrating Tablets (Greater than or equal to 1 in 1000 patients and less than 1 in 100 patients) 881
Abilify Discmelt Orally Disintegrating Tablets (Greater than or equal to 1 in 1000 patients and less than 1 in 100 patients) 2466
Abilify Tablets (Greater than or equal to 1 in 1000 patients and less than 1 in 100 patients) 881
Abilify Tablets (Greater than or equal to 1 in 1000 patients and less than 1 in 100 patients) 2466
Alinia for Oral Suspension (Less than 1%) 2677
Alinia Tablets (Less than 1%) 2677
Busulfex Injection 2477
Celexa (Frequent) 1160
Delatestryl Injection 1730
▲ Depakote ER Tablets (Greater than 1% to less than 5%) 423
Effexor XR Extended-Release Capsules (Infrequent) 3195
Emsam Transdermal System (Infrequent) 905
Estratest Tablets (Among most common) 3043
Estratest H.S. Tablets (Among most common) 3043
Evoxac Capsules (Less than 1%) 1013
Gabitril Tablets (Infrequent) 973
Geodon Capsules (Infrequent) 2520
▲ Intron A for Injection (Less than 5%) 2859
Invega Extended-Release Tablets 1748
▲ Kaletra (0% to 4%) 452
Lamictal (2%) 1488
Leukeran Tablets 1508
Lunesta Tablets (Infrequent) 2994
Luvox CR Extended-Release Capsules 1759
Lybrel Tablets 3204
Lyrica Capsules (0.1% to 1%) 2527
Mirapex Tablets 857
Mircette Tablets 1034
▲ Mirena Intrauterine System (20%) 779
Moban Tablets (Infrequent) 1116
MS Contin Tablets (Less frequent) 2585
Mustargen for Injection 2492
▲ Novantrone for Injection Concentrate (28% to 53%) 1100
NuvaRing 2897
Ortho-Cyclen Tablets 2449
Ortho Evra Transdermal System 2437
Ortho Micronor Tablets 2446
Ortho Tri-Cyclen Tablets 2449
Ortho Tri-Cyclen Lo Tablets 2458
OxyContin Tablets (Less than 1%) 2589
Paxil (Infrequent) 1535
Paxil CR Controlled-Release Tablets (Infrequent) 1544
Pentasa Capsules (Less than 1%) 3030
Premarin Intravenous 3217

Premarin Vaginal Cream ... 3228
Premphase Tablets ... 3232
Prempro Tablets ... 3232
Prometrium Capsules (100 mg, 200 mg) ... 3047
Prozac Weekly Capsules (Infrequent) ... 1852
Prozac Pulvules and Liquid (Infrequent) ... 1852
Remeron Tablets (Infrequent) ... 2924
RemeronSolTab Tablets (Infrequent) ... 2927
Requip Tablets (Infrequent) ... 1561
Rilutek Tablets (Rare) ... 2771
Risperdal Consta Long-Acting Injection (Frequent) ... 1753
Sandostatin Injection (Less than 1%) ... 2300
Seasonique Tablets ... 1046
Symbyax Capsules (Infrequent) ... 1871
▲ Taxotere Injection Concentrate (61.7%) ... 2773
Thioridazine Hydrochloride Tablets ... 2195
Thiothixene Capsules ... 2197
Venlafaxine Hydrochloride Tablets (Infrequent) ... 2199
Yaz Tablets (Greater than 1%) ... 805
Zonegran Capsules (Infrequent) ... 1089
Zyprexa Tablets (Infrequent) ... 1883
Zyprexa ZYDIS Orally Disintegrating Tablets (Infrequent) ... 1883

Amnesia

Aceon Tablets (2 mg, 4 mg, 8 mg) (0.3% to 1%) ... 3038
Actiq (Less than 1%) ... 959
Aggrenox Capsules (2.4%) ... 819
▲ Agrylin Capsules (1% to less than 5%) ... 3017
Ambien Tablets (1%) ... 2692
▲ Ambien CR Tablets (1% to 3%) ... 2696
AndroGel (Less than 1%) ... 3159
▲ Arranon Injection (0% to 3%) ... 1319
Avelox (Less than 0.1%) ... 2803
▲ Avinza Capsules (Less than 5%) ... 1772
Campral Tablets (Frequent) ... 1158
Cardizem LA Extended Release Tablets (Less than 2%) ... 421
Celexa (Frequent) ... 1160
Chantix Tablets (Infrequent) ... 2511
Copaxone for Injection (At least 2%) ... 3110
Coreg Tablets (Less than or equal to 0.1%) ... 1387
Coreg CR Extended-Release Capsules (Less than or equal to 0.1%) ... 1393
▲ Depakote ER Tablets (4% to 7%) ... 423
Didronel Tablets ... 2583
Duragesic Transdermal System (1% or greater) ... 2405
Effexor XR Extended-Release Capsules (Frequent) ... 3195
Emsam Transdermal System (Frequent) ... 905
▲ Equetro Extended-Release Capsules (8%) ... 3174
Evoxac Capsules ... 1013
Exelon Capsules (Infrequent) ... 2229
Exelon Oral Solution (Infrequent) ... 2229
Exforge Tablets (Less than or equal to 0.1%) ... 2238
Frova Tablets (Infrequent) ... 1111
Geodon Capsules (Frequent) ... 2520
▲ Gliadel Wafer (1% to 9%) ... 1076
Intelence Tablets (Less than 2%) ... 3119
▲ Intron A for Injection (Up to 14%) ... 2859
Kaletra (Less than 2%) ... 452
Keppra Injection (2%) ... 3137
Keppra Oral Solution (2%) ... 3131
Keppra Tablets (2%) ... 3131
Klonopin ... 2639
▲ Lamictal (Greater than 1% to less than 5%) ... 1488
Lexapro Oral Suspension (Infrequent) ... 1174
Lexapro Tablets (Infrequent) ... 1174
Lipitor Tablets (Less than 2%) ... 2501
Luvox CR Extended-Release Capsules (Frequent) ... 1759
▲ Lyrica Capsules (1% to 6%) ... 2527
Marinol Capsules (Greater than 1%) ... 3163
Meridia Capsules ... 475
▲ Mirapex Tablets (4% to 6%) ... 857
Namenda (Infrequent) ... 1180
Norvir (Less than 2%) ... 489
OxyContin Tablets (Less than 1%) ... 2589
Paxil (2%) ... 1535
Paxil CR Controlled-Release Tablets (2%) ... 1544
▲ Prograf Capsules and Injection (3% to 15%) ... 622
Provigil Tablets (1%) ... 977
Prozac Weekly Capsules (Rare) ... 1852
Prozac Pulvules and Liquid (Frequent) ... 1852
Remeron Tablets (Frequent) ... 2924
RemeronSolTab Tablets (Frequent) ... 2927
▲ Requip Tablets (Infrequent to 3%) ... 1561
Rilutek Tablets (Infrequent) ... 2771
Risperdal Consta Long-Acting Injection (Infrequent) ... 1753
Sandostatin Injection (Less than 1%) ... 2300
Sular Extended Release Tablets (Less than or equal to 1%) ... 2975
Sustiva Capsules (Less than 2%) ... 930
Sustiva Tablets (Less than 2%) ... 930
▲ Symbyax Capsules (1% to 3%) ... 1871
▲ Temodar Capsules (4% to 10%) ... 2931
Valium Tablets ... 2658
Viadur Implant (Less than 2%) ... 802
Wellbutrin SR Sustained-Release Tablets (Rare) ... 1653
Wellbutrin XL Extended-Release Tablets (Rare) ... 1659
Zomig Tablets (Rare) ... 694
Zomig Nasal Spray (Infrequent) ... 689
Zomig-ZMT Tablets (Rare) ... 694
Zyban Sustained-Release Tablets (Rare) ... 1692
▲ Zyprexa Tablets (5%) ... 1883
▲ Zyprexa ZYDIS Orally Disintegrating Tablets (5%) ... 1883
Zyrtec Chewable Tablets (Less than 2%) ... 1920
Zyrtec Syrup (Less than 2%) ... 1920
Zyrtec Tablets (Less than 2%) ... 1920
Zyrtec-D 12 Hour Extended Release Tablets (Less than 2%) ... 1923

Amnesia, transient global

Levitra Tablets ... 2876

Amyloidosis, cardiac

Velcade for Injection ... 2168

ANA, positive

Aceon Tablets (2 mg, 4 mg, 8 mg) ... 3038
Advicor Tablets ... 402
Captopril Tablets ... 2182
▲ Enbrel for Injection (11%) ... 569
▲ Humira Injection (12%) ... 442
Lescol Capsules (Rare) ... 2268
Lescol XL Tablets ... 2268
Mevacor Tablets (Rare) ... 2063
Prinivil Tablets (0.3% to 1%) ... 2087
Prinzide Tablets ... 2092
Rythmol Tablets (0.7%) ... 1586
Vytorin 10/10 Tablets ... 2149
Vytorin 10/10 Tablets ... 2939
Vytorin 10/20 Tablets ... 2149
Vytorin 10/20 Tablets ... 2939
Vytorin 10/40 Tablets ... 2149
Vytorin 10/40 Tablets ... 2939
Vytorin 10/80 Tablets ... 2149
Vytorin 10/80 Tablets ... 2939
Zocor Tablets (Rare) ... 2136

Analgesia, decrease in

Lortab 5/500 Tablets ... 3143
Lortab 7.5/500 Tablets ... 3144
Lortab 10/500 Tablets ... 3144

Anaphylactic reactions

Abilify Injection ... 881
Abilify Injection (Rare) ... 2466
Abilify Oral Solution ... 881
Abilify Oral Solution (Rare) ... 2466
Abilify Discmelt Orally Disintegrating Tablets ... 881
Abilify Discmelt Orally Disintegrating Tablets (Rare) ... 2466
Abilify Tablets ... 881
Abilify Tablets (Rare) ... 2466
Aceon Tablets (2 mg, 4 mg, 8 mg) (0.3% to 1%) ... 3038
▲ Acetadote Injection (14% to 19%) ... 1001
Activella Tablets ... 2347
Advair Diskus 100/50 ... 1276
Advair Diskus 250/50 ... 1276
Advair Diskus 500/50 ... 1276
Ambien Tablets ... 2692
Amoxil Capsules ... 1305
Amoxil Chewable Tablets ... 1305
Amoxil Pediatric Drops for Oral Suspension ... 1305
Amoxil Powder for Oral Suspension ... 1305
Amoxil Tablets ... 1305
Antivenin (Black Widow Spider Antivenin) ... 1951
Anzemet Injection (Rare) ... 2701
Anzemet Tablets (Rare) ... 2704
Atacand HCT ... 642
Atrovent HFA Inhalation Aerosol ... 839
Atrovent Nasal Spray 0.06% ... 836
Augmentin ... 1323
Augmentin Tablets ... 1327
Augmentin ES-600 Powder for Oral Suspension ... 1329
Avalide Tablets ... 892
Avalide Tablets ... 2713
Avandamet Tablets ... 1336
Avandaryl Tablets ... 1344
Avandia Tablets ... 1351
Avelox ... 2803
Beconase AQ Nasal Spray ... 1369
Bexxar ... 1371
Boostrix (Rarely) ... 1377
Brovana Inhalation Solution ... 2990
Byetta Injection ... 600
Celebrex Capsules (Less than 0.1%) ... 2979
Cipro I.V. (1% or less) ... 2817
Cipro ... 2810
Cipro XR Tablets ... 2823
Climara Transdermal System ... 763
Climara Pro Transdermal System ... 768
Combivent Inhalation Aerosol ... 845
Concerta Extended-Release Tablets ... 1925
Coreg CR Extended-Release Capsules (Less than or equal to 0.1%) ... 1393
Cozaar Tablets ... 1973
Cymbalta Delayed-Release Capsules ... 1801
Dacogen Injection ... 1066
Digibind for Injection ... 1403
Divigel ... 3167
Doribax Injection ... 2400
Elidel Cream 1% ... 2221
Elspar for Injection ... 1990
Elspar for Injection ... 2488
Emend for Injection ... 1999
Enjuvia Tablets ... 1029
Flebogamma 5% DIF ... 1718
Flovent HFA (Very rare) ... 1440
Fluarix Vaccine ... 1446
FluMist Vaccine ... 1945
Foradil Aerolizer (Rare) ... 2849
Fortaz ... 1450
Gammagard Liquid ... 730
Gammagard S/D (A remote possibility) ... 734
Gamunex ... 3094
Gardasil Injection ... 2019
Humalog-Pen and KwikPen (Less common) ... 1829
Humalog Mix 50/50-Pen and KwikPen ... 1833
Humalog Mix 75/25-Pen and KwikPen ... 1835
Indapamide Tablets ... 2188
Infanrix Vaccine ... 1479
InnoPran XL Extended Release Capsules ... 1484
Intravenous Sodium Diuril ... 2490
Invega Extended-Release Tablets ... 1748
Iquix Ophthalmic Solution ... 3183
Kogenate FS ... 746
Levaquin ... 2416
Levaquin in 5% Dextrose Injection ... 2416
Levitra Tablets (Less than 2%) ... 2876
Lovenox Injection ... 2756
Luvox CR Extended-Release Capsules ... 1759
Lybrel Tablets ... 3204
Meruvax II ... 2061
Micardis HCT Tablets ... 854
Nabi-HB (Rare) ... 815
Neupro Transdermal System ... 3149
Nexium Delayed-Release Capsules (Rare) ... 645
Nexium I.V. (Rare) ... 652
Nexium Delayed-Release Oral Suspension (Rare) ... 645
Nimbex Injection ... 484
Noroxin Tablets (Occasional) ... 2069
NovoSeven ... 2367
NovoSeven RT ... 2370
Orthoclone OKT3 Sterile Solution ... 2387
OxyContin Tablets (Less than 1%) ... 2589
Pediarix Vaccine (Rare) ... 1552
Pred Mild Ophthalmic Suspension ... ⊙ 230
Premarin Vaginal Cream ... 3228
Prevnar ... 3241
Primaxin I.M. ... 2080
Primaxin I.V. ... 2083
Prinzide Tablets ... 2092
Prograf Capsules and Injection (A few patients) ... 622
ProQuad (Greater than or equal to 0.2% to less than 1%) ... 2099
Rapamune ... 3260
Refludan for Injection ... 795
Risperdal Consta Long-Acting Injection ... 1753
Sanctura XR Capsules ... 557
Sandimmune I.V. Ampuls for Infusion (Rare) ... 2296
Seasonique Tablets ... 1046
Suprax for Oral Suspension (Less than 2%) ... 1891
Suprax Tablets (Less than 2%) ... 1891
Tamiflu Capsules ... 2649
Tamiflu Oral Suspension ... 2649
Tekturna HCT Tablets ... 2324
Teveten HCT Tablets ... 517
Timentin ADD-Vantage ... 1606
Timentin Injection Galaxy Container ... 1609
Timentin IV Infusion ... 1603
Timentin Pharmacy Bulk Package ... 1613
Trasylol Injection (Less than 0.5%) ... 799
Traumeel Injection Solution (Rare) ... 1725
Treanda for Injection ... 983
Treximet Tablets ... 1616
Vicoprofen Tablets ... 533
Voltaren Tablets (Rarely) ... 2334
Voltaren-XR Tablets (Rarely) ... 2337
Yaz Tablets ... 805
Zeel Injection Solution ... 1726
Zemuron Injection ... 2947
Zometa for Intravenous Infusion (Very rare) ... 2341
Zostavax Injection ... 2145
Zosyn for Injection (Occasional) ... 3284

Anaphylactic shock

Ambien Tablets (Rare) ... 2692
Ambien CR Tablets (Rare) ... 2696
Avelox ... 2803
Bicillin L-A Injection ... 1777
Campath Ampules ... 761
Cipro ... 2810
Cipro XR Tablets ... 2823
Eloxatin for Injection ... 2731
Levaquin ... 2416
Levaquin in 5% Dextrose Injection ... 2416
Meridia Capsules ... 475
Miacalcin Injection (A few cases) ... 2273
Nexium Delayed-Release Capsules ... 645
Nexium I.V. ... 652
Nexium Delayed-Release Oral Suspension ... 645
Orthoclone OKT3 Sterile Solution ... 2387
Pentacel ... 2792
Protonix for Delayed-Release Oral Suspension ... 3254
Protonix Delayed-Release Tablets ... 3254
Protonix I.V. ... 3257
Sandostatin Injection ... 2300
Sandostatin LAR Depot ... 2302
Suprax for Oral Suspension (Less than 2%) ... 1891
Suprax Tablets (Less than 2%) ... 1891
Taxotere Injection Concentrate (Rare) ... 2773
Trasylol Injection ... 799
Varivax ... 2133
Wellbutrin Tablets (Rare) ... 1648
Wellbutrin SR Sustained-Release Tablets (Rare) ... 1653
Wellbutrin XL Extended-Release Tablets (Rare) ... 1659
Zometa for Intravenous Infusion (Very rare) ... 2341
Zosyn for Injection (1% or less) ... 3284
Zyban Sustained-Release Tablets (Rare) ... 1692

Anaphylactoid reactions

Abelcet Injection ... 1134
Activase I.V. (Very rare) ... 1188
Activella Tablets ... 2347
Amerge Tablets ... 1301
Amoxil Capsules (Occasional) ... 1305
Amoxil Chewable Tablets (Occasional) ... 1305
Amoxil Pediatric Drops for Oral Suspension (Occasional) ... 1305
Amoxil Powder for Oral Suspension (Occasional) ... 1305
Amoxil Tablets (Occasional) ... 1305
Anaprox Tablets (Less than 1%) ... 2632
Anaprox DS Tablets (Less than 1%) ... 2632
Angeliq Tablets ... 751
Attenuvax ... 1951
Beconase AQ Nasal Spray ... 1369
Captopril Tablets ... 2182
Cerezyme for Injection ... 1238
Climara Transdermal System ... 763
Climara Pro Transdermal System ... 768
Copaxone for Injection (Rare) ... 3110
Crixivan Capsules ... 1979

Delatestryl Injection 1730
Digibind for Injection 1403
Divigel 3167
Doxil Injection (Less than 1%) 2378
EC-Naprosyn Delayed-Release Tablets (Less than 1%) 2632
Engerix-B Vaccine 1409
Enjuvia Tablets 1029
Epogen for Injection 576
Erbitux 912
Estratest Tablets (Rare) 3043
Estratest H.S. Tablets (Rare) 3043
Fansidar Tablets 2636
Feiba VH 728
Flector Patch 561
Flonase Nasal Spray 1431
Fluarix Vaccine 1446
Fortaz 1450
Fragmin Injection (Few cases) 1070
Gardasil Injection 2019
Gemzar for Injection (Rare) 1820
Havrix Injection Vaccine 1454
Hyalgan Solution 2742
Hycamtin for Injection (Rare) 1459
Imitrex Injection (Rare) 1465
Imitrex Nasal Spray 1470
Imitrex Tablets (Rare) 1474
Invanz for Injection (Very rare) 2029
Kinrix Injection Vaccine 1486
Levaquin 2416
Levaquin in 5% Dextrose Injection 2416
Lovenox Injection 2756
Lupron Depot 3.75 mg (Rare) 462
Lupron Depot–3 Month 11.25 mg 462
Lupron Depot-PED 7.5 mg, 11.25 mg and 15 mg (Rare) 471
Lybrel Tablets 3204
Lyrica Capsules (Rare) 2527
Mavik Tablets 472
Maxalt Tablets 2056
Maxalt-MLT Orally Disintegrating Tablets 2056
Mephyton Tablets 700
Meridia Capsules 475
Meruvax II 2061
M-M-R II 2054
Mobic Oral Suspension (Less than 0.1%) 863
Mobic Tablets (Less than 0.1%) 863
Mumpsvax 2068
Mycamine for Injection 616
Naprosyn Suspension (Less than 1%) 2632
Naprosyn Tablets (Less than 1%) 2632
Nimbex Injection 484
Nitro-Dur Transdermal Infusion System (A few reports) 2887
Noroxin Tablets 2069
Novantrone for Injection Concentrate 1100
Orencia Powder for Intravenous Infusion (2 cases) 921
Orthoclone OKT3 Sterile Solution 2387
OxyContin Tablets (Less than 1%) 2589
Percocet Tablets 1127
Plavix Tablets (Very rare) 926
Plavix Tablets (Very rare) 2767
Pneumovax 23 2078
Prandin Tablets (Less than or equal to 1%) 2971
Premarin Vaginal Cream 3228
Premphase Tablets 3232
Prempro Tablets 3232
Prevnar 3241
Prinivil Tablets (0.3% to 1%) 2087
Prinzide Tablets 2092
Procrit for Injection 2391
Prometrium Capsules (100 mg, 200 mg) 3047
ProQuad 2099
Protopic Ointment (Greater than or equal to 1%) 628
Provigil Tablets 977
Prozac Weekly Capsules 1852
Rapamune 3260
Rilutek Tablets 2771
Rituxan I.V. 1223
Sandostatin Injection 2300
Sandostatin LAR Depot 2302
Seasonique Tablets 1046
Skelaxin Tablets (Rare) 1784
Suprax for Oral Suspension (Less than 2%) 1891
Suprax Tablets (Less than 2%) 1891
Tamiflu Capsules 2649
Tamiflu Oral Suspension 2649
Trasylol Injection 799
Treanda for Injection 983
Treximet Tablets 1616
Twinrix Vaccine 1628
Tygacil for Injection 3276
Ultane Liquid for Inhalation (Less than 1%) 524
Velcade for Injection 2168
Wellbutrin Tablets 1648
Wellbutrin SR Sustained-Release Tablets 1653
Wellbutrin XL Extended-Release Tablets 1659
Yaz Tablets 805
Zemuron Injection 2947
Zofran Injection 1682
Zofran 1687
Zofran ODT Orally Disintegrating Tablets 1687
Zomig Tablets (Very rare) 694
Zomig Nasal Spray (Very rare) 689
Zomig-ZMT Tablets (Very rare) 694
Zosyn for Injection 3284
Zyban Sustained-Release Tablets 1692
Zyprexa Tablets 1883
Zyprexa ZYDIS Orally Disintegrating Tablets 1883

Anaphylaxis

Abelcet Injection (Less than 0.1%) 1134
Aciphex Tablets 1053
Adderall XR Capsules 3012
Advicor Tablets (Rare) 402
Aggrenox Capsules 819
Alferon N Injection 1726
Allegra Oral Solution (Rare) 2684
Allegra Tablets (Rare) 2684
Allegra-D 12 Hour Extended-Release Tablets (Rare) 2687
Allegra-D 24 Hour Extended-Release Tablets (Rare) 2690
Amerge Tablets 1301
Aminohippurate Sodium "PAH" Injection 1950
Amoxil Capsules 1305
Amoxil Chewable Tablets 1305
Amoxil Pediatric Drops for Oral Suspension 1305
Amoxil Powder for Oral Suspension 1305
Amoxil Tablets 1305
Amrix Capsules 966
Angiomax for Injection (Very rare) 1933
Antivenin (Black Widow Spider Antivenin) 1951
Arimidex Tablets (Very rare) 672
Atrovent HFA Inhalation Aerosol 839
Atrovent Nasal Spray 0.03% 834
Atrovent Nasal Spray 0.06% 836
Attenuvax 1951
Axid Capsules 1364
Azmacort Inhalation Aerosol 407
Bayer Aspirin 750
BeneFIX Vials 3191
Bentyl Capsules 703
Bentyl Injection 703
Bentyl Syrup 703
Bentyl Tablets 703
Betaseron for SC Injection 756
Bexxar 1371
Biaxin/Biaxin XL (Rare) 411
Bicillin C-R Injectable Suspension 1775
Bicillin L-A Injection 1777
Calcijex Injection 419
Cancidas for Injection 1953
Ceftin 1380
Celexa 1160
Cimzia 3127
Clarinex Syrup (Rare) 2828
Clarinex Tablets (Rare) 2828
Clarinex Reditabs Tablets (Rare) 2828
Clarinex-D 12-Hour Extended-Release Tablets (Rare) 2831
Clarinex-D 24-Hour Extended-Release Tablets 2834
Clinoril Tablets 1962
Combigan Ophthalmic Solution 553
Combivent Inhalation Aerosol (Rare) 845
Combivir Tablets 1384
Comvax 1966
Coreg Tablets (Less than or equal to 0.1%) 1387
Cosopt Sterile Ophthalmic Solution 1969
Cubicin for Injection 995
Cyanokit 5g Antidote 1021
Dantrium Capsules (Less frequent) 2580
Dantrium Intravenous (One case) 2582
Daraprim Tablets 1400
Daytrana Transdermal Patch 3022
Depakote ER Tablets 423
Digibind for Injection 1403
Diovan HCT Tablets (Less frequent) 2216
Donnatal Extentabs 2507
Doribax Injection 2400
Duac Topical Gel 3054
Dyazide Capsules 1405
Dyrenium Capsules 3189
E.E.S. 433
Effexor XR Extended-Release Capsules 3195
Elitek (Less than 1%) 2729
Eloxatin for Injection 2731
Elspar for Injection 1990
Elspar for Injection 2488
Engerix-B Vaccine 1409
Epivir 1412
Epivir-HBV 1417
Epzicom Tablets 1422
EryPed 431
Exjade Tablets 2244
Flebogamma 5% DIF 1718
Flonase Nasal Spray 1431
Fluarix Vaccine 1446
Flulaval Injection Vaccine 1448
Fluorescite Injection ⊙ 203
Fortaz (Very rare) 1450
Gammagard S/D 734
Gantrisin Pediatric Suspension 2638
Herceptin I.V. 1199
Humira Injection 442
Imitrex Injection (Rare) 1465
Imitrex Nasal Spray 1470
Imitrex Tablets (Rare) 1474
Indocin Capsules (Less than 1%) 2024
Indocin I.V. (Less than 1%) 2489
Indocin (Less than 1%) 2024
Integrilin Injection (One patient) 2855
Intron A for Injection (Rare) 2859
Invanz for Injection (Very rare) 2029
Ixempra Kit for Injection 915
Janumet Tablets 2041
Januvia Tablets 2048
Ketek Tablets (Rare) 2744
Kinrix Injection Vaccine 1486
Lamisil Oral Granules 2264
Lamisil Tablets (Rare) 2266
Lescol Capsules (Rare) 2268
Lescol XL Tablets 2268
Lexapro Oral Suspension (Infrequent) 1174
Lexapro Tablets (Infrequent) 1174
Lipitor Tablets 2501
Malarone Pediatric Tablets 1521
Malarone Tablets 1521
Maxalt Tablets 2056
Maxalt-MLT Orally Disintegrating Tablets 2056
Meruvax II 2061
Mevacor Tablets (Rare) 2063
Miacalcin Injection (One case) 2273
Miacalcin Nasal Spray (One case) 2274
M-M-R II 2054
MoviPrep Oral Solution 2679
Moxatag Tablets 2165
MS Contin Tablets (Extremely rare) 2585
Mumpsvax 2068
Mustargen for Injection 2492
Mycamine for Injection 616
Mylotarg for Injection 3212
Nalfon Capsules (Less than 1%) 2508
Nasonex Nasal Spray 2883
Neosporin Ophthalmic Solution Sterile (Rare) ⊙ 252
Neulasta Injection 587
Norvir (Rare) 489
Novantrone for Injection Concentrate 1100
Omnicef Capsules 497
Omnicef for Oral Suspension 497
Oncaspar Injection (Greater than or equal to 2%) 1138
Orencia Powder for Intravenous Infusion (2 cases) 921
Orthoclone OKT3 Sterile Solution 2387
OsmoPrep Tablets 2680
Paxil 1535
Paxil CR Controlled-Release Tablets 1544
Pentacel 2792
Pepcid Tablets (Infrequent) 2075
Percocet Tablets 1127
Premarin Tablets 3221
Premphase Tablets 3232
Prempro Tablets 3232
Prograf Capsules and Injection (A small percentage of patients) 622
Proleukin for Injection 2287
Prometrium Capsules (100 mg, 200 mg) 3047
ProQuad 2099
Protonix for Delayed-Release Oral Suspension 3254
Protonix Delayed-Release Tablets 3254
Protonix I.V. 3257
Provigil Tablets 977
Recombivax HB (Less than 1%) 2107
ReFacto Vials 3269
Relenza Inhalation Powder 1556
Remicade for IV Injection (Less than 1%) 950
ReoPro Vials 1860
Retrovir Capsules (One patient) 1574
Retrovir IV Infusion (One patient) 1579
Retrovir (One patient) 1574
Rocephin Injectable Vials, ADD-Vantage, Galaxy, Bulk (Less than 0.1%) 2642
St. Joseph 81 mg Aspirin Chewable and Enteric Coated Tablets 1903
Serevent Diskus 1594
Simulect for Injection 2306
Singulair 2114
Solodyn Extended Release Tablets 1938
Synagis Intramuscular Solution 1948
Tamiflu Capsules (Rare) 2649
Tamiflu Oral Suspension (Rare) 2649
Taxotere Injection Concentrate 2773
Temodar Capsules (Rare) 2931
Thiothixene Capsules (Rare) 2197
Timoptic Sterile Ophthalmic Solution 2121
Timoptic in Ocudose 2124
Timoptic-XE Sterile Ophthalmic Gel Forming Solution 2125
TNKase (Less than 0.1% to less than 1%) 1233
Torisel Injection 3272
Trasylol Injection 799
Trizivir Tablets 1622
Twinrix Vaccine 1628
Tygacil for Injection 3276
Valtrex Caplets 1635
Varivax 2133
Vectibix 597
Venlafaxine Hydrochloride Tablets 2199
Ventolin HFA Inhalation Aerosol 1638
Viramune Oral Suspension 873
Viramune Tablets 873
Vytorin 10/10 Tablets 2149
Vytorin 10/10 Tablets 2939
Vytorin 10/20 Tablets 2149
Vytorin 10/20 Tablets 2939
Vytorin 10/40 Tablets 2149
Vytorin 10/40 Tablets 2939
Vytorin 10/80 Tablets 2149
Vytorin 10/80 Tablets 2939
Vyvanse Capsules 3033
Xenical Capsules 2672
Xolair (0.1% to 0.2%) 1235
Xolair (0.1% to 0.2%) 2339
Xopenex Inhalation Solution 3001
Xopenex Inhalation Solution Concentrate 3005
Xopenex HFA Inhalation Aerosol 3009
Xyntha Vials 3280
Xyzal Oral Solution 2789
Xyzal Oral Solution 3155
Zantac 25 EFFERdose Tablets (Rare) 1670
Zantac Injection (Rare) 1666
Zantac Injection Pharmacy Bulk Package (Rare) 1668
Zantac Injection Premixed (Rare) 1666
Zantac (Rare) 1670
Zetia Tablets 2157
Zetia Tablets 2951
Ziagen 1673
Zinacef for Injection (Rare) 1678
Zinacef Injection (Rare) 1678
Zocor Tablets (Rare) 2136
Zofran Injection (Rare) 1682
Zofran (Rare) 1687
Zofran ODT Orally Disintegrating Tablets (Rare) 1687
Zomig Tablets (Very rare) 694
Zomig Nasal Spray (Very rare) 689
Zomig-ZMT Tablets (Very rare) 694
Zosyn for Injection (1% or less) 3284
Zovirax Capsules (Rare) 1690
Zovirax Cream 817
Zovirax (Rare) 1690
Zyrtec Chewable Tablets 1920
Zyrtec Syrup 1920
Zyrtec Tablets 1920
Zyrtec-D 12 Hour Extended Release Tablets (Rare) 1923
Zyvox 2552

Anasarca

▲ Gleevec Tablets (6.9% to 22%) 2255

Anastomotic disruption

Avastin IV (Rare) 1192
Rapamune 3260

Anastomotic leak

Invanz for Injection (1.5%) 2029

ANC, low

▲ Novantrone for Injection Concentrate (100%) ... 1100

Androgen excess, signs or symptoms of

▲ Lupron Depot 3.75 mg (Less than 5%) ... 462
▲ Lupron Depot–3 Month 11.25 mg (Less than 5%) ... 462

Anemia

▲ Abelcet Injection (4%) ... 1134
Accutane Capsules ... 2607
Aceon Tablets (2 mg, 4 mg, 8 mg) ... 3038
Actiq (Less than 1%) ... 959
Actonel with Calcium Tablets (2.4%) ... 2574
Actos Tablets (Less than or equal to 2%) ... 3077
Aggrenox Capsules (1.6%) ... 819
▲ Agrylin Capsules (1% to less than 5%) ... 3017
▲ Alimta for Injection (1% to 33%) ... 1786
Alinia for Oral Suspension (Less than 1%) ... 2677
Alinia Tablets (Less than 1%) ... 2677
Ambien Tablets (Rare) ... 2692
AmBisome for Injection (Less common) ... 606
Amerge Tablets (Rare) ... 1301
Amoxil Capsules ... 1305
Amoxil Chewable Tablets ... 1305
Amoxil Pediatric Drops for Oral Suspension ... 1305
Amoxil Powder for Oral Suspension ... 1305
Amoxil Tablets ... 1305
▲ Anaprox Tablets (1% to 10%) ... 2632
▲ Anaprox DS Tablets (1% to 10%) ... 2632
AndroGel (2.5%) ... 3159
Anzemet Injection (Infrequently) ... 2701
Anzemet Tablets (Rare) ... 2704
▲ Aptivus Capsules (3.3%) ... 823
▲ Aptivus Oral Solution (3.3%) ... 823
Aricept Tablets (Frequent) ... 1062
Aricept ODT Tablets (Frequent) ... 1062
▲ Arimidex Tablets (2% to 5%) ... 672
▲ Arixtra Injection (1.5% to 19.6%) ... 1313
▲ Arranon Injection (10% to 99%) ... 1319
Asacol Delayed-Release Tablets ... 2579
Atacand Tablets ... 639
Augmentin ... 1323
Augmentin Tablets ... 1327
Augmentin XR Extended Release Tablets ... 1333
Augmentin ES-600 Powder for Oral Suspension ... 1329
▲ Avandamet Tablets (7.1%) ... 1336
Avandaryl Tablets (1.9% to 2.3%) ... 1344
▲ Avandia Tablets (5%) ... 1351
Avelox (Less than 0.1%) ... 2803
▲ Avinza Capsules (Less than 5%) ... 1772
Axid Capsules (0.2%) ... 1364
Betaseron for SC Injection ... 756
Bexxar ... 1371
▲ Busulfex Injection (100%) ... 2477
▲ Campath Ampules (12% to 76%) ... 761
Campral Tablets (Infrequent) ... 1158
▲ Cancidas for Injection (0% to10.5%) ... 1953
Captopril Tablets ... 2182
Celebrex Capsules (0.1% to 1.9%) ... 2979
Celexa (Infrequent) ... 1160
▲ CellCept Capsules (25.6% to 43%) ... 2622
▲ CellCept Intravenous (25.6% to 43%) ... 2622
▲ CellCept Oral Suspension (25.6% to 43%) ... 2622
▲ CellCept Tablets (25.6% to 43%) ... 2622
Chantix Tablets (Infrequent) ... 2511
Cimzia ... 3127
Cipro I.V. (Rare) ... 2817
Cipro (Less than 0.1%) ... 2810
Cipro XR Tablets ... 2823
Clinoril Tablets (Less than 1%) ... 1962
Clolar for Intravenous Infusion ... 1239
Combivir Tablets (2.9%) ... 1384
▲ Coreg Tablets (Greater than 0.1% to greater than 3%) ... 1387
▲ Coreg CR Extended-Release Capsules (Greater than 3%) ... 1393
Cosmegen for Injection ... 2485
▲ Cozaar Tablets (Less than 1% to 14%) ... 1973
Crinone 4% Gel ... 992
Crinone 8% Gel ... 992
Crixivan Capsules (0.6%) ... 1979
▲ Cubicin for Injection (2.1% to 12.5%) ... 995
▲ Dacogen Injection (82%) ... 1066
Daytrana Transdermal Patch ... 3022
Demser Capsules (Rare) ... 1989
Depakote ER Tablets (Greater than 1%) ... 423
▲ DepoCyt Injection (1% to 18%) ... 1136
▲ DepoDur Injection (Greater than 10%) ... 1095
▲ Doribax Injection (2% to 10%) ... 2400
▲ Doxil Injection (5.8% to 52.6%) ... 2378
Duetact Tablets (Less than 2%) ... 3085
▲ EC-Naprosyn Delayed-Release Tablets (1% to 10%) ... 2632
Effexor XR Extended-Release Capsules (Infrequent) ... 3195
Eldepryl Capsules ... 3052
Elmiron Capsules (Less than or equal to 1%) ... 2435
▲ Eloxatin for Injection (1% to 81%) ... 2731
Emend Capsules (Greater than 0.5%) ... 1992
Emend for Injection (Greater than 0.5%) ... 1999
Emsam Transdermal System (Infrequent) ... 905
▲ Emtriva Capsules (7%) ... 1246
▲ Emtriva Oral Solution (7%) ... 1246
Enbrel for Injection ... 569
▲ Entereg Capsules (5.2% to 5.4%) ... 3293
Epivir ... 1412
Epivir-HBV ... 1417
Epogen for Injection ... 576
Epzicom Tablets ... 1422
▲ Evoxac Capsules (1% to 3%) ... 1013
Exelon Capsules (Frequent) ... 2229
Exelon Oral Solution (Frequent) ... 2229
Exelon Patch (Frequent) ... 2233
▲ Fabrazyme for Intravenous Infusion (14%) ... 1241
▲ Faslodex Injection (4.5%) ... 682
Fenoglide Tablets ... 2960
▲ Fentora Tablets (1% to 32%) ... 968
Flector Patch ... 561
Flolan for Injection ... 1426
Focalin XR Capsules ... 2251
Furosemide Tablets ... 2186
Gabitril Tablets (Infrequent) ... 973
Gantrisin Pediatric Suspension ... 2638
▲ Gemzar for Injection (45% to 86%) ... 1820
Gengraf Capsules (1% to less than 3%) ... 435
Geodon Capsules (Infrequent) ... 2520
▲ Gleevec Tablets (0% to 42%) ... 2255
▲ Herceptin I.V. (4%) ... 1199
▲ Hexalen Capsules (33%) ... 1078
▲ Hycamtin Capsules (94% to 98%) ... 1456
▲ Hycamtin for Injection (40% to 95%) ... 1459
Imitrex Injection ... 1465
Imitrex Nasal Spray ... 1470
Imitrex Tablets (Rare) ... 1474
Indocin Capsules (Less than 1%) ... 2024
Indocin I.V. (Less than 1%) ... 2489
Indocin (Less than 1%) ... 2024
Intelence Tablets (Less than 2%) ... 3119
▲ Intron A for Injection (Less than 5% to 22%) ... 2859
▲ Invanz for Injection (5.7%) ... 2029
▲ Ionsys Transdermal System (3%) ... 2410
Isentress Tablets ... 2036
▲ Ixempra Kit for Injection (2% to 40%) ... 915
Kaletra (Less than 2%) ... 452
Klonopin ... 2639
Kogenate FS ... 746
Kogenate FS with Bio-Set ... 748
Lamictal (Rare) ... 1488
Lamisil Oral Granules ... 2264
Leukeran Tablets ... 1508
▲ Leustatin Injection (37%) ... 2384
Levaquin (0.1% to 1%) ... 2416
Levaquin in 5% Dextrose Injection (0.1% to 1%) ... 2416
Lexapro Oral Suspension (Infrequent) ... 1174
Lexapro Tablets (Infrequent) ... 1174
Lipitor Tablets (Less than 2%) ... 2501
▲ Lovenox Injection (Less than 2% to 16%) ... 2756
▲ Lucentis Injection (3% to 8%) ... 1205
Lunesta Tablets (Infrequent) ... 2994
Luvox CR Extended-Release Capsules (Infrequent) ... 1759
Lyrica Capsules (0.1% to 1%) ... 2527
Malarone Pediatric Tablets (Rare) ... 1521
Malarone Tablets (Rare) ... 1521
▲ Megace ES Oral Suspension (0% to 5%) ... 2499
▲ Mepron Suspension (4% to 6%) ... 1526
Meridia Capsules ... 475
▲ Merrem I.V. (Greater than 0.1% to 5.5%) ... 684
Metadate CD Capsules ... 3146
Miacalcin Nasal Spray (Less than 1%) ... 2274
▲ Mobic Oral Suspension (0% to 4.1%) ... 863
▲ Mobic Tablets (0% to 4.1%) ... 863
Moxatag Tablets ... 2165
▲ Mycamine for Injection (2.5% to 35.5%) ... 616
▲ Myfortic Tablets (3% to 21.6%) ... 2276
Myleran Tablets ... 1530
▲ Mylotarg for Injection (22%) ... 3212
Namenda (Frequent) ... 1180
▲ Naprosyn Suspension (1% to 10%) ... 2632
▲ Naprosyn Tablets (1% to 10%) ... 2632
Natrecor for Injection (Greater than or equal to 1%) ... 2977
▲ NeoProfen Injection (32%) ... 2496
Neoral Oral Solution (1% to less than 3%) ... 2280
Neoral Soft Gelatin Capsules (1% to less than 3%) ... 2280
▲ Neupogen for Injection (Approximately 10%) ... 589
▲ Nexavar Tablets (2% to 44%) ... 784
Nexium Delayed-Release Capsules (Less than 1%) ... 645
Nexium I.V. (Less than 1%) ... 652
Nexium Delayed-Release Oral Suspension (Less than 1%) ... 645
Nimotop Capsules (Less than 1%) ... 790
Norvir (Less than 2%) ... 489
▲ Novantrone for Injection Concentrate (5% to 9%) ... 1100
▲ Noxafil Oral Suspension (Less than 1% to 25%) ... 2889
▲ Ontak Vials (18%) ... 1079
ParaGard T 380A Intrauterine Copper Contraceptive ... 1041
Parnate Tablets ... 1532
Paxil (Infrequent) ... 1535
Paxil CR Controlled-Release Tablets (Infrequent) ... 1544
PegIntron Powder for Injection ... 2903
Pentasa Capsules ... 3030
▲ Photofrin for Injection (32%) ... 708
Plavix Tablets (1% to 2.5%) ... 926
Plavix Tablets (1% to 2.5%) ... 2767
Pletal Tablets (Less than 2%) ... 2481
Prandin Tablets (Rare) ... 2971
Prinivil Tablets ... 2087
▲ Prograf Capsules and Injection (5% to 47%) ... 622
▲ Proleukin for Injection (Less than 1% to 29%) ... 2287
Protonix for Delayed-Release Oral Suspension (Less than 1%) ... 3254
Protonix Delayed-Release Tablets (Less than 1%) ... 3254
Protonix I.V. (Less than 1%) ... 3257
Protopic Ointment (0.2% to less than 1%) ... 628
Provigil Tablets (At least 1%) ... 977
Prozac Weekly Capsules (Infrequent) ... 1852
Prozac Pulvules and Liquid (Infrequent) ... 1852
▲ Rapamune (23% to 33%) ... 3260
Raptiva for Injection ... 1218
▲ Rebetol (12% to 17%) ... 2917
▲ Rebif Prefilled Syringe for Injection (3% to 5%) ... 1107
▲ Refludan for Injection (12.4%) ... 795
Remeron Tablets (Rare) ... 2924
RemeronSolTab Tablets (Rare) ... 2927
Remicade for IV Injection (Greater than or equal to 0.2%) ... 950
ReoPro Vials (1.2%) ... 1860
Requip Tablets (Infrequent to greater than 1%) ... 1561
▲ Retrovir Capsules (1.1% to 29%) ... 1574
▲ Retrovir IV Infusion (1.1% to 29%) ... 1579
▲ Retrovir (1.1% to 29%) ... 1574
Rilutek Tablets (Infrequent) ... 2771
Risperdal Consta Long-Acting Injection (Frequent) ... 1753
▲ Rituxan I.V. (3% to 35%) ... 1223
Rocephin Injectable Vials, ADD-Vantage, Galaxy, Bulk (Less than 1%) ... 2642
Rythmol Tablets (Less than 1%) ... 1586
Rythmol SR Capsules ... 1590
Sandimmune (2% or less) ... 2296
Sandostatin Injection (Less than 1%) ... 2300
▲ Sandostatin LAR Depot (15.3%) ... 2302
▲ Simulect for Injection (Greater than or equal to 10%) ... 2306
▲ Somatuline Depot Injection (3% to 14%) ... 3102
Stromectol Tablets (One patient) ... 2120
Sular Extended Release Tablets (Less than or equal to 1%) ... 2975
▲ Sutent Capsules (2% to 26%) ... 2540
Symbyax Capsules (Infrequent) ... 1871
Synagis Intramuscular Solution (More than 1%) ... 1948
Tabloid Tablets ... 1601
Tamiflu Capsules (Less than 1%) ... 2649
Tamiflu Oral Suspension (Less than 1%) ... 2649
▲ Targretin Capsules (6% to 24.5%) ... 1084
▲ Tasigna Capsules (8% to 23%) ... 2316
▲ Taxotere Injection Concentrate (4.3% to 97%) ... 2773
Tekturna Tablets (0.1% to 0.3%) ... 2321
Temodar Capsules (Very rare) ... 2931
Teveten Tablets (Less than 1%) ... 515
Teveten HCT Tablets (Less than 1%) ... 517
Thioridazine Hydrochloride Tablets ... 2195
Tice BCG (Less than or equal to 1%) ... 2936
▲ Torisel Injection (Greater than or equal to 30%) ... 3272
▲ Tracleer Tablets (3%) ... 3289
Trasylol Injection (2%) ... 799
▲ Treanda for Injection (3% to 19%) ... 983
Treximet Tablets (Rare) ... 1616
Tricor Tablets ... 520
▲ Trisenox Injection (20%) ... 986
Trizivir Tablets (2.9%) ... 1622
▲ Tygacil for Injection (4.2%) ... 3276
▲ Valcyte Tablets (1% to 31%) ... 2654
Valstar Sterile Solution for Intravesical Instillation (2%) ... 1735
Valtrex Caplets (Up to 0.8%) ... 1635
Vantas (Less than 2%) ... 1737
▲ Vaprisol (3.8% to 6%) ... 632
▲ Velcade for Injection (26% to 43%) ... 2168
Venlafaxine Hydrochloride Tablets (Infrequent) ... 2199
Viadur Implant (2.3%) ... 802
Vicoprofen Tablets ... 533
▲ Viramune Oral Suspension (7.3%) ... 873
▲ Viramune Tablets (7.3%) ... 873
▲ Visudyne for Injection (1% to 10%) ... 2332
▲ Voltaren Tablets (1% to 10%) ... 2334
▲ Voltaren-XR Tablets (1% to 10%) ... 2337
Vytorin 10/10 Tablets ... 2149
Vytorin 10/10 Tablets ... 2939
Vytorin 10/20 Tablets ... 2149
Vytorin 10/20 Tablets ... 2939
Vytorin 10/40 Tablets ... 2149
Vytorin 10/40 Tablets ... 2939
Vytorin 10/80 Tablets ... 2149
Vytorin 10/80 Tablets ... 2939
Wellbutrin Tablets (Rare) ... 1648
Wellbutrin SR Sustained-Release Tablets ... 1653
Wellbutrin XL Extended-Release Tablets ... 1659
▲ Xeloda Tablets (1% to 80%) ... 2662
Ziagen (0% to less than 1%) ... 1673
Zocor Tablets ... 2136
▲ Zolinza Capsules (2.3% to 14%) ... 2142
▲ Zometa for Intravenous Infusion (22% to 33%) ... 2341
Zonegran Capsules (Infrequent) ... 1089
Zosyn for Injection (1% or less) ... 3284
Zovirax ... 1690
Zyban Sustained-Release Tablets ... 1692
Zyprexa Tablets (Infrequent) ... 1883
Zyprexa ZYDIS Orally Disintegrating Tablets (Infrequent) ... 1883
▲ Zyvox (0% to 5.6%) ... 2552

Anemia, aplastic

Aceon Tablets (2 mg, 4 mg, 8 mg) ... 3038
Aggrenox Capsules ... 819
Albenza Tablets ... 1297
Anaprox Tablets (Less than 1%) ... 2632
Anaprox DS Tablets (Less than 1%) ... 2632
Asacol Delayed-Release Tablets (Rare) ... 2579
Atacand HCT ... 642
Avalide Tablets ... 892
Avalide Tablets ... 2713
Avandaryl Tablets ... 1344
Avelox ... 2803
Campath Ampules ... 761
Carbatrol Capsules ... 3019
Ceftin ... 1380
Cimzia (Rare) ... 3127
Cipro I.V. (Rare) ... 2817
Cipro ... 2810
Cipro XR Tablets ... 2823
Clinoril Tablets (Less than 1 in 100) ... 1962
Clorpres Tablets ... 2185
Coreg Tablets (Rare) ... 1387
Cosmegen for Injection ... 2485
Cuprimine Capsules ... 1986
Dantrium Capsules (Less frequent) ... 2580
Dantrium Intravenous ... 2582
Dapsone Tablets USP ... 1746

Depakote ER Tablets 423
Diovan HCT Tablets 2216
Duetact Tablets 3085
Dyazide Capsules 1405
EC-Naprosyn Delayed-Release Tablets (Less than 1%) 2632
Effexor XR Extended-Release Capsules 3195
Enbrel for Injection 569
Epzicom Tablets 1422
Equetro Extended-Release Capsules 3174
Fansidar Tablets 2636
Fortaz 1450
Furosemide Tablets 2186
Gantrisin Pediatric Suspension 2638
Gleevec Tablets (Rare) 2255
Humira Injection 442
Indapamide Tablets 2188
Indocin Capsules (Less than 1%) 2024
Indocin I.V. (Less than 1%) 2489
Indocin (Less than 1%) 2024
Intravenous Sodium Diuril 2490
Intron A for Injection (Very rare) 2859
Lamictal (Rare) 1488
Leustatin Injection (Some reports) 2384
Levaquin 2416
Levaquin in 5% Dextrose Injection 2416
Luvox CR Extended-Release Capsules 1759
Micardis HCT Tablets 854
Myleran Tablets 1530
Nalfon Capsules (Less than 1%) 2508
Naprosyn Suspension (Less than 1%) 2632
Naprosyn Tablets (Less than 1%) 2632
Noroxin Tablets 2069
Omnicef Capsules 497
Omnicef for Oral Suspension 497
Orthoclone OKT3 Sterile Solution 2387
Paxil 1535
Paxil CR Controlled-Release Tablets 1544
Pentasa Capsules 3030
Plavix Tablets (Less than 1%) 926
Plavix Tablets (Less than 1%) 2767
Pletal Tablets 2481
Prinzide Tablets 2092
Prozac Weekly Capsules 1852
Prozac Pulvules and Liquid 1852
Rebetol 2917
Retrovir Capsules 1574
Retrovir IV Infusion 1579
Retrovir 1574
Rilutek Tablets (Rare) 2771
Rituxan I.V. 1223
Rocephin Injectable Vials, ADD-Vantage, Galaxy, Bulk 2642
Suprax for Oral Suspension 1891
Suprax Tablets 1891
Tekturna HCT Tablets 2324
Temodar Capsules 2931
Teveten HCT Tablets 517
Thioridazine Hydrochloride Tablets 2195
Trizivir Tablets 1622
Trusopt Sterile Ophthalmic Solution (Rare) 2128
▲ Valcyte Tablets (Less than 5%) 2654
Valtrex Caplets 1635
Venlafaxine Hydrochloride Tablets 2199
Voltaren Tablets (Rarely) 2334
Voltaren-XR Tablets (Rarely) 2337
Zantac 25 EFFERdose Tablets (Rare) 1670
Zantac Injection (Rare) 1666
Zantac Injection Pharmacy Bulk Package (Rare) 1668
Zantac Injection Premixed (Rare) 1666
Zantac (Rare) 1670
Zinacef for Injection 1678
Zinacef Injection 1678
Zonegran Capsules (Rare) 1089

Anemia, dilutional
Prolastin 3099

Anemia, hemolytic
Aceon Tablets (2 mg, 4 mg, 8 mg) 3038
Aciphex Tablets 1053
Aczone Gel 5% 3296
Advicor Tablets 402
Alphanate 1709
Amoxil Capsules 1305
Amoxil Chewable Tablets 1305
Amoxil Pediatric Drops for Oral Suspension 1305
Amoxil Powder for Oral Suspension 1305
Amoxil Tablets 1305
Anaprox Tablets (Less than 1%) 2632
Anaprox DS Tablets (Less than 1%) 2632
Aricept Tablets (Rare) 1062
Aricept ODT Tablets (Rare) 1062
Atacand HCT 642
Augmentin 1323
Augmentin Tablets 1327
Augmentin XR Extended Release Tablets 1333
Augmentin ES-600 Powder for Oral Suspension 1329
Avalide Tablets 892
Avalide Tablets 2713
Avandaryl Tablets 1344
Avelox 2803
Bicillin C-R Injectable Suspension 1775
Bicillin L-A Injection 1777
Campath Ampules 761
Captopril Tablets 2182
Cardizem LA Extended Release Tablets (Infrequent) 421
Ceftin 1380
Celexa 1160
Cipro I.V. (Rare) 2817
Cipro 2810
Cipro XR Tablets 2823
Clinoril Tablets (Less than 1 in 100) 1962
Crixivan Capsules 1979
Cuprimine Capsules 1986
Diovan HCT Tablets 2216
Duetact Tablets 3085
Dyazide Capsules 1405
EC-Naprosyn Delayed-Release Tablets (Less than 1%) 2632
Fansidar Tablets 2636
Fortaz (Rare) 1450
Furosemide Tablets 2186
Gamunex (Very rare) 3094
Gantrisin Pediatric Suspension 2638
Gengraf Capsules 435
Imitrex Injection 1465
Imitrex Tablets 1474
Indocin Capsules (Less than 1%) 2024
Indocin I.V. (Less than 1%) 2489
Indocin (Less than 1%) 2024
Intelence Tablets (Less than 2%) 3119
Intravenous Sodium Diuril 2490
▲ Intron A for Injection (Less than 5%) 2859
Lamictal 1488
Lescol Capsules (Rare) 2268
Lescol XL Tablets 2268
Leustatin Injection (Some reports) 2384
Levaquin 2416
Levaquin in 5% Dextrose Injection 2416
Lexapro Oral Suspension 1174
Lexapro Tablets 1174
Merrem I.V. 684
Mevacor Tablets (Rare) 2063
Micardis HCT Tablets 854
Moxatag Tablets 2165
Mustargen for Injection (Rare) 2492
Mycamine for Injection 616
Nalfon Capsules (Less than 1%) 2508
Naprosyn Suspension (Less than 1%) 2632
Naprosyn Tablets (Less than 1%) 2632
Neoral Oral Solution 2280
Neoral Soft Gelatin Capsules 2280
Noroxin Tablets (Rare) 2069
Omnicef Capsules 497
Omnicef for Oral Suspension 497
Orthoclone OKT3 Sterile Solution 2387
Paser Granules 1747
Paxil 1535
Paxil CR Controlled-Release Tablets 1544
PegIntron Powder for Injection 2903
Percocet Tablets 1127
Pneumovax 23 2078
PrandiMet Tablets 2967
Prandin Tablets (Rare) 2971
Primaxin I.M. 2080
Primaxin I.V. 2083
Prinivil Tablets (Rare) 2087
Prinzide Tablets 2092
Prograf Capsules and Injection 622
Pylera Capsules 714
Raptiva for Injection 1218
▲ Rebetol (10%) 2917
Remicade for IV Injection (Greater than or equal to 0.2%) 950
ReoPro Vials (0.3%) 1860
Retrovir Capsules 1574
Retrovir IV Infusion 1579
Retrovir 1574
Rituxan I.V. 1223
Rocephin Injectable Vials, ADD-Vantage, Galaxy, Bulk (Less than 1%) 2642
Skelaxin Tablets (Most frequent) 1784
Solodyn Extended Release Tablets 1938
Stalevo Tablets 2309
Sulfamylon Cream 2194
Sulfamylon for 5% Topical Solution 2194
Suprax for Oral Suspension 1891
Suprax Tablets 1891
Tekturna HCT Tablets 2324
Teveten HCT Tablets 517
Thiothixene Capsules 2197
Voltaren Tablets (Rarely) 2334
Voltaren-XR Tablets (Rarely) 2337
Vytorin 10/10 Tablets 2149
Vytorin 10/10 Tablets 2939
Vytorin 10/20 Tablets 2149
Vytorin 10/20 Tablets 2939
Vytorin 10/40 Tablets 2149
Vytorin 10/40 Tablets 2939
Vytorin 10/80 Tablets 2149
Vytorin 10/80 Tablets 2939
Zinacef for Injection 1678
Zinacef Injection 1678
Zocor Tablets (Rare) 2136
Zosyn for Injection 3284
Zyrtec Chewable Tablets 1920
Zyrtec Syrup 1920
Zyrtec Tablets 1920
Zyrtec-D 12 Hour Extended Release Tablets (Rare) 1923

Anemia, hemolytic, autoimmune
Fluarix Vaccine 1446

Anemia, hemolytic, immune
Eloxatin for Injection 2731
Prozac Weekly Capsules 1852
Prozac Pulvules and Liquid 1852
Zantac 25 EFFERdose Tablets (Exceedingly rare) 1670
Zantac Injection (Exceedingly rare) 1666
Zantac Injection Pharmacy Bulk Package (Rare) 1668
Zantac Injection Premixed (Exceedingly rare) 1666
Zantac (Exceedingly rare) 1670

Anemia, hypochromic
Celexa (Rare) 1160
CellCept Capsules 2622
CellCept Intravenous 2622
▲ CellCept Oral Suspension (24.6%) 2622
CellCept Tablets 2622
▲ Doxil Injection (5.2% to 9.8%) 2378
Evoxac Capsules (Less than 1%) 1013
Exelon Capsules (Infrequent) 2229
Exelon Oral Solution (Infrequent) 2229
Geodon Capsules (Rare) 2520
Lovenox Injection (2%) 2756
Lyrica Capsules (0.1% to 1%) 2527
Merrem I.V. (Greater than 0.1%) 684
Nexium Delayed-Release Capsules (Less than 1%) 645
Nexium I.V. (Less than 1%) 652
Nexium Delayed-Release Oral Suspension (Less than 1%) 645
Paxil (Rare) 1535
Paxil CR Controlled-Release Tablets (Rare) 1544
Plavix Tablets (Less than 1%) 926
Plavix Tablets (Less than 1%) 2767
▲ Prograf Capsules and Injection (3% to 15%) 622
Protonix for Delayed-Release Oral Suspension (Less than 1%) 3254
Protonix Delayed-Release Tablets (Less than 1%) 3254
Protonix I.V. (Less than 1%) 3257
Prozac Weekly Capsules (Rare) 1852
Prozac Pulvules and Liquid (Rare) 1852
Requip Tablets (Infrequent) 1561
Rilutek Tablets (Rare) 2771
▲ Targretin Capsules (3.6% to 13.2%) 1084

Anemia, iron deficiency
Aricept Tablets (Infrequent) 1062
Aricept ODT Tablets (Infrequent) 1062
Lamictal (Rare) 1488
Paxil (Rare) 1535
Paxil CR Controlled-Release Tablets (Rare) 1544
Percodan Tablets 1130
Pletal Tablets (Less than 2%) 2481
Protonix for Delayed-Release Oral Suspension (Less than 1%) 3254
Protonix Delayed-Release Tablets (Less than 1%) 3254
Protonix I.V. (Less than 1%) 3257
Prozac Weekly Capsules (Rare) 1852
Rilutek Tablets (Rare) 2771
Viadur Implant (Less than 2%) 802
Zyprexa IntraMuscular 1883

Anemia, macrocytic
Ambien Tablets (Rare) 2692
Ambien CR Tablets (Rare) 2696
Azilect Tablets (Infrequent) 3106
Depakote ER Tablets 423
Lamictal (Rare) 1488

Anemia, megaloblastic
Daraprim Tablets 1400
Dyazide Capsules 1405
Dyrenium Capsules (Rare) 3189
Fansidar Tablets 2636
Nembutal Sodium Solution, USP 2494
Phenytek Capsules 2192

Anemia, microangiopathic hemolytic
Gengraf Capsules 435
Plavix Tablets 926
Plavix Tablets 2767
Sandimmune (Occasional) 2296

Anemia, microcytic
Paxil (Rare) 1535
Paxil CR Controlled-Release Tablets (Rare) 1544
Zonegran Capsules (Rare) 1089

Anemia, nonhemolytic
Stalevo Tablets 2309

Anemia, normocytic
Paxil (Rare) 1535
Paxil CR Controlled-Release Tablets (Rare) 1544
Zyprexa Tablets (Infrequent) 1883
Zyprexa ZYDIS Orally Disintegrating Tablets (Infrequent) 1883

Anemia, sideroblastic
Cuprimine Capsules 1986

Anemia with thrombocytopenia, hemolytic, microangiopathic
Tarceva Tablets (0.8%) 1228

Anesthesia, local
Denavir Cream (0.9%) 2205

Anetoderma
Cuprimine Capsules (Rare) 1986

Aneurysm
Mirapex Tablets 857
Requip Tablets (Infrequent) 1561
Sandostatin LAR Depot 2302
Vivitrol 988

Aneurysm, aortic
Effexor XR Extended-Release Capsules (Rare) 3195
Imitrex Nasal Spray (Rare) 1470
Venlafaxine Hydrochloride Tablets (Rare) 2199

Anger
Abilify Injection (Greater than or equal to 1 in 1000 patients and less than 1 in 100 patients) 2466
Abilify Oral Solution (Greater than or equal to 1 in 1000 patients and less than 1 in 100 patients) 881
Abilify Oral Solution (Greater than or equal to 1 in 1000 patients and less than 1 in 100 patients) 2466
Abilify Discmelt Orally Disintegrating Tablets (Greater than or equal to 1 in 1000 patients and less than 1 in 100 patients) 881
Abilify Discmelt Orally Disintegrating Tablets (Greater than or equal to 1 in 1000 patients and less than 1 in 100 patients) 2466
Abilify Tablets (Greater than or equal to 1 in 1000 patients and less than 1 in 100 patients) 881
Abilify Tablets (Greater than or equal to 1 in 1000 patients and less than 1 in 100 patients) 2466
Concerta Extended-Release Tablets 1925
Cymbalta Delayed-Release Capsules 1801
▲ Keppra Injection (12.7% to 13.3%) 3137
Keppra Oral Solution 3131
Keppra Tablets 3131
Lexapro Oral Suspension 1174
Lexapro Tablets 1174
Meridia Capsules 475

Angiitis
Indocin Capsules (Less than 1%) 2024

Indocin I.V. (Less than 1%) 2489
Indocin (Less than 1%) 2024

Angina
Amerge Tablets 1301
▲ Avandaryl Tablets (5%) 1344
▲ Avandia Tablets (1.9% to 5%) 1351
Azor Tablets 1005
Brovana Inhalation Solution 2990
Cardizem LA Extended Release Tablets (Less than 2%) 421
Combivent Inhalation Aerosol (Less than 2%) 845
Concerta Extended-Release Tablets 1925
Daytrana Transdermal Patch 3022
Exforge Tablets 2238
Femara Tablets (Less than or equal to 2%) 2246
Focalin XR Capsules 2251
Foradil Aerolizer 2849
Imitrex Nasal Spray 1470
Imitrex Tablets (Rare) 1474
▲ Intron A for Injection (Less than 5%) 2859
Levothroid Tablets 1170
Levoxyl Tablets 1780
▲ Lupron Depot 7.5 mg (Less than 5%) 469
Metadate CD Capsules 3146
OptiPranolol Metipranolol Ophthalmic Solution 0.3% (A small number of patients) ⊙ 245
Orthoclone OKT3 Sterile Solution (Less than 1%) 2387
PegIntron Powder for Injection (Less than or equal to 1%) 2903
Perforomist Inhalation Solution 1025
PrandiMet Tablets (1.8%) 2967
Prandin Tablets (1.8%) 2971
Proventil HFA Inhalation Aerosol 2914
Rituxan I.V. 1223
▲ Rythmol Tablets (1% to 5%) 1586
Tarka Tablets (0.3% or more) 511
Tricor Tablets 520
Ventolin HFA Inhalation Aerosol 1638
Zofran Injection (Rare) 1682
Zofran (Rare) 1687
Zofran ODT Orally Disintegrating Tablets (Rare) 1687

Angina, crescendo
Nitro-Dur Transdermal Infusion System (Uncommon) 2887

Angina, increased
Azor Tablets 1005
Exforge Tablets 2238
Nitro-Dur Transdermal Infusion System (2%) 2887

Angina, Prinzmetal's, episodes of
Imitrex Injection 1465
Imitrex Nasal Spray 1470

Angina, unstable
Celebrex Capsules (Greater than or equal to 0.1% to less than 1%) 2979
Requip Tablets (Infrequent) 1561
Rythmol SR Capsules 1590
Selzentry Tablets 2534
Tamiflu Capsules (Less than 1%) 2649
Tamiflu Oral Suspension (Less than 1%) 2649
▲ Taxotere Injection Concentrate (8.1%) 2773
Vivitrol 988

Angina pectoris
Abilify Injection (Greater than or equal to 1 in 1000 patients and less than 1 in 100 patients) 2466
Abilify Oral Solution (Greater than or equal to 1 in 1000 patients and less than 1 in 100 patients) 881
Abilify Oral Solution (Greater than or equal to 1 in 1000 patients and less than 1 in 100 patients) 2466
Abilify Discmelt Orally Disintegrating Tablets (Greater than or equal to 1 in 1000 patients and less than 1 in 100 patients) 881
Abilify Discmelt Orally Disintegrating Tablets (Greater than or equal to 1 in 1000 patients and less than 1 in 100 patients) 2466
Abilify Tablets (Greater than or equal to 1 in 1000 patients and less than 1 in 100 patients) 881
Abilify Tablets (Greater than or equal to 1 in 1000 patients and less than 1 in 100 patients) 2466
Actiq (Less than 1%) 959
Actonel with Calcium Tablets (2.5%) 2574
Aggrenox Capsules 819
▲ Agrylin Capsules (1% to less than 5%) 3017
Ambien Tablets (Rare) 2692
Ambien CR Tablets (Rare) 2696
▲ Angiomax for Injection (5.3%) 1933
▲ Aranesp for Injection (8%) 564
Argatroban Injection (1.8%) 1308
Aricept Tablets (Infrequent) 1062
Aricept ODT Tablets (Infrequent) 1062
Arimidex Tablets 672
Atacand Tablets (Less frequently) 639
Atacand HCT (Less than 0.5%) 642
Avalide Tablets 892
Avalide Tablets 2713
Avapro Tablets (Less than 1%) 897
Avapro Tablets (Less than 1%) 2718
Azilect Tablets (Greater than 1%) 3106
Campral Tablets (Infrequent) 1158
Captopril Tablets (2 to 3 of 1000 patients) 2182
Cardene I.V. (Rare) 1093
Celebrex Capsules (0.1% to 1.9%) 2979
Celexa (Infrequent) 1160
▲ CellCept Capsules (3% to less than 20%) 2622
▲ CellCept Intravenous (3% to less than 20%) 2622
▲ CellCept Oral Suspension (3% to less than 20%) 2622
▲ CellCept Tablets (3% to less than 20%) 2622
Chantix Tablets (Infrequent) 2511
Cialis Tablets (Less than 2%) 1792
Cimzia 3127
Cipro I.V. (1% or less) 2817
Cipro (Less than 1%) 2810
Cipro XR Tablets 2823
Concerta Extended-Release Tablets 1925
▲ Coreg Tablets (2% to 6%) 1387
▲ Coreg CR Extended-Release Capsules (2% to 6%) 1393
Cosopt Sterile Ophthalmic Solution 1969
Cozaar Tablets (Less than 1%) 1973
Crixivan Capsules 1979
Doxil Injection (Less than 1%) 2378
Effexor XR Extended-Release Capsules (Infrequent) 3195
Eldepryl Capsules 3052
Evoxac Capsules (Less than 1%) 1013
Exelon Capsules (Frequent) 2229
Exelon Oral Solution (Frequent) 2229
Exelon Patch (Infrequent) 2233
Exubera Inhalation Powder (0.7%) 2515
▲ Flolan for Injection (19%) 1426
Forteo for Injection (2.5%) 1816
Gabitril Tablets (Infrequent) 973
Geodon Capsules (Infrequent) 2520
Imitrex Injection 1465
Imitrex Tablets 1474
Intelence Tablets (Less than 2%) 3119
Ixempra Kit for Injection 915
Lamictal (Rare) 1488
Levitra Tablets (Less than 2%) 2876
▲ Lexiscan Injection (12%) 614
Lipitor Tablets (Less than 2%) 2501
▲ Lovaza Capsules (1.3% to 3%) 1520
Luvox CR Extended-Release Capsules (Infrequent) 1759
Maxalt Tablets (Rare) 2056
Maxalt-MLT Orally Disintegrating Tablets (Rare) 2056
Meridia Capsules 475
▲ Miacalcin Nasal Spray (1% to 3%) 2274
Micardis Tablets (More than 0.3%) 852
Micardis HCT Tablets 854
Mobic Oral Suspension (Less than 2%) 863
Mobic Tablets (Less than 2%) 863
Namenda (Infrequent) 1180
▲ Natrecor for Injection (2% to 6%) 2977
NovoSeven 2367
NovoSeven RT 2370
Ortho-Cyclen/Ortho Tri-Cyclen 2449
Ortho Tri-Cyclen Lo Tablets 2458
Paxil (Rare) 1535
Paxil CR Controlled-Release Tablets (Rare) 1544
Persantine Tablets (Rare) 869
Photofrin for Injection 708
Pletal Tablets (2% or greater) 2481
Prinivil Tablets (Greater than 1%) 2087
Prinzide Tablets 2092
▲ Prograf Capsules and Injection (3% to 15%) 622
▲ Prometrium Capsules (100 mg, 200 mg) (Less than 5%) 3047
Protonix for Delayed-Release Oral Suspension (Less than 1%) 3254
Protonix Delayed-Release Tablets (Less than 1%) 3254
Protonix I.V. (Less than 1%) 3257
Protopic Ointment (Greater than or equal to 1%) 628
Prozac Weekly Capsules (Infrequent) 1852
Prozac Pulvules and Liquid (Infrequent) 1852
ReFacto Vials 3269
Remeron Tablets (Infrequent) 2924
RemeronSolTab Tablets (Infrequent) 2927
Requip Tablets (Infrequent) 1561
Rilutek Tablets (Infrequent) 2771
Risperdal Consta Long-Acting Injection (Infrequent) 1753
Rythmol SR Capsules (2%) 1590
Salagen Tablets (Less than 1%) 1082
▲ Simulect for Injection (3% to 10%) 2306
▲ Spiriva HandiHaler (1% to 3%) 870
Symbyax Capsules (Rare) 1871
Targretin Capsules 1084
Tasigna Capsules (0.1% to 1%) 2316
Teveten Tablets (Less than 1%) 515
Teveten HCT Tablets (Less than 1%) 517
▲ Travatan Z Ophthalmic Solution (1% to 5%) 547
Tricor Tablets 520
Uroxatral Tablets 2786
Velcade for Injection 2168
Venlafaxine Hydrochloride Tablets (Infrequent) 2199
Vivitrol 988
Zomig Tablets (Rare) 694
Zomig Nasal Spray (Rare) 689
Zomig-ZMT Tablets (Rare) 694

Angina pectoris, aggravation
Combigan Ophthalmic Solution 553
▲ Coreg Tablets (Greater than 1% to 3%) 1387
▲ Coreg CR Extended-Release Capsules (Greater than 1% to less than or equal to 3%) 1393
Eldepryl Capsules 3052
▲ Spiriva HandiHaler (1% to 3%) 870
Timoptic Sterile Ophthalmic Solution (Less frequent) 2121
Timoptic in Ocudose (Less frequent) 2124
Timoptic-XE Sterile Ophthalmic Gel Forming Solution 2125

Angina pectoris, exacerbation of, post-abrupt discontinuation
InnoPran XL Extended Release Capsules 1484
Toprol-XL Tablets 666

Angioedema
(*see also under* Edema, angioneurotic)
Abilify Injection 881
Abilify Injection (Greater than or equal to 1 in 1000 patients and less than 1 in 100 patients) 2466
Abilify Oral Solution (Less than 1 in 1000 patients) 881
Abilify Oral Solution (Greater than or equal to 1 in 1000 patients and less than 1 in 100 patients) 2466
Abilify Discmelt Orally Disintegrating Tablets (Less than 1 in 1000 patients) 881
Abilify Discmelt Orally Disintegrating Tablets (Greater than or equal to 1 in 1000 patients and less than 1 in 100 patients) 2466
Abilify Tablets (Less than 1 in 1000 patients) 881
Abilify Tablets (Greater than or equal to 1 in 1000 patients and less than 1 in 100 patients) 2466
Aceon Tablets (2 mg, 4 mg, 8 mg) (0.1%) 3038
▲ Acetadote Injection (1.62% to 7.73%) 1001
Aciphex Tablets 1053
Actonel Tablets (Rare) 2568
Actonel with Calcium Tablets (Very rare) 2574
Adderall XR Capsules 3012
Advair Diskus 100/50 (2%) 1276
Advair Diskus 250/50 1276
Advair Diskus 500/50 1276
Advair HFA 45/21 Inhalation Aerosol (Rare) 1288
Advair HFA 115/21 Inhalation Aerosol (Rare) 1288
Advair HFA 230/21 Inhalation Aerosol (Rare) 1288
Advicor Tablets (Rare) 402
Aldara Cream, 5% 1699
Allegra Oral Solution (Rare) 2684
Allegra Tablets (Rare) 2684
Allegra-D 12 Hour Extended-Release Tablets (Rare) 2687
Allegra-D 24 Hour Extended-Release Tablets (Rare) 2690
Ambien CR Tablets (Rare) 2696
AmBisome for Injection (Infrequent) 606
Amevive 611
Aminohippurate Sodium "PAH" Injection 1950
Amrix Capsules 966
Angeliq Tablets 751
Arimidex Tablets (Very rare) 672
Atacand Tablets (Less frequently) 639
Atacand HCT (Less than 0.5%) 642
Atrovent HFA Inhalation Aerosol 839
Atrovent Nasal Spray 0.03% 834
Augmentin 1323
Augmentin Tablets 1327
Augmentin XR Extended Release Tablets 1333
Augmentin ES-600 Powder for Oral Suspension 1329
Avalide Tablets (Rare) 892
Avalide Tablets (Rare) 2713
Avandamet Tablets 1336
Avandaryl Tablets (Rare) 1344
Avandia Tablets 1351
Avapro Tablets (Rare) 897
Avapro Tablets (Rare) 2718
Avelox 2803
Avodart Soft Gelatin Capsules 1359
Azor Tablets 1005
Bayer Aspirin 750
Beconase AQ Nasal Spray (Rare) 1369
BeneFIX Vials 3191
Benicar Tablets 1009
Benicar HCT Tablets (Rare) 1010
Brovana Inhalation Solution 2990
Bystolic Tablets (Rare) 1155
Campath Ampules 761
Captopril Tablets (Approximately 1 in 1000 patients) 2182
Cardizem LA Extended Release Tablets (Infrequent) 421
Catapres Tablets 841
Ceftin 1380
Celebrex Capsules (Less than 0.1%) 2979
Celexa 1160
▲ Cerezyme for Injection (Approximately 6.6%) 1238
Cimzia (Rare) 3127
Cipro I.V. (1% or less) 2817
Cipro (Less than 1%) 2810
Cipro XR Tablets 2823
Climara Transdermal System 763
Combigan Ophthalmic Solution 553
Combivent Inhalation Aerosol (Rare) 845
Comvax 1966
Concerta Extended-Release Tablets 1925
Copaxone for Injection (Infrequent) 3110
Coreg CR Extended-Release Capsules 1393
Cosopt Sterile Ophthalmic Solution 1969
Cozaar Tablets (Rare) 1973
Crestor Tablets 677
Daytrana Transdermal Patch 3022
Demadex Injection 2630
Demadex Tablets 2630
Didronel Tablets 2583
Diovan Tablets 2212
Diovan HCT Tablets (Rare to less frequent) 2216
Divigel 3167
DynaCirc CR Controlled Release Tablets 1407
Eloxatin for Injection 2731
Emend Capsules (One patient) 1992
Emend for Injection (One patient) 1999
Enablex Extended-Release Tablets 2225
Enbrel for Injection 569
Enjuvia Tablets 1029
Erbitux 912
Estratest Tablets 3043
Estratest H.S. Tablets 3043

Exforge Tablets (Rare to less than 1%) 2238
Exjade Tablets 2244
Faslodex Injection (Less than 1%) 682
Flomax Capsules 848
Flovent Diskus 50 mcg (Rare) 1435
Flovent HFA 1440
Fluarix Vaccine 1446
Foradil Aerolizer (Rare) 2849
Fortaz (Very rare) 1450
Fosamax (Rare) 2005
Fosamax Plus D Tablets (Rarely) 2013
Gantrisin Pediatric Suspension 2638
Geodon (Rare) 2520
Gleevec Tablets (Rare) 2255
Herceptin I.V. 1199
Hycamtin for Injection (Rare) 1459
Indocin (Less than 1%) 2024
Janumet Tablets 2041
Januvia Tablets 2048
Ketek Tablets (Rare) 2744
Kinrix Injection Vaccine 1486
Lamisil Oral Granules 2264
Lamisil Tablets (Rare) 2266
Levaquin 2416
Levaquin in 5% Dextrose Injection 2416
Levothroid Tablets 1170
Levoxyl Tablets 1780
Lexapro Oral Suspension 1174
Lexapro Tablets 1174
Lexiva Oral Suspension 1510
Lexiva Tablets 1510
Luvox CR Extended-Release Capsules 1759
Lyrica Capsules (Rare) 2527
Maxalt Tablets 2056
Maxalt-MLT Orally Disintegrating Tablets 2056
Mepron Suspension 1526
Merrem I.V. 684
Micardis Tablets (Single case) 852
Micardis HCT Tablets 854
Mobic Oral Suspension (Less than 2%) 863
Mobic Tablets (Less than 2%) 863
Nalfon Capsules (Less than 1%) 2508
Nasonex Nasal Spray 2883
Nembutal Sodium Solution, USP 2494
Neulasta Injection 587
Nexium Delayed-Release Capsules (Less than 1%) 645
Nexium I.V. (Less than 1%) 652
Nexium Delayed-Release Oral Suspension (Less than 1%) 645
Noroxin Tablets 2069
Ortho-Cyclen Tablets 2449
Ortho Evra Transdermal System 2437
Ortho Tri-Cyclen Tablets 2449
Pediarix Vaccine 1552
Pentasa Capsules 3030
Percocet Tablets 1127
Persantine Tablets (Rare) 869
Plavix Tablets 926
Plavix Tablets 2767
Premarin Intravenous 3217
Premarin Tablets 3221
Premarin Vaginal Cream 3228
Premphase Tablets 3232
Prempro Tablets 3232
Prinivil Tablets (0.1% to 1%) 2087
Protonix for Delayed-Release Oral Suspension 3254
Protonix Delayed-Release Tablets 3254
Protonix I.V. 3257
Protopic Ointment (Greater than or equal to 1%) 628
Provigil Tablets 977
Prozac Weekly Capsules 1852
Pulmicort Flexhaler 654
Qvar Inhalation Aerosol (Rare) 3116
Rapamune 3260
Recombivax HB (Less than 1%) 2107
Risperdal Consta Long-Acting Injection 1753
▲ Rituxan I.V. (1% to 11%) 1223
St. Joseph 81 mg Aspirin Chewable and Enteric Coated Tablets 1903
Seasonique Tablets 1046
Singulair 2114
Spiriva HandiHaler (Less than 1%) 870
Stalevo Tablets 2309
Suprax for Oral Suspension (Less than 2%) 1891
Suprax Tablets (Less than 2%) 1891
Synagis Intramuscular Solution 1948
Tekturna Tablets (0.06%) 2321
Tekturna HCT Tablets (0.6%) 2324
Timoptic Sterile Ophthalmic Solution 2121
Timoptic in Ocudose 2124
Timoptic-XE Sterile Ophthalmic Gel Forming Solution 2125
TNKase (Less than 1%) 1233
Trusopt Sterile Ophthalmic Solution 2128
Twinrix Vaccine 1628
Uroxatral Tablets 2786
Valtrex Caplets 1635
Velcade for Injection 2168
Ventolin HFA Inhalation Aerosol 1638
Viramune Oral Suspension 873
Viramune Tablets 873
Voltaren Tablets (Rarely) 2334
Voltaren-XR Tablets (Rarely) 2337
Vytorin 10/10 Tablets 2149
Vytorin 10/10 Tablets 2939
Vytorin 10/20 Tablets 2149
Vytorin 10/20 Tablets 2939
Vytorin 10/40 Tablets 2149
Vytorin 10/40 Tablets 2939
Vytorin 10/80 Tablets 2149
Vytorin 10/80 Tablets 2939
Vyvanse Capsules 3033
Xenical Capsules 2672
Xopenex Inhalation Solution 3001
Xopenex Inhalation Solution Concentrate 3005
Xopenex HFA Inhalation Aerosol 3009
Yaz Tablets 805
Zetia Tablets 2157
Zetia Tablets 2951
Zinacef for Injection 1678
Zinacef Injection 1678
Zocor Tablets (Rare) 2136
Zofran Injection 1682
Zofran 1687
Zofran ODT Orally Disintegrating Tablets 1687
Zometa for Intravenous Infusion 2341
Zyprexa Tablets 1883
Zyprexa ZYDIS Orally Disintegrating Tablets 1883
Zyrtec Chewable Tablets (Less than 2%) 1920
Zyrtec Syrup (Less than 2%) 1920
Zyrtec Tablets (Less than 2%) 1920
Zyrtec-D 12 Hour Extended Release Tablets (Less than 2%) 1923
Zyvox 2552

Angioedema, cutaneous
Xolair 1235
Xolair 2339

Angioedema, extremities
Aceon Tablets (2 mg, 4 mg, 8 mg) (0.1%) 3038
Captopril Tablets (Approximately 1 in 1000 patients) 2182
Mavik Tablets 472
▲ Neupro Transdermal System (7%) 3149
Prinivil Tablets (0.1%) 2087
Prinzide Tablets (Rare) 2092
Tekturna Tablets 2321
Tekturna HCT Tablets 2324

Angioedema, eyes
▲ Advair HFA 45/21 Inhalation Aerosol (1% to 3%) 1288
▲ Advair HFA 115/21 Inhalation Aerosol (1% to 3%) 1288
▲ Advair HFA 230/21 Inhalation Aerosol (1% to 3%) 1288
Captopril Tablets 2182
Ofloxacin Ophthalmic Solution 0.3% ⊙243

Angioedema, face
Aceon Tablets (2 mg, 4 mg, 8 mg) (0.1%) 3038
Atrovent HFA Inhalation Aerosol 839
Atrovent Nasal Spray 0.03% 834
Atrovent Nasal Spray 0.06% 836
Avalide Tablets (Rare) 892
Avalide Tablets (Rare) 2713
Avapro Tablets (Rare) 897
Avapro Tablets (Rare) 2718
Captopril Tablets (Approximately 1 in 1000 patients) 2182
Catapres-TTS (2 of 3,539 patients) 842
Combivent Inhalation Aerosol 845
Cozaar Tablets (Rare) 1973
Flomax Capsules 848
Levaquin 2416
Levaquin in 5% Dextrose Injection 2416
Mavik Tablets (0.13%) 472
Ofloxacin Ophthalmic Solution 0.3% ⊙243
Prinivil Tablets 2087
Prinzide Tablets (Rare) 2092
Tekturna HCT Tablets 2324

Angioedema, glottis
Aceon Tablets (2 mg, 4 mg, 8 mg) (0.1%) 3038
Ambien Tablets 2692
Captopril Tablets (Approximately 1 in 1000 patients) 2182
Cozaar Tablets (Rare) 1973
Mavik Tablets (0.3% to 1%) 472
Prinivil Tablets 2087
Prinzide Tablets (Rare) 2092
Tarka Tablets 511
Tekturna HCT Tablets 2324

Angioedema, intestinal
Aceon Tablets (2 mg, 4 mg, 8 mg) 3038
Captopril Tablets 2182
Mavik Tablets 472
Prinivil Tablets (Rare) 2087
Prinzide Tablets (Rare) 2092

Angioedema, larynx
Aceon Tablets (2 mg, 4 mg, 8 mg) (0.1%) 3038
Activase I.V. 1188
Ambien Tablets 2692
Captopril Tablets (Approximately 1 in 1000 patients) 2182
Levaquin 2416
Levaquin in 5% Dextrose Injection 2416
Mavik Tablets 472
Prinivil Tablets 2087
Prinzide Tablets (Rare) 2092
Tekturna HCT Tablets 2324

Angioedema, lips
Aceon Tablets (2 mg, 4 mg, 8 mg) (0.1%) 3038
Atrovent HFA Inhalation Aerosol 839
Atrovent Nasal Spray 0.03% 834
Atrovent Nasal Spray 0.06% 836
Avalide Tablets (Rare) 892
Avalide Tablets (Rare) 2713
Avapro Tablets (Rare) 897
Avapro Tablets (Rare) 2718
Captopril Tablets (Approximately 1 in 1000 patients) 2182
Combivent Inhalation Aerosol 845
Cozaar Tablets (Rare) 1973
Flomax Capsules 848
Mavik Tablets 472
Prinivil Tablets 2087
Prinzide Tablets (Rare) 2092
Tekturna HCT Tablets 2324

Angioedema, mucous membranes of the mouth
Activase I.V. 1188
Captopril Tablets 2182

Angioedema, oropharyngeal
Avalide Tablets (Rare) 892
Avalide Tablets (Rare) 2713
Avapro Tablets (Rare) 897
Avapro Tablets (Rare) 2718
Cozaar Tablets (Rare) 1973

Angioedema, throat
Atrovent Nasal Spray 0.03% 834
Atrovent Nasal Spray 0.06% 836
Levaquin 2416
Levaquin in 5% Dextrose Injection 2416
Xolair 1235
Xolair 2339

Angioedema, tongue
Aceon Tablets (2 mg, 4 mg, 8 mg) (0.1%) 3038
Ambien Tablets 2692
Atrovent HFA Inhalation Aerosol 839
Atrovent Nasal Spray 0.03% 834
Atrovent Nasal Spray 0.06% 836
Avalide Tablets (Rare) 892
Avalide Tablets (Rare) 2713
Avapro Tablets (Rare) 897
Avapro Tablets (Rare) 2718
Captopril Tablets (Approximately 1 in 1000 patients) 2182
Catapres-TTS (One case) 842
Combivent Inhalation Aerosol 845
Cozaar Tablets (Rare) 1973
Flomax Capsules 848
Levaquin 2416
Levaquin in 5% Dextrose Injection 2416
Mavik Tablets 472
Prinivil Tablets 2087
Prinzide Tablets (Rare) 2092
Tekturna Tablets 2321
Tekturna HCT Tablets 2324
Xolair 1235
Xolair 2339

Angiomyolipoma
Requip Tablets (Infrequent) 1561

Angiopathy
Mirapex Tablets 857

Angitis, necrotizing
Tekturna HCT Tablets 2324

Angulation, penile
▲ Edex Injection (7%) 2957

Anisocoria
Lyrica Capsules (Rare) 2527
Paxil (Rare) 1535
Paxil CR Controlled-Release Tablets (Rare) 1544

Anorexia
Abelcet Injection 1134
Abilify Injection (Greater than or equal to 1 in 1000 patients and less than 1 in 100 patients) 2466
Abilify Oral Solution (Greater than or equal to 1 in 1000 patients and less than 1 in 100 patients) 881
Abilify Oral Solution (Greater than or equal to 1 in 1000 patients and less than 1 in 100 patients) 2466
Abilify Discmelt Orally Disintegrating Tablets (Greater than or equal to 1 in 1000 patients and less than 1 in 100 patients) 881
Abilify Discmelt Orally Disintegrating Tablets (Greater than or equal to 1 in 1000 patients and less than 1 in 100 patients) 2466
Abilify Tablets (Greater than or equal to 1 in 1000 patients and less than 1 in 100 patients) 881
Abilify Tablets (Greater than or equal to 1 in 1000 patients and less than 1 in 100 patients) 2466
▲ Actimmune (3%) 1743
Actiq (Less than 1%) 959
▲ Adderall XR Capsules (2.9% to 33%) 3012
Advicor Tablets 402
Aggrenox Capsules (1.2%) 819
▲ Agrylin Capsules (7.7%) 3017
▲ Alferon N Injection (1% to 68%) 1726
▲ Alimta for Injection (1% to 62%) 1786
Alinia for Oral Suspension (Less than 1%) 2677
Alinia Tablets (Less than 1%) 2677
Aloxi Injection (Less than 1%) 1059
Ambien Tablets (Infrequent) 2692
AmBisome for Injection (Less common) 606
Amitiza Capsules (Less than 1%) 3082
Amrix Capsules 966
Anzemet Injection (Rare) 2701
Anzemet Tablets 2704
Aptivus Capsules (Less than 2%) 823
Aptivus Oral Solution (Less than 2%) 823
▲ Aricept Tablets (2% to 8%) 1062
▲ Aricept ODT Tablets (2% to 8%) 1062
▲ Arimidex Tablets (5% to 8%) 672
▲ Arranon Injection (0% to 9%) 1319
Asacol Delayed-Release Tablets 2579
Asmanex Twisthaler (1% to less than 3%) 2797
Atacand HCT 642
Atripla Tablets (Greater than or equal to 2%) 938
▲ Avastin IV (35% to 43%) 1192
Avelox (Greater than or equal to 0.1% to less than 2%) 2803
▲ Avinza Capsules (5% to 10%) 1772
Axid Capsules (1.2%) 1364
▲ Azilect Tablets (5%) 3106
Bentyl Capsules 703
Bentyl Injection 703
Bentyl Syrup 703
Bentyl Tablets 703
Betaseron for SC Injection 756
▲ Bexxar (0% to 14%) 1371
Biaxin/Biaxin XL 411
▲ Busulfex Injection (21% to 85%) 2477
Calcijex Injection 419
▲ Campral Tablets (2% to 5%) 1158
Cancidas for Injection 1953
Captopril Tablets (About 0.5% to 2%) 2182
Carbatrol Capsules 3019
Cardizem LA Extended Release Tablets (Less than 2%) 421
Catapres Tablets (About 1 in 100 patients) 841
Catapres-TTS (0.5% or less) 842
Ceftin Tablets (0.1% to 1%) 1380
Celebrex Capsules (0.1% to 1.9%) 2979
▲ Celexa (4%) 1160

▲ CellCept Capsules (3% to 25.3%) 2622
▲ CellCept Intravenous (3% to 25.3%) 2622
▲ CellCept Oral Suspension (3% to 25.3%) 2622
▲ CellCept Tablets (3% to 25.3%) 2622
Chantix Tablets (1% to 2%) 2511
Cipro I.V. (1% or less) 2817
Cipro (Less than 1%) 2810
Cipro XR Tablets (Less than 1%) 2823
▲ Clarinex Syrup (4.5%) 2828
Clarinex-D 12-Hour Extended-Release Tablets (2%) 2831
Clarinex-D 24-Hour Extended-Release Tablets (2%) 2834
Clinoril Tablets (Greater than 1%) 1962
▲ Clolar for Intravenous Infusion (31%) 1239
Clorpres Tablets (About 1%) 2185
Combigan Ophthalmic Solution 553
▲ Combivir Tablets (10%) 1384
▲ Comvax (0.8% to 3.9%) 1966
▲ Concerta Extended-Release Tablets (1.7%) 1925
▲ Copaxone for Injection (8%) 3110
Cosmegen for Injection 2485
Cosopt Sterile Ophthalmic Solution 1969
Cozaar Tablets (Less than 1%) 1973
Crixivan Capsules (2.7%) 1979
▲ Cuprimine Capsules (17%) 1986
▲ Cymbalta Delayed-Release Capsules (3% to 10%) 1801
▲ Dacogen Injection (16%) 1066
Dantrium Capsules (Rare) 2580
Daraprim Tablets 1400
▲ Daytrana Transdermal Patch (4% to 46%) 3022
▲ Depakote ER Tablets (4% to 12%) 423
▲ DepoCyt Injection (3% to 5%) 1136
Dexedrine 1401
Diovan Tablets 2212
Diovan HCT Tablets (Less frequent) 2216
▲ Doxil Injection (1% to 20.1%) 2378
▲ Duragesic Transdermal System (3% to 10%) 2405
Edecrin 698
E.E.S. (Among most frequent) 433
▲ Effexor XR Extended-Release Capsules (5% to 17%) 3195
Eldepryl Capsules 3052
Elmiron Capsules (Less than or equal to 1%) 2435
▲ Eloxatin for Injection (1% to 35%) 2731
Elspar for Injection 1990
▲ Emend Capsules (4.3% to 10.1%) 1992
▲ Emend for Injection (4.3% to 10.1%) 1999
Emsam Transdermal System (Frequent) 905
Enbrel for Injection 569
Engerix-B Vaccine (Less than 1%) 1409
▲ Epivir (10%) 1412
Equetro Extended-Release Capsules 3174
EryPed (Among most frequent) 431
▲ Evoxac Capsules (1% to 3%) 1013
▲ Exelon Capsules (6% to 17%) 2229
▲ Exelon Oral Solution (6% to 17%) 2229
▲ Exelon Patch (3% to 9%) 2233
Exforge Tablets (Greater than 0.1% to less than 1%) 2238
▲ Faslodex Injection (9%) 682
▲ Femara Tablets (3% to 5%) 2246
▲ Fentora Tablets (1% to 11%) 968
▲ Flolan for Injection (25% to 66%) 1426
Flumadine (1.6%) 1167
Focalin XR Capsules 2251
Frova Tablets (Infrequent) 1111
Furosemide Tablets 2186
Gabitril Tablets (1% or more) 973
Gantrisin Pediatric Suspension 2638
▲ Gemzar for Injection (16%) 1820
▲ Gengraf Capsules (Less than 2% to 3%) 435
Geodon (2% to frequent) 2520
▲ Gleevec Tablets (7% to 17%) 2255
▲ Havrix Injection Vaccine (1% to 10%) 1454
▲ Herceptin I.V. (14%) 1199
Hexalen Capsules (1%) 1078
▲ Hycamtin Capsules (7% to 14%) 1456
▲ Hycamtin for Injection (Up to 19%) 1459
▲ Indapamide Tablets (Less than 5%) 2188
Indocin (Less than 1%) 2024
Intelence Tablets (Less than 2%) 3119
Intravenous Sodium Diuril 2490
▲ Intron A for Injection (1% to 69%) 2859
Invanz for Injection (Greater than 0.1%) 2029
▲ Ixempra Kit for Injection (19% to greater than or equal to 20%) 915
▲ Kaletra (1% to 3%) 452
▲ Keppra Injection (3%) 3137
▲ Keppra Oral Solution (3% to 13%) 3131
▲ Keppra Tablets (3% to 13%) 3131
Ketek Tablets (Greater than or equal to 0.2% to less than 2%) 2744
Klonopin 2639
Lamictal (2%) 1488
Lamisil Tablets 2266
Lanoxin Injection (Common) 1498
Lanoxin Injection Pediatric 1502
Lanoxin Tablets 1505
Lescol Capsules 2268
Lescol XL Tablets 2268
▲ Leukine (13% to 54%) 774
Levaquin (0.1% to 1%) 2416
Levaquin in 5% Dextrose Injection (0.1% to 1%) 2416
Lexapro Oral Suspension 1174
Lexapro Tablets 1174
Lipitor Tablets (Less than 2%) 2501
Lovaza Capsules 1520
Lunesta Tablets (Infrequent) 2994
▲ Lupron Depot 7.5 mg (Less than 5%) 469
▲ Luvox CR Extended-Release Capsules (2% to 14%) 1759
▲ Malarone Pediatric Tablets (5%) 1521
▲ Malarone Tablets (5%) 1521
Marinol Capsules (Less than 1%) 3163
Maxair Autohaler 1705
Maxalt Tablets (Rare) 2056
Maxalt-MLT Orally Disintegrating Tablets (Rare) 2056
▲ Mepron Suspension (7%) 1526
▲ Meridia Capsules (13%) 475
Merrem I.V. (Greater than 0.1% to 1%) 684
▲ Metadate CD Capsules (9%) 3146
Mevacor Tablets (Rare) 2063
Miacalcin Nasal Spray (Less than 1%) 2274
▲ Mirapex Tablets (Greater than or equal to 1% to 4%) 857
MS Contin Tablets (Less frequent) 2585
Mustargen for Injection 2492
▲ Mycamine for Injection (6.2% to 27.3%) 616
Myleran Tablets 1530
▲ Mylotarg for Injection (22% to 27%) 3212
Nadolol Tablets (1 to 5 of 1000 patients) 2191
Nalfon Capsules (Less than 1%) 2508
Namenda (Greater than or equal to 2%) 1180
▲ Neoral Oral Solution (2% or less to 3%) 2280
▲ Neoral Soft Gelatin Capsules (2% or less to 3%) 2280
▲ Neulasta Injection (15% to 72%) 587
▲ Neupogen for Injection (9%) 589
▲ Neupro Transdermal System (3%) 3149
▲ Nexavar Tablets (16% to 29%) 784
Nexium Delayed-Release Capsules (Less than 1%) 645
Nexium I.V. (Less than 1%) 652
Nexium Delayed-Release Oral Suspension (Less than 1%) 645
Noroxin Tablets (Less frequent) 2069
▲ Norvir (1.7% to 7.8%) 489
▲ Novantrone for Injection Concentrate (22% to 25%) 1100
▲ Noxafil Oral Suspension (1% to 19%) 2889
Omnicef Capsules (0.3%) 497
Omnicef for Oral Suspension (0.3%) 497
▲ Ontak Vials (36%) 1079
Ortho-Cyclen/Ortho Tri-Cyclen 2449
Ortho Tri-Cyclen Lo Tablets 2458
Orthoclone OKT3 Sterile Solution (Less than 1%) 2387
▲ OxyContin Tablets (Between 1% and 5%) 2589
Parnate Tablets 1532
Paser Granules (Less frequent) 1747
Pediarix Vaccine 1552
▲ PegIntron Powder for Injection (20%) 2903
Pentasa Capsules (Less than 1% to 1.1%) 3030
Pepcid Tablets (Infrequent) 2075
Percodan Tablets 1130
PhosLo GelCaps 1184
▲ Photofrin for Injection (4% to 8%) 708
Pletal Tablets (Less than 2%) 2481
Potaba (Infrequent) 1698
Prinivil Tablets (Greater than 1%) 2087
Prinzide Tablets 2092
Proglycem Capsules (Frequent) 1185
Proglycem Suspension (Frequent) 1185
▲ Prograf Capsules and Injection (3% to 34%) 622
▲ Proleukin for Injection (20%) 2287
Prometrium Capsules (100 mg, 200 mg) 3047
ProQuad (Greater than or equal to 0.2% to less than 1%) 2099
Protonix for Delayed-Release Oral Suspension (Less than 1%) 3254
Protonix Delayed-Release Tablets (Less than 1%) 3254
Protonix I.V. (Less than 1%) 3257
Protopic Ointment (Greater than or equal to 1%) 628
▲ Provigil Tablets (4%) 977
▲ Prozac Weekly Capsules (4% to 17%) 1852
▲ Prozac Pulvules and Liquid (8% to 17%) 1852
▲ Rebetol (21% to 51%) 2917
Reclast Injection (1%) 2291
ReFacto Vials 3269
▲ Relenza Inhalation Powder (2% to 4%) 1556
Remeron Tablets (Frequent) 2924
RemeronSolTab Tablets (Frequent) 2927
▲ Requip Tablets (Infrequent to 4%) 1561
▲ Retrovir Capsules (11% to 20.1%) 1574
▲ Retrovir IV Infusion (11% to 20.1%) 1579
▲ Retrovir (11% to 20.1%) 1574
▲ Rilutek Tablets (3.8% to 8.6%) 2771
Risperdal Consta Long-Acting Injection (Infrequent) 1753
Rocaltrol Capsules 1150
Rocaltrol Oral Solution 1150
Rythmol Tablets (2%) 1586
Rythmol SR Capsules 1590
Salagen Tablets (Less than 1%) 1082
Sandimmune (2% or less) 2296
▲ Sensipar Tablets (6%) 594
▲ Soriatane Capsules (1% to 10%) 3062
Stalevo Tablets 2309
▲ Strattera Capsules (3%) 1864
Stromectol Tablets (0.9%) 2120
Sular Extended Release Tablets (Less than or equal to 1%) 2975
Sustiva Capsules (Less than 1% to 2%) 930
Sustiva Tablets (Less than 1% to 2%) 930
▲ Sutent Capsules (1% to 33%) 2540
Tabloid Tablets (Less frequent) 1601
▲ Tarceva Tablets (Less than 1% to 52%) 1228
▲ Targretin Capsules (2.4% to 22.6%) 1084
▲ Tasigna Capsules (1% to 10%) 2316
▲ Taxotere Injection Concentrate (0.6% to 50.7%) 2773
▲ Temodar Capsules (1% to 27%) 2931
Teveten Tablets (Less than 1%) 515
Teveten HCT Tablets (Less than 1%) 517
Thioridazine Hydrochloride Tablets 2195
Thiothixene Capsules 2197
Tice BCG (2%) 2936
Timoptic Sterile Ophthalmic Solution (Less frequent) 2121
Timoptic in Ocudose (Less frequent) 2124
Timoptic-XE Sterile Ophthalmic Gel Forming Solution 2125
▲ Torisel Injection (3% to 32%) 3272
Tricor Tablets 520
▲ Trisenox Injection (23%) 986
▲ Trizivir Tablets (15%) 1622
Twinrix Vaccine (Less than 1%) 1628
Tygacil for Injection (0.2% to less than 2%) 3276
▲ Ultram ER Extended-Release Tablets (0.7% to 5.9%) 2428
Valtrex Caplets (Less than 1% to 2%) 1635
Vaqta (1.2%) 2130
▲ Velcade for Injection (23% to 36%) 2168
▲ Venlafaxine Hydrochloride Tablets (10% to 17%) 2199
▲ Vesanoid Capsules (17%) 2660
Vicoprofen Tablets (Less than 3%) 533
Viramune Oral Suspension 873
Viramune Tablets 873
▲ Viread Tablets (3% to 4%) 1268
▲ Vivitrol (6% to 20%) 988
▲ Vyvanse Capsules (5%) 3033
▲ Wellbutrin Tablets (18.3%) 1648
▲ Wellbutrin SR Sustained-Release Tablets (3% to greater than or equal to 5%) 1653
▲ Wellbutrin XL Extended-Release Tablets (3% to greater than or equal to 5%) 1659
▲ Xeloda Tablets (1% to 13%) 2662
Xifaxan Tablets (Less than 2%) 2682
Xyrem Oral Solution (Frequent) 1766
▲ Zolinza Capsules (21% to 24.4%) 2142
▲ Zometa for Intravenous Infusion (9% to 22%) 2341
Zomig Tablets (Rare) 694
Zomig-ZMT Tablets (Rare) 694
▲ Zonegran Capsules (13%) 1089
▲ Zyban Sustained-Release Tablets (1% to 3%) 1692
Zyprexa Tablets 1883
Zyprexa ZYDIS Orally Disintegrating Tablets 1883
Zyrtec Chewable Tablets (Less than 2%) 1920
Zyrtec Syrup (Less than 2%) 1920
Zyrtec Tablets (Less than 2%) 1920
Zyrtec-D 12 Hour Extended Release Tablets (Less than 2%) 1923

Anorgasmia

Abilify Injection (Greater than or equal to 1 in 1000 patients and less than 1 in 100 patients) 2466
Abilify Oral Solution (Greater than or equal to 1 in 1000 patients and less than 1 in 100 patients) 881
Abilify Oral Solution (Greater than or equal to 1 in 1000 patients and less than 1 in 100 patients) 2466
Abilify Discmelt Orally Disintegrating Tablets (Greater than or equal to 1 in 1000 patients and less than 1 in 100 patients) 881
Abilify Discmelt Orally Disintegrating Tablets (Greater than or equal to 1 in 1000 patients and less than 1 in 100 patients) 2466
Abilify Tablets (Greater than or equal to 1 in 1000 patients and less than 1 in 100 patients) 881
Abilify Tablets (Greater than or equal to 1 in 1000 patients and less than 1 in 100 patients) 2466
▲ Cymbalta Delayed-Release Capsules (Frequent to 3%) 1801
▲ Duragesic Transdermal System (4%) 2405
▲ Effexor XR Extended-Release Capsules (3% to 17%) 3195
Eldepryl Capsules 3052
Emsam Transdermal System (0.2%) 905
Geodon Capsules (Infrequent) 2520
Lamictal (Rare) 1488
▲ Lexapro Oral Suspension (2% to 6%) 1174
▲ Lexapro Tablets (2% to 6%) 1174
▲ Luvox CR Extended-Release Capsules (4% to 5%) 1759
Lyrica Capsules (Greater than or equal to 1%) 2527
▲ Paxil (2% to 10%) 1535
▲ Paxil CR Controlled-Release Tablets (2% to 17%) 1544
▲ Pristiq Extended-Release Tablets (0% to 8%) 3247
Prozac Weekly Capsules (Infrequent) 1852
Prozac Pulvules and Liquid (Infrequent) 1852
▲ Symbyax Capsules (1% to 3%) 1871

Anosmia

▲ Aerobid/Aerobid-M (3% to 9%) 1153
Beconase AQ Nasal Spray (Rare) 1369
Cipro I.V. (1% or less) 2817
Cipro 2810
Cipro XR Tablets 2823
Flonase Nasal Spray 1431
Levaquin 2416
Levaquin in 5% Dextrose Injection 2416

Anotia, fetal

Accutane Capsules 2607

Antibodies, development of

Elspar for Injection 1990
Elspar for Injection 2488
Genotropin Lyophilized Powder (1.9%) 2547
NovoLog Injection 2359
NovoSeven RT 2370
▲ Sandostatin LAR Depot (25%) 2302
▲ Somatuline Depot Injection (Less than 1% to 4%) 3102
Xyntha Vials 3280

Anticholinergic syndrome

Mirapex Tablets 857

Antidiuretic effect

MS Contin Tablets (Less frequent) 2585

Antisocial reaction

Prozac Weekly Capsules (Rare) 1852

Prozac Pulvules and Liquid (Rare) 1852
Zyprexa Tablets (Infrequent) 1883
Zyprexa ZYDIS Orally Disintegrating Tablets (Infrequent) 1883

Antithrombin, decrease

Elspar for Injection 2488
Estratest Tablets 3043
Estratest H.S. Tablets 3043
Ortho-Cyclen/Ortho Tri-Cyclen 2449
Premarin Tablets 3221

Anuria

Abelcet Injection 1134
Effexor XR Extended-Release Capsules (Rare) 3195
Fansidar Tablets 2636
Flebogamma 5% 1715
Flebogamma 5% DIF 1718
Gammagard S/D (Some patients) 734
Gantrisin Pediatric Suspension 2638
Invanz for Injection (Greater than 0.1%) 2029
Luvox CR Extended-Release Capsules (Infrequent) 1759
Mycamine for Injection 616
Nalfon Capsules (Less than 1%) 2508
Orthoclone OKT3 Sterile Solution (Less than 1%) 2387
Primaxin I.M. 2080
Primaxin I.V. (2.2%) 2083
Prinivil Tablets (0.3% to 1%) 2087
Prinzide Tablets 2092
▲ Proleukin for Injection (5%) 2287
Venlafaxine Hydrochloride Tablets (Rare) 2199

Anuria, neonatal

Aceon Tablets (2 mg, 4 mg, 8 mg) 3038
Avalide Tablets 2713
Avapro Tablets 897
Avapro Tablets 2718
Captopril Tablets 2182
Cozaar Tablets 1973
Prinivil Tablets 2087
Prinzide Tablets 2092

Anxiety

▲ Abilify Injection (4%) 881
▲ Abilify Injection (4% to 17%) 2466
▲ Abilify Oral Solution (4% to 17%) 881
▲ Abilify Oral Solution (4% to 17%) 2466
▲ Abilify Discmelt Orally Disintegrating Tablets (4% to 17%) 881
▲ Abilify Discmelt Orally Disintegrating Tablets (4% to 17%) 2466
▲ Abilify Tablets (4% to 17%) 881
▲ Abilify Tablets (4% to 17%) 2466
Aceon Tablets (2 mg, 4 mg, 8 mg) (0.3% to 1%) 3038
▲ Actonel with Calcium Tablets (0.6% to 4.7%) 2574
▲ Adderall XR Capsules (8%) 3012
Advair HFA 45/21 Inhalation Aerosol 1288
Advair HFA 115/21 Inhalation Aerosol 1288
Advair HFA 230/21 Inhalation Aerosol 1288
Advicor Tablets 402
▲ Aerobid/Aerobid-M (1% to 3%) 1153
Aldara Cream, 5% (1%) 1699
Allegra-D 12 Hour Extended-Release Tablets (1.4%) 2687
Allegra-D 24 Hour Extended-Release Tablets (1.4%) 2690
Aloxi Injection (1%) 1059
Ambien Tablets (Infrequent) 2692
▲ Ambien CR Tablets (2% to 3%) 2696
▲ AmBisome for Injection (7.4% to 13.7%) 606
Amerge Tablets (Infrequent) 1301
Amitiza Capsules (Less than 1%) 3082
Amoxil Capsules (Rare) 1305
Amoxil Chewable Tablets (Rare) 1305
Amoxil Pediatric Drops for Oral Suspension (Rare) 1305
Amoxil Powder for Oral Suspension (Rare) 1305
Amoxil Tablets (Rare) 1305
Anaprox Tablets (Less than 1%) 2632
Anaprox DS Tablets (Less than 1%) 2632
AndroGel (Less than 1%) 3159
▲ Angiomax for Injection (6%) 1933
Anzemet Injection (Infrequently) 2701
Anzemet Tablets (Rare) 2704
Aricept Tablets (Frequent) 1062
Aricept ODT Tablets (Frequent) 1062
▲ Arimidex Tablets (2% to 6%) 672
Arixtra Injection (0.8%) 1313
Asacol Delayed-Release Tablets (2% or greater) 2579
Atacand Tablets (0.5% or greater) 639
Atacand HCT (0.5% or greater) 642
▲ Atripla Tablets (5%) 938
Augmentin (Rare) 1323
Augmentin Tablets (Rare) 1327
Augmentin XR Extended Release Tablets (Rare) 1333
Augmentin ES-600 Powder for Oral Suspension (Rare) 1329
Avalide Tablets (1% or greater) 892
Avalide Tablets (1% or greater) 2713
Avapro Tablets (Less than 1%) 897
Avapro Tablets (Less than 1%) 2718
Avelox (Greater than or equal to 0.1% to less than 2%) 2803
▲ Avinza Capsules (Less than 5%) 1772
Axert Tablets (Infrequent) 2431
Axid Capsules (1.6%) 1364
Azilect Tablets (Frequent) 3106
▲ Betaseron for SC Injection (10%) 756
Biaxin/Biaxin XL 411
Bicillin C-R Injectable Suspension 1775
Bicillin L-A Injection 1777
▲ BOTOX Purified Neurotoxin Complex (3% to 10%) 550
▲ Busulfex Injection (72% to 75%) 2477
▲ Campath Ampules (8%) 761
▲ Campral Tablets (5% to 8%) 1158
Cancidas for Injection 1953
Catapres Tablets 841
Catapres-TTS (0.5% or less) 842
Celebrex Capsules (0.1% to 1.9%) 2979
▲ Celexa (4%) 1160
▲ CellCept Capsules (3% to less than 28.4%) 2622
▲ CellCept Intravenous (3% to less than 28.4%) 2622
▲ CellCept Oral Suspension (3% to less than 28.4%) 2622
▲ CellCept Tablets (3% to less than 28.4%) 2622
Chantix Tablets (Frequent) 2511
Cimzia 3127
Cipro I.V. (1% or less) 2817
Cipro 2810
Cipro XR Tablets 2823
▲ Clolar for Intravenous Infusion (22%) 1239
Clorpres Tablets 2185
Combigan Ophthalmic Solution 553
Comtan Tablets (2%) 2208
▲ Concerta Extended-Release Tablets (0.8% to 8.2%) 1925
▲ Copaxone for Injection (23%) 3110
Cosopt Sterile Ophthalmic Solution 1969
Cozaar Tablets (Less than 1%) 1973
Crixivan Capsules (Less than 2%) 1979
▲ Cubicin for Injection (1% to 5%) 995
Cuprimine Capsules 1986
▲ Cymbalta Delayed-Release Capsules (3%) 1801
▲ Dacogen Injection (11%) 1066
Delatestryl Injection 1730
Demser Capsules 1989
▲ Depakote ER Tablets (Greater than 1% to less than 5%) 423
▲ DepoCyt Injection (3% to 7%) 1136
▲ DepoDur Injection (2% to 5%) 1095
Diovan Tablets (Greater than 0.2%) 2212
Diovan HCT Tablets (Greater than 0.2%) 2216
▲ Doxil Injection (Less than 1% to 10%) 2378
▲ Duragesic Transdermal System (3% to 10%) 2405
EC-Naprosyn Delayed-Release Tablets (Less than 1%) 2632
Effexor XR Extended-Release Capsules (1%) 3195
Eldepryl Capsules (1 of 49 patients) 3052
▲ Eloxatin for Injection (2% to 6%) 2731
Emend Capsules (Greater than 0.5%) 1992
Emend for Injection (Greater than 0.5%) 1999
Emsam Transdermal System 905
EpiPen 1024
▲ Epogen for Injection (2% to 7%) 576
▲ Epzicom Tablets (3% to 5%) 1422
▲ Equetro Extended-Release Capsules (7%) 3174
▲ Erbitux (2% to 14%) 912
Estratest Tablets 3043
Estratest H.S. Tablets 3043
Evoxac Capsules (1.3%) 1013
▲ Exelon Capsules (4% to 5%) 2229
▲ Exelon Oral Solution (4% to 5%) 2229
▲ Exelon Patch (3%) 2233
Exforge Tablets (Greater than or equal to 0.2%) 2238
Exjade Tablets (0.1% to 1%) 2244
▲ Fabrazyme for Intravenous Infusion (8%) 1241
▲ Faslodex Injection (5%) 682
Femara Tablets (Less frequent) 2246
Flebogamma 5% 1715
Flebogamma 5% DIF 1718
▲ Flolan for Injection (7% to 21%) 1426
▲ Focalin XR Capsules (5% to 11%) 2251
Foradil Aerolizer (1.5%) 2849
Frova Tablets (Frequent) 1111
Gabitril Tablets (1% or more) 973
Gantrisin Pediatric Suspension 2638
Gengraf Capsules (1% to less than 3%) 435
▲ Geodon (5%) 2520
▲ Gleevec Tablets (7% to 12%) 2255
▲ Gliadel Wafer (7%) 1076
Humulin 50/50, 100 Units 1843
Humulin 70/30 Vial 1844
Humulin N Vial 1846
Humulin R 1849
Imitrex Injection (Frequent) 1465
Imitrex Nasal Spray (Infrequent) 1470
Imitrex Tablets 1474
▲ Indapamide Tablets (Greater than or equal to 5%) 2188
Indocin (Less than 1%) 2024
▲ Infanrix Vaccine (3.3% to 9.2%) 1479
Intelence Tablets (Less than 2%) 3119
▲ Intron A for Injection (Up to 5%) 2859
Invanz for Injection (0.8% to 1.1%) 2029
▲ Ionsys Transdermal System (1% to less than 10%) 2410
Kaletra (Less than 2%) 452
▲ Keppra Injection (2% to 13.3%) 3137
Keppra Oral Solution (2%) 3131
Keppra Tablets (2%) 3131
Ketek Tablets (Less than 0.2%) 2744
Klonopin (Infrequent) 2639
▲ Lamictal (4% to 5%) 1488
Lanoxin Injection 1498
Lanoxin Injection Pediatric 1502
Lanoxin Tablets 1505
Lescol Capsules 2268
Lescol XL Tablets 2268
▲ Leukine (11%) 774
Levaquin (0.1% to 1%) 2416
Levaquin in 5% Dextrose Injection (0.1% to 1%) 2416
Levothroid Tablets 1170
Levoxyl Tablets 1780
Lexapro Oral Suspension (At least 2%) 1174
Lexapro Tablets (At least 2%) 1174
Lortab 5/500 Tablets 3143
Lortab 7.5/500 Tablets 3144
Lortab 10/500 Tablets 3144
▲ Lucentis Injection (0% to 7%) 1205
Lunesta Tablets (Infrequent) 2994
▲ Lupron Depot 3.75 mg (3%) 462
▲ Lupron Depot–3 Month 11.25 mg (Less than 5%) 462
▲ Luvox CR Extended-Release Capsules (2% to 8%) 1759
Lyrica Capsules (Greater than or equal to 1% to 2%) 2527
Malarone Pediatric Tablets (Less than 1%) 1521
Malarone Tablets (Less than 1%) 1521
Marinol Capsules (Greater than 1%) 3163
Marplan Tablets (0% to 2%) 3177
Mavik Tablets (0.3% to 1%) 472
Maxair Autohaler 1705
Maxalt Tablets (Infrequent) 2056
Maxalt-MLT Orally Disintegrating Tablets (Infrequent) 2056
▲ Mepron Suspension (7%) 1526
▲ Meridia Capsules (4.5%) 475
Merrem I.V. (Greater than 0.1% to 1%) 684
Mevacor Tablets (0.5% to 1%) 2063
Miacalcin Nasal Spray (Less than 1%) 2274
Micardis Tablets (More than 0.3%) 852
Micardis HCT Tablets 854
Mirapex Tablets (1% or more) 857
Mobic Oral Suspension (Less than 2%) 863
Mobic Tablets (Less than 2%) 863
Moxatag Tablets 2165
▲ Mycamine for Injection (6.4% to 22.4%) 616
▲ Myfortic Tablets (3% to less than 20%) 2276
▲ Mylotarg for Injection (7% to 10%) 3212
Namenda (Greater than or equal to 2%) 1180
Naprosyn Suspension (Less than 1%) 2632
Naprosyn Tablets (Less than 1%) 2632
▲ Natrecor for Injection (2% to 3%) 2977
Nembutal Sodium Solution, USP (Less than 1%) 2494
Neoral Oral Solution (1% to less than 3%) 2280
Neoral Soft Gelatin Capsules (1% to less than 3%) 2280
Neupro Transdermal System (Greater than or equal to 2%) 3149
Noroxin Tablets (Less frequent) 2069
Norvir (0% to 1.7%) 489
▲ Novantrone for Injection Concentrate (5%) 1100
▲ Noxafil Oral Suspension (9%) 2889
▲ Opana Tablets (1% to less than 10%) 1117
▲ Opana ER Tablets (1% to less than 10%) 1121
OptiPranolol Metipranolol Ophthalmic Solution 0.3% (A small number of patients) ⊙245
▲ OxyContin Tablets (Between 1% and 5%) 2589
Parnate Tablets 1532
▲ Paxil (1% to 5.9%) 1535
▲ Paxil CR Controlled-Release Tablets (1% to 5.9%) 1544
▲ PegIntron Powder for Injection (28%) 2903
Pepcid Tablets (Infrequent) 2075
Percocet Tablets 1127
Percodan Tablets 1130
▲ Photofrin for Injection (3% to 7%) 708
Plavix Tablets (1% to 2.5%) 926
Plavix Tablets (1% to 2.5%) 2767
Pletal Tablets (Less than 2%) 2481
▲ Premphase Tablets (2% to 5%) 3232
▲ Prempro Tablets (2% to 5%) 3232
▲ Pristiq Extended-Release Tablets (Greater than or equal to 3%) 3247
ProAir HFA Inhalation Aerosol (Less than 3%) 3113
ProAmatine Tablets (Less frequent) 3032
▲ Procrit for Injection (2% to 11%) 2391
Proglycem Capsules (Infrequent) 1185
Proglycem Suspension (Infrequent) 1185
▲ Prograf Capsules and Injection (3% to 15%) 622
▲ Proleukin for Injection (12%) 2287
▲ Prometrium Capsules (100 mg, 200 mg) (Less than 5%) 3047
Protonix for Delayed-Release Oral Suspension (Greater than or equal to 1%) 3254
Protonix Delayed-Release Tablets (Greater than or equal to 1%) 3254
Protonix I.V. (Greater than or equal to 1%) 3257
Proventil HFA Inhalation Aerosol (Less than 3%) 2914
▲ Provigil Tablets (5%) 977
▲ Prozac Weekly Capsules (1% to 16%) 1852
▲ Prozac Pulvules and Liquid (4% to 17%) 1852
Pulmicort Flexhaler 654
▲ Rebetol (47%) 2917
Relenza Inhalation Powder 1556
Remeron Tablets (Frequent) 2924
RemeronSolTab Tablets (Frequent) 2927
ReoPro Vials (1.7%) 1860
Requip Tablets (Frequent to greater than or equal to 1%) 1561
Requip XL Tablets (2%) 1568
Retrovir Capsules 1574
Retrovir IV Infusion 1579
Retrovir 1574
Risperdal Consta Long-Acting Injection (Frequent) 1753
▲ Rituxan I.V. (1% to 5%) 1223
▲ Romazicon Injection (3% to 9%) 2646
Rythmol Tablets (2%) 1586
▲ Rythmol SR Capsules (10% to 13%) 1590
Salagen Tablets (Less than 1%) 1082
Sandimmune (Rare) 2296
Sandostatin Injection (Less than 1%) 2300
Serevent Diskus (1% to less than 3%) 1594
▲ Simulect for Injection (3% to 10%) 2306
Singulair 2114
Soriatane Capsules (Less than 1%) 3062
Stalevo Tablets (2%) 2309
▲ Suboxone Tablets (12%) 2601
▲ Subutex Tablets (12%) 2601
Sular Extended Release Tablets (Less than or equal to 1%) 2975
▲ Sustiva Capsules (2% to 13%) 930
▲ Sustiva Tablets (2% to 13%) 930
Symbyax Capsules 1871
Tamiflu Capsules 2649
Tamiflu Oral Suspension 2649

▲ Tarceva Tablets (0% to 13%) 1228
Tarka Tablets (0.3% or more).......... 511
Tasigna Capsules (0.1% to 1%)........ 2316
▲ Temodar Capsules (1% to 7%) 2931
Teveten Tablets (Less than 1%)........ 515
Teveten HCT Tablets (Less than 1%).. 517
Timoptic Sterile Ophthalmic Solution (Less frequent)............... 2121
Timoptic in Ocudose (Less frequent).. 2124
Timoptic-XE Sterile Ophthalmic Gel Forming Solution 2125
Toprol-XL Tablets 666
Trasylol Injection (1% to 2%)........... 799
▲ Travatan Z Ophthalmic Solution (1% to 5%).. 547
Treximet Tablets (Infrequent)........... 1616
Tricor Tablets..................................... 520
▲ Trisenox Injection (30%) 986
▲ Truvada Tablets (Greater than or equal to 5%) 1262
Tussionex Pennkinetic Extended-Release Suspension 3154
▲ Ultram ER Extended-Release Tablets (1% to less than 5%) 2428
▲ Velcade for Injection (10%) 2168
▲ Venlafaxine Hydrochloride Tablets (2% to 11.2%) 2199
▲ Vesanoid Capsules (17%) 2660
Viadur Implant (Less than 2%) 802
Vicodin Tablets 529
Vicodin ES Tablets 530
Vicodin HP Tablets 531
▲ Vicoprofen Tablets (3% to 9%) 533
▲ Viread Tablets (6%) 1268
▲ Vivitrol (8% to 12%) 988
Voltaren Tablets (Occasionally) 2334
Voltaren-XR Tablets (Occasionally) 2337
▲ Vyvanse Capsules (6%) 3033
▲ Wellbutrin Tablets (3.1%) 1648
▲ Wellbutrin SR Sustained-Release Tablets (5% to 6%) 1653
▲ Wellbutrin XL Extended-Release Tablets (5% to 7%) 1659
▲ Xenical Capsules (2.8% to 4.4%) 2672
Xopenex Inhalation Solution (2.7%) .. 3001
Xopenex Inhalation Solution Concentrate (2.7%) 3005
Xopenex HFA Inhalation Aerosol (2.7%) 3009
▲ Ziagen (5%) 1673
▲ Zofran Injection (2% to 6%) 1682
▲ Zofran (6%) 1687
▲ Zofran ODT Orally Disintegrating Tablets (6%) 1687
▲ Zometa for Intravenous Infusion (11% to 14%) 2341
Zomig Tablets (Infrequent) 694
Zomig Nasal Spray (Infrequent) 689
Zomig-ZMT Tablets (Infrequent) 694
▲ Zonegran Capsules (3%) 1089
▲ Zosyn for Injection (1.2% to 3.2%) .. 3284
▲ Zyban Sustained-Release Tablets (8%) 1692
Zydone Tablets 1132
▲ Zyprexa Tablets (9%) 1883
Zyprexa IntraMuscular 1883
▲ Zyprexa ZYDIS Orally Disintegrating Tablets (9%) 1883
Zyrtec Chewable Tablets (Less than 2%) 1920
Zyrtec Syrup (Less than 2%) 1920
Zyrtec Tablets (Less than 2%) 1920
Zyrtec-D 12 Hour Extended Release Tablets (Less than 2%) 1923

Anxiety, paradoxical

Valium Tablets 2658

Aortic valve incompetence

Celebrex Capsules (Greater than or equal to 0.1% to less than 1%) 2979
Somatuline Depot Injection 3102

Apathy

Ambien Tablets (Rare) 2692
Ambien CR Tablets (1%) 2696
Aricept Tablets (Infrequent) 1062
Aricept ODT Tablets (Infrequent) 1062
Azilect Tablets (Rare) 3106
Campral Tablets (Infrequent) 1158
Celexa (Infrequent) 1160
Cymbalta Delayed-Release Capsules (Infrequent) 1801
Effexor XR Extended-Release Capsules (Infrequent) 3195
Eldepryl Capsules 3052
Evoxac Capsules 1013
Exelon Capsules (Infrequent) 2229
Exelon Oral Solution (Infrequent) 2229
Exforge Tablets (Less than or equal to 0.1%) 2238
Fansidar Tablets 2636
Gabitril Tablets (Infrequent)............. 973
Gantrisin Pediatric Suspension......... 2638
Imitrex Injection 1465
Imitrex Nasal Spray (Rare)............... 1470
Imitrex Tablets (Rare)...................... 1474
▲ Intron A for Injection (Less than 5%)... 2859
▲ Keppra Injection (12.7% to 13.3%).. 3137
Keppra Oral Solution........................ 3131
Keppra Tablets 3131
Klonopin (Infrequent)........................ 2639
Lamictal (Infrequent)......................... 1488
Lanoxin Injection.............................. 1498
Lanoxin Injection Pediatric 1502
Lanoxin Tablets................................ 1505
Lexapro Oral Suspension (Infrequent)..................................... 1174
Lexapro Tablets (Infrequent)............ 1174
Lunesta Tablets 2994
▲ Luvox CR Extended-Release Capsules (3%) 1759
Lyrica Capsules (0.1% to 1%) 2527
Mirapex Tablets (1% or more) 857
Myfortic Tablets 2276
Namenda (Infrequent) 1180
Nexium Delayed-Release Capsules (Less than 1%) 645
Nexium I.V. (Less than 1%) 652
Nexium Delayed-Release Oral Suspension (Less than 1%) 645
ProQuad 2099
Prozac Weekly Capsules (Infrequent) 1852
Prozac Pulvules and Liquid (Infrequent) 1852
Remeron Tablets (Frequent) 2924
RemeronSolTab Tablets (Frequent) ... 2927
Requip Tablets (Infrequent) 1561
Rilutek Tablets (Infrequent) 2771
Risperdal Consta Long-Acting Injection (Frequent) 1753
Rocaltrol Capsules 1150
Rocaltrol Oral Solution 1150
Sustiva Capsules (Less than 2%) 930
Sustiva Tablets (Less than 2%) 930
Venlafaxine Hydrochloride Tablets (Infrequent) 2199
Zomig Tablets (Rare) 694
Zomig Nasal Spray (Rare) 689
Zomig-ZMT Tablets (Rare) 694
▲ Zyprexa Tablets (4%) 1883
▲ Zyprexa ZYDIS Orally Disintegrating Tablets (4%) 1883

Aphasia

Amerge Tablets (Rare) 1301
Aricept Tablets (Frequent) 1062
Aricept ODT Tablets (Frequent) 1062
Arranon Injection (1%) 1319
Avelox (Less than 0.1%) 2803
Azilect Tablets (Infrequent) 3106
Duragesic Transdermal System (Less than 1%) 2405
Effexor XR Extended-Release Capsules (Rare) 3195
Evoxac Capsules 1013
Exelon Capsules (Infrequent) 2229
Exelon Oral Solution (Infrequent) 2229
▲ Gliadel Wafer (9% to 18%) 1076
▲ Intron A for Injection (Less than 5%) 2859
Lamictal (Infrequent) 1488
Lyrica Capsules (0.1% to 1%) 2527
Mirapex Tablets 857
Namenda (Infrequent) 1180
Norvir (Less than 2%) 489
Orthoclone OKT3 Sterile Solution (Less than 1%) 2387
Paxil (Rare) 1535
Paxil CR Controlled-Release Tablets (Rare) 1544
Remeron Tablets (Rare) 2924
RemeronSolTab Tablets (Rare) 2927
Requip Tablets (Infrequent) 1561
Salagen Tablets (Less than 1%) 1082
Sandostatin LAR Depot 2302
Symbyax Capsules (Rare) 1871
Treximet Tablets (Rare) 1616
Venlafaxine Hydrochloride Tablets (Rare) 2199
▲ Vesanoid Capsules (3%) 2660
Wellbutrin Tablets (Rare) 1648
Wellbutrin SR Sustained-Release Tablets 1653
Wellbutrin XL Extended-Release Tablets 1659
Zyban Sustained-Release Tablets 1692

Aphonia

Advair HFA 45/21 Inhalation Aerosol 1288
Advair HFA 115/21 Inhalation Aerosol 1288
Advair HFA 230/21 Inhalation Aerosol 1288
Flovent Diskus 50 mcg 1435
Flovent HFA 1440
Klonopin 2639

Aphthous stomatitis

(*see under* Stomatitis, ulcerative)

Aplasia, bone marrow

Campath Ampules 761
Paxil 1535
Paxil CR Controlled-Release Tablets 1544

Aplasia, red cell

Aranesp for Injection 564
Campath Ampules 761
Combivir Tablets 1384
Cuprimine Capsules 1986
Epivir 1412
Epivir-HBV 1417
▲ Epogen for Injection (4 to 11%) 576
Intron A for Injection 2859
Lamictal (Rare) 1488
PegIntron Powder for Injection 2903
Rebetol 2917
Retrovir Capsules 1574
Retrovir IV Infusion 1579
Retrovir 1574
Trizivir Tablets 1622

Aplastic anemia

(*see under* Anemia, aplastic)

Apnea

Actiq 959
Alphagan P Ophthalmic Solution 549
Aricept Tablets (Infrequent) 1062
Aricept ODT Tablets (Infrequent) 1062
Bentyl Capsules 703
Bentyl Injection 703
Bentyl Syrup 703
Bentyl Tablets 703
Bicillin C-R Injectable Suspension 1775
Bicillin L-A Injection 1777
▲ CellCept Capsules (3% to less than 20%) 2622
▲ CellCept Intravenous (3% to less than 20%) 2622
▲ CellCept Oral Suspension (3% to less than 20%) 2622
▲ CellCept Tablets (3% to less than 20%) 2622
Combigan Ophthalmic Solution 553
DepoDur Injection 1095
▲ Doxil Injection (1% to 10%) 2378
▲ Duragesic Transdermal System (3% to 10%) 2405
Effexor XR Extended-Release Capsules (Rare) 3195
Evoxac Capsules 1013
Exelon Capsules (Infrequent) 2229
Exelon Oral Solution (Infrequent) 2229
Flebogamma 5% 1715
Flebogamma 5% DIF 1718
Gabitril Tablets (Infrequent) 973
Gammagard Liquid 730
Gammagard S/D (Rare) 734
Gamunex (Rare) 3094
Indocin I.V. (Less than 3%) 2489
▲ Infasurf Intratracheal Suspension (61% to 76%) 1168
Ionsys Transdermal System (.1% to less than 1%) 2410
Kinrix Injection Vaccine 1486
Lamictal 1488
Luvox CR Extended-Release Capsules (Rare) 1759
Lyrica Capsules (Rare) 2527
Merrem I.V. (1.3%) 684
Mirapex Tablets 857
MS Contin Tablets 2585
Mycamine for Injection 616
Namenda (Infrequent) 1180
Natrecor for Injection (Greater than or equal to 1%) 2977
Nembutal Sodium Solution, USP (Less than 1%) 2494
▲ NeoProfen Injection (28%) 2496
Orthoclone OKT3 Sterile Solution (Less than 1%) 2387
OxyContin Tablets 2589
Pentacel 2792
Percocet Tablets 1127
Proleukin for Injection (1%) 2287
Prozac Weekly Capsules (Rare) 1852
Prozac Pulvules and Liquid (Rare) 1852
Pulmozyme Inhalation Solution 1217
Rilutek Tablets (More than 2%) 2771
Risperdal Consta Long-Acting Injection 1753
Rythmol Tablets (Less than 1%)........ 1586
Symbyax Capsules (Infrequent)........ 1871
Synagis Intramuscular Solution (More than 1%)........................... 1948
▲ Trasylol Injection (3%) 799
Ultane Liquid for Inhalation (Less than 1% to 2%) 524
Xyrem Oral Solution (Infrequent)....... 1766
Zomig Tablets (Rare)........................ 694
Zomig-ZMT Tablets (Rare)................ 694
Zonegran Capsules (Rare)................ 1089
Zyprexa Tablets (Infrequent)............. 1883
Zyprexa ZYDIS Orally Disintegrating Tablets (Infrequent)................................... 1883
Zyvox (0% to 2.3%)......................... 2552

Apnea, sleep

AndroGel 3159
Venlafaxine Hydrochloride Tablets (Rare) 2199

Apocrine gland disorders

▲ Selzentry Tablets (4.5%) 2534

Appendicitis

Amevive 611
Effexor XR Extended-Release Capsules (Rare) 3195
Enbrel for Injection 569
Evoxac Capsules (Less than 1%) 1013
Gardasil Injection (0.02%) 2019
Mirapex Tablets 857
Requip Tablets (Infrequent) 1561
Sandostatin Injection (Less than 1%) 2300
Sandostatin LAR Depot 2302
Ultram ER Extended-Release Tablets (0.5% to less than 1%) 2428
Venlafaxine Hydrochloride Tablets (Rare) 2199

Appetite, changes

Activella Tablets 2347
Anaprox Tablets (Less than 1%) 2632
Anaprox DS Tablets (Less than 1%) .. 2632
EC-Naprosyn Delayed-Release Tablets (Less than 1%) 2632
▲ Effexor XR Extended-Release Capsules (1% to 6%) 3195
Eldepryl Capsules 3052
Gleevec Tablets (Infrequent) 2255
Lupron Depot 3.75 mg (2%) 462
▲ Lupron Depot–3 Month 11.25 mg (Less than 5%) 462
Mircette Tablets 1034
Naprosyn Suspension (Less than 1%) 2632
Naprosyn Tablets (Less than 1%) 2632
NuvaRing 2897
Ortho-Cyclen Tablets 2449
Ortho Evra Transdermal System 2437
Ortho Tri-Cyclen Tablets 2449
Ortho Tri-Cyclen Lo Tablets 2458
Premphase Tablets 3232
Prempro Tablets 3232
Seasonique Tablets 1046
▲ Sutent Capsules (9%) 2540
Voltaren Tablets (Rarely) 2334
Voltaren-XR Tablets (Rarely) 2337
▲ Wellbutrin Tablets (3.7%) 1648
Yaz Tablets 805

Appetite, decreased

Abilify Oral Solution (Greater than or equal to 1 in 100 patients) 881
Abilify Discmelt Orally Disintegrating Tablets (Greater than or equal to 1 in 100 patients) 881
Abilify Tablets (Greater than or equal to 1 in 100 patients) 881
▲ Adderall XR Capsules (22% to 36%) 3012
▲ Aerobid/Aerobid-M (3% to 9%) 1153
Aloxi Injection (Less than 1%) 1059
Amitiza Capsules (Less than 1%) 3082
Aptivus Capsules (Less than 2%) 823
Aptivus Oral Solution (Less than 2%) 823
▲ Byetta Injection (Greater than or equal to 1% to less than 5%) 600
Cancidas for Injection 1953
Chantix Tablets (1% to 2%) 2511
▲ Clolar for Intravenous Infusion (11%) 1239
▲ Combivir Tablets (10%) 1384
▲ Concerta Extended-Release Tablets (0.7% to 25.3%) 1925
Crinone 4% Gel 992
Crinone 8% Gel 992
Cubicin for Injection (Less than 1% to 2%) 995

▲ Cymbalta Delayed-Release Capsules (3% to 11%) 1801
▲ Dacogen Injection (16%) 1066
▲ Daytrana Transdermal Patch (26%) 3022
▲ DepoCyt Injection (11% to 12%) 1136
DynaCirc CR Controlled Release Tablets (0.5% to 1%) 1407
Emend Capsules (Greater than 0.5%) 1992
Emend for Injection (Greater than 0.5%) 1999
▲ Epivir (10%) 1412
▲ Exelon Patch (3% to 9%) 2233
▲ Femara Tablets (4%) 2246
Fentora Tablets (Greater than 1%) 968
▲ FluMist Vaccine (13% to 21%) 1945
▲ Focalin XR Capsules (30%) 2251
Imitrex Injection (Rare) 1465
Imitrex Nasal Spray (Rare) 1470
Imitrex Tablets (Rare) 1474
Klonopin (1%) 2639
▲ Leustatin Injection (17%) 2384
▲ Lexapro Oral Suspension (3%) 1174
▲ Lexapro Tablets (3%) 1174
Mirapex Tablets 857
▲ Mycamine for Injection (20.5%) 616
▲ Nexavar Tablets (1% to less than 10%) 784
Opana Tablets (Less than 1%) 1117
Opana ER Tablets (2.9%) 1121
▲ Paxil (2% to 9%) 1535
▲ Paxil CR Controlled-Release Tablets (2% to 9%) 1544
Pentacel 2792
▲ Prevnar (0% to 30%) 3241
▲ Pristiq Extended-Release Tablets (5% to 10%) 3247
Recombivax HB (Greater than 1%) 2107
▲ Relenza Inhalation Powder (2% to 4%) 1556
Requip Tablets (Infrequent) 1561
▲ Strattera Capsules (11% to 16%) 1864
Tasigna Capsules (0.1% to 1%) 2316
▲ Trisenox Injection (15%) 986
▲ Ultram ER Extended-Release Tablets (1% to less than 5%) 2428
▲ Valcyte Tablets (Less than 5%) 2654
▲ Velcade for Injection (34% to 36%) 2168
▲ Vivitrol (6% to 20%) 988
▲ Vyvanse Capsules (27% to 39%) 3033
Wellbutrin SR Sustained-Release Tablets 1653
▲ Wellbutrin XL Extended-Release Tablets (4%) 1659
Xyrem Oral Solution (Infrequent) 1766
▲ Zometa for Intravenous Infusion (13%) 2341

Appetite, increased

▲ Abilify Injection (3% to 4%) 881
▲ Abilify Injection (3% to 4%) 2466
▲ Abilify Oral Solution (3% to 4%) 881
▲ Abilify Oral Solution (3% to 4%) 2466
▲ Abilify Discmelt Orally Disintegrating Tablets (3% to 4%) 881
▲ Abilify Discmelt Orally Disintegrating Tablets (3% to 4%) 2466
▲ Abilify Tablets (3% to 4%) 881
▲ Abilify Tablets (3% to 4%) 2466
Aceon Tablets (2 mg, 4 mg, 8 mg) (0.3% to 1%) 3038
▲ Aerobid/Aerobid-M (1% to 3%) 1153
Alinia for Oral Suspension (Less than 1%) 2677
Alinia Tablets (Less than 1%) 2677
Ambien Tablets (Rare) 2692
Aricept Tablets (Infrequent) 1062
Aricept ODT Tablets (Infrequent) 1062
Asacol Delayed-Release Tablets 2579
Campral Tablets (Frequent) 1158
Celebrex Capsules (0.1% to 1.9%) 2979
Celexa (Frequent) 1160
▲ Chantix Tablets (3% to 4%) 2511
▲ Clarinex Syrup (3.1%) 2828
Copaxone for Injection (Infrequent) 3110
▲ Crinone 4% Gel (5%) 992
▲ Crinone 8% Gel (8%) 992
Crixivan Capsules (2.1%) 1979
▲ Depakote ER Tablets (Greater than 1% to 6%) 423
Diovan HCT Tablets (Less than frequent) 2216
Doxil Injection (Less than 1%) 2378
DynaCirc CR Controlled Release Tablets (0.5% to 1%) 1407
Emsam Transdermal System (Infrequent) 905
Evoxac Capsules (Less than 1%) 1013
Exforge Tablets (Less than or equal to 0.1%) 2238
Gabitril Tablets (2%) 973
Gengraf Capsules (1% to less than 3%) 435
Genotropin Lyophilized Powder 2547
▲ Intron A for Injection (Less than 5%) 2859
Kaletra (Less than 2%) 452
Klonopin (Infrequent) 2639
Lamictal (Infrequent) 1488
Levothroid Tablets 1170
Levoxyl Tablets 1780
Lexapro Oral Suspension (Frequent) 1174
Lexapro Tablets (Frequent) 1174
Lipitor Tablets (Less than 2%) 2501
Lovaza Capsules 1520
Lunesta Tablets (Infrequent) 2994
▲ Lyrica Capsules (1% to 7%) 2527
Maxalt Tablets (Rare) 2056
Maxalt-MLT Orally Disintegrating Tablets (Rare) 2056
▲ Meridia Capsules (8.7%) 475
Miacalcin Nasal Spray (Less than 1%) 2274
Mirapex Tablets 857
Mobic Oral Suspension (Less than 2%) 863
Mobic Tablets (Less than 2%) 863
Namenda (Infrequent) 1180
Neoral Oral Solution (1% to less than 3%) 2280
Neoral Soft Gelatin Capsules (1% to less than 3%) 2280
Neupro Transdermal System 3149
Nexium Delayed-Release Capsules (Less than 1%) 645
Nexium I.V. (Less than 1%) 652
Nexium Delayed-Release Oral Suspension (Less than 1%) 645
OxyContin Tablets (Less than 1%) 2589
▲ Paxil (4%) 1535
▲ Paxil CR Controlled-Release Tablets (4%) 1544
▲ Prograf Capsules and Injection (3% to 15%) 622
Prometrium Capsules (100 mg, 200 mg) 3047
Protonix for Delayed-Release Oral Suspension (Less than 1%) 3254
Protonix Delayed-Release Tablets (Less than 1%) 3254
Protonix I.V. (Less than 1%) 3257
Provigil Tablets (At least 1%) 977
Prozac Weekly Capsules (Frequent) 1852
Prozac Pulvules and Liquid (Frequent) 1852
▲ Relenza Inhalation Powder (2% to 4%) 1556
▲ Remeron Tablets (17% to 49%) 2924
▲ RemeronSolTab Tablets (17% to 49%) 2927
Rilutek Tablets (Infrequent) 2771
Risperdal Consta Long-Acting Injection (Infrequent) 1753
Salagen Tablets (Less than 1%) 1082
▲ Soriatane Capsules (1% to 10%) 3062
Sular Extended Release Tablets (Less than or equal to 1%) 2975
▲ Symbyax Capsules (Greater than or equal to 5% to 16%) 1871
Tasigna Capsules (0.1% to 1%) 2316
Testim 1% Gel (Less than 1%) 701
Thiothixene Capsules 2197
Tricor Tablets 520
Vantas (Less than 2%) 1737
Vivitrol 988
Wellbutrin SR Sustained-Release Tablets (At least 1%) 1653
▲ Wellbutrin XL Extended-Release Tablets (4%) 1659
Xyrem Oral Solution (Infrequent) 1766
Yaz Tablets (Greater than 1%) 805
▲ Zolinza Capsules (12% to 14%) 2142
Zomig Tablets (Infrequent) 694
Zomig Nasal Spray (Rare) 689
Zomig-ZMT Tablets (Infrequent) 694
Zyban Sustained-Release Tablets (2%) 1692
▲ Zyprexa Tablets (2% to 24%) 1883
▲ Zyprexa ZYDIS Orally Disintegrating Tablets (2% to 24%) 1883
Zyrtec Chewable Tablets (Less than 2%) 1920
Zyrtec Syrup (Less than 2%) 1920
Zyrtec Tablets (Less than 2%) 1920
Zyrtec-D 12 Hour Extended Release Tablets (Less than 2%) 1923

Appetite, loss of

(*see also under* Anorexia)

▲ Chemet Capsules (12% to 20.9%) 2484
Focalin XR Capsules 2251
▲ Infanrix Vaccine (6% to 27.8%) 1479
▲ Kinrix Injection Vaccine (15.5%) 1486
Metadate CD Capsules 3146
Miacalcin Injection 2273
▲ Pediarix Vaccine (21.6% or less) 1552
▲ Rotarix Oral Suspension (21% to 25%) 1582
▲ Sutent Capsules (2% to 38%) 2540
Varivax (Greater than or equal to 1%) 2133
Ziagen 1673

Appetite disorder, unspecified

Ambien CR Tablets (1%) 2696
▲ Selzentry Tablets (7.3%) 2534
▲ Vivitrol (6% to 20%) 988

Application site discharge

Daytrana Transdermal Patch 3022

Application site rash

▲ AndroGel (3% to 5.6%) 3159
Authia Cream (Occasional) 3190
Daytrana Transdermal Patch 3022
▲ Targretin Gel 1% (14%) 1088

Application site reaction, unspecified

▲ Aczone Gel 5% (18%) 3296
▲ Aldara Cream, 5% (28% to 33%) 1699
AndroGel 3159
▲ Climara Pro Transdermal System (40.6%) 768
▲ Daytrana Transdermal Patch (6%) 3022
▲ Duragesic Transdermal System (3% to 10%) 2405
▲ Elidel Cream 1% (2.1% to 14.6%) 2221
▲ Emsam Transdermal System (24%) 905
▲ Erbitux (0% to 18%) 912
Evoclin Foam, 1% (1%) 3056
▲ Extina Foam, 2% (6%) 3057
▲ Flector Patch (4%) 561
▲ Neupro Transdermal System (5% to 46%) 3149
Olux-E Foam (1.6%) 3059
Vanos Cream (0.4% to 1.4%) 1941
Verdeso Foam (1%) 3069

Application site ulcer

Daytrana Transdermal Patch 3022
Fentora Tablets (Greater than 1%) 968

Apprehension

Adenocard IV Injection (Less than 1%) 603
Edecrin 698
EpiPen 1024
Lidoderm Patch 1114
Maxalt Tablets (Rare) 2056
Maxalt-MLT Orally Disintegrating Tablets (Rare) 2056
MS Contin Tablets (Less frequent) 2585

Apraxia

Eldepryl Capsules 3052
Exelon Capsules (Infrequent) 2229
Exelon Oral Solution (Infrequent) 2229
Risperdal Consta Long-Acting Injection (Infrequent) 1753

Arachnoiditis

▲ DepoCyt Injection (42%) 1136

Areflexia

▲ Ixempra Kit for Injection (62%) 915

Arm, stiffness of

Engerix-B Vaccine (Less than 1%) 1409

Arm circumference, increase

▲ Kinrix Injection Vaccine (36%) 1486
▲ Pentacel (0.5% to 33.6%) 2792

Arrhythmia, exacerbation of

Toprol-XL Tablets (Greater than 1%) 666

Arrhythmia, nodal

Anzemet Tablets 2704
Mirapex Tablets 857
Pletal Tablets (Less than 2%) 2481
ReoPro Vials (0.2%) 1860
Rythmol SR Capsules 1590

Arrhythmias

Abelcet Injection (Rare) 1134
Activase I.V. 1188
Actonel Tablets (2%) 2568
Adenocard IV Injection 603
Adenoscan (1%) 605
▲ Advair HFA 45/21 Inhalation Aerosol (1% to 3%) 1288
▲ Advair HFA 115/21 Inhalation Aerosol (1% to 3%) 1288
▲ Advair HFA 230/21 Inhalation Aerosol (1% to 3%) 1288
Advicor Tablets 402
Aggrenox Capsules (Less than 1%) 819
▲ Agrylin Capsules (1% to less than 5%) 3017
Aldara Cream, 5% 1699
Allegra-D 12 Hour Extended-Release Tablets 2687
Allegra-D 24 Hour Extended-Release Tablets 2690
Ambien Tablets (Rare) 2692
Ambien CR Tablets (Rare) 2696
AmBisome for Injection (Less common) 606
Amrix Capsules 966
Anaprox Tablets (Less than 1%) 2632
Anaprox DS Tablets (Less than 1%) 2632
▲ Aranesp for Injection (8%) 564
Avalide Tablets 892
Avalide Tablets 2713
Avapro Tablets (Less than 1%) 897
Avapro Tablets (Less than 1%) 2718
Bayer Aspirin 750
Betimol Ophthalmic Solution 3181
Brovana Inhalation Solution 2990
▲ Busulfex Injection (5%) 2477
Calcijex Injection 419
▲ Campath Ampules (14%) 761
Cancidas for Injection 1953
Carbatrol Capsules 3019
Cardizem LA Extended Release Tablets (Less than 2%) 421
Catapres Tablets (Rare) 841
Catapres-TTS (0.5% or less) 842
▲ CellCept Capsules (3% to less than 20%) 2622
▲ CellCept Intravenous (3% to less than 20%) 2622
▲ CellCept Oral Suspension (3% to less than 20%) 2622
▲ CellCept Tablets (3% to less than 20%) 2622
Chantix Tablets (Infrequent) 2511
Chemet Capsules (Up to 1.8%) 2484
Cimzia 3127
Cipro I.V. (1% or less) 2817
Cipro XR Tablets 2823
Clinoril Tablets (Rare) 1962
Clorpres Tablets (Rare) 2185
Combigan Ophthalmic Solution 553
Combivent Inhalation Aerosol (Less than 2%) 845
Concerta Extended-Release Tablets 1925
Copaxone for Injection 3110
Cosopt Sterile Ophthalmic Solution 1969
Cozaar Tablets (Less than 1%) 1973
Daytrana Transdermal Patch 3022
Depakote ER Tablets (Greater than 1%) 423
Doxil Injection (Less than 1%) 2378
Duragesic Transdermal System (1% or greater) 2405
Dyazide Capsules 1405
EC-Naprosyn Delayed-Release Tablets (Less than 1%) 2632
Effexor XR Extended-Release Capsules (Infrequent) 3195
Eldepryl Capsules 3052
Elitek (Less than or equal to 1%) 2729
EpiPen 1024
Equetro Extended-Release Capsules 3174
Evoxac Capsules (Less than 1%) 1013
Exelon Patch (Infrequent) 2233
Exforge Tablets (Greater than 0.1% to less than 1%) 2238
Fleet Enema 1143
Fleet Enema Extra 1143
Fleet Enema for Children 1143
Fleet Pedia-Lax Enema 1143
▲ Flolan for Injection (27%) 1426
Focalin XR Capsules 2251
Foradil Aerolizer 2849
Furosemide Tablets 2186
Gemzar for Injection (2%) 1820
Gengraf Capsules (2%) 435
Herceptin I.V. 1199
▲ Humira Injection (Less than 5%) 442
Imitrex Injection (Rare) 1465
Imitrex Nasal Spray (Infrequent) 1470
Imitrex Tablets (Rare to infrequent) 1474
Indocin Capsules (Less than 1%) 2024
Indocin I.V. (Less than 1%) 2489
Indocin (Less than 1%) 2024
▲ Intron A for Injection (Less than 5%) 2859
Invanz for Injection (Greater than 0.1%) 2029
Ionsys Transdermal System (.1% to less than 1%) 2410
Lanoxin Injection 1498

Lanoxin Injection Pediatric ... 1502
Leukine ... 774
Levaquin (0.1% to 1%) ... 2416
Levaquin in 5% Dextrose Injection (0.1% to 1%) ... 2416
Levothroid Tablets ... 1170
Levoxyl Tablets ... 1780
Lipitor Tablets (Less than 2%) ... 2501
Lovaza Capsules ... 1520
Maxalt Tablets (Infrequent) ... 2056
Maxalt-MLT Orally Disintegrating Tablets (Infrequent) ... 2056
Metadate CD Capsules ... 3146
Mirapex Tablets (Less than 1%) ... 857
Moban Tablets ... 1116
Mobic Oral Suspension (Less than 2%) ... 863
Mobic Tablets (Less than 2%) ... 863
Mycamine for Injection ... 616
Naprosyn Suspension (Less than 1%) ... 2632
Naprosyn Tablets (Less than 1%) ... 2632
Neoral Oral Solution (2%) ... 2280
Neoral Soft Gelatin Capsules (2%) ... 2280
▲ Neupogen for Injection (11 of 375 cancer patients) ... 589
Nexavar Tablets (0.1% to less than 1%) ... 784
Niaspan Extended-Release Tablets ... 480
▲ Novantrone for Injection Concentrate (3% to 18%) ... 1100
▲ Ontak Vials (6%) ... 1079
Orthoclone OKT3 Sterile Solution (Less than 1%) ... 2387
OsmoPrep Tablets (Rare) ... 2680
Paxil (Rare) ... 1535
Paxil CR Controlled-Release Tablets (Rare) ... 1544
Pepcid Tablets (Infrequent) ... 2075
Percocet Tablets ... 1127
Perforomist Inhalation Solution ... 1025
PrandiMet Tablets (Less than or equal to 1%) ... 2967
Prandin Tablets (Less than or equal to 1%) ... 2971
Prinivil Tablets (0.3% to 1%) ... 2087
Prinzide Tablets ... 2092
Prograf Capsules and Injection ... 622
▲ Proleukin for Injection (10%) ... 2287
Protonix for Delayed-Release Oral Suspension (Less than 1%) ... 3254
Protonix Delayed-Release Tablets (Less than 1%) ... 3254
Protonix I.V. (Less than 1%) ... 3257
Protopic Ointment (Greater than or equal to 1%) ... 628
Provigil Tablets (1%) ... 977
Prozac Weekly Capsules (Infrequent) ... 1852
Prozac Pulvules and Liquid (Infrequent) ... 1852
Relenza Inhalation Powder ... 1556
Remicade for IV Injection (Greater than or equal to 0.2%) ... 950
Rituxan I.V. ... 1223
Rocaltrol Capsules ... 1150
Rocaltrol Oral Solution ... 1150
Romazicon Injection (Less than 1%) ... 2646
Rythmol SR Capsules ... 1590
Salagen Tablets (Less than 1%) ... 1082
▲ Sandostatin Injection (9%) ... 2300
▲ Sandostatin LAR Depot (3% to 9%) ... 2302
Serevent Diskus ... 1594
Symbyax Capsules (Infrequent) ... 1871
Tamiflu Capsules ... 2649
Tamiflu Oral Suspension ... 2649
▲ Taxotere Injection Concentrate (0.3% to 7.9) ... 2773
Thiothixene Capsules ... 2197
Timoptic Sterile Ophthalmic Solution (Less frequent) ... 2121
Timoptic in Ocudose (Less frequent) ... 2124
Timoptic-XE Sterile Ophthalmic Gel Forming Solution ... 2125
TNKase ... 1233
▲ Trasylol Injection (4%) ... 799
Tricor Tablets ... 520
Ultane Liquid for Inhalation (Less than 1%) ... 524
Uniphyl Tablets ... 2595
Venlafaxine Hydrochloride Tablets (Infrequent) ... 2199
Ventolin HFA Inhalation Aerosol ... 1638
▲ Vesanoid Capsules (23%) ... 2660
Vicoprofen Tablets (Less than 1%) ... 533
Voltaren Tablets (Rarely) ... 2334
Voltaren-XR Tablets (Rarely) ... 2337
▲ Wellbutrin Tablets (5.3%) ... 1648
▲ Wellbutrin XL Extended-Release Tablets (5%) ... 1659
Xopenex Inhalation Solution ... 3001
Xopenex Inhalation Solution Concentrate ... 3005
Xopenex HFA Inhalation Aerosol ... 3009
Zantac 25 EFFERdose Tablets (Rare) ... 1670
Zantac Injection (Rare) ... 1666
Zantac Injection Pharmacy Bulk Package (Rare) ... 1668
Zantac Injection Premixed (Rare) ... 1666
Zantac (Rare) ... 1670
Zemuron Injection (Less than 1%) ... 2947
Zofran Injection ... 1682
Zomig Tablets (Infrequent) ... 694
Zomig Nasal Spray (Infrequent) ... 689
Zomig-ZMT Tablets (Infrequent) ... 694
Zosyn for Injection (1% or less) ... 3284
Zyrtec-D 12 Hour Extended Release Tablets ... 1923

Arrhythmias, sinus

Aloxi Injection (Less than 1%) ... 1059
Anzemet Injection ... 2701
Anzemet Tablets ... 2704
Imitrex Injection (Infrequent) ... 1465
Imitrex Nasal Spray ... 1470
Imitrex Tablets ... 1474
Invega Extended-Release Tablets (Less than 1% to 2%) ... 1748
Mirapex Tablets ... 857
Rythmol SR Capsules ... 1590

Arrhythmias, supraventricular

Anzemet Injection (Rare) ... 2701
Anzemet Tablets (Rare) ... 2704
Cubicin for Injection (Less than 1%) ... 995
Cymbalta Delayed-Release Capsules ... 1801
Intron A for Injection (Rare) ... 2859
Ixempra Kit for Injection ... 915
Leukine (Occasional) ... 774
Mirapex Tablets ... 857
PegIntron Powder for Injection (Less than or equal to 1%) ... 2903
Rituxan I.V. ... 1223

Arrhythmias, ventricular

Adenoscan (Less than 1%) ... 605
Anzemet Injection (Rare) ... 2701
Anzemet Tablets (Rare) ... 2704
Biaxin/Biaxin XL ... 411
Celexa ... 1160
Doxil Injection (Less than 1%) ... 2378
E.E.S. (Rare) ... 433
EryPed (Rare) ... 431
Lanoxin Injection ... 1498
Lanoxin Injection Pediatric (Less common) ... 1502
Lanoxin Tablets (Less common) ... 1505
Levaquin (0.1% to 1%) ... 2416
Levaquin in 5% Dextrose Injection (0.1% to 1%) ... 2416
Lexapro Oral Suspension ... 1174
Lexapro Tablets ... 1174
Lexiscan Injection ... 614
Neupro Transdermal System ... 3149
Noroxin Tablets (Rare) ... 2069
Prozac Weekly Capsules (Rare) ... 1852
Prozac Pulvules and Liquid (Rare) ... 1852
Remeron Tablets ... 2924
RemeronSolTab Tablets ... 2927
ReoPro Vials (0.3%) ... 1860
▲ Rythmol Tablets (4.7%) ... 1586
Rythmol SR Capsules ... 1590
Trasylol Injection (1% to 2%) ... 799
Zofran Injection ... 1682
Zofran ... 1687
Zofran ODT Orally Disintegrating Tablets ... 1687

Arterial carbon dioxide, decrease

Sulfamylon Cream ... 2194

Arterial insufficiency

Combigan Ophthalmic Solution ... 553
Cosopt Sterile Ophthalmic Solution ... 1969
InnoPran XL Extended Release Capsules ... 1484
Timoptic Sterile Ophthalmic Solution ... 2121
Timoptic in Ocudose ... 2124
Timoptic-XE Sterile Ophthalmic Gel Forming Solution ... 2125
Toprol-XL Tablets (About 1 of 100 patients) ... 666

Arterial occlusion

Follistim AQ Cartridge ... 2844

Arteriosclerosis

Brovana Inhalation Solution (Less than 2%) ... 2990
Mirapex Tablets ... 857

Arteriospasm

Fortaz ... 1450

Arteritis

Ambien Tablets (Rare) ... 2692
Ambien CR Tablets (Rare) ... 2696
Aricept Tablets (Infrequent) ... 1062
Aricept ODT Tablets (Infrequent) ... 1062
Effexor XR Extended-Release Capsules (Rare) ... 3195
Gantrisin Pediatric Suspension ... 2638
Venlafaxine Hydrochloride Tablets (Rare) ... 2199
Zyprexa Tablets (Rare) ... 1883
Zyprexa ZYDIS Orally Disintegrating Tablets (Rare) ... 1883

Arteritis, temporal

Imitrex Nasal Spray ... 1470
Imitrex Tablets ... 1474
Orthoclone OKT3 Sterile Solution (Less than 1%) ... 2387

Arthralgia

Abelcet Injection ... 1134
▲ Abilify Injection (2% to 4%) ... 881
▲ Abilify Injection (2% to 5%) ... 2466
▲ Abilify Oral Solution (2% to 4%) ... 881
▲ Abilify Oral Solution (2% to 5%) ... 2466
▲ Abilify Discmelt Orally Disintegrating Tablets (2% to 4%) ... 881
▲ Abilify Discmelt Orally Disintegrating Tablets (2% to 5%) ... 2466
▲ Abilify Tablets (2% to 4%) ... 881
▲ Abilify Tablets (2% to 5%) ... 2466
Accutane Capsules ... 2607
Aceon Tablets (2 mg, 4 mg, 8 mg) (0.3% to 1.1%) ... 3038
Aciphex Tablets ... 1053
Actimmune (2%) ... 1743
Actiq (1% or greater) ... 959
Activella Tablets ... 2347
▲ Actonel Tablets (11.5% to 32.8%) ... 2568
▲ Actonel with Calcium Tablets (11.5% to 23.7%) ... 2574
▲ Advair Diskus 100/50 (Greater than or equal to 3%) ... 1276
Advair Diskus 250/50 ... 1276
Advair Diskus 500/50 ... 1276
▲ Advair HFA 45/21 Inhalation Aerosol (1% to 3%) ... 1288
▲ Advair HFA 115/21 Inhalation Aerosol (1% to 3%) ... 1288
▲ Advair HFA 230/21 Inhalation Aerosol (1% to 3%) ... 1288
▲ Advate (23.3%) ... 721
Advicor Tablets ... 402
▲ Aggrenox Capsules (5.5%) ... 819
▲ Agrylin Capsules (1% to less than 5%) ... 3017
▲ Alferon N Injection (3% to 10%) ... 1726
▲ Alimta for Injection (Up to 8%) ... 1786
Aloxi Injection (Less than 1%) ... 1059
Alphanate ... 1709
▲ Alvesco Inhalation Aerosol (0.9% to greater than or equal to 3%) ... 2985
Ambien Tablets (Frequent) ... 2692
Ambien CR Tablets (2%) ... 2696
AmBisome for Injection (Less common) ... 606
Amerge Tablets (Infrequent) ... 1301
Angeliq Tablets ... 751
Anzemet Injection (Rare) ... 2701
Anzemet Tablets (Rare) ... 2704
Aptivus Oral Solution ... 823
▲ Aranesp for Injection (9% to 13%) ... 564
Aricept Tablets (Infrequent) ... 1062
Aricept ODT Tablets (Infrequent) ... 1062
▲ Arimidex Tablets (2% to 36%) ... 672
▲ Arranon Injection (0% to 9%) ... 1319
▲ Asacol Delayed-Release Tablets (5%) ... 2579
▲ Asmanex Twisthaler (13%) ... 2797
Atacand Tablets (More than 1%) ... 639
Atacand HCT (0.5% or greater) ... 642
▲ Atripla Tablets (Greater than or equal to 5%) ... 938
Attenuvax ... 1951
Augmentin ... 1323
Augmentin Tablets ... 1327
Augmentin XR Extended Release Tablets ... 1333
Augmentin ES-600 Powder for Oral Suspension ... 1329
▲ Avandamet Tablets (5%) ... 1336
Avapro Tablets (Less than 1%) ... 897
Avapro Tablets (Less than 1%) ... 2718
Avelox (Greater than or equal to 0.1% to less than 2%) ... 2803
Axert Tablets (Rare) ... 2431
▲ Azilect Tablets (7% to 8%) ... 3106
Azmacort Inhalation Aerosol ... 407
Beconase AQ Nasal Spray ... 1369
Benicar Tablets (Greater than 0.5%) ... 1009
Benicar HCT Tablets (Greater than 1%) ... 1010
▲ Betaseron for SC Injection (31%) ... 756
▲ Bexxar (1% to 10%) ... 1371
Bicillin C-R Injectable Suspension ... 1775
Bicillin L-A Injection ... 1777
▲ Boniva Injection (3.5% to 5.6%) ... 2614
▲ Boniva Tablets (3.5% to 5.6%) ... 2618
Boostrix ... 1377
Brovana Inhalation Solution (Less than 2%) ... 2990
▲ Busulfex Injection (13%) ... 2477
Campral Tablets (Frequent) ... 1158
Cancidas for Injection ... 1953
▲ Captopril Tablets (About 4 to 7 of 100 patients) ... 2182
Carbatrol Capsules ... 3019
Catapres Tablets (About 6 in 1,000 patients) ... 841
Catapres-TTS (0.5% or less) ... 842
Ceftin for Oral Suspension (0.1% to 1%) ... 1380
▲ Celebrex Capsules (0.1% to 7%) ... 2979
Celexa (2%) ... 1160
▲ CellCept Capsules (3% to less than 20%) ... 2622
▲ CellCept Intravenous (3% to less than 20%) ... 2622
▲ CellCept Oral Suspension (3% to less than 20%) ... 2622
▲ CellCept Tablets (3% to less than 20%) ... 2622
Chantix Tablets (Frequent) ... 2511
Cialis Tablets (Less than 2%) ... 1792
▲ Cimzia (6%) ... 3127
Cipro I.V. (1% or less) ... 2817
Cipro (Less than 1%) ... 2810
Cipro XR Tablets ... 2823
▲ Climara Transdermal System (1% to 5%) ... 763
▲ Climara Pro Transdermal System (4.2%) ... 768
Clinoril Tablets (Less than 1 in 100) ... 1962
▲ Clolar for Intravenous Infusion (11%) ... 1239
Clorpres Tablets (About 6 in 1,000) ... 2185
Combigan Ophthalmic Solution ... 553
Combivent Inhalation Aerosol (Less than 2%) ... 845
▲ Combivir Tablets (5%) ... 1384
Comvax ... 1966
Concerta Extended-Release Tablets ... 1925
▲ Copaxone for Injection (24%) ... 3110
▲ Coreg Tablets (1% to 6%) ... 1387
▲ Coreg CR Extended-Release Capsules (1% to 6%) ... 1393
Cosopt Sterile Ophthalmic Solution ... 1969
Cozaar Tablets (Less than 1%) ... 1973
▲ Crestor Tablets (10.1%) ... 677
▲ Crinone 8% Gel (8%) ... 992
Crixivan Capsules ... 1979
▲ Cubicin for Injection (0.9% to 3.3%) ... 995
Cuprimine Capsules ... 1986
▲ Dacogen Injection (20%) ... 1066
Daytrana Transdermal Patch ... 3022
Demadex Injection (1.8%) ... 2630
Demadex Tablets (1.8%) ... 2630
▲ Depakote ER Tablets (Greater than 1% to less than 5%) ... 423
▲ DepoCyt Injection (9% to 11%) ... 1136
Didronel Tablets (Infrequent) ... 2583
▲ Diovan Tablets (1% to 3%) ... 2212
Diovan HCT Tablets (Greater than 0.2%) ... 2216
Divigel ... 3167
▲ Doxil Injection (1% to 10%) ... 2378
DynaCirc CR Controlled Release Tablets (0.5% to 1%) ... 1407
Effexor XR Extended-Release Capsules ... 3195
Elidel Cream 1% (0% to 1.5%) ... 2221
Eligard 7.5 mg (Less than 2%) ... 2724
▲ Eligard 22.5 mg (Less than 2% to 3.4%) ... 2724
Eligard 30 mg (Less than 2%) ... 2724
Eligard 45 mg (Less than 2%) ... 2724
▲ Eloxatin for Injection (5% to 10%) ... 2731
Elspar for Injection ... 1990
Emend Capsules (Greater than 0.5%) ... 1992
Emend for Injection (Greater than 0.5%) ... 1999

Emsam Transdermal System (Infrequent) 905
▲ Emtriva Capsules (3% to 5%) 1246
▲ Emtriva Oral Solution (3% to 5%) 1246
Enablex Extended-Release Tablets (Greater than or equal to 1%) 2225
Enbrel for Injection 569
Engerix-B Vaccine (Less than 1%) 1409
Enjuvia Tablets 1029
▲ Epivir (5%) 1412
▲ Epivir-HBV (7%) 1417
Epogen for Injection (Rare) 576
Equetro Extended-Release Capsules 3174
Estratest Tablets 3043
Estratest H.S. Tablets 3043
▲ Evista Tablets (10.7% to 15.5%) 1810
▲ Evoxac Capsules (3.7%) 1013
Exelon Capsules (2% or more) 2229
Exelon Oral Solution (2% or more) 2229
Exelon Patch (Infrequent) 2233
Exforge Tablets (Greater than or equal to 0.2%) 2238
▲ Exjade Tablets (7.4%) 2244
Fansidar Tablets 2636
▲ Femara Tablets (1% to 22%) 2246
Fenoglide Tablets 2960
▲ Fentora Tablets (0% to 8%) 968
Flebogamma 5% 1715
Flebogamma 5% DIF 1718
▲ Flolan for Injection (6% to 84%) 1426
▲ Flovent Diskus 50 mcg (1% to 17%) 1435
▲ Fluarix Vaccine (6.4% to 11%) 1446
▲ Flulaval Injection Vaccine (1% to 8%) 1448
Focalin XR Capsules 2251
Follistim AQ Cartridge 2844
▲ Forteo for Injection (10.1%) 1816
▲ Fosamax (0.4% to approximately 6%) 2005
▲ Fosamax Plus D Tablets (0.4% to 4.1%) 2013
Frova Tablets (Infrequent) 1111
▲ Gamunex (4%) 3094
Gantrisin Pediatric Suspension 2638
Gardasil Injection (1.2%) 2019
▲ Gengraf Capsules (1% to 6%) 435
▲ Genotropin Lyophilized Powder (4.2% to 17.3%) 2547
Geodon Capsules 2520
▲ Gleevec Tablets (11% to 40%) 2255
Havrix Injection Vaccine (Less than 1%) 1454
▲ Herceptin I.V. (6% to 31%) 1199
▲ Humatrope Vials and Cartridges (10.8% to 17.3%) 1838
Hycamtin for Injection (0.2% to 0.9%) 1459
Imitrex Injection (Infrequent) 1465
▲ Increlex Injection (Greater than or equal to 5%) 3100
▲ Intron A for Injection (Up to 19%) 2859
Invanz for Injection (Greater than 0.5%) 2029
▲ Ixempra Kit for Injection (49%) 915
Kaletra (Less than 2%) 452
▲ Kepivance (10%) 583
Keppra Oral Solution (1% or more) 3131
Keppra Tablets (1% or more) 3131
▲ Kineret Injection (6%) 585
Klonopin (Infrequent) 2639
K-Phos Original (Sodium Free) Tablets (Less frequent) 814
K-Phos Neutral Tablets 813
▲ Lamictal (Greater than 1% to less than 5%) 1488
Lamisil Oral Granules 2264
Lamisil Tablets 2266
▲ Lescol Capsules (4%) 2268
Lescol XL Tablets (1.3%) 2268
▲ Leukine (11% to 21%) 774
▲ Leustatin Injection (5%) 2384
Levaquin (0.1% to 0.9%) 2416
Levaquin in 5% Dextrose Injection (0.1% to 0.9%) 2416
Levitra Tablets (Less than 2%) 2876
Levothroid Tablets 1170
Levoxyl Tablets 1780
Lexapro Oral Suspension (Frequent) 1174
Lexapro Tablets (Frequent) 1174
Lialda Tablets (Infrequent) 3029
▲ Lipitor Tablets (Up to 5.1%) 2501
Lovaza Capsules 1520
▲ Lucentis Injection (3% to 11%) 1205
Lunesta Tablets (Infrequent) 2994
Lupron Depot 7.5 mg 469
Lupron Depot–3 Month 11.25 mg 462
Luvox CR Extended-Release Capsules (Infrequent) 1759
▲ Lyrica Capsules (Greater than or equal to 1% to 6%) 2527
Maxalt Tablets (Infrequent) 2056
Maxalt-MLT Orally Disintegrating Tablets (Infrequent) 2056
▲ Meridia Capsules (5.9%) 475
Meruvax II 2061
Metadate CD Capsules 3146
Mevacor Tablets (0.5% to 1%) 2063
▲ Miacalcin Nasal Spray (3.8%) 2274
Micardis Tablets (More than 0.3%) 852
Micardis HCT Tablets 854
Mirapex Tablets (Greater than or equal to 1%) 857
M-M-R II 2054
▲ Mobic Oral Suspension (0% to 5.3%) 863
▲ Mobic Tablets (0% to 5.3%) 863
Mycamine for Injection 616
▲ Myfortic Tablets (3% to less than 20%) 2276
Namenda (Greater than or equal to 2%) 1180
Nasonex Nasal Spray (Greater than or equal to 2%) 2883
▲ Neoral Oral Solution (1% to 6%) 2280
▲ Neoral Soft Gelatin Capsules (1% to 6%) 2280
▲ Neulasta Injection (15% to 72%) 587
Neupogen for Injection (Infrequent) 589
▲ Neupro Transdermal System (4%) 3149
▲ Nexavar Tablets (10%) 784
Nexium Delayed-Release Capsules (Less than 1%) 645
Nexium I.V. (Less than 1%) 652
Nexium Delayed-Release Oral Suspension (Less than 1%) 645
▲ Norditropin Cartridges (19%) 2354
Noroxin Tablets 2069
Norvir (0% to 1.7%) 489
▲ Novantrone for Injection Concentrate (5%) 1100
NovoSeven 2367
NovoSeven RT 2370
▲ Noxafil Oral Suspension (11%) 2889
▲ Nutropin for Injection (0.1% to 27%) 1208
▲ Nutropin AQ Injection (0.1% to 27%) 1212
▲ Nutropin AQ NuSpin Injection (0.1% to 27%) 1212
▲ Nutropin AQ Pen (0.1% to 27%) 1212
▲ Nutropin AQ Pen Cartridge (0.1% to 27%) 1212
▲ Ontak Vials (8%) 1079
Orthoclone OKT3 Sterile Solution (Less than 1%) 2387
Paxil (Frequent) 1535
Paxil CR Controlled-Release Tablets (Frequent) 1544
Pediarix Vaccine 1552
▲ PegIntron Powder for Injection (23%) 2903
Pentasa Capsules (Less than 1%) 3030
Pepcid Tablets (Infrequent) 2075
Phenytek Capsules 2192
▲ Photofrin for Injection (31%) 708
▲ Plavix Tablets (6.3%) 926
▲ Plavix Tablets (6.3%) 2767
Pletal Tablets (Less than 2%) 2481
Pneumovax 23 2078
▲ Prandin Tablets (3% to 6%) 2971
Premarin Intravenous 3217
▲ Premarin Tablets (7% to 14%) 3221
Premarin Vaginal Cream 3228
▲ Premphase Tablets (7% to 13%) 3232
▲ Prempro Tablets (7% to 13%) 3232
Prinivil Tablets (0.3% to 1%) 2087
Prinzide Tablets 2092
▲ Procrit for Injection (Rare to 11%) 2391
▲ Prograf Capsules and Injection (3% to 25%) 622
▲ Prometrium Capsules (100 mg, 200 mg) (20%) 3047
ProQuad 2099
Protonix for Delayed-Release Oral Suspension (Greater than or equal to 1%) 3254
Protonix Delayed-Release Tablets (Greater than or equal to 1%) 3254
Protonix I.V. (Greater than or equal to 1%) 3257
▲ Protopic Ointment (Greater than or equal to 1% to 3%) 628
Provigil Tablets (At least 1%) 977
Prozac Weekly Capsules 1852
Prozac Pulvules and Liquid 1852
▲ Pulmicort Flexhaler (6%) 654
▲ Rapamune (25% to 31%) 3260
Raptiva for Injection 1218
▲ Rebetol (15% to 34%) 2917
▲ Reclast Injection (17.9% to 23.8%) 2291
Recombivax HB (Less than 1%) 2107
Relenza Inhalation Powder (Less than 1% to 2%) 1556
Remeron Tablets (Frequent) 2924
RemeronSolTab Tablets (Frequent) 2927
▲ Remicade for IV Injection (8%) 950
▲ Requip Tablets (4% to 7%) 1561
Retrovir Capsules 1574
Retrovir IV Infusion 1579
Retrovir 1574
Reyataz Capsules 3299
▲ Rilutek Tablets (1.6% to 5.1%) 2771
Risperdal Consta Long-Acting Injection (Frequent) 1753
▲ Rituxan I.V. (1% to 12%) 1223
Rozerem Tablets (2%) 3091
Rythmol Tablets (1%) 1586
Salagen Tablets (Less than 1%) 1082
Sandimmune (Rare) 2296
▲ Sandostatin Injection (1% to 4%) 2300
Serevent Diskus (1% to 2%) 1594
▲ Simulect for Injection (3% to 10%) 2306
Singulair 2114
Solodyn Extended Release Tablets (1%) 1938
▲ Somatuline Depot Injection (7% to 10%) 3102
▲ Soriatane Capsules (10% to 25%) 3062
▲ Stromectol Tablets (9.3%) 2120
Sular Extended Release Tablets (Less than or equal to 1%) 2975
Sustiva Capsules (Less than 2%) 930
Sustiva Tablets (Less than 2%) 930
▲ Sutent Capsules (1% to 28%) 2540
▲ Symbyax Capsules (3% to 5%) 1871
Targretin Capsules 1084
Tarka Tablets (0.3% to 1.7%) 511
▲ Tasigna Capsules (16% to 18%) 2316
▲ Taxotere Injection Concentrate (0% to 19.4%) 2773
Tekturna HCT Tablets (1%) 2324
▲ Temodar Capsules (Less than 1% to 6%) 2931
Teveten Tablets (2%) 515
Teveten HCT Tablets (Less than 1%) 517
▲ Tice BCG (3%) 2936
Timentin ADD-Vantage 1606
Timentin Injection Galaxy Container 1609
Timentin IV Infusion 1603
Timentin Pharmacy Bulk Package 1613
Timoptic Sterile Ophthalmic Solution 2121
Timoptic in Ocudose 2124
Timoptic-XE Sterile Ophthalmic Gel Forming Solution 2125
Toprol-XL Tablets 666
▲ Torisel Injection (1% to 18%) 3272
Trasylol Injection (1% to 2%) 799
Treximet Tablets (Infrequent) 1616
Tricor Tablets 520
▲ Trisenox Injection (33%) 986
▲ Trizivir Tablets (5%) 1622
▲ Truvada Tablets (Greater than or equal to 5%) 1262
Twinrix Vaccine (Less than 1%) 1628
▲ Tyzeka Tablets (Less than 1% to 4%) 2328
▲ Ultram ER Extended-Release Tablets (1% to less than 5%) 2428
Uroqid-Acid No. 2 Tablets 814
▲ Valcyte Tablets (Less than 5%) 2654
▲ Valtrex Caplets (Less than 1% to 6%) 1635
Vantas (Less than 2%) 1737
Varivax (Greater than or equal to 1%) 2133
▲ Velcade for Injection (11% to 17%) 2168
Veramyst Nasal Spray 1643
Vicoprofen Tablets (Less than 1%) 533
Viramune Oral Suspension 873
Viramune Tablets 873
▲ Viread Tablets (5%) 1268
▲ Visudyne for Injection (1% to 10%) 2332
▲ Vivitrol (4% to 12%) 988
Vytorin 10/10 Tablets 2149
Vytorin 10/10 Tablets 2939
Vytorin 10/20 Tablets 2149
Vytorin 10/20 Tablets 2939
Vytorin 10/40 Tablets 2149
Vytorin 10/40 Tablets 2939
Vytorin 10/80 Tablets 2149
Vytorin 10/80 Tablets 2939
Wellbutrin Tablets 1648
▲ Wellbutrin SR Sustained-Release Tablets (1% to 4%) 1653
▲ Wellbutrin XL Extended-Release Tablets (1% to 4%) 1659
WinRho SDF 741
Xifaxan Tablets (Less than 2%) 2682
▲ Xolair (8%) 1235
▲ Xolair (8%) 2339
Xyrem Oral Solution (Frequent) 1766
Yaz Tablets (Greater than 1%) 805
Zantac 25 EFFERdose Tablets (Rare) 1670
Zantac Injection (Rare) 1666
Zantac Injection Pharmacy Bulk Package (Rare) 1668
Zantac Injection Premixed (Rare) 1666
Zantac (Rare) 1670
▲ Zetia Tablets (3%) 2157
▲ Zetia Tablets (0.3% to 3%) 2951
Ziagen 1673
Zocor Tablets 2136
Zofran Injection (2%) 1682
▲ Zometa for Intravenous Infusion (5% to 21%) 2341
Zomig Tablets (Infrequent) 694
Zomig Nasal Spray (Infrequent) 689
Zomig-ZMT Tablets (Infrequent) 694
Zonegran Capsules (Infrequent) 1089
Zosyn for Injection (1% or less) 3284
▲ Zyban Sustained-Release Tablets (4% to 5%) 1692
▲ Zyprexa Tablets (5%) 1883
▲ Zyprexa ZYDIS Orally Disintegrating Tablets (5%) 1883
Zyrtec Chewable Tablets (Less than 2%) 1920
Zyrtec Syrup (Less than 2%) 1920
Zyrtec Tablets (Less than 2%) 1920
Zyrtec-D 12 Hour Extended Release Tablets (Less than 2%) 1923

Arthralgia, monoarticular

Recombivax HB (Less than 1%) 2107

Arthritis

Accutane Capsules 2607
Aceon Tablets (2 mg, 4 mg, 8 mg) (1%) 3038
Actiq (Less than 1%) 959
▲ Actonel Tablets (9.6%) 2568
▲ Actonel with Calcium Tablets (4.1% to 4.8%) 2574
Advicor Tablets 402
Aggrenox Capsules (2.1%) 819
Ambien Tablets (Infrequent) 2692
Ambien CR Tablets (Infrequent) 2696
Aricept Tablets (Frequent) 1062
Aricept ODT Tablets (Frequent) 1062
▲ Arimidex Tablets (17% to 36%) 672
Asacol Delayed-Release Tablets (1% to 2%) 2579
Atacand HCT (0.5% or greater) 642
Augmentin 1323
Augmentin Tablets 1327
Augmentin XR Extended Release Tablets 1333
Augmentin ES-600 Powder for Oral Suspension 1329
Avalide Tablets 892
Avalide Tablets 2713
Avapro Tablets (Less than 1%) 897
Avapro Tablets (Less than 1%) 2718
Avelox (Less than 0.1%) 2803
Axert Tablets (Rare) 2431
Azilect Tablets (2%) 3106
Benicar Tablets (Greater than 0.5%) 1009
Benicar HCT Tablets (Greater than 1%) 1010
▲ Boniva Injection (3.2%) 2614
▲ Boniva Tablets (3.2%) 2618
Brovana Inhalation Solution (Less than 2%) 2990
Celexa (Infrequent) 1160
Chantix Tablets (Infrequent) 2511
Clinoril Tablets (Less than 1 in 100) 1962
Comvax 1966
Copaxone for Injection (Infrequent) 3110
▲ Coreg Tablets (Greater than 1% to 3%) 1387
▲ Coreg CR Extended-Release Capsules (Greater than 1% to less than or equal to 3%) 1393
Cozaar Tablets (Less than 1%) 1973
Demadex Injection 2630
Demadex Tablets 2630
Didronel Tablets 2583
Effexor XR Extended-Release Capsules (Infrequent) 3195
Emsam Transdermal System (Infrequent) 905
Engerix-B Vaccine (Less than 1%) 1409
Evoxac Capsules (Less than 1%) 1013
Exelon Capsules (Frequent) 2229
Exelon Oral Solution (Frequent) 2229
Faslodex Injection (2.8%) 682
▲ Femara Tablets (0.4% to 21.1%) 2246
▲ Flolan for Injection (52%) 1426
Flulaval Injection Vaccine 1448
Gabitril Tablets (Infrequent) 973
Gardasil Injection (0.04%) 2019
▲ Humira Injection (Less than 5%) 442
Imitrex Nasal Spray (Infrequent) 1470
Imitrex Tablets 1474

▲ Intron A for Injection (Less than 5%) 2859
Lamictal (Infrequent) 1488
Lescol Capsules (2.1%) 2268
Lescol XL Tablets (1.3%) 2268
Levaquin (0.1% to 0.9%) 2416
Levaquin in 5% Dextrose Injection (0.1% to 0.9%) 2416
Lexapro Oral Suspension (Infrequent) 1174
Lexapro Tablets (Infrequent) 1174
Lipitor Tablets (Greater than or equal to 2%) 2501
Lovaza Capsules 1520
Lunesta Tablets (Infrequent) 2994
Luvox CR Extended-Release Capsules (Infrequent) 1759
Meridia Capsules (Greater than or equal to 1%) 475
Meruvax II (Rare) 2061
Mevacor Tablets (Rare) 2063
Miacalcin Nasal Spray (Less than 1%) 2274
Micardis Tablets (More than 0.3%) 852
Micardis HCT Tablets 854
▲ Mirapex Tablets (3%) 857
M-M-R II 2054
Noroxin Tablets 2069
Nutropin for Injection (0.1%) 1208
Nutropin AQ Injection (0.1%) 1212
Nutropin AQ NuSpin Injection (0.1%) 1212
Nutropin AQ Pen (0.1%) 1212
Nutropin AQ Pen Cartridge (0.1%) 1212
OptiPranolol Metipranolol Ophthalmic Solution 0.3% (A small number of patients) ⊙ 245
Orthoclone OKT3 Sterile Solution (Less than 1%) 2387
Paxil (Infrequent) 1535
Paxil CR Controlled-Release Tablets (Infrequent) 1544
Persantine Tablets (Rare) 869
Plavix Tablets (1% to 2.5%) 926
Plavix Tablets (1% to 2.5%) 2767
Pletal Tablets (2% or greater) 2481
Pneumovax 23 2078
Prinivil Tablets (0.3% to 1%) 2087
Prinzide Tablets 2092
▲ Prometrium Capsules (100 mg, 200 mg) (Less than 5%) 3047
ProQuad 2099
Protonix for Delayed-Release Oral Suspension (Less than 1%) 3254
Protonix Delayed-Release Tablets (Less than 1%) 3254
Protonix I.V. (Less than 1%) 3257
Protopic Ointment (Greater than or equal to 1%) 628
Provigil Tablets (At least 1%) 977
Prozac Weekly Capsules (Infrequent) 1852
Prozac Pulvules and Liquid (Infrequent) 1852
Raptiva for Injection 1218
Recombivax HB (Greater than 1%) 2107
Remeron Tablets (Infrequent) 2924
RemeronSolTab Tablets (Infrequent) 2927
Requip Tablets (Infrequent to greater than or equal to 1%) 1561
Risperdal Consta Long-Acting Injection (Infrequent) 1753
Rythmol SR Capsules 1590
Salagen Tablets (Less than 1%) 1082
Sandostatin Injection (Less than 1%) 2300
Sandostatin LAR Depot 2302
▲ Soriatane Capsules (1% to 10%) 3062
▲ Spiriva HandiHaler (Greater than or equal to 3%) 870
Sular Extended Release Tablets (Less than or equal to 1%) 2975
Symbyax Capsules (Infrequent) 1871
Tasigna Capsules 2316
Teveten Tablets (Less than 1%) 515
Teveten HCT Tablets (Less than 1%) 517
▲ Tice BCG (3%) 2936
▲ Travatan Z Ophthalmic Solution (1% to 5%) 547
Tricor Tablets 520
Twinrix Vaccine 1628
Venlafaxine Hydrochloride Tablets (Infrequent) 2199
Viadur Implant (Less than 2%) 802
▲ Vivitrol (4% to 12%) 988
Vytorin 10/10 Tablets 2149
Vytorin 10/10 Tablets 2939
Vytorin 10/20 Tablets 2149
Vytorin 10/20 Tablets 2939
Vytorin 10/40 Tablets 2149
Vytorin 10/40 Tablets 2939
Vytorin 10/80 Tablets 2149
Vytorin 10/80 Tablets 2939
▲ Wellbutrin Tablets (3.1%) 1648
Wellbutrin SR Sustained-Release Tablets (Up to 2%) 1653
Wellbutrin XL Extended-Release Tablets (0% to 2%) 1659
▲ Xeloda Tablets (Less than 5%) 2662
▲ Xenical Capsules (5.4%) 2672
Xyrem Oral Solution (Infrequent) 1766
Zocor Tablets (Rare) 2136
Zomig Tablets (Rare) 694
Zomig-ZMT Tablets (Rare) 694
Zonegran Capsules (Infrequent) 1089
Zyban Sustained-Release Tablets 1692
Zyprexa Tablets (Infrequent) 1883
Zyprexa ZYDIS Orally Disintegrating Tablets (Infrequent) 1883
Zyrtec Chewable Tablets (Less than 2%) 1920
Zyrtec Syrup (Less than 2%) 1920
Zyrtec Tablets (Less than 2%) 1920
Zyrtec-D 12 Hour Extended Release Tablets (Less than 2%) 1923

Arthritis, exacerbation of

Bicillin C-R Injectable Suspension 1775
Bicillin L-A Injection 1777
Evoxac Capsules (Less than 1%) 1013
Nexium Delayed-Release Capsules (Less than 1%) 645
Nexium I.V. (Less than 1%) 652
Nexium Delayed-Release Oral Suspension (Less than 1%) 645
Proleukin for Injection 2287
Teveten Tablets (Less than 1%) 515
Teveten HCT Tablets (Less than 1%) 517

Arthritis, inflammatory

Raptiva for Injection (0.4%) 1218

Arthritis, polyarticular

Rituxan I.V. 1223

Arthritis, psoriatic

Raptiva for Injection 1218

Arthritis, pyogenic

▲ Humira Injection (Less than 5%) 442

Arthritis, septic

Elidel Cream 1% 2221
Enbrel for Injection 569
▲ Humira Injection (Less than 5%) 442
Raptiva for Injection 1218

Arthritis, tuberculous

Enbrel for Injection 569

Arthropathy, unspecified

Didronel Tablets 2583
Evoxac Capsules (Less than 1%) 1013
▲ Gengraf Capsules (4%) 435
▲ Lescol XL Tablets (3.2%) 2268
Lexapro Oral Suspension (Infrequent) 1174
Lexapro Tablets (Infrequent) 1174
▲ Neoral Oral Solution (4%) 2280
▲ Neoral Soft Gelatin Capsules (4%) 2280
Nexium Delayed-Release Capsules (Less than 1%) 645
Nexium I.V. (Less than 1%) 652
Nexium Delayed-Release Oral Suspension (Less than 1%) 645
Risperdal Consta Long-Acting Injection (Infrequent) 1753
▲ Sandostatin LAR Depot (8% to 19.2%) 2302
▲ Simulect for Injection (3% to 10%) 2306
▲ Starlix Tablets (3.3%) 2314

Arthrosis

Aggrenox Capsules (1.1%) 819
Ambien Tablets (Rare) 2692
Ambien CR Tablets (Rare) 2696
Aricept Tablets (Infrequent) 1062
Aricept ODT Tablets (Infrequent) 1062
▲ Arimidex Tablets (7% to 36%) 672
Atacand HCT (0.5% or greater) 642
Azilect Tablets (Rare) 3106
Celebrex Capsules (0.1% to 1.9%) 2979
Cipro 2810
Depakote ER Tablets (Greater than 1%) 423
Effexor XR Extended-Release Capsules (Infrequent) 3195
Emsam Transdermal System (Infrequent) 905
Exforge Tablets (Greater than 0.1% to less than 1%) 2238
Frova Tablets (Infrequent) 1111
Gabitril Tablets (Infrequent) 973
▲ Humatrope Vials and Cartridges (10.8%) 1838
▲ Intron A for Injection (Less than 5%) 2859
Kaletra (Less than 2%) 452
Lunesta Tablets (Rare) 2994
▲ Luvox CR Extended-Release Capsules (Rare) 1759
Lyrica Capsules (0.1% to 1%) 2527
Meridia Capsules 475
▲ Miacalcin Nasal Spray (1% to 3%) 2274
Norvir (Less than 2%) 489
NovoSeven (1%) 2367
NovoSeven RT (1%) 2370
Paxil (Rare) 1535
Paxil CR Controlled-Release Tablets (Rare) 1544
Plavix Tablets (1% to 2.5%) 926
Plavix Tablets (1% to 2.5%) 2767
Protonix for Delayed-Release Oral Suspension (Less than 1%) 3254
Protonix Delayed-Release Tablets (Less than 1%) 3254
Protonix I.V. (Less than 1%) 3257
Protopic Ointment (0.2% to less than 1%) 628
Prozac Weekly Capsules (Rare) 1852
Prozac Pulvules and Liquid (Rare) 1852
Requip Tablets (1% or more) 1561
Rilutek Tablets (Infrequent) 2771
Risperdal Consta Long-Acting Injection (Infrequent) 1753
▲ Soriatane Capsules (1% to 10%) 3062
Symbyax Capsules (Rare) 1871
Targretin Capsules 1084
Teveten Tablets (Less than 1%) 515
Teveten HCT Tablets (Less than 1%) 517
Tricor Tablets 520
Venlafaxine Hydrochloride Tablets (Infrequent) 2199
▲ Visudyne for Injection (1% to 10%) 2332
Zyprexa Tablets (Infrequent) 1883
Zyprexa ZYDIS Orally Disintegrating Tablets (Infrequent) 1883
Zyrtec Chewable Tablets (Less than 2%) 1920
Zyrtec Syrup (Less than 2%) 1920
Zyrtec Tablets (Less than 2%) 1920
Zyrtec-D 12 Hour Extended Release Tablets (Less than 2%) 1923

Ascites

Actiq (1% or greater) 959
Campral Tablets (Rare) 1158
▲ CellCept Capsules (24.2%) 2622
▲ CellCept Intravenous (24.2%) 2622
▲ CellCept Oral Suspension (24.2%) 2622
▲ CellCept Tablets (24.2%) 2622
Cosmegen for Injection 2485
▲ Dacogen Injection (10%) 1066
▲ Doxil Injection (1% to 10%) 2378
▲ Eloxatin for Injection (2% to less than 5%) 2731
▲ Flolan for Injection (12% to 23%) 1426
Follistim AQ Cartridge 2844
▲ Gleevec Tablets (6.9% to 22%) 2255
▲ Intron A for Injection (Less than 5%) 2859
Lyrica Capsules (Rare) 2527
Mirapex Tablets 857
Mylotarg for Injection (Observed in 8 out of 274 patients) 3212
▲ Prograf Capsules and Injection (7% to 27%) 622
Requip Tablets (Rare) 1561
Sandostatin LAR Depot 2302
Tabloid Tablets 1601
▲ Taxotere Injection Concentrate (6.5%) 2773
▲ Valcyte Tablets (Less than 5%) 2654
Velcade for Injection 2168
▲ Vesanoid Capsules (3%) 2660
▲ Xeloda Tablets (Less than 5%) 2662

Aseptic meningitis syndrome

Clinoril Tablets (Less than 1 in 100) 1962
Gammagard Liquid (Infrequent) 730
Orthoclone OKT3 Sterile Solution (Less than 1%) 2387

Aspartate aminotransferase levels, changes in

▲ Eloxatin for Injection (0% to 54%) 2731
Prozac Pulvules and Liquid (Infrequent) 1852
Selzentry Tablets (Greater than or equal to 2%) 2534
▲ Sutent Capsules (2% to 39%) 2540
▲ Tykerb Tablets (Less than 1% to 49%) 1631
▲ Zyvox (1.7% to 5%) 2552

Aspartate aminotransferase levels, elevation of

Abelcet Injection 1134
Accutane Capsules 2607
Aceon Tablets (2 mg, 4 mg, 8 mg) (0.3% to 1%) 3038
▲ Alimta for Injection (Less than 1% to 8%) 1786
Aloxi Injection (Less than 1%) 1059
Ambien Tablets (Rare) 2692
Ambien CR Tablets (Rare) 2696
▲ AmBisome for Injection (12.8%) 606
Amevive (1.7%) 611
Amitiza Capsules (Less than 1%) 3082
Amoxil Capsules 1305
Amoxil Chewable Tablets 1305
Amoxil Pediatric Drops for Oral Suspension 1305
Amoxil Powder for Oral Suspension 1305
Amoxil Tablets 1305
Anaprox Tablets (1%) 2632
Anaprox DS Tablets (1%) 2632
AndroGel 3159
Anzemet Injection 2701
Anzemet Tablets (Less than 1%) 2704
▲ Aptivus Capsules (1.6% to 26%) 823
▲ Aptivus Oral Solution (1.6% to 26%) 823
▲ Aralast (11.1%) 726
Aricept Tablets (Infrequent) 1062
Aricept ODT Tablets (Infrequent) 1062
▲ Arimidex Tablets (Greater than or equal to 1% to less than 10%) 672
Arixtra Injection (0.2% to 2.6%) 1313
▲ Arranon Injection (1% to 6%) 1319
Asacol Delayed-Release Tablets 2579
▲ Atripla Tablets (3%) 938
Augmentin (Infrequent) 1323
Augmentin Tablets (Infrequent) 1327
Augmentin XR Extended Release Tablets (Infrequent) 1333
Augmentin ES-600 Powder for Oral Suspension 1329
Axid Capsules 1364
▲ Baraclude (5%) 900
BeneFIX Vials (1.6%) 3191
Benicar HCT Tablets (Greater than 1%) 1010
▲ Betaseron for SC Injection (4%) 756
Biaxin/Biaxin XL (Less than 1%) 411
Bicillin C-R Injectable Suspension 1775
Bicillin L-A Injection 1777
Bystolic Tablets 1155
Calcijex Injection 419
Campral Tablets (Infrequent) 1158
▲ Cancidas for Injection (1.8% to 15.8%) 1953
Cardizem LA Extended Release Tablets (Less than 2%) 421
Ceftin (0.1% to 1%) 1380
Celebrex Capsules (0.1% to 1.9%) 2979
▲ CellCept Capsules (3% to less than 20%) 2622
▲ CellCept Intravenous (3% to less than 20%) 2622
▲ CellCept Oral Suspension (3% to less than 20%) 2622
▲ CellCept Tablets (3% to less than 20%) 2622
▲ Chemet Capsules (4.2% to 10.4%) 2484
Cipro I.V. (Among most frequent) 2817
Cipro (1.7%) 2810
Cipro XR Tablets 2823
▲ Clolar for Intravenous Infusion (38%) 1239
Combivir Tablets 1384
▲ Coreg Tablets (Greater than 1% to 3%) 1387
▲ Coreg CR Extended-Release Capsules (Greater than 1% to less than or equal to 3%) 1393
Crestor Tablets 677
▲ Crixivan Capsules (3.7%) 1979
Cubicin for Injection (Less than 1%) 995
Cymbalta Delayed-Release Capsules 1801
▲ Dacogen Injection (10%) 1066
Demser Capsules (Rare) 1989
Doribax Injection (1% to 2%) 2400
EC-Naprosyn Delayed-Release Tablets (1%) 2632
Effexor XR Extended-Release Capsules (Infrequent) 3195
Elspar for Injection 1990
▲ Emend Capsules (3%) 1992
▲ Emend for Injection (3%) 1999
Emsam Transdermal System (Infrequent) 905
▲ Emtriva Capsules (3% to 6%) 1246
▲ Emtriva Oral Solution (3% to 6%) 1246

▲ Epivir (1.7% to 4%) 1412
Evoxac Capsules (Less than 1%) 1013
Femara Tablets 2246
▲ Fenoglide Tablets (3.4%) 2960
▲ Flebogamma 5% DIF (6.5%) 1718
Flector Patch (1%) 561
▲ Fortaz (1 in 16) 1450
Gamunex 3094
▲ Gemzar for Injection (52% to 78%) 1820
▲ Gleevec Tablets (0% to 4.7%) 2255
▲ Humatrope Vials and Cartridges (6.67% to 12.50%) 1838
Humira Injection 442
▲ Hycamtin for Injection (Less than 1% to 5%) 1459
Increlex Injection 3100
▲ Intron A for Injection (Up to 63% of patients) 2859
▲ Invanz for Injection (3.8% to 8.4%) 2029
▲ Isentress Tablets (0.4% to 9.1%) 2036
▲ Kaletra (5% to 11%) 452
▲ Lexiva Oral Suspension (Less than or equal to 1% to 8%) 1510
▲ Lexiva Tablets (Less than or equal to 1% to 8%) 1510
Lovaza Capsules 1520
▲ Lovenox Injection (Up to 3.9%) 2756
Lupron Depot 3.75 mg (One patient) 462
▲ Lupron Depot 7.5 mg (Greater than or equal to 5%) 469
Malarone Pediatric Tablets 1521
Malarone Tablets 1521
Marinol Capsules (Less than 1%) 3163
▲ Mepron Suspension (4%) 1526
Meridia Capsules (1.6%) 475
Merrem I.V. (Greater than 0.2%) 684
Mevacor Tablets 2063
Mobic Oral Suspension (Less than 2%) 863
Mobic Tablets (Less than 2%) 863
Moxatag Tablets 2165
▲ Mycamine for Injection (2.7% to 5.6%) 616
▲ Mylotarg for Injection (18%) 3212
Nabi-HB (2%) 815
Nalfon Capsules (Less than 1%) 2508
Namenda 1180
Naprosyn Suspension (1%) 2632
Naprosyn Tablets (1%) 2632
Nexium Delayed-Release Capsules (Less than 1%) 645
Nexium I.V. (Less than 1%) 652
Nexium Delayed-Release Oral Suspension (Less than 1%) 645
Niaspan Extended-Release Tablets 480
Noroxin Tablets (1.4% to 1.6%) 2069
▲ Norvir (6.4% to 9.5%) 489
▲ Novantrone for Injection Concentrate (8% to 15%) 1100
▲ Noxafil Oral Suspension (1% to 17%) 2889
Omnicef Capsules (0.4%) 497
Omnicef for Oral Suspension (0.2%) 497
▲ Oncaspar Injection (Greater than or equal to 2% to 11%) 1138
Orthoclone OKT3 Sterile Solution (Less than 1%) 2387
Paxil (Infrequent) 1535
Paxil CR Controlled-Release Tablets (Infrequent) 1544
Pentasa Capsules (Less than 1%) 3030
Precose Tablets 792
Primaxin I.M. 2080
Primaxin I.V. 2083
Proglycem Capsules (Infrequent) 1185
Proglycem Suspension (Infrequent) 1185
▲ Prograf Capsules and Injection (3% to 15%) 622
▲ Proleukin for Injection (1% to 23%) 2287
Protonix for Delayed-Release Oral Suspension (Less than 1%) 3254
Protonix Delayed-Release Tablets (Less than 1%) 3254
Protonix I.V. (Greater than or equal to 1%) 3257
Protopic Ointment (Greater than or equal to 1%) 628
Provigil Tablets (At least 1%) 977
Rapamune 3260
▲ Rebif Prefilled Syringe for Injection (10% to 17%) 1107
Remicade for IV Injection 950
Risperdal Consta Long-Acting Injection (Rare) 1753
Rocaltrol Capsules 1150
Rocaltrol Oral Solution 1150
▲ Rocephin Injectable Vials, ADD-Vantage, Galaxy, Bulk (3.1%) 2642
Rythmol SR Capsules 1590
Singulair (1.6%) 2114
▲ Soriatane Capsules (Approximately 1 in 3 patients) 3062
Stromectol Tablets (2%) 2120
Suprax for Oral Suspension (Less than 2%) 1891
Suprax Tablets (Less than 2%) 1891
Sustiva Capsules (2%) 930
Sustiva Tablets (2%) 930
Symbyax Capsules (2%) 1871
▲ Synagis Intramuscular Solution (4.9%) 1948
Tarceva Tablets 1228
Targretin Capsules 1084
Tarka Tablets 511
▲ Tasigna Capsules (1% to 10%) 2316
▲ Taxotere Injection Concentrate (4.3% to 18.9%) 2773
Teveten Tablets (Less than 1%) 515
Teveten HCT Tablets (Less than 1%) 517
Timentin ADD-Vantage 1606
Timentin Injection Galaxy Container 1609
Timentin IV Infusion 1603
Timentin Pharmacy Bulk Package 1613
▲ Torisel Injection (2% to 38%) 3272
▲ Tracleer Tablets (11%) 3289
Treximet Tablets (1%) 1616
▲ Tricor Tablets (3.4%) 520
▲ Trisenox Injection (13%) 986
Trizivir Tablets (1.7%) 1622
▲ Truvada Tablets (3%) 1262
▲ Tygacil for Injection (4.3%) 3276
▲ Tyzeka Tablets (3%) 2328
Ultane Liquid for Inhalation (Less than 1%) 524
Ultram ER Extended-Release Tablets (0.5% to less than 1%) 2428
▲ Valtrex Caplets (1% to 16%) 1635
Vantas (Less than 2%) 1737
Venlafaxine Hydrochloride Tablets (Infrequent) 2199
Vicoprofen Tablets (1%) 533
▲ Viramune Oral Suspension (3.7% to 7.6%) 873
▲ Viramune Tablets (3.7% to 7.6%) 873
▲ Viread Tablets (3% to 4%) 1268
Vivitrol (1.5%) 988
Vytorin 10/10 Tablets 2149
Vytorin 10/20 Tablets 2149
Vytorin 10/40 Tablets 2149
Vytorin 10/80 Tablets 2149
Xifaxan Tablets (Less than 2%) 2682
▲ Ziagen (6%) 1673
Zinacef for Injection (1 in 25 patients) 1678
Zinacef Injection (1 in 25 patients) 1678
Zocor Tablets 2136
▲ Zofran Injection (Approximately 5% of patients) 1682
Zofran (Approximately 1% to 2%) 1687
Zofran ODT Orally Disintegrating Tablets (Approximately 1% to 2%) 1687
Zonegran Capsules (Rare) 1089
Zosyn for Injection (1.1%) 3284
Zyprexa Tablets 1883
Zyprexa IntraMuscular 1883
Zyprexa ZYDIS Orally Disintegrating Tablets 1883

Aspartate transaminase, increased

Lamictal (Infrequent) 1488

Aspergillosis, bronchopulmonary

Dacogen Injection 1066

Asphyxia

Abilify Injection (Less than 1 in 1000 patients) 881
Abilify Injection (Less than 1 in 1000 patients) 2466
Abilify Oral Solution (Less than 1 in 1000 patients) 881
Abilify Oral Solution (Less than 1 in 1000 patients) 2466
Abilify Discmelt Orally Disintegrating Tablets (Less than 1 in 1000 patients) 881
Abilify Discmelt Orally Disintegrating Tablets (Less than 1 in 1000 patients) 2466
Abilify Tablets (Less than 1 in 1000 patients) 881
Abilify Tablets (Less than 1 in 1000 patients) 2466
Bentyl Capsules 703
Bentyl Injection 703
Bentyl Syrup 703
Bentyl Tablets 703

Aspiration

Abilify Injection 881
Abilify Injection 2466
Abilify Oral Solution 881
Abilify Oral Solution 2466
Abilify Discmelt Orally Disintegrating Tablets 881
Abilify Discmelt Orally Disintegrating Tablets 2466
Abilify Tablets 881
Abilify Tablets 2466
Invega Extended-Release Tablets 1748
Mirapex Tablets 857
Percocet Tablets 1127
Percodan Tablets 1130
Risperdal Consta Long-Acting Injection 1753

AST elevation

(*see under* Aspartate aminotransferase levels, elevation of)

Asterixis

Depakote ER Tablets 423
Fortaz 1450
Orthoclone OKT3 Sterile Solution (Less than 1%) 2387
Phenytek Capsules (Rare) 2192
▲ Vesanoid Capsules (3%) 2660

Asthenia

Abilify Injection (Greater than or equal to 1 in 1000 patients and less than 1 in 100 patients) 881
Abilify Injection (Less than 1 in 1000 patients) 2466
Abilify Oral Solution (Greater than or equal to 1 in 1000 patients and less than 1 in 100 patients) 881
Abilify Oral Solution (Less than 1 in 1000 patients) 2466
Abilify Discmelt Orally Disintegrating Tablets (Greater than or equal to 1 in 1000 patients and less than 1 in 100 patients) 881
Abilify Discmelt Orally Disintegrating Tablets (Less than 1 in 1000 patients) 2466
Abilify Tablets (Greater than or equal to 1 in 100 patients) 881
Abilify Tablets (Less than 1 in 1000 patients) 2466
Accolate Tablets (1.8%) 669
Accutane Capsules 2607
▲ Aceon Tablets (2 mg, 4 mg, 8 mg) (7.9%) 3038
▲ Actiq (4% to 38%) 959
▲ Actonel Tablets (5.4%) 2568
▲ Actonel with Calcium Tablets (3.5% to 5.4%) 2574
▲ Adderall XR Capsules (2% to 6%) 3012
Adenoscan (Less than 1%) 605
▲ Advicor Tablets (5%) 402
▲ Aerobid/Aerobid-M (1% to 3%) 1153
Aggrenox Capsules (1.8%) 819
▲ Agrylin Capsules (23.1%) 3017
Alinia for Oral Suspension (Less than 1%) 2677
Alinia Tablets (Less than 1%) 2677
Allegra-D 12 Hour Extended-Release Tablets 2687
Allegra-D 24 Hour Extended-Release Tablets 2690
Aloxi Injection (1%) 1059
▲ Alphagan P Ophthalmic Solution (1% to 4%) 549
Ambien Tablets (Frequent) 2692
Ambien CR Tablets (1%) 2696
▲ AmBisome for Injection (6.2% to 13.1%) 606
Amitiza Capsules 3082
Anaprox Tablets (Less than 1%) 2632
Anaprox DS Tablets (Less than 1%) 2632
AndroGel (0% to 3%) 3159
▲ Aranesp for Injection (5%) 564
Aricept Tablets (Frequent) 1062
Aricept ODT Tablets (Frequent) 1062
▲ Arimidex Tablets (13% to 19%) 672
▲ Arranon Injection (0% to 17%) 1319
▲ Asacol Delayed-Release Tablets (7%) 2579
Atacand Tablets (0.5% or greater) 639
Atacand HCT (0.5% or greater) 642
Atripla Tablets 938
Avalide Tablets 892
Avalide Tablets 2713
Avandaryl Tablets (1.6%) 1344
Avapro Tablets (1% or greater) 897
Avapro Tablets (1% or greater) 2718
▲ Avastin IV (10% to 74%) 1192
Avelox (Greater than or equal to 0.1% to less than 2%) 2803
▲ Avinza Capsules (5% to 10%) 1772
Axert Tablets (Infrequent) 2431
▲ Axid Capsules (3.1%) 1364
Azilect Tablets (Frequent) 3106
Azor Tablets 1005
Benicar Tablets 1009
Benicar HCT Tablets (Rare) 1010
▲ Bentyl Capsules (7%) 703
▲ Bentyl Injection (7%) 703
▲ Bentyl Syrup (7%) 703
▲ Bentyl Tablets (7%) 703
▲ Betaseron for SC Injection (53%) 756
▲ Betimol Ophthalmic Solution (1% to 5%) 3181
▲ Bexxar (2% to 46%) 1371
Bicillin C-R Injectable Suspension 1775
Bicillin L-A Injection 1777
▲ Boniva Injection (3.5%) 2614
▲ Boniva Tablets (3.5%) 2618
▲ BOTOX Purified Neurotoxin Complex (2% to 10%) 550
Brovana Inhalation Solution 2990
▲ Busulfex Injection (2% to 51%) 2477
▲ Byetta Injection (Greater than or equal to 1% to less than 5%) 600
Bystolic Tablets (Greater than or equal to 1%) 1155
Calcijex Injection 419
▲ Campral Tablets (5% to 7%) 1158
Cancidas for Injection 1953
Captopril Tablets 2182
Cardene I.V. (0.7%) 1093
Cardizem LA Extended Release Tablets (2.6%) 421
▲ Catapres Tablets (About 10 in 100 patients) 841
Catapres-TTS (0.5% or less) 842
Cathflo Activase (2%) 1198
Celebrex Capsules (0.1% to 1.9%) 2979
Celexa (At least 2%) 1160
▲ CellCept Capsules (35.4% to 43.3%) 2622
▲ CellCept Intravenous (35.4% to 43.3%) 2622
▲ CellCept Oral Suspension (35.4% to 43.3%) 2622
▲ CellCept Tablets (35.4% to 43.3%) 2622
▲ Chantix Tablets (4% to 7%) 2511
Cialis Tablets (Less than 2%) 1792
Cipro I.V. (1% or less) 2817
Cipro (Less than 1%) 2810
Cipro XR Tablets (Less than 1%) 2823
Clinoril Tablets (Less than 1 in 100) 1962
▲ Clorpres Tablets (About 10%) 2185
▲ Combigan Ophthalmic Solution (1% to 5%) 553
Combivent Inhalation Aerosol 845
Combivir Tablets 1384
Comtan Tablets (2%) 2208
▲ Copaxone for Injection (41%) 3110
▲ Coreg Tablets (7% to 11%) 1387
▲ Coreg CR Extended-Release Capsules (7% to 11%) 1393
Cosopt Sterile Ophthalmic Solution 1969
Cozaar Tablets (1% or greater) 1973
▲ Crestor Tablets (0.9% to 4.7%) 677
Crinone 4% Gel 992
Crinone 8% Gel 992
Crixivan Capsules (2.1%) 1979
▲ Cubicin for Injection (Less than 1% to 5%) 995
Cuprimine Capsules 1986
▲ Cymbalta Delayed-Release Capsules (2% to 10%) 1801
Dacogen Injection 1066
Dantrium Capsules (Among most frequent) 2580
Dapsone Tablets USP 1746
Demadex Injection (2%) 2630
Demadex Tablets (2%) 2630
▲ Depakote ER Tablets (6% to 27%) 423
▲ DepoCyt Injection (5% to 40%) 1136
Diclofenac Sodium Ophthalmic Solution ⊙ 240
Diovan Tablets (Greater than 0.2%) 2212
Diovan HCT Tablets (Greater than 0.2%) 2216
Donnatal Extentabs 2507
▲ Doxil Injection (6.5% to 40.2%) 2378
Duetact Tablets (1.6%) 3085
▲ Duragesic Transdermal System (10% or more) 2405
Dyazide Capsules 1405
DynaCirc CR Controlled Release Tablets 1407
Dyrenium Capsules (Rare) 3189

EC-Naprosyn Delayed-Release Tablets (Less than 1%) 2632
▲ Effexor XR Extended-Release Capsules (1% to 19%) 3195
Eldepryl Capsules 3052
Eligard 7.5 mg (Less than 2%) 2724
Eligard 22.5 mg 2724
Eligard 30 mg 2724
▲ Eligard 45 mg (3.6%) 2724
▲ Eloxatin for Injection (2% to less than 5%) 2731
▲ Emend Capsules (3.4% to 17.8%) 1992
▲ Emend for Injection (3.4% to 17.8%) 1999
Emsam Transdermal System 905
▲ Emtriva Capsules (Greater than or equal to 10%) 1246
▲ Emtriva Oral Solution (Greater than or equal to 10%) 1246
Enablex Extended-Release Tablets (1.5% to 2.7%) 2225
▲ Enbrel for Injection (5% to 11%) 569
Engerix-B Vaccine (Less than 1%) 1409
EpiPen 1024
Epivir 1412
Epivir-HBV 1417
▲ Epogen for Injection (7% to 13%) 576
Epzicom Tablets 1422
▲ Equetro Extended-Release Capsules (8%) 3174
▲ Erbitux (4% to 73%) 912
Evoxac Capsules (0.5%) 1013
▲ Exelon Capsules (2% to 6%) 2229
▲ Exelon Oral Solution (2% to 6%) 2229
▲ Exelon Patch (2% to 3%) 2233
Exforge Tablets (Greater than or equal to 0.2%) 2238
Fansidar Tablets 2636
▲ Faslodex Injection (22.7%) 682
▲ Femara Tablets (0.2% to 33.6%) 2246
Fenoglide Tablets 2960
▲ Fentora Tablets (1% to 16%) 968
▲ Flolan for Injection (87% to 100%) 1426
▲ Flomax Capsules (7.8% to 8.5%) 848
Fluarix Vaccine 1446
Flulaval Injection Vaccine 1448
Flumadine (1.4%) 1167
▲ FluMist Vaccine (26%) 1945
▲ Forteo for Injection (8.7%) 1816
Fosamax 2005
Fosamax Plus D Tablets 2013
Frova Tablets (Infrequent) 1111
Furosemide Tablets 2186
▲ Gabitril Tablets (18% to 23%) 973
▲ Gamunex (4% to 10%) 3094
Gantrisin Pediatric Suspension 2638
Gardasil Injection 2019
Gemzar for Injection (Common) 1820
Gengraf Capsules (Rare) 435
▲ Geodon (5% to 6%) 2520
▲ Gleevec Tablets (15% to 21%) 2255
▲ Gliadel Wafer (1% to 22%) 1076
▲ Hepsera Tablets (13%) 1253
▲ Herceptin I.V. (42%) 1199
▲ Humatrope Vials and Cartridges (3.33% to 6.25%) 1838
▲ Hycamtin Capsules (3% to 7%) 1456
▲ Hycamtin for Injection (Less than 1% to 25%) 1459
▲ Imitrex Injection (5%) 1465
Imitrex Nasal Spray (Infrequent) 1470
Imitrex Tablets (Less than 1% to 2%) 1474
▲ Indapamide Tablets (Less than 5%) 2188
InnoPran XL Extended Release Capsules 1484
Intravenous Sodium Diuril 2490
▲ Intron A for Injection (Up to 40%) 2859
Invanz for Injection (1.2%) 2029
Invega Extended-Release Tablets (Less than 1% to 2%) 1748
Ionsys Transdermal System (.1% to less than 1%) 2410
Isentress Tablets (1% to less than 2%) 2036
▲ Ixempra Kit for Injection (56%) 915
▲ Janumet Tablets (Greater than 5%) 2041
▲ Kaletra (3% to 9%) 452
▲ Keppra Injection (1.3% to 15%) 3137
▲ Keppra Oral Solution (8.9% to 15%) 3131
▲ Keppra Tablets (8.9% to 15%) 3131
K-Phos Neutral Tablets 813
▲ Lamictal (2% to 8%) 1488
Lanoxin Injection 1498
Lanoxin Injection Pediatric 1502
Lanoxin Tablets 1505
Lescol Capsules (Rare) 2268
Lescol XL Tablets 2268
▲ Leukine (17% to 66%) 774
▲ Leustatin Injection (9%) 2384
Levitra Tablets (Less than 2%) 2876
Levothroid Tablets 1170
Lexapro Oral Suspension (Infrequent) 1174
Lexapro Tablets (Infrequent) 1174
Lialda Tablets (Infrequent) 3029
Lidoderm Patch 1114
▲ Lipitor Tablets (Up to 3.8%) 2501
Lovaza Capsules 1520
▲ Lumigan Ophthalmic Solution (1% to 5%) 556
Lunesta Tablets 2994
▲ Lupron Depot 3.75 mg (9%) 462
▲ Lupron Depot 7.5 mg (Less than 5%) 469
▲ Lupron Depot–3 Month 11.25 mg (9%) 462
▲ Luvox CR Extended-Release Capsules (2% to 26%) 1759
▲ Lyrica Capsules (2% to 7%) 2527
▲ Malarone Pediatric Tablets (3% to 8%) 1521
▲ Malarone Tablets (3% to 8%) 1521
Marinol Capsules (Greater than 1%) 3163
▲ Mavik Tablets (3.3%) 472
Maxair Autohaler 1705
▲ Maxalt Tablets (4% to 7%) 2056
▲ Maxalt-MLT Orally Disintegrating Tablets (4% to 7%) 2056
▲ Megace ES Oral Suspension (2% to 6%) 2499
▲ Mepron Suspension (8% to 31%) 1526
▲ Meridia Capsules (5.9%) 475
Merrem I.V. (Greater than 0.1% to 1%) 684
Mevacor Tablets (1.2% to 1.7%) 2063
Micardis Tablets 852
Micardis HCT Tablets 854
▲ Mirapex Tablets (10% to 14%) 857
MS Contin Tablets (Less frequent) 2585
Mustargen for Injection 2492
Myleran Tablets 1530
▲ Mylotarg for Injection (37%) 3212
▲ Nalfon Capsules (5.4%) 2508
Namenda 1180
Naprosyn Suspension (Less than 1%) 2632
Naprosyn Tablets (Less than 1%) 2632
Neoral Oral Solution (Rare) 2280
Neoral Soft Gelatin Capsules (Rare) 2280
▲ Neulasta Injection (15% to 72%) 587
▲ Neupogen for Injection (4%) 589
Neupro Transdermal System (Greater than or equal to 2%) 3149
▲ Nexavar Tablets (Greater than or equal to 10%) 784
Nexium Delayed-Release Capsules (Less than 1%) 645
Nexium I.V. (Less than 1%) 652
Nexium Delayed-Release Oral Suspension (Less than 1%) 645
Niaspan Extended-Release Tablets 480
Nitrolingual Pumpspray 2965
Noroxin Tablets (Less frequent) 2069
▲ Norvir (10.3% to 15.3%) 489
▲ Novantrone for Injection Concentrate (24%) 1100
▲ Noxafil Oral Suspension (1% to 13%) 2889
Omnicef Capsules (0.2%) 497
Omnicef for Oral Suspension (0.2%) 497
▲ Ontak Vials (66%) 1079
Opana Tablets (Less than 1%) 1117
Opana ER Tablets (Less than 1%) 1121
OptiPranolol Metipranolol Ophthalmic Solution 0.3% (A small number of patients) ⊙ 245
Ortho-Cyclen Tablets 2449
Ortho Evra Transdermal System 2437
Ortho Tri-Cyclen Tablets 2449
Ortho Tri-Cyclen Lo Tablets 2458
Orthoclone OKT3 Sterile Solution (Less than 1%) 2387
▲ OxyContin Tablets (6%) 2589
Parnate Tablets 1532
▲ Pataday Ophthalmic Solution (Less than or equal to 5%) 543
▲ Patanol Ophthalmic Solution (Less than 5%) 546
▲ Paxil (1.6% to 22%) 1535
▲ Paxil CR Controlled-Release Tablets (1.6% to 22%) 1544
Pediarix Vaccine 1552
▲ PegIntron Powder for Injection (52%) 2903
Pentasa Capsules (Less than 1%) 3030
Pepcid Tablets (Infrequent) 2075
Percocet Tablets 1127
Percodan Tablets 1130
▲ Photofrin for Injection (6%) 708
Plavix Tablets (1% to 2.5%) 926
Plavix Tablets (1% to 2.5%) 2767
Pletal Tablets (2% or greater) 2481
Pneumovax 23 2078
▲ Premarin Tablets (7% to 8%) 3221
▲ Premphase Tablets (6% to 10%) 3232
▲ Prempro Tablets (6% to 10%) 3232
Primaxin I.M. 2080
Primaxin I.V. (Less than 0.2%) 2083
Prinivil Tablets (Greater than 1%) 2087
Prinzide Tablets (1.8%) 2092
Pristiq Extended-Release Tablets (1% to 2%) 3247
ProAmatine Tablets (Rare) 3032
▲ Procrit for Injection (7% to 13%) 2391
Proglycem Capsules (Frequent) 1185
Proglycem Suspension (Frequent) 1185
▲ Prograf Capsules and Injection (11% to 52%) 622
▲ Proleukin for Injection (23%) 2287
Prometrium Capsules (100 mg, 200 mg) 3047
Protonix for Delayed-Release Oral Suspension (Greater than or equal to 1%) 3254
Protonix Delayed-Release Tablets (Greater than or equal to 1%) 3254
Protonix I.V. (Greater than or equal to 1%) 3257
▲ Protopic Ointment (1% to 3%) 628
Provigil Tablets (At least 1%) 977
▲ Prozac Weekly Capsules (7% to 21%) 1852
▲ Prozac Pulvules and Liquid (7% to 21%) 1852
▲ Pulmicort Flexhaler (9%) 654
Pulmozyme Inhalation Solution 1217
Raptiva for Injection 1218
▲ Rebetol (5% to 66%) 2917
▲ Reclast Injection (2% to 5.3%) 2291
Recombivax HB (Equal to or greater than 1%) 2107
ReFacto Vials 3269
▲ Remeron Tablets (8%) 2924
▲ RemeronSolTab Tablets (8%) 2927
ReoPro Vials (0.7%) 1860
Requip Tablets (Infrequent to frequent) 1561
▲ Retrovir Capsules (8.6% to 69%) 1574
▲ Retrovir IV Infusion (8.6% to 69%) 1579
▲ Retrovir (8.6% to 69%) 1574
▲ Rilutek Tablets (14.8% to 20.1%) 2771
Risperdal Consta Long-Acting Injection (Frequent) 1753
▲ Rituxan I.V. (1% to 26%) 1223
Rocaltrol Capsules 1150
Rocaltrol Oral Solution 1150
▲ Romazicon Injection (1% to 3%) 2646
▲ Rythmol Tablets (2% to 3%) 1586
▲ Rythmol SR Capsules (3% to 4%) 1590
▲ Salagen Tablets (2% to 12%) 1082
Sandimmune (Rare) 2296
▲ Sandostatin Injection (1% to 4%) 2300
▲ Sensipar Tablets (7%) 594
▲ Simulect for Injection (3% to 10%) 2306
Singulair (1.8%) 2114
Stalevo Tablets (2%) 2309
Stromectol Tablets (0.9%) 2120
▲ Suboxone Tablets (6.5% to 14%) 2601
▲ Subutex Tablets (4.9% to 14%) 2601
Sustiva Capsules (Less than 2%) 930
Sustiva Tablets (Less than 2%) 930
▲ Sutent Capsules (5% to 22%) 2540
▲ Symbyax Capsules (Up to 15%) 1871
▲ Targretin Capsules (20.2% to 45.3%) 1084
▲ Targretin Gel 1% (6%) 1088
Tarka Tablets (0.3% or more) 511
▲ Tasigna Capsules (12% to 14%) 2316
▲ Taxotere Injection Concentrate (0% to 80.8%) 2773
Tekturna HCT Tablets (1.2%) 2324
▲ Temodar Capsules (6% to 13%) 2931
Teveten Tablets (Less than 1%) 515
Teveten HCT Tablets (Less than 1%) 517
Thiothixene Capsules 2197
Thyrogen for Injection (1.5%) 1244
Timoptic Sterile Ophthalmic Solution (Less frequent) 2121
Timoptic in Ocudose (Less frequent) 2124
Timoptic-XE Sterile Ophthalmic Gel Forming Solution 2125
▲ Torisel Injection (11% to 51%) 3272
Trasylol Injection (2%) 799
▲ Treanda for Injection (0% to 8%) 983
Treximet Tablets (Infrequent to greater than 1%) 1616
Tricor Tablets (2.1%) 520
▲ Trisenox Injection (10%) 986
▲ Trizivir Tablets (Greater than or equal to 5%) 1622
Trusopt Sterile Ophthalmic Solution (Infrequent) 2128
▲ Truvada Tablets (Greater than 5%) 1262
Twinrix Vaccine (Less than 1%) 1628
Tygacil for Injection (2.5%) 3276
Ultane Liquid for Inhalation (Less than 1%) 524
▲ Ultram ER Extended-Release Tablets (3.5% to 6.5%) 2428
Uroqid-Acid No. 2 Tablets 814
▲ Urso 250 Tablets (11.7%) 720
▲ Urso Forte Tablets (11.7%) 720
▲ Valcyte Tablets (Less than 5%) 2654
Valium Tablets 2658
▲ Valstar Sterile Solution for Intravesical Instillation (4%) 1735
▲ Valtrex Caplets (1% to 4%) 1635
Vantas (Less than 2%) 1737
▲ Vaqta (3.9%) 2130
▲ Velcade for Injection (21% to 72%) 2168
▲ Venlafaxine Hydrochloride Tablets (2% to 16.9%) 2199
Vesanoid Capsules 2660
▲ Viadur Implant (7.6%) 802
▲ Vicoprofen Tablets (3% to 9%) 533
▲ Viread Tablets (6% to 11%) 1268
▲ Visudyne for Injection (1% to 10%) 2332
▲ Vivitrol (12% to 23%) 988
▲ Voltaren Ophthalmic Solution (Less than or equal to 3%) 2336
Voltaren Tablets (Occasionally) 2334
Voltaren-XR Tablets (Occasionally) 2337
Vytorin 10/10 Tablets 2149
Vytorin 10/10 Tablets 2939
Vytorin 10/20 Tablets 2149
Vytorin 10/20 Tablets 2939
Vytorin 10/40 Tablets 2149
Vytorin 10/40 Tablets 2939
Vytorin 10/80 Tablets 2149
Vytorin 10/80 Tablets 2939
▲ WelChol Tablets (3.6%) 1015
▲ Wellbutrin SR Sustained-Release Tablets (2% to 4%) 1653
▲ Wellbutrin XL Extended-Release Tablets (2% to 4%) 1659
WinRho SDF 741
▲ Xeloda Tablets (Less than 1% to 26%) 2662
Xifaxan Tablets (Less than 2%) 2682
▲ Xopenex Inhalation Solution (3%) 3001
▲ Xopenex Inhalation Solution Concentrate (3%) 3005
▲ Xopenex HFA Inhalation Aerosol (3%) 3009
▲ Xyntha Vials (5%) 3280
▲ Xyrem Oral Solution (3% to 5.9%) 1766
Xyzal Oral Solution 2789
Xyzal Oral Solution 3155
Xyzal Tablets 2789
Xyzal Tablets 3155
Yaz Tablets (Greater than 1%) 805
▲ Zemplar Capsules (3%) 536
▲ Zemplar Injection (3%) 538
Zocor Tablets 2136
Zofran (Up to 2%) 1687
Zofran ODT Orally Disintegrating Tablets (Up to 2%) 1687
Zolinza Capsules 2142
▲ Zometa for Intravenous Infusion (5% to 24%) 2341
▲ Zomig Tablets (Common) 694
▲ Zomig Nasal Spray (0% to 3%) 689
Zomig-ZMT Tablets (Common) 694
Zonegran Capsules (Frequent) 1089
Zostavax Injection (1%) 2145
Zyban Sustained-Release Tablets (Frequent) 1692
▲ Zyprexa Tablets (8% to 20%) 1883
Zyprexa IntraMuscular (2%) 1883
▲ Zyprexa ZYDIS Orally Disintegrating Tablets (8% to 20%) 1883
Zyrtec Chewable Tablets (Less than 2%) 1920
Zyrtec Syrup (Less than 2%) 1920
Zyrtec Tablets (Less than 2%) 1920
Zyrtec-D 12 Hour Extended Release Tablets (Less than 2%) 1923

Asthenopia

Ambien CR Tablets (1%) 2696
▲ Lumigan Ophthalmic Solution (1% to 3%) 556

Asthma, allergic

Abelcet Injection 1134
Bicillin C-R Injectable Suspension 1775
Fluarix Vaccine 1446

Asthma, bronchial

Advair HFA 45/21 Inhalation Aerosol 1288
Advair HFA 115/21 Inhalation Aerosol 1288
Advair HFA 230/21 Inhalation Aerosol 1288
▲ Agrylin Capsules (1% to less than 5%) 3017
Aralast (Greater than or equal to 0.2%) 726

BeneFIX Vials (1.6%) 3191
▲ Busulfex Injection (8%) 2477
▲ CellCept Capsules (3% to less than 20%) 2622
▲ CellCept Intravenous (3% to less than 20%) 2622
▲ CellCept Oral Suspension (3% to less than 20%) 2622
▲ CellCept Tablets (3% to less than 20%) 2622
Chantix Tablets (Infrequent) 2511
Cipro I.V. (1.8%) 2817
Combivent Inhalation Aerosol 845
Coreg Tablets (Greater than 0.1% to 1%) 1387
Crinone 4% Gel 992
Crinone 8% Gel 992
Cuprimine Capsules (Rare) 1986
Doxil Injection (Less than 1%) 2378
Emsam Transdermal System (Infrequent) 905
▲ Gamunex (3% to 29%) 3094
Kaletra (Less than 2%) 452
Lipitor Tablets (Less than 2%) 2501
Mirapex Tablets 857
Norvir (Less than 2%) 489
Percocet Tablets 1127
Prinivil Tablets (0.3% to 1%) 2087
Proleukin for Injection (Less than 1%) 2287
Prozac Weekly Capsules (Infrequent) 1852
Prozac Pulvules and Liquid (Infrequent) 1852
Sular Extended Release Tablets (Less than or equal to 1%) 2975
Vaqta (Less than 1%) 2130
Venlafaxine Hydrochloride Tablets (Frequent) 2199
▲ Vesanoid Capsules (3%) 2660
Vicoprofen Tablets (Less than 1%) 533
Voltaren Tablets (Occasionally) 2334
Voltaren-XR Tablets (Occasionally) 2337
Xyrem Oral Solution (Infrequent) 1766

Asthma, worsening of

Activella Tablets 2347
Advair Diskus 100/50 1276
Advair Diskus 250/50 1276
Advair Diskus 500/50 1276
Advair HFA 45/21 Inhalation Aerosol 1288
Advair HFA 115/21 Inhalation Aerosol 1288
Advair HFA 230/21 Inhalation Aerosol 1288
Angeliq Tablets 751
Aricept Tablets (Infrequent) 1062
Aricept ODT Tablets (Infrequent) 1062
▲ Asacol Delayed-Release Tablets (5% or greater) 2579
Climara Transdermal System 763
Climara Pro Transdermal System 768
Divigel 3167
▲ Elidel Cream 1% (0% to 3.9%) 2221
Enjuvia Tablets 1029
Estratest Tablets 3043
Estratest H.S. Tablets 3043
Finacea Gel (Rare) 1742
▲ Flebogamma 5% (18%) 1715
▲ Flebogamma 5% DIF (Greater than 15%) 1718
Flovent Diskus 50 mcg 1435
Flovent HFA 1440
Foradil Aerolizer 2849
Nexium Delayed-Release Capsules (Less than 1%) 645
Nexium I.V. (Less than 1%) 652
Nexium Delayed-Release Oral Suspension (Less than 1%) 645
Premarin Intravenous 3217
Premarin Tablets 3221
Premarin Vaginal Cream 3228
Premphase Tablets 3232
Prempro Tablets 3232
▲ Qvar Inhalation Aerosol (Up to 4%) 3116
Stromectol Tablets 2120
Vaqta 2130
▲ Voltaren Ophthalmic Solution (Less than or equal to 3%) 2336
▲ Xopenex Inhalation Solution (9%) 3001
▲ Xopenex Inhalation Solution Concentrate (9%) 3005
▲ Xopenex HFA Inhalation Aerosol (9%) 3009

Asthmatic episodes

Actiq (Less than 1%) 959
Aggrenox Capsules (Less than 1%) 819
AmBisome for Injection (Less common) 606
Amerge Tablets (Rare) 1301
Anaprox Tablets (Less than 1%) 2632
Anaprox DS Tablets (Less than 1%) 2632
Avelox (Less than 0.1%) 2803
Azilect Tablets (Greater than 1%) 3106
Bayer Aspirin 750
Campral Tablets (Infrequent) 1158
Celexa (Rare) 1160
Cipro (1.8%) 2810
Copaxone for Injection (Infrequent) 3110
Coreg CR Extended-Release Capsules (0.1% to less than or equal to 1%) 1393
Doxil Injection (Less than 1%) 2378
Duragesic Transdermal System (Less than 1%) 2405
EC-Naprosyn Delayed-Release Tablets (Less than 1%) 2632
Effexor XR Extended-Release Capsules (Infrequent) 3195
Eldepryl Capsules 3052
▲ Elidel Cream 1% (0.7% to 3.7%) 2221
Engerix-B Vaccine 1409
Evoxac Capsules (Less than 1%) 1013
Exubera Inhalation Powder (1.3% to 2%) 2515
▲ Flonase Nasal Spray (3.3% to 7.2%) 1431
Fluarix Vaccine 1446
FluMist Vaccine 1945
Gabitril Tablets (Infrequent) 973
Gardasil Injection (2 cases) 2019
Gengraf Capsules (1% to less than 3%) 435
▲ Humira Injection (Less than 5%) 442
Imitrex Injection 1465
Imitrex Nasal Spray (Rare) 1470
Imitrex Tablets (Infrequent) 1474
Indocin Capsules (Less than 1%) 2024
Indocin I.V. (Less than 1%) 2489
Indocin (Less than 1%) 2024
Invanz for Injection (Greater than 0.1%) 2029
Ionsys Transdermal System (.1% to less than 1%) 2410
Keppra Oral Solution (2%) 3131
Keppra Tablets (2%) 3131
Klonopin (Infrequent) 2639
Lexapro Oral Suspension (Infrequent) 1174
Lexapro Tablets (Infrequent) 1174
Lovaza Capsules 1520
Lunesta Tablets (Infrequent) 2994
Lupron Depot 3.75 mg (Rare) 462
Lupron Depot–3 Month 11.25 mg 462
Lupron Depot-PED 7.5 mg, 11.25 mg and 15 mg (Rare) 471
Luvox CR Extended-Release Capsules (Infrequent) 1759
Merrem I.V. (Greater than 0.1% to 1%) 684
Micardis Tablets (More than 0.3%) 852
Micardis HCT Tablets 854
Mobic Oral Suspension (Less than 2%) 863
Mobic Tablets (Less than 2%) 863
Motrin IB Tablets and Caplets 1900
Children's Motrin Oral Suspension 1901
Children's Motrin Non-Staining Dye-Free Oral Suspension 1901
Children's Motrin Cold Oral Suspension 1899
Infants' Motrin Concentrated Drops 1901
Infants' Motrin Non-Staining Dye-Free Concentrated Drops 1901
Junior Strength Motrin Caplets and Chewable Tablets 1901
Namenda (Infrequent) 1180
Naprosyn Suspension (Less than 1%) 2632
Naprosyn Tablets (Less than 1%) 2632
Nasacort AQ Nasal Spray 2765
Nasonex Nasal Spray (Greater than or equal to 2%) 2883
Neupro Transdermal System 3149
Omnicef Capsules 497
Omnicef for Oral Suspension 497
Paxil (Infrequent) 1535
Paxil CR Controlled-Release Tablets (Infrequent) 1544
Pentacel 2792
Pletal Tablets (Less than 2%) 2481
Pred Mild Ophthalmic Suspension ⊙230
Prevnar 3241
Prinzide Tablets 2092
▲ Prograf Capsules and Injection (3% to 15%) 622
Protonix for Delayed-Release Oral Suspension (Less than 1%) 3254
Protonix Delayed-Release Tablets (Less than 1%) 3254
Protonix I.V. (Less than 1%) 3257
▲ Protopic Ointment (4% to 16%) 628
Provigil Tablets (1%) 977
Raptiva for Injection 1218
Relenza Inhalation Powder (Less than 1%) 1556
Remeron Tablets (Infrequent) 2924
RemeronSolTab Tablets (Infrequent) 2927
Requip Tablets (Infrequent to frequent) 1561
Rilutek Tablets (Infrequent) 2771
St. Joseph 81 mg Aspirin Chewable and Enteric Coated Tablets 1903
▲ Serevent Diskus (3% to 4%) 1594
Sustiva Capsules (Less than 2%) 930
Sustiva Tablets (Less than 2%) 930
Symbyax Capsules (Infrequent) 1871
Synagis Intramuscular Solution (More than 1%) 1948
▲ Tamiflu Capsules (1% to 3%) 2649
▲ Tamiflu Oral Suspension (1% to 3%) 2649
Teveten Tablets (Less than 1%) 515
Teveten HCT Tablets (Less than 1%) 517
Thioridazine Hydrochloride Tablets 2195
Trasylol Injection (2%) 799
Treximet Tablets (Infrequent) 1616
Tricor Tablets 520
Twinrix Vaccine 1628
Vaqta 2130
Verdeso Foam (1%) 3069
Viokase 721
▲ Xeloda Tablets (Less than 5%) 2662
Zemuron Injection (Less than 1%) 2947
Zyprexa Tablets (Infrequent) 1883
Zyprexa ZYDIS Orally Disintegrating Tablets (Infrequent) 1883

Asystole

Adenocard IV Injection 603
Cardizem LA Extended Release Tablets (Infrequent) 421
Invanz for Injection (Greater than 0.1%) 2029
Lanoxin Injection 1498
Lanoxin Injection Pediatric 1502
Lanoxin Tablets 1505
Zantac Injection (Rare) 1666
Zantac Injection Pharmacy Bulk Package (Rare) 1668
Zantac Injection Premixed (Rare) 1666

Ataxia

Actiq (Less than 1%) 959
Ambien Tablets (Frequent) 2692
Ambien CR Tablets (1%) 2696
Anzemet Injection (Rare) 2701
Anzemet Tablets (Rare) 2704
Aricept Tablets (Infrequent) 1062
Aricept ODT Tablets (Infrequent) 1062
▲ Arranon Injection (0% to 9%) 1319
Atripla Tablets 938
Attenuvax (Rare) 1951
Avelox (Less than 0.1%) 2803
▲ Avinza Capsules (Less than 5%) 1772
Axert Tablets (Rare) 2431
▲ Azilect Tablets (3%) 3106
▲ Betaseron for SC Injection (17%) 756
Captopril Tablets 2182
Celebrex Capsules (Less than 0.1%) 2979
Celexa (Infrequent) 1160
Cipro I.V. (1% or less) 2817
Cipro (Less than 1%) 2810
Cipro XR Tablets (Less than 1%) 2823
Copaxone for Injection (At least 2%) 3110
Cozaar Tablets (Less than 1%) 1973
▲ Depakote ER Tablets (8%) 423
Doxil Injection (Less than 1%) 2378
Effexor XR Extended-Release Capsules (Infrequent) 3195
▲ Eloxatin for Injection (2% to less than 5%) 2731
Emsam Transdermal System (Rare) 905
▲ Equetro Extended-Release Capsules (5% to 15%) 3174
Exelon Capsules (Frequent) 2229
Exelon Oral Solution (Frequent) 2229
Exforge Tablets (Less than or equal to 0.1%) 2238
Fansidar Tablets 2636
Flumadine (0.3% to 1%) 1167
Frova Tablets (Infrequent) 1111
▲ Gabitril Tablets (5%) 973
Gantrisin Pediatric Suspension 2638
Geodon Capsules (Frequent) 2520
▲ Gliadel Wafer (2% to 6%) 1076
Hexalen Capsules 1078
Imitrex Tablets (Infrequent) 1474
▲ Intron A for Injection (Less than 5%) 2859
Kaletra (Less than 2%) 452
▲ Keppra Injection (3%) 3137
▲ Keppra Oral Solution (2% to 3%) 3131
▲ Keppra Tablets (2% to 3%) 3131
▲ Klonopin (30%) 2639
▲ Lamictal (11% to 22%) 1488
Leukeran Tablets (Rare) 1508
Lexapro Oral Suspension 1174
Lexapro Tablets 1174
Lunesta Tablets (Infrequent) 2994
Luvox CR Extended-Release Capsules (Infrequent) 1759
▲ Lyrica Capsules (1% to 20%) 2527
Marinol Capsules (Greater than 1%) 3163
Marplan Tablets 3177
Maxalt Tablets (Infrequent) 2056
Maxalt-MLT Orally Disintegrating Tablets (Infrequent) 2056
Mirapex Tablets (1% or more) 857
M-M-R II (Rare) 2054
Myfortic Tablets 2276
Namenda (Frequent) 1180
Nembutal Sodium Solution, USP (Less than 1%) 2494
Neupro Transdermal System 3149
Noroxin Tablets 2069
Norvir (Less than 2%) 489
Parnate Tablets 1532
Paxil (Rare to infrequent) 1535
Paxil CR Controlled-Release Tablets (Rare to infrequent) 1544
Phenytek Capsules (Among most common) 2192
Prinivil Tablets (0.3% to 1%) 2087
Prinzide Tablets 2092
Pristiq Extended-Release Tablets 3247
▲ Prograf Capsules and Injection (3% to 15%) 622
ProQuad 2099
Proventil HFA Inhalation Aerosol (Less than 3%) 2914
Provigil Tablets (1%) 977
Prozac Weekly Capsules (Infrequent) 1852
Prozac Pulvules and Liquid (Infrequent) 1852
Remeron Tablets (Infrequent) 2924
RemeronSolTab Tablets (Infrequent) 2927
Requip Tablets (Infrequent) 1561
Rilutek Tablets (Infrequent) 2771
Risperdal Consta Long-Acting Injection (Infrequent) 1753
▲ Romazicon Injection (10%) 2646
Rythmol Tablets (2%) 1586
Rythmol SR Capsules 1590
Soma Tablets 1931
Stalevo Tablets 2309
Sular Extended Release Tablets (Less than or equal to 1%) 2975
Sustiva Capsules 930
Sustiva Tablets 930
Symbyax Capsules (Infrequent) 1871
Targretin Capsules 1084
▲ Temodar Capsules (2% to 8%) 2931
Teveten Tablets (Less than 1%) 515
Teveten HCT Tablets (Less than 1%) 517
Treximet Tablets 1616
Valcyte Tablets 2654
Valium Tablets (Among most common) 2658
Valtrex Caplets 1635
Varivax 2133
Velcade for Injection 2168
Venlafaxine Hydrochloride Tablets (Infrequent) 2199
Wellbutrin Tablets (Frequent) 1648
Wellbutrin SR Sustained-Release Tablets (Rare) 1653
Wellbutrin XL Extended-Release Tablets (Rare) 1659
▲ Xeloda Tablets (Less than 5%) 2662
Zomig Tablets (Rare) 694
Zomig Nasal Spray (Infrequent) 689
Zomig-ZMT Tablets (Rare) 694
▲ Zonegran Capsules (6%) 1089
Zovirax 1690
Zyban Sustained-Release Tablets (Rare) 1692
Zyprexa Tablets (2%) 1883
Zyprexa ZYDIS Orally Disintegrating Tablets (2%) 1883
Zyrtec Chewable Tablets (Less than 2%) 1920
Zyrtec Syrup (Less than 2%) 1920
Zyrtec Tablets (Less than 2%) 1920

Zyrtec-D 12 Hour Extended Release Tablets (Less than 2%) 1923
Zyvox 2552

Ataxia, cerebellar
Vaqta (Very rare) 2130

Ataxia, vestibular
Mirapex Tablets 857

Atelectasis
AmBisome for Injection (Less common) 606
Busulfex Injection (2%) 2477
▲ CellCept Capsules (3% to less than 20%) 2622
▲ CellCept Intravenous (3% to less than 20%) 2622
▲ CellCept Oral Suspension (3% to less than 20%) 2622
▲ CellCept Tablets (3% to less than 20%) 2622
Effexor XR Extended-Release Capsules (Rare) 3195
Evoxac Capsules 1013
Follistim AQ Cartridge 2844
▲ Invanz for Injection (3.4%) 2029
Ionsys Transdermal System (.1% to less than 1%) 2410
Lyrica Capsules (Rare) 2527
▲ NeoProfen Injection (4%) 2496
▲ Prograf Capsules and Injection (5% to 28%) 622
Prozac Weekly Capsules (Rare) 1852
Prozac Pulvules and Liquid (Rare) 1852
Rythmol SR Capsules 1590
▲ Trasylol Injection (5%) 799
Velcade for Injection 2168
Venlafaxine Hydrochloride Tablets (Rare) 2199
Zyprexa Tablets (Rare) 1883
Zyprexa ZYDIS Orally Disintegrating Tablets (Rare) 1883

Atherosclerosis
Imitrex Injection 1465
Imitrex Nasal Spray 1470
Requip Tablets (Infrequent) 1561

Atrial arrhythmias
Ketek Tablets 2744
Proleukin for Injection (Less than 1%) 2287
Remeron Tablets (Rare) 2924
RemeronSolTab Tablets (Rare) 2927
Romazicon Injection (Less than 1%) 2646
Symbyax Capsules (Rare) 1871
Thyrogen for Injection 1244
▲ Trasylol Injection (3%) 799
Ultane Liquid for Inhalation (Less than 1%) 524

Atrial contractions, premature
Adenocard IV Injection 603
▲ Lexiscan Injection (7%) 614

Atrial fibrillations
Abilify Injection 881
Abilify Injection (Greater than or equal to 1 in 1000 patients and less than 1 in 100 patients) 2466
Abilify Oral Solution 881
Abilify Oral Solution (Greater than or equal to 1 in 1000 patients and less than 1 in 100 patients) 2466
Abilify Discmelt Orally Disintegrating Tablets 881
Abilify Discmelt Orally Disintegrating Tablets (Greater than or equal to 1 in 1000 patients and less than 1 in 100 patients) 2466
Abilify Tablets 881
Abilify Tablets (Greater than or equal to 1 in 1000 patients and less than 1 in 100 patients) 2466
Adenocard IV Injection 603
Advair Diskus 100/50 (1%) 1276
Advair Diskus 250/50 1276
Advair Diskus 500/50 1276
Advair HFA 45/21 Inhalation Aerosol 1288
Advair HFA 115/21 Inhalation Aerosol 1288
Advair HFA 230/21 Inhalation Aerosol 1288
Advicor Tablets 402
Agrylin Capsules 3017
Aldara Cream, 5% (1%) 1699
AmBisome for Injection (Less common) 606
Amerge Tablets (Infrequent) 1301
Anzemet Injection 2701
Anzemet Tablets 2704
▲ Argatroban Injection (3%) 1308
Aricept Tablets (Infrequent) 1062
Aricept ODT Tablets (Infrequent) 1062
Atrovent HFA Inhalation Aerosol (0.5%) 839
Atrovent Nasal Spray 0.03% 834
Atrovent Nasal Spray 0.06% 836
Avelox (Less than 0.1%) 2803
Busulfex Injection (2%) 2477
Cancidas for Injection 1953
Celexa (Rare) 1160
▲ CellCept Capsules (3% to less than 20%) 2622
▲ CellCept Intravenous (3% to less than 20%) 2622
▲ CellCept Oral Suspension (3% to less than 20%) 2622
▲ CellCept Tablets (3% to less than 20%) 2622
Chantix Tablets (Rare) 2511
▲ Cleviprex (21%) 1936
Combivent Inhalation Aerosol (0.5%) 845
Copaxone for Injection (Infrequent) 3110
Cozaar Tablets (Less than 1%) 1973
Cubicin for Injection (Less than 1%) 995
Dacogen Injection (Greater than or equal to 1%) 1066
Demadex Injection 2630
Demadex Tablets 2630
DynaCirc CR Controlled Release Tablets (0.5% to 1%) 1407
Effexor XR Extended-Release Capsules 3195
Emsam Transdermal System (Infrequent) 905
Exelon Capsules (Frequent) 2229
Exelon Oral Solution (Frequent) 2229
Exelon Patch (Infrequent) 2233
Exforge Tablets (Greater than 0.1% but less than 1%) 2238
Geodon Capsules (Infrequent) 2520
▲ Humira Injection (Less than 5%) 442
Imitrex Injection (Extremely rare) 1465
Imitrex Nasal Spray 1470
Imitrex Tablets (Rare) 1474
Intelence Tablets (Less than 2%) 3119
▲ Intron A for Injection (Less than 5%) 2859
Invanz for Injection (Greater than 0.1%) 2029
Ionsys Transdermal System (.1% to less than 1%) 2410
Kaletra (Less than 2%) 452
Lamictal (Rare) 1488
Lexapro Oral Suspension 1174
Lexapro Tablets 1174
Lovenox Injection (0.7%) 2756
▲ Lucentis Injection (0% to 5%) 1205
Meridia Capsules 475
Micardis Tablets 852
Micardis HCT Tablets 854
Mirapex Tablets (Less than 1%) 857
▲ Mycamine for Injection (2.5% to 5%) 616
Nalfon Capsules (Less than 1%) 2508
Namenda (Infrequent) 1180
Natrecor for Injection (Greater than or equal to 1%) 2977
Neupro Transdermal System 3149
Niaspan Extended-Release Tablets 480
OptiPranolol Metipranolol Ophthalmic Solution 0.3% (A small number of patients) ..... ⊙245
Paxil (Rare) 1535
Paxil CR Controlled-Release Tablets (Rare) 1544
▲ Photofrin for Injection (10%) 708
Plavix Tablets (1% to 2.5%) 926
Plavix Tablets (1% to 2.5%) 2767
Pletal Tablets (Less than 2%) 2481
Prinivil Tablets (0.3% to 1%) 2087
Prinzide Tablets 2092
Prograf Capsules and Injection 622
Protonix for Delayed-Release Oral Suspension (Less than 1%) 3254
Protonix Delayed-Release Tablets (Less than 1%) 3254
Protonix I.V. (Less than 1%) 3257
Prozac Weekly Capsules (Rare) 1852
Prozac Pulvules and Liquid (Rare) 1852
▲ ReoPro Vials (3.5%) 1860
Requip Tablets (2%) 1561
Rilutek Tablets (Infrequent) 2771
Risperdal Consta Long-Acting Injection 1753
Rythmol Tablets (1%) 1586
Sandostatin LAR Depot 2302
Serevent Diskus 1594
▲ Simulect for Injection (3% to 10%) 2306
Spiriva HandiHaler (Less than 1%) 870
Sular Extended Release Tablets (Less than or equal to 1%) 2975
Symbyax Capsules (Rare) 1871
Tasigna Capsules (0.1% to 1%) 2316
Taxotere Injection Concentrate 2773
Teveten Tablets (Less than 1%) 515
Teveten HCT Tablets (Less than 1%) 517
▲ Trasylol Injection (21%) 799
Tricor Tablets 520
Ultane Liquid for Inhalation (Less than 1%) 524
▲ Vaprisol (2.7% to 7%) 632
Velcade for Injection 2168
Venlafaxine Hydrochloride Tablets 2199
Ventolin HFA Inhalation Aerosol 1638
▲ Visudyne for Injection (1% to 10%) 2332
Vivitrol 988
Vytorin 10/10 Tablets 2149
Vytorin 10/10 Tablets 2939
Vytorin 10/20 Tablets 2149
Vytorin 10/20 Tablets 2939
Vytorin 10/40 Tablets 2149
Vytorin 10/40 Tablets 2939
Vytorin 10/80 Tablets 2149
Vytorin 10/80 Tablets 2939
▲ Xeloda Tablets (Less than 5%) 2662
Xopenex Inhalation Solution 3001
Xopenex Inhalation Solution Concentrate 3005
Xopenex HFA Inhalation Aerosol 3009
▲ Zocor Tablets (5.7%) 2136
Zofran Injection 1682
Zomig Tablets (Rare) 694
Zomig Nasal Spray (Rare) 689
Zomig-ZMT Tablets (Rare) 694
Zonegran Capsules (Rare) 1089
Zosyn for Injection (1% or less) 3284
Zyprexa Tablets (Infrequent) 1883
Zyprexa ZYDIS Orally Disintegrating Tablets (Infrequent) 1883

Atrial flutter
Abilify Injection (Less than 1 in 1000 patients) 881
Abilify Injection (Less than 1 in 1000 patients) 2466
Abilify Oral Solution (Less than 1 in 1000 patients) 881
Abilify Oral Solution (Less than 1 in 1000 patients) 2466
Abilify Discmelt Orally Disintegrating Tablets (Less than 1 in 1000 patients) 881
Abilify Discmelt Orally Disintegrating Tablets (Less than 1 in 1000 patients) 2466
Abilify Tablets (Less than 1 in 1000 patients) 881
Abilify Tablets (Less than 1 in 1000 patients) 2466
Amerge Tablets (Infrequent) 1301
Anzemet Injection 2701
Anzemet Tablets 2704
Brovana Inhalation Solution (Less than 2%) 2990
▲ CellCept Capsules (3% to less than 20%) 2622
▲ CellCept Intravenous (3% to less than 20%) 2622
▲ CellCept Oral Suspension (3% to less than 20%) 2622
▲ CellCept Tablets (3% to less than 20%) 2622
Cipro I.V. (1% or less) 2817
Cipro (Less than 1%) 2810
Cipro XR Tablets 2823
Cubicin for Injection (Less than 1%) 995
Ixempra Kit for Injection 915
Pletal Tablets (Less than 2%) 2481
Prograf Capsules and Injection 622
Protonix for Delayed-Release Oral Suspension (Less than 1%) 3254
Protonix Delayed-Release Tablets (Less than 1%) 3254
Protonix I.V. (Less than 1%) 3257
▲ ReoPro Vials (3.5%) 1860
Rythmol Tablets (Less than 1%) 1586
Rythmol SR Capsules 1590
▲ Taxotere Injection Concentrate (8.1%) 2773
▲ Trasylol Injection (6%) 799
Uniphyl Tablets 2595
Velcade for Injection 2168

Atrial hypertrophy
Rythmol SR Capsules 1590

Atrial tachycardia
Lanoxin Injection 1498
Lanoxin Injection Pediatric 1502
Lanoxin Tablets 1505
Prinivil Tablets (0.3% to 1%) 2087
Prinzide Tablets 2092
Uniphyl Tablets 2595

Atrioventricular dissociation
Lanoxin Injection (Common) 1498
Lanoxin Tablets (Common) 1505
Rythmol Tablets (Less than 1%) 1586
Tarka Tablets 511

Atrophy, cutaneous
Cuprimine Capsules (Rare) 1986

Atrophy, testicular
AndroGel 3159
▲ Eligard 7.5 mg (5%) 2724
Eligard 22.5 mg 2724
▲ Eligard 30 mg (4.4%) 2724
▲ Eligard 45 mg (7.2%) 2724
▲ Vantas (5.3%) 1737

Atrophy at application site
▲ Flector Patch (4%) 561
Olux-E Foam (1.9%) 3059
Verdeso Foam (1%) 3069

Atrophy at injection site
Bicillin C-R Injectable Suspension 1775
Bicillin L-A Injection 1777

Attention, disturbance in
▲ Abilify Injection (3%) 881
▲ Abilify Injection (3%) 2466
▲ Abilify Oral Solution (3%) 881
▲ Abilify Oral Solution (3%) 2466
▲ Abilify Discmelt Orally Disintegrating Tablets (3%) 881
▲ Abilify Discmelt Orally Disintegrating Tablets (3%) 2466
▲ Abilify Tablets (3%) 881
▲ Abilify Tablets (3%) 2466
Ambien CR Tablets (2%) 2696
Amrix Capsules 966
Arranon Injection (1%) 1319
Chantix Tablets (Frequent) 2511
Cymbalta Delayed-Release Capsules (Infrequent) 1801
▲ Lyrica Capsules (4% to 6%) 2527
Mirapex Tablets 857
Pristiq Extended-Release Tablets (Less than 1% to 2%) 3247
Requip Tablets (Infrequent) 1561
Treximet Tablets (Infrequent) 1616
Ultram ER Extended-Release Tablets (0.5% to less than 1%) 2428
Vivitrol 988
▲ Xyrem Oral Solution (2.9% to 8.6%) 1766

Atypical measles
Attenuvax 1951
ProQuad 2099

Auditory acuity, decrease
▲ Capastat Sulfate for Injection (Approximately 11%) 1791

Auditory canals, small or absent, fetal
Accutane Capsules 2607

Auditory disturbances
▲ Wellbutrin Tablets (5.3%) 1648

Autoimmune disorders
Cimzia 3127
Intron A for Injection 2859
Ionsys Transdermal System (.1% to less than 1%) 2410
PegIntron Powder for Injection 2903
Proleukin for Injection 2287
Remicade for IV Injection 950

A-V block
Activase I.V. 1188
Adenocard IV Injection 603
Anzemet Injection 2701
Anzemet Tablets 2704
Brovana Inhalation Solution (Less than 2%) 2990
Bystolic Tablets 1155
Carbatrol Capsules 3019
Cardene I.V. (Rare) 1093
Catapres Tablets (Rare) 841
Catapres-TTS (0.5% or less) 842
Clorpres Tablets (Rare) 2185
▲ Coreg Tablets (Greater than 1% to 3%) 1387
▲ Coreg CR Extended-Release Capsules (Greater than 1% to less than or equal to 3%) 1393
Equetro Extended-Release Capsules 3174
Exelon Capsules (Infrequent) 2229
Exelon Oral Solution (Infrequent) 2229
Exelon Patch (Infrequent) 2233

Lanoxin Injection 1498
Lanoxin Injection Pediatric (Common) 1502
Lanoxin Tablets 1505
Luvox CR Extended-Release Capsules (Rare) 1759
Namenda 1180
Neupro Transdermal System 3149
Pepcid Tablets (Infrequent) 2075
ReoPro Vials (1.3%) 1860
Risperdal Consta Long-Acting Injection (Infrequent) 1753
Rythmol SR Capsules 1590
Salagen Tablets 1082
TNKase 1233
Ultane Liquid for Inhalation (Less than 1%) 524
Wellbutrin SR Sustained-Release Tablets 1653
Wellbutrin XL Extended-Release Tablets 1659
Zantac 25 EFFERdose Tablets (Rare) 1670
Zantac Injection (Rare) 1666
Zantac Injection Pharmacy Bulk Package (Rare) 1668
Zantac Injection Premixed (Rare) 1666
Zantac (Rare) 1670
Zyban Sustained-Release Tablets 1692
Zyprexa IntraMuscular (Infrequent) 1883

A-V block, complete
Abilify Injection (Greater than or equal to 1 in 1000 patients and less than 1 in 100 patients) 881
Abilify Injection (Greater than or equal to 1 in 1000 patients and less than 1 in 100 patients) 2466
Abilify Oral Solution (Greater than or equal to 1 in 1000 patients and less than 1 in 100 patients) 881
Abilify Oral Solution (Greater than or equal to 1 in 1000 patients and less than 1 in 100 patients) 2466
Abilify Discmelt Orally Disintegrating Tablets (Greater than or equal to 1 in 1000 patients and less than 1 in 100 patients) 881
Abilify Discmelt Orally Disintegrating Tablets (Greater than or equal to 1 in 1000 patients and less than 1 in 100 patients) 2466
Abilify Tablets (Greater than or equal to 1 in 1000 patients and less than 1 in 100 patients) 881
Abilify Tablets (Greater than or equal to 1 in 1000 patients and less than 1 in 100 patients) 2466
Azilect Tablets (Rare) 3106
Coreg CR Extended-Release Capsules (Less than or equal to 0.1%) 1393
Velcade for Injection 2168

A-V block, first-degree
Abilify Injection (Greater than or equal to 1 in 1000 patients and less than 1 in 100 patients) 2466
Abilify Oral Solution (Greater than or equal to 1 in 1000 patients and less than 1 in 100 patients) 2466
Abilify Discmelt Orally Disintegrating Tablets (Greater than or equal to 1 in 1000 patients and less than 1 in 100 patients) 2466
Abilify Tablets (Greater than or equal to 1 in 1000 patients and less than 1 in 100 patients) 2466
Adenocard IV Injection 603
▲ Adenoscan (2.9% to 3%) 605
Aricept Tablets (Infrequent) 1062
Aricept ODT Tablets (Infrequent) 1062
▲ Cardizem LA Extended Release Tablets (2.4% to 3.2%) 421
Cathflo Activase (1.2%) 1198
Effexor XR Extended-Release Capsules (Rare) 3195
Geodon Capsules (Rare) 2520
Invega Extended-Release Tablets (0% to 2%) 1748
Lanoxin Injection 1498
Lanoxin Injection Pediatric 1502
Lanoxin Tablets 1505
▲ Lexiscan Injection (3%) 614
Mavik Tablets (0.3% to 1%) 472
Mirapex Tablets 857
▲ Reyataz Capsules (5% to 5.9%) 3299
▲ Rythmol Tablets (2% to 5%) 1586
▲ Rythmol SR Capsules (2% to 3%) 1590
Sular Extended Release Tablets (Less than or equal to 1%) 2975
▲ Tarka Tablets (3.9%) 511
Venlafaxine Hydrochloride Tablets (Rare) 2199

A-V block, intensification of
InnoPran XL Extended Release Capsules 1484
Nadolol Tablets (Single instance) 2191
Toprol-XL Tablets 666

A-V block, second-degree
Adenocard IV Injection 603
Adenoscan (2.6% to 3%) 605
Azilect Tablets (Rare) 3106
Bystolic Tablets 1155
Cardizem LA Extended Release Tablets (Less than 2%) 421
Cozaar Tablets (Less than 1%) 1973
Lanoxin Injection 1498
Lanoxin Injection Pediatric 1502
Lanoxin Tablets 1505
Lexiscan Injection (0.1%) 614
Mirapex Tablets 857
Proleukin for Injection (Less than 1%) 2287
Reyataz Capsules (2%) 3299
Rythmol Tablets (0.6% to 1%) 1586
Tarka Tablets (Less frequent) 511
Ultane Liquid for Inhalation (Less than 1%) 524

A-V block, third-degree
Adenocard IV Injection 603
Adenoscan (0.8%; less than 1%) 605
Bystolic Tablets 1155
Cardizem LA Extended Release Tablets (Less than 2%) 421
Coreg Tablets (Less than or equal to 0.1%) 1387
Lanoxin Injection 1498
Lanoxin Injection Pediatric 1502
Lanoxin Tablets 1505
Lexiscan Injection 614
Reyataz Capsules 3299
Rythmol Tablets (0.2%) 1586
Tarka Tablets 511
Wellbutrin Tablets 1648

A-V conduction changes, unspecified
Lexiscan Injection (0.1%) 614
Natrecor for Injection (Greater than or equal to 1%) 2977
Nimotop Capsules 790

A-V shunt, thrombosis of
(*see under* Thrombosis of vascular access)

Avitaminosis
Campral Tablets (Infrequent) 1158
Kaletra (Less than 2%) 452
Norvir (Less than 2%) 489

Awareness, altered
Neupro Transdermal System 3149

Awareness, heightened
Imitrex Tablets (Rare) 1474
▲ Marinol Capsules (8% to 24%) 3163

Azoospermia
AndroGel 3159
Mustargen for Injection 2492
Rapamune 3260

Azotemia
Avalide Tablets 892
Avalide Tablets 2713
Carbatrol Capsules 3019
Demadex Injection 2630
Demadex Tablets 2630
Dyrenium Capsules (Rare) 3189
Effexor XR Extended-Release Capsules (Rare) 3195
Elspar for Injection (Frequent) 1990
Elspar for Injection (Frequent) 2488
Equetro Extended-Release Capsules 3174
Furosemide Tablets 2186
▲ Indocin I.V. (41% of infants) 2489
Intravenous Sodium Diuril 2490
Nalfon Capsules (Less than 1%) 2508
Prinivil Tablets (0.3% to 1%) 2087
Prinzide Tablets 2092
Proglycem Capsules (Infrequent) 1185
Proglycem Suspension (Infrequent) 1185
Requip Tablets (Rare) 1561
Teveten HCT Tablets 517
Tygacil for Injection 3276
Venlafaxine Hydrochloride Tablets (Rare) 2199

B

Back strain
Prinzide Tablets (0.3% to 1%) 2092

Backache
Accolate Tablets (1.5%) 669
▲ Aceon Tablets (2 mg, 4 mg, 8 mg) (0% to 5.8%) 3038
Actimmune (2%) 1743
Actiq (1% or greater) 959
▲ Activella Tablets (3% to 10%) 2347
▲ Actonel Tablets (17.8% to 28%) 2568
▲ Actonel with Calcium Tablets (8.7% to 26.1%) 2574
Adenocard IV Injection (Less than 1%) 603
Adenoscan (Less than 1%) 605
▲ Advair Diskus 250/50 (Greater than 5%) 1276
Advair HFA 45/21 Inhalation Aerosol 1288
Advair HFA 115/21 Inhalation Aerosol 1288
Advair HFA 230/21 Inhalation Aerosol 1288
▲ Advicor Tablets (5%) 402
▲ Aggrenox Capsules (4.6%) 819
▲ Agrylin Capsules (5.9%) 3017
▲ Alamast Ophthalmic Solution (Less than 5%) 3181
Aldara Cream, 5% (1% to 4%) 1699
▲ Alferon N Injection (Up to 4%) 1726
Allegra Oral Solution (2.2% to 2.8%) 2684
Allegra Tablets (2.1% to 2.5%) 2684
Allegra-D 12 Hour Extended-Release Tablets (1.9%) 2687
Allegra-D 24 Hour Extended-Release Tablets (1.9%) 2690
▲ Alvesco Inhalation Aerosol (0.6% to greater than or equal to 3%) 2985
▲ Ambien Tablets (3%) 2692
▲ AmBisome for Injection (12%) 606
▲ Angeliq Tablets (7%) 751
▲ Angiomax for Injection (9.2% to 42%) 1933
Aralast (Greater than or equal to 0.2%) 726
▲ Aranesp for Injection (7%) 564
▲ Argatroban Injection (8%) 1308
▲ Aricept Tablets (3%) 1062
▲ Aricept ODT Tablets (3%) 1062
▲ Arimidex Tablets (10% to 12%) 672
Arixtra Injection (1.3%) 1313
▲ Arranon Injection (0% to 8%) 1319
▲ Asacol Delayed-Release Tablets (7%) 2579
▲ Asmanex Twisthaler (3% to 6%) 2797
▲ Atacand Tablets (3%) 639
▲ Atacand HCT (3.3%) 642
▲ Atripla Tablets (Greater than or equal to 5%) 938
▲ Atrovent HFA Inhalation Aerosol (2% to 7%) 839
▲ Avandamet Tablets (5%) 1336
▲ Avandia Tablets (4% to 5.1%) 1351
▲ Avinza Capsules (5% to 10%) 1772
Axert Tablets (Infrequent) 2431
▲ Azmacort Inhalation Aerosol (2% to 4%) 407
Benicar HCT Tablets (Greater than 1%) 1010
▲ Bexxar (1% to 8%) 1371
▲ Boniva Injection (4.3% to 13.5%) 2614
▲ Boniva Tablets (4.3% to 13.5%) 2618
Boostrix 1377
▲ BOTOX Purified Neurotoxin Complex (2% to 10%) 550
▲ Brovana Inhalation Solution (6%) 2990
▲ Busulfex Injection (23%) 2477
Campral Tablets (Frequent) 1158
Carafate Suspension (Less than 0.5%) 706
Carafate Tablets (Less than 0.5%) 707
Celebrex Capsules (2.8%) 2979
Celexa (At least 2%) 1160
▲ Cerezyme for Injection (Approximately 6.5%) 1238
Chantix Tablets (Frequent) 2511
▲ Chemet Capsules (5.2% to 15.7%) 2484
▲ Cialis Tablets (2% to 6%) 1792
Cipro I.V. (1% or less) 2817
▲ Climara Transdermal System (4% to 9%) 763
▲ Climara Pro Transdermal System (6.1%) 768
▲ Clolar for Intravenous Infusion (13%) 1239
Comtan Tablets (2%) 2208
▲ Copaxone for Injection (16%) 3110
▲ Cosopt Sterile Ophthalmic Solution (1% to 5%) 1969
▲ Cozaar Tablets (2% to 12%) 1973
▲ Crinone 4% Gel (8%) 992
▲ Crinone 8% Gel (3%) 992
▲ Crixivan Capsules (8.4%) 1979
▲ Cubicin for Injection (1% to 6.7%) 995
▲ Dacogen Injection (17%) 1066
Dantrium Capsules (Less frequent) 2580
▲ Depakote ER Tablets (Greater than 1% to 8%) 423
▲ DepoCyt Injection (7% to 24%) 1136
▲ Diovan Tablets (0.2% to 3%) 2212
Diovan HCT Tablets (Greater than 0.2%) 2216
▲ Doxil Injection (6.8% to 11.7%) 2378
Duragesic Transdermal System (Greater than or equal to 1%) 2405
DynaCirc CR Controlled Release Tablets (0.5% to 1%) 1407
Edex Injection (2%) 2957
Effexor XR Extended-Release Capsules 3195
Eldepryl Capsules (1 of 49 patients) 3052
Eligard 7.5 mg (Less than 2%) 2724
Eligard 22.5 mg (Less than 2%) 2724
Eligard 30 mg (Less than 2%) 2724
Eligard 45 mg (Less than 2%) 2724
Emend Capsules (Greater than 0.5%) 1992
Emend for Injection (Greater than 0.5%) 1999
Emsam Transdermal System 905
Engerix-B Vaccine (Less than 1%) 1409
▲ Equetro Extended-Release Capsules (5%) 3174
▲ Evoxac Capsules (4.5%) 1013
Exelon Capsules (2% or more) 2229
Exelon Oral Solution (2% or more) 2229
▲ Exjade Tablets (5.7%) 2244
▲ Fabrazyme for Intravenous Infusion (5% to 16%) 1241
▲ Faslodex Injection (14.4%) 682
▲ Femara Tablets (0.3% to 22%) 2246
▲ Fenoglide Tablets (3.4%) 2960
▲ Fentora Tablets (0% to 11%) 968
Flebogamma 5% 1715
Flebogamma 5% DIF 1718
▲ Flolan for Injection (2% to 13%) 1426
▲ Flomax Capsules (7% to 8.3%) 848
▲ Flulaval Injection Vaccine (1% to 6%) 1448
▲ Foradil Aerolizer (4.2%) 2849
Frova Tablets (Infrequent) 1111
Gabitril Tablets (1% or more) 973
Gammagard Liquid 730
Gammagard S/D (Occasional) 734
▲ Gamunex (6%) 3094
▲ Genotropin Lyophilized Powder (2.8% to 5%) 2547
Geodon for Injection (Up to 1%) 2520
▲ Gleevec Tablets (23% to 26%) 2255
▲ Gliadel Wafer (1% to 7%) 1076
▲ Herceptin I.V. (22%) 1199
▲ Humatrope Vials and Cartridges (9.1% to 9.6%) 1838
▲ Humira Injection (6%) 442
▲ Hycamtin for Injection (2% to 23%) 1459
Imitrex Injection (Rare) 1465
Imitrex Nasal Spray (Infrequent) 1470
Imitrex Tablets 1474
▲ Indapamide Tablets (Greater than or equal to 5%) 2188
▲ Intron A for Injection (Up to 19%) 2859
Ionsys Transdermal System (2%) 2410
Kaletra (Less than 2%) 452
Klonopin (Infrequent) 2639
▲ Lamictal (8%) 1488
▲ Lescol Capsules (5.7%) 2268
▲ Lescol XL Tablets (4.7%) 2268
▲ Leukine (9%) 774
Lexapro Oral Suspension (At least 2%) 1174
Lexapro Tablets (At least 2%) 1174
Lialda Tablets (Infrequent) 3029
▲ Lipitor Tablets (Up to 3.8%) 2501
▲ Lovaza Capsules (2.2% to 5%) 1520
Lunesta Tablets 2994
▲ Lyrica Capsules (1% to 4%) 2527
▲ Meridia Capsules (8.2%) 475
Merrem I.V. (Greater than 0.1% to 1%) 684
▲ Miacalcin Nasal Spray (5%) 2274
▲ Micardis Tablets (3%) 852
Micardis HCT Tablets (Less than 2%) 854
Mirapex Tablets (2% or more) 857
▲ Mirena Intrauterine System (5% or more) 779
▲ Mobic Oral Suspension (0.4% to 3%) 863
▲ Mobic Tablets (0.4% to 3%) 863
▲ Myfortic Tablets (3% to less than 20%) 2276

▲ Mylotarg for Injection (12% to 16%) 3212
▲ Namenda (3%) 1180
▲ Natrecor for Injection (1% to 4%) 2977
▲ Neupro Transdermal System (6%) 3149
Nexium Delayed-Release Capsules (Less than 1%) 645
Nexium I.V. (Less than 1%) 652
Nexium Delayed-Release Oral Suspension (Less than 1%) 645
Noroxin Tablets (0.3% to 1%) 2069
Norvir (Less than 2%) 489
▲ Novantrone for Injection Concentrate (6% to 8%) 1100
▲ Orencia Powder for Intravenous Infusion (7%) 921
ParaGard T 380A Intrauterine Copper Contraceptive 1041
▲ Pataday Ophthalmic Solution (Less than or equal to 5%) 543
▲ Paxil (3%) 1535
▲ Paxil CR Controlled-Release Tablets (3%) 1544
▲ Photofrin fpr Injection (5% to 11%) 708
▲ Plavix Tablets (5.8%) 926
▲ Plavix Tablets (5.8%) 2767
▲ Pletal Tablets (6% to 7%) 2481
▲ Premarin Tablets (13% to 14%) 3221
▲ Premphase Tablets (13% to 16%) 3232
▲ Prempro Tablets (13% to 16%) 3232
Prinivil Tablets (0.3% to greater than 1%) 2087
Prinzide Tablets (0.3% to 1%) 2092
ProAmatine Tablets (Rare) 3032
▲ Prograf Capsules and Injection (17% to 30%) 622
▲ Prometrium Capsules (100 mg, 200 mg) (8%) 3047
Protonix for Delayed-Release Oral Suspension (Greater than or equal to 1%) 3254
Protonix Delayed-Release Tablets (Greater than or equal to 1%) 3254
Protonix I.V. (Greater than or equal to 1%) 3257
▲ Protopic Ointment (1% to 3%) 628
▲ Proventil HFA Inhalation Aerosol (4%) 2914
▲ Provigil Tablets (6%) 977
Prozac Pulvules and Liquid 1852
▲ Pulmicort Flexhaler (Greater than or equal to 3%) 654
▲ Qvar Inhalation Aerosol (Less than 1% to 4%) 3116
▲ Raptiva for Injection (4%) 1218
▲ Rebif Prefilled Syringe for Injection (23% to 25%) 1107
▲ Reclast Injection (4%) 2291
Recombivax HB (Less than 1%) 2107
Remeron Tablets (2%) 2924
RemeronSolTab Tablets (2%) 2927
▲ Remicade for IV Injection (8%) 950
Requip Tablets (1% or more) 1561
▲ Requip XL Tablets (3%) 1568
Retrovir Capsules 1574
Retrovir IV Infusion 1579
Retrovir 1574
▲ Rilutek Tablets (1.7% to 4.1%) 2771
Risperdal Consta Long-Acting Injection (Frequent) 1753
▲ Rituxan I.V. (1% to 10%) 1223
Sanctura XR Capsules (Less than 1%) 557
▲ Sandostatin Injection (1% to 4%) 2300
▲ Simulect for Injection (3% to 10%) 2306
▲ Soriatane Capsules (1% to 10%) 3062
▲ Stalevo Tablets (2% to 4%) 2309
Stromectol Tablets 2120
▲ Suboxone Tablets (3.7% to 14%) 2601
▲ Subutex Tablets (7.8% to 14%) 2601
▲ Sutent Capsules (1% to 17%) 2540
▲ Symbicort 80/4.5 Inhalation Aerosol (3.2%) 659
Symbicort 160/4.5 Inhalation Aerosol (1.6%) 659
▲ Targretin Capsules (2.4% to 11.3%) 1084
Tarka Tablets (2.2%) 511
Tekturna Tablets (Greater than 1%) 2321
▲ Temodar Capsules (3% to 8%) 2931
Teveten Tablets (Less than 1%) 515
Teveten HCT Tablets (2.6%) 517
▲ Torisel Injection (3% to 20%) 3272
▲ Travatan Z Ophthalmic Solution (1% to 5%) 547
Treximet Tablets (Infrequent) 1616
▲ Tricor Tablets (3.4%) 520
▲ Trisenox Injection (18%) 986
▲ Truvada Tablets (Greater than or equal to 5%) 1262
Twinrix Vaccine (Less than 1%) 1628
Tygacil for Injection (1.2%) 3276
▲ Tykerb Tablets (0% to 11%) 1631
▲ Tyzeka Tablets (2% to 4%) 2328
▲ Ultram ER Extended-Release Tablets (1% to less than 5%) 2428
▲ Vagifem Tablets (7%) 2375
▲ Valcyte Tablets (Less than 5%) 2654
▲ Valstar Sterile Solution for Intravesical Instillation (3%) 1735
Vantas (Less than 2%) 1737
Vaqta (1.1%) 2130
Veramyst Nasal Spray (1%) 1643
▲ Viread Tablets (3% to 9%) 1268
▲ Visudyne for Injection (1% to 10%) 2332
▲ Vivitrol (4% to 7%) 988
Wellbutrin SR Sustained-Release Tablets (At least 1%) 1653
Wellbutrin XL Extended-Release Tablets (At least 1%) 1659
WinRho SDF 741
▲ Xeloda Tablets (Less than 1% to 12%) 2662
▲ Xenical Capsules (13.9%) 2672
▲ Xyrem Oral Solution (5.7% to 6.1%) 1766
Yaz Tablets (Greater than 1%) 805
▲ Zometa for Intravenous Infusion (15%) 2341
Zomig Tablets (Infrequent) 694
Zomig Nasal Spray (Infrequent) 689
Zomig-ZMT Tablets (Infrequent) 694
Zosyn for Injection (1% or less) 3284
Zyban Sustained-Release Tablets (Infrequent) 1692
▲ Zyprexa Tablets (4% to 8%) 1883
▲ Zyprexa ZYDIS Orally Disintegrating Tablets (4% to 8%) 1883

Bacteremia
▲ Aranesp for Injection (27%) 564
Bexxar 1371
▲ Clolar for Intravenous Infusion (10%) 1239
Crixivan Capsules 1979
▲ Cubicin for Injection (5%) 995
▲ Dacogen Injection (5%) 1066
Enbrel for Injection 569
▲ Mycamine for Injection (5% to 15.5%) 616
Noxafil Oral Suspension (18%) 2889
Retrovir Capsules (1.6%) 1574
Retrovir IV Infusion (2%) 1579
Retrovir (1.6%) 1574
Velcade for Injection 2168
Venlafaxine Hydrochloride Tablets (Rare) 2199

Bacteriuria
Celebrex Capsules 2979
Primaxin I.M. 2080

Bad breath
(*see under* Halitosis)

Balance, loss of
(*see also under* Equilibrium dysfunction)
Eldepryl Capsules 3052
Rythmol Tablets (1%) 1586
Rythmol SR Capsules 1590
Tarka Tablets (Less frequent) 511
Venlafaxine Hydrochloride Tablets 2199

Balance disorder
Ambien CR Tablets (2%) 2696
Arranon Injection (0% to 2%) 1319
Chantix Tablets (Rare) 2511
Effexor XR Extended-Release Capsules 3195
Fentora Tablets (Greater than 1%) 968
▲ Lyrica Capsules (2% to 9%) 2527
Mirapex Tablets 857
Requip Tablets (Infrequent) 1561
Xyrem Oral Solution (Frequent) 1766

Balanitis
Doxil Injection (Less than 1%) 2378
Effexor XR Extended-Release Capsules (Rare) 3195
▲ Lupron Depot 7.5 mg (Less than 5%) 469
Lyrica Capsules (Rare) 2527
Protonix for Delayed-Release Oral Suspension (Less than 1%) 3254
Protonix Delayed-Release Tablets (Less than 1%) 3254
Protonix I.V. (Less than 1%) 3257
Solodyn Extended Release Tablets 1938
Venlafaxine Hydrochloride Tablets (Rare) 2199

Balanoposthitis
Requip Tablets (Infrequent) 1561

Baldness, male pattern
(*see under* Alopecia hereditaria)

Barrett's esophagus
Nexium Delayed-Release Capsules (Less than 1%) 645
Nexium I.V. (Less than 1%) 652
Nexium Delayed-Release Oral Suspension (Less than 1%) 645

Bartter's syndrome
Capastat Sulfate for Injection (1 patient) 1791

Basophils, decreased
Avelox (Greater than or equal to 2%) 2803

Basophils, increase
Effexor XR Extended-Release Capsules (Rare) 3195
Geodon Capsules (Rare) 2520
Paxil (Rare) 1535
Paxil CR Controlled-Release Tablets (Rare) 1544
Primaxin I.M. 2080
Primaxin I.V. 2083
Rocephin Injectable Vials, ADD-Vantage, Galaxy, Bulk (Less than 0.1%) 2642
Venlafaxine Hydrochloride Tablets (Rare) 2199
Vesanoid Capsules (Isolated cases) 2660

Behavior, abnormal
Ambien Tablets 2692
Ambien CR Tablets (Rare) 2696
Humulin 50/50, 100 Units 1843
Humulin 70/30 Vial 1844
Humulin N Vial 1846
Humulin R 1849
▲ Keppra Injection (11.4% to 13.3%) 3137
Keppra Oral Solution 3131
Keppra Tablets 3131
Mirapex Tablets 857
Relenza Inhalation Powder 1556
Tamiflu Capsules 2649
Tamiflu Oral Suspension 2649

Behavior, hostile
Focalin XR Capsules 2251

Behavior, inappropriate
Pristiq Extended-Release Tablets 3247
Tessalon Capsules (Isolated instances) 1183
Tessalon Perles (Isolated instances) 1183
Valium Tablets 2658

Behavior, schizophrenic
Zonegran Capsules (2%) 1089

Behavior, violent
Accutane Capsules 2607
Invanz for Injection (Greater than 0.1%) 2029
Prozac Weekly Capsules 1852
Prozac Pulvules and Liquid 1852
Venlafaxine Hydrochloride Tablets 2199
Zovirax 1690

Behavioral changes
▲ Advair Diskus 100/50 (Greater than or equal to 3%) 1276
Advair Diskus 250/50 1276
Advair Diskus 500/50 1276
Advair HFA 45/21 Inhalation Aerosol (Very Rare) 1288
Advair HFA 115/21 Inhalation Aerosol (Very Rare) 1288
Advair HFA 230/21 Inhalation Aerosol (Very Rare) 1288
Ambien Tablets 2692
Amoxil Capsules (Rare) 1305
Amoxil Chewable Tablets (Rare) 1305
Amoxil Pediatric Drops for Oral Suspension (Rare) 1305
Amoxil Powder for Oral Suspension (Rare) 1305
Amoxil Tablets (Rare) 1305
Augmentin (Rare) 1323
Augmentin Tablets (Rare) 1327
Augmentin XR Extended Release Tablets (Rare) 1333
Augmentin ES-600 Powder for Oral Suspension (Rare) 1329
Biaxin/Biaxin XL 411
Catapres Tablets 841
Catapres-TTS (0.5% or less) 842
Celexa 1160
Chantix Tablets 2511
Clorpres Tablets 2185
Combigan Ophthalmic Solution 553
Cosopt Sterile Ophthalmic Solution 1969
Cymbalta Delayed-Release Capsules 1801
Effexor XR Extended-Release Capsules 3195
Eldepryl Capsules 3052
▲ Keppra Oral Solution (5% to 37.6%) 3131
▲ Keppra Tablets (5% to 37.6%) 3131
▲ Klonopin (5% to 25%) 2639
Lexapro Oral Suspension 1174
Lexapro Tablets 1174
Luvox CR Extended-Release Capsules 1759
Moxatag Tablets 2165
Nadolol Tablets (6 of 1000 patients) 2191
Paxil 1535
Paxil CR Controlled-Release Tablets 1544
Pristiq Extended-Release Tablets 3247
Prozac Weekly Capsules 1852
Remeron Tablets 2924
RemeronSolTab Tablets 2927
Symbyax Capsules 1871
Thioridazine Hydrochloride Tablets 2195
Timoptic Sterile Ophthalmic Solution (Less frequent) 2121
Timoptic in Ocudose (Less frequent) 2124
Timoptic-XE Sterile Ophthalmic Gel Forming Solution 2125
Uniphyl Tablets 2595
Valtrex Caplets 1635
Wellbutrin Tablets 1648
Wellbutrin SR Sustained-Release Tablets 1653
Wellbutrin XL Extended-Release Tablets 1659
Zyban Sustained-Release Tablets 1692
Zyprexa Tablets 1883
Zyprexa ZYDIS Orally Disintegrating Tablets 1883

Behavioral deterioration
Depakote ER Tablets 423

Behavioral disturbances, exacerbation of
Focalin XR Capsules 2251

Belching
Lexapro Oral Suspension (Infrequent) 1174
Lexapro Tablets (Infrequent) 1174

Bell's palsy
Comvax 1966
Engerix-B Vaccine 1409
FluMist Vaccine 1945
▲ Intron A for Injection (Less than 5%) 2859
Mevacor Tablets (0.5% to 1%) 2063
ProQuad 2099
Recombivax HB 2107
Sandostatin Injection (Less than 1%) 2300
Sandostatin LAR Depot 2302
▲ Soriatane Capsules (Less than 5%) 3062
Twinrix Vaccine 1628
Varivax 2133

Benign prostatic hyperplasia
Exelon Patch (Infrequent) 2233

Benzyl alcohol, sensitivity to
Epogen for Injection 576
Herceptin I.V. 1199
Leukine 774
Leustatin Injection 2384
Nimbex Injection 484
Nutropin for Injection 1208
Procrit for Injection 2391

Bezoar
Carafate Suspension 706
Carafate Tablets 707
St. Joseph 81 mg Aspirin Chewable and Enteric Coated Tablets 1903

Bigeminy
Azilect Tablets (Rare) 3106
Effexor XR Extended-Release Capsules (Rare) 3195
Ionsys Transdermal System (.1% to less than 1%) 2410
Lanoxin Injection 1498
Lanoxin Injection Pediatric 1502
Lanoxin Tablets 1505

Remeron Tablets (Rare) 2924
RemeronSolTab Tablets (Rare) 2927
Ultane Liquid for Inhalation (Less than 1%) 524
Venlafaxine Hydrochloride Tablets (Rare) 2199

Bile duct obstruction
Salagen Tablets 1082
Sandostatin LAR Depot 2302

Bile duct sludge, presence of metabolites
Clinoril Tablets (Rare) 1962

Biliary duct dilation
▲ Sandostatin LAR Depot (12%) 2302

Biliary lithiasis
Rocephin Injectable Vials, ADD-Vantage, Galaxy, Bulk (Less than 0.1%) 2642

Biliary sludge
Rocephin Injectable Vials, ADD-Vantage, Galaxy, Bulk (Less than 0.1%) 2642
Sandostatin Injection (Frequent) 2300
▲ Sandostatin LAR Depot (24%) 2302
▲ Somatuline Depot Injection (20%) 3102

Biliary stasis
Thioridazine Hydrochloride Tablets 2195
Thiothixene Capsules 2197

Biliary tract abnormalities
▲ Sandostatin LAR Depot (52%) 2302
▲ Somatuline Depot Injection (4% to 26%) 3102

Bilirubin, conjugated, increased
▲ Cancidas for Injection (5.1% to 7.9%) 1953

Bilirubin, indirect, changes
▲ Sutent Capsules (0% to 15%) 2540

Bilirubin, total, decrease
▲ Avastin IV (1% to 6%) 1192
Avelox (Greater than or euqal to 2%) 2803
▲ Dacogen Injection (5%) 1066

Bilirubin, total, increase
Aloxi Injection (Less than 1%) 1059
▲ Arranon Injection (2% to 10%) 1319
▲ Atripla Tablets (Up to 3%) 938
▲ Baraclude (2% to 3%) 900
Crestor Tablets 677
Epzicom Tablets 1422
▲ Noxafil Oral Suspension (3% to 9%) 2889
Selzentry Tablets (Greater than or equal to 2%) 2534
▲ Tasigna Capsules (9% to 10%) 2316
▲ Torisel Injection (1% to 8%) 3272
Tricor Tablets 520
▲ Truvada Tablets (Less than or equal to 3%) 1262

Bilirubinemia
▲ Abelcet Injection (4%) 1134
Ambien Tablets (Rare) 2692
Ambien CR Tablets (Rare) 2696
▲ AmBisome for Injection (11.1% to 18.1%) 606
Aricept Tablets (Infrequent) 1062
Aricept ODT Tablets (Infrequent) 1062
Asacol Delayed-Release Tablets 2579
Campral Tablets (Infrequent) 1158
Celexa (Rare) 1160
▲ CellCept Capsules (3% to less than 20%) 2622
▲ CellCept Intravenous (3% to less than 20%) 2622
▲ CellCept Oral Suspension (3% to less than 20%) 2622
▲ CellCept Tablets (3% to less than 20%) 2622
Coreg Tablets (Greater than 0.1% to 1%) 1387
Coreg CR Extended-Release Capsules (0.1% to less than or equal to 1%) 1393
Doxil Injection (Less than 1%) 2378
Effexor XR Extended-Release Capsules (Rare) 3195
Emsam Transdermal System (Rare) 905
Gengraf Capsules (1% to less than 3%) 435
▲ Intron A for Injection (Less than 5%) 2859
Lamictal (Rare) 1488
Lexapro Oral Suspension 1174
Lexapro Tablets 1174
Mobic Oral Suspension (Less than 2%) 863
Mobic Tablets (Less than 2%) 863
▲ Mylotarg for Injection (11% to 13%) 3212
Neoral Oral Solution (1% to less than 3%) 2280
Neoral Soft Gelatin Capsules (1% to less than 3%) 2280
Nexium Delayed-Release Capsules (Less than 1%) 645
Nexium I.V. (Less than 1%) 652
Nexium Delayed-Release Oral Suspension (Less than 1%) 645
Niaspan Extended-Release Tablets 480
▲ Noxafil Oral Suspension (1% to 10%) 2889
Paxil (Rare) 1535
Paxil CR Controlled-Release Tablets (Rare) 1544
Percocet Tablets 1127
Plavix Tablets (Less than 1%) 926
Plavix Tablets (Less than 1%) 2767
▲ Prograf Capsules and Injection (3% to 15%) 622
▲ Proleukin for Injection (2% to 40%) 2287
Protonix for Delayed-Release Oral Suspension (Less than 1%) 3254
Protonix Delayed-Release Tablets (Less than 1%) 3254
Protonix I.V. (Less than 1%) 3257
Protopic Ointment (Greater than or equal to 1%) 628
▲ Rebif Prefilled Syringe for Injection (2% to 3%) 1107
ReFacto Vials 3269
Requip Tablets (Infrequent) 1561
Risperdal Consta Long-Acting Injection (Rare) 1753
Salagen Tablets (Less than 1%) 1082
Symbyax Capsules (Rare) 1871
Tygacil for Injection (2.3%) 3276
Ultane Liquid for Inhalation (Less than 1%) 524
Venlafaxine Hydrochloride Tablets (Rare) 2199
Zyprexa Tablets (Infrequent) 1883
Zyprexa ZYDIS Orally Disintegrating Tablets (Infrequent) 1883

Bilirubinuria
Primaxin I.M. 2080
Primaxin I.V. 2083
Viramune Oral Suspension 873
Viramune Tablets 873

Binge eating, unspecified
Ambien CR Tablets (1%) 2696

Bipolar illness
Cimzia 3127

Birth, premature
Accutane Capsules 2607
Paxil CR Controlled-Release Tablets 1544
Sandimmune 2296

Birth defects, increased risk of
Depakote ER Tablets 423
Klonopin 2639
Phenytek Capsules 2192
Premarin Intravenous 3217
Premarin Vaginal Cream 3228
Premphase Tablets 3232
Prempro Tablets 3232
Rebetol 2917
Soriatane Capsules 3062
Tracleer Tablets 3289

Birth weight, low
Adderall XR Capsules 3012
Aggrenox Capsules 819
Bayer Aspirin 750
Dexedrine 1401
Percodan Tablets 1130
St. Joseph 81 mg Aspirin Chewable and Enteric Coated Tablets 1903
Sandimmune 2296

Births, multiple
Follistim AQ Cartridge 2844

Black stools
Pylera Capsules 714

Bladder, contracted
Tice BCG (Less than or equal to 1%) 2936

Bladder, hypertonic
Requip Tablets (Infrequent) 1561

Bladder, neurogenic
Bicillin C-R Injectable Suspension 1775
Bicillin L-A Injection 1777
Exelon Capsules (Infrequent) 2229
Exelon Oral Solution (Infrequent) 2229
Mirapex Tablets 857

Bladder, spasms
Furosemide Tablets 2186
▲ Myfortic Tablets (3% to less than 20%) 2276
▲ Valstar Sterile Solution for Intravesical Instillation (31%) 1735
Velcade for Injection 2168

Bladder disorders
▲ Novantrone for Injection Concentrate (5%) 1100
▲ Selzentry Tablets (4.5%) 2534

Bladder dysfunction
Aricept Tablets (Infrequent) 1062
Aricept ODT Tablets (Infrequent) 1062
DepoCyt Injection 1136
Invanz for Injection (Greater than 0.1%) 2029

Blanching
Catapres-TTS (1 of 101 patients) 842

Blebs, filtering (ocular)
FML Ophthalmic Ointment ⊙ 223
FML Ophthalmic Suspension ⊙ 224
FML Forte Ophthalmic Suspension ⊙ 222
Pred Forte Ophthalmic Suspension ⊙ 227
Pred Mild Ophthalmic Suspension ⊙ 230

Bleeding
Accolate Tablets 669
Activase I.V. (Most common complication) 1188
▲ Aggrenox Capsules (3.2%) 819
▲ Agrylin Capsules (1% to less than 5%) 3017
Aldara Cream, 5% (More than 1%) 1699
Alphanate 1709
AmBisome for Injection (Less common) 606
▲ Angiomax for Injection (0.6% to 13.6%) 1933
▲ Aptivus Capsules (7.5% to 12%) 823
▲ Aptivus Oral Solution (7.5% to 12%) 823
▲ Arixtra Injection (0% to 3.4%) 1313
▲ Avastin IV (4% to 5%) 1192
Azilect Tablets (2%) 3106
Bexxar 1371
Busulfex Injection 2477
Byetta Injection 600
Cathflo Activase (Among most frequent) 1198
Ceftin 1380
▲ CellCept Capsules (3% to less than 20%) 2622
▲ CellCept Intravenous (3% to less than 20%) 2622
▲ CellCept Oral Suspension (3% to less than 20%) 2622
▲ CellCept Tablets (3% to less than 20%) 2622
Cimzia 3127
Crixivan Capsules 1979
Delatestryl Injection 1730
Depakote ER Tablets 423
▲ Doxil Injection (1% to 5%) 2378
Effexor XR Extended-Release Capsules 3195
Elitek (Less than or equal to 1%) 2729
Elspar for Injection 1990
Elspar for Injection 2488
Emend Capsules (Greater than 0.5%) 1992
Emend for Injection (Greater than 0.5%) 1999
▲ Flolan for Injection (11%) 1426
Flulaval Injection Vaccine 1448
Fortaz 1450
▲ Fragmin Injection (0.43% to 3.6%) 1070
Gabitril Tablets (Infrequent) 973
▲ Gamunex (29%) 3094
▲ Gemzar for Injection (Up to 17%) 1820
▲ Gleevec Tablets (26% to 53%) 2255
▲ Gliadel Wafer (7%) 1076
▲ Hycamtin for Injection (Rare to 15%) 1459
▲ Integrilin Injection (10.5% to 14.2%) 2855
▲ Intron A for Injection (8%) 2859
Invanz for Injection (Greater than 0.1%) 2029
Ionsys Transdermal System (.1% to less than 1%) 2410
Ixempra Kit for Injection 915
Lamictal (2%) 1488
Leukeran Tablets 1508
▲ Leukine (23% to 29%) 774
Lexiva Oral Suspension 1510
Lexiva Tablets 1510
▲ Lovenox Injection (1% to 13%) 2756
Meridia Capsules 475
Mustargen for Injection 2492
▲ Mylotarg for Injection (9% to 13%) 3212
Nalfon Capsules (Less than 1%) 2508
▲ NeoProfen Injection (6% to 32%) 2496
▲ Nexavar Tablets (0% to 18%) 784
Norvir (Less than 2%) 489
▲ Novantrone for Injection Concentrate (5% to 37%) 1100
NovoSeven (Greater than or equal to 2%) 2367
NovoSeven RT (Greater than or equal to 2%) 2370
Omnicef Capsules 497
Omnicef for Oral Suspension 497
Percodan Tablets 1130
Pletal Tablets (Less than 2%) 2481
▲ Prograf Capsules and Injection (3% to 15%) 622
Proleukin for Injection (Less than 1%) 2287
Protonix for Delayed-Release Oral Suspension (Less than 1%) 3254
Protonix Delayed-Release Tablets (Less than 1%) 3254
Protonix I.V. (Less than 1%) 3257
Prozac Weekly Capsules (Frequent) 1852
Prozac Pulvules and Liquid (Frequent) 1852
ReFacto Vials 3269
▲ ReoPro Vials (10.6% to 16.8%) 1860
Rilutek Tablets (Rare) 2771
Rocephin Injectable Vials, ADD-Vantage, Galaxy, Bulk 2642
Rythmol SR Capsules 1590
▲ Simulect for Injection (3% to 10%) 2306
Soriatane Capsules (Less than 1%) 3062
Suprax for Oral Suspension (Less than 2%) 1891
Suprax Tablets (Less than 2%) 1891
▲ Sutent Capsules (1% to 30%) 2540
Symbyax Capsules 1871
Targretin Capsules 1084
Taxotere Injection Concentrate 2773
▲ TNKase (1.3% to 21.8%) 1233
Trasylol Injection (1% to 2%) 799
▲ Trisenox Injection (8%) 986
Ultane Liquid for Inhalation (Less than 1%) 524
▲ Valcyte Tablets (Less than 5%) 2654
Venlafaxine Hydrochloride Tablets 2199
▲ Vesanoid Capsules (60%) 2660
▲ Xeloda Tablets (Less than 5%) 2662
Xigris Powder for Intravenous Infusion (Most common) 1880
Zinacef for Injection 1678
Zinacef Injection 1678
Zosyn for Injection (1% or less) 3284
Zyprexa Tablets (Infrequent) 1883
Zyprexa ZYDIS Orally Disintegrating Tablets (Infrequent) 1883

Bleeding, abnormal
Cymbalta Delayed-Release Capsules 1801
Pristiq Extended-Release Tablets 3247
Venlafaxine Hydrochloride Tablets 2199

Bleeding, antepartum
Aggrenox Capsules 819
Bayer Aspirin 750
Percodan Tablets 1130
St. Joseph 81 mg Aspirin Chewable and Enteric Coated Tablets 1903

Bleeding, at invaded sites
Fragmin Injection (3 cases) 1070

Bleeding, at site of administration
▲ Aldara Cream, 5% (2% to 3%) 1699
▲ Aranesp for Injection (7%) 564
▲ Copaxone for Injection (5%) 3110
Dacogen Injection 1066
Daytrana Transdermal Patch 3022
Doxil Injection (Less than 1%) 2378
Enbrel for Injection 569
▲ Flolan for Injection (11%) 1426
▲ Intron A for Injection (Less than 5%) 2859
Kogenate FS with Bio-Set 748
ReoPro Vials (1 to 50 events) 1860

Bleeding, breakthrough
Activella Tablets 2347
Angeliq Tablets 751
Climara Transdermal System 763

Climara Pro Transdermal System 768
Divigel 3167
Enjuvia Tablets 1029
Estratest Tablets 3043
Estratest H.S. Tablets 3043
Mircette Tablets 1034
NuvaRing 2897
Ortho-Cyclen Tablets 2449
Ortho Evra Transdermal System 2437
Ortho Tri-Cyclen Tablets 2449
Ortho Tri-Cyclen Lo Tablets 2458
Premarin Intravenous 3217
Premarin Tablets 3221
Premarin Vaginal Cream 3228
Premphase Tablets 3232
Prempro Tablets 3232
Prometrium Capsules (100 mg, 200 mg) 3047
Seasonique Tablets 1046
Yaz Tablets 805

Bleeding, central nervous system
Xigris Powder for Intravenous Infusion 1880

Bleeding, dental
Accutane Capsules 2607
Actiq (Less than 1%) 959
Activase I.V. (Less than 1%) 1188
Aggrenox Capsules (Less than 1%) 819
AmBisome for Injection (Less common) 606
▲ Avastin IV (6%) 1192
▲ Clolar for Intravenous Infusion (15%) 1239
Copaxone for Injection (Infrequent) 3110
Crixivan Capsules (Less than 2%) 1979
▲ Dacogen Injection (8%) 1066
Depakote ER Tablets (Greater than 1%) 423
Doxil Injection (Less than 1%) 2378
Effexor XR Extended-Release Capsules (Rare) 3195
Gengraf Capsules (1% to less than 3%) 435
Geodon Capsules (Rare) 2520
▲ Intron A for Injection (Less than 5%) 2859
Lamictal (Rare) 1488
Lipitor Tablets (Less than 2%) 2501
Mustargen for Injection 2492
Neoral Oral Solution (1% to less than 3%) 2280
Neoral Soft Gelatin Capsules (1% to less than 3%) 2280
Pletal Tablets (Less than 2%) 2481
Prozac Pulvules and Liquid (Infrequent) 1852
Remeron Tablets (Infrequent) 2924
RemeronSolTab Tablets (Infrequent) 2927
Retrovir Capsules 1574
Retrovir IV Infusion 1579
Retrovir 1574
Rilutek Tablets (Infrequent) 2771
Rythmol SR Capsules 1590
▲ Soriatane Capsules (1% to 10%) 3062
Sutent Capsules 2540
Wellbutrin SR Sustained-Release Tablets 1653
Wellbutrin XL Extended-Release Tablets 1659
Zonegran Capsules (Infrequent) 1089
Zyban Sustained-Release Tablets 1692

Bleeding, duodenal ulcer
Emend Capsules (Isolated cases) 1992
Emend for Injection (Isolated cases) 1999

Bleeding, excessive
Proglycem Capsules (Infrequent) 1185
Proglycem Suspension (Infrequent) 1185
Reyataz Capsules 3299

Bleeding, gastrointestinal
▲ Abelcet Injection (4%) 1134
Abilify Injection (Greater than or equal to 1 in 1000 patients and less than 1 in 100 patients) 2466
Abilify Oral Solution (Greater than or equal to 1 in 1000 patients and less than 1 in 100 patients) 2466
Abilify Discmelt Orally Disintegrating Tablets (Greater than or equal to 1 in 1000 patients and less than 1 in 100 patients) 2466
Abilify Tablets (Greater than or equal to 1 in 1000 patients and less than 1 in 100 patients) 2466
Actimmune (Rare) 1743
Actiq (1% or greater) 959
▲ Activase I.V. (5%) 1188
▲ Actonel Tablets (39%) 2568
▲ Aggrenox Capsules (1.2% to 4.1%) 819
▲ Agrylin Capsules (1% to less than 5%) 3017
▲ AmBisome for Injection (9.9%) 606
▲ Anaprox Tablets (Less than 1% to 10%) 2632
▲ Anaprox DS Tablets (Less than 1% to 10%) 2632
▲ Argatroban Injection (2.3% to 14.4%) 1308
Aricept Tablets (Frequent) 1062
Aricept ODT Tablets (Frequent) 1062
▲ Asacol Delayed-Release Tablets (2% to 5%) 2579
▲ Avastin IV (19% to 24%) 1192
Azilect Tablets (Frequent) 3106
Bayer Aspirin 750
Campral Tablets (Infrequent) 1158
Cathflo Activase 1198
Celebrex Capsules (Less than 0.1%) 2979
▲ CellCept Capsules (1.7% to less than 20%) 2622
▲ CellCept Intravenous (1.7% to less than 20%) 2622
▲ CellCept Oral Suspension (1.7% to less than 20%) 2622
▲ CellCept Tablets (1.7% to less than 20%) 2622
Chantix Tablets (Infrequent) 2511
Cipro I.V. (Less than 1%) 2817
Cipro (Less than 1%) 2810
Cipro XR Tablets 2823
Clinoril Tablets (Less than 1%) 1962
Coreg Tablets (Less than or equal to 0.1%) 1387
Coreg CR Extended-Release Capsules (Less than or equal to 0.1%) 1393
Cubicin for Injection (1.7%) 995
Dacogen Injection 1066
Dantrium Capsules (Rare) 2580
Demadex Injection 2630
Demadex Tablets 2630
Doxil Injection (Less than 1%) 2378
▲ EC-Naprosyn Delayed-Release Tablets (Less than 1% to 10%) 2632
Edecrin 698
Effexor XR Extended-Release Capsules (Rare) 3195
Eldepryl Capsules 3052
Eloxatin for Injection (0.2%) 2731
Enbrel for Injection (Infrequent) 569
Evoxac Capsules (Less than 1%) 1013
Exelon Capsules (Infrequent) 2229
Exelon Oral Solution (Infrequent) 2229
Flector Patch 561
Fosamax (Occasional) 2005
Fragmin Injection (1 case) 1070
Gabitril Tablets (Infrequent) 973
Gantrisin Pediatric Suspension 2638
Gengraf Capsules (1% to less than 3%) 435
▲ Gleevec Tablets (1.6% to 8%) 2255
Gliadel Wafer (1%) 1076
▲ Humira Injection (Less than 5%) 442
Imitrex Injection 1465
Imitrex Nasal Spray (Rare) 1470
Imitrex Tablets (Rare) 1474
Indocin Capsules (Less than 1%) 2024
▲ Indocin I.V. (3% to 9%) 2489
Indocin (Less than 1%) 2024
Integrilin Injection 2855
▲ Intron A for Injection (Less than 5%) 2859
Invanz for Injection (Greater than 0.1%) 2029
Ionsys Transdermal System (.1% to less than 1%) 2410
Ixempra Kit for Injection 915
Lamictal (Rare) 1488
▲ Leukine (11% to 27%) 774
Lexapro Oral Suspension 1174
Lexapro Tablets 1174
Limbrel Capsules (1 case) 2561
Luvox CR Extended-Release Capsules (Infrequent) 1759
Lyrica Capsules (0.1% to 1%) 2527
Meridia Capsules 475
Merrem I.V. (0.5%) 684
Mirapex Tablets 857
Mobic Oral Suspension (Less than 2%) 863
Mobic Tablets (Less than 2%) 863
Motrin IB Tablets and Caplets 1900
Children's Motrin Oral Suspension 1901
Children's Motrin Non-Staining Dye-Free Oral Suspension 1901
Children's Motrin Cold Oral Suspension 1899
Infants' Motrin Concentrated Drops 1901
Infants' Motrin Non-Staining Dye-Free Concentrated Drops 1901
Junior Strength Motrin Caplets and Chewable Tablets 1901
Mustargen for Injection 2492
Myfortic Tablets 2276
Mylotarg for Injection 3212
Nalfon Capsules (Less than 1%) 2508
Namenda (Infrequent) 1180
▲ Naprosyn Suspension (Less than 1% to 10%) 2632
▲ Naprosyn Tablets (Less than 1% to 10%) 2632
Neoral Oral Solution (1% to less than 3%) 2280
Neoral Soft Gelatin Capsules (1% to less than 3%) 2280
Nexavar Tablets (Greater than or equal to 10%) 784
Nexium Delayed-Release Capsules (Less than 1%) 645
Nexium I.V. (Less than 1%) 652
Nexium Delayed-Release Oral Suspension (Less than 1%) 645
Nimotop Capsules (Less than 1%) 790
Norvir (Less than 2%) 489
▲ Novantrone for Injection Concentrate (2% to 16%) 1100
NovoSeven 2367
▲ NovoSeven RT (4.7%) 2370
Omnicef Capsules 497
Omnicef for Oral Suspension 497
Orthoclone OKT3 Sterile Solution (Less than 1%) 2387
Pentasa Capsules (Less than 1%) 3030
Percodan Tablets 1130
Plavix Tablets (1% to 2.5%) 926
Plavix Tablets (1% to 2.5%) 2767
Pletal Tablets 2481
▲ Prograf Capsules and Injection (3% to 15%) 622
Proleukin for Injection (Less than 1%) 2287
Protonix for Delayed-Release Oral Suspension (Less than 1%) 3254
Protonix Delayed-Release Tablets (Less than 1%) 3254
Protonix I.V. (Less than 1%) 3257
Prozac Weekly Capsules (Rare) 1852
Prozac Pulvules and Liquid (Rare) 1852
▲ Refludan for Injection (5.3%) 795
Remicade for IV Injection (Greater than or equal to 0.2%) 950
ReoPro Vials (11 events) 1860
Requip Tablets (Infrequent) 1561
Rilutek Tablets (Infrequent) 2771
St. Joseph 81 mg Aspirin Chewable and Enteric Coated Tablets 1903
Salonpas Arthritis Pain Patches 608
Salonpas Pain Relief Patch 608
Sandimmune (Rare) 2296
Sandostatin Injection (Less than 1%) 2300
Sandostatin LAR Depot 2302
▲ Simulect for Injection (3% to 10%) 2306
Stalevo Tablets 2309
Sutent Capsules 2540
Symbyax Capsules (Rare) 1871
Tamiflu Capsules 2649
Tamiflu Oral Suspension 2649
Tarceva Tablets (Infrequent) 1228
Tasigna Capsules (0.1% to 1%) 2316
▲ Taxotere Injection Concentrate (.4% to 5.2%) 2773
TNKase (1% to 1.9%) 1233
Trasylol Injection (1% to 2%) 799
▲ Treximet Tablets (1% to 4%) 1616
▲ Trisenox Injection (8%) 986
Velcade for Injection 2168
Venlafaxine Hydrochloride Tablets (Rare) 2199
▲ Vesanoid Capsules (34%) 2660
Vicoprofen Tablets 533
Vivitrol 988
Voltaren Tablets (Occasionally) 2334
Voltaren-XR Tablets (Occasionally) 2337
Wellbutrin Tablets (Rare) 1648
Wellbutrin SR Sustained-Release Tablets 1653
Wellbutrin XL Extended-Release Tablets 1659
▲ Xeloda Tablets (1% to 6%) 2662
▲ Xigris Powder for Intravenous Infusion (5%) 1880
▲ Zemplar Capsules (5%) 536
▲ Zemplar Injection (5%) 538
Zyban Sustained-Release Tablets 1692
Zyprexa IntraMuscular 1883
Zyvox (0% to 2.3%) 2552

Bleeding, genital
Sutent Capsules 2540

Bleeding, genitourinary tract
▲ Activase I.V. (4%) 1188
Argatroban Injection (1.8%) 1308
Premphase Tablets 3232
Prempro Tablets 3232
ReoPro Vials (5 to 8 events) 1860
Xigris Powder for Intravenous Infusion (2%) 1880

Bleeding, gingival
(*see under* Bleeding, dental)

Bleeding, gums
Elmiron Capsules (Less than or equal to 1%) 2435
▲ Mylotarg for Injection (5% to 14%) 3212
Raptiva for Injection 1218
Symbyax Capsules (Rare) 1871

Bleeding, intermenstrual
Evoxac Capsules (Less than 1%) 1013
Imitrex Injection 1465
Imitrex Nasal Spray 1470
Imitrex Tablets (Infrequent) 1474
▲ Trisenox Injection (8%) 986
Yaz Tablets (Greater than 1%) 805
Zyrtec Chewable Tablets (Less than 2%) 1920
Zyrtec Syrup (Less than 2%) 1920
Zyrtec Tablets (Less than 2%) 1920
Zyrtec-D 12 Hour Extended Release Tablets (Less than 2%) 1923

Bleeding, internal
Activase I.V. 1188

Bleeding, intra-abdominal
Xigris Powder for Intravenous Infusion (2%) 1880

Bleeding, intracerebral
Torisel Injection 3272
Velcade for Injection 2168

Bleeding, intracranial
Activase I.V. (0.4% to 1.3%) 1188
Aggrenox Capsules (0.6% to less than 1%) 819
Angiomax for Injection (Less than 0.1% to 0.6%) 1933
▲ Argatroban Injection (1% to 4.3%) 1308
Aricept Tablets (Infrequent) 1062
Aricept ODT Tablets (Infrequent) 1062
Arranon Injection (1%) 1319
Bayer Aspirin 750
Elspar for Injection 1990
Exelon Capsules (Infrequent) 2229
Exelon Oral Solution (Infrequent) 2229
▲ Indocin I.V. (3% to 9%) 2489
▲ Infasurf Intratracheal Suspension (29% to 36%) 1168
Integrilin Injection (Rare) 2855
Lovenox Injection (0.8%) 2756
Mylotarg for Injection (1%) 3212
Namenda 1180
Percodan Tablets 1130
Plavix Tablets (Less than 1%) 926
Plavix Tablets (Less than 1%) 2767
Pletal Tablets 2481
Refludan for Injection (0.6%) 795
ReoPro Vials (1 to 3 events) 1860
St. Joseph 81 mg Aspirin Chewable and Enteric Coated Tablets 1903
Xigris Powder for Intravenous Infusion (2%) 1880

Bleeding, intra-thoracic
▲ Xigris Powder for Intravenous Infusion (4%) 1880

Bleeding, menstrual, prolonged
ParaGard T 380A Intrauterine Copper Contraceptive 1041

Bleeding, mouth
Evoxac Capsules (Less than 1%) 1013
▲ Intron A for Injection (Less than 5%) 2859
ReoPro Vials (4 events) 1860

Bleeding, mucosal
Venlafaxine Hydrochloride Tablets (Rare) 2199

Bleeding, nasal
(*see under* Epistaxis)

Bleeding, oropharyngeal
Integrilin Injection 2855

Bleeding, otic
Relenza Inhalation Powder (Less than 1%) 1556
ReoPro Vials (9 to 11 events) 1860

Bleeding, pericardial
Activase I.V. 1188

Bleeding, pharyngeal
Nexavar Tablets (2.4%) 784
▲ TNKase (3.1%) 1233

Bleeding, postmenopausal
▲ Activella Tablets (5% to 11%) 2347

Bleeding, postoperative
▲ Advair HFA 45/21 Inhalation Aerosol (1% to 3%) 1288
▲ Advair HFA 115/21 Inhalation Aerosol (1% to 3%) 1288
▲ Advair HFA 230/21 Inhalation Aerosol (1% to 3%) 1288
▲ Arixtra Injection (4.3%) 1313
Dacogen Injection 1066
Ionsys Transdermal System (.1% to less than 1%) 2410
Persantine Tablets (Rare) 869

Bleeding, postpartum
Percodan Tablets 1130

Bleeding, puncture site
Capastat Sulfate for Injection 1791
TNKase (Less than 1% to 3.6%) 1233

Bleeding, renal-pelvic
Cipro I.V. (1% or less) 2817

Bleeding, respiratory tract
▲ Nexavar Tablets (Greater than or equal to 10%) 784
TNKase (Less than 1%) 1233

Bleeding, retroperitoneal
Activase I.V. (Less than 1%) 1188
Angiomax for Injection (0.2% to 1.3%) 1933
Argatroban Injection (0.9%) 1308
Integrilin Injection 2855
Lovenox Injection 2756
▲ NovoSeven RT (4.7%) 2370
Plavix Tablets (Less than 1%) 926
Plavix Tablets (Less than 1%) 2767
Pletal Tablets (Less than 2%) 2481
ReoPro Vials (2 to 12 events) 1860
Tasigna Capsules 2316
TNKase (Less than 1%) 1233
▲ Xigris Powder for Intravenous Infusion (3%) 1880

Bleeding, sheath site
Angiomax for Injection (0.9%) 1933

Bleeding, skin and soft tissues
Xigris Powder for Intravenous Infusion (1%) 1880

Bleeding, subcutaneous
Imitrex Injection 1465

Bleeding, subdural
Bayer Aspirin 750

Bleeding, superficial
Activase I.V. 1188

Bleeding, upper GI
(*see under* Bleeding, gastrointestinal)

Bleeding, urethral
Ceftin Tablets (0.1% to 1%) 1380
Cipro (Less than 1%) 2810
Cipro XR Tablets 2823
Dacogen Injection 1066
Klonopin (Infrequent) 2639

Bleeding, urinary tract
Amerge Tablets (Rare) 1301
▲ TNKase (Less than 1% to 3.7%) 1233

Bleeding, uterine
Aggrenox Capsules (Less than 1%) 819
Climara Transdermal System 763
Effexor XR Extended-Release Capsules (Infrequent) 3195
Estrastest Tablets 3043
Estratest H.S. Tablets 3043
Evoxac Capsules (Less than 1%) 1013
Gengraf Capsules (1% to less than 3%) 435
Geodon Capsules (Rare) 2520
▲ Intron A for Injection (Less than 5%) 2859
Lipitor Tablets (Less than 2%) 2501
Lunesta Tablets 2994
Neoral Oral Solution (1% to less than 3%) 2280
Neoral Soft Gelatin Capsules (1% to less than 3%) 2280
Premarin Intravenous 3217
Premarin Vaginal Cream 3228
Premphase Tablets 3232
Prempro Tablets 3232
Prozac Pulvules and Liquid (Rare) 1852
Requip Tablets (Rare) 1561
Rilutek Tablets (Rare) 2771

Bleeding, vaginal
Actiq (Less than 1%) 959
▲ Activella Tablets (26%) 2347
AmBisome for Injection (Less common) 606
▲ Angeliq Tablets (9.3%) 751
▲ Arimidex Tablets (1% to 5%) 672
▲ Avastin IV (6%) 1192
Celebrex Capsules (0.1% to 1.9%) 2979
Climara Transdermal System 763
▲ Climara Pro Transdermal System (36.8%) 768
Clinoril Tablets (Less than 1%) 1962
▲ Doxil Injection (1% to 10%) 2378
Effexor XR Extended-Release Capsules (Infrequent) 3195
Emsam Transdermal System (Infrequent) 905
Enjuvia Tablets 1029
Estratest Tablets 3043
Estratest H.S. Tablets 3043
▲ Evista Tablets (2.5% to 6.2%) 1810
Evoxac Capsules (Less than 1%) 1013
Faslodex Injection (Less than 1%) 682
Gabitril Tablets (Infrequent) 973
Geodon Capsules (Rare) 2520
Indocin Capsules (Less than 1%) 2024
Indocin I.V. (Less than 1%) 2489
Indocin (Less than 1%) 2024
Lipitor Tablets (Less than 2%) 2501
Lunesta Tablets (Infrequent) 2994
Lupron Depot-PED 7.5 mg, 11.25 mg and 15 mg (2%) 471
Luvox CR Extended-Release Capsules (Infrequent) 1759
▲ Mylotarg for Injection (4% to 13%) 3212
Ortho-Cyclen/Ortho Tri-Cyclen 2449
Ortho Tri-Cyclen Lo Tablets 2458
Paxil (Rare) 1535
Paxil CR Controlled-Release Tablets (Rare) 1544
Pletal Tablets (Less than 2%) 2481
▲ Premarin Tablets (2% to 14%) 3221
▲ Premphase Tablets (1% to 6%) 3232
▲ Prempro Tablets (1% to 6%) 3232
Prozac Weekly Capsules 1852
Prozac Pulvules and Liquid (Infrequent) 1852
Refludan for Injection (1.8%) 795
Requip Tablets (Infrequent) 1561
Symbyax Capsules (Infrequent) 1871
▲ Trisenox Injection (13%) 986
Wellbutrin SR Sustained-Release Tablets (Up to 2%) 1653
Wellbutrin XL Extended-Release Tablets (0% to 2%) 1659
Xyrem Oral Solution (Infrequent) 1766

Bleeding, wound
▲ Fragmin Injection (0.1% to 3.4%) 1070
▲ Ionsys Transdermal System (1% to less than 10%) 2410
Sutent Capsules 2540

Bleeding at injection site
▲ Amevive (4%) 611
Bicillin C-R Injectable Suspension 1775
Bicillin L-A Injection 1777
▲ BOTOX Purified Neurotoxin Complex (3% to 10%) 550
▲ Edex Injection (15%) 2957
Forteo for Injection (Less than 1/30 patients) 1816
Genotropin Lyophilized Powder (Infrequent) 2547
▲ Humira Injection (20%) 442
▲ Lovenox Injection (3% to 5%) 2756
▲ Lucentis Injection (0% to 5%) 1205
ProQuad 2099
▲ Visudyne for Injection (10% to 30%) 2332

Bleeding diathesis
Cipro I.V. (Rare) 2817
Cipro (Less than 0.1%) 2810
Cipro XR Tablets 2823

Bleeding irregularities
Climara Transdermal System 763
Climara Pro Transdermal System 768
Lybrel Tablets 3204
Mirena Intrauterine System 779
Ortho Micronor Tablets 2446
Plavix Tablets (1% to 2.5%) 926
Plavix Tablets (1% to 2.5%) 2767
Premphase Tablets 3232
Prempro Tablets 3232

Bleeding secondary to eczema
Bactroban Cream (One report) 1366

Bleeding tendency, increased
Pletal Tablets 2481
Singulair 2114

Bleeding time, prolongation
Actiq (Less than 1%) 959
Advate (0.6%) 721
▲ Anaprox Tablets (1% to 10%) 2632
▲ Anaprox DS Tablets (1% to 10%) 2632
Cardizem LA Extended Release Tablets (Infrequent) 421
Depakote ER Tablets (Greater than 1%) 423
▲ EC-Naprosyn Delayed-Release Tablets (1% to 10%) 2632
Elmiron Capsules 2435
Flector Patch 561
▲ Naprosyn Suspension (1% to 10%) 2632
▲ Naprosyn Tablets (1% to 10%) 2632
Paxil (Rare) 1535
Paxil CR Controlled-Release Tablets (Rare) 1544
Rythmol Tablets (Less than 1%) 1586
Soriatane Capsules (Less than 1%) 3062
Timentin ADD-Vantage 1606
Timentin Injection Galaxy Container 1609
Timentin IV Infusion 1603
Timentin Pharmacy Bulk Package 1613
Venlafaxine Hydrochloride Tablets (Rare) 2199
Vicoprofen Tablets 533
▲ Voltaren Tablets (1% to 10%) 2334
▲ Voltaren-XR Tablets (1% to 10%) 2337
Zosyn for Injection 3284

Blepharitis
▲ Alphagan P Ophthalmic Solution (1% to 4%) 549
Aricept Tablets (Infrequent) 1062
Aricept ODT Tablets (Infrequent) 1062
▲ Azopt Ophthalmic Suspension (1% to 5%) 540
Bactroban Nasal (Less than 1%) 1367
▲ Betimol Ophthalmic Solution (1% to 5%) 3181
▲ Combigan Ophthalmic Solution (1% to 5%) 553
▲ Cosopt Sterile Ophthalmic Solution (1% to 5%) 1969
Doxil Injection (Less than 1%) 2378
▲ Durezol Ophthalmic Emulsion (5% to 15%) ⊙275
Effexor XR Extended-Release Capsules (Rare) 3195
Evoxac Capsules (Less than 1%) 1013
Exelon Capsules (Infrequent) 2229
Exelon Oral Solution (Infrequent) 2229
Gabitril Tablets (Infrequent) 973
Geodon Capsules (Infrequent) 2520
▲ Lucentis Injection (3% to 36%) 1205
▲ Lumigan Ophthalmic Solution (3% to 10%) 556
Lyrica Capsules (0.1% to 1%) 2527
Mirapex Tablets 857
Namenda (Infrequent) 1180
Norvir (Less than 2%) 489
OptiPranolol Metipranolol Ophthalmic Solution 0.3% (A small number of patients) ⊙245
Paxil (Rare) 1535
Paxil CR Controlled-Release Tablets (Rare) 1544
Protopic Ointment (0.2% to less than 1%) 628
Prozac Weekly Capsules (Rare) 1852
Prozac Pulvules and Liquid (Rare) 1852
Remeron Tablets (Rare) 2924
RemeronSolTab Tablets (Rare) 2927
Requip Tablets (Infrequent) 1561
Rilutek Tablets (Rare) 2771
▲ Soriatane Capsules (Less than 5%) 3062
Sular Extended Release Tablets (Less than or equal to 1%) 2975
Targretin Capsules 1084
Tasigna Capsules 2316
Timoptic Sterile Ophthalmic Solution (Less frequent) 2121
Timoptic in Ocudose (Less frequent) 2124
Timoptic-XE Sterile Ophthalmic Gel Forming Solution 2125
▲ Travatan Z Ophthalmic Solution (1% to 4%) 547
Venlafaxine Hydrochloride Tablets (Rare) 2199
▲ Visudyne for Injection (1% to 10%) 2332
Zyprexa Tablets (Infrequent) 1883
Zyprexa ZYDIS Orally Disintegrating Tablets (Infrequent) 1883

Blepharoconjunctivitis
▲ Alphagan P Ophthalmic Solution (1% to 4%) 549
Combigan Ophthalmic Solution (0.1% to 0.2%) 553
▲ Flovent Diskus 50 mcg (1% to 3%) 1435

Blepharoptosis
(*see also under* Ptosis, eyelids)
Betimol Ophthalmic Solution 3181

Blepharospasm
Eldepryl Capsules 3052
Exelon Capsules (Infrequent) 2229
Exelon Oral Solution (Infrequent) 2229
Mirapex Tablets 857
Requip Tablets (Infrequent) 1561
Stalevo Tablets 2309

Blindness
Bicillin C-R Injectable Suspension 1775
Bicillin L-A Injection 1777
DepoCyt Injection 1136
Doxil Injection (Less than 1%) 2378
Gabitril Tablets (Infrequent) 973
Imitrex Nasal Spray 1470
Imitrex Tablets 1474
Lyrica Capsules (Rare) 2527
Neoral Oral Solution 2280
Neoral Soft Gelatin Capsules 2280
Ortho-Cyclen/Ortho Tri-Cyclen (Rare) 2449
Orthoclone OKT3 Sterile Solution (Less than 1%) 2387
PegIntron Powder for Injection (Less than or equal to 1%) 2903
Pletal Tablets (Less than 2%) 2481
Prograf Capsules and Injection 622
Proleukin for Injection 2287
Sandimmune 2296
Treximet Tablets 1616
Zofran (Rare) 1687
Zofran ODT Orally Disintegrating Tablets (Rare) 1687
Zyrtec Chewable Tablets (Less than 2%) 1920
Zyrtec Syrup (Less than 2%) 1920
Zyrtec Tablets (Less than 2%) 1920
Zyrtec-D 12 Hour Extended Release Tablets (Less than 2%) 1923

Blindness, cortical
Prograf Capsules and Injection 622
Sutent Capsules 2540

Blindness, night
(*see under* Nyctalopia)

Blindness, transient
Chantix Tablets (Rare) 2511
Imitrex Tablets 1474
Proleukin for Injection 2287
Treximet Tablets 1616
Zofran Injection 1682
Zofran 1687
Zofran ODT Orally Disintegrating Tablets 1687

Blistering
Accolate Tablets 669
Avelox 2803
Cipro I.V. 2817
Levaquin 2416
Levaquin in 5% Dextrose Injection 2416
Lotrisone 2881
Motrin IB Tablets and Caplets 1900
Children's Motrin Oral Suspension 1901
Children's Motrin Non-Staining Dye-Free Oral Suspension 1901
Children's Motrin Cold Oral Suspension 1899
Infants' Motrin Concentrated Drops 1901
Infants' Motrin Non-Staining Dye-Free Concentrated Drops 1901
Junior Strength Motrin Caplets and Chewable Tablets 1901
Noroxin Tablets 2069
Reyataz Capsules 3299
Sulfamylon Cream 2194
Sulfamylon for 5% Topical Solution 2194
▲ Sutent Capsules (7%) 2540
Treximet Tablets (Rare) 1616
Viramune Oral Suspension 873
Viramune Tablets 873

Blisters at application site
Lidoderm Patch 1114

Bloating
(*see under* Abdominal bloating)

Blood clotting, mechanisms, disorders of
NovoSeven RT (1%) 2370
Plavix Tablets (Less than 1%) 926
Plavix Tablets (Less than 1%) 2767

Blood disorders, unspecified
▲ Cancidas for Injection (1.8% to 14.9%) 1953
▲ Mycamine for Injection (14.6% to 96%) 616
Patanase Nasal Spray 544

Blood dyscrasias
Abelcet Injection 1134
Asacol Delayed-Release Tablets 2579
Dapsone Tablets USP 1746
Furosemide Tablets 2186
Lamictal 1488
▲ Leukine (25%) 774
Prozac Weekly Capsules (Rare) 1852
Prozac Pulvules and Liquid (Rare) 1852
Thiothixene Capsules 2197
Trusopt Sterile Ophthalmic Solution (Rare) 2128
Zonegran Capsules (Rare) 1089

Blood glucose, elevation
(*see under* Hyperglycinemia)

Blood glucose, reduction
(*see under* Hypoglycemia)

Blood glucose levels, changes in
Abilify Injection (Rare) 2466
Abilify Oral Solution (Rare) 2466
Abilify Discmelt Orally Disintegrating Tablets (Rare) 2466
Abilify Tablets (Rare) 2466
Brovana Inhalation Solution (Infrequent) 2990
Ortho-Cyclen/Ortho Tri-Cyclen 2449

Blood loss, increase
(*see under* Bleeding)

Blood pressure, changes
Abilify Injection 881
Abilify Injection 2466
Abilify Oral Solution 881
Abilify Oral Solution 2466
Abilify Discmelt Orally Disintegrating Tablets 881
Abilify Discmelt Orally Disintegrating Tablets 2466
Abilify Tablets 881
Abilify Tablets 2466
Brovana Inhalation Solution 2990
Dantrium Capsules (Less frequent) 2580
Evoxac Capsules 1013
Flebogamma 5% 1715
Flebogamma 5% DIF 1718
Focalin XR Capsules 2251
Gammagard Liquid 730
Moban Tablets 1116
Premphase Tablets 3232
Prempro Tablets (Occasional) 3232
Pristiq Extended-Release Tablets 3247
Proleukin for Injection (1%) 2287
Rythmol SR Capsules 1590
Sandimmune 2296
Thiothixene Capsules 2197
Treximet Tablets 1616
Ventolin HFA Inhalation Aerosol 1638
Visudyne for Injection 2332

Blood pressure, elevation
(*see also under* Hypertension)
▲ Fabrazyme for Intravenous Infusion (10%) 1241

Blood pressure, reduction
(*see under* Hypotension)

Blood urea levels, increase
Abilify Injection (Less than 1 in 1000 patients) 881
Abilify Injection (Greater than or equal to 1 in 1000 patients and less than 1 in 100 patients) 2466
Abilify Oral Solution (Less than 1 in 1000 patients) 881
Abilify Oral Solution (Greater than or equal to 1 in 1000 patients and less than 1 in 100 patients) 2466
Abilify Discmelt Orally Disintegrating Tablets (Less than 1 in 1000 patients) 881
Abilify Discmelt Orally Disintegrating Tablets (Greater than or equal to 1 in 1000 patients and less than 1 in 100 patients) 2466
Abilify Tablets (Less than 1 in 1000 patients) 881
Abilify Tablets (Greater than or equal to 1 in 1000 patients and less than 1 in 100 patients) 2466
▲ Cancidas for Injection (3.9% to 8.8%) 1953
▲ Dacogen Injection (10%) 1066
Diovan HCT Tablets (Greater than 0.2%) 2216
Fortaz (Occasional) 1450
Rythmol SR Capsules 1590
Tasigna Capsules (0.1% to 1%) 2316

Blood urea nitrogen levels, increase
(*see under* BUN levels, elevation)

Blood urine
Patanase Nasal Spray 544
Requip Tablets (Infrequent) 1561
Xyrem Oral Solution (Infrequent) 1766

Blurred vision
(*see under* Vision, blurred)

Body fat accumulation
Intelence Tablets 3119
Lexiva Oral Suspension 1510
Lexiva Tablets 1510
Truvada Tablets 1262
Viramune Oral Suspension 873
Viramune Tablets 873

Body odor
Authia Cream 3190
Emsam Transdermal System (Rare) 905
Lovaza Capsules 1520
▲ Lupron Depot 3.75 mg (Less than 5%) 462
▲ Lupron Depot–3 Month 11.25 mg (Less than 5%) 462
Lupron Depot-PED 7.5 mg, 11.25 mg and 15 mg (Less than 2%) 471
Retrovir Capsules 1574
Retrovir IV Infusion 1579
Retrovir 1574
Salagen Tablets (Less than 1%) 1082
Wellbutrin Tablets (Rare) 1648

Bone, abnormal growth of
Nutropin for Injection 1208
Nutropin AQ Injection 1212
Nutropin AQ NuSpin Injection 1212
Nutropin AQ Pen 1212
Nutropin AQ Pen Cartridge 1212

Bone density, changes
Lupron Depot 3.75 mg 462
Lupron Depot–3 Month 11.25 mg 462
Proglycem Capsules (Infrequent) 1185
Proglycem Suspension (Infrequent) 1185
Viadur Implant (Less than 2%) 802

Bone density, decreased
Arimidex Tablets 672
Lupron Depot 7.5 mg 469
Truvada Tablets 1262
Vantas 1737

Bone disorders
Accutane Capsules 2607
▲ Actonel with Calcium Tablets (4%) 2574
Brovana Inhalation Solution (Less than 2%) 2990
Celebrex Capsules (0.1% to 1.9%) 2979
Evoxac Capsules (Less than 1%) 1013
▲ Humatrope Vials and Cartridges (9.6%) 1838
▲ Humira Injection (Less than 5%) 442
Protonix for Delayed-Release Oral Suspension (Less than 1%) 3254
Protonix Delayed-Release Tablets (Less than 1%) 3254
Protonix I.V. (Less than 1%) 3257
Protopic Ointment (0.2% to less than 1%) 628
Salagen Tablets (Less than 1%) 1082
Soriatane Capsules (Less than 1%) 3062
Symbyax Capsules (Infrequent) 1871
▲ Vesanoid Capsules (3%) 2660

Bone fractures
▲ Actonel with Calcium Tablets (5% to 6.4%) 2574
▲ ActoPlus Met Tablets (1.7% to 5.1%) 3071
Actos Tablets 3077
Alinia for Oral Suspension (Less than 1%) 2677
Alinia Tablets (Less than 1%) 2677
Aricept Tablets (Infrequent) 1062
Aricept ODT Tablets (Infrequent) 1062
▲ Arimidex Tablets (10%) 672
Avandamet Tablets 1336
▲ Avandaryl Tablets (9.3%) 1344
▲ Avandia Tablets (9.3%) 1351
Didronel Tablets 2583
Duetact Tablets 3085
Gengraf Capsules (1% to less than 3%) 435
▲ Humira Injection (Less than 5%) 442
Namenda (More than one patient) 1180
Neoral Oral Solution (1% to less than 3%) 2280
Neoral Soft Gelatin Capsules (1% to less than 3%) 2280
▲ Pulmicort Flexhaler (Greater than or equal to 1% to 3%) 654
▲ Remicade for IV Injection (7%) 950
Salagen Tablets (Less than 1%) 1082
Velcade for Injection 2168

Bone marrow depression
Carbatrol Capsules 3019
Cipro I.V. 2817
Cipro 2810
Cipro XR Tablets 2823
Clinoril Tablets (Less than 1%) 1962
Cuprimine Capsules 1986
Doxil Injection 2378
Elspar for Injection (Rare) 1990
Equetro Extended-Release Capsules 3174
Indocin Capsules (Less than 1%) 2024
Indocin I.V. (Less than 1%) 2489
Indocin (Less than 1%) 2024
Mavik Tablets (Rare) 472
Primaxin I.M. 2080
Primaxin I.V. 2083
Prinivil Tablets (Rare) 2087
Prinzide Tablets (Rare) 2092
Sulfamylon Cream (A single case) 2194
Sulfamylon for 5% Topical Solution 2194
▲ Valcyte Tablets (Less than 5%) 2654

Bone marrow hypoplasia
Captopril Tablets 2182
Retrovir Capsules 1574
Retrovir IV Infusion 1579
Retrovir 1574
Rituxan I.V. 1223
Zantac 25 EFFERdose Tablets (Rare) 1670
Zantac Injection (Sometimes) 1666
Zantac Injection Pharmacy Bulk Package (Rare) 1668
Zantac Injection Premixed (Sometimes) 1666
Zantac (Rare) 1670

Bone marrow suppression
Albenza Tablets 1297
Depakote ER Tablets 423
Doxil Injection 2378
Hycamtin Capsules 1456
Hycamtin for Injection 1459
Intron A for Injection 2859
Keppra Injection 3137
Keppra Oral Solution 3131
Keppra Tablets 3131
Leukeran Tablets (Frequent) 1508
Leustatin Injection (Common) 2384
Phenytek Capsules 2192
Tabloid Tablets 1601
Taxotere Injection Concentrate 2773

Bone mineral density, decreased
Accutane Capsules 2607
Advair Diskus 100/50 1276
Advair Diskus 250/50 1276
Advair Diskus 500/50 1276
Azmacort Inhalation Aerosol 407
Levothroid Tablets 1170

Bone spur
Requip Tablets (Infrequent) 1561
Venlafaxine Hydrochloride Tablets (Infrequent) 2199

Bowel, perforation of
▲ Indocin I.V. (1% to 3%) 2489
Proleukin for Injection 2287
Rituxan I.V. 1223
Torisel Injection (1%) 3272

Bowel disease, inflammatory, exacerbation of
Accutane Capsules 2607
Anaprox Tablets (Less than 1%) 2632
Anaprox DS Tablets (Less than 1%) 2632
Asacol Delayed-Release Tablets 2579
EC-Naprosyn Delayed-Release Tablets (Less than 1%) 2632
Naprosyn Suspension (Less than 1%) 2632
Naprosyn Tablets (Less than 1%) 2632

Bowel dysfunction
DepoCyt Injection 1136

Bowel frequency, increase
Klonopin (Infrequent) 2639

Bowel habits, changes
Evoxac Capsules 1013
Frova Tablets (Rare) 1111
Nexium Delayed-Release Capsules (Less than 1%) 645
Nexium I.V. (Less than 1%) 652
Nexium Delayed-Release Oral Suspension (Less than 1%) 645

Bowel infarction
Activase I.V. 1188
Orthoclone OKT3 Sterile Solution (Less than 1%) 2387

Bowel movements, frequent
Ambien CR Tablets (1%) 2696
Amitiza Capsules (Less than 1%) 3082
▲ Suprax for Oral Suspension (6%) 1891
▲ Suprax Tablets (6%) 1891
Tyzeka Tablets (Less than 1%) 2328
▲ Vivitrol (12% to 13%) 988

Bowel movements, light-colored
Levaquin 2416
Levaquin in 5% Dextrose Injection 2416

Bowel obstruction
Atrovent Nasal Spray 0.03% 834
Atrovent Nasal Spray 0.06% 836
Rituxan I.V. 1223

Bowel sounds, abnormal
Emend Capsules (Less than or equal to 0.5%) 1992
Emend for Injection (Less than or equal to 0.5%) 1999

Bowel syndrome, irritable
Evoxac Capsules (Less than 1%) 1013
Mirapex Tablets 857
Requip Tablets (Infrequent) 1561
Risperdal Consta Long-Acting Injection (Infrequent) 1753
Treximet Tablets (Rare) 1616

Bowel urgency
Copaxone for Injection (Frequent) 3110

Bowen's disease
Selzentry Tablets 2534

Brachial plexus neuropathies
BOTOX Purified Neurotoxin Complex 550
Fluarix Vaccine 1446
Flulaval Injection Vaccine 1448

Bradyarrhythmias
Janumet Tablets 2041

Bradycardia
Abilify Injection (Greater than or equal to 1 in 1000 patients and less than 1 in 100 patients) 881
Abilify Injection (Greater than or equal to 1 in 1000 patients and less than 1 in 100 patients) 2466
Abilify Oral Solution (Greater than or equal to 1 in 1000 patients and less than 1 in 100 patients) 881
Abilify Oral Solution (Greater than or equal to 1 in 1000 patients and less than 1 in 100 patients) 2466
Abilify Discmelt Orally Disintegrating Tablets (Greater than or equal to 1 in 1000 patients and less than 1 in 100 patients) 881
Abilify Discmelt Orally Disintegrating Tablets (Greater than or equal to 1 in 1000 patients and less than 1 in 100 patients) 2466
Abilify Tablets (Greater than or equal to 1 in 1000 patients and less than 1 in 100 patients) 881

Abilify Tablets (Greater than or equal to 1 in 1000 patients and less than 1 in 100 patients) 2466
Adenocard IV Injection 603
Adenoscan (Less than 1%) 605
▲ Aloxi Injection (4%) 1059
Alphagan P Ophthalmic Solution 549
AmBisome for Injection (Less common) 606
Amerge Tablets (Rare) 1301
▲ Angiomax for Injection (5%) 1933
▲ Anzemet Injection (5.1%) 2701
▲ Anzemet Tablets (Rare to 5.1%) 2704
▲ Argatroban Injection (4.5%) 1308
Aricept Tablets (Frequent) 1062
Aricept ODT Tablets (Frequent) 1062
Atacand HCT (0.5% or greater) 642
▲ Avinza Capsules (Less than 5%) 1772
Betimol Ophthalmic Solution 3181
Bystolic Tablets (0% to 1%) 1155
Cancidas for Injection 1953
▲ Cardizem LA Extended Release Tablets (1.7% to 3.6%) 421
Catapres Tablets (About 5 in 1,000 patients) 841
Catapres-TTS (0.5% or less) 842
Celexa (Infrequent) 1160
▲ CellCept Capsules (3% to less than 20%) 2622
▲ CellCept Intravenous (3% to less than 20%) 2622
▲ CellCept Oral Suspension (3% to less than 20%) 2622
▲ CellCept Tablets (3% to less than 20%) 2622
Chantix Tablets (Infrequent) 2511
Cipro XR Tablets (Less than 1%) 2823
Clorpres Tablets (About 5 in 1,000) 2185
Combigan Ophthalmic Solution 553
Concerta Extended-Release Tablets 1925
Copaxone for Injection (Infrequent) 3110
▲ Coreg Tablets (2% to 10%) 1387
▲ Coreg CR Extended-Release Capsules (2% to 10%) 1393
Cosopt Sterile Ophthalmic Solution (Less than 1%) 1969
Depakote ER Tablets 423
▲ DepoDur Injection (2% to 5%) 1095
Doxil Injection (Less than 1%) 2378
Duragesic Transdermal System (Less than 1%) 2405
Effexor XR Extended-Release Capsules (Rare) 3195
Emend Capsules (Isolated cases) 1992
Emend for Injection (Isolated cases) 1999
Exelon Capsules (Frequent) 2229
Exelon Oral Solution (Frequent) 2229
Exelon Patch (Infrequent) 2233
Exforge Tablets (Greater than 0.1% to less than 1%) 2238
▲ Fabrazyme for Intravenous Infusion (Greater than or equal to 5%) 1241
▲ Flolan for Injection (5% to 15%) 1426
Frova Tablets (Rare) 1111
Geodon Capsules (Infrequent) 2520
Imitrex Injection (Infrequent) 1465
Imitrex Nasal Spray (Rare) 1470
Imitrex Tablets (Rare) 1474
Indocin I.V. (Less than 3%) 2489
▲ Infasurf Intratracheal Suspension (34%) 1168
InnoPran XL Extended Release Capsules 1484
▲ Intron A for Injection (Less than 5%) 2859
Invanz for Injection (Greater than 0.1%) 2029
Invega Extended-Release Tablets 1748
Ionsys Transdermal System (.1% to less than 1%) 2410
Ketek Tablets (Less than 0.2%) 2744
Lexapro Oral Suspension (Infrequent) 1174
Lexapro Tablets (Infrequent) 1174
Lidoderm Patch 1114
Luvox CR Extended-Release Capsules (Frequent) 1759
▲ Mavik Tablets (0.3% to 4.7%) 472
Maxalt Tablets (Infrequent) 2056
Maxalt-MLT Orally Disintegrating Tablets (Infrequent) 2056
Merrem I.V. (Greater than 0.1% to 1%) 684
Mirapex Tablets 857
Mirena Intrauterine System 779
MS Contin Tablets (Less frequent) 2585
▲ Mycamine for Injection (2.5% to 5%) 616
Mylotarg for Injection 3212
Nadolol Tablets (Common) 2191
Namenda (Infrequent) 1180
▲ Natrecor for Injection (1% to 5%) 2977
Nembutal Sodium Solution, USP (Less than 1%) 2494
Nimbex Injection (0.4%) 484
Nimotop Capsules (Up to 1%) 790
NovoSeven (1%) 2367
NovoSeven RT (1%) 2370
Opana Tablets (Less than 1%) 1117
Opana ER Tablets (Less than 1%) 1121
OptiPranolol Metipranolol Ophthalmic Solution 0.3% (A small number of patients) ⊙245
Orthoclone OKT3 Sterile Solution (Less than 1%) 2387
Paxil (Infrequent) 1535
Paxil CR Controlled-Release Tablets (Infrequent) 1544
Percocet Tablets 1127
Percodan Tablets 1130
Photofrin for Injection 708
Prinivil Tablets (0.3% to 1%) 2087
Prinzide Tablets 2092
Proleukin for Injection (Less than 1%) 2287
Provigil Tablets (At least 1%) 977
Prozac Weekly Capsules (Rare) 1852
Prozac Pulvules and Liquid (Rare) 1852
Remeron Tablets (Infrequent) 2924
RemeronSolTab Tablets (Infrequent) 2927
Remicade for IV Injection (Greater than or equal to 0.2%) 950
▲ ReoPro Vials (5.2%) 1860
Requip Tablets (Infrequent) 1561
Requip XL Tablets 1568
Rilutek Tablets (Rare) 2771
Risperdal Consta Long-Acting Injection (Infrequent) 1753
Romazicon Injection (Less than 1%) 2646
Rythmol Tablets (1.5% to 2%) 1586
▲ Rythmol SR Capsules (3% to 4%) 1590
Salagen Tablets (Less than 1%) 1082
▲ Somatuline Depot Injection (2.8% to 18%) 3102
Symbyax Capsules (Infrequent) 1871
Tarka Tablets (1.8%) 511
Tasigna Capsules (0.1% to 1%) 2316
Teveten Tablets (Less than 1%) 515
Teveten HCT Tablets (Less than 1%) 517
Timoptic Sterile Ophthalmic Solution (Less frequent) 2121
Timoptic in Ocudose (Less frequent) 2124
Timoptic-XE Sterile Ophthalmic Gel Forming Solution 2125
Toprol-XL Tablets (1.5% to approximately 3 of 100 patients) 666
Trasylol Injection (1% to 2%) 799
▲ Travatan Z Ophthalmic Solution (1% to 5%) 547
Tygacil for Injection (0.2% to less than 2%) 3276
▲ Ultane Liquid for Inhalation (5%) 524
Velcade for Injection 2168
Venlafaxine Hydrochloride Tablets (Rare) 2199
▲ Xeloda Tablets (Less than 5%) 2662
Zantac 25 EFFERdose Tablets (Rare) 1670
Zantac Injection (Rare) 1666
Zantac Injection Pharmacy Bulk Package (Rare) 1668
Zantac Injection Premixed (Rare) 1666
Zantac (Rare) 1670
Zofran Injection (Rare) 1682
▲ Zofran (6%) 1687
▲ Zofran ODT Orally Disintegrating Tablets (6%) 1687
Zometa for Intravenous Infusion 2341
Zomig Tablets (Rare) 694
Zomig Nasal Spray (Rare) 689
Zomig-ZMT Tablets (Rare) 694
Zonegran Capsules (Infrequent) 1089
Zosyn for Injection (1% or less) 3284
Zyprexa Tablets (Infrequent) 1883
Zyprexa IntraMuscular 1883
Zyprexa ZYDIS Orally Disintegrating Tablets (Infrequent) 1883

Bradycardia, symptomatic
Nadolol Tablets (2 of 100 patients) 2191

Bradykinesia
Abilify Injection (Less than 1 in 1000 patients) 881
Abilify Injection (Greater than or equal to 1 in 1000 patients and less than 1 in 100 patients) 2466
Abilify Oral Solution (Less than 1 in 1000 patients) 881
Abilify Oral Solution (Greater than or equal to 1 in 1000 patients and less than 1 in 100 patients) 2466
Abilify Discmelt Orally Disintegrating Tablets (Less than 1 in 1000 patients) 881
Abilify Discmelt Orally Disintegrating Tablets (Greater than or equal to 1 in 1000 patients and less than 1 in 100 patients) 2466
Abilify Tablets (Less than 1 in 1000 patients) 881
Abilify Tablets (Greater than or equal to 1 in 1000 patients and less than 1 in 100 patients) 2466
Effexor XR Extended-Release Capsules (Rare) 3195
Eldepryl Capsules 3052
Exelon Capsules (Frequent) 2229
▲ Exelon Oral Solution (Frequent) 2229
Invega Extended-Release Tablets 1748
Maxalt Tablets (Rare) 2056
Maxalt-MLT Orally Disintegrating Tablets (Rare) 2056
Paxil 1535
Paxil CR Controlled-Release Tablets 1544
Risperdal Consta Long-Acting Injection (Infrequent) 1753
Venlafaxine Hydrochloride Tablets (Rare) 2199
▲ Wellbutrin Tablets (8%) 1648

Bradykinetic episodes
Stalevo Tablets 2309

Bradylogia
Imitrex Tablets (Rare) 1474

Bradyphrenia
Mirapex Tablets 857

Brain abscess
▲ Gliadel Wafer (4% to 5%) 1076

Brain damage
Rythmol SR Capsules 1590

Brain syndrome, acute
Actiq (Less than 1%) 959
Doxil Injection (Less than 1%) 2378
Prozac Weekly Capsules (Infrequent) 1852
Prozac Pulvules and Liquid (Infrequent) 1852
Rilutek Tablets (Rare) 2771
Symbyax Capsules (Rare) 1871

Breast, redistribution/accumulation of body fat
Retrovir 1574

Breast abscess
Lamictal (Rare) 1488
Rilutek Tablets (Rare) 2771

Breast atrophy
Paxil (Rare) 1535
Paxil CR Controlled-Release Tablets (Rare) 1544

Breast changes, fibrocystic
Activella Tablets 2347
Premarin Intravenous 3217

Breast changes, unspecified
▲ Lupron Depot 3.75 mg (3%) 462
▲ Lupron Depot–3 Month 11.25 mg (3%) 462
Lupron Depot-PED 7.5 mg, 11.25 mg and 15 mg (Less than 2%) 471
Lybrel Tablets 3204
Ortho-Cyclen Tablets 2449
▲ Ortho Evra Transdermal System (9% to 22%) 2437
Ortho Tri-Cyclen Tablets 2449
Ortho Tri-Cyclen Lo Tablets 2458
Premphase Tablets 3232
Prempro Tablets 3232

Breast discharge
Climara Transdermal System 763
Climara Pro Transdermal System 768
Divigel 3167
Effexor XR Extended-Release Capsules (Rare) 3195
Premarin Intravenous 3217
Premarin Tablets 3221
Premphase Tablets 3232
Prempro Tablets 3232
Venlafaxine Hydrochloride Tablets (Rare) 2199

Breast engorgement
Copaxone for Injection (Infrequent) 3110
Effexor XR Extended-Release Capsules (Rare) 3195
Prozac Weekly Capsules (Rare) 1852
Prozac Pulvules and Liquid (Rare) 1852
Remeron Tablets (Rare) 2924
RemeronSolTab Tablets (Rare) 2927
Symbyax Capsules (Rare) 1871
Thioridazine Hydrochloride Tablets 2195
Venlafaxine Hydrochloride Tablets (Rare) 2199

Breast enlargement
Activella Tablets 2347
Angeliq Tablets 751
Aptivus Capsules 823
Aptivus Oral Solution 823
Atripla Tablets 938
Catapres-TTS (0.5% or less) 842
Celexa (Infrequent) 1160
Climara Transdermal System 763
Climara Pro Transdermal System 768
Combivir Tablets 1384
Copaxone for Injection (Infrequent) 3110
▲ Crinone 8% Gel (40%) 992
Crixivan Capsules 1979
Depakote ER Tablets 423
Divigel 3167
Effexor XR Extended-Release Capsules (Rare) 3195
Emtriva Capsules 1246
Emtriva Oral Solution 1246
Enjuvia Tablets 1029
Estratest Tablets 3043
Estratest H.S. Tablets 3043
Gabitril Tablets (Infrequent) 973
Gleevec Tablets (Infrequent) 2255
Imitrex Nasal Spray 1470
Indocin Capsules (Less than 1%) 2024
Indocin I.V. (Less than 1%) 2489
Indocin (Less than 1%) 2024
Intelence Tablets 3119
Lexiva Oral Suspension 1510
Lexiva Tablets 1510
Lipitor Tablets (Less than 2%) 2501
Lunesta Tablets (Infrequent) 2994
▲ Lupron Depot 7.5 mg (Less than 5%) 469
Lybrel Tablets 3204
Mircette Tablets 1034
Norvir 489
Ortho-Cyclen Tablets 2449
Ortho Evra Transdermal System 2437
Ortho Tri-Cyclen Tablets 2449
Ortho Tri-Cyclen Lo Tablets 2458
Paxil (Rare) 1535
Paxil CR Controlled-Release Tablets (Rare) 1544
Premarin Intravenous 3217
Premarin Tablets 3221
Premarin Vaginal Cream 3228
▲ Premphase Tablets (2% to 5%) 3232
▲ Prempro Tablets (2% to 5%) 3232
Prometrium Capsules (100 mg, 200 mg) 3047
Propecia Tablets (0.5% to 1.8%) 2095
Proscar Tablets (0.5% to 1.8%) 2102
Prozac Weekly Capsules (Infrequent) 1852
Prozac Pulvules and Liquid (Infrequent) 1852
Requip Tablets (Rare) 1561
Seasonique Tablets 1046
Symbyax Capsules (Infrequent) 1871
Thiothixene Capsules 2197
Trizivir Tablets 1622
Truvada Tablets 1262
Venlafaxine Hydrochloride Tablets (Rare) 2199
▲ Viadur Implant (6.9%) 802
Viramune Oral Suspension 873
Viramune Tablets 873
Viread Tablets 1268
Yaz Tablets 805
Ziagen 1673
Zyprexa Tablets (Rare) 1883
Zyprexa ZYDIS Orally Disintegrating Tablets (Rare) 1883

Breast fibroadenosis
Ambien Tablets (Rare) 2692
Ambien CR Tablets (Rare) 2696
Aricept Tablets (Infrequent) 1062
Aricept ODT Tablets (Infrequent) 1062
Celebrex Capsules (0.1% to 1.9%) 2979
Gengraf Capsules (1% to less than 3%) 435
Neoral Oral Solution (1% to less than 3%) 2280

Neoral Soft Gelatin Capsules (1% to less than 3%) 2280

Breast fibrocystic

Angeliq Tablets 751
Aricept Tablets (Infrequent) 1062
Aricept ODT Tablets (Infrequent) 1062
Climara Transdermal System 763
Climara Pro Transdermal System 768
Copaxone for Injection (Infrequent) 3110
Effexor XR Extended-Release Capsules (Rare) 3195
Enjuvia Tablets 1029
Estratest Tablets 3043
Estratest H.S. Tablets 3043
Gabitril Tablets (Infrequent) 973
Lipitor Tablets (Less than 2%) 2501
Ortho-Cyclen/Ortho Tri-Cyclen 2449
Ortho Tri-Cyclen Lo Tablets 2458
Paxil (Rare) 1535
Paxil CR Controlled-Release Tablets (Rare) 1544
Premarin Tablets 3221
Premarin Vaginal Cream 3228
Premphase Tablets 3232
Prempro Tablets 3232
Prozac Weekly Capsules (Infrequent) 1852
Prozac Pulvules and Liquid (Infrequent) 1852
Symbyax Capsules (Infrequent) 1871
Venlafaxine Hydrochloride Tablets (Rare) 2199
Zomig Tablets (Rare) 694
Zomig Nasal Spray (Rare) 689
Zomig-ZMT Tablets (Rare) 694

Breast lumps

Amerge Tablets (Rare) 1301
Imitrex Nasal Spray 1470
Ortho-Cyclen Tablets 2449
Ortho Evra Transdermal System 2437
Ortho Tri-Cyclen Tablets 2449
Ortho Tri-Cyclen Lo Tablets 2458
Proglycem Capsules (Infrequent) 1185
Proglycem Suspension (Infrequent) 1185

Breast milk, maternal, excreted in

Accolate Tablets 669
Aczone Gel 5% 3296
Adderall XR Capsules 3012
Advicor Tablets 402
Aggrenox Capsules 819
Ambien Tablets 2692
Anaprox Tablets 2632
Anaprox DS Tablets 2632
Asacol Delayed-Release Tablets 2579
Augmentin 1323
Augmentin Tablets 1327
Augmentin XR Extended Release Tablets 1333
Augmentin ES-600 Powder for Oral Suspension 1329
Avalide Tablets 892
Avalide Tablets 2713
Avinza Capsules 1772
Captopril Tablets 2182
Carbatrol Capsules 3019
Catapres Tablets 841
Catapres-TTS 842
Ceftin Tablets 1380
Celexa 1160
Cipro I.V. 2817
Cipro 2810
Clarinex Tablets 2828
Clarinex Reditabs Tablets 2828
Clorpres Tablets 2185
Cosopt Sterile Ophthalmic Solution 1969
Dapsone Tablets USP 1746
Daraprim Tablets 1400
Depakote ER Tablets 423
Dexedrine 1401
Diovan HCT Tablets 2216
Duragesic Transdermal System 2405
Dyazide Capsules 1405
Dyrenium Capsules 3189
EC-Naprosyn Delayed-Release Tablets 2632
E.E.S. 433
Effexor XR Extended-Release Capsules 3195
EryPed 431
Fluorescite Injection ⊙ 203
Fortaz 1450
Furosemide Tablets 2186
Gengraf Capsules 435
Imitrex Injection 1465
Imitrex Nasal Spray 1470
Imitrex Tablets 1474
Indocin 2024
Intravenous Sodium Diuril 2490
Invanz for Injection 2029
Keppra Oral Solution 3131
Keppra Tablets 3131
Lamictal 1488
Lamisil Tablets 2266
Lanoxin Injection 1498
Lanoxin Injection Pediatric 1502
Lanoxin Tablets 1505
Lescol Capsules 2268
Lescol XL Tablets 2268
Levoxyl Tablets 1780
Lexapro Oral Suspension 1174
Lexapro Tablets 1174
Lortab 5/500 Tablets 3143
Lortab 7.5/500 Tablets 3144
Lortab 10/500 Tablets 3144
Marinol Capsules 3163
Meruvax II 2061
MS Contin Tablets 2585
Naprosyn Suspension 2632
Naprosyn Tablets 2632
Nembutal Sodium Solution, USP 2494
Neoral Oral Solution 2280
Neoral Soft Gelatin Capsules 2280
Niaspan Extended-Release Tablets 480
Nimotop Capsules 790
Ortho-Cyclen Tablets 2449
Ortho Evra Transdermal System 2437
Ortho Micronor Tablets 2446
Ortho Tri-Cyclen Tablets 2449
Ortho Tri-Cyclen Lo Tablets 2458
OxyContin Tablets 2589
OxyIR Capsules 2593
Paxil 1535
Paxil CR Controlled-Release Tablets 1544
Pentasa Capsules 3030
Pepcid Tablets 2075
Persantine Tablets 869
Phenytek Capsules 2192
Premphase Tablets 3232
Prempro Tablets 3232
Prinzide Tablets 2092
Prograf Capsules and Injection 622
Protopic Ointment 628
Qvar Inhalation Aerosol 3116
Retrovir Capsules 1574
Retrovir IV Infusion 1579
Retrovir 1574
Risperdal Consta Long-Acting Injection 1753
Rocaltrol Capsules 1150
Rocaltrol Oral Solution 1150
Rocephin Injectable Vials, ADD-Vantage, Galaxy, Bulk 2642
St. Joseph 81 mg Aspirin Chewable and Enteric Coated Tablets 1903
Sandimmune 2296
Stromectol Tablets 2120
Symbicort 80/4.5 Inhalation Aerosol 659
Symbicort 160/4.5 Inhalation Aerosol 659
Synthroid Tablets 507
Tarka Tablets 511
Timoptic Sterile Ophthalmic Solution 2121
Timoptic in Ocudose 2124
Timoptic-XE Sterile Ophthalmic Gel Forming Solution 2125
Toprol-XL Tablets 666
Trisenox Injection 986
Trizivir Tablets 1622
Tylenol with Codeine Tablets 2427
Uniphyl Tablets 2595
Uroqid-Acid No. 2 Tablets 814
Vicodin Tablets 529
Vicodin ES Tablets 530
Vicodin HP Tablets 531
Viramune Oral Suspension 873
Viramune Tablets 873
Wellbutrin SR Sustained-Release Tablets 1653
Wellbutrin XL Extended-Release Tablets 1659
Zantac 25 EFFERdose Tablets 1670
Zantac Injection 1666
Zantac 1670
Zinacef for Injection 1678
Zinacef Injection 1678
Zosyn for Injection 3284
Zovirax 1690
Zyban Sustained-Release Tablets 1692
Zyrtec Chewable Tablets 1920
Zyrtec Syrup 1920
Zyrtec Tablets 1920

Breast pain

Abilify Injection (Greater than or equal to 1 in 1000 patients and less than 1 in 100 patients) 881
Abilify Injection (Greater than or equal to 1 in 1000 patients and less than 1 in 100 patients) 2466
Abilify Oral Solution (Greater than or equal to 1 in 1000 patients and less than 1 in 100 patients) 881
Abilify Oral Solution (Greater than or equal to 1 in 1000 patients and less than 1 in 100 patients) 2466
Abilify Discmelt Orally Disintegrating Tablets (Greater than or equal to 1 in 1000 patients and less than 1 in 100 patients) 881
Abilify Discmelt Orally Disintegrating Tablets (Greater than or equal to 1 in 1000 patients and less than 1 in 100 patients) 2466
Abilify Tablets (Greater than or equal to 1 in 1000 patients and less than 1 in 100 patients) 881
Abilify Tablets (Greater than or equal to 1 in 1000 patients and less than 1 in 100 patients) 2466
Actiq (1% or greater) 959
▲ Activella Tablets (17% to 24%) 2347
Ambien Tablets (Rare) 2692
▲ AndroGel (1% to 3%) 3159
▲ Angeliq Tablets (18.9%) 751
▲ Arimidex Tablets (2% to 8%) 672
Celebrex Capsules (0.1% to 1.9%) 2979
Celexa (Infrequent) 1160
Cipro I.V. (1% or less) 2817
Cipro (Less than 1%) 2810
Cipro XR Tablets 2823
▲ Climara Transdermal System (5% to 29%) 763
▲ Climara Pro Transdermal System (18.9%) 768
Copaxone for Injection (At least 2%) 3110
▲ Crinone 8% Gel (13%) 992
Divigel 3167
Doxil Injection (Less than 1%) 2378
Effexor XR Extended-Release Capsules (Infrequent) 3195
Emsam Transdermal System (Infrequent) 905
▲ Enjuvia Tablets (0% to 14%) 1029
Estratest Tablets 3043
Estratest H.S. Tablets 3043
▲ Evista Tablets (4.4%) 1810
Evoxac Capsules (Less than 1%) 1013
Exelon Capsules (Infrequent) 2229
Exelon Oral Solution (Infrequent) 2229
▲ Femara Tablets (7%) 2246
▲ Follistim AQ Cartridge (15%) 2844
Gabitril Tablets (Infrequent) 973
Gengraf Capsules (1% to less than 3%) 435
Klonopin (Infrequent) 2639
Lamictal (Infrequent) 1488
Lunesta Tablets (Infrequent) 2994
▲ Lupron Depot 3.75 mg (3%) 462
▲ Lupron Depot–3 Month 11.25 mg (3%) 462
Luvox CR Extended-Release Capsules (Infrequent) 1759
Lybrel Tablets 3204
Mirapex Tablets 857
▲ Mirena Intrauterine System (5% or more) 779
Neoral Oral Solution (1% to less than 3%) 2280
Neoral Soft Gelatin Capsules (1% to less than 3%) 2280
Paxil (Infrequent) 1535
Paxil CR Controlled-Release Tablets (Infrequent) 1544
Pentasa Capsules (Less than 1%) 3030
Premarin Intravenous 3217
▲ Premarin Tablets (7% to 12%) 3221
▲ Premphase Tablets (13% to 38%) 3232
▲ Prempro Tablets (13% to 38%) 3232
Prinivil Tablets (0.3% to 1%) 2087
Prinzide Tablets 2092
▲ Prometrium Capsules (100 mg, 200 mg) (6% to 16%) 3047
Protonix for Delayed-Release Oral Suspension (Less than 1%) 3254
Protonix Delayed-Release Tablets (Less than 1%) 3254
Protonix I.V. (Less than 1%) 3257
Protopic Ointment (Greater than or equal to 1%) 628
Prozac Weekly Capsules (Infrequent) 1852
Prozac Pulvules and Liquid (Infrequent) 1852
Remeron Tablets (Infrequent) 2924
RemeronSolTab Tablets (Infrequent) 2927
Rilutek Tablets (Rare) 2771
Risperdal Consta Long-Acting Injection (Infrequent) 1753
Rythmol SR Capsules 1590
Salagen Tablets (Less than 1%) 1082
Soriatane Capsules (Less than 1%) 3062
Symbyax Capsules (Frequent) 1871
Targretin Capsules 1084
Tasigna Capsules (0.1% to 1%) 2316
▲ Temodar Capsules (6%) 2931
Vantas (Less than 2%) 1737
Venlafaxine Hydrochloride Tablets (Infrequent) 2199
▲ Viadur Implant (3.1%) 802
Yaz Tablets (Greater than 1%) 805
Zyprexa Tablets (Infrequent) 1883
Zyprexa ZYDIS Orally Disintegrating Tablets (Infrequent) 1883
Zyrtec Chewable Tablets (Less than 2%) 1920
Zyrtec Syrup (Less than 2%) 1920
Zyrtec Tablets (Less than 2%) 1920
Zyrtec-D 12 Hour Extended Release Tablets (Less than 2%) 1923

Breast secretion

Amerge Tablets (Rare) 1301
Estratest Tablets 3043
Estratest H.S. Tablets 3043
Imitrex Nasal Spray 1470
Imitrex Tablets (Rare) 1474
Lybrel Tablets 3204
Mircette Tablets 1034
Ortho-Cyclen Tablets 2449
Ortho Evra Transdermal System 2437
Ortho Tri-Cyclen Tablets 2449
Ortho Tri-Cyclen Lo Tablets 2458
Premarin Intravenous 3217
Premarin Vaginal Cream 3228
Seasonique Tablets 1046
Yaz Tablets 805

Breast soreness

Eligard 7.5 mg (Less than 2%) 2724
Eligard 22.5 mg (Less than 2%) 2724
Eligard 30 mg (Less than 2%) 2724
Eligard 45 mg (Less than 2%) 2724

Breast tenderness

Activella Tablets 2347
Angeliq Tablets 751
Avodart Soft Gelatin Capsules (0.3% to 1.1%) 1359
Climara Transdermal System 763
Climara Pro Transdermal System 768
▲ Divigel (2.5% to 8.8%) 3167
Eligard 7.5 mg (Less than 2%) 2724
Eligard 22.5 mg (Less than 2%) 2724
Eligard 30 mg (Less than 2%) 2724
Eligard 45 mg (Less than 2%) 2724
Enjuvia Tablets 1029
Estratest Tablets 3043
Estratest H.S. Tablets 3043
Follistim AQ Cartridge 2844
Imitrex Nasal Spray 1470
Imitrex Tablets (Infrequent) 1474
Indocin Capsules (Less than 1%) 2024
Indocin I.V. (Less than 1%) 2489
Indocin (Less than 1%) 2024
▲ Lupron Depot 3.75 mg (3%) 462
▲ Lupron Depot–3 Month 11.25 mg (3%) 462
Lybrel Tablets 3204
Mircette Tablets 1034
NuvaRing 2897
Ortho-Cyclen Tablets 2449
Ortho Evra Transdermal System 2437
Ortho Micronor Tablets 2446
Ortho Tri-Cyclen Tablets 2449
Ortho Tri-Cyclen Lo Tablets 2458
▲ Plan B Tablets (10.7%) 1044
Premarin Intravenous 3217
Premarin Tablets 3221
Premarin Vaginal Cream 3228
Premphase Tablets 3232
Prempro Tablets 3232
▲ Prometrium Capsules (100 mg, 200 mg) (27%) 3047
Propecia Tablets (0.4% to 0.7%) 2095
Proscar Tablets (0.4% to 0.7%) 2102
Seasonique Tablets 1046
Supprelin LA Implant 1731
Vantas (Less than 2%) 1737
Yaz Tablets 805

Breath sounds, abnormal

▲ Dacogen Injection (10%) 1066
Epivir 1412

Epivir-HBV ... 1417
▲ Trisenox Injection (10%) ... 986
Trizivir Tablets ... 1622

Breathholding
▲ Ultane Liquid for Inhalation (2% to 5%) ... 524

Breathing, difficult
(*see under* Dyspnea)

Breathing, irregular
Imitrex Nasal Spray ... 1470
Lortab 5/500 Tablets ... 3143
Lortab 7.5/500 Tablets ... 3144
Lortab 10/500 Tablets ... 3144
▲ Selzentry Tablets (3.3%) ... 2534
Stalevo Tablets ... 2309
Vicodin Tablets ... 529
Vicodin ES Tablets ... 530
Vicoprofen Tablets ... 533
Zydone Tablets ... 1132

Breathing, labored
(*see under* Dyspnea)

Breathing, shallow
(*see under* Hypopnea)

Breathing, stertorous
Duragesic Transdermal System (Less than 1%) ... 2405

Breathing sound, abnormal
Combivir Tablets ... 1384
Epzicom Tablets ... 1422
Fentora Tablets (Greater than 1%) ... 968

Bromsulphalein retention, increase
(*see under* BSP retention, increase)

Bronchial anastomotic dehiscence
Rapamune ... 3260

Bronchial constriction
Salagen Tablets ... 1082
Vaqta (Less than 1%) ... 2130

Bronchial obstruction
Combigan Ophthalmic Solution ... 553
Cosopt Sterile Ophthalmic Solution ... 1969
▲ Selzentry Tablets (21%) ... 2534
Timoptic Sterile Ophthalmic Solution ... 2121
Timoptic in Ocudose ... 2124
Timoptic-XE Sterile Ophthalmic Gel Forming Solution ... 2125

Bronchial secretions, increase
Mirapex Tablets ... 857
Salagen Tablets ... 1082

Bronchiectasis
Pulmozyme Inhalation Solution ... 1217

Bronchiolitis
Comvax (Two vaccinees) ... 1966
Lyrica Capsules (Rare) ... 2527
Mirapex Tablets ... 857
Pentacel ... 2792
Prevnar ... 3241
RotaTeq (0.6% to 1.4%) ... 2110
Synagis Intramuscular Solution (More than 1%) ... 1948
Vaqta ... 2130

Bronchiolitis, obliterative
Cuprimine Capsules (Rare) ... 1986
PegIntron Powder for Injection (Less than or equal to 1%) ... 2903
Pentasa Capsules (One case) ... 3030
Rituxan I.V. ... 1223
Tarceva Tablets (0.7%) ... 1228

Bronchiolitis obliterans
Limbrel Capsules (1 case) ... 2561
Raptiva for Injection (1 case) ... 1218

Bronchiolitis obliterans organizing pneumonia
Rapamune ... 3260

Bronchitis
Aceon Tablets (2 mg, 4 mg, 8 mg) (0.3% to 1%) ... 3038
Actiq (1% or greater) ... 959
▲ Actonel Tablets (10%) ... 2568
▲ Actonel with Calcium Tablets (2.3% to 4.9%) ... 2574
Advair Diskus 100/50 ... 1276
▲ Advair Diskus 250/50 (Greater than or equal to 3% to 8%) ... 1276
▲ Advair Diskus 500/50 (Greater than or equal to 3%) ... 1276
▲ Aerobid/Aerobid-M (1% to 3%) ... 1153
▲ Agrylin Capsules (1% to less than 5%) ... 3017
▲ Alamast Ophthalmic Solution (Less than 5%) ... 3181
▲ Alphagan P Ophthalmic Solution (1% to 4%) ... 549
Ambien Tablets (Infrequent) ... 2692
Ambien CR Tablets (Infrequent) ... 2696
Amerge Tablets (Infrequent) ... 1301
Aralast (Greater than or equal to 0.2%) ... 726
▲ Aranesp for Injection (5%) ... 564
Aricept Tablets (Frequent) ... 1062
Aricept ODT Tablets (Frequent) ... 1062
▲ Arimidex Tablets (2% to 5%) ... 672
Asacol Delayed-Release Tablets (2% or greater) ... 2579
Atacand Tablets (More than 1%) ... 639
Atacand HCT (0.5% or greater) ... 642
▲ Atrovent HFA Inhalation Aerosol (10% to 23%) ... 839
Axert Tablets (Infrequent) ... 2431
Bexxar ... 1371
▲ Boniva Injection (2.5% to 10%) ... 2614
▲ Boniva Tablets (2.5% to 10%) ... 2618
Brovana Inhalation Solution ... 2990
Campral Tablets (Frequent) ... 1158
Celebrex Capsules (0.1% to 1.9%) ... 2979
Celexa (Infrequent) ... 1160
▲ CellCept Capsules (3% to less than 20%) ... 2622
▲ CellCept Intravenous (3% to less than 20%) ... 2622
▲ CellCept Oral Suspension (3% to less than 20%) ... 2622
▲ CellCept Tablets (3% to less than 20%) ... 2622
Cialis Tablets (0% to 2%) ... 1792
▲ Clarinex Syrup (6.1%) ... 2828
▲ Climara Pro Transdermal System (4.2%) ... 768
Combigan Ophthalmic Solution (0.1% to 0.2%) ... 553
▲ Combivent Inhalation Aerosol (12.3%) ... 845
▲ Copaxone for Injection (9%) ... 3110
▲ Coreg Tablets (5%) ... 1387
▲ Cosopt Sterile Ophthalmic Solution (1% to 5%) ... 1969
▲ Cozaar Tablets (Less than 1% to 10%) ... 1973
▲ Depakote ER Tablets (5%) ... 423
Diovan HCT Tablets (Greater than 0.2%) ... 2216
Doxil Injection (Less than 1%) ... 2378
Duragesic Transdermal System (Greater than or equal to 1%) ... 2405
▲ Elidel Cream 1% (0.4% to 10.7%) ... 2221
Emsam Transdermal System (Frequent) ... 905
Enablex Extended-Release Tablets (Greater than or equal to 1%) ... 2225
Enbrel for Injection ... 569
▲ Enjuvia Tablets (0% to 7%) ... 1029
Epivir-HBV (Among most common) ... 1417
▲ Equetro Extended-Release Capsules (Less than 5%) ... 3174
▲ Evoxac Capsules (4.1%) ... 1013
Exelon Capsules (2% or more) ... 2229
Exelon Oral Solution (2% or more) ... 2229
Exforge Tablets (Greater than or equal to 0.2%) ... 2238
▲ Exjade Tablets (9.1%) ... 2244
▲ Exubera Inhalation Powder (3.2% to 5.4%) ... 2515
▲ Fabrazyme for Intravenous Infusion (8%) ... 1241
▲ Flebogamma 5% (20%) ... 1715
▲ Flebogamma 5% DIF (Greater than 15%) ... 1718
▲ Flonase Nasal Spray (1% to 3%) ... 1431
▲ Flovent Diskus 50 mcg (3%) ... 1435
Flovent HFA (2%) ... 1440
▲ Foradil Aerolizer (4.6%) ... 2849
▲ Fosrenol Chewable Tablets (5%) ... 3027
Gabitril Tablets (Frequent) ... 973
Gengraf Capsules (1%) ... 435
▲ Humira Injection (Less than 5%) ... 442
Imitrex Nasal Spray ... 1470
▲ Intron A for Injection (Less than or equal to 5%) ... 2859
Kaletra (Up to 2%) ... 452
Keppra Oral Solution (1% or more) ... 3131
Keppra Tablets (1% or more) ... 3131
Klonopin (1%) ... 2639
▲ Lamictal (7%) ... 1488
Lescol Capsules (1.8%) ... 2268
Lescol XL Tablets (2.6%) ... 2268
Lexapro Oral Suspension (Frequent) ... 1174
Lexapro Tablets (Frequent) ... 1174
Lipitor Tablets (Greater than or equal to 2%) ... 2501
Lovaza Capsules ... 1520
▲ Lucentis Injection (3% to 10%) ... 1205
Lunesta Tablets (Infrequent) ... 2994
Luvox CR Extended-Release Capsules (Infrequent to 2%) ... 1759
▲ Lyrica Capsules (1% to 3%) ... 2527
Meridia Capsules (Greater than or equal to 1%) ... 475
Miacalcin Nasal Spray (Less than 1%) ... 2274
Micardis Tablets (More than 0.3%) ... 852
Micardis HCT Tablets (Less than 2%) ... 854
Mirapex Tablets ... 857
Namenda (Greater than or equal to 2%) ... 1180
Nasonex Nasal Spray (Greater than or equal to 2%) ... 2883
Neoral Oral Solution (1%) ... 2280
Neoral Soft Gelatin Capsules (1%) ... 2280
▲ Norditropin Cartridges (9%) ... 2354
OptiPranolol Metipranolol Ophthalmic Solution 0.3% (A small number of patients) ... ⊙ 245
Orencia Powder for Intravenous Infusion (0.1% to 0.5%) ... 921
Paxil (Infrequent) ... 1535
Paxil CR Controlled-Release Tablets (Infrequent) ... 1544
Pediarix Vaccine ... 1552
▲ Photofrin for Injection (4%) ... 708
▲ Plavix Tablets (3.7%) ... 926
▲ Plavix Tablets (3.7%) ... 2767
Pletal Tablets (2% or greater) ... 2481
▲ Prandin Tablets (2% to 6%) ... 2971
Prinivil Tablets (0.3% to 1%) ... 2087
Prinzide Tablets (0.3% to 1%) ... 2092
▲ Prograf Capsules and Injection (3% to 17%) ... 622
▲ Prometrium Capsules (100 mg, 200 mg) (Less than 5%) ... 3047
ProQuad ... 2099
Protonix for Delayed-Release Oral Suspension (Greater than or equal to 1%) ... 3254
Protonix Delayed-Release Tablets (Greater than or equal to 1%) ... 3254
Protonix I.V. (Greater than or equal to 1%) ... 3257
▲ Protopic Ointment (2% to 6%) ... 628
Provigil Tablets (At least 1%) ... 977
Pulmozyme Inhalation Solution ... 1217
Raptiva for Injection ... 1218
Relenza Inhalation Powder (2%) ... 1556
Remeron Tablets (Infrequent) ... 2924
RemeronSolTab Tablets (Infrequent) ... 2927
▲ Remicade for IV Injection (10%) ... 950
ReoPro Vials (0.3%) ... 1860
▲ Requip Tablets (Frequent to 3%) ... 1561
Rilutek Tablets (More than 2%) ... 2771
Rituxan I.V. ... 1223
Salagen Tablets (Less than 1%) ... 1082
▲ Selzentry Tablets (5.9%) ... 2534
▲ Serevent Diskus (4% to 7%) ... 1594
▲ Simulect for Injection (3% to 10%) ... 2306
Singulair (Greater than or equal to 2%) ... 2114
Starlix Tablets (2.7%) ... 2314
Symbyax Capsules (Frequent) ... 1871
Synagis Intramuscular Solution (More than 1%) ... 1948
Tamiflu Capsules (1% to 2%) ... 2649
Tamiflu Oral Suspension (1% to 2%) ... 2649
Targretin Capsules ... 1084
Tarka Tablets (1.5%) ... 511
Tasigna Capsules ... 2316
Teveten Tablets (1% or greater) ... 515
Teveten HCT Tablets (Less than 1%) ... 517
▲ Travatan Z Ophthalmic Solution (1% to 5%) ... 547
Tricor Tablets ... 520
▲ Ultram ER Extended-Release Tablets (1% to less than 5%) ... 2428
Uroxatral Tablets (1% to 2%) ... 2786
▲ Vagifem Tablets (3% to 5%) ... 2375
▲ Velcade for Injection (13%) ... 2168
Venlafaxine Hydrochloride Tablets (Frequent) ... 2199
Vicoprofen Tablets (Less than 1%) ... 533
Vivitrol ... 988
Vytorin 10/10 Tablets ... 2149
Vytorin 10/10 Tablets ... 2939
Vytorin 10/20 Tablets ... 2149
Vytorin 10/20 Tablets ... 2939
Vytorin 10/40 Tablets ... 2149
Vytorin 10/40 Tablets ... 2939
Vytorin 10/80 Tablets ... 2149
Vytorin 10/80 Tablets ... 2939
Wellbutrin Tablets (Infrequent) ... 1648
Wellbutrin SR Sustained-Release Tablets (At least 1%) ... 1653
Wellbutrin XL Extended-Release Tablets (At least 1%) ... 1659
▲ Xeloda Tablets (Less than 5%) ... 2662
Xyrem Oral Solution (Frequent) ... 1766
Yaz Tablets (Greater than 1%) ... 805
▲ Ziagen (4%) ... 1673
▲ Zocor Tablets (6.6%) ... 2136
Zomig Tablets (Infrequent) ... 694
Zomig Nasal Spray (Infrequent) ... 689
Zomig-ZMT Tablets (Infrequent) ... 694
Zyban Sustained-Release Tablets (2%) ... 1692
Zyrtec Chewable Tablets (Less than 2%) ... 1920
Zyrtec Syrup (Less than 2%) ... 1920
Zyrtec Tablets (Less than 2%) ... 1920
Zyrtec-D 12 Hour Extended Release Tablets (Less than 2%) ... 1923

Bronchitis, bacterial
Selzentry Tablets ... 2534

Bronchitis, acute
Elidel Cream 1% (0% to 1.5%) ... 2221
Exforge Tablets (Greater than or equal to 0.2%) ... 2238
Requip Tablets (Infrequent) ... 1561
Selzentry Tablets ... 2534

Bronchoconstriction
Intron A for Injection (Rare) ... 2859
Invanz for Injection (Greater than 0.1%) ... 2029
▲ Lexiscan Injection (4% to 12%) ... 614
Zometa for Intravenous Infusion (Rare) ... 2341

Bronchopneumonia
Mirapex Tablets ... 857
Selzentry Tablets ... 2534
▲ Xeloda Tablets (Less than 5%) ... 2662

Bronchopulmonary dysplasia
Busulfex Injection (Rare) ... 2477
Myleran Tablets ... 1530

Bronchospasm
Abelcet Injection (Rare) ... 1134
Accutane Capsules ... 2607
▲ Acetadote Injection (1.23% to 5.85%) ... 1001
Actimmune (Rare) ... 1743
Adenocard IV Injection ... 603
▲ Advair Diskus 100/50 (3%) ... 1276
Advair Diskus 250/50 ... 1276
Advair Diskus 500/50 ... 1276
Advair HFA 45/21 Inhalation Aerosol (Rare) ... 1288
Advair HFA 115/21 Inhalation Aerosol (Rare) ... 1288
Advair HFA 230/21 Inhalation Aerosol (Rare) ... 1288
Aggrenox Capsules (Less than 1%) ... 819
Ambien Tablets (Rare) ... 2692
Ambien CR Tablets (Rare) ... 2696
Anzemet Injection (Rare) ... 2701
Anzemet Tablets (Rare) ... 2704
Atrovent HFA Inhalation Aerosol ... 839
Atrovent Nasal Spray 0.03% ... 834
Atrovent Nasal Spray 0.06% (Rare) ... 836
Attenuvax ... 1951
Axid Capsules ... 1364
Bayer Aspirin ... 750
Beconase AQ Nasal Spray (Rare) ... 1369
Betaseron for SC Injection ... 756
▲ Betimol Ophthalmic Solution (More than 5%) ... 3181
Bexxar ... 1371
Brovana Inhalation Solution ... 2990
Bystolic Tablets ... 1155
Campath Ampules ... 761
Cancidas for Injection ... 1953
Captopril Tablets ... 2182
Celebrex Capsules (0.1% to 1.9%) ... 2979
Celexa (Rare) ... 1160
Cipro I.V. (1% or less) ... 2817
Cipro (Less than 1%) ... 2810
Cipro XR Tablets ... 2823
Clinoril Tablets (Less than 1 in 100) ... 1962
Combigan Ophthalmic Solution ... 553
Combivent Inhalation Aerosol (0.3%) ... 845
Coreg Tablets (Less than or equal to 0.1%) ... 1387
Coreg CR Extended-Release Capsules (Less than or equal to 0.1%) ... 1393

Cosopt Sterile Ophthalmic Solution ... 1969
Diovan HCT Tablets (Less frequent) ... 2216
Elitek ... 2729
Eloxatin for Injection ... 2731
Engerix-B Vaccine ... 1409
Erbitux ... 912
Evoxac Capsules (Less than 1%) ... 1013
Exelon Capsules (Infrequent) ... 2229
Exelon Oral Solution (Infrequent) ... 2229
Exelon Patch (Infrequent) ... 2233
Flebogamma 5% ... 1715
Flebogamma 5% DIF ... 1718
Flonase Nasal Spray ... 1431
Flovent HFA ... 1440
Fluarix Vaccine ... 1446
Flulaval Injection Vaccine ... 1448
Flumadine (Less than 0.3%) ... 1167
Fluorescite Injection ... ⊙203
Fortaz (Very rare) ... 1450
Gammagard Liquid ... 730
Gammagard S/D ... 734
Gamunex ... 3094
Gardasil Injection (1 case) ... 2019
Gemzar for Injection (Less than 2%) ... 1820
▲ Gengraf Capsules (1% to 5%) ... 435
Herceptin I.V. ... 1199
▲ Humira Injection (Less than 5%) ... 442
Imitrex Injection ... 1465
Imitrex Nasal Spray ... 1470
InnoPran XL Extended Release Capsules ... 1484
Intelence Tablets (Less than 2%) ... 3119
▲ Intron A for Injection (Less than or equal to 5%) ... 2859
Lamictal (2%) ... 1488
Levaquin ... 2416
Levaquin in 5% Dextrose Injection ... 2416
Mepron Suspension ... 1526
Meruvax II ... 2061
Miacalcin Injection (A few cases) ... 2273
▲ Miacalcin Nasal Spray (1% to 3%) ... 2274
M-M-R II ... 2054
Mobic Oral Suspension (Less than 2%) ... 863
Mobic Tablets (Less than 2%) ... 863
Mumpsvax ... 2068
Nadolol Tablets (1 of 1000 patients) ... 2191
▲ Neoral Oral Solution (1% to 5%) ... 2280
▲ Neoral Soft Gelatin Capsules (1% to 5%) ... 2280
Nexium Delayed-Release Capsules ... 645
Nexium I.V. ... 652
Nexium Delayed-Release Oral Suspension ... 645
Nimbex Injection (0.2%) ... 484
Norvir ... 489
▲ Oncaspar Injection (Less than 1% to greater than 5%) ... 1138
Orthoclone OKT3 Sterile Solution (Less than 1%) ... 2387
OsmoPrep Tablets ... 2680
Pepcid Tablets (Infrequent) ... 2075
Percocet Tablets ... 1127
Percodan Tablets ... 1130
Persantine Tablets (Rare) ... 869
Photofrin for Injection ... 708
Plavix Tablets (Very rare) ... 926
Plavix Tablets (Very rare) ... 2767
Prevnar ... 3241
Prinivil Tablets (0.3% to 1.0%) ... 2087
Prinzide Tablets ... 2092
ProQuad ... 2099
Proventil HFA Inhalation Aerosol (Rare) ... 2914
Provigil Tablets ... 977
Prozac Weekly Capsules ... 1852
Pulmicort Flexhaler ... 654
Qvar Inhalation Aerosol (Rare) ... 3116
Recombivax HB (Less than 1%) ... 2107
Refludan for Injection (Common) ... 795
Relenza Inhalation Powder ... 1556
Remicade for IV Injection ... 950
ReoPro Vials (0.3%) ... 1860
▲ Rituxan I.V. (1% to 8%) ... 1223
Rocephin Injectable Vials, ADD-Vantage, Galaxy, Bulk (Less than 0.1%) ... 2642
RotaTeq (1.1%) ... 2110
St. Joseph 81 mg Aspirin Chewable and Enteric Coated Tablets ... 1903
▲ Selzentry Tablets (21%) ... 2534
▲ Simulect for Injection (3% to 10%) ... 2306
Taxotere Injection Concentrate ... 2773
Tessalon Capsules ... 1183
Tessalon Perles ... 1183
Timoptic Sterile Ophthalmic Solution (Less frequent) ... 2121
Timoptic in Ocudose (Less frequent) ... 2124
Timoptic-XE Sterile Ophthalmic Gel Forming Solution ... 2125
Toprol-XL Tablets (About 1 of 100 patients) ... 666
Trusopt Sterile Ophthalmic Solution ... 2128
Twinrix Vaccine ... 1628
Ultane Liquid for Inhalation (Less than 1%) ... 524
Vectibix ... 597
Ventolin HFA Inhalation Aerosol ... 1638
Wellbutrin SR Sustained-Release Tablets (Rare) ... 1653
Wellbutrin XL Extended-Release Tablets (Rare) ... 1659
Xolair ... 1235
Xolair ... 2339
Zantac 25 EFFERdose Tablets (Rare) ... 1670
Zantac Injection ... 1666
Zantac Injection Pharmacy Bulk Package (Rare) ... 1668
Zantac Injection Premixed ... 1666
Zantac (Rare) ... 1670
Zemuron Injection (Less than 1%) ... 2947
Zofran Injection (Rare to less than 1%) ... 1682
Zofran (Rare) ... 1687
Zofran ODT Orally Disintegrating Tablets (Rare) ... 1687
Zomig Tablets (Infrequent) ... 694
Zomig-ZMT Tablets (Infrequent) ... 694
Zosyn for Injection (1% or less) ... 3284
Zyban Sustained-Release Tablets (Rare) ... 1692
▲ Zyrtec Chewable Tablets (1.9% to 3.1%) ... 1920
▲ Zyrtec Syrup (1.9% to 3.1%) ... 1920
▲ Zyrtec Tablets (1.9% to 3.1%) ... 1920

Bronchospasm, exacerbation of

Celebrex Capsules (0.1% to 1.9%) ... 2979
Didronel Tablets (Rare) ... 2583
Serevent Diskus ... 1594

Bronchospasm, paradoxical

▲ Advair Diskus 100/50 (Greater than or equal to 3%) ... 1276
Advair Diskus 250/50 ... 1276
Advair Diskus 500/50 ... 1276
Advair HFA 45/21 Inhalation Aerosol ... 1288
Advair HFA 115/21 Inhalation Aerosol ... 1288
Advair HFA 230/21 Inhalation Aerosol ... 1288
Brovana Inhalation Solution ... 2990
Combivent Inhalation Aerosol ... 845
Flovent Diskus 50 mcg ... 1435
Flovent HFA ... 1440
Proventil HFA Inhalation Aerosol ... 2914
Serevent Diskus ... 1594
Ventolin HFA Inhalation Aerosol ... 1638
Xopenex Inhalation Solution ... 3001
Xopenex Inhalation Solution Concentrate ... 3005
Xopenex HFA Inhalation Aerosol ... 3009

Browache

OptiPranolol Metipranolol Ophthalmic Solution 0.3% (A small number of patients) ... ⊙245

Bruise, tendency to

Cymbalta Delayed-Release Capsules (Infrequent) ... 1801

Bruising

Accolate Tablets ... 669
Accutane Capsules ... 2607
Arixtra Injection (1%) ... 1313
Azmacort Inhalation Aerosol ... 407
Carbatrol Capsules ... 3019
Depakote ER Tablets ... 423
Eligard 7.5 mg (2.5%) ... 2724
Eligard 22.5 mg (1.7%) ... 2724
Eligard 30 mg ... 2724
Eligard 45 mg (Less than 1% to 2.3%) ... 2724
Elocon Cream 0.1% (1 in 97 patients) ... 2840
Enbrel for Injection ... 569
▲ Gleevec Tablets (0% to 27%) ... 2255
Hycamtin for Injection ... 1459
Imitrex Injection ... 1465
▲ Increlex Injection (Greater than or equal to 5%) ... 3100
Lexapro Oral Suspension (Infrequent) ... 1174
Lexapro Tablets (Infrequent) ... 1174
Maxair Autohaler (0.6%) ... 1705
Nalfon Capsules (Less than 1%) ... 2508
▲ Novantrone for Injection Concentrate (6%) ... 1100
Raptiva for Injection ... 1218
ReFacto Vials ... 3269
Rythmol Tablets (Less than 1%) ... 1586
▲ Sandostatin Injection (1% to 4%) ... 2300
Singulair ... 2114
Tarka Tablets ... 511

Bruising at application site

Daytrana Transdermal Patch ... 3022
Lidoderm Patch ... 1114

Bruising at injection site

Flulaval Injection Vaccine ... 1448
Forteo for Injection (Less than 1/30 patients) ... 1816
PegIntron Powder for Injection ... 2903
▲ Vantas (7.2%) ... 1737
Xolair ... 1235
Xolair ... 2339

Bruising at insertion site

▲ Supprelin LA Implant (51.1%) ... 1731
▲ Vantas (7.2%) ... 1737

Bruxism

Concerta Extended-Release Tablets (1.7%) ... 1925
Cymbalta Delayed-Release Capsules (Infrequent) ... 1801
Effexor XR Extended-Release Capsules (Infrequent) ... 3195
Eldepryl Capsules ... 3052
Lexapro Oral Suspension (Infrequent) ... 1174
Lexapro Tablets (Infrequent) ... 1174
Mirapex Tablets ... 857
Paxil (Infrequent) ... 1535
Paxil CR Controlled-Release Tablets (Infrequent) ... 1544
Requip Tablets (Infrequent) ... 1561
Stalevo Tablets ... 2309
Venlafaxine Hydrochloride Tablets (Infrequent) ... 2199
Wellbutrin Tablets (Infrequent) ... 1648
Wellbutrin SR Sustained-Release Tablets (Infrequent) ... 1653
Wellbutrin XL Extended-Release Tablets (Infrequent) ... 1659
Zyban Sustained-Release Tablets (Infrequent) ... 1692

BSP retention

Capastat Sulfate for Injection ... 1791

BSP retention, increase

Estratest Tablets ... 3043
Estratest H.S. Tablets ... 3043

Buccal-lingual-masticatory syndrome

Prozac Weekly Capsules ... 1852

Buccoglossal syndrome

Effexor XR Extended-Release Capsules (Rare) ... 3195
Geodon Capsules (Frequent) ... 2520
Prozac Weekly Capsules (Infrequent) ... 1852
Prozac Pulvules and Liquid (Infrequent) ... 1852
Symbyax Capsules (Infrequent) ... 1871
Venlafaxine Hydrochloride Tablets (Rare) ... 2199
Zyprexa Tablets (1% to 2%) ... 1883
Zyprexa ZYDIS Orally Disintegrating Tablets (1% to 2%) ... 1883

Budd-Chiari syndrome

Lybrel Tablets ... 3204
Mircette Tablets ... 1034
Mylotarg for Injection ... 3212
NuvaRing ... 2897
Ortho-Cyclen Tablets ... 2449
Ortho Evra Transdermal System ... 2437
Ortho Tri-Cyclen Tablets ... 2449
Ortho Tri-Cyclen Lo Tablets ... 2458
Seasonique Tablets ... 1046
Yaz Tablets ... 805

Buffalo hump

(*see under* Dorsocervical fat enlargement)

Bulbus oculi, perforation

Alrex Ophthalmic Suspension 0.2% ... ⊙236
FML Ophthalmic Ointment ... ⊙223
FML Ophthalmic Suspension ... ⊙224
FML Forte Ophthalmic Suspension ... ⊙222
Lotemax Ophthalmic Suspension 0.5% ... ⊙241
Pred Forte Ophthalmic Suspension ... ⊙227
Pred Mild Ophthalmic Suspension ... ⊙230

Bulimia

Paxil (Rare) ... 1535
Paxil CR Controlled-Release Tablets (Rare) ... 1544

BUN, increased

Ambien Tablets (Rare) ... 2692
Ambien CR Tablets (Rare) ... 2696
Aricept Tablets (Infrequent) ... 1062
Aricept ODT Tablets (Infrequent) ... 1062
Avalide Tablets (2.3%) ... 2713
Bystolic Tablets (Greater than or equal to 1%) ... 1155
▲ CellCept Capsules (34.6%) ... 2622
▲ CellCept Intravenous (34.6%) ... 2622
▲ CellCept Oral Suspension (34.6%) ... 2622
▲ CellCept Tablets (34.6%) ... 2622
Cipro (0.9%) ... 2810
Cipro XR Tablets ... 2823
▲ Coreg CR Extended-Release Capsules (Less than or equal to 0.1% to 6%) ... 1393
Demadex Injection ... 2630
Demadex Tablets ... 2630
Mycamine for Injection ... 616
Neupro Transdermal System ... 3149
OsmoPrep Tablets ... 2680
Proleukin for Injection (Less than 1%) ... 2287
Prozac Weekly Capsules (Rare) ... 1852
Pylera Capsules ... 714
▲ Tekturna HCT Tablets (11.8%) ... 2324
Venlafaxine Hydrochloride Tablets (Rare) ... 2199

BUN levels, abnormal

▲ Hexalen Capsules (9%) ... 1078
▲ Novantrone for Injection Concentrate (22%) ... 1100
Zyvox (0.2% to 2.1%) ... 2552

BUN levels, changes

▲ Intron A for Injection (Up to 12%) ... 2859
Moban Tablets ... 1116

BUN levels, decrease

Cipro I.V. (Infrequent) ... 2817
Cipro XR Tablets ... 2823

BUN levels, elevation

Aceon Tablets (2 mg, 4 mg, 8 mg) ... 3038
Aggrenox Capsules ... 819
▲ AmBisome for Injection (21%) ... 606
Asacol Delayed-Release Tablets ... 2579
Atacand Tablets (Infrequent) ... 639
Atacand HCT (0.5% or greater) ... 642
Avalide Tablets ... 892
Avapro Tablets (Less than 0.7%) ... 897
Avapro Tablets (Less than 0.7%) ... 2718
Bayer Aspirin ... 750
Benicar HCT Tablets (1.3%) ... 1010
▲ Biaxin/Biaxin XL (4%) ... 411
Bicillin C-R Injectable Suspension ... 1775
Bicillin L-A Injection ... 1777
▲ Busulfex Injection (2% to 3%) ... 2477
Calcijex Injection ... 419
▲ Capastat Sulfate for Injection (36%) ... 1791
Captopril Tablets ... 2182
Carbatrol Capsules ... 3019
Ceftin ... 1380
Celebrex Capsules (0.1% to 1.9%) ... 2979
Cipro I.V. ... 2817
▲ Coreg Tablets (Less than or equal to 1% to 6%) ... 1387
Cozaar Tablets (Less than 0.1%) ... 1973
▲ Diovan Tablets (16.6%) ... 2212
▲ Diovan HCT Tablets (15%) ... 2216
Doxil Injection (Less than 1%) ... 2378
Dyazide Capsules ... 1405
Dyrenium Capsules (Rare) ... 3189
Effexor XR Extended-Release Capsules (Rare) ... 3195
▲ Emend Capsules (4.4% to 4.7%) ... 1992
▲ Emend for Injection (4.4% to 4.7%) ... 1999
Equetro Extended-Release Capsules ... 3174
Evoxac Capsules (Less than 1%) ... 1013
Fansidar Tablets ... 2636
Flebogamma 5% ... 1715
Flebogamma 5% DIF ... 1718
Fortaz (Occasional) ... 1450
Gammagard S/D ... 734
Gantrisin Pediatric Suspension ... 2638
▲ Gemzar for Injection (8% to 16%) ... 1820

Gengraf Capsules (1% to less than 3%) 435
Geodon Capsules (Rare) 2520
▲ Indapamide Tablets (Less than 5%) 2188
Indocin Capsules (Less than 1%) 2024
▲ Indocin I.V. (41% of infants) 2489
Indocin (Less than 1%) 2024
▲ Intron A for Injection (Less than 5%) 2859
Invanz for Injection (0.1% to 1%) 2029
▲ Leukine (23%) 774
▲ Lupron Depot 7.5 mg (Greater than or equal to 5%) 469
▲ Mavik Tablets (0.6% to 9%) 472
Mepron Suspension (1%) 1526
Merrem I.V. (Greater than 0.2%) 684
Micardis HCT Tablets 854
Mobic Oral Suspension (Less than 2%) 863
Mobic Tablets (Less than 2%) 863
▲ NeoProfen Injection (1% to 7%) 2496
Neoral Oral Solution (1% to less than 3%) 2280
Neoral Soft Gelatin Capsules (1% to less than 3%) 2280
Noroxin Tablets (Less frequent) 2069
Omnicef Capsules (0.3%) 497
Omnicef for Oral Suspension (0.2%) 497
Paxil (Rare) 1535
Paxil CR Controlled-Release Tablets (Rare) 1544
Pletal Tablets 2481
Primaxin I.M. 2080
Primaxin I.V. 2083
▲ Prinivil Tablets (2% to 11.6%) 2087
Prinzide Tablets 2092
▲ Prograf Capsules and Injection (3% to 15%) 622
Prozac Pulvules and Liquid (Rare) 1852
Requip Tablets (Frequent) 1561
Rocaltrol Capsules 1150
Rocaltrol Oral Solution 1150
Rocephin Injectable Vials, ADD-Vantage, Galaxy, Bulk (1.2%) 2642
St. Joseph 81 mg Aspirin Chewable and Enteric Coated Tablets 1903
Sandimmune 2296
Sular Extended Release Tablets (Less than or equal to 1%) 2975
Suprax for Oral Suspension (Less than 2%) 1891
Suprax Tablets (Less than 2%) 1891
▲ Tekturna Tablets (Less than 7%) 2321
Teveten Tablets (0.6%) 515
Teveten HCT Tablets (1.3%) 517
Timentin ADD-Vantage 1606
Timentin Injection Galaxy Container 1609
Timentin IV Infusion 1603
Timentin Pharmacy Bulk Package 1613
Tricor Tablets 520
Tygacil for Injection (2.1%) 3276
Ultane Liquid for Inhalation (Less than 1%) 524
Zinacef for Injection 1678
Zinacef Injection 1678
Zonegran Capsules 1089
Zosyn for Injection 3284
Zovirax 1690

Bundle branch block
Abilify Injection (Greater than or equal to 1 in 1000 patients and less than 1 in 100 patients) 2466
Abilify Oral Solution (Greater than or equal to 1 in 1000 patients and less than 1 in 100 patients) 2466
Abilify Discmelt Orally Disintegrating Tablets (Greater than or equal to 1 in 1000 patients and less than 1 in 100 patients) 2466
Abilify Tablets (Greater than or equal to 1 in 1000 patients and less than 1 in 100 patients) 2466
Anzemet Injection 2701
Anzemet Tablets 2704
Azilect Tablets (Frequent) 3106
Cardizem LA Extended Release Tablets (Less than 2%) 421
Celexa (Rare) 1160
Coreg Tablets (Less than or equal to 0.1%) 1387
Coreg CR Extended-Release Capsules (Less than or equal to 0.1%) 1393
Doxil Injection (Less than 1%) 2378
Effexor XR Extended-Release Capsules (Infrequent) 3195
Evoxac Capsules 1013
Exelon Capsules (Infrequent) 2229
Exelon Oral Solution (Infrequent) 2229
Geodon Capsules (Rare) 2520
▲ Invega Extended-Release Tablets (Less than 1% to 3%) 1748
Lexapro Oral Suspension 1174
Lexapro Tablets 1174
Miacalcin Nasal Spray (Less than 1%) 2274
Mirapex Tablets 857
Neupro Transdermal System 3149
Paxil (Rare) 1535
Paxil CR Controlled-Release Tablets (Rare) 1544
Rilutek Tablets (Infrequent) 2771
Risperdal Consta Long-Acting Injection (Infrequent) 1753
Rythmol Tablets (1% to 2%) 1586
Rythmol SR Capsules (Greater than or equal to 2%) 1590
Symbyax Capsules (Rare) 1871
Tarka Tablets (Less frequent) 511
Trasylol Injection (1% to 2%) 799
Venlafaxine Hydrochloride Tablets (Rare) 2199

Bundle branch block, left
Anzemet Tablets 2704
Reyataz Capsules 3299

Bundle branch block, right
Anzemet Tablets 2704

Burn wound infection
Amevive 611

Burning
Analpram-HC 1140
Bactroban Nasal (2%) 1367
Bactroban Ointment (1.5%) 1368
Catapres-TTS (3 of 101 patients) 842
Elocon Cream 0.1% (1.6%) 2840
Elocon Lotion 0.1% (4 in 209 patients) 2841
▲ Elocon Ointment 0.1% (4.8%) 2842
Evoxac Capsules (Less than 1%) 1013
▲ Finacea Gel (4% to 16%) 1742
Fleet Bisacodyl Laxatives 1143
▲ Naftin Gel (5%) 2164
Noroxin Tablets 2069
Olux Foam (Less than 2%) 3061
Panafil Ointment (Occasional) 1723
Panafil SE Spray Emulsion 1724
▲ Panretin Gel 0.1% (0% to 34%) 1081
Pramosone 1141
Pred-G Ophthalmic Suspension ⊙ 228
Vanos Cream 1941
Zantac Injection 1666
Zantac Injection Pharmacy Bulk Package (Frequent) 1668
Zantac Injection Premixed 1666
▲ Zovirax Ointment (28.3%) 819

Burning, local
▲ Aldara Cream, 5% (6%) 1699
▲ Alphagan P Ophthalmic Solution (Approximately 5% to 9%) 549
▲ Bactroban Cream (Less than 1% to 3.6%) 1366
Diprolene Lotion 0.05% 2838
Mentax Cream (Approximately 1%) 2190
Mumpsvax 2068
▲ Naftin Cream (6%) 2164
Sulfamylon for 5% Topical Solution 2194
▲ Valstar Sterile Solution for Intravesical Instillation (5%) 1735

Burning at application site
Aczone Gel 5% (1%) 3296
▲ Aldara Cream, 5% (6% to 26%) 1699
Daytrana Transdermal Patch 3022
▲ Elidel Cream 1% (1.5% to 26%) 2221
▲ Evoclin Foam, 1% (6%) 3056
Flector Patch (Less than 1%) 561
Ionsys Transdermal System (.1% to less than 1%) 2410
Lidoderm Patch 1114
Premarin Vaginal Cream 3228
▲ Vanos Cream (1.8% to 6.6%) 1941
▲ Verdeso Foam (3%) 3069
▲ Ziana Gel (2% to 4%) 1942

Burning at injection site
Aloxi Injection (Very rare) 1059
Anzemet Injection 2701
Attenuvax 1951
Cerezyme for Injection (Less than 1%) 1238
Cipro I.V. (1% or less) 2817
▲ Eligard 7.5 mg (34.6%) 2724
▲ Eligard 22.5 mg (21.7%) 2724
▲ Eligard 30 mg (20%) 2724
▲ Eligard 45 mg (16%) 2724
▲ Extina Foam, 2% (10%) 3057
Genotropin Lyophilized Powder (Infrequent) 2547
▲ Intron A for Injection (Less than 5%) 2859
Invanz for Injection (1.3%) 2029
Meruvax II 2061
M-M-R II 2054
Mumpsvax 2068
Novantrone for Injection Concentrate 1100
ProQuad 2099
Timentin ADD-Vantage 1606
Timentin Injection Galaxy Container 1609
Timentin IV Infusion 1603
Timentin Pharmacy Bulk Package 1613
Xolair 1235
Xolair 2339
▲ Zofran Injection (4%) 1682

Burning sensation
Accuzyme Debriding Ointment (A small percentage) 1723
Accuzyme SE Spray Emulsion (Small Percentage) 1723
Adenocard IV Injection (Less than 1%) 603
Amerge Tablets (Infrequent) 1301
Arranon Injection (1%) 1319
BeneFIX Vials (1.5%) 3191
Copaxone for Injection (Infrequent) 3110
Doxil Injection 2378
▲ Fabrazyme for Intravenous Infusion (6%) 1241
Fleet Babylax Suppositories 1142
Fleet Glycerin Laxatives 1142
Fleet Glycerin Suppositories 1142
Fleet Pedia-Lax Suppositories 1142
▲ Imitrex Injection (7%) 1465
Imitrex Nasal Spray (0.4% to 1.4%) 1470
Imitrex Tablets (Frequent) 1474
▲ Ixempra Kit for Injection (62%) 915
Levaquin 2416
Levaquin in 5% Dextrose Injection 2416
▲ Olux Foam (10%) 3061
Requip Tablets (Infrequent) 1561
Reyataz Capsules 3299
▲ Sulfamylon Cream (One of two most frequent) 2194
Treximet Tablets (Infrequent) 1616

Bursitis
▲ Actonel with Calcium Tablets (1.3% to 3%) 2574
Avalide Tablets 892
Avalide Tablets 2713
Avapro Tablets (Less than 1%) 897
Avapro Tablets (Less than 1%) 2718
▲ Azmacort Inhalation Aerosol (1% to 3%) 407
Celexa (Rare) 1160
Copaxone for Injection (Infrequent) 3110
Effexor XR Extended-Release Capsules (Infrequent) 3195
Enbrel for Injection (Infrequent) 569
Evoxac Capsules (Less than 1%) 1013
Gabitril Tablets (Infrequent) 973
Gengraf Capsules (1% to less than 3%) 435
Lamictal (Rare) 1488
Lipitor Tablets (Less than 2%) 2501
Lunesta Tablets (Infrequent) 2994
Luvox CR Extended-Release Capsules (Infrequent) 1759
Meridia Capsules 475
Mirapex Tablets (2%) 857
Neoral Oral Solution (1% to less than 3%) 2280
Neoral Soft Gelatin Capsules (1% to less than 3%) 2280
Noroxin Tablets (Less frequent) 2069
Paxil (Rare) 1535
Paxil CR Controlled-Release Tablets (Rare) 1544
Pletal Tablets (Less than 2%) 2481
Protonix for Delayed-Release Oral Suspension (Less than 1%) 3254
Protonix Delayed-Release Tablets (Less than 1%) 3254
Protonix I.V. (Less than 1%) 3257
Protopic Ointment (0.2% to less than 1%) 628
Prozac Weekly Capsules (Infrequent) 1852
Prozac Pulvules and Liquid (Infrequent) 1852
Requip Tablets (Infrequent) 1561
Rythmol SR Capsules 1590
Symbyax Capsules (Rare) 1871
Tricor Tablets 520
Venlafaxine Hydrochloride Tablets (Infrequent) 2199
Zyprexa Tablets (Rare) 1883
Zyprexa ZYDIS Orally Disintegrating Tablets (Rare) 1883

C

Cachexia
Actiq (1% or greater) 959
Aricept Tablets (Infrequent) 1062
Aricept ODT Tablets (Infrequent) 1062
▲ Doxil Injection (1% to 10%) 2378
Exelon Capsules (Infrequent) 2229
Exelon Oral Solution (Infrequent) 2229
▲ Intron A for Injection (Less than or equal to 5%) 2859
Mirapex Tablets 857
Norvir (Less than 2%) 489
▲ Xeloda Tablets (Less than 5%) 2662

Calcification, ectopic
Calcijex Injection 419
Rocaltrol Capsules 1150
Rocaltrol Oral Solution 1150

Calcification, soft tissue
Rocaltrol Capsules 1150
Rocaltrol Oral Solution 1150

Calcium crystalluria
Brovana Inhalation Solution (Less than 2%) 2990
Venlafaxine Hydrochloride Tablets (Rare) 2199

Calcium retention
Delatestryl Injection 1730
Estratest Tablets 3043
Estratest H.S. Tablets 3043

Calf muscles, need to flex
Imitrex Injection (Rare) 1465

Cancer, anal
Selzentry Tablets 2534

Cancer, breast
Climara Pro Transdermal System 768
Mirapex Tablets 857
Premarin Tablets 3221
Premarin Vaginal Cream 3228
Propecia Tablets (Four cases) 2095
Proscar Tablets (Four cases) 2102

Cancer, cervical
Estratest Tablets 3043
Estratest H.S. Tablets 3043
Ortho-Cyclen/Ortho Tri-Cyclen 2449
Ortho Tri-Cyclen Lo Tablets 2458
Premarin Intravenous 3217
Premarin Vaginal Cream 3228

Cancer, lip
Mirapex Tablets 857

Cancer, oral cavity
Mirapex Tablets 857

Cancer, progression of
▲ Zometa for Intravenous Infusion (16%) 2341

Cancer, skin, non-melanoma
▲ CellCept Capsules (1.6% to 4.2%) 2622
▲ CellCept Intravenous (1.6% to 4.2%) 2622
▲ CellCept Oral Suspension (1.6% to 4.2%) 2622
▲ CellCept Tablets (1.6% to 4.2%) 2622
Myfortic Tablets (0.9% to 1.8%) 2276
Raptiva for Injection 1218
Remicade for IV Injection 950
Xolair 1235
Xolair 2339

Cancer, vaginal
Estratest Tablets 3043
Estratest H.S. Tablets 3043
Premarin Intravenous 3217
Premarin Vaginal Cream 3228

Candidiasis
▲ Advair Diskus 250/50 (Greater than 5%) 1276
▲ Advair HFA 45/21 Inhalation Aerosol (1% to 3%) 1288
▲ Advair HFA 115/21 Inhalation Aerosol (1% to 3%) 1288
▲ Advair HFA 230/21 Inhalation Aerosol (1% to 3%) 1288
▲ Aerobid/Aerobid-M (3% to 9%) 1153
Augmentin 1323
Augmentin Tablets 1327
Augmentin XR Extended Release Tablets 1333
Augmentin ES-600 Powder for Oral Suspension (1.4%) 1329

Avelox (Greater than or equal to 0.1% to less than 2%) 2803
Biaxin/Biaxin XL 411
Ceftin for Oral Suspension (0.1% to 1%) 1380
Celebrex Capsules (0.1% to 1.9%) 2979
▲ Chemet Capsules (5.2% to 15.7%) 2484
Cipro I.V. (1% or less) 2817
▲ Doxil Injection (23.5%) 2378
Elocon Cream 0.1% (1 in 182 patients) 2840
Emend Capsules (Greater than 0.5%) 1992
Emend for Injection (Greater than 0.5%) 1999
Emsam Transdermal System (Rare) 905
▲ Evoxac Capsules (1% to 3%) 1013
Fortaz (Less than 1%) 1450
▲ Intron A for Injection (Up to 17%) 2859
Invanz for Injection (Greater than 0.1%) 2029
Klonopin (Infrequent) 2639
Levaquin (0.1% to 1%) 2416
Levaquin in 5% Dextrose Injection (0.1% to 1%) 2416
Lybrel Tablets 3204
▲ Megace ES Oral Suspension (1% to 3%) 2499
▲ Myfortic Tablets (Less than or equal to 5.6%) 2276
Norvir (Less than 2%) 489
Omnicef Capsules (0.2%) 497
Omnicef for Oral Suspension (1%) 497
Paxil (Infrequent) 1535
Paxil CR Controlled-Release Tablets (Infrequent) 1544
Pentasa Capsules (Less than 1%) 3030
▲ Photofrin for Injection (9%) 708
Primaxin I.M. 2080
Primaxin I.V. (Less than 0.2%) 2083
ProQuad 2099
Protonix for Delayed-Release Oral Suspension (Less than 1%) 3254
Protonix Delayed-Release Tablets (Less than 1%) 3254
Protonix I.V. (Less than 1%) 3257
Protopic Ointment (0.2% to less than 1%) 628
RemeronSolTab Tablets (Rare) 2927
▲ Remicade for IV Injection (5%) 950
Requip Tablets (Infrequent) 1561
Rilutek Tablets (0.4% to 1.2%) 2771
Salagen Tablets (Less than 1%) 1082
Seasonique Tablets 1046
▲ Simulect for Injection (3% to 10%) 2306
Soriatane Capsules (Less than 1%) 3062
Spiriva HandiHaler 870
Suprax for Oral Suspension (Less than 2%) 1891
Suprax Tablets (Less than 2%) 1891
Symbyax Capsules (Infrequent) 1871
Targretin Capsules 1084
Tasigna Capsules 2316
Venlafaxine Hydrochloride Tablets (Infrequent) 2199
▲ Xeloda Tablets (Less than 5%) 2662
Yaz Tablets (Greater than 1%) 805
▲ Zometa for Intravenous Infusion (12%) 2341
Zosyn for Injection (1.6%) 3284
Zyprexa Tablets (Infrequent) 1883
Zyprexa ZYDIS Orally Disintegrating Tablets (Infrequent) 1883

Candidiasis, cutaneous
Cipro (Less than 1%) 2810
Cipro XR Tablets 2823
Omnicef for Oral Suspension (0.9%) 497
Protopic Ointment (0.2% to less than 1%) 628

Candidiasis, esophageal
Selzentry Tablets 2534

Candidiasis, gastrointestinal
Nexium Delayed-Release Capsules 645
Nexium I.V. 652
Nexium Delayed-Release Oral Suspension 645
Protonix for Delayed-Release Oral Suspension (Less than 1%) 3254
Protonix Delayed-Release Tablets (Less than 1%) 3254
Protonix I.V. (Less than 1%) 3257

Candidiasis, genital
(*see also under* Vaginal candidiasis)
▲ Azmacort Inhalation Aerosol (1% to 3%) 407
Celebrex Capsules (0.1% to 1.9%) 2979
▲ Crinone 8% Gel (5%) 992
Effexor XR Extended-Release Capsules 3195
Evoxac Capsules (Less than 1%) 1013
Lamictal (Infrequent) 1488
Levaquin (0.1% to 1%) 2416
Levaquin in 5% Dextrose Injection (0.1% to 1%) 2416
Nexium Delayed-Release Capsules (Less than 1%) 645
Nexium I.V. (Less than 1%) 652
Nexium Delayed-Release Oral Suspension (Less than 1%) 645
Paxil (Rare) 1535
Paxil CR Controlled-Release Tablets (Rare) 1544
Requip Tablets (Infrequent) 1561
Rilutek Tablets (Rare) 2771
Rocephin Injectable Vials, ADD-Vantage, Galaxy, Bulk (Less than 1%) 2642
▲ Vagifem Tablets (5%) 2375

Candidiasis, mouth
(*see under* Candidiasis, oral)

Candidiasis, mucocutaneous
Amoxil Capsules 1305
Amoxil Chewable Tablets 1305
Amoxil Pediatric Drops for Oral Suspension 1305
Amoxil Powder for Oral Suspension 1305
Amoxil Tablets 1305
▲ CellCept Capsules (15.3% to 18.4%) 2622
▲ CellCept Intravenous (15.3% to 18.4%) 2622
▲ CellCept Oral Suspension (15.3% to 18.4%) 2622
▲ CellCept Tablets (15.3% to 18.4%) 2622
Moxatag Tablets 2165

Candidiasis, nasal
Nasonex Nasal Spray (Rare) 2883

Candidiasis, oral
Actiq (Less than 1%) 959
▲ Advair Diskus 100/50 (4%) 1276
▲ Advair Diskus 250/50 (3% to 10%) 1276
▲ Advair Diskus 500/50 (Greater than or equal to 3%) 1276
▲ Advair HFA 45/21 Inhalation Aerosol (1% to 3%) 1288
▲ Advair HFA 115/21 Inhalation Aerosol (1% to 3%) 1288
▲ Advair HFA 230/21 Inhalation Aerosol (1% to 3%) 1288
▲ Alvesco Inhalation Aerosol (Less than 1% to greater than or equal to 3%) 2985
▲ Asmanex Twisthaler (4% to 22%) 2797
Augmentin ES-600 Powder for Oral Suspension 1329
Azmacort Inhalation Aerosol (A few cases) 407
Brovana Inhalation Solution 2990
Cipro I.V. (1% or less) 2817
Cipro (Less than 1%) 2810
Cipro XR Tablets 2823
▲ Clolar for Intravenous Infusion (13%) 1239
Comvax (0.2% to 0.8%) 1966
Copaxone for Injection (Frequent) 3110
Cubicin for Injection (Less than 1%) 995
▲ Dacogen Injection (6%) 1066
Doribax Injection (1%) 2400
▲ Doxil Injection (1% to 10%) 2378
Effexor XR Extended-Release Capsules (Infrequent) 3195
Fentora Tablets (Greater than 1%) 968
▲ Flovent Diskus 50 mcg (9% to 31%) 1435
▲ Flovent HFA (4%) 1440
Fortaz (Less than 1%) 1450
Gris-PEG Tablets (Occasional) 2507
Invanz for Injection (0.1% to 1%) 2029
Ketek Tablets (Greater than or equal to 0.2% to less than 2%) 2744
▲ Megace ES Oral Suspension (1% to 3%) 2499
▲ Mepron Suspension (5% to 10%) 1526
Merrem I.V. (Greater than 0.1% to 1%) 684
Mirapex Tablets 857
▲ Myfortic Tablets (3% to less than 20%) 2276
Nasonex Nasal Spray (Rare) 2883
▲ Noxafil Oral Suspension (1% to 12%) 2889
Prevnar 3241
▲ Prograf Capsules and Injection (3% to 15%) 622
Protonix for Delayed-Release Oral Suspension (Less than 1%) 3254
Protonix Delayed-Release Tablets (Less than 1%) 3254
Protonix I.V. (Less than 1%) 3257
Protopic Ointment (0.2% to less than 1%) 628
▲ Pulmicort Flexhaler (1.3% to 10%) 654
Serevent Diskus (1% to less than 3%) 1594
Spiriva HandiHaler 870
Symbicort 80/4.5 Inhalation Aerosol (1.4%) 659
▲ Symbicort 160/4.5 Inhalation Aerosol (3.2%) 659
Synagis Intramuscular Solution (More than 1%) 1948
▲ Trisenox Injection (5%) 986
Vaprisol (2.2%) 632
Velcade for Injection 2168
▲ Xeloda Tablets (Less than 1% to 7%) 2662
▲ Zosyn for Injection (3.9%) 3284
Zyprexa Tablets (Infrequent) 1883
Zyprexa ZYDIS Orally Disintegrating Tablets (Infrequent) 1883
Zyvox (0% to 1.1%) 2552

Candidiasis, pharynx
▲ Advair Diskus 100/50 (4%) 1276
▲ Advair Diskus 250/50 (10%) 1276
Advair Diskus 500/50 1276
▲ Advair HFA 45/21 Inhalation Aerosol (1% to 3%) 1288
▲ Advair HFA 115/21 Inhalation Aerosol (1% to 3%) 1288
▲ Advair HFA 230/21 Inhalation Aerosol (1% to 3%) 1288
Azmacort Inhalation Aerosol 407
Serevent Diskus (1% to less than 3%) 1594

Candidiasis, urinary tract
Nexium Delayed-Release Capsules (Less than 1%) 645
Nexium I.V. (Less than 1%) 652
Nexium Delayed-Release Oral Suspension (Less than 1%) 645

Candidiasis, vaginal
Activella Tablets 2347
Cipro 2810
Divigel 3167
▲ Doxil Injection (1% to 10%) 2378
Enjuvia Tablets 1029
Invanz for Injection (Greater than 0.1%) 2029
Mirapex Tablets 857
Requip Tablets (Infrequent) 1561

Candiduria
Cipro I.V. 2817
Cipro 2810
Cipro XR Tablets 2823
Noroxin Tablets 2069
Zosyn for Injection (1% or less) 3284

Cannula site reaction
▲ Vaprisol (5.5%) 632

Capillary fragility
▲ Aerobid/Aerobid-M (1% to 3%) 1153
Lotrisone 2881
Venlafaxine Hydrochloride Tablets (Rare) 2199

Capillary leak syndrome
Aldara Cream, 5% 1699
Betaseron for SC Injection 756
Busulfex Injection 2477
Clolar for Intravenous Infusion 1239
Leukine 774
Neupogen for Injection (One event) 589
Orthoclone OKT3 Sterile Solution (Less than 1%) 2387
Simulect for Injection 2306

Carbohydrate and lipid effects
Lybrel Tablets 3204

Carbohydrate craving
Lexapro Oral Suspension (Infrequent) 1174
Lexapro Tablets (Infrequent) 1174

Carbohydrate tolerance, decrease
Abilify Injection (Greater than or equal to 1 in 1000 patients and less than 1 in 100 patients) 2466
Abilify Oral Solution (Greater than or equal to 1 in 1000 patients and less than 1 in 100 patients) 881
Abilify Oral Solution (Greater than or equal to 1 in 1000 patients and less than 1 in 100 patients) 2466
Abilify Discmelt Orally Disintegrating Tablets (Greater than or equal to 1 in 1000 patients and less than 1 in 100 patients) 881
Abilify Discmelt Orally Disintegrating Tablets (Greater than or equal to 1 in 1000 patients and less than 1 in 100 patients) 2466
Abilify Tablets (Greater than or equal to 1 in 1000 patients and less than 1 in 100 patients) 881
Abilify Tablets (Greater than or equal to 1 in 1000 patients and less than 1 in 100 patients) 2466
Angeliq Tablets 751
Climara Transdermal System 763
Climara Pro Transdermal System 768
Estratest Tablets 3043
Estratest H.S. Tablets 3043
Mircette Tablets 1034
NuvaRing 2897
Ortho-Cyclen Tablets 2449
Ortho Evra Transdermal System 2437
Ortho Tri-Cyclen Tablets 2449
Ortho Tri-Cyclen Lo Tablets 2458
Premphase Tablets 3232
Prempro Tablets 3232
Yaz Tablets 805

Carbohydrate tolerance, reduced
Activella Tablets 2347
Divigel 3167
Enjuvia Tablets 1029

Carcinoma
Aranesp for Injection 564
Emsam Transdermal System (Infrequent) 905
Lovaza Capsules 1520
Mirapex Tablets 857
Myfortic Tablets 2276
Nutropin for Injection 1208
Nutropin AQ Injection 1212
Nutropin AQ NuSpin Injection 1212
Nutropin AQ Pen 1212
Nutropin AQ Pen Cartridge 1212
Venlafaxine Hydrochloride Tablets (Rare) 2199

Carcinoma, basal cell
Amevive (Less than 0.1%) 611
Elidel Cream 1% 2221
Evoxac Capsules (Less than 1%) 1013
Mirapex Tablets 857
Neoral Oral Solution (0.4%) 2280
Neoral Soft Gelatin Capsules (0.4%) 2280
Protopic Ointment 628
Rapamune (0.7% to less than 2.2%) 3260
Requip Tablets (Infrequent to greater than or equal to 1%) 1561
Sandostatin Injection (Less than 1%) 2300

Carcinoma, bile duct
▲ Humira Injection (Less than 5%) 442

Carcinoma, bladder
ActoPlus Met Tablets (0.16%) 3071
Actos Tablets (0.16%) 3077
Bexxar 1371
Mirapex Tablets 857
Requip Tablets (Infrequent) 1561

Carcinoma, breast
Actiq (1% or greater) 959
Activella Tablets 2347
Angeliq Tablets 751
Bexxar 1371
Celebrex Capsules (0.1% to 1.9%) 2979
Climara Transdermal System 763
Enbrel for Injection 569
Enjuvia Tablets 1029
Estratest Tablets 3043
Estratest H.S. Tablets 3043
▲ Humira Injection (Less than 5%) 442
Imitrex Nasal Spray 1470
Lamictal (Rare) 1488
Lybrel Tablets 3204
Ortho-Cyclen/Ortho Tri-Cyclen 2449
Ortho Tri-Cyclen Lo Tablets 2458

Paxil (Rare) ... 1535
Paxil CR Controlled-Release Tablets (Rare) ... 1544
Premarin Intravenous ... 3217
Premphase Tablets ... 3232
Prempro Tablets ... 3232
Prometrium Capsules (100 mg, 200 mg) (2%) ... 3047
Requip Tablets (Infrequent) ... 1561
Sandostatin LAR Depot ... 2302
Symbyax Capsules (Rare) ... 1871
Zomig Tablets (Rare) ... 694
Zomig Nasal Spray (Rare) ... 689
Zomig-ZMT Tablets (Rare) ... 694

Carcinoma, cervix
Copaxone for Injection (Infrequent) ... 3110
▲ Humira Injection (Less than 5%) ... 442

Carcinoma, CNS
Lovaza Capsules ... 1520

Carcinoma, colon
Enbrel for Injection ... 569
▲ Humira Injection (Less than 5%) ... 442

Carcinoma, colorectal
Bexxar ... 1371
Mirapex Tablets ... 857

Carcinoma, endometrial
Activella Tablets ... 2347
Angeliq Tablets ... 751
Arimidex Tablets (0.2%) ... 672
Climara Transdermal System ... 763
Climara Pro Transdermal System ... 768
Divigel ... 3167
Enjuvia Tablets ... 1029
Estratest Tablets ... 3043
Estratest H.S. Tablets ... 3043
Femara Tablets (0.2%) ... 2246
Lovaza Capsules ... 1520
Mirapex Tablets ... 857
Premarin Intravenous ... 3217
Premarin Tablets ... 3221
Premarin Vaginal Cream ... 3228
Premphase Tablets ... 3232
Prempro Tablets ... 3232

Carcinoma, esophageal
Requip Tablets (Infrequent) ... 1561
Selzentry Tablets ... 2534

Carcinoma, gallbladder
▲ Humira Injection (Less than 5%) ... 442
Mirapex Tablets ... 857

Carcinoma, gastric
Bexxar ... 1371
Mirapex Tablets ... 857
Requip Tablets (Infrequent) ... 1561

Carcinoma, gastrointestinal
Copaxone for Injection (Infrequent) ... 3110
▲ Humira Injection (Less than 5%) ... 442
Protonix for Delayed-Release Oral Suspension (Less than 1%) ... 3254
Protonix Delayed-Release Tablets (Less than 1%) ... 3254
Protonix I.V. (Less than 1%) ... 3257
▲ Visudyne for Injection (1% to 10%) ... 2332
Zomig Tablets (Rare) ... 694
Zomig Nasal Spray (Rare) ... 689
Zomig-ZMT Tablets (Rare) ... 694

Carcinoma, head and neck
Bexxar ... 1371

Carcinoma, hepatocellular
Ortho-Cyclen/Ortho Tri-Cyclen (Rare) ... 2449
Ortho Tri-Cyclen Lo Tablets ... 2458
Testim 1% Gel ... 701

Carcinoma, liver
Campral Tablets (Rare) ... 1158

Carcinoma, lung
Bexxar ... 1371
Brovana Inhalation Solution (Less than 2%) ... 2990
Enbrel for Injection ... 569
Exubera Inhalation Powder ... 2515
Orencia Powder for Intravenous Infusion (8 cases) ... 921
Prinivil Tablets (0.3% to 1%) ... 2087
Rilutek Tablets (Infrequent) ... 2771

Carcinoma, lung, non-small cell
Emend Capsules (Greater than 0.5%) ... 1992
Emend for Injection (Greater than 0.5%) ... 1999

Carcinoma, metastatic lung
Mirapex Tablets ... 857

Carcinoma, ovarian
Activella Tablets ... 2347
Angeliq Tablets ... 751
Climara Transdermal System ... 763
Climara Pro Transdermal System ... 768
Divigel ... 3167
Enjuvia Tablets ... 1029
Estratest Tablets ... 3043
Estratest H.S. Tablets ... 3043
Mirapex Tablets ... 857
Premarin Intravenous ... 3217
Premarin Tablets ... 3221
Premarin Vaginal Cream ... 3228
Premphase Tablets ... 3232
Prempro Tablets ... 3232

Carcinoma, papillary, enlargement of
Thyrogen for Injection ... 1244

Carcinoma, prostate
AndroGel (1.2%) ... 3159
Enbrel for Injection ... 569
▲ Humira Injection (Less than 5%) ... 442
Mirapex Tablets (Less than 1%) ... 857
Paxil (Rare) ... 1535
Paxil CR Controlled-Release Tablets (Rare) ... 1544
▲ Propecia Tablets (6.4%) ... 2095
▲ Proscar Tablets (6.4%) ... 2102
Requip Tablets (Infrequent) ... 1561
Rilutek Tablets (Infrequent) ... 2771
Testim 1% Gel ... 701

Carcinoma, rectal
▲ Humira Injection (Less than 5%) ... 442
Requip Tablets (Infrequent) ... 1561

Carcinoma, reproductive organs
Lybrel Tablets ... 3204

Carcinoma, skin
Actonel with Calcium Tablets (2%) ... 2574
Azilect Tablets (Greater than 1%) ... 3106
Bexxar ... 1371
▲ CellCept Capsules (3% to less than 20%) ... 2622
▲ CellCept Intravenous (3% to less than 20%) ... 2622
▲ CellCept Oral Suspension (3% to less than 20%) ... 2622
▲ CellCept Tablets (3% to less than 20%) ... 2622
Copaxone for Injection (Infrequent) ... 3110
Gabitril Tablets (Infrequent) ... 973
▲ Humira Injection (Less than 5%) ... 442
Mirapex Tablets ... 857
Orthoclone OKT3 Sterile Solution ... 2387
▲ Prograf Capsules and Injection (One of the two most common forms) ... 622
Rapamune (0% to 1.1%) ... 3260
Sandimmune ... 2296

Carcinoma, skin, benign
Copaxone for Injection (Infrequent) ... 3110
Gabitril Tablets (Infrequent) ... 973
Kaletra (Less than 2%) ... 452
▲ Protopic Ointment (1% to 3%) ... 628

Carcinoma, squamous
▲ Aldara Cream, 5% (4%) ... 1699
Amevive (Less than 0.1%) ... 611
Evoxac Capsules (Less than 1%) ... 1013
Protopic Ointment ... 628
▲ Zolinza Capsules (3.5%) ... 2142

Carcinoma, squamous cell
Elidel Cream 1% ... 2221
Mirapex Tablets ... 857
Nexavar Tablets (0.1% to less than 1%) ... 784
▲ Rapamune (0.4% to less than 20%) ... 3260
Requip Tablets (Infrequent) ... 1561
Selzentry Tablets ... 2534

Carcinoma, thyroid
Requip Tablets (Infrequent) ... 1561
Solodyn Extended Release Tablets ... 1938

Carcinoma, tongue
Selzentry Tablets ... 2534

Carcinoma, unspecified
▲ Actonel with Calcium Tablets (0.8% to 3.3%) ... 2574
Aggrenox Capsules (1.7%) ... 819
Brovana Inhalation Solution (Less than 2%) ... 2990
Effexor XR Extended-Release Capsules (Rare) ... 3195
Gabitril Tablets (Infrequent) ... 973
Gengraf Capsules ... 435
▲ Humira Injection (Less than 5%) ... 442
▲ Lupron Depot 7.5 mg (Less than 5%) ... 469
Neoral Oral Solution (1% to less than 3%) ... 2280
Neoral Soft Gelatin Capsules (1% to less than 3%) ... 2280
Paxil (Infrequent) ... 1535
Paxil CR Controlled-Release Tablets (Infrequent) ... 1544
Protonix for Delayed-Release Oral Suspension (Less than 1%) ... 3254
Protonix Delayed-Release Tablets (Less than 1%) ... 3254
Protonix I.V. (Less than 1%) ... 3257
Rilutek Tablets (Infrequent) ... 2771
Zomig Tablets (Rare to infrequent) ... 694
Zomig Nasal Spray (Rare to infrequent) ... 689
Zomig-ZMT Tablets (Rare to infrequent) ... 694

Carcinoma, uterine
▲ Humira Injection (Less than 5%) ... 442
Requip Tablets (Rare) ... 1561

Cardiac abnormalities
Accolate Tablets (Rare) ... 669
Flovent Diskus 50 mcg ... 1435
▲ Leukine (23%) ... 774
Rythmol SR Capsules ... 1590
Vyvanse Capsules ... 3033

Cardiac anomalies
Stalevo Tablets ... 2309

Cardiac arrest
▲ Abelcet Injection (6%) ... 1134
Aceon Tablets (2 mg, 4 mg, 8 mg) ... 3038
Activase I.V. ... 1188
Adenoscan ... 605
AmBisome for Injection (Less common) ... 606
Anzemet Injection ... 2701
Anzemet Tablets (Rare) ... 2704
▲ Aranesp for Injection (8%) ... 564
▲ Argatroban Injection (5.8%) ... 1308
Avelox ... 2803
Betimol Ophthalmic Solution ... 3181
Bicillin C-R Injectable Suspension ... 1775
Bicillin L-A Injection ... 1777
Campath Ampules ... 761
Cancidas for Injection ... 1953
Captopril Tablets ... 2182
Celexa (Rare) ... 1160
▲ CellCept Capsules (3% to less than 20%) ... 2622
▲ CellCept Intravenous (3% to less than 20%) ... 2622
▲ CellCept Oral Suspension (3% to less than 20%) ... 2622
▲ CellCept Tablets (3% to less than 20%) ... 2622
Cleviprex (Less than 1%) ... 1936
Combigan Ophthalmic Solution ... 553
Combivent Inhalation Aerosol ... 845
Cosopt Sterile Ophthalmic Solution ... 1969
Cubicin for Injection (Less than 1%) ... 995
DepoDur Injection ... 1095
▲ Doxil Injection (1% to 10%) ... 2378
Effexor XR Extended-Release Capsules (Rare) ... 3195
Elitek (Less than or equal to 1%) ... 2729
Erbitux ... 912
Exelon Capsules (Infrequent) ... 2229
Exelon Oral Solution (Infrequent) ... 2229
Flebogamma 5% ... 1715
Flebogamma 5% DIF ... 1718
Fleet Enema ... 1143
Fleet Enema Extra ... 1143
Fleet Enema for Children ... 1143
Fluorescite Injection ... ⊙ 203
Gammagard Liquid ... 730
Gammagard S/D (Rare) ... 734
Gamunex (Rare) ... 3094
▲ Humira Injection (Less than 5%) ... 442
Imitrex Injection ... 1465
Imitrex Tablets ... 1474
Invanz for Injection (Greater than 0.1%) ... 2029
Lanoxin Injection ... 1498
Lanoxin Injection Pediatric ... 1502
Lanoxin Tablets ... 1505
Levaquin (0.1% to 1%) ... 2416
Levaquin in 5% Dextrose Injection (0.1% to 1%) ... 2416
Levothroid Tablets ... 1170
Levoxyl Tablets ... 1780
Lexapro Oral Suspension ... 1174
Lexapro Tablets ... 1174
Lexiscan Injection ... 614
Lidoderm Patch ... 1114
Lovaza Capsules ... 1520
Meridia Capsules ... 475
Merrem I.V. (Greater than 0.1% to 1%) ... 684
Mirapex Tablets ... 857
MS Contin Tablets ... 2585
Mycamine for Injection ... 616
Namenda (Infrequent) ... 1180
Orthoclone OKT3 Sterile Solution (Less than 1%) ... 2387
Pletal Tablets (Less than 2%) ... 2481
Prinivil Tablets (0.3% to 1.0%) ... 2087
Prinzide Tablets ... 2092
Prograf Capsules and Injection ... 622
Proleukin for Injection (Less than or equal to 1%) ... 2287
Prozac Weekly Capsules (Rare) ... 1852
Prozac Pulvules and Liquid (Rare) ... 1852
Pulmozyme Inhalation Solution ... 1217
Remicade for IV Injection (Greater than or equal to 0.2%) ... 950
Requip Tablets (Infrequent) ... 1561
Rilutek Tablets (More than 2%) ... 2771
Rythmol Tablets (Less than 1%) ... 1586
Rythmol SR Capsules ... 1590
Sandostatin LAR Depot ... 2302
Thioridazine Hydrochloride Tablets ... 2195
Timoptic Sterile Ophthalmic Solution (Less frequent) ... 2121
Timoptic in Ocudose (Less frequent) ... 2124
Timoptic-XE Sterile Ophthalmic Gel Forming Solution ... 2125
TNKase ... 1233
Trasylol Injection (1% to 2%) ... 799
Velcade for Injection ... 2168
Venlafaxine Hydrochloride Tablets (Rare) ... 2199
▲ Vesanoid Capsules (3%) ... 2660
Zosyn for Injection (1% or less) ... 3284
Zyprexa Tablets (Rare) ... 1883
Zyprexa ZYDIS Orally Disintegrating Tablets (Rare) ... 1883

Cardiac arrhythmias
(*see under* Arrhythmias)

Cardiac asystole
(*see under* Asystole)

Cardiac collapse
BOTOX Purified Neurotoxin Complex (2 patients) ... 550

Cardiac death
Cialis Tablets ... 1792
Exelon Capsules (Infrequent) ... 2229
Exelon Oral Solution (Infrequent) ... 2229

Cardiac disorders, unspecified
▲ Cancidas for Injection (12.5% 26.3%) ... 1953
▲ Mycamine for Injection (17.5% to 34.6%) ... 616
▲ Novantrone for Injection Concentrate (18%) ... 1100
▲ Rituxan I.V. (29%) ... 1223
Tice BCG (2%) ... 2936
▲ Velcade for Injection (15%) ... 2168
Xolair ... 2339

Cardiac dysrhythmias
(*see under* Arrhythmias)

Cardiac failure
(*see also under* Heart failure)
Cimzia ... 3127
Combigan Ophthalmic Solution ... 553
Exelon Patch (Infrequent) ... 2233
Exforge Tablets (Less than or equal to 0.1%) ... 2238
Requip Tablets (Infrequent) ... 1561
Tasigna Capsules (0.1% to 1%) ... 2316
Zyrtec Chewable Tablets (Less than 2%) ... 1920
Zyrtec Syrup (Less than 2%) ... 1920
Zyrtec Tablets (Less than 2%) ... 1920
Zyrtec-D 12 Hour Extended Release Tablets (Less than 2%) ... 1923

Cardiac failure, acute
Selzentry Tablets ... 2534

Cardiac flutter
Tasigna Capsules ... 2316

Treximet Tablets (Rare) 1616

Cardiac insufficiency
Campath Ampules 761

Cardiac murmur
Aceon Tablets (2 mg, 4 mg, 8 mg) (0.3% to 1%) 3038
Amerge Tablets (Rare) 1301
Avalide Tablets 892
Avalide Tablets 2713
Avapro Tablets (Less than 1%) 897
Avapro Tablets (Less than 1%) 2718
Cipro I.V. (1% or less) 2817
Cipro XR Tablets 2823
Concerta Extended-Release Tablets 1925
Copaxone for Injection (Infrequent) 3110
▲ Dacogen Injection (16%) 1066
Evoxac Capsules (Less than 1%) 1013
▲ Increlex Injection (Greater than or equal to 5%) 3100
Invanz for Injection (Greater than 0.1%) 2029
▲ Rythmol SR Capsules (2% to 4%) 1590
Tasigna Capsules (0.1% to 1%) 2316
▲ Vesanoid Capsules (3%) 2660

Cardiac output, decrease
Digibind for Injection (Few instances) 1403
Paxil (Rare) 1535
Paxil CR Controlled-Release Tablets (Rare) 1544

Cardiac rhythms, disturbances
Captopril Tablets 2182
Daraprim Tablets 1400
Lanoxin Injection 1498
Lanoxin Injection Pediatric 1502
Lanoxin Tablets 1505
Nadolol Tablets (1 of 100 patients) 2191
Prinzide Tablets 2092
▲ Somatuline Depot Injection (6% to 21%) 3102

Cardiac tamponade
Activase I.V. 1188
Busulfex Injection 2477
Gleevec Tablets 2255
Myleran Tablets (A small number of patients) 1530
▲ Taxotere Injection Concentrate (6.5%) 2773
TNKase 1233
Velcade for Injection 2168

Cardiac toxicity, unspecified
Doxil Injection 2378
Lanoxin Injection 1498
Lanoxin Injection Pediatric 1502
Lanoxin Tablets 1505

Cardiac valve disorder, unspecified
Adipex-P 1185
Neupro Transdermal System 3149
Protopic Ointment (0.2% to less than 1%) 628

Cardialgia
(*see under* Heartburn)

Cardiodynia
(*see under* Heartburn)

Cardiomegaly
Agrylin Capsules 3017
AmBisome for Injection (Less common) 606
Aricept Tablets (Infrequent) 1062
Aricept ODT Tablets (Infrequent) 1062
▲ Busulfex Injection (5%) 2477
Doxil Injection (Less than 1%) 2378
Evoxac Capsules 1013
Geodon Capsules (Rare) 2520
Mirapex Tablets 857
Remeron Tablets (Rare) 2924
RemeronSolTab Tablets (Rare) 2927
Requip Tablets (Infrequent) 1561
Tasigna Capsules (0.1% to 1%) 2316

Cardiomyopathy
Abelcet Injection 1134
Adderall XR Capsules (Isolated cases) 3012
Agrylin Capsules 3017
Aldara Cream, 5% 1699
Betaseron for SC Injection 756
Campath Ampules 761
Campral Tablets (Rare) 1158
Combivir Tablets 1384
Dacogen Injection 1066
Dexedrine (Isolated reports) 1401
▲ Doxil Injection (1% to 5%) 2378
Herceptin I.V. 1199
Imitrex Injection 1465
Imitrex Nasal Spray 1470
Imitrex Tablets 1474
▲ Intron A for Injection (Less than 5%) 2859
Ixempra Kit for Injection 915
Luvox CR Extended-Release Capsules (Infrequent) 1759
▲ Megace ES Oral Suspension (1% to 3%) 2499
PegIntron Powder for Injection (Less than or equal to 1%) 2903
Proleukin for Injection 2287
Retrovir Capsules (0.8%) 1574
Retrovir IV Infusion (1%) 1579
Retrovir (0.8%) 1574
Trizivir Tablets 1622
Vyvanse Capsules 3033

Cardiopulmonary arrest
Abilify Injection (Greater than or equal to 1 in 1000 patients and less than 1 in 100 patients) 881
Abilify Injection (Greater than or equal to 1 in 1000 patients and less than 1 in 100 patients) 2466
Abilify Oral Solution (Greater than or equal to 1 in 1000 patients and less than 1 in 100 patients) 881
Abilify Oral Solution (Greater than or equal to 1 in 1000 patients and less than 1 in 100 patients) 2466
Abilify Discmelt Orally Disintegrating Tablets (Greater than or equal to 1 in 1000 patients and less than 1 in 100 patients) 881
Abilify Discmelt Orally Disintegrating Tablets (Greater than or equal to 1 in 1000 patients and less than 1 in 100 patients) 2466
Abilify Tablets (Greater than or equal to 1 in 1000 patients and less than 1 in 100 patients) 881
Abilify Tablets (Greater than or equal to 1 in 1000 patients and less than 1 in 100 patients) 2466
Cipro I.V. (1% or less) 2817
Cipro (Less than 1%) 2810
Cipro XR Tablets 2823
Erbitux (2%) 912
Fortaz 1450
Pulmozyme Inhalation Solution 1217
Risperdal Consta Long-Acting Injection 1753
Zofran Injection 1682
Zofran 1687
Zofran ODT Orally Disintegrating Tablets 1687

Cardiopulmonary failure
Abilify Injection (Greater than or equal to 1 in 1000 patients and less than 1 in 100 patients) 2466
Abilify Oral Solution (Greater than or equal to 1 in 1000 patients and less than 1 in 100 patients) 2466
Abilify Discmelt Orally Disintegrating Tablets (Greater than or equal to 1 in 1000 patients and less than 1 in 100 patients) 2466
Abilify Tablets (Greater than or equal to 1 in 1000 patients and less than 1 in 100 patients) 2466

Cardiorespiratory arrest
Alphanate 1709
Avalide Tablets 892
Avalide Tablets 2713
Avapro Tablets (Less than 1%) 897
Avapro Tablets (Less than 1%) 2718
Dacogen Injection (Greater than or equal to 1%) 1066
Orthoclone OKT3 Sterile Solution 2387

Cardiospasm
Paxil (Rare) 1535
Paxil CR Controlled-Release Tablets (Rare) 1544
Protonix for Delayed-Release Oral Suspension (Less than 1%) 3254
Protonix Delayed-Release Tablets (Less than 1%) 3254
Protonix I.V. (Less than 1%) 3257

Cardiovascular abnormalities, fetal
Accutane Capsules 2607
Clinoril Tablets 1962

Cardiovascular collapse
Allegra-D 12 Hour Extended-Release Tablets 2687
Allegra-D 24 Hour Extended-Release Tablets 2690
Avelox 2803
Carbatrol Capsules 3019
Cipro I.V. (1% or less) 2817
Cipro 2810
Cipro XR Tablets 2823
Clarinex-D 24-Hour Extended-Release Tablets 2834
Equetro Extended-Release Capsules 3174
Levaquin 2416
Levaquin in 5% Dextrose Injection 2416
Lidoderm Patch 1114
Noroxin Tablets 2069
Orthoclone OKT3 Sterile Solution 2387
Tessalon Capsules 1183
Tessalon Perles 1183
Vantas 1737
Zyrtec-D 12 Hour Extended Release Tablets 1923

Cardiovascular death
▲ Avandia Tablets (5%) 1351

Cardiovascular disorders
Actonel with Calcium Tablets (2.5%) 2574
▲ Agrylin Capsules (1% to less than 5%) 3017
Allegra-D 12 Hour Extended-Release Tablets (Rare) 2687
Allegra-D 24 Hour Extended-Release Tablets (Rare) 2690
Argatroban Injection (2.3%) 1308
▲ Brovana Inhalation Solution (6.9%) 2990
▲ CellCept Capsules (3% to less than 25.6%) 2622
▲ CellCept Intravenous (3% to less than 25.6%) 2622
▲ CellCept Oral Suspension (3% to less than 25.6%) 2622
▲ CellCept Tablets (3% to less than 25.6%) 2622
Crixivan Capsules 1979
Evoxac Capsules (Less than 1%) 1013
▲ Humira Injection (Less than 5%) 442
▲ Hycamtin for Injection (25%) 1459
Luvox CR Extended-Release Capsules (Infrequent) 1759
▲ Neoral Oral Solution (28%) 2280
▲ Neoral Soft Gelatin Capsules (28%) 2280
▲ Novantrone for Injection Concentrate (11% to 26%) 1100
▲ Proleukin for Injection (11%) 2287
Protonix for Delayed-Release Oral Suspension (Less than 1%) 3254
Protonix Delayed-Release Tablets (Less than 1%) 3254
Protonix I.V. (Less than 1%) 3257
Requip Tablets (Infrequent) 1561
Singulair 2114
Tricor Tablets 520
Venlafaxine Hydrochloride Tablets (Rare) 2199
Zostavax Injection (0.4% to 0.6%) 2145
Zyban Sustained-Release Tablets 1692

Cardiovascular events
Aranesp for Injection 564
Cialis Tablets 1792
Epogen for Injection 576
▲ PrandiMet Tablets (4%) 2967
▲ Prandin Tablets (Less than or equal to 1% to 4%) 2971
Procrit for Injection 2391
Rituxan I.V. (1.7%) 1223
Somatuline Depot Injection 3102
Ventolin HFA Inhalation Aerosol 1638

Cardiovascular toxicity, unspecified
Sutent Capsules (1 patient) 2540

Carnitine concentrations, decreased
Depakote ER Tablets 423

Carotid artery occlusion
Mirapex Tablets 857

Carotid bruit
Rythmol SR Capsules 1590

Carpal tunnel syndrome
Arimidex Tablets 672
Evoxac Capsules (Less than 1%) 1013
Exforge Tablets (Greater than or equal to 0.2%) 2238
Genotropin Lyophilized Powder (2%) 2547
Humatrope Vials and Cartridges (Rare) 1838
▲ Intron A for Injection (Less than 5%) 2859
Lexapro Oral Suspension (Infrequent) 1174
Lexapro Tablets (Infrequent) 1174
Mirapex Tablets 857
Namenda (More than one patient) 1180
Norditropin Cartridges 2354
▲ Nutropin for Injection (27%) 1208
▲ Nutropin AQ Injection (27%) 1212
▲ Nutropin AQ NuSpin Injection (27%) 1212
▲ Nutropin AQ Pen (27%) 1212
▲ Nutropin AQ Pen Cartridge (27%) 1212
Prograf Capsules and Injection 622
Prozac Weekly Capsules 1852
Prozac Pulvules and Liquid 1852
Requip Tablets (Infrequent) 1561

Cartilage trauma
Cipro 2810

Cataplexy
Provigil Tablets (Greater than or equal to 1%) 977
▲ Xyrem Oral Solution (8.6%) 1766

Cataracts
Accutane Capsules 2607
▲ Actonel Tablets (6.5%) 2568
▲ Actonel with Calcium Tablets (1.9% to 5.9%) 2574
▲ Advair Diskus 100/50 (5%) 1276
Advair Diskus 250/50 1276
Advair Diskus 500/50 1276
Advair HFA 45/21 Inhalation Aerosol 1288
Advair HFA 115/21 Inhalation Aerosol 1288
Advair HFA 230/21 Inhalation Aerosol 1288
▲ Alphagan P Ophthalmic Solution (1% to 4%) 549
Aricept Tablets (Frequent) 1062
Aricept ODT Tablets (Frequent) 1062
▲ Arimidex Tablets (6%) 672
Azmacort Inhalation Aerosol 407
Beconase AQ Nasal Spray (Rare) 1369
▲ Betimol Ophthalmic Solution (1% to 5%) 3181
Celebrex Capsules (0.1% to 1.9%) 2979
Celexa (Rare) 1160
▲ CellCept Capsules (3% to less than 20%) 2622
▲ CellCept Intravenous (3% to less than 20%) 2622
▲ CellCept Oral Suspension (3% to less than 20%) 2622
▲ CellCept Tablets (3% to less than 20%) 2622
Chantix Tablets (Rare) 2511
Combigan Ophthalmic Solution (0.1% to 0.2%) 553
Copaxone for Injection (Infrequent) 3110
▲ Cozaar Tablets (7%) 1973
Effexor XR Extended-Release Capsules (Infrequent) 3195
Evoxac Capsules (Less than 1%) 1013
Exelon Capsules (Frequent) 2229
Exelon Oral Solution (Frequent) 2229
Exelon Patch (infrequent) 2233
Exjade Tablets (0.1% to 1%) 2244
Flonase Nasal Spray 1431
Flovent Diskus 50 mcg 1435
Flovent HFA 1440
Gengraf Capsules (1% to less than 3%) 435
Geodon Capsules (Infrequent) 2520
▲ Humira Injection (Less than 5%) 442
Lescol Capsules 2268
Lescol XL Tablets 2268
Levaquin 2416
Levaquin in 5% Dextrose Injection 2416
Lovaza Capsules 1520
▲ Lucentis Injection (5% to 20%) 1205
▲ Lumigan Ophthalmic Solution (3% to 10%) 556
Lybrel Tablets 3204
Mircette Tablets 1034
Myleran Tablets (Rare) 1530
Namenda (Frequent) 1180
Neoral Oral Solution (1% to less than 3%) 2280
Neoral Soft Gelatin Capsules (1% to less than 3%) 2280
NuvaRing 2897
Omnaris Nasal Spray (Rare) 2998
Ortho-Cyclen Tablets 2449
Ortho Evra Transdermal System 2437
Ortho Tri-Cyclen Tablets 2449
Ortho Tri-Cyclen Lo Tablets 2458

Paxil (Rare) ... 1535
Paxil CR Controlled-Release Tablets (Rare) ... 1544
Photofrin for Injection ... 708
Plavix Tablets (1% to 2.5%) ... 926
Plavix Tablets (1% to 2.5%) ... 2767
Protonix for Delayed-Release Oral Suspension (Less than 1%) ... 3254
Protonix Delayed-Release Tablets (Less than 1%) ... 3254
Protonix I.V. (Less than 1%) ... 3257
Protopic Ointment (0.2% to less than 1%) ... 628
Prozac Weekly Capsules ... 1852
Prozac Pulvules and Liquid ... 1852
Pulmicort Flexhaler ... 654
Qvar Inhalation Aerosol (Rare) ... 3116
Rilutek Tablets (Rare) ... 2771
Salagen Tablets (Less than 1%) ... 1082
Seasonique Tablets ... 1046
▲ Spiriva HandiHaler (1% to 3%) ... 870
▲ Travatan Z Ophthalmic Solution (1% to 4%) ... 547
Treximet Tablets (Rare) ... 1616
Tricor Tablets ... 520
▲ Triesence Injectable Suspension (20% to 60%) ... ⊙ 209
Venlafaxine Hydrochloride Tablets (Infrequent) ... 2199
Veramyst Nasal Spray ... 1643
▲ Visudyne for Injection (1% to 10%) ... 2332
Yaz Tablets ... 805
Zyprexa Tablets (Infrequent) ... 1883
Zyprexa ZYDIS Orally Disintegrating Tablets (Infrequent) ... 1883

Cataracts, posterior subcapsular
Alrex Ophthalmic Suspension 0.2% ... ⊙ 236
▲ Cosopt Sterile Ophthalmic Solution (1% to 5%) ... 1969
FML Ophthalmic Ointment (Infrequent) ... ⊙ 223
FML Ophthalmic Suspension ... ⊙ 224
FML Forte Ophthalmic Suspension (Infrequent) ... ⊙ 222
Lotemax Ophthalmic Suspension 0.5% ... ⊙ 241
Pred Forte Ophthalmic Suspension ... ⊙ 227
Pred Mild Ophthalmic Suspension (Infrequent) ... ⊙ 230
Pred-G Ophthalmic Ointment ... ⊙ 229
Pred-G Ophthalmic Suspension ... ⊙ 228
▲ Soriatane Capsules (1% to 5%) ... 3062

Cataracts, transient
Proglycem Capsules (Infrequent) ... 1185
Proglycem Suspension (Infrequent) ... 1185

Cataracts, traumatic, iatrogenic
Lucentis Injection (Less than 0.1%) .. 1205

Catatonia
Abilify Injection (Less than 1 in 1000 patients) ... 881
Abilify Injection (Less than 1 in 1000 patients) ... 2466
Abilify Oral Solution (Less than 1 in 1000 patients) ... 881
Abilify Oral Solution (Less than 1 in 1000 patients) ... 2466
Abilify Discmelt Orally Disintegrating Tablets (Less than 1 in 1000 patients) ... 881
Abilify Discmelt Orally Disintegrating Tablets (Less than 1 in 1000 patients) ... 2466
Abilify Tablets (Less than 1 in 1000 patients) ... 881
Abilify Tablets (Less than 1 in 1000 patients) ... 2466
Celexa (Rare) ... 1160
Combigan Ophthalmic Solution ... 553
Cosopt Sterile Ophthalmic Solution ... 1969
Effexor XR Extended-Release Capsules ... 3195
InnoPran XL Extended Release Capsules ... 1484
Nadolol Tablets ... 2191
Timoptic Sterile Ophthalmic Solution ... 2121
Timoptic in Ocudose ... 2124
Timoptic-XE Sterile Ophthalmic Gel Forming Solution ... 2125
Toprol-XL Tablets ... 666
Venlafaxine Hydrochloride Tablets ... 2199

CD4 count, decreased
Truvada Tablets ... 1262

Cellulitis
Actiq (1% or greater) ... 959
AmBisome for Injection (Less common) ... 606
Aricept Tablets (Infrequent) ... 1062
Aricept ODT Tablets (Infrequent) ... 1062
Bactroban Cream (Less than 1%) ... 1366
BeneFIX Vials (1.5%) ... 3191
Celebrex Capsules (0.1% to 1.9%) ... 2979
Celexa (Rare) ... 1160
▲ CellCept Capsules (3% to less than 20%) ... 2622
▲ CellCept Intravenous (3% to less than 20%) ... 2622
▲ CellCept Oral Suspension (3% to less than 20%) ... 2622
▲ CellCept Tablets (3% to less than 20%) ... 2622
▲ Clolar for Intravenous Infusion (11%) ... 1239
Copaxone for Injection (Infrequent) .. 3110
▲ Cozaar Tablets (7%) ... 1973
Cubicin for Injection (1% to 2%) ... 995
▲ Dacogen Injection (12%) ... 1066
Doxil Injection (Less than 1%) ... 2378
Effexor XR Extended-Release Capsules (Rare) ... 3195
Elitek (Less than or equal to 1%) ... 2729
Enbrel for Injection ... 569
Evoxac Capsules (Less than 1%) ... 1013
Exelon Capsules (Infrequent) ... 2229
Exelon Oral Solution (Infrequent) ... 2229
Fentora Tablets (Greater than 1%) ... 968
Flulaval Injection Vaccine ... 1448
Gabitril Tablets (Infrequent) ... 973
Gemzar for Injection (Rare) ... 1820
Gengraf Capsules (1% to less than 3%) ... 435
▲ Humira Injection (Less than 5%) ... 442
Infanrix Vaccine ... 1479
▲ Intron A for Injection (Less than 5%) ... 2859
Invanz for Injection (1.5%) ... 2029
Kineret Injection ... 585
Klonopin (Infrequent) ... 2639
Lunesta Tablets (Infrequent) ... 2994
▲ Lupron Depot 7.5 mg (Less than 5%) ... 469
Lyrica Capsules (0.1% to 1%) ... 2527
Mirapex Tablets ... 857
Namenda (Infrequent) ... 1180
Neoral Oral Solution (1% to less than 3%) ... 2280
Neoral Soft Gelatin Capsules (1% to less than 3%) ... 2280
Orencia Powder for Intravenous Infusion (0.2% to 0.5%) ... 921
Paxil (Rare) ... 1535
Paxil CR Controlled-Release Tablets (Rare) ... 1544
Pediarix Vaccine ... 1552
PegIntron Powder for Injection (Less than or equal to 1%) ... 2903
▲ Prograf Capsules and Injection (3% to 15%) ... 622
Proleukin for Injection ... 2287
ProQuad ... 2099
Protopic Ointment (Greater than or equal to 1%) ... 628
Raptiva for Injection ... 1218
Rebif Prefilled Syringe for Injection ... 1107
Remeron Tablets (Rare) ... 2924
RemeronSolTab Tablets (Rare) ... 2927
Remicade for IV Injection (Greater than or equal to 0.2%) ... 950
ReoPro Vials (0.3%) ... 1860
Requip Tablets (Infrequent) ... 1561
Rilutek Tablets (Infrequent) ... 2771
Sandostatin Injection (Less than 1%) ... 2300
Sandostatin LAR Depot ... 2302
Sular Extended Release Tablets (Less than or equal to 1%) ... 2975
Symbyax Capsules (Infrequent) ... 1871
Targretin Capsules ... 1084
Ultram ER Extended-Release Tablets (0.5% to less than 1%) ... 2428
Varivax ... 2133
Venlafaxine Hydrochloride Tablets (Rare) ... 2199
▲ Vesanoid Capsules (8%) ... 2660
Vivitrol ... 988
Xyrem Oral Solution (Infrequent) ... 1766
Zomig Tablets (Rare) ... 694
Zomig Nasal Spray (Rare) ... 689
Zomig-ZMT Tablets (Rare) ... 694

Cellulitis, injection site
Bicillin C-R Injectable Suspension ... 1775
Bicillin L-A Injection ... 1777
Fluarix Vaccine ... 1446
Pneumovax 23 ... 2078

Cellulitis, pre-septal
Amevive ... 611

Cellulitis-like reactions
Pneumovax 23 (Rare) ... 2078

Central obesity
Viramune Oral Suspension ... 873
Viramune Tablets ... 873

Central/peripheral nervous system disorders
▲ Femara Tablets (2.5% to 33.7%) ... 2246
▲ Novantrone for Injection Concentrate (11% to 34%) ... 1100

Centrilobular sinusoidal fibrosis
Myleran Tablets ... 1530

Cephalin flocculation test, positive
Cuprimine Capsules ... 1986

Cerebellar dysfunction
Taxotere Injection Concentrate (0.1% to 2.4%) ... 2773

Cerebellar malformation, fetal
Accutane Capsules ... 2607

Cerebellar syndrome, acute
Lamictal (Rare) ... 1488
Lyrica Capsules (Rare) ... 2527

Cerebral abnormalities, fetal
Accutane Capsules ... 2607

Cerebral arterial insufficiency, symptoms
Carbatrol Capsules ... 3019
Equetro Extended-Release Capsules ... 3174

Cerebral arteritis
Daytrana Transdermal Patch ... 3022
Focalin XR Capsules ... 2251
Metadate CD Capsules (Isolated cases) ... 3146

Cerebral artery embolism
Mirapex Tablets ... 857

Cerebral atrophy
Depakote ER Tablets (Greater than 1%) ... 423

Cerebral bleeding
(*see under* Cerebral hemorrhage)

Cerebral embolism
Prozac Weekly Capsules (Rare) ... 1852
Prozac Pulvules and Liquid (Rare) ... 1852
Rilutek Tablets (Rare) ... 2771
Trasylol Injection (1% to 2%) ... 799

Cerebral hemorrhage
Aggrenox Capsules (Less than 1%) .. 819
Aricept Tablets (Infrequent) ... 1062
Aricept ODT Tablets (Infrequent) ... 1062
Arranon Injection (1%) ... 1319
Azilect Tablets (Rare) ... 3106
Busulfex Injection (One patient) ... 2477
Gleevec Tablets (0% to 1%) ... 2255
Gliadel Wafer (Less than 1%) ... 1076
Imitrex Injection ... 1465
Imitrex Tablets ... 1474
Ixempra Kit for Injection ... 915
Lybrel Tablets ... 3204
Mircette Tablets ... 1034
Mylotarg for Injection (2%) ... 3212
Namenda (Infrequent) ... 1180
Nexavar Tablets (0.1% to less than 1%) ... 784
NuvaRing ... 2897
Ortho-Cyclen Tablets ... 2449
Ortho Evra Transdermal System ... 2437
Ortho Tri-Cyclen Tablets ... 2449
Ortho Tri-Cyclen Lo Tablets ... 2458
Pletal Tablets ... 2481
Proleukin for Injection ... 2287
Rilutek Tablets (Infrequent) ... 2771
Seasonique Tablets ... 1046
Treximet Tablets ... 1616
Velcade for Injection ... 2168
▲ Vesanoid Capsules (9%) ... 2660
Yaz Tablets ... 805

Cerebral herniation
Activase I.V. ... 1188

Cerebral infarction
Activase I.V. ... 1188
Amerge Tablets ... 1301
Aricept Tablets (Infrequent) ... 1062
Aricept ODT Tablets (Infrequent) ... 1062
Arimidex Tablets ... 672
Brovana Inhalation Solution (Less than 2%) ... 2990
Celebrex Capsules (Greater than or equal to 0.1% to less than 1%) ... 2979
Geodon Capsules (Rare) ... 2520
Gliadel Wafer (Less than 1%) ... 1076
Kaletra (Less than 2%) ... 452
Mirapex Tablets ... 857
Namenda ... 1180
NovoSeven ... 2367
NovoSeven RT ... 2370
Pletal Tablets (Less than 2%) ... 2481
Prograf Capsules and Injection ... 622
Remicade for IV Injection (Greater than or equal to 0.2%) ... 950

Cerebral ischemia
(*see under* Ischemia, cerebral)

Cerebral lesions
Proleukin for Injection ... 2287

Cerebral occlusion
Daytrana Transdermal Patch ... 3022
Focalin XR Capsules ... 2251
Metadate CD Capsules (Isolated cases) ... 3146

Cerebral sinus thrombosis
Lamictal (Rare) ... 1488

Cerebral thrombosis
Cipro I.V. (1% or less) ... 2817
Cipro (Less than 1%) ... 2810
Cipro XR Tablets ... 2823
Lamictal (Rare) ... 1488
Lybrel Tablets ... 3204
Mircette Tablets ... 1034
NuvaRing ... 2897
Ortho-Cyclen Tablets ... 2449
Ortho Evra Transdermal System ... 2437
Ortho Tri-Cyclen Tablets ... 2449
Ortho Tri-Cyclen Lo Tablets ... 2458
Seasonique Tablets ... 1046
Trasylol Injection (0.5%) ... 799
Yaz Tablets ... 805

Cerebral vasculitis
Proleukin for Injection ... 2287

Cerebrospinal fluid leak
▲ Gliadel Wafer (5%) ... 1076

Cerebrospinal fluid proteins, changes
Thiothixene Capsules ... 2197

Cerebrovascular accident
Abelcet Injection ... 1134
Abilify Injection (Greater than or equal to 1 in 1000 patients and less than 1 in 100 patients) ... 881
Abilify Injection (Greater than or equal to 1 in 1000 patients and less than 1 in 100 patients) ... 2466
Abilify Oral Solution (Greater than or equal to 1 in 1000 patients and less than 1 in 100 patients) ... 881
Abilify Oral Solution (Greater than or equal to 1 in 1000 patients and less than 1 in 100 patients) ... 2466
Abilify Discmelt Orally Disintegrating Tablets (Greater than or equal to 1 in 1000 patients and less than 1 in 100 patients) ... 881
Abilify Discmelt Orally Disintegrating Tablets (Greater than or equal to 1 in 1000 patients and less than 1 in 100 patients) ... 2466
Abilify Tablets (Greater than or equal to 1 in 1000 patients and less than 1 in 100 patients) ... 881
Abilify Tablets (Greater than or equal to 1 in 1000 patients and less than 1 in 100 patients) ... 2466
Aceon Tablets (2 mg, 4 mg, 8 mg) (0.2%) ... 3038
▲ Agrylin Capsules (1% to less than 5%) ... 3017
Aldara Cream, 5% ... 1699
Amerge Tablets ... 1301
Aricept Tablets (Infrequent) ... 1062
Aricept ODT Tablets (Infrequent) ... 1062
Arimidex Tablets ... 672
Avalide Tablets ... 892
Avalide Tablets ... 2713
Avapro Tablets (Less than 1%) ... 897

Avapro Tablets (Less than 1%) 2718
Betimol Ophthalmic Solution 3181
Bicillin C-R Injectable Suspension 1775
Bicillin L-A Injection 1777
Captopril Tablets 2182
Catapres-TTS (0.5% or less) 842
Celebrex Capsules (Less than 0.1%) 2979
Celexa (Infrequent) 1160
Chantix Tablets (Rare) 2511
Combigan Ophthalmic Solution 553
▲ Coreg Tablets (Greater than 1% to 3%) 1387
▲ Coreg CR Extended-Release Capsules (Greater than 1% to less than or equal to 3%) 1393
Cosopt Sterile Ophthalmic Solution (Less than 1%) 1969
Cozaar Tablets (Less than 1%) 1973
Effexor XR Extended-Release Capsules (Rare) 3195
Epogen for Injection (0.4%) 576
▲ Flolan for Injection (4%) 1426
Gammagard S/D 734
Gemzar for Injection (2%) 1820
Geodon Capsules (Rare) 2520
Imitrex Injection 1465
Imitrex Nasal Spray 1470
Imitrex Tablets 1474
Invega Extended-Release Tablets 1748
Kinrix Injection Vaccine (0.1%) 1486
Lamictal (Rare) 1488
Luvox CR Extended-Release Capsules (Rare) 1759
Maxalt Tablets (Very rare) 2056
Maxalt-MLT Orally Disintegrating Tablets (Very rare) 2056
Meridia Capsules 475
Miacalcin Nasal Spray (Less than 1%) 2274
Namenda (Frequent) 1180
Orthoclone OKT3 Sterile Solution 2387
Paxil (Rare) 1535
Paxil CR Controlled-Release Tablets (Rare) 1544
Pletal Tablets 2481
Prinivil Tablets (0.3% to 1%) 2087
Prinzide Tablets 2092
▲ Procrit for Injection (0.4% to 3.2%) 2391
ProQuad 2099
Protopic Ointment (Greater than or equal to 1%) 628
Prozac Weekly Capsules (Rare) 1852
Prozac Pulvules and Liquid (Rare) 1852
Risperdal Consta Long-Acting Injection 1753
Rythmol SR Capsules 1590
Selzentry Tablets 2534
Sular Extended Release Tablets (Less than or equal to 1%) 2975
Tarceva Tablets (2.3%) 1228
Targretin Capsules 1084
Tarka Tablets 511
Timoptic Sterile Ophthalmic Solution (Less frequent) 2121
Timoptic in Ocudose (Less frequent) 2124
Timoptic-XE Sterile Ophthalmic Gel Forming Solution 2125
Trasylol Injection (1% to 2%) 799
Varivax 2133
Velcade for Injection 2168
Venlafaxine Hydrochloride Tablets (Rare) 2199
Vesanoid Capsules 2660
Zonegran Capsules (Infrequent) 1089
Zosyn for Injection (1% or less) 3284
Zyprexa Tablets (Infrequent) 1883
Zyprexa ZYDIS Orally Disintegrating Tablets (Infrequent) 1883

Cerebrovascular disorders
Ambien Tablets (Infrequent) 2692
Ambien CR Tablets (Infrequent) 2696
Coreg Tablets (Less than or equal to 0.1%) 1387
Coreg CR Extended-Release Capsules (Less than or equal to 0.1%) 1393
Crixivan Capsules 1979
Elitek (Less than or equal to 1%) 2729
Femara Tablets (1.1%) 2246
Flumadine (Less than 0.3%) 1167
Micardis Tablets (More than 0.3%) 852
Micardis HCT Tablets (More than 0.3%) 854
Ortho-Cyclen/Ortho Tri-Cyclen 2449
Ortho Tri-Cyclen Lo Tablets 2458
Risperdal Consta Long-Acting Injection 1753
Sandostatin LAR Depot 2302
Toprol-XL Tablets (Greater than 1%) 666

Cerebrovascular events
PegIntron Powder for Injection 2903
Symbyax Capsules 1871
Treximet Tablets 1616

Cerebrovascular insufficiency
Captopril Tablets 2182

Cerumen, increased
Norvir (Less than 2%) 489

Cervical disorders
(*see under* Cervical irregularities)

Cervical ectropion, changes
(*see also under* Cervical erosion, changes; Cervical eversion, changes in)
Activella Tablets 2347
Angeliq Tablets 751
Climara Transdermal System 763
Climara Pro Transdermal System 768
Divigel 3167
Enjuvia Tablets 1029
Premarin Tablets 3221
Seasonique Tablets 1046

Cervical erosion, changes
(*see also under* Cervical ectropion, changes; Cervical eversion, changes in)
Estratest Tablets 3043
Estratest H.S. Tablets 3043
Mircette Tablets 1034
NuvaRing 2897
Ortho-Cyclen/Ortho Tri-Cyclen 2449
Ortho Tri-Cyclen Lo Tablets 2458
Premarin Intravenous 3217
Premarin Vaginal Cream 3228
Premphase Tablets 3232
Prempro Tablets 3232
Yaz Tablets 805

Cervical eversion, changes in
(*see also under* Cervical ectropion, changes; Cervical erosion, changes)
Lybrel Tablets 3204

Cervical irregularities
Lupron Depot-PED 7.5 mg, 11.25 mg and 15 mg (Less than 2%) 471
▲ Premphase Tablets (4% to 5%) 3232
▲ Prempro Tablets (4% to 5%) 3232

Cervical secretion, changes
Activella Tablets 2347
Angeliq Tablets 751
Climara Transdermal System 763
Climara Pro Transdermal System 768
Divigel 3167
Enjuvia Tablets 1029
Estratest Tablets 3043
Estratest H.S. Tablets 3043
Lybrel Tablets 3204
Mircette Tablets 1034
Ortho-Cyclen/Ortho Tri-Cyclen 2449
Ortho Tri-Cyclen Lo Tablets 2458
Premarin Intravenous 3217
Premarin Tablets 3221
Premarin Vaginal Cream 3228
Premphase Tablets 3232
Prempro Tablets 3232
Prometrium Capsules (100 mg, 200 mg) 3047
Seasonique Tablets 1046
Yaz Tablets 805

Cervical smear test, abnormal
Yaz Tablets (Greater than 1%) 805
Zomig Tablets (Rare) 694
Zomig Nasal Spray (Rare) 689
Zomig-ZMT Tablets (Rare) 694

Cervical smear test, positive
Evoxac Capsules (Less than 1%) 1013

Cervicitis
Effexor XR Extended-Release Capsules (Rare) 3195
Lyrica Capsules (Rare) 2527
Venlafaxine Hydrochloride Tablets (Rare) 2199

Cerviocobrachial syndrome
Exforge Tablets (Greater than or equal to 0.2%) 2238

Cervix disorder, unspecified
Lovaza Capsules 1520

Chalazion
Soriatane Capsules (Less than 1%) 3062

Changes, retinal
Lamisil Oral Granules 2264

Character changes
Seromycin Capsules 1864

Charcot's syndrome
▲ Mavik Tablets (3.8%) 472
ReoPro Vials (0.4%) 1860
Risperdal Consta Long-Acting Injection (Rare) 1753
Soriatane Capsules (Less than 1%) 3062

Cheek puffing
Moban Tablets 1116
Thiothixene Capsules 2197

Cheilitis
Accutane Capsules 2607
Actiq (Less than 1%) 959
Cosmegen for Injection 2485
Effexor XR Extended-Release Capsules (Rare) 3195
Frova Tablets (Rare) 1111
Lipitor Tablets (Less than 2%) 2501
Mirapex Tablets 857
Norvir (Less than 2%) 489
Protopic Ointment (Greater than or equal to 1%) 628
Rilutek Tablets (Rare) 2771
▲ Soriatane Capsules (More than 75%) 3062
Targretin Capsules 1084
Venlafaxine Hydrochloride Tablets (Rare) 2199

Cheilosis
Cuprimine Capsules 1986

Chemosis
▲ Alrex Ophthalmic Suspension 0.2% (5% to 15%) ⊙236
Iquix Ophthalmic Solution (Less than 1%) 3183
▲ Lotemax Ophthalmic Suspension 0.5% (5% to 15%) ⊙241

Chest, pressure
Imitrex Injection (2%) 1465
▲ Imitrex Nasal Spray (2% to 3%) 1470
▲ Imitrex Tablets (2% to 3%) 1474
Meridia Capsules 475

Chest congestion
▲ Advair Diskus 100/50 (Greater than or equal to 3%) 1276
Advair Diskus 250/50 1276
Advair Diskus 500/50 1276
Advair HFA 45/21 Inhalation Aerosol 1288
Advair HFA 115/21 Inhalation Aerosol 1288
Advair HFA 230/21 Inhalation Aerosol 1288
▲ Aerobid/Aerobid-M (3% to 9%) 1153
▲ Azmacort Inhalation Aerosol (1% to 3%) 407
Brovana Inhalation Solution (Less than 2%) 2990
Effexor XR Extended-Release Capsules (Infrequent) 3195
Klonopin 2639
Venlafaxine Hydrochloride Tablets (Infrequent) 2199

Chest numbness
Tessalon Capsules 1183
Tessalon Perles 1183

Chest pain, atypical
▲ CellCept Capsules (26.3%) 2622
▲ CellCept Intravenous (26.3%) 2622
▲ CellCept Oral Suspension (26.3%) 2622
▲ CellCept Tablets (26.3%) 2622
Neupro Transdermal System (Greater than or equal to 2%) 3149

Chest pain, musculoskeletal
▲ Alvesco Inhalation Aerosol (Greater than or equal to 3%) 2985
Exforge Tablets (Greater than or equal to 0.2%) 2238
▲ Tasigna Capsules (1% to 10%) 2316
Tyzeka Tablets (2%) 2328
Wellbutrin SR Sustained-Release Tablets (Infrequent) 1653
▲ Wellbutrin XL Extended-Release Tablets (3% to 4%) 1659

Chest pain, substernal
Effexor XR Extended-Release Capsules (Frequent) 3195
▲ Intron A for Injection (Less than 5%) 2859
Kaletra (Less than 2%) 452
Nexium Delayed-Release Capsules (Less than 1%) 645
Nexium I.V. (Less than 1%) 652
Nexium Delayed-Release Oral Suspension (Less than 1%) 645
Norvir (Less than 2%) 489
▲ Photofrin for Injection (5%) 708
Protonix for Delayed-Release Oral Suspension (Less than 1%) 3254
Protonix Delayed-Release Tablets (Less than 1%) 3254
Protonix I.V. (Less than 1%) 3257
Remeron Tablets (Rare) 2924
RemeronSolTab Tablets (Rare) 2927
Venlafaxine Hydrochloride Tablets (Frequent) 2199

Chest sound, abnormalities
Gengraf Capsules (1% to less than 3%) 435
▲ Leustatin Injection (9%) 2384
Neoral Oral Solution (1% to less than 3%) 2280
Neoral Soft Gelatin Capsules (1% to less than 3%) 2280
Orthoclone OKT3 Sterile Solution 2387
Prinivil Tablets (Greater than 1%) 2087
Prinzide Tablets 2092
▲ Simulect for Injection (3% to 10%) 2306

Chest tightness
Acetadote Injection (1%) 1001
▲ Adenocard IV Injection (7%) 603
Advair Diskus 100/50 1276
Advair Diskus 250/50 1276
Advair Diskus 500/50 1276
Advair HFA 45/21 Inhalation Aerosol 1288
Advair HFA 115/21 Inhalation Aerosol 1288
Advair HFA 230/21 Inhalation Aerosol 1288
▲ Aerobid/Aerobid-M (1% to 3%) 1153
Alferon N Injection 1726
Allegra Oral Solution (Rare) 2684
Allegra Tablets (Rare) 2684
Allegra-D 12 Hour Extended-Release Tablets (Rare) 2687
Allegra-D 24 Hour Extended-Release Tablets (Rare) 2690
Alphanate 1709
Amitiza Capsules 3082
BeneFIX Vials (1.5%) 3191
Ceftin Tablets (0.1% to 1%) 1380
Cyanokit 5g Antidote 1021
▲ Doxil Injection (Approximately 6.8%) 2378
Elitek 2729
Erbitux 912
Flebogamma 5% 1715
Flebogamma 5% DIF 1718
Flovent Diskus 50 mcg 1435
Flovent HFA 1440
▲ Flulaval Injection Vaccine (1% to 3%) 1448
Gammagard Liquid 730
▲ Imitrex Injection (3%) 1465
Imitrex Nasal Spray (Infrequent) 1470
Imitrex Tablets (Frequent) 1474
Lexapro Oral Suspension (Infrequent) 1174
Lexapro Tablets (Infrequent) 1174
Maxair Autohaler (1.3%) 1705
▲ Maxalt Tablets (Less than 2% to 3%) 2056
▲ Maxalt-MLT Orally Disintegrating Tablets (Less than 2% to 3%) 2056
Meridia Capsules 475
MoviPrep Oral Solution 2679
Ortho-Cyclen/Ortho Tri-Cyclen 2449
Ortho Tri-Cyclen Lo Tablets 2458
Orthoclone OKT3 Sterile Solution 2387
▲ Rituxan I.V. (7%) 1223
Sular Extended Release Tablets (Very rare) 2975
Taxotere Injection Concentrate 2773
Tussionex Pennkinetic Extended-Release Suspension (Occasional) 3154
Vivitrol 988
Xolair 1235
Xolair 2339
Xyntha Vials 3280
▲ Zomig Tablets (Common) 694

Zomig Nasal Spray (1% to less than 2%) 689
Zomig-ZMT Tablets (Common) 694

Chewing movements
Moban Tablets 1116
Thioridazine Hydrochloride Tablets 2195
Thiothixene Capsules 2197

CHF
(*see under* Congestive heart failure)

Chills
▲ Abelcet Injection (18%) 1134
Aceon Tablets (2 mg, 4 mg, 8 mg) (0.3% to 1%) 3038
▲ Actimmune (14%) 1743
Actiq (1% or greater) 959
Advicor Tablets 402
▲ Aerobid/Aerobid-M (1% to 3%) 1153
▲ Agrylin Capsules (1% to less than 5%) 3017
Albutein 5% 1707
Albutein 25% 1708
▲ Alferon N Injection (14% to 87%) 1726
Alinia for Oral Suspension (Less than 1%) 2677
Alinia Tablets (Less than 1%) 2677
Alphanate 1709
AlphaNine SD 1713
▲ AmBisome for Injection (40% to 48.1%) 606
Amerge Tablets (Infrequent) 1301
▲ Amevive (6%) 611
Anaprox Tablets (Less than 1%) 2632
Anaprox DS Tablets (Less than 1%) 2632
Anzemet Injection (2%) 2701
Anzemet Tablets (1.3%) 2704
Aralast (0.1%) 726
Aricept Tablets (Infrequent) 1062
Aricept ODT Tablets (Infrequent) 1062
▲ Asacol Delayed-Release Tablets (3%) 2579
Avalide Tablets 892
Avalide Tablets 2713
Avapro Tablets (Less than 1%) 897
Avapro Tablets (Less than 1%) 2718
Axert Tablets (Infrequent) 2431
Azilect Tablets (Infrequent) 3106
BeneFIX Vials (1.6%) 3191
▲ Betaseron for SC Injection (21%) 756
▲ Bexxar (1% to 18%) 1371
Bicillin C-R Injectable Suspension 1775
Bicillin L-A Injection 1777
▲ Busulfex Injection (46%) 2477
▲ Campath Ampules (10% to 53%) 761
Campral Tablets (Frequent) 1158
▲ Cancidas for Injection (8.8% to 22.5%) 1953
Carbatrol Capsules 3019
Ceftin Tablets (0.1% to 1%) 1380
▲ CellCept Capsules (3% to less than 20%) 2622
▲ CellCept Intravenous (3% to less than 20%) 2622
▲ CellCept Oral Suspension (3% to less than 20%) 2622
▲ CellCept Tablets (3% to less than 20%) 2622
▲ Cerezyme for Injection (Approximately 6.5%) 1238
Chantix Tablets (Infrequent) 2511
▲ Chemet Capsules (5.2% to 15.7%) 2484
Cipro I.V. (1% or less) 2817
Cipro (Less than 1%) 2810
Cipro XR Tablets 2823
Clinoril Tablets (Less than 1 in 100) 1962
▲ Combivir Tablets (10%) 1384
▲ Copaxone for Injection (4%) 3110
Cymbalta Delayed-Release Capsules (Frequent) 1801
Dantrium Capsules (Less frequent) 2580
Depakote ER Tablets (Greater than 1%) 423
Diclofenac Sodium Ophthalmic Solution ⊙ 240
▲ Doxil Injection (1% to 5%) 2378
EC-Naprosyn Delayed-Release Tablets (Less than 1%) 2632
Edecrin 698
Effexor XR Extended-Release Capsules (Frequent) 3195
Eldepryl Capsules 3052
Elspar for Injection 1990
Emsam Transdermal System (Infrequent) 905
Engerix-B Vaccine (Less than 1%) 1409
▲ Epivir (7%) 1412
▲ Epivir-HBV (7%) 1417
Equetro Extended-Release Capsules 3174
▲ Erbitux (0% to 16%) 912
▲ Fabrazyme for Intravenous Infusion (43%) 1241
Fansidar Tablets 2636
Fentora Tablets (Greater than 1%) 968
Flebogamma 5% 1715
Flebogamma 5% DIF 1718
Flexbumin 25% I.V. (Occasional) 729
▲ Flolan for Injection (13% to 25%) 1426
Fluarix Vaccine 1446
▲ Flulaval Injection Vaccine (2% to 5%) 1448
▲ FluMist Vaccine (2% to 9%) 1945
Follistim AQ Cartridge 2844
Gabitril Tablets (Frequent) 973
▲ Gammagard Liquid (1.69% to 13.1%) 730
Gammagard S/D (Occasional) 734
Gantrisin Pediatric Suspension 2638
Gemzar for Injection (Common) 1820
Geodon Capsules (Frequent) 2520
Hemofil M (Extremely rare) 737
▲ Herceptin I.V. (32%) 1199
Human Albumin Grifols 25% 1706
▲ Hycamtin for Injection (69%) 1459
Imitrex Injection (Infrequent) 1465
Imitrex Nasal Spray (Infrequent) 1470
▲ Imitrex Tablets (2% to 3%) 1474
▲ Intron A for Injection (Up to 54%) 2859
Invanz for Injection (Greater than 0.1%) 2029
Ionsys Transdermal System (.1% to less than 1%) 2410
Ixempra Kit for Injection 915
Kaletra (Up to 2%) 452
Lamictal (Infrequent) 1488
Lescol Capsules (Rare) 2268
Lescol XL Tablets 2268
▲ Leukine (19% to 25%) 774
▲ Leustatin Injection (9%) 2384
Lexapro Oral Suspension (Infrequent) 1174
Lexapro Tablets (Infrequent) 1174
Lovaza Capsules 1520
Lyrica Capsules (0.1% to 1%) 2527
Marinol Capsules (Less than 1%) 3163
Marplan Tablets (0% to 2%) 3177
Maxalt Tablets (Infrequent) 2056
Maxalt-MLT Orally Disintegrating Tablets (Infrequent) 2056
Merrem I.V. (Greater than 0.1% to 1%) 684
Mevacor Tablets (Rare) 2063
Mirapex Tablets 857
MS Contin Tablets (Less frequent) 2585
▲ Mylotarg for Injection (64% to 68%) 3212
Nabi-HB 815
Naprosyn Suspension (Less than 1%) 2632
Naprosyn Tablets (Less than 1%) 2632
Niaspan Extended-Release Tablets 480
Noroxin Tablets (Less frequent) 2069
Norvir (Less than 2%) 489
▲ Novantrone for Injection Concentrate (5%) 1100
▲ Ontak Vials (81%) 1079
▲ Orthoclone OKT3 Sterile Solution (59%) 2387
▲ OxyContin Tablets (Between 1% and 5%) 2589
Parnate Tablets 1532
Paxil (2%) 1535
Paxil CR Controlled-Release Tablets (2%) 1544
Pletal Tablets (Less than 2%) 2481
Pneumovax 23 (Common) 2078
Prinivil Tablets (0.3% to 1%) 2087
Prinzide Tablets 2092
▲ Pristiq Extended-Release Tablets (1% to 4%) 3247
▲ ProAmatine Tablets (4.9%) 3032
Profilnine SD Solvent Detergent 1721
▲ Prograf Capsules and Injection (3% to 15%) 622
Prolastin (Occasional) 3099
▲ Proleukin for Injection (52%) 2287
Protonix for Delayed-Release Oral Suspension (Less than 1%) 3254
Protonix Delayed-Release Tablets (Less than 1%) 3254
Protonix I.V. (Less than 1%) 3257
Protopic Ointment (Greater than or equal to 1%) 628
Provigil Tablets (1%) 977
Prozac Weekly Capsules (Frequent) 1852
Prozac Pulvules and Liquid (Frequent) 1852
▲ Raptiva for Injection (13%) 1218
Recombinate (Extremely rare) 738
Recombivax HB (Less than 1%) 2107
ReFacto Vials 3269
Refludan for Injection (Uncommon) 795
▲ Relenza Inhalation Powder (5% to 9%) 1556
Remeron Tablets (Infrequent) 2924
RemeronSolTab Tablets (Infrequent) 2927
Retrovir Capsules 1574
Retrovir IV Infusion 1579
Retrovir 1574
Rilutek Tablets (Infrequent) 2771
▲ Rituxan I.V. (3% to 33%) 1223
Rocephin Injectable Vials, ADD-Vantage, Galaxy, Bulk (Less than 1%) 2642
▲ Salagen Tablets (3% to 15%) 1082
▲ Suboxone Tablets (6% to 7.5%) 2601
▲ Subutex Tablets (6% to 7.8%) 2601
Sular Extended Release Tablets (Less than or equal to 1%) 2975
▲ Sutent Capsules (1% to 11%) 2540
Symbyax Capsules (Frequent) 1871
▲ Targretin Capsules (9.5% to 13.2%) 1084
Tasigna Capsules (0.1% to 1%) 2316
Taxotere Injection Concentrate 2773
Tessalon Capsules 1183
Tessalon Perles 1183
Thyrogen for Injection (1%) 1244
▲ Tice BCG (9%) 2936
Timentin ADD-Vantage 1606
Timentin Injection Galaxy Container 1609
Timentin IV Infusion 1603
Timentin Pharmacy Bulk Package 1613
▲ Torisel Injection (1% to 8%) 3272
▲ Treanda for Injection (0% to 6%) 983
▲ Trizivir Tablets (20%) 1622
Tygacil for Injection (0.2% to less than 2%) 3276
Varivax (Greater than or equal to 1%) 2133
Vectibix 597
▲ Venlafaxine Hydrochloride Tablets (2.2% to 6.8%) 2199
Viadur Implant (Less than 2%) 802
▲ Voltaren Ophthalmic Solution (Less than or equal to 3%) 2336
Vytorin 10/10 Tablets 2149
Vytorin 10/10 Tablets 2939
Vytorin 10/20 Tablets 2149
Vytorin 10/20 Tablets 2939
Vytorin 10/40 Tablets 2149
Vytorin 10/40 Tablets 2939
Vytorin 10/80 Tablets 2149
Vytorin 10/80 Tablets 2939
Wellbutrin Tablets (1.2%) 1648
Wellbutrin SR Sustained-Release Tablets (Infrequent) 1653
Wellbutrin XL Extended-Release Tablets (Infrequent) 1659
WinRho SDF (Less than 2%) 741
Xopenex Inhalation Solution (Less than 2%) 3001
Xopenex Inhalation Solution Concentrate (Less than 2%) 3005
Xopenex HFA Inhalation Aerosol (Less than 2%) 3009
▲ Zemplar Capsules (5%) 536
▲ Zemplar Injection (5%) 538
▲ Ziagen (6% to 9 %) 1673
Zocor Tablets (Rare) 2136
▲ Zolinza Capsules (14% to 16.3%) 2142
Zometa for Intravenous Infusion 2341
Zomig Tablets (Infrequent) 694
Zomig Nasal Spray (Infrequent) 689
Zomig-ZMT Tablets (Infrequent) 694
Zyban Sustained-Release Tablets (Infrequent) 1692
Zyprexa Tablets (Infrequent) 1883
Zyprexa ZYDIS Orally Disintegrating Tablets (Infrequent) 1883

Chloasma
Activella Tablets 2347
Angeliq Tablets 751
Climara Transdermal System 763
Climara Pro Transdermal System 768
Divigel 3167
Enjuvia Tablets 1029
Estratest Tablets 3043
Estratest H.S. Tablets 3043
Mircette Tablets 1034
NuvaRing 2897
Ortho-Cyclen Tablets 2449
Ortho Evra Transdermal System 2437
Ortho Tri-Cyclen Tablets 2449
Ortho Tri-Cyclen Lo Tablets 2458
Premarin Intravenous 3217
Premarin Vaginal Cream 3228
Premphase Tablets 3232
Prempro Tablets 3232
Prometrium Capsules (100 mg, 200 mg) 3047

Chloasma, possibly persistent
Lybrel Tablets 3204
Seasonique Tablets 1046

Chloride retention
Delatestryl Injection 1730
Estratest Tablets 3043
Estratest H.S. Tablets 3043

Choking sensation
Advair Diskus 100/50 1276
Advair Diskus 250/50 1276
Advair Diskus 500/50 1276
Advair HFA 45/21 Inhalation Aerosol 1288
Advair HFA 115/21 Inhalation Aerosol 1288
Advair HFA 230/21 Inhalation Aerosol 1288
Dantrium Intravenous 2582
Evoxac Capsules (Less than 1%) 1013
Mirapex Tablets 857
Risperdal Consta Long-Acting Injection (Infrequent) 1753
Serevent Diskus (Rare) 1594

Cholangiocarcinoma
Selzentry Tablets 2534

Cholangitis
Abelcet Injection 1134
▲ CellCept Capsules (3% to less than 20%) 2622
▲ CellCept Intravenous (3% to less than 20%) 2622
▲ CellCept Oral Suspension (3% to less than 20%) 2622
▲ CellCept Tablets (3% to less than 20%) 2622
Kaletra (Less than 2%) 452
Norvir (Less than 2%) 489
▲ Prograf Capsules and Injection (3% to 15%) 622
Salagen Tablets 1082
Sandostatin LAR Depot 2302
Zonegran Capsules (Rare) 1089

Cholangitis, sclerosing
Doxil Injection (Less than 1%) 2378

Cholecystectomy
Prometrium Capsules (100 mg, 200 mg) (2%) 3047
Zetia Tablets (1.7%) 2951

Cholecystitis
Abelcet Injection 1134
Abilify Injection (Greater than or equal to 1 in 1000 patients and less than 1 in 100 patients) 2466
Abilify Oral Solution (Greater than or equal to 1 in 1000 patients and less than 1 in 100 patients) 2466
Abilify Discmelt Orally Disintegrating Tablets (Greater than or equal to 1 in 1000 patients and less than 1 in 100 patients) 2466
Abilify Tablets (Greater than or equal to 1 in 1000 patients and less than 1 in 100 patients) 2466
Amevive 611
Aricept Tablets 1062
Aricept ODT Tablets 1062
Asacol Delayed-Release Tablets 2579
Campral Tablets (Rare) 1158
Celexa (Rare) 1160
Copaxone for Injection (Infrequent) 3110
Dacogen Injection 1066
Effexor XR Extended-Release Capsules (Rare) 3195
Enbrel for Injection (Infrequent) 569
Evoxac Capsules 1013
Exelon Capsules (Infrequent) 2229
Exelon Oral Solution (Infrequent) 2229
Exelon Patch (Infrequent) 2233
▲ Flovent Diskus 50 mcg (1% to 3%) 1435
Gabitril Tablets (Infrequent) 973
▲ Humira Injection (Less than 5%) 442
Kaletra (Less than 2%) 452
Luvox CR Extended-Release Capsules (Rare) 1759
Lyrica Capsules (0.1% to 1%) 2527
Meridia Capsules 475
Mirapex Tablets 857
Proleukin for Injection 2287
Protonix for Delayed-Release Oral Suspension (Less than 1%) 3254
Protonix Delayed-Release Tablets (Less than 1%) 3254

Protonix I.V. (Less than 1%) 3257
Prozac Weekly Capsules (Rare) 1852
Prozac Pulvules and Liquid (Rare) 1852
Remeron Tablets (Infrequent) 2924
RemeronSolTab Tablets (Infrequent) 2927
Remicade for IV Injection (Greater than or equal to 0.2%) 950
Requip Tablets (Infrequent) 1561
Reyataz Capsules 3299
Rilutek Tablets (Rare) 2771
Salagen Tablets 1082
Tricor Tablets 520
Ultram ER Extended-Release Tablets (0.5% to less than 1%) 2428
Venlafaxine Hydrochloride Tablets (Rare) 2199
Vivitrol 988
Vytorin 10/10 Tablets 2149
Vytorin 10/10 Tablets 2939
Vytorin 10/20 Tablets 2149
Vytorin 10/20 Tablets 2939
Vytorin 10/40 Tablets 2149
Vytorin 10/40 Tablets 2939
Vytorin 10/80 Tablets 2149
Vytorin 10/80 Tablets 2939
Zetia Tablets 2157
Zetia Tablets 2951
Zolinza Capsules 2142
Zonegran Capsules (Rare) 1089

Cholecystitis, acute
Sandostatin LAR Depot 2302

Cholecystitis, chronic
Mirapex Tablets 857

Cholelithiasis
Abilify Injection (Greater than or equal to 1 in 1000 patients and less than 1 in 100 patients) 2466
Abilify Oral Solution (Greater than or equal to 1 in 1000 patients and less than 1 in 100 patients) 2466
Abilify Discmelt Orally Disintegrating Tablets (Greater than or equal to 1 in 1000 patients and less than 1 in 100 patients) 2466
Abilify Tablets (Greater than or equal to 1 in 1000 patients and less than 1 in 100 patients) 2466
Aggrenox Capsules (Less than 1%) 819
Aricept Tablets (Infrequent) 1062
Aricept ODT Tablets (Infrequent) 1062
Celebrex Capsules (Less than 0.1%) 2979
Celexa (Rare) 1160
Effexor XR Extended-Release Capsules (Rare) 3195
Evoxac Capsules (Less than 1%) 1013
Exjade Tablets (0.1% to 1%) 2244
Fenoglide Tablets 2960
Gabitril Tablets (Infrequent) 973
▲ Humira Injection (Less than 5%) 442
Invanz for Injection (Greater than 0.1%) 2029
Lunesta Tablets (Infrequent) 2994
Luvox CR Extended-Release Capsules (Rare) 1759
Lyrica Capsules (0.1% to 1%) 2527
Meridia Capsules 475
Miacalcin Nasal Spray (Less than 1%) 2274
Mirapex Tablets 857
Namenda 1180
Paxil (Rare) 1535
Paxil CR Controlled-Release Tablets (Rare) 1544
Persantine Tablets (Rare) 869
Pletal Tablets (Less than 2%) 2481
Protonix for Delayed-Release Oral Suspension (Less than 1%) 3254
Protonix Delayed-Release Tablets (Less than 1%) 3254
Protonix I.V. (Less than 1%) 3257
Prozac Weekly Capsules (Infrequent) 1852
Prozac Pulvules and Liquid (Infrequent) 1852
Remicade for IV Injection (Greater than or equal to 0.2%) 950
Requip Tablets (Infrequent) 1561
Reyataz Capsules 3299
Salagen Tablets (Less than 1%) 1082
▲ Sandostatin LAR Depot (13.4% to 38.2%) 2302
▲ Somatuline Depot Injection (Greater than 5% to 27%) 3102
Symbyax Capsules (Infrequent) 1871
Tricor Tablets 520
Ultram ER Extended-Release Tablets (0.5% to less than 1%) 2428
Venlafaxine Hydrochloride Tablets (Rare) 2199
Vivitrol 988
Vytorin 10/10 Tablets 2149
Vytorin 10/10 Tablets 2939
Vytorin 10/20 Tablets 2149
Vytorin 10/20 Tablets 2939
Vytorin 10/40 Tablets 2149
Vytorin 10/40 Tablets 2939
Vytorin 10/80 Tablets 2149
Vytorin 10/80 Tablets 2939
Zetia Tablets 2157
Zetia Tablets 2951
Zonegran Capsules (Infrequent) 1089

Cholestasis
Amrix Capsules 966
Avandaryl Tablets 1344
Azor Tablets 1005
Captopril Tablets (Rare) 2182
Ceftin 1380
Clinoril Tablets (Less than 1%) 1962
Exforge Tablets 2238
Fortaz 1450
Malarone Pediatric Tablets 1521
Malarone Tablets 1521
NeoProfen Injection 2496
Noxafil Oral Suspension (Rare) 2889
Omnicef Capsules 497
Omnicef for Oral Suspension 497
Remicade for IV Injection 950
Reyataz Capsules 3299
Rocephin Injectable Vials, ADD-Vantage, Galaxy, Bulk 2642
Rythmol Tablets (0.1%) 1586
Suprax for Oral Suspension 1891
Suprax Tablets 1891
Velcade for Injection 2168
Xyzal Oral Solution 2789
Xyzal Oral Solution 3155
Zinacef for Injection 1678
Zinacef Injection 1678
Zyrtec Chewable Tablets 1920
Zyrtec Syrup 1920
Zyrtec Tablets 1920
Zyrtec-D 12 Hour Extended Release Tablets (Rare) 1923

Cholestasis, intrahepatic
Amoxil Capsules 1305
Amoxil Chewable Tablets 1305
Amoxil Pediatric Drops for Oral Suspension 1305
Amoxil Powder for Oral Suspension 1305
Amoxil Tablets 1305
Cuprimine Capsules (Rare) 1986
Moxatag Tablets 2165

Cholestatic hepatic injury
Axid Capsules 1364
Rythmol Tablets 1586
Uroxatral Tablets 2786

Cholinergic reactions
Evoxac Capsules 1013

Choluria
Xifaxan Tablets (Less than 2%) 2682

Chondrodystrophy
Lyrica Capsules (Rare) 2527
Prozac Weekly Capsules (Rare) 1852
Prozac Pulvules and Liquid (Rare) 1852

Chorea
Activella Tablets 2347
Angeliq Tablets 751
Climara Transdermal System 763
Climara Pro Transdermal System 768
Divigel 3167
Eldepryl Capsules 3052
Enjuvia Tablets 1029
Estratest Tablets 3043
Estratest H.S. Tablets 3043
Klonopin 2639
Mirapex Tablets 857
Phenytek Capsules (Rare) 2192
Premarin Intravenous 3217
Premarin Tablets 3221
Premarin Vaginal Cream 3228
Premphase Tablets 3232
Prempro Tablets 3232

Chorea, exacerbation of
Lybrel Tablets 3204
Premarin Intravenous 3217
Premarin Vaginal Cream 3228
Seasonique Tablets 1046
Yaz Tablets 805

Choreoathetosis
Abilify Injection (Less than 1 in 1000 patients) 2466
Abilify Oral Solution (Less than 1 in 1000 patients) 2466
Abilify Discmelt Orally Disintegrating Tablets (Less than 1 in 1000 patients) 2466
Abilify Tablets (Less than 1 in 1000 patients) 2466
Celexa 1160
Gabitril Tablets (Infrequent) 973
Geodon Capsules (Frequent) 2520
Lexapro Oral Suspension 1174
Lexapro Tablets 1174
Requip Tablets (Infrequent) 1561

Choreoathetotic movements
Lamictal (Rare) 1488
Paxil (Rare) 1535
Paxil CR Controlled-Release Tablets (Rare) 1544
Thioridazine Hydrochloride Tablets 2195
Zyprexa Tablets (1% to 2%) 1883
Zyprexa ZYDIS Orally Disintegrating Tablets (1% to 2%) 1883

Chorioretinitis
Stromectol Tablets 2120

Choroidal detachment, post-filtration procedures
Combigan Ophthalmic Solution 553
Cosopt Sterile Ophthalmic Solution 1969
Timoptic Sterile Ophthalmic Solution 2121
Timoptic in Ocudose 2124
Timoptic-XE Sterile Ophthalmic Gel Forming Solution 2125
Trusopt Sterile Ophthalmic Solution 2128

Choroiditis
Stromectol Tablets 2120

Chromatopsia
Cipro I.V. (1% or less) 2817
Cipro (Less than 1%) 2810
Cipro XR Tablets 2823
Effexor XR Extended-Release Capsules (Rare) 3195
Levitra Tablets (Less than 2%) 2876
Venlafaxine Hydrochloride Tablets (Rare) 2199

Chromaturia
▲ Cyanokit 5g Antidote (100%) 1021
Mirapex Tablets 857
Xyrem Oral Solution (Infrequent) 1766

Chromosomal abnormalities
Mustargen for Injection 2492

Churg-Strauss syndrome
Accolate Tablets (Rare) 669
Advair Diskus 100/50 1276
Advair Diskus 250/50 1276
Advair Diskus 500/50 1276
Flovent Diskus 50 mcg (Rare) 1435
Flovent HFA (Rare) 1440
Singulair 2114

Circulatory collapse
Amerge Tablets 1301
Furosemide Tablets 2186
Mirapex Tablets 857
Requip Tablets (Infrequent) 1561
Zometa for Intravenous Infusion 2341

Circulatory collapse, peripheral
▲ Intron A for Injection (Less than or equal to 5%) 2859

Circulatory depression
Actiq 959
MS Contin Tablets 2585
OxyContin Tablets 2589
Percocet Tablets 1127
Venlafaxine Hydrochloride Tablets (Rare) 2199

Circulatory failure
Ambien Tablets (Rare) 2692
Ambien CR Tablets (Rare) 2696
Remicade for IV Injection (Greater than or equal to 0.2%) 950
Trasylol Injection 799
Zosyn for Injection (1% or less) 3284

Circulatory overload
Albutein 5% 1707
Albutein 25% 1708

Circulatory symptoms, severe reaction
Lybrel Tablets 3204

Cirrhosis, hepatic
(*see under* Cirrhosis of liver)

Cirrhosis of liver
Advicor Tablets (Rare) 402
Campral Tablets (Infrequent) 1158
Fenoglide Tablets 2960
Lescol Capsules (Rare) 2268
Lescol XL Tablets (Rare) 2268
Mevacor Tablets (Rare) 2063
Pentasa Capsules 3030
Remeron Tablets (Rare) 2924
RemeronSolTab Tablets (Rare) 2927
Selzentry Tablets 2534
Tracleer Tablets (Rare) 3289

Clamminess
Eligard 7.5 mg (Less than 2%) 2724
Eligard 22.5 mg (Less than 2%) 2724
▲ Eligard 30 mg (Less than 2% to 4.4%) 2724
Eligard 45 mg (Less than 2%) 2724
Evoxac Capsules (Less than 1%) 1013
Exelon Capsules (Infrequent) 2229
Exelon Oral Solution (Infrequent) 2229
▲ Intron A for Injection (Less than 5%) 2859
Opana Tablets (Less than 1%) 1117
Opana ER Tablets (Less than 1%) 1121
Ultram ER Extended-Release Tablets (0.5% to less than 1%) 2428
Xifaxan Tablets (Less than 2%) 2682

Claudication
Bystolic Tablets 1155
Combigan Ophthalmic Solution 553
Cosopt Sterile Ophthalmic Solution 1969
Namenda (More than one patient) 1180
Tarka Tablets 511
Timoptic Sterile Ophthalmic Solution 2121
Timoptic in Ocudose 2124
Timoptic-XE Sterile Ophthalmic Gel Forming Solution 2125

Claudication, intermittent
(*see under* Charcot's syndrome)

Cleft palate, neonatal
Accutane Capsules 2607

Clitoral hypertrophy
Delatestryl Injection 1730

Clitoris, enlargement
(*see under* Clitoromegaly)

Clitoromegaly
Estratest Tablets 3043
Estratest H.S. Tablets 3043

Clotting disorder, intravascular
Cosmegen for Injection 2485

Clotting time, prolongation
Testim 1% Gel (Less than 1%) 701
Zosyn for Injection 3284

CNS, unresponsiveness, unspecified
Ambien CR Tablets 2696
Cipro I.V. 2817
DepoDur Injection 1095

CNS abnormalities, fetal
Accutane Capsules 2607

CNS depression
Ambien Tablets 2692
Depakote ER Tablets 423
DepoDur Injection 1095
Klonopin (Most frequent) 2639
Lamictal (Infrequent) 1488
Lidoderm Patch 1114
Luvox CR Extended-Release Capsules (Infrequent) 1759
Nembutal Sodium Solution, USP (Less than 1%) 2494
Opana Tablets (Less than 1%) 1117
Opana ER Tablets (Less than 1%) 1121
Prozac Weekly Capsules (Infrequent) 1852
Prozac Pulvules and Liquid (Infrequent) 1852
Rilutek Tablets (Rare) 2771
Skelaxin Tablets 1784
▲ Vesanoid Capsules (3%) 2660

CNS reactions
Attenuvax 1951
Cipro 2810
▲ Intron A for Injection (Less than 5%) 2859

Lanoxin Injection........ 1498
Lanoxin Injection Pediatric........ 1502
Lanoxin Tablets........ 1505
▲ Leukine (11%)........ 774
Noroxin Tablets........ 2069
Orthoclone OKT3 Sterile Solution........ 2387
Stalevo Tablets........ 2309

CNS stimulation
Adipex-P........ 1185
Axert Tablets (Infrequent)........ 2431
Cipro I.V........ 2817
Clarinex-D 24-Hour Extended-Release Tablets........ 2834
Combivent Inhalation Aerosol........ 845
Effexor XR Extended-Release Capsules (Infrequent)........ 3195
Lamictal (Rare)........ 1488
Lidoderm Patch........ 1114
Meridia Capsules (1.5%)........ 475
Noroxin Tablets........ 2069
Paxil (Frequent)........ 1535
Paxil CR Controlled-Release Tablets (Frequent)........ 1544
Proventil HFA Inhalation Aerosol........ 2914
Prozac Weekly Capsules (Infrequent)........ 1852
Prozac Pulvules and Liquid (Infrequent)........ 1852
Venlafaxine Hydrochloride Tablets (Infrequent)........ 2199
Ventolin HFA Inhalation Aerosol........ 1638
Wellbutrin SR Sustained-Release Tablets (1% to 2%)........ 1653
Wellbutrin XL Extended-Release Tablets (1% to 2%)........ 1659
Zyban Sustained-Release Tablets (Infrequent)........ 1692
Zyprexa Tablets (Infrequent)........ 1883
Zyprexa ZYDIS Orally Disintegrating Tablets (Infrequent)........ 1883
Zyrtec-D 12 Hour Extended Release Tablets........ 1923

CNS toxicity
DepoCyt Injection........ 1136

Coagulation defects, neonatal
Phenytek Capsules........ 2192

Coagulation dysfunction
Abelcet Injection........ 1134
AmBisome for Injection (Less common)........ 606
Celexa (Rare)........ 1160
▲ CellCept Capsules (3% to less than 20%)........ 2622
▲ CellCept Intravenous (3% to less than 20%)........ 2622
▲ CellCept Oral Suspension (3% to less than 20%)........ 2622
▲ CellCept Tablets (3% to less than 20%)........ 2622
Depakote ER Tablets........ 423
Elspar for Injection........ 1990
Elspar for Injection........ 2488
Estratest Tablets........ 3043
Estratest H.S. Tablets........ 3043
▲ Leukine (19%)........ 774
Nimotop Capsules (Less than 1%)........ 790
NovoSeven (1%)........ 2367
Omnicef Capsules........ 497
Omnicef for Oral Suspension........ 497
Orthoclone OKT3 Sterile Solution........ 2387
Plavix Tablets (1% to 2.5%)........ 926
Plavix Tablets (1% to 2.5%)........ 2767
Premarin Intravenous........ 3217
Premarin Vaginal Cream........ 3228
▲ Prograf Capsules and Injection (3% to 15%)........ 622
Symbyax Capsules (Rare)........ 1871
▲ Xeloda Tablets (Less than 5%)........ 2662

Coagulation tests, altered results
Zosyn for Injection........ 3284

Coagulopathy
Aggrenox Capsules........ 819
Bayer Aspirin........ 750
Cancidas for Injection........ 1953
Enbrel for Injection........ 569
Ixempra Kit for Injection........ 915
Mycamine for Injection........ 616
NovoSeven........ 2367
NovoSeven RT........ 2370
▲ Oncaspar Injection (Greater than or equal to 2% to 7%)........ 1138
Proleukin for Injection (1%)........ 2287
St. Joseph 81 mg Aspirin Chewable and Enteric Coated Tablets........ 1903

Tice BCG (Less than or equal to 1%)........ 2936

Coccidioidomycosis, disseminated
Remicade for IV Injection........ 950

Cognition, decreased
Ambien Tablets (Infrequent)........ 2692
Ambien CR Tablets (Infrequent)........ 2696

Cognitive dysfunction
Abilify Injection........ 881
Abilify Injection........ 2466
Abilify Oral Solution........ 881
Abilify Oral Solution........ 2466
Abilify Discmelt Orally Disintegrating Tablets........ 881
Abilify Discmelt Orally Disintegrating Tablets........ 2466
Abilify Tablets........ 881
Abilify Tablets........ 2466
Amerge Tablets (Infrequent)........ 1301
Anaprox Tablets (Less than 1%)........ 2632
Anaprox DS Tablets (Less than 1%)........ 2632
EC-Naprosyn Delayed-Release Tablets (Less than 1%)........ 2632
Ixempra Kit for Injection........ 915
Mirapex Tablets........ 857
Myfortic Tablets........ 2276
Naprosyn Suspension (Less than 1%)........ 2632
Naprosyn Tablets (Less than 1%)........ 2632
Orthoclone OKT3 Sterile Solution........ 2387
Prozac Weekly Capsules........ 1852
Symbyax Capsules........ 1871
Zyvox........ 2552

Cogwheel rigidity
Abilify Injection (Greater than or equal to 1 in 1000 patients and less than 1 in 100 patients)........ 881
Abilify Injection (Greater than or equal to 1 in 1000 patients and less than 1 in 100 patients)........ 2466
Abilify Oral Solution (Greater than or equal to 1 in 1000 patients and less than 1 in 100 patients)........ 881
Abilify Oral Solution (Greater than or equal to 1 in 1000 patients and less than 1 in 100 patients)........ 2466
Abilify Discmelt Orally Disintegrating Tablets (Greater than or equal to 1 in 1000 patients and less than 1 in 100 patients)........ 881
Abilify Discmelt Orally Disintegrating Tablets (Greater than or equal to 1 in 1000 patients and less than 1 in 100 patients)........ 2466
Abilify Tablets (Greater than or equal to 1 in 1000 patients and less than 1 in 100 patients)........ 881
Abilify Tablets (Greater than or equal to 1 in 1000 patients and less than 1 in 100 patients)........ 2466
Geodon (Frequent)........ 2520
Invega Extended-Release Tablets........ 1748
Lyrica Capsules (Rare)........ 2527
Paxil........ 1535
Paxil CR Controlled-Release Tablets........ 1544
Symbyax Capsules (Infrequent)........ 1871
Thioridazine Hydrochloride Tablets........ 2195
▲ Zyprexa Tablets (8% to 20%)........ 1883
▲ Zyprexa IntraMuscular (2% to 4%)........ 1883
▲ Zyprexa ZYDIS Orally Disintegrating Tablets (8% to 20%)........ 1883

Cold feeling
Cymbalta Delayed-Release Capsules (Infrequent)........ 1801
▲ Fabrazyme for Intravenous Infusion (10%)........ 1241
Mirapex Tablets........ 857
Requip Tablets (Infrequent)........ 1561
Supprelin LA Implant........ 1731

Cold sensations
Aceon Tablets (2 mg, 4 mg, 8 mg) (0.3% to 1%)........ 3038
Aricept Tablets (Infrequent)........ 1062
Aricept ODT Tablets (Infrequent)........ 1062
▲ Frova Tablets (3%)........ 1111
Imitrex Injection (Rare)........ 1465
▲ Imitrex Nasal Spray (2% to 3%)........ 1470
▲ Imitrex Tablets (2% to 3%)........ 1474
Prograf Capsules and Injection........ 622
Xyrem Oral Solution (Infrequent)........ 1766
Zofran Injection (2%)........ 1682

Cold sore, non-herpetic
▲ Intron A for Injection (Less than 5%)........ 2859
Varivax (Greater than or equal to 1%)........ 2133

Cold symptoms, unspecified
▲ Aerobid/Aerobid-M (15%)........ 1153
▲ Alamast Ophthalmic Solution (10% to 25%)........ 3181
Carac Cream 0.5% (2.3%)........ 2722
▲ Elestat Ophthalmic Solution (Approximately 10%)........ 1741
▲ Geodon Capsules (8%)........ 2520
▲ Pataday Ophthalmic Solution (10%)........ 543
▲ Patanol Ophthalmic Solution (Less than 5%)........ 546
Paxil........ 1535
Paxil CR Controlled-Release Tablets........ 1544
Prinivil Tablets (1.1%)........ 2087
▲ Sandostatin Injection (1% to 4%)........ 2300
▲ Trizivir Tablets (Greater than or equal to 5%)........ 1622

Cold/flu syndrome
▲ Travatan Z Ophthalmic Solution (1% to 5%)........ 547

Coldness of extremities
Combigan Ophthalmic Solution........ 553
Cosopt Sterile Ophthalmic Solution........ 1969
Cymbalta Delayed-Release Capsules (Infrequent)........ 1801
Effexor XR Extended-Release Capsules (Infrequent)........ 3195
Gleevec Tablets (Infrequent)........ 2255
Luvox CR Extended-Release Capsules (Infrequent)........ 1759
Maxalt Tablets (Infrequent)........ 2056
Maxalt-MLT Orally Disintegrating Tablets (Infrequent)........ 2056
Metadate CD Capsules........ 3146
ReoPro Vials (0.2%)........ 1860
Rythmol SR Capsules........ 1590
Strattera Capsules........ 1864
Timoptic Sterile Ophthalmic Solution........ 2121
Timoptic in Ocudose........ 2124
Timoptic-XE Sterile Ophthalmic Gel Forming Solution........ 2125
Toprol-XL Tablets (About 1 of 100 patients)........ 666
Treximet Tablets (Rare)........ 1616
Xyrem Oral Solution (Infrequent)........ 1766

Colds, susceptibility
▲ Betimol Ophthalmic Solution (1% to 5%)........ 3181
Combigan Ophthalmic Solution (0.1% to 0.2%)........ 553
Prinzide Tablets (0.3% to 1%)........ 2092

Colic
Prevnar........ 3241

Colic, biliary
Mirapex Tablets........ 857
Treximet Tablets (Rare)........ 1616

Colitis
Accutane Capsules........ 2607
Actonel with Calcium Tablets (0.8% to 2.5%)........ 2574
Alimta for Injection (Rare)........ 1786
Anaprox Tablets (Less than 1%)........ 2632
Anaprox DS Tablets (Less than 1%)........ 2632
▲ Avastin IV (1% to 6%)........ 1192
Azilect Tablets (Infrequent)........ 3106
Benzaclin Topical Gel........ 2721
Biaxin/Biaxin XL........ 411
Bicillin C-R Injectable Suspension........ 1775
Campral Tablets (Rare)........ 1158
Canasa Rectal Suppositories (1.2%)........ 705
Celebrex Capsules (Less than 0.1%)........ 2979
Celexa (Rare)........ 1160
CellCept Capsules........ 2622
CellCept Intravenous........ 2622
CellCept Oral Suspension........ 2622
CellCept Tablets........ 2622
Clinoril Tablets (Less than 1%)........ 1962
Copaxone for Injection (Infrequent)........ 3110
Doxil Injection (Less than 1%)........ 2378
Duac Topical Gel........ 3054
EC-Naprosyn Delayed-Release Tablets (Less than 1%)........ 2632
Effexor XR Extended-Release Capsules (Infrequent)........ 3195
Eligard 7.5 mg (2.5%)........ 2724
Eligard 22.5 mg........ 2724
Eligard 30 mg........ 2724
Eligard 45 mg........ 2724
Elmiron Capsules (Less than or equal to 1%)........ 2435
▲ Eloxatin for Injection (2% to less than 5%)........ 2731
Emsam Transdermal System (Infrequent)........ 905
Evoclin Foam, 1% (Rarely)........ 3056
Exelon Capsules (Infrequent)........ 2229
Exelon Oral Solution (Infrequent)........ 2229
Exforge Tablets (Greater than or equal to 0.2%)........ 2238
Fortaz........ 1450
Gleevec Tablets (Rare)........ 2255
▲ Imitrex Nasal Spray (2% to 3%)........ 1470
Imitrex Tablets........ 1474
Invanz for Injection (1.7%)........ 2029
Ixempra Kit for Injection........ 915
Lipitor Tablets (Less than 2%)........ 2501
Lovaza Capsules........ 1520
Lunesta Tablets (Rare)........ 2994
Luvox CR Extended-Release Capsules (Infrequent)........ 1759
Lybrel Tablets........ 3204
Lyrica Capsules (0.1% to 1%)........ 2527
Mirapex Tablets........ 857
Mircette Tablets........ 1034
Mobic Oral Suspension (Less than 2%)........ 863
Mobic Tablets (Less than 2%)........ 863
Myfortic Tablets........ 2276
Namenda........ 1180
Naprosyn Suspension (Less than 1%)........ 2632
Naprosyn Tablets (Less than 1%)........ 2632
Norvir (Less than 2%)........ 489
NuvaRing........ 2897
Ortho-Cyclen Tablets........ 2449
Ortho Evra Transdermal System........ 2437
Ortho Tri-Cyclen Tablets........ 2449
Ortho Tri-Cyclen Lo Tablets........ 2458
Paxil (Rare)........ 1535
Paxil CR Controlled-Release Tablets (Rare)........ 1544
Plavix Tablets........ 926
Plavix Tablets........ 2767
Pletal Tablets (Less than 2%)........ 2481
Prevnar........ 3241
Prograf Capsules and Injection........ 622
Proleukin for Injection........ 2287
Protonix for Delayed-Release Oral Suspension (Less than 1%)........ 3254
Protonix Delayed-Release Tablets (Less than 1%)........ 3254
Protonix I.V. (Less than 1%)........ 3257
Protopic Ointment (0.2% to less than 1%)........ 628
Prozac Weekly Capsules (Infrequent)........ 1852
Prozac Pulvules and Liquid (Infrequent)........ 1852
Remeron Tablets (Infrequent)........ 2924
RemeronSolTab Tablets (Infrequent)........ 2927
Requip Tablets (Infrequent)........ 1561
Risperdal Consta Long-Acting Injection (Infrequent)........ 1753
Rocephin Injectable Vials, ADD-Vantage, Galaxy, Bulk (Less than 0.1%)........ 2642
Salagen Tablets (Less than 1%)........ 1082
Seasonique Tablets........ 1046
Sular Extended Release Tablets (Less than or equal to 1%)........ 2975
Suprax for Oral Suspension........ 1891
Suprax Tablets........ 1891
Symbyax Capsules (Infrequent)........ 1871
Targretin Capsules........ 1084
Taxotere Injection Concentrate........ 2773
Treximet Tablets (Rare)........ 1616
Tricor Tablets........ 520
Tygacil for Injection........ 3276
Venlafaxine Hydrochloride Tablets (Infrequent)........ 2199
Vivitrol........ 988
Voltaren Tablets (Rarely)........ 2334
Voltaren-XR Tablets (Rarely)........ 2337
Wellbutrin Tablets (Rare)........ 1648
Wellbutrin SR Sustained-Release Tablets........ 1653
Wellbutrin XL Extended-Release Tablets........ 1659
Yaz Tablets........ 805
Zinacef for Injection........ 1678
Zinacef Injection........ 1678
Zomig Tablets (Rare)........ 694
Zomig Nasal Spray (Rare)........ 689
Zomig-ZMT Tablets (Rare)........ 694
Zonegran Capsules (Rare)........ 1089
Zyban Sustained-Release Tablets........ 1692
Zyvox........ 2552

Colitis, C. difficile-associated
Cipro 2810
Doribax Injection 2400
Levaquin (0.1% to 1%) 2416
Levaquin in 5% Dextrose Injection (0.1% to 1%) 2416
Selzentry Tablets 2534
Suprax for Oral Suspension 1891
Suprax Tablets 1891
Zosyn for Injection 3284

Colitis, hemorrhagic
Amoxil Capsules 1305
Amoxil Chewable Tablets 1305
Amoxil Pediatric Drops for Oral Suspension 1305
Amoxil Powder for Oral Suspension 1305
Amoxil Tablets 1305
Augmentin ES-600 Powder for Oral Suspension 1329
Moxatag Tablets 2165
PegIntron Powder for Injection 2903
Tamiflu Capsules 2649
Tamiflu Oral Suspension 2649

Colitis, ischemic
Combigan Ophthalmic Solution 553
Cosopt Sterile Ophthalmic Solution 1969
Imitrex Injection 1465
Imitrex Nasal Spray 1470
Imitrex Tablets 1474
InnoPran XL Extended Release Capsules 1484
Nadolol Tablets 2191
PegIntron Powder for Injection 2903
Premarin Intravenous 3217
Premarin Tablets 3221
Premarin Vaginal Cream 3228
Taxotere Injection Concentrate 2773
Timoptic-XE Sterile Ophthalmic Gel Forming Solution 2125
Zomig Tablets (Very rare) 694
Zomig Nasal Spray (Very rare) 689
Zomig-ZMT Tablets (Very rare) 694

Colitis, lymphocytic
Plavix Tablets 926
Plavix Tablets 2767

Colitis, neutropenic
Hycamtin for Injection 1459

Colitis, pseudomembranous
Amoxil Capsules 1305
Amoxil Chewable Tablets 1305
Amoxil Pediatric Drops for Oral Suspension 1305
Amoxil Powder for Oral Suspension 1305
Amoxil Tablets 1305
Augmentin 1323
Augmentin Tablets 1327
Augmentin XR Extended Release Tablets 1333
Augmentin ES-600 Powder for Oral Suspension 1329
Avelox (Less than 0.1%) 2803
Benzaclin Topical Gel 2721
Bicillin L-A Injection 1777
Ceftin 1380
Cipro I.V. (1% or less) 2817
Cipro 2810
Cipro XR Tablets 2823
Duac Topical Gel 3054
E.E.S. 433
EryPed 431
Evoclin Foam, 1% (Rarely) 3056
Fortaz (Less frequent) 1450
Gantrisin Pediatric Suspension 2638
Invanz for Injection 2029
Levaquin (0.1% to 1%) 2416
Levaquin in 5% Dextrose Injection (0.1% to 1%) 2416
Moxatag Tablets 2165
Noroxin Tablets 2069
Omnicef Capsules 497
Omnicef for Oral Suspension 497
Primaxin I.M. 2080
Primaxin I.V. (Less than 0.2%) 2083
Rocephin Injectable Vials, ADD-Vantage, Galaxy, Bulk 2642
Suprax for Oral Suspension 1891
Suprax Tablets 1891
Tamiflu Capsules (Less than 1%) 2649
Tamiflu Oral Suspension (Less than 1%) 2649
Timentin ADD-Vantage 1606
Timentin Injection Galaxy Container 1609
Timentin IV Infusion 1603
Timentin Pharmacy Bulk Package 1613
Zinacef for Injection 1678
Zinacef Injection 1678
Zosyn for Injection (One patient) 3284

Colitis, ulcerative
Evoxac Capsules (Less than 1%) 1013
Indocin (Less than 1%) 2024
Mirapex Tablets 857
PegIntron Powder for Injection 2903
Plavix Tablets 926
Plavix Tablets 2767
Protonix for Delayed-Release Oral Suspension (Less than 1%) 3254
Protonix Delayed-Release Tablets (Less than 1%) 3254
Protonix I.V. (Less than 1%) 3257

Colitis, ulcerative, worsening of
Anaprox Tablets (Less than 1%) 2632
Anaprox DS Tablets (Less than 1%) 2632
▲ Asacol Delayed-Release Tablets (3%) 2579
EC-Naprosyn Delayed-Release Tablets (Less than 1%) 2632
Naprosyn Suspension (Less than 1%) 2632
Naprosyn Tablets (Less than 1%) 2632
Pentasa Capsules (0.4%) 3030

Collagen disease, unspecified
▲ Flolan for Injection (82%) 1426
Rythmol SR Capsules 1590

Collapse
Carbatrol Capsules 3019
Kinrix Injection Vaccine 1486
Nitrolingual Pumpspray 2965
▲ Xeloda Tablets (Less than 5%) 2662

Colon, cancer of
Mirapex Tablets 857

Colon, irritable
Aricept Tablets (Infrequent) 1062
Aricept ODT Tablets (Infrequent) 1062

Colon obstruction
VESIcare Tablets 636

Colonic strictures
Creon 5 Capsules 3041
Creon 10 Capsules 3042
Creon 20 Capsules 3042
Ultrase Capsules 718
Ultrase MT Capsules 719

Color perception, disturbed
Cipro (Less than 1%) 2810
Cipro XR Tablets 2823

Color vision, changes
Cialis Tablets (Less than 2%) 1792
Levitra Tablets (Less than 2%) 2876

Coma
Aciphex Tablets 1053
Aggrenox Capsules (Less than 1%) 819
AmBisome for Injection (Less common) 606
Anaprox Tablets (Less than 1%) 2632
Anaprox DS Tablets (Less than 1%) 2632
Arranon Injection (1%) 1319
▲ Avinza Capsules (Less than 5%) 1772
Bayer Aspirin 750
Bicillin C-R Injectable Suspension 1775
Bicillin L-A Injection 1777
Busulfex Injection (One patient) 2477
Celexa 1160
Copaxone for Injection (Infrequent) 3110
Depakote ER Tablets 423
EC-Naprosyn Delayed-Release Tablets (Less than 1%) 2632
Effexor XR Extended-Release Capsules 3195
Elspar for Injection 1990
Elspar for Injection 2488
Evoxac Capsules (Less than 1%) 1013
Flebogamma 5% 1715
Flebogamma 5% DIF 1718
Fortaz 1450
Gabitril Tablets (Infrequent) 973
Gammagard Liquid 730
Gammagard S/D (Rare) 734
Gamunex (Rare) 3094
▲ Gliadel Wafer (1% to 4%) 1076
Indocin Capsules (Less than 1%) 2024
Indocin I.V. (Less than 1%) 2489
Indocin (Less than 1%) 2024
▲ Intron A for Injection (Less than 5%) 2859
Klonopin 2639
Lexapro Oral Suspension 1174
Lexapro Tablets 1174
Luvox CR Extended-Release Capsules (Rare) 1759
Lyrica Capsules (Rare) 2527
Marplan Tablets 3177
Mirapex Tablets 857
Namenda 1180
Naprosyn Suspension (Less than 1%) 2632
Naprosyn Tablets (Less than 1%) 2632
Orthoclone OKT3 Sterile Solution 2387
Percodan Tablets 1130
PhosLo GelCaps 1184
Pristiq Extended-Release Tablets 3247
Prograf Capsules and Injection 622
Proleukin for Injection (2%) 2287
Prozac Weekly Capsules (Rare) 1852
Prozac Pulvules and Liquid (Rare) 1852
Remeron Tablets 2924
RemeronSolTab Tablets 2927
ReoPro Vials (0.4%) 1860
Requip Tablets (Infrequent) 1561
Rilutek Tablets (Infrequent) 2771
Rythmol Tablets (Less than 1%) 1586
St. Joseph 81 mg Aspirin Chewable and Enteric Coated Tablets 1903
Seromycin Capsules 1864
Stromectol Tablets 2120
Symbyax Capsules (Infrequent) 1871
Treximet Tablets 1616
▲ Trisenox Injection (5%) 986
Valtrex Caplets 1635
Velcade for Injection 2168
▲ Vesanoid Capsules (3%) 2660
Vicoprofen Tablets 533
Voltaren Tablets (Rarely) 2334
Voltaren-XR Tablets (Rarely) 2337
Wellbutrin Tablets 1648
Wellbutrin SR Sustained-Release Tablets 1653
Wellbutrin XL Extended-Release Tablets 1659
Zomig Tablets 694
Zomig Nasal Spray 689
Zomig-ZMT Tablets 694
Zovirax 1690
Zyban Sustained-Release Tablets 1692
Zyprexa Tablets (Rare) 1883
Zyprexa ZYDIS Orally Disintegrating Tablets (Rare) 1883

Coma, hepatic
Daytrana Transdermal Patch 3022
Focalin XR Capsules 2251
Metadate CD Capsules 3146
Prinzide Tablets 2092
▲ Xeloda Tablets (Less than 5%) 2662

Coma, hyperosmolar
Invega Extended-Release Tablets 1748
Proglycem Capsules (Infrequent) 1185
Proglycem Suspension (Infrequent) 1185
Risperdal Consta Long-Acting Injection 1753

Coma, hypoglycemic
Percocet Tablets 1127

Combativeness
Orthoclone OKT3 Sterile Solution 2387
Zosyn for Injection (1% or less) 3284

Complement activation
Visudyne for Injection (Less than 1%) 2332

Complication, catheter related
Velcade for Injection 2168

Complications, anesthesia
▲ NovoSeven RT (4.7%) 2370

Compulsive behaviors
Requip Tablets 1561

Concentration, impaired
Ambien Tablets (Infrequent) 2692
Ambien CR Tablets (Infrequent) 2696
Anaprox Tablets (Less than 1%) 2632
Anaprox DS Tablets (Less than 1%) 2632
Atripla Tablets (Greater than or equal to 2%) 938
Combigan Ophthalmic Solution 553
Coreg Tablets (Greater than 0.1% to 1%) 1387
Coreg CR Extended-Release Capsules (0.1% to less than or equal to 1%) 1393
EC-Naprosyn Delayed-Release Tablets (Less than 1%) 2632
Effexor XR Extended-Release Capsules 3195
Humulin 50/50, 100 Units 1843
Humulin 70/30 Vial 1844
Humulin N Vial 1846
Humulin R 1849
Imitrex Injection (Rare) 1465
Lunesta Tablets (Infrequent) 2994
Naprosyn Suspension (Less than 1%) 2632
Naprosyn Tablets (Less than 1%) 2632
▲ PegIntron Powder for Injection (10%) 2903
▲ Rebetol (5% to 21%) 2917
Risperdal Consta Long-Acting Injection (Infrequent) 1753
Symbyax Capsules 1871
Wellbutrin Tablets 1648
Wellbutrin SR Sustained-Release Tablets 1653
Wellbutrin XL Extended-Release Tablets 1659
Zyrtec Chewable Tablets (Less than 2%) 1920
Zyrtec Syrup (Less than 2%) 1920
Zyrtec Tablets (Less than 2%) 1920
Zyrtec-D 12 Hour Extended Release Tablets (Less than 2%) 1923

Concussion
Requip Tablets (Infrequent) 1561
Xyrem Oral Solution (Infrequent) 1766

Condition aggravated
Denavir Cream 2205

Conduct disorder
▲ Keppra Injection (11.4%) 3137
Keppra Oral Solution 3131
Keppra Tablets 3131

Conduction delay, intraventricular
▲ Rythmol Tablets (1% to 4%) 1586

Conduction disturbances
Aceon Tablets (2 mg, 4 mg, 8 mg) (0.3% to 1%) 3038
Avalide Tablets 892
Avalide Tablets 2713
Avapro Tablets (Less than 1%) 897
Avapro Tablets (Less than 1%) 2718
Catapres-TTS 842
Clorpres Tablets (Rare) 2185
Lanoxin Injection (Among most common) 1498
Lanoxin Injection Pediatric (Among most common) 1502
Lanoxin Tablets (Among most common) 1505
▲ Lexiscan Injection (6% to 26%) 614
Luvox CR Extended-Release Capsules (Infrequent) 1759
Nadolol Tablets (1 of 100 patients) 2191
Paxil (Infrequent) 1535
Paxil CR Controlled-Release Tablets (Infrequent) 1544
Reyataz Capsules 3299
Rythmol SR Capsules (Greater than or equal to 2%) 1590
▲ Sandostatin LAR Depot (9% to 10%) 2302

Condyloma acuminatum
Selzentry Tablets (2.1%) 2534

Confusion
Actimmune (Rare) 1743
▲ Actiq (1% to 6%) 959
Aggrenox Capsules (1.1%) 819
▲ Agrylin Capsules (1% to less than 5%) 3017
▲ Alferon N Injection (One patient to 3%) 1726
Ambien Tablets (Frequent) 2692
Ambien CR Tablets (Frequent) 2696
▲ AmBisome for Injection (8.6% to 12.9%) 606
Amerge Tablets (Rare) 1301
Amoxil Capsules (Rare) 1305
Amoxil Chewable Tablets (Rare) 1305
Amoxil Pediatric Drops for Oral Suspension (Rare) 1305
Amoxil Powder for Oral Suspension (Rare) 1305
Amoxil Tablets (Rare) 1305
Anaprox Tablets (Less than 1%) 2632
Anaprox DS Tablets (Less than 1%) 2632
Angiomax for Injection (Greater than 0.1% to less than 1%) 1933
Anzemet Injection (Infrequently) 2701
Anzemet Tablets (Rare) 2704
Aricept Tablets (2%) 1062
Aricept ODT Tablets (2%) 1062
▲ Arimidex Tablets (2% to 5%) 672
▲ Arixtra Injection (1.2% to 3.1%) 1313
▲ Arranon Injection (0% to 8%) 1319
Asacol Delayed-Release Tablets 2579

Augmentin (Rare) 1323
Augmentin Tablets (Rare) 1327
Augmentin XR Extended Release Tablets (Rare) 1333
Augmentin ES-600 Powder for Oral Suspension (Rare) 1329
Avalide Tablets 892
Avalide Tablets 2713
▲ Avastin IV (1% to 6%) 1192
Avelox (Less than 0.1%) 2803
▲ Avinza Capsules (Less than 5%) 1772
Axid Capsules 1364
Bayer Aspirin 750
Bentyl Capsules 703
Bentyl Injection 703
Bentyl Syrup 703
Bentyl Tablets 703
Betaseron for SC Injection 756
Biaxin/Biaxin XL 411
Bicillin C-R Injectable Suspension 1775
Bicillin L-A Injection 1777
▲ Busulfex Injection (11%) 2477
Campral Tablets (Infrequent) 1158
Cancidas for Injection 1953
Captopril Tablets 2182
Carbatrol Capsules 3019
Cardene I.V. (Rare) 1093
Celexa (Frequent) 1160
▲ CellCept Capsules (3% to less than 20%) 2622
▲ CellCept Intravenous (3% to less than 20%) 2622
▲ CellCept Oral Suspension (3% to less than 20%) 2622
▲ CellCept Tablets (3% to less than 20%) 2622
Cipro I.V. (1% or less) 2817
Cipro 2810
Cipro XR Tablets 2823
Combigan Ophthalmic Solution 553
Concerta Extended-Release Tablets (1.2%) 1925
Copaxone for Injection (2%) 3110
Cosopt Sterile Ophthalmic Solution 1969
Cozaar Tablets (Less than 1%) 1973
Cubicin for Injection (1% to 2%) 995
Cymbalta Delayed-Release Capsules (Infrequent) 1801
▲ Dacogen Injection (12%) 1066
Dantrium Capsules (Less frequent) 2580
Daytrana Transdermal Patch 3022
Demser Capsules 1989
▲ Depakote ER Tablets (Greater than 1% to less than 5%) 423
▲ DepoCyt Injection (4% to 36%) 1136
DepoDur Injection 1095
Didronel Tablets 2583
Diovan HCT Tablets 2216
▲ Doxil Injection (1% to 10%) 2378
▲ Duragesic Transdermal System (10% or more) 2405
Dyazide Capsules 1405
EC-Naprosyn Delayed-Release Tablets (Less than 1%) 2632
Edecrin 698
Effexor XR Extended-Release Capsules (Frequent) 3195
▲ Eldepryl Capsules (3 of 49 patients) 3052
Elspar for Injection 1990
Emend Capsules (Greater than 0.5%) 1992
Emend for Injection (Greater than 0.5%) 1999
Emsam Transdermal System (Infrequent) 905
Enablex Extended-Release Tablets 2225
Equetro Extended-Release Capsules 3174
▲ Erbitux (6% to 15%) 912
Evoxac Capsules (Less than 1%) 1013
▲ Exelon Capsules (8%) 2229
▲ Exelon Oral Solution (8%) 2229
▲ Fentora Tablets (1% to 16%) 968
▲ Flolan for Injection (6%) 1426
Flovent HFA 1440
Flumadine (Less than 0.3%) 1167
Frova Tablets (Infrequent) 1111
▲ Gabitril Tablets (5%) 973
Gengraf Capsules (1% to less than 3%) 435
Geodon Capsules (Frequent) 2520
Gleevec Tablets (Rare) 2255
▲ Gliadel Wafer (10% to 23%) 1076
Gris-PEG Tablets (Occasional) 2507
▲ Humira Injection (Less than 5%) 442
Imitrex Injection (Infrequent) 1465
Imitrex Nasal Spray (Infrequent) 1470
Imitrex Tablets (Infrequent) 1474
Indocin (Less than 1%) 2024
Intelence Tablets (Less than 2%) 3119
Intravenous Sodium Diuril 2490
▲ Intron A for Injection (Up to 12%) 2859
▲ Invanz for Injection (3.3% to 5.1%) 2029
Invega Extended-Release Tablets 1748
Ionsys Transdermal System (.1% to less than 1%) 2410
Kaletra (Less than 2%) 452
Keppra Oral Solution (1% to 2%) 3131
Keppra Tablets (1% to 2%) 3131
Klonopin (1%) 2639
K-Phos Original (Sodium Free) Tablets (Less frequent) 814
K-Phos Neutral Tablets 813
Lamictal (Frequent) 1488
Lanoxin Injection 1498
Lanoxin Injection Pediatric 1502
Lanoxin Tablets 1505
Leukeran Tablets (Rare) 1508
Levaquin (0.1% to 1%) 2416
Levaquin in 5% Dextrose Injection (0.1% to 1%) 2416
Lexapro Oral Suspension (Infrequent) 1174
Lexapro Tablets (Infrequent) 1174
Lidoderm Patch 1114
Lortab 5/500 Tablets 3143
Lortab 7.5/500 Tablets 3144
Lortab 10/500 Tablets 3144
Lovenox Injection (2.2%) 2756
▲ Lunesta Tablets (0% to 3%) 2994
Lupron Depot 3.75 mg 462
▲ Lyrica Capsules (1% to 10%) 2527
Marinol Capsules (Greater than 1%) 3163
Maxair Autohaler 1705
Maxalt Tablets (Infrequent) 2056
Maxalt-MLT Orally Disintegrating Tablets (Infrequent) 2056
▲ Megace ES Oral Suspension (1% to 3%) 2499
Meridia Capsules 475
Merrem I.V. (Greater than 0.1% to 1%) 684
▲ Mirapex Tablets (4% to 10%) 857
Mobic Oral Suspension (Less than 2%) 863
Mobic Tablets (Less than 2%) 863
Moxatag Tablets 2165
Myfortic Tablets 2276
Nalfon Capsules (1.4%) 2508
▲ Namenda (6%) 1180
Naprosyn Suspension (Less than 1%) 2632
Naprosyn Tablets (Less than 1%) 2632
Natrecor for Injection (Greater than or equal to 1%) 2977
Nembutal Sodium Solution, USP (Less than 1%) 2494
Neoral Oral Solution (1% to less than 3%) 2280
Neoral Soft Gelatin Capsules (1% to less than 3%) 2280
Neupro Transdermal System 3149
Nexium Delayed-Release Capsules (Less than 1%) 645
Nexium I.V. (Less than 1%) 652
Nexium Delayed-Release Oral Suspension (Less than 1%) 645
Noroxin Tablets 2069
Norvir (0.6% to 0.9%) 489
▲ Ontak Vials (8%) 1079
Opana Tablets (2.7%) 1117
Orthoclone OKT3 Sterile Solution 2387
▲ OxyContin Tablets (Between 1% and 5%) 2589
Parnate Tablets 1532
Paxil (1%) 1535
Paxil CR Controlled-Release Tablets (1%) 1544
Pepcid Tablets (Infrequent) 2075
Percocet Tablets 1127
Percodan Tablets 1130
Phenytek Capsules (Among most common) 2192
PhosLo GelCaps 1184
▲ Photofrin for Injection (8%) 708
Plavix Tablets 926
Plavix Tablets 2767
Primaxin I.M. 2080
Primaxin I.V. (Less than 0.2%) 2083
Prinivil Tablets (0.3% to 1%) 2087
Prinzide Tablets 2092
Pristiq Extended-Release Tablets 3247
ProAmatine Tablets (Less frequent) 3032
▲ Prograf Capsules and Injection (3% to 15%) 622
▲ Proleukin for Injection (1% to 34%) 2287
▲ Prometrium Capsules (100 mg, 200 mg) (Less than 5%) 3047
Protonix for Delayed-Release Oral Suspension (Less than 1%) 3254
Protonix Delayed-Release Tablets (Less than 1%) 3254
Protonix I.V. (Less than 1%) 3257
Provigil Tablets (1%) 977
Prozac Weekly Capsules (Rare) 1852
Prozac Pulvules and Liquid (Frequent) 1852
Relenza Inhalation Powder 1556
Remeron Tablets (2%) 2924
RemeronSolTab Tablets (2%) 2927
Remicade for IV Injection (Greater than or equal to 0.2%) 950
ReoPro Vials (0.6%) 1860
▲ Requip Tablets (Infrequent to 5%) 1561
Retrovir Capsules 1574
Retrovir IV Infusion 1579
Retrovir 1574
Rilutek Tablets (Infrequent) 2771
Risperdal Consta Long-Acting Injection (Infrequent) 1753
Romazicon Injection (Less than 1%) 2646
Rythmol Tablets (Less than 1%) 1586
St. Joseph 81 mg Aspirin Chewable and Enteric Coated Tablets 1903
Salagen Tablets (Less than 1%) 1082
Sandimmune (2% or less) 2296
Seromycin Capsules 1864
Stalevo Tablets 2309
Stromectol Tablets 2120
Sular Extended Release Tablets (Less than or equal to 1%) 2975
Sustiva Capsules (Less than 2%) 930
Sustiva Tablets (Less than 2%) 930
Symbyax Capsules (Infrequent) 1871
Tamiflu Capsules 2649
Tamiflu Oral Suspension 2649
Targretin Capsules 1084
Tarka Tablets 511
Tasigna Capsules 2316
Taxotere Injection Concentrate 2773
▲ Temodar Capsules (1% to 5%) 2931
Tessalon Capsules 1183
Tessalon Perles 1183
Timoptic Sterile Ophthalmic Solution (Less frequent) 2121
Timoptic in Ocudose (Less frequent) 2124
Timoptic-XE Sterile Ophthalmic Gel Forming Solution 2125
Toprol-XL Tablets 666
Transderm Scōp Transdermal Therapeutic System (Infrequent) 2206
▲ Trasylol Injection (4%) 799
Tricor Tablets 520
▲ Trisenox Injection (5%) 986
Ultane Liquid for Inhalation (Less than 1%) 524
▲ Ultram ER Extended-Release Tablets (1% to greater than 5%) 2428
Uroqid-Acid No. 2 Tablets 814
▲ Valcyte Tablets (Less than 5%) 2654
Valium Tablets (Infrequent) 2658
Valtrex Caplets 1635
▲ Vaprisol (0% to 5%) 632
Velcade for Injection 2168
Venlafaxine Hydrochloride Tablets (2%) 2199
▲ Vesanoid Capsules (14%) 2660
Vicodin Tablets 529
Vicodin ES Tablets 530
Vicodin HP Tablets 531
Vicoprofen Tablets (Less than 3%) 533
Voltaren Tablets (Occasionally) 2334
Voltaren-XR Tablets (Occasionally) 2337
▲ Wellbutrin Tablets (8.4%) 1648
Wellbutrin SR Sustained-Release Tablets 1653
▲ Wellbutrin XL Extended-Release Tablets (8%) 1659
▲ Xeloda Tablets (Less than 5%) 2662
▲ Xyrem Oral Solution (Less than 1% to 5.9%) 1766
Zantac 25 EFFERdose Tablets (Rare) 1670
Zantac Injection (Rare) 1666
Zantac Injection Pharmacy Bulk Package (Rare) 1668
Zantac Injection Premixed (Rare) 1666
Zantac (Rare) 1670
▲ Zometa for Intravenous Infusion (7% to 13%) 2341
Zomig Tablets (Infrequent) 694
Zomig Nasal Spray (Infrequent) 689
Zomig-ZMT Tablets (Infrequent) 694
▲ Zonegran Capsules (6%) 1089
Zosyn for Injection (1% or less) 3284
Zovirax 1690
Zyban Sustained-Release Tablets (Infrequent) 1692
▲ Zyprexa Tablets (4%) 1883
Zyprexa IntraMuscular (Infrequent) 1883
▲ Zyprexa ZYDIS Orally Disintegrating Tablets (4%) 1883
Zyrtec Chewable Tablets (Less than 2%) 1920
Zyrtec Syrup (Less than 2%) 1920
Zyrtec Tablets (Less than 2%) 1920
Zyrtec-D 12 Hour Extended Release Tablets (Less than 2%) 1923

Confusion, mental
(*see under* Confusion)

Confusion, nocturnal
Thioridazine Hydrochloride Tablets (Extremely rare) 2195

Confusional state
(*see under* Confusion)

Congelation
Eldepryl Capsules 3052

Congenital anomalies
Depakote ER Tablets 423
Effexor XR Extended-Release Capsules 3195
Follistim AQ Cartridge 2844
Havrix Injection Vaccine 1454
Lescol Capsules (Rare) 2268
Lescol XL Tablets 2268
Mevacor Tablets (Rare) 2063
Premarin Intravenous 3217
Retrovir Capsules 1574
Retrovir IV Infusion 1579
Retrovir 1574
Twinrix Vaccine 1628
Venlafaxine Hydrochloride Tablets 2199
Zocor Tablets 2136

Congenital malformation
Carbatrol Capsules 3019
CellCept Capsules 2622
CellCept Intravenous 2622
CellCept Oral Suspension 2622
CellCept Tablets 2622
Mirapex Tablets 857
Phenytek Capsules 2192
Singulair (Rare) 2114
Valium Tablets 2658

Congestion
▲ Advair HFA 45/21 Inhalation Aerosol (1% to 3%) 1288
▲ Advair HFA 115/21 Inhalation Aerosol (1% to 3%) 1288
▲ Advair HFA 230/21 Inhalation Aerosol (1% to 3%) 1288
Avalide Tablets 892
Avalide Tablets 2713
Avapro Tablets (Less than 1%) 897
Avapro Tablets (Less than 1%) 2718
Tricor Tablets 520

Congestion, nasal
(*see under* Nasal congestion)

Congestion, sinus
▲ Aerobid/Aerobid-M (3% to 9%) 1153
▲ Asmanex Twisthaler (9%) 2797
Cardizem LA Extended Release Tablets (1% to 2%) 421
Coreg CR Extended-Release Capsules (1%) 1393
Diovan HCT Tablets (Greater than 0.2%) 2216
Elidel Cream 1% (0.6% to 1.1%) 2221
Exforge Tablets (Greater than or equal to 0.2%) 2238
Lexapro Oral Suspension (Frequent) 1174
Lexapro Tablets (Frequent) 1174
Mirapex Tablets 857
▲ Myfortic Tablets (3% to less than 20%) 2276
Requip Tablets (Infrequent) 1561
▲ Serevent Diskus (9%) 1594
▲ Ultram ER Extended-Release Tablets (1% to less than 5%) 2428
Vivitrol 988
Xyrem Oral Solution (Frequent) 1766

Congestion, upper respiratory tract
Luvox CR Extended-Release Capsules (Rare) 1759
Mirapex Tablets 857
Xyrem Oral Solution (Infrequent) 1766

Congestive heart failure
ActoPlus Met Tablets 3071
Actos Tablets (1.1%) 3077
Agrylin Capsules 3017

Aminohippurate Sodium "PAH" Injection 1950
Anaprox Tablets (Less than 1%) 2632
Anaprox DS Tablets (Less than 1%) 2632
AndroGel 3159
▲ Aranesp for Injection (5%) 564
Aricept Tablets (Infrequent) 1062
Aricept ODT Tablets (Infrequent) 1062
Avandamet Tablets 1336
Avandaryl Tablets 1344
Avandia Tablets 1351
Avastin IV 1192
Brovana Inhalation Solution (Less than 2%) 2990
Captopril Tablets (2 to 3 of 1000 patients) 2182
Carbatrol Capsules 3019
Cardizem LA Extended Release Tablets (Less than 2%) 421
Catapres Tablets (Rare) 841
Catapres-TTS (0.5% or less) 842
Celebrex Capsules (Less than 0.1%) 2979
▲ CellCept Capsules (3% to less than 20%) 2622
▲ CellCept Intravenous (3% to less than 20%) 2622
▲ CellCept Oral Suspension (3% to less than 20%) 2622
▲ CellCept Tablets (3% to less than 20%) 2622
Cimzia 3127
Clinoril Tablets (Less than 1%) 1962
Clorpres Tablets (Rare) 2185
Dacogen Injection 1066
Digibind for Injection (Few instances) 1403
▲ Doxil Injection (1% to 5%) 2378
Duetact Tablets 3085
EC-Naprosyn Delayed-Release Tablets (Less than 1%) 2632
Effexor XR Extended-Release Capsules (Infrequent) 3195
Enbrel for Injection 569
Equetro Extended-Release Capsules 3174
Gemzar for Injection (Very rare) 1820
▲ Herceptin I.V. (7%) 1199
▲ Humira Injection (Less than 5%) 442
Indocin Capsules (Less than 1%) 2024
Indocin I.V. (Less than 1%) 2489
Indocin (Less than 1%) 2024
InnoPran XL Extended Release Capsules 1484
▲ Lupron Depot 7.5 mg (Less than 5%) 469
Meridia Capsules 475
Micardis Tablets 852
Micardis HCT Tablets 854
Mirapex Tablets 857
Naprosyn Suspension (Less than 1%) 2632
Naprosyn Tablets (Less than 1%) 2632
Nexavar Tablets (0.1% to less than 1%) 784
Nimotop Capsules (Less than 1%) 790
▲ Novantrone for Injection Concentrate (5%) 1100
Paxil (Rare) 1535
Paxil CR Controlled-Release Tablets (Rare) 1544
Pletal Tablets (Less than 2%) 2481
Prevnar 3241
Procrit for Injection 2391
Proglycem Capsules (Frequent) 1185
Proglycem Suspension (Frequent) 1185
Proleukin for Injection 2287
Protonix for Delayed-Release Oral Suspension (Less than 1%) 3254
Protonix Delayed-Release Tablets (Less than 1%) 3254
Protonix I.V. (Less than 1%) 3257
Prozac Weekly Capsules (Infrequent) 1852
Prozac Pulvules and Liquid (Infrequent) 1852
Remicade for IV Injection 950
Retrovir Capsules (0.8%) 1574
Retrovir IV Infusion (1%) 1579
Retrovir (0.8%) 1574
Rilutek Tablets (Infrequent) 2771
▲ Rythmol Tablets (0.9% to 4%) 1586
Rythmol SR Capsules (1% to 2%) 1590
Sandostatin Injection (Less than 1%) 2300
Seromycin Capsules 1864
Sular Extended Release Tablets (Less than or equal to 1%) 2975
Symbyax Capsules (Rare) 1871
Tarka Tablets 511
Taxotere Injection Concentrate (2.3%) 2773
Toprol-XL Tablets (About 1 of 100 patients) 666
Trasylol Injection (1% to 2%) 799
Treximet Tablets (Rare) 1616
▲ Velcade for Injection (5%) 2168
Venlafaxine Hydrochloride Tablets (Rare) 2199
Vivitrol 988
Voltaren Tablets (Occasionally) 2334
Voltaren-XR Tablets (Occasionally) 2337
Zostavax Injection (0.3% to 1.5%) 2145
Zyprexa Tablets (Infrequent) 1883
Zyprexa ZYDIS Orally Disintegrating Tablets (Infrequent) 1883

Congestive heart failure, worsening of

▲ Avandia Tablets (6%) 1351
Rythmol Tablets (0.9%) 1586
Sandostatin LAR Depot 2302
Velcade for Injection 2168

Conjunctival chemosis

Natacyn Antifungal Ophthalmic Suspension (One case) ⊙204

Conjunctival follicles

▲ Cosopt Sterile Ophthalmic Solution (1% to 5%) 1969

Conjunctival hemorrhage

Celebrex Capsules (Greater than or equal to 0.1% to less than 1%) 2979
Combigan Ophthalmic Solution (0.1% to 0.2%) 553
Requip Tablets (Infrequent) 1561

Conjunctival hyperemia

▲ Lumigan Ophthalmic Solution (15% to 45%) 556

Conjunctival injection

▲ Betimol Ophthalmic Solution (More than 5%) 3181
▲ Cosopt Sterile Ophthalmic Solution (1% to 5%) 1969
Fansidar Tablets 2636
Gantrisin Pediatric Suspension 2638
▲ Lotemax Ophthalmic Suspension 0.5% (5% to 15%) ⊙241
Pepcid Tablets (Infrequent) 2075
▲ Visudyne for Injection (1% to 10%) 2332

Conjunctival microhemorrhage

▲ Lucentis Injection (43% to 77%) 1205

Conjunctivitis

Accutane Capsules 2607
Aceon Tablets (2 mg, 4 mg, 8 mg) (0.3% to 1%) 3038
Actiq (1% or greater) 959
▲ Actonel with Calcium Tablets (3.1%) 2574
▲ Advair HFA 45/21 Inhalation Aerosol (1% to 3%) 1288
▲ Advair HFA 115/21 Inhalation Aerosol (1% to 3%) 1288
▲ Advair HFA 230/21 Inhalation Aerosol (1% to 3%) 1288
▲ Alphagan P Ophthalmic Solution (1% to 4%) 549
▲ Alrex Ophthalmic Suspension 0.2% (Less than 5%) ⊙236
▲ Alvesco Inhalation Aerosol (Greater than or equal to 3%) 2985
Ambien Tablets (Rare) 2692
AmBisome for Injection (Less common) 606
Anaprox Tablets (Less than 1%) 2632
Anaprox DS Tablets (Less than 1%) 2632
Aricept Tablets (Infrequent) 1062
Aricept ODT Tablets (Infrequent) 1062
Asacol Delayed-Release Tablets (1% to 2%) 2579
Atacand HCT (0.5% or greater) 642
Atrovent Nasal Spray 0.03% (Less than 2%) 834
Atrovent Nasal Spray 0.06% (Less than 1%) 836
Attenuvax 1951
Avalide Tablets 892
Avalide Tablets 2713
Avapro Tablets (Less than 1%) 897
Avapro Tablets (Less than 1%) 2718
Axert Tablets (Rare) 2431
▲ Azilect Tablets (3%) 3106
Azopt Ophthalmic Suspension (Less than 1%) 540
Betimol Ophthalmic Solution 3181
Carbatrol Capsules 3019
Cardene I.V. (Rare) 1093
Celebrex Capsules (0.1% to 1.9%) 2979
Celexa (Infrequent) 1160
▲ CellCept Capsules (3% to less than 20%) 2622
▲ CellCept Intravenous (3% to less than 20%) 2622
▲ CellCept Oral Suspension (3% to less than 20%) 2622
▲ CellCept Tablets (3% to less than 20%) 2622
Chantix Tablets (Infrequent) 2511
Cialis Tablets (Less than 2%) 1792
Clinoril Tablets (Less than 1 in 100) 1962
Combigan Ophthalmic Solution (0.1% to 0.2%) 553
Comvax 1966
Copaxone for Injection (At least 2%) 3110
▲ Cosopt Sterile Ophthalmic Solution (1% to 5%) 1969
Cozaar Tablets (Less than 1%) 1973
Crinone 4% Gel 992
Crinone 8% Gel 992
▲ Depakote ER Tablets (Greater than 1% to less than 5%) 423
▲ Diclofenac Sodium Ophthalmic Solution (Less than or equal to 5%) ⊙240
▲ Doxil Injection (1% to 10%) 2378
EC-Naprosyn Delayed-Release Tablets (Less than 1%) 2632
Effexor XR Extended-Release Capsules (Infrequent) 3195
▲ Elidel Cream 1% (0.7% to 3%) 2221
Elmiron Capsules (Less than or equal to 1%) 2435
Emend Capsules (Greater than 0.5%) 1992
Emend for Injection (Greater than 0.5%) 1999
Emsam Transdermal System (Infrequent) 905
Engerix-B Vaccine 1409
Equetro Extended-Release Capsules 3174
▲ Erbitux (Less than 1% to 14%) 912
▲ Evoxac Capsules (4.3%) 1013
Exelon Capsules (Infrequent) 2229
Exelon Oral Solution (Infrequent) 2229
Exforge Tablets (Greater than 0.1% to less than 1%) 2238
Flonase Nasal Spray 1431
▲ Flovent Diskus 50 mcg (1% to 3%) 1435
Fluarix Vaccine 1446
Flulaval Injection Vaccine 1448
FML Ophthalmic Ointment (Occasional) ⊙223
FML Ophthalmic Suspension (Occasional) ⊙224
FML Forte Ophthalmic Suspension (Occasional) ⊙222
Frova Tablets (Infrequent) 1111
Gabitril Tablets (1% or more) 973
Gengraf Capsules (1% to less than 3%) 435
Geodon Capsules (Infrequent) 2520
Gleevec Tablets (Less common) 2255
Imitrex Injection 1465
Imitrex Nasal Spray 1470
▲ Indapamide Tablets (Less than 5%) 2188
▲ Intron A for Injection (Less than 5%) 2859
▲ Keppra Oral Solution (3%) 3131
▲ Keppra Tablets (3%) 3131
Lamictal (Infrequent) 1488
Levitra Tablets (Less than 2%) 2876
Lexapro Oral Suspension (Infrequent) 1174
Lexapro Tablets (Infrequent) 1174
▲ Lotemax Ophthalmic Suspension 0.5% (Less than 5%) ⊙241
Lunesta Tablets (Infrequent) 2994
▲ Lupron Depot 3.75 mg (Less than 5%) 462
▲ Lupron Depot–3 Month 11.25 mg (Less than 5%) 462
Luvox CR Extended-Release Capsules (Infrequent) 1759
Luxíq Foam (One patient) 3058
Lyrica Capsules (Greater than or equal to 1%) 2527
Marinol Capsules (0.3% to 1%) 3163
Meruvax II 2061
▲ Miacalcin Nasal Spray (1% to 3%) 2274
Micardis Tablets (More than 0.3%) 852
Micardis HCT Tablets 854
Mirapex Tablets (1% or more) 857
M-M-R II 2054
Mobic Oral Suspension (Less than 2%) 863
Mobic Tablets (Less than 2%) 863
Mumpsvax 2068
Namenda (Frequent) 1180
Naprosyn Suspension (Less than 1%) 2632
Naprosyn Tablets (Less than 1%) 2632
Nasonex Nasal Spray (Greater than or equal to 2%) 2883
Neoral Oral Solution (1% to less than 3%) 2280
Neoral Soft Gelatin Capsules (1% to less than 3%) 2280
Nexium Delayed-Release Capsules (Less than 1%) 645
Nexium I.V. (Less than 1%) 652
Nexium Delayed-Release Oral Suspension (Less than 1%) 645
▲ Novantrone for Injection Concentrate (5%) 1100
Omnicef Capsules 497
Omnicef for Oral Suspension 497
OptiPranolol Metipranolol Ophthalmic Solution 0.3% (A small number of patients) ⊙245
Orthoclone OKT3 Sterile Solution 2387
▲ Pataday Ophthalmic Solution (Less than or equal to 5%) 543
Paxil (Infrequent) 1535
Paxil CR Controlled-Release Tablets (Infrequent) 1544
▲ PegIntron Powder for Injection (4%) 2903
Pentasa Capsules (Less than 1%) 3030
Plavix Tablets (1% to 2.5%) 926
Plavix Tablets (1% to 2.5%) 2767
Pletal Tablets (Less than 2%) 2481
Pred Forte Ophthalmic Suspension (Occasional) ⊙227
Pred Mild Ophthalmic Suspension (Occasional) ⊙230
Prevnar 3241
▲ Protopic Ointment (2% to 4%) 628
Provigil Tablets (Greater than or equal to 1%) 977
Prozac Weekly Capsules (Frequent) 1852
Prozac Pulvules and Liquid (Infrequent) 1852
▲ Pulmozyme Inhalation Solution (1% to 5%) 1217
▲ Rebetol (4% to 5%) 2917
Reclast Injection 2291
Recombivax HB 2107
Remeron Tablets (Infrequent) 2924
RemeronSolTab Tablets (Infrequent) 2927
Requip Tablets (Infrequent) 1561
Reyataz Capsules 3299
Risperdal Consta Long-Acting Injection (Infrequent) 1753
Rocaltrol Capsules 1150
Rocaltrol Oral Solution 1150
Salagen Tablets (Less than 1% to 2%) 1082
Sandimmune (2% or less) 2296
Serevent Diskus (1% to less than 3%) 1594
▲ Simulect for Injection (3% to 10%) 2306
Singulair (Greater than or equal to 2%) 2114
▲ Soriatane Capsules (1% to 10%) 3062
▲ Strattera Capsules (1% to 3%) 1864
Stromectol Tablets 2120
Sular Extended Release Tablets (Less than or equal to 1%) 2975
Symbyax Capsules (Infrequent) 1871
Synagis Intramuscular Solution (More than 1%) 1948
Tamiflu Capsules (1%) 2649
Tamiflu Oral Suspension (1%) 2649
▲ Tarceva Tablets (0% to 12%) 1228
Targretin Capsules 1084
Tasigna Capsules (0.1% to 1%) 2316
▲ Taxotere Injection Concentrate (0% to 5.1%) 2773
Teveten Tablets (Less than 1%) 515
Teveten HCT Tablets (Less than 1%) 517
Timoptic Sterile Ophthalmic Solution (Less frequent) 2121
Timoptic in Ocudose (Less frequent) 2124
▲ Timoptic-XE Sterile Ophthalmic Gel Forming Solution (1% to 5%) 2125
▲ Torisel Injection (7%) 3272
▲ Travatan Z Ophthalmic Solution (1% to 4%) 547
Treximet Tablets (Infrequent) 1616
Tricor Tablets 520
Trizivir Tablets 1622
▲ Trusopt Sterile Ophthalmic Solution (Approximately 1% to 5%) 2128
Twinrix Vaccine 1628

Ultane Liquid for Inhalation (Less than 1%) 524
Vaqta (1.3%) 2130
▲ Vectibix (4%) 597
Venlafaxine Hydrochloride Tablets (Infrequent) 2199
▲ Vigamox Ophthalmic Solution (1% to 6%) 548
Viramune Oral Suspension 873
Viramune Tablets 873
▲ Visudyne for Injection (1% to 10%) 2332
Vivitrol 988
▲ Voltaren Ophthalmic Solution (Less than or equal to 5%) 2336
Voltaren Tablets (Rarely) 2334
Voltaren-XR Tablets (Rarely) 2337
▲ Xeloda Tablets (Less than 5%) 2662
Xyrem Oral Solution (Infrequent) 1766
Ziagen 1673
Zomig Tablets (Rare) 694
Zomig Nasal Spray (Rare) 689
Zomig-ZMT Tablets (Rare) 694
Zonegran Capsules (Infrequent) 1089
Zyprexa Tablets 1883
Zyprexa ZYDIS Orally Disintegrating Tablets 1883
Zyrtec Chewable Tablets (Less than 2%) 1920
Zyrtec Syrup (Less than 2%) 1920
Zyrtec Tablets (Less than 2%) 1920
Zyrtec-D 12 Hour Extended Release Tablets (Less than 2%) 1923

Conjunctivitis, allergic
▲ Alphagan P Ophthalmic Solution (Approximately 10% to 20%) 549
▲ Combigan Ophthalmic Solution (5% to 15%) 553
▲ Lumigan Ophthalmic Solution (1% to 3%) 556

Conjunctivitis, calcific
Calcijex Injection 419

Conjunctivitis, chemical
Ofloxacin Ophthalmic Solution 0.3% ⊙ 243

Conjunctivitis, follicular
▲ Alphagan P Ophthalmic Solution (Approximately 5% to 9%) 549
Combigan Ophthalmic Solution (0.1% to 0.2%) 553

Conjunctivitis, hemorrhagic
▲ Alphagan P Ophthalmic Solution (1% to 4%) 549

Connective tissue symptoms, unspecified
▲ Cancidas for Injection (11.3% to 14.3%) 1953
▲ Mycamine for Injection (18.8%) 616
▲ Selzentry Tablets (8.7%) 2534
▲ Somatuline Depot Injection (7% to 10%) 3102

Consciousness, decreased
▲ Arranon Injection (0% to 6%) 1319
Mirapex Tablets 857
Namenda 1180
Opana Tablets (Less than 1%) 1117
Opana ER Tablets (Less than 1%) 1121
Pentacel 2792
Percocet Tablets 1127
Xyrem Oral Solution (Infrequent) 1766

Consciousness, disorders of
Amerge Tablets (Rare) 1301
Comtan Tablets 2208
Hexalen Capsules 1078
▲ Intron A for Injection (Less than 5%) 2859
Neoral Oral Solution 2280
Neoral Soft Gelatin Capsules 2280
Sandimmune 2296
▲ Selzentry Tablets (3.8%) 2534
Tamiflu Capsules 2649
Tamiflu Oral Suspension 2649
Valtrex Caplets 1635
Zovirax 1690

Consciousness, loss of
Adenocard IV Injection 603
Arranon Injection (1%) 1319
Avelox 2803
Cipro I.V. (1% or less) 2817
Cipro 2810
Cipro XR Tablets 2823
Effexor XR Extended-Release Capsules (Rare) 3195
Erbitux 912
Flebogamma 5% 1715
Flebogamma 5% DIF 1718
Gammagard Liquid 730
Gammagard S/D (Rare) 734
Gamunex (Rare) 3094
Humulin 50/50, 100 Units 1843
Humulin 70/30 Vial 1844
Humulin N Vial 1846
Humulin R 1849
Ketek Tablets 2744
Levaquin 2416
Levaquin in 5% Dextrose Injection 2416
Lidoderm Patch 1114
Mirapex Tablets 857
Namenda 1180
Noroxin Tablets 2069
Omnicef Capsules 497
Omnicef for Oral Suspension 497
Orthoclone OKT3 Sterile Solution 2387
PegIntron Powder for Injection (Less than or equal to 1%) 2903
Requip Tablets (Infrequent) 1561
Tasigna Capsules 2316
Taxotere Injection Concentrate (Rare) 2773
Venlafaxine Hydrochloride Tablets (Rare) 2199
▲ Vesanoid Capsules (3%) 2660
▲ Xeloda Tablets (Less than 5%) 2662

Constipation
▲ Abilify Injection (5% to 11%) 881
▲ Abilify Injection (2% to 11%) 2466
▲ Abilify Oral Solution (5% to 11%) 881
▲ Abilify Oral Solution (2% to 11%) 2466
▲ Abilify Discmelt Orally Disintegrating Tablets (5% to 11%) 881
▲ Abilify Discmelt Orally Disintegrating Tablets (2% to 11%) 2466
▲ Abilify Tablets (5% to 11%) 881
▲ Abilify Tablets (2% to 11%) 2466
Aceon Tablets (2 mg, 4 mg, 8 mg) (0.3% to 1%) 3038
Aciphex Tablets (2%) 1053
▲ Actiq (1% to 4%) 959
▲ Actonel Tablets (6.5% to 12.6%) 2568
▲ Actonel with Calcium Tablets (12.2% to 12.5%) 2574
▲ Adderall XR Capsules (2% to 4%) 3012
Adipex-P 1185
▲ Advair HFA 45/21 Inhalation Aerosol (1% to 3%) 1288
▲ Advair HFA 115/21 Inhalation Aerosol (1% to 3%) 1288
▲ Advair HFA 230/21 Inhalation Aerosol (1% to 3%) 1288
Advicor Tablets 402
▲ Aerobid/Aerobid-M (1% to 3%) 1153
▲ Agrylin Capsules (1% to less than 5%) 3017
Alferon N Injection (One patient) 1726
▲ Alimta for Injection (Up to 44%) 1786
Alinia for Oral Suspension (Less than 1%) 2677
Alinia Tablets (Less than 1%) 2677
▲ Aloxi Injection (5%) 1059
Ambien Tablets (Infrequent to 2%) 2692
Ambien CR Tablets (2%) 2696
AmBisome for Injection (Less common) 606
Amerge Tablets (Infrequent) 1301
Amitiza Capsules (Less than 1%) 3082
Amrix Capsules 966
▲ Anaprox Tablets (3% to 9%) 2632
▲ Anaprox DS Tablets (3% to 9%) 2632
Anzemet Injection (Rare) 2701
Anzemet Tablets 2704
▲ Aranesp for Injection (5% to 18%) 564
Aricept Tablets (Frequent) 1062
Aricept ODT Tablets (Frequent) 1062
▲ Arimidex Tablets (7% to 9%) 672
▲ Arixtra Injection (1.8% to 8.5%) 1313
▲ Arranon Injection (0% to 21%) 1319
▲ Asacol Delayed-Release Tablets (5%) 2579
Atacand HCT 642
Atripla Tablets 938
Atrovent HFA Inhalation Aerosol 839
Atrovent Nasal Spray 0.03% 834
Atrovent Nasal Spray 0.06% 836
Avalide Tablets 892
Avalide Tablets 2713
▲ Avandamet Tablets (5%) 1336
Avapro Tablets (Less than 1%) 897
Avapro Tablets (Less than 1%) 2718
▲ Avastin IV (4%) 1192
Avelox (Greater than or equal to 0.1% to less than 2%) 2803
▲ Avinza Capsules (Greater than 10%) 1772
Axid Capsules (2.5%) 1364
▲ Azilect Tablets (9%) 3106
Bentyl Capsules 703
Bentyl Injection 703
Bentyl Syrup 703
Bentyl Tablets 703
▲ Betaseron for SC Injection (20%) 756
▲ Bexxar (1% to 6%) 1371
▲ Boniva Injection (2.5% to 4%) 2614
▲ Boniva Tablets (2.5% to 4%) 2618
Brovana Inhalation Solution (Less than 2%) 2990
▲ Busulfex Injection (35% to 38%) 2477
Byetta Injection 600
Calcijex Injection 419
Campral Tablets (Frequent) 1158
Cancidas for Injection 1953
Captopril Tablets (About 0.5% to 2%) 2182
Carafate Suspension (2%) 706
Carafate Tablets (2%) 707
Carbatrol Capsules 3019
Cardizem LA Extended Release Tablets (Less than 2%) 421
▲ Catapres Tablets (About 10 in 100 patients) 841
Catapres-TTS (1 of 101 patients) 842
Celebrex Capsules (0.1% to 1.9%) 2979
Celexa (At least 2%) 1160
▲ CellCept Capsules (18.5% to 41.2%) 2622
▲ CellCept Intravenous (18.5% to 41.2%) 2622
▲ CellCept Oral Suspension (18.5% to 41.2%) 2622
▲ CellCept Tablets (18.5% to 41.2%) 2622
▲ Chantix Tablets (Greater than 5% to 8%) 2511
Cipro I.V. (1% or less) 2817
Cipro 2810
Cipro XR Tablets (Less than 1%) 2823
▲ Clinoril Tablets (3% to 9%) 1962
▲ Clolar for Intravenous Infusion (21%) 1239
▲ Clorpres Tablets (About 10%) 2185
Combivent Inhalation Aerosol 845
▲ Comtan Tablets (6%) 2208
Copaxone for Injection (At least 2%) 3110
Cozaar Tablets (Less than 1%) 1973
Creon 5 Capsules (Among most frequent) 3041
Creon 10 Capsules (Among most frequent) 3042
Creon 20 Capsules (Among most frequent) 3042
▲ Crestor Tablets (2.1% to 4.7%) 677
▲ Crinone 8% Gel (27%) 992
▲ Cubicin for Injection (6.2% to 10.8%) 995
▲ Cymbalta Delayed-Release Capsules (5% to 15%) 1801
▲ Dacogen Injection (35%) 1066
Dantrium Capsules (Less frequent) 2580
Demadex Injection (1.8%) 2630
Demadex Tablets (1.8%) 2630
▲ Depakote ER Tablets (Greater than 1% to less than 5%) 423
▲ DepoCyt Injection (7% to 24%) 1136
▲ DepoDur Injection (Greater than 10%) 1095
Dexedrine 1401
Diovan Tablets (Greater than 0.2%) 2212
Diovan HCT Tablets (Less frequent) 2216
Donnatal Extentabs 2507
▲ Doxil Injection (1% to 30.1%) 2378
▲ Duragesic Transdermal System (10% or more) 2405
Dyazide Capsules 1405
▲ DynaCirc CR Controlled Release Tablets (1.2% to 3.8%) 1407
▲ EC-Naprosyn Delayed-Release Tablets (3% to 9%) 2632
▲ Effexor XR Extended-Release Capsules (5% to 10%) 3195
Eldepryl Capsules 3052
▲ Elidel Cream 1% (0% to 3.7%) 2221
Eligard 7.5 mg (Less than 2%) 2724
Eligard 22.5 mg (Less than 2%) 2724
Eligard 30 mg (Less than 2%) 2724
Eligard 45 mg (Less than 2%) 2724
▲ Elitek (20%) 2729
Elmiron Capsules (Less than or equal to 1%) 2435
▲ Eloxatin for Injection (2% to 32%) 2731
▲ Emend Capsules (10.3% to 12.3%) 1992
▲ Emend for Injection (10.3% to 12.3%) 1999
Emsam Transdermal System (Frequent) 905
▲ Enablex Extended-Release Tablets (14.8% to 21.3%) 2225
Engerix-B Vaccine (Less than 1%) 1409
▲ Entereg Capsules (4% to 9.7%) 3293
▲ Epogen for Injection (42% to 43%) 576
▲ Equetro Extended-Release Capsules (5%) 3174
▲ Erbitux (4% to 46%) 912
▲ Evoxac Capsules (1% to 3%) 1013
▲ Exelon Capsules (5%) 2229
▲ Exelon Oral Solution (5%) 2229
Exelon Patch (Frequent) 2233
Exforge Tablets (Greater than or equal to 0.2%) 2238
▲ Faslodex Injection (12%) 682
▲ Femara Tablets (0.1% to 11.3%) 2246
Fenoglide Tablets (2.1%) 2960
▲ Fentora Tablets (1% to 26%) 968
Ferralet 90 Tablets 2175
▲ Flector Patch (3%) 561
▲ Flolan for Injection (4% to 6%) 1426
Flomax Capsules (Infrequent) 848
Flumadine 1167
▲ Follistim AQ Cartridge (5%) 2844
▲ Forteo for Injection (5.4%) 1816
▲ Fosamax (Up to 3.1%) 2005
▲ Fosamax Plus D Tablets (0% to 3.1%) 2013
▲ Fosrenol Chewable Tablets (6% to 14%) 3027
▲ Fosteum Capsules (2.8% to 5.3%) 2963
Frova Tablets (Infrequent) 1111
Furosemide Tablets 2186
Gabitril Tablets (1% or more) 973
▲ Gemzar for Injection (10% to 42%) 1820
Gengraf Capsules (1% to less than 3%) 435
▲ Geodon (9%) 2520
▲ Gleevec Tablets (9% to 16%) 2255
▲ Gliadel Wafer (2% to 19%) 1076
▲ Hycamtin for Injection (Less than 1% to 39%) 1459
Imitrex Nasal Spray (Infrequent) 1470
Imitrex Tablets (Infrequent) 1474
▲ Indapamide Tablets (Less than 5%) 2188
Indocin Capsules (Greater than 1%) 2024
▲ Indocin I.V. (1% to 3%) 2489
Indocin (Greater than 1%) 2024
▲ InnoPran XL Extended Release Capsules (1% to 3%) 1484
Intelence Tablets (Less than 2%) 3119
Intravenous Sodium Diuril 2490
▲ Intron A for Injection (Up to 10%) 2859
▲ Invanz for Injection (2.3% to 4%) 2029
▲ Ionsys Transdermal System (1% to less than 10%) 2410
▲ Ixempra Kit for Injection (16% to greater than or equal to 20%) 915
Kaletra (Less than 2%) 452
▲ Keppra Oral Solution (1% to 3%) 3131
▲ Keppra Tablets (1% to 3%) 3131
Ketek Tablets (Greater than or equal to 0.2% to less than 2%) 2744
Klonopin (2%) 2639
Kogenate FS 746
Kogenate FS with Bio-Set 748
▲ Lamictal (4% to 5%) 1488
▲ Lescol Capsules (3.1%) 2268
Lescol XL Tablets (2.3%) 2268
▲ Letairis Tablets (4%) 1258
▲ Leukine (8%) 774
▲ Leustatin Injection (9%) 2384
▲ Levaquin (3%) 2416
▲ Levaquin in 5% Dextrose Injection (3%) 2416
▲ Lexapro Oral Suspension (3% to 6%) 1174
▲ Lexapro Tablets (3% to 6%) 1174
Lipitor Tablets (Up to 2.5%) 2501
Lortab 5/500 Tablets 3143
Lortab 7.5/500 Tablets 3144
Lortab 10/500 Tablets 3144
Lovaza Capsules 1520
▲ Luvox CR Extended-Release Capsules (4% to 6%) 1759
▲ Lyrica Capsules (1% to 7%) 2527
▲ Marplan Tablets (4% to 7%) 3177
Mavik Tablets (0.3% to 1%) 472
Maxalt Tablets (Infrequent) 2056
Maxalt-MLT Orally Disintegrating Tablets (Infrequent) 2056
▲ Megace ES Oral Suspension (1% to 3%) 2499
▲ Mepron Suspension (3%) 1526
▲ Meridia Capsules (11.5%) 475
▲ Merrem I.V. (1.4% to 7%) 684
▲ Mevacor Tablets (2% to 4.9%) 2063
▲ Miacalcin Nasal Spray (1% to 3%) 2274
Micardis Tablets (More than 0.3%) 852
Micardis HCT Tablets 854
▲ Mirapex Tablets (4% to 10%) 857
Moban Tablets 1116
Mobic Oral Suspension (0.8% to 2.6%) 863
Mobic Tablets (0.8% to 2.6%) 863
MS Contin Tablets (Less frequent to among most frequent) 2585
▲ Mycamine for Injection (11.1% to 30.4%) 616
▲ Myfortic Tablets (3% to 38%) 2276

▲ Mylotarg for Injection (23%) 3212
Nadolol Tablets (1 to 5 of 1000 patients).. 2191
▲ Nalfon Capsules (7%) 2508
▲ Namenda (5%) 1180
▲ Naprosyn Suspension (3% to 9%) 2632
▲ Naprosyn Tablets (3% to 9%) 2632
Nembutal Sodium Solution, USP (Less than 1%)............................... 2494
Neoral Oral Solution (1% to less than 3%).. 2280
Neoral Soft Gelatin Capsules (1% to less than 3%)........................... 2280
▲ Neulasta Injection (15% to 72%) 587
▲ Neupogen for Injection (5%) 589
▲ Neupro Transdermal System (5%) 3149
▲ Nexavar Tablets (14% to 15%) 784
Nexium Delayed-Release Capsules (Greater than or equal to 1%)....... 645
Nexium I.V. (Greater than or equal to 1%).. 652
Nexium Delayed-Release Oral Suspension (Greater than or equal to 1%) 645
Noroxin Tablets (0.3% to 1%) 2069
Norvir (0% to 0.7%) 489
▲ Novantrone for Injection Concentrate (7% to16%) 1100
▲ Noxafil Oral Suspension (Less than 1% to 21%) 2889
Omnicef Capsules (0.3%) 497
Omnicef for Oral Suspension (0.3%) 497
▲ Ontak Vials (9%) 1079
▲ Opana Tablets (4.1%) 1117
▲ Opana ER Tablets (5.7% to 27.6%).. 1121
▲ OxyContin Tablets (23%) 2589
OxyIR Capsules 2593
Parnate Tablets 1532
▲ Paxil (1.1% to 16%) 1535
▲ Paxil CR Controlled-Release Tablets (1.1% to 16%) 1544
PegIntron Powder for Injection (1%) 2903
Pentasa Capsules (Less than 1%) 3030
Pepcid Tablets (1.2%) 2075
Percocet Tablets 1127
Percodan Tablets 1130
Phenytek Capsules 2192
PhosLo GelCaps 1184
▲ Photofrin for Injection (17% to 24%) 708
Plavix Tablets (1% to 2.5%) 926
Plavix Tablets (1% to 2.5%) 2767
▲ Prandin Tablets (2% to 3%) 2971
Prinivil Tablets (0.3% to 1%) 2087
Prinzide Tablets (0.3% to 1%) 2092
▲ Pristiq Extended-Release Tablets (5% to 14%) 3247
▲ Procrit for Injection (42% to 53%) ... 2391
▲ Prograf Capsules and Injection (23% to 35%) 622
▲ Prometrium Capsules (100 mg, 200 mg) (Less than 5%) 3047
Protonix for Delayed-Release Oral Suspension (Greater than or equal to 1%) 3254
Protonix Delayed-Release Tablets (Greater than or equal to 1%) 3254
Protonix I.V. (Greater than or equal to 1%) 3257
Protopic Ointment (Greater than or equal to 1%) 628
Provigil Tablets (2%) 977
▲ Prozac Weekly Capsules (5%) 1852
▲ Prozac Pulvules and Liquid (5%) 1852
▲ Rapamune (Greater than or equal to 30% to 38%) 3260
▲ Rebetol (5%) 2917
▲ Reclast Injection (6%) 2291
Recombivax HB 2107
ReFacto Vials 3269
▲ Remeron Tablets (13%) 2924
▲ RemeronSolTab Tablets (13%) 2927
Remicade for IV Injection (Greater than or equal to 0.2%) 950
ReoPro Vials (0.3%) 1860
▲ Requip Tablets (6%) 1561
▲ Requip XL Tablets (Greater than or equal to 5%) 1568
▲ Retrovir Capsules (6.4%) 1574
▲ Retrovir IV Infusion (6.4%) 1579
▲ Retrovir (6.4%) 1574
Rilutek Tablets (More than 2%) 2771
▲ Risperdal Consta Long-Acting Injection (5% to 7%) 1753
Rocaltrol Capsules 1150
Rocaltrol Oral Solution 1150
▲ Rythmol Tablets (4% to 8%) 1586
▲ Rythmol SR Capsules (8% to 14%) .. 1590
Salagen Tablets (1% to 2%) 1082
▲ Sanctura XR Capsules (8.5% to 9%) 557
Sandimmune (Rare) 2296
▲ Sandostatin Injection (Less than 10%) 2300
▲ Sandostatin LAR Depot (15% to 21%) 2302
▲ Selzentry Tablets (5.4%) 2534
Simcor Tablets (2.3%) 502
▲ Simulect for Injection (Greater than or equal to 10%)................... 2306
▲ Somatuline Depot Injection (Greater than 5 to 8%) 3102
Soriatane Capsules (Less than 1%).. 3062
▲ Spiriva HandiHaler (1% to 4%) 870
▲ Stalevo Tablets (6%) 2309
▲ Strattera Capsules (0.1% to 9%) 1864
Stromectol Tablets (0.9%)................ 2120
▲ Suboxone Tablets (11% to 12.1%) .. 2601
▲ Subutex Tablets (7.8% to 11%) 2601
Sustiva Capsules 930
Sustiva Tablets 930
▲ Sutent Capsules (0% to 34%) 2540
▲ Tarceva Tablets (1% to 31%) 1228
Targretin Capsules 1084
▲ Tarka Tablets (3.3%) 511
▲ Tasigna Capsules (Greater than 10% to 21%) 2316
▲ Taxotere Injection Concentrate (0.6% to 33.9%) 2773
▲ Temodar Capsules (1% to 33%) 2931
Tessalon Capsules 1183
Tessalon Perles 1183
Teveten Tablets (Less than 1%) 515
Teveten HCT Tablets (Less than 1%) 517
Thioridazine Hydrochloride Tablets .. 2195
Thiothixene Capsules (Infrequently) .. 2197
Toprol-XL Tablets (About 1 of 100 patients) 666
▲ Torisel Injection (0% to 20%) 3272
▲ Trasylol Injection (4%) 799
Treanda for Injection 983
Treximet Tablets (Infrequent) 1616
Tricor Tablets (2.1%) 520
▲ Trisenox Injection (28%) 986
Tussionex Pennkinetic Extended-Release Suspension 3154
Twinrix Vaccine (Less than 1%) 1628
Tygacil for Injection (2.8%) 3276
Tylenol with Codeine Tablets 2427
▲ Ultram ER Extended-Release Tablets (12.2% to 29.7%) 2428
Uroxatral Tablets (1% to 2%) 2786
▲ Valcyte Tablets (Less than 5%) 2654
Valium Tablets (Infrequent) 2658
▲ Valtrex Caplets (Less than 1% to 4%) 1635
▲ Vantas (3.5%) 1737
▲ Vaprisol (4.9% to 8%) 632
Varivax (Greater than or equal to 1%) 2133
▲ Vectibix (3% to 21%) 597
▲ Velcade for Injection (37% to 42%) 2168
▲ Venlafaxine Hydrochloride Tablets (15%) 2199
▲ Vesanoid Capsules (17%) 2660
▲ VESIcare Tablets (5.4% to 13.4%) ... 636
Viadur Implant (Less than 2%) 802
Vicodin Tablets 529
Vicodin ES Tablets 530
Vicodin HP Tablets 531
▲ Vicoprofen Tablets (22%) 533
▲ Visudyne for Injection (1% to 10%) .. 2332
Vivitrol 988
▲ Voltaren Tablets (1% to 10%) 2334
▲ Voltaren-XR Tablets (1% to 10%) 2337
Vytorin 10/10 Tablets 2149
Vytorin 10/10 Tablets 2939
Vytorin 10/20 Tablets 2149
Vytorin 10/20 Tablets 2939
Vytorin 10/40 Tablets 2149
Vytorin 10/40 Tablets 2939
Vytorin 10/80 Tablets 2149
Vytorin 10/80 Tablets 2939
Vyvanse Capsules 3033
▲ WelChol Tablets (8.7% to 11%) 1015
▲ Wellbutrin Tablets (26%) 1648
▲ Wellbutrin SR Sustained-Release Tablets (5% to 10%) 1653
▲ Wellbutrin XL Extended-Release Tablets (5% to 10%) 1659
▲ Xeloda Tablets (1% to 14%) 2662
▲ Xifaxan Tablets (3.8%) 2682
Xyrem Oral Solution (Frequent) 1766
Zantac 25 EFFERdose Tablets 1670
Zantac Injection 1666
Zantac Injection Pharmacy Bulk Package (Frequent) 1668
Zantac Injection Premixed 1666
Zantac 1670
Zemplar Injection 538
▲ Zocor Tablets (2.2% to 6.6%) 2136
▲ Zofran Injection (11%) 1682
▲ Zofran (6% to 9%) 1687
▲ Zofran ODT Orally Disintegrating Tablets (6% to 9%) 1687
▲ Zolinza Capsules (13% to 15.1%) 2142
▲ Zometa for Intravenous Infusion (27% to 31%)................................ 2341
Zomig Tablets (Rare) 694
Zomig Nasal Spray (Rare)................. 689
Zomig-ZMT Tablets (Rare) 694
Zonegran Capsules (2%) 1089
▲ Zosyn for Injection (1.1% to 8.4%) ... 3284
▲ Zyban Sustained-Release Tablets (8%) 1692
Zydone Tablets 1132
▲ Zyprexa Tablets (6% to 11%) 1883
▲ Zyprexa ZYDIS Orally Disintegrating Tablets (6% to 11%) 1883
Zyrtec Chewable Tablets (Less than 2%) 1920
Zyrtec Syrup (Less than 2%) 1920
Zyrtec Tablets (Less than 2%) 1920
Zyrtec-D 12 Hour Extended Release Tablets (Less than 2%) 1923
Zyvox (2.2%) 2552

Constipation, aggravation of

Nexium Delayed-Release Capsules (Less than 1%) 645
Nexium I.V. (Less than 1%) 652
Nexium Delayed-Release Oral Suspension (Less than 1%) 645
Sanctura XR Capsules (1.2% to less than 2%) 557
Ultram ER Extended-Release Tablets (0.5% to less than 1%) 2428

Constitutional symptoms, unspecified

▲ Alimta for Injection (1% to 11%) 1786

Constriction, pupillary

(*see under* Miosis)

Constriction, pupils

(*see under* Miosis)

Contact lenses, intolerance

Accutane Capsules 2607
Activella Tablets 2347
Angeliq Tablets 751
Climara Transdermal System 763
Climara Pro Transdermal System 768
Divigel 3167
Enjuvia Tablets 1029
Estratest Tablets 3043
Estratest H.S. Tablets 3043
Lybrel Tablets 3204
Mircette Tablets 1034
NuvaRing 2897
Ortho-Cyclen Tablets 2449
Ortho Evra Transdermal System 2437
Ortho Tri-Cyclen Tablets 2449
Ortho Tri-Cyclen Lo Tablets 2458
Premarin Intravenous 3217
Premarin Tablets 3221
Premarin Vaginal Cream 3228
Premphase Tablets 3232
Prempro Tablets 3232
Seasonique Tablets 1046
Yaz Tablets 805

Contusions

Advair HFA 45/21 Inhalation Aerosol 1288
Advair HFA 115/21 Inhalation Aerosol 1288
Advair HFA 230/21 Inhalation Aerosol 1288
Ambien CR Tablets (1%) 2696
▲ Clolar for Intravenous Infusion (11%) 1239
▲ DepoCyt Injection (2% to 3%) 1136
▲ Flovent Diskus 50 mcg (1% to 3%) 1435
▲ Gleevec Tablets (0% to 27%) 2255
▲ Myfortic Tablets (3% to less than 20%) 2276
Ultram ER Extended-Release Tablets (0.5% to less than 1%) 2428
Vantas (Less than 2%) 1737
Xyrem Oral Solution (Frequent) 1766

Convulsions

Abelcet Injection 1134
Abilify Injection (0.1%) 881
Abilify Injection (0% to 0.2%) 2466
Abilify Oral Solution (0.1%) 881
Abilify Oral Solution (0% to 0.2%) 2466
Abilify Discmelt Orally Disintegrating Tablets (0.1%) 881
Abilify Discmelt Orally Disintegrating Tablets (0% to 0.2%) 2466
Abilify Tablets (0.1%) 881
Abilify Tablets (0% to 0.2%) 2466
Aggrenox Capsules (1.7%) 819
Aldara Cream, 5%............................ 1699
AmBisome for Injection (Less common)....................................... 606
Amerge Tablets (Rare)...................... 1301
Anaprox Tablets (Less than 1%) 2632
Anaprox DS Tablets (Less than 1%).. 2632
Aranesp for Injection (0.6%)............. 564
Aricept Tablets (Frequent)................ 1062
Aricept ODT Tablets (Frequent) 1062
▲ Arranon Injection (0% to 4%) 1319
Atripla Tablets................................ 938
Attenuvax (Rare) 1951
Augmentin (Rare)............................ 1323
Augmentin Tablets (Rare)................. 1327
Augmentin XR Extended Release Tablets (Rare)............................. 1333
Augmentin ES-600 Powder for Oral Suspension (Rare)............... 1329
Avelox (Less than 0.1%)................... 2803
▲ Avinza Capsules (Less than 5%) 1772
Azilect Tablets (Infrequent) 3106
Betaseron for SC Injection 756
Biaxin/Biaxin XL 411
Boostrix 1377
Campral Tablets (Infrequent) 1158
Cancidas for Injection 1953
Ceftin for Oral Suspension 1380
▲ CellCept Capsules (3% to less than 20%) 2622
▲ CellCept Intravenous (3% to less than 20%) 2622
▲ CellCept Oral Suspension (3% to less than 20%) 2622
▲ CellCept Tablets (3% to less than 20%) 2622
Chantix Tablets (Rare) 2511
Cipro I.V. 2817
Cipro 2810
Cipro XR Tablets 2823
Clarinex-D 24-Hour Extended-Release Tablets 2834
Clinoril Tablets (Less than 1%) 1962
Concerta Extended-Release Tablets 1925
Coreg Tablets (Less than or equal to 0.1%) 1387
Coreg CR Extended-Release Capsules (Less than or equal to 0.1%) 1393
Daytrana Transdermal Patch 3022
Doxil Injection (Less than 1%) 2378
Duragesic Transdermal System (1% or greater) 2405
EC-Naprosyn Delayed-Release Tablets (Less than 1%) 2632
E.E.S. 433
Effexor XR Extended-Release Capsules (Infrequent) 3195
Elitek (Less than or equal to 1%) 2729
Eloxatin for Injection 2731
Epivir 1412
Epzicom Tablets 1422
EryPed (Rare) 431
Evoxac Capsules 1013
Exelon Capsules (Frequent) 2229
Exelon Oral Solution (Frequent) 2229
Fansidar Tablets 2636
▲ Flolan for Injection (4%) 1426
Fluarix Vaccine 1446
Flulaval Injection Vaccine 1448
Flumadine (Less than 0.3%) 1167
Fluorescite Injection .... ⊙ 203
Gabitril Tablets 973
Gantrisin Pediatric Suspension 2638
▲ Gengraf Capsules (1% to 5%) 435
Gleevec Tablets (Rare) 2255
▲ Gliadel Wafer (19% to 33.3%) 1076
Havrix Injection Vaccine 1454
Imitrex Injection (Rare) 1465
Imitrex Tablets (Rare) 1474
▲ Increlex Injection (Greater than or equal to 5%) 3100
Indocin Capsules (Less than 1%) 2024
Indocin I.V. (Less than 1%) 2489
Indocin (Less than 1%) 2024
Infanrix Vaccine 1479
Intelence Tablets (Less than 2%) 3119
Intravenous Sodium Diuril 2490
▲ Intron A for Injection (Less than 5%) 2859
Kaletra (Less than 2%) 452
Keppra Oral Solution (1% to greater than or equal to 2%) 3131
Keppra Tablets (1% to greater than or equal to 2%) 3131
Kinrix Injection Vaccine 1486
Lamictal (2%) 1488
Levaquin (0.1% to 1%) 2416
Levaquin in 5% Dextrose Injection (0.1% to 1%) 2416
Lexapro Oral Suspension 1174
Lexapro Tablets 1174

Lidoderm Patch ... 1114
Luvox CR Extended-Release Capsules (Infrequent) ... 1759
▲ Megace ES Oral Suspension (1% to 3%) ... 2499
Meridia Capsules (0.1%) ... 475
Mirapex Tablets ... 857
Mobic Oral Suspension (Less than 2%) ... 863
Mobic Tablets (Less than 2%) ... 863
Moxatag Tablets ... 2165
Mycamine for Injection ... 616
Namenda (Infrequent) ... 1180
Naprosyn Suspension (Less than 1%) ... 2632
Naprosyn Tablets (Less than 1%) ... 2632
NeoProfen Injection ... 2496
▲ Neoral Oral Solution (1% to 5%) ... 2280
▲ Neoral Soft Gelatin Capsules (1% to 5%) ... 2280
Neupro Transdermal System ... 3149
Noroxin Tablets ... 2069
Norvir (Less than 2%) ... 489
Paxil (0.1%) ... 1535
Paxil CR Controlled-Release Tablets (0.1%) ... 1544
Pediarix Vaccine ... 1552
Pepcid Tablets ... 2075
▲ Primaxin I.V. (5.9%) ... 2083
Pristiq Extended-Release Tablets (Less than 2%) ... 3247
▲ Prograf Capsules and Injection (3% to 15%) ... 622
Proleukin for Injection (Less than 1%) ... 2287
ProQuad (Greater than or equal to 0.2% to less than 1%) ... 2099
Protonix for Delayed-Release Oral Suspension (Less than 1%) ... 3254
Protonix Delayed-Release Tablets (Less than 1%) ... 3254
Protonix I.V. (Less than 1%) ... 3257
Prozac Weekly Capsules (0.1% to 0.2%) ... 1852
Prozac Pulvules and Liquid (0.1% to 0.2%) ... 1852
▲ Rebif Prefilled Syringe for Injection (4% to 5%) ... 1107
Remicade for IV Injection (Less than 1%) ... 950
Requip Tablets (Infrequent) ... 1561
Rilutek Tablets (Infrequent) ... 2771
Risperdal Consta Long-Acting Injection (Infrequent) ... 1753
Romazicon Injection ... 2646
▲ Sandimmune (1% to 5%) ... 2296
Sandostatin LAR Depot ... 2302
Seromycin Capsules ... 1864
Stalevo Tablets ... 2309
Sustiva Capsules (Less than 2%) ... 930
Sustiva Tablets (Less than 2%) ... 930
Symbyax Capsules ... 1871
▲ Temodar Capsules (5% to 23%) ... 2931
Timentin ADD-Vantage ... 1606
Timentin Injection Galaxy Container ... 1609
Timentin IV Infusion ... 1603
Timentin Pharmacy Bulk Package ... 1613
Trasylol Injection (1% to 2%) ... 799
▲ Trisenox Injection (8%) ... 986
Twinrix Vaccine ... 1628
▲ Valcyte Tablets (Less than 5%) ... 2654
Valtrex Caplets ... 1635
▲ Vesanoid Capsules (3%) ... 2660
Vivitrol ... 988
Voltaren Tablets (Rarely) ... 2334
Voltaren-XR Tablets (Rarely) ... 2337
Xyzal Oral Solution ... 2789
Xyzal Oral Solution ... 3155
Zomig Tablets (Rare) ... 694
Zomig Nasal Spray (Rare) ... 689
Zomig-ZMT Tablets (Rare) ... 694
Zonegran Capsules (Frequent) ... 1089
Zosyn for Injection (1% or less) ... 3284
Zyrtec Chewable Tablets ... 1920
Zyrtec Syrup ... 1920
Zyrtec Tablets ... 1920
Zyrtec-D 12 Hour Extended Release Tablets (Rare) ... 1923
Zyvox (0% to 2.8%) ... 2552

Convulsions, clonic
Seromycin Capsules ... 1864
Uniphyl Tablets (A few isolated reports) ... 2595

Convulsions, drug withdrawal
Keppra Injection ... 3137

Convulsions, grand mal
Abilify Injection (Less than 1 in 1000 patients) ... 881
Abilify Injection (Less than 1 in 1000 patients) ... 2466
Abilify Oral Solution (Less than 1 in 1000 patients) ... 881
Abilify Oral Solution (Less than 1 in 1000 patients) ... 2466
Abilify Discmelt Orally Disintegrating Tablets (Less than 1 in 1000 patients) ... 881
Abilify Discmelt Orally Disintegrating Tablets (Less than 1 in 1000 patients) ... 2466
Abilify Tablets (Less than 1 in 1000 patients) ... 881
Abilify Tablets (Less than 1 in 1000 patients) ... 2466
Aranesp for Injection (0.6%) ... 564
Aricept Tablets (Infrequent) ... 1062
Aricept ODT Tablets (Infrequent) ... 1062
Arranon Injection (0% to 1%) ... 1319
Celexa ... 1160
Cipro (Less than 1%) ... 2810
Cipro XR Tablets ... 2823
▲ Gliadel Wafer (5%) ... 1076
Keppra Oral Solution (1% or more) ... 3131
Keppra Tablets (1% or more) ... 3131
Lamictal (Rare) ... 1488
Lexapro Oral Suspension ... 1174
Lexapro Tablets ... 1174
Mirapex Tablets ... 857
Namenda ... 1180
Norvir (Less than 2%) ... 489
Paxil (Rare) ... 1535
Paxil CR Controlled-Release Tablets (Rare) ... 1544
Proleukin for Injection (Less than 1%) ... 2287
Remeron Tablets (Rare) ... 2924
RemeronSolTab Tablets (Rare) ... 2927
Requip Tablets (Rare) ... 1561
Velcade for Injection ... 2168

Convulsions, local
Aranesp for Injection (0.6%) ... 564
▲ Temodar Capsules (6%) ... 2931

Convulsions, major
Seromycin Capsules ... 1864

Convulsions, tonic generalized
Uniphyl Tablets (A few isolated reports) ... 2595

Convulsive threshold, lowering
Adderall XR Capsules ... 3012

Coombs' test, positive
Catapres Tablets ... 841
Ceftin (0.1% to 1%) ... 1380
Clorpres Tablets ... 2185
Flebogamma 5% ... 1715
Flebogamma 5% DIF ... 1718
▲ Fortaz (1 in 23) ... 1450
Gammagard Liquid ... 730
Gammagard S/D ... 734
Gamunex ... 3094
Merrem I.V. (Greater than 0.2%) ... 684
Paser Granules ... 1747
Primaxin I.M. ... 2080
Primaxin I.V. ... 2083
Rilutek Tablets (Infrequent) ... 2771
Rocephin Injectable Vials, ADD-Vantage, Galaxy, Bulk ... 2642
Suprax for Oral Suspension ... 1891
Suprax Tablets ... 1891
Zinacef for Injection (Fewer than 1 in 250 patients) ... 1678
Zinacef Injection (Fewer than 1 in 250 patients) ... 1678
Zosyn for Injection ... 3284

Coordination, cerebellar, disturbances
Sustiva Capsules ... 930
Sustiva Tablets ... 930

Coordination, disturbed
(*see under* Coordination, impaired)

Coordination, impaired
Abilify Injection (Greater than or equal to 1 in 100 patients) ... 881
Abilify Injection (Greater than or equal to 1 in 100 patients) ... 2466
Abilify Oral Solution (Greater than or equal to 1 in 100 patients) ... 881
Abilify Oral Solution (Greater than or equal to 1 in 100 patients) ... 2466
Abilify Discmelt Orally Disintegrating Tablets (Greater than or equal to 1 in 100 patients) ... 881
Abilify Discmelt Orally Disintegrating Tablets (Greater than or equal to 1 in 100 patients) ... 2466
Abilify Tablets (Greater than or equal to 1 in 100 patients) ... 881
Abilify Tablets (Greater than or equal to 1 in 100 patients) ... 2466
Amerge Tablets (Rare) ... 1301
Arranon Injection (1%) ... 1319
Atripla Tablets ... 938
Carbatrol Capsules ... 3019
Celexa (Rare) ... 1160
Combivent Inhalation Aerosol ... 845
Duragesic Transdermal System (1% or greater) ... 2405
Effexor XR Extended-Release Capsules ... 3195
Equetro Extended-Release Capsules ... 3174
Evoxac Capsules (Less than 1%) ... 1013
▲ Intron A for Injection (Less than 5%) ... 2859
Ixempra Kit for Injection ... 915
▲ Keppra Injection (3.4%) ... 3137
▲ Keppra Oral Solution (3.4%) ... 3131
▲ Keppra Tablets (3.4%) ... 3131
▲ Klonopin (6%) ... 2639
▲ Lamictal (6% to 7%) ... 1488
Lexapro Oral Suspension (Infrequent) ... 1174
Lexapro Tablets (Infrequent) ... 1174
Marinol Capsules ... 3163
Mirapex Tablets ... 857
Namenda (Infrequent) ... 1180
Phenytek Capsules (Among most common) ... 2192
ProQuad (Greater than or equal to 0.2% to less than 1%) ... 2099
▲ Rebif Prefilled Syringe for Injection (4% to 5%) ... 1107
Remeron Tablets (Infrequent) ... 2924
RemeronSolTab Tablets (Infrequent) ... 2927
Requip Tablets (Infrequent) ... 1561
Rilutek Tablets (Infrequent) ... 2771
▲ Temodar Capsules (1% to 11%) ... 2931
Venlafaxine Hydrochloride Tablets ... 2199
Wellbutrin SR Sustained-Release Tablets (Infrequent) ... 1653
Wellbutrin XL Extended-Release Tablets (Infrequent) ... 1659
Xyrem Oral Solution (Infrequent) ... 1766
Zomig Tablets (Infrequent) ... 694
Zomig Nasal Spray (Infrequent) ... 689
Zomig-ZMT Tablets (Infrequent) ... 694
Zyban Sustained-Release Tablets (Infrequent) ... 1692
Zyrtec Chewable Tablets (Less than 2%) ... 1920
Zyrtec Syrup (Less than 2%) ... 1920
Zyrtec Tablets (Less than 2%) ... 1920
Zyrtec-D 12 Hour Extended Release Tablets (Less than 2%) ... 1923

Coordination, lack of
(*see under* Ataxia)

Coordination difficulty
(*see under* Coordination, impaired)

Cor pulmonale
Chantix Tablets (Rare) ... 2511
Pulmozyme Inhalation Solution ... 1217

Cornea, opacities
Accutane Capsules ... 2607
Imitrex Injection ... 1465
Imitrex Tablets ... 1474

Corneal changes
▲ Lotemax Ophthalmic Suspension 0.5% (Less than 5%) ... ⊙241

Corneal clouding
▲ Chemet Capsules (1% to 3.7%) ... 2484

Corneal curvature, steepening
Climara Transdermal System ... 763
Climara Pro Transdermal System ... 768
Estratest Tablets ... 3043
Estratest H.S. Tablets ... 3043
Lybrel Tablets ... 3204
Mircette Tablets ... 1034
NuvaRing ... 2897
Ortho-Cyclen Tablets ... 2449
Ortho Evra Transdermal System ... 2437
Ortho Tri-Cyclen Tablets ... 2449
Ortho Tri-Cyclen Lo Tablets ... 2458
Premarin Vaginal Cream ... 3228
Premphase Tablets ... 3232
Prempro Tablets ... 3232
Seasonique Tablets ... 1046
Yaz Tablets ... 805

Corneal deposits
▲ Diclofenac Sodium Ophthalmic Solution (Less than or equal to 5%) ... ⊙240
Indocin (Less than 1%) ... 2024
Thioridazine Hydrochloride Tablets ... 2195
▲ Voltaren Ophthalmic Solution (Less than or equal to 5%) ... 2336

Corneal discharge
▲ Diclofenac Sodium Ophthalmic Solution (Less than or equal to 5%) ... ⊙240

Corneal epithelial breakdown
Diclofenac Sodium Ophthalmic Solution ... ⊙240
Voltaren Ophthalmic Solution (0.1%) ... 2336

Corneal infiltrate
Diclofenac Sodium Ophthalmic Solution ... ⊙240
Voltaren Ophthalmic Solution (0.1%) ... 2336

Corneal opacity
Anaprox Tablets (Less than 1%) ... 2632
Anaprox DS Tablets (Less than 1%) ... 2632
▲ Diclofenac Sodium Ophthalmic Solution (Less than or equal to 5%) ... ⊙240
EC-Naprosyn Delayed-Release Tablets (Less than 1%) ... 2632
Evoxac Capsules (Less than 1%) ... 1013
Namenda (Infrequent) ... 1180
Naprosyn Suspension (Less than 1%) ... 2632
Naprosyn Tablets (Less than 1%) ... 2632
▲ Voltaren Ophthalmic Solution (Less than or equal to 5%) ... 2336

Corneal sensitivity, decrease
Betimol Ophthalmic Solution ... 3181
Combigan Ophthalmic Solution ... 553
Cosopt Sterile Ophthalmic Solution ... 1969
Timoptic Sterile Ophthalmic Solution (Less frequent) ... 2121
Timoptic in Ocudose (Less frequent) ... 2124
Timoptic-XE Sterile Ophthalmic Gel Forming Solution ... 2125

Corneal staining
▲ Betimol Ophthalmic Solution (1% to 5%) ... 3181
▲ Travatan Z Ophthalmic Solution (1% to 4%) ... 547

Corneal thinning
Diclofenac Sodium Ophthalmic Solution ... ⊙240
Myleran Tablets ... 1530
Pred-G Ophthalmic Ointment ... ⊙229
Voltaren Ophthalmic Solution (0.1%) ... 2336

Corneal ulceration
Ambien Tablets (Rare) ... 2692
Ambien CR Tablets (Rare) ... 2696
BOTOX Purified Neurotoxin Complex ... 550
Diclofenac Sodium Ophthalmic Solution ... ⊙240
Evoxac Capsules (Less than 1%) ... 1013
Luvox CR Extended-Release Capsules (Infrequent) ... 1759
Paxil (Rare) ... 1535
Paxil CR Controlled-Release Tablets (Rare) ... 1544
Pred Forte Ophthalmic Suspension (Occasional) ... ⊙227
Pred Mild Ophthalmic Suspension (Occasional) ... ⊙230
Soriatane Capsules (Less than 1%) ... 3062
Tarceva Tablets ... 1228
Voltaren Ophthalmic Solution (0.1%) ... 2336

Coronary artery disease, aggravation
Carbatrol Capsules ... 3019
Equetro Extended-Release Capsules ... 3174

Coronary artery disease, unspecified
Amevive (Less than 1%) ... 611
Celebrex Capsules (0.1% to 1.9%) ... 2979
Chantix Tablets (Rare) ... 2511

Effexor XR Extended-Release Capsules (Rare) 3195
▲ Humira Injection (Less than 5%) 442
▲ Intron A for Injection (Less than 5%) 2859
Luvox CR Extended-Release Capsules (Rare) 1759
Proleukin for Injection (Less than 1%) 2287
Requip Tablets (Infrequent) 1561
Rythmol SR Capsules 1590
Selzentry Tablets 2534
Tasigna Capsules (0.1% to 1%) 2316
Testim 1% Gel 701
Toprol-XL Tablets (Greater than 1%) 666
Tricor Tablets 520
Venlafaxine Hydrochloride Tablets (Rare) 2199

Coronary artery occlusion

Selzentry Tablets 2534

Coronary heart disease

Duetact Tablets 3085
Premarin Tablets 3221

Coronary occlusion

Mirapex Tablets 857
Pristiq Extended-Release Tablets 3247
Trasylol Injection (1% to 2%) 799

Coronary syndrome, acute

Actos Tablets 3077
Chantix Tablets (Rare) 2511
Duetact Tablets 3085
Requip Tablets (Infrequent) 1561
Treximet Tablets (Rare) 1616

Corpuscular volume, mean, elevation

Avelox (Greater than or equal to 2%) 2803

Cortical lens opacities, scattered punctate

Carbatrol Capsules 3019
Equetro Extended-Release Capsules 3174

Corticosteroid binding globulin, elevated

Premphase Tablets 3232
Prempro Tablets 3232

Costochondritis

Evoxac Capsules (Less than 1%) 1013
Rythmol SR Capsules 1590

Cough

▲ Abilify Injection (3%) 881
▲ Abilify Injection (3%) 2466
▲ Abilify Oral Solution (3%) 881
▲ Abilify Oral Solution (3%) 2466
▲ Abilify Discmelt Orally Disintegrating Tablets (3%) 881
▲ Abilify Discmelt Orally Disintegrating Tablets (3%) 2466
▲ Abilify Tablets (3%) 881
▲ Abilify Tablets (3%) 2466
▲ Aceon Tablets (2 mg, 4 mg, 8 mg) (6% to 12%) 3038
▲ Acetadote Injection (0.88% to 4.22%) 1001
Actiq (1% or greater) 959
▲ Actonel with Calcium Tablets (2.5% to 3.1%) 2574
Aczone Gel 5% (2%) 3296
Adenoscan (Less than 1%) 605
▲ Advair Diskus 100/50 (12%) 1276
▲ Advair Diskus 250/50 (Greater than or equal to 3% to 6%) 1276
▲ Advair Diskus 500/50 (Greater than or equal to 3%) 1276
Advair HFA 45/21 Inhalation Aerosol 1288
Advair HFA 115/21 Inhalation Aerosol 1288
Advair HFA 230/21 Inhalation Aerosol 1288
▲ Advate (15.3%) 721
▲ Aerobid/Aerobid-M (3% to 9%) 1153
Aggrenox Capsules (1.5%) 819
▲ Agrylin Capsules (6.3%) 3017
▲ Alamast Ophthalmic Solution (Less than 5%) 3181
Aldara Cream, 5% (2%) 1699
Alferon N Injection (One patient to 1%) 1726
▲ Allegra Oral Solution (3.8%) 2684
▲ Allegra Tablets (3.8%) 2684
▲ Alphagan P Ophthalmic Solution (1% to 4%) 549
Alvesco Inhalation Aerosol (Less than 1%) 2985
Ambien Tablets (Infrequent) 2692
Ambien CR Tablets (Infrequent) 2696
▲ AmBisome for Injection (17.8%) 606
Amerge Tablets (Infrequent) 1301
Amevive (Common) 611
Amitiza Capsules (Less than 1%) 3082
▲ Aptivus Oral Solution (5.5%) 823
▲ Aranesp for Injection (9%) 564
Argatroban Injection (2.8%) 1308
Arixtra Injection (2.1%) 1313
▲ Arranon Injection (0% to 25%) 1319
Asacol Delayed-Release Tablets (1% to 2%) 2579
Atacand Tablets (More than 1%) 639
Atacand HCT (0.5% or greater) 642
▲ Atrovent HFA Inhalation Aerosol (3% to 5%) 839
Atrovent Nasal Spray 0.03% (Less than 2%) 834
Atrovent Nasal Spray 0.06% (Less than 1%) 836
Attenuvax 1951
Avalide Tablets (1% or greater) 892
Avalide Tablets (1% or greater) 2713
Avapro Tablets (2.8%) 897
Avapro Tablets (2.8%) 2718
Azmacort Inhalation Aerosol 407
Bactroban Nasal (2%) 1367
BeneFIX Vials (1.5%) 3191
Benicar HCT Tablets (Greater than 1%) 1010
▲ BOTOX Purified Neurotoxin Complex (2% to 10%) 550
▲ Busulfex Injection (28%) 2477
▲ Cancidas for Injection (6.1% to 10.6%) 1953
Captopril Tablets (0.5% to 2%) 2182
Cardizem LA Extended Release Tablets (2%) 421
Ceftin for Oral Suspension (0.1% to 1%) 1380
▲ Celebrex Capsules (0.1% to 7%) 2979
Celexa (Frequent) 1160
▲ Cerezyme for Injection (Approximately 6.6%) 1238
▲ Chemet Capsules (0.7% to 3.7%) 2484
Cialis Tablets (2% to 4%) 1792
▲ Clarinex Syrup (10.6% to 10.8%) 2828
▲ Clolar for Intravenous Infusion (19%) 1239
Combigan Ophthalmic Solution (0.1% to 0.2%) 553
▲ Combivent Inhalation Aerosol (4.2%) 845
▲ Combivir Tablets (18%) 1384
Comvax (0.2% to 0.9%) 1966
Concerta Extended-Release Tablets (1.9%) 1925
Copaxone for Injection (At least 2%) 3110
▲ Coreg Tablets (5% to 8%) 1387
▲ Cosopt Sterile Ophthalmic Solution (1% to 5%) 1969
Cozaar Tablets (1% or greater) 1973
Crixivan Capsules (1.5%) 1979
▲ Cubicin for Injection (1% to 3.3%) 995
▲ Cymbalta Delayed-Release Capsules (3% to 6%) 1801
▲ Dacogen Injection (40%) 1066
Demadex Injection (2%) 2630
Demadex Tablets (2%) 2630
▲ Depakote ER Tablets (Greater than 1% to less than 5%) 423
▲ DepoCyt Injection (7% to 9%) 1136
Diovan Tablets (0.6% to 2.6%) 2212
Diovan HCT Tablets (Greater than 0.2%) 2216
▲ Doxil Injection (Less than 1% to 9.6%) 2378
Duragesic Transdermal System (1% or greater) 2405
DynaCirc CR Controlled Release Tablets (0.5% to 1%) 1407
▲ Effexor XR Extended-Release Capsules (3%) 3195
▲ Elidel Cream 1% (2.4% to 15.8%) 2221
▲ Eloxatin for Injection (0% to 43%) 2731
Emend Capsules (Greater than 0.5%) 1992
Emend for Injection (Greater than 0.5%) 1999
Emsam Transdermal System (Frequent) 905
▲ Enbrel for Injection (5% to 6%) 569
▲ Epivir (15% to 18%) 1412
Epivir-HBV (Among most common) 1417
▲ Epogen for Injection (18%) 576
▲ Erbitux (2% to 29%) 912
▲ Evista Tablets (6% to 9.3%) 1810
▲ Evoxac Capsules (6.1%) 1013
Exelon Capsules (2% or more) 2229
Exelon Oral Solution (2% or more) 2229
▲ Exforge Tablets (0.2% to 20%) 2238
▲ Exjade Tablets (13.9%) 2244
▲ Fabrazyme for Intravenous Infusion (33%) 1241
▲ Faslodex Injection (10.4%) 682
▲ Femara Tablets (5% to 13%) 2246
▲ Fentora Tablets (1% to 9%) 968
▲ Flebogamma 5% (25%) 1715
▲ Flebogamma 5% DIF (Greater than 15%) 1718
▲ Flolan for Injection (38% to 82%) 1426
▲ Flomax Capsules (3.4% to 4.5%) 848
▲ Flonase Nasal Spray (3.6% to 3.8%) 1431
▲ Flovent Diskus 50 mcg (5% to 9%) 1435
▲ Flovent HFA (4%) 1440
Fluarix Vaccine 1446
▲ Flulaval Injection Vaccine (2% to 15%) 1448
Flumadine (Less than 0.3%) 1167
▲ FluMist Vaccine (14%) 1945
▲ Forteo for Injection (6.4%) 1816
▲ Gabitril Tablets (4%) 973
▲ Gammagard Liquid (0.61% to 8.2%) 730
Gantrisin Pediatric Suspension 2638
Gardasil Injection (2%) 2019
Gemzar for Injection (Common) 1820
▲ Gengraf Capsules (4% to 5%) 435
▲ Gleevec Tablets (14% to 27%) 2255
▲ Humatrope Vials and Cartridges (Up to 6.25%) 1838
▲ Hycamtin for Injection (1% to 15%) 1459
Imitrex Nasal Spray (Infrequent) 1470
Imitrex Tablets (Infrequent) 1474
▲ Indapamide Tablets (Less than 5%) 2188
▲ Intron A for Injection (Up to 31%) 2859
▲ Invanz for Injection (1.3% to 4.4%) 2029
Ixempra Kit for Injection (2%) 915
Klonopin (2%) 2639
▲ Lamictal (8%) 1488
▲ Lamisil Oral Granules (6%) 2264
Lescol Capsules (2.4%) 2268
Lescol XL Tablets (1.9%) 2268
Leukeran Tablets 1508
▲ Leustatin Injection (7% to 10%) 2384
Lexapro Oral Suspension (Frequent) 1174
Lexapro Tablets (Frequent) 1174
▲ Lucentis Injection (3% to 10%) 1205
▲ Malarone Pediatric Tablets (Less than 1% to 10%) 1521
▲ Malarone Tablets (Less than 1% to 10%) 1521
Marinol Capsules (Less than 1%) 3163
▲ Mavik Tablets (0.3% to 35%) 472
Maxair Autohaler (1.2%) 1705
Maxalt Tablets (Rare) 2056
Maxalt-MLT Orally Disintegrating Tablets (Rare) 2056
▲ Megace ES Oral Suspension (1% to 3%) 2499
▲ Mepron Suspension (25%) 1526
▲ Meridia Capsules (3.8%) 475
Meruvax II 2061
Miacalcin Nasal Spray (Less than 1%) 2274
Micardis Tablets (1% to 1.6%) 852
Micardis HCT Tablets (2% or greater) 854
Mirapex Tablets (1% or more) 857
M-M-R II 2054
Mobic Oral Suspension (0.2% to 2.4%) 863
Mobic Tablets (0.2% to 2.4%) 863
Mumpsvax 2068
▲ Mycamine for Injection (8.1% to 23.1%) 616
▲ Myfortic Tablets (3% to less than 20%) 2276
▲ Mylotarg for Injection (16% to 18%) 3212
Nadolol Tablets (1 to 5 of 1000 patients) 2191
▲ Namenda (4%) 1180
Nasacort AQ Nasal Spray (2.1%) 2765
▲ Nasonex Nasal Spray (7% to 13%) 2883
▲ Neoral Oral Solution (4% to 5%) 2280
▲ Neoral Soft Gelatin Capsules (4% to 5%) 2280
▲ Neupogen for Injection (6%) 589
Neupro Transdermal System (Greater than or equal to 2%) 3149
Nexium Delayed-Release Capsules (Less than 1%) 645
Nexium I.V. (Less than 1%) 652
Nexium Delayed-Release Oral Suspension (Less than 1%) 645
Norvir (Less than 2%) 489
▲ Novantrone for Injection Concentrate (5% to 13%) 1100
▲ Noxafil Oral Suspension (3% to 25%) 2889
▲ Ontak Vials (26%) 1079
OptiPranolol Metipranolol Ophthalmic Solution 0.3% (A small number of patients) ⊙245
▲ Orencia Powder for Intravenous Infusion (8%) 921
OxyContin Tablets (Less than 1%) 2589
Patanase Nasal Spray (1.4%) 544
Paxil (Frequent) 1535
Paxil CR Controlled-Release Tablets (Frequent) 1544
▲ PegIntron Powder for Injection (8%) 2903
Pentacel 2792
▲ Photofrin for Injection (7% to 9%) 708
▲ Plavix Tablets (3.1%) 926
▲ Plavix Tablets (3.1%) 2767
▲ Pletal Tablets (3% to 4%) 2481
▲ Prinivil Tablets (1% to 3.5%) 2087
▲ Prinzide Tablets (3.9%) 2092
▲ Procrit for Injection (18%) 2391
▲ Prograf Capsules and Injection (3% to 18%) 622
▲ Prometrium Capsules (100 mg, 200 mg) (8%) 3047
ProQuad (Greater than or equal to 0.2% to less than 1%) 2099
Protonix for Delayed-Release Oral Suspension (Greater than or equal to 1%) 3254
Protonix Delayed-Release Tablets (Greater than or equal to 1%) 3254
Protonix I.V. (Greater than or equal to 1%) 3257
▲ Protopic Ointment (1% to 15%) 628
Provigil Tablets (At least 1%) 977
Prozac Pulvules and Liquid 1852
Pulmozyme Inhalation Solution 1217
▲ Rebetol (16% to 23%) 2917
Recombivax HB (Less than 1%) 2107
ReFacto Vials 3269
Refludan for Injection (Common) 795
▲ Relenza Inhalation Powder (Less than 1% to 17%) 1556
Remeron Tablets (Frequent) 2924
RemeronSolTab Tablets (Frequent) 2927
▲ Remicade for IV Injection (12%) 950
▲ Requip Tablets (1% to 3%) 1561
Requip XL Tablets 1568
Retrovir Capsules 1574
Retrovir IV Infusion 1579
Retrovir 1574
▲ Reyataz Capsules (21%) 3299
▲ Rilutek Tablets (2.1% to 3.7%) 2771
Risperdal Consta Long-Acting Injection (2%) 1753
▲ Rotarix Oral Suspension (28% to 31%) 1582
Rythmol SR Capsules 1590
▲ Selzentry Tablets (12.7%) 2534
▲ Serevent Diskus (Greater than 3%) 1594
▲ Simulect for Injection (Greater than or equal to 10%) 2306
Singulair (1% to 2.7%) 2114
Soriatane Capsules (Less than 1%) 3062
▲ Spiriva HandiHaler (Greater than or equal to 3%) 870
Stalevo Tablets 2309
Starlix Tablets (2.4%) 2314
▲ Suboxone Tablets (4%) 2601
▲ Subutex Tablets (4%) 2601
Sular Extended Release Tablets (Less than or equal to 1%) 2975
▲ Sustiva Capsules (25%) 930
▲ Sustiva Tablets (25%) 930
▲ Sutent Capsules (0% to 18%) 2540
Synagis Intramuscular Solution (More than 1%) 1948
▲ Tamiflu Capsules (1% to 5%) 2649
▲ Tamiflu Oral Suspension (1% to 5%) 2649
▲ Tarceva Tablets (0% to 33%) 1228
Targretin Capsules 1084
▲ Tarka Tablets (4.6%) 511
▲ Tasigna Capsules (1% to 10%) 2316
▲ Taxotere Injection Concentrate (0% to 13.7%) 2773
Tekturna Tablets (1.1%) 2321
Tekturna HCT Tablets (Less than 1% to 1.3%) 2324
▲ Temodar Capsules (Less than 1% to 8%) 2931
▲ Teveten Tablets (4%) 515
Teveten HCT Tablets (Less than 1%) 517
Timoptic Sterile Ophthalmic Solution (Less frequent) 2121
Timoptic in Ocudose (Less frequent) 2124
Timoptic-XE Sterile Ophthalmic Gel Forming Solution 2125
▲ Torisel Injection (1% to 26%) 3272
▲ Treanda for Injection (Less than 1% to 4%) 983
Treximet Tablets (Infrequent) 1616

▲ Trisenox Injection (65%) 986
▲ Trizivir Tablets (18%) 1622
▲ Tyzeka Tablets (Less than 1% to 7%) 2328
▲ Ultram ER Extended-Release Tablets (1% to less than 5%) 2428
▲ Valcyte Tablets (Less than 5%) 2654
▲ Vaqta (1% to 5.1%) 2130
Varivax (Greater than or equal to 1%) 2133
▲ Vectibix (Less than 1% to 14%) 597
▲ Velcade for Injection (20% to 21%) 2168
▲ Ventolin HFA Inhalation Aerosol (3% to 5%) 1638
▲ Veramyst Nasal Spray (3% to 4%) 1643
▲ Verdeso Foam (4%) 3069
VESIcare Tablets (0.2% to 1.1%) 636
Vicoprofen Tablets (Less than 1%) 533
▲ Vigamox Ophthalmic Solution (1% to 4%) ⊙213
▲ Visudyne for Injection (1% to 10%) 2332
▲ Voltaren Ophthalmic Solution (Less than or equal to 3%) 2336
Wellbutrin SR Sustained-Release Tablets (1% to 2%) 1653
Wellbutrin XL Extended-Release Tablets (1% to 2%) 1659
▲ Xeloda Tablets (Less than 5%) 2662
Xolair 1235
Xolair 2339
▲ Xopenex Inhalation Solution (1.4% to 4.1%) 3001
▲ Xopenex Inhalation Solution Concentrate (1.4% to 4.1%) 3005
▲ Xopenex HFA Inhalation Aerosol (1.4% to 4.1%) 3009
Xyrem Oral Solution (Frequent) 1766
▲ Xyzal Oral Solution (3%) 2789
▲ Xyzal Oral Solution (3%) 3155
▲ Xyzal Tablets (Less than 1% to 3%) 2789
▲ Xyzal Tablets (Less than 1% to 3%) 3155
Yaz Tablets (Greater than 1%) 805
Ziagen 1673
Ziana Gel (1%) 1942
▲ Zolinza Capsules (9% to 10.5%) 2142
▲ Zometa for Intravenous Infusion (12% to 22%) 2341
Zosyn for Injection (1% or less) 3284
▲ Zyban Sustained-Release Tablets (3%) 1692
▲ Zyprexa Tablets (5%) 1883
▲ Zyprexa ZYDIS Orally Disintegrating Tablets (5%) 1883
▲ Zyrtec Chewable Tablets (2.8% to 4.4%) 1920
▲ Zyrtec Syrup (2.8% to 4.4%) 1920
▲ Zyrtec Tablets (2.8% to 4.4%) 1920
Zyvox 2552

Cough, increased
▲ Actonel Tablets (5.9%) 2568
Aralast (0.1% to 0.6%) 726
Aricept Tablets (Frequent) 1062
Aricept ODT Tablets (Frequent) 1062
▲ Arimidex Tablets (7% to 11%) 672
▲ Atripla Tablets (Greater than or equal to 5%) 938
Axid Capsules (2%) 1364
▲ Bexxar (1% to 21%) 1371
Campral Tablets (Frequent) 1158
▲ CellCept Capsules (31.1%) 2622
▲ CellCept Intravenous (31.1%) 2622
▲ CellCept Oral Suspension (31.1%) 2622
▲ CellCept Tablets (31.1%) 2622
▲ Coreg CR Extended-Release Capsules (5% to 8%) 1393
▲ Elestat Ophthalmic Solution (1% to 3%) 1741
▲ Emtriva Capsules (Greater than or equal to 10%) 1246
▲ Emtriva Oral Solution (Greater than or equal to 10%) 1246
▲ Exubera Inhalation Powder (21.9% to 29.5%) 2515
▲ Gamunex (1.7% to 54%) 3094
▲ Geodon Capsules (3%) 2520
▲ Herceptin I.V. (26%) 1199
Ionsys Transdermal System (.1% to less than 1%) 2410
Keppra Injection (2%) 3137
▲ Keppra Oral Solution (2% to 11%) 3131
▲ Keppra Tablets (2% to 11%) 3131
Lovaza Capsules 1520
Luvox CR Extended-Release Capsules (Frequent) 1759
Merrem I.V. (Greater than 0.1% to 1%) 684
Natrecor for Injection (Greater than or equal to 1%) 2977
▲ Pataday Ophthalmic Solution (Less than or equal to 5%) 543
▲ Premarin Tablets (4% to 7%) 3221
▲ Premphase Tablets (5% to 8%) 3232
▲ Prempro Tablets (5% to 8%) 3232
▲ Proleukin for Injection (11%) 2287
▲ Pulmicort Flexhaler (6%) 654
▲ Rituxan I.V. (1% to 13%) 1223
Salagen Tablets (1% to 2%) 1082
▲ Targretin Gel 1% (6%) 1088
Tricor Tablets 520
▲ Truvada Tablets (Greater than or equal to 5%) 1262
▲ Tygacil for Injection (3.7%) 3276
▲ Ultane Liquid for Inhalation (5% to 11%) 524
▲ Vigamox Ophthalmic Solution (1% to 4%) 548
Zomig Tablets (Infrequent) 694
Zomig Nasal Spray (Infrequent) 689
Zomig-ZMT Tablets (Infrequent) 694

Cough, productive
Exforge Tablets (Greater than or equal to 0.2%) 2238
▲ Flebogamma 5% (25%) 1715
▲ Flebogamma 5% DIF (Greater than 15%) 1718
Mirapex Tablets 857

Cough reflex, depression
Lortab 5/500 Tablets 3143
Lortab 7.5/500 Tablets 3144
Lortab 10/500 Tablets 3144
Prozac Weekly Capsules (Rare) 1852
Prozac Pulvules and Liquid (Rare) 1852
Vicodin Tablets 529

CPK, elevation
(*see under* Creatine kinase, increase)

Cramping
Alferon N Injection (One patient) 1726
Aminohippurate Sodium "PAH" Injection 1950
Asacol Delayed-Release Tablets 2579
Atacand HCT 642
Avalide Tablets 892
Avalide Tablets 2713
Clinoril Tablets (Greater than 1%) 1962
Clorpres Tablets 2185
▲ Crinone 4% Gel (19%) 992
▲ Crinone 8% Gel (15% to 26%) 992
Diovan HCT Tablets 2216
Dulcolax Suppositories ▣602
Dulcolax Tablets ▣602
Exelon Capsules (Infrequent) 2229
Exelon Oral Solution (Infrequent) 2229
Fleet Bisacodyl Laxatives 1143
▲ Gengraf Capsules (1% to 4%) 435
Intravenous Sodium Diuril 2490
▲ Neoral Oral Solution (1% to 4%) 2280
▲ Neoral Soft Gelatin Capsules (1% to 4%) 2280
Nexium Delayed-Release Capsules (Less than 1%) 645
Nexium I.V. (Less than 1%) 652
Nexium Delayed-Release Oral Suspension (Less than 1%) 645
ParaGard T 380A Intrauterine Copper Contraceptive 1041
Prinzide Tablets 2092
Protopic Ointment (0.2% to less than 1%) 628
▲ Sandimmune (Up to 4%) 2296
Tekturna HCT Tablets 2324
Teveten HCT Tablets 517
▲ Tice BCG (4%) 2936

Cramping, abdominal
(*see under* Abdominal pain/cramps)

Cramping, legs
Activella Tablets 2347
Ambien Tablets (Infrequent) 2692
Angeliq Tablets 751
▲ CellCept Capsules (3% to less than 20%) 2622
▲ CellCept Intravenous (3% to less than 20%) 2622
▲ CellCept Oral Suspension (3% to less than 20%) 2622
▲ CellCept Tablets (3% to less than 20%) 2622
Crinone 4% Gel 992
Crinone 8% Gel 992
Divigel 3167
Emsam Transdermal System (Infrequent) 905
Ionsys Transdermal System (.1% to less than 1%) 2410
Premarin Intravenous 3217
Prozac Weekly Capsules (Infrequent) 1852
Risperdal Consta Long-Acting Injection (Infrequent) 1753
Salagen Tablets (Less than 1%) 1082
Venlafaxine Hydrochloride Tablets (Infrequent) 2199
Zomig Tablets (Infrequent) 694
Zomig-ZMT Tablets (Infrequent) 694
Zyrtec Chewable Tablets (Less than 2%) 1920
Zyrtec Syrup (Less than 2%) 1920
Zyrtec Tablets (Less than 2%) 1920
Zyrtec-D 12 Hour Extended Release Tablets (Less than 2%) 1923

Cramping, muscular
▲ Advair Diskus 250/50 (3%) 1276
▲ Advair HFA 45/21 Inhalation Aerosol (1% to 3%) 1288
▲ Advair HFA 115/21 Inhalation Aerosol (1% to 3%) 1288
▲ Advair HFA 230/21 Inhalation Aerosol (1% to 3%) 1288
Advicor Tablets 402
Alferon N Injection (1%) 1726
Ambien CR Tablets (2%) 2696
Amerge Tablets (Infrequent) 1301
Amitiza Capsules (Less than 1%) 3082
Antivenin (Black Widow Spider Antivenin) 1951
Aptivus Capsules (Less than 2%) 823
Aptivus Oral Solution (Less than 2%) 823
▲ Aricept Tablets (3% to 8%) 1062
▲ Aricept ODT Tablets (3% to 8%) 1062
Asacol Delayed-Release Tablets 2579
Avalide Tablets (1% or greater) 892
Avalide Tablets (1% or greater) 2713
Avapro Tablets (Less than 1%) 897
Avapro Tablets (Less than 1%) 2718
Boniva Injection (1.8% to 2%) 2614
Boniva Tablets (1.8% to 2%) 2618
Brovana Inhalation Solution (Less than 2%) 2990
Cardizem LA Extended Release Tablets (Less than 2%) 421
Ceftin Tablets (0.1% to 1%) 1380
Chantix Tablets (Frequent) 2511
Climara Transdermal System 763
▲ Coreg Tablets (Greater than 1% to 3%) 1387
▲ Coreg CR Extended-Release Capsules (Greater than 1% to less than or equal to 3%) 1393
Cozaar Tablets (1%) 1973
Cubicin for Injection (Less than 1%) 995
▲ Cymbalta Delayed-Release Capsules (4% to 5%) 1801
Diovan Tablets (Greater than 0.2%) 2212
Diovan HCT Tablets (Greater than 0.2%) 2216
Divigel 3167
Dyazide Capsules 1405
Eldepryl Capsules 3052
Exforge Tablets (Greater than 0.1% to less than 1%) 2238
Flebogamma 5% 1715
Flebogamma 5% DIF 1718
Foradil Aerolizer (1.7%) 2849
▲ Fosamax (Up to approximately 6%) 2005
Fosamax Plus D Tablets (0% to 1.1%) 2013
Furosemide Tablets 2186
Gammagard Liquid 730
▲ Gleevec Tablets (28% to 62%) 2255
▲ Humira Injection (Less than 5%) 442
Imitrex Injection (Frequent) 1465
Imitrex Nasal Spray (Rare) 1470
Imitrex Tablets (Infrequent) 1474
▲ Indapamide Tablets (Greater than or equal to 5%) 2188
Intravenous Sodium Diuril 2490
Ketek Tablets 2744
Klonopin (Infrequent) 2639
K-Phos Original (Sodium Free) Tablets (Less frequent) 814
K-Phos Neutral Tablets 813
Lescol Capsules 2268
Lescol XL Tablets 2268
Lexapro Oral Suspension (Infrequent) 1174
Lexapro Tablets (Infrequent) 1174
Mavik Tablets (0.3% to 1%) 472
Maxalt Tablets (Infrequent) 2056
Maxalt-MLT Orally Disintegrating Tablets (Infrequent) 2056
Mevacor Tablets (0.6% to 1.1%) 2063
Micardis Tablets 852
Micardis HCT Tablets 854
▲ Myfortic Tablets (3% to less than 20%) 2276
Nimotop Capsules (Up to 1.4%) 790
Norvir (Less than 2%) 489
Pepcid Tablets (Infrequent) 2075
Perforomist Inhalation Solution 1025
Prinivil Tablets (Greater than 1%) 2087
Prinzide Tablets (2%) 2092
▲ Prograf Capsules and Injection (3% to 15%) 622
Prozac Pulvules and Liquid (Infrequent) 1852
▲ Requip Tablets (3%) 1561
Rythmol Tablets (Less than 1%) 1586
Rythmol SR Capsules 1590
▲ Serevent Diskus (3%) 1594
▲ Simulect for Injection (3% to 10%) 2306
Singulair 2114
Stalevo Tablets 2309
Teveten Tablets (Less than 1%) 515
Tyzeka Tablets (2%) 2328
Ultram ER Extended-Release Tablets (0.5% to less than 1%) 2428
Uroqid-Acid No. 2 Tablets 814
▲ Valcyte Tablets (Less than 5%) 2654
▲ Velcade for Injection (11% to 12%) 2168
Ventolin HFA Inhalation Aerosol 1638
▲ Vivitrol (2% to 8%) 988
Vytorin 10/10 Tablets 2149
Vytorin 10/10 Tablets 2939
Vytorin 10/20 Tablets 2149
Vytorin 10/20 Tablets 2939
Vytorin 10/40 Tablets 2149
Vytorin 10/40 Tablets 2939
Vytorin 10/80 Tablets 2149
Vytorin 10/80 Tablets 2939
Zocor Tablets 2136
Zometa for Intravenous Infusion 2341

Cramps, abdominal
(*see under* Abdominal pain/cramps)

Cramps, bladder
▲ Tice BCG (8%) 2936

Cramps, lower limbs
Actiq (1% or greater) 959
▲ Agrylin Capsules (1% to less than 5%) 3017
Alinia for Oral Suspension (Less than 1%) 2677
Alinia Tablets (Less than 1%) 2677
Aricept Tablets (Frequent) 1062
Aricept ODT Tablets (Frequent) 1062
Atacand HCT (0.5% or greater) 642
▲ Betaseron for SC Injection (4%) 756
▲ Brovana Inhalation Solution (4%) 2990
Campral Tablets (Frequent) 1158
Carbatrol Capsules 3019
Catapres Tablets (About 3 in 1,000) 841
Catapres-TTS (0.5% or less) 842
Celebrex Capsules (0.1% to 1.9%) 2979
Celexa (Infrequent) 1160
Climara Transdermal System 763
Climara Pro Transdermal System 768
Clorpres Tablets (About 3 in 1,000) 2185
▲ Depakote ER Tablets (Greater than 1% to less than 5%) 423
Didronel Tablets 2583
DynaCirc CR Controlled Release Tablets (0.5% to 1%) 1407
Effexor XR Extended-Release Capsules (Infrequent) 3195
Enjuvia Tablets 1029
Equetro Extended-Release Capsules 3174
Estratest H.S. Tablets 3043
▲ Evista Tablets (5.9% to 7%) 1810
▲ Evoxac Capsules (1% to 3%) 1013
Exelon Capsules (Frequent) 2229
Exelon Oral Solution (Frequent) 2229
Foradil Aerolizer (1.7%) 2849
Forteo for Injection (2.6%) 1816
Frova Tablets (Infrequent) 1111
Gabitril Tablets (Infrequent) 973
Gammagard S/D (Occasional) 734
▲ Gengraf Capsules (12%) 435
▲ Intron A for Injection (Less than 5%) 2859
Klonopin (Infrequent) 2639
Lamictal (Infrequent) 1488
Lipitor Tablets (Less than 2%) 2501
Lunesta Tablets (Infrequent) 2994
Lyrica Capsules (Greater than or equal to 1%) 2527
Meridia Capsules (Greater than or equal to 1%) 475
Micardis Tablets (More than 0.3%) 852
Micardis HCT Tablets 854
Mirapex Tablets (1% or more) 857
Natrecor for Injection (Greater than or equal to 1%) 2977
▲ Neoral Oral Solution (12%) 2280

▲ Neoral Soft Gelatin Capsules (12%) 2280
Pentasa Capsules (Less than 1%) 3030
Plavix Tablets (1% to 2.5%) 926
Plavix Tablets (1% to 2.5%) 2767
Pletal Tablets (2% or greater) 2481
▲ Premarin Tablets (3% to 7%) 3221
Premarin Vaginal Cream 3228
▲ Premphase Tablets (3% to 7%) 3232
▲ Prempro Tablets (3% to 7%) 3232
ProAmatine Tablets (Rare) 3032
▲ Prograf Capsules and Injection (3% to 15%) 622
▲ Prometrium Capsules (100 mg, 200 mg) (Less than 5%) 3047
Protonix for Delayed-Release Oral Suspension (Less than 1%) 3254
Protonix Delayed-Release Tablets (Less than 1%) 3254
Protonix I.V. (Less than 1%) 3257
Proventil HFA Inhalation Aerosol (Less than 3%) 2914
Provigil Tablets (At least 1%) 977
Prozac Pulvules and Liquid (Infrequent) 1852
Requip Tablets (1% or more) 1561
Rilutek Tablets (Infrequent) 2771
Risperdal Consta Long-Acting Injection (Infrequent) 1753
Sular Extended Release Tablets (Less than or equal to 1%) 2975
Symbyax Capsules (Infrequent) 1871
Teveten HCT Tablets (Less than 1%) 517
Tricor Tablets 520
Wellbutrin SR Sustained-Release Tablets (Infrequent) 1653
Wellbutrin XL Extended-Release Tablets (Infrequent) 1659
Xopenex Inhalation Solution (2.7%) 3001
Xopenex Inhalation Solution Concentrate (2.7%) 3005
Xopenex HFA Inhalation Aerosol (2.7%) 3009
Zonegran Capsules (Infrequent) 1089
Zyban Sustained-Release Tablets (Infrequent) 1692
Zyprexa Tablets (Infrequent) 1883
Zyprexa ZYDIS Orally Disintegrating Tablets (Infrequent) 1883

Cranial nerve, dysfunction
Advicor Tablets 402
Lescol Capsules 2268
Lescol XL Tablets 2268

Cranial nerve, paralysis of
Amerge Tablets (Rare) 1301

Cranial nerve deficit, fetal
Accutane Capsules 2607

Craniofacial deformities
Captopril Tablets 2182
Cozaar Tablets 1973
Prinivil Tablets 2087
Prinzide Tablets 2092

Craniosynostosis
Synthroid Tablets 507

Creatine kinase, increase
Accutane Capsules 2607
Actos Tablets 3077
Advicor Tablets 402
Atacand Tablets (0.5% or greater) 639
Atacand HCT (0.5% or greater) 642
▲ Atripla Tablets (9%) 938
Axert Tablets (Infrequent) 2431
Cardizem LA Extended Release Tablets (Less than 2%) 421
Combivir Tablets 1384
Comtan Tablets 2208
▲ Cubicin for Injection (2.8% to 6.7%) 995
Effexor XR Extended-Release Capsules 3195
▲ Emtriva Capsules (9% to 12%) 1246
▲ Emtriva Oral Solution (9% to 12%) 1246
Epivir 1412
▲ Epivir-HBV (9%) 1417
Evoxac Capsules 1013
Isentress Tablets (2.2% to 2.4%) 2036
Levitra Tablets (2%) 2876
▲ Mevacor Tablets (11%) 2063
Noroxin Tablets (Rare) 2069
Paxil (Rare) 1535
Paxil CR Controlled-Release Tablets (Rare) 1544
ReFacto Vials 3269
Retrovir IV Infusion 1579
Sandostatin Injection (Less than 1%) 2300
Sandostatin LAR Depot 2302
Selzentry Tablets 2534
Tekturna Tablets (1%) 2321
Teveten Tablets (Less than 1%) 515
Teveten HCT Tablets (Less than 1%) 517
▲ Tricor Tablets (3%) 520
Trizivir Tablets 1622
▲ Truvada Tablets (9%) 1262
Twinrix Vaccine 1628
▲ Tyzeka Tablets (9% to 72%) 2328
Ultane Liquid for Inhalation 524
▲ Viread Tablets (2% to 12%) 1268
Vytorin 10/10 Tablets (0.2%) 2149
Vytorin 10/20 Tablets (0.2%) 2149
Vytorin 10/40 Tablets (0.2%) 2149
Vytorin 10/80 Tablets (0.2%) 2149
Ziagen 1673
Zocor Tablets 2136

Creatine phosphokinase, increase
Abilify Injection (Greater than or equal to 1 in 100) 881
Abilify Injection (Greater than or equal to 1 in 100) 2466
Abilify Oral Solution (Greater than or equal to 1 in 100) 881
Abilify Oral Solution (Greater than or equal to 1 in 100) 2466
Abilify Discmelt Orally Disintegrating Tablets (Greater than or equal to 1 in 100) 881
Abilify Discmelt Orally Disintegrating Tablets (Greater than or equal to 1 in 100) 2466
Abilify Tablets (Greater than or equal to 1 in 100) 881
Abilify Tablets (Greater than or equal to 1 in 100) 2466
Altabax Ointment (Less than 1%) 1299
▲ Aptivus Capsules (11%) 823
▲ Aptivus Oral Solution (11%) 823
Cymbalta Delayed-Release Capsules 1801
Emtriva Capsules (2 patients) 1246
Emtriva Oral Solution (2 patients) 1246
▲ Fenoglide Tablets (3%) 2960
Patanase Nasal Spray (0.9%) 544
Prozac Weekly Capsules (Rare) 1852
Relenza Inhalation Powder (Less than 1.5%) 1556
Venlafaxine Hydrochloride Tablets 2199
▲ Vivitrol (11% to 16%) 988
Vytorin 10/10 Tablets 2149
Vytorin 10/20 Tablets 2149
Vytorin 10/40 Tablets 2149
Vytorin 10/80 Tablets 2149
Zetia Tablets 2157
Zetia Tablets 2951

Creatinine, increase
(*see under* Serum creatinine, elevation)

Creatinine clearance, decrease
▲ Alimta for Injection (Up to 5%) 1786
▲ NeoProfen Injection (3%) 2496
Proglycem Capsules (Infrequent) 1185
Proglycem Suspension (Infrequent) 1185
▲ Valcyte Tablets (Less than 5%) 2654
Vantas (Less than 2%) 1737
Zinacef for Injection 1678
Zinacef Injection 1678

Crepitations
▲ Dacogen Injection (5%) 1066
▲ Trisenox Injection (10%) 986

Crohn's disease
Fleet Prep Kits 1149

Crohn's disease, exacerbation
Anaprox Tablets (Less than 1%) 2632
Anaprox DS Tablets (Less than 1%) 2632
EC-Naprosyn Delayed-Release Tablets (Less than 1%) 2632
Naprosyn Suspension (Less than 1%) 2632
Naprosyn Tablets (Less than 1%) 2632
Proleukin for Injection 2287

Croup
(*see under* Laryngotracheobronchitis)

Crusting
Durezol Ophthalmic Emulsion (Less than 1%) ⊙ 275
▲ Panretin Gel 0.1% (1% to 8%) 1081

Crying
Aricept Tablets (Frequent) 1062
Aricept ODT Tablets (Frequent) 1062
▲ Comvax (0.2% to 10.6%) 1966
Daytrana Transdermal Patch 3022
▲ Infanrix Vaccine (2.2% to 3.9%) 1479
Lexapro Oral Suspension (Infrequent) 1174
Lexapro Tablets (Infrequent) 1174
Namenda (Infrequent) 1180
Paxil 1535
Paxil CR Controlled-Release Tablets 1544
▲ Pediarix Vaccine (1.4% to 24.9%) 1552
▲ Pentacel (0.9% to 59.3%) 2792
Prevnar 3241
ProQuad (Greater than or equal to 0.2% to less than 1%) 2099
Recombivax HB (Greater than 1%) 2107
▲ Romazicon Injection (1% to 3%) 2646
Ultane Liquid for Inhalation (Less than 1%) 524
Vaqta (1.8%) 2130
Xyrem Oral Solution (Infrequent) 1766

Crying, abnormal
Crinone 4% Gel 992
Crinone 8% Gel 992

Cryptococcosis
▲ CellCept Capsules (Less than 4%) 2622
▲ CellCept Intravenous (Less than 4%) 2622
▲ CellCept Oral Suspension (Less than 4%) 2622
▲ CellCept Tablets (Less than 4%) 2622
Doxil Injection (Less than 1%) 2378

Crystalluria
Amoxil Capsules 1305
Amoxil Chewable Tablets 1305
Amoxil Pediatric Drops for Oral Suspension 1305
Amoxil Powder for Oral Suspension 1305
Amoxil Tablets 1305
Augmentin 1323
Augmentin Tablets 1327
Augmentin XR Extended Release Tablets 1333
Cardizem LA Extended Release Tablets (Less than 2%) 421
Cipro I.V. (1% or less) 2817
Cipro (Rare) 2810
Cipro XR Tablets 2823
Clinoril Tablets (Less than 1 in 100) 1962
Crixivan Capsules 1979
Dantrium Capsules (Less frequent) 2580
Demser Capsules (Few patients) 1989
Effexor XR Extended-Release Capsules (Rare) 3195
Fansidar Tablets 2636
Gantrisin Pediatric Suspension 2638
Levaquin 2416
Levaquin in 5% Dextrose Injection 2416
Lyrica Capsules (Rare) 2527
Moxatag Tablets 2165
Noroxin Tablets 2069
Paser Granules 1747

Cushingoid appearance
▲ Advair Diskus 100/50 (Greater than or equal to 3%) 1276
Advair Diskus 250/50 1276
Advair Diskus 500/50 1276
Advair HFA 45/21 Inhalation Aerosol 1288
Advair HFA 115/21 Inhalation Aerosol 1288
Advair HFA 230/21 Inhalation Aerosol 1288
Aptivus Capsules 823
Aptivus Oral Solution 823
Atripla Tablets 938
Crixivan Capsules 1979
Emtriva Capsules 1246
Emtriva Oral Solution 1246
Intelence Tablets 3119
Lexiva Oral Suspension 1510
Lexiva Tablets 1510
Omnaris Nasal Spray (Very rare) 2998
Retrovir 1574
Truvada Tablets 1262
Viramune Oral Suspension 873
Viramune Tablets 873

Cushingoid state
(*see under* Cushing's syndrome)

Cushing's syndrome
▲ Advair Diskus 100/50 (5%) 1276
Advair Diskus 250/50 1276
Advair Diskus 500/50 1276
Advair HFA 45/21 Inhalation Aerosol 1288
Advair HFA 115/21 Inhalation Aerosol 1288
Advair HFA 230/21 Inhalation Aerosol 1288
▲ CellCept Capsules (3% to less than 20%) 2622
▲ CellCept Intravenous (3% to less than 20%) 2622
▲ CellCept Oral Suspension (3% to less than 20%) 2622
▲ CellCept Tablets (3% to less than 20%) 2622
Copaxone for Injection (Infrequent) 3110
Diprolene Lotion 0.05% 2838
Diprolene AF Cream 0.05% (Some patients) 2837
Elocon Cream 0.1% 2840
Elocon Lotion 0.1% 2841
Elocon Ointment 0.1% 2842
Flovent Diskus 50 mcg 1435
Flovent HFA 1440
▲ Gliadel Wafer (3%) 1076
Kaletra (Less than 2%) 452
Lotrisone 2881
▲ Myfortic Tablets (3% to less than 20%) 2276
Olux Foam 3061
Olux-E Foam 3059
▲ Prograf Capsules and Injection (3% to 15%) 622
Vanos Cream 1941
Verdeso Foam 3069

Cushing's syndrome, manifestations of
Diprolene Ointment 0.05% 2839

Cutaneous reactions, severe
Celexa (Rare) 1160
Relenza Inhalation Powder 1556
▲ Taxotere Injection Concentrate (0% to 16.7%) 2773
Viramune Oral Suspension 873
Viramune Tablets 873

Cutaneous reactions, unspecified
Flebogamma 5% 1715
Flebogamma 5% DIF 1718
Lotrisone Cream 2881
Malarone Pediatric Tablets 1521
Malarone Tablets 1521
▲ Taxotere Injection Concentrate (1% to 61.1%) 2773
Treanda for Injection 983
Valium Tablets 2658

Cyanosis
AmBisome for Injection (Infrequent) 606
BeneFIX Vials 3191
Bicillin C-R Injectable Suspension 1775
Bicillin L-A Injection 1777
▲ Cerezyme for Injection (Approximately 6.6%) 1238
Copaxone for Injection (Infrequent) 3110
Effexor XR Extended-Release Capsules (Rare) 3195
Elitek (Less than or equal to 1%) 2729
Flebogamma 5% 1715
Flebogamma 5% DIF 1718
▲ Flolan for Injection (31% to 54%) 1426
Gammagard Liquid 730
Gammagard S/D 734
Gamunex 3094
Gantrisin Pediatric Suspension 2638
Imitrex Injection 1465
Imitrex Nasal Spray 1470
Imitrex Tablets 1474
Infanrix Vaccine 1479
▲ Infasurf Intratracheal Suspension (65%) 1168
▲ Intron A for Injection (Less than or equal to 5%) 2859
Mephyton Tablets (Rare) 700
Mirapex Tablets 857
Mycamine for Injection 616
Pediarix Vaccine 1552
Pentacel 2792
Primaxin I.M. 2080
Primaxin I.V. (Less than 0.2%) 2083
Rilutek Tablets (Rare) 2771
Soriatane Capsules (Less than 1%) 3062
Synagis Intramuscular Solution 1948
Venlafaxine Hydrochloride Tablets (Rare) 2199
Zomig Tablets (Rare) 694
Zomig Nasal Spray (Infrequent) 689
Zomig-ZMT Tablets (Rare) 694
Zyprexa Tablets (Infrequent) 1883
Zyprexa ZYDIS Orally Disintegrating Tablets (Infrequent) 1883

Cyanosis, hand
▲ Intron A for Injection (Less than 5%) 2859

Cycloplegia
Bentyl Capsules 703
Bentyl Injection 703
Bentyl Syrup 703
Bentyl Tablets 703
Donnatal Extentabs 2507

Cylindruria
Cipro I.V. (1% or less) 2817
Cipro 2810
Cipro XR Tablets 2823
Levaquin 2416
Levaquin in 5% Dextrose Injection 2416
Noroxin Tablets 2069

Cyst, breast
Requip Tablets (Infrequent) 1561

Cyst, infected
Requip Tablets (Infrequent) 1561

Cyst, renal
Mirapex Tablets 857

Cyst, synovial
Gengraf Capsules (1% to less than 3%) 435
Neoral Oral Solution (1% to less than 3%) 2280
Neoral Soft Gelatin Capsules (1% to less than 3%) 2280

Cyst, unspecified
Actiq (Less than 1%) 959
▲ Arimidex Tablets (5%) 672
▲ CellCept Capsules (3% to 20%) 2622
▲ CellCept Intravenous (3% to 20%) 2622
▲ CellCept Oral Suspension (3% to 20%) 2622
▲ CellCept Tablets (3% to 20%) 2622
Copaxone for Injection (2%) 3110
Crinone 4% Gel 992
Crinone 8% Gel 992
Emsam Transdermal System (Infrequent) 905
Gabitril Tablets (Frequent) 973
Imitrex Injection 1465
Luvox CR Extended-Release Capsules (Rare) 1759
Protonix for Delayed-Release Oral Suspension (Less than 1%) 3254
Protonix Delayed-Release Tablets (Less than 1%) 3254
Protonix I.V. (Less than 1%) 3257
▲ Protopic Ointment (Up to 3%) 628
Salagen Tablets (Less than 1%) 1082
▲ Simulect for Injection (3% to 10%) 2306
Soriatane Capsules (Less than 1%) 3062
Symbyax Capsules (Infrequent) 1871
Tricor Tablets 520
Xyrem Oral Solution (Infrequent) 1766
Zomig Tablets (Infrequent) 694
Zomig Nasal Spray (Infrequent) 689
Zomig-ZMT Tablets (Infrequent) 694

Cystitis
▲ Actonel with Calcium Tablets (4.1%) 2574
Ambien Tablets (Infrequent) 2692
Ambien CR Tablets (Infrequent) 2696
Anaprox Tablets (Less than 1%) 2632
Anaprox DS Tablets (Less than 1%) 2632
Aricept Tablets (Frequent) 1062
Aricept ODT Tablets (Frequent) 1062
Atacand HCT (0.5% or greater) 642
▲ Azmacort Inhalation Aerosol (1% to 3%) 407
Brovana Inhalation Solution (Less than 2%) 2990
Celebrex Capsules (0.1% to 1.9%) 2979
Copaxone for Injection (At least 2%) 3110
Crinone 4% Gel 992
Crinone 8% Gel 992
Depakote ER Tablets (Greater than 1%) 423
▲ Doxil Injection (Less than 1% to 10%) 2378
EC-Naprosyn Delayed-Release Tablets (Less than 1%) 2632
Effexor XR Extended-Release Capsules (Infrequent) 3195
Emsam Transdermal System (Infrequent) 905
Estratest Tablets 3043
Estratest H.S. Tablets 3043
▲ Evista Tablets (3.3% to 4.6%) 1810
▲ Evoxac Capsules (1% to 3%) 1013
Exelon Capsules (Infrequent) 2229
Exelon Oral Solution (Infrequent) 2229
Gabitril Tablets (Infrequent) 973
▲ Humira Injection (Less than 5%) 442
▲ Intron A for Injection (Less than 5%) 2859
Klonopin (Infrequent) 2639
Lamictal (Rare) 1488
Leukeran Tablets 1508
Lipitor Tablets (Less than 2%) 2501
Lunesta Tablets (Infrequent) 2994
Luvox CR Extended-Release Capsules (Infrequent) 1759
▲ Miacalcin Nasal Spray (1% to 3%) 2274
Micardis Tablets (More than 0.3%) 852
Micardis HCT Tablets 854
Mirapex Tablets 857
Nalfon Capsules (Less than 1%) 2508
Naprosyn Suspension (Less than 1%) 2632
Naprosyn Tablets (Less than 1%) 2632
Nexium Delayed-Release Capsules (Less than 1%) 645
Nexium I.V. (Less than 1%) 652
Nexium Delayed-Release Oral Suspension (Less than 1%) 645
Ortho-Cyclen Tablets 2449
Ortho Evra Transdermal System 2437
Ortho Tri-Cyclen Tablets 2449
Ortho Tri-Cyclen Lo Tablets 2458
Paxil (Infrequent) 1535
Paxil CR Controlled-Release Tablets (Infrequent) 1544
Plavix Tablets (1% to 2.5%) 926
Plavix Tablets (1% to 2.5%) 2767
Pletal Tablets (Less than 2%) 2481
Premarin Intravenous 3217
Premarin Vaginal Cream 3228
Premphase Tablets 3232
Prempro Tablets 3232
▲ Prograf Capsules and Injection (3% to 15%) 622
Protonix for Delayed-Release Oral Suspension (Less than 1%) 3254
Protonix Delayed-Release Tablets (Less than 1%) 3254
Protonix I.V. (Less than 1%) 3257
Protopic Ointment (0.2% to less than 1%) 628
Provigil Tablets (At least 1%) 977
Prozac Weekly Capsules (Infrequent) 1852
Prozac Pulvules and Liquid (Infrequent) 1852
Remeron Tablets (Infrequent) 2924
RemeronSolTab Tablets (Infrequent) 2927
Requip Tablets (Infrequent) 1561
Symbyax Capsules (Infrequent) 1871
Teveten Tablets (Less than 1%) 515
Teveten HCT Tablets (Less than 1%) 517
▲ Tice BCG (6%) 2936
Tricor Tablets 520
▲ Valstar Sterile Solution for Intravesical Instillation (15%) 1735
Venlafaxine Hydrochloride Tablets (Infrequent) 2199
Vicoprofen Tablets (Less than 1%) 533
Voltaren Tablets (Occasionally) 2334
Voltaren-XR Tablets (Occasionally) 2337
Wellbutrin Tablets (Rare) 1648
Wellbutrin SR Sustained-Release Tablets 1653
Wellbutrin XL Extended-Release Tablets 1659
Yaz Tablets (Greater than 1%) 805
Zomig Tablets (Infrequent) 694
Zomig-ZMT Tablets (Infrequent) 694
Zyban Sustained-Release Tablets 1692
Zyprexa Tablets (Infrequent) 1883
Zyprexa ZYDIS Orally Disintegrating Tablets (Infrequent) 1883
Zyrtec Chewable Tablets (Less than 2%) 1920
Zyrtec Syrup (Less than 2%) 1920
Zyrtec Tablets (Less than 2%) 1920
Zyrtec-D 12 Hour Extended Release Tablets (Less than 2%) 1923

Cystitis, hemorrhagic
AmBisome for Injection (Infrequent) 606
▲ Busulfex Injection (7%) 2477
Cipro I.V. (1% or less) 2817
Cipro XR Tablets 2823
Prograf Capsules and Injection 622
▲ Tice BCG (9%) 2936
Velcade for Injection 2168

Cystitis, viral
Retrovir Capsules (0.8%) 1574
Retrovir IV Infusion (1%) 1579
Retrovir (0.8%) 1574

Cystitis-like syndrome
Activella Tablets 2347
Lybrel Tablets 3204
Mircette Tablets 1034
NuvaRing 2897
Seasonique Tablets 1046
Yaz Tablets 805

Cytokine Released Syndrome
Orthoclone OKT3 Sterile Solution (Occasional) 2387
Simulect for Injection 2306

Cytopenia, unspecified
Bexxar 1371
Campath Ampules 761
Exjade Tablets 2244
Humira Injection (Infrequent) 442
Intron A for Injection 2859
▲ Rituxan I.V. (48%) 1223

D

Darcyostenosis, acquired
Mirapex Tablets 857

D-dimer levels, high
NovoSeven RT 2370

Deafness
Abelcet Injection 1134
Actiq (Less than 1%) 959
Aggrenox Capsules (Less than 1%) 819
Campral Tablets (Infrequent) 1158
Celebrex Capsules (0.1% to 1.9%) 2979
▲ CellCept Capsules (3% to less than 20%) 2622
▲ CellCept Intravenous (3% to less than 20%) 2622
▲ CellCept Oral Suspension (3% to less than 20%) 2622
▲ CellCept Tablets (3% to less than 20%) 2622
Chantix Tablets (Rare) 2511
Copaxone for Injection (At least 2%) 3110
Depakote ER Tablets (Greater than 1%) 423
DepoCyt Injection 1136
Edecrin 698
Effexor XR Extended-Release Capsules (Rare) 3195
Eloxatin for Injection 2731
Evoxac Capsules (Less than 1%) 1013
Gabitril Tablets (Infrequent) 973
Gengraf Capsules (1% to less than 3%) 435
Imitrex Injection 1465
Imitrex Nasal Spray 1470
Imitrex Tablets 1474
Indocin Capsules (Less than 1%) 2024
Indocin I.V. (Less than 1%) 2489
Indocin (Less than 1%) 2024
Lamictal (Rare) 1488
Lipitor Tablets (Less than 2%) 2501
Luvox CR Extended-Release Capsules (Infrequent) 1759
Mirapex Tablets 857
Neoral Oral Solution (1% to less than 3%) 2280
Neoral Soft Gelatin Capsules (1% to less than 3%) 2280
Paxil (Rare) 1535
Paxil CR Controlled-Release Tablets (Rare) 1544
Prograf Capsules and Injection 622
ProQuad 2099
Protonix for Delayed-Release Oral Suspension (Less than 1%) 3254
Protonix Delayed-Release Tablets (Less than 1%) 3254
Protonix I.V. (Less than 1%) 3257
Prozac Weekly Capsules (Rare) 1852
Remeron Tablets (Infrequent) 2924
RemeronSolTab Tablets (Infrequent) 2927
Rilutek Tablets (Rare) 2771
Risperdal Consta Long-Acting Injection (Infrequent) 1753
Salagen Tablets (Less than 1%) 1082
Sandostatin LAR Depot 2302
Soriatane Capsules (Less than 1%) 3062
Symbyax Capsules (Infrequent) 1871
Velcade for Injection 2168
Venlafaxine Hydrochloride Tablets (Rare) 2199
Wellbutrin SR Sustained-Release Tablets 1653
Wellbutrin XL Extended-Release Tablets 1659
Zonegran Capsules (Infrequent) 1089
Zyban Sustained-Release Tablets 1692
Zyprexa Tablets (Infrequent) 1883
Zyprexa ZYDIS Orally Disintegrating Tablets (Infrequent) 1883
Zyrtec Chewable Tablets (Less than 2%) 1920
Zyrtec Syrup (Less than 2%) 1920
Zyrtec Tablets (Less than 2%) 1920
Zyrtec-D 12 Hour Extended Release Tablets (Less than 2%) 1923

Deafness, transient
Actiq (Less than 1%) 959
Remeron Tablets (Rare) 2924
RemeronSolTab Tablets (Rare) 2927

Death
Gemzar for Injection (Rare) 1820
Symbyax Capsules (Rare) 1871
Voltaren Tablets (Rarely) 2334
Voltaren-XR Tablets (Rarely) 2337
Zolinza Capsules 2142

Death, fetal
Aceon Tablets (2 mg, 4 mg, 8 mg) 3038
Atacand Tablets 639
Atacand HCT 642
Avalide Tablets 892
Avalide Tablets 2713
Avapro Tablets 897
Avapro Tablets 2718
Captopril Tablets 2182
Cozaar Tablets 1973
Doxil Injection 2378
Prinivil Tablets 2087
Prinzide Tablets 2092
Prometrium Capsules (100 mg, 200 mg) (Rare) 3047
Tekturna HCT Tablets 2324

Death, sudden
Adderall XR Capsules 3012
Campral Tablets (Rare) 1158
Celebrex Capsules (Less than 0.1%) 2979
Gabitril Tablets (Infrequent) 973
Imitrex Tablets 1474
Meridia Capsules 475
Namenda 1180
Prozac Pulvules and Liquid 1852
Thioridazine Hydrochloride Tablets 2195
Zyprexa Tablets (Rare) 1883
Zyprexa ZYDIS Orally Disintegrating Tablets (Rare) 1883

Deep tendon reflexes, loss
Eloxatin for Injection 2731

Defecate, desire to
Aminohippurate Sodium "PAH" Injection 1950

Defecation, increased
▲ Xenical Capsules (2.8% to 10.8%) 2672

Defect, atrial septal
Mirapex Tablets 857

Deglutition disorder
Emend Capsules (Greater than 0.5%) 1992
Emend for Injection (Greater than 0.5%) 1999

Dehydration
Actiq (1% or greater) 959
Aggrenox Capsules 819
▲ Agrylin Capsules (1% to less than 5%) 3017
▲ Alimta for Injection (Up to 9%) 1786
Amerge Tablets (Infrequent) 1301
Aptivus Capsules (2.1%) 823
Aptivus Oral Solution (2.1%) 823
▲ Aranesp for Injection (5%) 564
Aricept Tablets (2%) 1062
Aricept ODT Tablets (2%) 1062
▲ Arranon Injection (1% to 7%) 1319
▲ Avastin IV (3.3%) 1192
Bayer Aspirin 750
Bexxar 1371
Brovana Inhalation Solution (Less than 2%) 2990
Byetta Injection 600
Captopril Tablets 2182
Celexa (Rare) 1160
▲ CellCept Capsules (3% to less than 20%) 2622
▲ CellCept Intravenous (3% to less than 20%) 2622
▲ CellCept Oral Suspension (3% to less than 20%) 2622
▲ CellCept Tablets (3% to less than 20%) 2622

Cymbalta Delayed-Release Capsules (Infrequent) 1801
▲ Dacogen Injection (6%) 1066
Demadex Injection 2630
Demadex Tablets 2630
▲ DepoCyt Injection (13% to 18%) 1136
Diovan HCT Tablets (Less frequent) 2216
▲ Doxil Injection (1% to 10%) 2378
Effexor XR Extended-Release Capsules (Rare) 3195
Elitek (Less than or equal to 1%) 2729
Elmiron Capsules 2435
▲ Eloxatin for Injection (3% to 14%) 2731
▲ Emend Capsules (5.9%) 1992
▲ Emend for Injection (5.9%) 1999
Emsam Transdermal System (Infrequent) 905
Epivir 1412
▲ Erbitux (6% to 25%) 912
Evoxac Capsules (Less than 1%) 1013
Exelon Capsules (2% to Frequent) 2229
Exelon Oral Solution (2% to Frequent) 2229
Exelon Patch (Frequent) 2233
▲ Fentora Tablets (0% to 21%) 968
Fleet Enema 1143
Fleet Enema Extra 1143
Fleet Enema for Children 1143
Fleet Pedia-Lax Enema 1143
Fleet Phospho-soda 1145
Fleet Phospho-soda EZ-PREP 1147
Fleet Prep Kits 1149
Frova Tablets (Infrequent) 1111
Furosemide Tablets 2186
Gabitril Tablets (Infrequent) 973
Geodon Capsules (Infrequent) 2520
Gleevec Tablets (Infrequent) 2255
▲ Humira Injection (Less than 5%) 442
Imitrex Injection (Rare) 1465
Imitrex Nasal Spray 1470
Imitrex Tablets 1474
▲ Intron A for Injection (Less than or equal to 5%) 2859
Invanz for Injection (Greater than 0.1%) 2029
Ionsys Transdermal System (.1% to less than 1%) 2410
Ixempra Kit for Injection (2%) 915
Kaletra (Less than 2%) 452
Keppra Oral Solution (2%) 3131
Keppra Tablets (2%) 3131
Kinrix Injection Vaccine (0.1%) 1486
Klonopin 2639
Lunesta Tablets (Rare) 2994
Luvox CR Extended-Release Capsules (Infrequent) 1759
Maxalt Tablets (Infrequent) 2056
Maxalt-MLT Orally Disintegrating Tablets (Infrequent) 2056
Mirapex Tablets 857
Mobic Oral Suspension (Less than 2%) 863
Mobic Tablets (Less than 2%) 863
▲ Myfortic Tablets (3% to less than 20%) 2276
Namenda (Infrequent) 1180
Nexavar Tablets (0.1% to less than 1%) 784
Norvir (Less than 2%) 489
▲ Noxafil Oral Suspension (1% to 11%) 2889
▲ Ontak Vials (9%) 1079
Opana Tablets (Less than 1%) 1117
Opana ER Tablets (Less than 1%) 1121
OxyContin Tablets (Less than 1%) 2589
Paxil (Rare) 1535
Paxil CR Controlled-Release Tablets (Rare) 1544
Pentacel 2792
Percocet Tablets 1127
Percodan Tablets 1130
▲ Photofrin for Injection (7% to 10%) 708
Prinivil Tablets (0.3% to 1%) 2087
Prinzide Tablets 2092
▲ Prograf Capsules and Injection (3% to 15%) 622
Protonix for Delayed-Release Oral Suspension 3254
Protonix Delayed-Release Tablets 3254
Protonix I.V. 3257
Protopic Ointment (Greater than or equal to 1%) 628
Prozac Weekly Capsules (Infrequent) 1852
Prozac Pulvules and Liquid (Infrequent) 1852
Remeron Tablets (Infrequent) 2924
RemeronSolTab Tablets (Infrequent) 2927
Remicade for IV Injection (Greater than or equal to 0.2%) 950
Requip Tablets (Infrequent) 1561
Risperdal Consta Long-Acting Injection (Infrequent) 1753
Rocaltrol Capsules 1150
Rocaltrol Oral Solution 1150
Rythmol SR Capsules 1590
St. Joseph 81 mg Aspirin Chewable and Enteric Coated Tablets 1903
Salagen Tablets 1082
▲ Simulect for Injection (3% to 10%) 2306
▲ Sutent Capsules (3% to 11%) 2540
Symbyax Capsules (Infrequent) 1871
Tasigna Capsules (0.1% to 1%) 2316
Taxotere Injection Concentrate 2773
▲ Valcyte Tablets (Less than 5%) 2654
▲ Vaprisol (2.2% to 6%) 632
Vaqta 2130
Vectibix 597
▲ Velcade for Injection (3% to 10%) 2168
Venlafaxine Hydrochloride Tablets (Infrequent) 2199
Vivitrol 988
▲ Xeloda Tablets (2% to 10%) 2662
Xifaxan Tablets (Less than 2%) 2682
▲ Zometa for Intravenous Infusion (5% to 14%) 2341
Zomig Tablets (Rare) 694
Zomig Nasal Spray (Rare) 689
Zomig-ZMT Tablets (Rare) 694
Zonegran Capsules (Infrequent) 1089
Zyprexa Tablets (Infrequent) 1883
Zyprexa IntraMuscular (Infrequent) 1883
Zyprexa ZYDIS Orally Disintegrating Tablets (Infrequent) 1883
Zyrtec Chewable Tablets (Less than 2%) 1920
Zyrtec Syrup (Less than 2%) 1920
Zyrtec Tablets (Less than 2%) 1920
Zyrtec-D 12 Hour Extended Release Tablets (Less than 2%) 1923

Delirium

Abilify Injection (Greater than or equal to 1 in 1000 patients and less than 1 in 100 patients) 881
Abilify Injection (Greater than or equal to 1 in 1000 patients and less than 1 in 100 patients) 2466
Abilify Oral Solution (Greater than or equal to 1 in 1000 patients and less than 1 in 100 patients) 881
Abilify Oral Solution (Greater than or equal to 1 in 1000 patients and less than 1 in 100 patients) 2466
Abilify Discmelt Orally Disintegrating Tablets (Greater than or equal to 1 in 1000 patients and less than 1 in 100 patients) 881
Abilify Discmelt Orally Disintegrating Tablets (Greater than or equal to 1 in 1000 patients and less than 1 in 100 patients) 2466
Abilify Tablets (Greater than or equal to 1 in 1000 patients and less than 1 in 100 patients) 881
Abilify Tablets (Greater than or equal to 1 in 1000 patients and less than 1 in 100 patients) 2466
Aciphex Tablets 1053
▲ Avinza Capsules (Less than 5%) 1772
Azilect Tablets (Rare) 3106
Busulfex Injection (2%) 2477
Catapres Tablets 841
Catapres-TTS (0.5% or less) 842
Celexa 1160
▲ CellCept Capsules (3% to less than 20%) 2622
▲ CellCept Intravenous (3% to less than 20%) 2622
▲ CellCept Oral Suspension (3% to less than 20%) 2622
▲ CellCept Tablets (3% to less than 20%) 2622
Cipro I.V. 2817
Cipro 2810
Cipro XR Tablets 2823
Clorpres Tablets 2185
Effexor XR Extended-Release Capsules 3195
Evoxac Capsules 1013
Exelon Capsules (Infrequent) 2229
Exelon Oral Solution (Infrequent) 2229
Geodon Capsules (Frequent) 2520
Lamictal (Rare) 1488
Lanoxin Injection 1498
Lanoxin Injection Pediatric 1502
Lanoxin Tablets 1505
Lexapro Oral Suspension 1174
Lexapro Tablets 1174
Luvox CR Extended-Release Capsules (Infrequent) 1759
Lyrica Capsules (Rare) 2527
Merrem I.V. (Greater than 0.1% to 1%) 684
Mirapex Tablets 857
Mycamine for Injection 616
Namenda (Infrequent) 1180
Orthoclone OKT3 Sterile Solution (Less than 1%) 2387
Paxil (Rare) 1535
Paxil CR Controlled-Release Tablets (Rare) 1544
PhosLo GelCaps 1184
Prograf Capsules and Injection 622
Proleukin for Injection (Less than 1%) 2287
Relenza Inhalation Powder 1556
Remeron Tablets (Infrequent) 2924
RemeronSolTab Tablets (Infrequent) 2927
Requip Tablets (Infrequent) 1561
Rilutek Tablets (Infrequent) 2771
Risperdal Consta Long-Acting Injection (Infrequent) 1753
Romazicon Injection (Less than 1%) 2646
Sanctura XR Capsules 557
Tamiflu Capsules 2649
Tamiflu Oral Suspension 2649
Venlafaxine Hydrochloride Tablets 2199
Vivitrol 988
Wellbutrin Tablets 1648
Wellbutrin SR Sustained-Release Tablets 1653
Wellbutrin XL Extended-Release Tablets 1659
Zovirax 1690
Zyban Sustained-Release Tablets 1692
Zyprexa Tablets (Infrequent) 1883
Zyprexa ZYDIS Orally Disintegrating Tablets (Infrequent) 1883

Delivery complications, unspecified

Bayer Aspirin 750
Epivir 1412
Motrin IB Tablets and Caplets 1900
St. Joseph 81 mg Aspirin Chewable and Enteric Coated Tablets 1903

Delusional disorder persecutory type

Mirapex Tablets 857

Delusional thinking

Strattera Capsules (0.2%) 1864
Vyvanse Capsules (0.1%) 3033

Delusions

Ambien Tablets (Rare) 2692
Ambien CR Tablets (Rare) 2696
Aricept Tablets (Infrequent) 1062
Aricept ODT Tablets (Infrequent) 1062
Atripla Tablets 938
Azilect Tablets (Infrequent) 3106
Celexa (Rare) 1160
Effexor XR Extended-Release Capsules (Rare) 3195
Eldepryl Capsules 3052
Evoxac Capsules 1013
Exelon Capsules (2% or more) 2229
Exelon Oral Solution (2% or more) 2229
Exelon Patch (Infrequent) 2233
Gabitril Tablets (Infrequent) 973
Lamictal (Rare) 1488
Lexapro Oral Suspension 1174
Lexapro Tablets 1174
Lupron Depot 3.75 mg (Among most frequent) 462
▲ Lupron Depot–3 Month 11.25 mg (Less than 5%) 462
Luvox CR Extended-Release Capsules (Infrequent) 1759
Lyrica Capsules (Rare) 2527
Mirapex Tablets (1%) 857
Namenda (Infrequent) 1180
Paxil (Rare) 1535
Paxil CR Controlled-Release Tablets (Rare) 1544
Provigil Tablets 977
Prozac Weekly Capsules (Rare) 1852
Prozac Pulvules and Liquid (Rare) 1852
Relenza Inhalation Powder 1556
Remeron Tablets (Infrequent) 2924
RemeronSolTab Tablets (Infrequent) 2927
Requip Tablets (Infrequent) 1561
Rilutek Tablets (Infrequent) 2771
Risperdal Consta Long-Acting Injection (Frequent) 1753
Stalevo Tablets 2309
Sustiva Capsules 930
Sustiva Tablets 930
Tamiflu Capsules 2649
Tamiflu Oral Suspension 2649
Valium Tablets 2658
Venlafaxine Hydrochloride Tablets (Rare) 2199
Wellbutrin Tablets (1.2%) 1648
Wellbutrin SR Sustained-Release Tablets 1653
Wellbutrin XL Extended-Release Tablets 1659
Zyban Sustained-Release Tablets 1692
Zyprexa Tablets (Frequent) 1883

Dementia

Activella Tablets 2347
Ambien Tablets (Rare) 2692
Ambien CR Tablets (Rare) 2696
Angeliq Tablets 751
Aricept Tablets (Infrequent) 1062
Aricept ODT Tablets (Infrequent) 1062
Azilect Tablets (Infrequent) 3106
Depakote ER Tablets 423
Divigel 3167
Effexor XR Extended-Release Capsules (Rare) 3195
Enjuvia Tablets 1029
Estratest Tablets (1.8%) 3043
Estratest H.S. Tablets (1.8%) 3043
Evoxac Capsules 1013
Exelon Capsules (Infrequent) 2229
Exelon Oral Solution (Infrequent) 2229
Mirapex Tablets 857
Premarin Intravenous 3217
Premarin Tablets 3221
Premarin Vaginal Cream 3228
Premphase Tablets 3232
Prempro Tablets 3232
Remeron Tablets (Rare) 2924
RemeronSolTab Tablets (Rare) 2927
Requip Tablets (Infrequent) 1561
Rilutek Tablets (Rare) 2771
Risperdal Consta Long-Acting Injection (Infrequent) 1753
Rythmol SR Capsules 1590
Stalevo Tablets 2309
Venlafaxine Hydrochloride Tablets (Rare) 2199
▲ Vesanoid Capsules (3%) 2660
Zyprexa Tablets (Infrequent) 1883
Zyprexa ZYDIS Orally Disintegrating Tablets (Infrequent) 1883

Demyelinating disease

Cimzia (Rare) 3127

Demyelinating disorders, peripheral

Remicade for IV Injection 950

Demyelination

Infanrix Vaccine 1479
Proleukin for Injection 2287
Remicade for IV Injection 950

Dental caries

Actiq (Less than 1%) 959
Ambien Tablets (Rare) 2692
Ambien CR Tablets (Rare) 2696
Copaxone for Injection (Frequent) 3110
Emsam Transdermal System (Infrequent) 905
Gabitril Tablets (Infrequent) 973
Mirapex Tablets 857
Paxil (Rare) 1535
Paxil CR Controlled-Release Tablets (Rare) 1544
Protopic Ointment (0.2% to less than 1%) 628
Symbyax Capsules (Infrequent) 1871
Xyrem Oral Solution (Infrequent) 1766
Zyrtec-D 12 Hour Extended Release Tablets (Less than 2%) 1923

Dental disorders, unspecified

PegIntron Powder for Injection 2903
Rebetol 2917

Dependence, drug

Actiq 959
Adderall XR Capsules 3012
Adipex-P 1185
Ambien Tablets (Rare) 2692
Avinza Capsules 1772
Celexa (Infrequent) 1160
Daytrana Transdermal Patch 3022
DepoDur Injection 1095
Dexedrine 1401
Donnatal Extentabs 2507
Duragesic Transdermal System 2405

Lortab 5/500 Tablets 3143
Lortab 7.5/500 Tablets 3144
Lortab 10/500 Tablets 3144
Luvox CR Extended-Release Capsules (Infrequent) 1759
MS Contin Tablets 2585
Nembutal Sodium Solution, USP 2494
OxyIR Capsules 2593
Parnate Tablets 1532
Paxil (Rare) 1535
Paxil CR Controlled-Release Tablets (Rare) 1544
Percocet Tablets 1127
Percodan Tablets 1130
Remeron Tablets (Rare) 2924
RemeronSolTab Tablets (Rare) 2927
Soma Tablets 1931
Tylenol with Codeine Tablets 2427
Valium Tablets 2658
Vicodin Tablets 529
Vicodin ES Tablets 530
Vicodin HP Tablets 531
Vicoprofen Tablets 533

Dependence, physical

Dexedrine 1401
Donnatal Extentabs 2507
Duragesic Transdermal System 2405
Klonopin 2639
Lortab 5/500 Tablets 3143
Lortab 7.5/500 Tablets 3144
Lortab 10/500 Tablets 3144
Marinol Capsules (Uncommon) 3163
MS Contin Tablets 2585
OxyContin Tablets 2589
Percocet Tablets 1127
Percodan Tablets 1130
Vicodin HP Tablets 531
Vicoprofen Tablets 533
Xyrem Oral Solution 1766

Dependence, psychic

(*see under* Dependence, psychological)

Dependence, psychological

Adderall XR Capsules 3012
Avinza Capsules 1772
Concerta Extended-Release Tablets 1925
Dexedrine 1401
Donnatal Extentabs 2507
Duragesic Transdermal System 2405
Klonopin 2639
Lortab 5/500 Tablets 3143
Lortab 7.5/500 Tablets 3144
Lortab 10/500 Tablets 3144
Marinol Capsules (Uncommon) 3163
MS Contin Tablets (Very rare) 2585
Nembutal Sodium Solution, USP 2494
OxyContin Tablets 2589
OxyIR Capsules 2593
Percocet Tablets 1127
Percodan Tablets 1130
Tussionex Pennkinetic Extended-Release Suspension 3154
Vicodin Tablets 529
Vicodin ES Tablets 530
Vicodin HP Tablets 531
Vicoprofen Tablets 533
Xyrem Oral Solution 1766
Zydone Tablets 1132

Depersonalization

Ambien Tablets (Rare) 2692
Ambien CR Tablets (1%) 2696
Anzemet Injection (Infrequently) 2701
Anzemet Tablets 2704
Avelox (Less than 0.1%) 2803
Betaseron for SC Injection 756
Biaxin/Biaxin XL 411
Campral Tablets (Rare) 1158
Celexa (Infrequent) 1160
Cipro I.V. (1% or less) 2817
Cipro (Less than 1%) 2810
Cipro XR Tablets (Less than 1%) 2823
Copaxone for Injection (Infrequent) 3110
Duragesic Transdermal System (Less than 1%) 2405
Effexor XR Extended-Release Capsules (Frequent) 3195
Emsam Transdermal System (Infrequent) 905
▲ Equetro Extended-Release Capsules (Less than 5%) 3174
Evoxac Capsules (Less than 1%) 1013
Exelon Capsules (Infrequent) 2229
Exelon Oral Solution (Infrequent) 2229
Exforge Tablets (Greater than 0.1% to less than 1%) 2238
Frova Tablets (Infrequent) 1111
Gabitril Tablets (Frequent) 973
Indocin (Less than 1%) 2024
▲ Keppra Injection (13.3%) 3137
Keppra Oral Solution 3131
Keppra Tablets 3131
Klonopin (Infrequent) 2639
Kogenate FS 746
Kogenate FS with Bio-Set (1 case) 748
Lamictal (Infrequent) 1488
Lexapro Oral Suspension (Infrequent) 1174
Lexapro Tablets (Infrequent) 1174
Luvox CR Extended-Release Capsules (Infrequent) 1759
Lyrica Capsules (Greater than or equal to 1%) 2527
Marinol Capsules (Greater than 1%) 3163
Maxalt Tablets (Rare) 2056
Maxalt-MLT Orally Disintegrating Tablets (Rare) 2056
Namenda (Infrequent) 1180
OxyContin Tablets (Less than 1%) 2589
Paxil (Infrequent) 1535
Paxil CR Controlled-Release Tablets (Infrequent) 1544
Pristiq Extended-Release Tablets (Less than 2%) 3247
Prozac Weekly Capsules (Infrequent) 1852
Prozac Pulvules and Liquid (Infrequent) 1852
Remeron Tablets (Infrequent) 2924
RemeronSolTab Tablets (Infrequent) 2927
Requip Tablets (Infrequent) 1561
Rilutek Tablets (Infrequent) 2771
Risperdal Consta Long-Acting Injection (Infrequent) 1753
▲ Romazicon Injection (1% to 3%) 2646
Symbyax Capsules (Infrequent) 1871
Venlafaxine Hydrochloride Tablets (1%) 2199
Wellbutrin Tablets (Infrequent) 1648
Wellbutrin SR Sustained-Release Tablets (Infrequent) 1653
Wellbutrin XL Extended-Release Tablets (Infrequent) 1659
Zomig Tablets (Infrequent) 694
Zomig Nasal Spray (Infrequent) 689
Zomig-ZMT Tablets (Infrequent) 694
Zyban Sustained-Release Tablets (Infrequent) 1692
Zyprexa Tablets (Infrequent) 1883
Zyprexa ZYDIS Orally Disintegrating Tablets (Infrequent) 1883
Zyrtec Chewable Tablets (Less than 2%) 1920
Zyrtec Syrup (Less than 2%) 1920
Zyrtec Tablets (Less than 2%) 1920
Zyrtec-D 12 Hour Extended Release Tablets (Less than 2%) 1923

Depigmentation

Finacea Gel (Rare) 1742
▲ Intron A for Injection (Less than 5%) 2859

Depigmentation at application site

Lidoderm Patch 1114

Depressed mood

▲ Concerta Extended-Release Tablets (3.9%) 1925
Daytrana Transdermal Patch 3022
▲ Keppra Injection (1.7% to 6.7%) 3137
Strattera Capsules 1864

Depression

Accutane Capsules 2607
Aceon Tablets (2 mg, 4 mg, 8 mg) (2%) 3038
▲ Actimmune (3%) 1743
Activella Tablets 2347
▲ Actonel Tablets (6.8%) 2568
▲ Actonel with Calcium Tablets (2.3% to 6.8%) 2574
Aczone Gel 5% 3296
Adderall XR Capsules (0.7%) 3012
Advair Diskus 100/50 1276
Advair Diskus 250/50 1276
Advair Diskus 500/50 1276
Advair HFA 45/21 Inhalation Aerosol 1288
Advair HFA 115/21 Inhalation Aerosol 1288
Advair HFA 230/21 Inhalation Aerosol 1288
▲ Aerobid/Aerobid-M (1% to 3%) 1153
▲ Agrylin Capsules (1% to less than 5%) 3017
Aldara Cream, 5% 1699
▲ Alferon N Injection (One patient to 3%) 1726
▲ Alimta for Injection (Up to 14%) 1786
Alphagan P Ophthalmic Solution ⊙ 549
Ambien Tablets (2%) 2692
Ambien CR Tablets (1% to 2%) 2696
AmBisome for Injection (Less common) 606
Amerge Tablets (Infrequent) 1301
Amitiza Capsules (Less than 1%) 3082
Anaprox Tablets (Less than 1%) 2632
Anaprox DS Tablets (Less than 1%) 2632
AndroGel (0% to 1%) 3159
Angeliq Tablets 751
Aricept Tablets (2%) 1062
Aricept ODT Tablets (2%) 1062
▲ Arimidex Tablets (2% to 13%) 672
▲ Arranon Injection (0% to 6%) 1319
Asacol Delayed-Release Tablets 2579
▲ Asmanex Twisthaler (11%) 2797
Atacand Tablets (0.5% or greater) 639
Atacand HCT (0.5% or greater) 642
▲ Atripla Tablets (Greater than or equal to 10%) 938
Avalide Tablets 892
Avalide Tablets 2713
Avapro Tablets (Less than 1%) 897
Avapro Tablets (Less than 1%) 2718
Avelox (Less than 0.1%) 2803
Axert Tablets (Rare) 2431
▲ Azilect Tablets (5%) 3106
Azmacort Inhalation Aerosol 407
Beconase AQ Nasal Spray 1369
▲ Betaseron for SC Injection (30%) 756
Betimol Ophthalmic Solution 3181
▲ Busulfex Injection (23%) 2477
▲ Campral Tablets (4% to 8%) 1158
Cancidas for Injection 1953
Captopril Tablets 2182
Carbatrol Capsules 3019
Cardizem LA Extended Release Tablets (Less than 2%) 421
Catapres Tablets (About 1 in 100 patients) 841
Catapres-TTS (0.5% or less) 842
Celebrex Capsules (0.1% to 1.9%) 2979
Celexa (Frequent) 1160
▲ CellCept Capsules (3% to less than 20%) 2622
▲ CellCept Intravenous (3% to less than 20%) 2622
▲ CellCept Oral Suspension (3% to less than 20%) 2622
▲ CellCept Tablets (3% to less than 20%) 2622
Cipro I.V. (1% or less) 2817
Cipro (Less than 1%) 2810
Cipro XR Tablets (Less than 1%) 2823
▲ Climara Transdermal System (1% to 8%) 763
▲ Climara Pro Transdermal System (5.7%) 768
Clinoril Tablets (Less than 1%) 1962
▲ Clolar for Intravenous Infusion (11%) 1239
Clorpres Tablets (About 1%) 2185
▲ Combigan Ophthalmic Solution (1% to 5%) ⊙ 553
Concerta Extended-Release Tablets (1.7%) 1925
Copaxone for Injection (At least 2%) 3110
▲ Coreg Tablets (Greater than 1% to 3%) 1387
▲ Coreg CR Extended-Release Capsules (Greater than 1% to less than or equal to 3%) 1393
Cosopt Sterile Ophthalmic Solution (Less than 1%) 1969
Cozaar Tablets (Less than 1%) 1973
▲ Crinone 4% Gel (19%) 992
▲ Crinone 8% Gel (11% to 15%) 992
Crixivan Capsules 1979
Dacogen Injection (Greater than or equal to 1%) 1066
Dantrium Capsules (Less frequent) 2580
Daytrana Transdermal Patch 3022
Delatestryl Injection 1730
Demser Capsules 1989
▲ Depakote ER Tablets (1% to 5%) 423
▲ DepoCyt Injection (8% to 18%) 1136
Didronel Tablets 2583
Diovan HCT Tablets (Less frequent) 2216
▲ Doxil Injection (Less than 1% to 10%) 2378
▲ Duragesic Transdermal System (3% to 10%) 2405
DynaCirc CR Controlled Release Tablets (0.5% to 1%) 1407
EC-Naprosyn Delayed-Release Tablets (Less than 1%) 2632
▲ Effexor XR Extended-Release Capsules (3% to 5%) 3195
Eldepryl Capsules 3052
Eligard 7.5 mg (Less than 2%) 2724
Eligard 22.5 mg (Less than 2%) 2724
Eligard 30 mg (Less than 2%) 2724
Eligard 45 mg (Less than 2%) 2724
Elmiron Capsules 2435
▲ Eloxatin for Injection (2% to 9%) 2731
Elspar for Injection 1990
Emend Capsules (Greater than 0.5%) 1992
Emend for Injection (Greater than 0.5%) 1999
▲ Emtriva Capsules (Greater than or equal to 10%) 1246
▲ Emtriva Oral Solution (Greater than or equal to 10%) 1246
Enbrel for Injection (Infrequent) 569
Enjuvia Tablets 1029
▲ Epzicom Tablets (7%) 1422
▲ Equetro Extended-Release Capsules (7%) 3174
▲ Erbitux (1% to 13%) 912
Estratest Tablets 3043
Estratest H.S. Tablets 3043
▲ Evista Tablets (6.4%) 1810
▲ Evoxac Capsules (1% to 3%) 1013
▲ Exelon Capsules (6%) 2229
▲ Exelon Oral Solution (6%) 2229
▲ Exelon Patch (4%) 2233
Exforge Tablets (Greater than or equal to 0.2%) 2238
▲ Fabrazyme for Intravenous Infusion (6%) 1241
Fansidar Tablets 2636
▲ Faslodex Injection (5.7%) 682
Femara Tablets (Less frequent) 2246
▲ Fentora Tablets (3% to 11%) 968
▲ Flolan for Injection (13% to 37%) 1426
Flovent Diskus 50 mcg 1435
Flovent HFA 1440
Flumadine (0.3% to 1%) 1167
Focalin XR Capsules 2251
▲ Forteo for Injection (4.1%) 1816
Frova Tablets (Infrequent) 1111
▲ Gabitril Tablets (3%) 973
Gantrisin Pediatric Suspension 2638
Gengraf Capsules (Rare) 435
Geodon Capsules 2520
▲ Gleevec Tablets (14.9%) 2255
▲ Gliadel Wafer (3% to 16%) 1076
▲ Herceptin I.V. (6%) 1199
Humulin 50/50, 100 Units 1843
Humulin 70/30 Vial 1844
Humulin N Vial 1846
Humulin R 1849
Imitrex Injection (Rare) 1465
Imitrex Nasal Spray (Infrequent) 1470
Imitrex Tablets (Infrequent) 1474
▲ Indapamide Tablets (Less than 5%) 2188
Indocin (Greater than 1%) 2024
InnoPran XL Extended Release Capsules 1484
▲ Intron A for Injection (2% to 40%) 2859
Invanz for Injection (Greater than 0.1%) 2029
Kaletra (Up to 2%) 452
▲ Keppra Injection (1.7% to 13.3%) 3137
▲ Keppra Oral Solution (3% to 5%) 3131
▲ Keppra Tablets (3% to 5%) 3131
▲ Klonopin (4% to 7%) 2639
▲ Lamictal (Greater than 1% to less than 5%) 1488
Lanoxin Injection 1498
Lanoxin Injection Pediatric 1502
Lanoxin Tablets 1505
Lescol Capsules 2268
Lescol XL Tablets 2268
Levaquin (0.1% to 1%) 2416
Levaquin in 5% Dextrose Injection (0.1% to 1%) 2416
Lexapro Oral Suspension (Infrequent) 1174
Lexapro Tablets (Infrequent) 1174
Lipitor Tablets (Less than 2%) 2501
Lovaza Capsules 1520
▲ Lunesta Tablets (1% to 4%) 2994
▲ Lupron Depot 3.75 mg (16%) 462
▲ Lupron Depot–3 Month 11.25 mg (16%) 462
Luvox CR Extended-Release Capsules (1%) 1759
Lybrel Tablets 3204
Lyrica Capsules (2%) 2527
Malarone Pediatric Tablets (Less than 1%) 1521
Malarone Tablets (Less than 1%) 1521
Marinol Capsules (Less than 1%) 3163
Maxair Autohaler 1705
Maxalt Tablets (Infrequent) 2056
Maxalt-MLT Orally Disintegrating Tablets (Infrequent) 2056
▲ Megace ES Oral Suspension (1% to 3%) 2499
▲ Meridia Capsules (4.3%) 475

Merrem I.V. (Greater than 0.1% to 1%) 684
Metadate CD Capsules 3146
Mevacor Tablets (0.5% to 1%) 2063
▲ Miacalcin Nasal Spray (1% to 3%) 2274
Micardis Tablets (More than 0.3%) 852
Micardis HCT Tablets 854
Mirapex Tablets (1% or more) 857
Mircette Tablets 1034
▲ Mirena Intrauterine System (5% or more) 779
Moban Tablets (Less frequent) 1116
Mobic Oral Suspension (Less than 2%) 863
Mobic Tablets (Less than 2%) 863
MS Contin Tablets (Less frequent) 2585
▲ Myfortic Tablets (3% to less than 20%) 2276
▲ Mylotarg for Injection (8% to 10%) 3212
Nadolol Tablets 2191
Nalfon Capsules (Less than 1%) 2508
Namenda (Greater than or equal to 2%) 1180
Naprosyn Suspension (Less than 1%) 2632
Naprosyn Tablets (Less than 1%) 2632
Nembutal Sodium Solution, USP 2494
Neoral Oral Solution (1%) 2280
Neoral Soft Gelatin Capsules (1%) 2280
Neupro Transdermal System (Greater than or equal to 2%) 3149
▲ Nexavar Tablets (1% to less than 10%) 784
Nexium Delayed-Release Capsules 645
Nexium I.V. (Rare) 652
Nexium Delayed-Release Oral Suspension 645
Nimotop Capsules (Up to 1.4%) 790
Noroxin Tablets (Less frequent) 2069
Norvir (1.7%) 489
▲ Novantrone for Injection Concentrate (5%) 1100
NuvaRing 2897
Opana Tablets (Less than 1%) 1117
Opana ER Tablets (Less than 1%) 1121
OptiPranolol Metipranolol Ophthalmic Solution 0.3% (A small number of patients) ⊙ 245
Ortho-Cyclen Tablets 2449
Ortho Evra Transdermal System 2437
Ortho Tri-Cyclen Tablets 2449
Ortho Tri-Cyclen Lo Tablets 2458
OxyContin Tablets (Less than 1%) 2589
Paxil (Frequent) 1535
Paxil CR Controlled-Release Tablets (Frequent) 1544
▲ PegIntron Powder for Injection (Less than or equal to 1% to 29%) 2903
Pentasa Capsules (Less than 1%) 3030
Pepcid Tablets (Infrequent) 2075
Percocet Tablets 1127
Percodan Tablets 1130
▲ Plavix Tablets (3.6%) 926
▲ Plavix Tablets (3.6%) 2767
Premarin Intravenous 3217
▲ Premarin Tablets (5% to 8%) 3221
Premarin Vaginal Cream 3228
▲ Premphase Tablets (6% to 11%) 3232
▲ Prempro Tablets (6% to 11%) 3232
Prinivil Tablets (Greater than 1%) 2087
Prinzide Tablets (0.3% to 1%) 2092
▲ Prograf Capsules and Injection (3% to 15%) 622
Proleukin for Injection (Less than 1%) 2287
▲ Prometrium Capsules (100 mg, 200 mg) (5% to 19%) 3047
Protonix for Delayed-Release Oral Suspension (Less than 1%) 3254
Protonix Delayed-Release Tablets (Less than 1%) 3254
Protonix I.V. (Less than 1%) 3257
Protopic Ointment (Greater than or equal to 1% to 2%) 628
Proventil HFA Inhalation Aerosol (Less than 3%) 2914
Provigil Tablets (2%) 977
Prozac Pulvules and Liquid 1852
Pulmicort Flexhaler 654
▲ Rebetol (13% to 36%) 2917
▲ Rebif Prefilled Syringe for Injection (25%) 1107
Remeron Tablets (Frequent) 2924
RemeronSolTab Tablets (Frequent) 2927
Requip Tablets (Frequent to greater than 1%) 1561
Retrovir Capsules 1574
Retrovir IV Infusion 1579
Retrovir 1574
Reyataz Capsules (2%) 3299
▲ Rilutek Tablets (4.2% to 6.1%) 2771
Risperdal Consta Long-Acting Injection (Frequent) 1753
▲ Romazicon Injection (1% to 3%) 2646
Rozerem Tablets (2%) 3091
Rythmol Tablets (Less than 1%) 1586
▲ Rythmol SR Capsules (1% to 3%) 1590
Salagen Tablets (Less than 1%) 1082
Sandimmune (Rare) 2296
▲ Sandostatin Injection (1% to 4%) 2300
Seasonique Tablets 1046
▲ Simulect for Injection (3% to 10%) 2306
Singulair 2114
▲ Soriatane Capsules (1% to 10%) 3062
▲ Spiriva HandiHaler (1% to 3%) 870
Stalevo Tablets 2309
▲ Strattera Capsules (4% to 7%) 1864
▲ Suboxone Tablets (11%) 2601
▲ Subutex Tablets (11%) 2601
Sular Extended Release Tablets (Less than or equal to 1%) 2975
▲ Sustiva Capsules (2% to 19%) 930
▲ Sustiva Tablets (2% to 19%) 930
▲ Sutent Capsules (8%) 2540
▲ Tarceva Tablets (0% to 19%) 1228
Targretin Capsules 1084
Tasigna Capsules (0.1% to 1%) 2316
▲ Temodar Capsules (6%) 2931
Testim 1% Gel 701
Teveten Tablets (1%) 515
Teveten HCT Tablets (Less than 1%) 517
Timoptic Sterile Ophthalmic Solution (Less frequent) 2121
Timoptic in Ocudose (Less frequent) 2124
Timoptic-XE Sterile Ophthalmic Gel Forming Solution 2125
▲ Toprol-XL Tablets (About 5 of 100 patients) 666
▲ Torisel Injection (0% to 4%) 3272
▲ Travatan Z Ophthalmic Solution (1% to 5%) 547
Treximet Tablets (Infrequent) 1616
Tricor Tablets 520
▲ Trisenox Injection (20%) 986
▲ Trizivir Tablets (9%) 1622
▲ Truvada Tablets (Greater than or equal to 10%) 1262
▲ Ultram ER Extended-Release Tablets (1% to less than 5%) 2428
▲ Valcyte Tablets (Less than 5%) 2654
Valium Tablets (Infrequent) 2658
▲ Valtrex Caplets (Less than 1% to 7%) 1635
Vantas (Less than 2%) 1737
Venlafaxine Hydrochloride Tablets (1%) 2199
Veramyst Nasal Spray 1643
▲ Vesanoid Capsules (14%) 2660
VESIcare Tablets (0.8% to 1.2%) 636
▲ Viadur Implant (5.3%) 802
Vicoprofen Tablets (Less than 1%) 533
▲ Viread Tablets (4% to 11%) 1268
▲ Vivitrol (3% to 8%) 988
Voltaren Tablets (Occasionally) 2334
Voltaren-XR Tablets (Occasionally) 2337
Vytorin 10/10 Tablets 2149
Vytorin 10/10 Tablets 2939
Vytorin 10/20 Tablets 2149
Vytorin 10/20 Tablets 2939
Vytorin 10/40 Tablets 2149
Vytorin 10/40 Tablets 2939
Vytorin 10/80 Tablets 2149
Vytorin 10/80 Tablets 2939
Vyvanse Capsules 3033
Wellbutrin Tablets (Frequent) 1648
Wellbutrin SR Sustained-Release Tablets 1653
Wellbutrin XL Extended-Release Tablets 1659
▲ Xeloda Tablets (Less than 5%) 2662
▲ Xenical Capsules (3.4%) 2672
▲ Xyrem Oral Solution (5.9%) 1766
Yaz Tablets (Greater than 1%) 805
Zantac 25 EFFERdose Tablets (Rare) 1670
Zantac Injection (Rare) 1666
Zantac Injection Pharmacy Bulk Package (Rare) 1668
Zantac Injection Premixed (Rare) 1666
Zantac (Rare) 1670
Zetia Tablets 2157
Zetia Tablets 2951
Zocor Tablets 2136
▲ Zometa for Intravenous Infusion (14%) 2341
Zomig Tablets (Infrequent) 694
Zomig Nasal Spray (Infrequent) 689
Zomig-ZMT Tablets (Infrequent) 694
▲ Zonegran Capsules (6%) 1089
Zosyn for Injection (1.0% or less) 3284
Zyban Sustained-Release Tablets (Frequent) 1692
▲ Zyprexa Tablets (18%) 1883
▲ Zyprexa ZYDIS Orally Disintegrating Tablets (18%) 1883
Zyrtec Chewable Tablets (Less than 2%) 1920
Zyrtec Syrup (Less than 2%) 1920
Zyrtec Tablets (Less than 2%) 1920
Zyrtec-D 12 Hour Extended Release Tablets (Less than 2%) 1923

Depression, aggravation of
Celexa (Frequent) 1160
Coreg Tablets (Greater than 0.1% to 1%) 1387
Coreg CR Extended-Release Capsules (0.1% to less than or equal to 1%) 1393
Evoxac Capsules (Less than 1%) 1013
Frova Tablets (Rare) 1111
▲ Intron A for Injection (Less than 5%) 2859
Lexapro Oral Suspension (Infrequent) 1174
Lexapro Tablets (Infrequent) 1174
Lupron Depot 3.75 mg 462
Lupron Depot–3 Month 11.25 mg (Possible) 462
Meridia Capsules 475
Nexium Delayed-Release Capsules (Less than 1%) 645
Nexium I.V. (Less than 1%) 652
Nexium Delayed-Release Oral Suspension (Less than 1%) 645
Sustiva Capsules (Less than 2%) 930
Sustiva Tablets (Less than 2%) 930
Wellbutrin Tablets 1648
Wellbutrin SR Sustained-Release Tablets 1653
Wellbutrin XL Extended-Release Tablets 1659
Ziagen (5 patients) 1673

Depression, major
Strattera Capsules 1864

Depression, manic
Azilect Tablets (Rare) 3106

Depression, mood
(*see under* Depression)

Depression, psychotic
Azilect Tablets (Rare) 3106
Celexa (Infrequent) 1160
Copaxone for Injection (Infrequent) 3110
Effexor XR Extended-Release Capsules (Infrequent) 3195
Keppra Injection 3137
Keppra Oral Solution 3131
Keppra Tablets 3131
Lyrica Capsules (Rare) 2527
Paxil (Rare) 1535
Paxil CR Controlled-Release Tablets (Rare) 1544
Remeron Tablets (Rare) 2924
RemeronSolTab Tablets (Rare) 2927
Rilutek Tablets (Rare) 2771
Risperdal Consta Long-Acting Injection (Infrequent) 1753
Venlafaxine Hydrochloride Tablets (Rare) 2199

Depression, respiratory, neonatal
Lortab 5/500 Tablets 3143
Lortab 7.5/500 Tablets 3144
Lortab 10/500 Tablets 3144
MS Contin Tablets 2585
Percocet Tablets 1127
Tussionex Pennkinetic Extended-Release Suspension 3154
Vicodin Tablets 529
Vicodin ES Tablets 530

Depression, worsening
Cymbalta Delayed-Release Capsules 1801
Luvox CR Extended-Release Capsules 1759
Paxil 1535
Paxil CR Controlled-Release Tablets 1544
Pristiq Extended-Release Tablets 3247
Prozac Weekly Capsules 1852
Remeron Tablets 2924
RemeronSolTab Tablets 2927
Symbyax Capsules 1871
Venlafaxine Hydrochloride Tablets 2199

Depressive reactions
▲ Combivir Tablets (9%) 1384
▲ Epivir (9%) 1412
▲ Selzentry Tablets (3.5%) 2534
Soma Tablets 1931
Truvada Tablets 1262
▲ Ziagen (6%) 1673

Depressive symptoms
Strattera Capsules 1864

Derealization
Wellbutrin SR Sustained-Release Tablets (Rare) 1653
Wellbutrin XL Extended-Release Tablets (Rare) 1659
Zyban Sustained-Release Tablets (Rare) 1692

Dermal cyst
Mirapex Tablets 857

Dermatitis
▲ Advair HFA 45/21 Inhalation Aerosol (1% to 3%) 1288
▲ Advair HFA 115/21 Inhalation Aerosol (1% to 3%) 1288
▲ Advair HFA 230/21 Inhalation Aerosol (1% to 3%) 1288
Ambien Tablets (Rare) 2692
Ambien CR Tablets (Rare) 2696
Amerge Tablets (Rare) 1301
Aricept Tablets (Infrequent) 1062
Aricept ODT Tablets (Infrequent) 1062
Atacand HCT (0.5% or greater) 642
Avalide Tablets 892
Avalide Tablets 2713
Avapro Tablets (Less than 1%) 897
Avapro Tablets (Less than 1%) 2718
Axert Tablets (Rare) 2431
▲ Azopt Ophthalmic Suspension (1% to 5%) 540
Bactroban Cream (Less than 1%) 1366
Celebrex Capsules (0.1% to 1.9%) 2979
Celexa (Infrequent) 1160
Chantix Tablets (Infrequent) 2511
Cimzia 3127
▲ Clolar for Intravenous Infusion (41%) 1239
Copaxone for Injection (Infrequent) 3110
Cosopt Sterile Ophthalmic Solution 1969
Cozaar Tablets (Less than 1%) 1973
Evoxac Capsules (Less than 1%) 1013
Exelon Patch (Infrequent) 2233
Exforge Tablets (Less than or equal to 0.1%) 2238
▲ Flovent Diskus 50 mcg (1% to 3%) 1435
Gengraf Capsules (1% to less than 3%) 435
▲ Hycamtin for Injection (Rare to 16%) 1459
▲ Intron A for Injection (Up to 8%) 2859
Invanz for Injection (1%) 2029
Lexapro Oral Suspension (Infrequent) 1174
Lexapro Tablets (Infrequent) 1174
▲ Lupron Depot 7.5 mg (Less than 5%) 469
Maxair Autohaler 1705
Meridia Capsules 475
Micardis Tablets (More than 0.3%) 852
Micardis HCT Tablets 854
Mirapex Tablets 857
Namenda (Infrequent) 1180
Neoral Oral Solution (1% to less than 3%) 2280
Neoral Soft Gelatin Capsules (1% to less than 3%) 2280
Nexium Delayed-Release Capsules (Less than 1%) 645
Nexium I.V. (Less than 1%) 652
Nexium Delayed-Release Oral Suspension (Less than 1%) 645
Opana Tablets (Less than 1%) 1117
Opana ER Tablets (Less than 1%) 1121
▲ Panretin Gel 0.1% (25% to 77%) 1081
Pediarix Vaccine 1552
Phenytek Capsules (Rare) 2192
Prevnar 3241
Prinzide Tablets (0.3% to 1%) 2092
Requip Tablets (Infrequent) 1561
Risperdal Consta Long-Acting Injection (Infrequent) 1753
Rythmol SR Capsules 1590
▲ Selzentry Tablets (3.1%) 2534
▲ Soriatane Capsules (1% to 10%) 3062
▲ Strattera Capsules (2% to 4%) 1864
Tamiflu Capsules (1%) 2649
Tamiflu Oral Suspension (1%) 2649
Targretin Gel 1% 1088
Thioridazine Hydrochloride Tablets (Infrequent) 2195
▲ Trisenox Injection (43%) 986
▲ Ultram ER Extended-Release Tablets (1% to less than 5%) 2428
▲ Valcyte Tablets (Less than 5%) 2654
Vaqta (Less than 1%) 2130
Varivax (Greater than or equal to 1%) 2133

▲ Xeloda Tablets (1% to 37%) 2662
Xolair (2%) 1235
Xolair (2%) 2339
▲ Zometa for Intravenous Infusion (11%) 2341
Zyrtec Chewable Tablets (Less than 2%) 1920
Zyrtec Syrup (Less than 2%) 1920
Zyrtec Tablets (Less than 2%) 1920
Zyrtec-D 12 Hour Extended Release Tablets (Less than 2%) 1923

Dermatitis, acneiform
Abilify Injection (Greater than or equal to 1 in 100 patients) 2466
Abilify Oral Solution (Greater than or equal to 1 in 100 patients) 2466
Abilify Discmelt Orally Disintegrating Tablets (Greater than or equal to 1 in 100 patients) 2466
Abilify Tablets (Greater than or equal to 1 in 100 patients) 2466
Tykerb Tablets (Less than 1%) 1631
▲ Vectibix (7% to 57%) 597

Dermatitis, allergic
Abilify Injection (Greater than or equal to 1 in 100 patients) 2466
Abilify Oral Solution (Greater than or equal to 1 in 100 patients) 881
Abilify Oral Solution (Greater than or equal to 1 in 100 patients) 2466
Abilify Discmelt Orally Disintegrating Tablets (Greater than or equal to 1 in 100 patients) 881
Abilify Discmelt Orally Disintegrating Tablets (Greater than or equal to 1 in 100 patients) 2466
Abilify Tablets (Greater than or equal to 1 in 100 patients) 881
Abilify Tablets (Greater than or equal to 1 in 100 patients) 2466
Aloxi Injection (Less than 1%) 1059
Cimzia 3127
▲ Doribax Injection (1% to 5%) 2400
Geodon (Rare) 2520
Requip Tablets (Infrequent) 1561
Rocephin Injectable Vials, ADD-Vantage, Galaxy, Bulk 2642
Xifaxan Tablets 2682

Dermatitis, allergic contact
Analpram-HC 1140
▲ Catapres-TTS (About 19 in 100) 842
Daytrana Transdermal Patch 3022
Diprolene Lotion 0.05% (Infrequent) 2838
Diprolene Ointment 0.05% 2839
Diprolene AF Cream 0.05% (Infrequent) 2837
Elocon Cream 0.1% (Infrequent) 2840
Elocon Lotion 0.1% (Infrequent) 2841
Elocon Ointment 0.1% (Infrequent) 2842
Lotrisone 2881
Luxíq Foam 3058
Olux Foam 3061
Olux-E Foam 3059
Pramosone 1141
Vanos Cream 1941
Verdeso Foam 3069

Dermatitis, application site
Daytrana Transdermal Patch 3022
Exelon Patch (Infrequent) 2233
Flector Patch (2%) 561
Lidoderm Patch 1114
Verdeso Foam (1%) 3069

Dermatitis, atopic
Invanz for Injection (Greater than 0.5%) 2029
Singulair (Greater than or equal to 2%) 2114

Dermatitis, bullous
Aciphex Tablets 1053
Anaprox Tablets (Less than 1%) 2632
Anaprox DS Tablets (Less than 1%) 2632
▲ Doribax Injection (1% to 5%) 2400
EC-Naprosyn Delayed-Release Tablets (Less than 1%) 2632
Flebogamma 5% 1715
Flebogamma 5% DIF 1718
Gammagard Liquid 730
Gammagard S/D (Rare) 734
Gamunex (Rare) 3094
Mirapex Tablets 857
Naprosyn Suspension (Less than 1%) 2632
Naprosyn Tablets (Less than 1%) 2632
Phenytek Capsules 2192
Rituxan I.V. 1223

Dermatitis, contact
Abilify Injection (Greater than or equal to 1 in 100 patients) 2466
Abilify Oral Solution (Greater than or equal to 1 in 100 patients) 881
Abilify Oral Solution (Greater than or equal to 1 in 100 patients) 2466
Abilify Discmelt Orally Disintegrating Tablets (Greater than or equal to 1 in 100 patients) 881
Abilify Discmelt Orally Disintegrating Tablets (Greater than or equal to 1 in 100 patients) 2466
Abilify Tablets (Greater than or equal to 1 in 100 patients) 881
Abilify Tablets (Greater than or equal to 1 in 100 patients) 2466
Advair HFA 45/21 Inhalation Aerosol 1288
Advair HFA 115/21 Inhalation Aerosol 1288
Advair HFA 230/21 Inhalation Aerosol 1288
Altabax Ointment (Less than 1%) 1299
▲ Augmentin ES-600 Powder for Oral Suspension (3.5%) 1329
AzaSite Ophthalmic Drops (Less than 1%) 1740
Bactroban Ointment (Less than 1%) 1368
▲ Catapres-TTS (About 8 to 34 in 100 patients) 842
Celebrex Capsules (0.1% to 1.9%) 2979
Copaxone for Injection (Infrequent) 3110
Cosopt Sterile Ophthalmic Solution 1969
Cymbalta Delayed-Release Capsules (Infrequent) 1801
Daytrana Transdermal Patch 3022
Doxil Injection (Less than 1%) 2378
Effexor XR Extended-Release Capsules (Infrequent) 3195
Emsam Transdermal System (Infrequent) 905
Evoxac Capsules (Less than 1%) 1013
Exelon Capsules (Infrequent) 2229
Exelon Oral Solution (Infrequent) 2229
▲ Fabrazyme for Intravenous Infusion (5%) 1241
Finacea Gel (1% or less) 1742
Gabitril Tablets (Infrequent) 973
Geodon Capsules (Infrequent) 2520
Klonopin (Infrequent) 2639
▲ Lamictal (2% to 5%) 1488
Lipitor Tablets (Less than 2%) 2501
Lunesta Tablets (Infrequent) 2994
Mentax Cream (Less than 2%) 2190
Mirapex Tablets 857
Neupro Transdermal System 3149
Nitro-Dur Transdermal Infusion System (Uncommon) 2887
Norvir (Less than 2%) 489
Omnaris Nasal Spray 2998
Paxil (Rare) 1535
Paxil CR Controlled-Release Tablets (Rare) 1544
Protonix for Delayed-Release Oral Suspension (Less than 1%) 3254
Protonix Delayed-Release Tablets (Less than 1%) 3254
Protonix I.V. (Less than 1%) 3257
▲ Protopic Ointment (1% to 3%) 628
Prozac Weekly Capsules (Infrequent) 1852
Prozac Pulvules and Liquid (Infrequent) 1852
Pulmicort Flexhaler 654
Requip Tablets (Infrequent) 1561
Rilutek Tablets (Rare) 2771
Salagen Tablets (Less than 1%) 1082
▲ Serevent Diskus (1% to 3%) 1594
Symbyax Capsules (Infrequent) 1871
▲ Targretin Gel 1% (8% to 14%) 1088
Thioridazine Hydrochloride Tablets 2195
Thiothixene Capsules 2197
Tricor Tablets 520
Trusopt Sterile Ophthalmic Solution 2128
Varivax (Greater than or equal to 1%) 2133
Venlafaxine Hydrochloride Tablets (Infrequent) 2199
Verdeso Foam (1%) 3069
Xyrem Oral Solution (Infrequent) 1766
Zovirax Cream 817
Zyprexa Tablets (Infrequent) 1883
Zyprexa ZYDIS Orally Disintegrating Tablets (Infrequent) 1883

Dermatitis, exfoliative
Abelcet Injection 1134
Abilify Injection (Greater than or equal to 1 in 100 patients) 2466
Abilify Oral Solution (Greater than or equal to 1 in 100 patients) 881
Abilify Oral Solution (Greater than or equal to 1 in 100 patients) 2466
Abilify Discmelt Orally Disintegrating Tablets (Greater than or equal to 1 in 100 patients) 881
Abilify Discmelt Orally Disintegrating Tablets (Greater than or equal to 1 in 100 patients) 2466
Abilify Tablets (Greater than or equal to 1 in 100 patients) 881
Abilify Tablets (Greater than or equal to 1 in 100 patients) 2466
Aceon Tablets (2 mg, 4 mg, 8 mg) 3038
Actiq (Less than 1%) 959
Aldara Cream, 5% 1699
Amoxil Capsules 1305
Amoxil Chewable Tablets 1305
Amoxil Pediatric Drops for Oral Suspension 1305
Amoxil Powder for Oral Suspension 1305
Amoxil Tablets 1305
Anaprox Tablets (Less than 1%) 2632
Anaprox DS Tablets (Less than 1%) 2632
Atacand HCT 642
Augmentin (Occasional case) 1323
Augmentin Tablets (Occasional) 1327
Augmentin XR Extended Release Tablets (Occasional) 1333
Augmentin ES-600 Powder for Oral Suspension (Occasional) 1329
Avalide Tablets 892
Avalide Tablets 2713
▲ Avastin IV (3% to 19%) 1192
Axid Capsules 1364
Bicillin C-R Injectable Suspension 1775
Bicillin L-A Injection 1777
▲ Busulfex Injection (5%) 2477
Campral Tablets (Infrequent) 1158
Captopril Tablets 2182
Carbatrol Capsules 3019
Cardizem LA Extended Release Tablets (Infrequent) 421
Celebrex Capsules (Less than 0.1%) 2979
Cialis Tablets 1792
Cipro I.V. (1% or less) 2817
Cipro 2810
Cipro XR Tablets 2823
Clinoril Tablets 1962
Concerta Extended-Release Tablets 1925
Coreg Tablets (Less than or equal to 0.1%) 1387
Coreg CR Extended-Release Capsules (Less than or equal to 0.%) 1393
Cuprimine Capsules 1986
Daytrana Transdermal Patch 3022
Diovan HCT Tablets 2216
▲ Doxil Injection (Less than 1% to 10%) 2378
Duragesic Transdermal System (Less than 1%) 2405
EC-Naprosyn Delayed-Release Tablets (Less than 1%) 2632
Effexor XR Extended-Release Capsules (Rare) 3195
Equetro Extended-Release Capsules 3174
Erbitux 912
Fansidar Tablets 2636
Flector Patch 561
Focalin XR Capsules 2251
Furosemide Tablets 2186
Gabitril Tablets (Infrequent) 973
Gantrisin Pediatric Suspension 2638
Geodon Capsules (Infrequent) 2520
Gleevec Tablets (Infrequent) 2255
Imitrex Tablets (Rare) 1474
Indocin Capsules (Less than 1%) 2024
Indocin I.V. (Less than 1%) 2489
Indocin (Less than 1%) 2024
Intravenous Sodium Diuril 2490
Kaletra (Less than 2%) 452
Lamictal (Rare) 1488
Luvox CR Extended-Release Capsules (Infrequent) 1759
Lyrica Capsules (Rare) 2527
Metadate CD Capsules 3146
Micardis HCT Tablets 854
Mobic Oral Suspension 863
Mobic Tablets 863
Moxatag Tablets 2165
Nalfon Capsules (Less than 1%) 2508
Naprosyn Suspension (Less than 1%) 2632
Naprosyn Tablets (Less than 1%) 2632
Nembutal Sodium Solution, USP 2494
▲ Nexavar Tablets (1% to less than 10%) 784
Nitrolingual Pumpspray 2965
Noroxin Tablets 2069
Omnicef Capsules 497
Omnicef for Oral Suspension 497
OxyContin Tablets (Less than 1%) 2589
▲ Panretin Gel 0.1% (3% to 9%) 1081
Paser Granules 1747
Paxil (Rare) 1535
Paxil CR Controlled-Release Tablets (Rare) 1544
Phenytek Capsules 2192
Prinzide Tablets 2092
▲ Prograf Capsules and Injection (3% to 15%) 622
▲ Proleukin for Injection (18%) 2287
▲ Protopic Ointment (Up to 3%) 628
Prozac Weekly Capsules 1852
Prozac Pulvules and Liquid 1852
Pylera Capsules 714
Rapamune 3260
Remeron Tablets (Infrequent) 2924
RemeronSolTab Tablets (Infrequent) 2927
Rilutek Tablets (Up to 1.2%) 2771
Salagen Tablets (Less than 1%) 1082
Sular Extended Release Tablets (Less than or equal to 1%) 2975
▲ Sustiva Capsules (Up to 3.5%) 930
▲ Sustiva Tablets (Up to 3.5%) 930
Symbyax Capsules (Rare) 1871
▲ Targretin Capsules (9.5% to 28.3%) 1084
▲ Targretin Gel 1% (6%) 1088
Tekturna HCT Tablets 2324
Teveten HCT Tablets 517
Thioridazine Hydrochloride Tablets 2195
Thiothixene Capsules 2197
Treximet Tablets 1616
Venlafaxine Hydrochloride Tablets (Rare) 2199
Vicoprofen Tablets 533
Voltaren Tablets (Rarely) 2334
Voltaren-XR Tablets (Rarely) 2337
Wellbutrin Tablets 1648
Wellbutrin SR Sustained-Release Tablets 1653
Wellbutrin XL Extended-Release Tablets 1659
Xifaxan Tablets 2682
Zolinza Capsules 2142
Zyban Sustained-Release Tablets 1692

Dermatitis, eyelid
OptiPranolol Metipranolol Ophthalmic Solution 0.3% (A small number of patients) ⊙245

Dermatitis, fungal
Aricept Tablets (Infrequent) 1062
Aricept ODT Tablets (Infrequent) 1062
▲ CellCept Capsules (3% to less than 20%) 2622
▲ CellCept Intravenous (3% to less than 20%) 2622
▲ CellCept Oral Suspension (3% to less than 20%) 2622
▲ CellCept Tablets (3% to less than 20%) 2622
Copaxone for Injection (Infrequent) 3110
▲ Doxil Injection (1% to 10%) 2378
Emsam Transdermal System (Infrequent) 905
Geodon Capsules (2%) 2520
Lamictal (Rare) 1488
Paxil (Rare) 1535
Paxil CR Controlled-Release Tablets (Rare) 1544
▲ Prograf Capsules and Injection (3% to 15%) 622
Protonix for Delayed-Release Oral Suspension (Less than 1%) 3254
Protonix Delayed-Release Tablets (Less than 1%) 3254
Protonix I.V. (Less than 1%) 3257
▲ Protopic Ointment (1% to 6%) 628
Requip Tablets (Infrequent) 1561
Rilutek Tablets (Infrequent) 2771
Sular Extended Release Tablets (Less than or equal to 1%) 2975
Synagis Intramuscular Solution (More than 1%) 1948
Tricor Tablets 520

Dermatitis, herpes simplex
Elidel Cream 1% (0% to 1.5%) 2221
▲ Mylotarg for Injection (21%) 3212

Dermatitis, lichenoides
Effexor XR Extended-Release Capsules (Rare) 3195
Evoxac Capsules (Less than 1%) 1013
▲ Intron A for Injection (Less than 5%) 2859
Lyrica Capsules (Rare) 2527
Protonix for Delayed-Release Oral Suspension (Less than 1%) 3254
Protonix Delayed-Release Tablets (Less than 1%) 3254
Protonix I.V. (Less than 1%) 3257
Rituxan I.V. 1223
Venlafaxine Hydrochloride Tablets (Rare) 2199

Dermatitis, maculopapular
Bicillin C-R Injectable Suspension 1775
Bicillin L-A Injection 1777

Dermatitis, monilial
Proglycem Capsules (Infrequent) 1185
Proglycem Suspension (Infrequent) 1185

Dermatitis, perioral
Analpram-HC 1140
Diprolene Lotion 0.05% (Infrequent) 2838
Diprolene Ointment 0.05% 2839
Diprolene AF Cream 0.05% (Infrequent) 2837
Elocon Cream 0.1% (Infrequent) 2840
Elocon Lotion 0.1% (Infrequent) 2841
Elocon Ointment 0.1% (Infrequent) 2842
Lotrisone 2881
Luxíq Foam 3058
Olux Foam 3061
Olux-E Foam 3059
Pramosone 1141
Vanos Cream 1941
Verdeso Foam 3069

Dermatitis, photosensitive
Amerge Tablets (Rare) 1301
Anaprox Tablets (Less than 1%) 2632
Anaprox DS Tablets (Less than 1%) 2632
EC-Naprosyn Delayed-Release Tablets (Less than 1%) 2632
▲ Flovent Diskus 50 mcg (1% to 3%) 1435
Naprosyn Suspension (Less than 1%) 2632
Naprosyn Tablets (Less than 1%) 2632

Dermatitis, purpuric
Phenytek Capsules 2192

Dermatitis, radiation recall
▲ Erbitux (23% to 86%) 912

Dermatitis, vesicular bullous
(*see under* Dermatitis, bullous)

Dermatitis seborrhic
Abilify Injection (Greater than or equal to 1 in 100 patients) 2466
Abilify Oral Solution (Greater than or equal to 1 in 100 patients) 881
Abilify Oral Solution (Greater than or equal to 1 in 100 patients) 2466
Abilify Discmelt Orally Disintegrating Tablets (Greater than or equal to 1 in 100 patients) 881
Abilify Discmelt Orally Disintegrating Tablets (Greater than or equal to 1 in 100 patients) 2466
Abilify Tablets (Greater than or equal to 1 in 100 patients) 881
Abilify Tablets (Greater than or equal to 1 in 100 patients) 2466
Imitrex Injection 1465
Imitrex Nasal Spray 1470

Dermatologic reactions, unspecified
Aceon Tablets (2 mg, 4 mg, 8 mg) 3038
Aciphex Tablets 1053
Avelox 2803
Captopril Tablets 2182
Cipro 2810
Cipro XR Tablets 2823
Clinoril Tablets (Less than 1 in 100) 1962
Equetro Extended-Release Capsules 3174
▲ Erbitux (1% to 27%) 912
Follistim AQ Cartridge 2844
▲ Hycamtin for Injection (48%) 1459
Nexium Delayed-Release Capsules (Rare) 645
Nexium I.V. (Rare) 652
Nexium Delayed-Release Oral Suspension (Rare) 645
Prinivil Tablets (0.3% to 1%) 2087
Prinzide Tablets 2092
Protonix for Delayed-Release Oral Suspension 3254
Protonix Delayed-Release Tablets 3254
Protonix I.V. 3257

Dermatomyositis
Cuprimine Capsules (Rare) 1986
Mevacor Tablets 2063
Vytorin 10/10 Tablets 2149
Vytorin 10/10 Tablets 2939
Vytorin 10/20 Tablets 2149
Vytorin 10/20 Tablets 2939
Vytorin 10/40 Tablets 2149
Vytorin 10/40 Tablets 2939
Vytorin 10/80 Tablets 2149
Vytorin 10/80 Tablets 2939
Zocor Tablets (Rare) 2136

Dermatomyositis, exacerbation of
Actimmune (Rare) 1743

Dermatosis
▲ Advair HFA 45/21 Inhalation Aerosol (1% to 3%) 1288
▲ Advair HFA 115/21 Inhalation Aerosol (1% to 3%) 1288
▲ Advair HFA 230/21 Inhalation Aerosol (1% to 3%) 1288
Amerge Tablets (Rare) 1301
▲ Flovent Diskus 50 mcg (1% to 3%) 1435

Desquamation
▲ Alimta for Injection (Up to 22%) 1786
Avastin IV (2.5%) 1192
Doxil Injection (Some patients) 2378
Herceptin I.V. 1199
Invanz for Injection (Greater than 0.1%) 2029
▲ Nexavar Tablets (19% to 40%) 784
▲ Sustiva Capsules (16.7% to 24.5%) 930
▲ Sustiva Tablets (16.7% to 24.5%) 930
▲ Taxotere Injection Concentrate (0% to 6%) 2773
Xeloda Tablets 2662
Zovirax Cream (Less than 1%) 817

Detachment
Ambien Tablets (Infrequent) 2692

Deterioration, general
▲ Gliadel Wafer (82%) 1076
▲ Vectibix (8% to 11%) 597

Deterioration, lung function
Advair Diskus 100/50 1276
Advair Diskus 250/50 1276
Advair Diskus 500/50 1276

Diabetes
(*see under* Diabetes mellitus)

Diabetes, aggravation of
Activella Tablets 2347
▲ ActoPlus Met Tablets (5.1%) 3071
Climara Transdermal System 763
▲ Duetact Tablets (At least 5%) 3085
Enjuvia Tablets 1029
Geodon 2520
Lexiva Oral Suspension 1510
Lexiva Tablets 1510
Namenda (Infrequent) 1180
Premarin Tablets 3221
Premphase Tablets 3232
Prempro Tablets 3232
Proleukin for Injection 2287
Risperdal Consta Long-Acting Injection 1753
Tamiflu Capsules 2649
Tamiflu Oral Suspension 2649

Diabetes insipidus
Sandostatin LAR Depot 2302

Diabetes insipidus, nephrogenic
Atripla Tablets 938
Truvada Tablets 1262
Viread Tablets 1268

Diabetes mellitus
Abilify Injection (Greater than or equal to 1 in 1000 patients and less than 1 in 100 patients) 881
Abilify Injection (Greater than or equal to 1 in 1000 patients and less than 1 in 100 patients) 2466
Abilify Oral Solution (Greater than or equal to 1 in 1000 patients and less than 1 in 100 patients) 881
Abilify Oral Solution (Greater than or equal to 1 in 1000 patients and less than 1 in 100 patients) 2466
Abilify Discmelt Orally Disintegrating Tablets (Greater than or equal to 1 in 1000 patients and less than 1 in 100 patients) 881
Abilify Discmelt Orally Disintegrating Tablets (Greater than or equal to 1 in 1000 patients and less than 1 in 100 patients) 2466
Abilify Tablets (Greater than or equal to 1 in 1000 patients and less than 1 in 100 patients) 881
Abilify Tablets (Greater than or equal to 1 in 1000 patients and less than 1 in 100 patients) 2466
Accutane Capsules 2607
Aptivus Capsules (Less than 2%) 823
Aptivus Oral Solution (Less than 2%) 823
Aricept Tablets (Infrequent) 1062
Aricept ODT Tablets (Infrequent) 1062
Boostrix 1377
Brovana Inhalation Solution 2990
Campral Tablets (Infrequent) 1158
Celebrex Capsules (0.1% to 1.9%) 2979
▲ CellCept Capsules (3% to less than 20%) 2622
▲ CellCept Intravenous (3% to less than 20%) 2622
▲ CellCept Oral Suspension (3% to less than 20%) 2622
▲ CellCept Tablets (3% to less than 20%) 2622
Chantix Tablets (Infrequent) 2511
▲ Coreg Tablets (Greater than 1% to 3%) 1387
▲ Coreg CR Extended-Release Capsules (Greater than 1% to less than or equal to 3%) 1393
Crixivan Capsules 1979
Doxil Injection (Less than 1%) 2378
Dyazide Capsules 1405
Effexor XR Extended-Release Capsules (Infrequent) 3195
Emend Capsules (Greater than 0.5%) 1992
Emend for Injection (Greater than 0.5%) 1999
Evoxac Capsules (Less than 1%) 1013
Exelon Capsules (Infrequent) 2229
Exelon Oral Solution (Infrequent) 2229
Gengraf Capsules (1% to less than 3%) 435
Genotropin Lyophilized Powder (0.4%) 2547
Geodon 2520
▲ Gliadel Wafer (5%) 1076
Havrix Injection Vaccine 1454
Intelence Tablets (Less than 2%) 3119
Invega Extended-Release Tablets 1748
Kaletra (Less than 2%) 452
Lexiva Oral Suspension 1510
Lexiva Tablets 1510
Lupron Depot 7.5 mg 469
Luvox CR Extended-Release Capsules (Rare) 1759
Micardis Tablets (More than 0.3%) 852
Micardis HCT Tablets 854
Mirapex Tablets 857
M-M-R II 2054
Mumpsvax 2068
▲ Myfortic Tablets (3% to less than 20%) 2276
Neoral Oral Solution (1% to less than 3%) 2280
Neoral Soft Gelatin Capsules (1% to less than 3%) 2280
▲ Norditropin Cartridges (5%) 2354
Norvir (Less than 2%) 489
Nutropin for Injection (0.1%) 1208
Nutropin AQ Injection (0.1%) 1212
Nutropin AQ NuSpin Injection (0.1%) 1212
Nutropin AQ Pen (0.1%) 1212
Nutropin AQ Pen Cartridge (0.1%) 1212
Paxil (Rare) 1535
Paxil CR Controlled-Release Tablets (Rare) 1544
Pletal Tablets (Less than 2%) 2481
Prinivil Tablets (0.3% to 1%) 2087
Prinzide Tablets 2092
▲ Prograf Capsules and Injection (3% to 24%) 622
Proleukin for Injection 2287
Protonix for Delayed-Release Oral Suspension (Less than 1%) 3254
Protonix Delayed-Release Tablets (Less than 1%) 3254
Protonix I.V. (Less than 1%) 3257
Proventil HFA Inhalation Aerosol (Less than 3%) 2914
Prozac Weekly Capsules (Rare) 1852
Prozac Pulvules and Liquid (Rare) 1852
Pulmozyme Inhalation Solution 1217
Remeron Tablets (Rare) 2924
RemeronSolTab Tablets (Rare) 2927
ReoPro Vials (0.1%) 1860
Requip Tablets (Infrequent) 1561
Reyataz Capsules 3299
Rilutek Tablets (Infrequent) 2771
Risperdal Consta Long-Acting Injection (Infrequent) 1753
Rythmol SR Capsules 1590
Sandostatin Injection (Less than 1%) 2300
Sandostatin LAR Depot 2302
▲ Simulect for Injection (3% to 10%) 2306
▲ Somatuline Depot Injection (7%) 3102
Sular Extended Release Tablets (Less than or equal to 1%) 2975
Tasigna Capsules 2316
Teveten Tablets (Less than 1%) 515
Teveten HCT Tablets (Less than 1%) 517
Toprol-XL Tablets (Greater than 1%) 666
Treximet Tablets (Rare) 1616
Tricor Tablets 520
Venlafaxine Hydrochloride Tablets (Rare) 2199
Vytorin 10/10 Tablets 2939
Vytorin 10/20 Tablets 2939
Vytorin 10/40 Tablets 2939
Vytorin 10/80 Tablets 2939
▲ Zocor Tablets (4.2%) 2136
Zyprexa Tablets (Infrequent) 1883
Zyprexa ZYDIS Orally Disintegrating Tablets (Infrequent) 1883
Zyrtec Chewable Tablets (Less than 2%) 1920
Zyrtec Syrup (Less than 2%) 1920
Zyrtec Tablets (Less than 2%) 1920
Zyrtec-D 12 Hour Extended Release Tablets (Less than 2%) 1923

Diabetes mellitus, increase
▲ Actos Tablets (5.1%) 3077
Toprol-XL Tablets (Greater than 1%) 666

Diabetes mellitus, insulin-dependent, post-transplant
▲ Prograf Capsules and Injection (20%) 622

Diabetes mellitus, precipitation of latent
Furosemide Tablets 2186
▲ Intron A for Injection (Less than 5%) 2859
Prinzide Tablets 2092

Diabetes mellitus, type I
Abilify Injection (Greater than or equal to 1 in 1000 patients and less than 1 in 100 patients) 2466
Abilify Oral Solution (Greater than or equal to 1 in 1000 patients and less than 1 in 100 patients) 2466
Abilify Discmelt Orally Disintegrating Tablets (Greater than or equal to 1 in 1000 patients and less than 1 in 100 patients) 2466
Abilify Tablets (Greater than or equal to 1 in 1000 patients and less than 1 in 100 patients) 2466
Enbrel for Injection 569

Diabetes mellitus, type II
Abilify Injection (Greater than or equal to 1 in 1000 patients and less than 1 in 100 patients) 2466
Abilify Oral Solution (Greater than or equal to 1 in 1000 patients and less than 1 in 100 patients) 2466
Abilify Discmelt Orally Disintegrating Tablets (Greater than or equal to 1 in 1000 patients and less than 1 in 100 patients) 2466
Abilify Tablets (Greater than or equal to 1 in 1000 patients and less than 1 in 100 patients) 2466

Exforge Tablets (Greater than or equal to 0.2%) 2238

Diabetic acidosis
Prozac Weekly Capsules (Rare) 1852
Prozac Pulvules and Liquid (Rare) 1852
Zyprexa Tablets (Rare) 1883
Zyprexa ZYDIS Orally Disintegrating Tablets (Rare) 1883

Diabetic ketoacidosis
Abilify Injection (Less than 1 in 1000 patients) 2466
Abilify Oral Solution (Less than 1 in 1000 patients) 881
Abilify Oral Solution (Less than 1 in 1000 patients) 2466
Abilify Discmelt Orally Disintegrating Tablets (Less than 1 in 1000 patients) 881
Abilify Discmelt Orally Disintegrating Tablets (Less than 1 in 1000 patients) 2466
Abilify Tablets (Less than 1 in 1000 patients) 881
Abilify Tablets (Less than 1 in 1000 patients) 2466
Aptivus Capsules 823
Aptivus Oral Solution 823
Reyataz Capsules 3299
Risperdal Consta Long-Acting Injection 1753

Diabetic retinopathy
Genotropin Lyophilized Powder 2547
Norditropin Cartridges 2354

Dialysis graft complication
▲ Fosrenol Chewable Tablets (3% to 26%) 3027

Dialysis graft occlusion
▲ Fosrenol Chewable Tablets (4% to 21%) 3027

Diaphoresis
Abilify Injection 881
Abilify Injection 2466
Abilify Oral Solution 881
Abilify Oral Solution 2466
Abilify Discmelt Orally Disintegrating Tablets 881
Abilify Discmelt Orally Disintegrating Tablets 2466
Abilify Tablets 881
Abilify Tablets 2466
Accutane Capsules 2607
Aceon Tablets (2 mg, 4 mg, 8 mg) (0.3% to 1%) 3038
Acetadote Injection (0.29% to 1.41%) 1001
Actiq (1% to 2%) 959
▲ Adderall XR Capsules (2% to 4%) 3012
Adenocard IV Injection (Less than 1%) 603
Adenoscan (Less than 1%) 605
Advicor Tablets 402
▲ Aerobid/Aerobid-M (1% to 3%) 1153
▲ Alferon N Injection (One patient to 3%) 1726
Alinia for Oral Suspension (Less than 1%) 2677
Alinia Tablets (Less than 1%) 2677
▲ AmBisome for Injection (7%) 606
Amerge Tablets (Infrequent) 1301
Anaprox Tablets (Less than 3%) 2632
Anaprox DS Tablets (Less than 3%) 2632
AndroGel (Less than 1%) 3159
Anzemet Injection (Rare) 2701
Aricept Tablets (Frequent) 1062
Aricept ODT Tablets (Frequent) 1062
▲ Arimidex Tablets (1% to 5%) 672
▲ Asacol Delayed-Release Tablets (3%) 2579
Atacand Tablets (0.5% or greater) 639
Atacand HCT (0.5% or greater) 642
Avelox (Greater than or equal to 0.1% to less than 2%) 2803
▲ Avinza Capsules (5% to 10%) 1772
Axert Tablets (Rare) 2431
Axid Capsules 1364
▲ Azilect Tablets (3%) 3106
▲ Betaseron for SC Injection (8%) 756
▲ Bexxar (Less than 1% to 8%) 1371
Bicillin C-R Injectable Suspension 1775
Bicillin L-A Injection 1777
▲ Campral Tablets (2% to 3%) 1158
Captopril Tablets 2182
Carbatrol Capsules 3019
Cardene I.V. (1.4%) 1093
Celebrex Capsules (0.1% to 1.9%) 2979
▲ Celexa (11%) 1160
▲ CellCept Capsules (3% to less than 20%) 2622
▲ CellCept Intravenous (3% to less than 20%) 2622
▲ CellCept Oral Suspension (3% to less than 20%) 2622
▲ CellCept Tablets (3% to less than 20%) 2622
Cialis Tablets (Less than 2%) 1792
Cipro I.V. (1% or less) 2817
Cipro (Less than 1%) 2810
Cipro XR Tablets 2823
Clinoril Tablets (Less than 1 in 100) 1962
Combigan Ophthalmic Solution 553
Comtan Tablets (2%) 2208
▲ Copaxone for Injection (15%) 3110
Coreg Tablets (Greater than 0.1% to 1%) 1387
Cosopt Sterile Ophthalmic Solution 1969
Cozaar Tablets (Less than 1%) 1973
Crinone 4% Gel 992
Crinone 8% Gel 992
▲ Cubicin for Injection (5%) 995
Dantrium Capsules (Less frequent) 2580
Depakote ER Tablets (Greater than 1%) 423
▲ Doxil Injection (1% to 10%) 2378
▲ Duragesic Transdermal System (10% or more) 2405
Dyazide Capsules 1405
EC-Naprosyn Delayed-Release Tablets (Less than 3%) 2632
▲ Effexor XR Extended-Release Capsules (1% to 14%) 3195
Eldepryl Capsules 3052
▲ Eligard 7.5 mg (25% to 56.7%) 2724
▲ Eligard 22.5 mg (56.4%) 2724
▲ Eligard 30 mg (73.3%) 2724
▲ Eligard 45 mg (57.7%) 2724
▲ Eloxatin for Injection (5% to 12%) 2731
Emend Capsules (Greater than 0.5%) 1992
Emend for Injection (Greater than 0.5%) 1999
Emsam Transdermal System (Frequent) 905
Engerix-B Vaccine (Less than 1%) 1409
Equetro Extended-Release Capsules 3174
Erbitux 912
▲ Evista Tablets (2.5% to 3.1%) 1810
▲ Evoxac Capsules (18.7%) 1013
▲ Exelon Capsules (4%) 2229
▲ Exelon Oral Solution (4%) 2229
▲ Faslodex Injection (5%) 682
▲ Femara Tablets (Less than 0.1% to 24.2%) 2246
▲ Flolan for Injection (1% to 41%) 1426
▲ Fluarix Vaccine (1% to 10%) 1446
Flulaval Injection Vaccine 1448
Flumadine 1167
▲ Forteo for Injection (4.2%) 1816
Frova Tablets (Frequent) 1111
Gabitril Tablets (Frequent) 973
Gemzar for Injection (Infrequent) 1820
Gengraf Capsules (1% to less than 3%) 435
Geodon for Injection (Up to 2%) 2520
Humalog-Pen and KwikPen (Less common) 1829
Humalog Mix 50/50-Pen and KwikPen 1833
Humalog Mix 75/25-Pen and KwikPen (Less common) 1835
Humulin 50/50, 100 Units 1843
Humulin 70/30 Vial 1844
Humulin N Vial 1846
Humulin R 1849
Humulin R (U-500) (Less common) 1850
▲ Hycamtin for Injection (69%) 1459
Imitrex Injection (2%) 1465
Imitrex Nasal Spray (Infrequent) 1470
Imitrex Tablets (Infrequent) 1474
Indocin (Less than 1%) 2024
▲ Intron A for Injection (1% to 21%) 2859
Invanz for Injection (Greater than 0.1%) 2029
▲ Ionsys Transdermal System (1% to less than 10%) 2410
Kaletra (Less than 2%) 452
▲ Lamictal (2% to 5%) 1488
▲ Leukine (6%) 774
▲ Leustatin Injection (9%) 2384
Levitra Tablets (Less than 2%) 2876
Levoxyl Tablets 1780
▲ Lexapro Oral Suspension (3% to 8%) 1174
▲ Lexapro Tablets (3% to 8%) 1174
Lipitor Tablets (Less than 2%) 2501
Lovaza Capsules 1520
Lunesta Tablets 2994
▲ Lupron Depot 3.75 mg (50%) 462
▲ Lupron Depot 7.5 mg (57.1%) 469
▲ Lupron Depot–3 Month 11.25 mg (50%) 462
▲ Luvox CR Extended-Release Capsules (6% to 7%) 1759
Marinol Capsules (Less than 1%) 3163
Marplan Tablets (2%) 3177
Maxalt Tablets (Infrequent) 2056
Maxalt-MLT Orally Disintegrating Tablets (Infrequent) 2056
▲ Megace ES Oral Suspension (1% to 3%) 2499
Mephyton Tablets (Rare) 700
▲ Mepron Suspension (10%) 1526
Meridia Capsules (2.5%) 475
Merrem I.V. (Greater than 0.1% to 1%) 684
Micardis Tablets (More than 0.3%) 852
Micardis HCT Tablets 854
Mirapex Tablets (1% or more) 857
Moban Tablets 1116
Mobic Oral Suspension (Less than 2%) 863
Mobic Tablets (Less than 2%) 863
MS Contin Tablets (Less frequent to among most frequent) 2585
Nadolol Tablets (1 to 5 of 1000 patients) 2191
Naprosyn Suspension (Less than 3%) 2632
Naprosyn Tablets (Less than 3%) 2632
Natrecor for Injection (Greater than or equal to 1%) 2977
Neoral Oral Solution (1% to less than 3%) 2280
Neoral Soft Gelatin Capsules (1% to less than 3%) 2280
Nexium Delayed-Release Capsules (Less than 1%) 645
Nexium I.V. (Less than 1%) 652
Nexium Delayed-Release Oral Suspension (Less than 1%) 645
Niaspan Extended-Release Tablets 480
Nimotop Capsules (Less than 1%) 790
Nitrolingual Pumpspray 2965
Norvir (1.7% to 2.6%) 489
▲ Novantrone for Injection Concentrate (9%) 1100
▲ Ontak Vials (10%) 1079
Orthoclone OKT3 Sterile Solution (Less than 1%) 2387
▲ OxyContin Tablets (5%) 2589
▲ Paxil (1.1% to 19.2%) 1535
▲ Paxil CR Controlled-Release Tablets (1.1% to 19.2%) 1544
▲ PegIntron Powder for Injection (6%) 2903
Pentasa Capsules (Less than 1%) 3030
Percocet Tablets 1127
Prinivil Tablets (0.3% to 1%) 2087
Prinzide Tablets (0.3% to 1%) 2092
▲ Prograf Capsules and Injection (3% to 15%) 622
Prometrium Capsules (100 mg, 200 mg) 3047
Protonix for Delayed-Release Oral Suspension (Less than 1%) 3254
Protonix Delayed-Release Tablets (Less than 1%) 3254
Protonix I.V. (Less than 1%) 3257
Protopic Ointment (Greater than or equal to 1%) 628
Proventil HFA Inhalation Aerosol (Less than 3%) 2914
Provigil Tablets (1%) 977
▲ Prozac Weekly Capsules (2% to 8%) 1852
▲ Prozac Pulvules and Liquid (2% to 8%) 1852
▲ Rebetol (7% to 11%) 2917
Recombivax HB (Less than 1%) 2107
ReFacto Vials 3269
Remeron Tablets 2924
RemeronSolTab Tablets 2927
Remicade for IV Injection (Greater than or equal to 0.2%) 950
ReoPro Vials (1%) 1860
▲ Requip Tablets (6% to 7%) 1561
▲ Retrovir Capsules (5%) 1574
▲ Retrovir IV Infusion (5%) 1579
▲ Retrovir (5%) 1574
Rocephin Injectable Vials, ADD-Vantage, Galaxy, Bulk (Less than 1%) 2642
▲ Romazicon Injection (1% to 9%) 2646
Rythmol Tablets (1%) 1586
▲ Salagen Tablets (29% to 68%) 1082
▲ Soriatane Capsules (1% to 10%) 3062
▲ Suboxone Tablets (12% to 14%) 2601
▲ Subutex Tablets (12% to 12.6%) 2601
Sular Extended Release Tablets (Less than or equal to 1%) 2975
Sustiva Capsules (1% to 2%) 930
Sustiva Tablets (1% to 2%) 930
▲ Targretin Gel 1% (6%) 1088
Tarka Tablets 511
Teveten Tablets (Less than 1%) 515
Teveten HCT Tablets (Less than 1%) 517
Thiothixene Capsules 2197
▲ Tice BCG (3%) 2936
Timoptic Sterile Ophthalmic Solution 2121
Timoptic in Ocudose 2124
Timoptic-XE Sterile Ophthalmic Gel Forming Solution 2125
Tricor Tablets 520
Twinrix Vaccine (Less than 1%) 1628
Tygacil for Injection (2.3%) 3276
▲ Venlafaxine Hydrochloride Tablets (2% to 19.3%) 2199
▲ Vesanoid Capsules (20%) 2660
▲ Viadur Implant (5.3%) 802
▲ Vicoprofen Tablets (3% to 9%) 533
▲ Viread Tablets (3%) 1268
Vivitrol 988
▲ Wellbutrin Tablets (22.3%) 1648
▲ Wellbutrin SR Sustained-Release Tablets (5% to 6%) 1653
▲ Wellbutrin XL Extended-Release Tablets (5% to 6%) 1659
WinRho SDF 741
▲ Xeloda Tablets (Less than 5%) 2662
Xopenex Inhalation Solution 3001
Xopenex Inhalation Solution Concentrate 3005
Xopenex HFA Inhalation Aerosol 3009
Zomig Tablets (Infrequent) 694
Zomig Nasal Spray (Infrequent) 689
Zomig-ZMT Tablets (Infrequent) 694
Zonegran Capsules (Infrequent) 1089
Zosyn for Injection (1% or less) 3284
Zyban Sustained-Release Tablets (Frequent) 1692
▲ Zyprexa Tablets (3%) 1883
Zyprexa IntraMuscular (Infrequent) 1883
▲ Zyprexa ZYDIS Orally Disintegrating Tablets (3%) 1883

Diaphoresis, nocturnal
Sandimmune (Rare) 2296

Diaphragmatic hernia
(*see under* Hernia, hiatal)

Diarrhea
▲ Abelcet Injection (6%) 1134
▲ Abilify Injection (2% to 3%) 881
▲ Abilify Injection (2% to 3%) 2466
▲ Abilify Oral Solution (3%) 881
▲ Abilify Oral Solution (2% to 3%) 2466
▲ Abilify Discmelt Orally Disintegrating Tablets (3%) 881
▲ Abilify Discmelt Orally Disintegrating Tablets (2% to 3%) 2466
▲ Abilify Tablets (3%) 881
▲ Abilify Tablets (2% to 3%) 2466
Accolate Tablets (2.8%) 669
Accutane Capsules 2607
▲ Aceon Tablets (2 mg, 4 mg, 8 mg) (4.3%) 3038
▲ Aciphex Tablets (4.5%) 1053
▲ Actimmune (14%) 1743
Actiq (1% or greater) 959
▲ Activella Tablets (6%) 2347
▲ Actonel Tablets (4.9% to 19.7%) 2568
▲ Actonel with Calcium Tablets (4.9% to 10.6%) 2574
▲ ActoPlus Met Tablets (4.8% to 5.8%) 3071
▲ Adderall XR Capsules (2% to 6%) 3012
Adipex-P 1185
Advair Diskus 100/50 1276
Advair Diskus 250/50 (2%) 1276
Advair Diskus 500/50 1276
Advate (0.6%) 721
▲ Advicor Tablets (6%) 402
▲ Aerobid/Aerobid-M (10%) 1153
▲ Aggrenox Capsules (12.7%) 819
▲ Agrylin Capsules (25.7%) 3017
▲ Aldara Cream, 5% (3%) 1699
▲ Alferon N Injection (2% to 6%) 1726
▲ Alimta for Injection (Up to 26%) 1786
Alinia for Oral Suspension (2.1%) 2677
Alinia Tablets (2.1%) 2677
▲ Allegra Oral Solution (2.8% to 3.7%) 2684
▲ Allegra Tablets (2.8% to 3.7%) 2684
Aloxi Injection (1%) 1059
Altabax Ointment (1.4% to 1.7%) 1299
▲ Ambien Tablets (1% to 3%) 2692
Ambien CR Tablets (Frequent) 2696
▲ AmBisome for Injection (15.3% to 30.3%) 606
Amerge Tablets (Infrequent) 1301
▲ Amitiza Capsules (7% to 12%) 3082
▲ Amoxil Capsules (8%) 1305
▲ Amoxil Chewable Tablets (8%) 1305
▲ Amoxil Pediatric Drops for Oral Suspension (8%) 1305

▲ Amoxil Powder for Oral Suspension (8%)........................ 1305
▲ Amoxil Tablets (8%) 1305
Amrix Capsules.............................. 966
Anaprox Tablets (Less than 3%).......... 2632
Anaprox DS Tablets (Less than 3%).. 2632
▲ Anzemet Injection (12.4%) 2701
▲ Anzemet Tablets (2.1% to 5.3%) 2704
▲ Aptivus Capsules (3.6% to 15%) 823
▲ Aptivus Oral Solution (3.6% to 15%)... 823
▲ Aranesp for Injection (14% to 22%)... 564
▲ Argatroban Injection (6.2%) 1308
▲ Aricept Tablets (2% to 10%) 1062
▲ Aricept ODT Tablets (2% to 10%) 1062
▲ Arimidex Tablets (7% to 9%) 672
Arixtra Injection (1.9% to 2.5%)........ 1313
▲ Arranon Injection (0% to 22%) 1319
▲ Asacol Delayed-Release Tablets (7%)... 2579
Atacand Tablets (More than 1%)....... 639
Atacand HCT (0.5% or greater)........ 642
▲ Atripla Tablets (Greater than or equal to 10%)............................ 938
Atrovent HFA Inhalation Aerosol........ 839
Atrovent Nasal Spray 0.03%............ 834
Atrovent Nasal Spray 0.06%........... 836
Attenuvax (Rare)............................ 1951
▲ Augmentin (9%) 1323
▲ Augmentin Tablets (9%) 1327
▲ Augmentin XR Extended Release Tablets (14.4% to 15.6%).............. 1333
Augmentin ES-600 Powder for Oral Suspension (2.9%)............... 1329
Avalide Tablets (1% or greater)........ 892
Avalide Tablets (1% or greater)........ 2713
▲ Avandamet Tablets (12.7% to 14%)... 1336
Avandaryl Tablets (Less than 1%)..... 1344
Avandia Tablets (1% to 2.5%)........... 1351
▲ Avapro Tablets (3%) 897
▲ Avapro Tablets (3%) 2718
▲ Avastin IV (4.7%) 1192
▲ Avelox (5%) 2803
▲ Avinza Capsules (5% to 10%) 1772
Axert Tablets (Infrequent)................ 2431
▲ Axid Capsules (7.2%) 1364
▲ Azilect Tablets (5%) 3106
▲ Azmacort Inhalation Aerosol (1% to 3%).................................... 407
Azopt Ophthalmic Suspension (Less than 1%)............................ 540
Bactroban Nasal (Less than 1%)....... 1367
Baraclude (Less than or equal to 1%)... 900
BeneFIX Vials (1.5% to 1.6%)........... 3191
Benicar HCT Tablets (Greater than 1%)... 1010
Benzaclin Topical Gel...................... 2721
▲ Betaseron for SC Injection (19%) 756
Betimol Ophthalmic Solution............ 3181
▲ Bexxar (1% to 12%) 1371
▲ Biaxin/Biaxin XL (3% to 6%) 411
Bicillin C-R Injectable Suspension..... 1775
▲ Boniva Injection (4.1% to 6.8%) 2614
▲ Boniva Tablets (4.1% to 6.8%) 2618
▲ Boostrix (3% to 26%) 1377
▲ Brovana Inhalation Solution (6%) 2990
▲ Busulfex Injection (5% to 84%) 2477
▲ Byetta Injection (13%) 600
▲ Bystolic Tablets (2% to 3%) 1155
▲ Campath Ampules (10%) 761
▲ Campral Tablets (10% to 17%) 1158
▲ Canasa Rectal Suppositories (3.1%)... 705
▲ Cancidas for Injection (7.1% to 26.5%)...................................... 1953
Captopril Tablets (About 0.5% to 2%)... 2182
Carafate Suspension (Less than 0.5%)...................................... 706
Carafate Tablets (Less than 0.5%).... 707
Carbatrol Capsules......................... 3019
Cardizem LA Extended Release Tablets (Less than 2%)................ 421
▲ Ceftin (8.6%) 1380
▲ Celebrex Capsules (4% to 10.5%) ... 2979
▲ Celexa (8%) 1160
▲ CellCept Capsules (31% to 51.3%)..................................... 2622
▲ CellCept Intravenous (31% to 51.3%)..................................... 2622
▲ CellCept Oral Suspension (31% to 51.3%)..................................... 2622
▲ CellCept Tablets (31% to 51.3%) 2622
▲ Cerezyme for Injection (Approximately 6.5%)................... 1238
Cervidil Vaginal Insert (Less than 1%)... 1165
Chantix Tablets (Frequent)............... 2511
▲ Chemet Capsules (12% to 20.9%) ... 2484
Cialis Tablets (1% to 2%)................. 1792
Cimzia.. 3127
▲ Cipro I.V. (Greater than 1% to 4.8%)... 2817
▲ Cipro (1.6% to 4.8%) 2810
Cipro XR Tablets (2%)..................... 2823
▲ Clarinex Syrup (15.4% to 19.7%) 2828
▲ Clinoril Tablets (3% to 9%) 1962
▲ Clolar for Intravenous Infusion (53%).. 1239
Clorpres Tablets............................ 2185
Combigan Ophthalmic Solution........ 553
Combivent Inhalation Aerosol (Less than 2%)........................... 845
▲ Combivir Tablets (18%) 1384
▲ Comtan Tablets (10%) 2208
Comvax (0.8% to 2.2%)................... 1966
Concerta Extended-Release Tablets (Less than 1%)............... 1925
▲ Copaxone for Injection (12%) 3110
▲ Coreg Tablets (2% to 12%) 1387
▲ Coreg CR Extended-Release Capsules (1% to 12%)................. 1393
Cosmegen for Injection.................. 2485
Cosopt Sterile Ophthalmic Solution (Less than 1%)............. 1969
Cozaar Tablets (1% or greater)........ 1973
Creon 5 Capsules (Among most frequent).................................... 3041
Creon 10 Capsules (Among most frequent).................................... 3042
Creon 20 Capsules (Among most frequent).................................... 3042
▲ Crinone 8% Gel (8%) 992
▲ Crixivan Capsules (3.3%) 1979
▲ Cubicin for Injection (5.2% to 11.7%)...................................... 995
▲ Cuprimine Capsules (17%) 1986
Cyanokit 5g Antidote..................... 1021
▲ Cymbalta Delayed-Release Capsules (7% to 13%)................. 1801
▲ Dacogen Injection (34%) 1066
Dantrium Capsules (Among most frequent).................................... 2580
Demadex Injection (2%).................. 2630
Demadex Tablets (2%).................... 2630
▲ Demser Capsules (10%) 1989
▲ Depakote ER Tablets (6% to 23%) ... 423
▲ DepoCyt Injection (12% to 17%) 1136
Dexedrine.................................... 1401
▲ Didronel Tablets (About 1 patient in 15; possibly 2 or 3 in 10).......... 2583
▲ Diovan Tablets (1% to 5%) 2212
Diovan HCT Tablets (Greater than 0.2%).. 2216
▲ Doribax Injection (6% to 11%) 2400
▲ Doxil Injection (5.2% to 20.9%) 2378
Duac Topical Gel........................... 3054
▲ Duetact Tablets (4.3% to 6%) 3085
▲ Duragesic Transdermal System (3% to 10%)................................ 2405
Dyazide Capsules.......................... 1405
DynaCirc CR Controlled Release Tablets (0.5% to 1%).................... 1407
Dyrenium Capsules (Rare)............... 3189
EC-Naprosyn Delayed-Release Tablets (Less than 3%)............... 2632
Edecrin....................................... 698
E.E.S. (Among most frequent).......... 433
▲ Effexor XR Extended-Release Capsules (8%)............................ 3195
Eldepryl Capsules (1 of 49 patients)..................................... 3052
▲ Elidel Cream 1% (0.6% to 7.7%) 2221
▲ Elitek (20%) 2729
▲ Elmiron Capsules (4%) 2435
▲ Eloxatin for Injection (3% to 76%) 2731
▲ Emend Capsules (5.5% to 10.3%) ... 1992
▲ Emend for Injection (5.5% to 10.3%)...................................... 1999
▲ Emsam Transdermal System (9%) ... 905
▲ Emtriva Capsules (Greater than or equal to 10%)............................ 1246
▲ Emtriva Oral Solution (Greater than or equal to 10%)................. 1246
Enablex Extended-Release Tablets (0.9% to 2.1%)........................... 2225
Enbrel for Injection........................ 569
Engerix-B Vaccine (Less than 1%)..... 1409
▲ Epivir (8% to 18%) 1412
▲ Epivir-HBV (14%) 1417
▲ Epogen for Injection (0.11% to 21%)... 576
▲ Epzicom Tablets (5% to 6%) 1422
▲ Equetro Extended-Release Capsules (10%)........................... 3174
▲ Erbitux (2% to 72%) 912
EryPed (Among most frequent)......... 431
Evoclin Foam, 1% (Rarely)............... 3056
▲ Evoxac Capsules (10.3%) 1013
▲ Exelon Capsules (7% to 19%) 2229
▲ Exelon Oral Solution (7% to 19%) 2229
▲ Exelon Patch (6% to 10%) 2233
Exforge Tablets (Greater than or equal to 0.2%)........................... 2238
Exjade Tablets (11.8%).................... 2244
▲ Fabrazyme for Intravenous Infusion (Greater than or equal to 5%)....................................... 1241
Fansidar Tablets........................... 2636
▲ Faslodex Injection (12.3%) 682
▲ Femara Tablets (0.5% to 8%) 2246
▲ Fentora Tablets (1% to 16%) 968
Ferralet 90 Tablets........................ 2175
▲ Flebogamma 5% (20%) 1715
▲ Flebogamma 5% DIF (Greater than 15%)................................... 1718
▲ Flector Patch (3%) 561
▲ Flolan for Injection (37% to 50%) 1426
▲ Flomax Capsules (4.3% to 6.2%) 848
▲ Flonase Nasal Spray (1% to 3%) 1431
▲ Flovent Diskus 50 mcg (1% to 3%)... 1435
▲ Flovent HFA (1% to 3%) 1440
Fluarix Vaccine (1.6%).................... 1446
▲ Flulaval Injection Vaccine (1% to 5%)... 1448
Flumadine (0.3% to 1%).................. 1167
FluMist Vaccine 1945
Fortaz (1 in 78 patients) 1450
▲ Forteo for Injection (5.1%) 1816
▲ Fosamax (0.6% to 3.1%) 2005
▲ Fosamax Plus D Tablets (0% to 3.1%)....................................... 2013
▲ Fosrenol Chewable Tablets (13% to 23%)..................................... 3027
Frova Tablets (Frequent) 1111
Furosemide Tablets 2186
▲ Gabitril Tablets (2% to 10%) 973
▲ Gammagard Liquid (0.85% to 8.2%)....................................... 730
▲ Gamunex (28%) 3094
Gantrisin Pediatric Suspension 2638
▲ Gardasil Injection (3.6%) 2019
▲ Gemzar for Injection (19% to 31%)....................................... 1820
▲ Gengraf Capsules (3% to 13%) 435
▲ Geodon (5%) 2520
▲ Gleevec Tablets (25% to 70%) 2255
▲ Gliadel Wafer (2% to 5%) 1076
Gris-PEG Tablets (Occasional) 2507
Havrix Injection Vaccine (Less than 1%)... 1454
▲ Hepsera Tablets (3%) 1253
▲ Herceptin I.V. (25%) 1199
▲ Hycamtin Capsules (14% to 22%) ... 1456
▲ Hycamtin for Injection (Less than 1% to 42%)................................ 1459
Imitrex Injection (Infrequent) 1465
Imitrex Nasal Spray (Infrequent) 1470
Imitrex Tablets (Frequent) 1474
▲ Indapamide Tablets (Less than 5%)... 2188
Indocin Capsules (Greater than 1%)... 2024
▲ Indocin I.V. (1% to 3%) 2489
Indocin (Greater than 1%) 2024
▲ Infanrix Vaccine (3.8% to 4.3%) 1479
InnoPran XL Extended Release Capsules 1484
▲ Intelence Tablets (5.2%) 3119
Intravenous Sodium Diuril 2490
▲ Intron A for Injection (2% to 45%) ... 2859
▲ Invanz for Injection (9.2% to 11.7%)...................................... 2029
Ionsys Transdermal System (.1% to less than 1%).......................... 2410
Iquix Ophthalmic Solution (1% to 2%)... 3183
▲ Isentress Tablets (3.7% to 16.6%) ... 2036
▲ Ixempra Kit for Injection (22%) 915
▲ Janumet Tablets (2.4% to greater than 5%)................................... 2041
▲ Januvia Tablets (3%) 2048
▲ Kaletra (5% to 28%) 452
▲ Keppra Injection (8%) 3137
▲ Keppra Oral Solution (1% to 8%) 3131
▲ Keppra Tablets (1% to 8%) 3131
▲ Ketek Tablets (10% to 10.8%) 2744
▲ Kineret Injection (7%) 585
Klonopin 2639
K-Phos Original (Sodium Free) Tablets 814
K-Phos Neutral Tablets 813
Kristalose for Oral Solution 1004
▲ Lamictal (6%) 1488
▲ Lamisil Oral Granules (3% to 6%) 2264
▲ Lamisil Tablets (5.6%) 2266
Lanoxin Injection (Less common) 1498
Lanoxin Injection Pediatric 1502
Lanoxin Tablets (Less common) 1505
▲ Lescol Capsules (4.9%) 2268
▲ Lescol XL Tablets (3.3%) 2268
Leukeran Tablets (Infrequent) 1508
▲ Leukine (52% to 89%) 774
▲ Leustatin Injection (10%) 2384
▲ Levaquin (5%) 2416
▲ Levaquin in 5% Dextrose Injection (5%) 2416
Levitra Tablets (Less than 2%) 2876
Levothroid Tablets 1170
Levoxyl Tablets 1780
▲ Lexapro Oral Suspension (6% to 14%)...................................... 1174
▲ Lexapro Tablets (6% to 14%) 1174
▲ Lexiva Oral Suspension (5% to 13%)...................................... 1510
▲ Lexiva Tablets (5% to 13%) 1510
Lialda Tablets (Infrequent)............... 3029
▲ Limbrel Capsules (5% to 8%) 2561
▲ Lipitor Tablets (Up to 5.3%) 2501
Lovenox Injection (2.2%)................. 2756
▲ Lunesta Tablets (2% to 4%) 2994
▲ Luvox CR Extended-Release Capsules (2% to 18%)................. 1759
Lyrica Capsules............................ 2527
▲ Malarone Pediatric Tablets (1% to 8%)... 1521
▲ Malarone Tablets (1% to 8%) 1521
Marinol Capsules (0.3% to 1%)......... 3163
Marplan Tablets (0% to 2%)............. 3177
Mavik Tablets (0.3% to 1%).............. 472
Maxair Autohaler (1.3%).................. 1705
Maxalt Tablets (Frequent) 2056
Maxalt-MLT Orally Disintegrating Tablets (Frequent) 2056
▲ Megace ES Oral Suspension (6% to 15%) 2499
▲ Mepron Suspension (2.1% to 42%) 1526
Meridia Capsules (Greater than or equal to 1%) 475
▲ Merrem I.V. (3.5% to 7%) 684
Meruvax II 2061
▲ Mevacor Tablets (2.2% to 5.5%) 2063
▲ Miacalcin Nasal Spray (1% to 3%) ... 2274
▲ Micardis Tablets (3%) 852
▲ Micardis HCT Tablets (3%) 854
▲ Mirapex Tablets (1% to 7%) 857
M-M-R II 2054
▲ Mobic Oral Suspension (1.9% to 7.8%) 863
▲ Mobic Tablets (1.9% to 7.8%) 863
Moxatag Tablets (1.7%) 2165
MS Contin Tablets (Less frequent) 2585
Mumpsvax 2068
Mustargen for Injection 2492
▲ Mycamine for Injection (7.5% to 71.1%) 616
▲ Myfortic Tablets (21.4% to 23.5%) 2276
▲ Mylotarg for Injection (30% to 36%) 3212
▲ Nabi-HB (3%) 815
Nadolol Tablets (1 to 5 of 1000 patients) 2191
Nalfon Capsules (1.8%) 2508
Namenda (Greater than or equal to 2%) 1180
Naprosyn Suspension (Less than 3%) 2632
Naprosyn Tablets (Less than 3%) 2632
Nasonex Nasal Spray (Greater than or equal to 2%) 2883
▲ Neoral Oral Solution (3% to 13%) 2280
▲ Neoral Soft Gelatin Capsules (3% to 13%) 2280
▲ Neulasta Injection (15% to 72%) 587
▲ Neupogen for Injection (14%) 589
Neupro Transdermal System (Greater than or equal to 2%) 3149
▲ Nexavar Tablets (43% to 55%) 784
▲ Nexium Delayed-Release Capsules (Greater than or equal to 1% to 9.2%) 645
▲ Nexium I.V. (Greater than or equal to 1% to 9.2%) 652
▲ Nexium Delayed-Release Oral Suspension (Greater than or equal to 1% to 9.2%) 645
▲ Niaspan Extended-Release Tablets (6% to 8%) 480
▲ Nimotop Capsules (Up to 4.2%) 790
Noroxin Tablets (0.3% to 1%) 2069
▲ Norvir (15.4% to 23.3%) 489
▲ Novantrone for Injection Concentrate (14% to 47%) 1100
▲ NovoLog Injection (5%) 2359
▲ Noxafil Oral Suspension (3% to 42%) 2889
▲ Omnicef Capsules (15%) 497
▲ Omnicef for Oral Suspension (8%) ... 497
▲ Ontak Vials (29%) 1079
Opana Tablets (Less than 1%) 1117
▲ Opana ER Tablets (4.3%) 1121
▲ Orthoclone OKT3 Sterile Solution (14%) 2387
▲ OxyContin Tablets (Between 1% and 5%) 2589
Parnate Tablets 1532
Paser Granules (Among most common) 1747
Patanase Nasal Spray 544
▲ Paxil (1% to 12%) 1535
▲ Paxil CR Controlled-Release Tablets (1% to 12%) 1544
Pediarix Vaccine 1552
Liquid PedvaxHIB (One case) 2073

▲ PegIntron Powder for Injection (18%) ... 2903
Pentacel ... 2792
▲ Pentasa Capsules (3.4% to 3.5%) ... 3030
Pepcid Tablets (1.7%) ... 2075
Percocet Tablets ... 1127
Percodan Tablets ... 1130
▲ Perforomist Inhalation Solution (4.9%) ... 1025
Persantine Tablets ... 869
▲ Photofrin for Injection (5% to 9%) ... 708
▲ Plan B Tablets (5%) ... 1044
▲ Plavix Tablets (4.5%) ... 926
▲ Plavix Tablets (4.5%) ... 2767
▲ Pletal Tablets (12% to 19%) ... 2481
▲ PrandiMet Tablets (Greater than 5% to 19%) ... 2967
▲ Prandin Tablets (4% to 5%) ... 2971
▲ Precose Tablets (31%) ... 792
▲ Premarin Tablets (6% to 7%) ... 3221
▲ Premphase Tablets (5% to 7%) ... 3232
▲ Prempro Tablets (5% to 7%) ... 3232
▲ Prevnar (8.3% to 13.7%) ... 3241
Primaxin I.M. (0.6%) ... 2080
▲ Primaxin I.V. (1.8% to 3.9%) ... 2083
▲ Prinivil Tablets (3.7%) ... 2087
Prinzide Tablets (2.5%) ... 2092
▲ Pristiq Extended-Release Tablets (5% to 11%) ... 3247
ProAir HFA Inhalation Aerosol (Less than 3%) ... 3113
▲ Procrit for Injection (0.11% to 21%) ... 2391
Proglycem Capsules (Frequent) ... 1185
Proglycem Suspension (Frequent) ... 1185
▲ Prograf Capsules and Injection (37% to 72%) ... 622
▲ Proleukin for Injection (2% to 67%) ... 2287
▲ Prometrium Capsules (100 mg, 200 mg) (7%) ... 3047
ProQuad (1.2%) ... 2099
▲ Protonix for Delayed-Release Oral Suspension (4% to 6%) ... 3254
▲ Protonix Delayed-Release Tablets (4% to 6%) ... 3254
Protonix I.V. (Greater than 1%) ... 3257
▲ Protopic Ointment (3% to 6%) ... 628
▲ Provigil Tablets (6%) ... 977
▲ Prozac Weekly Capsules (Infrequent to 18%) ... 1852
▲ Prozac Pulvules and Liquid (8% to 18%) ... 1852
▲ Rapamune (25% to 35%) ... 3260
▲ Rebetol (17% to 22%) ... 2917
▲ Reclast Injection (5.2% to 6%) ... 2291
Recombivax HB (Greater than 1%) ... 2107
ReFacto Vials ... 3269
▲ Relenza Inhalation Powder (2% to 3%) ... 1556
▲ Relistor Injection (5.5%) ... 3310
▲ Remicade for IV Injection (12%) ... 950
ReoPro Vials (1.1%) ... 1860
▲ Requip Tablets (1% to 5%) ... 1561
▲ Requip XL Tablets (3%) ... 1568
▲ Retrovir Capsules (0.8% to 12%) ... 1574
▲ Retrovir IV Infusion (1% to 12%) ... 1579
▲ Retrovir (0.8% to 12%) ... 1574
▲ Reyataz Capsules (1% to 8%) ... 3299
▲ Rilutek Tablets (5.5% to 9%) ... 2771
Risperdal Consta Long-Acting Injection (1%) ... 1753
▲ Rituxan I.V. (1% to 10%) ... 1223
Rocephin Injectable Vials, ADD-Vantage, Galaxy, Bulk (2.7%) ... 2642
▲ Rotarix Oral Suspension (3% to 4%) ... 1582
▲ RotaTeq (3.7% to 24.1%) ... 2110
Rozerem Tablets (2%) ... 3091
▲ Rythmol Tablets (1% to 6%) ... 1586
▲ Rythmol SR Capsules (2% to 4%) ... 1590
▲ Salagen Tablets (4% to 7%) ... 1082
▲ Sandimmune (3% to 8%) ... 2296
▲ Sandostatin Injection (22% to 61%) ... 2300
▲ Sandostatin LAR Depot (14% to 47.4%) ... 2302
Selzentry Tablets ... 2534
▲ Sensipar Tablets (21%) ... 594
▲ Simcor Tablets (2.9% to 3%) ... 502
▲ Simulect for Injection (Greater than or equal to 10%) ... 2306
Singulair (Greater than or equal to 2%) ... 2114
▲ Somatuline Depot Injection (Greater than 5% to 65%) ... 3102
▲ Soriatane Capsules (1% to 10%) ... 3062
▲ Stalevo Tablets (5% to 10%) ... 2309
▲ Starlix Tablets (3.2%) ... 2314
Stromectol Tablets (1.8%) ... 2120
▲ Suboxone Tablets (3.7% to 5%) ... 2601
▲ Subutex Tablets (4.9% to 5%) ... 2601
Sular Extended Release Tablets (Less than or equal to 1%) ... 2975
▲ Suprax for Oral Suspension (16%) ... 1891
▲ Suprax Tablets (16%) ... 1891
▲ Sustiva Capsules (2% to 39%) ... 930
▲ Sustiva Tablets (2% to 39%) ... 930
▲ Sutent Capsules (4% to 58%) ... 2540
▲ Symbyax Capsules (8% to 19%) ... 1871
Synagis Intramuscular Solution (More than 1%) ... 1948
▲ Tamiflu Capsules (1% to 10%) ... 2649
▲ Tamiflu Oral Suspension (1% to 10%) ... 2649
▲ Tarceva Tablets (Less than 1% to 54%) ... 1228
▲ Targretin Capsules (7.1% to 41.5%) ... 1084
Tarka Tablets (1.5%) ... 511
▲ Tasigna Capsules (Greater than 10% to 22%) ... 2316
▲ Taxotere Injection Concentrate (2.1% to 77.8%) ... 2773
Tekturna Tablets (2% to 2.3%) ... 2321
Tekturna HCT Tablets (1.6% to 2.3%) ... 2324
▲ Temodar Capsules (2% to 16%) ... 2931
Teveten Tablets (1% or greater) ... 515
Teveten HCT Tablets (Less than 1%) ... 517
Thioridazine Hydrochloride Tablets .. 2195
Thiothixene Capsules ... 2197
Thyrogen for Injection (1.2%) ... 1244
Tice BCG (Less than or equal to 1%) ... 2936
Timentin ADD-Vantage ... 1606
Timentin Injection Galaxy Container ... 1609
Timentin IV Infusion ... 1603
Timentin Pharmacy Bulk Package ... 1613
Timoptic Sterile Ophthalmic Solution (Less frequent) ... 2121
Timoptic in Ocudose (Less frequent) ... 2124
Timoptic-XE Sterile Ophthalmic Gel Forming Solution ... 2125
▲ Toprol-XL Tablets (About 5 of 100 patients) ... 666
▲ Torisel Injection (1% to 27%) ... 3272
▲ Trasylol Injection (3%) ... 799
Treximet Tablets (Infrequent) ... 1616
Tricor Tablets (2.3%) ... 520
▲ Trisenox Injection (53%) ... 986
▲ Trizivir Tablets (12% to 26%) ... 1622
▲ Truvada Tablets (Greater than or equal to 10%) ... 1262
▲ Twinrix Vaccine (4% to 6%) ... 1628
▲ Tygacil for Injection (12.7%) ... 3276
▲ Tykerb Tablets (1% to 65%) ... 1631
▲ Tyzeka Tablets (Less than 1% to 7%) ... 2328
▲ Ultram ER Extended-Release Tablets (3.7% to 8.5%) ... 2428
Ultrase Capsules ... 718
▲ Ultrase MT Capsules (0.2% to 3.6%) ... 719
Uniphyl Tablets ... 2595
Urocit-K Tablets (Some patients) ... 2176
Uroqid-Acid No. 2 Tablets ... 814
Uroxatral Tablets ... 2786
Urso 250 Tablets (1%) ... 720
Urso Forte Tablets (1%) ... 720
▲ Valcyte Tablets (16% to 41%) ... 2654
▲ Valstar Sterile Solution for Intravesical Instillation (3%) ... 1735
Valtrex Caplets ... 1635
▲ Vaprisol (5.5% to 7%) ... 632
▲ Vaqta (1% to 5.9%) ... 2130
Varivax (Greater than or equal to 1%) ... 2133
▲ Vectibix (2% to 21%) ... 597
▲ Velcade for Injection (5% to 57%) ... 2168
▲ Venlafaxine Hydrochloride Tablets (8%) ... 2199
Ventolin HFA Inhalation Aerosol (Less than 3%) ... 1638
▲ Vesanoid Capsules (23%) ... 2660
Viadur Implant (2.3%) ... 802
▲ Vicoprofen Tablets (3% to 9%) ... 533
Viokase ... 721
Viramune Oral Suspension (0.2% to 2%) ... 873
Viramune Tablets (0.2% to 2%) ... 873
▲ Viread Tablets (5% to 16%) ... 1268
▲ Vivitrol (12% to 13%) ... 988
▲ Voltaren Tablets (1% to 10%) ... 2334
▲ Voltaren-XR Tablets (1% to 10%) ... 2337
Vytorin 10/10 Tablets (2.8%) ... 2149
Vytorin 10/10 Tablets (2.8%) ... 2939
Vytorin 10/20 Tablets (2.8%) ... 2149
Vytorin 10/20 Tablets (2.8%) ... 2939
Vytorin 10/40 Tablets (2.8%) ... 2149
Vytorin 10/40 Tablets (2.8%) ... 2939
Vytorin 10/80 Tablets (2.8%) ... 2149
Vytorin 10/80 Tablets (2.8%) ... 2939
▲ Vyvanse Capsules (7%) ... 3033
▲ Wellbutrin Tablets (6.8%) ... 1648
▲ Wellbutrin SR Sustained-Release Tablets (5% to 7%) ... 1653
▲ Wellbutrin XL Extended-Release Tablets (5% to 7%) ... 1659
WinRho SDF ... 741
▲ Xeloda Tablets (2% to 55%) ... 2662
Xifaxan Tablets (Less than 2%) ... 2682
▲ Xopenex Inhalation Solution (6%) ... 3001
▲ Xopenex Inhalation Solution Concentrate (1.5% to 6%) ... 3005
▲ Xopenex HFA Inhalation Aerosol (6%) ... 3009
▲ Xyntha Vials (5%) ... 3280
▲ Xyrem Oral Solution (6.1% to 8.6%) ... 1766
Yaz Tablets (Greater than 1%) ... 805
Zantac 25 EFFERdose Tablets ... 1670
Zantac Injection ... 1666
Zantac Injection Pharmacy Bulk Package (Frequent) ... 1668
Zantac Injection Premixed ... 1666
Zantac ... 1670
▲ Zetia Tablets (4.1%) ... 2157
▲ Zetia Tablets (2.5% to 4.1%) ... 2951
▲ Ziagen (0% to 7%) ... 1673
Zinacef for Injection (1 in 220 patients) ... 1678
Zinacef Injection (1 in 220 patients) ... 1678
Zocor Tablets ... 2136
▲ Zofran Injection (2% to 16%) ... 1682
▲ Zofran (4% to 6%) ... 1687
▲ Zofran ODT Orally Disintegrating Tablets (4% to 6%) ... 1687
▲ Zolinza Capsules (45% to 52.3%) ... 2142
▲ Zometa for Intravenous Infusion (7% to 24%) ... 2341
Zomig Tablets (Infrequent) ... 694
Zomig Nasal Spray (Infrequent) ... 689
Zomig-ZMT Tablets (Infrequent) ... 694
▲ Zonegran Capsules (5%) ... 1089
Zostavax Injection (1.5%) ... 2145
▲ Zosyn for Injection (7% to 20%) ... 3284
▲ Zovirax (2.4% to 3.2%) ... 1690
▲ Zyban Sustained-Release Tablets (4%) ... 1692
Zyprexa Tablets ... 1883
Zyprexa IntraMuscular (Infrequent) ... 1883
Zyprexa ZYDIS Orally Disintegrating Tablets ... 1883
▲ Zyrtec Chewable Tablets (1.9% to 3.1%) ... 1920
▲ Zyrtec Syrup (1.9% to 3.1%) ... 1920
▲ Zyrtec Tablets (1.9% to 3.1%) ... 1920
▲ Zyvox (3.8% to 10.8%) ... 2552

Diarrhea, bloody

Asacol Delayed-Release Tablets ... 2579
Augmentin Tablets ... 1327
Augmentin XR Extended Release Tablets ... 1333
Augmentin ES-600 Powder for Oral Suspension ... 1329
Benzaclin Topical Gel ... 2721
Canasa Rectal Suppositories ... 705
Ceftin ... 1380
Duac Topical Gel ... 3054
Evoclin Foam, 1% (Rarely) ... 3056
Imitrex Tablets ... 1474
Norvir (Less than 2%) ... 489
Omnicef Capsules ... 497
Omnicef for Oral Suspension ... 497
Paxil (Rare) ... 1535
Paxil CR Controlled-Release Tablets (Rare) ... 1544
Pentasa Capsules (0.9%) ... 3030
Proleukin for Injection (Less than 1%) ... 2287
Prozac Weekly Capsules (Rare) ... 1852
Prozac Pulvules and Liquid (Rare) ... 1852
Treximet Tablets ... 1616
▲ Trisenox Injection (8%) ... 986
Zomig Tablets (Rare) ... 694
Zomig Nasal Spray (Very rare) ... 689
Zomig-ZMT Tablets (Rare) ... 694
Zosyn for Injection (1.1%) ... 3284

Diarrhea, C. difficile-associated

Augmentin ... 1323
Augmentin Tablets ... 1327
Augmentin XR Extended Release Tablets ... 1333
Augmentin ES-600 Powder for Oral Suspension ... 1329
Avelox ... 2803
Biaxin/Biaxin XL ... 411
Bicillin C-R Injectable Suspension ... 1775
Ceftin ... 1380
Cipro I.V. ... 2817
Cipro ... 2810
Cipro XR Tablets ... 2823
Doribax Injection ... 2400
Eloxatin for Injection ... 2731
EryPed ... 431
Fortaz ... 1450
Invanz for Injection (Greater than 0.1%) ... 2029
Ketek Tablets ... 2744
Levaquin ... 2416
Levaquin in 5% Dextrose Injection ... 2416
Merrem I.V. ... 684
Moxatag Tablets ... 2165
Noroxin Tablets ... 2069
Omnicef Capsules ... 497
Omnicef for Oral Suspension ... 497
Primaxin I.M. ... 2080
Primaxin I.V. ... 2083
Suprax for Oral Suspension ... 1891
Suprax Tablets ... 1891
Timentin ADD-Vantage ... 1606
Timentin Injection Galaxy Container ... 1609
Timentin IV Infusion ... 1603
Timentin Pharmacy Bulk Package ... 1613
Tygacil for Injection ... 3276
Zinacef for Injection ... 1678
Zinacef Injection ... 1678
Zosyn for Injection ... 3284
Zyvox ... 2552

Diarrhea, infectious

Requip Tablets (Infrequent) ... 1561
▲ Xenical Capsules (5.3%) ... 2672

Diastolic blood pressure, decreased

Agrylin Capsules ... 3017
▲ Lexiscan Injection (4%) ... 614
Testim 1% Gel (1% or less) ... 701

Diastolic blood pressure changes

Focalin XR Capsules ... 2251
Pristiq Extended-Release Tablets (0.7% to 2.3%) ... 3247
Venlafaxine Hydrochloride Tablets ... 2199

Difficulty in walking

Rebif Prefilled Syringe for Injection ... 1107
Treximet Tablets (Rare) ... 1616

Digestive disorders, unspecified

CellCept Capsules ... 2622
CellCept Intravenous ... 2622
CellCept Oral Suspension ... 2622
CellCept Tablets ... 2622

Dilation, biliary

Sandostatin LAR Depot ... 2302

Dim vision

Levitra Tablets (Less than 2%) ... 2876

Diplegia

Imitrex Injection (Rare) ... 1465
Imitrex Nasal Spray (Rare) ... 1470
Imitrex Tablets ... 1474

Diplopia

Abelcet Injection ... 1134
Abilify Injection (Greater than or equal to 1 in 1000 patients and less than 1 in 100 patients) ... 881
Abilify Injection (Greater than or equal to 1 in 1000 patients and less than 1 in 100 patients) ... 2466
Abilify Oral Solution (Greater than or equal to 1 in 1000 patients and less than 1 in 100 patients) ... 881
Abilify Oral Solution (Greater than or equal to 1 in 1000 patients and less than 1 in 100 patients) ... 2466
Abilify Discmelt Orally Disintegrating Tablets (Greater than or equal to 1 in 1000 patients and less than 1 in 100 patients) ... 881
Abilify Discmelt Orally Disintegrating Tablets (Greater than or equal to 1 in 1000 patients and less than 1 in 100 patients) ... 2466
Abilify Tablets (Greater than or equal to 1 in 1000 patients and less than 1 in 100 patients) ... 881
Abilify Tablets (Greater than or equal to 1 in 1000 patients and less than 1 in 100 patients) ... 2466
▲ Agrylin Capsules (1% to less than 5%) ... 3017
Ambien Tablets (Frequent) ... 2692
Ambien CR Tablets (Frequent) ... 2696
Axert Tablets (Rare) ... 2431
Azopt Ophthalmic Suspension (Less than 1%) ... 540
Bentyl Capsules ... 703
Bentyl Injection ... 703
Bentyl Syrup ... 703

Bentyl Tablets 703
Betimol Ophthalmic Solution 3181
BOTOX Purified Neurotoxin Complex (Rare) 550
Campral Tablets (Rare) 1158
Carbatrol Capsules 3019
Celexa (Rare) 1160
Cipro I.V. (1% or less) 2817
Cipro (Less than 1%) 2810
Cipro XR Tablets (Less than 1%) 2823
Combigan Ophthalmic Solution 553
Concerta Extended-Release Tablets 1925
Copaxone for Injection (At least 2%) 3110
Cosopt Sterile Ophthalmic Solution 1969
Cymbalta Delayed-Release Capsules (Infrequent) 1801
Dantrium Capsules (Less frequent) 2580
▲ Depakote ER Tablets (16%) 423
Effexor XR Extended-Release Capsules (Infrequent) 3195
Eldepryl Capsules 3052
▲ Equetro Extended-Release Capsules (Less than 5%) 3174
Evoxac Capsules (Less than 1%) 1013
Exelon Capsules (Infrequent) 2229
Exelon Oral Solution (Infrequent) 2229
Exforge Tablets (Greater than 0.1% to less than 1%) 2238
Gabitril Tablets (1% or more) 973
Geodon Capsules (Frequent) 2520
Gliadel Wafer (1%) 1076
Indocin (Less than 1%) 2024
▲ Intron A for Injection (Less than 5%) 2859
Iquix Ophthalmic Solution (Less than 1%) 3183
Keppra Injection (1.7% to 2%) 3137
Keppra Oral Solution (2%) 3131
Keppra Tablets (2%) 3131
Ketek Tablets (Greater than or equal to 0.2% to less than 2%) 2744
Klonopin (Infrequent) 2639
▲ Lamictal (5% to 49%) 1488
Levaquin 2416
Levaquin in 5% Dextrose Injection 2416
Lexapro Oral Suspension 1174
Lexapro Tablets 1174
Lidoderm Patch 1114
Luvox CR Extended-Release Capsules (Infrequent) 1759
▲ Lyrica Capsules (2% to 12%) 2527
Mirapex Tablets (1% or more) 857
MS Contin Tablets (Less frequent) 2585
Nalfon Capsules (Less than 1%) 2508
Namenda (Infrequent) 1180
Noroxin Tablets 2069
Norvir (Less than 2%) 489
Ortho-Cyclen/Ortho Tri-Cyclen (Rare) 2449
Ortho Tri-Cyclen Lo Tablets 2458
Orthoclone OKT3 Sterile Solution 2387
Paxil (Rare) 1535
Paxil CR Controlled-Release Tablets (Rare) 1544
Photofrin for Injection 708
Pletal Tablets (Less than 2%) 2481
Premphase Tablets 3232
Prempro Tablets 3232
Prinivil Tablets (0.3% to 1%) 2087
Prinzide Tablets 2092
Proglycem Capsules (Infrequent) 1185
Proglycem Suspension (Infrequent) 1185
Protonix for Delayed-Release Oral Suspension (Less than 1%) 3254
Protonix Delayed-Release Tablets (Less than 1%) 3254
Protonix I.V. (Less than 1%) 3257
Prozac Weekly Capsules (Rare) 1852
Prozac Pulvules and Liquid (Rare) 1852
Remeron Tablets (Rare) 2924
RemeronSolTab Tablets (Rare) 2927
ReoPro Vials (0.1%) 1860
Requip Tablets (2%) 1561
Rilutek Tablets (Rare) 2771
▲ Romazicon Injection (1% to 3%) 2646
▲ Soriatane Capsules (1% to 5%) 3062
Stalevo Tablets 2309
Sustiva Capsules (Less than 2%) 930
Sustiva Tablets (Less than 2%) 930
Symbyax Capsules (Infrequent) 1871
Tasigna Capsules 2316
▲ Temodar Capsules (5%) 2931
Timoptic Sterile Ophthalmic Solution (Less frequent) 2121
Timoptic in Ocudose (Less frequent) 2124
Timoptic-XE Sterile Ophthalmic Gel Forming Solution 2125
Valium Tablets (Infrequent) 2658
Velcade for Injection 2168
Venlafaxine Hydrochloride Tablets (Infrequent) 2199
▲ Visudyne for Injection (1% to 10%) 2332
Wellbutrin Tablets (Rare) 1648
▲ Wellbutrin SR Sustained-Release Tablets (2% to 3%) 1653
▲ Wellbutrin XL Extended-Release Tablets (2% to 3%) 1659
Zomig Tablets (Rare) 694
Zomig-ZMT Tablets (Rare) 694
▲ Zonegran Capsules (6%) 1089
Zyban Sustained-Release Tablets (Frequent) 1692
Zyprexa Tablets (Infrequent) 1883
Zyprexa ZYDIS Orally Disintegrating Tablets (Infrequent) 1883

Dipsesis
Abilify Oral Solution (Less than 1 in 1000 patients) 881
Abilify Discmelt Orally Disintegrating Tablets (Less than 1 in 1000 patients) 881
Abilify Tablets (Less than 1 in 1000 patients) 881
Actiq (Less than 1%) 959
Aggrenox Capsules (Less than 1%) 819
Alferon N Injection (1%) 1726
Alinia for Oral Suspension (Less than 1%) 2677
Alinia Tablets (Less than 1%) 2677
Ambien Tablets (Infrequent) 2692
Ambien CR Tablets (Infrequent) 2696
Amerge Tablets (Infrequent) 1301
Amrix Capsules 966
Anaprox Tablets (Less than 3%) 2632
Anaprox DS Tablets (Less than 3%) 2632
Aricept Tablets (Infrequent) 1062
Aricept ODT Tablets (Infrequent) 1062
Atrovent Nasal Spray 0.06% (Less than 1%) 836
Avalide Tablets 892
▲ Avinza Capsules (Less than 5%) 1772
Axert Tablets (Rare) 2431
Bayer Aspirin 750
Campral Tablets (Infrequent) 1158
Cardizem LA Extended Release Tablets (Less than 2%) 421
Ceftin Tablets (0.1% to 1%) 1380
Celexa (Infrequent) 1160
▲ CellCept Capsules (3% to less than 20%) 2622
▲ CellCept Intravenous (3% to less than 20%) 2622
▲ CellCept Oral Suspension (3% to less than 20%) 2622
▲ CellCept Tablets (3% to less than 20%) 2622
Chantix Tablets (Frequent) 2511
Cipro XR Tablets (Less than 1%) 2823
Crinone 4% Gel 992
Crinone 8% Gel 992
Cymbalta Delayed-Release Capsules (Infrequent) 1801
Demadex Injection 2630
Demadex Tablets 2630
Dyazide Capsules 1405
EC-Naprosyn Delayed-Release Tablets (Less than 3%) 2632
Effexor XR Extended-Release Capsules (Infrequent) 3195
Emsam Transdermal System (Infrequent) 905
Evoxac Capsules (Less than 1%) 1013
Exelon Capsules (Infrequent) 2229
Exelon Oral Solution (Infrequent) 2229
Exforge Tablets (Greater than 0.1% to less than 1%) 2238
Fleet Phospho-soda EZ-PREP 1147
Frova Tablets (Infrequent) 1111
Furosemide Tablets 2186
Gabitril Tablets (Infrequent) 973
Geodon Capsules (Infrequent) 2520
Imitrex Injection (Infrequent) 1465
Imitrex Nasal Spray (Infrequent) 1470
Imitrex Tablets (Infrequent) 1474
▲ Intron A for Injection (Less than or equal to 5%) 2859
Klonopin (Infrequent) 2639
K-Phos Neutral Tablets 813
Lamictal (Rare) 1488
Lexapro Oral Suspension (Infrequent) 1174
Lexapro Tablets (Infrequent) 1174
Lunesta Tablets (Infrequent) 2994
Lupron Depot 3.75 mg (Among most frequent) 462
▲ Lupron Depot–3 Month 11.25 mg (Less than 5%) 462
Maxalt Tablets (Infrequent) 2056
Maxalt-MLT Orally Disintegrating Tablets (Infrequent) 2056
Meridia Capsules (1.7%) 475
Miacalcin Nasal Spray (Less than 1%) 2274
Mirapex Tablets (Less than 1%) 857
▲ MoviPrep Oral Solution (47.3%) 2679
Naprosyn Suspension (Less than 3%) 2632
Naprosyn Tablets (Less than 3%) 2632
Nexium Delayed-Release Capsules (Less than 1%) 645
Nexium I.V. (Less than 1%) 652
Nexium Delayed-Release Oral Suspension (Less than 1%) 645
Norvir (Less than 2%) 489
OxyContin Tablets (Less than 1%) 2589
Patanase Nasal Spray 544
Paxil (Infrequent) 1535
Paxil CR Controlled-Release Tablets (Infrequent) 1544
Pentasa Capsules (Less than 1%) 3030
Percocet Tablets 1127
Percodan Tablets 1130
Prinzide Tablets 2092
Protonix for Delayed-Release Oral Suspension (Less than 1%) 3254
Protonix Delayed-Release Tablets (Less than 1%) 3254
Protonix I.V. (Less than 1%) 3257
Provigil Tablets (1%) 977
Prozac Weekly Capsules (Infrequent to greater than or equal to 2%) 1852
Prozac Pulvules and Liquid (Infrequent to greater than or equal to 2%) 1852
Requip Tablets (Infrequent) 1561
Rilutek Tablets (Infrequent) 2771
St. Joseph 81 mg Aspirin Chewable and Enteric Coated Tablets 1903
Singulair 2114
▲ Soriatane Capsules (1% to 10%) 3062
Symbyax Capsules (Frequent) 1871
Treximet Tablets (Infrequent) 1616
Uroqid-Acid No. 2 Tablets 814
▲ Vaprisol (3% to 6%) 632
Venlafaxine Hydrochloride Tablets (Infrequent) 2199
Vicoprofen Tablets (Less than 3%) 533
Wellbutrin SR Sustained-Release Tablets (Infrequent) 1653
Wellbutrin XL Extended-Release Tablets (Infrequent) 1659
▲ Xeloda Tablets (Less than 5%) 2662
Zomig Tablets (Infrequent) 694
Zomig Nasal Spray (Infrequent) 689
Zomig-ZMT Tablets (Infrequent) 694
Zonegran Capsules (Infrequent) 1089
Zosyn for Injection (1% or less) 3284
Zyban Sustained-Release Tablets (Less than 1%) 1692
▲ Zyprexa Tablets (8%) 1883
▲ Zyprexa ZYDIS Orally Disintegrating Tablets (8%) 1883
Zyrtec Chewable Tablets (Less than 2%) 1920
Zyrtec Syrup (Less than 2%) 1920
Zyrtec Tablets (Less than 2%) 1920
Zyrtec-D 12 Hour Extended Release Tablets (Less than 2%) 1923

Discharge, nipple
Activella Tablets 2347
Angeliq Tablets 751
Enjuvia Tablets 1029

Discoloration, application site
Daytrana Transdermal Patch 3022
▲ Flector Patch (4%) 561
Lidoderm Patch 1114

Discoloration, injection site
Novantrone for Injection Concentrate 1100
ProQuad 2099
▲ Visudyne for Injection (10% to 30%) 2332

Discomfort, anal
▲ MoviPrep Oral Solution (51.5%) 2679

Discomfort, application site
Daytrana Transdermal Patch 3022
Iquix Ophthalmic Solution (1% to 2%) 3183

Discomfort, arm
▲ Adenoscan (4%) 605
Imitrex Injection 1465

Discomfort, chest
▲ Adenoscan (40%) 605
Alvesco Inhalation Aerosol (Less than 1 %) 2985
Ambien CR Tablets (1%) 2696
Amerge Tablets (Frequent) 1301
▲ Amitiza Capsules (0% to 3%) 3082
▲ Cerezyme for Injection (Approximately 6.6%) 1238
Chantix Tablets (Infrequent) 2511
Concerta Extended-Release Tablets 1925
Cyanokit 5g Antidote 1021
▲ Dacogen Injection (7%) 1066
▲ Fabrazyme for Intravenous Infusion (5%) 1241
▲ Imitrex Injection (5%) 1465
Imitrex Nasal Spray (Infrequent) 1470
Imitrex Tablets (Frequent) 1474
▲ Lexiscan Injection (13%) 614
Mirapex Tablets 857
▲ Photofrin for Injection (11%) 708
Primaxin I.M. 2080
Primaxin I.V. (Less than 0.2%) 2083
Prinivil Tablets (0.3% to 1%) 2087
Prinzide Tablets (0.3% to 1%) 2092
Recombivax HB (Less than 1%) 2107
Requip Tablets (Infrequent) 1561
Timentin ADD-Vantage 1606
Timentin Injection Galaxy Container 1609
Timentin IV Infusion 1603
Timentin Pharmacy Bulk Package 1613
▲ Treximet Tablets (3%) 1616
▲ Vesanoid Capsules (32%) 2660
Xyrem Oral Solution (Infrequent) 1766
Zomig Tablets (Infrequent) 694
Zomig Nasal Spray (Infrequent) 689
Zomig-ZMT Tablets (Infrequent) 694

Discomfort, general
Cubicin for Injection (Less than 1%) 995
▲ Selzentry Tablets (3.5%) 2534
Xyrem Oral Solution (Infrequent) 1766
Zovirax Ointment 819

Discomfort, head
Requip Tablets (Infrequent) 1561
Xyrem Oral Solution (Infrequent) 1766

Discomfort, jaw
▲ Adenoscan (15%) 605
Imitrex Injection (2%) 1465
Zomig Tablets (Rare) 694
Zomig Nasal Spray (Rare) 689
Zomig-ZMT Tablets (Rare) 694

Discomfort, local
▲ Betimol Ophthalmic Solution (More than 5%) 3181
OptiPranolol Metipranolol Ophthalmic Solution 0.3% (A small number of patients) ⊙245
▲ Supprelin LA Implant (51.1%) 1731

Discomfort, lower extremities
Adenoscan (Less than 1%) 605

Discomfort, musculoskeletal
▲ Dacogen Injection (6%) 1066
Xyrem Oral Solution (Infrequent) 1766

Discomfort, nasal
Amerge Tablets (Frequent) 1301
Imitrex Injection (2%) 1465
▲ Imitrex Nasal Spray (2.8% to 3.8%) 1470
▲ Imitrex Tablets (5% to 7%) 1474
Omnaris Nasal Spray 2998
Sudafed OM Sinus Cold Moisturizing Nasal Spray 1906
Sudafed OM Sinus Congestion Moisturizing Nasal Spray 1906
▲ Zomig Tablets (1% to 3%) 694
▲ Zomig Nasal Spray (1% to 3%) 689
▲ Zomig-ZMT Tablets (1% to 3%) 694

Discomfort, neck
▲ Adenoscan (15%) 605

Discomfort, sinus
Imitrex Injection (2%) 1465
▲ Imitrex Nasal Spray (2.8% to 3.8%) 1470

Discomfort, throat
▲ Adenoscan (15%) 605
▲ Imitrex Injection (3%) 1465
Imitrex Nasal Spray (0.8% to 2.4%) 1470
▲ Relenza Inhalation Powder (8% to 19%) 1556

Discomfort, upper extremities
▲ Adenoscan (4%) 605

Discomfort at injection site
Aloxi Injection (Very rare) 1059

Nutropin AQ Injection 1212
Nutropin AQ NuSpin Injection 1212
Nutropin AQ Pen 1212
Nutropin AQ Pen Cartridge 1212

Discontinuation syndrome
Catapres-TTS 842
Clorpres Tablets (About 1%) 2185
Luvox CR Extended-Release Capsules (Rare) 1759
Pristiq Extended-Release Tablets 3247

Disease progression, unspecified
Supprelin LA Implant 1731

Disinhibition
Ambien Tablets 2692
Ambien CR Tablets (1%) 2696

Disorder, pupillary
Proleukin for Injection (Less than 1%) 2287

Disorder, soft tissue, oral
▲ Dacogen Injection (6%) 1066

Disorientation
Aciphex Tablets 1053
Actimmune (Rare) 1743
Alferon N Injection (1%) 1726
▲ Ambien CR Tablets (3%) 2696
Asacol Delayed-Release Tablets 2579
Biaxin/Biaxin XL 411
BOTOX Purified Neurotoxin Complex 550
Chantix Tablets (Infrequent) 2511
Combigan Ophthalmic Solution 553
Concerta Extended-Release Tablets 1925
Cosopt Sterile Ophthalmic Solution 1969
Cymbalta Delayed-Release Capsules (Infrequent) 1801
Demser Capsules 1989
Eldepryl Capsules 3052
Eloxatin for Injection 2731
Emend Capsules (Isolated cases) 1992
Emend for Injection (Isolated cases) 1999
Fentora Tablets (Greater than 1%) 968
Gantrisin Pediatric Suspension 2638
Humulin 50/50, 100 Units 1843
Humulin 70/30 Vial 1844
Humulin N Vial 1846
Humulin R 1849
Intelence Tablets (Less than 2%) 3119
▲ Invanz for Injection (3.3% to 5.1%) 2029
Lexapro Oral Suspension (Infrequent) 1174
Lexapro Tablets (Infrequent) 1174
Lidoderm Patch 1114
Maxalt Tablets (Infrequent) 2056
Maxalt-MLT Orally Disintegrating Tablets (Infrequent) 2056
Mirapex Tablets 857
MS Contin Tablets (Less frequent) 2585
Nalfon Capsules (Less than 1%) 2508
Opana Tablets (Less than 1%) 1117
Opana ER Tablets (Less than 1%) 1121
Orthoclone OKT3 Sterile Solution 2387
Parnate Tablets 1532
Requip Tablets (Infrequent) 1561
Seromycin Capsules 1864
Stalevo Tablets 2309
Tasigna Capsules 2316
Timoptic Sterile Ophthalmic Solution (Less frequent) 2121
Timoptic in Ocudose (Less frequent) 2124
Timoptic-XE Sterile Ophthalmic Gel Forming Solution 2125
Transderm Scōp Transdermal Therapeutic System (Infrequent) 2206
Treximet Tablets (Rare) 1616
▲ Ultram ER Extended-Release Tablets (0.5% to less than 1%) 2428
▲ Xyrem Oral Solution (2.9% to 8.6%) 1766

Disorientation, place
Combigan Ophthalmic Solution 553
Cosopt Sterile Ophthalmic Solution 1969
InnoPran XL Extended Release Capsules 1484
Nadolol Tablets 2191
Timoptic Sterile Ophthalmic Solution 2121
Timoptic in Ocudose 2124
Timoptic-XE Sterile Ophthalmic Gel Forming Solution 2125
Toprol-XL Tablets 666

Disorientation, time
Combigan Ophthalmic Solution 553
Cosopt Sterile Ophthalmic Solution 1969
InnoPran XL Extended Release Capsules 1484
Nadolol Tablets 2191
Timoptic Sterile Ophthalmic Solution 2121
Timoptic in Ocudose 2124
Timoptic-XE Sterile Ophthalmic Gel Forming Solution 2125
Toprol-XL Tablets 666

Dissociation
Chantix Tablets (Infrequent) 2511
Mirapex Tablets 857

Distention, abdominal
(*see under* Abdominal distention)

Distress, abdominal
▲ Abilify Injection (2% to 3%) 2466
▲ Abilify Oral Solution (2% to 3%) 2466
▲ Abilify Discmelt Orally Disintegrating Tablets (2% to 3%) 2466
▲ Abilify Tablets (2% to 3%) 2466
▲ Advair HFA 45/21 Inhalation Aerosol (1% to 3%) 1288
▲ Advair HFA 115/21 Inhalation Aerosol (1% to 3%) 1288
▲ Advair HFA 230/21 Inhalation Aerosol (1% to 3%) 1288
Augmentin (Less frequent) 1323
Augmentin Tablets (Less frequent) 1327
Imitrex Injection (Frequent) 1465
Imitrex Tablets 1474
Indocin (Greater than 1%) 2024
▲ Persantine Tablets (6.1%) 869
Pylera Capsules 714
Stalevo Tablets 2309
Ultrase MT Capsules (0.2%) 719
Zantac Injection 1666

Distress, epigastric
Abelcet Injection 1134
Aricept Tablets (Frequent) 1062
Aricept ODT Tablets (Frequent) 1062
Cipro I.V. (1% or less) 2817
Cipro XR Tablets 2823
Clorpres Tablets 2185
Cubicin for Injection (Less than 1%) 995
▲ Cuprimine Capsules (17%) 1986
▲ Emend Capsules (4%) 1992
▲ Emend for Injection (4%) 1999
Fosteum Capsules 2963
Gris-PEG Tablets (Occasional) 2507
▲ Indocin (3% to 9%) 2024
InnoPran XL Extended Release Capsules 1484
Nexium Delayed-Release Capsules (Less than 1%) 645
Nexium I.V. (Less than 1%) 652
Nexium Delayed-Release Oral Suspension (Less than 1%) 645
▲ Novantrone for Injection Concentrate (14%) 1100
Sandostatin Injection (Rare) 2300
Sandostatin LAR Depot 2302
Soma Tablets 1931
Timentin ADD-Vantage 1606
Timentin Injection Galaxy Container 1609
Timentin IV Infusion 1603
Timentin Pharmacy Bulk Package 1613
Toprol-XL Tablets (About 1 of 100 patients) 666

Distress, gastric
(*see under* Distress, gastrointestinal)

Distress, gastrointestinal
▲ Abilify Injection (3%) 2466
▲ Abilify Oral Solution (3%) 2466
▲ Abilify Discmelt Orally Disintegrating Tablets (3%) 2466
▲ Abilify Tablets (3%) 2466
▲ Adenoscan (13%) 605
Advair Diskus 100/50 1276
Advair Diskus 250/50 (1%) 1276
Advair Diskus 500/50 1276
▲ Agrylin Capsules (1% to less than 5%) 3017
Alferon N Injection (One patient) 1726
Amitiza Capsules (0% to 1%) 3082
Appearex Tablets 2163
Atrovent HFA Inhalation Aerosol 839
Atrovent Nasal Spray 0.03% 834
Atrovent Nasal Spray 0.06% 836
Bios Life Drink Mix 3158
Carafate Suspension (Less than 0.5%) 706
Carafate Tablets (Less than 0.5%) 707
Carbatrol Capsules 3019
CardioEssentials Capsules 3159
▲ Clinoril Tablets (10%) 1962
CM Plex Softgels 3159
Combivent Inhalation Aerosol 845
Emend Capsules (Less than or equal to 0.5%) 1992
Emend for Injection (Less than or equal to 0.5%) 1999
Equetro Extended-Release Capsules 3174
Evoclin Foam, 1% 3056
Fentora Tablets (Greater than 1%) 968
▲ Flovent HFA (1% to 3%) 1440
Fluorescite Injection ⊙ 203
Fosteum Capsules 2963
Imitrex Tablets (Frequent) 1474
Januvia Tablets 2048
▲ Lupron Depot–3 Month 11.25 mg (3% to 7%) 462
ProAmatine Tablets (Rare) 3032
Timoptic Sterile Ophthalmic Solution 2121
Timoptic in Ocudose 2124
Valium Tablets 2658
Visutein Capsules 3159
▲ Vivitrol (11% to 16%) 988
Xifaxan Tablets (Less than 2%) 2682
Zovirax 1690

Distress, precordial
(*see under* Distress, epigastric)

Distress, stomach
(*see under* Distress, gastrointestinal)

Distress, upper GI
(*see under* Distress, epigastric)

Disturbances, emotional
(*see under* Emotional disturbances)

Disturbances, gastrointestinal
(*see under* Distress, gastrointestinal)

Disulfiram-like reactions
Avandaryl Tablets 1344

Diuresis
Amerge Tablets (Infrequent) 1301
Gantrisin Pediatric Suspension 2638

Diuresis, potentiation of
Uniphyl Tablets 2595

Diverticulitis
Aricept Tablets (Infrequent) 1062
Aricept ODT Tablets (Infrequent) 1062
Celebrex Capsules (0.1% to 1.9%) 2979
Celexa (Rare) 1160
Evoxac Capsules (Less than 1%) 1013
Exelon Capsules (Infrequent) 2229
Exelon Oral Solution (Infrequent) 2229
Exelon Patch (Infrequent) 2233
Gleevec Tablets (Rare) 2255
▲ Humira Injection (Less than 5%) 442
Mirapex Tablets 857
Namenda (Infrequent) 1180
Orencia Powder for Intravenous Infusion (0.2% to 0.5%) 921
Requip Tablets (Infrequent) 1561
Treximet Tablets (Rare) 1616

Dizziness
▲ Abilify Injection (4% to 11%) 881
▲ Abilify Injection (4% to 10%) 2466
▲ Abilify Oral Solution (4% to 11%) 881
▲ Abilify Oral Solution (4% to 10%) 2466
▲ Abilify Discmelt Orally Disintegrating Tablets (4% to 11%) 881
▲ Abilify Discmelt Orally Disintegrating Tablets (4% to 10%) 2466
▲ Abilify Tablets (4% to 11%) 881
▲ Abilify Tablets (4% to 10%) 2466
Accolate Tablets (1.6%) 669
Accutane Capsules 2607
Aciphex Tablets 1053
▲ Actiq (6% to 17%) 959
Activella Tablets 2347
▲ Actonel Tablets (6.6% to 7.1%) 2568
▲ Actonel with Calcium Tablets (4.9% to 6.4%) 2574
▲ ActoPlus Met Tablets (4.8% to 5.4%) 3071
▲ Adderall XR Capsules (2% to 7%) 3012
Adenocard IV Injection (1%) 603
▲ Adenoscan (12%) 605
Adipex-P 1185
▲ Advair Diskus 250/50 (4% to less than 5%) 1276
▲ Advair HFA 45/21 Inhalation Aerosol (1% to 4%) 1288
▲ Advair HFA 115/21 Inhalation Aerosol (1% to 4%) 1288
▲ Advair HFA 230/21 Inhalation Aerosol (1% to 4%) 1288
Advate (2%) 721
Advicor Tablets 402
▲ Aerobid/Aerobid-M (3% to 9%) 1153
Aggrenox Capsules (Less than 1%) 819
▲ Agrylin Capsules (15.4%) 3017
Albenza Tablets (Less than 1% to 1.2%) 1297
Aldara Cream, 5% (1%) 1699
▲ Alferon N Injection (9%) 1726
Alinia for Oral Suspension (Less than 1%) 2677
Alinia Tablets (Less than 1%) 2677
Allegra Oral Solution (2.2%) 2684
Allegra Tablets (2.1%) 2684
Allegra-D 12 Hour Extended-Release Tablets (1.9%) 2687
Allegra-D 24 Hour Extended-Release Tablets (1.9%) 2690
Aloxi Injection (1%) 1059
▲ Alphagan P Ophthalmic Solution (1% to 4%) 549
▲ Alvesco Inhalation Aerosol (Greater than or equal to 3%) 2985
▲ Ambien Tablets (1% to 5%) 2692
▲ Ambien CR Tablets (1% to 12%) 2696
AmBisome for Injection (Less common) 606
Amerge Tablets (1% to 2%) 1301
Amevive (Common) 611
▲ Amitiza Capsules (3%) 3082
Amoxil Capsules (Rare) 1305
Amoxil Chewable Tablets (Rare) 1305
Amoxil Pediatric Drops for Oral Suspension (Rare) 1305
Amoxil Powder for Oral Suspension (Rare) 1305
Amoxil Tablets (Rare) 1305
Amrix Capsules 966
▲ Anaprox Tablets (3% to 9%) 2632
▲ Anaprox DS Tablets (3% to 9%) 2632
AndroGel (Less than 1%) 3159
Angeliq Tablets 751
▲ Anzemet Injection (2.2% to 5.5%) 2701
▲ Anzemet Tablets (1.3% to 4.4%) 2704
Aptivus Capsules (Less than 2%) 823
Aptivus Oral Solution (Less than 2%) 823
Aralast (Greater than or equal to 0.02% to 0.1%) 726
▲ Aranesp for Injection (7% to 14%) 564
Aricept Tablets (2%) 1062
Aricept ODT Tablets (2%) 1062
▲ Arimidex Tablets (5% to 8%) 672
▲ Arixtra Injection (0.6% to 3.6%) 1313
▲ Arranon Injection (0% to 21%) 1319
▲ Asacol Delayed-Release Tablets (8%) 2579
▲ Atacand Tablets (4%) 639
Atacand HCT (2.9%) 642
▲ Atripla Tablets (Greater than or equal to 10%) 938
▲ Atrovent HFA Inhalation Aerosol (3%) 839
Atrovent Nasal Spray 0.03% (Less than 2%) 834
Atrovent Nasal Spray 0.06% (Less than 1%) 836
Attenuvax 1951
Augmentin (Rare) 1323
Augmentin Tablets (Rare) 1327
Augmentin XR Extended Release Tablets (Rare) 1333
Augmentin ES-600 Powder for Oral Suspension 1329
▲ Avalide Tablets (4.3% to 8%) 892
▲ Avalide Tablets (3% to 8%) 2713
▲ Avandamet Tablets (8%) 1336
Avandaryl Tablets (1.7%) 1344
Avandia Tablets 1351
▲ Avapro Tablets (5.4% to 6%) 897
▲ Avapro Tablets (5.4% to 10.2%) 2718
▲ Avastin IV (19% to 26%) 1192
Avelox (2%) 2803
Avodart Soft Gelatin Capsules (0% to 1.1%) 1359
Axert Tablets (Frequent) 2431
▲ Axid Capsules (4.6%) 1364
Azilect Tablets (Greater than 1%) 3106
Azopt Ophthalmic Suspension (Less than 1%) 540
▲ Azor Tablets (1.5% to 3.4%) 1005
Bactroban Cream (Less than 1%) 1366
Baraclude (Less than 1%) 900
Bayer Aspirin 750

▲ BeneFIX Vials (7.7%) 3191
▲ Benicar Tablets (3%) 1009
▲ Benicar HCT Tablets (9%) 1010
▲ Bentyl Capsules (29%) 703
▲ Bentyl Injection (29%) 703
▲ Bentyl Syrup (29%) 703
▲ Bentyl Tablets (29%) 703
▲ Betaseron for SC Injection (24%) 756
▲ Betimol Ophthalmic Solution (1% to 5%) 3181
▲ Bexxar (0% to 5%) 1371
Biaxin/Biaxin XL 411
Bicillin C-R Injectable Suspension 1775
Bicillin L-A Injection 1777
▲ Boniva Injection (1% to 3.7%) 2614
▲ Boniva Tablets (1% to 3.7%) 2618
▲ BOTOX Purified Neurotoxin Complex (2% to 10%) 550
Brovana Inhalation Solution (Less than 2%) 2990
▲ Busulfex Injection (30%) 2477
▲ Byetta Injection (9%) 600
▲ Bystolic Tablets (2% to 4%) 1155
▲ Campral Tablets (3% to 4%) 1158
▲ Canasa Rectal Suppositories (3%) 705
Cancidas for Injection 1953
Captopril Tablets (About 0.5% to 2%) 2182
Carafate Suspension (Less than 0.5%) 706
Carafate Tablets (Less than 0.5%) 707
Carbatrol Capsules (Among most frequent) 3019
Cardene I.V. (1.4%) 1093
▲ Cardizem LA Extended Release Tablets (3.5% to 6.4%) 421
▲ Catapres Tablets (About 16 in 100 patients) 841
Catapres-TTS (2 of 101 patients) 842
Ceftin Tablets (0.1% to 1%) 1380
Celebrex Capsules (1% to 2%) 2979
Celexa (At least 2%) 1160
▲ CellCept Capsules (28.7%) 2622
▲ CellCept Intravenous (28.7%) 2622
▲ CellCept Oral Suspension (28.7%) 2622
▲ CellCept Tablets (28.7%) 2622
▲ Cerezyme for Injection (Approximately 6.5%) 1238
Chantix Tablets (Frequent) 2511
▲ Chemet Capsules (1% to 12.7%) 2484
Cialis Tablets (Less than 2%) 1792
Cipro I.V. (1% or less) 2817
Cipro (Less than 1%) 2810
Cipro XR Tablets (1% to 2%) 2823
▲ Clarinex Tablets (4%) 2828
▲ Clarinex Reditabs Tablets (4%) 2828
▲ Clarinex-D 12-Hour Extended-Release Tablets (3%) 2831
Clarinex-D 24-Hour Extended-Release Tablets (2%) 2834
Climara Transdermal System 763
Climara Pro Transdermal System 768
▲ Clinoril Tablets (3% to 9%) 1962
▲ Clolar for Intravenous Infusion (16%) 1239
▲ Clorpres Tablets (About 16%) 2185
Combigan Ophthalmic Solution (0.1% to 0.2%) 553
Combivent Inhalation Aerosol (Less than 2%) 845
▲ Combivir Tablets (10%) 1384
▲ Comtan Tablets (8%) 2208
▲ Concerta Extended-Release Tablets (1.9% to 6.7%) 1925
Copaxone for Injection (At least 2%) 3110
▲ Coreg Tablets (6% to 32%) 1387
▲ Coreg CR Extended-Release Capsules (2% to 32%) 1393
▲ Cosopt Sterile Ophthalmic Solution (1% to 5%) 1969
▲ Cozaar Tablets (3%) 1973
▲ Crestor Tablets (4%) 677
▲ Crinone 8% Gel (5%) 992
▲ Crixivan Capsules (3%) 1979
▲ Cubicin for Injection (2.2% to 5.8%) 995
Cyanokit 5g Antidote 1021
▲ Cymbalta Delayed-Release Capsules (6% to 17%) 1801
▲ Dacogen Injection (18%) 1066
Dantrium Capsules (Among most frequent) 2580
Daytrana Transdermal Patch 3022
▲ Demadex Injection (3.2%) 2630
▲ Demadex Tablets (3.2%) 2630
▲ Depakote ER Tablets (Greater than 1% to 25%) 423
▲ DepoCyt Injection (18% to 21%) 1136
▲ DepoDur Injection (Greater than 10%) 1095
Dexedrine 1401
Diclofenac Sodium Ophthalmic Solution .... ⊙240
▲ Diovan Tablets (2% to 17%) 2212
Diovan HCT Tablets (Greater than 0.2%) 2216
Divigel 3167
Donnatal Extentabs 2507
▲ Doxil Injection (1% to 10%) 2378
Duetact Tablets (1.7%) 3085
▲ Duragesic Transdermal System (3% to 10%) 2405
Dyazide Capsules 1405
▲ DynaCirc CR Controlled Release Tablets (3.7% to 6.4%) 1407
Dyrenium Capsules (Rare) 3189
▲ EC-Naprosyn Delayed-Release Tablets (3% to 9%) 2632
Edex Injection (Less than 1%) 2957
▲ Effexor XR Extended-Release Capsules (2% to 20%) 3195
▲ Eldepryl Capsules (7 of 49 patients) 3052
▲ Eligard 7.5 mg (3.3%) 2724
Eligard 22.5 mg 2724
▲ Eligard 30 mg (4.4%) 2724
Eligard 45 mg 2724
Elmiron Capsules (1%) 2435
▲ Eloxatin for Injection (8% to 13%) 2731
▲ Emend Capsules (3.4% to 6.6%) 1992
▲ Emend for Injection (3.4% to 6.6%) 1999
Emsam Transdermal System 905
▲ Emtriva Capsules (Greater than or equal to 10%) 1246
▲ Emtriva Oral Solution (Greater than or equal to 10%) 1246
Enablex Extended-Release Tablets (0.9% to 2.1%) 2225
▲ Enbrel for Injection (7% to 8%) 569
▲ Engerix-B Vaccine (1% to 10%) 1409
▲ Enjuvia Tablets (1% to 7%) 1029
EpiPen 1024
▲ Epivir (10%) 1412
▲ Epogen for Injection (5% to 21%) 576
▲ Epzicom Tablets (6%) 1422
▲ Equetro Extended-Release Capsules (16% to 44%) 3174
Estratest Tablets 3043
Estratest H.S. Tablets 3043
▲ Evoxac Capsules (4.1%) 1013
▲ Exelon Capsules (6% to 21%) 2229
▲ Exelon Oral Solution (6% to 21%) 2229
▲ Exelon Patch (2% to 7%) 2233
Exforge Tablets (2.1%) 2238
Exjade Tablets (0.1% to 1%) 2244
▲ Fabrazyme for Intravenous Infusion (21%) 1241
▲ Faslodex Injection (6.9%) 682
▲ Femara Tablets (Less than 0.1% to 14.2%) 2246
▲ Fentora Tablets (1% to 32%) 968
Flector Patch (1%) 561
Fleet Phospho-soda 1145
Fleet Phospho-soda EZ-PREP 1147
Fleet Prep Kits 1149
▲ Flolan for Injection (8% to 83%) 1426
▲ Flomax Capsules (14.9% to 17.1%) 848
▲ Flonase Nasal Spray (1% to 3%) 1431
▲ Flovent Diskus 50 mcg (1% to 3%) 1435
▲ Flovent HFA (1% to 3%) 1440
Fluarix Vaccine 1446
Flumadine (0.7% to 1.9%) 1167
▲ Focalin XR Capsules (6%) 2251
Follistim AQ Cartridge 2844
Foradil Aerolizer (1.6%) 2849
Fortaz (Less than 1%) 1450
▲ Forteo for Injection (8%) 1816
Fosamax 2005
Fosamax Plus D Tablets 2013
▲ Frova Tablets (8%) 1111
Furosemide Tablets 2186
▲ Gabitril Tablets (27% to 31%) 973
▲ Gammagard Liquid (0.85% to 9.8%) 730
Gamunex (2%) 3094
Gantrisin Pediatric Suspension 2638
▲ Gardasil Injection (2.8% to 4%) 2019
▲ Gengraf Capsules (1% to 8%) 435
▲ Geodon (8% to 16%) 2520
▲ Gleevec Tablets (11% to 19.4%) 2255
▲ Gliadel Wafer (2% to 5%) 1076
Gris-PEG Tablets (Occasional) 2507
Havrix Injection Vaccine 1454
▲ Herceptin I.V. (13%) 1199
Hexalen Capsules 1078
Humulin 50/50, 100 Units 1843
Humulin 70/30 Vial 1844
Humulin N Vial 1846
Humulin R 1849
▲ Imitrex Injection (12%) 1465
Imitrex Nasal Spray (1% to 1.7%) 1470
Imitrex Tablets (Greater than 1%) 1474
Imodium A-D Liquid, Caplets, and EZ Chews 1898
▲ Increlex Injection (Greater than or equal to 5%) 3100
▲ Indapamide Tablets (Greater than or equal to 5%) 2188
▲ Indocin (3% to 9%) 2024
▲ InnoPran XL Extended Release Capsules (4% to 7%) 1484
Intravenous Sodium Diuril 2490
▲ Intron A for Injection (7% to 24%) 2859
Invanz for Injection (1.5% to 2.1%) 2029
▲ Invega Extended-Release Tablets (4% to 6%) 1748
▲ Ionsys Transdermal System (3%) 2410
Isentress Tablets (1% to less than 2%) 2036
▲ Ixempra Kit for Injection (7%) 915
Kaletra (Less than 2%) 452
▲ Keppra Injection (1.4% to 9%) 3137
▲ Keppra Oral Solution (5% to 9%) 3131
▲ Keppra Tablets (5% to 9%) 3131
▲ Ketek Tablets (2.8% to 3.7%) 2744
▲ Klonopin (1% to 8%) 2639
Kogenate FS 746
Kogenate FS with Bio-Set (2 cases) 748
K-Phos Original (Sodium Free) Tablets (Less frequent) 814
K-Phos Neutral Tablets 813
▲ Lamictal (7% to 54%) 1488
Lanoxin Injection 1498
Lanoxin Injection Pediatric 1502
Lanoxin Tablets 1505
Lescol Capsules (2.2%) 2268
Lescol XL Tablets (1.9%) 2268
▲ Leustatin Injection (9%) 2384
▲ Levaquin (3%) 2416
▲ Levaquin in 5% Dextrose Injection (3%) 2416
Levitra Tablets (2%) 2876
▲ Lexapro Oral Suspension (4% to 7%) 1174
▲ Lexapro Tablets (4% to 7%) 1174
▲ Lexiscan Injection (8%) 614
Lialda Tablets (Infrequent) 3029
Lidoderm Patch 1114
Lipitor Tablets (Greater than or equal to 2%) 2501
Lortab 5/500 Tablets (Among most frequent) 3143
Lortab 7.5/500 Tablets (Among most frequent) 3144
Lortab 10/500 Tablets (Among most frequent) 3144
Lovaza Capsules 1520
▲ Lunesta Tablets (1% to 7%) 2994
▲ Lupron Depot 3.75 mg (8%) 462
▲ Lupron Depot–3 Month 11.25 mg (8%) 462
▲ Luvox CR Extended-Release Capsules (3% to 15%) 1759
Lybrel Tablets 3204
▲ Lyrica Capsules (6% to 45%) 2527
▲ Malarone Pediatric Tablets (2% to 5%) 1521
▲ Malarone Tablets (2% to 5%) 1521
▲ Marinol Capsules (3% to 10%) 3163
▲ Marplan Tablets (15% to 29%) 3177
▲ Mavik Tablets (1.3% to 23%) 472
Maxair Autohaler (0.6% to 1.2%) 1705
▲ Maxalt Tablets (4% to 9%) 2056
▲ Maxalt-MLT Orally Disintegrating Tablets (4% to 9%) 2056
Mephyton Tablets (Rare) 700
▲ Mepron Suspension (3% to 8%) 1526
▲ Meridia Capsules (7%) 475
Merrem I.V. (Greater than 0.1% to 1%) 684
Meruvax II 2061
Metadate CD Capsules 3146
Mevacor Tablets (0.5% to 2%) 2063
▲ Miacalcin Nasal Spray (1% to 3%) 2274
Micardis Tablets (1%) 852
▲ Micardis HCT Tablets (4% to 7%) 854
▲ Mirapex Tablets (2% or more to 26%) 857
Mircette Tablets 1034
M-M-R II 2054
▲ Mobic Oral Suspension (0.4% to 3.8%) 863
▲ Mobic Tablets (0.4% to 3.8%) 863
▲ MoviPrep Oral Solution (6.5%) 2679
Moxatag Tablets 2165
MS Contin Tablets (Among most frequent) 2585
▲ Mycamine for Injection (12.9%) 616
▲ Myfortic Tablets (3% to less than 20%) 2276
▲ Mylotarg for Injection (10% to 15%) 3212
Nadolol Tablets (2 of 100 patients) 2191
▲ Nalfon Capsules (6.5%) 2508
▲ Namenda (7%) 1180
▲ Naprosyn Suspension (3% to 9%) 2632
▲ Naprosyn Tablets (3% to 9%) 2632
▲ Natrecor for Injection (3% to 6%) 2977
Nembutal Sodium Solution, USP (Less than 1%) 2494
▲ Neoral Oral Solution (1% to 8%) 2280
▲ Neoral Soft Gelatin Capsules (1% to 8%) 2280
▲ Neulasta Injection (15% to 72%) 587
▲ Neupro Transdermal System (5% to 22%) 3149
Nexium Delayed-Release Capsules (Less than 1%) 645
Nexium I.V. (Less than 1%) 652
Nexium Delayed-Release Oral Suspension (Less than 1%) 645
Niaspan Extended-Release Tablets 480
Nimotop Capsules (Less than 1%) 790
Nitrolingual Pumpspray (Occasional) 2965
Noroxin Tablets (1.7% to 2.6%) 2069
▲ Norvir (2.6% to 3.9%) 489
▲ Noxafil Oral Suspension (1% to 11%) 2889
NuvaRing 2897
Ofloxacin Ophthalmic Solution 0.3% (Rare) .... ⊙243
Omnicef Capsules (0.3%) 497
Omnicef for Oral Suspension (0.2%) 497
▲ Ontak Vials (22%) 1079
▲ Opana Tablets (6.5%) 1117
▲ Opana ER Tablets (0% to 17.8%) 1121
OptiPranolol Metipranolol Ophthalmic Solution 0.3% (A small number of patients) .... ⊙245
▲ Orencia Powder for Intravenous Infusion (9%) 921
Ortho-Cyclen Tablets 2449
Ortho Evra Transdermal System 2437
Ortho Micronor Tablets 2446
Ortho Tri-Cyclen Tablets 2449
Ortho Tri-Cyclen Lo Tablets 2458
Orthoclone OKT3 Sterile Solution 2387
OsmoPrep Tablets (Less frequent) 2680
▲ OxyContin Tablets (13%) 2589
OxyIR Capsules (Among most frequent) 2593
Parnate Tablets 1532
Patanase Nasal Spray 544
▲ Paxil (1% to 14%) 1535
▲ Paxil CR Controlled-Release Tablets (1% to 14%) 1544
▲ PegIntron Powder for Injection (12%) 2903
Pentasa Capsules (Less than 1%) 3030
Pepcid Tablets (1.3%) 2075
Percocet Tablets (Among most frequent) 1127
Percodan Tablets (Among most frequent) 1130
Perforomist Inhalation Solution (2.4%) 1025
▲ Persantine Tablets (13.6%) 869
Phenytek Capsules 2192
▲ Plan B Tablets (11.2%) 1044
▲ Plavix Tablets (6.2%) 926
▲ Plavix Tablets (6.2%) 2767
▲ Pletal Tablets (9% to 10%) 2481
Premarin Intravenous 3217
▲ Premarin Tablets (4% to 6%) 3221
Premarin Vaginal Cream 3228
▲ Premphase Tablets (3% to 5%) 3232
▲ Prempro Tablets (3% to 5%) 3232
Primaxin I.M. 2080
Primaxin I.V. (0.3%) 2083
▲ Prinivil Tablets (5.4% to 11.8%) 2087
▲ Prinzide Tablets (7.5%) 2092
▲ Pristiq Extended-Release Tablets (2% to 16%) 3247
▲ ProAir HFA Inhalation Aerosol (3%) 3113
ProAmatine Tablets (Rare) 3032
▲ Procrit for Injection (5% to 21%) 2391
Proglycem Capsules (Infrequent) 1185
Proglycem Suspension (Infrequent) 1185
▲ Prograf Capsules and Injection (3% to 19%) 622
Prolastin (0.19%) 3099
▲ Proleukin for Injection (11%) 2287
▲ Prometrium Capsules (100 mg, 200 mg) (15% to 24%) 3047
ProQuad 2099
Protonix for Delayed-Release Oral Suspension (Greater than or equal to 1%) 3254
Protonix Delayed-Release Tablets (Greater than or equal to 1%) 3254
Protonix I.V. (Greater than 1%) 3257
Protopic Ointment (Greater than or equal to 1%) 628
Proventil HFA Inhalation Aerosol (Less than 3%) 2914
▲ Provigil Tablets (5%) 977
▲ Prozac Weekly Capsules (9%) 1852
▲ Prozac Pulvules and Liquid (9%) 1852
Pylera Capsules 714
▲ Rebetol (7% to 26%) 2917
▲ Reclast Injection (2% to 9%) 2291
ReFacto Vials 3269

Relenza Inhalation Powder (1% to 2%)........ 1556
▲ Relistor Injection (7.3%)........ 3310
▲ Remeron Tablets (7%)........ 2924
▲ RemeronSolTab Tablets (7%)........ 2927
Remicade for IV Injection (Greater than or equal to 0.2%)........ 950
ReoPro Vials (2.9%)........ 1860
▲ Requip Tablets (11% to 40%)........ 1561
▲ Requip XL Tablets (Greater than or equal to 5%)........ 1568
▲ Retrovir Capsules (6% to 17.9%)........ 1574
▲ Retrovir IV Infusion (6% to 17.9%)........ 1579
▲ Retrovir (6% to 17.9%)........ 1574
Reyataz Capsules (Less than 1% to 2%)........ 3299
▲ Rilutek Tablets (5.1% to 12.7%)........ 2771
▲ Risperdal Consta Long-Acting Injection (11%)........ 1753
▲ Rituxan I.V. (1% to 10%)........ 1223
Rocephin Injectable Vials, ADD-Vantage, Galaxy, Bulk (Less than 1%)........ 2642
▲ Romazicon Injection (1% to 9%)........ 2646
▲ Rozerem Tablets (5%)........ 3091
▲ Rythmol Tablets (7% to 15%)........ 1586
▲ Rythmol SR Capsules (21% to 23%)........ 1590
St. Joseph 81 mg Aspirin Chewable and Enteric Coated Tablets........ 1903
▲ Salagen Tablets (5% to 12%)........ 1082
▲ Sandostatin Injection (5%)........ 2300
▲ Sandostatin LAR Depot (11.5% to 20%)........ 2302
Seasonique Tablets........ 1046
▲ Selzentry Tablets (8.2%)........ 2534
▲ Sensipar Tablets (10%)........ 594
▲ Serevent Diskus (4%)........ 1594
▲ Simulect for Injection (Greater than or equal to 10%)........ 2306
Singulair (1.9%)........ 2114
Skelaxin Tablets (Most frequent)........ 1784
▲ Solodyn Extended Release Tablets (9%)........ 1938
▲ Soma Tablets (7% to 8%)........ 1931
Soriatane Capsules (Less than 1%)........ 3062
▲ Stalevo Tablets (8%)........ 2309
▲ Starlix Tablets (3.6%)........ 2314
▲ Strattera Capsules (5% to 6%)........ 1864
Stromectol Tablets (2.8%)........ 2120
▲ Suboxone Tablets (4%)........ 2601
▲ Subutex Tablets (4%)........ 2601
▲ Sular Extended Release Tablets (5%)........ 2975
Suprax for Oral Suspension (Less than 2%)........ 1891
Suprax Tablets (Less than 2%)........ 1891
▲ Sustiva Capsules (2% to 10%)........ 930
▲ Sustiva Tablets (2% to 10%)........ 930
▲ Sutent Capsules (2% to 16%)........ 2540
Tamiflu Capsules (1% to 2%)........ 2649
Tamiflu Oral Suspension (1% to 2%)........ 2649
▲ Tarceva Tablets (0% to 15%)........ 1228
Targretin Capsules........ 1084
▲ Tarka Tablets (3.1%)........ 511
▲ Tasigna Capsules (1% to 10%)........ 2316
▲ Taxotere Injection Concentrate (4.5% to 15.8%)........ 2773
Tekturna Tablets (Greater than 1%)........ 2321
Tekturna HCT Tablets (Greater than 1% to 2.3%)........ 2324
▲ Temodar Capsules (1% to 12%)........ 2931
Tessalon Capsules........ 1183
Tessalon Perles........ 1183
Teveten Tablets (1% or greater)........ 515
▲ Teveten HCT Tablets (4.1%)........ 517
Thyrogen for Injection (2.5%)........ 1244
Tice BCG (2%)........ 2936
Timentin ADD-Vantage........ 1606
Timentin Injection Galaxy Container........ 1609
Timentin IV Infusion........ 1603
Timentin Pharmacy Bulk Package........ 1613
Timoptic Sterile Ophthalmic Solution (Less frequent)........ 2121
Timoptic in Ocudose (Less frequent)........ 2124
▲ Timoptic-XE Sterile Ophthalmic Gel Forming Solution (1% to 5%)........ 2125
▲ Toprol-XL Tablets (1.8% to about 10 of 100 patients)........ 666
▲ Transderm Scōp Transdermal Therapeutic System (12%)........ 2206
Trasylol Injection (1% to 2%)........ 799
▲ Treximet Tablets (4%)........ 1616
Tricor Tablets........ 520
▲ Trisenox Injection (23%)........ 986
▲ Trizivir Tablets (10%)........ 1622
Trusopt Sterile Ophthalmic Solution........ 2128
▲ Truvada Tablets (Greater than or equal to 10%)........ 1262
Tussionex Pennkinetic Extended-Release Suspension........ 3154
Twinrix Vaccine (Less than 1%)........ 1628
▲ Tygacil for Injection (3.5%)........ 3276
Tylenol with Codeine Tablets........ 2427
Tylenol Allergy Multi-Symptom Nighttime Caplets with Cool Burst........ 1916
Tylenol Cold Severe Congestion Daytime Caplets with Cool Burst........ 1912
Tylenol Sinus Congestion & Pain Daytime Caplets with Cool Burst and Gelcaps........ 1917
Tylenol Sinus Congestion & Pain Nighttime Caplets with Cool Burst........ 1917
Tylenol Sinus Congestion & Pain Severe Caplets with Cool Burst........ 1917
Tylenol Sinus Severe Congestion Caplets with Cool Burst........ 1917
▲ Tyzeka Tablets (4%)........ 2328
▲ Ultane Liquid for Inhalation (4%)........ 524
▲ Ultram ER Extended-Release Tablets (15.9% to 28.2%)........ 2428
Uroqid-Acid No. 2 Tablets........ 814
▲ Uroxatral Tablets (5.7%)........ 2786
Valcyte Tablets........ 2654
Valium Tablets........ 2658
▲ Valstar Sterile Solution for Intravesical Instillation (3%)........ 1735
▲ Valtrex Caplets (2% to 4%)........ 1635
Vantas (Less than 2%)........ 1737
Varivax........ 2133
▲ Velcade for Injection (14% to 17%)........ 2168
▲ Venlafaxine Hydrochloride Tablets (3% to 23.9%)........ 2199
Ventolin HFA Inhalation Aerosol (Less than 3%)........ 1638
▲ Vesanoid Capsules (20%)........ 2660
VESIcare Tablets (1.8% to 1.9%)........ 636
Viadur Implant (Less than 2%)........ 802
Vicks NyQuil LiquiCaps........ 2567
Vicks NyQuil Liquid........ 2567
Vicks NyQuil Multi-Symptom Cold/Flu Relief........ 2567
Vicodin Tablets........ 529
Vicodin ES Tablets (Among most frequent)........ 530
Vicodin HP Tablets (Among most frequent)........ 531
▲ Vicoprofen Tablets (14%)........ 533
▲ Viread Tablets (1% to 8%)........ 1268
Visudyne for Injection........ 2332
▲ Vivitrol (13% to 16%)........ 988
▲ Voltaren Ophthalmic Solution (Less than or equal to 3%)........ 2336
▲ Voltaren Tablets (1% to 10%)........ 2334
▲ Voltaren-XR Tablets (1% to 10%)........ 2337
Vytorin 10/10 Tablets........ 2149
Vytorin 10/10 Tablets........ 2939
Vytorin 10/20 Tablets........ 2149
Vytorin 10/20 Tablets........ 2939
Vytorin 10/40 Tablets........ 2149
Vytorin 10/40 Tablets........ 2939
Vytorin 10/80 Tablets........ 2149
Vytorin 10/80 Tablets........ 2939
▲ Vyvanse Capsules (5%)........ 3033
▲ Wellbutrin Tablets (22.3%)........ 1648
▲ Wellbutrin SR Sustained-Release Tablets (5% to 11%)........ 1653
▲ Wellbutrin XL Extended-Release Tablets (6% to 11%)........ 1659
WinRho SDF........ 741
▲ Xeloda Tablets (1% to 12%)........ 2662
▲ Xenical Capsules (5.2%)........ 2672
Xifaxan Tablets (Less than 2%)........ 2682
▲ Xolair (3%)........ 1235
▲ Xolair (3%)........ 2339
Xopenex Inhalation Solution (1.4% to 2.7%)........ 3001
Xopenex Inhalation Solution Concentrate (1.4% to 2.7%)........ 3005
Xopenex HFA Inhalation Aerosol (1.4% to 2.7%)........ 3009
▲ Xyrem Oral Solution (2% to 37.1%)........ 1766
Yaz Tablets (Greater than 1%)........ 805
Zantac 25 EFFERdose Tablets (Rare)........ 1670
Zantac Injection (Rare)........ 1666
Zantac Injection Pharmacy Bulk Package (Rare)........ 1668
Zantac Injection Premixed (Rare)........ 1666
Zantac (Rare)........ 1670
Zetia Tablets........ 2157
Zetia Tablets (0.2%)........ 2951
▲ Ziagen (6%)........ 1673
Zocor Tablets........ 2136
▲ Zofran Injection (12%)........ 1682
▲ Zofran (4% to 7%)........ 1687
▲ Zofran ODT Orally Disintegrating Tablets (4% to 7%)........ 1687
▲ Zolinza Capsules (13% to 15.1%)........ 2142
▲ Zometa for Intravenous Infusion (18%)........ 2341
Zomig Tablets (Common)........ 694
▲ Zomig Nasal Spray (2% to 6%)........ 689
Zomig-ZMT Tablets (Common)........ 694
▲ Zonegran Capsules (13%)........ 1089
Zosyn for Injection (1.4%)........ 3284
Zovirax........ 1690
▲ Zyban Sustained-Release Tablets (8% to 10%)........ 1692
Zydone Tablets (Among most frequent)........ 1132
▲ Zyprexa Tablets (11% to 18%)........ 1883
▲ Zyprexa IntraMuscular (4%)........ 1883
▲ Zyprexa ZYDIS Orally Disintegrating Tablets (11% to 18%)........ 1883
Zyrtec Chewable Tablets (2%)........ 1920
Zyrtec Syrup (2%)........ 1920
Zyrtec Tablets (2%)........ 1920
Zyrtec-D 12 Hour Extended Release Tablets (1.1% to 2%)........ 1923
Zyrtec-D Allergy & Congestion Extended-Release Tablets........ 1923
Zyvox (2%)........ 2552

Dizziness, aggravated

Ultram ER Extended-Release Tablets (0.5% to less than 1%)........ 2428

Dizziness, postural

Abilify Injection (0.5% to 0.6%)........ 881
Abilify Injection (0.5% to 0.6%)........ 2466
Abilify Oral Solution (0.2% to 0.5%)........ 881
Abilify Oral Solution (0.5% to 0.6%)........ 2466
Abilify Discmelt Orally Disintegrating Tablets (0.2% to 0.5%)........ 881
Abilify Discmelt Orally Disintegrating Tablets (0.5% to 0.6%)........ 2466
Abilify Tablets (0.2% to 0.5%)........ 881
Abilify Tablets (0.5% to 0.6%)........ 2466
Avalide Tablets (1%)........ 892
Avalide Tablets (1%)........ 2713
Cimzia........ 3127
Diovan HCT Tablets (Greater than 0.2%)........ 2216
Exforge Tablets (Less than 1%)........ 2238
Mirapex Tablets........ 857
▲ Neupro Transdermal System (22%)........ 3149
Requip Tablets (Infrequent)........ 1561
▲ Selzentry Tablets (8.2%)........ 2534
Xyrem Oral Solution (Infrequent)........ 1766

Dorsocervical fat enlargement

Aptivus Capsules........ 823
Aptivus Oral Solution........ 823
Combivir Tablets........ 1384
Crixivan Capsules........ 1979
Emtriva Capsules........ 1246
Emtriva Oral Solution........ 1246
Epivir........ 1412
Intelence Tablets........ 3119
Lexiva Oral Suspension........ 1510
Lexiva Tablets........ 1510
Norvir........ 489
Retrovir........ 1574
Reyataz Capsules........ 3299
Sustiva Capsules........ 930
Sustiva Tablets........ 930
Trizivir Tablets........ 1622
Truvada Tablets........ 1262
Viramune Oral Suspension........ 873
Viramune Tablets........ 873
Viread Tablets........ 1268
Ziagen........ 1673

Drainage

Panretin Gel 0.1%........ 1081

Dreaming

Amerge Tablets (Rare)........ 1301
▲ Malarone Pediatric Tablets (2% to 7%)........ 1521
▲ Malarone Tablets (2% to 7%)........ 1521
MS Contin Tablets (Less frequent)........ 2585

Dreaming, vivid

Chantix Tablets........ 2511
InnoPran XL Extended Release Capsules........ 1484

Dreaming abnormalities

Actiq (Less than 1%)........ 959
Ambien Tablets (1%)........ 2692
Anaprox Tablets (Less than 1%)........ 2632
Anaprox DS Tablets (Less than 1%)........ 2632
Anzemet Injection (Infrequently)........ 2701
Anzemet Tablets (Rare)........ 2704
Aricept Tablets (Infrequent)........ 1062
Aricept ODT Tablets (Infrequent)........ 1062
Atripla Tablets (Greater than or equal to 2%)........ 938
Avelox (Less than 0.1%)........ 2803
▲ Avinza Capsules (Less than 5%)........ 1772
Axert Tablets (Rare)........ 2431
Axid Capsules (1.9%)........ 1364
▲ Azilect Tablets (4%)........ 3106
Campral Tablets (Infrequent)........ 1158
Cardizem LA Extended Release Tablets (Less than 2%)........ 421
Catapres Tablets........ 841
Catapres-TTS (0.5% or less)........ 842
▲ Chantix Tablets (0.3% to 13%)........ 2511
Cipro XR Tablets (Less than 1%)........ 2823
Clorpres Tablets........ 2185
Copaxone for Injection (Frequent)........ 3110
Cozaar Tablets (Less than 1%)........ 1973
▲ Cymbalta Delayed-Release Capsules (Frequent to 3%)........ 1801
▲ Depakote ER Tablets (Greater than 1% to less than 5%)........ 423
Duragesic Transdermal System (1% or greater)........ 2405
EC-Naprosyn Delayed-Release Tablets (Less than 1%)........ 2632
▲ Effexor XR Extended-Release Capsules (3% to 7%)........ 3195
▲ Eldepryl Capsules (2 of 49 patients)........ 3052
▲ Emtriva Capsules (Greater than or equal to 10%)........ 1246
▲ Emtriva Oral Solution (Greater than or equal to 10%)........ 1246
▲ Epzicom Tablets (4% to 5%)........ 1422
Evoxac Capsules (Less than 1%)........ 1013
Exelon Capsules (Infrequent)........ 2229
Exelon Oral Solution (Infrequent)........ 2229
Exforge Tablets (Greater than 0.1% to less than 1%)........ 2238
Frova Tablets (Rare)........ 1111
Gabitril Tablets (Infrequent)........ 973
Intelence Tablets (Less than 2%)........ 3119
▲ Intron A for Injection (Less than 5%)........ 2859
Ionsys Transdermal System (.1% to less than 1%)........ 2410
Kaletra (Less than 2%)........ 452
Klonopin (Infrequent)........ 2639
Lamictal (Infrequent)........ 1488
Levaquin (0.1% to 1%)........ 2416
Levaquin in 5% Dextrose Injection (0.1% to 1%)........ 2416
▲ Lexapro Oral Suspension (3%)........ 1174
▲ Lexapro Tablets (3%)........ 1174
Lipitor Tablets (Less than 2%)........ 2501
▲ Lunesta Tablets (1% to 3%)........ 2994
▲ Luvox CR Extended-Release Capsules (3%)........ 1759
Lyrica Capsules (0.1% to 1%)........ 2527
Maxalt Tablets (Infrequent)........ 2056
Maxalt-MLT Orally Disintegrating Tablets (Infrequent)........ 2056
Meridia Capsules........ 475
▲ Mirapex Tablets (11%)........ 857
Mobic Oral Suspension (Less than 2%)........ 863
Mobic Tablets (Less than 2%)........ 863
Naprosyn Suspension (Less than 1%)........ 2632
Naprosyn Tablets (Less than 1%)........ 2632
▲ Neupro Transdermal System (2% to 7%)........ 3149
Norvir (Less than 2%)........ 489
▲ OxyContin Tablets (Between 1% and 5%)........ 2589
▲ Paxil (3% to 4%)........ 1535
▲ Paxil CR Controlled-Release Tablets (3% to 4%)........ 1544
Pristiq Extended-Release Tablets (Greater than or equal to 2%)........ 3247
▲ Prograf Capsules and Injection (3% to 15%)........ 622
ProQuad........ 2099
Protonix for Delayed-Release Oral Suspension (Less than 1%)........ 3254
Protonix Delayed-Release Tablets (Less than 1%)........ 3254
Protonix I.V. (Less than 1%)........ 3257
▲ Prozac Weekly Capsules (1% to 5%)........ 1852
▲ Prozac Pulvules and Liquid (1% to 5%)........ 1852
▲ Remeron Tablets (4%)........ 2924
▲ RemeronSolTab Tablets (4%)........ 2927
▲ Requip Tablets (Infrequent to 11%)........ 1561
Rilutek Tablets (Rare)........ 2771
Rythmol Tablets (Less than 1%)........ 1586
Salagen Tablets (Less than 1%)........ 1082
Singulair (Very rare)........ 2114
Stalevo Tablets........ 2309
Sular Extended Release Tablets (Less than or equal to 1%)........ 2975
▲ Sustiva Capsules (1% to 4%)........ 930
▲ Sustiva Tablets (1% to 4%)........ 930
Thioridazine Hydrochloride Tablets........ 2195

▲ Truvada Tablets (Greater than or equal to 10%) **1262**
Ultram ER Extended-Release Tablets (0.5% to less than 1%) **2428**
▲ Venlafaxine Hydrochloride Tablets (4%) **2199**
Vicoprofen Tablets (Less than 1%) **533**
Vivitrol **988**
Voltaren Tablets (Occasionally) **2334**
Voltaren-XR Tablets (Occasionally) **2337**
Wellbutrin Tablets **1648**
Wellbutrin SR Sustained-Release Tablets (At least 1%) **1653**
▲ Wellbutrin XL Extended-Release Tablets (At least 1% to 3%) **1659**
Xifaxan Tablets (Less than 2%) **2682**
Xyrem Oral Solution (Frequent) **1766**
Zomig Tablets (Rare) **694**
Zomig Nasal Spray (Rare) **689**
Zomig-ZMT Tablets (Rare) **694**
Zonegran Capsules (Infrequent) **1089**
▲ Zyban Sustained-Release Tablets (5%) **1692**
Zyprexa Tablets **1883**
Zyprexa ZYDIS Orally Disintegrating Tablets **1883**

Drooling

Aricept Tablets **1062**
Aricept ODT Tablets **1062**
Dantrium Capsules (Less frequent) **2580**
▲ Demser Capsules (10%) **1989**
Invega Extended-Release Tablets **1748**
Thioridazine Hydrochloride Tablets **2195**

Drowsiness

▲ Abilify Injection (5% to 23%) **881**
▲ Abilify Injection (5% to 23%) **2466**
▲ Abilify Oral Solution (5% to 23%) **881**
▲ Abilify Oral Solution (5% to 23%) **2466**
▲ Abilify Discmelt Orally Disintegrating Tablets (5% to 23%) **881**
▲ Abilify Discmelt Orally Disintegrating Tablets (5% to 23%) **2466**
▲ Abilify Tablets (5% to 23%) **881**
▲ Abilify Tablets (5% to 23%) **2466**
Accutane Capsules **2607**
Aceon Tablets (2 mg, 4 mg, 8 mg) (1.3%) **3038**
Actifed Cold & Allergy Tablets **1895**
▲ Actiq (9% to 20%) **959**
▲ Adderall XR Capsules (2% to 4%) **3012**
Adenoscan (Less than 1%) **605**
Aggrenox Capsules (1.2%) **819**
▲ Agrylin Capsules (1% to less than 5%) **3017**
▲ Alferon N Injection (3% to 10%) **1726**
Alinia for Oral Suspension (Less than 1%) **2677**
Alinia Tablets (Less than 1%) **2677**
Allegra Oral Solution (0.7% to 2.8%) **2684**
Allegra Tablets (0.9% to 2.8%) **2684**
Allegra-D 12 Hour Extended-Release Tablets **2687**
Allegra-D 24 Hour Extended-Release Tablets **2690**
Aloxi Injection (Less than 1%) **1059**
▲ Alphagan P Ophthalmic Solution (1% to 4%) **549**
Alphanate **1709**
▲ Ambien Tablets (Infrequent to 8%) **2692**
▲ Ambien CR Tablets (6% to 15%) **2696**
AmBisome for Injection (Less common) **606**
Amerge Tablets (1% to 2%) **1301**
Amrix Capsules **966**
▲ Anaprox Tablets (1% to 9%) **2632**
▲ Anaprox DS Tablets (1% to 9%) **2632**
Anzemet Injection (2.4%) **2701**
Aptivus Capsules (Less than 2%) **823**
Aptivus Oral Solution (Less than 2%) **823**
Aralast (Greater than or equal to 0.2% to 0.3%) **726**
Aricept Tablets (2%) **1062**
Aricept ODT Tablets (2%) **1062**
▲ Arimidex Tablets (2% to 5%) **672**
▲ Arranon Injection (0% to 23%) **1319**
Asacol Delayed-Release Tablets **2579**
Atacand Tablets (0.5% or greater) **639**
Atacand HCT **642**
Atripla Tablets (Greater than or equal to 2%) **938**
Avalide Tablets **892**
Avalide Tablets **2713**
Avapro Tablets (Less than 1%) **897**
Avapro Tablets (Less than 1%) **2718**
Avelox (Greater than or equal to 0.1% to less than 2%) **2803**
▲ Avinza Capsules (Greater than 10%) **1772**
Axert Tablets (Frequent) **2431**
Axid Capsules (1.9%) **1364**
▲ Azilect Tablets (6%) **3106**
Azor Tablets (0.3% to 1.6%) **1005**
Baraclude (Less than 1%) **900**
Benadryl Allergy & Cold Kapgels **1895**
Benadryl Allergy & Sinus Headache Kapgels **1895**
Benadryl Severe Allergy & Sinus Headache Caplets **1897**
Benadryl Dye-Free Allergy Liqui-gels Softgels **1897**
Benadryl Allergy Kapgels **1895**
Benadryl Allergy Quick Dissolve Strips **1896**
Benadryl Allergy Ultratab Tablets **1896**
Children's Benadryl Dye-Free Allergy Liquid **1897**
Children's Benadryl Allergy Fastmelts **1897**
Children's Benadryl Allergy Liquid **1898**
Children's Benadryl Allergy Perfect Measure **1896**
Children's Benadryl-D Allergy & Sinus Liquid **1896**
Benadryl-D Allergy & Sinus Tablet **1896**
BeneFIX Vials (1.5%) **3191**
▲ Bentyl Capsules (9%) **703**
▲ Bentyl Injection (9%) **703**
▲ Bentyl Syrup (9%) **703**
▲ Bentyl Tablets (9%) **703**
▲ Bexxar (0% to 5%) **1371**
Bicillin C-R Injectable Suspension **1775**
Bicillin L-A Injection **1777**
▲ BOTOX Purified Neurotoxin Complex (2% to 10%) **550**
Brovana Inhalation Solution (Less than 2%) **2990**
Byetta Injection **600**
Bystolic Tablets **1155**
Calcijex Injection **419**
Campral Tablets (Frequent) **1158**
Cancidas for Injection **1953**
Captopril Tablets **2182**
Carafate Suspension (Less than 0.5%) **706**
Carafate Tablets (Less than 0.5%) **707**
Carbatrol Capsules (Among most frequent) **3019**
Cardizem LA Extended Release Tablets (Less than 2%) **421**
▲ Catapres Tablets (About 33 in 100 patients) **841**
▲ Catapres-TTS (12 of 101 patients) **842**
Ceftin Tablets (0.1% to 1%) **1380**
Celebrex Capsules (0.1% to 1.9%) **2979**
▲ Celexa (18%) **1160**
▲ CellCept Capsules (3% to less than 20%) **2622**
▲ CellCept Intravenous (3% to less than 20%) **2622**
▲ CellCept Oral Suspension (3% to less than 20%) **2622**
▲ CellCept Tablets (3% to less than 20%) **2622**
▲ Chantix Tablets (3%) **2511**
▲ Chemet Capsules (1% to 12.7%) **2484**
Cialis Tablets (Less than 2%) **1792**
Cipro I.V. (1% or less) **2817**
Cipro (Less than 1%) **2810**
Cipro XR Tablets (Less than 1%) **2823**
▲ Clarinex Syrup (9.1%) **2828**
Clarinex Tablets (2.1%) **2828**
Clarinex Reditabs Tablets (2.1%) **2828**
▲ Clarinex-D 12-Hour Extended-Release Tablets (3%) **2831**
▲ Clarinex-D 24-Hour Extended-Release Tablets (3%) **2834**
Clinoril Tablets (Less than 1%) **1962**
▲ Clolar for Intravenous Infusion (10%) **1239**
▲ Clorpres Tablets (About 33%) **2185**
▲ Combigan Ophthalmic Solution (1% to 5%) **553**
Combivent Inhalation Aerosol **845**
Comtan Tablets (2%) **2208**
▲ Comvax (21.1% to 49.5%) **1966**
Concerta Extended-Release Tablets **1925**
Copaxone for Injection (At least 2%) **3110**
▲ Coreg Tablets (Greater than 1% to 3%) **1387**
▲ Coreg CR Extended-Release Capsules (Greater than 1% to less than or equal to 3%) **1393**
Cozaar Tablets (Less than 1%) **1973**
▲ Crinone 8% Gel (27%) **992**
Crixivan Capsules (2.4%) **1979**
▲ Cymbalta Delayed-Release Capsules (7% to 21%) **1801**
Dantrium Capsules (Among most frequent) **2580**
Daytrana Transdermal Patch **3022**
Demadex Injection **2630**
Demadex Tablets **2630**
▲ Depakote ER Tablets (7% to 30%) **423**
▲ DepoCyt Injection (4% to 12%) **1136**
▲ DepoDur Injection (2% to 5%) **1095**
Dibenzyline Capsules **3188**
Diovan Tablets (Greater than 0.2%) **2212**
Diovan HCT Tablets **2216**
Donnatal Extentabs **2507**
▲ Doxil Injection (1% to 10%) **2378**
Dramamine Chewable Tablets **1898**
Dramamine Less Drowsy Tablets **1898**
Dramamine Original Tablets **1898**
▲ Duragesic Transdermal System (10% or more) **2405**
Dyazide Capsules **1405**
DynaCirc CR Controlled Release Tablets (0.5% to 1%) **1407**
▲ EC-Naprosyn Delayed-Release Tablets (1% to 9%) **2632**
▲ Effexor XR Extended-Release Capsules (2% to 20%) **3195**
Eldepryl Capsules **3052**
▲ Eloxatin for Injection (2% to less than 5%) **2731**
Elspar for Injection **1990**
Emsam Transdermal System **905**
Engerix-B Vaccine (Less than 1%) **1409**
▲ Equetro Extended-Release Capsules (12% to 32%) **3174**
Evoxac Capsules (Less than 1%) **1013**
▲ Exelon Capsules (4% to 5%) **2229**
▲ Exelon Oral Solution (4% to 5%) **2229**
Exforge Tablets (Greater than or equal to 0.2%) **2238**
▲ Fabrazyme for Intravenous Infusion (Greater than or equal to 5%) **1241**
▲ Femara Tablets (2% to 4%) **2246**
▲ Fentora Tablets (0% to 15%) **968**
Flector Patch (1%) **561**
▲ Flolan for Injection (4%) **1426**
▲ Flomax Capsules (3% to 4.3%) **848**
Flulaval Injection Vaccine **1448**
Flumadine (0.3% to 1%) **1167**
Focalin XR Capsules **2251**
Frova Tablets (Greater than or equal to 2%) **1111**
Furosemide Tablets **2186**
▲ Gabitril Tablets (18%) **973**
Gantrisin Pediatric Suspension **2638**
▲ Gemzar for Injection (5% to 11%) **1820**
Gengraf Capsules (1% to less than 3%) **435**
▲ Geodon (14% to 31%) **2520**
Gleevec Tablets (Infrequent) **2255**
▲ Gliadel Wafer (11% to 14%) **1076**
▲ Havrix Injection Vaccine (13% to 34%) **1454**
Humulin 50/50, 100 Units **1843**
Humulin 70/30 Vial **1844**
Humulin N Vial **1846**
Humulin R **1849**
▲ Imitrex Injection (3%) **1465**
Imitrex Nasal Spray (Infrequent) **1470**
Imitrex Tablets (Greater than 1%) **1474**
Imodium A-D Liquid, Caplets, and EZ Chews **1898**
▲ Indapamide Tablets (Less than 5%) **2188**
Indocin (Less than 1%) **2024**
▲ Infanrix Vaccine (6.6% to 54%) **1479**
Intelence Tablets (Less than 2%) **3119**
Intravenous Sodium Diuril **2490**
▲ Intron A for Injection (Up to 14%) **2859**
▲ Invanz for Injection (Greater than 0.5% to 5.1%) **2029**
▲ Invega Extended-Release Tablets (Greater than 2% to 11%) **1748**
▲ Ionsys Transdermal System (1% to less than 10%) **2410**
Janumet Tablets **2041**
Kaletra (Less than 2%) **452**
▲ Keppra Injection (1.7% to 45%) **3137**
▲ Keppra Oral Solution (5% to 45%) **3131**
▲ Keppra Tablets (5% to 45%) **3131**
Ketek Tablets (Greater than or equal to 0.2% to less than 2%) **2744**
▲ Kinrix Injection Vaccine (19.1%) **1486**
▲ Klonopin (7% to 50%) **2639**
▲ Lamictal (9% to 17%) **1488**
Levaquin (0.1% to 1%) **2416**
Levaquin in 5% Dextrose Injection (0.1% to 1%) **2416**
Levitra Tablets (Less than 2%) **2876**
▲ Lexapro Oral Suspension (4% to 13%) **1174**
▲ Lexapro Tablets (4% to 13%) **1174**
Lidoderm Patch **1114**
Lipitor Tablets (Less than 2%) **2501**
Lortab 5/500 Tablets **3143**
Lortab 7.5/500 Tablets **3144**
Lortab 10/500 Tablets **3144**
▲ Lunesta Tablets (8% to 10%) **2994**
Lupron Depot-PED 7.5 mg, 11.25 mg and 15 mg (Less than 2%) **471**
▲ Luvox CR Extended-Release Capsules (4% to 27%) **1759**
▲ Lyrica Capsules (3% to 28%) **2527**
▲ Marinol Capsules (3% to 10%) **3163**
▲ Marplan Tablets (0% to 4%) **3177**
Mavik Tablets (0.3% to 1%) **472**
▲ Maxalt Tablets (4% to 8%) **2056**
▲ Maxalt-MLT Orally Disintegrating Tablets (4% to 8%) **2056**
Meridia Capsules (1.7%) **475**
Merrem I.V. (Greater than 0.1% to 1%) **684**
Metadate CD Capsules **3146**
Micardis Tablets (More than 0.3%) **852**
Micardis HCT Tablets **854**
▲ Mirapex Tablets (6% to 22%) **857**
Moban Tablets (Most frequent) **1116**
Mobic Oral Suspension (Less than 2%) **863**
Mobic Tablets (Less than 2%) **863**
▲ Nalfon Capsules (8.5%) **2508**
▲ Namenda (3%) **1180**
▲ Naprosyn Suspension (1% to 9%) **2632**
▲ Naprosyn Tablets (1% to 9%) **2632**
Natrecor for Injection (Greater than or equal to 1%) **2977**
▲ Nembutal Sodium Solution, USP (1% to 3%) **2494**
Neoral Oral Solution (1% to less than 3%) **2280**
Neoral Soft Gelatin Capsules (1% to less than 3%) **2280**
▲ Neupro Transdermal System (3% to 25%) **3149**
Nexium Delayed-Release Capsules (Less than 1% to 1.9%) **645**
Nexium I.V. (Less than 1%) **652**
Nexium Delayed-Release Oral Suspension (Less than 1% to 1.9%) **645**
Noroxin Tablets (0.3% to 1%) **2069**
Norvir (2.4% to 2.6%) **489**
Noxafil Oral Suspension (1%) **2889**
Omnicef Capsules (0.2%) **497**
Omnicef for Oral Suspension (0.2%) **497**
▲ Opana Tablets (9.3%) **1117**
▲ Opana ER Tablets (1.9% to 17.2%) **1121**
OptiPranolol Metipranolol Ophthalmic Solution 0.3% (A small number of patients) .... ⊙ **245**
▲ OxyContin Tablets (23%) **2589**
Parnate Tablets **1532**
Patanase Nasal Spray (0.9%) **544**
▲ Paxil (1.9% to 24%) **1535**
▲ Paxil CR Controlled-Release Tablets (1.9% to 24%) **1544**
PediaCare Children's Allergy & Cold Liquid **1902**
PediaCare Children's Allergy Liquid **1902**
Pediarix Vaccine **1552**
Liquid PedvaxHIB (Among most frequent) **2073**
Pentacel **2792**
Pentasa Capsules (Less than 1%) **3030**
Pepcid Tablets (Infrequent) **2075**
Percocet Tablets (Among most frequent) **1127**
Percodan Tablets **1130**
Premphase Tablets **3232**
Prempro Tablets **3232**
▲ Prevnar (11% to 40.7%) **3241**
Primaxin I.M. **2080**
Primaxin I.V. (0.2%) **2083**
Prinivil Tablets (0.3% to 1%) **2087**
Prinzide Tablets (0.3% to 1%) **2092**
▲ Pristiq Extended-Release Tablets (4% to 12%) **3247**
ProAmatine Tablets (Rare) **3032**
Profilnine SD Solvent Detergent **1721**
▲ Prograf Capsules and Injection (3% to 15%) **622**
▲ Proleukin for Injection (Less than 1% to 22%) **2287**
▲ Prometrium Capsules (100 mg, 200 mg) (Less than 5%) **3047**
ProQuad (Greater than or equal to 0.2% to less than 1%) **2099**
Protonix for Delayed-Release Oral Suspension (Less than 1%) **3254**
Protonix Delayed-Release Tablets (Less than 1%) **3254**
Protonix I.V. (Less than 1%) **3257**
Proventil HFA Inhalation Aerosol (Less than 3%) **2914**
Provigil Tablets (2%) **977**
▲ Prozac Weekly Capsules (5% to 17%) **1852**

▲ Prozac Pulvules and Liquid (5% to 17%) 1852
▲ Rebif Prefilled Syringe for Injection (4% to 5%) 1107
Recombivax HB 2107
ReFacto Vials 3269
▲ Remeron Tablets (10.4% to 54%) 2924
▲ RemeronSolTab Tablets (10.4% to 54%) 2927
▲ Requip Tablets (12% to 40%) 1561
▲ Requip XL Tablets (Greater than or equal to 5%) 1568
▲ Retrovir Capsules (8%) 1574
▲ Retrovir IV Infusion (8%) 1579
▲ Retrovir (8%) 1574
▲ Rilutek Tablets (0.8% to 4.1%) 2771
▲ Risperdal Consta Long-Acting Injection (5% to 6%) 1753
Rocaltrol Capsules 1150
Rocaltrol Oral Solution 1150
Romazicon Injection (Less than 1%) 2646
▲ Rozerem Tablets (5%) 3091
Rythmol Tablets (1%) 1586
▲ Rythmol SR Capsules (1% to 3%) 1590
Salagen Tablets (1% to 2%) 1082
Sanctura XR Capsules (Less than 1%) 557
Seromycin Capsules 1864
Singulair 2114
Skelaxin Tablets (Most frequent) 1784
Sleep-Tite Caplets ■ 640
Solodyn Extended Release Tablets (2%) 1938
▲ Soma Tablets (13% to 17%) 1931
▲ Soriatane Capsules (1% to 10%) 3062
Stalevo Tablets (2%) 2309
▲ Strattera Capsules (0.3% to 11%) 1864
Stromectol Tablets (0.9%) 2120
▲ Suboxone Tablets (5%) 2601
▲ Subutex Tablets (5%) 2601
Sudafed PE Nighttime Cold Caplets 1907
Sudafed PE Severe Cold Caplets 1908
Sudafed PE Sinus & Allergy Tablets 1908
Sular Extended Release Tablets (Less than or equal to 1%) 2975
▲ Sustiva Capsules (2% to 3%) 930
▲ Sustiva Tablets (2% to 3%) 930
▲ Symbyax Capsules (Up to 22%) 1871
Tarka Tablets (0.3% or more) 511
▲ Temodar Capsules (3% to 9%) 2931
Teveten Tablets (Less than 1%) 515
Teveten HCT Tablets (Less than 1%) 517
Thioridazine Hydrochloride Tablets (Occasional) 2195
Thiothixene Capsules 2197
Timoptic Sterile Ophthalmic Solution (Less frequent) 2121
Timoptic in Ocudose (Less frequent) 2124
Timoptic-XE Sterile Ophthalmic Gel Forming Solution 2125
Toprol-XL Tablets 666
Transderm Scōp Transdermal Therapeutic System (Less than one-sixth) 2206
Treanda for Injection 983
▲ Treximet Tablets (3%) 1616
Tricor Tablets 520
▲ Trisenox Injection (8%) 986
Tussionex Pennkinetic Extended-Release Suspension 3154
Twinrix Vaccine (Less than 1%) 1628
Tygacil for Injection (0.2% to less than 2%) 3276
Extra Strength Tylenol PM Caplets, Geltabs, Liquid, and Rapid Release Gels 1915
Tylenol with Codeine Tablets 2427
Tylenol Allergy Multi-Symptom Caplets with Cool Burst and Rapid Release Gelcaps 1916
Tylenol Allergy Multi-Symptom Nighttime Caplets with Cool Burst 1916
Tylenol Severe Allergy Caplets 1916
Children's Tylenol Plus Cold Suspension Liquid 1912
Children's Tylenol Plus Cold & Allergy Suspension Liquid 1914
Children's Tylenol Plus Cough & Runny Nose Suspension Liquid 1912
Children's Tylenol Plus Flu Suspension Liquid 1914
Children's Tylenol Plus Multi-Symptom Cold Suspension Liquid 1912
Tylenol Cold Head Congestion Nighttime Caplets with Cool Burst 1910
Tylenol Cold Multi-Symptom Nighttime Caplets with Cool Burst 1913
Tylenol Cold Multi-Symptom Nighttime Liquid with Cool Burst 1913
Tylenol Cough & Sore Throat Nighttime Liquid with Cool Burst 1918
Tylenol Sinus Congestion & Pain Nighttime Caplets with Cool Burst 1917
Tylenol Sore Throat Nighttime Liquid with Cool Burst 1918
▲ Ultane Liquid for Inhalation (9%) 524
▲ Ultram ER Extended-Release Tablets (7.3% to 20.3%) 2428
Valium Tablets (Among most common) 2658
▲ Venlafaxine Hydrochloride Tablets (3% to 26.1%) 2199
▲ Vesanoid Capsules (3%) 2660
Vicks NyQuil Cold & Flu Multi-Symptom Relief ■ 617
Vicks NyQuil LiquiCaps 2567
Vicks NyQuil Liquid 2567
Vicks NyQuil Multi-Symptom Cold/Flu Relief 2567
Vicodin Tablets 529
Vicodin ES Tablets 530
Vicodin HP Tablets 531
▲ Vicoprofen Tablets (22%) 533
Viramune Oral Suspension 873
Viramune Tablets 873
▲ Vivitrol (4% to 12%) 988
Voltaren Tablets (Occasionally) 2334
Voltaren-XR Tablets (Occasionally) 2337
Vyvanse Capsules (2%) 3033
▲ Wellbutrin SR Sustained-Release Tablets (2% to 3%) 1653
▲ Wellbutrin XL Extended-Release Tablets (2% to 3%) 1659
WinRho SDF 741
▲ Xyrem Oral Solution (Less than 1% to 14.3%) 1766
▲ Xyzal Oral Solution (3% to 6%) 2789
▲ Xyzal Oral Solution (3% to 6%) 3155
▲ Xyzal Tablets (Less than 1% to 6%) 2789
▲ Xyzal Tablets (Less than 1% to 6%) 3155
Zantac 25 EFFERdose Tablets (Rare) 1670
Zantac Injection 1666
Zantac Injection Pharmacy Bulk Package (Rare) 1668
Zantac Injection Premixed 1666
Zantac (Rare) 1670
Zemplar Injection 538
▲ Zofran Injection (5% to 8%) 1682
▲ Zofran (20%) 1687
▲ Zofran ODT Orally Disintegrating Tablets (20%) 1687
▲ Zometa for Intravenous Infusion (5% to less than 10%) 2341
▲ Zomig Tablets (Common) 694
▲ Zomig Nasal Spray (0% to 4%) 689
Zomig-ZMT Tablets (Common) 694
▲ Zonegran Capsules (17%) 1089
Zovirax 1690
Zyban Sustained-Release Tablets (2%) 1692
Zydone Tablets 1132
▲ Zyprexa Tablets (6% to 52%) 1883
▲ Zyprexa IntraMuscular (6%) 1883
▲ Zyprexa ZYDIS Orally Disintegrating Tablets (6% to 52%) 1883
Zyrtec Allergy Tablets 1919
▲ Zyrtec Chewable Tablets (1.9% to 13.7%) 1920
Children's Zyrtec Allergy Syrup 1920
Children's Zyrtec Allergy Chewable Tablets 1922
Children's Zyrtec Hives Relief Syrup 1920
▲ Zyrtec Syrup (1.9% to 13.7%) 1920
▲ Zyrtec Tablets (1.9% to 13.7%) 1920
▲ Zyrtec-D 12 Hour Extended Release Tablets (1.9% to 14%) 1923
Zyrtec-D Allergy & Congestion Extended-Release Tablets 1923

Drug abuse

DepoDur Injection 1095
Percocet Tablets 1127
Prozac Weekly Capsules 1852
Soma Tablets 1931
Tylenol with Codeine Tablets 2427
Vicodin Tablets 529
Vicodin ES Tablets 530
Vicodin HP Tablets 531
Vicoprofen Tablets 533

Drug administration site reactions, unspecified

Abelcet Injection 1134
▲ Cancidas for Injection (44.8% to 58.9%) 1953
Denavir Cream (1.3%) 2205
Doxil Injection 2378
Duragesic Transdermal System (1% or greater) 2405
Engerix-B Vaccine 1409
▲ Epogen for Injection (7% to 25%) 576
Fortaz (Among most common) 1450
▲ Imitrex Injection (58.7%) 1465
▲ Intron A for Injection (Less than 5%) 2859
Leukine 774
▲ Leustatin Injection (9% to 19%) 2384
Lupron Depot 3.75 mg (1%) 462
Lupron Depot–3 Month 11.25 mg (1%) 462
▲ Lupron Depot-PED 7.5 mg, 11.25 mg and 15 mg (5%) 471
Merrem I.V. (1.1%) 684
▲ Mycamine for Injection (20% to 96.5%) 616
Neupogen for Injection (Infrequent) 589
▲ Ontak Vials (8%) 1079
▲ Ortho Evra Transdermal System (1% to 22%) 2437
▲ Procrit for Injection (7% to 29%) 2391
Retrovir IV Infusion (Infrequent) 1579
Rilutek Tablets (Infrequent) 2771
▲ Rocephin Injectable Vials, ADD-Vantage, Galaxy, Bulk (5% to 17%) 2642
▲ Somatuline Depot Injection (Greater than 5% to 30%) 3102
▲ Testim 1% Gel (2% to 4%) 701
▲ Vesanoid Capsules (17%) 2660
Zosyn for Injection (0.5%) 3284
▲ Zyban Sustained-Release Tablets (11%) 1692

Drug effect, unspecified, diminished

Concerta Extended-Release Tablets 1925

Drug fever

DynaCirc CR Controlled Release Tablets (0.5% to 1%) 1407
Fansidar Tablets 2636
Leukeran Tablets 1508
Primaxin I.M. 2080
Primaxin I.V. (Less than 0.2%) 2083
Rocephin Injectable Vials, ADD-Vantage, Galaxy, Bulk 2642
Suprax for Oral Suspension (Less than 2%) 1891
Suprax Tablets (Less than 2%) 1891
Taxotere Injection Concentrate 2773
Timentin ADD-Vantage 1606
Timentin Injection Galaxy Container 1609
Timentin IV Infusion 1603
Timentin Pharmacy Bulk Package 1613
Zinacef for Injection (Rare) 1678
Zinacef Injection (Rare) 1678

Drug idiosyncrasies

(*see under* Allergic reactions)

Drug overdose

Campral Tablets (Infrequent) 1158
Emsam Transdermal System (Infrequent) 905
Luvox CR Extended-Release Capsules (Infrequent) 1759
Lyrica Capsules (0.1% to 1%) 2527
Percocet Tablets 1127
Prozac Pulvules and Liquid (Infrequent) 1852
▲ Reyataz Capsules (Less than 3%) 3299
Symbyax Capsules (Infrequent) 1871

Dry mouth

(*see under* Xerostomia)

Dry skin

(*see under* Xerosis cutis)

Dry sockets

Celebrex Capsules 2979

Dryness

Analpram-HC 1140
Elocon Lotion 0.1% (Infrequent) 2841
Extina Foam, 2% (Less than or equal to 1%) 3057
▲ Naftin Cream (3%) 2164
Ofloxacin Ophthalmic Solution 0.3% ⊙ 243
Olux Foam (Less than 1%) 3061
Pramosone 1141
ProQuad 2099
Vanos Cream 1941

Dryness, mucous membrane

Advicor Tablets 402
Myleran Tablets (Rare) 1530
▲ Vesanoid Capsules (77%) 2660
Vytorin 10/10 Tablets 2149
Vytorin 10/10 Tablets 2939
Vytorin 10/20 Tablets 2149
Vytorin 10/20 Tablets 2939
Vytorin 10/40 Tablets 2149
Vytorin 10/40 Tablets 2939
Vytorin 10/80 Tablets 2149
Vytorin 10/80 Tablets 2939
Zocor Tablets 2136

Dryness, nose

(*see under* Xeromycteria)

Dryness, vaginal

Crinone 4% Gel 992
Crinone 8% Gel 992
Effexor XR Extended-Release Capsules (Rare) 3195
▲ Femara Tablets (5.3%) 2246
Venlafaxine Hydrochloride Tablets (Rare) 2199

Dryness, vulvovaginal

Ambien CR Tablets (1%) 2696

Dryness at application site

▲ Aczone Gel 5% (Less than 1% to 16%) 3296
Daytrana Transdermal Patch 3022
Evoclin Foam, 1% (1%) 3056
▲ Flector Patch (4%) 561
Ionsys Transdermal System (.1% to less than 1%) 2410

Duodenitis

Actonel Tablets (1%) 2568
Actonel with Calcium Tablets (0.1% to 1%) 2574
Effexor XR Extended-Release Capsules (Rare) 3195
Evoxac Capsules (Less than 1%) 1013
Invanz for Injection (Greater than 0.1%) 2029
Nexium Delayed-Release Capsules (Less than 1%) 645
Nexium I.V. (Less than 1%) 652
Nexium Delayed-Release Oral Suspension (Less than 1%) 645
Paxil (Rare) 1535
Paxil CR Controlled-Release Tablets (Rare) 1544
Pletal Tablets (Less than 2%) 2481
Protonix for Delayed-Release Oral Suspension (Less than 1%) 3254
Protonix Delayed-Release Tablets (Less than 1%) 3254
Protonix I.V. (Less than 1%) 3257
Requip Tablets (Infrequent) 1561
Rythmol SR Capsules 1590
Velcade for Injection 2168
Venlafaxine Hydrochloride Tablets (Rare) 2199
Zonegran Capsules (Rare) 1089

Dupuytren's contracture

Requip Tablets (Rare) 1561

Dypnea

▲ Clolar for Intravenous Infusion (13%) 1239
Ionsys Transdermal System (.1% to less than 1%) 2410
Ultane Liquid for Inhalation (Less than 1%) 524

Dysarthria

Ambien Tablets (Infrequent) 2692
Ambien CR Tablets (Infrequent) 2696
Aricept Tablets (Infrequent) 1062
Aricept ODT Tablets (Infrequent) 1062
Arranon Injection (1%) 1319
Azilect Tablets (Infrequent) 3106
Chantix Tablets (Rare) 2511
Cymbalta Delayed-Release Capsules (Infrequent) 1801
Depakote ER Tablets (Greater than 1%) 423
Eloxatin for Injection 2731
Emend Capsules (Less than or equal to 0.5%) 1992
Emend for Injection (Less than or equal to 0.5%) 1999
Gabitril Tablets (Frequent) 973
Geodon Capsules (Frequent) 2520
Imitrex Injection (Rare) 1465
Imitrex Nasal Spray (Infrequent) 1470
Imitrex Tablets (Infrequent) 1474
Indocin Capsules (Less than 1%) 2024
Indocin I.V. (Less than 1%) 2489
Indocin (Less than 1%) 2024
Klonopin (2%) 2639
Lamictal (Infrequent) 1488

Lexapro Oral Suspension 1174
Lexapro Tablets 1174
Lyrica Capsules (0.1% to 1%) 2527
Maxalt Tablets (Infrequent) 2056
Maxalt-MLT Orally Disintegrating Tablets (Infrequent) 2056
Mirapex Tablets 857
Paxil (Rare) 1535
Paxil CR Controlled-Release Tablets (Rare) 1544
Protonix for Delayed-Release Oral Suspension (Less than 1%) 3254
Protonix Delayed-Release Tablets (Less than 1%) 3254
Protonix I.V. (Less than 1%) 3257
Prozac Weekly Capsules (Rare) 1852
Prozac Pulvules and Liquid (Rare) 1852
Remeron Tablets (Infrequent) 2924
RemeronSolTab Tablets (Infrequent) 2927
Rilutek Tablets (Infrequent) 2771
Seromycin Capsules 1864
Symbyax Capsules (Infrequent) 1871
Valium Tablets (Infrequent) 2658
Valtrex Caplets 1635
Velcade for Injection 2168
▲ Vesanoid Capsules (3%) 2660
Wellbutrin Tablets (Infrequent) 1648
Wellbutrin SR Sustained-Release Tablets 1653
Wellbutrin XL Extended-Release Tablets 1659
▲ Xeloda Tablets (Less than 5%) 2662
Xyrem Oral Solution (Infrequent) 1766
Zonegran Capsules (Infrequent) 1089
Zovirax 1690
Zyban Sustained-Release Tablets 1692
Zyprexa Tablets (Infrequent) 1883
Zyprexa ZYDIS Orally Disintegrating Tablets (Infrequent) 1883

Dysautonomia
Azilect Tablets (Infrequent) 3106
Lyrica Capsules (Rare) 2527
Velcade for Injection 2168

Dyscrasias, blood
(*see under* Blood dyscrasias)

Dysdiadochokinesia
Klonopin 2639

Dysentery
Xifaxan Tablets (Less than 2%) 2682

Dysesthesia
AmBisome for Injection (Less common) 606
Avelox 2803
Azilect Tablets (Infrequent) 3106
Cipro 2810
Copaxone for Injection (At least 2%) 3110
Eloxatin for Injection (1% to 2%) 2731
Evoxac Capsules (Less than 1%) 1013
Frova Tablets (Frequent) 1111
Imitrex Injection (Rare) 1465
Imitrex Nasal Spray (Rare) 1470
Imitrex Tablets (Rare) 1474
▲ Ixempra Kit for Injection (62%) 915
▲ Kepivance (12%) 583
Levaquin 2416
Levaquin in 5% Dextrose Injection 2416
Maxalt Tablets (Rare) 2056
Maxalt-MLT Orally Disintegrating Tablets (Rare) 2056
Prinivil Tablets (0.3% to 1%) 2087
Prinzide Tablets 2092
▲ Selzentry Tablets (4.7%) 2534
▲ Taxotere Injection Concentrate (5.5%) 2773
▲ Velcade for Injection (22% to 27%) 2168

Dysgeusia
Advate (2.6%) 721
Amitiza Capsules (Less than 1%) 3082
Amrix Capsules 966
▲ Arranon Injection (0% to 3%) 1319
AzaSite Ophthalmic Drops (Less than 1%) 1740
Byetta Injection 600
Captopril Tablets (Approximately 2 to 4 of 100 patients) 2182
Cardizem LA Extended Release Tablets (Less than 2%) 421
▲ Chantix Tablets (5% to 8%) 2511
Cozaar Tablets 1973
▲ Cymbalta Delayed-Release Capsules (Frequent to 3%) 1801
Emend Capsules (Greater than 0.5%) 1992
Emend for Injection (Greater than 0.5%) 1999
Fentora Tablets (Greater than 1%) 968
Flector Patch (2%) 561
Havrix Injection Vaccine (Less than 1%) 1454
Ketek Tablets (1.5% to 1.6%) 2744
Levaquin 2416
Levaquin in 5% Dextrose Injection 2416
▲ Lexiscan Injection (5%) 614
Maxalt Tablets 2056
Maxalt-MLT Orally Disintegrating Tablets 2056
Mevacor Tablets (0.8%) 2063
Noroxin Tablets 2069
Pristiq Extended-Release Tablets (1% to 2%) 3247
Requip Tablets (Infrequent) 1561
Rocephin Injectable Vials, ADD-Vantage, Galaxy, Bulk (Less than 1%) 2642
Rozerem Tablets (2%) 3091
▲ Sutent Capsules (Less than 1% to 44%) 2540
▲ Torisel Injection (0% to 20%) 3272
Treximet Tablets (Infrequent) 1616
Twinrix Vaccine (Less than 1%) 1628
Velcade for Injection 2168
Vivitrol 988
Xyrem Oral Solution (Infrequent) 1766
▲ Zolinza Capsules (24% to 27.9%) 2142

Dysgraphia
Mirapex Tablets 857

Dyskinesia
Abilify Injection (Greater than or equal to 1 in 1000 patients and less than or equal to 1 in 100 patients) 881
Abilify Injection (Greater than or equal to 1 in 1000 patients and less than 1 in 100 patients) 2466
Abilify Oral Solution (Greater than or equal to 1 in 1000 patients and less than or equal to 1 in 100 patients) 881
Abilify Oral Solution (Greater than or equal to 1 in 1000 patients and less than 1 in 100 patients) 2466
Abilify Discmelt Orally Disintegrating Tablets (Greater than or equal to 1 in 1000 patients and less than or equal to 1 in 100 patients) 881
Abilify Discmelt Orally Disintegrating Tablets (Greater than or equal to 1 in 1000 patients and less than 1 in 100 patients) 2466
Abilify Tablets (Greater than or equal to 1 in 1000 patients and less than or equal to 1 in 100 patients) 881
Abilify Tablets (Greater than or equal to 1 in 1000 patients and less than 1 in 100 patients) 2466
Adderall XR Capsules 3012
▲ Azilect Tablets (18%) 3106
Bentyl Capsules 703
Bentyl Injection 703
Bentyl Syrup 703
Bentyl Tablets 703
Celexa 1160
▲ Comtan Tablets (25%) 2208
Concerta Extended-Release Tablets 1925
Cubicin for Injection (Less than 1%) 995
Cymbalta Delayed-Release Capsules (Infrequent) 1801
Daytrana Transdermal Patch 3022
Dexedrine 1401
Effexor XR Extended-Release Capsules 3195
▲ Eldepryl Capsules (2 of 49 patients) 3052
Evoxac Capsules (Less than 1%) 1013
Exelon Capsules (Frequent) 2229
▲ Exelon Oral Solution (Frequent) 2229
Focalin XR Capsules 2251
▲ Geodon Capsules (14%) 2520
▲ Invega Extended-Release Tablets (3% to 9%) 1748
Kaletra (Less than 2%) 452
Lamictal (Infrequent) 1488
Lexapro Oral Suspension 1174
Lexapro Tablets 1174
Luvox CR Extended-Release Capsules (Infrequent) 1759
Lyrica Capsules (Rare) 2527
Metadate CD Capsules 3146
▲ Mirapex Tablets (47%) 857
Namenda 1180
Neupro Transdermal System (0.5%) 3149
Paxil (Rare) 1535
Paxil CR Controlled-Release Tablets (Rare) 1544
Phenytek Capsules (Rare) 2192
Provigil Tablets (1%) 977
Prozac Weekly Capsules 1852
Prozac Pulvules and Liquid 1852
Remeron Tablets (Infrequent) 2924
RemeronSolTab Tablets (Infrequent) 2927
Requip Tablets (Infrequent to greater than or equal to 1%) 1561
▲ Requip XL Tablets (Greater than or equal to 5%) 1568
Risperdal Consta Long-Acting Injection (Infrequent) 1753
▲ Stalevo Tablets (5% to 25%) 2309
Venlafaxine Hydrochloride Tablets 2199
Vyvanse Capsules 3033
Wellbutrin Tablets (Frequent) 1648
Wellbutrin SR Sustained-Release Tablets 1653
Wellbutrin XL Extended-Release Tablets 1659
Xyrem Oral Solution (Infrequent) 1766
Zonegran Capsules 1089
Zyban Sustained-Release Tablets 1692
Zyprexa Tablets (1% to 2%) 1883
Zyprexa ZYDIS Orally Disintegrating Tablets (1% to 2%) 1883

Dyskinesia, orofacial
Provigil Tablets (At least 1%) 977
Xyzal Oral Solution 2789
Xyzal Oral Solution 3155
Zyrtec Chewable Tablets 1920
Zyrtec Syrup 1920
Zyrtec Tablets 1920
Zyrtec-D 12 Hour Extended Release Tablets (Rare) 1923

Dyskinesia, tardive
(*see under* Tardive dyskinesia)

Dyslipidemia
Cymbalta Delayed-Release Capsules (Rare) 1801
Intelence Tablets (Less than 2%) 3119

Dysmenorrhea
Activella Tablets 2347
▲ Adderall XR Capsules (2% to 4%) 3012
▲ Advair Diskus 100/50 (3%) 1276
Advair Diskus 250/50 1276
Advair Diskus 500/50 1276
Advair HFA 45/21 Inhalation Aerosol 1288
Advair HFA 115/21 Inhalation Aerosol 1288
Advair HFA 230/21 Inhalation Aerosol 1288
▲ Alamast Ophthalmic Solution (Less than 5%) 3181
Allegra Oral Solution (1.5%) 2684
Allegra Tablets (1.5%) 2684
Angeliq Tablets 751
▲ Asacol Delayed-Release Tablets (3%) 2579
▲ Asmanex Twisthaler (4% to 9%) 2797
Axert Tablets (Infrequent) 2431
▲ Betaseron for SC Injection (7%) 756
Celebrex Capsules (0.1% to 1.9%) 2979
▲ Celexa (3%) 1160
Cipro XR Tablets (Less than 1%) 2823
Clarinex Tablets (2.1%) 2828
Clarinex Reditabs Tablets (2.1%) 2828
▲ Copaxone for Injection (6%) 3110
Crinone 4% Gel 992
Crinone 8% Gel 992
Depakote ER Tablets (Greater than 1%) 423
Divigel 3167
▲ Effexor XR Extended-Release Capsules (6%) 3195
Elidel Cream 1% (1.1% to 1.5%) 2221
Emsam Transdermal System (Frequent) 905
▲ Enjuvia Tablets (1% to 8%) 1029
Estratest Tablets 3043
Estratest H.S. Tablets 3043
Evoxac Capsules (Less than 1%) 1013
Fluarix Vaccine (1.3%) 1446
Gabitril Tablets (Frequent) 973
Geodon for Injection (Up to 2%) 2520
▲ Hycamtin for Injection (59%) 1459
Imitrex Injection (Rare) 1465
Imitrex Nasal Spray (Infrequent) 1470
Imitrex Tablets (Infrequent) 1474
▲ Intron A for Injection (Less than 5%) 2859
▲ Klonopin (3%) 2639
▲ Lamictal (5% to 7%) 1488
▲ Lunesta Tablets (0% to 3%) 2994
Lybrel Tablets 3204
Lyrica Capsules (0.1% to 1%) 2527
▲ Meridia Capsules (3.5%) 475
Mirapex Tablets 857
▲ Mirena Intrauterine System (5% or more) 779
▲ Nasonex Nasal Spray (1% to 5%) 2883
Nexium Delayed-Release Capsules (Less than 1%) 645
Nexium I.V. (Less than 1%) 652
Nexium Delayed-Release Oral Suspension (Less than 1%) 645
Noroxin Tablets (Less frequent) 2069
ParaGard T 380A Intrauterine Copper Contraceptive 1041
Paxil (Infrequent) 1535
Paxil CR Controlled-Release Tablets (Infrequent) 1544
Premarin Intravenous 3217
Premarin Tablets 3221
Premarin Vaginal Cream 3228
▲ Premphase Tablets (3% to 13%) 3232
▲ Prempro Tablets (3% to 13%) 3232
Protonix for Delayed-Release Oral Suspension (Less than 1%) 3254
Protonix Delayed-Release Tablets (Less than 1%) 3254
Protonix I.V. (Less than 1%) 3257
▲ Protopic Ointment (Up to 4%) 628
Provigil Tablets (At least 1%) 977
Prozac Pulvules and Liquid 1852
▲ Qvar Inhalation Aerosol (1% to 3%) 3116
Remeron Tablets (Infrequent) 2924
RemeronSolTab Tablets (Infrequent) 2927
Requip Tablets (Infrequent) 1561
Risperdal Consta Long-Acting Injection (Infrequent) 1753
Seasonique Tablets 1046
▲ Strattera Capsules (5% or 7%) 1864
Supprelin LA Implant 1731
▲ Valtrex Caplets (Less than 1% to 8%) 1635
Wellbutrin SR Sustained-Release Tablets (At least 1%) 1653
Wellbutrin XL Extended-Release Tablets (At least 1% to 2%) 1659
Yaz Tablets (Greater than 1%) 805
Zomig Tablets (Rare) 694
Zomig Nasal Spray (Rare) 689
Zomig-ZMT Tablets (Rare) 694
Zyprexa Tablets (2%) 1883
Zyprexa ZYDIS Orally Disintegrating Tablets (2%) 1883
Zyrtec Chewable Tablets (Less than 2%) 1920
Zyrtec Syrup (Less than 2%) 1920
Zyrtec Tablets (Less than 2%) 1920
Zyrtec-D 12 Hour Extended Release Tablets (Less than 2%) 1923

Dysmotility, esophageal
Abilify Injection 881
Abilify Injection 2466
Abilify Oral Solution 881
Abilify Oral Solution 2466
Abilify Discmelt Orally Disintegrating Tablets 881
Abilify Discmelt Orally Disintegrating Tablets 2466
Abilify Tablets 881
Abilify Tablets 2466
Invega Extended-Release Tablets 1748
Risperdal Consta Long-Acting Injection 1753

Dyspareunia
▲ Crinone 8% Gel (6%) 992
▲ Hycamtin for Injection (59%) 1459
Lyrica Capsules (Rare) 2527
ParaGard T 380A Intrauterine Copper Contraceptive 1041
Wellbutrin Tablets (Rare) 1648
Wellbutrin SR Sustained-Release Tablets 1653
Wellbutrin XL Extended-Release Tablets 1659
Zyban Sustained-Release Tablets 1692

Dyspepsia
Abelcet Injection 1134
▲ Abilify Injection (9%) 881
▲ Abilify Injection (9%) 2466
▲ Abilify Oral Solution (9%) 881
▲ Abilify Oral Solution (9%) 2466
▲ Abilify Discmelt Orally Disintegrating Tablets (9%) 881
▲ Abilify Discmelt Orally Disintegrating Tablets (9%) 2466
▲ Abilify Tablets (9%) 881
▲ Abilify Tablets (9%) 2466

Accolate Tablets (1.5%) 669
Aceon Tablets (2 mg, 4 mg, 8 mg) (0.3% to 1.9%) 3038
Acetadote Injection (0.24% to 1.17%) 1001
Actiq (1% or greater) 959
▲ Actonel Tablets (6.9% to 10.8%) 2568
▲ Actonel with Calcium Tablets (6.9% to 7.6%) 2574
Adderall XR Capsules (2%) 3012
Advair Diskus 100/50 1276
Advair Diskus 500/50 1276
Advair HFA 45/21 Inhalation Aerosol 1288
Advair HFA 115/21 Inhalation Aerosol 1288
Advair HFA 230/21 Inhalation Aerosol 1288
▲ Advicor Tablets (3%) 402
▲ Aerobid/Aerobid-M (1% to 3%) 1153
▲ Aggrenox Capsules (18.4%) 819
▲ Agrylin Capsules (5.2%) 3017
Aldara Cream, 5% (2%) 1699
▲ Alferon N Injection (3%) 1726
Alinia for Oral Suspension (Less than 1%) 2677
Alinia Tablets (Less than 1%) 2677
Allegra Oral Solution (1.3%) 2684
Allegra-D 12 Hour Extended-Release Tablets (2.8%) 2687
Allegra-D 24 Hour Extended-Release Tablets (2.8%) 2690
Aloxi Injection (Less than 1%) 1059
▲ Alphagan P Ophthalmic Solution (1% to 4%) 549
Ambien Tablets (Frequent) 2692
Ambien CR Tablets (Frequent) 2696
AmBisome for Injection (Less common) 606
Amerge Tablets (Infrequent) 1301
Amitiza Capsules (0% to 2.5%) 3082
Amrix Capsules 966
Anaprox Tablets (Less than 3%) 2632
Anaprox DS Tablets (Less than 3%) 2632
▲ Angiomax for Injection (5%) 1933
▲ Anzemet Injection (3%) 2701
▲ Anzemet Tablets (3%) 2704
Aptivus Capsules (Less than 2%) 823
Aptivus Oral Solution (Less than 2%) 823
Aricept Tablets (Frequent) 1062
Aricept ODT Tablets (Frequent) 1062
▲ Arimidex Tablets (7%) 672
Arixtra Injection (0.3% to 2.4%) 1313
▲ Asacol Delayed-Release Tablets (6%) 2579
▲ Asmanex Twisthaler (3% to 5%) 2797
Atacand Tablets (0.5% or greater) 639
Atacand HCT (0.5% or greater) 642
Atripla Tablets (Greater than or equal to 2%) 938
▲ Atrovent HFA Inhalation Aerosol (1% to 5%) 839
Avalide Tablets (2%) 892
Avalide Tablets (2%) 2713
▲ Avandamet Tablets (10%) 1336
Avapro Tablets (2%) 897
Avapro Tablets (2%) 2718
▲ Avastin IV (17% to 24%) 1192
Avelox (Greater than or equal to 0.1% to less than 2%) 2803
▲ Avinza Capsules (Less than 5%) 1772
Axert Tablets (Infrequent) 2431
▲ Axid Capsules (3.6%) 1364
▲ Azilect Tablets (5% to 7%) 3106
Azopt Ophthalmic Suspension (Less than 1%) 540
Baraclude (Less than or equal to 1%) 900
Bayer Aspirin 750
Benicar Tablets (Greater than 0.5%) 1009
Benicar HCT Tablets (Greater than 1%) 1010
▲ Betaseron for SC Injection (14%) 756
▲ Bexxar (Less than 1% to 6%) 1371
Biaxin/Biaxin XL (2%) 411
▲ Boniva Injection (5.6% to 11.9%) 2614
▲ Boniva Tablets (5.6% to 11.9%) 2618
▲ Busulfex Injection (44%) 2477
▲ Byetta Injection (6%) 600
Campral Tablets (Frequent) 1158
Cancidas for Injection 1953
Captopril Tablets 2182
Cardene I.V. (Rare) 1093
Ceftin Tablets (0.1% to 1%) 1380
▲ Celebrex Capsules (8.8%) 2979
▲ Celexa (5%) 1160
▲ CellCept Capsules (22.4%) 2622
▲ CellCept Intravenous (22.4%) 2622
▲ CellCept Oral Suspension (22.4%) 2622
▲ CellCept Tablets (22.4%) 2622
▲ Chantix Tablets (5%) 2511
▲ Cialis Tablets (1% to 10%) 1792
Cipro I.V. (2.7%) 2817
Cipro (2.7%) 2810
Cipro XR Tablets (1%) 2823
▲ Clarinex Tablets (3%) 2828
▲ Clarinex Reditabs Tablets (3%) 2828
▲ Clinoril Tablets (3% to 9%) 1962
Combigan Ophthalmic Solution (0.1% to 0.2%) 553
Combivent Inhalation Aerosol (Less than 2%) 845
▲ Combivir Tablets (5%) 1384
Comtan Tablets (2%) 2208
Concerta Extended-Release Tablets (2.2%) 1925
Copaxone for Injection (At least 2%) 3110
▲ Cosopt Sterile Ophthalmic Solution (1% to 5%) 1969
Cozaar Tablets (1% or greater) 1973
Crinone 4% Gel 992
Crinone 8% Gel 992
Crixivan Capsules (1.5%) 1979
▲ Cubicin for Injection (0.9% to 4.2%) 995
Cyanokit 5g Antidote 1021
▲ Cymbalta Delayed-Release Capsules (4% to 5%) 1801
▲ Dacogen Injection (12%) 1066
Demadex Injection (1.6%) 2630
Demadex Tablets (1.6%) 2630
▲ Depakote ER Tablets (7% to 23%) 423
▲ DepoDur Injection (2% to 5%) 1095
Diovan Tablets (Greater than 0.2%) 2212
Diovan HCT Tablets (Greater than 0.2%) 2216
▲ Doxil Injection (Less than 1% to 12.1%) 2378
▲ Duragesic Transdermal System (3% to 10%) 2405
EC-Naprosyn Delayed-Release Tablets (Less than 3%) 2632
Effexor XR Extended-Release Capsules (At least 2%) 3195
Eligard 7.5 mg (Less than 2%) 2724
Eligard 22.5 mg (Less than 2%) 2724
Eligard 30 mg (Less than 2%) 2724
Eligard 45 mg (Less than 2%) 2724
Elmiron Capsules (2%) 2435
▲ Eloxatin for Injection (5% to 14%) 2731
▲ Emend Capsules (8.4%) 1992
▲ Emend for Injection (8.4%) 1999
▲ Emsam Transdermal System (4%) 905
▲ Emtriva Capsules (4% to 8%) 1246
▲ Emtriva Oral Solution (4% to 8%) 1246
▲ Enablex Extended-Release Tablets (2.7% to 8.4%) 2225
▲ Enbrel for Injection (4% to 11%) 569
Engerix-B Vaccine 1409
▲ Entereg Capsules (5.9% to 7%) 3293
▲ Epivir (5%) 1412
▲ Epogen for Injection (9% to 11%) 576
▲ Equetro Extended-Release Capsules (10%) 3174
▲ Erbitux (0% to 14%) 912
▲ Evista Tablets (5.9%) 1810
▲ Evoxac Capsules (7.8%) 1013
▲ Exelon Capsules (9%) 2229
▲ Exelon Oral Solution (9%) 2229
Exforge Tablets (Greater than or equal to 0.2%) 2238
▲ Femara Tablets (3% to 4%) 2246
Fentora Tablets (Greater than 1%) 968
Flector Patch (1%) 561
Flolan for Injection (1%) 1426
Flumadine (0.3% to 1%) 1167
▲ Focalin XR Capsules (5% to 9%) 2251
▲ Forteo for Injection (5.2%) 1816
▲ Fosamax (1.1% to 3.6%) 2005
▲ Fosamax Plus D Tablets (1.1% to 3.6%) 2013
▲ Fosteum Capsules (1.1% to 4.7%) 2963
Frova Tablets (2%) 1111
Gabitril Tablets (1% or more) 973
▲ Gengraf Capsules (2.2% to 8%) 435
▲ Geodon (8%) 2520
▲ Gleevec Tablets (12% to 27%) 2255
▲ Hepsera Tablets (3%) 1253
Imitrex Nasal Spray 1470
▲ Indapamide Tablets (Less than 5%) 2188
▲ Indocin (3% to 9%) 2024
▲ Intron A for Injection (Up to 8%) 2859
Invanz for Injection (1% to 1.1%) 2029
▲ Ionsys Transdermal System (1% to less than 10%) 2410
Iquix Ophthalmic Solution (1% to 2%) 3183
▲ Kaletra (1% to 5%) 452
Keppra Oral Solution (1% or more) 3131
Keppra Tablets (1% or more) 3131
Ketek Tablets (Greater than or equal to 0.2% to less than 2%) 2744
Klonopin (Infrequent) 2639
▲ Lamictal (2% to 7%) 1488
▲ Lamisil Oral Granules (4%) 2264
▲ Lamisil Tablets (4.3%) 2266
▲ Lescol Capsules (7.9%) 2268
▲ Lescol XL Tablets (3.5%) 2268
▲ Leukine (17%) 774
Levaquin (2%) 2416
Levaquin in 5% Dextrose Injection (2%) 2416
▲ Levitra Tablets (4%) 2876
Lexapro Oral Suspension (Infrequent) 1174
Lexapro Tablets (Infrequent) 1174
Lipitor Tablets (1.3% to 2.8%) 2501
▲ Lovaza Capsules (3.1% to 7%) 1520
▲ Lunesta Tablets (2% to 6%) 2994
▲ Luvox CR Extended-Release Capsules (2% to 10%) 1759
▲ Malarone Pediatric Tablets (1% to 3%) 1521
▲ Malarone Tablets (1% to 3%) 1521
▲ Mavik Tablets (0.3% to 6.4%) 472
Maxalt Tablets (Infrequent) 2056
Maxalt-MLT Orally Disintegrating Tablets (Infrequent) 2056
▲ Megace ES Oral Suspension (0% to 4%) 2499
▲ Mepron Suspension (5%) 1526
▲ Meridia Capsules (5%) 475
Merrem I.V. (Greater than 0.1% to 1%) 684
▲ Mevacor Tablets (1% to 3.9%) 2063
▲ Miacalcin Nasal Spray (1% to 3%) 2274
Micardis Tablets (1%) 852
Micardis HCT Tablets (Less than 2%) 854
Mirapex Tablets (4%) 857
▲ Mobic Oral Suspension (3.8% to 9.5%) 863
▲ Mobic Tablets (3.8% to 9.5%) 863
MoviPrep Oral Solution (2.8%) 2679
MS Contin Tablets (Less frequent) 2585
▲ Mycamine for Injection (5.7% to 24.5%) 616
▲ Myfortic Tablets (3% to 22.5%) 2276
▲ Mylotarg for Injection (8% to 27%) 3212
▲ Nalfon Capsules (10.3%) 2508
Naprosyn Suspension (Less than 3%) 2632
Naprosyn Tablets (Less than 3%) 2632
Nasonex Nasal Spray (Greater than or equal to 2%) 2883
▲ Neoral Oral Solution (2.2% to 8%) 2280
▲ Neoral Soft Gelatin Capsules (2.2% to 8%) 2280
▲ Neulasta Injection (15% to 72%) 587
▲ Neupro Transdermal System (4%) 3149
▲ Nexavar Tablets (1% to less than 10%) 784
Nexium Delayed-Release Capsules (Less than 1%) 645
Nexium I.V. (Less than 1%) 652
Nexium Delayed-Release Oral Suspension (Less than 1%) 645
Noroxin Tablets (0.3% to 1%) 2069
▲ Norvir (0% to 5.9%) 489
▲ Noxafil Oral Suspension (1% to 10%) 2889
Omnicef Capsules (0.7%) 497
Omnicef for Oral Suspension (0.2%) 497
▲ Ontak Vials (7%) 1079
Opana Tablets (Less than 1%) 1117
Opana ER Tablets (Less than 1%) 1121
▲ Orencia Powder for Intravenous Infusion (6%) 921
▲ OxyContin Tablets (Between 1% and 5%) 2589
▲ Paxil (2% to 5%) 1535
▲ Paxil CR Controlled-Release Tablets (2% to 5%) 1544
▲ PegIntron Powder for Injection (6%) 2903
Pentasa Capsules (1.6%) 3030
Percocet Tablets 1127
Percodan Tablets 1130
Persantine Tablets (Rare) 869
▲ Photofrin for Injection (6%) 708
▲ Plavix Tablets (5.2%) 926
▲ Plavix Tablets (5.2%) 2767
▲ Pletal Tablets (6%) 2481
▲ Prandin Tablets (2% to 4%) 2971
▲ Premarin Tablets (9% to 11%) 3221
▲ Premphase Tablets (5% to 8%) 3232
▲ Prempro Tablets (5% to 8%) 3232
Prinivil Tablets (0.3% to 1%) 2087
Prinzide Tablets (1.3%) 2092
▲ Procrit for Injection (7% to 11%) 2391
▲ Prograf Capsules and Injection (3% to 28%) 622
▲ Prometrium Capsules (100 mg, 200 mg) (Less than 5%) 3047
Protonix for Delayed-Release Oral Suspension (Greater than or equal to 1%) 3254
Protonix Delayed-Release Tablets (Greater than or equal to 1%) 3254
Protonix I.V. (Greater than 1%) 3257
▲ Protopic Ointment (1% to 4%) 628
▲ Provigil Tablets (5%) 977
▲ Prozac Weekly Capsules (6% to 10%) 1852
▲ Prozac Pulvules and Liquid (6% to 10%) 1852
▲ Pulmicort Flexhaler (8%) 654
▲ Pulmozyme Inhalation Solution (3%) 1217
▲ Rebetol (Less than 1% to 16%) 2917
▲ Reclast Injection (1.7% to 5%) 2291
Recombivax HB (Less than 1%) 2107
ReFacto Vials 3269
▲ Remicade for IV Injection (10%) 950
ReoPro Vials (2.1%) 1860
▲ Requip Tablets (4% to 10%) 1561
▲ Retrovir Capsules (5% to 6%) 1574
▲ Retrovir IV Infusion (5% to 6%) 1579
▲ Retrovir (5% to 6%) 1574
▲ Rilutek Tablets (2.5% to 6.1%) 2771
▲ Risperdal Consta Long-Acting Injection (5% to 7%) 1753
▲ Rituxan I.V. (Less than 1% to 3%) 1223
Rocephin Injectable Vials, ADD-Vantage, Galaxy, Bulk (Less than 0.1%) 2642
▲ Rythmol Tablets (2% to 3%) 1586
Rythmol SR Capsules 1590
St. Joseph 81 mg Aspirin Chewable and Enteric Coated Tablets 1903
▲ Salagen Tablets (7%) 1082
Sanctura XR Capsules (1.2% to less than 2%) 557
▲ Sandostatin LAR Depot (4% to 6%) 2302
Serevent Diskus (1% to less than 3%) 1594
▲ Simulect for Injection (Greater than or equal to 10%) 2306
Singulair (2.1%) 2114
Soriatane Capsules (Less than 1%) 3062
▲ Spiriva HandiHaler (1% to 6%) 870
Stalevo Tablets (2%) 2309
▲ Strattera Capsules (4% to 8%) 1864
▲ Suboxone Tablets (3%) 2601
▲ Subutex Tablets (3%) 2601
Sular Extended Release Tablets (Less than or equal to 1%) 2975
▲ Suprax for Oral Suspension (3%) 1891
▲ Suprax Tablets (3%) 1891
▲ Sustiva Capsules (1% to 4%) 930
▲ Sustiva Tablets (1% to 4%) 930
▲ Sutent Capsules (1% to 46%) 2540
Tamiflu Capsules (Less than 1%) 2649
Tamiflu Oral Suspension (Less than 1%) 2649
▲ Tarceva Tablets (0% to 17%) 1228
Targretin Capsules 1084
Tarka Tablets (0.3% or more) 511
▲ Tasigna Capsules (1% to 10%) 2316
Tekturna Tablets 2321
Tekturna HCT Tablets 2324
Teveten Tablets (1% or greater) 515
Teveten HCT Tablets (Less than 1%) 517
Timoptic Sterile Ophthalmic Solution 2121
Timoptic in Ocudose (Less frequent) 2124
Timoptic-XE Sterile Ophthalmic Gel Forming Solution 2125
▲ Tracleer Tablets (4%) 3289
Trasylol Injection (1% to 2%) 799
▲ Travatan Z Ophthalmic Solution (1% to 5%) 547
Treximet Tablets (2%) 1616
Tricor Tablets 520
▲ Trisenox Injection (10%) 986
▲ Trizivir Tablets (5%) 1622
▲ Truvada Tablets (Greater than or equal to 5%) 1262
Twinrix Vaccine 1628
Tygacil for Injection (2.9%) 3276
▲ Tykerb Tablets (0% to 11%) 1631
▲ Tyzeka Tablets (3%) 2328
▲ Ultram ER Extended-Release Tablets (1% to less than 5%) 2428
Uroxatral Tablets (1% to 2%) 2786
▲ Urso 250 Tablets (10%) 720
▲ Urso Forte Tablets (10%) 720
▲ Vagifem Tablets (3% to 5%) 2375
▲ Valcyte Tablets (Less than 5%) 2654
▲ Velcade for Injection (11%) 2168
▲ Venlafaxine Hydrochloride Tablets (4.5% to 6.7%) 2199
▲ Vesanoid Capsules (14%) 2660
▲ VESIcare Tablets (1.4% to 3.9%) 636
▲ Vicoprofen Tablets (12%) 533
▲ Viread Tablets (3% to 4%) 1268
▲ Voltaren Tablets (1% to 10%) 2334
▲ Voltaren-XR Tablets (1% to 10%) 2337
Vytorin 10/10 Tablets 2149
Vytorin 10/10 Tablets 2939

Vytorin 10/20 Tablets 2149
Vytorin 10/20 Tablets 2939
Vytorin 10/40 Tablets 2149
Vytorin 10/40 Tablets 2939
Vytorin 10/80 Tablets 2149
Vytorin 10/80 Tablets 2939
▲ WelChol Tablets (3.9% to 8.3%) 1015
▲ Wellbutrin Tablets (3.1%) 1648
Wellbutrin SR Sustained-Release Tablets (At least 1%) 1653
▲ Wellbutrin XL Extended-Release Tablets (3%) 1659
Xopenex Inhalation Solution (1.4% to 2.7%) 3001
Xopenex Inhalation Solution Concentrate (1.4% to 2.7%) 3005
Xopenex HFA Inhalation Aerosol (1.4% to 2.7%) 3009
▲ Xyrem Oral Solution (2.9% to 9.1%) 1766
Yaz Tablets (Greater than 1%) 805
Zocor Tablets 2136
▲ Zometa for Intravenous Infusion (10%) 2341
Zomig Tablets (Infrequent) 694
Zomig Nasal Spray (Infrequent) 689
Zomig-ZMT Tablets (Infrequent) 694
▲ Zonegran Capsules (3%) 1089
▲ Zosyn for Injection (1.9% to 3.3%) 3284
Zyban Sustained-Release Tablets (Frequent) 1692
▲ Zyprexa Tablets (7% to 11%) 1883
▲ Zyprexa ZYDIS Orally Disintegrating Tablets (7% to 11%) 1883
Zyrtec Chewable Tablets (Less than 2%) 1920
Zyrtec Syrup (Less than 2%) 1920
Zyrtec Tablets (Less than 2%) 1920
Zyrtec-D 12 Hour Extended Release Tablets (Less than 2%) 1923
Zyvox 2552

Dyspeptic symptoms

Selzentry Tablets (2.8%) 2534

Dysphagia

Abilify Injection (Greater than or equal to 1 in 1000 patients and less than 1 in 100 patients) 881
Abilify Injection (Greater than or equal to 1 in 1000 patients and less than 1 in 100 patients) 2466
Abilify Oral Solution (Greater than or equal to 1 in 1000 patients and less than 1 in 100 patients) 881
Abilify Oral Solution (Greater than or equal to 1 in 1000 patients and less than 1 in 100 patients) 2466
Abilify Discmelt Orally Disintegrating Tablets (Greater than or equal to 1 in 1000 patients and less than 1 in 100 patients) 881
Abilify Discmelt Orally Disintegrating Tablets (Greater than or equal to 1 in 1000 patients and less than 1 in 100 patients) 2466
Abilify Tablets (Greater than or equal to 1 in 1000 patients and less than 1 in 100 patients) 881
Abilify Tablets (Greater than or equal to 1 in 1000 patients and less than 1 in 100 patients) 2466
Actiq (1% or greater) 959
Actonel Tablets 2568
Actonel with Calcium Tablets 2574
▲ Alimta for Injection (Up to 6%) 1786
Ambien Tablets (Infrequent) 2692
Ambien CR Tablets (Rare) 2696
AmBisome for Injection (Less common) 606
Avelox (Less than 0.1%) 2803
▲ Avinza Capsules (Less than 5%) 1772
▲ BOTOX Purified Neurotoxin Complex (19%) 550
Campral Tablets (Infrequent) 1158
Celebrex Capsules (0.1% to 1.9%) 2979
Celexa (Infrequent) 1160
▲ CellCept Capsules (3% to less than 20%) 2622
▲ CellCept Intravenous (3% to less than 20%) 2622
▲ CellCept Oral Suspension (3% to less than 20%) 2622
▲ CellCept Tablets (3% to less than 20%) 2622
Chantix Tablets (Infrequent) 2511
Cialis Tablets (Less than 2%) 1792
Cipro I.V. (1% or less) 2817
Cipro (Less than 1%) 2810
Cipro XR Tablets 2823
Copaxone for Injection (At least 2%) 3110
Cosmegen for Injection 2485
Cyanokit 5g Antidote 1021
▲ Dacogen Injection (6%) 1066
Depakote ER Tablets (Greater than 1%) 423
▲ DepoCyt Injection (8% to 9%) 1136
▲ Doxil Injection (1% to 10%) 2378
Edecrin 698
Effexor XR Extended-Release Capsules (Infrequent) 3195
Eldepryl Capsules 3052
▲ Eloxatin for Injection (3% to 5%) 2731
Emend Capsules (Greater than 0.5%) 1992
Emend for Injection (Greater than 0.5%) 1999
Emsam Transdermal System (Infrequent) 905
Evoxac Capsules (Less than 1%) 1013
Exelon Capsules (Infrequent) 2229
Exelon Oral Solution (Infrequent) 2229
Exforge Tablets (Greater than 0.1% but less than 1%) 2238
Fentora Tablets (Greater than 1%) 968
Flulaval Injection Vaccine 1448
Flumadine 1167
Fosamax (0.1% to 1%) 2005
Fosamax Plus D Tablets (0.1% to 1%) 2013
Frova Tablets (Infrequent) 1111
Gabitril Tablets (Infrequent) 973
Gengraf Capsules (1% to less than 3%) 435
Geodon Capsules (2%) 2520
Gliadel Wafer (1%) 1076
Imitrex Injection (Frequent) 1465
Imitrex Nasal Spray (Infrequent) 1470
Imitrex Tablets (Infrequent) 1474
▲ Intron A for Injection (Less than 5%) 2859
Invanz for Injection (Greater than 0.1%) 2029
Invega Extended-Release Tablets 1748
Ixempra Kit for Injection 915
Kaletra (0% to 2%) 452
Lamictal (Infrequent) 1488
▲ Leukine (11%) 774
Levitra Tablets (Less than 2%) 2876
Lipitor Tablets (Less than 2%) 2501
Lovaza Capsules 1520
Lunesta Tablets (Rare) 2994
▲ Lupron Depot 7.5 mg (Less than 5%) 469
Lupron Depot-PED 7.5 mg, 11.25 mg and 15 mg (Less than 2%) 471
Lyrica Capsules (0.1% to 1%) 2527
Maxalt Tablets (Infrequent) 2056
Maxalt-MLT Orally Disintegrating Tablets (Infrequent) 2056
Mirapex Tablets (2%) 857
Namenda 1180
Neoral Oral Solution (1% to less than 3%) 2280
Neoral Soft Gelatin Capsules (1% to less than 3%) 2280
▲ Nexavar Tablets (1% to less than 10%) 784
Nexium Delayed-Release Capsules (Less than 1%) 645
Nexium I.V. (Less than 1%) 652
Nexium Delayed-Release Oral Suspension (Less than 1%) 645
Noroxin Tablets 2069
Norvir (Less than 2%) 489
▲ Ontak Vials (6%) 1079
OxyContin Tablets (Less than 1%) 2589
Paxil (Infrequent) 1535
Paxil CR Controlled-Release Tablets (Infrequent) 1544
Pentasa Capsules (Less than 1%) 3030
▲ Photofrin for Injection (10% to 24%) 708
▲ Prograf Capsules and Injection (3% to 15%) 622
Protonix for Delayed-Release Oral Suspension (Less than 1%) 3254
Protonix Delayed-Release Tablets (Less than 1%) 3254
Protonix I.V. (Less than 1%) 3257
Provigil Tablets 977
Prozac Weekly Capsules (Infrequent) 1852
Prozac Pulvules and Liquid (Infrequent) 1852
Remicade for IV Injection 950
Requip Tablets (Infrequent) 1561
Retrovir Capsules 1574
Retrovir IV Infusion 1579
Retrovir 1574
Rilutek Tablets (More than 2%) 2771
Risperdal Consta Long-Acting Injection (Infrequent) 1753
Rythmol SR Capsules 1590
Salagen Tablets (1% to 2%) 1082
Solodyn Extended Release Tablets 1938
Spiriva HandiHaler 870
Stalevo Tablets 2309
Sular Extended Release Tablets (Less than or equal to 1%) 2975
Symbyax Capsules 1871
▲ Taxotere Injection Concentrate (1.1% to 25.1%) 2773
Treximet Tablets (Infrequent) 1616
Velcade for Injection 2168
Venlafaxine Hydrochloride Tablets (Infrequent) 2199
Vicoprofen Tablets (Less than 1%) 533
Wellbutrin Tablets (Infrequent) 1648
Wellbutrin SR Sustained-Release Tablets (Up to 2%) 1653
Wellbutrin XL Extended-Release Tablets (0% to 2%) 1659
▲ Xeloda Tablets (Less than 5%) 2662
Xyrem Oral Solution (Infrequent) 1766
▲ Zometa for Intravenous Infusion (5% to less than 10%) 2341
Zomig Tablets (1% to less than 2%) 694
Zomig Nasal Spray (1% to less than 2%) 689
Zomig-ZMT Tablets (1% to less than 2%) 694
Zonegran Capsules (Infrequent) 1089
Zyban Sustained-Release Tablets (Infrequent) 1692
Zyprexa Tablets (Infrequent) 1883
Zyprexa ZYDIS Orally Disintegrating Tablets (Infrequent) 1883

Dysphasia

Ambien Tablets (Rare) 2692
Aricept Tablets (Infrequent) 1062
Aricept ODT Tablets (Infrequent) 1062
Cipro I.V. (1% or less) 2817
Cipro XR Tablets 2823
Imitrex Injection 1465
Imitrex Nasal Spray 1470
▲ Temodar Capsules (1% to 7%) 2931
▲ Xeloda Tablets (Less than 5%) 2662

Dysphonia

▲ Advair Diskus 100/50 (Greater than or equal to 3%) 1276
▲ Advair Diskus 250/50 (2% to greater than 5%) 1276
▲ Advair Diskus 500/50 (Greater than or equal to 3%) 1276
▲ Advair HFA 45/21 Inhalation Aerosol (1% to 3%) 1288
▲ Advair HFA 115/21 Inhalation Aerosol (1% to 3%) 1288
▲ Advair HFA 230/21 Inhalation Aerosol (1% to 3%) 1288
Alvesco Inhalation Aerosol (Less than 1%) 2985
Combivent Inhalation Aerosol (Less than 2%) 845
Evoxac Capsules (Less than 1%) 1013
Exelon Capsules (Infrequent) 2229
Exelon Oral Solution (Infrequent) 2229
Exforge Tablets (Greater than or equal to 0.2%) 2238
▲ Flovent Diskus 50 mcg (1% to 9%) 1435
Flovent HFA (2%) 1440
Flulaval Injection Vaccine 1448
Foradil Aerolizer (1%) 2849
▲ Intron A for Injection (Less than 5%) 2859
Ixempra Kit for Injection 915
Mirapex Tablets 857
Proventil HFA Inhalation Aerosol (Less than 3%) 2914
▲ Qvar Inhalation Aerosol (Up to 4%) 3116
ReoPro Vials (0.3%) 1860
Requip Tablets (Infrequent) 1561
Romazicon Injection (Less than 1%) 2646
Soriatane Capsules (Less than 1%) 3062
▲ Spiriva HandiHaler (1% to 3%) 870
▲ Tasigna Capsules (1% to 10%) 2316
Zyrtec Chewable Tablets (Less than 2%) 1920
Zyrtec Syrup (Less than 2%) 1920
Zyrtec Tablets (Less than 2%) 1920
Zyrtec-D 12 Hour Extended Release Tablets (Less than 2%) 1923

Dysphoria

▲ Abilify Injection (12%) 881
▲ Abilify Injection (2% to 6%) 2466
▲ Abilify Oral Solution (2% to 12%) 881
▲ Abilify Oral Solution (2% to 6%) 2466
▲ Abilify Discmelt Orally Disintegrating Tablets (2% to 12%) 881
▲ Abilify Discmelt Orally Disintegrating Tablets (2% to 6%) 2466
▲ Abilify Tablets (2% to 12%) 881
▲ Abilify Tablets (2% to 6%) 2466
Acetadote Injection (0.39% to 1.87%) 1001
Actiq 959
Adderall XR Capsules 3012
Adipex-P 1185
▲ Advair Diskus 100/50 (27%) 1276
Advair Diskus 250/50 1276
Advair Diskus 500/50 1276
Advair HFA 45/21 Inhalation Aerosol 1288
Advair HFA 115/21 Inhalation Aerosol 1288
Advair HFA 230/21 Inhalation Aerosol 1288
Allegra-D 12 Hour Extended-Release Tablets 2687
Allegra-D 24 Hour Extended-Release Tablets 2690
Amerge Tablets (Rare) 1301
Aricept Tablets (Infrequent) 1062
Aricept ODT Tablets (Infrequent) 1062
Atacand HCT 642
Axert Tablets (Infrequent) 2431
Catapres Tablets 841
Catapres-TTS (0.5% or less) 842
Chantix Tablets (Frequent) 2511
Cipro I.V. (Greater than 1%) 2817
Cipro (Less than 1%) 2810
Cipro XR Tablets 2823
Clorpres Tablets 2185
▲ Concerta Extended-Release Tablets (3.1%) 1925
Cyanokit 5g Antidote 1021
▲ Cymbalta Delayed-Release Capsules (5%) 1801
Demadex Tablets 2630
Dexedrine 1401
Effexor XR Extended-Release Capsules 3195
Eldepryl Capsules 3052
Exelon Capsules (Frequent) 2229
Exelon Oral Solution (Frequent) 2229
Flovent Diskus 50 mcg 1435
Flovent HFA 1440
Furosemide Tablets 2186
Humulin 50/50, 100 Units 1843
Humulin 70/30 Vial 1844
Humulin N Vial 1846
▲ Infanrix Vaccine (8.6% to 15.9%) 1479
Intravenous Sodium Diuril 2490
Lamictal (Rare) 1488
Lexapro Oral Suspension (Infrequent) 1174
Lexapro Tablets (Infrequent) 1174
Lortab 5/500 Tablets 3143
Lortab 7.5/500 Tablets 3144
Lortab 10/500 Tablets 3144
Micardis HCT Tablets 854
Mirapex Tablets 857
MS Contin Tablets (Among most frequent) 2585
Namenda 1180
Nitrolingual Pumpspray 2965
Noroxin Tablets 2069
Opana Tablets (Less than 1%) 1117
Opana ER Tablets (Less than 1%) 1121
OxyIR Capsules 2593
Parnate Tablets 1532
Percocet Tablets 1127
Percodan Tablets 1130
Prinzide Tablets 2092
Pristiq Extended-Release Tablets 3247
Prozac Weekly Capsules 1852
▲ Romazicon Injection (1% to 3%) 2646
Singulair (Very rare) 2114
Strattera Capsules 1864
Tekturna HCT Tablets 2324
Teveten HCT Tablets 517
Thioridazine Hydrochloride Tablets (Extremely rare) 2195
Thiothixene Capsules 2197
Thyrogen for Injection 1244
Transderm Scōp Transdermal Therapeutic System (Infrequent) 2206
Tussionex Pennkinetic Extended-Release Suspension 3154
Tylenol with Codeine Tablets 2427
▲ Ultram ER Extended-Release Tablets (1% to less than 5%) 2428
Uniphyl Tablets 2595
Valium Tablets 2658
Venlafaxine Hydrochloride Tablets 2199
Vicodin Tablets 529
Vicodin ES Tablets 530

Vicodin HP Tablets 531
▲ Vyvanse Capsules (3%) 3033
Wellbutrin Tablets (Infrequent) 1648
Wellbutrin SR Sustained-Release Tablets (Infrequent) 1653
Wellbutrin XL Extended-Release Tablets (Infrequent) 1659
Xyrem Oral Solution (Infrequent) 1766
Zyban Sustained-Release Tablets (Less than 1%) 1692
Zydone Tablets 1132
Zyrtec-D 12 Hour Extended Release Tablets 1923

Dysplasia, gastrointestinal

Nexium Delayed-Release Capsules (Less than 1%) 645
Nexium I.V. (Less than 1%) 652
Nexium Delayed-Release Oral Suspension (Less than 1%) 645

Dyspnea

▲ Abelcet Injection (7%) 1134
Abilify Injection (Greater than or equal to 1 in 100 patients) 881
Abilify Injection (Greater than or equal to 1 in 100 patients) 2466
Abilify Oral Solution (Greater than or equal to 1 in 100 patients) 881
Abilify Oral Solution (Greater than or equal to 1 in 100 patients) 2466
Abilify Discmelt Orally Disintegrating Tablets (Greater than or equal to 1 in 100 patients) 881
Abilify Discmelt Orally Disintegrating Tablets (Greater than or equal to 1 in 100 patients) 2466
Abilify Tablets (Greater than or equal to 1 in 100 patients) 881
Abilify Tablets (Greater than or equal to 1 in 100 patients) 2466
Aceon Tablets (2 mg, 4 mg, 8 mg) (0.3% to 1%) 3038
Acetadote Injection (0.54% to 2.58%) 1001
▲ Actiq (2% to 6%) 959
▲ Actonel with Calcium Tablets (3.8%) 2574
Actos Tablets 3077
▲ Adderall XR Capsules (2% to 4%) 3012
▲ Adenocard IV Injection (12%) 603
▲ Adenoscan (Approximately 28%) 605
▲ Advair Diskus 100/50 (Greater than or equal to 3%) 1276
Advair Diskus 250/50 1276
Advair Diskus 500/50 1276
Advair HFA 45/21 Inhalation Aerosol 1288
Advair HFA 115/21 Inhalation Aerosol 1288
Advair HFA 230/21 Inhalation Aerosol 1288
Advate (0.6%) 721
Advicor Tablets 402
▲ Aerobid/Aerobid-M (1% to 3%) 1153
Aggrenox Capsules 819
▲ Agrylin Capsules (11.9%) 3017
Aldara Cream, 5% 1699
▲ Alimta for Injection (1% to 72%) 1786
Allegra Oral Solution (Rare) 2684
Allegra Tablets (Rare) 2684
Allegra-D 12 Hour Extended-Release Tablets (Rare) 2687
Allegra-D 24 Hour Extended-Release Tablets (Rare) 2690
▲ Alphagan P Ophthalmic Solution (1% to 4%) 549
Ambien Tablets (Infrequent) 2692
Ambien CR Tablets (Rare) 2696
▲ AmBisome for Injection (17.6% to 23%) 606
Amerge Tablets 1301
▲ Amitiza Capsules (2% to 3%) 3082
▲ Anaprox Tablets (3% to 9%) 2632
▲ Anaprox DS Tablets (3% to 9%) 2632
AndroGel 3159
Anzemet Injection (Rare) 2701
Anzemet Tablets (Rare) 2704
Aptivus Capsules (2.1%) 823
Aptivus Oral Solution (2.1%) 823
Aralast (0.1%) 726
▲ Aranesp for Injection (10%) 564
▲ Argatroban Injection (8.1%) 1308
Aricept Tablets (Infrequent) 1062
Aricept ODT Tablets (Infrequent) 1062
▲ Arimidex Tablets (8% to 11%) 672
▲ Arranon Injection (2% to 20%) 1319
Atacand Tablets (0.5% or greater) 639
Atacand HCT (0.5% or greater) 642
Atripla Tablets 938
▲ Atrovent HFA Inhalation Aerosol (7% to 8%) 839
Avalide Tablets 892
Avalide Tablets 2713
▲ Avandia Tablets (26%) 1351
Avapro Tablets (Less than 1%) 897
Avapro Tablets (Less than 1%) 2718
▲ Avastin IV (25% to 26%) 1192
Avelox (Less than 0.1%) 2803
▲ Avinza Capsules (5% to 10%) 1772
Axert Tablets (Infrequent) 2431
▲ Azilect Tablets (3%) 3106
Azopt Ophthalmic Suspension (Less than 1%) 540
▲ BeneFIX Vials (3.2%) 3191
Bentyl Capsules 703
Bentyl Injection 703
Bentyl Syrup 703
Bentyl Tablets 703
▲ Betaseron for SC Injection (6%) 756
Betimol Ophthalmic Solution 3181
▲ Bexxar (3% to 11%) 1371
Bicillin C-R Injectable Suspension 1775
Bicillin L-A Injection 1777
Boostrix (Rarely) 1377
BOTOX Purified Neurotoxin Complex (Rare) 550
▲ Brovana Inhalation Solution (4%) 2990
▲ Busulfex Injection (2% to 25%) 2477
Bystolic Tablets (0% to 1%) 1155
▲ Campath Ampules (10% to 35%) 761
Campral Tablets (Frequent) 1158
▲ Cancidas for Injection (9.2%) 1953
Captopril Tablets (About 0.5% to 2%) 2182
Carbatrol Capsules 3019
Cardene I.V. (0.7%) 1093
Cardizem LA Extended Release Tablets (Less than 2%) 421
Celebrex Capsules (0.1% to 2.8%) 2979
Celexa (Infrequent) 1160
▲ CellCept Capsules (31% to 36.7%) 2622
▲ CellCept Intravenous (31% to 36.7%) 2622
▲ CellCept Oral Suspension (31% to 36.7%) 2622
▲ CellCept Tablets (31% to 36.7%) 2622
▲ Cerezyme for Injection (Approximately 6.6%) 1238
Chantix Tablets (1% to 2%) 2511
Cialis Tablets (Less than 2%) 1792
Cimzia (Rare) 3127
Cipro I.V. (1% or less) 2817
Cipro (Less than 1%) 2810
Cipro XR Tablets 2823
Clarinex Syrup (Rare) 2828
Clarinex Tablets (Rare) 2828
Clarinex Reditabs Tablets (Rare) 2828
Clarinex-D 12-Hour Extended-Release Tablets (Rare) 2831
Clarinex-D 24-Hour Extended-Release Tablets 2834
Cleviprex (Less than 1%) 1936
Clinoril Tablets (Less than 1%) 1962
Combigan Ophthalmic Solution (0.1% to 0.2%) 553
▲ Combivent Inhalation Aerosol (4.5%) 845
▲ Comtan Tablets (3%) 2208
Comvax 1966
Concerta Extended-Release Tablets 1925
▲ Copaxone for Injection (19%) 3110
▲ Coreg Tablets (Greater than 3%) 1387
▲ Coreg CR Extended-Release Capsules (Greater than 3%) 1393
Cosopt Sterile Ophthalmic Solution (Less than 1%) 1969
Cozaar Tablets (Less than 1%) 1973
Crinone 4% Gel 992
Crinone 8% Gel 992
Crixivan Capsules 1979
▲ Cubicin for Injection (2.1% to 3.3%) 995
Cyanokit 5g Antidote 1021
Dacogen Injection 1066
▲ Depakote ER Tablets (1% to 5%) 423
▲ DepoCyt Injection (10% to 12%) 1136
▲ DepoDur Injection (2% to 5%) 1095
Diovan Tablets (Greater than 0.2%) 2212
Diovan HCT Tablets (Greater than 0.2%) 2216
▲ Doxil Injection (1% to 15.1%) 2378
▲ Duragesic Transdermal System (3% to 10%) 2405
DynaCirc CR Controlled Release Tablets (0.5% to 1%) 1407
▲ EC-Naprosyn Delayed-Release Tablets (3% to 9%) 2632
Effexor XR Extended-Release Capsules (Frequent) 3195
Elidel Cream 1% (0% to 1.8%) 2221
Elitek 2729
Elmiron Capsules (Less than or equal to 1%) 2435
▲ Eloxatin for Injection (Less than 1% to 43%) 2731
Emend Capsules (Greater than 0.5%) 1992
Emend for Injection (Greater than 0.5%) 1999
Emsam Transdermal System (Infrequent) 905
Enbrel for Injection (Infrequent) 569
Equetro Extended-Release Capsules 3174
▲ Erbitux (16% to 48%) 912
Evoxac Capsules (Less than 1%) 1013
Exelon Capsules (Frequent) 2229
Exelon Oral Solution (Frequent) 2229
Exelon Patch (Infrequent) 2233
Exforge Tablets (Greater than 0.1% to less than 1%) 2238
▲ Exubera Inhalation Powder (3.6% to 4.4%) 2515
Fabrazyme for Intravenous Infusion (8%) 1241
▲ Faslodex Injection (14.9%) 682
▲ Femara Tablets (0.8% to 18%) 2246
▲ Fentora Tablets (0% to 19%) 968
Flebogamma 5% 1715
Flebogamma 5% DIF 1718
▲ Flolan for Injection (2% to 100%) 1426
▲ Flonase Nasal Spray (1% to 3%) 1431
Flovent Diskus 50 mcg 1435
Flovent HFA 1440
Fluarix Vaccine 1446
Flulaval Injection Vaccine 1448
Flumadine (0.3% to 1%) 1167
Follistim AQ Cartridge 2844
Foradil Aerolizer (2.1%) 2849
▲ Forteo for Injection (3.6%) 1816
Frova Tablets (Infrequent) 1111
Gabitril Tablets (Frequent) 973
Gammagard Liquid 730
Gammagard S/D 734
Gamunex 3094
▲ Gemzar for Injection (3% to 23%) 1820
▲ Gengraf Capsules (1% to 5%) 435
Geodon Capsules (2%) 2520
▲ Gleevec Tablets (12% to 21%) 2255
▲ Gliadel Wafer (3%) 1076
Havrix Injection Vaccine 1454
▲ Herceptin I.V. (22%) 1199
▲ Humira Injection (Less than 5%) 442
▲ Hycamtin for Injection (1.8% to 22%) 1459
Imitrex Injection (Infrequent) 1465
Imitrex Nasal Spray (Infrequent) 1470
Imitrex Tablets (Frequent) 1474
Indocin Capsules (Less than 1%) 2024
Indocin I.V. (Less than 1%) 2489
Indocin (Less than 1%) 2024
Infanrix Vaccine 1479
▲ Intron A for Injection (Up to 34%) 2859
Invanz for Injection (1% to 2.6%) 2029
▲ Ixempra Kit for Injection (9%) 915
Januvia Tablets 2048
Kaletra (Less than 2%) 452
Klonopin (Infrequent) 2639
K-Phos Original (Sodium Free) Tablets (Less frequent) 814
K-Phos Neutral Tablets 813
Lamictal (1.1%) 1488
Lescol Capsules (Rare) 2268
Lescol XL Tablets 2268
▲ Letairis Tablets (4%) 1258
▲ Leukine (15% to 28%) 774
▲ Leustatin Injection (11%) 2384
Levaquin (1%) 2416
Levaquin in 5% Dextrose Injection (1%) 2416
Levitra Tablets (Less than 2%) 2876
Levothroid Tablets 1170
Levoxyl Tablets 1780
▲ Lexiscan Injection (28%) 614
Lipitor Tablets (Less than 2%) 2501
Lortab 5/500 Tablets 3143
Lortab 7.5/500 Tablets 3144
Lortab 10/500 Tablets 3144
Lovaza Capsules 1520
▲ Lovenox Injection (3.3%) 2756
▲ Lucentis Injection (0% to 5%) 1205
Lunesta Tablets (Infrequent) 2994
▲ Lyrica Capsules (2% to 3%) 2527
Mavik Tablets (0.3% to 1%) 472
Maxalt Tablets (Frequent) 2056
Maxalt-MLT Orally Disintegrating Tablets (Frequent) 2056
▲ Megace ES Oral Suspension (1% to 3%) 2499
Mephyton Tablets (Rare) 700
▲ Mepron Suspension (15% to 21%) 1526
Meridia Capsules (Greater than or equal to 1%) 475
Merrem I.V. (Greater than 0.1% to 1%) 684
Mevacor Tablets (Rare) 2063
Miacalcin Nasal Spray (Less than 1%) 2274
Micardis Tablets (More than 0.3%) 852
Micardis HCT Tablets 854
▲ Mirapex Tablets (Greater than or equal to 1% to 4%) 857
Moban Tablets 1116
Mobic Oral Suspension (Less than 2%) 863
Mobic Tablets (Less than 2%) 863
MoviPrep Oral Solution 2679
▲ Mycamine for Injection (5.9% to 12.7%) 616
▲ Myfortic Tablets (3% to less than 20%) 2276
▲ Mylotarg for Injection (26%) 3212
Nalfon Capsules (2.8%) 2508
Namenda (2%) 1180
▲ Naprosyn Suspension (3% to 9%) 2632
▲ Naprosyn Tablets (3% to 9%) 2632
▲ Neoral Oral Solution (1% to 5%) 2280
▲ Neoral Soft Gelatin Capsules (1% to 5%) 2280
▲ Neupogen for Injection (9%) 589
▲ Nexavar Tablets (14%) 784
Nexium Delayed-Release Capsules (Less than 1%) 645
Nexium I.V. (Less than 1%) 652
Nexium Delayed-Release Oral Suspension (Less than 1%) 645
Niaspan Extended-Release Tablets 480
Nimotop Capsules (Up to 1.2%) 790
Noroxin Tablets 2069
Norvir (Less than 2%) 489
▲ Novantrone for Injection Concentrate (6% to 18%) 1100
▲ Noxafil Oral Suspension (1% to 20%) 2889
▲ Ontak Vials (29%) 1079
Opana Tablets (Less than 1%) 1117
Opana ER Tablets (Less than 1%) 1121
OptiPranolol Metipranolol Ophthalmic Solution 0.3% (A small number of patients) .... ⊙ 245
Orencia Powder for Intravenous Infusion (Greater than 0.1% and less than or equal to 1%) 921
▲ Orthoclone OKT3 Sterile Solution (21%) 2387
OsmoPrep Tablets 2680
▲ OxyContin Tablets (Between 1% and 5%) 2589
Paxil (Infrequent) 1535
Paxil CR Controlled-Release Tablets (Infrequent) 1544
Pediarix Vaccine (Rare) 1552
▲ PegIntron Powder for Injection (4%) 2903
Pentasa Capsules (One case) 3030
Percocet Tablets 1127
Percodan Tablets 1130
▲ Photofrin for Injection (6% to 20%) 708
▲ Plavix Tablets (4.5%) 926
▲ Plavix Tablets (4.5%) 2767
Pletal Tablets (2% or greater) 2481
Prevnar 3241
Primaxin I.M. 2080
Primaxin I.V. (Less than 0.2%) 2083
Prinivil Tablets (Greater than 1%) 2087
Prinzide Tablets (0.3% to 1%) 2092
ProAir HFA Inhalation Aerosol (Less than 3%) 3113
▲ Prograf Capsules and Injection (5% to 29%) 622
Prolastin (Occasional) 3099
▲ Proleukin for Injection (Less than 1% to 43%) 2287
Protonix for Delayed-Release Oral Suspension (Greater than or equal to 1%) 3254
Protonix Delayed-Release Tablets (Greater than or equal to 1%) 3254
Protonix I.V. (Greater than or equal to 1%) 3257
Protopic Ointment (Greater than or equal to 1%) 628
Provigil Tablets (Greater than or equal to 1%) 977
Prozac Weekly Capsules 1852
▲ Pulmozyme Inhalation Solution (17%) 1217
Raptiva for Injection 1218
▲ Rebetol (5% to 26%) 2917
▲ Reclast Injection (5%) 2291
Recombivax HB (Less than 1%) 2107
ReFacto Vials 3269
Refludan for Injection (Common) 795
Relenza Inhalation Powder 1556
Remeron Tablets (1%) 2924
RemeronSolTab Tablets (1%) 2927

Remicade for IV Injection (1%).......... 950
▲ Requip Tablets (Infrequent to 3%) 1561
▲ Retrovir Capsules (5%) 1574
▲ Retrovir IV Infusion (5%) 1579
▲ Retrovir (5%) 1574
Reyataz Capsules.......................... 3299
Rilutek Tablets (More than 2%)......... 2771
Risperdal Consta Long-Acting Injection (Frequent) 1753
▲ Rituxan I.V. (1% to 7%) 1223
▲ Romazicon Injection (3% to 9%) 2646
▲ Rythmol Tablets (2% to 5%) 1586
▲ Rythmol SR Capsules (13% to 17%).. 1590
Salagen Tablets (Less than 1%)........ 1082
Sandimmune 2296
▲ Simulect for Injection (Greater than or equal to 10%)................... 2306
▲ Stalevo Tablets (3%) 2309
Stromectol Tablets 2120
Sular Extended Release Tablets (Less than or equal to 1%) 2975
Sustiva Capsules 930
Sustiva Tablets 930
▲ Sutent Capsules (0% to 28%) 2540
Symbyax Capsules (1% to 2%) 1871
Synagis Intramuscular Solution (More than 1%) 1948
▲ Tarceva Tablets (Less than 1% to 41%).. 1228
Targretin Capsules 1084
Tarka Tablets (1.3%) 511
▲ Tasigna Capsules (1% to 11%) 2316
▲ Taxotere Injection Concentrate (2.7% to 15.1%) 2773
▲ Temodar Capsules (Less than 1% to 5%) 2931
Thiothixene Capsules 2197
Thyrogen for Injection 1244
Timoptic Sterile Ophthalmic Solution (Less frequent) 2121
Timoptic in Ocudose (Less frequent) 2124
Timoptic-XE Sterile Ophthalmic Gel Forming Solution 2125
Toprol-XL Tablets (Greater than 1%) 666
▲ Torisel Injection (9% to 28%) 3272
▲ Trasylol Injection (4%) 799
Treximet Tablets (Infrequent) 1616
Tricor Tablets 520
▲ Trisenox Injection (53%) 986
Trizivir Tablets 1622
Trusopt Sterile Ophthalmic Solution 2128
Truvada Tablets 1262
Twinrix Vaccine 1628
Tygacil for Injection (2.9%) 3276
▲ Tykerb Tablets (0% to 12%) 1631
▲ Ultram ER Extended-Release Tablets (1% to less than 5%) 2428
Uroqid-Acid No. 2 Tablets 814
▲ Valcyte Tablets (Less than 5%) 2654
Valtrex Caplets 1635
Vectibix 597
▲ Velcade for Injection (3% to 21%) 2168
Venlafaxine Hydrochloride Tablets (Frequent) 2199
▲ Vesanoid Capsules (60%) 2660
Viadur Implant (2.3%) 802
Vicoprofen Tablets (Less than 3%) ... 533
Viread Tablets 1268
Visudyne for Injection 2332
Vivitrol 988
▲ Voltaren Ophthalmic Solution (Less than or equal to 3%) 2336
Voltaren Tablets (Occasionally) 2334
Voltaren-XR Tablets (Occasionally) 2337
Vytorin 10/10 Tablets 2149
Vytorin 10/10 Tablets 2939
Vytorin 10/20 Tablets 2149
Vytorin 10/20 Tablets 2939
Vytorin 10/40 Tablets 2149
Vytorin 10/40 Tablets 2939
Vytorin 10/80 Tablets 2149
Vytorin 10/80 Tablets 2939
Vyvanse Capsules (2%) 3033
Wellbutrin Tablets (Infrequent) 1648
Wellbutrin SR Sustained-Release Tablets 1653
Wellbutrin XL Extended-Release Tablets 1659
▲ Xeloda Tablets (Less than 5%) 2662
Xifaxan Tablets (Less than 2%) 2682
Xolair 1235
Xolair 2339
Xopenex Inhalation Solution 3001
Xopenex Inhalation Solution Concentrate 3005
Xopenex HFA Inhalation Aerosol 3009
Xyrem Oral Solution (Less than 1%) 1766
Xyzal Oral Solution 2789
Xyzal Oral Solution 3155
Ziagen 1673
Zocor Tablets (Rare) 2136
▲ Zometa for Intravenous Infusion (22% to 27%)................................ 2341
Zomig Tablets (Infrequent)................ 694
Zomig Nasal Spray (Infrequent)......... 689
Zomig-ZMT Tablets (Infrequent) 694
Zonegran Capsules (Infrequent) 1089
Zostavax Injection 2145
Zyban Sustained-Release Tablets (1%).. 1692
▲ Zyprexa Tablets (3%) 1883
▲ Zyprexa ZYDIS Orally Disintegrating Tablets (3%) 1883
Zyrtec Chewable Tablets (Less than 2%).................................... 1920
Zyrtec Syrup (Less than 2%)............. 1920
Zyrtec Tablets (Less than 2%)........... 1920
Zyrtec-D 12 Hour Extended Release Tablets (Less than 2%)..... 1923
Zyvox 2552

Dyspnea, aggravation of

Toprol-XL Tablets (Greater than 1%) 666

Dyspnea, exertional

▲ Arranon Injection (0% to 7%) 1319
Fentora Tablets (Greater than 1%) 968
▲ Gleevec Tablets (16.7%) 2255
Intelence Tablets (Less than 2%) 3119
Mirapex Tablets 857
▲ Myfortic Tablets (3% to less than 20%) 2276
▲ Tasigna Capsules (1% to 10%) 2316
Vantas (Less than 2%) 1737
Velcade for Injection 2168

Dyspnea, nocturnal

Prinivil Tablets (0.3% to 1%) 2087
Prinzide Tablets 2092
Xyrem Oral Solution (Infrequent) 1766

Dyspnea, worsening of

▲ Avandia Tablets (26%) 1351

Dysrhythmia

Percodan Tablets 1130
St. Joseph 81 mg Aspirin Chewable and Enteric Coated Tablets 1903
▲ Taxotere Injection Concentrate (1.7% to 8.1%) 2773

Dysstasia

Xyrem Oral Solution (Infrequent) 1766

Dystonia

Abilify Injection (2%) 881
Abilify Injection (2%) 2466
Abilify Oral Solution (2%) 881
Abilify Oral Solution (2%) 2466
Abilify Discmelt Orally Disintegrating Tablets (2%) 881
Abilify Discmelt Orally Disintegrating Tablets (2%) 2466
Abilify Tablets (2%) 881
Abilify Tablets (2%) 2466
AmBisome for Injection (Less common) 606
▲ Azilect Tablets (3%) 3106
Celexa (Infrequent) 1160
Cuprimine Capsules 1986
Effexor XR Extended-Release Capsules (Rare) 3195
Eldepryl Capsules 3052
Exelon Capsules (Infrequent) 2229
Exelon Oral Solution (Infrequent) 2229
Gabitril Tablets (Infrequent) 973
▲ Geodon Capsules (4% to 14%) 2520
Imitrex Injection (Rare) 1465
Imitrex Tablets (Rare) 1474
▲ Invega Extended-Release Tablets (1% to 5%) 1748
Lamictal (Rare) 1488
Lexapro Oral Suspension 1174
Lexapro Tablets 1174
Luvox CR Extended-Release Capsules (Infrequent) 1759
Lyrica Capsules (Rare) 2527
▲ Mirapex Tablets (2% to 8%) 857
Moban Tablets (Infrequent) 1116
Paxil (Infrequent) 1535
Paxil CR Controlled-Release Tablets (Infrequent) 1544
Phenytek Capsules (Rare) 2192
Prozac Weekly Capsules (Rare) 1852
Prozac Pulvules and Liquid (Rare) 1852
Remeron Tablets (Infrequent) 2924
RemeronSolTab Tablets (Infrequent) 2927
Requip Tablets (1% or more) 1561
Risperdal Consta Long-Acting Injection (Frequent) 1753
Symbyax Capsules (Less than 1%) ... 1871
Thioridazine Hydrochloride Tablets... 2195
Venlafaxine Hydrochloride Tablets (Rare) 2199
Wellbutrin Tablets (Frequent)........... 1648
Wellbutrin SR Sustained-Release Tablets 1653
Wellbutrin XL Extended-Release Tablets 1659
Zofran Injection 1682
Zofran 1687
Zofran ODT Orally Disintegrating Tablets 1687
Zomig Tablets (Rare) 694
Zomig-ZMT Tablets (Rare) 694
Zonegran Capsules (Rare)................ 1089
Zyban Sustained-Release Tablets 1692
▲ Zyprexa Tablets (Les than 1% to 3%).. 1883
▲ Zyprexa IntraMuscular (Less than 1% to 3%)................................... 1883
▲ Zyprexa ZYDIS Orally Disintegrating Tablets (Less than 1% to 3%) 1883

Dystonia, tardive

Thioridazine Hydrochloride Tablets... 2195

Dystonic reactions

(*see under* Dystonia)

Dystrophy

Rocaltrol Capsules.......................... 1150
Rocaltrol Oral Solution.................... 1150

Dysuria

Abelcet Injection 1134
Actiq (Less than 1%)........................ 959
▲ Agrylin Capsules (1% to less than 5%).. 3017
Alferon N Injection (1%).................. 1726
Alinia for Oral Suspension (Less than 1%)....................................... 2677
Alinia Tablets (Less than 1%)........... 2677
Allegra-D 12 Hour Extended-Release Tablets............ 2687
Allegra-D 24 Hour Extended-Release Tablets............ 2690
Ambien Tablets (Rare)..................... 2692
Ambien CR Tablets (1%).................. 2696
AmBisome for Injection (Less common)..................................... 606
Anaprox Tablets (Less than 1%)....... 2632
Anaprox DS Tablets (Less than 1%).. 2632
Anzemet Injection (Rare)................. 2701
Anzemet Tablets (Rare)................... 2704
Aricept Tablets (Infrequent)............. 1062
Aricept ODT Tablets (Infrequent)....... 1062
Asacol Delayed-Release Tablets....... 2579
▲ Avinza Capsules (Less than 5%) 1772
▲ Busulfex Injection (7%) 2477
Ceftin Tablets (0.1% to 1%).............. 1380
Celebrex Capsules (0.1% to 1.9%)... 2979
Celexa (Infrequent).......................... 1160
▲ CellCept Capsules (3% to less than 20%)...................................... 2622
▲ CellCept Intravenous (3% to less than 20%)...................................... 2622
▲ CellCept Oral Suspension (3% to less than 20%)............................. 2622
▲ CellCept Tablets (3% to less than 20%).. 2622
Clinoril Tablets................................ 1962
Clorpres Tablets (Rare).................... 2185
Combivent Inhalation Aerosol (Less than 2%)............................ 845
Copaxone for Injection (At least 2%)... 3110
Crinone 4% Gel............................... 992
Crixivan Capsules (1.5%)................. 1979
Cymbalta Delayed-Release Capsules (Infrequent)................... 1801
▲ Dacogen Injection (6%) 1066
Demser Capsules (Few patients)....... 1989
Depakote ER Tablets (Greater than or equal to 1%)............................ 423
Diovan HCT Tablets (Less Frequent)...................................... 2216
▲ Doxil Injection (1% to 10%) 2378
DynaCirc CR Controlled Release Tablets (0.5% to 1%).................... 1407
EC-Naprosyn Delayed-Release Tablets (Less than 1%)................. 2632
▲ Eloxatin for Injection (1% to 6%) 2731
Emend Capsules (Greater than 0.5%).. 1992
Emend for Injection (Greater than 0.5%).. 1999
Emsam Transdermal System (Infrequent).................................... 905
Evoxac Capsules (Less than 1%)...... 1013
Exelon Capsules (Infrequent)............ 2229
Exelon Oral Solution (Infrequent)...... 2229
Exforge Tablets (Less than equal to 0.1%).. 2238
Gabitril Tablets (Frequent)................ 973
Gengraf Capsules (1%).................... 435
Imitrex Injection (Rare).................... 1465
Imitrex Nasal Spray (Infrequent)....... 1470
Imitrex Tablets (Up to 2%)............... 1474
▲ Intron A for Injection (Less than 5%)... 2859
Invanz for Injection (1.1%)............... 2029
Ionsys Transdermal System (.1% to less than 1%)........................... 2410
Klonopin (Infrequent)....................... 2639
Lamictal (Rare)............................... 1488
Lexapro Oral Suspension (Infrequent)................................... 1174
Lexapro Tablets (Infrequent)............. 1174
Lipitor Tablets (Less than 2%).......... 2501
Lunesta Tablets (Infrequent)............. 2994
Lupron Depot 3.75 mg (Among most frequent)............................. 462
▲ Lupron Depot–3 Month 11.25 mg (Less than 5%)............................ 462
Luvox CR Extended-Release Capsules (Infrequent) 1759
Lyrica Capsules (0.1% to 1%) 2527
Marplan Tablets 3177
Maxalt Tablets (Rare) 2056
Maxalt-MLT Orally Disintegrating Tablets (Rare) 2056
Merrem I.V. (Greater than 0.1% to 1%) 684
Mirapex Tablets 857
▲ Myfortic Tablets (3% to less than 20%) 2276
Nalfon Capsules (Less than 1%) 2508
Namenda (Infrequent) 1180
Naprosyn Suspension (Less than 1%) 2632
Naprosyn Tablets (Less than 1%) 2632
Neoral Oral Solution (1%) 2280
Neoral Soft Gelatin Capsules (1%) 2280
Nexium Delayed-Release Capsules (Less than 1%) 645
Nexium I.V. (Less than 1%) 652
Nexium Delayed-Release Oral Suspension (Less than 1%) 645
Norvir (Less than 2%) 489
OxyContin Tablets (Less than 1%) 2589
Paxil (Infrequent) 1535
Paxil CR Controlled-Release Tablets (Infrequent) 1544
Prinivil Tablets (0.3% to 1%) 2087
Prinzide Tablets 2092
▲ ProAmatine Tablets (13.4%) 3032
▲ Prograf Capsules and Injection (3% to 15%) 622
Protonix for Delayed-Release Oral Suspension (Less than 1%) 3254
Protonix Delayed-Release Tablets (Less than 1%) 3254
Protonix I.V. (Less than 1%) 3257
Prozac Weekly Capsules (Infrequent) 1852
Prozac Pulvules and Liquid (Infrequent) 1852
Recombivax HB (Less than 1%) 2107
Remeron Tablets (Infrequent) 2924
RemeronSolTab Tablets (Infrequent) 2927
ReoPro Vials (0.4%) 1860
Requip Tablets (Infrequent) 1561
Retrovir Capsules 1574
Retrovir IV Infusion 1579
Retrovir 1574
Rilutek Tablets (Up to 1.2%) 2771
Rythmol SR Capsules 1590
Salagen Tablets (Less than 1%) 1082
▲ Simulect for Injection (3% to 10%) ... 2306
Soriatane Capsules (Less than 1%) .. 3062
Sular Extended Release Tablets (Less than or equal to 1%) 2975
Symbyax Capsules (Infrequent) 1871
Tasigna Capsules (0.1% to 1%) 2316
▲ Tice BCG (52% to 60%) 2936
Ultram ER Extended-Release Tablets (0.5% to less than 1%) 2428
Uroqid-Acid No. 2 Tablets (Occasional) 814
▲ Valcyte Tablets (Less than 5%) 2654
▲ Valstar Sterile Solution for Intravesical Instillation (56%) 1735
Vantas (Less than 2%) 1737
Venlafaxine Hydrochloride Tablets (Infrequent) 2199
▲ Vesanoid Capsules (9%) 2660
Viadur Implant (Less than 2%) 802
Voltaren Tablets (Occasionally) 2334
Voltaren-XR Tablets (Occasionally) 2337
Wellbutrin Tablets (Rare) 1648
Wellbutrin SR Sustained-Release Tablets 1653
Wellbutrin XL Extended-Release Tablets 1659

Xifaxan Tablets (Less than 2%)........ 2682
Zofran Injection (2%)........ 1682
Zonegran Capsules (Infrequent)........ 1089
Zosyn for Injection (1% or less)........ 3284
Zyban Sustained-Release Tablets........ 1692
Zyprexa Tablets (Infrequent)........ 1883
Zyprexa ZYDIS Orally Disintegrating Tablets (Infrequent)........ 1883
Zyrtec Chewable Tablets (Less than 2%)........ 1920
Zyrtec Syrup (Less than 2%)........ 1920
Zyrtec Tablets (Less than 2%)........ 1920
Zyrtec-D 12 Hour Extended Release Tablets (Less than 2%)........ 1923

Dyuria
Targretin Capsules........ 1084
Tricor Tablets........ 520

E

Ear, discomfort
Adenoscan (Less than 1%)........ 605
▲ Aerobid/Aerobid-M (1% to 3%)........ 1153
▲ Ciprodex Otic Suspension (3%)........ 541
Xyrem Oral Solution (Infrequent)........ 1766

Ear, disorders of
▲ Advair HFA 45/21 Inhalation Aerosol (1% to 3%)........ 1288
▲ Advair HFA 115/21 Inhalation Aerosol (1% to 3%)........ 1288
▲ Advair HFA 230/21 Inhalation Aerosol (1% to 3%)........ 1288
▲ Busulfex Injection (3%)........ 2477
▲ CellCept Capsules (3% to less than 20%)........ 2622
▲ CellCept Intravenous (3% to less than 20%)........ 2622
▲ CellCept Oral Suspension (3% to less than 20%)........ 2622
▲ CellCept Tablets (3% to less than 20%)........ 2622
Ciprodex Otic Suspension (1 patient)........ 541
▲ Imitrex Nasal Spray (2.5% to 3.8%)........ 1470
Meridia Capsules (1.7%)........ 475
ProAir HFA Inhalation Aerosol (Less than 3%)........ 3113
▲ Risperdal Consta Long-Acting Injection (3%)........ 1753
Salagen Tablets (Less than 1%)........ 1082

Ear, drainage
▲ Epivir (7%)........ 1412

Ear, external abnormalities, fetal
Accutane Capsules........ 2607
CellCept Capsules........ 2622
CellCept Intravenous........ 2622
CellCept Oral Suspension........ 2622
CellCept Tablets........ 2622

Ear congestion
Ciprodex Otic Suspension (0.4%)........ 541

Ear debris
Ciprodex Otic Suspension (0.6%)........ 541

Ear disease, unspecified
Actiq (1% or greater)........ 959
Asacol Delayed-Release Tablets (2% or greater)........ 2579
Avapro Tablets (Less than 1%)........ 897
Avapro Tablets (Less than 1%)........ 2718
Cardene I.V. (Rare)........ 1093
Celebrex Capsules (0.1% to 1.9%)........ 2979
Exubera Inhalation Powder (1.3%)........ 2515
Gengraf Capsules (1%)........ 435
▲ Humatrope Vials and Cartridges (11.8%)........ 1838
Lamictal (2%)........ 1488
Neoral Oral Solution (1%)........ 2280
Neoral Soft Gelatin Capsules (1%)........ 2280
Protopic Ointment (0.2% to less than 1%)........ 628
Provigil Tablets (At least 1%)........ 977
Tamiflu Capsules (2%)........ 2649
Tamiflu Oral Suspension (2%)........ 2649
▲ Vesanoid Capsules (6%)........ 2660

Ear precipitate
Ciprodex Otic Suspension (0.5%)........ 541

Earache
Aceon Tablets (2 mg, 4 mg, 8 mg) (0.3% to 1%)........ 3038
Advair HFA 45/21 Inhalation Aerosol........ 1288
Advair HFA 115/21 Inhalation Aerosol........ 1288
Advair HFA 230/21 Inhalation Aerosol........ 1288
Elidel Cream 1% (0% to 2.9%)........ 2221
▲ Hycamtin for Injection (59%)........ 1459
Risperdal Consta Long-Acting Injection (Infrequent)........ 1753
Twinrix Vaccine........ 1628
Xolair (2%)........ 2339
Zyrtec Chewable Tablets (Less than 2%)........ 1920
Zyrtec Syrup (Less than 2%)........ 1920
Zyrtec Tablets (Less than 2%)........ 1920
Zyrtec-D 12 Hour Extended Release Tablets (Less than 2%)........ 1923

Early morning awakening
Requip Tablets (Infrequent)........ 1561

Ears, blocked
Asacol Delayed-Release Tablets........ 2579
▲ Chemet Capsules (1% to 3.7%)........ 2484
Orthoclone OKT3 Sterile Solution........ 2387

Ears, ringing
(*see under* Tinnitus)

Ebriety, feeling of
▲ Intron A for Injection (Less than 5%)........ 2859

Ecchymoses
Abilify Injection (Greater than or equal to 1 in 1000 patients and less than 1 in 100 patients)........ 2466
Abilify Oral Solution (Greater than or equal to 1 in 1000 patients and less than 1 in 100 patients)........ 2466
Abilify Discmelt Orally Disintegrating Tablets (Greater than or equal to 1 in 1000 patients and less than 1 in 100 patients)........ 2466
Abilify Tablets (Greater than or equal to 1 in 1000 patients and less than 1 in 100 patients)........ 2466
Aceon Tablets (2 mg, 4 mg, 8 mg) (0.3% to 1%)........ 3038
Actiq (1% or greater)........ 959
Activase I.V. (1%)........ 1188
▲ Actonel with Calcium Tablets (4.3%)........ 2574
▲ Advair Diskus 100/50 (7%)........ 1276
Advair Diskus 250/50........ 1276
Advair Diskus 500/50........ 1276
Advair HFA 45/21 Inhalation Aerosol........ 1288
Advair HFA 115/21 Inhalation Aerosol........ 1288
Advair HFA 230/21 Inhalation Aerosol........ 1288
▲ Agrylin Capsules (1% to less than 5%)........ 3017
▲ Anaprox Tablets (3% to 9%)........ 2632
▲ Anaprox DS Tablets (3% to 9%)........ 2632
▲ Aricept Tablets (5%)........ 1062
▲ Aricept ODT Tablets (5%)........ 1062
Avapro Tablets (Less than 1%)........ 897
Avapro Tablets (Less than 1%)........ 2718
▲ Azilect Tablets (2% to 5%)........ 3106
Campral Tablets (Infrequent)........ 1158
Cardizem LA Extended Release Tablets (Less than 2%)........ 421
Celebrex Capsules (0.1% to 1.9%)........ 2979
Celexa........ 1160
Clinoril Tablets (Less than 1%)........ 1962
Comvax........ 1966
▲ Copaxone for Injection (8%)........ 3110
Cozaar Tablets (Less than 1%)........ 1973
▲ Dacogen Injection (22%)........ 1066
▲ Depakote ER Tablets (Greater than 1% to less than 5%)........ 423
▲ Doxil Injection (1% to 10%)........ 2378
▲ EC-Naprosyn Delayed-Release Tablets (3% to 9%)........ 2632
Effexor XR Extended-Release Capsules (Frequent)........ 3195
Elmiron Capsules (Less than or equal to 1%)........ 2435
Engerix-B Vaccine (Less than 1%)........ 1409
Flovent Diskus 50 mcg........ 1435
Flovent HFA........ 1440
▲ Gabitril Tablets (1% to 6%)........ 973
▲ Gamunex (40%)........ 3094
Geodon Capsules (Infrequent)........ 2520
▲ Hyalgan Solution (14%)........ 2742
Indocin Capsules (Less than 1%)........ 2024
Indocin I.V. (Less than 1%)........ 2489
Indocin (Less than 1%)........ 2024
Lamictal (Infrequent)........ 1488
Lexapro Oral Suspension........ 1174
Lexapro Tablets........ 1174
Lipitor Tablets (Less than 2%)........ 2501
Lotrisone........ 2881
▲ Lovenox Injection (Up to 3%)........ 2756
Lupron Depot 3.75 mg (Among most frequent)........ 462
▲ Lupron Depot 7.5 mg (Less than 5%)........ 469
▲ Lupron Depot–3 Month 11.25 mg (Less than 5%)........ 462
Meridia Capsules (0.7%)........ 475
▲ Mylotarg for Injection (9% to 11%)........ 3212
Nabi-HB (2%)........ 815
▲ Naprosyn Suspension (3% to 9%)........ 2632
▲ Naprosyn Tablets (3% to 9%)........ 2632
Norvir (Less than 2%)........ 489
▲ Novantrone for Injection Concentrate (7% to 11%)........ 1100
Paxil (Infrequent)........ 1535
Paxil CR Controlled-Release Tablets (Infrequent)........ 1544
Pentasa Capsules (Less than 1%)........ 3030
Pletal Tablets (Less than 2%)........ 2481
▲ Prograf Capsules and Injection (3% to 15%)........ 622
Protonix for Delayed-Release Oral Suspension (Less than 1%)........ 3254
Protonix Delayed-Release Tablets (Less than 1%)........ 3254
Protonix I.V. (Less than 1%)........ 3257
Protopic Ointment (Greater than or equal to 1%)........ 628
Provigil Tablets (At least 1%)........ 977
Prozac Weekly Capsules (Infrequent)........ 1852
Prozac Pulvules and Liquid (Infrequent)........ 1852
Rilutek Tablets (Infrequent)........ 2771
▲ Rythmol SR Capsules (2% to 4%)........ 1590
Sular Extended Release Tablets (Less than or equal to 1%)........ 2975
Tarka Tablets........ 511
Tricor Tablets........ 520
▲ Trisenox Injection (20%)........ 986
Twinrix Vaccine (Less than 1%)........ 1628
Vaqta (1%)........ 2130
▲ Viadur Implant (4.6%)........ 802
Voltaren Tablets (Occasionally)........ 2334
Voltaren-XR Tablets (Occasionally)........ 2337
Wellbutrin Tablets........ 1648
Wellbutrin SR Sustained-Release Tablets (Infrequent)........ 1653
Wellbutrin XL Extended-Release Tablets (Infrequent)........ 1659
Zomig Tablets (Rare)........ 694
Zomig Nasal Spray (Rare)........ 689
Zomig-ZMT Tablets (Rare)........ 694
Zonegran Capsules (2%)........ 1089
Zyban Sustained-Release Tablets (Infrequent)........ 1692
▲ Zyprexa Tablets (5%)........ 1883
▲ Zyprexa ZYDIS Orally Disintegrating Tablets (5%)........ 1883

Ecchymosis, injection site
Bicillin C-R Injectable Suspension........ 1775
Bicillin L-A Injection........ 1777
▲ Edex Injection (4%)........ 2957
▲ Fluarix Vaccine (1% to 10%)........ 1446
ProQuad (1.5%)........ 2099
▲ Vivitrol (4% to 7%)........ 988

Ecchymosis, soft eyelid tissue
BOTOX Purified Neurotoxin Complex........ 550

Ecchymosis, unspecified
▲ CellCept Capsules (3% to less than 20%)........ 2622
▲ CellCept Intravenous (3% to less than 20%)........ 2622
▲ CellCept Oral Suspension (3% to less than 20%)........ 2622
▲ CellCept Tablets (3% to less than 20%)........ 2622
Cymbalta Delayed-Release Capsules (Rare)........ 1801
Elmiron Capsules........ 2435
Emsam Transdermal System (Frequent)........ 905
▲ Keppra Oral Solution (1% to 4%)........ 3131
▲ Keppra Tablets (1% to 4%)........ 3131
▲ Luvox CR Extended-Release Capsules (4%)........ 1759
Lyrica Capsules (Greater than or equal to 1%)........ 2527
Mirapex Tablets........ 857
Percodan Tablets........ 1130
Pristiq Extended-Release Tablets........ 3247
▲ Pulmicort Flexhaler (Greater than or equal to 1% to 3%)........ 654
Symbyax Capsules (Frequent)........ 1871
Tasigna Capsules (0.1% to 1%)........ 2316
Treximet Tablets (Rare)........ 1616
Venlafaxine Hydrochloride Tablets (Frequent)........ 2199
Zomig Tablets (Infrequent)........ 694
Zomig-ZMT Tablets (Infrequent)........ 694

Eccrine gland disorders
▲ Selzentry Tablets (4.5%)........ 2534

ECG changes
(*see under* EKG changes)

Eclampsia
Paxil........ 1535
Paxil CR Controlled-Release Tablets........ 1544

Ectopy, ventricular
Cipro (Less than 1%)........ 2810
Cipro XR Tablets........ 2823

Ectropion
BOTOX Purified Neurotoxin Complex (Less than 1%)........ 550
Soriatane Capsules (Less than 1%)........ 3062

Eczema
Accutane Capsules........ 2607
▲ Advair HFA 45/21 Inhalation Aerosol (1% to 3%)........ 1288
▲ Advair HFA 115/21 Inhalation Aerosol (1% to 3%)........ 1288
▲ Advair HFA 230/21 Inhalation Aerosol (1% to 3%)........ 1288
▲ Aerobid/Aerobid-M (3% to 9%)........ 1153
Aldara Cream, 5% (2%)........ 1699
Altabax Ointment (1%)........ 1299
▲ Aricept Tablets (3%)........ 1062
▲ Aricept ODT Tablets (3%)........ 1062
Atacand HCT (0.5% or greater)........ 642
Celexa (Infrequent)........ 1160
Chantix Tablets (Infrequent)........ 2511
Copaxone for Injection (Frequent)........ 3110
Cubicin for Injection (Less than 1%)........ 995
Dantrium Capsules (Less frequent)........ 2580
Daytrana Transdermal Patch........ 3022
Effexor XR Extended-Release Capsules (Infrequent)........ 3195
Emsam Transdermal System (Rare)........ 905
Engerix-B Vaccine........ 1409
Evoxac Capsules (Less than 1%)........ 1013
Exelon Capsules (Frequent)........ 2229
Exelon Oral Solution (Frequent)........ 2229
Exelon Patch (Infrequent)........ 2233
Exforge Tablets (Greater than or equal to 0.2%)........ 2238
▲ Flolan for Injection (25%)........ 1426
▲ Flovent Diskus 50 mcg (1% to 3%)........ 1435
Gabitril Tablets (Infrequent)........ 973
Gengraf Capsules (1% to less than 3%)........ 435
Geodon Capsules (Infrequent)........ 2520
Imitrex Injection........ 1465
Imitrex Nasal Spray........ 1470
▲ Intron A for Injection (Less than 5%)........ 2859
Kaletra (Less than 2%)........ 452
Ketek Tablets (Less than 0.2%)........ 2744
Lamictal (2%)........ 1488
Lexapro Oral Suspension (Infrequent)........ 1174
Lexapro Tablets (Infrequent)........ 1174
Lipitor Tablets (Less than 2%)........ 2501
Lovaza Capsules........ 1520
Lunesta Tablets (Infrequent)........ 2994
Luvox CR Extended-Release Capsules (Infrequent)........ 1759
Lyrica Capsules (0.1% to 1%)........ 2527
Miacalcin Nasal Spray (Less than 1%)........ 2274
Micardis Tablets (More than 0.3%)........ 852
Micardis HCT Tablets........ 854
Mirapex Tablets........ 857
Namenda (Infrequent)........ 1180
Neoral Oral Solution (1% to less than 3%)........ 2280
Neoral Soft Gelatin Capsules (1% to less than 3%)........ 2280
Nexavar Tablets (0.1% to less than 1%)........ 784
Norditropin Cartridges........ 2354
Norvir (Less than 2%)........ 489
Olux Foam (One case)........ 3061
Paxil (Infrequent)........ 1535
Paxil CR Controlled-Release Tablets (Infrequent)........ 1544
Pentasa Capsules (Less than 1%)........ 3030
Plavix Tablets (1% to 2.5%)........ 926
Plavix Tablets (1% to 2.5%)........ 2767
Protonix for Delayed-Release Oral Suspension (Less than 1%)........ 3254
Protonix Delayed-Release Tablets (Less than 1%)........ 3254
Protonix I.V. (Less than 1%)........ 3257
▲ Protopic Ointment (Up to 3%)........ 628
Prozac Weekly Capsules (Infrequent)........ 1852

Prozac Pulvules and Liquid (Infrequent) 1852
Recombivax HB 2107
Requip Tablets (Infrequent) 1561
Rilutek Tablets (0.8% to 1.6%) 2771
Risperdal Consta Long-Acting Injection (Infrequent) 1753
Salagen Tablets (Less than 1%) 1082
▲ Selzentry Tablets (3.1%) 2534
▲ Serevent Diskus (1% to 3%) 1594
Singulair (Greater than or equal to 2%) 2114
Soriatane Capsules (Less than 1%) .. 3062
Sustiva Capsules (Less than 2%) 930
Sustiva Tablets (Less than 2%) 930
Symbyax Capsules (Infrequent) 1871
Synagis Intramuscular Solution (More than 1%) 1948
Tamiflu Capsules 2649
Tamiflu Oral Suspension 2649
▲ Tasigna Capsules (1% to 10%) 2316
Teveten Tablets (Less than 1%) 515
Teveten HCT Tablets (Less than 1%) 517
Tricor Tablets 520
Twinrix Vaccine 1628
Varivax (Greater than or equal to 1%) 2133
Venlafaxine Hydrochloride Tablets (Infrequent) 2199
▲ Visudyne for Injection (1% to 10%) .. 2332
▲ Voltaren Ophthalmic Solution (Less than or equal to 3%) 2336
Vytorin 10/10 Tablets 2939
Vytorin 10/20 Tablets 2939
Vytorin 10/40 Tablets 2939
Vytorin 10/80 Tablets 2939
Xopenex Inhalation Solution 3001
Xopenex Inhalation Solution Concentrate 3005
Xopenex HFA Inhalation Aerosol 3009
▲ Zocor Tablets (4.5%) 2136
Zomig Tablets (Rare) 694
Zomig Nasal Spray (Rare) 689
Zomig-ZMT Tablets (Rare) 694
Zonegran Capsules (Infrequent) 1089
▲ Zosyn for Injection (4.2%) 3284
Zovirax Cream 817
Zyprexa Tablets (Infrequent) 1883
Zyprexa ZYDIS Orally Disintegrating Tablets (Infrequent) 1883
Zyrtec Chewable Tablets (Less than 2%) 1920
Zyrtec Syrup (Less than 2%) 1920
Zyrtec Tablets (Less than 2%) 1920
Zyrtec-D 12 Hour Extended Release Tablets (Less than 2%) 1923

Eczema at injection site
ProQuad 2099

Eczema herpeticum
Protopic Ointment (Up to 2%) 628

Eczematous reactions
(*see under* Eczema)

Edema
Accolate Tablets 669
Accutane Capsules 2607
▲ Aceon Tablets (2 mg, 4 mg, 8 mg) (0.3% to 3.9%) 3038
Actiq (Less than 1%) 959
Activella Tablets 2347
▲ ActoPlus Met Tablets (4.8% to 6%) 3071
▲ Actos Tablets (4.8% to 7.2%) 3077
Advair Diskus 100/50 1276
Advair Diskus 250/50 1276
Advair Diskus 500/50 1276
Advicor Tablets 402
▲ Aerobid/Aerobid-M (3% to 9%) 1153
▲ Agrylin Capsules (20.6%) 3017
▲ Aldara Cream, 5% (Up to 49%) 1699
Alferon N Injection (One patient) 1726
▲ Alimta for Injection (Up to 19%) 1786
Ambien Tablets (Infrequent) 2692
Ambien CR Tablets (Infrequent) 2696
▲ AmBisome for Injection (12.3% to 14.3%) 606
Amerge Tablets (Infrequent) 1301
Amevive (2%) 611
▲ Amitiza Capsules (0% to 3%) 3082
▲ Anaprox Tablets (3% to 9%) 2632
▲ Anaprox DS Tablets (3% to 9%) 2632
AndroGel 3159
Angeliq Tablets 751
Anzemet Injection (Rare) 2701
Anzemet Tablets (Rare) 2704
▲ Aranesp for Injection (6% to 21%) 564
Aricept Tablets (Frequent) 1062
Aricept ODT Tablets (Frequent) 1062
▲ Arimidex Tablets (7% to 11%) 672
▲ Arixtra Injection (0.9% to 8.7%) 1313
▲ Arranon Injection (0% to 11%) 1319
Asacol Delayed-Release Tablets 2579
Atrovent Nasal Spray 0.03% 834
Atrovent Nasal Spray 0.06% 836
▲ Avalide Tablets (3%) 892
▲ Avalide Tablets (3%) 2713
▲ Avandamet Tablets (2% to 14.7%) ... 1336
▲ Avandaryl Tablets (1% to 4.8%) 1344
▲ Avandia Tablets (4.8% to 25%) 1351
Avapro Tablets (1% or greater) 897
Avapro Tablets (1% or greater) 2718
Avelox 2803
▲ Avinza Capsules (Less than 5%) 1772
▲ Azor Tablets (1.8% to 14.6%) 1005
Bicillin C-R Injectable Suspension 1775
Bicillin L-A Injection 1777
▲ Busulfex Injection (28% to 79%) 2477
Cancidas for Injection 1953
Captopril Tablets 2182
Carbatrol Capsules 3019
▲ Cardizem LA Extended Release Tablets (Up to 4.6%) 421
Catapres-TTS (3 of 101 patients) 842
Celebrex Capsules (0.1% to 1.9%) 2979
Chantix Tablets (Frequent) 2511
Cipro I.V. 2817
Clarinex Syrup (Rare) 2828
Clarinex Tablets (Rare) 2828
Clarinex Reditabs Tablets (Rare) 2828
Clarinex-D 12-Hour Extended-Release Tablets (Rare) ... 2831
Clarinex-D 24-Hour Extended-Release Tablets 2834
▲ Climara Transdermal System (0.5% to 13%) 763
▲ Climara Pro Transdermal System (3.8%) 768
Clinoril Tablets (Greater than 1%) 1962
▲ Clolar for Intravenous Infusion (20%) 1239
Combigan Ophthalmic Solution 553
Combivent Inhalation Aerosol (Less than 2%) 845
Comvax 1966
▲ Copaxone for Injection (3%) 3110
▲ Coreg Tablets (5% to 6%) 1387
Cozaar Tablets (1% or greater) 1973
Crinone 4% Gel 992
Crinone 8% Gel 992
▲ Cubicin for Injection (1% to 6.7%) 995
▲ Dacogen Injection (18%) 1066
Daytrana Transdermal Patch 3022
Delatestryl Injection 1730
Demadex Injection (1.1%) 2630
Demadex Tablets (1.1%) 2630
▲ Depakote ER Tablets (Greater than 1% to less than 5%) 423
▲ DepoCyt Injection (2% to 3%) 1136
Diovan Tablets (0.2% to greater than 1%) 2212
Divigel 3167
▲ Doxil Injection (1% to 10%) 2378
▲ Duetact Tablets (Greater than 5%) ... 3085
Duragesic Transdermal System (1% or greater) 2405
▲ DynaCirc CR Controlled Release Tablets (8.9% to 35.9%) 1407
▲ EC-Naprosyn Delayed-Release Tablets (3% to 9%) 2632
Effexor XR Extended-Release Capsules (Frequent) 3195
▲ Eloxatin for Injection (1% to 15%) 2731
Emend Capsules (Greater than 0.5%) 1992
Emend for Injection (Greater than 0.5%) 1999
Emsam Transdermal System (Infrequent) 905
Enjuvia Tablets 1029
▲ Epogen for Injection (6% to 17%) 576
▲ Equetro Extended-Release Capsules (Less than 5%) 3174
Estratest Tablets 3043
Estratest H.S. Tablets 3043
▲ Evoxac Capsules (1% to 3%) 1013
Exelon Capsules (Frequent) 2229
Exelon Oral Solution (Frequent) 2229
Exforge Tablets (Greater than or equal to 0.2%) 2238
Exjade Tablets (0.1% to 1%) 2244
▲ Femara Tablets (0.1% to 18.4%) 2246
Finacea Gel (1% or less) 1742
Flebogamma 5% 1715
Flebogamma 5% DIF 1718
Flector Patch 561
▲ Flolan for Injection (60% to 79%) 1426
▲ Flovent Diskus 50 mcg (1% to 3%) 1435
Gabitril Tablets (Frequent) 973
Gantrisin Pediatric Suspension 2638
▲ Gemzar for Injection (Less than 1% to 13%) 1820
▲ Gengraf Capsules (10%) 435
▲ Gleevec Tablets (61.7% to 81%) 2255
▲ Herceptin I.V. (8%) 1199
▲ Humatrope Vials and Cartridges (2.5% to 21.2%) 1838
Imitrex Nasal Spray (Infrequent) 1470
Imitrex Tablets (Rare to infrequent) ... 1474
Indocin Capsules (Less than 1%) 2024
Indocin I.V. (Less than 1%) 2489
Indocin (Less than 1%) 2024
▲ Intron A for Injection (Less than or equal to 5%) 2859
▲ Invanz for Injection (2.9% to 3.4%) 2029
Invega Extended-Release Tablets 1748
Ionsys Transdermal System (.1% to less than 1%) 2410
▲ Ixempra Kit for Injection (9%) 915
Kaletra (Less than 2%) 452
▲ Kepivance (28%) 583
Klonopin (Infrequent) 2639
Lamictal (2%) 1488
▲ Leukine (13% to 34%) 774
▲ Leustatin Injection (6%) 2384
Levaquin (1%) 2416
Levaquin in 5% Dextrose Injection (1%) 2416
Lipitor Tablets (Less than 2%) 2501
Lotrisone (Less than 1%) 2881
Lovenox Injection (2%) 2756
▲ Lupron Depot 3.75 mg (5.4%) 462
▲ Lupron Depot 7.5 mg (14.3%) 469
▲ Lupron Depot–3 Month 11.25 mg (5.4% to 7%) 462
Luvox CR Extended-Release Capsules (Frequent) 1759
Lybrel Tablets 3204
▲ Lyrica Capsules (1% to 6%) 2527
Mavik Tablets (0.3% to 1%) 472
Maxair Autohaler 1705
Maxalt Tablets (Rare) 2056
Maxalt-MLT Orally Disintegrating Tablets (Rare) 2056
▲ Megace ES Oral Suspension (1% to 3%) 2499
Meridia Capsules (1.2%) 475
Micardis Tablets 852
Micardis HCT Tablets 854
▲ Mirapex Tablets (4% to 5%) 857
Mircette Tablets 1034
Mobic Oral Suspension (0.6% to 2.4%) 863
Mobic Tablets (0.6% to 2.4%) 863
MS Contin Tablets (Less frequent) 2585
▲ Mycamine for Injection (16.2%) 616
▲ Myfortic Tablets (3% to less than 20%) 2276
▲ Naprosyn Suspension (3% to 9%) 2632
▲ Naprosyn Tablets (3% to 9%) 2632
▲ NeoProfen Injection (4%) 2496
▲ Neoral Oral Solution (2% to 10%) 2280
▲ Neoral Soft Gelatin Capsules (2% to 10%) 2280
Neupro Transdermal System 3149
Nexium Delayed-Release Capsules (Less than 1%) 645
Nexium I.V. (Less than 1%) 652
Nexium Delayed-Release Oral Suspension (Less than 1%) 645
Niaspan Extended-Release Tablets ... 480
Nimotop Capsules (Up to 1.2%) 790
▲ Norditropin Cartridges (25%) 2354
Noroxin Tablets (Less frequent) 2069
Norvir (Less than 2%) 489
▲ Novantrone for Injection Concentrate (10% to 30%) 1100
NovoSeven (1%) 2367
NovoSeven RT (1%) 2370
▲ Noxafil Oral Suspension (9%) 2889
▲ Nutropin for Injection (41%) 1208
▲ Nutropin AQ Injection (41%) 1212
▲ Nutropin AQ NuSpin Injection (41%) 1212
▲ Nutropin AQ Pen (41%) 1212
▲ Nutropin AQ Pen Cartridge (41%) 1212
NuvaRing 2897
▲ Ontak Vials (47%) 1079
Opana Tablets (Less than 1%) 1117
Opana ER Tablets (Less than 1%) 1121
OptiPranolol Metipranolol Ophthalmic Solution 0.3% (A small number of patients) .... ⊙ 245
Ortho-Cyclen Tablets 2449
Ortho Evra Transdermal System 2437
Ortho Tri-Cyclen Tablets 2449
Ortho Tri-Cyclen Lo Tablets 2458
OxyContin Tablets (Less than 1%) 2589
▲ Panretin Gel 0.1% (3% to 8%) 1081
Parnate Tablets 1532
Paxil (Frequent) 1535
Paxil CR Controlled-Release Tablets (Frequent) 1544
Pediarix Vaccine 1552
Pentasa Capsules (Less than 1%) 3030
▲ Photofrin for Injection (5% to 18%) 708
▲ Plavix Tablets (4.1%) 926
▲ Plavix Tablets (4.1%) 2767
Pletal Tablets (Less than 2%) 2481
Precose Tablets (Rare) 792
Premarin Intravenous 3217
Premarin Tablets 3221
Premarin Vaginal Cream 3228
Premphase Tablets 3232
Prempro Tablets 3232
Prinivil Tablets (0.3% to 1%) 2087
Prinzide Tablets 2092
▲ Procrit for Injection (6% to 17%) 2391
Proglycem Capsules (Frequent) 1185
Proglycem Suspension (Frequent) 1185
▲ Prograf Capsules and Injection (3% to 18%) 622
▲ Proleukin for Injection (15%) 2287
▲ Prometrium Capsules (100 mg, 200 mg) (Less than 5%) 3047
Protonix for Delayed-Release Oral Suspension (Less than 1%) 3254
Protonix Delayed-Release Tablets (Less than 1%) 3254
Protonix I.V. (Less than 1%) 3257
Protopic Ointment (Greater than or equal to 1%) 628
Proventil HFA Inhalation Aerosol (Less than 3%) 2914
Provigil Tablets (1%) 977
Prozac Weekly Capsules 1852
Prozac Pulvules and Liquid (Infrequent) 1852
▲ Rapamune (18% to 20%) 3260
Recombivax HB (Less than 1%) 2107
Remeron Tablets (1%) 2924
RemeronSolTab Tablets (1%) 2927
Remicade for IV Injection (Greater than or equal to 0.2%) 950
ReoPro Vials (0.3%) 1860
▲ Requip Tablets (Infrequent) 1561
Retrovir Capsules (0.8%) 1574
Retrovir IV Infusion (1%) 1579
Retrovir (0.8%) 1574
Reyataz Capsules 3299
Rilutek Tablets (Rare to frequent) 2771
Rocephin Injectable Vials, ADD-Vantage, Galaxy, Bulk 2642
Rythmol Tablets (1%) 1586
▲ Rythmol SR Capsules (5% to 13%) .. 1590
▲ Salagen Tablets (1% to 5%) 1082
Sandimmune (2% or less) 2296
▲ Sandostatin Injection (1% to 4%) 2300
Sandostatin LAR Depot 2302
Seasonique Tablets 1046
Selzentry Tablets 2534
▲ Serevent Diskus (1% to 3%) 1594
▲ Simulect for Injection (Greater than or equal to 10%) 2306
Singulair 2114
▲ Soriatane Capsules (1% to 10%) 3062
Stalevo Tablets 2309
▲ Symbyax Capsules (Greater than or equal to 5%) 1871
▲ Tarceva Tablets (Less than 1% to 37%) 1228
▲ Targretin Gel 1% (10%) 1088
Tarka Tablets (0.3% to 1.3%) 511
▲ Taxotere Injection Concentrate (0% to 66.7%) 2773
Thioridazine Hydrochloride Tablets ... 2195
▲ Thyrogen for Injection (4 patients out of 55) 1244
Timoptic Sterile Ophthalmic Solution 2121
Timoptic in Ocudose 2124
Timoptic-XE Sterile Ophthalmic Gel Forming Solution 2125
▲ Torisel Injection (3% to 35%) 3272
▲ Tracleer Tablets (4%) 3289
Tricor Tablets 520
▲ Trisenox Injection (40%) 986
Trizivir Tablets 1622
Uroxatral Tablets 2786
▲ Valcyte Tablets (Less than 5%) 2654
Vantas (Less than 2%) 1737
Vaqta (Less than 1%) 2130
▲ Velcade for Injection (23%) 2168
Venlafaxine Hydrochloride Tablets (Frequent) 2199
▲ Vesanoid Capsules (29% to 32%) 2660
Viadur Implant (Less than 2%) 802
▲ Vicoprofen Tablets (3% to 9%) 533
▲ Voltaren Tablets (1% to 10%) 2334
▲ Voltaren-XR Tablets (1% to 10%) 2337
Vytorin 10/10 Tablets 2149
Vytorin 10/10 Tablets 2939
Vytorin 10/20 Tablets 2149
Vytorin 10/20 Tablets 2939
Vytorin 10/40 Tablets 2149
Vytorin 10/40 Tablets 2939

Vytorin 10/80 Tablets 2149
Vytorin 10/80 Tablets 2939
Wellbutrin Tablets (Frequent) 1648
Wellbutrin SR Sustained-Release Tablets (Infrequent) 1653
Wellbutrin XL Extended-Release Tablets (Infrequent) 1659
▲ Xeloda Tablets (1% to 9%) 2662
Xyrem Oral Solution (Infrequent) 1766
Yaz Tablets 805
▲ Zemplar Capsules (7%) 536
▲ Zemplar Injection (7%) 538
Ziagen 1673
Zocor Tablets (2.7%) 2136
Zomig Tablets (Infrequent) 694
Zomig-ZMT Tablets (Infrequent) 694
Zonegran Capsules (Infrequent) 1089
Zosyn for Injection (0.1% to 1.9%) 3284
Zyban Sustained-Release Tablets (Infrequent) 1692
Zyprexa Tablets (2%) 1883
Zyprexa ZYDIS Orally Disintegrating Tablets (2%) 1883
Zyvox (0% to 2.3%) 2552

Edema, aggravated
▲ Gleevec Tablets (6.9% to 22%) 2255

Edema, allergic, face
Flulaval Injection Vaccine 1448

Edema, allergic, mouth
Flulaval Injection Vaccine 1448

Edema, allergic, throat
Flulaval Injection Vaccine 1448

Edema, angioneurotic
Accolate Tablets 669
Anaprox Tablets (Less than 1%) 2632
Anaprox DS Tablets (Less than 1%) 2632
Atrovent Nasal Spray 0.06% (Rare) 836
Augmentin 1323
Augmentin Tablets 1327
Augmentin XR Extended Release Tablets 1333
Bexxar 1371
Byetta Injection 600
Carafate Suspension 706
Carafate Tablets 707
Catapres Tablets (About 5 in 1,000 patients) 841
Catapres-TTS (0.5% or less) 842
Ceftin 1380
Climara Transdermal System 763
Climara Pro Transdermal System 768
Clinoril Tablets (Less than 1 in 100) 1962
Clorpres Tablets (About 5 in 1,000) 2185
Comvax (Rare) 1966
Cozaar Tablets (Rare) 1973
Cyanokit 5g Antidote 1021
Cymbalta Delayed-Release Capsules 1801
Diovan HCT Tablets (Less frequent) 2216
EC-Naprosyn Delayed-Release Tablets (Less than 1%) 2632
Elidel Cream 1% 2221
Engerix-B Vaccine 1409
Flonase Nasal Spray 1431
Fluarix Vaccine 1446
Gengraf Capsules (1% to less than 3%) 435
Gris-PEG Tablets (Rare) 2507
Havrix Injection Vaccine 1454
Humira Injection 442
Imitrex Injection 1465
Imitrex Nasal Spray 1470
Imitrex Tablets 1474
Intelence Tablets (Less than or equal to 0.5%) 3119
Intron A for Injection (Rare) 2859
Lamictal (Rare) 1488
Lescol Capsules (Rare) 2268
Lescol XL Tablets 2268
Leukeran Tablets 1508
Levaquin 2416
Levaquin in 5% Dextrose Injection 2416
Lipitor Tablets 2501
Lybrel Tablets 3204
Malarone Pediatric Tablets 1521
Malarone Tablets 1521
Mavik Tablets (0.13%) 472
Meridia Capsules 475
Mevacor Tablets (Rare) 2063
Micardis Tablets 852
Micardis HCT Tablets 854
M-M-R II 2054
Naprosyn Suspension (Less than 1%) 2632
Naprosyn Tablets (Less than 1%) 2632
Neoral Oral Solution (1% to less than 3%) 2280
Neoral Soft Gelatin Capsules (1% to less than 3%) 2280
Niaspan Extended-Release Tablets 480
Noroxin Tablets 2069
Norvir 489
Orthoclone OKT3 Sterile Solution 2387
Paxil (Rare) 1535
Paxil CR Controlled-Release Tablets (Rare) 1544
Liquid PedvaxHIB (Rare) 2073
Pepcid Tablets (Infrequent) 2075
Pneumovax 23 2078
Premarin Vaginal Cream 3228
Prevnar 3241
Primaxin I.M. 2080
Primaxin I.V. (Less than 0.2%) 2083
Prinzide Tablets (Rare) 2092
ProQuad 2099
Proventil HFA Inhalation Aerosol (Rare) 2914
Raptiva for Injection 1218
Rilutek Tablets (Rare) 2771
Solodyn Extended Release Tablets 1938
▲ Stromectol Tablets (22.7%) 2120
Sular Extended Release Tablets (Very rare) 2975
Tarka Tablets (0.15%) 511
Thioridazine Hydrochloride Tablets 2195
Tracleer Tablets 3289
Trusopt Sterile Ophthalmic Solution 2128
Varivax 2133
Xyzal Oral Solution 3155
VESIcare Tablets 636
Vivitrol 988
Wellbutrin Tablets 1648
Wellbutrin SR Sustained-Release Tablets 1653
Wellbutrin XL Extended-Release Tablets 1659
Xifaxan Tablets 2682
Xyzal Oral Solution 2789
Zantac 25 EFFERdose Tablets (Rare) 1670
Zantac Injection (Rare) 1666
Zantac Injection Pharmacy Bulk Package (Rare) 1668
Zantac Injection Premixed (Rare) 1666
Zantac (Rare) 1670
Zofran Injection (Rare) 1682
Zolinza Capsules 2142
Zomig Tablets (Rare) 694
Zomig Nasal Spray (Rare) 689
Zomig-ZMT Tablets (Rare) 694
Zovirax Cream 817
Zyban Sustained-Release Tablets 1692

Edema, aphakic cystoid macular
Cosopt Sterile Ophthalmic Solution 1969
Timoptic Sterile Ophthalmic Solution (Less frequent) 2121
Timoptic in Ocudose (Less frequent) 2124
Timoptic-XE Sterile Ophthalmic Gel Forming Solution 2125

Edema, brain
▲ Gliadel Wafer (4% to 22.5%) 1076
Mirapex Tablets 857
Tasigna Capsules 2316

Edema, cerebral
Activase I.V. 1188
Aggrenox Capsules 819
Bayer Aspirin 750
Gleevec Tablets (Rare) 2255
Orthoclone OKT3 Sterile Solution 2387
Percocet Tablets 1127
Percodan Tablets 1130
Proleukin for Injection 2287
St. Joseph 81 mg Aspirin Chewable and Enteric Coated Tablets 1903
Thiothixene Capsules 2197
▲ Vesanoid Capsules (3%) 2660

Edema, conjunctival
▲ Alphagan P Ophthalmic Solution (1% to 4%) 549
Cipro (Less than 1%) 2810
Cipro XR Tablets 2823
Combigan Ophthalmic Solution (0.1% to 0.2%) 553
▲ Cosopt Sterile Ophthalmic Solution (1% to 5%) 1969
Effexor XR Extended-Release Capsules (Rare) 3195
▲ Gliadel Wafer (7%) 1076
▲ Lumigan Ophthalmic Solution (1% to 3%) 556
▲ Nevanac Ophthalmic Suspension 0.1% (1% to 5%) ⊙ 205
▲ Patanol Ophthalmic Solution (Less than 5%) 546
Paxil (Rare) 1535
Paxil CR Controlled-Release Tablets (Rare) 1544
Protopic Ointment (0.2% to less than 1%) 628
Venlafaxine Hydrochloride Tablets (Rare) 2199

Edema, corneal
▲ Diclofenac Sodium Ophthalmic Solution (Less than or equal to 5%) ⊙ 240
▲ Durezol Ophthalmic Emulsion (5% to 15%) ⊙ 275
▲ Nevanac Ophthalmic Suspension 0.1% (1% to 5%) ⊙ 205
▲ Voltaren Ophthalmic Solution (Less than or equal to 5%) 2336

Edema, cystoid macular
Advicor Tablets 402
Combigan Ophthalmic Solution 553
Lumigan Ophthalmic Solution 556
Niaspan Extended-Release Tablets 480

Edema, dependent
▲ Coreg Tablets (4%) 1387
▲ Coreg CR Extended-Release Capsules (4%) 1393
Micardis Tablets (More than 0.3%) 852
Micardis HCT Tablets 854
▲ Mobic Oral Suspension (0.6% to 4.5%) 863
▲ Mobic Tablets (0.6% to 4.5%) 863
▲ Requip Tablets (6%) 1561
▲ Simulect for Injection (3% to 10%) 2306
▲ Spiriva HandiHaler (3% to 5%) 870
Tasigna Capsules (0.1% to 1%) 2316
Teveten Tablets (1% or greater) 515
Teveten HCT Tablets (Less than 1%) 517

Edema, ear
▲ Epivir (7%) 1412

Edema, esophageal
▲ Photofrin for Injection (8%) 708

Edema, extremities
Celexa (Infrequent) 1160
Cipro I.V. (1% or less) 2817
Depakote ER Tablets 423
Imitrex Injection (Rare) 1465
Lexapro Oral Suspension (Infrequent) 1174
Lexapro Tablets (Infrequent) 1174
Tarka Tablets 511
Taxotere Injection Concentrate 2773

Edema, eye
▲ Gleevec Tablets (33.3%) 2255

Edema, eyelid
Abilify Injection (Greater than or equal to 1 in 1000 patients and less than 1 in 100 patients) 881
Abilify Injection (Greater than or equal to 1 in 1000 patients and less than 1 in 100 patients) 2466
Abilify Oral Solution (Greater than or equal to 1 in 1000 patients and less than 1 in 100 patients) 881
Abilify Oral Solution (Greater than or equal to 1 in 1000 patients and less than 1 in 100 patients) 2466
Abilify Discmelt Orally Disintegrating Tablets (Greater than or equal to 1 in 1000 patients and less than 1 in 100 patients) 881
Abilify Discmelt Orally Disintegrating Tablets (Greater than or equal to 1 in 1000 patients and less than 1 in 100 patients) 2466
Abilify Tablets (Greater than or equal to 1 in 1000 patients and less than 1 in 100 patients) 881
Abilify Tablets (Greater than or equal to 1 in 1000 patients and less than 1 in 100 patients) 2466
▲ Combigan Ophthalmic Solution (1% to 5%) 553
Iquix Ophthalmic Solution (Less than 1%) 3183
Mirapex Tablets 857
▲ Pataday Ophthalmic Solution (Less than or equal to 5%) 543
ProQuad 2099

Edema, face
Abilify Injection (Greater than or equal to 1 in 1000 patients and less than 1 in 100 patients) 881
Abilify Injection (Greater than or equal to 1 in 1000 patients and less than 1 in 100 patients) 2466
Abilify Oral Solution (Greater than or equal to 1 in 1000 patients and less than 1 in 100 patients) 881
Abilify Oral Solution (Greater than or equal to 1 in 1000 patients and less than 1 in 100 patients) 2466
Abilify Discmelt Orally Disintegrating Tablets (Greater than or equal to 1 in 1000 patients and less than 1 in 100 patients) 881
Abilify Discmelt Orally Disintegrating Tablets (Greater than or equal to 1 in 1000 patients and less than 1 in 100 patients) 2466
Abilify Tablets (Greater than or equal to 1 in 1000 patients and less than 1 in 100 patients) 881
Abilify Tablets (Greater than or equal to 1 in 1000 patients and less than 1 in 100 patients) 2466
Alphanate 1709
▲ Alvesco Inhalation Aerosol (Greater than or equal to 3%) 2985
Ambien CR Tablets (Rare) 2696
Cialis Tablets (Less than 2%) 1792
Cipro XR Tablets 2823
Emsam Transdermal System (Infrequent) 905
▲ Fabrazyme for Intravenous Infusion (Greater than or equal to 5%) 1241
Forteo for Injection (Less than 1/1000 patients) 1816
▲ Gleevec Tablets (16.7%) 2255
▲ Gliadel Wafer (6%) 1076
Mirapex Tablets 857
Prozac Weekly Capsules (Infrequent) 1852
Salagen Tablets (1% to 2%) 1082
Tekturna HCT Tablets (0.4%) 2324
Velcade for Injection 2168
Venlafaxine Hydrochloride Tablets (Infrequent) 2199

Edema, facial
Aceon Tablets (2 mg, 4 mg, 8 mg) (0.3% to 1%) 3038
Actiq (Less than 1%) 959
▲ Advair Diskus 100/50 (4%) 1276
Advair Diskus 250/50 1276
Advair Diskus 500/50 1276
Advair HFA 45/21 Inhalation Aerosol 1288
Advair HFA 115/21 Inhalation Aerosol 1288
Advair HFA 230/21 Inhalation Aerosol 1288
Ambien Tablets (Rare) 2692
AmBisome for Injection (Less common) 606
Amrix Capsules 966
Anzemet Injection (Rare) 2701
Anzemet Tablets (Rare) 2704
Aricept Tablets (Infrequent) 1062
Aricept ODT Tablets (Infrequent) 1062
Asacol Delayed-Release Tablets 2579
Attenuvax 1951
Avalide Tablets 892
Avalide Tablets 2713
Avapro Tablets (Less than 1%) 897
Avapro Tablets (Less than 1%) 2718
Avelox (Less than 0.1%) 2803
Azilect Tablets (Infrequent) 3106
▲ Azmacort Inhalation Aerosol (1% to 3%) 407
Benicar Tablets (Five patients) 1009
Benicar HCT Tablets (2 out of 1,243 patients) 1010
Bexxar 1371
Campral Tablets (Rare) 1158
▲ Carac Cream 0.5% (35.4%) 2722
Celebrex Capsules (0.1% to 1.9%) 2979
Celexa (Rare) 1160
▲ CellCept Capsules (3% to less than 20%) 2622
▲ CellCept Intravenous (3% to less than 20%) 2622
▲ CellCept Oral Suspension (3% to less than 20%) 2622
▲ CellCept Tablets (3% to less than 20%) 2622
Cipro I.V. (1% or less) 2817
Cipro (Less than 1%) 2810
Cipro XR Tablets 2823

▲ Copaxone for Injection (6%) 3110
Cozaar Tablets (Rare) 1973
Crinone 4% Gel 992
Crinone 8% Gel 992
Depakote ER Tablets (Greater than or equal to 1%) 423
Diclofenac Sodium Ophthalmic Solution ⊙240
Doxil Injection (Less than 1%) 2378
Effexor XR Extended-Release Capsules (Infrequent) 3195
Elidel Cream 1% 2221
Evoxac Capsules (Less than 1%) 1013
Exelon Capsules (Infrequent) 2229
Exelon Oral Solution (Infrequent) 2229
Flonase Nasal Spray 1431
Flovent HFA 1440
FluMist Vaccine 1945
Gabitril Tablets (Infrequent) 973
Geodon Capsules (Frequent) 2520
Humatrope Vials and Cartridges (1.4%) 1838
Imitrex Nasal Spray 1470
Imitrex Tablets 1474
▲ Intron A for Injection (Up to 10%) 2859
Invanz for Injection (Greater than 0.1%) 2029
Kaletra (Less than 2%) 452
Keppra Oral Solution (2%) 3131
Keppra Tablets (2%) 3131
Ketek Tablets 2744
Klonopin 2639
Lamictal (2%) 1488
Levitra Tablets (Less than 2%) 2876
Lialda Tablets (Infrequent) 3029
Lipitor Tablets (Less than 2%) 2501
Lunesta Tablets (Infrequent) 2994
Lupron Depot–3 Month 11.25 mg 462
▲ Lyrica Capsules (1% to 3%) 2527
Maxalt Tablets (Infrequent) 2056
Maxalt-MLT Orally Disintegrating Tablets (Infrequent) 2056
Meridia Capsules 475
Meruvax II 2061
Micardis Tablets 852
Micardis HCT Tablets 854
M-M-R II 2054
Mobic Oral Suspension (Less than 2%) 863
Mobic Tablets (Less than 2%) 863
Mumpsvax 2068
Neupogen for Injection 589
Nexium Delayed-Release Capsules (Less than 1%) 645
Nexium I.V. (Less than 1%) 652
Nexium Delayed-Release Oral Suspension (Less than 1%) 645
Noroxin Tablets 2069
Norvir (Less than 2%) 489
Omnicef Capsules 497
Omnicef for Oral Suspension 497
OxyContin Tablets (Less than 1%) 2589
Paxil (Infrequent) 1535
Paxil CR Controlled-Release Tablets (Infrequent) 1544
Pepcid Tablets (Infrequent) 2075
Pletal Tablets (Less than 2%) 2481
Prevnar 3241
Primaxin I.V. (Less than 0.2%) 2083
Prinivil Tablets (0.3% to 1%) 2087
Prinzide Tablets 2092
Propecia Tablets 2095
ProQuad 2099
Protonix for Delayed-Release Oral Suspension (Less than 1%) 3254
Protonix Delayed-Release Tablets (Less than 1%) 3254
Protonix I.V. (Less than 1%) 3257
Protopic Ointment (1% to 3%) 628
Prozac Pulvules and Liquid (Infrequent) 1852
Relenza Inhalation Powder 1556
Remeron Tablets (Infrequent) 2924
RemeronSolTab Tablets (Infrequent) 2927
Remicade for IV Injection 950
Requip Tablets (Infrequent) 1561
Rilutek Tablets (Infrequent) 2771
Sandostatin LAR Depot 2302
▲ Simulect for Injection (3% to 10%) 2306
Stromectol Tablets (1.2%) 2120
Sular Extended Release Tablets (Less than or equal to 1%) 2975
Sulfamylon Cream 2194
Sulfamylon for 5% Topical Solution 2194
Suprax for Oral Suspension (Less than 2%) 1891
Suprax Tablets (Less than 2%) 1891
Tarka Tablets 511
Tasigna Capsules (0.1% to 1%) 2316
Tekturna Tablets (0.4%) 2321
Teveten HCT Tablets (Less than 1%) 517
Treximet Tablets (Infrequent) 1616
Tricor Tablets 520
▲ Trisenox Injection (8%) 986
Valtrex Caplets 1635
Varivax 2133
▲ Vesanoid Capsules (6%) 2660
Viramune Oral Suspension 873
Viramune Tablets 873
▲ Voltaren Ophthalmic Solution (Less than or equal to 3%) 2336
Wellbutrin SR Sustained-Release Tablets (Infrequent) 1653
Wellbutrin XL Extended-Release Tablets (Infrequent) 1659
Zemplar Injection 538
Zomig Tablets (Infrequent) 694
Zomig Nasal Spray (Infrequent) 689
Zomig-ZMT Tablets (Infrequent) 694
Zonegran Capsules (Infrequent) 1089
Zyban Sustained-Release Tablets (Less than 1%) 1692
Zyprexa Tablets (Infrequent) 1883
Zyprexa ZYDIS Orally Disintegrating Tablets (Infrequent) 1883
Zyrtec Chewable Tablets (Less than 2%) 1920
Zyrtec Syrup (Less than 2%) 1920
Zyrtec Tablets (Less than 2%) 1920
Zyrtec-D 12 Hour Extended Release Tablets (Less than 2%) 1923

Edema, generalized

▲ Cancidas for Injection (2.6% to 3.6%) 1953
▲ CellCept Capsules (3% to less than 28.2%) 2622
▲ CellCept Intravenous (3% to less than 28.2%) 2622
▲ CellCept Oral Suspension (3% to less than 28.2%) 2622
▲ CellCept Tablets (3% to less than 28.2%) 2622
▲ Coreg CR Extended-Release Capsules (5% to 6%) 1393
Lovaza Capsules 1520
Prozac Weekly Capsules (Infrequent) 1852
Symbyax Capsules (Frequent) 1871
Tekturna Tablets (0.4%) 2321
Tekturna HCT Tablets (0.4%) 2324
Zyrtec Chewable Tablets (Less than 2%) 1920
Zyrtec Syrup (Less than 2%) 1920
Zyrtec Tablets (Less than 2%) 1920
Zyrtec-D 12 Hour Extended Release Tablets (Less than 2%) 1923

Edema, genital

Doxil Injection (Less than 1%) 2378
▲ Simulect for Injection (3% to 10%) 2306

Edema, hand

Cipro (Less than 1%) 2810
Cipro XR Tablets 2823
Remicade for IV Injection 950
Tekturna Tablets (0.4%) 2321
Tekturna HCT Tablets (0.4%) 2324

Edema, heart failure

(*see under* Congestive heart failure)

Edema, injection site

Betaseron for SC Injection (2%) 756
Bicillin C-R Injectable Suspension 1775
Bicillin L-A Injection 1777
Eloxatin for Injection 2731
Ionsys Transdermal System (.1% to less than 1%) 2410
Merrem I.V. (0.2%) 684
Premarin Intravenous 3217
▲ Trisenox Injection (10%) 986
Tygacil for Injection (0% to less than 2%) 3276
▲ Visudyne for Injection (10% to 30%) 2332
Zemuron Injection (Less than 1%) 2947

Edema, labia

Alinia for Oral Suspension (Less than 1%) 2677
Alinia Tablets (Less than 1%) 2677

Edema, laryngeal

Activase I.V. (Very rare) 1188
Aggrenox Capsules 819
Avelox 2803
Axid Capsules 1364
Bayer Aspirin 750
BeneFIX Vials 3191
Bicillin C-R Injectable Suspension 1775
Bicillin L-A Injection 1777
Cipro I.V. (1% or less) 2817
Cipro (Less than 1%) 2810
Cipro XR Tablets 2823
Effexor XR Extended-Release Capsules (Rare) 3195
Fortaz 1450
Levitra Tablets (Less than 2%) 2876
Nexium Delayed-Release Capsules (Less than 1%) 645
Nexium I.V. (Less than 1%) 652
Nexium Delayed-Release Oral Suspension (Less than 1%) 645
Omnicef Capsules 497
Omnicef for Oral Suspension 497
Oncaspar Injection 1138
Orthoclone OKT3 Sterile Solution 2387
Percocet Tablets 1127
Percodan Tablets 1130
Persantine Tablets (Rare) 869
Prinivil Tablets (0.3% to 1%) 2087
Prinzide Tablets (Rare) 2092
Prozac Weekly Capsules (Rare) 1852
Prozac Pulvules and Liquid (Rare) 1852
Remicade for IV Injection 950
St. Joseph 81 mg Aspirin Chewable and Enteric Coated Tablets 1903
Tarka Tablets 511
Thioridazine Hydrochloride Tablets 2195
Thyrogen for Injection (1 patient out of 55) 1244
TNKase (Less than 1%) 1233
Velcade for Injection 2168
Venlafaxine Hydrochloride Tablets (Rare) 2199
▲ Vesanoid Capsules (3%) 2660
Zofran Injection 1682
Zofran 1687
Zofran ODT Orally Disintegrating Tablets 1687
Zomig Tablets (Infrequent) 694
Zomig Nasal Spray (Infrequent) 689
Zomig-ZMT Tablets (Infrequent) 694

Edema, laryngotracheal

Photofrin for Injection 708

Edema, legs

▲ Duetact Tablets (5.7% to 12.3%) 3085
▲ Noxafil Oral Suspension (15%) 2889
▲ Zometa for Intravenous Infusion (5% to less than 10%) 2341
Zyrtec Chewable Tablets (Less than 2%) 1920
Zyrtec Syrup (Less than 2%) 1920
Zyrtec Tablets (Less than 2%) 1920
Zyrtec-D 12 Hour Extended Release Tablets (Less than 2%) 1923

Edema, lips

Cipro I.V. (1% or less) 2817
Cipro (Less than 1%) 2810
Cipro XR Tablets 2823
Cozaar Tablets (Rare) 1973
Imitrex Tablets 1474
Orthoclone OKT3 Sterile Solution 2387
Propecia Tablets 2095
Remicade for IV Injection 950
Retrovir Capsules 1574
Retrovir IV Infusion 1579
Retrovir 1574
Tarka Tablets 511

Edema, local

Avodart Soft Gelatin Capsules 1359
Denavir Cream 2205
Havrix Injection Vaccine 1454
Lidoderm Patch 1114
Mirapex Tablets 857
Thyrogen for Injection 1244
Zovirax Ointment 819

Edema, lower extremities

▲ ActoPlus Met Tablets (2.9% to 11.3%) 3071
Advate (0.6%) 721
▲ Cardizem LA Extended Release Tablets (5% to 8%) 421
Cipro XR Tablets 2823
▲ Coreg Tablets (Greater than 1% to 3%) 1387
▲ Coreg CR Extended-Release Capsules (Greater than 1% to less than or equal to 3%) 1393
Eldepryl Capsules 3052
▲ Femara Tablets (5%) 2246
Miacalcin Injection 2273
Micardis Tablets (More than 0.3%) 852
Micardis HCT Tablets 854
▲ Mobic Oral Suspension (0.6% to 4.5%) 863
▲ Mobic Tablets (0.6% to 4.5%) 863
▲ Myfortic Tablets (3% to less than 20%) 2276
Nexium Delayed-Release Capsules (Less than 1%) 645
Nexium I.V. (Less than 1%) 652
Nexium Delayed-Release Oral Suspension (Less than 1%) 645
▲ Norditropin Cartridges (15%) 2354
▲ Requip Tablets (6%) 1561
▲ Simulect for Injection (Greater than or equal to 10%) 2306
▲ Tracleer Tablets (8%) 3289
Ultram ER Extended-Release Tablets (0.5% to less than 1%) 2428
▲ Velcade for Injection (11%) 2168
VESIcare Tablets (0.3% to 1.1%) 636
Xenical Capsules (2.8%) 2672
▲ Zometa for Intravenous Infusion (21%) 2341
Zyprexa Tablets (1%) 1883
Zyprexa ZYDIS Orally Disintegrating Tablets (1%) 1883

Edema, lung

Angiomax for Injection (Greater than 0.1% to less than 1%) 1933
▲ CellCept Capsules (3% to less than 20%) 2622
▲ CellCept Intravenous (3% to less than 20%) 2622
▲ CellCept Oral Suspension (3% to less than 20%) 2622
▲ CellCept Tablets (3% to less than 20%) 2622
▲ Coreg CR Extended-Release Capsules (Less than or equal to 0.1% to greater than 3%) 1393
Merrem I.V. (0.1% to 1%) 684
Proleukin for Injection (Less than 1%) 2287
Prozac Weekly Capsules (Rare) 1852

Edema, macular

ActoPlus Met Tablets 3071
Actos Tablets 3077
Avandamet Tablets 1336
Avandaryl Tablets (Very rare) 1344
Avandia Tablets 1351
Duetact Tablets 3085
Durezol Ophthalmic Emulsion (Less than 1%) ⊙275
Gleevec Tablets (Rare) 2255
Intron A for Injection 2859
Lumigan Ophthalmic Solution 556
PegIntron Powder for Injection 2903
Retrovir Capsules (A single case) 1574
Retrovir IV Infusion (A single case) 1579
Retrovir (A single case) 1574

Edema, mouth

Evoxac Capsules (Less than 1%) 1013
Frova Tablets (Rare) 1111
Zemplar Injection 538

Edema, nasal

▲ Atrovent Nasal Spray 0.03% (3.1) 834

Edema, neck

Cipro (Less than 1%) 2810
Cipro XR Tablets 2823

Edema, non-specific

(*see under* Edema)

Edema, orofacial

Forteo for Injection (Less than 1/1000 patients) 1816
Geodon (Rare) 2520

Edema, oropharyngeal

▲ Advair Diskus 100/50 (Greater than or equal to 3%) 1276
Advair Diskus 250/50 1276
Advair Diskus 500/50 1276
Advair HFA 45/21 Inhalation Aerosol 1288
Advair HFA 115/21 Inhalation Aerosol 1288
Advair HFA 230/21 Inhalation Aerosol 1288
Atrovent HFA Inhalation Aerosol 839
Atrovent Nasal Spray 0.03% 834
Atrovent Nasal Spray 0.06% (Rare) 836
Cipro I.V. (1% or less) 2817
Combivent Inhalation Aerosol (Rare) 845
Denavir Cream 2205
Flovent HFA 1440
Proventil HFA Inhalation Aerosol (Rare) 2914
Relenza Inhalation Powder 1556
Treximet Tablets (Infrequent) 1616
Ventolin HFA Inhalation Aerosol (Less than 3%) 1638

Edema, palpebral

Cipro I.V. (1% or less) 2817

Imitrex Nasal Spray 1470
Imitrex Tablets................................ 1474
Maxalt Tablets (Infrequent).............. 2056
Maxalt-MLT Orally Disintegrating Tablets (Infrequent)...................... 2056
Orthoclone OKT3 Sterile Solution..... 2387
Prinzide Tablets............................. 2092
Viroptic Ophthalmic Solution (2.8%).. ⊙253

Edema, periorbital

(*see under* Edema, peripheral)

Edema, peripheral

Abilify Injection (Greater than or equal to 1 in 100 patients)........... 881
Abilify Injection (Greater than or equal to 1 in 100 patients)........... 2466
Abilify Oral Solution (Greater than or equal to 1 in 100 patients)........ 881
Abilify Oral Solution (Greater than or equal to 1 in 100 patients)........ 2466
Abilify Discmelt Orally Disintegrating Tablets (Greater than or equal to 1 in 100 patients).. 881
Abilify Discmelt Orally Disintegrating Tablets (Greater than or equal to 1 in 100 patients).. 2466
Abilify Tablets (Greater than or equal to 1 in 100 patients)........... 881
Abilify Tablets (Greater than or equal to 1 in 100 patients)........... 2466
Aciphex Tablets 1053
Actiq (1% or greater)........................ 959
▲ Actonel Tablets (7.7% to 8.2%) 2568
▲ Actonel with Calcium Tablets (1.6% to 4.2%)................................. 2574
▲ ActoPlus Met Tablets (6%) 3071
▲ Aerobid/Aerobid-M (1% to 3%) 1153
▲ Agrylin Capsules (8.9%) 3017
Ambien Tablets (Rare)....................... 2692
Ambien CR Tablets (Rare)................... 2696
▲ AmBisome for Injection (14.6%) 606
Anaprox Tablets (Some patients)...... 2632
Anaprox DS Tablets (Some patients).. 2632
AndroGel (Less than 1%).................. 3159
Angeliq Tablets (1.8%)..................... 751
Anzemet Injection (Rare).................. 2701
Anzemet Tablets (Rare)..................... 2704
Aralast (Greater than or equal to 0.2%).. 726
▲ Aranesp for Injection (10%) 564
Aricept Tablets (Frequent).............. 1062
Aricept ODT Tablets (Frequent)........ 1062
▲ Arimidex Tablets (5% to 10%) 672
▲ Arranon Injection (0% to 15%) 1319
▲ Asacol Delayed-Release Tablets (3%).. 2579
Atacand HCT (0.5% or greater)........ 642
Attenuvax....................................... 1951
Avandamet Tablets........................... 1336
Avelox (Less than 0.1%)................... 2803
▲ Avinza Capsules (5% to 10%) 1772
Benicar Tablets (Greater than 0.5%).. 1009
Benicar HCT Tablets (Greater than 1%).. 1010
▲ Betaseron for SC Injection (12%) 756
▲ Betimol Ophthalmic Solution (1% to 5%).. 3181
▲ Bexxar (0% to 9%) 1371
▲ Brovana Inhalation Solution (Less than 2% to 3%)............................ 2990
Bystolic Tablets (1%)....................... 1155
Campral Tablets (Frequent).............. 1158
▲ Cancidas for Injection (6% to 10.6%)..................................... 1953
Cardene I.V. (Rare).......................... 1093
Celebrex Capsules (2.1%)................ 2979
▲ CellCept Capsules (27% to 64%) 2622
▲ CellCept Intravenous (27% to 64%).. 2622
▲ CellCept Oral Suspension (27% to 64%).. 2622
▲ CellCept Tablets (27% to 64%) 2622
Cerezyme for Injection.................... 1238
Cimzia... 3127
▲ Copaxone for Injection (7%) 3110
▲ Coreg Tablets (2% to 7%) 1387
▲ Coreg CR Extended-Release Capsules (1% to 7%)..................... 1393
▲ Cubicin for Injection (6.7%) 995
Cyanokit 5g Antidote....................... 1021
▲ Dacogen Injection (25%) 1066
Demser Capsules (Rare).................. 1989
▲ Depakote ER Tablets (Greater than 1% to 8%)............................. 423
▲ DepoCyt Injection (7% to 18%) 1136
Diovan HCT Tablets (Greater than 0.2%).. 2216
▲ Doxil Injection (1% to 11.3%) 2378
▲ Duetact Tablets (Greater than 5%) ... 3085
EC-Naprosyn Delayed-Release Tablets (Some patients)............... 2632
Eldepryl Capsules........................... 3052
▲ Eloxatin for Injection (5% to 10%) 2731
Emsam Transdermal System (Frequent)...................................... 905
Enablex Extended-Release Tablets (Greater than or equal to 1%)........ 2225
▲ Enbrel for Injection (2% to 8%) 569
▲ Equetro Extended-Release Capsules (Less than 5%).............. 3174
▲ Evista Tablets (3.3% to 5.2%) 1810
▲ Evoxac Capsules (Less than 1% to 3%).. 1013
Exelon Capsules (2% or more)......... 2229
Exelon Oral Solution (2% or more).... 2229
Exelon Patch (Infrequent)................ 2233
▲ Exforge Tablets (0.4% to 5.4%) 2238
▲ Fabrazyme for Intravenous Infusion (21%) 1241
Fansidar Tablets 2636
▲ Faslodex Injection (9%) 682
▲ Femara Tablets (5%) 2246
▲ Fentora Tablets (1% to 32%) 968
▲ Flolan for Injection (79%) 1426
Flulaval Injection Vaccine 1448
Gabitril Tablets (Frequent) 973
Gantrisin Pediatric Suspension 2638
▲ Gemzar for Injection (20%) 1820
▲ Genotropin Lyophilized Powder (0% to 10.8%) 2547
Geodon Capsules (Infrequent) 2520
▲ Gleevec Tablets (28.6% to 33.3%) .. 2255
▲ Gliadel Wafer (2% to 9%) 1076
▲ Herceptin I.V. (10%) 1199
▲ Humatrope Vials and Cartridges (11.5% to 18.2%) 1838
▲ Humira Injection (Less than 5%) 442
Imitrex Nasal Spray 1470
Imitrex Tablets 1474
▲ Indapamide Tablets (Less than 5%) 2188
▲ Intron A for Injection (Less than or equal to 5%) 2859
Ionsys Transdermal System (.1% to less than 1%) 2410
Kaletra (Less than 2%) 452
Klonopin (Infrequent) 2639
Lamictal (Infrequent) 1488
▲ Letairis Tablets (17%) 1258
▲ Leukine (11% to 15%) 774
Lipitor Tablets (Greater than or equal to 2%) 2501
▲ Lovenox Injection (Up to 6%) 2756
Lunesta Tablets (Frequent) 2994
Lupron Depot-PED 7.5 mg, 11.25 mg and 15 mg (Less than 2%) 471
▲ Lyrica Capsules (3% to 12%) 2527
▲ Megace ES Oral Suspension (1% to 3%) 2499
Meridia Capsules (Greater than or equal to 1%) 475
Merrem I.V. (Greater than 0.1% to 1%) 684
Meruvax II 2061
Miacalcin Nasal Spray (Less than 1%) 2274
Micardis Tablets (1%) 852
Micardis HCT Tablets (1%) 854
▲ Mirapex Tablets (2% to 5%) 857
M-M-R II 2054
▲ Mobic Oral Suspension (0.6% to 4.5%) 863
▲ Mobic Tablets (0.6% to 4.5%) 863
Mumpsvax 2068
▲ Mycamine for Injection (5.5% to 20.7%) 616
▲ Myfortic Tablets (3% to less than 20%) 2276
▲ Mylotarg for Injection (8% to 19%) ... 3212
▲ Nalfon Capsules (5%) 2508
Namenda (Greater than or equal to 2%) 1180
Naprosyn Suspension (Some patients) 2632
Naprosyn Tablets (Some patients) ... 2632
▲ Neulasta Injection (15% to 72%) 587
Neupro Transdermal System 3149
Nexium Delayed-Release Capsules (Less than 1%) 645
Nexium I.V. (Less than 1%) 652
Nexium Delayed-Release Oral Suspension (Less than 1%) 645
Niaspan Extended-Release Tablets ... 480
▲ Norditropin Cartridges (42%) 2354
Norvir (Less than 2%) 489
NovoLog Injection 2359
▲ Nutropin for Injection (41%) 1208
▲ Nutropin AQ Injection (41%) 1212
▲ Nutropin AQ NuSpin Injection (41%) 1212
▲ Nutropin AQ Pen (41%) 1212
▲ Nutropin AQ Pen Cartridge (41%) 1212
OxyContin Tablets (Less than 1%).... 2589
Paxil (Infrequent)............................. 1535
Paxil CR Controlled-Release Tablets (Infrequent)...................... 1544
Pepcid Tablets (Infrequent).............. 2075
▲ Photofrin for Injection (7%) 708
▲ Pletal Tablets (7% to 9%) 2481
Pneumovax 23 2078
▲ Premphase Tablets (3% to 4%) 3232
▲ Prempro Tablets (3% to 4%) 3232
Prinivil Tablets (0.3% to 1%)............ 2087
Prinzide Tablets 2092
▲ Prograf Capsules and Injection (12% to 36%)................................. 622
▲ Proleukin for Injection (28%) 2287
▲ Prometrium Capsules (100 mg, 200 mg) (Less than 5%).............. 3047
ProQuad 2099
Protonix for Delayed-Release Oral Suspension (Less than 1%).......... 3254
Protonix Delayed-Release Tablets (Less than 1%) 3254
Protonix I.V. (Less than 1%) 3257
▲ Protopic Ointment (1% to 4%) 628
Provigil Tablets (At least 1%) 977
Prozac Weekly Capsules (Infrequent) 1852
Prozac Pulvules and Liquid (Infrequent) 1852
▲ Rapamune (Greater than or equal to 30% to 58%) 3260
Raptiva for Injection 1218
▲ Reclast Injection (3% to 5.5%) 2291
Remeron Tablets (2%) 2924
RemeronSolTab Tablets (2%) 2927
ReoPro Vials (1.6%) 1860
Requip Tablets (Infrequent) 1561
▲ Requip XL Tablets (4%) 1568
▲ Rilutek Tablets (3.3% to 4.2%) 2771
▲ Risperdal Consta Long-Acting Injection (3%) 1753
▲ Rituxan I.V. (0% to 8%) 1223
Salagen Tablets (Less than 1%) 1082
▲ Simulect for Injection (Greater than or equal to 10%) 2306
▲ Stromectol Tablets (3.2%) 2120
▲ Sular Extended Release Tablets (22%) 2975
Sustiva Capsules (Less than 2%) 930
Sustiva Tablets (Less than 2%) 930
▲ Sutent Capsules (1% to 17%) 2540
▲ Symbyax Capsules (5% to 8%) 1871
▲ Targretin Capsules (4.8% to 11.3%) 1084
▲ Targretin Gel 1% (6%) 1088
▲ Tasigna Capsules (0.1% to 11%) 2316
▲ Taxotere Injection Concentrate (0.4% to 26.9%) 2773
Tekturna Tablets (0.06%) 2321
Tekturna HCT Tablets (0.6%) 2324
▲ Temodar Capsules (1% to 11%) 2931
Teveten Tablets (Less than 1%) 515
Teveten HCT Tablets (Less than 1%) 517
Thioridazine Hydrochloride Tablets .. 2195
Thiothixene Capsules 2197
Toprol-XL Tablets (About 1 of 100 patients) 666
▲ Trasylol Injection (5%) 799
Treximet Tablets (Infrequent) 1616
▲ Tygacil for Injection (3.3%) 3276
▲ Urso 250 Tablets (8.3%) 720
▲ Urso Forte Tablets (8.3%) 720
▲ Valcyte Tablets (Less than 5%) 2654
Valstar Sterile Solution for Intravesical Instillation (1%) 1735
Vantas (Less than 2%) 1737
▲ Vaprisol (3% to 8%) 632
Varivax 2133
▲ Vectibix (1% to 12%) 597
▲ Velcade for Injection (20%) 2168
▲ Vesanoid Capsules (52%) 2660
▲ Viadur Implant (3.1%) 802
Wellbutrin SR Sustained-Release Tablets (Infrequent) 1653
Wellbutrin XL Extended-Release Tablets (Infrequent) 1659
▲ Zolinza Capsules (11% to 12.8%) 2142
Zomig Tablets (Rare) 694
Zomig Nasal Spray (Rare) 689
Zomig-ZMT Tablets (Rare) 694
Zonegran Capsules (Infrequent) 1089
Zovirax 1690
Zyban Sustained-Release Tablets (Infrequent) 1692
▲ Zyprexa Tablets (2% to 6%) 1883
▲ Zyprexa ZYDIS Orally Disintegrating Tablets (2% to 6%) 1883
Zyrtec Chewable Tablets (Less than 2%) 1920
Zyrtec Syrup (Less than 2%) 1920
Zyrtec Tablets (Less than 2%) 1920
Zyrtec-D 12 Hour Extended Release Tablets (Less than 2%) 1923

Edema, pharyngeal

Atacand Tablets (More than 1%)....... 639
Avelox 2803
Cipro 2810
Cipro XR Tablets 2823
Cozaar Tablets (Rare)...................... 1973
Demser Capsules (Rare)................... 1989
Maxalt Tablets (Rare)....................... 2056
Maxalt-MLT Orally Disintegrating Tablets (Rare)........................... 2056
Noroxin Tablets............................... 2069
OsmoPrep Tablets 2680
Remicade for IV Injection 950
Xolair.. 1235

Edema, pitting

Exforge Tablets (Greater than or equal to 0.2%)............................ 2238
Mirapex Tablets............................... 857

Edema, pulmonary

Abelcet Injection............................. 1134
Activase I.V..................................... 1188
Aggrenox Capsules (Less than 1%) .. 819
Albutein 5% 1707
Albutein 25% 1708
Aldara Cream, 5% 1699
Ambien Tablets (Rare) 2692
Ambien CR Tablets (Rare) 2696
AmBisome for Injection (Less common) 606
Anaprox Tablets (Less than 1%) 2632
Anaprox DS Tablets (Less than 1%) .. 2632
Argatroban Injection (0.9%) 1308
Atacand HCT 642
Avalide Tablets 892
Avalide Tablets 2713
Avandamet Tablets 1336
Avandaryl Tablets 1344
Avandia Tablets 1351
Bayer Aspirin 750
Bystolic Tablets 1155
Cancidas for Injection 1953
Cipro I.V. (1% or less) 2817
Cipro (Less than 1%) 2810
Cipro XR Tablets 2823
Clolar for Intravenous Infusion 1239
Combigan Ophthalmic Solution 553
▲ Coreg Tablets (Less than or equal to 0.1% to greater than 3%) 1387
Cosopt Sterile Ophthalmic Solution 1969
▲ Dacogen Injection (6%) 1066
Dantrium Intravenous (Rare) 2582
Diovan HCT Tablets 2216
Dyazide Capsules 1405
EC-Naprosyn Delayed-Release Tablets (Less than 1%) 2632
Elitek (Less than or equal to 1%) 2729
Flebogamma 5% 1715
Flebogamma 5% DIF 1718
▲ Flolan for Injection (4%) 1426
Gammagard Liquid 730
Gammagard S/D 734
Gamunex 3094
▲ Gleevec Tablets (6.9% to 22%) 2255
Herceptin I.V. 1199
Human Albumin Grifols 25% 1706
Indocin Capsules (Less than 1%) 2024
Indocin I.V. (Less than 1%) 2489
Indocin (Less than 1%) 2024
Intravenous Sodium Diuril 2490
Ixempra Kit for Injection 915
Kaletra (Less than 2%) 452
Lovenox Injection (0.7%) 2756
▲ Lupron Depot 7.5 mg (Less than 5%) 469
Lyrica Capsules (Rare) 2527
Micardis HCT Tablets 854
Mirapex Tablets 857
Nalfon Capsules (Less than 1%) 2508
Namenda (Infrequent) 1180
Naprosyn Suspension (Less than 1%) 2632
Naprosyn Tablets (Less than 1%) 2632
Orthoclone OKT3 Sterile Solution (Less than 2%) 2387
Paxil (Rare) 1535
Paxil CR Controlled-Release Tablets (Rare) 1544
Percocet Tablets 1127
Percodan Tablets 1130
Photofrin for Injection 708
Prinivil Tablets (Greater than 1%) 2087
Prinzide Tablets 2092
▲ Prograf Capsules and Injection (3% to 15%) 622
Proleukin for Injection (Less than 1%) 2287
Prozac Pulvules and Liquid (Rare) 1852
Remicade for IV Injection (Greater than or equal to 0.2%) 950
ReoPro Vials (1.5%) 1860

Edema, retinal

Edema, scrotal

Edema, skin

(*see under* Edema, angioneurotic)

Edema, stromal

Edema, superficial

Edema, tongue

Edema, turbinate

Edema, upper extremities

Edema, worsening of

EEG changes

Efficacy, lack of

Effusion, middle ear

Ejaculate volume, decreased

Ejaculation, delayed

Ejaculation, inhibition

Ejaculation, premature

Ejaculation, retrograde

Ejaculation decreased

Ejaculation disturbances

Ejaculation failure

Ejection fraction reduction

EKG, abnormal

EKG changes

EKG changes, axis shifts

EKG changes, early R wave progression

EKG changes, early repolarization

EKG changes, low voltage

EKG changes, non-specific ST-T wave changes

EKG changes, PR prolongation

EKG changes, QRS interval prolonged

EKG changes, QT interval prolonged

Abilify Discmelt Orally Disintegrating Tablets (Greater than or equal to 1 in 1000 patients and less than 1 in 100 patients) 2466
Abilify Tablets (Greater than or equal to 1 in 1000 patients and less than 1 in 100 patients) 881
Abilify Tablets (Greater than or equal to 1 in 1000 patients and less than 1 in 100 patients) 2466
▲ Aloxi Injection (1% to 5%) 1059
Amerge Tablets (Infrequent) 1301
Avelox (Greater than or equal to 0.1% to less than 2%) 2803
Brovana Inhalation Solution (Less than 2%) 2990
Celexa 1160
Cipro 2810
Combivent Inhalation Aerosol 845
E.E.S. 433
Effexor XR Extended-Release Capsules (Rare) 3195
EryPed 431
Exelon Patch (Infrequent) 2233
Fleet Enema 1143
Fleet Enema Extra 1143
Fleet Enema for Children 1143
Fleet Pedia-Lax Enema 1143
Geodon Capsules 2520
Imitrex Injection (Infrequent) 1465
Invega Extended-Release Tablets 1748
Levaquin 2416
Levaquin in 5% Dextrose Injection 2416
Levitra Tablets 2876
Lexapro Oral Suspension 1174
Lexapro Tablets 1174
Namenda 1180
Noroxin Tablets (Rare) 2069
▲ Noxafil Oral Suspension (4%) 2889
OsmoPrep Tablets 2680
Pletal Tablets 2481
Prograf Capsules and Injection 622
Prozac Weekly Capsules 1852
Prozac Pulvules and Liquid 1852
Risperdal Consta Long-Acting Injection 1753
Rythmol SR Capsules 1590
Sandostatin LAR Depot 2302
Strattera Capsules 1864
▲ Sutent Capsules (11%) 2540
Symbyax Capsules (Infrequent) 1871
▲ Tasigna Capsules (1% to 10%) 2316
Thioridazine Hydrochloride Tablets 2195
▲ Trisenox Injection (40%) 986
Tykerb Tablets 1631
Velcade for Injection 2168
Venlafaxine Hydrochloride Tablets 2199
Ventolin HFA Inhalation Aerosol 1638
VESIcare Tablets 636
Zofran Injection (Rare) 1682
Zofran (Rare) 1687
Zofran ODT Orally Disintegrating Tablets (Rare) 1687
Zolinza Capsules 2142
Zomig Tablets (Rare) 694
Zomig-ZMT Tablets (Rare) 694

EKG changes, ST section
▲ Adenoscan (3%) 605
Amerge Tablets (Infrequent) 1301
Anzemet Injection 2701
Anzemet Tablets 2704
Brovana Inhalation Solution 2990
Cardene I.V. (Rare) 1093
Imitrex Injection (Infrequent) 1465
Imitrex Tablets 1474
Lanoxin Injection 1498
Lanoxin Injection Pediatric 1502
Lanoxin Tablets 1505
Luvox CR Extended-Release Capsules (Infrequent) 1759
OxyContin Tablets (Less than 1%) 2589
Tarka Tablets (0.3% or more) 511

EKG changes, ST segment depression
Combivent Inhalation Aerosol 845
▲ Lexiscan Injection (12%) 614
Ventolin HFA Inhalation Aerosol 1638
Zofran Injection 1682
Zofran 1687
Zofran ODT Orally Disintegrating Tablets 1687

EKG changes, T-wave
Adenoscan (Less than 1%) 605
Amerge Tablets (Infrequent) 1301
Anzemet Injection 2701
Anzemet Tablets 2704
Brovana Inhalation Solution (Less than 2%) 2990
Cardene I.V. (Rare) 1093
Combivent Inhalation Aerosol 845
Evoxac Capsules (Less than 1%) 1013
Imitrex Injection (Infrequent) 1465
Imitrex Tablets 1474
Moban Tablets (Rare) 1116
Pentasa Capsules (Infrequent) 3030
Prograf Capsules and Injection 622
Provigil Tablets 977
Pylera Capsules 714
Sular Extended Release Tablets (Less than or equal to 1%) 2975
Symbyax Capsules (Rare) 1871
Tarka Tablets (0.3% or more) 511
Ventolin HFA Inhalation Aerosol 1638

EKG changes, R/S transition
Sandostatin LAR Depot 2302

Elastosis perforans, serpiginosa
Cuprimine Capsules (Rare) 1986

Elation
▲ Marinol Capsules (8% to 24%) 3163

Electrocardiogram, abnormal
Cyanokit 5g Antidote 1021
PrandiMet Tablets (Less than or equal to 1%) 2967
Provigil Tablets (Greater than or equal to 1%) 977
Rythmol SR Capsules 1590
Salagen Tablets (Less than 1%) 1082
Symbyax Capsules (Infrequent) 1871
▲ Vaprisol (5%) 632
Zemuron Injection (Less than 1%) 2947

Electrocardiographic changes
(*see under* EKG changes)

Electroencephalographic changes
(*see under* EEG changes)

Electrolyte disturbances
(*see under* Electrolyte imbalance)

Electrolyte imbalance
Aloxi Injection (Less than 1%) 1059
AndroGel 3159
Avalide Tablets 892
Avalide Tablets 2713
Benicar HCT Tablets 1010
Capastat Sulfate for Injection (1 patient) 1791
Cubicin for Injection (Less than 1%) 995
Delatestryl Injection 1730
Diovan HCT Tablets 2216
Dyazide Capsules 1405
Epivir 1412
Fleet Enema 1143
Fleet Enema Extra 1143
Fleet Pedia-Lax Enema 1143
Fleet Phospho-soda 1145
Fleet Phospho-soda EZ-PREP 1147
Fleet Prep Kits 1149
Follistim AQ Cartridge 2844
Indapamide Tablets 2188
Intravenous Sodium Diuril 2490
OsmoPrep Tablets 2680
Prinzide Tablets 2092
Teveten HCT Tablets 517
Zosyn for Injection 3284

Electrolytes, loss of
Vectibix 597

Electromechanical dissociation
TNKase 1233

Electro-oculogram, abnormal
Norvir (Less than 2%) 489

Electroretinogram, abnormal
Norvir (Less than 2%) 489

Elevated bilirubin levels
(*see under* Hyperbilirubinemia)

Elevated mood
Mobic Oral Suspension 863
Mobic Tablets 863

Embolism
Activase I.V. 1188
▲ Alimta for Injection (1% to 7%) 1786
Furosemide Tablets 2186
Gleevec Tablets (Rare) 2255
Ixempra Kit for Injection 915
Luvox CR Extended-Release Capsules (Rare) 1759
Mirapex Tablets 857
NuvaRing 2897
Ortho-Cyclen/Ortho Tri-Cyclen 2449
Ortho Tri-Cyclen Lo Tablets 2458
TNKase 1233
Trasylol Injection (1% to 2%) 799
Velcade for Injection 2168
Zosyn for Injection (1% or less) 3284

Embolism, arterial
Rythmol SR Capsules 1590

Embolism, cholesterol
Activase I.V. (Rare) 1188
TNKase (Rare) 1233

Embolism, limb
ReoPro Vials (0.3%) 1860
Requip Tablets (Rare) 1561

Embolism, lower extremities
Rilutek Tablets (Infrequent) 2771

Embolism, pulmonary
Abelcet Injection 1134
Abilify Injection (Greater than or equal to 1 in 1000 patients and less than 1 in 100 patients) 881
Abilify Injection (Less than 1 in 1000 patients) 2466
Abilify Oral Solution (Greater than or equal to 1 in 1000 patients and less than 1 in 100 patients) 881
Abilify Oral Solution (Less than 1 in 1000 patients) 2466
Abilify Discmelt Orally Disintegrating Tablets (Greater than or equal to 1 in 1000 patients and less than 1 in 100 patients) 881
Abilify Discmelt Orally Disintegrating Tablets (Less than 1 in 1000 patients) 2466
Abilify Tablets (Greater than or equal to 1 in 1000 patients and less than 1 in 100 patients) 881
Abilify Tablets (Less than 1 in 1000 patients) 2466
Actimmune (Rare) 1743
Activella Tablets 2347
Alphanate 1709
Ambien Tablets (Rare) 2692
Ambien CR Tablets (Rare) 2696
Angeliq Tablets 751
Aranesp for Injection (1.3%) 564
▲ Avastin IV (16%) 1192
Betaseron for SC Injection 756
Bicillin C-R Injectable Suspension 1775
Bicillin L-A Injection 1777
Campral Tablets (Rare) 1158
Cathflo Activase 1198
Celebrex Capsules (Less than 0.1%) 2979
Celexa (Rare) 1160
Chantix Tablets (Rare) 2511
Cipro I.V. (1% or less) 2817
Cipro (Less than 1%) 2810
Cipro XR Tablets 2823
Climara Transdermal System 763
Climara Pro Transdermal System 768
Dacogen Injection 1066
Effexor XR Extended-Release Capsules (Rare) 3195
Emend Capsules (Greater than 0.5%) 1992
Emend for Injection (Greater than 0.5%) 1999
Enbrel for Injection (Infrequent) 569
Enjuvia Tablets 1029
Epogen for Injection (Rare) 576
Erbitux 912
Estratest Tablets 3043
Estratest H.S. Tablets 3043
Evista Tablets 1810
Evoxac Capsules (Less than 1%) 1013
Exelon Capsules (Infrequent) 2229
Exelon Oral Solution (Infrequent) 2229
Femara Tablets (Less than or equal to 2%) 2246
Fenoglide Tablets 2960
Follistim AQ Cartridge 2844
Gammagard S/D 734
Geodon Capsules (Rare) 2520
▲ Gliadel Wafer (8%) 1076
Imitrex Nasal Spray 1470
Imitrex Tablets 1474
Ionsys Transdermal System (.1% to less than 1%) 2410
Lexapro Oral Suspension 1174
Lexapro Tablets 1174
Lupron Depot 7.5 mg 469
Lupron Depot–3 Month 11.25 mg 462
Lybrel Tablets 3204
Megace ES Oral Suspension 2499
Merrem I.V. (Greater than 0.1% to 1%) 684
Mirapex Tablets (Less than 1%) 857
Mircette Tablets 1034
Mycamine for Injection 616
Namenda (Infrequent) 1180
NovoSeven 2367
NovoSeven RT 2370
Noxafil Oral Suspension (Rare) 2889
NuvaRing 2897
Ortho-Cyclen Tablets 2449
Ortho Evra Transdermal System 2437
Ortho Tri-Cyclen Tablets 2449
Ortho Tri-Cyclen Lo Tablets 2458
Paxil (Rare) 1535
Paxil CR Controlled-Release Tablets (Rare) 1544
Premarin Intravenous 3217
Premarin Tablets 3221
Premarin Vaginal Cream 3228
Premphase Tablets (1.3%) 3232
Prempro Tablets (1.3%) 3232
Prinivil Tablets (0.3% to 1%) 2087
Prinzide Tablets 2092
▲ Procrit for Injection (3.2%) 2391
Proleukin for Injection (Less than 1%) 2287
Prozac Weekly Capsules 1852
Prozac Pulvules and Liquid 1852
▲ Rapamune (Greater than or equal to 3% to less than 20%) 3260
Remeron Tablets (Rare) 2924
RemeronSolTab Tablets (Rare) 2927
Remicade for IV Injection (Greater than or equal to 0.2%) 950
ReoPro Vials (0.3%) 1860
Requip Tablets (Rare) 1561
Risperdal Consta Long-Acting Injection (Rare) 1753
Sandostatin LAR Depot 2302
Seasonique Tablets 1046
Sutent Capsules (2 patients) 2540
▲ Taxotere Injection Concentrate (2.3% to 3.6%) 2773
Torisel Injection (2%) 3272
Trasylol Injection (1% to 2%) 799
Tricor Tablets 520
Vectibix 597
Velcade for Injection 2168
Venlafaxine Hydrochloride Tablets (Rare) 2199
Vivitrol 988
Wellbutrin Tablets (Rare) 1648
Wellbutrin SR Sustained-Release Tablets 1653
Wellbutrin XL Extended-Release Tablets 1659
▲ Xeloda Tablets (Less than 5%) 2662
Yaz Tablets 805
▲ Zolinza Capsules (4.7%) 2142
Zonegran Capsules (Rare) 1089
Zosyn for Injection (1% or less) 3284
Zyban Sustained-Release Tablets 1692
Zyprexa Tablets 1883
Zyprexa ZYDIS Orally Disintegrating Tablets 1883

Emesis
(*see under* Vomiting)

Emotional distress
Mirapex Tablets 857

Emotional disturbances
Accutane Capsules 2607
Avalide Tablets 892
Avalide Tablets 2713
Avapro Tablets (Less than 1%) 897
Avapro Tablets (Less than 1%) 2718
Chantix Tablets (Frequent) 2511
Depakote ER Tablets 423
Imitrex Nasal Spray (Rare) 1470
Paxil (Infrequent) 1535
Paxil CR Controlled-Release Tablets (Infrequent) 1544
Rythmol SR Capsules 1590
Xyrem Oral Solution (Infrequent) 1766

Emotional lability
Accutane Capsules 2607
Actiq (Less than 1%) 959
▲ Activella Tablets (0% to 6%) 2347
▲ Adderall XR Capsules (1% to 9%) 3012
Adenoscan (Less than 1%) 605
Ambien Tablets (Infrequent) 2692
Ambien CR Tablets (Infrequent) 2696
▲ AndroGel (0% to 3%) 3159
Aricept Tablets (2%) 1062
Aricept ODT Tablets (2%) 1062
Asacol Delayed-Release Tablets 2579
Atripla Tablets 938
Avelox (Less than 0.1%) 2803
Azilect Tablets (Infrequent) 3106

Betaseron for SC Injection 756
Celexa (Infrequent) 1160
▲ CellCept Capsules (3% to less than 20%) 2622
▲ CellCept Intravenous (3% to less than 20%) 2622
▲ CellCept Oral Suspension (3% to less than 20%) 2622
▲ CellCept Tablets (3% to less than 20%) 2622
▲ Clarinex Syrup (3.1%) 2828
Combigan Ophthalmic Solution 553
Copaxone for Injection (At least 2%) 3110
Coreg Tablets (Greater than 0.1% to 1%) 1387
Coreg CR Extended-Release Capsules (0.1% to less than or equal to 1%) 1393
Cosopt Sterile Ophthalmic Solution 1969
▲ Depakote ER Tablets (6%) 423
▲ Doxil Injection (1% to 5%) 2378
Effexor XR Extended-Release Capsules (Infrequent) 3195
Elmiron Capsules 2435
Emsam Transdermal System (Infrequent) 905
Evoxac Capsules (Less than 1%) 1013
Exelon Capsules (Infrequent) 2229
Exelon Oral Solution (Infrequent) 2229
Frova Tablets (Infrequent) 1111
▲ Gabitril Tablets (3%) 973
Gengraf Capsules (1% to less than 3%) 435
InnoPran XL Extended Release Capsules 1484
▲ Intron A for Injection (Less than 5%) 2859
Kaletra (Less than 2%) 452
▲ Keppra Injection (2% to 13.3%) 3137
▲ Keppra Oral Solution (2% to 6%) 3131
▲ Keppra Tablets (2% to 6%) 3131
Klonopin (1%) 2639
▲ Lamictal (Greater than 1% to 5%) 1488
Levothroid Tablets 1170
Levoxyl Tablets 1780
Lexapro Oral Suspension (Infrequent) 1174
Lexapro Tablets (Infrequent) 1174
Lipitor Tablets (Less than 2%) 2501
Lovaza Capsules 1520
Lunesta Tablets (Infrequent) 2994
▲ Lupron Depot 3.75 mg (16%) 462
▲ Lupron Depot–3 Month 11.25 mg (16%) 462
Lupron Depot-PED 7.5 mg, 11.25 mg and 15 mg (Less than 2%) 471
Luvox CR Extended-Release Capsules (Infrequent) 1759
Meridia Capsules (1.3%) 475
Nadolol Tablets 2191
Namenda (Infrequent) 1180
Neoral Oral Solution (1% to less than 3%) 2280
Neoral Soft Gelatin Capsules (1% to less than 3%) 2280
Norvir (Less than 2%) 489
Ortho Evra Transdermal System (1% to 2.4%) 2437
OxyContin Tablets (Less than 1%) 2589
Paxil (Frequent) 1535
Paxil CR Controlled-Release Tablets (Frequent) 1544
▲ PegIntron Powder for Injection (28%) 2903
Pristiq Extended-Release Tablets 3247
▲ Prograf Capsules and Injection (3% to 15%) 622
▲ Prometrium Capsules (100 mg, 200 mg) (6%) 3047
Protonix for Delayed-Release Oral Suspension (Less than 1%) 3254
Protonix Delayed-Release Tablets (Less than 1%) 3254
Protonix I.V. (Less than 1%) 3257
Provigil Tablets (1%) 977
Prozac Weekly Capsules (Rare) 1852
Prozac Pulvules and Liquid (Frequent) 1852
▲ Rebetol (7% to 47%) 2917
Remeron Tablets (Infrequent) 2924
RemeronSolTab Tablets (Infrequent) 2927
Requip Tablets (Infrequent) 1561
Retrovir Capsules 1574
Retrovir IV Infusion 1579
Retrovir 1574
Rilutek Tablets (Infrequent) 2771
Risperdal Consta Long-Acting Injection (Infrequent) 1753
Romazicon Injection (1% to 3%) 2646
Salagen Tablets (Less than 1%) 1082
Sustiva Capsules (Less than 2%) 930
Sustiva Tablets (Less than 2%) 930
Symbyax Capsules (Infrequent) 1871
Timoptic Sterile Ophthalmic Solution 2121
Timoptic in Ocudose 2124
Timoptic-XE Sterile Ophthalmic Gel Forming Solution 2125
Toprol-XL Tablets 666
Venlafaxine Hydrochloride Tablets (Infrequent) 2199
Wellbutrin SR Sustained-Release Tablets (Infrequent) 1653
Wellbutrin XL Extended-Release Tablets (Infrequent) 1659
Yaz Tablets (Greater than 1%) 805
Zomig Tablets (Infrequent) 694
Zomig-ZMT Tablets (Infrequent) 694
Zyban Sustained-Release Tablets (Infrequent) 1692
Zyprexa Tablets 1883
Zyprexa IntraMuscular (Infrequent) 1883
Zyprexa ZYDIS Orally Disintegrating Tablets 1883
Zyrtec Chewable Tablets (Less than 2%) 1920
Zyrtec Syrup (Less than 2%) 1920
Zyrtec Tablets (Less than 2%) 1920
Zyrtec-D 12 Hour Extended Release Tablets (Less than 2%) 1923

Emphysema
▲ Lupron Depot 7.5 mg (Less than 5%) 469
Paxil (Rare) 1535
Paxil CR Controlled-Release Tablets (Rare) 1544
PegIntron Powder for Injection (Less than or equal to 1%) 2903
Prozac Weekly Capsules (Rare) 1852
Prozac Pulvules and Liquid (Rare) 1852
Symbyax Capsules (Rare) 1871

Enanthema
Gengraf Capsules (1% to less than 3%) 435
Neoral Oral Solution (1% to less than 3%) 2280
Neoral Soft Gelatin Capsules (1% to less than 3%) 2280

Encephalitis
Attenuvax 1951
Boostrix 1377
M-M-R II (Rare) 2054
Mumpsvax (Very rare) 2068
Orthoclone OKT3 Sterile Solution (Less than 1%) 2387
Pentacel 2792
ProQuad 2099
Recombivax HB 2107
Vaqta (Very rare) 2130
Varivax 2133

Encephalitis, measles inclusion body
Attenuvax 1951
M-M-R II 2054

Encephalomyelitis
Fluarix Vaccine 1446

Encephalomyopathy, mitochondrial, exacerbation of
FluMist Vaccine 1945

Encephalopathy
Abelcet Injection 1134
Arranon Injection (1%) 1319
Attenuvax 1951
Busulfex Injection (2%) 2477
Campral Tablets (Rare) 1158
Depakote ER Tablets 423
Fluarix Vaccine 1446
Flulaval Injection Vaccine 1448
Fortaz 1450
Gabitril Tablets (Infrequent) 973
Gengraf Capsules 435
Havrix Injection Vaccine 1454
Infanrix Vaccine 1479
Intron A for Injection 2859
Kaletra (Less than 2%) 452
Levaquin 2416
Levaquin in 5% Dextrose Injection 2416
Lyrica Capsules (Rare) 2527
M-M-R II (Rare) 2054
Mycamine for Injection 616
Namenda 1180
Neoral Oral Solution 2280
Neoral Soft Gelatin Capsules 2280
Orthoclone OKT3 Sterile Solution (Less than 1%) 2387
Paser Granules 1747
Pediarix Vaccine 1552
PegIntron Powder for Injection 2903
Pentacel 2792
Primaxin I.M. 2080
Primaxin I.V. (Less than 0.2%) 2083
▲ Prograf Capsules and Injection (3% to 15%) 622
Proleukin for Injection 2287
ProQuad 2099
Sandimmune 2296
Stromectol Tablets 2120
Twinrix Vaccine 1628
Valtrex Caplets 1635
Velcade for Injection 2168
▲ Vesanoid Capsules (3%) 2660
▲ Xeloda Tablets (Less than 5%) 2662
Zonegran Capsules (Rare) 1089
Zovirax 1690
Zyprexa Tablets (Rare) 1883
Zyprexa ZYDIS Orally Disintegrating Tablets (Rare) 1883

Encephalopathy, hepatic
Aciphex Tablets 1053
Intron A for Injection (Very rare) 2859
Nexium Delayed-Release Capsules 645
Nexium I.V. 652
Nexium Delayed-Release Oral Suspension 645
Viramune Oral Suspension 873
Viramune Tablets 873

Encephalopathy, hypertensive
Catapres-TTS (Rare) 842
Clorpres Tablets 2185
Epogen for Injection (On occasion) 576
▲ Humira Injection (Less than 5%) 442
Procrit for Injection (Occasional) 2391

Endocardial fibrosis
Myleran Tablets (One case) 1530

Endocarditis
Proleukin for Injection (Less than 1%) 2287

Endocarditis, infectious
CellCept Capsules 2622
CellCept Intravenous 2622
CellCept Oral Suspension 2622
CellCept Tablets 2622
Myfortic Tablets (Occasionally) 2276

Endocrine disturbances
Elocon Lotion 0.1% (1 in 65 patients) 2841
▲ Hycamtin for Injection (6%) 1459
Imitrex Nasal Spray 1470
▲ Novantrone for Injection Concentrate (6%) 1100

Endodontic procedure
Xyrem Oral Solution (Infrequent) 1766

Endometrial carcinoma
(*see under* Carcinoma, endometrial)

Endometrial disorder, unspecified
Angeliq Tablets (1.8%) 751
Evista Tablets 1810
Evoxac Capsules (Less than 1%) 1013
Femara Tablets (Less than 0.1%) 2246
Symbyax Capsules (Rare) 1871

Endometrial hyperplasia
Activella Tablets 2347
Angeliq Tablets 751
Climara Transdermal System 763
Climara Pro Transdermal System 768
Divigel 3167
Estratest Tablets 3043
Estratest H.S. Tablets 3043
Premarin Intravenous 3217
Premarin Tablets 3221
Premarin Vaginal Cream 3228
Premphase Tablets 3232
Prempro Tablets 3232

Endometrial proliferation disorders, unspecified
Femara Tablets (Less than 0.1% to 0.3%) 2246

Endometrial thickening
▲ Activella Tablets (10%) 2347

Endometriosis
Effexor XR Extended-Release Capsules (Rare) 3195
Imitrex Injection 1465
Imitrex Nasal Spray (Rare) 1470
Imitrex Tablets 1474
Tarka Tablets (Less frequent) 511
Venlafaxine Hydrochloride Tablets (Rare) 2199

Endometriosis, exacerbation of
Activella Tablets 2347
Enjuvia Tablets 1029
Premarin Tablets 3221

Endometrium disorders, unspecified
Amerge Tablets (Rare) 1301

Endophthalmitis
Lucentis Injection (Less than 0.1%) 1205
Triesence Injectable Suspension (2%) ⊙ 209

Endotracheal tube, reflux into
▲ Infasurf Intratracheal Suspension (21%) 1168

Energy, high
Eldepryl Capsules 3052

Energy, loss of
▲ Gabitril Tablets (20%) 973
Ortho-Cyclen/Ortho Tri-Cyclen 2449
Ortho Tri-Cyclen Lo Tablets 2458

Enteritis
Ambien Tablets (Rare) 2692
Ambien CR Tablets (Rare) 2696
Kaletra (Less than 2%) 452
Lipitor Tablets (Less than 2%) 2501
Micardis Tablets (Greater than 0.3%) 852
Micardis HCT Tablets 854
Mirapex Tablets 857
Paxil (Rare) 1535
Paxil CR Controlled-Release Tablets (Rare) 1544
Protonix for Delayed-Release Oral Suspension (Less than 1%) 3254
Protonix Delayed-Release Tablets (Less than 1%) 3254
Protonix I.V. (Less than 1%) 3257
Prozac Weekly Capsules (Rare) 1852
Prozac Pulvules and Liquid (Rare) 1852
Taxotere Injection Concentrate 2773
Zyprexa Tablets (Rare) 1883
Zyprexa ZYDIS Orally Disintegrating Tablets (Rare) 1883

Enterocolitis
Augmentin 1323
Augmentin Tablets 1327
Augmentin XR Extended Release Tablets 1333
Augmentin ES-600 Powder for Oral Suspension 1329
Chantix Tablets (Infrequent) 2511
Evoxac Capsules (Less than 1%) 1013
Indocin I.V. (Less than 3%) 2489
Ixempra Kit for Injection 915
Kaletra (Less than 2%) 452
Omnicef Capsules 497
Omnicef for Oral Suspension 497
Prograf Capsules and Injection 622
Solodyn Extended Release Tablets 1938

Enterocolitis, necrotizing
Indocin I.V. 2489
▲ Infasurf Intratracheal Suspension (5% to 17%) 1168
NeoProfen Injection 2496
▲ Xeloda Tablets (Less than 5%) 2662

Enterocolitis, neutropenic
Taxotere Injection Concentrate 2773

Enterocolitis, non-necrotizing
▲ NeoProfen Injection (22%) 2496

Entropion
BOTOX Purified Neurotoxin Complex (Less than 1%) 550

Enuresis
Aricept Tablets 1062
Aricept ODT Tablets 1062
Depakote ER Tablets 423
Geodon (Rare) 2520
Klonopin (Infrequent) 2639
Wellbutrin Tablets (Rare) 1648
▲ Xyrem Oral Solution (3% to 17.1%) 1766
Zonegran Capsules (Rare) 1089

Eosinophil count, decreased
Avelox (Greater than or equal to 0.1% to less than 2%) 2803

Eosinophil count increased
Cipro XR Tablets 2823

Merrem I.V. (Greater than 0.2%) 684

Eosinophilia
Abelcet Injection 1134
Accolate Tablets (Rare) 669
Aceon Tablets (2 mg, 4 mg, 8 mg) 3038
▲ Advair Diskus 100/50 (4%) 1276
Advair Diskus 250/50 1276
Advair Diskus 500/50 1276
Advicor Tablets 402
Amoxil Capsules 1305
Amoxil Chewable Tablets 1305
Amoxil Pediatric Drops for Oral Suspension 1305
Amoxil Powder for Oral Suspension 1305
Amoxil Tablets 1305
Anaprox Tablets (Less than 1%) 2632
Anaprox DS Tablets (Less than 1%) 2632
Aricept Tablets (Infrequent) 1062
Aricept ODT Tablets (Infrequent) 1062
Asacol Delayed-Release Tablets 2579
Augmentin 1323
Augmentin Tablets 1327
Augmentin XR Extended Release Tablets 1333
Augmentin ES-600 Powder for Oral Suspension 1329
Avelox (Greater than or equal to 0.1% to less than 2%) 2803
Axid Capsules 1364
Bicillin C-R Injectable Suspension 1775
Bicillin L-A Injection 1777
Campral Tablets (Infrequent) 1158
Capastat Sulfate for Injection (Majority of patients) 1791
▲ Captopril Tablets (About 4 to 7 of 100 patients) 2182
Carbatrol Capsules 3019
Ceftin (0.1% to 1%) 1380
Chemet Capsules (0.5% to 1.5%) 2484
Cipro I.V. (Greater than 1%) 2817
Cipro (0.6%) 2810
Clinoril Tablets (Less than 1 in 100) 1962
Copaxone for Injection (Infrequent) 3110
Cubicin for Injection (Less than 1% to 1.7%) 995
Cuprimine Capsules 1986
Demser Capsules (Rare) 1989
Depakote ER Tablets 423
Doxil Injection (Less than 1%) 2378
EC-Naprosyn Delayed-Release Tablets (Less than 1%) 2632
Effexor XR Extended-Release Capsules (Rare) 3195
Equetro Extended-Release Capsules 3174
Evoxac Capsules (Less than 1%) 1013
Fansidar Tablets 2636
Flovent Diskus 50 mcg 1435
▲ Fortaz (1 in 13) 1450
Gantrisin Pediatric Suspension 2638
Geodon Capsules (Infrequent) 2520
Invanz for Injection (1.1% to 2.1%) 2029
Kineret Injection 585
Klonopin 2639
Lamictal (Rare) 1488
Lescol Capsules (Rare) 2268
Lescol XL Tablets 2268
Leukine 774
Levaquin 2416
Levaquin in 5% Dextrose Injection 2416
Lyrica Capsules (0.1% to 1%) 2527
Mevacor Tablets 2063
Moxatag Tablets 2165
Naprosyn Suspension (Less than 1%) 2632
Naprosyn Tablets (Less than 1%) 2632
Noroxin Tablets (0.6% to 1.5%) 2069
Omnicef Capsules (0.7%) 497
Omnicef for Oral Suspension (1%) 497
Orthoclone OKT3 Sterile Solution (Less than 1%) 2387
▲ Paser Granules (55% of 38 patients with drug-induced hepatitis) 1747
Paxil (Rare) 1535
Paxil CR Controlled-Release Tablets (Rare) 1544
Pentasa Capsules 3030
Phenytek Capsules 2192
Primaxin I.M. 2080
Primaxin I.V. 2083
Prinivil Tablets (0.3% to 1%) 2087
Prinzide Tablets 2092
Proglycem Capsules (Infrequent) 1185
Proglycem Suspension (Infrequent) 1185
Protonix for Delayed-Release Oral Suspension (Less than 1%) 3254
Protonix Delayed-Release Tablets (Less than 1%) 3254
Protonix I.V. (Less than 1%) 3257
Provigil Tablets (1%) 977
Pylera Capsules 714
Requip Tablets (Infrequent) 1561
▲ Rocephin Injectable Vials, ADD-Vantage, Galaxy, Bulk (6%) 2642
Rythmol SR Capsules 1590
Singulair (Rare) 2114
Solodyn Extended Release Tablets 1938
▲ Stromectol Tablets (3%) 2120
Sulfamylon Cream 2194
Sulfamylon for 5% Topical Solution 2194
Suprax for Oral Suspension (Less than 2%) 1891
Suprax Tablets (Less than 2%) 1891
Targretin Capsules 1084
Thioridazine Hydrochloride Tablets 2195
Thiothixene Capsules 2197
Timentin ADD-Vantage 1606
Timentin Injection Galaxy Container 1609
Timentin IV Infusion 1603
Timentin Pharmacy Bulk Package 1613
Tricor Tablets 520
Tygacil for Injection (0% to less than 2%) 3276
Vaqta (Isolated reports) 2130
Venlafaxine Hydrochloride Tablets (Rare) 2199
Viramune Oral Suspension 873
Viramune Tablets 873
Voltaren Tablets (Occasionally) 2334
Voltaren-XR Tablets (Occasionally) 2337
Vytorin 10/10 Tablets 2149
Vytorin 10/10 Tablets 2939
Vytorin 10/20 Tablets 2149
Vytorin 10/20 Tablets 2939
Vytorin 10/40 Tablets 2149
Vytorin 10/40 Tablets 2939
Vytorin 10/80 Tablets 2149
Vytorin 10/80 Tablets 2939
Xolair 2339
Zantac 25 EFFERdose Tablets (Rare) 1670
Zantac Injection 1666
Zantac Injection Pharmacy Bulk Package (Rare) 1668
Zantac Injection Premixed 1666
Zantac (Rare) 1670
Zinacef for Injection (1 in 14 patients) 1678
Zinacef Injection (1 in 14 patients) 1678
Zocor Tablets (Rare) 2136
Zomig Tablets (Rare) 694
Zomig-ZMT Tablets (Rare) 694
Zosyn for Injection 3284
Zyvox (0.4% to 1.4%) 2552

Eosinophilia, myoclonus
Carbatrol Capsules (One case) 3019

Eosinophilia, peripheral
Carbatrol Capsules (One case) 3019

Eosinophilia, pulmonary
Dapsone Tablets USP 1746
Daraprim Tablets (Rare) 1400
Effexor XR Extended-Release Capsules 3195
Venlafaxine Hydrochloride Tablets 2199

Eosinophilic pneumonitis
(*see under* Pneumonitis, eosinophilic)

Epicondylitis
Celebrex Capsules (Greater than or equal to 0.1% to less than 1%) 2979
Exforge Tablets (Greater than or equal to 0.2%) 2238
Mirapex Tablets 857

Epidermal necrolysis
(*see under* Necrolysis, epidermal, toxic)

Epidermolysis
Flebogamma 5% 1715
Flebogamma 5% DIF 1718
Gammagard Liquid 730
Gamunex (Rare) 3094

Epidermolysis bullosa
Anaprox Tablets (Less than 1%) 2632
Anaprox DS Tablets (Less than 1%) 2632
EC-Naprosyn Delayed-Release Tablets (Less than 1%) 2632
Gammagard S/D (Rare) 734
Naprosyn Suspension (Less than 1%) 2632
Naprosyn Tablets (Less than 1%) 2632

Epididymitis
Asacol Delayed-Release Tablets 2579
Evoxac Capsules (Less than 1%) 1013
Lamictal (Rare) 1488
Lipitor Tablets (Less than 2%) 2501
Lovaza Capsules 1520
Lyrica Capsules (Rare) 2527
Mirapex Tablets 857
M-M-R II 2054
Paxil (Rare) 1535
Paxil CR Controlled-Release Tablets (Rare) 1544
ProQuad 2099
Protonix for Delayed-Release Oral Suspension (Less than 1%) 3254
Protonix Delayed-Release Tablets (Less than 1%) 3254
Protonix I.V. (Less than 1%) 3257
Requip Tablets (Infrequent) 1561
Tice BCG (Less than or equal to 1%) 2936

Epigastric pain
(*see under* Distress, epigastric)

Epilepsy
Exelon Patch 2233

Epilepsy, aggravation
Angeliq Tablets 751
Climara Transdermal System 763
Climara Pro Transdermal System 768
Enjuvia Tablets 1029
Estratest Tablets 3043
Estratest H.S. Tablets 3043
Exelon Capsules (Infrequent) 2229
Exelon Oral Solution (Infrequent) 2229
Indocin Capsules (Less than 1%) 2024
Indocin I.V. (Less than 1%) 2489
Indocin (Less than 1%) 2024
Premarin Intravenous 3217
Premphase Tablets 3232
Prempro Tablets 3232

Epilepsy, exacerbation of
Activella Tablets 2347
Climara Transdermal System 763
Divigel 3167
Premarin Tablets 3221
Premarin Vaginal Cream 3228

Epiphora
▲ Alphagan P Ophthalmic Solution (1% to 4%) 549
▲ Alrex Ophthalmic Suspension 0.2% (5% to 15%) ⊙236
▲ Betimol Ophthalmic Solution (1% to 5%) 3181
▲ Combigan Ophthalmic Solution (1% to 5%) 553
▲ Lotemax Ophthalmic Suspension 0.5% (5% to 15%) ⊙241
▲ Restasis Ophthalmic Emulsion (1% to 5%) 557

Epiphyseal closure, premature
Accutane Capsules 2607
Estratest Tablets 3043
Estratest H.S. Tablets 3043

Episcleritis
Durezol Ophthalmic Emulsion (Less than 1%) ⊙275
Fosamax 2005
Fosamax Plus D Tablets (Rarely) 2013
Zometa for Intravenous Infusion 2341

Epistaxis
Accutane Capsules 2607
Aceon Tablets (2 mg, 4 mg, 8 mg) (0.3% to 1%) 3038
Actiq (1% or greater) 959
Activase I.V. (Less than 1%) 1188
▲ Advair HFA 45/21 Inhalation Aerosol (1% to 3%) 1288
▲ Advair HFA 115/21 Inhalation Aerosol (1% to 3%) 1288
▲ Advair HFA 230/21 Inhalation Aerosol (1% to 3%) 1288
▲ Aerobid/Aerobid-M (1% to 3%) 1153
Aggrenox Capsules (2.4%) 819
▲ Agrylin Capsules (1% to less than 5%) 3017
Alferon N Injection (1%) 1726
Alinia for Oral Suspension (Less than 1%) 2677
Alinia Tablets (Less than 1%) 2677
Ambien Tablets (Rare) 2692
Ambien CR Tablets (Rare) 2696
▲ AmBisome for Injection (8.6% to 14.9%) 606
Amerge Tablets (Rare) 1301
Anzemet Injection (Rare) 2701
Anzemet Tablets (Rare) 2704
▲ Aptivus Capsules (3.7%) 823
▲ Aptivus Oral Solution (3.7%) 823
Aricept Tablets (Infrequent) 1062
Aricept ODT Tablets (Infrequent) 1062
Arixtra Injection (1.3%) 1313
▲ Arranon Injection (0% to 8%) 1319
Asmanex Twisthaler (1% to less than 3%) 2797
Atacand Tablets (0.5% or greater) 639
Atacand HCT (0.5% or greater) 642
▲ Atrovent Nasal Spray 0.03% (7% to 9%) 834
▲ Atrovent Nasal Spray 0.06% (8.2%) 836
Avalide Tablets 892
Avalide Tablets 2713
Avapro Tablets (Less than 1%) 897
Avapro Tablets (Less than 1%) 2718
▲ Avastin IV (32% to 35%) 1192
Axert Tablets (Infrequent) 2431
Bactroban Nasal (Less than 1%) 1367
Beconase AQ Nasal Spray (Fewer than 3 per 100 patients) 1369
▲ Busulfex Injection (25%) 2477
Campral Tablets (Infrequent) 1158
Cancidas for Injection 1953
Cardizem LA Extended Release Tablets (Less than 2%) 421
Celebrex Capsules (0.1% to 1.9%) 2979
Celexa (Infrequent) 1160
▲ CellCept Capsules (3% to less than 20%) 2622
▲ CellCept Intravenous (3% to less than 20%) 2622
▲ CellCept Oral Suspension (3% to less than 20%) 2622
▲ CellCept Tablets (3% to less than 20%) 2622
Chantix Tablets (Frequent) 2511
Cialis Tablets (Less than 2%) 1792
Cipro I.V. (1% or less) 2817
Cipro (Less than 1%) 2810
Cipro XR Tablets 2823
▲ Clarinex Syrup (3.1%) 2828
Clinoril Tablets (Less than 1%) 1962
▲ Clolar for Intravenous Infusion (31%) 1239
Copaxone for Injection (Infrequent) 3110
Cosopt Sterile Ophthalmic Solution 1969
Cozaar Tablets (Less than 1%) 1973
▲ Depakote ER Tablets (1% to 5%) 423
Diovan HCT Tablets (Less frequent) 2216
▲ Doxil Injection (1% to 10%) 2378
DynaCirc CR Controlled Release Tablets (0.5% to 1%) 1407
Effexor XR Extended-Release Capsules (Infrequent) 3195
▲ Elidel Cream 1% (0% to 3.3%) 2221
Elmiron Capsules (Less than or equal to 1%) 2435
▲ Eloxatin for Injection (2% to 16%) 2731
Emsam Transdermal System (Infrequent) 905
▲ Evoxac Capsules (1% to 3%) 1013
Exelon Capsules (Frequent) 2229
Exelon Oral Solution (Frequent) 2229
Exforge Tablets (Greater than or equal to 0.2%) 2238
Exubera Inhalation Powder (1.2% to 1.3%) 2515
▲ Flolan for Injection (4% to 9%) 1426
▲ Flonase Nasal Spray (6% to 6.9%) 1431
▲ Flovent Diskus 50 mcg (1% to 3%) 1435
FluMist Vaccine 1945
Frova Tablets (Infrequent) 1111
Gabitril Tablets (Frequent) 973
▲ Gamunex (23%) 3094
Gengraf Capsules (1% to less than 3%) 435
Geodon Capsules (Infrequent) 2520
▲ Gleevec Tablets (0% to 27%) 2255
Imitrex Nasal Spray 1470
Indocin Capsules (Less than 1%) 2024
Indocin I.V. (Less than 1%) 2489
Indocin (Less than 1%) 2024
▲ Intron A for Injection (Less than or equal to 5%) 2859
Invanz for Injection (Greater than 0.1%) 2029
Keppra Oral Solution (Greater than or equal to 2%) 3131
Keppra Tablets (Greater than or equal to 2%) 3131
Klonopin (Infrequent) 2639
Lamictal (Infrequent) 1488
▲ Leukine (17%) 774
▲ Leustatin Injection (5%) 2384
Levaquin (0.1% to 1%) 2416

Levaquin in 5% Dextrose Injection (0.1% to 1%) 2416
Levitra Tablets (Less than 2%) 2876
Lexapro Oral Suspension (Infrequent) 1174
Lexapro Tablets (Infrequent) 1174
Lipitor Tablets (Less than 2%) 2501
Lovaza Capsules 1520
Lunesta Tablets (Infrequent) 2994
Lupron Depot-PED 7.5 mg, 11.25 mg and 15 mg (Less than 2%) 471
Luvox CR Extended-Release Capsules (2%) 1759
Mavik Tablets (0.3% to 1%) 472
Maxalt Tablets (Infrequent) 2056
Maxalt-MLT Orally Disintegrating Tablets (Infrequent) 2056
Meridia Capsules 475
Merrem I.V. (0.2%) 684
▲ Miacalcin Nasal Spray (3.5%) 2274
Micardis Tablets (More than 0.3%) 852
Micardis HCT Tablets 854
Mirapex Tablets 857
▲ Mycamine for Injection (5.6% to 11.5%) 616
▲ Mylotarg for Injection (3% to 34%) 3212
Nasacort AQ Nasal Spray (2.7%) 2765
▲ Nasonex Nasal Spray (8% to 11%) 2883
Neoral Oral Solution (1% to less than 3%) 2280
Neoral Soft Gelatin Capsules (1% to less than 3%) 2280
▲ Neupogen for Injection (9% to 15%) 589
Nexium Delayed-Release Capsules (Less than 1%) 645
Nexium I.V. (Less than 1%) 652
Nexium Delayed-Release Oral Suspension (Less than 1%) 645
Norvir (Less than 2%) 489
▲ Noxafil Oral Suspension (14%) 2889
▲ Omnaris Nasal Spray (1% to 4.9%) 2998
OptiPranolol Metipranolol Ophthalmic Solution 0.3% (A small number of patients) ⊙ 245
▲ Patanase Nasal Spray (3.2% to 19%) 544
Paxil (Infrequent) 1535
Paxil CR Controlled-Release Tablets (Infrequent) 1544
Plavix Tablets (2.9%) 926
Plavix Tablets (2.9%) 2767
Pletal Tablets (Less than 2%) 2481
Prinivil Tablets (0.3% to 1%) 2087
Prinzide Tablets 2092
Pristiq Extended-Release Tablets (Less than 2%) 3247
ProQuad 2099
Protonix for Delayed-Release Oral Suspension (Less than 1%) 3254
Protonix Delayed-Release Tablets (Less than 1%) 3254
Protonix I.V. (Less than 1%) 3257
Protopic Ointment (Greater than or equal to 1%) 628
Provigil Tablets (1%) 977
Prozac Weekly Capsules (Infrequent to greater than or equal to 2%) 1852
Prozac Pulvules and Liquid (Infrequent to greater than or equal to 2%) 1852
▲ Rapamune (Greater than or equal to 3% to less than 20%) 3260
Recombinate 738
▲ Refludan for Injection (4.4%) 795
Relenza Inhalation Powder (Less than 1%) 1556
Remeron Tablets (Infrequent) 2924
RemeronSolTab Tablets (Infrequent) 2927
ReoPro Vials (9 to 11 events) 1860
Requip Tablets (Infrequent) 1561
Retrovir Capsules 1574
Retrovir IV Infusion 1579
Retrovir 1574
Rilutek Tablets (Infrequent) 2771
Risperdal Consta Long-Acting Injection (Infrequent) 1753
Rocephin Injectable Vials, ADD-Vantage, Galaxy, Bulk (Less than 0.1%) 2642
Rythmol SR Capsules 1590
Salagen Tablets (1% to 2%) 1082
Sandostatin Injection (Less than 1%) 2300
Sandostatin LAR Depot 2302
Singulair (Greater than or equal to 1%) 2114
▲ Spiriva HandiHaler (1% to 4%) 870
Sular Extended Release Tablets (Less than or equal to 1%) 2975
Supprelin LA Implant 1731
Sutent Capsules 2540
Symbyax Capsules (Infrequent) 1871
▲ Tamiflu Capsules (1% to 3%) 2649
▲ Tamiflu Oral Suspension (1% to 3%) 2649
Tarka Tablets (Less frequent) 511
Tasigna Capsules (0.1% to 1%) 2316
▲ Taxotere Injection Concentrate (0.3% to 5.7%) 2773
Teveten Tablets (Less than 1%) 515
Teveten HCT Tablets (Less than 1%) 517
TNKase (1.5%) 1233
▲ Torisel Injection (0% to 12%) 3272
Treximet Tablets (Rare) 1616
Tricor Tablets 520
▲ Trisenox Injection (25%) 986
Trusopt Sterile Ophthalmic Solution 2128
Velcade for Injection 2168
Venlafaxine Hydrochloride Tablets (Infrequent) 2199
▲ Veramyst Nasal Spray (4% to 6%) 1643
Wellbutrin Tablets (Rare) 1648
▲ Xeloda Tablets (Less than 5%) 2662
Xyzal Oral Solution (2%) 2789
Xyzal Oral Solution (2%) 3155
Xyzal Tablets (Less than 1% to 2%) 2789
Xyzal Tablets (Less than 1% to 2%) 3155
Zomig Tablets (Infrequent) 694
Zomig Nasal Spray (Infrequent) 689
Zomig-ZMT Tablets (Infrequent) 694
Zosyn for Injection (1% or less) 3284
Zyban Sustained-Release Tablets (2%) 1692
Zyprexa Tablets (Infrequent) 1883
Zyprexa ZYDIS Orally Disintegrating Tablets (Infrequent) 1883
▲ Zyrtec Chewable Tablets (1.9% to 3.7%) 1920
▲ Zyrtec Syrup (1.9% to 3.7%) 1920
▲ Zyrtec Tablets (1.9% to 3.7%) 1920
Zyrtec-D 12 Hour Extended Release Tablets (1.1%) 1923

Equilibrium dysfunction
Amerge Tablets (Infrequent) 1301
Lexapro Oral Suspension (Infrequent) 1174
Lexapro Tablets (Infrequent) 1174
Sustiva Capsules 930
Sustiva Tablets 930
Transderm Scōp Transdermal Therapeutic System (Few patients) 2206
▲ Xeloda Tablets (Less than 5%) 2662

Erectile disturbances, unspeficied
▲ Strattera Capsules (7%) 1864

Erectile dysfunction
Abilify Injection (Greater than or equal to 1 in 1000 patients and less than 1 in 100 patients) 881
Abilify Injection (Greater than or equal to 1 in 1000 patients and less than 1 in 100 patients) 2466
Abilify Oral Solution (Greater than or equal to 1 in 1000 patients and less than 1 in 100 patients) 881
Abilify Oral Solution (Greater than or equal to 1 in 1000 patients and less than 1 in 100 patients) 2466
Abilify Discmelt Orally Disintegrating Tablets (Greater than or equal to 1 in 1000 patients and less than 1 in 100 patients) 881
Abilify Discmelt Orally Disintegrating Tablets (Greater than or equal to 1 in 1000 patients and less than 1 in 100 patients) 2466
Abilify Tablets (Greater than or equal to 1 in 1000 patients and less than 1 in 100 patients) 881
Abilify Tablets (Greater than or equal to 1 in 1000 patients and less than 1 in 100 patients) 2466
Bystolic Tablets 1155
Chantix Tablets (Infrequent) 2511
▲ Cymbalta Delayed-Release Capsules (0% to 5%) 1801
Eligard 7.5 mg (Less than 2%) 2724
Eligard 22.5 mg (Less than 2%) 2724
Eligard 30 mg (Less than 2%) 2724
Eligard 45 mg (Less than 2%) 2724
Exforge Tablets (Greater than or equal to 0.2%) 2238
▲ Nexavar Tablets (1% to less than 10%) 784
▲ Pristiq Extended-Release Tablets (3% to 11%) 3247
Requip Tablets (Frequent) 1561
Tasigna Capsules (0.1% to 1%) 2316

Erection disturbances, unspecified
(*see also under* Impotence)
Advicor Tablets 402
Dantrium Capsules (Less frequent) 2580
Effexor XR Extended-Release Capsules (Rare) 3195
Lescol Capsules 2268
Lescol XL Tablets 2268
Mevacor Tablets (0.5% to 1%) 2063
Micardis Tablets 852
▲ Paxil (3.7% to 10%) 1535
▲ Paxil CR Controlled-Release Tablets (3.7% to 10%) 1544
Propecia Tablets (1.3%) 2095
▲ Vantas (3.5%) 1737
Wellbutrin Tablets (Infrequent) 1648
Wellbutrin SR Sustained-Release Tablets 1653
Wellbutrin XL Extended-Release Tablets 1659
Zyban Sustained-Release Tablets 1692

Erosion, corneal
Alphagan P Ophthalmic Solution (Less than 1%) 549
AzaSite Ophthalmic Drops (Less than 1%) 1740
▲ Combigan Ophthalmic Solution (1% to 5%) 553
Diclofenac Sodium Ophthalmic Solution ⊙ 240
Iquix Ophthalmic Solution (Less than 1%) 3183
Voltaren Ophthalmic Solution (0.1%) 2336

Erosion, skin
▲ Aldara Cream, 5% (2% to 48%) 1699
Daytrana Transdermal Patch 3022

Eructation
Actiq (Less than 1%) 959
▲ Agrylin Capsules (1% to less than 5%) 3017
Ambien Tablets (Rare) 2692
Ambien CR Tablets (Rare) 2696
AmBisome for Injection (Less common) 606
Amitiza Capsules (Less than 1%) 3082
Anaprox Tablets (Less than 1%) 2632
Anaprox DS Tablets (Less than 1%) 2632
Aricept Tablets (Infrequent) 1062
Aricept ODT Tablets (Infrequent) 1062
▲ Asacol Delayed-Release Tablets (16%) 2579
Byetta Injection 600
Campral Tablets (Infrequent) 1158
Celebrex Capsules (0.1% to 1.9%) 2979
Celexa (Infrequent) 1160
Chantix Tablets (Infrequent) 2511
Crinone 4% Gel 992
Crinone 8% Gel 992
Cymbalta Delayed-Release Capsules (Infrequent) 1801
Depakote ER Tablets (Greater than 1%) 423
Doxil Injection (Less than 1%) 2378
EC-Naprosyn Delayed-Release Tablets (Less than 1%) 2632
Effexor XR Extended-Release Capsules (Infrequent) 3195
Emend Capsules (Greater than 0.5%) 1992
Emend for Injection (Greater than 0.5%) 1999
Emsam Transdermal System (Infrequent) 905
▲ Evoxac Capsules (1% to 3%) 1013
Exelon Capsules (2%) 2229
Exelon Oral Solution (2%) 2229
Frova Tablets (Rare) 1111
Gabitril Tablets (Infrequent) 973
Gengraf Capsules (1% to less than 3%) 435
Imitrex Injection (Rare) 1465
Imitrex Nasal Spray (Rare) 1470
Imitrex Tablets 1474
▲ Intron A for Injection (Less than 5%) 2859
Kaletra (Less than 2%) 452
Lamictal (Infrequent) 1488
Lipitor Tablets (Less than 2%) 2501
▲ Lovaza Capsules (4.9% to 11%) 1520
▲ Lupron Depot 7.5 mg (Less than 5%) 469
Luvox CR Extended-Release Capsules (Infrequent) 1759
Maxalt Tablets (Rare) 2056
Maxalt-MLT Orally Disintegrating Tablets (Rare) 2056
Meridia Capsules 475
Mirapex Tablets 857
Mobic Oral Suspension (Less than 2%) 863
Mobic Tablets (Less than 2%) 863
Naprosyn Suspension (Less than 1%) 2632
Naprosyn Tablets (Less than 1%) 2632
Neoral Oral Solution (1% to less than 3%) 2280
Neoral Soft Gelatin Capsules (1% to less than 3%) 2280
Nexium Delayed-Release Capsules (Less than 1%) 645
Nexium I.V. (Less than 1%) 652
Nexium Delayed-Release Oral Suspension (Less than 1%) 645
Niaspan Extended-Release Tablets 480
Norvir (Less than 2%) 489
OxyContin Tablets (Less than 1%) 2589
Paxil (Infrequent) 1535
Paxil CR Controlled-Release Tablets (Infrequent) 1544
Pentasa Capsules (Less than 1%) 3030
Percodan Tablets 1130
▲ Photofrin for Injection (5%) 708
Protonix for Delayed-Release Oral Suspension (1%) 3254
Protonix Delayed-Release Tablets (1%) 3254
Protonix I.V. (Greater than or equal to 1%) 3257
Proventil HFA Inhalation Aerosol (Less than 3%) 2914
Prozac Weekly Capsules (Infrequent) 1852
Prozac Pulvules and Liquid (Infrequent) 1852
Remeron Tablets (Infrequent) 2924
RemeronSolTab Tablets (Infrequent) 2927
Requip Tablets (Infrequent) 1561
Retrovir Capsules 1574
Retrovir IV Infusion 1579
Retrovir 1574
Rythmol SR Capsules 1590
Salagen Tablets (Less than 1%) 1082
Symbyax Capsules (Infrequent) 1871
Tricor Tablets 520
Venlafaxine Hydrochloride Tablets (Frequent) 2199
Voltaren Tablets (Rarely) 2334
Voltaren-XR Tablets (Rarely) 2337
Xyrem Oral Solution (Infrequent) 1766
Zomig Tablets (Rare) 694
Zomig Nasal Spray (Rare) 689
Zomig-ZMT Tablets (Rare) 694
Zyprexa Tablets (Rare) 1883
Zyprexa ZYDIS Orally Disintegrating Tablets (Rare) 1883
Zyrtec Chewable Tablets (Less than 2%) 1920
Zyrtec Syrup (Less than 2%) 1920
Zyrtec Tablets (Less than 2%) 1920
Zyrtec-D 12 Hour Extended Release Tablets (Less than 2%) 1923

Eruptions
Abilify Injection (Greater than or equal to 1 in 100 patients) 2466
Abilify Oral Solution (Greater than or equal to 1 in 100 patients) 2466
Abilify Discmelt Orally Disintegrating Tablets (Greater than or equal to 1 in 100 patients) 2466
Abilify Tablets (Greater than or equal to 1 in 100 patients) 2466
Concerta Extended-Release Tablets 1925
Meridia Capsules 475
Raptiva for Injection 1218
Solodyn Extended Release Tablets 1938

Eruptions, acneiform
(*see under* Acneiform eruptions)

Eruptions, bullous
Ambien Tablets (Rare) 2692
Ambien CR Tablets (Rare) 2696
▲ Argatroban Injection (1% to 10%) 1308
▲ Arixtra Injection (0% to 3.1%) 1313
Evoxac Capsules (Less than 1%) 1013
Fragmin Injection (Rare) 1070
Frova Tablets (Infrequent) 1111
Gemzar for Injection (Very rare) 1820

Gengraf Capsules (1%) 435
Gleevec Tablets (Infrequent) 2255
▲ Hycamtin for Injection (Less than 1% to 16%) 1459
Indapamide Tablets 2188
Levaquin 2416
Levaquin in 5% Dextrose Injection 2416
Luvox CR Extended-Release Capsules 1759
Mobic Oral Suspension (Less than 2%) 863
Mobic Tablets (Less than 2%) 863
Neoral Oral Solution (1%) 2280
Neoral Soft Gelatin Capsules (1%) 2280
Plavix Tablets (Less than 1%) 926
Plavix Tablets (Less than 1%) 2767
ReoPro Vials (0.1%) 1860
▲ Soriatane Capsules (1% to 10%) 3062
Taxotere Injection Concentrate (Rare) 2773
Viramune Oral Suspension 873
Viramune Tablets 873
Zyrtec Chewable Tablets (Less than 2%) 1920
Zyrtec Syrup (Less than 2%) 1920
Zyrtec Tablets (Less than 2%) 1920
Zyrtec-D 12 Hour Extended Release Tablets (Less than 2%) 1923

Eruptions, eczematoid
(*see under* Eczema)

Eruptions, erythematous
Percocet Tablets 1127

Eruptions, fixed
Cipro 2810
Cipro XR Tablets 2823

Eruptions, fixed drug
Anaprox Tablets (Less than 1%) 2632
Anaprox DS Tablets (Less than 1%) 2632
Cipro I.V. 2817
Cuprimine Capsules 1986
EC-Naprosyn Delayed-Release Tablets (Less than 1%) 2632
Naprosyn Suspension (Less than 1%) 2632
Naprosyn Tablets (Less than 1%) 2632
Nitro-Dur Transdermal Infusion System (Uncommon) 2887
Xyzal Oral Solution 2789
Xyzal Oral Solution 3155

Eruptions, hemorrhagic
Activella Tablets 2347
Angeliq Tablets 751
Climara Transdermal System 763
Climara Pro Transdermal System 768
Divigel 3167
Enjuvia Tablets 1029
Estratest Tablets 3043
Estratest H.S. Tablets 3043
Lybrel Tablets 3204
Mircette Tablets 1034
NuvaRing 2897
Ortho-Cyclen Tablets 2449
Ortho Evra Transdermal System 2437
Ortho Tri-Cyclen Tablets 2449
Ortho Tri-Cyclen Lo Tablets 2458
Premarin Intravenous 3217
Premarin Tablets 3221
Premarin Vaginal Cream 3228
Premphase Tablets 3232
Prempro Tablets 3232
Seasonique Tablets 1046
Yaz Tablets 805

Eruptions, herpetic
▲ Chemet Capsules (2.6% to 11.2%) 2484

Eruptions, maculopapular
Avandaryl Tablets (Less than 1%) 1344
▲ Doribax Injection (1% to 5%) 2400
Duetact Tablets (Less than 1%) 3085
Mustargen for Injection (Occasional) 2492
Reyataz Capsules 3299

Eruptions, morbilliform
Avandaryl Tablets (Less than 1%) 1344
Duetact Tablets (Less than 1%) 3085

Eruptions, mucocutaneous
▲ Chemet Capsules (2.6% to 11.2%) 2484

Eruptions, psoriasis form
Lamisil Oral Granules 2264

Erysipelas
▲ Humira Injection (Less than 5%) 442

Erythema
Abilify Injection (Greater than or equal to 1 in 100 patients) 881
Abilify Injection (Greater than or equal to 1 in 1000 patients and less than 1 in 100 patients) 2466
Abilify Oral Solution (Greater than or equal to 1 in 100 patients) 881
Abilify Oral Solution (Greater than or equal to 1 in 1000 patients and less than 1 in 100 patients) 2466
Abilify Discmelt Orally Disintegrating Tablets (Greater than or equal to 1 in 100 patients) 881
Abilify Discmelt Orally Disintegrating Tablets (Greater than or equal to 1 in 1000 patients and less than 1 in 100 patients) 2466
Abilify Tablets (Greater than or equal to 1 in 100 patients) 881
Abilify Tablets (Greater than or equal to 1 in 1000 patients and less than 1 in 100 patients) 2466
Accutane Capsules 2607
Aceon Tablets (2 mg, 4 mg, 8 mg) (0.3% to 1%) 3038
▲ Aldara Cream, 5% (2% to 100%) 1699
Alphagan P Ophthalmic Solution 549
Altabax Ointment (Less than 1%) 1299
AmBisome for Injection (Infrequent) 606
Amerge Tablets (Infrequent) 1301
Amitiza Capsules (Less than 1%) 3082
Aricept Tablets (Infrequent) 1062
Aricept ODT Tablets (Infrequent) 1062
Avandaryl Tablets (Less than 1%) 1344
Avelox 2803
Axert Tablets (Rare) 2431
Bactroban Ointment (Less than 1%) 1368
Benzaclin Topical Gel (2%) 2721
Brevoxyl-4 Creamy Wash 3054
Brevoxyl-4 Gel 3054
Brevoxyl-8 Creamy Wash 3054
Brevoxyl-8 Gel 3054
▲ Campath Ampules (4%) 761
▲ Cancidas for Injection (3.5% to 8.9%) 1953
▲ Carac Cream 0.5% (93.4%) 2722
▲ Catapres-TTS (26 of 101 patients) 842
Ceftin Tablets (0.1% to 1%) 1380
Chantix Tablets (Infrequent) 2511
Cipro I.V. (1% or less) 2817
Ciprodex Otic Suspension (0.4%) 541
▲ Clarinex Syrup (3%) 2828
Climara Transdermal System 763
▲ Clolar for Intravenous Infusion (18%) 1239
Combigan Ophthalmic Solution 553
▲ Copaxone for Injection (4%) 3110
Cosmegen for Injection 2485
Cozaar Tablets (Less than 1%) 1973
▲ Cubicin for Injection (5%) 995
▲ Cyanokit 5g Antidote (94% to 100%) 1021
Cymbalta Delayed-Release Capsules (Infrequent) 1801
▲ Dacogen Injection (14%) 1066
Dantrium Intravenous (Rare) 2582
Digibind for Injection (One patient) 1403
Diprolene Lotion 0.05% (Less than 1%) 2838
Diprolene Ointment 0.05% (Less than 1%) 2839
▲ Doribax Injection (1% to 5%) 2400
▲ Doxil Injection (3.4%) 2378
▲ Duac Topical Gel (0% to 26%) 3054
Duetact Tablets (Less than 1%) 3085
Duragesic Transdermal System (1% or greater) 2405
Eligard 7.5 mg (2.6%) 2724
Eligard 22.5 mg (0.9%) 2724
Eligard 30 mg (1.1%) 2724
Eligard 45 mg 2724
Eloxatin for Injection 2731
Emsam Transdermal System 905
Engerix-B Vaccine (Less than 1%) 1409
Exelon Patch (Infrequent) 2233
Exforge Tablets (Greater than or equal to 0.2%) 2238
Extina Foam, 2% (Less than or equal to 1%) 3057
Finacea Gel (Less than 1% to 2%) 1742
Fluarix Vaccine 1446
Follistim AQ Cartridge 2844
Fosamax (Rare) 2005
Hycamtin for Injection 1459
Imitrex Injection (Infrequent) 1465
Imitrex Nasal Spray 1470
Imitrex Tablets (Infrequent) 1474
Infanrix Vaccine 1479
▲ Intron A for Injection (Less than 5%) 2859
Invanz for Injection (1.2% to 1.6%) 2029
▲ Kepivance (32%) 583
Lamictal (Rare) 1488
▲ Leustatin Injection (6%) 2384
Levaquin 2416
Levaquin in 5% Dextrose Injection 2416
Lotrisone 2881
Lovenox Injection 2756
Maxalt Tablets (Infrequent) 2056
Maxalt-MLT Orally Disintegrating Tablets (Infrequent) 2056
Mentax Cream (Less than 2%) 2190
Meruvax II 2061
▲ Miacalcin Nasal Spray (10.6%) 2274
Micardis Tablets 852
Mirapex Tablets 857
M-M-R II 2054
▲ Mycamine for Injection (11.3%) 616
▲ Nabi-HB (12%) 815
Naftin Cream (2%) 2164
Naftin Gel (0.5%) 2164
Neulasta Injection 587
▲ Nexavar Tablets (Greater than or equal to 10%) 784
Noroxin Tablets (Less frequent) 2069
Olux Foam (Less than 2%) 3061
▲ Oncaspar Injection (Greater than 5%) 1138
Orthoclone OKT3 Sterile Solution (Less than 1%) 2387
▲ Panretin Gel 0.1% (25% to 77%) 1081
▲ Pediarix Vaccine (0.6% to 41.9%) 1552
Pentacel 2792
Percocet Tablets 1127
▲ Photofrin for Injection (Approximately 20%) 708
▲ Prevnar (0% to 48.3%) 3241
Prinivil Tablets (0.3% to 1%) 2087
Prinzide Tablets 2092
▲ Protopic Ointment (9% to 28%) 628
Prozac Pulvules and Liquid 1852
Recombivax HB (Equal to or greater than 1%) 2107
Rythmol SR Capsules 1590
Sulfamylon Cream 2194
Sulfamylon for 5% Topical Solution 2194
▲ Sustiva Capsules (8.8% to 9.9%) 930
▲ Sustiva Tablets (8.8% to 9.9%) 930
▲ Targretin Gel 1% (56% to 72%) 1088
▲ Tasigna Capsules (1% to 10%) 2316
Taxotere Injection Concentrate 2773
▲ Temodar Capsules (5%) 2931
Thioridazine Hydrochloride Tablets 2195
Transderm Scōp Transdermal Therapeutic System (Infrequent) 2206
▲ Trisenox Injection (13%) 986
Twinrix Vaccine (Less than 1%) 1628
Vaprisol (2.7%) 632
Vaqta (Less than 1%) 2130
▲ Vectibix (5% to 65%) 597
Vivitrol 988
▲ Voltaren Ophthalmic Solution (Less than or equal to 3%) 2336
Xeloda Tablets 2662
▲ Ziana Gel (26% to 35%) 1942
Zomig Tablets (Rare) 694
Zomig Nasal Spray (Rare) 689
Zomig-ZMT Tablets (Rare) 694

Erythema, application site
▲ Aczone Gel 5% (Less than 1% to 13%) 3296
AndroGel 3159
▲ Dacogen Injection (5%) 1066
Elidel Cream 1% (0% to 2.2%) 2221
▲ Flector Patch (4%) 561
▲ Humira Injection (20%) 442
▲ Ionsys Transdermal System (14%) 2410
Lidoderm Patch 1114
Neupro Transdermal System 3149

Erythema, conjunctival
Neosporin Ophthalmic Solution Sterile ⊙252

Erythema, eyelid
▲ Combigan Ophthalmic Solution (1% to 5%) 553

Erythema, eyelids
▲ Alphagan P Ophthalmic Solution (1% to 4%) 549
▲ Alrex Ophthalmic Suspension 0.2% (Less than 5%) ⊙236
▲ Betimol Ophthalmic Solution (More than 5%) 3181
Iquix Ophthalmic Solution (Less than 1%) 3183
▲ Lotemax Ophthalmic Suspension 0.5% (Less than 5%) ⊙241
▲ Lumigan Ophthalmic Solution (3% to 10%) 556

Erythema, facial
Acetadote Injection (0.24% to 1.17%) 1001
Avalide Tablets 892
Avalide Tablets 2713
Avapro Tablets (Less than 1%) 897
Avapro Tablets (Less than 1%) 2718
▲ Carac Cream 0.5% (89.4% to 96.5%) 2722

Erythema, hemorrhagic exudative
(*see under* Henoch-Schönlein purpura)

Erythema, insertion site
Supprelin LA Implant 1731
Vantas (2.8%) 1737

Erythema, palmar
Acetadote Injection (0.29% to 1.41%) 1001

Erythema at injection site
▲ Actimmune (14%) 1743
Attenuvax 1951
Cimzia 3127
▲ Comvax (22.4% to 27.2%) 1966
Cubicin for Injection (2.5%) 995
Daytrana Transdermal Patch 3022
Edex Injection (2%) 2957
▲ Enbrel for Injection (37%) 569
▲ Engerix-B Vaccine (1% to 10%) 1409
▲ Flulaval Injection Vaccine (1% to 5%) 1448
Forteo for Injection (Less than 1/30 patients) 1816
▲ Gardasil Injection (0.2% to 24.6%) 2019
Humalog-Pen and KwikPen 1829
▲ Invanz for Injection (3.9%) 2029
▲ Leustatin Injection (9%) 2384
Neulasta Injection 587
Novantrone for Injection Concentrate 1100
Pediarix Vaccine 1552
Liquid PedvaxHIB (0.4% to 2.2%) 2073
Pneumovax 23 (Common) 2078
Primaxin I.V. (0.4%) 2083
▲ ProQuad (14.4%) 2099
▲ Trisenox Injection (13%) 986
▲ Vaprisol (0% to 6%) 632
▲ Vaqta (0.8% to 13.1%) 2130
▲ Varivax (19.3% to 32.5%) 2133
Velcade for Injection 2168
▲ Zostavax Injection (33.7%) 2145

Erythema multiforme
Abelcet Injection 1134
Aciphex Tablets 1053
Activella Tablets 2347
Advicor Tablets 402
Albenza Tablets 1297
Aldara Cream, 5% 1699
Amoxil Capsules 1305
Amoxil Chewable Tablets 1305
Amoxil Pediatric Drops for Oral Suspension 1305
Amoxil Powder for Oral Suspension 1305
Amoxil Tablets 1305
Anaprox Tablets (Less than 1%) 2632
Anaprox DS Tablets (Less than 1%) 2632
Angeliq Tablets 751
Arimidex Tablets (Very rare) 672
Atacand HCT 642
Atripla Tablets 938
Attenuvax (Rare) 1951
Augmentin 1323
Augmentin Tablets 1327
Augmentin XR Extended Release Tablets 1333
Augmentin ES-600 Powder for Oral Suspension 1329
Avalide Tablets 892
Avalide Tablets 2713
Cancidas for Injection 1953
Captopril Tablets 2182
Carbatrol Capsules 3019
Cardizem LA Extended Release Tablets (Infrequent) 421
Ceftin 1380
Celebrex Capsules (Less than 0.1%) 2979
Celexa (At least 3 patients) 1160
Cimzia 3127
Cipro I.V. (1% or less) 2817
Cipro 2810
Cipro XR Tablets 2823
Climara Transdermal System 763
Climara Pro Transdermal System 768
Clinoril Tablets (Less than 1%) 1962
Combivir Tablets 1384
Comvax 1966

Crixivan Capsules........................... 1979
Cymbalta Delayed-Release Capsules.................................. 1801
Daraprim Tablets........................... 1400
Daytrana Transdermal Patch........... 3022
Depakote ER Tablets....................... 423
Diovan HCT Tablets......................... 2216
Divigel.. 3167
▲ Doribax Injection (1% to 5%) 2400
Doxil Injection (Less than 1%)........... 2378
EC-Naprosyn Delayed-Release Tablets (Less than 1%)................. 2632
E.E.S. (Rare)...................................... 433
Effexor XR Extended-Release Capsules.. 3195
Enbrel for Injection............................ 569
Engerix-B Vaccine (Less than 1%)..... 1409
Enjuvia Tablets.................................. 1029
Epzicom Tablets................................. 1422
Equetro Extended-Release Capsules.. 3174
EryPed (Rare) 431
Estratest Tablets 3043
Estratest H.S. Tablets 3043
Exforge Tablets (Greater than 0.1% to less than 1%) 2238
Fansidar Tablets 2636
Flebogamma 5% 1715
Flebogamma 5% DIF 1718
Fluarix Vaccine 1446
Focalin XR Capsules 2251
Fortaz 1450
Furosemide Tablets 2186
Gammagard Liquid 730
Gammagard S/D (Rare) 734
Gamunex (Rare) 3094
Gleevec Tablets 2255
Gris-PEG Tablets (Occasional) 2507
Havrix Injection Vaccine 1454
Indocin Capsules (Less than 1%) 2024
Indocin I.V. (Less than 1%) 2489
Indocin (Less than 1%) 2024
Intelence Tablets (Less than 0.1%) ... 3119
Intravenous Sodium Diuril 2490
Intron A for Injection 2859
Ixempra Kit for Injection 915
Ketek Tablets (Less than 0.2%) 2744
Lamictal (Rare) 1488
Lescol Capsules (Rare) 2268
Lescol XL Tablets 2268
Leukeran Tablets (Rare) 1508
Levaquin 2416
Levaquin in 5% Dextrose Injection 2416
Lexapro Oral Suspension 1174
Lexapro Tablets 1174
Lipitor Tablets 2501
Lunesta Tablets (Rare) 2994
Lupron Depot-PED 7.5 mg, 11.25 mg and 15 mg (2%) 471
Lybrel Tablets 3204
Malarone Pediatric Tablets (Rare) 1521
Malarone Tablets (Rare) 1521
Mepron Suspension 1526
Merrem I.V. 684
Meruvax II (Rare) 2061
Metadate CD Capsules 3146
Mevacor Tablets (Rare) 2063
Micardis HCT Tablets 854
Mircette Tablets 1034
M-M-R II (Rare) 2054
Mobic Oral Suspension (Less than 0.1%) 863
Mobic Tablets (Less than 0.1%) 863
Moxatag Tablets 2165
Mumpsvax (Rare) 2068
Mustargen for Injection 2492
Mycamine for Injection 616
Myleran Tablets (Rare) 1530
Naprosyn Suspension (Less than 1%) 2632
Naprosyn Tablets (Less than 1%) 2632
Nexavar Tablets (0.1% to less than 1%) 784
Nexium Delayed-Release Capsules .. 645
Nexium I.V. 652
Nexium Delayed-Release Oral Suspension 645
Noroxin Tablets 2069
NuvaRing 2897
Omnicef Capsules 497
Omnicef for Oral Suspension 497
Ortho-Cyclen Tablets 2449
Ortho Evra Transdermal System 2437
Ortho Tri-Cyclen Tablets 2449
Ortho Tri-Cyclen Lo Tablets 2458
Paxil (Rare) 1535
Paxil CR Controlled-Release Tablets (Rare) 1544
Pediarix Vaccine 1552
PegIntron Powder for Injection 2903
Plavix Tablets 926
Plavix Tablets.................................... 2767
Premarin Intravenous........................ 3217
Premarin Tablets............................... 3221
Premarin Vaginal Cream 3228
Premphase Tablets........................... 3232
Prempro Tablets............................... 3232
Prevnar 3241
Primaxin I.M...................................... 2080
Primaxin I.V. (Less than 0.2%).......... 2083
Prinzide Tablets................................ 2092
ProAmatine Tablets (Rare)................ 3032
ProQuad 2099
Protonix for Delayed-Release Oral Suspension 3254
Protonix Delayed-Release Tablets..... 3254
Protonix I.V....................................... 3257
Provigil Tablets (Rare)...................... 977
Prozac Weekly Capsules................... 1852
Raptiva for Injection......................... 1218
Remicade for IV Injection 950
Reyataz Capsules............................. 3299
Rilutek Tablets (Rare)....................... 2771
Rocaltrol Capsules (One case)......... 1150
Rocaltrol Oral Solution (One case).... 1150
Rocephin Injectable Vials, ADD-Vantage, Galaxy, Bulk............ 2642
Seasonique Tablets 1046
Solodyn Extended Release Tablets... 1938
Suprax for Oral Suspension (Less than 2%).. 1891
Suprax Tablets (Less than 2%)......... 1891
▲ Sustiva Capsules (Up to 3.3%) 930
▲ Sustiva Tablets (Up to 3.3%) 930
Tamiflu Capsules (Rare)................... 2649
Tamiflu Oral Suspension (Rare)......... 2649
Tarka Tablets.................................... 511
Taxotere Injection Concentrate (Rare).. 2773
Tekturna HCT Tablets....................... 2324
Temodar Capsules (Rare)................. 2931
Teveten HCT Tablets........................ 517
Timentin ADD-Vantage 1606
Timentin Injection Galaxy Container 1609
Timentin IV Infusion......................... 1603
Timentin Pharmacy Bulk Package.... 1613
Trizivir Tablets.................................. 1622
Twinrix Vaccine................................ 1628
Valtrex Caplets................................. 1635
Varivax.. 2133
Venlafaxine Hydrochloride Tablets.... 2199
Voltaren Tablets (Rarely).................. 2334
Voltaren-XR Tablets (Rarely)............ 2337
Vytorin 10/10 Tablets....................... 2149
Vytorin 10/10 Tablets....................... 2939
Vytorin 10/20 Tablets....................... 2149
Vytorin 10/20 Tablets....................... 2939
Vytorin 10/40 Tablets....................... 2149
Vytorin 10/40 Tablets....................... 2939
Vytorin 10/80 Tablets....................... 2149
Vytorin 10/80 Tablets....................... 2939
Wellbutrin Tablets (Rare).................. 1648
Wellbutrin SR Sustained-Release Tablets (Rare)................................ 1653
Wellbutrin XL Extended-Release Tablets (Rare)................................ 1659
Yaz Tablets....................................... 805
Zantac 25 EFFERdose Tablets (Rare)... 1670
Zantac Injection (Rare)..................... 1666
Zantac (Rare).................................... 1670
Ziagen... 1673
Zinacef for Injection (Rare)............... 1678
Zinacef Injection (Rare).................... 1678
Zocor Tablets (Rare)......................... 2136
Zomig Tablets (Rare)......................... 694
Zomig Nasal Spray (Rare)................. 689
Zomig-ZMT Tablets (Rare)................ 694
Zosyn for Injection (Rare)................. 3284
Zovirax.. 1690
Zyban Sustained-Release Tablets (Rare)... 1692

Erythema nodosum
Accutane Capsules........................... 2607
Activella Tablets............................... 2347
Anaprox Tablets (Less than 1%)....... 2632
Anaprox DS Tablets (Less than 1%).. 2632
Angeliq Tablets................................. 751
Asacol Delayed-Release Tablets....... 2579
Busulfex Injection (2%).................... 2477
Carbatrol Capsules........................... 3019
Cimzia... 3127
Cipro I.V. (1% or less)...................... 2817
Cipro (Less than 1%)........................ 2810
Cipro XR Tablets.............................. 2823
Climara Transdermal System........... 763
Climara Pro Transdermal System..... 768
Copaxone for Injection (Infrequent).... 3110
Depakote ER Tablets (Greater than 1%).. 423
Divigel.. 3167
Doxil Injection (Less than 1%)........... 2378
EC-Naprosyn Delayed-Release Tablets (Less than 1%)................. 2632
Effexor XR Extended-Release Capsules (Rare)............................. 3195
Engerix-B Vaccine (Less than 1%)..... 1409
Enjuvia Tablets................................. 1029
Estratest Tablets.............................. 3043
Estratest H.S. Tablets....................... 3043
Indocin Capsules (Less than 1%)...... 2024
Indocin I.V. (Less than 1%).............. 2489
Indocin (Less than 1%)..................... 2024
▲ Intron A for Injection (Less than 5%).. 2859
Lybrel Tablets................................... 3204
Mircette Tablets................................ 1034
Myleran Tablets (Rare)..................... 1530
Naprosyn Suspension (Less than 1%).. 2632
Naprosyn Tablets (Less than 1%)..... 2632
Neupogen for Injection (One event) .. 589
NuvaRing.. 2897
Omnicef Capsules 497
Omnicef for Oral Suspension 497
Ortho-Cyclen/Ortho Tri-Cyclen 2449
Ortho Tri-Cyclen Lo Tablets 2458
Paxil (Rare) 1535
Paxil CR Controlled-Release Tablets (Rare) 1544
Pentasa Capsules (Less than 1%) 3030
Premarin Intravenous 3217
Premarin Tablets 3221
Premarin Vaginal Cream 3228
Premphase Tablets 3232
Prempro Tablets 3232
Prozac Weekly Capsules 1852
Recombivax HB (Less than 1%) 2107
Salagen Tablets (Less than 1%) 1082
Seasonique Tablets 1046
Singulair 2114
Tasigna Capsules 2316
Twinrix Vaccine 1628
Venlafaxine Hydrochloride Tablets (Rare) 2199
Vesanoid Capsules (Isolated cases) 2660
Yaz Tablets 805

Erythrocytes, abnormal
Gabitril Tablets (Infrequent) 973
Paxil (Rare) 1535
Paxil CR Controlled-Release Tablets (Rare) 1544
▲ Somatuline Depot Injection (5% to 14%) 3102

Erythrocytosis
Moban Tablets 1116

Erythrocyturia
Emend Capsules (Greater than 0.5%) 1992
Emend for Injection (Greater than 0.5%) 1999

Erythroderma
Cozaar Tablets 1973

Erythromelalgia
Gammagard S/D 734

Erythropenia
Accutane Capsules 2607
Aricept Tablets (Infrequent) 1062
Aricept ODT Tablets (Infrequent) 1062
Moban Tablets 1116
Mustargen for Injection 2492
Primaxin I.M. 2080

Escharotic effect
▲ Panretin Gel 0.1% (1% to 8%) 1081

Esophageal disease, unspecified
Myleran Tablets 1530
Nexium Delayed-Release Capsules (Less than 1%) 645
Nexium I.V. (Less than 1%) 652
Nexium Delayed-Release Oral Suspension (Less than 1%) 645

Esophageal erosions
Fosamax 2005
Fosamax Plus D Tablets 2013

Esophageal irration
Pylera Capsules 714

Esophageal perforation
Celebrex Capsules (Less than 0.1%) 2979
Fosamax (Rare) 2005
Fosamax Plus D Tablets (Rarely) 2013

Esophageal rupture
Exelon Capsules (One case) 2229
Exelon Oral Solution (One case)....... 2229

Esophageal stenosis
Actiq (Less than 1%)....................... 959
Mirapex Tablets................................ 857
Rilutek Tablets (Infrequent).............. 2771

Esophageal stricture
Evoxac Capsules (Less than 1%)...... 1013
Fosamax (Rare)................................ 2005
Fosamax Plus D Tablets (Rarely)....... 2013
Nexium Delayed-Release Capsules (Less than 1%)............................ 645
Nexium I.V. (Less than 1%).............. 652
Nexium Delayed-Release Oral Suspension (Less than 1%)........... 645
▲ Photofrin for Injection (6% to 38%).. 708

Esophageal ulceration
Accutane Capsules.......................... 2607
Actonel with Calcium Tablets........... 2574
Azilect Tablets (Infrequent) 3106
Fosamax Plus D Tablets (0.1% to 1.5%) 2013
Pylera Capsules 714

Esophagitis
Abilify Injection (Greater than or equal to 1 in 1000 patients and less than 1 in 100 patients) 881
Abilify Injection (Greater than or equal to 1 in 1000 patients and less than 1 in 100 patients) 2466
Abilify Oral Solution (Greater than or equal to 1 in 1000 patients and less than 1 in 100 patients) 881
Abilify Oral Solution (Greater than or equal to 1 in 1000 patients and less than 1 in 100 patients) 2466
Abilify Discmelt Orally Disintegrating Tablets (Greater than or equal to 1 in 1000 patients and less than 1 in 100 patients) 881
Abilify Discmelt Orally Disintegrating Tablets (Greater than or equal to 1 in 1000 patients and less than 1 in 100 patients) 2466
Abilify Tablets (Greater than or equal to 1 in 1000 patients and less than 1 in 100 patients) 881
Abilify Tablets (Greater than or equal to 1 in 1000 patients and less than 1 in 100 patients) 2466
Accutane Capsules 2607
Actiq (Less than 1%) 959
Actonel Tablets 2568
Actonel with Calcium Tablets 2574
▲ Alimta for Injection (Up to 6%) 1786
Amerge Tablets (Rare) 1301
Anaprox Tablets (Less than 1%) 2632
Anaprox DS Tablets (Less than 1%) .. 2632
Azilect Tablets (Infrequent) 3106
Busulfex Injection (2%) 2477
Campral Tablets (Infrequent) 1158
Celebrex Capsules (0.1% to 1.9%) ... 2979
Celexa (Infrequent) 1160
▲ CellCept Capsules (3% to less than 20%) 2622
▲ CellCept Intravenous (3% to less than 20%) 2622
▲ CellCept Oral Suspension (3% to less than 20%) 2622
▲ CellCept Tablets (3% to less than 20%) 2622
Chantix Tablets (Infrequent) 2511
Cialis Tablets (Less than 2%) 1792
Copaxone for Injection (Infrequent) .. 3110
Cosmegen for Injection 2485
Didronel Tablets 2583
▲ Doxil Injection (1% to 10%) 2378
EC-Naprosyn Delayed-Release Tablets (Less than 1%) 2632
Effexor XR Extended-Release Capsules (Infrequent) 3195
Elmiron Capsules (Less than or equal to 1%) 2435
Enbrel for Injection 569
Evoxac Capsules (Less than 1%) 1013
Exelon Capsules (Infrequent) 2229
Exelon Oral Solution (Infrequent) 2229
Fosamax 2005
Fosamax Plus D Tablets 2013
Gabitril Tablets (Infrequent) 973
Gengraf Capsules (1% to less than 3%) 435
▲ Humira Injection (Less than 5%) 442
▲ Intron A for Injection (Less than 5%) 2859
Invanz for Injection (Greater than 0.1%) 2029
Ixempra Kit for Injection 915

Kaletra (Less than 2%) 452
Lamictal 1488
Levaquin (0.1% to 1%) 2416
Levaquin in 5% Dextrose Injection (0.1% to 1%) 2416
Levitra Tablets (Less than 2%) 2876
Lipitor Tablets (Less than 2%) 2501
Luvox CR Extended-Release Capsules (Infrequent) 1759
Lyrica Capsules (0.1% to 1%) 2527
Mirapex Tablets 857
Mobic Oral Suspension (Less than 2%) 863
Mobic Tablets (Less than 2%) 863
Myfortic Tablets 2276
Naprosyn Suspension (Less than 1%) 2632
Naprosyn Tablets (Less than 1%) 2632
Neoral Oral Solution (1% to less than 3%) 2280
Neoral Soft Gelatin Capsules (1% to less than 3%) 2280
Nexium Delayed-Release Capsules (Less than 1%) 645
Nexium I.V. (Less than 1%) 652
Nexium Delayed-Release Oral Suspension (Less than 1%) 645
Norvir (Less than 2%) 489
Paxil (Rare) 1535
Paxil CR Controlled-Release Tablets (Rare) 1544
▲ Photofrin for Injection (5%) 708
Pletal Tablets (Less than 2%) 2481
▲ Prograf Capsules and Injection (3% to 15%) 622
Protonix for Delayed-Release Oral Suspension (Less than 1%) 3254
Protonix Delayed-Release Tablets (Less than 1%) 3254
Protonix I.V. (Less than 1%) 3257
Prozac Weekly Capsules (Infrequent) 1852
Prozac Pulvules and Liquid (Infrequent) 1852
Pylera Capsules 714
Requip Tablets (Infrequent) 1561
Rythmol Tablets (2%) 1586
Salagen Tablets (Less than 1%) 1082
▲ Simulect for Injection (3% to 10%) 2306
Soriatane Capsules (Less than 1%) 3062
Symbyax Capsules (Infrequent) 1871
▲ Taxotere Injection Concentrate (1.1% to 25.1%) 2773
Teveten Tablets (Less than 1%) 515
Teveten HCT Tablets (Less than 1%) 517
Tricor Tablets 520
Venlafaxine Hydrochloride Tablets (Infrequent) 2199
Vicoprofen Tablets (Less than 1%) 533
Voltaren Tablets (Occasionally) 2334
Voltaren-XR Tablets (Occasionally) 2337
Wellbutrin Tablets 1648
Wellbutrin SR Sustained-Release Tablets 1653
Wellbutrin XL Extended-Release Tablets 1659
Xeloda Tablets 2662
Zomig Tablets (Infrequent) 694
Zomig-ZMT Tablets (Infrequent) 694
Zonegran Capsules (Rare) 1089
Zyban Sustained-Release Tablets 1692
Zyprexa Tablets (Infrequent) 1883
Zyprexa ZYDIS Orally Disintegrating Tablets (Infrequent) 1883

Esophagitis, reflux
Requip Tablets (Infrequent) 1561
▲ Sutent Capsules (11%) 2540

Esophagitis, ulcerative
Indocin I.V. (Less than 1%) 2489
Tasigna Capsules 2316

Esophagospasm
Ambien Tablets (Rare) 2692
Ambien CR Tablets (Rare) 2696
Effexor XR Extended-Release Capsules (Rare) 3195
Frova Tablets (Infrequent) 1111
Mirapex Tablets 857
Venlafaxine Hydrochloride Tablets (Rare) 2199

ESR, elevation
Accutane Capsules 2607
Aceon Tablets (2 mg, 4 mg, 8 mg) 3038
Advicor Tablets 402
Ambien Tablets (Rare) 2692
Ambien CR Tablets (Rare) 2696
Captopril Tablets 2182
Cipro I.V. (Rare) 2817
Comvax 1966
Lescol Capsules (Rare) 2268
Lescol XL Tablets 2268
Mevacor Tablets (Rare) 2063
Prinivil Tablets (0.3% to 1%) 2087
Prinzide Tablets 2092
Recombivax HB 2107
Vytorin 10/10 Tablets 2149
Vytorin 10/10 Tablets 2939
Vytorin 10/20 Tablets 2149
Vytorin 10/20 Tablets 2939
Vytorin 10/40 Tablets 2149
Vytorin 10/40 Tablets 2939
Vytorin 10/80 Tablets 2149
Vytorin 10/80 Tablets 2939
Zocor Tablets (Rare) 2136

Euphoria
Actiq (Less than 1%) 959
Adderall XR Capsules 3012
Adipex-P 1185
Ambien Tablets (Frequent) 2692
Aricept Tablets (Infrequent) 1062
Aricept ODT Tablets (Infrequent) 1062
▲ Avinza Capsules (Less than 5%) 1772
Axert Tablets (Rare) 2431
Bicillin C-R Injectable Suspension 1775
Bicillin L-A Injection 1777
Celexa (Infrequent) 1160
Chantix Tablets (Rare) 2511
Copaxone for Injection (At least 2%) 3110
Dexedrine 1401
▲ Duragesic Transdermal System (3% to 10%) 2405
Effexor XR Extended-Release Capsules (Infrequent) 3195
Eldepryl Capsules 3052
Emsam Transdermal System (Infrequent) 905
Flumadine (Less than 0.3%) 1167
Frova Tablets (Infrequent) 1111
Gabitril Tablets (Frequent) 973
Imitrex Injection (Infrequent) 1465
Imitrex Nasal Spray (Infrequent) 1470
Imitrex Tablets (Infrequent) 1474
Lamictal (Infrequent) 1488
Lidoderm Patch 1114
Lunesta Tablets (Rare) 2994
Luvox CR Extended-Release Capsules (Infrequent) 1759
▲ Lyrica Capsules (2% to 7%) 2527
▲ Marinol Capsules (3% to 10%) 3163
Marplan Tablets 3177
Maxalt Tablets (Frequent) 2056
Maxalt-MLT Orally Disintegrating Tablets (Frequent) 2056
Moban Tablets (Less frequent) 1116
MS Contin Tablets (Among most frequent) 2585
Norvir (Less than 2%) 489
Opana Tablets (Less than 1%) 1117
Opana ER Tablets (Less than 1%) 1121
▲ OxyContin Tablets (Between 1% and 5%) 2589
OxyIR Capsules 2593
Paxil (Rare) 1535
Paxil CR Controlled-Release Tablets (Rare) 1544
Percocet Tablets 1127
Percodan Tablets 1130
Prozac Weekly Capsules (Infrequent) 1852
Prozac Pulvules and Liquid (Among Most Frequent) 1852
Remeron Tablets (Infrequent) 2924
RemeronSolTab Tablets (Infrequent) 2927
Requip Tablets (Infrequent) 1561
Rilutek Tablets (Rare) 2771
Risperdal Consta Long-Acting Injection (Infrequent) 1753
▲ Romazicon Injection (1% to 3%) 2646
Stalevo Tablets 2309
Sustiva Capsules (Less than 2%) 930
Sustiva Tablets (Less than 2%) 930
Symbyax Capsules (Infrequent) 1871
Tussionex Pennkinetic Extended-Release Suspension 3154
Tylenol with Codeine Tablets 2427
Ultram ER Extended-Release Tablets (0.5% to less than 1%) 2428
Venlafaxine Hydrochloride Tablets (Infrequent) 2199
Vicoprofen Tablets (Less than 1%) 533
Vivitrol 988
Vyvanse Capsules 3033
Wellbutrin Tablets (1.2%) 1648
Wellbutrin SR Sustained-Release Tablets 1653
Wellbutrin XL Extended-Release Tablets 1659
Xyrem Oral Solution (Infrequent) 1766
Zomig Tablets (Rare) 694
Zomig Nasal Spray (Rare) 689
Zomig-ZMT Tablets (Rare) 694
Zonegran Capsules (Infrequent) 1089
Zyban Sustained-Release Tablets 1692
▲ Zyprexa Tablets (2% to 3%) 1883
▲ Zyprexa ZYDIS Orally Disintegrating Tablets (2% to 3%) 1883
Zyrtec Chewable Tablets (Less than 2%) 1920
Zyrtec Syrup (Less than 2%) 1920
Zyrtec Tablets (Less than 2%) 1920
Zyrtec-D 12 Hour Extended Release Tablets (Less than 2%) 1923

Euphoric mood
Ambien CR Tablets (1%) 2696
Fentora Tablets (Greater than 1%) 968
Mirapex Tablets 857

Exanthema
Aptivus Capsules (Less than 2%) 823
Aptivus Oral Solution (Less than 2%) 823
Boostrix 1377
Copaxone for Injection (Infrequent) 3110
Exforge Tablets (Greater than or equal to 0.2%) 2238
Requip Tablets (Infrequent) 1561
Rocephin Injectable Vials, ADD-Vantage, Galaxy, Bulk 2642
Tarka Tablets 511

Exanthema, bullous
Treanda for Injection 983

Exanthema, viral
ProQuad (1.2%) 2099
Vaqta (1%) 2130

Excitability
Abilify Injection (Greater than or equal to 1 in 1000 patients and less than 1 in 100 patients) 2466
Abilify Oral Solution (Greater than or equal to 1 in 1000 patients and less than 1 in 100 patients) 2466
Abilify Discmelt Orally Disintegrating Tablets (Greater than or equal to 1 in 1000 patients and less than 1 in 100 patients) 2466
Abilify Tablets (Greater than or equal to 1 in 1000 patients and less than 1 in 100 patients) 2466
Actifed Cold & Allergy Tablets 1895
Benadryl Allergy & Cold Kapgels 1895
Benadryl Allergy & Sinus Headache Kapgels 1895
Benadryl Severe Allergy & Sinus Headache Caplets 1897
Benadryl Dye-Free Allergy Liqui-gels Softgels 1897
Benadryl Allergy Kapgels 1895
Benadryl Allergy Quick Dissolve Strips 1896
Benadryl Allergy Ultratab Tablets 1896
Children's Benadryl Dye-Free Allergy Liquid 1897
Children's Benadryl Allergy Fastmelts 1897
Children's Benadryl Allergy Liquid 1898
Children's Benadryl Allergy Perfect Measure 1896
Children's Benadryl-D Allergy & Sinus Liquid 1896
Benadryl-D Allergy & Sinus Tablet 1896
Bentyl Capsules 703
Bentyl Injection 703
Bentyl Syrup 703
Bentyl Tablets 703
Donnatal Extentabs 2507
Klonopin (Infrequent) 2639
Lexapro Oral Suspension (Infrequent) 1174
Lexapro Tablets (Infrequent) 1174
Nembutal Sodium Solution, USP 2494
PediaCare Children's Allergy & Cold Liquid 1902
PediaCare Children's Allergy Liquid 1902
Sudafed PE Nighttime Cold Caplets 1907
Sudafed PE Severe Cold Caplets 1908
Sudafed PE Sinus & Allergy Tablets 1908
Tylenol Allergy Multi-Symptom Caplets with Cool Burst and Rapid Release Gelcaps 1916
Tylenol Severe Allergy Caplets 1916
Children's Tylenol Plus Cold Suspension Liquid 1912
Children's Tylenol Plus Cold & Allergy Suspension Liquid 1914
Children's Tylenol Plus Cough & Runny Nose Suspension Liquid 1912
Children's Tylenol Plus Flu Suspension Liquid 1914
Children's Tylenol Plus Multi-Symptom Cold Suspension Liquid 1912
Tylenol Cold Head Congestion Daytime Caplets with Cool Burst 1910
Tylenol Cold Head Congestion Nighttime Caplets with Cool Burst 1910
Tylenol Cold Head Congestion Severe Daytime Caplets with Cool Burst 1910
Tylenol Cold Multi-Symptom Nighttime Caplets with Cool Burst 1913
Tylenol Cold Multi-Symptom Nighttime Liquid with Cool Burst 1913
Tylenol Cough & Sore Throat Nighttime Liquid with Cool Burst 1918
Tylenol Sinus Congestion & Pain Nighttime Caplets with Cool Burst 1917
Tylenol Sore Throat Nighttime Liquid with Cool Burst 1918
Vicks NyQuil Cold & Flu Multi-Symptom Relief ▣ 617
Vicks NyQuil LiquiCaps 2567
Vicks NyQuil Liquid 2567
Vicks NyQuil Multi-Symptom Cold/Flu Relief 2567
Zyrtec-D 12 Hour Extended Release Tablets 1923

Excitement, paradoxical
Valium Tablets 2658

Excoriation
Catapres-TTS (3 of 101 patients) 842
Daytrana Transdermal Patch 3022
▲ Fabrazyme for Intravenous Infusion (9%) 1241
▲ Panretin Gel 0.1% (1% to 8%) 1081
▲ Strattera Capsules (2% to 4%) 1864
Sulfamylon Cream (Rare) 2194
▲ Targretin Gel 1% (18% to 26%) 1088

Exercise tolerance, decreased
Combigan Ophthalmic Solution 553
Cosopt Sterile Ophthalmic Solution 1969
Timoptic Sterile Ophthalmic Solution (Less frequent) 2121
Timoptic in Ocudose (Less frequent) 2124
Timoptic-XE Sterile Ophthalmic Gel Forming Solution 2125

Exophthalmos
Effexor XR Extended-Release Capsules (Rare) 3195
Lyrica Capsules (Rare) 2527
Paxil (Rare) 1535
Paxil CR Controlled-Release Tablets (Rare) 1544
Prozac Weekly Capsules (Rare) 1852
Prozac Pulvules and Liquid (Rare) 1852
Triesence Injectable Suspension (2%) ⊙ 209
Venlafaxine Hydrochloride Tablets (Rare) 2199

Extraocular movement, impairment of
Lescol Capsules 2268
Lescol XL Tablets 2268

Extrapyramidal disorder
▲ Abilify Injection (2% to 20%) 881
▲ Abilify Injection (2% to 20%) 2466
▲ Abilify Oral Solution (2% to 20%) 881
▲ Abilify Oral Solution (2% to 20%) 2466
▲ Abilify Discmelt Orally Disintegrating Tablets (2% to 20%) 881
▲ Abilify Discmelt Orally Disintegrating Tablets (2% to 20%) 2466
▲ Abilify Tablets (2% to 20%) 881
▲ Abilify Tablets (2% to 20%) 2466
Cymbalta Delayed-Release Capsules 1801
▲ Invega Extended-Release Tablets (2% to 7%) 1748
Lexapro Oral Suspension 1174
Lexapro Tablets 1174
Namenda (Infrequent) 1180
Pristiq Extended-Release Tablets (Less than 2%) 3247
Symbyax Capsules (Infrequent) 1871

Extrapyramidal symptoms
Abelcet Injection 1134
▲ Abilify Injection (2% to 21.6%) 881
▲ Abilify Injection (2% to 21.6%) 2466
▲ Abilify Oral Solution (2% to 20%) 881
▲ Abilify Oral Solution (2% to 21.6%) 2466
▲ Abilify Discmelt Orally Disintegrating Tablets (2% to 20%) 881
▲ Abilify Discmelt Orally Disintegrating Tablets (2% to 21.6%) 2466
▲ Abilify Tablets (2% to 20%) 881
▲ Abilify Tablets (2% to 21.6%) 2466
Cardizem LA Extended Release Tablets (Infrequent) 421
Celexa (Infrequent) 1160
▲ Demser Capsules (10%) 1989
Effexor XR Extended-Release Capsules 3195
▲ Equetro Extended-Release Capsules (Less than 5%) 3174
▲ Geodon (14% to 31%) 2520
▲ Intron A for Injection (Less than 5%) 2859
Invega Extended-Release Tablets 1748
Lamictal (Rare) 1488
▲ Mirapex Tablets (Greater than or equal to 1% to 28%) 857
Moban Tablets 1116
Paxil (Rare) 1535
Paxil CR Controlled-Release Tablets (Rare) 1544
Proglycem Capsules (Infrequent) 1185
Proglycem Suspension (Infrequent) 1185
Prozac Pulvules and Liquid (Rare) 1852
Remeron Tablets (Infrequent) 2924
RemeronSolTab Tablets (Infrequent) 2927
Requip Tablets (Infrequent) 1561
Rilutek Tablets (Infrequent) 2771
Risperdal Consta Long-Acting Injection 1753
Stalevo Tablets 2309
Thioridazine Hydrochloride Tablets (Infrequent) 2195
Thiothixene Capsules 2197
Venlafaxine Hydrochloride Tablets 2199
Wellbutrin SR Sustained-Release Tablets 1653
Wellbutrin XL Extended-Release Tablets 1659
Zofran Injection (Rare) 1682
Zofran (Rare) 1687
Zofran ODT Orally Disintegrating Tablets (Rare) 1687
Zyban Sustained-Release Tablets 1692
▲ Zyprexa Tablets (8% to 32%) 1883
▲ Zyprexa IntraMuscular (2% to 4%) 1883
▲ Zyprexa ZYDIS Orally Disintegrating Tablets (8% to 32%) 1883

Extrapyramidal syndrome
Aricept Tablets (Infrequent) 1062
Aricept ODT Tablets (Infrequent) 1062
Luvox CR Extended-Release Capsules (Infrequent) 1759
Lyrica Capsules (Rare) 2527
Proleukin for Injection 2287
Prozac Weekly Capsules (Rare) 1852

Extrasystoles
Abilify Injection (Greater than or equal to 1 in 1000 patients and less than 1 in 100 patients) 2466
Abilify Oral Solution (Greater than or equal to 1 in 1000 patients and less than 1 in 100 patients) 881
Abilify Oral Solution (Greater than or equal to 1 in 1000 patients and less than 1 in 100 patients) 2466
Abilify Discmelt Orally Disintegrating Tablets (Greater than or equal to 1 in 1000 patients and less than 1 in 100 patients) 881
Abilify Discmelt Orally Disintegrating Tablets (Greater than or equal to 1 in 1000 patients and less than 1 in 100 patients) 2466
Abilify Tablets (Greater than or equal to 1 in 1000 patients and less than 1 in 100 patients) 881
Abilify Tablets (Greater than or equal to 1 in 1000 patients and less than 1 in 100 patients) 2466
▲ Advair Diskus 100/50 (4%) 1276
Advair Diskus 250/50 1276
Advair Diskus 500/50 1276
Advair HFA 45/21 Inhalation Aerosol 1288
Advair HFA 115/21 Inhalation Aerosol 1288
Advair HFA 230/21 Inhalation Aerosol 1288
Aloxi Injection (Less than 1%) 1059
Ambien Tablets (Rare) 2692
Ambien CR Tablets (Rare) 2696
Anzemet Injection 2701
Anzemet Tablets 2704
Atacand HCT (0.5% or greater) 642
Cardene I.V. (0.7%) 1093
Celexa (Infrequent) 1160
▲ CellCept Capsules (3% to less than 20%) 2622
▲ CellCept Intravenous (3% to less than 20%) 2622
▲ CellCept Oral Suspension (3% to less than 20%) 2622
▲ CellCept Tablets (3% to less than 20%) 2622
Concerta Extended-Release Tablets 1925
Effexor XR Extended-Release Capsules (Infrequent) 3195
Evoxac Capsules (Less than 1%) 1013
Exelon Capsules (Infrequent) 2229
Exelon Oral Solution (Infrequent) 2229
Exforge Tablets (Less than or equal to 0.1%) 2238
▲ Intron A for Injection (Less than 5%) 2859
Mirapex Tablets 857
Prozac Weekly Capsules (Rare) 1852
Prozac Pulvules and Liquid (Rare) 1852
Requip Tablets (2%) 1561
Rythmol SR Capsules 1590
Serevent Diskus 1594
Tasigna Capsules 2316
Teveten Tablets (Less than 1%) 515
Teveten HCT Tablets (Less than 1%) 517
Tricor Tablets 520
Venlafaxine Hydrochloride Tablets (Infrequent) 2199
Ventolin HFA Inhalation Aerosol (Less than 3%) 1638
Wellbutrin SR Sustained-Release Tablets 1653
Wellbutrin XL Extended-Release Tablets 1659
▲ Xeloda Tablets (Less than 5%) 2662
Xopenex Inhalation Solution 3001
Xopenex Inhalation Solution Concentrate 3005
Xopenex HFA Inhalation Aerosol 3009
Zomig Tablets (Rare) 694
Zomig-ZMT Tablets (Rare) 694
Zyban Sustained-Release Tablets 1692

Extrasystoles, supraventricular
Aloxi Injection (Less than 1%) 1059
Aricept Tablets (Infrequent) 1062
Aricept ODT Tablets (Infrequent) 1062
▲ CellCept Capsules (3% to less than 20%) 2622
▲ CellCept Intravenous (3% to less than 20%) 2622
▲ CellCept Oral Suspension (3% to less than 20%) 2622
▲ CellCept Tablets (3% to less than 20%) 2622
Exelon Patch (Infrequent) 2233
Luvox CR Extended-Release Capsules (Rare) 1759
Mirapex Tablets 857
Rythmol SR Capsules 1590
Ultane Liquid for Inhalation (Less than 1%) 524

Extravasation
Cosmegen for Injection 2485
Doxil Injection 2378
Fluorescite Injection ⊙ 203
Gemzar for Injection (Infrequent) 1820
Novantrone for Injection Concentrate 1100
ProQuad 2099
Romazicon Injection 2646
Taxotere Injection Concentrate 2773
▲ Visudyne for Injection (10% to 30%) 2332

Extroversion
Ambien Tablets 2692
Ambien CR Tablets (Rare) 2696

Exudate, increased
Bactroban Ointment (Less than 1%) 1368

Exudation
Avelox 2803
Cipro I.V. 2817
Levaquin 2416
Levaquin in 5% Dextrose Injection 2416
Noroxin Tablets 2069

Eye abnormalities, fetal
Accutane Capsules 2607

Eye abnormality, unspecified
Vyvanse Capsules 3033

Eye discharge
AzaSite Ophthalmic Drops (Less than 1%) 1740
▲ Azopt Ophthalmic Suspension (1% to 5%) 540
▲ Combigan Ophthalmic Solution (1% to 5%) 553
▲ Voltaren Ophthalmic Solution (Less than or equal to 5%) 2336

Eye disorder, unspecified
▲ Celebrex Capsules (5%) 2979
▲ Gliadel Wafer (3%) 1076
Lyrica Capsules (1% to 2%) 2527
▲ Novantrone for Injection Concentrate (2% to 7%) 1100
Salagen Tablets (Less than 1%) 1082
▲ Travatan Z Ophthalmic Solution (1% to 4%) 547
▲ Vectibix (Less than 1% to 15%) 597

Eye fatigue
Azopt Ophthalmic Suspension (Less than 1%) 540

Eye globe, perforation
(*see under* Bulbus oculi, perforation)

Eye movements, abnormal
Klonopin 2639
Mevacor Tablets (0.5% to 1%) 2063

Eye swelling
▲ Advair HFA 45/21 Inhalation Aerosol (1% to 3%) 1288
▲ Advair HFA 115/21 Inhalation Aerosol (1% to 3%) 1288
▲ Advair HFA 230/21 Inhalation Aerosol (1% to 3%) 1288
Fluarix Vaccine 1446
Provigil Tablets 977
Tasigna Capsules 2316
Xyrem Oral Solution (Infrequent) 1766

Eyeball, perforation
(*see under* Bulbus oculi, perforation)

Eyelash darkening
▲ Lumigan Ophthalmic Solution (3% to 10%) 556

Eyelashes, increase in growth
▲ Lumigan Ophthalmic Solution (15% to 45%) 556
▲ Vectibix (0% to 6%) 597

Eyelashes, matting of
Lacrisert Sterile Ophthalmic Insert ⊙ 233

Eyelid crusting
Cosopt Sterile Ophthalmic Solution 1969
Trusopt Sterile Ophthalmic Solution 2128

Eyelid disorder, unspecified
Combigan Ophthalmic Solution (0.1% to 0.2%) 553

Eyelid skin darkening
▲ Lumigan Ophthalmic Solution (3% to 10%) 556

Eyelid swelling
Cialis Tablets (Less than 2%) 1792
▲ Diclofenac Sodium Ophthalmic Solution (Less than or equal to 5%) ⊙ 240
Fluarix Vaccine 1446
▲ Voltaren Ophthalmic Solution (Less than or equal to 5%) 2336

Eyelids, deposits in
▲ Soriatane Capsules (Less than 5%) 3062

Eyelids, edema of
▲ Alphagan P Ophthalmic Solution (1% to 4%) 549
BOTOX Purified Neurotoxin Complex (2 cases) 550
Lacrisert Sterile Ophthalmic Insert ⊙ 233
Quixin Ophthalmic Solution (Less than 1%) 3184
Stromectol Tablets 2120
▲ Trisenox Injection (5%) 986

Eyes, burning of
▲ Alamast Ophthalmic Solution (Less than 5%) 3181
▲ Alrex Ophthalmic Suspension 0.2% (5% to 15%) ⊙ 236
AzaSite Ophthalmic Drops (Less than 1%) 1740
▲ Betimol Ophthalmic Solution (1 in 8 patients) 3181
Bleph-10 Ophthalmic Solution 10% ⊙ 215
▲ Carac Cream 0.5% (5.4%) 2722
Catapres Tablets 841
Catapres-TTS (0.5% or less) 842
Clorpres Tablets 2185
▲ Combigan Ophthalmic Solution (5% to 15%) 553
▲ Cosopt Sterile Ophthalmic Solution (Up to 30%) 1969
Cozaar Tablets (Less than 1%) 1973
▲ Diclofenac Sodium Ophthalmic Solution (15%) ⊙ 240
▲ Elestat Ophthalmic Solution (1% to 10%) 1741
FML Ophthalmic Suspension ⊙ 224
FML Forte Ophthalmic Suspension ⊙ 222
▲ Lotemax Ophthalmic Suspension 0.5% (5% to 15%) ⊙ 241
▲ Lumigan Ophthalmic Solution (3% to 10%) 556
Maxalt Tablets (Infrequent) 2056
Maxalt-MLT Orally Disintegrating Tablets (Infrequent) 2056
Muro 128 Ophthalmic Solution 2% and 5% ⊙ 242
Ofloxacin Ophthalmic Solution 0.3% ⊙ 243
▲ Pataday Ophthalmic Solution (Less than or equal to 5%) 543
▲ Patanol Ophthalmic Solution (Less than 5%) 546
Pred Forte Ophthalmic Suspension ⊙ 227
Pred Mild Ophthalmic Suspension ⊙ 230
▲ Quixin Ophthalmic Solution (1% to 3%) 3184
▲ Restasis Ophthalmic Emulsion (17%) 557
Tessalon Capsules 1183
Tessalon Perles 1183
▲ Timoptic Sterile Ophthalmic Solution (Approximately 1 in 8 patients) 2121
▲ Timoptic in Ocudose (Approximately 1 in 8 patients) 2124
▲ Timoptic-XE Sterile Ophthalmic Gel Forming Solution (1 in 8 patients) 2125
▲ Trusopt Sterile Ophthalmic Solution (Approximately one-third of patients) 2128
▲ Viroptic Ophthalmic Solution (4.6%) ⊙ 253
▲ Voltaren Ophthalmic Solution (15%) 2336

Eyes, cotton wool spots
Intron A for Injection 2859
PegIntron Powder for Injection 2903

Eyes, dilatation of pupil
(*see under* Mydriasis)

Eyes, discoloration
Alinia for Oral Suspension (Less than 1%) 2677
Alinia Tablets (Less than 1%) 2677

Eyes, disorders of
▲ Aerobid/Aerobid-M (1% to 3%) 1153
▲ Alphagan P Ophthalmic Solution (1% to 4%) 549
Avapro Tablets (Less than 1%) 897
Avapro Tablets (Less than 1%) 2718
Carbatrol Capsules 3019
Clinoril Tablets (Less than 1%) 1962
▲ Copaxone for Injection (4%) 3110
Depakote ER Tablets (Greater than 1%) 423
Kaletra (Less than 2%) 452
Lupron Depot 3.75 mg (Among most frequent) 462
Luvox CR Extended-Release Capsules (Infrequent) 1759
Protopic Ointment (Greater than or equal to 1%) 628
▲ Requip Tablets (3%) 1561
▲ Soriatane Capsules (1% to 10%) 3062
Stromectol Tablets 2120
Tricor Tablets 520
Varivax (Greater than or equal to 1%) 2133
▲ Vesanoid Capsules (17%) 2660

Eyes, dry
(*see under* Xerophthalmia)

Eyes, irritation of
Advicor Tablets 402
Aloxi Injection (Less than 1%) 1059
▲ Alphagan P Ophthalmic Solution (1% to 4%) 549
▲ Alrex Ophthalmic Suspension 0.2% (Less than 5%) ⊙236
Ambien Tablets (Infrequent) 2692
Aricept Tablets (Frequent) 1062
Aricept ODT Tablets (Frequent) 1062
Atrovent Nasal Spray 0.06% 836
AzaSite Ophthalmic Drops (Less than 1% to 2%) 1740
Bleph-10 Ophthalmic Solution 10% ⊙215
▲ BOTOX Purified Neurotoxin Complex (10%) 550
▲ Carac Cream 0.5% (5.4%) 2722
Cardizem LA Extended Release Tablets (Less than 2%) 421
Chantix Tablets (Infrequent) 2511
▲ Combigan Ophthalmic Solution (1% to 5%) 553
Cubicin for Injection (Less than 1%) 995
Cyanokit 5g Antidote 1021
Flonase Nasal Spray 1431
Fluarix Vaccine 1446
FML Ophthalmic Suspension ⊙224
FML Forte Ophthalmic Suspension ⊙222
Imitrex Injection (Infrequent) 1465
Imitrex Nasal Spray (Infrequent) 1470
Imitrex Tablets (Up to 2%) 1474
Klonopin (Infrequent) 2639
Lacrisert Sterile Ophthalmic Insert ⊙233
Lexapro Oral Suspension (Infrequent) 1174
Lexapro Tablets (Infrequent) 1174
▲ Lotemax Ophthalmic Suspension 0.5% (Less than 5%) ⊙241
▲ Lucentis Injection (4% to 19%) 1205
▲ Lumigan Ophthalmic Solution (3% to 10%) 556
Maxalt Tablets (Infrequent) 2056
Maxalt-MLT Orally Disintegrating Tablets (Infrequent) 2056
Mevacor Tablets (0.5% to 1%) 2063
Mirapex Tablets 857
Muro 128 Ophthalmic Solution 2% and 5% ⊙242
Neosporin Ophthalmic Solution Sterile ⊙252
Pred Forte Ophthalmic Suspension ⊙227
Pred Mild Ophthalmic Suspension ⊙230
ProQuad 2099
Requip Tablets (Infrequent) 1561
Rythmol Tablets (Less than 1%) 1586
▲ Soriatane Capsules (1% to 10%) 3062
Tasigna Capsules (0.1% to 1%) 2316
Timoptic Sterile Ophthalmic Solution (Less frequent) 2121
Timoptic in Ocudose (Less frequent) 2124
Timoptic-XE Sterile Ophthalmic Gel Forming Solution 2125
▲ Trisenox Injection (10%) 986
Vaqta (Less than 1%) 2130
Vectibix (1%) 597
Velcade for Injection 2168
▲ Xeloda Tablets (13%) 2662
Xyrem Oral Solution (Infrequent) 1766

Eyes, redness of
Ambien CR Tablets (2%) 2696
Cyanokit 5g Antidote 1021
Fluarix Vaccine 1446
▲ Flulaval Injection Vaccine (3% to 6%) 1448
Levitra Tablets (Less than 2%) 2876
Ofloxacin Ophthalmic Solution 0.3% ⊙243
Percocet Tablets 1127
Percodan Tablets 1130
Stromectol Tablets 2120
Transderm Scōp Transdermal Therapeutic System (Infrequent) 2206
Trusopt Sterile Ophthalmic Solution 2128
▲ Voltaren Ophthalmic Solution (Less than or equal to 5%) 2336
Xyrem Oral Solution (Infrequent) 1766

Eyes, "spots" before the
Aricept Tablets (Infrequent) 1062
Aricept ODT Tablets (Infrequent) 1062
Depakote ER Tablets 423

Eyes, stinging
AzaSite Ophthalmic Drops (Less than 1%) 1740
▲ Combigan Ophthalmic Solution (5% to 15%) 553
▲ Diclofenac Sodium Ophthalmic Solution (15%) ⊙240
Ofloxacin Ophthalmic Solution 0.3% ⊙243
▲ Pataday Ophthalmic Solution (Less than or equal to 5%) 543
▲ Restasis Ophthalmic Emulsion (1% to 5%) 557
▲ Viroptic Ophthalmic Solution (4.6%) ⊙253
▲ Voltaren Ophthalmic Solution (15%) 2336

Eyes, swollen
Cyanokit 5g Antidote 1021

Eyes, tearing
▲ Alphagan P Ophthalmic Solution (1% to 4%) 549
Beconase AQ Nasal Spray (Fewer than 3 per 100 patients) 1369
▲ Carac Cream 0.5% (5.4%) 2722
▲ Chemet Capsules (1% to 3.7%) 2484
Combigan Ophthalmic Solution (0.1% to 0.2%) 553
Cosopt Sterile Ophthalmic Solution 1969
Dantrium Capsules (Less frequent) 2580
Keppra Oral Solution 3131
Keppra Tablets 3131
▲ Lumigan Ophthalmic Solution (1% to 3%) 556
Ofloxacin Ophthalmic Solution 0.3% ⊙243
▲ Suboxone Tablets (5%) 2601
▲ Subutex Tablets (5%) 2601
Timoptic Sterile Ophthalmic Solution (Less frequent) 2121
Timoptic in Ocudose (Less frequent) 2124
▲ Timoptic-XE Sterile Ophthalmic Gel Forming Solution (1% to 5%) 2125

Eyes, watering
Levitra Tablets (Less than 2%) 2876

Eyes, yellowing
Levaquin 2416
Levaquin in 5% Dextrose Injection 2416

F

Face, rhythmical involuntary movements
Moban Tablets 1116
Thiothixene Capsules 2197

Facial dehiscence
Rapamune 3260

Facial droop
Geodon (Rare) 2520

Facial dysmorphia, fetal
Accutane Capsules 2607

Facial features, coarsening
Phenytek Capsules 2192

Facial wasting
Aptivus Capsules (Less than 2%) 823
Aptivus Oral Solution (Less than 2%) 823
Atripla Tablets 938
Combivir Tablets 1384
Crixivan Capsules 1979
Emtriva Capsules 1246
Emtriva Oral Solution 1246
Lexiva Oral Suspension 1510
Lexiva Tablets 1510
Norvir 489
Retrovir 1574
Reyataz Capsules 3299
Truvada Tablets 1262
Viramune Oral Suspension 873
Viramune Tablets 873
Viread Tablets 1268

Facies, mask-like
▲ Zyprexa Tablets (8% to 20%) 1883
▲ Zyprexa IntraMuscular (2% to 4%) 1883
▲ Zyprexa ZYDIS Orally Disintegrating Tablets (8% to 20%) 1883

Factor VIII decrease
Advate (0.6%) 721

Factors II, V, VII, X, decrease
Estratest Tablets 3043
Estratest H.S. Tablets 3043

Factors VII, VIII, IX, X, increase
Estratest Tablets 3043
Estratest H.S. Tablets 3043
Ortho-Cyclen/Ortho Tri-Cyclen 2449

Fainting
(*see under* Syncope)

Faintness
BeneFIX Vials 3191
Dulcolax Suppositories ▣602
Dulcolax Tablets ▣602

Falling
Abilify Injection (Greater than or equal to 1 in 100 patients) 881
Abilify Injection (Greater than or equal to 1 in 100 patients) 2466
Abilify Oral Solution (Greater than or equal to 1 in 100 patients) 881
Abilify Oral Solution (Greater than or equal to 1 in 100 patients) 2466
Abilify Discmelt Orally Disintegrating Tablets (Greater than or equal to 1 in 100 patients) 881
Abilify Discmelt Orally Disintegrating Tablets (Greater than or equal to 1 in 100 patients) 2466
Abilify Tablets (Greater than or equal to 1 in 100 patients) 881
Abilify Tablets (Greater than or equal to 1 in 100 patients) 2466
Aceon Tablets (2 mg, 4 mg, 8 mg) 3038
▲ Advate (12.7%) 721
Ambien Tablets (Infrequent) 2692
Ambien CR Tablets (Infrequent) 2696
▲ Azilect Tablets (5% to 11%) 3106
▲ Dacogen Injection (8%) 1066
▲ DepoCyt Injection (5%) 1136
Eldepryl Capsules 3052
Evoxac Capsules (Less than 1%) 1013
Exelon Patch (Frequent) 2233
▲ Fabrazyme for Intravenous Infusion (6%) 1241
Fentora Tablets (Greater than 1%) 968
Geodon Capsules (Frequent) 2520
Klonopin (Infrequent) 2639
Lexapro Oral Suspension (Infrequent) 1174
Lexapro Tablets (Infrequent) 1174
Mobic Oral Suspension (0% to 2.6%) 863
Mobic Tablets (0% to 2.6%) 863
Namenda (Greater than or equal to 2%) 1180
Neupro Transdermal System (Greater than or equal to 2%) 3149
Requip Tablets (1% or more) 1561
Requip XL Tablets (2%) 1568
▲ Ultram ER Extended-Release Tablets (1% to less than 5%) 2428
Xyrem Oral Solution (Frequent) 1766

Fanconi syndrome
Atripla Tablets 938
Depakote ER Tablets 423
Hepsera Tablets 1253
Truvada Tablets 1262
Viread Tablets 1268

Fasciculations
Amerge Tablets (Rare) 1301
Aricept Tablets (Infrequent) 1062
Aricept ODT Tablets (Infrequent) 1062
Cymbalta Delayed-Release Capsules (Infrequent) 1801
Effexor XR Extended-Release Capsules 3195
Eldepryl Capsules 3052
Eloxatin for Injection 2731
Leukeran Tablets (Rare) 1508
MS Contin Tablets (Less frequent) 2585
Parnate Tablets 1532
Paxil (Rare) 1535
Paxil CR Controlled-Release Tablets (Rare) 1544
ReoPro Vials (0.4%) 1860
Retrovir 1574
Stalevo Tablets 2309
▲ Ultram ER Extended-Release Tablets (0.5% to greater than 5%) 2428
Uniphyl Tablets 2595
Venlafaxine Hydrochloride Tablets 2199
▲ Vivitrol (2% to 8%) 988
Xyrem Oral Solution (Infrequent) 1766

Fasciitis
Mirapex Tablets 857

Fasciitis, necrotizing
Raptiva for Injection 1218

Fasciitis, necrotizing fulminant
Clinoril Tablets (Rare) 1962
Indocin (Rare) 2024

Fasting glucose, impaired
Norditropin Cartridges 2354

Fat redistribution, unspecified
Aptivus Capsules 823
Aptivus Oral Solution 823
Atripla Tablets 938
Crixivan Capsules (2.1%) 1979
Emtriva Capsules 1246
Emtriva Oral Solution 1246
Epzicom Tablets 1422
Intelence Tablets 3119
Truvada Tablets 1262
Viramune Oral Suspension 873
Viramune Tablets 873
Viread Tablets 1268

Fatigue
▲ Abilify Injection (2% to 11%) 881
▲ Abilify Injection (2% to 11%) 2466
▲ Abilify Oral Solution (2% to 11%) 881
▲ Abilify Oral Solution (2% to 11%) 2466
▲ Abilify Discmelt Orally Disintegrating Tablets (2% to 11%) 881
▲ Abilify Discmelt Orally Disintegrating Tablets (2% to 11%) 2466
▲ Abilify Tablets (2% to 11%) 881
▲ Abilify Tablets (2% to 11%) 2466
Accutane Capsules 2607
▲ Actimmune (14%) 1743
Activella Tablets 2347
▲ Advair Diskus 250/50 (3%) 1276
▲ Aerobid/Aerobid-M (1% to 3%) 1153
▲ Aggrenox Capsules (5.8%) 819
Agrylin Capsules 3017
Aldara Cream, 5% (1% to 2%) 1699
▲ Alferon N Injection (6% to 14%) 1726
▲ Alimta for Injection (Up to 87%) 1786
Allegra Oral Solution (1.3%) 2684
Allegra Tablets (0.9% to 2.8%) 2684
Aloxi Injection (Less than 1%) 1059
▲ Alphagan P Ophthalmic Solution (1% to 4%) 549
▲ Alvesco Inhalation Aerosol (Greater than or equal to 3%) 2985
Ambien Tablets (Infrequent) 2692
▲ Ambien CR Tablets (3%) 2696
Amerge Tablets (2%) 1301
Amitiza Capsules (0% to 2%) 3082
Amrix Capsules 966
▲ Anzemet Injection (3.6%) 2701
▲ Anzemet Tablets (2.6% to 5.7%) 2704
▲ Aptivus Capsules (5.7%) 823
▲ Aptivus Oral Solution (5.7%) 823
▲ Aranesp for Injection (9% to 33%) 564
▲ Aricept Tablets (3% to 8%) 1062
▲ Aricept ODT Tablets (3% to 8%) 1062
▲ Arimidex Tablets (19%) 672
▲ Arranon Injection (2% to 50%) 1319
▲ Asmanex Twisthaler (2% to 7%) 2797
Atacand Tablets (More than 1%) 639
Atacand HCT (0.5% or greater) 642
▲ Atripla Tablets (Greater than or equal to 10%) 938
▲ Avalide Tablets (7%) 892
▲ Avalide Tablets (7%) 2713
▲ Avandamet Tablets (6.2%) 1336
▲ Avandia Tablets (3.6%) 1351
▲ Avapro Tablets (4%) 897
▲ Avapro Tablets (4%) 2718
▲ Avastin IV (10.7%) 1192
Axert Tablets (Infrequent) 2431
Azmacort Inhalation Aerosol 407
▲ Baraclude (1% to 3%) 900
Benicar Tablets (Greater than 0.5%) 1009
Bicillin C-R Injectable Suspension 1775
Bicillin L-A Injection 1777
▲ Boostrix (3.7% to 37%) 1377
Brovana Inhalation Solution 2990
Busulfex Injection (2%) 2477
▲ Bystolic Tablets (2% to 5%) 1155
Cancidas for Injection 1953
Captopril Tablets (About 0.5% to 2%) 2182
Carbatrol Capsules 3019
▲ Cardizem LA Extended Release Tablets (4.8%) 421
▲ Catapres Tablets (About 4 in 100 patients) 841
▲ Catapres-TTS (6 of 101 patients) 842
Celebrex Capsules (0.1% to 1.9%) 2979
▲ Celexa (5%) 1160
▲ Cerezyme for Injection (Approximately 6.5%) 1238
▲ Chantix Tablets (4% to 7%) 2511
▲ Chemet Capsules (5.2% to 15.7%) 2484
Cialis Tablets (Less than 2%) 1792
▲ Clarinex Tablets (2.1% to 5%) 2828

▲ Clarinex Reditabs Tablets (2.1% to 5%) 2828
▲ Clarinex-D 12-Hour Extended-Release Tablets (4%) 2831
▲ Clarinex-D 24-Hour Extended-Release Tablets (3%) 2834
Clinoril Tablets (Less than 1 in 100) 1962
▲ Clolar for Intravenous Infusion (36%) 1239
▲ Clorpres Tablets (About 4%) 2185
Combigan Ophthalmic Solution (0.1% to 0.2%) 553
Combivent Inhalation Aerosol (Less than 2%) 845
▲ Combivir Tablets (10%) 1384
▲ Comtan Tablets (6%) 2208
Concerta Extended-Release Tablets 1925
▲ Coreg Tablets (24%) 1387
▲ Coreg CR Extended-Release Capsules (24%) 1393
Cosmegen for Injection 2485
Cosopt Sterile Ophthalmic Solution 1969
Cozaar Tablets (1% or greater) 1973
▲ Crinone 4% Gel (21%) 992
▲ Crinone 8% Gel (22%) 992
Crixivan Capsules (2.7%) 1979
Cubicin for Injection (Less than 1%) 995
▲ Cymbalta Delayed-Release Capsules (2% to 15%) 1801
Dantrium Capsules (Among most frequent) 2580
Dibenzyline Capsules 3188
▲ Diovan Tablets (2% to 3%) 2212
Diovan HCT Tablets (Greater than 0.2%) 2216
Doxil Injection 2378
▲ Duragesic Transdermal System (3% to 10%) 2405
Dyazide Capsules 1405
▲ DynaCirc CR Controlled Release Tablets (2.5% to 7.6%) 1407
Dyrenium Capsules (Rare) 3189
Edecrin 698
Effexor XR Extended-Release Capsules 3195
Eldepryl Capsules 3052
▲ Eligard 7.5 mg (17.5%) 2724
▲ Eligard 22.5 mg (6%) 2724
▲ Eligard 30 mg (13.3%) 2724
▲ Eligard 45 mg (11.7%) 2724
▲ Eloxatin for Injection (4% to 70%) 2731
Elspar for Injection 1990
▲ Emend Capsules (17.8% to 21.9%) 1992
▲ Emend for Injection (17.8% to 21.9%) 1999
▲ Emtriva Capsules (Greater than or equal to 10%) 1246
▲ Emtriva Oral Solution (Greater than or equal to 10%) 1246
Enbrel for Injection 569
▲ Engerix-B Vaccine (14%) 1409
▲ Epivir (27%) 1412
▲ Epivir-HBV (24%) 1417
▲ Epogen for Injection (9% to 25%) 576
▲ Epzicom Tablets (6% to 8%) 1422
Equetro Extended-Release Capsules 3174
▲ Erbitux (33% to 89%) 912
▲ Evoxac Capsules (3.3%) 1013
▲ Exelon Capsules (4% to 9%) 2229
▲ Exelon Oral Solution (4% to 9%) 2229
Exelon Patch (2%) 2233
Exforge Tablets (Greater than or equal to 0.2%) 2238
▲ Exjade Tablets (0.1% to 6.1%) 2244
▲ Fabrazyme for Intravenous Infusion (25%) 1241
Fansidar Tablets 2636
▲ Femara Tablets (0.2% to 13%) 2246
▲ Fentora Tablets (1% to 20%) 968
Flebogamma 5% 1715
Flebogamma 5% DIF 1718
Flolan for Injection 1426
▲ Flovent Diskus 50 mcg (1% to 16%) 1435
▲ Fluarix Vaccine (12.2% to 19.7%) 1446
▲ Flulaval Injection Vaccine (1% to 17%) 1448
Flumadine (1%) 1167
▲ FluMist Vaccine (26%) 1945
Foradil Aerolizer 2849
▲ Frova Tablets (5%) 1111
Gabitril Tablets 973
▲ Gammagard Liquid (2.18% to 16.4%) 730
Gammagard S/D (Occasional) 734
Gantrisin Pediatric Suspension 2638
Gardasil Injection 2019
▲ Gemzar for Injection (40%) 1820
▲ Gengraf Capsules (3%) 435
▲ Genotropin Lyophilized Powder (1.7% to 6.3%) 2547
▲ Gleevec Tablets (28.6% to 53%) 2255
Gris-PEG Tablets 2507
▲ Havrix Injection Vaccine (1% to 10%) 1454
Herceptin I.V. 1199
Hexalen Capsules (1%) 1078
▲ Hycamtin Capsules (11% to 19%) 1456
▲ Hycamtin for Injection (Up to 37%) 1459
Imitrex Injection (1.1%) 1465
▲ Imitrex Tablets (2% to 3%) 1474
Imodium A-D Liquid, Caplets, and EZ Chews 1898
▲ Indapamide Tablets (Greater than or equal to 5%) 2188
Indocin (Greater than 1%) 2024
▲ InnoPran XL Extended Release Capsules (5% to 7%) 1484
▲ Intelence Tablets (3.3%) 3119
▲ Intron A for Injection (4% to 96%) 2859
Invanz for Injection (1.2%) 2029
Invega Extended-Release Tablets (1% to 2%) 1748
Isentress Tablets (1% to less than 2%) 2036
▲ Ixempra Kit for Injection (56%) 915
▲ Keppra Injection (10%) 3137
▲ Keppra Oral Solution (5% to 10%) 3131
▲ Keppra Tablets (5% to 10%) 3131
Ketek Tablets (Greater than or equal to 0.2% to less than 2%) 2744
▲ Klonopin (7%) 2639
K-Phos Original (Sodium Free) Tablets (Less frequent) 814
K-Phos Neutral Tablets 813
▲ Lamictal (8%) 1488
Lamisil Oral Granules 2264
Lamisil Tablets 2266
Lescol Capsules (2.7%) 2268
Lescol XL Tablets (1.6%) 2268
▲ Leustatin Injection (11% to 45%) 2384
Levaquin 2416
Levaquin in 5% Dextrose Injection 2416
Levothroid Tablets 1170
Levoxyl Tablets 1780
▲ Lexapro Oral Suspension (2% to 8%) 1174
▲ Lexapro Tablets (2% to 8%) 1174
▲ Lexiva Oral Suspension (2% to 4%) 1510
▲ Lexiva Tablets (2% to 4%) 1510
Lialda Tablets (Infrequent) 3029
▲ Lyrica Capsules (5% to 8%) 2527
Mavik Tablets (More than 1%) 472
Maxair Autohaler 1705
▲ Maxalt Tablets (4% to 7%) 2056
▲ Maxalt-MLT Orally Disintegrating Tablets (4% to 7%) 2056
▲ Miacalcin Nasal Spray (1% to 3%) 2274
Micardis Tablets (1%) 852
▲ Micardis HCT Tablets (3%) 854
Mobic Oral Suspension (Less than 2%) 863
Mobic Tablets (Less than 2%) 863
▲ Mycamine for Injection (6.4% to 29.6%) 616
▲ Myfortic Tablets (3% to less than 20%) 2276
Myleran Tablets 1530
Nabi-HB 815
Nadolol Tablets (2 of 100 patients) 2191
Nalfon Capsules (1.7%) 2508
Namenda (2%) 1180
▲ Neoral Oral Solution (3%) 2280
▲ Neoral Soft Gelatin Capsules (3%) 2280
▲ Neulasta Injection (15% to 72%) 587
▲ Neupogen for Injection (11%) 589
▲ Neupro Transdermal System (8%) 3149
▲ Nexavar Tablets (37% to 46%) 784
Nexium Delayed-Release Capsules (Less than 1%) 645
Nexium I.V. (Less than 1%) 652
Nexium Delayed-Release Oral Suspension (Less than 1%) 645
▲ Novantrone for Injection Concentrate (34% to 39%) 1100
▲ Noxafil Oral Suspension (1% to 17%) 2889
Opana Tablets (Less than 1%) 1117
▲ Opana ER Tablets (3.9%) 1121
Ortho-Cyclen Tablets 2449
Ortho Evra Transdermal System 2437
Ortho Tri-Cyclen Tablets 2449
Ortho Tri-Cyclen Lo Tablets 2458
Orthoclone OKT3 Sterile Solution 2387
Patanase Nasal Spray (0.9%) 544
▲ PegIntron Powder for Injection (52%) 2903
Pepcid Tablets (Infrequent) 2075
Percocet Tablets 1127
Perforomist Inhalation Solution 1025
Persantine Tablets (Rare) 869
▲ Photofrin for Injection (4%) 708
▲ Plan B Tablets (16.9%) 1044
▲ Plavix Tablets (3.3%) 926
▲ Plavix Tablets (3.3%) 2767
Premphase Tablets 3232
Prempro Tablets 3232
Prinivil Tablets (2.5%) 2087
▲ Prinzide Tablets (3.7%) 2092
▲ Pristiq Extended-Release Tablets (5% to 11%) 3247
▲ Procrit for Injection (9% to 25%) 2391
▲ Prometrium Capsules (100 mg, 200 mg) (8% to 9%) 3047
▲ Rebetol (58% to 70%) 2917
▲ Rebif Prefilled Syringe for Injection (33% to 41%) 1107
▲ Reclast Injection (2.1% to 8%) 2291
Recombinate 738
Recombivax HB (Greater than 1%) 2107
▲ Relenza Inhalation Powder (Less than 1.5% to 8%) 1556
▲ Remicade for IV Injection (9%) 950
▲ Requip Tablets (8% to 11%) 1561
▲ Risperdal Consta Long-Acting Injection (5% to 7%) 1753
Romazicon Injection (1% to 3%) 2646
▲ Rozerem Tablets (4%) 3091
▲ Rythmol Tablets (4% to 6%) 1586
▲ Rythmol SR Capsules (11% to 13%) 1590
▲ Sandostatin Injection (1% to 4%) 2300
▲ Sandostatin LAR Depot (8% to 31.8%) 2302
▲ Simulect for Injection (3% to 10%) 2306
Singulair (1.8%) 2114
▲ Solodyn Extended Release Tablets (9%) 1938
▲ Soriatane Capsules (1% to 10%) 3062
▲ Stalevo Tablets (6%) 2309
Strattera Capsules 1864
Stromectol Tablets (0.9%) 2120
▲ Sustiva Capsules (2% to 8%) 930
▲ Sustiva Tablets (2% to 8%) 930
▲ Sutent Capsules (8% to 74%) 2540
▲ Tamiflu Capsules (1% to 8%) 2649
▲ Tamiflu Oral Suspension (1% to 8%) 2649
▲ Tarceva Tablets (2% to 73%) 1228
Tarka Tablets (2.8%) 511
▲ Tasigna Capsules (Greater than 10% to 28%) 2316
▲ Taxotere Injection Concentrate (4.5% to 53.3%) 2773
Tekturna Tablets (Greater than 1%) 2321
Tekturna HCT Tablets (Greater than 1%) 2324
▲ Temodar Capsules (13% to 34%) 2931
Teveten Tablets (2%) 515
Teveten HCT Tablets (1.9%) 517
Thiothixene Capsules 2197
▲ Thyrogen for Injection (3.3%) 1244
▲ Tice BCG (7%) 2936
Timoptic Sterile Ophthalmic Solution (Less frequent) 2121
Timoptic in Ocudose (Less frequent) 2124
Timoptic-XE Sterile Ophthalmic Gel Forming Solution 2125
▲ Toprol-XL Tablets (About 10 of 100 patients) 666
▲ Tracleer Tablets (4%) 3289
▲ Treanda for Injection (1% to 9%) 983
Treximet Tablets (Frequent) 1616
▲ Tricor Tablets (5%) 520
▲ Trisenox Injection (63%) 986
▲ Trizivir Tablets (44%) 1622
Trusopt Sterile Ophthalmic Solution (Infrequent) 2128
▲ Truvada Tablets (Greater than or equal to 10%) 1262
▲ Twinrix Vaccine (11% to 14%) 1628
▲ Tyzeka Tablets (1% to 12%) 2328
Uroqid-Acid No. 2 Tablets 814
Uroxatral Tablets (2.7%) 2786
▲ Valcyte Tablets (Less than 5%) 2654
Valium Tablets (Among most common) 2658
▲ Valtrex Caplets (8%) 1635
▲ Vantas (9.9%) 1737
▲ Vaqta (3.9%) 2130
Varivax (Greater than or equal to 1%) 2133
▲ Vectibix (4% to 26%) 597
▲ Velcade for Injection (29% to 64%) 2168
Venlafaxine Hydrochloride Tablets 2199
Vesanoid Capsules 2660
VESIcare Tablets (1% to 2.1%) 636
Viadur Implant (Rare) 802
Vicoprofen Tablets 533
▲ Viramune Oral Suspension (0.2% to 4.7%) 873
▲ Viramune Tablets (0.2% to 4.7%) 873
▲ Viread Tablets (Greater than 5%) 1268
▲ Vivitrol (12% to 23%) 988
Vytorin 10/10 Tablets 2149
Vytorin 10/10 Tablets 2939
Vytorin 10/20 Tablets 2149
Vytorin 10/20 Tablets 2939
Vytorin 10/40 Tablets 2149
Vytorin 10/40 Tablets 2939
Vytorin 10/80 Tablets 2149
Vytorin 10/80 Tablets 2939
▲ Wellbutrin Tablets (5%) 1648
▲ Xeloda Tablets (4% to 42%) 2662
▲ Xenical Capsules (3.1% to 7.2%) 2672
Xifaxan Tablets (Less than 2%) 2682
▲ Xolair (3%) 1235
▲ Xolair (3%) 2339
Xyrem Oral Solution (Frequent) 1766
▲ Xyzal Oral Solution (1% to 4%) 2789
▲ Xyzal Oral Solution (1% to 4%) 3155
▲ Xyzal Tablets (1% to 4%) 2789
▲ Xyzal Tablets (1% to 4%) 3155
Zetia Tablets (2.4%) 2157
Zetia Tablets (2% to 2.4%) 2951
▲ Ziagen (12%) 1673
▲ Zofran Injection (5%) 1682
▲ Zofran (9% to 13%) 1687
▲ Zofran ODT Orally Disintegrating Tablets (9% to 13%) 1687
▲ Zolinza Capsules (45% to 52.3%) 2142
▲ Zometa for Intravenous Infusion (39%) 2341
▲ Zonegran Capsules (8%) 1089
▲ Zyrtec Chewable Tablets (5.9%) 1920
▲ Zyrtec Syrup (5.9%) 1920
▲ Zyrtec Tablets (5.9%) 1920
▲ Zyrtec-D 12 Hour Extended Release Tablets (2.4% to 5.9%) 1923

Fatigue, muscular

Dyazide Capsules 1405
Furosemide Tablets 2186
Imitrex Injection (Rare) 1465
Prinzide Tablets 2092

Fear

Lortab 5/500 Tablets 3143
Lortab 7.5/500 Tablets 3144
Lortab 10/500 Tablets 3144
Romazicon Injection 2646
Tussionex Pennkinetic Extended-Release Suspension 3154
Vicodin Tablets 529
Vicodin ES Tablets 530
Vicodin HP Tablets 531
Xyrem Oral Solution (Infrequent) 1766
Zydone Tablets 1132
Zyrtec-D 12 Hour Extended Release Tablets 1923

Febrile reactions

Capastat Sulfate for Injection 1791
Digibind for Injection 1403
Follistim AQ Cartridge 2844
▲ Leustatin Injection (11%) 2384
Liquid PedvaxHIB 2073
Varivax (Less than 0.1%) 2133

Fecal fat, increase

(*see under* Steatorrhea)

Fecal impaction

Actiq (Less than 1%) 959
Doxil Injection (Less than 1%) 2378
Geodon Capsules (Rare) 2520
Paxil (Rare) 1535
Paxil CR Controlled-Release Tablets (Rare) 1544
Rilutek Tablets (Infrequent) 2771
Velcade for Injection 2168
VESIcare Tablets 636
Zyprexa Tablets (Infrequent) 1883
Zyprexa ZYDIS Orally Disintegrating Tablets (Infrequent) 1883

Fecal urgency

Amitiza Capsules (Less than 1%) 3082
▲ Xenical Capsules (2.8% to 22.1%) 2672
▲ Xifaxan Tablets (5.9%) 2682

Fecaloma

Exelon Capsules (Infrequent) 2229
Exelon Oral Solution (Infrequent) 2229

Feces, discoloration

Ortho Evra Transdermal System 2437
▲ Sandostatin LAR Depot (4% to 6%) 2302

Feces, hard

Sanctura XR Capsules (Less than 1%) 557

Feces abnormal

Xifaxan Tablets (Less than 2%) 2682

Feeding Problems

NeoProfen Injection 2496
▲ Relenza Inhalation Powder (2% to 4%) 1556

Feeling, abnormal

Ambien CR Tablets (Rare) 2696

Cymbalta Delayed-Release Capsules (Infrequent) 1801
▲ Lyrica Capsules (1% to 3%) 2527
Strattera Capsules (0.1%) 1864

Feeling, drugged
▲ Ambien Tablets (3%) 2692
Ambien CR Tablets (Frequent) 2696
Paxil (2%) 1535
Paxil CR Controlled-Release Tablets (2%) 1544

Feeling, intoxicated
(*see also under* Inebriated feeling)
Ambien Tablets (Rare) 2692
Ambien CR Tablets (Rare) 2696
Effexor XR Extended-Release Capsules (Rare) 3195
Imitrex Injection (Rare) 1465
Lyrica Capsules (1% to 2%) 2527
Venlafaxine Hydrochloride Tablets (Rare) 2199

Feeling, strange
Ambien Tablets (Rare) 2692
Amerge Tablets (Infrequent) 1301
Imitrex Injection (2%) 1465
Imitrex Nasal Spray (Infrequent) 1470
Imitrex Tablets 1474
Lexapro Oral Suspension (Infrequent) 1174
Lexapro Tablets (Infrequent) 1174
MS Contin Tablets (Less frequent) 2585

Feet, cold
Combigan Ophthalmic Solution 553
Venlafaxine Hydrochloride Tablets (Infrequent) 2199

Fertility, impairment of
Intron A for Injection 2859
Levothroid Tablets 1170

Fertility, male, decrease
Tricor Tablets 520

Festination
Eldepryl Capsules 3052

Fetal death
(*see under* Death, fetal)

Fetal defects
Accutane Capsules 2607
Climara Transdermal System 763
Nembutal Sodium Solution, USP 2494

Fetal harm
Accutane Capsules 2607
Advicor Tablets 402
Albenza Tablets 1297
Arimidex Tablets 672
Atacand Tablets 639
Atacand HCT 642
Avalide Tablets 892
Avalide Tablets 2713
Avapro Tablets 897
Avapro Tablets 2718
Benicar Tablets 1009
Captopril Tablets 2182
Carac Cream 0.5% 2722
Carbatrol Capsules 3019
Cosmegen for Injection 2485
Cozaar Tablets 1973
Eloxatin for Injection 2731
Estratest Tablets 3043
Estratest H.S. Tablets 3043
Evista Tablets 1810
Exforge Tablets 2238
Faslodex Injection 682
Femara Tablets 2246
Gemzar for Injection 1820
Hycamtin for Injection 1459
Lescol Capsules 2268
Lescol XL Tablets 2268
Leukeran Tablets 1508
Mavik Tablets 472
Mevacor Tablets 2063
Micardis Tablets 852
Micardis HCT Tablets 854
Mustargen for Injection 2492
Myleran Tablets 1530
Mylotarg for Injection 3212
Nembutal Sodium Solution, USP 2494
Nexavar Tablets 784
Premarin Intravenous 3217
Prinivil Tablets 2087
Prinzide Tablets 2092
Rebetol 2917
ReoPro Vials 1860
Tabloid Tablets 1601
Targretin Capsules 1084
Taxotere Injection Concentrate 2773
▲ Temodar Capsules (5%) 2931
Teveten HCT Tablets 517
Tracleer Tablets 3289
Tygacil for Injection 3276
Vesanoid Capsules 2660
Viadur Implant 802
Xeloda Tablets 2662
Zocor Tablets 2136

Fetal hydantoin syndrome
Phenytek Capsules 2192

Fetal problems, unspecified
Bayer Aspirin 750
Cipro I.V. 2817

Fever
▲ Abelcet Injection (14%) 1134
Abilify Injection 881
▲ Abilify Injection (3%) 2466
Abilify Oral Solution 881
▲ Abilify Oral Solution (3%) 2466
Abilify Discmelt Orally Disintegrating Tablets 881
▲ Abilify Discmelt Orally Disintegrating Tablets (3%) 2466
Abilify Tablets 881
▲ Abilify Tablets (3%) 2466
Accolate Tablets (1.6%) 669
Aceon Tablets (2 mg, 4 mg, 8 mg) (0.3% to 1.5%) 3038
▲ Actimmune (52%) 1743
Actiq (1% or greater) 959
Activase I.V. 1188
Actonel Tablets (0% to 0.6%) 2568
Aczone Gel 5% (1%) 3296
▲ Adderall XR Capsules (5%) 3012
▲ Advair Diskus 250/50 (4%) 1276
Advair HFA 45/21 Inhalation Aerosol 1288
Advair HFA 115/21 Inhalation Aerosol 1288
Advair HFA 230/21 Inhalation Aerosol 1288
▲ Advate (16.7%) 721
Advicor Tablets 402
▲ Aerobid/Aerobid-M (3% to 9%) 1153
Aggrenox Capsules (Less than 1%) 819
▲ Agrylin Capsules (8.9%) 3017
▲ Alamast Ophthalmic Solution (Less than 5%) 3181
Albenza Tablets (Up to 1%) 1297
Albutein 5% 1707
Albutein 25% 1708
Aldara Cream, 5% (1% to 2%) 1699
▲ Alferon N Injection (18% to 81%) 1726
▲ Alimta for Injection (Up to 26%) 1786
Alinia for Oral Suspension (Less than 1%) 2677
Alinia Tablets (Less than 1%) 2677
Allegra Oral Solution (2.4%) 2684
Allegra Tablets (2.4%) 2684
Aloxi Injection (Less than 1%) 1059
Alphanate 1709
Altabax Ointment (1.2%) 1299
Ambien Tablets (Infrequent) 2692
Ambien CR Tablets (1%) 2696
Amerge Tablets (Infrequent) 1301
Anaprox Tablets (Less than 1%) 2632
Anaprox DS Tablets (Less than 1%) 2632
▲ Angiomax for Injection (Greater than 0.1% to 5%) 1933
▲ Anzemet Injection (4.3%) 2701
▲ Anzemet Tablets (3.5%) 2704
▲ Aptivus Capsules (6.4% to 7.5%) 823
▲ Aptivus Oral Solution (6.4% to 7.5%) 823
Aralast (0.1%) 726
▲ Aranesp for Injection (7% to 19%) 564
▲ Argatroban Injection (3.6% to 6.9%) 1308
Aricept Tablets (2%) 1062
Aricept ODT Tablets (2%) 1062
▲ Arimidex Tablets (2% to 5%) 672
▲ Arixtra Injection (0.3% to 13.6%) 1313
▲ Arranon Injection (0% to 23%) 1319
▲ Asacol Delayed-Release Tablets (6%) 2579
Asmanex Twisthaler (1% to less than 3%) 2797
Atacand Tablets (0.5% or greater) 639
▲ Atripla Tablets (Greater than or equal to 5%) 938
Attenuvax (Occasional) 1951
Augmentin (Frequent) 1323
Augmentin Tablets (Frequent) 1327
Augmentin XR Extended Release Tablets (Frequent) 1333
Augmentin ES-600 Powder for Oral Suspension 1329
Avalide Tablets 892
Avalide Tablets 2713
Avapro Tablets (Less than 1%) 897
Avapro Tablets (Less than 1%) 2718
Avelox 2803
▲ Avinza Capsules (5% to 10%) 1772
Axert Tablets (Rare) 2431
Axid Capsules (1.6%) 1364
▲ Azilect Tablets (3%) 3106
Bayer Aspirin 750
▲ BeneFIX Vials (3.1%) 3191
▲ Betaseron for SC Injection (31%) 756
▲ Bexxar (2% to 37%) 1371
Bicillin C-R Injectable Suspension 1775
Bicillin L-A Injection 1777
▲ Boostrix (1% to 13.5%) 1377
▲ BOTOX Purified Neurotoxin Complex (2% to 10%) 550
Brovana Inhalation Solution 2990
▲ Busulfex Injection (3% to 80%) 2477
▲ Campath Ampules (10% to 69%) 761
Campral Tablets (Infrequent) 1158
Canasa Rectal Suppositories (1.2%) 705
▲ Cancidas for Injection (13.2% to 30.4%) 1953
▲ Captopril Tablets (About 4 to 7 of 100) 2182
Carbatrol Capsules 3019
Cardene I.V. (Rare) 1093
Catapres Tablets 841
Catapres-TTS (0.5% or less) 842
Cathflo Activase 1198
Ceftin for Oral Suspension (0.1% to 1%) 1380
▲ Celebrex Capsules (0.1% to 9%) 2979
Celexa (2%) 1160
▲ CellCept Capsules (3% to 52.3%) 2622
▲ CellCept Intravenous (3% to 52.3%) 2622
▲ CellCept Oral Suspension (3% to 52.3%) 2622
▲ CellCept Tablets (3% to 52.3%) 2622
▲ Cerezyme for Injection (Approximately 6.5%) 1238
Cervidil Vaginal Insert (Less than 1%) 1165
Chantix Tablets (Infrequent) 2511
▲ Chemet Capsules (5.2% to 15.7%) 2484
Cimzia 3127
Cipro I.V. (1% or less to 2.1%) 2817
Cipro (Less than 1% to 2.1%) 2810
Cipro XR Tablets 2823
▲ Clarinex Syrup (5.5% to 16.9%) 2828
Clinoril Tablets (Less than 1%) 1962
▲ Clolar for Intravenous Infusion (41%) 1239
Clorpres Tablets 2185
Combigan Ophthalmic Solution 553
▲ Combivir Tablets (10%) 1384
Comtan Tablets 2208
▲ Comvax (0.8% to 14.2%) 1966
Concerta Extended-Release Tablets (2.2%) 1925
▲ Copaxone for Injection (8%) 3110
▲ Coreg Tablets (Greater than 1% to 3%) 1387
▲ Coreg CR Extended-Release Capsules (Greater than 1% to less than or equal to 3%) 1393
Cosmegen for Injection 2485
Cosopt Sterile Ophthalmic Solution 1969
Cozaar Tablets (Less than 1%) 1973
Crinone 4% Gel 992
Crinone 8% Gel 992
Crixivan Capsules (1.5%) 1979
▲ Cubicin for Injection (1.9% to 6.7%) 995
Cuprimine Capsules (Rare) 1986
▲ Cymbalta Delayed-Release Capsules (1% to 3%) 1801
▲ Dacogen Injection (53%) 1066
Dantrium Capsules (Less frequent) 2580
Dapsone Tablets USP 1746
Daytrana Transdermal Patch 3022
▲ Depakote ER Tablets (6%) 423
▲ DepoCyt Injection (4% to 45%) 1136
▲ DepoDur Injection (Greater than 10%) 1095
Diclofenac Sodium Ophthalmic Solution ⊙ 240
Diovan HCT Tablets 2216
Donnatal Extentabs 2507
▲ Doxil Injection (6.9% to 21.3%) 2378
▲ Duragesic Transdermal System (35%) 2405
EC-Naprosyn Delayed-Release Tablets (Less than 1%) 2632
Edecrin 698
Effexor XR Extended-Release Capsules (Frequent) 3195
▲ Elidel Cream 1% (1.2% to 12.5%) 2221
▲ Elitek (46%) 2729
▲ Eloxatin for Injection (1% to 29%) 2731
Elspar for Injection 1990
Emend Capsules (2.9%) 1992
Emend for Injection (2.9%) 1999
Emsam Transdermal System (Infrequent) 905
▲ Emtriva Capsules (18%) 1246
▲ Emtriva Oral Solution (18%) 1246
Enbrel for Injection 569
▲ Engerix-B Vaccine (1% to 10%) 1409
▲ Epivir (10% to 25%) 1412
▲ Epivir-HBV (7%) 1417
▲ Epogen for Injection (29% to 51%) 576
▲ Epzicom Tablets (3% to 5%) 1422
Equetro Extended-Release Capsules 3174
▲ Erbitux (1% to 30%) 912
▲ Evista Tablets (3.1% to 3.9%) 1810
▲ Evoxac Capsules (1% to 3%) 1013
Exelon Capsules (Frequent) 2229
Exelon Oral Solution (Frequent) 2229
Exelon Patch (Infrequent) 2233
Exforge Tablets (Greater than or equal to 0.2%) 2238
▲ Exjade Tablets (0.1% to 18.9%) 2244
▲ Fabrazyme for Intravenous Infusion (36%) 1241
▲ Faslodex Injection (6.4%) 682
Fentora Tablets (Greater than 1%) 968
▲ Flebogamma 5% (27%) 1715
▲ Flebogamma 5% DIF (Greater than 15%) 1718
Flexbumin 25% I.V. (Occasional) 729
▲ Flolan for Injection (13% to 25%) 1426
▲ Flonase Nasal Spray (1% to 3%) 1431
▲ Flovent Diskus 50 mcg (7%) 1435
▲ Flovent HFA (1% to 3%) 1440
Fluarix Vaccine (0.4% to 1.7%) 1446
▲ Flulaval Injection Vaccine (1% to 11%) 1448
Flumadine 1167
▲ FluMist Vaccine (1% to 9%) 1945
Focalin XR Capsules 2251
Follistim AQ Cartridge 2844
Foradil Aerolizer (2.2%) 2849
Fortaz (2%) 1450
Fosamax (Rare) 2005
Fosamax Plus D Tablets (Rarely) 2013
Fragmin Injection (Rare) 1070
Frova Tablets (Infrequent) 1111
Furosemide Tablets 2186
Gabitril Tablets (1% or more) 973
▲ Gammagard Liquid (2.3% to 21.3%) 730
Gammagard S/D (Occasional) 734
▲ Gamunex (0.1% to 28%) 3094
Gantrisin Pediatric Suspension 2638
▲ Gardasil Injection (10.3% to 13%) 2019
▲ Gemzar for Injection (16% to 41%) 1820
▲ Gengraf Capsules (3%) 435
Genotropin Lyophilized Powder 2547
Geodon Capsules (Frequent) 2520
▲ Gleevec Tablets (16% to 41%) 2255
▲ Gliadel Wafer (12% to 18%) 1076
▲ Havrix Injection Vaccine (1% to 10%) 1454
Hemofil M (Extremely rare) 737
▲ Herceptin I.V. (36%) 1199
Human Albumin Grifols 25% 1706
▲ Humira Injection (Less than 5%) 442
Hyalgan Solution (Seven cases) 2742
▲ Hycamtin Capsules (5% to 7%) 1456
▲ Hycamtin for Injection (Less than 1% to 34%) 1459
Imitrex Injection (Rare) 1465
Imitrex Nasal Spray (Infrequent) 1470
Imitrex Tablets (Infrequent) 1474
Indapamide Tablets 2188
▲ Infanrix Vaccine (Up to 19.8%) 1479
InnoPran XL Extended Release Capsules 1484
Intravenous Sodium Diuril 2490
▲ Intron A for Injection (3% to 86%) 2859
▲ Invanz for Injection (2.3% to 5%) 2029
▲ Ionsys Transdermal System (9%) 2410
Iquix Ophthalmic Solution (1% to 2%) 3183
▲ Isentress Tablets (4.9%) 2036
▲ Ixempra Kit for Injection (8%) 915
Kaletra (1% to 2%) 452
▲ Kepivance (39%) 583
Keppra Oral Solution (1% to greater than or equal to 2%) 3131
Keppra Tablets (1% to greater than or equal to 2%) 3131
▲ Kinrix Injection Vaccine (0.1% to 16%) 1486
Klonopin (Infrequent) 2639
▲ Lamictal (1% to 15%) 1488
▲ Lamisil Oral Granules (7%) 2264
Lescol Capsules (Rare) 2268
Lescol XL Tablets 2268
Leukeran Tablets 1508
▲ Leukine (77% to 95%) 774
▲ Leustatin Injection (11% to 69%) 2384
Levaquin 2416

Levaquin in 5% Dextrose Injection 2416
Levothroid Tablets 1170
Levoxyl Tablets 1780
Lexapro Oral Suspension (Frequent) 1174
Lexapro Tablets (Frequent) 1174
Lialda Tablets (Infrequent) 3029
Lipitor Tablets (Less than 2%) 2501
Lovaza Capsules 1520
▲ Lovenox Injection (8%) 2756
Lunesta Tablets (Infrequent) 2994
▲ Lupron Depot 7.5 mg (Less than 5%) 469
Lupron Depot-PED 7.5 mg, 11.25 mg and 15 mg (Less than 2%) 471
Lyrica Capsules (Greater than or equal to 1%) 2527
▲ Malarone Pediatric Tablets (Less than 1% to 6%) 1521
▲ Malarone Tablets (Less than 1% to 6%) 1521
Maxalt Tablets (Rare) 2056
Maxalt-MLT Orally Disintegrating Tablets (Rare) 2056
▲ Megace ES Oral Suspension (1% to 6%) 2499
▲ Mepron Suspension (0.6% to 40%) 1526
Meridia Capsules (Greater than or equal to 1%) 475
Merrem I.V. (Greater than 0.1% to 1%) 684
Meruvax II 2061
Metadate CD Capsules 3146
Mevacor Tablets (Rare) 2063
Miacalcin Nasal Spray (Less than 1%) 2274
Micardis Tablets (More than 0.3%) 852
Micardis HCT Tablets 854
M-M-R II 2054
Moban Tablets 1116
Mobic Oral Suspension (Less than 2%) 863
Mobic Tablets (Less than 2%) 863
Mumpsvax (Uncommon) 2068
▲ Mycamine for Injection (7% to 44.9%) 616
▲ Myfortic Tablets (3% to less than 20%) 2276
▲ Mylotarg for Injection (78% to 88%) 3212
Nadolol Tablets 2191
Nalfon Capsules (Less than 1%) 2508
Naprosyn Suspension (Less than 1%) 2632
Naprosyn Tablets (Less than 1%) 2632
Natrecor for Injection (Greater than or equal to 1%) 2977
Nembutal Sodium Solution, USP 2494
Neoral Oral Solution (1% to less than 3%) 2280
Neoral Soft Gelatin Capsules (1% to less than 3%) 2280
▲ Neulasta Injection (15% to 72%) 587
▲ Neupogen for Injection (12%) 589
Neupro Transdermal System 3149
▲ Nexavar Tablets (1% to less than 10%) 784
Nexium Delayed-Release Capsules (Less than 1%) 645
Nexium I.V. (Less than 1%) 652
Nexium Delayed-Release Oral Suspension (Less than 1%) 645
Noroxin Tablets (0.3% to 1%) 2069
▲ Norvir (0.9% to 5%) 489
▲ Novantrone for Injection Concentrate (6% to 78%) 1100
NovoSeven (Greater than or equal to 2%) 2367
NovoSeven RT (Greater than or equal to 2%) 2370
▲ Noxafil Oral Suspension (2% to 45%) 2889
Omnicef Capsules 497
Omnicef for Oral Suspension 497
▲ Ontak Vials (81%) 1079
▲ Opana Tablets (14.2%) 1117
Ortho-Cyclen Tablets 2449
Ortho Evra Transdermal System 2437
Ortho Tri-Cyclen Tablets 2449
Ortho Tri-Cyclen Lo Tablets 2458
▲ Orthoclone OKT3 Sterile Solution (89% to 90%) 2387
▲ OxyContin Tablets (Between 1% and 5%) 2589
Panhematin for Injection 2497
Paser Granules 1747
Paxil (2%) 1535
Paxil CR Controlled-Release Tablets (2%) 1544
▲ Pediarix Vaccine (31.3% or less) 1552
▲ Liquid PedvaxHIB (0.5% to 18.1%) 2073
▲ PegIntron Powder for Injection (22%) 2903
▲ Pentacel (0% to 16.3%) 2792
Pentasa Capsules (0.9%) 3030
Pepcid Tablets (Infrequent) 2075
Percocet Tablets 1127
Percodan Tablets 1130
Phenytek Capsules 2192
▲ Photofrin for Injection (19% to 31%) 708
Plavix Tablets (1% to 2.5%) 926
Plavix Tablets (1% to 2.5%) 2767
Pletal Tablets (Less than 2%) 2481
Pneumovax 23 (Common) 2078
Potaba (Infrequent) 1698
Premphase Tablets 3232
Prempro Tablets 3232
▲ Prevnar (0% to 36.7%) 3241
Primaxin I.M. 2080
Primaxin I.V. (0.5%) 2083
Prinivil Tablets (0.3% to 1.1%) 2087
Prinzide Tablets (0.3% to 1%) 2092
▲ Procrit for Injection (29% to 51%) 2391
Profilnine SD Solvent Detergent 1721
Proglycem Capsules (Infrequent) 1185
Proglycem Suspension (Infrequent) 1185
▲ Prograf Capsules and Injection (19% to 48%) 622
Prolastin (0.77%) 3099
▲ Proleukin for Injection (1% to 29%) 2287
▲ Prometrium Capsules (100 mg, 200 mg) (Less than 5%) 3047
▲ ProQuad (21.5%) 2099
Protonix for Delayed-Release Oral Suspension (Less than 1%) 3254
Protonix Delayed-Release Tablets (Less than 1%) 3254
Protonix I.V. (Less than 1%) 3257
▲ Protopic Ointment (1% to 18%) 628
▲ Proventil HFA Inhalation Aerosol (6%) 2914
Provigil Tablets (At least 1%) 977
Prozac Weekly Capsules (Infrequent to 2%) 1852
Prozac Pulvules and Liquid (2%) 1852
▲ Pulmicort Flexhaler (Greater than or equal to 3%) 654
▲ Pulmozyme Inhalation Solution (32%) 1217
Pylera Capsules 714
▲ Quixin Ophthalmic Solution (1% to 3%) 3184
▲ Rapamune (23% to 34%) 3260
▲ Raptiva for Injection (7%) 1218
▲ Rebetol (32% to 61%) 2917
▲ Rebif Prefilled Syringe for Injection (25% to 28%) 1107
▲ Reclast Injection (7% to 18%) 2291
Recombinate (Extremely rare) 738
Recombivax HB (Greater than 1%) 2107
ReFacto Vials 3269
▲ Refludan for Injection (4.4%) 795
▲ Relenza Inhalation Powder (Less than 1.5% to 9%) 1556
Remeron Tablets (Infrequent) 2924
RemeronSolTab Tablets (Infrequent) 2927
▲ Remicade for IV Injection (7%) 950
Requip Tablets (Infrequent) 1561
Requip XL Tablets 1568
▲ Retrovir Capsules (3.2% to 16%) 1574
▲ Retrovir IV Infusion (4% to 16%) 1579
▲ Retrovir (3.2% to 16%) 1574
▲ Reyataz Capsules (2% to 19%) 3299
Risperdal Consta Long-Acting Injection (1%) 1753
▲ Rituxan I.V. (1% to 56%) 1223
Rocephin Injectable Vials, ADD-Vantage, Galaxy, Bulk (Less than 1%) 2642
▲ Rotarix Oral Suspension (25% to 31%) 1582
RotaTeq (0.1%) 2110
Rythmol Tablets (2%) 1586
Rythmol SR Capsules 1590
St. Joseph 81 mg Aspirin Chewable and Enteric Coated Tablets 1903
Salagen Tablets (1% to 2%) 1082
Sandimmune (2% or less) 2296
Sandostatin LAR Depot 2302
▲ Selzentry Tablets (12%) 2534
▲ Serevent Diskus (1% to 3%) 1594
Singulair (1.5% to greater than or equal to 2%) 2114
Soriatane Capsules (Less than 1%) 3062
▲ Stromectol Tablets (22.6%) 2120
▲ Suboxone Tablets (3%) 2601
▲ Subutex Tablets (3%) 2601
Sular Extended Release Tablets (Less than or equal to 1%) 2975
▲ Sustiva Capsules (21%) 930
▲ Sustiva Tablets (21%) 930
▲ Sutent Capsules (1% to 18%) 2540
▲ Symbyax Capsules (3% to 4%) 1871
Synagis Intramuscular Solution (More than 1%) 1948
Tamiflu Capsules (Less than 1%) 2649
Tamiflu Oral Suspension (Less than 1%) 2649
▲ Tarceva Tablets (0% to 36%) 1228
▲ Targretin Capsules (4.8% to 17%) 1084
Tarka Tablets (Several cases) 511
▲ Tasigna Capsules (1% to 24%) 2316
▲ Taxotere Injection Concentrate (0.6% to 46.5%) 2773
Tekturna HCT Tablets 2324
▲ Temodar Capsules (2% to 13%) 2931
Teveten Tablets (Less than 1%) 515
Teveten HCT Tablets (Less than 1%) 517
Thioridazine Hydrochloride Tablets 2195
Thiothixene Capsules 2197
Thyrogen for Injection 1244
▲ Tice BCG (17% to 20%) 2936
Timoptic Sterile Ophthalmic Solution 2121
Timoptic in Ocudose 2124
Timoptic-XE Sterile Ophthalmic Gel Forming Solution 2125
TNKase 1233
Toprol-XL Tablets 666
▲ Torisel Injection (1% to 24%) 3272
Tracleer Tablets 3289
▲ Trasylol Injection (15%) 799
▲ Treanda for Injection (1% to 24%) 983
Treximet Tablets (Infrequent) 1616
Tricor Tablets 520
▲ Trisenox Injection (63%) 986
▲ Trizivir Tablets (20%) 1622
▲ Truvada Tablets (Greater than or equal to 5%) 1262
▲ Twinrix Vaccine (2% to 4%) 1628
▲ Tygacil for Injection (7.1%) 3276
▲ Tyzeka Tablets (1% to 4%) 2328
Ultane Liquid for Inhalation (1%) 524
▲ Ultram ER Extended-Release Tablets (1% to less than 5%) 2428
Urso 250 Tablets 720
Urso Forte Tablets 720
▲ Valcyte Tablets (13% to 31%) 2654
Valstar Sterile Solution for Intravesical Instillation (2%) 1735
▲ Vaprisol (3.8% to 11%) 632
▲ Vaqta (2.7% to 11.3%) 2130
▲ Varivax (10.2% to 14.7%) 2133
Vectibix 597
▲ Velcade for Injection (6% to 37%) 2168
Ventolin HFA Inhalation Aerosol 1638
▲ Veramyst Nasal Spray (4% to 5%) 1643
▲ Vesanoid Capsules (83%) 2660
Vicoprofen Tablets (Rare; less than 3%) 533
▲ Vigamox Ophthalmic Solution (1% to 4%) 548
Viramune Oral Suspension 873
Viramune Tablets 873
▲ Viread Tablets (2% to 8%) 1268
▲ Visudyne for Injection (1% to 10%) 2332
Vivitrol 988
▲ Voltaren Ophthalmic Solution (Less than or equal to 3%) 2336
Voltaren Tablets (Occasionally) 2334
Voltaren-XR Tablets (Occasionally) 2337
Vytorin 10/10 Tablets 2149
Vytorin 10/10 Tablets 2939
Vytorin 10/20 Tablets 2149
Vytorin 10/20 Tablets 2939
Vytorin 10/40 Tablets 2149
Vytorin 10/40 Tablets 2939
Vytorin 10/80 Tablets 2149
Vytorin 10/80 Tablets 2939
Vyvanse Capsules (2%) 3033
Wellbutrin Tablets (1.2%) 1648
Wellbutrin SR Sustained-Release Tablets (1% to 2%) 1653
Wellbutrin XL Extended-Release Tablets (1% to 2%) 1659
WinRho SDF (1%) 741
▲ Xeloda Tablets (1% to 12%) 2662
▲ Xifaxan Tablets (3.1%) 2682
▲ Xopenex Inhalation Solution (3%) 3001
▲ Xopenex Inhalation Solution Concentrate (3% to 9.1%) 3005
▲ Xopenex HFA Inhalation Aerosol (3%) 3009
▲ Xyntha Vials (5% to 41%) 3280
Xyrem Oral Solution (Frequent) 1766
▲ Xyzal Oral Solution (4%) 2789
▲ Xyzal Oral Solution (4%) 3155
▲ Xyzal Tablets (2% to 4%) 2789
▲ Xyzal Tablets (2% to 4%) 3155
Yaz Tablets (Greater than 1%) 805
Zantac 25 EFFERdose Tablets (Rare) 1670
Zantac Injection 1666
Zantac Injection Pharmacy Bulk Package (Rare) 1668
Zantac Injection Premixed 1666
Zantac (Rare) 1670
▲ Zemplar Capsules (5%) 536
▲ Zemplar Injection (5%) 538
▲ Ziagen (6% to 9%) 1673
Zocor Tablets (Rare) 2136
▲ Zofran Injection (2% to 8%) 1682
▲ Zofran (8%) 1687
▲ Zofran ODT Orally Disintegrating Tablets (8%) 1687
▲ Zolinza Capsules (9% to 10.5%) 2142
▲ Zometa for Intravenous Infusion (32% to 44%) 2341
Zomig Tablets (Infrequent) 694
Zomig Nasal Spray (Rare) 689
Zomig-ZMT Tablets (Infrequent) 694
Zostavax Injection (1.8%) 2145
▲ Zosyn for Injection (2.4% to 4.8%) 3284
Zovirax 1690
Zyban Sustained-Release Tablets (Frequent) 1692
▲ Zyprexa Tablets (6%) 1883
Zyprexa IntraMuscular (Infrequent) 1883
▲ Zyprexa ZYDIS Orally Disintegrating Tablets (6%) 1883
Zyrtec Chewable Tablets (Less than 2%) 1920
Zyrtec Syrup (Less than 2%) 1920
Zyrtec Tablets (Less than 2%) 1920
Zyrtec-D 12 Hour Extended Release Tablets (Less than 2%) 1923
▲ Zyvox (0% to 14.1%) 2552

Fever, intermittent
▲ Dacogen Injection (6%) 1066

Fever, neutropenic
▲ Mylotarg for Injection (15% to 19%) 3212
▲ Neulasta Injection (15% to 72%) 587
▲ Neupogen for Injection (13%) 589
▲ Xeloda Tablets (3% to 16%) 2662

Fever blisters
Aceon Tablets (2 mg, 4 mg, 8 mg) (0.3% to 1%) 3038

Fibrillations
Luvox CR Extended-Release Capsules (Rare) 1759

Fibrillations, ventricular
Abelcet Injection 1134
Adenocard IV Injection (Rare) 603
Angiomax for Injection (Greater than 0.1% to less than 1%) 1933
Azilect Tablets (Rare) 3106
Celebrex Capsules (Less than 0.1%) 2979
DynaCirc CR Controlled Release Tablets (0.5% to 1%) 1407
Effexor XR Extended-Release Capsules (Rare) 3195
Frova Tablets 1111
Imitrex Injection (Rare) 1465
Imitrex Tablets (Rare) 1474
Lanoxin Injection 1498
Lanoxin Injection Pediatric 1502
Lanoxin Tablets 1505
Levaquin 2416
Levaquin in 5% Dextrose Injection 2416
Lyrica Capsules (Rare) 2527
Meridia Capsules 475
Mirapex Tablets 857
Paxil 1535
Paxil CR Controlled-Release Tablets 1544
Prograf Capsules and Injection 622
Prozac Weekly Capsules (Rare) 1852
Prozac Pulvules and Liquid (Rare) 1852
Refludan for Injection 795
Rilutek Tablets (Rare) 2771
Rituxan I.V. 1223
▲ Rythmol Tablets (1.9% to 4%) 1586
Trasylol Injection (2%) 799
Venlafaxine Hydrochloride Tablets 2199
Zomig Tablets 694
Zomig Nasal Spray 689
Zomig-ZMT Tablets 694
Zosyn for Injection (1% or less) 3284

Fibrinolysis increased
NovoSeven (1%) 2367
NovoSeven RT (1%) 2370

Fibromyalgia
Amitiza Capsules (Less than 1%) 3082
Cozaar Tablets (Less than 1%) 1973
Lupron Depot 7.5 mg 469
Lupron Depot–3 Month 11.25 mg 462
Nexium Delayed-Release Capsules (Less than 1%) 645
Nexium I.V. (Less than 1%) 652
Nexium Delayed-Release Oral Suspension (Less than 1%) 645

Tyzeka Tablets (2%)........ 2328

Fibrosing colonopathy
Creon 5 Capsules........ 3041
Creon 10 Capsules........ 3042
Creon 20 Capsules........ 3042
Ultrase Capsules........ 718
Ultrase MT Capsules........ 719

Fibrosis
Copaxone for Injection (Infrequent)... 3110
Genotropin Lyophilized Powder (Infrequent)........ 2547
▲ Xeloda Tablets (Less than 5%)........ 2662

Fibrosis, cavernous body
Edex Injection (2%)........ 2957

Fibrosis, hepatic
▲ Xeloda Tablets (Less than 5%)........ 2662

Fibrosis, interstitial pulmonary
(*see under* Fibrosis, pulmonary)

Fibrosis, penile
▲ Edex Injection (5%)........ 2957

Fibrosis, perisinusoidal
Eloxatin for Injection........ 2731

Fibrosis, pleural
▲ Intron A for Injection (Less than or equal to 5%)........ 2859
Mirapex Tablets (Rare)........ 857

Fibrosis, pulmonary
Aceon Tablets (2 mg, 4 mg, 8 mg) (Less than 0.1%)........ 3038
Agrylin Capsules........ 3017
Busulfex Injection (Rare)........ 2477
CellCept Capsules........ 2622
CellCept Intravenous........ 2622
CellCept Oral Suspension........ 2622
CellCept Tablets........ 2622
Cuprimine Capsules (Rare)........ 1986
Eloxatin for Injection (Less than 1%)........ 2731
Evoxac Capsules (Less than 1%)........ 1013
Gleevec Tablets (Rare)........ 2255
Herceptin I.V........ 1199
Humira Injection........ 442
Leukeran Tablets........ 1508
Lyrica Capsules (Rare)........ 2527
Mirapex Tablets (Rare)........ 857
Myfortic Tablets (Rare)........ 2276
Myleran Tablets (Rare)........ 1530
Paxil (Rare)........ 1535
Paxil CR Controlled-Release Tablets (Rare)........ 1544
Pentasa Capsules (One case)........ 3030
Prozac Weekly Capsules........ 1852
Rapamune........ 3260
Remicade for IV Injection........ 950
Tarceva Tablets (0.7%)........ 1228
Taxotere Injection Concentrate (Rare)........ 2773
Vectibix (Less than 1%)........ 597

Fibrosis, retroperitoneal
Lyrica Capsules (Rare)........ 2527
Neupro Transdermal System........ 3149

Fingernails, brittle
Gengraf Capsules (2% or less)........ 435
Neoral Oral Solution (2% or less)...... 2280
Neoral Soft Gelatin Capsules (2% or less)........ 2280
Sandimmune (2% or less)........ 2296

Fissuring, unspecified
Olux Foam (Less than 2%)........ 3061
▲ Soriatane Capsules (1% to 10%)..... 3062

Fistula, arteriovenous
ReoPro Vials (0.4%)........ 1860

Fistula, biliary
Avastin IV........ 1192

Fistula, bladder
Avastin IV........ 1192

Fistula, bronchopleural
Avastin IV........ 1192

Fistula, tracheo-esophageal
Avastin IV........ 1192
▲ Photofrin for Injection (6%)........ 708
Proleukin for Injection........ 2287

Fistula, vagina
Avastin IV........ 1192

Flare
Humira Injection (0.7%)........ 442
▲ Travatan Z Ophthalmic Solution (1% to 4%)........ 547

Flare, postinjection
Attenuvax (Rare)........ 1951
Meruvax II........ 2061
M-M-R II........ 2054
Mumpsvax (Rare)........ 2068

Flare at injection site
ProQuad........ 2099

Flatulence
Aceon Tablets (2 mg, 4 mg, 8 mg) (1%)........ 3038
▲ Aciphex Tablets (3%)........ 1053
Actiq (1% or greater)........ 959
Activella Tablets........ 2347
▲ Actonel with Calcium Tablets (3.1% to 4.6%)........ 2574
▲ Advair HFA 45/21 Inhalation Aerosol (1% to 3%)........ 1288
▲ Advair HFA 115/21 Inhalation Aerosol (1% to 3%)........ 1288
▲ Advair HFA 230/21 Inhalation Aerosol (1% to 3%)........ 1288
Advicor Tablets........ 402
▲ Aerobid/Aerobid-M (1% to 3%)........ 1153
▲ Agrylin Capsules (10.2%)........ 3017
Alinia for Oral Suspension (Less than 1%)........ 2677
Alinia Tablets (Less than 1%)........ 2677
Aloxi Injection (Less than 1%)........ 1059
Ambien Tablets (Infrequent)........ 2692
Ambien CR Tablets (1%)........ 2696
AmBisome for Injection (Less common)........ 606
▲ Amitiza Capsules (3% to 6%)........ 3082
Amrix Capsules........ 966
▲ Anaprox Tablets (1% to 10%)........ 2632
▲ Anaprox DS Tablets (1% to 10%)..... 2632
Aptivus Capsules (Less than 2%)........ 823
Aptivus Oral Solution (Less than 2%)........ 823
Aricept Tablets (Infrequent)........ 1062
Aricept ODT Tablets (Infrequent)........ 1062
▲ Asacol Delayed-Release Tablets (3% to 5%)........ 2579
Augmentin (Less frequent)........ 1323
Augmentin Tablets (Less frequent)... 1327
Avalide Tablets........ 892
Avalide Tablets........ 2713
Avapro Tablets (Less than 1%)........ 897
Avapro Tablets (Less than 1%)........ 2718
▲ Avastin IV (11% to 19%)........ 1192
Avelox (Greater than or equal to 0.1% to less than 2%)........ 2803
▲ Axid Capsules (4.9%)........ 1364
Bios Life Drink Mix........ 3158
Byetta Injection........ 600
▲ Campral Tablets (1% to 4%)........ 1158
▲ Canasa Rectal Suppositories (5.2%)........ 705
Carafate Suspension (Less than 0.5%)........ 706
Carafate Tablets (Less than 0.5%).... 707
Ceftin (0.1% to 1%)........ 1380
Celebrex Capsules (2.2%)........ 2979
Celexa (Frequent)........ 1160
▲ CellCept Capsules (3% to less than 20%)........ 2622
▲ CellCept Intravenous (3% to less than 20%)........ 2622
▲ CellCept Oral Suspension (3% to less than 20%)........ 2622
▲ CellCept Tablets (3% to less than 20%)........ 2622
▲ Chantix Tablets (Greater than 5% to 9%)........ 2511
Cipro I.V. (1% or less)........ 2817
Cipro........ 2810
Cipro XR Tablets (Less than 1%)........ 2823
▲ Climara Transdermal System (1% to 7%)........ 763
▲ Climara Pro Transdermal System (3.8%)........ 768
▲ Clinoril Tablets (1% to 3%)........ 1962
Comtan Tablets (2%)........ 2208
Copaxone for Injection (At least 2%)........ 3110
Cozaar Tablets (Less than 1%)........ 1973
Crinone 4% Gel........ 992
Crinone 8% Gel........ 992
Cubicin for Injection (Less than 1%)........ 995
Cymbalta Delayed-Release Capsules (Frequent)........ 1801
▲ Depakote ER Tablets (Greater than 1% to less than 5%)........ 423
▲ DepoDur Injection (5% to 10%)........ 1095
Diovan Tablets (Greater than 0.2%).. 2212
Diovan HCT Tablets (Greater than 0.2%)........ 2216
▲ Doxil Injection (1% to 10%)........ 2378
Duragesic Transdermal System (1% or greater)........ 2405
▲ EC-Naprosyn Delayed-Release Tablets (1% to 10%)........ 2632
▲ Effexor XR Extended-Release Capsules (4% to 5%)........ 3195
Eligard 7.5 mg (Less than 2%)........ 2724
Eligard 22.5 mg (Less than 2%)........ 2724
Eligard 30 mg (Less than 2%)........ 2724
Eligard 45 mg (Less than 2%)........ 2724
Elmiron Capsules (Less than or equal to 1%)........ 2435
▲ Eloxatin for Injection (2% to 9%)...... 2731
Emend Capsules (Greater than 0.5%)........ 1992
Emend for Injection (Greater than 0.5%)........ 1999
Emsam Transdermal System (Frequent)........ 905
▲ Enjuvia Tablets (4% to 7%)........ 1029
▲ Entereg Capsules (3.1% to 8.7%).... 3293
▲ Evista Tablets (3.1%)........ 1810
▲ Evoxac Capsules (1% to 3%)........ 1013
▲ Exelon Capsules (4%)........ 2229
▲ Exelon Oral Solution (4%)........ 2229
▲ Flolan for Injection (5%)........ 1426
▲ Follistim AQ Cartridge (27%)........ 2844
▲ Fosamax (Up to 4.1%)........ 2005
▲ Fosamax Plus D Tablets (0% to 4.1%)........ 2013
Frova Tablets (Infrequent)........ 1111
Gabitril Tablets (1% or more)........ 973
Gantrisin Pediatric Suspension........ 2638
▲ Gengraf Capsules (4%)........ 435
▲ Gleevec Tablets (0% to 34%)........ 2255
▲ Hepsera Tablets (4%)........ 1253
Imitrex Injection (Rare)........ 1465
Imitrex Nasal Spray (Rare)........ 1470
Imitrex Tablets........ 1474
Indocin Capsules (Less than 1%)...... 2024
Indocin I.V. (Less than 1%)........ 2489
Indocin (Less than 1%)........ 2024
Intelence Tablets (Less than 2%)...... 3119
▲ Intron A for Injection (Less than 5%)........ 2859
Invanz for Injection (Greater than 0.1%)........ 2029
▲ Ionsys Transdermal System (1% to less than 10%)........ 2410
▲ Janumet Tablets (Greater than 5%)........ 2041
Kaletra (1% to 2%)........ 452
Ketek Tablets (Greater than or equal to 0.2% to less than 2%)........ 2744
Klonopin (Infrequent)........ 2639
Kristalose for Oral Solution........ 1004
▲ Lamictal (More than 1% to less than 5%)........ 1488
Lamisil Tablets (2.2%)........ 2266
Lescol Capsules (2.6%)........ 2268
Lescol XL Tablets (1.4%)........ 2268
Lexapro Oral Suspension (2%)........ 1174
Lexapro Tablets (2%)........ 1174
▲ Lialda Tablets (2.8% to 4%)........ 3029
▲ Limbrel Capsules (5% to 8%)........ 2561
Lipitor Tablets (1.1% to 2.8%)........ 2501
▲ Lyrica Capsules (1% to 3%)........ 2527
Maxalt Tablets (Infrequent)........ 2056
Maxalt-MLT Orally Disintegrating Tablets (Infrequent)........ 2056
▲ Megace ES Oral Suspension (0% to 10%)........ 2499
Meridia Capsules (Greater than or equal to 1%)........ 475
Merrem I.V. (Greater than 0.1% to 1%)........ 684
▲ Mevacor Tablets (3.7% to 6.4%)...... 2063
Miacalcin Nasal Spray (Less than 1%)........ 2274
Micardis Tablets (More than 0.3%)... 852
Micardis HCT Tablets........ 854
Mirapex Tablets (Greater than or equal to 1%)........ 857
▲ Mobic Oral Suspension (0.5% to 4.5%)........ 863
▲ Mobic Tablets (0.5% to 4.5%)........ 863
▲ Myfortic Tablets (3% to less than 20%)........ 2276
Nadolol Tablets (1 to 5 of 1000 patients)........ 2191
Nalfon Capsules (Less than 1%)........ 2508
▲ Naprosyn Suspension (1% to 10%)........ 2632
▲ Naprosyn Tablets (1% to 10%)........ 2632
▲ Neoral Oral Solution (4%)........ 2280
▲ Neoral Soft Gelatin Capsules (4%)..... 2280
Nexium Delayed-Release Capsules (Greater than or equal to 1%)........ 645
Nexium I.V. (Greater than or equal to 1%)........ 652
Nexium Delayed-Release Oral Suspension (Greater than or equal to 1%)........ 645
Niaspan Extended-Release Tablets.... 480
Noroxin Tablets (0.3% to 1%)........ 2069
Norvir (0.9% to 1.7%)........ 489
▲ Noxafil Oral Suspension (1% to 5%)........ 2889
Omnicef Capsules (0.7%)........ 497
Omnicef for Oral Suspension (0.6%)........ 497
▲ Opana Tablets (1% to less than 10%)........ 1117
▲ Opana ER Tablets (1% to less than 10%)........ 1121
OxyContin Tablets (Less than 1%).... 2589
▲ Paxil (4%)........ 1535
▲ Paxil CR Controlled-Release Tablets (4%)........ 1544
Percocet Tablets........ 1127
▲ Pletal Tablets (2% to 3%)........ 2481
▲ Precose Tablets (74%)........ 792
▲ Premarin Tablets (6% to 7%)........ 3221
▲ Premphase Tablets (5% to 9%)........ 3232
▲ Prempro Tablets (5% to 9%)........ 3232
Prinivil Tablets (0.3% to 1%)........ 2087
Prinzide Tablets........ 2092
ProAmatine Tablets (Rare)........ 3032
▲ Prograf Capsules and Injection (3% to 15%)........ 622
ProQuad........ 2099
▲ Protonix for Delayed-Release Oral Suspension (2% to 4%)........ 3254
▲ Protonix Delayed-Release Tablets (2% to 4%)........ 3254
Protonix I.V. (Greater than or equal to 1%)........ 3257
Proventil HFA Inhalation Aerosol (Less than 3%)........ 2914
Provigil Tablets (1%)........ 977
▲ Prozac Weekly Capsules (3%)........ 1852
▲ Prozac Pulvules and Liquid (3%)...... 1852
▲ Relistor Injection (13.3%)........ 3310
▲ Requip Tablets (Infrequent to 3%).... 1561
Requip XL Tablets........ 1568
Retrovir Capsules........ 1574
Retrovir IV Infusion........ 1579
Retrovir........ 1574
Rilutek Tablets (2% to 2.5%)........ 2771
Risperdal Consta Long-Acting Injection (Infrequent)........ 1753
Rocephin Injectable Vials, ADD-Vantage, Galaxy, Bulk (Less than 0.1%)........ 2642
Rotarix Oral Suspension (2.2%)........ 1582
Rythmol Tablets (1% to 2%)........ 1586
Rythmol SR Capsules (1% to 2%)...... 1590
Salagen Tablets (1% to 2%)........ 1082
Sanctura XR Capsules (1.6%)........ 557
▲ Sandostatin Injection (Less than 10%)........ 2300
▲ Sandostatin LAR Depot (9.1% to 38%)........ 2302
Simcor Tablets (1.9%)........ 502
▲ Simulect for Injection (3% to 10%)... 2306
▲ Somatuline Depot Injection (Greater than 5% to 14%)........ 3102
Stalevo Tablets (2%)........ 2309
Strattera Capsules (2%)........ 1864
Sular Extended Release Tablets (Less than or equal to 1%)........ 2975
▲ Suprax for Oral Suspension (4%)...... 1891
▲ Suprax Tablets (4%)........ 1891
Sustiva Capsules (1% to 2%)........ 930
Sustiva Tablets (1% to 2%)........ 930
▲ Sutent Capsules (0% to 14%)........ 2540
▲ Tarceva Tablets (0% to 13%)........ 1228
Targretin Capsules........ 1084
▲ Tasigna Capsules (1% to 10%)........ 2316
Teveten Tablets (Less than 1%)........ 515
Teveten HCT Tablets (Less than 1%)........ 517
Timentin ADD-Vantage........ 1606
Timentin Injection Galaxy Container........ 1609
Timentin IV Infusion........ 1603
Timentin Pharmacy Bulk Package..... 1613
Toprol-XL Tablets (About 1 of 100 patients)........ 666
Treximet Tablets (Infrequent)........ 1616
▲ Tricor Tablets (3%)........ 520
Ultram ER Extended-Release Tablets (0.5% to less than 1%)...... 2428
Ultrase MT Capsules (1.5%)........ 719
Valstar Sterile Solution for Intravesical Instillation (1%)........ 1735
▲ Venlafaxine Hydrochloride Tablets (3%)........ 2199
▲ Vicoprofen Tablets (3% to 9%)........ 533
▲ Viread Tablets (3% to 4%)........ 1268
Vivitrol........ 988
▲ Voltaren Tablets (1% to 10%)........ 2334
▲ Voltaren-XR Tablets (1% to 10%)........ 2337
Vytorin 10/10 Tablets........ 2149
Vytorin 10/10 Tablets........ 2939
Vytorin 10/20 Tablets........ 2149
Vytorin 10/20 Tablets........ 2939
Vytorin 10/40 Tablets........ 2149

Vytorin 10/40 Tablets 2939
Vytorin 10/80 Tablets 2149
Vytorin 10/80 Tablets 2939
Wellbutrin SR Sustained-Release Tablets (At least 1%) 1653
▲ Wellbutrin XL Extended-Release Tablets (At least 1% to 6%) 1659
▲ Xifaxan Tablets (11.3%) 2682
Xyrem Oral Solution (Infrequent) 1766
Zocor Tablets 2136
Zonegran Capsules (Infrequent) 1089
Zosyn for Injection (1% or less to 1.3%) 3284
Zyban Sustained-Release Tablets (Frequent) 1692
Zyprexa Tablets (Frequent) 1883
Zyprexa ZYDIS Orally Disintegrating Tablets (Frequent) ... 1883
Zyrtec Chewable Tablets (Less than 2%) 1920
Zyrtec Syrup (Less than 2%) 1920
Zyrtec Tablets (Less than 2%) 1920
Zyrtec-D 12 Hour Extended Release Tablets (Less than 2%) 1923

Flatus with discharge

▲ Xenical Capsules (2.1% to 23.9%) ... 2672

Floating feeling

MS Contin Tablets (Less frequent) 2585

Flu Syndrome

▲ Actonel with Calcium Tablets (7.1% to 8.7%) 2574
Alinia for Oral Suspension (Less than 1%) 2677
Alinia Tablets (Less than 1%) 2677
Aricept Tablets (Frequent) 1062
Aricept ODT Tablets (Frequent) 1062
▲ Arimidex Tablets (2% to 7%) 672
▲ Brovana Inhalation Solution (3%) 2990
Campral Tablets (Frequent) 1158
▲ CellCept Capsules (3% to less than 20%) 2622
▲ CellCept Intravenous (3% to less than 20%) 2622
▲ CellCept Oral Suspension (3% to less than 20%) 2622
▲ CellCept Tablets (3% to less than 20%) 2622
▲ Climara Pro Transdermal System (4.7%) 768
Combigan Ophthalmic Solution (0.1% to 0.2%) 553
▲ Coreg CR Extended-Release Capsules (Greater than 1% to less than or equal to 3%) 1393
▲ Depakote ER Tablets (Greater than 1% to less than 5%) 423
▲ Enablex Extended-Release Tablets (1% to 3%) 2225
▲ Enjuvia Tablets (4% to 7%) 1029
▲ Humira Injection (7%) 442
▲ Keppra Oral Solution (1% to 3%) 3131
▲ Keppra Tablets (1% to 3%) 3131
▲ Levitra Tablets (3%) 2876
▲ Lovaza Capsules (3.5% to 8%) 1520
Lunesta Tablets 2994
Mirapex Tablets (Greater than or equal to 1%) 857
▲ Pataday Ophthalmic Solution (Less than or equal to 5%) 543
▲ Premphase Tablets (8% to 13%) 3232
▲ Prempro Tablets (8% to 13%) 3232
▲ Prozac Weekly Capsules (3% to 10%) 1852
Pulmicort Flexhaler 654
▲ Raptiva for Injection (7%) 1218
▲ Salagen Tablets (9%) 1082
Yaz Tablets (Greater than 1%) 805
Zomig Tablets (Infrequent) 694
Zomig Nasal Spray (Infrequent) 689
Zomig-ZMT Tablets (Infrequent) 694

Fluid depletion

Captopril Tablets 2182
Kristalose for Oral Solution 1004

Fluid imbalance

Benicar HCT Tablets 1010
Imitrex Nasal Spray 1470
Photofrin for Injection 708
Prinzide Tablets 2092
▲ Vesanoid Capsules (6%) 2660

Fluid overload

AmBisome for Injection (Less common) 606
▲ Aranesp for Injection (6%) 564
Cancidas for Injection 1953
▲ Coreg Tablets (Greater than 1% to 3%) 1387
▲ Coreg CR Extended-Release Capsules (Greater than 1% to less than or equal to 3%) 1393
▲ Mycamine for Injection (5% to 17.4%) 616
▲ Myfortic Tablets (3% to less than 20%) 2276
Orthoclone OKT3 Sterile Solution 2387
Prinivil Tablets (0.3% to 1%) 2087
▲ Simulect for Injection (3% to 10%) ... 2306
Zosyn for Injection (1.9%) 3284

Fluid retention

(*see under* Edema)

Flu-like symptoms

Actimmune (Most common) 1743
Actiq (Less than 1%) 959
▲ Actonel Tablets (9.8% to 10.5%) 2568
▲ Advicor Tablets (6%) 402
▲ Aerobid/Aerobid-M (10%) 1153
▲ Agrylin Capsules (1% to less than 5%) 3017
▲ Alamast Ophthalmic Solution (10% to 25%) 3181
▲ Aldara Cream, 5% (1% to 3%) 1699
▲ Alferon N Injection (30%) 1726
Allegra Oral Solution (2.5%) 2684
Aloxi Injection (Less than 1%) 1059
▲ Alphagan P Ophthalmic Solution (1% to 4%) 549
Ambien Tablets (2%) 2692
AmBisome for Injection (Less common) 606
▲ Angeliq Tablets (7%) 751
▲ Aranesp for Injection (6%) 564
Aricept Tablets (Frequent) 1062
Aricept ODT Tablets (Frequent) 1062
▲ Asacol Delayed-Release Tablets (3% to 5%) 2579
Asmanex Twisthaler (1% to less than 3%) 2797
Atacand HCT (2.5%) 642
▲ Atrovent HFA Inhalation Aerosol (4% to 8%) 839
Avapro Tablets (1% or greater) 897
Avapro Tablets (1% or greater) 2718
▲ Avinza Capsules (5% to 10%) 1772
▲ Azilect Tablets (5%) 3106
▲ Azmacort Inhalation Aerosol (2% to 5%) 407
▲ Betaseron for SC Injection (57%) 756
Bexxar 1371
▲ Boniva Injection (0.8% to 3.3%) 2614
▲ Boniva Tablets (0.8% to 3.3%) 2618
▲ BOTOX Purified Neurotoxin Complex (2% to 10%) 550
Celebrex Capsules (0.1% to 1.9%) ... 2979
Celexa (Infrequent) 1160
▲ Chemet Capsules (5.2% to 15.7%) 2484
▲ Copaxone for Injection (19%) 3110
▲ Coreg Tablets (Greater than 1% to 3%) 1387
▲ Cozaar Tablets (10%) 1973
▲ Depakote ER Tablets (12%) 423
Doxil Injection (Less than 1%) 2378
▲ Duragesic Transdermal System (3% to 10%) 2405
▲ Effexor XR Extended-Release Capsules (6%) 3195
Emsam Transdermal System 905
Enbrel for Injection 569
Engerix-B Vaccine (Less than 1%) 1409
Epogen for Injection (Rare) 576
▲ Evista Tablets (13.5% to 14.6%) 1810
▲ Evoxac Capsules (1% to 3%) 1013
▲ Exelon Capsules (3%) 2229
▲ Exelon Oral Solution (3%) 2229
▲ Faslodex Injection (7.1%) 682
▲ Femara Tablets (6%) 2246
▲ Flolan for Injection (13% to 25%) 1426
▲ Flonase Nasal Spray (1% to 3%) 1431
Fluarix Vaccine (1.6%) 1446
Flulaval Injection Vaccine 1448
Follistim AQ Cartridge 2844
Fosamax 2005
▲ Gabitril Tablets (1% to 9%) 973
▲ Gemzar for Injection (19%) 1820
Gengraf Capsules (2%) 435
Geodon (Frequent) 2520
▲ Herceptin I.V. (10%) 1199
▲ Humatrope Vials and Cartridges (3.9% to 22.9%) 1838
Imitrex Injection (Rare) 1465
Imitrex Nasal Spray 1470
Imitrex Tablets 1474
▲ Indapamide Tablets (Less than 5%) 2188
▲ Intron A for Injection (Up to 79%) 2859
Kaletra (Less than 2%) 452
▲ Kineret Injection (6%) 585
▲ Klonopin (4%) 2639
▲ Lamictal (5% to 7%) 1488
▲ Lescol Capsules (5.1%) 2268
▲ Lescol XL Tablets (7.1%) 2268
▲ Lexapro Oral Suspension (5%) 1174
▲ Lexapro Tablets (5%) 1174
▲ Lipitor Tablets (Up to 3.2%) 2501
▲ Lupron Depot 3.75 mg (Less than 5%) 462
▲ Lupron Depot–3 Month 11.25 mg (Less than 5%) 462
Lyrica Capsules (1% to 2%) 2527
▲ Meridia Capsules (8.2%) 475
▲ Miacalcin Nasal Spray (1% to 3%) ... 2274
Micardis Tablets (1%) 852
Micardis HCT Tablets (2%) 854
▲ Mobic Oral Suspension (5.8%) 863
▲ Mobic Tablets (5.8%) 863
Namenda (Greater than or equal to 2%) 1180
Nasonex Nasal Spray (Greater than or equal to 2%) 2883
▲ Neoral Oral Solution (3% to 9.9%) ... 2280
▲ Neoral Soft Gelatin Capsules (3% to 9.9%) 2280
Nexium Delayed-Release Capsules (Less than 1%) 645
Nexium I.V. (Less than 1%) 652
Nexium Delayed-Release Oral Suspension (Less than 1%) 645
▲ Norditropin Cartridges (8%) 2354
Norvir (Less than 2%) 489
▲ Ontak Vials (8%) 1079
Orthoclone OKT3 Sterile Solution 2387
Paxil (Infrequent) 1535
Paxil CR Controlled-Release Tablets (Infrequent) 1544
▲ PegIntron Powder for Injection (46%) 2903
▲ Plavix Tablets (7.9%) 926
▲ Plavix Tablets (7.5%) 2767
Pletal Tablets (2% or greater) 2481
▲ Premarin Tablets (10% to 11%) 3221
Prevnar 3241
Prinivil Tablets (0.3%) 2087
Prinzide Tablets (0.3% to 1%) 2092
Procrit for Injection (Rare) 2391
▲ Prograf Capsules and Injection (3% to 15%) 622
Prolastin (Occasional) 3099
Protonix for Delayed-Release Oral Suspension (Greater than or equal to 1%) 3254
Protonix Delayed-Release Tablets (Greater than or equal to 1%) 3254
Protonix I.V. (Greater than or equal to 1%) 3257
▲ Protopic Ointment (22% to 35%) 628
▲ Provigil Tablets (4%) 977
▲ Prozac Pulvules and Liquid (3% to 10%) 1852
Pulmozyme Inhalation Solution 1217
▲ Rebetol (13% to 31%) 2917
▲ Rebif Prefilled Syringe for Injection (56% to 59%) 1107
Recombivax HB (Less than 1%) 2107
▲ Remeron Tablets (5%) 2924
▲ RemeronSolTab Tablets (5%) 2927
Requip Tablets (Infrequent) 1561
Retrovir Capsules 1574
Retrovir IV Infusion 1579
Retrovir 1574
Rilutek Tablets (More than 2%) 2771
▲ Sandostatin Injection (1% to 4%) 2300
▲ Serevent Diskus (5%) 1594
Soriatane Capsules (Less than 1%) .. 3062
▲ Spiriva HandiHaler (Greater than or equal to 3%) 870
▲ Starlix Tablets (3.6%) 2314
▲ Suboxone Tablets (6%) 2601
▲ Subutex Tablets (6%) 2601
Sular Extended Release Tablets (Less than or equal to 1%) 2975
Synagis Intramuscular Solution (More than 1%) 1948
▲ Targretin Capsules (3.6% to 13.2%) 1084
Teveten Tablets (Less than 1%) 515
Teveten HCT Tablets (Less than 1%) 517
Thyrogen for Injection 1244
▲ Tice BCG (24%) 2936
Tricor Tablets (2.1%) 520
Twinrix Vaccine (Less than 1%) 1628
▲ Tyzeka Tablets (7%) 2328
Ultram ER Extended-Release Tablets (0.2% to 2%) 2428
Vicoprofen Tablets (Less than 3%) ... 533
Viramune Oral Suspension 873
Viramune Tablets 873
▲ Visudyne for Injection (1% to 10%) .. 2332
▲ WelChol Tablets (3.2%) 1015
Wellbutrin Tablets (Frequent) 1648
Wellbutrin SR Sustained-Release Tablets (At least 1%) 1653
Wellbutrin XL Extended-Release Tablets (At least 1%) 1659
▲ Xeloda Tablets (Less than 5%) 2662
▲ Xenical Capsules (39.7%) 2672
▲ Xopenex Inhalation Solution (1.4% to 4.2%) 3001
▲ Xopenex Inhalation Solution Concentrate (1.4% to 4.2%) 3005
▲ Xopenex HFA Inhalation Aerosol (1.4% to 4.2%) 3009
Xyrem Oral Solution (Frequent) 1766
▲ Zemplar Capsules (5%) 536
▲ Zemplar Injection (5%) 538
▲ Zonegran Capsules (4%) 1089
Zostavax Injection (1.7%) 2145
Zyprexa Tablets (Frequent) 1883
Zyprexa ZYDIS Orally Disintegrating Tablets (Frequent) ... 1883

Flu-like syndrome

Rebif Prefilled Syringe for Injection ... 1107
Reyataz Capsules 3299
▲ Tice BCG (33%) 2936
▲ Zometa for Intravenous Infusion (Less than 15%) 2341

Fluorosis

Ultane Liquid for Inhalation (Less than 1%) 524

Flushing

Accutane Capsules 2607
▲ Acetadote Injection (2% to 4%) 1001
▲ Adenoscan (44%) 605
▲ Advicor Tablets (71%) 402
Aggrenox Capsules (Less than 1%) .. 819
Allegra Oral Solution (Rare) 2684
Allegra Tablets (Rare) 2684
Allegra-D 12 Hour Extended-Release Tablets (Rare) ... 2687
Allegra-D 24 Hour Extended-Release Tablets (Rare) ... 2690
Alphanate 1709
Ambien Tablets (Rare) 2692
Ambien CR Tablets (Rare) 2696
AmBisome for Injection (Less common) 606
Aminohippurate Sodium "PAH" Injection 1950
AndroGel 3159
Anzemet Injection (Infrequently) 2701
Anzemet Tablets 2704
Atripla Tablets 938
Avalide Tablets 892
Avalide Tablets 2713
Avapro Tablets (Less than 1%) 897
Avapro Tablets (Less than 1%) 2718
▲ Azor Tablets (0.7% to 4.5%) 1005
▲ BeneFIX Vials (3.1%) 3191
▲ Busulfex Injection (25%) 2477
Cancidas for Injection 1953
Captopril Tablets (2 to 5 of 1000 patients) 2182
Cardizem LA Extended Release Tablets (1.4%) 421
Celexa (Infrequent) 1160
▲ Cerezyme for Injection (Approximately 6.6%) 1238
▲ Cialis Tablets (1% to 3%) 1792
Cipro I.V. (1% or less) 2817
Cipro (Less than 1%) 2810
Cipro XR Tablets 2823
Clinoril Tablets (Less than 1 in 100) 1962
▲ Clolar for Intravenous Infusion (18%) 1239
Combivent Inhalation Aerosol 845
Cozaar Tablets (Less than 1%) 1973
Cubicin for Injection (Less than 1%) 995
Cymbalta Delayed-Release Capsules (Infrequent) 1801
Diovan HCT Tablets (Less frequent) 2216
▲ Doxil Injection (Approximately 6.8%) 2378
Duragesic Transdermal System (1% or greater) 2405
▲ DynaCirc CR Controlled Release Tablets (1.2% to 3.8%) 1407
▲ Eloxatin for Injection (5% to 10%) 2731
Emend Capsules (Greater than 0.5%) 1992
Emend for Injection (Greater than 0.5%) 1999
Enbrel for Injection 569
Engerix-B Vaccine (Less than 1%) 1409
Erbitux 912
Evoxac Capsules (0.3%) 1013
Exelon Capsules (Infrequent) 2229
Exelon Oral Solution (Infrequent) 2229
Exforge Tablets (Greater than or equal to 0.2%) 2238
Fabrazyme for Intravenous Infusion 1241
▲ Femara Tablets (0.1% to 49.7%) 2246
▲ Flolan for Injection (23% to 58%) 1426
Flulaval Injection Vaccine 1448
▲ Frova Tablets (4%) 1111
Gammagard Liquid 730
Gammagard S/D (Occasional) 734

Gantrisin Pediatric Suspension 2638
▲ Gengraf Capsules (Less than 1% to 5%) 435
Gleevec Tablets (Infrequent) 2255
▲ Imitrex Injection (7%) 1465
Imitrex Nasal Spray (Infrequent) 1470
▲ Imitrex Tablets (Up to 4%) 1474
▲ Indapamide Tablets (Less than 5%) 2188
Indocin Capsules (Less than 1%) 2024
Indocin I.V. (Less than 1%) 2489
Indocin (Less than 1%) 2024
▲ Intron A for Injection (Less than 5%) 2859
Invanz for Injection (Greater than 0.1%) 2029
Ketek Tablets (Less than 0.2%) 2744
Klonopin (Infrequent) 2639
Lamictal (Infrequent) 1488
Lescol Capsules (Rare) 2268
Lescol XL Tablets 2268
▲ Letairis Tablets (4%) 1258
Leukine 774
▲ Levitra Tablets (11%) 2876
Levothroid Tablets 1170
Levoxyl Tablets 1780
Lexapro Oral Suspension (Infrequent) 1174
Lexapro Tablets (Infrequent) 1174
▲ Lexiscan Injection (16%) 614
Lidoderm Patch 1114
Marinol Capsules (0.3% to 1%) 3163
Mavik Tablets (0.3% to 1%) 472
Maxair Autohaler 1705
Maxalt Tablets (Frequent) 2056
Maxalt-MLT Orally Disintegrating Tablets (Frequent) 2056
Mephyton Tablets 700
Mevacor Tablets (Rare) 2063
Miacalcin Nasal Spray (Less than 1%) 2274
Micardis Tablets (More than 0.3%) 852
Micardis HCT Tablets 854
▲ Mycamine for Injection (11.1%) 616
▲ Neoral Oral Solution (1% to 5%) 2280
▲ Neoral Soft Gelatin Capsules (1% to 5%) 2280
Neupro Transdermal System 3149
▲ Nexavar Tablets (1% to less than 10%) 784
Nexium Delayed-Release Capsules (Less than 1%) 645
Nexium I.V. (Less than 1%) 652
Nexium Delayed-Release Oral Suspension (Less than 1%) 645
Niaspan Extended-Release Tablets (Among most common) 480
Nimbex Injection (0.2%) 484
Nimotop Capsules (Less than 1% to 2.1%) 790
Nitrolingual Pumpspray 2965
Opana Tablets (Less than 1%) 1117
Opana ER Tablets (Less than 1%) 1121
Orencia Powder for Intravenous Infusion (Greater than 0.1% and less than or equal to 1%) 921
Orthoclone OKT3 Sterile Solution 2387
▲ PegIntron Powder for Injection (6%) 2903
Pepcid Tablets (Infrequent) 2075
Percocet Tablets 1127
Percodan Tablets 1130
Persantine Tablets 869
Pletal Tablets 2481
Primaxin I.M. 2080
Primaxin I.V. (Less than 0.2%) 2083
Prinivil Tablets (0.3% to 1%) 2087
Prinzide Tablets (0.3% to 1%) 2092
Profilnine SD Solvent Detergent 1721
Prograf Capsules and Injection 622
Pylera Capsules 714
▲ Rebetol (3% to 4%) 2917
Recombinate 738
Recombivax HB (Less than 1%) 2107
ReFacto Vials 3269
Refludan for Injection (Uncommon) 795
Remeron Tablets 2924
RemeronSolTab Tablets 2927
▲ Remicade for IV Injection (9%) 950
▲ Requip Tablets (Infrequent to 3%) 1561
Risperdal Consta Long-Acting Injection (Rare) 1753
▲ Rituxan I.V. (0% to 5%) 1223
Rocephin Injectable Vials, ADD-Vantage, Galaxy, Bulk (Less than 1%) 2642
▲ Romazicon Injection (1% to 3%) 2646
Rythmol Tablets (Less than 1%) 1586
Rythmol SR Capsules 1590
▲ Salagen Tablets (8% to 13%) 1082
▲ Sandimmune (Less than 1% to 4%) 2296
▲ Sandostatin Injection (1% to 4%) 2300
▲ Soriatane Capsules (1% to 10%) 3062
Stalevo Tablets 2309
Strattera Capsules 1864
Sustiva Capsules (Less than 2%) 930
Sustiva Tablets (Less than 2%) 930
Tarka Tablets (0.3% or more) 511
▲ Tasigna Capsules (1% to 10%) 2316
Taxotere Injection Concentrate 2773
Thyrogen for Injection 1244
Torisel Injection 3272
▲ Tracleer Tablets (9%) 3289
Treximet Tablets (Infrequent) 1616
▲ Trisenox Injection (10%) 986
Twinrix Vaccine (Less than 1%) 1628
▲ Ultram ER Extended-Release Tablets (7.7% to 15.8%) 2428
Uroxatral Tablets 2786
Vantas (Less than 2%) 1737
Venlafaxine Hydrochloride Tablets 2199
▲ Vesanoid Capsules (23%) 2660
Visudyne for Injection 2332
Vytorin 10/10 Tablets 2149
Vytorin 10/10 Tablets 2939
Vytorin 10/20 Tablets 2149
Vytorin 10/20 Tablets 2939
Vytorin 10/40 Tablets 2149
Vytorin 10/40 Tablets 2939
Vytorin 10/80 Tablets 2149
Vytorin 10/80 Tablets 2939
Wellbutrin Tablets (Rare) 1648
▲ Wellbutrin SR Sustained-Release Tablets (1% to 4%) 1653
▲ Wellbutrin XL Extended-Release Tablets (1% to 4%) 1659
▲ Xeloda Tablets (5%) 2662
Zocor Tablets (Rare) 2136
Zofran Injection 1682
Zofran 1687
Zofran ODT Orally Disintegrating Tablets 1687
Zometa for Intravenous Infusion 2341
Zosyn for Injection (1% or less) 3284
Zyban Sustained-Release Tablets (Infrequent) 1692
Zyrtec Chewable Tablets (Less than 2%) 1920
Zyrtec Syrup (Less than 2%) 1920
Zyrtec Tablets (Less than 2%) 1920
Zyrtec-D 12 Hour Extended Release Tablets (Less than 2%) 1923

Flushing, cutaneous
Elidel Cream 1% 2221
Nitrolingual Pumpspray 2965

Flushing, facial
▲ Adenocard IV Injection (18%) 603
Alferon N Injection (One patient) 1726
Doxil Injection 2378
Eloxatin for Injection 2731
Imitrex Nasal Spray 1470
Imitrex Tablets 1474
Marinol Capsules (Greater than 1%) 3163
▲ Miacalcin Injection (About 2% to 5%) 2273
MS Contin Tablets (Less frequent) 2585
ProAmatine Tablets (Less frequent) 3032
Sandimmune 2296
Soma Tablets 1931

Flushing, generalized
Neulasta Injection 587

Flushing, hands
▲ Miacalcin Injection (About 2% to 5%) 2273

Flushing, upper thorax
Sandimmune 2296

Focal segmental glomerulosclerosis
Rapamune 3260

Folliculitis
Amerge Tablets (Rare) 1301
Analpram-HC 1140
Didronel Tablets 2583
Diprolene Lotion 0.05% (Less than 1% to 2%) 2838
Diprolene Ointment 0.05% (Less than 1%) 2839
Diprolene AF Cream 0.05% (Infrequent) 2837
▲ Elidel Cream 1% (0.9% to 6.1%) 2221
Elocon Cream 0.1% (Infrequent) 2840
Elocon Lotion 0.1% (4 in 156 subjects) 2841
Elocon Ointment 0.1% (Infrequent) 2842
Evoclin Foam, 1% 3056
▲ Flovent Diskus 50 mcg (1% to 3%) 1435
Gengraf Capsules (1% to less than 3%) 435
▲ Intron A for Injection (Less than 5%) 2859
Lexapro Oral Suspension (Infrequent) 1174
Lexapro Tablets (Infrequent) 1174
Lotrisone 2881
Luxiq Foam 3058
Mirapex Tablets 857
Neoral Oral Solution (1% to less than 3%) 2280
Neoral Soft Gelatin Capsules (1% to less than 3%) 2280
Nexavar Tablets (0.1% to less than 1%) 784
Norvir (Less than 2%) 489
Olux Foam (Less than 2%) 3061
Olux-E Foam 3059
Pramosone 1141
▲ Protopic Ointment (4% to 11%) 628
Requip Tablets (Infrequent) 1561
▲ Selzentry Tablets (3.3%) 2534
Sustiva Capsules (Less than 2%) 930
Sustiva Tablets (Less than 2%) 930
Vanos Cream 1941
Verdeso Foam 3069

Folliculosis
▲ Elestat Ophthalmic Solution (1% to 10%) 1741

Folliculosis, conjunctival
▲ Combigan Ophthalmic Solution (5% to 15%) 553

Fontanels, bulging
Pylera Capsules 714
Solodyn Extended Release Tablets 1938

Food craving
Vantas (Less than 2%) 1737

Foot drop
Actiq (Less than 1%) 959
Azilect Tablets (Infrequent) 3106
▲ Copaxone for Injection (3%) 3110
Prozac Weekly Capsules (Rare) 1852
Prozac Pulvules and Liquid (Rare) 1852

Foreign body reaction
▲ Alamast Ophthalmic Solution (Less than 5%) 3181
▲ Alphagan P Ophthalmic Solution (1% to 4%) 549
▲ Alrex Ophthalmic Suspension 0.2% (5% to 15%) ⊙ 236
▲ Lumigan Ophthalmic Solution (3% to 10%) 556

Foreign body sensation
▲ Combigan Ophthalmic Solution (1% to 5%) 553
Xyrem Oral Solution (Infrequent) 1766

Forgetfulness
Crinone 4% Gel 992
Crinone 8% Gel 992
Lexapro Oral Suspension (Infrequent) 1174
Lexapro Tablets (Infrequent) 1174
Marplan Tablets (2%) 3177

Fracture, ankle
Xyrem Oral Solution (Infrequent) 1766

Fracture, humerus
Tamiflu Capsules (Less than 1%) 2649
Tamiflu Oral Suspension (Less than 1%) 2649

Fracture, lower limb
Requip Tablets (Infrequent) 1561

Fracture, pathological
Actiq (Less than 1%) 959
▲ Arimidex Tablets (2% to 5%) 672
▲ Doxil Injection (1% to 10%) 2378
Effexor XR Extended-Release Capsules (Rare) 3195
Emsam Transdermal System (Frequent) 905
Lamictal (Rare) 1488
Luvox CR Extended-Release Capsules (Rare) 1759
Remeron Tablets (Rare) 2924
RemeronSolTab Tablets (Rare) 2927
Salagen Tablets (Less than 1%) 1082
Venlafaxine Hydrochloride Tablets (Rare) 2199

Fracture, traumatic bone
▲ Actonel Tablets (9.3%) 2568

Fractures, unspecified
Celebrex Capsules (0.1% to 1.9%) 2979
Exelon Capsules (2% or more) 2229
Exelon Oral Solution (2% or more) 2229
▲ Femara Tablets (1.9% to 5.6%) 2246
Genotropin Lyophilized Powder 2547
Klonopin (Infrequent) 2639
Lovaza Capsules 1520
Nutropin for Injection 1208
Nutropin AQ Injection 1212
Nutropin AQ NuSpin Injection 1212
Nutropin AQ Pen 1212
Nutropin AQ Pen Cartridge 1212
▲ Simulect for Injection (3% to 10%) 2306
Xolair (2%) 1235
Xolair (2%) 2339

Free T3 resin uptake, decrease
(*see under* T3, decrease)

Freezing phenomenon
Exelon Capsules (Infrequent) 2229
Exelon Oral Solution (Infrequent) 2229

Frequent blinking
Abilify Injection (Less than 1 in 1000 patients) 2466
Abilify Oral Solution (Less than 1 in 1000 patients) 2466
Abilify Discmelt Orally Disintegrating Tablets (Less than 1 in 1000 patients) 2466
Abilify Tablets (Less than 1 in 1000 patients) 2466

Fretfulness
(*see under* Anxiety)

Frigidity, unspecified
Wellbutrin Tablets (Infrequent) 1648

Fullness, abdominal
(*see under* Abdominal bloating)

Fungal invasion
FML Ophthalmic Ointment (Possibility) ⊙ 223
FML Ophthalmic Suspension (Possibility) ⊙ 224
FML Forte Ophthalmic Suspension (Possibility) ⊙ 222
Pred Mild Ophthalmic Suspension ⊙ 230
Pred-G Ophthalmic Ointment ⊙ 229
Pred-G Ophthalmic Suspension ⊙ 228

Fungemia
▲ CellCept Capsules (Less than 4%) 2622
▲ CellCept Intravenous (Less than 4%) 2622
▲ CellCept Oral Suspension (Less than 4%) 2622
▲ CellCept Tablets (Less than 4%) 2622
Cubicin for Injection (Less than 1%) 995

Furuncle
Mirapex Tablets 857

Furunculosis
Ambien Tablets (Rare) 2692
Ambien CR Tablets (Rare) 2696
Copaxone for Injection (Infrequent) 3110
Depakote ER Tablets (Greater than 1%) 423
▲ Doxil Injection (1% to 10%) 2378
Effexor XR Extended-Release Capsules (Rare) 3195
▲ Elocon Cream 0.1% (Approximately 7%) 2840
▲ Elocon Ointment 0.1% (4.8% to approximately 7%) 2842
Evoxac Capsules (Less than 1%) 1013
Gabitril Tablets (Infrequent) 973
Geodon for Injection (Up to 2%) 2520
▲ Intron A for Injection (Less than 5%) 2859
Kaletra (Less than 2%) 452
Lexapro Oral Suspension (Infrequent) 1174
Lexapro Tablets (Infrequent) 1174
Lunesta Tablets (Rare) 2994
Luvox CR Extended-Release Capsules (Infrequent) 1759
Paxil (Infrequent) 1535
Paxil CR Controlled-Release Tablets (Infrequent) 1544
Pletal Tablets (Less than 2%) 2481
Protopic Ointment (Greater than or equal to 1%) 628
Prozac Weekly Capsules (Rare) 1852
Prozac Pulvules and Liquid (Rare) 1852
Requip Tablets (Infrequent) 1561
Rilutek Tablets (Rare) 2771
Soriatane Capsules (Less than 1%) 3062
Teveten Tablets (Less than 1%) 515

Teveten HCT Tablets (Less than 1%) 517
Venlafaxine Hydrochloride Tablets (Rare) 2199
Zyrtec Chewable Tablets (Less than 2%) 1920
Zyrtec Syrup (Less than 2%) 1920
Zyrtec Tablets (Less than 2%) 1920
Zyrtec-D 12 Hour Extended Release Tablets (Less than 2%) 1923

Fussiness
▲ Pentacel (4% to 76.9%) 2792
▲ Prevnar (16.7% to 54.1%) 3241
▲ Rotarix Oral Suspension (42% to 52%) 1582

G

Gagging
Lexapro Oral Suspension (Infrequent) 1174
Lexapro Tablets (Infrequent) 1174

Gait, abnormal
Acetadote Injection (0.24% to 1.17%) 1001
Actimmune (Rare) 1743
▲ Actiq (1% to 4%) 959
Ambien Tablets (Rare) 2692
Ambien CR Tablets (Rare) 2696
Aricept Tablets (Frequent) 1062
Aricept ODT Tablets (Frequent) 1062
▲ Arranon Injection (0% to 6%) 1319
▲ Avastin IV (1% to 5%) 1192
▲ Avinza Capsules (Less than 5%) 1772
Azilect Tablets (Frequent) 3106
Cardizem LA Extended Release Tablets (Less than 2%) 421
Celexa (Infrequent) 1160
Cipro I.V. (1% or less) 2817
Cipro (Less than 1%) 2810
Cipro XR Tablets 2823
Copaxone for Injection (At least 2%) 3110
Cymbalta Delayed-Release Capsules (Rare) 1801
▲ Depakote ER Tablets (Greater than 1% to less than 5%) 423
▲ DepoCyt Injection (1% to 23%) 1136
Duragesic Transdermal System (1% or greater) 2405
Effexor XR Extended-Release Capsules (Rare) 3195
Evoxac Capsules 1013
Exelon Capsules (Frequent) 2229
Exelon Oral Solution (Frequent) 2229
Flulaval Injection Vaccine 1448
Flumadine (Less than 0.3%) 1167
Frova Tablets (Infrequent) 1111
▲ Gabitril Tablets (3%) 973
Geodon Capsules (Frequent) 2520
▲ Gliadel Wafer (5%) 1076
▲ Intron A for Injection (Less than 5%) 2859
Keppra Injection 3137
Keppra Oral Solution 3131
Keppra Tablets 3131
▲ Lamictal (4%) 1488
Levaquin (0.1% to 1%) 2416
Levaquin in 5% Dextrose Injection (0.1% to 1%) 2416
Lexapro Oral Suspension 1174
Lexapro Tablets 1174
Lunesta Tablets (Rare) 2994
Luvox CR Extended-Release Capsules (Infrequent) 1759
▲ Lyrica Capsules (1% to 8%) 2527
Maxalt Tablets (Infrequent) 2056
Maxalt-MLT Orally Disintegrating Tablets (Infrequent) 2056
Meridia Capsules 475
▲ Mirapex Tablets (Greater than or equal to 1% to 7%) 857
Namenda (Greater than or equal to 2%) 1180
Neupro Transdermal System 3149
Norvir (Less than 2%) 489
OxyContin Tablets (Less than 1%) 2589
Paxil (Rare) 1535
Paxil CR Controlled-Release Tablets (Rare) 1544
Prozac Weekly Capsules (Infrequent) 1852
Prozac Pulvules and Liquid (Infrequent) 1852
Requip Tablets (Infrequent) 1561
Rilutek Tablets (Infrequent) 2771
Risperdal Consta Long-Acting Injection (Infrequent) 1753
Rythmol SR Capsules 1590
Soriatane Capsules (Less than 1%) 3062
Stalevo Tablets 2309
Symbyax Capsules (Infrequent) 1871
▲ Temodar Capsules (1% to 6%) 2931
Venlafaxine Hydrochloride Tablets (Rare) 2199
▲ Vesanoid Capsules (3%) 2660
▲ Xeloda Tablets (Less than 5%) 2662
Xyrem Oral Solution (Infrequent) 1766
Zantac Injection 1666
Zantac 150 Tablets 1670
Zonegran Capsules (Frequent) 1089
▲ Zyprexa Tablets (6%) 1883
Zyprexa IntraMuscular (Infrequent) 1883
▲ Zyprexa ZYDIS Orally Disintegrating Tablets (6%) 1883

Galactorrhea
Abilify Injection (Less than 1 in 1000 patients) 2466
Abilify Oral Solution (Less than 1 in 1000 patients) 2466
Abilify Discmelt Orally Disintegrating Tablets (Less than 1 in 1000 patients) 2466
Abilify Tablets (Less than 1 in 1000 patients) 2466
Activella Tablets 2347
Angeliq Tablets 751
Celexa (Infrequent) 1160
Climara Transdermal System 763
Climara Pro Transdermal System 768
Demser Capsules (Infrequent) 1989
Depakote ER Tablets 423
Enjuvia Tablets 1029
Estratest Tablets 3043
Estratest H.S. Tablets 3043
Geodon (Rare) 2520
Imitrex Injection 1465
Imitrex Nasal Spray (Rare) 1470
Imitrex Tablets (Rare) 1474
Invega Extended-Release Tablets 1748
Moban Tablets (Infrequent) 1116
Paxil 1535
Paxil CR Controlled-Release Tablets 1544
Premarin Intravenous 3217
Premarin Tablets 3221
Premphase Tablets 3232
Prempro Tablets 3232
Proglycem Capsules (Infrequent) 1185
Proglycem Suspension (Infrequent) 1185
Sandostatin Injection (Less than 1%) 2300
Sandostatin LAR Depot 2302
Tarka Tablets 511
Thioridazine Hydrochloride Tablets 2195

Gallbladder, sonographic abnormalities
Rocephin Injectable Vials, ADD-Vantage, Galaxy, Bulk 2642

Gallbladder disease
Activella Tablets 2347
Angeliq Tablets 751
Chantix Tablets (Infrequent) 2511
Climara Transdermal System 763
Climara Pro Transdermal System 768
Divigel 3167
Enjuvia Tablets 1029
Estratest Tablets 3043
Estratest H.S. Tablets 3043
Lybrel Tablets 3204
Mircette Tablets 1034
NuvaRing 2897
Ortho-Cyclen Tablets 2449
Ortho Evra Transdermal System 2437
Ortho Tri-Cyclen Tablets 2449
Ortho Tri-Cyclen Lo Tablets 2458
Premarin Intravenous 3217
Premarin Tablets 3221
Premarin Vaginal Cream 3228
Premphase Tablets 3232
Prempro Tablets 3232
Pulmozyme Inhalation Solution 1217
Reyataz Capsules 3299
Rocephin Injectable Vials, ADD-Vantage, Galaxy, Bulk 2642
Sandostatin Injection (Frequent) 2300
Sandostatin LAR Depot 2302
Seasonique Tablets 1046
Yaz Tablets 805

Gallstones
Imitrex Injection (Rare) 1465
Imitrex Nasal Spray 1470
Imitrex Tablets 1474
▲ Intron A for Injection (Less than 5%) 2859
Reyataz Capsules 3299
Sandostatin Injection (Frequent) 2300
▲ Sandostatin LAR Depot (24% to 27%) 2302

Gambling, pathological
Requip Tablets 1561

Gamma-glutamyl transferase, increase
Cipro (Less than 0.1%) 2810
Emtriva Capsules (1 patient) 1246
Emtriva Oral Solution (1 patient) 1246
Ixempra Kit for Injection 915
▲ Novantrone for Injection Concentrate (3% to 15%) 1100
▲ Tasigna Capsules (1% to 10%) 2316
Zetia Tablets 2157
Zetia Tablets (0.2%) 2951
Zosyn for Injection 3284

Gamma-glutamyl transpeptidase, elevation
Abilify Injection (Greater than or equal to 1 in 100 patients) 881
Abilify Injection (Less than 1 in 1000 patients) 2466
Abilify Oral Solution (Greater than or equal to 1 in 100 patients) 881
Abilify Oral Solution (Less than 1 in 1000 patients) 2466
Abilify Discmelt Orally Disintegrating Tablets (Greater than or equal to 1 in 100 patients) 881
Abilify Discmelt Orally Disintegrating Tablets (Less than 1 in 1000 patients) 2466
Abilify Tablets (Greater than or equal to 1 in 100 patients) 881
Abilify Tablets (Less than 1 in 1000 patients) 2466
Accutane Capsules 2607
Advicor Tablets 402
Anzemet Tablets (Rare) 2704
Aptivus Capsules (2%) 823
Aptivus Oral Solution (2%) 823
Aricept Tablets (Infrequent) 1062
Aricept ODT Tablets (Infrequent) 1062
▲ Arimidex Tablets (Greater than 0.1% to less than or equal to 5%) 672
Asacol Delayed-Release Tablets 2579
Avelox (Greater than or equal to 0.1% to less than 2%) 2803
Axert Tablets (Rare) 2431
Benicar HCT Tablets (Greater than 1%) 1010
Betaseron for SC Injection 756
Biaxin/Biaxin XL (Less than 1%) 411
▲ CellCept Capsules (3% to less than 20%) 2622
▲ CellCept Intravenous (3% to less than 20%) 2622
▲ CellCept Oral Suspension (3% to less than 20%) 2622
▲ CellCept Tablets (3% to less than 20%) 2622
Cialis Tablets (Less than 2%) 1792
Cipro I.V. (Infrequent) 2817
Cipro XR Tablets 2823
▲ Coreg Tablets (Greater than 1% to 3%) 1387
▲ Coreg CR Extended-Release Capsules (Greater than 1% to less than or equal to 3%) 1393
Crestor Tablets 677
Effexor XR Extended-Release Capsules 3195
Elmiron Capsules (1.2%) 2435
Epzicom Tablets 1422
Evoxac Capsules (Less than 1%) 1013
Exelon Capsules (Infrequent) 2229
Exelon Oral Solution (Infrequent) 2229
▲ Fortaz (1 in 19) 1450
Gemzar for Injection (Rare) 1820
Geodon Capsules (Rare) 2520
▲ Kaletra (10%) 452
Lescol Capsules 2268
Lescol XL Tablets 2268
Levitra Tablets (Less than 2%) 2876
Meridia Capsules (1.6%) 475
Mevacor Tablets 2063
Mobic Oral Suspension (Less than 2%) 863
Mobic Tablets (Less than 2%) 863
Neupro Transdermal System 3149
▲ Noxafil Oral Suspension (2% to 3%) 2889
Omnicef Capsules (1%) 497
Pentasa Capsules (Less than 1%) 3030
▲ Prograf Capsules and Injection (3% to 15%) 622
Protonix for Delayed-Release Oral Suspension (Less than 1%) 3254
Protonix Delayed-Release Tablets (Less than 1%) 3254
Protonix I.V. (Less than 1%) 3257
Provigil Tablets (At least 1%) 977
Rilutek Tablets (Infrequent) 2771
Risperdal Consta Long-Acting Injection (Rare) 1753
Rythmol SR Capsules 1590
▲ Soriatane Capsules (Approximately 1 in 3 patients) 3062
Tricor Tablets 520
Truvada Tablets 1262
Venlafaxine Hydrochloride Tablets 2199
Viramune Oral Suspension 873
Viramune Tablets 873
Vytorin 10/10 Tablets 2149
Vytorin 10/10 Tablets 2939
Vytorin 10/20 Tablets 2149
Vytorin 10/20 Tablets 2939
Vytorin 10/40 Tablets 2149
Vytorin 10/40 Tablets 2939
Vytorin 10/80 Tablets 2149
Vytorin 10/80 Tablets 2939
Ziagen 1673
Zocor Tablets 2136
Zyprexa Tablets 1883
Zyprexa ZYDIS Orally Disintegrating Tablets 1883

Gangrene
Bicillin C-R Injectable Suspension 1775
Bicillin L-A Injection 1777
Gemzar for Injection (Very rare) 1820
Mirapex Tablets 857
Requip Tablets (Rare) 1561

Gangrene, peripheral
Celebrex Capsules (Less than 0.1%) 2979
Proleukin for Injection (Less than 1%) 2287
Requip Tablets (Infrequent) 1561

Gastralgia
▲ Novantrone for Injection Concentrate (14%) 1100

Gastric acid, regurgitation
Crixivan Capsules (2.7%) 1979
▲ Fosamax (Up to 4.1%) 2005
▲ Fosamax Plus D Tablets (0% to 4.2%) 2013

Gastric discomfort
(*see under* Distress, gastrointestinal)

Gastric disorder
(*see under* Distress, gastrointestinal)

Gastric emptying, impaired
Donnatal Extentabs 2507
Ixempra Kit for Injection 915
Prograf Capsules and Injection 622

Gastric regurgitation
Wellbutrin SR Sustained-Release Tablets (Infrequent) 1653
Wellbutrin XL Extended-Release Tablets (Infrequent) 1659

Gastric ulcer, nonsteroidal anti-inflammatory drug-induced
Percodan Tablets 1130

Gastritis
Actonel Tablets (2.7%) 2568
Actonel with Calcium Tablets (2.5%) 2574
Aggrenox Capsules (Less than 1%) 819
▲ Agrylin Capsules (1% to less than 5%) 3017
Ambien Tablets (Rare) 2692
Ambien CR Tablets (Rare) 2696
Amerge Tablets (Rare) 1301
Amitiza Capsules (Less than 1%) 3082
Amrix Capsules 966
Anaprox Tablets (Less than 1%) 2632
Anaprox DS Tablets (Less than 1%) 2632
Aricept Tablets (Infrequent) 1062
Aricept ODT Tablets (Infrequent) 1062
Asacol Delayed-Release Tablets 2579
Atacand HCT (0.5% or greater) 642
Augmentin 1323
Augmentin Tablets 1327
Augmentin XR Extended Release Tablets 1333
Augmentin ES-600 Powder for Oral Suspension 1329
Avelox (Less than 0.1%) 2803
Axert Tablets (Rare) 2431
Boniva Injection (2.2%) 2614
Boniva Tablets (2.2%) 2618

Brovana Inhalation Solution (Less than 2%) 2990
Campral Tablets (Infrequent) 1158
Celebrex Capsules (0.1% to 1.9%) 2979
Celexa (Infrequent) 1160
▲ CellCept Capsules (3% to less than 20%) 2622
▲ CellCept Intravenous (3% to less than 20%) 2622
▲ CellCept Oral Suspension (3% to less than 20%) 2622
▲ CellCept Tablets (3% to less than 20%) 2622
Chantix Tablets (Infrequent) 2511
Cialis Tablets (Less than 2%) 1792
Clinoril Tablets (Less than 1%) 1962
Comtan Tablets (1%) 2208
Copaxone for Injection (At least 2%) 3110
▲ Cozaar Tablets (Less than 1% to 5%) 1973
Crinone 4% Gel 992
Crinone 8% Gel 992
Cymbalta Delayed-Release Capsules (Infrequent) 1801
Didronel Tablets 2583
Doxil Injection (Less than 1%) 2378
EC-Naprosyn Delayed-Release Tablets (Less than 1%) 2632
Effexor XR Extended-Release Capsules (Infrequent) 3195
Elmiron Capsules (Less than or equal to 1%) 2435
▲ Emend Capsules (4.2%) 1992
▲ Emend for Injection (4.2%) 1999
Emsam Transdermal System (Infrequent) 905
Enbrel for Injection 569
Evoxac Capsules (Less than 1%) 1013
Exelon Capsules (Frequent) 2229
Exelon Oral Solution (Frequent) 2229
Exelon Patch (Frequent) 2233
Exforge Tablets (Less than or equal to 0.1% to greater than 0.2%) 2238
Exjade Tablets (0.1% to 1%) 2244
▲ Flector Patch (3%) 561
▲ Flolan for Injection (61%) 1426
Fosamax (0.2% to 1.1%) 2005
Fosamax Plus D Tablets (0.2% to 1.1%) 2013
Gabitril Tablets (Infrequent) 973
Gengraf Capsules (1% to less than 3%) 435
Gleevec Tablets (Infrequent) 2255
▲ Humatrope Vials and Cartridges (Up to 6.67%) 1838
Imitrex Injection 1465
Imitrex Nasal Spray 1470
Intelence Tablets (Less than 2%) 3119
▲ Intron A for Injection (Less than 5%) 2859
Invanz for Injection (Greater than 0.1%) 2029
Isentress Tablets 2036
Ixempra Kit for Injection 915
Kaletra (Less than 2%) 452
Ketek Tablets (Greater than or equal to 0.2% to less than 2%) 2744
Klonopin 2639
Lamictal (Infrequent) 1488
Levaquin (0.1% to 1%) 2416
Levaquin in 5% Dextrose Injection (0.1% to 1%) 2416
Levitra Tablets (Less than 2%) 2876
Lexapro Oral Suspension (Infrequent) 1174
Lexapro Tablets (Infrequent) 1174
Lipitor Tablets (Less than 2%) 2501
Lovaza Capsules 1520
Lunesta Tablets (Rare) 2994
Luvox CR Extended-Release Capsules (Infrequent) 1759
Lyrica Capsules (0.1% to 1%) 2527
▲ Malarone Pediatric Tablets (2% to 3%) 1521
▲ Malarone Tablets (2% to 3%) 1521
▲ Mavik Tablets (4.2%) 472
Maxalt Tablets (Rare) 2056
Maxalt-MLT Orally Disintegrating Tablets (Rare) 2056
Meridia Capsules (1.7%) 475
Miacalcin Nasal Spray (Less than 1%) 2274
Micardis Tablets (More than 0.3%) 852
Micardis HCT Tablets 854
Mobic Oral Suspension (Less than 2%) 863
Mobic Tablets (Less than 2%) 863
Nalfon Capsules (Less than 1%) 2508
Namenda 1180
Naprosyn Suspension (Less than 1%) 2632
Naprosyn Tablets (Less than 1%) 2632
NeoProfen Injection 2496
Neoral Oral Solution (1% to less than 3%) 2280
Neoral Soft Gelatin Capsules (1% to less than 3%) 2280
Nexavar Tablets (0.1% to less than 1%) 784
Norvir (Less than 2%) 489
▲ OxyContin Tablets (Between 1% and 5%) 2589
Plavix Tablets 926
Plavix Tablets 2767
Pletal Tablets (Less than 2%) 2481
Prinivil Tablets (0.3% to 1%) 2087
Prinzide Tablets 2092
▲ Prograf Capsules and Injection (3% to 15%) 622
Proleukin for Injection 2287
Protopic Ointment (Greater than or equal to 1%) 628
Prozac Weekly Capsules (Infrequent) 1852
Prozac Pulvules and Liquid (Infrequent) 1852
ReFacto Vials 3269
Remeron Tablets (Rare) 2924
RemeronSolTab Tablets (Rare) 2927
Requip Tablets (Infrequent) 1561
Rilutek Tablets (Infrequent) 2771
Risperdal Consta Long-Acting Injection (Infrequent) 1753
Rythmol SR Capsules 1590
Salagen Tablets (Less than 1%) 1082
Sanctura XR Capsules 557
Sandimmune (2% or less) 2296
Soriatane Capsules (Less than 1%) 3062
Stalevo Tablets (1%) 2309
Sular Extended Release Tablets (Less than or equal to 1%) 2975
Symbyax Capsules (Infrequent) 1871
Teveten Tablets (Less than 1%) 515
Teveten HCT Tablets (Less than 1%) 517
Treximet Tablets (Infrequent) 1616
Tricor Tablets 520
Tyzeka Tablets (Less than 1%) 2328
Venlafaxine Hydrochloride Tablets (Infrequent) 2199
Vicoprofen Tablets (Less than 3%) 533
Voltaren Tablets (Occasionally) 2334
Voltaren-XR Tablets (Occasionally) 2337
Vytorin 10/10 Tablets 2149
Vytorin 10/10 Tablets 2939
Vytorin 10/20 Tablets 2149
Vytorin 10/20 Tablets 2939
Vytorin 10/40 Tablets 2149
Vytorin 10/40 Tablets 2939
Vytorin 10/80 Tablets 2149
Vytorin 10/80 Tablets 2939
Xeloda Tablets 2662
▲ Zocor Tablets (4.9%) 2136
Zomig Tablets (Rare) 694
Zomig Nasal Spray (Rare) 689
Zomig-ZMT Tablets (Rare) 694
Zonegran Capsules (Infrequent) 1089
Zosyn for Injection (1% or less) 3284
Zyprexa Tablets (Infrequent) 1883
Zyprexa ZYDIS Orally Disintegrating Tablets (Infrequent) 1883
Zyrtec Chewable Tablets (Less than 2%) 1920
Zyrtec Syrup (Less than 2%) 1920
Zyrtec Tablets (Less than 2%) 1920
Zyrtec-D 12 Hour Extended Release Tablets (Less than 2%) 1923

Gastritis, atrophic

Protonix for Delayed-Release Oral Suspension 3254
Protonix Delayed-Release Tablets 3254

Gastritis, hemorrhagic

Azilect Tablets (Rare) 3106
Plavix Tablets (Less than 1%) 926
Plavix Tablets (Less than 1%) 2767
Requip Tablets (Rare) 1561
Velcade for Injection 2168

Gastroenteritis

Aceon Tablets (2 mg, 4 mg, 8 mg) (0.3% to 1%) 3038
Actiq (Less than 1%) 959
▲ Activella Tablets (0% to 6%) 2347
▲ Actonel with Calcium Tablets (3.5% to 3.8%) 2574
▲ Alvesco Inhalation Aerosol (Greater than or equal to 3%) 2985
Ambien Tablets (Infrequent) 2692
Ambien CR Tablets (1%) 2696
Amerge Tablets (Infrequent) 1301
Amevive 611
Aricept Tablets (Frequent) 1062
Aricept ODT Tablets (Frequent) 1062
Asacol Delayed-Release Tablets (2% or greater) 2579
Atacand Tablets (0.5% or greater) 639
Atacand HCT (0.5% or greater) 642
Avalide Tablets 892
Avalide Tablets 2713
Avapro Tablets (Less than 1%) 897
Avapro Tablets (Less than 1%) 2718
▲ Avinza Capsules (Less than 5%) 1772
Axert Tablets (Rare) 2431
▲ Azilect Tablets (3%) 3106
Benicar Tablets (Greater than 0.5%) 1009
Benicar HCT Tablets (Greater than 1%) 1010
Campral Tablets (Infrequent) 1158
Celebrex Capsules (0.1% to 1.9%) 2979
Celexa (Infrequent) 1160
▲ CellCept Capsules (3% to less than 20%) 2622
▲ CellCept Intravenous (3% to less than 20%) 2622
▲ CellCept Oral Suspension (3% to less than 20%) 2622
▲ CellCept Tablets (3% to less than 20%) 2622
Clinoril Tablets (Less than 1%) 1962
▲ Copaxone for Injection (3%) 3110
Cymbalta Delayed-Release Capsules (Infrequent) 1801
Depakote ER Tablets (Greater than 1%) 423
Diovan HCT Tablets (Greater than 0.2%) 2216
Effexor XR Extended-Release Capsules (Infrequent) 3195
▲ Elidel Cream 1% (0% to 7.4%) 2221
Eligard 7.5 mg (2.5%) 2724
Eligard 22.5 mg 2724
Eligard 30 mg (2.5%) 2724
Eligard 45 mg 2724
Emsam Transdermal System (Frequent) 905
▲ Emtriva Capsules (11%) 1246
▲ Emtriva Oral Solution (11%) 1246
Enbrel for Injection 569
Epivir 1412
Evista Tablets (2.6%) 1810
Evoxac Capsules (Less than 1%) 1013
Exelon Capsules (Infrequent) 2229
Exelon Oral Solution (Infrequent) 2229
Exforge Tablets (Greater than or equal to 0.2%) 2238
▲ Flovent Diskus 50 mcg (1% to 3%) 1435
Gabitril Tablets (1% or more) 973
Gardasil Injection (0.03%) 2019
Gengraf Capsules (1% to less than 3%) 435
Genotropin Lyophilized Powder 2547
Gleevec Tablets (Infrequent) 2255
▲ Humira Injection (Less than 5%) 442
Imitrex Injection 1465
Imitrex Nasal Spray (Rare) 1470
Indocin Capsules (Less than 1%) 2024
Indocin I.V. (Less than 1%) 2489
Indocin (Less than 1%) 2024
▲ Intron A for Injection (Less than 5%) 2859
Kaletra (Less than 2%) 452
▲ Keppra Oral Solution (1% to 4%) 3131
▲ Keppra Tablets (1% to 4%) 3131
Ketek Tablets (Greater than or equal to 0.2% to less than 2%) 2744
Kinrix Injection Vaccine (0.1%) 1486
Kogenate FS 746
Kogenate FS with Bio-Set 748
Levaquin (0.1% to 1%) 2416
Levaquin in 5% Dextrose Injection (0.1% to 1%) 2416
Lexapro Oral Suspension (Frequent) 1174
Lexapro Tablets (Frequent) 1174
Lipitor Tablets (Less than 2%) 2501
Lovaza Capsules 1520
Luvox CR Extended-Release Capsules (Infrequent) 1759
Lyrica Capsules (Greater than or equal to 1%) 2527
Meridia Capsules (Greater than or equal to 1%) 475
Micardis Tablets (More than 0.3%) 852
Micardis HCT Tablets 854
Namenda (Infrequent) 1180
Neoral Oral Solution (1% to less than 3%) 2280
Neoral Soft Gelatin Capsules (1% to less than 3%) 2280
Nexium Delayed-Release Capsules (Less than 1%) 645
Nexium I.V. (Less than 1%) 652
Nexium Delayed-Release Oral Suspension (Less than 1%) 645
▲ Norditropin Cartridges (8%) 2354
Norvir (Less than 2%) 489
Paxil (Rare) 1535
Paxil CR Controlled-Release Tablets (Rare) 1544
PegIntron Powder for Injection (Less than or equal to 1%) 2903
Pentacel 2792
Pletal Tablets (Less than 2%) 2481
Prevnar 3241
Primaxin I.M. 2080
Primaxin I.V. (Less than 0.2%) 2083
Prograf Capsules and Injection 622
▲ Prometrium Capsules (100 mg, 200 mg) (Less than 5%) 3047
Protonix for Delayed-Release Oral Suspension (Greater than or equal to 1%) 3254
Protonix Delayed-Release Tablets (Greater than or equal to 1%) 3254
Protonix I.V. (Greater than or equal to 1%) 3257
▲ Protopic Ointment (2% to 4%) 628
Provigil Tablets (At least 1%) 977
Prozac Weekly Capsules (Infrequent) 1852
Prozac Pulvules and Liquid (Infrequent) 1852
Raptiva for Injection 1218
ReFacto Vials 3269
Remeron Tablets (Rare) 2924
RemeronSolTab Tablets (Rare) 2927
Requip Tablets (Frequent) 1561
RotaTeq (0.2%) 2110
Rythmol Tablets (Less than 1% to 2%) 1586
Salagen Tablets (Less than 1%) 1082
▲ Simulect for Injection (3% to 10%) 2306
Singulair (Greater than or equal to 2%) 2114
Soriatane Capsules (Less than 1%) 3062
Symbyax Capsules (Infrequent) 1871
Synagis Intramuscular Solution (More than 1%) 1948
Targretin Capsules 1084
Tasigna Capsules (0.1% to 1%) 2316
Teveten Tablets (Less than 1%) 515
Teveten HCT Tablets (Less than 1%) 517
Tricor Tablets 520
Trizivir Tablets 1622
Ultram ER Extended-Release Tablets (0.5% to less than 1%) 2428
Vaqta 2130
Velcade for Injection 2168
Venlafaxine Hydrochloride Tablets (Infrequent) 2199
Vicoprofen Tablets (Less than 1%) 533
Vivitrol 988
▲ Xeloda Tablets (Less than 5%) 2662
Xopenex Inhalation Solution 3001
Xopenex Inhalation Solution Concentrate 3005
Xopenex HFA Inhalation Aerosol 3009
Xyrem Oral Solution (Infrequent) 1766
Yaz Tablets (Greater than 1%) 805
Zomig Tablets (Infrequent) 694
Zomig-ZMT Tablets (Infrequent) 694
Zonegran Capsules (Infrequent) 1089
Zyprexa Tablets (Infrequent) 1883
Zyprexa ZYDIS Orally Disintegrating Tablets (Infrequent) 1883

Gastroenteritis, infectious

Singulair (1.5%) 2114

Gastroenteritis, viral

▲ Cialis Tablets (3% to 5%) 1792
Cymbalta Delayed-Release Capsules (2%) 1801
▲ Flovent Diskus 50 mcg (3%) 1435
▲ Lucentis Injection (0% to 4%) 1205
Pulmicort Flexhaler (1.8%) 654
Requip Tablets (Frequent) 1561
▲ Ultram ER Extended-Release Tablets (1% to less than 5%) 2428
▲ Xyrem Oral Solution (6.1%) 1766

Gastroesophageal reflux

Abilify Injection (Greater than or equal to 1 in 1000 patients and less than 1 in 100 patients) 881
Abilify Injection (Greater than or equal to 1 in 1000 patients and less than 1 in 100 patients) 2466
Abilify Oral Solution (Greater than or equal to 1 in 1000 patients and less than 1 in 100 patients) 881
Abilify Oral Solution (Greater than or equal to 1 in 1000 patients and less than 1 in 100 patients) 2466

Abilify Discmelt Orally Disintegrating Tablets (Greater than or equal to 1 in 1000 patients and less than 1 in 100 patients) ... 881
Abilify Discmelt Orally Disintegrating Tablets (Greater than or equal to 1 in 1000 patients and less than 1 in 100 patients) ... 2466
Abilify Tablets (Greater than or equal to 1 in 1000 patients and less than 1 in 100 patients) ... 881
Abilify Tablets (Greater than or equal to 1 in 1000 patients and less than 1 in 100 patients) ... 2466
Ambien CR Tablets (1%) ... 2696
Amerge Tablets (Rare) ... 1301
Amitiza Capsules (Less than 1%) ... 3082
Aptivus Capsules (Less than 2%) ... 823
Aptivus Oral Solution (Less than 2%) ... 823
Axert Tablets (Rare) ... 2431
▲ Byetta Injection (Greater than or equal to 1% to less than 5%) ... 600
▲ Celebrex Capsules (0.1% to 4.7%) ... 2979
Celexa (Rare) ... 1160
Chantix Tablets (1%) ... 2511
▲ Cialis Tablets (1% to 3%) ... 1792
▲ Dacogen Injection (5%) ... 1066
Emend Capsules (Greater than 0.5%) ... 1992
Emend for Injection (Greater than 0.5%) ... 1999
▲ Evoxac Capsules (1% to 3%) ... 1013
Exelon Capsules (Infrequent) ... 2229
Exelon Oral Solution (Infrequent) ... 2229
Exelon Patch (Infrequent) ... 2233
Fentora Tablets (Greater than 1%) ... 968
▲ Flolan for Injection (61%) ... 1426
Fosamax (0.7% to 2.8%) ... 2005
Fosamax Plus D Tablets (0.7% to 2.8%) ... 2013
Frova Tablets (Rare) ... 1111
Gleevec Tablets (Less common) ... 2255
Imitrex Injection (Infrequent) ... 1465
Imitrex Nasal Spray (Infrequent) ... 1470
Imitrex Tablets (Infrequent) ... 1474
Intelence Tablets (Less than 2%) ... 3119
▲ Ixempra Kit for Injection (6%) ... 915
Levitra Tablets (Less than 2%) ... 2876
Lexapro Oral Suspension (Frequent) ... 1174
Lexapro Tablets (Frequent) ... 1174
Micardis Tablets (More than 0.3%) ... 852
Micardis HCT Tablets ... 854
Mirapex Tablets ... 857
Mobic Oral Suspension (Less than 2%) ... 863
Mobic Tablets (Less than 2%) ... 863
▲ Myfortic Tablets (3% to less than 20%) ... 2276
Namenda ... 1180
NeoProfen Injection ... 2496
Prograf Capsules and Injection ... 622
ReoPro Vials (0.1%) ... 1860
Requip Tablets (Infrequent to frequent) ... 1561
Risperdal Consta Long-Acting Injection (Infrequent) ... 1753
Rythmol SR Capsules ... 1590
▲ Spiriva HandiHaler (1% to 3%) ... 870
▲ Sutent Capsules (11%) ... 2540
Tasigna Capsules (0.1% to 1%) ... 2316
Tekturna Tablets ... 2321
Tekturna HCT Tablets ... 2324
Treximet Tablets (Infrequent) ... 1616
Velcade for Injection ... 2168
Vivitrol ... 988
Xyrem Oral Solution (Infrequent) ... 1766

Gastrointestinal anomaly, unspecified
Vyvanse Capsules ... 3033

Gastrointestinal bleeding
(*see under* Bleeding, gastrointestinal)

Gastrointestinal disorders, unspecified
Accutane Capsules ... 2607
Actonel with Calcium Tablets (1.9% to 2.5%) ... 2574
Adderall XR Capsules ... 3012
▲ Adenoscan (13%) ... 605
Adipex-P ... 1185
▲ Advair HFA 45/21 Inhalation Aerosol (1% to 3%) ... 1288
▲ Advair HFA 115/21 Inhalation Aerosol (1% to 3%) ... 1288
▲ Advair HFA 230/21 Inhalation Aerosol (1% to 3%) ... 1288
▲ Aerobid/Aerobid-M (1% to 10%) ... 1153
▲ Alphagan P Ophthalmic Solution (1% to 4%) ... 549
▲ Amerge Tablets (6% to 7%) ... 1301
Anaprox Tablets ... 2632
Anaprox DS Tablets ... 2632
Argatroban Injection (0.9%) ... 1308
▲ Arimidex Tablets (4% to 34%) ... 672
Avelox (Less than 0.1%) ... 2803
Axid Capsules (1.1%) ... 1364
▲ Boostrix (3% to 26%) ... 1377
▲ Cancidas for Injection (39.5% to 57.8%) ... 1953
Captopril Tablets ... 2182
▲ Celebrex Capsules (24% to 26%) ... 2979
▲ CellCept Capsules (3% to less than 20%) ... 2622
▲ CellCept Intravenous (3% to less than 20%) ... 2622
▲ CellCept Oral Suspension (3% to less than 20%) ... 2622
▲ CellCept Tablets (3% to less than 20%) ... 2622
▲ Chemet Capsules (About 10%) ... 2484
▲ Cipro (15%) ... 2810
▲ Clinoril Tablets (3% to 9%) ... 1962
Combigan Ophthalmic Solution (0.1% to 0.2%) ... 553
Comtan Tablets (1%) ... 2208
▲ Copaxone for Injection (5%) ... 3110
Cosopt Sterile Ophthalmic Solution ... 1969
Creon 5 Capsules (Among most frequent) ... 3041
Depakote ER Tablets ... 423
Dexedrine ... 1401
Didronel Tablets ... 2583
Dyazide Capsules ... 1405
EC-Naprosyn Delayed-Release Tablets ... 2632
▲ Erbitux (10% to 23%) ... 912
▲ Evista Tablets (3.3%) ... 1810
Exjade Tablets (0.1% to 1%) ... 2244
▲ Femara Tablets (1.7% to 28.3%) ... 2246
▲ Flector Patch (3%) ... 561
▲ Flovent Diskus 50 mcg (4%) ... 1435
▲ Flovent HFA (1% to 3%) ... 1440
▲ Focalin XR Capsules (28% to 44%) ... 2251
Follistim AQ Cartridge ... 2844
Fortaz (Among most common) ... 1450
Forteo for Injection (2.3%) ... 1816
Furosemide Tablets ... 2186
▲ Gengraf Capsules (4% to 19.8%) ... 435
▲ Humira Injection (Less than 5%) ... 442
▲ Hyalgan Solution (29%) ... 2742
▲ Hycamtin for Injection (63%) ... 1459
Ionsys Transdermal System (.1% to less than 1%) ... 2410
Kaletra (Less than 2%) ... 452
Ketek Tablets (Greater than or equal to 0.2% to less than 2%) ... 2744
Klonopin (Infrequent) ... 2639
K-Phos Neutral Tablets ... 813
Lamisil Oral Granules ... 2264
Leukeran Tablets (Infrequent) ... 1508
▲ Leukine (37%) ... 774
Lialda Tablets ... 3029
Lovaza Capsules ... 1520
Lupron Depot 3.75 mg (2%) ... 462
▲ Lupron Depot 7.5 mg (14.3%) ... 469
Lupron Depot–3 Month 11.25 mg (2%) ... 462
Lybrel Tablets ... 3204
Meribin Capsules ... 2163
Merrem I.V. (Greater than 1%) ... 684
Micardis Tablets (More than 0.3%) ... 852
Micardis HCT Tablets ... 854
Mircette Tablets ... 1034
▲ Mycamine for Injection (32.3% to 99.1%) ... 616
Naprosyn Suspension ... 2632
Naprosyn Tablets ... 2632
▲ Neoral Oral Solution (4% to 19.8%) ... 2280
▲ Neoral Soft Gelatin Capsules (4% to 19.8%) ... 2280
Nexium Delayed-Release Capsules (Less than 1%) ... 645
Nexium I.V. (Less than 1%) ... 652
Nexium Delayed-Release Oral Suspension (Less than 1%) ... 645
Nimotop Capsules (Up to 2.4%) ... 790
Norvir (Less than 2%) ... 489
▲ Novantrone for Injection Concentrate (14% to 88%) ... 1100
NuvaRing ... 2897
Omnicef Capsules ... 497
Omnicef for Oral Suspension ... 497
Ortho-Cyclen/Ortho Tri-Cyclen ... 2449
Ortho Tri-Cyclen Lo Tablets ... 2458
OxyContin Tablets (Less than 1%) ... 2589
Percocet Tablets ... 1127
▲ Plavix Tablets (About 27.1%) ... 926
▲ Plavix Tablets (About 27.1%) ... 2767
▲ PrandiMet Tablets (Greater than 5% to 33%) ... 2967
Precose Tablets (Among most common) ... 792
Prinzide Tablets (0.3% to 1%) ... 2092
Proglycem Capsules (Frequent) ... 1185
Proglycem Suspension (Frequent) ... 1185
Proleukin for Injection (Less than 1%) ... 2287
Protonix for Delayed-Release Oral Suspension (Greater than or equal to 1%) ... 3254
Protonix Delayed-Release Tablets (Greater than or equal to 1%) ... 3254
Protonix I.V. (Greater than or equal to 1%) ... 3257
Protopic Ointment (0.2% to less than 1%) ... 628
Provigil Tablets (At least 1%) ... 977
Requip Tablets (Infrequent) ... 1561
▲ Retrovir Capsules (20%) ... 1574
▲ Retrovir IV Infusion (20%) ... 1579
▲ Retrovir (20%) ... 1574
St. Joseph 81 mg Aspirin Chewable and Enteric Coated Tablets ... 1903
Salagen Tablets (Less than 1%) ... 1082
Seasonique Tablets ... 1046
▲ Simulect for Injection (3% to 10%) ... 2306
Skelaxin Tablets (Most frequent) ... 1784
▲ Somatuline Depot Injection (Greater than 5% to 73%) ... 3102
▲ Spiriva HandiHaler (1% to 3%) ... 870
Stalevo Tablets (1%) ... 2309
▲ Suprax for Oral Suspension (30%) ... 1891
▲ Suprax Tablets (30%) ... 1891
Tekturna HCT Tablets ... 2324
Tessalon Capsules ... 1183
Tessalon Perles ... 1183
Timoptic-XE Sterile Ophthalmic Gel Forming Solution ... 2125
Toprol-XL Tablets ... 666
▲ Travatan Z Ophthalmic Solution (1% to 5%) ... 547
Tricor Tablets ... 520
▲ Ultrase Capsules (Most frequent) ... 718
Uroqid-Acid No. 2 Tablets ... 814
▲ Urso 250 Tablets (5%) ... 720
▲ Urso Forte Tablets (5%) ... 720
▲ Vesanoid Capsules (26%) ... 2660
Viokase ... 721
▲ Vivitrol (12% to 13%) ... 988
▲ Xenical Capsules (Among most frequent) ... 2672
Yaz Tablets ... 805
Zinacef for Injection (1 in 150 patients) ... 1678
Zinacef Injection (1 in 150 patients) ... 1678
Zocor Tablets ... 2136
Zomig Tablets (Infrequent) ... 694
Zomig Nasal Spray (Infrequent) ... 689
Zomig-ZMT Tablets (Infrequent) ... 694
Zosyn for Injection ... 3284

Gastrointestinal fistula
Avastin IV ... 1192

Gastrointestinal infarction
Zomig Tablets (Very rare) ... 694
Zomig Nasal Spray (Very rare) ... 689
Zomig-ZMT Tablets (Very rare) ... 694

Gastrointestinal inflammation
Flector Patch ... 561
Mobic Oral Suspension ... 863
Mobic Tablets ... 863
Treximet Tablets ... 1616
Vicoprofen Tablets ... 533
Voltaren Tablets ... 2334

Gastrointestinal motility, decreased
Enablex Extended-Release Tablets ... 2225

Gastrointestinal neoplasm, benign
Mirapex Tablets ... 857

Gastrointestinal obstruction
Invega Extended-Release Tablets ... 1748
Sandostatin Injection (Rare) ... 2300

Gastrointestinal reactions
(*see under* Gastrointestinal disorders, unspecified)

Gastrointestinal reflux
Nexavar Tablets (0.1% to less than 1%) ... 784

Gastrointestinal symptoms
(*see under* Gastrointestinal disorders, unspecified)

Gastrointestinal toxicity
Anaprox Tablets ... 2632
Anaprox DS Tablets ... 2632
Busulfex Injection (Frequent) ... 2477
EC-Naprosyn Delayed-Release Tablets ... 2632
Naprosyn Suspension ... 2632
Naprosyn Tablets ... 2632

Gastrointestinal upset
(*see under* Gastrointestinal disorders, unspecified)

Genital abnormalities
Vesanoid Capsules ... 2660

Genital moniliasis
▲ Activella Tablets (0% to 6%) ... 2347
Augmentin XR Extended Release Tablets (2.1%) ... 1333
Levaquin (0.1% to 0.9%) ... 2416
Levaquin in 5% Dextrose Injection (0.1% to 0.9%) ... 2416

Genitalia, male, external, abnormalities of
Propecia Tablets ... 2095
Proscar Tablets ... 2102

Genitourinary disturbances
▲ Hycamtin for Injection (36%) ... 1459
▲ Leukine (50%) ... 774
▲ Paxil (3%) ... 1535
▲ Paxil CR Controlled-Release Tablets (3%) ... 1544

Germinal aplasia
Mustargen for Injection ... 2492

GGTP, elevation
(*see under* Gamma-glutamyl transpeptidase, elevation)

Giddiness
(*see under* Dizziness)

Gingival disorder, unspecified
Cubicin for Injection (Less than 1%) ... 995
Xenical Capsules (2%) ... 2672
Xifaxan Tablets (Less than 2%) ... 2682

Gingival hyperplasia
Cardizem LA Extended Release Tablets (Infrequent) ... 421
▲ CellCept Capsules (3% to less than 20%) ... 2622
▲ CellCept Intravenous (3% to less than 20%) ... 2622
▲ CellCept Oral Suspension (3% to less than 20%) ... 2622
▲ CellCept Tablets (3% to less than 20%) ... 2622
Evoxac Capsules ... 1013
Exforge Tablets (Greater than 0.1% to less than 1%) ... 2238
Gabitril Tablets (Infrequent) ... 973
▲ Gengraf Capsules (4% to 16%) ... 435
▲ Intron A for Injection (Less than 5%) ... 2859
Lamictal (Rare) ... 1488
▲ Myfortic Tablets (3% to less than 20%) ... 2276
▲ Neoral Oral Solution (3.8% to 16%) ... 2280
▲ Neoral Soft Gelatin Capsules (3.8% to 16%) ... 2280
Phenytek Capsules ... 2192
▲ Sandimmune (4% to 16%) ... 2296
▲ Simulect for Injection (3% to 10%) ... 2306
Soriatane Capsules (Less than 1%) ... 3062
Sular Extended Release Tablets (Less than or equal to 1%) ... 2975
Tarka Tablets ... 511
Zonegran Capsules (Infrequent) ... 1089

Gingival infection
Mirapex Tablets ... 857

Gingival pain
Fentora Tablets (Greater than 1%) ... 968

Gingivitis
Accutane Capsules ... 2607
Actiq (1% or greater) ... 959
Aricept Tablets (Infrequent) ... 1062
Aricept ODT Tablets (Infrequent) ... 1062
Azilect Tablets (2%) ... 3106
Celexa (Infrequent) ... 1160
▲ CellCept Capsules (3% to less than 20%) ... 2622

▲ CellCept Intravenous (3% to less than 20%) 2622
▲ CellCept Oral Suspension (3% to less than 20%) 2622
▲ CellCept Tablets (3% to less than 20%) 2622
Chantix Tablets (Frequent) 2511
Copaxone for Injection (At least 2%) 3110
▲ Doxil Injection (1% to 10%) 2378
Effexor XR Extended-Release Capsules (Infrequent) 3195
▲ Eloxatin for Injection (2% to less than 5%) 2731
Evoxac Capsules (Less than 1%) 1013
Exelon Capsules (Infrequent) 2229
Exelon Oral Solution (Infrequent) 2229
Gabitril Tablets (Frequent) 973
Gengraf Capsules 435
▲ Intron A for Injection (Up to 14%) 2859
Keppra Oral Solution (1% or more) 3131
Keppra Tablets (1% or more) 3131
Klonopin 2639
Lamictal (Infrequent) 1488
Lupron Depot-PED 7.5 mg, 11.25 mg and 15 mg (Less than 2%) 471
Luvox CR Extended-Release Capsules (2%) 1759
Mirapex Tablets 857
Neoral Oral Solution 2280
Neoral Soft Gelatin Capsules 2280
Norvir (Less than 2%) 489
Paxil (Rare) 1535
Paxil CR Controlled-Release Tablets (Rare) 1544
Protonix for Delayed-Release Oral Suspension (Less than 1%) 3254
Protonix Delayed-Release Tablets (Less than 1%) 3254
Protonix I.V. (Less than 1%) 3257
Provigil Tablets (1%) 977
Requip Tablets (1% or more) 1561
Risperdal Consta Long-Acting Injection (Infrequent) 1753
Salagen Tablets (Less than 1%) 1082
▲ Soriatane Capsules (1% to 10%) 3062
Symbyax Capsules (Infrequent) 1871
Targretin Capsules 1084
Teveten Tablets (Less than 1%) 515
Teveten HCT Tablets (Less than 1%) 517
Venlafaxine Hydrochloride Tablets (Infrequent) 2199
Wellbutrin SR Sustained-Release Tablets (Infrequent) 1653
Wellbutrin XL Extended-Release Tablets (Infrequent) 1659
Zomig Tablets (Rare) 694
Zomig Nasal Spray (Rare) 689
Zomig-ZMT Tablets (Rare) 694
Zonegran Capsules (Infrequent) 1089
Zyban Sustained-Release Tablets (Infrequent) 1692
Zyprexa Tablets (Infrequent) 1883
Zyprexa ZYDIS Orally Disintegrating Tablets (Infrequent) 1883

Gingivostomatitis
Cuprimine Capsules 1986

Glassy-eyed appearance
Klonopin 2639

Glaucoma
(*see also under* IOP, elevation of)
▲ Advair Diskus 100/50 (Greater than or equal to 3%) 1276
Advair Diskus 250/50 1276
Advair Diskus 500/50 1276
Advair HFA 45/21 Inhalation Aerosol 1288
Advair HFA 115/21 Inhalation Aerosol 1288
Advair HFA 230/21 Inhalation Aerosol 1288
Ambien Tablets (Rare) 2692
Ambien CR Tablets (Rare) 2696
Aricept Tablets (Infrequent) 1062
Aricept ODT Tablets (Infrequent) 1062
Azmacort Inhalation Aerosol 407
Beconase AQ Nasal Spray (Rare) 1369
Brovana Inhalation Solution (Less than 2%) 2990
Celebrex Capsules (0.1% to 1.9%) 2979
Celexa 1160
Cymbalta Delayed-Release Capsules 1801
Effexor XR Extended-Release Capsules (Rare) 3195
Evoxac Capsules (Less than 1%) 1013
Exelon Capsules (Infrequent) 2229
Exelon Oral Solution (Infrequent) 2229
Exelon Patch (Infrequent) 2233
Flonase Nasal Spray 1431
FML Forte Ophthalmic Suspension .... ⊙222
Levitra Tablets (Less than 2%) 2876
Lipitor Tablets (Less than 2%) 2501
▲ Lucentis Injection (8% to 25%) 1205
Namenda (Infrequent) 1180
Omnaris Nasal Spray (Rare) 2998
Pred-G Ophthalmic Ointment .... ⊙229
Pred-G Ophthalmic Suspension .... ⊙228
Protonix for Delayed-Release Oral Suspension (Less than 1%) 3254
Protonix Delayed-Release Tablets (Less than 1%) 3254
Protonix I.V. (Less than 1%) 3257
Prozac Weekly Capsules (Rare) 1852
Prozac Pulvules and Liquid (Rare) 1852
Pulmicort Flexhaler 654
Qvar Inhalation Aerosol (Rare) 3116
Remeron Tablets (Infrequent) 2924
RemeronSolTab Tablets (Infrequent) 2927
Requip Tablets (Infrequent) 1561
Rilutek Tablets (Rare) 2771
Salagen Tablets (Less than 1%) 1082
Sandostatin LAR Depot 2302
Spiriva HandiHaler 870
Sular Extended Release Tablets (Less than or equal to 1%) 2975
Triesence Injectable Suspension (2%) .... ⊙209
Venlafaxine Hydrochloride Tablets (Rare) 2199
Veramyst Nasal Spray 1643
Viroptic Ophthalmic Solution .... ⊙253
Wellbutrin Tablets 1648
Wellbutrin SR Sustained-Release Tablets 1653
Zonegran Capsules (Infrequent) 1089
Zyban Sustained-Release Tablets 1692
Zyprexa Tablets (Rare) 1883
Zyprexa ZYDIS Orally Disintegrating Tablets (Rare) 1883
Zyrtec Chewable Tablets (Less than 2%) 1920
Zyrtec Syrup (Less than 2%) 1920
Zyrtec Tablets (Less than 2%) 1920
Zyrtec-D 12 Hour Extended Release Tablets (Less than 2%) 1923

Glaucoma, angle closure precipitation
Atrovent Nasal Spray 0.06% 836
BOTOX Purified Neurotoxin Complex (One report) 550
Transderm Scōp Transdermal Therapeutic System (Infrequent) 2206
Venlafaxine Hydrochloride Tablets 2199

Glaucoma, corticosteroid-induced
FML Ophthalmic Ointment .... ⊙223
FML Ophthalmic Suspension .... ⊙224
FML Forte Ophthalmic Suspension .... ⊙222
Pred Forte Ophthalmic Suspension .... ⊙227
Pred Mild Ophthalmic Suspension .... ⊙230
Pred-G Ophthalmic Suspension .... ⊙228

Glaucoma, narrow-angle
Atrovent HFA Inhalation Aerosol 839
Atrovent Nasal Spray 0.03% 834
Combivent Inhalation Aerosol 845

Glaucoma, worsening of narrow angle
Atrovent HFA Inhalation Aerosol 839
Atrovent Nasal Spray 0.03% 834
Atrovent Nasal Spray 0.06% 836
Combivent Inhalation Aerosol 845

Globus hystericus
Imitrex Injection (Rare) 1465

Glomerular filtration rate, decrease
Captopril Tablets 2182
Rapamune 3260

Glomerulitis
Lyrica Capsules (Rare) 2527

Glomerulonephritis
Accutane Capsules 2607
Anaprox Tablets (Less than 1%) 2632
Anaprox DS Tablets (Less than 1%) 2632
Cuprimine Capsules (Rare) 1986
EC-Naprosyn Delayed-Release Tablets (Less than 1%) 2632
Naprosyn Suspension (Less than 1%) 2632
Naprosyn Tablets (Less than 1%) 2632
Orthoclone OKT3 Sterile Solution 2387
Proleukin for Injection 2287
Velcade for Injection 2168
Xyzal Oral Solution 2789
Xyzal Oral Solution 3155
Zyrtec Chewable Tablets 1920
Zyrtec Syrup 1920
Zyrtec Tablets 1920
Zyrtec-D 12 Hour Extended Release Tablets (Rare) 1923

Glomerulonephropathy, membranous
Enbrel for Injection (Infrequent) 569

Glomerulopathy
Cuprimine Capsules 1986
Herceptin I.V. 1199
Plavix Tablets 926
Plavix Tablets 2767

Glossitis
Actiq (1% or greater) 959
Actonel Tablets (1%) 2568
Actonel with Calcium Tablets (0.1% to 1%) 2574
▲ Aerobid/Aerobid-M (1% to 3%) 1153
Anaprox Tablets (Less than 1%) 2632
Anaprox DS Tablets (Less than 1%) 2632
Augmentin 1323
Augmentin Tablets 1327
Augmentin XR Extended Release Tablets 1333
Augmentin ES-600 Powder for Oral Suspension 1329
Avelox (Greater than or equal to 0.1% to less than 2%) 2803
Biaxin/Biaxin XL 411
Captopril Tablets 2182
Carbatrol Capsules 3019
Celexa (Rare) 1160
Clinoril Tablets (Less than 1%) 1962
Cuprimine Capsules 1986
Daraprim Tablets 1400
Depakote ER Tablets (Greater than 1%) 423
Didronel Tablets 2583
▲ Doxil Injection (1% to 5%) 2378
EC-Naprosyn Delayed-Release Tablets (Less than 1%) 2632
Effexor XR Extended-Release Capsules (Infrequent) 3195
Emsam Transdermal System (Infrequent) 905
Equetro Extended-Release Capsules 3174
Evoxac Capsules (Less than 1%) 1013
Exelon Capsules (Infrequent) 2229
Exelon Oral Solution (Infrequent) 2229
Fansidar Tablets 2636
Gabitril Tablets (Infrequent) 973
Gantrisin Pediatric Suspension 2638
Gengraf Capsules (1% to less than 3%) 435
Ketek Tablets (Greater than or equal to 0.2% to less than 2%) 2744
Lamictal (Rare) 1488
Levaquin (0.1% to 1%) 2416
Levaquin in 5% Dextrose Injection (0.1% to 1%) 2416
Lipitor Tablets (Less than 2%) 2501
Lupron Depot 3.75 mg 462
Lupron Depot–3 Month 11.25 mg 462
Luvox CR Extended-Release Capsules (Infrequent) 1759
Maxair Autohaler 1705
Merrem I.V. (1.0%) 684
Naprosyn Suspension (Less than 1%) 2632
Naprosyn Tablets (Less than 1%) 2632
Neoral Oral Solution (1% to less than 3%) 2280
Neoral Soft Gelatin Capsules (1% to less than 3%) 2280
Paxil (Infrequent) 1535
Paxil CR Controlled-Release Tablets (Infrequent) 1544
Primaxin I.M. 2080
Primaxin I.V. (Less than 0.2%) 2083
ProAir HFA Inhalation Aerosol (Less than 3%) 3113
Protonix for Delayed-Release Oral Suspension (Less than 1%) 3254
Protonix Delayed-Release Tablets (Less than 1%) 3254
Protonix I.V. (Less than 1%) 3257
Prozac Weekly Capsules (Infrequent) 1852
Prozac Pulvules and Liquid (Infrequent) 1852
Pylera Capsules 714
Remeron Tablets (Infrequent) 2924
RemeronSolTab Tablets (Infrequent) 2927
Requip Tablets (Infrequent) 1561
Rilutek Tablets (Infrequent) 2771
Rocephin Injectable Vials, ADD-Vantage, Galaxy, Bulk 2642
Rythmol SR Capsules 1590
Salagen Tablets (1% to 2%) 1082
Solodyn Extended Release Tablets 1938
Soriatane Capsules (Less than 1%) 3062
▲ Spiriva HandiHaler (1% to 3%) 870
Sular Extended Release Tablets (Less than or equal to 1%) 2975
Venlafaxine Hydrochloride Tablets (Infrequent) 2199
Vicoprofen Tablets (Less than 1%) 533
Voltaren Tablets (Occasionally) 2334
Voltaren-XR Tablets (Occasionally) 2337
Wellbutrin Tablets (Rare) 1648
Wellbutrin SR Sustained-Release Tablets (Infrequent) 1653
Wellbutrin XL Extended-Release Tablets (Infrequent) 1659
Zonegran Capsules (Infrequent) 1089
Zyban Sustained-Release Tablets (Infrequent) 1692
Zyprexa Tablets (Infrequent) 1883
Zyprexa ZYDIS Orally Disintegrating Tablets (Infrequent) 1883

Glossodynia
Adenoscan (Less than 1%) 605
▲ Dacogen Injection (5%) 1066
Fentora Tablets (Greater than 1%) 968
▲ Imitrex Injection (4.9%) 1465
Imitrex Tablets 1474
▲ Nexavar Tablets (1% to less than 10%) 784
Rythmol SR Capsules 1590
▲ Sutent Capsules (0% to 15%) 2540

Glossoncus
Abilify Injection (Greater than or equal to 1 in 1000 patients and less than 1 in 100 patients) 2466
Abilify Oral Solution (Greater than or equal to 1 in 1000 patients and less than 1 in 100 patients) 2466
Abilify Discmelt Orally Disintegrating Tablets (Greater than or equal to 1 in 1000 patients and less than 1 in 100 patients) 2466
Abilify Tablets (Greater than or equal to 1 in 1000 patients and less than 1 in 100 patients) 2466
Avalide Tablets (Rare) 2713
Ceftin Tablets (0.1% to 1%) 1380
Fluarix Vaccine 1446
Geodon (Rare) 2520
Invega Extended-Release Tablets 1748
Janumet Tablets 2041
Januvia Tablets 2048
Lyrica Capsules 2527
Maxalt Tablets 2056
Maxalt-MLT Orally Disintegrating Tablets 2056
Miacalcin Injection (A few cases) 2273
Miacalcin Nasal Spray (Few reports) 2274
Provigil Tablets 977
Romazicon Injection (Less than 1%) 2646
Tamiflu Capsules 2649
Tamiflu Oral Suspension 2649
Treximet Tablets (Rare) 1616
Xifaxan Tablets 2682

Glossotrichia
Amoxil Capsules 1305
Amoxil Chewable Tablets 1305
Amoxil Pediatric Drops for Oral Suspension 1305
Amoxil Powder for Oral Suspension 1305
Amoxil Tablets 1305
Augmentin 1323
Augmentin Tablets 1327
Augmentin XR Extended Release Tablets 1333
Augmentin ES-600 Powder for Oral Suspension 1329
Klonopin (Infrequent) 2639

Glucocorticoids, decreased
Elocon Cream 0.1% (2 in 182 subjects) 2840
▲ Elocon Lotion 0.1% (4 in 65 subjects) 2841
Elocon Ointment 0.1% (1 in 63 patients) 2842

Glucocorticoids, increased
Evoxac Capsules (Less than 1%) 1013

Glucose intolerance
Elspar for Injection 2488
Genotropin Lyophilized Powder 2547
Premarin Intravenous 3217
Premarin Tablets 3221
Torisel Injection 3272

Glucose tolerance, changes
Celexa (Infrequent) 1160
Estratest Tablets 3043
Estratest H.S. Tablets 3043
Furosemide Tablets 2186
Oncaspar Injection 1138
Premarin Intravenous 3217

Glucose tolerance, decreased
Brovana Inhalation Solution (Less than 2%) 2990
Kaletra (Less than 2%) 452
Lyrica Capsules (Rare) 2527
Niaspan Extended-Release Tablets 480
Nutropin for Injection 1208
Nutropin AQ Injection 1212
Nutropin AQ NuSpin Injection 1212
Nutropin AQ Pen 1212
Nutropin AQ Pen Cartridge 1212
Ortho-Cyclen/Ortho Tri-Cyclen 2449
Ortho Tri-Cyclen Lo Tablets 2458
Premarin Intravenous 3217
Premarin Vaginal Cream 3228

Glucose tolerance, impaired
Abilify Injection (Greater than or equal to 1 in 1000 patients and less than 1 in 100 patients) 2466
Abilify Oral Solution (Greater than or equal to 1 in 1000 patients and less than 1 in 100 patients) 881
Abilify Oral Solution (Greater than or equal to 1 in 1000 patients and less than 1 in 100 patients) 2466
Abilify Discmelt Orally Disintegrating Tablets (Greater than or equal to 1 in 1000 patients and less than 1 in 100 patients) 881
Abilify Discmelt Orally Disintegrating Tablets (Greater than or equal to 1 in 1000 patients and less than 1 in 100 patients) 2466
Abilify Tablets (Greater than or equal to 1 in 1000 patients and less than 1 in 100 patients) 881
Abilify Tablets (Greater than or equal to 1 in 1000 patients and less than 1 in 100 patients) 2466
Activella Tablets 2347
AndroGel 3159
Megace ES Oral Suspension 2499
▲ Norditropin Cartridges (6%) 2354
Premarin Tablets 3221
Premphase Tablets 3232
Prempro Tablets 3232

Glucose urine present
Abilify Injection (Greater than or equal to 1 in 1000 patients and less than 1 in 100 patients) 2466
Abilify Oral Solution (Greater than or equal to 1 in 1000 patients and less than 1 in 100 patients) 2466
Abilify Discmelt Orally Disintegrating Tablets (Greater than or equal to 1 in 1000 patients and less than 1 in 100 patients) 2466
Abilify Tablets (Greater than or equal to 1 in 1000 patients and less than 1 in 100 patients) 2466

Glucosuria
Abilify Injection (Greater than or equal to 1 in 1000 patients and less than 1 in 100 patients) 2466
Abilify Oral Solution (Greater than or equal to 1 in 1000 patients and less than 1 in 100 patients) 2466
Abilify Discmelt Orally Disintegrating Tablets (Greater than or equal to 1 in 1000 patients and less than 1 in 100 patients) 2466
Abilify Tablets (Greater than or equal to 1 in 1000 patients and less than 1 in 100 patients) 2466
Clorpres Tablets (Rare) 2185
Diprolene Lotion 0.05% 2838
Diprolene Ointment 0.05% (Some patients) 2839
Diprolene AF Cream 0.05% (Some patients) 2837
Elspar for Injection (Low) 1990
Humatrope Vials and Cartridges (Infrequent) 1838
Lotrisone 2881
Olux Foam 3061
Olux-E Foam 3059
Vanos Cream 1941
Verdeso Foam 3069

Glycosuria
Abilify Injection (Greater than or equal to 1 in 1000 patients and less than 1 in 100 patients) 2466
Abilify Oral Solution (Greater than or equal to 1 in 1000 patients and less than 1 in 100 patients) 881
Abilify Oral Solution (Greater than or equal to 1 in 1000 patients and less than 1 in 100 patients) 2466
Abilify Discmelt Orally Disintegrating Tablets (Greater than or equal to 1 in 1000 patients and less than 1 in 100 patients) 881
Abilify Discmelt Orally Disintegrating Tablets (Greater than or equal to 1 in 1000 patients and less than 1 in 100 patients) 2466
Abilify Tablets (Greater than or equal to 1 in 1000 patients and less than 1 in 100 patients) 881
Abilify Tablets (Greater than or equal to 1 in 1000 patients and less than 1 in 100 patients) 2466
Aloxi Injection (Less than 1%) 1059
Amerge Tablets (Rare) 1301
Atripla Tablets (Less than 1%) 938
Avalide Tablets 892
Avalide Tablets 2713
▲ Baraclude (4%) 900
Brovana Inhalation Solution (Less than 2%) 2990
Carbatrol Capsules 3019
Clorpres Tablets 2185
▲ Coreg Tablets (Greater than 1% to 3%) 1387
▲ Coreg CR Extended-Release Capsules (Greater than 1% to less than or equal to 3%) 1393
Diovan HCT Tablets 2216
Doxil Injection (Less than 1%) 2378
Dyazide Capsules 1405
Effexor XR Extended-Release Capsules (Infrequent) 3195
Elocon Cream 0.1% 2840
Elocon Lotion 0.1% 2841
Elocon Ointment 0.1% 2842
Emtriva Capsules (Less than 1%) 1246
Emtriva Oral Solution (Less than 1%) 1246
Equetro Extended-Release Capsules 3174
Evoxac Capsules 1013
Exjade Tablets 2244
Furosemide Tablets 2186
Geodon Capsules (Infrequent) 2520
▲ Indapamide Tablets (Less than 5%) 2188
Indocin Capsules (Less than 1%) 2024
Indocin I.V. (Less than 1%) 2489
Indocin (Less than 1%) 2024
Intravenous Sodium Diuril 2490
Micardis HCT Tablets 854
Mirapex Tablets 857
Nexium Delayed-Release Capsules (Less than 1%) 645
Nexium I.V. (Less than 1%) 652
Nexium Delayed-Release Oral Suspension (Less than 1%) 645
Noroxin Tablets (Less frequent) 2069
Norvir (Less than 2%) 489
Proglycem Capsules (Frequent) 1185
Proglycem Suspension (Frequent) 1185
Prograf Capsules and Injection 622
Protonix for Delayed-Release Oral Suspension (Less than 1%) 3254
Protonix Delayed-Release Tablets (Less than 1%) 3254
Protonix I.V. (Less than 1%) 3257
Prozac Weekly Capsules (Rare) 1852
Prozac Pulvules and Liquid (Rare) 1852
Requip Tablets (Infrequent) 1561
Risperdal Consta Long-Acting Injection (Infrequent) 1753
Rocephin Injectable Vials, ADD-Vantage, Galaxy, Bulk (Less than 0.1%) 2642
Rythmol SR Capsules 1590
Symbyax Capsules (Infrequent) 1871
Tekturna HCT Tablets 2324
Teveten Tablets (Less than 1%) 515
Teveten HCT Tablets (Less than 1%) 517
Thiothixene Capsules 2197
▲ Truvada Tablets (Less than 1%) 1262
Ultane Liquid for Inhalation (Less than 1%) 524
Venlafaxine Hydrochloride Tablets (Rare) 2199
Vicoprofen Tablets (Less than 1%) 533
Wellbutrin Tablets (Rare) 1648
Wellbutrin SR Sustained-Release Tablets 1653
Wellbutrin XL Extended-Release Tablets 1659
Zyban Sustained-Release Tablets 1692

Glycosylated hemoglobin, increased
Abilify Injection (Greater than or equal to 1 in 100 patients) 881
Abilify Injection (Less than 1 in 1000 patients) 2466
Abilify Oral Solution (Greater than or equal to 1 in 100 patients) 881
Abilify Oral Solution (Less than 1 in 1000 patients) 2466
Abilify Discmelt Orally Disintegrating Tablets (Greater than or equal to 1 in 100 patients) 881
Abilify Discmelt Orally Disintegrating Tablets (Less than 1 in 1000 patients) 2466
Abilify Tablets (Greater than or equal to 1 in 100 patients) 881
Abilify Tablets (Less than 1 in 1000 patients) 2466

Goiter
Aricept Tablets (Infrequent) 1062
Aricept ODT Tablets (Infrequent) 1062
Campral Tablets (Rare) 1158
Celexa (Rare) 1160
Copaxone for Injection (Infrequent) 3110
Effexor XR Extended-Release Capsules (Rare) 3195
Evoxac Capsules (Less than 1%) 1013
Exelon Capsules (Infrequent) 2229
Exelon Oral Solution (Infrequent) 2229
Gabitril Tablets (Infrequent) 973
Gantrisin Pediatric Suspension 2638
Gengraf Capsules (1% to less than 3%) 435
Lamictal (Rare) 1488
Luvox CR Extended-Release Capsules (Rare) 1759
Meridia Capsules 475
Miacalcin Nasal Spray (Less than 1%) 2274
Mirapex Tablets 857
Neoral Oral Solution (1% to less than 3%) 2280
Neoral Soft Gelatin Capsules (1% to less than 3%) 2280
Nexium Delayed-Release Capsules (Less than 1%) 645
Nexium I.V. (Less than 1%) 652
Nexium Delayed-Release Oral Suspension (Less than 1%) 645
Paxil (Rare) 1535
Paxil CR Controlled-Release Tablets (Rare) 1544
Protonix for Delayed-Release Oral Suspension (Less than 1%) 3254
Protonix Delayed-Release Tablets (Less than 1%) 3254
Protonix I.V. (Less than 1%) 3257
Remeron Tablets (Rare) 2924
RemeronSolTab Tablets (Rare) 2927
Requip Tablets (Infrequent) 1561
▲ Sandostatin Injection (6%) 2300
▲ Sandostatin LAR Depot (2% to 8%) 2302
Treximet Tablets (Rare) 1616
Venlafaxine Hydrochloride Tablets (Rare) 2199
Zyprexa Tablets (Infrequent) 1883
Zyprexa ZYDIS Orally Disintegrating Tablets (Infrequent) 1883

Goiter, euthyroid
Zomig Tablets (Rare) 694
Zomig Nasal Spray (Rare) 689
Zomig-ZMT Tablets (Rare) 694

Goiter production
(*see under* Goiter)

Gonadotropin secretion, increase
Supprelin LA Implant 1731

Gonadotropin secretion, inhibition
Delatestryl Injection 1730
Estratest Tablets (Among most common) 3043
Estratest H.S. Tablets (Among most common) 3043

Goodpasture's syndrome
Campath Ampules 761
Cuprimine Capsules (Rare) 1986

Goosebumps
(*see under* Piloerection)

Gout
Aceon Tablets (2 mg, 4 mg, 8 mg) (0.3% to 1%) 3038
Advicor Tablets 402
Ambien Tablets (Rare) 2692
Ambien CR Tablets (Rare) 2696
Aricept Tablets (Infrequent) 1062
Aricept ODT Tablets (Infrequent) 1062
Asacol Delayed-Release Tablets 2579
Avalide Tablets 892
Avalide Tablets 2713
Avapro Tablets (Less than 1%) 897
Avapro Tablets (Less than 1%) 2718
Brovana Inhalation Solution (Less than 2%) 2990
Campral Tablets (Infrequent) 1158
▲ CellCept Capsules (3% to less than 20%) 2622
▲ CellCept Intravenous (3% to less than 20%) 2622
▲ CellCept Oral Suspension (3% to less than 20%) 2622
▲ CellCept Tablets (3% to less than 20%) 2622
Cipro I.V. (1% or less) 2817
Clorpres Tablets 2185
Copaxone for Injection (Infrequent) 3110
▲ Coreg Tablets (Greater than 1% to 3%) 1387
▲ Coreg CR Extended-Release Capsules (Greater than 1% to less than or equal to 3%) 1393
Cozaar Tablets (Less than 1%) 1973
Demadex Injection 2630
Demadex Tablets 2630
Diovan HCT Tablets (Less frequent) 2216
Edecrin 698
Effexor XR Extended-Release Capsules (Rare) 3195
Evoxac Capsules 1013
Exelon Capsules (Infrequent) 2229
Exelon Oral Solution (Infrequent) 2229
Exforge Tablets (Greater than or equal to 0.2%) 2238
Furosemide Tablets 2186
Geodon Capsules (Rare) 2520
Gleevec Tablets (Infrequent) 2255
Invanz for Injection (Greater than 0.1%) 2029
Klonopin (Infrequent) 2639
Lexapro Oral Suspension (Infrequent) 1174
Lexapro Tablets (Infrequent) 1174
Lipitor Tablets (Less than 2%) 2501
Lunesta Tablets (Rare) 2994
Mavik Tablets (0.3% to 1%) 472
Micardis Tablets (More than 0.3%) 852
Micardis HCT Tablets 854
Niaspan Extended-Release Tablets 480
Norvir (Less than 2%) 489
Paxil (Rare) 1535
Paxil CR Controlled-Release Tablets (Rare) 1544
PegIntron Powder for Injection (Less than or equal to 1%) 2903
Plavix Tablets (1% to 2.5%) 926
Plavix Tablets (1% to 2.5%) 2767
Pletal Tablets (Less than 2%) 2481
Prinivil Tablets (0.3% to 1%) 2087
Prinzide Tablets 2092
Proglycem Capsules (Infrequent) 1185
Proglycem Suspension (Infrequent) 1185
Protonix for Delayed-Release Oral Suspension (Less than 1%) 3254
Protonix Delayed-Release Tablets (Less than 1%) 3254
Protonix I.V. (Less than 1%) 3257

Prozac Weekly Capsules (Infrequent) ... 1852
Prozac Pulvules and Liquid (Infrequent) ... 1852
Remeron Tablets (Rare) ... 2924
RemeronSolTab Tablets (Rare) ... 2927
Requip Tablets (Infrequent to greater than or equal to 1%) ... 1561
Rilutek Tablets (Infrequent) ... 2771
Rythmol SR Capsules ... 1590
Sular Extended Release Tablets (Less than or equal to 1%) ... 2975
Symbyax Capsules (Rare) ... 1871
Tarka Tablets (Less frequent) ... 511
Tekturna Tablets (0.2%) ... 2321
Tekturna HCT Tablets (0.2%) ... 2324
Teveten Tablets (Less than 1%) ... 515
Teveten HCT Tablets (Less than 1%) ... 517
Tricor Tablets ... 520
Venlafaxine Hydrochloride Tablets (Rare) ... 2199
Zyprexa Tablets (Rare) ... 1883
Zyprexa ZYDIS Orally Disintegrating Tablets (Rare) ... 1883

Gout, exacerbation of
Cipro (Less than 1%) ... 2810
Cipro XR Tablets ... 2823

Graft dysfunction, primary
Prograf Capsules and Injection ... 622

Graft loss
▲ Rapamune (22%) ... 3260

Graft versus host reaction
▲ Busulfex Injection (18%) ... 2477
▲ Cancidas for Injection (0.9% to 3.6%) ... 1953
▲ Valcyte Tablets (24%) ... 2654

Granulocytopenia
Albenza Tablets (Rare) ... 1297
Anaprox Tablets (Less than 1%) ... 2632
Anaprox DS Tablets (Less than 1%) ... 2632
▲ Busulfex Injection (100%) ... 2477
Celexa (Rare) ... 1160
EC-Naprosyn Delayed-Release Tablets (Less than 1%) ... 2632
Eloxatin for Injection ... 2731
Evoxac Capsules (Less than 1%) ... 1013
Gris-PEG Tablets ... 2507
▲ Humira Injection (Less than 5%) ... 442
▲ Intron A for Injection (Less than 5%) ... 2859
Levaquin (0.1% to 1%) ... 2416
Levaquin in 5% Dextrose Injection (0.1% to 1%) ... 2416
Mustargen for Injection ... 2492
Naprosyn Suspension (Less than 1%) ... 2632
Naprosyn Tablets (Less than 1%) ... 2632
▲ Neulasta Injection (15% to 72%) ... 587
▲ Novantrone for Injection Concentrate (6% to 79%) ... 1100
Omnicef Capsules ... 497
Omnicef for Oral Suspension ... 497
Pentasa Capsules ... 3030
Phenytek Capsules (Occasional) ... 2192
Plavix Tablets (Less than 1%) ... 926
Plavix Tablets (Less than 1%) ... 2767
Pletal Tablets ... 2481
▲ Retrovir Capsules (1.8% to 47%) ... 1574
▲ Retrovir IV Infusion (1.8% to 47%) ... 1579
▲ Retrovir (1.8% to 47%) ... 1574
Risperdal Consta Long-Acting Injection (Rare) ... 1753
Rythmol Tablets (Less than 1%) ... 1586
Viramune Oral Suspension (0.4% to 1.8%) ... 873
Viramune Tablets (0.4% to 1.8%) ... 873
▲ Xeloda Tablets (2% to 86%) ... 2662
Zantac 25 EFFERdose Tablets (A few patients) ... 1670
Zantac Injection (Few patients) ... 1666
Zantac Injection Pharmacy Bulk Package (Infrequent) ... 1668
Zantac Injection Premixed (Few patients) ... 1666
Zantac (A few patients) ... 1670
▲ Zometa for Intravenous Infusion (5% to less than 10%) ... 2341

Granuloma, hepatic
Tice BCG (Less than or equal to 1%) ... 2936

Granuloma, subcutaneous
Fluorescite Injection ... ⊙ 203

Granuloma, unspecified
Actiq (Less than 1%) ... 959
Effexor XR Extended-Release Capsules (Rare) ... 3195
Lyrica Capsules (Rare) ... 2527

Granulomatosis, Wegener's
Accutane Capsules ... 2607

Grave's Disease
Campath Ampules ... 761

Growth, abnormal
Nutropin for Injection ... 1208
Nutropin AQ Injection ... 1212
Nutropin AQ NuSpin Injection ... 1212
Nutropin AQ Pen ... 1212
Nutropin AQ Pen Cartridge ... 1212

Growth, temporary slowing in
Adderall XR Capsules ... 3012
Concerta Extended-Release Tablets ... 1925

Growth rate, decrease
▲ Advair Diskus 100/50 (Greater than or equal to 3% to 13%) ... 1276
Advair Diskus 250/50 ... 1276
Advair Diskus 500/50 ... 1276
Advair HFA 45/21 Inhalation Aerosol ... 1288
Advair HFA 115/21 Inhalation Aerosol ... 1288
Advair HFA 230/21 Inhalation Aerosol ... 1288
Azmacort Inhalation Aerosol ... 407
Flovent HFA ... 1440
Rocaltrol Capsules ... 1150
Rocaltrol Oral Solution ... 1150
▲ Sandostatin Injection (37%) ... 2300
Venlafaxine Hydrochloride Tablets ... 2199

Growth retardation
Cosmegen for Injection ... 2485
Elocon Cream 0.1% ... 2840
Elocon Lotion 0.1% ... 2841
Elocon Ointment 0.1% ... 2842
Lotrisone Cream ... 2881
Phenytek Capsules ... 2192
Veramyst Nasal Spray ... 1643
Verdeso Foam ... 3069

Growth retardation, intrauterine
Captopril Tablets ... 2182
Cozaar Tablets ... 1973
Prinivil Tablets ... 2087
Prinzide Tablets ... 2092

Growth suppression
Azmacort Inhalation Aerosol ... 407
Beconase AQ Nasal Spray ... 1369
Flonase Nasal Spray ... 1431
Flovent Diskus 50 mcg ... 1435
Flovent HFA ... 1440
Focalin XR Capsules ... 2251
Omnaris Nasal Spray ... 2998
Qvar Inhalation Aerosol ... 3116
Vyvanse Capsules ... 3033

Guillain-Barré syndrome
Asacol Delayed-Release Tablets (Rare) ... 2579
Attenuvax (Rare) ... 1951
Boostrix ... 1377
Campath Ampules ... 761
Comvax ... 1966
Cuprimine Capsules ... 1986
Effexor XR Extended-Release Capsules (Rare) ... 3195
Engerix-B Vaccine (Less than 1%) ... 1409
Fluarix Vaccine ... 1446
Flulaval Injection Vaccine ... 1448
FluMist Vaccine ... 1945
Gardasil Injection ... 2019
Havrix Injection Vaccine ... 1454
Infanrix Vaccine ... 1479
Lyrica Capsules (Rare) ... 2527
Meruvax II (Isolated reports) ... 2061
M-M-R II (Rare) ... 2054
Mumpsvax ... 2068
Noroxin Tablets ... 2069
Paxil ... 1535
Paxil CR Controlled-Release Tablets ... 1544
Pediarix Vaccine ... 1552
Liquid PedvaxHIB ... 2073
Pentacel ... 2792
Pneumovax 23 ... 2078
ProQuad ... 2099
Recombivax HB ... 2107
Remicade for IV Injection ... 950
Twinrix Vaccine ... 1628
Vaqta (Very rare) ... 2130
Varivax ... 2133
Venlafaxine Hydrochloride Tablets (Rare) ... 2199
Zolinza Capsules ... 2142

Gum line erosion
Actiq ... 959

Gums, sore
Rythmol SR Capsules ... 1590
Wellbutrin Tablets (Infrequent) ... 1648

Gustatory disturbances
▲ Wellbutrin XL Extended-Release Tablets (3%) ... 1659

Gustatory sensation
▲ Wellbutrin Tablets (3.1%) ... 1648

Gynecological disorders, unspecified
▲ Zofran (7%) ... 1687
▲ Zofran ODT Orally Disintegrating Tablets (7%) ... 1687

Gynecomastia
Abilify Injection (Greater than or equal to 1 in 100 patients) ... 881
Abilify Injection (Less than 1 in 1000 patients) ... 2466
Abilify Oral Solution (Greater than or equal to 1 in 100 patients) ... 881
Abilify Oral Solution (Less than 1 in 1000 patients) ... 2466
Abilify Discmelt Orally Disintegrating Tablets (Greater than or equal to 1 in 100 patients) ... 881
Abilify Discmelt Orally Disintegrating Tablets (Less than 1 in 1000 patients) ... 2466
Abilify Tablets (Greater than or equal to 1 in 100 patients) ... 881
Abilify Tablets (Less than 1 in 1000 patients) ... 2466
Advicor Tablets ... 402
▲ AndroGel (0% to 3%) ... 3159
Atripla Tablets ... 938
Avodart Soft Gelatin Capsules (0.3% to 1.1%) ... 1359
Axid Capsules ... 1364
Azor Tablets (Infrequent) ... 1005
Captopril Tablets ... 2182
Cardizem LA Extended Release Tablets (Less than 2%) ... 421
Catapres Tablets (About 1 in 1,000 patients) ... 841
Catapres-TTS (0.5% or less) ... 842
Celexa (Rare) ... 1160
Cipro I.V. (1% or less) ... 2817
Cipro XR Tablets ... 2823
Clinoril Tablets (Rare) ... 1962
Clorpres Tablets (About 1 in 1,000) ... 2185
Delatestryl Injection ... 1730
Effexor XR Extended-Release Capsules (Rare) ... 3195
Eligard 7.5 mg (Less than 2%) ... 2724
Eligard 22.5 mg (Less than 2%) ... 2724
Eligard 30 mg (Less than 2%) ... 2724
▲ Eligard 45 mg (3.6%) ... 2724
Exforge Tablets (Infrequent) ... 2238
▲ Gengraf Capsules (Less than 1% to 4%) ... 435
Genotropin Lyophilized Powder (Rare) ... 2547
Geodon Capsules (Rare) ... 2520
▲ Humatrope Vials and Cartridges (Rare to 5.4%) ... 1838
Indocin Capsules (Less than 1%) ... 2024
Indocin I.V. (Less than 1%) ... 2489
Indocin (Less than 1%) ... 2024
Intelence Tablets (Less than 2%) ... 3119
▲ Intron A for Injection (Less than 5%) ... 2859
Invega Extended-Release Tablets ... 1748
Kaletra (Less than 2%) ... 452
Lanoxin Injection (Occasional) ... 1498
Lanoxin Injection Pediatric (Occasional) ... 1502
Lanoxin Tablets (Occasional) ... 1505
Lescol Capsules ... 2268
Lescol XL Tablets ... 2268
▲ Lunesta Tablets (0% to 3%) ... 2994
Lupron Depot-PED 7.5 mg, 11.25 mg and 15 mg (Less than 2%) ... 471
▲ Megace ES Oral Suspension (1% to 3%) ... 2499
Mevacor Tablets (0.5% to 1%) ... 2063
Mirapex Tablets ... 857
Moban Tablets (Infrequent) ... 1116
Myleran Tablets (Rare) ... 1530
▲ Neoral Oral Solution (Less than 1% to 4%) ... 2280
▲ Neoral Soft Gelatin Capsules (Less than 1% to 4%) ... 2280
Nexavar Tablets (0.1% to less than 1%) ... 784
Nexium Delayed-Release Capsules ... 645
Nexium I.V. ... 652
Nexium Delayed-Release Oral Suspension ... 645
Norditropin Cartridges ... 2354
Nutropin for Injection (0.1%) ... 1208
Nutropin AQ Injection (0.1%) ... 1212
Nutropin AQ NuSpin Injection (0.1%) ... 1212
Nutropin AQ Pen (0.1%) ... 1212
Nutropin AQ Pen Cartridge (0.1%) ... 1212
Pepcid Tablets (Rare) ... 2075
Prozac Weekly Capsules ... 1852
Prozac Pulvules and Liquid ... 1852
Requip Tablets (Infrequent) ... 1561
Retrovir Capsules ... 1574
Retrovir IV Infusion ... 1579
Retrovir ... 1574
Reyataz Capsules (Less than 3%) ... 3299
Risperdal Consta Long-Acting Injection (Infrequent) ... 1753
▲ Sandimmune (Less than 1% to 4%) ... 2296
Sandostatin Injection (Less than 1%) ... 2300
Sandostatin LAR Depot ... 2302
Sular Extended Release Tablets ... 2975
Supprelin LA Implant ... 1731
Sustiva Capsules ... 930
Sustiva Tablets ... 930
Symbyax Capsules (Rare) ... 1871
Tarka Tablets ... 511
Tasigna Capsules (0.1% to 1%) ... 2316
Testim 1% Gel (1% or less) ... 701
Thioridazine Hydrochloride Tablets ... 2195
Thiothixene Capsules ... 2197
Tricor Tablets ... 520
Trizivir Tablets ... 1622
▲ Vantas (4.1%) ... 1737
Venlafaxine Hydrochloride Tablets (Rare) ... 2199
▲ Viadur Implant (6.9%) ... 802
Wellbutrin Tablets (Infrequent) ... 1648
Wellbutrin SR Sustained-Release Tablets ... 1653
Wellbutrin XL Extended-Release Tablets ... 1659
Zantac 25 EFFERdose Tablets (Occasional) ... 1670
Zantac Injection ... 1666
Zantac Injection Pharmacy Bulk Package (Infrequent) ... 1668
Zantac Injection Premixed ... 1666
Zantac (Occasional) ... 1670
Zonegran Capsules (Rare) ... 1089
Zyban Sustained-Release Tablets ... 1692
Zyprexa Tablets (Infrequent) ... 1883
Zyprexa ZYDIS Orally Disintegrating Tablets (Infrequent) ... 1883

Gynecomastia, aggravated
Vantas (Less than 2%) ... 1737

H

Haematemesis
Mirapex Tablets ... 857

Haematochezia
Mirapex Tablets ... 857

Haemophilus B disease
Liquid PedvaxHIB ... 2073

Haemoptysis
Mirapex Tablets ... 857

Hair, abnormal growth
(*see under* Hirsutism)

Hair, dry brittle
Gengraf Capsules (Rare) ... 435
Neoral Oral Solution (Rare) ... 2280
Neoral Soft Gelatin Capsules (Rare) ... 2280
Sandimmune (Rare) ... 2296

Hair discoloration
AndroGel (Less than 1%) ... 3159
Effexor XR Extended-Release Capsules (Rare) ... 3195
Soriatane Capsules (Less than 1%) ... 3062
▲ Sutent Capsules (0% to 17%) ... 2540
Venlafaxine Hydrochloride Tablets (Rare) ... 2199
Wellbutrin Tablets (Rare) ... 1648

Hair loss
(*see under* Alopecia)

Hair problems, unspecified
Accutane Capsules ... 2607

Advicor Tablets ... 402
Lescol Capsules ... 2268
Lescol XL Tablets ... 2268
Lupron Depot 3.75 mg (Among most frequent) ... 462
▲ Lupron Depot 7.5 mg (Less than 5%) ... 469
▲ Lupron Depot–3 Month 11.25 mg (Less than 5%) ... 462
Mevacor Tablets ... 2063
▲ Vectibix (0% to 9%) ... 597
Vytorin 10/10 Tablets ... 2149
Vytorin 10/10 Tablets ... 2939
Vytorin 10/20 Tablets ... 2149
Vytorin 10/20 Tablets ... 2939
Vytorin 10/40 Tablets ... 2149
Vytorin 10/40 Tablets ... 2939
Vytorin 10/80 Tablets ... 2149
Vytorin 10/80 Tablets ... 2939
Zocor Tablets ... 2136
Zomig Tablets (Rare) ... 694
Zomig Nasal Spray (Rare) ... 689
Zomig-ZMT Tablets (Rare) ... 694

Hair texture, abnormal

▲ Intron A for Injection (Less than 5%) ... 2859
▲ Soriatane Capsules (1% to 10%) ... 3062

Hair thinning

Accutane Capsules ... 2607
▲ Arimidex Tablets (2% to 5%) ... 672
Clorpres Tablets ... 2185
Fansidar Tablets ... 2636
Intron A for Injection ... 2859

Halitosis

Cymbalta Delayed-Release Capsules (Infrequent) ... 1801
Emsam Transdermal System (Rare) ... 905
Exelon Capsules (Infrequent) ... 2229
Exelon Oral Solution (Infrequent) ... 2229
Gabitril Tablets (Infrequent) ... 973
▲ Intron A for Injection (Less than 5%) ... 2859
Lamictal (Infrequent) ... 1488
Lunesta Tablets (Infrequent) ... 2994
Protonix for Delayed-Release Oral Suspension (Less than 1%) ... 3254
Protonix Delayed-Release Tablets (Less than 1%) ... 3254
Protonix I.V. (Less than 1%) ... 3257
Rythmol SR Capsules ... 1590

Hallucinations

Actimmune (Rare) ... 1743
Actiq (1% to 2%) ... 959
Allegra-D 12 Hour Extended-Release Tablets ... 2687
Allegra-D 24 Hour Extended-Release Tablets ... 2690
▲ Ambien Tablets (Infrequent to 7.4%) ... 2692
AmBisome for Injection (Less common) ... 606
Amerge Tablets (Rare) ... 1301
Anaprox Tablets (Less than 1%) ... 2632
Anaprox DS Tablets (Less than 1%) .. 2632
▲ Aricept Tablets (3%) ... 1062
▲ Aricept ODT Tablets (3%) ... 1062
Avelox (Less than 0.1%) ... 2803
▲ Avinza Capsules (Less than 5%) ... 1772
▲ Azilect Tablets (4%) ... 3106
Biaxin/Biaxin XL ... 411
▲ Busulfex Injection (5%) ... 2477
Campral Tablets (Infrequent) ... 1158
Cardizem LA Extended Release Tablets (Less than 2%) ... 421
Catapres Tablets ... 841
Celexa (Infrequent) ... 1160
▲ CellCept Capsules (3% to less than 20%) ... 2622
▲ CellCept Intravenous (3% to less than 20%) ... 2622
▲ CellCept Oral Suspension (3% to less than 20%) ... 2622
▲ CellCept Tablets (3% to less than 20%) ... 2622
Chantix Tablets (Rare) ... 2511
Cipro I.V. (1% or less) ... 2817
Cipro (Less than 1%) ... 2810
Cipro XR Tablets ... 2823
Combigan Ophthalmic Solution ... 553
Comtan Tablets ... 2208
Copaxone for Injection (Infrequent) .. 3110
Cosopt Sterile Ophthalmic Solution ... 1969
Crestor Tablets ... 677
Cubicin for Injection (Less than 1%) ... 995
Cymbalta Delayed-Release Capsules ... 1801
Demser Capsules ... 1989
Depakote ER Tablets (Greater than 1%) ... 423
Didronel Tablets ... 2583
▲ Duragesic Transdermal System (3% to 10%) ... 2405
EC-Naprosyn Delayed-Release Tablets (Less than 1%) ... 2632
Effexor XR Extended-Release Capsules (Infrequent) ... 3195
▲ Eldepryl Capsules (3 of 49 patients) ... 3052
Elspar for Injection ... 1990
Elspar for Injection ... 2488
Enablex Extended-Release Tablets ... 2225
Equetro Extended-Release Capsules ... 3174
Evoxac Capsules (Less than 1%) ... 1013
▲ Exelon Capsules (4%) ... 2229
▲ Exelon Oral Solution (4%) ... 2229
Fansidar Tablets ... 2636
Fentora Tablets (Greater than 1%) ... 968
Flumadine (Less than 0.3%) ... 1167
Gabitril Tablets (Frequent) ... 973
Gantrisin Pediatric Suspension ... 2638
▲ Gliadel Wafer (5%) ... 1076
Imitrex Injection ... 1465
Imitrex Tablets (Rare) ... 1474
InnoPran XL Extended Release Capsules ... 1484
Intron A for Injection ... 2859
Invanz for Injection (Very rare) ... 2029
Keppra Injection ... 3137
Keppra Oral Solution ... 3131
Keppra Tablets ... 3131
Klonopin ... 2639
Lamictal (Infrequent) ... 1488
Lanoxin Injection ... 1498
Lanoxin Injection Pediatric ... 1502
Lanoxin Tablets ... 1505
Leukeran Tablets (Rare) ... 1508
Levaquin (0.1% to 1%) ... 2416
Levaquin in 5% Dextrose Injection (0.1% to 1%) ... 2416
▲ Lunesta Tablets (1% to 3%) ... 2994
Luvox CR Extended-Release Capsules (Infrequent) ... 1759
Lyrica Capsules (0.1% to 1%) ... 2527
Marinol Capsules (Greater than 1%) ... 3163
Marplan Tablets ... 3177
Merrem I.V. (Greater than 0.1% to 1%) ... 684
▲ Mirapex Tablets (9% to 17%) ... 857
MS Contin Tablets (Less frequent) ... 2585
Nadolol Tablets ... 2191
Namenda ... 1180
Naprosyn Suspension (Less than 1%) ... 2632
Naprosyn Tablets (Less than 1%) ... 2632
Nembutal Sodium Solution, USP (Less than 1%) ... 2494
▲ Neupro Transdermal System (2% to 3%) ... 3149
Nexium Delayed-Release Capsules ... 645
Nexium I.V. ... 652
Nexium Delayed-Release Oral Suspension ... 645
Noroxin Tablets ... 2069
Norvir (Less than 2%) ... 489
Opana Tablets (Less than 1%) ... 1117
Opana ER Tablets (Less than 1%) ... 1121
OxyContin Tablets (Less than 1%) ... 2589
Paxil (Infrequent) ... 1535
Paxil CR Controlled-Release Tablets (Infrequent) ... 1544
Pepcid Tablets (Infrequent) ... 2075
Percocet Tablets ... 1127
Percodan Tablets ... 1130
Plavix Tablets ... 926
Plavix Tablets ... 2767
Primaxin I.M. ... 2080
Primaxin I.V. ... 2083
Pristiq Extended-Release Tablets ... 3247
▲ Prograf Capsules and Injection (3% to 15%) ... 622
Protonix for Delayed-Release Oral Suspension (Less than 1%) ... 3254
Protonix Delayed-Release Tablets (Less than 1%) ... 3254
Protonix I.V. (Less than 1%) ... 3257
Provigil Tablets (At least 1%) ... 977
Prozac Weekly Capsules (Infrequent) ... 1852
Prozac Pulvules and Liquid (Infrequent) ... 1852
Relenza Inhalation Powder ... 1556
Remeron Tablets (Infrequent) ... 2924
RemeronSolTab Tablets (Infrequent) ... 2927
▲ Requip Tablets (5% to 10%) ... 1561
Requip XL Tablets (Greater than or equal to 5%) ... 1568
Rilutek Tablets (Infrequent) ... 2771
▲ Risperdal Consta Long-Acting Injection (6%) ... 1753
Sanctura XR Capsules ... 557
Singulair ... 2114
▲ Stalevo Tablets (4%) ... 2309
Strattera Capsules ... 1864
Sustiva Capsules (Less than 2%) ... 930
Sustiva Tablets (Less than 2%) ... 930
Symbyax Capsules ... 1871
Tamiflu Capsules ... 2649
Tamiflu Oral Suspension ... 2649
Timoptic Sterile Ophthalmic Solution (Less frequent) ... 2121
Timoptic in Ocudose (Less frequent) ... 2124
Timoptic-XE Sterile Ophthalmic Gel Forming Solution ... 2125
Toprol-XL Tablets ... 666
Transderm Scōp Transdermal Therapeutic System (Infrequent) ... 2206
Treximet Tablets ... 1616
▲ Valcyte Tablets (Less than 5%) ... 2654
Valium Tablets ... 2658
Venlafaxine Hydrochloride Tablets (Infrequent) ... 2199
▲ Vesanoid Capsules (6%) ... 2660
Voltaren Tablets (Rarely) ... 2334
Voltaren-XR Tablets (Rarely) ... 2337
Vyvanse Capsules (1%) ... 3033
Wellbutrin Tablets (Frequent) ... 1648
Wellbutrin SR Sustained-Release Tablets ... 1653
Wellbutrin XL Extended-Release Tablets ... 1659
Xyzal Oral Solution ... 2789
Xyzal Oral Solution ... 3155
Zantac 25 EFFERdose Tablets (Rare) ... 1670
Zantac Injection ... 1666
Zantac Injection Pharmacy Bulk Package (Rare) ... 1668
Zantac Injection Premixed ... 1666
Zantac (Rare) ... 1670
Zomig Tablets (Rare) ... 694
Zomig Nasal Spray ... 689
Zomig-ZMT Tablets (Rare) ... 694
Zosyn for Injection (1% or less) ... 3284
Zovirax ... 1690
Zyban Sustained-Release Tablets ... 1692
Zyprexa Tablets ... 1883
Zyprexa ZYDIS Orally Disintegrating Tablets ... 1883
Zyrtec Chewable Tablets ... 1920
Zyrtec Syrup ... 1920
Zyrtec Tablets ... 1920
Zyrtec-D 12 Hour Extended Release Tablets ... 1923

Hallucinations, auditory

Ambien Tablets ... 2692
Ambien CR Tablets (Infrequent) ... 2696
Bicillin C-R Injectable Suspension ... 1775
Bicillin L-A Injection ... 1777
Catapres Tablets (Rare) ... 841
Catapres-TTS (0.5% or less) ... 842
Clorpres Tablets ... 2185
Concerta Extended-Release Tablets ... 1925
Keppra Injection ... 3137
Keppra Oral Solution ... 3131
Keppra Tablets ... 3131
Lexapro Oral Suspension (Infrequent) ... 1174
Lexapro Tablets (Infrequent) ... 1174
Mirapex Tablets ... 857
Namenda ... 1180
Orthoclone OKT3 Sterile Solution ... 2387
Provigil Tablets ... 977
Valtrex Caplets ... 1635
Xyrem Oral Solution (Infrequent) ... 1766

Hallucinations, hypnagogic

Xyrem Oral Solution (Infrequent) ... 1766

Hallucinations, mixed

▲ Ambien CR Tablets (4%) ... 2696

Hallucinations, visual

Ambien Tablets ... 2692
Ambien CR Tablets (Infrequent) ... 2696
Bicillin C-R Injectable Suspension ... 1775
Bicillin L-A Injection ... 1777
Carbatrol Capsules ... 3019
Catapres Tablets (Rare) ... 841
Catapres-TTS (0.5% or less) ... 842
Clorpres Tablets ... 2185
Concerta Extended-Release Tablets ... 1925
Lexapro Oral Suspension ... 1174
Lexapro Tablets ... 1174
Mirapex Tablets ... 857
Namenda ... 1180
Orthoclone OKT3 Sterile Solution ... 2387
Tessalon Capsules ... 1183
Tessalon Perles ... 1183
Valtrex Caplets ... 1635

Halos

Atrovent Nasal Spray 0.06% ... 836

Hand-foot syndrome

(*see under* Palmar-plantar erythrodysesthesia syndrome)

Hands, cold

Combigan Ophthalmic Solution ... 553
Venlafaxine Hydrochloride Tablets (Infrequent) ... 2199

Hangover

▲ Advair HFA 45/21 Inhalation Aerosol (0% to 3%) ... 1288
▲ Advair HFA 115/21 Inhalation Aerosol (0% to 3%) ... 1288
▲ Advair HFA 230/21 Inhalation Aerosol (0% to 3%) ... 1288
Effexor XR Extended-Release Capsules (Infrequent) ... 3195
Lyrica Capsules (Rare) ... 2527
Maxalt Tablets (Infrequent) ... 2056
Maxalt-MLT Orally Disintegrating Tablets (Infrequent) ... 2056
Xyrem Oral Solution (Infrequent) ... 1766
Zyprexa Tablets (Infrequent) ... 1883
Zyprexa ZYDIS Orally Disintegrating Tablets (Infrequent) ... 1883

HDL, decrease

AndroGel ... 3159
Bystolic Tablets (Greater than or equal to 1%) ... 1155
Coreg Tablets (Less than or equal to 0.1%) ... 1387
Coreg CR Extended-Release Capsules (Less than or equal to 0.1%) ... 1393
Enjuvia Tablets ... 1029
Premphase Tablets ... 3232
Prempro Tablets ... 3232
Targretin Capsules ... 1084

HDL, increase

AndroGel ... 3159
Enjuvia Tablets ... 1029
Equetro Extended-Release Capsules ... 3174
Premarin Tablets ... 3221
Premphase Tablets ... 3232
Prempro Tablets ... 3232

Head, tight feeling

Adenocard IV Injection (Less than 1%) ... 603
Aricept Tablets (Infrequent) ... 1062
Aricept ODT Tablets (Infrequent) ... 1062
Imitrex Injection (2.2%) ... 1465
Imitrex Tablets (Infrequent) ... 1474
Klonopin (Infrequent) ... 2639
ProAmatine Tablets (Less frequent) ... 3032

Headache

▲ Abelcet Injection (6%) ... 1134
▲ Abilify Injection (12% to 27%) ... 881
▲ Abilify Injection (10% to 27%) ... 2466
▲ Abilify Oral Solution (12% to 27%) ... 881
▲ Abilify Oral Solution (10% to 27%) ... 2466
▲ Abilify Discmelt Orally Disintegrating Tablets (12% to 27%) ... 881
▲ Abilify Discmelt Orally Disintegrating Tablets (10% to 27%) ... 2466
▲ Abilify Tablets (12% to 27%) ... 881
▲ Abilify Tablets (10% to 27%) ... 2466
▲ Accolate Tablets (4.5% to 12.9%) ... 669
Accutane Capsules ... 2607
▲ Aceon Tablets (2 mg, 4 mg, 8 mg) (23.8%) ... 3038
▲ Aciphex Tablets (5.4% to 9.9%) ... 1053
▲ Actimmune (33%) ... 1743
▲ Actiq (3% to 6%) ... 959
▲ Activella Tablets (11% to 22%) ... 2347
▲ Actonel Tablets (9.9% to 18%) ... 2568
▲ Actonel with Calcium Tablets (7.2% to 7.3%) ... 2574
▲ ActoPlus Met Tablets (4.6% to 5.3%) ... 3071
▲ Actos Tablets (9.1%) ... 3077
▲ Aczone Gel 5% (4%) ... 3296
▲ Adderall XR Capsules (26%) ... 3012
Adenocard IV Injection (2%) ... 603
▲ Adenoscan (18%) ... 605
Adipex-P ... 1185
▲ Advair Diskus 100/50 (Greater than or equal to 3%) ... 1276

▲ Advair Diskus 250/50 (3% to 16%) 1276
▲ Advair Diskus 500/50 (Greater than or equal to 3%) 1276
▲ Advair HFA 45/21 Inhalation Aerosol (15% to 21%) 1288
▲ Advair HFA 115/21 Inhalation Aerosol (15% to 21%) 1288
▲ Advair HFA 230/21 Inhalation Aerosol (15% to 21%) 1288
▲ Advate (29.3%) 721
▲ Advicor Tablets (9%) 402
▲ Aerobid/Aerobid-M (25%) 1153
▲ Aggrenox Capsules (39.2%) 819
▲ Agrylin Capsules (43.5%) 3017
▲ Alamast Ophthalmic Solution (10% to 25%) 3181
▲ Albenza Tablets (1.3% to 11%) 1297
▲ Aldara Cream, 5% (4% to 8%) 1699
▲ Alferon N Injection (3% to 31%) 1726
Alinia for Oral Suspension (1.1%) 2677
Alinia Tablets (1.1%) 2677
▲ Allegra Oral Solution (7.2% to 10.6%) 2684
▲ Allegra Tablets (4.8% to 10.3%) 2684
▲ Allegra-D 12 Hour Extended-Release Tablets (13.8%) 2687
▲ Allegra-D 24 Hour Extended-Release Tablets (13.8%) 2690
▲ Aloxi Injection (9%) 1059
▲ Alphagan P Ophthalmic Solution (1% to 4%) 549
Alphanate 1709
Altabax Ointment (1.2% to 2%) 1299
▲ Alvesco Inhalation Aerosol (3% to 11%) 2985
▲ Ambien Tablets (Frequent to 12.5%) 2692
▲ Ambien CR Tablets (14% to 19%) 2696
▲ AmBisome for Injection (9.4% to 19.8%) 606
Amevive (0.2%) 611
▲ Amitiza Capsules (3% to 11%) 3082
▲ Amoxil Capsules (7%) 1305
▲ Amoxil Chewable Tablets (7%) 1305
▲ Amoxil Pediatric Drops for Oral Suspension (7%) 1305
▲ Amoxil Powder for Oral Suspension (7%) 1305
▲ Amoxil Tablets (7%) 1305
Amrix Capsules 966
▲ Anaprox Tablets (3% to 9%) 2632
▲ Anaprox DS Tablets (3% to 9%) 2632
▲ AndroGel (0% to 4%) 3159
▲ Angeliq Tablets (5.3%) 751
▲ Angiomax for Injection (2.6% to 12%) 1933
▲ Anzemet Injection (9.4% to 24.3%) 2701
▲ Anzemet Tablets (7% to 22.9%) 2704
▲ Aptivus Capsules (5.2%) 823
▲ Aptivus Oral Solution (5.2%) 823
Aralast (0.3% to 0.7%) 726
▲ Aranesp for Injection (12% to 15%) 564
▲ Argatroban Injection (5.4%) 1308
▲ Aricept Tablets (4%) 1062
▲ Aricept ODT Tablets (4%) 1062
▲ Arimidex Tablets (9% to 18%) 672
▲ Arixtra Injection (0% to 4.5%) 1313
▲ Arranon Injection (0% to 17%) 1319
▲ Asacol Delayed-Release Tablets (35%) 2579
▲ Asmanex Twisthaler (17% to 22%) 2797
Atacand Tablets (More than 1%) 639
▲ Atripla Tablets (Greater than or equal to 10%) 938
▲ Atrovent HFA Inhalation Aerosol (6% to 7%) 839
▲ Atrovent Nasal Spray 0.03% (9.8%) 834
Attenuvax 1951
Augmentin (Less frequent) 1323
Augmentin Tablets (Less frequent) 1327
▲ Augmentin XR Extended Release Tablets (3.5%) 1333
Avalide Tablets (1% or greater) 892
▲ Avalide Tablets (1% to 5.5%) 2713
▲ Avandamet Tablets (6.5% to 11%) 1336
▲ Avandaryl Tablets (3.1% to 6%) 1344
▲ Avandia Tablets (5.9% to 17.2%) 1351
Avapro Tablets (1% or greater) 897
Avapro Tablets (1% or greater) 2718
▲ Avastin IV (3% to 26%) 1192
Avelox (Greater than or equal to 0.1% to less than 2%) 2803
▲ Avinza Capsules (Greater than 10%) 1772
Axert Tablets (Frequent) 2431
▲ Axid Capsules (16.6%) 1364
▲ Azilect Tablets (11% to 14%) 3106
▲ Azmacort Inhalation Aerosol (7% to 21%) 407
▲ Azopt Ophthalmic Suspension (1% to 5%) 540
▲ Bactroban Cream (1.7% to 3.6%) 1366
▲ Bactroban Nasal (9%) 1367
▲ Baraclude (2% to 4%) 900
Bayer Aspirin 750
Beconase AQ Nasal Spray (Fewer than 5 per 100 patients) 1369
▲ BeneFIX Vials (10.8%) 3191
Benicar HCT Tablets (Greater than 2%) 1010
Bentyl Capsules 703
Bentyl Injection 703
Bentyl Syrup 703
Bentyl Tablets 703
▲ Betaseron for SC Injection (50%) 756
▲ Betimol Ophthalmic Solution (More than 5%) 3181
▲ Bexxar (0% to 16%) 1371
Biaxin/Biaxin XL (2%) 411
Bicillin C-R Injectable Suspension 1775
Bicillin L-A Injection 1777
▲ Boniva Injection (3.3% to 6.5%) 2614
▲ Boniva Tablets (3.3% to 6.5%) 2618
▲ Boostrix (3.7% to 43.1%) 1377
▲ BOTOX Purified Neurotoxin Complex (3% to 11%) 550
Brovana Inhalation Solution 2990
▲ Busulfex Injection (5% to 69%) 2477
▲ Byetta Injection (9%) 600
▲ Bystolic Tablets (7% to 9%) 1155
Calcijex Injection 419
▲ Campath Ampules (14%) 761
Campral Tablets (Frequent) 1158
▲ Canasa Rectal Suppositories (14.4%) 705
▲ Cancidas for Injection (5.2% to 14.5%) 1953
Captopril Tablets (About 0.5% to 2%) 2182
▲ Carac Cream 0.5% (3.1%) 2722
Carafate Suspension (Less than 0.5%) 706
Carafate Tablets (Less than 0.5%) 707
Carbatrol Capsules 3019
▲ Cardene I.V. (14.6%) 1093
▲ Cardizem LA Extended Release Tablets (Up to 4.6%) 421
Catapres Tablets (About 1 in 100 patients) 841
▲ Catapres-TTS (5 of 101 patients) 842
Ceftin Tablets (0.1% to 1%) 1380
▲ Celebrex Capsules (15.8%) 2979
Celexa (At least 2%) 1160
▲ CellCept Capsules (16.1% to 54.3%) 2622
▲ CellCept Intravenous (16.1% to 54.3%) 2622
▲ CellCept Oral Suspension (16.1% to 54.3%) 2622
▲ CellCept Tablets (16.1% to 54.3%) 2622
▲ Cerezyme for Injection (Approximately 6.5%) 1238
▲ Chantix Tablets (0.6% to 19%) 2511
▲ Chemet Capsules (5.2% to 15.7%) 2484
▲ Cialis Tablets (3% to 15%) 1792
Cipro I.V. (Greater than 1%) 2817
Cipro (Less than 1%) 2810
▲ Cipro XR Tablets (1% to 3%) 2823
▲ Clarinex Tablets (14%) 2828
▲ Clarinex Reditabs Tablets (14%) 2828
▲ Clarinex-D 12-Hour Extended-Release Tablets (8%) 2831
▲ Clarinex-D 24-Hour Extended-Release Tablets (6%) 2834
▲ Cleviprex (6.3%) 1936
▲ Climara Transdermal System (5% to 18%) 763
▲ Climara Pro Transdermal System (5.2%) 768
▲ Clinoril Tablets (3% to 9%) 1962
▲ Clolar for Intravenous Infusion (46%) 1239
Clorpres Tablets (About 1 in 100) 2185
▲ Combigan Ophthalmic Solution (1% to 5%) 553
▲ Combivent Inhalation Aerosol (5.6%) 845
▲ Combivir Tablets (35%) 1384
▲ Concerta Extended-Release Tablets (0.3% to 22.2%) 1925
Copaxone for Injection (At least 2%) 3110
▲ Coreg Tablets (5% to 8%) 1387
▲ Coreg CR Extended-Release Capsules (5% to 8%) 1393
▲ Cosopt Sterile Ophthalmic Solution (1% to 5%) 1969
Cozaar Tablets (1% or greater) 1973
▲ Crestor Tablets (3.1% to 8.5%) 677
▲ Crinone 4% Gel (19%) 992
▲ Crinone 8% Gel (13% to 17%) 992
▲ Crixivan Capsules (5.4%) 1979
▲ Cubicin for Injection (5.4% to 6.7%) 995
▲ Cyanokit 5g Antidote (6% to 33%) 1021
▲ Cymbalta Delayed-Release Capsules (13% to 20%) 1801
▲ Dacogen Injection (28%) 1066
Dantrium Capsules (Less frequent) 2580
Dapsone Tablets USP 1746
▲ Daytrana Transdermal Patch (28%) 3022
Delatestryl Injection 1730
▲ Demadex Injection (7.3%) 2630
▲ Demadex Tablets (7.3%) 2630
Demser Capsules (Infrequent) 1989
Denavir Cream 2205
▲ Depakote ER Tablets (31%) 423
▲ DepoCyt Injection (18% to 56%) 1136
▲ DepoDur Injection (Greater than 10%) 1095
Dexedrine 1401
Diclofenac Sodium Ophthalmic Solution ⊙240
Didronel Tablets 2583
Diovan Tablets (More than 1%) 2212
Diovan HCT Tablets 2216
Divigel 3167
Donnatal Extentabs 2507
▲ Doribax Injection (4% to 16%) 2400
▲ Doxil Injection (Approximately 5.3% to 10.5%) 2378
▲ Duetact Tablets (4% to 7.1%) 3085
▲ Duragesic Transdermal System (3% to 10%) 2405
Dyazide Capsules 1405
▲ DynaCirc CR Controlled Release Tablets (10.3% to 18.3%) 1407
Dyrenium Capsules (Rare) 3189
▲ EC-Naprosyn Delayed-Release Tablets (3% to 9%) 2632
Edecrin 698
Edex Injection (2%) 2957
▲ Effexor XR Extended-Release Capsules (2% to 38%) 3195
▲ Eldepryl Capsules (2 of 49 patients) 3052
▲ Elestat Ophthalmic Solution (1% to 3%) 1741
▲ Elidel Cream 1% (7% to 25.4%) 2221
▲ Elitek (26%) 2729
▲ Elmiron Capsules (3%) 2435
▲ Eloxatin for Injection (9% to 17%) 2731
Elspar for Injection 1990
▲ Emend Capsules (5% to 16.4%) 1992
▲ Emend for Injection (3% to 16.4%) 1999
▲ Emsam Transdermal System (18%) 905
▲ Emtriva Capsules (Greater than or equal to 10%) 1246
▲ Emtriva Oral Solution (Greater than or equal to 10%) 1246
▲ Enablex Extended-Release Tablets (6.7%) 2225
▲ Enbrel for Injection (17% to 24%) 569
▲ Engerix-B Vaccine (1% to 10%) 1409
▲ Enjuvia Tablets (15% to 25%) 1029
EpiPen 1024
▲ Epivir (35%) 1412
▲ Epivir-HBV (21%) 1417
▲ Epogen for Injection (0.4% to 19%) 576
▲ Epzicom Tablets (6% to 7%) 1422
▲ Equetro Extended-Release Capsules (22%) 3174
▲ Erbitux (Less than 1% to 33%) 912
Estratest Tablets 3043
Estratest H.S. Tablets 3043
▲ Evoclin Foam, 1% (3%) 3056
▲ Evoxac Capsules (14.4%) 1013
▲ Exelon Capsules (4% to 17%) 2229
▲ Exelon Oral Solution (4% to 17%) 2229
▲ Exelon Patch (3% to 4%) 2233
Exforge Tablets (Greater than or equal to 0.2%) 2238
▲ Exjade Tablets (15.9%) 2244
▲ Fabrazyme for Intravenous Infusion (39%) 1241
Fansidar Tablets 2636
▲ Faslodex Injection (15.4%) 682
▲ Femara Tablets (0.3% to 20%) 2246
▲ Fenoglide Tablets (3.2%) 2960
▲ Fentora Tablets (1% to 15%) 968
▲ Flebogamma 5% (53%) 1715
▲ Flebogamma 5% DIF (Greater than 15%) 1718
Flector Patch (1%) 561
Fleet Phospho-soda 1145
Fleet Phospho-soda EZ-PREP 1147
Fleet Prep Kits 1149
▲ Flolan for Injection (49% to 83%) 1426
▲ Flomax Capsules (19.3% to 21.1%) 848
▲ Flonase Nasal Spray (6.6% to 16.1%) 1431
▲ Flovent Diskus 50 mcg (12%) 1435
▲ Flovent HFA (11%) 1440
▲ Fluarix Vaccine (14.3% to 19.3%) 1446
▲ Flulaval Injection Vaccine (7% to 18%) 1448
Flumadine (1.4%) 1167
▲ FluMist Vaccine (3% to 40%) 1945
Fluorescite Injection ⊙203
▲ Focalin XR Capsules (25% to 39%) 2251
▲ Follistim AQ Cartridge (5%) 2844
Foradil Aerolizer 2849
Fortaz (Less than 1%) 1450
▲ Forteo for Injection (7.5%) 1816
Fosamax (Up to 2.6%) 2005
Fosamax Plus D Tablets (0% to 2.6%) 2013
▲ Fosrenol Chewable Tablets (5% to 21%) 3027
▲ Frova Tablets (4%) 1111
Furosemide Tablets 2186
Gabitril Tablets (1% or more) 973
▲ Gammagard Liquid (6.9% to 36.1%) 730
Gammagard S/D (Occasional) 734
▲ Gamunex (0.8% to 58%) 3094
Gantrisin Pediatric Suspension 2638
Gardasil Injection (0.03%) 2019
Gemzar for Injection (Common) 1820
▲ Gengraf Capsules (2% to 25%) 435
▲ Genotropin Lyophilized Powder (0% to 9.9%) 2547
▲ Geodon (18%) 2520
▲ Gleevec Tablets (27% to 39%) 2255
▲ Gliadel Wafer (15% to 28%) 1076
Gris-PEG Tablets (Occasional) 2507
▲ Havrix Injection Vaccine (Less than 9% to 14%) 1454
▲ Hepsera Tablets (9%) 1253
▲ Herceptin I.V. (22%) 1199
Human Albumin Grifols 25% 1706
▲ Humatrope Vials and Cartridges (6.07% to 9.38%) 1838
▲ Humira Injection (12%) 442
Humulin 50/50, 100 Units 1843
Humulin 70/30 Vial 1844
Humulin N Vial 1846
Humulin R 1849
▲ Hyalgan Solution (18%) 2742
▲ Hycamtin for Injection (0.2% to 21%) 1459
Imitrex Injection (2%) 1465
Imitrex Tablets (Greater than 1%) 1474
▲ Increlex Injection (Greater than or equal to 5%) 3100
▲ Indapamide Tablets (Greater than or equal to 5%) 2188
▲ Indocin (11.7%) 2024
Intelence Tablets (2.7%) 3119
Intravenous Sodium Diuril 2490
▲ Intron A for Injection (4% to 62%) 2859
▲ Invanz for Injection (4.4% to 6.8%) 2029
▲ Invega Extended-Release Tablets (11% to 14%) 1748
▲ Ionsys Transdermal System (9%) 2410
▲ Iquix Ophthalmic Solution (8% to 10%) 3183
▲ Isentress Tablets (2.4% to 9.7%) 2036
▲ Ixempra Kit for Injection (11%) 915
▲ Janumet Tablets (1.1% to 6.9%) 2041
▲ Januvia Tablets (1.1% to 5.9%) 2048
▲ Kaletra (2% to 3%) 452
▲ Keppra Injection (14%) 3137
▲ Keppra Oral Solution (2% to 14%) 3131
▲ Keppra Tablets (2% to 14%) 3131
▲ Ketek Tablets (2% to 5.5%) 2744
▲ Kineret Injection (12%) 585
Klonopin 2639
K-Phos Neutral Tablets 813
▲ Lamictal (29.1%) 1488
▲ Lamisil Oral Granules (7%) 2264
▲ Lamisil Tablets (12.9%) 2266
Lanoxin Injection 1498
Lanoxin Injection Pediatric 1502
Lanoxin Tablets 1505
▲ Lescol Capsules (8.9%) 2268
▲ Lescol XL Tablets (4.7%) 2268
▲ Letairis Tablets (15%) 1258
▲ Leukine (26% to 36%) 774
▲ Leustatin Injection (7% to 22%) 2384
▲ Levaquin (6%) 2416
▲ Levaquin in 5% Dextrose Injection (6%) 2416
▲ Levitra Tablets (15%) 2876
Levothroid Tablets 1170
Levoxyl Tablets 1780
▲ Lexapro Oral Suspension (24%) 1174
▲ Lexapro Tablets (24%) 1174
▲ Lexiscan Injection (26%) 614
▲ Lexiva Oral Suspension (Less than or equal to 1% to 3%) 1510
▲ Lexiva Tablets (Less than or equal to 1% to 3%) 1510
▲ Lialda Tablets (3.4% to 5.6%) 3029
Lidoderm Patch 1114
▲ Lipitor Tablets (2.5% to 16.7%) 2501
▲ Lotemax Ophthalmic Suspension 0.5% (Less than 15%) ⊙241
▲ Lucentis Injection (2% to 15%) 1205
▲ Lumigan Ophthalmic Solution (1% to 5%) 556
▲ Lunesta Tablets (13% to 21%) 2994

▲ Lupron Depot 3.75 mg (33%) 462
▲ Lupron Depot 7.5 mg (Less than 5%) 469
▲ Lupron Depot–3 Month 11.25 mg (33%) 462
Lupron Depot-PED 7.5 mg, 11.25 mg and 15 mg (Less than 2%) 471
▲ Luvox CR Extended-Release Capsules (3% to 35%) 1759
Lybrel Tablets 3204
▲ Lyrica Capsules (5% to 14%) 2527
▲ Malarone Pediatric Tablets (3% to 22%) 1521
▲ Malarone Tablets (3% to 22%) 1521
Marinol Capsules (Less than 1%) 3163
▲ Marplan Tablets (6% to 15%) 3177
Mavik Tablets (More than 1%) 472
Maxair Autohaler (1.3% to 2%) 1705
Maxalt Tablets (Less than 2%) 2056
Maxalt-MLT Orally Disintegrating Tablets (Less than 2%) 2056
▲ Megace ES Oral Suspension (1% to 10%) 2499
▲ Mepron Suspension (16% to 31%) 1526
▲ Meridia Capsules (30.3%) 475
▲ Merrem I.V. (2.3% to 7.8%) 684
Meruvax II 2061
▲ Metadate CD Capsules (12%) 3146
▲ Mevacor Tablets (2.1% to 9.3%) 2063
▲ Miacalcin Nasal Spray (3.2%) 2274
Micardis Tablets (1%) 852
Micardis HCT Tablets (2% or greater) 854
▲ Mirapex Tablets (16%) 857
Mircette Tablets 1034
▲ Mirena Intrauterine System (5% or more) 779
M-M-R II 2054
▲ Mobic Oral Suspension (2.4% to 10.2%) 863
▲ Mobic Tablets (2.4% to 10.2%) 863
MoviPrep Oral Solution (1.8%) 2679
Moxatag Tablets (1%) 2165
MS Contin Tablets (Less frequent) 2585
▲ Mycamine for Injection (2% to 42.1%) 616
▲ Myfortic Tablets (3% to less than 20%) 2276
▲ Mylotarg for Injection (27% to 50%) 3212
▲ Nabi-HB (14%) 815
Nadolol Tablets (1 to 5 of 1000 patients) 2191
▲ Nalfon Capsules (8.7%) 2508
▲ Namenda (6%) 1180
▲ Naprosyn Suspension (3% to 9%) 2632
▲ Naprosyn Tablets (3% to 9%) 2632
Nasacort AQ Nasal Spray (2% or greater) 2765
▲ Nasonex Nasal Spray (17% to 26%) 2883
▲ Natrecor for Injection (7% to 9%) 2977
Nembutal Sodium Solution, USP 2494
▲ Neoral Oral Solution (2% to 25%) 2280
▲ Neoral Soft Gelatin Capsules (2% to 25%) 2280
▲ Neulasta Injection (15% to 72%) 587
▲ Neupogen for Injection (7%) 589
▲ Neupro Transdermal System (5% to 14%) 3149
▲ Nexavar Tablets (10%) 784
▲ Nexium Delayed-Release Capsules (1.9% to 8.1%) 645
▲ Nexium I.V. (3.8% to 5.5%) 652
▲ Nexium Delayed-Release Oral Suspension (1.9% to 8.1%) 645
▲ Niaspan Extended-Release Tablets (5% to 11%) 480
Nimotop Capsules (Up to 4.1%) 790
▲ Nitro-Dur Transdermal Infusion System (63%) 2887
▲ Nitrolingual Pumpspray (50%) 2965
▲ Norditropin Cartridges (Small number of patients -9%) 2354
Noroxin Tablets (2% to 2.8%) 2069
▲ Norvir (6% to 6.5%) 489
▲ Novantrone for Injection Concentrate (6% to 13%) 1100
▲ NovoLog Injection (5% to 12%) 2359
NovoSeven (1%) 2367
NovoSeven RT (1%) 2370
▲ Noxafil Oral Suspension (1% to 28%) 2889
Nutropin for Injection (A small number of patients) 1208
Nutropin AQ Injection (A small number of patients) 1212
Nutropin AQ NuSpin Injection (A small number of patients) 1212
Nutropin AQ Pen (A small number of patients) 1212
Nutropin AQ Pen Cartridge (A small number of patients) 1212
▲ NuvaRing (5% to 14%) 2897
▲ Omnaris Nasal Spray (6% to 6.6%) 2998
Omnicef Capsules (2%) 497
Omnicef for Oral Suspension (2%) 497
▲ Ontak Vials (26%) 1079
▲ Opana Tablets (7.9%) 1117
▲ Opana ER Tablets (2.9% to 12.2%) 1121
OptiPranolol Metipranolol Ophthalmic Solution 0.3% (A small number of patients) .... ⊙ 245
▲ Orencia Powder for Intravenous Infusion (18%) 921
Ortho-Cyclen Tablets 2449
▲ Ortho Evra Transdermal System (9% to 22%) 2437
Ortho Micronor Tablets 2446
Ortho Tri-Cyclen Tablets 2449
Ortho Tri-Cyclen Lo Tablets 2458
▲ Orthoclone OKT3 Sterile Solution (11% to 44%) 2387
OsmoPrep Tablets (Less frequent) 2680
▲ OxyContin Tablets (7%) 2589
Parnate Tablets 1532
▲ Pataday Ophthalmic Solution (Less than or equal to 5%) 543
▲ Patanase Nasal Spray (4.4%) 544
▲ Patanol Ophthalmic Solution (7%) 546
▲ Paxil (17% to 18%) 1535
▲ Paxil CR Controlled-Release Tablets (17% to 18%) 1544
Pediarix Vaccine 1552
▲ PegIntron Powder for Injection (56%) 2903
Pentasa Capsules (2% to 2.2%) 3030
▲ Pepcid Tablets (4.7%) 2075
Percocet Tablets 1127
Percodan Tablets 1130
Perforomist Inhalation Solution 1025
Persantine Tablets (2.3%) 869
Phenytek Capsules 2192
▲ Photofrin for Injection (6%) 708
▲ Plan B Tablets (16.8%) 1044
▲ Plavix Tablets (7.6%) 926
▲ Plavix Tablets (7.6%) 2767
▲ Pletal Tablets (27% to 34%) 2481
Pneumovax 23 2078
▲ PrandiMet Tablets (22%) 2967
▲ Prandin Tablets (9% to 11%) 2971
Premarin Intravenous 3217
▲ Premarin Tablets (26% to 32%) 3221
Premarin Vaginal Cream 3228
▲ Premphase Tablets (28% to 37%) 3232
▲ Prempro Tablets (28% to 37%) 3232
Primaxin I.M. 2080
Primaxin I.V. (Less than 0.2%) 2083
▲ Prinivil Tablets (4.4% to 5.7%) 2087
▲ Prinzide Tablets (5.2%) 2092
▲ Pristiq Extended-Release Tablets (2% to 29%) 3247
▲ ProAir HFA Inhalation Aerosol (7%) 3113
ProAmatine Tablets (Less frequent) 3032
▲ Procrit for Injection (0.4% to 19%) 2391
Profilnine SD Solvent Detergent 1721
Proglycem Capsules (Frequent) 1185
Proglycem Suspension (Frequent) 1185
▲ Prograf Capsules and Injection (37% to 64%) 622
▲ Prometrium Capsules (100 mg, 200 mg) (10% to 31%) 3047
ProQuad 2099
▲ Protonix for Delayed-Release Oral Suspension (5% to 9%) 3254
▲ Protonix Delayed-Release Tablets (5% to 9%) 3254
Protonix I.V. (Greater than 1%) 3257
▲ Protopic Ointment (10% to 20%) 628
Proventil HFA Inhalation Aerosol 2914
▲ Provigil Tablets (34%) 977
▲ Prozac Weekly Capsules (21%) 1852
▲ Prozac Pulvules and Liquid (21%) 1852
▲ Pulmicort Flexhaler (Greater than or equal to 3% to 12%) 654
Pylera Capsules 714
▲ Quixin Ophthalmic Solution (1% to 3%) 3184
▲ Qvar Inhalation Aerosol (8% to 25%) 3116
▲ Rapamune (Greater than or equal to 30% to 34%) 3260
▲ Raptiva for Injection (32%) 1218
▲ Rebetol (58% to 69%) 2917
▲ Rebif Prefilled Syringe for Injection (65% to 70%) 1107
▲ Reclast Injection (3.9% to 22%) 2291
Recombivax HB (Greater than or equal to 1%) 2107
ReFacto Vials 3269
▲ Relenza Inhalation Powder (2% to 24%) 1556
▲ Remicade for IV Injection (18%) 950
Requip Tablets (1% or more) 1561
Requip XL Tablets (Greater than or equal to 5%) 1568
▲ Retrovir Capsules (1.6% to 62.5%) 1574
▲ Retrovir IV Infusion (2% to 62.5%) 1579
▲ Retrovir (1.6% to 62.5%) 1574
▲ Reyataz Capsules (1% to 7%) 3299
▲ Rilutek Tablets (7% to 8%) 2771
▲ Risperdal Consta Long-Acting Injection (22%) 1753
▲ Rituxan I.V. (1% to 19%) 1223
Rocaltrol Capsules 1150
Rocaltrol Oral Solution 1150
Rocephin Injectable Vials, ADD-Vantage, Galaxy, Bulk (Less than 1%) 2642
▲ Romazicon Injection (1% to 9%) 2646
▲ Rozerem Tablets (7%) 3091
▲ Rythmol Tablets (2% to 6%) 1586
▲ Rythmol SR Capsules (6% to 10%) 1590
St. Joseph 81 mg Aspirin Chewable and Enteric Coated Tablets 1903
▲ Salagen Tablets (11% to 13%) 1082
▲ Sandimmune (2% to 15%) 2296
▲ Sandostatin Injection (6%) 2300
▲ Sandostatin LAR Depot (10.5% to 30%) 2302
Seasonique Tablets 1046
▲ Serevent Diskus (13% to 17%) 1594
Seromycin Capsules 1864
▲ Simcor Tablets (3.5% to 4.6%) 502
▲ Simulect for Injection (Greater than or equal to 10%) 2306
▲ Singulair (1% to 18.4%) 2114
Skelaxin Tablets (Most frequent) 1784
▲ Solodyn Extended Release Tablets (23%) 1938
▲ Soma Tablets (3% to 5%) 1931
▲ Somatuline Depot Injection (5% to 7%) 3102
▲ Soriatane Capsules (1% to 10%) 3062
Stalevo Tablets 2309
▲ Strattera Capsules (0.1% to 19%) 1864
Stromectol Tablets (0.2%) 2120
▲ Suboxone Tablets (30% to 36.4%) 2601
▲ Subutex Tablets (29.1% to 30%) 2601
▲ Sular Extended Release Tablets (22%) 2975
Supprelin LA Implant 1731
Suprax for Oral Suspension (Less than 2%) 1891
Suprax Tablets (Less than 2%) 1891
▲ Sustiva Capsules (5% to 11%) 930
▲ Sustiva Tablets (5% to 11%) 930
▲ Sutent Capsules (1% to 25%) 2540
▲ Symbicort 80/4.5 Inhalation Aerosol (6.5%) 659
▲ Symbicort 160/4.5 Inhalation Aerosol (11.3%) 659
Symbyax Capsules 1871
▲ Tamiflu Capsules (2% to 18%) 2649
▲ Tamiflu Oral Suspension (2% to 18%) 2649
▲ Tarceva Tablets (0% to 15%) 1228
▲ Targretin Capsules (29.8% to 41.5%) 1084
▲ Targretin Gel 1% (14%) 1088
▲ Tarka Tablets (8.9%) 511
▲ Tasigna Capsules (Greater than 10% to 31%) 2316
Tekturna Tablets (Greater than 1%) 2321
Tekturna HCT Tablets (Greater than 1%) 2324
▲ Temodar Capsules (5% to 56%) 2931
Tessalon Capsules 1183
Tessalon Perles 1183
Testim 1% Gel (1%) 701
Teveten Tablets (1% or greater) 515
▲ Teveten HCT Tablets (3.4%) 517
Tev-Tropin for Injection (Infrequently) 1187
Thioridazine Hydrochloride Tablets (Extremely rare) 2195
▲ Thyrogen for Injection (7.3%) 1244
Tice BCG (2%) 2936
Timentin ADD-Vantage 1606
Timentin Injection Galaxy Container 1609
Timentin IV Infusion 1603
Timentin Pharmacy Bulk Package 1613
Timoptic Sterile Ophthalmic Solution (Less frequent) 2121
Timoptic in Ocudose (Less frequent) 2124
▲ Timoptic-XE Sterile Ophthalmic Gel Forming Solution (1% to 5%) 2125
Toprol-XL Tablets 666
▲ Torisel Injection (1% to 15%) 3272
▲ Tracleer Tablets (22%) 3289
Transderm Scōp Transdermal Therapeutic System (Few patients) 2206
▲ Travatan Z Ophthalmic Solution (1% to 5%) 547
Treanda for Injection 983
▲ Tricor Tablets (3.2%) 520
▲ Trisenox Injection (60%) 986
▲ Trizivir Tablets (28%) 1622
Trusopt Sterile Ophthalmic Solution (Infrequent) 2128
▲ Truvada Tablets (Greater than or equal to 10%) 1262
▲ Twinrix Vaccine (13% to 22%) 1628
▲ Tygacil for Injection (5.9%) 3276
▲ Tyzeka Tablets (1% to 11%) 2328
Ultane Liquid for Inhalation (1%) 524
▲ Ultram ER Extended-Release Tablets (11.5% to 15.8%) 2428
Uniphyl Tablets 2595
Uroqid-Acid No. 2 Tablets 814
▲ Uroxatral Tablets (3%) 2786
▲ Vagifem Tablets (9% to 10%) 2375
▲ Valcyte Tablets (9% to 22%) 2654
Valium Tablets (Infrequent) 2658
▲ Valstar Sterile Solution for Intravesical Instillation (4%) 1735
▲ Valtrex Caplets (13% to 38%) 1635
▲ Vanos Cream (2.8% to 4%) 1941
Vantas (2.9%) 1737
▲ Vaprisol (8% to 12%) 632
▲ Vaqta (0.4% to 16%) 2130
Varivax (Greater than or equal to 1%) 2133
▲ Velcade for Injection (14% to 26%) 2168
▲ Venlafaxine Hydrochloride Tablets (3% to 25%) 2199
Ventolin HFA Inhalation Aerosol 1638
▲ Veramyst Nasal Spray (8% to 9%) 1643
Verdeso Foam (2%) 3069
▲ Vesanoid Capsules (86%) 2660
▲ Viadur Implant (4.6%) 802
▲ Vicoprofen Tablets (27%) 533
▲ Viramune Oral Suspension (0.7% to 3.6%) 873
▲ Viramune Tablets (0.7% to 3.6%) 873
▲ Viread Tablets (5% to 14%) 1268
Visudyne for Injection 2332
▲ Vivitrol (16% to 36%) 988
▲ Voltaren Ophthalmic Solution (Less than or equal to 3%) 2336
▲ Voltaren Tablets (1% to 10%) 2334
▲ Voltaren-XR Tablets (1% to 10%) 2337
▲ Vytorin 10/10 Tablets (5.8%) 2149
▲ Vytorin 10/10 Tablets (5.8%) 2939
▲ Vytorin 10/20 Tablets (5.8%) 2149
▲ Vytorin 10/20 Tablets (5.8%) 2939
▲ Vytorin 10/40 Tablets (5.8%) 2149
▲ Vytorin 10/40 Tablets (5.8%) 2939
▲ Vytorin 10/80 Tablets (5.8%) 2149
▲ Vytorin 10/80 Tablets (5.8%) 2939
Vyvanse Capsules 3033
▲ Wellbutrin SR Sustained-Release Tablets (25% to 26%) 1653
▲ Wellbutrin XL Extended-Release Tablets (25% to 34%) 1659
WinRho SDF (2%) 741
▲ Xeloda Tablets (1% to 9%) 2662
▲ Xenical Capsules (30.6%) 2672
▲ Xifaxan Tablets (9.7%) 2682
▲ Xolair (15%) 1235
▲ Xolair (15%) 2339
▲ Xopenex Inhalation Solution (11.9%) 3001
▲ Xopenex Inhalation Solution Concentrate (7.6% to 11.9%) 3005
▲ Xopenex HFA Inhalation Aerosol (11.9%) 3009
▲ Xyntha Vials (9% to 24%) 3280
▲ Xyrem Oral Solution (8.8% to 37.1%) 1766
Yaz Tablets (Greater than 1%) 805
Zantac 25 EFFERdose Tablets 1670
Zantac Injection 1666
Zantac Injection Pharmacy Bulk Package (Frequent) 1668
Zantac Injection Premixed 1666
Zantac 1670
Zemplar Injection 538
▲ Ziagen (1% to 13%) 1673
▲ Zocor Tablets (2.5% to 7.4%) 2136
▲ Zofran Injection (17% to 25%) 1682
▲ Zofran (9% to 27%) 1687
▲ Zofran ODT Orally Disintegrating Tablets (9% to 27%) 1687
▲ Zolinza Capsules (10% to 11.6%) 2142
▲ Zometa for Intravenous Infusion (5% to 19%) 2341
Zomig Tablets (Rare) 694
Zomig Nasal Spray (Rare to less than 2%) 689
Zomig-ZMT Tablets (Rare) 694
▲ Zonegran Capsules (10%) 1089
Zostavax Injection (1.4%) 2145
▲ Zosyn for Injection (4.5% to 7.7%) 3284
Zovirax (2.2%) 1690
Zyban Sustained-Release Tablets (Frequent) 1692
▲ Zyprexa Tablets (17%) 1883
Zyprexa IntraMuscular 1883
▲ Zyprexa ZYDIS Orally Disintegrating Tablets (17%) 1883

Zyrtec Chewable Tablets (Greater than 2%)...... 1920
Zyrtec Syrup (Greater than 2%)...... 1920
Zyrtec Tablets (Greater than 2%)...... 1920
Zyrtec-D 12 Hour Extended Release Tablets (Greater than 2%)...... 1923
▲ Zyvox (0% to 6.5%)...... 2552

Headache, exacerbation of
Treximet Tablets...... 1616

Headache, migraine
(*see under* Migraine)

Headache, sinus
Arranon Injection (1%)...... 1319
Exforge Tablets (Greater than or equal to 0.2%)...... 2238
▲ Flebogamma 5% (53%)...... 1715
▲ Flebogamma 5% DIF (Greater than 15%)...... 1718
Lexapro Oral Suspension (Frequent)...... 1174
Lexapro Tablets (Frequent)...... 1174
Requip Tablets (Infrequent)...... 1561
▲ Serevent Diskus (1% to 3%)...... 1594
▲ Strattera Capsules (3%)...... 1864
Tyzeka Tablets (1%)...... 2328
▲ Vivitrol (16% to 36%)...... 988
Xyrem Oral Solution (Infrequent)...... 1766

Headache, tension
Concerta Extended-Release Tablets (1.2%)...... 1925
Mirapex Tablets...... 857
Requip Tablets (Infrequent)...... 1561
Tyzeka Tablets (1%)...... 2328
Xyrem Oral Solution (Infrequent)...... 1766

Headache, vascular
Meridia Capsules...... 475
Paxil...... 1535
Paxil CR Controlled-Release Tablets...... 1544
Prozac Weekly Capsules (Infrequent)...... 1852
Prozac Pulvules and Liquid (Infrequent)...... 1852

Healing, abnormal
▲ CellCept Capsules (3% to less than 20%)...... 2622
▲ CellCept Intravenous (3% to less than 20%)...... 2622
▲ CellCept Oral Suspension (3% to less than 20%)...... 2622
▲ CellCept Tablets (3% to less than 20%)...... 2622
▲ Gliadel Wafer (14% to 16%)...... 1076
▲ Humira Injection (Less than 5%)...... 442
Ionsys Transdermal System (.1% to less than 1%)...... 2410
▲ Prograf Capsules and Injection (3% to 15%)...... 622
▲ Rapamune (Greater than or equal to 3% to less than 20%)...... 3260
Soriatane Capsules (Less than 1%)...... 3062
▲ Tygacil for Injection (3.5%)...... 3276
Venlafaxine Hydrochloride Tablets (Rare)...... 2199

Hearing, decreased
Aricept Tablets (Infrequent)...... 1062
Aricept ODT Tablets (Infrequent)...... 1062
Cialis Tablets (Less than 2%)...... 1792
Ciprodex Otic Suspension (1 patient)...... 541
Clinoril Tablets (Less than 1%)...... 1962
Coreg CR Extended-Release Capsules (Less than or equal to 0.1%)...... 1393
Evoxac Capsules (Less than 1%)...... 1013
Levitra Tablets (Less than 2%)...... 2876
Nalfon Capsules (1.6%)...... 2508
Namenda (Infrequent)...... 1180
Risperdal Consta Long-Acting Injection (Infrequent)...... 1753
Solodyn Extended Release Tablets...... 1938
▲ Visudyne for Injection (1% to 10%)...... 2332

Hearing, impaired
Accutane Capsules...... 2607
Anaprox Tablets (Less than 1%)...... 2632
Anaprox DS Tablets (Less than 1%)...... 2632
EC-Naprosyn Delayed-Release Tablets (Less than 1%)...... 2632
Lortab 5/500 Tablets...... 3143
Lortab 7.5/500 Tablets...... 3144
Lortab 10/500 Tablets...... 3144
Mirapex Tablets...... 857
Mustargen for Injection...... 2492
Naprosyn Suspension (Less than 1%)...... 2632
Naprosyn Tablets (Less than 1%)...... 2632
Norvir (Less than 2%)...... 489
PegIntron Powder for Injection...... 2903
Requip Tablets (Infrequent)...... 1561
Rythmol SR Capsules...... 1590
Tasigna Capsules...... 2316
Velcade for Injection...... 2168
Vesanoid Capsules (Less than 1%)...... 2660
Vicodin Tablets (Very rare)...... 529
Vicodin ES Tablets (Very rare)...... 530
Vicodin HP Tablets (Very rare)...... 531
Voltaren Tablets (Rarely)...... 2334
Voltaren-XR Tablets (Rarely)...... 2337

Hearing, loss of
Abelcet Injection...... 1134
Aggrenox Capsules...... 819
Bayer Aspirin...... 750
▲ Capastat Sulfate for Injection (3%)...... 1791
Cialis Tablets (Less than 2%)...... 1792
Cipro I.V. (1% or less)...... 2817
Cipro (Less than 1%)...... 2810
Cipro XR Tablets...... 2823
Coreg Tablets (Less than or equal to 0.1%)...... 1387
Demadex Injection...... 2630
Demadex Tablets...... 2630
Depakote ER Tablets...... 423
Exjade Tablets (0.1% to 1%)...... 2244
Furosemide Tablets...... 2186
Gantrisin Pediatric Suspension...... 2638
Gengraf Capsules (2% or less)...... 435
Imitrex Nasal Spray...... 1470
Intron A for Injection...... 2859
Levitra Tablets (Less than 2%)...... 2876
Lortab 5/500 Tablets...... 3143
Lortab 7.5/500 Tablets...... 3144
Lortab 10/500 Tablets...... 3144
Miacalcin Nasal Spray (Less than 1%)...... 2274
Neoral Oral Solution (2% or less)...... 2280
Neoral Soft Gelatin Capsules (2% or less)...... 2280
Orthoclone OKT3 Sterile Solution...... 2387
PegIntron Powder for Injection...... 2903
Percocet Tablets...... 1127
Percodan Tablets...... 1130
Primaxin I.M....... 2080
Primaxin I.V. (Less than 0.2%)...... 2083
Prograf Capsules and Injection...... 622
Prozac Pulvules and Liquid (Rare)...... 1852
Raptiva for Injection (1 case)...... 1218
Retrovir Capsules...... 1574
Retrovir IV Infusion...... 1579
Retrovir...... 1574
St. Joseph 81 mg Aspirin Chewable and Enteric Coated Tablets...... 1903
Sandimmune (2% or less)...... 2296
Sandostatin Injection (Less than 1%)...... 2300
Taxotere Injection Concentrate (Rare)...... 2773
▲ Vesanoid Capsules (6%)...... 2660
Vicodin Tablets...... 529
Vicodin ES Tablets...... 530
Vicodin HP Tablets...... 531
Zinacef for Injection (A few pediatric patients)...... 1678
Zinacef Injection (A few pediatric patients)...... 1678

Hearing disturbances
Amerge Tablets (Infrequent)...... 1301
Anaprox Tablets (Less than 3%)...... 2632
Anaprox DS Tablets (Less than 3%)...... 2632
Avalide Tablets...... 892
Avalide Tablets...... 2713
Avapro Tablets (Less than 1%)...... 897
Avapro Tablets (Less than 1%)...... 2718
EC-Naprosyn Delayed-Release Tablets (Less than 3%)...... 2632
Imitrex Nasal Spray (Infrequent)...... 1470
Imitrex Tablets (Infrequent)...... 1474
Indocin Capsules (Less than 1%)...... 2024
Indocin I.V. (Less than 1%)...... 2489
Indocin (Less than 1%)...... 2024
▲ Intron A for Injection (Less than 5%)...... 2859
Naprosyn Suspension (Less than 3%)...... 2632
Naprosyn Tablets (Less than 3%)...... 2632
Rebetol...... 2917
▲ Taxotere Injection Concentrate (Rare to 12.7%)...... 2773

Hearing loss, reversible
Depakote ER Tablets...... 423
E.E.S. (Isolated reports)...... 433
EryPed (Isolated reports)...... 431
Romazicon Injection (Less than 1%)...... 2646

Heart beat, irregular
Adenocard IV Injection...... 603
▲ Indapamide Tablets (Less than 5%)...... 2188
K-Phos Original (Sodium Free) Tablets (Less frequent)...... 814
K-Phos Neutral Tablets...... 813
Children's Motrin Oral Suspension...... 1901
Children's Motrin Non-Staining Dye-Free Oral Suspension...... 1901
Infants' Motrin Concentrated Drops...... 1901
Infants' Motrin Non-Staining Dye-Free Concentrated Drops...... 1901
Junior Strength Motrin Caplets and Chewable Tablets...... 1901
Rythmol SR Capsules...... 1590
Uroqid-Acid No. 2 Tablets...... 814

Heart beats, ectopic
Imitrex Injection (Infrequent)...... 1465
Imitrex Nasal Spray...... 1470
Imitrex Tablets...... 1474

Heart block
(*see also under* Sinoatrial block)
Actimmune (Rare)...... 1743
Adenocard IV Injection...... 603
Agrylin Capsules...... 3017
Aricept Tablets...... 1062
Aricept ODT Tablets...... 1062
Betimol Ophthalmic Solution...... 3181
Brovana Inhalation Solution (Less than 2%)...... 2990
Combigan Ophthalmic Solution...... 553
Imitrex Nasal Spray...... 1470
Imitrex Tablets (Rare)...... 1474
Lanoxin Injection...... 1498
Lanoxin Injection Pediatric...... 1502
Lanoxin Tablets...... 1505
Paxil (Rare)...... 1535
Paxil CR Controlled-Release Tablets (Rare)...... 1544
Prozac Weekly Capsules (Rare)...... 1852
Prozac Pulvules and Liquid (Rare)...... 1852
Timoptic Sterile Ophthalmic Solution (Less frequent)...... 2121
Timoptic in Ocudose (Less frequent)...... 2124
Trasylol Injection (1% to 2%)...... 799
Zyprexa IntraMuscular (Infrequent)...... 1883

Heart block, second degree
Toprol-XL Tablets...... 666
Zofran Injection...... 1682

Heart block, third degree
Busulfex Injection (2%)...... 2477
Nadolol Tablets (Single instance)...... 2191
Toprol-XL Tablets...... 666
Wellbutrin Tablets...... 1648

Heart disease
Cimzia...... 3127

Heart failure
Abelcet Injection...... 1134
Actimmune (Rare)...... 1743
Activase I.V....... 1188
ActoPlus Met Tablets...... 3071
▲ Actos Tablets (5.7%)...... 3077
Aggrenox Capsules (1.6%)...... 819
▲ Agrylin Capsules (1% to less than 5%)...... 3017
Aldara Cream, 5%...... 1699
Aricept Tablets (Frequent)...... 1062
Aricept ODT Tablets (Frequent)...... 1062
Avalide Tablets...... 892
Avalide Tablets...... 2713
Avapro Tablets (Less than 1%)...... 897
Avapro Tablets (Less than 1%)...... 2718
Azilect Tablets (Infrequent)...... 3106
Betimol Ophthalmic Solution...... 3181
Busulfex Injection (2%)...... 2477
Campral Tablets (Rare)...... 1158
Celexa (Infrequent)...... 1160
▲ CellCept Capsules (3% to less than 20%)...... 2622
▲ CellCept Intravenous (3% to less than 20%)...... 2622
▲ CellCept Oral Suspension (3% to less than 20%)...... 2622
▲ CellCept Tablets (3% to less than 20%)...... 2622
Cimzia...... 3127
Coreg Tablets...... 1387
Coreg CR Extended-Release Capsules...... 1393
Cosopt Sterile Ophthalmic Solution (Less than 1%)...... 1969
Cubicin for Injection (1% to 2%)...... 995
Dantrium Capsules (Less frequent)...... 2580
Dantrium Intravenous...... 2582
Doxil Injection (Less than 1%)...... 2378
Duetact Tablets...... 3085
DynaCirc CR Controlled Release Tablets (0.5% to 1%)...... 1407
Elitek (Less than or equal to 1%)...... 2729
Enbrel for Injection (Infrequent)...... 569
Exelon Capsules (Frequent)...... 2229
Exelon Oral Solution (Frequent)...... 2229
Exelon Patch (Infrequent)...... 2233
▲ Flolan for Injection (11%)...... 1426
Flumadine (Less than 0.3%)...... 1167
Gengraf Capsules (1% to less than 3%)...... 435
Gleevec Tablets (Infrequent)...... 2255
Herceptin I.V....... 1199
▲ Intron A for Injection (Less than 5%)...... 2859
Invanz for Injection (Greater than 0.1%)...... 2029
Levothroid Tablets...... 1170
Levoxyl Tablets...... 1780
Lovenox Injection (0.95%)...... 2756
Luvox CR Extended-Release Capsules (Infrequent)...... 1759
Lyrica Capsules (0.1% to 1%)...... 2527
Merrem I.V. (Greater than 0.1% to 1%)...... 684
Mirapex Tablets (Less than 1%)...... 857
Mobic Oral Suspension (Less than 2%)...... 863
Mobic Tablets (Less than 2%)...... 863
Nadolol Tablets (1 of 100 patients)...... 2191
Namenda (Frequent)...... 1180
NeoProfen Injection...... 2496
Neoral Oral Solution (1% to less than 3%)...... 2280
Neoral Soft Gelatin Capsules (1% to less than 3%)...... 2280
Neupro Transdermal System...... 3149
Omnicef Capsules...... 497
Omnicef for Oral Suspension...... 497
Orthoclone OKT3 Sterile Solution...... 2387
▲ Photofrin for Injection (7%)...... 708
Plavix Tablets (1% to 2.5%)...... 926
Plavix Tablets (1% to 2.5%)...... 2767
Pulmozyme Inhalation Solution...... 1217
Refludan for Injection (1.8%)...... 795
Remeron Tablets (Rare)...... 2924
RemeronSolTab Tablets (Rare)...... 2927
Requip Tablets (Infrequent)...... 1561
Rilutek Tablets (Infrequent)...... 2771
Rituxan I.V....... 1223
▲ Simulect for Injection (3% to 10%)...... 2306
Targretin Capsules...... 1084
▲ Taxotere Injection Concentrate (8.1%)...... 2773
Timoptic Sterile Ophthalmic Solution (Less frequent)...... 2121
Timoptic in Ocudose (Less frequent)...... 2124
Timoptic-XE Sterile Ophthalmic Gel Forming Solution...... 2125
TNKase...... 1233
Toprol-XL Tablets...... 666
▲ Trasylol Injection (5%)...... 799
▲ Velcade for Injection (5%)...... 2168
▲ Vesanoid Capsules (6%)...... 2660
Zonegran Capsules (Rare)...... 1089
Zosyn for Injection (1% or less)...... 3284
Zyprexa Tablets...... 1883
Zyprexa ZYDIS Orally Disintegrating Tablets...... 1883

Heart failure, congestive
(*see under* Congestive heart failure)

Heart failure, right ventricular
Treximet Tablets (Rare)...... 1616

Heart failure, worsening of
Avandaryl Tablets...... 1344
▲ Avandia Tablets (6%)...... 1351
Cimzia...... 3127
Cleviprex...... 1936
Prinivil Tablets (Greater than 1%)...... 2087
Prinzide Tablets...... 2092
Sensipar Tablets (2%)...... 594
Toprol-XL Tablets...... 666

Heart rate, abnormal
▲ Somatuline Depot Injection (6% to 21%)...... 3102

Heart rate, changes
Abilify Injection...... 881
Abilify Injection...... 2466
Abilify Oral Solution...... 881
Abilify Oral Solution...... 2466
Abilify Discmelt Orally Disintegrating Tablets...... 881
Abilify Discmelt Orally Disintegrating Tablets...... 2466
Abilify Tablets...... 881
Abilify Tablets...... 2466
Requip XL Tablets...... 1568

Transderm Scōp Transdermal Therapeutic System 2206
Visudyne for Injection 2332

Heart rate, decrease
Meridia Capsules 475
ProAmatine Tablets 3032
Requip Tablets (Infrequent) 1561

Heart rate, increased
Amitiza Capsules 3082
Concerta Extended-Release Tablets 1925
Cyanokit 5g Antidote 1021
Daytrana Transdermal Patch 3022
Levothroid Tablets 1170
Meridia Capsules 475
▲ Neupro Transdermal System (9%) 3149
Pristiq Extended-Release Tablets 3247
Ultram ER Extended-Release Tablets (0.5% to less than 1%) 2428
▲ Xopenex Inhalation Solution (0.8% to 6%) 3001
▲ Xopenex Inhalation Solution Concentrate (0.8% to 6%) 3005
▲ Xopenex HFA Inhalation Aerosol (0.8% to 6%) 3009
Xyrem Oral Solution (Infrequent) 1766

Heart sounds, abnormal
Gengraf Capsules (1% to less than 3%) 435
Neoral Oral Solution (1% to less than 3%) 2280
Neoral Soft Gelatin Capsules (1% to less than 3%) 2280
Rythmol SR Capsules 1590
▲ Simulect for Injection (3% to 10%) 2306

Heart spasms
(*see under* Cardiospasm)

Heartburn
▲ Aerobid/Aerobid-M (3% to 9%) 1153
Aggrenox Capsules 819
▲ Alferon N Injection (3%) 1726
▲ Anaprox Tablets (3% to 9%) 2632
▲ Anaprox DS Tablets (3% to 9%) 2632
Avalide Tablets (2%) 892
Avalide Tablets (2%) 2713
Avapro Tablets (2%) 897
Avapro Tablets (2%) 2718
Bayer Aspirin 750
Combivent Inhalation Aerosol 845
▲ EC-Naprosyn Delayed-Release Tablets (3% to 9%) 2632
Eldepryl Capsules 3052
▲ Emend Capsules (5.3%) 1992
▲ Emend for Injection (5.3%) 1999
▲ Indocin (3% to 9%) 2024
Klonopin (Infrequent) 2639
Lexapro Oral Suspension (Frequent) 1174
Lexapro Tablets (Frequent) 1174
Mevacor Tablets (1.6%) 2063
▲ Naprosyn Suspension (3% to 9%) 2632
▲ Naprosyn Tablets (3% to 9%) 2632
Noroxin Tablets (0.3% to 1%) 2069
Primaxin I.M. 2080
Primaxin I.V. (Less than 0.2%) 2083
Prinivil Tablets (0.3% to 1%) 2087
Prinzide Tablets (0.3% to 1%) 2092
ProAmatine Tablets (Rare) 3032
St. Joseph 81 mg Aspirin Chewable and Enteric Coated Tablets 1903
Stalevo Tablets 2309
▲ Taxotere Injection Concentrate (0% to 12.7%) 2773
Toprol-XL Tablets (About 1 of 100 patients) 666
▲ Voltaren Tablets (1% to 10%) 2334
▲ Voltaren-XR Tablets (1% to 10%) 2337

Heat intolerance
Alferon N Injection (1%) 1726
Imitrex Tablets 1474
Levothroid Tablets 1170
Levoxyl Tablets 1780
Treximet Tablets (Infrequent) 1616

Heat sensations
Prograf Capsules and Injection 622

Heat stroke
Abilify Injection (Less than 1 in 1000 patients) 881
Abilify Injection (Less than 1 in 1000 patients) 2466
Abilify Oral Solution (Less than 1 in 1000 patients) 881
Abilify Oral Solution (Less than 1 in 1000 patients) 2466
Abilify Discmelt Orally Disintegrating Tablets (Less than 1 in 1000 patients) 881
Abilify Discmelt Orally Disintegrating Tablets (Less than 1 in 1000 patients) 2466
Abilify Tablets (Less than 1 in 1000 patients) 881
Abilify Tablets (Less than 1 in 1000 patients) 2466
Donnatal Extentabs 2507
Emsam Transdermal System (Rare) 905
Evoxac Capsules (Less than 1%) 1013
Lunesta Tablets (Infrequent) 2994
Protonix for Delayed-Release Oral Suspension (Less than 1%) 3254
Protonix Delayed-Release Tablets (Less than 1%) 3254
Protonix I.V. (Less than 1%) 3257
Vivitrol 988

Heaviness
▲ Imitrex Injection (7%) 1465
Xyrem Oral Solution (Infrequent) 1766

Heavy feeling, unspecified
Marplan Tablets 3177
Treximet Tablets (Infrequent) 1616

Heavy sensation, arms
Adenocard IV Injection (Less than 1%) 603

Heavy sensation, legs
Eldepryl Capsules 3052
K-Phos Original (Sodium Free) Tablets (Less frequent) 814
K-Phos Neutral Tablets 813

Hemangioma
Mirapex Tablets 857

Hemarthrosis
Kaletra 452
NovoSeven (Greater than or equal to 2%) 2367
NovoSeven RT (Greater than or equal to 2%) 2370
Reyataz Capsules 3299

Hematemesis
Aggrenox Capsules 819
AmBisome for Injection (Less common) 606
Anaprox Tablets (Less than 1%) 2632
Anaprox DS Tablets (Less than 1%) 2632
Angiomax for Injection (1.3%) 1933
Argatroban Injection (2.6%) 1308
Azilect Tablets (Rare) 3106
Busulfex Injection (2%) 2477
Campral Tablets (Infrequent) 1158
Copaxone for Injection (Infrequent) 3110
Depakote ER Tablets (Greater than 1%) 423
EC-Naprosyn Delayed-Release Tablets (Less than 1%) 2632
Effexor XR Extended-Release Capsules (Rare) 3195
Exelon Capsules (Infrequent) 2229
Exelon Oral Solution (Infrequent) 2229
Exelon Patch (Infrequent) 2233
Geodon Capsules (Rare) 2520
Imitrex Injection 1465
Imitrex Nasal Spray (Rare) 1470
Imitrex Tablets (Rare) 1474
Intelence Tablets (Less than 2%) 3119
Lamictal (Rare) 1488
▲ Leukine (13%) 774
Luvox CR Extended-Release Capsules (Rare) 1759
Mobic Oral Suspension (Less than 2%) 863
Mobic Tablets (Less than 2%) 863
Naprosyn Suspension (Less than 1%) 2632
Naprosyn Tablets (Less than 1%) 2632
Paxil (Rare) 1535
Paxil CR Controlled-Release Tablets (Rare) 1544
▲ Photofrin for Injection (8%) 708
Pletal Tablets (Less than 2%) 2481
Proleukin for Injection (Less than 1%) 2287
Protonix for Delayed-Release Oral Suspension (Less than 1%) 3254
Protonix Delayed-Release Tablets (Less than 1%) 3254
Protonix I.V. (Less than 1%) 3257
Prozac Weekly Capsules (Rare) 1852
Prozac Pulvules and Liquid (Rare) 1852
ReoPro Vials (5 to 11 events) 1860
Requip Tablets (Infrequent to rare) 1561
Rilutek Tablets (Rare) 2771
Tarceva Tablets 1228
Tasigna Capsules 2316
Tricor Tablets 520
Velcade for Injection 2168
Venlafaxine Hydrochloride Tablets (Rare) 2199
Voltaren Tablets (Occasionally) 2334
Voltaren-XR Tablets (Occasionally) 2337
Xeloda Tablets 2662
Zomig Tablets (Rare) 694
Zomig-ZMT Tablets (Rare) 694
Zonegran Capsules (Rare) 1089

Hematochezia
Avelox 2803
Biaxin/Biaxin XL 411
Bicillin C-R Injectable Suspension 1775
Bicillin L-A Injection 1777
Cipro 2810
Cyanokit 5g Antidote 1021
Cymbalta Delayed-Release Capsules (Rare) 1801
Exelon Patch (Infrequent) 2233
▲ Gleevec Tablets (0% to 27%) 2255
Nalfon Capsules (Less than 1%) 2508
Omnicef Capsules 497
Omnicef for Oral Suspension 497
Primaxin I.M. 2080
Primaxin I.V. 2083
ProQuad 2099
▲ Remicade for IV Injection (10%) 950
Rotarix Oral Suspension 1582
RotaTeq (Less than 0.1% to 0.6%) 2110
Tarceva Tablets 1228
Torisel Injection 3272
Tygacil for Injection 3276
Xifaxan Tablets (Less than 2%) 2682

Hematocrit, decrease
Aceon Tablets (2 mg, 4 mg, 8 mg) 3038
ActoPlus Met Tablets 3071
▲ Actos Tablets (2% to 4%) 3077
Advate (0.6%) 721
Aggrenox Capsules 819
Alphanate 1709
▲ Argatroban Injection (10.4%) 1308
Atacand Tablets 639
Atacand HCT 642
Avandamet Tablets 1336
Avandaryl Tablets 1344
Avandia Tablets 1351
Azor Tablets 1005
Benicar Tablets 1009
Benicar HCT Tablets (One patient) 1010
▲ Cancidas for Injection (13.2% to 18.1%) 1953
Celebrex Capsules 2979
Cipro I.V. (Among most frequent) 2817
Cipro XR Tablets 2823
▲ DepoDur Injection (2% to 5%) 1095
Diovan Tablets (0.8%) 2212
Diovan HCT Tablets (Less than 0.1%) 2216
Eligard 7.5 mg (Less than 2%) 2724
Eligard 22.5 mg (Less than 2%) 2724
Eligard 30 mg (Less than 2%) 2724
Eligard 45 mg (Less than 2%) 2724
Fenoglide Tablets 2960
Fentora Tablets (Greater than 1%) 968
▲ Invanz for Injection (3% to 3.4%) 2029
Keppra Injection 3137
Keppra Oral Solution 3131
Keppra Tablets 3131
Letairis Tablets 1258
▲ Lupron Depot 7.5 mg (Greater than or equal to 5%) 469
Merrem I.V. (Greater than 0.2%) 684
Micardis HCT Tablets (0.6%) 854
Noroxin Tablets (Less frequent) 2069
Omnicef for Oral Suspension (0.2%) 497
Panhematin for Injection 2497
Precose Tablets 792
Primaxin I.M. 2080
Primaxin I.V. 2083
Prinivil Tablets (Frequent) 2087
Prinzide Tablets (Frequent) 2092
Proglycem Capsules (Infrequent) 1185
Proglycem Suspension (Infrequent) 1185
ReoPro Vials (7 to 11 events) 1860
Tekturna Tablets 2321
Tekturna HCT Tablets (Less than 0.1%) 2324
Teveten HCT Tablets (0.1%) 517
Timentin ADD-Vantage 1606
Timentin Injection Galaxy Container 1609
Timentin IV Infusion 1603
Timentin Pharmacy Bulk Package 1613
Tracleer Tablets 3289
Zinacef for Injection (1 in 10 patients) 1678
Zinacef Injection (1 in 10 patients) 1678
Zosyn for Injection 3284

Hematocrit, increase
AndroGel 3159
Epogen for Injection 576
Procrit for Injection 2391
Testim 1% Gel (1% to 2%) 701

Hematologic abnormalities
Avelox 2803
Cipro I.V. (Rare) 2817
Cipro 2810
Cipro XR Tablets 2823
Depakote ER Tablets 423
Keppra Oral Solution 3131
Keppra Tablets 3131
Levaquin 2416
Levaquin in 5% Dextrose Injection 2416
Marplan Tablets 3177

Hematologic reactions
Dapsone Tablets USP 1746
Daraprim Tablets 1400
Lamictal 1488
Malarone Pediatric Tablets 1521
Malarone Tablets 1521
Rebif Prefilled Syringe for Injection 1107

Hematologic toxicity
Bexxar 1371
Doxil Injection 2378
Retrovir IV Infusion 1579

Hematoma
Aceon Tablets (2 mg, 4 mg, 8 mg) (0.3% to 1%) 3038
Advate (0.6%) 721
Aggrenox Capsules (Less than 1%) 819
Angiomax for Injection (1.3%) 1933
Anzemet Injection (Infrequently) 2701
Anzemet Tablets (Rare) 2704
▲ Argatroban Injection (3.6%) 1308
Arixtra Injection (2.1% to 2.8%) 1313
Copaxone for Injection (Infrequent) 3110
▲ Dacogen Injection (5%) 1066
Depakote ER Tablets 423
Eldepryl Capsules 3052
Emend Capsules (Greater than 0.5%) 1992
Emend for Injection (Greater than 0.5%) 1999
Evoxac Capsules (Less than 1%) 1013
Exelon Capsules (Infrequent) 2229
Exelon Oral Solution (Infrequent) 2229
▲ Flovent Diskus 50 mcg (1% to 3%) 1435
Flulaval Injection Vaccine 1448
Havrix Injection Vaccine (Less than 1%) 1454
Imitrex Injection 1465
Imitrex Tablets (Rare) 1474
Invanz for Injection (Greater than 0.1%) 2029
Lexapro Oral Suspension (Infrequent) 1174
Lexapro Tablets (Infrequent) 1174
Lovenox Injection 2756
Mirapex Tablets 857
Nimotop Capsules (Less than 1%) 790
Paxil (Infrequent) 1535
Paxil CR Controlled-Release Tablets (Infrequent) 1544
Plavix Tablets (1% to 2.5%) 926
Plavix Tablets (1% to 2.5%) 2767
Pristiq Extended-Release Tablets 3247
Prozac Weekly Capsules 1852
ReFacto Vials 3269
▲ Refludan for Injection (10.6%) 795
ReoPro Vials 1860
Requip Tablets (Infrequent) 1561
Risperdal Consta Long-Acting Injection (Rare) 1753
Rythmol SR Capsules 1590
▲ Sandostatin Injection (1% to 4%) 2300
▲ Simulect for Injection (3% to 10%) 2306
Symbyax Capsules 1871
Tasigna Capsules (0.1% to 1%) 2316
▲ TNKase (1.7% to 12.3%) 1233
Vantas (Less than 2%) 1737
▲ Varivax (24.4% to 32.5%) 2133

Hematoma, extradural
Pletal Tablets 2481

Hematoma, spinal-epidural
Fragmin Injection (9 cases) 1070

Hematoma, splenic
NovoSeven 2367
▲ NovoSeven RT (4.7%) 2370

Hematoma, subdural
Actiq (Less than 1%) 959
Exelon Patch (Infrequent) 2233

▲ Humira Injection (Less than 5%) 442
NovoSeven 2367
NovoSeven RT 2370
Pletal Tablets 2481
Rilutek Tablets (Infrequent) 2771
Velcade for Injection 2168

Hematoma at injection site

▲ Edex Injection (5%) 2957
▲ Fragmin Injection (0.2% to 4.7%) 1070
ProQuad 2099
Zostavax Injection (1.4%) 2145

Hematopoietic depression

Cosmegen for Injection 2485
Mustargen for Injection (Occasional) 2492

Hematospermia

Luvox CR Extended-Release Capsules (Rare) 1759

Hematuria

Accutane Capsules 2607
Aceon Tablets (2 mg, 4 mg, 8 mg) (0.3% to 1%) 3038
Actiq (Less than 1%) 959
Aggrenox Capsules (Less than 1%) 819
▲ Agrylin Capsules (1% to less than 5%) 3017
▲ AmBisome for Injection (14%) 606
Anaprox Tablets (Less than 1%) 2632
Anaprox DS Tablets (Less than 1%) 2632
Angiomax for Injection (1.3%) 1933
Anzemet Injection (Rare) 2701
Anzemet Tablets (Rare) 2704
▲ Argatroban Injection (0.9% to 11.8%) 1308
Aricept Tablets (Frequent) 1062
Aricept ODT Tablets (Frequent) 1062
Asacol Delayed-Release Tablets 2579
Atacand Tablets (0.5% or greater) 639
Atacand HCT (0.5% or greater) 642
Atripla Tablets (3%) 938
Augmentin (Rare) 1323
Augmentin Tablets (Rare) 1327
Augmentin XR Extended Release Tablets (Rare) 1333
Augmentin ES-600 Powder for Oral Suspension (Rare) 1329
▲ Baraclude (9%) 900
Benicar HCT Tablets (Greater than 1%) 1010
Bicillin C-R Injectable Suspension 1775
Bicillin L-A Injection 1777
Brovana Inhalation Solution (Less than 2%) 2990
Campral Tablets (Rare) 1158
▲ Cancidas for Injection (9.6%) 1953
Cardene I.V. (0.7%) 1093
Celebrex Capsules (0.1% to 1.9%) 2979
Celexa (Rare) 1160
▲ CellCept Capsules (3% to less than 20%) 2622
▲ CellCept Intravenous (3% to less than 20%) 2622
▲ CellCept Oral Suspension (3% to less than 20%) 2622
▲ CellCept Tablets (3% to less than 20%) 2622
Cipro I.V. (1% or less) 2817
Cipro 2810
Cipro XR Tablets (Less than 1%) 2823
Clinoril Tablets (Less than 1%) 1962
▲ Clolar for Intravenous Infusion (17%) 1239
▲ Coreg Tablets (Greater than 1% to 3%) 1387
▲ Coreg CR Extended-Release Capsules (Greater than 1% to less than or equal to 3%) 1393
Crestor Tablets 677
▲ Crixivan Capsules (Approximately 12.4%) 1979
Cuprimine Capsules 1986
Dantrium Capsules (Less frequent) 2580
Daraprim Tablets 1400
Demser Capsules (Few patients) 1989
▲ Doxil Injection (1% to 10%) 2378
EC-Naprosyn Delayed-Release Tablets (Less than 1%) 2632
Edecrin 698
Effexor XR Extended-Release Capsules (Infrequent) 3195
▲ Eloxatin for Injection (0% to 6%) 2731
Emsam Transdermal System (Infrequent) 905
Emtriva Capsules (3%) 1246
Emtriva Oral Solution (3%) 1246
Evoxac Capsules (Less than 1%) 1013
Exelon Capsules (Frequent) 2229
Exelon Oral Solution (Frequent) 2229
Exelon Patch (Infrequent) 2233
Exforge Tablets (Greater than or equal to 0.2%) 2238
▲ Flolan for Injection (5%) 1426
Fragmin Injection (2.9%) 1070
Gabitril Tablets (Infrequent) 973
Gantrisin Pediatric Suspension 2638
▲ Gemzar for Injection (Up to 35%) 1820
Gengraf Capsules (1% to less than 3%) 435
Genotropin Lyophilized Powder (Infrequent) 2547
Geodon Capsules (Infrequent) 2520
▲ Gleevec Tablets (0% to 27%) 2255
▲ Humira Injection (5%) 442
Imitrex Nasal Spray 1470
Imitrex Tablets (Rare) 1474
Indocin Capsules (Less than 1%) 2024
Indocin I.V. (Less than 1%) 2489
Indocin (Less than 1%) 2024
Intravenous Sodium Diuril (1 case) 2490
▲ Intron A for Injection (Less than 5%) 2859
Invanz for Injection (Greater than 0.1%) 2029
Ionsys Transdermal System (.1% to less than 1%) 2410
Lamictal (Infrequent) 1488
▲ Leukine (9%) 774
Lexapro Oral Suspension (Infrequent) 1174
Lexapro Tablets (Infrequent) 1174
Lipitor Tablets (Less than 2%) 2501
Lovenox Injection (Less than 1% to 2%) 2756
Lunesta Tablets (Infrequent) 2994
Luvox CR Extended-Release Capsules (Infrequent) 1759
Lyrica Capsules (0.1% to 1%) 2527
Meridia Capsules 475
Miacalcin Nasal Spray (Less than 1%) 2274
Mobic Oral Suspension (Less than 2%) 863
Mobic Tablets (Less than 2%) 863
▲ Myfortic Tablets (3% to less than 20%) 2276
▲ Mylotarg for Injection (1% to 37%) 3212
Nalfon Capsules (Less than 1%) 2508
Namenda (Infrequent) 1180
Naprosyn Suspension (Less than 1%) 2632
Naprosyn Tablets (Less than 1%) 2632
NeoProfen Injection (1%) 2496
Neoral Oral Solution (1% to less than 3%) 2280
Neoral Soft Gelatin Capsules (1% to less than 3%) 2280
Neupogen for Injection (Infrequent) 589
Nexium Delayed-Release Capsules (Less than 1%) 645
Nexium I.V. (Less than 1%) 652
Nexium Delayed-Release Oral Suspension (Less than 1%) 645
Noroxin Tablets 2069
Norvir (Less than 2%) 489
▲ Novantrone for Injection Concentrate (11%) 1100
▲ Ontak Vials (10%) 1079
OxyContin Tablets (Less than 1%) 2589
Paxil (Infrequent) 1535
Paxil CR Controlled-Release Tablets (Infrequent) 1544
Pentasa Capsules (Less than 1%) 3030
Plavix Tablets (Less than 1%) 926
Plavix Tablets (Less than 1%) 2767
Pletal Tablets (2% or greater) 2481
Primaxin I.M. 2080
Primaxin I.V. 2083
Proglycem Capsules (Infrequent) 1185
Proglycem Suspension (Infrequent) 1185
▲ Prograf Capsules and Injection (3% to 15%) 622
Protonix for Delayed-Release Oral Suspension (Less than 1%) 3254
Protonix Delayed-Release Tablets (Less than 1%) 3254
Protonix I.V. (Less than 1%) 3257
Provigil Tablets (1%) 977
Prozac Weekly Capsules (Infrequent) 1852
Prozac Pulvules and Liquid (Infrequent) 1852
▲ Refludan for Injection (4.4%) 795
Remeron Tablets (Infrequent) 2924
RemeronSolTab Tablets (Infrequent) 2927
ReoPro Vials (4 events) 1860
Requip Tablets (Infrequent) 1561
Retrovir Capsules (0.8%) 1574
Retrovir IV Infusion (1%) 1579
Retrovir (0.8%) 1574
Rilutek Tablets (Infrequent) 2771
Risperdal Consta Long-Acting Injection (Infrequent) 1753
Rocephin Injectable Vials, ADD-Vantage, Galaxy, Bulk (Less than 0.1%) 2642
▲ Rythmol SR Capsules (1% to 3%) 1590
Salagen Tablets (Less than 1%) 1082
Sandimmune (Rare) 2296
Sandostatin Injection (Less than 1%) 2300
Sandostatin LAR Depot 2302
▲ Simulect for Injection (3% to 10%) 2306
Sular Extended Release Tablets (Less than or equal to 1%) 2975
Sustiva Capsules (Up to 1%) 930
Sustiva Tablets (Up to 1%) 930
Symbyax Capsules (Infrequent) 1871
Targretin Capsules 1084
Tarka Tablets (Less frequent) 511
Tasigna Capsules 2316
Teveten Tablets (Less than 1%) 515
Teveten HCT Tablets (Less than 1%) 517
▲ Tice BCG (26% to 38%) 2936
▲ Truvada Tablets (3%) 1262
Ultram ER Extended-Release Tablets (0.5% to less than 1%) 2428
Uroqid-Acid No. 2 Tablets (Rare) 814
▲ Vagifem Tablets (3% to 5%) 2375
▲ Valstar Sterile Solution for Intravesical Instillation (1% to 29%) 1735
Vaprisol (2.2%) 632
Velcade for Injection 2168
Venlafaxine Hydrochloride Tablets (Infrequent) 2199
▲ Viread Tablets (3% to 7%) 1268
Voltaren Tablets (Occasionally) 2334
Voltaren-XR Tablets (Occasionally) 2337
Xifaxan Tablets (Less than 2%) 2682
Xyrem Oral Solution (Infrequent) 1766
Zometa for Intravenous Infusion 2341
Zomig Tablets (Infrequent) 694
Zomig-ZMT Tablets (Infrequent) 694
Zonegran Capsules (Infrequent) 1089
Zosyn for Injection (1% or less) 3284
Zovirax 1690
Zyprexa Tablets (Infrequent) 1883
Zyprexa ZYDIS Orally Disintegrating Tablets (Infrequent) 1883
Zyrtec Chewable Tablets (Less than 2%) 1920
Zyrtec Syrup (Less than 2%) 1920
Zyrtec Tablets (Less than 2%) 1920
Zyrtec-D 12 Hour Extended Release Tablets (Less than 2%) 1923

Hematuria, aggravated

Vantas (Less than 2%) 1737

Hematuria, microscopic

▲ Crixivan Capsules (Approximately 12.4%) 1979
▲ Ontak Vials (Less than 5%) 1079

Hemiparesis

Arranon Injection (1%) 1319
Exelon Capsules (Infrequent) 2229
Exelon Oral Solution (Infrequent) 2229
Femara Tablets (Less than or equal to 2%) 2246
Klonopin 2639
Myfortic Tablets 2276
Orthoclone OKT3 Sterile Solution 2387
Prograf Capsules and Injection 622
Requip Tablets (Rare) 1561
Sandostatin LAR Depot 2302
▲ Temodar Capsules (6% to 18%) 2931
▲ Thyrogen for Injection (4 patients out of 55) 1244

Hemiplegia

Actiq (Less than 1%) 959
Aricept Tablets (Infrequent) 1062
Aricept ODT Tablets (Infrequent) 1062
Azilect Tablets (Infrequent) 3106
DepoCyt Injection 1136
Doxil Injection (Less than 1%) 2378
Gabitril Tablets (Infrequent) 973
▲ Gliadel Wafer (19% to 41%) 1076
Imitrex Injection (Rare) 1465
Imitrex Tablets 1474
Lamictal (Rare) 1488
Luvox CR Extended-Release Capsules (Infrequent) 1759
Mirapex Tablets 857
Namenda (Infrequent) 1180
Orthoclone OKT3 Sterile Solution 2387
Requip Tablets (Rare) 1561
Rilutek Tablets (Infrequent) 2771
▲ Thyrogen for Injection (4 patients out of 55) 1244
▲ Vesanoid Capsules (3%) 2660

Hemochromatosis

Effexor XR Extended-Release Capsules (Rare) 3195
Venlafaxine Hydrochloride Tablets (Rare) 2199

Hemoconcentration

Follistim AQ Cartridge 2844

Hemoglobin, decrease

Aceon Tablets (2 mg, 4 mg, 8 mg) 3038
ActoPlus Met Tablets 3071
▲ Actos Tablets (2% to 4%) 3077
Aggrenox Capsules 819
Angiomax for Injection (0.6% to 1.9%) 1933
▲ Argatroban Injection (10.4%) 1308
Atacand Tablets 639
Atacand HCT 642
Avandamet Tablets 1336
Avandaryl Tablets 1344
Avandia Tablets 1351
Avapro Tablets (Less than 0.2%) 897
Avapro Tablets (Less than 0.2%) 2718
Avelox (Greater than or equal to 2%) 2803
Azor Tablets 1005
Benicar Tablets 1009
▲ Cancidas for Injection (5.4% to 20.5%) 1953
Celebrex Capsules 2979
Cipro I.V. (Among most frequent) 2817
Cipro (Less than 0.1%) 2810
Cipro XR Tablets 2823
Crixivan Capsules (0.6%) 1979
Dapsone Tablets USP (Almost all patients) 1746
Diovan HCT Tablets (Greater than 0.1%) 2216
Eligard 7.5 mg (Less than 2%) 2724
Eligard 22.5 mg (Less than 2%) 2724
Eligard 30 mg (Less than 2%) 2724
Eligard 45 mg (Less than 2%) 2724
▲ Emend Capsules (3.8%) 1992
▲ Emend for Injection (3.8%) 1999
Emtriva Capsules (1 patient) 1246
Emtriva Oral Solution (1 patient) 1246
▲ Epivir (2.2% to 4%) 1412
Fenoglide Tablets 2960
Fentora Tablets (Greater than 1%) 968
▲ Invanz for Injection (4.5% to 4.9%) 2029
Keppra Injection 3137
Keppra Oral Solution 3131
Keppra Tablets 3131
▲ Letairis Tablets (7%) 1258
▲ Lupron Depot 7.5 mg (Greater than or equal to 5%) 469
Merrem I.V. (Greater than 0.2%) 684
Micardis Tablets 852
Micardis HCT Tablets (1.2%) 854
Mustargen for Injection 2492
▲ Myfortic Tablets (3% to less than 20%) 2276
▲ Neupro Transdermal System (4% to 8%) 3149
Noroxin Tablets (0.6%) 2069
▲ Novantrone for Injection Concentrate (43% to 75%) 1100
Omnicef Capsules (0.3%) 497
Omnicef for Oral Suspension (0.4%) 497
▲ PegIntron Powder for Injection (30%) 2903
Primaxin I.M. 2080
Primaxin I.V. 2083
Prinivil Tablets (Frequent) 2087
Prinzide Tablets (Frequent) 2092
Proglycem Capsules (Infrequent) 1185
Proglycem Suspension (Infrequent) 1185
Rebetol 2917
Refludan for Injection 795
ReoPro Vials (7 to 11 events) 1860
Requip Tablets (Infrequent) 1561
Rythmol SR Capsules 1590
Tekturna Tablets 2321
Tekturna HCT Tablets (0.1%) 2324
▲ Temodar Capsules (51%) 2931
Teveten Tablets (0.1%) 515
Teveten HCT Tablets (0.1%) 517
Timentin ADD-Vantage 1606
Timentin Injection Galaxy Container 1609
Timentin IV Infusion 1603
Timentin Pharmacy Bulk Package 1613
▲ Torisel Injection (20% to 94%) 3272
Tracleer Tablets 3289
▲ Treanda for Injection (13% to 89%) 983
Valtrex Caplets (Up to 0.8%) 1635

▲ Viramune Oral Suspension (0% to 3.2%) 873
▲ Viramune Tablets (0% to 3.2%) 873
WinRho SDF 741
Xeloda Tablets (1%) 2662
Zinacef for Injection (1 in 10 patients) 1678
Zinacef Injection (1 in 10 patients) 1678
Zosyn for Injection 3284

Hemoglobin, increase
AndroGel 3159
Testim 1% Gel (1% to 2%) 701

Hemoglobin abnormalities, unspecified
▲ Tykerb Tablets (0% to 56%) 1631

Hemoglobin content, deviation
Amerge Tablets (Rare) 1301
Diovan Tablets (0.4%) 2212
▲ Intron A for Injection (Up to 32%) 2859

Hemoglobinemia
Stromectol Tablets (1%) 2120

Hemoglobinuria
Mycamine for Injection 616
Raptiva for Injection 1218
WinRho SDF 741

Hemolysis
Aczone Gel 5% 3296
Cozaar Tablets 1973
Dapsone Tablets USP (Most common) 1746
▲ Doxil Injection (1% to 5%) 2378
Elitek (Less than 1%) 2729
Flebogamma 5% 1715
Flebogamma 5% DIF 1718
Gammagard Liquid 730
Gammagard S/D 734
Gamunex 3094
Mycamine for Injection 616
Trasylol Injection (0.3%) 799

Hemolysis, intravascular
Alphanate 1709
Mycamine for Injection 616

Hemolysis, neonatal
Dapsone Tablets USP 1746
Mephyton Tablets 700

Hemolytic icterus
(*see under* Jaundice)

Hemolytic-uremic syndrome
Eloxatin for Injection 2731
Gemzar for Injection (Rare) 1820
Gengraf Capsules 435
Lybrel Tablets 3204
Mircette Tablets 1034
Neoral Oral Solution 2280
Neoral Soft Gelatin Capsules 2280
Noxafil Oral Suspension (Rare) 2889
NuvaRing 2897
Ortho-Cyclen Tablets 2449
Ortho Evra Transdermal System 2437
Ortho Tri-Cyclen Tablets 2449
Ortho Tri-Cyclen Lo Tablets 2458
Prograf Capsules and Injection 622
▲ Rapamune (Greater than or equal to 3% to less than 20%) 3260
Seasonique Tablets 1046
Valtrex Caplets 1635
Yaz Tablets 805

Hemopericardium
Cardene I.V. (0.7%) 1093

Hemoperitoneum
Follistim AQ Cartridge 2844
Merrem I.V. (0.2%) 684
Trasylol Injection (1% to 2%) 799

Hemophilus
▲ Intron A for Injection (Less than 5%) 2859

Hemoptysis
Abelcet Injection 1134
Actiq (Less than 1%) 959
Aggrenox Capsules (Less than 1%) 819
AmBisome for Injection (Less common) 606
Argatroban Injection (2.9%) 1308
▲ Busulfex Injection (3%) 2477
▲ CellCept Capsules (3% to less than 20%) 2622
▲ CellCept Intravenous (3% to less than 20%) 2622
▲ CellCept Oral Suspension (3% to less than 20%) 2622
▲ CellCept Tablets (3% to less than 20%) 2622
Cipro I.V. (1% or less) 2817
Cipro (Less than 1%) 2810
Cipro XR Tablets 2823
Dacogen Injection 1066
Duragesic Transdermal System (1% or greater) 2405
Effexor XR Extended-Release Capsules (Rare) 3195
▲ Eloxatin for Injection (2% to less than 5%) 2731
Evoxac Capsules (Less than 1%) 1013
Gabitril Tablets (Infrequent) 973
▲ Intron A for Injection (Less than or equal to 5%) 2859
Invanz for Injection (Greater than 0.1%) 2029
▲ Lupron Depot 7.5 mg (Less than 5%) 469
Luvox CR Extended-Release Capsules (Rare) 1759
Namenda (Infrequent) 1180
Natrecor for Injection (Greater than or equal to 1%) 2977
Neupogen for Injection 589
Paxil (Rare) 1535
Paxil CR Controlled-Release Tablets (Rare) 1544
Photofrin for Injection (One patient) 708
Plavix Tablets (Less than 1%) 926
Plavix Tablets (Less than 1%) 2767
Pletal Tablets (Less than 2%) 2481
Prinivil Tablets (0.3% to 1%) 2087
Prinzide Tablets 2092
Proleukin for Injection (Less than 1%) 2287
Prozac Weekly Capsules (Rare) 1852
Prozac Pulvules and Liquid (Rare) 1852
Pulmozyme Inhalation Solution 1217
ReoPro Vials (9 to 11 events) 1860
Requip Tablets (Infrequent) 1561
Rilutek Tablets (Infrequent) 2771
Risperdal Consta Long-Acting Injection (Infrequent) 1753
Rythmol SR Capsules 1590
Symbyax Capsules (Rare) 1871
Targretin Capsules 1084
▲ Trisenox Injection (8%) 986
Velcade for Injection 2168
Venlafaxine Hydrochloride Tablets (Rare) 2199
▲ Xeloda Tablets (Less than 5%) 2662
Zolinza Capsules 2142
Zonegran Capsules (Rare) 1089
Zyprexa Tablets (Infrequent) 1883
Zyprexa ZYDIS Orally Disintegrating Tablets (Infrequent) 1883

Hemorrhage
(*see under* Bleeding)

Hemorrhage, alveolar
Neupogen for Injection 589

Hemorrhage, cerebral
(*see under* Cerebral hemorrhage)

Hemorrhage, CNS
Elspar for Injection 2488
▲ Gleevec Tablets (0% to 9%) 2255

Hemorrhage, colon
Actiq (Less than 1%) 959
Prozac Weekly Capsules (Rare) 1852
Prozac Pulvules and Liquid (Rare) 1852

Hemorrhage, conjunctival
Exelon Capsules (Infrequent) 2229
Exelon Oral Solution (Infrequent) 2229
▲ Gleevec Tablets (0% to 27%) 2255
Namenda (Infrequent) 1180
Plavix Tablets 926
Plavix Tablets 2767
Stromectol Tablets 2120
Treximet Tablets (Rare) 1616
Triesence Injectable Suspension (2%) ⊙209

Hemorrhage, ear
Imitrex Nasal Spray 1470
Relenza Inhalation Powder (Less than 1%) 1556

Hemorrhage, esophageal
Demadex Injection 2630
Demadex Tablets 2630
Pletal Tablets (Less than 2%) 2481
Protonix for Delayed-Release Oral Suspension (Less than 1%) 3254
Protonix Delayed-Release Tablets (Less than 1%) 3254
Protonix I.V. (Less than 1%) 3257

Hemorrhage, eye, anterior chamber
Evoxac Capsules (Less than 1%) 1013

Hemorrhage, eyes
Actiq (Less than 1%) 959
AmBisome for Injection (Less common) 606
Amerge Tablets (Rare) 1301
▲ CellCept Capsules (3% to less than 20%) 2622
▲ CellCept Intravenous (3% to less than 20%) 2622
▲ CellCept Oral Suspension (3% to less than 20%) 2622
▲ CellCept Tablets (3% to less than 20%) 2622
Effexor XR Extended-Release Capsules 3195
Imitrex Nasal Spray 1470
▲ Leukine (11%) 774
Lipitor Tablets (Less than 2%) 2501
Lyrica Capsules (0.1% to 1%) 2527
Mirapex Tablets 857
Paxil (Rare) 1535
Paxil CR Controlled-Release Tablets (Rare) 1544
Plavix Tablets 926
Plavix Tablets 2767
Pletal Tablets (Less than 2%) 2481
Prozac Weekly Capsules (Rare) 1852
Prozac Pulvules and Liquid (Rare) 1852
ReoPro Vials (9 to 11 events) 1860
Rythmol SR Capsules 1590
Salagen Tablets (Less than 1%) 1082
Soriatane Capsules (Less than 1%) 3062
Symbyax Capsules (Rare) 1871
Tasigna Capsules (0.1% to 1%) 2316
Venlafaxine Hydrochloride Tablets 2199
Zyprexa Tablets (Infrequent) 1883
Zyprexa ZYDIS Orally Disintegrating Tablets (Infrequent) 1883
Zyrtec-D 12 Hour Extended Release Tablets (Less than 2%) 1923

Hemorrhage, focal
▲ Thyrogen for Injection (4 patients out of 55) 1244
Voltaren Ophthalmic Solution 2336

Hemorrhage, gastrointestinal
(*see under* Bleeding, gastrointestinal)

Hemorrhage, gum
Elmiron Capsules 2435
Lamictal (Rare) 1488
Prozac Weekly Capsules (Infrequent) 1852
Venlafaxine Hydrochloride Tablets (Rare) 2199

Hemorrhage, hepatic
Velcade for Injection 2168

Hemorrhage, intra-alveolar
▲ Busulfex Injection (5%) 2477
Cuprimine Capsules (Rare) 1986

Hemorrhage, intracerebral
(*see under* Bleeding, intracerebral)

Hemorrhage, intracranial
Aptivus Capsules (Less than 2%) 823
Aptivus Oral Solution (Less than 2%) 823
Cardene I.V. (0.7%) 1093
Dacogen Injection (Greater than or equal to 1%) 1066
Mycamine for Injection 616
NovoSeven RT 2370
Salagen Tablets (Less than 1%) 1082
Sandostatin LAR Depot 2302
Tasigna Capsules (0.1% to 1%) 2316

Hemorrhage, intraventricular
▲ NeoProfen Injection (15% to 29%) 2496

Hemorrhage, ocular
Zyrtec Chewable Tablets (Less than 2%) 1920
Zyrtec Syrup (Less than 2%) 1920
Zyrtec Tablets (Less than 2%) 1920

Hemorrhage, post-menopausal
Requip Tablets (Infrequent) 1561

Hemorrhage, postpartum
Aggrenox Capsules 819
Bayer Aspirin 750
St. Joseph 81 mg Aspirin Chewable and Enteric Coated Tablets 1903

Hemorrhage, post-procedural
▲ Fabrazyme for Intravenous Infusion (5%) 1241
▲ Gleevec Tablets (0% to 27%) 2255
Requip Tablets (Infrequent) 1561

Hemorrhage, pulmonary
Mylotarg for Injection 3212
Photofrin for Injection 708
Plavix Tablets (Less than 1%) 926
Plavix Tablets (Less than 1%) 2767
Pletal Tablets 2481
Rapamune 3260
ReoPro Vials (9 to 11 events) 1860
Sutent Capsules (2 patients) 2540

Hemorrhage, purpuric
Carbatrol Capsules 3019

Hemorrhage, rectal
Ambien Tablets (Rare) 2692
Ambien CR Tablets (Rare) 2696
Amitiza Capsules (Less than 1%) 3082
Aricept Tablets (Infrequent) 1062
Aricept ODT Tablets (Infrequent) 1062
Brovana Inhalation Solution (Less than 2%) 2990
Campral Tablets (Infrequent) 1158
Demadex Injection 2630
Demadex Tablets 2630
▲ Elmiron Capsules (6.3%) 2435
▲ Eloxatin for Injection (2% to less than 5%) 2731
Emsam Transdermal System (Rare) 905
Luvox CR Extended-Release Capsules (Infrequent) 1759
Lyrica Capsules (0.1% to 1%) 2527
Mirapex Tablets 857
Prozac Weekly Capsules (Rare) 1852
Prozac Pulvules and Liquid (Rare) 1852
Requip Tablets (Infrequent) 1561
Risperdal Consta Long-Acting Injection (Infrequent) 1753
Sutent Capsules 2540
Tricor Tablets 520
Venlafaxine Hydrochloride Tablets (Infrequent) 2199
Zyrtec Chewable Tablets (Less than 2%) 1920
Zyrtec Syrup (Less than 2%) 1920
Zyrtec Tablets (Less than 2%) 1920
Zyrtec-D 12 Hour Extended Release Tablets (Less than 2%) 1923

Hemorrhage, retinal
Aricept Tablets (Infrequent) 1062
Aricept ODT Tablets (Infrequent) 1062
Cimzia 3127
Effexor XR Extended-Release Capsules (Rare) 3195
Elitek (Less than or equal to 1%) 2729
Elmiron Capsules (Less than or equal to 1%) 2435
Gleevec Tablets (Rare) 2255
Intron A for Injection (Rare) 2859
Namenda (Infrequent) 1180
Paxil (Rare) 1535
Paxil CR Controlled-Release Tablets (Rare) 1544
PegIntron Powder for Injection 2903
Plavix Tablets 926
Plavix Tablets 2767
Pletal Tablets (Less than 2%) 2481
Venlafaxine Hydrochloride Tablets (Rare) 2199
▲ Visudyne for Injection (1% to 10%) 2332

Hemorrhage, retroperitoneal
Proleukin for Injection 2287

Hemorrhage, subarachnoid
Aggrenox Capsules (Less than 1%) 819
Amerge Tablets 1301
Imitrex Injection 1465
Imitrex Nasal Spray 1470
Imitrex Tablets 1474
Orthoclone OKT3 Sterile Solution 2387
Requip Tablets (Rare) 1561
Rilutek Tablets (Rare) 2771
Symbyax Capsules (Rare) 1871
Treximet Tablets 1616
Zyprexa Tablets (Rare) 1883
Zyprexa ZYDIS Orally Disintegrating Tablets (Rare) 1883

Hemorrhage, subconjunctival
Effexor XR Extended-Release Capsules (Rare) 3195
Proglycem Capsules (Infrequent) 1185

Proglycem Suspension (Infrequent) 1185
▲ Travatan Z Ophthalmic Solution (1% to 4%) 547
Venlafaxine Hydrochloride Tablets (Rare) 2199
▲ Vigamox Ophthalmic Solution (1% to 6%) 548
▲ Visudyne for Injection (1% to 10%) 2332

Hemorrhage, subcutaneous
Mustargen for Injection 2492
Pletal Tablets 2481

Hemorrhage, throat
Imitrex Nasal Spray 1470
Relenza Inhalation Powder (Less than 1%) 1556

Hemorrhage, tumor
▲ Gleevec Tablets (1% to 4%) 2255
Zolinza Capsules 2142

Hemorrhage, uterine
Mirapex Tablets 857
Prozac Weekly Capsules (Rare) 1852
Prozac Pulvules and Liquid (Rare) 1852
Venlafaxine Hydrochloride Tablets (Rare) 2199

Hemorrhage, vaginal
▲ Eloxatin for Injection (2% to less than 5%) 2731
▲ Femara Tablets (Less than 0.1% to 4.8%) 2246
Mirapex Tablets 857
▲ Noxafil Oral Suspension (10%) 2889
Prozac Weekly Capsules (Infrequent) 1852
Salagen Tablets (Less than 1%) 1082
Venlafaxine Hydrochloride Tablets (Infrequent) 2199

Hemorrhage, vitreous
Gleevec Tablets (Rare) 2255
▲ Visudyne for Injection (1% to 10%) 2332

Hemorrhagic colitis
Amoxil Capsules 1305
Amoxil Chewable Tablets 1305
Amoxil Pediatric Drops for Oral Suspension 1305
Amoxil Powder for Oral Suspension 1305
Amoxil Tablets 1305
Augmentin 1323
Augmentin Tablets 1327
Augmentin XR Extended Release Tablets 1333
Kaletra (Less than 2%) 452
Lamictal (Rare) 1488
Omnicef Capsules 497
Omnicef for Oral Suspension 497
Primaxin I.M. 2080
Primaxin I.V. (Less than 0.2%) 2083

Hemorrhagic complications
Lovenox Injection (Low incidence) 2756
Zolinza Capsules 2142

Hemorrhagic eruptions
(*see under* Eruptions, hemorrhagic)

Hemorrhagic tendency
Mustargen for Injection 2492

Hemorrhoids
Aggrenox Capsules (1%) 819
Ambien Tablets (Rare) 2692
Ambien CR Tablets (Rare) 2696
AmBisome for Injection (Less common) 606
Amerge Tablets (Rare) 1301
Aricept Tablets (Infrequent) 1062
Aricept ODT Tablets (Infrequent) 1062
Celebrex Capsules (0.1% to 1.9%) 2979
Celexa (Infrequent) 1160
▲ Chemet Capsules (12% to 20.9%) 2484
▲ Dacogen Injection (8%) 1066
▲ DepoCyt Injection (3%) 1136
Effexor XR Extended-Release Capsules (Infrequent) 3195
▲ Eloxatin for Injection (2% to less than 5%) 2731
Evoxac Capsules (Less than 1%) 1013
Exelon Capsules (Infrequent) 2229
Exelon Oral Solution (Infrequent) 2229
Invanz for Injection (Greater than 0.1%) 2029
Klonopin (Infrequent) 2639
Lexapro Oral Suspension (Infrequent) 1174
Lexapro Tablets (Infrequent) 1174
Luvox CR Extended-Release Capsules (Infrequent) 1759
Micardis Tablets (More than 0.3%) 852
Micardis HCT Tablets 854
Mirapex Tablets 857
Requip Tablets (Infrequent) 1561
Risperdal Consta Long-Acting Injection (Infrequent) 1753
Sandostatin Injection (Less than 1%) 2300
Soriatane Capsules (Less than 1%) 3062
Venlafaxine Hydrochloride Tablets (Infrequent) 2199
Vivitrol 988
Zyrtec Chewable Tablets (Less than 2%) 1920
Zyrtec Syrup (Less than 2%) 1920
Zyrtec Tablets (Less than 2%) 1920
Zyrtec-D 12 Hour Extended Release Tablets (Less than 2%) 1923

Hemothorax
Plavix Tablets (Less than 1%) 926
Plavix Tablets (Less than 1%) 2767
Refludan for Injection 795

Henoch-Schönlein purpura
Aldara Cream, 5% 1699
Boostrix 1377
Cozaar Tablets 1973
Exjade Tablets 2244
Fluarix Vaccine 1446
Luvox CR Extended-Release Capsules 1759
Paxil 1535
Paxil CR Controlled-Release Tablets 1544
ProQuad 2099
Stalevo Tablets 2309
Varivax 2133

Hepatic adenoma
Estratest Tablets (Rare) 3043
Estratest H.S. Tablets (Rare) 3043
Lybrel Tablets 3204
Mircette Tablets 1034
Ortho-Cyclen Tablets 2449
Ortho Evra Transdermal System 2437
Ortho Tri-Cyclen Tablets 2449
Ortho Tri-Cyclen Lo Tablets 2458
Premarin Intravenous 3217
Premarin Vaginal Cream 3228
Seasonique Tablets 1046
Yaz Tablets 805

Hepatic artery thrombosis
▲ Rapamune (7%) 3260

Hepatic dysfunction
Accolate Tablets 669
Actimmune (Rare) 1743
Advicor Tablets 402
Aggrenox Capsules (Less than 1%) 819
▲ Albenza Tablets (Less than 1% to 15.6%) 1297
Aldara Cream, 5% 1699
Ambien Tablets (Infrequent) 2692
Ambien CR Tablets (Infrequent) 2696
AmBisome for Injection (Less common) 606
Amerge Tablets (Rare) 1301
Amoxil Capsules 1305
Amoxil Chewable Tablets 1305
Amoxil Pediatric Drops for Oral Suspension 1305
Amoxil Powder for Oral Suspension 1305
Amoxil Tablets 1305
Amrix Capsules 966
Anaprox Tablets (Less than 1%) 2632
Anaprox DS Tablets (Less than 1%) 2632
▲ Anzemet Injection (3.6%) 2701
Aptivus Capsules 823
Aptivus Oral Solution 823
Arixtra Injection (0.4%) 1313
Atacand Tablets 639
Atacand HCT 642
Augmentin (Infrequent) 1323
Augmentin Tablets (Infrequent) 1327
Augmentin XR Extended Release Tablets (Infrequent) 1333
Augmentin ES-600 Powder for Oral Suspension (Infrequently) 1329
Avandaryl Tablets 1344
▲ Avinza Capsules (Less than 5%) 1772
Biaxin/Biaxin XL (Infrequent) 411
Bystolic Tablets 1155
Cancidas for Injection 1953
Capastat Sulfate for Injection 1791
Captopril Tablets 2182
Carbatrol Capsules 3019
Catapres Tablets 841
Ceftin 1380
Celebrex Capsules (0.1% to 1.9%) 2979
Cipro I.V. (Among most frequent) 2817
Clinoril Tablets (Less than 1 in 100) 1962
Concerta Extended-Release Tablets 1925
Cosmegen for Injection 2485
Crixivan Capsules 1979
Cuprimine Capsules 1986
Dantrium Capsules 2580
Daytrana Transdermal Patch 3022
Depakote ER Tablets 423
Diovan Tablets 2212
Doxil Injection 2378
Dyazide Capsules 1405
EC-Naprosyn Delayed-Release Tablets (Less than 1%) 2632
Edecrin (Rare) 698
E.E.S. 433
Effexor XR Extended-Release Capsules 3195
Engerix-B Vaccine 1409
Epivir 1412
EryPed 431
Estratest Tablets 3043
Estratest H.S. Tablets 3043
Evoxac Capsules (Less than 1%) 1013
Exelon Capsules (Infrequent) 2229
Exelon Oral Solution (Infrequent) 2229
Flebogamma 5% 1715
Flebogamma 5% DIF 1718
Fleet Phospho-soda 1145
Focalin XR Capsules 2251
Fortaz 1450
Gabitril Tablets (Infrequent) 973
Gammagard Liquid 730
Gammagard S/D 734
Gamunex 3094
Hepsera Tablets 1253
▲ Hycamtin for Injection (24%) 1459
Imitrex Injection (Infrequent) 1465
Imitrex Nasal Spray 1470
Imitrex Tablets 1474
▲ Intron A for Injection (Less than 5%) 2859
Kaletra 452
Ketek Tablets 2744
Lamictal (Infrequent) 1488
▲ Lamisil Tablets (3.3%) 2266
Leukine 774
Levaquin (0.1% to 1%) 2416
Levaquin in 5% Dextrose Injection (0.1% to 1%) 2416
Lipitor Tablets (Less than 2%) 2501
▲ Lumigan Ophthalmic Solution (1% to 5%) 556
Metadate CD Capsules 3146
Mevacor Tablets 2063
Moban Tablets (Rare) 1116
Moxatag Tablets 2165
Mycamine for Injection 616
Naprosyn Suspension (Less than 1%) 2632
Naprosyn Tablets (Less than 1%) 2632
Neupro Transdermal System 3149
▲ Nexavar Tablets (11%) 784
Nexium Delayed-Release Capsules (Less than 1%) 645
Nexium I.V. (Less than 1%) 652
Nexium Delayed-Release Oral Suspension (Less than 1%) 645
Niaspan Extended-Release Tablets 480
Nimotop Capsules (Up to 1.2%) 790
Norvir (Less than 2%) 489
NovoLog Injection 2359
Noxafil Oral Suspension (0% to 1%) 2889
Omnicef Capsules 497
Omnicef for Oral Suspension 497
Patanase Nasal Spray 544
Paxil 1535
Paxil CR Controlled-Release Tablets 1544
Pediarix Vaccine 1552
Persantine Tablets (Rare) 869
Phenytek Capsules 2192
Plavix Tablets 926
Plavix Tablets 2767
PrandiMet Tablets 2967
Prandin Tablets (Rare) 2971
Premarin Vaginal Cream 3228
▲ Prograf Capsules and Injection (5% to 36%) 622
Protopic Ointment (Greater than or equal to 1%) 628
▲ Provigil Tablets (2% to 3%) 977
Prozac Pulvules and Liquid (Infrequent) 1852
▲ Rebif Prefilled Syringe for Injection (4% to 18%) 1107
▲ Refludan for Injection (5.3%) 795
Remeron Tablets (Infrequent) 2924
RemeronSolTab Tablets (Infrequent) 2927
Remicade for IV Injection (Rare) 950
Reyataz Capsules 3299
Rilutek Tablets (Infrequent) 2771
Rocephin Injectable Vials, ADD-Vantage, Galaxy, Bulk 2642
Soriatane Capsules (Less than 1%) 3062
Strattera Capsules 1864
Sular Extended Release Tablets (Less than or equal to 1%) 2975
Suprax for Oral Suspension 1891
Suprax Tablets 1891
Synagis Intramuscular Solution (More than 1%) 1948
Tabloid Tablets (Occasional) 1601
▲ Tracleer Tablets (8%) 3289
▲ Trasylol Injection (3%) 799
Ultane Liquid for Inhalation (Less than 1%) 524
▲ Valcyte Tablets (Less than 5%) 2654
Valtrex Caplets 1635
Vantas (Less than 2%) 1737
Vaqta (Isolated reports) 2130
▲ Vesanoid Capsules (50% to 60%) 2660
Vicoprofen Tablets 533
Vytorin 10/10 Tablets 2939
Vytorin 10/20 Tablets 2939
Vytorin 10/40 Tablets 2939
Vytorin 10/80 Tablets 2939
Wellbutrin SR Sustained-Release Tablets (Infrequent) 1653
Wellbutrin XL Extended-Release Tablets (Infrequent) 1659
Zinacef for Injection 1678
Zinacef Injection 1678
Zofran Injection 1682
Zofran 1687
Zofran ODT Orally Disintegrating Tablets 1687
Zovirax 1690
Zyban Sustained-Release Tablets (Infrequent) 1692
Zyrtec Chewable Tablets (Less than 2%) 1920
Zyrtec Syrup (Less than 2%) 1920
Zyrtec Tablets (Less than 2%) 1920
Zyrtec-D 12 Hour Extended Release Tablets (Less than 2%) 1923
Zyvox (0.4% to 1.3%) 2552

Hepatic enzymes, elevation
(*see also under* Serum transaminase, elevation)
Accolate Tablets (Rare) 669
Accutane Capsules 2607
Aggrenox Capsules 819
Agrylin Capsules (2 of 551 patients) 3017
▲ Albenza Tablets (16%) 1297
▲ Anaprox Tablets (1% to 10%) 2632
▲ Anaprox DS Tablets (1% to 10%) 2632
Arixtra Injection (0.3%) 1313
Asacol Delayed-Release Tablets 2579
Atacand Tablets (Infrequent) 639
Atacand HCT 642
Avandamet Tablets 1336
Avandia Tablets 1351
Avapro Tablets 897
Avapro Tablets (Very rare) 2718
Azor Tablets 1005
Benicar Tablets (Infrequently) 1009
Betaseron for SC Injection 756
Biaxin/Biaxin XL (Infrequent) 411
Canasa Rectal Suppositories 705
Captopril Tablets 2182
Ceftin for Oral Suspension (0.1% to 1%) 1380
Celexa (Infrequent) 1160
Clarinex Syrup (Rare) 2828
Clarinex Tablets (Rare) 2828
Clarinex Reditabs Tablets (Rare) 2828
Comvax 1966
Coreg Tablets (Greater than 0.1% to 1%) 1387
Crestor Tablets 677
Dantrium Capsules 2580
Depakote ER Tablets 423
Diovan Tablets 2212
Diovan HCT Tablets 2216
Dyazide Capsules 1405
DynaCirc CR Controlled Release Tablets (0.5% to 1%) 1407
Dyrenium Capsules (Rare) 3189
▲ EC-Naprosyn Delayed-Release Tablets (1% to 10%) 2632
EryPed 431
Evoxac Capsules (Less than 1%) 1013
▲ Hycamtin for Injection (Less than 1% to 8%) 1459
Imitrex Nasal Spray 1470
Imitrex Tablets 1474

Ketek Tablets (Greater than or equal to 0.2% to less than 2%) 2744
Lescol Capsules 2268
Lescol XL Tablets 2268
Micardis HCT Tablets 854
MS Contin Tablets (Less frequent) 2585
Nadolol Tablets 2191
▲ Naprosyn Suspension (1% to 10%) 2632
▲ Naprosyn Tablets (1% to 10%) 2632
Niaspan Extended-Release Tablets 480
Noroxin Tablets 2069
Paxil 1535
Paxil CR Controlled-Release Tablets 1544
Percodan Tablets 1130
Persantine Tablets 869
Plavix Tablets (1% to 2.5%) 926
Plavix Tablets (1% to 2.5%) 2767
Prinivil Tablets (Rare) 2087
Prinzide Tablets (Rare) 2092
Provigil Tablets (At least 1%) 977
Rebif Prefilled Syringe for Injection 1107
Recombivax HB 2107
Risperdal Consta Long-Acting Injection (Frequent) 1753
St. Joseph 81 mg Aspirin Chewable and Enteric Coated Tablets 1903
Sandostatin Injection (Less than 1%) 2300
Sustiva Capsules 930
Sustiva Tablets 930
Tabloid Tablets (Occasional) 1601
Tarka Tablets (2.8%) 511
Trizivir Tablets 1622
▲ Vicoprofen Tablets (Up to 15%) 533
▲ Visudyne for Injection (1% to 10%) 2332
▲ Voltaren Tablets (1% to 10%) 2334
▲ Voltaren-XR Tablets (1% to 10%) 2337
Zovirax 1690

Hepatic enzymes, increased
Abilify Injection (Greater than or equal to 1 in 1000 patients and less than 1 in 100 patients) 881
Abilify Injection (Greater than or equal to 1 in 1000 patients and less than 1 in 100 patients) 2466
Abilify Oral Solution (Greater than or equal to 1 in 1000 patients and less than 1 in 100 patients) 881
Abilify Oral Solution (Greater than or equal to 1 in 1000 patients and less than 1 in 100 patients) 2466
Abilify Discmelt Orally Disintegrating Tablets (Greater than or equal to 1 in 1000 patients and less than 1 in 100 patients) 881
Abilify Discmelt Orally Disintegrating Tablets (Greater than or equal to 1 in 1000 patients and less than 1 in 100 patients) 2466
Abilify Tablets (Greater than or equal to 1 in 1000 patients and less than 1 in 100 patients) 881
Abilify Tablets (Greater than or equal to 1 in 1000 patients and less than 1 in 100 patients) 2466
Aciphex Tablets 1053
Aptivus Capsules (Less than 2%) 823
Aptivus Oral Solution (Less than 2%) 823
Atripla Tablets 938
Coreg CR Extended-Release Capsules (0.1% to less than or equal to 1%) 1393
Doribax Injection (1% to 2%) 2400
Exforge Tablets 2238
Levaquin (0.1% to 1%) 2416
Levaquin in 5% Dextrose Injection (0.1% to 1%) 2416
Lexapro Oral Suspension (Infrequent) 1174
Lexapro Tablets (Infrequent) 1174
MS Contin Tablets (Less frequent) 2585
▲ Noxafil Oral Suspension (Less than 1% to 3%) 2889
OxyContin Tablets (Less than 1%) 2589

Hepatic eosinophilic infiltration
Singulair (Very rare) 2114

Hepatic failure
Abelcet Injection 1134
Accolate Tablets (Rare) 669
Aceon Tablets (2 mg, 4 mg, 8 mg) 3038
Aggrenox Capsules 819
Anaprox Tablets (Less than 1%) 2632
Anaprox DS Tablets (Less than 1%) 2632
Aptivus Capsules (Less than 2%) 823
Aptivus Oral Solution (Less than 2%) 823
Asacol Delayed-Release Tablets (Rare) 2579
Atripla Tablets 938
Avelox 2803
Biaxin/Biaxin XL (Very rare) 411
Cancidas for Injection 1953
Captopril Tablets (Rare) 2182
Celebrex Capsules (Less than 0.1%) 2979
Cipro I.V. (Rare) 2817
Cipro 2810
Cipro XR Tablets 2823
Clinoril Tablets (Less than 1 in 100) 1962
Cosmegen for Injection 2485
Crixivan Capsules 1979
Cuprimine Capsules 1986
Depakote ER Tablets 423
Doxil Injection (Less than 1%) 2378
EC-Naprosyn Delayed-Release Tablets (Less than 1%) 2632
Effexor XR Extended-Release Capsules 3195
Elspar for Injection 1990
Elspar for Injection 2488
Exjade Tablets 2244
Flolan for Injection 1426
Gemzar for Injection (Rare) 1820
Gleevec Tablets (Rare) 2255
Intron A for Injection (Very rare) 2859
Ixempra Kit for Injection 915
Keppra Injection 3137
Keppra Oral Solution 3131
Keppra Tablets 3131
Lamisil Oral Granules 2264
Lamisil Tablets (Rare) 2266
Levaquin 2416
Levaquin in 5% Dextrose Injection 2416
Lexapro Oral Suspension 1174
Lexapro Tablets 1174
Malarone Pediatric Tablets 1521
Malarone Tablets 1521
Mavik Tablets (Rare) 472
Merrem I.V. (Greater than 0.1% to 1%) 684
Mobic Oral Suspension (Less than 0.1%) 863
Mobic Tablets (Less than 0.1%) 863
Mycamine for Injection 616
Mylotarg for Injection 3212
Namenda 1180
Naprosyn Suspension (Less than 1%) 2632
Naprosyn Tablets (Less than 1%) 2632
Nexium Delayed-Release Capsules 645
Nexium I.V. 652
Nexium Delayed-Release Oral Suspension 645
Noxafil Oral Suspension (Rare) 2889
Omnicef Capsules 497
Omnicef for Oral Suspension 497
Pentasa Capsules 3030
Percocet Tablets 1127
Persantine Tablets 869
Primaxin I.M. 2080
Primaxin I.V. 2083
Prinivil Tablets (Rare) 2087
Prinzide Tablets (Rare) 2092
Proleukin for Injection (Less than 1%) 2287
Protonix for Delayed-Release Oral Suspension 3254
Protonix Delayed-Release Tablets 3254
Protonix I.V. 3257
Prozac Weekly Capsules 1852
Prozac Pulvules and Liquid 1852
Pylera Capsules 714
Rebif Prefilled Syringe for Injection (Very rare) 1107
Remicade for IV Injection 950
Rituxan I.V. 1223
Selzentry Tablets 2534
Solodyn Extended Release Tablets 1938
Sustiva Capsules 930
Sustiva Tablets 930
Sutent Capsules (Less than 1%) 2540
Targretin Capsules 1084
Tracleer Tablets 3289
Trasylol Injection (1% to 2%) 799
Trizivir Tablets 1622
Velcade for Injection 2168
Venlafaxine Hydrochloride Tablets 2199
Vicoprofen Tablets 533
Viramune Oral Suspension 873
Viramune Tablets 873
Voltaren Tablets (Rarely) 2334
Voltaren-XR Tablets (Rarely) 2337
Vytorin 10/10 Tablets 2149
Vytorin 10/10 Tablets 2939
Vytorin 10/20 Tablets 2149
Vytorin 10/20 Tablets 2939
Vytorin 10/40 Tablets 2149
Vytorin 10/40 Tablets 2939
Vytorin 10/80 Tablets 2149
Vytorin 10/80 Tablets 2939
▲ Xeloda Tablets (Less than 5%) 2662
Zantac 25 EFFERdose Tablets (Rare) 1670
Zantac Injection (Rare) 1666
Zantac Injection Pharmacy Bulk Package (Rare) 1668
Zantac Injection Premixed (Rare) 1666
Zantac (Rare) 1670
Ziagen 1673
Zocor Tablets 2136
Zofran Injection 1682
Zofran 1687
Zofran ODT Orally Disintegrating Tablets 1687

Hepatic failure, fatal
Cymbalta Delayed-Release Capsules 1801
Mepron Suspension 1526
Noroxin Tablets 2069

Hepatic failure, fulminant
Elspar for Injection 1990
Elspar for Injection 2488
Zofran Injection Premixed 1682

Hepatic function tests, impaired
(*see under* Hepatic dysfunction)

Hepatic hemangioma, exacerbation of
Activella Tablets 2347
Climara Transdermal System 763
Enjuvia Tablets 1029
Premarin Tablets 3221

Hepatic hemangioma, enlargement
Activella Tablets 2347
Angeliq Tablets 751
Divigel 3167
Enjuvia Tablets 1029
Premarin Intravenous 3217
Premarin Vaginal Cream 3228
Premphase Tablets 3232
Prempro Tablets 3232

Hepatic necrosis
Aceon Tablets (2 mg, 4 mg, 8 mg) (Rare) 3038
Advicor Tablets 402
Asacol Delayed-Release Tablets (Rare) 2579
Avelox 2803
Cancidas for Injection 1953
Captopril Tablets (Rare) 2182
Celebrex Capsules (Rare) 2979
Celexa 1160
Cipro I.V. (1% or less) 2817
Cipro 2810
Cipro XR Tablets 2823
Effexor XR Extended-Release Capsules 3195
Fansidar Tablets 2636
Gantrisin Pediatric Suspension 2638
▲ Humira Injection (Less than 5%) 442
Lescol Capsules (Rare) 2268
Lescol XL Tablets 2268
Levaquin 2416
Levaquin in 5% Dextrose Injection 2416
Lexapro Oral Suspension 1174
Lexapro Tablets 1174
Mavik Tablets (Rare) 472
Mevacor Tablets (Rare) 2063
Myleran Tablets 1530
Niaspan Extended-Release Tablets 480
Noroxin Tablets 2069
Paxil 1535
Paxil CR Controlled-Release Tablets 1544
Pentasa Capsules 3030
Percocet Tablets 1127
Prinivil Tablets (Rare) 2087
Prinzide Tablets (Rare) 2092
Prograf Capsules and Injection 622
Prozac Weekly Capsules 1852
Rapamune 3260
Tabloid Tablets 1601
Tarka Tablets (Rare) 511
Treximet Tablets 1616
Trusopt Sterile Ophthalmic Solution (Rare) 2128
Venlafaxine Hydrochloride Tablets 2199
Vicoprofen Tablets 533
Viramune Oral Suspension 873
Viramune Tablets 873
Zonegran Capsules (Rare) 1089

Hepatic reaction
Noxafil Oral Suspension 2889
▲ Viramune Oral Suspension (4%) 873
▲ Viramune Tablets (4%) 873

Hepatic veno-occlusive disease
Abelcet Injection 1134
AmBisome for Injection (Less common) 606
▲ Busulfex Injection (8%) 2477
Cosmegen for Injection 2485
Eloxatin for Injection 2731
Myleran Tablets 1530
▲ Mylotarg for Injection (5%) 3212
Tabloid Tablets 1601

Hepatitis
Abelcet Injection 1134
Abilify Injection (Less than 1 in 1000 patients) 881
Abilify Injection (Less than 1 in 1000 patients) 2466
Abilify Oral Solution (Less than 1 in 1000 patients) 881
Abilify Oral Solution (Less than 1 in 1000 patients) 2466
Abilify Discmelt Orally Disintegrating Tablets (Less than 1 in 1000 patients) 881
Abilify Discmelt Orally Disintegrating Tablets (Less than 1 in 1000 patients) 2466
Abilify Tablets (Less than 1 in 1000 patients) 881
Abilify Tablets (Less than 1 in 1000 patients) 2466
Accutane Capsules 2607
Aciphex Tablets 1053
Advicor Tablets 402
Aggrenox Capsules 819
Albenza Tablets 1297
Amevive (1 case) 611
Amrix Capsules 966
Anaprox Tablets (Less than 1%) 2632
Anaprox DS Tablets (Less than 1%) 2632
Aptivus Capsules (Less than 2%) 823
Aptivus Oral Solution (Less than 2%) 823
Aricept Tablets 1062
Aricept ODT Tablets 1062
Arimidex Tablets (Greater than or equal to 0.1% to less than 1%) 672
Asacol Delayed-Release Tablets (Rare) 2579
Atacand Tablets 639
Atacand HCT 642
Atripla Tablets 938
Augmentin (Rare) 1323
Augmentin Tablets (Rare) 1327
Augmentin XR Extended Release Tablets 1333
Augmentin ES-600 Powder for Oral Suspension 1329
Avalide Tablets 892
Avandamet Tablets 1336
Avandaryl Tablets 1344
Avandia Tablets 1351
Avapro Tablets 897
Avapro Tablets (Very rare) 2718
Avelox 2803
Axid Capsules 1364
Azor Tablets 1005
Bayer Aspirin 750
Betaseron for SC Injection 756
Campral Tablets (Infrequent) 1158
Cancidas for Injection 1953
Captopril Tablets 2182
Carbatrol Capsules 3019
Catapres Tablets (Rare) 841
Ceftin 1380
Celebrex Capsules (Less than 0.1%) 2979
Celexa (Rare) 1160
▲ CellCept Capsules (3% to less than 20%) 2622
▲ CellCept Intravenous (3% to less than 20%) 2622
▲ CellCept Oral Suspension (3% to less than 20%) 2622
▲ CellCept Tablets (3% to less than 20%) 2622
Cimzia 3127
Cipro I.V. (1% or less) 2817
Cipro (Less than 1%) 2810
Cipro XR Tablets 2823
Clarinex Syrup (Very rare) 2828
Clarinex Tablets (Very rare) 2828
Clarinex Reditabs Tablets (Very rare) 2828
Clarinex-D 12-Hour Extended-Release Tablets (Very rare) 2831

Clarinex-D 24-Hour Extended-Release Tablets (Very rare) 2834
Clinoril Tablets (Less than 1%) 1962
Clorpres Tablets (Rare) 2185
Cosmegen for Injection 2485
Cozaar Tablets (Rare) 1973
Crestor Tablets 677
Crixivan Capsules 1979
Dantrium Capsules (Less frequent) 2580
Depakote ER Tablets 423
Diovan Tablets 2212
Diovan HCT Tablets (Very rare) 2216
Doxil Injection (Less than 1%) 2378
Duetact Tablets (Rare) 3085
EC-Naprosyn Delayed-Release Tablets (Less than 1%) 2632
E.E.S. 433
Effexor XR Extended-Release Capsules (Rare) 3195
Enbrel for Injection 569
Equetro Extended-Release Capsules 3174
EryPed 431
Exforge Tablets 2238
Fansidar Tablets 2636
Fenoglide Tablets 2960
Gantrisin Pediatric Suspension 2638
Gleevec Tablets (Infrequent) 2255
Havrix Injection Vaccine 1454
Intelence Tablets (Less than 2%) 3119
Isentress Tablets 2036
Keppra Injection 3137
Keppra Oral Solution 3131
Keppra Tablets 3131
Ketek Tablets (Greater than or equal to 0.2% to less than 2%) 2744
Lamictal (Rare) 1488
Lescol Capsules 2268
Lescol XL Tablets 2268
Levaquin 2416
Levaquin in 5% Dextrose Injection 2416
Lexapro Oral Suspension 1174
Lexapro Tablets 1174
Lipitor Tablets (Less than 2%) 2501
Lunesta Tablets (Rare) 2994
Luvox CR Extended-Release Capsules 1759
Malarone Pediatric Tablets (Rare) 1521
Malarone Tablets (Rare) 1521
Mepron Suspension (Rare) 1526
Mevacor Tablets 2063
Miacalcin Nasal Spray (Less than 1%) 2274
Mobic Oral Suspension (Less than 2%) 863
Mobic Tablets (Less than 2%) 863
Mycamine for Injection 616
Namenda 1180
Naprosyn Suspension (Less than 1%) 2632
Naprosyn Tablets (Less than 1%) 2632
Nexium Delayed-Release Capsules 645
Nexium I.V. (Very rare) 652
Nexium Delayed-Release Oral Suspension 645
Nimotop Capsules (Less than 1%) 790
Noroxin Tablets 2069
Norvir (Less than 2%) 489
Noxafil Oral Suspension (1% to 2%) 2889
Omnicef Capsules 497
Omnicef for Oral Suspension 497
Orthoclone OKT3 Sterile Solution 2387
Parnate Tablets (Rare) 1532
Paser Granules 1747
Paxil (Rare) 1535
Paxil CR Controlled-Release Tablets (Rare) 1544
Pentasa Capsules (Infrequent) 3030
Percocet Tablets 1127
Percodan Tablets 1130
Persantine Tablets (Rare) 869
Plavix Tablets 926
Plavix Tablets 2767
PrandiMet Tablets 2967
Prandin Tablets (Rare) 2971
Primaxin I.M. 2080
Primaxin I.V. (Less than 0.2%) 2083
Prinivil Tablets (0.3% to 1%) 2087
Prinzide Tablets 2092
▲ Prograf Capsules and Injection (3% to 15%) 622
Proleukin for Injection 2287
Prometrium Capsules (100 mg, 200 mg) 3047
Protonix for Delayed-Release Oral Suspension (Less than 1%) 3254
Protonix Delayed-Release Tablets (Less than 1%) 3254
Protonix I.V. (Less than 1%) 3257
Prozac Weekly Capsules (Rare) 1852
Prozac Pulvules and Liquid (Rare) 1852
Rebif Prefilled Syringe for Injection (Rare) 1107
Remicade for IV Injection 950
Retrovir Capsules (Rare) 1574
Retrovir IV Infusion (Rare) 1579
Retrovir (Rare) 1574
Rilutek Tablets (Infrequent) 2771
Risperdal Consta Long-Acting Injection (Rare) 1753
Rituxan I.V. 1223
Rythmol Tablets 1586
St. Joseph 81 mg Aspirin Chewable and Enteric Coated Tablets 1903
Salagen Tablets (Less than 1%) 1082
Sandostatin Injection (Less than 1%) 2300
Sandostatin LAR Depot 2302
Solodyn Extended Release Tablets 1938
Soriatane Capsules (Less than 1%) 3062
Suprax for Oral Suspension (Less than 2%) 1891
Suprax Tablets (Less than 2%) 1891
Sustiva Capsules (Less than 2%) 930
Sustiva Tablets (Less than 2%) 930
Symbyax Capsules (Rare) 1871
Tamiflu Capsules 2649
Tamiflu Oral Suspension 2649
Tasigna Capsules (0.1% to 1%) 2316
Taxotere Injection Concentrate (Rare) 2773
Tice BCG (Less than or equal to 1%) 2936
Timentin ADD-Vantage (Rare) 1606
Timentin Injection Galaxy Container (Rare) 1609
Timentin IV Infusion (Rare) 1603
Timentin Pharmacy Bulk Package (Rare) 1613
Toprol-XL Tablets 666
Tricor Tablets 520
Truvada Tablets 1262
Twinrix Vaccine 1628
Ultane Liquid for Inhalation (Less than 1%) 524
Valtrex Caplets 1635
Velcade for Injection 2168
Venlafaxine Hydrochloride Tablets (Rare) 2199
▲ Vesanoid Capsules (3%) 2660
Viramune Oral Suspension 873
Viramune Tablets 873
Voltaren Tablets (Occasionally) 2334
Voltaren-XR Tablets (Occasionally) 2337
Vytorin 10/10 Tablets 2149
Vytorin 10/10 Tablets 2939
Vytorin 10/20 Tablets 2149
Vytorin 10/20 Tablets 2939
Vytorin 10/40 Tablets 2149
Vytorin 10/40 Tablets 2939
Vytorin 10/80 Tablets 2149
Vytorin 10/80 Tablets 2939
Wellbutrin Tablets 1648
Wellbutrin SR Sustained-Release Tablets 1653
Wellbutrin XL Extended-Release Tablets 1659
▲ Xeloda Tablets (Less than 5%) 2662
Xyzal Oral Solution 2789
Xyzal Oral Solution 3155
Zantac 25 EFFERdose Tablets (Occasional) 1670
Zantac Injection 1666
Zantac Injection Pharmacy Bulk Package (Infrequent) 1668
Zantac Injection Premixed 1666
Zantac (Occasional) 1670
Zetia Tablets 2157
Zetia Tablets 2951
Zocor Tablets 2136
Zosyn for Injection 3284
Zovirax 1690
Zyban Sustained-Release Tablets 1692
Zyprexa Tablets (Infrequent) 1883
Zyprexa ZYDIS Orally Disintegrating Tablets (Infrequent) 1883
Zyrtec Chewable Tablets (Rare) 1920
Zyrtec Syrup (Rare) 1920
Zyrtec Tablets (Rare) 1920
Zyrtec-D 12 Hour Extended Release Tablets (Rare) 1923

Hepatitis, acute
Levaquin 2416
Levaquin in 5% Dextrose Injection 2416

Hepatitis, autoimmune
Enbrel for Injection 569
Remicade for IV Injection 950

Hepatitis, cholestatic
Avelox 2803
Biaxin/Biaxin XL (Infrequent) 411
EryPed 431
Estratest Tablets 3043
Estratest H.S. Tablets 3043
Ketek Tablets 2744
Lamisil Tablets (Rare) 2266
Nalfon Capsules (Less than 1%) 2508
Sandostatin LAR Depot 2302
Singulair (Rare) 2114
Starlix Tablets 2314
Symbyax Capsules (Very rare) 1871
Viramune Oral Suspension 873
Viramune Tablets 873
▲ Xeloda Tablets (Less than 5%) 2662
Zantac 25 EFFERdose Tablets (Occasional) 1670
Zantac Injection (Occasional) 1666
Zantac Injection Pharmacy Bulk Package (Infrequent) 1668
Zantac Injection Premixed (Occasional) 1666
Zantac (Occasional) 1670
Zosyn for Injection 3284

Hepatitis, cytolytic
Amoxil Capsules 1305
Amoxil Chewable Tablets 1305
Amoxil Pediatric Drops for Oral Suspension 1305
Amoxil Powder for Oral Suspension 1305
Amoxil Tablets 1305
Aptivus Capsules (Less than 2%) 823
Aptivus Oral Solution (Less than 2%) 823
Intelence Tablets (Less than 2%) 3119
Moxatag Tablets 2165
Prograf Capsules and Injection 622

Hepatitis, fulminant
Celebrex Capsules (Less than 0.1%) 2979
Lexapro Oral Suspension 1174
Lexapro Tablets 1174
Omnicef Capsules 497
Omnicef for Oral Suspension 497
Precose Tablets (Few cases) 792
Primaxin I.M. (0.2%) 2080
Primaxin I.V. (0.2%) 2083
Rituxan I.V. 1223
Rythmol Tablets 1586
Treximet Tablets 1616
Vicoprofen Tablets 533
Viramune Oral Suspension 873
Viramune Tablets 873

Hepatitis, hepatocellular
Ketek Tablets 2744

Hepatitis, idiopathic
Raptiva for Injection (1 case) 1218

Hepatitis, infectious
Plavix Tablets (Less than 1%) 926
Plavix Tablets (Less than 1%) 2767

Hepatitis, ischemic
Requip Tablets (Infrequent) 1561

Hepatitis, post-treatment exacerbations of
Combivir Tablets 1384
Emtriva Capsules 1246
Emtriva Oral Solution 1246
Epivir 1412
Epivir-HBV 1417
Epzicom Tablets 1422
▲ Hepsera Tablets (Less than or equal to 25%) 1253
Trizivir Tablets 1622
Truvada Tablets 1262

Hepatitis, reactivation
Cimzia 3127
Emtriva Capsules 1246
Emtriva Oral Solution 1246
Enbrel for Injection 569
Humira Injection 442
Remicade for IV Injection 950
Rituxan I.V. 1223

Hepatitis, symptomatic
Accolate Tablets (Rare) 669

Hepatitis, toxic
Aptivus Capsules (Less than 2%) 823
Aptivus Oral Solution (Less than 2%) 823
Cuprimine Capsules (Rare) 1986
Dapsone Tablets USP 1746
Indocin Capsules (Less than 1%) 2024
Indocin I.V. (Less than 1%) 2489
Indocin (Less than 1%) 2024
Phenytek Capsules 2192

Hepatitis, viral
Evoxac Capsules (Less than 1%) 1013
Prolastin 3099

Hepatobiliary dysfunction
Lamisil Tablets (Rare) 2266
▲ Somatuline Depot Injection (24% to 31%) 3102

Hepatocellular atrophy
Myleran Tablets 1530

Hepatocellular damage
Mycamine for Injection 616
Risperdal Consta Long-Acting Injection (Rare) 1753
Rythmol Tablets 1586
Uroxatral Tablets 2786

Hepatomas
Advicor Tablets 402
Concerta Extended-Release Tablets 1925
Lescol Capsules (Rare) 2268
Lescol XL Tablets 2268
Lybrel Tablets 3204
Mevacor Tablets (Rare) 2063
NuvaRing 2897
Premarin Intravenous 3217
Premarin Vaginal Cream 3228

Hepatomas, benign
Mircette Tablets 1034
Ortho-Cyclen/Ortho Tri-Cyclen (Rare) 2449
Ortho Tri-Cyclen Lo Tablets 2458
Seasonique Tablets 1046
Yaz Tablets 805

Hepatomegaly
Abelcet Injection 1134
AmBisome for Injection (Less common) 606
Atripla Tablets 938
▲ Busulfex Injection (6%) 2477
Cancidas for Injection 1953
▲ Clolar for Intravenous Infusion (15%) 1239
Combigan Ophthalmic Solution 553
Combivir Tablets 1384
Copaxone for Injection (Infrequent) 3110
Cosmegen for Injection 2485
Cosopt Sterile Ophthalmic Solution 1969
Emtriva Capsules 1246
Emtriva Oral Solution 1246
▲ Epivir (11%) 1412
Epivir-HBV 1417
Epzicom Tablets 1422
Gabitril Tablets (Infrequent) 973
Geodon Capsules (Rare) 2520
Hepsera Tablets 1253
Intelence Tablets (Less than 2%) 3119
Klonopin 2639
Lunesta Tablets (Rare) 2994
▲ Megace ES Oral Suspension (1% to 3%) 2499
Mycamine for Injection 616
Neupogen for Injection (Infrequent) 589
Norvir (Less than 2%) 489
▲ Noxafil Oral Suspension (0% to 3%) 2889
Orthoclone OKT3 Sterile Solution 2387
Paser Granules 1747
▲ PegIntron Powder for Injection (6%) 2903
▲ Rebetol (4%) 2917
Retrovir Capsules (Rare) 1574
Retrovir IV Infusion (Rare) 1579
Retrovir (Rare) 1574
Risperdal Consta Long-Acting Injection (Infrequent) 1753
Rythmol SR Capsules 1590
Sular Extended Release Tablets (Less than or equal to 1%) 2975
Symbyax Capsules (Infrequent) 1871
Tabloid Tablets 1601
Tasigna Capsules 2316
Timoptic Sterile Ophthalmic Solution 2121
Timoptic in Ocudose 2124
Timoptic-XE Sterile Ophthalmic Gel Forming Solution 2125
Tricor Tablets 520
Trizivir Tablets 1622
Truvada Tablets 1262
Viramune Oral Suspension 873
Viramune Tablets 873
Viread Tablets 1268

Hepatorenal syndrome, unspecified
Actiq (Less than 1%) 959

Depakote ER Tablets 423

Hepatosplenomegaly

Doxil Injection (Less than 1%) 2378
Mylotarg for Injection 3212
Proleukin for Injection 2287
▲ Vesanoid Capsules (9%) 2660

Hepatotoxicity

Accutane Capsules 2607
Advicor Tablets 402
Asacol Delayed-Release Tablets (Rare) 2579
Avandaryl Tablets 1344
Benadryl Allergy & Cold Kapgels 1895
Benadryl Allergy & Sinus Headache Kapgels 1895
Benadryl Severe Allergy & Sinus Headache Caplets 1897
Busulfex Injection 2477
Cancidas for Injection 1953
Carbatrol Capsules 3019
▲ CellCept Capsules (3% to less than 20%) 2622
▲ CellCept Intravenous (3% to less than 20%) 2622
▲ CellCept Oral Suspension (3% to less than 20%) 2622
▲ CellCept Tablets (3% to less than 20%) 2622
Combivir Tablets 1384
Cosmegen for Injection 2485
Cymbalta Delayed-Release Capsules 1801
Dantrium Capsules 2580
Depakote ER Tablets 423
Effexor XR Extended-Release Capsules 3195
▲ Eloxatin for Injection (42% to 57%) 2731
Estratest Tablets 3043
Estratest H.S. Tablets 3043
Furosemide Tablets 2186
Gemzar for Injection (Rare) 1820
▲ Gengraf Capsules (Less than 1% to 7%) 435
▲ Gleevec Tablets (6% to 12%) 2255
Hexalen Capsules 1078
Intron A for Injection (Rare) 2859
Lamisil Oral Granules 2264
Lamisil Tablets 2266
Letairis Tablets 1258
Leukeran Tablets 1508
▲ Leukine (13%) 774
Levaquin 2416
Levaquin in 5% Dextrose Injection 2416
Lunesta Tablets (Rare) 2994
Mylotarg for Injection 3212
Nembutal Sodium Solution, USP 2494
▲ Neoral Oral Solution (Less than 1% to 7%) 2280
▲ Neoral Soft Gelatin Capsules (Less than 1% to 7%) 2280
Norvir (Less than 2%) 489
Pentasa Capsules 3030
Percocet Tablets 1127
Percodan Tablets 1130
Phenytek Capsules 2192
▲ Prograf Capsules and Injection (3% to 15%) 622
Pylera Capsules 714
Rapamune 3260
▲ Sandimmune (Less than 1% to 7%) 2296
Soriatane Capsules 3062
Sudafed PE Cold & Cough Caplets 1907
Sudafed PE Nighttime Cold Caplets 1907
Sudafed PE Severe Cold Caplets 1908
Sudafed PE Sinus Headache Caplets 1908
Tasigna Capsules 2316
Thiothixene Capsules 2197
Trasylol Injection (0.5%) 799
Tykerb Tablets 1631
Regular Strength Tylenol Tablets 1915
Tylenol 8 Hour Extended Release Caplets 1915
Extra Strength Tylenol Caplets, Cool Caplets, and EZ Tabs 1915
Extra Strength Tylenol Adult Rapid Blast Liquid 1915
Extra Strength Tylenol PM Caplets, Geltabs, Liquid, and Rapid Release Gels 1915
Extra Strength Tylenol Rapid Release Gels 1915
Tylenol Allergy Multi-Symptom Caplets with Cool Burst and Rapid Release Gelcaps 1916
Tylenol Allergy Multi-Symptom Nighttime Caplets with Cool Burst 1916
Tylenol Severe Allergy Caplets 1916
Tylenol Arthritis Pain Extended Release Geltabs/Caplets 1915
Tylenol Chest Congestion Caplets with Cool Burst 1910
Tylenol Chest Congestion Liquid with Cool Burst 1910
Tylenol Cold Severe Congestion Daytime Caplets with Cool Burst 1912
Tylenol Cold Head Congestion Daytime Caplets with Cool Burst 1910
Tylenol Cold Head Congestion Nighttime Caplets with Cool Burst 1910
Tylenol Cold Head Congestion Severe Daytime Caplets with Cool Burst 1910
Tylenol Cold Multi-Symptom Daytime Caplets with Cool Burst and Rapid Release Gels 1913
Tylenol Cold Multi-Symptom Daytime Liquid with Citrus Burst 1913
Tylenol Cold Multi-Symptom Nighttime Caplets with Cool Burst 1913
Tylenol Cold Multi-Symptom Nighttime Liquid with Cool Burst 1913
Tylenol Cold Multi-Symptom Severe Caplets with Cool Burst 1913
Tylenol Cold Multi-Symptom Severe Daytime Liquid with Citrus Burst 1913
Tylenol Cough & Sore Throat Daytime Liquid with Cool Burst 1918
Tylenol Cough & Sore Throat Nighttime Liquid with Cool Burst 1918
Tylenol Sinus Congestion & Pain Daytime Caplets with Cool Burst and Gelcaps 1917
Tylenol Sinus Congestion & Pain Nighttime Caplets with Cool Burst 1917
Tylenol Sinus Congestion & Pain Severe Caplets with Cool Burst 1917
Tylenol Sinus Severe Congestion Caplets with Cool Burst 1917
Tylenol Sore Throat Daytime Liquid with Cool Burst 1918
Tylenol Sore Throat Nighttime Liquid with Cool Burst 1918
Women's Tylenol Menstrual Relief Caplets 1919
Venlafaxine Hydrochloride Tablets 2199
Vicks DayQuil Cold & Flu Multi-Symptom Relief ◙ 616
Vicks DayQuil LiquiCaps 2567
Vicks DayQuil Liquid 2567
Vicks DayQuil Multi-Symptom Cold/Flu Relief 2567
Vicks NyQuil LiquiCaps 2567
Vicks NyQuil Liquid 2567
Vicks NyQuil Multi-Symptom Cold/Flu Relief 2567
Viramune Oral Suspension 873
Viramune Tablets 873
Wellbutrin Tablets (Infrequent) 1648
Wellbutrin SR Sustained-Release Tablets 1653
Wellbutrin XL Extended-Release Tablets 1659
▲ Xeloda Tablets (Less than 5%) 2662
Zyban Sustained-Release Tablets 1692

Hernia, hiatal

Aricept Tablets (Infrequent) 1062
Aricept ODT Tablets (Infrequent) 1062
Celebrex Capsules (0.1% to 1.9%) 2979
Mirapex Tablets 857
▲ Prometrium Capsules (100 mg, 200 mg) (Less than 5%) 3047
Remicade for IV Injection (Greater than or equal to 0.2%) 950
Requip Tablets (Infrequent) 1561

Hernia, incisional

Rapamune 3260

Hernia, inguinal

Edex Injection (1%) 2957
Mirapex Tablets 857
NeoProfen Injection 2496
Prevnar 3241
Xifaxan Tablets (Less than 2%) 2682
Zyban Sustained-Release Tablets (Infrequent) 1692

Hernia, umbilical

Mirapex Tablets 857

Hernia, unspecified

Actonel with Calcium Tablets (2.9%) 2574
Aricept Tablets (Infrequent) 1062
Aricept ODT Tablets (Infrequent) 1062
Azilect Tablets (2%) 3106
Campral Tablets (Infrequent) 1158
▲ CellCept Capsules (3% to less than 20%) 2622
▲ CellCept Intravenous (3% to less than 20%) 2622
▲ CellCept Oral Suspension (3% to less than 20%) 2622
▲ CellCept Tablets (3% to less than 20%) 2622
Effexor XR Extended-Release Capsules 3195
Emsam Transdermal System (Infrequent) 905
Exelon Capsules (Infrequent) 2229
Exelon Oral Solution (Infrequent) 2229
Gabitril Tablets (Infrequent) 973
Lunesta Tablets (Infrequent) 2994
Nexium Delayed-Release Capsules (Less than 1%) 645
Nexium I.V. (Less than 1%) 652
Nexium Delayed-Release Oral Suspension (Less than 1%) 645
Plavix Tablets (1% to 2.5%) 926
Plavix Tablets (1% to 2.5%) 2767
▲ Prograf Capsules and Injection (3% to 15%) 622
Protonix for Delayed-Release Oral Suspension (Less than 1%) 3254
Protonix Delayed-Release Tablets (Less than 1%) 3254
Protonix I.V. (Less than 1%) 3257
Protopic Ointment (Greater than or equal to 1%) 628
Rilutek Tablets (Infrequent) 2771
▲ Simulect for Injection (3% to 10%) 2306
Symbyax Capsules (Infrequent) 1871
▲ Synagis Intramuscular Solution (6.3%) 1948
Tricor Tablets 520

Herpes, meningoencephalitis

Velcade for Injection 2168

Herpes, unspecified

Bexxar 1371
Imitrex Nasal Spray (Rare) 1470
▲ Megace ES Oral Suspension (1% to 3%) 2499
▲ Selzentry Tablets (6.8%) 2534
Velcade for Injection 2168

Herpes labialis

Alferon N Injection (1%) 1726
Finacea Gel (Rare) 1742

Herpes ophthalmic

Selzentry Tablets 2534
Velcade for Injection 2168

Herpes simplex

Alrex Ophthalmic Suspension 0.2% ⊙ 236
Ambien Tablets (Rare) 2692
AmBisome for Injection (Less common) 606
Amevive 611
Aptivus Capsules (Less than 2%) 823
Aricept Tablets (Infrequent) 1062
Aricept ODT Tablets (Infrequent) 1062
Brovana Inhalation Solution (Less than 2%) 2990
Celebrex Capsules (0.1% to 1.9%) 2979
▲ Clolar for Intravenous Infusion (11%) 1239
▲ Copaxone for Injection (4%) 3110
▲ Doxil Injection (1% to 10%) 2378
Effexor XR Extended-Release Capsules 3195
▲ Elidel Cream 1% (0.4% to 4%) 2221
Emend Capsules (Greater than 0.5%) 1992
Emend for Injection (Greater than 0.5%) 1999
Emsam Transdermal System (Infrequent) 905
Evoxac Capsules (Less than 1%) 1013
Exelon Capsules (Infrequent) 2229
Exelon Oral Solution (Infrequent) 2229
FML Ophthalmic Ointment ⊙ 223
Gabitril Tablets (Infrequent) 973
Gengraf Capsules (1% to less than 3%) 435
Gleevec Tablets (Infrequent) 2255
Herceptin I.V. (2%) 1199
▲ Intron A for Injection (Up to 5%) 2859
Invanz for Injection (1%) 2029
Isentress Tablets 2036
Klonopin (Infrequent) 2639
Lotemax Ophthalmic Suspension 0.5% ⊙ 241
Meridia Capsules (1.3%) 475
▲ Myfortic Tablets (1.3% to less than 20%) 2276
▲ Mylotarg for Injection (2% to 25%) 3212
Neoral Oral Solution (1% to less than 3%) 2280
Neoral Soft Gelatin Capsules (1% to less than 3%) 2280
▲ Orencia Powder for Intravenous Infusion (Less than 5%) 921
Paxil (Rare) 1535
Paxil CR Controlled-Release Tablets (Rare) 1544
▲ Prograf Capsules and Injection (3% to 15%) 622
▲ Prometrium Capsules (100 mg, 200 mg) (Less than 5%) 3047
ProQuad 2099
Protonix for Delayed-Release Oral Suspension (Less than 1%) 3254
Protonix Delayed-Release Tablets (Less than 1%) 3254
Protonix I.V. (Less than 1%) 3257
▲ Protopic Ointment (4% to 12%) 628
Provigil Tablets (1%) 977
▲ Rapamune (Greater than or equal to 3% to less than 20%) 3260
Remeron Tablets (Infrequent) 2924
RemeronSolTab Tablets (Infrequent) 2927
Requip Tablets (Infrequent) 1561
Salagen Tablets (Less than 1%) 1082
Selzentry Tablets 2534
▲ Simulect for Injection (3% to 10%) 2306
Soriatane Capsules (Less than 1%) 3062
Sular Extended Release Tablets (Less than or equal to 1%) 2975
Tasigna Capsules 2316
Teveten Tablets (Less than 1%) 515
Teveten HCT Tablets (Less than 1%) 517
▲ Treanda for Injection (0% to 3%) 983
Tricor Tablets 520
▲ Trisenox Injection (13%) 986
▲ Velcade for Injection (2% to 8%) 2168
Xyrem Oral Solution (Infrequent) 1766

Herpes simplex, disseminated

Accutane Capsules 2607

Herpes virus

Selzentry Tablets 2534

Herpes zoster

Actiq (Less than 1%) 959
Ambien Tablets (Rare) 2692
Aptivus Capsules (Less than 2%) 823
Aricept Tablets (Infrequent) 1062
Aricept ODT Tablets (Infrequent) 1062
Brovana Inhalation Solution (Less than 2%) 2990
Celebrex Capsules (0.1% to 1.9%) 2979
▲ CellCept Capsules (Less than 4% to 10.7%) 2622
▲ CellCept Intravenous (Less than 4% to 10.7%) 2622
▲ CellCept Oral Suspension (Less than 4% to 10.7%) 2622
▲ CellCept Tablets (Less than 4% to 10.7%) 2622
Copaxone for Injection (Frequent) 3110
▲ Doxil Injection (Less than 1% to 10%) 2378
Effexor XR Extended-Release Capsules 3195
Emsam Transdermal System (Infrequent) 905
Engerix-B Vaccine 1409
Evoxac Capsules (Less than 1%) 1013
Gabitril Tablets (Infrequent) 973
Gengraf Capsules (1% to less than 3%) 435
Gleevec Tablets (Infrequent) 2255
▲ Humira Injection (Less than 5%) 442
▲ Intron A for Injection (Less than 5%) 2859
Lamictal (Rare) 1488
Leustatin Injection (8 episodes) 2384
Lunesta Tablets (Rare) 2994
Mirapex Tablets 857
Mustargen for Injection 2492
▲ Myfortic Tablets (1.9% to less than 20%) 2276
Neoral Oral Solution (1% to less than 3%) 2280
Neoral Soft Gelatin Capsules (1% to less than 3%) 2280
Orencia Powder for Intravenous Infusion (0.7%) 921
Paxil (Rare) 1535
Paxil CR Controlled-Release Tablets (Rare) 1544
Prinivil Tablets (0.3% to 1%) 2087
Prinzide Tablets 2092

ProQuad 2099
Protonix for Delayed-Release Oral Suspension (Less than 1%) 3254
Protonix Delayed-Release Tablets (Less than 1%) 3254
Protonix I.V. (Less than 1%) 3257
▲ Protopic Ointment (Up to 3%) 628
Prozac Weekly Capsules (Rare) 1852
Prozac Pulvules and Liquid (Rare) 1852
▲ Rapamune (Greater than or equal to 3% to less than 20%) 3260
Recombivax HB 2107
Remeron Tablets (Rare) 2924
RemeronSolTab Tablets (Rare) 2927
Remicade for IV Injection 950
Requip Tablets (Infrequent) 1561
▲ Simulect for Injection (3% to 10%) 2306
▲ Spiriva HandiHaler (1% to 3%) 870
Sular Extended Release Tablets (Less than or equal to 1%) 2975
Tricor Tablets 520
▲ Trisenox Injection (8%) 986
Twinrix Vaccine 1628
Varivax 2133
▲ Velcade for Injection (3% to 17%) 2168
Xyrem Oral Solution (Infrequent) 1766

Herxheimer's reaction

Bicillin L-A Injection 1777
▲ Ceftin Tablets (5.6%) 1380

Hiccups

Actiq (Less than 1%) 959
Aloxi Injection (Less than 1%) 1059
Ambien Tablets (Frequent) 2692
Ambien CR Tablets (Frequent) 2696
AmBisome for Injection (Less common) 606
▲ Avinza Capsules (Less than 5%) 1772
▲ Busulfex Injection (18%) 2477
Celexa (Rare) 1160
▲ CellCept Capsules (3% to less than 20%) 2622
▲ CellCept Intravenous (3% to less than 20%) 2622
▲ CellCept Oral Suspension (3% to less than 20%) 2622
▲ CellCept Tablets (3% to less than 20%) 2622
Cipro I.V. (1% or less) 2817
Cipro (Less than 1%) 2810
Cipro XR Tablets 2823
Depakote ER Tablets (Greater than 1%) 423
Doxil Injection (Less than 1%) 2378
Duragesic Transdermal System (1% or greater) 2405
▲ Eloxatin for Injection (1% to 5%) 2731
▲ Emend Capsules (10.8%) 1992
▲ Emend for Injection (10.8%) 1999
▲ Evoxac Capsules (1% to 3%) 1013
Frova Tablets (Rare) 1111
Gabitril Tablets (Infrequent) 973
Gengraf Capsules (2% or less) 435
Imitrex Injection (Rare) 1465
Imitrex Nasal Spray 1470
Imitrex Tablets (Rare) 1474
Invanz for Injection (Greater than 0.1%) 2029
Ionsys Transdermal System (.1% to less than 1%) 2410
Lamictal (Rare) 1488
Lunesta Tablets (Infrequent) 2994
Luvox CR Extended-Release Capsules (Rare) 1759
Lyrica Capsules (Rare) 2527
Maxalt Tablets (Rare) 2056
Maxalt-MLT Orally Disintegrating Tablets (Rare) 2056
Mirapex Tablets 857
Neoral Oral Solution (2% or less) 2280
Neoral Soft Gelatin Capsules (2% or less) 2280
Nexium Delayed-Release Capsules (Less than 1%) 645
Nexium I.V. (Less than 1%) 652
Nexium Delayed-Release Oral Suspension (Less than 1%) 645
Norvir (Less than 2%) 489
▲ OxyContin Tablets (Between 1% and 5%) 2589
Paxil (Rare) 1535
Paxil CR Controlled-Release Tablets (Rare) 1544
▲ Photofrin for Injection (6%) 708
Protonix for Delayed-Release Oral Suspension (Less than 1%) 3254
Protonix Delayed-Release Tablets (Less than 1%) 3254
Protonix I.V. (Less than 1%) 3257
Prozac Weekly Capsules (Infrequent) 1852
Prozac Pulvules and Liquid (Infrequent) 1852
Remeron Tablets (Rare) 2924
RemeronSolTab Tablets (Rare) 2927
Requip Tablets (Infrequent) 1561
Rilutek Tablets (Infrequent) 2771
Romazicon Injection (Less than 1%) 2646
Salagen Tablets (Less than 1%) 1082
Sandimmune (2% or less) 2296
Stalevo Tablets 2309
Symbyax Capsules (Infrequent) 1871
Ultane Liquid for Inhalation (Less than 1%) 524
Vicoprofen Tablets (Less than 3%) 533
Xyrem Oral Solution (Infrequent) 1766
Zemuron Injection (Less than 1%) 2947
Zofran Injection 1682
Zofran 1687
Zofran ODT Orally Disintegrating Tablets 1687
Zomig Tablets (Infrequent) 694
Zomig Nasal Spray (Rare) 689
Zomig-ZMT Tablets (Infrequent) 694
Zosyn for Injection (1% or less to 2.6%) 3284
Zyprexa Tablets (Rare) 1883
Zyprexa ZYDIS Orally Disintegrating Tablets (Rare) 1883

Hip fracture

Arimidex Tablets (1%) 672
Exelon Patch (Infrequent) 2233

Hirsutism

Abilify Injection (Greater than or equal to 1 in 1000 patients and less than 1 in 100 patients) 881
Abilify Injection (Greater than or equal to 1 in 1000 patients and less than 1 in 100 patients) 2466
Abilify Oral Solution (Greater than or equal to 1 in 1000 patients and less than 1 in 100 patients) 881
Abilify Oral Solution (Greater than or equal to 1 in 1000 patients and less than 1 in 100 patients) 2466
Abilify Discmelt Orally Disintegrating Tablets (Greater than or equal to 1 in 1000 patients and less than 1 in 100 patients) 881
Abilify Discmelt Orally Disintegrating Tablets (Greater than or equal to 1 in 1000 patients and less than 1 in 100 patients) 2466
Abilify Tablets (Greater than or equal to 1 in 1000 patients and less than 1 in 100 patients) 881
Abilify Tablets (Greater than or equal to 1 in 1000 patients and less than 1 in 100 patients) 2466
Accutane Capsules 2607
Activella Tablets 2347
AndroGel (Less than 1%) 3159
Angeliq Tablets 751
Aricept Tablets (Infrequent) 1062
Aricept ODT Tablets (Infrequent) 1062
Carbatrol Capsules (Isolated cases) 3019
▲ CellCept Capsules (3% to less than 20%) 2622
▲ CellCept Intravenous (3% to less than 20%) 2622
▲ CellCept Oral Suspension (3% to less than 20%) 2622
▲ CellCept Tablets (3% to less than 20%) 2622
Climara Transdermal System 763
Climara Pro Transdermal System 768
Dantrium Capsules (Less frequent) 2580
Delatestryl Injection 1730
Divigel 3167
Effexor XR Extended-Release Capsules (Rare) 3195
Eldepryl Capsules 3052
Enjuvia Tablets 1029
Equetro Extended-Release Capsules 3174
Estratest Tablets 3043
Estratest H.S. Tablets 3043
Gabitril Tablets (Infrequent) 973
▲ Gengraf Capsules (21% to 45%) 435
▲ Intron A for Injection (Less than 5%) 2859
Klonopin 2639
Lamictal (Infrequent) 1488
▲ Lumigan Ophthalmic Solution (1% to 5%) 556
Lunesta Tablets (Rare) 2994
Lupron Depot–3 Month 11.25 mg (0.6% to 1%) 462
Lybrel Tablets 3204
Lyrica Capsules (0.1% to 1%) 2527
Mircette Tablets 1034
▲ Myfortic Tablets (3% to less than 20%) 2276
▲ Neoral Oral Solution (21% to 45%) 2280
▲ Neoral Soft Gelatin Capsules (21% to 45%) 2280
NuvaRing 2897
Ortho-Cyclen Tablets 2449
Ortho Evra Transdermal System 2437
Ortho Micronor Tablets (Rare) 2446
Ortho Tri-Cyclen Tablets 2449
Ortho Tri-Cyclen Lo Tablets 2458
Paxil (Rare) 1535
Paxil CR Controlled-Release Tablets (Rare) 1544
Photofrin for Injection 708
Premarin Intravenous 3217
Premarin Tablets 3221
Premarin Vaginal Cream 3228
Premphase Tablets 3232
Prempro Tablets 3232
Proglycem Capsules (Frequent) 1185
Proglycem Suspension (Frequent) 1185
▲ Prograf Capsules and Injection (3% to 15%) 622
Prozac Weekly Capsules (Rare) 1852
Prozac Pulvules and Liquid (Rare) 1852
▲ Sandimmune (21% to 45%) 2296
Seasonique Tablets 1046
Venlafaxine Hydrochloride Tablets (Rare) 2199
Viadur Implant (Less than 2%) 802
Wellbutrin Tablets (Rare) 1648
Wellbutrin SR Sustained-Release Tablets 1653
Wellbutrin XL Extended-Release Tablets 1659
Yaz Tablets 805
Zonegran Capsules (Infrequent) 1089
Zyban Sustained-Release Tablets 1692
Zyprexa Tablets (Infrequent) 1883
Zyprexa ZYDIS Orally Disintegrating Tablets (Infrequent) 1883

Histoplasmosis

Remicade for IV Injection 950

Hives

(*see also under* Urticaria)
BeneFIX Vials 3191
Follistim AQ Cartridge 2844
Janumet Tablets 2041
Xyntha Vials 3280

Hives at injection site

Prevnar 3241
Xolair 1235
Xolair 2339

Hoarseness

Aceon Tablets (2 mg, 4 mg, 8 mg) (0.3% to 1%) 3038
Advair Diskus 100/50 1276
▲ Advair Diskus 250/50 (2% to 5%) 1276
Advair Diskus 500/50 1276
▲ Aerobid/Aerobid-M (3% to 9%) 1153
▲ Alvesco Inhalation Aerosol (Greater than or equal to 3%) 2985
Atrovent Nasal Spray 0.03% (Less than 2%) 834
Atrovent Nasal Spray 0.06% (Less than 1%) 836
Azmacort Inhalation Aerosol 407
Captopril Tablets 2182
Combivent Inhalation Aerosol 845
Erbitux 912
Flonase Nasal Spray 1431
▲ Flovent Diskus 50 mcg (1% to 9%) 1435
Flovent HFA (2%) 1440
Klonopin (Infrequent) 2639
Levaquin 2416
Levaquin in 5% Dextrose Injection 2416
Luvox CR Extended-Release Capsules (Infrequent) 1759
Maxalt Tablets (Rare) 2056
Maxalt-MLT Orally Disintegrating Tablets (Rare) 2056
▲ Nexavar Tablets (1% to less than 10%) 784
Provigil Tablets 977
Requip Tablets (Infrequent) 1561
Retrovir Capsules 1574
Retrovir IV Infusion 1579
Retrovir 1574
Spiriva HandiHaler 870
Stalevo Tablets 2309
Ventolin HFA Inhalation Aerosol 1638
Vicoprofen Tablets (Less than 1%) 533
▲ Xeloda Tablets (Less than 5%) 2662

Hodgkin's disease

Phenytek Capsules 2192

Hoigne's syndrome

Bicillin C-R Injectable Suspension 1775
Bicillin L-A Injection 1777

Homicidal ideation

Abilify Injection (Greater than or equal to 1 in 1000 patients and less than 1 in 100 patients) 881
Abilify Injection (Greater than or equal to 1 in 1000 patients and less than 1 in 100 patients) 2466
Abilify Oral Solution (Greater than or equal to 1 in 1000 patients and less than 1 in 100 patients) 881
Abilify Oral Solution (Greater than or equal to 1 in 1000 patients and less than 1 in 100 patients) 2466
Abilify Discmelt Orally Disintegrating Tablets (Greater than or equal to 1 in 1000 patients and less than 1 in 100 patients) 881
Abilify Discmelt Orally Disintegrating Tablets (Greater than or equal to 1 in 1000 patients and less than 1 in 100 patients) 2466
Abilify Tablets (Greater than or equal to 1 in 1000 patients and less than 1 in 100 patients) 881
Abilify Tablets (Greater than or equal to 1 in 1000 patients and less than 1 in 100 patients) 2466

Hordeolum

Alphagan P Ophthalmic Solution (Less than 1%) 549
Combigan Ophthalmic Solution (0.1% to 0.2%) 553
Mirapex Tablets 857

Hormonal imbalance

Norvir (Less than 2%) 489
Wellbutrin Tablets (Rare) 1648

Horner's syndrome

Stalevo Tablets 2309

Hostility

Abilify Injection (Greater than or equal to 1 in 1000 patients and less than 1 in 100 patients) 881
Abilify Injection (Greater than or equal to 1 in 1000 patients and less than 1 in 100 patients) 2466
Abilify Oral Solution (Greater than or equal to 1 in 1000 patients and less than 1 in 100 patients) 881
Abilify Oral Solution (Greater than or equal to 1 in 1000 patients and less than 1 in 100 patients) 2466
Abilify Discmelt Orally Disintegrating Tablets (Greater than or equal to 1 in 1000 patients and less than 1 in 100 patients) 881
Abilify Discmelt Orally Disintegrating Tablets (Greater than or equal to 1 in 1000 patients and less than 1 in 100 patients) 2466
Abilify Tablets (Greater than or equal to 1 in 1000 patients and less than 1 in 100 patients) 881
Abilify Tablets (Greater than or equal to 1 in 1000 patients and less than 1 in 100 patients) 2466
Adderall XR Capsules 3012
Amerge Tablets (Rare) 1301
AndroGel (Less than 1%) 3159
▲ Aricept Tablets (3%) 1062
▲ Aricept ODT Tablets (3%) 1062
Azilect Tablets (Rare) 3106
Campral Tablets (Infrequent) 1158
Copaxone for Injection (Infrequent) 3110
Depakote ER Tablets 423
Duragesic Transdermal System (Less than 1%) 2405
Effexor XR Extended-Release Capsules (Infrequent) 3195
Emsam Transdermal System (Infrequent) 905
Gabitril Tablets (2%) 973
Geodon Capsules (Frequent) 2520
▲ Keppra Injection (2% to 13.3%) 3137
▲ Keppra Oral Solution (2% to 12%) 3131
▲ Keppra Tablets (2% to 12%) 3131
Klonopin 2639
Lamictal (Infrequent) 1488
Lunesta Tablets (Infrequent) 2994
Luvox CR Extended-Release Capsules (Infrequent) 1759
Lyrica Capsules (0.1% to 1%) 2527

Paxil (Infrequent) 1535
Paxil CR Controlled-Release Tablets (Infrequent) 1544
Pristiq Extended-Release Tablets 3247
Prozac Weekly Capsules (Infrequent) 1852
Prozac Pulvules and Liquid (Infrequent) 1852
Remeron Tablets (Infrequent) 2924
RemeronSolTab Tablets (Infrequent) 2927
Rilutek Tablets (Frequent) 2771
Strattera Capsules 1864
Symbyax Capsules (Infrequent) 1871
Venlafaxine Hydrochloride Tablets (Infrequent) 2199
▲ Wellbutrin Tablets (5.6%) 1648
Wellbutrin SR Sustained-Release Tablets (Infrequent) 1653
Wellbutrin XL Extended-Release Tablets (Infrequent) 1659
Zyban Sustained-Release Tablets (Infrequent) 1692
▲ Zyprexa Tablets (15%) 1883
▲ Zyprexa ZYDIS Orally Disintegrating Tablets (15%) 1883

Hot feeling

Cymbalta Delayed-Release Capsules (Infrequent) 1801
Fabrazyme for Intravenous Infusion 1241
▲ Lexiscan Injection (5%) 614
Mirapex Tablets 857
Requip Tablets (Infrequent) 1561
Treximet Tablets (Greater than 1%) 1616
▲ Ultram ER Extended-Release Tablets (1% to less than 5%) 2428

Hot flashes

Advate (1.3%) 721
Alferon N Injection (1%) 1726
Aloxi Injection (Less than 1%) 1059
Ambien Tablets (Rare) 2692
Ambien CR Tablets (Rare) 2696
Aricept Tablets (Frequent) 1062
Aricept ODT Tablets (Frequent) 1062
▲ Arimidex Tablets (11% to 36%) 672
▲ Busulfex Injection (25%) 2477
Celebrex Capsules (0.1% to 1.9%) 2979
Celexa (Infrequent) 1160
Cymbalta Delayed-Release Capsules (Frequent) 1801
▲ Effexor XR Extended-Release Capsules (4%) 3195
▲ Eligard 7.5 mg (25% to 56.7%) 2724
▲ Eligard 22.5 mg (56.4%) 2724
▲ Eligard 30 mg (73.3%) 2724
▲ Eligard 45 mg (57.7%) 2724
Elitek (Less than or equal to 1%) 2729
▲ Eloxatin for Injection (2% to less than 5%) 2731
▲ Evista Tablets (9.7% to 24.6%) 1810
Evoxac Capsules (2.4%) 1013
Exelon Capsules (Frequent) 2229
Exelon Oral Solution (Frequent) 2229
▲ Femara Tablets (5% to 33.7%) 2246
Fluarix Vaccine 1446
Frova Tablets (Infrequent) 1111
Gengraf Capsules (1% to less than 3%) 435
Herceptin I.V. 1199
▲ Intron A for Injection (Less than 5%) 2859
Lamictal (Infrequent) 1488
Lexapro Oral Suspension (Frequent) 1174
Lexapro Tablets (Frequent) 1174
▲ Lupron Depot 3.75 mg (50%) 462
▲ Lupron Depot 7.5 mg (57.1%) 469
▲ Lupron Depot–3 Month 11.25 mg (58% to 98%) 462
Maxalt Tablets (Frequent) 2056
Maxalt-MLT Orally Disintegrating Tablets (Frequent) 2056
Mobic Oral Suspension (Less than 2%) 863
Mobic Tablets (Less than 2%) 863
Neoral Oral Solution (1% to less than 3%) 2280
Neoral Soft Gelatin Capsules (1% to less than 3%) 2280
Nexium I.V. (Less than 1%) 652
Opana Tablets (Less than 1%) 1117
Opana ER Tablets (Less than 1%) 1121
▲ Prometrium Capsules (100 mg, 200 mg) (11%) 3047
Requip Tablets (1% or more) 1561
▲ Romazicon Injection (1% to 3%) 2646
Rythmol Tablets (Less than 1%) 1586
▲ Soriatane Capsules (1% to 10%) 3062
Stalevo Tablets 2309
Sustiva Capsules (Less than 2%) 930
Sustiva Tablets (Less than 2%) 930
Testim 1% Gel (1% or less) 701
Teveten Tablets (Less than 1%) 515
Teveten HCT Tablets (Less than 1%) 517
▲ Ultram ER Extended-Release Tablets (1% to less than 5%) 2428
▲ Vagifem Tablets (3% to 5%) 2375
▲ Vantas (65.5%) 1737
▲ Wellbutrin SR Sustained-Release Tablets (1% to 3%) 1653
▲ Wellbutrin XL Extended-Release Tablets (6%) 1659
▲ Xeloda Tablets (Less than 5%) 2662
Xifaxan Tablets (Less than 2%) 2682
Zyban Sustained-Release Tablets (1%) 1692
Zyrtec Chewable Tablets (Less than 2%) 1920
Zyrtec Syrup (Less than 2%) 1920
Zyrtec Tablets (Less than 2%) 1920
Zyrtec-D 12 Hour Extended Release Tablets (Less than 2%) 1923

Hot flushes

▲ Arimidex Tablets (2% to 26%) 672
Chantix Tablets (Frequent) 2511
Cimzia 3127
Crinone 4% Gel 992
Crinone 8% Gel 992
Cyanokit 5g Antidote 1021
▲ Cymbalta Delayed-Release Capsules (2% to 3%) 1801
▲ Emend Capsules (3%) 1992
▲ Emend for Injection (3%) 1999
Exforge Tablets (Greater than 0.1% to less than 1%) 2238
▲ Ixempra Kit for Injection (6%) 915
Mirapex Tablets 857
Neupro Transdermal System 3149
Nexium Delayed-Release Capsules (Less than 1%) 645
Nexium Delayed-Release Oral Suspension (Less than 1%) 645
Pristiq Extended-Release Tablets (1% to 2%) 3247
Prograf Capsules and Injection 622
Requip Tablets (Frequent) 1561
Treximet Tablets (Infrequent) 1616
Vivitrol 988

HPA axis suppression

(*see also under* Adrenal suppression)

Diprolene Lotion 0.05% 2838
Diprolene Ointment 0.05% (Some patients) 2839
Diprolene AF Cream 0.05% (Some patients) 2837
▲ Elocon Cream 0.1% (16%) 2840
Elocon Lotion 0.1% 2841
▲ Elocon Ointment 0.1% (27%) 2842
Lotrisone 2881
▲ Olux Foam (5 of 13 patients) 3061
Olux-E Foam 3059
Qvar Inhalation Aerosol 3116
Vanos Cream 1941
Veramyst Nasal Spray 1643
Verdeso Foam 3069

HPA function suppression

Azmacort Inhalation Aerosol 407

Hunger

Humulin 50/50, 100 Units 1843
Humulin 70/30 Vial 1844
Humulin N Vial 1846
Humulin R 1849
Imitrex Injection (Rare) 1465
Imitrex Nasal Spray (Rare) 1470
Imitrex Tablets (Rare) 1474
Klonopin (Infrequent) 2639
▲ MoviPrep Oral Solution (30.2%) 2679
Requip Tablets (Infrequent) 1561

Hydrocephalus

Arranon Injection (1%) 1319
DepoCyt Injection 1136
▲ Gliadel Wafer (3%) 1076

Hydrocephalus, fetal

Accutane Capsules 2607

Hydronephrosis

Actiq (1% or greater) 959
▲ CellCept Capsules (3% to less than 20%) 2622
▲ CellCept Intravenous (3% to less than 20%) 2622
▲ CellCept Oral Suspension (3% to less than 20%) 2622
▲ CellCept Tablets (3% to less than 20%) 2622
Crixivan Capsules (2.8%) 1979
Doxil Injection (Less than 1%) 2378
▲ Myfortic Tablets (3% to less than 20%) 2276
▲ Prograf Capsules and Injection (3% to 15%) 622
Velcade for Injection 2168

Hydrothorax

Follistim AQ Cartridge 2844

Hyoacusis

▲ DepoCyt Injection (6% to 18%) 1136

Hypalgesia

Lyrica Capsules (Rare) 2527

Hyperactivity

Advair Diskus 100/50 1276
Advair Diskus 250/50 1276
Advair Diskus 500/50 1276
Advair HFA 45/21 Inhalation Aerosol (Very Rare) 1288
Advair HFA 115/21 Inhalation Aerosol (Very Rare) 1288
Advair HFA 230/21 Inhalation Aerosol (Very Rare) 1288
▲ Aerobid/Aerobid-M (1% to 3%) 1153
Amerge Tablets (Rare) 1301
Amoxil Capsules (Rare) 1305
Amoxil Chewable Tablets (Rare) 1305
Amoxil Pediatric Drops for Oral Suspension (Rare) 1305
Amoxil Powder for Oral Suspension (Rare) 1305
Amoxil Tablets (Rare) 1305
Augmentin (Rare) 1323
Augmentin Tablets (Rare) 1327
Augmentin XR Extended Release Tablets (Rare) 1333
Augmentin ES-600 Powder for Oral Suspension (Rare) 1329
Ceftin for Oral Suspension (0.1% to 1%) 1380
Clarinex-D 24-Hour Extended-Release Tablets (2%) 2834
Depakote ER Tablets 423
Exjade Tablets 2244
Klonopin (Infrequent) 2639
Levothroid Tablets 1170
Levoxyl Tablets 1780
Marplan Tablets (0% to 2%) 3177
Moban Tablets (Less frequent) 1116
Moxatag Tablets 2165
Rocephin Injectable Vials, ADD-Vantage, Galaxy, Bulk 2642
Thioridazine Hydrochloride Tablets (Extremely rare) 2195
Ventolin HFA Inhalation Aerosol 1638

Hyperactivity, psychomotor

Chantix Tablets (Infrequent) 2511
Clarinex Syrup (Rare) 2828
Clarinex Tablets (Rare) 2828
Clarinex Reditabs Tablets (Rare) 2828
Concerta Extended-Release Tablets 1925
Mirapex Tablets 857
Singulair 2114
Vyvanse Capsules 3033
Xyrem Oral Solution (Infrequent) 1766

Hyperacusis

Axert Tablets (Infrequent) 2431
Carbatrol Capsules 3019
Effexor XR Extended-Release Capsules (Rare) 3195
Equetro Extended-Release Capsules 3174
Frova Tablets (Infrequent) 1111
Gabitril Tablets (Infrequent) 973
Lunesta Tablets (Rare) 2994
Lyrica Capsules (0.1% to 1%) 2527
Maxalt Tablets (Rare) 2056
Maxalt-MLT Orally Disintegrating Tablets (Rare) 2056
Paxil (Rare) 1535
Paxil CR Controlled-Release Tablets (Rare) 1544
Prozac Weekly Capsules (Rare) 1852
Prozac Pulvules and Liquid (Rare) 1852
Remeron Tablets (Infrequent) 2924
RemeronSolTab Tablets (Infrequent) 2927
Rilutek Tablets (Rare) 2771
Romazicon Injection (Less than 1%) 2646
Venlafaxine Hydrochloride Tablets (Infrequent) 2199
Zomig Tablets (Infrequent) 694
Zomig-ZMT Tablets (Infrequent) 694

Hyperaesthesia

Mirapex Tablets 857
Xyrem Oral Solution (Infrequent) 1766

Hyperalbuminemia

Avelox (Greater than or equal to 2%) 2803

Hyperalgesia

Lamictal (Rare) 1488
Lyrica Capsules (0.1% to 1%) 2527
Paxil (Rare) 1535
Paxil CR Controlled-Release Tablets (Rare) 1544
Retrovir Capsules 1574
Retrovir IV Infusion 1579
Retrovir 1574

Hyperammonemia

Aciphex Tablets 1053
Depakote ER Tablets 423

Hyperammonemic encephalopathy

Depakote ER Tablets 423

Hyperamylasemia

Aptivus Capsules (Less than 2%) 823
Aptivus Oral Solution (Less than 2%) 823

Hyperbilirubinemia

Abelcet Injection 1134
Abilify Injection (Greater than or equal to 1 in 1000 patients and less than 1 in 100 patients) 881
Abilify Injection (Greater than or equal to 1 in 1000 patients and less than 1 in 100 patients) 2466
Abilify Oral Solution (Greater than or equal to 1 in 1000 patients and less than 1 in 100 patients) 881
Abilify Oral Solution (Greater than or equal to 1 in 1000 patients and less than 1 in 100 patients) 2466
Abilify Discmelt Orally Disintegrating Tablets (Greater than or equal to 1 in 1000 patients and less than 1 in 100 patients) 881
Abilify Discmelt Orally Disintegrating Tablets (Greater than or equal to 1 in 1000 patients and less than 1 in 100 patients) 2466
Abilify Tablets (Greater than or equal to 1 in 1000 patients and less than 1 in 100 patients) 881
Abilify Tablets (Greater than or equal to 1 in 1000 patients and less than 1 in 100 patients) 2466
Accolate Tablets (Rare) 669
Advicor Tablets 402
AndroGel 3159
Anzemet Injection (Less than 1%) 2701
Anzemet Tablets (Less than 1%) 2704
Aptivus Capsules (Less than 2%) 823
Aptivus Oral Solution (Less than 2%) 823
Arimidex Tablets (Greater than or equal to 0.1% to less than 1%) 672
Atacand Tablets (Infrequent) 639
Atacand HCT 642
Augmentin (Infrequent) 1323
Augmentin Tablets (Infrequent) 1327
Augmentin XR Extended Release Tablets (Infrequent) 1333
Augmentin ES-600 Powder for Oral Suspension (Infrequently) 1329
Avelox (Greater than or equal to 2%) 2803
Benicar Tablets (Infrequently) 1009
Biaxin/Biaxin XL (Less than 1%) 411
▲ Busulfex Injection (30% to 49%) 2477
Bystolic Tablets 1155
▲ Cancidas for Injection (6.4% to 13.2%) 1953
Captopril Tablets 2182
Ceftin 1380
Cipro I.V. (Among most frequent) 2817
Cipro (0.3%) 2810
Cipro XR Tablets 2823
Clarinex Tablets (Rare) 2828
Clarinex Reditabs Tablets (Rare) 2828
Clarinex-D 12-Hour Extended-Release Tablets (Rare) 2831
Clarinex-D 24-Hour Extended-Release Tablets 2834
▲ Clolar for Intravenous Infusion (15%) 1239
Concerta Extended-Release Tablets 1925
▲ Crixivan Capsules (11.9% to 14%) 1979
▲ Dacogen Injection (14%) 1066
Dapsone Tablets USP 1746

Depakote ER Tablets 423
▲ Doxil Injection (1% to 5%) 2378
▲ Eloxatin for Injection (4% to 20%) 2731
Elspar for Injection 1990
Elspar for Injection 2488
Emend Capsules (Greater than 0.5%) 1992
Emend for Injection (Greater than 0.5%) 1999
Emtriva Capsules (Less than or equal to 1%) 1246
Emtriva Oral Solution (Less than or equal to 1%) 1246
Epivir (0.8%) 1412
Fortaz 1450
▲ Gemzar for Injection (13% to 26%) 1820
Gengraf Capsules (1% to less than 3%) 435
▲ Gleevec Tablets (0% to 3.8%) 2255
Hycamtin for Injection (Less than 3%) 1459
Invanz for Injection (0.6% to 1.7%) ... 2029
▲ Isentress Tablets (0.8% to 5.3%) 2036
Kaletra (Up to 1%) 452
Ketek Tablets (Less than 0.2%) 2744
Lescol Capsules 2268
Lescol XL Tablets 2268
▲ Leukine (30%) 774
Leustatin Injection 2384
Lexapro Oral Suspension (Infrequent) 1174
Lexapro Tablets (Infrequent) 1174
Lialda Tablets (Infrequent) 3029
Mavik Tablets (0.2% of patients) 472
Mephyton Tablets (Rare) 700
Meridia Capsules (1.6%) 475
Merrem I.V. (Greater than 0.2%) 684
Mevacor Tablets 2063
Micardis HCT Tablets (Occasional) ... 854
Mycamine for Injection 616
Myleran Tablets 1530
▲ Mylotarg for Injection (29%) 3212
Neoral Oral Solution (1% to less than 3%) 2280
Neoral Soft Gelatin Capsules (1% to less than 3%) 2280
Nexavar Tablets (0.1% to less than 1%) 784
Omnicef Capsules (0.2%) 497
Omnicef for Oral Suspension (0.2%) 497
Oncaspar Injection (1% to greater than or equal to 2%) 1138
▲ PegIntron Powder for Injection (10% to 14%) 2903
Pentasa Capsules 3030
Primaxin I.M. 2080
Primaxin I.V. 2083
Prinivil Tablets (Rare) 2087
Prinzide Tablets (Rare) 2092
▲ Prograf Capsules and Injection (12% to 30%) 622
Protonix for Delayed-Release Oral Suspension (Less than 1%) 3254
Protonix Delayed-Release Tablets (Less than 1%) 3254
▲ Rebetol (10% to 14%) 2917
Retrovir Capsules (Rare) 1574
Retrovir IV Infusion (Rare) 1579
Retrovir (Rare) 1574
▲ Reyataz Capsules (49%) 3299
Rocephin Injectable Vials, ADD-Vantage, Galaxy, Bulk (Less than 1%) 2642
Rythmol SR Capsules 1590
Strattera Capsules 1864
Stromectol Tablets 2120
Suprax for Oral Suspension (Less than 2%) 1891
Suprax Tablets (Less than 2%) 1891
Tarceva Tablets 1228
Tarka Tablets 511
▲ Tasigna Capsules (1% to 10%) 2316
▲ Taxotere Injection Concentrate (8.9%) 2773
Timentin ADD-Vantage 1606
Timentin Injection Galaxy Container 1609
Timentin IV Infusion 1603
Timentin Pharmacy Bulk Package 1613
Tracleer Tablets 3289
Trizivir Tablets (0.8%) 1622
▲ Truvada Tablets (Less than or equal to 3%) 1262
Tyzeka Tablets (Less than 1%) 2328
Velcade for Injection 2168
Viramune Oral Suspension (1.7%) 873
Viramune Tablets (1.7%) 873
▲ Xeloda Tablets (2% to 22%) 2662
Xyzal Oral Solution (Less than 1%) ... 2789
Xyzal Oral Solution (Less than 1%) ... 3155
Xyzal Tablets (Less than 1%) 2789
Xyzal Tablets (Less than 1%) 3155
Zinacef for Injection (1 in 500 patients) 1678
Zinacef Injection (1 in 500 patients) 1678
Zosyn for Injection 3284
Zovirax 1690
Zyrtec Chewable Tablets 1920
Zyrtec Syrup 1920
Zyrtec Tablets 1920
Zyrtec-D 12 Hour Extended Release Tablets 1923

Hypercalcemia

Abelcet Injection 1134
Actiq (Less than 1%) 959
Activella Tablets 2347
Avelox (Greater than or equal to 2%) 2803
Benicar HCT Tablets 1010
Calcijex Injection 419
Cancidas for Injection 1953
▲ CellCept Capsules (3% to less than 20%) 2622
▲ CellCept Intravenous (3% to less than 20%) 2622
▲ CellCept Oral Suspension (3% to less than 20%) 2622
▲ CellCept Tablets (3% to less than 20%) 2622
Cipro I.V. (Infrequent) 2817
Cipro XR Tablets 2823
Climara Transdermal System 763
▲ Doxil Injection (1% to 10%) 2378
Dyazide Capsules 1405
Estratest Tablets 3043
Estratest H.S. Tablets 3043
Evoxac Capsules (Less than 1%) 1013
Femara Tablets (Less frequent) 2246
Fentora Tablets (Greater than 1%) 968
▲ Flolan for Injection (48%) 1426
▲ Forteo for Injection (6% to 11.1%) ... 1816
▲ Fosrenol Chewable Tablets (0% to 4%) 3027
▲ Intron A for Injection (Less than or equal to 5%) 2859
Micardis HCT Tablets 854
▲ Myfortic Tablets (3% to less than 20%) 2276
Paxil (Rare) 1535
Paxil CR Controlled-Release Tablets (Rare) 1544
PhosLo GelCaps 1184
Premarin Intravenous 3217
Premarin Vaginal Cream 3228
Premphase Tablets 3232
Prempro Tablets 3232
Prinzide Tablets 2092
▲ Prograf Capsules and Injection (3% to 15%) 622
Rilutek Tablets (Rare) 2771
▲ Rocaltrol Capsules (1 in 3) 1150
▲ Rocaltrol Oral Solution (1 in 3) 1150
▲ Simulect for Injection (3% to 10%) ... 2306
Tasigna Capsules 2316
Vantas (Less than 2%) 1737
Velcade for Injection (2%) 2168
Vesanoid Capsules (Isolated cases) 2660
Xeloda Tablets (1.1%) 2662
Zemplar Capsules 536
Zemplar Injection 538
Zosyn for Injection 3284

Hypercalciuria

Calcijex Injection 419
Effexor XR Extended-Release Capsules (Rare) 3195
▲ Rocaltrol Capsules (1 in 7) 1150
▲ Rocaltrol Oral Solution (1 in 7) 1150
Venlafaxine Hydrochloride Tablets (Rare) 2199

Hypercapnia

▲ DepoDur Injection (2% to 5%) 1095

Hyperchloremia

Avelox (Greater than or equal to 2%) 2803
Demadex Injection 2630
Demadex Tablets 2630
Geodon Capsules (Rare) 2520
Primaxin I.M. 2080
Primaxin I.V. 2083
Sulfamylon Cream 2194
Sulfamylon for 5% Topical Solution .. 2194

Hyperchlorhydria

Effexor XR Extended-Release Capsules (Rare) 3195
Mirapex Tablets 857
Prozac Weekly Capsules (Infrequent) 1852
Prozac Pulvules and Liquid (Infrequent) 1852
Venlafaxine Hydrochloride Tablets (Rare) 2199

Hypercholesterolemia

Accutane Capsules 2607
Aceon Tablets (2 mg, 4 mg, 8 mg) (0.3% to 1%) 3038
▲ Alphagan P Ophthalmic Solution (1% to 4%) 549
Ambien Tablets (Rare) 2692
Ambien CR Tablets (Rare) 2696
Amerge Tablets (Rare) 1301
AndroGel 3159
▲ Aptivus Capsules (1% to 17.7%) 823
▲ Aptivus Oral Solution (1% to 17.7%) 823
Aricept Tablets (Infrequent) 1062
Aricept ODT Tablets (Infrequent) 1062
▲ Arimidex Tablets (2% to 9%) 672
▲ Atripla Tablets (22%) 938
Axert Tablets (Rare) 2431
Benicar Tablets (Greater than 0.5%) 1009
Benicar HCT Tablets (Greater than 0.5%) 1010
▲ Boniva Injection (4.8%) 2614
▲ Boniva Tablets (4.8%) 2618
Bystolic Tablets (Greater than or equal to 1%) 1155
Calcijex Injection 419
Carbatrol Capsules (Occasional) 3019
Celebrex Capsules (0.1% to 1.9%) ... 2979
▲ CellCept Capsules (3% to 41.2%) 2622
▲ CellCept Intravenous (3% to 41.2%) 2622
▲ CellCept Oral Suspension (3% to 41.2%) 2622
▲ CellCept Tablets (3% to 41.2%) 2622
▲ Chemet Capsules (4.2% to 10.4%) 2484
Cipro I.V. (Infrequent) 2817
Cipro 2810
Cipro XR Tablets 2823
Combigan Ophthalmic Solution (0.1% to 0.2%) 553
▲ Coreg Tablets (1% to 4%) 1387
▲ Coreg CR Extended-Release Capsules (1% to 4%) 1393
Crixivan Capsules (0.9%) 1979
Cymbalta Delayed-Release Capsules (Infrequent) 1801
Delatestryl Injection 1730
Edex Injection (1%) 2957
▲ Effexor XR Extended-Release Capsules (5.3%) 3195
▲ Emsam Transdermal System (Infrequent) 905
▲ Emtriva Capsules (22%) 1246
▲ Emtriva Oral Solution (22%) 1246
Equetro Extended-Release Capsules 3174
Estratest Tablets 3043
Estratest H.S. Tablets 3043
Evoxac Capsules (Less than 1%) 1013
Exelon Capsules (Infrequent) 2229
Exelon Oral Solution (Infrequent) 2229
Exforge Tablets (Greater than or equal to 0.2%) 2238
▲ Femara Tablets (Less than 0.1% to 15.6%) 2246
Gabitril Tablets (Infrequent) 973
Gengraf Capsules (Less than 3%) 435
Geodon Capsules (Infrequent) 2520
▲ Humira Injection (6%) 442
▲ Kaletra (9% to 39%) 452
▲ Leukine (17%) 774
Lexapro Oral Suspension (Infrequent) 1174
Lexapro Tablets (Infrequent) 1174
▲ Lucentis Injection (1% to 8%) 1205
Lunesta Tablets (Infrequent) 2994
▲ Lupron Depot 3.75 mg (7%) 462
▲ Lupron Depot 7.5 mg (Greater than or equal to 5%) 469
Luvox CR Extended-Release Capsules (Infrequent) 1759
Micardis Tablets (More than 0.3%) 852
Micardis HCT Tablets 854
Mirapex Tablets 857
▲ Myfortic Tablets (3% to less than 20%) 2276
Neoral Oral Solution (Less than 3%) 2280
Neoral Soft Gelatin Capsules (Less than 3%) 2280
Noroxin Tablets 2069
▲ Norvir (36.5% to 44.8%) 489
Patanase Nasal Spray 544
Paxil (Rare) 1535
Paxil CR Controlled-Release Tablets (Rare) 1544
▲ Plavix Tablets (4%) 926
▲ Plavix Tablets (4%) 2767
Prinzide Tablets 2092
▲ Pristiq Extended-Release Tablets (3% to 10%) 3247
▲ Prograf Capsules and Injection (3% to 15%) 622
Protopic Ointment (0.2% to less than 1%) 628
Prozac Weekly Capsules (Infrequent) 1852
Prozac Pulvules and Liquid (Infrequent) 1852
▲ Rapamune (Greater than or equal to 30% to 46%) 3260
▲ Remeron Tablets (Greater than or equal to 20%) 2924
▲ RemeronSolTab Tablets (Greater than or equal to 20%) 2927
Requip Tablets (Infrequent) 1561
Rilutek Tablets (Rare) 2771
Risperdal Consta Long-Acting Injection (Infrequent) 1753
Rocaltrol Capsules 1150
Rocaltrol Oral Solution 1150
Rythmol SR Capsules 1590
▲ Spiriva HandiHaler (1% to 3%) 870
Sustiva Capsules 930
Sustiva Tablets 930
▲ Targretin Capsules (32.1% to 62.3%) 1084
Teveten Tablets (Less than 1%) 515
Teveten HCT Tablets (Less than 1%) 517
▲ Torisel Injection (2% to 87%) 3272
▲ Travatan Z Ophthalmic Solution (1% to 5%) 547
▲ Truvada Tablets (22%) 1262
Vantas (Less than 2%) 1737
▲ Venlafaxine Hydrochloride Tablets (Infrequent to 5.3%) 2199
▲ Vesanoid Capsules (Up to 60%) 2660
▲ Viread Tablets (19% to 22%) 1268
Vivitrol 988
Xyrem Oral Solution (Infrequent) 1766
Zyprexa Tablets (Rare) 1883
Zyprexa ZYDIS Orally Disintegrating Tablets (Rare) 1883

Hypercorticism

▲ Advair Diskus 100/50 (Greater than or equal to 3%) 1276
Advair Diskus 250/50 1276
Advair Diskus 500/50 1276
Advair HFA 45/21 Inhalation Aerosol 1288
Advair HFA 115/21 Inhalation Aerosol 1288
Advair HFA 230/21 Inhalation Aerosol 1288
Beconase AQ Nasal Spray 1369
FML Ophthalmic Ointment (Rare) ..... ⊙ 223
FML Ophthalmic Suspension (Rare) .... ⊙ 224
Omnaris Nasal Spray (Very rare) 2998
Pred Forte Ophthalmic Suspension (Rare) .... ⊙ 227
Pred Mild Ophthalmic Suspension (Rare) .... ⊙ 230
Qvar Inhalation Aerosol 3116
Veramyst Nasal Spray 1643

Hyperdipsia

(*see under* Dipsesis)

Hyperemia

▲ Azopt Ophthalmic Suspension (1% to 5%) 540
▲ Elestat Ophthalmic Solution (1% to 10%) 1741
Iquix Ophthalmic Solution (Less than 1%) 3183
Lacrisert Sterile Ophthalmic Insert .... ⊙ 233
▲ Pataday Ophthalmic Solution (Less than or equal to 5%) 543
▲ Patanol Ophthalmic Solution (Less than 5%) 546
Viroptic Ophthalmic Solution .... ⊙ 253

Hyperemia, conjunctival

▲ Alphagan P Ophthalmic Solution (Approximately 10% to 20%) 549
Cialis Tablets (Less than 2%) 1792
▲ Combigan Ophthalmic Solution (5% to 15%) 553
▲ Cosopt Sterile Ophthalmic Solution (5% to 30%) 1969
▲ Durezol Ophthalmic Emulsion (5% to 15%) .... ⊙ 275
FML Ophthalmic Ointment (Occasional) .... ⊙ 223
FML Ophthalmic Suspension (Occasional) .... ⊙ 224
FML Forte Ophthalmic Suspension (Occasional) .... ⊙ 222
▲ Lucentis Injection (0% to 12.6%) 1205

▲ Lumigan Ophthalmic Solution (15% to 45%) 556
Natacyn Antifungal Ophthalmic Suspension (One case) ⊙204
Pred Forte Ophthalmic Suspension (Occasional) ⊙227
Pred Mild Ophthalmic Suspension (Occasional) ⊙230
▲ Restasis Ophthalmic Emulsion (1% to 5%) 557
▲ Vigamox Ophthalmic Solution (1% to 6%) 548

Hyperemia, subconjunctival

▲ Travatan Z Ophthalmic Solution (3%) 547

Hypereosinophilia

Ketek Tablets (Less than 0.2%) 2744
Leustatin Injection 2384
Vivitrol 988
Zyprexa Tablets (0.3%) 1883
Zyprexa IntraMuscular (0.3%) 1883
Zyprexa ZYDIS Orally Disintegrating Tablets (0.3%) 1883

Hyperesthesia

Amerge Tablets (Rare) 1301
Asacol Delayed-Release Tablets 2579
Axert Tablets (Infrequent) 2431
Celexa (Rare) 1160
Cipro I.V. 2817
Cipro 2810
Cipro XR Tablets 2823
▲ Dacogen Injection (11%) 1066
Diprolene Lotion 0.05% (Less than 1%) 2838
Doxil Injection (Less than 1%) 2378
Effexor XR Extended-Release Capsules (Frequent) 3195
Emsam Transdermal System (Infrequent) 905
Evoxac Capsules 1013
▲ Flolan for Injection (5% to 12%) 1426
Frova Tablets (Frequent) 1111
Gengraf Capsules 435
Imitrex Injection (Rare) 1465
Imitrex Tablets (Rare) 1474
▲ Intron A for Injection (Less than 5%) 2859
▲ Ixempra Kit for Injection (62%) 915
▲ Kepivance (12%) 583
Lamictal (Rare) 1488
Lidoderm Patch 1114
Lunesta Tablets (Rare) 2994
Lyrica Capsules (0.1% to 1%) 2527
Maxalt Tablets (Infrequent) 2056
Maxalt-MLT Orally Disintegrating Tablets (Infrequent) 2056
Neoral Oral Solution 2280
Neoral Soft Gelatin Capsules 2280
Neupro Transdermal System 3149
Norvir (Less than 2%) 489
Pletal Tablets (2% or greater) 2481
ProAmatine Tablets (Rare) 3032
▲ Protopic Ointment (Up to 7%) 628
Prozac Weekly Capsules (Rare) 1852
Prozac Pulvules and Liquid (Rare) 1852
▲ Requip Tablets (Infrequent to 4%) 1561
▲ Soriatane Capsules (10% to 25%) 3062
Targretin Capsules 1084
Tasigna Capsules (0.1% to 1%) 2316
Venlafaxine Hydrochloride Tablets (Infrequent) 2199
Zometa for Intravenous Infusion 2341
Zomig Tablets (Infrequent) 694
▲ Zomig Nasal Spray (0% to 5%) 689
Zomig-ZMT Tablets (Infrequent) 694
Zonegran Capsules (Rare) 1089
Zyrtec Chewable Tablets (Less than 2%) 1920
Zyrtec Syrup (Less than 2%) 1920
Zyrtec Tablets (Less than 2%) 1920
Zyrtec-D 12 Hour Extended Release Tablets (Less than 2%) 1923

Hyperesthesia, tongue

Alferon N Injection (1%) 1726

Hyperexcitability, paradoxical

Valium Tablets 2658

Hyperfibrinogenemia

Alphanate 1709
Premarin Tablets 3221
Premphase Tablets 3232
Prempro Tablets 3232

Hyperglycemia

Abelcet Injection 1134
Abilify Injection (Greater than or equal to 1 in 1000 patients and less than 1 in 100 patients) 881
Abilify Injection (Greater than or equal to 1 in 1000 patients and less than 1 in 100 patients) 2466
Abilify Oral Solution (Greater than or equal to 1 in 1000 patients and less than 1 in 100 patients) 881
Abilify Oral Solution (Greater than or equal to 1 in 1000 patients and less than 1 in 100 patients) 2466
Abilify Discmelt Orally Disintegrating Tablets (Greater than or equal to 1 in 1000 patients and less than 1 in 100 patients) 881
Abilify Discmelt Orally Disintegrating Tablets (Greater than or equal to 1 in 1000 patients and less than 1 in 100 patients) 2466
Abilify Tablets (Greater than or equal to 1 in 1000 patients and less than 1 in 100 patients) 881
Abilify Tablets (Greater than or equal to 1 in 1000 patients and less than 1 in 100 patients) 2466
Accutane Capsules 2607
Aceon Tablets (2 mg, 4 mg, 8 mg) (0.3% to 1%) 3038
Actimmune (Rare) 1743
Actiq (1% or greater) 959
Advair Diskus 100/50 1276
Advair Diskus 250/50 1276
Advair Diskus 500/50 1276
Advair HFA 45/21 Inhalation Aerosol 1288
Advair HFA 115/21 Inhalation Aerosol 1288
Advair HFA 230/21 Inhalation Aerosol 1288
▲ Advicor Tablets (4%) 402
Aggrenox Capsules (Less than 1%) 819
Aloxi Injection (Less than 1%) 1059
Ambien Tablets (Infrequent) 2692
Ambien CR Tablets (Infrequent) 2696
▲ AmBisome for Injection (8.2% to 23%) 606
Amerge Tablets (Rare) 1301
Anaprox Tablets (Less than 1%) 2632
Anaprox DS Tablets (Less than 1%) 2632
AndroGel 3159
Aptivus Capsules (Less than 2%) 823
Aptivus Oral Solution (Less than 2%) 823
Aricept Tablets (Infrequent) 1062
Aricept ODT Tablets (Infrequent) 1062
▲ Arranon Injection (0% to 6%) 1319
Atacand Tablets (0.5% or greater) 639
Atacand HCT (0.5% or greater) 642
Atripla Tablets (2%) 938
Avalide Tablets 892
Avalide Tablets 2713
▲ Avandamet Tablets (5.9%) 1336
▲ Avandia Tablets (3.9%) 1351
Avelox (Less than 0.1%) 2803
Axert Tablets (Infrequent) 2431
Baraclude (2%) 900
Bayer Aspirin 750
Benicar HCT Tablets (Greater than 1%) 1010
Brovana Inhalation Solution (Less than 2%) 2990
▲ Busulfex Injection (15% to 67%) 2477
Campral Tablets (Infrequent) 1158
▲ Cancidas for Injection (6.4%) 1953
Cardizem LA Extended Release Tablets (Less than 2%) 421
Catapres Tablets (Rare) 841
Celebrex Capsules (0.1% to 1.9%) 2979
▲ CellCept Capsules (43.7% to 46.7%) 2622
▲ CellCept Intravenous (43.7% to 46.7%) 2622
▲ CellCept Oral Suspension (43.7% to 46.7%) 2622
▲ CellCept Tablets (43.7% to 46.7%) 2622
Cipro I.V. (Among most frequent) 2817
Cipro 2810
Cipro XR Tablets (Less than 1%) 2823
Clinoril Tablets (Rare) 1962
Clorpres Tablets 2185
Combigan Ophthalmic Solution 553
Combivir Tablets 1384
▲ Coreg Tablets (5% to 12%) 1387
▲ Coreg CR Extended-Release Capsules (5% to 12%) 1393
Cosopt Sterile Ophthalmic Solution 1969
Crixivan Capsules 1979
Cubicin for Injection (1% to 2%) 995
Cymbalta Delayed-Release Capsules 1801
▲ Dacogen Injection (33%) 1066
Demadex Injection 2630
Demadex Tablets 2630
Diovan HCT Tablets 2216
Diprolene Lotion 0.05% 2838
Diprolene Ointment 0.05% (Some patients) 2839
Diprolene AF Cream 0.05% (Some patients) 2837
▲ Doxil Injection (1% to 10%) 2378
Dyazide Capsules 1405
EC-Naprosyn Delayed-Release Tablets (Less than 1%) 2632
Edecrin 698
Edex Injection (1%) 2957
Effexor XR Extended-Release Capsules (Infrequent) 3195
Elocon Cream 0.1% 2840
Elocon Lotion 0.1% 2841
Elocon Ointment 0.1% 2842
▲ Eloxatin for Injection (2% to 14%) 2731
Elspar for Injection (Low) 1990
Elspar for Injection (Low) 2488
Emend Capsules (Greater than 0.5%) 1992
Emend for Injection (Greater than 0.5%) 1999
Emsam Transdermal System (Infrequent) 905
Emtriva Capsules (2%) 1246
Emtriva Oral Solution (2%) 1246
Epivir 1412
Epivir-HBV 1417
Epzicom Tablets 1422
Evoxac Capsules (Less than 1%) 1013
Exelon Capsules (Infrequent) 2229
Exelon Oral Solution (Infrequent) 2229
Exforge Tablets (Greater than 0.1% to less than 1%) 2238
Flovent Diskus 50 mcg 1435
Flovent HFA 1440
Foradil Aerolizer 2849
Furosemide Tablets 2186
Gabitril Tablets (Infrequent) 973
Gengraf Capsules (2% or less) 435
Genotropin Lyophilized Powder (Infrequent) 2547
Geodon Capsules (Infrequent) 2520
▲ Gliadel Wafer (3%) 1076
Humatrope Vials and Cartridges (Infrequent) 1838
Imitrex Injection 1465
Imitrex Nasal Spray 1470
Imitrex Tablets (Rare) 1474
▲ Indapamide Tablets (Less than 5%) 2188
Indocin Capsules (Less than 1%) 2024
Indocin I.V. (Less than 1%) 2489
Indocin (Less than 1%) 2024
Intravenous Sodium Diuril 2490
▲ Intron A for Injection (Less than or equal to 5%) 2859
Invanz for Injection (1.2% to 1.7%) 2029
Invega Extended-Release Tablets 1748
Ionsys Transdermal System (.1% to less than 1%) 2410
▲ Kaletra (1% to 5%) 452
Lamictal (Rare) 1488
▲ Leukine (25% to 41%) 774
Levaquin (0.1% to 1%) 2416
Levaquin in 5% Dextrose Injection (0.1% to 1%) 2416
Lexapro Oral Suspension (Infrequent) 1174
Lexapro Tablets (Infrequent) 1174
Lexiva Oral Suspension (2%) 1510
Lexiva Tablets (2%) 1510
Lipitor Tablets (Less than 2%) 2501
Lotrisone 2881
Lovaza Capsules 1520
▲ Lupron Depot 7.5 mg (Greater than or equal to 5%) 469
Luvox CR Extended-Release Capsules (Rare) 1759
▲ Megace ES Oral Suspension (0% to 6%) 2499
▲ Mepron Suspension (9%) 1526
Meridia Capsules 475
Micardis HCT Tablets 854
Mirapex Tablets 857
▲ Mycamine for Injection (5.6% to 16%) 616
▲ Myfortic Tablets (3% to less than 20%) 2276
▲ Mylotarg for Injection (10% to 11%) 3212
Namenda 1180
Naprosyn Suspension (Less than 1%) 2632
Naprosyn Tablets (Less than 1%) 2632
NeoProfen Injection 2496
Neoral Oral Solution (2% or less) 2280
Neoral Soft Gelatin Capsules (2% or less) 2280
Niaspan Extended-Release Tablets 480
Nimotop Capsules (0.8%; rare) 790
Norditropin Cartridges 2354
Noroxin Tablets 2069
Norvir 489
▲ Noxafil Oral Suspension (11%) 2889
Olux Foam 3061
Olux-E Foam 3059
Omnicef Capsules (0.9%) 497
Omnicef for Oral Suspension (0.9%) 497
▲ Oncaspar Injection (Greater than or equal to 2% to 5%) 1138
Paxil (Infrequent) 1535
Paxil CR Controlled-Release Tablets (Infrequent) 1544
PegIntron Powder for Injection (Less than or equal to 1%) 2903
Percocet Tablets 1127
Percodan Tablets 1130
Perforomist Inhalation Solution 1025
Phenytek Capsules 2192
Pletal Tablets 2481
Prandin Tablets 2971
Prinzide Tablets 2092
Proglycem Capsules (Frequent) 1185
Proglycem Suspension (Frequent) 1185
▲ Prograf Capsules and Injection (Many patients; 13% to 47%) 622
Proleukin for Injection 2287
Protonix for Delayed-Release Oral Suspension (Less than or equal to 1%) 3254
Protonix Delayed-Release Tablets (Less than or equal to 1%) 3254
Protonix I.V. (Less than or equal to 1%) 3257
Protopic Ointment (Greater than or equal to 1%) 628
Provigil Tablets (Greater than or equal to 1%) 977
Prozac Weekly Capsules 1852
Rapamune 3260
Requip Tablets (1% or more) 1561
Reyataz Capsules 3299
Risperdal Consta Long-Acting Injection (Infrequent) 1753
▲ Rituxan I.V. (1% to 9%) 1223
Rythmol Tablets (Less than 1%) 1586
Rythmol SR Capsules 1590
St. Joseph 81 mg Aspirin Chewable and Enteric Coated Tablets 1903
Sandimmune (2% or less) 2296
▲ Sandostatin Injection (3% to 16%) 2300
▲ Sandostatin LAR Depot (15% to 27%) 2302
Serevent Diskus (1% to less than 3%) 1594
▲ Simulect for Injection (Greater than or equal to 10%) 2306
▲ Somatuline Depot Injection (7%) 3102
▲ Spiriva HandiHaler (1% to 3%) 870
Symbyax Capsules 1871
Targretin Capsules 1084
▲ Tasigna Capsules (1% to 11%) 2316
Tekturna HCT Tablets 2324
Teveten Tablets (Less than 1%) 515
Teveten HCT Tablets (Less than 1%) 517
Thiothixene Capsules 2197
Timoptic Sterile Ophthalmic Solution 2121
Timoptic in Ocudose 2124
Timoptic-XE Sterile Ophthalmic Gel Forming Solution 2125
▲ Torisel Injection (16% to 89%) 3272
Trasylol Injection (1% to 2%) 799
▲ Trisenox Injection (45%) 986
Trizivir Tablets 1622
▲ Truvada Tablets (Less than or equal to 3%) 1262
Tygacil for Injection (1.8%) 3276
Ultane Liquid for Inhalation (Less than 1%) 524
Ultram ER Extended-Release Tablets (0.5% to less than 1%) 2428
Urso 250 Tablets (1%) 720
Urso Forte Tablets (1%) 720
▲ Valcyte Tablets (Less than 5%) 2654
Valstar Sterile Solution for Intravesical Instillation (1%) 1735
Vanos Cream 1941
Vantas (Less than 2%) 1737
Vaprisol (2.7%) 632
Venlafaxine Hydrochloride Tablets (Infrequent) 2199
Verdeso Foam 3069
▲ Viread Tablets (2% to 3%) 1268
Voltaren Tablets (Rarely) 2334
Voltaren-XR Tablets (Rarely) 2337

Wellbutrin Tablets 1648
Wellbutrin SR Sustained-Release Tablets 1653
Wellbutrin XL Extended-Release Tablets 1659
▲ Xopenex Inhalation Solution (2.6% to 5.2%) 3001
▲ Xopenex Inhalation Solution Concentrate (2.6% to 5.2%) 3005
▲ Xopenex HFA Inhalation Aerosol (2.6% to 5.2%) 3009
Xyrem Oral Solution (Infrequent) 1766
Ziagen (Less than 1%) 1673
▲ Zolinza Capsules (8.1%) 2142
Zomig Tablets (Rare) 694
Zomig-ZMT Tablets (Rare) 694
Zosyn for Injection 3284
Zyprexa Tablets (Infrequent) 1883
Zyprexa ZYDIS Orally Disintegrating Tablets (Infrequent) 1883

Hyperglycinemia

Abilify Injection (Infrequent) 2466
Abilify Oral Solution (Infrequent) 2466
Abilify Discmelt Orally Disintegrating Tablets (Infrequent) 2466
Abilify Tablets (Infrequent) 2466
Atripla Tablets (1%) 938
Depakote ER Tablets 423
Fentora Tablets (Greater than 1%) 968
Moban Tablets 1116
▲ Novantrone for Injection Concentrate (10% to 31%) 1100
Rythmol SR Capsules 1590
▲ Tasigna Capsules (1% to 10%) 2316

Hyperhemoglobinemia

Ambien Tablets (Rare) 2692
Ambien CR Tablets (Rare) 2696
Evoxac Capsules 1013

Hyperheparinemia

Mustargen for Injection (Rare) 2492

Hyperhidrosis

Abilify Injection (Greater than or equal to 1 in 100 patients) 881
Abilify Injection (Greater than or equal to 1 in 100 patients) 2466
Abilify Oral Solution (Greater than or equal to 1 in 100 patients) 881
Abilify Oral Solution (Greater than or equal to 1 in 100 patients) 2466
Abilify Discmelt Orally Disintegrating Tablets (Greater than or equal to 1 in 100 patients) 881
Abilify Discmelt Orally Disintegrating Tablets (Greater than or equal to 1 in 100 patients) 2466
Abilify Tablets (Greater than or equal to 1 in 100 patients) 881
Abilify Tablets (Greater than or equal to 1 in 100 patients) 2466
Accutane Capsules 2607
Amitiza Capsules (Less than 1%) 3082
Byetta Injection (Greater than or equal to 1% to less than 5%) 600
▲ Celexa (11%) 1160
Chantix Tablets (Frequent) 2511
▲ Concerta Extended-Release Tablets (5.1%) 1925
▲ Cymbalta Delayed-Release Capsules (6% to 8%) 1801
Diovan HCT Tablets (Greater than 0.2%) 2216
DynaCirc CR Controlled Release Tablets (0.5% to 1%) 1407
Exforge Tablets (Greater than or equal to 0.2%) 2238
Fentora Tablets (Greater than 1%) 968
Havrix Injection Vaccine 1454
Intelence Tablets (Less than 2%) 3119
Miacalcin Nasal Spray (Less than 1%) 2274
Nexium Delayed-Release Capsules 645
Nexium I.V. 652
Nexium Delayed-Release Oral Suspension 645
Noroxin Tablets (0.3% to 1%) 2069
Primaxin I.M. 2080
Primaxin I.V. (Less than 0.2%) 2083
Prinivil Tablets 2087
Prinzide Tablets (0.3% to 1%) 2092
▲ Pristiq Extended-Release Tablets (5% to 21%) 3247
▲ Requip Tablets (3%) 1561
▲ Tasigna Capsules (1% to 10%) 2316
Treximet Tablets (Infrequent) 1616
Twinrix Vaccine 1628
▲ Vyvanse Capsules (3%) 3033
▲ Xyrem Oral Solution (2.9% to 5.7%) 1766

Hyperhidrosis, application site

▲ Flector Patch (4%) 561

Hyperhistaminemia

▲ Vesanoid Capsules (3%) 2660

Hyperirritability

Seromycin Capsules 1864

Hyperirritability, neuromuscular

Timentin ADD-Vantage 1606
Timentin Injection Galaxy Container 1609
Timentin IV Infusion 1603
Timentin Pharmacy Bulk Package 1613

Hyperkalemia

Abelcet Injection 1134
Aceon Tablets (2 mg, 4 mg, 8 mg) (1.4%) 3038
Aggrenox Capsules 819
Aloxi Injection (1%) 1059
AmBisome for Injection (Less common) 606
Anaprox Tablets (Less than 1%) 2632
Anaprox DS Tablets (Less than 1%) 2632
Atacand Tablets 639
Atacand HCT (Very rare) 642
Avalide Tablets 892
Avalide Tablets (Rare to 1.2%) 2713
▲ Avapro Tablets (18.6%) 897
▲ Avapro Tablets (18.6%) 2718
Azor Tablets 1005
Bayer Aspirin 750
Benicar Tablets 1009
Benicar HCT Tablets 1010
Brovana Inhalation Solution 2990
Cancidas for Injection (0% to 2.6%) 1953
Captopril Tablets 2182
Celebrex Capsules (Greater than or equal to 0.1% to less than 1%) 2979
▲ CellCept Capsules (22%) 2622
▲ CellCept Intravenous (22%) 2622
▲ CellCept Oral Suspension (22%) 2622
▲ CellCept Tablets (22%) 2622
Chantix Tablets (Rare) 2511
Cipro I.V. (Infrequent) 2817
Cipro 2810
Cipro XR Tablets 2823
Clinoril Tablets (Less than 1 in 100) 1962
▲ Coreg Tablets (Greater than 1% to 3%) 1387
▲ Coreg CR Extended-Release Capsules (Greater than 1% to less than or equal to 3%) 1393
▲ Cozaar Tablets (7%) 1973
▲ Cubicin for Injection (5%) 995
▲ Dacogen Injection (13%) 1066
Delatestryl Injection 1730
Demadex Injection 2630
Demadex Tablets 2630
Diovan Tablets (2%) 2212
Diovan HCT Tablets (0.4%) 2216
Doxil Injection (Less than 1%) 2378
Dyazide Capsules 1405
Dyrenium Capsules (Rare) 3189
EC-Naprosyn Delayed-Release Tablets (Less than 1%) 2632
Effexor XR Extended-Release Capsules (Rare) 3195
Epogen for Injection (Approximately 0.11%) 576
Estratest Tablets 3043
Estratest H.S. Tablets 3043
Evoxac Capsules 1013
Exforge Tablets 2238
▲ Flolan for Injection (4%) 1426
Gengraf Capsules (1% to less than 3%) 435
Geodon Capsules (Rare) 2520
Gleevec Tablets (Rare) 2255
Indocin Capsules (Less than 1%) 2024
Indocin I.V. (Less than 1%) 2489
Indocin (Less than 1%) 2024
Invanz for Injection (0.5% to 1.3%) 2029
Levaquin (0.1% to 1%) 2416
Levaquin in 5% Dextrose Injection (0.1% to 1%) 2416
Lovenox Injection 2756
▲ Mavik Tablets (0.3% to 5.3%) 472
Micardis Tablets 852
▲ Mycamine for Injection (4% to 5%) 616
▲ Myfortic Tablets (3% to less than 20%) 2276
Naprosyn Suspension (Less than 1%) 2632
Naprosyn Tablets (Less than 1%) 2632
Neoral Oral Solution (1% to less than 3%) 2280
Neoral Soft Gelatin Capsules (1% to less than 3%) 2280
Noroxin Tablets 2069
Omnicef Capsules (0.2%) 497
Omnicef for Oral Suspension (0.2%) 497
Paxil (Rare) 1535
Paxil CR Controlled-Release Tablets (Rare) 1544
Percocet Tablets 1127
Percodan Tablets 1130
Primaxin I.M. 2080
Primaxin I.V. 2083
▲ Prinivil Tablets (Approximately 2.2% to 4.8%) 2087
Prinzide Tablets (Approximately 1.4%) 2092
Procrit for Injection (0.11%) 2391
▲ Prograf Capsules and Injection (13% to 45%) 622
Prozac Weekly Capsules (Rare) 1852
Prozac Pulvules and Liquid (Rare) 1852
ReoPro Vials (0.1%) 1860
Requip Tablets (Infrequent) 1561
Rituxan I.V. 1223
St. Joseph 81 mg Aspirin Chewable and Enteric Coated Tablets 1903
Sandimmune (Occasional) 2296
▲ Simulect for Injection (Greater than or equal to 10%) 2306
▲ Sutent Capsules (6%) 2540
Symbyax Capsules (Rare) 1871
Targretin Capsules 1084
Tarka Tablets 511
▲ Tasigna Capsules (1% to 10%) 2316
▲ Tekturna Tablets (0.9% to 5.5%) 2321
Tekturna HCT Tablets (0.8%) 2324
Teveten Tablets (Less than 1%) 515
Teveten HCT Tablets (Less than 1%) 517
▲ Trisenox Injection (18%) 986
Ultane Liquid for Inhalation 524
▲ Valcyte Tablets (Less than 5%) 2654
Velcade for Injection 2168
Venlafaxine Hydrochloride Tablets (Rare) 2199
Zometa for Intravenous Infusion 2341
Zosyn for Injection 3284
Zyprexa Tablets (Infrequent) 1883
Zyprexa IntraMuscular (Infrequent) 1883
Zyprexa ZYDIS Orally Disintegrating Tablets (Infrequent) 1883

Hyperkalemia, neonatal

Prograf Capsules and Injection 622

Hyperkeratosis

Aricept Tablets (Infrequent) 1062
Aricept ODT Tablets (Infrequent) 1062
Evoxac Capsules (Less than 1%) 1013
Mirapex Tablets 857
Requip Tablets (Infrequent) 1561
Soriatane Capsules (Less than 1%) 3062
Tarka Tablets 511
Zyrtec Chewable Tablets (Less than 2%) 1920
Zyrtec Syrup (Less than 2%) 1920
Zyrtec Tablets (Less than 2%) 1920
Zyrtec-D 12 Hour Extended Release Tablets (Less than 2%) 1923

Hyperkinesia

AndroGel (One patient) 3159
Azilect Tablets (Frequent) 3106
Campral Tablets (Rare) 1158
Celexa (Infrequent) 1160
▲ Comtan Tablets (10%) 2208
Effexor XR Extended-Release Capsules (Infrequent) 3195
Elmiron Capsules 2435
Emsam Transdermal System (Infrequent) 905
Evoxac Capsules (Less than 1%) 1013
Exelon Capsules (Infrequent) 2229
Exelon Oral Solution (Infrequent) 2229
Flector Patch (1%) 561
▲ Flolan for Injection (7%) 1426
Flumadine (Less than 0.3%) 1167
Gabitril Tablets (Frequent) 973
Geodon Capsules (Frequent) 2520
▲ Intron A for Injection (Less than 5%) 2859
▲ Invega Extended-Release Tablets (3% to 10%) 1748
Keppra Oral Solution (Greater than or equal to 2%) 3131
Keppra Tablets (Greater than or equal to 2%) 3131
Lamictal (Infrequent) 1488
Levaquin (0.1% to 1%) 2416
Levaquin in 5% Dextrose Injection (0.1% to 1%) 2416
Lipitor Tablets (Less than 2%) 2501
Luvox CR Extended-Release Capsules (Frequent) 1759
Lyrica Capsules (0.1% to 1%) 2527
Maxair Autohaler 1705
Maxalt Tablets (Rare) 2056
Maxalt-MLT Orally Disintegrating Tablets (Rare) 2056
Mirapex Tablets 857
Namenda (Infrequent) 1180
Nembutal Sodium Solution, USP (Less than 1%) 2494
Omnicef for Oral Suspension (0.2%) 497
OxyContin Tablets (Less than 1%) 2589
Paxil (Infrequent) 1535
Paxil CR Controlled-Release Tablets (Infrequent) 1544
Protonix for Delayed-Release Oral Suspension (Less than 1%) 3254
Protonix Delayed-Release Tablets (Less than 1%) 3254
Protonix I.V. (Less than 1%) 3257
Proventil HFA Inhalation Aerosol (Less than 3%) 2914
Provigil Tablets (1%) 977
Prozac Weekly Capsules (Infrequent to greater than or equal to 2%) 1852
Prozac Pulvules and Liquid (At least 2%) 1852
Remeron Tablets (Frequent) 2924
RemeronSolTab Tablets (Frequent) 2927
Requip Tablets (2%) 1561
Salagen Tablets (Less than 1%) 1082
▲ Stalevo Tablets (5% to 10%) 2309
Symbyax Capsules (1% to 2%) 1871
Venlafaxine Hydrochloride Tablets (Infrequent) 2199
Wellbutrin SR Sustained-Release Tablets (Infrequent) 1653
Wellbutrin XL Extended-Release Tablets (Infrequent) 1659
WinRho SDF 741
Zomig Tablets (Rare) 694
Zomig-ZMT Tablets (Rare) 694
Zonegran Capsules (Infrequent) 1089
Zyban Sustained-Release Tablets (Infrequent) 1692
▲ Zyprexa Tablets (5% to 11%) 1883
Zyprexa IntraMuscular (2%) 1883
▲ Zyprexa ZYDIS Orally Disintegrating Tablets (5% to 11%) 1883
Zyrtec Chewable Tablets (Less than 2%) 1920
Zyrtec Syrup (Less than 2%) 1920
Zyrtec Tablets (Less than 2%) 1920
Zyrtec-D 12 Hour Extended Release Tablets (Less than 2%) 1923

Hyperlactemia

Abilify Injection (Greater than or equal to 1 in 1000 patients and less than 1 in 100 patients) 2466
Abilify Oral Solution (Greater than or equal to 1 in 1000 patients and less than 1 in 100 patients) 2466
Abilify Discmelt Orally Disintegrating Tablets (Greater than or equal to 1 in 1000 patients and less than 1 in 100 patients) 2466
Abilify Tablets (Greater than or equal to 1 in 1000 patients and less than 1 in 100 patients) 2466

Hyperlipemia

Aricept Tablets (2%) 1062
Aricept ODT Tablets (2%) 1062
Benicar HCT Tablets (Greater than 1%) 1010
▲ CellCept Capsules (3% to less than 20%) 2622
▲ CellCept Intravenous (3% to less than 20%) 2622
▲ CellCept Oral Suspension (3% to less than 20%) 2622
▲ CellCept Tablets (3% to less than 20%) 2622
Lovaza Capsules 1520
Lunesta Tablets (Rare) 2994
Prozac Weekly Capsules (Infrequent) 1852
Prozac Pulvules and Liquid (Infrequent) 1852
Risperdal Consta Long-Acting Injection (Infrequent) 1753
Symbyax Capsules (Infrequent) 1871
▲ Targretin Gel 1% (10%) 1088

Venlafaxine Hydrochloride Tablets (Infrequent) 2199

Hyperlipidemia

Abilify Injection (Greater than or equal to 1 in 1000 patients and less than 1 in 100 patients) 881
Abilify Injection (Greater than or equal to 1 in 1000 patients and less than 1 in 100 patients) 2466
Abilify Oral Solution (Greater than or equal to 1 in 1000 patients and less than 1 in 100 patients) 881
Abilify Oral Solution (Greater than or equal to 1 in 1000 patients and less than 1 in 100 patients) 2466
Abilify Discmelt Orally Disintegrating Tablets (Greater than or equal to 1 in 1000 patients and less than 1 in 100 patients) 881
Abilify Discmelt Orally Disintegrating Tablets (Greater than or equal to 1 in 1000 patients and less than 1 in 100 patients) 2466
Abilify Tablets (Greater than or equal to 1 in 1000 patients and less than 1 in 100 patients) 881
Abilify Tablets (Greater than or equal to 1 in 1000 patients and less than 1 in 100 patients) 2466
Ambien Tablets (Rare) 2692
Ambien CR Tablets (Rare) 2696
Amerge Tablets (Rare) 1301
AndroGel 3159
Aptivus Capsules (2.5%) 823
Aptivus Oral Solution (2.5%) 823
Avelox (Less than 0.1%) 2803
Benicar Tablets (Greater than 0.5%) 1009
Brovana Inhalation Solution (Less than 2%) 2990
Chantix Tablets (Infrequent) 2511
Cymbalta Delayed-Release Capsules (Infrequent) 1801
Doxil Injection (Less than 1%) 2378
Effexor XR Extended-Release Capsules (Infrequent) 3195
Evoxac Capsules (Less than 1%) 1013
Exelon Capsules (Infrequent) 2229
Exelon Oral Solution (Infrequent) 2229
Exelon Patch (Infrequent) 2233
Gabitril Tablets (Infrequent) 973
Geodon Capsules (Rare) 2520
▲ Humatrope Vials and Cartridges (8.1%) 1838
▲ Humira Injection (7%) 442
Lovenox Injection (Rare) 2756
Luvox CR Extended-Release Capsules (Rare) 1759
Mirapex Tablets 857
▲ Myfortic Tablets (3% to less than 20%) 2276
Namenda (More than one patient) 1180
Norvir (1.7% to 4.1%) 489
Pletal Tablets (Less than 2%) 2481
▲ Prograf Capsules and Injection (3% to 31%) 622
Protonix for Delayed-Release Oral Suspension (Greater than or equal to 1%) 3254
Protonix Delayed-Release Tablets (Greater than or equal to 1%) 3254
Protonix I.V. (Greater than or equal to 1%) 3257
Rythmol SR Capsules 1590
Sandimmune 2296
▲ Targretin Capsules (76.6% to 79.2%) 1084
▲ Torisel Injection (Greater than or equal to 30%) 3272
Yaz Tablets 805
Zyprexa Tablets (Rare) 1883
Zyprexa ZYDIS Orally Disintegrating Tablets (Rare) 1883

Hypermagnesemia

Doxil Injection (Less than 1%) 2378
▲ Zometa for Intravenous Infusion (12%) 2341

Hypernatremia

▲ AmBisome for Injection (4.1%) 606
Celebrex Capsules (Greater than or equal to 0.1% to less than 1%) 2979
Demadex Injection 2630
Demadex Tablets 2630
Doxil Injection (Less than 1%) 2378
Fleet Enema 1143
Fleet Enema Extra 1143
Fleet Enema for Children 1143
Fleet Pedia-Lax Enema 1143
Fleet Phospho-soda 1145
Fleet Phospho-soda EZ-PREP 1147
Fleet Prep Kits 1149
Invanz for Injection (0.1% to 1%) 2029
▲ Kaletra (3%) 452
Kinrix Injection Vaccine (0.1%) 1486
Kristalose for Oral Solution 1004
▲ Mycamine for Injection (4% to 6.4%) 616
▲ NeoProfen Injection (7%) 2496
▲ Sutent Capsules (0% to 10%) 2540
Timentin ADD-Vantage 1606
Timentin Injection Galaxy Container 1609
Timentin IV Infusion 1603
Timentin Pharmacy Bulk Package 1613
Velcade for Injection 2168
Xyrem Oral Solution (Infrequent) 1766
Zometa for Intravenous Infusion 2341
Zosyn for Injection 3284
Zyprexa Tablets (Rare) 1883
Zyprexa ZYDIS Orally Disintegrating Tablets (Rare) 1883

Hyperostosis, skeletal

Accutane Capsules 2607
▲ Soriatane Capsules (Less than 1% to 25%) 3062

Hyperparathyroidism

Nutropin for Injection 1208
Nutropin AQ Injection 1212
Nutropin AQ NuSpin Injection 1212
Nutropin AQ Pen 1212
Nutropin AQ Pen Cartridge 1212
Prinzide Tablets 2092

Hyperphenylalaninemia

Daraprim Tablets (Rare) 1400

Hyperphosphatemia

AmBisome for Injection (Less common) 606
▲ CellCept Capsules (3% to less than 20%) 2622
▲ CellCept Intravenous (3% to less than 20%) 2622
▲ CellCept Oral Suspension (3% to less than 20%) 2622
▲ CellCept Tablets (3% to less than 20%) 2622
Delatestryl Injection 1730
Didronel Tablets 2583
Effexor XR Extended-Release Capsules (Rare) 3195
Estratest Tablets 3043
Estratest H.S. Tablets 3043
Fleet Enema 1143
Fleet Enema Extra 1143
Fleet Enema for Children 1143
Fleet Pedia-Lax Enema 1143
Fleet Phospho-soda 1145
Fleet Phospho-soda EZ-PREP 1147
Fleet Prep Kits 1149
▲ Myfortic Tablets (3% to less than 20%) 2276
Paxil (Rare) 1535
Paxil CR Controlled-Release Tablets (Rare) 1544
▲ Prograf Capsules and Injection (3% to 15%) 622
Requip Tablets (Infrequent) 1561
Rituxan I.V. 1223
Tasigna Capsules 2316
Venlafaxine Hydrochloride Tablets (Rare) 2199

Hyperpigmentation

Accutane Capsules 2607
Advicor Tablets 402
Aldara Cream, 5% 1699
▲ Catapres-TTS (5 of 101 patients) 842
Cipro I.V. (1% or less) 2817
Cipro (Less than 1%) 2810
Cipro XR Tablets 2823
Combigan Ophthalmic Solution 553
Crixivan Capsules 1979
Daytrana Transdermal Patch 3022
▲ Emtriva Capsules (32%) 1246
▲ Emtriva Oral Solution (32%) 1246
▲ Myleran Tablets (5% to 10%) 1530
Niaspan Extended-Release Tablets 480
Taxotere Injection Concentrate 2773
▲ Trisenox Injection (8%) 986

Hyperpigmentation, nail beds

Taxotere Injection Concentrate 2773

Hyperplasia, endometrial

Enjuvia Tablets 1029
Premarin Tablets 3221

Hyperplasia, gingival

(*see under* Gingival hyperplasia)

Hyperplasia, mammary

Cuprimine Capsules (Rare) 1986

Hyperplasia, nodular, focal

Eloxatin for Injection 2731
Lybrel Tablets 3204

Hyperpnea

Aggrenox Capsules (Less than 1%) 819
Bayer Aspirin 750
Percocet Tablets 1127
Percodan Tablets 1130

Hyperprolactinemia

Abilify Injection (Greater than or equal to 1 in 1000 patients and less than 1 in 100 patients) 881
Abilify Injection (Greater than or equal to 1 in 1000 patients and less than 1 in 100 patients) 2466
Abilify Oral Solution (Greater than or equal to 1 in 1000 patients and less than 1 in 100 patients) 881
Abilify Oral Solution (Greater than or equal to 1 in 1000 patients and less than 1 in 100 patients) 2466
Abilify Discmelt Orally Disintegrating Tablets (Greater than or equal to 1 in 1000 patients and less than 1 in 100 patients) 881
Abilify Discmelt Orally Disintegrating Tablets (Greater than or equal to 1 in 1000 patients and less than 1 in 100 patients) 2466
Abilify Tablets (Greater than or equal to 1 in 1000 patients and less than 1 in 100 patients) 881
Abilify Tablets (Greater than or equal to 1 in 1000 patients and less than 1 in 100 patients) 2466
Celexa 1160
Effexor XR Extended-Release Capsules 3195
Invega Extended-Release Tablets 1748
Lexapro Oral Suspension 1174
Lexapro Tablets 1174
Moban Tablets 1116
Paxil 1535
Paxil CR Controlled-Release Tablets 1544
Pristiq Extended-Release Tablets (Less than 2%) 3247
Prozac Weekly Capsules 1852
Prozac Pulvules and Liquid 1852
Risperdal Consta Long-Acting Injection (Infrequent) 1753
Rythmol SR Capsules 1590
Symbyax Capsules 1871
Tarka Tablets 511
Thiothixene Capsules 2197
Venlafaxine Hydrochloride Tablets 2199
Zyprexa Tablets 1883
Zyprexa IntraMuscular 1883
Zyprexa ZYDIS Orally Disintegrating Tablets 1883

Hyperproteinemia

Evoxac Capsules 1013

Hyperprothrombinemia

AmBisome for Injection (Less common) 606
▲ Doxil Injection (1% to 10%) 2378
Estratest Tablets 3043
Estratest H.S. Tablets 3043
Rythmol SR Capsules 1590

Hyperpyrexia

(*see under* Fever)

Hyperreflexia

Celexa 1160
Depakote ER Tablets (Greater than 1%) 423
Effexor XR Extended-Release Capsules (Rare) 3195
Exelon Capsules (Infrequent) 2229
Exelon Oral Solution (Infrequent) 2229
Gabitril Tablets (Infrequent) 973
Geodon Capsules (Rare) 2520
Keppra Oral Solution (2%) 3131
Keppra Tablets (2%) 3131
Lexapro Oral Suspension (Infrequent) 1174
Lexapro Tablets (Infrequent) 1174
Mirapex Tablets 857
Orthoclone OKT3 Sterile Solution 2387
Paxil (Rare) 1535
Paxil CR Controlled-Release Tablets (Rare) 1544
Pristiq Extended-Release Tablets 3247
Prozac Weekly Capsules (Rare) 1852
Prozac Pulvules and Liquid (Rare) 1852
Remeron Tablets (Infrequent) 2924
RemeronSolTab Tablets (Infrequent) 2927
Seromycin Capsules 1864
Thiothixene Capsules 2197
Treximet Tablets 1616
Venlafaxine Hydrochloride Tablets (Rare) 2199
Zonegran Capsules (Infrequent) 1089
Zyvox 2552

Hypersalivation

(*see also under* Sialism)

Exelon Patch (Infrequent) 2233
Luvox CR Extended-Release Capsules (Infrequent) 1759
▲ Salagen Tablets (3%) 1082
Valium Tablets 2658
Zyrtec Chewable Tablets (Less than 2%) 1920
Zyrtec Syrup (Less than 2%) 1920
Zyrtec Tablets (Less than 2%) 1920

Hypersecretion

Klonopin 2639

Hypersecretion, salivary

▲ Abilify Injection (4% to 8.1%) 881
▲ Abilify Injection (4%) 2466
▲ Abilify Oral Solution (4% to 8.1%) 881
▲ Abilify Oral Solution (4%) 2466
▲ Abilify Discmelt Orally Disintegrating Tablets (4% to 8.1%) 881
▲ Abilify Discmelt Orally Disintegrating Tablets (4%) 2466
▲ Abilify Tablets (4% to 8.1%) 881
▲ Abilify Tablets (4%) 2466
Exelon Patch (Infrequent) 2233
▲ Invega Extended-Release Tablets (0% to 4%) 1748

Hypersensitivity

Abilify Oral Solution (Greater than or equal to 1 in 1000 patients and less than 1 in 100 patients) 881
Abilify Discmelt Orally Disintegrating Tablets (Greater than or equal to 1 in 1000 patients and less than 1 in 100 patients) 881
Abilify Tablets (Greater than or equal to 1 in 1000 patients and less than 1 in 100 patients) 881
▲ Alimta for Injection (Up to 8%) 1786
Aloxi Injection (Very rare) 1059
Amoxil Capsules 1305
Amoxil Chewable Tablets 1305
Amoxil Pediatric Drops for Oral Suspension 1305
Amoxil Powder for Oral Suspension 1305
Amoxil Tablets 1305
Aptivus Capsules (Less than 2%) 823
Aptivus Oral Solution (Less than 2%) 823
Avalide Tablets 2713
Avelox 2803
Axid Capsules 1364
Bleph-10 Ophthalmic Solution 10% ⊙215
Chantix Tablets (Infrequent) 2511
Cipro 2810
Cipro XR Tablets 2823
Clinoril Tablets (Less than 1%) 1962
Cubicin for Injection (Less than 1%) 995
Cymbalta Delayed-Release Capsules 1801
Dacogen Injection 1066
▲ Elidel Cream 1% (3.4% to 5.1%) 2221
▲ Eloxatin for Injection (1% to 12%) 2731
▲ Elspar for Injection (32.5% to 75%) 1990
Enablex Extended-Release Tablets 2225
Estratest Tablets (Rare) 3043
Estratest H.S. Tablets (Rare) 3043
Exforge Tablets (Greater than or equal to 0.2%) 2238
Fluarix Vaccine 1446
Fluorescite Injection ⊙203
Fortaz (Immediate in 1 in 285 patients) 1450
Human Albumin Grifols 25% 1706
Imitrex Injection (Infrequent) 1465
Imitrex Nasal Spray (Rare) 1470
Imitrex Tablets (Frequent) 1474
Indocin (Less than 1%) 2024
Lacrisert Sterile Ophthalmic Insert ⊙233
Lamictal 1488
Leukeran Tablets 1508
Lyrica Capsules 2527
Micardis Tablets 852
Mirapex Tablets 857

Moxatag Tablets 2165
Mustargen for Injection 2492
Mycamine for Injection 616
Nembutal Sodium Solution, USP 2494
Noroxin Tablets (A few patients) 2069
NovoSeven RT 2370
Opana Tablets (Less than 1%) 1117
Opana ER Tablets (Less than 1%) 1121
▲ Pataday Ophthalmic Solution (Less than or equal to 5%) 543
Patanase Nasal Spray 544
Pediarix Vaccine 1552
Pentacel 2792
Percocet Tablets 1127
Premarin Vaginal Cream 3228
Prinzide Tablets 2092
Pristiq Extended-Release Tablets (Less than 2%) 3247
Proleukin for Injection 2287
Pulmicort Flexhaler 654
Rapamune 3260
Recombivax HB 2107
Requip Tablets (Infrequent) 1561
Rocephin Injectable Vials, ADD-Vantage, Galaxy, Bulk 2642
Sensipar Tablets 594
Seromycin Capsules 1864
Solodyn Extended Release Tablets 1938
Starlix Tablets 2314
Thyrogen for Injection 1244
Timoptic Sterile Ophthalmic Solution (Less frequent) 2121
Timoptic in Ocudose (Less frequent) 2124
Tracleer Tablets 3289
▲ Treanda for Injection (1% to 5%) 983
Velcade for Injection 2168
Ventolin HFA Inhalation Aerosol 1638
Viramune Oral Suspension 873
Viramune Tablets 873
Vytorin 10/10 Tablets 2149
Vytorin 10/10 Tablets 2939
Vytorin 10/20 Tablets 2149
Vytorin 10/20 Tablets 2939
Vytorin 10/40 Tablets 2149
Vytorin 10/40 Tablets 2939
Vytorin 10/80 Tablets 2149
Vytorin 10/80 Tablets 2939
Vyvanse Capsules 3033
Xyntha Vials 3280
Xyrem Oral Solution (Infrequent) 1766
Xyzal Oral Solution 2789
Xyzal Oral Solution 3155
Zantac 25 EFFERdose Tablets (Rare) 1670
Zantac Injection (Rare) 1666
Zantac Injection Pharmacy Bulk Package (Rare) 1668
Zantac Injection Premixed (Rare) 1666
Zantac (Rare) 1670
Zetia Tablets 2951
Zinacef for Injection (Fewer than 1%) 1678
Zinacef Injection (Fewer than 1%) 1678
Zomig Tablets (Rare) 694
Zomig-ZMT Tablets (Rare) 694

Hypersensitivity, cutaneous

Nexavar Tablets (0.1% to less than 1%) 784

Hypersensitivity, drug

Chantix Tablets (Rare) 2511

Hypersensitivity, immune complex mediated

Velcade for Injection 2168

Hypersensitivity at injection site

Aloxi Injection (Very rare) 1059
Amevive (Less than 1%) 611
▲ Betaseron for SC Injection (4%) 756
Bexxar 1371
Bicillin C-R Injectable Suspension 1775
Bicillin L-A Injection 1777

Hypersensitivity reactions, Arthus-type

Boostrix 1377
Pediarix Vaccine 1552

Hypersensitivity reactions, general

Abilify Injection (Greater than or equal to 1 in 1000 patients and less than 1 in 100 patients) 2466
Abilify Oral Solution (Greater than or equal to 1 in 1000 patients and less than 1 in 100 patients) 2466
Abilify Discmelt Orally Disintegrating Tablets (Greater than or equal to 1 in 1000 patients and less than 1 in 100 patients) 2466
Abilify Tablets (Greater than or equal to 1 in 1000 patients and less than 1 in 100 patients) 2466
Accolate Tablets 669
Actonel Tablets (Rare) 2568
Actonel with Calcium Tablets (Very rare) 2574
Adderall XR Capsules 3012
Advair Diskus 100/50 1276
Advair Diskus 250/50 1276
Advair Diskus 500/50 1276
Advair HFA 45/21 Inhalation Aerosol (Rare) 1288
Advair HFA 115/21 Inhalation Aerosol (Rare) 1288
Advair HFA 230/21 Inhalation Aerosol (Rare) 1288
Albenza Tablets (Less than 1%) 1297
Alferon N Injection 1726
Allegra Oral Solution (Rare) 2684
Allegra Tablets (Rare) 2684
Aminohippurate Sodium "PAH" Injection 1950
Angiomax for Injection 1933
Antivenin (Black Widow Spider Antivenin) 1951
Asacol Delayed-Release Tablets (Some patients) 2579
Atrovent HFA Inhalation Aerosol 839
Augmentin 1323
Augmentin Tablets 1327
Augmentin XR Extended Release Tablets 1333
Augmentin ES-600 Powder for Oral Suspension 1329
Avodart Soft Gelatin Capsules 1359
Beconase AQ Nasal Spray (Rare) 1369
Benicar HCT Tablets 1010
▲ Betimol Ophthalmic Solution (More than 5%) 3181
Bexxar 1371
Bystolic Tablets 1155
Calcijex Injection 419
Carafate Suspension 706
Carafate Tablets 707
Ceftin 1380
Cialis Tablets 1792
Cimzia (Rare) 3127
Cipro I.V. (Rare) 2817
Clarinex Syrup (Rare) 2828
Clarinex Tablets (Rare) 2828
Clarinex Reditabs Tablets (Rare) 2828
Clarinex-D 12-Hour Extended-Release Tablets (Rare) 2831
Clarinex-D 24-Hour Extended-Release Tablets 2834
Combivent Inhalation Aerosol 845
Comvax 1966
Concerta Extended-Release Tablets 1925
Cozaar Tablets 1973
Crestor Tablets 677
Daytrana Transdermal Patch 3022
Demser Capsules (Rare) 1989
Depakote ER Tablets 423
Didronel Tablets 2583
Digibind for Injection 1403
Doribax Injection (Less than 1%) 2400
▲ Eloxatin for Injection (2% to 3%) 2731
Emend for Injection 1999
Faslodex Injection (Less than 1%) 682
Fenoglide Tablets (Rare) 2960
Fleet Phospho-soda (Rare) 1145
Fleet Phospho-soda EZ-PREP (Rare) 1147
Fleet Prep Kits 1149
Flovent HFA (Rare) 1440
FluMist Vaccine 1945
Focalin XR Capsules 2251
Fosamax 2005
Fosamax Plus D Tablets 2013
Furosemide Tablets 2186
Gammagard Liquid 730
▲ Humira Injection (6%) 442
Infanrix Vaccine 1479
Intelence Tablets (Less than 0.1%) 3119
Iquix Ophthalmic Solution 3183
Isentress Tablets 2036
▲ Ixempra Kit for Injection (5%) 915
Janumet Tablets 2041
Januvia Tablets 2048
Lescol Capsules (Rare) 2268
Lescol XL Tablets (Rare) 2268
Levaquin 2416
Levaquin in 5% Dextrose Injection 2416
Levothroid Tablets 1170
Maxalt Tablets 2056
Maxalt-MLT Orally Disintegrating Tablets 2056
Mephyton Tablets 700
Mepron Suspension 1526
Mevacor Tablets (Rare) 2063
MoviPrep Oral Solution 2679
Mylotarg for Injection 3212
Neosporin Ophthalmic Solution Sterile (Rare) ⊙ 252
Nimbex Injection 484
Norditropin Cartridges 2354
NovoSeven 2367
Noxafil Oral Suspension (Rare) 2889
Omnaris Nasal Spray 2998
Oncaspar Injection 1138
Orencia Powder for Intravenous Infusion (Greater than 0.1% and less than or equal to 1%) 921
Orthoclone OKT3 Sterile Solution 2387
Plavix Tablets 926
Plavix Tablets 2767
Prevnar 3241
Propecia Tablets 2095
Proscar Tablets 2102
Provigil Tablets 977
▲ Raptiva for Injection (8%) 1218
Remicade for IV Injection 950
ReoPro Vials 1860
Rocaltrol Capsules 1150
Rocaltrol Oral Solution 1150
Singulair 2114
Skelaxin Tablets (Most frequent) 1784
Sular Extended Release Tablets (Very rare) 2975
Synagis Intramuscular Solution 1948
▲ Taxotere Injection Concentrate (0% to 21%) 2773
Tessalon Capsules 1183
Tessalon Perles 1183
Tice BCG 2936
Timoptic-XE Sterile Ophthalmic Gel Forming Solution 2125
▲ Torisel Injection (9%) 3272
Trasylol Injection 799
▲ Trizivir Tablets (Greater than or equal to 5%) 1622
▲ Valcyte Tablets (Less than 5%) 2654
Viroptic Ophthalmic Solution ⊙ 253
Visudyne for Injection (Less than 1%) 2332
Vivitrol 988
▲ Xeloda Tablets (Less than 5%) 2662
Xifaxan Tablets 2682
Zetia Tablets 2157
▲ Ziagen (2% to 9%) 1673
Zocor Tablets (Rare) 2136
Zofran Injection (Rare) 1682
Zometa for Intravenous Infusion (Rare) 2341
Zomig Tablets (Rare) 694
Zomig Nasal Spray (Rare) 689
Zomig-ZMT Tablets (Rare) 694
Zostavax Injection 2145
Zosyn for Injection (1% or less) 3284

Hypersensitivity reactions, multi-organ

▲ Epzicom Tablets (2% to 9%) 1422
Janumet Tablets 2041
Provigil Tablets 977

Hypersexuality

Requip Tablets 1561

Hypersomnia

Aloxi Injection (Less than 1%) 1059
▲ Cymbalta Delayed-Release Capsules (7%) 1801
Intelence Tablets (Less than 2%) 3119
Keppra Injection (1.7%) 3137
Keppra Oral Solution 3131
Keppra Tablets 3131
Luvox CR Extended-Release Capsules (Infrequent) 1759
Maxalt Tablets (Rare) 2056
Maxalt-MLT Orally Disintegrating Tablets (Rare) 2056
Prinivil Tablets (0.3% to 1%) 2087
Prinzide Tablets 2092
ProQuad 2099
Requip Tablets (Infrequent) 1561

Hypersplenism

Flolan for Injection 1426

Hypertension

▲ Abelcet Injection (5%) 1134
Abilify Injection (2%) 881
Abilify Injection (Greater than or equal to 1 in 100 patients) 2466
Abilify Oral Solution (Greater than or equal to 1 in 100 patients) 881
Abilify Oral Solution (Greater than or equal to 1 in 100 patients) 2466
Abilify Discmelt Orally Disintegrating Tablets (Greater than or equal to 1 in 100 patients) 881
Abilify Discmelt Orally Disintegrating Tablets (Greater than or equal to 1 in 100 patients) 2466
Abilify Tablets (Greater than or equal to 1 in 100 patients) 881
Abilify Tablets (Greater than or equal to 1 in 100 patients) 2466
Actiq (Less than 1%) 959
Activase I.V. 1188
Activella Tablets 2347
▲ Actonel Tablets (10.5%) 2568
▲ Actonel with Calcium Tablets (4.9% to 10%) 2574
▲ Adderall XR Capsules (12% to 35%) 3012
Adenocard IV Injection 603
Adenoscan (Less than 1%) 605
Adipex-P 1185
Advair HFA 45/21 Inhalation Aerosol 1288
Advair HFA 115/21 Inhalation Aerosol 1288
Advair HFA 230/21 Inhalation Aerosol 1288
▲ Aerobid/Aerobid-M (1% to 3%) 1153
▲ Agrylin Capsules (1% to less than 5%) 3017
▲ Alimta for Injection (3% to 11%) 1786
Alinia for Oral Suspension (Less than 1%) 2677
Alinia Tablets (Less than 1%) 2677
Aloxi Injection (Less than 1%) 1059
▲ Alphagan P Ophthalmic Solution (Approximately 5% to 9%) 549
Ambien Tablets (Infrequent) 2692
Ambien CR Tablets (Infrequent to 1%) 2696
▲ AmBisome for Injection (7.9% to 19.8%) 606
Amerge Tablets (Infrequent) 1301
Anaprox Tablets (Less than 1%) 2632
Anaprox DS Tablets (Less than 1%) 2632
▲ AndroGel (0% to 3%) 3159
Angeliq Tablets 751
▲ Angiomax for Injection (6%) 1933
Anzemet Injection (2.9%) 2701
Anzemet Tablets (2.2%) 2704
▲ Aranesp for Injection (3.7% to 20%) 564
Aricept Tablets (Infrequent) 1062
▲ Aricept ODT Tablets (3%) 1062
▲ Arimidex Tablets (2% to 13%) 672
Arixtra Injection (2.4%) 1313
Avalide Tablets 892
Avalide Tablets 2713
▲ Avandaryl Tablets (2.3% to greater than or equal to 5%) 1344
Avapro Tablets (Less than 1%) 897
Avapro Tablets (Less than 1%) 2718
▲ Avastin IV (8% to 34%) 1192
Avelox (Less than 0.1%) 2803
▲ Avinza Capsules (Less than 5%) 1772
Axert Tablets (Rare) 2431
▲ Betaseron for SC Injection (6%) 756
▲ Betimol Ophthalmic Solution (1% to 5%) 3181
▲ Boniva Injection (6.3% to 7.3%) 2614
▲ Boniva Tablets (6.3% to 7.3%) 2618
▲ Busulfex Injection (7% to 36%) 2477
Calcijex Injection 419
▲ Campath Ampules (14%) 761
Campral Tablets (Frequent) 1158
▲ Cancidas for Injection (8.9% to 9.6%) 1953
Carbatrol Capsules 3019
Cardene I.V. (0.7%) 1093
Catapres-TTS (0.5% or less) 842
▲ Celebrex Capsules (12.5%) 2979
Celexa (Infrequent) 1160
▲ CellCept Capsules (28.2% to 77.5%) 2622
▲ CellCept Intravenous (28.2% to 77.5%) 2622
▲ CellCept Oral Suspension (28.2% to 77.5%) 2622
▲ CellCept Tablets (28.2% to 77.5%) 2622
Chantix Tablets (Frequent) 2511
▲ Cialis Tablets (1% to 3%) 1792
Cipro I.V. (1% or less) 2817
Cipro (Less than 1%) 2810
Cipro XR Tablets 2823
Climara Transdermal System 763
▲ Climara Pro Transdermal System (3.3%) 768
Clinoril Tablets (Less than 1%) 1962

▲ Clolar for Intravenous Infusion (11%) ... 1239
▲ Combigan Ophthalmic Solution (1% to 5%) ... 553
Combivent Inhalation Aerosol (Less than 2%) ... 845
Concerta Extended-Release Tablets ... 1925
Copaxone for Injection (Frequent) ... 3110
▲ Coreg Tablets (Greater than 1% to 3%) ... 1387
▲ Coreg CR Extended-Release Capsules (Greater than 1% to less than or equal to 3%) ... 1393
▲ Cosopt Sterile Ophthalmic Solution (1% to 5%) ... 1969
▲ Cubicin for Injection (1.1% to 5.8%) ... 995
▲ Cyanokit 5g Antidote (18% to 28%) ... 1021
Daytrana Transdermal Patch ... 3022
▲ Depakote ER Tablets (Greater than 1% to less than 5%) ... 423
▲ DepoCyt Injection (6% to 15%) ... 1136
▲ DepoDur Injection (2% to 5%) ... 1095
Dexedrine ... 1401
Divigel ... 3167
Doxil Injection (Less than 1%) ... 2378
▲ Duragesic Transdermal System (1% to 3%) ... 2405
EC-Naprosyn Delayed-Release Tablets (Less than 1%) ... 2632
Edex Injection (2%) ... 2957
▲ Effexor XR Extended-Release Capsules (4% to 5%) ... 3195
Eldepryl Capsules ... 3052
Eligard 7.5 mg (Less than 2%) ... 2724
Eligard 22.5 mg (Less than 2%) ... 2724
Eligard 30 mg (Less than 2%) ... 2724
Eligard 45 mg (Less than 2%) ... 2724
▲ Eloxatin for Injection (2% to less than 5%) ... 2731
Emend Capsules (Greater than 0.5%) ... 1992
Emend for Injection (Greater than 0.5%) ... 1999
Emsam Transdermal System (Frequent) ... 905
Enablex Extended-Release Tablets (Greater than or equal to 1%) ... 2225
Enbrel for Injection (Infrequent) ... 569
Enjuvia Tablets ... 1029
▲ Epogen for Injection (0.75% to 24%) ... 576
Equetro Extended-Release Capsules ... 3174
Erbitux ... 912
Estratest Tablets (Common) ... 3043
Estratest H.S. Tablets (Common) ... 3043
Evoxac Capsules (Less than 1%) ... 1013
▲ Exelon Capsules (3%) ... 2229
▲ Exelon Oral Solution (3%) ... 2229
▲ Fabrazyme for Intravenous Infusion (5%) ... 1241
▲ Femara Tablets (5% to 8%) ... 2246
Fentora Tablets (Greater than 1%) ... 968
Flector Patch ... 561
Flumadine (Less than 0.3%) ... 1167
Focalin XR Capsules ... 2251
Foradil Aerolizer ... 2849
▲ Forteo for Injection (7.1%) ... 1816
Gabitril Tablets (Frequent) ... 973
Gammagard S/D (Occasional) ... 734
Gemzar for Injection (2%) ... 1820
▲ Gengraf Capsules (25% to 50%) ... 435
▲ Geodon (3%) ... 2520
Gleevec Tablets (Infrequent) ... 2255
▲ Gliadel Wafer (3%) ... 1076
Herceptin I.V. ... 1199
▲ Humatrope Vials and Cartridges (2.7% to 7.7%) ... 1838
▲ Humira Injection (5%) ... 442
Imitrex Injection (Infrequent) ... 1465
Imitrex Nasal Spray (Infrequent) ... 1470
Imitrex Tablets (Infrequent) ... 1474
Indocin Capsules (Less than 1%) ... 2024
Indocin I.V. (Less than 1%) ... 2489
Indocin (Less than 1%) ... 2024
Intelence Tablets (2.8%) ... 3119
▲ Intron A for Injection (Less than 5% to 9%) ... 2859
Invanz for Injection (0.7% to 1.6%) ... 2029
▲ Ionsys Transdermal System (1% to less than 10%) ... 2410
Kaletra (Less than 2%) ... 452
▲ Kepivance (7% to 14%) ... 583
Kogenate FS ... 746
Kogenate FS with Bio-Set (1 case) ... 748
Lamictal (Infrequent) ... 1488
▲ Leukine (25% to 34%) ... 774
Levitra Tablets (Less than 2%) ... 2876
Levothroid Tablets ... 1170
Levoxyl Tablets ... 1780
Lexapro Oral Suspension (Frequent) ... 1174
Lexapro Tablets (Frequent) ... 1174
Lialda Tablets (Infrequent) ... 3029
Lipitor Tablets (Less than 2%) ... 2501
Lovaza Capsules ... 1520
Lunesta Tablets (Frequent) ... 2994
Luvox CR Extended-Release Capsules (Frequent to 2%) ... 1759
Lybrel Tablets ... 3204
Maxalt Tablets (Infrequent) ... 2056
Maxalt-MLT Orally Disintegrating Tablets (Infrequent) ... 2056
▲ Megace ES Oral Suspension (0% to 8%) ... 2499
Meridia Capsules (2.1%) ... 475
Merrem I.V. (Greater than 0.1% to 1%) ... 684
Metadate CD Capsules ... 3146
▲ Miacalcin Nasal Spray (1% to 3%) ... 2274
Micardis Tablets (1%) ... 852
Micardis HCT Tablets ... 854
Mirapex Tablets (1% or more) ... 857
Mircette Tablets ... 1034
▲ Mirena Intrauterine System (5% or more) ... 779
Mobic Oral Suspension (Less than 2%) ... 863
Mobic Tablets (Less than 2%) ... 863
MS Contin Tablets (Less frequent) ... 2585
▲ Mycamine for Injection (6.9% to 24.3%) ... 616
▲ Myfortic Tablets (3% to less than 20%) ... 2276
▲ Mylotarg for Injection (13% to 17%) ... 3212
▲ Namenda (4%) ... 1180
Naprosyn Suspension (Less than 1%) ... 2632
Naprosyn Tablets (Less than 1%) ... 2632
▲ Neoral Oral Solution (Approximately 25% to 50% most patients) ... 2280
▲ Neoral Soft Gelatin Capsules (25% to 50%) ... 2280
▲ Neupogen for Injection (4%) ... 589
▲ Nevanac Ophthalmic Suspension 0.1% (1% to 4%) ... ⊙ 205
▲ Nexavar Tablets (4% to 17%) ... 784
Nexium Delayed-Release Capsules (Less than 1%) ... 645
Nexium I.V. (Less than 1%) ... 652
Nexium Delayed-Release Oral Suspension (Less than 1%) ... 645
Nimotop Capsules (Less than 1%) ... 790
▲ Norditropin Cartridges (8%) ... 2354
▲ Novantrone for Injection Concentrate (4%) ... 1100
NovoSeven (Greater than or equal to 2%) ... 2367
NovoSeven RT (Greater than or equal to 2%) ... 2370
▲ Noxafil Oral Suspension (1% to 18%) ... 2889
NuvaRing ... 2897
Omnicef Capsules ... 497
Omnicef for Oral Suspension ... 497
▲ Ontak Vials (6%) ... 1079
Opana Tablets (Less than 1%) ... 1117
Opana ER Tablets (Less than 1%) ... 1121
OptiPranolol Metipranolol Ophthalmic Solution 0.3% (A small number of patients) ... ⊙ 245
▲ Orencia Powder for Intravenous Infusion (7%) ... 921
Ortho-Cyclen Tablets ... 2449
Ortho Evra Transdermal System ... 2437
Ortho Tri-Cyclen Tablets ... 2449
Ortho Tri-Cyclen Lo Tablets ... 2458
▲ Orthoclone OKT3 Sterile Solution (8%) ... 2387
Paxil (Frequent) ... 1535
Paxil CR Controlled-Release Tablets (Frequent) ... 1544
Percocet Tablets ... 1127
Perforomist Inhalation Solution ... 1025
▲ Photofrin for Injection (0% to 6%) ... 708
▲ Plavix Tablets (4.3%) ... 926
▲ Plavix Tablets (4.3%) ... 2767
Pletal Tablets (2% or greater) ... 2481
PrandiMet Tablets (Less than or equal to 1%) ... 2967
Prandin Tablets (Less than or equal to 1%) ... 2971
Premarin Intravenous ... 3217
Premarin Tablets ... 3221
Premarin Vaginal Cream ... 3228
Premphase Tablets ... 3232
Prempro Tablets ... 3232
Pristiq Extended-Release Tablets (1% to 2%) ... 3247
▲ Procrit for Injection (0.75% to 24%) ... 2391
▲ Prograf Capsules and Injection (Common; 38% to 62%) ... 622
Prolastin (Rare) ... 3099
Proleukin for Injection ... 2287
▲ Prometrium Capsules (100 mg, 200 mg) (Less than 5%) ... 3047
Protonix for Delayed-Release Oral Suspension (Less than 1%) ... 3254
Protonix Delayed-Release Tablets (Less than 1%) ... 3254
Protonix I.V. (Less than 1%) ... 3257
Protopic Ointment (Greater than or equal to 1% to 2%) ... 628
Proventil HFA Inhalation Aerosol ... 2914
▲ Provigil Tablets (3%) ... 977
Prozac Weekly Capsules (Frequent) ... 1852
Prozac Pulvules and Liquid (Frequent) ... 1852
▲ Rapamune (Greater than or equal to 30% to 49%) ... 3260
Remeron Tablets (Frequent) ... 2924
RemeronSolTab Tablets (Frequent) ... 2927
▲ Remicade for IV Injection (7%) ... 950
▲ Requip Tablets (Infrequent to 5%) ... 1561
▲ Requip XL Tablets (3%) ... 1568
▲ Rilutek Tablets (3.3% to 6.8%) ... 2771
▲ Risperdal Consta Long-Acting Injection (3%) ... 1753
▲ Rituxan I.V. (1% to 6%) ... 1223
Rocaltrol Capsules ... 1150
Rocaltrol Oral Solution ... 1150
Romazicon Injection (Less than 1%) ... 2646
Rythmol SR Capsules ... 1590
St. Joseph 81 mg Aspirin Chewable and Enteric Coated Tablets ... 1903
▲ Salagen Tablets (1% to 3%) ... 1082
▲ Sandimmune (13% to 53%) ... 2296
Sandostatin Injection (Less than 1%) ... 2300
▲ Sandostatin LAR Depot (12.6%) ... 2302
Seasonique Tablets ... 1046
▲ Sensipar Tablets (7%) ... 594
▲ Serevent Diskus (4%) ... 1594
▲ Simulect for Injection (Greater than or equal to 10%) ... 2306
▲ Somatuline Depot Injection (5% to 7%) ... 3102
Stalevo Tablets ... 2309
Strattera Capsules ... 1864
Sular Extended Release Tablets (Less than or equal to 1%) ... 2975
▲ Sutent Capsules (4% to 28%) ... 2540
Symbyax Capsules (2%) ... 1871
Targretin Capsules ... 1084
▲ Tasigna Capsules (1% to 10%) ... 2316
▲ Taxotere Injection Concentrate (8.1%) ... 2773
Tekturna Tablets (2.2%) ... 2321
Testim 1% Gel (1%) ... 701
Timoptic Sterile Ophthalmic Solution (Less frequent) ... 2121
Timoptic in Ocudose (Less frequent) ... 2124
Timoptic-XE Sterile Ophthalmic Gel Forming Solution ... 2125
▲ Torisel Injection (7%) ... 3272
▲ Trasylol Injection (4%) ... 799
▲ Travatan Z Ophthalmic Solution (1% to 5%) ... 547
Treximet Tablets (Infrequent) ... 1616
Tricor Tablets ... 520
▲ Trisenox Injection (10%) ... 986
▲ Tygacil for Injection (4.9%) ... 3276
Ultane Liquid for Inhalation (2%) ... 524
Ultram ER Extended-Release Tablets (0.5% to less than 1%) ... 2428
▲ Urso 250 Tablets (8.3%) ... 720
▲ Urso Forte Tablets (8.3%) ... 720
▲ Valcyte Tablets (18%) ... 2654
Valtrex Caplets ... 1635
▲ Vaprisol (5.5% to 8%) ... 632
▲ Velcade for Injection (13%) ... 2168
▲ Venlafaxine Hydrochloride Tablets (1.1% to 13%) ... 2199
Ventolin HFA Inhalation Aerosol ... 1638
Verdeso Foam (2%) ... 3069
▲ Vesanoid Capsules (11%) ... 2660
VESIcare Tablets (0.5% to 1.4%) ... 636
Viadur Implant (Rare) ... 802
▲ Visudyne for Injection (1% to 10%) ... 2332
Vivitrol ... 988
Voltaren Tablets (Occasionally) ... 2334
Voltaren-XR Tablets (Occasionally) ... 2337
▲ Vyvanse Capsules (3%) ... 3033
WelChol Tablets (2.8%) ... 1015
▲ Wellbutrin Tablets (4.3%) ... 1648
Wellbutrin SR Sustained-Release Tablets (At least 1%) ... 1653
▲ Wellbutrin XL Extended-Release Tablets (2% to 4%) ... 1659
WinRho SDF ... 741
Xeloda Tablets ... 2662
Xopenex Inhalation Solution ... 3001
Xopenex Inhalation Solution Concentrate ... 3005
Xopenex HFA Inhalation Aerosol ... 3009
▲ Xyrem Oral Solution (6.1%) ... 1766
Yaz Tablets ... 805
Zemuron Injection (0.1% to 2%) ... 2947
Zolinza Capsules ... 2142
Zometa for Intravenous Infusion ... 2341
Zomig Tablets (Infrequent) ... 694
Zomig Nasal Spray (Infrequent) ... 689
Zomig-ZMT Tablets (Infrequent) ... 694
Zonegran Capsules (Infrequent) ... 1089
Zosyn for Injection (1.3% to 1.6%) ... 3284
Zyban Sustained-Release Tablets (1% to 2.5%) ... 1692
Zyprexa Tablets (2%) ... 1883
Zyprexa IntraMuscular ... 1883
Zyprexa ZYDIS Orally Disintegrating Tablets (2%) ... 1883
Zyrtec Chewable Tablets (Less than 2%) ... 1920
Zyrtec Syrup (Less than 2%) ... 1920
Zyrtec Tablets (Less than 2%) ... 1920
Zyrtec-D 12 Hour Extended Release Tablets (Less than 2%) ... 1923
Zyvox ... 2552

Hypertension, aggravation

Ambien Tablets (Rare) ... 2692
Ambien CR Tablets (Rare) ... 2696
Carbatrol Capsules ... 3019
Celebrex Capsules (0.1% to 1.9%) ... 2979
Equetro Extended-Release Capsules ... 3174
Evoxac Capsules (Less than 1%) ... 1013
Flector Patch ... 561
Micardis Tablets ... 852
▲ Myfortic Tablets (3% to less than 20%) ... 2276
Ultram ER Extended-Release Tablets (0.5% to less than 1%) ... 2428

Hypertension, intracranial

Diprolene Lotion 0.05% ... 2838
Diprolene Ointment 0.05% ... 2839
Elocon Cream 0.1% ... 2840
Elocon Ointment 0.1% ... 2842
Gantrisin Pediatric Suspension ... 2638
Genotropin Lyophilized Powder ... 2547
▲ Gliadel Wafer (4% to 9%) ... 1076
Humatrope Vials and Cartridges ... 1838
Increlex Injection (3 subjects) ... 3100
Lotrisone Cream ... 2881
Lyrica Capsules (Rare) ... 2527
Nutropin for Injection ... 1208
Nutropin AQ Injection ... 1212
Nutropin AQ NuSpin Injection ... 1212
Nutropin AQ Pen ... 1212
Nutropin AQ Pen Cartridge ... 1212
Requip Tablets (Infrequent) ... 1561
Verdeso Foam ... 3069
▲ Vesanoid Capsules (9%) ... 2660

Hypertension, portal

Myleran Tablets ... 1530
Tabloid Tablets ... 1601

Hypertension, rebound

Cleviprex ... 1936
Nitro-Dur Transdermal Infusion System (Uncommon) ... 2887

Hypertension, supine

▲ ProAmatine Tablets (7.3%) ... 3032

Hypertension, transient

Proglycem Capsules (Infrequent) ... 1185
Proglycem Suspension (Infrequent) ... 1185
Prolastin (Rare) ... 3099

Hypertensive crises

Avalide Tablets ... 892
Avalide Tablets ... 2713
Avapro Tablets (Less than 1%) ... 897
Avapro Tablets (Less than 1%) ... 2718
Avastin IV ... 1192
Cymbalta Delayed-Release Capsules ... 1801
Imitrex Injection (Rare) ... 1465
Mirapex Tablets ... 857
Nexavar Tablets (0.1% to less than 1%) ... 784
Parnate Tablets ... 1532
Rythmol SR Capsules ... 1590
Sanctura XR Capsules ... 557
Tasigna Capsules (0.1% to 1%) ... 2316

Hyperthermia

Calcijex Injection ... 419
Celexa ... 1160
Elspar for Injection ... 1990

▲ Fabrazyme for Intravenous Infusion (6%) 1241
Lexapro Oral Suspension 1174
Lexapro Tablets 1174
Neupro Transdermal System 3149
Pristiq Extended-Release Tablets 3247
Remeron Tablets 2924
RemeronSolTab Tablets 2927
Risperdal Consta Long-Acting Injection 1753
Rocaltrol Capsules 1150
Rocaltrol Oral Solution 1150
Treximet Tablets 1616
Zomig Tablets 694
Zomig Nasal Spray 689
Zomig-ZMT Tablets 694

Hyperthyroidism

▲ Advair Diskus 100/50 (Greater than or equal to 3%) 1276
Advair Diskus 250/50 1276
Advair Diskus 500/50 1276
Betaseron for SC Injection 756
Copaxone for Injection (Infrequent) 3110
Cytomel Tablets 1778
Effexor XR Extended-Release Capsules (Rare) 3195
Flolan for Injection 1426
▲ Intron A for Injection (Less than 5%) 2859
Levoxyl Tablets 1780
Meridia Capsules 475
Miacalcin Nasal Spray (Less than 1%) 2274
Mirapex Tablets 857
Naturethroid Tablets 2605
▲ Ontak Vials (Less than 5%) 1079
Paxil (Rare) 1535
Paxil CR Controlled-Release Tablets (Rare) 1544
PegIntron Powder for Injection (Less than or equal to 1%) 2903
Proleukin for Injection 2287
Requip Tablets (Infrequent) 1561
▲ Sutent Capsules (4%) 2540
Synthroid Tablets (Rare) 507
Tasigna Capsules (0.1% to 1%) 2316
Venlafaxine Hydrochloride Tablets (Rare) 2199
Zomig Tablets (Rare) 694
Zomig Nasal Spray (Rare) 689
Zomig-ZMT Tablets (Rare) 694

Hyperthyroidism, drug-induced

Thyrogen for Injection 1244

Hyperthyroidism, exacerbation of

InnoPran XL Extended Release Capsules 1484

Hypertonia

Abilify Injection (Greater than or equal to 1 in 1000 patients and less than 1 in 100 patients) 881
Abilify Injection (Greater than or equal to 1 in 1000 patients and less than 1 in 100 patients) 2466
Abilify Oral Solution (Greater than or equal to 1 in 1000 patients and less than 1 in 100 patients) 881
Abilify Oral Solution (Greater than or equal to 1 in 1000 patients and less than 1 in 100 patients) 2466
Abilify Discmelt Orally Disintegrating Tablets (Greater than or equal to 1 in 1000 patients and less than 1 in 100 patients) 881
Abilify Discmelt Orally Disintegrating Tablets (Greater than or equal to 1 in 1000 patients and less than 1 in 100 patients) 2466
Abilify Tablets (Greater than or equal to 1 in 1000 patients and less than 1 in 100 patients) 881
Abilify Tablets (Greater than or equal to 1 in 1000 patients and less than 1 in 100 patients) 2466
Aceon Tablets (2 mg, 4 mg, 8 mg) (0.2% to 2.7%) 3038
Actonel with Calcium Tablets (2.2%) 2574
Aricept Tablets (Infrequent) 1062
Aricept ODT Tablets (Infrequent) 1062
▲ Arimidex Tablets (3%) 672
Arranon Injection (1%) 1319
▲ Asacol Delayed-Release Tablets (5%) 2579
Avelox (Less than 0.1%) 2803
Axert Tablets (Rare) 2431
Azilect Tablets (Frequent) 3106
Azopt Ophthalmic Suspension (Less than 1%) 540
▲ Betaseron for SC Injection (40%) 756
▲ BOTOX Purified Neurotoxin Complex (2% to 10%) 550
Cardene I.V. (Rare) 1093
Celebrex Capsules (0.1% to 1.9%) 2979
Celexa (Infrequent) 1160
▲ CellCept Capsules (3% to less than 20%) 2622
▲ CellCept Intravenous (3% to less than 20%) 2622
▲ CellCept Oral Suspension (3% to less than 20%) 2622
▲ CellCept Tablets (3% to less than 20%) 2622
Cipro I.V. 2817
Cipro 2810
Cipro XR Tablets (Less than 1%) 2823
▲ Copaxone for Injection (22%) 3110
▲ Depakote ER Tablets (Greater than 1% to less than 5%) 423
▲ Doxil Injection (1% to 10%) 2378
Duragesic Transdermal System (Less than 1%) 2405
Effexor XR Extended-Release Capsules (Infrequent) 3195
Emsam Transdermal System (Infrequent) 905
▲ Evoxac Capsules (1% to 3%) 1013
Exelon Capsules (Infrequent) 2229
Exelon Oral Solution (Infrequent) 2229
Exforge Tablets (Less than or equal to 0.1%) 2238
Frova Tablets (Rare) 1111
Gabitril Tablets (Frequent) 973
▲ Geodon (3% to 14%) 2520
Havrix Injection Vaccine (Less than 1%) 1454
▲ Indapamide Tablets (Less than 5%) 2188
▲ Intron A for Injection (Less than 5%) 2859
▲ Invega Extended-Release Tablets (1% to 4%) 1748
▲ Ionsys Transdermal System (1% to less than 10%) 2410
Kaletra (Less than 2%) 452
Klonopin (Infrequent) 2639
Lamictal (Infrequent) 1488
Levaquin (0.1% to 1%) 2416
Levaquin in 5% Dextrose Injection (0.1% to 1%) 2416
Levitra Tablets (Less than 2%) 2876
Lexapro Oral Suspension (Infrequent) 1174
Lexapro Tablets (Infrequent) 1174
Lipitor Tablets (Less than 2%) 2501
Lunesta Tablets (Infrequent) 2994
Luvox CR Extended-Release Capsules (2%) 1759
▲ Lyrica Capsules (Greater than or equal to 1% to 3%) 2527
Meridia Capsules (Greater than or equal to 1%) 475
▲ Mirapex Tablets (7%) 857
Namenda (Infrequent) 1180
Nexium Delayed-Release Capsules (Less than 1%) 645
Nexium I.V. (Less than 1%) 652
Nexium Delayed-Release Oral Suspension (Less than 1%) 645
OxyContin Tablets (Less than 1%) 2589
Paxil (Infrequent) 1535
Paxil CR Controlled-Release Tablets (Infrequent) 1544
▲ PegIntron Powder for Injection (5%) 2903
▲ Premphase Tablets (3%) 3232
▲ Prempro Tablets (3% to 4%) 3232
▲ Prograf Capsules and Injection (3% to 15%) 622
▲ Prometrium Capsules (100 mg, 200 mg) (Less than 5%) 3047
Protonix for Delayed-Release Oral Suspension (Greater than or equal to 1%) 3254
Protonix Delayed-Release Tablets (Greater than or equal to 1%) 3254
Protonix I.V. (Greater than or equal to 1%) 3257
Protopic Ointment (0.2% to less than 1%) 628
Provigil Tablets (1%) 977
Prozac Weekly Capsules (Infrequent) 1852
Prozac Pulvules and Liquid (Infrequent) 1852
▲ Pulmicort Flexhaler (Greater than or equal to 1% to 3%) 654
▲ Rebif Prefilled Syringe for Injection (6% to 7%) 1107
ReoPro Vials (0.2%) 1860
Requip Tablets (Infrequent) 1561
▲ Rilutek Tablets (5.3% to 5.9%) 2771
Risperdal Consta Long-Acting Injection (Frequent) 1753
Rocephin Injectable Vials, ADD-Vantage, Galaxy, Bulk 2642
Rythmol SR Capsules 1590
▲ Soriatane Capsules (1% to 10%) 3062
Sular Extended Release Tablets (Less than or equal to 1%) 2975
Tricor Tablets 520
Ultane Liquid for Inhalation (Less than 1%) 524
▲ Venlafaxine Hydrochloride Tablets (3%) 2199
Vicoprofen Tablets (Less than 3%) 533
Wellbutrin SR Sustained-Release Tablets (Infrequent) 1653
Wellbutrin XL Extended-Release Tablets (Infrequent) 1659
Zomig Tablets (Rare) 694
Zomig Nasal Spray (Rare to infrequent) 689
Zomig-ZMT Tablets (Rare) 694
Zonegran Capsules (Infrequent) 1089
Zyban Sustained-Release Tablets (Infrequent) 1692
▲ Zyprexa Tablets (4% to 20%) 1883
▲ Zyprexa IntraMuscular (2% to 4%) 1883
▲ Zyprexa ZYDIS Orally Disintegrating Tablets (4% to 20%) 1883
Zyrtec Chewable Tablets (Less than 2%) 1920
Zyrtec Syrup (Less than 2%) 1920
Zyrtec Tablets (Less than 2%) 1920
Zyrtec-D 12 Hour Extended Release Tablets (Less than 2%) 1923

Hypertrichosis

Analpram-HC 1140
Celexa (Rare) 1160
Diprolene Lotion 0.05% (Infrequent) 2838
Diprolene Ointment 0.05% 2839
Diprolene AF Cream 0.05% (Infrequent) 2837
Elocon Cream 0.1% (Infrequent) 2840
Elocon Lotion 0.1% (Infrequent) 2841
Elocon Ointment 0.1% (Infrequent) 2842
Finacea Gel (Rare) 1742
▲ Gengraf Capsules (6.6% to 15%) 435
Lotrisone 2881
▲ Neoral Oral Solution (6.6% to 15%) 2280
▲ Neoral Soft Gelatin Capsules (6.6% to 15%) 2280
Olux Foam 3061
Phenytek Capsules 2192
Pramosone 1141
▲ Simulect for Injection (3% to 10%) 2306
Soriatane Capsules (Less than 1%) 3062
Vanos Cream 1941
Zyrtec Chewable Tablets (Less than 2%) 1920
Zyrtec Syrup (Less than 2%) 1920
Zyrtec Tablets (Less than 2%) 1920
Zyrtec-D 12 Hour Extended Release Tablets (Less than 2%) 1923

Hypertriglyceridemia

Accutane Capsules 2607
Aceon Tablets (2 mg, 4 mg, 8 mg) (1.3%) 3038
Activella Tablets 2347
AndroGel 3159
Angeliq Tablets 751
▲ Aptivus Capsules (3.9% to 49%) 823
▲ Aptivus Oral Solution (3.9% to 49%) 823
Atacand Tablets (0.5% or greater) 639
Atacand HCT 642
▲ Atripla Tablets (4%) 938
Benicar HCT Tablets 1010
Betaseron for SC Injection 756
Bystolic Tablets (Greater than or equal to 1%) 1155
Carbatrol Capsules (Occasional) 3019
Cipro I.V. (Among most frequent) 2817
Cipro 2810
Cipro XR Tablets 2823
Climara Transdermal System 763
Climara Pro Transdermal System 768
Coreg Tablets (Greater than 0.1% to 1%) 1387
Coreg CR Extended-Release Capsules (1%) 1393
Crixivan Capsules 1979
Divigel 3167
Edex Injection (2%) 2957
▲ Emtriva Capsules (4% to 10%) 1246
▲ Emtriva Oral Solution (4% to 10%) 1246
Enjuvia Tablets 1029
Epzicom Tablets 1422
Equetro Extended-Release Capsules 3174
Estratest Tablets 3043
Estratest H.S. Tablets 3043
Evoxac Capsules (Less than 1%) 1013
▲ Gengraf Capsules (About 15%) 435
▲ Intron A for Injection (Less than 5%) 2859
▲ Kaletra (1% to 36%) 452
▲ Lexiva Oral Suspension (0% to 11%) 1510
▲ Lexiva Tablets (0% to 11%) 1510
Lovenox Injection 2756
▲ Lupron Depot 3.75 mg (12%) 462
▲ Lupron Depot–3 Month 11.25 mg (32%) 462
▲ Neoral Oral Solution (About 15%) 2280
▲ Neoral Soft Gelatin Capsules (About 15%) 2280
Noroxin Tablets 2069
▲ Norvir (1.3% to 33.6%) 489
Ortho-Cyclen/Ortho Tri-Cyclen 2449
Ortho Tri-Cyclen Lo Tablets 2458
PegIntron Powder for Injection 2903
Premarin Intravenous 3217
Premarin Tablets 3221
Premarin Vaginal Cream 3228
Premphase Tablets 3232
Prempro Tablets 3232
Prinzide Tablets 2092
▲ Pristiq Extended-Release Tablets (1% to 6%) 3247
▲ Rapamune (Greater than or equal to 30% to 57%) 3260
Rythmol SR Capsules 1590
▲ Simulect for Injection (3% to 10%) 2306
Soriatane Capsules (Less common) 3062
Sustiva Capsules 930
Sustiva Tablets 930
▲ Targretin Capsules (Approximately 70%) 1084
Teveten Tablets (1%) 515
Teveten HCT Tablets (Less than 1%) 517
▲ Torisel Injection (44% to 83%) 3272
Trizivir Tablets 1622
▲ Truvada Tablets (4%) 1262
▲ Vesanoid Capsules (Up to 60%) 2660
▲ Viread Tablets (1% to 11%) 1268
▲ WelChol Tablets (18% to 22%) 1015
▲ Xeloda Tablets (Less than 5%) 2662
▲ Ziagen (2% to 6%) 1673
Zyprexa Tablets (Rare) 1883
Zyprexa IntraMuscular (Rare) 1883
Zyprexa ZYDIS Orally Disintegrating Tablets (Rare) 1883

Hypertrophic papillae of the tongue

Primaxin I.M. 2080
Primaxin I.V. (Less than 0.2%) 2083

Hypertrophy, endometrial

Exelon Capsules (Infrequent) 2229
Exelon Oral Solution (Infrequent) 2229

Hypertrophy, thymus

▲ Increlex Injection (Greater than or equal to 5%) 3100

Hypertrophy, tonsillar

▲ Increlex Injection (Greater than or equal to 5%) 3100

Hypertrophy, unspecified

Kaletra (Less than 2%) 452

Hyperuricemia

Abelcet Injection 1134
Accutane Capsules 2607
Aceon Tablets (2 mg, 4 mg, 8 mg) (0.3% to 1%) 3038
Advicor Tablets 402
Atacand Tablets (0.6%) 639
Atacand HCT (0.5% or greater) 642
Avalide Tablets 892
Avalide Tablets 2713
Avelox (Less than 0.1%) 2803
Axid Capsules 1364
Benicar Tablets (Greater than 0.5%) 1009
▲ Benicar HCT Tablets (4%) 1010
Betaseron for SC Injection 756
Bystolic Tablets (Greater than or equal to 1%) 1155
Campral Tablets (Infrequent) 1158
Cardizem LA Extended Release Tablets (Less than 2%) 421
Celebrex Capsules 2979
▲ CellCept Capsules (3% to less than 20%) 2622
▲ CellCept Intravenous (3% to less than 20%) 2622

▲ CellCept Oral Suspension (3% to less than 20%) 2622
▲ CellCept Tablets (3% to less than 20%) 2622
Cipro I.V. (Among most frequent) 2817
Cipro (Less than 0.1%) 2810
Cipro XR Tablets 2823
Clorpres Tablets 2185
▲ Coreg Tablets (Greater than 1% to 3%) 1387
▲ Coreg CR Extended-Release Capsules (Greater than 1% to less than or equal to 3%) 1393
Creon 5 Capsules 3041
Creon 10 Capsules 3042
Creon 20 Capsules 3042
Demadex Injection 2630
Demadex Tablets 2630
Diovan HCT Tablets 2216
▲ Doxil Injection (1% to 5%) 2378
Dyazide Capsules 1405
Edecrin 698
Effexor XR Extended-Release Capsules (Infrequent) 3195
Evoxac Capsules (Less than 1%) 1013
Furosemide Tablets 2186
Gengraf Capsules (1% to less than 3%) 435
Geodon Capsules (Rare) 2520
▲ Indapamide Tablets (Less than 5%) 2188
Intravenous Sodium Diuril 2490
▲ Kaletra (0% to 5%) 452
▲ Lupron Depot 7.5 mg (Greater than or equal to 5%) 469
▲ Mavik Tablets (15%) 472
Micardis HCT Tablets 854
Mirapex Tablets 857
▲ Myfortic Tablets (3% to less than 20%) 2276
Myleran Tablets 1530
Neoral Oral Solution (1% to less than 3%) 2280
Neoral Soft Gelatin Capsules (1% to less than 3%) 2280
▲ Neulasta Injection (8%) 587
▲ Neupogen for Injection (27% to 58%) 589
Nexium Delayed-Release Capsules (Less than 1%) 645
Nexium I.V. (Less than 1%) 652
Nexium Delayed-Release Oral Suspension (Less than 1%) 645
▲ Norvir (3.8%) 489
▲ PegIntron Powder for Injection (33% to 38%) 2903
Plavix Tablets (1% to 2.5%) 926
Plavix Tablets (1% to 2.5%) 2767
Pletal Tablets (Less than 2%) 2481
Prinzide Tablets 2092
Proglycem Capsules (Frequent) 1185
Proglycem Suspension (Frequent) 1185
▲ Prograf Capsules and Injection (3% to 15%) 622
Proleukin for Injection (Less than 1%) 2287
Prozac Weekly Capsules (Rare) 1852
Prozac Pulvules and Liquid (Rare) 1852
▲ Rebetol (33% to 38%) 2917
Requip Tablets (Infrequent) 1561
Risperdal Consta Long-Acting Injection (Infrequent) 1753
▲ Rituxan I.V. (1.5% to 3%) 1223
Rythmol SR Capsules 1590
St. Joseph 81 mg Aspirin Chewable and Enteric Coated Tablets 1903
Sandimmune (Occasional) 2296
▲ Simulect for Injection (Greater than or equal to 10%) 2306
Starlix Tablets 2314
▲ Sutent Capsules (10%) 2540
Tabloid Tablets (Frequent) 1601
Tekturna Tablets (0.4%) 2321
Tekturna HCT Tablets (0.4% to 2.2%) 2324
Teveten HCT Tablets 517
▲ Treanda for Injection (2% to 7%) 983
Tricor Tablets 520
Ultrase Capsules 718
Ultrase MT Capsules 719
Velcade for Injection 2168
Venlafaxine Hydrochloride Tablets (Rare) 2199
Viokase 721
Xyrem Oral Solution (Infrequent) 1766
Zyprexa Tablets (Infrequent) 1883
Zyprexa ZYDIS Orally Disintegrating Tablets (Infrequent) 1883

Hyperuricosuria
Creon 5 Capsules 3041
Creon 10 Capsules 3042
Creon 20 Capsules 3042
Myleran Tablets 1530
Ultrase Capsules 718
Ultrase MT Capsules 719

Hyperuricuria
Viokase 721

Hyperventilation
Actiq (Less than 1%) 959
Adenocard IV Injection (Less than 1%) 603
AmBisome for Injection (Less common) 606
Aricept Tablets (Infrequent) 1062
Aricept ODT Tablets (Infrequent) 1062
Axert Tablets (Rare) 2431
▲ Busulfex Injection (2% to 3%) 2477
▲ CellCept Capsules (3% to less than 20%) 2622
▲ CellCept Intravenous (3% to less than 20%) 2622
▲ CellCept Oral Suspension (3% to less than 20%) 2622
▲ CellCept Tablets (3% to less than 20%) 2622
Copaxone for Injection (Frequent) 3110
Crinone 4% Gel 992
Crinone 8% Gel 992
Doxil Injection (Less than 1%) 2378
Effexor XR Extended-Release Capsules (Infrequent) 3195
Frova Tablets (Infrequent) 1111
Gabitril Tablets (Infrequent) 973
Ionsys Transdermal System (.1% to less than 1%) 2410
Lamictal (Infrequent) 1488
Luvox CR Extended-Release Capsules (Infrequent) 1759
Mirapex Tablets 857
Orthoclone OKT3 Sterile Solution 2387
Paxil (Infrequent) 1535
Paxil CR Controlled-Release Tablets (Infrequent) 1544
Primaxin I.M. 2080
Primaxin I.V. (Less than 0.2%) 2083
Proleukin for Injection (Less than 1%) 2287
Prozac Weekly Capsules (Infrequent) 1852
Prozac Pulvules and Liquid (Infrequent) 1852
Rilutek Tablets (Infrequent) 2771
▲ Romazicon Injection (3% to 9%) 2646
Sulfamylon Cream 2194
Sulfamylon for 5% Topical Solution 2194
Symbyax Capsules (Infrequent) 1871
Ultane Liquid for Inhalation (Less than 1%) 524
Venlafaxine Hydrochloride Tablets (Infrequent) 2199
Xyrem Oral Solution (Infrequent) 1766
Zomig Tablets (Rare) 694
Zomig Nasal Spray (Rare) 689
Zomig-ZMT Tablets (Rare) 694
Zyprexa Tablets (Infrequent) 1883
Zyprexa ZYDIS Orally Disintegrating Tablets (Infrequent) 1883
Zyrtec Chewable Tablets (Less than 2%) 1920
Zyrtec Syrup (Less than 2%) 1920
Zyrtec Tablets (Less than 2%) 1920
Zyrtec-D 12 Hour Extended Release Tablets (Less than 2%) 1923

Hypervigilance
Concerta Extended-Release Tablets 1925

Hyperviscosity syndrome
Rituxan I.V. 1223

Hypervolemia
▲ AmBisome for Injection (8.2% to 12.2%) 606
Busulfex Injection 2477
▲ CellCept Capsules (3% to less than 20%) 2622
▲ CellCept Intravenous (3% to less than 20%) 2622
▲ CellCept Oral Suspension (3% to less than 20%) 2622
▲ CellCept Tablets (3% to less than 20%) 2622
▲ Coreg Tablets (Greater than 1% to 3%) 1387
▲ Coreg CR Extended-Release Capsules (Greater than 1% to less than or equal to 3%) 1393
Merrem I.V. (Greater than 0.1% to 1%) 684
▲ Prograf Capsules and Injection (3% to 15%) 622
Trasylol Injection (1% to 2%) 799

Hypesthesia
(*see also under* Hypoesthesia)
Ionsys Transdermal System (.1% to less than 1%) 2410

Hyphema
Voltaren Ophthalmic Solution 2336

Hypoactivity
▲ Aerobid/Aerobid-M (1% to 3%) 1153

Hypoacusis
▲ Fabrazyme for Intravenous Infusion (5%) 1241
▲ Increlex Injection (Greater than or equal to 5%) 3100
Levaquin 2416
Levaquin in 5% Dextrose Injection 2416
Mirapex Tablets 857

Hypoadrenalism
Sandostatin Injection (Less than 1%) 2300
Sandostatin LAR Depot 2302

Hypoadrenalism, neonatal
Azmacort Inhalation Aerosol 407

Hypoaesthesia
▲ DepoCyt Injection (10% to 12%) 1136
Exforge Tablets (Greater than or equal to 0.2%) 2238
▲ Fabrazyme for Intravenous Infusion (9%) 1241
Lexapro Oral Suspension 1174
Lexapro Tablets 1174

Hypoalbuminemia
▲ Arranon Injection (1% to 10%) 1319
Baraclude (0% to less than 1%) 900
▲ Cancidas for Injection (7.4%) 1953
Cipro XR Tablets 2823
▲ Dacogen Injection (24%) 1066
Dapsone Tablets USP 1746
▲ Eloxatin for Injection (0% to 9%) 2731
Emend Capsules (Greater than 0.5%) 1992
Emend for Injection (Greater than 0.5%) 1999
Evista Tablets 1810
Fentora Tablets (Greater than 1%) 968
▲ Gleevec Tablets (0% to 4%) 2255
▲ Leukine (27%) 774
▲ Lupron Depot 7.5 mg (Greater than or equal to 5%) 469
Neupro Transdermal System 3149
▲ Nexavar Tablets (59%) 784
▲ Ontak Vials (83%) 1079
Tasigna Capsules (1%) 2316
Zosyn for Injection 3284

Hypoalbuminuria
Elspar for Injection 1990
Invanz for Injection (0.9% to 1.7%) 2029

Hypocalcemia
Abelcet Injection 1134
Actiq (Less than 1%) 959
Activella Tablets 2347
▲ Actonel Tablets (0.2% to 4.5%) 2568
Actonel with Calcium Tablets (0.8%) 2574
▲ AmBisome for Injection (4.9% to 18.4%) 606
Angeliq Tablets 751
▲ Arranon Injection (1% to 8%) 1319
Azilect Tablets (Infrequent) 3106
Betaseron for SC Injection 756
▲ Busulfex Injection (3% to 49%) 2477
Capastat Sulfate for Injection 1791
▲ CellCept Capsules (3% to 30%) 2622
▲ CellCept Intravenous (3% to 30%) 2622
▲ CellCept Oral Suspension (3% to 30%) 2622
▲ CellCept Tablets (3% to 30%) 2622
Climara Transdermal System 763
Climara Pro Transdermal System 768
Cosmegen for Injection 2485
Divigel 3167
▲ Doxil Injection (1% to 5%) 2378
▲ Eloxatin for Injection (4% to 7%) 2731
Enjuvia Tablets 1029
Equetro Extended-Release Capsules 3174
Estratest Tablets 3043
Estratest H.S. Tablets 3043
Evista Tablets 1810
Fleet Enema 1143
Fleet Enema Extra 1143
Fleet Enema for Children 1143
Fleet Pedia-Lax Enema 1143
Fleet Phospho-soda 1145
Fleet Phospho-soda EZ-PREP 1147
Fleet Prep Kits 1149
▲ Fosamax (Approximately 18%) 2005
▲ Fosamax Plus D Tablets (18%) 2013
Frova Tablets (Rare) 1111
Furosemide Tablets 2186
Geodon Capsules (Rare) 2520
Ionsys Transdermal System (.1% to less than 1%) 2410
Leukine (2%) 774
▲ Mavik Tablets (4.7%) 472
Mirapex Tablets 857
▲ Mycamine for Injection (6.5% to 16.9%) 616
▲ Myfortic Tablets (3% to less than 20%) 2276
▲ Mylotarg for Injection (10% to 12%) 3212
▲ NeoProfen Injection (12%) 2496
▲ Novantrone for Injection Concentrate (10%) 1100
▲ Noxafil Oral Suspension (9%) 2889
Omnicef for Oral Suspension (0.5%) 497
▲ Ontak Vials (17%) 1079
OsmoPrep Tablets 2680
Paxil (Rare) 1535
Paxil CR Controlled-Release Tablets (Rare) 1544
Precose Tablets 792
Premarin Intravenous 3217
Premarin Tablets 3221
Premarin Vaginal Cream 3228
Premphase Tablets 3232
Prempro Tablets 3232
▲ Prograf Capsules and Injection (3% to 15%) 622
▲ Proleukin for Injection (Less than 1% to 11%) 2287
Prozac Weekly Capsules (Rare) 1852
Prozac Pulvules and Liquid (Rare) 1852
▲ Reclast Injection (3% to 22%) 2291
Rituxan I.V. 1223
▲ Sensipar Tablets (80%) 594
▲ Simulect for Injection (3% to 10%) 2306
Targretin Capsules 1084
▲ Tasigna Capsules (0.1% to 4%) 2316
▲ Trisenox Injection (10%) 986
Tygacil for Injection (0% to less than 2%) 3276
▲ Valcyte Tablets (Less than 5%) 2654
Vectibix 597
Velcade for Injection 2168
Xeloda Tablets (2.3%) 2662
Xyrem Oral Solution (Infrequent) 1766
▲ Zometa for Intravenous Infusion (Less than 15%) 2341
Zosyn for Injection 3284

Hypochloremia
▲ CellCept Capsules (3% to less than 20%) 2622
▲ CellCept Intravenous (3% to less than 20%) 2622
▲ CellCept Oral Suspension (3% to less than 20%) 2622
▲ CellCept Tablets (3% to less than 20%) 2622
Demadex Injection 2630
Demadex Tablets 2630
Doxil Injection (Less than 1%) 2378
Dyazide Capsules 1405
Geodon Capsules (Rare) 2520
▲ Indapamide Tablets (Less than 5%) 2188
Requip Tablets (Rare) 1561

Hypochloremic alkalosis
Furosemide Tablets 2186
Intravenous Sodium Diuril 2490
Prinzide Tablets 2092
Teveten HCT Tablets 517

Hypocholesterolemia
Bystolic Tablets (Greater than or equal to 1%) 1155
Evista Tablets 1810
Geodon Capsules (Rare) 2520
▲ Simulect for Injection (Greater than or equal to 10%) 2306
Venlafaxine Hydrochloride Tablets (Rare) 2199

Hypochondriasis
Luvox CR Extended-Release Capsules (Infrequent) 1759

Hypoesthesia
Actiq (1% or greater) 959
Alinia for Oral Suspension (Less than 1%) 2677
Alinia Tablets (Less than 1%) 2677
Ambien Tablets (Infrequent) 2692
Ambien CR Tablets (2%) 2696
Amerge Tablets (Rare) 1301
▲ Arranon Injection (0% to 17%) 1319
Atacand HCT (0.5% or greater) 642
Atripla Tablets 938
Avelox (Less than 0.1%) 2803
Azilect Tablets (Infrequent) 3106

Campral Tablets (Infrequent) 1158
Cardene I.V. (0.7%) 1093
Celebrex Capsules (0.1% to 1.9%) 2979
Celexa (Infrequent) 1160
▲ CellCept Capsules (3% to less than 20%) 2622
▲ CellCept Intravenous (3% to less than 20%) 2622
▲ CellCept Oral Suspension (3% to less than 20%) 2622
▲ CellCept Tablets (3% to less than 20%) 2622
Cialis Tablets (Less than 2%) 1792
Cipro I.V. 2817
Cipro 2810
Cipro XR Tablets 2823
Copaxone for Injection (At least 2%) 3110
▲ Coreg Tablets (Greater than 1% to 3%) 1387
▲ Coreg CR Extended-Release Capsules (Greater than 1% to less than or equal to 3%) 1393
▲ Cozaar Tablets (Less than 1% to 5%) 1973
Cymbalta Delayed-Release Capsules (Frequent) 1801
Denavir Cream (0.9%) 2205
Depakote ER Tablets 423
▲ DepoDur Injection (2% to 5%) 1095
Eloxatin for Injection 2731
Emend Capsules (Greater than 0.5%) 1992
Emend for Injection (Greater than 0.5%) 1999
Engerix-B Vaccine 1409
▲ Evoxac Capsules (1% to 3%) 1013
Exelon Capsules (Infrequent) 2229
Exelon Oral Solution (Infrequent) 2229
▲ Fabrazyme for Intravenous Infusion (9%) 1241
Fentora Tablets (Greater than 1%) 968
Flector Patch (1%) 561
▲ Flolan for Injection (1% to 12%) 1426
Fluarix Vaccine 1446
Flumadine 1167
Frova Tablets (Infrequent) 1111
Gabitril Tablets (Frequent) 973
Gengraf Capsules (1% to less than 3%) 435
Genotropin Lyophilized Powder 2547
Geodon Capsules (2%) 2520
▲ Gliadel Wafer (6%) 1076
▲ Humatrope Vials and Cartridges (Up to 6.25%) 1838
Intelence Tablets (Less than 2%) 3119
▲ Intron A for Injection (Up to 10%) 2859
Invanz for Injection (Greater than 0.1%) 2029
▲ Ixempra Kit for Injection (62%) 915
▲ Kepivance (12%) 583
Klonopin (Infrequent) 2639
▲ Lamictal (Greater than 1% to less than 5%) 1488
Levaquin (0.1% to 0.9%) 2416
Levaquin in 5% Dextrose Injection (0.1% to 0.9%) 2416
Levitra Tablets (Less than 2%) 2876
Lidoderm Patch 1114
Lipitor Tablets (Less than 2%) 2501
Lunesta Tablets (Infrequent) 2994
Lupron Depot 3.75 mg 462
Lupron Depot–3 Month 11.25 mg 462
Lyrica Capsules (Greater than or equal to 1%) 2527
Maxalt Tablets (Frequent) 2056
Maxalt-MLT Orally Disintegrating Tablets (Frequent) 2056
▲ Megace ES Oral Suspension (1% to 3%) 2499
Meridia Capsules 475
Micardis Tablets (More than 0.3%) 852
Micardis HCT Tablets 854
▲ Mirapex Tablets (Greater than or equal to 1% to 3%) 857
Namenda (Infrequent) 1180
Neoral Oral Solution (1% to less than 3%) 2280
Neoral Soft Gelatin Capsules (1% to less than 3%) 2280
Neupro Transdermal System 3149
Nexium Delayed-Release Capsules (Less than 1%) 645
Nexium I.V. (Less than 1%) 652
Nexium Delayed-Release Oral Suspension (Less than 1%) 645
Noroxin Tablets 2069
OxyContin Tablets (Less than 1%) 2589
Paxil (Infrequent) 1535
Paxil CR Controlled-Release Tablets (Infrequent) 1544
Percocet Tablets 1127
Plavix Tablets (1% to 2.5%) 926
Plavix Tablets (1% to 2.5%) 2767
Protonix for Delayed-Release Oral Suspension (Less than 1%) 3254
Protonix Delayed-Release Tablets (Less than 1%) 3254
Protonix I.V. (Less than 1%) 3257
Prozac Weekly Capsules (Infrequent) 1852
Prozac Pulvules and Liquid (Infrequent) 1852
Rebif Prefilled Syringe for Injection 1107
Recombivax HB 2107
Remeron Tablets (Frequent) 2924
RemeronSolTab Tablets (Frequent) 2927
ReoPro Vials (0.3%) 1860
Requip Tablets (Infrequent to frequent) 1561
Rilutek Tablets (Infrequent) 2771
▲ Romazicon Injection (1% to 3%) 2646
Salagen Tablets (Less than 1%) 1082
▲ Simulect for Injection (3% to 10%) 2306
Singulair 2114
Soriatane Capsules (Less than 1%) 3062
Sular Extended Release Tablets (Less than or equal to 1%) 2975
Sustiva Capsules (1% to 2%) 930
Sustiva Tablets (1% to 2%) 930
Symbyax Capsules (Infrequent) 1871
Targretin Capsules 1084
Tarka Tablets (Less frequent) 511
Tasigna Capsules (0.1% to 1%) 2316
▲ Ultram ER Extended-Release Tablets (1% to les than 5%) 2428
▲ Visudyne for Injection (1% to 10%) 2332
Wellbutrin SR Sustained-Release Tablets (Infrequent) 1653
Wellbutrin XL Extended-Release Tablets (Infrequent) 1659
▲ Xeloda Tablets (Less than 1% to 4%) 2662
Xopenex Inhalation Solution 3001
Xopenex Inhalation Solution Concentrate 3005
Xopenex HFA Inhalation Aerosol 3009
▲ Xyrem Oral Solution (Less than 1% to 5.9%) 1766
▲ Zometa for Intravenous Infusion (12%) 2341
Zyban Sustained-Release Tablets (Infrequent) 1692
Zyprexa Tablets (Infrequent) 1883
Zyprexa ZYDIS Orally Disintegrating Tablets (Infrequent) 1883
Zyrtec Chewable Tablets (Less than 2%) 1920
Zyrtec Syrup (Less than 2%) 1920
Zyrtec Tablets (Less than 2%) 1920
Zyrtec-D 12 Hour Extended Release Tablets (Less than 2%) 1923

Hypoestrogeneism

Lupron Depot 3.75 mg (Among most frequent) 462
Lupron Depot–3 Month 11.25 mg 462

Hypofibrinogenemia

Depakote ER Tablets 423
Elspar for Injection 1990
Elspar for Injection 2488
Gantrisin Pediatric Suspension 2638
Lamictal (Rare) 1488
NovoSeven (Greater than or equal to 2%) 2367
NovoSeven RT (Greater than or equal to 2%) 2370
Oncaspar Injection 1138
Panhematin for Injection 2497

Hypogeusia

▲ Sutent Capsules (Less than 1% to 44%) 2540

Hypoglycemia

Abelcet Injection 1134
Actiq (Less than 1%) 959
▲ Actos Tablets (8% to 15%) 3077
Aggrenox Capsules 819
Anaprox Tablets (Less than 1%) 2632
Anaprox DS Tablets (Less than 1%) 2632
Apidra Injection 2706
Aricept Tablets (Infrequent) 1062
Aricept ODT Tablets (Infrequent) 1062
▲ Arranon Injection (0% to 6%) 1319
▲ Avandamet Tablets (3%) 1336
▲ Avandaryl Tablets (Less than 1% to 5.5%) 1344
Avandia Tablets (0.6% to 2.9%) 1351
Avelox (Greater than or equal to 2%) 2803
Bayer Aspirin 750
Biaxin/Biaxin XL (Rare) 411
Brovana Inhalation Solution (Less than 2%) 2990
▲ Byetta Injection (3.3% to 35.7%) 600
Celebrex Capsules (Less than 0.1%) 2979
Celexa (Rare) 1160
▲ CellCept Capsules (3% to less than 20%) 2622
▲ CellCept Intravenous (3% to less than 20%) 2622
▲ CellCept Oral Suspension (3% to less than 20%) 2622
▲ CellCept Tablets (3% to less than 20%) 2622
Chantix Tablets (Rare) 2511
Cipro I.V. (Rare) 2817
Cipro (Less than 0.1%) 2810
Cipro XR Tablets 2823
Combigan Ophthalmic Solution 553
▲ Coreg Tablets (5% to 12%) 1387
▲ Coreg CR Extended-Release Capsules (Greater than 1% to less than or equal to 3%) 1393
Cosopt Sterile Ophthalmic Solution 1969
▲ Cozaar Tablets (14%) 1973
Cubicin for Injection (1% to 2%) 995
Cuprimine Capsules (Rare) 1986
▲ DepoCyt Injection (6% to 12%) 1136
Doxil Injection (Less than 1%) 2378
▲ Duetact Tablets (13.4% to 15.7%) 3085
EC-Naprosyn Delayed-Release Tablets (Less than 1%) 2632
Edecrin (In 2 uremic patients) 698
Effexor XR Extended-Release Capsules (Infrequent) 3195
▲ Emtriva Capsules (3%) 1246
▲ Emtriva Oral Solution (3%) 1246
Epivir 1412
Evoxac Capsules (Less than 1%) 1013
Exelon Capsules (Infrequent) 2229
Exelon Oral Solution (Infrequent) 2229
Exubera Inhalation Powder 2515
Frova Tablets (Rare) 1111
Gabitril Tablets (Infrequent) 973
Gantrisin Pediatric Suspension 2638
Gengraf Capsules (1% to less than 3%) 435
Geodon Capsules (Rare) 2520
Humalog-Pen and KwikPen (Most common) 1829
Humalog Mix 50/50-Pen and KwikPen 1833
Humalog Mix 75/25-Pen and KwikPen 1835
Humulin 50/50, 100 Units 1843
Humulin 70/30 Vial 1844
Humulin N Vial 1846
Humulin R 1849
Humulin R (U-500) 1850
Imitrex Nasal Spray 1470
Imitrex Tablets (Rare) 1474
▲ Increlex Injection (5% to 42%) 3100
▲ Indocin I.V. (1% to 3%) 2489
▲ Janumet Tablets (16.4%) 2041
▲ Januvia Tablets (0.6% to 12.2%) 2048
Lantus Injection 2749
Levaquin (0.1% to 1%) 2416
Levaquin in 5% Dextrose Injection (0.1% to 1%) 2416
Levemir Injection 2352
Lexapro Oral Suspension 1174
Lexapro Tablets 1174
Lipitor Tablets (Less than 2%) 2501
Luvox CR Extended-Release Capsules (Rare) 1759
▲ Lyrica Capsules (1% to 3%) 2527
Mepron Suspension (1%) 1526
Meridia Capsules 475
Merrem I.V. (Greater than 1%) 684
Mirapex Tablets 857
Moban Tablets 1116
▲ Mycamine for Injection (6% to 6.9%) 616
Namenda 1180
Naprosyn Suspension (Less than 1%) 2632
Naprosyn Tablets (Less than 1%) 2632
▲ NeoProfen Injection (12%) 2496
Neoral Oral Solution (1% to less than 3%) 2280
Neoral Soft Gelatin Capsules (1% to less than 3%) 2280
▲ Neupro Transdermal System (7%) 3149
Noroxin Tablets 2069
NovoLog Mix 70/30 2364
Omnicef Capsules (0.2%) 497
Omnicef for Oral Suspension (0.2%) 497
Paser Granules 1747
Paxil (Rare) 1535
Paxil CR Controlled-Release Tablets (Rare) 1544
Percocet Tablets 1127
Percodan Tablets 1130
▲ PrandiMet Tablets (Greater than 5% to 33%) 2967
▲ Prandin Tablets (7% to 31%) 2971
Precose Tablets 792
Prinivil Tablets 2087
▲ Prograf Capsules and Injection (3% to 15%) 622
Protopic Ointment (Greater than or equal to 1%) 628
Prozac Weekly Capsules 1852
Prozac Pulvules and Liquid 1852
Requip Tablets (Infrequent) 1561
St. Joseph 81 mg Aspirin Chewable and Enteric Coated Tablets 1903
Salagen Tablets (Less than 1%) 1082
▲ Sandostatin Injection (3% to 16%) 2300
▲ Sandostatin LAR Depot (2% to 4%) 2302
▲ Somatuline Depot Injection (7%) 3102
Starlix Tablets (2.4%) 2314
Symbyax Capsules (Infrequent) 1871
Tasigna Capsules (0.1% to 1%) 2316
Thiothixene Capsules 2197
Timoptic-XE Sterile Ophthalmic Gel Forming Solution 2125
Treximet Tablets (Rare) 1616
Tricor Tablets 520
▲ Trisenox Injection (8%) 986
▲ Truvada Tablets (Less than or equal to 3%) 1262
Tygacil for Injection (0% to less than 2%) 3276
▲ Vaprisol (3.3%) 632
Venlafaxine Hydrochloride Tablets (Rare) 2199
▲ WelChol Tablets (3%) 1015
Wellbutrin Tablets 1648
Wellbutrin SR Sustained-Release Tablets 1653
Wellbutrin XL Extended-Release Tablets 1659
Zonegran Capsules (Rare) 1089
Zosyn for Injection (1% or less) 3284
Zyprexa Tablets (Infrequent) 1883
Zyprexa ZYDIS Orally Disintegrating Tablets (Infrequent) 1883

Hypoglycemia, masked symptoms of

Betimol Ophthalmic Solution 3181
Combigan Ophthalmic Solution 553
InnoPran XL Extended Release Capsules 1484
Timoptic in Ocudose (Less frequent) 2124
Timoptic-XE Sterile Ophthalmic Gel Forming Solution 2125

Hypoglycemic reactions

Emsam Transdermal System (Rare) 905
Symbyax Capsules (Rare) 1871

Hypogonadism, male

Kaletra (Up to 2%) 452

Hypohidrosis

Bentyl Capsules 703
Bentyl Injection 703
Bentyl Syrup 703
Bentyl Tablets 703
Celexa (Rare) 1160
Donnatal Extentabs 2507
Paxil (Rare) 1535
Paxil CR Controlled-Release Tablets (Rare) 1544
Zonegran Capsules 1089

Hypokalemia

▲ Abelcet Injection (5%) 1134
Abilify Injection (Greater than or equal to 1 in 1000 patients and less than 1 in 100 patients) 2466
Abilify Oral Solution (Greater than or equal to 1 in 1000 patients and less than 1 in 100 patients) 881
Abilify Oral Solution (Greater than or equal to 1 in 1000 patients and less than 1 in 100 patients) 2466
Abilify Discmelt Orally Disintegrating Tablets (Greater than or equal to 1 in 1000 patients and less than 1 in 100 patients) 881
Abilify Discmelt Orally Disintegrating Tablets (Greater than or equal to 1 in 1000 patients and less than 1 in 100 patients) 2466
Abilify Tablets (Greater than or equal to 1 in 1000 patients and less than 1 in 100 patients) 881

Abilify Tablets (Greater than or equal to 1 in 1000 patients and less than 1 in 100 patients) 2466
Aceon Tablets (2 mg, 4 mg, 8 mg) (0.3% to 1%) 3038
Actiq (1% or greater) 959
▲ Advair Diskus 100/50 (4%) 1276
Advair Diskus 250/50 1276
Advair Diskus 500/50 1276
Aggrenox Capsules 819
▲ AmBisome for Injection (37.6% to 43.2%) 606
AndroGel 3159
Apidra Injection 2706
Aricept Tablets (Infrequent) 1062
Aricept ODT Tablets (Infrequent) 1062
▲ Arixtra Injection (0% to 4.2%) 1313
▲ Arranon Injection (2% to 11%) 1319
Atacand HCT (0.5% or greater) 642
Avalide Tablets 892
▲ Avalide Tablets (0.6% to 7.5%) 2713
▲ Avastin IV (12% to 16%) 1192
Benicar HCT Tablets 1010
Brovana Inhalation Solution 2990
▲ Busulfex Injection (2% to 64%) 2477
▲ Cancidas for Injection (6.4% to 22.8%) 1953
Capastat Sulfate for Injection 1791
Cardene I.V. (0.7%) 1093
Celebrex Capsules (0.1% to 1.9%) 2979
Celexa (Rare) 1160
▲ CellCept Capsules (31.8% to 37.2%) 2622
▲ CellCept Intravenous (31.8% to 37.2%) 2622
▲ CellCept Oral Suspension (31.8% to 37.2%) 2622
▲ CellCept Tablets (31.8% to 37.2%) 2622
Chantix Tablets (Infrequent) 2511
Cipro I.V. (Infrequent) 2817
Cipro XR Tablets 2823
Clorpres Tablets 2185
Combivent Inhalation Aerosol 845
▲ Coreg Tablets (Greater than 1% to 3%) 1387
Coreg CR Extended-Release Capsules (0.1% to less than or equal to 1%) 1393
▲ Cubicin for Injection (1% to 9.2%) 995
▲ Dacogen Injection (22%) 1066
Demadex Injection 2630
Demadex Tablets 2630
▲ DepoCyt Injection (7% to 15%) 1136
▲ DepoDur Injection (2% to 5%) 1095
Digibind for Injection 1403
▲ Diovan HCT Tablets (3%) 2216
▲ Doxil Injection (1% to 10%) 2378
Dyazide Capsules (Uncommon) 1405
Dyrenium Capsules (Rare) 3189
Effexor XR Extended-Release Capsules (Infrequent) 3195
▲ Eloxatin for Injection (1% to 11%) 2731
Emend Capsules (Greater than 0.5%) 1992
Emend for Injection (Greater than 0.5%) 1999
▲ Entereg Capsules (6.9% to 9.5%) 3293
Evoxac Capsules (Less than 1%) 1013
Exelon Capsules (Frequent) 2229
Exelon Oral Solution (Frequent) 2229
Exelon Patch (Infrequent) 2233
▲ Fentora Tablets (0% to 15%) 968
Fleet Enema 1143
Fleet Enema Extra 1143
Fleet Enema for Children 1143
Fleet Pedia-Lax Enema 1143
Fleet Phospho-soda 1145
Fleet Phospho-soda EZ-PREP 1147
Fleet Prep Kits 1149
▲ Flolan for Injection (6%) 1426
Foradil Aerolizer 2849
Furosemide Tablets 2186
Gabitril Tablets (Infrequent) 973
Geodon Capsules (Infrequent) 2520
▲ Gleevec Tablets (6% to 13%) 2255
Gliadel Wafer (1%) 1076
Humalog-Pen and KwikPen 1829
Humalog Mix 50/50-Pen and KwikPen 1833
Humalog Mix 75/25-Pen and KwikPen 1835
▲ Indapamide Tablets (3% to 7%) 2188
Intravenous Sodium Diuril 2490
Invanz for Injection (1.7% to 1.8%) 2029
▲ Ionsys Transdermal System (1% to less than 10%) 2410
Ixempra Kit for Injection 915
Kristalose for Oral Solution 1004
Levaquin (0.1% to 1%) 2416
Levaquin in 5% Dextrose Injection (0.1% to 1%) 2416
Lexapro Oral Suspension 1174
Lexapro Tablets 1174
Lunesta Tablets (Rare) 2994
Luvox CR Extended-Release Capsules (Rare) 1759
Merrem I.V. (Greater than 0.2%) 684
Micardis HCT Tablets (Less than 2%) 854
Mirapex Tablets 857
▲ Mycamine for Injection (14% to 49.2%) 616
▲ Myfortic Tablets (3% to less than 20%) 2276
▲ Mylotarg for Injection (24% to 29%) 3212
▲ Novantrone for Injection Concentrate (7% to 10%) 1100
NovoLog Mix 70/30 2364
NovoLog Injection 2359
▲ Noxafil Oral Suspension (1% to 30%) 2889
▲ Ontak Vials (6%) 1079
OsmoPrep Tablets 2680
Paxil (Rare) 1535
Paxil CR Controlled-Release Tablets (Rare) 1544
Perforomist Inhalation Solution 1025
Prinzide Tablets 2092
▲ Prograf Capsules and Injection (13% to 29%) 622
Proventil HFA Inhalation Aerosol (Some patients) 2914
Prozac Weekly Capsules (Infrequent) 1852
Prozac Pulvules and Liquid (Infrequent) 1852
▲ Rapamune (Greater than or equal to 3% to less than 20%) 3260
Requip Tablets (Infrequent) 1561
Rilutek Tablets (Infrequent) 2771
Risperdal Consta Long-Acting Injection (Infrequent) 1753
Rythmol SR Capsules 1590
▲ Simulect for Injection (Greater than or equal to 10%) 2306
Sular Extended Release Tablets (Less than or equal to 1%) 2975
▲ Sutent Capsules (1% to 12%) 2540
Symbyax Capsules (Infrequent) 1871
▲ Tasigna Capsules (0.1% to 5%) 2316
Tekturna HCT Tablets (2.2%) 2324
Teveten Tablets (Less than 1%) 515
Teveten HCT Tablets (Less than 1%) 517
Timentin ADD-Vantage (Rare) 1606
Timentin Injection Galaxy Container 1609
Timentin IV Infusion (Rare) 1603
Timentin Pharmacy Bulk Package (Rare) 1613
▲ Torisel Injection (5% to 21%) 3272
Trasylol Injection (1% to 2%) 799
▲ Trisenox Injection (50%) 986
Tygacil for Injection (2.1%) 3276
▲ Valcyte Tablets (Less than 5%) 2654
▲ Vaprisol (9.8% to 22%) 632
▲ Velcade for Injection (13%) 2168
Venlafaxine Hydrochloride Tablets (Infrequent) 2199
Ventolin HFA Inhalation Aerosol 1638
▲ Xeloda Tablets (Less than 5%) 2662
Xopenex Inhalation Solution 3001
Xopenex Inhalation Solution Concentrate 3005
Xopenex HFA Inhalation Aerosol 3009
Zofran Injection (Rare) 1682
Zofran (Rare) 1687
Zofran ODT Orally Disintegrating Tablets (Rare) 1687
Zolinza Capsules 2142
Zometa for Intravenous Infusion (Less than 15%) 2341
Zosyn for Injection 3284
Zyprexa Tablets (Infrequent) 1883
Zyprexa ZYDIS Orally Disintegrating Tablets (Infrequent) 1883
Zyvox (0% to 2.8%) 2552

Hypokinesia

Abilify Injection (Greater than or equal to 1 in 1000 patients and less than 1 in 100 patients) 881
Abilify Injection (Greater than or equal to 1 in 1000 patients and less than 1 in 100 patients) 2466
Abilify Oral Solution (Greater than or equal to 1 in 1000 patients and less than 1 in 100 patients) 881
Abilify Oral Solution (Greater than or equal to 1 in 1000 patients and less than 1 in 100 patients) 2466
Abilify Discmelt Orally Disintegrating Tablets (Greater than or equal to 1 in 1000 patients and less than 1 in 100 patients) 881
Abilify Discmelt Orally Disintegrating Tablets (Greater than or equal to 1 in 1000 patients and less than 1 in 100 patients) 2466
Abilify Tablets (Greater than or equal to 1 in 1000 patients and less than 1 in 100 patients) 881
Abilify Tablets (Greater than or equal to 1 in 1000 patients and less than 1 in 100 patients) 2466
Actiq (1% or greater) 959
Ambien Tablets (Rare) 2692
Ambien CR Tablets (Rare) 2696
Aricept Tablets (Infrequent) 1062
Aricept ODT Tablets (Infrequent) 1062
Brovana Inhalation Solution (Less than 2%) 2990
Celexa (Infrequent) 1160
▲ Comtan Tablets (9%) 2208
Copaxone for Injection (Infrequent) 3110
Coreg Tablets (Greater than 0.1% to 1%) 1387
Coreg CR Extended-Release Capsules (0.1% to less than or equal to 1%) 1393
Depakote ER Tablets (Greater than 1%) 423
Doxil Injection (Less than 1%) 2378
Effexor XR Extended-Release Capsules (Rare) 3195
Exelon Capsules (Infrequent) 2229
Exelon Oral Solution (Infrequent) 2229
Gabitril Tablets (Frequent) 973
▲ Geodon Capsules (14%) 2520
Gliadel Wafer (2%) 1076
▲ Intron A for Injection (Less than 5%) 2859
Invega Extended-Release Tablets 1748
Lamictal (Rare) 1488
Lunesta Tablets (Rare) 2994
Lyrica Capsules (0.1% to 1%) 2527
Mirapex Tablets (1% or more) 857
Namenda (Frequent) 1180
Paxil (Rare) 1535
Paxil CR Controlled-Release Tablets (Rare) 1544
Protonix I.V. 3257
Remeron Tablets (Frequent) 2924
RemeronSolTab Tablets (Frequent) 2927
Rilutek Tablets (Infrequent) 2771
Risperdal Consta Long-Acting Injection (Infrequent) 1753
▲ Stalevo Tablets (9%) 2309
Symbyax Capsules (Infrequent) 1871
Venlafaxine Hydrochloride Tablets (Rare) 2199
Wellbutrin SR Sustained-Release Tablets 1653
Wellbutrin XL Extended-Release Tablets 1659
Zonegran Capsules (Rare) 1089
Zyban Sustained-Release Tablets 1692
▲ Zyprexa Tablets (8% to 20%) 1883
▲ Zyprexa IntraMuscular (2% to 4%) 1883
▲ Zyprexa ZYDIS Orally Disintegrating Tablets (8% to 20%) 1883

Hypomagnesemia

Abelcet Injection 1134
Actiq (1% or greater) 959
▲ AmBisome for Injection (15.3% to 25.9%) 606
▲ Arranon Injection (0% to 6%) 1319
Avalide Tablets 892
Avalide Tablets 2713
Benicar HCT Tablets 1010
▲ Busulfex Injection (77%) 2477
▲ Cancidas for Injection (7.1%) 1953
Capastat Sulfate for Injection 1791
▲ CellCept Capsules (39%) 2622
▲ CellCept Intravenous (39%) 2622
▲ CellCept Oral Suspension (39%) 2622
▲ CellCept Tablets (39%) 2622
Cubicin for Injection (Less than 1%) 995
▲ Dacogen Injection (24%) 1066
Diovan HCT Tablets 2216
Doxil Injection (Less than 1%) 2378
▲ Erbitux (55%) 912
Fentora Tablets (Greater than 1%) 968
Furosemide Tablets 2186
Gengraf Capsules 435
Geodon Capsules (Rare) 2520
Intravenous Sodium Diuril 2490
Ionsys Transdermal System (.1% to less than 1%) 2410
▲ Leukine (15%) 774
Micardis HCT Tablets 854
▲ Mycamine for Injection (5.5% to 50.4%) 616
▲ Myfortic Tablets (3% to less than 20%) 2276
▲ Mylotarg for Injection (3% to 10%) 3212
▲ Neoral Oral Solution (6%) 2280
▲ Neoral Soft Gelatin Capsules (6%) 2280
▲ Noxafil Oral Suspension (18%) 2889
Prinzide Tablets 2092
▲ Prograf Capsules and Injection (16% to 48%) 622
▲ Proleukin for Injection (12%) 2287
Sandimmune (In some patients) 2296
▲ Simulect for Injection (3% to 10%) 2306
▲ Tasigna Capsules (1% to 10%) 2316
▲ Trisenox Injection (45%) 986
▲ Valcyte Tablets (Less than 5%) 2654
▲ Vaprisol (2% to 5%) 632
▲ Vectibix (2% to 38%) 597
▲ Xeloda Tablets (Less than 5%) 2662
▲ Zometa for Intravenous Infusion (Less that 1% to 11%) 2341

Hypomania

Celexa 1160
Cymbalta Delayed-Release Capsules 1801
Effexor XR Extended-Release Capsules (0.3%) 3195
Geodon (Rare) 2520
▲ Lamictal (5%) 1488
Lexapro Oral Suspension 1174
Luvox CR Extended-Release Capsules 1759
Parnate Tablets 1532
Paxil (Approximately 1%) 1535
Paxil CR Controlled-Release Tablets (Approximately 1%) 1544
Pristiq Extended-Release Tablets (Less than 2%) 3247
Prozac Weekly Capsules (0.1% to 1.8%) 1852
Prozac Pulvules and Liquid (0.1% to 1.8%) 1852
Remeron Tablets (Approximately 0.2%) 2924
RemeronSolTab Tablets (Approximately 0.2%) 2927
Symbyax Capsules 1871
Venlafaxine Hydrochloride Tablets (0.5%) 2199
Wellbutrin Tablets (Frequent) 1648
Wellbutrin SR Sustained-Release Tablets (Rare) 1653
Wellbutrin XL Extended-Release Tablets (Rare) 1659
Zyban Sustained-Release Tablets (Rare) 1692

Hypomenorrhea

Effexor XR Extended-Release Capsules (Rare) 3195
Pentasa Capsules (Less than 1%) 3030
Prozac Weekly Capsules (Rare) 1852
Prozac Pulvules and Liquid (Rare) 1852
Symbyax Capsules (Infrequent) 1871
Venlafaxine Hydrochloride Tablets (Rare) 2199

Hyponatremia

Abilify Injection (Greater than or equal to 1 in 1000 patients and less than 1 in 100 patients) 2466
Abilify Oral Solution (Greater than or equal to 1 in 1000 patients and less than 1 in 100 patients) 881
Abilify Oral Solution (Greater than or equal to 1 in 1000 patients and less than 1 in 100 patients) 2466
Abilify Discmelt Orally Disintegrating Tablets (Greater than or equal to 1 in 1000 patients and less than 1 in 100 patients) 881
Abilify Discmelt Orally Disintegrating Tablets (Greater than or equal to 1 in 1000 patients and less than 1 in 100 patients) 2466
Abilify Tablets (Greater than or equal to 1 in 1000 patients and less than 1 in 100 patients) 881
Abilify Tablets (Greater than or equal to 1 in 1000 patients and less than 1 in 100 patients) 2466
Aceon Tablets (2 mg, 4 mg, 8 mg) 3038
Actimmune (Rare) 1743
Actiq (Less than 1%) 959
AmBisome for Injection (Less common) 606
Aricept Tablets (Infrequent) 1062
Aricept ODT Tablets (Infrequent) 1062

Atacand Tablets ... 639
Atacand HCT (Very rare) ... 642
Avandaryl Tablets ... 1344
▲ Avastin IV (4%) ... 1192
Benicar HCT Tablets ... 1010
Busulfex Injection (2%) ... 2477
Campral Tablets (Rare) ... 1158
Captopril Tablets ... 2182
Carbatrol Capsules ... 3019
Celebrex Capsules (Less than 0.1%) ... 2979
Celexa (Several cases) ... 1160
▲ CellCept Capsules (3% to less than 20%) ... 2622
▲ CellCept Intravenous (3% to less than 20%) ... 2622
▲ CellCept Oral Suspension (3% to less than 20%) ... 2622
▲ CellCept Tablets (3% to less than 20%) ... 2622
Coreg Tablets (Greater than 1% to 3%) ... 1387
▲ Coreg CR Extended-Release Capsules (Greater than 1% to less than or equal to 3%) ... 1393
Cozaar Tablets ... 1973
Cymbalta Delayed-Release Capsules ... 1801
▲ Dacogen Injection (19%) ... 1066
Demadex Injection ... 2630
Demadex Tablets ... 2630
Depakote ER Tablets ... 423
▲ DepoCyt Injection (7% to 12%) ... 1136
▲ Doxil Injection (1% to 10%) ... 2378
Duetact Tablets ... 3085
Dyazide Capsules ... 1405
Effexor XR Extended-Release Capsules ... 3195
▲ Eloxatin for Injection (1% to 8%) ... 2731
Emend Capsules (Greater than 0.5%) ... 1992
Emend for Injection (Greater than 0.5%) ... 1999
Emsam Transdermal System (Infrequent) ... 905
Equetro Extended-Release Capsules ... 3174
Evoxac Capsules (Less than 1%) ... 1013
Exelon Capsules (Infrequent) ... 2229
Exelon Oral Solution (Infrequent) ... 2229
Exelon Patch (Infrequent) ... 2233
Fentora Tablets (Greater than 1%) ... 968
Furosemide Tablets ... 2186
Gabitril Tablets (Infrequent) ... 973
Geodon Capsules (Rare) ... 2520
Gleevec Tablets (Rare) ... 2255
▲ Gliadel Wafer (3%) ... 1076
▲ Indapamide Tablets (Less than 5%) ... 2188
▲ Indocin I.V. (3% to 9%) ... 2489
Intravenous Sodium Diuril ... 2490
Ionsys Transdermal System (.1% to less than 1%) ... 2410
Ixempra Kit for Injection ... 915
▲ Kaletra (3%) ... 452
Lexapro Oral Suspension (One case) ... 1174
Lexapro Tablets (One case) ... 1174
Luvox CR Extended-Release Capsules ... 1759
Malarone Pediatric Tablets ... 1521
Malarone Tablets ... 1521
Mavik Tablets (0.3% to 1%) ... 472
▲ Mepron Suspension (7% to 10%) ... 1526
Mirapex Tablets ... 857
Mycamine for Injection ... 616
Namenda (Infrequent) ... 1180
Nexavar Tablets (0.1% to less than 1%) ... 784
Nexium Delayed-Release Capsules (Less than 1%) ... 645
Nexium I.V. (Less than 1%) ... 652
Nexium Delayed-Release Oral Suspension (Less than 1%) ... 645
Nimotop Capsules (Less than 1%) ... 790
▲ Novantrone for Injection Concentrate (9%) ... 1100
OsmoPrep Tablets ... 2680
OxyContin Tablets (Less than 1%) ... 2589
Paxil (Rare) ... 1535
Paxil CR Controlled-Release Tablets (Rare) ... 1544
Primaxin I.M. ... 2080
Primaxin I.V. ... 2083
Prinivil Tablets ... 2087
Prinzide Tablets ... 2092
Pristiq Extended-Release Tablets ... 3247
▲ Prograf Capsules and Injection (3% to 15%) ... 622
Prozac Weekly Capsules ... 1852
Prozac Pulvules and Liquid ... 1852
Requip Tablets (Infrequent) ... 1561
Rilutek Tablets (Infrequent) ... 2771
Risperdal Consta Long-Acting Injection (Infrequent) ... 1753
Rythmol Tablets (Less than 1%) ... 1586
Rythmol SR Capsules ... 1590
▲ Sutent Capsules (6%) ... 2540
Symbyax Capsules ... 1871
Tarka Tablets ... 511
▲ Tasigna Capsules (0.1% to 3%) ... 2316
Teveten Tablets (Less than 1%) ... 515
Teveten HCT Tablets (Less than 1%) ... 517
Tygacil for Injection (0% to less than 2%) ... 3276
▲ Vaprisol (3.3% to 8%) ... 632
Velcade for Injection ... 2168
Venlafaxine Hydrochloride Tablets (Rare) ... 2199
Zolinza Capsules ... 2142
Zonegran Capsules (Rare) ... 1089
Zosyn for Injection ... 3284
Zyprexa Tablets (Infrequent) ... 1883
Zyprexa ZYDIS Orally Disintegrating Tablets (Infrequent) ... 1883

Hyponatremia, dilutional
Intravenous Sodium Diuril ... 2490
Prinzide Tablets ... 2092

Hypoparathyroidism
▲ Rocaltrol Capsules (1 in 3) ... 1150
▲ Rocaltrol Oral Solution (1 in 3) ... 1150

Hypophosphatemia
Abelcet Injection ... 1134
▲ Actonel Tablets (2.6% to 3.8%) ... 2568
Advicor Tablets ... 402
AmBisome for Injection (Less common) ... 606
Atripla Tablets ... 938
▲ Busulfex Injection (17%) ... 2477
Cardene I.V. (Rare) ... 1093
▲ CellCept Capsules (3% to less than 20%) ... 2622
▲ CellCept Intravenous (3% to less than 20%) ... 2622
▲ CellCept Oral Suspension (3% to less than 20%) ... 2622
▲ CellCept Tablets (3% to less than 20%) ... 2622
Doxil Injection (Less than 1%) ... 2378
Evista Tablets ... 1810
▲ Fosamax (Approximately 10%) ... 2005
▲ Fosamax Plus D Tablets (10%) ... 2013
Gleevec Tablets (Infrequent) ... 2255
Hepsera Tablets ... 1253
Ionsys Transdermal System (.1% to less than 1%) ... 2410
▲ Myfortic Tablets (3% to less than 20%) ... 2276
▲ Mylotarg for Injection (6% to 10%) ... 3212
▲ Nexavar Tablets (11% to 45%) ... 784
Niaspan Extended-Release Tablets ... 480
▲ Prograf Capsules and Injection (3% to 49%) ... 622
Rapamune ... 3260
▲ Rituxan I.V. (12% to 23%) ... 1223
▲ Simulect for Injection (Greater than or equal to 10%) ... 2306
▲ Sutent Capsules (9% to 10%) ... 2540
▲ Tasigna Capsules (0.1% to 10%) ... 2316
▲ Torisel Injection (Greater than or equal to 30%) ... 3272
Truvada Tablets ... 1262
Tygacil for Injection ... 3276
Ultane Liquid for Inhalation (Less than 1%) ... 524
▲ Valcyte Tablets (Less than 5%) ... 2654
Venlafaxine Hydrochloride Tablets (Rare) ... 2199
Viread Tablets ... 1268
▲ Zometa for Intravenous Infusion (Less than 1% to 51%) ... 2341

Hypopigmentation
Accutane Capsules ... 2607
Aldara Cream, 5% (More than 1%) ... 1699
Analpram-HC ... 1140
Catapres-TTS (0.5% or less) ... 842
Daytrana Transdermal Patch ... 3022
Diprolene Lotion 0.05% (Infrequent) ... 2838
Diprolene Ointment 0.05% ... 2839
Diprolene AF Cream 0.05% (Infrequent) ... 2837
Elocon Cream 0.1% (Infrequent) ... 2840
Elocon Lotion 0.1% (Infrequent) ... 2841
Elocon Ointment 0.1% (Infrequent) ... 2842
Lotrisone ... 2881
Luxíq Foam ... 3058
Olux Foam ... 3061
Olux-E Foam ... 3059
Pramosone ... 1141
Vanos Cream ... 1941
Verdeso Foam ... 3069

Hypopigmentation, nail beds
Taxotere Injection Concentrate ... 2773

Hypoplasia, enamel
Pylera Capsules ... 714

Hypoplasia, erythroid
Captopril Tablets ... 2182

Hypoplasia, myeloid
(*see under* Bone marrow hypoplasia)

Hypoplasia, unspecified
Campath Ampules ... 761

Hypoplastic anemia
(*see under* Anemia, hypoplastic)

Hypopnea
Vicoprofen Tablets (Less than 1%) ... 533

Hypoproteinemia
Actiq (Less than 1%) ... 959
AmBisome for Injection (Less common) ... 606
Aricept Tablets (Infrequent) ... 1062
Aricept ODT Tablets (Infrequent) ... 1062
▲ CellCept Capsules (3% to less than 20%) ... 2622
▲ CellCept Intravenous (3% to less than 20%) ... 2622
▲ CellCept Oral Suspension (3% to less than 20%) ... 2622
▲ CellCept Tablets (3% to less than 20%) ... 2622
Cipro I.V. ... 2817
Cipro XR Tablets ... 2823
▲ Dacogen Injection (5%) ... 1066
Depakote ER Tablets (Greater than 1%) ... 423
Doxil Injection (Less than 1%) ... 2378
Effexor XR Extended-Release Capsules (Rare) ... 3195
Elspar for Injection ... 2488
Evista Tablets ... 1810
Geodon Capsules (Rare) ... 2520
▲ Lupron Depot 7.5 mg (Greater than or equal to 5%) ... 469
▲ Prograf Capsules and Injection (3% to 15%) ... 622
▲ Simulect for Injection (3% to 10%) ... 2306
Targretin Capsules ... 1084
▲ Tygacil for Injection (4.5%) ... 3276
Venlafaxine Hydrochloride Tablets (Rare) ... 2199
Zosyn for Injection ... 3284
Zyprexa Tablets (Rare) ... 1883
Zyprexa ZYDIS Orally Disintegrating Tablets (Rare) ... 1883

Hypoprothrombinemia
AmBisome for Injection (Less common) ... 606
Arixtra Injection (1.3%) ... 1313
Celexa ... 1160
Cipro I.V. (Rare) ... 2817
Cipro XR Tablets (Less than 1%) ... 2823
▲ Coreg Tablets (Greater than 1% to 3%) ... 1387
▲ Coreg CR Extended-Release Capsules (Greater than 1% to less than or equal to 3%) ... 1393
Fansidar Tablets ... 2636
Gantrisin Pediatric Suspension ... 2638
Lexapro Oral Suspension ... 1174
Lexapro Tablets ... 1174
Lyrica Capsules (Rare) ... 2527
Merrem I.V. (Greater than 0.2%) ... 684
NovoSeven (1%) ... 2367
NovoSeven RT (1%) ... 2370
Paser Granules ... 1747
▲ Prograf Capsules and Injection (3% to 15%) ... 622
Rocephin Injectable Vials, ADD-Vantage, Galaxy, Bulk ... 2642
Rythmol SR Capsules ... 1590

Hypoptyalism
▲ Advair HFA 45/21 Inhalation Aerosol (1% to 3%) ... 1288
▲ Advair HFA 115/21 Inhalation Aerosol (1% to 3%) ... 1288
▲ Advair HFA 230/21 Inhalation Aerosol (1% to 3%) ... 1288
Amerge Tablets (Frequent) ... 1301
Demser Capsules (Infrequent) ... 1989
▲ Flovent HFA (1% to 3%) ... 1440
Imitrex Injection ... 1465
Imitrex Nasal Spray ... 1470
Imitrex Tablets (Greater than 1%) ... 1474
Serevent Diskus (1% to less than 3%) ... 1594

Hypopyon
Triesence Injectable Suspension (2%) ... ⊙209

Hyporeflexia
Arranon Injection (1%) ... 1319
Axert Tablets (Rare) ... 2431
▲ Evoxac Capsules (1% to 3%) ... 1013
Gabitril Tablets (Frequent) ... 973
▲ Ixempra Kit for Injection (62%) ... 915
Lunesta Tablets (Infrequent) ... 2994
Maxalt Tablets (Rare) ... 2056
Maxalt-MLT Orally Disintegrating Tablets (Rare) ... 2056
Mirapex Tablets ... 857
▲ NovoLog Injection (11%) ... 2359
Paxil (Rare) ... 1535
Paxil CR Controlled-Release Tablets (Rare) ... 1544
Protonix for Delayed-Release Oral Suspension (Less than 1%) ... 3254
Protonix Delayed-Release Tablets (Less than 1%) ... 3254
Protonix I.V. (Less than 1%) ... 3257
Prozac Weekly Capsules (Rare) ... 1852
Prozac Pulvules and Liquid (Rare) ... 1852
▲ Retrovir Capsules (5.6%) ... 1574
▲ Retrovir IV Infusion (7%) ... 1579
▲ Retrovir (5.6%) ... 1574
Venlafaxine Hydrochloride Tablets (Rare) ... 2199
▲ Vesanoid Capsules (3%) ... 2660

Hyposalivation
(*see under* Hypoptyalism)

Hypospadias
Prometrium Capsules (100 mg, 200 mg) ... 3047

Hypotaxia
▲ Vesanoid Capsules (3%) ... 2660

Hypotension
▲ Abelcet Injection (8%) ... 1134
Abilify Injection (Greater than or equal to 1 in 1000 patients and less than or equal to 1 in 100 patients) ... 881
Abilify Injection (Greater than or equal to 1 in 1000 patients and less than 1 in 100 patients) ... 2466
Abilify Oral Solution (Greater than or equal to 1 in 1000 patients and less than or equal to 1 in 100 patients) ... 881
Abilify Oral Solution (Greater than or equal to 1 in 1000 patients and less than 1 in 100 patients) ... 2466
Abilify Discmelt Orally Disintegrating Tablets (Greater than or equal to 1 in 1000 patients and less than or equal to 1 in 100 patients) ... 881
Abilify Discmelt Orally Disintegrating Tablets (Greater than or equal to 1 in 1000 patients and less than 1 in 100 patients) ... 2466
Abilify Tablets (Greater than or equal to 1 in 1000 patients and less than or equal to 1 in 100 patients) ... 881
Abilify Tablets (Greater than or equal to 1 in 1000 patients and less than 1 in 100 patients) ... 2466
Aceon Tablets (2 mg, 4 mg, 8 mg) (0.3% to 1%) ... 3038
▲ Acetadote Injection (0.78% to 3.75%) ... 1001
Actimmune (Rare) ... 1743
Actiq (Less than 1%) ... 959
Activase I.V. ... 1188
Adenocard IV Injection (Less than 1%) ... 603
Adenoscan (2%) ... 605
Advicor Tablets ... 402
Aggrenox Capsules (Less than 1%) ... 819
Albutein 5% ... 1707
Albutein 25% ... 1708
▲ Alferon N Injection (6%) ... 1726
Allegra-D 12 Hour Extended-Release Tablets ... 2687
Allegra-D 24 Hour Extended-Release Tablets ... 2690
Aloxi Injection (1%) ... 1059
Alphagan P Ophthalmic Solution ... 549
Ambien Tablets (Rare) ... 2692
Ambien CR Tablets (Rare) ... 2696
▲ AmBisome for Injection (7.4% to 14.3%) ... 606
Amerge Tablets (Infrequent) ... 1301
Amrix Capsules ... 966
Anaprox Tablets (Less than 1%) ... 2632

Anaprox DS Tablets (Less than 1%) 2632
▲ Angiomax for Injection (Greater than 0.1% to 12%) 1933
Anzemet Injection (Infrequently) 2701
▲ Anzemet Tablets (5.3%) 2704
▲ Aranesp for Injection (20%) 564
▲ Argatroban Injection (7.2% to 10.7%) 1308
Aricept Tablets (Frequent) 1062
Aricept ODT Tablets (Frequent) 1062
▲ Arixtra Injection (0.3% to 3.5%) 1313
▲ Arranon Injection (1% to 8%) 1319
Atacand Tablets 639
Atacand HCT (Rare) 642
Atrovent HFA Inhalation Aerosol 839
Avalide Tablets 892
Avalide Tablets (0.6% to 1%) 2713
Avapro Tablets (0.4%) 897
Avapro Tablets (0.4%) 2718
▲ Avastin IV (7% to 15%) 1192
Avelox (Less than 0.1%) 2803
▲ Avinza Capsules (Less than 5%) 1772
Azor Tablets 1005
Bayer Aspirin 750
BeneFIX Vials 3191
Benicar Tablets 1009
Betimol Ophthalmic Solution 3181
▲ Bexxar (1% to 7%) 1371
Bicillin C-R Injectable Suspension 1775
Bicillin L-A Injection 1777
Boostrix (Rarely) 1377
▲ Busulfex Injection (3% to 11%) 2477
▲ Campath Ampules (10% to 35%) 761
Campral Tablets (Infrequent) 1158
▲ Cancidas for Injection (6.2% to 20.3%) 1953
Captopril Tablets (Rare) 2182
Carbatrol Capsules 3019
▲ Cardene I.V. (5.6%) 1093
Cardizem LA Extended Release Tablets (Less than 2%) 421
Celexa (Frequent) 1160
▲ CellCept Capsules (3% to 32.5%) 2622
▲ CellCept Intravenous (3% to 32.5%) 2622
▲ CellCept Oral Suspension (3% to 32.5%) 2622
▲ CellCept Tablets (3% to 32.5%) 2622
▲ Cerezyme for Injection (Approximately 6.6%) 1238
Chantix Tablets (Infrequent) 2511
Cialis Tablets (Less than 2%) 1792
Cimzia (Rare) 3127
Cipro I.V. (1% or less) 2817
Cipro (Less than 1%) 2810
Cipro XR Tablets 2823
Cleviprex 1936
Clinoril Tablets (Less than 1 in 100) 1962
▲ Clolar for Intravenous Infusion (29%) 1239
Combigan Ophthalmic Solution (0.1% to 0.2%) 553
Combivent Inhalation Aerosol 845
Comtan Tablets 2208
Comvax 1966
Copaxone for Injection (Infrequent) 3110
▲ Coreg Tablets (9% to 14%) 1387
▲ Coreg CR Extended-Release Capsules (9% to 14%) 1393
Cosopt Sterile Ophthalmic Solution (Less than 1%) 1969
▲ Cozaar Tablets (Less than 1% to 7%) 1973
▲ Cubicin for Injection (2.4% to 5%) 995
▲ Dacogen Injection (6%) 1066
Daytrana Transdermal Patch 3022
Demadex Injection 2630
Demadex Tablets 2630
Depakote ER Tablets (Greater than 1%) 423
▲ DepoCyt Injection (8% to 18%) 1136
▲ DepoDur Injection (Greater than 10%) 1095
▲ Diovan Tablets (1.4% to 7%) 2212
Diovan HCT Tablets (Greater than 0.2%) 2216
▲ Doxil Injection (1% to 10%) 2378
▲ Duragesic Transdermal System (1% to 3%) 2405
Dyazide Capsules 1405
DynaCirc CR Controlled Release Tablets (0.5% to 1%) 1407
EC-Naprosyn Delayed-Release Tablets (Less than 1%) 2632
Edex Injection 2957
Effexor XR Extended-Release Capsules (Infrequent) 3195
Eldepryl Capsules 3052
Eligard 7.5 mg (Less than 2%) 2724
Eligard 22.5 mg (Less than 2%) 2724
Eligard 30 mg (Less than 2%) 2724
Eligard 45 mg (Less than 2%) 2724
Elitek 2729
Eloxatin for Injection (0.6%) 2731
Emend Capsules (Greater than 0.5%) 1992
Emend for Injection (Greater than 0.5%) 1999
▲ Emsam Transdermal System (3% to 6.2%) 905
Enbrel for Injection (Infrequent) 569
Engerix-B Vaccine (Less than 1%) 1409
Equetro Extended-Release Capsules 3174
Erbitux 912
Evoxac Capsules (Less than 1%) 1013
Exelon Capsules (Frequent) 2229
Exelon Oral Solution (Frequent) 2229
Exelon Patch (Infrequent) 2233
Exforge Tablets (Greater than or equal to 0.2% to 0.4%) 2238
▲ Fabrazyme for Intravenous Infusion (Greater than or equal to 5%) 1241
Fentora Tablets (Greater than 1%) 968
Flebogamma 5% 1715
Flebogamma 5% DIF 1718
▲ Flolan for Injection (13% to 27%) 1426
Flomax Capsules (Infrequent) 848
Fluorescite Injection ⊙ 203
Focalin XR Capsules 2251
Foradil Aerolizer (Rare) 2849
Fortaz (Very rare) 1450
▲ Fosrenol Chewable Tablets (8% to 16%) 3027
Furosemide Tablets 2186
Gabitril Tablets (Infrequent) 973
Gammagard Liquid 730
Gammagard S/D 734
Gamunex 3094
Gleevec Tablets (Infrequent) 2255
Gliadel Wafer (1%) 1076
Glucagon for Injection Vials and Emergency Kit 1827
Herceptin I.V. 1199
Humalog-Pen and KwikPen (Less common) 1829
Humalog Mix 50/50-Pen and KwikPen 1833
Humalog Mix 75/25-Pen and KwikPen (Less common) 1835
Human Albumin Grifols 25% 1706
Humulin 50/50, 100 Units 1843
Humulin 70/30 Vial (Less common) 1844
Humulin N Vial (Less common) 1846
Humulin R 1849
Humulin R (U-500) (Less common) 1850
Imitrex Injection (Infrequent) 1465
Imitrex Nasal Spray (Rare) 1470
Imitrex Tablets (Infrequent) 1474
Indocin Capsules (Less than 1%) 2024
Indocin I.V. (Less than 1%) 2489
Indocin (Less than 1%) 2024
Infanrix Vaccine 1479
InnoPran XL Extended Release Capsules 1484
▲ Integrilin Injection (7%) 2855
Intravenous Sodium Diuril 2490
▲ Intron A for Injection (Less than 5%) 2859
Invanz for Injection (1% to 2%) 2029
Ionsys Transdermal System (2%) 2410
Ixempra Kit for Injection 915
Janumet Tablets 2041
Ketek Tablets (Less than 0.2%) 2744
Kogenate FS (Very rare) 746
▲ Leukine (13%) 774
Levaquin 2416
Levaquin in 5% Dextrose Injection 2416
Levitra Tablets (Less than 2%) 2876
Lexapro Oral Suspension 1174
Lexapro Tablets 1174
Lexiscan Injection 614
Lialda Tablets (Infrequent) 3029
Lidoderm Patch 1114
Lupron Depot 3.75 mg 462
Lupron Depot 7.5 mg 469
Lupron Depot–3 Month 11.25 mg 462
Lupron Depot-PED 7.5 mg, 11.25 mg and 15 mg 471
Luvox CR Extended-Release Capsules (Frequent) 1759
Lyrica Capsules (0.1% to 1%) 2527
Marinol Capsules (0.3 to 1%) 3163
▲ Mavik Tablets (0.3% to 11%) 472
Maxair Autohaler 1705
Mephyton Tablets (Rare) 700
Mepron Suspension (1%) 1526
Merrem I.V. (Greater than 0.1% to 1%) 684
Metadate CD Capsules 3146
Micardis Tablets 852
Mirapex Tablets (Greater than or equal to 1%) 857
Moban Tablets (Rare) 1116
Mobic Oral Suspension (Less than 2%) 863
Mobic Tablets (Less than 2%) 863
MS Contin Tablets (Less frequent) 2585
▲ Mycamine for Injection (5.9% to 18.6%) 616
▲ Myfortic Tablets (3% to less than 20%) 2276
▲ Mylotarg for Injection (18% to 23%) 3212
Nadolol Tablets (2 of 100 patients) 2191
Namenda (Infrequent) 1180
Naprosyn Suspension (Less than 1%) 2632
Naprosyn Tablets (Less than 1%) 2632
▲ Natrecor for Injection (4% to 35%) 2977
Nembutal Sodium Solution, USP (Less than 1%) 2494
NeoProfen Injection 2496
Neupogen for Injection (7 of 176 patients) 589
▲ Neupro Transdermal System (3%) 3149
Niaspan Extended-Release Tablets 480
Nimbex Injection (0.2%) 484
▲ Nimotop Capsules (1.2% to 50%) 790
▲ Nitro-Dur Transdermal Infusion System (4%) 2887
Nitrolingual Pumpspray 2965
Norvir (Less than 2%) 489
Novantrone for Injection Concentrate 1100
NovoLog Injection 2359
NovoSeven (1%) 2367
NovoSeven RT (1%) 2370
▲ Noxafil Oral Suspension (14%) 2889
▲ Oncaspar Injection (Greater than 1% but less than 5%) 1138
▲ Ontak Vials (36%) 1079
▲ Opana Tablets (1% to less than 10%) 1117
▲ Opana ER Tablets (1% to less than 10%) 1121
Orencia Powder for Intravenous Infusion (Greater than 0.1% and less than or equal to 1%) 921
Orthoclone OKT3 Sterile Solution 2387
OxyContin Tablets 2589
OxyIR Capsules 2593
Parnate Tablets 1532
Paxil (Infrequent) 1535
Paxil CR Controlled-Release Tablets (Infrequent) 1544
Pediarix Vaccine (Rare) 1552
Percocet Tablets 1127
Percodan Tablets 1130
Perforomist Inhalation Solution 1025
Persantine Tablets (Rare) 869
▲ Photofrin for Injection (7%) 708
Plavix Tablets 926
Plavix Tablets 2767
Pletal Tablets (Less than 2%) 2481
Premarin Intravenous 3217
Primaxin I.M. 2080
Primaxin I.V. (0.4%) 2083
▲ Prinivil Tablets (0.3% to 4.4%; rare) 2087
Prinzide Tablets (1.4%) 2092
Proglycem Capsules (Infrequent) 1185
Proglycem Suspension (Infrequent) 1185
▲ Prograf Capsules and Injection (3% to 15%) 622
Prolastin (Rare) 3099
▲ Proleukin for Injection (3% to 71%) 2287
Prometrium Capsules (100 mg, 200 mg) (Rare) 3047
Protonix for Delayed-Release Oral Suspension (Less than 1%) 3254
Protonix Delayed-Release Tablets (Less than 1%) 3254
Protonix I.V. (Less than 1%) 3257
Provigil Tablets (Greater than or equal to 1%) 977
Prozac Weekly Capsules (Infrequent) 1852
Prozac Pulvules and Liquid (Infrequent) 1852
Recombivax HB (Less than 1%) 2107
ReFacto Vials 3269
Refludan for Injection 795
Remeron Tablets (Infrequent) 2924
RemeronSolTab Tablets (Infrequent) 2927
Remicade for IV Injection (Greater than or equal to 0.2%) 950
▲ ReoPro Vials (21.1%) 1860
Requip Tablets (Frequent to 2%) 1561
Requip XL Tablets (2%) 1568
Rilutek Tablets (Infrequent) 2771
Risperdal Consta Long-Acting Injection (Frequent) 1753
▲ Rituxan I.V. (1% to 10%) 1223
Rythmol Tablets (1%) 1586
Rythmol SR Capsules (Greater than or equal to 2%) 1590
St. Joseph 81 mg Aspirin Chewable and Enteric Coated Tablets 1903
Salagen Tablets (Less than 1%) 1082
▲ Sensipar Tablets (7%) 594
▲ Simulect for Injection (3% to 10%) 2306
Stalevo Tablets 2309
Sular Extended Release Tablets (Less than or equal to 1%; very rare) 2975
Symbyax Capsules (Infrequent) 1871
Tarka Tablets (0.3% to 0.6%) 511
Tasigna Capsules 2316
Taxotere Injection Concentrate (0% to 2.8%) 2773
Tekturna Tablets (0.1% and less than 1%) 2321
Tekturna HCT Tablets (Less than 1%) 2324
Teveten Tablets (Less than 1%) 515
Teveten HCT Tablets (Less than 1%) 517
Thioridazine Hydrochloride Tablets 2195
Thiothixene Capsules 2197
Timoptic Sterile Ophthalmic Solution (Less frequent) 2121
Timoptic in Ocudose (Less frequent) 2124
Timoptic-XE Sterile Ophthalmic Gel Forming Solution 2125
TNKase 1233
Toprol-XL Tablets (About 1 of 100 patients) 666
▲ Tracleer Tablets (7%) 3289
▲ Trasylol Injection (8%) 799
▲ Travatan Z Ophthalmic Solution (1% to 5%) 547
Tricor Tablets 520
▲ Trisenox Injection (25%) 986
Trizivir Tablets 1622
Twinrix Vaccine (Less than 1%) 1628
Tygacil for Injection (2.3%) 3276
▲ Ultane Liquid for Inhalation (4% to 11%) 524
▲ Valcyte Tablets (Less than 5%) 2654
Valium Tablets (Infrequent) 2658
▲ Vaprisol (2.7% to 8%) 632
Vectibix 597
▲ Velcade for Injection (2% to 15%) 2168
Venlafaxine Hydrochloride Tablets (Infrequent) 2199
▲ Vesanoid Capsules (14%; occasional) 2660
Vicoprofen Tablets (Less than 1%) 533
Voltaren Tablets (Rarely) 2334
Voltaren-XR Tablets (Rarely) 2337
Wellbutrin Tablets (2.5%) 1648
Wellbutrin SR Sustained-Release Tablets 1653
Wellbutrin XL Extended-Release Tablets 1659
WinRho SDF 741
Xeloda Tablets 2662
▲ Xolair (14%) 1235
▲ Xolair (14%) 2339
Xopenex Inhalation Solution 3001
Xopenex Inhalation Solution Concentrate 3005
Xopenex HFA Inhalation Aerosol 3009
Xyntha Vials 3280
Xyrem Oral Solution (Infrequent) 1766
Xyzal Oral Solution 2789
Xyzal Oral Solution 3155
Zantac Injection 1666
Zemuron Injection (0.1% to 2%) 2947
Ziagen 1673
Zofran Injection (Rare) 1682
▲ Zofran (5%) 1687
▲ Zofran ODT Orally Disintegrating Tablets (5%) 1687
▲ Zometa for Intravenous Infusion (11%) 2341
Zonegran Capsules (Infrequent) 1089
Zosyn for Injection (1% or less to 1.3%) 3284
Zyban Sustained-Release Tablets 1692
Zyprexa Tablets (2%) 1883
Zyprexa IntraMuscular (2%) 1883
Zyprexa ZYDIS Orally Disintegrating Tablets (2%) 1883
Zyrtec Chewable Tablets 1920
Zyrtec Syrup 1920
Zyrtec Tablets 1920

Hypotension, neonatal

Aceon Tablets (2 mg, 4 mg, 8 mg) 3038
Avalide Tablets 2713
Captopril Tablets 2182
Cozaar Tablets 1973

Prinivil Tablets 2087
Prinzide Tablets 2092

Hypotension, orthostatic

▲ Abilify Injection (0% to 5%) 881
▲ Abilify Injection (0% to 5%) 2466
Abilify Oral Solution (Greater than or equal to 1 in 1000 patients and less than 1 in 100 patients) 881
▲ Abilify Oral Solution (0% to 5%) 2466
Abilify Discmelt Orally Disintegrating Tablets (Greater than or equal to 1 in 1000 patients and less than 1 in 100 patients) 881
▲ Abilify Discmelt Orally Disintegrating Tablets (0% to 5%) 2466
Abilify Tablets (Greater than or equal to 1 in 1000 patients and less than 1 in 100 patients) 881
▲ Abilify Tablets (0% to 5%) 2466
Aceon Tablets (2 mg, 4 mg, 8 mg) (0.3% to 1%) 3038
Actiq (Less than 1%) 959
Advicor Tablets 402
▲ Agrylin Capsules (1% to less than 5%) 3017
Alphanate 1709
AmBisome for Injection (Less common) 606
Anzemet Injection (Rare) 2701
Anzemet Tablets (Rare) 2704
Aricept Tablets (Infrequent) 1062
Aricept ODT Tablets (Infrequent) 1062
Atacand HCT 642
Avalide Tablets 892
Avalide Tablets 2713
▲ Avapro Tablets (5.4%) 897
▲ Avapro Tablets (5.4%) 2718
▲ Azilect Tablets (9%) 3106
Campral Tablets (Infrequent) 1158
Captopril Tablets 2182
Cardene I.V. (1.4%) 1093
Catapres-TTS (0.5% or less) 842
Celexa (Frequent) 1160
Cipro I.V. 2817
▲ Clorpres Tablets (About 3 in 100) 2185
Comtan Tablets 2208
Copaxone for Injection (Infrequent) 3110
▲ Coreg Tablets (1% to 3%) 1387
▲ Coreg CR Extended-Release Capsules (Greater than 1% to less than or equal to 3%) 1393
▲ Cozaar Tablets (4%) 1973
Cymbalta Delayed-Release Capsules (Infrequent) 1801
Depakote ER Tablets (Greater than 1%) 423
Dibenzyline Capsules 3188
Diovan Tablets (2%) 2212
Diovan HCT Tablets (Less than 0.1%) 2216
Doxil Injection (Less than 1%) 2378
Dyazide Capsules 1405
Effexor XR Extended-Release Capsules (Infrequent) 3195
Eldepryl Capsules 3052
▲ Emsam Transdermal System (9.8%) 905
Evoxac Capsules 1013
Exelon Capsules (Frequent) 2229
Exelon Oral Solution (Frequent) 2229
Exforge Tablets (Less than 1%) 2238
Flomax Capsules (0.2% to 0.4%) 848
Furosemide Tablets 2186
Gabitril Tablets (Infrequent) 973
Geodon (Rare) 2520
▲ Indapamide Tablets (Less than 5%) 2188
Intravenous Sodium Diuril 2490
▲ Intron A for Injection (Less than 5%) 2859
▲ Invega Extended-Release Tablets (1% to 4%) 1748
Ionsys Transdermal System (.1% to less than 1%) 2410
Kaletra (Less than 2%) 452
Klonopin (Infrequent) 2639
Lamictal (Infrequent) 1488
Lexapro Oral Suspension 1174
Lexapro Tablets 1174
Lipitor Tablets (Less than 2%) 2501
Lyrica Capsules (0.1% to 1%) 2527
▲ Marplan Tablets (4%) 3177
Micardis Tablets 852
Micardis HCT Tablets (Less than 2%) 854
▲ Mirapex Tablets (53%) 857
MS Contin Tablets 2585
Namenda (Infrequent) 1180
▲ Neupro Transdermal System (3% to 6%) 3149
Niaspan Extended-Release Tablets 480
Nitrolingual Pumpspray (Occasional) 2965
Noroxin Tablets 2069
Norvir (Less than 2%) 489
Opana Tablets (Less than 1%) 1117
Opana ER Tablets (Less than 1%) 1121
▲ OxyContin Tablets (Between 1% and 5%) 2589
Paxil (1.2%) 1535
Paxil CR Controlled-Release Tablets (1.2%) 1544
Percocet Tablets 1127
Percodan Tablets 1130
Pletal Tablets (Less than 2%) 2481
Prinivil Tablets (0.3% to 1.2%) 2087
Prinzide Tablets (0.5% to 1%) 2092
Pristiq Extended-Release Tablets (Less than 2%) 3247
▲ Prograf Capsules and Injection (3% to 15%) 622
Prometrium Capsules (100 mg, 200 mg) (Rare) 3047
Prozac Pulvules and Liquid (Infrequent) 1852
▲ Requip Tablets (6%) 1561
▲ Requip XL Tablets (Greater than or equal to 5%) 1568
Rilutek Tablets (0.8% to 1.6%) 2771
Risperdal Consta Long-Acting Injection (2%) 1753
Sandostatin Injection (Less than 1%) 2300
Sandostatin LAR Depot 2302
Stalevo Tablets 2309
Strattera Capsules (0.2% to 1.8%) 1864
Stromectol Tablets (1.1%) 2120
Sular Extended Release Tablets (Less than or equal to 1%) 2975
Symbyax Capsules 1871
Teveten Tablets (Less than 1%) 515
Teveten HCT Tablets (Less than 1%) 517
▲ Ultram ER Extended-Release Tablets (1.7% to 5.4%) 2428
Uroxatral Tablets (0.4%) 2786
▲ Vaprisol (5.5% to 14%) 632
▲ Velcade for Injection (13%) 2168
Wellbutrin Tablets 1648
Wellbutrin SR Sustained-Release Tablets (Infrequent) 1653
Wellbutrin XL Extended-Release Tablets (Infrequent) 1659
▲ Xeloda Tablets (Less than 5%) 2662
Zomig Tablets (Rare) 694
Zomig-ZMT Tablets (Rare) 694
Zyban Sustained-Release Tablets (Infrequent) 1692
▲ Zyprexa Tablets (3% to 5%) 1883
Zyprexa IntraMuscular (1%) 1883
▲ Zyprexa ZYDIS Orally Disintegrating Tablets (3% to 5%) 1883

Hypotension, postural

(*see also under* Hypotension, orthostatic)

Ambien Tablets (Infrequent) 2692
Ambien CR Tablets (Infrequent) 2696
▲ CellCept Capsules (3% to less than 20%) 2622
▲ CellCept Intravenous (3% to less than 20%) 2622
▲ CellCept Oral Suspension (3% to less than 20%) 2622
▲ CellCept Tablets (3% to less than 20%) 2622
Cialis Tablets (Less than 2%) 1792
Cipro 2810
Cipro XR Tablets 2823
Exforge Tablets (Greater than 0.1% less than 1%) 2238
Levitra Tablets (Less than 2%) 2876
Prozac Weekly Capsules (Infrequent) 1852
Requip XL Tablets 1568
Risperdal Consta Long-Acting Injection (Infrequent) 1753
Soma Tablets 1931
▲ Velcade for Injection (13%) 2168
Venlafaxine Hydrochloride Tablets (1%) 2199

Hypotension, symptomatic

Aceon Tablets (2 mg, 4 mg, 8 mg) 3038
Benicar HCT Tablets 1010
Cozaar Tablets 1973
Mavik Tablets (Rare; 0.6%) 472
Neupro Transdermal System 3149
Prinivil Tablets 2087
Tarka Tablets 511
Tekturna HCT Tablets 2324

Hypotensive crisis

Hyalgan Solution (One case) 2742

Hypothermia

Abilify Injection (Less than 1 in 1000 patients) 881
Abilify Injection (Less than 1 in 1000 patients) 2466
Abilify Oral Solution (Less than 1 in 1000 patients) 881
Abilify Oral Solution (Less than 1 in 1000 patients) 2466
Abilify Discmelt Orally Disintegrating Tablets (Less than 1 in 1000 patients) 881
Abilify Discmelt Orally Disintegrating Tablets (Less than 1 in 1000 patients) 2466
Abilify Tablets (Less than 1 in 1000 patients) 881
Abilify Tablets (Less than 1 in 1000 patients) 2466
Aggrenox Capsules 819
Alphagan P Ophthalmic Solution 549
Bayer Aspirin 750
Combigan Ophthalmic Solution 553
Depakote ER Tablets 423
Doxil Injection (Less than 1%) 2378
Emend Capsules (Greater than 0.5%) 1992
Emend for Injection (Greater than 0.5%) 1999
Exelon Capsules (Infrequent) 2229
Exelon Oral Solution (Infrequent) 2229
Geodon Capsules (Frequent) 2520
Invanz for Injection (1.6%) 2029
Ionsys Transdermal System (.1% to less than 1%) 2410
Janumet Tablets 2041
Namenda (Infrequent) 1180
Norvir (Less than 2%) 489
Percocet Tablets 1127
Percodan Tablets 1130
Proleukin for Injection (Less than 1%) 2287
Provigil Tablets (At least 1%) 977
Prozac Weekly Capsules (Rare) 1852
Prozac Pulvules and Liquid (Rare) 1852
Rilutek Tablets (Rare) 2771
Risperdal Consta Long-Acting Injection 1753
St. Joseph 81 mg Aspirin Chewable and Enteric Coated Tablets 1903
Salagen Tablets (Less than 1%) 1082
Ultane Liquid for Inhalation (1%) 524
Venlafaxine Hydrochloride Tablets 2199
▲ Vesanoid Capsules (3%) 2660

Hypothesia

Rythmol SR Capsules 1590

Hypothyroidism

Amerge Tablets (Rare) 1301
Betaseron for SC Injection 756
▲ Bexxar (0% to 7%) 1371
Campral Tablets (Rare) 1158
Celexa (Rare) 1160
▲ CellCept Capsules (3% to less than 20%) 2622
▲ CellCept Intravenous (3% to less than 20%) 2622
▲ CellCept Oral Suspension (3% to less than 20%) 2622
▲ CellCept Tablets (3% to less than 20%) 2622
Climara Transdermal System 763
Copaxone for Injection (Infrequent) 3110
Cymbalta Delayed-Release Capsules (Infrequent) 1801
Effexor XR Extended-Release Capsules (Rare) 3195
Evoxac Capsules (Less than 1%) 1013
Exelon Capsules (Infrequent) 2229
Exelon Oral Solution (Infrequent) 2229
Gabitril Tablets (Infrequent) 973
Genotropin Lyophilized Powder (Infrequent) 2547
▲ Humatrope Vials and Cartridges (11% to 13.5%) 1838
Imitrex Injection 1465
Imitrex Nasal Spray (Rare) 1470
Imitrex Tablets (Rare) 1474
▲ Intron A for Injection (Less than 5%) 2859
Kaletra (Less than 2%) 452
Lamictal (Rare) 1488
Luvox CR Extended-Release Capsules (Infrequent) 1759
Meridia Capsules 475
Mirapex Tablets 857
Norditropin Cartridges 2354
▲ Ontak Vials (Less than 5%) 1079
Paxil (Rare) 1535
Paxil CR Controlled-Release Tablets (Rare) 1544
▲ PegIntron Powder for Injection (Less than or equal to 1% to 5%) 2903
Premarin Tablets 3221
Proleukin for Injection 2287
Protopic Ointment (0.2% to less than 1%) 628
Prozac Weekly Capsules (Infrequent) 1852
Prozac Pulvules and Liquid (Infrequent) 1852
▲ Rebetol (4% to 5%) 2917
Remeron Tablets (Rare) 2924
RemeronSolTab Tablets (Rare) 2927
Requip Tablets (Infrequent) 1561
Risperdal Consta Long-Acting Injection (Infrequent) 1753
▲ Sandostatin Injection (12%) 2300
▲ Sandostatin LAR Depot (2% to 12%) 2302
▲ Sutent Capsules (4% to 7%) 2540
Symbyax Capsules (Infrequent) 1871
▲ Targretin Capsules (28.6% to 52.8%) 1084
Tasigna Capsules 2316
Treximet Tablets (Rare) 1616
Venlafaxine Hydrochloride Tablets (Rare) 2199

Hypotonia

Abilify Injection (Greater than or equal to 1 in 1000 patients and less than 1 in 100 patients) 881
Abilify Injection (Greater than or equal to 1 in 1000 patients and less than 1 in 100 patients) 2466
Abilify Oral Solution (Greater than or equal to 1 in 1000 patients and less than 1 in 100 patients) 881
Abilify Oral Solution (Greater than or equal to 1 in 1000 patients and less than 1 in 100 patients) 2466
Abilify Discmelt Orally Disintegrating Tablets (Greater than or equal to 1 in 1000 patients and less than 1 in 100 patients) 881
Abilify Discmelt Orally Disintegrating Tablets (Greater than or equal to 1 in 1000 patients and less than 1 in 100 patients) 2466
Abilify Tablets (Greater than or equal to 1 in 1000 patients and less than 1 in 100 patients) 881
Abilify Tablets (Greater than or equal to 1 in 1000 patients and less than 1 in 100 patients) 2466
Alphagan P Ophthalmic Solution 549
Ambien Tablets (Rare) 2692
Ambien CR Tablets (Rare) 2696
Combigan Ophthalmic Solution 553
▲ Coreg Tablets (Greater than 1% to 3%) 1387
▲ Coreg CR Extended-Release Capsules (Greater than 1% to less than or equal to 3%) 1393
Doxil Injection (Less than 1%) 2378
Duragesic Transdermal System (Less than 1%) 2405
Effexor XR Extended-Release Capsules (Infrequent) 3195
Frova Tablets (Rare) 1111
Gabitril Tablets (Frequent) 973
Geodon Capsules (Frequent) 2520
Infanrix Vaccine 1479
Klonopin 2639
Lamictal (Rare) 1488
Luvox CR Extended-Release Capsules (Infrequent) 1759
Lyrica Capsules (0.1% to 1%) 2527
Mirapex Tablets 857
Orthoclone OKT3 Sterile Solution (Less than 1%) 2387
OxyContin Tablets (Less than 1%) 2589
Pediarix Vaccine 1552
Remeron Tablets (Rare) 2924
RemeronSolTab Tablets (Rare) 2927
Requip Tablets (Infrequent) 1561
Rilutek Tablets (Rare) 2771
Synagis Intramuscular Solution 1948
Venlafaxine Hydrochloride Tablets (Infrequent) 2199
Zomig Tablets (Rare) 694
Zomig-ZMT Tablets (Rare) 694
Zonegran Capsules (Infrequent) 1089
Zyprexa Tablets (Infrequent) 1883
Zyprexa ZYDIS Orally Disintegrating Tablets (Infrequent) 1883

Hypotonic-hyporesponsive episode
Infanrix Vaccine 1479
Kinrix Injection Vaccine 1486
Pentacel 2792

Hypotrichosis
Vantas (Less than 2%) 1737

Hypouresis
▲ Chemet Capsules (Up to 3.7%) 2484
Fleet Phospho-soda EZ-PREP 1147
▲ Indocin I.V. (41% of infants) 2489
K-Phos Neutral Tablets 813
▲ NeoProfen Injection (3%) 2496
Proglycem Capsules (Infrequent) 1185
Proglycem Suspension (Infrequent) 1185
Prograf Capsules and Injection 622
Uroqid-Acid No. 2 Tablets 814

Hypouricemia
Cipro I.V. (Infrequent) 2817
Timentin ADD-Vantage 1606
Timentin Injection Galaxy Container 1609
Timentin IV Infusion 1603
Timentin Pharmacy Bulk Package 1613

Hypoventilation
Actiq 959
▲ Avinza Capsules (Less than 5%) 1772
Copaxone for Injection (Infrequent) 3110
▲ Duragesic Transdermal System (2% to 10%) 2405
Effexor XR Extended-Release Capsules (Rare) 3195
Ionsys Transdermal System (.1% to less than 1%) 2410
Nembutal Sodium Solution, USP (Less than 1%) 2494
Norvir (Less than 2%) 489
Percocet Tablets 1127
Percodan Tablets 1130
Proleukin for Injection (Less than 1%) 2287
Prozac Weekly Capsules (Rare) 1852
Prozac Pulvules and Liquid (Rare) 1852
Rilutek Tablets (Infrequent) 2771
Ultane Liquid for Inhalation (Less than 1%) 524
Venlafaxine Hydrochloride Tablets (Rare) 2199
Zyprexa Tablets (Rare) 1883
Zyprexa ZYDIS Orally Disintegrating Tablets (Rare) 1883

Hypovitaminosis
Mirapex Tablets 857

Hypovolemia
▲ CellCept Capsules (3% to less than 20%) 2622
▲ CellCept Intravenous (3% to less than 20%) 2622
▲ CellCept Oral Suspension (3% to less than 20%) 2622
▲ CellCept Tablets (3% to less than 20%) 2622
▲ Coreg Tablets (Greater than 1% to 3%) 1387
▲ Coreg CR Extended-Release Capsules (Greater than 1% to less than or equal to 3%) 1393
Demadex Injection 2630
Demadex Tablets 2630
Emend Capsules (Greater than 0.5%) 1992
Emend for Injection (Greater than 0.5%) 1999
Estratest Tablets 3043
Estratest H.S. Tablets 3043
Fleet Enema 1143
Fleet Enema Extra 1143
Fleet Enema for Children 1143
Fleet Pedia-Lax Enema 1143
Fleet Phospho-soda 1145
Follistim AQ Cartridge 2844
Ixempra Kit for Injection 915

Hypoxemia
Flebogamma 5% 1715
Flebogamma 5% DIF 1718
Gammagard Liquid 730
Gammagard S/D 734
Gamunex 3094
Invanz for Injection (Greater than 0.1%) 2029
Orthoclone OKT3 Sterile Solution 2387

Hypoxia
Ambien Tablets (Rare) 2692
Ambien CR Tablets (Rare) 2696
▲ AmBisome for Injection (6.2% to 7.5%) 606
Aricept Tablets (Infrequent) 1062
Aricept ODT Tablets (Infrequent) 1062
BeneFIX Vials (1.5%) 3191
Bicillin C-R Injectable Suspension 1775
Bicillin L-A Injection 1777
Busulfex Injection (2%) 2477
Carbatrol Capsules 3019
▲ CellCept Capsules (3% to less than 20%) 2622
▲ CellCept Intravenous (3% to less than 20%) 2622
▲ CellCept Oral Suspension (3% to less than 20%) 2622
▲ CellCept Tablets (3% to less than 20%) 2622
Combivent Inhalation Aerosol 845
▲ Dacogen Injection (10%) 1066
▲ DepoDur Injection (5% to 10%) 1095
Effexor XR Extended-Release Capsules (Rare) 3195
Elitek 2729
▲ Eloxatin for Injection (2% to 43%) 2731
Emend Capsules (Greater than 0.5%) 1992
Emend for Injection (Greater than 0.5%) 1999
▲ Flolan for Injection (55%) 1426
Herceptin I.V. 1199
▲ Ionsys Transdermal System (1% to less than 10%) 2410
Ixempra Kit for Injection 915
Leukine 774
Merrem I.V. (Greater than 0.1% to 1%) 684
Mycamine for Injection 616
▲ Mylotarg for Injection (5%) 3212
Neulasta Injection (Single case) 587
▲ Opana Tablets (1% to less than 10%) 1117
▲ Opana ER Tablets (1% to less than 10%) 1121
Orthoclone OKT3 Sterile Solution 2387
Proleukin for Injection (Less than 1%) 2287
Protopic Ointment (Greater than or equal to 1%) 628
Prozac Weekly Capsules (Rare) 1852
Prozac Pulvules and Liquid (Rare) 1852
Pulmozyme Inhalation Solution 1217
Rilutek Tablets (Infrequent) 2771
Rituxan I.V. (0.3%) 1223
Targretin Capsules 1084
Torisel Injection 3272
Trasylol Injection (2%) 799
▲ Trisenox Injection (23%) 986
Ultane Liquid for Inhalation (Less than 1%) 524
Velcade for Injection 2168
Venlafaxine Hydrochloride Tablets (Rare) 2199
▲ Zofran (9%) 1687
▲ Zofran ODT Orally Disintegrating Tablets (9%) 1687
Zyprexa Tablets (Infrequent) 1883
Zyprexa ZYDIS Orally Disintegrating Tablets (Infrequent) 1883

Hysteria
Ambien Tablets (Rare) 2692
Ambien CR Tablets (Rare) 2696
Imitrex Injection (Rare) 1465
Imitrex Tablets (Rare) 1474
Klonopin 2639
Luvox CR Extended-Release Capsules (Infrequent) 1759
Paxil (Rare) 1535
Paxil CR Controlled-Release Tablets (Rare) 1544

I

Ichthyosis
Tricor Tablets 520

Icterus
(*see under* Jaundice)

Idiosyncrasy
Furosemide Tablets 2186

Idiosyncratic reactions
(*see under* Idiosyncrasy)

Idioventricular rhythms
Activase I.V. 1188

Ileitis, regional
Accutane Capsules 2607
Effexor XR Extended-Release Capsules (Rare) 3195
Indocin (Less than 1%) 2024
Norvir (Less than 2%) 489
Paxil (Rare) 1535
Paxil CR Controlled-Release Tablets (Rare) 1544
Venlafaxine Hydrochloride Tablets (Rare) 2199

Ileus
Aricept Tablets (Infrequent) 1062
Aricept ODT Tablets (Infrequent) 1062
▲ Avastin IV (4% to 5%) 1192
▲ Busulfex Injection (2% to 8%) 2477
Celebrex Capsules (Less than 0.1%) 2979
▲ CellCept Capsules (3% to less than 20%) 2622
▲ CellCept Intravenous (3% to less than 20%) 2622
▲ CellCept Oral Suspension (3% to less than 20%) 2622
▲ CellCept Tablets (3% to less than 20%) 2622
Cipro I.V. (1% or less) 2817
Cipro XR Tablets 2823
▲ Doxil Injection (1% to 10%) 2378
Effexor XR Extended-Release Capsules 3195
Elitek (Less than or equal to 1%) 2729
Eloxatin for Injection 2731
Evoxac Capsules (Less than 1%) 1013
▲ Indocin I.V. (1% to 3%) 2489
Invanz for Injection (Greater than 0.1%) 2029
▲ Ionsys Transdermal System (1% to less than 10%) 2410
Ixempra Kit for Injection 915
Luvox CR Extended-Release Capsules 1759
Merrem I.V. (Greater than 0.1% to 1%) 684
Mirapex Tablets 857
MS Contin Tablets (Less frequent) 2585
Myfortic Tablets 2276
Namenda 1180
NeoProfen Injection 2496
Nimotop Capsules (Rare) 790
Omnicef Capsules 497
Omnicef for Oral Suspension 497
Opana Tablets (Less than 1%) 1117
Opana ER Tablets (Less than 1%) 1121
OxyContin Tablets (Less than 1%) 2589
Paxil (Rare) 1535
Paxil CR Controlled-Release Tablets (Rare) 1544
Percocet Tablets 1127
Percodan Tablets 1130
▲ Photofrin for Injection (Less than 5%) 708
Proglycem Capsules (Frequent) 1185
Proglycem Suspension (Frequent) 1185
▲ Prograf Capsules and Injection (3% to 15%) 622
Remicade for IV Injection (Greater than or equal to 0.2%) 950
ReoPro Vials (0.3%) 1860
Rilutek Tablets (Rare) 2771
Taxotere Injection Concentrate 2773
Velcade for Injection 2168
▲ Xeloda Tablets (1% to 6%) 2662
Zosyn for Injection (1% or less) 3284
Zyprexa Tablets (Rare) 1883
Zyprexa ZYDIS Orally Disintegrating Tablets (Rare) 1883

Ileus, adynamic
Thiothixene Capsules 2197

Ileus, paralytic
▲ DepoDur Injection (2% to 5%) 1095
Spiriva HandiHaler 870
Tarka Tablets (Infrequent) 511
Thioridazine Hydrochloride Tablets 2195
Velcade for Injection 2168
Vivitrol 988

Illusion, unspecified
Ambien Tablets (Infrequent) 2692
Evoxac Capsules 1013
Klonopin (Infrequent) 2639

Immobility
Moban Tablets 1116
Remicade for IV Injection 950

Immune reconstitution syndrome
Aptivus Capsules 823
Aptivus Oral Solution 823
Atripla Tablets 938
Emtriva Capsules 1246
Emtriva Oral Solution 1246
Epivir 1412
Epzicom Tablets 1422
Intelence Tablets 3119
Isentress Tablets 2036
Lexiva Oral Suspension 1510
Lexiva Tablets 1510
Norvir 489
Retrovir Capsules 1574
Retrovir IV Infusion 1579
Retrovir 1574
Viramune Oral Suspension 873
Viramune Tablets 873
Viread Tablets 1268
Ziagen 1673

Immune system disorders
▲ Cancidas for Injection (7% to 7.1%) 1953
Vyvanse Capsules 3033

Immunogenicity
Avastin IV 1192
▲ Betaseron for SC Injection (16.5% to 45%) 756
▲ Bexxar (1% to 7%) 1371
▲ Campath Ampules (1.9% to 8.3%) 761
▲ Cimzia (8%) 3127
Elspar for Injection 2488
▲ Enbrel for Injection (6%) 569
Epogen for Injection 576
▲ Erbitux (5%) 912
Fabrazyme for Intravenous Infusion 1241
Forteo for Injection (2.8%) 1816
NovoLog Injection 2359
Orencia Powder for Intravenous Infusion (1.7%) 921
PegIntron Powder for Injection 2903
Procrit for Injection 2391
▲ Raptiva for Injection (6.3%) 1218
Remicade for IV Injection 950
▲ Rituxan I.V. (1.1% to 11%) 1223
Synagis Intramuscular Solution 1948
▲ Vectibix (Less than 1% to 4.6%) 597
Xolair (Less than 0.1%) 2339
▲ Xyntha Vials (2.2% to 4.17%) 3280

Immunoglobulin, abnormalities
Phenytek Capsules 2192
Rilutek Tablets (Infrequent) 2771
Xolair 1235

Immunoglobulin G, decreased
Proglycem Capsules (Infrequent) 1185
Proglycem Suspension (Infrequent) 1185

Immunosuppression
Campath Ampules 761
Cimzia 3127
Torisel Injection 3272
Veramyst Nasal Spray 1643

Immunosuppression, progressive
Lamictal 1488

Impetigo
▲ Elidel Cream 1% (1.9% to 4%) 2221
ProQuad 2099
Varivax 2133

Impetigo, bullous
Protopic Ointment 628

Impotence
(*see also under* Sexual dysfunction)
Abelcet Injection 1134
▲ Adderall XR Capsules (2% to 4%) 3012
Adipex-P 1185
Advicor Tablets 402
Ambien Tablets (Rare) 2692
Ambien CR Tablets (Rare) 2696
Atacand HCT 642
▲ Avinza Capsules (Less than 5%) 1772
▲ Avodart Soft Gelatin Capsules (0.3% to 5.5%) 1359
Axid Capsules 1364
Azilect Tablets (Greater than 1%) 3106
▲ Betaseron for SC Injection (8%) 756
Betimol Ophthalmic Solution 3181
Bicillin C-R Injectable Suspension 1775
Bicillin L-A Injection 1777
Campral Tablets (Frequent) 1158
Captopril Tablets 2182
Carbatrol Capsules 3019
Cardizem LA Extended Release Tablets (Less than 2%) 421
▲ Catapres Tablets (About 3 in 100 patients) 841
Catapres-TTS (2 of 101 patients) 842
▲ Celexa (3%) 1160
▲ CellCept Capsules (3% to less than 20%) 2622
▲ CellCept Intravenous (3% to less than 20%) 2622
▲ CellCept Oral Suspension (3% to less than 20%) 2622

▲ CellCept Tablets (3% to less than 20%) 2622
▲ Clorpres Tablets (About 3%) 2185
Combigan Ophthalmic Solution 553
▲ Coreg Tablets (Greater than 1% to 3%) 1387
▲ Coreg CR Extended-Release Capsules (Greater than 1% to less than or equal to 3%) 1393
Cosopt Sterile Ophthalmic Solution 1969
Cozaar Tablets (Less than 1%) 1973
Demadex Injection 2630
Demadex Tablets 2630
Demser Capsules (Infrequent) 1989
Dexedrine 1401
Diovan Tablets (Greater than 0.2%) 2212
Donnatal Extentabs 2507
Dyazide Capsules 1405
DynaCirc CR Controlled Release Tablets (0.5% to 1%) 1407
▲ Effexor XR Extended-Release Capsules (3% to 10%) 3195
Eligard 7.5 mg (Less than 2%) 2724
Eligard 22.5 mg (Less than 2%) 2724
Eligard 30 mg (Less than 2%) 2724
Eligard 45 mg (Less than 2%) 2724
Emsam Transdermal System (0.7%) 905
Equetro Extended-Release Capsules 3174
Evoxac Capsules 1013
Exelon Capsules (Infrequent) 2229
Exelon Oral Solution (Infrequent) 2229
Exforge Tablets (Greater than 0.2%) 2238
Gabitril Tablets (Infrequent) 973
Geodon Capsules (Infrequent) 2520
▲ Indapamide Tablets (Less than 5%) 2188
InnoPran XL Extended Release Capsules 1484
Intravenous Sodium Diuril 2490
▲ Intron A for Injection (Less than 5%) 2859
Invega Extended-Release Tablets 1748
Klonopin (1%) 2639
▲ Lamictal (13%) 1488
▲ Lexapro Oral Suspension (Less than 1% to 3%) 1174
▲ Lexapro Tablets (Less than 1% to 3%) 1174
Lipitor Tablets (Less than 2%) 2501
Lovaza Capsules 1520
▲ Lupron Depot 7.5 mg (5.4%) 469
Luvox CR Extended-Release Capsules (2%) 1759
Lyrica Capsules (Greater than or equal to 1%) 2527
Marplan Tablets (0% to 2%) 3177
Mavik Tablets (0.3% to 1%) 472
▲ Megace ES Oral Suspension (4% to 14%) 2499
Meridia Capsules 475
Micardis Tablets (More than 0.3%) 852
Micardis HCT Tablets 854
Mirapex Tablets (2%) 857
MS Contin Tablets (Less frequent) 2585
Nadolol Tablets (1 to 5 of 1000 patients) 2191
Namenda (More than one patient) 1180
Neupro Transdermal System 3149
Nexium Delayed-Release Capsules (Less than 1%) 645
Nexium I.V. (Less than 1%) 652
Nexium Delayed-Release Oral Suspension (Less than 1%) 645
Norvir (Less than 2%) 489
▲ Novantrone for Injection Concentrate (7%) 1100
OxyContin Tablets (Less than 1%) 2589
Parnate Tablets 1532
▲ Paxil (4% to 10%) 1535
▲ Paxil CR Controlled-Release Tablets (4% to 10%) 1544
Pepcid Tablets (Rare) 2075
Prinivil Tablets (1%) 2087
Prinzide Tablets (1.2%) 2092
▲ Propecia Tablets (5.1% to 8.1%) 2095
▲ Proscar Tablets (5.15 to 8.1%) 2102
Protonix for Delayed-Release Oral Suspension (Less than 1%) 3254
Protonix Delayed-Release Tablets (Less than 1%) 3254
Protonix I.V. (Less than 1%) 3257
▲ Prozac Weekly Capsules (1% to 7%) 1852
Prozac Pulvules and Liquid (Less than 1%) 1852
Remeron Tablets (Infrequent) 2924
RemeronSolTab Tablets (Infrequent) 2927
▲ Requip Tablets (3%) 1561
Rilutek Tablets (Infrequent) 2771
Risperdal Consta Long-Acting Injection (Infrequent) 1753
Rythmol Tablets (Less than 1%) 1586
Rythmol SR Capsules 1590
▲ Simulect for Injection (3% to 10%) 2306
▲ Strattera Capsules (3%) 1864
▲ Symbyax Capsules (2% to 4%) 1871
Tarka Tablets (0.3% or more) 511
Teveten HCT Tablets 517
Thiothixene Capsules (Infrequently) 2197
Timoptic Sterile Ophthalmic Solution (Less frequent) 2121
Timoptic in Ocudose (Less frequent) 2124
Timoptic-XE Sterile Ophthalmic Gel Forming Solution 2125
Toprol-XL Tablets 666
Uroxatral Tablets (1% to 2%) 2786
▲ Venlafaxine Hydrochloride Tablets (2.1% to 6%) 2199
Viadur Implant (2.3%) 802
Vicoprofen Tablets (Less than 1%) 533
Vyvanse Capsules 3033
▲ Wellbutrin Tablets (3.4%) 1648
Wellbutrin SR Sustained-Release Tablets (Infrequent) 1653
Wellbutrin XL Extended-Release Tablets (Infrequent) 1659
Zantac 25 EFFERdose Tablets (Occasional) 1670
Zantac Injection 1666
Zantac Injection Pharmacy Bulk Package (Infrequent) 1668
Zantac Injection Premixed 1666
Zantac (Occasional) 1670
Zonegran Capsules (Infrequent) 1089
Zyban Sustained-Release Tablets (Infrequent) 1692
Zyprexa Tablets (Infrequent) 1883
Zyprexa ZYDIS Orally Disintegrating Tablets (Infrequent) 1883

Impulse control, impaired
Effexor XR Extended-Release Capsules 3195
Parnate Tablets 1532
Paxil 1535
Paxil CR Controlled-Release Tablets 1544
Pristiq Extended-Release Tablets 3247
Prozac Pulvules and Liquid 1852
Requip Tablets 1561
Symbyax Capsules 1871
Venlafaxine Hydrochloride Tablets (Rare) 2199
Wellbutrin Tablets 1648
Wellbutrin SR Sustained-Release Tablets 1653
Wellbutrin XL Extended-Release Tablets 1659
Zyban Sustained-Release Tablets 1692

Impulsive behavior
Luvox CR Extended-Release Capsules 1759
Prozac Weekly Capsules 1852
Remeron Tablets 2924
RemeronSolTab Tablets 2927
Venlafaxine Hydrochloride Tablets 2199

Incontinence
▲ DepoCyt Injection (7% to 9%) 1136
Eligard 7.5 mg (Less than 2%) 2724
Eligard 22.5 mg (Less than 2%) 2724
Eligard 30 mg (Less than 2%) 2724
Eligard 45 mg (Less than 2%) 2724
Marplan Tablets 3177
Namenda (Greater than or equal to 2%) 1180
▲ Tice BCG (4%) 2936
Valium Tablets (Infrequent) 2658

Incontinence, fecal
Actiq (Less than 1%) 959
AmBisome for Injection (Less common) 606
Amitiza Capsules (Less than 1%) 3082
Aricept Tablets (Frequent) 1062
Aricept ODT Tablets (Frequent) 1062
Azilect Tablets (Infrequent) 3106
Copaxone for Injection (At least 2%) 3110
Depakote ER Tablets (Greater than 1%) 423
Exelon Capsules (Frequent) 2229
Exelon Oral Solution (Frequent) 2229
Gabitril Tablets (Infrequent) 973
Gliadel Wafer (1%) 1076
Kaletra (Less than 2%) 452
Klonopin 2639
Lovaza Capsules 1520
Luvox CR Extended-Release Capsules (Rare) 1759
Marinol Capsules (Less than 1%) 3163
Mirapex Tablets 857
Paxil (Rare) 1535
Paxil CR Controlled-Release Tablets (Rare) 1544
Pentasa Capsules (Less than 1%) 3030
Prozac Weekly Capsules (Rare) 1852
Prozac Pulvules and Liquid (Rare) 1852
Requip Tablets (Infrequent) 1561
Rilutek Tablets (Infrequent) 2771
Risperdal Consta Long-Acting Injection (Infrequent) 1753
Stromectol Tablets 2120
Symbyax Capsules (Rare) 1871
▲ Trisenox Injection (8%) 986
▲ Xenical Capsules (1.8% to 7.7%) 2672
Xyrem Oral Solution (Infrequent) 1766
Zonegran Capsules (Rare) 1089
Zyprexa Tablets (Infrequent) 1883
Zyprexa ZYDIS Orally Disintegrating Tablets (Infrequent) 1883

Incoordination
(*see under* Ataxia)

Indigestion
Asacol Delayed-Release Tablets 2579
Augmentin 1323
Augmentin Tablets 1327
Augmentin XR Extended Release Tablets 1333
Augmentin ES-600 Powder for Oral Suspension 1329
Carafate Suspension (Less than 0.5%) 706
Carafate Tablets (Less than 0.5%) 707
Ceftin Tablets (0.1% to 1%) 1380
Depakote ER Tablets 423
▲ Indocin (3% to 9%) 2024
▲ Janumet Tablets (Greater than 5%) 2041
▲ Lexapro Oral Suspension (2% to 6%) 1174
▲ Lexapro Tablets (2% to 6%) 1174
Nadolol Tablets (1 to 5 of 1000 patients) 2191

Induration at application site
Daytrana Transdermal Patch 3022

Induration at injection site
▲ Aldara Cream, 5% (0% to 7%) 1699
Aloxi Injection (Very rare) 1059
Boostrix 1377
Capastat Sulfate for Injection 1791
▲ Comvax (27.2% to 27.6%) 1966
▲ Copaxone for Injection (13%) 3110
Daytrana Transdermal Patch 3022
Eligard 7.5 mg (0.4%) 2724
Eligard 22.5 mg 2724
Eligard 30 mg 2724
Eligard 45 mg 2724
Emend for Injection (1.5%) 1999
▲ Engerix-B Vaccine (1% to 10 %) 1409
▲ Fluarix Vaccine (1% to 10%) 1446
▲ Havrix Injection Vaccine (1% to 10%) 1454
Imitrex Injection 1465
Invanz for Injection (1%) 2029
Lupron Depot 3.75 mg 462
Lupron Depot 7.5 mg 469
Lupron Depot–3 Month 11.25 mg 462
Lupron Depot-PED 7.5 mg, 11.25 mg and 15 mg 471
Meruvax II 2061
M-M-R II 2054
Neulasta Injection 587
Liquid PedvaxHIB 2073
Pneumovax 23 (Common) 2078
▲ Prevnar (0% to 48.3%) 3241
Primaxin I.V. (0.2%) 2083
ProQuad 2099
Risperdal Consta Long-Acting Injection (1%) 1753
Rocephin Injectable Vials, ADD-Vantage, Galaxy, Bulk (1%) 2642
▲ Somatuline Depot Injection (4.8% to 17%) 3102
Timentin ADD-Vantage 1606
Timentin Injection Galaxy Container 1609
Timentin IV Infusion 1603
Timentin Pharmacy Bulk Package 1613
▲ Twinrix Vaccine (1% to 10%) 1628
▲ Varivax (19.35% to 32.5%) 2133
▲ Vivitrol (25% to 35%) 988
Xolair 1235
Xolair 2339

Inebriated feeling
Klonopin (Infrequent) 2639
▲ Xyrem Oral Solution (8.6%) 1766

Infection, access site
▲ Aranesp for Injection (6%) 564
▲ Dacogen Injection (8%) 1066
▲ Sensipar Tablets (5%) 594
Velcade for Injection 2168

Infection, application site
Aldara Cream, 5% (1%) 1699
Daytrana Transdermal Patch 3022

Infection, aspergillus
▲ Cancidas for Injection (13%) 1953
▲ CellCept Capsules (Less than 4%) 2622
▲ CellCept Intravenous (Less than 4%) 2622
▲ CellCept Oral Suspension (Less than 4%) 2622
▲ CellCept Tablets (Less than 4%) 2622
Myfortic Tablets (Rare) 2276
Velcade for Injection 2168

Infection, bacterial
Actiq (Less than 1%) 959
Advair Diskus 100/50 1276
Advair Diskus 250/50 1276
Advair Diskus 500/50 1276
▲ Advair HFA 45/21 Inhalation Aerosol (1% to 3%) 1288
▲ Advair HFA 115/21 Inhalation Aerosol (1% to 3%) 1288
▲ Advair HFA 230/21 Inhalation Aerosol (1% to 3%) 1288
▲ Campath Ampules (16%) 761
Celebrex Capsules (0.1% to 1.9%) 2979
Cimzia 3127
Comtan Tablets (1%) 2208
▲ Copaxone for Injection (5%) 3110
Elidel Cream 1% (1.1% to 1.8%) 2221
Elocon Cream 0.1% (1 in 182 patients) 2840
Elocon Ointment 0.1% (1 in 63 patients) 2842
Emsam Transdermal System (Infrequent) 905
Enbrel for Injection 569
▲ Equetro Extended-Release Capsules (Less than 5%) 3174
Evoxac Capsules (Less than 1%) 1013
▲ Flovent Diskus 50 mcg (1% to 3%) 1435
Gengraf Capsules (1% to less than 3%) 435
▲ Humira Injection (Less than 5%) 442
▲ Intron A for Injection (Less than 5%) 2859
Ixempra Kit for Injection 915
Kaletra (Less than 2%) 452
▲ Leustatin Injection (42%) 2384
Neoral Oral Solution (1% to less than 3%) 2280
Neoral Soft Gelatin Capsules (1% to less than 3%) 2280
Orthoclone OKT3 Sterile Solution 2387
▲ Remicade for IV Injection (6%) 950
Requip Tablets (Infrequent) 1561
▲ Rituxan I.V. (19%) 1223
Stalevo Tablets (1%) 2309
▲ Targretin Capsules (1.2% to 13.2%) 1084
Tice BCG 2936
▲ Trisenox Injection (8%) 986
Varivax 2133

Infection, bladder
Advate (0.6%) 721
Requip Tablets (Infrequent) 1561
Xyrem Oral Solution (Infrequent) 1766

Infection, bone
Tice BCG 2936

Infection, bone marrow
Tice BCG 2936

Infection, C. diff
Invanz for Injection (1.7%) 2029

Infection, candida albicans
Aerobid/Aerobid-M 1153
▲ CellCept Capsules (Less than 4% to 22.4%) 2622
▲ CellCept Intravenous (Less than 4% to 22.4%) 2622
▲ CellCept Oral Suspension (Less than 4% to 22.4%) 2622
▲ CellCept Tablets (Less than 4% to 22.4%) 2622
Cubicin for Injection (1% to 2%) 995
▲ Dacogen Injection (10%) 1066
Myfortic Tablets (0.6% to 2.3%) 2276
Veramyst Nasal Spray 1643
Zosyn for Injection (1% or less) 3284

Infection, central line
▲ Cancidas for Injection (0.9% to 8.9%) 1953
Dacogen Injection (Greater than or equal to 1%) 1066

Infection, conjunctiva
Velcade for Injection 2168

Infection, corneal, fungal
Pred Forte Ophthalmic Suspension ⊙ 227
Pred Mild Ophthalmic Suspension ⊙ 230
Pred-G Ophthalmic Suspension ⊙ 228

Infection, cryptococcus
Myfortic Tablets (Rare) 2276
Orthoclone OKT3 Sterile Solution (1.6%) 2387

Infection, cytomegalovirus
▲ Campath Ampules (6% to 16%) 761
▲ CellCept Capsules (5.8% to 14.1%) 2622
▲ CellCept Intravenous (5.8% to 14.1%) 2622
▲ CellCept Oral Suspension (5.8% to 14.1%) 2622
▲ CellCept Tablets (5.8% to 14.1%) 2622
▲ Doxil Injection (20.1%) 2378
▲ Gengraf Capsules (4.8%) 435
▲ Myfortic Tablets (1.9% to 21.6%) 2276
▲ Neoral Oral Solution (4.8%) 2280
▲ Neoral Soft Gelatin Capsules (4.8%) 2280
▲ Noxafil Oral Suspension (14%) 2889
▲ Orthoclone OKT3 Sterile Solution (3% to 19%) 2387
Rapamune (Less than 3%) 3260
Remicade for IV Injection 950
Rituxan I.V. 1223
▲ Sandimmune (4.8% to 12.3%) 2296
▲ Simulect for Injection (14%) 2306

Infection, decreased resistance
Orthoclone OKT3 Sterile Solution 2387
Prograf Capsules and Injection 622
Sandimmune 2296

Infection, dental
Xyrem Oral Solution (Infrequent) 1766

Infection, ears
Aceon Tablets (2 mg, 4 mg, 8 mg) (0% to 1.3%) 3038
Advair Diskus 100/50 1276
Advair Diskus 250/50 1276
Advair Diskus 500/50 1276
▲ Aerobid/Aerobid-M (3% to 9%) 1153
Amerge Tablets (Frequent) 1301
Avalide Tablets 892
Avalide Tablets 2713
Avapro Tablets (Less than 1%) 897
Avapro Tablets (Less than 1%) 2718
Ciprodex Otic Suspension (0.6%) 541
▲ Elidel Cream 1% (0.6% to 5.7%) 2221
▲ Epivir-HBV (25%) 1417
▲ Exjade Tablets (5.4%) 2244
Flovent HFA 1440
Imitrex Nasal Spray (Infrequent) 1470
Invanz for Injection (Greater than 0.5%) 2029
Mirapex Tablets 857
Liquid PedvaxHIB (Among most frequent) 2073
▲ Relenza Inhalation Powder (1% to 5%) 1556
Requip Tablets (Infrequent) 1561
▲ Trizivir Tablets (Greater than or equal to 5%) 1622
Ultram ER Extended-Release Tablets (0.5% to less than 1%) 2428
Xyrem Oral Solution (Infrequent) 1766
▲ Ziagen (5%) 1673

Infection, Epstein-Barr virus
Campath Ampules 761
Rapamune (Less than 3%) 3260

Infection, eyes
Advair Diskus 250/50 1276
▲ Aerobid/Aerobid-M (1% to 3%) 1153
Elidel Cream 1% (0% to 1.1%) 2221
▲ Evoxac Capsules (1% to 3%) 1013
Lexapro Oral Suspension (Infrequent) 1174
Lexapro Tablets (Infrequent) 1174
Mirapex Tablets 857

Infection, fungal
Actiq (1% or greater) 959
Aricept Tablets (Frequent) 1062
Aricept ODT Tablets (Frequent) 1062
▲ Campath Ampules (6%) 761
Celebrex Capsules (0.1% to 1.9%) 2979
Cimzia 3127
Cubicin for Injection (2.6%) 995
Dacogen Injection 1066
▲ Depakote ER Tablets (Greater than 1% to less than 5%) 423
Emsam Transdermal System (Infrequent) 905
Enbrel for Injection 569
▲ Equetro Extended-Release Capsules (Less than 5%) 3174
▲ Evoxac Capsules (1% to 3%) 1013
▲ Fabrazyme for Intravenous Infusion (5%) 1241
FML Ophthalmic Ointment ⊙ 223
FML Ophthalmic Suspension ⊙ 224
FML Forte Ophthalmic Suspension ⊙ 222
Gengraf Capsules (1% to less than 3%) 435
Humira Injection 442
▲ Intron A for Injection (Less than 5%) 2859
Keppra Oral Solution (1% or more) 3131
Keppra Tablets (1% or more) 3131
Klonopin (Infrequent) 2639
▲ Leustatin Injection (20%) 2384
Lovaza Capsules 1520
Micardis Tablets (More than 0.3%) 852
Micardis HCT Tablets 854
Mirapex Tablets 857
▲ Myfortic Tablets (2.5% to 10.8%) 2276
Neoral Oral Solution (1% to less than 3%) 2280
Neoral Soft Gelatin Capsules (1% to less than 3%) 2280
▲ Novantrone for Injection Concentrate (9% to 15%) 1100
▲ Orthoclone OKT3 Sterile Solution (4% to 34%) 2387
PegIntron Powder for Injection (Less than 1%) 2903
▲ Rebetol (1% to 6%) 2917
Remicade for IV Injection 950
Requip Tablets (Infrequent) 1561
Rituxan I.V. (1%) 1223
Soriatane Capsules (Less than 1%) 3062
▲ Xeloda Tablets (Less than 5%) 2662
Xyrem Oral Solution (Infrequent) 1766
Zyvox (0.1% to 1.5%) 2552

Infection, fungal, local
▲ Aldara Cream, 5% (2% to 11%) 1699
Doxil Injection (Less than 1%) 2378
▲ Gengraf Capsules (7.5%) 435
▲ Neoral Oral Solution (7.5%) 2280
▲ Neoral Soft Gelatin Capsules (7.5%) 2280
▲ Sandimmune (7.5% to 9.6%) 2296

Infection, fungal, systemic
Gengraf Capsules (2.2%) 435
Neoral Oral Solution (2.2%) 2280
Neoral Soft Gelatin Capsules (2.2%) 2280
▲ Sandimmune (2.2% to 3.9%) 2296

Infection, gastrointestinal
▲ Advair HFA 45/21 Inhalation Aerosol (1% to 4%) 1288
▲ Advair HFA 115/21 Inhalation Aerosol (1% to 4%) 1288
▲ Advair HFA 230/21 Inhalation Aerosol (1% to 4%) 1288
Ceftin for Oral Suspension (0.1% to 1%) 1380
▲ Flovent Diskus 50 mcg (1% to 3%) 1435
FluMist Vaccine 1945
Requip Tablets (Infrequent) 1561
Serevent Diskus (1% to less than 3%) 1594

Infection, gastrointestinal, viral
Advair Diskus 100/50 1276
Advair Diskus 250/50 1276
Advair Diskus 500/50 1276

Infection, genitourinary
Tice BCG 2936

Infection, gram-negative bacteria
▲ Orthoclone OKT3 Sterile Solution (1.6% to 7.5%) 2387

Infection, gram-positive bacteria
▲ Orthoclone OKT3 Sterile Solution (9.0%) 2387
Zolinza Capsules 2142

Infection, helminthic
▲ Xolair (53%) 1235
▲ Xolair (53%) 2339

Infection, herpes simplex
▲ CellCept Capsules (10.1% to 20.8%) 2622
▲ CellCept Intravenous (10.1% to 20.8%) 2622
▲ CellCept Oral Suspension (10.1% to 20.8%) 2622
▲ CellCept Tablets (10.1% to 20.8%) 2622
▲ Noxafil Oral Suspension (3% to 15%) 2889
▲ Orthoclone OKT3 Sterile Solution (5% to 31%) 2387
Proglycem Capsules (Infrequent) 1185
Proglycem Suspension (Infrequent) 1185
Rituxan I.V. 1223

Infection, increased susceptibility to
Myfortic Tablets 2276

Infection, kidney
Tice BCG 2936
Treximet Tablets (Rare) 1616

Infection, Legionella
Orthoclone OKT3 Sterile Solution (0.7% to 1.6%) 2387
Raptiva for Injection 1218

Infection, liver
Tice BCG 2936

Infection, localized
▲ Flolan for Injection (21%) 1426
Omnaris Nasal Spray (Rare) 2998
Orencia Powder for Intravenous Infusion (0.2%) 921
Requip Tablets (Infrequent) 1561
▲ Valcyte Tablets (Less than 5%) 2654
Vantas (2 patients) 1737
Xyrem Oral Solution (Infrequent) 1766

Infection, lower respiratory tract
Advair Diskus 100/50 1276
Advair Diskus 250/50 1276
Advair Diskus 500/50 1276
▲ Advair HFA 45/21 Inhalation Aerosol (3% to 5%) 1288
▲ Advair HFA 115/21 Inhalation Aerosol (3% to 5%) 1288
▲ Advair HFA 230/21 Inhalation Aerosol (3% to 5%) 1288
Ambien CR Tablets (1%) 2696
▲ Aralast (96.3%) 726
Emend Capsules (Greater than 0.5%) 1992
Emend for Injection (Greater than 0.5%) 1999
▲ Fabrazyme for Intravenous Infusion (11%) 1241
▲ Flovent Diskus 50 mcg (1% to 3%) 1435
Foradil Aerolizer (2.1%) 2849
Imitrex Injection 1465
Imitrex Tablets 1474
Ixempra Kit for Injection 915
Remicade for IV Injection (Greater than or equal to 0.2%) 950
Requip Tablets (Frequent) 1561
▲ Velcade for Injection (15%) 2168
▲ Xenical Capsules (7.8%) 2672

Infection, lung
Tice BCG 2936

Infection, lymph nodes
Tice BCG 2936

Infection, masking signs of
FML Ophthalmic Ointment ⊙ 223
FML Ophthalmic Suspension ⊙ 224
FML Forte Ophthalmic Suspension ⊙ 222
Pred Forte Ophthalmic Suspension ⊙ 227
Pred Mild Ophthalmic Suspension ⊙ 230

Infection, mononucleosis-like syndrome
Klonopin (Infrequent) 2639
Paser Granules 1747

Infection, mycobacterial
CellCept Capsules 2622
CellCept Intravenous 2622
CellCept Oral Suspension 2622
CellCept Tablets 2622
Dacogen Injection (Greater than or equal to 1%) 1066
Myfortic Tablets 2276
Rapamune (Less than 3%) 3260
Remicade for IV Injection 950

Infection, mycobacterium tuberculosis
Rapamune (Less than 3%) 3260

Infection, nail
Mirapex Tablets 857

Infection, nasal
Advair Diskus 100/50 1276
Advair Diskus 250/50 1276
Advair Diskus 500/50 1276
Amerge Tablets (Frequent) 1301
▲ Epivir-HBV (25%) 1417
▲ Miacalcin Nasal Spray (1% to 10.6%) 2274
▲ Relenza Inhalation Powder (1% to 5%) 1556
▲ Trizivir Tablets (Greater than or equal to 5%) 1622
▲ Ziagen (5%) 1673

Infection, neutropenic
▲ Avastin IV (9.1%) 1192
Ixempra Kit for Injection 915
▲ Taxotere Injection Concentrate (11.7% to 13.9%) 2773

Infection, ocular, secondary
Iquix Ophthalmic Solution (1% to 2%) 3183

Infection, ophthalmic, fungal
Pred-G Ophthalmic Ointment ⊙ 229

Infection, ophthalmic, viral
Pred-G Ophthalmic Ointment ⊙ 229
Selzentry Tablets 2534

Infection, opportunistic
Campath Ampules 761
CellCept Capsules 2622
CellCept Intravenous 2622
CellCept Oral Suspension 2622
CellCept Tablets 2622
▲ Doxil Injection (50.4%) 2378
Humira Injection 442
Kineret Injection (Rare) 585
Leustatin Injection 2384

Infection, parasitic
▲ Clarinex Syrup (3.1%) 2828
Emsam Transdermal System (Rare) 905
▲ Intron A for Injection (Less than 5%) 2859

Infection, parovirus B-19
Rituxan I.V. 1223

Infection, pelvis
ParaGard T 380A Intrauterine Copper Contraceptive 1041
Wellbutrin Tablets (Rare) 1648

Infection, pharyngeal
▲ Epivir-HBV (25%) 1417

Infection, Pneumocystis carinii
(*see under* Pneumocystis carinii, susceptibility)

Infection, post-operative
Emend Capsules (Greater than 0.5%) 1992
Emend for Injection (Greater than 0.5%) 1999
Invanz for Injection (2.3%) 2029
Requip Tablets (Infrequent) 1561

Infection, post-surgical
Amevive 611
Humira Injection 442

Infection, prostate
Tice BCG 2936

Infection, prosthetic
Humira Injection 442
▲ Myfortic Tablets (3% to less than 20%) 2276

Infection, protozoan
Enbrel for Injection 569
Orthoclone OKT3 Sterile Solution 2387
Remicade for IV Injection 950

Infection, pseudomonal, lung
Dacogen Injection 1066

Infection, respiratory
Accutane Capsules 2607
▲ Alphagan P Ophthalmic Solution (1% to 4%) 549
▲ Betimol Ophthalmic Solution (1% to 5%) 3181
▲ CellCept Capsules (22% to 37%) 2622
▲ CellCept Intravenous (22% to 37%) 2622
▲ CellCept Oral Suspension (22% to 37%) 2622
▲ CellCept Tablets (22% to 37%) 2622
Combigan Ophthalmic Solution (0.1% to 0.2%) 553
▲ Depakote ER Tablets (12% to 20%) 423
Epivir 1412

Epivir-HBV (Among most common)... 1417
▲ Exjade Tablets (9.5%) ... 2244
▲ Flovent Diskus 50 mcg (5%) ... 1435
FluMist Vaccine ... 1945
▲ Geodon Capsules (8%) ... 2520
Gliadel Wafer (2%) ... 1076
Imitrex Nasal Spray (Infrequent) ... 1470
Infanrix Vaccine ... 1479
▲ NeoProfen Injection (19%) ... 2496
Pediarix Vaccine ... 1552
ProQuad ... 2099
▲ Pulmicort Flexhaler (Greater than or equal to 3% to 32%) ... 654
Remicade for IV Injection ... 950
Requip Tablets (Infrequent) ... 1561
Selzentry Tablets ... 2534
Xifaxan Tablets (Less than 2%) ... 2682

Infection, respiratory tract, viral

Advair Diskus 100/50 ... 1276
▲ Advair Diskus 250/50 (3% to 6%) ... 1276
▲ Advair Diskus 500/50 (Greater than or equal to 3%) ... 1276
▲ Fabrazyme for Intravenous Infusion (6%) ... 1241
▲ Relenza Inhalation Powder (3% to 13%) ... 1556
Selzentry Tablets ... 2534
▲ Ventolin HFA Inhalation Aerosol (7%) ... 1638

Infection, secondary

Alrex Ophthalmic Suspension 0.2% ... ⊙ 236
Analpram-HC ... 1140
Bactroban Cream (Less than 1%) ... 1366
Diprolene Lotion 0.05% (Infrequent) ... 2838
Diprolene Ointment 0.05% ... 2839
Diprolene AF Cream 0.05% (Infrequent) ... 2837
Elocon Cream 0.1% (Infrequent) ... 2840
Elocon Lotion 0.1% (Infrequent) ... 2841
Elocon Ointment 0.1% (Infrequent) ... 2842
EryPed 200 & EryPed 400 Oral Suspension ... 431
FML Ophthalmic Ointment ... ⊙ 223
FML Ophthalmic Suspension ... ⊙ 224
FML Forte Ophthalmic Suspension ... ⊙ 222
Lotemax Ophthalmic Suspension 0.5% ... ⊙ 241
Lotrisone (Less than 1%) ... 2881
Luxíq Foam ... 3058
Olux Foam ... 3061
Olux-E Foam ... 3059
Pramosone ... 1141
Pred Forte Ophthalmic Suspension ... ⊙ 227
Pred Mild Ophthalmic Suspension ... ⊙ 230
Pred-G Ophthalmic Ointment ... ⊙ 229
Pred-G Ophthalmic Suspension ... ⊙ 228
Vanos Cream ... 1941
Varivax ... 2133
Verdeso Foam ... 3069

Infection, serious

CellCept Capsules ... 2622
CellCept Intravenous ... 2622
CellCept Oral Suspension ... 2622
CellCept Tablets ... 2622
Raptiva for Injection (0.4%) ... 1218

Infection, serratia

Orthoclone OKT3 Sterile Solution (1.6%) ... 2387

Infection, sinus

▲ Alphagan P Ophthalmic Solution (1% to 4%) ... 549
Combigan Ophthalmic Solution (0.1% to 0.2%) ... 553
▲ Flovent Diskus 50 mcg (10% to 33%) ... 1435
▲ Flovent HFA (1% to 6%) ... 1440

Infection, skin

Accutane Capsules ... 2607
Aceon Tablets (2 mg, 4 mg, 8 mg) (0.3% to 1%) ... 3038
Bexxar ... 1371
▲ Elidel Cream 1% (2.2% to 6.4%) ... 2221
▲ Flovent HFA (1% to 3%) ... 1440
▲ Gengraf Capsules (7%) ... 435
Mirapex Tablets ... 857
▲ Neoral Oral Solution (7%) ... 2280
▲ Neoral Soft Gelatin Capsules (7%) ... 2280
▲ Novantrone for Injection Concentrate (5%) ... 1100
Prinivil Tablets (0.3% to 1%) ... 2087
Prinzide Tablets ... 2092
ProQuad ... 2099
▲ Sandimmune (7% to 10.1%) ... 2296
Singulair (Greater than or equal to 2%) ... 2114

Infection, skin and soft tissue

Celebrex Capsules (0.1% to 1.9%) ... 2979
Enbrel for Injection ... 569
▲ Flovent Diskus 50 mcg (1% to 3%) ... 1435
▲ Gengraf Capsules (7%) ... 435
▲ Protopic Ointment (5% to 12%) ... 628
Varivax ... 2133

Infection, staphylococcal

Elidel Cream 1% (0% to 2.1%) ... 2221
Treximet Tablets (Rare) ... 1616

Infection, staphylococcus epidermidis

▲ Clolar for Intravenous Infusion (13%) ... 1239
▲ Dacogen Injection (7%) ... 1066
▲ Orthoclone OKT3 Sterile Solution (4.8%) ... 2387

Infection, systemic

▲ Novantrone for Injection Concentrate (10%) ... 1100

Infection, throat

Advair Diskus 100/50 ... 1276
Advair Diskus 250/50 ... 1276
Advair Diskus 500/50 ... 1276
▲ Novantrone for Injection Concentrate (19%) ... 1100
▲ Relenza Inhalation Powder (1% to 5%) ... 1556
▲ Trizivir Tablets (Greater than or equal to 5%) ... 1622
▲ Ziagen (5%) ... 1673

Infection, tooth

Mirapex Tablets ... 857
Requip Tablets (Infrequent) ... 1561
Singulair (Greater than or equal to 2%) ... 2114

Infection, unspecified

▲ Abelcet Injection (5%) ... 1134
▲ Accolate Tablets (3.5%) ... 669
Actiq (1% or greater) ... 959
▲ Actonel Tablets (31.1%) ... 2568
▲ Actonel with Calcium Tablets (19% to 29.9%) ... 2574
▲ Adderall XR Capsules (2% to 4%) ... 3012
▲ Advicor Tablets (20%) ... 402
▲ Alimta for Injection (Less than 1% to 23%) ... 1786
Alinia for Oral Suspension (Less than 1%) ... 2677
Alinia Tablets (Less than 1%) ... 2677
Ambien Tablets (Infrequent) ... 2692
▲ AmBisome for Injection (11.1%) ... 606
Amevive (0.7% to 1.5%) ... 611
Anaprox Tablets (Less than 1%) ... 2632
Anaprox DS Tablets (Less than 1%) ... 2632
Angiomax for Injection (Greater than 0.1% to less than 1%) ... 1933
▲ Aranesp for Injection (24%) ... 564
▲ Argatroban Injection (3.7%) ... 1308
▲ Aricept Tablets (11%) ... 1062
▲ Aricept ODT Tablets (11%) ... 1062
▲ Arimidex Tablets (2% to 9%) ... 672
▲ Arranon Injection (1% to 9%) ... 1319
Asacol Delayed-Release Tablets (2% or greater) ... 2579
Asmanex Twisthaler (1% to less than 3%) ... 2797
Atacand HCT (0.5% or greater) ... 642
▲ Avastin IV (7%) ... 1192
▲ Avinza Capsules (5% to 10%) ... 1772
Axid Capsules (1.7%) ... 1364
▲ Azilect Tablets (3%) ... 3106
▲ Bexxar (Less than 1% to 21%) ... 1371
▲ Boniva Injection (4.3%) ... 2614
▲ Boniva Tablets (4.3%) ... 2618
▲ BOTOX Purified Neurotoxin Complex (3% to 10%) ... 550
▲ Busulfex Injection (51%) ... 2477
▲ Campath Ampules (50% to 74%) ... 761
Campral Tablets (Frequent) ... 1158
▲ Cancidas for Injection (30.4% to 48.2%) ... 1953
▲ Celebrex Capsules (20% to 25%) ... 2979
▲ CellCept Capsules (3% to 27.1%) ... 2622
▲ CellCept Intravenous (3% to 27.1%) ... 2622
▲ CellCept Oral Suspension (3% to 27.1%) ... 2622
▲ CellCept Tablets (3% to 27.1%) ... 2622
Cimzia ... 3127
▲ Climara Pro Transdermal System (3.3%) ... 768
▲ Clolar for Intravenous Infusion (85%) ... 1239
Combigan Ophthalmic Solution (0.1% to 0.2%) ... 553
▲ Copaxone for Injection (50%) ... 3110
Cosmegen for Injection ... 2485
▲ Cozaar Tablets (5%) ... 1973
Crinone 4% Gel ... 992
Crinone 8% Gel ... 992
▲ Depakote ER Tablets (15%) ... 423
▲ Doxil Injection (1% to 11.7%) ... 2378
EC-Naprosyn Delayed-Release Tablets (Less than 1%) ... 2632
Edex Injection (2%) ... 2957
▲ Effexor XR Extended-Release Capsules (10%) ... 3195
▲ Elestat Ophthalmic Solution (Approximately 10%) ... 1741
Elitek (Less than or equal to 1%) ... 2729
▲ Eloxatin for Injection (1% to 25%) ... 2731
Emsam Transdermal System ... 905
▲ Emtriva Capsules (44%) ... 1246
▲ Emtriva Oral Solution (44%) ... 1246
▲ Enbrel for Injection (35% to 64%) ... 569
▲ Equetro Extended-Release Capsules (12%) ... 3174
▲ Erbitux (1% to 35%) ... 912
▲ Evista Tablets (15.1%) ... 1810
▲ Evoxac Capsules (1% to 3%) ... 1013
Exelon Capsules (2% or more) ... 2229
Exelon Oral Solution (2% or more) ... 2229
Exjade Tablets ... 2244
▲ Femara Tablets (1.6% to 6.5%) ... 2246
▲ Flolan for Injection (21%) ... 1426
▲ Flomax Capsules (9% to 10.8%) ... 848
▲ Gabitril Tablets (1% to 19%) ... 973
▲ Gemzar for Injection (3% to 16%) ... 1820
▲ Gengraf Capsules (1% to 24.7%) ... 435
▲ Gliadel Wafer (1% to 18%) ... 1076
▲ Herceptin I.V. (20%) ... 1199
▲ Hycamtin for Injection (26% to 28%) ... 1459
▲ Indapamide Tablets (Greater than or equal to 5%) ... 2188
▲ Intron A for Injection (Less than 5%) ... 2859
Ionsys Transdermal System (.1% to less than 1%) ... 2410
Iquix Ophthalmic Solution (1% to 2%) ... 3183
Ixempra Kit for Injection ... 915
▲ Keppra Oral Solution (2% to 13%) ... 3131
▲ Keppra Tablets (2% to 13%) ... 3131
▲ Kineret Injection (39%) ... 585
▲ Lamictal (5% to 20%) ... 1488
Lescol Capsules ... 2268
Lescol XL Tablets ... 2268
▲ Leukine (65%) ... 774
▲ Leustatin Injection (28%) ... 2384
▲ Lipitor Tablets (2.8% to 10.3%) ... 2501
▲ Lovaza Capsules (4.4% to 10%) ... 1520
▲ Lunesta Tablets (5% to 10%) ... 2994
▲ Lupron Depot 7.5 mg (5.4%) ... 469
Lupron Depot-PED 7.5 mg, 11.25 mg and 15 mg (Less than 2%) ... 471
▲ Lyrica Capsules (3% to 14%) ... 2527
▲ Megace ES Oral Suspension (1% to 3%) ... 2499
▲ Mepron Suspension (18% to 22%) ... 1526
▲ Miacalcin Nasal Spray (1% to 3%) ... 2274
Micardis Tablets (More than 0.3%) ... 852
Micardis HCT Tablets ... 854
Mirapex Tablets (Greater than or equal to 1%) ... 857
▲ Mycamine for Injection (33.5% to 41.9%) ... 616
Myleran Tablets ... 1530
▲ Mylotarg for Injection (3% to 10%) ... 3212
Naprosyn Suspension (Less than 1%) ... 2632
Naprosyn Tablets (Less than 1%) ... 2632
Nasacort AQ Nasal Spray ... 2765
NeoProfen Injection ... 2496
▲ Neoral Oral Solution (1% to 24.7%) ... 2280
▲ Neoral Soft Gelatin Capsules (1% to 24.7%) ... 2280
Nexavar Tablets (0.1% to less than 1%) ... 784
▲ Norditropin Cartridges (13%) ... 2354
▲ Novantrone for Injection Concentrate (17% to 85%) ... 1100
▲ Ontak Vials (48%) ... 1079
Panhematin for Injection ... 2497
▲ Pataday Ophthalmic Solution (Less than or equal to 5%) ... 543
▲ Paxil (5% to 6%) ... 1535
▲ Paxil CR Controlled-Release Tablets (5% to 6%) ... 1544
PegIntron Powder for Injection (Less than or equal to 1%) ... 2903
▲ Pletal Tablets (10% to 14%) ... 2481
▲ Premarin Tablets (18% to 23%) ... 3221
▲ Premphase Tablets (16% to 18%) ... 3232
▲ Prempro Tablets (16% to 18%) ... 3232
ProAir HFA Inhalation Aerosol (Less than 3%) ... 3113
▲ Prograf Capsules and Injection (45%) ... 622
▲ Proleukin for Injection (1% to 13%) ... 2287
ProQuad ... 2099
Protonix for Delayed-Release Oral Suspension (Greater than or equal to 1%) ... 3254
Protonix Delayed-Release Tablets (Greater than or equal to 1%) ... 3254
Protonix I.V. (Greater than or equal to 1%) ... 3257
▲ Protopic Ointment (1% to 14%) ... 628
Provigil Tablets (At least 1%) ... 977
Prozac Pulvules and Liquid ... 1852
Rapamune ... 3260
▲ Raptiva for Injection (29%) ... 1218
Refludan for Injection (1.8%) ... 795
Remeron Tablets ... 2924
RemeronSolTab Tablets ... 2927
▲ Remicade for IV Injection (56%) ... 950
Reyataz Capsules ... 3299
▲ Rituxan I.V. (2% to 39%) ... 1223
▲ Simulect for Injection (3% to 10%) ... 2306
▲ Soriatane Capsules (1% to 10%) ... 3062
▲ Spiriva HandiHaler (1% to 4%) ... 870
▲ Suboxone Tablets (5.6% to 20%) ... 2601
▲ Subutex Tablets (11.7% to 20%) ... 2601
Sutent Capsules ... 2540
Symbyax Capsules (Frequent) ... 1871
▲ Tarceva Tablets (0% to 33%) ... 1228
▲ Targretin Capsules (13.1% to 22.6%) ... 1084
▲ Targretin Gel 1% (18%) ... 1088
▲ Taxotere Injection Concentrate (0% to 39.4%) ... 2773
▲ Trasylol Injection (6%) ... 799
▲ Travatan Z Ophthalmic Solution (1% to 5%) ... 547
▲ Treanda for Injection (2% to 6%) ... 983
Tricor Tablets ... 520
▲ Tygacil for Injection (8.3%) ... 3276
▲ Valcyte Tablets (Less than 5%) ... 2654
Vectibix ... 597
▲ Venlafaxine Hydrochloride Tablets (2.2% to 6%) ... 2199
▲ Verdeso Foam (20%) ... 3069
▲ Vesanoid Capsules (58%) ... 2660
▲ Vicoprofen Tablets (3% to 9%) ... 533
▲ Vigamox Ophthalmic Solution (1% to 4%) ... 548
Voltaren Tablets (Occasionally) ... 2334
Voltaren-XR Tablets (Occasionally) ... 2337
Wellbutrin Tablets (Rare) ... 1648
▲ Wellbutrin SR Sustained-Release Tablets (8% to 9%) ... 1653
▲ Wellbutrin XL Extended-Release Tablets (8% to 9%) ... 1659
Yaz Tablets (Greater than 1%) ... 805
Zolinza Capsules ... 2142
▲ Zometa for Intravenous Infusion (5% to less than 10%) ... 2341
Zomig Tablets (Infrequent) ... 694
Zomig Nasal Spray (Infrequent) ... 689
Zomig-ZMT Tablets (Infrequent) ... 694

Infection, upper respiratory tract

▲ Abilify Injection (6%) ... 881
▲ Abilify Injection (6%) ... 2466
▲ Abilify Oral Solution (6%) ... 881
▲ Abilify Oral Solution (6%) ... 2466
▲ Abilify Discmelt Orally Disintegrating Tablets (6%) ... 881
▲ Abilify Discmelt Orally Disintegrating Tablets (6%) ... 2466
▲ Abilify Tablets (6%) ... 881
▲ Abilify Tablets (6%) ... 2466
▲ Aceon Tablets (2 mg, 4 mg, 8 mg) (8.6%) ... 3038
▲ Activella Tablets (10% to 18%) ... 2347
▲ ActoPlus Met Tablets (12.4% to 13.5%) ... 3071
▲ Actos Tablets (13.2%) ... 3077
▲ Aczone Gel 5% (3%) ... 3296
Advair Diskus 100/50 ... 1276
▲ Advair Diskus 250/50 (3% to 21%) ... 1276
▲ Advair Diskus 500/50 (Greater than or equal to 3%) ... 1276
▲ Advair HFA 45/21 Inhalation Aerosol (16% to 24%) ... 1288
▲ Advair HFA 115/21 Inhalation Aerosol (16% to 24%) ... 1288
▲ Advair HFA 230/21 Inhalation Aerosol (16% to 24%) ... 1288
▲ Aerobid/Aerobid-M (25%) ... 1153
Aggrenox Capsules (1%) ... 819
▲ Aldara Cream, 5% (3% to 15%) ... 1699
▲ Allegra Oral Solution (0.9% to 4.3%) ... 2684
Allegra Tablets (2.9%) ... 2684
Allegra-D 12 Hour Extended-Release Tablets (1.4%) ... 2687
Allegra-D 24 Hour Extended-Release Tablets (1.4%) ... 2690
▲ Alvesco Inhalation Aerosol (4.1% to 8.7%) ... 2985

Ambien Tablets (Frequent) 2692
Ambien CR Tablets (1%) 2696
▲ Angeliq Tablets (18.9%) 751
▲ Aralast (96.3%) 726
▲ Aranesp for Injection (15%) 564
▲ Asmanex Twisthaler (8% to 15%) 2797
▲ Atacand Tablets (6%) 639
▲ Atacand HCT (3.6%) 642
▲ Atripla Tablets (8%) 938
▲ Atrovent HFA Inhalation Aerosol (9% to 34%) 839
▲ Atrovent Nasal Spray 0.03% (9.8%) 834
Avalide Tablets (1% or greater) 892
Avalide Tablets (1% or greater) 2713
▲ Avandamet Tablets (9% to 16%) 1336
▲ Avandaryl Tablets (Greater than or equal to 5%) 1344
▲ Avandia Tablets (4.3% to 9.9%) 1351
▲ Avapro Tablets (9%) 897
▲ Avapro Tablets (9%) 2718
▲ Avastin IV (40% to 47%) 1192
▲ Benicar HCT Tablets (7%) 1010
Bexxar 1371
▲ Boniva Injection (2% to 33.7%) 2614
▲ Boniva Tablets (2% to 33.7%) 2618
▲ BOTOX Purified Neurotoxin Complex (12%) 550
Ceftin for Oral Suspension (0.1% to 1%) 1380
▲ Celebrex Capsules (8.1%) 2979
▲ Celexa (5%) 1160
▲ Cialis Tablets (3% to 4%) 1792
▲ Cimzia (20%) 3127
▲ Clarinex Syrup (10.8% to 21.2%) 2828
▲ Climara Transdermal System (6% to 17%) 763
▲ Climara Pro Transdermal System (13.2%) 768
▲ Combivent Inhalation Aerosol (10.9%) 845
Comvax (0.5% to 1.3%) 1966
Concerta Extended-Release Tablets (2.2%) 1925
▲ Cosopt Sterile Ophthalmic Solution (1% to 5%) 1969
▲ Cozaar Tablets (8%) 1973
▲ Crinone 4% Gel (5%) 992
▲ Crinone 8% Gel (8%) 992
Crixivan Capsules 1979
▲ Cymbalta Delayed-Release Capsules (7%) 1801
Dacogen Injection 1066
Diovan Tablets (More than 1%) 2212
Diovan HCT Tablets (Greater than 0.2%) 2216
▲ Divigel (1.6% to 5.7%) 3167
▲ Duetact Tablets (12.3% to 14.8%) 3085
▲ Duragesic Transdermal System (3% to 10%) 2405
▲ Edex Injection (5%) 2957
▲ Elestat Ophthalmic Solution (Approximately 10%) 1741
▲ Elidel Cream 1% (4.3% to 19.4%) 2221
▲ Eloxatin for Injection (7% to 10%) 2731
Emend Capsules (Greater than 0.5%) 1992
Emend for Injection (Greater than 0.5%) 1999
▲ Emtriva Capsules (8%) 1246
▲ Emtriva Oral Solution (8%) 1246
▲ Enbrel for Injection (12% to 31%) 569
▲ Epogen for Injection (11%) 576
▲ Evoxac Capsules (11.4%) 1013
Exelon Capsules (2% or more) 2229
Exelon Oral Solution (2% or more) 2229
Exforge Tablets (2.9%) 2238
▲ Exubera Inhalation Powder (29.2% to 43.3%) 2515
▲ Fabrazyme for Intravenous Infusion (19%) 1241
Fentora Tablets (Greater than 1%) 968
▲ Flebogamma 5% (33%) 1715
▲ Flebogamma 5% DIF (Greater than 15%) 1718
▲ Flovent Diskus 50 mcg (18% to 31%) 1435
▲ Flovent HFA (18%) 1440
▲ Fluarix Vaccine (3.9%) 1446
▲ Flulaval Injection Vaccine (1% to 9%) 1448
▲ Follistim AQ Cartridge (5%) 2844
▲ Foradil Aerolizer (7.4%) 2849
Gardasil Injection (1.5%) 2019
▲ Gengraf Capsules (7.7%) 435
▲ Genotropin Lyophilized Powder (13.1% to 15.9%) 2547
▲ Gleevec Tablets (3% to 21.2%) 2255
Havrix Injection Vaccine (Less than 1%) 1454
Herceptin I.V. 1199
▲ Humira Injection (17%) 442
Invanz for Injection (2.3%) 2029
Ionsys Transdermal System (.1% to less than 1%) 2410
▲ Ixempra Kit for Injection (6%) 915
Janumet Tablets 2041
▲ Januvia Tablets (4.5%) 2048
▲ Kineret Injection (14%) 585
▲ Klonopin (8%) 2639
▲ Lamisil Oral Granules (5%) 2264
▲ Lescol Capsules (16.2%) 2268
▲ Lescol XL Tablets (12.5%) 2268
Levaquin Tablets (0.1% to 0.9%) 2416
Lexapro Oral Suspension (At least 2%) 1174
Lexapro Tablets (At least 2%) 1174
▲ Lucentis Injection (2% to 15%) 1205
▲ Lumigan Ophthalmic Solution (Approximately 10%) 556
Mavik Tablets (0.3% to 1%) 472
Maxalt Tablets (Infrequent) 2056
Maxalt-MLT Orally Disintegrating Tablets (Infrequent) 2056
▲ Miacalcin Nasal Spray (1% to 3%) 2274
▲ Micardis Tablets (7%) 852
▲ Micardis HCT Tablets (8%) 854
Mirapex Tablets 857
▲ Mirena Intrauterine System (5% or more) 779
▲ Mobic Oral Suspension (0% to 7.5%) 863
▲ Mobic Tablets (0% to 7.5%) 863
▲ Myfortic Tablets (3% to less than 20%) 2276
Nalfon Capsules (1.5%) 2508
Namenda (Greater than or equal to 2%) 1180
▲ Nasonex Nasal Spray (5% to 7%) 2883
▲ Neoral Oral Solution (7.7% to 13%) 2280
▲ Neoral Soft Gelatin Capsules (7.7% to 13%) 2280
Neupro Transdermal System (Greater than or equal to 2%) 3149
Norditropin Cartridges 2354
▲ Novantrone for Injection Concentrate (51% to 53%) 1100
▲ Noxafil Oral Suspension (7%) 2889
▲ NuvaRing (5% to 14%) 2897
▲ Orencia Powder for Intravenous Infusion (5% to 13%) 921
▲ Ortho Evra Transdermal System (9% to 22%) 2437
Liquid PedvaxHIB (Among most frequent) 2073
▲ Plavix Tablets (8.7%) 926
▲ Plavix Tablets (8.7%) 2767
▲ PrandiMet Tablets (11%) 2967
▲ Prandin Tablets (10% to 16%) 2971
▲ Premarin Tablets (9% to 12%) 3221
▲ Premphase Tablets (9% to 11%) 3232
▲ Prempro Tablets (9% to 11%) 3232
Prinivil Tablets (1.2% to 1.5%) 2087
Prinzide Tablets (2.2%) 2092
▲ Procrit for Injection (11%) 2391
▲ Prometrium Capsules (100 mg, 200 mg) (5%) 3047
ProQuad (1.3%) 2099
Protonix for Delayed-Release Oral Suspension (Greater than or equal to 1%) 3254
Protonix Delayed-Release Tablets (Greater than or equal to 1%) 3254
Protonix I.V. (Greater than or equal to 1%) 3257
▲ Proventil HFA Inhalation Aerosol (21%) 2914
Pulmicort Flexhaler (2.2%) 654
▲ Qvar Inhalation Aerosol (5% to 11%) 3116
Recombivax HB (Equal to or greater than 1%) 2107
ReFacto Vials 3269
▲ Remicade for IV Injection (32%) 950
Requip Tablets (1% or more) 1561
Rituxan I.V. 1223
▲ Rozerem Tablets (3%) 3091
▲ Rythmol SR Capsules (8% to 12%) 1590
▲ Sandostatin LAR Depot (10% to 23.1%) 2302
▲ Selzentry Tablets (20%) 2534
▲ Serevent Diskus (Greater than 3%) 1594
Simcor Tablets (2.1%) 502
▲ Simulect for Injection (Greater than or equal to 10%) 2306
Singulair (1% to 1.9%) 2114
▲ Spiriva HandiHaler (41% to 43%) 870
Stalevo Tablets 2309
▲ Starlix Tablets (10.5%) 2314
▲ Symbicort 80/4.5 Inhalation Aerosol (7.6%) 659
▲ Symbicort 160/4.5 Inhalation Aerosol (10.5%) 659
▲ Synagis Intramuscular Solution (52.6%) 1948
Tamiflu Capsules (Less than 1%) 2649
▲ Tarka Tablets (0.3% to 5.4%) 511
Tekturna Tablets (Greater than 1%) 2321
Tekturna HCT Tablets (Greater than 1%) 2324
▲ Temodar Capsules (8%) 2931
▲ Teveten Tablets (8%) 515
Teveten HCT Tablets (0.4%) 517
Timoptic Sterile Ophthalmic Solution (Less frequent) 2121
Timoptic in Ocudose (Less frequent) 2124
▲ Timoptic-XE Sterile Ophthalmic Gel Forming Solution (1% to 5%) 2125
▲ Torisel Injection (7%) 3272
▲ Trisenox Injection (13%) 986
▲ Truvada Tablets (8%) 1262
▲ Twinrix Vaccine (1% to 10%) 1628
▲ Tyzeka Tablets (14%) 2328
▲ Ultram ER Extended-Release Tablets (1% to less than 5%) 2428
▲ Uroxatral Tablets (3%) 2786
▲ Vagifem Tablets (5% to 11%) 2375
▲ Valcyte Tablets (Less than 5%) 2654
Valtrex Caplets 1635
▲ Vaqta (1.1% to 10.1%) 2130
▲ Velcade for Injection (12%) 2168
Ventolin HFA Inhalation Aerosol 1638
▲ Verdeso Foam (10%) 3069
▲ Viread Tablets (8%) 1268
▲ Vivitrol (12% to 13%) 988
▲ Vytorin 10/10 Tablets (3.6%) 2149
▲ Vytorin 10/10 Tablets (3.6%) 2939
▲ Vytorin 10/20 Tablets (3.6%) 2149
▲ Vytorin 10/20 Tablets (3.6%) 2939
▲ Vytorin 10/40 Tablets (3.6%) 2149
▲ Vytorin 10/40 Tablets (3.6%) 2939
▲ Vytorin 10/80 Tablets (3.6%) 2149
▲ Vytorin 10/80 Tablets (3.6%) 2939
▲ Wellbutrin XL Extended-Release Tablets (9%) 1659
▲ Xeloda Tablets (4%) 2662
▲ Xenical Capsules (26.1% to 38.1%) 2672
Xifaxan Tablets (Less than 2%) 2682
▲ Xolair (20%) 1235
▲ Xolair (20%) 2339
▲ Xyrem Oral Solution (2.9% to 6.1%) 1766
Yaz Tablets (Greater than 1%) 805
▲ Zetia Tablets (4.3%) 2157
▲ Zetia Tablets (2.9% to 4.3%) 2951
▲ Zocor Tablets (9%) 2136
▲ Zolinza Capsules (9% to 10.5%) 2142
▲ Zometa for Intravenous Infusion (10%) 2341
Zostavax Injection (1.9%) 2145
Zyrtec Chewable Tablets (Less than 2%) 1920
Zyrtec Syrup (Less than 2%) 1920
Zyrtec Tablets (Less than 2%) 1920
Zyrtec-D 12 Hour Extended Release Tablets (Less than 2%) 1923
▲ Zyvox (3.7% to 4.2%) 2552

Infection, upper respiratory tract, viral

Elidel Cream 1% (0.3% to 1.5%) 2221

Infection, urinary tract

Aceon Tablets (2 mg, 4 mg, 8 mg) (2.8%) 3038
Actiq (Less than 1%) 959
▲ Actonel Tablets (11.1%) 2568
▲ Actonel with Calcium Tablets (2.9% to 10.9%) 2574
▲ ActoPlus Met Tablets (5.3% to 5.8%) 3071
▲ Adderall XR Capsules (5%) 3012
▲ Advair HFA 45/21 Inhalation Aerosol (1% to 3%) 1288
▲ Advair HFA 115/21 Inhalation Aerosol (1% to 3%) 1288
▲ Advair HFA 230/21 Inhalation Aerosol (1% to 3%) 1288
Aldara Cream, 5% (1%) 1699
Ambien Tablets (Frequent) 2692
Ambien CR Tablets (Frequent) 2696
Amitiza Capsules (Less than 1%) 3082
▲ Argatroban Injection (4.6%) 1308
Aricept Tablets (2%) 1062
Aricept ODT Tablets (2%) 1062
▲ Arimidex Tablets (2% to 8%) 672
▲ Arixtra Injection (2.3% to 4%) 1313
Asmanex Twisthaler (2%) 2797
Atacand HCT (0.5% or greater) 642
▲ Atrovent HFA Inhalation Aerosol (2% to 10%) 839
Avalide Tablets (1% or greater) 892
Avalide Tablets (1% or greater) 2713
Avapro Tablets (1% or greater) 897
Avapro Tablets (1% or greater) 2718
▲ Avinza Capsules (5% to 10%) 1772
▲ Azmacort Inhalation Aerosol (1% to 3%) 407
Benicar Tablets (Greater than 0.5%) 1009
Benicar HCT Tablets (Greater than 2%) 1010
Betaseron for SC Injection 756
▲ Boniva Injection (1.8% to 5.5%) 2614
▲ Boniva Tablets (1.8% to 5.5%) 2618
Campral Tablets (Infrequent) 1158
Cancidas for Injection 1953
Ceftin for Oral Suspension (0.1% to 1%) 1380
Celebrex Capsules (0.1% to 1.9%) 2979
▲ CellCept Capsules (Less than 4% to 37.2%) 2622
▲ CellCept Intravenous (Less than 4% to 37.2%) 2622
▲ CellCept Oral Suspension (Less than 4% to 37.2%) 2622
▲ CellCept Tablets (Less than 4% to 37.2%) 2622
Cialis Tablets (0% to 2%) 1792
▲ Cimzia (7%) 3127
▲ Clarinex Syrup (3.6%) 2828
▲ Climara Pro Transdermal System (3.3%) 768
Combivent Inhalation Aerosol (Less than 2%) 845
▲ Cosopt Sterile Ophthalmic Solution (1% to 5%) 1969
▲ Cozaar Tablets (Less than 1% to 16%) 1973
Crinone 4% Gel 992
Crinone 8% Gel 992
▲ Cubicin for Injection (2.4% to 6.7%) 995
▲ Cymbalta Delayed-Release Capsules (3%) 1801
▲ Dacogen Injection (7%) 1066
▲ Depakote ER Tablets (Greater than 1% to less than 5%) 423
▲ DepoCyt Injection (14% to 18%) 1136
Diovan HCT Tablets (Greater than 0.2%) 2216
▲ Doxil Injection (1% to 10%) 2378
▲ Duetact Tablets (5.7% to 6.8%) 3085
Emend Capsules (Greater than 0.5%) 1992
Emend for Injection (Greater than 0.5%) 1999
Emsam Transdermal System (Frequent) 905
▲ Enablex Extended-Release Tablets (3.7% to 4.7%) 2225
Enbrel for Injection 569
Epivir 1412
▲ Epogen for Injection (3% to 12%) 576
▲ Equetro Extended-Release Capsules (Less than 5%) 3174
▲ Evista Tablets (4%) 1810
▲ Evoxac Capsules (6.1%) 1013
▲ Exelon Capsules (7%) 2229
▲ Exelon Oral Solution (7%) 2229
Exelon Patch (2%) 2233
▲ Faslodex Injection (6.1%) 682
▲ Femara Tablets (6%) 2246
Fentora Tablets (Greater than 1%) 968
▲ Flolan for Injection (7%) 1426
▲ Flovent Diskus 50 mcg (1% to 3%) 1435
▲ Flovent HFA (1% to 3%) 1440
Gabitril Tablets (1% or more) 973
▲ Gengraf Capsules (3% to 21.1%) 435
▲ Gliadel Wafer (8% to 21%) 1076
▲ Herceptin I.V. (5%) 1199
▲ Humira Injection (8%) 442
Imitrex Injection 1465
Imitrex Nasal Spray 1470
▲ Intron A for Injection (Less than 5% to 15%) 2859
▲ Invanz for Injection (3.8%) 2029
Ionsys Transdermal System (.1% to less than 1%) 2410
Ixempra Kit for Injection 915
Keppra Oral Solution (1% or more) 3131
Keppra Tablets (1% or more) 3131
Klonopin (1%) 2639
▲ Lamictal (3%) 1488
Lescol Capsules (1.6%) 2268
Lescol XL Tablets (2.7%) 2268
Lexapro Oral Suspension (Frequent) 1174
Lexapro Tablets (Frequent) 1174
Lipitor Tablets (Greater than or equal to 2%) 2501
▲ Lucentis Injection (4% to 12%) 1205
▲ Lunesta Tablets (0% to 3%) 2994
▲ Lupron Depot 7.5 mg (Less than 5%) 469
Luvox CR Extended-Release Capsules (2%) 1759
▲ Megace ES Oral Suspension (1% to 3%) 2499
Meridia Capsules (2.3%) 475
Micardis Tablets (1%) 852
Micardis HCT Tablets (2% or greater) 854
▲ Mirapex Tablets (Greater than or equal to 1% to 4%) 857
▲ Mobic Oral Suspension (0.3% to 6.9%) 863
▲ Mobic Tablets (0.3% to 6.9%) 863
▲ Myfortic Tablets (29.1%) 2276

Namenda (Greater than or equal to 2%) 1180
▲ NeoProfen Injection (9%) 2496
▲ Neoral Oral Solution (3% to 21.1%) 2280
▲ Neoral Soft Gelatin Capsules (3% to 21.1%) 2280
▲ Neupro Transdermal System (3%) 3149
▲ Novantrone for Injection Concentrate (7% to 32%) 1100
▲ NovoLog Injection (8%) 2359
▲ Orencia Powder for Intravenous Infusion (0.2% to 13%) 921
Patanase Nasal Spray (1.2%) 544
Paxil (2%) 1535
Paxil CR Controlled-Release Tablets (2%) 1544
▲ Photofrin for Injection (7%) 708
▲ Plavix Tablets (3.1%) 926
▲ Plavix Tablets (3.1%) 2767
Pletal Tablets (2% or greater) 2481
▲ Prandin Tablets (2% to 3%) 2971
Prevnar 3241
Prinivil Tablets (0.3% to 1%) 2087
Prinzide Tablets (0.3% to 1%) 2092
ProAir HFA Inhalation Aerosol (Less than 3%) 3113
▲ Procrit for Injection (3% to 12%) 2391
▲ Prograf Capsules and Injection (16% to 34%) 622
▲ Prometrium Capsules (100 mg, 200 mg) (Less than 5%) 3047
Protonix for Delayed-Release Oral Suspension (Greater than or equal to 1%) 3254
Protonix Delayed-Release Tablets (Greater than or equal to 1%) 3254
Protonix I.V. (Greater than or equal to 1%) 3257
Protopic Ointment (1% to 2%) 628
▲ Proventil HFA Inhalation Aerosol (3%) 2914
Provigil Tablets (At least 1%) 977
▲ Rapamune (26% to 33%) 3260
Remeron Tablets (Frequent) 2924
RemeronSolTab Tablets (Frequent) 2927
▲ Remicade for IV Injection (8%) 950
ReoPro Vials (1.9%) 1860
▲ Requip Tablets (Frequent to 5%) 1561
▲ Rilutek Tablets (2.5% to 4.5%) 2771
Rituxan I.V. 1223
Rocaltrol Capsules 1150
Rocaltrol Oral Solution 1150
RotaTeq (0.1%) 2110
Salagen Tablets (1% to 2%) 1082
▲ Sanctura XR Capsules (1.2% to 7.3%) 557
▲ Sandimmune (20.2% to 21.1%) 2296
▲ Sandostatin Injection (1% to 4%) 2300
▲ Simulect for Injection (Greater than or equal to 10%) 2306
▲ Spiriva HandiHaler (4% to 7%) 870
Stalevo Tablets 2309
Symbyax Capsules (Frequent) 1871
Targretin Capsules 1084
Tasigna Capsules (0.1% to 1%) 2316
▲ Temodar Capsules (8%) 2931
Testim 1% Gel 701
Teveten Tablets (1%) 515
Teveten HCT Tablets (Less than 1%) 517
Tice BCG (2%) 2936
▲ Torisel Injection (1% to 15%) 3272
Trasylol Injection (2%) 799
▲ Travatan Z Ophthalmic Solution (1% to 5%) 547
▲ Ultram ER Extended-Release Tablets (1% to lees than 5%) 2428
▲ Valcyte Tablets (Less than 5%) 2654
▲ Valstar Sterile Solution for Intravesical Instillation (15%) 1735
▲ Vaprisol (3.3% to 5%) 632
Velcade for Injection 2168
▲ VESIcare Tablets (2.8% to 4.8%) 636
Viadur Implant (Less than 2%) 802
Vivitrol 988
Vytorin 10/10 Tablets 2149
Vytorin 10/10 Tablets 2939
Vytorin 10/20 Tablets 2149
Vytorin 10/20 Tablets 2939
Vytorin 10/40 Tablets 2149
Vytorin 10/40 Tablets 2939
Vytorin 10/80 Tablets 2149
Vytorin 10/80 Tablets 2939
Wellbutrin Tablets (Infrequent) 1648
Wellbutrin SR Sustained-Release Tablets (Up to 1%) 1653
Wellbutrin XL Extended-Release Tablets (0% to 1%) 1659
▲ Xeloda Tablets (Less than 1% to 6%) 2662
▲ Xenical Capsules (5.9% to 7.5%) 2672
Xyrem Oral Solution (Frequent) 1766
Yaz Tablets (Greater than 1%) 805
▲ Zocor Tablets (3.2%) 2136
▲ Zometa for Intravenous Infusion (12% to 14%) 2341
Zomig Tablets (Rare) 694
Zomig Nasal Spray (Rare) 689
Zomig-ZMT Tablets (Rare) 694
Zyprexa Tablets (2%) 1883
Zyprexa ZYDIS Orally Disintegrating Tablets (2%) 1883
Zyrtec Chewable Tablets (Less than 2%) 1920
Zyrtec Syrup (Less than 2%) 1920
Zyrtec Tablets (Less than 2%) 1920
Zyrtec-D 12 Hour Extended Release Tablets (Less than 2%) 1923

Infection, urinary tract, fungal
Cubicin for Injection (Less than 1%) 995
Nexium Delayed-Release Capsules (Less than 1%) 645
Nexium I.V. (Less than 1%) 652
Nexium Delayed-Release Oral Suspension (Less than 1%) 645

Infection, vaginal
Mirapex Tablets 857
Ortho-Cyclen Tablets 2449
Ortho Evra Transdermal System 2437
Ortho Tri-Cyclen Tablets 2449
Ortho Tri-Cyclen Lo Tablets 2458
Requip Tablets (Infrequent) 1561
Xyrem Oral Solution (Infrequent) 1766

Infection, varicella zoster
Rituxan I.V. 1223

Infection, viral
▲ Aceon Tablets (2 mg, 4 mg, 8 mg) (0.3% to 3.4%) 3038
Actiq (1% or greater) 959
▲ Activella Tablets (0% to 6%) 2347
Adderall XR Capsules (2%) 3012
Advair Diskus 100/50 1276
Advair Diskus 250/50 1276
Advair Diskus 500/50 1276
▲ Advair HFA 45/21 Inhalation Aerosol (2% to 5%) 1288
▲ Advair HFA 115/21 Inhalation Aerosol (2% to 5%) 1288
▲ Advair HFA 230/21 Inhalation Aerosol (2% to 5%) 1288
Aldara Cream, 5% (1%) 1699
Allegra Oral Solution (2.5%) 2684
Aralast (Greater than or equal to 0.2%) 726
Atacand HCT (0.5% or greater) 642
▲ Avandamet Tablets (5%) 1336
Bexxar 1371
▲ Campath Ampules (4%) 761
Celebrex Capsules (0.1% to 1.9%) 2979
Cimzia 3127
Clarinex-D 12-Hour Extended-Release Tablets (2%) 2831
▲ Daytrana Transdermal Patch (28%) 3022
▲ Depakote ER Tablets (Greater than 1% to less than 5%) 423
Diclofenac Sodium Ophthalmic Solution ⊙240
▲ Diovan Tablets (3%) 2212
Diovan HCT Tablets (Less frequent) 2216
▲ Elidel Cream 1% (0% to 6.6%) 2221
Emsam Transdermal System (Infrequent) 905
Enbrel for Injection 569
Epivir-HBV (Among most common) 1417
▲ Equetro Extended-Release Capsules (Less than 5%) 3174
Evoxac Capsules (Less than 1%) 1013
▲ Fabrazyme for Intravenous Infusion (5%) 1241
▲ Femara Tablets (5% to 6%) 2246
▲ Flovent Diskus 50 mcg (2% to 9%) 1435
▲ Flovent HFA (1% to 3%) 1440
FML Ophthalmic Ointment ⊙223
FML Ophthalmic Suspension ⊙224
FML Forte Ophthalmic Suspension ⊙222
▲ Foradil Aerolizer (17.2%) 2849
▲ Gengraf Capsules (1% to 15.9%) 435
Humira Injection 442
▲ Intron A for Injection (Less than 5% to 7%) 2859
Kaletra (Less than 2%) 452
Keppra Oral Solution (2%) 3131
Keppra Tablets (2%) 3131
Klonopin (Infrequent) 2639
▲ Leustatin Injection (20%) 2384
Lovaza Capsules 1520
▲ Lunesta Tablets (3%) 2994
Luvox CR Extended-Release Capsules (2%) 1759
Mirapex Tablets 857
▲ Nasonex Nasal Spray (8% to 14%) 2883
▲ Neoral Oral Solution (1% to 15.9%) 2280
▲ Neoral Soft Gelatin Capsules (1% to 15.9%) 2280
Orthoclone OKT3 Sterile Solution (1.5%) 2387
▲ PegIntron Powder for Injection (11%) 2903
Pentacel 2792
Prinivil Tablets (0.3% to 1%) 2087
Prinzide Tablets (0.3% to 1%) 2092
Prolastin 3099
▲ Prometrium Capsules (100 mg, 200 mg) (7% to 12%) 3047
ProQuad (Greater than or equal to 0.2% to less than 1%) 2099
Provigil Tablets (Greater than or equal to 1%) 977
▲ Rebetol (12%) 2917
▲ Remicade for IV Injection (8%) 950
▲ Requip Tablets (Infrequent to 11%) 1561
▲ Rituxan I.V. (10%) 1223
Salagen Tablets (Less than 1%) 1082
▲ Sandimmune (15.9% to 18.4%) 2296
▲ Simulect for Injection (Greater than or equal to 10%) 2306
Singulair (Greater than or equal to 2%) 2114
Synagis Intramuscular Solution (More than 1%) 1948
▲ Temodar Capsules (11%) 2931
Teveten Tablets (2%) 515
Teveten HCT Tablets (Less than 1%) 517
Ultram ER Extended-Release Tablets (0.5% to less than 1%) 2428
Verdeso Foam (2%) 3069
▲ Voltaren Ophthalmic Solution (Less than or equal to 3%) 2336
▲ Xolair (23%) 1235
▲ Xolair (23%) 2339
▲ Xopenex Inhalation Solution (6.9% to 12.3%) 3001
▲ Xopenex Inhalation Solution Concentrate (6.9% to 12.3%) 3005
▲ Xopenex HFA Inhalation Aerosol (6.9% to 12.3%) 3009
▲ Ziagen (5%) 1673

Infection, vulvomycotic
Doribax Injection (1% to 2%) 2400
Moxatag Tablets (2%) 2165

Infection, West Nile virus
Rituxan I.V. 1223

Infection at injection site
Busulfex Injection 2477
Rebif Prefilled Syringe for Injection 1107
▲ Valcyte Tablets (3%) 2654

Infection with grade 3/4 neutropenia
▲ Alimta for Injection (Up to 6%) 1786

Infection/febrile neutropenia
▲ Alimta for Injection (Up to 6%) 1786
▲ Eloxatin for Injection (1% to 12%) 2731

Infections, unspecified
Aciphex Tablets (2%) 1053
▲ Keppra Injection (13%) 3137
Lamisil Oral Granules 2264
Salagen Tablets (2%) 1082
Tice BCG 2936
▲ Torisel Injection (3% to 20%) 3272

Infectious disorders, life-threatening, aggravation of
Bicillin C-R Injectable Suspension 1775
Bicillin L-A Injection 1777

Infectious-mononucleosis-like syndrome
Dapsone Tablets USP 1746

Infertility
Anaprox Tablets (Less than 1%) 2632
Anaprox DS Tablets (Less than 1%) 2632
EC-Naprosyn Delayed-Release Tablets (Less than 1%) 2632
Leukeran Tablets 1508
Levoxyl Tablets 1780
Naprosyn Suspension (Less than 1%) 2632
Naprosyn Tablets (Less than 1%) 2632

Infertility, male
Dapsone Tablets USP 1746

Infertility, temporary
Lybrel Tablets 3204
Mircette Tablets 1034
NuvaRing 2897
Ortho-Cyclen Tablets 2449
Ortho Evra Transdermal System 2437
Ortho Tri-Cyclen Tablets 2449
Ortho Tri-Cyclen Lo Tablets 2458
Seasonique Tablets 1046

Inflammation, eye
Actonel Tablets 2568
▲ Durezol Ophthalmic Emulsion (1% to 5%) ⊙275

Inflammation, eye, anterior chamber
▲ Durezol Ophthalmic Emulsion (5% to 15%) ⊙275
Triesence Injectable Suspension (2%) ⊙209

Inflammation, genital
Tice BCG (2%) 2936

Inflammation, mucosal
▲ Cancidas for Injection (3.6% to 10.4%) 1953
▲ Clolar for Intravenous Infusion (18%) 1239
Dacogen Injection 1066
Emend Capsules (2.5%) 1992
Emend for Injection (2.5%) 1999
Fentora Tablets (Greater than 1%) 968
▲ Mycamine for Injection (14.2% to 75.8%) 616
Treanda for Injection 983
▲ Tykerb Tablets (0% to 15%) 1631
▲ Vectibix (Less than 1% to 6%) 597

Inflammation, nasal
Imitrex Nasal Spray 1470
Relenza Inhalation Powder (1%) 1556

Inflammation, ocular
Enbrel for Injection 569
Rilutek Tablets (Infrequent) 2771
Rythmol SR Capsules 1590
Zometa for Intravenous Infusion 2341
Zyprexa Tablets (Infrequent) 1883
Zyprexa ZYDIS Orally Disintegrating Tablets (Infrequent) 1883

Inflammation, oral
(*see under* Stomatitis)

Inflammation, unspecified
▲ Advair HFA 45/21 Inhalation Aerosol (1% to 3%) 1288
▲ Advair HFA 115/21 Inhalation Aerosol (1% to 3%) 1288
▲ Advair HFA 230/21 Inhalation Aerosol (1% to 3%) 1288
Klonopin (Infrequent) 2639
▲ Panretin Gel 0.1% (3% to 8%) 1081
ProQuad 2099
ReoPro Vials (0.1%) 1860

Inflammation, upper respiratory tract
Advair Diskus 100/50 1276
▲ Advair Diskus 250/50 (6%) 1276
▲ Advair Diskus 500/50 (6%) 1276
▲ Advair HFA 45/21 Inhalation Aerosol (4%) 1288
▲ Advair HFA 115/21 Inhalation Aerosol (4%) 1288
▲ Advair HFA 230/21 Inhalation Aerosol (4%) 1288
Amerge Tablets (Infrequent) 1301
▲ Flovent Diskus 50 mcg (5%) 1435
Flovent HFA (2%) 1440
Imitrex Nasal Spray 1470
▲ Ventolin HFA Inhalation Aerosol (5%) 1638

Inflammation, wound
Ionsys Transdermal System (.1% to less than 1%) 2410

Inflammation at application site
Aldara Cream, 5% 1699
Daytrana Transdermal Patch 3022
Zovirax Cream 817

Inflammation at injection site
Abelcet Injection 1134
Ambien Tablets (Rare) 2692
AmBisome for Injection (Less common) 606
▲ Amevive (4% to common) 611
▲ Betaseron for SC Injection (42%) 756
Bicillin C-R Injectable Suspension 1775
Bicillin L-A Injection 1777
Boostrix 1377
▲ Busulfex Injection (25%) 2477
▲ Copaxone for Injection (49%) 3110

Delatestryl Injection ... 1730
Doxil Injection (Less than 1%) ... 2378
Estratest Tablets ... 3043
Estratest H.S. Tablets ... 3043
Flulaval Injection Vaccine ... 1448
Fortaz (1 in 69 patients) ... 1450
Genotropin Lyophilized Powder (Infrequent) ... 2547
▲ Havrix Injection Vaccine (1% to 10%) ... 1454
Humalog-Pen and KwikPen ... 1829
Humulin 50/50, 100 Units ... 1843
Humulin 70/30 Vial ... 1844
Humulin N Vial ... 1846
Humulin R (U-500) ... 1850
Imitrex Injection ... 1465
▲ Infanrix Vaccine (1% to 39.5%) ... 1479
▲ Intron A for Injection (Up to 5%) ... 2859
Lovenox Injection ... 2756
Merrem I.V. (2.4%) ... 684
▲ Miacalcin Injection (About 10%) ... 2273
▲ PegIntron Powder for Injection (47%) ... 2903
Pentacel ... 2792
Romazicon Injection ... 2646
Taxotere Injection Concentrate ... 2773
Tygacil for Injection (0% to less than 2%) ... 3276
Varivax (Less than 0.05%) ... 2133
▲ Visudyne for Injection (10% to 30%) ... 2332
Xolair ... 1235
Xolair ... 2339
▲ Zofran Injection (4%) ... 1682
Zosyn for Injection (0.2% to 1.3%) ... 3284

Inflammation at insertion site
Vantas (2 patients) ... 1737

Influenza
Aczone Gel 5% (1%) ... 3296
Advair HFA 45/21 Inhalation Aerosol ... 1288
Advair HFA 115/21 Inhalation Aerosol ... 1288
Advair HFA 230/21 Inhalation Aerosol ... 1288
▲ Alvesco Inhalation Aerosol (Greater than or equal to 3%) ... 2985
▲ Ambien CR Tablets (1% to 3%) ... 2696
Amitiza Capsules (Less than 1%) ... 3082
▲ Avalide Tablets (3%) ... 892
▲ Avalide Tablets (3%) ... 2713
Avandamet Tablets (1%) ... 1336
▲ Boniva Injection (3.8% to 4%) ... 2614
▲ Boniva Tablets (3.8% to 4%) ... 2618
▲ Cialis Tablets (2% to 5%) ... 1792
Combivent Inhalation Aerosol (1.4%) ... 845
Cymbalta Delayed-Release Capsules (2%) ... 1801
Diovan HCT Tablets (Greater than 0.2%) ... 2216
▲ Elidel Cream 1% (3% to 13.2%) ... 2221
▲ Exjade Tablets (10.8%) ... 2244
Fentora Tablets (Greater than 1%) ... 968
Genotropin Lyophilized Powder ... 2547
▲ Gleevec Tablets (0.8% to 13.8%) ... 2255
▲ Keppra Injection (5%) ... 3137
Lamisil Oral Granules (2%) ... 2264
Lescol Capsules ... 2268
Lescol XL Tablets ... 2268
▲ Lucentis Injection (2% to 10%) ... 1205
▲ Myfortic Tablets (3% to less than 20%) ... 2276
▲ Orencia Powder for Intravenous Infusion (5% to 13%) ... 921
Patanase Nasal Spray (0.9%) ... 544
ProQuad ... 2099
▲ Reclast Injection (7%) ... 2291
▲ Requip Tablets (3%) ... 1561
Rozerem Tablets (1%) ... 3091
Sanctura XR Capsules (2.2%) ... 557
Selzentry Tablets (1.6%) ... 2534
▲ Singulair (4.2%) ... 2114
▲ Symbicort 80/4.5 Inhalation Aerosol (3.2%) ... 659
Symbicort 160/4.5 Inhalation Aerosol (2.4%) ... 659
Tekturna HCT Tablets (2.3%) ... 2324
▲ Tyzeka Tablets (7%) ... 2328
▲ Ultram ER Extended-Release Tablets (1% to less than 5%) ... 2428
VESIcare Tablets (0.9% to 2.2%) ... 636
Vivitrol ... 988
Vytorin 10/10 Tablets (2.3%) ... 2149
Vytorin 10/10 Tablets (2.3%) ... 2939
Vytorin 10/20 Tablets (2.3%) ... 2149
Vytorin 10/20 Tablets (2.3%) ... 2939
Vytorin 10/40 Tablets (2.3%) ... 2149
Vytorin 10/40 Tablets (2.3%) ... 2939
Vytorin 10/80 Tablets (2.3%) ... 2149
Vytorin 10/80 Tablets (2.3%) ... 2939
Xyrem Oral Solution (Frequent) ... 1766
Zetia Tablets (2%) ... 2157
Zetia Tablets (2% to 2.2%) ... 2951

Influenza-like illness
Actonel Tablets (0% to 0.6%) ... 2568
Ambien Tablets (2%) ... 2692
Aptivus Capsules (Less than 2%) ... 823
Aptivus Oral Solution (Less than 2%) ... 823
▲ Aranesp for Injection (6%) ... 564
Chantix Tablets (Frequent) ... 2511
Crinone 4% Gel ... 992
Crinone 8% Gel ... 992
▲ Edex Injection (3%) ... 2957
Elidel Cream 1% (0.4% to 1.8%) ... 2221
Mirapex Tablets ... 857
Neupro Transdermal System (Greater than or equal to 2%) ... 3149
▲ Nexavar Tablets (1% to less than 10%) ... 784
▲ Reclast Injection (0.8% to 11%) ... 2291
▲ Sandostatin LAR Depot (19.9%) ... 2302
Selzentry Tablets ... 2534
Supprelin LA Implant ... 1731
Tasigna Capsules (0.1% to 1%) ... 2316
Thyrogen for Injection ... 1244
▲ Ultram ER Extended-Release Tablets (1% to less than 5%) ... 2428

Infusion reaction
▲ Campath Ampules (10% to 35%) ... 761
▲ Cancidas for Injection (20.2%) ... 1953
Doxil Injection ... 2378
▲ Erbitux (2% to 21%) ... 912
Fabrazyme for Intravenous Infusion ... 1241
Herceptin I.V. ... 1199
Orencia Powder for Intravenous Infusion ... 921
▲ Remicade for IV Injection (18%) ... 950
▲ Rituxan I.V. (9% to 32%) ... 1223
Treanda for Injection ... 983
▲ Vectibix (1% to 4%) ... 597

Inhalation site sensation
▲ Proventil HFA Inhalation Aerosol (6%) ... 2914

Initial insomnia
▲ Concerta Extended-Release Tablets (4.3%) ... 1925
▲ Cymbalta Delayed-Release Capsules (10%) ... 1801
Mirapex Tablets ... 857
▲ Vyvanse Capsules (4%) ... 3033

Injection site sterile abscess
Flulaval Injection Vaccine ... 1448
Pentacel ... 2792
Vivitrol ... 988

Injury, accidental
▲ Activella Tablets (3% to 17%) ... 2347
▲ Actonel Tablets (16.9%) ... 2568
▲ Advate (17.3%) ... 721
▲ Angeliq Tablets (5.7%) ... 751
▲ Arimidex Tablets (2% to 10%) ... 672
▲ Azilect Tablets (12%) ... 3106
▲ Climara Pro Transdermal System (3.3%) ... 768
▲ Concerta Extended-Release Tablets (6%) ... 1925
▲ Duetact Tablets (Greater than 5%) ... 3085
▲ Effexor XR Extended-Release Capsules (4%) ... 3195
Emsam Transdermal System ... 905
▲ Equetro Extended-Release Capsules (7%) ... 3174
▲ Herceptin I.V. (6%) ... 1199
▲ Humira Injection (10%) ... 442
▲ Lunesta Tablets (0% to 3%) ... 2994
▲ Luvox CR Extended-Release Capsules (5%) ... 1759
▲ Lyrica Capsules (2% to 11%) ... 2527
▲ Meridia Capsules (5.9%) ... 475
▲ Mirapex Tablets (17%) ... 857
▲ Premarin Tablets (6% to 12%) ... 3221
▲ Premphase Tablets (4% to 5%) ... 3232
▲ Prempro Tablets (4% to 5%) ... 3232
ProAir HFA Inhalation Aerosol (Less than 3%) ... 3113
Prozac Pulvules and Liquid ... 1852
Salagen Tablets (1% to 2%) ... 1082
▲ Suboxone Tablets (3%) ... 2601
▲ Subutex Tablets (3%) ... 2601
▲ Symbyax Capsules (3% to 5%) ... 1871
▲ Travatan Z Ophthalmic Solution (1% to 5%) ... 547
Yaz Tablets (Greater than 1%) ... 805
▲ Zyprexa Tablets (4% to 12%) ... 1883
▲ Zyprexa ZYDIS Orally Disintegrating Tablets (4% to 12%) ... 1883

Injury, back
Xyrem Oral Solution (Infrequent) ... 1766

Injury, head
Xyrem Oral Solution (Infrequent) ... 1766

Injury, intentional
Campral Tablets (Infrequent) ... 1158
Emsam Transdermal System (Infrequent) ... 905
Lyrica Capsules (Rare) ... 2527
Prozac Weekly Capsules (Rare) ... 1852
Symbyax Capsules (Infrequent) ... 1871
Tamiflu Capsules ... 2649
Tamiflu Oral Suspension ... 2649
Zyprexa Tablets (Infrequent) ... 1883
Zyprexa ZYDIS Orally Disintegrating Tablets (Infrequent) ... 1883

Injury, limb
▲ Advate (34.7%) ... 721
Exforge Tablets (Greater than or equal to 0.2%) ... 2238
Xyrem Oral Solution (Infrequent) ... 1766

Injury, tooth
Xyrem Oral Solution (Infrequent) ... 1766

INR, abnormal
Avelox (Less than 0.1%) ... 2803
Nexavar Tablets (0.1% to less than 1%) ... 784

INR, increase
Avelox (Greater than or equal to 0.1% to less than 2%) ... 2803
Cubicin for Injection (1.7%) ... 995
Eloxatin for Injection ... 2731
Levaquin ... 2416
Levaquin in 5% Dextrose Injection ... 2416
Lexapro Oral Suspension ... 1174
Lexapro Tablets ... 1174
Namenda ... 1180
▲ Nexavar Tablets (4% to 42%) ... 784
Stromectol Tablets ... 2120
Tygacil for Injection (0% to less than 2%) ... 3276

Insomnia
▲ Abilify Injection (8% to 18%) ... 881
▲ Abilify Injection (8% to 18%) ... 2466
▲ Abilify Oral Solution (8% to 18%) ... 881
▲ Abilify Oral Solution (8% to 18%) ... 2466
▲ Abilify Discmelt Orally Disintegrating Tablets (8% to 18%) ... 881
▲ Abilify Discmelt Orally Disintegrating Tablets (8% to 18%) ... 2466
▲ Abilify Tablets (8% to 18%) ... 881
▲ Abilify Tablets (8% to 18%) ... 2466
Accolate Tablets ... 669
Accutane Capsules ... 2607
Actiq (1% to 2%) ... 959
▲ Activella Tablets (0% to 6%) ... 2347
▲ Actonel Tablets (5%) ... 2568
▲ Actonel with Calcium Tablets (4.3%) ... 2574
▲ Adderall XR Capsules (1.5% to 27%) ... 3012
Adipex-P ... 1185
Advicor Tablets ... 402
▲ Aerobid/Aerobid-M (1% to 3%) ... 1153
▲ Agrylin Capsules (1% to less than 5%) ... 3017
Aldara Cream, 5% ... 1699
Alferon N Injection (2%) ... 1726
Alinia for Oral Suspension (Less than 1%) ... 2677
Alinia Tablets (Less than 1%) ... 2677
Allegra Oral Solution (Less than 1%) ... 2684
Allegra Tablets (Rare) ... 2684
▲ Allegra-D 12 Hour Extended-Release Tablets (12.6%) ... 2687
▲ Allegra-D 24 Hour Extended-Release Tablets (12.6%) ... 2690
Aloxi Injection (Less than 1%) ... 1059
▲ Alphagan P Ophthalmic Solution (1% to 4%) ... 549
Ambien Tablets (Frequent) ... 2692
Ambien CR Tablets (Frequent) ... 2696
Amoxil Capsules (Rare) ... 1305
Amoxil Chewable Tablets (Rare) ... 1305
Amoxil Pediatric Drops for Oral Suspension (Rare) ... 1305
Amoxil Powder for Oral Suspension (Rare) ... 1305
Amoxil Tablets (Rare) ... 1305
Amrix Capsules ... 966
Anaprox Tablets (Less than 1%) ... 2632
Anaprox DS Tablets (Less than 1%) ... 2632
AndroGel ... 3159
▲ Angiomax for Injection (7%) ... 1933
Aptivus Capsules (1.7%) ... 823
Aptivus Oral Solution (1.7%) ... 823
▲ Aricept Tablets (5%) ... 1062
▲ Aricept ODT Tablets (5%) ... 1062
▲ Arimidex Tablets (2% to 10%) ... 672
▲ Arixtra Injection (0.9% to 5%) ... 1313
▲ Arranon Injection (0% to 7%) ... 1319
Asacol Delayed-Release Tablets (2%) ... 2579
Atacand HCT (0.5% or greater) ... 642
▲ Atripla Tablets (Greater than or equal to 10%) ... 938
Augmentin (Rare) ... 1323
Augmentin Tablets (Rare) ... 1327
Augmentin XR Extended Release Tablets (Rare) ... 1333
Augmentin ES-600 Powder for Oral Suspension (Rare) ... 1329
Avelox (Greater than or equal to 0.1% to less than 2%) ... 2803
▲ Avinza Capsules (5% to 10%) ... 1772
Axert Tablets (Infrequent) ... 2431
Axid Capsules (2.7%) ... 1364
Baraclude (Less than 1%) ... 900
Benicar Tablets (Greater than 0.5%) ... 1009
Bentyl Capsules ... 703
Bentyl Injection ... 703
Bentyl Syrup ... 703
Bentyl Tablets ... 703
▲ Betaseron for SC Injection (21%) ... 756
Biaxin/Biaxin XL ... 411
Boniva Injection (0.8% to 2%) ... 2614
Boniva Tablets (0.8% to 2%) ... 2618
Brovana Inhalation Solution ... 2990
▲ Busulfex Injection (84%) ... 2477
Bystolic Tablets (1%) ... 1155
▲ Campath Ampules (10%) ... 761
▲ Campral Tablets (6% to 9%) ... 1158
Cancidas for Injection ... 1953
Captopril Tablets (About 0.5 to 2%) ... 2182
Carafate Suspension (Less than 0.5%) ... 706
Carafate Tablets (Less than 0.5%) ... 707
Cardizem LA Extended Release Tablets (Less than 2%) ... 421
Catapres Tablets (About 5 in 1,000 patients) ... 841
Catapres-TTS (2 of 101 patients) ... 842
Celebrex Capsules (2.3%) ... 2979
▲ Celexa (3% to 15%) ... 1160
▲ CellCept Capsules (40.8% to 52.3%) ... 2622
▲ CellCept Intravenous (40.8% to 52.3%) ... 2622
▲ CellCept Oral Suspension (40.8% to 52.3%) ... 2622
▲ CellCept Tablets (40.8% to 52.3%) ... 2622
▲ Chantix Tablets (1.2% to 19%) ... 2511
Cialis Tablets (Less than 2%) ... 1792
Cipro I.V. (1% or less) ... 2817
Cipro (Less than 1%) ... 2810
Cipro XR Tablets (Less than 1%) ... 2823
▲ Clarinex Syrup (4.5%) ... 2828
▲ Clarinex-D 12-Hour Extended-Release Tablets (10%) ... 2831
▲ Clarinex-D 24-Hour Extended-Release Tablets (5%) ... 2834
Clinoril Tablets (Less than 1%) ... 1962
Clorpres Tablets (About 5 in 1,000) ... 2185
Combigan Ophthalmic Solution (0.1% to 0.2%) ... 553
Combivent Inhalation Aerosol (Less than 2%) ... 845
▲ Combivir Tablets (11%) ... 1384
▲ Concerta Extended-Release Tablets (1.3% to 12.3%) ... 1925
Copaxone for Injection (At least 2%) ... 3110
Coreg Tablets (2%) ... 1387
Coreg CR Extended-Release Capsules (1% to 2%) ... 1393
Cosopt Sterile Ophthalmic Solution ... 1969
Cozaar Tablets (1% or greater) ... 1973
Crinone 4% Gel ... 992
Crinone 8% Gel ... 992
▲ Cubicin for Injection (4.5% to 11.2%) ... 995
▲ Cymbalta Delayed-Release Capsules (8% to 16%) ... 1801
▲ Dacogen Injection (28%) ... 1066
Dantrium Capsules (Less frequent) ... 2580
Dapsone Tablets USP ... 1746
▲ Daytrana Transdermal Patch (4% to 30%) ... 3022
Demadex Injection (1.2%) ... 2630
Demadex Tablets (1.2%) ... 2630
▲ Depakote ER Tablets (Greater than 1% to less than 5%) ... 423
▲ DepoCyt Injection (14% to 18%) ... 1136
▲ DepoDur Injection (5% to 10%) ... 1095
Dexedrine ... 1401

Diclofenac Sodium Ophthalmic Solution ⊙ 240
Diovan Tablets (Greater than 0.2%) 2212
Diovan HCT Tablets (Greater than 0.2%) 2216
Donnatal Extentabs 2507
▲ Doxil Injection (Less than 1% to 10%) 2378
▲ Duragesic Transdermal System (3% to 10%) 2405
DynaCirc CR Controlled Release Tablets (0.5% to 1%) 1407
EC-Naprosyn Delayed-Release Tablets (Less than 1%) 2632
▲ Effexor XR Extended-Release Capsules (3% to 24%) 3195
Eldepryl Capsules (1 of 49 patients) 3052
Eligard 7.5 mg (Less than 2%) 2724
Eligard 22.5 mg (Less than 2%) 2724
Eligard 30 mg (Less than 2%) 2724
Eligard 45 mg (Less than 2%) 2724
Elmiron Capsules 2435
▲ Eloxatin for Injection (11% to 13%) 2731
▲ Emend Capsules (2.1% to 4.1%) 1992
▲ Emend for Injection (2.1% to 4.1%) 1999
▲ Emsam Transdermal System (12%) 905
▲ Emtriva Capsules (Greater than or equal to 10%) 1246
▲ Emtriva Oral Solution (Greater than or equal to 10%) 1246
Engerix-B Vaccine (Less than 1%) 1409
▲ Epivir (11%) 1412
▲ Epogen for Injection (13% to 21%) 576
▲ Epzicom Tablets (7% to 9%) 1422
▲ Equetro Extended-Release Capsules (Less than 5%) 3174
▲ Erbitux (1% to 30%) 912
▲ Evista Tablets (5.5%) 1810
Evoxac Capsules (2.4%) 1013
▲ Exelon Capsules (3% to 9%) 2229
▲ Exelon Oral Solution (3% to 9%) 2229
▲ Exelon Patch (1% to 4%) 2233
Exforge Tablets (Greater than or equal to 0.2%) 2238
Exjade Tablets 2244
▲ Fabrazyme for Intravenous Infusion (9%) 1241
Fansidar Tablets 2636
▲ Faslodex Injection (6.9%) 682
▲ Femara Tablets (Less than 0.1% to 7%) 2246
▲ Fentora Tablets (1% to 11%) 968
▲ Flolan for Injection (4% to 9%) 1426
Flomax Capsules (1.4% to 2.4%) 848
Flulaval Injection Vaccine 1448
Flumadine (2.1% to 3.4%) 1167
Focalin XR Capsules 2251
Foradil Aerolizer (1.5%) 2849
▲ Forteo for Injection (4.3%) 1816
Frova Tablets (Frequent) 1111
▲ Gabitril Tablets (6%) 973
Gantrisin Pediatric Suspension 2638
Gardasil Injection (1.2%) 2019
Gemzar for Injection (Infrequent) 1820
Gengraf Capsules (1% to less than 3%) 435
Geodon (Rare) 2520
▲ Gleevec Tablets (10% to 19%) 2255
▲ Gliadel Wafer (2% to 5%) 1076
Gris-PEG Tablets (Occasional) 2507
Havrix Injection Vaccine (Less than 1%) 1454
▲ Herceptin I.V. (14%) 1199
▲ Indapamide Tablets (Less than 5%) 2188
Indocin (Less than 1%) 2024
InnoPran XL Extended Release Capsules 1484
Intelence Tablets (Less than 2%) 3119
▲ Intron A for Injection (Up to 12%) 2859
▲ Invanz for Injection (3% to 3.2%) 2029
▲ Ionsys Transdermal System (3%) 2410
▲ Ixempra Kit for Injection (5%) 915
Kaletra (Up to 2%) 452
Keppra Injection (1.7%) 3137
Keppra Oral Solution (1% to greater than or equal to 2%) 3131
Keppra Tablets (1% to greater than or equal to 2%) 3131
Ketek Tablets (Greater than or equal to 0.2% to less than 2%) 2744
Klonopin (Infrequent) 2639
▲ Lamictal (5% to 10%) 1488
Lescol Capsules (2.7%) 2268
Lescol XL Tablets (0.8%) 2268
▲ Leukine (11%) 774
▲ Leustatin Injection (7%) 2384
▲ Levaquin (4%) 2416
▲ Levaquin in 5% Dextrose Injection (4%) 2416
Levitra Tablets (Less than 2%) 2876
Levothroid Tablets 1170
Levoxyl Tablets 1780
▲ Lexapro Oral Suspension (1% to 14%) 1174
▲ Lexapro Tablets (1% to 14%) 1174
Lipitor Tablets (Greater than or equal to 2%) 2501
Lovaza Capsules 1520
Lunesta Tablets (Infrequent) 2994
▲ Lupron Depot 3.75 mg (16%) 462
▲ Lupron Depot 7.5 mg (Less than 5%) 469
▲ Lupron Depot–3 Month 11.25 mg (16%) 462
▲ Luvox CR Extended-Release Capsules (5% to 35%) 1759
▲ Malarone Pediatric Tablets (2% to 3%) 1521
▲ Malarone Tablets (2% to 3%) 1521
▲ Marplan Tablets (4% to 6%) 3177
Mavik Tablets (0.3% to 1%) 472
Maxair Autohaler 1705
Maxalt Tablets (Infrequent) 2056
Maxalt-MLT Orally Disintegrating Tablets (Infrequent) 2056
▲ Megace ES Oral Suspension (0% to 6%) 2499
▲ Mepron Suspension (10% to 19%) 1526
▲ Meridia Capsules (10.7%) 475
Merrem I.V. (Greater than 0.1% to 1%) 684
▲ Metadate CD Capsules (5%) 3146
Mevacor Tablets (0.5% to 1%) 2063
Miacalcin Nasal Spray (Less than 1%) 2274
Micardis Tablets (More than 0.3%) 852
Micardis HCT Tablets 854
▲ Mirapex Tablets (13% to 27%) 857
▲ Mobic Oral Suspension (0% to 3.6%) 863
▲ Mobic Tablets (0% to 3.6%) 863
Moxatag Tablets 2165
MS Contin Tablets (Less frequent) 2585
▲ Mycamine for Injection (3.5% to 35.8%) 616
▲ Myfortic Tablets (23.5%) 2276
▲ Mylotarg for Injection (11% to 13%) 3212
Nalfon Capsules (Less than 1%) 2508
Namenda (Greater than or equal to 2%) 1180
Naprosyn Suspension (Less than 1%) 2632
Naprosyn Tablets (Less than 1%) 2632
▲ Natrecor for Injection (2% to 6%) 2977
Nembutal Sodium Solution, USP (Less than 1%) 2494
▲ Neoral Oral Solution (1% to 3%) 2280
▲ Neoral Soft Gelatin Capsules (1% to 3%) 2280
▲ Neulasta Injection (15% to 72%) 587
▲ Neupro Transdermal System (5% to 14%) 3149
Nexium Delayed-Release Capsules (Less than 1%) 645
Nexium I.V. (Less than 1%) 652
Nexium Delayed-Release Oral Suspension (Less than 1%) 645
Niaspan Extended-Release Tablets 480
Noroxin Tablets (Less frequent) 2069
Norvir (2% to 2.6%) 489
▲ Noxafil Oral Suspension (1% to 17%) 2889
Omnicef Capsules (0.2%) 497
Omnicef for Oral Suspension (0.2%) 497
▲ Ontak Vials (9%) 1079
Opana Tablets (Less than 1%) 1117
▲ Opana ER Tablets (4%) 1121
Ortho-Cyclen/Ortho Tri-Cyclen 2449
Ortho Tri-Cyclen Lo Tablets 2458
▲ OxyContin Tablets (Between 1% and 5%) 2589
Parnate Tablets 1532
▲ Paxil (1.3% to 24%) 1535
▲ Paxil CR Controlled-Release Tablets (1.3% to 24%) 1544
▲ PegIntron Powder for Injection (23%) 2903
Pentasa Capsules (Less than 1%) 3030
Pepcid Tablets (Infrequent) 2075
Percocet Tablets 1127
Perforomist Inhalation Solution (2.4%) 1025
Phenytek Capsules 2192
▲ Photofrin for Injection (4% to 14%) 708
Plavix Tablets (1% to 2.5%) 926
Plavix Tablets (1% to 2.5%) 2767
Pletal Tablets (Less than 2%) 2481
▲ Premarin Tablets (6% to 7%) 3221
▲ Premphase Tablets (6% to 7%) 3232
▲ Prempro Tablets (6% to 7%) 3232
Prinivil Tablets (0.3% to 1%) 2087
Prinzide Tablets 2092
▲ Pristiq Extended-Release Tablets (5% to 15%) 3247
ProAmatine Tablets (Rare) 3032
▲ Procrit for Injection (13% to 21%) 2391
Proglycem Capsules (Infrequent) 1185
Proglycem Suspension (Infrequent) 1185
▲ Prograf Capsules and Injection (32% to 64%) 622
Proleukin for Injection 2287
▲ Prometrium Capsules (100 mg, 200 mg) (Less than 5%) 3047
ProQuad (Greater than or equal to 0.2% to less than 1%) 2099
Protonix for Delayed-Release Oral Suspension (Less than or equal to 1%) 3254
Protonix Delayed-Release Tablets (Less than or equal to 1%) 3254
Protonix I.V. (Greater than or equal to 1%) 3257
▲ Protopic Ointment (Up to 4%) 628
Proventil HFA Inhalation Aerosol 2914
▲ Provigil Tablets (5%) 977
▲ Prozac Weekly Capsules (2% to 33%) 1852
▲ Prozac Pulvules and Liquid (10% to 33%) 1852
▲ Pulmicort Flexhaler (Greater than or equal to 1% to 3%) 654
▲ Rebetol (14% to 41%) 2917
Recombivax HB (Less to greater than 1%) 2107
ReFacto Vials 3269
Remeron Tablets 2924
RemeronSolTab Tablets 2927
ReoPro Vials (0.3%) 1860
Requip Tablets (1% or more) 1561
Requip XL Tablets 1568
▲ Retrovir Capsules (2.4% to 5%) 1574
▲ Retrovir IV Infusion (3% to 5%) 1579
▲ Retrovir (2.4% to 5%) 1574
▲ Reyataz Capsules (Less than 1% to 3%) 3299
Rilutek Tablets (2.1% to 2.9%) 2771
▲ Risperdal Consta Long-Acting Injection (13%) 1753
▲ Romazicon Injection (3% to 9%) 2646
▲ Rozerem Tablets (3%) 3091
Rythmol Tablets (2%) 1586
Rythmol SR Capsules 1590
Salagen Tablets (Less than 1%) 1082
▲ Simulect for Injection (Greater than or equal to 10%) 2306
Singulair 2114
Soma Tablets 1931
▲ Soriatane Capsules (1% to 10%) 3062
Stalevo Tablets 2309
▲ Strattera Capsules (0.9% to 15%) 1864
▲ Suboxone Tablets (14% to 25%) 2601
▲ Subutex Tablets (21.4% to 25%) 2601
Sular Extended Release Tablets (Less than or equal to 1%) 2975
▲ Sustiva Capsules (1% to 7%) 930
▲ Sustiva Tablets (1% to 7%) 930
▲ Sutent Capsules (Less than 1% to 11%) 2540
Symbyax Capsules 1871
Tamiflu Capsules (1%) 2649
Tamiflu Oral Suspension (1%) 2649
▲ Tarceva Tablets (0% to 15%) 1228
▲ Targretin Capsules (4.8% to 11.3%) 1084
Tarka Tablets (Less frequent) 511
▲ Tasigna Capsules (1% to 10%) 2316
▲ Temodar Capsules (4% to 10%) 2931
Testim 1% Gel (1% or less) 701
Teveten Tablets (Less than 1%) 515
Teveten HCT Tablets (Less than 1%) 517
Thiothixene Capsules 2197
Thyrogen for Injection (1.5%) 1244
Timoptic Sterile Ophthalmic Solution 2121
Timoptic in Ocudose (Less frequent) 2124
Timoptic-XE Sterile Ophthalmic Gel Forming Solution 2125
Toprol-XL Tablets 666
▲ Torisel Injection (1% to 12%) 3272
▲ Trasylol Injection (3%) 799
Treximet Tablets (Infrequent) 1616
Tricor Tablets 520
▲ Trisenox Injection (43%) 986
▲ Trizivir Tablets (7% to 13%) 1622
▲ Truvada Tablets (Greater than or equal to 10%) 1262
Twinrix Vaccine (Less than 1%) 1628
Tygacil for Injection (2.3%) 3276
▲ Tykerb Tablets (0% to 10%) 1631
Tylenol Cold Severe Congestion Daytime Caplets with Cool Burst 1912
Tylenol Sinus Congestion & Pain Daytime Caplets with Cool Burst and Gelcaps 1917
Tylenol Sinus Congestion & Pain Nighttime Caplets with Cool Burst 1917
Tylenol Sinus Congestion & Pain Severe Caplets with Cool Burst 1917
Tylenol Sinus Severe Congestion Caplets with Cool Burst 1917
▲ Tyzeka Tablets (3%) 2328
Ultane Liquid for Inhalation (Less than 1%) 524
▲ Ultram ER Extended-Release Tablets (6.5% to 10.9%) 2428
Uniphyl Tablets 2595
▲ Vagifem Tablets (3% to 5%) 2375
▲ Valcyte Tablets (16% to 20%) 2654
Valium Tablets 2658
Vantas (2.9%) 1737
▲ Vaprisol (3.3% to 5%) 632
▲ Velcade for Injection (18% to 20%) 2168
▲ Venlafaxine Hydrochloride Tablets (3% to 22.5%) 2199
Ventolin HFA Inhalation Aerosol 1638
▲ Vesanoid Capsules (14%) 2660
▲ Vicoprofen Tablets (3% to 9%) 533
▲ Viread Tablets (3% to 5%) 1268
▲ Vivitrol (8% to 14%) 988
▲ Voltaren Ophthalmic Solution (Less than or equal to 3%) 2336
Voltaren Tablets (Occasionally) 2334
Voltaren-XR Tablets (Occasionally) 2337
Vytorin 10/10 Tablets 2149
Vytorin 10/10 Tablets 2939
Vytorin 10/20 Tablets 2149
Vytorin 10/20 Tablets 2939
Vytorin 10/40 Tablets 2149
Vytorin 10/40 Tablets 2939
Vytorin 10/80 Tablets 2149
Vytorin 10/80 Tablets 2939
▲ Vyvanse Capsules (19% to 27%) 3033
▲ Wellbutrin Tablets (18.6%) 1648
▲ Wellbutrin SR Sustained-Release Tablets (5% to 16%) 1653
▲ Wellbutrin XL Extended-Release Tablets (11% to 20%) 1659
▲ Xeloda Tablets (Less than 5%) 2662
Xifaxan Tablets (Less than 2%) 2682
Xopenex Inhalation Solution 3001
Xopenex Inhalation Solution Concentrate 3005
Xopenex HFA Inhalation Aerosol 3009
Xyrem Oral Solution (Frequent) 1766
Zantac 25 EFFERdose Tablets (Rare) 1670
Zantac Injection 1666
Zantac Injection Pharmacy Bulk Package (Rare) 1668
Zantac Injection Premixed 1666
Zantac (Rare) 1670
Zocor Tablets 2136
▲ Zometa for Intravenous Infusion (15% to 16%) 2341
Zomig Tablets (Infrequent) 694
Zomig Nasal Spray (Infrequent to less than 2%) 689
Zomig-ZMT Tablets (Infrequent) 694
▲ Zonegran Capsules (6%) 1089
▲ Zosyn for Injection (4.5% to 6.6%) 3284
▲ Zyban Sustained-Release Tablets (31% to 40%) 1692
▲ Zyprexa Tablets (12% to 20%) 1883
Zyprexa IntraMuscular 1883
▲ Zyprexa ZYDIS Orally Disintegrating Tablets (12% to 20%) 1883
Zyrtec Chewable Tablets (Less than 2%) 1920
Zyrtec Syrup (Less than 2%) 1920
Zyrtec Tablets (Less than 2%) 1920
▲ Zyrtec-D 12 Hour Extended Release Tablets (Less than 2% to 4%) 1923
Zyrtec-D Allergy & Congestion Extended-Release Tablets 1923
Zyvox (2.5%) 2552

Insomnia, early morning
▲ Cymbalta Delayed-Release Capsules (10%) 1801

Insomnia, mania middle
▲ Cymbalta Delayed-Release Capsules (10%) 1801
Mirapex Tablets 857

Instability, autonomic
Neupro Transdermal System 3149
Pristiq Extended-Release Tablets 3247
Remeron Tablets 2924
RemeronSolTab Tablets 2927
Thiothixene Capsules 2197
Treximet Tablets 1616

Instability, postural
Invega Extended-Release Tablets 1748

Insulin, blood, increased
Abilify Injection (Greater than or equal to 1 in 1000 patients and less than 1 in 100 patients) 881
Abilify Injection (Greater than or equal to 1 in 1000 patients and less than 1 in 100 patients) 2466
Abilify Oral Solution (Greater than or equal to 1 in 1000 patients and less than 1 in 100 patients) 881
Abilify Oral Solution (Greater than or equal to 1 in 1000 patients and less than 1 in 100 patients) 2466
Abilify Discmelt Orally Disintegrating Tablets (Greater than or equal to 1 in 1000 patients and less than 1 in 100 patients) 881
Abilify Discmelt Orally Disintegrating Tablets (Greater than or equal to 1 in 1000 patients and less than 1 in 100 patients) 2466
Abilify Tablets (Greater than or equal to 1 in 1000 patients and less than 1 in 100 patients) 881
Abilify Tablets (Greater than or equal to 1 in 1000 patients and less than 1 in 100 patients) 2466

Insulin reaction
▲ Torisel Injection (89%) 3272

Insulin requirement, changes
Prinzide Tablets 2092

Intentional self injury
Abilify Injection (Greater than or equal to 1 in 1000 patients and less than 1 in 100 patients) 881
Abilify Injection (Greater than or equal to 1 in 1000 patients and less than 1 in 100 patients) 2466
Abilify Oral Solution (Greater than or equal to 1 in 1000 patients and less than 1 in 100 patients) 881
Abilify Oral Solution (Greater than or equal to 1 in 1000 patients and less than 1 in 100 patients) 2466
Abilify Discmelt Orally Disintegrating Tablets (Greater than or equal to 1 in 1000 patients and less than 1 in 100 patients) 881
Abilify Discmelt Orally Disintegrating Tablets (Greater than or equal to 1 in 1000 patients and less than 1 in 100 patients) 2466
Abilify Tablets (Greater than or equal to 1 in 1000 patients and less than 1 in 100 patients) 881
Abilify Tablets (Greater than or equal to 1 in 1000 patients and less than 1 in 100 patients) 2466
Tamiflu Capsules 2649

Interstitial lung disease
Agrylin Capsules 3017
CellCept Capsules 2622
CellCept Intravenous 2622
CellCept Oral Suspension 2622
CellCept Tablets 2622
Effexor XR Extended-Release Capsules (Rare) 3195
Eloxatin for Injection 2731
Erbitux (Less than 0.5%) 912
Humira Injection 442
Myfortic Tablets (Rare) 2276
Pristiq Extended-Release Tablets 3247
Rapamune 3260
Requip Tablets (Infrequent) 1561
Tarceva Tablets (0.7%) 1228
Tasigna Capsules (0.1% to 1%) 2316
Torisel Injection (2%) 3272
Tykerb Tablets 1631
Venlafaxine Hydrochloride Tablets 2199

Intervertebral disc degeneration
Requip Tablets (Infrequent) 1561

Intervertebral disc protrusion
Mirapex Tablets 857
Requip Tablets (Infrequent) 1561

Intervertebral discitis
Mirapex Tablets 857

Intervertebral disk disorder, unspecified
Imitrex Nasal Spray (Rare) 1470
Mirapex Tablets 857

Intervertebral disk herniation
Remicade for IV Injection (Greater than or equal to 0.2%) 950

Intestinal functional disorder, unspecified
Amitiza Capsules (Less than 1%) 3082

Intestinal obstruction
Ambien Tablets (Rare) 2692
Ambien CR Tablets (Rare) 2696
Avastin IV (Rare) 1192
Azilect Tablets (Infrequent) 3106
Celebrex Capsules (Less than 0.1%) 2979
Chantix Tablets (Rare) 2511
Cimzia 3127
Dantrium Capsules (Rare) 2580
▲ Doxil Injection (11.3%) 2378
Effexor XR Extended-Release Capsules (Rare) 3195
Elitek (Less than or equal to 1%) 2729
▲ Eloxatin for Injection (2% to less than 5%) 2731
Evoxac Capsules 1013
Exelon Capsules (Infrequent) 2229
Exelon Oral Solution (Infrequent) 2229
Gleevec Tablets (Rare) 2255
▲ Hycamtin for Injection (1.1% to 4.5%) 1459
Imitrex Injection 1465
Imitrex Nasal Spray (Rare) 1470
Imitrex Tablets 1474
Invanz for Injection (2.1%) 2029
Lovaza Capsules 1520
Luvox CR Extended-Release Capsules (Rare) 1759
Meridia Capsules 475
Merrem I.V. (Greater than 0.1% to 1%) 684
Mirapex Tablets 857
MS Contin Tablets (Less frequent) 2585
Paxil (Rare) 1535
Paxil CR Controlled-Release Tablets (Rare) 1544
Percocet Tablets 1127
Percodan Tablets 1130
Proleukin for Injection 2287
Prozac Weekly Capsules (Rare) 1852
Prozac Pulvules and Liquid (Rare) 1852
Pulmozyme Inhalation Solution 1217
Remeron Tablets (Rare) 2924
RemeronSolTab Tablets (Rare) 2927
Remicade for IV Injection (Greater than or equal to 0.2%) 950
Requip Tablets (Infrequent) 1561
Rilutek Tablets (Infrequent) 2771
Risperdal Consta Long-Acting Injection 1753
Rythmol SR Capsules 1590
Sandostatin Injection (Rare) 2300
Sandostatin LAR Depot 2302
Spiriva HandiHaler 870
Symbyax Capsules (Rare) 1871
Taxotere Injection Concentrate 2773
Velcade for Injection 2168
Venlafaxine Hydrochloride Tablets (Rare) 2199
VESIcare Tablets 636
Xeloda Tablets 2662
Zomig Tablets (Rare) 694
Zomig Nasal Spray (Rare) 689
Zomig-ZMT Tablets (Rare) 694
Zyprexa Tablets (Rare) 1883
Zyprexa ZYDIS Orally Disintegrating Tablets (Rare) 1883

Intestinal obstruction, paralytic
Velcade for Injection 2168

Intestinal obstruction, pseudo
Catapres Tablets (Rare) 841
Nimotop Capsules (Rare) 790

Intestinal perforation
Azilect Tablets (Rare) 3106
Celebrex Capsules (Less than 0.1%) 2979
Cipro I.V. (Less than 1%) 2817
Cipro (Less than 1%) 2810
Cipro XR Tablets 2823
Enbrel for Injection 569
Flector Patch 561
Mobic Oral Suspension (Less than 2%) 863
Mobic Tablets (Less than 2%) 863
Myfortic Tablets 2276
Percodan Tablets 1130
Proleukin for Injection (Less than 1%) 2287
Remicade for IV Injection (Greater than or equal to 0.2%) 950
Tabloid Tablets 1601
Taxotere Injection Concentrate 2773
Treximet Tablets 1616
Velcade for Injection 2168
Wellbutrin Tablets (Rare) 1648
Wellbutrin SR Sustained-Release Tablets 1653
Wellbutrin XL Extended-Release Tablets 1659
Zyban Sustained-Release Tablets 1692

Intestinal strictures
Clinoril Tablets (Rare) 1962
Indocin Capsules (Less than 1%) 2024
Indocin I.V. (Less than 1%) 2489

Intestinal villous atrophy
CellCept Capsules 2622
CellCept Intravenous 2622
CellCept Oral Suspension 2622
CellCept Tablets 2622

Intestines, hemorrhagic necrosis of
Lanoxin Injection 1498
Lanoxin Injection Pediatric 1502
Lanoxin Tablets 1505

Intoxication, state of
▲ Advair HFA 45/21 Inhalation Aerosol (0% to 3%) 1288
▲ Advair HFA 115/21 Inhalation Aerosol (0% to 3%) 1288
▲ Advair HFA 230/21 Inhalation Aerosol (0% to 3%) 1288

Intracranial hypertension with papilledema
Gengraf Capsules 435
Neoral Oral Solution 2280
Neoral Soft Gelatin Capsules 2280
Norditropin Cartridges (Small number of patients) 2354
Nutropin for Injection (A small number of patients) 1208
Nutropin AQ Injection (A small number of patients) 1212
Nutropin AQ NuSpin Injection (A small number of patients) 1212
Nutropin AQ Pen (A small number of patients) 1212
Nutropin AQ Pen Cartridge (A small number of patients) 1212
Tev-Tropin for Injection (Small number of patients) 1187

Intracranial pressure, increase
Albenza Tablets (Up to 1.5%) 1297
Cipro I.V. 2817
Cipro XR Tablets 2823
Gleevec Tablets (Rare) 2255
Levaquin 2416
Levaquin in 5% Dextrose Injection 2416
MS Contin Tablets (Less frequent) 2585
Noroxin Tablets 2069

Intraocular disorders
Amerge Tablets (Rare) 1301
Imitrex Tablets 1474

Intraocular pressure, increase
(*see also under* Glaucoma)
Advair Diskus 100/50 1276
Advair Diskus 250/50 1276
Advair Diskus 500/50 1276
Atrovent Nasal Spray 0.06% 836
▲ Diclofenac Sodium Ophthalmic Solution (Less than or equal to 5% to 15%) .... ⊙240
▲ Nevanac Ophthalmic Suspension 0.1% (5% to 10%) .... ⊙205
Omnaris Nasal Spray (Rare) 2998
▲ Triesence Injectable Suspension (20% to 60%) .... ⊙209
▲ Voltaren Ophthalmic Solution (Less than or equal to 5% to 15%) 2336

Intraoperative floppy iris syndrome
Uroxatral Tablets 2786

Intravascular coagulation, disseminated
Aggrenox Capsules 819
AlphaNine SD 1713
Bayer Aspirin 750
Celebrex Capsules 2979
Clinoril Tablets (Less than 1 in 100) 1962
Indocin Capsules (Less than 1%) 2024
Indocin I.V. 2489
Indocin (Less than 1%) 2024
Lamictal 1488
Mylotarg for Injection (1%) 3212
NovoSeven 2367
▲ NovoSeven RT (1% to 4.7%) 2370
Omnicef Capsules 497
Omnicef for Oral Suspension 497
Percodan Tablets 1130
Profilnine SD Solvent Detergent 1721
Prograf Capsules and Injection 622
St. Joseph 81 mg Aspirin Chewable and Enteric Coated Tablets 1903
Sulfamylon Cream 2194
Sulfamylon for 5% Topical Solution... 2194
Taxotere Injection Concentrate 2773
Trasylol Injection (1% to 2%) 799
▲ Trisenox Injection (8%) 986
Velcade for Injection 2168
▲ Vesanoid Capsules (26%) 2660

Intussusception
Rotarix Oral Suspension 1582
RotaTeq 2110

Intussusception, gastrointestinal
Infanrix Vaccine 1479
Pediarix Vaccine 1552

Involuntary movements, abnormal
Carbatrol Capsules 3019
Effexor XR Extended-Release Capsules 3195
Eldepryl Capsules 3052
▲ Equetro Extended-Release Capsules (Less than 5%) 3174
Moban Tablets 1116
Omnicef Capsules 497
Omnicef for Oral Suspension 497
Venlafaxine Hydrochloride Tablets 2199

Involuntary movements, extremities
Moban Tablets 1116
Thiothixene Capsules 2197

IOP, elevation of
Alrex Ophthalmic Suspension 0.2% (2%) .... ⊙236
Beconase AQ Nasal Spray (Rare) 1369
Celexa 1160
Flonase Nasal Spray 1431
FML Ophthalmic Ointment .... ⊙223
FML Ophthalmic Suspension .... ⊙224
FML Forte Ophthalmic Suspension .... ⊙222
Gleevec Tablets (Rare) 2255
Lexapro Oral Suspension 1174
Lexapro Tablets 1174
Lotemax Ophthalmic Suspension 0.5% .... ⊙241
Meridia Capsules 475
Paxil (Rare) 1535
Paxil CR Controlled-Release Tablets (Rare) 1544
Pred Forte Ophthalmic Suspension .... ⊙227
Pred Mild Ophthalmic Suspension ... ⊙230
Pred-G Ophthalmic Suspension .... ⊙228
Sandostatin Injection (Less than 1%) 2300

Iridocyclitis
(*see also under* Iritis)
Cosopt Sterile Ophthalmic Solution (Less than 1%) 1969
Trusopt Sterile Ophthalmic Solution (Rare) 2128

Iris, discoloration
▲ Travatan Z Ophthalmic Solution (1% to 4%) 547

Iris pigmentation, increase in
▲ Lumigan Ophthalmic Solution (1% to 3%) 556

Iritis
(*see also under* Uveitis)
Actonel Tablets (Rare) 2568
Actonel with Calcium Tablets (Very rare) 2574
Alphagan P Ophthalmic Solution 549
Combigan Ophthalmic Solution 553
▲ Diclofenac Sodium Ophthalmic Solution (Less than or equal to 5%) .... ⊙240
▲ Durezol Ophthalmic Emulsion (1% to 5%) .... ⊙275
Lumigan Ophthalmic Solution (Less than 1%) 556
Lunesta Tablets (Rare) 2994
Lyrica Capsules (Rare) 2527
Norvir (Less than 2%) 489

Prozac Weekly Capsules (Rare) 1852
Prozac Pulvules and Liquid (Rare) 1852
▲ Voltaren Ophthalmic Solution (Less than or equal to 5%) 2336
Zonegran Capsules (Rare) 1089

Iron deficiency
Epogen for Injection 576
Prozac Pulvules and Liquid (Rare) 1852
Requip Tablets (Infrequent) 1561
Sandostatin Injection (Less than 1%) 2300

Irritability
Abilify Injection (Greater than or equal to 1 in 100 patients) 881
Abilify Injection (Greater than or equal to 1 in 100 patients) 2466
Abilify Oral Solution (Greater than or equal to 1 in 100 patients) 881
Abilify Oral Solution (Greater than or equal to 1 in 100 patients) 2466
Abilify Discmelt Orally Disintegrating Tablets (Greater than or equal to 1 in 100 patients) 881
Abilify Discmelt Orally Disintegrating Tablets (Greater than or equal to 1 in 100 patients) 2466
Abilify Tablets (Greater than or equal to 1 in 100 patients) 881
Abilify Tablets (Greater than or equal to 1 in 100 patients) 2466
Activella Tablets 2347
Advair Diskus 100/50 1276
Advair Diskus 250/50 1276
Advair Diskus 500/50 1276
Advair HFA 45/21 Inhalation Aerosol (Very Rare) 1288
Advair HFA 115/21 Inhalation Aerosol (Very Rare) 1288
Advair HFA 230/21 Inhalation Aerosol (Very Rare) 1288
▲ Aerobid/Aerobid-M (3% to 9%) 1153
Angeliq Tablets 751
Aricept Tablets (Frequent) 1062
Aricept ODT Tablets (Frequent) 1062
Attenuvax 1951
Catapres-TTS (0.5% or less) 842
Ceftin for Oral Suspension (0.1% to 1%) 1380
Chantix Tablets (Frequent) 2511
Cipro I.V. (1% or less) 2817
Cipro (Less than 1%) 2810
Ciprodex Otic Suspension (0.5%) 541
▲ Clarinex Syrup (12.1%) 2828
Climara Transdermal System 763
Climara Pro Transdermal System 768
▲ Clolar for Intravenous Infusion (11%) 1239
▲ Comvax (32.2% to 57%) 1966
▲ Concerta Extended-Release Tablets (0.8% to 5.8%) 1925
Cymbalta Delayed-Release Capsules (Infrequent) 1801
Daytrana Transdermal Patch 3022
Divigel 3167
Effexor XR Extended-Release Capsules 3195
Eldepryl Capsules 3052
Elspar for Injection 1990
Engerix-B Vaccine (Less than 1%) 1409
Enjuvia Tablets 1029
Estratest Tablets 3043
Estratest H.S. Tablets 3043
▲ FluMist Vaccine (12% to 21%) 1945
▲ Gabitril Tablets (10%) 973
▲ Havrix Injection Vaccine (24% to 36%) 1454
Humulin 50/50, 100 Units 1843
Humulin 70/30 Vial 1844
Humulin N Vial 1846
Humulin R 1849
▲ Indapamide Tablets (Greater than or equal to 5%) 2188
▲ Infanrix Vaccine (28.8% to 61.5%) 1479
▲ Intron A for Injection (Up to 16%) 2859
▲ Keppra Injection (1.7% to 13.3%) 3137
▲ Keppra Oral Solution (6% to 6.3%) 3131
▲ Keppra Tablets (6% to 6.3%) 3131
▲ Lamictal (3%) 1488
Levothroid Tablets 1170
Levoxyl Tablets 1780
Lexapro Oral Suspension (Frequent) 1174
Lexapro Tablets (Frequent) 1174
Luvox CR Extended-Release Capsules 1759
Maxalt Tablets (Infrequent) 2056
Maxalt-MLT Orally Disintegrating Tablets (Infrequent) 2056
Meruvax II 2061
M-M-R II 2054
Mumpsvax 2068
Paxil Tablets 1535
Paxil CR Controlled-Release Tablets 1544
▲ Pediarix Vaccine (1.7% to 63.8%) 1552
Liquid PedvaxHIB 2073
▲ PegIntron Powder for Injection (28%) 2903
Premarin Tablets 3221
Premarin Vaginal Cream 3228
Premphase Tablets 3232
Prempro Tablets 3232
▲ Prevnar (44.2% to 58.7%) 3241
Prinivil Tablets (0.3% to 1%) 2087
Prinzide Tablets 2092
Pristiq Extended-Release Tablets (Greater than or equal to 2%) 3247
▲ Prometrium Capsules (100 mg, 200 mg) (5% to 8%) 3047
▲ ProQuad (6.7%) 2099
Prozac Weekly Capsules 1852
Prozac Pulvules and Liquid 1852
Pulmicort Flexhaler 654
▲ Rebetol (10% to 47%) 2917
Recombivax HB (Greater than 1%) 2107
Remeron Tablets 2924
RemeronSolTab Tablets 2927
Requip Tablets (Frequent) 1561
Retrovir Capsules (1.6%) 1574
Retrovir IV Infusion (2%) 1579
Retrovir (1.6%) 1574
▲ Rotarix Oral Suspension (11.4% to 52%) 1582
▲ RotaTeq (2.9% to 8.1%) 2110
Singulair (Very rare) 2114
Skelaxin Tablets (Most frequent) 1784
Soma Tablets 1931
▲ Strattera Capsules (0.3% to 6%) 1864
Symbyax Capsules 1871
Treximet Tablets (Infrequent) 1616
Twinrix Vaccine (Less than 1%) 1628
Ultram ER Extended-Release Tablets (0.5% to less than 1%) 2428
Uniphyl Tablets 2595
Valium Tablets 2658
Vantas (Less than 2%) 1737
▲ Vaqta (10.8%) 2130
Varivax (Greater than or equal to 1%) 2133
Venlafaxine Hydrochloride Tablets 2199
Verdeso Foam (1%) 3069
Vivitrol 988
▲ Vyvanse Capsules (10%) 3033
▲ Wellbutrin SR Sustained-Release Tablets (2% to 3%) 1653
▲ Wellbutrin XL Extended-Release Tablets (2% to 3%) 1659
▲ Xeloda Tablets (Less than 5%) 2662
Zomig Tablets (Rare) 694
Zomig Nasal Spray (Rare) 689
Zomig-ZMT Tablets (Rare) 694
▲ Zonegran Capsules (9%) 1089
Zyban Sustained-Release Tablets (Frequent) 1692

Irritation
Analpram-HC 1140
Bleph-10 Ophthalmic Solution 10% ⊙ 215
Climara Pro Transdermal System 768
Combivent Inhalation Aerosol 845
Diprolene Lotion 0.05% (Less than 1%) 2838
Extina Foam, 2% (Less than or equal to 1%) 3057
Lotrisone 2881
Olux Foam (Less than 2%) 3061
Olux-E Foam 3059
Panretin Gel 0.1% 1081
Pramosone 1141
Pred-G Ophthalmic Suspension ⊙ 228
▲ Targretin Gel 1% (56% to 72%) 1088
Vanos Cream 1941
Velcade for Injection 2168
Viroptic Ophthalmic Solution ⊙ 253

Irritation, anal
Fleet Babylax Suppositories 1142
Fleet Glycerin Laxatives 1142
Fleet Glycerin Suppositories 1142
Fleet Pedia-Lax Suppositories 1142
Zosyn for Injection (1% or less) 3284

Irritation, application site
Altabax Ointment (1.4% to 1.6%) 1299
Daytrana Transdermal Patch 3022
▲ Elidel Cream 1% (0.4% to 6.4%) 2221
Exelon Patch (Infrequent) 2233
Fentora Tablets (Greater than 1%) 968
▲ Flector Patch (4%) 561
Iquix Ophthalmic Solution (1% to 2%) 3183
▲ Spiriva HandiHaler (1% to 3%) 870

Irritation, eyelid
Vectibix (1%) 597

Irritation, gastric
Atacand HCT 642
Avalide Tablets 892
Avalide Tablets 2713
Captopril Tablets (About 0.5% to 2%) 2182
Clorpres Tablets 2185
Dantrium Capsules (Rare) 2580
Diovan HCT Tablets 2216
Furosemide Tablets 2186
▲ Indapamide Tablets (Less than 5%) 2188
Intravenous Sodium Diuril 2490
Micardis HCT Tablets 854
Prinzide Tablets 2092
Tekturna HCT Tablets 2324
Teveten HCT Tablets 517

Irritation, gastrointestinal
Actonel Tablets 2568
Dibenzyline Capsules 3188
Ferralet 90 Tablets 2175
Urocit-K Tablets (Some patients) 2176

Irritation, glossal
(*see under* Irritation, oral)

Irritation, local
Aldara Cream, 5% (2%) 1699
Arixtra Injection 1313
Bentyl Injection 703
Bleph-10 Ophthalmic Solution 10% ⊙ 215
▲ Carac Cream 0.5% (94.6%) 2722
Climara Transdermal System 763
Edecrin Sodium Intravenous (Occasionally) 698
Finacea Gel (Less than 1% to 2%) 1742
Lidoderm Patch 1114
Lovenox Injection 2756
Mentax Cream (Less than 2%) 2190
Mirapex Tablets 857
Naftin Cream (2%) 2164
▲ NeoProfen Injection (16%) 2496
Nitro-Dur Transdermal Infusion System 2887
Ortho Evra Transdermal System 2437
Rosac Wash 3062
Valstar Sterile Solution for Intravesical Instillation (Less than 1%) 1735
Xyrem Oral Solution (Infrequent) 1766

Irritation, nasal
▲ Aerobid/Aerobid-M (1% to 3%) 1153
Asmanex Twisthaler (1% to less than 3%) 2797
Atrovent Nasal Spray 0.03% (2%) 834
Beconase AQ Nasal Spray 1369
▲ Flonase Nasal Spray (1% to 3%) 1431
Maxalt Tablets (Infrequent) 2056
Maxalt-MLT Orally Disintegrating Tablets (Infrequent) 2056
▲ Miacalcin Nasal Spray (10.6%) 2274
Nasonex Nasal Spray (Greater than or equal to 2%) 2883
Xifaxan Tablets (Less than 2%) 2682

Irritation, nasopharyngeal
Advair Diskus 100/50 1276
Advair Diskus 250/50 1276
Advair Diskus 500/50 1276
▲ Beconase AQ Nasal Spray (24% of patients) 1369

Irritation, ocular
Atrovent Nasal Spray 0.03% (Less than 2%) 834
Combivent Inhalation Aerosol 845
▲ Diclofenac Sodium Ophthalmic Solution (Less than or equal to 5%) ⊙ 240
Elidel Cream 1% 2221
Pred-G Ophthalmic Ointment ⊙ 229
▲ Voltaren Ophthalmic Solution (Less than or equal to 5%) 2336

Irritation, oral
▲ Aerobid/Aerobid-M (1% to 3%) 1153
Amerge Tablets (Rare) 1301
Axert Tablets (Rare) 2431
Furosemide Tablets 2186
Imitrex Nasal Spray 1470
Sandimmune (Rare) 2296

Irritation, oropharynx
Proventil HFA Inhalation Aerosol 2914
▲ Serevent Diskus (7%) 1594
Ventolin HFA Inhalation Aerosol 1638

Irritation, perianal
(*see under* Irritation, anal)

Irritation, skin
(*see under* Irritation, local)

Irritation, vaginal
Ceftin for Oral Suspension (0.1% to 1%) 1380
▲ Femara Tablets (0.2% to 3.5%) 2246

Irritation, vulvovaginal
(*see under* Irritation, vaginal)

Irritation at injection site
▲ Gammagard S/D (16%) 734
Nembutal Sodium Solution, USP 2494
PegIntron Powder for Injection 2903
Retrovir IV Infusion (Infrequent) 1579
Romazicon Injection 2646

Ischemia
Aldara Cream, 5% 1699
▲ Avandia Tablets (9%) 1351
Gammagard S/D 734
Invega Extended-Release Tablets 1748
▲ PrandiMet Tablets (4%) 2967
▲ Prandin Tablets (4%) 2971
Sandostatin Injection (Less than 1%) 2300
Selzentry Tablets 2534
▲ Vesanoid Capsules (3%) 2660

Ischemia, arteria basilaris
Fluorescite Injection ⊙ 203

Ischemia, cerebral
Actiq (Less than 1%) 959
Angiomax for Injection (Greater than 0.1% to less than 1%) 1933
Aricept Tablets (Infrequent) 1062
Aricept ODT Tablets (Infrequent) 1062
Arimidex Tablets 672
Betimol Ophthalmic Solution 3181
Combigan Ophthalmic Solution 553
Cosopt Sterile Ophthalmic Solution 1969
Effexor XR Extended-Release Capsules (Rare) 3195
Enbrel for Injection (Infrequent) 569
Gabitril Tablets (Infrequent) 973
Imitrex Injection 1465
Imitrex Nasal Spray 1470
Imitrex Tablets (Rare) 1474
Mirapex Tablets 857
Nitrolingual Pumpspray (Occasional) 2965
NovoSeven 2367
NovoSeven RT 2370
Paxil (Rare) 1535
Paxil CR Controlled-Release Tablets (Rare) 1544
Pletal Tablets (Less than 2%) 2481
Prozac Weekly Capsules (Rare) 1852
Prozac Pulvules and Liquid (Rare) 1852
Remeron Tablets (Rare) 2924
RemeronSolTab Tablets (Rare) 2927
ReoPro Vials (0.3%) 1860
Rilutek Tablets (Rare) 2771
Sular Extended Release Tablets (Less than or equal to 1%) 2975
Symbyax Capsules (Infrequent) 1871
Timoptic Sterile Ophthalmic Solution (Less frequent) 2121
Timoptic in Ocudose 2124
Timoptic-XE Sterile Ophthalmic Gel Forming Solution 2125
Venlafaxine Hydrochloride Tablets (Rare) 2199
Zomig Tablets (Rare) 694
Zomig-ZMT Tablets (Rare) 694

Ischemia, colonic
Imitrex Tablets 1474
Treximet Tablets 1616

Ischemia, gastrointestinal
Zomig Tablets (Rare) 694
Zomig Nasal Spray (Very rare) 689
Zomig-ZMT Tablets (Rare) 694

Ischemia, intestinal
Amerge Tablets 1301
Imitrex Nasal Spray 1470
Lanoxin Injection 1498
Lanoxin Injection Pediatric 1502
Lanoxin Tablets 1505

Ischemia, myocardial
Abilify Injection (Greater than or equal to 1 in 1000 patients and less than 1 in 100 patients) 2466

Abilify Oral Solution (Greater than or equal to 1 in 1000 patients and less than 1 in 100 patients) 881
Abilify Oral Solution (Greater than or equal to 1 in 1000 patients and less than 1 in 100 patients) 2466
Abilify Discmelt Orally Disintegrating Tablets (Greater than or equal to 1 in 1000 patients and less than 1 in 100 patients) 881
Abilify Discmelt Orally Disintegrating Tablets (Greater than or equal to 1 in 1000 patients and less than 1 in 100 patients) 2466
Abilify Tablets (Greater than or equal to 1 in 1000 patients and less than 1 in 100 patients) 881
Abilify Tablets (Greater than or equal to 1 in 1000 patients and less than 1 in 100 patients) 2466
▲ Alimta for Injection (1% to 3%) 1786
Aloxi Injection (Less than 1%) 1059
Anzemet Injection (Rare) 2701
Anzemet Tablets (Rare) 2704
Argatroban Injection (1.8%) 1308
Arimidex Tablets 672
Avandia Tablets 1351
Cimzia 3127
Coreg Tablets (Less than or equal to 0.1%) 1387
Coreg CR Extended-Release Capsules (Less than or equal to 0.1%) 1393
Enbrel for Injection (Infrequent) 569
Femara Tablets (Less than or equal to 2%) 2246
Flolan for Injection (2%) 1426
Frova Tablets 1111
Imitrex Injection (Extremely rare) 1465
Imitrex Nasal Spray 1470
Imitrex Tablets (Rare) 1474
Ixempra Kit for Injection 915
Levitra Tablets (Less than 2%) 2876
Lovaza Capsules 1520
Maxalt Tablets (Very rare) 2056
Maxalt-MLT Orally Disintegrating Tablets (Very rare) 2056
▲ Novantrone for Injection Concentrate (5%) 1100
NovoSeven 2367
NovoSeven RT 2370
Paxil (Rare) 1535
Paxil CR Controlled-Release Tablets (Rare) 1544
PegIntron Powder for Injection 2903
Pletal Tablets (Less than 2%) 2481
PrandiMet Tablets (1.4%) 2967
Pristiq Extended-Release Tablets 3247
Prograf Capsules and Injection 622
Proleukin for Injection (Less than 1%) 2287
Protonix for Delayed-Release Oral Suspension (Less than 1%) 3254
Protonix Delayed-Release Tablets (Less than 1%) 3254
Protonix I.V. (Less than 1%) 3257
Rilutek Tablets (Infrequent) 2771
Risperdal Consta Long-Acting Injection (Infrequent) 1753
Sutent Capsules (2 patients) 2540
Tarceva Tablets (2.3%) 1228
Taxotere Injection Concentrate (0% to 1.7%) 2773
TNKase 1233
Trasylol Injection (1% to 2%) 799
Velcade for Injection 2168
Zomig Tablets 694
Zomig Nasal Spray 689
Zomig-ZMT Tablets 694

Ischemia, peripheral
Anzemet Injection (Rare) 2701
Anzemet Tablets (Rare) 2704
Bystolic Tablets 1155
Chantix Tablets (Infrequent) 2511
Coreg Tablets (Greater than 0.1% to 1%) 1387
Coreg CR Extended-Release Capsules (0.1% to less than or equal to 1%) 1393
Evoxac Capsules (Less than 1%) 1013
Exelon Capsules (Infrequent) 2229
Exelon Oral Solution (Infrequent) 2229
Exforge Tablets (Greater than 0.1% to less than 1%) 2238
Gengraf Capsules (1% to less than 3%) 435
Imitrex Tablets 1474
▲ Intron A for Injection (Less than 5%) 2859
Maxalt Tablets 2056
Maxalt-MLT Orally Disintegrating Tablets 2056
Neoral Oral Solution (1% to less than 3%) 2280
Neoral Soft Gelatin Capsules (1% to less than 3%) 2280
▲ Requip Tablets (3%) 1561
Soriatane Capsules (Less than 1%) .. 3062
Teveten Tablets (Less than 1%) 515
Teveten HCT Tablets (Less than 1%) 517
Ultram ER Extended-Release Tablets (0.5% to less than 1%) 2428
Zomig Tablets 694
Zomig Nasal Spray 689
Zomig-ZMT Tablets 694

Ischemia, recurrent
Activase I.V. 1188
TNKase 1233

Ischemia, retinal
PegIntron Powder for Injection (Less than or equal to 1%) 2903

Ischemia, transient
Imitrex Tablets 1474
Velcade for Injection 2168

Ischemic attacks, transient
Actimmune (Rare) 1743
Aggrenox Capsules (2%) 819
Amerge Tablets 1301
Aranesp for Injection (Less than or equal to 1%) 564
Aricept Tablets (Infrequent) 1062
Aricept ODT Tablets (Infrequent) 1062
Avalide Tablets 892
Avalide Tablets 2713
Avapro Tablets (Less than 1%) 897
Avapro Tablets (Less than 1%) 2718
Celexa (Rare) 1160
Chantix Tablets (Rare) 2511
DynaCirc CR Controlled Release Tablets (0.5% to 1%) 1407
Epogen for Injection (0.4%) 576
Exelon Capsules (Frequent) 2229
Exelon Oral Solution (Frequent) 2229
▲ Femara Tablets (6.8%) 2246
Gammagard S/D 734
Imitrex Injection 1465
Invega Extended-Release Tablets 1748
Lybrel Tablets 3204
Meridia Capsules 475
Namenda (Frequent) 1180
Orthoclone OKT3 Sterile Solution (Less than 1%) 2387
PegIntron Powder for Injection (Less than or equal to 1%) 2903
Prinivil Tablets (0.3% to 1%) 2087
Prinzide Tablets 2092
Procrit for Injection (0.4%) 2391
Proleukin for Injection 2287
Requip Tablets (Infrequent) 1561
Risperdal Consta Long-Acting Injection 1753
Treximet Tablets 1616

Ischemic colitis
Imitrex Injection 1465
Imitrex Nasal Spray 1470
Imitrex Tablets 1474
Timoptic Sterile Ophthalmic Solution 2121
Timoptic in Ocudose 2124
Velcade for Injection 2168
Zomig Tablets (Rare) 694
Zomig-ZMT Tablets (Rare) 694

Itching
(*see under* Pruritus)

Itching, eyes
(*see also under* Pruritus, ocular)
▲ Diclofenac Sodium Ophthalmic Solution (Less than or equal to 5%) .... ⊙240
Transderm Scōp Transdermal Therapeutic System 2206

Itching, vulvovaginal
Ceftin Tablets (0.1% to 1%) 1380

Itching at application site
▲ Supprelin LA Implant (51.1%) 1731
▲ Ziana Gel (4% to 10%) 1942

Itching at injection site
Humalog Mix 50/50-Pen and KwikPen 1833
▲ Humira Injection (20%) 442
Humulin R (Occasionally) 1849
PegIntron Powder for Injection 2903
Xolair 1235
Xolair 2339

IUD, expulsion (complete)
ParaGard T 380A Intrauterine Copper Contraceptive 1041

IUD, expulsion (partial)
ParaGard T 380A Intrauterine Copper Contraceptive 1041

J

Jarisch-Herxheimer's reaction
(*see under* Herxheimer's reaction)

Jaundice
Abelcet Injection 1134
Abilify Injection (Less than 1 in 1000 patients) 881
Abilify Injection (Less than 1 in 1000 patients) 2466
Abilify Oral Solution (Less than 1 in 1000 patients) 881
Abilify Oral Solution (Less than 1 in 1000 patients) 2466
Abilify Discmelt Orally Disintegrating Tablets (Less than 1 in 1000 patients) 881
Abilify Discmelt Orally Disintegrating Tablets (Less than 1 in 1000 patients) 2466
Abilify Tablets (Less than 1 in 1000 patients) 881
Abilify Tablets (Less than 1 in 1000 patients) 2466
Aceon Tablets (2 mg, 4 mg, 8 mg) 3038
Aciphex Tablets 1053
Actiq (1% or greater) 959
Advicor Tablets 402
Aggrenox Capsules (Less than 1%) .. 819
Amrix Capsules 966
Anaprox Tablets (Rare; less than 1%) 2632
Anaprox DS Tablets (Rare; less than 1%) 2632
Aricept Tablets (Infrequent) 1062
Aricept ODT Tablets (Infrequent) 1062
Asacol Delayed-Release Tablets (Rare) 2579
Atacand HCT 642
Avalide Tablets 892
Avalide Tablets 2713
Avandaryl Tablets 1344
Avapro Tablets 897
Avapro Tablets (Very rare) 2718
Avelox (Less than 0.1%) 2803
Axid Capsules 1364
Azilect Tablets (Rare) 3106
Azor Tablets 1005
Biaxin/Biaxin XL (Infrequent) 411
▲ Busulfex Injection (12%) 2477
Cancidas for Injection 1953
Captopril Tablets 2182
Ceftin 1380
Celebrex Capsules 2979
Celexa (Rare) 1160
▲ CellCept Capsules (3% to less than 20%) 2622
▲ CellCept Intravenous (3% to less than 20%) 2622
▲ CellCept Oral Suspension (3% to less than 20%) 2622
▲ CellCept Tablets (3% to less than 20%) 2622
Cipro I.V. (1% or less) 2817
Cipro 2810
Cipro XR Tablets 2823
Clinoril Tablets (Less than 1%) 1962
▲ Clolar for Intravenous Infusion (15%) 1239
Clorpres Tablets 2185
Crestor Tablets 677
Crixivan Capsules (1.5%) 1979
Cubicin for Injection (Less than 1%) 995
Dantrium Capsules 2580
Dapsone Tablets USP 1746
Diovan HCT Tablets 2216
Doxil Injection (Less than 1%) 2378
Duetact Tablets (Rare) 3085
Dyazide Capsules 1405
Dyrenium Capsules (Rare) 3189
EC-Naprosyn Delayed-Release Tablets (Rare; less than 1%) 2632
Edecrin (Rare) 698
Effexor XR Extended-Release Capsules (Rare) 3195
Epivir 1412
EryPed 431
Exforge Tablets 2238
Fentora Tablets (Greater than 1%) 968
Fortaz 1450
Furosemide Tablets 2186
Gantrisin Pediatric Suspension 2638
Geodon Capsules (Rare) 2520
Havrix Injection Vaccine 1454
Indapamide Tablets 2188
Indocin Capsules (Less than 1%) 2024
Indocin I.V. (Less than 1%) 2489
Indocin (Less than 1%) 2024
▲ Intron A for Injection (Less than 5%) 2859
Invanz for Injection (Greater than 0.1%) 2029
Ixempra Kit for Injection 915
Kaletra (Less than 2%) 452
Lamisil Tablets 2266
Leukeran Tablets 1508
Levaquin 2416
Levaquin in 5% Dextrose Injection 2416
Limbrel Capsules 2561
Luvox CR Extended-Release Capsules (Rare) 1759
Mavik Tablets (Rare) 472
Merrem I.V. (Greater than 0.1% to 1%) 684
Micardis HCT Tablets 854
Mobic Oral Suspension (Less than 0.1%) 863
Mobic Tablets (Less than 0.1%) 863
Mustargen for Injection (Infrequent) .. 2492
Mycamine for Injection 616
Mylotarg for Injection 3212
Nalfon Capsules (Less than 1%) 2508
Naprosyn Suspension (Rare; less than 1%) 2632
Naprosyn Tablets (Rare; less than 1%) 2632
NeoProfen Injection 2496
Nexium Delayed-Release Capsules (Rare) 645
Nexium I.V. (Very rare) 652
Nexium Delayed-Release Oral Suspension (Rare) 645
Niaspan Extended-Release Tablets ... 480
Nimotop Capsules (Less than 1%) 790
Noroxin Tablets 2069
Norvir 489
▲ Novantrone for Injection Concentrate (3% to 7%) 1100
Noxafil Oral Suspension (0% to 2%) 2889
Omnicef Capsules 497
Omnicef for Oral Suspension 497
Ortho-Cyclen Tablets 2449
Ortho Evra Transdermal System 2437
Ortho Tri-Cyclen Tablets 2449
Ortho Tri-Cyclen Lo Tablets 2458
Paser Granules 1747
Paxil (Rare) 1535
Paxil CR Controlled-Release Tablets (Rare) 1544
Pediarix Vaccine 1552
Pentasa Capsules 3030
Percocet Tablets 1127
▲ Photofrin for Injection (Less than 5%) 708
Pletal Tablets 2481
PrandiMet Tablets 2967
Prandin Tablets (Rare) 2971
Precose Tablets 792
Primaxin I.M. 2080
Primaxin I.V. (Less than 0.2%) 2083
Prinivil Tablets 2087
Prinzide Tablets 2092
▲ Prograf Capsules and Injection (3% to 15%) 622
Protonix for Delayed-Release Oral Suspension 3254
Protonix Delayed-Release Tablets 3254
Protonix I.V. 3257
Raptiva for Injection 1218
Rebif Prefilled Syringe for Injection (Rare) 1107
Remicade for IV Injection 950
Retrovir IV Infusion 1579
▲ Reyataz Capsules (7% to 13%) 3299
Rilutek Tablets (Infrequent) 2771
Risperdal Consta Long-Acting Injection (Rare) 1753
Rocephin Injectable Vials, ADD-Vantage, Galaxy, Bulk (Less than 0.1%) 2642
Sandostatin Injection (Less than 1%) 2300
Sandostatin LAR Depot 2302
Skelaxin Tablets (Most frequent) 1784
Soriatane Capsules (2 of 525 patients) 3062
Starlix Tablets 2314
Suprax for Oral Suspension (Less than 2%) 1891
Suprax Tablets (Less than 2%) 1891

Tabloid Tablets (A few cases) 1601
Tasigna Capsules 2316
Tekturna HCT Tablets 2324
Teveten HCT Tablets 517
Thioridazine Hydrochloride Tablets 2195
Thiothixene Capsules 2197
Tracleer Tablets 3289
Trasylol Injection (1% to 2%) 799
Treximet Tablets 1616
Tricor Tablets 520
Twinrix Vaccine 1628
Tygacil for Injection (0% to less than 2%) 3276
Ultane Liquid for Inhalation (Less than 1%) 524
Uroxatral Tablets 2786
Valium Tablets (Isolated reports) 2658
Venlafaxine Hydrochloride Tablets (Rare) 2199
Vicoprofen Tablets 533
Viramune Oral Suspension 873
Viramune Tablets 873
Voltaren Tablets (Occasionally) 2334
Voltaren-XR Tablets (Occasionally) 2337
Vytorin 10/10 Tablets 2149
Vytorin 10/10 Tablets 2939
Vytorin 10/20 Tablets 2149
Vytorin 10/20 Tablets 2939
Vytorin 10/40 Tablets 2149
Vytorin 10/40 Tablets 2939
Vytorin 10/80 Tablets 2149
Vytorin 10/80 Tablets 2939
Wellbutrin Tablets (Infrequent) 1648
Wellbutrin SR Sustained-Release Tablets (Infrequent) 1653
Wellbutrin XL Extended-Release Tablets (Infrequent) 1659
▲ Xeloda Tablets (Less than 5%) 2662
Zantac 25 EFFERdose Tablets (Occasional) 1670
Zantac Injection 1666
Zantac Injection Pharmacy Bulk Package (Infrequent) 1668
Zantac Injection Premixed 1666
Zantac (Occasional) 1670
Zocor Tablets 2136
Zomig Tablets (Rare) 694
Zomig Nasal Spray (Rare) 689
Zomig-ZMT Tablets (Rare) 694
Zovirax 1690
Zyban Sustained-Release Tablets (Infrequent) 1692

Jaundice, cholestatic

Aceon Tablets (2 mg, 4 mg, 8 mg) (Rare) 3038
Activella Tablets 2347
Amoxil Capsules 1305
Amoxil Chewable Tablets 1305
Amoxil Pediatric Drops for Oral Suspension 1305
Amoxil Powder for Oral Suspension 1305
Amoxil Tablets 1305
Angeliq Tablets 751
Asacol Delayed-Release Tablets (Rare) 2579
Augmentin 1323
Augmentin Tablets 1327
Augmentin XR Extended Release Tablets 1333
Augmentin ES-600 Powder for Oral Suspension 1329
Avelox (Less than 0.1%) 2803
Captopril Tablets (Rare) 2182
Carbatrol Capsules 3019
Ceftin 1380
▲ CellCept Capsules (3% to less than 20%) 2622
▲ CellCept Intravenous (3% to less than 20%) 2622
▲ CellCept Oral Suspension (3% to less than 20%) 2622
▲ CellCept Tablets (3% to less than 20%) 2622
Cipro (Less than 1%) 2810
Cipro XR Tablets 2823
Climara Transdermal System 763
Climara Pro Transdermal System 768
Dapsone Tablets USP 1746
Delatestryl Injection 1730
Divigel 3167
Doxil Injection (Less than 1%) 2378
Duetact Tablets (Rare) 3085
Enjuvia Tablets 1029
Equetro Extended-Release Capsules 3174
Estratest Tablets 3043
Estratest H.S. Tablets 3043
Geodon Capsules (Rare) 2520
Lescol Capsules 2268
Lescol XL Tablets 2268
Lipitor Tablets (Less than 2%) 2501
Lybrel Tablets 3204
Mavik Tablets (Rare) 472
Merrem I.V. (Greater than 0.1% to 1%) 684
Mevacor Tablets 2063
Mircette Tablets 1034
Moxatag Tablets 2165
Myleran Tablets (Rare) 1530
Noroxin Tablets 2069
NuvaRing 2897
Ortho-Cyclen Tablets 2449
Ortho Evra Transdermal System 2437
Ortho Tri-Cyclen Tablets 2449
Ortho Tri-Cyclen Lo Tablets 2458
Pentasa Capsules 3030
Pepcid Tablets (Infrequent) 2075
Premarin Intravenous 3217
Premarin Tablets 3221
Premarin Vaginal Cream 3228
Premphase Tablets 3232
Prempro Tablets 3232
Prinivil Tablets (0.3% to 1%) 2087
Prinzide Tablets (Rare) 2092
▲ Prograf Capsules and Injection (3% to 15%) 622
Prometrium Capsules (100 mg, 200 mg) 3047
Protonix for Delayed-Release Oral Suspension (Less than 1%) 3254
Protonix Delayed-Release Tablets (Less than 1%) 3254
Protonix I.V. (Less than 1%) 3257
Prozac Weekly Capsules 1852
Prozac Pulvules and Liquid 1852
Seasonique Tablets 1046
Selzentry Tablets 2534
Tarka Tablets (Rare) 511
Timentin ADD-Vantage (Rare) 1606
Timentin Injection Galaxy Container (Rare) 1609
Timentin IV Infusion (Rare) 1603
Timentin Pharmacy Bulk Package (Rare) 1613
Yaz Tablets 805
Zonegran Capsules (Rare) 1089
Zosyn for Injection 3284

Jaundice, fetal

Avalide Tablets 2713
Intravenous Sodium Diuril 2490

Jaundice, hepatocellular

Aceon Tablets (2 mg, 4 mg, 8 mg) 3038
Augmentin 1323
Augmentin Tablets 1327
Augmentin XR Extended Release Tablets 1333
Augmentin ES-600 Powder for Oral Suspension 1329
Biaxin/Biaxin XL (Infrequent) 411
Carbatrol Capsules 3019
Equetro Extended-Release Capsules 3174
Prinivil Tablets (0.3% to 1%) 2087
Prinzide Tablets 2092
Zantac (Occasional) 1670

Jaundice, intrahepatic cholestatic

Atacand HCT 642
Augmentin 1323
Augmentin Tablets 1327
Augmentin XR Extended Release Tablets 1333
Augmentin ES-600 Powder for Oral Suspension 1329
Avalide Tablets 892
Avalide Tablets 2713
Clorpres Tablets 2185
Diovan HCT Tablets 2216
Furosemide Tablets 2186
Indapamide Tablets 2188
Intravenous Sodium Diuril 2490
Micardis HCT Tablets 854
Prinzide Tablets 2092
Teveten HCT Tablets 517

Jaundice, neonatal

Dyazide Capsules 1405
Intravenous Sodium Diuril 2490
Mephyton Tablets 700
Prinzide Tablets 2092

Jaw tightness

Imitrex Injection (Relatively common) 1465
▲ Imitrex Tablets (Less than 1% to 3%) 1474
Lexapro Oral Suspension (Infrequent) 1174
Lexapro Tablets (Infrequent) 1174
▲ Treximet Tablets (3%) 1616
Zomig Tablets (Infrequent) 694
Zomig Nasal Spray (Infrequent) 689
Zomig-ZMT Tablets (Infrequent) 694

Jerks

(*see under* Twitching)

Jitteriness

▲ Byetta Injection (9%) 600
Cubicin for Injection (Less than 1%) 995
▲ Focalin XR Capsules (12%) 2251
Lexapro Oral Suspension (Infrequent) 1174
Lexapro Tablets (Infrequent) 1174
Opana Tablets (Less than 1%) 1117
Opana ER Tablets (Less than 1%) 1121
Prograf Capsules and Injection 622
Ultram ER Extended-Release Tablets (0.5% to less than 1%) 2428
▲ Wellbutrin XL Extended-Release Tablets (3%) 1659
Xyrem Oral Solution (Infrequent) 1766

Jittery feeling

▲ Abilify Injection (3%) 881
▲ Abilify Injection (3%) 2466
▲ Abilify Oral Solution (3%) 881
▲ Abilify Oral Solution (3%) 2466
▲ Abilify Discmelt Orally Disintegrating Tablets (3%) 881
▲ Abilify Discmelt Orally Disintegrating Tablets (3%) 2466
▲ Abilify Tablets (3%) 881
▲ Abilify Tablets (3%) 2466
Concerta Extended-Release Tablets 1925
▲ Cymbalta Delayed-Release Capsules (5%) 1801
Mirapex Tablets 857
▲ Pristiq Extended-Release Tablets (1% to 3%) 3247
Treximet Tablets (Infrequent) 1616
▲ Vyvanse Capsules (4%) 3033

Joint dislocation

Evoxac Capsules (Less than 1%) 1013

Joint disorder, unspecified

Actiq (1% or greater) 959
▲ Actonel Tablets (7%) 2568
▲ Actonel with Calcium Tablets (6.8%) 2574
▲ Arimidex Tablets (6% to 36%) 672
Asacol Delayed-Release Tablets (2% or greater) 2579
Bicillin C-R Injectable Suspension 1775
Bicillin L-A Injection 1777
▲ Boniva Injection (3.6%) 2614
▲ Boniva Tablets (3.6%) 2618
▲ CellCept Capsules (3% to less than 20%) 2622
▲ CellCept Intravenous (3% to less than 20%) 2622
▲ CellCept Oral Suspension (3% to less than 20%) 2622
▲ CellCept Tablets (3% to less than 20%) 2622
▲ Cipro (9.3%) 2810
▲ Humatrope Vials and Cartridges (2.3% to 5.8%) 1838
▲ Humira Injection (Less than 5%) 442
Imitrex Nasal Spray (Infrequent) 1470
Lamictal (Rare) 1488
Lunesta Tablets (Infrequent) 2994
▲ Lupron Depot 3.75 mg (7.8%) 462
▲ Lupron Depot–3 Month 11.25 mg (7.8% to 8%) 462
Meridia Capsules (1.1%) 475
Mobic Oral Suspension (1.5% to 2.3%) 863
Mobic Tablets (1.5% to 2.3%) 863
Norvir (Less than 2%) 489
▲ Prograf Capsules and Injection (3% to 15%) 622
Protonix for Delayed-Release Oral Suspension (Less than 1%) 3254
Protonix Delayed-Release Tablets (Less than 1%) 3254
Protonix I.V. (Less than 1%) 3257
Protopic Ointment (0.2% to less than 1%) 628
Provigil Tablets (1%) 977
Rythmol SR Capsules 1590
Symbyax Capsules (1% to 2%) 1871
Tricor Tablets 520
Xenical Capsules (2.3%) 2672
Zomig Tablets (Infrequent) 694
Zomig Nasal Spray (Infrequent) 689
Zomig-ZMT Tablets (Infrequent) 694
Zyprexa IntraMuscular (Infrequent) 1883

Joint disturbances

Imitrex Injection (Infrequent) 1465

Joint effusion

Mirapex Tablets 857
Sandostatin Injection (Less than 1%) 2300
Sandostatin LAR Depot 2302

Joint pain

(*see under* Arthralgia)

Joint range of motion decreased

Cipro 2810

Joint related symptoms, unspecified

▲ Selzentry Tablets (6.1%) 2534

Joint sprain

Aczone Gel 5% (1%) 3296
Cipro 2810
Exforge Tablets (Greater than or equal to 0.2%) 2238
Ultram ER Extended-Release Tablets (0.5% to less than 1%) 2428
Xyrem Oral Solution (Infrequent) 1766

Joint stiffness

Amerge Tablets (Infrequent) 1301
Aptivus Capsules 823
Aptivus Oral Solution 823
Arimidex Tablets 672
Avalide Tablets 892
Avalide Tablets 2713
Avapro Tablets (Less than 1%) 897
Avapro Tablets (Less than 1%) 2718
Cipro I.V. (1% or less) 2817
Cipro (Less than 1%) 2810
Cipro XR Tablets 2823
Gleevec Tablets (Infrequent) 2255
Imitrex Injection (Infrequent) 1465
Lexapro Oral Suspension (Infrequent) 1174
Lexapro Tablets (Infrequent) 1174
Lunesta Tablets (Infrequent) 2994
Mirapex Tablets 857
Nabi-HB (2%) 815
Requip Tablets (Infrequent) 1561
Ultram ER Extended-Release Tablets (0.5% to less than 1%) 2428
▲ Vivitrol (4% to 12%) 988
Xeloda Tablets 2662
Xyrem Oral Solution (Infrequent) 1766
Zyprexa Tablets 1883
Zyprexa ZYDIS Orally Disintegrating Tablets 1883

Joints, swollen

Remicade for IV Injection 950

Judgement impaired

Abilify Injection 881
▲ Abilify Injection (11% to 21%) 2466
Abilify Oral Solution 881
▲ Abilify Oral Solution (11% to 21%) 2466
Abilify Discmelt Orally Disintegrating Tablets 881
▲ Abilify Discmelt Orally Disintegrating Tablets (11% to 21%) 2466
Abilify Tablets 881
▲ Abilify Tablets (11% to 21%) 2466
Invega Extended-Release Tablets 1748
Risperdal Consta Long-Acting Injection 1753

K

Kaposi's sarcoma, disease progression of

Rituxan I.V. 1223

Kawasaki-like syndrome

Asacol Delayed-Release Tablets (One case) 2579
Pentasa Capsules (Less than 1%) 3030

Kawasaki's disease

Havrix Injection Vaccine 1454
Rotarix Oral Suspension 1582
RotaTeq 2110

Keloids

▲ Supprelin LA Implant (6.4%) 1731

Keratitis

▲ Alphagan P Ophthalmic Solution (1% to 4%) 549
▲ Azopt Ophthalmic Suspension (1% to 5%) 540
▲ Betimol Ophthalmic Solution (1% to 5%) 3181
BOTOX Purified Neurotoxin Complex (Less than 1%) 550
Celexa (Rare) 1160
Combigan Ophthalmic Solution (0.1% to 0.2%) 553

▲ Diclofenac Sodium Ophthalmic Solution (Less than or equal to 28%) ⊙ 240
Effexor XR Extended-Release Capsules (Rare) 3195
Engerix-B Vaccine 1409
Evoxac Capsules (Less than 1%) 1013
▲ Flovent Diskus 50 mcg (1% to 3%) 1435
FML Ophthalmic Ointment (Occasional) ⊙ 223
FML Ophthalmic Suspension (Occasional) ⊙ 224
FML Forte Ophthalmic Suspension (Occasional) ⊙ 222
Geodon Capsules (Rare) 2520
Imitrex Injection 1465
Imitrex Nasal Spray 1470
Lyrica Capsules (Rare) 2527
Mirapex Tablets 857
Ofloxacin Ophthalmic Solution 0.3% ⊙ 243
▲ Pataday Ophthalmic Solution (Less than or equal to 5%) 543
▲ Patanol Ophthalmic Solution (Less than 5%) 546
Pred Forte Ophthalmic Suspension (Occasional) ⊙ 227
Pred Mild Ophthalmic Suspension (Occasional) ⊙ 230
Serevent Diskus (1% to less than 3%) 1594
Stromectol Tablets 2120
Tarceva Tablets (Infrequent) 1228
Targretin Capsules 1084
Timoptic Sterile Ophthalmic Solution (Less frequent) 2121
Timoptic-XE Sterile Ophthalmic Gel Forming Solution 2125
▲ Travatan Z Ophthalmic Solution (1% to 4%) 547
Twinrix Vaccine 1628
Venlafaxine Hydrochloride Tablets (Rare) 2199
▲ Vigamox Ophthalmic Solution (1% to 6%) 548
▲ Voltaren Ophthalmic Solution (28%) 2336

Keratitis, bacterial
Trusopt Sterile Ophthalmic Solution 2128

Keratitis, punctate
AzaSite Ophthalmic Drops (Less than 1%) 1740
▲ Cosopt Sterile Ophthalmic Solution (5% to 30%) 1969
▲ Durezol Ophthalmic Emulsion (1% to 5%) ⊙ 275
▲ Lumigan Ophthalmic Solution (3% to 10%) 556
Pred-G Ophthalmic Ointment ⊙ 229
Pred-G Ophthalmic Suspension (Occasional) ⊙ 228

Keratitis, superficial punctate
▲ Combigan Ophthalmic Solution (1% to 5%) 553
Diclofenac Sodium Ophthalmic Solution ⊙ 240
▲ Trusopt Sterile Ophthalmic Solution (10% to 15%) 2128
Voltaren Ophthalmic Solution (0.1%) 2336

Keratitis nigricans
Timoptic in Ocudose (Less frequent) 2124

Keratitis sicca
Viroptic Ophthalmic Solution ⊙ 253

Keratoconjunctivitis
▲ Alrex Ophthalmic Suspension 0.2% (Less than 5%) ⊙ 236
Azopt Ophthalmic Suspension (Less than 1%) 540
Evoxac Capsules (Less than 1%) 1013
Gabitril Tablets (Infrequent) 973
Geodon Capsules (Rare) 2520
▲ Lotemax Ophthalmic Suspension 0.5% (Less than 5%) ⊙ 241
Lyrica Capsules (Rare) 2527
Paxil (Rare) 1535
Paxil CR Controlled-Release Tablets (Rare) 1544
Remeron Tablets (Infrequent) 2924
RemeronSolTab Tablets (Infrequent) 2927
Sular Extended Release Tablets (Less than or equal to 1%) 2975
▲ Xeloda Tablets (Less than 5%) 2662
Xyrem Oral Solution (Infrequent) 1766
Zyprexa Tablets (Rare) 1883
Zyprexa ZYDIS Orally Disintegrating Tablets (Rare) 1883

Keratoconjunctivitis sicca
Alphagan P Ophthalmic Solution (Less than 1%) 549
Combigan Ophthalmic Solution 553
Requip Tablets (Infrequent) 1561
▲ Tarceva Tablets (0% to 12%) 1228

Keratopathy
▲ Alphagan P Ophthalmic Solution (1% to 4%) 549

Keratopathy, epithelial
Viroptic Ophthalmic Solution ⊙ 253

Keratopathy, superficial punctate
Viroptic Ophthalmic Solution ⊙ 253

Keratopathy, vortex
Mepron Suspension 1526

Keratosis
Gengraf Capsules (1% to less than 3%) 435
Neoral Oral Solution (1% to less than 3%) 2280
Neoral Soft Gelatin Capsules (1% to less than 3%) 2280

Keratosis pilaris
Finacea Gel (Rare) 1742

Ketoacidosis
Brovana Inhalation Solution 2990
Invega Extended-Release Tablets 1748
Proglycem Capsules (Infrequent) 1185
Proglycem Suspension (Infrequent) 1185
Risperdal Consta Long-Acting Injection 1753

Ketoniuria
Amerge Tablets (Rare) 1301

Ketosis
Doxil Injection (Less than 1%) 2378
Geodon Capsules (Rare) 2520
▲ Humira Injection (Less than 5%) 442
Paxil (Rare) 1535
Paxil CR Controlled-Release Tablets (Rare) 1544
Zyprexa Tablets (Infrequent) 1883
Zyprexa ZYDIS Orally Disintegrating Tablets (Infrequent) 1883

Kidney calculus
Brovana Inhalation Solution (Less than 2%) 2990
▲ Humira Injection (Less than 5%) 442
Luvox CR Extended-Release Capsules (Rare) 1759
Lyrica Capsules (0.1% to 1%) 2527
Velcade for Injection 2168
Venlafaxine Hydrochloride Tablets (Rare) 2199

Kidney damage
Furosemide Tablets 2186

Kidney failure, acute
▲ CellCept Capsules (3% to less than 20%) 2622
▲ CellCept Intravenous (3% to less than 20%) 2622
▲ CellCept Oral Suspension (3% to less than 20%) 2622
▲ CellCept Tablets (3% to less than 20%) 2622
Lamictal (Rare) 1488
Lyrica Capsules (Rare) 2527
Proleukin for Injection (1%) 2287

Kidney function, abnormal
Avelox (Less than 0.1%) 2803
▲ CellCept Capsules (21.8% to 25.6%) 2622
▲ CellCept Intravenous (21.8% to 25.6%) 2622
▲ CellCept Oral Suspension (21.8% to 25.6%) 2622
▲ CellCept Tablets (21.8% to 25.6%) 2622
Proleukin for Injection (Less than 1%) 2287
Tricor Tablets 520
Venlafaxine Hydrochloride Tablets (Rare) 2199

Kidney pain
(*see under* Pain, renal)

Kidney stones
(*see under* Nephrolithiasis)

L

Lab test, abnormal, unspecified
Avelox (Less than 0.1%) 2803
▲ CellCept Capsules (3% to less than 20%) 2622
▲ CellCept Intravenous (3% to less than 20%) 2622
▲ CellCept Oral Suspension (3% to less than 20%) 2622
▲ CellCept Tablets (3% to less than 20%) 2622
▲ Humira Injection (8%) 442

Labor, prolonged
Bayer Aspirin 750
Percodan Tablets 1130

Labor, slowing
Aggrenox Capsules 819

Labor pneumonia
Selzentry Tablets 2534

Laboratory abnormalities, unspecified
Avelox 2803
▲ Hycamtin for Injection (39%) 1459
Salagen Tablets (1% to 2%) 1082
Zomig Tablets (Infrequent) 694
Zomig Nasal Spray (Infrequent) 689
Zomig-ZMT Tablets (Infrequent) 694

Labyrinth disorder
▲ Intron A for Injection (Less than 5%) 2859

Labyrinthitis
Ambien CR Tablets (1%) 2696
Amerge Tablets (Rare) 1301
Celebrex Capsules (Greater than or equal to 0.1% to less than 1%) 2979
Effexor XR Extended-Release Capsules (Rare) 3195
Venlafaxine Hydrochloride Tablets (Rare) 2199

Laceration
▲ Advair HFA 45/21 Inhalation Aerosol (1% to 3%) 1288
▲ Advair HFA 115/21 Inhalation Aerosol (1% to 3%) 1288
▲ Advair HFA 230/21 Inhalation Aerosol (1% to 3%) 1288
Elidel Cream 1% (0% to 1.5%) 2221
▲ Flovent Diskus 50 mcg (1% to 3%) 1435
Xyrem Oral Solution (Infrequent) 1766

Lacrimal duct, stenosis
Xeloda Tablets 2662

Lacrimal gland, disorders
▲ Intron A for Injection (Less than 5%) 2859

Lacrimation
▲ Avastin IV (6% to 18%) 1192
Azopt Ophthalmic Suspension (Less than 1%) 540
▲ BOTOX Purified Neurotoxin Complex (10%) 550
Durezol Ophthalmic Emulsion (Less than 1%) ⊙ 275
Elmiron Capsules 2435
▲ Eloxatin for Injection (1% to 9%) 2731
Imitrex Injection (Infrequent) 1465
Imitrex Nasal Spray (Infrequent) 1470
Imitrex Tablets (Infrequent) 1474
Maxalt Tablets (Infrequent) 2056
Maxalt-MLT Orally Disintegrating Tablets (Infrequent) 2056
OptiPranolol Metipranolol Ophthalmic Solution 0.3% (A small number of patients) ⊙ 245
Proglycem Capsules (Infrequent) 1185
Proglycem Suspension (Infrequent) 1185
▲ Salagen Tablets (6%) 1082
Testim 1% Gel (1% or less) 701
▲ Trusopt Sterile Ophthalmic Solution (Approximately 1% to 5%) 2128
▲ Vigamox Ophthalmic Solution (1% to 6%) 548
▲ Voltaren Ophthalmic Solution (Less than or equal to 5% to 30%) 2336
Zomig Tablets (Rare) 694
Zomig-ZMT Tablets (Rare) 694

Lacrimation, abnormal
Ambien Tablets (Rare) 2692
Ambien CR Tablets (Rare) 2696
Celexa (Infrequent) 1160
Flumadine 1167
Frova Tablets (Infrequent) 1111
Lamictal (Rare) 1488
▲ Miacalcin Nasal Spray (1% to 3%) 2274
Mirapex Tablets (Greater than or equal to 1%) 857
Namenda (Infrequent) 1180
Remeron Tablets (Infrequent) 2924
RemeronSolTab Tablets (Infrequent) 2927
Requip Tablets (Infrequent) 1561
▲ Romazicon Injection (1% to 3%) 2646
Soriatane Capsules (Less than 1%) 3062
▲ Visudyne for Injection (1% to 10%) 2332
Zomig Tablets (Infrequent) 694
Zomig Nasal Spray (Infrequent) 689
Zomig-ZMT Tablets (Infrequent) 694

Lacrimation, increased
Cialis Tablets (Less than 2%) 1792
▲ Gleevec Tablets (16% to 25%) 2255
▲ Ixempra Kit for Injection (4%) 915
▲ Lucentis Injection (3% to 17%) 1205
▲ Sutent Capsules (6%) 2540
Vectibix (2%) 597

Lacrimation disorder, unspecified
Aricept Tablets (Infrequent) 1062
Aricept ODT Tablets (Infrequent) 1062
▲ CellCept Capsules (3% to less than 20%) 2622
▲ CellCept Intravenous (3% to less than 20%) 2622
▲ CellCept Oral Suspension (3% to less than 20%) 2622
▲ CellCept Tablets (3% to less than 20%) 2622
▲ Diclofenac Sodium Ophthalmic Solution (Less than or equal to 5% to 30%) ⊙ 240
Salagen Tablets (Less than 1%) 1082
▲ Taxotere Injection Concentrate (0.1% to 11.3%) 2773

Lactate dehydrogenase, increased
Luvox CR Extended-Release Capsules (Rare) 1759
Tasigna Capsules (0.1% to 1%) 2316
Tricor Tablets 520

Lactation
Effexor XR Extended-Release Capsules (Rare) 3195
Geodon Capsules (Infrequent) 2520
Lamictal (Rare) 1488
Lupron Depot 3.75 mg (Among most frequent) 462
▲ Lupron Depot–3 Month 11.25 mg (Less than 5%) 462
Paxil (Rare) 1535
Paxil CR Controlled-Release Tablets (Rare) 1544
Prozac Pulvules and Liquid (Infrequent) 1852
Symbyax Capsules (Infrequent) 1871
Thioridazine Hydrochloride Tablets 2195
Thiothixene Capsules 2197
Zyprexa Tablets (Infrequent) 1883
Zyprexa ZYDIS Orally Disintegrating Tablets (Infrequent) 1883

Lactation, female
Lunesta Tablets (Infrequent) 2994
Luvox CR Extended-Release Capsules (Infrequent) 1759
Lyrica Capsules (Rare) 2527
Prozac Weekly Capsules (Infrequent) 1852
Venlafaxine Hydrochloride Tablets (Rare) 2199

Lactation, non-puerperal
Flumadine (Less than 0.3%) 1167
Risperdal Consta Long-Acting Injection (Infrequent) 1753

Lactation, possible diminution
Lybrel Tablets 3204
Mircette Tablets 1034
NuvaRing 2897
Ortho-Cyclen Tablets 2449
Ortho Evra Transdermal System 2437

Ortho Tri-Cyclen Tablets 2449
Ortho Tri-Cyclen Lo Tablets 2458
Seasonique Tablets 1046
Yaz Tablets 805

Lactation, suppression
Bentyl Capsules 703
Bentyl Injection 703
Bentyl Syrup 703
Bentyl Tablets 703
Donnatal Extentabs 2507

Lactic acidosis
ActoPlus Met Tablets 3071
Atripla Tablets 938
Combivir Tablets 1384
Emtriva Capsules 1246
Emtriva Oral Solution 1246
Epivir 1412
Epivir-HBV 1417
Epzicom Tablets 1422
Hepsera Tablets 1253
Janumet Tablets 2041
Kaletra (Less than 2%) 452
PrandiMet Tablets 2967
Retrovir Capsules (Rare) 1574
Retrovir IV Infusion (Rare) 1579
Retrovir (Rare) 1574
Reyataz Capsules 3299
Trizivir Tablets 1622
Truvada Tablets 1262
Viread Tablets 1268
Ziagen 1673
Zyvox 2552

Lactic dehydrogenase increased
Abilify Injection (Less than 1 in 1000 patients) 881
Abilify Injection (Less than 1 in 1000 patients) 2466
Abilify Oral Solution (Less than 1 in 1000 patients) 881
Abilify Oral Solution (Less than 1 in 1000 patients) 2466
Abilify Discmelt Orally Disintegrating Tablets (Less than 1 in 1000 patients) 881
Abilify Discmelt Orally Disintegrating Tablets (Less than 1 in 1000 patients) 2466
Abilify Tablets (Less than 1 in 1000 patients) 881
Abilify Tablets (Less than 1 in 1000 patients) 2466
Aricept Tablets (Frequent) 1062
Aricept ODT Tablets (Frequent) 1062
Avelox (Greater than or equal to 0.1% to less than 2%) 2803
Campral Tablets (Rare) 1158
▲ CellCept Capsules (3% to 23.2%) 2622
▲ CellCept Intravenous (3% to 23.2%) 2622
▲ CellCept Oral Suspension (3% to 23.2%) 2622
▲ CellCept Tablets (3% to 23.2%) 2622
Cuprimine Capsules 1986
▲ Dacogen Injection (8%) 1066
Elmiron Capsules (1.2%) 2435
Emsam Transdermal System (Infrequent) 905
▲ Rapamune (Greater than or equal to 3% to less than 20%) 3260
▲ Tygacil for Injection (4%) 3276

Lagophthalmos
BOTOX Purified Neurotoxin Complex 550

Laryngismus
Axert Tablets (Infrequent) 2431
Bexxar 1371
Campral Tablets (Rare) 1158
▲ Copaxone for Injection (5%) 3110
Effexor XR Extended-Release Capsules (Infrequent) 3195
Emsam Transdermal System (Infrequent) 905
Luvox CR Extended-Release Capsules (Rare) 1759
Lyrica Capsules (Rare) 2527
Paxil 1535
Paxil CR Controlled-Release Tablets 1544
Salagen Tablets (Less than 1%) 1082
Symbyax Capsules (Rare) 1871
Venlafaxine Hydrochloride Tablets (Infrequent) 2199

Laryngitis
▲ Advair HFA 45/21 Inhalation Aerosol (1% to 3%) 1288
▲ Advair HFA 115/21 Inhalation Aerosol (1% to 3%) 1288
▲ Advair HFA 230/21 Inhalation Aerosol (1% to 3%) 1288
▲ Aerobid/Aerobid-M (1% to 3%) 1153
Ambien Tablets (Rare) 2692
Ambien CR Tablets (Rare) 2696
Axert Tablets (Rare) 2431
Celebrex Capsules (0.1% to 1.9%) 2979
Celexa (Rare) 1160
Copaxone for Injection (At least 2%) 3110
Cymbalta Delayed-Release Capsules (Infrequent) 1801
Doxil Injection (Less than 1%) 2378
Effexor XR Extended-Release Capsules (Infrequent) 3195
Emsam Transdermal System (Infrequent) 905
Evista Tablets (2.2%) 1810
Evoxac Capsules (Less than 1%) 1013
Exelon Capsules (Infrequent) 2229
Exelon Oral Solution (Infrequent) 2229
Exubera Inhalation Powder (0.5% to 1.1%) 2515
▲ Flovent Diskus 50 mcg (1% to 3%) 1435
▲ Flovent HFA (1% to 3%) 1440
Flulaval Injection Vaccine 1448
Frova Tablets (Infrequent) 1111
Gabitril Tablets (Infrequent) 973
Ixempra Kit for Injection 915
Lexapro Oral Suspension (Infrequent) 1174
Lexapro Tablets (Infrequent) 1174
Lovaza Capsules 1520
Lunesta Tablets (Infrequent) 2994
Lupron Depot–3 Month 11.25 mg 462
▲ Luvox CR Extended-Release Capsules (3%) 1759
Meridia Capsules (1.3%) 475
Mirapex Tablets 857
▲ Norditropin Cartridges (6%) 2354
Prinivil Tablets (0.3% to 1%) 2087
Prinzide Tablets 2092
Protonix for Delayed-Release Oral Suspension (Less than 1%) 3254
Protonix Delayed-Release Tablets (Less than 1%) 3254
Protonix I.V. (Less than 1%) 3257
Protopic Ointment (Greater than or equal to 1%) 628
▲ Pulmozyme Inhalation Solution (3% to 4%) 1217
Remeron Tablets (Rare) 2924
RemeronSolTab Tablets (Rare) 2927
Requip Tablets (Infrequent) 1561
Rilutek Tablets (Infrequent) 2771
Salagen Tablets (Less than 1%) 1082
Selzentry Tablets 2534
Singulair (Greater than or equal to 2%) 2114
Soriatane Capsules (Less than 1%) 3062
▲ Spiriva HandiHaler (1% to 3%) 870
Sular Extended Release Tablets (Less than or equal to 1%) 2975
Symbyax Capsules (Infrequent) 1871
Tricor Tablets 520
Venlafaxine Hydrochloride Tablets (Infrequent) 2199
Ventolin HFA Inhalation Aerosol (Less than 3%) 1638
▲ Vivitrol (12% to 13%) 988
▲ Xeloda Tablets (Less than 5%) 2662
Xyrem Oral Solution (Infrequent) 1766
Zomig Tablets (Infrequent) 694
Zomig Nasal Spray (Rare) 689
Zomig-ZMT Tablets (Infrequent) 694
Zyprexa Tablets (Rare) 1883
Zyprexa ZYDIS Orally Disintegrating Tablets (Rare) 1883

Laryngopharyngitis
Selzentry Tablets 2534

Laryngospasm
Abilify Injection (Rare) 881
Abilify Injection (Rare) 2466
Abilify Oral Solution (Rare) 881
Abilify Oral Solution (Rare) 2466
Abilify Discmelt Orally Disintegrating Tablets (Rare) 881
Abilify Discmelt Orally Disintegrating Tablets (Rare) 2466
Abilify Tablets (Rare) 881
Abilify Tablets (Rare) 2466
Advair Diskus 100/50 1276
Advair Diskus 250/50 1276
Advair Diskus 500/50 1276
Atrovent HFA Inhalation Aerosol 839
Atrovent Nasal Spray 0.03% 834
Atrovent Nasal Spray 0.06% 836
Carafate Suspension 706
Carafate Tablets 707
Combigan Ophthalmic Solution 553
Combivent Inhalation Aerosol 845
Cosopt Sterile Ophthalmic Solution 1969
InnoPran XL Extended Release Capsules 1484
Mirapex Tablets 857
MS Contin Tablets (Less frequent) 2585
Nadolol Tablets 2191
Orthoclone OKT3 Sterile Solution (Less than 1%) 2387
Prozac Weekly Capsules 1852
Raptiva for Injection 1218
Serevent Diskus (Rare) 1594
Tessalon Capsules 1183
Tessalon Perles 1183
Timoptic Sterile Ophthalmic Solution 2121
Timoptic in Ocudose 2124
Timoptic-XE Sterile Ophthalmic Gel Forming Solution 2125
Toprol-XL Tablets 666
▲ Ultane Liquid for Inhalation (2% to 8%) 524
Zofran Injection 1682
Zofran 1687
Zofran ODT Orally Disintegrating Tablets 1687

Laryngotracheobronchitis
Prevnar 3241
Synagis Intramuscular Solution (More than 1%) 1948
Vaqta (1.2%) 2130

Larynx, swelling
Provigil Tablets 977

Lassitude
Azmacort Inhalation Aerosol 407
Beconase AQ Nasal Spray 1369
Dexedrine 1401
Gantrisin Pediatric Suspension 2638
InnoPran XL Extended Release Capsules 1484
Veramyst Nasal Spray 1643

Laughing, easy
▲ Marinol Capsules (8% to 24%) 3163

Laxative effect
Beelith Tablets 813

LDH abnormalities
Ceftin Tablets (1.0%) 1380
Nimotop Capsules (0.4%; rare) 790
Zyvox (0.2% to 1.8%) 2552

LDH increase
Abelcet Injection 1134
Accutane Capsules 2607
Advicor Tablets 402
AmBisome for Injection (Less common) 606
Aricept Tablets (Infrequent) 1062
Aricept ODT Tablets (Infrequent) 1062
Asacol Delayed-Release Tablets 2579
Biaxin/Biaxin XL (Less than 1%) 411
Cardizem LA Extended Release Tablets (Less than 2%) 421
Cipro I.V. (Among most frequent) 2817
Cipro (0.4%) 2810
Cipro XR Tablets 2823
Cubicin for Injection (Less than 1%) 995
Depakote ER Tablets 423
Doxil Injection (Less than 1%) 2378
Effexor XR Extended-Release Capsules 3195
Evoxac Capsules 1013
▲ Fortaz (1 in 18) 1450
Geodon Capsules (Infrequent) 2520
Gleevec Tablets (Infrequent) 2255
Increlex Injection 3100
▲ Intron A for Injection (Less than 5%) 2859
▲ Lupron Depot 3.75 mg (Approximately 5% to 8%) 462
▲ Lupron Depot 7.5 mg (Greater than or equal to 5%) 469
▲ Megace ES Oral Suspension (1% to 3%) 2499
Meridia Capsules (1.6%) 475
Merrem I.V. (Greater than 0.2%) 684
▲ Mylotarg for Injection (14% to 18%) 3212
Nalfon Capsules (Less than 1%) 2508
▲ Neulasta Injection (19%) 587
▲ Neupogen for Injection (27% to 58%) 589
Niaspan Extended-Release Tablets 480
Noroxin Tablets (Less frequent) 2069
Omnicef Capsules (0.2%) 497
Omnicef for Oral Suspension (1%) 497
Paxil (Rare) 1535
Paxil CR Controlled-Release Tablets (Rare) 1544
Pentasa Capsules (Less than 1%) 3030
Primaxin I.M. 2080
Primaxin I.V. 2083
▲ Prograf Capsules and Injection (3% to 15%) 622
Requip Tablets (Infrequent) 1561
Retrovir IV Infusion 1579
Rilutek Tablets (Rare) 2771
▲ Rituxan I.V. (0% to 66%) 1223
Rocephin Injectable Vials, ADD-Vantage, Galaxy, Bulk 2642
Rythmol SR Capsules 1590
▲ Soriatane Capsules (Approximately 1 in 3 patients) 3062
Suprax for Oral Suspension 1891
Suprax Tablets 1891
▲ Targretin Capsules (7.1% to 13.2%) 1084
Tarka Tablets 511
Timentin ADD-Vantage 1606
Timentin Injection Galaxy Container 1609
Timentin IV Infusion 1603
Timentin Pharmacy Bulk Package 1613
Toprol-XL Tablets 666
Ultane Liquid for Inhalation (Less than 1%) 524
Venlafaxine Hydrochloride Tablets 2199
WinRho SDF 741
Zinacef for Injection (1 in 75 patients) 1678
Zinacef Injection (1 in 75 patients) 1678
Zonegran Capsules (Rare) 1089

LDL, decrease
Enjuvia Tablets 1029
Premarin Tablets 3221
Premphase Tablets 3232
Prempro Tablets 3232

LDL, increase
Enjuvia Tablets 1029
Premphase Tablets 3232
Prempro Tablets 3232
Pristiq Extended-Release Tablets (0% to 2%) 3247

LE cells test positive
(*see under* Lupus erythematosus)

Lead, increased excretion
Cuprimine Capsules (Rare) 1986

Left ventricular dysfunction
▲ Clolar for Intravenous Infusion (27%) 1239
Herceptin I.V. 1199
Ixempra Kit for Injection 915
Novantrone for Injection Concentrate 1100
Orthoclone OKT3 Sterile Solution (Less than 1%) 2387
▲ Taxotere Injection Concentrate (0.3% to 9.6%) 2773

Left ventricular ejection fraction, asymptomatic declines in
Novantrone for Injection Concentrate 1100

Left ventricular ejection fraction, decrease
▲ Novantrone for Injection Concentrate (5%) 1100
▲ Sutent Capsules (1% to 15%) 2540
Tykerb Tablets (1 to 3 patients) 1631
Velcade for Injection 2168

Left ventricular failure
Mirapex Tablets 857

Leg cramps, nocturnal
▲ Actonel with Calcium Tablets (3.5%) 2574
Ambien CR Tablets (Infrequent) 2696
Niaspan Extended-Release Tablets 480

Legs, heaviness
Uroqid-Acid No. 2 Tablets 814

Legs, restless
Ambien Tablets (Rare) 2692
Lexapro Oral Suspension (Infrequent) 1174
Lexapro Tablets (Infrequent) 1174

Leiomyoma
(*see* Uterine fibroids)

LE-like reactions
(*see under* Lupus erythematosus)

Lens, pigmentation
Zyprexa Tablets (Rare) 1883
Zyprexa ZYDIS Orally Disintegrating Tablets (Rare) 1883

Lens changes, unspecified
Lamisil Oral Granules 2264
Myleran Tablets 1530

Lens opacities, changes
▲ Cosopt Sterile Ophthalmic Solution (1% to 5%) 1969
Lamisil Tablets 2266
Lescol Capsules 2268
Lescol XL Tablets 2268
Levaquin 2416
Levaquin in 5% Dextrose Injection 2416
Mevacor Tablets 2063

Lens opacities, irregular
Thioridazine Hydrochloride Tablets 2195

Lenticular deposits
Thioridazine Hydrochloride Tablets 2195

Lesions, bullous
Stalevo Tablets 2309

Lesions, cerebrovascular
Imitrex Nasal Spray 1470

Lesions, corneal
▲ Diclofenac Sodium Ophthalmic Solution (Less than or equal to 5%) ⊙240
Effexor XR Extended-Release Capsules (Infrequent) 3195
▲ Soriatane Capsules (1% to 5%) 3062
Targretin Capsules 1084
Venlafaxine Hydrochloride Tablets (Infrequent) 2199
▲ Voltaren Ophthalmic Solution (Less than or equal to 5%) 2336
Zyprexa Tablets (Rare) 1883
Zyprexa ZYDIS Orally Disintegrating Tablets (Rare) 1883

Lesions, nerve root
Boniva Injection (2.2%) 2614
Boniva Tablets (2.2%) 2618

Lesions, neuro-ocular
Premphase Tablets 3232
Prempro Tablets 3232

Lesions, oral
Advair Diskus 100/50 1276
Advair Diskus 250/50 1276
Advair Diskus 500/50 1276
Avapro Tablets (Less than 1%) 897
Avapro Tablets (Less than 1%) 2718
▲ Trisenox Injection (8%) 986
Viramune Oral Suspension 873
Viramune Tablets 873

Lesions, punctiform
Fleet Phospho-soda 1145
Fleet Phospho-soda EZ-PREP 1147

Lesions, rectal mucosal
Fleet Prep Kits 1149

Lesions, retinal vascular
Ortho-Cyclen/Ortho Tri-Cyclen 2449
Ortho Tri-Cyclen Lo Tablets 2458
Premphase Tablets 3232
Prempro Tablets 3232

Lethargy
▲ Abilify Injection (5%) 881
▲ Abilify Injection (5%) 2466
▲ Abilify Oral Solution (5%) 881
▲ Abilify Oral Solution (5%) 2466
▲ Abilify Discmelt Orally Disintegrating Tablets (5%) 881
▲ Abilify Discmelt Orally Disintegrating Tablets (5%) 2466
▲ Abilify Tablets (5%) 881
▲ Abilify Tablets (5%) 2466
Accutane Capsules 2607
Alphanate 1709
▲ Ambien Tablets (3%) 2692
Ambien CR Tablets (Frequent) 2696
Amitiza Capsules (Less than 1%) 3082
Arimidex Tablets (1%) 672
Arranon Injection (1%) 1319
Asacol Delayed-Release Tablets 2579
Avalide Tablets 892
▲ Avinza Capsules (Less than 5%) 1772
Bayer Aspirin 750
BeneFIX Vials 3191
Bentyl Capsules 703
Bentyl Injection 703
Bentyl Syrup 703
Bentyl Tablets 703
▲ Busulfex Injection (7%) 2477
Catapres-TTS (3 of 101 patients) 842
Cathflo Activase 1198
Celebrex Capsules 2979
Chantix Tablets (1% to 2%) 2511
Cipro I.V. (1% or less) 2817
Cipro (Less than 1%) 2810
Cipro XR Tablets 2823
▲ Clolar for Intravenous Infusion (11%) 1239
Concerta Extended-Release Tablets 1925
Cosmegen for Injection 2485
Cymbalta Delayed-Release Capsules (Frequent) 1801
▲ Dacogen Injection (12%) 1066
Demadex Injection 2630
Demadex Tablets 2630
Depakote ER Tablets 423
▲ DepoCyt Injection (12% to 16%) 1136
DepoDur Injection 1095
Diovan HCT Tablets 2216
Dyazide Capsules 1405
DynaCirc CR Controlled Release Tablets (0.5% to 1%) 1407
Eldepryl Capsules (1 of 49 patients) 3052
Eligard 7.5 mg (Less than 2%) 2724
Eligard 22.5 mg (Less than 2%) 2724
Eligard 30 mg (Less than 2%) 2724
Eligard 45 mg (Less than 2%) 2724
▲ Femara Tablets (0.2% to 8.4%) 2246
Fentora Tablets (Greater than 1%) 968
▲ FluMist Vaccine (6% to 14%) 1945
Furosemide Tablets 2186
Gengraf Capsules (Rare) 435
▲ Hycamtin for Injection (69%) 1459
InnoPran XL Extended Release Capsules 1484
Intravenous Sodium Diuril 2490
Ixempra Kit for Injection 915
▲ Lexapro Oral Suspension (3%) 1174
▲ Lexapro Tablets (3%) 1174
Lortab 5/500 Tablets 3143
Lortab 7.5/500 Tablets 3144
Lortab 10/500 Tablets 3144
Lyrica Capsules (1% to 2%) 2527
Marplan Tablets (2%) 3177
Mirapex Tablets 857
Namenda 1180
Neoral Oral Solution (Rare) 2280
Neoral Soft Gelatin Capsules (Rare) 2280
Opana Tablets (Less than 1%) 1117
Opana ER Tablets (Less than 1%) 1121
Orthoclone OKT3 Sterile Solution (Less than 1%) 2387
Pediarix Vaccine 1552
▲ Pentacel (0.2% to 45.8%) 2792
Percocet Tablets 1127
Percodan Tablets 1130
Prinzide Tablets 2092
Pristiq Extended-Release Tablets 3247
Profilnine SD Solvent Detergent 1721
Prozac Weekly Capsules 1852
▲ Reclast Injection (5%) 2291
ReFacto Vials 3269
Requip Tablets (Infrequent) 1561
St. Joseph 81 mg Aspirin Chewable and Enteric Coated Tablets 1903
Sandimmune (Rare) 2296
Stromectol Tablets 2120
▲ Taxotere Injection Concentrate (3.4% to 62.9%) 2773
Thioridazine Hydrochloride Tablets (Extremely rare) 2195
Tice BCG 2936
Tracleer Tablets 3289
Treximet Tablets (Infrequent) 1616
Trizivir Tablets 1622
Tussionex Pennkinetic Extended-Release Suspension 3154
▲ Ultram ER Extended-Release Tablets (1% to less than 5%) 2428
Vantas (Less than 2%) 1737
Venlafaxine Hydrochloride Tablets 2199
Vicodin Tablets 529
Vicodin ES Tablets 530
Vicodin HP Tablets 531
Vicoprofen Tablets 533
▲ Vivitrol (12% to 23%) 988
▲ Xeloda Tablets (Up to 7%) 2662
▲ Xyrem Oral Solution (5.9%) 1766
Ziagen 1673
Zolinza Capsules 2142
Zydone Tablets 1132

Leucocytosis
Ultane Liquid for Inhalation (Less than 1%) 524

Leukemia, acute
Busulfex Injection (Four cases) 2477
Leukeran Tablets 1508
Novantrone for Injection Concentrate 1100

Leukemia, chronic lymphocytic
Mirapex Tablets 857

Leukemia, lymphocytic
Mustargen for Injection 2492

Leukemia, myelogenous
Temodar Capsules 2931

Leukemia, myeloid
Taxotere Injection Concentrate (Rare) 2773

Leukemia, secondary
Bexxar 1371

Leukemia, unspecified
Genotropin Lyophilized Powder 2547
Humatrope Vials and Cartridges 1838
Indocin (Rare) 2024
Norditropin Cartridges (A small number of children) 2354
Nutropin for Injection (A small number of patients) 1208
Nutropin AQ Injection (A small number of patients) 1212
Nutropin AQ NuSpin Injection (A small number of patients) 1212
Nutropin AQ Pen (A small number of patients) 1212
Nutropin AQ Pen Cartridge (A small number of patients) 1212
Plavix Tablets (Less than 1%) 926
Plavix Tablets (Less than 1%) 2767
Tev-Tropin for Injection 1187

Leukocyte count, abnormal
Cipro XR Tablets 2823
▲ Zyvox (0.2% to 12.4%) 2552

Leukocyte count, elevated
Agrylin Capsules 3017
Vivitrol 988

Leukocytosis
Abelcet Injection 1134
Aceon Tablets (2 mg, 4 mg, 8 mg) 3038
Alinia for Oral Suspension (Less than 1%) 2677
Alinia Tablets (Less than 1%) 2677
Amerge Tablets (Infrequent) 1301
Aricept Tablets (Frequent) 1062
Aricept ODT Tablets (Frequent) 1062
Attenuvax 1951
Brovana Inhalation Solution 2990
Capastat Sulfate for Injection 1791
Carbatrol Capsules 3019
Celexa (Infrequent) 1160
▲ CellCept Capsules (22.4% to 40.5%) 2622
▲ CellCept Intravenous (22.4% to 40.5%) 2622
▲ CellCept Oral Suspension (22.4% to 40.5%) 2622
▲ CellCept Tablets (22.4% to 40.5%) 2622
Chantix Tablets (Rare) 2511
Cipro I.V. (Rare) 2817
Cipro (Less than 0.1%) 2810
Cipro XR Tablets 2823
Clinoril Tablets (Less than 1 in 100) 1962
Cubicin for Injection (Less than 1%) 995
Cuprimine Capsules 1986
Effexor XR Extended-Release Capsules (Infrequent) 3195
Emend Capsules (Greater than 0.5%) 1992
Emend for Injection (Greater than 0.5%) 1999
Emsam Transdermal System (Rare) 905
Equetro Extended-Release Capsules 3174
Evoxac Capsules (Less than 1%) 1013
Exelon Capsules (Infrequent) 2229
Exelon Oral Solution (Infrequent) 2229
Geodon Capsules (Infrequent) 2520
Gliadel Wafer (1%) 1076
Ionsys Transdermal System (.1% to less than 1%) 2410
Lamictal (Rare) 1488
Luvox CR Extended-Release Capsules (Infrequent) 1759
Lyrica Capsules (0.1% to 1%) 2527
Merrem I.V. (Greater than 0.2%) 684
Meruvax II 2061
M-M-R II 2054
Moban Tablets 1116
Mumpsvax 2068
Neulasta Injection (Less than 1%) 587
Neupogen for Injection (Approximately 2%) 589
Nexium Delayed-Release Capsules (Less than 1%) 645
Nexium I.V. (Less than 1%) 652
Nexium Delayed-Release Oral Suspension (Less than 1%) 645
Omnicef Capsules (0.7%) 497
Omnicef for Oral Suspension (0.3%) 497
Orthoclone OKT3 Sterile Solution (Less than 1%) 2387
Panhematin for Injection 2497
▲ Paser Granules (79% of 38 patients with drug-induced hepatitis) 1747
Paxil (Rare) 1535
Paxil CR Controlled-Release Tablets (Rare) 1544
Pneumovax 23 2078
Primaxin I.V. 2083
Prinivil Tablets (0.3% to 1%) 2087
Prinzide Tablets 2092
▲ Prograf Capsules and Injection (3% to 32%) 622
Prolastin 3099
Proleukin for Injection (Less than 1%) 2287
Protonix for Delayed-Release Oral Suspension (Less than 1%) 3254
Protonix Delayed-Release Tablets (Less than 1%) 3254
Protonix I.V. (Less than 1%) 3257
Protopic Ointment (Greater than or equal to 1%) 628
Provigil Tablets (At least 1%) 977
Prozac Weekly Capsules 1852
Prozac Pulvules and Liquid 1852
▲ Raptiva for Injection (26%) 1218
ReoPro Vials (1%) 1860
Requip Tablets (Infrequent) 1561
Rilutek Tablets (Infrequent) 2771
Risperdal Consta Long-Acting Injection (Rare) 1753
Rocephin Injectable Vials, ADD-Vantage, Galaxy, Bulk (Less than 0.1%) 2642
Symbyax Capsules (Infrequent) 1871
Tasigna Capsules 2316
Thiothixene Capsules (Occasional) 2197
Trasylol Injection (1% to 2%) 799
▲ Trisenox Injection (50%) 986
▲ Tygacil for Injection (3.7%) 3276
Venlafaxine Hydrochloride Tablets (Infrequent) 2199
▲ Vesanoid Capsules (About 40%) 2660
Wellbutrin Tablets 1648
Wellbutrin SR Sustained-Release Tablets 1653
Wellbutrin XL Extended-Release Tablets 1659
Zyban Sustained-Release Tablets 1692
Zyprexa Tablets (Infrequent) 1883
Zyprexa ZYDIS Orally Disintegrating Tablets (Infrequent) 1883

Leukocyturia
Crixivan Capsules 1979
Emend Capsules (Greater than 0.5%) 1992
Emend for Injection (Greater than 0.5%) 1999
Omnicef Capsules (2%) 497
Primaxin I.M. 2080
Primaxin I.V. 2083

Leukoderma
Effexor XR Extended-Release Capsules (Rare) 3195
Lamictal (Rare) 1488
Protopic Ointment (0.2% to less than 1%) 628
Venlafaxine Hydrochloride Tablets (Rare) 2199

Leukoencephalopathy
Arranon Injection (1%) 1319

Leukoencephalopathy, multifocal, progressive
Campath Ampules 761
CellCept Capsules 2622
CellCept Intravenous 2622
CellCept Oral Suspension 2622
CellCept Tablets 2622

Myfortic Tablets 2276
Rituxan I.V. 1223

Leukoencephalopathy, posterior

Avastin IV 1192
Nexavar Tablets (0.1% to less than 1%) 784
Sutent Capsules (Less than 1%) 2540
Velcade for Injection 2168

Leukoencephalopathy, unspecified

Prograf Capsules and Injection 622

Leukopenia

▲ Abelcet Injection (4%) 1134
Abilify Injection (Greater than or equal to 1 in 1000 patients and less than 1 in 100 patients) 881
Abilify Injection (Greater than or equal to 1 in 1000 patients and less than 1 in 100 patients) 2466
Abilify Oral Solution (Greater than or equal to 1 in 1000 patients and less than 1 in 100 patients) 881
Abilify Oral Solution (Greater than or equal to 1 in 1000 patients and less than 1 in 100 patients) 2466
Abilify Discmelt Orally Disintegrating Tablets (Greater than or equal to 1 in 1000 patients and less than 1 in 100 patients) 881
Abilify Discmelt Orally Disintegrating Tablets (Greater than or equal to 1 in 1000 patients and less than 1 in 100 patients) 2466
Abilify Tablets (Greater than or equal to 1 in 1000 patients and less than 1 in 100 patients) 881
Abilify Tablets (Greater than or equal to 1 in 1000 patients and less than 1 in 100 patients) 2466
Accutane Capsules 2607
Aceon Tablets (2 mg, 4 mg, 8 mg) (0.1%) 3038
Aciphex Tablets 1053
Actiq (Less than 1%) 959
Advicor Tablets 402
Albenza Tablets (Less than 1%) 1297
Aldara Cream, 5% 1699
▲ Alferon N Injection (11%) 1726
▲ Alimta for Injection (Less than 1% to 55%) 1786
Ambien Tablets (Rare) 2692
Ambien CR Tablets (Rare) 2696
Amoxil Capsules 1305
Amoxil Chewable Tablets 1305
Amoxil Pediatric Drops for Oral Suspension 1305
Amoxil Powder for Oral Suspension 1305
Amoxil Tablets 1305
Anaprox Tablets (Less than 1%) 2632
Anaprox DS Tablets (Less than 1%) 2632
▲ Arimidex Tablets (2% to 5%) 672
▲ Arranon Injection (7% to 38%) 1319
Asacol Delayed-Release Tablets 2579
Atacand Tablets (Very rare) 639
Atacand HCT 642
Augmentin 1323
Augmentin Tablets 1327
Augmentin XR Extended Release Tablets 1333
Augmentin ES-600 Powder for Oral Suspension 1329
Avalide Tablets 892
Avalide Tablets 2713
Avandaryl Tablets 1344
▲ Avastin IV (37%) 1192
Avelox (Greater than or equal to 0.1% to less than 2%) 2803
Azilect Tablets (Greater than 1%) 3106
▲ Betaseron for SC Injection (6% to 18%) 756
Biaxin/Biaxin XL (Less than 1%) 411
Bicillin C-R Injectable Suspension 1775
Bicillin L-A Injection 1777
Campral Tablets (Rare) 1158
Canasa Rectal Suppositories (One patient) 705
Capastat Sulfate for Injection 1791
Carbatrol Capsules 3019
Cardizem LA Extended Release Tablets (Infrequent) 421
Ceftin 1380
Celexa (Infrequent) 1160
▲ CellCept Capsules (23.2% to 45.8%) 2622
▲ CellCept Intravenous (23.2% to 45.8%) 2622
▲ CellCept Oral Suspension (23.2% to 45.8%) 2622
▲ CellCept Tablets (23.2% to 45.8%) 2622
Cimzia (Infrequent) 3127
Cipro I.V. (Rare to Infrequent) 2817
Cipro (0.4%) 2810
Cipro XR Tablets 2823
Clinoril Tablets (Less than 1%) 1962
Clolar for Intravenous Infusion 1239
Clorpres Tablets 2185
Concerta Extended-Release Tablets (Less than 1%) 1925
Copaxone for Injection (Infrequent) 3110
Coreg Tablets (Greater than 0.1 to 1%) 1387
Coreg CR Extended-Release Capsules (0.1% to less than or equal to 1%) 1393
Cosmegen for Injection 2485
▲ Cuprimine Capsules (2% to 5%) 1986
▲ Dacogen Injection (28%) 1066
Dantrium Capsules (Less frequent) 2580
Dantrium Intravenous 2582
Daraprim Tablets 1400
Daytrana Transdermal Patch 3022
Depakote ER Tablets (Greater than 1%) 423
Didronel Tablets (One report) 2583
Diovan HCT Tablets 2216
▲ Doxil Injection (About 42.2% to 60%) 2378
Duetact Tablets 3085
Dyazide Capsules 1405
DynaCirc CR Controlled Release Tablets (0.5% to 1%) 1407
EC-Naprosyn Delayed-Release Tablets (Less than 1%) 2632
Effexor XR Extended-Release Capsules (Infrequent) 3195
Elmiron Capsules (Less than or equal to 1%) 2435
▲ Eloxatin for Injection (0% to 85%) 2731
Elspar for Injection 1990
Emsam Transdermal System (Rare) 905
Enbrel for Injection 569
▲ Equetro Extended-Release Capsules (Up to 5%) 3174
▲ Erbitux (17%) 912
Evoxac Capsules (Less than 1%) 1013
Exforge Tablets (Greater than 0.1% to less than 1%) 2238
Fansidar Tablets 2636
Faslodex Injection (Less than 1%) 682
Fentora Tablets (Greater than 1%) 968
Flebogamma 5% 1715
Flebogamma 5% DIF 1718
Focalin XR Capsules 2251
Fortaz (Very rare) 1450
Furosemide Tablets 2186
Gabitril Tablets (Infrequent) 973
Gammagard Liquid 730
Gammagard S/D (Rare) 734
Gamunex (Rare) 3094
Gantrisin Pediatric Suspension 2638
▲ Gemzar for Injection (15% to 86%) 1820
▲ Gengraf Capsules (1% to 6%) 435
Geodon Capsules (Infrequent) 2520
Gris-PEG Tablets (Rare) 2507
▲ Herceptin I.V. (3%) 1199
▲ Hexalen Capsules (5%) 1078
▲ Humira Injection (Less than 5%) 442
▲ Hycamtin Capsules (86% to 90%) 1456
▲ Hycamtin for Injection (32% to 98%) 1459
Indapamide Tablets 2188
Indocin Capsules (Less than 1%) 2024
Indocin I.V. (Less than 1%) 2489
Indocin (Less than 1%) 2024
Intravenous Sodium Diuril 2490
▲ Intron A for Injection (Less than 5% to 68%) 2859
▲ Ixempra Kit for Injection (13% to greater than 40%) 915
Kaletra (Less than 2%) 452
Keppra Injection 3137
Keppra Oral Solution 3131
Keppra Tablets 3131
Klonopin 2639
Lamictal (Infrequent) 1488
Lescol Capsules (Rare) 2268
Lescol XL Tablets 2268
▲ Leukine (17%) 774
Levaquin 2416
Levaquin in 5% Dextrose Injection 2416
▲ Lupron Depot 7.5 mg (Greater than or equal to 5%) 469
Luvox CR Extended-Release Capsules (Rare) 1759
Lyrica Capsules (0.1% to 1%) 2527
Mavik Tablets (Rare) 472
▲ Megace ES Oral Suspension (1% to 3%) 2499
▲ Mepron Suspension (4%) 1526
Meridia Capsules 475
Merrem I.V. (Greater than 0.2%) 684
Metadate CD Capsules 3146
Mevacor Tablets (Rare) 2063
Micardis HCT Tablets 854
Moban Tablets 1116
Mobic Oral Suspension (Less than 2%) 863
Mobic Tablets (Less than 2%) 863
Moxatag Tablets 2165
▲ Myfortic Tablets (3% to less than 20%) 2276
Myleran Tablets 1530
▲ Mylotarg for Injection (43% to 52%) 3212
Namenda (Infrequent) 1180
Naprosyn Suspension (Less than 1%) 2632
Naprosyn Tablets (Less than 1%) 2632
▲ Neoral Oral Solution (1% to 6%) 2280
▲ Neoral Soft Gelatin Capsules (1% to 6%) 2280
▲ Nexavar Tablets (Greater than or equal to 10%) 784
Nexium Delayed-Release Capsules (Less than 1%) 645
Nexium I.V. (Less than 1%) 652
Nexium Delayed-Release Oral Suspension (Less than 1%) 645
Noroxin Tablets 2069
▲ Norvir (0.9% to 36.9%) 489
▲ Novantrone for Injection Concentrate (9% to 19%) 1100
Omnicef Capsules (0.9%) 497
Omnicef for Oral Suspension (0.3%) 497
▲ Ontak Vials (6%) 1079
Orthoclone OKT3 Sterile Solution (Less than 1%) 2387
Parnate Tablets 1532
Paser Granules 1747
Paxil (Infrequent) 1535
Paxil CR Controlled-Release Tablets (Infrequent) 1544
▲ PegIntron Powder for Injection (4%) 2903
Pentasa Capsules 3030
Pepcid Tablets (Rare) 2075
Percodan Tablets 1130
Phenytek Capsules (Occasional) 2192
Plavix Tablets (Less than 1%) 926
Plavix Tablets (Less than 1%) 2767
Pletal Tablets 2481
Prandin Tablets (Less than or equal to 1%) 2971
Primaxin I.M. 2080
Primaxin I.V. (Less than 0.2%) 2083
Prinivil Tablets (Rare) 2087
Prinzide Tablets 2092
▲ Prograf Capsules and Injection (3% to 15%) 622
▲ Proleukin for Injection (Less than 1% to 16%) 2287
Protonix for Delayed-Release Oral Suspension (Less than 1%) 3254
Protonix Delayed-Release Tablets (Less than 1%) 3254
Protonix I.V. (Less than 1%) 3257
Protopic Ointment (Greater than or equal to 1%) 628
Prozac Weekly Capsules (Rare) 1852
Prozac Pulvules and Liquid (Rare) 1852
Pylera Capsules 714
▲ Rapamune (Greater than or equal to 3% to less than 20%) 3260
▲ Rebetol (5% to 6%) 2917
▲ Rebif Prefilled Syringe for Injection (6% to 36%) 1107
Remeron Tablets (Rare) 2924
RemeronSolTab Tablets (Rare) 2927
Remicade for IV Injection (Greater than or equal to 0.2%) 950
Requip Tablets (Infrequent) 1561
Retrovir Capsules 1574
Retrovir IV Infusion 1579
Retrovir 1574
Rilutek Tablets (Infrequent) 2771
Risperdal Consta Long-Acting Injection (Infrequent) 1753
▲ Rituxan I.V. (4% to 14%) 1223
Rocephin Injectable Vials, ADD-Vantage, Galaxy, Bulk (2.1%) 2642
Rythmol Tablets (Less than 1%) 1586
Salagen Tablets (Less than 1%) 1082
▲ Sandimmune (Up to 6%) 2296
▲ Simulect for Injection (3% to 10%) 2306
Skelaxin Tablets (Most frequent) 1784
Soma Tablets 1931
Stalevo Tablets 2309
Stromectol Tablets (One patient) 2120
Sular Extended Release Tablets (Less than or equal to 1%) 2975
Suprax for Oral Suspension (Less than 2%) 1891
Suprax Tablets (Less than 2%) 1891
▲ Sutent Capsules (0% to 7%) 2540
Symbyax Capsules (Rare) 1871
Tabloid Tablets 1601
▲ Targretin Capsules (16.7% to 47.2%) 1084
▲ Targretin Gel 1% (6%) 1088
Tarka Tablets (0.3% or more) 511
Tasigna Capsules 2316
▲ Taxotere Injection Concentrate (31.6% to 98.6%) 2773
Tekturna HCT Tablets 2324
▲ Temodar Capsules (55%) 2931
Teveten Tablets (0.3%) 515
Teveten HCT Tablets 517
Thioridazine Hydrochloride Tablets (Infrequent) 2195
Thiothixene Capsules (Occasional) 2197
Tice BCG (Less than or equal to 1%) 2936
Timentin ADD-Vantage 1606
Timentin Injection Galaxy Container 1609
Timentin IV Infusion 1603
Timentin Pharmacy Bulk Package 1613
▲ Torisel Injection (1% to 32%) 3272
▲ Treanda for Injection (15% to 61%) 983
Treximet Tablets (Rare) 1616
Tricor Tablets 520
Urso 250 Tablets (2%) 720
Urso Forte Tablets (2%) 720
▲ Valcyte Tablets (14%) 2654
Valtrex Caplets (0.7% to 1.3%) 1635
▲ Velcade for Injection (33%) 2168
Venlafaxine Hydrochloride Tablets (Infrequent) 2199
Voltaren Tablets (Occasionally) 2334
Voltaren-XR Tablets (Occasionally) 2337
Vytorin 10/10 Tablets 2149
Vytorin 10/10 Tablets 2939
Vytorin 10/20 Tablets 2149
Vytorin 10/20 Tablets 2939
Vytorin 10/40 Tablets 2149
Vytorin 10/40 Tablets 2939
Vytorin 10/80 Tablets 2149
Vytorin 10/80 Tablets 2939
Wellbutrin Tablets 1648
Wellbutrin SR Sustained-Release Tablets 1653
Wellbutrin XL Extended-Release Tablets 1659
▲ Xeloda Tablets (24% to 91%) 2662
Xyrem Oral Solution (Infrequent) 1766
Zantac 25 EFFERdose Tablets (A few patients) 1670
Zantac Injection (Few patients) 1666
Zantac Injection Pharmacy Bulk Package (Infrequent) 1668
Zantac Injection Premixed (Few patients) 1666
Zantac (A few patients) 1670
Ziagen (Less than 1%) 1673
Zinacef for Injection (1 in 750 patients) 1678
Zinacef Injection (1 in 750 patients) 1678
Zocor Tablets (Rare) 2136
Zolinza Capsules 2142
Zomig Tablets (Rare) 694
Zomig Nasal Spray (Rare) 689
Zomig-ZMT Tablets (Rare) 694
Zonegran Capsules (Infrequent) 1089
Zosyn for Injection 3284
Zovirax 1690
Zyban Sustained-Release Tablets 1692
Zyprexa Tablets (Infrequent) 1883
Zyprexa ZYDIS Orally Disintegrating Tablets (Infrequent) 1883

Leukoplakia, oral

Doxil Injection (Less than 1%) 2378
Geodon Capsules (Rare) 2520
▲ Intron A for Injection (Less than 5%) 2859

Leukorrhea

Angeliq Tablets (1.3%) 751
▲ Arimidex Tablets (2% to 3%) 672
▲ Climara Transdermal System (1% to 7%) 763
▲ Doxil Injection (1% to 10%) 2378
Effexor XR Extended-Release Capsules (Infrequent) 3195
▲ Evista Tablets (3.3%) 1810
Evoxac Capsules (Less than 1%) 1013
Gengraf Capsules (1%) 435

▲ Intron A for Injection (Less than 5%) 2859
Lyrica Capsules (0.1% to 1%) 2527
▲ Mirena Intrauterine System (5% or more) 779
Neoral Oral Solution (1%) 2280
Neoral Soft Gelatin Capsules (1%) 2280
Omnicef Capsules (0.2%) 497
Omnicef for Oral Suspension (0.2%) 497
ParaGard T 380A Intrauterine Copper Contraceptive 1041
Paxil (Rare) 1535
Paxil CR Controlled-Release Tablets (Rare) 1544
▲ Premarin Tablets (4% to 7%) 3221
▲ Premphase Tablets (3% to 9%) 3232
▲ Prempro Tablets (3% to 9%) 3232
▲ Prometrium Capsules (100 mg, 200 mg) (Less than 5%) 3047
Prozac Weekly Capsules (Infrequent) 1852
Prozac Pulvules and Liquid (Infrequent) 1852
Remeron Tablets (Infrequent) 2924
RemeronSolTab Tablets (Infrequent) 2927
Risperdal Consta Long-Acting Injection (Infrequent) 1753
Soriatane Capsules (Less than 1%) 3062
Symbyax Capsules (Infrequent) 1871
Tygacil for Injection (0% to less than 2%) 3276
Venlafaxine Hydrochloride Tablets (Infrequent) 2199
Yaz Tablets (Greater than 1%) 805
Zosyn for Injection (1% or less) 3284
Zyrtec Chewable Tablets (Less than 2%) 1920
Zyrtec Syrup (Less than 2%) 1920
Zyrtec Tablets (Less than 2%) 1920
Zyrtec-D 12 Hour Extended Release Tablets (Less than 2%) 1923

Lhermitte's sign
Copaxone for Injection (At least 2%) 3110
Eloxatin for Injection 2731

Libido, changes
Activella Tablets 2347
Adderall XR Capsules 3012
Adipex-P 1185
Avalide Tablets 892
Avalide Tablets 2713
Avapro Tablets (Less than 1%) 897
Avapro Tablets (Less than 1%) 2718
Climara Transdermal System 763
Climara Pro Transdermal System 768
Dexedrine 1401
Divigel 3167
Enjuvia Tablets 1029
Estratest Tablets 3043
Estratest H.S. Tablets 3043
▲ Lupron Depot 3.75 mg (16%) 462
▲ Lupron Depot–3 Month 11.25 mg (16%) 462
Lybrel Tablets 3204
Mircette Tablets 1034
▲ Novantrone for Injection Concentrate (7%) 1100
Ortho-Cyclen Tablets 2449
Ortho Evra Transdermal System 2437
Ortho Tri-Cyclen Tablets 2449
Ortho Tri-Cyclen Lo Tablets 2458
Premarin Intravenous 3217
Premarin Tablets 3221
Premarin Vaginal Cream 3228
Premphase Tablets 3232
Prempro Tablets 3232
Seasonique Tablets 1046
Thioridazine Hydrochloride Tablets 2195
Valium Tablets (Infrequent) 2658
Vyvanse Capsules 3033
Yaz Tablets 805

Libido, decreased
Abilify Injection (Greater than or equal to 1 in 1000 patients and less than 1 in 100 patients) 881
Abilify Injection (Greater than or equal to 1 in 1000 patients and less than 1 in 100 patients) 2466
Abilify Oral Solution (Greater than or equal to 1 in 1000 patients and less than 1 in 100 patients) 881
Abilify Oral Solution (Greater than or equal to 1 in 1000 patients and less than 1 in 100 patients) 2466
Abilify Discmelt Orally Disintegrating Tablets (Greater than or equal to 1 in 1000 patients and less than 1 in 100 patients) 881
Abilify Discmelt Orally Disintegrating Tablets (Greater than or equal to 1 in 1000 patients and less than 1 in 100 patients) 2466
Abilify Tablets (Greater than or equal to 1 in 1000 patients and less than 1 in 100 patients) 881
Abilify Tablets (Greater than or equal to 1 in 1000 patients and less than 1 in 100 patients) 2466
Actiq (Less than 1%) 959
▲ Adderall XR Capsules (2% to 4%) 3012
Ambien Tablets (Rare) 2692
Ambien CR Tablets (Rare) 2696
Amerge Tablets (Rare) 1301
▲ AndroGel (0% to 3%) 3159
Aricept Tablets (Infrequent) 1062
Aricept ODT Tablets (Infrequent) 1062
Asacol Delayed-Release Tablets 2579
▲ Avinza Capsules (Less than 5%) 1772
▲ Avodart Soft Gelatin Capsules (Less than 0.1% to 4.5%) 1359
Axid Capsules 1364
Azilect Tablets (Greater than 1%) 3106
Calcijex Injection 419
Campral Tablets (Frequent) 1158
Celexa (2%) 1160
Chantix Tablets (Infrequent) 2511
Combigan Ophthalmic Solution 553
Concerta Extended-Release Tablets (1.7%) 1925
Copaxone for Injection (Infrequent) 3110
Coreg Tablets (Greater than 0.1 to 1%) 1387
Coreg CR Extended-Release Capsules (0.1% to less than or equal to 1%) 1393
Cosopt Sterile Ophthalmic Solution 1969
Cozaar Tablets (Less than 1%) 1973
▲ Crinone 8% Gel (10%) 992
▲ Cymbalta Delayed-Release Capsules (2% to 4%) 1801
Delatestryl Injection 1730
Diovan HCT Tablets (Less frequent) 2216
Duragesic Transdermal System (Less than 1%) 2405
DynaCirc CR Controlled Release Tablets (0.5% to 1%) 1407
▲ Effexor XR Extended-Release Capsules (3% to 10%) 3195
Eligard 7.5 mg (Less than 2%) 2724
Eligard 22.5 mg (Less than 2%) 2724
▲ Eligard 30 mg (Less than 2% to 3.3%) 2724
Eligard 45 mg (Less than 2%) 2724
Emsam Transdermal System (0.7%) 905
Exelon Capsules (Infrequent) 2229
Exelon Oral Solution (Infrequent) 2229
Flomax Capsules (1% to 2%) 848
Gabitril Tablets (Infrequent) 973
Gengraf Capsules (1% to less than 3%) 435
▲ Indapamide Tablets (Less than 5%) 2188
▲ Intron A for Injection (Up to 5%) 2859
Kaletra (Up to 2%) 452
Klonopin (1%) 2639
Lamictal (Infrequent) 1488
▲ Lexapro Oral Suspension (3% to 7%) 1174
▲ Lexapro Tablets (3% to 7%) 1174
Lipitor Tablets (Less than 2%) 2501
▲ Lunesta Tablets (0% to 3%) 2994
▲ Lupron Depot 3.75 mg (Less than 5%) 462
▲ Lupron Depot 7.5 mg (5.4%) 469
▲ Lupron Depot–3 Month 11.25 mg (1.8% to 11%) 462
▲ Luvox CR Extended-Release Capsules (4% to 10%) 1759
Lyrica Capsules (Greater than or equal to 1%) 2527
Mavik Tablets (0.3% to 1%) 472
▲ Megace ES Oral Suspension (0% to 5%) 2499
Meridia Capsules 475
Mirapex Tablets (1%) 857
▲ Mirena Intrauterine System (5% or more) 779
MS Contin Tablets (Less frequent) 2585
Nadolol Tablets (1 to 5 of 1000 patients) 2191
Neoral Oral Solution (1% to less than 3%) 2280
Neoral Soft Gelatin Capsules (1% to less than 3%) 2280
Norvir (Less than 2%) 489
OxyContin Tablets (Less than 1%) 2589
▲ Paxil (3% to 9%) 1535
▲ Paxil CR Controlled-Release Tablets (3% to 9%) 1544
Pepcid Tablets (Infrequent) 2075
Prinivil Tablets (0.4%) 2087
Prinzide Tablets (0.3% to 1%) 2092
▲ Pristiq Extended-Release Tablets (3% to 6%) 3247
▲ Propecia Tablets (1.8% to 6.4%) 2095
▲ Proscar Tablets (2.6% to 6.4%) 2102
Protonix for Delayed-Release Oral Suspension (Less than 1%) 3254
Protonix Delayed-Release Tablets (Less than 1%) 3254
Protonix I.V. (Less than 1%) 3257
Provigil Tablets (At least 1%) 977
▲ Prozac Weekly Capsules (1% to 11%) 1852
▲ Prozac Pulvules and Liquid (1% to 11%) 1852
Requip Tablets (Infrequent) 1561
Rilutek Tablets (Infrequent) 2771
Risperdal Consta Long-Acting Injection (Infrequent) 1753
Rocaltrol Capsules 1150
Rocaltrol Oral Solution 1150
Rythmol SR Capsules 1590
Sandostatin Injection (Less than 1%) 2300
Sandostatin LAR Depot 2302
Soriatane Capsules (Less than 1%) 3062
▲ Strattera Capsules (5% to 6%) 1864
Sular Extended Release Tablets (Less than or equal to 1%) 2975
▲ Symbyax Capsules (2% to 4%) 1871
Tarka Tablets 511
Timoptic Sterile Ophthalmic Solution 2121
Timoptic in Ocudose 2124
Timoptic-XE Sterile Ophthalmic Gel Forming Solution 2125
Toprol-XL Tablets 666
Tricor Tablets 520
Ultram ER Extended-Release Tablets (0.5% to less than 1%) 2428
Vantas (2.3%) 1737
▲ Venlafaxine Hydrochloride Tablets (1.1% to 5.7%) 2199
Vicoprofen Tablets (Less than 1%) 533
Vivitrol 988
▲ Wellbutrin Tablets (3.1%) 1648
Wellbutrin SR Sustained-Release Tablets (Infrequent) 1653
▲ Wellbutrin XL Extended-Release Tablets (3%) 1659
Yaz Tablets (Greater than 1%) 805
Zantac Injection 1666
Zantac Injection Pharmacy Bulk Package (Infrequent) 1668
Zantac Injection Premixed 1666
Zonegran Capsules (Infrequent) 1089
Zyban Sustained-Release Tablets (Infrequent) 1692
Zyprexa Tablets (Infrequent) 1883
Zyprexa ZYDIS Orally Disintegrating Tablets (Infrequent) 1883
Zyrtec Chewable Tablets (Less than 2%) 1920
Zyrtec Syrup (Less than 2%) 1920
Zyrtec Tablets (Less than 2%) 1920
Zyrtec-D 12 Hour Extended Release Tablets (Less than 2%) 1923

Libido, increased
Abilify Injection (Greater than or equal to 1 in 1000 patients and less than 1 in 100 patients) 881
Abilify Injection (Greater than or equal to 1 in 1000 patients and less than 1 in 100 patients) 2466
Abilify Oral Solution (Greater than or equal to 1 in 1000 patients and less than 1 in 100 patients) 881
Abilify Oral Solution (Greater than or equal to 1 in 1000 patients and less than 1 in 100 patients) 2466
Abilify Discmelt Orally Disintegrating Tablets (Greater than or equal to 1 in 1000 patients and less than 1 in 100 patients) 881
Abilify Discmelt Orally Disintegrating Tablets (Greater than or equal to 1 in 1000 patients and less than 1 in 100 patients) 2466
Abilify Tablets (Greater than or equal to 1 in 1000 patients and less than 1 in 100 patients) 881
Abilify Tablets (Greater than or equal to 1 in 1000 patients and less than 1 in 100 patients) 2466
AndroGel (1 patient) 3159
Aricept Tablets (Frequent) 1062
Aricept ODT Tablets (Frequent) 1062
Campral Tablets (Infrequent) 1158
Celexa (Infrequent) 1160
Delatestryl Injection 1730
Effexor XR Extended-Release Capsules (Infrequent) 3195
Emsam Transdermal System (Infrequent) 905
Exelon Capsules (Infrequent) 2229
Exelon Oral Solution (Infrequent) 2229
Gabitril Tablets (Infrequent) 973
Gengraf Capsules (1% to less than 3%) 435
Klonopin (Infrequent) 2639
Lamictal (Rare) 1488
Luvox CR Extended-Release Capsules (Infrequent) 1759
Lyrica Capsules (0.1% to 1%) 2527
Meridia Capsules 475
Mirapex Tablets 857
Moban Tablets 1116
Namenda (Infrequent) 1180
Neoral Oral Solution (1% to less than 3%) 2280
Neoral Soft Gelatin Capsules (1% to less than 3%) 2280
Paxil (Rare) 1535
Paxil CR Controlled-Release Tablets (Rare) 1544
Prozac Weekly Capsules (Infrequent) 1852
Prozac Pulvules and Liquid (Infrequent) 1852
Remeron Tablets (Infrequent) 2924
RemeronSolTab Tablets (Infrequent) 2927
Requip Tablets (Infrequent) 1561
Rilutek Tablets (Infrequent) 2771
Stalevo Tablets 2309
Symbyax Capsules (Rare) 1871
Venlafaxine Hydrochloride Tablets (Infrequent) 2199
Wellbutrin Tablets (Frequent) 1648
Wellbutrin SR Sustained-Release Tablets 1653
Wellbutrin XL Extended-Release Tablets 1659
Xyrem Oral Solution (Infrequent) 1766
Zyban Sustained-Release Tablets 1692
Zyprexa Tablets 1883
Zyprexa ZYDIS Orally Disintegrating Tablets 1883

Libido, loss of
Advicor Tablets 402
Catapres Tablets (About 3 in 100 patients) 841
Catapres-TTS (0.5% or less) 842
▲ Clorpres Tablets (About 3%) 2185
▲ Cymbalta Delayed-Release Capsules (4%) 1801
Eligard 7.5 mg (Less than 2%) 2724
Eligard 22.5 mg (Less than 2%) 2724
Eligard 30 mg (Less than 2%) 2724
Eligard 45 mg (Less than 2%) 2724
Klonopin (Infrequent) 2639
Lescol Capsules 2268
Lescol XL Tablets 2268
Mevacor Tablets (0.5% to 1%) 2063
Requip Tablets (Infrequent) 1561
Zantac (Occasional) 1670

Lichen planus
Anaprox Tablets (Less than 1%) 2632
Anaprox DS Tablets (Less than 1%) 2632
Cuprimine Capsules (Rare) 1986
EC-Naprosyn Delayed-Release Tablets (Less than 1%) 2632
Evoxac Capsules (Less than 1%) 1013
Naprosyn Suspension (Less than 1%) 2632
Naprosyn Tablets (Less than 1%) 2632
Pentasa Capsules (Less than 1%) 3030
Plavix Tablets 926
Plavix Tablets 2767

Lid margin crusting
Azopt Ophthalmic Suspension (Less than 1%) 540
▲ Nevanac Ophthalmic Suspension 0.1% (1% to 5%) ⊙ 205
▲ Travatan Z Ophthalmic Solution (1% to 4%) 547

Ligaments, calcification of
Accutane Capsules 2607

Light-headedness
Adenocard IV Injection (2%) 603
▲ Adenoscan (12%) 605
▲ Alferon N Injection (One patient to 3%) 1726

Ambien Tablets (2%) 2692
Anaprox Tablets (Less than 3%) 2632
Anaprox DS Tablets (Less than 3%) 2632
Avelox 2803
Beconase AQ Nasal Spray (Fewer than 5 per 100 patients) 1369
Benicar HCT Tablets 1010
▲ Bentyl Capsules (11%) 703
▲ Bentyl Injection (11%) 703
▲ Bentyl Syrup (11%) 703
▲ Bentyl Tablets (11%) 703
Captopril Tablets 2182
Cipro I.V. (1% or less) 2817
Cipro (Less than 1%) 2810
Cipro XR Tablets 2823
Dantrium Capsules (Less frequent) 2580
Dantrium Intravenous 2582
Diovan HCT Tablets 2216
EC-Naprosyn Delayed-Release Tablets (Less than 3%) 2632
▲ Eldepryl Capsules (7 of 49 patients) 3052
Femara Tablets (Less than 0.1% to 2.4%) 2246
Flebogamma 5% DIF 1718
▲ Gabitril Tablets (27%) 973
Gammagard S/D (Occasional) 734
Humulin 50/50, 100 Units 1843
Humulin 70/30 Vial 1844
Humulin N Vial 1846
Humulin R 1849
▲ Indapamide Tablets (Less than 5%) 2188
Indocin (Less than 1%) 2024
InnoPran XL Extended Release Capsules 1484
Levaquin 2416
Levaquin in 5% Dextrose Injection 2416
Lexapro Oral Suspension (Frequent) 1174
Lexapro Tablets (Frequent) 1174
Lidoderm Patch 1114
Lortab 5/500 Tablets (Among most frequent) 3143
Lortab 7.5/500 Tablets (Among most frequent) 3144
Lortab 10/500 Tablets (Among most frequent) 3144
Mavik Tablets 472
Micardis HCT Tablets 854
MS Contin Tablets (Among most frequent) 2585
Naprosyn Suspension (Less than 3%) 2632
Naprosyn Tablets (Less than 3%) 2632
Nimotop Capsules (Less than 1%) 790
▲ Nitro-Dur Transdermal Infusion System (6%) 2887
Noroxin Tablets 2069
OxyIR Capsules (Among most frequent) 2593
Percocet Tablets (Among most frequent) 1127
Percodan Tablets (Among most frequent) 1130
Prinivil Tablets 2087
Prinzide Tablets 2092
Prolastin (0.19%) 3099
Raptiva for Injection 1218
Recombivax HB (Less than 1%) 2107
Thiothixene Capsules 2197
Tylenol with Codeine Tablets 2427
Vicodin Tablets (Among most frequent) 529
Vicodin ES Tablets (Among most frequent) 530
Vicodin HP Tablets (Among most frequent) 531
▲ Zemplar Capsules (5%) 536
▲ Zemplar Injection (5%) 538
Zydone Tablets (Among most frequent) 1132

Limb ischemia
Lovenox Injection 2756

Limb mobility, decreased
Pneumovax 23 2078

Limb reduction defects
Captopril Tablets 2182
Cozaar Tablets 1973
Prinivil Tablets 2087
Prinzide Tablets 2092

Limbitis
▲ Stromectol Tablets (3.5% to 5.5%) 2120

Lip abnormality
ProQuad 2099

Lipoatrophy
Aptivus Capsules (Less than 2%) 823
Aptivus Oral Solution (Less than 2%) 823
Genotropin Lyophilized Powder (Infrequent) 2547
Imitrex Injection (Rare) 1465
Norditropin Cartridges 2354

Lipodystrophy
Apidra Injection 2706
Aptivus Capsules (Less than 2%) 823
Aptivus Oral Solution (Less than 2%) 823
Humalog-Pen and KwikPen 1829
Humalog Mix 50/50-Pen and KwikPen 1833
Humalog Mix 75/25-Pen and KwikPen 1835
Humulin 50/50, 100 Units (Rare) 1843
Humulin 70/30 Vial (Rare) 1844
Humulin N Vial (Rare) 1846
Humulin R (Rare) 1849
Humulin R (U-500) (Rare) 1850
Intelence Tablets (Less than or equal to 0.5%) 3119
Isentress Tablets (1% to less than 2%) 2036
Lantus Injection 2749
Levemir Injection 2352
NovoLog Mix 70/30 2364
NovoLog Injection 2359
Selzentry Tablets (2.8%) 2534
Viread Tablets (1%) 1268

Lipohypertrophy
Aptivus Capsules (Less than 2%) 823
Aptivus Oral Solution (Less than 2%) 823
Humulin R (Rare) 1849
Imitrex Injection (Rare) 1465
▲ Increlex Injection (Greater than or equal to 5%) 3100
Intelence Tablets (Less than or equal to 0.5%) 3119

Lipoma
Copaxone for Injection (Infrequent) 3110
▲ Intron A for Injection (Less than 5%) 2859
Lexapro Oral Suspension (Infrequent) 1174
Lexapro Tablets (Infrequent) 1174
Requip Tablets (Infrequent) 1561

Lipoprotein levels, changes
Accutane Capsules 2607
Carbatrol Capsules (Occasional) 3019
▲ Soriatane Capsules (25% to 50%) 3062

Lipoproteins, electrophoretic abnormalities
Sandimmune 2296

Lipotrophy
Humulin 50/50, 100 Units (Rare) 1843
Humulin 70/30 Vial (Rare) 1844
Humulin N Vial (Rare) 1846
Humulin R (U-500) (Rare) 1850

Lips, cracked
Zovirax Cream (Less than 1%) 817

Lips, dry
(*see under* Xerochilia)

Lips, enlargement
Phenytek Capsules 2192

Lips, swelling
Janumet Tablets 2041
Januvia Tablets 2048
Levaquin 2416
Levaquin in 5% Dextrose Injection 2416
MoviPrep Oral Solution 2679
OsmoPrep Tablets 2680
Propecia Tablets 2095
Proscar Tablets 2102
Provigil Tablets 977
Rocaltrol Capsules 1150
Rocaltrol Oral Solution 1150

Listeriosis
Remicade for IV Injection 950
Velcade for Injection 2168

Listlessness
Aricept Tablets (Infrequent) 1062
Aricept ODT Tablets (Infrequent) 1062
Indocin (Greater than 1%) 2024

Livedo reticularis
Activase I.V. 1188
Mirapex Tablets 857

Liver, fatty
Advicor Tablets 402
Effexor XR Extended-Release Capsules 3195
Geodon Capsules (Rare) 2520
Lescol Capsules 2268
Lescol XL Tablets 2268
Plavix Tablets (Less than 1%) 926
Plavix Tablets (Less than 1%) 2767
Prograf Capsules and Injection 622
Prozac Pulvules and Liquid (Rare) 1852
Risperdal Consta Long-Acting Injection (Rare) 1753
Sandostatin LAR Depot 2302
Symbyax Capsules (Rare) 1871
Tricor Tablets 520
Venlafaxine Hydrochloride Tablets 2199
Zyprexa Tablets (Rare) 1883
Zyprexa ZYDIS Orally Disintegrating Tablets (Rare) 1883

Liver, metastases to
Selzentry Tablets 2534

Liver abnormalities
Catapres Tablets (About 1 in 100 patients) 841
Clorpres Tablets 2185
▲ Lamisil Oral Granules (3%) 2264
Pepcid Tablets (Infrequent) 2075
Rythmol Tablets 1586
▲ Tarka Tablets (3.2%) 511
Viramune Oral Suspension 873
Viramune Tablets 873
Ziagen 1673
Zomig Tablets (Infrequent) 694
Zomig-ZMT Tablets (Infrequent) 694

Liver damage
(*see under* Hepatotoxicity)

Liver disease, venoocclusive
Prograf Capsules and Injection 622

Liver disorders
Cosmegen for Injection 2485
▲ Leukine (77%) 774
Mycamine for Injection 616
▲ Novantrone for Injection Concentrate (8% to 14%) 1100
Percocet Tablets 1127
Pulmozyme Inhalation Solution 1217
▲ Somatuline Depot Injection (4% to 26%) 3102
▲ Vesanoid Capsules (3%) 2660

Liver dysfunction
(*see under* Hepatic dysfunction)

Liver enzymes, elevated
Atripla Tablets 938
Avandaryl Tablets (Rare) 1344
Bayer Aspirin 750
Cimzia 3127
Clarinex-D 12-Hour Extended-Release Tablets (Rare) 2831
Clarinex-D 24-Hour Extended-Release Tablets 2834
Crestor Tablets 677
Duetact Tablets (Rare) 3085
Fansidar Tablets 2636
Gantrisin Pediatric Suspension 2638
Limbrel Capsules (10 cases) 2561
Percocet Tablets 1127
Prandin Tablets (Less than or equal to 1%) 2971
Relenza Inhalation Powder (Less than 1.5%) 1556
Rythmol Tablets (0.2%) 1586
Sandostatin LAR Depot 2302
Starlix Tablets 2314
Strattera Capsules 1864
Stromectol Tablets 2120
Truvada Tablets 1262
Ultane Liquid for Inhalation (Less than 1%) 524
Velcade for Injection 2168
▲ Vicoprofen Tablets (15%) 533
Vytorin 10/10 Tablets 2939
Vytorin 10/20 Tablets 2939
Vytorin 10/40 Tablets 2939
Vytorin 10/80 Tablets 2939
Zetia Tablets 2951

Liver failure, acute
Albenza Tablets 1297
Plavix Tablets 926
Plavix Tablets 2767
Remicade for IV Injection 950
Velcade for Injection 2168

Liver fatty deposit
Prozac Weekly Capsules (Rare) 1852

Liver function, changes
(*see under* Hepatic dysfunction)

Liver function, impaired
(*see under* Hepatic dysfunction)

Liver function tests, abnormal
Actonel Tablets (Less than 0.1%) 2568
Advair Diskus 100/50 1276
Advair Diskus 250/50 1276
Advair Diskus 500/50 1276
Advair HFA 45/21 Inhalation Aerosol 1288
Advair HFA 115/21 Inhalation Aerosol 1288
Advair HFA 230/21 Inhalation Aerosol 1288
▲ Albenza Tablets (Less than 1% to 15.6%) 1297
Anaprox Tablets (Less than 1%) 2632
Anaprox DS Tablets (Less than 1%) 2632
AndroGel 3159
Aptivus Capsules (Less than 2%) 823
Aptivus Oral Solution (Less than 2%) 823
Aricept Tablets (Infrequent) 1062
Aricept ODT Tablets (Infrequent) 1062
Atripla Tablets 938
Avelox (Greater than or equal to 0.1% to less than 2%) 2803
Azilect Tablets (Greater than 1%) 3106
Campral Tablets (Infrequent) 1158
Cancidas for Injection 1953
Carbatrol Capsules 3019
Celebrex Capsules 2979
▲ CellCept Capsules (3% to 24.9%) 2622
▲ CellCept Intravenous (3% to 24.9%) 2622
▲ CellCept Oral Suspension (3% to 24.9%) 2622
▲ CellCept Tablets (3% to 24.9%) 2622
Chantix Tablets (Frequent) 2511
Cialis Tablets (Less than 2%) 1792
Cipro I.V. (Greater than 1% to 1.3%) 2817
Cipro (1.3%) 2810
Cipro XR Tablets (Less than 1%) 2823
Cosmegen for Injection 2485
▲ Cubicin for Injection (1.7% to 3%) 995
Dacogen Injection (Greater than or equal to 1%) 1066
Delatestryl Injection 1730
Depakote ER Tablets 423
EC-Naprosyn Delayed-Release Tablets (Less than 1%) 2632
Effexor XR Extended-Release Capsules 3195
Elmiron Capsules (1%) 2435
Emsam Transdermal System (Infrequent) 905
Epzicom Tablets 1422
▲ Equetro Extended-Release Capsules (Less than 5%) 3174
Exjade Tablets 2244
▲ Fenoglide Tablets (7.5%) 2960
Gliadel Wafer (1%) 1076
Keppra Injection (1.4%) 3137
Keppra Oral Solution (0.07% to 1.4%) 3131
Keppra Tablets (0.07% to 1.4%) 3131
Ketek Tablets (Greater than or equal to 0.2% to less than 2%) 2744
Lamictal (Infrequent) 1488
Levitra Tablets (Less than 2%) 2876
Luvox CR Extended-Release Capsules (2%) 1759
▲ Mycamine for Injection (4.2%) 616
▲ Myfortic Tablets (3% to less than 20%) 2276
▲ Mylotarg for Injection (20% to 29%) 3212
Naprosyn Suspension (Less than 1%) 2632
Naprosyn Tablets (Less than 1%) 2632
▲ Oncaspar Injection (5%) 1138
Plavix Tablets 926
Plavix Tablets 2767
Pletal Tablets 2481
Pristiq Extended-Release Tablets (Less than 2%) 3247
Proleukin for Injection (Less than 1%) 2287
Prozac Weekly Capsules (Infrequent) 1852
Rapamune 3260
Rythmol SR Capsules 1590
Salagen Tablets (Less than 1%) 1082
Tamiflu Capsules 2649
Tamiflu Oral Suspension 2649
Tarceva Tablets 1228
▲ Tricor Tablets (7.5%) 520
Twinrix Vaccine 1628

Ultram ER Extended-Release Tablets (0.5% to less than 1%) 2428
Venlafaxine Hydrochloride Tablets 2199
Xyrem Oral Solution (Infrequent) 1766
Zyvox (0.4% to 1.3%) 2552

Liver function tests, elevated
▲ Anaprox Tablets (1% to 10%) 2632
▲ Anaprox DS Tablets (1% to 10%) 2632
▲ EC-Naprosyn Delayed-Release Tablets (1% to 10%) 2632
▲ Elmiron Capsules (11.8%) 2435
▲ Flector Patch (Less than or equal to 15%) 561
Levothroid Tablets 1170
Malarone Pediatric Tablets 1521
Malarone Tablets 1521
Mepron Suspension 1526
▲ Naprosyn Suspension (1% to 10%) 2632
▲ Naprosyn Tablets (1% to 10%) 2632
Nexavar Tablets 784
▲ Raptiva for Injection (3.1%) 1218
Sutent Capsules 2540
Trizivir Tablets 1622
Zocor Tablets 2136

Liver injury
Axid Capsules 1364
Ketek Tablets 2744
Lamisil Oral Granules 2264
Remicade for IV Injection 950
Singulair (Rare) 2114
Strattera Capsules (Rare) 1864

Liver pain
▲ Hycamtin for Injection (59%) 1459

Liver tenderness
Actiq (Less than 1%) 959
Viramune Oral Suspension 873
Viramune Tablets 873

Liver transplant, need for
Lamisil Tablets 2266

Liver tumors
(*see under* Hepatomas)

Loffler's syndrome
Paser Granules 1747

Loss of balance
(*see under* Balance, loss of)

Lower respiratory signs and symptoms
▲ Advair HFA 45/21 Inhalation Aerosol (1% to 3%) 1288
▲ Advair HFA 115/21 Inhalation Aerosol (1% to 3%) 1288
▲ Advair HFA 230/21 Inhalation Aerosol (1% to 3%) 1288
Serevent Diskus (1% to less than 3%) 1594

Lumbago
Klonopin (Infrequent) 2639
Prinivil Tablets (0.3% to 1%) 2087
Prinzide Tablets 2092

Lump at injection site
Bicillin C-R Injectable Suspension 1775
Bicillin L-A Injection 1777
ProQuad 2099

Lung, metastases to
Mirapex Tablets 857

Lung crackles
▲ Dacogen Injection (14%) 1066

Lung development, hypoplastic
Captopril Tablets 2182
Cozaar Tablets 1973
Prinivil Tablets 2087
Prinzide Tablets 2092

Lung disorders, unspecified
Actiq (Less than 1%) 959
Alinia for Oral Suspension (Less than 1%) 2677
Alinia Tablets (Less than 1%) 2677
▲ AmBisome for Injection (13.6% to 17.8%) 606
BeneFIX Vials (1.5%) 3191
▲ Busulfex Injection (34%) 2477
▲ CellCept Capsules (3% to 30.1%) 2622
▲ CellCept Intravenous (3% to 30.1%) 2622
▲ CellCept Oral Suspension (3% to 30.1%) 2622
▲ CellCept Tablets (3% to 30.1%) 2622
▲ Humira Injection (Less than 5%) 442
Ionsys Transdermal System (.1% to less than 1%) 2410
▲ Leukine (20%) 774
▲ Megace ES Oral Suspension (1% to 3%) 2499
Norvir (Less than 2%) 489
▲ Ontak Vials (8%) 1079
▲ Prograf Capsules and Injection (3% to 15%) 622
▲ Proleukin for Injection (24%) 2287
Protonix for Delayed-Release Oral Suspension (Less than 1%) 3254
Protonix Delayed-Release Tablets (Less than 1%) 3254
Protonix I.V. (Less than 1%) 3257
Protopic Ointment (Greater than or equal to 1%) 628
Provigil Tablets (2%) 977
Pulmozyme Inhalation Solution 1217
▲ Rituxan I.V. (6% to 31%) 1223
Rythmol SR Capsules 1590
Symbyax Capsules (Frequent) 1871
▲ Trasylol Injection (7%) 799
Ventolin HFA Inhalation Aerosol (Less than 3%) 1638

Lung function, decreased
▲ Humira Injection (Less than 5%) 442

Lung infiltration
Dacogen Injection 1066
Prograf Capsules and Injection 622
Solodyn Extended Release Tablets 1938
Tarceva Tablets (0.7%) 1228
Velcade for Injection 2168

Lung injury, acute, infusion related
Gammagard Liquid 730

Lung injury, transfusion-associated
Flebogamma 5% 1715
Flebogamma 5% DIF 1718
Gammagard S/D (Rare) 734
Gamunex (Rare) 3094

Lung neoplasms, malignant
Mirapex Tablets 857
Prinzide Tablets 2092

Lupus erythematosus
Advicor Tablets 402
Carbatrol Capsules (Isolated cases) 3019
Cosopt Sterile Ophthalmic Solution 1969
Cuprimine Capsules 1986
Dapsone Tablets USP 1746
Depakote ER Tablets (Greater than 1%) 423
Evoxac Capsules (Less than 1%) 1013
Gantrisin Pediatric Suspension 2638
Gris-PEG Tablets 2507
▲ Humira Injection (Less than 5%) 442
InnoPran XL Extended Release Capsules 1484
Intron A for Injection 2859
Phenytek Capsules 2192
Recombivax HB 2107
Rythmol Tablets (Less than 1%) 1586
Taxotere Injection Concentrate (Rare) 2773
Timoptic Sterile Ophthalmic Solution (Less frequent) 2121
Timoptic in Ocudose (Less frequent) 2124
Timoptic-XE Sterile Ophthalmic Gel Forming Solution 2125
Zonegran Capsules (Rare) 1089

Lupus erythematosus, discoid
Enbrel for Injection 569

Lupus erythematosus, disseminated, aggravation of
Equetro Extended-Release Capsules 3174

Lupus erythematosus, systemic
Anaprox Tablets (Less than 1%) 2632
Anaprox DS Tablets (Less than 1%) 2632
Benicar HCT Tablets 1010
Combigan Ophthalmic Solution 553
Cosopt Sterile Ophthalmic Solution 1969
EC-Naprosyn Delayed-Release Tablets (Less than 1%) 2632
InnoPran XL Extended Release Capsules (Rare) 1484
Lamisil Tablets (Infrequently) 2266
Lybrel Tablets 3204
Naprosyn Suspension (Less than 1%) 2632
Naprosyn Tablets (Less than 1%) 2632
PegIntron Powder for Injection 2903
Pentasa Capsules 3030
Phenytek Capsules 2192
Recombivax HB 2107
Timoptic Sterile Ophthalmic Solution (Less frequent) 2121
Timoptic in Ocudose (Less frequent) 2124
Timoptic-XE Sterile Ophthalmic Gel Forming Solution 2125
Treximet Tablets (Rare) 1616

Lupus erythematosus, systemic, exacerbation of
Activella Tablets 2347
Climara Transdermal System 763
Enjuvia Tablets 1029
Premarin Tablets 3221
Seasonique Tablets 1046
Yaz Tablets 805

Lupus erythematosus, systemic, exacerbation or activation of
Avalide Tablets 2713
Carbatrol Capsules 3019
Dyazide Capsules 1405
Furosemide Tablets 2186
Lamisil Oral Granules 2264
Premphase Tablets 3232
Prempro Tablets 3232
Prinzide Tablets 2092
Solodyn Extended Release Tablets 1938

Lupus-like syndrome
Asacol Delayed-Release Tablets 2579
Cimzia 3127
Cuprimine Capsules 1986
Enbrel for Injection 569
Equetro Extended-Release Capsules 3174
Gris-PEG Tablets 2507
Humira Injection 442
Lamictal 1488
Lescol Capsules (Rare) 2268
Lescol XL Tablets 2268
Mevacor Tablets (Rare) 2063
PegIntron Powder for Injection (Less than or equal to 1%) 2903
Prozac Weekly Capsules 1852
Recombivax HB 2107
Remicade for IV Injection (Rare) 950
Rituxan I.V. 1223
Solodyn Extended Release Tablets 1938
Thiothixene Capsules 2197
Tricor Tablets 520
Vytorin 10/10 Tablets 2149
Vytorin 10/20 Tablets 2149
Vytorin 10/40 Tablets 2149
Vytorin 10/80 Tablets 2149
Zocor Tablets (Rare) 2136

Lyell's syndrome
(*see under* Necrolysis, epidermal, toxic)

Lymph nodes, tender
Stromectol Tablets (1.9%) 2120

Lymphadenitis
Boostrix 1377
▲ Intron A for Injection (Less than or equal to 5%) 2859
Pneumovax 23 2078
ProQuad 2099

Lymphadenopathy
Accutane Capsules 2607
Actiq (1% or greater) 959
▲ Aerobid/Aerobid-M (1% to 3%) 1153
Alferon N Injection (1%) 1726
Ambien Tablets (Rare) 2692
Ambien CR Tablets (Rare) 2696
Anaprox Tablets (Less than 1%) 2632
Anaprox DS Tablets (Less than 1%) 2632
Asacol Delayed-Release Tablets 2579
Attenuvax (Less common) 1951
▲ Betaseron for SC Injection (6%) 756
Bicillin C-R Injectable Suspension 1775
Bicillin L-A Injection 1777
Boostrix 1377
Campral Tablets (Rare) 1158
Carbatrol Capsules 3019
Celexa (Infrequent) 1160
Chantix Tablets (Infrequent) 2511
Cimzia 3127
Cipro I.V. (1% or less) 2817
Cipro (Less than 1%) 2810
Cipro XR Tablets 2823
Combivir Tablets 1384
Comvax 1966
▲ Copaxone for Injection (12%) 3110
Cubicin for Injection (Less than 1%) 995
Cuprimine Capsules 1986
▲ Dacogen Injection (12%) 1066
Depakote ER Tablets 423
Doxil Injection (Less than 1%) 2378
EC-Naprosyn Delayed-Release Tablets (Less than 1%) 2632
Effexor XR Extended-Release Capsules (Infrequent) 3195
Elidel Cream 1% (0.9%) 2221
Emsam Transdermal System (Infrequent) 905
Enbrel for Injection 569
Engerix-B Vaccine (Less than 1%) 1409
▲ Epivir (9%) 1412
Epivir-HBV 1417
Epzicom Tablets 1422
▲ Equetro Extended-Release Capsules (Less than 5%) 3174
Evoxac Capsules (Less than 1%) 1013
Exelon Capsules (Infrequent) 2229
Exelon Oral Solution (Infrequent) 2229
Exforge Tablets (Greater than or equal to 0.2%) 2238
Fluarix Vaccine 1446
Flulaval Injection Vaccine 1448
Gabitril Tablets (Frequent) 973
Gardasil Injection 2019
Gengraf Capsules (1% to less than 3%) 435
Geodon Capsules (Infrequent) 2520
Havrix Injection Vaccine 1454
Imitrex Nasal Spray (Rare) 1470
Imitrex Tablets (Rare) 1474
Infanrix Vaccine 1479
▲ Intron A for Injection (Less than or equal to 5%) 2859
Kaletra (Less than 2%) 452
Kinrix Injection Vaccine 1486
Klonopin 2639
Lamictal (2%) 1488
Lipitor Tablets (Less than 2%) 2501
Lovaza Capsules 1520
Lunesta Tablets (Infrequent) 2994
Lupron Depot 3.75 mg (Among most frequent) 462
▲ Lupron Depot–3 Month 11.25 mg (Less than 5%) 462
Luvox CR Extended-Release Capsules (Infrequent) 1759
Lyrica Capsules (0.1% to 1%) 2527
Meridia Capsules 475
Meruvax II 2061
▲ Miacalcin Nasal Spray (1% to 3%) 2274
M-M-R II 2054
Mumpsvax 2068
Nalfon Capsules (Less than 1%) 2508
Naprosyn Suspension (Less than 1%) 2632
Naprosyn Tablets (Less than 1%) 2632
Neoral Oral Solution (1% to less than 3%) 2280
Neoral Soft Gelatin Capsules (1% to less than 3%) 2280
Norvir (Less than 2%) 489
Orthoclone OKT3 Sterile Solution (Less than 1%) 2387
OxyContin Tablets (Less than 1%) 2589
▲ Paser Granules (46% of 38 patients with drug-induced hepatitis) 1747
Paxil (Infrequent) 1535
Paxil CR Controlled-Release Tablets (Infrequent) 1544
Pediarix Vaccine 1552
Liquid PedvaxHIB 2073
Phenytek Capsules 2192
Pneumovax 23 2078
Proglycem Capsules (Infrequent) 1185
Proglycem Suspension (Infrequent) 1185
▲ Prometrium Capsules (100 mg, 200 mg) (Less than 5%) 3047
▲ Protopic Ointment (1% to 3%) 628
Prozac Weekly Capsules 1852
Prozac Pulvules and Liquid 1852
▲ Rebif Prefilled Syringe for Injection (11% to 12%) 1107
Recombivax HB (Less than 1%) 2107
Remeron Tablets (Rare) 2924
RemeronSolTab Tablets (Rare) 2927
Remicade for IV Injection (Greater than or equal to 0.2%) 950
Requip Tablets (Infrequent) 1561
Retrovir Capsules 1574
Retrovir IV Infusion 1579
Retrovir 1574
Rilutek Tablets (Rare) 2771
Risperdal Consta Long-Acting Injection (Infrequent) 1753

Rythmol SR Capsules ... 1590
Salagen Tablets (Less than 1%) ... 1082
Symbyax Capsules (Infrequent) ... 1871
Tamiflu Capsules (1%) ... 2649
Tamiflu Oral Suspension (1%) ... 2649
▲ Targretin Gel 1% (6%) ... 1088
Treximet Tablets (Infrequent) ... 1616
Tricor Tablets ... 520
▲ Trisenox Injection (8%) ... 986
Trizivir Tablets ... 1622
Twinrix Vaccine (Less than 1%) ... 1628
Varivax (Greater than or equal to 1%) ... 2133
Venlafaxine Hydrochloride Tablets (Infrequent) ... 2199
Viramune Oral Suspension ... 873
Viramune Tablets ... 873
Vivitrol ... 988
Voltaren Tablets (Rarely) ... 2334
Voltaren-XR Tablets (Rarely) ... 2337
Wellbutrin Tablets (Rare) ... 1648
Wellbutrin SR Sustained-Release Tablets ... 1653
Wellbutrin XL Extended-Release Tablets ... 1659
Xopenex Inhalation Solution ... 3001
Xopenex Inhalation Solution Concentrate ... 3005
Xopenex HFA Inhalation Aerosol ... 3009
Xyrem Oral Solution (Infrequent) ... 1766
Ziagen ... 1673
Zomig Tablets (Rare) ... 694
Zomig Nasal Spray (Rare) ... 689
Zomig-ZMT Tablets (Rare) ... 694
Zonegran Capsules (Infrequent) ... 1089
Zovirax ... 1690
Zyban Sustained-Release Tablets ... 1692
Zyprexa Tablets (Infrequent) ... 1883
Zyprexa ZYDIS Orally Disintegrating Tablets (Infrequent) ... 1883
Zyrtec Chewable Tablets (Less than 2%) ... 1920
Zyrtec Syrup (Less than 2%) ... 1920
Zyrtec Tablets (Less than 2%) ... 1920
Zyrtec-D 12 Hour Extended Release Tablets (Less than 2%) ... 1923

Lymphadenopathy, cervical
Lexapro Oral Suspension (Infrequent) ... 1174
Lexapro Tablets (Infrequent) ... 1174
Nexium Delayed-Release Capsules (Less than 1%) ... 645
Nexium I.V. (Less than 1%) ... 652
Nexium Delayed-Release Oral Suspension (Less than 1%) ... 645
Risperdal Consta Long-Acting Injection (Infrequent) ... 1753

Lymphadenopathy, localized
▲ Aldara Cream, 5% (3%) ... 1699
Prevnar ... 3241
ProQuad ... 2099

Lymphadenopathy, post-cervical
Evoxac Capsules (Less than 1%) ... 1013

Lymphangitis, regional
Doxil Injection (Less than 1%) ... 2378

Lymphatic disorders, unspecified
▲ Cancidas for Injection (1.8% to 14.9%) ... 1953
▲ Mycamine for Injection (14.6% to 96%) ... 616

Lymphedema
Actiq (1% or greater) ... 959
▲ Arimidex Tablets (10%) ... 672
Copaxone for Injection (Infrequent) ... 3110
Doxil Injection (Less than 1%) ... 2378
Humatrope Vials and Cartridges ... 1838
Paxil (Rare) ... 1535
Paxil CR Controlled-Release Tablets (Rare) ... 1544
Prozac Weekly Capsules (Rare) ... 1852
Prozac Pulvules and Liquid (Rare) ... 1852
Rapamune ... 3260
Requip Tablets (Infrequent) ... 1561
▲ Taxotere Injection Concentrate (0% to 4.4%) ... 2773
▲ Xeloda Tablets (Less than 1% to 3%) ... 2662

Lymphedema, post-mastectomy
▲ Femara Tablets (7%) ... 2246

Lymphocele
▲ Myfortic Tablets (3% to less than 20%) ... 2276
▲ Rapamune (Greater than or equal to 3% to less than 20%) ... 3260

Lymphocytes, atypical
Cipro XR Tablets ... 2823
Coreg Tablets (Less than or equal to 0.1%) ... 1387
Coreg CR Extended-Release Capsules (Less than or equal to 0.1%) ... 1393

Lymphocytes, decrease
(*see under* Lymphocytopenia)

Lymphocytes, increase
(*see under* Lymphocytosis)

Lymphocytopenia
▲ Amevive (2% to 59%) ... 611
▲ Betaseron for SC Injection (88%) ... 756
Busulfex Injection ... 2477
▲ Cyanokit 5g Antidote (8% to 17%) ... 1021
Fosamax ... 2005
Keppra Oral Solution ... 3131
Keppra Tablets ... 3131
Lamisil Oral Granules (1.7%) ... 2264
Leukeran Tablets ... 1508
Mavik Tablets (0.3% to 1%) ... 472
Mustargen for Injection ... 2492
Nabi-HB (2%) ... 815
▲ Novantrone for Injection Concentrate (72% to 95%) ... 1100
Omnicef Capsules (1%) ... 497
Omnicef for Oral Suspension (0.8%) ... 497
Orthoclone OKT3 Sterile Solution (Less than 1%) ... 2387
Paxil (Rare) ... 1535
Paxil CR Controlled-Release Tablets (Rare) ... 1544
Requip Tablets (Infrequent) ... 1561
▲ Rituxan I.V. (40% to 48%) ... 1223
Rocephin Injectable Vials, ADD-Vantage, Galaxy, Bulk (Less than 1%) ... 2642
▲ Sutent Capsules (1% to 38%) ... 2540
Tarka Tablets ... 511
Temodar Capsules ... 2931
▲ Torisel Injection (16% to 53%) ... 3272
Trizivir Tablets ... 1622
▲ Xeloda Tablets (13% to 99%) ... 2662
Ziagen ... 1673

Lymphocytosis
Campral Tablets (Infrequent) ... 1158
Celexa (Rare) ... 1160
Cipro I.V. (Infrequent) ... 2817
Depakote ER Tablets ... 423
Evoxac Capsules ... 1013
Fortaz (Very rare) ... 1450
Geodon Capsules (Rare) ... 2520
▲ Intron A for Injection (Less than 5%) ... 2859
Lamictal (Rare) ... 1488
Norvir (Less than 2%) ... 489
Omnicef Capsules (0.2%) ... 497
Omnicef for Oral Suspension (2%) ... 497
Paxil (Rare) ... 1535
Paxil CR Controlled-Release Tablets (Rare) ... 1544
Primaxin I.M. ... 2080
Primaxin I.V. ... 2083
Prozac Weekly Capsules (Rare) ... 1852
Prozac Pulvules and Liquid (Rare) ... 1852
▲ Raptiva for Injection (40%) ... 1218
Remeron Tablets (Rare) ... 2924
RemeronSolTab Tablets (Rare) ... 2927
Requip Tablets (Infrequent) ... 1561
Rocephin Injectable Vials, ADD-Vantage, Galaxy, Bulk (Less than 0.1%) ... 2642
Targretin Capsules ... 1084
Venlafaxine Hydrochloride Tablets (Rare) ... 2199
Xifaxan Tablets (Less than 2%) ... 2682

Lymphoma
Aldara Cream, 5% ... 1699
Amevive (Less than 0.1%) ... 611
CellCept Capsules (0.4% to 1%) ... 2622
CellCept Intravenous (0.4% to 1%) ... 2622
CellCept Oral Suspension (0.4% to 1%) ... 2622
CellCept Tablets (0.4% to 1%) ... 2622
Cimzia ... 3127
▲ DepoCyt Injection (3%) ... 1136
Elidel Cream 1% ... 2221
▲ Enbrel for Injection (9%) ... 569
▲ Gengraf Capsules (Less than 1% to 6%) ... 435
▲ Humira Injection (Less than 5%) ... 442
Mirapex Tablets ... 857
Myfortic Tablets (0.9% to 1.3%) ... 2276
▲ Neoral Oral Solution (Less than 1% to 6%) ... 2280
▲ Neoral Soft Gelatin Capsules (Less than 1% to 6%) ... 2280
Orencia Powder for Intravenous Infusion (4 cases) ... 921
Orthoclone OKT3 Sterile Solution (Less than 1%) ... 2387
Phenytek Capsules ... 2192
Prograf Capsules and Injection ... 622
Protopic Ointment ... 628
▲ Rapamune (0.5% to 3.2%) ... 3260
Remicade for IV Injection (Greater than or equal to 0.2%) ... 950
▲ Sandimmune (Less than 1% to 6%) ... 2296
Selzentry Tablets ... 2534
Simulect for Injection (0.3%) ... 2306

Lymphoma, basal cell
Remicade for IV Injection (Greater than or equal to 0.2%) ... 950

Lymphoma, breast
Remicade for IV Injection (Greater than or equal to 0.2%) ... 950

Lymphoma, Hodgkin's
Raptiva for Injection ... 1218

Lymphoma, lymphocytic
Dantrium Capsules (Less frequent) ... 2580
Dantrium Intravenous ... 2582

Lymphoma, non-Hodgkin's
Raptiva for Injection ... 1218

Lymphoma, t-cell
Zolinza Capsules ... 2142

Lymphoma-like disorder
▲ Humira Injection (Less than 5%) ... 442
Paser Granules ... 1747

Lymphopenia
(*see also under* Lymphocytopenia)
Amevive ... 611
▲ Campath Ampules (97%) ... 761
▲ Eloxatin for Injection (2% to 6%) ... 2731
Ixempra Kit for Injection ... 915
▲ Nexavar Tablets (13% to 23%) ... 784
Relenza Inhalation Powder (Less than 1.5%) ... 1556
Risperdal Consta Long-Acting Injection (Rare) ... 1753
▲ Rituxan I.V. (40% to 48%) ... 1223
▲ Temodar Capsules (39% to 60%) ... 2931
▲ Treanda for Injection (7% to 68%) ... 983
▲ Velcade for Injection (24%) ... 2168

Lymphoproliferative disorder
CellCept Capsules (0.4% to 1%) ... 2622
CellCept Intravenous (0.4% to 1%) ... 2622
CellCept Oral Suspension (0.4% to 1%) ... 2622
CellCept Tablets (0.4% to 1%) ... 2622
Orthoclone OKT3 Sterile Solution ... 2387
▲ Rapamune (0.5% to 3.2%) ... 3260
Simulect for Injection ... 2306

M

Maceration, skin
Analpram-HC ... 1140
Diprolene Lotion 0.05% (Infrequent) ... 2838
Diprolene AF Cream 0.05% (Infrequent) ... 2837
Olux Foam ... 3061
Pramosone ... 1141
Sulfamylon for 5% Topical Solution ... 2194
Vanos Cream ... 1941

Macrocytosis
Depakote ER Tablets ... 423
Phenytek Capsules ... 2192
Retrovir Capsules ... 1574
Retrovir IV Infusion ... 1579
Retrovir ... 1574

Macroglobulinemia, Waldenstrom's, hyperviscosity syndrome in
Rituxan I.V. ... 1223

Macula lutea degeneration
Namenda (Infrequent) ... 1180

Maculae
Tarka Tablets ... 511

Macular degeneration
Mirapex Tablets ... 857

Macular hypopigmentation
Zyprexa Tablets (Rare) ... 1883
Zyprexa ZYDIS Orally Disintegrating Tablets (Rare) ... 1883

Maculopathy
Exjade Tablets (0.1% to 1%) ... 2244
▲ Lucentis Injection (3% to 10%) ... 1205

Malabsorption syndrome
Atripla Tablets ... 938
Elspar for Injection ... 1990
Sustiva Capsules ... 930
Sustiva Tablets ... 930

Maladministration
Rotarix Oral Suspension ... 1582

Malaise
Abelcet Injection ... 1134
Accolate Tablets ... 669
Accutane Capsules ... 2607
Aceon Tablets (2 mg, 4 mg, 8 mg) (0.3% to 1%) ... 3038
Actiq (1% or greater) ... 959
▲ Advair Diskus 250/50 (3%) ... 1276
Advicor Tablets ... 402
▲ Aerobid/Aerobid-M (1% to 3%) ... 1153
Aggrenox Capsules (1.6%) ... 819
▲ Agrylin Capsules (6.4%) ... 3017
▲ Alferon N Injection (9% to 65%) ... 1726
Alinia for Oral Suspension (Less than 1%) ... 2677
Alinia Tablets (Less than 1%) ... 2677
Ambien Tablets (Infrequent) ... 2692
Ambien CR Tablets (Infrequent) ... 2696
AmBisome for Injection (Less common) ... 606
Amerge Tablets (2%) ... 1301
Amitiza Capsules ... 3082
Amrix Capsules ... 966
Anaprox Tablets (Less than 1%) ... 2632
Anaprox DS Tablets (Less than 1%) ... 2632
AndroGel ... 3159
Aptivus Capsules (Less than 2%) ... 823
Aptivus Oral Solution (Less than 2%) ... 823
Aricept Tablets (Infrequent) ... 1062
Aricept ODT Tablets (Infrequent) ... 1062
▲ Arimidex Tablets (2% to 5%) ... 672
Asacol Delayed-Release Tablets (1% to 2%) ... 2579
Attenuvax ... 1951
Avelox (Greater than or equal to 0.1% to less than 2%) ... 2803
▲ Avinza Capsules (Less than 5%) ... 1772
Azilect Tablets (2%) ... 3106
▲ Betaseron for SC Injection (6%) ... 756
Brovana Inhalation Solution ... 2990
Campral Tablets (Infrequent) ... 1158
Captopril Tablets (0.5% to 2%) ... 2182
Catapres Tablets (About 1 in 100 patients) ... 841
Catapres-TTS (0.5% or less) ... 842
▲ CellCept Capsules (3% to less than 20%) ... 2622
▲ CellCept Intravenous (3% to less than 20%) ... 2622
▲ CellCept Oral Suspension (3% to less than 20%) ... 2622
▲ CellCept Tablets (3% to less than 20%) ... 2622
▲ Chantix Tablets (4% to 7%) ... 2511
Cimzia ... 3127
Cipro I.V. (1% or less) ... 2817
Cipro (Less than 1%) ... 2810
Cipro XR Tablets (Less than 1%) ... 2823
Clinoril Tablets (Less than 1 in 100) ... 1962
Clorpres Tablets (About 1%) ... 2185
▲ Combivir Tablets (27%) ... 1384
Copaxone for Injection (At least 2%) ... 3110
▲ Coreg Tablets (Greater than 1% to 3%) ... 1387
▲ Coreg CR Extended-Release Capsules (Greater than 1% to less than or equal to 3%) ... 1393
Cosmegen for Injection ... 2485
Crixivan Capsules (2.1%) ... 1979
Cymbalta Delayed-Release Capsules (Infrequent) ... 1801
▲ Dacogen Injection (5%) ... 1066
Dantrium Capsules (Among most frequent) ... 2580
Depakote ER Tablets (Greater than 1%) ... 423
▲ Doxil Injection (1% to 5%) ... 2378
EC-Naprosyn Delayed-Release Tablets (Less than 1%) ... 2632
Edecrin ... 698
Effexor XR Extended-Release Capsules (Infrequent) ... 3195
Eldepryl Capsules ... 3052
▲ Eligard 7.5 mg (17.5%) ... 2724
▲ Eligard 22.5 mg (6%) ... 2724
▲ Eligard 30 mg (13.3%) ... 2724

▲ Eligard 45 mg (11.7%) 2724
Emend Capsules (Greater than 0.5%) 1992
Emend for Injection (Greater than 0.5%) 1999
Emsam Transdermal System (Rare) 905
Engerix-B Vaccine (Less than 1%) 1409
▲ Epivir (27%) 1412
▲ Epivir-HBV (24%) 1417
▲ Erbitux (16% to 73%) 912
Evoxac Capsules (Less than 1%) 1013
▲ Exelon Capsules (5%) 2229
▲ Exelon Oral Solution (5%) 2229
Exforge Tablets (Greater than 0.1% to less than 1%) 2238
▲ Femara Tablets (0.2% to 8.4%) 2246
Flebogamma 5% 1715
Flebogamma 5% DIF 1718
▲ Flovent Diskus 50 mcg (1% to 16%) 1435
▲ Fluarix Vaccine (1% to 10%) 1446
▲ Flulaval Injection Vaccine (4% to 10%) 1448
Follistim AQ Cartridge 2844
Foradil Aerolizer 2849
Fosamax 2005
Fosamax Plus D Tablets 2013
Frova Tablets (Infrequent) 1111
Gabitril Tablets (Frequent) 973
Gardasil Injection (1.4%) 2019
Gemzar for Injection (Infrequent) 1820
Gengraf Capsules (1% to less than 3%) 435
▲ Havrix Injection Vaccine (1% to 10%) 1454
Hycamtin for Injection (0.5% to 1.8%) 1459
Imitrex Injection (1.1%) 1465
▲ Imitrex Tablets (2% to 3%) 1474
▲ Indapamide Tablets (Greater than or equal to 5%) 2188
Indocin (Greater than 1%) 2024
▲ Intron A for Injection (Up to 14%) 2859
Invanz for Injection (Greater than 0.1%) 2029
Janumet Tablets 2041
Kaletra (Less than 2%) 452
Klonopin (Infrequent) 2639
Lamictal (Infrequent) 1488
Lamisil Oral Granules 2264
Lamisil Tablets 2266
Lescol Capsules (Rare) 2268
▲ Lescol XL Tablets (3.8%) 2268
▲ Leukine (57%) 774
▲ Leustatin Injection (5% to 7%) 2384
Lexapro Oral Suspension (Infrequent) 1174
Lexapro Tablets (Infrequent) 1174
Lipitor Tablets (Less than 2%) 2501
Lovaza Capsules 1520
Lunesta Tablets (Infrequent) 2994
Luvox CR Extended-Release Capsules (Frequent) 1759
Lyrica Capsules (0.1% to 1%) 2527
Marinol Capsules (Less than 1%) 3163
Meruvax II 2061
Mevacor Tablets (Rare) 2063
Micardis Tablets (More than 0.3%) 852
Micardis HCT Tablets 854
▲ Mirapex Tablets (2% to 3%) 857
M-M-R II 2054
Mobic Oral Suspension (Less than 2%) 863
Mobic Tablets (Less than 2%) 863
▲ MoviPrep Oral Solution (19.4%) 2679
▲ Nabi-HB (6%) 815
Nalfon Capsules (Less than 1%) 2508
Namenda 1180
Naprosyn Suspension (Less than 1%) 2632
Naprosyn Tablets (Less than 1%) 2632
Neoral Oral Solution (1% to less than 3%) 2280
Neoral Soft Gelatin Capsules (1% to less than 3%) 2280
Neupro Transdermal System 3149
Nexium Delayed-Release Capsules (Less than 1%) 645
Nexium I.V. (Less than 1%) 652
Nexium Delayed-Release Oral Suspension (Less than 1%) 645
Norvir (0.7% to 1.7%) 489
▲ Novantrone for Injection Concentrate (34%) 1100
Orthoclone OKT3 Sterile Solution (Less than 1%) 2387
OxyContin Tablets (Less than 1%) 2589
Patanase Nasal Spray 544
Paxil (Frequent) 1535
Paxil CR Controlled-Release Tablets (Frequent) 1544
Pediarix Vaccine 1552
▲ PegIntron Powder for Injection (7%) 2903
Pentasa Capsules (Less than 1%) 3030
Percocet Tablets 1127
Percodan Tablets 1130
Perforomist Inhalation Solution 1025
Persantine Tablets (Rare) 869
Pletal Tablets (Less than 2%) 2481
Pneumovax 23 2078
Prinivil Tablets (0.3% to 1%) 2087
Prinzide Tablets 2092
Proglycem Capsules (Frequent) 1185
Proglycem Suspension (Frequent) 1185
▲ Proleukin for Injection (27%) 2287
ProQuad (Greater than or equal to 0.2% to less than 1%) 2099
Protonix for Delayed-Release Oral Suspension (Less than 1%) 3254
Protonix Delayed-Release Tablets (Less than 1%) 3254
Protonix I.V. (Less than 1%) 3257
Protopic Ointment (Greater than or equal to 1%) 628
Prozac Weekly Capsules (Infrequent) 1852
Prozac Pulvules and Liquid (Infrequent) 1852
Pulmozyme Inhalation Solution 1217
▲ Rebetol (4% to 6%) 2917
▲ Rebif Prefilled Syringe for Injection (4% to 5%) 1107
Recombivax HB (Equal to or greater than 1%) 2107
▲ Relenza Inhalation Powder (Less than 1.5% to 8%) 1556
Remeron Tablets (Frequent) 2924
RemeronSolTab Tablets (Frequent) 2927
▲ Requip Tablets (Infrequent to 3%) 1561
▲ Retrovir Capsules (8% to 53.2%) 1574
▲ Retrovir IV Infusion (8% to 53.2%) 1579
▲ Retrovir (8% to 53.2%) 1574
Reyataz Capsules 3299
Rilutek Tablets (0.4% to 1.2%) 2771
Risperdal Consta Long-Acting Injection (Infrequent) 1753
▲ Romazicon Injection (1% to 3%) 2646
Rythmol SR Capsules 1590
▲ Simulect for Injection (3% to 10%) 2306
▲ Solodyn Extended Release Tablets (4%) 1938
Soriatane Capsules (Less than 1%) 3062
Stalevo Tablets 2309
Sular Extended Release Tablets (Less than or equal to 1%) 2975
Sustiva Capsules (Less than 2%) 930
Sustiva Tablets (Less than 2%) 930
Symbyax Capsules (Infrequent) 1871
Tarka Tablets (0.3% or more) 511
Tasigna Capsules (0.1% to 1%) 2316
Teveten Tablets (Less than 1%) 515
Teveten HCT Tablets (Less than 1%) 517
▲ Tice BCG (7%) 2936
Treanda for Injection 983
Treximet Tablets (Infrequent) 1616
Tricor Tablets 520
▲ Trizivir Tablets (44%) 1622
▲ Tyzeka Tablets (1% to 12%) 2328
Ultram ER Extended-Release Tablets (0.5% to less than 1%) 2428
▲ Valstar Sterile Solution for Intravesical Instillation (4%) 1735
Vantas (Less than 2%) 1737
Varivax (Greater than or equal to 1%) 2133
▲ Velcade for Injection (64%) 2168
Venlafaxine Hydrochloride Tablets (Infrequent) 2199
▲ Vesanoid Capsules (66%) 2660
Viadur Implant (Less than 2%) 802
Viramune Oral Suspension 873
Viramune Tablets 873
Visudyne for Injection 2332
▲ Vivitrol (12% to 23%) 988
Voltaren Tablets (Occasionally) 2334
Voltaren-XR Tablets (Occasionally) 2337
Vytorin 10/10 Tablets 2149
Vytorin 10/10 Tablets 2939
Vytorin 10/20 Tablets 2149
Vytorin 10/20 Tablets 2939
Vytorin 10/40 Tablets 2149
Vytorin 10/40 Tablets 2939
Vytorin 10/80 Tablets 2149
Vytorin 10/80 Tablets 2939
Wellbutrin SR Sustained-Release Tablets (Rare) 1653
Wellbutrin XL Extended-Release Tablets (Rare) 1659
Xifaxan Tablets (Less than 2%) 2682
Xyrem Oral Solution (Frequent) 1766
Zantac 25 EFFERdose Tablets (Rare) 1670
Zantac Injection (Rare) 1666
Zantac Injection Pharmacy Bulk Package (Rare) 1668
Zantac Injection Premixed (Rare) 1666
Zantac (Rare) 1670
▲ Ziagen (12%) 1673
Zocor Tablets (Rare) 2136
▲ Zofran Injection (5%) 1682
▲ Zofran (9% to 13%) 1687
▲ Zofran ODT Orally Disintegrating Tablets (9% to 13%) 1687
Zomig Tablets (Infrequent) 694
Zomig-ZMT Tablets (Infrequent) 694
Zonegran Capsules (Infrequent) 1089
Zosyn for Injection (1% or less) 3284
▲ Zovirax (11.5%) 1690
Zyban Sustained-Release Tablets (Rare) 1692
Zyprexa Tablets (Infrequent) 1883
Zyprexa ZYDIS Orally Disintegrating Tablets (Infrequent) 1883
Zyrtec Chewable Tablets (Less than 2%) 1920
Zyrtec Syrup (Less than 2%) 1920
Zyrtec Tablets (Less than 2%) 1920
Zyrtec-D 12 Hour Extended Release Tablets (Less than 2%) 1923

Male pattern baldness

(*see under* Alopecia hereditaria)

Malformation, spine

Mirapex Tablets 857

Malignancies, secondary

Busulfex Injection 2477
Cimzia 3127
Eloxatin for Injection 2731
Leukeran Tablets 1508
Temodar Capsules 2931

Malignancies, various types

CellCept Capsules (0.7% to 2.1%) 2622
CellCept Intravenous (0.7% to 2.1%) 2622
CellCept Oral Suspension (0.7% to 2.1%) 2622
CellCept Tablets (0.7% to 2.1%) 2622
Cimzia 3127
Enbrel for Injection 569
Humira Injection 442
Kineret Injection (45 patients) 585
Remicade for IV Injection (18 of 1678 patients) 950
Xolair (0.5%) 1235

Malignancy

Amevive (1.3% to 1.8%) 611
Elidel Cream 1% 2221
Myfortic Tablets (0.5%) 2276
▲ Rapamune (1.1% to 3.2%) 3260
Raptiva for Injection 1218

Malignant hyperthermia

Proleukin for Injection (Less than 1%) 2287
Ultane Liquid for Inhalation (Less than 1%) 524

Malignant melanoma

Elidel Cream 1% 2221
Mirapex Tablets 857
Protopic Ointment 628
Raptiva for Injection 1218
Requip Tablets (Infrequent) 1561
Xolair (0.5%) 1235
Xolair 2339

Malignant neoplasms

Emend Capsules (Greater than 0.5%) 1992
Emend for Injection (Greater than 0.5%) 1999
Mirapex Tablets 857
Orthoclone OKT3 Sterile Solution (Less than 1%) 2387
Xolair (0.5%) 2339

Mania

Atripla Tablets 938
Concerta Extended-Release Tablets 1925
Cymbalta Delayed-Release Capsules 1801
Geodon (Rare) 2520
Luvox CR Extended-Release Capsules 1759
Parnate Tablets 1532
Paxil 1535
Paxil CR Controlled-Release Tablets 1544
Pristiq Extended-Release Tablets (0.1%) 3247
Provigil Tablets 977
Prozac Weekly Capsules (0.1% to 1.8%) 1852
Prozac Pulvules and Liquid 1852
Risperdal Consta Long-Acting Injection 1753
Rythmol Tablets (Less than 1%) 1586
Strattera Capsules 1864
Symbyax Capsules 1871
Venlafaxine Hydrochloride Tablets (0.5%) 2199
Vyvanse Capsules (0.1%) 3033

Manic behavior

Ambien Tablets (Rare) 2692
Campral Tablets (Rare) 1158
Celexa 1160
Cipro I.V. (1% or less) 2817
Copaxone for Injection (Infrequent) 3110
Effexor XR Extended-Release Capsules (0.5%) 3195
Evoxac Capsules (Less than 1%) 1013
▲ Intron A for Injection (Less than 5%) 2859
▲ Lamictal (5%) 1488
Orthoclone OKT3 Sterile Solution (Less than 1%) 2387
Parnate Tablets 1532
Paxil (Infrequent) 1535
Paxil CR Controlled-Release Tablets (Infrequent) 1544
Provigil Tablets 977
Remeron Tablets (Approximately 0.2%) 2924
RemeronSolTab Tablets (Approximately 0.2%) 2927
Requip Tablets (Infrequent) 1561
Retrovir IV Infusion 1579
Rilutek Tablets (Infrequent) 2771
Sustiva Capsules (0.2%) 930
Sustiva Tablets (0.2%) 930
Valtrex Caplets 1635
Wellbutrin Tablets (Frequent) 1648
Wellbutrin SR Sustained-Release Tablets 1653
Wellbutrin XL Extended-Release Tablets 1659
Zomig Tablets (Rare) 694
Zomig Nasal Spray (Rare) 689
Zomig-ZMT Tablets (Rare) 694
Zyban Sustained-Release Tablets 1692
Zyprexa Tablets (Frequent) 1883
Zyprexa ZYDIS Orally Disintegrating Tablets (Frequent) 1883

Manic reaction

Ambien CR Tablets (Rare) 2696
Azilect Tablets (Infrequent) 3106
Cipro (Less than 1%) 2810
Cipro XR Tablets 2823
▲ Equetro Extended-Release Capsules (Less than 5%) 3174
Lyrica Capsules (Rare) 2527
Meridia Capsules 475
Risperdal Consta Long-Acting Injection (Infrequent) 1753
Venlafaxine Hydrochloride Tablets (Infrequent) 2199

Manic symptoms

Concerta Extended-Release Tablets 1925

Manic-depressive reaction

Azilect Tablets (Rare) 3106
▲ Equetro Extended-Release Capsules (7%) 3174

Mass, abdominal

(*see under* Abdominal mass)

Mass, pulmonary

Dacogen Injection 1066

Mass at injection site

Amevive (1%) 611
Betaseron for SC Injection (2%) 756
Boostrix 1377
Fluarix Vaccine 1446
Pentacel 2792
▲ Somatuline Depot Injection (1.7% to 17%) 3102
Xolair 1235
Xolair 2339

Mastalgia

(*see under* Mastodynia)

Mastitis

Amerge Tablets (Rare) 1301
Aricept Tablets (Infrequent) 1062
Aricept ODT Tablets (Infrequent) 1062
Doxil Injection (Less than 1%) 2378
Effexor XR Extended-Release Capsules (Rare) 3195

▲ Intron A for Injection (Less than or equal to 5%) 2859
Lunesta Tablets (Infrequent) 2994
Paxil (Rare) 1535
Paxil CR Controlled-Release Tablets (Rare) 1544
Requip Tablets (Infrequent to rare) 1561
Salagen Tablets (Less than 1%) 1082
Venlafaxine Hydrochloride Tablets (Rare) 2199
Zonegran Capsules (Rare) 1089

Mastodynia
AndroGel 3159
Climara Transdermal System 763
Estratest Tablets 3043
Estratest H.S. Tablets 3043
Nalfon Capsules (Less than 1%) 2508
Premarin Intravenous 3217
Premarin Vaginal Cream 3228

Mazzotti reactions, worsening of
Stromectol Tablets 2120

Measles
ProQuad 2099

Mediastinal disorders, unspecified
Betaseron for SC Injection 756
▲ Cancidas for Injection (32.1% to 46.5%) 1953
▲ Focalin XR Capsules (9% to 16%) 2251
▲ Mycamine for Injection (35.9% to 68.5%) 616
▲ Verdeso Foam (7%) 3069

Megacolon, unspecified
Azilect Tablets (Rare) 3106

Megaloblastic anemia
(*see under* Anemia, megaloblastic)

Melancholia
Celexa (Rare) 1160

Melanocytic naevus
Mirapex Tablets 857

Melanoma, malignant, activation of
Stalevo Tablets 2309

Melanoma, skin
Paxil 1535
Paxil CR Controlled-Release Tablets 1544
▲ Rapamune (0% to less than 20%) 3260

Melanoma, unspecified
Bexxar 1371
▲ Humira Injection (Less than 5%) 442
Neupro Transdermal System 3149

Melanosis
Celexa (Rare) 1160
Copaxone for Injection (Infrequent) 3110
Humatrope Vials and Cartridges 1838
▲ Intron A for Injection (Less than 5%) 2859
Lyrica Capsules (Rare) 2527

Melasma
(*see also under* Chloasma)
Activella Tablets 2347
Ortho Tri-Cyclen Lo Tablets 2458

Melasma, possibly persistent
Estratest Tablets 3043
Estratest H.S. Tablets 3043
Premarin Tablets 3221
Premphase Tablets 3232
Prempro Tablets 3232
Seasonique Tablets 1046
Yaz Tablets 805

Melena
Abelcet Injection 1134
Aggrenox Capsules (1.9%) 819
▲ Agrylin Capsules (1% to less than 5%) 3017
Anaprox Tablets (Less than 1%) 2632
Anaprox DS Tablets (Less than 1%) 2632
Aricept Tablets (Infrequent) 1062
Aricept ODT Tablets (Infrequent) 1062
Azilect Tablets (Rare) 3106
Brovana Inhalation Solution (Less than 2%) 2990
Campral Tablets (Rare) 1158
Celebrex Capsules (0.1% to 1.9%) 2979
▲ CellCept Capsules (3% to less than 20%) 2622
▲ CellCept Intravenous (3% to less than 20%) 2622
▲ CellCept Oral Suspension (3% to less than 20%) 2622
▲ CellCept Tablets (3% to less than 20%) 2622
Copaxone for Injection (Infrequent) 3110
▲ Coreg Tablets (Greater than 1% to 3%) 1387
▲ Coreg CR Extended-Release Capsules (Greater than 1% to less than or equal to 3%) 1393
Cymbalta Delayed-Release Capsules (Rare) 1801
Doxil Injection (Less than 1%) 2378
EC-Naprosyn Delayed-Release Tablets (Less than 1%) 2632
Effexor XR Extended-Release Capsules (Infrequent) 3195
▲ Eloxatin for Injection (2% to less than 5%) 2731
Emsam Transdermal System (Infrequent) 905
Evoxac Capsules (Less than 1%) 1013
Exelon Capsules (Infrequent) 2229
Exelon Oral Solution (Infrequent) 2229
Fosamax (Up to 1.3%) 2005
Fosamax Plus D Tablets (0% to 1.3%) 2013
Gabitril Tablets (Infrequent) 973
Gantrisin Pediatric Suspension 2638
Geodon Capsules (Rare) 2520
Imitrex Injection 1465
Imitrex Nasal Spray (Rare) 1470
Imitrex Tablets (Rare) 1474
▲ Intron A for Injection (Less than 5%) 2859
Lamictal (Rare) 1488
Lipitor Tablets (Less than 2%) 2501
Lovaza Capsules 1520
Lunesta Tablets (Infrequent) 2994
Luvox CR Extended-Release Capsules (Infrequent) 1759
Lyrica Capsules (0.1% to 1%) 2527
Merrem I.V. (0.3%) 684
Mobic Oral Suspension (Less than 2%) 863
Mobic Tablets (Less than 2%) 863
Mylotarg for Injection (1%) 3212
Namenda (Infrequent) 1180
Naprosyn Suspension (Less than 1%) 2632
Naprosyn Tablets (Less than 1%) 2632
Nexium Delayed-Release Capsules (Less than 1%) 645
Nexium I.V. (Less than 1%) 652
Nexium Delayed-Release Oral Suspension (Less than 1%) 645
Omnicef Capsules 497
Omnicef for Oral Suspension 497
Paxil (Rare) 1535
Paxil CR Controlled-Release Tablets (Rare) 1544
▲ Photofrin for Injection (5%) 708
Pletal Tablets (Less than 2%) 2481
Protonix for Delayed-Release Oral Suspension (Less than 1%) 3254
Protonix Delayed-Release Tablets (Less than 1%) 3254
Protonix I.V. (Less than 1%) 3257
Prozac Weekly Capsules (Infrequent) 1852
Prozac Pulvules and Liquid (Infrequent) 1852
Requip Tablets (Infrequent) 1561
Rilutek Tablets (Rare) 2771
Risperdal Consta Long-Acting Injection (Infrequent) 1753
Rythmol SR Capsules 1590
Salagen Tablets (Less than 1%) 1082
▲ Simulect for Injection (3% to 10%) 2306
Soriatane Capsules (Less than 1%) 3062
Sular Extended Release Tablets (Less than or equal to 1%) 2975
Tarceva Tablets 1228
Targretin Capsules 1084
Tasigna Capsules (0.1% to 1%) 2316
Velcade for Injection 2168
Venlafaxine Hydrochloride Tablets (Infrequent) 2199
Vicoprofen Tablets (Less than 3%) 533
Voltaren Tablets (Occasionally) 2334
Voltaren-XR Tablets (Occasionally) 2337
Zomig Tablets (Rare) 694
Zomig-ZMT Tablets (Rare) 694
Zonegran Capsules (Infrequent) 1089
Zosyn for Injection (1% or less) 3284
Zyprexa Tablets (Infrequent) 1883
Zyprexa ZYDIS Orally Disintegrating Tablets (Infrequent) 1883
Zyrtec Chewable Tablets (Less than 2%) 1920
Zyrtec Syrup (Less than 2%) 1920
Zyrtec Tablets (Less than 2%) 1920
Zyrtec-D 12 Hour Extended Release Tablets (Less than 2%) 1923

Memory impairment
Abilify Injection (Greater than or equal to 1 in 1000 patients and less than 1 in 100 patients) 881
Abilify Injection (Greater than or equal to 1 in 1000 patients and less than 1 in 100 patients) 2466
Abilify Oral Solution (Greater than or equal to 1 in 1000 patients and less than 1 in 100 patients) 881
Abilify Oral Solution (Greater than or equal to 1 in 1000 patients and less than 1 in 100 patients) 2466
Abilify Discmelt Orally Disintegrating Tablets (Greater than or equal to 1 in 1000 patients and less than 1 in 100 patients) 881
Abilify Discmelt Orally Disintegrating Tablets (Greater than or equal to 1 in 1000 patients and less than 1 in 100 patients) 2466
Abilify Tablets (Greater than or equal to 1 in 1000 patients and less than 1 in 100 patients) 881
Abilify Tablets (Greater than or equal to 1 in 1000 patients and less than 1 in 100 patients) 2466
▲ Ambien CR Tablets (1% to 3%) 2696
AndroGel 3159
Combigan Ophthalmic Solution 553
Copaxone for Injection (Infrequent) 3110
Cozaar Tablets (Less than 1%) 1973
Cyanokit 5g Antidote 1021
▲ DepoCyt Injection (12% to 14%) 1136
Effexor XR Extended-Release Capsules 3195
Eldepryl Capsules 3052
Gleevec Tablets (Infrequent) 2255
Imitrex Nasal Spray (Rare) 1470
Imitrex Tablets (Rare) 1474
▲ Klonopin (4%) 2639
Lamictal (2.4%) 1488
Lunesta Tablets (Infrequent) 2994
Lupron Depot 3.75 mg (Among most frequent) 462
▲ Lupron Depot–3 Month 11.25 mg (Less than 5%) 462
▲ Lyrica Capsules (1% to 4%) 2527
Maxalt Tablets (Infrequent) 2056
Maxalt-MLT Orally Disintegrating Tablets (Infrequent) 2056
Mirapex Tablets 857
Prinivil Tablets (0.3% to 1%) 2087
Prinzide Tablets 2092
Requip Tablets (Infrequent) 1561
Rythmol Tablets (Less than 1%) 1586
Seromycin Capsules 1864
Stalevo Tablets 2309
Symbyax Capsules 1871
▲ Temodar Capsules (Less than 1% to 7%) 2931
Transderm Scōp Transdermal Therapeutic System (Infrequent) 2206
▲ Vesanoid Capsules (3%) 2660
Vytorin 10/10 Tablets 2149
Vytorin 10/10 Tablets 2939
Vytorin 10/20 Tablets 2149
Vytorin 10/20 Tablets 2939
Vytorin 10/40 Tablets 2149
Vytorin 10/40 Tablets 2939
Vytorin 10/80 Tablets 2149
Vytorin 10/80 Tablets 2939
Wellbutrin Tablets (Infrequent) 1648
▲ Wellbutrin SR Sustained-Release Tablets (Up to 3%) 1653
▲ Wellbutrin XL Extended-Release Tablets (3%) 1659
Xyrem Oral Solution (Frequent) 1766
Zocor Tablets 2136
▲ Zonegran Capsules (6%) 1089
Zyban Sustained-Release Tablets (Infrequent) 1692

Memory loss, short-term
▲ Ambien CR Tablets (1% to 3%) 2696
Cosopt Sterile Ophthalmic Solution 1969
Crestor Tablets 677
InnoPran XL Extended Release Capsules 1484
Lescol Capsules 2268
Lescol XL Tablets 2268
Meridia Capsules 475
Mevacor Tablets (0.5% to 1%) 2063
Nadolol Tablets 2191
Parnate Tablets 1532
PegIntron Powder for Injection 2903
Timoptic Sterile Ophthalmic Solution 2121
Timoptic in Ocudose 2124
Timoptic-XE Sterile Ophthalmic Gel Forming Solution 2125
Toprol-XL Tablets 666

Meniere's disease
Exelon Capsules (Infrequent) 2229
Exelon Oral Solution (Infrequent) 2229

Meniere's syndrome
Chantix Tablets (Rare) 2511
Imitrex Nasal Spray (Rare) 1470
Imitrex Tablets 1474

Meningioma
Norditropin Cartridges 2354

Meningioma, benign, growth potentiation of
Premarin Intravenous 3217
Premarin Vaginal Cream 3228

Meningism
Albenza Tablets (Up to 1%) 1297

Meningitis
CellCept Capsules 2622
CellCept Intravenous 2622
CellCept Oral Suspension 2622
CellCept Tablets 2622
▲ Gliadel Wafer (4% to 5%) 1076
Myfortic Tablets (Occasionally) 2276
Orthoclone OKT3 Sterile Solution (Less than 1%) 2387
Paxil (Rare) 1535
Paxil CR Controlled-Release Tablets (Rare) 1544
Pentacel 2792
Proleukin for Injection 2287
Remicade for IV Injection (Greater than or equal to 0.2%) 950
Voltaren Tablets (Rarely) 2334
Voltaren-XR Tablets (Rarely) 2337

Meningitis, aseptic
Anaprox Tablets (Less than 1%) 2632
Anaprox DS Tablets (Less than 1%) 2632
Carbatrol Capsules (One case) 3019
Celebrex Capsules (Less than 0.1%) 2979
Clinoril Tablets 1962
EC-Naprosyn Delayed-Release Tablets (Less than 1%) 2632
Gammagard Liquid 730
Gamunex (Very rare) 3094
Mumpsvax 2068
Naprosyn Suspension (Less than 1%) 2632
Naprosyn Tablets (Less than 1%) 2632
ProQuad 2099
Raptiva for Injection (1 case) 1218
Varivax 2133
Vicoprofen Tablets (Rare) 533

Meningitis, infectious
DepoCyt Injection 1136
Selzentry Tablets 2534

Menometrorrhagia
Mirapex Tablets 857

Menopausal symptoms, unspecified
Cymbalta Delayed-Release Capsules (Infrequent) 1801
Mirapex Tablets 857

Menopause
Effexor XR Extended-Release Capsules (Rare) 3195
Luvox CR Extended-Release Capsules (Infrequent) 1759
Symbyax Capsules (Infrequent) 1871
Venlafaxine Hydrochloride Tablets (Rare) 2199
Wellbutrin Tablets (Rare) 1648
Wellbutrin SR Sustained-Release Tablets 1653
Wellbutrin XL Extended-Release Tablets 1659
Zyban Sustained-Release Tablets 1692

Menorrhagia
Ambien CR Tablets (1%) 2696
Asacol Delayed-Release Tablets 2579
▲ Betaseron for SC Injection (8%) 756
Campral Tablets (Rare) 1158
Effexor XR Extended-Release Capsules (Infrequent) 3195

Emsam Transdermal System (Infrequent) 905
Evoxac Capsules (Less than 1%) 1013
Gabitril Tablets (Infrequent) 973
Geodon Capsules (Infrequent) 2520
Gleevec Tablets (Infrequent) 2255
▲ Intron A for Injection (Less than 5%) 2859
Lamictal (Infrequent) 1488
Lunesta Tablets (Infrequent) 2994
▲ Luvox CR Extended-Release Capsules (3%) 1759
Lyrica Capsules (0.1% to 1%) 2527
Mirapex Tablets 857
▲ Novantrone for Injection Concentrate (7%) 1100
Paxil (Infrequent) 1535
Paxil CR Controlled-Release Tablets (Infrequent) 1544
Pentasa Capsules (Less than 1%) 3030
Plavix Tablets (Less than 1%) 926
Plavix Tablets (Less than 1%) 2767
Prozac Weekly Capsules (Infrequent to greater than or equal to 2%) 1852
Prozac Pulvules and Liquid (At least 2%) 1852
Remeron Tablets (Rare) 2924
RemeronSolTab Tablets (Rare) 2927
Requip Tablets (Infrequent) 1561
Salagen Tablets (Less than 1%) 1082
Supprelin LA Implant 1731
Symbyax Capsules (Frequent) 1871
Venlafaxine Hydrochloride Tablets (Infrequent) 2199
Yaz Tablets 805
Zomig Tablets (Infrequent) 694
Zomig Nasal Spray (Infrequent) 689
Zomig-ZMT Tablets (Infrequent) 694
Zonegran Capsules (Rare) 1089
Zyprexa Tablets (Infrequent) 1883
Zyprexa ZYDIS Orally Disintegrating Tablets (Infrequent) 1883
Zyrtec Chewable Tablets (Less than 2%) 1920
Zyrtec Syrup (Less than 2%) 1920
Zyrtec Tablets (Less than 2%) 1920
Zyrtec-D 12 Hour Extended Release Tablets (Less than 2%) 1923

Menstrual cramps
Lexapro Oral Suspension (Frequent) 1174
Lexapro Tablets (Frequent) 1174
▲ Ortho Evra Transdermal System (9% to 22%) 2437
Strattera Capsules 1864

Menstrual disorders
Aceon Tablets (2 mg, 4 mg, 8 mg) (1.1%) 3038
▲ Advair HFA 45/21 Inhalation Aerosol (3% to 5%) 1288
▲ Advair HFA 115/21 Inhalation Aerosol (3% to 5%) 1288
▲ Advair HFA 230/21 Inhalation Aerosol (3% to 5%) 1288
▲ Aerobid/Aerobid-M (3% to 9%) 1153
Ambien Tablets (Infrequent) 2692
Ambien CR Tablets (Infrequent) 2696
Anaprox Tablets (Less than 1%) 2632
Anaprox DS Tablets (Less than 1%) 2632
Celebrex Capsules (0.1% to 1.9%) 2979
Chantix Tablets (Frequent) 2511
Cimzia 3127
Depakote ER Tablets (Greater than 1%) 423
EC-Naprosyn Delayed-Release Tablets (Less than 1%) 2632
Evoxac Capsules (Less than 1%) 1013
Gengraf Capsules (1%) 435
▲ Humira Injection (Less than 5%) 442
Lamictal (More than 1%) 1488
Lexapro Oral Suspension (2% to frequent) 1174
Lexapro Tablets (2% to frequent) 1174
Lupron Depot 3.75 mg (1%) 462
Lupron Depot–3 Month 11.25 mg (1%) 462
Maxalt Tablets (Infrequent) 2056
Maxalt-MLT Orally Disintegrating Tablets (Infrequent) 2056
Meridia Capsules (Greater than or equal to 1%) 475
Mustargen for Injection 2492
Naprosyn Suspension (Less than 1%) 2632
Naprosyn Tablets (Less than 1%) 2632
Neoral Oral Solution (1%) 2280
Neoral Soft Gelatin Capsules (1%) 2280
Nexium Delayed-Release Capsules (Less than 1%) 645
Nexium I.V. (Less than 1%) 652
Nexium Delayed-Release Oral Suspension (Less than 1%) 645
▲ Novantrone for Injection Concentrate (51% to 61%) 1100
▲ PegIntron Powder for Injection (4%) 2903
Provigil Tablets (At least 1%) 977
▲ Rebetol (6% to 7%) 2917
▲ Strattera Capsules (3%) 1864
Vaqta (1.1%) 2130
▲ Wellbutrin Tablets (4.7%) 1648
Yaz Tablets (Greater than 1%) 805

Menstrual flow, changes
Divigel 3167
Estratest Tablets 3043
Estratest H.S. Tablets 3043
Lybrel Tablets 3204
Moban Tablets 1116
NuvaRing 2897
Ortho-Cyclen Tablets 2449
Ortho Evra Transdermal System 2437
Ortho Tri-Cyclen Tablets 2449
Ortho Tri-Cyclen Lo Tablets 2458
▲ Plan B Tablets (12.5% to 13.8%) 1044
Premarin Intravenous 3217
Premarin Tablets 3221
Premarin Vaginal Cream 3228
Seasonique Tablets 1046
Tarka Tablets 511
Yaz Tablets 805

Menstrual irregularities
Accutane Capsules 2607
Advair HFA 45/21 Inhalation Aerosol 1288
Advair HFA 115/21 Inhalation Aerosol 1288
Advair HFA 230/21 Inhalation Aerosol 1288
Delatestryl Injection 1730
Estratest Tablets (Among most common) 3043
Estratest H.S. Tablets (Among most common) 3043
Imitrex Nasal Spray 1470
▲ Intron A for Injection (Less than 5%) 2859
Klonopin (Infrequent) 2639
Levothroid Tablets 1170
Levoxyl Tablets 1780
Mircette Tablets 1034
Omnaris Nasal Spray 2998
Ortho Micronor Tablets (Among most frequent) 2446
ParaGard T 380A Intrauterine Copper Contraceptive 1041
Premphase Tablets 3232
Prempro Tablets 3232
Prometrium Capsules (100 mg, 200 mg) 3047
Remicade for IV Injection (Greater than or equal to 0.2%) 950
Thioridazine Hydrochloride Tablets 2195
▲ Wellbutrin XL Extended-Release Tablets (5%) 1659
▲ Xenical Capsules (9.8%) 2672
Zyprexa Tablets (Infrequent) 1883
Zyprexa ZYDIS Orally Disintegrating Tablets (Infrequent) 1883

Menstruation, irregular
Abilify Injection (Greater than or equal to 1 in 1000 patients and less than 1 in 100 patients) 881
Abilify Injection (Greater than or equal to 1 in 1000 patients and less than 1 in 100 patients) 2466
Abilify Oral Solution (Greater than or equal to 1 in 1000 patients and less than 1 in 100 patients) 881
Abilify Oral Solution (Greater than or equal to 1 in 1000 patients and less than 1 in 100 patients) 2466
Abilify Discmelt Orally Disintegrating Tablets (Greater than or equal to 1 in 1000 patients and less than 1 in 100 patients) 881
Abilify Discmelt Orally Disintegrating Tablets (Greater than or equal to 1 in 1000 patients and less than 1 in 100 patients) 2466
Abilify Tablets (Greater than or equal to 1 in 1000 patients and less than 1 in 100 patients) 881
Abilify Tablets (Greater than or equal to 1 in 1000 patients and less than 1 in 100 patients) 2466
Luvox CR Extended-Release Capsules (Infrequent) 1759

Menstruation, painful
Asmanex Twisthaler 2797

Mental acuity, loss of
Retrovir Capsules 1574
Retrovir IV Infusion 1579
Retrovir 1574
Stalevo Tablets 2309

Mental clouding
Lortab 5/500 Tablets 3143
Lortab 7.5/500 Tablets 3144
Lortab 10/500 Tablets 3144
Tussionex Pennkinetic Extended-Release Suspension 3154
Vicodin Tablets 529
Vicodin ES Tablets 530
Vicodin HP Tablets 531
Zydone Tablets 1132

Mental confusion
(*see under* Confusion)

Mental depression
(*see also under* Depression)
Chantix Tablets (Frequent) 2511
Divigel 3167
▲ Sutent Capsules (8%) 2540

Mental disturbances, unspecified
Cuprimine Capsules 1986

Mental performance, impairment
Alferon N Injection (1%) 1726
Amerge Tablets (Infrequent) 1301
Arranon Injection (1%) 1319
Celexa (Frequent) 1160
Chantix Tablets (Rare) 2511
Copaxone for Injection (Infrequent) 3110
Cosopt Sterile Ophthalmic Solution 1969
Exelon Capsules (Infrequent) 2229
Exelon Oral Solution (Infrequent) 2229
Flumadine (0.3% to 2.1%) 1167
Frova Tablets (Infrequent) 1111
▲ Gabitril Tablets (6%) 973
Gengraf Capsules (1% to less than 3%) 435
Imitrex Injection (Rare) 1465
Imitrex Nasal Spray (Rare) 1470
Imitrex Tablets (Infrequent) 1474
▲ Intron A for Injection (Up to 14%) 2859
Klonopin (1% to 2%) 2639
Lamictal (1.7%) 1488
Lexapro Oral Suspension (Frequent) 1174
Lexapro Tablets (Frequent) 1174
Lortab 5/500 Tablets 3143
Lortab 7.5/500 Tablets 3144
Lortab 10/500 Tablets 3144
Maxalt Tablets (Frequent) 2056
Maxalt-MLT Orally Disintegrating Tablets (Infrequent) 2056
Meridia Capsules 475
MS Contin Tablets 2585
Neoral Oral Solution (1% to less than 3%) 2280
Neoral Soft Gelatin Capsules (1% to less than 3%) 2280
Opana Tablets (Less than 1%) 1117
Opana ER Tablets (Less than 1%) 1121
Paxil (Frequent) 1535
Paxil CR Controlled-Release Tablets (Frequent) 1544
Percocet Tablets 1127
Percodan Tablets 1130
▲ Prometrium Capsules (100 mg, 200 mg) (Less than 5%) 3047
Remeron Tablets 2924
RemeronSolTab Tablets 2927
Requip Tablets (Infrequent) 1561
Soma Tablets 1931
▲ Sustiva Capsules (1% to 9%) 930
▲ Sustiva Tablets (1% to 9%) 930
Sutent Capsules 2540
Tarka Tablets (Less frequent) 511
Timoptic Sterile Ophthalmic Solution 2121
Timoptic in Ocudose 2124
Timoptic-XE Sterile Ophthalmic Gel Forming Solution 2125
Treximet Tablets (Infrequent) 1616
Tussionex Pennkinetic Extended-Release Suspension 3154
Vicodin Tablets 529
Vicodin ES Tablets 530
Vicodin HP Tablets 531
Vivitrol 988
Xyrem Oral Solution (Infrequent) 1766
▲ Zonegran Capsules (6%) 1089
▲ Zyban Sustained-Release Tablets (9%) 1692
Zydone Tablets 1132

Mental slowness
▲ Zonegran Capsules (4%) 1089

Mental status, altered
Celexa 1160
Cubicin for Injection (Less than 1%) 995
Dacogen Injection 1066
Eldepryl Capsules 3052
▲ Invanz for Injection (3.3% to 5.1%) 2029
Lanoxin Injection 1498
Lanoxin Injection Pediatric 1502
Lanoxin Tablets 1505
Moban Tablets 1116
Opana Tablets (Less than 1%) 1117
Opana ER Tablets (Less than 1%) 1121
Orthoclone OKT3 Sterile Solution (Less than 1%) 2387
Patanase Nasal Spray 544
Pristiq Extended-Release Tablets 3247
▲ Prograf Capsules and Injection (Approximately 55%) 622
Remeron Tablets 2924
RemeronSolTab Tablets 2927
Stalevo Tablets 2309
Stromectol Tablets 2120
Thiothixene Capsules 2197
Treximet Tablets 1616
Vantas 1737
Velcade for Injection 2168

Mercury, increased excretion
Cuprimine Capsules (Rare) 1986

Mesenteric arterial thrombosis
Combigan Ophthalmic Solution 553
InnoPran XL Extended Release Capsules 1484
Rilutek Tablets (Rare) 2771
Timoptic Sterile Ophthalmic Solution 2121
Timoptic in Ocudose 2124

Metabolic acidosis
(*see under* Acidosis, metabolic)

Metabolic changes
Clinoril Tablets (Rare) 1962
▲ Hycamtin for Injection (39%) 1459
▲ Leukine (58%) 774
▲ Neoral Oral Solution (9.3%) 2280
▲ Neoral Soft Gelatin Capsules (9.3%) 2280
▲ Somatuline Depot Injection (16% to 25%) 3102

Metabolism disorders, unspecified
▲ Cancidas for Injection (10.7% to 21.7%) 1953
▲ Focalin XR Capsules (34%) 2251
▲ Mycamine for Injection (38.5% to 90.6%) 616

Methemoglobinemia
Cipro I.V. 2817
Cipro 2810
Cipro XR Tablets 2823
Elitek (Less than 1%) 2729
Fansidar Tablets 2636
Gantrisin Pediatric Suspension 2638
Mepron Suspension 1526
Nitro-Dur Transdermal Infusion System (Very rare) 2887

Metrorrhagia
Alinia for Oral Suspension (Less than 1%) 2677
Alinia Tablets (Less than 1%) 2677
Aricept Tablets (Infrequent) 1062
Aricept ODT Tablets (Infrequent) 1062
▲ Betaseron for SC Injection (9%) 756
Campral Tablets (Infrequent) 1158
Copaxone for Injection (At least 2%) 3110
▲ Depakote ER Tablets (Greater than 1% to less than 5%) 423
▲ Divigel (4.1% to 9.6%) 3167
Emsam Transdermal System (Frequent) 905
Gabitril Tablets (Frequent) 973
Geodon Capsules (Infrequent) 2520
Lipitor Tablets (Less than 2%) 2501
Lunesta Tablets (Infrequent) 2994
Luvox CR Extended-Release Capsules (Infrequent) 1759
Lyrica Capsules (0.1% to 1%) 2527
Meridia Capsules (1%) 475
▲ Mylotarg for Injection (2% to 10%) 3212
Paxil (Rare) 1535

Paxil CR Controlled-Release Tablets (Rare) 1544
Pentasa Capsules (Less than 1%) 3030
Prozac Pulvules and Liquid (Infrequent) 1852
Remeron Tablets (Rare) 2924
RemeronSolTab Tablets (Rare) 2927
Rilutek Tablets (Infrequent) 2771
Salagen Tablets (Less than 1%) 1082
Supprelin LA Implant 1731
Symbyax Capsules (Infrequent) 1871
Venlafaxine Hydrochloride Tablets (Frequent) 2199
Yaz Tablets (Greater than 1%) 805
Zomig Tablets (Rare) 694
Zomig Nasal Spray (Rare) 689
Zomig-ZMT Tablets (Rare) 694
Zyprexa Tablets (Infrequent) 1883
Zyprexa ZYDIS Orally Disintegrating Tablets (Infrequent) 1883

Metyrapone test, altered results

Estratest Tablets 3043
Estratest H.S. Tablets 3043
Premarin Tablets 3221
Premphase Tablets 3232
Prempro Tablets 3232

Microcephaly, fetal

Accutane Capsules 2607
Phenytek Capsules 2192

Microlithiasis, biliary

Sandostatin LAR Depot 2302

Microphthalmia, fetal

Accutane Capsules 2607

Micropinna, fetal

Accutane Capsules 2607

Micturition, difficulty

Catapres Tablets (About 2 in 1,000 patients) 841
Catapres-TTS (0.5% or less) 842
▲ Chemet Capsules (Up to 3.7%) 2484
Clorpres Tablets (About 2 in 1,000) 2185
Combigan Ophthalmic Solution 553
Cosopt Sterile Ophthalmic Solution 1969
Dantrium Capsules (Less frequent) 2580
Effexor XR Extended-Release Capsules (Frequent) 3195
Eligard 7.5 mg (Less than 2%) 2724
Eligard 22.5 mg (Less than 2%) 2724
Eligard 30 mg (Less than 2%) 2724
Eligard 45 mg (Less than 2%) 2724
OxyContin Tablets (Less than 1%) 2589
▲ Paxil (3%) 1535
▲ Paxil CR Controlled-Release Tablets (3%) 1544
Pristiq Extended-Release Tablets (Less than 1% to 2%) 3247
ProAmatine Tablets (Rare) 3032
▲ Prometrium Capsules (100 mg, 200 mg) (11%) 3047
Salagen Tablets (Less than 1%) 1082
Timoptic Sterile Ophthalmic Solution 2121
Timoptic in Ocudose 2124
Timoptic-XE Sterile Ophthalmic Gel Forming Solution 2125
Transderm Scōp Transdermal Therapeutic System (Infrequent) 2206
Ultram ER Extended-Release Tablets (0.5% to less than 1%) 2428
Uroqid-Acid No. 2 Tablets (Occasional) 814
Zonegran Capsules (Infrequent) 1089
Zyprexa Tablets (Infrequent) 1883
Zyprexa ZYDIS Orally Disintegrating Tablets (Infrequent) 1883

Micturition, frequent

Ambien Tablets (Rare) 2692
Ambien CR Tablets (Rare) 2696
Campral Tablets (Infrequent) 1158
▲ Doxil Injection (1% to 10%) 2378
Exforge Tablets (Greater than 0.1% but less thatn 1%) 2238
Namenda (Frequent) 1180
Neupro Transdermal System (Greater than or equal to 2%) 3149
Risperdal Consta Long-Acting Injection (Infrequent) 1753
Zyrtec Chewable Tablets (Less than 2%) 1920
Zyrtec Syrup (Less than 2%) 1920
Zyrtec Tablets (Less than 2%) 1920
Zyrtec-D 12 Hour Extended Release Tablets (Less than 2%) 1923

Micturition, painful

Uroqid-Acid No. 2 Tablets (Occasional) 814

Micturition, urgency

Cymbalta Delayed-Release Capsules (Infrequent) 1801
▲ Doxil Injection (1% to 10%) 2378
Tasigna Capsules (0.1% to 1%) 2316

Micturition disturbances

Aceon Tablets (2 mg, 4 mg, 8 mg) (0.3% to 1%) 3038
Aricept Tablets (2%) 1062
Aricept ODT Tablets (2%) 1062
Avalide Tablets (2%) 892
Avalide Tablets (2%) 2713
Captopril Tablets (Approximately 1 to 2 of 1000 patients) 2182
Carbatrol Capsules 3019
Cardene I.V. (Rare) 1093
Celebrex Capsules (0.1% to 1.9%) 2979
▲ Celexa (3%) 1160
▲ CellCept Capsules (3% to less than 20%) 2622
▲ CellCept Intravenous (3% to less than 20%) 2622
▲ CellCept Oral Suspension (3% to less than 20%) 2622
▲ CellCept Tablets (3% to less than 20%) 2622
Cipro I.V. (1% or less) 2817
Cipro XR Tablets 2823
Copaxone for Injection (At least 2%) 3110
Coreg CR Extended-Release Capsules (0.1% to less than or equal to 1%) 1393
Cozaar Tablets (Less than 1%) 1973
Crinone 4% Gel 992
Crinone 8% Gel 992
▲ Dacogen Injection (5%) 1066
Dantrium Capsules (Less frequent) 2580
Duragesic Transdermal System (Greater than 1%) 2405
Effexor XR Extended-Release Capsules (Frequent) 3195
Eldepryl Capsules 3052
Eligard 7.5 mg (Less than 2%) 2724
Eligard 22.5 mg (2.6%) 2724
Eligard 30 mg (2.2%) 2724
Eligard 45 mg 2724
▲ Eloxatin for Injection (1% to 5%) 2731
Equetro Extended-Release Capsules 3174
Evoxac Capsules (0.9%; less than 1%) 1013
Exelon Capsules (Infrequent) 2229
Exelon Oral Solution (Infrequent) 2229
Exforge Tablets (Greater than 0.1% to less than 1%) 2238
Flumadine 1167
Frova Tablets (Infrequent) 1111
Gabitril Tablets (1% or more) 973
Gengraf Capsules (1% to less than 3%) 435
Gleevec Tablets (Infrequent) 2255
Imitrex Injection (Rare) 1465
Imitrex Nasal Spray (Infrequent) 1470
Imitrex Tablets (Infrequent) 1474
▲ Indapamide Tablets (Less than 5%) 2188
Indocin (Rare) 2024
▲ Intron A for Injection (Less than 5%) 2859
Klonopin (1%) 2639
▲ Lamictal (Greater than 1% to less than 5%) 1488
Lexapro Oral Suspension (Frequent) 1174
Lexapro Tablets (Frequent) 1174
Lipitor Tablets (Less than 2%) 2501
Lunesta Tablets (Infrequent) 2994
Lyrica Capsules (Greater than or equal to 1%) 2527
Marplan Tablets (0% to 2%) 3177
Maxalt Tablets (Infrequent) 2056
Maxalt-MLT Orally Disintegrating Tablets (Infrequent) 2056
Megace ES Oral Suspension (0% to 2%) 2499
Meridia Capsules 475
Micardis Tablets (More than 0.3%) 852
Micardis HCT Tablets 854
▲ Mirapex Tablets (Greater than or equal to 1% to 6%) 857
Mobic Oral Suspension (0.1% to 2.4%) 863
Mobic Tablets (0.1% to 2.4%) 863
Neoral Oral Solution (1% to less than 3%) 2280
Neoral Soft Gelatin Capsules (1% to less than 3%) 2280
Nexium Delayed-Release Capsules (Less than 1%) 645
Nexium I.V. (Less than 1%) 652
Nexium Delayed-Release Oral Suspension (Less than 1%) 645
Norvir (Less than 2%) 489
Opana Tablets (Less than 1%) 1117
Opana ER Tablets (Less than 1%) 1121
Parnate Tablets 1532
▲ Paxil (3%) 1535
▲ Paxil CR Controlled-Release Tablets (3%) 1544
Pentasa Capsules (Less than 1%) 3030
Pletal Tablets (Less than 2%) 2481
ProAmatine Tablets (Among most frequent) 3032
▲ Prograf Capsules and Injection (3% to 15%) 622
Protonix for Delayed-Release Oral Suspension (Less than 1%) 3254
Protonix Delayed-Release Tablets (Less than 1%) 3254
Protonix I.V. (Less than 1%) 3257
Prozac Weekly Capsules (Frequent to greater than or equal to 2%) 1852
▲ Rebif Prefilled Syringe for Injection (2% to 7%) 1107
Remeron Tablets (2%) 2924
RemeronSolTab Tablets (2%) 2927
ReoPro Vials (0.1%) 1860
Requip Tablets (Infrequent) 1561
Retrovir Capsules 1574
Retrovir IV Infusion 1579
Retrovir 1574
Rythmol SR Capsules 1590
▲ Salagen Tablets (9% to 12%) 1082
▲ Simulect for Injection (3% to 10%) 2306
Symbyax Capsules (Frequent) 1871
Tarka Tablets 511
▲ Temodar Capsules (6%) 2931
Teveten Tablets (Less than 1%) 515
Teveten HCT Tablets (Less than 1%) 517
▲ Tice BCG (40% to 50%) 2936
Tricor Tablets 520
Ultram ER Extended-Release Tablets (0.5% to less than 1%) 2428
▲ Valstar Sterile Solution for Intravesical Instillation (61%) 1735
Vantas (Less than 2%) 1737
▲ Venlafaxine Hydrochloride Tablets (3%) 2199
▲ Vesanoid Capsules (3%) 2660
▲ Viadur Implant (3.8%) 802
Vicoprofen Tablets (Less than 3%) 533
Wellbutrin Tablets (2.5%) 1648
▲ Wellbutrin SR Sustained-Release Tablets (2% to 5%) 1653
▲ Wellbutrin XL Extended-Release Tablets (2% to 5%) 1659
Xifaxan Tablets (Less than 2%) 2682
Zomig Tablets (Infrequent) 694
Zomig Nasal Spray (Rare) 689
Zomig-ZMT Tablets (Infrequent) 694
Zyban Sustained-Release Tablets (Frequent) 1692
Zyprexa Tablets (Infrequent) 1883
Zyprexa ZYDIS Orally Disintegrating Tablets (Infrequent) 1883

Middle ear, fluid in

▲ Increlex Injection (Greater than or equal to 5%) 3100

Migraine

Aceon Tablets (2 mg, 4 mg, 8 mg) (0.3% to 1%) 3038
Actiq (1% or greater) 959
Activella Tablets 2347
▲ Advair HFA 45/21 Inhalation Aerosol (1% to 3%) 1288
▲ Advair HFA 115/21 Inhalation Aerosol (1% to 3%) 1288
▲ Advair HFA 230/21 Inhalation Aerosol (1% to 3%) 1288
Advicor Tablets 402
Aggrenox Capsules 819
▲ Agrylin Capsules (1% to less than 5%) 3017
Ambien Tablets (Infrequent) 2692
Ambien CR Tablets (Infrequent) 2696
Angeliq Tablets 751
Asacol Delayed-Release Tablets (2% or greater) 2579
Azilect Tablets (Infrequent) 3106
Campral Tablets (Infrequent) 1158
Celexa (Frequent) 1160
Chantix Tablets (Infrequent) 2511
Cialis Tablets 1792
Cipro I.V. (1% or less) 2817
Cipro (Less than 1%) 2810
Cipro XR Tablets (Less than 1%) 2823
Climara Pro Transdermal System 768
▲ Copaxone for Injection (5%) 3110
Coreg Tablets (Less than or equal to 0.1%) 1387
Coreg CR Extended-Release Capsules (Less than or equal to 0.1%) 1393
Cozaar Tablets (Less than 1%) 1973
Crinone 4% Gel 992
Crinone 8% Gel 992
▲ Cymbalta Delayed-Release Capsules (3%) 1801
Divigel 3167
Doxil Injection (Less than 1%) 2378
Effexor XR Extended-Release Capsules (Frequent) 3195
Eldepryl Capsules 3052
Emsam Transdermal System (Infrequent) 905
Engerix-B Vaccine 1409
Enjuvia Tablets 1029
▲ Epzicom Tablets (6% to 7%) 1422
Estratest Tablets 3043
Estratest H.S. Tablets 3043
Evista Tablets (2.4%) 1810
▲ Evoxac Capsules (1% to 3%) 1013
Exelon Capsules (Infrequent) 2229
Exelon Oral Solution (Infrequent) 2229
Exelon Patch (Infrequent) 2233
Exforge Tablets (Less than or equal to 0.1%) 2238
Fentora Tablets (Greater than 1%) 968
▲ Flovent Diskus 50 mcg (1% to 3%) 1435
▲ Flovent HFA (1% to 3%) 1440
Gabitril Tablets (Frequent) 973
▲ Gengraf Capsules (3%) 435
Gleevec Tablets (Infrequent) 2255
Imitrex Tablets 1474
▲ Intron A for Injection (Less than 5%) 2859
Ionsys Transdermal System (.1% to less than 1%) 2410
Kaletra (0% to 2%) 452
Klonopin (Infrequent) 2639
▲ Lamictal (1% to 5%) 1488
Lexapro Oral Suspension (Frequent) 1174
Lexapro Tablets (Frequent) 1174
Lipitor Tablets (Less than 2%) 2501
Lovaza Capsules 1520
Lunesta Tablets (Frequent) 2994
▲ Lupron Depot 3.75 mg (33%) 462
▲ Lupron Depot–3 Month 11.25 mg (33%) 462
Lybrel Tablets 3204
Maxair Autohaler 1705
Meridia Capsules (2.4%) 475
Miacalcin Nasal Spray (Less than 1%) 2274
Micardis Tablets (More than 0.3%) 852
Micardis HCT Tablets 854
Mirapex Tablets 857
Mircette Tablets 1034
▲ Neoral Oral Solution (3%) 2280
▲ Neoral Soft Gelatin Capsules (3%) 2280
Nexium Delayed-Release Capsules (Less than 1%) 645
Nexium I.V. (Less than 1%) 652
Nexium Delayed-Release Oral Suspension (Less than 1%) 645
Niaspan Extended-Release Tablets 480
Norvir (Less than 2%) 489
NuvaRing 2897
Ortho-Cyclen Tablets 2449
Ortho Evra Transdermal System 2437
Ortho Tri-Cyclen Tablets 2449
Ortho Tri-Cyclen Lo Tablets 2458
OxyContin Tablets (Less than 1%) 2589
Paxil (Infrequent) 1535
Paxil CR Controlled-Release Tablets (Infrequent) 1544
PegIntron Powder for Injection 2903
Premarin Intravenous 3217
Premarin Vaginal Cream 3228
Premphase Tablets 3232
Prempro Tablets 3232
Protonix for Delayed-Release Oral Suspension (Greater than or equal to 1%) 3254
Protonix Delayed-Release Tablets (Greater than or equal to 1%) 3254
Protonix I.V. (Greater than or equal to 1%) 3257
Protopic Ointment (Greater than or equal to 1%) 628
Provigil Tablets (At least 1%) 977
Prozac Weekly Capsules (Infrequent) 1852

Prozac Pulvules and Liquid (Infrequent) 1852
▲ Pulmicort Flexhaler (Greater than or equal to 1% to 3%) 654
Recombivax HB 2107
Remeron Tablets (Infrequent) 2924
RemeronSolTab Tablets (Infrequent) 2927
Requip Tablets (Infrequent to frequent) 1561
Rilutek Tablets (Infrequent) 2771
Risperdal Consta Long-Acting Injection (Infrequent) 1753
Rituxan I.V. (Less than 1% to 2%) 1223
Salagen Tablets (Less than 1%) 1082
Sandostatin LAR Depot 2302
Seasonique Tablets 1046
▲ Serevent Diskus (1% to 3%) 1594
Soriatane Capsules (Less than 1%) 3062
Sular Extended Release Tablets (Less than or equal to 1%) 2975
Supprelin LA Implant 1731
Sustiva Capsules (Less than 2%) 930
Sustiva Tablets (Less than 2%) 930
Symbyax Capsules (Frequent) 1871
Tasigna Capsules (0.1% to 1%) 2316
Teveten Tablets (Less than 1%) 515
Teveten HCT Tablets (Less than 1%) 517
Tricor Tablets 520
Tyzeka Tablets (1%) 2328
Ultram ER Extended-Release Tablets (0.5% to less than 1%) 2428
Venlafaxine Hydrochloride Tablets (Frequent) 2199
▲ Vivitrol (16% to 36%) 988
▲ Wellbutrin Tablets (25.7%) 1648
▲ Wellbutrin SR Sustained-Release Tablets (1% to 4%) 1653
▲ Wellbutrin XL Extended-Release Tablets (0% to 4%) 1659
▲ Xeloda Tablets (Less than 5%) 2662
Xifaxan Tablets (Less than 2%) 2682
Xopenex Inhalation Solution (2.7%) 3001
Xopenex Inhalation Solution Concentrate (2.7%) 3005
Xopenex HFA Inhalation Aerosol (2.7%) 3009
Xyrem Oral Solution (Infrequent) 1766
Yaz Tablets (Greater than 1%) 805
▲ Ziagen (7%) 1673
Zyban Sustained-Release Tablets (Infrequent) 1692
Zyprexa Tablets (Infrequent) 1883
Zyprexa ZYDIS Orally Disintegrating Tablets (Infrequent) 1883
Zyrtec Chewable Tablets (Less than 2%) 1920
Zyrtec Syrup (Less than 2%) 1920
Zyrtec Tablets (Less than 2%) 1920
Zyrtec-D 12 Hour Extended Release Tablets (Less than 2%) 1923

Migraine, aggravated
Activella Tablets 2347
Climara Transdermal System 763
Enjuvia Tablets 1029
Frova Tablets (Infrequent) 1111
Nexium Delayed-Release Capsules (Less than 1%) 645
Nexium I.V. (Less than 1%) 652
Nexium Delayed-Release Oral Suspension (Less than 1%) 645
Premarin Tablets 3221
Premphase Tablets 3232
Prempro Tablets 3232

Migration of implant
Viadur Implant (Rare) 802

Miliaria
Analpram-HC 1140
Diprolene Lotion 0.05% (Infrequent) 2838
Diprolene Ointment 0.05% 2839
Diprolene AF Cream 0.05% (Infrequent) 2837
Elocon Cream 0.1% (Infrequent) 2840
Elocon Lotion 0.1% (Infrequent) 2841
Elocon Ointment 0.1% (Infrequent) 2842
Lotrisone 2881
Luxíq Foam 3058
Olux Foam 3061
Olux-E Foam 3059
Pramosone 1141
Vanos Cream 1941
Verdeso Foam 3069

Miliaria ruba
ProQuad (Greater than or equal to 0.2% to less than 1%) 2099

Mind racing
Lamictal (Infrequent) 1488

Miosis
Actiq (Less than 1%) 959
Alphagan P Ophthalmic Solution 549
Combigan Ophthalmic Solution 553
Dibenzyline Capsules 3188
Effexor XR Extended-Release Capsules (Rare) 3195
Emend Capsules (Less than or equal to 0.5%) 1992
Emend for Injection (Less than or equal to 0.5%) 1999
Lyrica Capsules (Rare) 2527
MS Contin Tablets (Less frequent) 2585
Opana Tablets (Less than 1%) 1117
Opana ER Tablets (Less than 1%) 1121
Percocet Tablets 1127
Percodan Tablets 1130
Rythmol SR Capsules 1590
Symbyax Capsules (Infrequent) 1871
Thioridazine Hydrochloride Tablets 2195
Thiothixene Capsules 2197
Venlafaxine Hydrochloride Tablets (Rare) 2199
Xyrem Oral Solution (Infrequent) 1766
Zyprexa Tablets (Rare) 1883
Zyprexa ZYDIS Orally Disintegrating Tablets (Rare) 1883

Miscarriage
Limbrel Capsules 2561
Zomig Tablets (Rare) 694
Zomig-ZMT Tablets (Rare) 694

Mitochondrial toxicity
Aptivus Capsules (Less than 2%) 823
Aptivus Oral Solution (Less than 2%) 823

Mitral insufficiency
Requip Tablets (Infrequent) 1561

Mitral regurgitation
Activase I.V. 1188
Somatuline Depot Injection 3102
TNKase 1233

Mitral valve disease
Effexor XR Extended-Release Capsules (Rare) 3195
Venlafaxine Hydrochloride Tablets (Rare) 2199

Mitral valve prolapse
Effexor XR Extended-Release Capsules (Rare) 3195

Mobility disorders, non-site specific
Abilify Injection (Greater than or equal to 1 in 1000 patients and less than 1 in 100 patients) 881
Abilify Injection (Greater than or equal to 1 in 1000 patients and less than 1 in 100 patients) 2466
Abilify Oral Solution (Greater than or equal to 1 in 1000 patients and less than 1 in 100 patients) 881
Abilify Oral Solution (Greater than or equal to 1 in 1000 patients and less than 1 in 100 patients) 2466
Abilify Discmelt Orally Disintegrating Tablets (Greater than or equal to 1 in 1000 patients and less than 1 in 100 patients) 881
Abilify Discmelt Orally Disintegrating Tablets (Greater than or equal to 1 in 1000 patients and less than 1 in 100 patients) 2466
Abilify Tablets (Greater than or equal to 1 in 1000 patients and less than 1 in 100 patients) 881
Abilify Tablets (Greater than or equal to 1 in 1000 patients and less than 1 in 100 patients) 2466
Amerge Tablets (Rare) 1301

Molluscum contagiosum
Elidel Cream 1% (0% to 1.8%) 2221
Norvir (Less than 2%) 489

Moniliasis
(*see under* Candidiasis)

Moniliasis, gastrointestinal
▲ CellCept Capsules (3% to less than 20%) 2622
▲ CellCept Intravenous (3% to less than 20%) 2622
▲ CellCept Oral Suspension (3% to less than 20%) 2622
▲ CellCept Tablets (3% to less than 20%) 2622
Cipro 2810
Cipro XR Tablets 2823

Moniliasis, genital
(*see under* Candidiasis, genital)

Moniliasis, oral
(*see also under* Candidiasis, oral)
Avelox (Greater than or equal to 0.1% to less than 2%) 2803
▲ CellCept Capsules (3% to less than 20%) 2622
▲ CellCept Intravenous (3% to less than 20%) 2622
▲ CellCept Oral Suspension (3% to less than 20%) 2622
▲ CellCept Tablets (3% to less than 20%) 2622
Cipro 2810
Cipro XR Tablets 2823
Venlafaxine Hydrochloride Tablets (Infrequent) 2199

Moniliasis, vaginal
Avelox (Greater than or equal to 0.1% to less than 2%) 2803
Cipro 2810
Cipro XR Tablets (1% to 2%) 2823
Emsam Transdermal System (Infrequent) 905
Lamictal (Rare) 1488
Merrem I.V. (Greater than 0.1% to 1%) 684
▲ Omnicef Capsules (4%) 497
Omnicef for Oral Suspension (0.3%) 497
▲ Premarin Tablets (5% to 6%) 3221
▲ Premphase Tablets (4% to 8%) 3232
▲ Prempro Tablets (4% to 8%) 3232
Salagen Tablets (Less than 1%) 1082
Symbyax Capsules (Infrequent) 1871
Tricor Tablets 520
Tygacil for Injection (0% to less than 2%) 3276
Yaz Tablets (Greater than 1%) 805
Zyvox (1% to 1.6%) 2552

Monoarthritis
Mirapex Tablets 857
Requip Tablets (Infrequent) 1561

Monocytosis
Campral Tablets (Rare) 1158
Cipro (Less than 0.1%) 2810
Cipro XR Tablets 2823
Cuprimine Capsules 1986
Geodon Capsules (Rare) 2520
Paxil (Rare) 1535
Paxil CR Controlled-Release Tablets (Rare) 1544
Primaxin I.M. 2080
Primaxin I.V. 2083
Rocephin Injectable Vials, ADD-Vantage, Galaxy, Bulk (Less than 0.1%) 2642
Rythmol SR Capsules 1590
Xifaxan Tablets (Less than 2%) 2682

Mononeuropathy
Infanrix Vaccine 1479

Mononeuropathy, cranial
Pediarix Vaccine 1552

Mononeuropathy, peripheal
Pediarix Vaccine 1552

Mononucleosis, infectious
Daytrana Transdermal Patch 3022

Monoplegia
Gliadel Wafer (2%) 1076
Imitrex Injection (Rare) 1465
Imitrex Nasal Spray (Rare) 1470
Imitrex Tablets (Infrequent) 1474

Mood changes
Activella Tablets 2347
▲ Aerobid/Aerobid-M (1% to 3%) 1153
▲ Alimta for Injection (Up to 14%) 1786
Aloxi Injection (Less than 1%) 1059
Ambien CR Tablets (1%) 2696
Angeliq Tablets 751
▲ Arimidex Tablets (19%) 672
Chantix Tablets (Infrequent) 2511
Climara Transdermal System 763
Climara Pro Transdermal System 768
Concerta Extended-Release Tablets 1925
Cymbalta Delayed-Release Capsules (Infrequent) 1801
Divigel 3167
Eldepryl Capsules 3052
Enbrel for Injection 569
Enjuvia Tablets 1029
Estratest Tablets 3043
Estratest H.S. Tablets 3043
Genotropin Lyophilized Powder 2547
Hexalen Capsules 1078
▲ Keppra Injection (5% to 12.7%) 3137
▲ Keppra Oral Solution (5% to 6.7%) 3131
▲ Keppra Tablets (5% to 6.7%) 3131
Lortab 5/500 Tablets 3143
Lortab 7.5/500 Tablets 3144
Lortab 10/500 Tablets 3144
Lupron Depot 3.75 mg 462
Lybrel Tablets 3204
Marinol Capsules 3163
Meridia Capsules 475
Mirapex Tablets 857
Mobic Oral Suspension 863
Mobic Tablets 863
MS Contin Tablets (Less frequent) 2585
▲ Novantrone for Injection Concentrate (6%) 1100
Ortho-Cyclen Tablets 2449
Ortho Evra Transdermal System 2437
Ortho Tri-Cyclen Tablets 2449
Ortho Tri-Cyclen Lo Tablets 2458
Orthoclone OKT3 Sterile Solution 2387
Paxil 1535
Paxil CR Controlled-Release Tablets 1544
Premarin Tablets 3221
Premarin Vaginal Cream 3228
Premphase Tablets 3232
Prempro Tablets 3232
Requip Tablets (Infrequent) 1561
Seasonique Tablets 1046
▲ Solodyn Extended Release Tablets (3%) 1938
Strattera Capsules (0.4% to 2%) 1864
Supprelin LA Implant 1731
Testim 1% Gel (1% or less) 701
Tussionex Pennkinetic Extended-Release Suspension 3154
Vicodin Tablets 529
Vicodin ES Tablets 530
Vicodin HP Tablets 531
Vicoprofen Tablets (Less than 1%) 533
Wellbutrin Tablets (Infrequent) 1648
▲ Xeloda Tablets (5%) 2662
Xyrem Oral Solution (Infrequent) 1766
Yaz Tablets 805
Zydone Tablets 1132

Moon face
Copaxone for Injection (Infrequent) 3110

Motion sickness
Aloxi Injection (Less than 1%) 1059
Aricept Tablets 1062
Aricept ODT Tablets 1062
Evoxac Capsules (Less than 1%) 1013
Klonopin (Infrequent) 2639
Mirapex Tablets 857
Treximet Tablets (Rare) 1616
Xifaxan Tablets (Less than 2%) 2682

Motor and phonic tics, exacerbations
Adderall XR Capsules 3012
Dexedrine 1401
Vyvanse Capsules 3033

Motor disturbances, reversible involuntary
Zantac 25 EFFERdose Tablets (Rare) 1670
Zantac Injection (Rare) 1666
Zantac Injection Pharmacy Bulk Package (Rare) 1668
Zantac Injection Premixed (Rare) 1666
Zantac (Rare) 1670

Motor dysfunction
▲ Arranon Injection (0% to 4%) 1319
Velcade for Injection 2168

Motor function, loss of
Neoral Oral Solution 2280
Neoral Soft Gelatin Capsules 2280
Sandimmune 2296

Motor restlessness
Moban Tablets 1116
Paxil Tablets 1535
Paxil CR Controlled-Release Tablets 1544
▲ Pediarix Vaccine (0.6% to 41.4%) 1552
Thioridazine Hydrochloride Tablets 2195

Motor skills, impairment
▲ Abilify Injection (11% to 21%) 881
▲ Abilify Injection (11% to 21%) 2466
▲ Abilify Oral Solution (11% to 21%) 881
▲ Abilify Oral Solution (11% to 21%) 2466

▲ Abilify Discmelt Orally Disintegrating Tablets (11% to 21%) 881
▲ Abilify Discmelt Orally Disintegrating Tablets (11% to 21%) 2466
▲ Abilify Tablets (11% to 21%) 881
▲ Abilify Tablets (11% to 21%) 2466
Ambien Tablets 2692
Amerge Tablets (Rare) 1301
Dapsone Tablets USP 1746
Invega Extended-Release Tablets 1748
Moban Tablets 1116
Patanase Nasal Spray 544
▲ Prograf Capsules and Injection (Approximately 55%) 622
Prozac Weekly Capsules 1852
Remeron Tablets 2924
RemeronSolTab Tablets 2927
Risperdal Consta Long-Acting Injection 1753
Zyprexa Tablets 1883
Zyprexa IntraMuscular 1883
Zyprexa ZYDIS Orally Disintegrating Tablets 1883

Mottling
Bicillin C-R Injectable Suspension 1775
Bicillin L-A Injection 1777

Mouth, burning
Eldepryl Capsules 3052

Mouth, discoloration
▲ Kepivance (17%) 583

Mouth, dry
(*see under* Xerostomia)

Mouth, fissuring in corner of
Parnate Tablets 1532

Mouth, puckering
Moban Tablets 1116
Thiothixene Capsules 2197

Mouth, sore
Alferon N Injection (One patient) 1726
▲ Flovent Diskus 50 mcg (1% to 3%) 1435
Gengraf Capsules (Rare) 435
▲ Imitrex Injection (4.9%) 1465
Neoral Oral Solution (Rare) 2280
Neoral Soft Gelatin Capsules (Rare) 2280
Reyataz Capsules 3299

Mouth, thickening of
▲ Kepivance (17%) 583

Mouth ulceration
Azilect Tablets (Infrequent) 3106
▲ CellCept Capsules (3% to less than 20%) 2622
▲ CellCept Intravenous (3% to less than 20%) 2622
▲ CellCept Oral Suspension (3% to less than 20%) 2622
▲ CellCept Tablets (3% to less than 20%) 2622
Chantix Tablets (Infrequent) 2511
▲ Doxil Injection (1% to 10%) 2378
Fentora Tablets (Greater than 1%) 968
Lyrica Capsules (0.1% to 1%) 2527
Prograf Capsules and Injection 622
ProQuad 2099
Protopic Ointment (0.2% to less than 1%) 628
Prozac Weekly Capsules (Infrequent) 1852
▲ Spiriva HandiHaler (1% to 3%) 870
Tasigna Capsules (0.1% to 1%) 2316
Venlafaxine Hydrochloride Tablets (Infrequent) 2199

Movement, abnormal
Gabitril Tablets (Infrequent) 973
Lamictal (Infrequent) 1488
Neoral Oral Solution 2280
Neoral Soft Gelatin Capsules 2280
Orthoclone OKT3 Sterile Solution 2387
Prozac Pulvules and Liquid 1852
Sandimmune 2296
Zonegran Capsules (Infrequent) 1089
▲ Zyprexa Tablets (1% to 5%) 1883
▲ Zyprexa ZYDIS Orally Disintegrating Tablets (1% to 5%) 1883

Movement, unspecified
Ultane Liquid for Inhalation (1%) 524

Movement, unsteady
Humulin 50/50, 100 Units 1843
Humulin 70/30 Vial 1844
Humulin N Vial 1846
Humulin R 1849

Movement disorder
Prozac Weekly Capsules 1852
Symbyax Capsules (Infrequent) 1871
▲ Zyprexa IntraMuscular (2% to 4%) 1883

Mucocutaneous lymph node syndrome
(*see under* Kawasaki-like syndrome)

Mucocutaneous reactions
Rituxan I.V. 1223

Mucocutaneous toxicity
Rituxan I.V. 1223

Mucosal inflammation
Cancidas for Injection 1953
▲ DepoCyt Injection (3% to 12%) 1136
▲ Vectibix (Less than 1% to 6%) 597

Mucosal pigmentation, changes
▲ Intron A for Injection (Less than 5%) 2859

Mucositis
Alferon N Injection (One patient) 1726
AmBisome for Injection (Less common) 606
▲ Busulfex Injection (97%) 2477
▲ Elitek (2% to 15%) 2729
▲ Eloxatin for Injection (2% to 7%) 2731
Erbitux 912
Evoxac Capsules (Less than 1%) 1013
▲ Intron A for Injection (Less than 5%) 2859
▲ Ixempra Kit for Injection (29%) 915
Myleran Tablets 1530
▲ Mylotarg for Injection (25%) 3212
▲ Neulasta Injection (15% to 72%) 587
▲ Neupogen for Injection (12%) 589
▲ Nexavar Tablets (1% to less than 10%) 784
▲ Novantrone for Injection Concentrate (10% to 29%) 1100
▲ Noxafil Oral Suspension (2% to 17%) 2889
▲ Sutent Capsules (1% to 53%) 2540
▲ Torisel Injection (3% to 41%) 3272
▲ Vectibix (6%) 597
▲ Vesanoid Capsules (26%) 2660
▲ Zometa for Intravenous Infusion (5% to less than 10%) 2341

Mucous membrane, abnormalities
Aceon Tablets (2 mg, 4 mg, 8 mg) (0.3% to 1%) 3038
Actiq (Less than 1%) 959
Captopril Tablets (Approximately 1 in 1000 patients) 2182
Clinoril Tablets 1962
Emend Capsules (2.6%) 1992
Emend for Injection (2.6%) 1999
Lescol Capsules 2268
Lescol XL Tablets 2268
▲ Leukine (75%) 774
Mevacor Tablets 2063
Remeron Tablets 2924
RemeronSolTab Tablets 2927
Salagen Tablets (Less than 1%) 1082

Mucous membrane, irritation of
Vectibix 597

Mucus, blood-tinted
Atrovent Nasal Spray 0.03% (2%) 834
▲ Flonase Nasal Spray (1% to 3%) 1431

Multiorgan failure
Fleet Enema 1143
Fleet Enema Extra 1143
Fleet Enema for Children 1143
Fleet Pedia-Lax Enema 1143
Lamictal 1488
Prograf Capsules and Injection 622
Taxotere Injection Concentrate 2773

Multiorgan system failure
Clolar for Intravenous Infusion 1239
Cosmegen for Injection 2485
Lamictal 1488
Levaquin 2416
Levaquin in 5% Dextrose Injection 2416

Multiple sclerosis, acute exacerbations of
Aldara Cream, 5% 1699

Muscle, rupture
Levaquin 2416
Levaquin in 5% Dextrose Injection 2416

Muscle atrophy
Actiq (Less than 1%) 959
Azilect Tablets (Infrequent) 3106
Copaxone for Injection (Infrequent) 3110
Eligard 7.5 mg (Less than 2%) 2724
Eligard 22.5 mg (Less than 2%) 2724
Eligard 30 mg (Less than 2%) 2724
Eligard 45 mg (Less than 2%) 2724
Lamictal (Rare) 1488

Muscle contractions, abnormal, prolonged
Moban Tablets 1116
Thiothixene Capsules 2197

Muscle contractions, involuntary
Ambien CR Tablets (1%) 2696
▲ Eloxatin for Injection (2% to less than 5%) 2731
Lexapro Oral Suspension (Infrequent) 1174
Lexapro Tablets (Infrequent) 1174
Mirapex Tablets 857
Namenda (Infrequent) 1180
Risperdal Consta Long-Acting Injection (Infrequent) 1753

Muscle cramp
(*see under* Cramping, muscular)

Muscle enzyme increased
Chantix Tablets (Infrequent) 2511

Muscle hypertonia
Lexapro Oral Suspension (Infrequent) 1174
Lexapro Tablets (Infrequent) 1174

Muscle injury
Advair Diskus 100/50 1276
▲ Advair HFA 45/21 Inhalation Aerosol (0% to 3%) 1288
▲ Advair HFA 115/21 Inhalation Aerosol (0% to 3%) 1288
▲ Advair HFA 230/21 Inhalation Aerosol (0% to 3%) 1288
Levaquin 2416
Levaquin in 5% Dextrose Injection 2416
Ultram ER Extended-Release Tablets (0.5% to less than 1%) 2428

Muscle rigidity
Abilify Injection (Greater than or equal to 1 in 1000 patients and less than 1 in 100 patients) 881
Abilify Injection (Less than 1 in 100 patients) 2466
Abilify Oral Solution (Greater than or equal to 1 in 1000 patients and less than 1 in 100 patients) 881
Abilify Oral Solution (Less than 1 in 100 patients) 2466
Abilify Discmelt Orally Disintegrating Tablets (Greater than or equal to 1 in 1000 patients and less than 1 in 100 patients) 881
Abilify Discmelt Orally Disintegrating Tablets (Less than 1 in 100 patients) 2466
Abilify Tablets (Greater than or equal to 1 in 1000 patients and less than 1 in 100 patients) 881
Abilify Tablets (Less than 1 in 100 patients) 2466
Amerge Tablets (Infrequent) 1301
Ceftin Tablets (0.1% to 1%) 1380
Comtan Tablets 2208
Cozaar Tablets (Less than 1%) 1973
▲ Flovent HFA (1% to 3%) 1440
Imitrex Injection (Rare) 1465
Invega Extended-Release Tablets 1748
Lexapro Oral Suspension (Infrequent) 1174
Lexapro Tablets (Infrequent) 1174
Miacalcin Nasal Spray (Less than 1%) 2274
Mirapex Tablets 857
MS Contin Tablets (Less frequent) 2585
Neupro Transdermal System 3149
Orthoclone OKT3 Sterile Solution 2387
▲ Serevent Diskus (1% to 3%) 1594
Thioridazine Hydrochloride Tablets 2195
Thiothixene Capsules 2197
▲ Vivitrol (2% to 8%) 988
Wellbutrin Tablets 1648
Wellbutrin SR Sustained-Release Tablets 1653
Wellbutrin XL Extended-Release Tablets 1659
Zyban Sustained-Release Tablets 1692

Muscle spasms
Abilify Injection (2%) 881
Abilify Injection (Greater than or equal to 1 in 100 patients) 2466
Abilify Oral Solution (2%) 881
Abilify Oral Solution (Greater than or equal to 1 in 100 patients) 2466
Abilify Discmelt Orally Disintegrating Tablets (2%) 881
Abilify Discmelt Orally Disintegrating Tablets (Greater than or equal to 1 in 100 patients) 2466
Abilify Tablets (2%) 881
Abilify Tablets (Greater than or equal to 1 in 100 patients) 2466
▲ Advair Diskus 250/50 (3%) 1276
▲ Advair HFA 45/21 Inhalation Aerosol (1% to 3%) 1288
▲ Advair HFA 115/21 Inhalation Aerosol (1% to 3%) 1288
▲ Advair HFA 230/21 Inhalation Aerosol (1% to 3%) 1288
Amerge Tablets (Infrequent) 1301
Amitiza Capsules 3082
▲ Aranesp for Injection (17%) 564
Aricept Tablets (Infrequent) 1062
Aricept ODT Tablets (Infrequent) 1062
Atacand HCT 642
Avalide Tablets 892
Avalide Tablets 2713
Celexa 1160
Clorpres Tablets 2185
▲ Cymbalta Delayed-Release Capsules (4%) 1801
Diovan HCT Tablets 2216
Exelon Patch (Infrequent) 2233
Exforge Tablets (Greater than or equal to 0.2%) 2238
▲ Fabrazyme for Intravenous Infusion (5%) 1241
Fenoglide Tablets 2960
Fentora Tablets (Greater than 1%) 968
▲ Forteo for Injection (1% to 10%) 1816
Furosemide Tablets 2186
▲ Indapamide Tablets (Greater than or equal to 5%) 2188
Indocin I.V. (Less than 1%) 2489
Intravenous Sodium Diuril 2490
Invega Extended-Release Tablets 1748
Ixempra Kit for Injection 915
Lamictal (1%) 1488
Luvox CR Extended-Release Capsules (Infrequent) 1759
▲ Lyrica Capsules (2% to 4%) 2527
Maxalt Tablets (Infrequent) 2056
Maxalt-MLT Orally Disintegrating Tablets (Infrequent) 2056
Micardis HCT Tablets 854
Mirapex Tablets 857
Parnate Tablets 1532
Prinzide Tablets 2092
Rebif Prefilled Syringe for Injection 1107
Requip Tablets (Frequent to greater than or equal to 1%) 1561
Requip XL Tablets 1568
Retrovir Capsules 1574
Retrovir IV Infusion 1579
Retrovir 1574
Rythmol SR Capsules 1590
▲ Tasigna Capsules (11% to 14%) 2316
Tekturna HCT Tablets 2324
Teveten HCT Tablets 517
Ultram ER Extended-Release Tablets (0.5% to less than 1%) 2428
Valium Tablets 2658
▲ Vivitrol (2% to 8%) 988
Wellbutrin Tablets (1.9%) 1648
Xifaxan Tablets (Less than 2%) 2682
▲ Zolinza Capsules (17% to 19.8%) 2142

Muscle stiffness
Exelon Capsules (Infrequent) 2229
Exelon Oral Solution (Infrequent) 2229
▲ Flovent HFA (1% to 3%) 1440
Gleevec Tablets (Infrequent) 2255
Imitrex Injection (Rare) 1465
Requip Tablets (Frequent) 1561
▲ Vivitrol (2% to 8%) 988

Muscle tightness
Abilify Injection (Greater than or equal to 1 in 1000 patients and less than 1 in 100 patients) 881
Abilify Injection (Greater than or equal to 1 in 1000 patients and less than 1 in 100 patients) 2466
Abilify Oral Solution (Greater than or equal to 1 in 1000 patients and less than 1 in 100 patients) 881
Abilify Oral Solution (Greater than or equal to 1 in 1000 patients and less than 1 in 100 patients) 2466

Abilify Discmelt Orally Disintegrating Tablets (Greater than or equal to 1 in 1000 patients and less than 1 in 100 patients) 881
Abilify Discmelt Orally Disintegrating Tablets (Greater than or equal to 1 in 1000 patients and less than 1 in 100 patients) 2466
Abilify Tablets (Greater than or equal to 1 in 1000 patients and less than 1 in 100 patients) 881
Abilify Tablets (Greater than or equal to 1 in 1000 patients and less than 1 in 100 patients) 2466
Concerta Extended-Release Tablets (1.9%) 1925
Cymbalta Delayed-Release Capsules (Infrequent) 1801
Requip Tablets (Infrequent) 1561
Treximet Tablets (Greater than 1%) 1616
Xyrem Oral Solution (Infrequent) 1766

Muscle tiredness
Imitrex Injection (Rare) 1465

Muscle twitching
(*see also under* Fasciculations)
Concerta Extended-Release Tablets 1925
Invega Extended-Release Tablets 1748
Requip Tablets (Infrequent) 1561

Muscle weakness
(*see under* Myasthenia)

Muscle-related symptoms, unspecified
Tyzeka Tablets (2%) 2328

Muscular disturbances
Copaxone for Injection (Infrequent) 3110
▲ Gengraf Capsules (12%) 435
Lescol Capsules 2268
Lescol XL Tablets 2268
▲ Neoral Oral Solution (12%) 2280
▲ Neoral Soft Gelatin Capsules (12%) 2280
▲ Prometrium Capsules (100 mg, 200 mg) (Less than 5%) 3047
Zosyn for Injection (1% or less) 3284

Musculoskeletal aches
Avalide Tablets 2713
Follistim AQ Cartridge 2844
Viramune Oral Suspension 873
Viramune Tablets 873

Musculoskeletal contracture
Requip Tablets (Infrequent) 1561

Musculoskeletal dysfunction
▲ Cancidas for Injection (11.3% to 14.3%) 1953
▲ Mycamine for Injection (18.8%) 616
▲ Somatuline Depot Injection (17% to 26%) 3102
Vytorin 10/10 Tablets 2939
Vytorin 10/20 Tablets 2939
Vytorin 10/40 Tablets 2939
Vytorin 10/80 Tablets 2939

Musculoskeletal stiffness
▲ Abilify Injection (4%) 2466
▲ Abilify Oral Solution (4%) 881
▲ Abilify Oral Solution (4%) 2466
▲ Abilify Discmelt Orally Disintegrating Tablets (4%) 881
▲ Abilify Discmelt Orally Disintegrating Tablets (4%) 2466
▲ Abilify Tablets (4%) 881
▲ Abilify Tablets (4%) 2466
Invega Extended-Release Tablets 1748
Mirapex Tablets 857
Rebif Prefilled Syringe for Injection 1107
Reclast Injection (2%) 2291
Xyrem Oral Solution (Infrequent) 1766

Musculoskeletal symptoms, unspecified
Accutane Capsules 2607
Cipro 2810
▲ Epivir (12%) 1412
▲ Femara Tablets (2.8% to 38.2%) 2246
Flovent Diskus 50 mcg 1435
▲ Gengraf Capsules (13.2%) 435
▲ Hycamtin for Injection (14%) 1459
▲ Mobic Oral Suspension (1.7% to 3.8%) 863
▲ Mobic Tablets (1.7% to 3.8%) 863
▲ Neoral Oral Solution (13.2%) 2280
▲ Neoral Soft Gelatin Capsules (13.2%) 2280
▲ Selzentry Tablets (8.7%) 2534
Trasylol Injection (2%) 799

Musculoskeletal trauma
Avalide Tablets 892
Avalide Tablets 2713
Avapro Tablets (2%) 897
Avapro Tablets (2%) 2718

Mutism
Luvox CR Extended-Release Capsules (Rare) 1759
Prograf Capsules and Injection 622

Myalgia
Abelcet Injection 1134
▲ Abilify Injection (2% to 3%) 881
Abilify Injection (2%) 2466
▲ Abilify Oral Solution (2% to 3%) 881
Abilify Oral Solution (2%) 2466
▲ Abilify Discmelt Orally Disintegrating Tablets (2% to 3%) 881
Abilify Discmelt Orally Disintegrating Tablets (2%) 2466
▲ Abilify Tablets (2% to 3%) 881
Abilify Tablets (2%) 2466
Accolate Tablets (1.6%) 669
Aceon Tablets (2 mg, 4 mg, 8 mg) (0.3% to 1.1%) 3038
Aciphex Tablets 1053
▲ Actimmune (6%) 1743
Actiq (Less than 1%) 959
Activella Tablets 2347
▲ Actonel Tablets (4.6% to 6.7%) 2568
▲ Actonel with Calcium Tablets (4.6% to 6.6%) 2574
▲ ActoPlus Met Tablets (5.4%) 3071
▲ Actos Tablets (5.4%) 3077
▲ Advair HFA 45/21 Inhalation Aerosol (1% to 4%) 1288
▲ Advair HFA 115/21 Inhalation Aerosol (1% to 4%) 1288
▲ Advair HFA 230/21 Inhalation Aerosol (1% to 4%) 1288
▲ Advicor Tablets (3%) 402
Aggrenox Capsules (1.2%) 819
▲ Agrylin Capsules (1% to less than 5%) 3017
Aldara Cream, 5% (1%) 1699
▲ Alferon N Injection (One patient to 45%) 1726
▲ Alimta for Injection (Up to 13%) 1786
Alinia for Oral Suspension (Less than 1%) 2677
Alinia Tablets (Less than 1%) 2677
Ambien Tablets (Frequent) 2692
▲ Ambien CR Tablets (4%) 2696
AmBisome for Injection (Less common) 606
Amerge Tablets (Infrequent) 1301
Amevive (Common) 611
Amitiza Capsules (Less than 1%) 3082
Anaprox Tablets (Less than 1%) 2632
Anaprox DS Tablets (Less than 1%) 2632
Anzemet Injection (Rare) 2701
Anzemet Tablets (Rare) 2704
Aptivus Capsules (2.3%) 823
Aptivus Oral Solution (2.3%) 823
▲ Aranesp for Injection (8% to 21%) 564
Aricept Tablets (Infrequent) 1062
Aricept ODT Tablets (Infrequent) 1062
▲ Arimidex Tablets (2% to 6%) 672
▲ Arranon Injection (1% to 13%) 1319
▲ Asacol Delayed-Release Tablets (3%) 2579
▲ Asmanex Twisthaler (2% to 3%) 2797
Atacand Tablets (0.5% or greater) 639
Atacand HCT (0.5% or greater) 642
▲ Atripla Tablets (Greater than or equal to 5%) 938
Attenuvax 1951
Augmentin 1323
Augmentin Tablets 1327
Augmentin XR Extended Release Tablets 1333
Augmentin ES-600 Powder for Oral Suspension 1329
Avalide Tablets 892
Avapro Tablets (1% or greater) 897
Avapro Tablets (1% or greater) 2718
▲ Avastin IV (8% to 15%) 1192
Avelox (Greater than or equal to 0.1% to less than 2%) 2803
Axert Tablets (Infrequent) 2431
Axid Capsules (1.7%) 1364
▲ Azmacort Inhalation Aerosol (1% to 3%) 407
Beconase AQ Nasal Spray 1369
Benicar Tablets (Greater than 0.5%) 1009
Benicar HCT Tablets (Greater than 1%) 1010
▲ Betaseron for SC Injection (23%) 756
▲ Bexxar (Less than 1% to 13%) 1371
▲ Boniva Injection (0.8% to 5.7%) 2614
▲ Boniva Tablets (0.8% to 5.7%) 2618
Boostrix 1377
▲ Busulfex Injection (16%) 2477
Calcijex Injection 419
Campral Tablets (Frequent) 1158
Captopril Tablets 2182
Carbatrol Capsules 3019
Catapres Tablets (About 6 in 1,000 patients) 841
Catapres-TTS (0.5% or less) 842
Celebrex Capsules (0.1% to 1.9%) 2979
Celexa (2%) 1160
▲ CellCept Capsules (3% to less than 20%) 2622
▲ CellCept Intravenous (3% to less than 20%) 2622
▲ CellCept Oral Suspension (3% to less than 20%) 2622
▲ CellCept Tablets (3% to less than 20%) 2622
Chantix Tablets (Frequent) 2511
▲ Cialis Tablets (1% to 4%) 1792
Cipro I.V. (Rare) 2817
Cipro 2810
Cipro XR Tablets 2823
▲ Clarinex Tablets (2.1% to 3%) 2828
▲ Clarinex Reditabs Tablets (2.1% to 3%) 2828
Clinoril Tablets (Less than 1 in 100) 1962
▲ Clolar for Intravenous Infusion (14%) 1239
Clorpres Tablets (About 6 in 1,000) 2185
▲ Combivir Tablets (8%) 1384
Concerta Extended-Release Tablets 1925
Copaxone for Injection (At least 2%) 3110
Cosmegen for Injection 2485
Cozaar Tablets (1% or greater) 1973
▲ Crestor Tablets (1.9% to 12.7%) 677
Cubicin for Injection (Less than 1%) 995
▲ Cymbalta Delayed-Release Capsules (1% to 4%) 1801
▲ Dacogen Injection (5%) 1066
Dantrium Capsules (Less frequent) 2580
Demadex Injection (1.6%) 2630
Demadex Tablets (1.6%) 2630
▲ Depakote ER Tablets (Greater than 1% to less than 5%) 423
Didronel Tablets (Infrequent) 2583
Diovan Tablets (Greater than 0.2%) 2212
Diovan HCT Tablets (Greater than 0.2%) 2216
▲ Doxil Injection (Less than 1% to 10%) 2378
▲ Duetact Tablets (At least 5%) 3085
Dyazide Capsules 1405
EC-Naprosyn Delayed-Release Tablets (Less than 1%) 2632
▲ Effexor XR Extended-Release Capsules (4%) 3195
Eligard 7.5 mg (Less than 2%) 2724
Eligard 22.5 mg 2724
Eligard 30 mg (2.2%) 2724
▲ Eligard 45 mg (4.5%) 2724
▲ Eloxatin for Injection (2% to 14%) 2731
Emend Capsules (Greater than 0.5%) 1992
Emend for Injection (Greater than 0.5%) 1999
Emsam Transdermal System (Frequent) 905
▲ Emtriva Capsules (4% to 6%) 1246
▲ Emtriva Oral Solution (4% to 6%) 1246
Engerix-B Vaccine (Less than 1%) 1409
▲ Epivir (8%) 1412
▲ Epivir-HBV (14%) 1417
Epogen for Injection (Rare) 576
Equetro Extended-Release Capsules 3174
▲ Evista Tablets (7.7%) 1810
▲ Evoxac Capsules (1% to 3%) 1013
Exelon Capsules (Frequent) 2229
Exelon Oral Solution (Frequent) 2229
Exelon Patch (Infrequent) 2233
Exforge Tablets (Greater than or equal to 0.2%) 2238
▲ Fabrazyme for Intravenous Infusion (5% to 8%) 1241
Faslodex Injection (Less than 1%) 682
▲ Femara Tablets (0.3% to 6.7%) 2246
Fenoglide Tablets 2960
Fentora Tablets (Greater than 1%) 968
▲ Flolan for Injection (3% to 44%) 1426
▲ Flovent Diskus 50 mcg (1% to 12%) 1435
▲ Flovent HFA (1% to 3%) 1440
▲ Fluarix Vaccine (10.2% to 23%) 1446
▲ Flulaval Injection Vaccine (1% to 16%) 1448
▲ FluMist Vaccine (2% to 17%) 1945
▲ Fosamax (0.4% to approximately 6%) 2005
▲ Fosamax Plus D Tablets (0.4% to 4.1%) 2013
Frova Tablets (Infrequent) 1111
Furosemide Tablets 2186
▲ Gabitril Tablets (1% to 5%) 973
Gantrisin Pediatric Suspension 2638
Gardasil Injection (2%) 2019
Gemzar for Injection (Common) 1820
Gengraf Capsules (1% to less than 3%) 435
▲ Genotropin Lyophilized Powder (1.6% to 6.7%) 2547
Geodon Capsules (2% to frequent) 2520
▲ Gleevec Tablets (9% to 27%) 2255
Havrix Injection Vaccine (Less than 1%) 1454
Herceptin I.V. 1199
Humalog Mix 50/50-Pen and KwikPen 1833
▲ Humatrope Vials and Cartridges (9.1% to 24.3%) 1838
▲ Hycamtin for Injection (59%) 1459
Imitrex Injection (2%) 1465
Imitrex Nasal Spray (Infrequent) 1470
Imitrex Tablets (Frequent) 1474
▲ Intron A for Injection (3% to 75%) 2859
Ionsys Transdermal System (.1% to less than 1%) 2410
▲ Ixempra Kit for Injection (49%) 915
Janumet Tablets 2041
Kaletra (Up to 2%) 452
Klonopin (1%) 2639
▲ Lamictal (More than 1% to less than 5%) 1488
Lamisil Oral Granules 2264
Lamisil Tablets 2266
▲ Lescol Capsules (5%) 2268
▲ Lescol XL Tablets (3.8%) 2268
▲ Leukine (18%) 774
▲ Leustatin Injection (7%) 2384
Levaquin (0.1% to 1%) 2416
Levaquin in 5% Dextrose Injection (0.1% to 1%) 2416
Levitra Tablets (Less than 2%) 2876
Lexapro Oral Suspension (Frequent) 1174
Lexapro Tablets (Frequent) 1174
▲ Lipitor Tablets (Up to 5.6%) 2501
Lovaza Capsules 1520
Lunesta Tablets 2994
▲ Lupron Depot 3.75 mg (Less than 5%) 462
▲ Lupron Depot 7.5 mg (Less than 5%) 469
Lupron Depot–3 Month 11.25 mg (0.6% to 1%) 462
▲ Luvox CR Extended-Release Capsules (5%) 1759
Lyrica Capsules (Greater than or equal to 1%) 2527
Marinol Capsules (Less than 1%) 3163
▲ Mavik Tablets (4.7%) 472
Maxalt Tablets (Infrequent) 2056
Maxalt-MLT Orally Disintegrating Tablets (Infrequent) 2056
Meridia Capsules (1.9%) 475
Meruvax II 2061
Mevacor Tablets (1.8% to 2.4%) 2063
▲ Miacalcin Nasal Spray (1% to 3%) 2274
Micardis Tablets (1%) 852
Micardis HCT Tablets 854
Mirapex Tablets (Greater than or equal to 1%) 857
M-M-R II 2054
▲ Myfortic Tablets (3% to less than 20%) 2276
▲ Mylotarg for Injection (3% to 11%) 3212
▲ Nabi-HB (10%) 815
Naprosyn Suspension (Less than 1%) 2632
Naprosyn Tablets (Less than 1%) 2632
Nasonex Nasal Spray (Greater than or equal to 2%) 2883
Neoral Oral Solution (1% to less than 3%) 2280
Neoral Soft Gelatin Capsules (1% to less than 3%) 2280
▲ Neulasta Injection (15% to 72%) 587
Neupogen for Injection 589
▲ Neupro Transdermal System (2% to 3%) 3149
▲ Nexavar Tablets (Greater than or equal to 10%) 784
Nexium Delayed-Release Capsules (Rare) 645
Nexium I.V. (Rare) 652
Nexium Delayed-Release Oral Suspension (Rare) 645
Niaspan Extended-Release Tablets 480
Nimotop Capsules (Up to 1.4%) 790
▲ Norditropin Cartridges (15%) 2354
Noroxin Tablets 2069

Norvir (1.7% to 2.4.%) 489
▲ Novantrone for Injection Concentrate (5%) 1100
Noxafil Oral Suspension (Less than 1% to 2%) 2889
▲ Ontak Vials (17%) 1079
OptiPranolol Metipranolol Ophthalmic Solution 0.3% (A small number of patients) ⊙245
Orthoclone OKT3 Sterile Solution (Less than 1%) 2387
Paxil (2%) 1535
Paxil CR Controlled-Release Tablets (2%) 1544
▲ PegIntron Powder for Injection (54%) 2903
Pentasa Capsules (Less than 1%) 3030
Pepcid Tablets (Infrequent) 2075
Percocet Tablets 1127
Persantine Tablets (Rare) 869
Plavix Tablets 926
Plavix Tablets 2767
▲ Pletal Tablets (2% to 3%) 2481
Pneumovax 23 2078
▲ Premarin Tablets (5% to 9%) 3221
▲ Premphase Tablets (4% to 5%) 3232
▲ Prempro Tablets (4% to 5%) 3232
Prinivil Tablets (0.3% to greater than 1%) 2087
Prinzide Tablets (0.3% to 1%) 2092
Procrit for Injection (Rare) 2391
▲ Prograf Capsules and Injection (3% to 15%) 622
▲ Prometrium Capsules (100 mg, 200 mg) (Less than 5%) 3047
ProQuad 2099
Protonix for Delayed-Release Oral Suspension (Less than 1%) 3254
Protonix Delayed-Release Tablets (Less than 1%) 3254
Protonix I.V. (Less than 1%) 3257
▲ Protopic Ointment (Up to 3%) 628
Provigil Tablets (At least 1%) 977
Prozac Pulvules and Liquid 1852
▲ Pulmicort Flexhaler (Greater than or equal to 1% to 3%) 654
▲ Raptiva for Injection (8%) 1218
▲ Rebetol (32% to 64%) 2917
▲ Rebif Prefilled Syringe for Injection (25%) 1107
▲ Reclast Injection (4.9% to 11.7%) 2291
Recombivax HB (Less than 1%) 2107
ReFacto Vials 3269
▲ Relenza Inhalation Powder (Less than 1.5% to 8%) 1556
Remeron Tablets (2%) 2924
RemeronSolTab Tablets (2%) 2927
Remicade for IV Injection 950
ReoPro Vials (0.3%) 1860
Requip Tablets (Frequent to greater than or equal to 1%) 1561
Requip XL Tablets 1568
▲ Retrovir Capsules (8%) 1574
▲ Retrovir IV Infusion (8%) 1579
▲ Retrovir (8%) 1574
▲ Reyataz Capsules (4%) 3299
Risperdal Consta Long-Acting Injection (2%) 1753
▲ Rituxan I.V. (1% to 10%) 1223
Rocaltrol Capsules 1150
Rocaltrol Oral Solution 1150
Rozerem Tablets (2%) 3091
Rythmol SR Capsules 1590
Salagen Tablets (1% to 2%) 1082
Sandimmune (2% or less) 2296
Sandostatin Injection (Less than 1%) 2300
▲ Sandostatin LAR Depot (4% to 18.2%) 2302
Selzentry Tablets (2.8%) 2534
▲ Sensipar Tablets (15%) 594
▲ Serevent Diskus (1% to 3%) 1594
▲ Simulect for Injection (3% to 10%) 2306
Singulair 2114
Solodyn Extended Release Tablets (1%) 1938
▲ Soriatane Capsules (1% to 10%) 3062
▲ Spiriva HandiHaler (4%) 870
Stromectol Tablets (0.4%) 2120
Sular Extended Release Tablets (Less than or equal to 1%) 2975
Sustiva Capsules (Less than 2%) 930
Sustiva Tablets (Less than 2%) 930
▲ Sutent Capsules (1% to 17%) 2540
▲ Tarceva Tablets (0% to 21%) 1228
Targretin Capsules 1084
Tarka Tablets (0.3% or more) 511
▲ Tasigna Capsules (14%) 2316
▲ Taxotere Injection Concentrate (0% to 33.3%) 2773
▲ Temodar Capsules (5%) 2931
Teveten Tablets (1% or greater) 515
Teveten HCT Tablets (0.4%) 517
▲ Tice BCG (3%) 2936
Timentin ADD-Vantage 1606
Timentin Injection Galaxy Container 1609
Timentin IV Infusion 1603
Timentin Pharmacy Bulk Package 1613
Toprol-XL Tablets 666
▲ Torisel Injection (1% to 8%) 3272
Treximet Tablets (Infrequent) 1616
Tricor Tablets 520
▲ Trisenox Injection (25%) 986
▲ Trizivir Tablets (8%) 1622
▲ Truvada Tablets (Greater than or equal to 5%) 1262
Twinrix Vaccine (Less than 1%) 1628
▲ Tyzeka Tablets (2% to 3%) 2328
Ultram ER Extended-Release Tablets (0.5% to less than 1%) 2428
Valstar Sterile Solution for Intravesical Instillation (1%) 1735
Vantas (Less than 2%) 1737
Vaqta (1.9%) 2130
Varivax (Greater than or equal to 1%) 2133
▲ Velcade for Injection (12%) 2168
Veramyst Nasal Spray 1643
▲ Vesanoid Capsules (14%) 2660
Vicoprofen Tablets (Less than 1%) 533
Viramune Oral Suspension (0.2% to 1.2%) 873
Viramune Tablets (0.2% to 1.2%) 873
▲ Viread Tablets (3% to 4%) 1268
▲ Vytorin 10/10 Tablets (3.6%) 2149
▲ Vytorin 10/10 Tablets (0.6% to 3.6%) 2939
▲ Vytorin 10/20 Tablets (3.6%) 2149
▲ Vytorin 10/20 Tablets (0.6% to 3.6%) 2939
▲ Vytorin 10/40 Tablets (3.6%) 2149
▲ Vytorin 10/40 Tablets (0.6% to 3.6%) 2939
▲ Vytorin 10/80 Tablets (3.6%) 2149
▲ Vytorin 10/80 Tablets (0.6% to 3.6%) 2939
WelChol Tablets (2.1%) 1015
Wellbutrin Tablets 1648
▲ Wellbutrin SR Sustained-Release Tablets (2% to 6%) 1653
▲ Wellbutrin XL Extended-Release Tablets (2% to 6%) 1659
WinRho SDF 741
▲ Xeloda Tablets (Less than 5% to 9%) 2662
▲ Xenical Capsules (4.2%) 2672
Xifaxan Tablets (Less than 2%) 2682
Xopenex Inhalation Solution (1.5%) 3001
Xopenex Inhalation Solution Concentrate (1.5%) 3005
Xopenex HFA Inhalation Aerosol (1.5%) 3009
Xyrem Oral Solution (Frequent) 1766
Xyzal Oral Solution 2789
Xyzal Oral Solution 3155
Zantac 25 EFFERdose Tablets (Rare) 1670
Zantac Injection (Rare) 1666
Zantac Injection Pharmacy Bulk Package (Rare) 1668
Zantac Injection Premixed (Rare) 1666
Zantac (Rare) 1670
Zemplar Injection 538
Zetia Tablets 2157
▲ Zetia Tablets (3.2%) 2951
Ziagen 1673
▲ Zocor Tablets (3.7%) 2136
▲ Zofran Injection (10%) 1682
▲ Zometa for Intravenous Infusion (23%) 2341
Zomig Tablets (Infrequent) 694
Zomig Nasal Spray (Infrequent) 689
Zomig-ZMT Tablets (Infrequent) 694
Zonegran Capsules (Infrequent) 1089
Zosyn for Injection (1% or less) 3284
Zovirax 1690
▲ Zyban Sustained-Release Tablets (2% to 4%) 1692
Zyprexa Tablets 1883
Zyprexa ZYDIS Orally Disintegrating Tablets 1883
Zyrtec Chewable Tablets (Less than 2%) 1920
Zyrtec Syrup (Less than 2%) 1920
Zyrtec Tablets (Less than 2%) 1920
Zyrtec-D 12 Hour Extended Release Tablets (Less than 2%) 1923

Myasthenia

Actiq (Less than 1%) 959
Anaprox Tablets (Less than 1%) 2632
Anaprox DS Tablets (Less than 1%) 2632
Aricept Tablets (Infrequent) 1062
Aricept ODT Tablets (Infrequent) 1062
Avalide Tablets 892
Axert Tablets (Infrequent) 2431
Azilect Tablets (2%) 3106
▲ Betaseron for SC Injection (46%) 756
Celexa (Infrequent) 1160
▲ CellCept Capsules (3% to less than 20%) 2622
▲ CellCept Intravenous (3% to less than 20%) 2622
▲ CellCept Oral Suspension (3% to less than 20%) 2622
▲ CellCept Tablets (3% to less than 20%) 2622
Cipro I.V. 2817
Cipro XR Tablets 2823
Combivir Tablets 1384
Copaxone for Injection (At least 2%) 3110
Cozaar Tablets (Less than 1%) 1973
▲ Depakote ER Tablets (Greater than 1% to less than 5%) 423
Doxil Injection (Less than 1%) 2378
EC-Naprosyn Delayed-Release Tablets (Less than 1%) 2632
Effexor XR Extended-Release Capsules (Infrequent) 3195
Emend Capsules (Greater than 0.5%) 1992
Emend for Injection (Greater than 0.5%) 1999
Emsam Transdermal System (Infrequent) 905
Epivir 1412
Epzicom Tablets 1422
Evoxac Capsules (Less than 1%) 1013
Exelon Capsules (Infrequent) 2229
Exelon Oral Solution (Infrequent) 2229
Flulaval Injection Vaccine 1448
Frova Tablets (Infrequent) 1111
Gabitril Tablets (1%) 973
▲ Gliadel Wafer (4%) 1076
▲ Humira Injection (Less than 5%) 442
▲ Intron A for Injection (Less than 5%) 2859
Klonopin 2639
Lescol Capsules 2268
Lescol XL Tablets 2268
Levoxyl Tablets 1780
Lexapro Oral Suspension (Infrequent) 1174
Lexapro Tablets (Infrequent) 1174
Lunesta Tablets (Infrequent) 2994
Luvox CR Extended-Release Capsules (Infrequent) 1759
Lyrica Capsules (Greather than or equal to 1%) 2527
Mevacor Tablets 2063
Naprosyn Suspension (Less than 1%) 2632
Naprosyn Tablets (Less than 1%) 2632
Niaspan Extended-Release Tablets 480
Nimbex Injection 484
Norvir (Less than 2%) 489
Prozac Weekly Capsules (Rare) 1852
Prozac Pulvules and Liquid (Rare) 1852
Recombivax HB 2107
ReFacto Vials 3269
Requip Tablets (Infrequent) 1561
Retrovir Capsules 1574
Retrovir IV Infusion 1579
Retrovir 1574
▲ Rythmol SR Capsules (1% to 4%) 1590
Salagen Tablets (Less than 1%) 1082
Soriatane Capsules (Less than 1%) 3062
Sular Extended Release Tablets (Less than or equal to 1%) 2975
Symbyax Capsules (Rare) 1871
Targretin Capsules 1084
Tricor Tablets 520
Trizivir Tablets 1622
Venlafaxine Hydrochloride Tablets (Infrequent) 2199
▲ Visudyne for Injection (1% to 10%) 2332
Wellbutrin Tablets 1648
▲ Xeloda Tablets (Less than 5%) 2662
Zonegran Capsules (Infrequent) 1089

Myasthenia gravis

Abelcet Injection 1134
Captopril Tablets 2182
Cuprimine Capsules 1986
Ketek Tablets 2744
Lamictal (Infrequent) 1488
Lipitor Tablets (Less than 2%) 2501
Myleran Tablets (Rare) 1530
Paxil (1%) 1535
Paxil CR Controlled-Release Tablets (1%) 1544
▲ Prograf Capsules and Injection (3% to 15%) 622
Remeron Tablets (Frequent) 2924
RemeronSolTab Tablets (Frequent) 2927
Rilutek Tablets (Infrequent) 2771

Myasthenia gravis, exacerbation of

Cipro I.V. 2817
Cipro 2810
Cipro XR Tablets 2823
Combigan Ophthalmic Solution 553
Cosopt Sterile Ophthalmic Solution 1969
Ketek Tablets 2744
Noroxin Tablets 2069
Proleukin for Injection 2287
Rythmol Tablets 1586
Timoptic Sterile Ophthalmic Solution (Less frequent) 2121
Timoptic-XE Sterile Ophthalmic Gel Forming Solution 2125

Myasthenia gravis, increase

Betimol Ophthalmic Solution 3181
Combigan Ophthalmic Solution 553
Timoptic in Ocudose (Less frequent) 2124

Myasthenic syndrome

Pylera Capsules 714

Mycosis, cutaneous

▲ Novantrone for Injection Concentrate (10%) 1100

Mycosis, vaginal

▲ Divigel (0.8% to 6.4%) 3167
Requip Tablets (Infrequent) 1561

Mydriasis

Atrovent HFA Inhalation Aerosol 839
Atrovent Nasal Spray 0.03% 834
Atrovent Nasal Spray 0.06% 836
Bentyl Capsules 703
Bentyl Injection 703
Bentyl Syrup 703
Bentyl Tablets 703
Celexa (Rare) 1160
Combivent Inhalation Aerosol 845
Concerta Extended-Release Tablets 1925
Copaxone for Injection (Infrequent) 3110
Daytrana Transdermal Patch 3022
Donnatal Extentabs 2507
Effexor XR Extended-Release Capsules (Frequent) 3195
Emsam Transdermal System (Rare) 905
Evoxac Capsules (Less than 1%) 1013
FML Ophthalmic Ointment (Occasional) ⊙223
FML Ophthalmic Suspension (Occasional) ⊙224
FML Forte Ophthalmic Suspension (Occasional) ⊙222
Imitrex Nasal Spray 1470
Imitrex Tablets (Rare) 1474
Lexapro Oral Suspension (Infrequent) 1174
Lexapro Tablets (Infrequent) 1174
Lunesta Tablets (Rare) 2994
Luvox CR Extended-Release Capsules (Infrequent) 1759
Lyrica Capsules (Rare) 2527
Meridia Capsules 475
Paxil (Infrequent) 1535
Paxil CR Controlled-Release Tablets (Infrequent) 1544
Pred Forte Ophthalmic Suspension (Occasional) ⊙227
Pred Mild Ophthalmic Suspension (Occasional) ⊙230
▲ Pristiq Extended-Release Tablets (2% to 6%) 3247
Proleukin for Injection (Less than 1%) 2287
Prozac Weekly Capsules (Infrequent) 1852
Prozac Pulvules and Liquid (Infrequent) 1852
Stalevo Tablets 2309
Strattera Capsules (1% to 2%) 1864
Thioridazine Hydrochloride Tablets 2195
Thiothixene Capsules 2197
Transderm Scōp Transdermal Therapeutic System 2206
Venlafaxine Hydrochloride Tablets (2%) 2199
Vyvanse Capsules 3033
Wellbutrin Tablets (Infrequent) 1648
Wellbutrin SR Sustained-Release Tablets 1653
Wellbutrin XL Extended-Release Tablets 1659
Zyban Sustained-Release Tablets 1692
Zyprexa Tablets (Rare) 1883
Zyprexa ZYDIS Orally Disintegrating Tablets (Rare) 1883

Myelitis
Azilect Tablets (Rare) 3106
Fluarix Vaccine 1446
Havrix Injection Vaccine 1454
Paxil (Rare) 1535
Paxil CR Controlled-Release Tablets (Rare) 1544
Recombivax HB 2107
Twinrix Vaccine 1628
Zyrtec Chewable Tablets (Less than 2%) 1920
Zyrtec Syrup (Less than 2%) 1920
Zyrtec Tablets (Less than 2%) 1920
Zyrtec-D 12 Hour Extended Release Tablets (Less than 2%) 1923

Myelitis, transverse
Asacol Delayed-Release Tablets (Rare) 2579
Bicillin C-R Injectable Suspension 1775
Bicillin L-A Injection 1777
Enbrel for Injection (Rare) 569
Engerix-B Vaccine 1409
ProQuad 2099
Raptiva for Injection (1 case) 1218
Recombivax HB 2107
Remicade for IV Injection 950
Twinrix Vaccine 1628
Varivax 2133

Myelodysplastic syndrome
Bexxar 1371
Neupogen for Injection (Approximately 3%) 589
Taxotere Injection Concentrate (Rare) 2773
Temodar Capsules 2931

Myelofibrosis
Lyrica Capsules (Rare) 2527

Myeloma, multiple
Effexor XR Extended-Release Capsules (Rare) 3195
Mirapex Tablets 857
Venlafaxine Hydrochloride Tablets (Rare) 2199

Myelosuppression
▲ Busulfex Injection (100%, most frequent, occurring in all patients) 2477
Campath Ampules 761
Dacogen Injection 1066
Doxil Injection 2378
Gemzar for Injection 1820
Hexalen Capsules 1078
Ixempra Kit for Injection 915
Leukeran Tablets 1508
Leustatin Injection (Frequent) 2384
Myleran Tablets (Most frequent) 1530
Mylotarg for Injection 3212
Sutent Capsules 2540
Tabloid Tablets (Most frequent) 1601
Tasigna Capsules 2316
▲ Temodar Capsules (16% to 53%) 2931
Treanda for Injection 983

Myocardial hypertrophy
Prograf Capsules and Injection (Rare) 622

Myocardial infarction
▲ Abelcet Injection (3%) 1134
Abilify Injection (Greater than or equal to 1 in 1000 patients and less than 1 in 100 patients) 881
Abilify Injection (Greater than or equal to 1 in 1000 patients and less than 1 in 100 patients) 2466
Abilify Oral Solution (Greater than or equal to 1 in 1000 patients and less than 1 in 100 patients) 881
Abilify Oral Solution (Greater than or equal to 1 in 1000 patients and less than 1 in 100 patients) 2466
Abilify Discmelt Orally Disintegrating Tablets (Greater than or equal to 1 in 1000 patients and less than 1 in 100 patients) 881
Abilify Discmelt Orally Disintegrating Tablets (Greater than or equal to 1 in 1000 patients and less than 1 in 100 patients) 2466
Abilify Tablets (Greater than or equal to 1 in 1000 patients and less than 1 in 100 patients) 881
Abilify Tablets (Greater than or equal to 1 in 1000 patients and less than 1 in 100 patients) 2466
Aceon Tablets (2 mg, 4 mg, 8 mg) (0.3% to 1%) 3038
Actimmune (Rare) 1743
Activella Tablets 2347
▲ Actos Tablets (5%) 3077
Adderall XR Capsules 3012
Adenoscan (Less than 1%) 605
▲ Advair HFA 45/21 Inhalation Aerosol (1% to 3%) 1288
▲ Advair HFA 115/21 Inhalation Aerosol (1% to 3%) 1288
▲ Advair HFA 230/21 Inhalation Aerosol (1% to 3%) 1288
Agrylin Capsules 3017
Aldara Cream, 5% 1699
Ambien Tablets (Rare) 2692
Ambien CR Tablets (Rare) 2696
Amerge Tablets 1301
Amevive (Less than 1%) 611
Anaprox Tablets (Less than 1%) 2632
Anaprox DS Tablets (Less than 1%) 2632
Angeliq Tablets 751
Anzemet Injection 2701
Anzemet Tablets (Rare) 2704
Aranesp for Injection (2%) 564
▲ Argatroban Injection (3.6%) 1308
Aricept Tablets (Infrequent) 1062
Aricept ODT Tablets (Infrequent) 1062
Arimidex Tablets 672
Atacand Tablets (Less frequently) 639
Atacand HCT (Less than 0.5%) 642
Avalide Tablets 892
Avalide Tablets 2713
▲ Avandaryl Tablets (5%) 1344
▲ Avandia Tablets (5%) 1351
Avapro Tablets (Less than 1%) 897
Avapro Tablets (Less than 1%) 2718
Azilect Tablets (Infrequent) 3106
Azor Tablets 1005
Brovana Inhalation Solution (Less than 2%) 2990
Bystolic Tablets 1155
Campath Ampules 761
Campral Tablets (Infrequent) 1158
Cancidas for Injection 1953
Captopril Tablets (2 to 3 of 1000 patients) 2182
Carbatrol Capsules 3019
Cardene I.V. 1093
Cardizem LA Extended Release Tablets 421
Celebrex Capsules (0.1% to 1.9%) 2979
Celexa (Infrequent) 1160
Chantix Tablets (Infrequent) 2511
Cialis Tablets (Less than 2%) 1792
Cimzia 3127
Cipro I.V. (1% or less) 2817
Cipro (Less than 1%) 2810
Cipro XR Tablets 2823
Cleviprex (Less than 1%) 1936
Climara Transdermal System 763
Climara Pro Transdermal System 768
Coreg Tablets (0.1% to 1%) 1387
Cosopt Sterile Ophthalmic Solution (Less than 1%) 1969
Cozaar Tablets (Less than 1%) 1973
Crixivan Capsules 1979
Cymbalta Delayed-Release Capsules (Infrequent) 1801
Dacogen Injection 1066
Divigel 3167
Duetact Tablets 3085
DynaCirc CR Controlled Release Tablets (0.5% to 1%) 1407
EC-Naprosyn Delayed-Release Tablets (Less than 1%) 2632
Edex Injection (1%) 2957
Effexor XR Extended-Release Capsules (Infrequent) 3195
Elitek (Less than or equal to 1%) 2729
Emend Capsules (Greater than 0.5%) 1992
Emend for Injection (Greater than 0.5%) 1999
Emsam Transdermal System (Rare) 905
Enbrel for Injection (Infrequent) 569
Enjuvia Tablets 1029
Epogen for Injection (0.4%) 576
Estratest Tablets 3043
Estratest H.S. Tablets 3043
Evoxac Capsules (Less than 1%) 1013
Exelon Capsules (Frequent) 2229
Exelon Oral Solution (Frequent) 2229
Exelon Patch (Infrequent) 2233
Exforge Tablets 2238
Exubera Inhalation Powder (0.7%) 2515
Feiba VH 728
Femara Tablets (0.4% to less than or equal to 2%) 2246
Flector Patch 561
▲ Flolan for Injection (4%) 1426
Frova Tablets 1111
Gabitril Tablets (Infrequent) 973
Gammagard S/D 734
Gemzar for Injection (Very rare) 1820
Gengraf Capsules (1% to less than 3%) 435
▲ Humira Injection (Less than 5%) 442
Imitrex Injection (Extremely rare) 1465
Imitrex Nasal Spray 1470
Imitrex Tablets (Rare) 1474
Intelence Tablets (Less than 2%) 3119
Ionsys Transdermal System (.1% to less than 1%) 2410
Isentress Tablets 2036
Ixempra Kit for Injection 915
Lamictal (Rare) 1488
Levitra Tablets (Less than 2%) 2876
Levothroid Tablets 1170
Levoxyl Tablets 1780
Lexapro Oral Suspension 1174
Lexapro Tablets 1174
Lexiscan Injection 614
Lovaza Capsules 1520
Lupron Depot 7.5 mg 469
Luvox CR Extended-Release Capsules (Infrequent) 1759
Lybrel Tablets 3204
Maxalt Tablets (Very rare) 2056
Maxalt-MLT Orally Disintegrating Tablets (Very rare) 2056
Meridia Capsules 475
Merrem I.V. (Greater than 0.1% to 1%) 684
Miacalcin Nasal Spray (Less than 1%) 2274
Micardis Tablets 852
Micardis HCT Tablets 854
Mirapex Tablets (Less than 1%) 857
Mircette Tablets 1034
Mobic Oral Suspension (Less than 2%) 863
Mobic Tablets (Less than 2%) 863
Mycamine for Injection 616
Namenda (Infrequent) 1180
Naprosyn Suspension (Less than 1%) 2632
Naprosyn Tablets (Less than 1%) 2632
Neoral Oral Solution (1% to less than 3%) 2280
Neoral Soft Gelatin Capsules (1% to less than 3%) 2280
▲ Neupogen for Injection (11 of 375 cancer patients) 589
Nexavar Tablets (2.7% to 2.9%) 784
Noroxin Tablets (Less frequent) 2069
NovoSeven 2367
NovoSeven RT 2370
NuvaRing 2897
Omnicef Capsules 497
Omnicef for Oral Suspension 497
Ontak Vials (Two patients) 1079
OptiPranolol Metipranolol Ophthalmic Solution 0.3% (A small number of patients) ⊙245
Ortho-Cyclen Tablets 2449
Ortho Evra Transdermal System 2437
Ortho Tri-Cyclen Tablets 2449
Ortho Tri-Cyclen Lo Tablets 2458
Orthoclone OKT3 Sterile Solution (Less than 1%) 2387
Paxil (Rare) 1535
Paxil CR Controlled-Release Tablets (Rare) 1544
PegIntron Powder for Injection (Less than or equal to 1%) 2903
Photofrin for Injection 708
Pletal Tablets (Less than 2%) 2481
PrandiMet Tablets (Less than or equal to 1%) 2967
Prandin Tablets (Less than or equal to 1%) 2971
Premarin Intravenous 3217
Premarin Tablets 3221
Premarin Vaginal Cream 3228
Premphase Tablets 3232
Prempro Tablets 3232
Prinivil Tablets (0.3% to 1%) 2087
Prinzide Tablets 2092
Pristiq Extended-Release Tablets 3247
Procrit for Injection (0.4%) 2391
Prograf Capsules and Injection 622
Proleukin for Injection (Less than or equal to 1%) 2287
Protonix for Delayed-Release Oral Suspension (Less than 1%) 3254
Protonix Delayed-Release Tablets (Less than 1%) 3254
Protonix I.V. (Less than 1%) 3257
Prozac Weekly Capsules (Infrequent) 1852
Prozac Pulvules and Liquid (Infrequent) 1852
Rebetol 2917
Remeron Tablets (Infrequent) 2924
RemeronSolTab Tablets (Infrequent) 2927
Remicade for IV Injection (Greater than or equal to 0.2%) 950
Requip Tablets (Infrequent) 1561
Rilutek Tablets (Infrequent) 2771
Risperdal Consta Long-Acting Injection (Infrequent) 1753
Rituxan I.V. 1223
Rythmol SR Capsules 1590
Salagen Tablets (Less than 1%) 1082
Sandimmune (Rare) 2296
Sandostatin LAR Depot 2302
Seasonique Tablets 1046
Selzentry Tablets 2534
Soriatane Capsules 3062
Stalevo Tablets 2309
Strattera Capsules 1864
Sular Extended Release Tablets (Less than or equal to 1%) 2975
Sutent Capsules (1 patient) 2540
Symbyax Capsules (Rare) 1871
Tarka Tablets (Less frequent) 511
Tasigna Capsules 2316
Taxotere Injection Concentrate 2773
Thyrogen for Injection (One patient) 1244
Toprol-XL Tablets (Greater than 1%) 666
▲ Trasylol Injection (6%) 799
Tricor Tablets 520
Ultram ER Extended-Release Tablets (0.5% to less than 1%) 2428
Velcade for Injection 2168
Venlafaxine Hydrochloride Tablets (Rare) 2199
▲ Vesanoid Capsules (3%) 2660
Vicoprofen Tablets 533
Vivitrol 988
Voltaren Tablets (Rarely) 2334
Voltaren-XR Tablets (Rarely) 2337
Vyvanse Capsules 3033
Wellbutrin Tablets (Rare) 1648
Wellbutrin SR Sustained-Release Tablets 1653
Wellbutrin XL Extended-Release Tablets 1659
Yaz Tablets 805
Zolinza Capsules 2142
Zomig Tablets (Rare) 694
Zomig Nasal Spray (Rare) 689
Zomig-ZMT Tablets (Rare) 694
Zosyn for Injection (1% or less) 3284
Zyban Sustained-Release Tablets 1692

Myocardial infarction, acute
Aranesp for Injection (2%) 564
Tarceva Tablets (2.3%) 1228

Myocardial infarction, post-abrupt discontinuation
InnoPran XL Extended Release Capsules 1484

Myocardial insufficiency
Orthoclone OKT3 Sterile Solution 2387

Myocardial reinfarction
Activase I.V. 1188
TNKase 1233

Myocardial rupture
Activase I.V. 1188
TNKase 1233

Myocarditis
Asacol Delayed-Release Tablets (Rare) 2579
Boostrix 1377
Geodon Capsules (Rare) 2520
Pentasa Capsules (Infrequent) 3030
Proleukin for Injection 2287
▲ Vesanoid Capsules (3%) 2660
▲ Xeloda Tablets (Less than 5%) 2662

Myocarditis, allergic
Fansidar Tablets 2636
Gantrisin Pediatric Suspension 2638

Myocarditis, viral
Treximet Tablets (Rare) 1616

Myoclonia
Celexa 1160
Cipro I.V. 2817
Copaxone for Injection (Infrequent) 3110
Effexor XR Extended-Release Capsules (Infrequent) 3195
Eldepryl Capsules 3052
Fortaz 1450

Gabitril Tablets (Frequent) ... 973
Geodon Capsules (Rare) ... 2520
Imitrex Injection (Rare) ... 1465
Lamictal (Infrequent) ... 1488
Leukeran Tablets (Rare) ... 1508
Lexapro Oral Suspension ... 1174
Lexapro Tablets ... 1174
Mirapex Tablets (1%) ... 857
Noroxin Tablets ... 2069
Orthoclone OKT3 Sterile Solution ... 2387
▲ Paxil (3%) ... 1535
▲ Paxil CR Controlled-Release Tablets (3%) ... 1544
Primaxin I.M. ... 2080
Primaxin I.V. (Less than 0.2%) ... 2083
▲ Prograf Capsules and Injection (3% to 15%) ... 622
Remeron Tablets (Rare) ... 2924
RemeronSolTab Tablets (Rare) ... 2927
Rilutek Tablets (Infrequent) ... 2771
Symbyax Capsules (Infrequent) ... 1871
Wellbutrin Tablets (Frequent) ... 1648
Zonegran Capsules (Rare) ... 1089
▲ Zyprexa Tablets (1% to 5%) ... 1883
▲ Zyprexa ZYDIS Orally Disintegrating Tablets (1% to 5%) ... 1883

Myoclonic jerks
Marplan Tablets (0% to 2%) ... 3177

Myoclonus
Abilify Injection (Greater than or equal to 1 in 1000 patients and less than 1 in 100 patients) ... 881
Abilify Injection (Greater than or equal to 1 in 1000 patients and less than 1 in 100 patients) ... 2466
Abilify Oral Solution (Greater than or equal to 1 in 1000 patients and less than 1 in 100 patients) ... 881
Abilify Oral Solution (Greater than or equal to 1 in 1000 patients and less than 1 in 100 patients) ... 2466
Abilify Discmelt Orally Disintegrating Tablets (Greater than or equal to 1 in 1000 patients and less than 1 in 100 patients) ... 881
Abilify Discmelt Orally Disintegrating Tablets (Greater than or equal to 1 in 1000 patients and less than 1 in 100 patients) ... 2466
Abilify Tablets (Greater than or equal to 1 in 1000 patients and less than 1 in 100 patients) ... 881
Abilify Tablets (Greater than or equal to 1 in 1000 patients and less than 1 in 100 patients) ... 2466
Azilect Tablets (Infrequent) ... 3106
Cipro ... 2810
Cipro XR Tablets ... 2823
Cymbalta Delayed-Release Capsules (Infrequent) ... 1801
Emsam Transdermal System (Infrequent) ... 905
Exelon Capsules (Infrequent) ... 2229
Exelon Oral Solution (Infrequent) ... 2229
Luvox CR Extended-Release Capsules (Frequent) ... 1759
▲ Lyrica Capsules (0.1% to 4%) ... 2527
Namenda ... 1180
Prozac Weekly Capsules (Infrequent) ... 1852
Venlafaxine Hydrochloride Tablets (Infrequent) ... 2199
Xyrem Oral Solution (Infrequent) ... 1766
▲ Zyprexa IntraMuscular (2% to 4%) ... 1883

Myoglobinuria
Abilify Injection ... 881
Abilify Injection ... 2466
Abilify Oral Solution ... 881
Abilify Oral Solution ... 2466
Abilify Discmelt Orally Disintegrating Tablets ... 881
Abilify Discmelt Orally Disintegrating Tablets ... 2466
Abilify Tablets ... 881
Abilify Tablets ... 2466
Bicillin C-R Injectable Suspension ... 1775
Bicillin L-A Injection ... 1777
Ultane Liquid for Inhalation ... 524

Myolysis
Trizivir Tablets ... 1622
Ziagen ... 1673

Myopathy
Actiq (Less than 1%) ... 959
Advicor Tablets ... 402
Atripla Tablets ... 938
Axert Tablets (Rare) ... 2431
Campral Tablets (Frequent) ... 1158
Copaxone for Injection (Infrequent) ... 3110
Crestor Tablets ... 677
Effexor XR Extended-Release Capsules (Rare) ... 3195
Geodon Capsules (Rare) ... 2520
Hepsera Tablets ... 1253
Isentress Tablets ... 2036
Lescol Capsules (Occasional) ... 2268
Lescol XL Tablets ... 2268
Lunesta Tablets (Rare) ... 2994
Luvox CR Extended-Release Capsules (Rare) ... 1759
Mevacor Tablets ... 2063
Mirapex Tablets ... 857
Nimbex Injection ... 484
Paxil (2%) ... 1535
Paxil CR Controlled-Release Tablets (2%) ... 1544
Proleukin for Injection ... 2287
Prozac Weekly Capsules (Rare) ... 1852
Prozac Pulvules and Liquid (Rare) ... 1852
ReoPro Vials (0.4%) ... 1860
Retrovir Capsules ... 1574
Retrovir IV Infusion ... 1579
Retrovir ... 1574
Reyataz Capsules ... 3299
Soriatane Capsules ... 3062
Sustiva Capsules ... 930
Sustiva Tablets ... 930
Sutent Capsules (Rare) ... 2540
Symbyax Capsules (Rare) ... 1871
Trizivir Tablets ... 1622
Truvada Tablets ... 1262
Tyzeka Tablets (2%) ... 2328
Venlafaxine Hydrochloride Tablets (Rare) ... 2199
Vytorin 10/10 Tablets ... 2149
Vytorin 10/10 Tablets (0.02% to 0.53%) ... 2939
Vytorin 10/20 Tablets ... 2149
Vytorin 10/20 Tablets (0.02% to 0.53%) ... 2939
Vytorin 10/40 Tablets ... 2149
Vytorin 10/40 Tablets (0.02% to 0.53%) ... 2939
Vytorin 10/80 Tablets ... 2149
Vytorin 10/80 Tablets (0.02% to 0.53%) ... 2939
Zetia Tablets ... 2157
Zetia Tablets ... 2951
Zocor Tablets ... 2136
Zyprexa Tablets (Rare) ... 1883
Zyprexa ZYDIS Orally Disintegrating Tablets (Rare) ... 1883

Myopia
Evoxac Capsules (Less than 1%) ... 1013
Mirapex Tablets ... 857
Namenda (Infrequent) ... 1180
Singulair (Greater than or equal to 2%) ... 2114

Myopia, transient
Clorpres Tablets (Occasional) ... 2185
Cosopt Sterile Ophthalmic Solution ... 1969
Trusopt Sterile Ophthalmic Solution ... 2128

Myosis
Doxil Injection (Less than 1%) ... 2378

Myositis
Advair Diskus 100/50 ... 1276
Advair Diskus 250/50 ... 1276
Advair Diskus 500/50 ... 1276
Advair HFA 45/21 Inhalation Aerosol ... 1288
Advair HFA 115/21 Inhalation Aerosol ... 1288
Advair HFA 230/21 Inhalation Aerosol ... 1288
Chantix Tablets (Rare) ... 2511
Crestor Tablets (Less than 1%) ... 677
Intron A for Injection ... 2859
Lipitor Tablets (Less than 2%) ... 2501
Mirapex Tablets ... 857
Norvir (Less than 2%) ... 489
Paxil (Rare) ... 1535
Paxil CR Controlled-Release Tablets (Rare) ... 1544
PegIntron Powder for Injection ... 2903
Proleukin for Injection ... 2287
Prozac Weekly Capsules (Rare) ... 1852
Prozac Pulvules and Liquid (Rare) ... 1852
Raptiva for Injection ... 1218
Remeron Tablets (Rare) ... 2924
RemeronSolTab Tablets (Rare) ... 2927
Retrovir Capsules ... 1574
Retrovir IV Injection ... 1579
Retrovir ... 1574
Selzentry Tablets ... 2534
Sular Extended Release Tablets (Less than or equal to 1%) ... 2975
Tricor Tablets ... 520
Vesanoid Capsules (Isolated cases) ... 2660

N

Nail bed changes
▲ Novantrone for Injection Concentrate (11%) ... 1100

Nail discoloration
Evoxac Capsules (Less than 1%) ... 1013
Retrovir Capsules ... 1574
Retrovir IV Infusion ... 1579
Retrovir ... 1574

Nail disorders, unspecified
Atripla Tablets ... 938
▲ Avastin IV (2% to 8%) ... 1192
Celebrex Capsules (0.1% to 1.9%) ... 2979
▲ Erbitux (0% to 21%) ... 912
Evoxac Capsules (Less than 1%) ... 1013
Gleevec Tablets (Infrequent) ... 2255
▲ Ixempra Kit for Injection (9% to greater than or equal to 20%) ... 915
Kaletra (Less than 2%) ... 452
Rythmol SR Capsules ... 1590
Soriatane Capsules ... 3062
Sustiva Capsules ... 930
Sustiva Tablets ... 930
▲ Taxotere Injection Concentrate (0.4% to 18.5%) ... 2773
Tricor Tablets ... 520
▲ Vectibix (0% to 29%) ... 597
Zocor Tablets ... 2136

Nails, brittle
Venlafaxine Hydrochloride Tablets (Infrequent) ... 2199

Nails, changes of
Accutane Capsules ... 2607
Advicor Tablets ... 402
Copaxone for Injection (At least 2%) ... 3110
Effexor XR Extended-Release Capsules (Infrequent) ... 3195
▲ Eloxatin for Injection (2% to less than 5%) ... 2731
Gengraf Capsules (1% to less than 3%) ... 435
Herceptin I.V. ... 1199
▲ Intron A for Injection (Less than 5%) ... 2859
Lescol Capsules ... 2268
Lescol XL Tablets ... 2268
▲ Lupron Depot 3.75 mg (Less than 5%) ... 462
▲ Lupron Depot–3 Month 11.25 mg (Less than 5%) ... 462
Mevacor Tablets ... 2063
Neoral Oral Solution (1% to less than 3%) ... 2280
Neoral Soft Gelatin Capsules (1% to less than 3%) ... 2280
Pentasa Capsules (Less than 1%) ... 3030
Protopic Ointment (0.2% to less than 1%) ... 628
▲ Soriatane Capsules (25% to 50%) ... 3062
▲ Taxotere Injection Concentrate (0% to 40.5%) ... 2773
▲ Torisel Injection (0% to 14%) ... 3272
Vytorin 10/10 Tablets ... 2149
Vytorin 10/10 Tablets ... 2939
Vytorin 10/20 Tablets ... 2149
Vytorin 10/20 Tablets ... 2939
Vytorin 10/40 Tablets ... 2149
Vytorin 10/40 Tablets ... 2939
Vytorin 10/80 Tablets ... 2149
Vytorin 10/80 Tablets ... 2939
▲ Xeloda Tablets (Less than 5%) ... 2662

Narcolepsy
Mirapex Tablets ... 857

Nasal burning
Atrovent Nasal Spray 0.03% (2%) ... 834
Atrovent Nasal Spray 0.06% (Less than 1%) ... 836
▲ Flonase Nasal Spray (2.4% to 3.2%) ... 1431
Nasonex Nasal Spray ... 2883
Sudafed OM Sinus Cold Moisturizing Nasal Spray ... 1906
Sudafed OM Sinus Congestion Moisturizing Nasal Spray ... 1906

Nasal congestion
▲ Abilify Injection (Greater than or equal to 1 in 100 patients to 3%) ... 881
▲ Abilify Injection (Greater than or equal to 1 in 100 patients) ... 2466
▲ Abilify Oral Solution (Greater than or equal to 1 in 100 patients to 3%) ... 881
▲ Abilify Oral Solution (Greater than or equal to 1 in 100 patients) ... 2466
▲ Abilify Discmelt Orally Disintegrating Tablets (Greater than or equal to 1 in 100 patients to 3%) ... 881
▲ Abilify Discmelt Orally Disintegrating Tablets (Greater than or equal to 1 in 100 patients) ... 2466
▲ Abilify Tablets (Greater than or equal to 1 in 100 patients to 3%) ... 881
▲ Abilify Tablets (Greater than or equal to 1 in 100 patients) ... 2466
Adenoscan (Less than 1%) ... 605
▲ Advair Diskus 250/50 (>5%) ... 1276
▲ Advair HFA 45/21 Inhalation Aerosol (1% to 3%) ... 1288
▲ Advair HFA 115/21 Inhalation Aerosol (1% to 3%) ... 1288
▲ Advair HFA 230/21 Inhalation Aerosol (1% to 3%) ... 1288
▲ Aerobid/Aerobid-M (15%) ... 1153
▲ Alamast Ophthalmic Solution (Less than 5%) ... 3181
▲ Alvesco Inhalation Aerosol (1.8% to 5.5%) ... 2985
Asacol Delayed-Release Tablets ... 2579
▲ Atrovent Nasal Spray 0.03% (3.1%) ... 834
Atrovent Nasal Spray 0.06% (1.1%) ... 836
AzaSite Ophthalmic Drops (Less than 1%) ... 1740
Bentyl Capsules ... 703
Bentyl Injection ... 703
Bentyl Syrup ... 703
Bentyl Tablets ... 703
Betimol Ophthalmic Solution ... 3181
Cardizem LA Extended Release Tablets (Less than 2%) ... 421
▲ Chemet Capsules (0.7% to 3.7%) ... 2484
▲ Cialis Tablets (0% to 4%) ... 1792
Combigan Ophthalmic Solution ... 553
Combivent Inhalation Aerosol ... 845
Coreg CR Extended-Release Capsules (1%) ... 1393
▲ Cosopt Sterile Ophthalmic Solution (1% to 5%) ... 1969
Cozaar Tablets (2%) ... 1973
▲ Daytrana Transdermal Patch (6%) ... 3022
Dibenzyline Capsules ... 3188
Diovan HCT Tablets (Greater than 0.2%) ... 2216
DynaCirc CR Controlled Release Tablets (0.5% to 1%) ... 1407
Elidel Cream 1% (0.6% to 2.6%) ... 2221
▲ Epivir (8%) ... 1412
Exforge Tablets (Greater than or equal to 0.2%) ... 2238
▲ Fabrazyme for Intravenous Infusion (19%) ... 1241
▲ Flebogamma 5% (21%) ... 1715
▲ Flebogamma 5% DIF (Greater than 15%) ... 1718
▲ Flovent Diskus 50 mcg (16%) ... 1435
Fluarix Vaccine (2.2%) ... 1446
▲ Flulaval Injection Vaccine (1% to 5%) ... 1448
▲ FluMist Vaccine (9% to 58%) ... 1945
Gardasil Injection (1.1%) ... 2019
▲ Intron A for Injection (Up to 10%) ... 2859
Lamisil Oral Granules (2%) ... 2264
▲ Letairis Tablets (6%) ... 1258
Lexapro Oral Suspension (Frequent) ... 1174
Lexapro Tablets (Frequent) ... 1174
Maxalt Tablets (Infrequent) ... 2056
Maxalt-MLT Orally Disintegrating Tablets (Infrequent) ... 2056
Meridia Capsules ... 475
▲ Miacalcin Nasal Spray (10.6%) ... 2274
Orthoclone OKT3 Sterile Solution ... 2387
Prinivil Tablets (0.4%) ... 2087
Prinzide Tablets (0.3% to 1%) ... 2092
▲ Prometrium Capsules (100 mg, 200 mg) (Less than 5%) ... 3047
ProQuad (Greater than or equal to 0.2% to less than 1%) ... 2099
Pulmicort Flexhaler (2.7%) ... 654
Pylera Capsules ... 714
Requip Tablets (2%) ... 1561
▲ Serevent Diskus (4% to 9%) ... 1594
Singulair (1.6%) ... 2114
Symbicort 80/4.5 Inhalation Aerosol (2.5%) ... 659
▲ Symbicort 160/4.5 Inhalation Aerosol (3.2%) ... 659
Tessalon Capsules ... 1183
Tessalon Perles ... 1183
Thiothixene Capsules (Infrequently) ... 2197

Timoptic Sterile Ophthalmic Solution (Less frequent)...... 2121
Timoptic in Ocudose (Less frequent)...... 2124
Timoptic-XE Sterile Ophthalmic Gel Forming Solution...... 2125
▲ Ultram ER Extended-Release Tablets (1% to less than 5%)...... 2428
Vanos Cream (0% to 1.4%)...... 1941
Vaqta (1.2%)...... 2130
Xyrem Oral Solution (Frequent)...... 1766

Nasal discharge, increase
Emend Capsules (Greater than 0.5%)...... 1992
Emend for Injection (Greater than 0.5%)...... 1999
▲ Flovent Diskus 50 mcg (1% to 3%)...... 1435
▲ Miacalcin Nasal Spray (10.6%)...... 2274
Sudafed OM Sinus Cold Moisturizing Nasal Spray...... 1906
Sudafed OM Sinus Congestion Moisturizing Nasal Spray...... 1906

Nasal drainage
Alferon N Injection (2%)...... 1726

Nasal drip, posterior
Aceon Tablets (2 mg, 4 mg, 8 mg) (0.3% to 1%)...... 3038
Aricept Tablets (Infrequent)...... 1062
Aricept ODT Tablets (Infrequent)...... 1062
▲ Atrovent Nasal Spray 0.03% (3.1%)...... 834
▲ Dacogen Injection (5%)...... 1066
▲ Flovent HFA (1% to 3%)...... 1440
▲ Trisenox Injection (13%)...... 986

Nasal itching
(*see under* Pruritus, rhinal)

Nasal mucosa, dryness
(*see under* Xeromycteria)

Nasal mucosal disorder, unspecified
Requip Tablets (Infrequent)...... 1561

Nasal septum, perforation
Avastin IV (Rare)...... 1192
Beconase AQ Nasal Spray (Rare)...... 1369
Flonase Nasal Spray (Rare)...... 1431
Nasacort AQ Nasal Spray (One patient)...... 2765
Nasonex Nasal Spray (Rare)...... 2883
Omnaris Nasal Spray (Rare)...... 2998

Nasal stinging
Sudafed OM Sinus Cold Moisturizing Nasal Spray...... 1906
Sudafed OM Sinus Congestion Moisturizing Nasal Spray...... 1906

Nasal stuffiness
Beconase AQ Nasal Spray (Fewer than 3 per 100 patients)...... 1369
Demser Capsules (Infrequent)...... 1989
Nadolol Tablets (1 to 5 of 1000 patients)...... 2191
Thioridazine Hydrochloride Tablets...... 2195

Nasal symptoms
Atrovent Nasal Spray 0.03% (3.1%)...... 834
▲ Epivir (8% to 20%)...... 1412

Nasal ulceration
Beconase AQ Nasal Spray (Rare)...... 1369
Nasonex Nasal Spray (Rare)...... 2883
▲ Patanase Nasal Spray (9%)...... 544
Veramyst Nasal Spray (1%)...... 1643

Nasopharyngitis
▲ Abilify Injection (3% to 5%)...... 881
▲ Abilify Injection (3% to 4%)...... 2466
▲ Abilify Oral Solution (3% to 5%)...... 881
▲ Abilify Oral Solution (3% to 4%)...... 2466
▲ Abilify Discmelt Orally Disintegrating Tablets (3% to 5%)...... 881
▲ Abilify Discmelt Orally Disintegrating Tablets (3% to 4%)...... 2466
▲ Abilify Tablets (3% to 5%)...... 881
▲ Abilify Tablets (3% to 4%)...... 2466
▲ Activella Tablets (21%)...... 2347
▲ Aczone Gel 5% (5%)...... 3296
▲ Advair Diskus 250/50 (Greater than 5%)...... 1276
▲ Advate (14.7%)...... 721
Altabax Ointment (1.2% to 1.5%)...... 1299
▲ Alvesco Inhalation Aerosol (3% to 10.5%)...... 2985
▲ Ambien CR Tablets (6%)...... 2696
▲ Atripla Tablets (5%)...... 938
▲ Avandamet Tablets (6%)...... 1336
▲ Avandaryl Tablets (4% to greater than or equal to 5%)...... 1344
▲ Avandia Tablets (3% to 6.3%)...... 1351
▲ Boniva Injection (3.5% to 4.3%)...... 2614
▲ Boniva Tablets (3.5% to 4.3%)...... 2618
▲ Celebrex Capsules (5% to 6%)...... 2979
▲ Cialis Tablets (3% to 6%)...... 1792
Concerta Extended-Release Tablets (2.8%)...... 1925
▲ Coreg CR Extended-Release Capsules (4%)...... 1393
▲ Cymbalta Delayed-Release Capsules (7% to 9%)...... 1801
▲ Daytrana Transdermal Patch (5%)...... 3022
Diovan HCT Tablets (2.4%)...... 2216
▲ Divigel (4.1% to 5.7%)...... 3167
▲ Elidel Cream 1% (7.6% to 26.5%)...... 2221
▲ Emtriva Capsules (5%)...... 1246
▲ Emtriva Oral Solution (5%)...... 1246
Exelon Patch (Frequent)...... 2233
▲ Exforge Tablets (0.2% to 4.3%)...... 2238
▲ Exjade Tablets (13.2%)...... 2244
▲ Fabrazyme for Intravenous Infusion (28%)...... 1241
Fentora Tablets (Greater than 1%)...... 968
Flovent HFA...... 1440
▲ Fluarix Vaccine (2.5%)...... 1446
▲ Flulaval Injection Vaccine (1% to 7%)...... 1448
▲ Gardasil Injection (6.4%)...... 2019
Genotropin Lyophilized Powder...... 2547
▲ Gleevec Tablets (10% to 30.5%)...... 2255
Invanz for Injection (1.6%)...... 2029
▲ Janumet Tablets (Greater than or equal to 5%)...... 2041
▲ Januvia Tablets (6.3%)...... 2048
▲ Keppra Injection (14%)...... 3137
▲ Keppra Oral Solution (14%)...... 3131
▲ Keppra Tablets (14%)...... 3131
▲ Lamisil Oral Granules (10%)...... 2264
▲ Letairis Tablets (3%)...... 1258
▲ Lucentis Injection (5% to 16%)...... 1205
▲ Myfortic Tablets (3% to less than 20%)...... 2276
Nalfon Capsules (1.2%)...... 2508
▲ Omnaris Nasal Spray (3.7% to 6.6%)...... 2998
▲ Orencia Powder for Intravenous Infusion (12%)...... 921
Patanase Nasal Spray (0.9%)...... 544
▲ Perforomist Inhalation Solution (3.3%)...... 1025
▲ Pulmicort Flexhaler (9.3%)...... 654
▲ Requip Tablets (9%)...... 1561
Requip XL Tablets...... 1568
Rituxan I.V....... 1223
▲ RotaTeq (6.9%)...... 2110
Sanctura XR Capsules (2.9%)...... 557
Selzentry Tablets...... 2534
▲ Symbicort 80/4.5 Inhalation Aerosol (10.5%)...... 659
▲ Symbicort 160/4.5 Inhalation Aerosol (9.7%)...... 659
▲ Tasigna Capsules (11% to 16%)...... 2316
Tekturna Tablets (Greater than 1%)...... 2321
Tekturna HCT Tablets...... 2324
Thyrogen for Injection (1%)...... 1244
▲ Tracleer Tablets (11%)...... 3289
▲ Treanda for Injection (0% to 7%)...... 983
▲ Trisenox Injection (5%)...... 986
▲ Truvada Tablets (5%)...... 1262
▲ Tyzeka Tablets (11%)...... 2328
▲ Ultram ER Extended-Release Tablets (1% to less than 5%)...... 2428
Valtrex Caplets...... 1635
Vanos Cream (0.9% to 1.4%)...... 1941
▲ Velcade for Injection (11% to 14%)...... 2168
Ventolin HFA Inhalation Aerosol...... 1638
▲ Veramyst Nasal Spray (5%)...... 1643
▲ Viread Tablets (Greater than or equal to 5%)...... 1268
▲ Vivitrol (11% to 17%)...... 988
▲ WelChol Tablets (4.1%)...... 1015
▲ Wellbutrin XL Extended-Release Tablets (13%)...... 1659
Xifaxan Tablets (Less than 2%)...... 2682
▲ Xyrem Oral Solution (2.9% to 8%)...... 1766
▲ Xyzal Oral Solution (4% to 6%)...... 2789
▲ Xyzal Oral Solution (4% to 6%)...... 3155
▲ Xyzal Tablets (4% to 6%)...... 2789
▲ Xyzal Tablets (4% to 6%)...... 3155
▲ Zetia Tablets (3.7%)...... 2951
▲ Ziana Gel (4%)...... 1942

Nausea
▲ Abelcet Injection (9%)...... 1134
▲ Abilify Injection (8% to 15%)...... 881
▲ Abilify Injection (8% to 15%)...... 2466
▲ Abilify Oral Solution (8% to 15%)...... 881
▲ Abilify Oral Solution (8% to 15%)...... 2466
▲ Abilify Discmelt Orally Disintegrating Tablets (8% to 15%)...... 881
▲ Abilify Discmelt Orally Disintegrating Tablets (8% to 15%)...... 2466
▲ Abilify Tablets (8% to 15%)...... 881
▲ Abilify Tablets (8% to 15%)...... 2466
▲ Accolate Tablets (3.1%)...... 669
Accutane Capsules...... 2607
Aceon Tablets (2 mg, 4 mg, 8 mg) (2.3%)...... 3038
▲ Acetadote Injection (2% to 7%)...... 1001
▲ Aciphex Tablets (1.8% to 4.5%)...... 1053
▲ Actimmune (10%)...... 1743
▲ Actiq (11% to 23%)...... 959
Activase I.V....... 1188
▲ Activella Tablets (3% to 11%)...... 2347
▲ Actonel Tablets (9.8% to 10.5%)...... 2568
▲ Actonel with Calcium Tablets (6.2% to 10.9%)...... 2574
▲ ActoPlus Met Tablets (3.6% to 5.8%)...... 3071
▲ Adderall XR Capsules (5%)...... 3012
▲ Adenocard IV Injection (3%)...... 603
Advair Diskus 100/50...... 1276
▲ Advair Diskus 250/50 (3% to 6%)...... 1276
▲ Advair Diskus 500/50 (Greater than or equal to 3%)...... 1276
▲ Advair HFA 45/21 Inhalation Aerosol (3% to 5%)...... 1288
▲ Advair HFA 115/21 Inhalation Aerosol (3% to 5%)...... 1288
▲ Advair HFA 230/21 Inhalation Aerosol (3% to 5%)...... 1288
Advate (0.6%)...... 721
▲ Advicor Tablets (7%)...... 402
▲ Aerobid/Aerobid-M (25%)...... 1153
▲ Aggrenox Capsules (16%)...... 819
▲ Agrylin Capsules (17.1%)...... 3017
▲ Albenza Tablets (3.7% to 6.2%)...... 1297
Albutein 5%...... 1707
Albutein 25%...... 1708
Aldara Cream, 5% (1%)...... 1699
▲ Alferon N Injection (4% to 48%)...... 1726
▲ Alimta for Injection (Up to 84%)...... 1786
Alinia for Oral Suspension (Less than 1%)...... 2677
Alinia Tablets (Less than 1%)...... 2677
Allegra Oral Solution (1.6%)...... 2684
▲ Allegra-D 12 Hour Extended-Release Tablets (7.4%)...... 2687
▲ Allegra-D 24 Hour Extended-Release Tablets (7.4%)...... 2690
Alphanate...... 1709
AlphaNine SD...... 1713
Altabax Ointment (1.2%)...... 1299
Alvesco Inhalation Aerosol (Less than 1%)...... 2985
Ambien Tablets (Frequent)...... 2692
▲ Ambien CR Tablets (7%)...... 2696
▲ AmBisome for Injection (25.9% to 39.7%)...... 606
▲ Amerge Tablets (4% to 5%)...... 1301
Amevive (0.2% to common)...... 611
Aminohippurate Sodium "PAH" Injection...... 1950
▲ Amitiza Capsules (7% to 29%)...... 3082
Amoxil Capsules...... 1305
Amoxil Chewable Tablets...... 1305
Amoxil Pediatric Drops for Oral Suspension...... 1305
Amoxil Powder for Oral Suspension...... 1305
Amoxil Tablets...... 1305
Amrix Capsules...... 966
▲ Anaprox Tablets (3% to 9%)...... 2632
▲ Anaprox DS Tablets (3% to 9%)...... 2632
AndroGel...... 3159
Angeliq Tablets...... 751
▲ Angiomax for Injection (3% to 15%)...... 1933
▲ Aptivus Capsules (4.5% to 8.5%)...... 823
▲ Aptivus Oral Solution (4.5% to 8.5%)...... 823
▲ Aranesp for Injection (11%)...... 564
▲ Argatroban Injection (4.8% to 7.1%)...... 1308
▲ Aricept Tablets (2% to 6%)...... 1062
▲ Aricept ODT Tablets (2% to 6%)...... 1062
▲ Arimidex Tablets (11% to 20%)...... 672
▲ Arixtra Injection (0.3% to 11.3%)...... 1313
▲ Arranon Injection (0% to 41%)...... 1319
▲ Asacol Delayed-Release Tablets (13%)...... 2579
▲ Asmanex Twisthaler (1% to 3%)...... 2797
Atacand Tablets (More than 1%)...... 639
Atacand HCT (0.5% or greater)...... 642
▲ Atripla Tablets (Greater than or equal to 10%)...... 938
▲ Atrovent HFA Inhalation Aerosol (4%)...... 839
Atrovent Nasal Spray 0.03% (2.2%)...... 834
Atrovent Nasal Spray 0.06%...... 836
Attenuvax...... 1951
▲ Augmentin (3%)...... 1323
▲ Augmentin Tablets (3%)...... 1327
▲ Augmentin XR Extended Release Tablets (2.1% to 3.5%)...... 1333
Augmentin ES-600 Powder for Oral Suspension...... 1329
▲ Avalide Tablets (3%)...... 892
▲ Avalide Tablets (3%)...... 2713
▲ Avandamet Tablets (16%)...... 1336
Avandaryl Tablets (1.1%)...... 1344
▲ Avandia Tablets (4%)...... 1351
Avapro Tablets (1% or greater)...... 897
Avapro Tablets (1% or greater)...... 2718
▲ Avastin IV (4.1% to 12%)...... 1192
▲ Avelox (6%)...... 2803
▲ Avinza Capsules (Greater than 10%)...... 1772
Axert Tablets (1% to 2%)...... 2431
▲ Axid Capsules (1.2% to 5.4%)...... 1364
▲ Azilect Tablets (12%)...... 3106
Azopt Ophthalmic Suspension (Less than 1%)...... 540
▲ Bactroban Cream (1.1% to 4.9%)...... 1366
Bactroban Nasal (Less than 1%)...... 1367
Bactroban Ointment (Less than 1%)...... 1368
Baraclude (Less than 1%)...... 900
Bayer Aspirin...... 750
Beconase AQ Nasal Spray (Fewer than 5 in 100 patients)...... 1369
▲ BeneFIX Vials (6.2%)...... 3191
Benicar Tablets (Greater than 0.5%)...... 1009
▲ Benicar HCT Tablets (3%)...... 1010
▲ Bentyl Capsules (14%)...... 703
▲ Bentyl Injection (14%)...... 703
▲ Bentyl Syrup (14%)...... 703
▲ Bentyl Tablets (14%)...... 703
▲ Betaseron for SC Injection (27%)...... 756
▲ Betimol Ophthalmic Solution (1% to 5%)...... 3181
▲ Bexxar (3% to 36%)...... 1371
▲ Biaxin/Biaxin XL (3%)...... 411
Bicillin C-R Injectable Suspension...... 1775
Bicillin L-A Injection...... 1777
▲ Boniva Injection (4.8% to 5.1%)...... 2614
▲ Boniva Tablets (4.8% to 5.1%)...... 2618
▲ Boostrix (3% to 26%)...... 1377
Brovana Inhalation Solution...... 2990
▲ Busulfex Injection (7% to 98%)...... 2477
▲ Byetta Injection (44%)...... 600
▲ Bystolic Tablets (1% to 3%)...... 1155
Calcijex Injection...... 419
Campath Ampules...... 761
▲ Campral Tablets (3% to 4%)...... 1158
▲ Canasa Rectal Suppositories (3.1%)...... 705
▲ Cancidas for Injection (3.5% to 14.5%)...... 1953
Captopril Tablets (About 0.5% to 2%)...... 2182
Carafate Suspension (Less than 0.5%)...... 706
Carafate Tablets (Less than 0.5%)...... 707
Carbatrol Capsules (Among most frequent)...... 3019
▲ Cardene I.V. (4.9%)...... 1093
Cardizem LA Extended Release Tablets (1.4%)...... 421
▲ Catapres Tablets (About 5 in 100 patients)...... 841
Catapres-TTS (1 of 101 patients)...... 842
Ceftin (2.6%)...... 1380
▲ Celebrex Capsules (3.5% to 7%)...... 2979
▲ Celexa (4% to 21%)...... 1160
▲ CellCept Capsules (3% to 54.5%)...... 2622
▲ CellCept Intravenous (3% to 54.5%)...... 2622
▲ CellCept Oral Suspension (3% to 54.5%)...... 2622
▲ CellCept Tablets (3% to 54.5%)...... 2622
▲ Cerezyme for Injection (Approximately 6.5%)...... 1238
Cervidil Vaginal Insert (Less than 1%)...... 1165
▲ Chantix Tablets (3% to 30%)...... 2511
▲ Chemet Capsules (12% to 20.9%)...... 2484
Cialis Tablets (Less than 2%)...... 1792
Cipro I.V. (Greater than 1% to 2.7%)...... 2817
Cipro (2.5% to 2.7%)...... 2810
▲ Cipro XR Tablets (3% to 4%)...... 2823
▲ Clarinex Syrup (3%)...... 2828
▲ Clarinex Tablets (5%)...... 2828
▲ Clarinex Reditabs Tablets (5%)...... 2828
Clarinex-D 12-Hour Extended-Release Tablets (2%)...... 2831
Clarinex-D 24-Hour Extended-Release Tablets (2%)...... 2834
▲ Cleviprex (4.8% to 21%)...... 1936
▲ Climara Transdermal System (1% to 6%)...... 763
Climara Pro Transdermal System...... 768
▲ Clinoril Tablets (3% to 9%)...... 1962
▲ Clolar for Intravenous Infusion (75%)...... 1239
▲ Clorpres Tablets (About 5%)...... 2185
Combigan Ophthalmic Solution...... 553

Combivent Inhalation Aerosol (2%) ... 845
▲ Combivir Tablets (13% to 33%) ... 1384
▲ Comtan Tablets (14%) ... 2208
▲ Concerta Extended-Release Tablets (12.8%) ... 1925
▲ Copaxone for Injection (22%) ... 3110
▲ Coreg Tablets (4% to 9%) ... 1387
▲ Coreg CR Extended-Release Capsules (2% to 9%) ... 1393
Cosmegen for Injection (Common) ... 2485
▲ Cosopt Sterile Ophthalmic Solution (1% to 5%) ... 1969
Cozaar Tablets (1% or greater) ... 1973
Creon 5 Capsules (Among most frequent) ... 3041
Creon 10 Capsules (Among most frequent) ... 3042
Creon 20 Capsules (Among most frequent) ... 3042
▲ Crestor Tablets (0% to 6.3%) ... 677
▲ Crinone 4% Gel (8%) ... 992
▲ Crinone 8% Gel (6% to 22%) ... 992
▲ Crixivan Capsules (11.7%) ... 1979
▲ Cubicin for Injection (5.8% to 10%) ... 995
▲ Cuprimine Capsules (17%) ... 1986
▲ Cyanokit 5g Antidote (6% to 11%) ... 1021
▲ Cymbalta Delayed-Release Capsules (14% to 30%) ... 1801
▲ Dacogen Injection (42%) ... 1066
Dantrium Capsules (Rare) ... 2580
Dapsone Tablets USP ... 1746
▲ Daytrana Transdermal Patch (12%) ... 3022
Delatestryl Injection ... 1730
Demadex Injection (1.8%) ... 2630
Demadex Tablets (1.8%) ... 2630
Demser Capsules (Infrequent) ... 1989
▲ Depakote ER Tablets (9% to 48%) ... 423
▲ DepoCyt Injection (11% to 46%) ... 1136
▲ DepoDur Injection (Greater than 10%) ... 1095
Diclofenac Sodium Ophthalmic Solution ... ⊙ 240
▲ Didronel Tablets (About 1 patient in 15; possibly 2 or 3 in 10) ... 2583
Diovan Tablets (More than 1%) ... 2212
Diovan HCT Tablets (Greater than 0.2%) ... 2216
Divigel ... 3167
Donnatal Extentabs ... 2507
▲ Doribax Injection (4% to 12%) ... 2400
▲ Doxil Injection (16.9% to 46%) ... 2378
▲ Duetact Tablets (4% to 5.1%) ... 3085
▲ Duragesic Transdermal System (Greater than 10% to 24%) ... 2405
Dyazide Capsules ... 1405
DynaCirc CR Controlled Release Tablets ... 1407
Dyrenium Capsules (Rare) ... 3189
▲ EC-Naprosyn Delayed-Release Tablets (3% to 9%) ... 2632
Edecrin ... 698
E.E.S. (Among most frequent) ... 433
▲ Effexor XR Extended-Release Capsules (4% to 35%) ... 3195
▲ Eldepryl Capsules (10 of 49 patients) ... 3052
▲ Elidel Cream 1% (0.4% to 4%) ... 2221
Eligard 7.5 mg ... 2724
▲ Eligard 22.5 mg (3.4%) ... 2724
Eligard 30 mg (2.2%) ... 2724
Eligard 45 mg ... 2724
▲ Elitek (27%) ... 2729
▲ Elmiron Capsules (4%) ... 2435
▲ Eloxatin for Injection (4% to 83%) ... 2731
Elspar for Injection ... 1990
▲ Emend Capsules (7.1% to12.7%) ... 1992
▲ Emend for Injection (7.1% to12.7%) ... 1999
Emsam Transdermal System ... 905
▲ Emtriva Capsules (Greater than or equal to 10%) ... 1246
▲ Emtriva Oral Solution (Greater than or equal to 10%) ... 1246
▲ Enablex Extended-Release Tablets (1.5% to 4.1%) ... 2225
▲ Enbrel for Injection (9% to 15%) ... 569
Engerix-B Vaccine (Less than 1%) ... 1409
▲ Enjuvia Tablets (7% to 12%) ... 1029
EpiPen ... 1024
▲ Epivir (8% to 33%) ... 1412
▲ Epivir-HBV (15%) ... 1417
▲ Epogen for Injection (0.26% to 48%) ... 576
▲ Epzicom Tablets (5% to 6%) ... 1422
▲ Equetro Extended-Release Capsules (10% to 29%) ... 3174
▲ Erbitux (2% to 55%) ... 912
EryPed (Among most frequent) ... 431
Estratest Tablets ... 3043
Estratest H.S. Tablets ... 3043
▲ Evista Tablets (8.3% to 8.8%) ... 1810
▲ Evoxac Capsules (13.8%) ... 1013
▲ Exelon Capsules (29% to 47%) ... 2229
▲ Exelon Oral Solution (29% to 47%) ... 2229
▲ Exelon Patch (7% to 21%) ... 2233
Exforge Tablets (Greater than or equal to 0.2%) ... 2238
▲ Exjade Tablets (11%) ... 2244
▲ Fabrazyme for Intravenous Infusion (Greater than or equal to 5%) ... 1241
Fansidar Tablets ... 2636
▲ Faslodex Injection (26%) ... 682
▲ Femara Tablets (0.1% to 17%) ... 2246
Fenoglide Tablets (2.3%) ... 2960
▲ Fentora Tablets (1% to 42%) ... 968
Ferralet 90 Tablets ... 2175
Flebogamma 5% DIF ... 1718
▲ Flector Patch (3%) ... 561
Fleet Phospho-soda EZ-PREP ... 1147
Fleet Prep Kits ... 1149
Flexbumin 25% I.V. (Occasional) ... 729
▲ Flolan for Injection (32% to 67%) ... 1426
Flomax Capsules (2% to 3.9%) ... 848
▲ Flonase Nasal Spray (2.6% to 4.8%) ... 1431
▲ Flovent Diskus 50 mcg (4% to 9%) ... 1435
Fluarix Vaccine ... 1446
▲ Flulaval Injection Vaccine (1% to 5%) ... 1448
Flumadine (2.8%) ... 1167
FluMist Vaccine ... 1945
Fluorescite Injection ... ⊙ 203
Focalin XR Capsules ... 2251
▲ Follistim AQ Cartridge (17%) ... 2844
Foradil Aerolizer ... 2849
Fortaz (1 in 156 patients) ... 1450
▲ Forteo for Injection (8.5%) ... 1816
▲ Fosamax (Up to 3.6%) ... 2005
▲ Fosamax Plus D Tablets (0% to 3.6%) ... 2013
▲ Fosrenol Chewable Tablets (11% to 36%) ... 3027
Frova Tablets (Greater than or equal to 2%) ... 1111
Furosemide Tablets ... 2186
▲ Gabitril Tablets (11%) ... 973
▲ Gammagard Liquid (1.09% to 9.8%) ... 730
Gammagard S/D (Occasional) ... 734
▲ Gamunex (0.5% to 21%) ... 3094
Gantrisin Pediatric Suspension ... 2638
▲ Gardasil Injection (4.2% to 6.7%) ... 2019
▲ Gemzar for Injection (58% to 71%) ... 1820
▲ Gengraf Capsules (2% to 18%) ... 435
Genotropin Lyophilized Powder ... 2547
▲ Geodon (10%) ... 2520
▲ Gleevec Tablets (41.7% to 74%) ... 2255
▲ Gliadel Wafer (8% to 22%) ... 1076
Glucagon for Injection Vials and Emergency Kit (Occasional) ... 1827
Gris-PEG Tablets (Occasional) ... 2507
▲ Havrix Injection Vaccine (1% to 10%) ... 1454
Hemofil M (Extremely rare) ... 737
▲ Hepsera Tablets (5%) ... 1253
▲ Herceptin I.V. (8% to 33%) ... 1199
▲ Hexalen Capsules (33%) ... 1078
Human Albumin Grifols 25% ... 1706
Humatrope Vials and Cartridges ... 1838
▲ Humira Injection (9%) ... 442
▲ Hycamtin Capsules (27% to 33%) ... 1456
▲ Hycamtin for Injection (Less than 1% to 77%) ... 1459
▲ Imitrex Injection (4%) ... 1465
▲ Imitrex Nasal Spray (11% to 13.5%) ... 1470
Imitrex Tablets (Greater than 1%) ... 1474
Increlex Injection ... 3100
▲ Indapamide Tablets (Less than 5%) ... 2188
▲ Indocin (3% to 9%) ... 2024
InnoPran XL Extended Release Capsules ... 1484
▲ Intelence Tablets (4.7% to 13.9%) ... 3119
Intravenous Sodium Diuril ... 2490
▲ Intron A for Injection (1% to 66%) ... 2859
▲ Invanz for Injection (1.6% to 8.5%) ... 2029
▲ Ionsys Transdermal System (39%) ... 2410
Iquix Ophthalmic Solution (1% to 2%) ... 3183
▲ Isentress Tablets (2.2% to 9.9%) ... 2036
▲ Ixempra Kit for Injection (42%) ... 915
▲ Janumet Tablets (1.3% to greater than 5%) ... 2041
Januvia Tablets (1.4%) ... 2048
▲ Kaletra (5% to 16%) ... 452
Keppra Oral Solution (1% to greater than or equal to 2%) ... 3131
Keppra Tablets (1% to greater than or equal to 2%) ... 3131
▲ Ketek Tablets (7% to 7.9%) ... 2744
▲ Kineret Injection (8%) ... 585
Klonopin ... 2639
Kogenate FS ... 746
Kogenate FS with Bio-Set (1 case) ... 748
K-Phos Original (Sodium Free) Tablets ... 814
K-Phos Neutral Tablets ... 813
Kristalose for Oral Solution ... 1004
▲ Lamictal (2% to 19%) ... 1488
Lamisil Oral Granules (2%) ... 2264
Lamisil Tablets (2.6%) ... 2266
Lanoxin Injection ... 1498
Lanoxin Injection Pediatric ... 1502
Lanoxin Tablets (Common) ... 1505
▲ Lescol Capsules (3.2%) ... 2268
Lescol XL Tablets (2.5%) ... 2268
Leukeran Tablets (Infrequent) ... 1508
▲ Leukine (58% to 90%) ... 774
▲ Leustatin Injection (28%) ... 2384
▲ Levaquin (7%) ... 2416
▲ Levaquin in 5% Dextrose Injection (7%) ... 2416
Levitra Tablets (2%) ... 2876
Levothroid Tablets ... 1170
▲ Lexapro Oral Suspension (2% to 18%) ... 1174
▲ Lexapro Tablets (2% to 18%) ... 1174
▲ Lexiscan Injection (6%) ... 614
▲ Lexiva Oral Suspension (Less than or equal to 1% to 7%) ... 1510
▲ Lexiva Tablets (Less than or equal to 1% to 7%) ... 1510
Lidoderm Patch ... 1114
Limbrel Capsules ... 2561
Lipitor Tablets (Greater than or equal to 2%) ... 2501
Lortab 5/500 Tablets (Among most frequent) ... 3143
Lortab 7.5/500 Tablets (Among most frequent) ... 3144
Lortab 10/500 Tablets (Among most frequent) ... 3144
▲ Lovenox Injection (2.5% to 3%) ... 2756
▲ Lucentis Injection (2% to 9%) ... 1205
▲ Lunesta Tablets (4% to 5%) ... 2994
▲ Lupron Depot 3.75 mg (13%) ... 462
▲ Lupron Depot–3 Month 11.25 mg (4.8% to 13%) ... 462
Lupron Depot-PED 7.5 mg, 11.25 mg and 15 mg (Less than 2%) ... 471
▲ Luvox CR Extended-Release Capsules (6% to 39%) ... 1759
Lybrel Tablets ... 3204
▲ Malarone Pediatric Tablets (Less than 1% to 12%) ... 1521
▲ Malarone Tablets (Less than 1% to 12%) ... 1521
▲ Marinol Capsules (3% to 10%) ... 3163
▲ Marplan Tablets (4% to 6%) ... 3177
Maxair Autohaler (1.3% to 1.7%) ... 1705
▲ Maxalt Tablets (4% to 6%) ... 2056
▲ Maxalt-MLT Orally Disintegrating Tablets (4% to 6%) ... 2056
▲ Megace ES Oral Suspension (0% to 5%) ... 2499
▲ Mepron Suspension (2.5% to 32%) ... 1526
▲ Meridia Capsules (5.9%) ... 475
▲ Merrem I.V. (0.8% to 7.8%) ... 684
Meruvax II ... 2061
Metadate CD Capsules ... 3146
▲ Mevacor Tablets (1.9% to 4.7%) ... 2063
▲ Miacalcin Injection (About 10%) ... 2273
▲ Miacalcin Nasal Spray (1% to 3%) ... 2274
Micardis Tablets (1%) ... 852
Micardis HCT Tablets (2%) ... 854
▲ Mirapex Tablets (11% to 27%) ... 857
Mircette Tablets ... 1034
▲ Mirena Intrauterine System (5% or more) ... 779
M-M-R II ... 2054
Moban Tablets (Occasional) ... 1116
▲ Mobic Oral Suspension (2.4% to 7.2%) ... 863
▲ Mobic Tablets (2.4% to 7.2%) ... 863
▲ MoviPrep Oral Solution (14.4%) ... 2679
Moxatag Tablets (1.3%) ... 2165
MS Contin Tablets (Among most frequent) ... 2585
Mustargen for Injection ... 2492
▲ Mycamine for Injection (7.4% to 69.6%) ... 616
▲ Myfortic Tablets (24.5% to 29.1%) ... 2276
Myleran Tablets ... 1530
▲ Mylotarg for Injection (63% to 74%) ... 3212
▲ Nabi-HB (4%) ... 815
Nadolol Tablets (1 to 5 of 1000 patients) ... 2191
▲ Nalfon Capsules (7.7%) ... 2508
Namenda (Greater than or equal to 2%) ... 1180
▲ Naprosyn Suspension (3% to 9%) ... 2632
▲ Naprosyn Tablets (3% to 9%) ... 2632
Nasonex Nasal Spray (Greater than or equal to 2%) ... 2883
▲ Natrecor for Injection (4% to 13%) ... 2977
Nembutal Sodium Solution, USP (Less than 1%) ... 2494
▲ Neoral Oral Solution (2% to 18%) ... 2280
▲ Neoral Soft Gelatin Capsules (2% to 18%) ... 2280
▲ Neulasta Injection (15% to 72%) ... 587
▲ Neupogen for Injection (10% to 57%) ... 589
▲ Neupro Transdermal System (2% to 41%) ... 3149
▲ Nevanac Ophthalmic Suspension 0.1% (1% to 4%) ... ⊙ 205
▲ Nexavar Tablets (23% to 24%) ... 784
Nexium Delayed-Release Capsules (Greater than or equal to 1%) ... 645
Nexium I.V. (Greater than or equal to 1%) ... 652
Nexium Delayed-Release Oral Suspension (Greater than or equal to 1%) ... 645
▲ Niaspan Extended-Release Tablets (2% to 8%) ... 480
Nimotop Capsules (Up to 1.4%) ... 790
Nitrolingual Pumpspray (Uncommon) ... 2965
Norditropin Cartridges (Small number of patients) ... 2354
▲ Noroxin Tablets (2.6% to 4.2%) ... 2069
▲ Norvir (25.6% to 29.8%) ... 489
▲ Novantrone for Injection Concentrate (26% to 76%) ... 1100
▲ NovoLog Injection (7%) ... 2359
NovoSeven ... 2367
NovoSeven RT ... 2370
▲ Noxafil Oral Suspension (5% to 38%) ... 2889
Nutropin for Injection (A small number of patients) ... 1208
Nutropin AQ Injection (A small number of patients) ... 1212
Nutropin AQ NuSpin Injection (A small number of patients) ... 1212
Nutropin AQ Pen (A small number of patients) ... 1212
Nutropin AQ Pen Cartridge (A small number of patients) ... 1212
▲ NuvaRing (5% to 14%) ... 2897
Ofloxacin Ophthalmic Solution 0.3% (Rare) ... ⊙ 243
▲ Omnicef Capsules (3%) ... 497
Omnicef for Oral Suspension (0.2%) ... 497
▲ Ontak Vials (64%) ... 1079
▲ Opana Tablets (19%) ... 1117
▲ Opana ER Tablets (2.9% to 33.1%) ... 1121
OptiPranolol Metipranolol Ophthalmic Solution 0.3% (A small number of patients) ... ⊙ 245
Orencia Powder for Intravenous Infusion (Greater than 0.1% and less than or equal to 1%) ... 921
Ortho-Cyclen Tablets ... 2449
▲ Ortho Evra Transdermal System (9% to 22%) ... 2437
Ortho Micronor Tablets ... 2446
Ortho Tri-Cyclen Tablets ... 2449
Ortho Tri-Cyclen Lo Tablets ... 2458
▲ Orthoclone OKT3 Sterile Solution (19%) ... 2387
▲ OsmoPrep Tablets (26% to 37%) ... 2680
▲ OxyContin Tablets (Less than 1% to 23%) ... 2589
OxyIR Capsules (Among most frequent) ... 2593
Parnate Tablets ... 1532
Paser Granules (Among most common) ... 1747
▲ Pataday Ophthalmic Solution (Less than or equal to 5%) ... 543
Patanase Nasal Spray ... 544
▲ Patanol Ophthalmic Solution (Less than 5%) ... 546
▲ Paxil (1.9% to 36.3%) ... 1535
▲ Paxil CR Controlled-Release Tablets (1.9% to 36.3%) ... 1544
Pediarix Vaccine ... 1552
▲ PegIntron Powder for Injection (26%) ... 2903
▲ Pentasa Capsules (1.8% to 3.1%) ... 3030
Pepcid Tablets (Infrequent) ... 2075
Percocet Tablets (Among most frequent) ... 1127
Percodan Tablets (Among most frequent) ... 1130
▲ Perforomist Inhalation Solution (4.9%) ... 1025
Persantine Tablets (Rare) ... 869
Phenytek Capsules ... 2192
PhosLo GelCaps (Occasional) ... 1184
▲ Photofrin for Injection (24% to 39%) ... 708
▲ Plan B Tablets (23.1%) ... 1044
▲ Plavix Tablets (3.4%) ... 926

▲ Plavix Tablets (3.4%) 2767
▲ Pletal Tablets (6% to 7%) 2481
Pneumovax 23 2078
Potaba (Infrequent) 1698
▲ PrandiMet Tablets (Greater than 5% to 15%) 2967
▲ Prandin Tablets (3% to 5%) 2971
Premarin Intravenous 3217
▲ Premarin Tablets (6% to 9%) 3221
Premarin Vaginal Cream 3228
▲ Premphase Tablets (7% to 11%) 3232
▲ Prempro Tablets (7% to 11%) 3232
Primaxin I.M. (0.6%) 2080
Primaxin I.V. (2%) 2083
Prinivil Tablets (Greater than 1% to 2%) 2087
Prinzide Tablets (2.2%) 2092
▲ Pristiq Extended-Release Tablets (4% to 41%) 3247
ProAmatine Tablets (Rare) 3032
▲ Procrit for Injection (0.26% to 58%) 2391
Profilnine SD Solvent Detergent 1721
Proglycem Capsules (Frequent) 1185
Proglycem Suspension (Frequent) 1185
▲ Prograf Capsules and Injection (32% to 46%) 622
▲ Proleukin for Injection (Less than 1% to 35%) 2287
▲ Prometrium Capsules (100 mg, 200 mg) (8%) 3047
Protonix for Delayed-Release Oral Suspension (2%) 3254
Protonix Delayed-Release Tablets (2%) 3254
Protonix I.V. (Greater than 1%) 3257
▲ Protopic Ointment (1% to 3%) 628
▲ Proventil HFA Inhalation Aerosol (10%) 2914
▲ Provigil Tablets (11%) 977
▲ Prozac Weekly Capsules (Infrequent to 29%) 1852
▲ Prozac Pulvules and Liquid (12% to 22%) 1852
▲ Pulmicort Flexhaler (1.8% to 6%) 654
Pylera Capsules 714
Qvar Inhalation Aerosol (Less than 1% to 2%) 3116
▲ Rapamune (25% to 31%) 3260
▲ Raptiva for Injection (11%) 1218
▲ Rebetol (33% to 47%) 2917
▲ Reclast Injection (4.5% to 8.5%) 2291
Recombinate (Extremely rare) 738
Recombivax HB (Equal to or greater than 1%) 2107
ReFacto Vials 3269
▲ Relenza Inhalation Powder (Less than 1.5% to 3%) 1556
▲ Relistor Injection (11.5%) 3310
Remeron Tablets (1.5%) 2924
RemeronSolTab Tablets (1.5%) 2927
▲ Remicade for IV Injection (21%) 950
▲ ReoPro Vials (18.4%) 1860
▲ Requip Tablets (30% to 60%) 1561
▲ Requip XL Tablets (Greater than or equal to 5%) 1568
▲ Retrovir Capsules (0.8% to 61%) 1574
▲ Retrovir IV Infusion (1% to 61%) 1579
▲ Retrovir (0.8% to 61%) 1574
▲ Reyataz Capsules (3% to 14%) 3299
▲ Rilutek Tablets (12.2% to 20.5%) 2771
Risperdal Consta Long-Acting Injection (Frequent) 1753
▲ Rituxan I.V. (1% to 23%) 1223
Rocaltrol Capsules 1150
Rocaltrol Oral Solution 1150
Rocephin Injectable Vials, ADD-Vantage, Galaxy, Bulk (Less than 1%) 2642
▲ Romazicon Injection (11%) 2646
▲ Rozerem Tablets (3%) 3091
▲ Rythmol Tablets (3% to 11%) 1586
▲ Rythmol SR Capsules (9% to 17%) 1590
St. Joseph 81 mg Aspirin Chewable and Enteric Coated Tablets 1903
▲ Salagen Tablets (1% to 15%) 1082
Sanctura XR Capsules (1.4%) 557
▲ Sandimmune (2% to 10%) 2296
▲ Sandostatin Injection (34% to 61%) 2300
▲ Sandostatin LAR Depot (10.3% to 40.9%) 2302
Seasonique Tablets 1046
▲ Sensipar Tablets (31%) 594
▲ Serevent Diskus (1% to 3%) 1594
▲ Simcor Tablets (3.2% to 4.2%) 502
▲ Simulect for Injection (Greater than or equal to 10%) 2306
Singulair (Greater than or equal to 2%) 2114
Skelaxin Tablets (Most frequent) 1784
Soma Tablets 1931
▲ Somatuline Depot Injection (Greater than 5% to 11%) 3102
▲ Soriatane Capsules (1% to 10%) 3062
▲ Stalevo Tablets (5% to 14%) 2309
▲ Strattera Capsules (0.2% to 21%) 1864
Stromectol Tablets (1.8%) 2120
▲ Suboxone Tablets (10% to 15%) 2601
▲ Subutex Tablets (10% to 13.6%) 2601
Sular Extended Release Tablets (2%) 2975
▲ Suprax for Oral Suspension (7%) 1891
▲ Suprax Tablets (7%) 1891
▲ Sustiva Capsules (2% to 16%) 930
▲ Sustiva Tablets (2% to 16%) 930
▲ Sutent Capsules (2% to 54%) 2540
Symbyax Capsules (Infrequent) 1871
Tabloid Tablets (Less frequent) 1601
▲ Tamiflu Capsules (3% to 10%) 2649
▲ Tamiflu Oral Suspension (3% to 10%) 2649
▲ Tarceva Tablets (0% to 60%) 1228
▲ Targretin Capsules (7.5% to 15.5%) 1084
Tarka Tablets (0.3% to 1.5%) 511
▲ Tasigna Capsules (Greater than 10% to 31%) 2316
▲ Taxotere Injection Concentrate (0.6% to 80.5%) 2773
▲ Temodar Capsules (4% to 53%) 2931
Tessalon Capsules 1183
Tessalon Perles 1183
Teveten Tablets (Less than 1%) 515
Teveten HCT Tablets (Less than 1%) 517
Tev-Tropin for Injection (Small number of patients) 1187
Thioridazine Hydrochloride Tablets 2195
Thiothixene Capsules 2197
▲ Thyrogen for Injection (11.9%) 1244
▲ Tice BCG (3% to 7%) 2936
Timentin ADD-Vantage 1606
Timentin Injection Galaxy Container 1609
Timentin IV Infusion 1603
Timentin Pharmacy Bulk Package 1613
Timoptic Sterile Ophthalmic Solution (Less frequent) 2121
Timoptic in Ocudose (Less frequent) 2124
Timoptic-XE Sterile Ophthalmic Gel Forming Solution 2125
TNKase 1233
Toprol-XL Tablets (About 1 of 100 patients) 666
▲ Torisel Injection (2% to 37%) 3272
Tracleer Tablets 3289
Transderm Scōp Transdermal Therapeutic System (Few patients) 2206
▲ Trasylol Injection (11%) 799
▲ Treanda for Injection (Less than 1% to 20%) 983
▲ Treximet Tablets (3%) 1616
Tricor Tablets (2.3%) 520
▲ Trisenox Injection (75%) 986
▲ Trizivir Tablets (12% to 60%) 1622
Trusopt Sterile Ophthalmic Solution (Infrequent) 2128
▲ Truvada Tablets (Greater than or equal to 10%) 1262
Tussionex Pennkinetic Extended-Release Suspension 3154
▲ Twinrix Vaccine (2% to 4%) 1628
▲ Tygacil for Injection (25.3% to 35%) 3276
▲ Tykerb Tablets (0% to 44%) 1631
Tylenol with Codeine Tablets 2427
▲ Tyzeka Tablets (7%) 2328
▲ Ultane Liquid for Inhalation (25%) 524
▲ Ultram ER Extended-Release Tablets (15.1% to 26.2%) 2428
Uniphyl Tablets 2595
Urocit-K Tablets (Some patients) 2176
Uroqid-Acid No. 2 Tablets 814
Uroxatral Tablets (1% to 2%) 2786
▲ Urso 250 Tablets (8.3%) 720
▲ Urso Forte Tablets (8.3%) 720
▲ Valcyte Tablets (8% to 30%) 2654
Valium Tablets (Infrequent) 2658
▲ Valstar Sterile Solution for Intravesical Instillation (5%) 1735
▲ Valtrex Caplets (5% to 15%) 1635
Vantas (Less than 2%) 1737
▲ Vaprisol (3% to 5%) 632
Vaqta (2.3%) 2130
Varivax (Greater than or equal to 1%) 2133
▲ Vectibix (1% to 23%) 597
▲ Velcade for Injection (3% to 57%) 2168
▲ Venlafaxine Hydrochloride Tablets (6% to 58%) 2199
▲ Vesanoid Capsules (57%) 2660
▲ VESIcare Tablets (1.7% to 3.3%) 636
Viadur Implant (Less than 2%) 802
Vicodin Tablets (Among most frequent) 529
Vicodin ES Tablets (Among most frequent) 530
Vicodin HP Tablets (Among most frequent) 531
▲ Vicoprofen Tablets (21%) 533
▲ Viramune Oral Suspension (0.5% to 8.7%) 873
▲ Viramune Tablets (0.5% to 8.7%) 873
▲ Viread Tablets (8% to 11%) 1268
▲ Visudyne for Injection (1% to 10%) 2332
▲ Vivitrol (25% to 33%) 988
▲ Voltaren Ophthalmic Solution (Less than or equal to 3%) 2336
▲ Voltaren Tablets (1% to 10%) 2334
▲ Voltaren-XR Tablets (1% to 10%) 2337
Vytorin 10/10 Tablets 2149
Vytorin 10/20 Tablets 2149
Vytorin 10/40 Tablets 2149
Vytorin 10/80 Tablets 2149
▲ Vyvanse Capsules (6% to 7%) 3033
▲ WelChol Tablets (3% to 4.2%) 1015
▲ Wellbutrin Tablets (22.9%) 1648
▲ Wellbutrin SR Sustained-Release Tablets (5% to 18%) 1653
▲ Wellbutrin XL Extended-Release Tablets (0.8% to 18%) 1659
WinRho SDF 741
▲ Xeloda Tablets (4% to 43%) 2662
▲ Xenical Capsules (3.6% to 8.1%) 2672
▲ Xifaxan Tablets (5.3%) 2682
Xopenex Inhalation Solution 3001
Xopenex Inhalation Solution Concentrate 3005
Xopenex HFA Inhalation Aerosol 3009
▲ Xyntha Vials (6% to 9%) 3280
▲ Xyrem Oral Solution (2% to 40%) 1766
Xyzal Oral Solution 2789
Xyzal Oral Solution 3155
Yaz Tablets (Greater than 1%) 805
Zantac 25 EFFERdose Tablets 1670
Zantac Injection 1666
Zantac Injection Pharmacy Bulk Package (Frequent) 1668
Zantac Injection Premixed 1666
Zantac 1670
▲ Zemplar Capsules (13%) 536
▲ Zemplar Injection (13%) 538
Zemuron Injection (Less than 1%) 2947
Zetia Tablets 2157
Zetia Tablets 2951
▲ Ziagen (9% to 19%) 1673
Zinacef for Injection (1 in 440 patients) 1678
Zinacef Injection (1 in 440 patients) 1678
▲ Zocor Tablets (5.4%) 2136
▲ Zolinza Capsules (35% to 40.7%) 2142
▲ Zometa for Intravenous Infusion (29% to 46%) 2341
Zomig Tablets (Common) 694
▲ Zomig Nasal Spray (0% to 4%) 689
Zomig-ZMT Tablets (Common) 694
▲ Zonegran Capsules (9%) 1089
▲ Zosyn for Injection (5.8% to 6.9%) 3284
▲ Zovirax (2.4% to 4.8%) 1690
▲ Zyban Sustained-Release Tablets (9%) 1692
Zydone Tablets (Among most frequent) 1132
▲ Zyprexa Tablets (2% to 9%) 1883
Zyprexa IntraMuscular (Infrequent) 1883
▲ Zyprexa ZYDIS Orally Disintegrating Tablets (2% to 9%) 1883
Zyrtec Chewable Tablets (1.9% to greater than 2%) 1920
Zyrtec Syrup (1.9% to greater than 2%) 1920
Zyrtec Tablets (1.9% to greater than 2%) 1920
Zyrtec-D 12 Hour Extended Release Tablets (Greater than 2%) 1923
▲ Zyvox (1.4% to 6.2%) 2552

Neck, rigidity of

Amerge Tablets 1301
Axert Tablets (Infrequent) 2431
Cardizem LA Extended Release Tablets (Less than 2%) 421
Depakote ER Tablets (Greater than 1%) 423
Effexor XR Extended-Release Capsules (Infrequent) 3195
Eldepryl Capsules 3052
Emsam Transdermal System (Infrequent) 905
▲ Imitrex Injection (5%) 1465
Imitrex Nasal Spray 1470
Imitrex Tablets 1474
Lipitor Tablets (Less than 2%) 2501
Lunesta Tablets (Infrequent) 2994
Luvox CR Extended-Release Capsules (Infrequent) 1759
Lyrica Capsules (0.1% to 1%) 2527
Maxalt Tablets (Less than 2%) 2056
Maxalt-MLT Orally Disintegrating Tablets (Less than 2%) 2056
Norvir (Less than 2%) 489
Paxil (Rare) 1535
Paxil CR Controlled-Release Tablets (Rare) 1544
Pletal Tablets (Less than 2%) 2481
Protonix for Delayed-Release Oral Suspension (Less than 1%) 3254
Protonix Delayed-Release Tablets (Less than 1%) 3254
Protonix I.V. (Less than 1%) 3257
Provigil Tablets (1%) 977
Remeron Tablets (Infrequent) 2924
RemeronSolTab Tablets (Infrequent) 2927
Salagen Tablets (Less than 1%) 1082
Symbyax Capsules (Frequent) 1871
Varivax (Greater than or equal to 1%) 2133
Venlafaxine Hydrochloride Tablets (Infrequent) 2199
Zonegran Capsules (Infrequent) 1089
▲ Zyprexa Tablets (2% to 3%) 1883
▲ Zyprexa ZYDIS Orally Disintegrating Tablets (2% to 3%) 1883

Neck, spasms of

Geodon 2520
Moban Tablets 1116
Risperdal Consta Long-Acting Injection 1753
Symbyax Capsules (Less than 1%) 1871
Thiothixene Capsules 2197
Zyprexa Tablets (Less than 1%) 1883
Zyprexa IntraMuscular (Less than 1%) 1883
Zyprexa ZYDIS Orally Disintegrating Tablets (Less than 1%) 1883

Neck, stiffness of

▲ DepoCyt Injection (6% to 11%) 1136

Neck, redistribution/accumulation of body fat

Kaletra 452
Retrovir 1574

Neck tightness

Imitrex Injection (Relatively common) 1465
▲ Treximet Tablets (3%) 1616
Zomig Tablets (Common) 694
Zomig Nasal Spray (Infrequent) 689
Zomig-ZMT Tablets (Common) 694

Necrolysis, digitus

▲ Sustiva Capsules (Up to 3.5%) 930
▲ Sustiva Tablets (Up to 3.5%) 930

Necrolysis, epidermal

Celexa 1160
Luvox CR Extended-Release Capsules 1759
Prozac Weekly Capsules 1852
Prozac Pulvules and Liquid 1852

Necrolysis, epidermal, toxic

Aciphex Tablets 1053
Advicor Tablets 402
Amoxil Capsules 1305
Amoxil Chewable Tablets 1305
Amoxil Pediatric Drops for Oral Suspension 1305
Amoxil Powder for Oral Suspension 1305
Amoxil Tablets 1305
Anaprox Tablets (Less than 1%) 2632
Anaprox DS Tablets (Less than 1%) 2632
Atacand HCT 642
Augmentin (Occasional) 1323
Augmentin Tablets (Occasional) 1327
Augmentin XR Extended Release Tablets 1333
Augmentin ES-600 Powder for Oral Suspension 1329
Avalide Tablets 892
Avalide Tablets 2713
Avelox 2803
Biaxin/Biaxin XL 411
Carbatrol Capsules (1 to 6 in 10,000 users) 3019
Ceftin 1380
Celebrex Capsules (Less than 0.1%) 2979
Celexa (3 cases) 1160
Cimzia 3127
Cipro I.V. (1% or less) 2817
Cipro 2810
Cipro XR Tablets 2823
Clinoril Tablets (Less than 1%) 1962

Clorpres Tablets 2185
Cuprimine Capsules (Rare) 1986
Daraprim Tablets 1400
Depakote ER Tablets 423
Diovan HCT Tablets 2216
Doribax Injection 2400
▲ Duac Topical Gel (0% to 17%) 3054
EC-Naprosyn Delayed-Release Tablets (Less than 1%) 2632
E.E.S. (Rare) 433
Effexor XR Extended-Release Capsules 3195
Enbrel for Injection 569
Epzicom Tablets 1422
Equetro Extended-Release Capsules 3174
EryPed (Rare) 431
Fansidar Tablets 2636
Flector Patch 561
Fortaz 1450
Fosamax (Rare) 2005
Fosamax Plus D Tablets 2013
Gantrisin Pediatric Suspension 2638
Indocin Capsules (Less than 1%) 2024
Indocin I.V. (Less than 1%) 2489
Indocin (Less than 1%) 2024
Intravenous Sodium Diuril 2490
▲ Intron A for Injection (Less than 5%) 2859
Lamictal (Rare) 1488
Lamisil Oral Granules 2264
Lamisil Tablets (Isolated reports) 2266
Lescol Capsules (Rare) 2268
Lescol XL Tablets 2268
Leukeran Tablets (Rare) 1508
Leustatin Injection (Isolated cases) 2384
Levaquin 2416
Levaquin in 5% Dextrose Injection 2416
Lexapro Oral Suspension 1174
Lexapro Tablets 1174
Lipitor Tablets 2501
Maxalt Tablets 2056
Maxalt-MLT Orally Disintegrating Tablets 2056
Merrem I.V. 684
Mevacor Tablets (Rare) 2063
Micardis HCT Tablets 854
Mobic Oral Suspension (Less than 0.1%) 863
Mobic Tablets (Less than 0.1%) 863
Moxatag Tablets 2165
Nalfon Capsules (Less than 1%) 2508
Naprosyn Suspension (Less than 1%) 2632
Naprosyn Tablets (Less than 1%) 2632
Nexium Delayed-Release Capsules (Rare) 645
Nexium I.V. (Rare) 652
Nexium Delayed-Release Oral Suspension (Rare) 645
Noroxin Tablets 2069
Omnicef Capsules 497
Omnicef for Oral Suspension 497
Paxil 1535
Paxil CR Controlled-Release Tablets 1544
PegIntron Powder for Injection 2903
Pepcid Tablets (Very rare) 2075
Phenytek Capsules 2192
Plavix Tablets 926
Plavix Tablets 2767
Primaxin I.M. 2080
Primaxin I.V. (Less than 0.2%) 2083
Prinivil Tablets (Rare) 2087
Prinzide Tablets (Rare) 2092
Prograf Capsules and Injection 622
Protonix for Delayed-Release Oral Suspension 3254
Protonix Delayed-Release Tablets 3254
Protonix I.V. 3257
Provigil Tablets 977
Raptiva for Injection 1218
Remicade for IV Injection 950
Retrovir IV Infusion 1579
Rituxan I.V. 1223
Rocephin Injectable Vials, ADD-Vantage, Galaxy, Bulk 2642
Stromectol Tablets 2120
Suprax for Oral Suspension (Less than 2%) 1891
Suprax Tablets (Less than 2%) 1891
▲ Sustiva Capsules (Up to 3.5%) 930
▲ Sustiva Tablets (Up to 3.5%) 930
Tamiflu Capsules (Rare) 2649
Tamiflu Oral Suspension (Rare) 2649
Taxotere Injection Concentrate (Rare) 2773
Tekturna HCT Tablets 2324
Teveten HCT Tablets 517
Timentin ADD-Vantage 1606
Timentin Injection Galaxy Container 1609
Timentin IV Infusion 1603
Timentin Pharmacy Bulk Package 1613
Treximet Tablets 1616
Tricor Tablets (Rare) 520
Trizivir Tablets 1622
Trusopt Sterile Ophthalmic Solution (Rare) 2128
Velcade for Injection 2168
Venlafaxine Hydrochloride Tablets 2199
Viramune Oral Suspension 873
Viramune Tablets 873
Voltaren Tablets (Rarely) 2334
Voltaren-XR Tablets (Rarely) 2337
Vytorin 10/10 Tablets 2149
Vytorin 10/10 Tablets 2939
Vytorin 10/20 Tablets 2149
Vytorin 10/20 Tablets 2939
Vytorin 10/40 Tablets 2149
Vytorin 10/40 Tablets 2939
Vytorin 10/80 Tablets 2149
Vytorin 10/80 Tablets 2939
Vyvanse Capsules 3033
Ziagen 1673
Zinacef for Injection (Rare) 1678
Zinacef Injection (Rare) 1678
Zocor Tablets (Rare) 2136
Zonegran Capsules (Rare) 1089
Zosyn for Injection 3284
Zovirax 1690

Necrosis
Captopril Tablets (Rare) 2182
Fortaz 1450
Invanz for Injection (Greater than 0.1%) 2029
▲ Sustiva Capsules (Up to 3.5%) 930
▲ Sustiva Tablets (Up to 3.5%) 930
Zomig Tablets (Rare) 694
Zomig-ZMT Tablets (Rare) 694

Necrosis, aseptic
Requip Tablets (Infrequent) 1561

Necrosis, avascular
Gleevec Tablets (Rare) 2255

Necrosis, bone
Azilect Tablets (Infrequent) 3106
▲ Humira Injection (Less than 5%) 442
▲ Rapamune (Greater than or equal to 3% to less than 20%) 3260
Requip Tablets (Infrequent) 1561
Rilutek Tablets (Rare) 2771

Necrosis, bowel
Proleukin for Injection 2287

Necrosis, cutaneous
Doxil Injection (Less than 1%) 2378
Lovenox Injection 2756

Necrosis, femoral head avascular
Evoxac Capsules (Less than 1%) 1013
Nutropin for Injection 1208
Nutropin AQ Injection 1212
Nutropin AQ NuSpin Injection 1212
Nutropin AQ Pen 1212
Nutropin AQ Pen Cartridge 1212

Necrosis, gastrointestinal
Zomig Tablets (Very rare) 694
Zomig Nasal Spray (Very rare) 689
Zomig-ZMT Tablets (Very rare) 694

Necrosis, injection site
▲ Betaseron for SC Injection (4%) 756
Bicillin C-R Injectable Suspension 1775
Bicillin L-A Injection 1777
Intron A for Injection 2859
PegIntron Powder for Injection (Less than or equal to 1%) 2903
Proleukin for Injection 2287
▲ Rebif Prefilled Syringe for Injection (1% to 3%) 1107
Vivitrol 988

Necrosis, intestinal
Avastin IV (Rare) 1192
Bicillin L-A Injection 1777
Tabloid Tablets 1601

Necrosis, ischemic
Plavix Tablets (Less than 1%) 926
Plavix Tablets (Less than 1%) 2767

Necrosis, pancreatic
Proglycem Capsules (Infrequent) 1185
Proglycem Suspension (Infrequent) 1185

Necrosis, papillary
Aggrenox Capsules 819
Bayer Aspirin 750
Nalfon Capsules (Less than 1%) 2508
Percocet Tablets 1127
Percodan Tablets 1130
St. Joseph 81 mg Aspirin Chewable and Enteric Coated Tablets 1903

Necrosis, renal papillary
Anaprox Tablets (Less than 1%) 2632
Anaprox DS Tablets (Less than 1%) 2632
Dapsone Tablets USP 1746
EC-Naprosyn Delayed-Release Tablets (Less than 1%) 2632
Flector Patch 561
Mobic Oral Suspension 863
Mobic Tablets 863
Naprosyn Suspension (Less than 1%) 2632
Naprosyn Tablets (Less than 1%) 2632
Vicoprofen Tablets 533

Necrosis, renal tubular
Atripla Tablets 938
Capastat Sulfate for Injection 1791
▲ CellCept Capsules (3% to less than 20%) 2622
▲ CellCept Intravenous (3% to less than 20%) 2622
▲ CellCept Oral Suspension (3% to less than 20%) 2622
▲ CellCept Tablets (3% to less than 20%) 2622
Eloxatin for Injection 2731
Flebogamma 5% 1715
Flebogamma 5% DIF 1718
Gammagard S/D 734
Isentress Tablets 2036
Mycamine for Injection 616
▲ Myfortic Tablets (3% to less than 20%) 2276
OsmoPrep Tablets 2680
Percocet Tablets 1127
▲ Prograf Capsules and Injection (3% to 15%) 622
Proleukin for Injection (Less than 1%) 2287
▲ Simulect for Injection (3% to 10%) 2306
Trasylol Injection (1% to 2%) 799
Truvada Tablets 1262
▲ Vesanoid Capsules (3%) 2660

Necrosis, skin
Augmentin XR Extended Release Tablets 1333
Depakote ER Tablets 423
Fragmin Injection (Rare) 1070
Lyrica Capsules (Rare) 2527
Mycamine for Injection 616

Necrosis, tumor
Gleevec Tablets (Rare) 2255

Necrotizing angiitis
Atacand HCT 642
Avalide Tablets 892
Avalide Tablets 2713
Clorpres Tablets 2185
Diovan HCT Tablets 2216
Dyazide Capsules 1405
Furosemide Tablets 2186
Indapamide Tablets 2188
Intravenous Sodium Diuril 2490
Micardis HCT Tablets 854
Prinzide Tablets 2092
Teveten HCT Tablets 517

Necrotizing cellulitis
Amevive 611

Neonatal morbidity
Aceon Tablets (2 mg, 4 mg, 8 mg) 3038
Avalide Tablets 892
Avalide Tablets 2713
Avapro Tablets 897
Avapro Tablets 2718
Captopril Tablets 2182
Cozaar Tablets 1973
Exforge Tablets 2238
Mavik Tablets 472
Prinivil Tablets 2087
Prinzide Tablets 2092
Tekturna HCT Tablets 2324

Neonatal prematurity
Captopril Tablets 2182
Cozaar Tablets 1973
Prinivil Tablets 2087
Prinzide Tablets 2092

Neoplasia, gastrointestinal
Emsam Transdermal System (Rare) 905

Neoplasia, hepatic
Lybrel Tablets 3204
Mirapex Tablets 857

Neoplasm
(*see under* Carcinoma, unspecified)

Neoplasm, abdominal
Mirapex Tablets 857
Selzentry Tablets 2534

Neoplasm, bladder
Lyrica Capsules (Rare) 2527

Neoplasm, brain, benign
Requip Tablets (Infrequent) 1561

Neoplasm, breast
Ambien Tablets (Rare) 2692
Ambien CR Tablets (Rare) 2696
▲ Arimidex Tablets (5%) 672
Brovana Inhalation Solution (Less than 2%) 2990
Emsam Transdermal System (Infrequent) 905
Lamictal (Rare) 1488
Lunesta Tablets (Infrequent) 2994
Mirapex Tablets 857
Protopic Ointment (0.2% to less than 1%) 628

Neoplasm, breast malignant
Evoxac Capsules (Less than 1%) 1013
Symbyax Capsules (Infrequent) 1871
Xolair (0.5%) 1235
Xolair 2339

Neoplasm, hepatic, malignant
Mirapex Tablets 857

Neoplasm, laryngeal, malignant
Requip Tablets (Infrequent) 1561

Neoplasm, malignant
Estratest Tablets 3043
Estratest H.S. Tablets 3043
Orthoclone OKT3 Sterile Solution 2387

Neoplasm, malignant, aggravated
▲ Zometa for Intravenous Infusion (20%) 2341

Neoplasm, oral, benign
Mirapex Tablets 857

Neoplasm, ovarian
Follistim AQ Cartridge (Infrequent) 2844

Neoplasm, parotid, malignant
Xolair 1235
Xolair 2339

Neoplasm, prostate
Mirapex Tablets 857

Neoplasm, prostatic malignant
Xolair (0.5%) 1235
Xolair 2339

Neoplasm, renal
Mirapex Tablets 857

Neoplasm, skin
Mirapex Tablets 857

Neoplasm, skin, benign
▲ CellCept Capsules (3% to less than 20%) 2622
▲ CellCept Intravenous (3% to less than 20%) 2622
▲ CellCept Oral Suspension (3% to less than 20%) 2622
▲ CellCept Tablets (3% to less than 20%) 2622
Emsam Transdermal System (Infrequent) 905
Humatrope Vials and Cartridges 1838
Selzentry Tablets (2.6%) 2534

Neoplasm, thyroid
Mirapex Tablets 857

Neoplasm, unspecified
▲ Arimidex Tablets (5%) 672
▲ CellCept Capsules (3% to less than 20%) 2622
▲ CellCept Intravenous (3% to less than 20%) 2622
▲ CellCept Oral Suspension (3% to less than 20%) 2622
▲ CellCept Tablets (3% to less than 20%) 2622
Protopic Ointment (0.2% to less than 1%) 628

Neoplasm, urogenital
Zomig Tablets (Rare) 694

Zomig Nasal Spray (Rare) ... 689
Zomig-ZMT Tablets (Rare) ... 694

Neoplasms, hepatic

Delatestryl Injection ... 1730
Estratest Tablets (Rare) ... 3043
Estratest H.S. Tablets (Rare) ... 3043
Ortho-Cyclen/Ortho Tri-Cyclen ... 2449
Ortho Tri-Cyclen Lo Tablets ... 2458
Zomig Tablets (Rare) ... 694
Zomig Nasal Spray (Rare) ... 689
Zomig-ZMT Tablets (Rare) ... 694

Nephritis

Aceon Tablets (2 mg, 4 mg, 8 mg) ... 3038
Capastat Sulfate for Injection (1 patient) ... 1791
Cipro I.V. (1% or less) ... 2817
Cipro (Less than 1%) ... 2810
Cipro XR Tablets ... 2823
Depakote ER Tablets ... 423
Gantrisin Pediatric Suspension ... 2638
Kaletra (Less than 2%) ... 452
Lipitor Tablets (Less than 2%) ... 2501
Lyrica Capsules (0.1% to 1%) ... 2527
Paxil (Rare) ... 1535
Paxil CR Controlled-Release Tablets (Rare) ... 1544
Rilutek Tablets (Rare) ... 2771
Truvada Tablets ... 1262

Nephritis, interstitial

Aciphex Tablets ... 1053
Aggrenox Capsules ... 819
Anaprox Tablets (Less than 1%) ... 2632
Anaprox DS Tablets (Less than 1%) ... 2632
Asacol Delayed-Release Tablets ... 2579
Atacand HCT ... 642
Atripla Tablets ... 938
Augmentin (Rare) ... 1323
Augmentin Tablets (Rare) ... 1327
Augmentin XR Extended Release Tablets (Rare) ... 1333
Augmentin ES-600 Powder for Oral Suspension (Rare) ... 1329
Avalide Tablets ... 892
Avalide Tablets ... 2713
Avelox ... 2803
Bayer Aspirin ... 750
Biaxin/Biaxin XL ... 411
Captopril Tablets ... 2182
Celebrex Capsules (Less than 0.1%) ... 2979
Cipro I.V. (1% or less) ... 2817
Cipro (Less than 1%) ... 2810
Cipro XR Tablets ... 2823
Clinoril Tablets (Less than 1 in 100) ... 1962
Crixivan Capsules ... 1979
Diovan HCT Tablets ... 2216
Dyazide Capsules ... 1405
Dyrenium Capsules (Rare) ... 3189
EC-Naprosyn Delayed-Release Tablets (Less than 1%) ... 2632
Eloxatin for Injection ... 2731
Fansidar Tablets ... 2636
Furosemide Tablets ... 2186
Indocin (Less than 1%) ... 2024
Intravenous Sodium Diuril ... 2490
Levaquin ... 2416
Levaquin in 5% Dextrose Injection ... 2416
Meridia Capsules (One patient) ... 475
Micardis HCT Tablets ... 854
Mobic Oral Suspension (Less than 0.1%) ... 863
Mobic Tablets (Less than 0.1%) ... 863
Nalfon Capsules (Less than 1%) ... 2508
Naprosyn Suspension (Less than 1%) ... 2632
Naprosyn Tablets (Less than 1%) ... 2632
Nexium Delayed-Release Capsules ... 645
Nexium I.V. ... 652
Nexium Delayed-Release Oral Suspension ... 645
Noroxin Tablets ... 2069
Orthoclone OKT3 Sterile Solution ... 2387
PegIntron Powder for Injection (Less than or equal to 1%) ... 2903
Pentasa Capsules (Infrequent) ... 3030
Percocet Tablets ... 1127
Percodan Tablets ... 1130
Prinzide Tablets ... 2092
Protonix for Delayed-Release Oral Suspension ... 3254
Protonix Delayed-Release Tablets ... 3254
Protonix I.V. ... 3257
St. Joseph 81 mg Aspirin Chewable and Enteric Coated Tablets ... 1903
Tekturna HCT Tablets ... 2324
Teveten HCT Tablets ... 517
Truvada Tablets ... 1262
Voltaren Tablets (Occasionally) ... 2334
Voltaren-XR Tablets (Occasionally) ... 2337
Zinacef for Injection (Rare) ... 1678
Zinacef Injection (Rare) ... 1678
Zosyn for Injection (Rare) ... 3284

Nephrocalcinosis

Fleet Phospho-soda ... 1145
Fleet Phospho-soda EZ-PREP ... 1147
Fleet Prep Kits ... 1149
OsmoPrep Tablets ... 2680
Rocaltrol Capsules ... 1150
Rocaltrol Oral Solution ... 1150

Nephrolithiasis

Celebrex Capsules (0.1% to 1.9%) ... 2979
Celexa (Rare) ... 1160
Chantix Tablets (Infrequent) ... 2511
Cipro I.V. (1% or less) ... 2817
Clinoril Tablets ... 1962
Copaxone for Injection (Infrequent) ... 3110
▲ Crixivan Capsules (8.7% to 12.4%) ... 1979
Dyazide Capsules ... 1405
Dyrenium Capsules (Rare) ... 3189
Effexor XR Extended-Release Capsules (Infrequent) ... 3195
Emsam Transdermal System (Infrequent) ... 905
Evoxac Capsules (Less than 1%) ... 1013
Exelon Capsules (Infrequent) ... 2229
Exelon Oral Solution (Infrequent) ... 2229
Exforge Tablets (Greater than or equal to 0.2%) ... 2238
▲ Humira Injection (Less than 5%) ... 442
Imitrex Injection (Rare) ... 1465
Imitrex Nasal Spray ... 1470
Imitrex Tablets ... 1474
Ixempra Kit for Injection ... 915
Kaletra (Less than 2%) ... 452
Lexapro Oral Suspension (Infrequent) ... 1174
Lexapro Tablets (Infrequent) ... 1174
Lipitor Tablets (Less than 2%) ... 2501
Lunesta Tablets (Infrequent) ... 2994
Miacalcin Nasal Spray (Less than 1%) ... 2274
Mirapex Tablets ... 857
Norvir (Less than 2%) ... 489
Paxil (Rare) ... 1535
Paxil CR Controlled-Release Tablets (Rare) ... 1544
Protonix for Delayed-Release Oral Suspension (Less than 1%) ... 3254
Protonix Delayed-Release Tablets (Less than 1%) ... 3254
Protonix I.V. (Less than 1%) ... 3257
Remeron Tablets (Infrequent) ... 2924
RemeronSolTab Tablets (Infrequent) ... 2927
Remicade for IV Injection (Greater than or equal to 0.2%) ... 950
Requip Tablets (Infrequent) ... 1561
Reyataz Capsules ... 3299
Rilutek Tablets (Infrequent) ... 2771
Rocephin Injectable Vials, ADD-Vantage, Galaxy, Bulk (Less than 0.1%) ... 2642
Sandostatin Injection (Less than 1%) ... 2300
Sustiva Capsules (Up to 1%) ... 930
Sustiva Tablets (Up to 1%) ... 930
Symbyax Capsules (Rare) ... 1871
Teveten Tablets (Less than 1%) ... 515
Teveten HCT Tablets (Less than 1%) ... 517
Treximet Tablets (Infrequent) ... 1616
Tricor Tablets ... 520
Zonegran Capsules (Rare) ... 1089

Nephropathy

AmBisome for Injection (Less common) ... 606
Asacol Delayed-Release Tablets ... 2579
Bicillin C-R Injectable Suspension ... 1775
Bicillin L-A Injection ... 1777
Ceftin ... 1380
Fortaz ... 1450
Isentress Tablets ... 2036
Omnicef Capsules ... 497
Omnicef for Oral Suspension ... 497
Suprax for Oral Suspension ... 1891
Suprax Tablets ... 1891
Zinacef for Injection ... 1678
Zinacef Injection ... 1678

Nephropathy, proximal tubular

Flebogamma 5% ... 1715
Flebogamma 5% DIF ... 1718
Gammagard S/D ... 734

Nephropathy, toxic

Rocephin Injectable Vials, ADD-Vantage, Galaxy, Bulk ... 2642

Nephrosis, osmotic

Flebogamma 5% ... 1715
Flebogamma 5% DIF ... 1718
Gammagard S/D ... 734

Nephrosis, toxic

Evoxac Capsules (Less than 1%) ... 1013
Fansidar Tablets ... 2636
Gantrisin Pediatric Suspension ... 2638

Nephrosis, unspecified

Nalfon Capsules (Less than 1%) ... 2508

Nephrotic syndrome

Anaprox Tablets (Less than 1%) ... 2632
Anaprox DS Tablets (Less than 1%) ... 2632
Avastin IV ... 1192
Captopril Tablets (Approximately 1 to 2 of 1000 patients) ... 2182
Cimzia ... 3127
Clinoril Tablets (Less than 1 in 100) ... 1962
Cuprimine Capsules ... 1986
Dapsone Tablets USP ... 1746
EC-Naprosyn Delayed-Release Tablets (Less than 1%) ... 2632
Indocin (Less than 1%) ... 2024
Intron A for Injection ... 2859
Naprosyn Suspension (Less than 1%) ... 2632
Naprosyn Tablets (Less than 1%) ... 2632
Pentasa Capsules (Infrequent) ... 3030
Rapamune (2.2%) ... 3260
Rythmol Tablets (Less than 1%) ... 1586
Sutent Capsules (Rare) ... 2540

Nephrotic syndrome, reversible

Proglycem Capsules (Infrequent) ... 1185
Proglycem Suspension (Infrequent) ... 1185

Nephrotoxicity

Canasa Rectal Suppositories ... 705
Cancidas for Injection (2.6%) ... 1953
Capastat Sulfate for Injection ... 1791
Flector Patch ... 561
▲ Gengraf Capsules (25% to 38%) ... 435
Hepsera Tablets ... 1253
Leustatin Injection ... 2384
Levaquin ... 2416
Levaquin in 5% Dextrose Injection ... 2416
▲ Neoral Oral Solution (25% to 38%) ... 2280
▲ Neoral Soft Gelatin Capsules (25% to 38%) ... 2280
▲ Prograf Capsules and Injection (36% to 52%) ... 622
Rituxan I.V. ... 1223
▲ Sandimmune (25% to 38%) ... 2296
Vicoprofen Tablets ... 533
Zinacef for Injection ... 1678
Zinacef Injection ... 1678

Nerve compression, unspecified

Norditropin Cartridges ... 2354

Nerve deafness

M-M-R II ... 2054
Mumpsvax ... 2068

Nerve paralysis

Arranon Injection (1%) ... 1319

Nerve syndromes, compressed

Amerge Tablets (Rare) ... 1301
Norditropin Cartridges ... 2354

Nervous system disorders, unspecified

▲ Arranon Injection (0% to 4%) ... 1319
▲ Cancidas for Injection (13% to 25.4%) ... 1953
Flector Patch (1%) ... 561
▲ Focalin XR Capsules (30% to 50%) ... 2251
▲ Hycamtin for Injection (35%) ... 1459
▲ Mycamine for Injection (10.5% to 61.4%) ... 616
▲ Somatuline Depot Injection (19% to 20%) ... 3102
Verdeso Foam (2%) ... 3069

Nervousness

Accutane Capsules ... 2607
Aceon Tablets (2 mg, 4 mg, 8 mg) (1.1%) ... 3038
Actiq (1% to 2%) ... 959
Activella Tablets ... 2347
▲ Adderall XR Capsules (6%) ... 3012
Adenoscan (2%) ... 605
▲ Aerobid/Aerobid-M (3% to 9%) ... 1153
▲ Agrylin Capsules (1% to less than 5%) ... 3017
Alferon N Injection (1%) ... 1726
Allegra Oral Solution (Less than 1%) ... 2684
Allegra Tablets (Rare) ... 2684
Allegra-D 12 Hour Extended-Release Tablets (1.4%) ... 2687
Allegra-D 24 Hour Extended-Release Tablets (1.4%) ... 2690
Ambien Tablets (Infrequent) ... 2692
Ambien CR Tablets (Infrequent) ... 2696
AmBisome for Injection (Less common) ... 606
Anaprox Tablets (Less than 1%) ... 2632
Anaprox DS Tablets (Less than 1%) ... 2632
▲ AndroGel (0% to 3%) ... 3159
Angeliq Tablets ... 751
▲ Angiomax for Injection (5%) ... 1933
▲ Aricept Tablets (3%) ... 1062
▲ Aricept ODT Tablets (3%) ... 1062
▲ Arimidex Tablets (2% to 5%) ... 672
Asacol Delayed-Release Tablets (2% or greater) ... 2579
Atripla Tablets (Greater than or equal to 2%) ... 938
Avalide Tablets (1% or greater) ... 892
Avalide Tablets (1% or greater) ... 2713
Avapro Tablets (1% or greater) ... 897
Avapro Tablets (1% or greater) ... 2718
Avelox (Greater than or equal to 0.1% to less than 2%) ... 2803
▲ Avinza Capsules (Less than 5%) ... 1772
Axert Tablets (Rare) ... 2431
Axid Capsules (1.1%) ... 1364
▲ Bentyl Capsules (6%) ... 703
▲ Bentyl Injection (6%) ... 703
▲ Bentyl Syrup (6%) ... 703
▲ Bentyl Tablets (6%) ... 703
▲ Betaseron for SC Injection (7%) ... 756
Bicillin C-R Injectable Suspension ... 1775
Bicillin L-A Injection ... 1777
Brovana Inhalation Solution ... 2990
Captopril Tablets ... 2182
Cardizem LA Extended Release Tablets (Less than 2%) ... 421
Catapres Tablets (About 3 in 100 patients) ... 841
Catapres-TTS (1 of 101 patients) ... 842
Celebrex Capsules (0.1% to 1.9%) ... 2979
▲ CellCept Capsules (3% to less than 20%) ... 2622
▲ CellCept Intravenous (3% to less than 20%) ... 2622
▲ CellCept Oral Suspension (3% to less than 20%) ... 2622
▲ CellCept Tablets (3% to less than 20%) ... 2622
Cipro I.V. ... 2817
Cipro ... 2810
Clarinex-D 24-Hour Extended-Release Tablets (2%) ... 2834
Climara Transdermal System ... 763
Climara Pro Transdermal System ... 768
Clinoril Tablets (Greater than 1%) ... 1962
▲ Clorpres Tablets (About 3%) ... 2185
Combigan Ophthalmic Solution ... 553
Combivent Inhalation Aerosol (Less than 2%) ... 845
▲ Concerta Extended-Release Tablets (0.7% to 3.1%) ... 1925
Copaxone for Injection (2%) ... 3110
Coreg Tablets (Greater than 0.1% to 1%) ... 1387
Coreg CR Extended-Release Capsules (0.1% to less than or equal to 1%) ... 1393
Cosopt Sterile Ophthalmic Solution ... 1969
▲ Cozaar Tablets (Less than 1% to 4%) ... 1973
▲ Crinone 8% Gel (16%) ... 992
▲ Cymbalta Delayed-Release Capsules (5%) ... 1801
Dantrium Capsules (Less frequent) ... 2580
Daytrana Transdermal Patch ... 3022
Demadex Injection (1.1%) ... 2630
Demadex Tablets (1.1%) ... 2630
▲ Depakote ER Tablets (Greater than 1% to 11%) ... 423
Divigel ... 3167
Donnatal Extentabs ... 2507
Doxil Injection (Less than 1%) ... 2378
▲ Duragesic Transdermal System (3% to 10%) ... 2405
DynaCirc CR Controlled Release Tablets (0.5% to 1%) ... 1407
EC-Naprosyn Delayed-Release Tablets (Less than 1%) ... 2632
▲ Effexor XR Extended-Release Capsules (3% to 10%) ... 3195
Eldepryl Capsules ... 3052
▲ Eloxatin for Injection (2% to less than 5%) ... 2731

Emsam Transdermal System 905
Enjuvia Tablets 1029
EpiPen Jr. Auto-Injector 1024
▲ Equetro Extended-Release Capsules (Less than 5%) 3174
Estratest Tablets 3043
Estratest H.S. Tablets 3043
Exelon Capsules (2% or more) 2229
Exelon Oral Solution (2% or more) 2229
Exforge Tablets (Greater than 0.1% to less than 1%) 2238
Fansidar Tablets 2636
Fentora Tablets (Greater than 1%) 968
▲ Flolan for Injection (7% to 21%) 1426
Flumadine (1.3% to 2.1%) 1167
Focalin XR Capsules 2251
Foradil Aerolizer 2849
Frova Tablets (Infrequent) 1111
▲ Gabitril Tablets (10%) 973
Gengraf Capsules (1% to less than 3%) 435
▲ Indapamide Tablets (Less than 5%) 2188
Indocin (Less than 1%) 2024
Intelence Tablets (Less than 2%) 3119
▲ Intron A for Injection (Up to 3%) 2859
Invanz for Injection (Greater than 0.1%) 2029
Ionsys Transdermal System (.1% to less than 1%) 2410
Kaletra (Less than 2%) 452
▲ Keppra Injection (1.7% to 4%) 3137
▲ Keppra Oral Solution (4% to 10%) 3131
▲ Keppra Tablets (4% to 10%) 3131
▲ Klonopin (1% to 3%) 2639
Lamictal (2%) 1488
Levothroid Tablets 1170
Levoxyl Tablets 1780
Lexapro Oral Suspension (Infrequent) 1174
Lexapro Tablets (Infrequent) 1174
Lidoderm Patch 1114
▲ Lunesta Tablets (0% to 5%) 2994
▲ Lupron Depot 3.75 mg (4%) 462
▲ Lupron Depot–3 Month 11.25 mg (4%) 462
Lupron Depot-PED 7.5 mg, 11.25 mg and 15 mg (Less than 2%) 471
▲ Luvox CR Extended-Release Capsules (2% to 10%) 1759
Lybrel Tablets 3204
Lyrica Capsules (1% to greater than or equal to 2%) 2527
Marinol Capsules (Greater than 1%) 3163
▲ Maxair Autohaler (4.5% to 6.9%) 1705
Maxalt Tablets (Infrequent) 2056
Maxalt-MLT Orally Disintegrating Tablets (Infrequent) 2056
▲ Meridia Capsules (5.2%) 475
Merrem I.V. (Greater than 0.1% to 1%) 684
Metadate CD Capsules (Among most common) 3146
Micardis Tablets (Greater than 0.3%) 852
Micardis HCT Tablets 854
Mirapex Tablets (1% or more) 857
Mircette Tablets 1034
▲ Mirena Intrauterine System (5% or more) 779
Mobic Oral Suspension (Less than 2%) 863
Mobic Tablets (Less than 2%) 863
MS Contin Tablets (Less frequent) 2585
▲ Nalfon Capsules (5.7%) 2508
Namenda (Infrequent) 1180
Naprosyn Suspension (Less than 1%) 2632
Naprosyn Tablets (Less than 1%) 2632
Nembutal Sodium Solution, USP (Less than 1%) 2494
Neoral Oral Solution (1% to less than 3%) 2280
Neoral Soft Gelatin Capsules (1% to less than 3%) 2280
Nexium Delayed-Release Capsules (Less than 1%) 645
Nexium I.V. (Less than 1%) 652
Nexium Delayed-Release Oral Suspension (Less than 1%) 645
Niaspan Extended-Release Tablets 480
Norvir (Less than 2%) 489
NuvaRing 2897
▲ Ontak Vials (11%) 1079
Opana Tablets (Less than 1%) 1117
Opana ER Tablets (Less than 1%) 1121
OptiPranolol Metipranolol Ophthalmic Solution 0.3% (A small number of patients) ⊙ 245
Ortho-Cyclen Tablets 2449
Ortho Evra Transdermal System 2437
Ortho Tri-Cyclen Tablets 2449
Ortho Tri-Cyclen Lo Tablets 2458
▲ OxyContin Tablets (Between 1% and 5%) 2589
▲ Paxil (4% to 9%) 1535
▲ Paxil CR Controlled-Release Tablets (4% to 9%) 1544
▲ PegIntron Powder for Injection (4%) 2903
Percocet Tablets 1127
Percodan Tablets 1130
Perforomist Inhalation Solution 1025
Phenytek Capsules 2192
Premarin Intravenous 3217
▲ Premarin Tablets (2% to 5%) 3221
Premarin Vaginal Cream 3228
▲ Premphase Tablets (2% to 3%) 3232
▲ Prempro Tablets (2% to 3%) 3232
Prinivil Tablets (0.3% to 1%) 2087
Prinzide Tablets 2092
Pristiq Extended-Release Tablets (Less than 1% to 2%) 3247
ProAir HFA Inhalation Aerosol (Frequent) 3113
ProAmatine Tablets (Less frequent) 3032
▲ Prograf Capsules and Injection (3%) 622
Prometrium Capsules (100 mg, 200 mg) 3047
ProQuad 2099
Protonix for Delayed-Release Oral Suspension (Less than 1%) 3254
Protonix Delayed-Release Tablets (Less than 1%) 3254
Protonix I.V. (Less than 1%) 3257
▲ Proventil HFA Inhalation Aerosol (7%) 2914
▲ Provigil Tablets (7%) 977
▲ Prozac Weekly Capsules (1% to 16%) 1852
▲ Prozac Pulvules and Liquid (8% to 16%) 1852
▲ Rebetol (3% to 6%) 2917
Requip Tablets (Infrequent to greater than or equal to 1%) 1561
Retrovir Capsules (1.6%) 1574
Retrovir IV Infusion (2%) 1579
Retrovir (1.6%) 1574
Risperdal Consta Long-Acting Injection (Frequent) 1753
▲ Romazicon Injection (3% to 9%) 2646
Salagen Tablets (Less than 1%) 1082
Seasonique Tablets 1046
Skelaxin Tablets (Most frequent) 1784
Stalevo Tablets 2309
▲ Suboxone Tablets (6%) 2601
▲ Subutex Tablets (6%) 2601
Sular Extended Release Tablets (Less than or equal to 1%) 2975
▲ Sustiva Capsules (1% to 7%) 930
▲ Sustiva Tablets (1% to 7%) 930
Synagis Intramuscular Solution (More than 1%) 1948
Teveten Tablets (Less than 1%) 515
Teveten HCT Tablets (Less than 1%) 517
Timoptic Sterile Ophthalmic Solution (Less frequent) 2121
Timoptic in Ocudose (Less frequent) 2124
Timoptic-XE Sterile Ophthalmic Gel Forming Solution 2125
Toprol-XL Tablets 666
Treximet Tablets (Infrequent) 1616
Tricor Tablets 520
▲ Trizivir Tablets (Greater than or equal to 5%) 1622
Tylenol Cold Severe Congestion Daytime Caplets with Cool Burst 1912
Tylenol Sinus Congestion & Pain Daytime Caplets with Cool Burst and Gelcaps 1917
Tylenol Sinus Congestion & Pain Nighttime Caplets with Cool Burst 1917
Tylenol Sinus Congestion & Pain Severe Caplets with Cool Burst 1917
Tylenol Sinus Severe Congestion Caplets with Cool Burst 1917
Ultane Liquid for Inhalation (Less than 1%) 524
▲ Ultram ER Extended-Release Tablets (1% to less than 5%) 2428
Varivax (Greater than or equal to 1%) 2133
▲ Venlafaxine Hydrochloride Tablets (2% to 21.3%) 2199
▲ Vicoprofen Tablets (3% to 9%) 533
▲ Vivitrol (8% to 12%) 988
Voltaren Tablets (Occasionally) 2334
Voltaren-XR Tablets (Occasionally) 2337
Wellbutrin Tablets 1648
▲ Wellbutrin SR Sustained-Release Tablets (3% to 5%) 1653
▲ Wellbutrin XL Extended-Release Tablets (3% to 5%) 1659
▲ Xopenex Inhalation Solution (2.8% to 9.6%) 3001
▲ Xopenex Inhalation Solution Concentrate (2.8% to 9.6%) 3005
▲ Xopenex HFA Inhalation Aerosol (2.8% to 9.6%) 3009
Xyrem Oral Solution (Frequent) 1766
Yaz Tablets 805
Zomig Tablets (Infrequent) 694
Zomig Nasal Spray (Infrequent) 689
Zomig-ZMT Tablets (Infrequent) 694
Zonegran Capsules (2%) 1089
▲ Zyban Sustained-Release Tablets (4%) 1692
▲ Zyprexa Tablets (16%) 1883
Zyprexa IntraMuscular 1883
▲ Zyprexa ZYDIS Orally Disintegrating Tablets (16%) 1883
Zyrtec Chewable Tablets (Less than 2%) 1920
Zyrtec Syrup (Less than 2%) 1920
Zyrtec Tablets (Less than 2%) 1920
Zyrtec-D 12 Hour Extended Release Tablets 1923
Zyrtec-D Allergy & Congestion Extended-Release Tablets 1923

Neuralgia

▲ Actonel with Calcium Tablets (3.8%) 2574
Ambien Tablets (Rare) 2692
Ambien CR Tablets (Rare) 2696
Amerge Tablets (Rare) 1301
Aricept Tablets (Infrequent) 1062
Aricept ODT Tablets (Infrequent) 1062
Azilect Tablets (Rare) 3106
Campral Tablets (Infrequent) 1158
Celebrex Capsules (0.1% to 1.9%) 2979
Celexa (Infrequent) 1160
Coreg Tablets (Less than or equal to 0.1%) 1387
Coreg CR Extended-Release Capsules (Less than or equal to 0.1%) 1393
▲ Doxil Injection (1% to 10%) 2378
Effexor XR Extended-Release Capsules (Infrequent) 3195
▲ Eloxatin for Injection (0% to 5%) 2731
Evoxac Capsules (Less than 1%) 1013
Exelon Capsules (Infrequent) 2229
Exelon Oral Solution (Infrequent) 2229
Imitrex Injection 1465
Imitrex Nasal Spray (Infrequent) 1470
Imitrex Tablets (Rare) 1474
▲ Intron A for Injection (Less than 5%) 2859
▲ Ixempra Kit for Injection (62%) 915
Lamictal (Rare) 1488
▲ Lunesta Tablets (0% to 3%) 2994
Luvox CR Extended-Release Capsules (Infrequent) 1759
Lyrica Capsules (0.1% to 1%) 2527
Miacalcin Nasal Spray (Less than 1%) 2274
Mirapex Tablets 857
Namenda (Infrequent) 1180
Neupro Transdermal System 3149
Norvir (Less than 2%) 489
Paxil (Rare) 1535
Paxil CR Controlled-Release Tablets (Rare) 1544
Plavix Tablets (1% to 2.5%) 926
Plavix Tablets (1% to 2.5%) 2767
Pletal Tablets (Less than 2%) 2481
Proleukin for Injection 2287
Protonix for Delayed-Release Oral Suspension (Less than 1%) 3254
Protonix Delayed-Release Tablets (Less than 1%) 3254
Protonix I.V. (Less than 1%) 3257
Prozac Weekly Capsules (Infrequent) 1852
Prozac Pulvules and Liquid (Infrequent) 1852
Requip Tablets (Infrequent to frequent) 1561
Sustiva Capsules (Less than 2%) 930
Sustiva Tablets (Less than 2%) 930
Symbyax Capsules (Infrequent) 1871
Tricor Tablets 520
▲ Velcade for Injection (36%) 2168
Venlafaxine Hydrochloride Tablets (Infrequent) 2199
Vicoprofen Tablets (Less than 1%) 533
Wellbutrin SR Sustained-Release Tablets 1653
Wellbutrin XL Extended-Release Tablets 1659
Zyban Sustained-Release Tablets 1692
Zyprexa Tablets (Rare) 1883
Zyprexa ZYDIS Orally Disintegrating Tablets (Rare) 1883

Neuralgia, trigeminal

Nalfon Capsules (Less than 1%) 2508

Neuritis

Ambien Tablets (Rare) 2692
Ambien CR Tablets (Rare) 2696
Amerge Tablets (Rare) 1301
Azilect Tablets (Infrequent) 3106
Clinoril Tablets (Rare) 1962
Effexor XR Extended-Release Capsules (Rare) 3195
Fluarix Vaccine 1446
Fluorescite Injection ⊙ 203
Gabitril Tablets (Infrequent) 973
Infanrix Vaccine 1479
▲ Intron A for Injection (Less than 5%) 2859
▲ Ixempra Kit for Injection (62%) 915
Lunesta Tablets (Rare) 2994
Marplan Tablets 3177
Proleukin for Injection 2287
Protonix for Delayed-Release Oral Suspension (Less than 1%) 3254
Protonix Delayed-Release Tablets (Less than 1%) 3254
Protonix I.V. (Less than 1%) 3257
Protopic Ointment (Greater than or equal to 1%) 628
Prozac Weekly Capsules (Rare) 1852
Prozac Pulvules and Liquid (Rare) 1852
Remicade for IV Injection (Greater than or equal to 0.2%) 950
Sandostatin Injection (Less than 1%) 2300
Soriatane Capsules (Less than 1%) 3062
Teveten Tablets (Less than 1%) 515
Teveten HCT Tablets (Less than 1%) 517
Venlafaxine Hydrochloride Tablets (Rare) 2199

Neuritis, brachial

Boostrix 1377
Pediarix Vaccine 1552
Pentacel 2792

Neuritis, optic

Accutane Capsules 2607
Attenuvax 1951
Cimzia (Rare) 3127
Copaxone for Injection (Infrequent) 3110
Cuprimine Capsules 1986
▲ Doxil Injection (1% to 5%) 2378
Elmiron Capsules (Less than or equal to 1%) 2435
Eloxatin for Injection 2731
Enbrel for Injection 569
Engerix-B Vaccine 1409
Estratest Tablets 3043
Estratest H.S. Tablets 3043
Fluarix Vaccine 1446
Flulaval Injection Vaccine 1448
Intron A for Injection 2859
Lybrel Tablets 3204
Meruvax II 2061
M-M-R II (Infrequent) 2054
Mumpsvax 2068
Nalfon Capsules (Less than 1%) 2508
Ortho Evra Transdermal System 2437
Paser Granules 1747
Paxil 1535
Paxil CR Controlled-Release Tablets 1544
PegIntron Powder for Injection (Less than or equal to 1%) 2903
Premarin Intravenous 3217
Premarin Vaginal Cream 3228
Premphase Tablets 3232
Prempro Tablets 3232
Proleukin for Injection 2287
ProQuad 2099
Prozac Weekly Capsules 1852
Prozac Pulvules and Liquid 1852
Recombivax HB 2107
Remicade for IV Injection (Rare) 950
Rituxan I.V. 1223
Seasonique Tablets 1046
Tasigna Capsules 2316
Twinrix Vaccine 1628
Yaz Tablets 805

Neuritis, peripheral

▲ Atripla Tablets (Greater than or equal to 5%) 938
Carbatrol Capsules 3019
▲ Doxil Injection (1% to 10%) 2378
▲ Emtriva Capsules (4%) 1246
▲ Emtriva Oral Solution (4%) 1246
Equetro Extended-Release Capsules 3174

Fansidar Tablets 2636
Gabitril Tablets (Infrequent) 973
Gantrisin Pediatric Suspension 2638
Herceptin I.V. (2%) 1199
Kaletra (Less than 2%) 452
Lamictal (Rare) 1488
Lyrica Capsules (Rare) 2527
Paxil (Rare) 1535
Paxil CR Controlled-Release Tablets (Rare) 1544
Rilutek Tablets (Rare) 2771
▲ Truvada Tablets (Greater than or equal to 5%) 1262
▲ Viread Tablets (1% to 5%) 1268
Zonegran Capsules (Infrequent) 1089

Neuritis, retrobulbar
Anaprox Tablets (Less than 1%) 2632
Anaprox DS Tablets (Less than 1%) 2632
Attenuvax 1951
EC-Naprosyn Delayed-Release Tablets (Less than 1%) 2632
Meruvax II 2061
M-M-R II 2054
Mumpsvax (Infrequent) 2068
Naprosyn Suspension (Less than 1%) 2632
Naprosyn Tablets (Less than 1%) 2632
ProQuad 2099

Neuro-cortical, unspecified
▲ Taxotere Injection Concentrate (0.5% to 5.1%) 2773

Neurodermatitis
Abilify Injection (Greater than or equal to 1 in 100 patients) 2466
Abilify Oral Solution (Greater than or equal to 1 in 100 patients) 881
Abilify Oral Solution (Greater than or equal to 1 in 100 patients) 2466
Abilify Discmelt Orally Disintegrating Tablets (Greater than or equal to 1 in 100 patients) 881
Abilify Discmelt Orally Disintegrating Tablets (Greater than or equal to 1 in 100 patients) 2466
Abilify Tablets (Greater than or equal to 1 in 100 patients) 881
Abilify Tablets (Greater than or equal to 1 in 100 patients) 2466
Aricept Tablets (Infrequent) 1062
Aricept ODT Tablets (Infrequent) 1062

Neuroleptic malignant syndrome
Abilify Injection 881
Abilify Injection 2466
Abilify Oral Solution 881
Abilify Oral Solution 2466
Abilify Discmelt Orally Disintegrating Tablets 881
Abilify Discmelt Orally Disintegrating Tablets 2466
Abilify Tablets 881
Abilify Tablets 2466
Celexa 1160
Comtan Tablets 2208
Concerta Extended-Release Tablets (Very rare) 1925
Daytrana Transdermal Patch 3022
Effexor XR Extended-Release Capsules 3195
Focalin XR Capsules 2251
Geodon (Rare) 2520
Invega Extended-Release Tablets 1748
Lexapro Oral Suspension 1174
Lexapro Tablets 1174
Metadate CD Capsules (Very rare) 3146
Moban Tablets 1116
Namenda 1180
Neupro Transdermal System 3149
Paxil 1535
Paxil CR Controlled-Release Tablets 1544
Prozac Weekly Capsules (Rare) 1852
Prozac Pulvules and Liquid (Rare) 1852
Risperdal Consta Long-Acting Injection (Rare) 1753
Stalevo Tablets 2309
Symbyax Capsules 1871
Thioridazine Hydrochloride Tablets 2195
Thiothixene Capsules 2197
Venlafaxine Hydrochloride Tablets 2199
Zyprexa Tablets 1883
Zyprexa IntraMuscular 1883
Zyprexa ZYDIS Orally Disintegrating Tablets 1883

Neurological disability, unspecified
Abelcet Injection 1134
▲ Cipro (3%) 2810
Malarone Pediatric Tablets 1521
Malarone Tablets 1521
Proleukin for Injection 2287
Tice BCG (Less than or equal to 1%) 2936

Neuroma
Mirapex Tablets 857

Neuromotor, unspecified
▲ Novantrone for Injection Concentrate (7%) 1100
▲ Taxotere Injection Concentrate (0.4% to 19%) 2773

Neuromuscular block, inadequate
Nimbex Injection 484

Neuromuscular block, prolonged
Nimbex Injection 484
Zemuron Injection 2947

Neuromuscular blockade
Capastat Sulfate for Injection 1791

Neuromuscular disorders, unspecified
Lupron Depot 3.75 mg (1%) 462
▲ Lupron Depot 7.5 mg (Less than 5%) 469
Lupron Depot–3 Month 11.25 mg (1%) 462
Pristiq Extended-Release Tablets 3247

Neuromuscular excitability
Fortaz 1450
Zosyn for Injection 3284

Neuromuscular toxicity
▲ Ixempra Kit for Injection (10%) 915

Neuropathy
Accolate Tablets (Rare) 669
Actiq (Less than 1%) 959
Advair Diskus 100/50 1276
Advair Diskus 250/50 1276
Advair Diskus 500/50 1276
▲ Alimta for Injection (Up to 29%) 1786
Ambien Tablets (Rare) 2692
Ambien CR Tablets (Rare) 2696
▲ Arranon Injection (0% to 4%) 1319
▲ Atripla Tablets (Greater than or equal to 5%) 938
Axert Tablets (Rare) 2431
Azilect Tablets (Frequent) 3106
Bicillin C-R Injectable Suspension 1775
Bicillin L-A Injection 1777
Celebrex Capsules (0.1% to 1.9%) 2979
▲ CellCept Capsules (3% to less than 20%) 2622
▲ CellCept Intravenous (3% to less than 20%) 2622
▲ CellCept Oral Suspension (3% to less than 20%) 2622
▲ CellCept Tablets (3% to less than 20%) 2622
▲ Chemet Capsules (1% to 12.7%) 2484
Cipro 2810
▲ Combivir Tablets (12%) 1384
Cuprimine Capsules 1986
▲ DepoCyt Injection (3% to 9%) 1136
▲ Doxil Injection (1% to 10%) 2378
Effexor XR Extended-Release Capsules (Infrequent) 3195
Eloxatin for Injection 2731
▲ Emtriva Capsules (4%) 1246
▲ Emtriva Oral Solution (4%) 1246
Engerix-B Vaccine 1409
▲ Epivir (12%) 1412
Evoxac Capsules (Less than 1%) 1013
Fentora Tablets (Greater than 1%) 968
Flovent Diskus 50 mcg 1435
Fluarix Vaccine 1446
Gengraf Capsules (1% to less than 3%) 435
Geodon Capsules (Frequent) 2520
▲ Gliadel Wafer (7%) 1076
Havrix Injection Vaccine 1454
Herceptin I.V. (1%) 1199
▲ Hycamtin for Injection (3%) 1459
▲ Intron A for Injection (Less than 5%) 2859
▲ Ixempra Kit for Injection (62%) 915
Kaletra (Less than 2%) 452
Lunesta Tablets (Rare) 2994
Luvox CR Extended-Release Capsules 1759
▲ Lyrica Capsules (2% to 9%) 2527
▲ Megace ES Oral Suspension (1% to 3%) 2499
Mirapex Tablets 857
Namenda (Infrequent) 1180
Neoral Oral Solution (1% to less than 3%) 2280
Neoral Soft Gelatin Capsules (1% to less than 3%) 2280
▲ Nexavar Tablets (13%) 784
Nimotop Capsules (Less than 1%) 790
Norvir (Less than 2%) 489
Paxil (Rare) 1535
Paxil CR Controlled-Release Tablets (Rare) 1544
▲ Prograf Capsules and Injection (3%) 622
Proleukin for Injection (Less than 1%) 2287
Protonix for Delayed-Release Oral Suspension 3254
Protonix Delayed-Release Tablets 3254
Protonix I.V. (Less than 1%) 3257
Prozac Weekly Capsules (Infrequent) 1852
Prozac Pulvules and Liquid (Infrequent) 1852
ReFacto Vials 3269
▲ Simulect for Injection (3% to 10%) 2306
Singulair 2114
Sustiva Capsules 930
Sustiva Tablets 930
▲ Tarceva Tablets (Less than 1% to 13%) 1228
Targretin Capsules 1084
▲ Trizivir Tablets (12%) 1622
▲ Truvada Tablets (Greater than or equal to 5%) 1262
Twinrix Vaccine 1628
Venlafaxine Hydrochloride Tablets (Infrequent) 2199
Wellbutrin SR Sustained-Release Tablets 1653
Wellbutrin XL Extended-Release Tablets 1659
Xolair 2339
Zomig Tablets (Rare) 694
Zomig Nasal Spray (Rare) 689
Zomig-ZMT Tablets (Rare) 694
Zonegran Capsules (Infrequent) 1089
Zyban Sustained-Release Tablets 1692
Zyprexa Tablets (Rare) 1883
Zyprexa ZYDIS Orally Disintegrating Tablets (Rare) 1883

Neuropathy, motor
▲ Taxotere Injection Concentrate (0.1% to 7.2%) 2773

Neuropathy, motor, multifocal
▲ Ixempra Kit for Injection (10%) 915
Remicade for IV Injection 950

Neuropathy, optic
Campath Ampules 761
Fluarix Vaccine 1446
Imitrex Injection 1465
Imitrex Nasal Spray 1470
Imitrex Tablets 1474
Protonix for Delayed-Release Oral Suspension 3254
Protonix Delayed-Release Tablets 3254
Protonix I.V. 3257
Zyvox 2552

Neuropathy, optic, anterior ischemic, non-arteritic
Cialis Tablets 1792
Levitra Tablets (Rare) 2876

Neuropathy, peripheral
Abelcet Injection 1134
Advicor Tablets 402
Aptivus Capsules (1.5%) 823
Aptivus Oral Solution (1.5%) 823
▲ Arranon Injection (0% to 13%) 1319
Asacol Delayed-Release Tablets (Rare) 2579
▲ Atripla Tablets (Greater than or equal to 5%) 938
Cimzia (Rare) 3127
Cipro I.V. 2817
Cipro 2810
Cipro XR Tablets 2823
Combivir Tablets 1384
Cozaar Tablets (Less than 1%) 1973
Dapsone Tablets USP 1746
▲ DepoCyt Injection (4% to 12%) 1136
Emend Capsules (Greater than 0.5%) 1992
Emend for Injection (Greater than 0.5%) 1999
▲ Epivir (Less than 1% to 15%) 1412
Epivir-HBV 1417
Epzicom Tablets 1422
Exelon Capsules (Infrequent) 2229
Exelon Oral Solution (Infrequent) 2229
Exforge Tablets (Greater than 0.1% to less than 1%) 2238
Fentora Tablets (Greater than 1%) 968
Gleevec Tablets (Infrequent) 2255
Indocin Capsules (Less than 1%) 2024
Indocin I.V. (Less than 1%) 2489
Indocin (Less than 1%) 2024
Infanrix Vaccine 1479
Intelence Tablets (2.8%) 3119
▲ Ixempra Kit for Injection (62%) 915
Lescol Capsules 2268
Lescol XL Tablets 2268
Leukeran Tablets 1508
Levaquin 2416
Levaquin in 5% Dextrose Injection 2416
Lipitor Tablets (Less than 2%) 2501
Lupron Depot 3.75 mg 462
Lupron Depot 7.5 mg 469
Lupron Depot–3 Month 11.25 mg 462
Lupron Depot-PED 7.5 mg, 11.25 mg and 15 mg 471
Mevacor Tablets (0.5% to 1%) 2063
Noroxin Tablets 2069
Norvir (Less than 2%) 489
PegIntron Powder for Injection 2903
Prinivil Tablets (0.3% to 1%) 2087
Prinzide Tablets 2092
Pylera Capsules 714
Recombivax HB 2107
Remicade for IV Injection (Greater than or equal to 0.2%) 950
Requip Tablets (Infrequent) 1561
Rythmol SR Capsules 1590
▲ Selzentry Tablets (3.1%) 2534
Soriatane Capsules 3062
Stalevo Tablets 2309
Sustiva Capsules (Less than 2%) 930
Sustiva Tablets (Less than 2%) 930
▲ Sutent Capsules (10%) 2540
Tasigna Capsules 2316
Trizivir Tablets 1622
▲ Truvada Tablets (Greater than or equal to 5%) 1262
▲ Valcyte Tablets (9%) 2654
▲ Velcade for Injection (36% to 55%) 2168
▲ Viread Tablets (1% to 5%) 1268
Vytorin 10/10 Tablets 2149
Vytorin 10/10 Tablets 2939
Vytorin 10/20 Tablets 2149
Vytorin 10/20 Tablets 2939
Vytorin 10/40 Tablets 2149
Vytorin 10/40 Tablets 2939
Vytorin 10/80 Tablets 2149
Vytorin 10/80 Tablets 2939
▲ Xeloda Tablets (Less than 5%) 2662
Zocor Tablets 2136
Zyvox 2552

Neuropathy, peripheral motor
▲ Ixempra Kit for Injection (10%) 915
Velcade for Injection 2168

Neuropathy, peripheral sensorimotor
▲ Ixempra Kit for Injection (10%) 915

Neuropathy, peripheral sensory
Cuprimine Capsules 1986
▲ DepoCyt Injection (3% to 6%) 1136
▲ Eloxatin for Injection (0% to 92%) 2731
Emend Capsules (Greater than 0.5%) 1992
Emend for Injection (Greater than 0.5%) 1999
▲ Hexalen Capsules (31%) 1078
▲ Ixempra Kit for Injection (62%) 915
Norvir (Less than 2%) 489
Velcade for Injection 2168
▲ Xeloda Tablets (10%) 2662

Neuropathy, sensory
▲ Avastin IV (24.2%) 1192
▲ Gemzar for Injection (29%) 1820
▲ Taxotere Injection Concentrate (0% to 30.4%) 2773

Neuropsychiatric disorders
Chantix Tablets 2511

Neuropsychometrics performance, decrease
Combigan Ophthalmic Solution 553
Cosopt Sterile Ophthalmic Solution 1969
InnoPran XL Extended Release Capsules 1484
Nadolol Tablets 2191
Timoptic Sterile Ophthalmic Solution 2121
Timoptic in Ocudose 2124
Timoptic-XE Sterile Ophthalmic Gel Forming Solution 2125

Toprol-XL Tablets ... 666

Neurosensory, unspecified

▲ Alimta for Injection (Up to 29%) ... 1786
▲ Eloxatin for Injection (1% to 12%) ... 2731
▲ Taxotere Injection Concentrate (0% to 58.3%) ... 2773

Neurosis, unspecified

Ambien Tablets (Rare) ... 2692
Ambien CR Tablets (Rare) ... 2696
Atripla Tablets ... 938
Azilect Tablets (Infrequent) ... 3106
Campral Tablets (Infrequent) ... 1158
Emsam Transdermal System (Infrequent) ... 905
Evoxac Capsules ... 1013
Exelon Capsules (Infrequent) ... 2229
Exelon Oral Solution (Infrequent) ... 2229
Gabitril Tablets (Infrequent) ... 973
▲ Intron A for Injection (Less than 5%) ... 2859
Keppra Oral Solution ... 3131
Keppra Tablets ... 3131
Lamictal (Rare) ... 1488
Lunesta Tablets (Infrequent) ... 2994
▲ Luvox CR Extended-Release Capsules (3%) ... 1759
Namenda (Infrequent) ... 1180
Paxil (Infrequent) ... 1535
Paxil CR Controlled-Release Tablets (Infrequent) ... 1544
Prozac Weekly Capsules (Infrequent) ... 1852
Prozac Pulvules and Liquid (Infrequent) ... 1852
Remeron Tablets (Infrequent) ... 2924
RemeronSolTab Tablets (Infrequent) ... 2927
Requip Tablets (Infrequent) ... 1561
Rythmol SR Capsules ... 1590
Sustiva Capsules ... 930
Sustiva Tablets ... 930
Symbyax Capsules (Infrequent) ... 1871

Neurotoxicity

▲ Ixempra Kit for Injection (62%) ... 915
Leustatin Injection (Rare) ... 2384
▲ Prograf Capsules and Injection (Approximately 55%) ... 622
Taxotere Injection Concentrate ... 2773

Neurovascular episodes

Bicillin C-R Injectable Suspension ... 1775
Bicillin L-A Injection ... 1777

Neutropenia

Abilify Injection (Greater than or equal to 1 in 1000 patients and less than 1 in 100 patients) ... 881
Abilify Injection (Greater than or equal to 1 in 1000 patients and less than 1 in 100 patients) ... 2466
Abilify Oral Solution (Greater than or equal to 1 in 1000 patients and less than 1 in 100 patients) ... 881
Abilify Oral Solution (Greater than or equal to 1 in 1000 patients and less than 1 in 100 patients) ... 2466
Abilify Discmelt Orally Disintegrating Tablets (Greater than or equal to 1 in 1000 patients and less than 1 in 100 patients) ... 881
Abilify Discmelt Orally Disintegrating Tablets (Greater than or equal to 1 in 1000 patients and less than 1 in 100 patients) ... 2466
Abilify Tablets (Greater than or equal to 1 in 1000 patients and less than 1 in 100 patients) ... 881
Abilify Tablets (Greater than or equal to 1 in 1000 patients and less than 1 in 100 patients) ... 2466
Accutane Capsules ... 2607
Aceon Tablets (2 mg, 4 mg, 8 mg) (0.1%) ... 3038
Albenza Tablets ... 1297
▲ Alimta for Injection (2% to 58%) ... 1786
Aptivus Capsules (2%) ... 823
Aptivus Oral Solution (2%) ... 823
▲ Arranon Injection (14% to 94%) ... 1319
Asacol Delayed-Release Tablets ... 2579
Atacand Tablets (Very rare) ... 639
Atacand HCT ... 642
▲ Avastin IV (21% to 27%) ... 1192
Avelox (Greater than or equal to 2%) ... 2803
▲ Betaseron for SC Injection (13%) ... 756
Bexxar ... 1371
▲ Busulfex Injection (100%) ... 2477
▲ Campath Ampules (42% to 77%) ... 761
Captopril Tablets ... 2182
Ceftin ... 1380
▲ CellCept Capsules (2% to 3.6%) ... 2622
▲ CellCept Intravenous (2% to 3.6%) ... 2622
▲ CellCept Oral Suspension (2% to 3.6%) ... 2622
▲ CellCept Tablets (2% to 3.6%) ... 2622
Chemet Capsules (0.5% to 1.5%) ... 2484
Clinoril Tablets (Less than 1 in 100) ... 1962
▲ Clolar for Intravenous Infusion (10%) ... 1239
▲ Combivir Tablets (7.2%) ... 1384
Crixivan Capsules (1.1%) ... 1979
▲ Dacogen Injection (90%) ... 1066
Depakote ER Tablets ... 423
▲ DepoCyt Injection (8% to 36%) ... 1136
Diovan Tablets (1.9%) ... 2212
Diovan HCT Tablets (0.1%) ... 2216
Doribax Injection ... 2400
▲ Doxil Injection (12.1% to 45.9%) ... 2378
Edecrin ... 698
Effexor XR Extended-Release Capsules (Rare) ... 3195
Elitek (2%) ... 2729
▲ Eloxatin for Injection (0% to 81%) ... 2731
▲ Emend Capsules (3.1% to 8.9%) ... 1992
▲ Emend for Injection (3.1% to 8.9%) ... 1999
▲ Emtriva Capsules (3% to 5%) ... 1246
▲ Emtriva Oral Solution (3% to 5%) ... 1246
Enbrel for Injection ... 569
▲ Epivir (7.2% to 15%) ... 1412
Epivir-HBV ... 1417
Epzicom Tablets ... 1422
Exjade Tablets ... 2244
▲ Fentora Tablets (0% to 8%) ... 968
Fortaz (Very rare) ... 1450
▲ Gemzar for Injection (18% to 90%) ... 1820
▲ Gleevec Tablets (0% to 48%) ... 2255
Herceptin I.V. ... 1199
▲ Hycamtin Capsules (83% to 91%) ... 1456
▲ Hycamtin for Injection (26% to 98%) ... 1459
▲ Intron A for Injection (Less than 5% to 92%) ... 2859
▲ Invanz for Injection (1% to 5.8%) ... 2029
Isentress Tablets ... 2036
▲ Ixempra Kit for Injection (23% to greater than 40%) ... 915
▲ Kaletra (1% to 5%) ... 452
Keppra Injection (2.4%) ... 3137
Keppra Oral Solution ... 3131
Keppra Tablets ... 3131
Kineret Injection (0.4%) ... 585
Lamictal ... 1488
Lamisil Oral Granules ... 2264
Lamisil Tablets (Isolated case) ... 2266
Leukeran Tablets ... 1508
▲ Leustatin Injection (70%) ... 2384
▲ Lexiva Oral Suspension (3%) ... 1510
▲ Lexiva Tablets (3%) ... 1510
Malarone Pediatric Tablets ... 1521
Malarone Tablets ... 1521
Mavik Tablets (Rare) ... 472
▲ Mepron Suspension (5%) ... 1526
Merrem I.V. ... 684
▲ Mycamine for Injection (14.1% to 75.3%) ... 616
Mylotarg for Injection ... 3212
NeoProfen Injection ... 2496
▲ Nexavar Tablets (5% to 18%) ... 784
Noroxin Tablets (1.4%) ... 2069
▲ Norvir (6%) ... 489
▲ Noxafil Oral Suspension (2% to 23%) ... 2889
Omnicef Capsules ... 497
Omnicef for Oral Suspension ... 497
Orthoclone OKT3 Sterile Solution (Less than 1%) ... 2387
▲ PegIntron Powder for Injection (Less than or equal to 1% to 6%) ... 2903
Percocet Tablets ... 1127
Plavix Tablets (Less than 1%) ... 926
Plavix Tablets (Less than 1%) ... 2767
Primaxin I.M. ... 2080
Primaxin I.V. (Less than 0.2%) ... 2083
Prinivil Tablets (Rare) ... 2087
Prinzide Tablets (Rare) ... 2092
Prograf Capsules and Injection ... 622
Proleukin for Injection ... 2287
Pylera Capsules ... 714
Rapamune ... 3260
Raptiva for Injection ... 1218
▲ Rebetol (14% to 26%) ... 2917
Rebif Prefilled Syringe for Injection ... 1107
Relenza Inhalation Powder (Less than 1.5%) ... 1556
Remeron Tablets ... 2924
RemeronSolTab Tablets ... 2927
Remicade for IV Injection ... 950
Retrovir Capsules ... 1574
Retrovir IV Infusion ... 1579
Retrovir ... 1574
Rilutek Tablets (Three cases) ... 2771
▲ Rituxan I.V. (6% to 14%) ... 1223
Rocephin Injectable Vials, ADD-Vantage, Galaxy, Bulk (Less than 1%) ... 2642
Suprax for Oral Suspension (Less than 2%) ... 1891
Suprax Tablets (Less than 2%) ... 1891
▲ Sutent Capsules (1% to 53%) ... 2540
Tarka Tablets (Less frequent) ... 511
▲ Tasigna Capsules (28% to 37%) ... 2316
▲ Taxotere Injection Concentrate (32% to 100%) ... 2773
▲ Temodar Capsules (20% to 51%) ... 2931
Teveten Tablets (1.3%) ... 515
Teveten HCT Tablets ... 517
Timentin ADD-Vantage ... 1606
Timentin Injection Galaxy Container ... 1609
Timentin IV Infusion ... 1603
Timentin Pharmacy Bulk Package ... 1613
▲ Torisel Injection (5% to 19%) ... 3272
▲ Treanda for Injection (24% to 75%) ... 983
▲ Trisenox Injection (10%) ... 986
▲ Trizivir Tablets (7.2%) ... 1622
▲ Truvada Tablets (3%) ... 1262
Tyzeka Tablets (2%) ... 2328
▲ Valcyte Tablets (11% to 27%) ... 2654
Valium Tablets (Isolated reports) ... 2658
▲ Valtrex Caplets (18%) ... 1635
▲ Velcade for Injection (Less than 1% to 49%) ... 2168
Venlafaxine Hydrochloride Tablets ... 2199
▲ Viramune Oral Suspension (3.6% to 13.3%) ... 873
▲ Viramune Tablets (3.6% to 13.3%) ... 873
▲ Xeloda Tablets (2.2% to 86%) ... 2662
Xifaxan Tablets (Less than 2%) ... 2682
▲ Ziagen (2% to 5%) ... 1673
Zinacef for Injection (Fewer than 1 in 100) ... 1678
Zinacef Injection (Fewer than 1 in 100) ... 1678
Zolinza Capsules ... 2142
▲ Zometa for Intravenous Infusion (12%) ... 2341
Zosyn for Injection ... 3284

Neutropenia, aggravated

Noxafil Oral Suspension (0% to 2%) ... 2889

Neutropenia, febrile

▲ Alimta for Injection (Up to 9%) ... 1786
▲ Arranon Injection (1% to 12%) ... 1319
▲ Avastin IV (5%) ... 1192
▲ Campath Ampules (5% to 10%) ... 761
Cancidas for Injection ... 1953
▲ Clolar for Intravenous Infusion (57%) ... 1239
▲ Dacogen Injection (29%) ... 1066
▲ Elitek (4%) ... 2729
Emend Capsules (Greater than 0.5%) ... 1992
Emend for Injection (Greater than 0.5%) ... 1999
▲ Ixempra Kit for Injection (3%) ... 915
▲ Mycamine for Injection (6.1% to 36.5%) ... 616
▲ Noxafil Oral Suspension (20%) ... 2889
▲ Tasigna Capsules (1% to 10%) ... 2316
▲ Taxotere Injection Concentrate (0% to 33.3%) ... 2773
▲ Treanda for Injection (3%) ... 983
▲ Trisenox Injection (13%) ... 986
Velcade for Injection (Less than 1%) ... 2168

Neutropenia, transient

Proglycem Capsules (Frequent) ... 1185
Proglycem Suspension (Frequent) ... 1185

Neutrophil count, abnormal

Avelox (Greater than or equal to 2%) ... 2803
Selzentry Tablets (Greater than or equal to 2%) ... 2534
▲ Tykerb Tablets (Less than 1% to 22%) ... 1631
▲ Zyvox (0% to 5.9%) ... 2552

Neutrophil count, low

▲ Keppra Oral Solution (1.4% to 5%) ... 3131
▲ Keppra Tablets (1.4% to 5%) ... 3131
Rythmol SR Capsules ... 1590

Neutrophilia

▲ Atripla Tablets (3%) ... 938
▲ Avastin IV (5.8%) ... 1192

Neutrophils, decrease

(*see under* Neutropenia)

Nevi, pre-existing, increased growth of

▲ Humatrope Vials and Cartridges (10.8%) ... 1838
Nutropin for Injection (Rare) ... 1208
Nutropin AQ Injection (Rare) ... 1212
Nutropin AQ NuSpin Injection (Rare) ... 1212
Nutropin AQ Pen (Rare) ... 1212
Nutropin AQ Pen Cartridge (Rare) ... 1212

Nevus, pigmented

Genotropin Lyophilized Powder ... 2547
Requip Tablets (Infrequent) ... 1561

Night blindness

(*see under* Nyctalopia)

Night sweat

Aricept Tablets (Infrequent) ... 1062
Aricept ODT Tablets (Infrequent) ... 1062
Cymbalta Delayed-Release Capsules (Infrequent) ... 1801
Effexor XR Extended-Release Capsules (Rare) ... 3195
Gengraf Capsules (Rare) ... 435
▲ Gleevec Tablets (13% to 17%) ... 2255
Intelence Tablets (Less than 2%) ... 3119
Neoral Oral Solution (Rare) ... 2280
Neoral Soft Gelatin Capsules (Rare) ... 2280
▲ Prometrium Capsules (100 mg, 200 mg) (7%) ... 3047
Requip Tablets (Frequent) ... 1561
▲ Rituxan I.V. (1% to 15%) ... 1223
Sandimmune (Rare) ... 2296
▲ Tasigna Capsules (1% to 10%) ... 2316
▲ Trisenox Injection (8%) ... 986
Ultram ER Extended-Release Tablets (0.5% to less than 1%) ... 2428
Vantas (Less than 2%) ... 1737
Venlafaxine Hydrochloride Tablets ... 2199
Vivitrol ... 988
Xyrem Oral Solution (Infrequent) ... 1766

Nightmares

Avelox ... 2803
Axert Tablets (Rare) ... 2431
Biaxin/Biaxin XL ... 411
Catapres Tablets ... 841
Catapres-TTS (0.5% or less) ... 842
Chantix Tablets (1% to 2%) ... 2511
Cipro I.V. (1% or less) ... 2817
Cipro (Less than 1%) ... 2810
Cipro XR Tablets ... 2823
Clorpres Tablets ... 2185
Combigan Ophthalmic Solution ... 553
Cosopt Sterile Ophthalmic Solution ... 1969
Cymbalta Delayed-Release Capsules (2%) ... 1801
▲ Effexor XR Extended-Release Capsules (4% to 7%) ... 3195
Eldepryl Capsules ... 3052
Intelence Tablets (Less than 2%) ... 3119
Klonopin (Infrequent) ... 2639
Levaquin (0.1% to 1%) ... 2416
Levaquin in 5% Dextrose Injection (0.1% to 1%) ... 2416
Lexapro Oral Suspension ... 1174
Lexapro Tablets ... 1174
Marinol Capsules (Less than 1%) ... 3163
Meridia Capsules ... 475
Mirapex Tablets ... 857
Nembutal Sodium Solution, USP (Less than 1%) ... 2494
Requip Tablets (Infrequent) ... 1561
Rythmol SR Capsules ... 1590
Stalevo Tablets ... 2309
Tamiflu Capsules ... 2649
Tamiflu Oral Suspension ... 2649
Timoptic Sterile Ophthalmic Solution ... 2121
Timoptic in Ocudose ... 2124
Timoptic-XE Sterile Ophthalmic Gel Forming Solution ... 2125
Toprol-XL Tablets ... 666
Valium Tablets ... 2658
Venlafaxine Hydrochloride Tablets ... 2199
▲ Xyrem Oral Solution (2.9% to 6.1%) ... 1766

Nipples, sensitive

Testim 1% Gel (Less than 1%) ... 701

Nitrogen balance, changes
(*see under* BUN levels, changes)

NMS
(*see under* Neuroleptic malignant syndrome)

Nocardiosis
Remicade for IV Injection ... 950

Nocturia
Abilify Injection (Greater than or equal to 1 in 1000 patients and less than 1 in 100 patients) ... 881
Abilify Injection (Greater than or equal to 1 in 1000 patients and less than 1 in 100 patients) ... 2466
Abilify Oral Solution (Greater than or equal to 1 in 1000 patients and less than 1 in 100 patients) ... 881
Abilify Oral Solution (Greater than or equal to 1 in 1000 patients and less than 1 in 100 patients) ... 2466
Abilify Discmelt Orally Disintegrating Tablets (Greater than or equal to 1 in 1000 patients and less than 1 in 100 patients) ... 881
Abilify Discmelt Orally Disintegrating Tablets (Greater than or equal to 1 in 1000 patients and less than 1 in 100 patients) ... 2466
Abilify Tablets (Greater than or equal to 1 in 1000 patients and less than 1 in 100 patients) ... 881
Abilify Tablets (Greater than or equal to 1 in 1000 patients and less than 1 in 100 patients) ... 2466
Actiq (Less than 1%) ... 959
Ambien Tablets (Rare) ... 2692
Ambien CR Tablets (Rare) ... 2696
AndroGel ... 3159
Aricept Tablets (Frequent) ... 1062
Aricept ODT Tablets (Frequent) ... 1062
Brovana Inhalation Solution (Less than 2%) ... 2990
Calcijex Injection ... 419
Campral Tablets (Rare) ... 1158
Cardizem LA Extended Release Tablets (Less than 2%) ... 421
Catapres Tablets (About 1 in 100 patients) ... 841
▲ CellCept Capsules (3% to less than 20%) ... 2622
▲ CellCept Intravenous (3% to less than 20%) ... 2622
▲ CellCept Oral Suspension (3% to less than 20%) ... 2622
▲ CellCept Tablets (3% to less than 20%) ... 2622
Chantix Tablets (Infrequent) ... 2511
Clorpres Tablets (About 1%) ... 2185
Copaxone for Injection (Infrequent) ... 3110
Cozaar Tablets (Less than 1%) ... 1973
▲ Crinone 8% Gel (13%) ... 992
Cymbalta Delayed-Release Capsules (Infrequent) ... 1801
Dantrium Capsules (Less frequent) .. 2580
Doxil Injection (Less than 1%) ... 2378
DynaCirc CR Controlled Release Tablets (0.5% to 1%) ... 1407
Effexor XR Extended-Release Capsules (Infrequent) ... 3195
Eldepryl Capsules ... 3052
Eligard 7.5 mg (Less than 2%) ... 2724
Eligard 22.5 mg (Less than 2%) ... 2724
Eligard 30 mg (2.2%) ... 2724
Eligard 45 mg (Less than 2%) ... 2724
Evoxac Capsules (Less than 1%) ... 1013
Exelon Capsules (Infrequent) ... 2229
Exelon Oral Solution (Infrequent) ... 2229
Exelon Patch (Infrequent) ... 2233
Exforge Tablets (Greater than 0.1% to less than 1%) ... 2238
Frova Tablets (Rare) ... 1111
Gabitril Tablets (Infrequent) ... 973
Gengraf Capsules (1% to less than 3%) ... 435
Geodon Capsules (Rare) ... 2520
▲ Indapamide Tablets (Less than 5%) ... 2188
▲ Intron A for Injection (Less than 5%) ... 2859
Klonopin ... 2639
Lamictal (Rare) ... 1488
Lipitor Tablets (Less than 2%) ... 2501
Luvox CR Extended-Release Capsules (Infrequent) ... 1759
Miacalcin Injection ... 2273
Mirapex Tablets ... 857
Neoral Oral Solution (1% to less than 3%) ... 2280
Neoral Soft Gelatin Capsules (1% to less than 3%) ... 2280
Norvir (0% to 0.2%) ... 489
Paxil (Infrequent) ... 1535
Paxil CR Controlled-Release Tablets (Infrequent) ... 1544
▲ Prograf Capsules and Injection (3% to 15%) ... 622
Protonix for Delayed-Release Oral Suspension (Less than 1%) ... 3254
Protonix Delayed-Release Tablets (Less than 1%) ... 3254
Protonix I.V. (Less than 1%) ... 3257
Prozac Weekly Capsules (Infrequent) ... 1852
Prozac Pulvules and Liquid (Infrequent) ... 1852
Requip Tablets (Infrequent) ... 1561
Rilutek Tablets (Rare) ... 2771
Rocaltrol Capsules ... 1150
Rocaltrol Oral Solution ... 1150
Rythmol SR Capsules ... 1590
Sular Extended Release Tablets (Less than or equal to 1%) ... 2975
Tarka Tablets (Less frequent) ... 511
Tasigna Capsules (0.1% to 1%) ... 2316
▲ Tice BCG (5%) ... 2936
▲ Valstar Sterile Solution for Intravesical Instillation (7%) ... 1735
Venlafaxine Hydrochloride Tablets (Infrequent) ... 2199
▲ Viadur Implant (3.8%) ... 802
Wellbutrin Tablets (Frequent) ... 1648
Xeloda Tablets ... 2662
Zonegran Capsules (Infrequent) ... 1089

Nocturia, aggravated
Eligard 7.5 mg (Less than 2%) ... 2724
Eligard 22.5 mg (Less than 2%) ... 2724
Eligard 30 mg (Less than 2%) ... 2724
Eligard 45 mg (Less than 2%) ... 2724

Nodal rhythm
Lanoxin Injection (Common) ... 1498
Lanoxin Injection Pediatric (Common) ... 1502
Lanoxin Tablets (Common) ... 1505
Romazicon Injection (Less than 1%) ... 2646

Nodule, subcutaneous
Enbrel for Injection ... 569
Gabitril Tablets (Infrequent) ... 973
Lyrica Capsules (Rare) ... 2527

Nodule at injection site
Boostrix ... 1377
Genotropin Lyophilized Powder (Infrequent) ... 2547
Lovenox Injection ... 2756
▲ Somatuline Depot Injection (9% to 17%) ... 3102
▲ Vivitrol (8% to 32%) ... 988

Nodulosis
Advicor Tablets ... 402

Nonprotein nitrogen increase
Valstar Sterile Solution for Intravesical Instillation (Less than 1%) ... 1735

Nose, runny
▲ FluMist Vaccine (44% to 58%) ... 1945
▲ Rotarix Oral Suspension (28% to 31%) ... 1582

NPN elevation
Celebrex Capsules (0.1% to 1.9%) ... 2979
▲ Coreg Tablets (6%) ... 1387
▲ Coreg CR Extended-Release Capsules (6%) ... 1393
▲ Gengraf Capsules (18%) ... 435
▲ Neoral Oral Solution (18%) ... 2280
▲ Neoral Soft Gelatin Capsules (18%) ... 2280
Proleukin for Injection (Less than 1%) ... 2287

Nuchal rigidity
Mirapex Tablets ... 857

Numbness
Adenocard IV Injection (1%) ... 603
▲ Aerobid/Aerobid-M (1% to 3%) ... 1153
▲ Alferon N Injection (One patient to 3%) ... 1726
Aricept Tablets (Infrequent) ... 1062
Aricept ODT Tablets (Infrequent) ... 1062
Avalide Tablets ... 892
Avalide Tablets ... 2713
Avapro Tablets (Less than 1%) ... 897
Avapro Tablets (Less than 1%) ... 2718
Bentyl Capsules ... 703
Bentyl Injection ... 703
Bentyl Syrup ... 703
Bentyl Tablets ... 703
BOTOX Purified Neurotoxin Complex (Rare) ... 550
Catapres-TTS (0.5% or less) ... 842
DepoCyt Injection ... 1136
DynaCirc CR Controlled Release Tablets (0.5% to 1%) ... 1407
▲ Imitrex Injection (5%) ... 1465
Imitrex Nasal Spray (Infrequent) ... 1470
Imitrex Tablets (Frequent) ... 1474
K-Phos Original (Sodium Free) Tablets (Less frequent) ... 814
K-Phos Neutral Tablets ... 813
Levaquin ... 2416
Levaquin in 5% Dextrose Injection ... 2416
Parnate Tablets ... 1532
Reyataz Capsules ... 3299
Rythmol Tablets (Less than 1%) ... 1586
Stalevo Tablets ... 2309
Xeloda Tablets ... 2662

Numbness, buccal mucosa
Imitrex Injection ... 1465
Imitrex Nasal Spray (Infrequent) ... 1470
Rythmol SR Capsules ... 1590

Numbness, extremities
Bicillin C-R Injectable Suspension ... 1775
Bicillin L-A Injection ... 1777
▲ Indapamide Tablets (Greater than or equal to 5%) ... 2188
Maxair Autohaler ... 1705
Ortho-Cyclen Tablets ... 2449
Ortho Evra Transdermal System ... 2437
Ortho Tri-Cyclen Tablets ... 2449
Ortho Tri-Cyclen Lo Tablets ... 2458
Pylera Capsules ... 714

Numbness, feet
Uroqid-Acid No. 2 Tablets ... 814

Numbness, fingers
Alferon N Injection (One patient) ... 1726
Olux Foam (Less than 2%) ... 3061

Numbness, hands
Alferon N Injection (One patient) ... 1726
Uroqid-Acid No. 2 Tablets ... 814

Numbness, lips
K-Phos Original (Sodium Free) Tablets (Less frequent) ... 814
K-Phos Neutral Tablets ... 813
Uroqid-Acid No. 2 Tablets ... 814

Numbness, mouth
(*see under* Numbness, buccal mucosa)

Numbness/tingling, fingers and toes
Eldepryl Capsules ... 3052

Nutrition disorders, unspecified
▲ Cancidas for Injection (10.7% to 21.7%) ... 1953
▲ Focalin XR Capsules (34%) ... 2251
▲ Mycamine for Injection (38.5% to 90.6%) ... 616
▲ Somatuline Depot Injection (11% to 25%) ... 3102

Nyctalopia
Accutane Capsules ... 2607
Chantix Tablets (Rare) ... 2511
Lyrica Capsules (Rare) ... 2527
Paxil (Rare) ... 1535
Paxil CR Controlled-Release Tablets (Rare) ... 1544
▲ Soriatane Capsules (1% to 10%) ... 3062

Nystagmus
Aricept Tablets (Infrequent) ... 1062
Aricept ODT Tablets (Infrequent) ... 1062
Arranon Injection (1%) ... 1319
Axert Tablets (Rare) ... 2431
Carbatrol Capsules ... 3019
Celexa ... 1160
Chantix Tablets (Rare) ... 2511
Cipro I.V. (1% or less) ... 2817
Cipro ... 2810
Cipro XR Tablets ... 2823
▲ Depakote ER Tablets (1% to 8%) ... 423
Effexor XR Extended-Release Capsules (Rare) ... 3195
Elmiron Capsules ... 2435
Equetro Extended-Release Capsules ... 3174
Exelon Capsules (Infrequent) ... 2229
Exelon Oral Solution (Infrequent) ... 2229
Gabitril Tablets (2%) ... 973
Geodon Capsules (Rare) ... 2520
Klonopin ... 2639
Lamictal (1%) ... 1488
Lexapro Oral Suspension ... 1174
Lexapro Tablets ... 1174
Lunesta Tablets (Infrequent) ... 2994
Lyrica Capsules (Greater than or equal to 2%) ... 2527
Mirapex Tablets ... 857
MS Contin Tablets (Less frequent) ... 2585
Noroxin Tablets ... 2069
Paxil (Rare) ... 1535
Paxil CR Controlled-Release Tablets (Rare) ... 1544
Phenytek Capsules (Among most common) ... 2192
Remeron Tablets (Rare) ... 2924
RemeronSolTab Tablets (Rare) ... 2927
Venlafaxine Hydrochloride Tablets (Rare) ... 2199
▲ Zonegran Capsules (4%) ... 1089
Zyprexa Tablets (Rare) ... 1883
Zyprexa ZYDIS Orally Disintegrating Tablets (Rare) ... 1883

Nystagmus, horizontal
(*see under* Nystagmus)

O

Obesity
Aptivus Capsules ... 823
Aptivus Oral Solution ... 823
Atripla Tablets ... 938
Celexa (Rare) ... 1160
Crixivan Capsules ... 1979
Emtriva Capsules ... 1246
Emtriva Oral Solution ... 1246
Intelence Tablets ... 3119
Kaletra (Less than 2%) ... 452
Lexiva Oral Suspension ... 1510
Lexiva Tablets ... 1510
Reyataz Capsules (Less than 3%) ... 3299
Risperdal Consta Long-Acting Injection (Infrequent) ... 1753
Symbyax Capsules (Infrequent) ... 1871
Truvada Tablets ... 1262

Obsessive compulsive symptoms
Mirapex Tablets ... 857
▲ Vivitrol (8% to 12%) ... 988
Zyprexa Tablets (Infrequent) ... 1883
Zyprexa ZYDIS Orally Disintegrating Tablets (Infrequent) ... 1883

Obsessive thoughts
Luvox CR Extended-Release Capsules (Rare) ... 1759
Mirapex Tablets ... 857

Obstipation
Emend Capsules (Greater than 0.5%) ... 1992
Emend for Injection (Greater than 0.5%) ... 1999
Thioridazine Hydrochloride Tablets .. 2195

Obstructive airway disorder
Mirapex Tablets ... 857

Obtundation
Invega Extended-Release Tablets ... 1748
Orthoclone OKT3 Sterile Solution (Less than 1%) ... 2387
Risperdal Consta Long-Acting Injection ... 1753

Occlusion, unspecified
Lovaza Capsules ... 1520

Ocular, foreign body sensation
▲ Azopt Ophthalmic Suspension (1% to 5%) ... 540
▲ Betimol Ophthalmic Solution (More than 5%) ... 3181
▲ Cosopt Sterile Ophthalmic Solution (1% to 5%) ... 1969
▲ Lotemax Ophthalmic Suspension 0.5% (5% to 15%) ... ⊙ 241
▲ Lucentis Injection (6% to 19%) ... 1205
▲ Nevanac Ophthalmic Suspension 0.1% (5% to 10%) ... ⊙ 205
Ofloxacin Ophthalmic Solution 0.3% ... ⊙ 243
▲ Pataday Ophthalmic Solution (Less than or equal to 5%) ... 543
▲ Patanol Ophthalmic Solution (Less than 5%) ... 546
▲ Quixin Ophthalmic Solution (1% to 3%) ... 3184
▲ Restasis Ophthalmic Emulsion (1% to 5%) ... 557

Timoptic Sterile Ophthalmic Solution (Less frequent) 2121
Timoptic in Ocudose (Less frequent) 2124
▲ Timoptic-XE Sterile Ophthalmic Gel Forming Solution (1% to 5%) 2125
▲ Travatan Z Ophthalmic Solution (5% to 10%) 547

Ocular, foreign body sensation, decreased

Lacrisert Sterile Ophthalmic Insert ⊙233

Ocular, hyperemia

▲ Durezol Ophthalmic Emulsion (5% to 15%) ⊙275
▲ Lucentis Injection (5% to 12%) 1205
▲ Nevanac Ophthalmic Suspension 0.1% (1% to 5%) ⊙205
▲ Travatan Z Ophthalmic Solution (30% to 50%) 547
▲ Vectibix (3%) 597

Ocular, sticky sensation

▲ Nevanac Ophthalmic Suspension 0.1% (5% to 10%) ⊙205

Ocular allergy

▲ Diclofenac Sodium Ophthalmic Solution (Less than or equal to 5%) ⊙240
▲ Trusopt Sterile Ophthalmic Solution (Approximately 10%) 2128
▲ Voltaren Ophthalmic Solution (Less than or equal to 5%) 2336

Ocular discomfort

▲ Alamast Ophthalmic Solution (Less than 5%) 3181
Amerge Tablets (Rare) 1301
▲ Azopt Ophthalmic Suspension (1% to 5%) 540
▲ Evoxac Capsules (1% to 3%) 1013
Iquix Ophthalmic Solution (1% to 2%) 3183
Lacrisert Sterile Ophthalmic Insert ⊙233
▲ Lotemax Ophthalmic Suspension 0.5% (Less than 5%) ⊙241
▲ Lucentis Injection (0% to 8%) 1205
▲ Nevanac Ophthalmic Suspension 0.1% (1% to 5%) ⊙205
Ofloxacin Ophthalmic Solution 0.3% ⊙243
Photofrin for Injection 708
▲ Quixin Ophthalmic Solution (1% to 3%) 3184
▲ Trusopt Sterile Ophthalmic Solution (Approximately one-third of patients) 2128
▲ Vigamox Ophthalmic Solution (1% to 6%) 548

Ocular exudate

▲ Cosopt Sterile Ophthalmic Solution (1% to 5%) 1969
▲ Lucentis Injection (1% to 9%) 1205
▲ Restasis Ophthalmic Emulsion (1% to 5%) 557
Timoptic Sterile Ophthalmic Solution (Less frequent) 2121
Timoptic in Ocudose (Less frequent) 2124
▲ Timoptic-XE Sterile Ophthalmic Gel Forming Solution (1% to 5%) 2125

Ocular lesions

Lybrel Tablets 3204

Ocular palsies

Attenuvax (Rare) 1951
M-M-R II (Rare) 2054
Mumpsvax 2068
ProQuad 2099

Ocular tension, increase

Bentyl Capsules 703
Bentyl Injection 703
Bentyl Syrup 703
Bentyl Tablets 703
Donnatal Extentabs 2507

Ocular toxicity

▲ Vectibix (15%) 597

Ocular vascular disorder

Chantix Tablets (Rare) 2511

Oculogyration

Invega Extended-Release Tablets 1748

Oculogyric crisis

Geodon Capsules (Frequent) 2520
Paxil 1535
Paxil CR Controlled-Release Tablets 1544
Risperdal Consta Long-Acting Injection (Infrequent) 1753
Stalevo Tablets 2309
Thioridazine Hydrochloride Tablets 2195
Zofran Injection 1682
Zofran 1687
Zofran ODT Orally Disintegrating Tablets 1687
Zonegran Capsules (Rare) 1089
▲ Zyprexa Tablets (2% to 3%) 1883
▲ Zyprexa ZYDIS Orally Disintegrating Tablets (2% to 3%) 1883

Oculomotor disturbances

Carbatrol Capsules 3019
Equetro Extended-Release Capsules 3174

Odynophagia

▲ Alimta for Injection (Up to 6%) 1786
▲ Photofrin for Injection (5%) 708
▲ Taxotere Injection Concentrate (1.1% to 25.1%) 2773

Oiliness

▲ Aczone Gel 5% (Less than 1% to 14%) 3296

Oily evacuation

▲ Xenical Capsules (2.3% to 11.9%) 2672

Oligohydramnios

Aceon Tablets (2 mg, 4 mg, 8 mg) 3038
Avalide Tablets 892
Avalide Tablets 2713
Avapro Tablets 897
Avapro Tablets 2718
Captopril Tablets 2182
Clinoril Tablets 1962
Cozaar Tablets 1973
Prinivil Tablets 2087
Prinzide Tablets 2092

Oligomenorrhea

Mustargen for Injection 2492
Ortho-Cyclen/Ortho Tri-Cyclen 2449
Ortho Tri-Cyclen Lo Tablets 2458
Sandostatin Injection (Less than 1%) 2300

Oligospermia

AndroGel 3159
Avodart Soft Gelatin Capsules 1359
Delatestryl Injection 1730

Oliguria

Abelcet Injection 1134
Actiq (Less than 1%) 959
Anaprox Tablets (Less than 1%) 2632
Anaprox DS Tablets (Less than 1%) 2632
Angiomax for Injection (Greater than 0.1% to less than 1%) 1933
Anzemet Injection (2.6%) 2701
Anzemet Tablets (2.6%) 2704
▲ Avinza Capsules (Less than 5%) 1772
▲ Busulfex Injection (15%) 2477
Capastat Sulfate for Injection (1 patient) 1791
Captopril Tablets (Approximately 1 to 2 of 1000 patients) 2182
Carbatrol Capsules 3019
Celexa (Rare) 1160
▲ CellCept Capsules (3% to less than 20%) 2622
▲ CellCept Intravenous (3% to less than 20%) 2622
▲ CellCept Oral Suspension (3% to less than 20%) 2622
▲ CellCept Tablets (3% to less than 20%) 2622
Demadex Injection 2630
Demadex Tablets 2630
Depakote ER Tablets 423
▲ DepoDur Injection (2% to 5%) 1095
Diovan HCT Tablets 2216
Doxil Injection (Less than 1%) 2378
Duragesic Transdermal System (Less than 1%) 2405
Dyazide Capsules 1405
EC-Naprosyn Delayed-Release Tablets (Less than 1%) 2632
Equetro Extended-Release Capsules 3174
Evoxac Capsules 1013
Exelon Capsules (Infrequent) 2229
Exelon Oral Solution (Infrequent) 2229
Fansidar Tablets 2636
Flebogamma 5% 1715
Flebogamma 5% DIF 1718
Follistim AQ Cartridge 2844
Furosemide Tablets 2186
Gammagard S/D (Some patients) 734
Gantrisin Pediatric Suspension 2638
Geodon Capsules (Rare) 2520
Invanz for Injection (Greater than 0.1%) 2029
Ionsys Transdermal System (.1% to less than 1%) 2410
Lunesta Tablets (Rare) 2994
Luvox CR Extended-Release Capsules (Rare) 1759
Lyrica Capsules (0.1% to 1%) 2527
Mirapex Tablets 857
Mycamine for Injection 616
Nalfon Capsules (Less than 1%) 2508
Naprosyn Suspension (Less than 1%) 2632
Naprosyn Tablets (Less than 1%) 2632
Orthoclone OKT3 Sterile Solution (Less than 1%) 2387
Paxil (Rare) 1535
Paxil CR Controlled-Release Tablets (Rare) 1544
Primaxin I.M. 2080
Primaxin I.V. (2.2%) 2083
Prinivil Tablets (0.3% to 1%) 2087
Prinzide Tablets 2092
▲ Prograf Capsules and Injection (3% to 19%) 622
▲ Proleukin for Injection (6% to 63%) 2287
Prozac Weekly Capsules (Rare) 1852
Prozac Pulvules and Liquid (Rare) 1852
Rocephin Injectable Vials, ADD-Vantage, Galaxy, Bulk 2642
Rythmol SR Capsules 1590
▲ Simulect for Injection (3% to 10%) 2306
Symbyax Capsules (Infrequent) 1871
Trasylol Injection (1% to 2%) 799
▲ Trisenox Injection (5%) 986
Ultane Liquid for Inhalation (Less than 1%) 524
Venlafaxine Hydrochloride Tablets (Rare) 2199
Voltaren Tablets (Occasionally) 2334
Voltaren-XR Tablets (Occasionally) 2337
Zosyn for Injection (1% or less) 3284

Oliguria, neonatal

Captopril Tablets 2182

"On-off" phenomenon

Stalevo Tablets 2309

Onychia

Evoxac Capsules (Less than 1%) 1013

Onycholysis

Taxotere Injection Concentrate 2773
▲ Xeloda Tablets (1% to 5%) 2662

Onychomycosis

Evoxac Capsules (Less than 1%) 1013
Mirapex Tablets 857
▲ NovoLog Injection (10%) 2359

Oozing

Panretin Gel 0.1% 1081

Oozing at injection site

Lovenox Injection 2756

Opacification, posterior capsule

▲ Durezol Ophthalmic Emulsion (5% to 15%) ⊙275
▲ Lucentis Injection (0% to 8%) 1205

Opacity, capsular

▲ Nevanac Ophthalmic Suspension 0.1% (5% to 10%) ⊙205

Opacity, punctate

Stromectol Tablets (1.4% to 1.8%) 2120

Operation

▲ Gleevec Tablets (4% to 12%) 2255

Ophthalmitis

Campral Tablets (Rare) 1158

Ophthalmoplegia

Advicor Tablets 402
Lescol Capsules 2268
Lescol XL Tablets 2268
Lyrica Capsules (Rare) 2527
Mevacor Tablets 2063
Vantas 1737
Vytorin 10/10 Tablets 2149
Vytorin 10/20 Tablets 2149
Vytorin 10/40 Tablets 2149
Vytorin 10/80 Tablets 2149

Opisthotonos

Geodon Capsules (Rare) 2520
Thioridazine Hydrochloride Tablets 2195
▲ Zyprexa Tablets (2% to 3%) 1883
▲ Zyprexa ZYDIS Orally Disintegrating Tablets (2% to 3%) 1883

Optic atrophy

Lyrica Capsules (Rare) 2527

Optic nerve, damage

Alrex Ophthalmic Suspension 0.2% ⊙236
Dapsone Tablets USP 1746
FML Ophthalmic Ointment (Infrequent) ⊙223
FML Ophthalmic Suspension (Infrequent) ⊙224
FML Forte Ophthalmic Suspension (Infrequent) ⊙222
Lotemax Ophthalmic Suspension 0.5% ⊙241
Pred Forte Ophthalmic Suspension (Infrequent) ⊙227
Pred Mild Ophthalmic Suspension (Infrequent) ⊙230
Pred-G Ophthalmic Ointment ⊙229
Pred-G Ophthalmic Suspension (Infrequent) ⊙228

Optic nerve, metastases to

Thyrogen for Injection 1244

Orchitis

Effexor XR Extended-Release Capsules (Rare) 3195
Mirapex Tablets 857
M-M-R II 2054
Mumpsvax (Rare) 2068
ProQuad 2099
Tice BCG (Less than or equal to 1%) 2936
Venlafaxine Hydrochloride Tablets (Rare) 2199

Organomegaly

▲ Vesanoid Capsules (3%) 2660

Orgasm, abnormal

▲ Cymbalta Delayed-Release Capsules (Frequent to 3%) 1801
▲ Pristiq Extended-Release Tablets (0% to 3%) 3247
Strattera Capsules (2%) 1864
▲ Venlafaxine Hydrochloride Tablets (2% to 12.5%) 2199

Orgasmic dysfunction, female

▲ Effexor XR Extended-Release Capsules (2% to 8%) 3195
Prozac Weekly Capsules 1852

Oropharyngeal spasm

Abilify Injection (Rare) 881
Abilify Injection (Rare) 2466
Abilify Oral Solution (Rare) 881
Abilify Oral Solution (Rare) 2466
Abilify Discmelt Orally Disintegrating Tablets (Rare) 881
Abilify Discmelt Orally Disintegrating Tablets (Rare) 2466
Abilify Tablets (Rare) 881
Abilify Tablets (Rare) 2466

Oropharynx, dry

Atrovent Nasal Spray 0.03% 834
Atrovent Nasal Spray 0.06% 836
Proventil HFA Inhalation Aerosol 2914
Tussionex Pennkinetic Extended-Release Suspension 3154
Ventolin HFA Inhalation Aerosol 1638

Orthopnea

▲ Intron A for Injection (Less than or equal to 5%) 2859
Prinivil Tablets (0.3% to 1%) 2087
Prinzide Tablets 2092

Orthostatic circulatory disorders

Avalide Tablets 2713

Oscillopsia

Lamictal (Rare) 1488

Osteoarthritis

Exforge Tablets (Greater than or equal to 0.2%) 2238
Mirapex Tablets 857
Requip Tablets (Infrequent) 1561

Osteoarthritis, aggravated

Ultram ER Extended-Release Tablets (0.5% to less than 1%) 2428

Osteoarthritis, localized

▲ Boniva Injection (1.3% to 3%) 2614
▲ Boniva Tablets (1.3% to 3%) 2618

Osteoarthritis, spinal

Mirapex Tablets 857

Osteoarticular pain

Cardizem LA Extended Release Tablets (Less than 2%)........ 421

Osteomalacia

Atripla Tablets........ 938
Didronel Tablets........ 2583
Hepsera Tablets........ 1253
Phenytek Capsules........ 2192
Truvada Tablets........ 1262
Viread Tablets........ 1268

Osteomalacia, phosphate-induced

K-Phos Original (Sodium Free) Tablets........ 814
K-Phos Neutral Tablets........ 813
Uroqid-Acid No. 2 Tablets........ 814

Osteomyelitis

Copaxone for Injection (Infrequent)... 3110
▲ Cubicin for Injection (Less than 1% to 5%)........ 995
Enbrel for Injection........ 569
Evoxac Capsules (Less than 1%)........ 1013
Mirapex Tablets........ 857
Protopic Ointment (0.2% to less than 1%)........ 628
Prozac Weekly Capsules (Rare)........ 1852
Prozac Pulvules and Liquid (Rare)........ 1852

Osteomyelitis, vertebral

Raptiva for Injection........ 1218

Osteonecrosis

Boniva Injection........ 2614
Boniva Tablets........ 2618
Mirapex Tablets........ 857
Selzentry Tablets........ 2534

Osteonecrosis, hip

Gleevec Tablets (Rare)........ 2255

Osteonecrosis, jaw

Actonel Tablets (Rare)........ 2568
Actonel with Calcium Tablets (Very rare)........ 2574
Didronel Tablets........ 2583
Fosamax Tablets........ 2005
Fosamax Plus D Tablets (Rarely)........ 2013
Reclast Injection........ 2291
Zometa for Intravenous Infusion........ 2341

Osteoporosis

Advair Diskus 100/50........ 1276
Advair Diskus 250/50........ 1276
Advair Diskus 500/50........ 1276
Advair HFA 45/21 Inhalation Aerosol........ 1288
Advair HFA 115/21 Inhalation Aerosol........ 1288
Advair HFA 230/21 Inhalation Aerosol........ 1288
Aricept Tablets (Infrequent)........ 1062
Aricept ODT Tablets (Infrequent)........ 1062
▲ Arimidex Tablets (11%)........ 672
Azmacort Inhalation Aerosol........ 407
Celexa (Rare)........ 1160
▲ CellCept Capsules (3% to less than 20%)........ 2622
▲ CellCept Intravenous (3% to less than 20%)........ 2622
▲ CellCept Oral Suspension (3% to less than 20%)........ 2622
▲ CellCept Tablets (3% to less than 20%)........ 2622
Chantix Tablets (Infrequent)........ 2511
Effexor XR Extended-Release Capsules (Rare)........ 3195
Emsam Transdermal System (Rare)........ 905
Evoxac Capsules (Less than 1%)........ 1013
▲ Femara Tablets (0.2% to 6.9%)........ 2246
Flovent Diskus 50 mcg........ 1435
Flovent HFA........ 1440
Mirapex Tablets........ 857
Neupogen for Injection (Infrequent)........ 589
Paxil (Rare)........ 1535
Paxil CR Controlled-Release Tablets (Rare)........ 1544
▲ Prograf Capsules and Injection (3% to 15%)........ 622
Prozac Weekly Capsules (Rare)........ 1852
Prozac Pulvules and Liquid (Rare)........ 1852
Requip Tablets (Infrequent)........ 1561
Rilutek Tablets (Rare)........ 2771
Symbyax Capsules (Rare)........ 1871
Venlafaxine Hydrochloride Tablets (Rare)........ 2199
Zomig Tablets (Rare)........ 694
Zomig Nasal Spray (Rare)........ 689
Zomig-ZMT Tablets (Rare)........ 694
Zyprexa Tablets (Rare)........ 1883
Zyprexa ZYDIS Orally Disintegrating Tablets (Rare)........ 1883

Osteosclerosis

Effexor XR Extended-Release Capsules (Rare)........ 3195
Venlafaxine Hydrochloride Tablets (Rare)........ 2199

Otitis

Genotropin Lyophilized Powder........ 2547
ProQuad (Greater than or equal to 0.2% to less than 1%)........ 2099
Vaqta (1.8%)........ 2130

Otitis externa

Ambien Tablets (Rare)........ 2692
Ambien CR Tablets (1%)........ 2696
Aricept Tablets (Infrequent)........ 1062
Aricept ODT Tablets (Infrequent)........ 1062
Copaxone for Injection (Infrequent)... 3110
Effexor XR Extended-Release Capsules (Rare)........ 3195
Emsam Transdermal System (Rare)........ 905
Gabitril Tablets (Infrequent)........ 973
Imitrex Nasal Spray........ 1470
Lunesta Tablets (Infrequent)........ 2994
Meridia Capsules........ 475
Mirapex Tablets........ 857
Norditropin Cartridges........ 2354
Paxil (Rare)........ 1535
Paxil CR Controlled-Release Tablets (Rare)........ 1544
Protonix for Delayed-Release Oral Suspension (Less than 1%)........ 3254
Protonix Delayed-Release Tablets (Less than 1%)........ 3254
Protonix I.V. (Less than 1%)........ 3257
Protopic Ointment (0.2% to less than 1%)........ 628
Requip Tablets (Infrequent)........ 1561
Singulair (Greater than or equal to 2%)........ 2114
Soriatane Capsules (Less than 1%)... 3062
Targretin Capsules........ 1084
Teveten Tablets (Less than 1%)........ 515
Teveten HCT Tablets (Less than 1%)........ 517
Venlafaxine Hydrochloride Tablets (Rare)........ 2199
Xyrem Oral Solution (Infrequent)........ 1766

Otitis media

Actonel with Calcium Tablets (2.5%)........ 2574
▲ Advair HFA 45/21 Inhalation Aerosol (1% to 3%)........ 1288
▲ Advair HFA 115/21 Inhalation Aerosol (1% to 3%)........ 1288
▲ Advair HFA 230/21 Inhalation Aerosol (1% to 3%)........ 1288
▲ Allegra Oral Solution (2.4% to 3.8%)........ 2684
Allegra Tablets (2.4%)........ 2684
Ambien Tablets (Rare)........ 2692
Ambien CR Tablets (Rare)........ 2696
Aricept Tablets (Infrequent)........ 1062
Aricept ODT Tablets (Infrequent)........ 1062
Attenuvax........ 1951
Axert Tablets (Rare)........ 2431
Celebrex Capsules (0.1% to 1.9%)... 2979
▲ Chemet Capsules (1% to 3.7%)........ 2484
▲ Clarinex Syrup (6.1%)........ 2828
Comvax (0.5% to 2.7%)........ 1966
Depakote ER Tablets........ 423
Doxil Injection (Less than 1%)........ 2378
Effexor XR Extended-Release Capsules (Infrequent)........ 3195
▲ Elidel Cream 1% (0.6% to 3%)........ 2221
Emsam Transdermal System (Infrequent)........ 905
▲ Emtriva Capsules (23%)........ 1246
▲ Emtriva Oral Solution (23%)........ 1246
▲ Evoxac Capsules (1% to 3%)........ 1013
Exelon Capsules (Infrequent)........ 2229
Exelon Oral Solution (Infrequent)........ 2229
▲ Exubera Inhalation Powder (6.5%)... 2515
▲ Flovent Diskus 50 mcg (1% to 3%)........ 1435
Flovent HFA........ 1440
▲ FluMist Vaccine (3%)........ 1945
Gabitril Tablets (Frequent)........ 973
▲ Humatrope Vials and Cartridges (16.2% to 35.3%)........ 1838
▲ Increlex Injection (Greater than or equal to 5%)........ 3100
Kaletra (Less than 2%)........ 452
Keppra Oral Solution (1% to greater than or equal to 2%)........ 3131
Keppra Tablets (1% to greater than or equal to 2%)........ 3131
Klonopin (Infrequent)........ 2639
Kogenate FS with Bio-Set........ 748
Lunesta Tablets (Infrequent)........ 2994
Luvox CR Extended-Release Capsules (Infrequent)........ 1759
Lyrica Capsules (Greater than or equal to 1%)........ 2527
Meridia Capsules........ 475
Meruvax II........ 2061
Micardis Tablets (More than 0.3%)........ 852
Micardis HCT Tablets........ 854
Mirapex Tablets........ 857
M-M-R II........ 2054
Mumpsvax........ 2068
Namenda (More than one patient)........ 1180
Nasacort AQ Nasal Spray........ 2765
Nasonex Nasal Spray (Greater than or equal to 2%)........ 2883
Nexium Delayed-Release Capsules (Less than 1%)........ 645
Nexium I.V. (Less than 1%)........ 652
Nexium Delayed-Release Oral Suspension (Less than 1%)........ 645
▲ Norditropin Cartridges (69.6% to 86.4%)........ 2354
Orthoclone OKT3 Sterile Solution (Less than 1%)........ 2387
Paxil (Infrequent)........ 1535
Paxil CR Controlled-Release Tablets (Infrequent)........ 1544
Liquid PedvaxHIB (Among most frequent)........ 2073
Prevnar........ 3241
▲ Prograf Capsules and Injection (3% to 15%)........ 622
ProQuad (Greater than or equal to 0.2% to less than 1%)........ 2099
▲ Protopic Ointment (Up to 7%)........ 628
Pulmicort Flexhaler (1.3%)........ 654
Remeron Tablets (Rare)........ 2924
RemeronSolTab Tablets (Rare)........ 2927
Requip Tablets (Infrequent)........ 1561
▲ RotaTeq (14.5%)........ 2110
Sandostatin Injection (Less than 1%)........ 2300
Singulair (Greater than or equal to 2%)........ 2114
Soriatane Capsules (Less than 1%)... 3062
Sular Extended Release Tablets (Less than or equal to 1%)........ 2975
Symbyax Capsules (Up to 2%)........ 1871
▲ Synagis Intramuscular Solution (41.9%)........ 1948
▲ Tamiflu Capsules (2% to 9%)........ 2649
▲ Tamiflu Oral Suspension (2% to 9%)........ 2649
Teveten Tablets (Less than 1%)........ 515
Teveten HCT Tablets (Less than 1%)........ 517
Tricor Tablets........ 520
▲ Vaqta (7.6%)........ 2130
Varivax (Greater than or equal to 1%)........ 2133
Venlafaxine Hydrochloride Tablets (Infrequent)........ 2199
▲ Vigamox Ophthalmic Solution (1% to 4%)........ 548
▲ Xenical Capsules (2.9% to 4.3%)........ 2672

Otitis media, serous

Kogenate FS........ 746

Ototoxicity

Furosemide Tablets........ 2186
Taxotere Injection Concentrate (Rare)........ 2773
Zyrtec Chewable Tablets (Less than 2%)........ 1920
Zyrtec Syrup (Less than 2%)........ 1920
Zyrtec Tablets (Less than 2%)........ 1920
Zyrtec-D 12 Hour Extended Release Tablets (Less than 2%)........ 1923

Ovarian cyst

Activella Tablets........ 2347
Celebrex Capsules (Greater than or equal to 0.1% to less than 1%)........ 2979
Copaxone for Injection (Infrequent)... 3110
Effexor XR Extended-Release Capsules (Rare)........ 3195
Evoxac Capsules (Less than 1%)........ 1013
Mirapex Tablets........ 857
Venlafaxine Hydrochloride Tablets (Rare)........ 2199
Xyrem Oral Solution (Infrequent)........ 1766

Ovarian disorder, unspecified

Evoxac Capsules (Less than 1%)........ 1013
Lyrica Capsules (Rare)........ 2527
Salagen Tablets (Less than 1%)........ 1082
Symbyax Capsules (Infrequent)........ 1871
Wellbutrin Tablets (Rare)........ 1648

Ovarian enlargement

Follistim AQ Cartridge........ 2844

Ovarian hyperstimulation syndrome

▲ Follistim AQ Cartridge (5.3% to 9%)........ 2844

Overdose, intentional

Prozac Weekly Capsules (Infrequent)........ 1852

Oversedation

Vicodin Tablets........ 529
Vicodin ES Tablets........ 530
Vicodin HP Tablets........ 531

Overstimulation

Adderall XR Capsules........ 3012
Adipex-P........ 1185
Dexedrine........ 1401
Eldepryl Capsules........ 3052
Parnate Tablets........ 1532
Vyvanse Capsules........ 3033

Ovulation

ActoPlus Met Tablets........ 3071

Oxygen saturation, decreased

Avelox (Greater than or equal to 2%)........ 2803
▲ DepoDur Injection (Greater than 10%)........ 1095
Opana Tablets (Less than 1%)........ 1117
Opana ER Tablets (Less than 1%)........ 1121

P

Pain

▲ Abelcet Injection (5%)........ 1134
▲ Abilify Injection (3%)........ 881
▲ Abilify Injection (3%)........ 2466
▲ Abilify Oral Solution (3%)........ 881
▲ Abilify Oral Solution (3%)........ 2466
▲ Abilify Discmelt Orally Disintegrating Tablets (3%)........ 881
▲ Abilify Discmelt Orally Disintegrating Tablets (3%)........ 2466
▲ Abilify Tablets (3%)........ 881
▲ Abilify Tablets (3%)........ 2466
Accolate Tablets (1.9%)........ 669
Aceon Tablets (2 mg, 4 mg, 8 mg) (0.3% to 1%)........ 3038
▲ Aciphex Tablets (3%)........ 1053
Actiq (1% or greater)........ 959
▲ Actonel Tablets (14.1%)........ 2568
▲ Actonel with Calcium Tablets (7.7% to 13.6%)........ 2574
▲ Advair HFA 45/21 Inhalation Aerosol (1% to 3%)........ 1288
▲ Advair HFA 115/21 Inhalation Aerosol (1% to 3%)........ 1288
▲ Advair HFA 230/21 Inhalation Aerosol (1% to 3%)........ 1288
▲ Advicor Tablets (8%)........ 402
▲ Aggrenox Capsules (6.4%)........ 819
▲ Agrylin Capsules (15%)........ 3017
Aldara Cream, 5% (More than 1%)........ 1699
Alinia for Oral Suspension (Less than 1%)........ 2677
Alinia Tablets (Less than 1%)........ 2677
Allegra Oral Solution (2.4%)........ 2684
Alphanate........ 1709
Ambien Tablets (Rare)........ 2692
Ambien CR Tablets (Rare)........ 2696
▲ AmBisome for Injection (14%)........ 606
Amitiza Capsules (Less than 1%)........ 3082
▲ Angiomax for Injection (3.4% to 15%)........ 1933
Anzemet Injection (2.4%)........ 2701
▲ Anzemet Tablets (0% to 3.1%)........ 2704
Aralast (Greater than or equal to 0.2%)........ 726
▲ Argatroban Injection (4.6%)........ 1308
▲ Aricept Tablets (3%)........ 1062
▲ Aricept ODT Tablets (3%)........ 1062
▲ Arimidex Tablets (11% to 17%)........ 672
Arixtra Injection (0% to 1.7%)........ 1313
▲ Arranon Injection (0% to 11%)........ 1319
▲ Asacol Delayed-Release Tablets (14%)........ 2579
▲ Asmanex Twisthaler (1% to 3%)........ 2797
Atacand HCT (0.5% or greater)........ 642
▲ Atripla Tablets (Greater than or equal to 5%)........ 938
▲ Avastin IV (8% to 62%)........ 1192
Avelox (Greater than or equal to 0.1% to less than 2%)........ 2803
▲ Axid Capsules (4.2%)........ 1364
▲ Azmacort Inhalation Aerosol (1% to 3%)........ 407
Bactroban Ointment (1.5%)........ 1368
Benicar Tablets (Greater than 0.5%)........ 1009
▲ Betaseron for SC Injection (42%)........ 756
▲ Bexxar (1% to 19%)........ 1371
Bicillin C-R Injectable Suspension........ 1775
Bicillin L-A Injection........ 1777
▲ Brovana Inhalation Solution (8%)........ 2990

▲ Busulfex Injection (2% to 44%) 2477
▲ Campral Tablets (2% to 4%) 1158
Cardizem LA Extended Release Tablets (Less than 2%)................ 421
Celebrex Capsules (0.1% to 1.9%)... 2979
Cialis Tablets (Less than 2%)........... 1792
Cipro I.V. (1% or less)....................... 2817
Cipro (Less than 1%)......................... 2810
▲ Climara Transdermal System (1% to 11%).. 763
▲ Climara Pro Transdermal System (5.2%).. 768
▲ Clolar for Intravenous Infusion (19%).. 1239
Combivent Inhalation Aerosol (2.5%).. 845
▲ Combivir Tablets (12%) 1384
▲ Copaxone for Injection (28%) 3110
▲ Crinone 8% Gel (8%) 992
Crixivan Capsules.............................. 1979
▲ Dacogen Injection (13%) 1066
Denavir Cream.................................... 2205
▲ DepoCyt Injection (3% to 14%) 1136
Diclofenac Sodium Ophthalmic Solution.. ⊙240
▲ Doxil Injection (3.4% to 7.2%) 2378
DynaCirc CR Controlled Release Tablets (0.5% to 1%).................... 1407
▲ Eloxatin for Injection (1% to 14%) 2731
Emend Capsules (Greater than 0.5%).. 1992
Emend for Injection (Greater than 0.5%).. 1999
Emsam Transdermal System........... 905
Enablex Extended-Release Tablets (Greater than or equal to 1%)........ 2225
Enbrel for Injection........................... 569
▲ Enjuvia Tablets (10% to 19%) 1029
▲ Equetro Extended-Release Capsules (12%)............................ 3174
▲ Erbitux (16% to 51%) 912
▲ Evoxac Capsules (3.3%) 1013
Exelon Capsules (2% or more)............ 2229
Exelon Oral Solution (2% or more).... 2229
▲ Fabrazyme for Intravenous Infusion (16%)................................ 1241
▲ Faslodex Injection (18.9%) 682
▲ Femara Tablets (5%) 2246
Fentora Tablets (Greater than 1%).... 968
▲ Flebogamma 5% (16%) 1715
▲ Flonase Nasal Spray (1% to 3%) 1431
▲ Flovent Diskus 50 mcg (1% to 10%).. 1435
▲ Flovent HFA (1% to 3%) 1440
▲ Flulaval Injection Vaccine (24% to 31%).. 1448
Fluorescite Injection......................... ⊙203
▲ Forteo for Injection (21.3%) 1816
Frova Tablets (Frequent).................. 1111
▲ Gabitril Tablets (2% to 7%) 973
▲ Gemzar for Injection (7% to 48%) 1820
▲ Gengraf Capsules (6% to 13%) 435
▲ Gliadel Wafer (7% to 13%) 1076
▲ Herceptin I.V. (47%) 1199
▲ Humatrope Vials and Cartridges (6.25% to 13.6%)......................... 1838
Hyalgan Solution............................... 2742
▲ Hycamtin for Injection (1.1% to 23%).. 1459
Imitrex Tablets (1% to 2%)................ 1474
▲ Indapamide Tablets (Greater than or equal to 5%)............................ 2188
▲ Intron A for Injection (Up to 18%) 2859
Invanz for Injection (Greater than 0.1%).. 2029
▲ Ionsys Transdermal System (1% to less than 10%)........................ 2410
▲ Ixempra Kit for Injection (8%) 915
▲ Kepivance (16%) 583
▲ Keppra Injection (7%) 3137
▲ Keppra Oral Solution (6% to 7%) 3131
▲ Keppra Tablets (6% to 7%) 3131
Klonopin (Infrequent)........................ 2639
K-Phos Original (Sodium Free) Tablets (Less frequent)................. 814
K-Phos Neutral Tablets..................... 813
▲ Lamictal (5%) 1488
▲ Leukine (17%) 774
Levaquin.. 2416
Levaquin in 5% Dextrose Injection.... 2416
Levitra Tablets (Less than 2%).......... 2876
▲ Lovaza Capsules (1.8% to 4%) 1520
Lovenox Injection.............................. 2756
▲ Lunesta Tablets (4% to 5%) 2994
▲ Lupron Depot 3.75 mg (12%) 462
▲ Lupron Depot 7.5 mg (23.2%) 469
▲ Lupron Depot–3 Month 11.25 mg (12%).. 462
Lupron Depot-PED 7.5 mg, 11.25 mg and 15 mg (2%)............. 471
▲ Luvox CR Extended-Release Capsules (2% to 10%).................. 1759
▲ Lyrica Capsules (2% to 5%) 2527
▲ Megace ES Oral Suspension (0% to 6%).. 2499
▲ Mepron Suspension (10%) 1526
▲ Merrem I.V. (Greater than 0.1% to 5.1%).. 684
Micardis Tablets (1%)........................ 852
Micardis HCT Tablets (2% or greater)... 854
Mirapex Tablets (1% or more)........... 857
▲ Mobic Oral Suspension (0.9% to 5.2%).. 863
▲ Mobic Tablets (0.9% to 5.2%) 863
▲ Myfortic Tablets (3% to less than 20%).. 2276
▲ Mylotarg for Injection (18%) 3212
▲ Namenda (3%) 1180
▲ Neoral Oral Solution (4.4% to 13%).. 2280
▲ Neoral Soft Gelatin Capsules (4.4% to 13%).............................. 2280
Neupogen for Injection (2%)............. 589
Nexium Delayed-Release Capsules (Less than 1%)............................. 645
Nexium I.V. (Less than 1%)............... 652
Nexium Delayed-Release Oral Suspension (Less than 1%)........... 645
▲ Niaspan Extended-Release Tablets (1% to 5%)...................... 480
Norvir (1.7% to 2.2%)........................ 489
▲ Novantrone for Injection Concentrate (8% to 41%)............. 1100
NovoSeven (1%)................................ 2367
NovoSeven RT (1%)........................... 2370
▲ Noxafil Oral Suspension (1% to 11%).. 2889
▲ Ontak Vials (48%) 1079
Orthoclone OKT3 Sterile Solution (Less than 1%)............................. 2387
OxyContin Tablets (Less than 1%).... 2589
▲ Panretin Gel 0.1% (0% to 34%) 1081
ParaGard T 380A Intrauterine Copper Contraceptive 1041
▲ Pediarix Vaccine (0.3% to 30.5%) 1552
▲ Photofrin for Injection (8% to 22%).. 708
▲ Plavix Tablets (6.4%) 926
▲ Plavix Tablets (6.4%) 2767
Pletal Tablets.................................... 2481
▲ Premarin Tablets (17% to 20%) 3221
Premarin Vaginal Cream 3228
▲ Premphase Tablets (11% to 20%) 3232
▲ Prempro Tablets (11% to 20%) 3232
Prinivil Tablets (0.3% to 1%)............. 2087
Prinzide Tablets................................ 2092
▲ ProAir HFA Inhalation Aerosol (3%) ... 3113
▲ ProAmatine Tablets (4.9%) 3032
▲ Prograf Capsules and Injection (24% to 63%)................................ 622
▲ Proleukin for Injection (12%) 2287
Protonix for Delayed-Release Oral Suspension (Greater than or equal to 1%).............................. 3254
Protonix Delayed-Release Tablets (Greater than or equal to 1%)........ 3254
▲ Protopic Ointment (1% to 4%) 628
Prozac Pulvules and Liquid............... 1852
▲ Pulmicort Flexhaler (Greater than or equal to 3% to 10%)................ 654
▲ Qvar Inhalation Aerosol (1% to 5%).. 3116
▲ Rapamune (29% to 33%) 3260
▲ Raptiva for Injection (10%) 1218
▲ Reclast Injection (5%) 2291
ReFacto Vials.................................... 3269
▲ Remicade for IV Injection (8%) 950
▲ ReoPro Vials (3.4% to 5.4%) 1860
▲ Requip Tablets (Infrequent to 8%) 1561
▲ Risperdal Consta Long-Acting Injection (3%)............................... 1753
▲ Rituxan I.V. (1% to 12%) 1223
Rythmol Tablets (Less than 1%)........ 1586
Rythmol SR Capsules........................ 1590
▲ Salagen Tablets (4%) 1082
▲ Sandostatin LAR Depot (4% to 15.4%).. 2302
▲ Selzentry Tablets (3.5%) 2534
▲ Serevent Diskus (1% to 3%) 1594
▲ Simulect for Injection (Greater than or equal to 10%)................... 2306
▲ Soriatane Capsules (1% to 10%) 3062
▲ Suboxone Tablets (22.4% to 24%) .. 2601
▲ Subutex Tablets (18.4% to 24%) .. 2601
Sulfamylon for 5% Topical Solution... 2194
▲ Sustiva Capsules (2% to 14%) 930
▲ Sustiva Tablets (2% to 14%) 930
▲ Synagis Intramuscular Solution (8.5%).. 1948
Tamiflu Capsules (Less than 1%)...... 2649
Tamiflu Oral Suspension (Less than 1%)...................................... 2649
▲ Taxotere Injection Concentrate (5.5%).. 2773
Teveten Tablets (Less than 1%)........ 515
Teveten HCT Tablets (Less than 1%).. 517
▲ Thyrogen for Injection (4 patients out of 55)..................................... 1244
▲ Torisel Injection (5% to 28%) 3272
▲ Travatan Z Ophthalmic Solution (1% to 5%)................................... 547
Tricor Tablets.................................... 520
▲ Trisenox Injection (15%) 986
▲ Truvada Tablets (Greater than or equal to 5%)................................ 1262
▲ Tygacil for Injection (3.7%) 3276
Tyzeka Tablets (2%)......................... 2328
Ultane Liquid for Inhalation (Less than 1%)...................................... 524
▲ Ultram ER Extended-Release Tablets (1% to less than 5%)......... 2428
Uroxatral Tablets (1% to 2%)............ 2786
▲ Vagifem Tablets (3% to 5%) 2375
▲ Valcyte Tablets (Less than 5%) 2654
Vantas (Less than 2%)...................... 1737
Vaprisol (2.2%)................................. 632
▲ Vesanoid Capsules (37%) 2660
Viadur Implant (Less than 2%).......... 802
Vicoprofen Tablets (Less than 3%).... 533
▲ Viread Tablets (7% to 13%) 1268
▲ Voltaren Ophthalmic Solution (Less than or equal to 3%)........... 2336
▲ WelChol Tablets (6.7%) 1015
Wellbutrin Tablets (Infrequent)......... 1648
▲ Wellbutrin SR Sustained-Release Tablets (2% to 3%)...................... 1653
▲ Wellbutrin XL Extended-Release Tablets (2% to 3%)...................... 1659
▲ Xeloda Tablets (Less than 5%) 2662
Xifaxan Tablets (Less than 2%)......... 2682
▲ Xolair (7%) 1235
▲ Xolair (7%) 2339
Xopenex Inhalation Solution (1.4% to 2.8%).. 3001
▲ Xopenex Inhalation Solution Concentrate (1.4% to 3%)............ 3005
Xopenex HFA Inhalation Aerosol (1.4% to 2.8%)............................ 3009
Xyrem Oral Solution (2.9% to 5.7%).. 1766
Yaz Tablets (Greater than 1%).......... 805
Ziagen (Less than 1%)...................... 1673
Zomig Tablets (Common).................. 694
Zomig-ZMT Tablets (Common).......... 694
▲ Zosyn for Injection (1.7% to 3.2%) ... 3284
Zovirax Capsules.............................. 1690
Zovirax Ointment.............................. 819
Zovirax... 1690
Zyban Sustained-Release Tablets (Infrequent)................................. 1692
Zyrtec Chewable Tablets (Less than 2%)...................................... 1920
Zyrtec Syrup (Less than 2%)............ 1920
Zyrtec Tablets (Less than 2%).......... 1920
Zyrtec-D 12 Hour Extended Release Tablets (Less than 2%)..... 1923

Pain, abdominal
(*see under* Abdominal pain/cramps)

Pain, application site
▲ Aldara Cream, 5% (2% to 8%) 1699
Altabax Ointment (Less than 1%)...... 1299
Daytrana Transdermal Patch............ 3022
Fentora Tablets (Greater than 1%).... 968
▲ Sulfamylon Cream (One of two most frequent)............................ 2194
▲ Targretin Gel 1% (10% to 40%) 1088
Zovirax Ointment.............................. 819

Pain, arm
Cipro... 2810
Cipro XR Tablets............................... 2823
Cozaar Tablets (Less than 1%)......... 1973
▲ Femara Tablets (21% to 22%) 2246
Prinzide Tablets................................ 2092
Vaqta (1.3%).................................... 2130
Xolair (2%)....................................... 1235
Xolair (2%)....................................... 2339

Pain, back
(*see also under* Backache)
▲ Ambien CR Tablets (4%) 2696
Avelox (Less than 0.1%).................... 2803
Axid Capsules (2.4%)........................ 1364
▲ Cancidas for Injection (Up to 3.5%).. 1953
▲ CellCept Capsules (34.6% to 46.6%).. 2622
▲ CellCept Intravenous (34.6% to 46.6%).. 2622
▲ CellCept Oral Suspension (34.6% to 46.6%)..................................... 2622
▲ CellCept Tablets (34.6% to 46.6%).. 2622
Cipro (Less than 1%)........................ 2810
Cipro XR Tablets............................... 2823
▲ DepoDur Injection (2% to 5%) 1095
Elidel Cream 1% (0.3% to 1.8%)...... 2221
▲ Eloxatin for Injection (0% to 19%) 2731
Enablex Extended-Release Tablets (Greater than or equal to 1%)........ 2225
▲ Entereg Capsules (3.3% to 3.4%) 3293
Exforge Tablets (Greater than or equal to 0.2%)............................ 2238
▲ Fabrazyme for Intravenous Infusion (16%)................................ 1241
▲ Follistim AQ Cartridge (7%) 2844
Keppra Oral Solution (Greater than or equal to 1%)............................ 3131
Keppra Tablets (Greater than or equal to 1%)............................... 3131
Levitra Tablets (Less than or equal to 2%).. 2876
▲ Mycamine for Injection (5.4%) 616
▲ Noxafil Oral Suspension (10%) 2889
▲ Prandin Tablets (5% to 6%) 2971
Risperdal Consta Long-Acting Injection (Frequent)...................... 1753
Salagen Tablets (Less than 1% to 2%).. 1082
▲ Sandostatin LAR Depot (8% to 27.3%).. 2302
▲ Simcor Tablets (2.1% to 3.2%) 502
▲ Starlix Tablets (4%) 2314
▲ Tasigna Capsules (10% to 12%) 2316
Taxotere Injection Concentrate 2773
Tekturna HCT Tablets (Greater than 1%)...................................... 2324
▲ Velcade for Injection (13% to 17%).. 2168
Vytorin 10/10 Tablets........................ 2149
Vytorin 10/10 Tablets (0.4%)........... 2939
Vytorin 10/20 Tablets........................ 2149
Vytorin 10/20 Tablets (0.4%)........... 2939
Vytorin 10/40 Tablets........................ 2149
Vytorin 10/40 Tablets (0.4%)........... 2939
Vytorin 10/80 Tablets........................ 2149
Vytorin 10/80 Tablets (0.4%)........... 2939
Zetia Tablets (2.4%)......................... 2951
Zyrtec Chewable Tablets (Less than 2%)...................................... 1920
Zyrtec Syrup (Less than 2%)............ 1920
Zyrtec Tablets (Less than 2%).......... 1920
Zyrtec-D 12 Hour Extended Release Tablets (Less than 2%)..... 1923

Pain, biliary
▲ Avinza Capsules (Less than 5%) 1772
Lipitor Tablets (Less than 2%).......... 2501
Luvox CR Extended-Release Capsules (Rare)........................... 1759
Protonix for Delayed-Release Oral Suspension (Less than 1%)........... 3254
Protonix Delayed-Release Tablets (Less than 1%)............................. 3254
Protonix I.V. (Less than 1%)............. 3257
Prozac Weekly Capsules (Rare)......... 1852
Prozac Pulvules and Liquid (Rare)..... 1852
Remicade for IV Injection (Greater than or equal to 0.2%)................. 950
Requip Tablets (Rare)....................... 1561
Rilutek Tablets (Rare)....................... 2771

Pain, bone
Abelcet Injection.............................. 1134
Actiq (Less than 1%)........................ 959
▲ Actonel Tablets (5.3%) 2568
▲ Actonel with Calcium Tablets (1.4% to 4.6%)............................ 2574
▲ Advair HFA 45/21 Inhalation Aerosol (1% to 3%)...................... 1288
▲ Advair HFA 115/21 Inhalation Aerosol (1% to 3%)...................... 1288
▲ Advair HFA 230/21 Inhalation Aerosol (1% to 3%)...................... 1288
AmBisome for Injection (Less common)...................................... 606
Amerge Tablets (Rare)...................... 1301
▲ Aranesp for Injection (10%) 564
▲ Arimidex Tablets (6% to 12%) 672
▲ Avastin IV (3.9%) 1192
Benicar Tablets (Greater than 0.5%).. 1009
Boniva Injection............................... 2614
Boniva Tablets.................................. 2618
Calcijex Injection.............................. 419
Celexa (Infrequent)........................... 1160
Cipro... 2810
Copaxone for Injection (Infrequent)... 3110
Depakote ER Tablets........................ 423
▲ Didronel Tablets (About 1 patient in 10 to about 2 in 10)................. 2583
Doxil Injection (Less than 1%).......... 2378
Effexor XR Extended-Release Capsules (Infrequent).................... 3195
▲ Eloxatin for Injection (2% to less than 5%).. 2731
▲ Erbitux (3% to 15%) 912
▲ Faslodex Injection (15.8%) 682
▲ Femara Tablets (22%) 2246
▲ Fosamax (0.4% to approximately 6%).. 2005
▲ Fosamax Plus D Tablets (0.4% to 4.1%).. 2013
▲ Frova Tablets (3%) 1111

▲ Gleevec Tablets (11.3%) 2255
▲ Herceptin I.V. (7%) 1199
▲ Hycamtin for Injection (59%) 1459
▲ Intron A for Injection (Less than 5%) 2859
K-Phos Original (Sodium Free) Tablets (Less frequent) 814
K-Phos Neutral Tablets 813
▲ Leukine (21%) 774
Lexapro Oral Suspension (Frequent) 1174
Lexapro Tablets (Frequent) 1174
▲ Lupron Depot 7.5 mg (Less than 5%) 469
Mirapex Tablets 857
▲ Neulasta Injection (15% to 72%) 587
▲ Neupogen for Injection (22% to 33%) 589
▲ Nexavar Tablets (Greater than or equal to 10%) 784
Novantrone for Injection Concentrate 1100
Pletal Tablets (Less than 2%) 2481
Protonix for Delayed-Release Oral Suspension (Less than 1%) 3254
Protonix Delayed-Release Tablets (Less than 1%) 3254
Protonix I.V. (Less than 1%) 3257
Prozac Weekly Capsules (Infrequent) 1852
Prozac Pulvules and Liquid (Infrequent) 1852
▲ Reclast Injection (9%) 2291
Remeron Tablets (Rare) 2924
RemeronSolTab Tablets (Rare) 2927
Requip Tablets (Infrequent) 1561
Rocaltrol Capsules 1150
Rocaltrol Oral Solution 1150
▲ Serevent Diskus (1% to 3%) 1594
▲ Soriatane Capsules (1% to 10%) 3062
▲ Tarceva Tablets (Less than 1% to 31%) 1228
Targretin Capsules 1084
▲ Tasigna Capsules (11% to 13%) 2316
Teveten HCT Tablets (Less than 1%) 517
▲ Trisenox Injection (23%) 986
Uroqid-Acid No. 2 Tablets 814
Vantas (Less than 2%) 1737
▲ Velcade for Injection (11% to 16%) 2168
Venlafaxine Hydrochloride Tablets (Infrequent) 2199
▲ Vesanoid Capsules (77%) 2660
Viadur Implant (Less than 2%) 802
▲ Xeloda Tablets (Less than 5%) 2662
Zemplar Injection 538
▲ Zometa for Intravenous Infusion (55%) 2341
Zomig Tablets (Rare) 694
Zomig Nasal Spray (Rare) 689
Zomig-ZMT Tablets (Rare) 694
Zyprexa Tablets (Rare) 1883
Zyprexa ZYDIS Orally Disintegrating Tablets (Rare) 1883

Pain, cancer related

▲ Fentora Tablets (2% to 16%) 968
▲ Taxotere Injection Concentrate (4.6% to 20.7%) 2773

Pain, catheter

▲ Dacogen Injection (5%) 1066
Natrecor for Injection (Greater than or equal to 1%) 2977

Pain, chest

▲ Abelcet Injection (3%) 1134
Abilify Injection (Greater than or equal to 1 in 100 patients) 2466
Abilify Oral Solution (Greater than or equal to 1 in 100 patients) 881
Abilify Oral Solution (Greater than or equal to 1 in 100 patients) 2466
Abilify Discmelt Orally Disintegrating Tablets (Greater than or equal to 1 in 100 patients) 881
Abilify Discmelt Orally Disintegrating Tablets (Greater than or equal to 1 in 100 patients) 2466
Abilify Tablets (Greater than or equal to 1 in 100 patients) 881
Abilify Tablets (Greater than or equal to 1 in 100 patients) 2466
Accutane Capsules (Less frequent) 2607
Aceon Tablets (2 mg, 4 mg, 8 mg) (2.4%) 3038
Actiq (1% or greater) 959
▲ Actonel Tablets (5% to 6.6%) 2568
▲ Actonel with Calcium Tablets (2.3% to 5%) 2574
Adenocard IV Injection (Less than 1%) 603
Advate (0.6%) 721
Advicor Tablets 402
▲ Aerobid/Aerobid-M (3% to 9%) 1153
Aggrenox Capsules 819
▲ Agrylin Capsules (7.8%) 3017
Aldara Cream, 5% (1%) 1699
▲ Alferon N Injection (6% to 10%) 1726
▲ Alimta for Injection (Less than 1% to 40%) 1786
Ambien Tablets (1%) 2692
Ambien CR Tablets (Infrequent) 2696
▲ AmBisome for Injection (8.2% to 12%) 606
Angiomax for Injection (2.3%) 1933
Anzemet Injection (Rare) 2701
Anzemet Tablets (Rare) 2704
Aralast (0.1%) 726
▲ Aranesp for Injection (7% to 8%) 564
▲ Argatroban Injection (15.2%) 1308
Aricept Tablets (2%) 1062
Aricept ODT Tablets (2%) 1062
▲ Arimidex Tablets (5% to 7%) 672
Arixtra Injection (1.4%) 1313
▲ Arranon Injection (0% to 5%) 1319
▲ Asacol Delayed-Release Tablets (3%) 2579
Atacand Tablets (More than 1%) 639
Atacand HCT (0.5% or greater) 642
Avalide Tablets (2%) 892
Avalide Tablets (2%) 2713
Avapro Tablets (1% or greater) 897
Avapro Tablets (1% or greater) 2718
Avelox (Less than 0.1%) 2803
Axert Tablets (Infrequent) 2431
Axid Capsules (2.3%) 1364
Azilect Tablets (Greater than 1%) 3106
Azopt Ophthalmic Suspension (Less than 1%) 540
Benicar Tablets (Greater than 0.5%) 1009
Benicar HCT Tablets (Greater than 1%) 1010
▲ Betaseron for SC Injection (9%) 756
Betimol Ophthalmic Solution 3181
▲ Bexxar (0% to 7%) 1371
▲ Brovana Inhalation Solution (7%) 2990
▲ Busulfex Injection (26%) 2477
Byetta Injection 600
Bystolic Tablets (0% to 1%) 1155
Campral Tablets (Frequent) 1158
Captopril Tablets (Approximately 1 in 100 patients) 2182
Cardene I.V. (0.7%) 1093
Catapres-TTS (0.5% or less) 842
Ceftin Tablets (0.1% to 1%) 1380
Celebrex Capsules (0.1% to 1.9%) 2979
Celexa 1160
Chantix Tablets (Frequent) 2511
Cialis Tablets (Less than 2%) 1792
Cipro I.V. (1% or less) 2817
Cipro (Less than 1%) 2810
Cipro XR Tablets 2823
Clinoril Tablets (Less than 1 in 100) 1962
Combigan Ophthalmic Solution 553
Combivent Inhalation Aerosol (0.3%) 845
Concerta Extended-Release Tablets 1925
▲ Copaxone for Injection (21%) 3110
Coreg Tablets 1387
Cosopt Sterile Ophthalmic Solution (Less than 1%) 1969
Cozaar Tablets (1% or greater) 1973
▲ Cubicin for Injection (1% to 6.7%) 995
▲ Dacogen Injection (7%) 1066
Demadex Injection (1.2%) 2630
Demadex Tablets (1.2%) 2630
▲ Depakote ER Tablets (Greater than 1% to less than 5%) 423
Diovan Tablets (Greater than 0.2%) 2212
Diovan HCT Tablets (Less frequent to greater than 0.2%) 2216
▲ Doxil Injection (1% to 5%) 2378
Duragesic Transdermal System (1% or greater) 2405
DynaCirc CR Controlled Release Tablets (0.5% to 1%) 1407
Effexor XR Extended-Release Capsules (Frequent) 3195
Elitek (Less than or equal to 1%) 2729
▲ Eloxatin for Injection (1% to 8%) 2731
Emsam Transdermal System (Frequent) 905
Enbrel for Injection 569
▲ Epogen for Injection (7%) 576
▲ Equetro Extended-Release Capsules (5%) 3174
▲ Evista Tablets (4%) 1810
▲ Evoxac Capsules (1% to 3%) 1013
Exelon Capsules (2% or more) 2229
Exelon Oral Solution (2% or more) 2229
Exelon Patch (Infrequent) 2233
Exforge Tablets (Greater than 0.1% but less than 1%) 2238
▲ Exubera Inhalation Powder (4.7%) 2515
▲ Fabrazyme for Intravenous Infusion (Greater than or equal to 5%) 1241
▲ Faslodex Injection (7.1%) 682
▲ Femara Tablets (3% to 8%) 2246
Fentora Tablets (Greater than 1%) 968
▲ Flolan for Injection (11% to 67%) 1426
▲ Flomax Capsules (4% to 4.1%) 848
Fluarix Vaccine 1446
Flulaval Injection Vaccine 1448
▲ Foradil Aerolizer (3.2%) 2849
Forteo for Injection (Less than 1/1000 patients) 1816
Frova Tablets (2%) 1111
Gabitril Tablets (1% or more) 973
Gammagard Liquid 730
▲ Gengraf Capsules (6%) 435
▲ Geodon Capsules (3%) 2520
▲ Gleevec Tablets (7% to 11%) 2255
▲ Humira Injection (Less than 5%) 442
Hycamtin for Injection (2%) 1459
Imitrex Injection 1465
Imitrex Nasal Spray 1470
▲ Imitrex Tablets (2% to 3%) 1474
▲ Indapamide Tablets (Less than 5%) 2188
Indocin (Less than 1%) 2024
▲ Intron A for Injection (Up to 28%) 2859
Invanz for Injection (1% to 1.5%) 2029
Ionsys Transdermal System (.1% to less than 1%) 2410
▲ Ixempra Kit for Injection (5%) 915
Kaletra (Less than 2%) 452
Keppra Oral Solution (1% or more) 3131
Keppra Tablets (1% or more) 3131
Klonopin (Infrequent) 2639
▲ Lamictal (5%) 1488
▲ Leukine (15%) 774
Levaquin 2416
Levaquin in 5% Dextrose Injection 2416
Levitra Tablets (Less than 2%) 2876
Lexapro Oral Suspension (Frequent) 1174
Lexapro Tablets (Frequent) 1174
▲ Lexiscan Injection (7%) 614
Lipitor Tablets (Greater than or equal to 2%) 2501
Lovaza Capsules 1520
Lunesta Tablets (Frequent) 2994
▲ Luvox CR Extended-Release Capsules (3%) 1759
▲ Lyrica Capsules (1% to 4%) 2527
Mavik Tablets (0.3% to 1%) 472
Maxair Autohaler (1.3%) 1705
▲ Maxalt Tablets (Less than 2% to 3%) 2056
▲ Maxalt-MLT Orally Disintegrating Tablets (Less than 2% to 3%) 2056
▲ Megace ES Oral Suspension (1% to 3%) 2499
▲ Meridia Capsules (1.8%) 475
Merrem I.V. (Greater than 0.1% to 1%) 684
Mevacor Tablets (0.5% to 1%) 2063
Micardis Tablets (1%) 852
Micardis HCT Tablets 854
▲ Mirapex Tablets (Greater than or equal to 1% to 3%) 857
▲ Myfortic Tablets (3% to less than 20%) 2276
Namenda 1180
Nasonex Nasal Spray (Greater than or equal to 2%) 2883
▲ Neoral Oral Solution (6%) 2280
▲ Neoral Soft Gelatin Capsules (6%) 2280
▲ Neupogen for Injection (5%) 589
Noroxin Tablets (Less frequent) 2069
Norvir (Less than 2%) 489
Novantrone for Injection Concentrate 1100
▲ NovoLog Injection (5%) 2359
Omnicef Capsules 497
Omnicef for Oral Suspension 497
▲ Ontak Vials (24%) 1079
Ortho-Cyclen Tablets 2449
Ortho Evra Transdermal System 2437
Ortho Tri-Cyclen Tablets 2449
Ortho Tri-Cyclen Lo Tablets 2458
▲ Orthoclone OKT3 Sterile Solution (14%) 2387
OxyContin Tablets (Less than 1%) 2589
▲ Paxil (3%) 1535
▲ Paxil CR Controlled-Release Tablets (3%) 1544
▲ PegIntron Powder for Injection (6%) 2903
Pentasa Capsules (Infrequent) 3030
Percocet Tablets 1127
▲ Photofrin for Injection (22% to 35%) 708
▲ Plavix Tablets (8.3%) 926
▲ Plavix Tablets (8.3%) 2767
Pletal Tablets 2481
PrandiMet Tablets (1.8%) 2967
▲ Prandin Tablets (1.8% to 3%) 2971
▲ Prinivil Tablets (3.4%) 2087
Prinzide Tablets (0.3% to 1%) 2092
ProAir HFA Inhalation Aerosol (Less than 3%) 3113
▲ Procrit for Injection (7%) 2391
Proglycem Capsules (Infrequent) 1185
Proglycem Suspension (Infrequent) 1185
▲ Prograf Capsules and Injection (3% to 19%) 622
Prolastin (Rare) 3099
▲ Prometrium Capsules (100 mg, 200 mg) (5% to 7%) 3047
Protonix for Delayed-Release Oral Suspension (Greater than or equal to 1%) 3254
Protonix Delayed-Release Tablets (Greater than or equal to 1%) 3254
▲ Protonix I.V. (6%) 3257
Protopic Ointment (0.2% to less than 1%) 628
Proventil HFA Inhalation Aerosol (Less than 3%) 2914
▲ Provigil Tablets (3%) 977
Prozac Weekly Capsules (Frequent) 1852
Prozac Pulvules and Liquid (Frequent) 1852
▲ Pulmozyme Inhalation Solution (18% to 25%) 1217
▲ Rebetol (5% to 9%) 2917
▲ Rebif Prefilled Syringe for Injection (6% to 8%) 1107
Remicade for IV Injection (1%) 950
▲ Requip Tablets (Frequent to 4%) 1561
Retrovir Capsules 1574
Retrovir IV Infusion 1579
Retrovir 1574
Risperdal Consta Long-Acting Injection (Frequent) 1753
Romazicon Injection (Less than 1%) 2646
Rythmol Tablets (2%) 1586
Rythmol SR Capsules 1590
Salagen Tablets (Less than 1%) 1082
Sanctura XR Capsules 557
Sandimmune (Rare) 2296
Sandostatin Injection (Less than 1%) 2300
▲ Sensipar Tablets (6%) 594
▲ Simulect for Injection (3% to 10%) 2306
Soriatane Capsules (Less than 1%) 3062
▲ Spiriva HandiHaler (5% to 7%) 870
Stalevo Tablets 2309
Strattera Capsules (0.7%) 1864
Sular Extended Release Tablets (2%) 2975
Symbyax Capsules (Up to 1%) 1871
Targretin Capsules 1084
Tarka Tablets (0.3% to 2.2%) 511
Tasigna Capsules (0.1% to 1%) 2316
Taxotere Injection Concentrate 2773
Teveten Tablets (1% or greater) 515
Teveten HCT Tablets (Less than 1%) 517
Timoptic Sterile Ophthalmic Solution (Less frequent) 2121
Timoptic in Ocudose (Less frequent) 2124
Timoptic-XE Sterile Ophthalmic Gel Forming Solution 2125
Toprol-XL Tablets (Greater than 1%) 666
▲ Torisel Injection (1% to 16%) 3272
Trasylol Injection (2%) 799
▲ Travatan Z Ophthalmic Solution (1% to 5%) 547
▲ Treximet Tablets (3%) 1616
Tricor Tablets 520
▲ Trisenox Injection (25%) 986
▲ Ultram ER Extended-Release Tablets (1% to less than 5%) 2428
Uroxatral Tablets 2786
▲ Urso 250 Tablets (5%) 720
▲ Urso Forte Tablets (5%) 720
▲ Valstar Sterile Solution for Intravesical Instillation (3%) 1735
Venlafaxine Hydrochloride Tablets (2%) 2199
▲ Viread Tablets (3%) 1268
Visudyne for Injection (Less than 1%) 2332
Vivitrol 988
Wellbutrin Tablets (Infrequent) 1648
▲ Wellbutrin SR Sustained-Release Tablets (3% to 4%) 1653
▲ Wellbutrin XL Extended-Release Tablets (3% to 4%) 1659
▲ Xeloda Tablets (Less than 5%) 2662
Xifaxan Tablets (Less than 2%) 2682

Xopenex Inhalation Solution 3001
Xopenex Inhalation Solution Concentrate 3005
Xopenex HFA Inhalation Aerosol 3009
Xyrem Oral Solution (Frequent) 1766
Zofran Injection (Rare) 1682
Zofran (Rare) 1687
Zofran ODT Orally Disintegrating Tablets (Rare) 1687
Zolinza Capsules 2142
▲ Zometa for Intravenous Infusion (Rare to less than 10%) 2341
Zomig Tablets (Infrequent) 694
Zomig Nasal Spray (Infrequent) 689
Zomig-ZMT Tablets (Infrequent) 694
Zonegran Capsules (Infrequent) 1089
Zyban Sustained-Release Tablets (Less than 1%) 1692
▲ Zyprexa Tablets (3% to 4%) 1883
▲ Zyprexa ZYDIS Orally Disintegrating Tablets (3% to 4%) 1883
Zyrtec Chewable Tablets (Less than 2%) 1920
Zyrtec Syrup (Less than 2%) 1920
Zyrtec Tablets (Less than 2%) 1920
Zyrtec-D 12 Hour Extended Release Tablets (Less than 2%) 1923

Pain, chest wall

Fentora Tablets (Greater than 1%) 968
Xyrem Oral Solution (Infrequent) 1766

Pain, dental

▲ Advair HFA 45/21 Inhalation Aerosol (1% to 3%) 1288
▲ Advair HFA 115/21 Inhalation Aerosol (1% to 3%) 1288
▲ Advair HFA 230/21 Inhalation Aerosol (1% to 3%) 1288
▲ Azmacort Inhalation Aerosol (1% to 3%) 407
Cozaar Tablets (Less than 1%) 1973
▲ Evoxac Capsules (1% to 3%) 1013
▲ Flovent Diskus 50 mcg (1% to 3%) 1435
Frova Tablets (Rare) 1111
Gardasil Injection (1.5%) 2019
Imitrex Nasal Spray 1470
Klonopin (Infrequent) 2639
Lexapro Oral Suspension (Frequent) 1174
Lexapro Tablets (Frequent) 1174
Micardis Tablets (More than 0.3%) 852
Micardis HCT Tablets 854
Requip Tablets (Infrequent) 1561
Serevent Diskus (1% to less than 3%) 1594
Singulair (1.7%) 2114
Teveten Tablets (Less than 1%) 515
Teveten HCT Tablets (Less than 1%) 517
Wellbutrin Tablets (Infrequent) 1648
Zyprexa Tablets (Frequent) 1883
Zyprexa ZYDIS Orally Disintegrating Tablets (Frequent) 1883

Pain, ear

Aceon Tablets (2 mg, 4 mg, 8 mg) (0.3% to 1%) 3038
Acetadote Injection (1%) 1001
Actiq (Less than 1%) 959
Adenoscan (Less than 1%) 605
Alinia for Oral Suspension (Less than 1%) 2677
Alinia Tablets (Less than 1%) 2677
Aricept Tablets (Infrequent) 1062
Aricept ODT Tablets (Infrequent) 1062
Asacol Delayed-Release Tablets (2% or greater) 2579
Asmanex Twisthaler (1% to less than 3%) 2797
Avalide Tablets 892
Avalide Tablets 2713
Avapro Tablets (Less than 1%) 897
Avapro Tablets (Less than 1%) 2718
Axert Tablets (Infrequent) 2431
Bactroban Nasal (Less than 1%) 1367
Celebrex Capsules (0.1% to 1.9%) 2979
▲ CellCept Capsules (3% to less than 20%) 2622
▲ CellCept Intravenous (3% to less than 20%) 2622
▲ CellCept Oral Suspension (3% to less than 20%) 2622
▲ CellCept Tablets (3% to less than 20%) 2622
Ciprodex Otic Suspension (0.4% to 2.3%) 541
Cymbalta Delayed-Release Capsules (Infrequent) 1801
Depakote ER Tablets 423
▲ Doxil Injection (1% to 10%) 2378
Emsam Transdermal System (Infrequent) 905
Engerix-B Vaccine 1409
▲ Epivir (7%) 1412
▲ Equetro Extended-Release Capsules (Less than 5%) 3174
▲ Evoxac Capsules (1% to 3%) 1013
Exforge Tablets (Greater than or equal to 0.2%) 2238
▲ Exubera Inhalation Powder (3.9%) 2515
▲ Flovent Diskus 50 mcg (1% to 3%) 1435
Frova Tablets (Infrequent) 1111
Gabitril Tablets (Frequent) 973
▲ Gamunex (18%) 3094
Imitrex Nasal Spray (Rare) 1470
Imitrex Tablets (Infrequent) 1474
▲ Increlex Injection (Greater than or equal to 5%) 3100
Infanrix Vaccine 1479
▲ Intron A for Injection (Less than or equal to 5%) 2859
Keppra Oral Solution (2%) 3131
Keppra Tablets (2%) 3131
Klonopin (Infrequent) 2639
Lamictal (Infrequent) 1488
Lexapro Oral Suspension (Frequent) 1174
Lexapro Tablets (Frequent) 1174
Lialda Tablets (Infrequent) 3029
Lunesta Tablets (Infrequent) 2994
Lupron Depot–3 Month 11.25 mg 462
Luvox CR Extended-Release Capsules (Infrequent) 1759
Maxalt Tablets (Infrequent) 2056
Maxalt-MLT Orally Disintegrating Tablets (Infrequent) 2056
Meridia Capsules (1.1%) 475
Miacalcin Nasal Spray (Less than 1%) 2274
Micardis Tablets (More than 0.3%) 852
Micardis HCT Tablets 854
Mirapex Tablets 857
Nasonex Nasal Spray (Greater than or equal to 2%) 2883
Nexium I.V. (Less than 1%) 652
Norvir (Less than 2%) 489
Omnaris Nasal Spray (2.2%) 2998
Paxil (Infrequent) 1535
Paxil CR Controlled-Release Tablets (Infrequent) 1544
Pediarix Vaccine 1552
Pletal Tablets (Less than 2%) 2481
Prinzide Tablets (0.3% to 1%) 2092
ProAir HFA Inhalation Aerosol (Less than 3%) 3113
▲ Prograf Capsules and Injection (3% to 15%) 622
▲ Prometrium Capsules (100 mg, 200 mg) (Less than 5%) 3047
ProQuad 2099
Protonix for Delayed-Release Oral Suspension (Less than 1%) 3254
Protonix Delayed-Release Tablets (Less than 1%) 3254
Protonix I.V. (Less than 1%) 3257
Protopic Ointment (Greater than or equal to 1%) 628
Provigil Tablets (At least 1%) 977
Prozac Weekly Capsules (Frequent) 1852
Prozac Pulvules and Liquid (Frequent) 1852
Recombivax HB (Less than 1%) 2107
Remeron Tablets (Infrequent) 2924
RemeronSolTab Tablets (Infrequent) 2927
Requip Tablets (Infrequent) 1561
Rilutek Tablets (Rare) 2771
Risperdal Consta Long-Acting Injection (Infrequent) 1753
Salagen Tablets (Less than 1%) 1082
Singulair (Greater than or equal to 2%) 2114
▲ Soriatane Capsules (1% to 10%) 3062
Sular Extended Release Tablets (Less than or equal to 1%) 2975
Symbyax Capsules (1% to 2%) 1871
Targretin Capsules 1084
Tasigna Capsules 2316
Treximet Tablets (Infrequent) 1616
Tricor Tablets 520
▲ Trisenox Injection (8%) 986
Twinrix Vaccine 1628
▲ Vesanoid Capsules (23%) 2660
Xifaxan Tablets (Less than 2%) 2682
Xolair (2%) 1235
Xyrem Oral Solution (Infrequent) 1766
Zomig Tablets (Infrequent) 694
Zomig Nasal Spray (Infrequent) 689
Zomig-ZMT Tablets (Infrequent) 694
Zyprexa Tablets (Infrequent) 1883
Zyprexa ZYDIS Orally Disintegrating Tablets (Infrequent) 1883

Pain, epigastric

(*see under* Distress, epigastric)

Pain, esophageal

▲ Photofrin for Injection (8%) 708

Pain, exacerbation of

Lidoderm Patch 1114
Vantas (Less than 2%) 1737

Pain, extremities

▲ Abilify Injection (4%) 881
▲ Abilify Injection (4%) 2466
▲ Abilify Oral Solution (4%) 881
▲ Abilify Oral Solution (4%) 2466
▲ Abilify Discmelt Orally Disintegrating Tablets (4%) 881
▲ Abilify Discmelt Orally Disintegrating Tablets (4%) 2466
▲ Abilify Tablets (4%) 881
▲ Abilify Tablets (4%) 2466
▲ Activella Tablets (5%) 2347
Allegra Oral Solution (2.1%) 2684
Allegra Tablets (2.1%) 2684
▲ Alvesco Inhalation Aerosol (0.3% to 3.1%) 2985
▲ Angeliq Tablets (8.4%) 751
▲ Aranesp for Injection (8%) 564
▲ Arranon Injection (0% to 7%) 1319
▲ Betimol Ophthalmic Solution (1% to 5%) 3181
▲ Boniva Injection (1.3% to 7.8%) 2614
▲ Boniva Tablets (1.3% to 7.8%) 2618
Cancidas for Injection 1953
Cialis Tablets (1% to 2%) 1792
Cimzia 3127
Cipro I.V. (1% or less) 2817
Cipro (Less than 1%) 2810
Cipro XR Tablets 2823
Combigan Ophthalmic Solution 553
Cosopt Sterile Ophthalmic Solution 1969
▲ Cubicin for Injection (9.2%) 995
Exforge Tablets (Greater than or equal to 0.2%) 2238
▲ Fabrazyme for Intravenous Infusion (19%) 1241
Fentora Tablets (Greater than 1%) 968
Fluarix Vaccine 1446
▲ Gammagard Liquid (0.85% to 8.2%) 730
▲ Genotropin Lyophilized Powder (1.6% to 14.7%) 2547
▲ Humira Injection (Less than 5%) 442
▲ Increlex Injection (Greater than or equal to 5%) 3100
▲ Ionsys Transdermal System (1% to less than 10%) 2410
▲ Lucentis Injection (1% to 6%) 1205
Mavik Tablets (0.3% to 1%) 472
▲ Orencia Powder for Intravenous Infusion (3%) 921
Recombivax HB 2107
Tarka Tablets (1.1%) 511
▲ Tasigna Capsules (13% to 16%) 2316
Timoptic-XE Sterile Ophthalmic Gel Forming Solution 2125
▲ Tykerb Tablets (0% to 12%) 1631
Tyzeka Tablets (2%) 2328
Uroqid-Acid No. 2 Tablets 814
▲ Valcyte Tablets (Less than 5%) 2654
▲ Velcade for Injection (14%) 2168
▲ Viadur Implant (3.1%) 802
Vivitrol 988
Vytorin 10/10 Tablets (2.3%) 2149
Vytorin 10/10 Tablets (2.3%) 2939
Vytorin 10/20 Tablets (2.3%) 2149
Vytorin 10/20 Tablets (2.3%) 2939
Vytorin 10/40 Tablets (2.3%) 2149
Vytorin 10/40 Tablets (2.3%) 2939
Vytorin 10/80 Tablets (2.3%) 2149
Vytorin 10/80 Tablets (2.3%) 2939
▲ Wellbutrin XL Extended-Release Tablets (3%) 1659
Yaz Tablets (Greater than 1%) 805
Zetia Tablets (2.7%) 2157
Zetia Tablets (2.1% to 2.7%) 2951
▲ Zyprexa Tablets (4% to 5%) 1883
▲ Zyprexa ZYDIS Orally Disintegrating Tablets (4% to 5%) 1883

Pain, eye

Acetadote Injection (0.54% to 2.58%) 1001
▲ Alphagan P Ophthalmic Solution (1% to 4%) 549
▲ Alrex Ophthalmic Suspension 0.2% (Less than 5%) ⊙ 236
Ambien Tablets (Infrequent) 2692
Ambien CR Tablets (Infrequent) 2696
Amerge Tablets (Rare) 1301
Asacol Delayed-Release Tablets 2579
Atrovent HFA Inhalation Aerosol 839
Atrovent Nasal Spray 0.03% 834
Atrovent Nasal Spray 0.06% 836
▲ Avinza Capsules (Less than 5%) 1772
Axert Tablets (Rare) 2431
▲ Azopt Ophthalmic Suspension (1% to 5%) 540
▲ Betimol Ophthalmic Solution (1% to 5%) 3181
Celebrex Capsules (0.1% to 1.9%) 2979
Celexa (Infrequent) 1160
Chantix Tablets (Infrequent) 2511
Cialis Tablets (Less than 2%) 1792
Cipro I.V. (1% or less) 2817
Cipro (Less than 1%) 2810
Cipro XR Tablets 2823
▲ Combigan Ophthalmic Solution (1% to 5%) 553
Combivent Inhalation Aerosol 845
▲ Copaxone for Injection (7%) 3110
▲ Cosopt Sterile Ophthalmic Solution (1% to 5%) 1969
Depakote ER Tablets (Greater than 1%) 423
Doxil Injection (Less than 1%) 2378
▲ Durezol Ophthalmic Emulsion (5% to 15%) ⊙ 275
Effexor XR Extended-Release Capsules (Infrequent) 3195
Eldepryl Capsules 3052
Eloxatin for Injection 2731
Emsam Transdermal System (Infrequent) 905
▲ Evoxac Capsules (1% to 3%) 1013
Exelon Capsules 2229
Exelon Oral Solution 2229
Exforge Tablets (Greater than 0.1% to less than 1%) 2238
Fluarix Vaccine 1446
Flulaval Injection Vaccine 1448
Flumadine 1167
Frova Tablets (Infrequent) 1111
Gabitril Tablets (Infrequent) 973
Gengraf Capsules (1% to less than 3%) 435
Gliadel Wafer (1%) 1076
Imitrex Nasal Spray 1470
▲ Intron A for Injection (Less than 5%) 2859
Levitra Tablets (Less than 2%) 2876
▲ Lotemax Ophthalmic Suspension 0.5% (Less than 5%) ⊙ 241
▲ Lucentis Injection (17% to 37%) 1205
▲ Lumigan Ophthalmic Solution (3% to 10%) 556
Luvox CR Extended-Release Capsules (Infrequent) 1759
Maxalt Tablets (Infrequent) 2056
Maxalt-MLT Orally Disintegrating Tablets (Infrequent) 2056
Meridia Capsules 475
Miacalcin Injection 2273
Mirapex Tablets 857
Namenda (Infrequent) 1180
Neoral Oral Solution (1% to less than 3%) 2280
Neoral Soft Gelatin Capsules (1% to less than 3%) 2280
Norvir (Less than 2%) 489
Ofloxacin Ophthalmic Solution 0.3% ⊙ 243
Paxil (Infrequent) 1535
Paxil CR Controlled-Release Tablets (Infrequent) 1544
Photofrin for Injection 708
Protopic Ointment (Greater than or equal to 1%) 628
Provigil Tablets (1%) 977
▲ Quixin Ophthalmic Solution (1% to 3%) 3184
Remeron Tablets (Infrequent) 2924
RemeronSolTab Tablets (Infrequent) 2927
Requip Tablets (Infrequent) 1561
▲ Restasis Ophthalmic Emulsion (1% to 5%) 557
Risperdal Consta Long-Acting Injection (Infrequent) 1753
Salagen Tablets (Less than 1%) 1082
▲ Soriatane Capsules (1% to 10%) 3062
Symbyax Capsules (Infrequent) 1871
Tasigna Capsules 2316
Timoptic Sterile Ophthalmic Solution (Less frequent) 2121
Timoptic in Ocudose (Less frequent) 2124
▲ Timoptic-XE Sterile Ophthalmic Gel Forming Solution (1% to 5%) 2125
Trusopt Sterile Ophthalmic Solution 2128
Venlafaxine Hydrochloride Tablets (Infrequent) 2199
▲ Vigamox Ophthalmic Solution (1% to 6%) 548
Xyrem Oral Solution (Infrequent) 1766

Zomig Tablets (Infrequent) 694
Zomig-ZMT Tablets (Infrequent) 694
Zyprexa Tablets (Infrequent) 1883
Zyprexa ZYDIS Orally Disintegrating Tablets (Infrequent) 1883
Zyrtec Chewable Tablets (Less than 2%) 1920
Zyrtec Syrup (Less than 2%) 1920
Zyrtec Tablets (Less than 2%) 1920
Zyrtec-D 12 Hour Extended Release Tablets (Less than 2%) 1923

Pain, facial
▲ Carac Cream 0.5% (43.6%) 2722
Imitrex Injection (Infrequent) 1465
Imitrex Nasal Spray (Rare) 1470
Imitrex Tablets (Infrequent) 1474
Norvir (Less than 2%) 489

Pain, feet
Cipro XR Tablets 2823

Pain, flank
Aceon Tablets (2 mg, 4 mg, 8 mg) (0.3% to 1%) 3038
Actiq (Less than 1%) 959
Azilect Tablets (Infrequent) 3106
▲ Chemet Capsules (5.2% to 15.7%) 2484
Copaxone for Injection (Infrequent) 3110
Crixivan Capsules (Less than 2%) 1979
Emsam Transdermal System (Infrequent) 905
Geodon Capsules (Frequent) 2520
Invanz for Injection (Greater than 0.1%) 2029
Mirapex Tablets 857
Neupogen for Injection (Infrequent) 589
Prinivil Tablets (0.3% to 1%) 2087
Prinzide Tablets 2092
▲ Sutent Capsules (3% to 22%) 2540
▲ Vesanoid Capsules (9%) 2660
Zonegran Capsules (Infrequent) 1089

Pain, foot
Cipro (Less than 1%) 2810

Pain, gastrointestinal
Advair Diskus 100/50 1276
Advair Diskus 250/50 (1%) 1276
Advair Diskus 500/50 1276
Amrix Capsules 966
Avandaryl Tablets (Less than 1%) 1344
Combigan Ophthalmic Solution 553
▲ Coreg Tablets (Greater than 1% to 3%) 1387
▲ Coreg CR Extended-Release Capsules (Greater than 1% to less than or equal to 3%) 1393
▲ Cymbalta Delayed-Release Capsules (4%) 1801
Duetact Tablets (Less than 1%) 3085
Requip Tablets (Infrequent) 1561
▲ Selzentry Tablets (8.2%) 2534
Stalevo Tablets 2309
▲ Taxotere Injection Concentrate (0.6% to 14.7%) 2773

Pain, groin
Requip Tablets (Infrequent) 1561

Pain, hip
Cozaar Tablets (Less than 1%) 1973
Humatrope Vials and Cartridges (2.7%) 1838
Prinivil Tablets (0.3% to 1%) 2087
Prinzide Tablets 2092
ProQuad 2099
Zyprexa Tablets (Infrequent) 1883
Zyprexa ZYDIS Orally Disintegrating Tablets (Infrequent) 1883

Pain, infusion site
Cancidas for Injection 1953
▲ Emend for Injection (7.6%) 1999
▲ Vaprisol (0% to 5%) 632
▲ Visudyne for Injection (10% to 30%) 2332

Pain, jaw
Cipro I.V. (1% or less) 2817
Cipro XR Tablets 2823
▲ Flolan for Injection (54% to 75%) 1426
Klonopin (Infrequent) 2639
Rythmol SR Capsules 1590
Zomig Tablets (Infrequent) 694
Zomig Nasal Spray (Infrequent) 689
Zomig-ZMT Tablets (Infrequent) 694

Pain, knee
▲ Cozaar Tablets (Less than 1% to 5%) 1973
Klonopin (Infrequent) 2639
Prinivil Tablets (0.3% to 1%) 2087

Pain, leg
Arixtra Injection (1.4%) 1313
Avelox (Less than 0.1%) 2803
Cipro 2810
Crinone 4% Gel 992
Crinone 8% Gel 992
Edex Injection (1%) 2957
Neupro Transdermal System 3149
ProQuad 2099
Risperdal Consta Long-Acting Injection (1%) 1753
▲ Xolair (4%) 1235
▲ Xolair (4%) 2339

Pain, limb
▲ Cialis Tablets (1% to 3%) 1792
▲ Clolar for Intravenous Infusion (29%) 1239
Cubicin for Injection (1.5%) 995
▲ Dacogen Injection (19%) 1066
▲ DepoCyt Injection (12% to 15%) 1136
▲ Duetact Tablets (4% to 5.4%) 3085
Eligard 7.5 mg (Less than 2%) 2724
Eligard 22.5 mg 2724
Eligard 30 mg 2724
Eligard 45 mg (2.7%) 2724
▲ Femara Tablets (10%) 2246
Meridia Capsules 475
Stalevo Tablets 2309
▲ Sutent Capsules (1% to 18%) 2540
▲ Trisenox Injection (13%) 986
▲ Ultram ER Extended-Release Tablets (1% to less than 5%) 2428
Vantas (Less than 2%) 1737
▲ Velcade for Injection (15%) 2168
▲ Zometa for Intravenous Infusion (14%) 2341

Pain, localized
▲ Havrix Injection Vaccine (9.5% to 22.3%) 1454
▲ Zomig Tablets (0% to 4%) 694
▲ Zomig Nasal Spray (0% to 4%) 689
▲ Zomig-ZMT Tablets (0% to 4%) 694
Zyvox (0.9% to 2%) 2552

Pain, lower extremities
▲ Aceon Tablets (2 mg, 4 mg, 8 mg) (4.7%) 3038
▲ Chemet Capsules (Up to 3%) 2484
▲ Cozaar Tablets (1% to 5%) 1973
Diovan HCT Tablets (Greater than 0.2%) 2216
DynaCirc CR Controlled Release Tablets (0.5% to 1%) 1407
Eldepryl Capsules (1 of 49 patients) 3052
▲ Femara Tablets (21% to 22%) 2246
Frova Tablets (Rare) 1111
Invanz for Injection (0.4% to 1.1%) 2029
Klonopin (Infrequent) 2639
Lexapro Oral Suspension (Infrequent) 1174
Lexapro Tablets (Infrequent) 1174
Mevacor Tablets (0.5% to 1%) 2063
Micardis Tablets (More than 0.3%) 852
Micardis HCT Tablets 854
▲ Myfortic Tablets (3% to less than 20%) 2276
Ortho Evra Transdermal System 2437
Prinivil Tablets (0.3% to 1%) 2087
Prinzide Tablets (0.3% to 1%) 2092
▲ Simulect for Injection (3% to 10%) 2306
▲ Spiriva HandiHaler (1% to 3%) 870
Timoptic Sterile Ophthalmic Solution 2121
Timoptic in Ocudose 2124
▲ Xenical Capsules (10.8%) 2672

Pain, medullary bone
▲ Neulasta Injection (26%) 587
▲ Neupogen for Injection (33%) 589

Pain, mouth
Cipro XR Tablets 2823
Xyrem Oral Solution (Infrequent) 1766

Pain, muscle
(*see under* Myalgia)

Pain, musculoskeletal
▲ Abilify Injection (3%) 2466
▲ Abilify Oral Solution (3%) 2466
▲ Abilify Discmelt Orally Disintegrating Tablets (3%) 2466
▲ Abilify Tablets (3%) 2466
Advair Diskus 100/50 1276
▲ Advair Diskus 250/50 (2% to 9%) 1276
▲ Advair Diskus 500/50 (Greater than or equal to 3%) 1276
▲ Advair HFA 45/21 Inhalation Aerosol (5% to 7%) 1288
▲ Advair HFA 115/21 Inhalation Aerosol (5% to 7%) 1288
▲ Advair HFA 230/21 Inhalation Aerosol (5% to 7%) 1288
▲ Asmanex Twisthaler (4% to 22%) 2797
▲ Avalide Tablets (7%) 892
▲ Avalide Tablets (7%) 2713
Chantix Tablets (Frequent) 2511
Cipro 2810
▲ Cymbalta Delayed-Release Capsules (Frequent to 5%) 1801
Donnatal Extentabs 2507
Emend Capsules (Greater than 0.5%) 1992
Emend for Injection (Greater than 0.5%) 1999
Evoxac Capsules (2.8%) 1013
▲ Femara Tablets (21% to 22%) 2246
▲ Flovent Diskus 50 mcg (3%) 1435
▲ Flovent HFA (1% to 3%) 1440
▲ Fosamax (0.4% to approximately 6%) 2005
▲ Fosamax Plus D Tablets (0.4% to 4.1%) 2013
▲ Gleevec Tablets (30% to 49%) 2255
▲ Ixempra Kit for Injection (Greater than or equal to 20%) 915
Maxalt Tablets (Infrequent) 2056
Maxalt-MLT Orally Disintegrating Tablets (Infrequent) 2056
▲ Nasonex Nasal Spray (1% to 5%) 2883
▲ Noxafil Oral Suspension (16%) 2889
▲ PegIntron Powder for Injection (28%) 2903
▲ Prometrium Capsules (100 mg, 200 mg) (12%) 3047
ProQuad 2099
▲ Rebetol (19% to 28%) 2917
▲ Rebif Prefilled Syringe for Injection (10% to 15%) 1107
▲ Relenza Inhalation Powder (6%) 1556
▲ Sandostatin LAR Depot (5% to 15.4%) 2302
▲ Serevent Diskus (12%) 1594
▲ Spiriva HandiHaler (1% to 3%) 870
▲ Tasigna Capsules (1% to 10%) 2316
▲ Trizivir Tablets (12%) 1622
▲ Ventolin HFA Inhalation Aerosol (5%) 1638
Visudyne for Injection (Less than 1%) 2332
▲ Ziagen (5% to 6%) 1673

Pain, neck
(*see also under* Torticollis)
Ambien CR Tablets (1%) 2696
▲ CellCept Capsules (3% to less than 20%) 2622
▲ CellCept Intravenous (3% to less than 20%) 2622
▲ CellCept Oral Suspension (3% to less than 20%) 2622
▲ CellCept Tablets (3% to less than 20%) 2622
Cialis Tablets (Less than 2%) 1792
Cipro (Less than 1%) 2810
Cipro XR Tablets 2823
▲ Fabrazyme for Intravenous Infusion (5%) 1241
▲ Keppra Injection (8%) 3137
▲ Keppra Oral Solution (2% to 8%) 3131
▲ Keppra Tablets (2% to 8%) 3131
Levitra Tablets (Less than 2%) 2876
Luvox CR Extended-Release Capsules (Infrequent) 1759
Venlafaxine Hydrochloride Tablets (Frequent) 2199

Pain, neuropathic
Arranon Injection (1%) 1319
Ixempra Kit for Injection 915

Pain, ocular
Iquix Ophthalmic Solution (1% to 2%) 3183
▲ Nevanac Ophthalmic Suspension 0.1% (1% to 5%) ⊙205
▲ Pataday Ophthalmic Solution (Less than or equal to 5%) 543
▲ Travatan Z Ophthalmic Solution (5% to 10%) 547

Pain, oral mucosa
Cipro I.V. (1% or less) 2817
Cipro (Less than 1%) 2810
▲ Flovent Diskus 50 mcg (1% to 3%) 1435
▲ Nexavar Tablets (Greater than or equal to 10%) 784
▲ Sutent Capsules (6% to 10%) 2540

Pain, ovarian
▲ Follistim AQ Cartridge (5%) 2844

Pain, paranasal sinus
Advair HFA 45/21 Inhalation Aerosol 1288
Advair HFA 115/21 Inhalation Aerosol 1288
Advair HFA 230/21 Inhalation Aerosol 1288

Pain, pelvic
Actiq (1% or greater) 959
Alinia for Oral Suspension (Less than 1%) 2677
Alinia Tablets (Less than 1%) 2677
▲ Angiomax for Injection (6%) 1933
▲ Arimidex Tablets (5% to 7%) 672
Avelox (Less than 1%) 2803
▲ CellCept Capsules (3% to less than 20%) 2622
▲ CellCept Intravenous (3% to less than 20%) 2622
▲ CellCept Oral Suspension (3% to less than 20%) 2622
▲ CellCept Tablets (3% to less than 20%) 2622
▲ Doxil Injection (1% to 10%) 2378
Effexor XR Extended-Release Capsules (Infrequent) 3195
Emend Capsules (Greater than 0.5%) 1992
Emend for Injection (Greater than 0.5%) 1999
Emsam Transdermal System (Infrequent) 905
▲ Faslodex Injection (9.9%) 682
Follistim AQ Cartridge 2844
Gabitril Tablets (Infrequent) 973
▲ Humira Injection (Less than 5%) 442
▲ Intron A for Injection (Less than 5%) 2859
Klonopin (Infrequent) 2639
Luvox CR Extended-Release Capsules (Rare) 1759
Lyrica Capsules (0.1% to 1%) 2527
Merrem I.V. (Greater than 0.1% to 1%) 684
Paxil (Rare) 1535
Paxil CR Controlled-Release Tablets (Rare) 1544
Pletal Tablets (Less than 2%) 2481
Premarin Intravenous 3217
Premarin Tablets 3221
▲ Premphase Tablets (4% to 5%) 3232
▲ Prempro Tablets (4% to 5%) 3232
Prinivil Tablets (0.3% to 1%) 2087
Prinzide Tablets 2092
Prozac Weekly Capsules (Infrequent) 1852
Prozac Pulvules and Liquid (Infrequent) 1852
Symbyax Capsules (Infrequent) 1871
Valstar Sterile Solution for Intravesical Instillation (1%) 1735
Venlafaxine Hydrochloride Tablets (Infrequent) 2199
Yaz Tablets (Greater than 1%) 805
Zyprexa Tablets (Infrequent) 1883
Zyprexa ZYDIS Orally Disintegrating Tablets (Infrequent) 1883

Pain, penile
▲ Edex Injection (11% to 35%) 2957

Pain, perineal
▲ Crinone 8% Gel (17%) 992
Requip Tablets (Infrequent) 1561

Pain, peripheral
Celebrex Capsules (0.1% to 1.9%) 2979

Pain, pharyngeal
▲ Gammagard Liquid (0.61% to 6.5%) 730

Pain, pharyngolaryngeal
▲ Abilify Injection (3%) 881
▲ Abilify Injection (3%) 2466
▲ Abilify Oral Solution (3%) 881
▲ Abilify Oral Solution (3%) 2466
▲ Abilify Discmelt Orally Disintegrating Tablets (3%) 881
▲ Abilify Discmelt Orally Disintegrating Tablets (3%) 2466
▲ Abilify Tablets (3%) 881
▲ Abilify Tablets (3%) 2466
▲ Advate (11.3%) 721
▲ Alvesco Inhalation Aerosol (2.4% to 4.7%) 2985
Amitiza Capsules (Less than 1%) 3082
Concerta Extended-Release Tablets (1.2% to 1.7%) 1925
▲ Cubicin for Injection (8.3%) 995
▲ Cymbalta Delayed-Release Capsules (1% to 6%) 1801
Diovan HCT Tablets (Greater than 0.2%) 2216
▲ Emend Capsules (3%) 1992
▲ Emend for Injection (3%) 1999
Exforge Tablets (Greater than or equal to 0.2%) 2238

▲ Exjade Tablets (0.1% to 10.5%) 2244
▲ Fabrazyme for Intravenous Infusion (16%) 1241
Fentora Tablets (Greater than 1%) 968
▲ Flulaval Injection Vaccine (2% to 12%) 1448
▲ Focalin XR Capsules (4% to 7%) 2251
▲ Gleevec Tablets (7% to 18.1%) 2255
Ixempra Kit for Injection 915
Lamisil Oral Granules (2%) 2264
Lialda Tablets (Infrequent) 3029
▲ Lyrica Capsules (1% to 3%) 2527
Mirapex Tablets 857
▲ Myfortic Tablets (3% to less than 20%) 2276
▲ Omnaris Nasal Spray (3.4%) 2998
Patanase Nasal Spray (2.2%) 544
Requip Tablets (Frequent) 1561
▲ Spiriva HandiHaler (1% to 3%) 870
▲ Symbicort 80/4.5 Inhalation Aerosol (6.1%) 659
▲ Symbicort 160/4.5 Inhalation Aerosol (8.9%) 659
Tasigna Capsules (0.1% to 1%) 2316
▲ Tyzeka Tablets (5%) 2328
▲ Veramyst Nasal Spray (2% to 4%) 1643
Vivitrol 988
Xifaxan Tablets (Less than 2%) 2682
▲ Xyrem Oral Solution (2.9% to 9.1%) 1766
Ziana Gel (2%) 1942

Pain, pharynx
▲ Advate (11.3%) 721
Primaxin I.M. 2080
Primaxin I.V. (Less than 0.2%) 2083
Prinivil Tablets (0.3% to 1%) 2087
Prinzide Tablets (0.3% to 1%) 2092
Stalevo Tablets 2309

Pain, pleural
Invanz for Injection (Greater than 0.1%) 2029
Tasigna Capsules (0.1% to 1%) 2316

Pain, postoperative
▲ Advair HFA 45/21 Inhalation Aerosol (1% to 3%) 1288
▲ Advair HFA 115/21 Inhalation Aerosol (1% to 3%) 1288
▲ Advair HFA 230/21 Inhalation Aerosol (1% to 3%) 1288
▲ Evoxac Capsules (1% to 3%) 1013
▲ Myfortic Tablets (3% to 23.9%) 2276

Pain, post-procedure
Dacogen Injection 1066
▲ Fabrazyme for Intravenous Infusion (25%) 1241
▲ Supprelin LA Implant (4.3%) 1731
▲ Tyzeka Tablets (7%) 2328
▲ Xyrem Oral Solution (Infrequent to 5.7%) 1766
Zofran Injection (1%) 1682

Pain, precordium
Imitrex Tablets 1474

Pain, prostate
Lupron Depot 3.75 mg 462
Lupron Depot 7.5 mg 469
Lupron Depot–3 Month 11.25 mg 462
Lupron Depot-PED 7.5 mg, 11.25 mg and 15 mg 471

Pain, rectum
Canasa Rectal Suppositories (1.8%) 705
Noroxin Tablets (0.3% to 1%) 2069
▲ Xeloda Tablets (Less than 5%) 2662
▲ Xenical Capsules (3.3% to 5.2%) 2672

Pain, renal
Actiq (Less than 1%) 959
Alinia for Oral Suspension (Less than 1%) 2677
Alinia Tablets (Less than 1%) 2677
Ambien Tablets (Rare) 2692
Ambien CR Tablets (Rare) 2696
Azopt Ophthalmic Suspension (Less than 1%) 540
Ceftin Tablets (0.1% to 1%) 1380
Celexa (Rare) 1160
Copaxone for Injection (Infrequent) 3110
Effexor XR Extended-Release Capsules (Rare) 3195
Evoxac Capsules (Less than 1%) 1013
Frova Tablets (Rare) 1111
Lamictal (Rare) 1488
Lunesta Tablets (Infrequent) 2994
Norvir (Less than 2%) 489
Paxil (Rare) 1535
Paxil CR Controlled-Release Tablets (Rare) 1544
Protonix for Delayed-Release Oral Suspension (Less than 1%) 3254
Protonix Delayed-Release Tablets (Less than 1%) 3254
Protonix I.V. (Less than 1%) 3257
Prozac Weekly Capsules (Rare) 1852
Prozac Pulvules and Liquid (Rare) 1852
Rilutek Tablets (Infrequent) 2771
Risperdal Consta Long-Acting Injection (Infrequent) 1753
Valtrex Caplets 1635
Venlafaxine Hydrochloride Tablets (Rare) 2199
Zomig Tablets (Rare) 694
Zomig Nasal Spray (Rare) 689
Zomig-ZMT Tablets (Rare) 694
Zovirax 1690

Pain, retrosternal
Zofran Injection (2%) 1682

Pain, right upper quadrant
▲ Intron A for Injection (Less than 5% to 15%) 2859
Lamisil Tablets 2266
▲ PegIntron Powder for Injection (8%) 2903
▲ Rebetol (6% to 12%) 2917
Tarka Tablets (Several cases) 511

Pain, salivary gland
▲ Evoxac Capsules (1% to 3%) 1013
Frova Tablets (Rare) 1111

Pain, shoulder
Cozaar Tablets (Less than 1%) 1973
Engerix-B Vaccine (Less than 1%) 1409
Fentora Tablets (Greater than 1%) 968
Klonopin (Infrequent) 2639
▲ Lexapro Oral Suspension (3%) 1174
▲ Lexapro Tablets (3%) 1174
Mevacor Tablets (0.5% to 1%) 2063
Mirapex Tablets 857
Prinivil Tablets (0.3% to 1%) 2087
Prinzide Tablets (0.3% to 1%) 2092
Recombivax HB (Less than 1%) 2107
Stalevo Tablets 2309
Zofran Injection (2%) 1682

Pain, skeletal
▲ Advair HFA 45/21 Inhalation Aerosol (1% to 3%) 1288
▲ Advair HFA 115/21 Inhalation Aerosol (1% to 3%) 1288
▲ Advair HFA 230/21 Inhalation Aerosol (1% to 3%) 1288
Crinone 4% Gel 992
Crinone 8% Gel 992
▲ Hycamtin for Injection (23%) 1459
Levaquin (0.1% to 1%) 2416
Levaquin in 5% Dextrose Injection (0.1% to 1%) 2416
▲ Neulasta Injection (15% to 72%) 587
▲ Norditropin Cartridges (11%) 2354
Risperdal Consta Long-Acting Injection (Frequent) 1753
▲ Spiriva HandiHaler (1% to 3%) 870
▲ Zometa for Intravenous Infusion (12%) 2341

Pain, stomach
(*see also under* Stomachache)
Aggrenox Capsules 819
Cipro 2810

Pain, substernal
Evoxac Capsules (Less than 1%) 1013
Teveten Tablets (Less than 1%) 515
Teveten HCT Tablets (Less than 1%) 517

Pain, testicular
Edex Injection (1%) 2957
Eligard 7.5 mg (Less than 2%) 2724
Eligard 22.5 mg (Less than 2%) 2724
Eligard 30 mg (2.2%) 2724
Eligard 45 mg (Less than 2%) 2724
Propecia Tablets 2095
Proscar Tablets 2102
▲ Viadur Implant (3.8%) 802

Pain, thoracic spine
▲ Chemet Capsules (5.2% to 15.7%) 2484
Primaxin I.M. 2080
Primaxin I.V. (Less than 0.2%) 2083

Pain, thorax
▲ Humira Injection (Less than 5%) 442

Pain, throat
Amerge Tablets (1% to 2%) 1301
▲ Imitrex Tablets (Less than 1% to 3%) 1474
▲ Relenza Inhalation Powder (8% to 19%) 1556
▲ Zomig Tablets (1% to 4%) 694
▲ Zomig Nasal Spray (1% to 4%) 689
▲ Zomig-ZMT Tablets (1% to 4%) 694

Pain, tingling
▲ Supprelin LA Implant (51.1%) 1731

Pain, trauma activated
Xyrem Oral Solution (Frequent) 1766

Pain, trunk
▲ Epogen for Injection (3%) 576
▲ Leustatin Injection (6%) 2384
▲ Procrit for Injection (3%) 2391
Requip Tablets (Infrequent) 1561

Pain, tumor site
Herceptin I.V. 1199
▲ Nexavar Tablets (Greater than or equal to 10%) 784

Pain, unspecified
▲ CellCept Capsules (3% to 75.8%) 2622
▲ CellCept Intravenous (3% to 75.8%) 2622
▲ CellCept Oral Suspension (3% to 75.8%) 2622
▲ CellCept Tablets (3% to 75.8%) 2622
▲ Depakote ER Tablets (11%) 423
Edex Injection (2%) 2957
▲ Tice BCG (4% to 17%) 2936

Pain, upper extremities
Aceon Tablets (2 mg, 4 mg, 8 mg) (0.2% to 2.8%) 3038
Cipro I.V. (1% or less) 2817
Engerix-B Vaccine (Less than 1%) 1409
Prinivil Tablets (0.3% to 1%) 2087
Timoptic Sterile Ophthalmic Solution 2121
Timoptic in Ocudose 2124

Pain, urethral
Ceftin Tablets (0.1% to 1%) 1380
Protonix for Delayed-Release Oral Suspension (Less than 1%) 3254
Protonix Delayed-Release Tablets (Less than 1%) 3254
Protonix I.V. (Less than 1%) 3257
Salagen Tablets (Less than 1%) 1082
▲ Valstar Sterile Solution for Intravesical Instillation (3%) 1735

Pain, urinary bladder
Duragesic Transdermal System (Less than 1%) 2405
Effexor XR Extended-Release Capsules (Infrequent) 3195
ReoPro Vials (0.1%) 1860
▲ Valstar Sterile Solution for Intravesical Instillation (28%) 1735
Venlafaxine Hydrochloride Tablets (Infrequent) 2199
Zonegran Capsules (Rare) 1089

Pain, wrist
Cipro 2810

Pain at injection site
Actimmune 1743
Actiq (Less than 1%) 959
▲ Alferon N Injection (12%) 1726
Aloxi Injection (Very rare) 1059
▲ Amevive (7% to common) 611
▲ Angiomax for Injection (2.7% to 8%) 1933
Anzemet Injection 2701
▲ Aranesp for Injection (6%) 564
Attenuvax 1951
▲ Betaseron for SC Injection (16%) 756
Bicillin C-R Injectable Suspension 1775
Bicillin L-A Injection 1777
▲ Boostrix (4.6% to 75.3%) 1377
▲ BOTOX Purified Neurotoxin Complex (2% to 10%) 550
▲ Busulfex Injection (15%) 2477
Calcijex Injection (Occasional) 419
Capastat Sulfate for Injection 1791
Cardene I.V. (0.7%) 1093
Cimzia 3127
Cipro I.V. (1% or less) 2817
▲ Clolar for Intravenous Infusion (14%) 1239
▲ Comvax (23.9% to 34.5%) 1966
▲ Copaxone for Injection (73%) 3110
Delatestryl Injection 1730
Doxil Injection (Less than 1%) 2378
Edecrin Sodium Intravenous (Occasional) 698
▲ Eligard 7.5 mg (4.3%) 2724
▲ Eligard 22.5 mg (3.5%) 2724
Eligard 30 mg (2.3%) 2724
▲ Eligard 45 mg (4.6%) 2724
Eloxatin for Injection 2731
▲ Enbrel for Injection (34% to 37%) 569
Engerix-B Vaccine (Less than 1%) 1409
▲ Faslodex Injection (10.9%) 682
▲ Flolan for Injection (13%) 1426
▲ Fluarix Vaccine (12.2% to 54.7%) 1446
Fluorescite Injection ⊙ 203
Fortaz 1450
Forteo for Injection (Less than 1/30 patients) 1816
▲ Fragmin Injection (2% to 12%) 1070
▲ Gammagard S/D (16%) 734
▲ Gardasil Injection (0.9% to 83.9%) 2019
Genotropin Lyophilized Powder (Infrequent) 2547
▲ Geodon for Injection (7% to 9%) 2520
Humatrope Vials and Cartridges (Infrequent) 1838
▲ Humira Injection (12% to 20%) 442
▲ Hyalgan Solution (23%) 2742
Imitrex Injection 1465
▲ Infanrix Vaccine (0.9% to 10.5%) 1479
▲ Intron A for Injection (Less than 5%) 2859
▲ Invanz for Injection (7%) 2029
Ionsys Transdermal System (.1% to less than 1%) 2410
▲ Kinrix Injection Vaccine (57%) 1486
Lantus Injection (2.7%) 2749
▲ Leustatin Injection (9% to 19%) 2384
Lovenox Injection (2%) 2756
Merrem I.V. (0.4%) 684
Meruvax II 2061
▲ Nabi-HB (4%) 815
Neulasta Injection 587
Novantrone for Injection Concentrate 1100
Nutropin for Injection (Infrequent) 1208
Pediarix Vaccine 1552
Liquid PedvaxHIB 2073
▲ PegIntron Powder for Injection (2% to 3%) 2903
Pneumovax 23 2078
Premarin Intravenous 3217
Primaxin I.M. (1.2%) 2080
Primaxin I.V. (0.7%) 2083
▲ ProQuad (22%) 2099
Protonix I.V. (Greater than 1%) 3257
Reclast Injection 2291
Recombivax HB (Equal to or greater than 1%) 2107
ReoPro Vials (0.1%) 1860
Retrovir IV Infusion (Infrequent) 1579
Risperdal Consta Long-Acting Injection (Frequent) 1753
Rocephin Injectable Vials, ADD-Vantage, Galaxy, Bulk (1%) 2642
▲ Romazicon Injection (3% to 9%) 2646
▲ Sandostatin Injection (7.7%) 2300
▲ Sandostatin LAR Depot (2% to 50%) 2302
▲ Somatuline Depot Injection (4.1% to 17%) 3102
Timentin ADD-Vantage 1606
Timentin Injection Galaxy Container 1609
Timentin IV Infusion 1603
Timentin Pharmacy Bulk Package 1613
Traumeel Injection Solution 1725
▲ Trisenox Injection (20%) 986
Tygacil for Injection (0% to less than 2%) 3276
▲ Vaqta (1.2% to 51.1%) 2130
▲ Varivax (19.3% to 32.5%; less than 0.05%) 2133
Velcade for Injection 2168
▲ Vivitrol (10% to 17%) 988
Xolair 1235
Xolair 2339
Zantac Injection 1666
Zantac Injection Pharmacy Bulk Package (Frequent) 1668
Zantac Injection Premixed 1666
Zeel Injection Solution 1726
▲ Zofran Injection (4%) 1682
▲ Zostavax Injection (33.4%) 2145
▲ Zosyn for Injection (0.2%) 3284
Zyprexa IntraMuscular (Frequent) 1883

Pain at insertion site
▲ Supprelin LA Implant (4.3% to 51.1%) 1731
▲ Vantas (3.6%) 1737

Pain secondary to eczema
Bactroban Cream (One report) 1366

Pallanesthesia
▲ Ixempra Kit for Injection (62%) 915

Pallor
Advair HFA 45/21 Inhalation Aerosol 1288
Advair HFA 115/21 Inhalation Aerosol 1288
Advair HFA 230/21 Inhalation Aerosol 1288
Allegra-D 12 Hour Extended-Release Tablets 2687
Allegra-D 24 Hour Extended-Release Tablets 2690

- Ambien Tablets (Infrequent) 2692
- Ambien CR Tablets (Infrequent) 2696
- Bicillin C-R Injectable Suspension 1775
- Bicillin L-A Injection 1777
- Captopril Tablets (2 to 5 of 1000 patients) 2182
- Catapres Tablets 841
- Catapres-TTS (0.5% or less) 842
- ▲ CellCept Capsules (3% to less than 20%) 2622
- ▲ CellCept Intravenous (3% to less than 20%) 2622
- ▲ CellCept Oral Suspension (3% to less than 20%) 2622
- ▲ CellCept Tablets (3% to less than 20%) 2622
- Clorpres Tablets 2185
- ▲ Dacogen Injection (23%) 1066
- Dapsone Tablets USP 1746
- ▲ Doxil Injection (1% to 10%) 2378
- Effexor XR Extended-Release Capsules (Rare) 3195
- Enbrel for Injection 569
- EpiPen 1024
- Evoxac Capsules (Less than 1%) 1013
- ▲ Fabrazyme for Intravenous Infusion (Greater than or equal to 5%) 1241
- Fentora Tablets (Greater than 1%) 968
- ▲ Flolan for Injection (21% to 32%) 1426
- Flulaval Injection Vaccine 1448
- Flumadine (Less than 0.3%) 1167
- Gabitril Tablets (Infrequent) 973
- Imitrex Injection (Rare) 1465
- Imitrex Nasal Spray (Rare) 1470
- Imitrex Tablets (Infrequent) 1474
- Kogenate FS 746
- Kogenate FS with Bio-Set 748
- Luvox CR Extended-Release Capsules (Infrequent) 1759
- ▲ Miacalcin Nasal Spray (10.6%) 2274
- Mirapex Tablets 857
- Nitrolingual Pumpspray 2965
- Paxil (Rare) 1535
- Paxil CR Controlled-Release Tablets (Rare) 1544
- Pediarix Vaccine 1552
- Pentacel 2792
- Prozac Weekly Capsules (Rare) 1852
- Prozac Pulvules and Liquid (Rare) 1852
- ReoPro Vials (0.1%) 1860
- Rythmol SR Capsules 1590
- ▲ Serevent Diskus (9%) 1594
- Thioridazine Hydrochloride Tablets 2195
- ▲ Trisenox Injection (10%) 986
- Venlafaxine Hydrochloride Tablets (Rare) 2199
- ▲ Vesanoid Capsules (6%) 2660
- Wellbutrin Tablets (Rare) 1648
- WinRho SDF 741
- Zyprexa Tablets 1883
- Zyprexa ZYDIS Orally Disintegrating Tablets 1883
- Zyrtec Chewable Tablets (Less than 2%) 1920
- Zyrtec Syrup (Less than 2%) 1920
- Zyrtec Tablets (Less than 2%) 1920
- Zyrtec-D 12 Hour Extended Release Tablets (Less than 2%) 1923

Pallor, optic disc

- Triesence Injectable Suspension (2%) ⊙209

Palmar-plantar erythrodysesthesia syndrome

- ▲ Clolar for Intravenous Infusion (13%) 1239
- ▲ Doxil Injection (3.4% to 50.6%) 2378
- ▲ Ixempra Kit for Injection (8% to greater than or equal to 20%) 915
- ▲ Sutent Capsules (3% to 14%) 2540
- Taxotere Injection Concentrate 2773
- ▲ Tykerb Tablets (0% to 53%) 1631
- ▲ Xeloda Tablets (17% to 54%) 2662

Palpitations

- Abilify Injection (Greater than or equal to 1 in 1000 patients and less than 1 in 100 patients) 2466
- Abilify Oral Solution (Greater than or equal to 1 in 1000 patients and less than 1 in 100 patients) 881
- Abilify Oral Solution (Greater than or equal to 1 in 1000 patients and less than 1 in 100 patients) 2466
- Abilify Discmelt Orally Disintegrating Tablets (Greater than or equal to 1 in 1000 patients and less than 1 in 100 patients) 881
- Abilify Discmelt Orally Disintegrating Tablets (Greater than or equal to 1 in 1000 patients and less than 1 in 100 patients) 2466
- Abilify Tablets (Greater than or equal to 1 in 1000 patients and less than 1 in 100 patients) 881
- Abilify Tablets (Greater than or equal to 1 in 1000 patients and less than 1 in 100 patients) 2466
- Accutane Capsules 2607
- Aceon Tablets (2 mg, 4 mg, 8 mg) (0.9% to 1.1%) 3038
- Actiq (1% or greater) 959
- ▲ Adderall XR Capsules (2% to 4%) 3012
- Adenocard IV Injection (Less than 1%) 603
- Adenoscan (Less than 1%) 605
- Adipex-P 1185
- Advicor Tablets 402
- ▲ Aerobid/Aerobid-M (3% to 9%) 1153
- Aggrenox Capsules (Less than 1%) 819
- ▲ Agrylin Capsules (26.1%) 3017
- Aldara Cream, 5% 1699
- Allegra-D 12 Hour Extended-Release Tablets (1.9%) 2687
- Allegra-D 24 Hour Extended-Release Tablets (1.9%) 2690
- Ambien Tablets (2%) 2692
- Ambien CR Tablets (1%) 2696
- Amerge Tablets (Infrequent) 1301
- Amitiza Capsules (Less than 1%) 3082
- Amrix Capsules 966
- Anaprox Tablets (Less than 3%) 2632
- Anaprox DS Tablets (Less than 3%) 2632
- Anzemet Injection (Rare) 2701
- Anzemet Tablets (Rare) 2704
- Atacand Tablets (0.5% or greater) 639
- Atacand HCT (0.5% or greater) 642
- Atripla Tablets 938
- Atrovent Nasal Spray 0.03% 834
- Atrovent Nasal Spray 0.06% (Less than 1%) 836
- Avelox (Greater than or equal to 0.1% to less than 2%) 2803
- ▲ Avinza Capsules (Less than 5%) 1772
- Axert Tablets (Infrequent) 2431
- ▲ Azor Tablets (0.7% to 4.5%) 1005
- Bentyl Capsules 703
- Bentyl Injection 703
- Bentyl Syrup 703
- Bentyl Tablets 703
- ▲ Betaseron for SC Injection (4%) 756
- Betimol Ophthalmic Solution 3181
- Bicillin C-R Injectable Suspension 1775
- Bicillin L-A Injection 1777
- Brovana Inhalation Solution (Less than 2%) 2990
- Campral Tablets (Frequent) 1158
- Captopril Tablets (Approximately 1 of 100 patients) 2182
- Cardizem LA Extended Release Tablets (Less than 2%) 421
- Catapres Tablets (About 5 in 1,000 patients) 841
- Catapres-TTS (0.5% or less) 842
- Celebrex Capsules (0.1% to 1.9%) 2979
- Celexa (At least 2%) 1160
- ▲ CellCept Capsules (3% to less than 20%) 2622
- ▲ CellCept Intravenous (3% to less than 20%) 2622
- ▲ CellCept Oral Suspension (3% to less than 20%) 2622
- ▲ CellCept Tablets (3% to less than 20%) 2622
- Chantix Tablets (Infrequent) 2511
- Cialis Tablets (Less than 2%) 1792
- Cipro I.V. (1% or less) 2817
- Cipro (Less than 1%) 2810
- Cipro XR Tablets 2823
- Clarinex Syrup 2828
- Clarinex Tablets 2828
- Clarinex Reditabs Tablets 2828
- Clarinex-D 12-Hour Extended-Release Tablets 2831
- Clarinex-D 24-Hour Extended-Release Tablets 2834
- Clinoril Tablets (Less than 1 in 100) 1962
- Clorpres Tablets (About 5 in 1,000) 2185
- Combigan Ophthalmic Solution 553
- Combivent Inhalation Aerosol (Less than 2%) 845
- ▲ Concerta Extended-Release Tablets (3.1%) 1925
- ▲ Copaxone for Injection (17%) 3110
- ▲ Coreg Tablets (Greater than 1% to 3%) 1387
- ▲ Coreg CR Extended-Release Capsules (Greater than 1% to less than or equal to 3%) 1393
- Cosopt Sterile Ophthalmic Solution 1969
- Cozaar Tablets (Less than 1%) 1973
- Cymbalta Delayed-Release Capsules (Frequent to 2%) 1801
- Daytrana Transdermal Patch 3022
- Depakote ER Tablets (Greater than 1% to less than 5%) 423
- Dexedrine 1401
- Diovan Tablets 2212
- Diovan HCT Tablets (Greater than 0.2%) 2216
- Donnatal Extentabs 2507
- Doxil Injection (Less than 1%) 2378
- DynaCirc CR Controlled Release Tablets (1.2%) 1407
- EC-Naprosyn Delayed-Release Tablets (Less than 3%) 2632
- ▲ Effexor XR Extended-Release Capsules (3%) 3195
- Eldepryl Capsules (1 of 49 patients) 3052
- Emend Capsules (Greater than 0.5%) 1992
- Emend for Injection (Greater than 0.5%) 1999
- Emsam Transdermal System 905
- Enablex Extended-Release Tablets 2225
- Engerix-B Vaccine 1409
- EpiPen 1024
- ▲ Evoxac Capsules (1% to 3%) 1013
- Exelon Capsules (Frequent) 2229
- Exelon Oral Solution (Frequent) 2229
- Exforge Tablets (Greater than or equal to 0.2%) 2238
- Flebogamma 5% 1715
- Flebogamma 5% DIF 1718
- ▲ Flolan for Injection (63%) 1426
- Flomax Capsules (Infrequent) 848
- ▲ Flovent Diskus 50 mcg (1% to 3%) 1435
- Flumadine (Less than 0.3%) 1167
- Focalin XR Capsules 2251
- Foradil Aerolizer 2849
- Frova Tablets (Frequent) 1111
- Gabitril Tablets (Frequent) 973
- Gantrisin Pediatric Suspension 2638
- ▲ Humira Injection (Less than 5%) 442
- Humulin 50/50, 100 Units 1843
- Humulin 70/30 Vial 1844
- Humulin N Vial 1846
- Humulin R 1849
- Imitrex Injection (Infrequent) 1465
- Imitrex Nasal Spray (Infrequent) 1470
- Imitrex Tablets (Up to 2%) 1474
- ▲ Indapamide Tablets (Less than 5%) 2188
- Indocin (Less than 1%) 2024
- ▲ Intron A for Injection (Less than 5%) 2859
- Invega Extended-Release Tablets 1748
- Kaletra (Less than 2%) 452
- Ketek Tablets 2744
- Klonopin (Infrequent) 2639
- Lamictal (Infrequent) 1488
- Lanoxin Injection 1498
- Lanoxin Injection Pediatric 1502
- Lanoxin Tablets 1505
- ▲ Letairis Tablets (5%) 1258
- Levaquin (0.1% to 1%) 2416
- Levaquin in 5% Dextrose Injection (0.1% to 1%) 2416
- Levitra Tablets (Less than 2%) 2876
- Levothroid Tablets 1170
- Levoxyl Tablets 1780
- Lexapro Oral Suspension (Frequent) 1174
- Lexapro Tablets (Frequent) 1174
- Lipitor Tablets (Less than 2%) 2501
- Lupron Depot 3.75 mg (Among most frequent) 462
- ▲ Lupron Depot–3 Month 11.25 mg (Less than 5%) 462
- ▲ Luvox CR Extended-Release Capsules (3%) 1759
- Marinol Capsules (Greater than 1%) 3163
- Marplan Tablets (0% to 2%) 3177
- Mavik Tablets (0.3% to 1%) 472
- Maxair Autohaler (1.3% to 1.7%) 1705
- Maxalt Tablets (Frequent) 2056
- Maxalt-MLT Orally Disintegrating Tablets (Frequent) 2056
- ▲ Megace ES Oral Suspension (1% to 3%) 2499
- Meridia Capsules (2%) 475
- Metadate CD Capsules 3146
- Miacalcin Nasal Spray (Less than 1%) 2274
- Micardis Tablets (More than 0.3%) 852
- Micardis HCT Tablets 854
- Mirapex Tablets (Greater than or equal to 1%) 857
- Mobic Oral Suspension (Less than 2%) 863
- Mobic Tablets (Less than 2%) 863
- MS Contin Tablets (Less frequent) 2585
- Nalfon Capsules (2.5%) 2508
- Naprosyn Suspension (Less than 3%) 2632
- Naprosyn Tablets (Less than 3%) 2632
- Niaspan Extended-Release Tablets 480
- Nimotop Capsules (Less than 1%) 790
- Noroxin Tablets (Less frequent) 2069
- Norvir (Less than 2%) 489
- Opana Tablets (Less than 1%) 1117
- Opana ER Tablets (Less than 1%) 1121
- OptiPranolol Metipranolol Ophthalmic Solution 0.3% (A small number of patients) ⊙245
- OxyContin Tablets (Less than 1%) 2589
- Parnate Tablets 1532
- ▲ Paxil (2% to 3%) 1535
- ▲ Paxil CR Controlled-Release Tablets (2% to 3%) 1544
- Pentasa Capsules (Less than 1%) 3030
- Pepcid Tablets (Infrequent) 2075
- Percocet Tablets 1127
- Percodan Tablets 1130
- Perforomist Inhalation Solution 1025
- Persantine Tablets (Rare) 869
- Plavix Tablets (1% to 2.5%) 926
- Plavix Tablets (1% to 2.5%) 2767
- ▲ Pletal Tablets (5% to 10%) 2481
- PrandiMet Tablets (Less than or equal to 1%) 2967
- Prandin Tablets (Less than or equal to 1%) 2971
- Primaxin I.M. 2080
- Primaxin I.V. (Less than 0.2%) 2083
- Prinivil Tablets (0.3% to 1%) 2087
- Prinzide Tablets (0.3% to 1%) 2092
- ▲ Pristiq Extended-Release Tablets (1% to 3%) 3247
- Proglycem Capsules (Frequent) 1185
- Proglycem Suspension (Frequent) 1185
- ▲ Prometrium Capsules (100 mg, 200 mg) (Less than 5%) 3047
- Protonix for Delayed-Release Oral Suspension (Less than 1%) 3254
- Protonix Delayed-Release Tablets (Less than 1%) 3254
- Protonix I.V. (Less than 1%) 3257
- Protopic Ointment (Greater than or equal to 1%) 628
- Proventil HFA Inhalation Aerosol (Less than 3%) 2914
- Provigil Tablets (2%) 977
- Prozac Weekly Capsules (Frequent) 1852
- Prozac Pulvules and Liquid (Frequent) 1852
- Recombivax HB (Less than 1%) 2107
- ReFacto Vials 3269
- ReoPro Vials (0.7%) 1860
- ▲ Requip Tablets (Frequent to 3%) 1561
- Rilutek Tablets (0.4% to 1.2%) 2771
- Risperdal Consta Long-Acting Injection (Infrequent) 1753
- Rocephin Injectable Vials, ADD-Vantage, Galaxy, Bulk (Less than 0.1%) 2642
- ▲ Romazicon Injection (3% to 9%) 2646
- ▲ Rythmol Tablets (2% to 3%) 1586
- Rythmol SR Capsules 1590
- Salagen Tablets (Less than 1% to 2%) 1082
- Sanctura XR Capsules 557
- Sandostatin Injection (Less than 1%) 2300
- Singulair 2114
- Spiriva HandiHaler 870
- Stalevo Tablets 2309
- ▲ Strattera Capsules (0.7% to 4%) 1864
- ▲ Sular Extended Release Tablets (3%) 2975
- Sustiva Capsules (Less than 2%) 930
- Sustiva Tablets (Less than 2%) 930
- Tarka Tablets (0.3% or more) 511
- ▲ Tasigna Capsules (1% to 10%) 2316
- Teveten Tablets (Less than 1%) 515
- Teveten HCT Tablets (Less than 1%) 517
- Timoptic Sterile Ophthalmic Solution (Less frequent) 2121
- Timoptic in Ocudose (Less frequent) 2124
- Timoptic-XE Sterile Ophthalmic Gel Forming Solution 2125
- Toprol-XL Tablets (About 1 of 100 patients) 666
- ▲ Tracleer Tablets (5%) 3289

Treximet Tablets (Greater than 1%)... 1616
Tricor Tablets... 520
▲ Trisenox Injection (10%)... 986
Twinrix Vaccine... 1628
Ultram ER Extended-Release Tablets (0.5% to less than 1%)... 2428
Vantas (Less than 2%)... 1737
Ventolin HFA Inhalation Aerosol (Less than 3%)... 1638
Vicoprofen Tablets (Less than 3%)... 533
Vivitrol... 988
Voltaren Tablets (Rarely)... 2334
Voltaren-XR Tablets (Rarely)... 2337
Vyvanse Capsules... 3033
▲ Wellbutrin Tablets (3.7%)... 1648
▲ Wellbutrin SR Sustained-Release Tablets (2% to 6%)... 1653
▲ Wellbutrin XL Extended-Release Tablets (2% to 6%)... 1659
Xyzal Oral Solution... 2789
Xyzal Oral Solution... 3155
▲ Zemplar Capsules (3%)... 536
▲ Zemplar Injection (3%)... 538
Zofran Injection... 1682
Zomig Tablets (1% to 2%)... 694
Zomig Nasal Spray (1% to 2%)... 689
Zomig-ZMT Tablets (1% to 2%)... 694
Zonegran Capsules (Infrequent)... 1089
Zyban Sustained-Release Tablets (2%)... 1692
Zyprexa Tablets (Infrequent)... 1883
Zyprexa ZYDIS Orally Disintegrating Tablets (Infrequent)... 1883
Zyrtec Chewable Tablets (Less than 2%)... 1920
Zyrtec Syrup (Less than 2%)... 1920
Zyrtec Tablets (Less than 2%)... 1920
Zyrtec-D 12 Hour Extended Release Tablets (Less than 2%)... 1923

Palsy, cranial nerve

DepoCyt Injection... 1136
Eloxatin for Injection... 2731
Orthoclone OKT3 Sterile Solution (Less than 1%)... 2387
Velcade for Injection... 2168

Palsy, extraocular

Lyrica Capsules (Rare)... 2527
Protonix for Delayed-Release Oral Suspension (Less than 1%)... 3254
Protonix Delayed-Release Tablets (Less than 1%)... 3254
Protonix I.V. (Less than 1%)... 3257

Palsy, facial

Boostrix... 1377
Chantix Tablets (Rare)... 2511
Fluarix Vaccine... 1446
Mirapex Tablets... 857
PegIntron Powder for Injection (Less than or equal to 1%)... 2903
Treximet Tablets (Rare)... 1616

Palsy, nerve

PegIntron Powder for Injection (Less than or equal to 1%)... 2903

Palsy, oculomotor

PegIntron Powder for Injection (Less than or equal to 1%)... 2903

Palsy, peripheral nerve

Lescol Capsules... 2268
Lescol XL Tablets... 2268
Mevacor Tablets... 2063

Palsy, peroneal nerve

Arranon Injection (1%)... 1319

Pancolitis

Canasa Rectal Suppositories... 705

Pancreatic amylase, increased

▲ Truvada Tablets (Less than or equal to 3%)... 1262

Pancreatic disease, unspecified

Pulmozyme Inhalation Solution... 1217

Pancreatic enzymes, increased

▲ Atripla Tablets (Up to 3%)... 938
Emtriva Capsules (Less than 1% to 2%)... 1246
Emtriva Oral Solution (Less than 1% to 2%)... 1246
Sutent Capsules... 2540

Pancreatitis

Abilify Injection (Less than 1 in 1000 patients)... 881
Abilify Injection (Less than 1 in 1000 patients)... 2466
Abilify Oral Solution (Less than 1 in 1000 patients)... 881
Abilify Oral Solution (Less than 1 in 1000 patients)... 2466
Abilify Discmelt Orally Disintegrating Tablets (Less than 1 in 1000 patients)... 881
Abilify Discmelt Orally Disintegrating Tablets (Less than 1 in 1000 patients)... 2466
Abilify Tablets (Less than 1 in 1000 patients)... 881
Abilify Tablets (Less than 1 in 1000 patients)... 2466
Accutane Capsules... 2607
Actimmune (Rare)... 1743
Activase I.V.... 1188
Activella Tablets... 2347
Aczone Gel 5%... 3296
Advicor Tablets... 402
Aggrenox Capsules... 819
Agrylin Capsules... 3017
Anaprox Tablets (Less than 1%)... 2632
Anaprox DS Tablets (Less than 1%)... 2632
Angeliq Tablets... 751
Anzemet Injection (Rare)... 2701
Anzemet Tablets (Rare)... 2704
Aptivus Capsules (Less than 2%)... 823
Aptivus Oral Solution (Less than 2%)... 823
Aricept Tablets... 1062
Aricept ODT Tablets... 1062
Asacol Delayed-Release Tablets... 2579
Atacand HCT... 642
Atripla Tablets... 938
Avalide Tablets... 892
Avalide Tablets... 2713
Bayer Aspirin... 750
Betaseron for SC Injection... 756
Biaxin/Biaxin XL... 411
Busulfex Injection (2%)... 2477
Calcijex Injection... 419
Campral Tablets (Infrequent)... 1158
Canasa Rectal Suppositories... 705
Cancidas for Injection... 1953
Captopril Tablets... 2182
Carbatrol Capsules... 3019
Celebrex Capsules (Less than 0.1%)... 2979
Celexa... 1160
CellCept Capsules... 2622
CellCept Intravenous... 2622
CellCept Oral Suspension... 2622
CellCept Tablets... 2622
Cipro I.V. (1% or less)... 2817
Cipro... 2810
Cipro XR Tablets... 2823
Climara Transdermal System... 763
Climara Pro Transdermal System... 768
Clinoril Tablets (Less than 1 in 100)... 1962
Clorpres Tablets... 2185
Combivir Tablets (Less than 0.5%)... 1384
Copaxone for Injection (Infrequent)... 3110
Crestor Tablets... 677
Crixivan Capsules... 1979
Cuprimine Capsules... 1986
Dapsone Tablets USP... 1746
▲ Depakote ER Tablets (Greater than 1% to less than 5%)... 423
Diovan HCT Tablets... 2216
Divigel... 3167
Doxil Injection (Less than 1%)... 2378
Dyazide Capsules... 1405
EC-Naprosyn Delayed-Release Tablets (Less than 1%)... 2632
Edecrin (Rare)... 698
E.E.S.... 433
Effexor XR Extended-Release Capsules... 3195
Eloxatin for Injection... 2731
Elspar for Injection... 1990
Elspar for Injection (Rare)... 2488
Enbrel for Injection (Infrequent)... 569
Enjuvia Tablets... 1029
▲ Epivir (Less than 0.3% to 18%)... 1412
▲ Epivir-HBV (14% to 15%)... 1417
Epzicom Tablets... 1422
EryPed (Rare)... 431
Estratest Tablets... 3043
Estratest H.S. Tablets... 3043
Exelon Capsules (Infrequent)... 2229
Exelon Oral Solution (Infrequent)... 2229
Exelon Patch (Infrequent)... 2233
Exforge Tablets (Greater than 0.1% to less than 1%)... 2238
Fansidar Tablets... 2636
Fenoglide Tablets... 2960
Furosemide Tablets... 2186
Gantrisin Pediatric Suspension... 2638
Gengraf Capsules (Rare)... 435
Genotropin Lyophilized Powder (Rare)... 2547
Gleevec Tablets (Rare)... 2255
Humatrope Vials and Cartridges (Rare)... 1838
Imitrex Injection... 1465
Imitrex Nasal Spray (Rare)... 1470
Imitrex Tablets... 1474
Intelence Tablets (Less than 2%)... 3119
Intravenous Sodium Diuril... 2490
Intron A for Injection... 2859
Invanz for Injection (Greater than 0.1%)... 2029
Kaletra (Less than 2%)... 452
Keppra Injection... 3137
Keppra Oral Solution... 3131
Keppra Tablets... 3131
Ketek Tablets... 2744
Lamictal... 1488
Lescol Capsules... 2268
Lescol XL Tablets... 2268
Levaquin (0.1% to 1%)... 2416
Levaquin in 5% Dextrose Injection (0.1% to 1%)... 2416
Lexapro Oral Suspension... 1174
Lexapro Tablets... 1174
Lialda Tablets (Less than 1% to infrequent)... 3029
Lipitor Tablets (Less than 2%)... 2501
Lovaza Capsules... 1520
Luvox CR Extended-Release Capsules... 1759
Lybrel Tablets... 3204
Lyrica Capsules (0.1% to 1%)... 2527
Mavik Tablets (Rare)... 472
Mepron Suspension... 1526
Mevacor Tablets... 2063
Micardis HCT Tablets... 854
Mirapex Tablets... 857
M-M-R II... 2054
Mobic Oral Suspension (Less than 2%)... 863
Mobic Tablets (Less than 2%)... 863
Mumpsvax... 2068
Myfortic Tablets... 2276
Nalfon Capsules (Less than 1%)... 2508
Namenda... 1180
Naprosyn Suspension (Less than 1%)... 2632
Naprosyn Tablets (Less than 1%)... 2632
Neoral Oral Solution (Rare)... 2280
Neoral Soft Gelatin Capsules (Rare)... 2280
Nexavar Tablets (0.1% to less htan 1%)... 784
Nexium Delayed-Release Capsules (Rare)... 645
Nexium I.V. (Rare)... 652
Nexium Delayed-Release Oral Suspension (Rare)... 645
Norditropin Cartridges... 2354
Noroxin Tablets (Rare)... 2069
Norvir (Less than 2%)... 489
Nutropin for Injection (Rare)... 1208
Nutropin AQ Injection (Rare)... 1212
Nutropin AQ NuSpin Injection (Rare)... 1212
Nutropin AQ Pen (Rare)... 1212
Nutropin AQ Pen Cartridge (Rare)... 1212
Oncaspar Injection (Greater than or equal to 2%)... 1138
▲ Ontak Vials (Less than 5%)... 1079
Paxil... 1535
Paxil CR Controlled-Release Tablets... 1544
PegIntron Powder for Injection (Less than or equal to 1%)... 2903
Pentasa Capsules (Infrequent to less than 1%)... 3030
Percocet Tablets... 1127
Percodan Tablets... 1130
Plavix Tablets... 926
Plavix Tablets... 2767
PrandiMet Tablets... 2967
Prandin Tablets (Rare)... 2971
Premarin Intravenous... 3217
Premarin Tablets... 3221
Premarin Vaginal Cream... 3228
Premphase Tablets... 3232
Prempro Tablets... 3232
Prinivil Tablets (0.3% to 1%)... 2087
Prinzide Tablets... 2092
Prograf Capsules and Injection... 622
Proleukin for Injection (Less than 1%)... 2287
Protonix for Delayed-Release Oral Suspension... 3254
Protonix Delayed-Release Tablets... 3254
Protonix I.V.... 3257
Prozac Weekly Capsules (Rare)... 1852
Prozac Pulvules and Liquid (Rare)... 1852
Rapamune (Less than 3%)... 3260
Remeron Tablets (Rare)... 2924
RemeronSolTab Tablets (Rare)... 2927
Remicade for IV Injection (Greater than or equal to 0.2%)... 950
Requip Tablets (Infrequent)... 1561
Retrovir Capsules (Rare)... 1574
Retrovir IV Infusion (Rare)... 1579
Retrovir (Rare)... 1574
Reyataz Capsules... 3299
Rilutek Tablets (Infrequent)... 2771
Risperdal Consta Long-Acting Injection... 1753
Rocaltrol Capsules... 1150
Rocaltrol Oral Solution... 1150
Rocephin Injectable Vials, ADD-Vantage, Galaxy, Bulk (Rare)... 2642
Rythmol SR Capsules... 1590
St. Joseph 81 mg Aspirin Chewable and Enteric Coated Tablets... 1903
Salagen Tablets (Less than 1%)... 1082
Sandimmune (Rare)... 2296
Sandostatin Injection (Less than 1%)... 2300
Sandostatin LAR Depot... 2302
Seasonique Tablets... 1046
Singulair (Very rare)... 2114
Solodyn Extended Release Tablets... 1938
Soriatane Capsules... 3062
Sustiva Capsules (Less than 2%)... 930
Sustiva Tablets (Less than 2%)... 930
Sutent Capsules (Less than 1% to 1%)... 2540
Symbyax Capsules (Rare)... 1871
Targretin Capsules... 1084
Tarka Tablets... 511
Tasigna Capsules (0.1% to 1%)... 2316
Tekturna HCT Tablets... 2324
Teveten HCT Tablets... 517
Tricor Tablets... 520
Trizivir Tablets (3 of 656 patients)... 1622
Truvada Tablets... 1262
Tygacil for Injection... 3276
Ultram ER Extended-Release Tablets (0.5% to less than 1%)... 2428
Venlafaxine Hydrochloride Tablets... 2199
Vesanoid Capsules (Isolated cases)... 2660
Viread Tablets... 1268
Voltaren Tablets (Rarely)... 2334
Voltaren-XR Tablets (Rarely)... 2337
Vytorin 10/10 Tablets... 2149
Vytorin 10/10 Tablets... 2939
Vytorin 10/20 Tablets... 2149
Vytorin 10/20 Tablets... 2939
Vytorin 10/40 Tablets... 2149
Vytorin 10/40 Tablets... 2939
Vytorin 10/80 Tablets... 2149
Vytorin 10/80 Tablets... 2939
Wellbutrin SR Sustained-Release Tablets... 1653
Wellbutrin XL Extended-Release Tablets... 1659
Yaz Tablets... 805
Zantac 25 EFFERdose Tablets (Rare)... 1670
Zantac Injection (Rare)... 1666
Zantac Injection Pharmacy Bulk Package (Rare)... 1668
Zantac Injection Premixed (Rare)... 1666
Zantac (Rare)... 1670
Zetia Tablets... 2157
Zetia Tablets... 2951
Ziagen... 1673
Zocor Tablets... 2136
Zomig Tablets (Rare)... 694
Zomig-ZMT Tablets (Rare)... 694
Zyban Sustained-Release Tablets... 1692
Zyprexa Tablets... 1883
Zyprexa ZYDIS Orally Disintegrating Tablets... 1883

Pancreatitis, acute

Aceon Tablets (2 mg, 4 mg, 8 mg)... 3038
Byetta Injection... 600
Chantix Tablets (Rare)... 2511
Lamisil Oral Granules... 2264
Proglycem Capsules (Infrequent)... 1185
Proglycem Suspension (Infrequent)... 1185
Requip Tablets (Infrequent)... 1561
Tygacil for Injection... 3276
Velcade for Injection... 2168

Pancreatitis, hemorrhagic

Prograf Capsules and Injection... 622

Pancreatitis, necrotizing

Prograf Capsules and Injection... 622

Pancytopenia
Aceon Tablets (2 mg, 4 mg, 8 mg)... 3038
Aciphex Tablets ... 1053
Actiq (1% or greater) ... 959
Aggrenox Capsules ... 819
Albenza Tablets (Rare) ... 1297
Anaprox Tablets (Less than 1%) ... 2632
Anaprox DS Tablets (Less than 1%).. 2632
Asacol Delayed-Release Tablets ... 2579
Avandaryl Tablets ... 1344
Avastin IV (Rare) ... 1192
Avelox ... 2803
Captopril Tablets ... 2182
Carbatrol Capsules ... 3019
Ceftin ... 1380
▲ CellCept Capsules (3% to less than 20%) ... 2622
▲ CellCept Intravenous (3% to less than 20%) ... 2622
▲ CellCept Oral Suspension (3% to less than 20%) ... 2622
▲ CellCept Tablets (3% to less than 20%) ... 2622
Cimzia (Rare/Infrequent) ... 3127
Cipro I.V. (Rare) ... 2817
Cipro (0.1%) ... 2810
Cipro XR Tablets ... 2823
Concerta Extended-Release Tablets ... 1925
Copaxone for Injection (Infrequent) .. 3110
Coreg Tablets (Less than or equal to 0.1%) ... 1387
Coreg CR Extended-Release Capsules (Less than or equal to 0.1%) ... 1393
Cosmegen for Injection ... 2485
Daraprim Tablets ... 1400
Depakote ER Tablets ... 423
Didronel Tablets (Rare) ... 2583
Duetact Tablets ... 3085
EC-Naprosyn Delayed-Release Tablets (Less than 1%) ... 2632
Effexor XR Extended-Release Capsules (Rare) ... 3195
Elitek (Less than or equal to 1%) ... 2729
Enbrel for Injection (Rare) ... 569
Equetro Extended-Release Capsules ... 3174
Flebogamma 5% ... 1715
Flebogamma 5% DIF ... 1718
Flolan for Injection ... 1426
Fortaz ... 1450
Gammagard Liquid ... 730
Gammagard S/D (Rare) ... 734
Gamunex (Rare) ... 3094
Gleevec Tablets (Infrequent) ... 2255
▲ Humira Injection (Less than 5%) ... 442
Hycamtin for Injection ... 1459
Imitrex Injection ... 1465
Imitrex Nasal Spray ... 1470
Imitrex Tablets ... 1474
Keppra Injection ... 3137
Keppra Oral Solution ... 3131
Keppra Tablets ... 3131
Lamictal ... 1488
Lamisil Oral Granules ... 2264
Leukeran Tablets ... 1508
Leustatin Injection ... 2384
Levaquin ... 2416
Levaquin in 5% Dextrose Injection ... 2416
Mustargen for Injection ... 2492
Mycamine for Injection ... 616
Myleran Tablets ... 1530
Nalfon Capsules (Less than 1%) ... 2508
Naprosyn Suspension (Less than 1%) ... 2632
Naprosyn Tablets (Less than 1%) ... 2632
Nexium Delayed-Release Capsules .. 645
Nexium I.V. (Rare) ... 652
Nexium Delayed-Release Oral Suspension ... 645
Noroxin Tablets ... 2069
Omnicef Capsules ... 497
Omnicef for Oral Suspension ... 497
Orthoclone OKT3 Sterile Solution (Less than 1%) ... 2387
Paxil ... 1535
Paxil CR Controlled-Release Tablets ... 1544
Pentasa Capsules ... 3030
Pepcid Tablets (Rare) ... 2075
Percocet Tablets ... 1127
Phenytek Capsules (Occasional) ... 2192
Plavix Tablets ... 926
Plavix Tablets ... 2767
Pletal Tablets ... 2481
Primaxin I.M. ... 2080
Primaxin I.V. ... 2083
Prograf Capsules and Injection ... 622
Protonix for Delayed-Release Oral Suspension ... 3254
Protonix Delayed-Release Tablets ... 3254
Protonix I.V. ... 3257
Prozac Weekly Capsules ... 1852
Prozac Pulvules and Liquid ... 1852
Rapamune ... 3260
Remeron Tablets (Rare) ... 2924
RemeronSolTab Tablets (Rare) ... 2927
Remicade for IV Injection (Greater than or equal to 0.2%) ... 950
Retrovir Capsules ... 1574
Retrovir IV Infusion ... 1579
Retrovir ... 1574
Rituxan I.V. ... 1223
Sandostatin LAR Depot ... 2302
Soma Tablets ... 1931
Suprax for Oral Suspension ... 1891
Suprax Tablets ... 1891
Tabloid Tablets (Nearly all patients) .. 1601
▲ Tasigna Capsules (1% to 10%) ... 2316
Temodar Capsules (Very rare) ... 2931
Thioridazine Hydrochloride Tablets ... 2195
Thiothixene Capsules ... 2197
▲ Valcyte Tablets (Less than 5%) ... 2654
Venlafaxine Hydrochloride Tablets ... 2199
Voltaren Tablets (Rarely) ... 2334
Voltaren-XR Tablets (Rarely) ... 2337
Wellbutrin Tablets (Rare) ... 1648
Wellbutrin SR Sustained-Release Tablets ... 1653
Wellbutrin XL Extended-Release Tablets ... 1659
▲ Xeloda Tablets (Less than 5%) ... 2662
Zantac 25 EFFERdose Tablets (Rare) ... 1670
Zantac Injection (Rare) ... 1666
Zantac Injection Pharmacy Bulk Package (Rare) ... 1668
Zantac Injection Premixed (Rare) ... 1666
Zantac (Rare) ... 1670
Zinacef for Injection ... 1678
Zinacef Injection ... 1678
▲ Zometa for Intravenous Infusion (5% to less than 10%) ... 2341
Zosyn for Injection (1% or less) ... 3284
Zyban Sustained-Release Tablets ... 1692

Panencephalitis, sclerosing, subacute
Attenuvax ... 1951
M-M-R II ... 2054
ProQuad ... 2099

Panic attack
Ambien Tablets (Rare) ... 2692
Ambien CR Tablets (Rare) ... 2696
Amerge Tablets (Rare) ... 1301
Celexa (Infrequent) ... 1160
Cozaar Tablets (Less than 1%) ... 1973
Effexor XR Extended-Release Capsules ... 3195
Imitrex Injection ... 1465
Imitrex Nasal Spray ... 1470
Imitrex Tablets ... 1474
Lamictal (Infrequent) ... 1488
Lexapro Oral Suspension (Infrequent) ... 1174
Lexapro Tablets (Infrequent) ... 1174
Luvox CR Extended-Release Capsules ... 1759
Parnate Tablets ... 1532
Paxil Tablets ... 1535
Paxil CR Controlled-Release Tablets ... 1544
Pristiq Extended-Release Tablets ... 3247
Prozac Weekly Capsules ... 1852
Prozac Pulvules and Liquid ... 1852
Remeron Tablets ... 2924
RemeronSolTab Tablets ... 2927
Requip Tablets (Infrequent) ... 1561
Romazicon Injection ... 2646
Symbyax Capsules ... 1871
Treximet Tablets (Rare) ... 1616
Venlafaxine Hydrochloride Tablets ... 2199
▲ Vivitrol (8% to 12%) ... 988
Wellbutrin Tablets ... 1648
Wellbutrin SR Sustained-Release Tablets ... 1653
Wellbutrin XL Extended-Release Tablets ... 1659
Zyban Sustained-Release Tablets ... 1692

Panic disorder
Xyrem Oral Solution (Infrequent) ... 1766

Panic reaction
Mirapex Tablets ... 857
Venlafaxine Hydrochloride Tablets ... 2199

Panniculitis
Attenuvax ... 1951
M-M-R II ... 2054
ProQuad ... 2099

Papillae
▲ Lotemax Ophthalmic Suspension 0.5% (Less than 5%) ... ⊙241

Papilledema
Accutane Capsules ... 2607
Anaprox Tablets (Less than 1%) ... 2632
Anaprox DS Tablets (Less than 1%).. 2632
EC-Naprosyn Delayed-Release Tablets (Less than 1%) ... 2632
Effexor XR Extended-Release Capsules (Rare) ... 3195
Genotropin Lyophilized Powder ... 2547
Gleevec Tablets (Rare) ... 2255
Humatrope Vials and Cartridges ... 1838
Increlex Injection ... 3100
Intron A for Injection ... 2859
Lyrica Capsules (Rare) ... 2527
Naprosyn Suspension (Less than 1%) ... 2632
Naprosyn Tablets (Less than 1%) ... 2632
Neoral Oral Solution ... 2280
Neoral Soft Gelatin Capsules ... 2280
Ortho-Cyclen/Ortho Tri-Cyclen ... 2449
Ortho Tri-Cyclen Lo Tablets ... 2458
PegIntron Powder for Injection ... 2903
Premphase Tablets ... 3232
Prempro Tablets ... 3232
Soriatane Capsules (Less than 1%) .. 3062
Tasigna Capsules ... 2316
Venlafaxine Hydrochloride Tablets (Rare) ... 2199

Papilledema, exacerbation of
Intron A for Injection ... 2859

Papillitis
Anaprox Tablets (Less than 1%) ... 2632
Anaprox DS Tablets (Less than 1%) .. 2632
Attenuvax ... 1951
EC-Naprosyn Delayed-Release Tablets (Less than 1%) ... 2632
Meruvax II ... 2061
M-M-R II (Infrequent) ... 2054
Mumpsvax (Infrequent) ... 2068
Naprosyn Suspension (Less than 1%) ... 2632
Naprosyn Tablets (Less than 1%) ... 2632
ProQuad ... 2099

Papules
Catapres-TTS (1 of 101 patients) ... 842
Cuprimine Capsules (Rare) ... 1986
Duragesic Transdermal System (1% or greater) ... 2405

Papules, erythematous
(*see under* Erythema multiforme)

Papules at application site
Aldara Cream, 5% (2%) ... 1699
Daytrana Transdermal Patch ... 3022
Ionsys Transdermal System (.1% to less than 1%) ... 2410
Lidoderm Patch ... 1114

Paralysis
Arranon Injection (1%) ... 1319
Brovana Inhalation Solution (Less than 2%) ... 2990
Carbatrol Capsules ... 3019
Equetro Extended-Release Capsules ... 3174
Evoxac Capsules ... 1013
Gabitril Tablets (Infrequent) ... 973
▲ Geodon Capsules (14%) ... 2520
Imitrex Injection ... 1465
Imitrex Tablets (Rare) ... 1474
Lamictal (Rare) ... 1488
Lovenox Injection (Rare) ... 2756
Lupron Depot 7.5 mg ... 469
Lupron Depot-PED 7.5 mg, 11.25 mg and 15 mg ... 471
Luvox CR Extended-Release Capsules (Infrequent) ... 1759
Mirapex Tablets (1% or more) ... 857
Norvir (Less than 2%) ... 489
Paxil (Infrequent) ... 1535
Paxil CR Controlled-Release Tablets (Infrequent) ... 1544
Prozac Weekly Capsules (Rare) ... 1852
Prozac Pulvules and Liquid (Rare) ... 1852
Remeron Tablets (Rare) ... 2924
RemeronSolTab Tablets (Rare) ... 2927
Requip Tablets (Infrequent) ... 1561
Rythmol SR Capsules ... 1590
Velcade for Injection ... 2168
Xyrem Oral Solution (Infrequent) ... 1766
Zyprexa Tablets (Rare) ... 1883
Zyprexa ZYDIS Orally Disintegrating Tablets (Rare) ... 1883
Zyrtec Chewable Tablets (Less than 2%) ... 1920
Zyrtec Syrup (Less than 2%) ... 1920
Zyrtec Tablets (Less than 2%) ... 1920
Zyrtec-D 12 Hour Extended Release Tablets (Less than 2%) ... 1923

Paralysis, facial
Actiq (Less than 1%) ... 959
Angiomax for Injection (Greater than 0.1% to less than 1%) ... 1933
Azilect Tablets (Infrequent) ... 3106
Copaxone for Injection (Infrequent)... 3110
Effexor XR Extended-Release Capsules (Rare) ... 3195
Fluarix Vaccine ... 1446
Flulaval Injection Vaccine ... 1448
▲ Gliadel Wafer (7%) ... 1076
Imitrex Tablets (Rare) ... 1474
Kaletra (Less than 2%) ... 452
Lescol Capsules ... 2268
Lescol XL Tablets ... 2268
Lipitor Tablets (Less than 2%) ... 2501
Lovaza Capsules ... 1520
Rilutek Tablets (Infrequent) ... 2771
Venlafaxine Hydrochloride Tablets (Rare) ... 2199
▲ Vesanoid Capsules (3%) ... 2660
Zonegran Capsules (Rare) ... 1089
Zyprexa Tablets (Rare) ... 1883
Zyprexa ZYDIS Orally Disintegrating Tablets (Rare) ... 1883

Paralysis, facial, partial
Flulaval Injection Vaccine ... 1448

Paralysis, legs
(*see under* Paralysis, lower extremities)

Paralysis, limbs
Flulaval Injection Vaccine ... 1448

Paralysis, sleep
▲ Xyrem Oral Solution (2.9% to 14.3%) ... 1766

Paralysis, spinal cord
Lupron Depot 3.75 mg ... 462
Lupron Depot–3 Month 11.25 mg ... 462

Paralysis, tongue
Frova Tablets (Rare) ... 1111
Maxalt Tablets (Rare) ... 2056
Maxalt-MLT Orally Disintegrating Tablets (Rare) ... 2056

Paralysis agitans
(*see under* Parkinsonism)

Paranasal sinus disorders
Selzentry Tablets (2.1%) ... 2534

Paranoia
Allegra-D 12 Hour Extended-Release Tablets (Less than 1%) ... 2687
Allegra-D 24 Hour Extended-Release Tablets (Less than 1%) ... 2690
Aricept Tablets (Infrequent) ... 1062
Aricept ODT Tablets (Infrequent) ... 1062
Atripla Tablets ... 938
Avelox ... 2803
Celexa (Infrequent) ... 1160
Cipro I.V. (1% or less) ... 2817
Cipro ... 2810
Cipro XR Tablets ... 2823
Copaxone for Injection (Infrequent) .. 3110
Duragesic Transdermal System (1% or greater) ... 2405
Effexor XR Extended-Release Capsules (Infrequent) ... 3195
Evoxac Capsules ... 1013
Exelon Capsules (2% or more) ... 2229
Exelon Oral Solution (2% or more) ... 2229
Gabitril Tablets (Frequent) ... 973
Lamictal (Infrequent) ... 1488
Levaquin ... 2416
Levaquin in 5% Dextrose Injection ... 2416
Lexapro Oral Suspension ... 1174
Lexapro Tablets ... 1174
▲ Marinol Capsules (3% to 10%) ... 3163
Orthoclone OKT3 Sterile Solution (Less than 1%) ... 2387
Paxil (Infrequent) ... 1535
Paxil CR Controlled-Release Tablets (Infrequent) ... 1544
Prozac Pulvules and Liquid (Infrequent) ... 1852
Remeron Tablets (Infrequent) ... 2924
RemeronSolTab Tablets (Infrequent) ... 2927
Requip Tablets (Infrequent) ... 1561
Rilutek Tablets (Infrequent) ... 2771
▲ Romazicon Injection (1% to 3%) ... 2646

Sandostatin Injection (Less than 1%)........ 2300
Sandostatin LAR Depot........ 2302
Stalevo Tablets........ 2309
Sustiva Capsules (0.4%)........ 930
Sustiva Tablets (0.4%)........ 930
Wellbutrin Tablets (Infrequent)........ 1648
Wellbutrin SR Sustained-Release Tablets........ 1653
Wellbutrin XL Extended-Release Tablets........ 1659
Xyrem Oral Solution (Infrequent)........ 1766
Zyban Sustained-Release Tablets........ 1692
Zyprexa Tablets........ 1883
Zyprexa ZYDIS Orally Disintegrating Tablets........ 1883

Paraparesis
Leustatin Injection........ 2384
Orthoclone OKT3 Sterile Solution (Less than 1%)........ 2387

Paraplegia
Copaxone for Injection (Infrequent) .. 3110
Orthoclone OKT3 Sterile Solution 2387

Paraproteinemia
▲ Humira Injection (Less than 5%) 442

Parasomnia
Mirapex Tablets 857
Selzentry Tablets 2534

Parathyroid disorder, unspecified
▲ CellCept Capsules (3% to less than 20%) 2622
▲ CellCept Intravenous (3% to less than 20%) 2622
▲ CellCept Oral Suspension (3% to less than 20%) 2622
▲ CellCept Tablets (3% to less than 20%) 2622
▲ Humira Injection (Less than 5%) 442

Parathyroid hormone deficiency, fetal
Accutane Capsules 2607

Parathyroid hormone levels, compensatory increase
▲ Actonel Tablets (Less than 30%) 2568

Parathyroid neoplasm
Amerge Tablets (Rare) 1301

Paratracheal area, metastases to
Thyrogen for Injection 1244

Parenchymatous organs, toxic damage
Gemzar for Injection (Rare) 1820

Paresis
Aldara Cream, 5% 1699
Ambien Tablets (Rare) 2692
Ambien CR Tablets (Rare) 2696
Coreg Tablets (Less than or equal to 0.1%) 1387
Coreg CR Extended-Release Capsules (Less than or equal to 0.1%) 1393
Engerix-B Vaccine 1409
Exelon Capsules (Infrequent) 2229
Exelon Oral Solution (Infrequent) 2229
▲ Intron A for Injection (Less than 5%) 2859
Klonopin (Infrequent) 2639
Leukeran Tablets (Rare) 1508
▲ Requip Tablets (3%) 1561
Sandostatin LAR Depot 2302
Seromycin Capsules 1864
▲ Temodar Capsules (3% to 8%) 2931
Twinrix Vaccine 1628
Venlafaxine Hydrochloride Tablets (Rare) 2199

Paresis, facial
(*see also under* Bell's palsy)
Fluarix Vaccine 1446

Paresthesia
Accutane Capsules 2607
Aceon Tablets (2 mg, 4 mg, 8 mg) (2.3%) 3038
Actiq (Less than 1%) 959
Actonel with Calcium Tablets (2.1%) 2574
Adenoscan (2%) 605
Advair Diskus 100/50 1276
Advair Diskus 250/50 1276
Advair Diskus 500/50 1276
Advair HFA 45/21 Inhalation Aerosol 1288
Advair HFA 115/21 Inhalation Aerosol........ 1288
Advair HFA 230/21 Inhalation Aerosol........ 1288
Advicor Tablets........ 402
Aggrenox Capsules (Less than 1%).. 819
▲ Agrylin Capsules (5.9%) 3017
Aloxi Injection (Less than 1%)........ 1059
Alphanate........ 1709
Ambien Tablets (Infrequent)........ 2692
Ambien CR Tablets (1%)........ 2696
AmBisome for Injection (Less common)........ 606
Amerge Tablets (1% to 2%)........ 1301
Anaprox Tablets (Less than 1%)...... 2632
Anaprox DS Tablets (Less than 1%).. 2632
AndroGel (Less than 1%)........ 3159
Anzemet Injection (Infrequently)........ 2701
Anzemet Tablets........ 2704
Aricept Tablets (Frequent)........ 1062
Aricept ODT Tablets (Frequent)........ 1062
▲ Arimidex Tablets (5% to 7%) 672
▲ Arranon Injection (0% to 15%) 1319
Asacol Delayed-Release Tablets (2% or greater)........ 2579
Atacand Tablets (0.5% or greater).... 639
Atacand HCT (0.5% or greater)........ 642
▲ Atripla Tablets (Greater than or equal to 5%)........ 938
Avalide Tablets........ 892
Avalide Tablets........ 2713
Avapro Tablets (Less than 1%)........ 897
Avapro Tablets (Less than 1%)........ 2718
Avelox (Less than 0.1%)........ 2803
▲ Avinza Capsules (5% to 10%) 1772
Axert Tablets (1%)........ 2431
▲ Azilect Tablets (2% to 5%) 3106
Betaseron for SC Injection........ 756
Betimol Ophthalmic Solution........ 3181
Boostrix........ 1377
Bystolic Tablets (Greater than or equal to 1%)........ 1155
▲ Campral Tablets (2% to 3%) 1158
Captopril Tablets (About 0.5% to 2%)........ 2182
Carbatrol Capsules........ 3019
Cardene I.V. (0.7%)........ 1093
Cardizem LA Extended Release Tablets (Less than 2%)........ 421
Celebrex Capsules (0.1% to 1.9%)... 2979
Celexa (Frequent)........ 1160
▲ CellCept Capsules (3% to 20.8%) 2622
▲ CellCept Intravenous (3% to 20.8%)........ 2622
▲ CellCept Oral Suspension (3% to 20.8%)........ 2622
▲ CellCept Tablets (3% to 20.8%) 2622
▲ Chemet Capsules (1% to 12.7%) 2484
Cialis Tablets (Less than 2%)........ 1792
Cipro I.V. (1% or less)........ 2817
Cipro (Less than 1%)........ 2810
Cipro XR Tablets........ 2823
Clinoril Tablets (Less than 1%)........ 1962
Clorpres Tablets........ 2185
Combigan Ophthalmic Solution........ 553
Combivent Inhalation Aerosol (Less than 2%)........ 845
Combivir Tablets........ 1384
Concerta Extended-Release Tablets (1.2%)........ 1925
Copaxone for Injection (At least 2%)........ 3110
▲ Coreg Tablets (Greater than 1% to 3%)........ 1387
▲ Coreg CR Extended-Release Capsules (1% to less than or equal to 3%)........ 1393
▲ Cosopt Sterile Ophthalmic Solution (1% to 5%)........ 1969
Cozaar Tablets (Less than 1%)........ 1973
Cubicin for Injection (Less than 1%)........ 995
▲ Cymbalta Delayed-Release Capsules (Frequent to 4%)........ 1801
Delatestryl Injection........ 1730
Denavir Cream........ 2205
▲ Depakote ER Tablets (Greater than 1% to less than 5%)........ 423
DepoCyt Injection........ 1136
▲ DepoDur Injection (2% to 5%) 1095
Didronel Tablets........ 2583
Diovan Tablets (Greater than 0.2%).. 2212
Diovan HCT Tablets (Greater than 0.2%)........ 2216
▲ Doxil Injection (Less than 1% to 10%)........ 2378
Duragesic Transdermal System (1% or greater)........ 2405
Dyazide Capsules........ 1405
DynaCirc CR Controlled Release Tablets (0.5% to 1%)........ 1407
EC-Naprosyn Delayed-Release Tablets (Less than 1%)........ 2632
▲ Effexor XR Extended-Release Capsules (2% to 3%)........ 3195
Elitek (Less than or equal to 1%)...... 2729
Elocon Cream 0.1% (2 in 182 patients)........ 2840
Elocon Lotion 0.1% (2 in 65 patients)........ 2841
▲ Eloxatin for Injection (6% to 77%) 2731
Emsam Transdermal System (Frequent)........ 905
▲ Emtriva Capsules (5% to 6%) 1246
▲ Emtriva Oral Solution (5% to 6%) 1246
Enbrel for Injection........ 569
Engerix-B Vaccine........ 1409
▲ Enjuvia Tablets (0% to 6%) 1029
▲ Epivir (13%) 1412
Epivir-HBV........ 1417
▲ Epogen for Injection (11%) 576
Epzicom Tablets........ 1422
Equetro Extended-Release Capsules 3174
Estratest Tablets 3043
Estratest H.S. Tablets 3043
Evoxac Capsules (Less than 1%) 1013
Exelon Capsules (Frequent) 2229
Exelon Oral Solution (Frequent) 2229
Exforge Tablets (Greater than or equal to 0.2%) 2238
Extina Foam, 2% (Less than or equal to 1%) 3057
▲ Fabrazyme for Intravenous Infusion (31%) 1241
▲ Faslodex Injection (6.4%) 682
Fentora Tablets (Greater than 1%) 968
Flector Patch (1%) 561
▲ Flolan for Injection (1% to 12%) 1426
Fluarix Vaccine 1446
Fortaz (Less than 1%) 1450
▲ Frova Tablets (4%) 1111
Furosemide Tablets 2186
▲ Gabitril Tablets (3%) 973
Gantrisin Pediatric Suspension 2638
Gemzar for Injection (Less than 1%) 1820
▲ Gengraf Capsules (1% to 11%) 435
▲ Genotropin Lyophilized Powder (0% to 9.6%) 2547
Geodon (Frequent) 2520
Gleevec Tablets (Less common) 2255
▲ Gliadel Wafer (6%) 1076
Havrix Injection Vaccine 1454
▲ Herceptin I.V. (9%) 1199
▲ Humatrope Vials and Cartridges (13.6% to 17.3%) 1838
▲ Humira Injection (Less than 5%) 442
▲ Hycamtin for Injection (7% to 9%) 1459
Imitrex Injection (Infrequent) 1465
Imitrex Nasal Spray (Infrequent) 1470
▲ Imitrex Tablets (3% to 5%) 1474
Indapamide Tablets 2188
Indocin (Less than 1%) 2024
Intelence Tablets (Less than 2%) 3119
Intravenous Sodium Diuril 2490
▲ Intron A for Injection (1% to 21%) 2859
Invanz for Injection (Greater than 0.1%) 2029
Ionsys Transdermal System (.1% to less than 1%) 2410
▲ Ixempra Kit for Injection (62%) 915
Kaletra (Up to 2%) 452
▲ Kepivance (12%) 583
Keppra Injection (2%) 3137
Keppra Oral Solution (2%) 3131
Keppra Tablets (2%) 3131
Ketek Tablets (Less than 0.2%) 2744
Klonopin (Infrequent) 2639
Lamictal (Frequent) 1488
Lescol Capsules 2268
Lescol XL Tablets 2268
▲ Leukine (11%) 774
Levaquin (0.1% to 1%) 2416
Levaquin in 5% Dextrose Injection (0.1% to 1%) 2416
Levitra Tablets (Less than 2%) 2876
Lexapro Oral Suspension (2%) 1174
Lexapro Tablets (2%) 1174
Lidoderm Patch 1114
Lipitor Tablets (Less than 2%) 2501
Lotrisone (1.9%) 2881
Lunesta Tablets (Infrequent) 2994
▲ Lupron Depot 3.75 mg (Less than 5%) 462
▲ Lupron Depot–3 Month 11.25 mg (1.2% to 7%) 462
▲ Luvox CR Extended-Release Capsules (1% to 3%) 1759
Luxiq Foam (One patient) 3058
Lyrica Capsules (Greater than or equal to 2%) 2527
Marplan Tablets (0% to 2%) 3177
Mavik Tablets (0.3% to 1%) 472
▲ Maxalt Tablets (3% to 4%) 2056
▲ Maxalt-MLT Orally Disintegrating Tablets (3% to 4%)........ 2056
▲ Megace ES Oral Suspension (1% to 3%)........ 2499
Meridia Capsules (2%)........ 475
Merrem I.V. (Greater than 0.1% to 1%)........ 684
Meruvax II........ 2061
Mevacor Tablets (0.5% to 1%)........ 2063
▲ Miacalcin Nasal Spray (1% to 3%) .. 2274
Micardis Tablets (More than 0.3%).... 852
Micardis HCT Tablets........ 854
Mirapex Tablets (1% or more)........ 857
M-M-R II........ 2054
Mobic Oral Suspension (Less than 2%)........ 863
Mobic Tablets (Less than 2%)........ 863
MS Contin Tablets (Less frequent).... 2585
Nadolol Tablets (6 of 1000 patients)........ 2191
Namenda (Infrequent)........ 1180
Naprosyn Suspension (Less than 1%)........ 2632
Naprosyn Tablets (Less than 1%) 2632
Natrecor for Injection (Greater than or equal to 1%)........ 2977
▲ Neoral Oral Solution (1% to 11%) 2280
▲ Neoral Soft Gelatin Capsules (1% to 11%)........ 2280
Neupro Transdermal System 3149
Nexium Delayed-Release Capsules (Less than 1%) 645
Nexium I.V. (Less than 1%) 652
Nexium Delayed-Release Oral Suspension (Less than 1%) 645
Niaspan Extended-Release Tablets ... 480
▲ Norditropin Cartridges (11%) 2354
Noroxin Tablets 2069
▲ Norvir (2.6% to 3%) 489
▲ Ontak Vials (13%) 1079
OxyContin Tablets (Less than 1%) 2589
▲ Panretin Gel 0.1% (3% to 22%) 1081
Parnate Tablets 1532
▲ Paxil (1% to 5.9%) 1535
▲ Paxil CR Controlled-Release Tablets (1% to 5.9%) 1544
Pentasa Capsules (Less than 1%) 3030
Pepcid Tablets (Infrequent) 2075
Percocet Tablets 1127
Percodan Tablets 1130
Persantine Tablets (Rare) 869
Plavix Tablets (1% to 2.5%) 926
Plavix Tablets (1% to 2.5%) 2767
Pletal Tablets (2% or greater) 2481
Pneumovax 23 2078
▲ Prandin Tablets (2% to 3%) 2971
Primaxin I.M. 2080
Primaxin I.V. (Less than 0.2%) 2083
Prinivil Tablets (0.3% to 1%) 2087
Prinzide Tablets (1.5%) 2092
▲ Pristiq Extended-Release Tablets (1% to 3%) 3247
▲ ProAmatine Tablets (18.3%) 3032
▲ Procrit for Injection (11%) 2391
Proglycem Capsules (Infrequent) 1185
Proglycem Suspension (Infrequent) 1185
▲ Prograf Capsules and Injection (17% to 40%) 622
ProQuad 2099
Protonix for Delayed-Release Oral Suspension (Less than 1%) 3254
Protonix Delayed-Release Tablets (Less than 1%) 3254
Protonix I.V. (Less than 1%) 3257
▲ Protopic Ointment (Greater than or equal to 1% to 3%) 628
Provigil Tablets (2%) 977
Prozac Weekly Capsules 1852
Prozac Pulvules and Liquid 1852
Pylera Capsules 714
Rebif Prefilled Syringe for Injection ... 1107
Reclast Injection (2%) 2291
Remeron Tablets (Frequent) 2924
RemeronSolTab Tablets (Frequent) ... 2927
▲ Requip Tablets (3% to 5%) 1561
▲ Retrovir Capsules (6%) 1574
▲ Retrovir IV Infusion (6%) 1579
▲ Retrovir (6%) 1574
Risperdal Consta Long-Acting Injection (Infrequent) 1753
Rituxan I.V. (Less than 1% to 2%) 1223
▲ Romazicon Injection (1% to 3%) 2646
Rythmol Tablets (Less than 1%) 1586
Rythmol SR Capsules 1590
Salagen Tablets (Less than 1%) 1082
▲ Sandimmune (1% to 3%) 2296
▲ Selzentry Tablets (4.7%) 2534
▲ Serevent Diskus (1% to 3%) 1594
Seromycin Capsules 1864
▲ Simulect for Injection (3% to 10%) 2306
Singulair 2114
▲ Soriatane Capsules (10% to 25%) 3062
▲ Spiriva HandiHaler (1% to 3%) 870

Stalevo Tablets 2309
Sular Extended Release Tablets (Less than or equal to 1%) 2975
Sustiva Capsules (Less than 2%) 930
Sustiva Tablets (Less than 2%) 930
▲ Targretin Gel 1% (6%) 1088
Tarka Tablets (Less frequent) 511
▲ Tasigna Capsules (1% to 10%) 2316
▲ Taxotere Injection Concentrate (5.5%) 2773
▲ Temodar Capsules (1% to 9%) 2931
Teveten Tablets (Less than 1%) 515
Teveten HCT Tablets (Less than 1%) 517
Thyrogen for Injection (1.7%) 1244
Timoptic Sterile Ophthalmic Solution (Less frequent) 2121
Timoptic in Ocudose (Less frequent) 2124
Timoptic-XE Sterile Ophthalmic Gel Forming Solution 2125
Toprol-XL Tablets 666
Treximet Tablets (2%) 1616
Tricor Tablets 520
▲ Trisenox Injection (33%) 986
Trizivir Tablets 1622
Trusopt Sterile Ophthalmic Solution 2128
▲ Truvada Tablets (Greater than or equal to 5%) 1262
Twinrix Vaccine (Less than 1%) 1628
▲ Ultram ER Extended-Release Tablets (1% to less than 5%) 2428
▲ Valcyte Tablets (8%) 2654
Varivax 2133
▲ Velcade for Injection (13% to 27%) 2168
▲ Venlafaxine Hydrochloride Tablets (3%) 2199
▲ Vesanoid Capsules (17%) 2660
Viadur Implant (Less than 2%) 802
Vicoprofen Tablets (Less than 3%) 533
Viramune Oral Suspension 873
Viramune Tablets 873
Voltaren Tablets (Occasionally) 2334
Voltaren-XR Tablets (Occasionally) 2337
Vytorin 10/10 Tablets 2149
Vytorin 10/10 Tablets 2939
Vytorin 10/20 Tablets 2149
Vytorin 10/20 Tablets 2939
Vytorin 10/40 Tablets 2149
Vytorin 10/40 Tablets 2939
Vytorin 10/80 Tablets 2149
Vytorin 10/80 Tablets 2939
Wellbutrin Tablets 1648
Wellbutrin SR Sustained-Release Tablets (1% to 2%) 1653
Wellbutrin XL Extended-Release Tablets (1% to 2%) 1659
▲ Xeloda Tablets (1% to 21%) 2662
Xopenex Inhalation Solution 3001
Xopenex Inhalation Solution Concentrate 3005
Xopenex HFA Inhalation Aerosol 3009
Xyrem Oral Solution (Less than 1%) 1766
Zetia Tablets 2157
Zetia Tablets 2951
Ziagen 1673
Zocor Tablets 2136
Zofran Injection (2%) 1682
▲ Zometa for Intravenous Infusion (15%) 2341
Zomig Tablets (Common) 694
▲ Zomig Nasal Spray (5% to 10%) 689
Zomig-ZMT Tablets (Common) 694
▲ Zonegran Capsules (4%) 1089
Zovirax 1690
Zyban Sustained-Release Tablets (Infrequent) 1692
▲ Zyprexa Tablets (5%) 1883
▲ Zyprexa ZYDIS Orally Disintegrating Tablets (5%) 1883
Zyrtec Chewable Tablets (Less than 2%) 1920
Zyrtec Syrup (Less than 2%) 1920
Zyrtec Tablets (Less than 2%) 1920
Zyrtec-D 12 Hour Extended Release Tablets (Less than 2%) 1923

Paresthesia, application site
Altabax Ointment (1.4%) 1299
AndroGel 3159
Daytrana Transdermal Patch 3022

Paresthesia, circumoral
Azilect Tablets (Infrequent) 3106
Brovana Inhalation Solution (Less than 2%) 2990
Copaxone for Injection (Infrequent) 3110
Effexor XR Extended-Release Capsules (Infrequent) 3195
Emsam Transdermal System (Infrequent) 905
Gabitril Tablets (Infrequent) 973
Geodon Capsules (Rare) 2520
Lyrica Capsules (0.1% to 1%) 2527
▲ Norvir (3.4% to 6.7%) 489
Paxil (Rare) 1535
Paxil CR Controlled-Release Tablets (Rare) 1544
Prozac Weekly Capsules (Rare) 1852
Prozac Pulvules and Liquid (Rare) 1852
▲ Rilutek Tablets (1.3% to 3.3%) 2771
Venlafaxine Hydrochloride Tablets (Infrequent) 2199
Zomig Tablets (Infrequent) 694
Zomig Nasal Spray (Infrequent) 689
Zomig-ZMT Tablets (Infrequent) 694
Zonegran Capsules (Rare) 1089
Zyprexa Tablets (Rare) 1883
Zyprexa ZYDIS Orally Disintegrating Tablets (Rare) 1883

Paresthesia, extremities
Pylera Capsules 714

Paresthesia, feet
Gris-PEG Tablets (Rare) 2507

Paresthesia, hands
Gris-PEG Tablets (Rare) 2507
InnoPran XL Extended Release Capsules 1484

Paresthesia, lip
Fleet Phospho-soda (Rare) 1145
Fleet Phospho-soda EZ-PREP (Rare) 1147
Fleet Prep Kits 1149
OsmoPrep Tablets (Rare) 2680

Paresthesia, oral
Crixivan Capsules 1979

Paresthesia, peripheral
▲ Norvir (5% to 6%) 489

Parkinsonism
Abilify Injection (Greater than or equal to 1 in 1000 patients and less than 1 in 100 patients) 881
Abilify Injection (Greater than or equal to 1 in 1000 patients and less than 1 in 100 patients) 2466
Abilify Oral Solution (Greater than or equal to 1 in 1000 patients and less than 1 in 100 patients) 881
Abilify Oral Solution (Greater than or equal to 1 in 1000 patients and less than 1 in 100 patients) 2466
Abilify Discmelt Orally Disintegrating Tablets (Greater than or equal to 1 in 1000 patients and less than 1 in 100 patients) 881
Abilify Discmelt Orally Disintegrating Tablets (Greater than or equal to 1 in 1000 patients and less than 1 in 100 patients) 2466
Abilify Tablets (Greater than or equal to 1 in 1000 patients and less than 1 in 100 patients) 881
Abilify Tablets (Greater than or equal to 1 in 1000 patients and less than 1 in 100 patients) 2466
Demser Capsules 1989
Depakote ER Tablets 423
Exelon Capsules (2%) 2229
Exelon Oral Solution (2%) 2229
Exelon Patch (Infrequent) 2233
Indocin (Less than 1%) 2024
▲ Invega Extended-Release Tablets (0% to 15%) 1748
Namenda 1180
▲ Risperdal Consta Long-Acting Injection (5% to 10%) 1753
▲ Zyprexa Tablets (8% to 20%) 1883
▲ Zyprexa IntraMuscular (2% to 4%) 1883
▲ Zyprexa ZYDIS Orally Disintegrating Tablets (8% to 20%) 1883

Parkinsonism, aggravation of
Lamictal 1488
Requip Tablets (1% or more) 1561
Risperdal Consta Long-Acting Injection 1753

Parkinson-like symptoms
Actimmune (Rare) 1743
Elspar for Injection (Rare) 1990
Moban Tablets 1116

Parkinson's disease worsening
▲ Exelon Capsules (3%) 2229
▲ Exelon Oral Solution (3%) 2229

Paroniria
Allegra Oral Solution (Less than 1%) 2684
Allegra Tablets (Rare) 2684
Celexa (Infrequent) 1160
Coreg Tablets (Greater than 0.1% to 1%) 1387
Coreg CR Extended-Release Capsules (0.1% to less than or equal to 1%) 1393
Evoxac Capsules (Less than 1%) 1013
Gengraf Capsules (1% to less than 3%) 435
▲ Intron A for Injection (Less than 5%) 2859
Namenda (Infrequent) 1180
Neoral Oral Solution (1% to less than 3%) 2280
Neoral Soft Gelatin Capsules (1% to less than 3%) 2280
Risperdal Consta Long-Acting Injection (Infrequent) 1753
Zyrtec Chewable Tablets (Less than 2%) 1920
Zyrtec Syrup (Less than 2%) 1920
Zyrtec Tablets (Less than 2%) 1920
Zyrtec-D 12 Hour Extended Release Tablets (Less than 2%) 1923

Paronychia
Accutane Capsules 2607
Crixivan Capsules 1979
Evoxac Capsules (Less than 1%) 1013
Mirapex Tablets 857
▲ Soriatane Capsules (10% to 25%) 3062
▲ Vectibix (2% to 25%) 597

Parosmia
Ambien Tablets (Rare) 2692
Ambien CR Tablets (Rare) 2696
Avelox (Less than 0.1%) 2803
Axert Tablets (Rare) 2431
Chantix Tablets (Infrequent) 2511
Denavir Cream 2205
Doxil Injection (Less than 1%) 2378
Effexor XR Extended-Release Capsules (Infrequent) 3195
Emsam Transdermal System (Infrequent) 905
Evoxac Capsules (Less than 1%) 1013
Exforge Tablets (Less than or equal to 0.1%) 2238
Flumadine (Less than 0.3%) 1167
Gabitril Tablets (Infrequent) 973
▲ Intron A for Injection (Less than 5%) 2859
Lamictal (Rare) 1488
Levaquin (0.1% to 0.9%) 2416
Levaquin in 5% Dextrose Injection 2416
Lipitor Tablets (Less than 2%) 2501
Luvox CR Extended-Release Capsules (Infrequent) 1759
Lyrica Capsules (Rare) 2527
Miacalcin Nasal Spray (Less than 1%) 2274
Mirapex Tablets 857
Nexium Delayed-Release Capsules (Less than 1%) 645
Nexium I.V. (Less than 1%) 652
Nexium Delayed-Release Oral Suspension (Less than 1%) 645
Norvir (Less than 2%) 489
Paxil (Rare) 1535
Paxil CR Controlled-Release Tablets (Rare) 1544
Prozac Weekly Capsules (Rare) 1852
Prozac Pulvules and Liquid (Rare) 1852
Remeron Tablets (Rare) 2924
RemeronSolTab Tablets (Rare) 2927
Sustiva Capsules (Less than 2%) 930
Sustiva Tablets (Less than 2%) 930
Venlafaxine Hydrochloride Tablets (Infrequent) 2199
Zomig Tablets (Infrequent) 694
Zomig Nasal Spray (Infrequent) 689
Zomig-ZMT Tablets (Infrequent) 694
Zonegran Capsules (Infrequent) 1089
Zyrtec Chewable Tablets (Less than 2%) 1920
Zyrtec Syrup (Less than 2%) 1920
Zyrtec Tablets (Less than 2%) 1920
Zyrtec-D 12 Hour Extended Release Tablets (Less than 2%) 1923

Parotid gland enlargement
Alphanate 1709
Depakote ER Tablets 423
Salagen Tablets (Less than 1%) 1082
Thioridazine Hydrochloride Tablets (Rare) 2195

Parotitis
Catapres Tablets (Rare) 841
Clorpres Tablets (Rare) 2185
Effexor XR Extended-Release Capsules (Rare) 3195
M-M-R II 2054
Mumpsvax (Very low) 2068
ProQuad 2099
Venlafaxine Hydrochloride Tablets (Rare) 2199

Partial thromboplastin time, prolonged
Anzemet Tablets (Rare) 2704
Arixtra Injection 1313
Celebrex Capsules 2979
Elmiron Capsules (Less than or equal to 1%) 2435
Elspar for Injection 2488
Tygacil for Injection (0% to less than 2%) 3276
Viramune Oral Suspension 873
Viramune Tablets 873

Partial thromboplastin time, accelerated
Premphase Tablets 3232

Partial thromboplastin time, decrease
Merrem I.V. (Greater than 0.2%) 684
Prempro Tablets 3232

Patent ductus arteriosus
Captopril Tablets 2182
Cozaar Tablets 1973
▲ Infasurf Intratracheal Suspension (45% to 47%) 1168
Percodan Tablets 1130
Prinivil Tablets 2087
Prinzide Tablets 2092

PBI decrease
Dyazide Capsules 1405
Estratest Tablets 3043
Estratest H.S. Tablets 3043

Peeling, epidermal
Accutane Capsules 2607
Benzaclin Topical Gel (2%) 2721
▲ Brevoxyl-4 Creamy Wash (5 of 100 patients) 3054
▲ Brevoxyl-4 Gel (5 of 100 patients) 3054
▲ Brevoxyl-8 Creamy Wash (5 of 100 patients) 3054
▲ Brevoxyl-8 Gel (5 of 100 patients) 3054
Cozaar Tablets (One subject) 1973
▲ Duac Topical Gel (0% to 17%) 3054
Imitrex Injection (Rare) 1465
Imitrex Nasal Spray (Rare) 1470
Lotrisone 2881
▲ Panretin Gel 0.1% (3% to 9%) 1081
▲ Soriatane Capsules (50% to 75%) 3062

Peliosis hepatis
Delatestryl Injection 1730
Eloxatin for Injection 2731
Estratest Tablets 3043
Estratest H.S. Tablets 3043

Pelvic inflammation
Gardasil Injection (0.02%) 2019
Lexapro Oral Suspension (Infrequent) 1174
Lexapro Tablets (Infrequent) 1174

Pelvic inflammatory disease
Advair HFA 45/21 Inhalation Aerosol 1288
Advair HFA 115/21 Inhalation Aerosol 1288
Advair HFA 230/21 Inhalation Aerosol 1288
Mirena Intrauterine System 779

Pelvic peritoneal adhesions
Requip Tablets (Infrequent) 1561

Pemphigoid-like lesion
Captopril Tablets 2182
Timoptic Sterile Ophthalmic Solution 2121
Timoptic in Ocudose 2124
Timoptic-XE Sterile Ophthalmic Gel Forming Solution 2125

Pemphigus
Aceon Tablets (2 mg, 4 mg, 8 mg) 3038
Cuprimine Capsules 1986
Mavik Tablets (0.3% to 1%) 472
Prinivil Tablets (0.3% to 1%) 2087
Prinzide Tablets 2092
Rituxan I.V. 1223

Pemphigus, bullous
Aceon Tablets (2 mg, 4 mg, 8 mg) 3038
Captopril Tablets 2182

Proleukin for Injection ... 2287

Penile discharge, unspecified
Alferon N Injection (1%) ... 1726

Penile disorder, unspecified
AndroGel (Less than 1%) ... 3159
Cymbalta Delayed-Release Capsules (2%) ... 1801
▲ Edex Injection (3%) ... 2957
Eligard 7.5 mg (Less than 2%) ... 2724
Eligard 22.5 mg (Less than 2%) ... 2724
Eligard 30 mg (Less than 2%) ... 2724
Eligard 45 mg (Less than 2%) ... 2724
Lamictal (2%) ... 1488
Norvir (Less than 2%) ... 489
Requip Tablets (Infrequent) ... 1561
Soriatane Capsules (Less than 1%) .. 3062
Testim 1% Gel (1% or less) ... 701

Penile erection, increase
(*see under* Priapism)

Penile erection, prolonged or inappropriate
AndroGel ... 3159
Cialis Tablets ... 1792
▲ Edex Injection (Less than 1% to 4%) ... 2957
Levitra Tablets (Less than 2%) ... 2876
Venlafaxine Hydrochloride Tablets (Rare) ... 2199

Penile erection, spontaneous
Cialis Tablets (Less than 2%) ... 1792

Penis, decreased sensation
Eldepryl Capsules ... 3052

Penis, enlargement
▲ Intron A for Injection (Less than or equal to 5%) ... 2859

Penis, fibrotic plaques
(*see under* Peyronie's disease)

Penis, size decrease
Eligard 7.5 mg (Less than 2%) ... 2724
Eligard 22.5 mg (Less than 2%) ... 2724
Eligard 30 mg (Less than 2%) ... 2724
Eligard 45 mg (Less than 2%) ... 2724

Perforation, corneal
Diclofenac Sodium Ophthalmic Solution ... ⊙ 240
Voltaren Ophthalmic Solution (0.1%) ... 2336

Perforation, gastrointestinal
▲ Actonel Tablets (39%) ... 2568
Aggrenox Capsules (Less than 1%) .. 819
▲ Anaprox Tablets (1% to 10%) ... 2632
▲ Anaprox DS Tablets (1% to 10%) ... 2632
▲ Avastin IV (0% to 3.7%) ... 1192
Bayer Aspirin ... 750
Celebrex Capsules ... 2979
CellCept Capsules ... 2622
CellCept Intravenous ... 2622
CellCept Oral Suspension ... 2622
CellCept Tablets ... 2622
Clinoril Tablets ... 1962
▲ EC-Naprosyn Delayed-Release Tablets (1% to 10%) ... 2632
Flector Patch ... 561
Gleevec Tablets (Rare) ... 2255
Indocin Capsules (Approximately 1%) ... 2024
Indocin I.V. ... 2489
Indocin (Approximately 1%) ... 2024
Mobic Oral Suspension ... 863
Mobic Tablets ... 863
Nalfon Capsules ... 2508
▲ Naprosyn Suspension (1% to 10%) ... 2632
▲ Naprosyn Tablets (1% to 10%) ... 2632
NeoProfen Injection ... 2496
Nexavar Tablets (0.1% to less than 1%) ... 784
▲ Prograf Capsules and Injection (3%) ... 622
Proleukin for Injection (Less than 1%) ... 2287
St. Joseph 81 mg Aspirin Chewable and Enteric Coated Tablets ... 1903
Taxotere Injection Concentrate ... 2773
▲ Treximet Tablets (1% to 4%) ... 1616
Vicoprofen Tablets ... 533
▲ Voltaren Tablets (1% to 10%) ... 2334
▲ Voltaren-XR Tablets (1% to 10%) ... 2337

Perforation, gastrointestinal ulcer
Tasigna Capsules ... 2316

Perforation, uterine wall
ParaGard T 380A Intrauterine Copper Contraceptive ... 1041

Perforation, uterine wall (partial)
ParaGard T 380A Intrauterine Copper Contraceptive ... 1041

Perforation, uterine wall (total)
ParaGard T 380A Intrauterine Copper Contraceptive ... 1041

Periarteritis nodosum
Fansidar Tablets ... 2636
Gantrisin Pediatric Suspension ... 2638
Phenytek Capsules ... 2192

Pericardial effusion
Activase I.V. ... 1188
Agrylin Capsules ... 3017
Busulfex Injection (2%) ... 2477
▲ CellCept Capsules (3% to less than 20%) ... 2622
▲ CellCept Intravenous (3% to less than 20%) ... 2622
▲ CellCept Oral Suspension (3% to less than 20%) ... 2622
▲ CellCept Tablets (3% to less than 20%) ... 2622
Cimzia ... 3127
▲ Clolar for Intravenous Infusion (35%) ... 1239
▲ Doxil Injection (1% to 5%) ... 2378
▲ Gleevec Tablets (6.9% to 22%) ... 2255
▲ Humira Injection (Less than 5%) ... 442
▲ Leukine (25%) ... 774
PegIntron Powder for Injection (Less than or equal to 1%) ... 2903
▲ Prograf Capsules and Injection (15%) ... 622
Proleukin for Injection (Less than 1%) ... 2287
Rapamune ... 3260
Refludan for Injection ... 795
Remicade for IV Injection ... 950
ReoPro Vials (0.4%) ... 1860
Tasigna Capsules (0.1% to 1%) ... 2316
TNKase ... 1233
Trasylol Injection (1% to 2%) ... 799
Velcade for Injection ... 2168
Vesanoid Capsules ... 2660
▲ Xeloda Tablets (Less than 5%) ... 2662

Pericardial tamponade
Rapamune ... 3260

Pericarditis
Activase I.V. ... 1188
Agrylin Capsules ... 3017
Asacol Delayed-Release Tablets (Rare) ... 2579
Canasa Rectal Suppositories (Rare) ... 705
Cimzia ... 3127
Evoxac Capsules (Less than 1%) ... 1013
Gleevec Tablets (Rare) ... 2255
▲ Humira Injection (Less than 5%) ... 442
Luvox CR Extended-Release Capsules (Rare) ... 1759
Neupro Transdermal System ... 3149
Paser Granules ... 1747
Pentasa Capsules (Infrequent to less than 1%) ... 3030
Proleukin for Injection ... 2287
Rilutek Tablets (Infrequent) ... 2771
Rythmol SR Capsules ... 1590
Solodyn Extended Release Tablets .. 1938
Tasigna Capsules ... 2316
TNKase ... 1233
▲ Trasylol Injection (5%) ... 799
Velcade for Injection ... 2168
▲ Vesanoid Capsules (3%) ... 2660

Pericarditis, allergic
Fansidar Tablets ... 2636

Periodontal destruction
Evoxac Capsules (Less than 1%) ... 1013

Periodontal disorders, unspecified
PegIntron Powder for Injection ... 2903
Rebetol ... 2917

Periodontitis
Aricept Tablets (Infrequent) ... 1062
Aricept ODT Tablets (Infrequent) ... 1062
▲ Coreg Tablets (Greater than 1% to 3%) ... 1387
▲ Coreg CR Extended-Release Capsules (Greater than 1% to less than or equal to 3%) ... 1393
Effexor XR Extended-Release Capsules (Rare) ... 3195
Kaletra (Less than 2%) ... 452
Mirapex Tablets ... 857
Protonix for Delayed-Release Oral Suspension (Less than 1%) ... 3254
Protonix Delayed-Release Tablets (Less than 1%) ... 3254
Protonix I.V. (Less than 1%) ... 3257
Requip Tablets (Infrequent) ... 1561
Teveten Tablets (Less than 1%) ... 515
Teveten HCT Tablets (Less than 1%) ... 517
Venlafaxine Hydrochloride Tablets (Rare) ... 2199

Periostitis
Bicillin C-R Injectable Suspension ... 1775
Bicillin L-A Injection ... 1777

Peripheral nerve symptoms
▲ Reyataz Capsules (Less than 1% to 4%) ... 3299

Peripheral vascular disorder, unspecified
Actiq (Less than 1%) ... 959
Aricept Tablets (Infrequent) ... 1062
Aricept ODT Tablets (Infrequent) ... 1062
▲ Betaseron for SC Injection (6%) ... 756
▲ CellCept Capsules (3% to less than 20%) ... 2622
▲ CellCept Intravenous (3% to less than 20%) ... 2622
▲ CellCept Oral Suspension (3% to less than 20%) ... 2622
▲ CellCept Tablets (3% to less than 20%) ... 2622
▲ Coreg Tablets (Greater than 1% to 3%) ... 1387
▲ Coreg CR Extended-Release Capsules (Greater than 1% to less than or equal to 3%) ... 1393
Effexor XR Extended-Release Capsules (Infrequent) ... 3195
Emsam Transdermal System (Infrequent) ... 905
▲ Flolan for Injection (96%) ... 1426
Gabitril Tablets (Infrequent) ... 973
Lovaza Capsules ... 1520
Merrem I.V. (Greater than 1%) ... 684
Norvir (Less than 2%) ... 489
Paxil (Infrequent) ... 1535
Paxil CR Controlled-Release Tablets (Infrequent) ... 1544
▲ Prograf Capsules and Injection (3% to 15%) ... 622
Protopic Ointment (Greater than or equal to 1%) ... 628
Prozac Weekly Capsules (Rare) ... 1852
Prozac Pulvules and Liquid (Rare) ... 1852
Rilutek Tablets (Infrequent) ... 2771
Rythmol SR Capsules ... 1590
Symbyax Capsules (Rare) ... 1871
Tricor Tablets ... 520
Venlafaxine Hydrochloride Tablets (Infrequent) ... 2199
▲ Visudyne for Injection (1% to 10%) .. 2332

Peripheral wasting
Aptivus Capsules ... 823
Aptivus Oral Solution ... 823
Atripla Tablets ... 938
Combivir Tablets ... 1384
Crixivan Capsules ... 1979
Emtriva Capsules ... 1246
Emtriva Oral Solution ... 1246
Intelence Tablets ... 3119
Lexiva Oral Suspension ... 1510
Lexiva Tablets ... 1510
Norvir ... 489
Retrovir ... 1574
Reyataz Capsules ... 3299
Trizivir Tablets ... 1622
Truvada Tablets ... 1262
Viramune Oral Suspension ... 873
Viramune Tablets ... 873
Viread Tablets ... 1268
Ziagen ... 1673

Peritoneal, fibrosis
Mirapex Tablets (Rare) ... 857

Peritonitis
▲ Aranesp for Injection (27%) ... 564
▲ CellCept Capsules (3% to less than 20%) ... 2622
▲ CellCept Intravenous (3% to less than 20%) ... 2622
▲ CellCept Oral Suspension (3% to less than 20%) ... 2622
▲ CellCept Tablets (3% to less than 20%) ... 2622
Epogen for Injection ... 576
Exelon Capsules (Infrequent) ... 2229
Exelon Oral Solution (Infrequent) ... 2229
Neupogen for Injection (2%) ... 589
Paxil (Rare) ... 1535
Paxil CR Controlled-Release Tablets (Rare) ... 1544
▲ Photofrin for Injection (Less than 5%) ... 708
▲ Prograf Capsules and Injection (3% to 15%) ... 622
Remicade for IV Injection (Greater than or equal to 0.2%) ... 950
Rilutek Tablets (Infrequent) ... 2771
Velcade for Injection ... 2168

Personality changes
Cardizem LA Extended Release Tablets (Less than 2%) ... 421
▲ Depakote ER Tablets (Greater than 1% to less than 5%) ... 423
Eldepryl Capsules ... 3052
Enbrel for Injection ... 569
Evoxac Capsules ... 1013
Exelon Capsules (Infrequent) ... 2229
Exelon Oral Solution (Infrequent) ... 2229
Frova Tablets (Rare) ... 1111
Gabitril Tablets (Frequent) ... 973
Geodon for Injection (Up to 2%) ... 2520
Humulin 50/50, 100 Units ... 1843
Humulin 70/30 Vial ... 1844
Humulin N Vial ... 1846
Humulin R ... 1849
Imitrex Tablets (Rare) ... 1474
▲ Intron A for Injection (Less than 5%) ... 2859
Lamictal (Infrequent) ... 1488
Lupron Depot 3.75 mg (Among most frequent) ... 462
▲ Lupron Depot–3 Month 11.25 mg (Less than 5%) ... 462
Lupron Depot-PED 7.5 mg, 11.25 mg and 15 mg (Less than 2%) ... 471
Nalfon Capsules (Less than 1%) ... 2508
Namenda (Infrequent) ... 1180
Norvir (Less than 2%) ... 489
▲ Prometrium Capsules (100 mg, 200 mg) (Less than 5%) ... 3047
Prozac Pulvules and Liquid (At least 2%) ... 1852
Requip Tablets (Infrequent) ... 1561
Rilutek Tablets (Infrequent) ... 2771
▲ Zyprexa Tablets (8%) ... 1883
▲ Zyprexa ZYDIS Orally Disintegrating Tablets (8%) ... 1883

Personality disorder
Ambien Tablets (Rare) ... 2692
Ambien CR Tablets (Rare) ... 2696
Aricept Tablets (2%) ... 1062
Aricept ODT Tablets (2%) ... 1062
Azilect Tablets (Infrequent) ... 3106
▲ Gliadel Wafer (8%) ... 1076
▲ Keppra Oral Solution (8%) ... 3131
▲ Keppra Tablets (8%) ... 3131
Lamictal (Infrequent) ... 1488
Mirapex Tablets ... 857
Prozac Weekly Capsules (Infrequent to greater than or equal to 2%) ... 1852
Symbyax Capsules (1% to 2%) ... 1871

Perspiration
(*see under* Diaphoresis)

Petechia at application site
Lidoderm Patch ... 1114

Petechiae
AmBisome for Injection (Less common) ... 606
▲ Arranon Injection (0% to 12%) ... 1319
Cancidas for Injection ... 1953
Cardizem LA Extended Release Tablets (Less than 2%) ... 421
▲ CellCept Capsules (3% to less than 20%) ... 2622
▲ CellCept Intravenous (3% to less than 20%) ... 2622
▲ CellCept Oral Suspension (3% to less than 20%) ... 2622
▲ CellCept Tablets (3% to less than 20%) ... 2622
Cipro I.V. (1% or less) ... 2817
Cipro (Less than 1%) ... 2810
Cipro XR Tablets ... 2823
▲ Clolar for Intravenous Infusion (29%) ... 1239
▲ Dacogen Injection (39%) ... 1066
Depakote ER Tablets (Greater than 1%) ... 423
Doxil Injection (Less than 1%) ... 2378
Emsam Transdermal System (Rare) ... 905
Engerix-B Vaccine (Less than 1%) ... 1409
Gabitril Tablets (Infrequent) ... 973
▲ Gamunex (21%) ... 3094
▲ Gemzar for Injection (16%) ... 1820

Indocin Capsules (Less than 1%) 2024
Indocin I.V. (Less than 1%) 2489
Indocin (Less than 1%) 2024
Lamictal (Rare to infrequent) 1488
▲ Leukine (6%) 774
▲ Leustatin Injection (8%) 2384
Lipitor Tablets (Less than 2%) 2501
Meridia Capsules 475
Mirapex Tablets 857
Mustargen for Injection 2492
▲ Mylotarg for Injection (1% to 20%) 3212
▲ Neupogen for Injection (17%) 589
▲ Novantrone for Injection Concentrate (7% to 11%) 1100
▲ Noxafil Oral Suspension (11%) 2889
Pediarix Vaccine 1552
Pristiq Extended-Release Tablets 3247
Prozac Weekly Capsules (Rare) 1852
Prozac Pulvules and Liquid (Rare) 1852
Raptiva for Injection 1218
Recombivax HB 2107
Remeron Tablets (Rare) 2924
RemeronSolTab Tablets (Rare) 2927
ReoPro Vials (0.3%) 1860
Rilutek Tablets (Rare) 2771
Rythmol SR Capsules 1590
Sandostatin Injection (Less than 1%) 2300
Sandostatin LAR Depot 2302
Sular Extended Release Tablets (Less than or equal to 1%) 2975
Tasigna Capsules 2316
▲ Trisenox Injection (8%) 986
Twinrix Vaccine (Less than 1%) 1628
Zonegran Capsules (Rare) 1089

Petechiae, oral mucosal

▲ Dacogen Injection (13%) 1066
Velcade for Injection 2168

Petechial hemorrhage

Carbatrol Capsules 3019
Symbyax Capsules 1871

Peyronie's disease

Combigan Ophthalmic Solution 553
Cosopt Sterile Ophthalmic Solution 1969
Edex Injection (1%) 2957
InnoPran XL Extended Release Capsules 1484
Nadolol Tablets 2191
Phenytek Capsules 2192
Requip Tablets (Rare) 1561
Timoptic Sterile Ophthalmic Solution 2121
Timoptic in Ocudose 2124
Timoptic-XE Sterile Ophthalmic Gel Forming Solution 2125
Toprol-XL Tablets (Fewer than 1 of 100,000 patients) 666

Pharyngeal discomfort

Cozaar Tablets (Less than 1%) 1973
Invanz for Injection (Greater than 0.1%) 2029
Nexium I.V. (Less than 1%) 652
Prinzide Tablets (0.3% to 1%) 2092

Pharyngeal secretion, increase

Xyrem Oral Solution (Infrequent) 1766

Pharyngitis

▲ Aceon Tablets (2 mg, 4 mg, 8 mg) (3.3%) 3038
Acetadote Injection (1%) 1001
▲ Aciphex Tablets (3%) 1053
Actiq (1% or greater) 959
▲ Actonel Tablets (6%) 2568
▲ Actonel with Calcium Tablets (2.9% to 5.8%) 2574
▲ ActoPlus Met Tablets (5.1%) 3071
▲ Actos Tablets (5.1%) 3077
Aczone Gel 5% (2%) 3296
Advair Diskus 100/50 1276
▲ Advair Diskus 250/50 (Greater than or equal to 3% to 10%) 1276
▲ Advair Diskus 500/50 (Greater than or equal to 3%) 1276
▲ Aerobid/Aerobid-M (1% to 3%) 1153
▲ Agrylin Capsules (6.8%) 3017
Aldara Cream, 5% (1%) 1699
Alferon N Injection (1%) 1726
▲ Alimta for Injection (Up to 28%) 1786
Alinia for Oral Suspension (Less than 1%) 2677
Alinia Tablets (Less than 1%) 2677
▲ Alphagan P Ophthalmic Solution (1% to 4%) 549
Alphanate 1709
▲ Ambien Tablets (3%) 2692
AmBisome for Injection (Less common) 606
Amevive (Common) 611
Aralast (1.6%) 726
Aricept Tablets (Infrequent) 1062
Aricept ODT Tablets (Infrequent) 1062
▲ Arimidex Tablets (6% to 14%) 672
▲ Asacol Delayed-Release Tablets (11%) 2579
▲ Asmanex Twisthaler (8% to 13%) 2797
Atacand Tablets (2%) 639
Atacand HCT (0.5% or greater) 642
▲ Atrovent Nasal Spray 0.03% (8.1%) 834
Atrovent Nasal Spray 0.06% (Less than 1%) 836
Avalide Tablets (1% or greater) 892
Avalide Tablets (1% or greater) 2713
Avapro Tablets (1% or greater) 897
Avapro Tablets (1% or greater) 2718
Axert Tablets (Infrequent) 2431
▲ Axid Capsules (3.3%) 1364
▲ Azmacort Inhalation Aerosol (7% to 25%) 407
Azopt Ophthalmic Suspension (Less than 1%) 540
▲ Bactroban Nasal (0.5% to 4%) 1367
▲ Bexxar (0% to 12%) 1371
Boniva Injection (2.5%) 2614
Boniva Tablets (2.5%) 2618
▲ BOTOX Purified Neurotoxin Complex (3% to 10%) 550
▲ Busulfex Injection (18%) 2477
Campral Tablets (Frequent) 1158
Celebrex Capsules (2.3%) 2979
Celexa (At least 2%) 1160
▲ CellCept Capsules (3% to less than 20%) 2622
▲ CellCept Intravenous (3% to less than 20%) 2622
▲ CellCept Oral Suspension (3% to less than 20%) 2622
▲ CellCept Tablets (3% to less than 20%) 2622
Cialis Tablets (Less than 2%) 1792
▲ Clarinex Syrup (3.1% to 4.5%) 2828
▲ Clarinex Tablets (3% to 4.1%) 2828
▲ Clarinex Reditabs Tablets (3% to 4.1%) 2828
▲ Clarinex-D 12-Hour Extended-Release Tablets (3%) 2831
▲ Clarinex-D 24-Hour Extended-Release Tablets (3%) 2834
▲ Climara Transdermal System (0.5% to 7%) 763
Combigan Ophthalmic Solution (0.1% to 0.2%) 553
Combivent Inhalation Aerosol (2.2%) 845
Copaxone for Injection (At least 2%) 3110
Cosmegen for Injection 2485
▲ Cosopt Sterile Ophthalmic Solution (1% to 5%) 1969
Cozaar Tablets (1% or greater) 1973
Crinone 4% Gel 992
Crinone 8% Gel 992
Crixivan Capsules (Less than 2%) 1979
▲ Dacogen Injection (16%) 1066
▲ Depakote ER Tablets (2% to 8%) 423
Diovan Tablets (More than 1%) 2212
Diovan HCT Tablets (Less frequent to 2.4%) 2216
▲ Doxil Injection (Less than 1% to 15.9%) 2378
▲ Duetact Tablets (At least 5%) 3085
Duragesic Transdermal System (1% or greater) 2405
▲ Effexor XR Extended-Release Capsules (7%) 3195
▲ Elestat Ophthalmic Solution (1% to 3%) 1741
▲ Elidel Cream 1% (0.7% to 8.1%) 2221
Elmiron Capsules (Less than or equal to 1%) 2435
▲ Eloxatin for Injection (2% to 9%) 2731
Emend Capsules (Greater than 0.5%) 1992
Emend for Injection (Greater than 0.5%) 1999
▲ Emsam Transdermal System (3%) 905
Enablex Extended-Release Tablets (Greater than or equal to 1%) 2225
▲ Enbrel for Injection (6% to 7%) 569
Epogen for Injection 576
▲ Equetro Extended-Release Capsules (Less than 5%) 3174
▲ Erbitux (3% to 26%) 912
▲ Evista Tablets (5.3% to 7.6%) 1810
▲ Evoxac Capsules (5.2%) 1013
Exelon Capsules (2% or more) 2229
Exelon Oral Solution (2% or more) 2229
Exforge Tablets (Greater than or equal to 0.2%) 2238
▲ Exjade Tablets (7.8%) 2244
▲ Exubera Inhalation Powder (9.5% to 18.2%) 2515
▲ Fabrazyme for Intravenous Infusion (6%) 1241
▲ Faslodex Injection (16.1%) 682
▲ Flebogamma 5% DIF (Greater than 15%) 1718
▲ Flolan for Injection (5%) 1426
▲ Flomax Capsules (5.1% to 5.8%) 848
▲ Flonase Nasal Spray (6% to 7.8%) 1431
▲ Flovent HFA (1% to 3%) 1440
Fluarix Vaccine 1446
Flulaval Injection Vaccine 1448
▲ Foradil Aerolizer (3.5%) 2849
▲ Forteo for Injection (5.5%) 1816
Frova Tablets (Infrequent) 1111
▲ Gabitril Tablets (7%) 973
▲ Gamunex (0.8% to 41%) 3094
▲ Gemzar for Injection (22%) 1820
▲ Gengraf Capsules (4%) 435
▲ Geodon Capsules (3%) 2520
▲ Gleevec Tablets (10% to 15%) 2255
Havrix Injection Vaccine (Less than 1%) 1454
▲ Herceptin I.V. (12%) 1199
▲ Humatrope Vials and Cartridges (3.13% to 6.67%) 1838
▲ Hycamtin for Injection (6%) 1459
▲ Indapamide Tablets (Less than 5%) 2188
InnoPran XL Extended Release Capsules 1484
▲ Intron A for Injection (1% to 31%) 2859
Invanz for Injection (0.7% to 1.1%) 2029
▲ Ionsys Transdermal System (1% to less than 10%) 2410
Kaletra (Less than 2%) 452
▲ Keppra Injection (6% to 7%) 3137
▲ Keppra Oral Solution (6% to 10%) 3131
▲ Keppra Tablets (6% to 10%) 3131
Klonopin (2%) 2639
▲ Lamictal (5% to 14%) 1488
▲ Lescol Capsules (3.8%) 2268
Lescol XL Tablets (2.4%) 2268
▲ Leukine (23%) 774
Levitra Tablets (Less than 2%) 2876
Lexapro Oral Suspension (At least 2%) 1174
Lexapro Tablets (At least 2%) 1174
Lipitor Tablets (Up to 2.5%) 2501
▲ Lotemax Ophthalmic Suspension 0.5% (Less than 15%) ⊙ 241
Lovaza Capsules 1520
Lunesta Tablets 2994
▲ Luvox CR Extended-Release Capsules (6%) 1759
Maxalt Tablets (Infrequent) 2056
Maxalt-MLT Orally Disintegrating Tablets (Infrequent) 2056
▲ Megace ES Oral Suspension (1% to 3%) 2499
▲ Meridia Capsules (10%) 475
Merrem I.V. (Greater than 1%) 684
Miacalcin Nasal Spray (Less than 1%) 2274
Micardis Tablets (1%) 852
Micardis HCT Tablets (Less than 2%) 854
Mirapex Tablets (Greater than or equal to 1%) 857
▲ Mobic Oral Suspension (0.6% to 3.2%) 863
▲ Mobic Tablets (0.6% to 3.2%) 863
▲ Mylotarg for Injection (10% to 14%) 3212
▲ Nasacort AQ Nasal Spray (5.1%) 2765
▲ Nasonex Nasal Spray (10 % to 12%) 2883
▲ Neoral Oral Solution (4%) 2280
▲ Neoral Soft Gelatin Capsules (4%) 2280
Nexium Delayed-Release Capsules (Less than 1%) 645
Nexium I.V. (Less than 1%) 652
Nexium Delayed-Release Oral Suspension (Less than 1%) 645
Norvir (0.4% to 2.6%) 489
▲ Novantrone for Injection Concentrate (19%) 1100
▲ Noxafil Oral Suspension (12%) 2889
▲ Ontak Vials (17%) 1079
OxyContin Tablets (Less than 1%) 2589
▲ Pataday Ophthalmic Solution (10%) 543
▲ Patanol Ophthalmic Solution (Less than 5%) 546
Paxil (2.1%) 1535
Paxil CR Controlled-Release Tablets (2.1%) 1544
▲ PegIntron Powder for Injection (10%) 2903
▲ Photofrin for Injection (11%) 708
▲ Pletal Tablets (7% to 10%) 2481
▲ Premarin Tablets (10% to 12%) 3221
▲ Premphase Tablets (8% to 13%) 3232
▲ Prempro Tablets (8% to 13%) 3232
Prevnar 3241
Prinivil Tablets (0.3% to 1%) 2087
Prinzide Tablets 2092
▲ ProAir HFA Inhalation Aerosol (14%) 3113
▲ Prograf Capsules and Injection (3% to 15%) 622
▲ Prometrium Capsules (100 mg, 200 mg) (Less than 5%) 3047
ProQuad (Greater than or equal to 0.2% to less than 1%) 2099
Protonix for Delayed-Release Oral Suspension (Greater than or equal to 1%) 3254
Protonix Delayed-Release Tablets (Greater than or equal to 1%) 3254
Protonix I.V. (Greater than or equal to 1%) 3257
▲ Protopic Ointment (3% to 12%) 628
▲ Provigil Tablets (4%) 977
▲ Prozac Weekly Capsules (3% to 11%) 1852
▲ Prozac Pulvules and Liquid (3% to 11%) 1852
Pulmicort Flexhaler (2.7%) 654
▲ Pulmozyme Inhalation Solution (32% to 40%) 1217
▲ Quixin Ophthalmic Solution (1% to 3%) 3184
▲ Qvar Inhalation Aerosol (8% to 27%) 3116
▲ Rebetol (12% to 13%) 2917
Recombivax HB (Equal to or greater than 1%) 2107
ReFacto Vials 3269
▲ Remicade for IV Injection (12%) 950
▲ Requip Tablets (Infrequent to 6%) 1561
Retrovir Capsules 1574
Retrovir IV Infusion 1579
Retrovir 1574
▲ Salagen Tablets (2% to 3%) 1082
Selzentry Tablets 2534
▲ Serevent Diskus (3% to 6%) 1594
▲ Simulect for Injection (3% to 10%) 2306
Singulair (Greater than or equal to 2%) 2114
Soriatane Capsules (Less than 1%) 3062
▲ Spiriva HandiHaler (7% to 9%) 870
▲ Suboxone Tablets (4%) 2601
▲ Subutex Tablets (4%) 2601
Sular Extended Release Tablets (Less than 1% to 5%) 2975
▲ Symbyax Capsules (4% to 6%) 1871
Synagis Intramuscular Solution (2.6%) 1948
Targretin Capsules 1084
▲ Targretin Gel 1% (6%) 1088
Tasigna Capsules (0.1% to 1%) 2316
▲ Taxotere Injection Concentrate (0.9% to 19.6%) 2773
▲ Temodar Capsules (8%) 2931
▲ Teveten Tablets (4%) 515
Teveten HCT Tablets (Less than 1%) 517
▲ Torisel Injection (0% to 12%) 3272
Tricor Tablets 520
Trizivir Tablets 1622
Ultane Liquid for Inhalation (Less than 1%) 524
Uroxatral Tablets (1% to 2%) 2786
▲ Valcyte Tablets (Less than 5%) 2654
Vaqta (Up to 2.7%) 2130
Varivax 2133
Verdeso Foam (1%) 3069
VESIcare Tablets (0.3% to 1.1%) 636
Vicoprofen Tablets (Less than 3%) 533
▲ Vigamox Ophthalmic Solution (1% to 4%) 548
▲ Visudyne for Injection (1% to 10%) 2332
▲ Vivitrol (11% to 17%) 988
▲ WelChol Tablets (3.2%) 1015
▲ Wellbutrin SR Sustained-Release Tablets (3% to 11%) 1653
▲ Wellbutrin XL Extended-Release Tablets (3% to 11%) 1659
Xifaxan Tablets (Less than 2%) 2682
▲ Xolair (11%) 1235
▲ Xolair (11%) 2339
▲ Xopenex Inhalation Solution (10.4%) 3001
▲ Xopenex Inhalation Solution Concentrate (3% to 10.4%) 3005
▲ Xopenex HFA Inhalation Aerosol (10.4%) 3009
Xyrem Oral Solution (Infrequent) 1766
Xyzal Oral Solution (1% to 2%) 2789
Xyzal Oral Solution (1% to 2%) 3155
Xyzal Tablets (1% to 2%) 2789
Xyzal Tablets (1% to 2%) 3155
Yaz Tablets (Greater than 1%) 805
Ziagen 1673
Zomig Tablets (Infrequent) 694
Zomig Nasal Spray (Infrequent) 689
Zomig-ZMT Tablets (Infrequent) 694
Zonegran Capsules (Frequent) 1089
Zosyn for Injection (Less than 1% to 1.5%) 3284

▲ Zyban Sustained-Release Tablets (3%) ... 1692
▲ Zyprexa Tablets (5%) ... 1883
▲ Zyprexa ZYDIS Orally Disintegrating Tablets (5%) ... 1883
▲ Zyrtec Chewable Tablets (2% to 6.2%) ... 1920
▲ Zyrtec Syrup (2% to 6.2%) ... 1920
▲ Zyrtec Tablets (2% to 6.2%) ... 1920
Zyrtec-D 12 Hour Extended Release Tablets (1.7% to 2%) ... 1923
Zyvox (0.5% to 2.9%) ... 2552

Pharyngitis, streptococcal
▲ Elidel Cream 1% (0% to 3%) ... 2221
Verdeso Foam (1%) ... 3069
▲ Vivitrol (11% to 17%) ... 988

Pharyngotonsillitis
Exforge Tablets (Greater than or equal to 0.2%) ... 2238

Pharyngoxerosis
Carbatrol Capsules ... 3019

Pharynix, dryness of
Equetro Extended-Release Capsules ... 3174

Phlebitis
Abilify Injection (Greater than or equal to 1 in 1000 patients and less than 1 in 100 patients) ... 2466
Abilify Oral Solution (Greater than or equal to 1 in 1000 patients and less than 1 in 100 patients) ... 2466
Abilify Discmelt Orally Disintegrating Tablets (Greater than or equal to 1 in 1000 patients and less than 1 in 100 patients) ... 2466
Abilify Tablets (Greater than or equal to 1 in 1000 patients and less than 1 in 100 patients) ... 2466
Ambien Tablets (Rare) ... 2692
Ambien CR Tablets (Rare) ... 2696
Anzemet Injection (Rare) ... 2701
Anzemet Tablets (Rare) ... 2704
Avelox (Greater than or equal to 0.1% to less than 2%) ... 2803
Azilect Tablets (Infrequent) ... 3106
BeneFIX Vials (1.5%) ... 3191
Campral Tablets (Infrequent) ... 1158
▲ Cancidas for Injection (18.1%) ... 1953
Celexa (Rare) ... 1160
▲ CellCept Intravenous (4%) ... 2622
Cipro (Less than 1%) ... 2810
Cipro XR Tablets ... 2823
Dantrium Capsules (Less frequent) ... 2580
▲ Doribax Injection (4% to 8%) ... 2400
Doxil Injection (Less than 1%) ... 2378
Evoxac Capsules (Less than 1%) ... 1013
Fluorescite Injection ... ⊙ 203
Fortaz (1 in 69 patients) ... 1450
Gabitril Tablets (Infrequent) ... 973
Geodon Capsules (Rare) ... 2520
Imitrex Injection ... 1465
Imitrex Nasal Spray (Rare) ... 1470
Imitrex Tablets ... 1474
▲ Intron A for Injection (Less than or equal to 5%) ... 2859
Invanz for Injection (Greater than 0.5% to 1.9%) ... 2029
Leustatin Injection (2%) ... 2384
Levaquin (0.1% to 1%) ... 2416
Levaquin in 5% Dextrose Injection (0.1% to 1%) ... 2416
Lipitor Tablets (Less than 2%) ... 2501
Luvox CR Extended-Release Capsules (Rare) ... 1759
Merrem I.V. (0.8%) ... 684
Mirapex Tablets ... 857
▲ Mycamine for Injection (5.6% to 18.8%) ... 616
NovoSeven ... 2367
Panhematin for Injection ... 2497
Paxil (Rare) ... 1535
Paxil CR Controlled-Release Tablets (Rare) ... 1544
Premarin Intravenous ... 3217
▲ Primaxin I.V. (3.1%) ... 2083
▲ Prograf Capsules and Injection (3% to 15%) ... 622
Proleukin for Injection (Less than 1%) ... 2287
Prozac Weekly Capsules (Rare) ... 1852
Prozac Pulvules and Liquid (Rare) ... 1852
Remeron Tablets (Rare) ... 2924
RemeronSolTab Tablets (Rare) ... 2927
Requip Tablets (Infrequent) ... 1561
Retrovir Capsules (1.6%) ... 1574
Retrovir IV Infusion (2%) ... 1579
Retrovir (1.6%) ... 1574
Rilutek Tablets (0.4% to 0.8%) ... 2771
Risperdal Consta Long-Acting Injection (Infrequent) ... 1753
Rocephin Injectable Vials, ADD-Vantage, Galaxy, Bulk (Less than 1%) ... 2642
Stalevo Tablets ... 2309
Taxotere Injection Concentrate (0% to 1.2%) ... 2773
Trasylol Injection (1%) ... 799
Tricor Tablets ... 520
Tygacil for Injection (1.8%) ... 3276
▲ Vaprisol (4.9%) ... 632
Velcade for Injection ... 2168
▲ Vesanoid Capsules (11%) ... 2660
Wellbutrin Tablets (Rare) ... 1648
Wellbutrin SR Sustained-Release Tablets ... 1653
Wellbutrin XL Extended-Release Tablets ... 1659
▲ Xeloda Tablets (Less than 5%) ... 2662
Zosyn for Injection (1.3%) ... 3284
Zyban Sustained-Release Tablets ... 1692

Phlebitis, injection site
Novantrone for Injection Concentrate ... 1100
NovoSeven RT ... 2370
Tygacil for Injection (0% to less than 2%) ... 3276
▲ Vaprisol (15.8% to 51%) ... 632

Phobia, unspecified
Cipro (Less than 1%) ... 2810
Cipro XR Tablets ... 2823
Imitrex Injection ... 1465
Luvox CR Extended-Release Capsules (Infrequent) ... 1759

Phobic disorder
Cipro I.V. (1% or less) ... 2817
Imitrex Tablets (Rare) ... 1474
Zyprexa Tablets (Infrequent) ... 1883
Zyprexa ZYDIS Orally Disintegrating Tablets (Infrequent) ... 1883

Phonophobia
Imitrex Tablets (Frequent) ... 1474

Phospholipid concentration, increase
Estratest Tablets ... 3043
Estratest H.S. Tablets ... 3043

Phosphorus, decrease
Actonel with Calcium Tablets (2.7%) ... 2574
Omnicef Capsules (0.3%) ... 497
Omnicef for Oral Suspension (0.4%) ... 497
▲ Torisel Injection (18% to 49%) ... 3272

Photoallergenicity
▲ Extina Foam, 2% (17%) ... 3057

Photodermatitis
Advair Diskus 100/50 ... 1276
Advair Diskus 250/50 ... 1276
Advair Diskus 500/50 ... 1276
Advair HFA 45/21 Inhalation Aerosol ... 1288
Advair HFA 115/21 Inhalation Aerosol ... 1288
Advair HFA 230/21 Inhalation Aerosol ... 1288
Atripla Tablets ... 938
Serevent Diskus (1% to 2%) ... 1594

Photophobia
Abilify Injection (Greater than or equal to 1 in 1000 patients and less than 1 in 100 patients) ... 881
Abilify Injection (Greater than or equal to 1 in 1000 patients and less than 1 in 100 patients) ... 2466
Abilify Oral Solution (Greater than or equal to 1 in 1000 patients and less than 1 in 100 patients) ... 881
Abilify Oral Solution (Greater than or equal to 1 in 1000 patients and less than 1 in 100 patients) ... 2466
Abilify Discmelt Orally Disintegrating Tablets (Greater than or equal to 1 in 1000 patients and less than 1 in 100 patients) ... 881
Abilify Discmelt Orally Disintegrating Tablets (Greater than or equal to 1 in 1000 patients and less than 1 in 100 patients) ... 2466
Abilify Tablets (Greater than or equal to 1 in 1000 patients and less than 1 in 100 patients) ... 881
Abilify Tablets (Greater than or equal to 1 in 1000 patients and less than 1 in 100 patients) ... 2466
Accutane Capsules ... 2607
▲ Alphagan P Ophthalmic Solution (1% to 4%) ... 549
▲ Alrex Ophthalmic Suspension 0.2% (5% to 15%) ... ⊙ 236
Amerge Tablets (Frequent) ... 1301
Anzemet Tablets (Rare) ... 2704
▲ Betimol Ophthalmic Solution (More than 5%) ... 3181
BOTOX Purified Neurotoxin Complex ... 550
Calcijex Injection ... 419
Campral Tablets (Rare) ... 1158
Celexa (Infrequent) ... 1160
Chantix Tablets (Rare) ... 2511
Combigan Ophthalmic Solution (0.1% to 0.2%) ... 553
Copaxone for Injection (Infrequent) ... 3110
Cosopt Sterile Ophthalmic Solution (Less than 1%) ... 1969
Depakote ER Tablets (Greater than 1%) ... 423
▲ Durezol Ophthalmic Emulsion (5% to 15%) ... ⊙ 275
Effexor XR Extended-Release Capsules (Infrequent) ... 3195
Flulaval Injection Vaccine ... 1448
Gabitril Tablets (Infrequent) ... 973
Geodon Capsules (Infrequent) ... 2520
Havrix Injection Vaccine (Less than 1%) ... 1454
Imitrex Injection (Infrequent) ... 1465
Imitrex Tablets (Frequent) ... 1474
▲ Intron A for Injection (Less than 5%) ... 2859
Lacrisert Sterile Ophthalmic Insert ... ⊙ 233
Lamictal (Infrequent) ... 1488
Levitra Tablets (Less than 2%) ... 2876
▲ Lotemax Ophthalmic Suspension 0.5% (5% to 15%) ... ⊙ 241
▲ Lumigan Ophthalmic Solution (1% to 3%) ... 556
Lunesta Tablets (Rare) ... 2994
Luvox CR Extended-Release Capsules (Infrequent) ... 1759
Lyrica Capsules (0.1% to 1%) ... 2527
Maxalt Tablets (Rare) ... 2056
Maxalt-MLT Orally Disintegrating Tablets (Rare) ... 2056
Mirapex Tablets ... 857
▲ Nevanac Ophthalmic Suspension 0.1% (1% to 5%) ... ⊙ 205
Norvir (Less than 2%) ... 489
Ofloxacin Ophthalmic Solution 0.3% ... ⊙ 243
OptiPranolol Metipranolol Ophthalmic Solution 0.3% (A small number of patients) ... ⊙ 245
▲ Orthoclone OKT3 Sterile Solution (10%) ... 2387
Paxil (Rare) ... 1535
Paxil CR Controlled-Release Tablets (Rare) ... 1544
Photofrin for Injection ... 708
Prinivil Tablets (0.3% to 1%) ... 2087
Prinzide Tablets ... 2092
Prograf Capsules and Injection ... 622
Prozac Weekly Capsules (Infrequent) ... 1852
Prozac Pulvules and Liquid (Infrequent) ... 1852
▲ Quixin Ophthalmic Solution (1% to 3%) ... 3184
Requip Tablets (Infrequent) ... 1561
Retrovir Capsules ... 1574
Retrovir IV Infusion ... 1579
Retrovir ... 1574
Rilutek Tablets (Rare) ... 2771
Rocaltrol Capsules ... 1150
Rocaltrol Oral Solution ... 1150
▲ Soriatane Capsules (1% to 10%) ... 3062
Tasigna Capsules ... 2316
▲ Travatan Z Ophthalmic Solution (1% to 4%) ... 547
▲ Trusopt Sterile Ophthalmic Solution (Approximately 1% to 5%) ... 2128
Twinrix Vaccine (Less than 1%) ... 1628
Venlafaxine Hydrochloride Tablets (Infrequent) ... 2199
Zomig Tablets (Rare) ... 694
Zomig Nasal Spray (Rare) ... 689
Zomig-ZMT Tablets (Rare) ... 694
Zonegran Capsules (Rare) ... 1089
Zosyn for Injection (1% or less) ... 3284

Photopsia
Abilify Injection (Greater than or equal to 1 in 1000 patients and less than 1 in 100 patients) ... 881
Abilify Injection (Greater than or equal to 1 in 1000 patients and less than 1 in 100 patients) ... 2466
Abilify Oral Solution (Greater than or equal to 1 in 1000 patients and less than 1 in 100 patients) ... 881
Abilify Oral Solution (Greater than or equal to 1 in 1000 patients and less than 1 in 100 patients) ... 2466
Abilify Discmelt Orally Disintegrating Tablets (Greater than or equal to 1 in 1000 patients and less than 1 in 100 patients) ... 881
Abilify Discmelt Orally Disintegrating Tablets (Greater than or equal to 1 in 1000 patients and less than 1 in 100 patients) ... 2466
Abilify Tablets (Greater than or equal to 1 in 1000 patients and less than 1 in 100 patients) ... 881
Abilify Tablets (Greater than or equal to 1 in 1000 patients and less than 1 in 100 patients) ... 2466
Ambien Tablets (Rare) ... 2692
Ambien CR Tablets (Rare) ... 2696
Evoxac Capsules (Less than 1%) ... 1013
Maxalt Tablets (Rare) ... 2056
Maxalt-MLT Orally Disintegrating Tablets (Rare) ... 2056
Neupro Transdermal System ... 3149

Photosensitivity
Abilify Injection (Greater than or equal to 1 in 1000 patients and less than 1 in 100 patients) ... 881
Abilify Injection (Greater than or equal to 1 in 1000 patients and less than 1 in 100 patients) ... 2466
Abilify Oral Solution (Greater than or equal to 1 in 1000 patients and less than 1 in 100 patients) ... 881
Abilify Oral Solution (Greater than or equal to 1 in 1000 patients and less than 1 in 100 patients) ... 2466
Abilify Discmelt Orally Disintegrating Tablets (Greater than or equal to 1 in 1000 patients and less than 1 in 100 patients) ... 881
Abilify Discmelt Orally Disintegrating Tablets (Greater than or equal to 1 in 1000 patients and less than 1 in 100 patients) ... 2466
Abilify Tablets (Greater than or equal to 1 in 1000 patients and less than 1 in 100 patients) ... 881
Abilify Tablets (Greater than or equal to 1 in 1000 patients and less than 1 in 100 patients) ... 2466
Accutane Capsules ... 2607
▲ Agrylin Capsules (1% to less than 5%) ... 3017
Alferon N Injection (1%) ... 1726
Ambien CR Tablets (Rare) ... 2696
Amerge Tablets (Rare) ... 1301
Anaprox Tablets (Less than 1%) ... 2632
Anaprox DS Tablets (Less than 1%) ... 2632
Aptivus Oral Solution ... 823
Atacand HCT ... 642
Avalide Tablets ... 892
Avalide Tablets ... 2713
Axert Tablets (Rare) ... 2431
▲ Azmacort Inhalation Aerosol (1% to 3%) ... 407
Captopril Tablets ... 2182
Carbatrol Capsules ... 3019
Cardizem LA Extended Release Tablets (Less than 2%) ... 421
Celebrex Capsules (0.1% to 1.9%) ... 2979
Celexa (Infrequent) ... 1160
Cipro I.V. (1% or less) ... 2817
Cipro XR Tablets (Less than 1%) ... 2823
Clinoril Tablets (Less than 1 in 100) ... 1962
Clorpres Tablets ... 2185
Copaxone for Injection (Infrequent) ... 3110
Coreg Tablets (Greater than 0.1% to 1%) ... 1387
Cozaar Tablets (Less than 1%) ... 1973
Cyanokit 5g Antidote ... 1021
Dantrium Capsules ... 2580
Depakote ER Tablets ... 423
Diovan HCT Tablets ... 2216
Dyazide Capsules ... 1405
Dyrenium Capsules (Rare) ... 3189
EC-Naprosyn Delayed-Release Tablets (Less than 1%) ... 2632
Effexor XR Extended-Release Capsules (Infrequent) ... 3195

Eldepryl Capsules 3052
Elmiron Capsules (Less than or equal to 1%) 2435
Evoxac Capsules (Less than 1%) 1013
Fansidar Tablets 2636
Fosamax (Occasional) 2005
Furosemide Tablets 2186
Gabitril Tablets (Infrequent) 973
Gantrisin Pediatric Suspension 2638
Geodon Capsules (Frequent) 2520
Gleevec Tablets (Infrequent) 2255
Gris-PEG Tablets (Occasional) 2507
Imitrex Injection 1465
Imitrex Nasal Spray 1470
Imitrex Tablets 1474
Indapamide Tablets 2188
Intravenous Sodium Diuril 2490
▲ Intron A for Injection (Less than 5%) 2859
Lamictal (2%) 1488
Lescol Capsules (Rare) 2268
Lescol XL Tablets 2268
Lipitor Tablets (Less than 2%) 2501
Lunesta Tablets (Infrequent) 2994
Lupron Depot 3.75 mg 462
Lupron Depot 7.5 mg 469
Lupron Depot–3 Month 11.25 mg 462
Malarone Pediatric Tablets 1521
Malarone Tablets 1521
Marplan Tablets 3177
Maxalt Tablets (Infrequent) 2056
Maxalt-MLT Orally Disintegrating Tablets (Infrequent) 2056
Meridia Capsules 475
Mevacor Tablets (Rare) 2063
Micardis HCT Tablets 854
Mobic Oral Suspension (Less than 2%) 863
Mobic Tablets (Less than 2%) 863
Naprosyn Suspension (Less than 1%) 2632
Naprosyn Tablets (Less than 1%) 2632
Nexium Delayed-Release Capsules 645
Nexium I.V. 652
Nexium Delayed-Release Oral Suspension 645
Noroxin Tablets 2069
Norvir (Less than 2%) 489
Paxil (Rare) 1535
Paxil CR Controlled-Release Tablets (Rare) 1544
Pentasa Capsules (Less than 1%) 3030
▲ Photofrin for Injection (19% to 68%) 708
Prinivil Tablets (0.3% to 1%) 2087
Prinzide Tablets 2092
▲ Prograf Capsules and Injection (3% to 15%) 622
Protopic Ointment (Greater than or equal to 1%) 628
Prozac Pulvules and Liquid (Rare) 1852
Pylera Capsules 714
Remeron Tablets (Infrequent) 2924
RemeronSolTab Tablets (Infrequent) 2927
Requip Tablets (Infrequent) 1561
Rilutek Tablets (Infrequent) 2771
Solodyn Extended Release Tablets 1938
Soriatane Capsules (Less than 1%) 3062
Sular Extended Release Tablets (One case) 2975
Targretin Capsules 1084
Tasigna Capsules 2316
Tekturna HCT Tablets 2324
Teveten HCT Tablets 517
Thioridazine Hydrochloride Tablets (Extremely rare) 2195
Thiothixene Capsules 2197
Toprol-XL Tablets 666
Tricor Tablets 520
Tygacil for Injection 3276
Valtrex Caplets 1635
Vectibix 597
▲ Visudyne for Injection (1% to 10%) 2332
Voltaren Tablets (Occasionally) 2334
Voltaren-XR Tablets (Occasionally) 2337
Vytorin 10/10 Tablets 2149
Vytorin 10/10 Tablets 2939
Vytorin 10/20 Tablets 2149
Vytorin 10/20 Tablets 2939
Vytorin 10/40 Tablets 2149
Vytorin 10/40 Tablets 2939
Vytorin 10/80 Tablets 2149
Vytorin 10/80 Tablets 2939
Wellbutrin SR Sustained-Release Tablets (Infrequent) 1653
Wellbutrin XL Extended-Release Tablets (Infrequent) 1659
▲ Xeloda Tablets (Less than 5%) 2662
Zocor Tablets (Rare) 2136
Zomig Tablets (Infrequent) 694
Zomig-ZMT Tablets (Infrequent) 694
Zovirax 1690
Zyban Sustained-Release Tablets (Infrequent) 1692
Zyprexa Tablets (Infrequent) 1883
Zyprexa ZYDIS Orally Disintegrating Tablets (Infrequent) 1883

Photosensitivity, cutaneous

Agrylin Capsules 3017
Fosamax Plus D Tablets 2013

Photosensitivity reaction

▲ Adderall XR Capsules (2% to 4%) 3012
Ambien Tablets (Rare) 2692
Avandaryl Tablets 1344
Azilect Tablets (Infrequent) 3106
BeneFIX Vials (1.6%) 3191
Campral Tablets (Rare) 1158
Chantix Tablets (Rare) 2511
Cipro (Less than 1%) 2810
Coreg CR Extended-Release Capsules (0.1% to less than or equal to 1%) 1393
Cymbalta Delayed-Release Capsules (Infrequent) 1801
Duetact Tablets (Less than 1%) 3085
Emsam Transdermal System (Infrequent) 905
▲ Equetro Extended-Release Capsules (Less than 5%) 3174
Levaquin 2416
Levaquin in 5% Dextrose Injection 2416
Levitra Tablets (Less than 2%) 2876
Lexapro Oral Suspension 1174
Lexapro Tablets 1174
Lupron Depot-PED 7.5 mg, 11.25 mg and 15 mg 471
Luvox CR Extended-Release Capsules (Infrequent) 1759
Lyrica Capsules (0.1% to 1%) 2527
Mirapex Tablets 857
Protonix I.V. (Less than 1%) 3257
Prozac Weekly Capsules (Rare) 1852
Raptiva for Injection 1218
Risperdal Consta Long-Acting Injection (Infrequent) 1753
Salagen Tablets (Less than 1%) 1082
Symbyax Capsules (Frequent) 1871
Venlafaxine Hydrochloride Tablets (Infrequent) 2199
Zyrtec Chewable Tablets (Less than 2%) 1920
Zyrtec Syrup (Less than 2%) 1920
Zyrtec Tablets (Less than 2%) 1920
Zyrtec-D 12 Hour Extended Release Tablets (Less than 2%) 1923

Phototoxicity

Avelox (Less than 0.1%) 2803
Cipro I.V. 2817
Cipro (Less than 1%) 2810
Cipro XR Tablets (Less than 1%) 2823
Dapsone Tablets USP 1746
Levaquin 2416
Levaquin in 5% Dextrose Injection 2416
Noroxin Tablets 2069
PegIntron Powder for Injection (Less than or equal to 1%) 2903
Protonix for Delayed-Release Oral Suspension (Less than 1%) 3254
Protonix Delayed-Release Tablets (Less than 1%) 3254
Zyrtec-D 12 Hour Extended Release Tablets (Less than 2%) 1923

Physical performance, impairment

Adipex-P 1185
Gris-PEG Tablets (Occasional) 2507
Lortab 5/500 Tablets 3143
Lortab 7.5/500 Tablets 3144
Lortab 10/500 Tablets 3144
MS Contin Tablets 2585
Percocet Tablets 1127
Percodan Tablets 1130
Soma Tablets 1931
Thiothixene Capsules 2197
Tussionex Pennkinetic Extended-Release Suspension 3154
Vicodin Tablets 529
Vicodin ES Tablets 530
Vicodin HP Tablets 531
Zydone Tablets 1132

Pigmentary deposits, conjuctiva

▲ Eloxatin for Injection (2% to 9%) 2731

Pigmentation

Copaxone for Injection (Infrequent) 3110
Cosmegen for Injection 2485
Cosopt Sterile Ophthalmic Solution 1969
▲ Eloxatin for Injection (2% to less than 5%) 2731
Genotropin Lyophilized Powder (Infrequent) 2547
Solodyn Extended Release Tablets 1938
Timoptic Sterile Ophthalmic Solution 2121
Timoptic in Ocudose 2124
Timoptic-XE Sterile Ophthalmic Gel Forming Solution 2125

Pigmentation disorders

Accutane Capsules 2607
Carbatrol Capsules 3019
Equetro Extended-Release Capsules 3174
Exjade Tablets (0.1% to 1%) 2244
Gengraf Capsules (1% to less than 3%) 435
Gleevec Tablets (Infrequent) 2255
Neoral Oral Solution (1% to less than 3%) 2280
Neoral Soft Gelatin Capsules (1% to less than 3%) 2280
Retrovir Capsules 1574
Retrovir IV Infusion 1579
Retrovir 1574

Pill rolling motion

Thioridazine Hydrochloride Tablets 2195

Piloerection

▲ ProAmatine Tablets (13.4%) 3032
Ultram ER Extended-Release Tablets (0.5% to less than 1%) 2428

Pituitary apoplexy

Eligard 7.5 mg (Less than 2%) 2724
Eligard 22.5 mg 2724
Eligard 30 mg 2724
Eligard 45 mg 2724
Lupron Depot 3.75 mg (Rare) 462
Lupron Depot 7.5 mg 469
Sandostatin Injection (Less than 1%) 2300
Sandostatin LAR Depot 2302
Vantas 1737
Viadur Implant (Rare) 802

Pituitary tumors

Imitrex Nasal Spray (Rare) 1470
Supprelin LA Implant 1731

Plantar fasciitis

Effexor XR Extended-Release Capsules (Rare) 3195
Evoxac Capsules (Less than 1%) 1013
Venlafaxine Hydrochloride Tablets (Rare) 2199

Plasma testosterone level, reduction

Celebrex Capsules (Greater than or equal to 0.1% to less than 1%) 2979
Zocor Tablets 2136

Plasminogen, increase

Premarin Tablets 3221
Premphase Tablets 3232
Prempro Tablets 3232

Platelet, decrease

(*see under* Thrombocytopenia)

Platelet, increase

(*see under* Thrombocytosis)

Platelet aggregation decrease

Vicoprofen Tablets 533

Platelet aggregation time, decrease

Premarin Tablets 3221
Premphase Tablets 3232
Prempro Tablets 3232

Platelet disorder, unspecified

Salagen Tablets (Less than 1%) 1082
▲ Tykerb Tablets (0% to 18%) 1631

Pleural effusion

Abelcet Injection 1134
Actiq (Less than 1%) 959
Activase I.V. 1188
Agrylin Capsules 3017
▲ AmBisome for Injection (12.5%) 606
▲ Arranon Injection (1% to 10%) 1319
Avandamet Tablets 1336
Avandaryl Tablets 1344
Avandia Tablets 1351
Bexxar 1371
▲ Busulfex Injection (3%) 2477
▲ Cancidas for Injection (8.8%) 1953
▲ CellCept Capsules (3% to 34.3%) 2622
▲ CellCept Intravenous (3% to 34.3%) 2622
▲ CellCept Oral Suspension (3% to 34.3%) 2622
▲ CellCept Tablets (3% to 34.3%) 2622
Cipro I.V. (1% or less) 2817
Cipro XR Tablets 2823
Clinoril Tablets (Less than 1 in 100) 1962
▲ Clolar for Intravenous Infusion (10%) 1239
▲ Cubicin for Injection (5.8%) 995
Cyanokit 5g Antidote 1021
▲ Doxil Injection (1% to 10%) 2378
Evoxac Capsules (Less than 1%) 1013
Femara Tablets (Less frequent) 2246
Fentora Tablets (Greater than 1%) 968
▲ Flolan for Injection (4% to 7%) 1426
Follistim AQ Cartridge 2844
▲ Gleevec Tablets (6.9% to 22%) 2255
Herceptin I.V. 1199
▲ Humira Injection (Less than 5%) 442
Invanz for Injection (Greater than 0.1%) 2029
Leukine 774
Merrem I.V. (Greater than 0.1% to 1%) 684
Neupro Transdermal System 3149
PegIntron Powder for Injection (Less than 1%) 2903
▲ Photofrin for Injection (13% to 32%) 708
Prinivil Tablets (0.3% to 1%) 2087
Prinzide Tablets 2092
▲ Prograf Capsules and Injection (30% to 36%) 622
Rapamune 3260
Remicade for IV Injection (Greater than or equal to 0.2%) 950
ReoPro Vials (1.3%) 1860
Rilutek Tablets (Infrequent) 2771
Rythmol SR Capsules 1590
Sandostatin LAR Depot 2302
Stalevo Tablets (Rare) 2309
Sular Extended Release Tablets (Less than or equal to 1%) 2975
Targretin Capsules 1084
Tasigna Capsules (0.1% to 1%) 2316
▲ Taxotere Injection Concentrate (6.5%) 2773
▲ Trasylol Injection (7%) 799
▲ Trisenox Injection (20%) 986
▲ Valcyte Tablets (Less than 5%) 2654
Velcade for Injection 2168
▲ Vesanoid Capsules (20%) 2660
Xeloda Tablets (1% to 2%) 2662
Zosyn for Injection (1.3%) 3284

Pleural effusion with pericarditis

Dantrium Capsules (Less frequent) 2580

Pleural thickening

Neupro Transdermal System 3149
Stalevo Tablets (Rare) 2309

Pleuralgia

▲ Intron A for Injection (Less than 5%) 2859

Pleurisy

▲ Aerobid/Aerobid-M (1% to 3%) 1153
Aricept Tablets (Infrequent) 1062
Aricept ODT Tablets (Infrequent) 1062
Chantix Tablets (Rare) 2511
Effexor XR Extended-Release Capsules (Rare) 3195
Evoxac Capsules (Less than 1%) 1013
Klonopin (Infrequent) 2639
Mirapex Tablets 857
Remicade for IV Injection (Greater than or equal to 0.2%) 950
ReoPro Vials (1.3%) 1860
Requip Tablets (Infrequent) 1561
Tasigna Capsules (0.1% to 1%) 2316
Treximet Tablets (Infrequent) 1616
Venlafaxine Hydrochloride Tablets (Rare) 2199

Pleuritis

Amerge Tablets (Rare) 1301
Asacol Delayed-Release Tablets 2579
Rituxan I.V. 1223

Pneumocystis carinii

▲ CellCept Capsules (Less than 4%) 2622
▲ CellCept Intravenous (Less than 4%) 2622
▲ CellCept Oral Suspension (Less than 4%) 2622
▲ CellCept Tablets (Less than 4%) 2622

Pneumocystis carinii, susceptibility
▲ Doxil Injection (9.2%) 2378
▲ Orthoclone OKT3 Sterile Solution (3.1%) 2387

Pneumocytosis
Remicade for IV Injection 950

Pneumonia
Actiq (Less than 1%) 959
▲ Actonel with Calcium Tablets (0.8% to 3.1%) 2574
Advair Diskus 100/50 1276
▲ Advair Diskus 250/50 (3% to 16%) 1276
▲ Advair Diskus 500/50 (3% to 18%) 1276
Advair HFA 45/21 Inhalation Aerosol 1288
Advair HFA 115/21 Inhalation Aerosol 1288
Advair HFA 230/21 Inhalation Aerosol 1288
▲ Aerobid/Aerobid-M (1% to 3%) 1153
▲ Agrylin Capsules (1% to less than 5%) 3017
▲ Alvesco Inhalation Aerosol (Greater than or equal to 3%) 2985
Ambien Tablets (Rare) 2692
Ambien CR Tablets (Rare) 2696
AmBisome for Injection (Less common) 606
Amerge Tablets (Infrequent) 1301
Amevive 611
Anaprox Tablets (Less than 1%) 2632
Anaprox DS Tablets (Less than 1%) 2632
▲ Aranesp for Injection (27%) 564
▲ Argatroban Injection (3.3%) 1308
Aricept Tablets (Infrequent) 1062
Aricept ODT Tablets (Infrequent) 1062
Arixtra Injection (2.3%) 1313
▲ Arranon Injection (1% to 8%) 1319
▲ Atripla Tablets (Greater than or equal to 5%) 938
Betaseron for SC Injection 756
▲ Bexxar (0% to 6%) 1371
▲ Boniva Injection (5.9%) 2614
▲ Boniva Tablets (5.9%) 2618
Busulfex Injection 2477
Campral Tablets (Infrequent) 1158
▲ Cancidas for Injection (4.4% to 11.3%) 1953
Carbatrol Capsules 3019
Celebrex Capsules (0.1% to 1.9%) 2979
Celexa (Infrequent) 1160
▲ CellCept Capsules (3% to less than 20%) 2622
▲ CellCept Intravenous (3% to less than 20%) 2622
▲ CellCept Oral Suspension (3% to less than 20%) 2622
▲ CellCept Tablets (3% to less than 20%) 2622
Cimzia 3127
▲ Clolar for Intravenous Infusion (10%) 1239
Combivent Inhalation Aerosol (1.4%) 845
Comvax 1966
Copaxone for Injection (Infrequent) 3110
▲ Cubicin for Injection (3.3%) 995
▲ Dacogen Injection (22%) 1066
Depakote ER Tablets (Greater than 1% to less than 5%) 423
▲ DepoCyt Injection (6%) 1136
▲ Doxil Injection (1% to 10%) 2378
EC-Naprosyn Delayed-Release Tablets (Less than 1%) 2632
Effexor XR Extended-Release Capsules (Infrequent) 3195
Elidel Cream 1% (0% to 1.5%) 2221
Elitek (Less than or equal to 1%) 2729
▲ Eloxatin for Injection (2% to less than 5%) 2731
Emsam Transdermal System (Infrequent) 905
▲ Emtriva Capsules (15%) 1246
▲ Emtriva Oral Solution (15%) 1246
Enbrel for Injection 569
Equetro Extended-Release Capsules 3174
Evista Tablets (2.6%) 1810
▲ Evoxac Capsules (1% to 3%) 1013
Exelon Patch (Frequent) 2233
Exubera Inhalation Powder (0.9%) 2515
▲ Fentora Tablets (1% to 16%) 968
▲ Flolan for Injection (5%) 1426
Flovent Diskus 50 mcg 1435
Flovent HFA 1440
Fluarix Vaccine 1446
▲ Forteo for Injection (3.9%) 1816
Gabitril Tablets (Frequent) 973
▲ Gengraf Capsules (1% to 6.2%) 435
Geodon Capsules (Infrequent) 2520
▲ Gleevec Tablets (4% to 13%) 2255
▲ Gliadel Wafer (8%) 1076
▲ Humira Injection (Less than 5%) 442
Hycamtin for Injection (2%) 1459
Intron A for Injection (Rare) 2859
Invanz for Injection (2.1%) 2029
Ionsys Transdermal System (.1% to less than 1%) 2410
Ixempra Kit for Injection 915
Kineret Injection 585
Klonopin (Infrequent) 2639
Lamictal (Rare) 1488
▲ Leustatin Injection (6%) 2384
Lexapro Oral Suspension (Infrequent) 1174
Lexapro Tablets (Infrequent) 1174
Lipitor Tablets (Less than 2%) 2501
Lovaza Capsules 1520
Lovenox Injection (0.82%) 2756
Luvox CR Extended-Release Capsules (Rare) 1759
Megace ES Oral Suspension (0% to 2%) 2499
Merrem I.V. (Greater than 1%) 684
Miacalcin Nasal Spray (Less than 1%) 2274
M-M-R II 2054
▲ Mycamine for Injection (1.5% to 5.4%) 616
▲ Myfortic Tablets (3% to less than 20%) 2276
Myleran Tablets 1530
▲ Mylotarg for Injection (8% to 13%) 3212
Namenda (Frequent) 1180
Naprosyn Suspension (Less than 1%) 2632
Naprosyn Tablets (Less than 1%) 2632
▲ Neoral Oral Solution (1% to 6.2%) 2280
▲ Neoral Soft Gelatin Capsules (1% to 6.2%) 2280
▲ Novantrone for Injection Concentrate (9%) 1100
NovoSeven (1%) 2367
▲ NovoSeven RT (1% to 4.7%) 2370
▲ Noxafil Oral Suspension (3% to 10%) 2889
Omnicef Capsules 497
Omnicef for Oral Suspension 497
▲ Orencia Powder for Intravenous Infusion (0.2% to 3%) 921
Orthoclone OKT3 Sterile Solution 2387
Paxil (Infrequent) 1535
Paxil CR Controlled-Release Tablets (Infrequent) 1544
PegIntron Powder for Injection (Less than or equal to 1%) 2903
Pentacel 2792
▲ Photofrin for Injection (18%) 708
Plavix Tablets (1% to 2.5%) 926
Plavix Tablets (1% to 2.5%) 2767
Pletal Tablets (Less than 2%) 2481
Prevnar 3241
Prinivil Tablets (0.3% to 1%) 2087
Prinzide Tablets 2092
▲ Prograf Capsules and Injection (3% to 15%) 622
ProQuad 2099
Protonix for Delayed-Release Oral Suspension (Less than 1%) 3254
Protonix Delayed-Release Tablets (Less than 1%) 3254
Protonix I.V. (Less than 1%) 3257
Protopic Ointment (1% to 2%) 628
Provigil Tablets (At least 1%) 977
Pulmozyme Inhalation Solution 1217
▲ Rapamune (Greater than or equal to 3% to less than 20%) 3260
Raptiva for Injection 1218
Rebetol 2917
▲ Refludan for Injection (4.4%) 795
Remeron Tablets (Infrequent) 2924
RemeronSolTab Tablets (Infrequent) 2927
Remicade for IV Injection (Greater than or equal to 0.2%) 950
ReoPro Vials (1%) 1860
Requip Tablets (Infrequent) 1561
Rilutek Tablets (More than 2%) 2771
Risperdal Consta Long-Acting Injection (Infrequent) 1753
RotaTeq (0.2%) 2110
Salagen Tablets (Less than 1%) 1082
▲ Sandimmune (6.2% to 9.2%) 2296
Sandostatin Injection (Less than 1%) 2300
Sandostatin LAR Depot 2302
Selzentry Tablets (2.1%) 2534
▲ Simulect for Injection (3% to 10%) 2306
Singulair (Greater than or equal to 2%) 2114
Symbyax Capsules (Infrequent) 1871
Synagis Intramuscular Solution (More than 1%) 1948
Tamiflu Capsules (Less than 1% to 2%) 2649
Tamiflu Oral Suspension (Less than 1% to 2%) 2649
Tasigna Capsules (0.1% to 1%) 2316
Testim 1% Gel 701
Toprol-XL Tablets (Greater than 1%) 666
▲ Torisel Injection (8%) 3272
▲ Trasylol Injection (4%) 799
Treanda for Injection 983
Treximet Tablets (Rare) 1616
Tricor Tablets 520
▲ Truvada Tablets (Greater than or equal to 5%) 1262
Ultram ER Extended-Release Tablets (0.5% to less than 1%) 2428
Valstar Sterile Solution for Intravesical Instillation (1%) 1735
▲ Vaprisol (2.7% to 5%) 632
Vaqta 2130
Varivax 2133
▲ Velcade for Injection (4% to 16%) 2168
Venlafaxine Hydrochloride Tablets (Infrequent) 2199
▲ Vesanoid Capsules (14%) 2660
Vicoprofen Tablets (Less than 1%) 533
▲ Viread Tablets (2% to 5%) 1268
▲ Visudyne for Injection (1% to 10%) 2332
Vivitrol 988
Voltaren Tablets (Rarely) 2334
Voltaren-XR Tablets (Rarely) 2337
Wellbutrin Tablets (Rare) 1648
Wellbutrin SR Sustained-Release Tablets 1653
Wellbutrin XL Extended-Release Tablets 1659
▲ Xeloda Tablets (Less than 5%) 2662
Xyrem Oral Solution (Infrequent) 1766
Zantac 25 EFFERdose Tablets 1670
Zantac Injection 1666
Zantac Injection Pharmacy Bulk Package 1668
Zantac Injection Premixed 1666
Zantac 1670
▲ Zemplar Capsules (5%) 536
▲ Zemplar Injection (5%) 538
▲ Ziagen (4%) 1673
Zolinza Capsules 2142
Zomig Tablets (Rare) 694
Zomig Nasal Spray (Rare) 689
Zomig-ZMT Tablets (Rare) 694
Zyban Sustained-Release Tablets 1692
Zyrtec Chewable Tablets (Less than 2%) 1920
Zyrtec Syrup (Less than 2%) 1920
Zyrtec Tablets (Less than 2%) 1920
Zyrtec-D 12 Hour Extended Release Tablets (Less than 2%) 1923
Zyvox (0% to 2.8%) 2552

Pneumonia, aspiration
Abilify Injection (Greater than or equal to 1 in 1000 patients and less than 1 in 100 patients) 881
Abilify Injection (Greater than or equal to 1 in 1000 patients and less than 1 in 100 patients) 2466
Abilify Oral Solution (Greater than or equal to 1 in 100 patients) 881
Abilify Oral Solution (Greater than or equal to 1 in 1000 patients and less than 1 in 100 patients) 2466
Abilify Discmelt Orally Disintegrating Tablets (Greater than or equal to 1 in 100 patients) 881
Abilify Discmelt Orally Disintegrating Tablets (Greater than or equal to 1 in 1000 patients and less than 1 in 100 patients) 2466
Abilify Tablets (Greater than or equal to 1 in 100 patients) 881
Abilify Tablets (Greater than or equal to 1 in 1000 patients and less than 1 in 100 patients) 2466
Gliadel Wafer (1%) 1076
Mirapex Tablets 857
Namenda 1180
Velcade for Injection 2168

Pneumonia, bacterial
Proleukin for Injection 2287
Selzentry Tablets 2534

Pneumonia, eosinophilic
Agrylin Capsules 3017
▲ Asacol Delayed-Release Tablets (5% or greater) 2579
Effexor XR Extended-Release Capsules (Rare) 3195
Omnicef Capsules 497
Omnicef for Oral Suspension 497
Pristiq Extended-Release Tablets 3247
Prozac Weekly Capsules 1852
Prozac Pulvules and Liquid 1852

Pneumonia, fungal
Arranon Injection 1319
Proleukin for Injection 2287

Pneumonia, interstitial
Aciphex Tablets 1053
Doribax Injection 2400
Leukeran Tablets 1508
Norvir (Less than 2%) 489
Omnicef Capsules 497
Omnicef for Oral Suspension 497
Pepcid Tablets 2075
Pletal Tablets 2481
Tarceva Tablets (0.7%) 1228
Taxotere Injection Concentrate 2773
Velcade for Injection 2168

Pneumonia, lobar
Mirapex Tablets 857

Pneumonia, pneumocystis carinii
Temodar Capsules (Rare) 2931

Pneumonia, tuberculous
Raptiva for Injection 1218

Pneumonia, viral
Proleukin for Injection 2287

Pneumonitis
Atacand HCT 642
Attenuvax 1951
Avalide Tablets 892
Avalide Tablets 2713
▲ Avastin IV (5%) 1192
Carbatrol Capsules 3019
Celexa (Rare) 1160
Clinoril Tablets (Less than 1 in 100) 1962
Cosmegen for Injection 2485
Diovan HCT Tablets 2216
Doribax Injection 2400
Emend Capsules (Greater than 0.5%) 1992
Emend for Injection (Greater than 0.5%) 1999
Gantrisin Pediatric Suspension 2638
Herceptin I.V. 1199
Indapamide Tablets 2188
Intravenous Sodium Diuril 2490
Intron A for Injection (Rare) 2859
Ixempra Kit for Injection 915
Levaquin 2416
Levaquin in 5% Dextrose Injection 2416
Micardis HCT Tablets 854
M-M-R II 2054
Novantrone for Injection Concentrate 1100
Orthoclone OKT3 Sterile Solution 2387
PegIntron Powder for Injection (1%) 2903
Pentasa Capsules 3030
Photofrin for Injection 708
Prinzide Tablets 2092
▲ Prometrium Capsules (100 mg, 200 mg) (Less than 5%) 3047
ProQuad 2099
Rapamune 3260
Rebetol 2917
Rituxan I.V. 1223
Rocephin Injectable Vials, ADD-Vantage, Galaxy, Bulk 2642
Tarceva Tablets (0.7%) 1228
Taxotere Injection Concentrate (Rare) 2773
Tekturna HCT Tablets 2324
Teveten HCT Tablets 517
Tice BCG (Less than or equal to 1%) 2936
Tykerb Tablets 1631
Varivax (Less than 1%) 2133
Velcade for Injection 2168

Pneumonitis, allergic
Avelox 2803
Cipro I.V. (Rare) 2817
Cipro 2810
Cipro XR Tablets 2823
Dyazide Capsules 1405
Equetro Extended-Release Capsules 3174
Levaquin 2416
Levaquin in 5% Dextrose Injection 2416
Noroxin Tablets 2069
Rocephin Injectable Vials, ADD-Vantage, Galaxy, Bulk (Less than 0.1%) 2642

Pneumonitis, eosinophilic
Aceon Tablets (2 mg, 4 mg, 8 mg)... 3038
Anaprox Tablets (Less than 1%)....... 2632
Anaprox DS Tablets (Less than 1%).. 2632
Captopril Tablets 2182
EC-Naprosyn Delayed-Release Tablets (Less than 1%)...................... 2632
Naprosyn Suspension (Less than 1%).. 2632
Naprosyn Tablets (Less than 1%)..... 2632
Prinivil Tablets.................................. 2087
Prinzide Tablets................................ 2092
Raptiva for Injection........................ 1218

Pneumonitis, hypersensitivity
Byetta Injection................................. 600
Limbrel Capsules (3 cases).............. 2561
Pentasa Capsules (Infrequent).......... 3030
Tarceva Tablets (0.7%)..................... 1228

Pneumonitis, interstitial
Actimmune (Rare)............................. 1743
Agrylin Capsules............................... 3017
Alimta for Injection........................... 1786
Asacol Delayed-Release Tablets....... 2579
Cuprimine Capsules (Rare).............. 1986
Gleevec Tablets (Rare)...................... 2255
PegIntron Powder for Injection......... 2903
Plavix Tablets.................................... 926
Plavix Tablets.................................... 2767
Raptiva for Injection......................... 1218
Remicade for IV Injection.................. 950
Rituxan I.V. 1223

Pneumonitis, radiation
Tarceva Tablets (0.7%)..................... 1228
Taxotere Injection Concentrate (Rare)... 2773

Pneumothorax
Actiq (Less than 1%)........................ 959
Arranon Injection 1319
▲ CellCept Capsules (3% to less than 20%).. 2622
▲ CellCept Intravenous (3% to less than 20%).. 2622
▲ CellCept Oral Suspension (3% to less than 20%)............................... 2622
▲ CellCept Tablets (3% to less than 20%).. 2622
Doxil Injection (Less than 1%).......... 2378
▲ Flolan for Injection (4%) 1426
▲ Intron A for Injection (Less than or equal to 5%)................................ 2859
Mirapex Tablets.................................. 857
▲ Prograf Capsules and Injection (3% to 15%).................................. 622
Proleukin for Injection (Less than 1%)... 2287
Prozac Weekly Capsules (Rare)....... 1852
Prozac Pulvules and Liquid (Rare).... 1852
Pulmozyme Inhalation Solution......... 1217
Remeron Tablets (Rare).................... 2924
RemeronSolTab Tablets (Rare)......... 2927
Rilutek Tablets (Infrequent)............... 2771
Sandostatin LAR Depot..................... 2302
▲ Trasylol Injection (4%) 799
Zosyn for Injection (1.3%)................. 3284

Pollakiuria
Amitiza Capsules (Less than 1%)...... 3082
▲ Cymbalta Delayed-Release Capsules (1% to 5%)...................... 1801
Diovan HCT Tablets (Greater than 0.2%)... 2216
DynaCirc CR Controlled Release Tablets (0.5% to 1%).................... 1407
Exelon Patch (Infrequent).................. 2233
Exforge Tablets (Greater than or equal to 0.2%)............................ 2238
Mirapex Tablets.................................. 857
Requip Tablets (Infrequent)............... 1561
Tasigna Capsules (0.1% to 1%)........ 2316
▲ Vaprisol (6%) 632

Polyangitis, microscopic
Fluarix Vaccine 1446

Polyarteritis nodosa
▲ Intron A for Injection (Less than 5%)... 2859
Recombivax HB................................ 2107

Polyarthralgia
Primaxin I.M...................................... 2080
Primaxin I.V. (Less than 0.2%).......... 2083
Solodyn Extended Release Tablets... 1938

Polyarthralgia, migratory
Cuprimine Capsules.......................... 1986

Polyarthritis
Xyrem Oral Solution (Infrequent)....... 1766

Polycythemia
AndroGel... 3159
▲ CellCept Capsules (3% to less than 20%).. 2622
▲ CellCept Intravenous (3% to less than 20%).. 2622
▲ CellCept Oral Suspension (3% to less than 20%)............................... 2622
▲ CellCept Tablets (3% to less than 20%).. 2622
Delatestryl Injection........................... 1730
Estratest Tablets............................... 3043
Estratest H.S. Tablets....................... 3043
Geodon Capsules (Rare).................. 2520
▲ Humira Injection (Less than 5%) 442
Lyrica Capsules (Rare)..................... 2527
Pletal Tablets (Less than 2%)........... 2481
▲ Prograf Capsules and Injection (3% to 15%).................................. 622
▲ Simulect for Injection (3% to 10%) ... 2306

Polydipsia
Abilify Injection (Greater than or equal to 1 in 1000 patients and less than 1 in 100 patients) 881
Abilify Injection (Greater than or equal to 1 in 1000 patients and less than 1 in 100 patients) 2466
Abilify Oral Solution (Greater than or equal to 1 in 1000 patients and less than 1 in 100 patients) 881
Abilify Oral Solution (Greater than or equal to 1 in 1000 patients and less than 1 in 100 patients) 2466
Abilify Discmelt Orally Disintegrating Tablets (Greater than or equal to 1 in 1000 patients and less than 1 in 100 patients) 881
Abilify Discmelt Orally Disintegrating Tablets (Greater than or equal to 1 in 1000 patients and less than 1 in 100 patients) 2466
Abilify Tablets (Greater than or equal to 1 in 1000 patients and less than 1 in 100 patients) 881
Abilify Tablets (Greater than or equal to 1 in 1000 patients and less than 1 in 100 patients) 2466
Amerge Tablets (Infrequent) 1301
Aricept Tablets (Infrequent) 1062
Aricept ODT Tablets (Infrequent) 1062
Calcijex Injection 419
Imitrex Injection (Rare) 1465
Imitrex Nasal Spray 1470
Imitrex Tablets (Rare) 1474
Rocaltrol Capsules 1150
Rocaltrol Oral Solution 1150
Thiothixene Capsules 2197

Polymenorrhea
Sandostatin Injection (Less than 1%) 2300

Polymyalgia
Mirapex Tablets 857

Polymyalgia rheumatica
Advicor Tablets 402
Lescol Capsules (Rare) 2268
Lescol XL Tablets 2268
Mevacor Tablets (Rare) 2063
Miacalcin Nasal Spray (Less than 1%) 2274
Nexium Delayed-Release Capsules (Less than 1%) 645
Nexium I.V. (Less than 1%) 652
Nexium Delayed-Release Oral Suspension (Less than 1%) 645
Requip Tablets (Infrequent) 1561
Vytorin 10/10 Tablets 2149
Vytorin 10/10 Tablets 2939
Vytorin 10/20 Tablets 2149
Vytorin 10/20 Tablets 2939
Vytorin 10/40 Tablets 2149
Vytorin 10/40 Tablets 2939
Vytorin 10/80 Tablets 2149
Vytorin 10/80 Tablets 2939
Zocor Tablets (Rare) 2136

Polymyositis
Enbrel for Injection (Infrequent) 569

Polyneuritis
Fansidar Tablets 2636
Meruvax II 2061
M-M-R II 2054
Proglycem Capsules (Infrequent) 1185
Proglycem Suspension (Infrequent) 1185
ProQuad 2099

Polyneuropathy
▲ Intron A for Injection (Less than 5%) 2859
▲ Ixempra Kit for Injection (62%) 915
Levaquin... 2416
Levaquin in 5% Dextrose Injection.... 2416
Meruvax II (Isolated reports)............ 2061
M-M-R II... 2054
Phenytek Capsules........................... 2192
ProQuad... 2099
▲ Xeloda Tablets (Less than 5%) 2662

Polyneuropathy, axonal
Avelox.. 2803
Cipro.. 2810
Cipro XR Tablets.............................. 2823

Polyneuropathy, demyelinating, inflammatory
Remicade for IV Injection 950

Polyneuropathy, peripheral
Leustatin Injection........................... 2384

Polyneuropathy, toxic
▲ Ixempra Kit for Injection (62%) 915

Polyphagia
Abilify Injection................................. 881
Abilify Injection 2466
Abilify Oral Solution 881
Abilify Oral Solution 2466
Abilify Discmelt Orally Disintegrating Tablets 881
Abilify Discmelt Orally Disintegrating Tablets 2466
Abilify Tablets 881
Abilify Tablets 2466
Mirapex Tablets 857

Polyposis, gastric
Lexapro Oral Suspension (Infrequent) 1174
Lexapro Tablets (Infrequent) 1174

Polyps, gallbladder
Sandostatin Injection (Less than 1%) 2300
Sandostatin LAR Depot 2302

Polyps, gastric
Requip Tablets (Infrequent) 1561

Polyps, nasal
Atrovent Nasal Spray 0.03% 834
Mirapex Tablets 857
Pulmozyme Inhalation Solution 1217
Requip Tablets (Infrequent) 1561
Zyrtec Chewable Tablets (Less than 2%) 1920
Zyrtec Syrup (Less than 2%) 1920
Zyrtec Tablets (Less than 2%) 1920
Zyrtec-D 12 Hour Extended Release Tablets (Less than 2%) 1923

Polyps, rectal
Lialda Tablets (Infrequent) 3029

Polyradiculoneuropathy
Campath Ampules 761
Cuprimine Capsules 1986

Polyserositis
Avastin IV (Rare) 1192

Polyuria
Abilify Injection (Greater than or equal to 1 in 1000 patients and less than 1 in 100 patients) 881
Abilify Injection (Greater than or equal to 1 in 1000 patients and less than 1 in 100 patients) 2466
Abilify Oral Solution (Greater than or equal to 1 in 1000 patients and less than 1 in 100 patients) 881
Abilify Oral Solution (Greater than or equal to 1 in 1000 patients and less than 1 in 100 patients) 2466
Abilify Discmelt Orally Disintegrating Tablets (Greater than or equal to 1 in 1000 patients and less than 1 in 100 patients) 881
Abilify Discmelt Orally Disintegrating Tablets (Greater than or equal to 1 in 1000 patients and less than 1 in 100 patients) 2466
Abilify Tablets (Greater than or equal to 1 in 1000 patients and less than 1 in 100 patients) 881
Abilify Tablets (Greater than or equal to 1 in 1000 patients and less than 1 in 100 patients) 2466
Ambien Tablets (Rare) 2692
Ambien CR Tablets (Rare) 2696
Amerge Tablets (Infrequent) 1301
Anaprox Tablets (Less than 1%) 2632
Anaprox DS Tablets (Less than 1%) .. 2632
Anzemet Injection (Rare).................. 2701
Anzemet Tablets (Rare).................... 2704
Aricept Tablets (Infrequent).............. 1062
Aricept ODT Tablets (Infrequent)....... 1062
Atripla Tablets.................................. 938
▲ Avastin IV (3% to 6%) 1192
▲ Betaseron for SC Injection (7%) 756
Calcijex Injection.............................. 419
Campral Tablets (Rare)..................... 1158
Captopril Tablets (Approximately 1 to 2 of 1000 patients).................. 2182
Cardene I.V. (1.4%).......................... 1093
Cardizem LA Extended Release Tablets (Less than 2%)................. 421
Celexa (Frequent)............................. 1160
Chantix Tablets (Frequent)............... 2511
Cipro I.V. (1% or less)...................... 2817
Cipro (Less than 1%)........................ 2810
Cipro XR Tablets.............................. 2823
Coreg Tablets (Greater than 0.1% to 1%) 1387
Cymbalta Delayed-Release Capsules (Infrequent) 1801
EC-Naprosyn Delayed-Release Tablets (Less than 1%) 2632
Effexor XR Extended-Release Capsules (Infrequent) 3195
Elspar for Injection (Low) 1990
Emsam Transdermal System (Frequent) 905
Evoxac Capsules (0.1%) 1013
Exelon Capsules (Infrequent) 2229
Exelon Oral Solution (Infrequent) 2229
Exforge Tablets (Less than or equal to 0.1%)................................. 2238
Frova Tablets (Infrequent) 1111
Gabitril Tablets (Infrequent) 973
Gengraf Capsules (1% to less than 3%) 435
Geodon Capsules (Infrequent) 2520
▲ Indapamide Tablets (Less than 5%) 2188
▲ Intron A for Injection (Less than 5%) 2859
Klonopin (Infrequent) 2639
Lamictal (Infrequent) 1488
Luvox CR Extended-Release Capsules (2%) 1759
Maxalt Tablets (Infrequent) 2056
Maxalt-MLT Orally Disintegrating Tablets (Infrequent) 2056
Naprosyn Suspension (Less than 1%) 2632
Naprosyn Tablets (Less than 1%) 2632
Neoral Oral Solution (1% to less than 3%) 2280
Neoral Soft Gelatin Capsules (1% to less than 3%)............................ 2280
Nexium Delayed-Release Capsules (Less than 1%) 645
Nexium I.V. (Less than 1%) 652
Nexium Delayed-Release Oral Suspension (Less than 1%) 645
Norvir (Less than 2%) 489
OxyContin Tablets (Less than 1%) 2589
Paxil (Infrequent) 1535
Paxil CR Controlled-Release Tablets (Infrequent) 1544
Primaxin I.M. 2080
Primaxin I.V. (Less than 0.2%) 2083
Prozac Weekly Capsules (Infrequent) 1852
Prozac Pulvules and Liquid (At least 2%) 1852
▲ Rebif Prefilled Syringe for Injection (2% to 7%) 1107
Remeron Tablets (Rare) 2924
RemeronSolTab Tablets (Rare) 2927
Requip Tablets (Infrequent) 1561
Retrovir Capsules 1574
Retrovir IV Infusion 1579
Retrovir 1574
Rocaltrol Capsules 1150
Rocaltrol Oral Solution 1150
Stalevo Tablets 2309
Symbyax Capsules (Infrequent) 1871
Tarka Tablets (Less frequent) 511
Teveten Tablets (Less than 1%) 515
Teveten HCT Tablets (Less than 1%) 517
Tricor Tablets 520
Truvada Tablets 1262
▲ Vaprisol (4.9%) 632
Venlafaxine Hydrochloride Tablets (Infrequent) 2199
Voltaren Tablets (Occasionally) 2334
Voltaren-XR Tablets (Occasionally) 2337
Wellbutrin SR Sustained-Release Tablets (Infrequent) 1653
Wellbutrin XL Extended-Release Tablets (Infrequent) 1659
Xifaxan Tablets (Less than 2%) 2682

Zomig Tablets (Infrequent) 694
Zomig Nasal Spray (Infrequent) 689
Zomig-ZMT Tablets (Infrequent) 694
Zonegran Capsules (Infrequent) 1089
Zyban Sustained-Release Tablets (Infrequent) 1692
Zyprexa Tablets (Infrequent) 1883
Zyprexa ZYDIS Orally Disintegrating Tablets (Infrequent) 1883
Zyrtec Chewable Tablets (Less than 2%) 1920
Zyrtec Syrup (Less than 2%) 1920
Zyrtec Tablets (Less than 2%) 1920
Zyrtec-D 12 Hour Extended Release Tablets (Less than 2%) 1923

Porphyria
Luvox CR Extended-Release Capsules 1759
Mircette Tablets 1034
NuvaRing 2897
Ortho-Cyclen Tablets 2449
Ortho Evra Transdermal System 2437
Ortho Tri-Cyclen Tablets 2449
Ortho Tri-Cyclen Lo Tablets 2458
Paxil 1535
Paxil CR Controlled-Release Tablets 1544
Sulfamylon Cream (A single case) 2194
Sulfamylon for 5% Topical Solution 2194
Yaz Tablets 805

Porphyria, aggravation of
Activella Tablets 2347
Angeliq Tablets 751
Climara Transdermal System 763
Climara Pro Transdermal System 768
Divigel 3167
Enjuvia Tablets 1029
Epogen for Injection (Rare) 576
Estratest Tablets 3043
Estratest H.S. Tablets 3043
Phenytek Capsules (Isolated reports) 2192
Premarin Intravenous 3217
Premarin Vaginal Cream 3228
Premphase Tablets 3232
Prempro Tablets 3232
Procrit for Injection (Rare) 2391
Zantac 25 EFFERdose Tablets (Rare) 1670
Zantac Injection (Rare) 1666
Zantac (Rare) 1670

Porphyria, cutaneous, drug-induced
Photofrin for Injection 708

Porphyria, exacerbation of
Climara Transdermal System 763
Lybrel Tablets 3204
Premarin Tablets 3221
Seasonique Tablets 1046
Yaz Tablets 805

Porphyria, hepatic
Avandaryl Tablets 1344
Duetact Tablets 3085

Porphyria, intermittent, acute
Carbatrol Capsules 3019
Depakote ER Tablets 423
Equetro Extended-Release Capsules 3174

Porphyria cutanea tarda
Anaprox Tablets (Less than 1%) 2632
Anaprox DS Tablets (Less than 1%) 2632
Avandaryl Tablets 1344
Duetact Tablets (Less than 1%) 3085
EC-Naprosyn Delayed-Release Tablets (Less than 1%) 2632
Myleran Tablets (Rare) 1530
Naprosyn Suspension (Less than 1%) 2632
Naprosyn Tablets (Less than 1%) 2632

Postnasal drip
Mirapex Tablets 857
Patanase Nasal Spray (1.5%) 544

Potassium loss
(*see under* Hypokalemia)

Potassium retention
(*see under* Hyperkalemia)

Pre syncope
Rythmol Tablets (2%) 1586

Precocious puberty
Premarin Vaginal Cream 3228

Pregnancy, accidental
Emsam Transdermal System (Infrequent) 905
Tricor Tablets 520
Zomig Tablets (Rare) 694
Zomig Nasal Spray (Rare) 689
Zomig-ZMT Tablets (Rare) 694

Pregnancy, ectopic
Mirena Intrauterine System 779
ParaGard T 380A Intrauterine Copper Contraceptive 1041

Pregnancy, intrauterine
ParaGard T 380A Intrauterine Copper Contraceptive 1041

Pregnancy, prolonged
Aggrenox Capsules 819
Bayer Aspirin 750
Percodan Tablets 1130

Pregnancy tests, false positive
Thioridazine Hydrochloride Tablets 2195
Thiothixene Capsules 2197

Premature ventricular contractions
Imitrex Injection (Infrequent) 1465
Prinivil Tablets (0.3% to 1%) 2087
Prinzide Tablets 2092
Rythmol Tablets (0.7% to 2%) 1586
Tarka Tablets (0.3% or more) 511

Premenstrual syndrome
Requip Tablets (Infrequent) 1561

Premenstrual-like syndrome
Activella Tablets 2347
Estratest Tablets 3043
Estratest H.S. Tablets 3043
Lexapro Oral Suspension (Infrequent) 1174
Lexapro Tablets (Infrequent) 1174
Luvox CR Extended-Release Capsules (Infrequent) 1759
Lybrel Tablets 3204
Mircette Tablets 1034
NuvaRing 2897
Ortho-Cyclen Tablets 2449
Ortho Evra Transdermal System 2437
Ortho Tri-Cyclen Tablets 2449
Ortho Tri-Cyclen Lo Tablets 2458
Premarin Intravenous 3217
Premarin Vaginal Cream 3228
Premphase Tablets 3232
Prempro Tablets 3232
Seasonique Tablets 1046
Yaz Tablets 805
Zyprexa Tablets (2%) 1883
Zyprexa ZYDIS Orally Disintegrating Tablets (2%) 1883

Pressor response, paradoxical
Zyrtec-D 12 Hour Extended Release Tablets 1923

Priapism
Abilify Injection (Less than 1 in 1000 patients) 881
Abilify Injection (Less than 1 in 1000 patients) 2466
Abilify Oral Solution (Less than 1 in 1000 patients) 881
Abilify Oral Solution (Less than 1 in 1000 patients) 2466
Abilify Discmelt Orally Disintegrating Tablets (Less than 1 in 1000 patients) 881
Abilify Discmelt Orally Disintegrating Tablets (Less than 1 in 1000 patients) 2466
Abilify Tablets (Less than 1 in 1000 patients) 881
Abilify Tablets (Less than 1 in 1000 patients) 2466
AndroGel 3159
Bicillin C-R Injectable Suspension 1775
Bicillin L-A Injection 1777
Celexa 1160
Cialis Tablets (Less than 2%) 1792
Copaxone for Injection (Infrequent) 3110
▲ Edex Injection (Less than 1% to 4%) 2957
Effexor XR Extended-Release Capsules (Rare) 3195
Flomax Capsules (Rare) 848
Geodon (Rare) 2520
Invega Extended-Release Tablets 1748
Levitra Tablets (Less than 2%) 2876
Lexapro Oral Suspension 1174
Lexapro Tablets 1174
Luvox CR Extended-Release Capsules 1759
Mirapex Tablets 857
Moban Tablets 1116
Paxil 1535
Paxil CR Controlled-Release Tablets 1544
Prozac Weekly Capsules (Rare) 1852
Prozac Pulvules and Liquid (Rare) 1852
Rilutek Tablets (Infrequent) 2771
Risperdal Consta Long-Acting Injection (Rare) 1753
Stalevo Tablets 2309
Strattera Capsules (Rare) 1864
Testim 1% Gel (1% or less) 701
Thioridazine Hydrochloride Tablets 2195
Uroxatral Tablets 2786
Zyprexa Tablets 1883
Zyprexa ZYDIS Orally Disintegrating Tablets 1883

Proarrhythmia
▲ Rythmol Tablets (1% to 5%) 1586

Proctalgia
Remicade for IV Injection (Greater than or equal to 0.2%) 950

Proctitis
Cosmegen for Injection 2485
Doxil Injection (Less than 1%) 2378
Effexor XR Extended-Release Capsules (Rare) 3195
▲ Eloxatin for Injection (2% to less than 5%) 2731
Indocin Capsules (Less than 1%) 2024
Indocin I.V. (Less than 1%) 2489
Indocin (Less than 1%) 2024
Rilutek Tablets (Rare) 2771
Venlafaxine Hydrochloride Tablets (Rare) 2199

Proctitis, ulceration
Doxil Injection (Less than 1%) 2378

Proctitis herpes
Selzentry Tablets 2534

Prolactin levels, elevated
(*see under* Hyperprolactinemia)

Prolactinemia
Celexa 1160
Lexapro Oral Suspension 1174
Lexapro Tablets 1174

Proptosis
Ortho-Cyclen/Ortho Tri-Cyclen 2449
Ortho Tri-Cyclen Lo Tablets 2458
Premphase Tablets 3232
Prempro Tablets 3232

Prostate disorders, unspecified
▲ AndroGel (3% to 5%) 3159
Atrovent Nasal Spray 0.03% 834
Atrovent Nasal Spray 0.06% 836
Avalide Tablets 892
Avalide Tablets 2713
Avapro Tablets (Less than 1%) 897
Avapro Tablets (Less than 1%) 2718
▲ Betaseron for SC Injection (3%) 756
Celebrex Capsules (0.1% to 1.9%) 2979
▲ CellCept Capsules (3% to less than 20%) 2622
▲ CellCept Intravenous (3% to less than 20%) 2622
▲ CellCept Oral Suspension (3% to less than 20%) 2622
▲ CellCept Tablets (3% to less than 20%) 2622
Edex Injection (1%) 2957
Evoxac Capsules (Less than 1%) 1013
Protonix for Delayed-Release Oral Suspension (Less than 1%) 3254
Protonix Delayed-Release Tablets (Less than 1%) 3254
Protonix I.V. (Less than 1%) 3257
Requip Tablets (Infrequent) 1561
Testim 1% Gel (1%) 701
▲ Travatan Z Ophthalmic Solution (1% to 5%) 547
Tricor Tablets 520
Venlafaxine Hydrochloride Tablets (Frequent) 2199
Viadur Implant (Less than 2%) 802
▲ Visudyne for Injection (1% to 10%) 2332
Wellbutrin SR Sustained-Release Tablets (Infrequent) 1653
Wellbutrin XL Extended-Release Tablets (Infrequent) 1659
Zyban Sustained-Release Tablets 1692

Prostate enlargement
▲ AndroGel (11.7%) 3159
Venlafaxine Hydrochloride Tablets (Frequent) 2199

Prostate specific antigen decrease
▲ Avodart Soft Gelatin Capsules (Approximately 40% to 50%) 1359

Prostate specific antigen increase
Rythmol SR Capsules 1590

Prostatic acid phosphatase, decreased
▲ Lupron Depot 7.5 mg (Greater than or equal to 5%) 469

Prostatic acid phosphatase, increased
▲ Lupron Depot 7.5 mg (Greater than or equal to 5%) 469
Vantas (Less than 2%) 1737

Prostatic hypertrophy
Aricept Tablets (Infrequent) 1062
Aricept ODT Tablets (Infrequent) 1062
Eldepryl Capsules 3052
Testim 1% Gel (1% or less) 701
▲ Vesanoid Capsules (3%) 2660

Prostatism
Rythmol SR Capsules 1590

Prostatitis
Effexor XR Extended-Release Capsules (Infrequent) 3195
Mirapex Tablets 857
ReoPro Vials (0.1%) 1860
Requip Tablets (Infrequent) 1561
▲ Strattera Capsules (3%) 1864
Tice BCG (Less than or equal to 1%) 2936
Venlafaxine Hydrochloride Tablets (Frequent) 2199

Prostration
Bicillin C-R Injectable Suspension 1775
Bicillin L-A Injection 1777

Protein bound iodine, lowered
(*see under* PBI decrease)

Proteinuria
Accutane Capsules 2607
Aceon Tablets (2 mg, 4 mg, 8 mg) (1% to 1.5%) 3038
Aggrenox Capsules 819
Aldara Cream, 5% 1699
Anaprox Tablets (Less than 1%) 2632
Anaprox DS Tablets (Less than 1%) 2632
Atripla Tablets 938
▲ Avastin IV (3% to 36%) 1192
Bayer Aspirin 750
Bicillin C-R Injectable Suspension 1775
Bicillin L-A Injection 1777
Captopril Tablets (Approximately 1 of 100 patients) 2182
Celebrex Capsules 2979
Clinoril Tablets (Less than 1 in 100) 1962
Crestor Tablets 677
Cubicin for Injection (Less than 1%) 995
▲ Cuprimine Capsules (6%) 1986
EC-Naprosyn Delayed-Release Tablets (Less than 1%) 2632
Elspar for Injection (Infrequent) 1990
▲ Emend Capsules (6.8%) 1992
▲ Emend for Injection (6.8%) 1999
Exjade Tablets 2244
▲ Fabrazyme for Intravenous Infusion (5%) 1241
▲ Gemzar for Injection (2% to 45%) 1820
Gris-PEG Tablets (Rare) 2507
Indocin (Less than 1%) 2024
▲ Intron A for Injection (Less than 5%) 2859
Kepivance (9 patients) 583
Mirapex Tablets 857
Naprosyn Suspension (Less than 1%) 2632
Naprosyn Tablets (Less than 1%) 2632
Neupogen for Injection (Infrequent) 589
▲ Novantrone for Injection Concentrate (6%) 1100
Percocet Tablets 1127
Percodan Tablets 1130
Primaxin I.M. 2080
Primaxin I.V. 2083
▲ Pristiq Extended-Release Tablets (5% to 8%) 3247
Prozac Weekly Capsules 1852
Prozac Pulvules and Liquid 1852
▲ Rapamune (9.2%) 3260
Requip Tablets (Infrequent) 1561
Rythmol SR Capsules 1590

St. Joseph 81 mg Aspirin Chewable and Enteric Coated Tablets 1903
Sutent Capsules 2540
Tarka Tablets (Less frequent) 511
Truvada Tablets 1262
Vaqta (Isolated reports) 2130
Voltaren Tablets (Occasionally) 2334
Voltaren-XR Tablets (Occasionally) 2337
Xifaxan Tablets (Less than 2%) 2682
Xyrem Oral Solution (Infrequent) 1766
▲ Zolinza Capsules (51.4%) 2142
Zometa for Intravenous Infusion 2341
Zosyn for Injection 3284

Proteinuria, increased
▲ Chemet Capsules (Up to 3.7%) 2484
Noroxin Tablets (1%) 2069
Omnicef Capsules (2%) 497
Omnicef for Oral Suspension (1%) 497
Requip Tablets (Infrequent) 1561

Prothrombin, decrease
(*see under* Hypoprothrombinemia)

Prothrombin, increase
(*see under* Hyperprothrombinemia)

Prothrombin time, elevation
Advicor Tablets 402
St. Joseph 81 mg Aspirin Chewable and Enteric Coated Tablets 1903

Prothrombin time, increase
(*see under* Prothrombin time prolongation)

Prothrombin time prolongation
Aggrenox Capsules 819
Avelox (Greater than or equal to 0.1% to less than 2%) 2803
Bayer Aspirin 750
Biaxin/Biaxin XL (1%) 411
Busulfex Injection (2%) 2477
Ceftin 1380
▲ CellCept Capsules (3% to less than 20%) 2622
▲ CellCept Intravenous (3% to less than 20%) 2622
▲ CellCept Oral Suspension (3% to less than 20%) 2622
▲ CellCept Tablets (3% to less than 20%) 2622
Cipro I.V. 2817
Cipro 2810
Cipro XR Tablets 2823
Clinoril Tablets 1962
Cubicin for Injection (Less than 1%) 995
Elmiron Capsules (Less than or equal to 1%) 2435
▲ Eloxatin for Injection (2% to less than 5%) 2731
Elspar for Injection 2488
Fortaz 1450
Invanz for Injection (0.3% to 1.2%) 2029
Levaquin 2416
Levaquin in 5% Dextrose Injection 2416
Limbrel Capsules 2561
Niaspan Extended-Release Tablets 480
Noroxin Tablets 2069
Oncaspar Injection 1138
Ortho-Cyclen/Ortho Tri-Cyclen 2449
Ortho Tri-Cyclen Lo Tablets 2458
Panhematin for Injection 2497
Percodan Tablets 1130
Primaxin I.M. 2080
Primaxin I.V. 2083
Rocephin Injectable Vials, ADD-Vantage, Galaxy, Bulk (Less than 1%) 2642
Suprax for Oral Suspension (Rare) 1891
Suprax Tablets (Rare) 1891
Testim 1% Gel (1% or less) 701
Timentin ADD-Vantage 1606
Timentin Injection Galaxy Container 1609
Timentin IV Infusion 1603
Timentin Pharmacy Bulk Package 1613
Tygacil for Injection (0% to less than 2%) 3276
Zinacef for Injection 1678
Zinacef Injection 1678
Zosyn for Injection 3284

Prothrombin time, decrease
Avelox (Less than 0.1% to greater than or equal to 2%) 2803
Celexa 1160
Cipro I.V. 2817
Cipro 2810
Limbrel Capsules 2561
Premarin Tablets 3221
Premphase Tablets 3232
Prempro Tablets 3232

Protrusion, implant area
▲ Supprelin LA Implant (51.1%) 1731

Prurigo
Intelence Tablets (Less than 2%) 3119
Lialda Tablets (Infrequent) 3029

Pruritus
Abelcet Injection 1134
Abilify Injection (Greater than or equal to 1 in 1000 patients and less than 1 in 100 patients) 881
Abilify Injection (Greater than or equal to 1 in 1000 patients and less than 1 in 100 patients) 2466
Abilify Oral Solution (Greater than or equal to 1 in 1000 patients and less than 1 in 100 patients) 881
Abilify Oral Solution (Greater than or equal to 1 in 1000 patients and less than 1 in 100 patients) 2466
Abilify Discmelt Orally Disintegrating Tablets (Greater than or equal to 1 in 1000 patients and less than 1 in 100 patients) 881
Abilify Discmelt Orally Disintegrating Tablets (Greater than or equal to 1 in 1000 patients and less than 1 in 100 patients) 2466
Abilify Tablets (Greater than or equal to 1 in 1000 patients and less than 1 in 100 patients) 881
Abilify Tablets (Greater than or equal to 1 in 1000 patients and less than 1 in 100 patients) 2466
Accolate Tablets 669
Accutane Capsules 2607
Aceon Tablets (2 mg, 4 mg, 8 mg) (0.3% to 1%) 3038
▲ Acetadote Injection (0.2% to 20.8%) 1001
▲ Actiq (Up to 5%) 959
Activella Tablets 2347
▲ Actonel with Calcium Tablets (1.9% to 3%) 2574
Advair HFA 45/21 Inhalation Aerosol 1288
Advair HFA 115/21 Inhalation Aerosol 1288
Advair HFA 230/21 Inhalation Aerosol 1288
Advate (0.6%) 721
▲ Advicor Tablets (7%) 402
▲ Aerobid/Aerobid-M (3% to 9%) 1153
Aggrenox Capsules (Less than 1%) 819
▲ Agrylin Capsules (5.5%) 3017
Aldara Cream, 5% (More than 1%) 1699
Alferon N Injection (2%) 1726
Alinia for Oral Suspension (Less than 1%) 2677
Alinia Tablets (Less than 1%) 2677
Allegra Oral Solution (Rare) 2684
Allegra Tablets (Rare) 2684
Allegra-D 12 Hour Extended-Release Tablets (Rare) 2687
Allegra-D 24 Hour Extended-Release Tablets (Rare) 2690
Alphanate 1709
Altabax Ointment (1.5%) 1299
Ambien Tablets (Infrequent) 2692
▲ AmBisome for Injection (10.8%) 606
Amerge Tablets (Infrequent) 1301
Amevive (Common) 611
Amrix Capsules 966
Analpram-HC 1140
▲ Anaprox Tablets (3% to 9%) 2632
▲ Anaprox DS Tablets (3% to 9%) 2632
AndroGel (1.9%) 3159
Angeliq Tablets 751
▲ Anzemet Injection (3.1%) 2701
▲ Anzemet Tablets (3.1%) 2704
Apidra Injection 2706
Aptivus Capsules (Less than 2%) 823
Aptivus Oral Solution (Less than 2%) 823
Aralast (0.1%) 726
▲ Aranesp for Injection (8%) 564
Aricept Tablets (Frequent) 1062
Aricept ODT Tablets (Frequent) 1062
▲ Arimidex Tablets (2% to 5%) 672
▲ Asacol Delayed-Release Tablets (3%) 2579
Atacand Tablets 639
Atacand HCT (0.5% or greater) 642
Atripla Tablets (Greater than or equal to 2%) 938
Augmentin 1323
Augmentin Tablets 1327
Augmentin XR Extended Release Tablets 1333
Augmentin ES-600 Powder for Oral Suspension 1329
Avalide Tablets 892
Avalide Tablets 2713
Avandamet Tablets 1336
Avandaryl Tablets (Less than 1%) 1344
Avandia Tablets 1351
Avapro Tablets (Less than 1%) 897
Avapro Tablets (Less than 1%) 2718
Avelox (Greater than or equal to 0.1% to less than 2%) 2803
Avodart Soft Gelatin Capsules 1359
Axert Tablets (Rare) 2431
Axid Capsules (1.7%) 1364
Azor Tablets 1005
Bactroban Cream (Less than 1%) 1366
Bactroban Nasal (1%) 1367
Bactroban Ointment (1%) 1368
Benicar Tablets 1009
Benicar HCT Tablets (Rare) 1010
Bentyl Capsules 703
Bentyl Injection 703
Bentyl Syrup 703
Bentyl Tablets 703
▲ Benzaclin Topical Gel (12%) 2721
Betaseron for SC Injection 756
▲ Bexxar (0% to 10%) 1371
Bicillin C-R Injectable Suspension 1775
Bicillin L-A Injection 1777
▲ BOTOX Purified Neurotoxin Complex (3% to 10%) 550
▲ Busulfex Injection (28%) 2477
Byetta Injection 600
Bystolic Tablets 1155
Calcijex Injection 419
▲ Campral Tablets (3% to 4%) 1158
▲ Cancidas for Injection (5.4% to 7%) 1953
Captopril Tablets (About 2 of 100 patients) 2182
Carafate Suspension (Less than 0.5%) 706
Carafate Tablets (Less than 0.5%) 707
Cardizem LA Extended Release Tablets (Less than 2%) 421
Catapres Tablets (About 7 in 1,000 patients) 841
▲ Catapres-TTS (51 of 101 patients) 842
Ceftin (0.1% to 1%) 1380
Celebrex Capsules (0.1% to 1.9%) 2979
Celexa (Frequent) 1160
▲ CellCept Capsules (3% to less than 20%) 2622
▲ CellCept Intravenous (3% to less than 20%) 2622
▲ CellCept Oral Suspension (3% to less than 20%) 2622
▲ CellCept Tablets (3% to less than 20%) 2622
▲ Cerezyme for Injection (Approximately 6.6%) 1238
Chantix Tablets (0% to 1%) 2511
▲ Chemet Capsules (2.6% to 11.2%) 2484
Cialis Tablets (Less than 2%) 1792
Cipro I.V. (1% or less) 2817
Cipro (Less than 1%) 2810
Cipro XR Tablets 2823
Clarinex Syrup (Rare) 2828
Clarinex Tablets (Rare) 2828
Clarinex Reditabs Tablets (Rare) 2828
Clarinex-D 12-Hour Extended-Release Tablets (Rare) 2831
Clarinex-D 24-Hour Extended-Release Tablets 2834
▲ Climara Transdermal System (0.5% to 6%) 763
Climara Pro Transdermal System 768
Clinoril Tablets (Greater than 1%) 1962
Clorpres Tablets (About 7 in 1,000) 2185
Combigan Ophthalmic Solution 553
Combivent Inhalation Aerosol 845
Comvax 1966
Concerta Extended-Release Tablets 1925
▲ Copaxone for Injection (18%) 3110
Coreg Tablets (Greater than 0.1% to 1%) 1387
Coreg CR Extended-Release Capsules (0.1% to less than or equal to 1%) 1393
Cosopt Sterile Ophthalmic Solution 1969
Cozaar Tablets (Less than 1%) 1973
Crestor Tablets 677
Crinone 4% Gel 992
Crinone 8% Gel 992
▲ Crixivan Capsules (4.2%) 1979
▲ Cubicin for Injection (2.8% to 5.8%) 995
Cuprimine Capsules 1986
Cyanokit 5g Antidote 1021
▲ Cymbalta Delayed-Release Capsules (3%) 1801
▲ Dacogen Injection (11%) 1066
Dantrium Capsules (Less frequent) 2580
Denavir Cream 2205
▲ Depakote ER Tablets (Greater than 1% to 5%) 423
DepoCyt Injection (2%) 1136
▲ DepoDur Injection (Greater than 10%) 1095
Didronel Tablets 2583
Diovan Tablets (Greater than 0.2%) 2212
Diovan HCT Tablets (Less frequent) 2216
Diprolene Lotion 0.05% (Less than 1%) 2838
Diprolene Ointment 0.05% (Less than 1%) 2839
Diprolene AF Cream 0.05% (Infrequent) 2837
Divigel 3167
▲ Doribax Injection (Less than 1% to 3%) 2400
▲ Doxil Injection (1% to 10%) 2378
Duetact Tablets (Less than 1%) 3085
▲ Duragesic Transdermal System (1% to 10%) 2405
Durezol Ophthalmic Emulsion (Less than 1%) ⊙275
DynaCirc CR Controlled Release Tablets (0.5% to 1%) 1407
▲ EC-Naprosyn Delayed-Release Tablets (3% to 9%) 2632
Effexor XR Extended-Release Capsules (Frequent) 3195
Eligard 7.5 mg (1.4%) 2724
▲ Eligard 22.5 mg (0.4% to 2.6%) 2724
Eligard 30 mg 2724
Eligard 45 mg 2724
Elmiron Capsules (Less than or equal to 1%) 2435
▲ Elocon Cream 0.1% (1.6% to approximately 7%) 2840
Elocon Lotion 0.1% (1 in 209 patients) 2841
▲ Elocon Ointment 0.1% (4.8% to approximately 7%) 2842
▲ Eloxatin for Injection (2% to 6%) 2731
Emend Capsules 1992
Emend for Injection 1999
Emsam Transdermal System (Frequent) 905
▲ Emtriva Capsules (17% to 30%) 1246
▲ Emtriva Oral Solution (17% to 30%) 1246
Enablex Extended-Release Tablets (Greater than or equal to 1%) 2225
Enbrel for Injection 569
Engerix-B Vaccine (Less than 1%) 1409
Enjuvia Tablets 1029
▲ Epivir (Less than 1% to 15%) 1412
Epivir-HBV 1417
▲ Epogen for Injection (16% to 22%) 576
▲ Equetro Extended-Release Capsules (5% to 8%) 3174
▲ Erbitux (0% to 40%) 912
Estratest Tablets 3043
Estratest H.S. Tablets 3043
▲ Evoxac Capsules (1% to 3%) 1013
Exelon Patch (Frequent) 2233
Exforge Tablets (Greater than or equal to 0.2%) 2238
Extina Foam, 2% (Less than or equal to 1%) 3057
▲ Fabrazyme for Intravenous Infusion (8%) 1241
Fansidar Tablets 2636
Femara Tablets (1% to 2%) 2246
Fentora Tablets (Greater than 1%) 968
▲ Finacea Gel (1% to 6%) 1742
Fleet Phospho-soda (Rare) 1145
Fleet Phospho-soda EZ-PREP (Rare) 1147
Fleet Prep Kits 1149
▲ Flolan for Injection (4%) 1426
Flomax Capsules 848
Flonase Nasal Spray 1431
▲ Flovent Diskus 50 mcg (1% to 6%) 1435
Flovent HFA 1440
Fluarix Vaccine 1446
Flulaval Injection Vaccine 1448
Fluorescite Injection ⊙203
Foradil Aerolizer (1.5%) 2849
Fortaz (2%) 1450
Fosamax 2005

Fosamax Plus D Tablets 2013
Fragmin Injection (Rare) 1070
Frova Tablets (Infrequent) 1111
Furosemide Tablets 2186
Gabitril Tablets (2%) 973
▲ Gammagard Liquid (0.61% to 6.5%) 730
▲ Gamunex (4%) 3094
Gantrisin Pediatric Suspension 2638
▲ Gemzar for Injection (13%) 1820
Gengraf Capsules (1% to less than 3%) 435
▲ Gleevec Tablets (8% to 14%) 2255
Havrix Injection Vaccine (Less than 1%) 1454
Hepsera Tablets 1253
Hexalen Capsules 1078
Humalog-Pen and KwikPen (Less common) 1829
Humalog Mix 50/50-Pen and KwikPen 1833
Humalog Mix 75/25-Pen and KwikPen 1835
▲ Hyalgan Solution (7%) 2742
▲ Hycamtin for Injection (Rare to 16%) 1459
Imitrex Injection (Infrequent) 1465
Imitrex Nasal Spray (Infrequent) 1470
Imitrex Tablets (Infrequent) 1474
Indocin (Less than 1%) 2024
Infanrix Vaccine 1479
▲ Intron A for Injection (Up to 11%) 2859
Invanz for Injection (1% to 2%) 2029
▲ Ionsys Transdermal System (6%) 2410
▲ Ixempra Kit for Injection (6%) 915
Kaletra (Less than 2%) 452
▲ Kepivance (35%) 583
Keppra Oral Solution (2%) 3131
Keppra Tablets (2%) 3131
Ketek Tablets (Less than 0.2%) 2744
Kinrix Injection Vaccine 1486
Klonopin (Infrequent) 2639
Kogenate FS 746
Kogenate FS with Bio-Set (1 case) 748
▲ Lamictal (2% to 3%) 1488
▲ Lamisil Oral Granules (1% to 3%) 2264
Lamisil Tablets (2.8%) 2266
Lantus Injection 2749
Lescol Capsules 2268
Lescol XL Tablets 2268
▲ Leukine (23%) 774
▲ Leustatin Injection (6%) 2384
Levaquin (1%) 2416
Levaquin in 5% Dextrose Injection (1%) 2416
Levemir Injection 2352
Levitra Tablets (Less than 2%) 2876
Levothroid Tablets 1170
Levoxyl Tablets 1780
Lexapro Oral Suspension (Infrequent) 1174
Lexapro Tablets (Infrequent) 1174
▲ Lexiva Oral Suspension (Up to 8%) 1510
▲ Lexiva Tablets (Up to 8%) 1510
Lialda Tablets (0.6% to 1.1%) 3029
Lipitor Tablets (Less than 2%) 2501
Lortab 5/500 Tablets 3143
Lortab 7.5/500 Tablets 3144
Lortab 10/500 Tablets 3144
Lotrisone 2881
Lovaza Capsules 1520
Lovenox Injection 2756
▲ Lunesta Tablets (1% to 4%) 2994
▲ Luxiq Foam (2% to 44%) 3058
Lyrica Capsules (Greater than or equal to 1%) 2527
▲ Malarone Pediatric Tablets (1% to 6%) 1521
▲ Malarone Tablets (1% to 6%) 1521
Mavik Tablets (0.3% to 1%) 472
Maxair Autohaler 1705
Maxalt Tablets (Infrequent) 2056
Maxalt-MLT Orally Disintegrating Tablets (Infrequent) 2056
▲ Megace ES Oral Suspension (1% to 3%) 2499
▲ Mepron Suspension (5%) 1526
Meridia Capsules (Greater than or equal to 1%) 475
Merrem I.V. (1.2%) 684
Meruvax II 2061
▲ Mevacor Tablets (0.5% to 5.2%) 2063
Miacalcin Nasal Spray (Less than 1%) 2274
Micardis Tablets (More than 0.3%) 852
Micardis HCT Tablets (Less than 2%) 854
Mirapex Tablets 857
M-M-R II 2054
Mobic Oral Suspension (0% to 2.4%) 863
Mobic Tablets (0% to 2.4%) 863
MS Contin Tablets (Less frequent) 2585
▲ Mycamine for Injection (6.1% to 17.6%) 616
▲ Myfortic Tablets (3% to less than 20%) 2276
▲ Mylotarg for Injection (4% to 10%) 3212
Nadolol Tablets (1 to 5 of 1000 patients) 2191
Naftin Cream (2%) 2164
Naftin Gel (1%) 2164
▲ Nalfon Capsules (4.2%) 2508
Namenda (Infrequent) 1180
▲ Naprosyn Suspension (3% to 9%) 2632
▲ Naprosyn Tablets (3% to 9%) 2632
Natrecor for Injection (Greater than or equal to 1%) 2977
Neoral Oral Solution (1% to less than 3%) 2280
Neoral Soft Gelatin Capsules (1% to less than 3%) 2280
Neosporin Ophthalmic Solution Sterile ⊙ 252
Neupro Transdermal System 3149
▲ Nexavar Tablets (14% to 19%) 784
▲ Niaspan Extended-Release Tablets (1% to 6%) 480
Nimotop Capsules (Less than 1%) 790
Noroxin Tablets (0.3% to 1%) 2069
Norvir (Less than 2%) 489
NovoLog Injection 2359
NovoSeven (1%) 2367
NovoSeven RT (1%) 2370
▲ Noxafil Oral Suspension (1% to 11%) 2889
Olux Foam (Less than 2%) 3061
Omnicef Capsules (0.2%) 497
Omnicef for Oral Suspension (0.2%) 497
▲ Ontak Vials (20%) 1079
▲ Opana Tablets (9%) 1117
▲ Opana ER Tablets (0% to 15.2%) 1121
Orencia Powder for Intravenous Infusion (Greater than 0.1% and less than or equal to 1%) 921
Orthoclone OKT3 Sterile Solution 2387
OsmoPrep Tablets (Rare) 2680
▲ OxyContin Tablets (13%) 2589
OxyIR Capsules 2593
▲ Panretin Gel 0.1% (4% to 11%) 1081
▲ Patanol Ophthalmic Solution (Less than 5%) 546
Paxil (Frequent) 1535
Paxil CR Controlled-Release Tablets (Frequent) 1544
Pediarix Vaccine 1552
▲ PegIntron Powder for Injection (12%) 2903
Pentasa Capsules (Less than 1%) 3030
Pepcid Tablets (Infrequent) 2075
Percocet Tablets 1127
Percodan Tablets 1130
Persantine Tablets 869
PhosLo GelCaps (Isolated cases) 1184
▲ Photofrin for Injection (4%) 708
▲ Plavix Tablets (3.3%) 926
▲ Plavix Tablets (3.3%) 2767
Pletal Tablets 2481
Pramosone 1141
Premarin Intravenous 3217
▲ Premarin Tablets (4% to 5%) 3221
Premarin Vaginal Cream 3228
▲ Premphase Tablets (5% to 10%) 3232
▲ Prempro Tablets (5% to 10%) 3232
Prevnar 3241
Primaxin I.M. 2080
Primaxin I.V. (0.3%) 2083
Prinivil Tablets (Greater than 1%) 2087
Prinzide Tablets (0.3% to 1%) 2092
▲ ProAmatine Tablets (12.2%) 3032
▲ Procrit for Injection (14% to 22%) 2391
Proglycem Capsules (Infrequent) 1185
Proglycem Suspension (Infrequent) 1185
▲ Prograf Capsules and Injection (15% to 36%) 622
▲ Proleukin for Injection (24%) 2287
Prometrium Capsules (100 mg, 200 mg) 3047
ProQuad (Greater than or equal to 0.2% to less than 1%) 2099
Proscar Tablets 2102
Protonix for Delayed-Release Oral Suspension (Less than 1%) 3254
Protonix Delayed-Release Tablets (Less than 1%) 3254
▲ Protonix I.V. (4%) 3257
▲ Protopic Ointment (25% to 46%) 628
Provigil Tablets (At least 1%) 977
▲ Prozac Weekly Capsules (3%) 1852
▲ Prozac Pulvules and Liquid (3%) 1852
▲ Rebetol (12% to 29%) 2917
Recombivax HB (Less than 1%) 2107
ReFacto Vials 3269
Refludan for Injection (Uncommon) 795
Remeron Tablets (Frequent) 2924
RemeronSolTab Tablets (Frequent) 2927
▲ Remicade for IV Injection (7%) 950
ReoPro Vials (0.3%) 1860
Requip Tablets (Infrequent) 1561
Retrovir Capsules 1574
Retrovir IV Infusion 1579
Retrovir 1574
▲ Rilutek Tablets (2.5% to 3.8%) 2771
Risperdal Consta Long-Acting Injection (Infrequent) 1753
▲ Rituxan I.V. (1% to 14%) 1223
Rocaltrol Capsules 1150
Rocaltrol Oral Solution 1150
Rocephin Injectable Vials, ADD-Vantage, Galaxy, Bulk (Less than 1%) 2642
Rythmol Tablets (Less than 1%) 1586
Rythmol SR Capsules 1590
Salagen Tablets (1% to 2%) 1082
Sandimmune (Rare) 2296
▲ Sandostatin Injection (1% to 4%) 2300
▲ Sandostatin LAR Depot (18.2%) 2302
▲ Selzentry Tablets (3.8%) 2534
▲ Simcor Tablets (3.2%) 502
▲ Simulect for Injection (3% to 10%) 2306
Singulair 2114
Skelaxin Tablets (Most frequent) 1784
▲ Solodyn Extended Release Tablets (5%) 1938
▲ Soriatane Capsules (25% to 50%) 3062
Spiriva HandiHaler 870
Stalevo Tablets 2309
Starlix Tablets 2314
Strattera Capsules (1% to 2%) 1864
▲ Stromectol Tablets (2.8% to 27.5%) 2120
Sular Extended Release Tablets (Less than or equal to 1%) 2975
Sulfamylon Cream (2.8%) 2194
Sulfamylon for 5% Topical Solution (2.3%) 2194
Suprax for Oral Suspension (Less than 2%) 1891
Suprax Tablets (Less than 2%) 1891
Sustiva Capsules (Less than 1% to 2%) 930
Sustiva Tablets (Less than 1% to 2%) 930
Symbyax Capsules (Infrequent) 1871
Synagis Intramuscular Solution 1948
▲ Tarceva Tablets (0% to 13%) 1228
▲ Targretin Gel 1% (10% to 40%) 1088
Tarka Tablets (Less frequent) 511
▲ Tasigna Capsules (Greater than 10% to 29%) 2316
▲ Taxotere Injection Concentrate (0% to 19.9%) 2773
▲ Temodar Capsules (1% to 8%) 2931
Tessalon Capsules 1183
Tessalon Perles 1183
Teveten Tablets (Less than 1%) 515
Teveten HCT Tablets (Less than 1%) 517
Thiothixene Capsules 2197
Thyrogen for Injection 1244
Timentin ADD-Vantage 1606
Timentin Injection Galaxy Container 1609
Timentin IV Infusion 1603
Timentin Pharmacy Bulk Package 1613
Timoptic-XE Sterile Ophthalmic Gel Forming Solution 2125
▲ Toprol-XL Tablets (About 5 of 100 patients) 666
▲ Torisel Injection (1% to 19%) 3272
▲ Tracleer Tablets (4%) 3289
Trasylol Injection 799
▲ Treanda for Injection (0% to 5%) 983
Treximet Tablets (Infrequent) 1616
Tricor Tablets 520
▲ Trisenox Injection (33%) 986
Trusopt Sterile Ophthalmic Solution 2128
▲ Truvada Tablets (5%) 1262
Tussionex Pennkinetic Extended-Release Suspension 3154
Twinrix Vaccine (Less than 1%) 1628
Tygacil for Injection (2.6%) 3276
Tylenol with Codeine Tablets 2427
Ultane Liquid for Inhalation (Less than 1%) 524
▲ Ultram ER Extended-Release Tablets (6.2% to 11.9%) 2428
Uroxatral Tablets 2786
▲ Urso 250 Tablets (5%) 720
▲ Urso Forte Tablets (5%) 720
▲ Valcyte Tablets (Less than 5%) 2654
Valstar Sterile Solution for Intravesical Instillation (Less than 1%) 1735
Valtrex Caplets 1635
Vanos Cream 1941
Vantas (Less than 2%) 1737
▲ Vaprisol (1% to 5%) 632
Vaqta (Less than 1%) 2130
Varivax (Greater than or equal to 1%) 2133
▲ Vectibix (2% to 57%) 597
▲ Velcade for Injection (10%) 2168
Venlafaxine Hydrochloride Tablets (1%) 2199
▲ Vesanoid Capsules (20%) 2660
Viadur Implant (Less than 2%) 802
Vicodin Tablets 529
Vicodin ES Tablets 530
Vicodin HP Tablets 531
▲ Vicoprofen Tablets (3% to 9%) 533
Viramune Oral Suspension 873
Viramune Tablets 873
▲ Viread Tablets (5% to 18%) 1268
Visudyne for Injection 2332
Vivitrol 988
▲ Voltaren Ophthalmic Solution (Less than or equal to 3%) 2336
▲ Voltaren Tablets (1% to 10%) 2334
▲ Voltaren-XR Tablets (1% to 10%) 2337
Vytorin 10/10 Tablets 2149
Vytorin 10/10 Tablets 2939
Vytorin 10/20 Tablets 2149
Vytorin 10/20 Tablets 2939
Vytorin 10/40 Tablets 2149
Vytorin 10/40 Tablets 2939
Vytorin 10/80 Tablets 2149
Vytorin 10/80 Tablets 2939
Wellbutrin Tablets (2.2%) 1648
▲ Wellbutrin SR Sustained-Release Tablets (2% to 4%) 1653
▲ Wellbutrin XL Extended-Release Tablets (2% to 4%) 1659
WinRho SDF 741
▲ Xeloda Tablets (Less than 5%) 2662
Xenical Capsules 2672
Xifaxan Tablets 2682
Xolair (2%) 1235
Xolair (2%) 2339
Xyrem Oral Solution (Frequent) 1766
Xyzal Oral Solution 2789
Xyzal Oral Solution 3155
Zantac Injection 1666
Zemplar Injection 538
Zemuron Injection (Less than 1%) 2947
Zinacef for Injection (Fewer than 1 in 250 patients) 1678
Zinacef Injection (Fewer than 1 in 250 patients) 1678
Zocor Tablets 2136
Zofran Injection (2%) 1682
▲ Zofran (5%) 1687
▲ Zofran ODT Orally Disintegrating Tablets (5%) 1687
▲ Zolinza Capsules (10% to 11.6%) 2142
Zometa for Intravenous Infusion (Rare) 2341
Zomig Tablets (Infrequent) 694
Zomig Nasal Spray (Infrequent) 689
Zomig-ZMT Tablets (Infrequent) 694
Zonegran Capsules (Frequent) 1089
▲ Zosyn for Injection (3.1% to 3.2%) 3284
Zovirax Capsules 1690
Zovirax Cream 817
Zovirax Ointment 819
Zovirax 1690
▲ Zyban Sustained-Release Tablets (3%) 1692
Zyprexa Tablets 1883
Zyprexa ZYDIS Orally Disintegrating Tablets 1883
Zyrtec Chewable Tablets (Less than 2%) 1920
Zyrtec Syrup (Less than 2%) 1920
Zyrtec Tablets (Less than 2%) 1920
Zyrtec-D 12 Hour Extended Release Tablets (Less than 2%) 1923
Zyvox (0% to 0.4%) 2552

Pruritus, application site

Aczone Gel 5% (1%) 3296
Altabax Ointment (1.4% to 1.9%) 1299
AndroGel 3159
Daytrana Transdermal Patch 3022
▲ Elidel Cream 1% (0.6% to 5.5%) 2221
Evoclin Foam, 1% (1%) 3056
▲ Flector Patch (5%) 561
Ionsys Transdermal System (.1% to less than 1%) 2410
Lidoderm Patch 1114
Neupro Transdermal System 3149
▲ Somatuline Depot Injection (9% to 17%) 3102
▲ Targretin Gel 1% (Greater than or equal to 10%) 1088

Pruritus, ear

Ciprodex Otic Suspension (1.5%) 541

Pruritus, ear lobes

Miacalcin Injection 2273

Pruritus, eyelids
Alphagan P Ophthalmic Solution....... 549
▲ Combigan Ophthalmic Solution (1% to 5%)....... 553

Pruritus, genital
Ceftin Tablets (0.1% to 1%)....... 1380
Cipro I.V. (1%)....... 2817
Crinone 4% Gel (2%)....... 992
▲ Crinone 8% Gel (5% to 6%)....... 992
Evoxac Capsules (Less than 1%)....... 1013
Primaxin I.M....... 2080
Primaxin I.V. (Less than 0.2%)....... 2083
Suprax for Oral Suspension (Less than 2%)....... 1891
Suprax Tablets (Less than 2%)....... 1891
▲ Vagifem Tablets (6%)....... 2375
Zosyn for Injection (1% or less)....... 3284

Pruritus, genital, male
Vantas (Less than 2%)....... 1737

Pruritus, injection site
▲ Alferon N Injection (12%)....... 1726
Cancidas for Injection....... 1953
Cerezyme for Injection (Less than 1%)....... 1238
Cipro I.V. (1% or less)....... 2817
▲ Copaxone for Injection (40%)....... 3110
▲ Enbrel for Injection (37%)....... 569
Engerix-B Vaccine (Less than 1%)....... 1409
Forteo for Injection (Less than 1/30 patients)....... 1816
▲ Gardasil Injection (3.1%)....... 2019
Humalog-Pen and KwikPen....... 1829
Humulin 50/50, 100 Units....... 1843
Humulin 70/30 Vial....... 1844
Humulin N Vial....... 1846
Humulin R (U-500)....... 1850
▲ Intron A for Injection (Less than 5%)....... 2859
Invanz for Injection (Greater than 0.5%)....... 2029
Vaqta (Less than 1%)....... 2130
▲ Varivax (19.3% to 32.5%)....... 2133
▲ Vivitrol (6% to 10%)....... 988
▲ Zostavax Injection (6.6%)....... 2145

Pruritus, localized
▲ Aldara Cream, 5% (16% to 32%)....... 1699
Mentax Cream (Less than 2%)....... 2190

Pruritus, ocular
▲ Alphagan P Ophthalmic Solution (Approximately 10% to 20%)....... 549
▲ Alrex Ophthalmic Suspension 0.2% (5% to 15%)....... ⊙236
▲ Azopt Ophthalmic Suspension (1% to 5%)....... 540
▲ Betimol Ophthalmic Solution (More than 5%)....... 3181
▲ Carac Cream 0.5% (5.4%)....... 2722
Clorpres Tablets....... 2185
▲ Combigan Ophthalmic Solution (5% to 15%)....... 553
▲ Cosopt Sterile Ophthalmic Solution (5% to 15%)....... 1969
▲ Elestat Ophthalmic Solution (1% to 10%)....... 1741
Imitrex Nasal Spray....... 1470
▲ Lotemax Ophthalmic Suspension 0.5% (5% to 15%)....... ⊙241
▲ Lucentis Injection (0% to 13%)....... 1205
▲ Lumigan Ophthalmic Solution (15% to 45%)....... 556
Maxalt Tablets (Infrequent)....... 2056
Maxalt-MLT Orally Disintegrating Tablets (Infrequent)....... 2056
▲ Pataday Ophthalmic Solution (Less than or equal to 5%)....... 543
Quixin Ophthalmic Solution (Less than 1%)....... 3184
▲ Restasis Ophthalmic Emulsion (1% to 5%)....... 557
▲ Soriatane Capsules (1% to 5%)....... 3062
Timoptic Sterile Ophthalmic Solution....... 2121
Timoptic in Ocudose....... 2124
Timoptic-XE Sterile Ophthalmic Gel Forming Solution....... 2125
Transderm Scōp Transdermal Therapeutic System (Infrequent)....... 2206
▲ Travatan Z Ophthalmic Solution (5% to 10%)....... 547
Vaqta (Less than 1%)....... 2130
▲ Vigamox Ophthalmic Solution (1% to 6%)....... 548
▲ Visudyne for Injection (1% to 10%)....... 2332
▲ Voltaren Ophthalmic Solution (Less than or equal to 5%)....... 2336
Xopenex Inhalation Solution Concentrate (Less than 2%)....... 3005

Pruritus, oral
Imitrex Nasal Spray....... 1470
▲ Nevanac Ophthalmic Suspension 0.1% (1% to 5%)....... ⊙205
Ofloxacin Ophthalmic Solution 0.3%....... ⊙243

Pruritus, rhinal
Atrovent Nasal Spray 0.03% (2%)....... 834
▲ Miacalcin Nasal Spray (10.6%)....... 2274

Pruritus, vaginal
Cipro XR Tablets....... 2823
Invanz for Injection (Greater than 0.1%)....... 2029

Pruritus ani
Celexa (Rare)....... 1160
Nexium Delayed-Release Capsules (Less than 1%)....... 645
Nexium I.V. (Less than 1%)....... 652
Nexium Delayed-Release Oral Suspension (Less than 1%)....... 645
Noroxin Tablets (Less frequent)....... 2069

PSA increase
▲ AndroGel (18%)....... 3159
Brovana Inhalation Solution (Less than 2%)....... 2990

Pseudoaneurysm
ReoPro Vials (0.8%)....... 1860

Pseudohypoparathyroidism
▲ Rocaltrol Capsules (1 in 3)....... 1150
▲ Rocaltrol Oral Solution (1 in 3)....... 1150

Pseudolymphoma
Mirapex Tablets....... 857
Phenytek Capsules....... 2192

Pseudolymphoma, cutaneous
Prinivil Tablets....... 2087
Prinzide Tablets....... 2092

Pseudomembranous enterocolitis
Rilutek Tablets (Rare)....... 2771

Pseudoparkinsonism
Thioridazine Hydrochloride Tablets (Infrequent)....... 2195
Thiothixene Capsules....... 2197
Wellbutrin Tablets (1.5%)....... 1648

Pseudopemphigoid
Combigan Ophthalmic Solution....... 553

Pseudotumor cerebri
Accutane Capsules....... 2607
Levothroid Tablets....... 1170
Levoxyl Tablets....... 1780
Pylera Capsules....... 714
Solodyn Extended Release Tablets....... 1938
Soriatane Capsules (Less than 1%)....... 3062
Synthroid Tablets....... 507
Tygacil for Injection....... 3276
Vesanoid Capsules....... 2660

Psoriasis
Aceon Tablets (2 mg, 4 mg, 8 mg)....... 3038
Aricept Tablets (Infrequent)....... 1062
Aricept ODT Tablets (Infrequent)....... 1062
Asacol Delayed-Release Tablets (Rare)....... 2579
Bystolic Tablets....... 1155
Campral Tablets (Rare)....... 1158
Celexa (Infrequent)....... 1160
Chantix Tablets (Infrequent)....... 2511
Copaxone for Injection (Infrequent)....... 3110
Doxil Injection (Less than 1%)....... 2378
Effexor XR Extended-Release Capsules (Infrequent)....... 3195
Gabitril Tablets (Infrequent)....... 973
Gleevec Tablets (Infrequent)....... 2255
▲ Intron A for Injection (Less than 5%)....... 2859
Mirapex Tablets....... 857
Norvir (Less than 2%)....... 489
PegIntron Powder for Injection....... 2903
Provigil Tablets (At least 1%)....... 977
Prozac Weekly Capsules (Rare)....... 1852
Prozac Pulvules and Liquid (Rare)....... 1852
Raptiva for Injection (0.7%)....... 1218
Requip Tablets (Infrequent)....... 1561
Rilutek Tablets (Infrequent)....... 2771
Symbyax Capsules (Infrequent)....... 1871
Venlafaxine Hydrochloride Tablets (Infrequent)....... 2199

Psoriasis, exacerbation of
Cosopt Sterile Ophthalmic Solution....... 1969
▲ Intron A for Injection (Less than 5%)....... 2859
Lamisil Oral Granules....... 2264
Lamisil Tablets....... 2266
Neupogen for Injection (Infrequent)....... 589
PegIntron Powder for Injection (Less than or equal to 1%)....... 2903
Soriatane Capsules (Less than 1%)....... 3062
Timoptic Sterile Ophthalmic Solution....... 2121
Timoptic in Ocudose....... 2124
Timoptic-XE Sterile Ophthalmic Gel Forming Solution....... 2125
Toprol-XL Tablets....... 666

Psoriasis, plaque
Remicade for IV Injection....... 950

Psoriasis, pustular
Remicade for IV Injection....... 950

Psoriasis, worsening of
Combigan Ophthalmic Solution....... 553
Enbrel for Injection....... 569

Psychiatric disorders, unspecified
Cymbalta Delayed-Release Capsules....... 1801
▲ Femara Tablets (0.8% to 12.5%)....... 2246
▲ Mycamine for Injection (7.7% to 60.5%)....... 616
▲ Velcade for Injection (35%)....... 2168
Verdeso Foam (1%)....... 3069

Psychiatric disturbances
Accutane Capsules....... 2607
Advicor Tablets....... 402
Clinoril Tablets (Less than 1 in 100)....... 1962
Cosopt Sterile Ophthalmic Solution....... 1969
Didronel Tablets....... 2583
▲ Focalin XR Capsules (26% to 46%)....... 2251
▲ Gengraf Capsules (5%)....... 435
Indocin (Less than 1%)....... 2024
Lescol Capsules....... 2268
Lescol XL Tablets....... 2268
▲ Leukine (15%)....... 774
Nembutal Sodium Solution, USP (Less than 1%)....... 2494
Neoral Oral Solution....... 2280
Neoral Soft Gelatin Capsules....... 2280
Noroxin Tablets....... 2069
Pepcid Tablets (Infrequent)....... 2075
Primaxin I.M....... 2080
Primaxin I.V. (Less than 0.2%)....... 2083
Sandimmune....... 2296
Thioridazine Hydrochloride Tablets (Extremely rare)....... 2195
Timoptic Sterile Ophthalmic Solution (Less frequent)....... 2121
Timoptic in Ocudose (Less frequent)....... 2124
Timoptic-XE Sterile Ophthalmic Gel Forming Solution....... 2125

Psychic dependence
(*see under* Dependence, psychological)

Psychic disturbances
Combigan Ophthalmic Solution....... 553
Cuprimine Capsules....... 1986
Demser Capsules....... 1989

Psychomotor agitation
Abilify Injection....... 881
Abilify Injection (Less than 1 in 1000 patients)....... 2466
Abilify Oral Solution....... 881
Abilify Oral Solution (Less than 1 in 1000 patients)....... 2466
Abilify Discmelt Orally Disintegrating Tablets....... 881
Abilify Discmelt Orally Disintegrating Tablets (Less than 1 in 1000 patients)....... 2466
Abilify Tablets....... 881
Abilify Tablets (Less than 1 in 1000 patients)....... 2466
▲ Cymbalta Delayed-Release Capsules (5%)....... 1801
Valium Tablets....... 2658

Psychomotor retardation
Ambien CR Tablets (2%)....... 2696

Psychomotor skills, impaired
Abilify Injection (Greater than or equal to 1 in 1000 patients and less than 1 in 100 patients)....... 2466
Abilify Oral Solution (Greater than or equal to 1 in 1000 patients and less than 1 in 100 patients)....... 2466
Abilify Discmelt Orally Disintegrating Tablets (Greater than or equal to 1 in 1000 patients and less than 1 in 100 patients)....... 2466
Abilify Tablets (Greater than or equal to 1 in 1000 patients and less than 1 in 100 patients)....... 2466
Chantix Tablets (Rare)....... 2511
Treximet Tablets (Rare)....... 1616

Psychoses
Accutane Capsules....... 2607
Adderall XR Capsules....... 3012
Adipex-P....... 1185
Avelox....... 2803
Azilect Tablets (Infrequent)....... 3106
Biaxin/Biaxin XL....... 411
Campral Tablets (Rare)....... 1158
Celexa (Infrequent)....... 1160
Clinoril Tablets (Less than 1 in 100)....... 1962
Dapsone Tablets USP....... 1746
Depakote ER Tablets (Greater than 1%)....... 423
Dexedrine (Rare at recommended doses)....... 1401
Effexor XR Extended-Release Capsules (Infrequent)....... 3195
Exelon Capsules (Infrequent)....... 2229
Exelon Oral Solution (Infrequent)....... 2229
Gabitril Tablets (Infrequent)....... 973
Geodon for Injection (Up to 1%)....... 2520
Indocin (Less than 1%)....... 2024
Intron A for Injection....... 2859
Keppra Oral Solution (0.3%)....... 3131
Keppra Tablets (0.3%)....... 3131
Klonopin....... 2639
Lamictal (Infrequent)....... 1488
Lanoxin Injection....... 1498
Lanoxin Injection Pediatric....... 1502
Levaquin....... 2416
Levaquin in 5% Dextrose Injection....... 2416
Luvox CR Extended-Release Capsules (Frequent)....... 1759
Mirapex Tablets (Less than 1%)....... 857
Namenda (Infrequent)....... 1180
Noroxin Tablets....... 2069
Orthoclone OKT3 Sterile Solution....... 2387
Paxil (Rare)....... 1535
Paxil CR Controlled-Release Tablets (Rare)....... 1544
PegIntron Powder for Injection (Less than or equal to 1%)....... 2903
▲ Prograf Capsules and Injection (3% to 15%)....... 622
Provigil Tablets....... 977
Prozac Pulvules and Liquid (Infrequent)....... 1852
Rilutek Tablets (Rare)....... 2771
Rocaltrol Capsules (Rare)....... 1150
Rocaltrol Oral Solution (Rare)....... 1150
Seromycin Capsules....... 1864
Stalevo Tablets....... 2309
Sustiva Capsules (Less than 2%)....... 930
Sustiva Tablets (Less than 2%)....... 930
Tarka Tablets....... 511
▲ Valcyte Tablets (Less than 5%)....... 2654
Valium Tablets....... 2658
Valtrex Caplets....... 1635
Vyvanse Capsules....... 3033
Wellbutrin Tablets (Infrequent)....... 1648
Wellbutrin SR Sustained-Release Tablets....... 1653
Wellbutrin XL Extended-Release Tablets....... 1659
Zomig Tablets (Rare)....... 694
Zomig Nasal Spray (Rare)....... 689
Zomig-ZMT Tablets (Rare)....... 694
Zovirax....... 1690
Zyban Sustained-Release Tablets....... 1692

Psychoses, aggravation
Requip XL Tablets....... 1568
Thioridazine Hydrochloride Tablets....... 2195

Psychoses, toxic
Cipro I.V. (1% or less)....... 2817
Cipro....... 2810
Cipro XR Tablets....... 2823
Daytrana Transdermal Patch....... 3022
Focalin XR Capsules....... 2251
Metadate CD Capsules....... 3146

Psychosexual disorder
Aceon Tablets (2 mg, 4 mg, 8 mg) (0.3% to 1%)....... 3038

Psychosis, activation
Carbatrol Capsules....... 3019
Wellbutrin SR Sustained-Release Tablets....... 1653

Wellbutrin XL Extended-Release Tablets 1659
Zyban Sustained-Release Tablets 1692

Psychosis, overt
Calcijex Injection (Rare) 419

Psychosis, unspecified
Atripla Tablets 938
Bicillin C-R Injectable Suspension 1775
Bicillin L-A Injection 1777
▲ CellCept Capsules (3% to less than 20%) 2622
▲ CellCept Intravenous (3% to less than 20%) 2622
▲ CellCept Oral Suspension (3% to less than 20%) 2622
▲ CellCept Tablets (3% to less than 20%) 2622
Gantrisin Pediatric Suspension 2638
Keppra Injection (0.3%) 3137
Levaquin 2416
Levaquin in 5% Dextrose Injection 2416
Luvox CR Extended-Release Capsules (Infrequent) 1759
Neupro Transdermal System 3149
Proleukin for Injection (1%) 2287
Prozac Weekly Capsules (Infrequent) 1852
Pulmicort Flexhaler 654
Risperdal Consta Long-Acting Injection (Frequent) 1753
Rythmol Tablets (Less than 1%) 1586
Venlafaxine Hydrochloride Tablets (Infrequent) 2199

Psychotic disorder
Chantix Tablets (Rare) 2511
Mirapex Tablets 857
Requip XL Tablets 1568
Velcade for Injection 2168

Psychotic episodes
(*see under* Psychoses)

Psychotic symptoms
Betaseron for SC Injection 756
Keppra Injection (0.7%) 3137
Keppra Oral Solution (0.7%) 3131
Keppra Tablets (0.7%) 3131
Strattera Capsules 1864
Thiothixene Capsules (Infrequently) .. 2197

Ptosis
Combigan Ophthalmic Solution 553
Lunesta Tablets (Rare) 2994
Lyrica Capsules (Rare) 2527
Namenda (Infrequent) 1180
Zyrtec Chewable Tablets (Less than 2%) 1920
Zyrtec Syrup (Less than 2%) 1920
Zyrtec Tablets (Less than 2%) 1920
Zyrtec-D 12 Hour Extended Release Tablets (Less than 2%) 1923

Ptosis, eyelids
Betimol Ophthalmic Solution 3181
▲ BOTOX Purified Neurotoxin Complex (0.3% to 15.7%) 550
Celexa (Rare) 1160
Copaxone for Injection (Infrequent) .. 3110
Cosopt Sterile Ophthalmic Solution 1969
FML Ophthalmic Ointment (Occasional) .... ⊙ 223
FML Ophthalmic Suspension (Occasional) .... ⊙ 224
FML Forte Ophthalmic Suspension (Occasional) .... ⊙ 222
Lamictal (Rare) 1488
Lexapro Oral Suspension (Frequent) 1174
Lexapro Tablets (Frequent) 1174
Mirapex Tablets 857
Paxil (Rare) 1535
Paxil CR Controlled-Release Tablets (Rare) 1544
Pred Forte Ophthalmic Suspension (Occasional) .... ⊙ 227
Pred Mild Ophthalmic Suspension (Occasional) .... ⊙ 230
Rythmol SR Capsules 1590
Timoptic Sterile Ophthalmic Solution (Less frequent) 2121
Timoptic in Ocudose (Less frequent) 2124
Timoptic-XE Sterile Ophthalmic Gel Forming Solution 2125

Pulmonary allergy, unspecified
▲ Remicade for IV Injection (6%) 950

Pulmonary complications, unspecified
Follistim AQ Cartridge 2844
Prozac Weekly Capsules 1852

Pulmonary congestion
Aricept Tablets (Infrequent) 1062
Aricept ODT Tablets (Infrequent) 1062
Avalide Tablets 892
Avalide Tablets 2713
Avapro Tablets (Less than 1%) 897
Avapro Tablets (Less than 1%) 2718
Evoxac Capsules (Less than 1%) 1013
Prinzide Tablets 2092
Proleukin for Injection 2287
ProQuad 2099
Rythmol SR Capsules 1590
Vicoprofen Tablets (Less than 1%) 533

Pulmonary disease, acute diffuse infiltrative
Velcade for Injection 2168

Pulmonary disease, chronic obstructive
Brovana Inhalation Solution 2990
Exelon Patch (Infrequent) 2233
▲ Lucentis Injection (0% to 5%) 1205
Luvox CR Extended-Release Capsules (Rare) 1759
Mirapex Tablets 857
Rythmol SR Capsules 1590
Vivitrol 988

Pulmonary disease, chronic obstructive, exacerbation of
▲ Atrovent HFA Inhalation Aerosol (8% to 23%) 839
Combivent Inhalation Aerosol 845
Orencia Powder for Intravenous Infusion 921
Velcade for Injection 2168

Pulmonary disorder, unspecified
▲ Hycamtin for Injection (17%) 1459
▲ Novantrone for Injection Concentrate (5% to 43%) 1100
▲ Taxotere Injection Concentrate (21% to 40.9%) 2773

Pulmonary distress
Follistim AQ Cartridge 2844

Pulmonary edema
(*see under* Edema, pulmonary)

Pulmonary edema, acute
Taxotere Injection Concentrate 2773
▲ Velcade for Injection (5%) 2168

Pulmonary embolism
(*see under* Embolism, pulmonary)

Pulmonary emphysema, interstitial
▲ Infasurf Intratracheal Suspension (7% to 10%) 1168

Pulmonary events, unspecified
▲ Mylotarg for Injection (8% to 10%) 3212

Pulmonary function, changes
Intron A for Injection 2859
▲ Leukine (48%) 774
Proleukin for Injection 2287

Pulmonary function, decreased
▲ Rilutek Tablets (13.1% to 16%) 2771

Pulmonary hemorrhage
(*see under* Hemorrhage, pulmonary)

Pulmonary hypersensitivity
Carbatrol Capsules 3019
Equetro Extended-Release Capsules 3174

Pulmonary hypertension
Adipex-P (Rare) 1185
Agrylin Capsules 3017
Bicillin C-R Injectable Suspension 1775
Bicillin L-A Injection 1777
▲ CellCept Capsules (3% to less than 20%) 2622
▲ CellCept Intravenous (3% to less than 20%) 2622
▲ CellCept Oral Suspension (3% to less than 20%) 2622
▲ CellCept Tablets (3% to less than 20%) 2622
Elitek (Less than or equal to 1%) 2729
▲ Indocin I.V. (1% to 3%) 2489
Paxil 1535
Paxil CR Controlled-Release Tablets 1544
Prozac Weekly Capsules 1852
Prozac Pulvules and Liquid 1852
Sandostatin LAR Depot 2302
Tasigna Capsules 2316
Trasylol Injection (1% to 2%) 799
Velcade for Injection 2168
▲ Vesanoid Capsules (3%) 2660
Zemuron Injection 2947

Pulmonary infarction
Follistim AQ Cartridge 2844
Luvox CR Extended-Release Capsules (Rare) 1759
Prinivil Tablets (0.3% to 1%) 2087
Prinzide Tablets 2092

Pulmonary infiltrates
Agrylin Capsules 3017
▲ Avastin IV (5%) 1192
Campath Ampules 761
Cancidas for Injection 1953
Fansidar Tablets 2636
Gantrisin Pediatric Suspension 2638
Herceptin I.V. 1199
Intron A for Injection (Rare) 2859
Leustatin Injection 2384
Neupogen for Injection 589
Neupro Transdermal System 3149
PegIntron Powder for Injection 2903
Pentasa Capsules (Less than 1%) 3030
Prinivil Tablets (0.3% to 1%) 2087
Prinzide Tablets 2092
Proleukin for Injection 2287
Rebetol 2917
Rituxan I.V. 1223
Stalevo Tablets (Rare) 2309
Tarceva Tablets 1228
▲ Vesanoid Capsules (6%) 2660

Pulmonary insufficiency
Herceptin I.V. 1199

Pulmonary nodule
Sandostatin Injection (Less than 1%) 2300
Sandostatin LAR Depot 2302

Pulmonary physical finding
Tygacil for Injection (1.9%) 3276

Pulmonary reembolism
Activase I.V. 1188

Pulmonary symptoms, worsening
Accolate Tablets (Rare) 669
Advair Diskus 100/50 1276
Advair Diskus 250/50 1276
Advair Diskus 500/50 1276
Flovent Diskus 50 mcg 1435
Singulair 2114
Xolair 2339

Pulmonary toxicity, unspecified
Herceptin I.V. 1199
Myleran Tablets 1530

Pulse, fast
Humalog-Pen and KwikPen (Less common) 1829
Humalog Mix 50/50-Pen and KwikPen 1833
Humulin 50/50, 100 Units 1843
Humulin 70/30 Vial (Less common) 1844
Humulin N Vial (Less common) 1846
Humulin R 1849
Humulin R (U-500) 1850
Levoxyl Tablets 1780
Children's Motrin Oral Suspension 1901
Children's Motrin Non-Staining Dye-Free Oral Suspension 1901
Infants' Motrin Concentrated Drops 1901
Infants' Motrin Non-Staining Dye-Free Concentrated Drops 1901
Junior Strength Motrin Caplets and Chewable Tablets 1901

Pulse, irregular
Exforge Tablets (Less than or equal to 0.1%) 2238
Luvox CR Extended-Release Capsules (Infrequent) 1759
Rythmol SR Capsules 1590
Thiothixene Capsules 2197

Pulse changes
Concerta Extended-Release Tablets 1925
Focalin XR Capsules 2251
Imitrex Injection (Rare) 1465
Imitrex Nasal Spray 1470
Mephyton Tablets (Rare) 700
Metadate CD Capsules 3146
Moban Tablets 1116
Ventolin HFA Inhalation Aerosol 1638

Pulse rate, decreased
Daytrana Transdermal Patch 3022
Edex Injection 2957
Focalin XR Capsules 2251

Pulse rate, depression
Lanoxin Injection 1498
ReoPro Vials (1%) 1860

Pulse rate, increased
Agrylin Capsules 3017
Brovana Inhalation Solution 2990
Daytrana Transdermal Patch 3022
Edex Injection 2957
Focalin XR Capsules 2251
Pristiq Extended-Release Tablets 3247
Venlafaxine Hydrochloride Tablets 2199

Pupil enlargement
Clear Eyes Itchy Eye Relief .... ⊙ 255
Clear Eyes Triple Action Relief .... ⊙ 255

Pupillary atonia
Venlafaxine Hydrochloride Tablets (Rare) 2199

Purple toes syndrome
Activase I.V. 1188

Purpura
Aceon Tablets (2 mg, 4 mg, 8 mg) (0.3% to 1%) 3038
Advicor Tablets 402
Aggrenox Capsules (1.4%) 819
Ambien Tablets (Rare) 2692
Ambien CR Tablets (Rare) 2696
AmBisome for Injection (Less common) 606
Amerge Tablets (Rare) 1301
Anaprox Tablets (Less than 3%) 2632
Anaprox DS Tablets (Less than 3%) .. 2632
Anzemet Injection (Infrequently) 2701
Anzemet Tablets (Rare) 2704
▲ Arixtra Injection (0% to 3.5%) 1313
Attenuvax (Rare) 1951
Avalide Tablets 892
Avalide Tablets 2713
Azilect Tablets (Rare) 3106
Carbatrol Capsules 3019
Cardizem LA Extended Release Tablets (Infrequent) 421
Celexa (Infrequent) 1160
Cipro I.V. (1% or less) 2817
Cipro XR Tablets 2823
Clinoril Tablets (Less than 1 in 100) 1962
Clorpres Tablets (Few) 2185
Comtan Tablets (2%) 2208
▲ Coreg Tablets (Greater than 1% to 3%) 1387
▲ Coreg CR Extended-Release Capsules (Greater than 1% to less than or equal to 3%) 1393
Crinone 4% Gel 992
Crinone 8% Gel 992
Dapsone Tablets USP 1746
Diovan HCT Tablets 2216
Dyazide Capsules 1405
EC-Naprosyn Delayed-Release Tablets (Less than 3%) 2632
Effexor XR Extended-Release Capsules (Rare) 3195
▲ Eloxatin for Injection (2% to less than 5%) 2731
Engerix-B Vaccine 1409
Equetro Extended-Release Capsules 3174
Evoxac Capsules (Less than 1%) 1013
Exelon Capsules (Infrequent) 2229
Exelon Oral Solution (Infrequent) 2229
Exforge Tablets (Greater than 0.1% to less than 1%) 2238
Fansidar Tablets 2636
Frova Tablets (Rare) 1111
Furosemide Tablets 2186
▲ Gamunex (40%) 3094
Gantrisin Pediatric Suspension 2638
Gengraf Capsules (2%) 435
Gleevec Tablets (Infrequent) 2255
Indapamide Tablets 2188
Indocin Capsules (Less than 1%) 2024
Indocin I.V. (Less than 1%) 2489
Indocin (Less than 1%) 2024
Intravenous Sodium Diuril 2490
▲ Intron A for Injection (Less than or equal to 5%) 2859
Lescol Capsules (Rare) 2268

Lescol XL Tablets 2268
▲ Leustatin Injection (10%) 2384
Lovenox Injection 2756
Luvox CR Extended-Release Capsules (Rare) 1759
Lyrica Capsules (Rare) 2527
Meruvax II 2061
Mevacor Tablets (Rare) 2063
Micardis HCT Tablets 854
Mirapex Tablets 857
M-M-R II 2054
Mobic Oral Suspension (Less than 2%) 863
Mobic Tablets (Less than 2%) 863
Mumpsvax (Extremely rare) 2068
Nalfon Capsules (Less than 1%) 2508
Naprosyn Suspension (Less than 3%) 2632
Naprosyn Tablets (Less than 3%) 2632
Neoral Oral Solution (2%) 2280
Neoral Soft Gelatin Capsules (2%) 2280
Neupro Transdermal System 3149
NovoSeven (1%) 2367
NovoSeven RT (1%) 2370
Paxil (Infrequent) 1535
Paxil CR Controlled-Release Tablets (Infrequent) 1544
Percodan Tablets 1130
▲ Plavix Tablets (5.3%) 926
▲ Plavix Tablets (5.3%) 2767
Pletal Tablets (Less than 2%) 2481
Prinzide Tablets 2092
ProQuad 2099
Prozac Weekly Capsules (Rare) 1852
Prozac Pulvules and Liquid (Rare) 1852
Requip Tablets (Infrequent) 1561
Rilutek Tablets (Rare) 2771
Risperdal Consta Long-Acting Injection (Infrequent) 1753
Rythmol Tablets (Less than 1%) 1586
▲ Simulect for Injection (3% to 10%) 2306
▲ Soriatane Capsules (1% to 10%) 3062
Stalevo Tablets (2%) 2309
Symbyax Capsules (Rare) 1871
Tarka Tablets 511
Tekturna HCT Tablets 2324
Teveten Tablets (Less than 1%) 515
Teveten HCT Tablets (Less than 1%) 517
Venlafaxine Hydrochloride Tablets (Rare) 2199
Voltaren Tablets (Occasionally) 2334
Voltaren-XR Tablets (Occasionally) 2337
Vytorin 10/10 Tablets 2149
Vytorin 10/10 Tablets 2939
Vytorin 10/20 Tablets 2149
Vytorin 10/20 Tablets 2939
Vytorin 10/40 Tablets 2149
Vytorin 10/40 Tablets 2939
Vytorin 10/80 Tablets 2149
Vytorin 10/80 Tablets 2939
Zocor Tablets (Rare) 2136
Zosyn for Injection (1% or less) 3284
Zyrtec Chewable Tablets (Less than 2%) 1920
Zyrtec Syrup (Less than 2%) 1920
Zyrtec Tablets (Less than 2%) 1920
Zyrtec-D 12 Hour Extended Release Tablets (Less than 2%) 1923

Purpura, allergic
Plavix Tablets (Less than 1%) 926
Plavix Tablets (Less than 1%) 2767

Purpura, anaphylactoid
Solodyn Extended Release Tablets 1938

Purpura, nonthrombocytopenic
Combigan Ophthalmic Solution 553
Cosopt Sterile Ophthalmic Solution 1969
Edecrin (Rare) 698
InnoPran XL Extended Release Capsules 1484
Nadolol Tablets 2191
Timoptic Sterile Ophthalmic Solution 2121
Timoptic in Ocudose 2124
Timoptic-XE Sterile Ophthalmic Gel Forming Solution 2125
Toprol-XL Tablets 666

Purpura, thrombocytopenic
Amoxil Capsules 1305
Amoxil Chewable Tablets 1305
Amoxil Pediatric Drops for Oral Suspension 1305
Amoxil Powder for Oral Suspension 1305
Amoxil Tablets 1305
Augmentin 1323
Augmentin Tablets 1327
Augmentin XR Extended Release Tablets 1333
Augmentin ES-600 Powder for Oral Suspension 1329
Axid Capsules 1364
Combigan Ophthalmic Solution 553
Concerta Extended-Release Tablets 1925
Cosopt Sterile Ophthalmic Solution 1969
Daytrana Transdermal Patch 3022
Evoxac Capsules (Less than 1%) 1013
Focalin XR Capsules 2251
Indocin Capsules (Less than 1%) 2024
Indocin I.V. (Less than 1%) 2489
Indocin (Less than 1%) 2024
Infanrix Vaccine 1479
InnoPran XL Extended Release Capsules 1484
▲ Intron A for Injection (Less than 5%) 2859
Metadate CD Capsules 3146
Moxatag Tablets 2165
Nadolol Tablets 2191
Omnicef Capsules 497
Omnicef for Oral Suspension 497
Pediarix Vaccine 1552
PegIntron Powder for Injection (Less than or equal to 1%) 2903
Prograf Capsules and Injection 622
Prozac Weekly Capsules 1852
Prozac Pulvules and Liquid 1852
Pylera Capsules 714
Remicade for IV Injection 950
Thiothixene Capsules 2197
Timoptic Sterile Ophthalmic Solution 2121
Timoptic in Ocudose 2124
Timoptic-XE Sterile Ophthalmic Gel Forming Solution 2125
Toprol-XL Tablets 666
▲ Xeloda Tablets (Less than 5%) 2662

Purpura, thrombocytopenic, idiopathic
Abilify Injection (Less than 1 in 1000 patients) 2466
Abilify Oral Solution (Less than 1 in 1000 patients) 2466
Abilify Discmelt Orally Disintegrating Tablets (Less than 1 in 1000 patients) 2466
Abilify Tablets (Less than 1 in 1000 patients) 2466
Aldara Cream, 5% 1699
Intron A for Injection 2859
PegIntron Powder for Injection 2903
Remicade for IV Injection 950
Rotarix Oral Suspension 1582

Purpura, thrombocytopenic, thrombotic
Avelox 2803
Cipro I.V. (Rare) 2817
Cipro 2810
Cipro XR Tablets 2823
Cuprimine Capsules 1986
Intron A for Injection 2859
Levaquin 2416
Levaquin in 5% Dextrose Injection 2416
Mycamine for Injection 616
Noroxin Tablets 2069
Noxafil Oral Suspension (Rare) 2889
PegIntron Powder for Injection 2903
Plavix Tablets (Rare) 926
Plavix Tablets (Rare) 2767
Prograf Capsules and Injection 622
▲ Rapamune (Greater than or equal to 3% to less than 20%) 3260
Remicade for IV Injection 950
Risperdal Consta Long-Acting Injection 1753
Valtrex Caplets 1635

Pustules, unspecified
Duragesic Transdermal System (Less than 1%) 2405
Klonopin (Infrequent) 2639

Pustulosis, exanthematous
Amoxil Capsules 1305
Amoxil Chewable Tablets 1305
Amoxil Pediatric Drops for Oral Suspension 1305
Amoxil Powder for Oral Suspension 1305
Amoxil Tablets 1305
Augmentin 1323
Augmentin Tablets 1327
Augmentin XR Extended Release Tablets 1333
Augmentin ES-600 Powder for Oral Suspension 1329
Gleevec Tablets (Rare) 2255
Lamisil Oral Granules 2264
Lamisil Tablets 2266
Moxatag Tablets 2165

Pyelitis
Amerge Tablets (Rare) 1301

Pyelonephritis
Actiq (Less than 1%) 959
Ambien Tablets (Rare) 2692
Ambien CR Tablets (Rare) 2696
Aricept Tablets (Infrequent) 1062
Aricept ODT Tablets (Infrequent) 1062
Celexa (Rare) 1160
▲ CellCept Capsules (3% to less than 20%) 2622
▲ CellCept Intravenous (3% to less than 20%) 2622
▲ CellCept Oral Suspension (3% to less than 20%) 2622
▲ CellCept Tablets (3% to less than 20%) 2622
Cimzia 3127
Copaxone for Injection (Infrequent) 3110
Crixivan Capsules 1979
Effexor XR Extended-Release Capsules (Infrequent) 3195
Enbrel for Injection 569
Evoxac Capsules (Less than 1%) 1013
Gabitril Tablets (Infrequent) 973
Gengraf Capsules (1% to less than 3%) 435
▲ Humira Injection (Less than 5%) 442
Lunesta Tablets (Rare) 2994
Lupron Depot 3.75 mg 462
Lupron Depot–3 Month 11.25 mg 462
Lyrica Capsules (Rare) 2527
Miacalcin Nasal Spray (Less than 1%) 2274
Mirapex Tablets 857
Neoral Oral Solution (1% to less than 3%) 2280
Neoral Soft Gelatin Capsules (1% to less than 3%) 2280
Norvir (Less than 2%) 489
Orencia Powder for Intravenous Infusion (0.2% to 0.5%) 921
Prinivil Tablets (0.3% to 1%) 2087
Prinzide Tablets 2092
Protonix for Delayed-Release Oral Suspension (Less than 1%) 3254
Protonix Delayed-Release Tablets (Less than 1%) 3254
Protonix I.V. (Less than 1%) 3257
▲ Rapamune (Greater than or equal to 3% to less than 20%) 3260
Requip Tablets (Rare) 1561
Rilutek Tablets (Rare) 2771
Venlafaxine Hydrochloride Tablets (Rare) 2199
Zomig Tablets (Rare) 694
Zomig Nasal Spray (Rare) 689
Zomig-ZMT Tablets (Rare) 694

Pyloric stenosis
EryPed 431
Invanz for Injection (Greater than 0.1%) 2029

Pyoderma
Mirapex Tablets 857

Pyoderma gangrenosum
Asacol Delayed-Release Tablets (Rare) 2579

Pyogenic granuloma
Accutane Capsules 2607
▲ Soriatane Capsules (1% to 10%) 3062

Pyrexia
(*see under* Fever)

Pyrosis
(*see under* Heartburn)

Pyuria
Aricept Tablets (Infrequent) 1062
Aricept ODT Tablets (Infrequent) 1062
Brovana Inhalation Solution 2990
Effexor XR Extended-Release Capsules (Infrequent) 3195
Evoxac Capsules (Less than 1%) 1013
▲ Ontak Vials (10%) 1079
Paxil (Rare) 1535
Paxil CR Controlled-Release Tablets (Rare) 1544
▲ Prograf Capsules and Injection (3% to 15%) 622
Provigil Tablets (1%) 977
Requip Tablets (2%) 1561
Rythmol SR Capsules 1590
Salagen Tablets (Less than 1%) 1082
Singulair (1%) 2114
Tice BCG (Less than or equal to 1%) 2936
Zosyn for Injection 3284
Zyprexa Tablets (Infrequent) 1883
Zyprexa ZYDIS Orally Disintegrating Tablets (Infrequent) 1883

Q

Quadriplegia
Orthoclone OKT3 Sterile Solution 2387
Prograf Capsules and Injection 622

Quncke's edema
(*see also under* Angioedema)
Protonix for Delayed-Release Oral Suspension 3254
Protonix Delayed-Release Tablets 3254
Protonix I.V. 3257

R

Radiation recall
Alimta for Injection 1786

Radiation recall syndrome
Doxil Injection 2378
Taxotere Injection Concentrate 2773
▲ Xeloda Tablets (Less than 5%) 2662

Radiculoneuropathy
Imitrex Injection 1465
Imitrex Tablets (Rare) 1474
Pneumovax 23 2078
Recombivax HB 2107

Rage
Valium Tablets 2658

Rales
▲ Cancidas for Injection (6.9%) 1953
Combigan Ophthalmic Solution 553
▲ Coreg Tablets (4%) 1387
▲ Coreg CR Extended-Release Capsules (4%) 1393
Cosopt Sterile Ophthalmic Solution 1969
▲ Dacogen Injection (8%) 1066
Invanz for Injection (0.5% to 1.1%) 2029
Proleukin for Injection 2287
ReoPro Vials (0.4%) 1860
Rythmol SR Capsules (1% to 2%) 1590
Sular Extended Release Tablets (Less than or equal to 1%) 2975
Timoptic Sterile Ophthalmic Solution 2121
Timoptic in Ocudose 2124
Timoptic-XE Sterile Ophthalmic Gel Forming Solution 2125
▲ Trisenox Injection (10%) 986
▲ Vesanoid Capsules (14%) 2660

Rash
▲ Abelcet Injection (4%) 1134
Abilify Injection (1 in 100 patients to 2%) 881
Abilify Injection (Greater than or equal to 1 in 100 patients) 2466
Abilify Oral Solution (1 in 100 patients to 2%) 881
Abilify Oral Solution (Greater than or equal to 1 in 100 patients) 2466
Abilify Discmelt Orally Disintegrating Tablets (1 in 100 patients to 2%) 881
Abilify Discmelt Orally Disintegrating Tablets (Greater than or equal to 1 in 100 patients) 2466
Abilify Tablets (1 in 100 patients to 2%) 881
Abilify Tablets (Greater than or equal to 1 in 100 patients) 2466
Accolate Tablets 669
Accutane Capsules 2607
Aceon Tablets (2 mg, 4 mg, 8 mg) (2.3%) 3038
▲ Acetadote Injection (0.2% to 20.8%) 1001
▲ Actimmune (17%) 1743
Actiq (1% to 2%) 959
Activase I.V. (Very rare) 1188
Activella Tablets 2347
▲ Actonel Tablets (7.9% to 11.5%) 2568
▲ Actonel with Calcium Tablets (3.1% to 7.7%) 2574
Adderall XR Capsules 3012
Advair Diskus 100/50 1276
Advair Diskus 250/50 1276
Advair Diskus 500/50 1276
Advair HFA 45/21 Inhalation Aerosol (Rare) 1288

Advair HFA 115/21 Inhalation Aerosol (Rare) 1288
Advair HFA 230/21 Inhalation Aerosol (Rare) 1288
▲ Advicor Tablets (5%) 402
▲ Aerobid/Aerobid-M (3% to 9%) 1153
Aggrenox Capsules 819
▲ Agrylin Capsules (8.3%) 3017
Albenza Tablets (Less than 1%) 1297
Albutein 5% 1707
Albutein 25% 1708
▲ Alimta for Injection (Up to 22%) 1786
Alinia for Oral Suspension (Less than 1%) 2677
Alinia Tablets (Less than 1%) 2677
Allegra Oral Solution (Rare) 2684
Allegra Tablets (Rare) 2684
Allegra-D 12 Hour Extended-Release Tablets (Rare) 2687
Allegra-D 24 Hour Extended-Release Tablets (Rare) 2690
Aloxi Injection (Less than 1%) 1059
▲ Alphagan P Ophthalmic Solution (1% to 4%) 549
Alphanate 1709
Ambien Tablets (2%) 2692
Ambien CR Tablets (1%) 2696
▲ AmBisome for Injection (22.2% to 24.8%) 606
Amerge Tablets (Infrequent) 1301
Amitiza Capsules 3082
Amoxil Capsules 1305
Amoxil Chewable Tablets 1305
Amoxil Pediatric Drops for Oral Suspension 1305
Amoxil Powder for Oral Suspension 1305
Amoxil Tablets 1305
Amrix Capsules 966
▲ Anaprox Tablets (Less than 1% to 10%) 2632
▲ Anaprox DS Tablets (Less than 1% to 10%) 2632
Angeliq Tablets 751
Anzemet Injection (Rare) 2701
Anzemet Tablets 2704
Apidra Injection 2706
▲ Aptivus Capsules (3.1% to 21%) 823
▲ Aptivus Oral Solution (3.1% to 21%) 823
Aralast (0.1% to greater than or equal to 0.2%) 726
▲ Aranesp for Injection (7%) 564
▲ Argatroban Injection (1% to 10%) 1308
Aricept Tablets (Frequent) 1062
Aricept ODT Tablets (Frequent) 1062
▲ Arimidex Tablets (6% to 11%) 672
▲ Arixtra Injection (0.6% to 7.5%) 1313
▲ Asacol Delayed-Release Tablets (6%) 2579
Atacand Tablets (0.5% or greater) 639
Atacand HCT (0.5% or greater) 642
▲ Atripla Tablets (5% to 26%) 938
Atrovent HFA Inhalation Aerosol 839
Atrovent Nasal Spray 0.03% (Infrequent) 834
Atrovent Nasal Spray 0.06% (Rare) 836
Attenuvax (Occasional) 1951
▲ Augmentin (3%) 1323
▲ Augmentin Tablets (3%) 1327
Augmentin XR Extended Release Tablets 1333
Augmentin ES-600 Powder for Oral Suspension (1.1%) 1329
Avalide Tablets (1% or greater) 892
Avalide Tablets (1% or greater) 2713
Avandamet Tablets 1336
Avandaryl Tablets 1344
Avandia Tablets 1351
Avapro Tablets (1% or greater) 897
Avapro Tablets (1% or greater) 2718
Avastin IV (2.5%) 1192
Avelox (Greater than or equal to 0.1% to less than 2%) 2803
▲ Avinza Capsules (5% to 10%) 1772
Avodart Soft Gelatin Capsules 1359
Axert Tablets (Rare) 2431
Axid Capsules (1.9%) 1364
▲ Azilect Tablets (6%) 3106
▲ Azmacort Inhalation Aerosol (1% to 3%) 407
Bactroban Cream (1.1%) 1366
Bactroban Nasal (Less than 1%) 1367
Bactroban Ointment (Less than 1%) 1368
Beconase AQ Nasal Spray (Rare) 1369
▲ BeneFIX Vials (1.6% to 7.7%) 3191
Benicar Tablets (Greater than 0.5%) 1009
Benicar HCT Tablets (Greater than 1%) 1010
Bentyl Capsules 703
Bentyl Injection 703
Bentyl Syrup 703
Bentyl Tablets 703
▲ Betaseron for SC Injection (21%) 756
▲ Betimol Ophthalmic Solution (More than 5%) 3181
▲ Bexxar (Less than 1% to 17%) 1371
▲ Biaxin/Biaxin XL (3%) 411
Boniva Injection (1.3% to 2.3%) 2614
Boniva Tablets (1.3% to 2.3%) 2618
Boostrix 1377
BOTOX Purified Neurotoxin Complex (7 cases) 550
▲ Brovana Inhalation Solution (Up to 4%) 2990
▲ Busulfex Injection (57%) 2477
Bystolic Tablets (0% to 1%) 1155
▲ Campath Ampules (13%) 761
Campral Tablets (Frequent) 1158
Canasa Rectal Suppositories (1.2%) 705
▲ Cancidas for Injection (3.5% to 23.2%) 1953
▲ Captopril Tablets (About 4 to 7 of 100 patients) 2182
Carafate Suspension (Less than 0.5%) 706
Carafate Tablets (Less than 0.5%) 707
Carbatrol Capsules 3019
▲ Cardizem LA Extended Release Tablets (1% to 4%) 421
Catapres Tablets (About 1 in 100 patients) 841
Catapres-TTS (0.5% or less) 842
Ceftin (0.1% to 1%) 1380
Celebrex Capsules 2979
Celexa (Frequent) 1160
▲ CellCept Capsules (3% to 22.1%) 2622
▲ CellCept Intravenous (3% to 22.1%) 2622
▲ CellCept Oral Suspension (3% to 22.1%) 2622
▲ CellCept Tablets (3% to 22.1%) 2622
▲ Cerezyme for Injection (Approximately 6.5%) 1238
▲ Chantix Tablets (1% to 3%) 2511
▲ Chemet Capsules (2.6% to 11.2%) 2484
Cialis Tablets (Less than 2%) 1792
Cimzia (Rare) 3127
Cipro I.V. (Greater than or equal to 1%) 2817
Cipro (1% to 1.8%) 2810
Cipro XR Tablets 2823
Clarinex Syrup (Rare) 2828
Clarinex Tablets (Rare) 2828
Clarinex Reditabs Tablets (Rare) 2828
Clarinex-D 12-Hour Extended-Release Tablets (Rare) 2831
Clarinex-D 24-Hour Extended-Release Tablets 2834
Climara Transdermal System 763
Climara Pro Transdermal System (2.4%) 768
▲ Clinoril Tablets (3% to 9%) 1962
Clorpres Tablets (1%) 2185
Combigan Ophthalmic Solution (0.1% to 0.2%) 553
Combivent Inhalation Aerosol (Rare) 845
▲ Combivir Tablets (9%) 1384
Comvax (0.8% to 0.9%) 1966
Concerta Extended-Release Tablets 1925
▲ Copaxone for Injection (18%) 3110
▲ Cosopt Sterile Ophthalmic Solution (1% to 5%) 1969
Cozaar Tablets (Less than 1%) 1973
Crestor Tablets 677
Crinone 4% Gel 992
Crinone 8% Gel 992
Crixivan Capsules (1.2%) 1979
▲ Cubicin for Injection (4.3% to 6.7%) 995
▲ Cuprimine Capsules (5%) 1986
▲ Cyanokit 5g Antidote (20% to 44%) 1021
▲ Cymbalta Delayed-Release Capsules (4%) 1801
▲ Dacogen Injection (19%) 1066
Daytrana Transdermal Patch 3022
Demadex Injection 2630
Demadex Tablets 2630
▲ Depakote ER Tablets (Greater than 1% to less than 5%) 423
Diovan Tablets (Greater than or equal to 0.2%) 2212
Diovan HCT Tablets (Greater than 0.2%) 2216
Divigel 3167
▲ Doribax Injection (1% to 5%) 2400
▲ Doxil Injection (1% to 28.5%) 2378
Duragesic Transdermal System (1% or greater) 2405
Dyazide Capsules 1405
DynaCirc CR Controlled Release Tablets (1.3% to 2.6%) 1407
Dyrenium Capsules (Rare) 3189
▲ EC-Naprosyn Delayed-Release Tablets (Less than 1% to 10%) 2632
Edecrin 698
Effexor XR Extended-Release Capsules (Frequent) 3195
Eldepryl Capsules 3052
▲ Elitek (1% to 13%) 2729
▲ Elmiron Capsules (3%) 2435
▲ Eloxatin for Injection (5% to 11%) 2731
Elspar for Injection 1990
Emend Capsules (Greater than 0.5%) 1992
Emend for Injection (Greater than 0.5%) 1999
▲ Emsam Transdermal System (4%) 905
▲ Emtriva Capsules (Greater than or equal to 10%) 1246
▲ Emtriva Oral Solution (Greater than or equal to 10%) 1246
Enablex Extended-Release Tablets (Greater than or equal to 1%) 2225
▲ Enbrel for Injection (5% to 14%) 569
Engerix-B Vaccine (Less than 1%) 1409
Enjuvia Tablets 1029
▲ Epivir (9% to 12%) 1412
▲ Epivir-HBV (5%) 1417
▲ Epogen for Injection (16%) 576
▲ Epzicom Tablets (5%) 1422
▲ Equetro Extended-Release Capsules (13%) 3174
▲ Erbitux (12% to 89%) 912
Estratest Tablets 3043
Estratest H.S. Tablets 3043
▲ Evista Tablets (5.5%) 1810
▲ Evoxac Capsules (4.3%) 1013
Exelon Capsules (2% or more) 2229
Exelon Oral Solution (2% or more) 2229
Exelon Patch (Infrequent) 2233
Exforge Tablets (Greater than or equal to 0.2%) 2238
▲ Exjade Tablets (8.4%) 2244
Extina Foam, 2% (Less than or equal to 1%) 3057
▲ Fabrazyme for Intravenous Infusion (10%) 1241
▲ Faslodex Injection (7.3%) 682
Feiba VH 728
▲ Femara Tablets (4% to 5%) 2246
Fenoglide Tablets (Rare) 2960
Fentora Tablets (Greater than 1%) 968
Flebogamma 5% 1715
Flebogamma 5% DIF 1718
Fleet Phospho-soda (Rare) 1145
Fleet Phospho-soda EZ-PREP (Rare) 1147
Fleet Prep Kits 1149
▲ Flolan for Injection (10% to 25%) 1426
Flomax Capsules 848
Flonase Nasal Spray 1431
▲ Flovent Diskus 50 mcg (8%) 1435
Fluarix Vaccine 1446
Flulaval Injection Vaccine 1448
Flumadine (0.3% to 1%) 1167
FluMist Vaccine 1945
Focalin XR Capsules 2251
Foradil Aerolizer (1.1%) 2849
Fortaz (2%) 1450
▲ Forteo for Injection (4.9%) 1816
Fosamax (Rare) 2005
Fosamax Plus D Tablets 2013
Fragmin Injection (Rare) 1070
Furosemide Tablets 2186
▲ Gabitril Tablets (5%) 973
▲ Gamunex (6%) 3094
Gantrisin Pediatric Suspension 2638
▲ Gemzar for Injection (28% to 30%) 1820
▲ Gengraf Capsules (1% to 8%) 435
Genotropin Lyophilized Powder (Infrequent) 2547
▲ Geodon (4%) 2520
▲ Gleevec Tablets (25% to 53%) 2255
▲ Gliadel Wafer (2% to 12%) 1076
Gris-PEG Tablets (Rare) 2507
Havrix Injection Vaccine (Less than 1%) 1454
Hepsera Tablets 1253
▲ Herceptin I.V. (18%) 1199
Hexalen Capsules 1078
Humalog-Pen and KwikPen (Less common) 1829
Humalog Mix 50/50-Pen and KwikPen 1833
Humalog Mix 75/25-Pen and KwikPen 1835
Human Albumin Grifols 25% 1706
▲ Humira Injection (Less than 1% to 12%) 442
Humulin 50/50, 100 Units 1843
Humulin 70/30 Vial (Less common) 1844
Humulin N Vial (Less common) 1846
Humulin R 1849
Humulin R (U-500) 1850
▲ Hyalgan Solution (14%) 2742
▲ Hycamtin for Injection (Less than 1% to 16%) 1459
Imitrex Injection (Infrequent) 1465
Imitrex Nasal Spray (Infrequent) 1470
Imitrex Tablets (Rare to infrequent) 1474
Indocin Capsules (Less than 1%) 2024
Indocin I.V. (Less than 1%) 2489
Indocin (Less than 1%) 2024
Infanrix Vaccine 1479
▲ Intelence Tablets (9% to 16.9%) 3119
Intravenous Sodium Diuril 2490
▲ Intron A for Injection (Up to 25%) 2859
Invanz for Injection (2.3% to 2.9%) 2029
▲ Ionsys Transdermal System (1% to less than 10%) 2410
Isentress Tablets 2036
▲ Ixempra Kit for Injection (9%) 915
Janumet Tablets 2041
Januvia Tablets 2048
Kaletra (0% to 2%) 452
▲ Kepivance (Less than 1% to 62%) 583
Keppra Oral Solution (1% to greater than or equal to 2%) 3131
Keppra Tablets (1% to greater than or equal to 2%) 3131
Ketek Tablets (Greater than or equal to 0.2% to less than 2%) 2744
Klonopin 2639
Kogenate FS 746
Kogenate FS with Bio-Set 748
▲ Lamictal (10%) 1488
▲ Lamisil Oral Granules (2% to 6%) 2264
▲ Lamisil Tablets (5.6%) 2266
Lantus Injection 2749
Lescol Capsules (2.3%) 2268
Lescol XL Tablets (1.6%) 2268
Leukeran Tablets (Rare) 1508
▲ Leukine (44% to 70%) 774
▲ Leustatin Injection (10% to 27%) 2384
▲ Levaquin (2%) 2416
Levaquin in 5% Dextrose Injection (2%) 2416
Levemir Injection 2352
Levitra Tablets (Less than 2%) 2876
Levothroid Tablets 1170
Levoxyl Tablets 1780
Lexapro Oral Suspension (Frequent) 1174
Lexapro Tablets (Frequent) 1174
▲ Lexiva Oral Suspension (Less than or equal to 1% to 19%) 1510
▲ Lexiva Tablets (Less than or equal to 1% to 19%) 1510
Lialda Tablets (Infrequent) 3029
▲ Lipitor Tablets (1.1% to 3.9%) 2501
Lortab 5/500 Tablets 3143
Lortab 7.5/500 Tablets 3144
Lortab 10/500 Tablets 3144
Lotrisone Cream (Less than 1%) 2881
▲ Lovaza Capsules (1.8% to 4%) 1520
▲ Lunesta Tablets (3% to 4%) 2994
Lupron Depot 3.75 mg 462
Lupron Depot 7.5 mg 469
Lupron Depot–3 Month 11.25 mg 462
Lupron Depot-PED 7.5 mg, 11.25 mg and 15 mg 471
Lyrica Capsules 2527
Malarone Pediatric Tablets 1521
Malarone Tablets 1521
Mavik Tablets (0.3% to 1%) 472
Maxair Autohaler 1705
Maxalt Tablets (Infrequent) 2056
Maxalt-MLT Orally Disintegrating Tablets (Infrequent) 2056
▲ Megace ES Oral Suspension (2% to 12%) 2499
▲ Mepron Suspension (6.3% to 46%) 1526
▲ Meridia Capsules (3.8%) 475
▲ Merrem I.V. (1.6% to 3.1%) 684
Meruvax II 2061
Metadate CD Capsules 3146
▲ Mevacor Tablets (0.8% to 5.2%) 2063
Miacalcin Injection 2273
Micardis Tablets (More than 0.3%) 852
Micardis HCT Tablets (2% or greater) 854
Mirapex Tablets (Greater than or equal to 1%) 857
M-M-R II (Infrequent) 2054
Moban Tablets 1116
▲ Mobic Oral Suspension (0.3% to 3%) 863
▲ Mobic Tablets (0.3% to 3%) 863
Motrin IB Tablets and Caplets 1900
Children's Motrin Oral Suspension 1901

Children's Motrin Non-Staining Dye-Free Oral Suspension 1901
Children's Motrin Cold Oral Suspension 1899
Infants' Motrin Concentrated Drops 1901
Infants' Motrin Non-Staining Dye-Free Concentrated Drops 1901
Junior Strength Motrin Caplets and Chewable Tablets 1901
MoviPrep Oral Solution 2679
MS Contin Tablets (Less frequent) 2585
▲ Mycamine for Injection (5.4% to 25.9%) 616
▲ Myfortic Tablets (3% to less than 20%) 2276
▲ Mylotarg for Injection (18%) 3212
Nadolol Tablets (1 to 5 of 1000 patients) 2191
Naftin Gel (0.5%) 2164
▲ Nalfon Capsules (3.7%) 2508
Namenda (Frequent) 1180
▲ Naprosyn Suspension (Less than 1% to 10%) 2632
▲ Naprosyn Tablets (Less than 1% to 10%) 2632
Natrecor for Injection (Greater than or equal to 1%) 2977
Nembutal Sodium Solution, USP 2494
▲ Neoral Oral Solution (1% to 8%) 2280
▲ Neoral Soft Gelatin Capsules (1% to 8%) 2280
Neulasta Injection 587
▲ Neupogen for Injection (6% to 12%) 589
▲ Nexavar Tablets (19% to 40%) 784
Nexium Delayed-Release Capsules (Less than 1%) 645
Nexium I.V. (Less than 1%) 652
Nexium Delayed-Release Oral Suspension (Less than 1%) 645
▲ Niaspan Extended-Release Tablets (1% to 5%) 480
Nimbex Injection (0.1%) 484
Nimotop Capsules (Up to 2.4%) 790
Norditropin Cartridges 2354
Noroxin Tablets (0.3% to 1%) 2069
▲ Norvir (0% to 3.5%) 489
Novantrone for Injection Concentrate 1100
NovoLog Injection 2359
NovoSeven (1%) 2367
NovoSeven RT (1%) 2370
▲ Noxafil Oral Suspension (1% to 19%) 2889
NuvaRing 2897
Omnicef Capsules (0.9%) 497
▲ Omnicef for Oral Suspension (3%) 497
▲ Oncaspar Injection (Greater than 5%) 1138
▲ Ontak Vials (34%) 1079
OptiPranolol Metipranolol Ophthalmic Solution 0.3% (A small number of patients) ..... ⊙ 245
▲ Orencia Powder for Intravenous Infusion (4%) 921
Ortho-Cyclen/Ortho Tri-Cyclen 2449
Ortho Tri-Cyclen Lo Tablets 2458
Orthoclone OKT3 Sterile Solution 2387
OsmoPrep Tablets (Rare) 2680
▲ OxyContin Tablets (Between 1% and 5%) 2589
OxyIR Capsules 2593
▲ Panretin Gel 0.1% (25% to 77%) 1081
Parnate Tablets (Rare) 1532
Paser Granules (Among most common) 1747
▲ Paxil (2% to 3%) 1535
▲ Paxil CR Controlled-Release Tablets (2% to 3%) 1544
▲ PegIntron Powder for Injection (6%) 2903
Pentasa Capsules (1% to 1.3%) 3030
Pepcid Tablets (Infrequent) 2075
Percocet Tablets 1127
Percodan Tablets 1130
Persantine Tablets (2.3%) 869
Phenytek Capsules 2192
▲ Photofrin for Injection (7%) 708
▲ Plavix Tablets (4.2%) 926
▲ Plavix Tablets (4.2%) 2767
Pletal Tablets (2% or greater) 2481
Pneumovax 23 2078
Potaba (Infrequent) 1698
Precose Tablets (Rare) 792
Premarin Intravenous 3217
Premarin Tablets 3221
Premarin Vaginal Cream 3228
▲ Premphase Tablets (4% to 6%) 3232
▲ Prempro Tablets (4% to 6%) 3232
Primaxin I.M. (0.4%) 2080
Primaxin I.V. (1.5%) 2083
Prinivil Tablets (0.3% to 1.7%) 2087
Prinzide Tablets (1.2%) 2092
Pristiq Extended-Release Tablets (Less than 1% to 2%) 3247
ProAmatine Tablets (2.4%; Less frequent) 3032
▲ Procrit for Injection (Rare to 16%) 2391
Proglycem Capsules (Frequent) 1185
Proglycem Suspension (Frequent) 1185
▲ Prograf Capsules and Injection (10% to 24%) 622
Prolastin (Occasional) 3099
▲ Proleukin for Injection (42%) 2287
Propecia Tablets (0.5%) 2095
ProQuad (1.6%) 2099
Proscar Tablets (0.5%) 2102
Protonix for Delayed-Release Oral Suspension (Less than 1% to 2%) 3254
Protonix Delayed-Release Tablets (Less than 1% to 2%) 3254
▲ Protonix I.V. (6%) 3257
▲ Protopic Ointment (2% to 5%) 628
Proventil HFA Inhalation Aerosol (Less than 3%) 2914
Provigil Tablets (At least 1%) 977
▲ Prozac Weekly Capsules (1% to 6%) 1852
▲ Prozac Pulvules and Liquid (2% to 6%) 1852
Pulmicort Flexhaler 654
▲ Pulmozyme Inhalation Solution (3% to 12%) 1217
Qvar Inhalation Aerosol (Rare) 3116
▲ Rapamune Oral Solution (10% to 20%) 3260
▲ Rebetol (17% to 28%) 2917
▲ Reclast Injection (3%) 2291
Recombivax HB (Less than 1%) 2107
ReFacto Vials 3269
Refludan for Injection (Uncommon) 795
Remeron Tablets (Frequent) 2924
RemeronSolTab Tablets (Frequent) 2927
▲ Remicade for IV Injection (10%) 950
Requip Tablets (Infrequent to frequent) 1561
▲ Retrovir Capsules (17%) 1574
▲ Retrovir IV Infusion (17%) 1579
▲ Retrovir (17%) 1574
▲ Reyataz Capsules (5% to 21%) 3299
Risperdal Consta Long-Acting Injection (Frequent) 1753
▲ Rituxan I.V. (1% to 15%) 1223
Rocaltrol Capsules 1150
Rocaltrol Oral Solution 1150
Rocephin Injectable Vials, ADD-Vantage, Galaxy, Bulk (1.7%) 2642
▲ Romazicon Injection (1% to 3%) 2646
▲ Rythmol Tablets (3%) 1586
Salagen Tablets (1% to 2%) 1082
Sanctura XR Capsules (Less than 2%) 557
Sandostatin Injection (Less than 1%) 2300
▲ Sandostatin LAR Depot (3.8% to 15%) 2302
▲ Selzentry Tablets (9.6%) 2534
Sensipar Tablets 594
▲ Serevent Diskus (Less than 3% to 4%) 1594
Seromycin Capsules 1864
▲ Simulect for Injection (3% to 10%) 2306
Singulair (1.6% to 2% or greater) 2114
Skelaxin Tablets (Most frequent) 1784
▲ Soriatane Capsules (1% to 10%) 3062
▲ Spiriva HandiHaler (2% to 4%) 870
Starlix Tablets 2314
Strattera Capsules (2%) 1864
Stromectol Tablets (0.9%) 2120
Sular Extended Release Tablets (2%) 2975
▲ Sulfamylon Cream (4.6%) 2194
▲ Sulfamylon for 5% Topical Solution (4.6%) 2194
Suprax for Oral Suspension (Less than 2%) 1891
Suprax Tablets (Less than 2%) 1891
▲ Sustiva Capsules (5% to 46%) 930
▲ Sustiva Tablets (5% to 46%) 930
▲ Sutent Capsules (1% to 38%) 2540
▲ Synagis Intramuscular Solution (25.6%) 1948
Synthroid Tablets 507
Tamiflu Capsules 2649
Tamiflu Oral Suspension 2649
▲ Tarceva Tablets (0% to 69%) 1228
▲ Targretin Capsules (16.7% to 22.6%) 1084
▲ Targretin Gel 1% (10% to 78%) 1088
Tarka Tablets (0.3% or more) 511
▲ Tasigna Capsules (Greater than 10% to 33%) 2316
▲ Taxotere Injection Concentrate (0.3% to 19.9%) 2773
Tekturna Tablets (1%) 2321
Tekturna HCT Tablets (1%) 2324
▲ Temodar Capsules (1% to 19%) 2931
Teveten Tablets (Less than 1%) 515
Teveten HCT Tablets (Less than 1%) 517
Thiothixene Capsules 2197
Thyrogen for Injection 1244
▲ Tice BCG (Less than or equal to 1% to 3%) 2936
Timentin ADD-Vantage 1606
Timentin Injection Galaxy Container 1609
Timentin IV Infusion 1603
Timentin Pharmacy Bulk Package 1613
Timoptic Sterile Ophthalmic Solution (Less frequent) 2121
Timoptic in Ocudose (Less frequent) 2124
Timoptic-XE Sterile Ophthalmic Gel Forming Solution 2125
TNKase (Less than 1%) 1233
▲ Toprol-XL Tablets (About 5 of 100 patients) 666
▲ Torisel Injection (5% to 47%) 3272
Tracleer Tablets 3289
Transderm Scōp Transdermal Therapeutic System (Infrequent) 2206
Trasylol Injection (2%) 799
▲ Treanda for Injection (3% to 8%) 983
Treximet Tablets (Infrequent) 1616
▲ Tricor Tablets (1.4% to 6%) 520
▲ Trizivir Tablets (9%) 1622
Trusopt Sterile Ophthalmic Solution (Rare) 2128
▲ Truvada Tablets (Greater than or equal to 10%) 1262
Tussionex Pennkinetic Extended-Release Suspension 3154
Twinrix Vaccine (Less than 1%) 1628
Tygacil for Injection (2.4%) 3276
▲ Tykerb Tablets (0% to 28%) 1631
Tylenol with Codeine Tablets 2427
▲ Tyzeka Tablets (4%) 2328
Ultane Liquid for Inhalation (Less than 1%) 524
Uroqid-Acid No. 2 Tablets (Occasional) 814
Urso 250 Tablets (1%) 720
Urso Forte Tablets (1%) 720
Valium Tablets (Infrequent) 2658
▲ Valstar Sterile Solution for Intravesical Instillation (3%) 1735
▲ Valtrex Caplets (0.4% to 8%) 1635
▲ Vaqta (1% to 4.5%) 2130
Varivax (Greater than or equal to 1%) 2133
▲ Vectibix (1% to 22%) 597
▲ Velcade for Injection (18% to 19%) 2168
▲ Venlafaxine Hydrochloride Tablets (3%) 2199
Ventolin HFA Inhalation Aerosol 1638
▲ Vesanoid Capsules (54%) 2660
Viadur Implant (Less than 2%) 802
Vicodin Tablets 529
Vicodin ES Tablets 530
Vicodin HP Tablets 531
Vicoprofen Tablets (Less than 1%) 533
▲ Vigamox Ophthalmic Solution (1% to 4%) 548
▲ Viread Tablets (5% to 18%) 1268
▲ Visudyne for Injection (10% to 30%) 2332
▲ Vivitrol (5% to 12%) 988
▲ Voltaren Ophthalmic Solution (Less than or equal to 3%) 2336
Vytorin 10/10 Tablets 2149
Vytorin 10/10 Tablets 2939
Vytorin 10/20 Tablets 2149
Vytorin 10/20 Tablets 2939
Vytorin 10/40 Tablets 2149
Vytorin 10/40 Tablets 2939
Vytorin 10/80 Tablets 2149
Vytorin 10/80 Tablets 2939
▲ Vyvanse Capsules (1% to 3%) 3033
▲ Wellbutrin Tablets (8%) 1648
▲ Wellbutrin SR Sustained-Release Tablets (4% to greater than or equal to 5%) 1653
▲ Wellbutrin XL Extended-Release Tablets (0.9% to 3%) 1659
WinRho SDF 741
▲ Xenical Capsules (4.3%) 2672
Xifaxan Tablets (Less than 2%) 2682
▲ Xopenex Inhalation Solution (7.5%) 3001
▲ Xopenex Inhalation Solution Concentrate (7.5%) 3005
▲ Xopenex HFA Inhalation Aerosol (7.5%) 3009
Xyzal Oral Solution 2789
Xyzal Oral Solution 3155
Zantac 25 EFFERdose Tablets (Rare) 1670
Zantac Injection 1666
Zantac Injection Pharmacy Bulk Package (Rare) 1668
Zantac Injection Premixed 1666
Zantac (Rare) 1670
Zemplar Injection 538
Zemuron Injection (Less than 1%) 2947
Zetia Tablets 2157
Zetia Tablets 2951
▲ Ziagen (5% to 7%) 1673
Zinacef for Injection (1 in 125 patients) 1678
Zinacef Injection (1 in 125 patients) 1678
Zocor Tablets 2136
Zofran Injection (Approximately 1%) 1682
Zofran (Approximately 1%) 1687
Zofran ODT Orally Disintegrating Tablets (Approximately 1%) 1687
Zometa for Intravenous Infusion (Rare) 2341
Zomig Tablets (Infrequent) 694
Zomig Nasal Spray (Infrequent) 689
Zomig-ZMT Tablets (Infrequent) 694
▲ Zonegran Capsules (3%) 1089
Zostavax Injection 2145
▲ Zosyn for Injection (1.3% to 4.2%) 3284
Zovirax Capsules 1690
Zovirax Ointment 819
Zovirax 1690
▲ Zyban Sustained-Release Tablets (3% to 4%) 1692
Zyprexa Tablets 1883
Zyprexa ZYDIS Orally Disintegrating Tablets 1883
Zyrtec Chewable Tablets (Less than 2%) 1920
Zyrtec Syrup (Less than 2%) 1920
Zyrtec Tablets (Less than 2%) 1920
Zyrtec-D 12 Hour Extended Release Tablets (Less than 2%) 1923
▲ Zyvox (0.4% to 7%) 2552

Rash, allergic

Humira Injection 442
Lybrel Tablets 3204
Mircette Tablets 1034
Neupro Transdermal System 3149
Ortho-Cyclen Tablets 2449
Ortho Evra Transdermal System 2437
Ortho Tri-Cyclen Tablets 2449
Ortho Tri-Cyclen Lo Tablets 2458
Premphase Tablets 3232
Prempro Tablets 3232
Prometrium Capsules (100 mg, 200 mg) 3047
Relenza Inhalation Powder 1556
Seasonique Tablets 1046
Varivax (Greater than or equal to 1%) 2133
Yaz Tablets 805

Rash, bullous

Actonel with Calcium Tablets 2574
Exelon Capsules (Frequent) 2229
Exelon Oral Solution (Frequent) 2229
Lipitor Tablets 2501
▲ Zosyn for Injection (4.2%) 3284

Rash, diaper

▲ Augmentin ES-600 Powder for Oral Suspension (3.5%) 1329
▲ Ceftin for Oral Suspension (3.4%) 1380
Comvax (0.2% to 0.5%) 1966
▲ Invanz for Injection (4.7%) 2029

Rash, drug

Nitrolingual Pumpspray 2965

Rash, eczematous

Exelon Capsules (Frequent) 2229
Exelon Oral Solution (Frequent) 2229
▲ Ontak Vials (34%) 1079

Rash, erythematous

Abilify Injection (Greater than or equal to 1 in 100 patients) 2466
Abilify Oral Solution (Greater than or equal to 1 in 100 patients) 881
Abilify Oral Solution (Greater than or equal to 1 in 100 patients) 2466
Abilify Discmelt Orally Disintegrating Tablets (Greater than or equal to 1 in 100 patients) 881
Abilify Discmelt Orally Disintegrating Tablets (Greater than or equal to 1 in 100 patients) 2466
Abilify Tablets (Greater than or equal to 1 in 100 patients) 881
Abilify Tablets (Greater than or equal to 1 in 100 patients) 2466
Carbatrol Capsules 3019

Celebrex Capsules (0.1% to 1.9%) ... 2979
Combigan Ophthalmic Solution ... 553
Coreg Tablets (Greater than 0.1% to 1%) ... 1387
Coreg CR Extended-Release Capsules (0.1% to less than or equal to 1%) ... 1393
Cosopt Sterile Ophthalmic Solution ... 1969
Daytrana Transdermal Patch ... 3022
Denavir Cream (0.1%) ... 2205
Duragesic Transdermal System (1% or greater) ... 2405
▲ Eloxatin for Injection (2% to less than 5%) ... 2731
Equetro Extended-Release Capsules ... 3174
▲ Evoxac Capsules (1% to 3%) ... 1013
Exelon Capsules (Frequent) ... 2229
Exelon Oral Solution (Frequent) ... 2229
Exelon Patch (Infrequent) ... 2233
Exforge Tablets (Greater than 0.1% to less than 1%) ... 2238
▲ Femara Tablets (4% to 5%) ... 2246
▲ Hycamtin for Injection (Less than 1% to 16%) ... 1459
InnoPran XL Extended Release Capsules ... 1484
▲ Intron A for Injection (Less than 5%) ... 2859
Invanz for Injection (Greater than 0.5%) ... 2029
▲ Miacalcin Nasal Spray (1% to 3%) ... 2274
Mirapex Tablets ... 857
▲ Mobic Oral Suspension (0.3% to 3%) ... 863
▲ Mobic Tablets (0.3% to 3%) ... 863
Moxatag Tablets ... 2165
Namenda (Infrequent) ... 1180
▲ Neupro Transdermal System (2% to 6%) ... 3149
Nexium Delayed-Release Capsules (Less than 1%) ... 645
Nexium I.V. (Less than 1%) ... 652
Nexium Delayed-Release Oral Suspension (Less than 1%) ... 645
Plavix Tablets (Less than 1%) ... 926
Plavix Tablets (Less than 1%) ... 2767
Pylera Capsules ... 714
▲ Rebif Prefilled Syringe for Injection (5% to 7%) ... 1107
Remicade for IV Injection (Less than 1%) ... 950
Risperdal Consta Long-Acting Injection (Infrequent) ... 1753
Rocaltrol Capsules ... 1150
Rocaltrol Oral Solution ... 1150
▲ Soriatane Capsules (10% to 25%) ... 3062
Timoptic Sterile Ophthalmic Solution ... 2121
Timoptic in Ocudose ... 2124
Timoptic-XE Sterile Ophthalmic Gel Forming Solution ... 2125
▲ Xeloda Tablets (Less than 1% to 9%) ... 2662
▲ Zosyn for Injection (3.9%) ... 3284
Zyrtec Chewable Tablets (Less than 2%) ... 1920
Zyrtec Syrup (Less than 2%) ... 1920
Zyrtec Tablets (Less than 2%) ... 1920
Zyrtec-D 12 Hour Extended Release Tablets (Less than 2%) ... 1923

Rash, erythematous maculopapular
Amoxil Capsules ... 1305
Amoxil Chewable Tablets ... 1305
Amoxil Pediatric Drops for Oral Suspension ... 1305
Amoxil Powder for Oral Suspension ... 1305
Amoxil Tablets ... 1305
Mirapex Tablets ... 857
Moxatag Tablets ... 2165
Viramune Oral Suspension ... 873
Viramune Tablets ... 873

Rash, exfoliative
Abilify Injection (Greater than or equal to 1 in 100 patients) ... 2466
Abilify Oral Solution (Greater than or equal to 1 in 100 patients) ... 881
Abilify Oral Solution (Greater than or equal to 1 in 100 patients) ... 2466
Abilify Discmelt Orally Disintegrating Tablets (Greater than or equal to 1 in 100 patients) ... 881
Abilify Discmelt Orally Disintegrating Tablets (Greater than or equal to 1 in 100 patients) ... 2466
Abilify Tablets (Greater than or equal to 1 in 100 patients) ... 881
Abilify Tablets (Greater than or equal to 1 in 100 patients) ... 2466
▲ Atripla Tablets (Greater than or equal to 5%) ... 938
▲ Emtriva Capsules (7%) ... 1246
▲ Emtriva Oral Solution (7%) ... 1246
Exelon Capsules (Frequent) ... 2229
Exelon Oral Solution (Frequent) ... 2229
Tasigna Capsules (0.1% to 1%) ... 2316

Rash, extremities
Viramune Oral Suspension ... 873
Viramune Tablets ... 873

Rash, facial
Viramune Oral Suspension ... 873
Viramune Tablets ... 873

Rash, heat
Cubicin for Injection (Less than 1%) ... 995
▲ Vivitrol (5% to 12%) ... 988

Rash, herpetic
(*see under* Eruptions, herpetic)

Rash, injection site
Flulaval Injection Vaccine ... 1448
ProQuad (2.3%) ... 2099

Rash, lupus erythematosus
Evoxac Capsules (Less than 1%) ... 1013

Rash, macular
Abilify Injection (Greater than or equal to 1 in 100 patients) ... 2466
Abilify Oral Solution (Greater than or equal to 1 in 100 patients) ... 881
Abilify Oral Solution (Greater than or equal to 1 in 100 patients) ... 2466
Abilify Discmelt Orally Disintegrating Tablets (Greater than or equal to 1 in 100 patients) ... 881
Abilify Discmelt Orally Disintegrating Tablets (Greater than or equal to 1 in 100 patients) ... 2466
Abilify Tablets (Greater than or equal to 1 in 100 patients) ... 881
Abilify Tablets (Greater than or equal to 1 in 100 patients) ... 2466
Amerge Tablets (Rare) ... 1301
▲ Atripla Tablets (Greater than or equal to 5%) ... 938
Byetta Injection ... 600
Concerta Extended-Release Tablets ... 1925
▲ Emtriva Capsules (7%) ... 1246
▲ Emtriva Oral Solution (7%) ... 1246
Truvada Tablets ... 1262

Rash, maculopapular
Abelcet Injection ... 1134
Abilify Injection (Greater than or equal to 1 in 100 patients) ... 2466
Abilify Oral Solution (Greater than or equal to 1 in 100 patients) ... 881
Abilify Oral Solution (Greater than or equal to 1 in 100 patients) ... 2466
Abilify Discmelt Orally Disintegrating Tablets (Greater than or equal to 1 in 100 patients) ... 881
Abilify Discmelt Orally Disintegrating Tablets (Greater than or equal to 1 in 100 patients) ... 2466
Abilify Tablets (Greater than or equal to 1 in 100 patients) ... 881
Abilify Tablets (Greater than or equal to 1 in 100 patients) ... 2466
Actiq (Less than 1%) ... 959
Aptivus Capsules ... 823
Aptivus Oral Solution ... 823
▲ Atripla Tablets (Greater than or equal to 5%) ... 938
Avelox (Greater than or equal to 0.1% to less than 2%) ... 2803
▲ Busulfex Injection (8%) ... 2477
Campral Tablets (Infrequent) ... 1158
Capastat Sulfate for Injection ... 1791
Captopril Tablets ... 2182
Catapres-TTS ... 842
Celebrex Capsules (0.1% to 1.9%) ... 2979
Cipro XR Tablets (Less than 1%) ... 2823
▲ Clarinex Syrup (3.1%) ... 2828
Copaxone for Injection (Infrequent) ... 3110
Coreg Tablets (Greater than 0.1% to 1%) ... 1387
Coreg CR Extended-Release Capsules (0.1% to less than or equal to 1%) ... 1393
Depakote ER Tablets (Greater than 1%) ... 423
Didronel Tablets ... 2583
▲ Doxil Injection (Less than 1% to 10%) ... 2378
Effexor XR Extended-Release Capsules (Infrequent) ... 3195
Emsam Transdermal System (Infrequent) ... 905
▲ Emtriva Capsules (7% to 30%) ... 1246
▲ Emtriva Oral Solution (7% to 30%) ... 1246
Epivir ... 1412
Erbitux ... 912
Exelon Capsules (Frequent) ... 2229
Exelon Oral Solution (Frequent) ... 2229
Exforge Tablets (Greater than 0.1% to less than 1%) ... 2238
▲ Femara Tablets (4% to 5%) ... 2246
Gabitril Tablets (Infrequent) ... 973
Geodon Capsules (Infrequent) ... 2520
▲ Hycamtin for Injection (Less than 1% to 16%) ... 1459
▲ Intron A for Injection (Less than 5%) ... 2859
Kaletra (Less than 2%) ... 452
Lamictal (Infrequent) ... 1488
Lanoxin Injection (Rare) ... 1498
Lanoxin Injection Pediatric (Rare) ... 1502
Lanoxin Tablets (Rare) ... 1505
Lunesta Tablets (Rare) ... 2994
▲ Mobic Oral Suspension (0.3% to 3%) ... 863
▲ Mobic Tablets (0.3% to 3%) ... 863
Neupro Transdermal System ... 3149
Nexium Delayed-Release Capsules (Less than 1%) ... 645
Nexium I.V. (Less than 1%) ... 652
Nexium Delayed-Release Oral Suspension (Less than 1%) ... 645
Norvir (Less than 2%) ... 489
Omnicef for Oral Suspension (0.2%) ... 497
▲ Ontak Vials (34%) ... 1079
Paxil (Rare) ... 1535
Paxil CR Controlled-Release Tablets (Rare) ... 1544
Plavix Tablets (Less than 1%) ... 926
Plavix Tablets (Less than 1%) ... 2767
Protonix for Delayed-Release Oral Suspension (Less than 1%) ... 3254
Protonix Delayed-Release Tablets (Less than 1%) ... 3254
Protonix I.V. (Less than 1%) ... 3257
Protopic Ointment (2% to 4%) ... 628
Prozac Weekly Capsules (Infrequent) ... 1852
Prozac Pulvules and Liquid (Infrequent) ... 1852
Pylera Capsules ... 714
Raptiva for Injection ... 1218
▲ Rebif Prefilled Syringe for Injection (4% to 5%) ... 1107
Requip Tablets (Infrequent) ... 1561
Reyataz Capsules ... 3299
Sular Extended Release Tablets (Less than or equal to 1%) ... 2975
▲ Sustiva Capsules (16.7% to 24.5%) ... 930
▲ Sustiva Tablets (16.7% to 24.5%) ... 930
Symbyax Capsules (Rare) ... 1871
Targretin Capsules ... 1084
▲ Targretin Gel 1% (6%) ... 1088
Teveten Tablets (Less than 1%) ... 515
Teveten HCT Tablets (Less than 1%) ... 517
Tricor Tablets ... 520
Trizivir Tablets ... 1622
▲ Truvada Tablets (5%) ... 1262
Venlafaxine Hydrochloride Tablets (Infrequent) ... 2199
▲ Viread Tablets (5% to 18%) ... 1268
Wellbutrin SR Sustained-Release Tablets (Rare) ... 1653
Wellbutrin XL Extended-Release Tablets (Rare) ... 1659
Ziagen ... 1673
Zonegran Capsules (Infrequent) ... 1089
▲ Zosyn for Injection (4.2%) ... 3284
Zyban Sustained-Release Tablets (Rare) ... 1692
Zyprexa Tablets (Rare) ... 1883
Zyprexa ZYDIS Orally Disintegrating Tablets (Rare) ... 1883
Zyrtec Chewable Tablets (Less than 2%) ... 1920
Zyrtec Syrup (Less than 2%) ... 1920
Zyrtec Tablets (Less than 2%) ... 1920
Zyrtec-D 12 Hour Extended Release Tablets (Less than 2%) ... 1923

Rash, measles-like
▲ ProQuad (3%) ... 2099

Rash, morbilliform
Phenytek Capsules (Among most common) ... 2192

Rash, papular
Abilify Injection (Greater than or equal to 1 in 100 patients) ... 2466
Abilify Oral Solution (Greater than or equal to 1 in 100 patients) ... 881
Abilify Oral Solution (Greater than or equal to 1 in 100 patients) ... 2466
Abilify Discmelt Orally Disintegrating Tablets (Greater than or equal to 1 in 100 patients) ... 881
Abilify Discmelt Orally Disintegrating Tablets (Greater than or equal to 1 in 100 patients) ... 2466
Abilify Tablets (Greater than or equal to 1 in 100 patients) ... 881
Abilify Tablets (Greater than or equal to 1 in 100 patients) ... 2466
Byetta Injection ... 600
▲ Chemet Capsules (2.6% to 11.2%) ... 2484
Mirapex Tablets ... 857
▲ Stromectol Tablets (22.7%) ... 2120
▲ Vivitrol (5% to 12%) ... 988

Rash, papular, neck
Alferon N Injection (1%) ... 1726

Rash, pemphigoid
Nadolol Tablets ... 2191
Stalevo Tablets ... 2309

Rash, petechial
Effexor XR Extended-Release Capsules (Rare) ... 3195
Lamictal (Rare) ... 1488
Lyrica Capsules (Rare) ... 2527
▲ Ontak Vials (34%) ... 1079
Prozac Weekly Capsules (Rare) ... 1852
Prozac Pulvules and Liquid (Rare) ... 1852
Venlafaxine Hydrochloride Tablets (Rare) ... 2199

Rash, pruritic
Amerge Tablets (Rare) ... 1301
▲ Atripla Tablets (Greater than or equal to 5%) ... 938
▲ Captopril Tablets (About 4 to 7 of 100 patients) ... 2182
Carbatrol Capsules ... 3019
▲ Emtriva Capsules (7%) ... 1246
▲ Emtriva Oral Solution (7%) ... 1246
Equetro Extended-Release Capsules ... 3174
Premphase Tablets ... 3232
Prempro Tablets ... 3232
Requip Tablets (Infrequent) ... 1561
Skelaxin Tablets (Most frequent) ... 1784
Truvada Tablets ... 1262
Velcade for Injection ... 2168

Rash, psoriaform
Coreg Tablets (Less than or equal to 0.1% to 1%) ... 1387
Coreg CR Extended-Release Capsules (0.1% to less than or equal to 1%) ... 1393
Cosopt Sterile Ophthalmic Solution ... 1969
Exelon Capsules (Frequent) ... 2229
Exelon Oral Solution (Frequent) ... 2229
▲ Femara Tablets (4% to 5%) ... 2246
InnoPran XL Extended Release Capsules ... 1484
Lamisil Tablets ... 2266
Requip Tablets (Infrequent) ... 1561
▲ Soriatane Capsules (1% to 10%) ... 3062
Timoptic Sterile Ophthalmic Solution ... 2121
Timoptic in Ocudose ... 2124
Timoptic-XE Sterile Ophthalmic Gel Forming Solution ... 2125

Rash, psoriasiform
Combigan Ophthalmic Solution ... 553

Rash, purpuric
Avelox (Greater than or equal to 0.1% to less than 2%) ... 2803
Lyrica Capsules (Rare) ... 2527
Phenytek Capsules ... 2192
Prozac Weekly Capsules (Rare) ... 1852
Prozac Pulvules and Liquid (Rare) ... 1852

Rash, pustular
Anaprox Tablets (Less than 1%) ... 2632
Anaprox DS Tablets (Less than 1%) ... 2632
▲ Atripla Tablets (Greater than or equal to 5%) ... 938

Avelox (Greater than or equal to 0.1% to less than 2%) 2803
Copaxone for Injection (Frequent) 3110
Doxil Injection (Less than 1%) 2378
EC-Naprosyn Delayed-Release Tablets (Less than 1%) 2632
Effexor XR Extended-Release Capsules (Rare) 3195
▲ Emtriva Capsules (17% to 30%) 1246
▲ Emtriva Oral Solution (17% to 30%) 1246
Erbitux 912
Lamictal (Rare) 1488
Lyrica Capsules (Rare) 2527
Naprosyn Suspension (Less than 1%) 2632
Naprosyn Tablets (Less than 1%) 2632
▲ Protopic Ointment (3% to 8%) 628
Prozac Weekly Capsules (Rare) 1852
Prozac Pulvules and Liquid (Rare) 1852
▲ Stromectol Tablets (22.7%) 2120
Sular Extended Release Tablets (Less than or equal to 1%) 2975
Targretin Capsules 1084
Venlafaxine Hydrochloride Tablets (Rare) 2199
▲ Viread Tablets (5% to 18%) 1268
Zonegran Capsules (Infrequent) 1089
Zyprexa Tablets (Rare) 1883
Zyprexa ZYDIS Orally Disintegrating Tablets (Rare) 1883

Rash, rubella-like
ProQuad (Greater than or equal to 0.2% to less than 1%) 2099

Rash, scarlatiniform
Phenytek Capsules 2192

Rash, trunk
Viramune Oral Suspension 873
Viramune Tablets 873

Rash, unspecified
Follistim AQ Cartridge 2844
Uroxatral Tablets 2786
▲ Viramune Oral Suspension (5.1% to 6.7%) 873
▲ Viramune Tablets (5.1% to 6.7%) 873
▲ Voltaren Tablets (1% to 10%) 2334
▲ Voltaren-XR Tablets (1% to 10%) 2337

Rash, urticarial
Aptivus Capsules 823
Aptivus Oral Solution 823
Captopril Tablets (Rare) 2182
Daytrana Transdermal Patch 3022
▲ Ontak Vials (34%) 1079
Prevnar (0.4% to 1.4%) 3241
ProNutra Protein Supplement 1730
▲ Stromectol Tablets (22.7%) 2120
Trizivir Tablets 1622
Ziagen 1673
▲ Zosyn for Injection (4.2%) 3284

Rash, varicella-like
ProQuad (2.1%) 2099
▲ Varivax (0.9% to 5.5%) 2133

Rash, vasculitic
Accolate Tablets (Rare) 669
Advair Diskus 100/50 1276
Advair Diskus 250/50 1276
Advair Diskus 500/50 1276
Flovent Diskus 50 mcg 1435
Gleevec Tablets (Rare) 2255
Paxil 1535
Paxil CR Controlled-Release Tablets 1544
Singulair 2114
Xolair 2339

Rash, vesicular
▲ Atripla Tablets (Greater than or equal to 5%) 938
▲ Emtriva Capsules (7%) 1246
▲ Emtriva Oral Solution (7%) 1246
Truvada Tablets 1262

Rash, vesiculobullous
Actiq (Less than 1%) 959
AmBisome for Injection (Less common) 606
Aricept Tablets (Infrequent) 1062
Aricept ODT Tablets (Infrequent) 1062
▲ Atripla Tablets (Greater than or equal to 5%) 938
Azilect Tablets (Greater than 1%) 3106
▲ Busulfex Injection (10%) 2477
Campral Tablets (Infrequent) 1158
▲ CellCept Capsules (3% to less than 20%) 2622
▲ CellCept Intravenous (3% to less than 20%) 2622
▲ CellCept Oral Suspension (3% to less than 20%) 2622
▲ CellCept Tablets (3% to less than 20%) 2622
Copaxone for Injection (Infrequent) 3110
Depakote ER Tablets (Greater than 1%) 423
▲ Doxil Injection (Less than 1% to 10%) 2378
Effexor XR Extended-Release Capsules (Rare) 3195
Emsam Transdermal System (Infrequent) 905
▲ Emtriva Capsules (17% to 30%) 1246
▲ Emtriva Oral Solution (17% to 30%) 1246
Gabitril Tablets (Infrequent) 973
Geodon Capsules (Infrequent) 2520
Ionsys Transdermal System (.1% to less than 1%) 2410
Keppra Oral Solution (2%) 3131
Keppra Tablets (2%) 3131
Lamictal (Rare) 1488
Lovenox Injection 2756
Lunesta Tablets (Rare) 2994
Lyrica Capsules (0.1% to 1%) 2527
▲ Megace ES Oral Suspension (1% to 3%) 2499
Norvir (Less than 2%) 489
▲ Ontak Vials (34%) 1079
Paxil (Rare) 1535
Paxil CR Controlled-Release Tablets (Rare) 1544
▲ Protopic Ointment (2% to 3%) 628
Prozac Weekly Capsules (Infrequent) 1852
Prozac Pulvules and Liquid (Infrequent) 1852
Salagen Tablets (Less than 1%) 1082
Symbyax Capsules (Infrequent) 1871
Targretin Capsules 1084
Venlafaxine Hydrochloride Tablets (Rare) 2199
▲ Viread Tablets (5% to 18%) 1268
Zonegran Capsules (Infrequent) 1089
Zyprexa Tablets (2%) 1883
Zyprexa ZYDIS Orally Disintegrating Tablets (2%) 1883

Rash at injection site
Norditropin Cartridges 2354
ProQuad 2099

Raynaud's phenomenon
Bystolic Tablets 1155
Captopril Tablets (2 to 3 of 1000 patients) 2182
Catapres Tablets (Rare) 841
Catapres-TTS (0.5% or less) 842
Clorpres Tablets (Rare) 2185
Combigan Ophthalmic Solution 553
Concerta Extended-Release Tablets 1925
Cosopt Sterile Ophthalmic Solution 1969
Imitrex Injection (Rare) 1465
Imitrex Nasal Spray 1470
Imitrex Tablets 1474
Intron A for Injection 2859
Metadate CD Capsules 3146
Mirapex Tablets 857
Nadolol Tablets (2 of 100 patients) 2191
Sandostatin Injection (Less than 1%) 2300
Sandostatin LAR Depot 2302
Strattera Capsules (Very Rare) 1864
Timoptic Sterile Ophthalmic Solution 2121
Timoptic in Ocudose 2124
Timoptic-XE Sterile Ophthalmic Gel Forming Solution 2125
Toprol-XL Tablets (About 1 of 100 patients) 666

Reaction, aggravated
Lamictal (2%) 1488
Zomig Tablets (0% to 2%) 694
Zomig Nasal Spray (0% to 2%) 689
Zomig-ZMT Tablets (0% to 2%) 694

Reaction, local
Humalog Mix 50/50-Pen and KwikPen 1833
▲ Tygacil for Injection (9%) 3276

Reaction, paranoid
Azilect Tablets (Infrequent) 3106
Campral Tablets (Rare) 1158
Emsam Transdermal System (Infrequent) 905
Gliadel Wafer (1%) 1076
Luvox CR Extended-Release Capsules (Infrequent) 1759
Lyrica Capsules (Rare) 2527
Mirapex Tablets (2%) 857
Namenda (Infrequent) 1180
Neupro Transdermal System 3149
Proleukin for Injection (Less than 1%) 2287
Prozac Weekly Capsules (Infrequent) 1852
Risperdal Consta Long-Acting Injection (Frequent) 1753
Venlafaxine Hydrochloride Tablets (Rare) 2199
Wellbutrin SR Sustained-Release Tablets 1653
Wellbutrin XL Extended-Release Tablets 1659

Reaction, schizophrenic
Lyrica Capsules (Rare) 2527

Reaction at injection site
Abilify Injection (Greater than or equal to 1 in 100 patients) 881
Aloxi Injection (Very rare) 1059
▲ Amevive (2% to 16%) 611
▲ Apidra Injection (10.3%) 2706
▲ BeneFIX Vials (1.6% to 7.7%) 3191
▲ Betaseron for SC Injection (78%) 756
Bicillin L-A Injection 1777
Byetta Injection 600
Cardene I.V. (1.4%) 1093
Celebrex Capsules (0.1% to 1.9%) 2979
Cimzia 3127
Cipro I.V. (Greater than 1%) 2817
▲ Cubicin for Injection (5.8%) 995
▲ Eloxatin for Injection (0% to 32%) 2731
▲ Enbrel for Injection (7% to 37%) 569
▲ Flebogamma 5% DIF (Greater than 15%) 1718
▲ Follistim AQ Cartridge (5% to 10%) 2844
Forteo for Injection (Less than 1/30 patients) 1816
Fragmin Injection (Rare) 1070
▲ Gamunex (5%) 3094
Gemzar for Injection (Rare) 1820
Humalog Mix 50/50-Pen and KwikPen 1833
▲ Humira Injection (8% to 20%) 442
▲ Imitrex Injection (59%) 1465
Infanrix Vaccine 1479
Ionsys Transdermal System (.1% to less than 1%) 2410
▲ Kineret Injection (71%) 585
Kogenate FS with Bio-Set (2 cases) 748
▲ Levaquin Injection (19%) 2416
▲ Levaquin in 5% Dextrose Injection (19%) 2416
Levemir Injection 2352
Lovenox Injection 2756
▲ Lupron Depot 7.5 mg (Less than 5%) 469
▲ Lupron Depot–3 Month 11.25 mg (Less than 5%) 462
Merrem I.V. (0.9%) 684
Natrecor for Injection (Greater than or equal to 1%) 2977
NeoProfen Injection 2496
Neulasta Injection 587
Norditropin Cartridges 2354
▲ NovoLog Mix 70/30 (7%) 2364
NovoSeven 2367
NovoSeven RT (1%) 2370
Nutropin for Injection (0.3%) 1208
Nutropin AQ Injection (0.3%) 1212
Nutropin AQ NuSpin Injection (0.3%) 1212
Nutropin AQ Pen (0.3%) 1212
Nutropin AQ Pen Cartridge (0.3%) 1212
Pediarix Vaccine 1552
▲ PegIntron Powder for Injection (47%) 2903
Pentacel 2792
Pneumovax 23 (Common) 2078
▲ Rebif Prefilled Syringe for Injection (89% to 92%) 1107
Risperdal Consta Long-Acting Injection (Infrequent) 1753
Synagis Intramuscular Solution 1948
▲ Tev-Tropin for Injection (8 out of 164 patients) 1187
Tygacil for Injection (0% to less than 2%) 3276
Vaqta 2130
▲ Vivitrol (58% to 88%) 988
▲ Xolair (12% to 45%) 1235
▲ Xolair (12% to 45%) 2339
▲ Zyvox Injection (0% to 3.3%) 2552

Reactions, infusion site
Alphanate 1709
▲ Cyanokit 5g Antidote (6% to 39%) 1021
▲ Gammagard Liquid (0.97% to 13.1%) 730
▲ Taxotere Injection Concentrate (3.3% to 4.4%) 2773
▲ Vaprisol (19% to 52%) 632

Reactions, local, unspecified
Boostrix 1377
Lotrisone 2881
▲ Zosyn for Injection (3.3%) 3284

Rectal bleeding
Accutane Capsules 2607
Actiq (1% or greater) 959
Aggrenox Capsules (1.6%) 819
Anaprox Tablets (Less than 1%) 2632
Anaprox DS Tablets (Less than 1%) 2632
Asacol Delayed-Release Tablets (2% or greater) 2579
Celexa (Rare) 1160
Copaxone for Injection (Infrequent) 3110
▲ Doxil Injection (1% to 10%) 2378
EC-Naprosyn Delayed-Release Tablets (Less than 1%) 2632
Effexor XR Extended-Release Capsules (Infrequent) 3195
Eldepryl Capsules 3052
▲ Elmiron Capsules (6.3% to 15%) 2435
▲ Eloxatin for Injection (2% to less than 5%) 2731
Evoxac Capsules (Less than 1%) 1013
Exelon Capsules (Infrequent) 2229
Exelon Oral Solution (Infrequent) 2229
▲ Flolan for Injection (11%) 1426
Gabitril Tablets (Infrequent) 973
Gengraf Capsules (1%) 435
Geodon (Infrequent) 2520
Imitrex Nasal Spray 1470
Indocin Capsules (Less than 1%) 2024
Indocin I.V. (Less than 1%) 2489
Indocin (Less than 1%) 2024
▲ Intron A for Injection (Less than 5%) 2859
Lipitor Tablets (Less than 2%) 2501
Lunesta Tablets (Rare) 2994
Naprosyn Suspension (Less than 1%) 2632
Naprosyn Tablets (Less than 1%) 2632
Neoral Oral Solution (1%) 2280
Neoral Soft Gelatin Capsules (1%) 2280
Paxil (Infrequent) 1535
Paxil CR Controlled-Release Tablets (Infrequent) 1544
Pentasa Capsules (Less than 1%) 3030
Pletal Tablets (Less than 2%) 2481
▲ Prometrium Capsules (100 mg, 200 mg) (Less than 5%) 3047
Protonix for Delayed-Release Oral Suspension (Less than 1%) 3254
Protonix Delayed-Release Tablets (Less than 1%) 3254
Protonix I.V. (Greater than or equal to 1%) 3257
▲ Refludan for Injection (5.3%) 795
Requip Tablets (Infrequent) 1561
Retrovir Capsules 1574
Retrovir IV Infusion 1579
Retrovir 1574
Rythmol SR Capsules 1590
Sandostatin LAR Depot 2302
Tricor Tablets 520
Voltaren Tablets (Occasionally) 2334
Voltaren-XR Tablets (Occasionally) 2337
Xeloda Tablets 2662
Zonegran Capsules (Infrequent) 1089
Zyprexa Tablets (Infrequent) 1883
Zyprexa ZYDIS Orally Disintegrating Tablets (Infrequent) 1883

Rectal burning
Dulcolax Suppositories ▣ 602

Rectal discomfort
▲ Busulfex Injection (24%) 2477
Fleet Babylax Suppositories 1142
Fleet Glycerin Laxatives 1142
Fleet Glycerin Suppositories 1142
Fleet Pedia-Lax Suppositories 1142
▲ Xenical Capsules (3.3% to 5.2%) 2672

Rectal disorders, unspecified
Actiq (1% or greater) 959
Actonel with Calcium Tablets (2.2%) 2574
Asacol Delayed-Release Tablets (2% or greater) 2579
▲ Avinza Capsules (Less than 5%) 1772
▲ Busulfex Injection (25%) 2477
▲ CellCept Capsules (3% to less than 20%) 2622
▲ CellCept Intravenous (3% to less than 20%) 2622
▲ CellCept Oral Suspension (3% to less than 20%) 2622
▲ CellCept Tablets (3% to less than 20%) 2622
Evoxac Capsules (Less than 1%) 1013
Meridia Capsules (1.2%) 475

Nexium Delayed-Release Capsules (Less than 1%) 645
Nexium I.V. (Less than 1%) 652
Nexium Delayed-Release Oral Suspension (Less than 1%) 645
Norvir (Less than 2%) 489
▲ Prograf Capsules and Injection (3% to 15%) 622
Protonix for Delayed-Release Oral Suspension (Greater than or equal to 1%) 3254
Protonix Delayed-Release Tablets (Greater than or equal to 1%) 3254
Protonix I.V. (Greater than or equal to 1%) 3257
Protopic Ointment (0.2% to less than 1%) 628
Tricor Tablets 520
Wellbutrin Tablets (Rare) 1648

Rectal urgency
(*see under* Defecate, desire to)

Red blood cell, aplasia
Rituxan I.V. 1223

Red blood cell count, decrease
Aldara Cream, 5% 1699
Avelox (Greater than or equal to 2%) 2803
Eligard 7.5 mg (Less than 2%) 2724
Eligard 22.5 mg (Less than 2%) 2724
Eligard 30 mg (Less than 2%) 2724
Eligard 45 mg (Less than 2%) 2724
Keppra Injection 3137
Keppra Oral Solution 3131
Keppra Tablets 3131
▲ Norvir (18.6%) 489
Rythmol SR Capsules 1590

Red blood cells excretion, increase
Invanz for Injection (1.1% to 2.5%) 2029

Redness, local
▲ Flulaval Injection Vaccine (10% to 14%) 1448
▲ Havrix Injection Vaccine (16% to 41%) 1454
Ortho Evra Transdermal System 2437
Tylenol Chest Congestion Caplets with Cool Burst 1910
Tylenol Chest Congestion Liquid with Cool Burst 1910
Tylenol Cold Severe Congestion Daytime Caplets with Cool Burst 1912

Redness at injection site
Avelox (Greater than or equal to 0.1% to less than 2%) 2803
▲ Boostrix (1.7% to 47.7%) 1377
▲ Fluarix Vaccine (15.9% to 17.5%) 1446
Humalog Mix 50/50-Pen and KwikPen 1833
Humulin R (Occasionally) 1849
▲ Kinrix Injection Vaccine (36.6%) 1486
▲ Pentacel (0% to 17.3%) 2792
Reclast Injection 2291
Risperdal Consta Long-Acting Injection 1753
Traumeel Injection Solution 1725
▲ Twinrix Vaccine (8% to 11%) 1628
Xolair 1235
Xolair 2339
Zeel Injection Solution 1726

Reflexes, abnormal
▲ DepoCyt Injection (3%) 1136
Frova Tablets (Rare) 1111
Luvox CR Extended-Release Capsules (Rare) 1759

Reflexes, increased
(*see under* Hyperreflexia)

Reflux esophagitis
Mirapex Tablets 857
Sutent Capsules 2540

Refraction disorder, unspecified
Tricor Tablets 520

Refractive changes
Combigan Ophthalmic Solution 553

Regurgitation
Amerge Tablets (Rare) 1301
Invanz for Injection (1.1% to 1.6%) 2029
Maxalt Tablets (Infrequent) 2056
Maxalt-MLT Orally Disintegrating Tablets (Infrequent) 2056
Mevacor Tablets (0.5% to 1%) 2063
Zyban Sustained-Release Tablets (Infrequent) 1692

Rejection, acute
Rapamune 3260

Relaxation
Imitrex Injection (Infrequent) 1465

Renal agenesis, unilateral, neonatal
Leukeran Tablets 1508

Renal artery stenosis
Mirapex Tablets 857

Renal calculi
(*see under* Nephrolithiasis)

Renal colic
Crixivan Capsules (Less than 2%) 1979
Mirapex Tablets 857
Noroxin Tablets (Less frequent) 2069
Salagen Tablets 1082

Renal disease
Anaprox Tablets (Less than 1%) 2632
Anaprox DS Tablets (Less than 1%) .. 2632
EC-Naprosyn Delayed-Release Tablets (Less than 1%) 2632
Naprosyn Suspension (Less than 1%) 2632
Naprosyn Tablets (Less than 1%) 2632

Renal disorders, unspecified
▲ Femara Tablets (0.5% to 5.1%) 2246
▲ Novantrone for Injection Concentrate (5%) 1100
Somatuline Depot Injection 3102
Ziagen (Less than 1%) 1673

Renal dysfunction
(*see under* Renal impairment)

Renal failure
▲ Abelcet Injection (5%) 1134
Actiq (1% or greater) 959
Aggrenox Capsules (Less than 1%) .. 819
Agrylin Capsules (6 of 551 patients) 3017
Alimta for Injection (Up to 2%) 1786
AmBisome for Injection (Less common) 606
Anaprox Tablets (Less than 1%) 2632
Anaprox DS Tablets (Less than 1%) .. 2632
AndroGel 3159
Angiomax for Injection (Greater than 0.1% to less than 1%) 1933
Aranesp for Injection 564
Aricept Tablets (Infrequent) 1062
Aricept ODT Tablets (Infrequent) 1062
Atacand Tablets 639
Atacand HCT (Very rare) 642
Atripla Tablets 938
Avalide Tablets 892
Avalide Tablets 2713
Bayer Aspirin 750
Benicar Tablets 1009
Benicar HCT Tablets (Rare) 1010
Bicillin C-R Injectable Suspension 1775
Bicillin L-A Injection 1777
Bystolic Tablets 1155
Cancidas for Injection 1953
Captopril Tablets (Approximately 1 to 2 of 1000 patients) 2182
Carbatrol Capsules 3019
▲ CellCept Capsules (3% to less than 20%) 2622
▲ CellCept Intravenous (3% to less than 20%) 2622
▲ CellCept Oral Suspension (3% to less than 20%) 2622
▲ CellCept Tablets (3% to less than 20%) 2622
Cimzia 3127
Cipro I.V. (1% or less) 2817
Cipro (Less than 1%) 2810
Cipro XR Tablets 2823
Clinoril Tablets (Less than 1 in 100) 1962
▲ Cubicin for Injection (2.2% to 3.3%) 995
Cuprimine Capsules 1986
Dacogen Injection 1066
Diovan HCT Tablets 2216
Doribax Injection (Less than 1% to 1%) 2400
Dyrenium Capsules (One case) 3189
EC-Naprosyn Delayed-Release Tablets (Less than 1%) 2632
Effexor XR Extended-Release Capsules 3195
Elitek (Less than or equal to 1%) 2729
Equetro Extended-Release Capsules 3174
Erbitux (Less than 1%) 912
Exelon Patch (Infrequent) 2233
Fansidar Tablets 2636
Fenoglide Tablets 2960
Fentora Tablets (Greater than 1%) 968
Fleet Enema 1143
Fleet Enema Extra 1143
Fleet Enema for Children 1143
Fleet Pedia-Lax Enema 1143
Fleet Phospho-soda 1145
Fleet Phospho-soda EZ-PREP 1147
Fleet Prep Kits 1149
Gabitril Tablets (Infrequent) 973
Gemzar for Injection (Rare) 1820
Gleevec Tablets (Infrequent) 2255
Hepsera Tablets 1253
Indocin (Less than 1%) 2024
Intelence Tablets (Less than 2%) 3119
Intravenous Sodium Diuril 2490
Intron A for Injection 2859
Isentress Tablets 2036
Ixempra Kit for Injection 915
Lamictal (Rare) 1488
Merrem I.V. (Greater than 0.1% to 1%) 684
Micardis HCT Tablets 854
Mirapex Tablets 857
Mobic Oral Suspension (Less than 2%) 863
Mobic Tablets (Less than 2%) 863
Mylotarg for Injection 3212
Nalfon Capsules (Less than 1%) 2508
Namenda 1180
Naprosyn Suspension (Less than 1%) 2632
Naprosyn Tablets (Less than 1%) 2632
NeoProfen Injection (1%) 2496
Nexavar Tablets (Less than 1%) 784
Noroxin Tablets 2069
Norvir (Less than 2%) 489
▲ Novantrone for Injection Concentrate (8%) 1100
NuvaRing 2897
Orthoclone OKT3 Sterile Solution 2387
PegIntron Powder for Injection 2903
Percocet Tablets 1127
Percodan Tablets 1130
Prinzide Tablets 2092
▲ Prograf Capsules and Injection (3% to 15%) 622
Proleukin for Injection (Less than 1%) 2287
Prozac Weekly Capsules 1852
Prozac Pulvules and Liquid 1852
Remicade for IV Injection (Greater than or equal to 0.2%) 950
Rythmol Tablets (Less than 1%) 1586
Rythmol SR Capsules 1590
St. Joseph 81 mg Aspirin Chewable and Enteric Coated Tablets 1903
Sandostatin LAR Depot 2302
Solodyn Extended Release Tablets .. 1938
Sutent Capsules (Rare) 2540
Tasigna Capsules 2316
Tekturna HCT Tablets 2324
Teveten HCT Tablets 517
Torisel Injection 3272
Trasylol Injection (1% to 2%) 799
▲ Trisenox Injection (8%) 986
Trizivir Tablets 1622
Truvada Tablets 1262
Valtrex Caplets 1635
Velcade for Injection 2168
Venlafaxine Hydrochloride Tablets 2199
Viread Tablets 1268
Voltaren Tablets (Occasionally) 2334
Voltaren-XR Tablets (Occasionally) 2337
▲ Xeloda Tablets (Less than 5%) 2662
Ziagen 1673
Zolinza Capsules 2142
Zometa for Intravenous Infusion 2341
Zosyn for Injection 3284
Zovirax 1690

Renal failure, acute
Abelcet Injection 1134
Abilify Injection 881
Abilify Injection 2466
Abilify Oral Solution 881
Abilify Oral Solution 2466
Abilify Discmelt Orally Disintegrating Tablets 881
Abilify Discmelt Orally Disintegrating Tablets 2466
Abilify Tablets 881
Abilify Tablets 2466
Aceon Tablets (2 mg, 4 mg, 8 mg) 3038
Activase I.V. 1188
Albenza Tablets 1297
Ambien Tablets (Rare) 2692
Ambien CR Tablets (Rare) 2696
AmBisome for Injection (Less common) 606
Anzemet Injection (Rare) 2701
Anzemet Tablets (Rare) 2704
Atripla Tablets 938
Avelox 2803
Azor Tablets 1005
Byetta Injection 600
Celebrex Capsules (Less than 0.1%) 2979
Celexa 1160
Chantix Tablets (Rare) 2511
Cipro I.V. (Rare) 2817
Cipro 2810
Cipro XR Tablets 2823
▲ Cleviprex (9%) 1936
Crestor Tablets 677
Crixivan Capsules 1979
Dyazide Capsules 1405
Dyrenium Capsules 3189
Eloxatin for Injection 2731
Elspar for Injection 1990
Exelon Capsules (Infrequent) 2229
Exelon Oral Solution (Infrequent) 2229
Fenoglide Tablets 2960
Flebogamma 5% 1715
Flebogamma 5% DIF 1718
Gammagard S/D 734
Gantrisin Pediatric Suspension 2638
Imitrex Injection 1465
Imitrex Nasal Spray 1470
Imitrex Tablets 1474
Indocin I.V. (Less than 1%) 2489
Lamictal (Rare) 1488
Levaquin (0.1% to 1%) 2416
Levaquin in 5% Dextrose Injection (0.1% to 1%) 2416
Lexapro Oral Suspension 1174
Lexapro Tablets 1174
Lipitor Tablets (Rare) 2501
Luvox CR Extended-Release Capsules 1759
Mevacor Tablets 2063
Mycamine for Injection 616
Nexavar Tablets (0.1% to less than 1%) 784
▲ Noxafil Oral Suspension (0% to 3%) 2889
Omnicef Capsules 497
Omnicef for Oral Suspension 497
OsmoPrep Tablets 2680
Paxil 1535
Paxil CR Controlled-Release Tablets 1544
Pentasa Capsules 3030
Plavix Tablets (1% to 2.5%) 926
Plavix Tablets (1% to 2.5%) 2767
Primaxin I.M. 2080
Primaxin I.V. (Less than 0.2%) 2083
Prinivil Tablets (0.3% to 1.3%) 2087
Prinzide Tablets 2092
Prograf Capsules and Injection 622
Protopic Ointment 628
Requip Tablets (Rare) 1561
Rituxan I.V. 1223
Suprax for Oral Suspension (Less than 2%) 1891
Suprax Tablets (Less than 2%) 1891
Sutent Capsules (Rare) 2540
Tarceva Tablets 1228
Torisel Injection 3272
Trasylol Injection (1% to 2%) 799
Truvada Tablets 1262
Velcade for Injection 2168
▲ Vesanoid Capsules (3%) 2660
Zocor Tablets 2136

Renal failure, aggravated
Vantas (Less than 2%) 1737

Renal failure, chronic
Pentasa Capsules 3030
Velcade for Injection 2168

Renal failure, neonatal
Aceon Tablets (2 mg, 4 mg, 8 mg) 3038
Avalide Tablets 2713
Captopril Tablets 2182
Cozaar Tablets 1973
Prinivil Tablets 2087
Prinzide Tablets 2092

Renal failure, worsening of
Byetta Injection 600
▲ NovoSeven RT (4.7%) 2370

Renal failure secondary to TLS
Mylotarg for Injection 3212

Renal function impairment
(*see under* Renal impairment)

Renal impairment
Abelcet Injection 1134
Agrylin Capsules (10 of 551 patients) 3017

▲ Anaprox Tablets (1% to 10%) 2632
▲ Anaprox DS Tablets (1% to 10%) 2632
Argatroban Injection (2.8%)............. 1308
Asacol Delayed-Release Tablets....... 2579
Atacand Tablets.............................. 639
Atacand HCT (Very rare).................. 642
Avalide Tablets................................ 892
Avalide Tablets 2713
Azor Tablets 1005
Benicar HCT Tablets 1010
Byetta Injection.............................. 600
Cancidas for Injection..................... 1953
Ceftin 1380
Cipro XR Tablets (Less than 1%)....... 2823
Clinoril Tablets (Less than 1 in 100).. 1962
Cubicin for Injection (Less than 1%).. 995
Diovan Tablets................................ 2212
Diovan HCT Tablets......................... 2216
Doribax Injection (Less than 1% to 1%) 2400
Doxil Injection (Less than 1%) 2378
▲ EC-Naprosyn Delayed-Release Tablets (1% to 10%) 2632
Effexor XR Extended-Release Capsules (Rare) 3195
Evoxac Capsules (Less than 1%) 1013
Exforge Tablets 2238
Fortaz 1450
▲ Gengraf Capsules (25% to 38%) 435
Hepsera Tablets 1253
▲ Indocin I.V. (41% of infants) 2489
Intravenous Sodium Diuril 2490
Lescol Capsules 2268
Lescol XL Tablets 2268
▲ Leukine (8%) 774
Levaquin (0.1% to 1%) 2416
Levaquin in 5% Dextrose Injection (0.1% to 1%) 2416
Lybrel Tablets 3204
Mepron Suspension 1526
Micardis HCT Tablets 854
Mirapex Tablets 857
Mircette Tablets 1034
Mycamine for Injection 616
▲ Myfortic Tablets (3% to less than 20%) 2276
Mylotarg for Injection 3212
▲ Naprosyn Suspension (1% to 10%) 2632
▲ Naprosyn Tablets (1% to 10%) 2632
▲ NeoProfen Injection (6%) 2496
▲ Neoral Oral Solution (25% to 38%) 2280
▲ Neoral Soft Gelatin Capsules (25% to 38%) 2280
NovoLog Injection 2359
NovoSeven RT (1%) 2370
Omnicef Capsules 497
Omnicef for Oral Suspension 497
Ortho-Cyclen Tablets 2449
Ortho Evra Transdermal System 2437
Ortho Tri-Cyclen Tablets 2449
Ortho Tri-Cyclen Lo Tablets 2458
OsmoPrep Tablets 2680
Panhematin for Injection 2497
Paxil (Rare) 1535
Paxil CR Controlled-Release Tablets (Rare) 1544
Plavix Tablets 926
Plavix Tablets 2767
Prinivil Tablets (0.3% to 1%) 2087
Prinzide Tablets 2092
▲ Prograf Capsules and Injection (36% to 40%) 622
Protopic Ointment 628
▲ Rapamune (Greater than or equal to 3% to less than 20%) 3260
Reclast Injection 2291
Refludan for Injection (1.8%) 795
ReoPro Vials (0.3%) 1860
Rocephin Injectable Vials, ADD-Vantage, Galaxy, Bulk 2642
▲ Sandimmune (25% to 38%) 2296
Seasonique Tablets 1046
▲ Simulect for Injection (3% to 10%) ... 2306
Suprax for Oral Suspension 1891
Suprax Tablets 1891
Tekturna HCT Tablets 2324
Teveten HCT Tablets 517
▲ Trasylol Injection (5% to 30%) 799
Tricor Tablets 520
▲ Trisenox Injection (8%) 986
Truvada Tablets 1262
▲ Valcyte Tablets (Less than 5%) 2654
▲ Vantas (4.7%) 1737
Vicoprofen Tablets 533
Viramune Oral Suspension 873
Viramune Tablets 873
Yaz Tablets 805
▲ Zometa for Intravenous Infusion (8% to 40%) 2341

Renal infarct
BeneFIX Vials (1.5%)....................... 3191
Vesanoid Capsules 2660

Renal injury
Capastat Sulfate for Injection........... 1791
Flector Patch 561
Vicoprofen Tablets 533

Renal insufficiency
Aggrenox Capsules (Less than 1%).. 819
Aptivus Capsules (Less than 2%)...... 823
Aptivus Oral Solution (Less than 2%)... 823
Atripla Tablets................................. 938
Avelox 2803
Bayer Aspirin.................................. 750
Capastat Sulfate for Injection (1 patient).. 1791
Captopril Tablets (Approximately 1 to 2 of 1000 patients)................... 2182
Cipro I.V. (Rare).............................. 2817
Cipro 2810
Cipro XR Tablets 2823
▲ Coreg Tablets (Greater than 1% to 3%) 1387
▲ Coreg CR Extended-Release Capsules (Greater than 1% to less than or equal to 3%) 1393
Crixivan Capsules (Some cases) 1979
Elspar for Injection 1990
Emend Capsules (Greater than 0.5%) 1992
Emend for Injection (Greater than 0.5%) 1999
Indocin Capsules (Less than 1%) 2024
Indocin I.V. (Less than 1%) 2489
Indocin (Less than 1%) 2024
Intron A for Injection 2859
Invanz for Injection (Greater than 0.1%) 2029
Mobic Oral Suspension 863
Mobic Tablets 863
Namenda 1180
Neupogen for Injection (Two events) 589
Norvir 489
▲ Ontak Vials (Less than 5%) 1079
Orthoclone OKT3 Sterile Solution 2387
PegIntron Powder for Injection 2903
Percocet Tablets 1127
Percodan Tablets 1130
St. Joseph 81 mg Aspirin Chewable and Enteric Coated Tablets 1903
Sandostatin LAR Depot 2302
Tarceva Tablets 1228
Taxotere Injection Concentrate 2773
Treximet Tablets (Rare) 1616
Truvada Tablets 1262
▲ Vesanoid Capsules (11%) 2660
Viread Tablets 1268
▲ Voltaren Tablets (1% to 10%) 2334
▲ Voltaren-XR Tablets (1% to 10%) 2337

Renal insufficiency, reversible
Actimmune (Rare) 1743

Renal precipitation
Rocephin Injectable Vials, ADD-Vantage, Galaxy, Bulk (Less than 0.1%) 2642

Renal stones
Aceon Tablets (2 mg, 4 mg, 8 mg) (0.3% to 1%) 3038
Campral Tablets (Rare) 1158
Celebrex Capsules (0.1% to 1.9%) ... 2979
Cipro 2810
Cipro XR Tablets 2823
Clinoril Tablets 1962
Enbrel for Injection 569
Reyataz Capsules 3299
Tekturna Tablets (0.2%) 2321
Tekturna HCT Tablets (0.2%) 2324
Vantas (Less than 2%) 1737
▲ Zonegran Capsules (4%) 1089

Renal toxicity
(*see under* Nephrotoxicity)

Rencephalopathy, metabolic
Arranon Injection (1%) 1319

Reproductive disorders, female
Amerge Tablets (Rare) 1301
▲ Femara Tablets (0.4% to 11.8%) 2246
▲ Hycamtin for Injection (5%) 1459

Resistance mechanism
Moxatag Tablets 2165

Respiration, painful
Prinivil Tablets (0.3% to 1%) 2087
Prinzide Tablets 2092

Respiratory alkalosis
Aggrenox Capsules.......................... 819
AmBisome for Injection (Less common)....................................... 606
Coreg Tablets (Less than or equal to 0.1%)....................................... 1387
Geodon Capsules (Rare)................. 2520
Mirapex Tablets............................... 857
St. Joseph 81 mg Aspirin Chewable and Enteric Coated Tablets 1903

Respiratory arrest
Abilify Injection (Greater than or equal to 1 in 1000 to less than 1 in 100)... 881
Abilify Injection (Greater than or equal to 1 in 1000 to less than 1 in 100)... 2466
Abilify Oral Solution (Greater than or equal to 1 in 1000 patients and less than 1 in 100 patients) 881
Abilify Oral Solution (Greater than or equal to 1 in 1000 to less than 1 in 100) 2466
Abilify Discmelt Orally Disintegrating Tablets (Greater than or equal to 1 in 1000 patients and less than 1 in 100 patients)... 881
Abilify Discmelt Orally Disintegrating Tablets (Greater than or equal to 1 in 1000 to less than 1 in 100)........................ 2466
Abilify Tablets (Greater than or equal to 1 in 1000 patients and less than 1 in 100 patients) 881
Abilify Tablets (Greater than or equal to 1 in 1000 to less than 1 in 100) 2466
Actiq 959
Arranon Injection 1319
Campath Ampules 761
Cipro I.V. (1% or less) 2817
Cipro XR Tablets 2823
Dacogen Injection 1066
DepoDur Injection 1095
Effexor XR Extended-Release Capsules 3195
Lidoderm Patch 1114
MS Contin Tablets 2585
Orthoclone OKT3 Sterile Solution 2387
OxyContin Tablets 2589
Percocet Tablets 1127
Proleukin for Injection (Less than 1%) 2287
Symbyax Capsules 1871

Respiratory congestion, unspecified
Comvax (0.3% to 1.2%) 1966
Cozaar Tablets (Less than 1%) 1973
▲ Epogen for Injection (15%) 576
▲ Fabrazyme for Intravenous Infusion (8%) 1241
Maxalt Tablets (Infrequent) 2056
Maxalt-MLT Orally Disintegrating Tablets (Infrequent) 2056
▲ Procrit for Injection (15%) 2391
ProQuad (Greater than or equal to 0.2% to less than 1%) 2099
Requip Tablets (Infrequent) 1561
Vaqta (1.6%) 2130

Respiratory depression
Actiq 959
Anaprox Tablets (Less than 1%) 2632
Anaprox DS Tablets (Less than 1%) .. 2632
Dantrium Capsules (Less frequent) .. 2580
▲ DepoDur Injection (2% to 5%) 1095
EC-Naprosyn Delayed-Release Tablets (Less than 1%) 2632
Emend Capsules (Greater than 0.5%) 1992
Emend for Injection (Greater than 0.5%) 1999
Klonopin 2639
Lidoderm Patch 1114
Lortab 5/500 Tablets 3143
Lortab 7.5/500 Tablets 3144
Lortab 10/500 Tablets 3144
MS Contin Tablets 2585
Naprosyn Suspension (Less than 1%) 2632
Naprosyn Tablets (Less than 1%) 2632
Opana Tablets (Less than 1%) 1117
Opana ER Tablets (Less than 1%) 1121
OxyContin Tablets 2589
OxyIR Capsules 2593
Percocet Tablets 1127
Tussionex Pennkinetic Extended-Release Suspension...... 3154
Tylenol with Codeine Tablets........... 2427
Vicodin Tablets 529
Vicodin ES Tablets 530
Vicodin HP Tablets 531
Vicoprofen Tablets 533
Voltaren Tablets (Rarely).................. 2334
Voltaren-XR Tablets (Rarely)............. 2337
Zydone Tablets 1132

Respiratory depression, postoperative
▲ Advair HFA 45/21 Inhalation Aerosol (1% to 3%) 1288
▲ Advair HFA 115/21 Inhalation Aerosol (1% to 3%) 1288
▲ Advair HFA 230/21 Inhalation Aerosol (1% to 3%) 1288

Respiratory difficulty
▲ Abelcet Injection (4%) 1134
Allegra-D 12 Hour Extended-Release Tablets 2687
Allegra-D 24 Hour Extended-Release Tablets 2690
Ambien Tablets 2692
Carafate Suspension 706
Carafate Tablets 707
Cardene I.V. (Rare) 1093
EpiPen 1024
▲ Photofrin for Injection (10%) 708
Rilutek Tablets (More than 2%) 2771
Thyrogen for Injection 1244
▲ Trasylol Injection (3%) 799
▲ Vesanoid Capsules (26%) 2660
Zyrtec-D 12 Hour Extended Release Tablets 1923

Respiratory disorders, unspecified
Asmanex Twisthaler (1% to less than 3%) 2797
Brovana Inhalation Solution (Less than 2%) 2990
▲ Cancidas for Injection (0% to 46.5%) 1953
▲ Chantix Tablets (Frequent to 7%) 2511
Combivent Inhalation Aerosol (2.5%) 845
▲ Enbrel for Injection (5%) 569
Evoxac Capsules (Less than 1%) 1013
▲ Femara Tablets (1.2% to 10.9%) 2246
▲ Fenoglide Tablets (6.2%) 2960
▲ Flolan for Injection (7%) 1426
▲ Focalin XR Capsules (9% to 16%) 2251
Gabitril Tablets (Infrequent) 973
▲ Geodon Capsules (8%) 2520
▲ Intron A for Injection (Less than or equal to 5%) 2859
▲ Lupron Depot 7.5 mg (10.7%) 469
Meridia Capsules 475
Merrem I.V. (Greater than 0.1% to 1%) 684
▲ Mycamine for Injection (35.9% to 68.5%) 616
▲ Paxil (7%) 1535
▲ Paxil CR Controlled-Release Tablets (7%) 1544
▲ Proleukin for Injection (3% to 11%) 2287
▲ Proventil HFA Inhalation Aerosol (6%) 2914
Rituxan I.V. 1223
▲ Simulect for Injection (3% to 10%) ... 2306
Tice BCG (2%) 2936
▲ Tricor Tablets (6.2%) 520
▲ Verdeso Foam (7%) 3069
Wellbutrin SR Sustained-Release Tablets (At least 1%) 1653
▲ Wellbutrin XL Extended-Release Tablets (At least 1% to 4%) 1659
Xyrem Oral Solution (Infrequent) 1766
Zostavax Injection (1.1%) 2145
Zyrtec Chewable Tablets (Less than 2%) 1920
Zyrtec Syrup (Less than 2%) 1920
Zyrtec Tablets (Less than 2%) 1920
Zyrtec-D 12 Hour Extended Release Tablets (Less than 2%) 1923

Respiratory distress
Abilify Injection (Greater than or equal to 1 in 1000 patients and less than 1 in 100 patients) 881
Abilify Injection (Greater than or equal to 1 in 1000 patients and less than 1 in 100 patients) 2466
Abilify Oral Solution (Greater than or equal to 1 in 1000 patients and less than 1 in 100 patients) 881
Abilify Oral Solution (Greater than or equal to 1 in 1000 patients and less than 1 in 100 patients) 2466

Abilify Discmelt Orally Disintegrating Tablets (Greater than or equal to 1 in 1000 patients and less than 1 in 100 patients) 881
Abilify Discmelt Orally Disintegrating Tablets (Greater than or equal to 1 in 1000 patients and less than 1 in 100 patients) 2466
Abilify Tablets (Greater than or equal to 1 in 1000 patients and less than 1 in 100 patients) 881
Abilify Tablets (Greater than or equal to 1 in 1000 patients and less than 1 in 100 patients) 2466
▲ Agrylin Capsules (1% to less than 5%) 3017
Atacand HCT 642
Avalide Tablets 2713
Cancidas for Injection 1953
Cipro I.V. (1% or less) 2817
Cipro XR Tablets 2823
▲ Clolar for Intravenous Infusion (14%) 1239
Combigan Ophthalmic Solution 553
Comvax 1966
Cosopt Sterile Ophthalmic Solution 1969
Diovan HCT Tablets 2216
Duragesic Transdermal System (Less than 1%) 2405
Dyazide Capsules 1405
▲ Elitek (3%) 2729
Elspar for Injection 1990
Fluarix Vaccine 1446
Glucagon for Injection Vials and Emergency Kit 1827
Herceptin I.V. 1199
▲ Humatrope Vials and Cartridges (3.13% to 6.67%) 1838
Indapamide Tablets 2188
Indocin Capsules (Less than 1%) 2024
Indocin I.V. (Less than 1%) 2489
Indocin (Less than 1%) 2024
InnoPran XL Extended Release Capsules 1484
Intravenous Sodium Diuril 2490
Janumet Tablets 2041
Lamictal (More than 1%) 1488
Leukine 774
Levaquin 2416
Levaquin in 5% Dextrose Injection 2416
Micardis HCT Tablets 854
Mirapex Tablets 857
Nadolol Tablets 2191
Opana Tablets (Less than 1%) 1117
Opana ER Tablets (Less than 1%) 1121
Paxil 1535
Paxil CR Controlled-Release Tablets 1544
Prinzide Tablets 2092
▲ Prograf Capsules and Injection (3% to 15%) 622
Prozac Weekly Capsules 1852
Prozac Pulvules and Liquid 1852
Salagen Tablets 1082
Sandimmune 2296
Tekturna HCT Tablets 2324
Teveten HCT Tablets 517
Timoptic Sterile Ophthalmic Solution (Less frequent) 2121
Timoptic in Ocudose 2124
Timoptic-XE Sterile Ophthalmic Gel Forming Solution 2125
Toprol-XL Tablets 666
Velcade for Injection 2168
▲ Xeloda Tablets (Less than 5%) 2662

Respiratory distress syndrome
Campath Ampules 761
Flebogamma 5% 1715
Flebogamma 5% DIF 1718
Follistim AQ Cartridge 2844
Gammagard Liquid 730
Gammagard S/D (Rare) 734
Gamunex (Rare) 3094
Neulasta Injection 587
Neupogen for Injection 589
Prograf Capsules and Injection 622
Proleukin for Injection 2287
Remicade for IV Injection (Greater than or equal to 0.2%) 950
Rituxan I.V. 1223
Tarceva Tablets (0.7%) 1228
Taxotere Injection Concentrate 2773
Trizivir Tablets 1622
Velcade for Injection 2168
Ziagen 1673

Respiratory failure
▲ Abelcet Injection (8%) 1134
Actiq (Less than 1%) 959
AmBisome for Injection (Less common) 606
Betimol Ophthalmic Solution 3181
▲ Cancidas for Injection (10.5% to 20.3%) 1953
Combigan Ophthalmic Solution 553
Cosopt Sterile Ophthalmic Solution 1969
Gemzar for Injection (Very rare) 1820
Ixempra Kit for Injection 915
Mirapex Tablets 857
▲ NeoProfen Injection (10%) 2496
Omnicef Capsules 497
Omnicef for Oral Suspension 497
Orthoclone OKT3 Sterile Solution 2387
PegIntron Powder for Injection 2903
Photofrin for Injection 708
Prograf Capsules and Injection 622
Proleukin for Injection (Less than 1%) 2287
Pulmozyme Inhalation Solution 1217
Rythmol SR Capsules 1590
Simulect for Injection 2306
Synagis Intramuscular Solution 1948
Timoptic Sterile Ophthalmic Solution (Less frequent) 2121
Timoptic in Ocudose (Less frequent) 2124
Timoptic-XE Sterile Ophthalmic Gel Forming Solution 2125
Trizivir Tablets 1622
Velcade for Injection 2168
Ziagen 1673

Respiratory insufficiency
Emend Capsules (Greater than 0.5%) 1992
Emend for Injection (Greater than 0.5%) 1999
Remicade for IV Injection (Greater than or equal to 0.2%) 950
Velcade for Injection 2168

Respiratory moniliasis
▲ CellCept Capsules (3% to less than 20%) 2622
▲ CellCept Intravenous (3% to less than 20%) 2622
▲ CellCept Oral Suspension (3% to less than 20%) 2622
▲ CellCept Tablets (3% to less than 20%) 2622
Rilutek Tablets (Infrequent) 2771
Tricor Tablets 520

Respiratory rate, decreased
Opana Tablets (Less than 1%) 1117
Opana ER Tablets (Less than 1%) 1121

Respiratory rate, increased
Xyrem Oral Solution (Infrequent) 1766

Respiratory symptoms, severe reaction
Lybrel Tablets 3204

Respiratory symptoms, unspecified
Flomax Capsules 848
Thyrogen for Injection 1244

Respiratory tract disorders
▲ CellCept Capsules (3% to less than 20%) 2622
▲ CellCept Intravenous (3% to less than 20%) 2622
▲ CellCept Oral Suspension (3% to less than 20%) 2622
▲ CellCept Tablets (3% to less than 20%) 2622
▲ Exubera Inhalation Powder (6.1% to 7.4%) 2515
Selzentry Tablets (2.1%) 2534

Restless legs syndrome
Ambien CR Tablets (Rare) 2696
Chantix Tablets (Infrequent) 2511
Exelon Capsules (Infrequent) 2229
Exelon Oral Solution (Infrequent) 2229
Requip Tablets 1561
Xyrem Oral Solution (Infrequent) 1766

Restlessness
(*see also under* Dysphoria)
Humulin R 1849

Retching
Imitrex Injection (Rare) 1465
Imitrex Nasal Spray 1470
Imitrex Tablets 1474
Intelence Tablets (Less than 2%) 3119
Xyrem Oral Solution (Infrequent) 1766

Reticulocytopenia
Cosmegen for Injection 2485

Reticulocytosis
Dapsone Tablets USP (Almost all patients) 1746
Percodan Tablets 1130

Retinal artery occlusion
Activase I.V. 1188
Cialis Tablets 1792
Imitrex Nasal Spray 1470
Imitrex Tablets 1474
Risperdal Consta Long-Acting Injection 1753

Retinal atrophy
Clinoril Tablets 1962

Retinal damage
Dapsone Tablets USP 1746

Retinal degeneration
▲ Lucentis Injection (1% to 11%) 1205

Retinal detachment
▲ Lucentis Injection (Less than 0.1% to 11%) 1205
Luvox CR Extended-Release Capsules (Infrequent) 1759
Mirapex Tablets 857
Namenda (Infrequent) 1180
Sular Extended Release Tablets (Less than or equal to 1%) 2975
▲ Valcyte Tablets (15%) 2654
Visudyne for Injection (Less than 1%) 2332

Retinal disorder, unspecified
Evoxac Capsules (Less than 1%) 1013
Lamisil Tablets 2266
▲ Lucentis Injection (0% to 13%) 1205
Requip XL Tablets 1568
Rythmol SR Capsules 1590
Salagen Tablets (Less than 1%) 1082

Retinal pigmentation disorders
Ontak Vials 1079
Triesence Injectable Suspension (2%) ⊙ 209

Retinal vascular disorder
Betimol Ophthalmic Solution 3181
Climara Transdermal System 763
Climara Pro Transdermal System 768
Intron A for Injection (Rare) 2859
Lyrica Capsules (0.1% to 1%) 2527
Mirapex Tablets 857
Protonix for Delayed-Release Oral Suspension (Less than 1%) 3254
Protonix Delayed-Release Tablets (Less than 1%) 3254
Protonix I.V. (Less than 1%) 3257
Visudyne for Injection (Less than 1%) 2332

Retinal vein occlusion
Cialis Tablets 1792
Evista Tablets (Very rare) 1810
Levitra Tablets (Rare) 2876

Retinitis
Attenuvax (Infrequent) 1951
▲ Doxil Injection (1% to 5%) 2378
Indocin (Less than 1%) 2024
M-M-R II (Infrequent) 2054
ProQuad 2099

Retinoic-acid-APL syndrome
▲ Vesanoid Capsules (Up to 25%) 2660

Retinopathy
Cardizem LA Extended Release Tablets (Infrequent) 421
Clinoril Tablets 1962
Exelon Capsules (Infrequent) 2229
Exelon Oral Solution (Infrequent) 2229
Intron A for Injection 2859
PegIntron Powder for Injection 2903

Retinopathy, pigmentary
Thioridazine Hydrochloride Tablets 2195
Thiothixene Capsules 2197

Retrolental fibroplasia
▲ Indocin I.V. (3% to 9%) 2489

Retroperitoneal fibrosis
Combigan Ophthalmic Solution 553
Cosopt Sterile Ophthalmic Solution 1969
Stalevo Tablets (Rare) 2309
Timoptic Sterile Ophthalmic Solution (Less frequent) 2121
Timoptic in Ocudose (Less frequent) 2124
Timoptic-XE Sterile Ophthalmic Gel Forming Solution 2125

Retroperitoneum, redistribution/accumulation of body fat
Retrovir 1574

Reversible ischaemic neurological deficit
Metadate CD Capsules 3146

Reversible syndrome, acute
Combigan Ophthalmic Solution 553
InnoPran XL Extended Release Capsules 1484

Reye's Syndrome, potential for development of
Aggrenox Capsules 819
Bayer Aspirin 750
Pepto-Bismol Original Liquid, Original and Cherry Chewable Tablets & Caplets ▣ 613
Pepto-Bismol Original Liquid, Maximum Strength Liquid, Original and Cherry Tablets, Chewable Tablets and Easy-To-Swallow Caplets (Rare) 2564
Pepto-Bismol Maximum Strength Liquid (Rare) ▣ 613
Percodan Tablets 1130
St. Joseph 81 mg Aspirin Chewable and Enteric Coated Tablets 1903

Rhabdomyolysis
Abilify Injection (Less than 1 in 1000 patients) 881
Abilify Injection (Less than 1 in 1000 patients) 2466
Abilify Oral Solution (Less than 1 in 1000 patients) 881
Abilify Oral Solution (Less than 1 in 1000 patients) 2466
Abilify Discmelt Orally Disintegrating Tablets (Less than 1 in 1000 patients) 881
Abilify Discmelt Orally Disintegrating Tablets (Less than 1 in 1000 patients) 2466
Abilify Tablets (Less than 1 in 1000 patients) 881
Abilify Tablets (Less than 1 in 1000 patients) 2466
Accutane Capsules (Rare) 2607
Aciphex Tablets 1053
Activase I.V. 1188
Advicor Tablets 402
Aggrenox Capsules 819
Atacand Tablets 639
Atacand HCT (Rare) 642
Avalide Tablets 892
Avalide Tablets (Rare) 2713
Avapro Tablets (Rare) 897
Avapro Tablets (Rare) 2718
Azor Tablets 1005
Bayer Aspirin 750
Benicar Tablets 1009
Benicar HCT Tablets (Rare) 1010
Bicillin C-R Injectable Suspension 1775
Bicillin L-A Injection 1777
Celexa 1160
Combivir Tablets 1384
Comtan Tablets 2208
Cozaar Tablets (Rare) 1973
Crestor Tablets 677
Cubicin for Injection 995
Diovan Tablets 2212
Diovan HCT Tablets (Rare) 2216
Effexor XR Extended-Release Capsules 3195
Epivir 1412
Epivir-HBV 1417
Epzicom Tablets 1422
Exforge Tablets 2238
Fenoglide Tablets 2960
Intron A for Injection 2859
Isentress Tablets 2036
Lamictal 1488
Lamisil Oral Granules 2264
Lescol Capsules 2268
Lescol XL Tablets 2268
Levaquin 2416
Levaquin in 5% Dextrose Injection 2416
Lexapro Oral Suspension 1174
Lexapro Tablets 1174
Lipitor Tablets (Rare) 2501
Mevacor Tablets 2063
Micardis Tablets (Rare) 852
Mirapex Tablets (One case) 857
Neupro Transdermal System 3149
Omnicef Capsules 497
Omnicef for Oral Suspension 497
PegIntron Powder for Injection 2903

- Percocet Tablets 1127
- Percodan Tablets 1130
- Proleukin for Injection 2287
- Protonix for Delayed-Release Oral Suspension 3254
- Protonix Delayed-Release Tablets 3254
- Protonix I.V. 3257
- Retrovir IV Infusion 1579
- St. Joseph 81 mg Aspirin Chewable and Enteric Coated Tablets 1903
- Sanctura XR Capsules 557
- Selzentry Tablets 2534
- Stalevo Tablets (Rare) 2309
- Sutent Capsules (Rare) 2540
- Teveten Tablets (Rare) 515
- Tricor Tablets 520
- Trizivir Tablets 1622
- Venlafaxine Hydrochloride Tablets 2199
- Viramune Oral Suspension 873
- Viramune Tablets 873
- Vytorin 10/10 Tablets 2149
- Vytorin 10/10 Tablets (0.02% to 0.53%) 2939
- Vytorin 10/20 Tablets 2149
- Vytorin 10/20 Tablets (0.02% to 0.53%) 2939
- Vytorin 10/40 Tablets 2149
- Vytorin 10/40 Tablets (0.02% to 0.53%) 2939
- Vytorin 10/80 Tablets 2149
- Vytorin 10/80 Tablets (0.02% to 0.53%) 2939
- Wellbutrin Tablets 1648
- Wellbutrin SR Sustained-Release Tablets 1653
- Wellbutrin XL Extended-Release Tablets 1659
- Zetia Tablets 2157
- Zetia Tablets 2951
- Zocor Tablets 2136
- Zyban Sustained-Release Tablets 1692

Rheumatism, articular

- ▲ Advair HFA 45/21 Inhalation Aerosol (1% to 3%) 1288
- ▲ Advair HFA 115/21 Inhalation Aerosol (1% to 3%) 1288
- ▲ Advair HFA 230/21 Inhalation Aerosol (1% to 3%) 1288
- ▲ Flovent Diskus 50 mcg (1% to 17%) 1435
- Relenza Inhalation Powder (2%) 1556
- Serevent Diskus (1% to less than 3%) 1594

Rheumatoid arthritis

- Asacol Delayed-Release Tablets 2579
- Brovana Inhalation Solution (Less than 2%) 2990
- Campral Tablets (Frequent) 1158
- Effexor XR Extended-Release Capsules (Rare) 3195
- Evoxac Capsules (Less than 1%) 1013
- Gardasil Injection (2 cases) 2019
- Intron A for Injection 2859
- Lovaza Capsules 1520
- Mirapex Tablets 857
- PegIntron Powder for Injection (Less than or equal to 1%) 2903
- Prozac Weekly Capsules (Rare) 1852
- Prozac Pulvules and Liquid (Rare) 1852
- Rilutek Tablets (Rare) 2771
- Symbyax Capsules (Rare) 1871
- Venlafaxine Hydrochloride Tablets (Rare) 2199
- Zyprexa Tablets (Infrequent) 1883
- Zyprexa ZYDIS Orally Disintegrating Tablets (Infrequent) 1883

Rheumatoid arthritis, worsening of

- ▲ Kineret Injection (19%) 585

Rhinitis

- ▲ Aceon Tablets (2 mg, 4 mg, 8 mg) (4.8%) 3038
- Actiq (Less than 1%) 959
- ▲ Actonel Tablets (6.2%) 2568
- ▲ Actonel with Calcium Tablets (2.1% to 5.7%) 2574
- Advair HFA 45/21 Inhalation Aerosol 1288
- Advair HFA 115/21 Inhalation Aerosol 1288
- Advair HFA 230/21 Inhalation Aerosol 1288
- Advicor Tablets 402
- ▲ Aerobid/Aerobid-M (3% to 9%) 1153
- ▲ Agrylin Capsules (1% to less than 5%) 3017
- ▲ Alamast Ophthalmic Solution (10% to 25%) 3181
- ▲ Aldara Cream, 5% (3%) 1699
- Alinia for Oral Suspension (Less than 1%) 2677
- Alinia Tablets (Less than 1%) 2677
- ▲ Alphagan P Ophthalmic Solution (1% to 4%) 549
- Ambien Tablets (Infrequent) 2692
- ▲ AmBisome for Injection (11.1%) 606
- Amerge Tablets (Rare) 1301
- Aralast (Greater than or equal to 0.2%) 726
- Aricept Tablets (Infrequent) 1062
- Aricept ODT Tablets (Infrequent) 1062
- ▲ Arimidex Tablets (2% to 5%) 672
- ▲ Asacol Delayed-Release Tablets (5% or greater) 2579
- Atacand Tablets (2%) 639
- Atacand HCT (0.5% or greater) 642
- ▲ Atripla Tablets (Greater than or equal to 5%) 938
- ▲ Atrovent HFA Inhalation Aerosol (4% to 6%) 839
- Atrovent Nasal Spray 0.03% 834
- Attenuvax 1951
- Avalide Tablets (1% or greater) 892
- Avalide Tablets (1% or greater) 2713
- Avapro Tablets (1% or greater) 897
- Avapro Tablets (1% or greater) 2718
- Axert Tablets (Infrequent) 2431
- ▲ Axid Capsules (9.8%) 1364
- ▲ Azilect Tablets (3%) 3106
- ▲ Azopt Ophthalmic Suspension (1% to 5%) 540
- ▲ Bactroban Nasal (1% to 6%) 1367
- ▲ Bexxar (0% to 10%) 1371
- ▲ Busulfex Injection (44%) 2477
- Campral Tablets (Frequent) 1158
- Captopril Tablets 2182
- Carafate Suspension 706
- Carafate Tablets 707
- Cardizem LA Extended Release Tablets (Less than 2%) 421
- Celebrex Capsules (2%) 2979
- ▲ Celexa (5%) 1160
- ▲ CellCept Capsules (3% to less than 20%) 2622
- ▲ CellCept Intravenous (3% to less than 20%) 2622
- ▲ CellCept Oral Suspension (3% to less than 20%) 2622
- ▲ CellCept Tablets (3% to less than 20%) 2622
- ▲ Cipro I.V. (3%) 2817
- ▲ Cipro (3%) 2810
- ▲ Climara Transdermal System (2% to 6%) 763
- Combigan Ophthalmic Solution (0.1% to 0.2%) 553
- Combivent Inhalation Aerosol (1.1%) 845
- ▲ Copaxone for Injection (14%) 3110
- Cozaar Tablets (Less than 1%) 1973
- Crinone 4% Gel 992
- Crinone 8% Gel 992
- Demadex Injection (2.8%) 2630
- Demadex Tablets (2.8%) 2630
- ▲ Depakote ER Tablets (Greater than 1% to less than 5%) 423
- Diclofenac Sodium Ophthalmic Solution ⊙ 240
- Diovan Tablets (More than 1%) 2212
- ▲ Doxil Injection (Less than 1% to 10%) 2378
- Duragesic Transdermal System (1% or greater) 2405
- ▲ Effexor XR Extended-Release Capsules (8%) 3195
- ▲ Elestat Ophthalmic Solution (1% to 3%) 1741
- ▲ Elidel Cream 1% (0.4% to 4.4%) 2221
- Elmiron Capsules (Less than or equal to 1%) 2435
- ▲ Eloxatin for Injection (6% to 15%) 2731
- Emsam Transdermal System 905
- ▲ Emtriva Capsules (Greater than or equal to 10%) 1246
- ▲ Emtriva Oral Solution (Greater than or equal to 10%) 1246
- Enablex Extended-Release Tablets (Greater than or equal to 1%) 2225
- ▲ Enbrel for Injection (12% to 16%) 569
- ▲ Enjuvia Tablets (4% to 7%) 1029
- ▲ Equetro Extended-Release Capsules (Less than 5%) 3174
- ▲ Evoxac Capsules (11.2%) 1013
- ▲ Exelon Capsules (4%) 2229
- ▲ Exelon Oral Solution (4%) 2229
- Exforge Tablets (Less than or equal to 0.1%) 2238
- ▲ Exjade Tablets (6.1%) 2244
- ▲ Exubera Inhalation Powder (8.8% to 14.5%) 2515
- Fenoglide Tablets (2.3%) 2960
- ▲ Flolan for Injection (21%) 1426
- ▲ Flomax Capsules (13.1% to 17.9%) 848
- ▲ Flovent Diskus 50 mcg (3% to 13%) 1435
- ▲ Flovent HFA (1% to 3%) 1440
- Fluarix Vaccine 1446
- Flulaval Injection Vaccine 1448
- ▲ Forteo for Injection (9.6%) 1816
- ▲ Fosrenol Chewable Tablets (5% to 7%) 3027
- Frova Tablets (Frequent) 1111
- Gabitril Tablets (1% or more) 973
- ▲ Gamunex (51%) 3094
- Gemzar for Injection (Infrequent) 1820
- ▲ Gengraf Capsules (1% to 5%) 435
- ▲ Geodon (4%) 2520
- ▲ Gleevec Tablets (16.7%) 2255
- ▲ Herceptin I.V. (14%) 1199
- ▲ Humatrope Vials and Cartridges (6.25% to 13.5%) 1838
- ▲ Indapamide Tablets (Greater than or equal to 5%) 2188
- ▲ Intron A for Injection (Less than 5%) 2859
- Invanz for Injection (Greater than 0.5%) 2029
- Ionsys Transdermal System (.1% to less than 1%) 2410
- Kaletra (Less than 2%) 452
- ▲ Keppra Injection (4%) 3137
- ▲ Keppra Oral Solution (4% to 13%) 3131
- ▲ Keppra Tablets (4% to 13%) 3131
- Klonopin (2%) 2639
- Kogenate FS 746
- Kogenate FS with Bio-Set (1 case) 748
- ▲ Lamictal (7% to 14%) 1488
- ▲ Lescol Capsules (4.7%) 2268
- Lescol XL Tablets (1.5%) 2268
- ▲ Leukine (11%) 774
- ▲ Levitra Tablets (9%) 2876
- ▲ Lexapro Oral Suspension (2% to 5%) 1174
- ▲ Lexapro Tablets (2% to 5%) 1174
- Lipitor Tablets (Greater than or equal to 2%) 2501
- ▲ Lotemax Ophthalmic Suspension 0.5% (Less than 15%) ⊙ 241
- Lovaza Capsules 1520
- Lunesta Tablets 2994
- ▲ Lupron Depot 3.75 mg (Less than 5%) 462
- ▲ Lupron Depot–3 Month 11.25 mg (Less than 5%) 462
- Marinol Capsules (Less than 1%) 3163
- ▲ Mepron Suspension (5% to 24%) 1526
- ▲ Meridia Capsules (10.2%) 475
- Meruvax II 2061
- ▲ Miacalcin Nasal Spray (12%) 2274
- Micardis Tablets (More than 0.3%) 852
- Micardis HCT Tablets 854
- ▲ Mirapex Tablets (Greater than or equal to 1% to 3%) 857
- M-M-R II 2054
- Mumpsvax 2068
- ▲ Mylotarg for Injection (7% to 10%) 3212
- Nasacort AQ Nasal Spray (2% or greater) 2765
- Nasonex Nasal Spray (Greater than or equal to 2%) 2883
- ▲ Neoral Oral Solution (1% to 5%) 2280
- ▲ Neoral Soft Gelatin Capsules (1% to 5%) 2280
- Neupro Transdermal System (Greater than or equal to 2%) 3149
- Nexium Delayed-Release Capsules (Less than 1%) 645
- Nexium I.V. (Less than 1%) 652
- Nexium Delayed-Release Oral Suspension (Less than 1%) 645
- ▲ Niaspan Extended-Release Tablets (2% to 5%) 480
- Norvir (Less than 2%) 489
- ▲ Novantrone for Injection Concentrate (10%) 1100
- ▲ Ontak Vials (13%) 1079
- OptiPranolol Metipranolol Ophthalmic Solution 0.3% (A small number of patients) ⊙ 245
- ▲ Orencia Powder for Intravenous Infusion (Less than 5%) 921
- ▲ Pataday Ophthalmic Solution (Less than or equal to 5%) 543
- ▲ Patanol Ophthalmic Solution (Less than 5%) 546
- Paxil (Frequent) 1535
- Paxil CR Controlled-Release Tablets (Frequent) 1544
- PegIntron Powder for Injection (2%) 2903
- Pentacel 2792
- ▲ Plavix Tablets (4.2%) 926
- ▲ Plavix Tablets (4.2%) 2767
- ▲ Pletal Tablets (7% to 12%) 2481
- ▲ Prandin Tablets (3% to 7%) 2971
- ▲ Premarin Tablets (6% to 10%) 3221
- ▲ Premphase Tablets (6% to 10%) 3232
- ▲ Prempro Tablets (6% to 10%) 3232
- Prinivil Tablets (0.3% to 1%) 2087
- Prinzide Tablets (0.3% to 1%) 2092
- ▲ ProAir HFA Inhalation Aerosol (5%) 3113
- ▲ Prograf Capsules and Injection (3% to 15%) 622
- ▲ Proleukin for Injection (10%) 2287
- ProQuad 2099
- Protonix for Delayed-Release Oral Suspension (Greater than or equal to 1%) 3254
- Protonix Delayed-Release Tablets (Greater than or equal to 1%) 3254
- Protonix I.V. (Greater than 1%) 3257
- ▲ Protopic Ointment (3% to 5%) 628
- ▲ Proventil HFA Inhalation Aerosol (16%) 2914
- ▲ Provigil Tablets (7%) 977
- Prozac Pulvules and Liquid 1852
- ▲ Pulmicort Flexhaler (6%) 654
- ▲ Pulmozyme Inhalation Solution (30%) 1217
- ▲ Qvar Inhalation Aerosol (3% to 8%) 3116
- ▲ Rebetol (6% to 8%) 2917
- Recombivax HB (Greater than 1%) 2107
- ReFacto Vials 3269
- ▲ Remicade for IV Injection (8%) 950
- ▲ Requip Tablets (Frequent to 4%) 1561
- Retrovir Capsules 1574
- Retrovir IV Infusion 1579
- Retrovir 1574
- ▲ Rilutek Tablets (7.8% to 8.9%) 2771
- ▲ Risperdal Consta Long-Acting Injection (4%) 1753
- ▲ Rituxan I.V. (1% to 12%) 1223
- Rythmol SR Capsules 1590
- ▲ Salagen Tablets (5% to 14%) 1082
- Selzentry Tablets 2534
- ▲ Serevent Diskus (2% to 5%) 1594
- ▲ Simulect for Injection (3% to 10%) 2306
- Singulair (Greater than or equal to 2%) 2114
- ▲ Soriatane Capsules (25% to 50%) 3062
- ▲ Spiriva HandiHaler (3% to 6%) 870
- ▲ Suboxone Tablets (4.7% to 11%) 2601
- ▲ Subutex Tablets (9.7% to 11%) 2601
- Sular Extended Release Tablets (Less than or equal to 1%) 2975
- ▲ Synagis Intramuscular Solution (28.7%) 1948
- Targretin Capsules 1084
- ▲ Teveten Tablets (4%) 515
- Teveten HCT Tablets (Less than 1%) 517
- ▲ Torisel Injection (0% to 10%) 3272
- Tricor Tablets (2.3%) 520
- ▲ Truvada Tablets (Greater than or equal to 5%) 1262
- Uroxatral Tablets 2786
- Vicoprofen Tablets (Less than 3%) 533
- ▲ Vigamox Ophthalmic Solution (1% to 4%) 548
- ▲ Voltaren Ophthalmic Solution (Less than or equal to 3%) 2336
- ▲ WelChol Tablets (3.2%) 1015
- Wellbutrin SR Sustained-Release Tablets (At least 1%) 1653
- Wellbutrin XL Extended-Release Tablets (At least 1%) 1659
- Xifaxan Tablets (Less than 2%) 2682
- ▲ Xopenex Inhalation Solution (2.7% to 11.1%) 3001
- ▲ Xopenex Inhalation Solution Concentrate (2.7% to 11.1%) 3005
- ▲ Xopenex HFA Inhalation Aerosol (2.7% to 11.1%) 3009
- Xyrem Oral Solution (Infrequent) 1766
- Yaz Tablets (Greater than 1%) 805
- Zomig Tablets (Infrequent) 694
- Zomig Nasal Spray (Infrequent) 689
- Zomig-ZMT Tablets (Infrequent) 694
- Zonegran Capsules (2%) 1089
- Zostavax Injection (1.4%) 2145
- Zosyn for Injection (1.2%) 3284
- ▲ Zyban Sustained-Release Tablets (12%) 1692
- ▲ Zyprexa Tablets (7% to 10%) 1883
- ▲ Zyprexa ZYDIS Orally Disintegrating Tablets (7% to 10%) 1883
- Zyrtec Chewable Tablets (Less than 2%) 1920
- Zyrtec Syrup (Less than 2%) 1920
- Zyrtec Tablets (Less than 2%) 1920
- Zyrtec-D 12 Hour Extended Release Tablets (Less than 2%) 1923

Rhinitis, allergic

- ▲ Asmanex Twisthaler (11% to 20%) 2797
- ▲ BeneFIX Vials (4.6%) 3191
- ▲ Eloxatin for Injection (6% to 10%) 2731
- Imitrex Injection 1465
- Imitrex Nasal Spray 1470
- Mirapex Tablets 857
- Pulmicort Flexhaler (2.2%) 654

Xyrem Oral Solution (Infrequent) 1766

Rhinitis, ulcerative
Atrovent Nasal Spray 0.03% 834

Rhinorrhea
Aceon Tablets (2 mg, 4 mg, 8 mg) (0.3% to 1%) 3038
Acetadote Injection (1%) 1001
▲ Advair HFA 45/21 Inhalation Aerosol (1% to 3%) 1288
▲ Advair HFA 115/21 Inhalation Aerosol (1% to 3%) 1288
▲ Advair HFA 230/21 Inhalation Aerosol (1% to 3%) 1288
▲ Aerobid/Aerobid-M (3% to 9%) 1153
Allegra Oral Solution (0.9% to 2.1%) 2684
Allegra Tablets (0.9% to 2.1%) 2684
▲ Atrovent Nasal Spray 0.03% (3.1%) 834
Beconase AQ Nasal Spray (Fewer than 3 per 100 patients) 1369
Calcijex Injection 419
Chantix Tablets (0% to 1%) 2511
▲ Chemet Capsules (0.7% to 3.7%) 2484
▲ Clarinex Syrup (4.5%) 2828
Comvax (0.2% to 1.3%) 1966
Elidel Cream 1% (0% to 1.9%) 2221
▲ Flebogamma 5% (20%) 1715
▲ Flonase Nasal Spray (1% to 3%) 1431
▲ Flovent Diskus 50 mcg (1% to 3%) 1435
▲ Flovent HFA (1% to 3%) 1440
▲ Indapamide Tablets (Less than 5%) 2188
▲ Intron A for Injection (Less than 5%) 2859
Invanz for Injection (Greater than 0.5%) 2029
Klonopin 2639
Lamisil Oral Granules (2%) 2264
Maxalt Tablets (Rare) 2056
Maxalt-MLT Orally Disintegrating Tablets (Rare) 2056
Mirapex Tablets 857
Nexavar Tablets (0.1% to less than 1%) 784
Prinivil Tablets (0.3% to 1%) 2087
Prinzide Tablets 2092
ProQuad (Greater than or equal to 0.2% to less than 1%) 2099
Requip Tablets (Infrequent) 1561
Reyataz Capsules 3299
Rocaltrol Capsules 1150
Rocaltrol Oral Solution 1150
Singulair (Greater than or equal to 2%) 2114
Tamiflu Capsules (Less than 1%) 2649
Tamiflu Oral Suspension (Less than 1%) 2649
▲ Ultram ER Extended-Release Tablets (1% to less than 5%) 2428
▲ Valcyte Tablets (Less than 5%) 2654
▲ Vaqta (5.7%) 2130
▲ Xeloda Tablets (5%) 2662
Xifaxan Tablets (Less than 2%) 2682

Rhonchi
Acetadote Injection (1%) 1001
Invanz for Injection (0.5% to 1.1%) 2029
Orencia Powder for Intravenous Infusion 921
Proleukin for Injection 2287
ReoPro Vials (0.1%) 1860
▲ Trisenox Injection (8%) 986
Zemuron Injection (Less than 1%) 2947

Rigidity
Flumadine 1167
Gengraf Capsules (1% to less than 3%) 435
Imitrex Tablets (Rare) 1474
▲ Intron A for Injection (Up to 42%) 2859
Moban Tablets 1116
Neoral Oral Solution (1% to less than 3%) 2280
Neoral Soft Gelatin Capsules (1% to less than 3%) 2280
▲ Orthoclone OKT3 Sterile Solution (8%) 2387
Remeron Tablets 2924
RemeronSolTab Tablets 2927
Romazicon Injection (Less than 1%) 2646
▲ Soriatane Capsules (10% to 25%) 3062
Zosyn for Injection (1% or less) 3284

Rigors
Advate (0.6%) 721
Aldara Cream, 5% (1%) 1699
Alphanate 1709
Ambien Tablets (Rare) 2692
Ambien CR Tablets (Rare) 2696
AmBisome for Injection (Less common) 606
▲ Arranon Injection (0% to 8%) 1319
BeneFIX Vials (1.6%) 3191
Bexxar 1371
Campath Ampules 761
Celexa (Infrequent) 1160
▲ Clolar for Intravenous Infusion (38%) 1239
Cubicin for Injection (Less than 1%) 995
Cymbalta Delayed-Release Capsules (Frequent) 1801
▲ Dacogen Injection (22%) 1066
▲ DepoDur Injection (2% to 5%) 1095
Duragesic Transdermal System (Greater than or less than 1%) 2405
Eligard 7.5 mg (Less than 2%) 2724
Eligard 22.5 mg (Less than 2%) 2724
Eligard 30 mg (Less than 2%) 2724
Eligard 45 mg (Less than 2%) 2724
Elitek (Less than or equal to 1%) 2729
▲ Eloxatin for Injection (7% to 9%) 2731
Emend Capsules (Greater than 0.5%) 1992
Emend for Injection (Greater than 0.5%) 1999
Evoxac Capsules (1.3%) 1013
Exelon Capsules (Frequent) 2229
Exelon Oral Solution (Frequent) 2229
Exforge Tablets (Greater than 0.1% to less than 1%) 2238
Fabrazyme for Intravenous Infusion 1241
Flebogamma 5% 1715
Flebogamma 5% DIF 1718
Flulaval Injection Vaccine 1448
Frova Tablets (Infrequent) 1111
Gammagard Liquid 730
Gammagard S/D 734
Gamunex 3094
Gantrisin Pediatric Suspension 2638
▲ Gengraf Capsules (3%) 435
▲ Gleevec Tablets (10% to 12%) 2255
Herceptin I.V. 1199
▲ Hycamtin for Injection (69%) 1459
▲ Intron A for Injection (2% to 42%) 2859
▲ MoviPrep Oral Solution (33.7%) 2679
▲ Mycamine for Injection (9.1% to 26.4%) 616
▲ Neoral Oral Solution (3%) 2280
▲ Neoral Soft Gelatin Capsules (3%) 2280
Neupro Transdermal System 3149
Nexium Delayed-Release Capsules (Less than 1%) 645
Nexium I.V. (Less than 1%) 652
Nexium Delayed-Release Oral Suspension (Less than 1%) 645
▲ Noxafil Oral Suspension (Less than 1% to 20%) 2889
▲ PegIntron Powder for Injection (23%) 2903
Proventil HFA Inhalation Aerosol (Less than 3%) 2914
▲ Rebetol (25% to 48%) 2917
▲ Rebif Prefilled Syringe for Injection (6% to 13%) 1107
▲ Reclast Injection (8%) 2291
Requip Tablets (Greater than or equal to 1%) 1561
Rituxan I.V. 1223
Romazicon Injection (Less than 1%) 2646
▲ Simulect for Injection (3% to 10%) 2306
▲ Strattera Capsules (3%) 1864
▲ Tarceva Tablets (0% to 12%) 1228
Teveten Tablets (Less than 1%) 515
Teveten HCT Tablets (Less than 1%) 517
▲ Tice BCG (3%) 2936
▲ Trisenox Injection (38%) 986
▲ Ultram ER Extended-Release Tablets (1% to less than 5%) 2428
▲ Velcade for Injection (11%) 2168
Vivitrol 988
▲ Zometa for Intravenous Infusion (Less than 15%) 2341
Zyrtec Chewable Tablets (Less than 2%) 1920
Zyrtec Syrup (Less than 2%) 1920
Zyrtec Tablets (Less than 2%) 1920
Zyrtec-D 12 Hour Extended Release Tablets (Less than 2%) 1923

Rosacea
Elocon Cream 0.1% 2840
Elocon Ointment 0.1% 2842
Evoxac Capsules (Less than 1%) 1013
Mirapex Tablets 857
Protopic Ointment 628
Xyrem Oral Solution (Infrequent) 1766

Roseola
Prevnar 3241

Rotator cuff syndrome
Requip Tablets (Infrequent) 1561

Roughness, unspecified
ProQuad 2099

Rupture, Achilles tendon
Avelox 2803
Cipro 2810
Cipro XR Tablets 2823
Levaquin 2416
Levaquin in 5% Dextrose Injection 2416

Rupture, hand
Avelox 2803
Cipro 2810
Cipro XR Tablets 2823

Rupture, shoulder
Avelox 2803
Cipro 2810
Cipro XR Tablets 2823

S

S_3 gallop
(*see under* Ventricular gallop)

Sacrolitis
Requip Tablets (Infrequent) 1561

Saliva, discoloration
Stalevo Tablets 2309

Salivary gland enlargement
Alinia for Oral Suspension (Less than 1%) 2677
Alinia Tablets (Less than 1%) 2677
Copaxone for Injection (Frequent) 3110
▲ Evoxac Capsules (1% to 3%) 1013
Gantrisin Pediatric Suspension 2638
Gengraf Capsules (1% to less than 3%) 435
Imitrex Nasal Spray 1470
Neoral Oral Solution (1% to less than 3%) 2280
Neoral Soft Gelatin Capsules (1% to less than 3%) 2280
Prozac Weekly Capsules (Rare) 1852
Prozac Pulvules and Liquid (Rare) 1852
Remeron Tablets (Rare) 2924
RemeronSolTab Tablets (Rare) 2927
Rilutek Tablets (Rare) 2771
Salagen Tablets (Less than 1%) 1082

Salivation
(*see under* Sialism)

Salivation, change in
Valium Tablets 2658

Salivation, increase
(*see under* Sialism)

Salpingitis
Amerge Tablets (Rare) 1301
Effexor XR Extended-Release Capsules (Rare) 3195
Gabitril Tablets (Infrequent) 973
Salagen Tablets (Less than 1%) 1082
Venlafaxine Hydrochloride Tablets (Rare) 2199
Wellbutrin SR Sustained-Release Tablets 1653
Wellbutrin XL Extended-Release Tablets 1659
Zyban Sustained-Release Tablets 1692

Sarcoidosis
Enbrel for Injection 569
Intron A for Injection (Very rare) 2859
PegIntron Powder for Injection (Less than or equal to 1%) 2903
Rebetol 2917

Sarcoidosis, exacerbation of
Intron A for Injection (Very rare) 2859
Rebetol 2917

Sarcoma, unspecified
▲ Megace ES Oral Suspension (1% to 3%) 2499

Scabbing
▲ Aldara Cream, 5% (8% to 79%) 1699
Daytrana Transdermal Patch 3022
▲ Panretin Gel 0.1% (1% to 8%) 1081

Scalp hair, loss of
Activella Tablets 2347
Divigel 3167
Lybrel Tablets 3204
NuvaRing 2897
Ortho Tri-Cyclen Lo Tablets 2458
Proglycem Capsules (Infrequent) 1185
Proglycem Suspension (Infrequent) 1185

Scalp hair, thinning
Angeliq Tablets 751
Mircette Tablets 1034
Ortho Evra Transdermal System 2437
Seasonique Tablets 1046
Yaz Tablets 805

Scarring
▲ Supprelin LA Implant (6.4%) 1731

Schilling's test, abnormal
Sandostatin LAR Depot 2302

Schizophrenia, precipitation
Zyprexa Tablets 1883
Zyprexa ZYDIS Orally Disintegrating Tablets 1883

Schizophrenia, worsening of
Keppra Injection 3137
Keppra Oral Solution 3131
Keppra Tablets 3131

Sciatica
Ambien Tablets (Rare) 2692
Ambien CR Tablets (Rare) 2696
Arranon Injection (1%) 1319
Atacand HCT (0.5% or greater) 642
Exforge Tablets (Greater than or equal to 0.2%) 2238
Gleevec Tablets (Infrequent) 2255
Mirapex Tablets 857
Requip Tablets (Infrequent) 1561
Rythmol SR Capsules 1590
Wellbutrin Tablets (Rare) 1648

Scleral injection
Fansidar Tablets 2636
Gantrisin Pediatric Suspension 2638

Scleral thinning
Pred-G Ophthalmic Ointment ⊙229

Scleritis
Ambien Tablets (Infrequent) 2692
Ambien CR Tablets (Infrequent) 2696
Effexor XR Extended-Release Capsules (Rare) 3195
Evoxac Capsules (Less than 1%) 1013
Fosamax 2005
Fosamax Plus D Tablets (Rarely) 2013
Prozac Weekly Capsules (Rare) 1852
Prozac Pulvules and Liquid (Rare) 1852
Venlafaxine Hydrochloride Tablets (Rare) 2199
Zometa for Intravenous Infusion 2341

Scleroderma
Evoxac Capsules (Less than 1%) 1013
Proleukin for Injection 2287
Soriatane Capsules (Less than 1%) 3062

Sclerosis, multiple
Chantix Tablets (Rare) 2511
Enbrel for Injection 569
Engerix-B Vaccine (Less than 1%) 1409
Evoxac Capsules (Less than 1%) 1013
Havrix Injection Vaccine 1454
▲ Humira Injection (Less than 5%) 442
Recombivax HB 2107
Remicade for IV Injection 950
Twinrix Vaccine 1628

Sclerosis, skin
Parnate Tablets 1532

Scoliosis
▲ Humatrope Vials and Cartridges (18.9%) 1838
Nutropin for Injection (0.2%) 1208
Nutropin AQ Injection (0.2%) 1212
Nutropin AQ NuSpin Injection (0.2%) 1212
Nutropin AQ Pen (0.2%) 1212
Nutropin AQ Pen Cartridge (0.2%) 1212
Tev-Tropin for Injection 1187

Scoliosis, progression of
Genotropin Lyophilized Powder 2547
Norditropin Cartridges 2354

Scotoma
Mirapex Tablets 857
Proglycem Capsules (Infrequent) 1185
Proglycem Suspension (Infrequent) 1185
Sandostatin LAR Depot 2302
▲ Visudyne for Injection (10% to 30%) 2332

Scotomata
Adenoscan (Less than 1%) 605
Amerge Tablets (Rare) 1301

Emend for Injection (Greater than 0.5%) 1999
Emsam Transdermal System (Rare) 905
Emtriva Capsules (1%) 1246
Emtriva Oral Solution (1%) 1246
Evoxac Capsules 1013
Exelon Capsules (Infrequent) 2229
Exelon Oral Solution (Infrequent) 2229
▲ Fortaz (1 in 23) 1450
▲ Gemzar for Injection (55% to 77%) 1820
Geodon Capsules (Infrequent) 2520
▲ Gleevec Tablets (0% to 5.5%) 2255
▲ Hexalen Capsules (9%) 1078
▲ Humira Injection (5%) 442
▲ Intron A for Injection (Up to 13%) 2859
▲ Invanz for Injection (1.1% to 6.6%) 2029
Isentress Tablets (0.4% to 2%) 2036
Ixempra Kit for Injection 915
Ketek Tablets (Less than 0.2%) 2744
Klonopin 2639
Lamictal (Rare) 1488
Lescol Capsules 2268
Lescol XL Tablets 2268
▲ Leukine (8%) 774
Levaquin (0.1% to 1%) 2416
Levaquin in 5% Dextrose Injection (0.1% to 1%) 2416
▲ Mepron Suspension (5% to 8%) 1526
Meridia Capsules (1.6%) 475
Merrem I.V. (Greater than 0.2%) 684
Mevacor Tablets 2063
▲ Mycamine for Injection (3% to 7.9%) 616
▲ Mylotarg for Injection (5% to 10%) 3212
▲ Nabi-HB (4%) 815
Nalfon Capsules (Less than 1%) 2508
Namenda (Frequent) 1180
▲ Neulasta Injection (9%) 587
▲ Neupogen for Injection (21% to 58%) 589
Nexavar Tablets (0.1% to less than 1%) 784
Nexium Delayed-Release Capsules (Less than 1%) 645
Nexium I.V. (Less than 1%) 652
Nexium Delayed-Release Oral Suspension (Less than 1%) 645
Nimotop Capsules (0.2%; rare) 790
Noroxin Tablets (1.1%) 2069
NovoLog Mix 70/30 2364
▲ Noxafil Oral Suspension (1% to 13%) 2889
Nutropin for Injection 1208
Nutropin AQ Injection 1212
Nutropin AQ NuSpin Injection 1212
Nutropin AQ Pen 1212
Nutropin AQ Pen Cartridge 1212
Omnicef Capsules (0.3%) 497
Omnicef for Oral Suspension (1%) 497
Paxil (Rare) 1535
Paxil CR Controlled-Release Tablets (Rare) 1544
Pentasa Capsules (Less than 1%) 3030
Primaxin I.M. 2080
Primaxin I.V. 2083
Proglycem Capsules (Infrequent) 1185
Proglycem Suspension (Infrequent) 1185
▲ Prograf Capsules and Injection (3% to 15%) 622
▲ Proleukin for Injection (Less than 1% to 10%) 2287
Protonix for Delayed-Release Oral Suspension (Less than 1%) 3254
Protonix Delayed-Release Tablets (Less than 1%) 3254
Protonix I.V. (Less than 1%) 3257
Prozac Weekly Capsules (Rare) 1852
Prozac Pulvules and Liquid (Rare) 1852
▲ Raptiva for Injection (4%) 1218
Requip Tablets (Infrequent) 1561
Rilutek Tablets (Infrequent) 2771
Rocephin Injectable Vials, ADD-Vantage, Galaxy, Bulk (Less than 1%) 2642
Rythmol Tablets (0.2%) 1586
▲ Rythmol SR Capsules (3%) 1590
Suprax for Oral Suspension (Less than 2%) 1891
Suprax Tablets (Less than 2%) 1891
Symbyax Capsules 1871
Tabloid Tablets 1601
Tarka Tablets (2.8%) 511
▲ Tasigna Capsules (1% to 10%) 2316
▲ Taxotere Injection Concentrate (4.3% to 7.3%) 2773
Teveten Tablets 515
Teveten HCT Tablets 517
Thiothixene Capsules (Infrequently) 2197
Timentin ADD-Vantage 1606
Timentin Injection Galaxy Container 1609
Timentin IV Infusion 1603
Timentin Pharmacy Bulk Package 1613
Toprol-XL Tablets 666
▲ Torisel Injection (3% to 68%) 3272
Tricor Tablets 520
Truvada Tablets (1%) 1262
▲ Tygacil for Injection (3.5%) 3276
Ultane Liquid for Inhalation (Less than 1%) 524
Valium Tablets 2658
▲ Valtrex Caplets (4%) 1635
Venlafaxine Hydrochloride Tablets (Infrequent) 2199
Vytorin 10/10 Tablets 2149
Vytorin 10/10 Tablets 2939
Vytorin 10/20 Tablets 2149
Vytorin 10/20 Tablets 2939
Vytorin 10/40 Tablets 2149
Vytorin 10/40 Tablets 2939
Vytorin 10/80 Tablets 2149
Vytorin 10/80 Tablets 2939
Xyrem Oral Solution (Infrequent) 1766
Zinacef for Injection (1 in 50 patients) 1678
Zinacef Injection (1 in 50 patients) 1678
Zocor Tablets 2136
Zomig Tablets (Rare) 694
Zomig-ZMT Tablets (Rare) 694
Zonegran Capsules 1089
Zosyn for Injection 3284
Zyprexa Tablets (Infrequent) 1883
Zyprexa ZYDIS Orally Disintegrating Tablets (Infrequent) 1883

Serum aminotransferase, elevation
Arixtra Injection (1.7% to 2.6%) 1313
Lovenox Injection (Greater than 1%) 2756

Serum amylase, abnormal
▲ Sutent Capsules (5% to 17%) 2540
Zyvox (0.2% to 2.4%) 2552

Serum amylase, decreased
Avelox (Greater than or equal to 2%) 2803

Serum amylase, elevation
Abelcet Injection 1134
AmBisome for Injection (Less common) 606
▲ Aptivus Capsules (0.3% to 5.7%) 823
▲ Aptivus Oral Solution (0.3% to 5.7%) 823
▲ Atripla Tablets (8%) 938
Avelox (Greater than or equal to 0.1% to less than 2%) 2803
▲ Baraclude (2% to 3%) 900
Cipro I.V. (1% or less) 2817
Cipro (Less than 0.1% to less than 1%) 2810
Cipro XR Tablets 2823
Crixivan Capsules (2.1%) 1979
▲ Emtriva Capsules (2% to 8%) 1246
▲ Emtriva Oral Solution (2% to 8%) 1246
▲ Epivir (2.2% to 4%) 1412
Epivir-HBV (Less than 1%) 1417
Epzicom Tablets 1422
▲ Evoxac Capsules (1% to 3%) 1013
Exelon Patch (Infrequent) 2233
Isentress Tablets (0.2% to 1.4%) 2036
▲ Kaletra (2% to 8%) 452
▲ Kepivance (38% to 62%) 583
Malarone Pediatric Tablets 1521
Malarone Tablets 1521
▲ Mepron Suspension (1% to 8%) 1526
▲ Nexavar Tablets (1% to 40%) 784
Niaspan Extended-Release Tablets 480
Omnicef Capsules 497
Omnicef for Oral Suspension 497
Pentasa Capsules (Less than 1%) 3030
Prograf Capsules and Injection 622
Selzentry Tablets (Greater than or equal to 2%) 2534
▲ Sustiva Capsules (10%) 930
▲ Sustiva Tablets (10%) 930
▲ Sutent Capsules (1% to 5%) 2540
Targretin Capsules 1084
▲ Tasigna Capsules (1% to 10%) 2316
▲ Truvada Tablets (8%) 1262
▲ Tygacil for Injection (3.1%) 3276
Tylenol with Codeine Tablets 2427
Tyzeka Tablets (Less than 1%) 2328
▲ Viread Tablets (4% to 9%) 1268
▲ Ziagen (2% to 4%) 1673

Serum bicarbonate, decrease
▲ Dacogen Injection (5%) 1066
▲ Fabrazyme for Intravenous Infusion (9%) 1241
Omnicef Capsules (0.6%) 497
Omnicef for Oral Suspension (1%) 497

Serum bicarbonate, increase
Cubicin for Injection (Less than 1%) 995
▲ Dacogen Injection (6%) 1066

Serum bicarbonate content, variations
▲ Prograf Capsules and Injection (3% to 15%) 622

Serum bilirubin, elevation
(*see under* Hyperbilirubinemia)

Serum bilirubin, unconjugated, elevation
Tasigna Capsules 2316

Serum bilirubin levels, abnormalities
Amerge Tablets (Rare) 1301
AndroGel 3159
▲ Eloxatin for Injection (0% to 36%) 2731
▲ Sutent Capsules (1% to 16%) 2540
▲ Tykerb Tablets (0% to 45%) 1631
▲ Zyvox (0.2% to 6.3%) 2552

Serum calcium, depression
(*see under* Hypocalcemia)

Serum calcium decrease
(*see under* Hypocalcemia)

Serum chloride levels, decreased
▲ Dacogen Injection (6%) 1066

Serum cholesterol, increase
(*see under* Hypercholesterolemia)

Serum C-reactive protein, increased
Pneumovax 23 2078

Serum creatine phosphokinase, elevation
Abilify Injection (Greater than or equal to 1 in 100 patients) 881
Abilify Injection (Greater than or equal to 1 in 100 patients) 2466
Abilify Oral Solution (Greater than or equal to 1 in 100 patients) 881
Abilify Oral Solution (Greater than or equal to 1 in 100 patients) 2466
Abilify Discmelt Orally Disintegrating Tablets (Greater than or equal to 1 in 100 patients) 881
Abilify Discmelt Orally Disintegrating Tablets (Greater than or equal to 1 in 100 patients) 2466
Abilify Tablets (Greater than or equal to 1 in 100 patients) 881
Abilify Tablets (Greater than or equal to 1 in 100 patients) 2466
Accutane Capsules 2607
ActoPlus Met Tablets 3071
▲ Aricept Tablets (3%) 1062
▲ Aricept ODT Tablets (3%) 1062
Benicar HCT Tablets (Greater than 1%) 1010
Catapres Tablets (Rare) 841
Celebrex Capsules 2979
▲ CellCept Capsules (3% to less than 20%) 2622
▲ CellCept Intravenous (3% to less than 20%) 2622
▲ CellCept Oral Suspension (3% to less than 20%) 2622
▲ CellCept Tablets (3% to less than 20%) 2622
Cipro I.V. (Among most frequent) 2817
Cipro XR Tablets 2823
Clorpres Tablets (Rare) 2185
Crestor Tablets (2.6%) 677
Epzicom Tablets 1422
Exelon Patch (Infrequent) 2233
Geodon Capsules (Infrequent) 2520
Gleevec Tablets (Infrequent) 2255
Havrix Injection Vaccine (Less than 1%) 1454
Lipitor Tablets (Less than 2%) 2501
Mirapex Tablets (1% or more) 857
Norvir (0.9% to 3.4%) 489
Protonix for Delayed-Release Oral Suspension 3254
Protonix Delayed-Release Tablets 3254
Protonix I.V. 3257
Prozac Pulvules and Liquid (Rare) 1852
Requip Tablets (Infrequent) 1561
Sular Extended Release Tablets (Less than or equal to 1%) 2975
▲ Tasigna Capsules (1% to 10%) 2316
Trasylol Injection (2%) 799
Trizivir Tablets 1622
▲ Ultram ER Extended-Release Tablets (1% to less than 5%) 2428
Vytorin 10/10 Tablets 2939
Vytorin 10/20 Tablets 2939
Vytorin 10/40 Tablets 2939
Vytorin 10/80 Tablets 2939
▲ Ziagen (7% to 8%) 1673
Zyprexa Tablets 1883
Zyprexa IntraMuscular (Infrequent) 1883
Zyprexa ZYDIS Orally Disintegrating Tablets 1883

Serum creatinine, abnormal
▲ Novantrone for Injection Concentrate (13%) 1100
▲ Sutent Capsules (1% to 12%) 2540
Zometa for Intravenous Infusion (1% to 2%) 2341
Zyvox (0.4% to 2.4%) 2552

Serum creatinine, elevation
▲ Abelcet Injection (11%) 1134
Aceon Tablets (2 mg, 4 mg, 8 mg) (0.3% to 1%) 3038
Aggrenox Capsules 819
▲ Alimta for Injection (Up to 16%) 1786
Alinia for Oral Suspension (Less than 1%) 2677
Alinia Tablets (Less than 1%) 2677
▲ AmBisome for Injection (18.5% to 22.4%) 606
Anaprox Tablets (Less than 1%) 2632
Anaprox DS Tablets (Less than 1%) 2632
AndroGel 3159
▲ Arranon Injection (0% to 6%) 1319
Asacol Delayed-Release Tablets 2579
Atacand Tablets (Infrequent) 639
Avalide Tablets (1.1%) 892
Avapro Tablets (Less than 0.7%) 897
Avapro Tablets (Less than 0.7%) 2718
Azor Tablets 1005
Baraclude (0% to 2%) 900
Benicar Tablets 1009
Benicar HCT Tablets (Rare) 1010
Biaxin/Biaxin XL (Less than 1%) 411
Bicillin C-R Injectable Suspension 1775
Bicillin L-A Injection 1777
▲ Busulfex Injection (21%) 2477
Byetta Injection 600
Campral Tablets (Rare) 1158
Capastat Sulfate for Injection (A significant number of patients) 1791
Captopril Tablets 2182
Ceftin 1380
Celebrex Capsules (0.1% to 1.9%) 2979
▲ CellCept Capsules (39.4%) 2622
▲ CellCept Intravenous (39.4%) 2622
▲ CellCept Oral Suspension (39.4%) 2622
▲ CellCept Tablets (39.4%) 2622
Cipro I.V. (Among most frequent) 2817
Cipro (1.1%) 2810
Cipro XR Tablets 2823
▲ Clolar for Intravenous Infusion (6%) 1239
▲ Coreg Tablets (Greater than 1% to 3%) 1387
▲ Coreg CR Extended-Release Capsules (Greater than 1% to less than or equal to 3%) 1393
Cozaar Tablets (Less than 0.1%) 1973
Crixivan Capsules 1979
Didronel Tablets 2583
▲ Diovan Tablets (4.2%) 2212
Diovan HCT Tablets (2%) 2216
Doxil Injection (Less than 1%) 2378
Dyazide Capsules 1405
Dyrenium Capsules (Rare) 3189
EC-Naprosyn Delayed-Release Tablets (Less than 1%) 2632
Effexor XR Extended-Release Capsules (Infrequent) 3195
▲ Eloxatin for Injection (1% to 10%) 2731
▲ Emend Capsules (3.7%) 1992
▲ Emend for Injection (3.7%) 1999
▲ Exjade Tablets (2.4% to 38.2%) 2244
Fansidar Tablets 2636
Fenoglide Tablets 2960
Flebogamma 5% 1715
Flebogamma 5% DIF 1718
Fortaz (Occasional) 1450
Gammagard S/D 734
Gantrisin Pediatric Suspension 2638
▲ Gemzar for Injection (Up to 8%) 1820
▲ Gengraf Capsules (18% to 48%) 435
Geodon Capsules (Rare) 2520
▲ Gleevec Tablets (0% to 8%) 2255
▲ Hexalen Capsules (7%) 1078

▲ Indapamide Tablets (Less than 5%) 2188
Indocin I.V. 2489
▲ Intron A for Injection (Up to 3%) 2859
Invanz for Injection (0.9% to 1.1%) 2029
Lamictal (Rare) 1488
▲ Leukine (15%) 774
▲ Lupron Depot 7.5 mg (Greater than or equal to 5%) 469
▲ Mavik Tablets (1.1% to 4.7%) 472
Mepron Suspension (1%) 1526
Merrem I.V. (Greater than 0.2%) 684
Micardis Tablets 852
Mobic Oral Suspension (Less than 2%) 863
Mobic Tablets (Less than 2%) 863
Mycamine for Injection 616
▲ Myfortic Tablets (3% to less than 20%) 2276
Nabi-HB (2%) 815
Namenda 1180
Naprosyn Suspension (Less than 1%) 2632
Naprosyn Tablets (Less than 1%) 2632
Natrecor for Injection (Greater than or equal to 1%) 2977
▲ Neoral Oral Solution (18% to 48%) 2280
▲ Neoral Soft Gelatin Capsules (18% to 48%) 2280
Noroxin Tablets (Less frequent) 2069
▲ Ontak Vials (7%) 1079
OsmoPrep Tablets 2680
Plavix Tablets 926
Plavix Tablets 2767
Pletal Tablets (Less than 2%) 2481
Primaxin I.M. 2080
Primaxin I.V. 2083
▲ Prinivil Tablets (About 2% to approximately 11.6%) 2087
Prinzide Tablets 2092
▲ Prograf Capsules and Injection (24% to 45%) 622
▲ Proleukin for Injection (1% to 33%) 2287
Protopic Ointment (Greater than or equal to 1%) 628
▲ Rapamune Oral Solution (Greater than 3% to 40%) 3260
▲ Rocaltrol Capsules (1 in 6) 1150
▲ Rocaltrol Oral Solution (1 in 6) 1150
Rocephin Injectable Vials, ADD-Vantage, Galaxy, Bulk (Less than 1%) 2642
Rythmol SR Capsules 1590
Sandimmune 2296
Sandostatin LAR Depot 2302
Sular Extended Release Tablets (Less than or equal to 1%) 2975
Suprax for Oral Suspension (Less than 2%) 1891
Suprax Tablets (Less than 2%) 1891
Sutent Capsules 2540
Symbyax Capsules (Rare) 1871
Targretin Capsules 1084
Tasigna Capsules (Less than 1% to 1%) 2316
▲ Tekturna HCT Tablets (7%) 2324
Testim 1% Gel (Less than 1%) 701
Teveten Tablets (1.3%) 515
Teveten HCT Tablets (0.6%) 517
Timentin ADD-Vantage 1606
Timentin Injection Galaxy Container 1609
Timentin IV Infusion 1603
Timentin Pharmacy Bulk Package 1613
▲ Torisel Injection (3% to 57%) 3272
▲ Trasylol Injection (18% to 21%) 799
Tricor Tablets 520
Trizivir Tablets 1622
Truvada Tablets 1262
Tygacil for Injection (0% to less than 2%) 3276
Ultane Liquid for Inhalation (Less than 1%) 524
Urso 250 Tablets (1%) 720
Urso Forte Tablets (1%) 720
Valtrex Caplets (Up to 0.7%) 1635
Venlafaxine Hydrochloride Tablets (Rare) 2199
Viread Tablets 1268
▲ Visudyne for Injection (1% to 10%) 2332
▲ Vytorin 10/10 Tablets (Up to 5%) 2939
▲ Vytorin 10/20 Tablets (Up to 5%) 2939
▲ Vytorin 10/40 Tablets (Up to 5%) 2939
▲ Vytorin 10/80 Tablets (Up to 5%) 2939
Zantac 25 EFFERdose Tablets (Rare) 1670
Zantac Injection 1666
Zantac Injection Pharmacy Bulk Package (Rare) 1668
Zantac Injection Premixed 1666
Zantac (Rare) 1670
Ziagen 1673
Zinacef for Injection 1678
Zinacef Injection 1678
▲ Zolinza Capsules (14% to 46.5%) 2142
Zonegran Capsules 1089
Zosyn for Injection 3284
Zovirax 1690

Serum creatinine, increased
Abilify Injection (Greater than or equal to 1 in 1000 patients and less than 1 in 100 patients) 881
Abilify Injection (Greater than or equal to 1 in 1000 patients and less than 1 in 100 patients) 2466
Abilify Oral Solution (Greater than or equal to 1 in 1000 patients and less than 1 in 100 patients) 881
Abilify Oral Solution (Greater than or equal to 1 in 1000 patients and less than 1 in 100 patients) 2466
Abilify Discmelt Orally Disintegrating Tablets (Greater than or equal to 1 in 1000 patients and less than 1 in 100 patients) 881
Abilify Discmelt Orally Disintegrating Tablets (Greater than or equal to 1 in 1000 patients and less than 1 in 100 patients) 2466
Abilify Tablets (Greater than or equal to 1 in 1000 patients and less than 1 in 100 patients) 881
Abilify Tablets (Greater than or equal to 1 in 1000 patients and less than 1 in 100 patients) 2466
Avalide Tablets (1.1%) 2713
▲ Cancidas for Injection (3.4% to 11.4%) 1953
▲ Fabrazyme for Intravenous Infusion (9%) 1241
Hepsera Tablets 1253
Noxafil Oral Suspension (2%) 2889
▲ Rapamune Tablets (Greater than or equal to 3% to greater than or equal to 30%) 3260

Serum electrolyte changes
(*see under* Electrolyte imbalance)

Serum folate levels, decreased
Lybrel Tablets 3204
Seasonique Tablets 1046
Yaz Tablets 805

Serum gastrin levels, increased
Nexium Delayed-Release Capsules (Less than 1%) 645
Nexium I.V. (Less than 1%) 652
Nexium Delayed-Release Oral Suspension (Less than 1%) 645

Serum lipase, abnormal
▲ Sutent Capsules (10% to 25%) 2540
Zyvox (0.4% to 2.3%) 2552

Serum lipase, elevation
▲ Aptivus Capsules (Less than 2% to 7.5%) 823
▲ Aptivus Oral Solution (Less than 2% to 7.5%) 823
▲ Atripla Tablets (Up to 3%) 938
▲ Baraclude (7% to 8%) 900
Cipro I.V. (1% or less) 2817
Cipro (Less than 1%) 2810
Cipro XR Tablets 2823
Emtriva Capsules (Greater than or equal to 1%) 1246
Emtriva Oral Solution (Greater than or equal to 1%) 1246
▲ Epivir (3%) 1412
▲ Epivir-HBV (10%) 1417
Epzicom Tablets 1422
Exelon Patch (Infrequent) 2233
▲ Isentress Tablets (0.2% to 3.4%) 2036
▲ Kepivance (11% to 28%) 583
▲ Lexiva Oral Suspension (5% to 8%) 1510
▲ Lexiva Tablets (5% to 8%) 1510
▲ Nexavar Tablets (12% to 41%) 784
Pentasa Capsules (Less than 1%) 3030
Selzentry Tablets (Greater than or equal to 2%) 2534
▲ Sutent Capsules (2% to 16%) 2540
▲ Tasigna Capsules (Greater than or equal to 0.1% to 17%) 2316
▲ Truvada Tablets (Less than or equal to 3%) 1262
Tyzeka Tablets (2%) 2328

Serum lipids, changes in
Avandamet Tablets 1336
Avandia Tablets 1351
Reyataz Capsules 3299

Serum PBI levels, decrease
(*see under* PBI decrease)

Serum phosphorus, elevation
Cubicin for Injection (2.5%) 995
▲ Lupron Depot 3.75 mg (Approximately 5% to 8%) 462
▲ Lupron Depot 7.5 mg (Greater than or equal to 5%) 469
Nutropin for Injection 1208
Nutropin AQ Injection 1212
Nutropin AQ NuSpin Injection 1212
Nutropin AQ Pen 1212
Nutropin AQ Pen Cartridge 1212
Omnicef Capsules (0.6%) 497
Omnicef for Oral Suspension (0.9%) 497

Serum potassium, changes in
Brovana Inhalation Solution (Infrequent) 2990

Serum potassium, reduction
(*see under* Hypokalemia)

Serum proteins, changes
Premarin Tablets 3221
Premphase Tablets 3232
Prempro Tablets 3232

Serum sickness
Amoxil Capsules 1305
Amoxil Chewable Tablets 1305
Amoxil Pediatric Drops for Oral Suspension 1305
Amoxil Powder for Oral Suspension 1305
Amoxil Tablets 1305
Antivenin (Black Widow Spider Antivenin) 1951
Augmentin 1323
Augmentin Tablets 1327
Augmentin XR Extended Release Tablets 1333
Augmentin ES-600 Powder for Oral Suspension 1329
Avelox 2803
Bexxar 1371
Bicillin C-R Injectable Suspension 1775
Bicillin L-A Injection 1777
Campath Ampules 761
Ceftin 1380
Cimzia (Rare) 3127
Cipro I.V. (Rare) 2817
Cipro 2810
Cipro XR Tablets 2823
Copaxone for Injection (Infrequent) 3110
Engerix-B Vaccine (Less than 1%) 1409
Fansidar Tablets 2636
Fluarix Vaccine 1446
Gantrisin Pediatric Suspension 2638
Levaquin 2416
Levaquin in 5% Dextrose Injection 2416
Levothroid Tablets 1170
Levoxyl Tablets 1780
Noroxin Tablets 2069
Orthoclone OKT3 Sterile Solution 2387
Plavix Tablets 926
Plavix Tablets 2767
Pneumovax 23 2078
Prozac Weekly Capsules 1852
Recombivax HB (Less than 1%) 2107
Remicade for IV Injection (Greater than or equal to 0.2%) 950
Rituxan I.V. 1223
Rocephin Injectable Vials, ADD-Vantage, Galaxy, Bulk (Less than 0.1%) 2642
Twinrix Vaccine 1628
Wellbutrin Tablets 1648
Wellbutrin SR Sustained-Release Tablets 1653
Wellbutrin XL Extended-Release Tablets 1659

Serum sickness-like reaction
Augmentin Tablets 1327
Augmentin XR Extended Release Tablets 1333
Augmentin ES-600 Powder for Oral Suspension 1329
Axid Capsules 1364
Cipro 2810
Cipro XR Tablets 2823
Moxatag Tablets 2165
Raptiva for Injection (1 patient) 1218
Rocephin Injectable Vials, ADD-Vantage, Galaxy, Bulk 2642
Suprax for Oral Suspension (Less than 2%) 1891
Suprax Tablets (Less than 2%) 1891

Serum transaminase, elevation
Advicor Tablets 402
Aricept Tablets (Infrequent) 1062
Aricept ODT Tablets (Infrequent) 1062
▲ Arranon Injection (0% to 12%) 1319
Augmentin (Infrequent) 1323
Augmentin Tablets (Infrequent) 1327
Augmentin XR Extended Release Tablets (Infrequent) 1333
Augmentin ES-600 Powder for Oral Suspension (Infrequently) 1329
Benicar Tablets 1009
Captopril Tablets 2182
Celebrex Capsules 2979
▲ Chemet Capsules (6% to 10%) 2484
Crestor Tablets 677
Daytrana Transdermal Patch 3022
Depakote ER Tablets 423
Doribax Injection (1% to 2%) 2400
Elmiron Capsules (1.2%) 2435
▲ Eloxatin for Injection (2% to 57%) 2731
Elspar for Injection 2488
Enbrel for Injection 569
Exjade Tablets 2244
Fenoglide Tablets 2960
Focalin XR Capsules 2251
Gemzar for Injection (Approximately two-thirds) 1820
Geodon Capsules (Infrequent) 2520
▲ Intron A for Injection (Less than 5%) 2859
Ixempra Kit for Injection 915
Ketek Tablets (Greater than or equal to 0.2% to less than 2%) 2744
Klonopin 2639
Lescol Capsules 2268
Lescol XL Tablets 2268
Leustatin Injection 2384
▲ Lupron Depot–3 Month 11.25 mg (3%) 462
Marinol Capsules (Less than 1%) 3163
Mavik Tablets (0.8% of patients) 472
Metadate CD Capsules 3146
Mevacor Tablets (1.9%) 2063
Mylotarg for Injection (13 Patients) 3212
▲ Nexavar Tablets (Greater than or equal to 10%) 784
Niaspan Extended-Release Tablets 480
Norvir 489
▲ Novantrone for Injection Concentrate (20%) 1100
▲ Oncaspar Injection (Greater than or equal to 2% to 11%) 1138
▲ Ontak Vials (61%) 1079
Paxil 1535
Paxil CR Controlled-Release Tablets 1544
Precose Tablets 792
Prometrium Capsules (100 mg, 200 mg) 3047
Prozac Weekly Capsules 1852
Prozac Pulvules and Liquid 1852
Remicade for IV Injection 950
Rythmol Tablets (0.2%) 1586
Seromycin Capsules 1864
Thiothixene Capsules (Infrequently) 2197
Toprol-XL Tablets 666
▲ Trasylol Injection (5%) 799
Tricor Tablets 520
Valium Tablets 2658
Viramune Oral Suspension 873
Viramune Tablets 873
Vytorin 10/10 Tablets (1.7% to 1.8%) 2149
▲ Vytorin 10/10 Tablets (1.8% to 3.6%) 2939
Vytorin 10/20 Tablets (1.7% to 1.8%) 2149
▲ Vytorin 10/20 Tablets (1.8% to 3.6%) 2939
Vytorin 10/40 Tablets (1.7% to 1.8%) 2149
▲ Vytorin 10/40 Tablets (1.8% to 3.6%) 2939
▲ Vytorin 10/80 Tablets (2.6% to 3.6%) 2149
▲ Vytorin 10/80 Tablets (1.8% to 3.6%) 2939
Xyzal Oral Solution (Less than 1%) 2789
Xyzal Oral Solution (Less than 1%) 3155
Xyzal Tablets (Less than 1%) 2789
Xyzal Tablets (Less than 1%) 3155
Zetia Tablets 2157
Zetia Tablets (0.5% to 2.7%) 2951
Zocor Tablets 2136
Zofran 1687
Zofran ODT Orally Disintegrating Tablets 1687
Zyrtec Chewable Tablets 1920
Zyrtec Syrup 1920
Zyrtec Tablets 1920
Zyrtec-D 12 Hour Extended Release Tablets 1923

Serum triglyceride, elevation
(*see under* Hypertriglyceridemia)

Serum vitamin B_{12} levels, subnormal
▲ Avandamet Tablets (7%) 1336
▲ Janumet Tablets (7%) 2041
PrandiMet Tablets 2967
Sandostatin LAR Depot 2302

Sex hormone binding globulin, elevated
Prempro Tablets 3232

Sexual activity, decrease
Catapres Tablets (About 3 in 100 patients) 841
Catapres-TTS (0.5% or less) 842
▲ Clorpres Tablets (About 3%) 2185

Sexual dysfunction
Aceon Tablets (2 mg, 4 mg, 8 mg) (0.3% to 1.4%) 3038
Avalide Tablets 892
Avalide Tablets 2713
Avapro Tablets (Less than 1%) 897
Avapro Tablets (Less than 1%) 2718
Bentyl Capsules 703
Bentyl Injection 703
Bentyl Syrup 703
Bentyl Tablets 703
Campral Tablets (Infrequent) 1158
Cardizem LA Extended Release Tablets (Less than 2%) 421
Catapres-TTS (2 of 101 patients) 842
Celexa 1160
Chantix Tablets (Rare) 2511
Copaxone for Injection (Infrequent) 3110
Cymbalta Delayed-Release Capsules (Infrequent) 1801
Effexor XR Extended-Release Capsules 3195
Eldepryl Capsules 3052
Evoxac Capsules (Less than 1%) 1013
Exforge Tablets (Greater than 0.1% to less than 1%) 2238
Geodon Capsules (Infrequent) 2520
Gleevec Tablets (Infrequent) 2255
Lexapro Oral Suspension 1174
Lexapro Tablets 1174
▲ Luvox CR Extended-Release Capsules (2% to 4%) 1759
Marplan Tablets 3177
Micardis HCT Tablets 854
Mirapex Tablets 857
▲ Paxil (3.7% to 10%) 1535
▲ Paxil CR Controlled-Release Tablets (3.7% to 10%) 1544
▲ Pristiq Extended-Release Tablets (0% to greater than or equal to 5%) 3247
Strattera Capsules (2%) 1864
Vantas (Less than 2%) 1737
Wellbutrin Tablets (Frequent) 1648

Sexual maturity, accelerated
Lupron Depot-PED 7.5 mg, 11.25 mg and 15 mg (Less than 2%) 471

SGOT changes
(*see under* Aspartate aminotransferase levels, changes in)

SGOT elevation
(*see under* Aspartate aminotransferase levels, elevation of)

SGPT changes
(*see under* Alanine aminotransferase levels, changes in)

SGPT elevation
(*see under* Alanine aminotransferase levels, elevation of)

Shaking
(*see under* Tremors)

Shivering
(*see under* Tremors)

Shock
Abelcet Injection (Rare) 1134
Abilify Injection (Less than 1 in 1000 patients) 2466
Abilify Oral Solution (Less than 1 in 1000 patients) 2466
Abilify Discmelt Orally Disintegrating Tablets (Less than 1 in 1000 patients) 2466
Abilify Tablets (Less than 1 in 1000 patients) 2466
Actiq 959
Boostrix (Rarely) 1377
Campral Tablets (Rare) 1158
Doxil Injection (Less than 1%) 2378
Effexor XR Extended-Release Capsules 3195
Elitek 2729
▲ Flolan for Injection (5%) 1426
Fluarix Vaccine 1446
Fluorescite Injection ⊙ 203
Hyalgan Solution (One case) 2742
Imitrex Injection 1465
Imitrex Nasal Spray 1470
Imitrex Tablets 1474
Indocin Capsules (Less than 1%) 2024
Indocin I.V. (Less than 1%) 2489
Indocin (Less than 1%) 2024
Infanrix Vaccine 1479
Kinrix Injection Vaccine 1486
Levaquin 2416
Levaquin in 5% Dextrose Injection 2416
Lyrica Capsules (Rare) 2527
Merrem I.V. (1.2%) 684
Mirapex Tablets 857
Mobic Oral Suspension (Less than 0.1%) 863
Mobic Tablets (Less than 0.1%) 863
Motrin IB Tablets and Caplets 1900
Children's Motrin Oral Suspension 1901
Children's Motrin Non-Staining Dye-Free Oral Suspension 1901
Children's Motrin Cold Oral Suspension 1899
Infants' Motrin Concentrated Drops 1901
Infants' Motrin Non-Staining Dye-Free Concentrated Drops 1901
Junior Strength Motrin Caplets and Chewable Tablets 1901
MS Contin Tablets 2585
Mycamine for Injection 616
▲ Mylotarg for Injection (4%) 3212
Nexium I.V. (Rare) 652
NovoSeven 2367
NovoSeven RT 2370
Omnicef Capsules 497
Omnicef for Oral Suspension 497
Orthoclone OKT3 Sterile Solution (Less than 1%) 2387
OxyContin Tablets 2589
Pediarix Vaccine (Rare) 1552
Prevnar 3241
Proleukin for Injection (Less than 1%) 2287
Prozac Weekly Capsules (Rare) 1852
Prozac Pulvules and Liquid (Rare) 1852
Rilutek Tablets (Infrequent) 2771
Salagen Tablets 1082
Trasylol Injection (1% to 2%) 799
Zemuron Injection 2947
Zofran Injection (Rare) 1682
Zofran 1687
Zofran ODT Orally Disintegrating Tablets 1687

Shock, anaphylactic
(*see under* Anaphylactic shock)

Shock, cardiogenic
Activase I.V. 1188
▲ Mavik Tablets (3.8%) 472
Rituxan I.V. 1223
TNKase 1233
▲ Velcade for Injection (5%) 2168

Shock, hemorrhagic
Tasigna Capsules 2316

Shock, hypovolemic
Ixempra Kit for Injection 915

Shortness of breath
▲ Adenocard IV Injection (12%) 603
Aerobid/Aerobid-M (Less than 1%) 1153
Alphanate 1709
Ceftin Tablets (0.1% to 1%) 1380
Cubicin for Injection 995
▲ Doxil Injection (Approximately 6.8%) 2378
DynaCirc CR Controlled Release Tablets (0.5% to 1%) 1407
Eldepryl Capsules 3052
Eloxatin for Injection 2731
▲ Epogen for Injection (0.14% to 14%) 576
Gantrisin Pediatric Suspension 2638
Humalog-Pen and KwikPen (Less common) 1829
Humalog Mix 50/50-Pen and KwikPen 1833
Humalog Mix 75/25-Pen and KwikPen (Less common) 1835
Humulin 50/50, 100 Units 1843
Humulin 70/30 Vial (Less common) 1844
Humulin N Vial (Less common) 1846
Humulin R 1849
Humulin R (U-500) (Less common) 1850
Imitrex Injection 1465
Imitrex Nasal Spray 1470
Imitrex Tablets 1474
Klonopin 2639
K-Phos Original (Sodium Free) Tablets (Less frequent) 814
K-Phos Neutral Tablets 813
▲ Leustatin Injection (7%) 2384
Levaquin 2416
Levaquin in 5% Dextrose Injection 2416
Lexapro Oral Suspension (Infrequent) 1174
Lexapro Tablets (Infrequent) 1174
Lupron Depot 7.5 mg 469
Lupron Depot–3 Month 11.25 mg 462
Children's Motrin Oral Suspension 1901
Children's Motrin Non-Staining Dye-Free Oral Suspension 1901
Infants' Motrin Concentrated Drops 1901
Infants' Motrin Non-Staining Dye-Free Concentrated Drops 1901
Junior Strength Motrin Caplets and Chewable Tablets 1901
Niaspan Extended-Release Tablets 480
NovoLog Injection 2359
Ortho-Cyclen Tablets 2449
Ortho Evra Transdermal System 2437
Ortho Tri-Cyclen Tablets 2449
Ortho Tri-Cyclen Lo Tablets 2458
Orthoclone OKT3 Sterile Solution (Less than 1%) 2387
▲ Procrit for Injection (0.14% to 14%) 2391
Retrovir Capsules 1574
Retrovir IV Infusion 1579
Retrovir 1574
Sandostatin Injection (Less than 1%) 2300
Sular Extended Release Tablets (Very rare) 2975
▲ Toprol-XL Tablets (Approximately 3 of 100 patients) 666
Tylenol with Codeine Tablets 2427
Uroqid-Acid No. 2 Tablets 814
Wellbutrin Tablets (Infrequent) 1648
Ziagen 1673
Zofran Injection (Rare) 1682
Zofran 1687
Zofran ODT Orally Disintegrating Tablets 1687

SIADH secretion syndrome
(*see under* ADH syndrome, inappropriate)

Sialadenitis
Amerge Tablets (Rare) 1301
Atacand HCT 642
Avalide Tablets 892
Avalide Tablets 2713
Diovan HCT Tablets 2216
Dyazide Capsules 1405
▲ Evoxac Capsules (1% to 3%) 1013
Indapamide Tablets 2188
Intravenous Sodium Diuril 2490
Kaletra (Less than 2%) 452
Micardis HCT Tablets 854
Paxil (Rare) 1535
Paxil CR Controlled-Release Tablets (Rare) 1544
Prinzide Tablets 2092
Raptiva for Injection (1 case) 1218
Tekturna HCT Tablets 2324
Teveten HCT Tablets 517
Zomig Tablets (Rare) 694
Zomig Nasal Spray (Rare) 689
Zomig-ZMT Tablets (Rare) 694

Sialism
Alferon N Injection (1%) 1726
Ambien Tablets (Rare) 2692
Ambien CR Tablets (Rare) 2696
Aricept Tablets (Infrequent) 1062
Aricept ODT Tablets (Infrequent) 1062
Axert Tablets (Rare) 2431
Campral Tablets (Rare) 1158
Ceftin for Oral Suspension (0.1% to 1%) 1380
Celexa (Frequent) 1160
Doxil Injection (Less than 1%) 2378
Effexor XR Extended-Release Capsules 3195
Emend Capsules (Greater than 0.5%) 1992
Emend for Injection (Greater than 0.5%) 1999
Emsam Transdermal System (Infrequent) 905
Evoxac Capsules (2.2%) 1013
Exelon Capsules (Infrequent) 2229
Exelon Oral Solution (Infrequent) 2229
Frova Tablets (Infrequent) 1111
Gabitril Tablets (Infrequent) 973
▲ Geodon Capsules (4%) 2520
Imitrex Injection 1465
Imitrex Nasal Spray 1470
▲ Intron A for Injection (Less than 5%) 2859
Klonopin 2639
Lamictal (Infrequent) 1488
▲ Megace ES Oral Suspension (1% to 3%) 2499
Meridia Capsules 475
Mirapex Tablets (1% or more) 857
Moban Tablets (Occasional) 1116
Neupro Transdermal System 3149
Paxil (Infrequent) 1535
Paxil CR Controlled-Release Tablets (Infrequent) 1544
Primaxin I.M. 2080
Primaxin I.V. (Less than 0.2%) 2083
Prinivil Tablets (Greater than 1%) 2087
Prinzide Tablets 2092
Protonix for Delayed-Release Oral Suspension 3254
Protonix Delayed-Release Tablets 3254
Protonix I.V. 3257
Prozac Weekly Capsules (Infrequent) 1852
Prozac Pulvules and Liquid (Infrequent) 1852
Remeron Tablets (Rare) 2924
RemeronSolTab Tablets (Rare) 2927
Requip Tablets (1% or more) 1561
Risperdal Consta Long-Acting Injection (2%) 1753
▲ Soriatane Capsules (1% to 10%) 3062
Stalevo Tablets 2309
Symbyax Capsules (Frequent) 1871
Thiothixene Capsules (Infrequently) 2197
▲ Ultane Liquid for Inhalation (2% to 4%) 524
Valium Tablets (Infrequent) 2658
Venlafaxine Hydrochloride Tablets (Rare) 2199
▲ Wellbutrin Tablets (3.4%) 1648
Wellbutrin SR Sustained-Release Tablets (Infrequent) 1653
Wellbutrin XL Extended-Release Tablets (Infrequent) 1659
Xyrem Oral Solution (Infrequent) 1766
Zomig Tablets (Infrequent) 694
Zomig Nasal Spray (Infrequent) 689
Zomig-ZMT Tablets (Infrequent) 694
Zyban Sustained-Release Tablets 1692
▲ Zyprexa Tablets (6%) 1883
▲ Zyprexa ZYDIS Orally Disintegrating Tablets (6%) 1883
Zyrtec-D 12 Hour Extended Release Tablets (Less than 2%) 1923

Sialorrhea
(*see under* Sialism)

Sialosis
(*see under* Sialism)

Sickle cell crises
Neupogen for Injection 589

Sickle cell disease
Neulasta Injection 587

Sinoatrial block
Flumadine (Less than 0.3%) 1167
Rythmol SR Capsules 1590
Timoptic in Ocudose (Less frequent) 2124
Timoptic-XE Sterile Ophthalmic Gel Forming Solution 2125

Sinobronchitis
Selzentry Tablets 2534

Sinus arrest
Catapres Tablets (Rare) 841
Rythmol Tablets (Less than 1%) 1586
Rythmol SR Capsules 1590
Velcade for Injection 2168

Sinus bradycardia
Activase I.V. 1188
Adenocard IV Injection 603
Adenoscan 605

Catapres Tablets (Rare) 841
Catapres-TTS (0.5% or less) 842
Celebrex Capsules (Greater than or equal to 0.1% to less than 1%) 2979
Clorpres Tablets (Rare) 2185
Cozaar Tablets (Less than 1%) 1973
Eldepryl Capsules 3052
Lanoxin Injection 1498
Lanoxin Injection Pediatric 1502
Lanoxin Tablets 1505
Lexiscan Injection 614
Mirapex Tablets 857
Rythmol SR Capsules (Greater than 2%) 1590
▲ Sandostatin Injection (25%) 2300
▲ Sandostatin LAR Depot (19% to 25%) 2302
▲ Somatuline Depot Injection (3% to 17%) 3102

Sinus discomfort

▲ Aerobid/Aerobid-M (1% to 3%) 1153
Avalide Tablets 892
Avapro Tablets (1% or greater) 897
Avapro Tablets (1% or greater) 2718
Cozaar Tablets (1% or greater) 1973
Imitrex Injection (2.2%) 1465
Imitrex Nasal Spray (0.8% to 2.4%) 1470
Maxalt Tablets (Infrequent) 2056
Maxalt-MLT Orally Disintegrating Tablets (Infrequent) 2056

Sinus disorder

Avalide Tablets (Greater than or equal to 1%) 2713
Xyrem Oral Solution (Infrequent) 1766

Sinus drainage

▲ Aerobid/Aerobid-M (3% to 9%) 1153
Alferon N Injection (2%) 1726

Sinus exit block

Adenoscan (Less than 1%) 605

Sinus node dysfunction

Cardene I.V. 1093

Sinus pause

Adenoscan (Less than 1%) 605
Rythmol Tablets (Less than 1%) 1586

Sinus syndrome, sick

Exelon Capsules (Infrequent) 2229
Exelon Oral Solution (Infrequent) 2229
Photofrin for Injection 708
Requip Tablets (Infrequent) 1561
Rythmol Tablets (Less than 1%) 1586

Sinus tachycardia

Abilify Injection (Greater than or equal to 1 in 1000 patients and less than 1 in 100 patients) 881
Abilify Injection (Greater than or equal to 1 in 1000 patients and less than 1 in 100 patients) 2466
Abilify Oral Solution (Greater than or equal to 1 in 1000 patients and less than 1 in 100 patients) 881
Abilify Oral Solution (Greater than or equal to 1 in 1000 patients and less than 1 in 100 patients) 2466
Abilify Discmelt Orally Disintegrating Tablets (Greater than or equal to 1 in 1000 patients and less than 1 in 100 patients) 881
Abilify Discmelt Orally Disintegrating Tablets (Greater than or equal to 1 in 1000 patients and less than 1 in 100 patients) 2466
Abilify Tablets (Greater than or equal to 1 in 1000 patients and less than 1 in 100 patients) 881
Abilify Tablets (Greater than or equal to 1 in 1000 patients and less than 1 in 100 patients) 2466
Adenocard IV Injection 603
Aloxi Injection (Less than 1%) 1059
▲ Arranon Injection (0% to 8%) 1319
Mirapex Tablets 857
Strattera Capsules 1864
▲ Taxotere Injection Concentrate (8.1%) 2773

Sinusitis

▲ Aceon Tablets (2 mg, 4 mg, 8 mg) (0.6% to 5.2%) 3038
Actiq (1% or greater) 959
▲ Activella Tablets (7% to 15%) 2347
▲ Actonel Tablets (8.7%) 2568
▲ Actonel with Calcium Tablets (4.5% to 4.6%) 2574
▲ ActoPlus Met Tablets (4.4% to 5%) 3071
▲ Actos Tablets (6.3%) 3077
Aczone Gel 5% (2%) 3296
Advair Diskus 100/50 1276
▲ Advair Diskus 250/50 (3% to greater than 5%) 1276
Advair Diskus 500/50 1276
▲ Aerobid/Aerobid-M (3% to 9%) 1153
▲ Agrylin Capsules (1% to less than 5%) 3017
▲ Alamast Ophthalmic Solution (Less than 5%) 3181
▲ Aldara Cream, 5% (2% to 7%) 1699
Allegra Oral Solution (2.2%) 2684
▲ Alphagan P Ophthalmic Solution (1% to 4%) 549
▲ Alvesco Inhalation Aerosol (Greater than or equal to 3%) 2985
▲ Ambien Tablets (4%) 2692
Ambien CR Tablets (Frequent) 2696
AmBisome for Injection (Less common) 606
Amerge Tablets (Infrequent) 1301
▲ Angeliq Tablets (5.3%) 751
Aralast (Greater than or equal to 0.2%) 726
▲ Arimidex Tablets (2% to 6%) 672
▲ Arranon Injection (0% to 7%) 1319
Asacol Delayed-Release Tablets (2% or greater) 2579
▲ Asmanex Twisthaler (5% to 22%) 2797
Atacand Tablets (More than 1%) 639
Atacand HCT (0.5% or greater) 642
▲ Atripla Tablets (8%) 938
▲ Atrovent HFA Inhalation Aerosol (1% to 11%) 839
Atrovent Nasal Spray 0.03% 834
▲ Avandia Tablets (3.2%) 1351
Axert Tablets (Infrequent) 2431
Axid Capsules (2.4%) 1364
AzaSite Ophthalmic Drops (Less than 1%) 1740
▲ Azmacort Inhalation Aerosol (2% to 9%) 407
▲ Betimol Ophthalmic Solution (1% to 5%) 3181
▲ Brovana Inhalation Solution (5%) 2990
▲ Busulfex Injection (3%) 2477
Carac Cream 0.5% (1.6%) 2722
Ceftin for Oral Suspension (0.1% to 1%) 1380
▲ Celebrex Capsules (5%) 2979
▲ Celexa (3%) 1160
▲ CellCept Capsules (3% to 26%) 2622
▲ CellCept Intravenous (3% to 26%) 2622
▲ CellCept Oral Suspension (3% to 26%) 2622
▲ CellCept Tablets (3% to 26%) 2622
▲ Climara Transdermal System (4% to 5%) 763
▲ Climara Pro Transdermal System (3.8%) 768
Combigan Ophthalmic Solution (0.1% to 0.2%) 553
Combivent Inhalation Aerosol (2.3%) 845
Copaxone for Injection (At least 2%) 3110
▲ Cosopt Sterile Ophthalmic Solution (1% to 5%) 1969
▲ Cozaar Tablets (1% to 6%) 1973
Crinone 4% Gel 992
Crinone 8% Gel 992
▲ Dacogen Injection (5%) 1066
▲ Depakote ER Tablets (Greater than 1% to less than 5%) 423
Diovan Tablets (More than 1%) 2212
Diovan HCT Tablets (Greater than 0.2%) 2216
▲ Doxil Injection (1% to 10%) 2378
Duragesic Transdermal System (Greater than or less than 1%) 2405
Edex Injection (1%) 2957
Effexor XR Extended-Release Capsules (2%) 3195
▲ Elestat Ophthalmic Solution (1% to 3%) 1741
▲ Elidel Cream 1% (0.6% to 3.3%) 2221
▲ Emsam Transdermal System (3%) 905
▲ Emtriva Capsules (8%) 1246
▲ Emtriva Oral Solution (8%) 1246
Enablex Extended-Release Tablets (Greater than or equal to 1%) 2225
▲ Enbrel for Injection (3% to 5%) 569
▲ Enjuvia Tablets (3% to 7%) 1029
▲ Equetro Extended-Release Capsules (Less than 5%) 3174
▲ Evista Tablets (7.9% to 10.3%) 1810
▲ Evoxac Capsules (12.3%) 1013
Exforge Tablets (Greater than or equal to 0.2%) 2238
▲ Exubera Inhalation Powder (5.4% to 10.3%) 2515
▲ Fabrazyme for Intravenous Infusion (9%) 1241
Fentora Tablets (Greater than 1%) 968
▲ Flebogamma 5% (39%) 1715
▲ Flebogamma 5% DIF (Greater than 15%) 1718
▲ Flolan for Injection (4%) 1426
▲ Flomax Capsules (2.2% to 3.7%) 848
▲ Flovent Diskus 50 mcg (10% to 33%) 1435
▲ Flovent HFA (1% to 6%) 1440
▲ FluMist Vaccine (4%) 1945
▲ Follistim AQ Cartridge (5%) 2844
Foradil Aerolizer (2.7%) 2849
Frova Tablets (Frequent) 1111
Gabitril Tablets (1% or more) 973
Gengraf Capsules (Less than 1%) 435
Genotropin Lyophilized Powder 2547
▲ Gleevec Tablets (4% to 11.4%) 2255
▲ Herceptin I.V. (9%) 1199
▲ Humira Injection (11%) 442
Imitrex Nasal Spray 1470
▲ Indapamide Tablets (Less than 5%) 2188
▲ Intron A for Injection (Up to 21%) 2859
Ionsys Transdermal System (.1% to less than 1%) 2410
Kaletra (Less than 2%) 452
Keppra Injection (2%) 3137
Keppra Oral Solution (Greater than or equal to 2%) 3131
Keppra Tablets (Greater than or equal to 2%) 3131
▲ Kineret Injection (7%) 585
▲ Klonopin (4%) 2639
Lamictal (2%) 1488
Lescol Capsules (2.6%) 2268
▲ Lescol XL Tablets (3.5%) 2268
▲ Letairis Tablets (3%) 1258
▲ Levitra Tablets (3%) 2876
▲ Lexapro Oral Suspension (3%) 1174
▲ Lexapro Tablets (3%) 1174
▲ Lipitor Tablets (Up to 6.4%) 2501
Lovaza Capsules 1520
▲ Lucentis Injection (2% to 8%) 1205
Luvox CR Extended-Release Capsules (Frequent) 1759
▲ Lyrica Capsules (4% to 7%) 2527
Marinol Capsules (Less than 1%) 3163
▲ Mepron Suspension (7%) 1526
▲ Meridia Capsules (5%) 475
▲ Miacalcin Nasal Spray (1% to 3%) 2274
▲ Micardis Tablets (3%) 852
▲ Micardis HCT Tablets (4%) 854
Mirapex Tablets (1% or more) 857
▲ Mirena Intrauterine System (5% or more) 779
▲ Myfortic Tablets (3% to less than 20%) 2276
Nasacort AQ Nasal Spray 2765
▲ Nasonex Nasal Spray (4% to 5%) 2883
▲ Neoral Oral Solution (1% to 7%) 2280
▲ Neoral Soft Gelatin Capsules (1% to 7%) 2280
▲ Neupro Transdermal System (3%) 3149
▲ Nevanac Ophthalmic Suspension 0.1% (1% to 4%) ⊙ 205
Nexium Delayed-Release Capsules (Less than 1%) 645
Nexium I.V. (Less than 1%) 652
Nexium Delayed-Release Oral Suspension (Less than 1%) 645
▲ Novantrone for Injection Concentrate (3% to 6%) 1100
▲ NovoLog Injection (5%) 2359
▲ NuvaRing (5% to 14%) 2897
▲ Orencia Powder for Intravenous Infusion (5% to 13%) 921
▲ Pataday Ophthalmic Solution (Less than or equal to 5%) 543
▲ Patanol Ophthalmic Solution (Less than 5%) 546
▲ Paxil (Infrequent to 4%) 1535
▲ Paxil CR Controlled-Release Tablets (Infrequent to 4%) 1544
▲ PegIntron Powder for Injection (7%) 2903
▲ Photofrin for Injection (4%) 708
Plavix Tablets (1% to 2.5%) 926
Plavix Tablets (1% to 2.5%) 2767
Pletal Tablets (Less than 2%) 2481
▲ Prandin Tablets (3% to 6%) 2971
▲ Premarin Tablets (6% to 11%) 3221
▲ Premphase Tablets (7% to 10%) 3232
▲ Prempro Tablets (7% to 10%) 3232
Prinivil Tablets (0.3% to 1%) 2087
Prinzide Tablets (0.3% to 1%) 2092
▲ Prograf Capsules and Injection (3% to 15%) 622
▲ Prometrium Capsules (100 mg, 200 mg) (Less than 5%) 3047
ProQuad 2099
Protonix for Delayed-Release Oral Suspension (Greater than or equal to 1%) 3254
Protonix Delayed-Release Tablets (Greater than or equal to 1%) 3254
Protonix I.V. (Greater than or equal to 1%) 3257
▲ Protopic Ointment (2% to 7%) 628
Provigil Tablets (At least 1%) 977
▲ Prozac Weekly Capsules (1% to 6%) 1852
▲ Prozac Pulvules and Liquid (1% to 6%) 1852
▲ Pulmicort Flexhaler (Greater than or equal to 3% to 16%) 654
Pulmozyme Inhalation Solution 1217
▲ Qvar Inhalation Aerosol (Up to 3%) 3116
Raptiva for Injection 1218
▲ Rebetol (Less than 1% to 12%) 2917
ReFacto Vials 3269
▲ Relenza Inhalation Powder (2% to 3%) 1556
Remeron Tablets (Frequent) 2924
RemeronSolTab Tablets (Frequent) 2927
▲ Remicade for IV Injection (14%) 950
▲ Requip Tablets (4%) 1561
Retrovir Capsules 1574
Retrovir IV Infusion 1579
Retrovir 1574
Rilutek Tablets (0.4% to 1.6%) 2771
Risperdal Consta Long-Acting Injection (1%) 1753
▲ Rituxan I.V. (0% to 6%) 1223
▲ Salagen Tablets (1% to 4%) 1082
▲ Sandimmune (Less than 1% to 7%) 2296
▲ Sandostatin LAR Depot (5% to 15.4%) 2302
▲ Selzentry Tablets (6.3%) 2534
▲ Serevent Diskus (2% to greater than or equal to 3%) 1594
▲ Simulect for Injection (3% to 10%) 2306
Singulair (Greater than or equal to 1%) 2114
▲ Soriatane Capsules (1% to 10%) 3062
▲ Spiriva HandiHaler (3% to 11%) 870
▲ Sular Extended Release Tablets (3%) 2975
▲ Symbicort 80/4.5 Inhalation Aerosol (5.8%) 659
▲ Symbicort 160/4.5 Inhalation Aerosol (4.8%) 659
Synagis Intramuscular Solution (More than 1%) 1948
Tamiflu Capsules (2%) 2649
Tamiflu Oral Suspension (2%) 2649
▲ Temodar Capsules (6%) 2931
Teveten Tablets (1% or greater) 515
Teveten HCT Tablets 517
▲ Travatan Z Ophthalmic Solution (1% to 5%) 547
Tricor Tablets 520
▲ Trisenox Injection (20%) 986
▲ Truvada Tablets (8%) 1262
Twinrix Vaccine 1628
▲ Ultram ER Extended-Release Tablets (1% to less than 5%) 2428
Uroxatral Tablets (1% to 2%) 2786
▲ Vagifem Tablets (3% to 5%) 2375
Velcade for Injection 2168
Vicoprofen Tablets (Less than 1%) 533
▲ Viread Tablets (8%) 1268
▲ Vivitrol (12% to 13%) 988
Vytorin 10/10 Tablets 2149
Vytorin 10/10 Tablets 2939
Vytorin 10/20 Tablets 2149
Vytorin 10/20 Tablets 2939
Vytorin 10/40 Tablets 2149
Vytorin 10/40 Tablets 2939
Vytorin 10/80 Tablets 2149
Vytorin 10/80 Tablets 2939
▲ Wellbutrin SR Sustained-Release Tablets (1% to 3%) 1653
▲ Wellbutrin XL Extended-Release Tablets (1% to 5%) 1659
▲ Xolair (16%) 1235
▲ Xolair (16%) 2339
▲ Xopenex Inhalation Solution (1.4% to 4.2%) 3001
▲ Xopenex Inhalation Solution Concentrate (1.4% to 4.2%) 3005
▲ Xopenex HFA Inhalation Aerosol (1.4% to 4.2%) 3009
Xyrem Oral Solution (Frequent) 1766
Yaz Tablets (Greater than 1%) 805
Zetia Tablets (2.8%) 2157
▲ Zetia Tablets (2.8%) 2951
Ziana Gel (1%) 1942
Zocor Tablets (2.3%) 2136
Zomig Tablets (Infrequent) 694
Zomig Nasal Spray (Infrequent) 689
Zomig-ZMT Tablets (Infrequent) 694
Zyban Sustained-Release Tablets (2%) 1692
Zyrtec Chewable Tablets (Less than 2%) 1920
Zyrtec Syrup (Less than 2%) 1920
Zyrtec Tablets (Less than 2%) 1920

Zyrtec-D 12 Hour Extended Release Tablets (1% to less than 2%) 1923

Sinusitis, acute
Selzentry Tablets 2534

Sinusitis, allergic
Xyrem Oral Solution (Infrequent) 1766

Sinusitis, chronic
Selzentry Tablets 2534

Skin, anesthesia
(*see under* Numbness, skin)

Skin, burning of
Avelox 2803
Cipro I.V. 2817
Diprolene Lotion 0.05% (1%) 2838
Diprolene Ointment 0.05% 2839
Diprolene AF Cream 0.05% (Infrequent) 2837
▲ Duac Topical Gel (0% to 5%) 3054
Klonopin (Infrequent) 2639
Levaquin 2416
Levaquin in 5% Dextrose Injection 2416
Lotrisone (1.6%) 2881
▲ Luxíq Foam (2% to 44%) 3058
▲ Protopic Ointment (25% to 58%) 628
Zovirax Cream (Less than 1%) 817

Skin, clammy
Exforge Tablets (Greater than or equal to 0.1%) 2238

Skin, cold
Exforge Tablets (Greater than or equal to 0.1%) 2238

Skin, cracking
Olux Foam (Less than 2%) 3061
▲ Panretin Gel 0.1% (1% to 8%) 1081
Soriatane Capsules 3062

Skin, dryness of
(*see under* Xerosis cutis)

Skin, eruptions of
Aciphex Tablets 1053
▲ Anaprox Tablets (3% to 9%) 2632
▲ Anaprox DS Tablets (3% to 9%) 2632
Biaxin/Biaxin XL 411
Cosmegen for Injection 2485
▲ EC-Naprosyn Delayed-Release Tablets (3% to 9%) 2632
E.E.S. 433
Fansidar Tablets 2636
Imitrex Injection (Infrequent) 1465
Imitrex Nasal Spray (Infrequent) 1470
▲ Naprosyn Suspension (3% to 9%) 2632
▲ Naprosyn Tablets (3% to 9%) 2632
Norvir 489
Paser Granules 1747
Reyataz Capsules 3299
Tessalon Capsules 1183
Tessalon Perles 1183
Thioridazine Hydrochloride Tablets (Infrequent) 2195
Trasylol Injection 799

Skin, exfoliation
Cancidas for Injection 1953
Concerta Extended-Release Tablets 1925
Ixempra Kit for Injection (2%) 915
Mirapex Tablets 857
▲ Panretin Gel 0.1% (3% to 9%) 1081
▲ Trisenox Injection (5%) 986
▲ Vectibix (2% to 25%) 597

Skin, exfoliation, application site
▲ Aczone Gel 5% (Less than 1% to 13%) 3296
Daytrana Transdermal Patch 3022
Lidoderm Patch 1114

Skin, flakiness
▲ Panretin Gel 0.1% (3% to 9%) 1081
Zovirax Cream (Less than 1%) 817

Skin, fragile
Accutane Capsules 2607
Photofrin for Injection 708
Soriatane Capsules 3062

Skin, hyperpigmentation
▲ Emtriva Capsules (Greater than or equal to 10%) 1246
▲ Emtriva Oral Solution (Greater than or equal to 10%) 1246
Ixempra Kit for Injection (2%) 915
Mirapex Tablets 857

Skin, irritation of
Accuzyme Debriding Ointment (Occasional) 1723
Accuzyme SE Spray Emulsion (Occasional) 1723
Carac Cream 0.5% (1.2%) 2722
Combigan Ophthalmic Solution 553
Cosopt Sterile Ophthalmic Solution 1969
Diprolene Lotion 0.05% (Less than 1%) 2838
Diprolene Ointment 0.05% 2839
Diprolene AF Cream 0.05% (Infrequent) 2837
Elocon Cream 0.1% (Infrequent) 2840
Elocon Lotion 0.1% (Infrequent) 2841
Elocon Ointment 0.1% (Infrequent) 2842
Lotrisone 2881
Luxíq Foam 3058
Panafil Ointment (Occasional) 1723
Panafil SE Spray Emulsion (Occasional) 1724
Soriatane Capsules (Less than 1%) .. 3062
Timoptic Sterile Ophthalmic Solution 2121
Timoptic in Ocudose 2124
Timoptic-XE Sterile Ophthalmic Gel Forming Solution 2125

Skin, lesions non-specific
Cancidas for Injection 1953
▲ Dacogen Injection (11%) 1066
Invanz for Injection (Greater than 0.5%) 2029
▲ NeoProfen Injection (16%) 2496
Prinivil Tablets (0.3% to 1%) 2087
Prinzide Tablets 2092
Requip Tablets (Infrequent) 1561
▲ Trisenox Injection (8%) 986

Skin, reddening
Motrin IB Tablets and Caplets 1900
Children's Motrin Oral Suspension 1901
Children's Motrin Non-Staining Dye-Free Oral Suspension 1901
Children's Motrin Cold Oral Suspension 1899
Infants' Motrin Concentrated Drops 1901
Infants' Motrin Non-Staining Dye-Free Concentrated Drops 1901
Junior Strength Motrin Caplets and Chewable Tablets 1901

Skin, scaling of
▲ Finacea Gel (1% to 5%) 1742
▲ Panretin Gel 0.1% (25% to 77%) 1081
Targretin Gel 1% 1088
▲ Ziana Gel (13% to 17%) 1942

Skin, tenderness
Imitrex Injection (Rare) 1465
Imitrex Nasal Spray 1470
Imitrex Tablets (Infrequent) 1474
Naftin Gel (0.5%) 2164

Skin, wrinkling
Ambien CR Tablets (1%) 2696
Amerge Tablets (Rare) 1301
Cuprimine Capsules (Rare) 1986
Imitrex Nasal Spray 1470
Imitrex Tablets (Rare) 1474
Photofrin for Injection 708

Skin, yellowing
Levaquin 2416
Levaquin in 5% Dextrose Injection 2416

Skin atrophy
Analpram-HC 1140
Copaxone for Injection (Frequent) 3110
Diprolene Lotion 0.05% (Infrequent) 2838
Diprolene Ointment 0.05% 2839
Diprolene AF Cream 0.05% (Infrequent) 2837
Effexor XR Extended-Release Capsules (Rare) 3195
Elocon Cream 0.1% (1.6%) 2840
Elocon Lotion 0.1% (Infrequent) 2841
▲ Elocon Ointment 0.1% (4.8%) 2842
Lotrisone 2881
Luxíq Foam 3058
Lyrica Capsules (Rare) 2527
Olux Foam (Less than 2%) 3061
Pramosone 1141
Soriatane Capsules 3062
Vanos Cream 1941
Venlafaxine Hydrochloride Tablets (Rare) 2199

Skin burning sensation
Mirapex Tablets 857

Skin desquamation
Flomax Capsules (Infrequent) 848
Gemzar for Injection (Very rare) 1820
Mepron Suspension 1526
▲ Panretin Gel 0.1% (3% to 9%) 1081
Taxotere Injection Concentrate (0% to 1.8%) 2773

Skin discoloration
Actiq (Less than 1%) 959
AmBisome for Injection (Less common) 606
Aricept Tablets (Infrequent) 1062
Aricept ODT Tablets (Infrequent) 1062
Atripla Tablets 938
▲ Avastin IV (2% to 16%) 1192
Betaseron for SC Injection 756
Brovana Inhalation Solution (Less than 2%) 2990
▲ Busulfex Injection (8%) 2477
Carbatrol Capsules 3019
Celexa (Infrequent) 1160
Crinone 4% Gel 992
Crinone 8% Gel 992
Denavir Cream 2205
▲ Doxil Injection (Less than 1% to 10%) 2378
Effexor XR Extended-Release Capsules (Rare) 3195
Elidel Cream 1% 2221
Emtriva Capsules 1246
Emtriva Oral Solution 1246
Estratest Tablets 3043
Estratest H.S. Tablets 3043
Evoxac Capsules (Less than 1%) 1013
Exforge Tablets (Less than or equal to 0.1%) 2238
Fluorescite Injection .... ⊙203
Gabitril Tablets (Infrequent) 973
▲ Intron A for Injection (Less than 5%) 2859
Kaletra (Less than 2%) 452
Keppra Oral Solution (2%) 3131
Keppra Tablets (2%) 3131
Lamictal (Infrequent) 1488
Lescol Capsules 2268
Lescol XL Tablets 2268
Lunesta Tablets (Infrequent) 2994
Luvox CR Extended-Release Capsules (Infrequent) 1759
Mevacor Tablets 2063
Mirapex Tablets 857
Paxil (Rare) 1535
Paxil CR Controlled-Release Tablets (Rare) 1544
Pentacel 2792
Photofrin for Injection 708
▲ Prograf Capsules and Injection (3% to 15%) 622
Protopic Ointment (Greater than or equal to 1%) 628
Prozac Weekly Capsules (Infrequent) 1852
Prozac Pulvules and Liquid (Infrequent) 1852
Retrovir IV Infusion 1579
Sular Extended Release Tablets (Less than or equal to 1%) 2975
Sustiva Capsules 930
Sustiva Tablets 930
▲ Sutent Capsules (0% to 33%) 2540
Symbyax Capsules (Infrequent) 1871
Trasylol Injection (1% to 2%) 799
Truvada Tablets 1262
Venlafaxine Hydrochloride Tablets (Rare) 2199
Vytorin 10/10 Tablets 2149
Vytorin 10/10 Tablets 2939
Vytorin 10/20 Tablets 2149
Vytorin 10/20 Tablets 2939
Vytorin 10/40 Tablets 2149
Vytorin 10/40 Tablets 2939
Vytorin 10/80 Tablets 2149
Vytorin 10/80 Tablets 2939
Zocor Tablets 2136
Zyprexa Tablets (Infrequent) 1883
Zyprexa ZYDIS Orally Disintegrating Tablets (Infrequent) 1883

Skin disorder, unspecified
Advicor Tablets 402
▲ Agrylin Capsules (1% to less than 5%) 3017
AmBisome for Injection (Less common) 606
▲ Betaseron for SC Injection (10%) 756
Bystolic Tablets 1155
▲ Cancidas for Injection (25.4% to 42.2%) 1953
▲ Catapres-TTS (51 of 101 patients) 842
Celebrex Capsules (0.1% to 1.9%) .. 2979
▲ CellCept Capsules (3% to less than 20%) 2622
▲ CellCept Intravenous (3% to less than 20%) 2622
▲ CellCept Oral Suspension (3% to less than 20%) 2622
▲ CellCept Tablets (3% to less than 20%) 2622
Crinone 4% Gel 992
Crinone 8% Gel 992
▲ Doxil Injection (1% to 5%) 2378
Edex Injection (1%) 2957
Elocon Lotion 0.1% (1 in 65 patients) 2841
Elocon Ointment 0.1% (1 in 63 patients) 2842
▲ Eloxatin for Injection (2% to 35%) 2731
▲ Epogen for Injection (7% to 29%) 576
▲ Erbitux (4% to 15%) 912
EryPed 431
▲ Evoxac Capsules (1% to 3%) 1013
▲ Femara Tablets (0.7% to 32.4%) 2246
Klonopin (Infrequent) 2639
Lamisil Tablets (Isolated reports) 2266
Lanoxin Injection (Rare) 1498
Lanoxin Injection Pediatric (Rare) 1502
▲ Leukine (77%) 774
Levaquin (0.1% to 0.9%) 2416
Levaquin in 5% Dextrose Injection (0.1% to 0.9%) 2416
Lupron Depot 3.75 mg (2%) 462
▲ Lupron Depot 7.5 mg (Less than 5%) 469
Lupron Depot–3 Month 11.25 mg (2%) 462
▲ Megace ES Oral Suspension (1% to 3%) 2499
Mirapex Tablets (2%) 857
▲ Mirena Intrauterine System (5% or more) 779
▲ Mycamine for Injection (13% to 68.2%) 616
▲ Neoral Oral Solution (1% to 17.6%) 2280
▲ Neoral Soft Gelatin Capsules (1% to 17.6%) 2280
Panretin Gel 0.1% 1081
▲ Plavix Tablets (15.8%) 2767
Primaxin I.M. 2080
Primaxin I.V. (Less than 0.2%) 2083
Prinivil Tablets (Rare) 2087
Prinzide Tablets (Rare) 2092
▲ Prograf Capsules and Injection (3% to 15%) 622
Protonix for Delayed-Release Oral Suspension (Less than 1%) 3254
Protonix Delayed-Release Tablets (Less than 1%) 3254
Protonix I.V. (Less than 1%) 3257
Rilutek Tablets (Infrequent) 2771
Rocaltrol Capsules 1150
Rocaltrol Oral Solution 1150
▲ Romazicon Injection (1% to 3%) 2646
Soriatane Capsules (Less than 1%) .. 3062
▲ Targretin Gel 1% (18% to 26%) 1088
Tricor Tablets 520
▲ Vectibix (14% to 90%) 597
▲ Verdeso Foam (3%) 3069
▲ Vesanoid Capsules (14%) 2660
Yaz Tablets (Greater than 1%) 805
Zocor Tablets 2136
Zomig Tablets (Infrequent) 694
Zomig Nasal Spray (Infrequent) 689
Zomig-ZMT Tablets (Infrequent) 694
Zostavax Injection (1.1%) 2145
Zyrtec Chewable Tablets (Less than 2%) 1920
Zyrtec Syrup (Less than 2%) 1920
Zyrtec Tablets (Less than 2%) 1920
Zyrtec-D 12 Hour Extended Release Tablets (Less than 2%) 1923
Zyvox (0.9% to 2%) 2552

Skin eruptions
Bicillin C-R Injectable Suspension 1775
Bicillin L-A Injection 1777
Gantrisin Pediatric Suspension 2638
Imitrex Tablets 1474
Taxotere Injection Concentrate 2773

Skin fissures
Daytrana Transdermal Patch 3022
▲ Panretin Gel 0.1% (1% to 8%) 1081
▲ Vectibix (1% to 20%) 597

Skin friability, increased
Cuprimine Capsules (Rare) 1986

Skin hypertrophy
Brovana Inhalation Solution (Less than 2%) 2990
▲ CellCept Capsules (3% to less than 20%) 2622
▲ CellCept Intravenous (3% to less than 20%) 2622

▲ CellCept Oral Suspension (3% to less than 20%) 2622
▲ CellCept Tablets (3% to less than 20%) 2622
Copaxone for Injection (Infrequent) 3110
Effexor XR Extended-Release Capsules (Infrequent) 3195
Emsam Transdermal System (Infrequent) 905
Evoxac Capsules (Less than 1%) 1013
Humatrope Vials and Cartridges 1838
Mirapex Tablets 857
Olux Foam (One case) 3061
Paxil (Rare) 1535
Paxil CR Controlled-Release Tablets (Rare) 1544
Pletal Tablets (Less than 2%) 2481
Protopic Ointment (0.2% to less than 1%) 628
Remeron Tablets (Rare) 2924
RemeronSolTab Tablets (Rare) 2927
Soriatane Capsules (Less than 1%) .. 3062
Venlafaxine Hydrochloride Tablets (Infrequent) 2199

Skin nodule
Celebrex Capsules (0.1% to 1.9%) ... 2979
Copaxone for Injection (2%) 3110
Doxil Injection (Less than 1%) 2378
Gabitril Tablets (Infrequent) 973
Imitrex Nasal Spray 1470
Imitrex Tablets (Rare) 1474
Lescol Capsules 2268
Lescol XL Tablets 2268
Lexapro Oral Suspension (Infrequent) 1174
Lexapro Tablets (Infrequent) 1174
Lyrica Capsules (Rare) 2527
Mevacor Tablets 2063
Mirapex Tablets 857
Photofrin for Injection 708
Rilutek Tablets (Rare) 2771
Soriatane Capsules (Less than 1%) .. 3062
Targretin Capsules 1084
Vytorin 10/10 Tablets 2149
Vytorin 10/10 Tablets 2939
Vytorin 10/20 Tablets 2149
Vytorin 10/20 Tablets 2939
Vytorin 10/40 Tablets 2149
Vytorin 10/40 Tablets 2939
Vytorin 10/80 Tablets 2149
Vytorin 10/80 Tablets 2939
Zocor Tablets 2136
Zyrtec Chewable Tablets (Less than 2%) 1920
Zyrtec Syrup (Less than 2%) 1920
Zyrtec Tablets (Less than 2%) 1920
Zyrtec-D 12 Hour Extended Release Tablets (Less than 2%) 1923

Skin odor, abnormal
Mirapex Tablets 857
▲ Soriatane Capsules (1% to 10%) 3062

Skin papilloma
▲ Elidel Cream 1% (0% to 3.3%) 2221
Mirapex Tablets 857
Requip Tablets (Infrequent) 1561

Skin reactions, allergic
Duetact Tablets (Less than 1%) 3085

Skin reactions, hand and foot
▲ Eloxatin for Injection (0% to 11%) 2731
▲ Nexavar Tablets (21% to 30%) 784

Skin reactions, unspecified
Actonel Tablets (Rare) 2568
Actonel with Calcium Tablets (Very rare) 2574
Alphagan P Ophthalmic Solution 549
Combigan Ophthalmic Solution 553
Doribax Injection 2400
Duragesic Transdermal System (1% or greater) 2405
Fosamax Plus D Tablets (Rarely) 2013
▲ Gengraf Capsules (1% to 17.6%) 435
Lamisil Oral Granules 2264
Malarone Pediatric Tablets 1521
Malarone Tablets 1521
▲ Novantrone for Injection Concentrate (6%) 1100
▲ Protopic Ointment (1% to 4%) 628
Ultrase MT Capsules (0.2%) 719
Vicoprofen Tablets 533

Skin redness
▲ Panretin Gel 0.1% (25% to 77%) 1081
Targretin Gel 1% 1088
Taxotere Injection Concentrate 2773

Skin trauma
Nasonex Nasal Spray (Greater than or equal to 2%) 2883

Skull abnormalities, fetal
Accutane Capsules 2607
Aceon Tablets (2 mg, 4 mg, 8 mg) 3038
Avalide Tablets 2713
Captopril Tablets 2182
Cozaar Tablets 1973
Prinivil Tablets 2087
Prinzide Tablets 2092

Sleep, initiating of, disturbances
▲ Selzentry Tablets (7%) 2534

Sleep, maintaining of, disturbances
▲ Selzentry Tablets (7%) 2534

Sleep, sudden onset of
Neupro Transdermal System 3149
Xyrem Oral Solution (Infrequent) 1766

Sleep apnea syndrome
Requip Tablets (Infrequent) 1561
Risperdal Consta Long-Acting Injection 1753

Sleep apnoea syndrome
Mirapex Tablets 857

Sleep attacks
Xyrem Oral Solution (Infrequent) 1766

Sleep disturbances
Aceon Tablets (2 mg, 4 mg, 8 mg) (2.5%) 3038
▲ Advair HFA 45/21 Inhalation Aerosol (1% to 3%) 1288
▲ Advair HFA 115/21 Inhalation Aerosol (1% to 3%) 1288
▲ Advair HFA 230/21 Inhalation Aerosol (1% to 3%) 1288
Allegra Oral Solution (Rare) 2684
Allegra Tablets (Rare) 2684
Allegra-D 12 Hour Extended-Release Tablets (Less than 1%) 2687
Allegra-D 24 Hour Extended-Release Tablets (Less than 1%) 2690
Ambien Tablets (1%) 2692
Amerge Tablets (Infrequent) 1301
Anzemet Injection (Infrequently) 2701
Anzemet Tablets 2704
Aptivus Capsules (Less than 2%) 823
Aptivus Oral Solution (Less than 2%) 823
Avalide Tablets 892
Avalide Tablets 2713
Avapro Tablets (Less than 1%) 897
Avapro Tablets (Less than 1%) 2718
Avelox (Less than 0.1%) 2803
Celexa (At least 2%) 1160
▲ Chantix Tablets (2% to greater than 5%) 2511
Cipro 2810
▲ Combivir Tablets (11%) 1384
Concerta Extended-Release Tablets 1925
Copaxone for Injection (At least 2%) 3110
Coreg Tablets (Greater than 0.1% to 1%) 1387
Coreg CR Extended-Release Capsules (0.1% to less than or equal to 1%) 1393
Cozaar Tablets (Less than 1%) 1973
▲ Crinone 4% Gel (18%) 992
▲ Crinone 8% Gel (18%) 992
▲ Cymbalta Delayed-Release Capsules (Infrequent to 3%) 1801
Depakote ER Tablets (Greater than 1%) 423
Eldepryl Capsules 3052
▲ Epivir (11%) 1412
Exjade Tablets (0.1% to 1%) 2244
▲ Flovent Diskus 50 mcg (1% to 3%) 1435
Humulin 50/50, 100 Units 1843
Humulin 70/30 Vial 1844
Humulin N Vial 1846
Humulin R 1849
Imitrex Injection (Rare) 1465
Imitrex Nasal Spray (Infrequent) 1470
Imitrex Tablets (Rare to infrequent) ... 1474
Intelence Tablets (Less than 2%) 3119
Klonopin (Infrequent) 2639
Lamictal (1.4%) 1488
Levaquin (0.1% to 1%) 2416
Levaquin in 5% Dextrose Injection (0.1% to 1%) 2416
▲ Lupron Depot 3.75 mg (16%) 462
▲ Lupron Depot 7.5 mg (Less than 5%) 469
▲ Lupron Depot–3 Month 11.25 mg (16%) 462
Luvox CR Extended-Release Capsules (Infrequent) 1759
▲ Marplan Tablets (2% to 5%) 3177
Mirapex Tablets (Less than or equal to 1%) 857
▲ MoviPrep Oral Solution (39.1%) 2679
Nadolol Tablets 2191
Namenda (Infrequent) 1180
Nexium Delayed-Release Capsules (Less than 1%) 645
Nexium I.V. (Less than 1%) 652
Nexium Delayed-Release Oral Suspension (Less than 1%) 645
Noroxin Tablets (Less frequent) 2069
Ortho Evra Transdermal System 2437
▲ Pediarix Vaccine (0.4% to 46.7%) 1552
▲ Prevnar (15.3% to 25.2%) 3241
ProQuad (Greater than or equal to 0.2% to less than 1%) 2099
Protonix for Delayed-Release Oral Suspension (Less than 1%) 3254
Protonix Delayed-Release Tablets (Less than 1%) 3254
Protonix I.V. (Less than 1%) 3257
Provigil Tablets (At least 1%) 977
Prozac Weekly Capsules (Rare) 1852
Prozac Pulvules and Liquid (Frequent) 1852
Recombivax HB (Less than 1%) 2107
Requip Tablets (Frequent) 1561
Requip XL Tablets 1568
Reyataz Capsules 3299
Rythmol SR Capsules 1590
Selzentry Tablets 2534
▲ Serevent Diskus (1% to 3%) 1594
▲ Strattera Capsules (4%) 1864
Symbyax Capsules (1% to 2%) 1871
Tricor Tablets 520
▲ Trizivir Tablets (7% to 11%) 1622
Ultram ER Extended-Release Tablets (0.5% to less than 1%) 2428
Valium Tablets 2658
Varivax (Greater than or equal to 1%) 2133
▲ Visudyne for Injection (1% to 10%) .. 2332
▲ Wellbutrin Tablets (4%) 1648
▲ Wellbutrin XL Extended-Release Tablets (4%) 1659
▲ Xenical Capsules (3.9%) 2672
▲ Xyrem Oral Solution (2.9% to 6.1%) 1766
▲ Ziagen (10%) 1673
Zyrtec Chewable Tablets (Less than 2%) 1920
Zyrtec Syrup (Less than 2%) 1920
Zyrtec Tablets (Less than 2%) 1920
Zyrtec-D 12 Hour Extended Release Tablets (Less than 2%) 1923

Sleep driving
Ambien Tablets (1%) 2692
Ambien CR Tablets 2696

Sleep talking
Abilify Injection (Greater than or equal to 1 in 1000 patients and less than 1 in 100 patients) 881
Abilify Injection (Greater than or equal to 1 in 1000 patients and less than 1 in 100 patients) 2466
Abilify Oral Solution (Greater than or equal to 1 in 1000 patients and less than 1 in 100 patients) 881
Abilify Oral Solution (Greater than or equal to 1 in 1000 patients and less than 1 in 100 patients) 2466
Abilify Discmelt Orally Disintegrating Tablets (Greater than or equal to 1 in 1000 patients and less than 1 in 100 patients) 881
Abilify Discmelt Orally Disintegrating Tablets (Greater than or equal to 1 in 1000 patients and less than 1 in 100 patients) 2466
Abilify Tablets (Greater than or equal to 1 in 1000 patients and less than 1 in 100 patients) 881
Abilify Tablets (Greater than or equal to 1 in 1000 patients and less than 1 in 100 patients) 2466
Ambien Tablets (1%) 2692
Mirapex Tablets 857
Xyrem Oral Solution (Infrequent) 1766

Sleep walking
Abilify Injection (Less than 1 in 1000 patients) 881
Abilify Injection (Less than 1 in 1000 patients) 2466
Abilify Oral Solution (Less than 1 in 1000 patients) 881
Abilify Oral Solution (Less than 1 in 1000 patients) 2466
Abilify Discmelt Orally Disintegrating Tablets (Less than 1 in 1000 patients) 881
Abilify Discmelt Orally Disintegrating Tablets (Less than 1 in 1000 patients) 2466
Abilify Tablets (Less than 1 in 1000 patients) 881
Abilify Tablets (Less than 1 in 1000 patients) 2466
Mirapex Tablets 857
▲ Xyrem Oral Solution (5.7%) 1766

Sleepiness
(*see under* Drowsiness)

Sleeplessness
(*see under* Insomnia)

SLE-like syndrome
(*see under* Lupus erythematosus, systemic)

Slipped capital femoral epiphysis
Genotropin Lyophilized Powder 2547
Levothroid Tablets 1170
Norditropin Cartridges 2354
Nutropin for Injection 1208
Nutropin AQ Injection 1212
Nutropin AQ NuSpin Injection 1212
Nutropin AQ Pen 1212
Nutropin AQ Pen Cartridge 1212

Sloughing
Fluorescite Injection .... ⊙203

Sluggishness
Intelence Tablets (Less than 2%) 3119
Lexapro Oral Suspension (Infrequent) 1174
Lexapro Tablets (Infrequent) 1174
▲ Vivitrol (12% to 23%) 988
Xyrem Oral Solution (Infrequent) 1766

Smell, loss of the sense
(*see under* Anosmia)

Smell disturbances
Amerge Tablets (Infrequent) 1301
Beconase AQ Nasal Spray (Rare) 1369
Biaxin/Biaxin XL 411
Eligard 7.5 mg (Less than 2%) 2724
Eligard 22.5 mg (Less than 2%) 2724
Eligard 30 mg (Less than 2%) 2724
Eligard 45 mg (Less than 2%) 2724
Flonase Nasal Spray 1431
Imitrex Injection (Rare) 1465
Imitrex Nasal Spray (Infrequent) 1470
Imitrex Tablets (Infrequent) 1474
Maxair Autohaler (0.6%) 1705
Maxalt Tablets (Rare) 2056
Maxalt-MLT Orally Disintegrating Tablets (Rare) 2056
Nasonex Nasal Spray (Very rare) 2883
Rythmol Tablets (Less than 1%) 1586
▲ Taxotere Injection Concentrate (0% to 20.3%) 2773
Testim 1% Gel (1% or less) 701
Timentin ADD-Vantage 1606
Timentin Injection Galaxy Container 1609
Timentin IV Infusion 1603
Timentin Pharmacy Bulk Package 1613

Smoker's tongue
(*see under* Leukoplakia, oral)

Sneezing
Aceon Tablets (2 mg, 4 mg, 8 mg) (0.3% to 1%) 3038
▲ Aerobid/Aerobid-M (3% to 9%) 1153
▲ Alamast Ophthalmic Solution (Less than 5%) 3181
Atrovent Nasal Spray 0.03% 834
Axert Tablets (Rare) 2431
▲ Beconase AQ Nasal Spray (4%) 1369
Bentyl Capsules 703
Bentyl Injection 703
Bentyl Syrup 703
Bentyl Tablets 703
▲ Intron A for Injection (Less than or equal to 5%) 2859
Klonopin (Infrequent) 2639
Maxalt Tablets (Rare) 2056
Maxalt-MLT Orally Disintegrating Tablets (Rare) 2056
Mirapex Tablets 857
ProQuad 2099
Requip Tablets (Infrequent) 1561
Rituxan I.V. 1223
Simulect for Injection 2306

Sudafed OM Sinus Cold Moisturizing Nasal Spray ... 1906
Sudafed OM Sinus Congestion Moisturizing Nasal Spray ... 1906
▲ Ultram ER Extended-Release Tablets (1% to less than 5%) ... 2428
Vicks NyQuil Cold & Flu Multi-Symptom Relief ... ▣ 617
Vicks NyQuil LiquiCaps ... ▣ 617

Snoring
Aricept Tablets (Infrequent) ... 1062
Aricept ODT Tablets (Infrequent) ... 1062
▲ Increlex Injection (Greater than or equal to 5%) ... 3100
Mirapex Tablets ... 857
Xyrem Oral Solution (Infrequent) ... 1766

Social reaction, anti
(*see under* Sociopathy)

Sociopathy
Paxil (Rare) ... 1535
Paxil CR Controlled-Release Tablets (Rare) ... 1544
Zyprexa Tablets (Infrequent) ... 1883
Zyprexa ZYDIS Orally Disintegrating Tablets (Infrequent) ... 1883

Sodium depletion
(*see under* Hyponatremia)

Sodium loss
(*see under* Hyponatremia)

Sodium retention
Delatestryl Injection ... 1730
Estratest Tablets (Among most common) ... 3043
Estratest H.S. Tablets (Among most common) ... 3043
Proglycem Capsules (Frequent) ... 1185
Proglycem Suspension (Frequent) ... 1185

Somatization
Zyprexa Tablets (Infrequent) ... 1883
Zyprexa ZYDIS Orally Disintegrating Tablets (Infrequent) ... 1883

Somnambulism
Ambien Tablets (Rare) ... 2692
Ambien CR Tablets (Rare) ... 2696
Requip Tablets (Infrequent) ... 1561

Somnolence
(*see under* Drowsiness)

Sore throat
(*see also under* Throat soreness)
Yaz Tablets (Greater than 1%) ... 805

Soreness, injection site
▲ Alferon N Injection (10%) ... 1726
▲ Comvax (23.9% to 34.5%) ... 1966
▲ Engerix-B Vaccine (22%) ... 1409
▲ Havrix Injection Vaccine (21% to 56%) ... 1454
Pneumovax 23 (Common) ... 2078
▲ ProQuad (22%) ... 2099
▲ Twinrix Vaccine (35% to 41%) ... 1628
▲ Vaqta (1.2% to 3.5%) ... 2130
▲ Varivax (19.3% to 32.5%) ... 2133
WinRho SDF ... 741

Soreness, testicular
Eligard 7.5 mg (Less than 2%) ... 2724
Eligard 22.5 mg (Less than 2%) ... 2724
Eligard 30 mg (Less than 2%) ... 2724
Eligard 45 mg (Less than 2%) ... 2724

Soreness at insertion site
▲ Supprelin LA Implant (51.1%) ... 1731
▲ Vantas (3.6%) ... 1737

Spasm, biliary tract
MS Contin Tablets (Less frequent) ... 2585

Spasm, gastrointestinal
Salagen Tablets ... 1082

Spasm, generalized
Emsam Transdermal System (Infrequent) ... 905
Gabitril Tablets (Infrequent) ... 973
Lyrica Capsules (Rare) ... 2527
Paxil (Rare) ... 1535
Paxil CR Controlled-Release Tablets (Rare) ... 1544
Prinivil Tablets (0.3% to 1%) ... 2087
Prinzide Tablets ... 2092
▲ Prograf Capsules and Injection (3% to 15%) ... 622
Symbyax Capsules (Infrequent) ... 1871
▲ Zyprexa Tablets (2% to 3%) ... 1883
▲ Zyprexa ZYDIS Orally Disintegrating Tablets (2% to 3%) ... 1883

Spasm, jaw
Eloxatin for Injection ... 2731

Spasm, non-site specific
Amerge Tablets (Rare) ... 1301
Invanz for Injection (Greater than 0.1%) ... 2029

Spasm, tonic-clonic
Aczone Gel 5% ... 3296
OsmoPrep Tablets ... 2680
Tekturna Tablets (Greater than 1%) ... 2321

Spasm, urinary bladder
▲ DepoDur Injection (2% to 5%) ... 1095

Spasm, vesical sphincters
Lortab 5/500 Tablets ... 3143
Lortab 7.5/500 Tablets ... 3144
Lortab 10/500 Tablets ... 3144
Tussionex Pennkinetic Extended-Release Suspension ... 3154
Vicodin Tablets ... 529
Vicodin ES Tablets ... 530
Vicodin HP Tablets ... 531
Zydone Tablets ... 1132

Spasms, back
▲ Forteo for Injection (1% to 10%) ... 1816

Spasms, leg
▲ Forteo for Injection (1% to 10%) ... 1816

Spasticity
Valium Tablets ... 2658

Speech, slurring
Humulin 50/50, 100 Units ... 1843
Humulin 70/30 Vial ... 1844
Humulin N Vial ... 1846
Humulin R ... 1849
Klonopin ... 2639
Luvox CR Extended-Release Capsules (Rare) ... 1759
Nadolol Tablets (1 to 5 of 1000 patients) ... 2191
Phenytek Capsules (Among most common) ... 2192
Valium Tablets (Infrequent) ... 2658
Vicoprofen Tablets (Less than 1%) ... 533

Speech difficulties
▲ Demser Capsules (10%) ... 1989
Geodon for Injection (Up to 2%) ... 2520
Marinol Capsules (Less than 1%) ... 3163
▲ Zyprexa Tablets (2% to 7%) ... 1883
▲ Zyprexa ZYDIS Orally Disintegrating Tablets (2% to 7%) ... 1883

Speech disorder
Abilify Injection (Greater than or equal to 1 in 1000 patients and less than 1 in 100 patients) ... 881
Abilify Injection (Greater than or equal to 1 in 1000 patients and less than 1 in 100 patients) ... 2466
Abilify Oral Solution (Greater than or equal to 1 in 1000 patients and less than 1 in 100 patients) ... 881
Abilify Oral Solution (Greater than or equal to 1 in 1000 patients and less than 1 in 100 patients) ... 2466
Abilify Discmelt Orally Disintegrating Tablets (Greater than or equal to 1 in 1000 patients and less than 1 in 100 patients) ... 881
Abilify Discmelt Orally Disintegrating Tablets (Greater than or equal to 1 in 1000 patients and less than 1 in 100 patients) ... 2466
Abilify Tablets (Greater than or equal to 1 in 1000 patients and less than 1 in 100 patients) ... 881
Abilify Tablets (Greater than or equal to 1 in 1000 patients and less than 1 in 100 patients) ... 2466
Ambien Tablets (Infrequent) ... 2692
Ambien CR Tablets (Infrequent) ... 2696
Avelox (Less than 0.1%) ... 2803
▲ Gliadel Wafer (11%) ... 1076
▲ Lyrica Capsules (1% to 7%) ... 2527
Prograf Capsules and Injection ... 622
Salagen Tablets (Less than 1%) ... 1082

Speech disturbances
Actiq (Less than 1%) ... 959
▲ Adderall XR Capsules (2% to 4%) ... 3012
Arranon Injection (1%) ... 1319
Bentyl Capsules ... 703
Bentyl Injection ... 703
Bentyl Syrup ... 703
Bentyl Tablets ... 703
Carbatrol Capsules ... 3019
Copaxone for Injection (2%) ... 3110
Dantrium Capsules (Less frequent) ... 2580
Depakote ER Tablets (Greater than 1%) ... 423
Duragesic Transdermal System (1% or greater) ... 2405
Effexor XR Extended-Release Capsules (Infrequent) ... 3195
Eldepryl Capsules ... 3052
▲ Equetro Extended-Release Capsules (6%) ... 3174
Evoxac Capsules (Less than 1%) ... 1013
Frova Tablets (Infrequent) ... 1111
▲ Gabitril Tablets (4%) ... 973
Geodon Capsules (2%) ... 2520
Imitrex Injection ... 1465
▲ Intron A for Injection (Less than 5%) ... 2859
▲ Lamictal (3%) ... 1488
Meridia Capsules ... 475
Ortho-Cyclen Tablets ... 2449
Ortho Evra Transdermal System ... 2437
Ortho Tri-Cyclen Tablets ... 2449
Ortho Tri-Cyclen Lo Tablets ... 2458
OxyContin Tablets (Less than 1%) ... 2589
▲ Prometrium Capsules (100 mg, 200 mg) (Less than 5%) ... 3047
Protonix for Delayed-Release Oral Suspension ... 3254
Protonix Delayed-Release Tablets ... 3254
Protonix I.V. ... 3257
Romazicon Injection (Less than 1%) ... 2646
Rythmol Tablets (Less than 1%) ... 1586
Rythmol SR Capsules ... 1590
Symbyax Capsules (Up to 2%) ... 1871
Venlafaxine Hydrochloride Tablets (Infrequent) ... 2199
▲ Vesanoid Capsules (3%) ... 2660
Zomig Tablets (Infrequent) ... 694
Zomig Nasal Spray (Infrequent) ... 689
Zomig-ZMT Tablets (Infrequent) ... 694
▲ Zonegran Capsules (5%) ... 1089
▲ Zyprexa Tablets (2% to 7%) ... 1883
▲ Zyprexa ZYDIS Orally Disintegrating Tablets (2% to 7%) ... 1883

Spermatogenesis, defective
Mustargen for Injection ... 2492

Spermatogenesis, inhibition
Rythmol Tablets ... 1586

Spinal cord, compression
Velcade for Injection ... 2168

Spinal cord infarction
Activase I.V. ... 1188

Spinal cord injury
Zolinza Capsules ... 2142

Spinal fracture
Arimidex Tablets (1%) ... 672
Lupron Depot 3.75 mg ... 462
Lupron Depot 7.5 mg ... 469
Lupron Depot–3 Month 11.25 mg ... 462
Lupron Depot-PED 7.5 mg, 11.25 mg and 15 mg ... 471

Spleen disorder
Rythmol SR Capsules ... 1590

Spleenomegaly
Flolan for Injection ... 1426

Splenic infarction
Zomig Tablets (Rare) ... 694
Zomig Nasal Spray (Very rare) ... 689
Zomig-ZMT Tablets (Rare) ... 694

Splenic rupture
Neulasta Injection (Rare) ... 587
Neupogen for Injection (Rare) ... 589

Splenomegaly
Chantix Tablets (Rare) ... 2511
Combivir Tablets ... 1384
Copaxone for Injection (Infrequent) ... 3110
Dacogen Injection ... 1066
▲ Epivir (5%) ... 1412
Epivir-HBV ... 1417
Epzicom Tablets ... 1422
▲ Neupogen for Injection (Approximately 30%) ... 589
Orthoclone OKT3 Sterile Solution ... 2387
Retrovir IV Infusion ... 1579
Tabloid Tablets ... 1601
Trizivir Tablets ... 1622

Spotting
Activella Tablets ... 2347
Angeliq Tablets ... 751
Climara Transdermal System ... 763
Climara Pro Transdermal System ... 768
Divigel ... 3167
Enjuvia Tablets ... 1029
Estratest Tablets ... 3043
Estratest H.S. Tablets ... 3043
Lexapro Oral Suspension (Infrequent) ... 1174
Lexapro Tablets (Infrequent) ... 1174
Lybrel Tablets ... 3204
Mircette Tablets ... 1034
NuvaRing ... 2897
Ortho-Cyclen Tablets ... 2449
Ortho Evra Transdermal System ... 2437
Ortho Tri-Cyclen Tablets ... 2449
Ortho Tri-Cyclen Lo Tablets ... 2458
Premarin Intravenous ... 3217
Premarin Tablets ... 3221
Premarin Vaginal Cream ... 3228
Premphase Tablets ... 3232
Prempro Tablets ... 3232
Prometrium Capsules (100 mg, 200 mg) ... 3047
Seasonique Tablets ... 1046
Yaz Tablets ... 805

Spotting, oily
▲ Xenical Capsules (4.4% to 26.6%) ... 2672

Sputum increased
Actiq (Less than 1%) ... 959
▲ Aerobid/Aerobid-M (3% to 9%) ... 1153
Celexa (Rare) ... 1160
▲ CellCept Capsules (3% to less than 20%) ... 2622
▲ CellCept Intravenous (3% to less than 20%) ... 2622
▲ CellCept Oral Suspension (3% to less than 20%) ... 2622
▲ CellCept Tablets (3% to less than 20%) ... 2622
Combivent Inhalation Aerosol (Less than 2%) ... 845
▲ Exubera Inhalation Powder (2.8% to 3.9%) ... 2515
Foradil Aerolizer (1.5%) ... 2849
▲ Lupron Depot 7.5 mg (Less than 5%) ... 469
Paxil (Rare) ... 1535
Paxil CR Controlled-Release Tablets (Rare) ... 1544
Pulmozyme Inhalation Solution ... 1217
Rilutek Tablets (More than 2%) ... 2771
Salagen Tablets (Less than 1%) ... 1082
Soriatane Capsules (Less than 1%) ... 3062
Ultane Liquid for Inhalation (Less than 1%) ... 524
Zomig Tablets (Rare) ... 694
Zomig Nasal Spray (Rare) ... 689
Zomig-ZMT Tablets (Rare) ... 694
Zyrtec Chewable Tablets (Less than 2%) ... 1920
Zyrtec Syrup (Less than 2%) ... 1920
Zyrtec Tablets (Less than 2%) ... 1920
Zyrtec-D 12 Hour Extended Release Tablets (Less than 2%) ... 1923

S-T depressed
Lyrica Capsules (Rare) ... 2527
Ultane Liquid for Inhalation (Less than 1%) ... 524

ST section changes
(*see under* EKG changes, ST section)

Standing, difficulty in
Stromectol Tablets ... 2120

Status asthmaticus
Sandostatin Injection (Less than 1%) ... 2300
Sandostatin LAR Depot ... 2302

Status epilepticus
Arranon Injection (0% to 1%) ... 1319
Carbatrol Capsules ... 3019
Gabitril Tablets ... 973
Keppra Oral Solution (Greater than or equal to 2%) ... 3131
Keppra Tablets (Greater than or equal to 2%) ... 3131
Paxil ... 1535
Paxil CR Controlled-Release Tablets ... 1544

Steatorrhea
▲ Sandostatin Injection (22% to 35%) ... 2300
▲ Sandostatin LAR Depot (4% to 6%) ... 2302

Steatosis, hepatic
Aptivus Capsules (Less than 2%) ... 823

Aptivus Oral Solution (Less than 2%) 823
Atripla Tablets 938
Combivir Tablets 1384
Emtriva Capsules 1246
Emtriva Oral Solution 1246
Epivir 1412
Epivir-HBV 1417
Epzicom Tablets 1422
Hepsera Tablets 1253
Intelence Tablets (Less than 2%) 3119
Retrovir Capsules 1574
Retrovir IV Infusion (Rare) 1579
Retrovir 1574
Trizivir Tablets 1622
Truvada Tablets 1262
Viread Tablets 1268
Ziagen 1673

Stenosis, aortic
Argatroban Injection (0.9%) 1308

Stenosis, bile duct
Prograf Capsules and Injection 622

Stenosis, intestinal
Azilect Tablets (Rare) 3106
Remicade for IV Injection (Greater than or equal to 0.2%) 950

Sterility
▲ Novantrone for Injection Concentrate (3%) 1100

Stevens-Johnson syndrome
Aciphex Tablets 1053
Advicor Tablets 402
Aggrenox Capsules 819
Albenza Tablets 1297
Amoxil Capsules 1305
Amoxil Chewable Tablets 1305
Amoxil Pediatric Drops for Oral Suspension 1305
Amoxil Powder for Oral Suspension 1305
Amoxil Tablets 1305
Anaprox Tablets (Less than 1%) 2632
Anaprox DS Tablets (Less than 1%) 2632
Arimidex Tablets (Very rare) 672
Atacand HCT 642
Atripla Tablets 938
Attenuvax 1951
Augmentin (Rare) 1323
Augmentin Tablets (Rare) 1327
Augmentin XR Extended Release Tablets (Rare) 1333
Augmentin ES-600 Powder for Oral Suspension 1329
Avalide Tablets 892
Avalide Tablets 2713
Avandamet Tablets 1336
Avandia Tablets 1351
Avelox 2803
Biaxin/Biaxin XL (Rare) 411
Bleph-10 Ophthalmic Solution 10% (Isolated incident) ⊙215
Cancidas for Injection 1953
Captopril Tablets 2182
Carbatrol Capsules (1 to 6 in 10,000 users) 3019
Ceftin 1380
Celebrex Capsules (Less than 0.1%) 2979
Cialis Tablets 1792
Cimzia 3127
Cipro I.V. (1% or less) 2817
Cipro 2810
Cipro XR Tablets 2823
Clinoril Tablets (Less than 1 in 100) 1962
Combivir Tablets 1384
Comvax 1966
Crixivan Capsules 1979
Cymbalta Delayed-Release Capsules 1801
Daraprim Tablets 1400
Depakote ER Tablets 423
Didronel Tablets (A single case) 2583
Diovan HCT Tablets 2216
Doribax Injection 2400
EC-Naprosyn Delayed-Release Tablets (Less than 1%) 2632
E.E.S. (Rare) 433
Effexor XR Extended-Release Capsules 3195
Emend Capsules (One patient) 1992
Emend for Injection (One patient) 1999
Enbrel for Injection 569
Engerix-B Vaccine 1409
Epzicom Tablets 1422
Equetro Extended-Release Capsules 3174
EryPed (Rare) 431
Exelon Capsules 2229
Exelon Oral Solution 2229
Fansidar Tablets 2636
Flebogamma 5% 1715
Flebogamma 5% DIF 1718
Flector Patch 561
Fluarix Vaccine 1446
Fortaz 1450
Fosamax (Rare) 2005
Fosamax Plus D Tablets (Rarely) 2013
Gammagard Liquid 730
Gammagard S/D (Rare) 734
Gamunex (Rare) 3094
Gantrisin Pediatric Suspension 2638
Gleevec Tablets (Rare) 2255
Indapamide Tablets 2188
Indocin Capsules (Less than 1%) 2024
Indocin I.V. (Less than 1%) 2489
Indocin (Less than 1%) 2024
Intelence Tablets (Less than 0.1%) 3119
Intravenous Sodium Diuril 2490
Intron A for Injection 2859
Isentress Tablets 2036
Janumet Tablets 2041
Januvia Tablets 2048
Lamictal (Rare) 1488
Lamisil Oral Granules 2264
Lamisil Tablets (Isolated reports) 2266
Lescol Capsules (Rare) 2268
Lescol XL Tablets 2268
Leukeran Tablets (Rare) 1508
Leustatin Injection (Isolated cases) 2384
Levaquin 2416
Levaquin in 5% Dextrose Injection 2416
Lexapro Oral Suspension 1174
Lexapro Tablets 1174
Lexiva Oral Suspension (Less than 1%) 1510
Lexiva Tablets (Less than 1%) 1510
Lipitor Tablets 2501
Luvox CR Extended-Release Capsules 1759
Lyrica Capsules (Rare) 2527
Malarone Pediatric Tablets 1521
Malarone Tablets 1521
Mepron Suspension 1526
Merrem I.V. 684
Meruvax II 2061
Mevacor Tablets (Rare) 2063
Micardis HCT Tablets 854
M-M-R II 2054
Mobic Oral Suspension (Less than 0.1%) 863
Mobic Tablets (Less than 0.1%) 863
Moxatag Tablets 2165
Mumpsvax 2068
Nalfon Capsules (Less than 1%) 2508
Namenda 1180
Naprosyn Suspension (Less than 1%) 2632
Naprosyn Tablets (Less than 1%) 2632
Nexium Delayed-Release Capsules (Rare) 645
Nexium I.V. (Rare) 652
Nexium Delayed-Release Oral Suspension (Rare) 645
Noroxin Tablets 2069
Norvir (Rare) 489
Omnicef Capsules 497
Omnicef for Oral Suspension 497
Orthoclone OKT3 Sterile Solution 2387
PegIntron Powder for Injection 2903
Pepcid Tablets 2075
Phenytek Capsules 2192
Plavix Tablets 926
Plavix Tablets 2767
Pletal Tablets 2481
PrandiMet Tablets 2967
Prandin Tablets (Rare) 2971
Primaxin I.M. 2080
Primaxin I.V. 2083
Prinivil Tablets (Rare) 2087
Prinzide Tablets (Rare) 2092
Prograf Capsules and Injection 622
Proleukin for Injection 2287
ProQuad 2099
Protonix for Delayed-Release Oral Suspension 3254
Protonix Delayed-Release Tablets 3254
Protonix I.V. 3257
Provigil Tablets (Rare) 977
Prozac Weekly Capsules 1852
Prozac Pulvules and Liquid 1852
Recombivax HB 2107
Remicade for IV Injection 950
Retrovir IV Infusion 1579
Reyataz Capsules 3299
Rituxan I.V. 1223
Rocephin Injectable Vials, ADD-Vantage, Galaxy, Bulk 2642
Sanctura XR Capsules 557
Solodyn Extended Release Tablets 1938
Stromectol Tablets 2120
Suprax for Oral Suspension (Less than 2%) 1891
Suprax Tablets (Less than 2%) 1891
▲ Sustiva Capsules (Up to 3.5%) 930
▲ Sustiva Tablets (Up to 3.5%) 930
Tamiflu Capsules (Rare) 2649
Tamiflu Oral Suspension (Rare) 2649
Tarka Tablets 511
Taxotere Injection Concentrate (Rare) 2773
Tekturna HCT Tablets 2324
Teveten HCT Tablets 517
Timentin ADD-Vantage 1606
Timentin Injection Galaxy Container 1609
Timentin IV Infusion 1603
Timentin Pharmacy Bulk Package 1613
Treximet Tablets 1616
Tricor Tablets (Rare) 520
Trizivir Tablets 1622
Trusopt Sterile Ophthalmic Solution (Rare) 2128
Twinrix Vaccine 1628
Varivax 2133
Venlafaxine Hydrochloride Tablets 2199
Viramune Oral Suspension 873
Viramune Tablets 873
Voltaren Tablets (Rarely) 2334
Voltaren-XR Tablets (Rarely) 2337
Vytorin 10/10 Tablets 2149
Vytorin 10/10 Tablets 2939
Vytorin 10/20 Tablets 2149
Vytorin 10/20 Tablets 2939
Vytorin 10/40 Tablets 2149
Vytorin 10/40 Tablets 2939
Vytorin 10/80 Tablets 2149
Vytorin 10/80 Tablets 2939
Vyvanse Capsules 3033
Wellbutrin Tablets (Rare) 1648
Wellbutrin SR Sustained-Release Tablets (Rare) 1653
Wellbutrin XL Extended-Release Tablets (Rare) 1659
Ziagen 1673
Zinacef for Injection (Rare) 1678
Zinacef Injection (Rare) 1678
Zocor Tablets (Rare) 2136
Zonegran Capsules (Rare) 1089
Zosyn for Injection (Rare) 3284
Zovirax 1690
Zyban Sustained-Release Tablets 1692
Zyvox 2552

Stiffness, unspecified
▲ Genotropin Lyophilized Powder (0% to 7.9%) 2547
ProQuad 2099

Stillbirths
Aggrenox Capsules 819
Bayer Aspirin 750
Percodan Tablets 1130
St. Joseph 81 mg Aspirin Chewable and Enteric Coated Tablets 1903
Xyzal Oral Solution 2789
Xyzal Oral Solution 3155
Zyrtec Chewable Tablets 1920
Zyrtec Syrup 1920
Zyrtec Tablets 1920
Zyrtec-D 12 Hour Extended Release Tablets (Rare) 1923

Stimulation
Stalevo Tablets 2309
Valium Tablets 2658

Stinging
▲ Aldara Cream, 5% (3%) 1699
Attenuvax 1951
Bactroban Nasal (2%) 1367
Bactroban Ointment (1.5%) 1368
▲ Betimol Ophthalmic Solution (1 in 8 patients) 3181
Bleph-10 Ophthalmic Solution 10% ⊙215
▲ Cosopt Sterile Ophthalmic Solution (Up to 30%) 1969
Cozaar Tablets (Less than 1%) 1973
Diprolene AF Cream 0.05% (0.4%) 2837
Doxil Injection 2378
Elidel Cream 1% 2221
▲ Elocon Cream 0.1% (1.6% to approximately 7%) 2840
▲ Elocon Ointment 0.1% (4.8% to approximately 7%) 2842
▲ Finacea Gel (4% to 16%) 1742
FML Ophthalmic Suspension ⊙224
FML Forte Ophthalmic Suspension ⊙222
Imitrex Injection (Infrequent) 1465
Lotrisone (Less than 1%) 2881
▲ Luxiq Foam (2% to 44%) 3058
Mentax Cream (Approximately 1%) 2190
Meruvax II 2061
M-M-R II 2054
Mumpsvax 2068
▲ Naftin Cream (6%) 2164
▲ Naftin Gel (5%) 2164
Olux Foam (Less than 2%) 3061
▲ Panretin Gel 0.1% (3% to 22%) 1081
▲ Patanol Ophthalmic Solution (Less than 5%) 546
Pred Forte Ophthalmic Suspension ⊙227
Pred Mild Ophthalmic Suspension ⊙230
Pred-G Ophthalmic Suspension ⊙228
▲ Timoptic Sterile Ophthalmic Solution (Approximately 1 in 8 patients) 2121
▲ Timoptic in Ocudose (Approximately 1 in 8 patients) 2124
▲ Timoptic-XE Sterile Ophthalmic Gel Forming Solution (1 in 8 patients) 2125
▲ Trusopt Sterile Ophthalmic Solution (Approximately one-third of patients) 2128
▲ Zovirax Ointment (28.3%) 819

Stinging at application site
▲ Eligard 7.5 mg (34.6%) 2724
▲ Eligard 22.5 mg (21.7%) 2724
▲ Eligard 30 mg (20%) 2724
▲ Eligard 45 mg (16%) 2724
Ziana Gel (2%) 1942

Stinging at injection site
AlphaNine SD 1713
ProQuad 2099
Xolair 1235
Xolair 2339

Stomach burn
▲ Novantrone for Injection Concentrate (14%) 1100

Stomach complaints
Xyrem Oral Solution (Infrequent) 1766

Stomach discomfort
Allegra Oral Solution (2.1%) 2684
Allegra Tablets (2.1%) 2684
▲ Chantix Tablets (5% to 7%) 2511
Requip Tablets (Frequent) 1561

Stomachache
▲ Aerobid/Aerobid-M (10%) 1153
▲ Bayer Aspirin (14.5%) 750
▲ Chemet Capsules (5.2% to 15.7%) 2484
▲ Fabrazyme for Intravenous Infusion (6%) 1241
Klonopin (Infrequent) 2639
K-Phos Original (Sodium Free) Tablets 814
K-Phos Neutral Tablets 813
Ortho-Cyclen Tablets 2449
Ortho Evra Transdermal System 2437
Ortho Tri-Cyclen Tablets 2449
Ortho Tri-Cyclen Lo Tablets 2458
Rocaltrol Capsules 1150
Rocaltrol Oral Solution 1150
St. Joseph 81 mg Aspirin Chewable and Enteric Coated Tablets 1903
Uroqid-Acid No. 2 Tablets 814
Zofran Injection (2%) 1682

Stomatitis
Actiq (1% or greater) 959
▲ Alferon N Injection (6%) 1726
▲ Alimta for Injection (Up to 28%) 1786
AmBisome for Injection (Less common) 606
Anaprox Tablets (Less than 3%) 2632
Anaprox DS Tablets (Less than 3%) 2632
▲ Arranon Injection (0% to 8%) 1319
Asacol Delayed-Release Tablets 2579
Augmentin 1323
Augmentin Tablets 1327
Augmentin XR Extended Release Tablets 1333
Augmentin ES-600 Powder for Oral Suspension 1329
▲ Avastin IV (30% to 32%) 1192
Avelox (Greater than or equal to 0.1% to less than 2%) 2803
Azilect Tablets (Infrequent) 3106
Biaxin/Biaxin XL 411
▲ Busulfex Injection (26% to 97%) 2477
Carbatrol Capsules 3019
Celebrex Capsules (0.1% to 1.9%) 2979
Celexa (Infrequent) 1160
▲ CellCept Capsules (3% to less than 20%) 2622
▲ CellCept Intravenous (3% to less than 20%) 2622

▲ CellCept Oral Suspension (3% to less than 20%) 2622
▲ CellCept Tablets (3% to less than 20%) 2622
Clinoril Tablets (Less than 1 in 100) 1962
Combivir Tablets 1384
Copaxone for Injection (Infrequent) 3110
Cubicin for Injection (Less than 1%) 995
Cymbalta Delayed-Release Capsules (Infrequent) 1801
▲ Dacogen Injection (12%) 1066
▲ Depakote ER Tablets (Greater than 1% to less than 5%) 423
▲ Doxil Injection (5.2% to 41.4%) 2378
EC-Naprosyn Delayed-Release Tablets (Less than 3%) 2632
Effexor XR Extended-Release Capsules (Infrequent) 3195
▲ Eloxatin for Injection (0% to 42%) 2731
▲ Emend Capsules (5.3%) 1992
▲ Emend for Injection (5.3%) 1999
▲ Epivir (6%) 1412
Epivir-HBV 1417
Epzicom Tablets 1422
Equetro Extended-Release Capsules 3174
▲ Erbitux (1% to 25%) 912
Estratest Tablets 3043
Estratest H.S. Tablets 3043
Evoxac Capsules (Less than 1%) 1013
Fansidar Tablets 2636
Fentora Tablets (Greater than 1%) 968
Flumadine 1167
Frova Tablets (Rare) 1111
Gabitril Tablets (Frequent) 973
Gantrisin Pediatric Suspension 2638
▲ Gemzar for Injection (10% to 22%) 1820
▲ Gengraf Capsules (6%) 435
▲ Hycamtin for Injection (Less than 1% to 24%) 1459
Intelence Tablets (Less than 2%) 3119
▲ Intron A for Injection (Less than 5%) 2859
Invanz for Injection (Greater than 0.1%) 2029
▲ Ixempra Kit for Injection (29%) 915
Kaletra (Less than 2%) 452
Ketek Tablets (Greater than or equal to 0.2% to less than 2%) 2744
Lamictal (Rare) 1488
▲ Leukine (24% to 62%) 774
Levaquin (0.1% to 1%) 2416
Levaquin in 5% Dextrose Injection (0.1% to 1%) 2416
Lipitor Tablets (Less than 2%) 2501
Lunesta Tablets (Rare) 2994
Luvox CR Extended-Release Capsules (Infrequent) 1759
Malarone Pediatric Tablets 1521
Malarone Tablets 1521
Maxair Autohaler 1705
▲ Mylotarg for Injection (2% to 29%) 3212
Naprosyn Suspension (Less than 3%) 2632
Naprosyn Tablets (Less than 3%) 2632
▲ Neoral Oral Solution (6%) 2280
▲ Neoral Soft Gelatin Capsules (6%) 2280
▲ Neulasta Injection (15% to 72%) 587
▲ Neupogen for Injection (5%) 589
▲ Nexavar Tablets (1% to less than 10%) 784
Nexium Delayed-Release Capsules 645
Nexium I.V. 652
Nexium Delayed-Release Oral Suspension 645
Noroxin Tablets 2069
▲ Novantrone for Injection Concentrate (8% to 29%) 1100
Omnicef Capsules 497
Omnicef for Oral Suspension 497
OxyContin Tablets (Less than 1%) 2589
Paxil (Rare) 1535
Paxil CR Controlled-Release Tablets (Rare) 1544
PegIntron Powder for Injection 2903
Plavix Tablets 926
Plavix Tablets 2767
▲ Prograf Capsules and Injection (3% to 15%) 622
▲ Proleukin for Injection (Less than 1% to 22%) 2287
Protonix for Delayed-Release Oral Suspension (Less than 1%) 3254
Protonix Delayed-Release Tablets (Less than 1%) 3254
Protonix I.V. (Less than 1%) 3257
Protopic Ointment (0.2% to less than 1%) 628
Prozac Weekly Capsules (Infrequent) 1852
Prozac Pulvules and Liquid (Infrequent) 1852
Pylera Capsules 714
▲ Rapamune (Greater than or equal to 3% to less than 20%) 3260
Remeron Tablets (Infrequent) 2924
RemeronSolTab Tablets (Infrequent) 2927
Requip Tablets (Infrequent) 1561
Retrovir IV Infusion 1579
Rilutek Tablets (0.8% to 1.2%) 2771
Risperdal Consta Long-Acting Injection (Infrequent) 1753
Rocephin Injectable Vials, ADD-Vantage, Galaxy, Bulk 2642
Salagen Tablets (1% to 2%) 1082
▲ Soriatane Capsules (1% to 10%) 3062
▲ Spiriva HandiHaler (1% to 3%) 870
▲ Sutent Capsules (1% to 53%) 2540
Symbyax Capsules (Infrequent) 1871
Tabloid Tablets (Less frequent) 1601
▲ Tarceva Tablets (0% to 22%) 1228
Tasigna Capsules (0.1% to 1%) 2316
▲ Taxotere Injection Concentrate (0.6% to 69.4%) 2773
▲ Temodar Capsules (1% to 9%) 2931
Timentin ADD-Vantage 1606
Timentin Injection Galaxy Container 1609
Timentin IV Infusion 1603
Timentin Pharmacy Bulk Package 1613
Treanda for Injection 983
Trizivir Tablets 1622
▲ Tykerb Tablets (0% to 14%) 1631
▲ Vectibix (0% to 7%) 597
Velcade for Injection 2168
Venlafaxine Hydrochloride Tablets (Infrequent) 2199
Voltaren Tablets (Occasionally) 2334
Voltaren-XR Tablets (Occasionally) 2337
Wellbutrin Tablets (Frequent) 1648
Wellbutrin SR Sustained-Release Tablets (Infrequent) 1653
Wellbutrin XL Extended-Release Tablets (Infrequent) 1659
▲ Xeloda Tablets (2% to 25%) 2662
▲ Zometa for Intravenous Infusion (8%) 2341
Zomig Tablets (Rare) 694
Zomig Nasal Spray (Rare) 689
Zomig-ZMT Tablets (Rare) 694
Zonegran Capsules (Infrequent) 1089
Zyban Sustained-Release Tablets (Infrequent) 1692
Zyprexa Tablets (Infrequent) 1883
Zyprexa ZYDIS Orally Disintegrating Tablets (Infrequent) 1883
Zyrtec Chewable Tablets (Less than 2%) 1920
Zyrtec Syrup (Less than 2%) 1920
Zyrtec Tablets (Less than 2%) 1920
Zyrtec-D 12 Hour Extended Release Tablets (Less than 2%) 1923

Stomatitis, aphthous
Prozac Weekly Capsules (Infrequent) 1852

Stomatitis, ulcerative
▲ Agrylin Capsules (1% to less than 5%) 3017
AmBisome for Injection (Less common) 606
Anaprox Tablets (Less than 1%) 2632
Anaprox DS Tablets (Less than 1%) 2632
Bactroban Cream (Less than 1%) 1366
Copaxone for Injection (Frequent) 3110
Cosmegen for Injection 2485
▲ Doxil Injection (1% to 5%) 2378
EC-Naprosyn Delayed-Release Tablets (Less than 1%) 2632
▲ Evoxac Capsules (1% to 3%) 1013
Exelon Capsules (Infrequent) 2229
Exelon Oral Solution (Infrequent) 2229
Gabitril Tablets (Infrequent) 973
Indocin Capsules (Less than 1%) 2024
Indocin I.V. (Less than 1%) 2489
Indocin (Less than 1%) 2024
▲ Intron A for Injection (Less than 5%) 2859
Kaletra (Less than 2%) 452
Lipitor Tablets (Less than 2%) 2501
Lunesta Tablets (Infrequent) 2994
Lyrica Capsules (Rare) 2527
Mirapex Tablets 857
Mobic Oral Suspension (Less than 2%) 863
Mobic Tablets (Less than 2%) 863
Naprosyn Suspension (Less than 1%) 2632
Naprosyn Tablets (Less than 1%) 2632
Nexium Delayed-Release Capsules (Less than 1%) 645
Nexium I.V. (Less than 1%) 652
Nexium Delayed-Release Oral Suspension (Less than 1%) 645
▲ Novantrone for Injection Concentrate (10%) 1100
Paxil (Rare to infrequent) 1535
Paxil CR Controlled-Release Tablets (Rare to infrequent) 1544
PegIntron Powder for Injection 2903
Protonix for Delayed-Release Oral Suspension (Less than 1%) 3254
Protonix Delayed-Release Tablets (Less than 1%) 3254
Protonix I.V. (Less than 1%) 3257
Prozac Pulvules and Liquid (Infrequent) 1852
Remeron Tablets (Rare) 2924
RemeronSolTab Tablets (Rare) 2927
Requip Tablets (Infrequent) 1561
Risperdal Consta Long-Acting Injection (Infrequent) 1753
Selzentry Tablets (2.6%) 2534
▲ Simulect for Injection (3% to 10%) 2306
▲ Soriatane Capsules (1% to 10%) 3062
▲ Spiriva HandiHaler (1% to 3%) 870
Symbyax Capsules (Rare) 1871
Viramune Oral Suspension 873
Viramune Tablets 873
Zonegran Capsules (Infrequent) 1089
Zosyn for Injection (1% or less) 3284
Zyprexa Tablets (Infrequent) 1883
Zyprexa ZYDIS Orally Disintegrating Tablets (Infrequent) 1883
Zyrtec Chewable Tablets (Less than 2%) 1920
Zyrtec Syrup (Less than 2%) 1920
Zyrtec Tablets (Less than 2%) 1920
Zyrtec-D 12 Hour Extended Release Tablets (Less than 2%) 1923

Stool, bloody
(*see also under* Hematochezia)
Zyvox 2552

Stool, color changes
Lamisil Tablets 2266
Ortho-Cyclen/Ortho Tri-Cyclen 2449
Ortho Tri-Cyclen Lo Tablets 2458
Pepto-Bismol Original Liquid, Maximum Strength Liquid, Original and Cherry Tablets, Chewable Tablets and Easy-To-Swallow Caplets 2564

Stool, oily
▲ Xenical Capsules (5.5% to 20%) 2672

Stool frequency, increased
Lexapro Oral Suspension (Infrequent) 1174
Lexapro Tablets (Infrequent) 1174

Stools, abnormal
Asacol Delayed-Release Tablets (2% or greater) 2579
Effexor XR Extended-Release Capsules (Rare) 3195
Gabitril Tablets (Infrequent) 973
▲ Kaletra (Up to 6%) 452
Nexium Delayed-Release Capsules (Less than 1%) 645
Nexium I.V. (Less than 1%) 652
Nexium Delayed-Release Oral Suspension (Less than 1%) 645
Norvir (Less than 2%) 489
Omnicef Capsules (0.3%) 497
Omnicef for Oral Suspension (0.2%) 497
Pentasa Capsules (Less than 1%) 3030
▲ Pletal Tablets (12% to 15%) 2481
Protonix for Delayed-Release Oral Suspension (Less than 1%) 3254
Protonix Delayed-Release Tablets (Less than 1%) 3254
Protonix I.V. (Less than 1%) 3257
▲ Sandostatin Injection (Less than 10%) 2300
Tygacil for Injection (0% to less than 2%) 3276
Ultrase MT Capsules (1.5%) 719
Vicoprofen Tablets (Less than 1%) 533
Zosyn for Injection (1.9% to 2.4%) 3284
Zyban Sustained-Release Tablets 1692

Stools, dark
Ferralet 90 Tablets 2175
Pepto-Bismol Original Liquid, Original and Cherry Chewable Tablets & Caplets ▣ 613
Pepto-Bismol Maximum Strength Liquid ▣ 613

Stools, loose
▲ Amitiza Capsules (0% to 3%) 3082
▲ Augmentin (9%) 1323
▲ Augmentin Tablets (9%) 1327
Augmentin XR Extended Release Tablets (1.6%) 1333
▲ Avandamet Tablets (5%) 1336
Bios Life Drink Mix 3158
▲ Ceftin (8.6%) 1380
▲ Chemet Capsules (12% to 20.9%) 2484
Cialis Tablets (Less than 2%) 1792
▲ Cubicin for Injection (4.2%) 995
▲ Cymbalta Delayed-Release Capsules (2% to 3%) 1801
▲ Dacogen Injection (7%) 1066
Elidel Cream 1% (0% to 1.2%) 2221
Exforge Tablets (Less than or equal to 0.1%) 2238
▲ Gleevec Tablets (10% to 12%) 2255
▲ Intron A for Injection (Up to 10%) 2859
Invanz for Injection (2.1%) 2029
Ketek Tablets (Greater than or equal to 0.2% to less than 2%) 2744
▲ Myfortic Tablets (3% to less than 20%) 2276
Noroxin Tablets (0.3% to 1%) 2069
Requip Tablets (Infrequent) 1561
▲ Sandostatin Injection (34% to 61%) 2300
▲ Somatuline Depot Injection (Greater than 5% to 9%) 3102
▲ Suprax for Oral Suspension (6%) 1891
▲ Suprax Tablets (6%) 1891
▲ Sustiva Capsules (39%) 930
▲ Sustiva Tablets (39%) 930
▲ Trisenox Injection (10%) 986
Urocit-K Tablets (Some patients) 2176
Venlafaxine Hydrochloride Tablets (Rare) 2199
▲ Vivitrol (12% to 13%) 988
Zyvox (1.2% to 2.3%) 2552

Stools, watery
Augmentin Tablets 1327
Augmentin XR Extended Release Tablets 1333
Augmentin ES-600 Powder for Oral Suspension 1329
Avelox 2803
Biaxin/Biaxin XL 411
Ceftin 1380
Cipro 2810
Omnicef Capsules 497
Omnicef for Oral Suspension 497
Primaxin I.M. 2080
Primaxin I.V. 2083
Tygacil for Injection 3276
Zyvox 2552

Strabismus
Lamictal (Rare) 1488
Prozac Weekly Capsules (Rare) 1852
Prozac Pulvules and Liquid (Rare) 1852

Strain, muscle
Xyrem Oral Solution (Infrequent) 1766

Strangury
Evoxac Capsules (Less than 1%) 1013

Stress symptoms, unspecified
Ambien CR Tablets (1%) 2696
Requip Tablets (Infrequent) 1561
Xyrem Oral Solution (Infrequent) 1766

Striae
Analpram-HC 1140
Aricept Tablets (Infrequent) 1062
Aricept ODT Tablets (Infrequent) 1062
Copaxone for Injection (Infrequent) 3110
Diprolene Lotion 0.05% (Infrequent) 2838
Diprolene Ointment 0.05% 2839
Diprolene AF Cream 0.05% (Infrequent) 2837
Durezol Ophthalmic Emulsion (Less than 1%) ⊙ 275
Elocon Cream 0.1% (Infrequent) 2840
Elocon Lotion 0.1% (Infrequent) 2841
Elocon Ointment 0.1% (Infrequent) 2842
Lotrisone 2881
Lupron Depot-PED 7.5 mg, 11.25 mg and 15 mg (Less than 2%) 471
Luxíq Foam 3058
Olux Foam 3061
Olux-E Foam 3059
Pramosone 1141
Vanos Cream 1941
Venlafaxine Hydrochloride Tablets (Rare) 2199
Verdeso Foam 3069

Stridor
Advair Diskus 100/50 1276
Advair Diskus 250/50 1276
Advair Diskus 500/50 1276

Advair HFA 45/21 Inhalation Aerosol 1288
Advair HFA 115/21 Inhalation Aerosol 1288
Advair HFA 230/21 Inhalation Aerosol 1288
Erbitux 912
Fluarix Vaccine 1446
Fortaz 1450
Paxil (Rare) 1535
Paxil CR Controlled-Release Tablets (Rare) 1544
Photofrin for Injection 708
Prozac Weekly Capsules (Rare) 1852
Prozac Pulvules and Liquid (Rare) 1852
Refludan for Injection (Common) 795
Rilutek Tablets (Infrequent) 2771
Risperdal Consta Long-Acting Injection (Infrequent) 1753
Salagen Tablets (Less than 1%) 1082
Serevent Diskus (Rare) 1594
Thyrogen for Injection 1244
Ultane Liquid for Inhalation (Less than 1%) 524
Zofran Injection 1682
Zofran 1687
Zofran ODT Orally Disintegrating Tablets 1687
Zyprexa Tablets (Rare) 1883
Zyprexa ZYDIS Orally Disintegrating Tablets (Rare) 1883

Stroke

Accutane Capsules 2607
Activase I.V. (0.9%) 1188
Activella Tablets 2347
Actos Tablets 3077
Adderall XR Capsules 3012
Aggrenox Capsules (2%) 819
Amerge Tablets 1301
Angeliq Tablets 751
Aranesp for Injection (2%) 564
Avandia Tablets 1351
Cialis Tablets 1792
Climara Transdermal System 763
Climara Pro Transdermal System 768
Divigel 3167
Duetact Tablets 3085
DynaCirc CR Controlled Release Tablets (0.5% to 1%) 1407
Enbrel for Injection 569
Enjuvia Tablets 1029
Estratest Tablets 3043
Estratest H.S. Tablets 3043
Evista Tablets (Very rare) 1810
Flector Patch 561
Follistim AQ Cartridge 2844
Imitrex Injection 1465
Imitrex Tablets 1474
Integrilin Injection (0.5%) 2855
▲ Intron A for Injection (Less than 5%) 2859
Invega Extended-Release Tablets 1748
▲ Mavik Tablets (3.3%) 472
Maxalt Tablets 2056
Maxalt-MLT Orally Disintegrating Tablets 2056
Mobic Oral Suspension 863
Mobic Tablets 863
Ortho-Cyclen/Ortho Tri-Cyclen 2449
Premarin Intravenous 3217
▲ Premarin Tablets (45%) 3221
Premarin Vaginal Cream 3228
Premphase Tablets (1.55%) 3232
Prempro Tablets (1.55%) 3232
Prinivil Tablets (0.3% to 1%) 2087
Prinzide Tablets 2092
Procrit for Injection 2391
Proleukin for Injection (Less than 1%) 2287
Risperdal Consta Long-Acting Injection 1753
Soriatane Capsules 3062
Symbyax Capsules 1871
Treximet Tablets 1616
▲ Vesanoid Capsules (3%) 2660
Vicoprofen Tablets 533
Vyvanse Capsules 3033
Wellbutrin SR Sustained-Release Tablets (Infrequent) 1653
Wellbutrin XL Extended-Release Tablets (Infrequent) 1659
Zyban Sustained-Release Tablets (Infrequent) 1692

Stroke, hemorrhagic

Activase I.V. (0.7%) 1188
Femara Tablets (Less than or equal to 2%) 2246
Intelence Tablets (Less than or equal to 0.5%) 3119
Ortho-Cyclen/Ortho Tri-Cyclen 2449
Velcade for Injection 2168

Stroke, ischemic

▲ Premarin Tablets (38%) 3221

Stroke, new ischemic

Activase I.V. 1188
Vivitrol 988
Zolinza Capsules 2142

Stroke, thrombotic

Ortho-Cyclen/Ortho Tri-Cyclen 2449

Stuffiness, nasal

(*see under* Nasal congestion)

Stupor

Ambien Tablets (Infrequent) 2692
Ambien CR Tablets (Infrequent) 2696
Azilect Tablets 3106
Celexa (Rare) 1160
Copaxone for Injection (Frequent) 3110
Duragesic Transdermal System (Less than 1%) 2405
Effexor XR Extended-Release Capsules (Infrequent) 3195
Gabitril Tablets (Frequent) 973
▲ Gliadel Wafer (6%) 1076
▲ Invanz for Injection (3.3% to 5.1%) 2029
Lamictal (Infrequent) 1488
Lunesta Tablets (Rare) 2994
Luvox CR Extended-Release Capsules (Infrequent) 1759
Lyrica Capsules (Greater than or equal to 1%) 2527
Mirapex Tablets 857
Namenda (Infrequent) 1180
Orthoclone OKT3 Sterile Solution 2387
OxyContin Tablets (Less than 1%) 2589
Paxil (Rare) 1535
Paxil CR Controlled-Release Tablets (Rare) 1544
Percocet Tablets 1127
Percodan Tablets 1130
PhosLo GelCaps 1184
Proleukin for Injection (1%) 2287
Prozac Weekly Capsules (Rare) 1852
Prozac Pulvules and Liquid (Rare) 1852
Remeron Tablets (Rare) 2924
RemeronSolTab Tablets (Rare) 2927
Requip Tablets (Infrequent) 1561
Rilutek Tablets (Infrequent) 2771
Romazicon Injection (Less than 1%) 2646
Stromectol Tablets 2120
Venlafaxine Hydrochloride Tablets (Infrequent) 2199
Zyprexa Tablets (Infrequent) 1883
Zyprexa ZYDIS Orally Disintegrating Tablets (Infrequent) 1883

Stuttering

Zyprexa Tablets (Infrequent) 1883
Zyprexa ZYDIS Orally Disintegrating Tablets (Infrequent) 1883

Stye

▲ Intron A for Injection (Less than 5%) 2859
Klonopin (Infrequent) 2639

Subacute cutaneous lupus erythematosus-like reactions

Dyazide Capsules 1405
Lamisil Oral Granules 2264
Vytorin 10/10 Tablets 2939
Vytorin 10/20 Tablets 2939
Vytorin 10/40 Tablets 2939
Vytorin 10/80 Tablets 2939

Subcutaneous tissue disorders, unspecified

▲ Cancidas for Injection (25.4% to 42.2%) 1953
Lamisil Oral Granules 2264
▲ Mycamine for Injection (13% to 68.2%) 616
▲ Verdeso Foam (3%) 3069

Subdural effusion

▲ Gliadel Wafer (16%) 1076

Subgaleal effusion

▲ Gliadel Wafer (16%) 1076

Subileus

Tasigna Capsules 2316

Sudden Infant Death Syndrome

Infanrix Vaccine 1479
Pediarix Vaccine 1552

Suicidal ideation

Abilify Injection (Greater than or equal to 1 in 100 patients) 881
Abilify Injection (Greater than or equal to 1 in 100 patients) 2466
Abilify Oral Solution (Greater than or equal to 1 in 100 patients) 881
Abilify Oral Solution (Greater than or equal to 1 in 100 patients) 2466
Abilify Discmelt Orally Disintegrating Tablets (Greater than or equal to 1 in 100 patients) 881
Abilify Discmelt Orally Disintegrating Tablets (Greater than or equal to 1 in 100 patients) 2466
Abilify Tablets (Greater than or equal to 1 in 100 patients) 881
Abilify Tablets (Greater than or equal to 1 in 100 patients) 2466
Accutane Capsules 2607
Ambien CR Tablets (Rare) 2696
Avelox 2803
Betaseron for SC Injection 756
Campral Tablets (Infrequent) 1158
Chantix Tablets (Rare) 2511
Cipro 2810
Cipro XR Tablets 2823
Cymbalta Delayed-Release Capsules 1801
Effexor XR Extended-Release Capsules (Rare) 3195
Emsam Transdermal System 905
Exelon Capsules (Infrequent) 2229
Exelon Oral Solution (Infrequent) 2229
Intron A for Injection (Rare) 2859
▲ Keppra Injection (12.7%) 3137
Keppra Oral Solution 3131
Keppra Tablets 3131
Klonopin (Infrequent) 2639
Lamictal (Rare) 1488
Levaquin 2416
Levaquin in 5% Dextrose Injection 2416
Lexapro Oral Suspension (Infrequent) 1174
Lexapro Tablets (Infrequent) 1174
Lupron Depot 3.75 mg (Very rare) 462
Lupron Depot–3 Month 11.25 mg (Very rare) 462
Luvox CR Extended-Release Capsules 1759
Meridia Capsules 475
Namenda 1180
▲ Parnate Tablets (4%) 1532
Paxil 1535
Paxil CR Controlled-Release Tablets 1544
PegIntron Powder for Injection (Less than or equal to 1%) 2903
Pristiq Extended-Release Tablets 3247
Provigil Tablets 977
Prozac Weekly Capsules 1852
Prozac Pulvules and Liquid 1852
Rebetol 2917
Rebif Prefilled Syringe for Injection 1107
Remeron Tablets 2924
RemeronSolTab Tablets 2927
Seromycin Capsules 1864
Soriatane Capsules 3062
Stalevo Tablets 2309
Strattera Capsules (0.4%) 1864
Sustiva Capsules (0.7%) 930
Sustiva Tablets (0.7%) 930
Symbyax Capsules 1871
Velcade for Injection 2168
Venlafaxine Hydrochloride Tablets (Rare) 2199
Wellbutrin Tablets (Rare) 1648
Wellbutrin SR Sustained-Release Tablets (Infrequent) 1653
Wellbutrin XL Extended-Release Tablets (Infrequent) 1659
Xyzal Oral Solution 2789
Xyzal Oral Solution 3155
Zyban Sustained-Release Tablets (Infrequent) 1692
Zyrtec Chewable Tablets 1920
Zyrtec Syrup 1920
Zyrtec Tablets 1920

Suicidal tendency

Marplan Tablets 3177

Suicidality

Abilify Injection 881
Abilify Injection 2466
Abilify Oral Solution 881
Abilify Oral Solution 2466
Abilify Discmelt Orally Disintegrating Tablets 881
Abilify Discmelt Orally Disintegrating Tablets 2466
Abilify Tablets 881
Abilify Tablets 2466
Celexa 1160
Cymbalta Delayed-Release Capsules 1801
Effexor XR Extended-Release Capsules 3195
Emsam Transdermal System (Infrequent) 905
Keppra Injection 3137
Lexapro Oral Suspension 1174
Lexapro Tablets 1174
Marplan Tablets 3177
Paxil 1535
Paxil CR Controlled-Release Tablets 1544
Pristiq Extended-Release Tablets 3247
Prozac Weekly Capsules 1852
Prozac Pulvules and Liquid 1852
Remeron Tablets 2924
RemeronSolTab Tablets 2927
Singulair 2114
Symbyax Capsules 1871
Venlafaxine Hydrochloride Tablets 2199

Suicide

Abilify Injection (0.5%) 881
Abilify Injection (Greater than or equal to 1 in 1000 patients and less than 1 in 100 patients) 2466
Abilify Oral Solution (0.5%) 881
Abilify Oral Solution (Greater than or equal to 1 in 1000 patients and less than 1 in 100 patients) 2466
Abilify Discmelt Orally Disintegrating Tablets (0.5%) 881
Abilify Discmelt Orally Disintegrating Tablets (Greater than or equal to 1 in 1000 patients and less than 1 in 100 patients) 2466
Abilify Tablets (0.5%) 881
Abilify Tablets (Greater than or equal to 1 in 1000 patients and less than 1 in 100 patients) 2466
Aczone Gel 5% 3296
Aldara Cream, 5% 1699
Atripla Tablets 938
Chantix Tablets 2511
Cymbalta Delayed-Release Capsules (Rare) 1801
Intron A for Injection 2859
Keppra Injection 3137
Keppra Oral Solution 3131
Keppra Tablets 3131
Lovaza Capsules 1520
Lyrica Capsules (Rare) 2527
Meridia Capsules 475
Mirapex Tablets 857
Percocet Tablets 1127
Proleukin for Injection (Less than 1%) 2287
Singulair 2114
Zyrtec Chewable Tablets 1920
Zyrtec Syrup 1920
Zyrtec Tablets 1920

Suicide, attempt of

Abilify Injection (Greater than or equal to 1 in 1000 patients and less than 1 in 100 patients) 881
Abilify Injection (Greater than or equal to 1 in 1000 patients and less than 1 in 100 patients) 2466
Abilify Oral Solution (Greater than or equal to 1 in 1000 patients and less than 1 in 100 patients) 881
Abilify Oral Solution (Greater than or equal to 1 in 1000 patients and less than 1 in 100 patients) 2466
Abilify Discmelt Orally Disintegrating Tablets (Greater than or equal to 1 in 1000 patients and less than 1 in 100 patients) 881
Abilify Discmelt Orally Disintegrating Tablets (Greater than or equal to 1 in 1000 patients and less than 1 in 100 patients) 2466
Abilify Tablets (Greater than or equal to 1 in 1000 patients and less than 1 in 100 patients) 881
Abilify Tablets (Greater than or equal to 1 in 1000 patients and less than 1 in 100 patients) 2466
Accutane Capsules 2607
Ambien Tablets (Rare) 2692
Campral Tablets (Frequent) 1158
Celexa (Frequent) 1160

Cimzia 3127
Cipro 2810
Copaxone for Injection (Infrequent) 3110
Cymbalta Delayed-Release Capsules (Infrequent) 1801
Effexor XR Extended-Release Capsules (Infrequent) 3195
▲ Equetro Extended-Release Capsules (Less than 5%) 3174
Exelon Capsules (Infrequent) 2229
Exelon Oral Solution (Infrequent) 2229
Gabitril Tablets (Infrequent) 973
Imitrex Tablets (Rare) 1474
▲ Intron A for Injection (Rare; less than 5%) 2859
Keppra Injection (0.5%) 3137
Keppra Oral Solution (0.5%) 3131
Keppra Tablets (0.5%) 3131
Klonopin (Infrequent) 2639
Lamictal (Rare) 1488
Levaquin 2416
Levaquin in 5% Dextrose Injection 2416
Lexapro Oral Suspension (Infrequent) 1174
Lexapro Tablets (Infrequent) 1174
Lupron Depot 3.75 mg (Very rare) 462
Lupron Depot–3 Month 11.25 mg (Very rare) 462
Luvox CR Extended-Release Capsules (Infrequent) 1759
Lyrica Capsules (0.1% to 1%) 2527
Mirapex Tablets (Less than 1%) 857
Namenda (Infrequent) 1180
▲ Parnate Tablets (4%) 1532
Paxil 1535
Paxil CR Controlled-Release Tablets 1544
PegIntron Powder for Injection (Less than or equal to 1%) 2903
Prozac Weekly Capsules (Infrequent) 1852
Prozac Pulvules and Liquid (Infrequent) 1852
Rebif Prefilled Syringe for Injection 1107
Remicade for IV Injection (Greater than or equal to 0.2%) 950
Requip Tablets (Rare) 1561
Rilutek Tablets (Infrequent) 2771
▲ Risperdal Consta Long-Acting Injection (4%) 1753
Sandostatin LAR Depot 2302
Sustiva Capsules (0.5%) 930
Sustiva Tablets (0.5%) 930
Symbyax Capsules (Infrequent) 1871
Venlafaxine Hydrochloride Tablets (Infrequent) 2199
Zyprexa Tablets (Infrequent) 1883
Zyprexa ZYDIS Orally Disintegrating Tablets (Infrequent) 1883

Sulfhemoglobinemia
Gantrisin Pediatric Suspension 2638

Sulfite, sensitivity to
EpiPen 1024
Moban Tablets 1116
Pred Forte Ophthalmic Suspension ⊙ 227
Pred Mild Ophthalmic Suspension ⊙ 230
Tylenol with Codeine Tablets 2427

Sunburn
Accutane Capsules 2607
Benzaclin Topical Gel (1%) 2721
Diovan HCT Tablets (Less frequent) 2216
Mirapex Tablets 857
▲ Photofrin for Injection (4%) 708
ProQuad 2099
▲ Protopic Ointment (1% to 4%) 628
▲ Soriatane Capsules (1% to 10%) 3062
Xifaxan Tablets (Less than 2%) 2682

Sunburn, exacerbation of
Avelox 2803
Imitrex Injection 1465
Imitrex Nasal Spray 1470
Imitrex Tablets 1474

Sunburn reactions
Cipro I.V. 2817
Noroxin Tablets 2069

Superinfection
Augmentin 1323
Augmentin Tablets 1327
Augmentin XR Extended Release Tablets 1333
Ceftin 1380
Fortaz 1450
Iquix Ophthalmic Solution 3183
Moxatag Tablets 2165
Primaxin I.M. 2080
Rocephin Injectable Vials, ADD-Vantage, Galaxy, Bulk 2642
Suprax for Oral Suspension 1891
Suprax Tablets 1891
Zinacef for Injection 1678
Zinacef Injection 1678

Superior Vena Cava Syndrome
(*see under* SVC Syndrome)

Supraventricular contractions, premature
Paxil (Rare) 1535
Paxil CR Controlled-Release Tablets (Rare) 1544

Surgery
▲ Humira Injection (Less than 5%) 442
Yaz Tablets (Greater than 1%) 805

Surgical site reaction, unspecified
▲ Arixtra Injection (0.8% to 3.2%) 1313

Suture-related complications
▲ Supprelin LA Implant (6.4%) 1731

SVC Syndrome
BeneFIX Vials 3191

Swallowing, difficulty
Geodon 2520
Moban Tablets 1116
Provigil Tablets 977
Risperdal Consta Long-Acting Injection 1753
Symbyax Capsules 1871
Thiothixene Capsules 2197
Xifaxan Tablets 2682
Zostavax Injection 2145
Zyprexa Tablets 1883
Zyprexa IntraMuscular 1883
Zyprexa ZYDIS Orally Disintegrating Tablets 1883

Swallowing, impairment
Captopril Tablets 2182
Cubicin for Injection 995
Dantrium Capsules (Rare) 2580
Dantrium Intravenous 2582
Emend Capsules (Greater than 0.5%) 1992
Emend for Injection (Greater than 0.5%) 1999
Gengraf Capsules (Rare) 435
Imitrex Injection 1465
Imitrex Nasal Spray 1470
Januvia Tablets 2048
Levaquin 2416
Levaquin in 5% Dextrose Injection 2416
Lexapro Oral Suspension (Infrequent) 1174
Lexapro Tablets (Infrequent) 1174
Mavik Tablets 472
Neoral Oral Solution (Rare) 2280
Neoral Soft Gelatin Capsules (Rare) 2280
Orthoclone OKT3 Sterile Solution 2387
Prinivil Tablets 2087
Prinzide Tablets 2092
Sandimmune (Rare) 2296
Thioridazine Hydrochloride Tablets 2195

Sweat, cold
Amitiza Capsules (Less than 1%) 3082
Cymbalta Delayed-Release Capsules (Infrequent) 1801
Fentora Tablets (Greater than 1%) 968
Mirapex Tablets 857
Requip Tablets (Infrequent) 1561
Xyrem Oral Solution (Infrequent) 1766

Sweat discoloration
Stalevo Tablets 2309

Sweat gland disorder
Soriatane Capsules (Less than 1%) 3062

Sweating
(*see under* Diaphoresis)

Sweating, decreased
(*see under* Hypohidrosis)

Sweating, increased
Advate (0.6%) 721
Ambien CR Tablets (Infrequent) 2696
Anzemet Tablets 2704
Celebrex Capsules (0.1% to 1.9%) 2979
Cipro XR Tablets 2823
Coreg CR Extended-Release Capsules (0.1% to less than or equal to 1%) 1393
▲ DepoCyt Injection (2% to 3%) 1136
▲ DepoDur Injection (2% to 5%) 1095
Eligard 7.5 mg (Less than 2%) 2724
Eligard 22.5 mg (Less than 2%) 2724
Eligard 30 mg (Less than 2%) 2724
Eligard 45 mg (Less than 2%) 2724
Elmiron Capsules 2435
Exforge Tablets (Greater than 0.1% to less than 1%) 2238
Ketek Tablets (Greater than or equal to 0.2% to less than 2%) 2744
Levothroid Tablets 1170
▲ Lexapro Oral Suspension (3% to 8%) 1174
▲ Lexapro Tablets (3% to 8%) 1174
Mobic Oral Suspension (Less than 2%) 863
Mobic Tablets (Less than 2%) 863
▲ Nalfon Capsules (4.6%) 2508
▲ Neupro Transdermal System (4%) 3149
▲ Norditropin Cartridges (8%) 2354
▲ Noxafil Oral Suspension (2% to 10%) 2889
▲ Opana Tablets (1% to less than 10%) 1117
▲ Opana ER Tablets (8.6% to greater than or equal to 10%) 1121
Percodan Tablets 1130
Remicade for IV Injection (Greater than or equal to 0.2%) 950
Risperdal Consta Long-Acting Injection (Infrequent) 1753
Rythmol SR Capsules 1590
Stalevo Tablets (2%) 2309
▲ Strattera Capsules (4%) 1864
Toprol-XL Tablets 666
▲ Trisenox Injection (13%) 986
▲ Ultram ER Extended-Release Tablets (1.5% to 6.4%) 2428
Vantas (Less than 2%) 1737
Visudyne for Injection 2332
Voltaren Tablets (Occasionally) 2334
Voltaren-XR Tablets (Occasionally) 2337
Xifaxan Tablets (Less than 2%) 2682
Zometa for Intravenous Infusion 2341
Zyrtec Chewable Tablets (Less than 2%) 1920
Zyrtec Syrup (Less than 2%) 1920
Zyrtec Tablets (Less than 2%) 1920
Zyrtec-D 12 Hour Extended Release Tablets (Less than 2%) 1923

Sweating, non-axillary
▲ BOTOX Purified Neurotoxin Complex (3% to 10%) 550

Sweats, night
Eligard 7.5 mg (Less than 2%) 2724
Eligard 22.5 mg (Less than 2%) 2724
▲ Eligard 30 mg (Less than 2% to 3.3%) 2724
Eligard 45 mg (2.7%) 2724
Mirapex Tablets 857
Ultram ER Extended-Release Tablets (0.5% to less than 1%) 2428

Sweet's syndrome
Gleevec Tablets (Rare) 2255
Neulasta Injection 587
Neupogen for Injection 589
▲ Vesanoid Capsules (3%) 2660

Swelling, auricular
Concerta Extended-Release Tablets 1925

Swelling, breast
Demser Capsules (Infrequent) 1989

Swelling, edematous, ankles
Estratest Tablets 3043
Estratest H.S. Tablets 3043
Klonopin (Infrequent) 2639
Ortho-Cyclen/Ortho Tri-Cyclen 2449

Swelling, extremities
Avalide Tablets 892
Avalide Tablets 2713
Avapro Tablets (Less than 1%) 897
Avapro Tablets (Less than 1%) 2718
Imitrex Injection (Rare) 1465
Imitrex Nasal Spray (Rare) 1470
Infanrix Vaccine 1479
Noroxin Tablets (Less frequent) 2069
Pediarix Vaccine 1552

Swelling, facial
Aczone Gel 5% 3296
Cancidas for Injection 1953
Carafate Suspension 706
Carafate Tablets 707
▲ Dacogen Injection (6%) 1066
▲ Doxil Injection (Approximately 6.8%) 2378
Fluarix Vaccine 1446
Flulaval Injection Vaccine (1%) 1448
Imitrex Nasal Spray (Rare) 1470
Intelence Tablets (Less than or equal to 0.5%) 3119
Janumet Tablets 2041
Januvia Tablets 2048
Levaquin 2416
Levaquin in 5% Dextrose Injection 2416
Motrin IB Tablets and Caplets 1900
Children's Motrin Oral Suspension 1901
Children's Motrin Non-Staining Dye-Free Oral Suspension 1901
Children's Motrin Cold Oral Suspension 1899
Infants' Motrin Concentrated Drops 1901
Infants' Motrin Non-Staining Dye-Free Concentrated Drops 1901
Junior Strength Motrin Caplets and Chewable Tablets 1901
MoviPrep Oral Solution 2679
Mycamine for Injection 616
Nadolol Tablets (1 to 5 of 1000 patients) 2191
OsmoPrep Tablets 2680
Proscar Tablets 2102
Provigil Tablets 977
Reyataz Capsules 3299
Tamiflu Capsules 2649
Tamiflu Oral Suspension 2649
Tasigna Capsules (0.1% to 1%) 2316
Xifaxan Tablets 2682

Swelling, feet
K-Phos Neutral Tablets 813
▲ Prometrium Capsules (100 mg, 200 mg) (6%) 3047
Uroqid-Acid No. 2 Tablets 814

Swelling, hands
▲ Prometrium Capsules (100 mg, 200 mg) (6%) 3047

Swelling, joint
Advate (0.6%) 721
Amitiza Capsules (Less than 1%) 3082
Ceftin for Oral Suspension (0.1% to 1%) 1380
Cipro 2810
Cozaar Tablets (Less than 1%) 1973
Exforge Tablets (Greater than or equal to 0.2%) 2238
Fosamax 2005
Fosamax Plus D Tablets 2013
Gleevec Tablets (Less common) 2255
Imitrex Injection (Infrequent) 1465
Lunesta Tablets (Infrequent) 2994
Mirapex Tablets 857
Requip Tablets (Infrequent) 1561
Tasigna Capsules 2316
Ultram ER Extended-Release Tablets (0.5% to less than 1%) 2428
Xyrem Oral Solution (Infrequent) 1766

Swelling, legs
K-Phos Neutral Tablets 813
Uroqid-Acid No. 2 Tablets 814

Swelling, lower legs
(*see under* Swelling, legs)

Swelling, mouth
Boostrix (Rarely) 1377
Fluarix Vaccine 1446
Infanrix Vaccine 1479
Pediarix Vaccine (Rare) 1552

Swelling, non-site specific
Amerge Tablets (Infrequent) 1301
Bactroban Ointment (Less than 1%) 1368
Cancidas for Injection 1953
▲ Doxil Injection (3.4%) 2378
▲ Flulaval Injection Vaccine (6% to 10%) 1448
Oncaspar Injection 1138
▲ Panretin Gel 0.1% (3% to 8%) 1081
Recombivax HB (Equal to or greater than 1%) 2107
Serevent Diskus (1% to less than 3%) 1594
Sulfamylon Cream 2194
Sulfamylon for 5% Topical Solution 2194
Vaqta (Less than 1%) 2130

Swelling, oropharyngeal
Xyrem Oral Solution (Infrequent) 1766

Swelling, peripheral
▲ Genotropin Lyophilized Powder (0% to 17.5%) 2547
Ultram ER Extended-Release Tablets (0.5% to less than 1%) 2428

Swelling, unspecified
Advair Diskus 100/50 1276
Advair Diskus 250/50 1276

Advair Diskus 500/50 1276
Amitiza Capsules 3082
Erbitux 912
Neosporin Ophthalmic Solution Sterile ⊙252
▲ Pediarix Vaccine (1% to 22.3%) 1552
Pentacel 2792
ProQuad 2099
Tylenol Chest Congestion Caplets with Cool Burst 1910
Tylenol Chest Congestion Liquid with Cool Burst 1910
Tylenol Cold Severe Congestion Daytime Caplets with Cool Burst 1912
Vytorin 10/10 Tablets 2149
Vytorin 10/20 Tablets 2149
Vytorin 10/40 Tablets 2149
Vytorin 10/80 Tablets 2149

Swelling at application site

Daytrana Transdermal Patch 3022

Swelling at injection site

Attenuvax 1951
▲ Boostrix (0.5% to 38.9%) 1377
Cancidas for Injection 1953
Cerezyme for Injection (Less than 1%) 1238
Cipro I.V. (1% or less) 2817
▲ Comvax (27.2% to 27.6%) 1966
▲ Dacogen Injection (5%) 1066
Eloxatin for Injection 2731
▲ Enbrel for Injection (37%) 569
▲ Engerix-B Vaccine (1% to 10%) 1409
▲ Fluarix Vaccine (9.3% to 16.7%) 1446
Forteo for Injection (Less than 1/30 patients) 1816
▲ Gardasil Injection (0.6% to 25.4%) 2019
▲ Havrix Injection Vaccine (1% to 10%) 1454
Humalog-Pen and KwikPen 1829
Humalog Mix 50/50-Pen and KwikPen 1833
▲ Humira Injection (20%) 442
Humulin 50/50, 100 Units 1843
Humulin 70/30 Vial (Occasional) 1844
Humulin N Vial (Occasional) 1846
Humulin R (Occasionally) 1849
Humulin R (U-500) 1850
Hyalgan Solution (Common) 2742
Imitrex Injection 1465
▲ Infanrix Vaccine (0.7% to 32.9%) 1479
Invanz for Injection (1.8%) 2029
▲ Kinrix Injection Vaccine (26%) 1486
▲ Leustatin Injection (9% to 19%) 2384
M-M-R II 2054
Novantrone for Injection Concentrate 1100
Pediarix Vaccine 1552
Liquid PedvaxHIB (0.9% to 2.5%) 2073
▲ Pentacel (0% to 9.7%) 2792
Pneumovax 23 (Common) 2078
▲ ProQuad (8.4%) 2099
Risperdal Consta Long-Acting Injection (1%) 1753
Taxotere Injection Concentrate 2773
Timentin ADD-Vantage 1606
Timentin Injection Galaxy Container 1609
Timentin IV Infusion 1603
Timentin Pharmacy Bulk Package 1613
Traumeel Injection Solution 1725
▲ Twinrix Vaccine (4% to 6%) 1628
Vaprisol (2.7%) 632
▲ Vaqta (1.3% to 13.8%) 2130
▲ Varivax (19.3% to 32.5%) 2133
▲ Vivitrol (8% to 32%) 988
Zeel Injection Solution 1726
▲ Zostavax Injection (24.9%) 2145

Swelling at insertion site

▲ Supprelin LA Implant (51.1%) 1731
Vantas (0.7%) 1737

Syncope

Abilify Injection (0.3% to 0.5%) 881
Abilify Injection (0.3% to 0.6%) 2466
Abilify Oral Solution (0.3% to 0.5%) 881
Abilify Oral Solution (0.3% to 0.6%) 2466
Abilify Discmelt Orally Disintegrating Tablets (0.3% to 0.5%) 881
Abilify Discmelt Orally Disintegrating Tablets (0.3% to 0.6%) 2466
Abilify Tablets (0.3% to 0.5%) 881
Abilify Tablets (0.3% to 0.6%) 2466
Accutane Capsules 2607
Aceon Tablets (2 mg, 4 mg, 8 mg) (0.3% to 1%) 3038
▲ Acetadote Injection (0.64% to 3.04%) 1001
Actimmune (Rare) 1743
Actonel with Calcium Tablets (0.6% to 2.1%) 2574
Advair Diskus 100/50 1276
Advair Diskus 250/50 1276
Advair Diskus 500/50 1276
Advicor Tablets 402
▲ Aerobid/Aerobid-M (1% to 3%) 1153
Aggrenox Capsules (1%) 819
▲ Agrylin Capsules (1% to less than 5%) 3017
Aldara Cream, 5% 1699
Alinia for Oral Suspension (Less than 1%) 2677
Alinia Tablets (Less than 1%) 2677
Ambien Tablets (Infrequent) 2692
Ambien CR Tablets (Infrequent) 2696
Amerge Tablets (Infrequent) 1301
Amitiza Capsules (Less than 1%) 3082
Amrix Capsules 966
Anaprox Tablets (Less than 1%) 2632
Anaprox DS Tablets (Less than 1%) 2632
Angiomax for Injection (Greater than 0.1% to less than 1%) 1933
Anzemet Injection (Rare) 2701
Anzemet Tablets (Rare) 2704
Aricept Tablets (2%) 1062
Aricept ODT Tablets (2%) 1062
Attenuvax 1951
Avalide Tablets 892
Avalide Tablets 2713
Avapro Tablets 897
Avapro Tablets 2718
▲ Avastin IV (3%) 1192
Avelox (Less than 0.1%) 2803
▲ Avinza Capsules (Less than 5%) 1772
Axert Tablets (Rare) 2431
Azilect Tablets (Greater than 1%) 3106
Bentyl Capsules 703
Bentyl Injection 703
Bentyl Syrup 703
Bentyl Tablets 703
Betimol Ophthalmic Solution 3181
Bicillin C-R Injectable Suspension 1775
Bicillin L-A Injection 1777
Bystolic Tablets 1155
Campath Ampules 761
Campral Tablets (Frequent) 1158
Captopril Tablets 2182
Carbatrol Capsules 3019
Cardizem LA Extended Release Tablets (Less than 2%) 421
Catapres Tablets (Rare) 841
Catapres-TTS (0.5% or less) 842
Celebrex Capsules (Less than 0.1%) 2979
Celexa (Infrequent) 1160
▲ CellCept Capsules (3% to less than 20%) 2622
▲ CellCept Intravenous (3% to less than 20%) 2622
▲ CellCept Oral Suspension (3% to less than 20%) 2622
▲ CellCept Tablets (3% to less than 20%) 2622
Chantix Tablets (Infrequent) 2511
Cialis Tablets (Less than 2%) 1792
Cipro I.V. (1% or less) 2817
Cipro (Less than 1%) 2810
Cipro XR Tablets (Less than 1%) 2823
Cleviprex (Less than 1%) 1936
Clinoril Tablets (Less than 1%) 1962
Combigan Ophthalmic Solution 553
Comtan Tablets 2208
Comvax 1966
▲ Copaxone for Injection (5%) 3110
▲ Coreg Tablets (3% to 8%) 1387
▲ Coreg CR Extended-Release Capsules (3% to 8%) 1393
Cosopt Sterile Ophthalmic Solution 1969
Cozaar Tablets (Less than 1%) 1973
Crinone 4% Gel 992
Crinone 8% Gel 992
Cymbalta Delayed-Release Capsules 1801
Demadex Injection 2630
Demadex Tablets 2630
▲ DepoCyt Injection (3%) 1136
Diovan Tablets (Greater than 0.2%) 2212
Diovan HCT Tablets (Less frequent) 2216
Doxil Injection (Less than 1%) 2378
Duragesic Transdermal System (1% or greater) 2405
DynaCirc CR Controlled Release Tablets (0.5% to 1%) 1407
EC-Naprosyn Delayed-Release Tablets (Less than 1%) 2632
Edex Injection (Less than 1%) 2957
Effexor XR Extended-Release Capsules (Infrequent) 3195
▲ Eldepryl Capsules (7 of 49 patients) 3052
Eligard 7.5 mg (Less than 2%) 2724
Eligard 22.5 mg (Less than 2%) 2724
Eligard 30 mg (Less than 2%) 2724
Eligard 45 mg (Less than 2%) 2724
▲ Eloxatin for Injection (2% to less than 5%) 2731
Emend Capsules (Greater than 0.5%) 1992
Emend for Injection (Greater than 0.5%) 1999
Emsam Transdermal System (Infrequent) 905
Engerix-B Vaccine 1409
Equetro Extended-Release Capsules 3174
Evoxac Capsules (Less than 1%) 1013
▲ Exelon Capsules (3%) 2229
▲ Exelon Oral Solution (3%) 2229
Exforge Tablets (Greater than 0.1% to less than 1%) 2238
Fleet Bisacodyl Laxatives 1143
▲ Flolan for Injection (7%) 1426
Flomax Capsules (0.2% to 0.4%) 848
Flulaval Injection Vaccine 1448
Flumadine (Less than 0.3%) 1167
Fluorescite Injection ⊙203
Forteo for Injection (2.6%) 1816
Frova Tablets (Rare) 1111
Gabitril Tablets (Frequent) 973
Gantrisin Pediatric Suspension 2638
Gardasil Injection 2019
Geodon (0.6%) 2520
Gleevec Tablets (Infrequent) 2255
Havrix Injection Vaccine 1454
▲ Humira Injection (Less than 5%) 442
Imitrex Injection (Infrequent) 1465
Imitrex Nasal Spray (Infrequent) 1470
Imitrex Tablets (Rare to infrequent) 1474
Indocin (Less than 1%) 2024
Intelence Tablets (Less than 2%) 3119
▲ Intron A for Injection (Less than 5%) 2859
Invanz for Injection (Greater than 0.1%) 2029
Invega Extended-Release Tablets 1748
Ionsys Transdermal System (.1% to less than 1%) 2410
Ixempra Kit for Injection 915
Ketek Tablets 2744
Lamictal (Infrequent) 1488
Leukine 774
Levaquin (0.1% to 1%) 2416
Levaquin in 5% Dextrose Injection (0.1% to 1%) 2416
Levitra Tablets (Less than 2%) 2876
Lexapro Oral Suspension (Infrequent) 1174
Lexapro Tablets (Infrequent) 1174
Lipitor Tablets (Less than 2%) 2501
Lovaza Capsules 1520
Lupron Depot 3.75 mg (Among most frequent) 462
▲ Lupron Depot–3 Month 11.25 mg (Less than 5%) 462
Lupron Depot-PED 7.5 mg, 11.25 mg and 15 mg (Less than 2%) 471
Luvox CR Extended-Release Capsules (Frequent) 1759
Lyrica Capsules (0.1% to 1%) 2527
Marplan Tablets (0% to 2%) 3177
▲ Mavik Tablets (0.2% to 5.9%) 472
Maxair Autohaler 1705
Maxalt Tablets (Rare) 2056
Maxalt-MLT Orally Disintegrating Tablets (Rare) 2056
Meridia Capsules 475
Merrem I.V. (Greater than 0.1% to 1%) 684
Meruvax II 2061
Micardis Tablets 852
Micardis HCT Tablets 854
Mirapex Tablets (1% or more) 857
Mirena Intrauterine System 779
M-M-R II 2054
Mobic Oral Suspension (Less than 2%) 863
Mobic Tablets (Less than 2%) 863
MS Contin Tablets (Less frequent) 2585
Mumpsvax 2068
Namenda (Frequent) 1180
Naprosyn Suspension (Less than 1%) 2632
Naprosyn Tablets (Less than 1%) 2632
Nembutal Sodium Solution, USP (Less than 1%) 2494
Neupro Transdermal System 3149
Niaspan Extended-Release Tablets 480
▲ Nitro-Dur Transdermal Infusion System (4%) 2887
Norvir (0.6% to 1.7%) 489
Opana Tablets (Less than 1%) 1117
Opana ER Tablets (Less than 1%) 1121
Ortho-Cyclen Tablets 2449
Ortho Evra Transdermal System 2437
Ortho Tri-Cyclen Tablets 2449
OxyContin Tablets (Less than 1%) 2589
Paxil (Frequent) 1535
Paxil CR Controlled-Release Tablets (Frequent) 1544
Plavix Tablets (1% to 2.5%) 926
Plavix Tablets (1% to 2.5%) 2767
Pletal Tablets (Less than 2%) 2481
Prinivil Tablets (0.3% to 1%) 2087
Prinzide Tablets (0.8% to 0.1%) 2092
Pristiq Extended-Release Tablets (Less than 2%) 3247
Prograf Capsules and Injection 622
Proleukin for Injection (Less than 1%) 2287
Prometrium Capsules (100 mg, 200 mg) (Rare) 3047
ProQuad 2099
Protonix for Delayed-Release Oral Suspension (Less than 1%) 3254
Protonix Delayed-Release Tablets (Less than 1%) 3254
Protonix I.V. (Less than 1%) 3257
Protopic Ointment (0.2% to less than 1%) 628
Provigil Tablets (1%) 977
Prozac Weekly Capsules (Infrequent) 1852
Prozac Pulvules and Liquid (Infrequent) 1852
▲ Pulmicort Flexhaler (Greater than or equal to 1% to 3%) 654
Recombivax HB 2107
Relenza Inhalation Powder 1556
Remeron Tablets (Infrequent) 2924
RemeronSolTab Tablets (Infrequent) 2927
Remicade for IV Injection (Greater than or equal to 0.2%) 950
▲ Requip Tablets (3% to 12%) 1561
Requip XL Tablets 1568
Retrovir Capsules 1574
Retrovir IV Infusion 1579
Retrovir 1574
Reyataz Capsules 3299
Rilutek Tablets (Infrequent) 2771
Risperdal Consta Long-Acting Injection 1753
Rythmol Tablets (2%) 1586
Rythmol SR Capsules 1590
Salagen Tablets (Less than 1%) 1082
Sanctura XR Capsules 557
Sandostatin Injection (Less than 1%) 2300
Soma Tablets 1931
Stalevo Tablets (1.2%) 2309
▲ Strattera Capsules (0.8% to 3%) 1864
Sular Extended Release Tablets (Less than or equal to 1%) 2975
Sustiva Capsules (Less than 2%) 930
Sustiva Tablets (Less than 2%) 930
Symbyax Capsules 1871
Targretin Capsules 1084
Tarka Tablets (0.1% to 0.3% or more) 511
Taxotere Injection Concentrate (0.5% to 1.6%) 2773
Thiothixene Capsules 2197
Timoptic Sterile Ophthalmic Solution (Less frequent) 2121
Timoptic in Ocudose (Less frequent) 2124
Timoptic-XE Sterile Ophthalmic Gel Forming Solution 2125
Toprol-XL Tablets (Greater than 1%) 666
Twinrix Vaccine (Less than 1%) 1628
Ultane Liquid for Inhalation (Less than 1%) 524
▲ Ultram ER Extended-Release Tablets (1% to less than 5%) 2428
Uroxatral Tablets (0.2%) 2786
Venlafaxine Hydrochloride Tablets (Infrequent) 2199
Viadur Implant (Rare) 802
Visudyne for Injection (Less than 1%) 2332
▲ Vivitrol (13% to 16%) 988
Voltaren Tablets (Occasionally) 2334
Voltaren-XR Tablets (Occasionally) 2337
Wellbutrin Tablets (1.2%) 1648
Wellbutrin SR Sustained-Release Tablets (Rare) 1653
Wellbutrin XL Extended-Release Tablets (Rare) 1659
▲ Xeloda Tablets (Less than 5%) 2662
Xifaxan Tablets (Less than 2%) 2682
▲ Xolair (14%) 1235
▲ Xolair (14%) 2339

Xopenex Inhalation Solution 3001
Xopenex Inhalation Solution Concentrate 3005
Xopenex HFA Inhalation Aerosol 3009
Xyrem Oral Solution (Infrequent) 1766
Xyzal Oral Solution (0.2%) 2789
Xyzal Oral Solution (0.2%) 3155
Xyzal Tablets (0.2%) 2789
Xyzal Tablets (0.2%) 3155
Zofran Injection (Rare) 1682
Zolinza Capsules 2142
Zometa for Intravenous Infusion 2341
Zomig Tablets (Infrequent) 694
Zomig Nasal Spray (Infrequent) 689
Zomig-ZMT Tablets (Infrequent) 694
Zonegran Capsules (Infrequent) 1089
Zosyn for Injection (1% or less) 3284
Zyban Sustained-Release Tablets (Rare) 1692
Zyprexa Tablets (0.6%) 1883
Zyprexa IntraMuscular (Infrequent) 1883
Zyprexa ZYDIS Orally Disintegrating Tablets (0.6%) 1883
Zyrtec Chewable Tablets (Less than 2%) 1920
Zyrtec Syrup (Less than 2%) 1920
Zyrtec Tablets (Less than 2%) 1920
Zyrtec-D 12 Hour Extended Release Tablets (Less than 2%) 1923

Syncope, vasovagal

Cimzia 3127
Mirapex Tablets 857
Requip Tablets (Infrequent) 1561

Synovitis

Actiq (Less than 1%) 959
Celebrex Capsules (0.1% to 1.9%) 2979
Cuprimine Capsules 1986
Evoxac Capsules (Less than 1%) 1013
▲ Humira Injection (Less than 5%) 442
Requip Tablets (Infrequent) 1561
▲ Stromectol Tablets (9.3%) 2120

Systemic inflammatory response syndrome

Clolar for Intravenous Infusion 1239

Systolic blood pressure, decreased

Agrylin Capsules 3017
▲ Lexiscan Injection (7%) 614
▲ Neupro Transdermal System (5% to 7%) 3149

T

T3, decrease

Estratest Tablets 3043
Estratest H.S. Tablets 3043
Premarin Tablets 3221

T3, increase

Premphase Tablets 3232
Prempro Tablets 3232

T4, increase

Activella Tablets 2347
Enjuvia Tablets 1029
Estratest Tablets 3043
Estratest H.S. Tablets 3043
Ortho-Cyclen/Ortho Tri-Cyclen 2449
Premarin Tablets 3221
Premphase Tablets 3232
Prempro Tablets 3232

Tachyarrhythmia

Actimmune (Rare) 1743
Amerge Tablets (Infrequent) 1301

Tachyarrhythmia, ventricular

Avelox 2803
Frova Tablets 1111
Levaquin Oral Solution (0.1% to 0.9%) 2416

Tachyarrhythmias, supraventricular

Lanoxin Injection 1498
Lanoxin Injection Pediatric 1502
Lanoxin Tablets 1505

Tachycardia

Abilify Injection (2%) 881
Abilify Injection 2466
Abilify Oral Solution (2%) 881
Abilify Oral Solution 2466
Abilify Discmelt Orally Disintegrating Tablets (2%) 881
Abilify Discmelt Orally Disintegrating Tablets 2466
Abilify Tablets (2%) 881
Abilify Tablets 2466
Accutane Capsules 2607
▲ Acetadote Injection (3% to 5%) 1001
Actiq (Less than 1%) 959
▲ Adderall XR Capsules (6%) 3012
Adipex-P 1185
▲ Advair HFA 45/21 Inhalation Aerosol (1% to 3%) 1288
▲ Advair HFA 115/21 Inhalation Aerosol (1% to 3%) 1288
▲ Advair HFA 230/21 Inhalation Aerosol (1% to 3%) 1288
Advicor Tablets 402
▲ Aerobid/Aerobid-M (1% to 3%) 1153
Aggrenox Capsules (Less than 1%) 819
▲ Agrylin Capsules (7.5%) 3017
Albutein 5% 1707
Albutein 25% 1708
Aldara Cream, 5% 1699
Alinia for Oral Suspension (Less than 1%) 2677
Alinia Tablets (Less than 1%) 2677
Allegra-D 12 Hour Extended-Release Tablets 2687
Allegra-D 24 Hour Extended-Release Tablets 2690
Aloxi Injection (1%) 1059
Alphagan P Ophthalmic Solution 549
Ambien Tablets (Infrequent) 2692
Ambien CR Tablets (Infrequent) 2696
▲ AmBisome for Injection (9.4% to 18.5%) 606
Amrix Capsules 966
Anaprox Tablets (Less than 1%) 2632
Anaprox DS Tablets (Less than 1%) 2632
▲ Anzemet Injection (2.2% to 3.3%) 2701
▲ Anzemet Tablets (2.2% to 3.3%) 2704
Atacand Tablets (0.5% or greater) 639
Atacand HCT (0.5% or greater) 642
Atrovent HFA Inhalation Aerosol 839
Atrovent Nasal Spray 0.03% 834
Atrovent Nasal Spray 0.06% (Less than 1%) 836
Avalide Tablets (1%) 892
Avalide Tablets (1%) 2713
Avapro Tablets (1% or greater) 897
Avapro Tablets (1% or greater) 2718
Avelox (Greater than or equal to 0.1% to less than 2%) 2803
▲ Avinza Capsules (Less than 5%) 1772
Axert Tablets (Infrequent) 2431
Bayer Aspirin 750
BeneFIX Vials 3191
Benicar Tablets (Greater than 0.5%) 1009
Bentyl Capsules 703
Bentyl Injection 703
Bentyl Syrup 703
Bentyl Tablets 703
▲ Betaseron for SC Injection (4%) 756
Bicillin C-R Injectable Suspension 1775
Bicillin L-A Injection 1777
Brovana Inhalation Solution 2990
▲ Busulfex Injection (44%) 2477
▲ Campath Ampules (10%) 761
Campral Tablets (Infrequent) 1158
▲ Cancidas for Injection (3.5% to 10.7%) 1953
Captopril Tablets (Approximately 1 of 100 patients) 2182
▲ Cardene I.V. (3.5%) 1093
Cardizem LA Extended Release Tablets (Less than 2%) 421
Catapres Tablets (About 5 in 1,000 patients) 841
Catapres-TTS (0.5% or less) 842
Ceftin Tablets (0.1% to 1%) 1380
Celebrex Capsules (0.1% to 1.9%) 2979
Celexa (Frequent) 1160
▲ CellCept Capsules (3% to 22%) 2622
▲ CellCept Intravenous (3% to 22%) 2622
▲ CellCept Oral Suspension (3% to 22%) 2622
▲ CellCept Tablets (3% to 22%) 2622
▲ Cerezyme for Injection (Approximately 6.5%) 1238
Chantix Tablets (Infrequent) 2511
Cialis Tablets (Less than 2%) 1792
Cipro I.V. (1% or less) 2817
Cipro (Less than 1%) 2810
Cipro XR Tablets 2823
Clarinex Syrup 2828
Clarinex Tablets 2828
Clarinex Reditabs Tablets 2828
Clarinex-D 12-Hour Extended-Release Tablets 2831
Clarinex-D 24-Hour Extended-Release Tablets 2834
Clinoril Tablets (Less than 1 in 100) 1962
▲ Clolar for Intravenous Infusion (34%) 1239
Clorpres Tablets (About 5 in 1,000) 2185
Combigan Ophthalmic Solution 553
Combivent Inhalation Aerosol (Less than 2%) 845
Comvax 1966
▲ Concerta Extended-Release Tablets (4.8%) 1925
▲ Copaxone for Injection (5%) 3110
Coreg Tablets (Greater than 0.1% to 1%) 1387
Coreg CR Extended-Release Capsules (0.1% to less than or equal to 1%) 1393
Cozaar Tablets (Less than 1%) 1973
Cymbalta Delayed-Release Capsules (Infrequent) 1801
Dacogen Injection (Greater than or equal to 1%) 1066
Dantrium Capsules (Less frequent) 2580
Dapsone Tablets USP 1746
Daytrana Transdermal Patch 3022
Demadex Injection 2630
Demadex Tablets 2630
▲ Depakote ER Tablets (Greater than 1% to less than 5%) 423
▲ DepoCyt Injection (9%) 1136
▲ DepoDur Injection (5% to 10%) 1095
Dexedrine 1401
Dibenzyline Capsules 3188
Diovan HCT Tablets (Greater than 0.2%) 2216
Donnatal Extentabs 2507
▲ Doxil Injection (1% to 10%) 2378
Duragesic Transdermal System 2405
Dyazide Capsules 1405
DynaCirc CR Controlled Release Tablets (0.5% to 1%) 1407
EC-Naprosyn Delayed-Release Tablets (Less than 1%) 2632
Effexor XR Extended-Release Capsules (Frequent) 3195
Eldepryl Capsules 3052
▲ Eloxatin for Injection (2% to less than 5%) 2731
Emend Capsules (Greater than 0.5%) 1992
Emend for Injection (Greater than 0.5%) 1999
Emsam Transdermal System (Infrequent) 905
Engerix-B Vaccine 1409
EpiPen 1024
Epogen for Injection (0.31%) 576
Erbitux 912
Evoxac Capsules (Less than 1%) 1013
Exelon Capsules (Infrequent) 2229
Exelon Oral Solution (Infrequent) 2229
Exelon Patch (Infrequent) 2233
Exforge Tablets (Greater than or equal to 0.2%) 2238
▲ Fabrazyme for Intravenous Infusion (5%) 1241
Fentora Tablets (Greater than 1%) 968
Flebogamma 5% 1715
Flebogamma 5% DIF 1718
▲ Flolan for Injection (1% to 43%) 1426
Fluarix Vaccine 1446
Flumadine (Less than 0.3%) 1167
Focalin XR Capsules 2251
Follistim AQ Cartridge 2844
Foradil Aerolizer 2849
Frova Tablets (Infrequent) 1111
Furosemide Tablets 2186
Gabitril Tablets (Frequent) 973
Gantrisin Pediatric Suspension 2638
Geodon (Frequent) 2520
Gleevec Tablets (Infrequent) 2255
▲ Herceptin I.V. (5%) 1199
Human Albumin Grifols 25% 1706
▲ Humira Injection (Less than 5%) 442
Imitrex Injection (Infrequent) 1465
Imitrex Nasal Spray (Infrequent) 1470
Imitrex Tablets (Infrequent) 1474
Indocin Capsules (Less than 1%) 2024
Indocin I.V. (Less than 1%) 2489
Indocin (Less than 1%) 2024
▲ Intron A for Injection (Less than 5%) 2859
Invanz for Injection (1.3% to 1.6%) 2029
▲ Invega Extended-Release Tablets (12% to 14%) 1748
▲ Ionsys Transdermal System (1% to less than 10%) 2410
K-Phos Neutral Tablets 813
Lamictal (Infrequent) 1488
Lanoxin Injection 1498
Lanoxin Injection Pediatric 1502
Lanoxin Tablets 1505
▲ Leukine (11%) 774
▲ Leustatin Injection (6%) 2384
Levaquin 2416
Levaquin in 5% Dextrose Injection 2416
Levitra Tablets (Less than 2%) 2876
Levothroid Tablets 1170
Levoxyl Tablets 1780
Lexapro Oral Suspension (Infrequent) 1174
Lexapro Tablets (Infrequent) 1174
Lialda Tablets (Infrequent) 3029
Lovaza Capsules 1520
▲ Lupron Depot 3.75 mg (Less than 5%) 462
▲ Lupron Depot–3 Month 11.25 mg (Less than 5%) 462
Marinol Capsules (Greater than 1%) 3163
Maxair Autohaler (1.2% to 1.3%) 1705
Maxalt Tablets (Infrequent) 2056
Maxalt-MLT Orally Disintegrating Tablets (Infrequent) 2056
Meridia Capsules (2.6%) 475
Merrem I.V. (Greater than 0.1% to 1%) 684
Metadate CD Capsules 3146
Miacalcin Nasal Spray (Less than 1%) 2274
Micardis Tablets (More than 0.3%) 852
Micardis HCT Tablets (Less than 2%) 854
▲ Mirapex Tablets (Greater than or equal to 1%) 857
Moban Tablets 1116
Mobic Oral Suspension (Less than 2%) 863
Mobic Tablets (Less than 2%) 863
MS Contin Tablets (Less frequent) 2585
▲ Mycamine for Injection (3% to 24.7%) 616
▲ Myfortic Tablets (3% to less than 20%) 2276
▲ Mylotarg for Injection (9% to 11%) 3212
Nalfon Capsules (Less than 1%) 2508
Namenda 1180
Naprosyn Suspension (Less than 1%) 2632
Naprosyn Tablets (Less than 1%) 2632
Natrecor for Injection (Greater than or equal to 1%) 2977
NeoProfen Injection 2496
Neupogen for Injection 589
Nexium Delayed-Release Capsules (Less than 1%) 645
Nexium I.V. (Less than 1%) 652
Nexium Delayed-Release Oral Suspension (Less than 1%) 645
Niaspan Extended-Release Tablets 480
Nimotop Capsules (Up to 1.4%) 790
Norvir (Less than 2%) 489
Novantrone for Injection Concentrate 1100
▲ Noxafil Oral Suspension (12%) 2889
▲ Ontak Vials (12%) 1079
▲ Opana Tablets (1% to less than 10%) 1117
▲ Opana ER Tablets (1% to less than 10%) 1121
▲ Orthoclone OKT3 Sterile Solution (10%) 2387
Parnate Tablets 1532
Paxil (Frequent) 1535
Paxil CR Controlled-Release Tablets (Frequent) 1544
Percocet Tablets 1127
Percodan Tablets 1130
Perforomist Inhalation Solution 1025
Persantine Tablets (Rare) 869
▲ Photofrin for Injection (6%) 708
▲ Pletal Tablets (4%) 2481
Primaxin I.M. 2080
Primaxin I.V. (1.5%) 2083
Prinzide Tablets 2092
Pristiq Extended-Release Tablets (1% to 2%) 3247
▲ ProAir HFA Inhalation Aerosol (3%) 3113
Procrit for Injection (0.31%) 2391
Proglycem Capsules (Frequent) 1185
Proglycem Suspension (Frequent) 1185
▲ Prograf Capsules and Injection (3% to 15%) 622
Prolastin (Occasional) 3099
▲ Proleukin for Injection (23%) 2287
Protonix for Delayed-Release Oral Suspension (Less than 1%) 3254
Protonix Delayed-Release Tablets (Less than 1%) 3254
Protonix I.V. (Less than 1%) 3257
Protopic Ointment (0.2% to less than 1%) 628
▲ Proventil HFA Inhalation Aerosol (7%) 2914
Provigil Tablets (2%) 977
Prozac Weekly Capsules (Infrequent) 1852
Prozac Pulvules and Liquid (Infrequent) 1852
▲ Rapamune (Greater than or equal to 3% to less than 20%) 3260
Recombivax HB 2107

ReFacto Vials 3269
Remicade for IV Injection (Greater than or equal to 0.2%) 950
Requip Tablets (Infrequent to 2%) 1561
Rilutek Tablets (1.3% to 2%) 2771
Risperdal Consta Long-Acting Injection (Frequent) 1753
Rituxan I.V. 1223
Romazicon Injection (Less than 1%) 2646
St. Joseph 81 mg Aspirin Chewable and Enteric Coated Tablets 1903
Salagen Tablets (1% to 2%) 1082
Sanctura XR Capsules (Less than 2%) 557
Sandimmune 2296
Sandostatin Injection (Less than 1%) 2300
▲ Simulect for Injection (3% to 10%) 2306
Soma Tablets 1931
Spiriva HandiHaler 870
▲ Stromectol Tablets (3.5%) 2120
Sular Extended Release Tablets (Very rare) 2975
Sustiva Capsules (Less than 2%) 930
Sustiva Tablets (Less than 2%) 930
Symbyax Capsules (2%) 1871
Targretin Capsules 1084
Tarka Tablets (0.3% or more) 511
Taxotere Injection Concentrate 2773
Teveten Tablets (Less than 1%) 515
Teveten HCT Tablets (Less than 1%) 517
Thiothixene Capsules 2197
Trasylol Injection (2%) 799
Treximet Tablets (Infrequent) 1616
Tricor Tablets 520
▲ Trisenox Injection (55%) 986
Twinrix Vaccine 1628
Tygacil for Injection (0% to less than 2%) 3276
▲ Ultane Liquid for Inhalation (2% to 6%) 524
Uroqid-Acid No. 2 Tablets 814
Uroxatral Tablets 2786
Valtrex Caplets 1635
Venlafaxine Hydrochloride Tablets (2%) 2199
Ventolin HFA Inhalation Aerosol (Less than 3%) 1638
Vicoprofen Tablets (Less than 1%) 533
Voltaren Tablets (Occasionally) 2334
Voltaren-XR Tablets (Occasionally) 2337
Vyvanse Capsules (2%) 3033
▲ Wellbutrin Tablets (10.8%) 1648
Wellbutrin SR Sustained-Release Tablets (Infrequent) 1653
▲ Wellbutrin XL Extended-Release Tablets (11%) 1659
▲ Xeloda Tablets (Less than 5%) 2662
Xopenex Inhalation Solution (2.7%) 3001
Xopenex Inhalation Solution Concentrate (2.7%) 3005
Xopenex HFA Inhalation Aerosol (2.7%) 3009
Xyrem Oral Solution (Infrequent) 1766
Zantac 25 EFFERdose Tablets (Rare) 1670
Zantac Injection (Rare) 1666
Zantac Injection Pharmacy Bulk Package (Rare) 1668
Zantac Injection Premixed (Rare) 1666
Zantac (Rare) 1670
Zemuron Injection (Less than 1%) 2947
Zofran Injection (Rare) 1682
Zofran (Rare) 1687
Zofran ODT Orally Disintegrating Tablets (Rare) 1687
Zomig Tablets (Rare) 694
Zomig Nasal Spray (Infrequent) 689
Zomig-ZMT Tablets (Rare) 694
Zonegran Capsules (Infrequent) 1089
Zosyn for Injection (1% or less) 3284
Zyban Sustained-Release Tablets (Infrequent) 1692
▲ Zyprexa Tablets (3% to 4%) 1883
Zyprexa IntraMuscular 1883
▲ Zyprexa ZYDIS Orally Disintegrating Tablets (3% to 4%) 1883
Zyrtec Chewable Tablets (Less than 2%) 1920
Zyrtec Syrup (Less than 2%) 1920
Zyrtec Tablets (Less than 2%) 1920
Zyrtec-D 12 Hour Extended Release Tablets (Less than 2%) 1923

Tachycardia, junctional

Lanoxin Injection 1498
Lanoxin Injection Pediatric (Among most common) 1502
Lanoxin Tablets 1505
Romazicon Injection (1 of 446 patients) 2646

Tachycardia, reflex

Cleviprex 1936

Tachycardia, supraventricular

Abilify Injection (Less than 1 in 1000 patients) 881
Abilify Injection (Less than 1 in 1000 patients) 2466
Abilify Oral Solution (Less than 1 in 1000 patients) 881
Abilify Oral Solution (Less than 1 in 1000 patients) 2466
Abilify Discmelt Orally Disintegrating Tablets (Less than 1 in 1000 patients) 881
Abilify Discmelt Orally Disintegrating Tablets (Less than 1 in 1000 patients) 2466
Abilify Tablets (Less than 1 in 1000 patients) 881
Abilify Tablets (Less than 1 in 1000 patients) 2466
Advair Diskus 100/50 1276
Advair Diskus 250/50 1276
Advair Diskus 500/50 1276
Advair HFA 45/21 Inhalation Aerosol 1288
Advair HFA 115/21 Inhalation Aerosol 1288
Advair HFA 230/21 Inhalation Aerosol 1288
Aggrenox Capsules (Less than 1%) 819
Aricept Tablets (Infrequent) 1062
Aricept ODT Tablets (Infrequent) 1062
Atrovent HFA Inhalation Aerosol (0.5%) 839
Atrovent Nasal Spray 0.03% 834
Atrovent Nasal Spray 0.06% 836
Avelox (Less than 0.1%) 2803
Cardene I.V. (0.7%) 1093
▲ CellCept Capsules (3% to less than 20%) 2622
▲ CellCept Intravenous (3% to less than 20%) 2622
▲ CellCept Oral Suspension (3% to less than 20%) 2622
▲ CellCept Tablets (3% to less than 20%) 2622
Combivent Inhalation Aerosol (0.5%) 845
Concerta Extended-Release Tablets 1925
Dacogen Injection 1066
Effexor XR Extended-Release Capsules 3195
Evoxac Capsules (Less than 1%) 1013
Exelon Capsules (Infrequent) 2229
Exelon Oral Solution (Infrequent) 2229
▲ Flolan for Injection (8%) 1426
Meridia Capsules 475
Mirapex Tablets 857
Nalfon Capsules (Less than 1%) 2508
Namenda 1180
Photofrin for Injection 708
Pletal Tablets (Less than 2%) 2481
▲ Proleukin for Injection (1% to 12%) 2287
ReoPro Vials (1%) 1860
Requip Tablets (Infrequent) 1561
Rilutek Tablets (Rare) 2771
Rythmol Tablets (Less than 1% to 2.3%) 1586
Rythmol SR Capsules 1590
Sanctura XR Capsules 557
Serevent Diskus 1594
Spiriva HandiHaler (Less than 1%) 870
Sular Extended Release Tablets (Less than or equal to 1%) 2975
▲ Trasylol Injection (4%) 799
Venlafaxine Hydrochloride Tablets 2199
Ventolin HFA Inhalation Aerosol 1638
▲ Xeloda Tablets (Less than 5%) 2662
Xopenex Inhalation Solution 3001
Xopenex Inhalation Solution Concentrate 3005
Xopenex HFA Inhalation Aerosol 3009
Zofran Injection 1682
Zosyn for Injection (1% or less to 1.3%) 3284

Tachycardia, ventricular

Abilify Injection (Less than 1 in 1000 patients) 881
Abilify Injection (Less than 1 in 1000 patients) 2466
Abilify Oral Solution (Less than 1 in 1000 patients) 881
Abilify Oral Solution (Less than 1 in 1000 patients) 2466
Abilify Discmelt Orally Disintegrating Tablets (Less than 1 in 1000 patients) 881
Abilify Discmelt Orally Disintegrating Tablets (Less than 1 in 1000 patients) 2466
Abilify Tablets (Less than 1 in 1000 patients) 881
Abilify Tablets (Less than 1 in 1000 patients) 2466
Activase I.V. 1188
Adenocard IV Injection 603
Adenoscan 605
Advair Diskus 100/50 1276
Advair Diskus 250/50 1276
Advair Diskus 500/50 1276
Advair HFA 45/21 Inhalation Aerosol 1288
Advair HFA 115/21 Inhalation Aerosol 1288
Advair HFA 230/21 Inhalation Aerosol 1288
Ambien Tablets (Rare) 2692
Ambien CR Tablets (Rare) 2696
▲ Argatroban Injection (4.8%) 1308
Avelox (Less than 0.1%) 2803
Axid Capsules 1364
Azilect Tablets (Infrequent) 3106
Biaxin/Biaxin XL (Rare) 411
Cardene I.V. (0.7%) 1093
▲ CellCept Capsules (3% to less than 20%) 2622
▲ CellCept Intravenous (3% to less than 20%) 2622
▲ CellCept Oral Suspension (3% to less than 20%) 2622
▲ CellCept Tablets (3% to less than 20%) 2622
Cozaar Tablets (Less than 1%) 1973
Demadex Injection 2630
Demadex Tablets 2630
E.E.S. (Rare) 433
Effexor XR Extended-Release Capsules (Rare) 3195
EryPed (Rare) 431
Exforge Tablets (Greater than 0.1% but less than 1%) 2238
Imitrex Injection (Extremely rare) 1465
Imitrex Tablets (Rare) 1474
Invanz for Injection (Greater than 0.1%) 2029
Lanoxin Injection 1498
Lanoxin Injection Pediatric 1502
Lanoxin Tablets 1505
Levaquin (0.1% to 1%) 2416
Levaquin in 5% Dextrose Injection (0.1% to 1%) 2416
Lexapro Oral Suspension 1174
Lexapro Tablets 1174
Luvox CR Extended-Release Capsules 1759
Meridia Capsules 475
▲ Natrecor for Injection (2% to 10%) 2977
Neupro Transdermal System 3149
Paxil 1535
Paxil CR Controlled-Release Tablets 1544
Pletal Tablets (Less than 2%) 2481
Prinivil Tablets (0.3% to 1%) 2087
Prinzide Tablets 2092
Proleukin for Injection (1%) 2287
Prozac Weekly Capsules 1852
Prozac Pulvules and Liquid 1852
ReoPro Vials (1.4%) 1860
Requip Tablets (Rare) 1561
Rilutek Tablets (Rare) 2771
Romazicon Injection (1 of 446 patients) 2646
▲ Rythmol Tablets (1.9% to 4%) 1586
Thioridazine Hydrochloride Tablets 2195
Toprol-XL Tablets (Greater than 1%) 666
Trasylol Injection (1% to 2%) 799
Velcade for Injection 2168
Venlafaxine Hydrochloride Tablets 2199
Zofran Injection 1682
Zomig Tablets 694
Zomig Nasal Spray 689
Zomig-ZMT Tablets 694
Zosyn for Injection (1% or less) 3284

Tachyphylaxis

▲ Sandostatin Injection (35%) 2300

Tachypnea

Abelcet Injection 1134
Actimmune (Rare) 1743
Aggrenox Capsules 819
Bayer Aspirin 750
Cancidas for Injection (0.9%) 1953
Clolar for Intravenous Infusion 1239
Follistim AQ Cartridge 2844
Maxalt Tablets (Rare) 2056
Maxalt-MLT Orally Disintegrating Tablets (Rare) 2056
Mirapex Tablets 857
Orthoclone OKT3 Sterile Solution 2387
Percocet Tablets 1127
Percodan Tablets 1130
Retrovir Capsules 1574
Retrovir IV Infusion 1579
Retrovir 1574
Sulfamylon Cream 2194
Sulfamylon for 5% Topical Solution 2194
▲ Trisenox Injection (8%) 986

Talkativeness

Carbatrol Capsules 3019
Equetro Extended-Release Capsules 3174

Tardive dyskinesia

Abilify Injection (Greater than or equal to 1 in 1000 patients and less than 1 in 100 patients) 881
Abilify Injection (Greater than or equal to 1 in 1000 patients and less than 1 in 100 patients) 2466
Abilify Oral Solution (Greater than or equal to 1 in 1000 patients and less than 1 in 100 patients) 881
Abilify Oral Solution (Greater than or equal to 1 in 1000 patients and less than 1 in 100 patients) 2466
Abilify Discmelt Orally Disintegrating Tablets (Greater than or equal to 1 in 1000 patients and less than 1 in 100 patients) 881
Abilify Discmelt Orally Disintegrating Tablets (Greater than or equal to 1 in 1000 patients and less than 1 in 100 patients) 2466
Abilify Tablets (Greater than or equal to 1 in 1000 patients and less than 1 in 100 patients) 881
Abilify Tablets (Greater than or equal to 1 in 1000 patients and less than 1 in 100 patients) 2466
Depakote ER Tablets (Greater than 1%) 423
Effexor XR Extended-Release Capsules 3195
Eldepryl Capsules 3052
Geodon 2520
Invega Extended-Release Tablets 1748
Luvox CR Extended-Release Capsules (Rare) 1759
Moban Tablets 1116
Namenda 1180
Risperdal Consta Long-Acting Injection (0.6%) 1753
Symbyax Capsules 1871
Thioridazine Hydrochloride Tablets 2195
Thiothixene Capsules 2197
Venlafaxine Hydrochloride Tablets 2199
Wellbutrin Tablets 1648
Wellbutrin SR Sustained-Release Tablets 1653
Wellbutrin XL Extended-Release Tablets 1659
Zomig Tablets (Rare) 694
Zomig Nasal Spray (Rare) 689
Zomig-ZMT Tablets (Rare) 694
Zyban Sustained-Release Tablets 1692
Zyprexa Tablets (1% to 2%) 1883
Zyprexa ZYDIS Orally Disintegrating Tablets (1% to 2%) 1883

Tardive dyskinesia, unmasking of

Wellbutrin Tablets 1648

Tardive dystonia

(*see under* Dystonia, tardive)

Taste, altered

Actiq (Less than 1%) 959
Alferon N Injection (1%) 1726
Alphagan P Ophthalmic Solution (Less than 1%) 549
Ambien CR Tablets (Infrequent) 2696
Amerge Tablets (Rare) 1301
Anzemet Injection (Infrequently) 2701
Asacol Delayed-Release Tablets 2579
Atrovent HFA Inhalation Aerosol (0.9%) 839
Atrovent Nasal Spray 0.06% (Less than 1%) 836
▲ Avastin IV (14% to 21%) 1192
▲ Avinza Capsules (Less than 5%) 1772
Axert Tablets (Infrequent) 2431
▲ Bactroban Nasal (0.8% to 3%) 1367
▲ BeneFIX Vials (4.6%) 3191

▲ Biaxin/Biaxin XL (3%) 411
Bicillin C-R Injectable Suspension 1775
Bicillin L-A Injection 1777
Campral Tablets (Frequent) 1158
Captopril Tablets (Approximately 2 to 4 of 100 patients) 2182
Catapres-TTS (1 of 101 patients) 842
Celebrex Capsules (0.1% to 1.9%) 2979
Celexa (Frequent) 1160
Ciprodex Otic Suspension (0.5%) 541
Comtan Tablets (1%) 2208
Copaxone for Injection (At least 2%) 3110
▲ Cosopt Sterile Ophthalmic Solution (Up to 30%) 1969
Cozaar Tablets (Less than 1%) 1973
Crixivan Capsules (2.7%) 1979
Cubicin for Injection (Less than 1%) 995
Dantrium Capsules (Less frequent) 2580
Denavir Cream (0.2%) 2205
Depakote ER Tablets (Greater than 1%) 423
▲ Doxil Injection (Less than 1% to 10%) 2378
Effexor XR Extended-Release Capsules (Frequent) 3195
Eldepryl Capsules 3052
▲ Eloxatin for Injection (8% to 14%) 2731
Emend Capsules (Greater than 0.5%) 1992
Emend for Injection (Greater than 0.5%) 1999
Enbrel for Injection 569
Evoxac Capsules (Less than 1%) 1013
Exelon Capsules (Infrequent) 2229
Exelon Oral Solution (Infrequent) 2229
Flonase Nasal Spray 1431
Flumadine (Less than 0.3%) 1167
FML Ophthalmic Suspension ⊙ 224
FML Forte Ophthalmic Suspension ⊙ 222
Fosamax (0.1% to 0.5%) 2005
Fosamax Plus D Tablets (0.1% to 0.5%) 2013
Frova Tablets (Infrequent) 1111
Gabitril Tablets (Infrequent) 973
Gengraf Capsules (1% to less than 3%) 435
Imitrex Injection (Infrequent) 1465
▲ Imitrex Nasal Spray (13.5% to 24.5%) 1470
Imitrex Tablets 1474
▲ Intron A for Injection (Up to 24%) 2859
Invanz for Injection (Greater than 0.1%) 2029
Kaletra (Less than 2%) 452
▲ Kepivance (16%) 583
Kogenate FS 746
Lamictal (Infrequent) 1488
Lamisil Tablets (2.8%) 2266
Lescol Capsules 2268
Lescol XL Tablets 2268
Lexapro Oral Suspension (Infrequent) 1174
Lexapro Tablets (Infrequent) 1174
Lidoderm Patch 1114
Lipitor Tablets (Less than 2%) 2501
▲ Lovaza Capsules (2.7% to 6%) 1520
▲ Lupron Depot 3.75 mg (Less than 5%) 462
▲ Lupron Depot–3 Month 11.25 mg (Less than 5%) 462
Luvox CR Extended-Release Capsules (Infrequent) 1759
Lyrica Capsules (0.1% to 1%) 2527
Maxair Autohaler (0.6%) 1705
▲ Mepron Suspension (3%) 1526
Meridia Capsules (2.2%) 475
Mevacor Tablets 2063
Miacalcin Nasal Spray (Less than 1%) 2274
Mirapex Tablets (Greater than or equal to 1%) 857
Mobic Oral Suspension (Less than 2%) 863
Mobic Tablets (Less than 2%) 863
MS Contin Tablets (Less frequent) 2585
Nasonex Nasal Spray (Very rare) 2883
Neoral Oral Solution (1% to less than 3%) 2280
Neoral Soft Gelatin Capsules (1% to less than 3%) 2280
▲ Neulasta Injection (15% to 72%) 587
▲ Nexium Delayed-Release Capsules (Less than 1% to 6.6%) 645
▲ Nexium I.V. (Less than 1% to 6.6%) 652
▲ Nexium Delayed-Release Oral Suspension (Less than 1% to 6.6%) 645
▲ Norvir (7% to 11.1%) 489
OxyContin Tablets (Less than 1%) 2589
▲ Patanol Ophthalmic Solution (Less than 5%) 546
Paxil (2%) 1535
Paxil CR Controlled-Release Tablets (2%) 1544
PegIntron Powder for Injection (Less than 1%) 2903
Pepcid Tablets (Infrequent) 2075
Plavix Tablets 926
Plavix Tablets 2767
Primaxin I.M. 2080
Primaxin I.V. (Less than 0.2%) 2083
Prinivil Tablets 2087
Prinzide Tablets 2092
Protonix for Delayed-Release Oral Suspension (Less than 1%) 3254
Protonix Delayed-Release Tablets (Less than 1%) 3254
Protonix I.V. (Less than 1%) 3257
Protopic Ointment (Greater than or equal to 1%) 628
▲ Proventil HFA Inhalation Aerosol (4%) 2914
Provigil Tablets (1%) 977
Prozac Pulvules and Liquid (Frequent) 1852
▲ Rebetol (Less than 1% to 9%) 2917
ReFacto Vials 3269
▲ Retrovir Capsules (5%) 1574
▲ Retrovir IV Infusion (5%) 1579
▲ Retrovir (5%) 1574
▲ Rythmol SR Capsules (6% to 22%) 1590
▲ Soriatane Capsules (1% to 10%) 3062
Stalevo Tablets (1%) 2309
Sular Extended Release Tablets (Less than or equal to 1%) 2975
Sustiva Capsules (Less than 2%) 930
Sustiva Tablets (Less than 2%) 930
▲ Sutent Capsules (0% to 44%) 2540
Symbyax Capsules (Frequent) 1871
▲ Taxotere Injection Concentrate (0% to 20.3%) 2773
▲ Temodar Capsules (6%) 2931
Testim 1% Gel (1%) 701
Timentin ADD-Vantage 1606
Timentin Injection Galaxy Container 1609
Timentin IV Infusion 1603
Timentin Pharmacy Bulk Package 1613
Toprol-XL Tablets 666
Tygacil for Injection (0% to less than 2%) 3276
Ultane Liquid for Inhalation (Less than 1%) 524
Valstar Sterile Solution for Intravesical Instillation (Less than 1%) 1735
▲ Wellbutrin SR Sustained-Release Tablets (2% to 4%) 1653
▲ Wellbutrin XL Extended-Release Tablets (2% to 4%) 1659
Zemplar Capsules (Rare) 536
Zemplar Injection (Rare) 538
▲ Zomig Tablets (5% to 21%) 694
▲ Zomig Nasal Spray (5% to 21%) 689
▲ Zomig-ZMT Tablets (5% to 21%) 694
Zonegran Capsules (2%) 1089
Zosyn for Injection (1% or less) 3284
▲ Zyban Sustained-Release Tablets (2% to 3%) 1692
Zyprexa Tablets (Infrequent) 1883
Zyprexa ZYDIS Orally Disintegrating Tablets (Infrequent) 1883
Zyvox (0.9% to 1.8%) 2552

Taste, bad
Aricept Tablets (Infrequent) 1062
Aricept ODT Tablets (Infrequent) 1062
Cipro I.V. (1% or less) 2817
Cipro (Less than 1%) 2810
Fluorescite Injection ⊙ 203
Imitrex Injection 1465
▲ Imitrex Nasal Spray (13.5% to 24.5%) 1470
Imitrex Tablets 1474
Vicoprofen Tablets (Less than 1%) 533

Taste, bitter
▲ Azopt Ophthalmic Suspension (5% to 10%) 540
Ceftin Tablets 1380
Clinoril Tablets (Less than 1 in 100) 1962
▲ Cosopt Sterile Ophthalmic Solution (Up to 30%) 1969
Noroxin Tablets (Less frequent) 2069
▲ Patanase Nasal Spray (12.8%) 544
▲ Trusopt Sterile Ophthalmic Solution (Approximately one-quarter of patients) 2128

Taste, changes
(*see under* Taste, altered)

Taste, loss
(*see under* Ageusia)

Taste, metallic
Adenocard IV Injection (Less than 1%) 603
Adenoscan (Less than 1%) 605
Calcijex Injection 419
▲ Chemet Capsules (12% to 20.9%) 2484
Clinoril Tablets (Less than 1 in 100) 1962
Lexapro Oral Suspension (Infrequent) 1174
Lexapro Tablets (Infrequent) 1174
Lidoderm Patch 1114
Nalfon Capsules (Less than 1%) 2508
Pylera Capsules 714
Rocaltrol Capsules 1150
Rocaltrol Oral Solution 1150

Taste, perversion
Ambien Tablets (Infrequent) 2692
Anzemet Tablets 2704
Atrovent Nasal Spray 0.03% (Less than 2%) 834
Avelox (Greater than or equal to 0.1% to less than 2%) 2803
Cipro XR Tablets (Less than 1%) 2823
Combigan Ophthalmic Solution (0.1% to 0.2%) 553
Combivent Inhalation Aerosol (Less than 2%) 845
Emsam Transdermal System (Frequent) 905
Exforge Tablets (Less than or equal to 0.1%) 2238
Luvox CR Extended-Release Capsules (2%) 1759
Noxafil Oral Suspension (1%) 2889
▲ Pataday Ophthalmic Solution (Less than or equal to 5%) 543
Prozac Weekly Capsules (Frequent) 1852
▲ Pulmicort Flexhaler (Greater than or equal to 1% to 3%) 654
Salagen Tablets (Less than 1% to 2%) 1082
▲ Taxotere Injection Concentrate (0.6% to 27.8%) 2773
Venlafaxine Hydrochloride Tablets (2%) 2199
Zyrtec Chewable Tablets (Less than 2%) 1920
Zyrtec Syrup (Less than 2%) 1920
Zyrtec Tablets (Less than 2%) 1920
Zyrtec-D 12 Hour Extended Release Tablets (Less than 2%) 1923

Taste, salty
Miacalcin Injection 2273

Taste, unpleasant
Adderall XR Capsules 3012
Adipex-P 1185
▲ Aerobid/Aerobid-M (10%) 1153
▲ Azopt Ophthalmic Suspension (5% to 10%) 540
Beconase AQ Nasal Spray 1369
▲ Ceftin for Oral Suspension (5%) 1380
Dexedrine 1401
Flonase Nasal Spray (Less than 1%) 1431
Kogenate FS with Bio-Set (1 case) 748
▲ Lunesta Tablets (8% to 34%) 2994
Mephyton Tablets 700
Vyvanse Capsules 3033

Taste disturbances
Combigan Ophthalmic Solution (0.1% to 0.2%) 553
▲ Cuprimine Capsules (12%) 1986
Eligard 7.5 mg (Less than 2%) 2724
Eligard 22.5 mg (Less than 2%) 2724
Eligard 30 mg (Less than 2%) 2724
Eligard 45 mg (Less than 2%) 2724
▲ Gleevec Tablets (3% to 15%) 2255
▲ Iquix Ophthalmic Solution (8% to 10%) 3183
▲ Ixempra Kit for Injection (6%) 915
▲ Lamisil Oral Granules (3%) 2264
Nexium Delayed-Release Capsules 645
Nexium I.V. 652
Nexium Delayed-Release Oral Suspension 645
Percocet Tablets 1127
▲ Rythmol Tablets (7% to 23%) 1586
▲ Taxotere Injection Concentrate (0% to 18.4%) 2773
Zometa for Intravenous Infusion 2341

Tearing, ocular
▲ Nevanac Ophthalmic Suspension 0.1% (1% to 5%) ⊙ 205
Ofloxacin Ophthalmic Solution 0.3% ⊙ 243

Tearing, unspecified
Concerta Extended-Release Tablets 1925
▲ Taxotere Injection Concentrate (0% to 9.9%) 2773
▲ Travatan Z Ophthalmic Solution (1% to 4%) 547

Teeth, discoloration
Primaxin I.M. 2080
Primaxin I.V. (Less than 0.2%) 2083
Pylera Capsules 714

Teeth, mottling of enamel
(*see under* Teeth, discoloration)

Teeth grinding
Celexa (Infrequent) 1160

Telangiectasia
Diprolene AF Cream 0.05% 2837
Marplan Tablets 3177
Olux Foam (Less than 2%) 3061
Tricor Tablets 520
Verdeso Foam (1%) 3069

Temperature disturbances, cutaneous
Wellbutrin Tablets (1.9%) 1648
Xyrem Oral Solution (Infrequent) 1766

Temperature elevation
(*see also under* Hyperthermia)
▲ Fabrazyme for Intravenous Infusion (6%) 1241

Temperature regulation, disruption
Abilify Injection 881
Abilify Injection 2466
Abilify Oral Solution 881
Abilify Oral Solution 2466
Abilify Discmelt Orally Disintegrating Tablets 881
Abilify Discmelt Orally Disintegrating Tablets 2466
Abilify Tablets 881
Abilify Tablets 2466
Invega Extended-Release Tablets 1748
Risperdal Consta Long-Acting Injection 1753
Symbyax Capsules 1871

Tenderness
Aldara Cream, 5% (1% to 2%) 1699
Bactroban Ointment (Less than 1%) 1368
▲ Dacogen Injection (11%) 1066
Mevacor Tablets 2063
▲ Miacalcin Nasal Spray (10.6%) 2274
Recombivax HB (Equal to or greater than 1%) 2107
Tabloid Tablets 1601
Tyzeka Tablets (2%) 2328

Tenderness, right upper quadrant
Celebrex Capsules 2979
Levaquin 2416
Levaquin in 5% Dextrose Injection 2416

Tenderness at injection site
▲ Actimmune (14%) 1743
▲ Infanrix Vaccine (4% to 5.2%) 1479
M-M-R II 2054
▲ Pentacel (1.4% to 56.1%) 2792
▲ Prevnar (0.8% to 82.8%) 3241
▲ ProQuad (22%) 2099
Rocephin Injectable Vials, ADD-Vantage, Galaxy, Bulk (1%) 2642
▲ Vantas (3.6%) 1737
▲ Vaqta (1.7% to 52.7%) 2130
▲ Vivitrol (42% to 72%) 988
WinRho SDF 741
▲ Zostavax Injection (33.4%) 2145

Tendinitis
Ambien Tablets (Rare) 2692
Ambien CR Tablets (Rare) 2696
Celebrex Capsules (0.1% to 1.9%) 2979
Cipro I.V. 2817
Cipro 2810
Cipro XR Tablets 2823
Evoxac Capsules (Less than 1%) 1013
▲ Intron A for Injection (Less than 5%) 2859
Klonopin (Infrequent) 2639

Levaquin (0.1% to 1%) 2416
Levaquin in 5% Dextrose Injection (0.1% to 1%) 2416
Noroxin Tablets 2069
Requip Tablets (Infrequent to frequent) 1561
Risperdal Consta Long-Acting Injection (Infrequent) 1753
Teveten Tablets (Less than 1%) 515
Teveten HCT Tablets (Less than 1%) 517

Tendinous contracture

Brovana Inhalation Solution (Less than 2%) 2990
Gabitril Tablets (Infrequent) 973
Lamictal (Rare) 1488
Lipitor Tablets (Less than 2%) 2501
Luvox CR Extended-Release Capsules (Infrequent) 1759
Symbyax Capsules (Infrequent) 1871

Tendon disorder, unspecified

Actiq (Less than 1%) 959
▲ Actonel with Calcium Tablets (3%) 2574
Avelox (Less than 0.1%) 2803
Cipro I.V. 2817
Gengraf Capsules (1% to less than 3%) 435
▲ Humira Injection (Less than 5%) 442
Levaquin 2416
Levaquin in 5% Dextrose Injection 2416
Lovaza Capsules 1520
Neoral Oral Solution (1% to less than 3%) 2280
Neoral Soft Gelatin Capsules (1% to less than 3%) 2280
Protopic Ointment (0.2% to less than 1%) 628
Remicade for IV Injection (Greater than or equal to 0.2%) 950
Salagen Tablets (Less than 1%) 1082

Tendon rupture

Avelox 2803
Celebrex Capsules (Greater than or equal to 0.1% to less than 1%) 2979
Cipro I.V. 2817
Cipro 2810
Cipro XR Tablets 2823
Effexor XR Extended-Release Capsules (Rare) 3195
Levaquin 2416
Levaquin in 5% Dextrose Injection 2416
Lipitor Tablets 2501
Mirapex Tablets 857
Noroxin Tablets 2069
Remeron Tablets (Rare) 2924
RemeronSolTab Tablets (Rare) 2927
Venlafaxine Hydrochloride Tablets (Rare) 2199

Tendonitis

Accutane Capsules 2607
Mirapex Tablets 857
Rythmol SR Capsules 1590
Soriatane Capsules (Less than 1%) 3062
Xenical Capsules (2%) 2672
Xyrem Oral Solution (Infrequent) 1766

Tendons, calcification of

Accutane Capsules 2607

Tenesmus

Ambien Tablets (Rare) 2692
Ambien CR Tablets (Rare) 2696
Asacol Delayed-Release Tablets (2% or greater) 2579
Celebrex Capsules (0.1% to 1.9%) 2979
Copaxone for Injection (Infrequent) 3110
Doxil Injection (Less than 1%) 2378
▲ Eloxatin for Injection (2% to less than 5%) 2731
Evoxac Capsules (Less than 1%) 1013
Exelon Capsules (Infrequent) 2229
Exelon Oral Solution (Infrequent) 2229
Lipitor Tablets (Less than 2%) 2501
Lovaza Capsules 1520
Norvir (Less than 2%) 489
Rilutek Tablets (Infrequent) 2771
▲ Sandostatin LAR Depot (4% to 6%) 2302
Soriatane Capsules (Less than 1%) 3062
Valstar Sterile Solution for Intravesical Instillation (Less than 1%) 1735
▲ Xifaxan Tablets (7.2%) 2682

Tenosynovitis

▲ Azilect Tablets (3%) 3106
▲ Azmacort Inhalation Aerosol (1% to 3%) 407
Copaxone for Injection (Infrequent) 3110
Effexor XR Extended-Release Capsules (Infrequent) 3195
Emsam Transdermal System (Infrequent) 905
Evoxac Capsules (Less than 1%) 1013
Geodon Capsules (Infrequent) 2520
Lipitor Tablets (Less than 2%) 2501
Lupron Depot 3.75 mg 462
Lupron Depot 7.5 mg 469
Lupron Depot–3 Month 11.25 mg 462
Lupron Depot-PED 7.5 mg, 11.25 mg and 15 mg 471
Luvox CR Extended-Release Capsules (Infrequent) 1759
Meridia Capsules (1.2%) 475
Mirapex Tablets 857
Paxil (Rare) 1535
Paxil CR Controlled-Release Tablets (Rare) 1544
Protonix for Delayed-Release Oral Suspension (Less than 1%) 3254
Protonix Delayed-Release Tablets (Less than 1%) 3254
Protonix I.V. (Less than 1%) 3257
Prozac Weekly Capsules (Infrequent) 1852
Prozac Pulvules and Liquid (Infrequent) 1852
Remeron Tablets (Infrequent) 2924
RemeronSolTab Tablets (Infrequent) 2927
Salagen Tablets (Less than 1%) 1082
Sular Extended Release Tablets (Less than or equal to 1%) 2975
Symbyax Capsules (Infrequent) 1871
Tricor Tablets 520
Venlafaxine Hydrochloride Tablets (Infrequent) 2199
Zomig Tablets (Infrequent) 694
Zomig Nasal Spray (Rare) 689
Zomig-ZMT Tablets (Infrequent) 694

Tenseness

Allegra-D 12 Hour Extended-Release Tablets 2687
Allegra-D 24 Hour Extended-Release Tablets 2690
▲ Indapamide Tablets (Greater than or equal to 5%) 2188
Zyrtec-D 12 Hour Extended Release Tablets 1923

Tension

Concerta Extended-Release Tablets (1.2%) 1925
▲ Cymbalta Delayed-Release Capsules (5%) 1801
Requip Tablets (Infrequent) 1561

Tension, premenstrual

Crinone 4% Gel 992
Crinone 8% Gel 992

Teratogenicity

Nexavar Tablets 784

Testicular atrophy

AndroGel 3159
▲ Lupron Depot 7.5 mg (5.4%) 469
▲ Viadur Implant (3.8%) 802

Testicular disorder, unspecified

▲ AndroGel (0% to 3%) 3159

Testicular swelling

Wellbutrin Tablets (Infrequent) 1648

Testicular tenderness

AndroGel 3159

Testosterone serum levels, transient increase

▲ AndroGel (9.3%) 3159
Avodart Soft Gelatin Capsules 1359
Vantas (Less than 2%) 1737

Tetany

Ambien Tablets (Rare) 2692
Ambien CR Tablets (Rare) 2696
Fleet Enema 1143
Fleet Enema Extra 1143
Fleet Enema for Children 1143
Fleet Pedia-Lax Enema 1143
Furosemide Tablets 2186
Imitrex Injection 1465
Imitrex Nasal Spray (Rare) 1470
Imitrex Tablets (Rare) 1474
Paxil (Rare) 1535
Paxil CR Controlled-Release Tablets (Rare) 1544
Rilutek Tablets (Rare) 2771
Risperdal Consta Long-Acting Injection (Infrequent) 1753
Zomig Tablets (Rare) 694
Zomig-ZMT Tablets (Rare) 694

Therapeutic response, decreased

Concerta Extended-Release Tablets 1925
NovoSeven RT (1%) 2370
Pentacel 2792

Thickening, facial tissue

Increlex Injection (Several patients) 3100

Thinking, slowed

Invega Extended-Release Tablets 1748

Thinking abnormality

Abilify Injection 881
▲ Abilify Injection (11% to 21%) 2466
Abilify Oral Solution 881
▲ Abilify Oral Solution (11% to 21%) 2466
Abilify Discmelt Orally Disintegrating Tablets 881
▲ Abilify Discmelt Orally Disintegrating Tablets (11% to 21%) 2466
Abilify Tablets 881
▲ Abilify Tablets (11% to 21%) 2466
Actiq (1% to 2%) 959
Ambien Tablets (Rare) 2692
Ambien CR Tablets (Rare) 2696
AmBisome for Injection (Less common) 606
Avelox (Less than 0.1%) 2803
▲ Avinza Capsules (Less than 5%) 1772
Campral Tablets (Frequent) 1158
▲ CellCept Capsules (3% to less than 20%) 2622
▲ CellCept Intravenous (3% to less than 20%) 2622
▲ CellCept Oral Suspension (3% to less than 20%) 2622
▲ CellCept Tablets (3% to less than 20%) 2622
Chantix Tablets (Infrequent) 2511
Coreg Tablets (Greater than 0.1% to 1%) 1387
Coreg CR Extended-Release Capsules (0.1% to less than or equal to 1%) 1393
▲ Depakote ER Tablets (6%) 423
Doxil Injection (Less than 1%) 2378
Duragesic Transdermal System (1% or greater) 2405
Effexor XR Extended-Release Capsules (Frequent) 3195
Emsam Transdermal System (Frequent) 905
Evoxac Capsules (Less than 1%) 1013
Frova Tablets (Infrequent) 1111
▲ Gabitril Tablets (6%) 973
▲ Gliadel Wafer (2% to 6%) 1076
▲ Intron A for Injection (Less than 5%) 2859
Kaletra (Less than 2%) 452
Keppra Oral Solution (1% to greater than or equal to 2%) 3131
Keppra Tablets (1% to greater than or equal to 2%) 3131
▲ Lamictal (3%) 1488
Lunesta Tablets 2994
▲ Luvox CR Extended-Release Capsules (2% to 3%) 1759
▲ Lyrica Capsules (1% to 9%) 2527
▲ Marinol Capsules (3% to 10%) 3163
▲ Megace ES Oral Suspension (1% to 3%) 2499
Meridia Capsules (Greater than or equal to 1%) 475
▲ Mirapex Tablets (2% to 3%) 857
Namenda (Infrequent) 1180
Nembutal Sodium Solution, USP (Less than 1%) 2494
Norvir (0% to 0.9%) 489
▲ OxyContin Tablets (Between 1% and 5%) 2589
Paxil (Infrequent) 1535
Paxil CR Controlled-Release Tablets (Infrequent) 1544
ProAmatine Tablets (Less frequent) 3032
▲ Prograf Capsules and Injection (3% to 15%) 622
Protonix for Delayed-Release Oral Suspension (Less than 1%) 3254
Protonix Delayed-Release Tablets (Less than 1%) 3254
Protonix I.V. (Less than 1%) 3257
Protopic Ointment (0.2% to less than 1%) 628
Provigil Tablets (At least 1%) 977
Prozac Weekly Capsules (2%) 1852
Prozac Pulvules and Liquid (2%) 1852
▲ Remeron Tablets (3%) 2924
▲ RemeronSolTab Tablets (3%) 2927
ReoPro Vials (2.1%) 1860
Rilutek Tablets (Infrequent) 2771
▲ Risperdal Consta Long-Acting Injection (3%) 1753
Salagen Tablets (Less than 1%) 1082
Sular Extended Release Tablets (Less than or equal to 1%) 2975
▲ Symbyax Capsules (Greater than or equal to 5% to 6%) 1871
Venlafaxine Hydrochloride Tablets (2%) 2199
Vicoprofen Tablets (Less than 3%) 533
Wellbutrin Tablets (Infrequent) 1648
Zomig Tablets (Infrequent) 694
Zomig Nasal Spray (Infrequent) 689
Zomig-ZMT Tablets (Infrequent) 694
Zyban Sustained-Release Tablets (1%) 1692
Zyprexa Tablets 1883
Zyprexa ZYDIS Orally Disintegrating Tablets 1883
Zyrtec Chewable Tablets (Less than 2%) 1920
Zyrtec Syrup (Less than 2%) 1920
Zyrtec Tablets (Less than 2%) 1920
Zyrtec-D 12 Hour Extended Release Tablets (Less than 2%) 1923

Thirst

(*see under* Dipsesis)

Thoracic disorders, unspecified

Betaseron for SC Injection 756
▲ Cancidas for Injection (32.1% to 46.5%) 1953
▲ Focalin XR Capsules (9% to 16%) 2251
▲ Mycamine for Injection (35.9% to 68.5%) 616
▲ Verdeso Foam (7%) 3069

Thought disorders, exacerbation of

Focalin XR Capsules 2251

Throat, aching

Zomig Tablets (Infrequent) 694
Zomig Nasal Spray (Infrequent) 689
Zomig-ZMT Tablets (Infrequent) 694

Throat, burning

Eldepryl Capsules 3052

Throat, congestion

Bentyl Capsules 703
Bentyl Injection 703
Bentyl Syrup 703
Bentyl Tablets 703

Throat, dryness of

▲ Aerobid/Aerobid-M (1% to 3%) 1153
▲ Alvesco Inhalation Aerosol (Less than 1%) 2985
Ambien CR Tablets (1%) 2696
Amrix Capsules 966
Asmanex Twisthaler (1% to less than 3%) 2797
Atrovent Nasal Spray 0.06% (1.4%) 836
Azmacort Inhalation Aerosol 407
Beconase AQ Nasal Spray 1369
Catapres-TTS (2 of 101 patients) 842
Cyanokit 5g Antidote 1021
Flonase Nasal Spray 1431
Maxalt Tablets (Infrequent) 2056
Maxalt-MLT Orally Disintegrating Tablets (Infrequent) 2056
Mirapex Tablets 857
Requip Tablets (Infrequent) 1561
Rythmol SR Capsules 1590
Xifaxan Tablets (Less than 2%) 2682
Xopenex Inhalation Solution 3001
Xopenex Inhalation Solution Concentrate 3005
Xopenex HFA Inhalation Aerosol 3009
Xyrem Oral Solution (Infrequent) 1766

Throat, swelling of

Fluarix Vaccine 1446
Janumet Tablets 2041
Januvia Tablets 2048
Miacalcin Injection (A few cases) 2273
Miacalcin Nasal Spray (Few reports) 2274

Throat closing

Ambien CR Tablets (Rare) 2696

Throat disorder, unspecified

Aceon Tablets (2 mg, 4 mg, 8 mg) (0.3% to 1%) 3038

Throat irritation

Advair Diskus 100/50 1276
▲ Advair Diskus 250/50 (3% to 8%) 1276

▲ Advair Diskus 500/50 (Greater than or equal to 3%) 1276
▲ Advair HFA 45/21 Inhalation Aerosol (7% to 9%) 1288
▲ Advair HFA 115/21 Inhalation Aerosol (7% to 9%) 1288
▲ Advair HFA 230/21 Inhalation Aerosol (7% to 9%) 1288
▲ Aerobid/Aerobid-M (1% to 3%) 1153
Allegra Oral Solution (Greater than 1%) 2684
Allegra-D 12 Hour Extended-Release Tablets (2.3%) 2687
Allegra-D 24 Hour Extended-Release Tablets (2.3%) 2690
Ambien CR Tablets (1%) 2696
Azmacort Inhalation Aerosol 407
Cosopt Sterile Ophthalmic Solution 1969
▲ Epivir-HBV (13%) 1417
Flonase Nasal Spray 1431
▲ Flovent Diskus 50 mcg (10% to 13%) 1435
▲ Flovent HFA (8%) 1440
Iquix Ophthalmic Solution (1% to 2%) 3183
Norvir (1.7% to 2.8%) 489
Patanase Nasal Spray (0.9%) 544
Paxil (2%) 1535
Paxil CR Controlled-Release Tablets (2%) 1544
▲ Rituxan I.V. (0% to 9%) 1223
Spiriva HandiHaler 870
Tasigna Capsules (0.1% to 1%) 2316
Trusopt Sterile Ophthalmic Solution 2128
▲ Ventolin HFA Inhalation Aerosol (10%) 1638

Throat soreness

Aceon Tablets (2 mg, 4 mg, 8 mg) 3038
Advair HFA 45/21 Inhalation Aerosol 1288
Advair HFA 115/21 Inhalation Aerosol 1288
Advair HFA 230/21 Inhalation Aerosol 1288
▲ Aerobid/Aerobid-M (20%) 1153
Aricept Tablets (Frequent) 1062
Aricept ODT Tablets (Frequent) 1062
Captopril Tablets 2182
Carbatrol Capsules 3019
▲ Chemet Capsules (0.7% to 3.7%) 2484
▲ Clolar for Intravenous Infusion (14%) 1239
Combigan Ophthalmic Solution 553
Cosopt Sterile Ophthalmic Solution 1969
Cubicin for Injection (1% to 2%) 995
Dapsone Tablets USP 1746
Demadex Injection (1.6%) 2630
Demadex Tablets (1.6%) 2630
▲ Elidel Cream 1% (3.4% to 8.1%) 2221
▲ Flebogamma 5% (20%) 1715
Flovent Diskus 50 mcg 1435
Flovent HFA 1440
▲ Flulaval Injection Vaccine (5% to 9%) 1448
▲ FluMist Vaccine (5% to 28%) 1945
▲ Imitrex Injection (3.3%) 1465
InnoPran XL Extended Release Capsules 1484
Mavik Tablets (0.3% to 1%) 472
Maxair Autohaler 1705
Meruvax II 2061
M-M-R II 2054
▲ Myfortic Tablets (3% to less than 20%) 2276
Nadolol Tablets 2191
▲ Neupogen for Injection (4%) 589
Prinivil Tablets 2087
Prinzide Tablets 2092
ProQuad 2099
Remeron Tablets 2924
RemeronSolTab Tablets 2927
Remicade for IV Injection 950
Rythmol SR Capsules 1590
Timoptic Sterile Ophthalmic Solution 2121
Timoptic in Ocudose 2124
Timoptic-XE Sterile Ophthalmic Gel Forming Solution 2125
Toprol-XL Tablets 666
▲ Trisenox Injection (35%) 986
▲ Ultram ER Extended-Release Tablets (1% to less than 5%) 2428
Wellbutrin SR Sustained-Release Tablets 1653
Wellbutrin XL Extended-Release Tablets 1659
▲ Xeloda Tablets (2% to 12%) 2662
▲ Zometa for Intravenous Infusion (8%) 2341

Throat tightness

Acetadote Injection (1%) 1001
Adenocard IV Injection (Less than 1%) 603
Alferon N Injection (1%) 1726
Ambien Tablets 2692
Amitiza Capsules 3082
Aptivus Capsules 823
Aptivus Oral Solution 823
Cyanokit 5g Antidote 1021
Cymbalta Delayed-Release Capsules (Infrequent) 1801
▲ Doxil Injection (Approximately 6.8%) 2378
▲ Fabrazyme for Intravenous Infusion (Greater than or equal to 5%) 1241
Fleet Phospho-soda (Rare) 1145
Fleet Phospho-soda EZ-PREP (Rare) 1147
Fleet Prep Kits 1149
Flulaval Injection Vaccine 1448
Geodon 2520
▲ Imitrex Tablets (Less than 1% to 3%) 1474
Levaquin 2416
Levaquin in 5% Dextrose Injection 2416
Maxalt Tablets (Less than 2%) 2056
Maxalt-MLT Orally Disintegrating Tablets (Less than 2%) 2056
Mepron Suspension 1526
Moban Tablets 1116
MoviPrep Oral Solution 2679
OsmoPrep Tablets (Rare) 2680
Paxil (2%) 1535
Paxil CR Controlled-Release Tablets (2%) 1544
Risperdal Consta Long-Acting Injection 1753
Rythmol SR Capsules 1590
Symbyax Capsules 1871
Thiothixene Capsules 2197
▲ Treximet Tablets (3%) 1616
Zomig Tablets (0% to 2%) 694
Zomig Nasal Spray (0% to 2%) 689
Zomig-ZMT Tablets (0% to 2%) 694
Zyprexa Tablets 1883
Zyprexa IntraMuscular 1883
Zyprexa ZYDIS Orally Disintegrating Tablets 1883

Throbbing, localized

Catapres-TTS (1 of 101 patients) 842

Thrombocythemia

(*see also under* Thrombocytosis)

▲ Tygacil for Injection (6.1%) 3276

Thrombocytopenia

▲ Abelcet Injection (5%) 1134
Abilify Injection (Greater than or equal to 1 in 1000 patients and less than 1 in 100 patients) 881
Abilify Injection (Less than 1 in 1000 patients) 2466
Abilify Oral Solution (Greater than or equal to 1 in 1000 patients and less than 1 in 100 patients) 881
Abilify Oral Solution (Less than 1 in 1000 patients) 2466
Abilify Discmelt Orally Disintegrating Tablets (Greater than or equal to 1 in 1000 patients and less than 1 in 100 patients) 881
Abilify Discmelt Orally Disintegrating Tablets (Less than 1 in 1000 patients) 2466
Abilify Tablets (Greater than or equal to 1 in 1000 patients and less than 1 in 100 patients) 881
Abilify Tablets (Less than 1 in 1000 patients) 2466
Accutane Capsules 2607
Aceon Tablets (2 mg, 4 mg, 8 mg) 3038
Aciphex Tablets 1053
Actiq (1% or greater) 959
Advicor Tablets 402
Aggrenox Capsules 819
▲ Agrylin Capsules (1% to less than 5%) 3017
Albenza Tablets (Rare) 1297
Aldara Cream, 5% 1699
▲ Alimta for Injection (Up to 27%) 1786
AmBisome for Injection (Less common) 606
Amerge Tablets (Rare) 1301
Amoxil Capsules 1305
Amoxil Chewable Tablets 1305
Amoxil Pediatric Drops for Oral Suspension 1305
Amoxil Powder for Oral Suspension 1305
Amoxil Tablets 1305
Anaprox Tablets (Less than 1%) 2632
Anaprox DS Tablets (Less than 1%) 2632
Angiomax for Injection (0.3% to 0.7%) 1933
Anzemet Injection (Infrequently) 2701
Anzemet Tablets (Rare) 2704
Aptivus Capsules (Less than 2%) 823
Aptivus Oral Solution (Less than 2%) 823
Aricept Tablets (Infrequent) 1062
Aricept ODT Tablets (Infrequent) 1062
Arixtra Injection (2.9%) 1313
▲ Arranon Injection (22% to 88%) 1319
Asacol Delayed-Release Tablets 2579
Atacand Tablets 639
Atacand HCT 642
Attenuvax (Rare) 1951
Augmentin 1323
Augmentin Tablets 1327
Augmentin XR Extended Release Tablets 1333
Augmentin ES-600 Powder for Oral Suspension 1329
Avalide Tablets 892
Avalide Tablets 2713
Avandaryl Tablets 1344
▲ Avastin IV (5%) 1192
Avelox (Less than 0.1%) 2803
▲ Avinza Capsules (Less than 5%) 1772
Axid Capsules 1364
Baraclude (Less than 1%) 900
Bayer Aspirin 750
Betaseron for SC Injection 756
Bexxar 1371
Bicillin C-R Injectable Suspension 1775
Bicillin L-A Injection 1777
▲ Busulfex Injection (100%) 2477
Bystolic Tablets (Greater than or equal to 1%) 1155
▲ Campath Ampules (2% to 71%) 761
Campral Tablets (Infrequent) 1158
Canasa Rectal Suppositories (One patient) 705
Cancidas for Injection 1953
Capastat Sulfate for Injection (Rare) 1791
Captopril Tablets 2182
Carbatrol Capsules 3019
Cardene I.V. (Rare) 1093
Cardizem LA Extended Release Tablets (Infrequent) 421
Catapres Tablets (Rare) 841
Cathflo Activase 1198
Ceftin 1380
Celebrex Capsules (0.1% to 1.9%) 2979
Celexa 1160
▲ CellCept Capsules (23.5% to 38.3%) 2622
▲ CellCept Intravenous (23.5% to 38.3%) 2622
▲ CellCept Oral Suspension (23.5% to 38.3%) 2622
▲ CellCept Tablets (23.5% to 38.3%) 2622
Chantix Tablets (Rare) 2511
Cimzia (Infrequent) 3127
Cipro I.V. (Among most frequent) 2817
Cipro (0.1%) 2810
Cipro XR Tablets 2823
Clinoril Tablets (Less than 1 in 100) 1962
Clolar for Intravenous Infusion 1239
Clorpres Tablets 2185
Combivir Tablets (0.4%) 1384
Comvax 1966
Concerta Extended-Release Tablets 1925
▲ Coreg Tablets (1% to 3%) 1387
▲ Coreg CR Extended-Release Capsules (1% to less than or equal to 3%) 1393
Cosmegen for Injection 2485
Cozaar Tablets (Rare) 1973
Crixivan Capsules (0.9%) 1979
Cubicin for Injection (Less than 1%) 995
▲ Cuprimine Capsules (4% to 5%) 1986
▲ Dacogen Injection (89%) 1066
Dantrium Capsules (Less frequent) 2580
Daraprim Tablets 1400
Demser Capsules (Rare) 1989
▲ Depakote ER Tablets (24%) 423
▲ DepoCyt Injection (3% to 24%) 1136
Diovan Tablets (Very rare) 2212
Diovan HCT Tablets 2216
▲ Doxil Injection (1.3% to 24.2%) 2378
Duetact Tablets 3085
Dyazide Capsules 1405
Dyrenium Capsules (Rare) 3189
EC-Naprosyn Delayed-Release Tablets (Less than 1%) 2632
Edecrin (Rare) 698
Elmiron Capsules (Less than or equal to 1%) 2435
▲ Eloxatin for Injection (2% to 77%) 2731
Emend Capsules (Greater than 0.5%) 1992
Emend for Injection (Greater than 0.5%) 1999
Enbrel for Injection 569
Engerix-B Vaccine 1409
Epivir (0.4% to 2.8%) 1412
▲ Epivir-HBV (4%) 1417
Epzicom Tablets 1422
Equetro Extended-Release Capsules 3174
Evoxac Capsules (Less than 1%) 1013
Exelon Capsules (Infrequent) 2229
Exelon Oral Solution (Infrequent) 2229
Exforge Tablets (Rare to less than 1%) 2238
Exjade Tablets 2244
Fansidar Tablets 2636
Fentora Tablets (Greater than 1%) 968
▲ Flolan for Injection (4%) 1426
Fluarix Vaccine 1446
Fortaz (Very rare) 1450
Fragmin Injection (Rare) 1070
Furosemide Tablets 2186
Gabitril Tablets (Infrequent) 973
▲ Gamunex (15%) 3094
Gantrisin Pediatric Suspension 2638
▲ Gemzar for Injection (15% to 78%) 1820
Gengraf Capsules (2% or less) 435
Geodon Capsules (Rare) 2520
▲ Gleevec Tablets (0% to 33%) 2255
Gliadel Wafer (1%) 1076
▲ Hexalen Capsules (9%) 1078
Humira Injection (Infrequent) 442
▲ Hycamtin Capsules (81%) 1456
▲ Hycamtin for Injection (26% to 69%) 1459
Imitrex Injection 1465
Imitrex Nasal Spray 1470
Imitrex Tablets 1474
Indapamide Tablets 2188
▲ Indocin I.V. (1% to 3%) 2489
Infanrix Vaccine 1479
Integrilin Injection 2855
Intravenous Sodium Diuril 2490
▲ Intron A for Injection (Less than 5% to 15%) 2859
Invanz for Injection (1.1% to 1.3%) 2029
▲ Ixempra Kit for Injection (2% to greater than 40%) 915
▲ Kaletra (4%) 452
Keppra Injection 3137
Keppra Oral Solution 3131
Keppra Tablets 3131
Kinrix Injection Vaccine 1486
Klonopin 2639
Lamictal (Rare) 1488
Lamisil Oral Granules 2264
Lamisil Tablets (Rare) 2266
Lescol Capsules (Rare) 2268
Lescol XL Tablets 2268
Leukeran Tablets 1508
▲ Leukine (19%) 774
▲ Leustatin Injection (12%) 2384
Levaquin (0.1% to 1%) 2416
Levaquin in 5% Dextrose Injection (0.1% to 1%) 2416
Lexapro Oral Suspension 1174
Lexapro Tablets 1174
Lialda Tablets (Infrequent) 3029
Lipitor Tablets (Less than 2%) 2501
Lortab 5/500 Tablets 3143
Lortab 7.5/500 Tablets 3144
Lortab 10/500 Tablets 3144
Lovenox Injection (1.5% to 2.8%) 2756
Luvox CR Extended-Release Capsules (Infrequent) 1759
Lyrica Capsules (0.1% to 1%) 2527
Mavik Tablets (0.3% to 1%) 472
Mepron Suspension 1526
Meridia Capsules 475
Merrem I.V. (Greater than 0.2%) 684
Meruvax II 2061
Mevacor Tablets (Rare) 2063
Micardis HCT Tablets 854
M-M-R II 2054
Mobic Oral Suspension (Less than 2%) 863
Mobic Tablets (Less than 2%) 863
Moxatag Tablets 2165
Mumpsvax 2068
Mustargen for Injection 2492
▲ Mycamine for Injection (4% to 72.2%) 616
▲ Myfortic Tablets (3% to less than 20%) 2276
Myleran Tablets 1530
▲ Mylotarg for Injection (49% to 52%) 3212

Nalfon Capsules (Less than 1%) 2508
Namenda (More than one patient) 1180
Naprosyn Suspension (Less than 1%) 2632
Naprosyn Tablets (Less than 1%) 2632
NeoProfen Injection 2496
Neoral Oral Solution (2% or less) 2280
Neoral Soft Gelatin Capsules (2% or less) 2280
▲ Neupogen for Injection (Fewer than 6% to 12%) 589
Neupro Transdermal System 3149
▲ Nexavar Tablets (1% to 46%) 784
Nexium Delayed-Release Capsules (Less than 1%) 645
Nexium I.V. (Less than 1%) 652
Nexium Delayed-Release Oral Suspension (Less than 1%) 645
Niaspan Extended-Release Tablets ... 480
Nimotop Capsules (0.3%; rare) 790
Noroxin Tablets (1%) 2069
Norvir (Less than 2%) 489
▲ Novantrone for Injection Concentrate (335 to 39%) 1100
▲ Noxafil Oral Suspension (1% to 29%) 2889
Omnicef Capsules 497
Omnicef for Oral Suspension 497
▲ Ontak Vials (8%) 1079
Orthoclone OKT3 Sterile Solution 2387
Panhematin for Injection 2497
Parnate Tablets 1532
Paser Granules 1747
Paxil 1535
Paxil CR Controlled-Release Tablets 1544
Pediarix Vaccine 1552
Liquid PedvaxHIB (One child) 2073
▲ PegIntron Powder for Injection (7%) 2903
Pentasa Capsules (Less than 1%) 3030
Pepcid Tablets (Rare) 2075
Percocet Tablets 1127
Percodan Tablets 1130
Persantine Tablets (Rare) 869
Phenytek Capsules (Occasional) 2192
Plavix Tablets (1% to 2.5%) 926
Plavix Tablets (1% to 2.5%) 2767
Pletal Tablets 2481
Pneumovax 23 2078
Prandin Tablets (Less than or equal to 1%) 2971
Primaxin I.M. 2080
Primaxin I.V. (Less than 0.2%) 2083
Prinivil Tablets (Rare) 2087
Prinzide Tablets (Rare) 2092
Proglycem Capsules (Frequent) 1185
Proglycem Suspension (Frequent) 1185
▲ Prograf Capsules and Injection (3% to 24%) 622
▲ Proleukin for Injection (1% to 37%) 2287
ProQuad 2099
Protonix for Delayed-Release Oral Suspension (Less than 1%) 3254
Protonix Delayed-Release Tablets (Less than 1%) 3254
Protonix I.V. (Less than 1%) 3257
Prozac Weekly Capsules (Rare) 1852
Prozac Pulvules and Liquid (Rare) 1852
Pylera Capsules 714
▲ Rapamune (14% to greater than or equal to 30%) 3260
Raptiva for Injection (0.3%) 1218
Rebetol (2%) 2917
▲ Rebif Prefilled Syringe for Injection (2% to 8%) 1107
Recombivax HB 2107
Remeron Tablets (Rare) 2924
RemeronSolTab Tablets (Rare) 2927
Remicade for IV Injection (Greater than or equal to 0.2%) 950
ReoPro Vials (0.7% to 5.2%) 1860
Requip Tablets (Infrequent) 1561
▲ Retrovir Capsules (12%) 1574
▲ Retrovir IV Infusion (12%) 1579
▲ Retrovir (12%) 1574
Risperdal Consta Long-Acting Injection (Rare) 1753
▲ Rituxan I.V. (2% to 12%) 1223
Rocephin Injectable Vials, ADD-Vantage, Galaxy, Bulk (Less than 1%) 2642
Rythmol Tablets (Less than 1%) 1586
Rythmol SR Capsules 1590
St. Joseph 81 mg Aspirin Chewable and Enteric Coated Tablets 1903
Salagen Tablets (Less than 1%) 1082
Sandimmune (2% or less; occasional) 2296
Sandostatin LAR Depot 2302
▲ Simulect for Injection (3% to 10%) ... 2306
Solodyn Extended Release Tablets ... 1938
Stalevo Tablets 2309
▲ Sutent Capsules (0% to 38%) 2540
Synagis Intramuscular Solution 1948
Tabloid Tablets 1601
Targretin Capsules 1084
Tarka Tablets 511
▲ Tasigna Capsules (28% to 37%) 2316
▲ Taxotere Injection Concentrate (0.6% to 44.4%) 2773
Tekturna HCT Tablets 2324
▲ Temodar Capsules (4% to 58%) 2931
Teveten Tablets (0.3%) 515
Teveten HCT Tablets 517
Thioridazine Hydrochloride Tablets ... 2195
Thiothixene Capsules 2197
Tice BCG (Less than or equal to 1%) 2936
Timentin ADD-Vantage 1606
Timentin Injection Galaxy Container 1609
Timentin IV Infusion 1603
Timentin Pharmacy Bulk Package 1613
Toprol-XL Tablets 666
▲ Torisel Injection (1% to 40%) 3272
Tracleer Tablets 3289
Trasylol Injection (2%) 799
▲ Treanda for Injection (11% to 77%) 983
Tricor Tablets (Rare) 520
▲ Trisenox Injection (18%) 986
Trizivir Tablets (0.4%) 1622
Twinrix Vaccine 1628
Tygacil for Injection (0% to less than 2%) 3276
Tylenol with Codeine Tablets 2427
Tyzeka Tablets (Less than 1%) 2328
Ultane Liquid for Inhalation (Less than 1%) 524
Urso 250 Tablets 720
Urso Forte Tablets 720
▲ Valcyte Tablets (0% to 18%) 2654
▲ Valtrex Caplets (0.1% to 3%) 1635
Vaqta (Very rare) 2130
Varivax 2133
▲ Velcade for Injection (3% to 52%) 2168
Vicodin Tablets 529
Vicodin ES Tablets 530
Vicodin HP Tablets 531
Viramune Oral Suspension (0.4% to 1.3%) 873
Viramune Tablets (0.4% to 1.3%) 873
Vivitrol 988
Voltaren Tablets (Occasionally) 2334
Voltaren-XR Tablets (Occasionally) 2337
Vytorin 10/10 Tablets 2149
Vytorin 10/10 Tablets 2939
Vytorin 10/20 Tablets 2149
Vytorin 10/20 Tablets 2939
Vytorin 10/40 Tablets 2149
Vytorin 10/40 Tablets 2939
Vytorin 10/80 Tablets 2149
Vytorin 10/80 Tablets 2939
Wellbutrin Tablets 1648
Wellbutrin SR Sustained-Release Tablets 1653
Wellbutrin XL Extended-Release Tablets 1659
▲ Xeloda Tablets (1% to 41%) 2662
Xolair 1235
Xolair 2339
Zantac 25 EFFERdose Tablets (A few patients) 1670
Zantac Injection (Few patients) 1666
Zantac Injection Pharmacy Bulk Package (Infrequent) 1668
Zantac Injection Premixed (Few patients) 1666
Zantac (A few patients) 1670
Zetia Tablets 2157
Zetia Tablets 2951
Ziagen (1%) 1673
Zinacef for Injection (Rare) 1678
Zinacef Injection (Rare) 1678
Zocor Tablets (Rare) 2136
▲ Zolinza Capsules (22% to 25.6%) 2142
▲ Zometa for Intravenous Infusion (5% to 10%) 2341
Zomig Tablets (Rare) 694
Zomig-ZMT Tablets (Rare) 694
Zonegran Capsules (Rare) 1089
Zosyn for Injection 3284
Zovirax 1690
Zyban Sustained-Release Tablets 1692
Zyrtec Chewable Tablets 1920
Zyrtec Syrup 1920
Zyrtec Tablets 1920
Zyrtec-D 12 Hour Extended Release Tablets (Rare) 1923
▲ Zyvox (0% to 4.7%) 2552

Thrombocytopenia, immune

PegIntron Powder for Injection (Less than or equal to 1%) 2903

Thrombocytopenia, immuno-allergic

Eloxatin for Injection 2731

Thrombocytopenia, neonatal

Avalide Tablets 2713
Dyazide Capsules (Rare) 1405
Prinzide Tablets 2092

Thrombocytopenia, transient

Suprax for Oral Suspension (Less than 2%) 1891
Suprax Tablets (Less than 2%) 1891

Thrombocytopenic purpura

(*see under* Purpura, thrombocytopenic)

Thrombocytosis

Accutane Capsules 2607
Aggrenox Capsules 819
Aricept Tablets (Infrequent) 1062
Aricept ODT Tablets (Infrequent) 1062
Augmentin (Less than 1%) 1323
Augmentin Tablets (Less than 1%) 1327
▲ Augmentin XR Extended Release Tablets (3.6%) 1333
Avelox (Greater than or equal to 0.1% to less than 2%) 2803
Azilect Tablets (Rare) 3106
Celebrex Capsules (0.1% to 1.9%) ... 2979
Chemet Capsules (0.5% to 1.5%) 2484
Cipro I.V. (Among most frequent) 2817
Cipro (0.1%) 2810
Cipro XR Tablets 2823
Cubicin for Injection (Less than 1%) 995
Cuprimine Capsules 1986
▲ Dacogen Injection (5%) 1066
Demser Capsules (Rare) 1989
Estratest Tablets 3043
Estratest H.S. Tablets 3043
Evoxac Capsules (Less than 1%) 1013
Fortaz (1 in 45) 1450
Geodon Capsules (Rare) 2520
▲ Invanz for Injection (4.3% to 6.5%) 2029
Ketek Tablets (Greater than or equal to 0.2% to less than 2%) 2744
Lovenox Injection 2756
▲ Lupron Depot 7.5 mg (Greater than or equal to 5%) 469
Lyrica Capsules (Rare) 2527
Omnicef Capsules (0.2%) 497
Omnicef for Oral Suspension (1%) 497
Paxil (Rare) 1535
Paxil CR Controlled-Release Tablets (Rare) 1544
Pentasa Capsules (Less than 1%) 3030
Premarin Tablets 3221
Primaxin I.M. 2080
Primaxin I.V. 2083
Prozac Weekly Capsules (Rare) 1852
Prozac Pulvules and Liquid (Rare) 1852
▲ Rocephin Injectable Vials, ADD-Vantage, Galaxy, Bulk (5.1%) 2642
Salagen Tablets (Less than 1%) 1082
Symbyax Capsules (Rare) 1871
Targretin Capsules 1084
Tasigna Capsules 2316
▲ Tygacil for Injection (6.1%) 3276
Venlafaxine Hydrochloride Tablets (Infrequent) 2199
Vesanoid Capsules 2660
Zosyn for Injection (1% or less) 3284
Zyprexa Tablets (Rare) 1883
Zyprexa ZYDIS Orally Disintegrating Tablets (Rare) 1883
Zyvox (0% to 2.8%) 2552

Thromboembolic complications

▲ Arimidex Tablets (4% to 13%) 672
Estratest Tablets 3043
Estratest H.S. Tablets 3043
Faslodex Injection (Less than 1%) 682
Femara Tablets (Less than or equal to 2%) 2246
Lybrel Tablets 3204
NovoSeven 2367
Ortho-Cyclen/Ortho Tri-Cyclen 2449
Ortho Tri-Cyclen Lo Tablets 2458
Premarin Intravenous 3217
Premarin Vaginal Cream 3228
Premphase Tablets 3232
Prempro Tablets 3232

Thromboembolic disease

(*see under* Thromboembolic complications)

Thromboembolic events

Alphanate 1709
Follistim AQ Cartridge 2844
NovoSeven RT 2370
Procrit for Injection 2391

Thromboembolism

Activase I.V. 1188
▲ Aranesp for Injection (5.6%) 564
▲ Eloxatin for Injection (1% to 9%) 2731
Equetro Extended-Release Capsules 3174
Estratest Tablets 3043
Estratest H.S. Tablets 3043
Flebogamma 5% 1715
Flebogamma 5% DIF 1718
Gammagard Liquid 730
Gammagard S/D 734
Gamunex 3094
Nexavar Tablets (0.1% to less than 1%) 784
Ortho-Cyclen/Ortho Tri-Cyclen 2449
Ortho Tri-Cyclen Lo Tablets 2458
Premarin Vaginal Cream 3228
Soriatane Capsules 3062

Thromboembolism, arterial

▲ Avastin IV (3%) 1192
▲ Lucentis Injection (2.1% to 3%) 1205
Lybrel Tablets 3204
Mircette Tablets 1034
NuvaRing 2897
Ortho-Cyclen Tablets 2449
Ortho Evra Transdermal System 2437
Ortho Tri-Cyclen Tablets 2449
Ortho Tri-Cyclen Lo Tablets 2458
Seasonique Tablets 1046
Yaz Tablets 805

Thromboembolism, venous

▲ Avastin IV (5% to 15.1%) 1192
Mircette Tablets 1034
Ortho Evra Transdermal System 2437
Premarin Intravenous 3217
Premphase Tablets 3232
▲ Sutent Capsules (2% to 3%) 2540

Thrombopenia

(*see under* Thrombocytopenia)

Thrombophilia

Cimzia 3127

Thrombophlebitis

Abelcet Injection 1134
Abilify Injection (Less than 1 in 1000 patients) 2466
Abilify Oral Solution (Less than 1 in 1000 patients) 2466
Abilify Discmelt Orally Disintegrating Tablets (Less than 1 in 1000 patients) 2466
Abilify Tablets (Less than 1 in 1000 patients) 2466
Actiq (Less than 1%) 959
Activella Tablets 2347
Angeliq Tablets 751
Anzemet Injection (Rare) 2701
Anzemet Tablets (Rare) 2704
▲ Aranesp for Injection (5.6%) 564
▲ Arimidex Tablets (2% to 5%) 672
Campral Tablets (Rare) 1158
Carbatrol Capsules 3019
Celebrex Capsules (Less than 0.1%) 2979
Cipro I.V. (1% or less) 2817
Climara Transdermal System 763
Climara Pro Transdermal System 768
Cuprimine Capsules (Rare) 1986
Dantrium Intravenous 2582
Divigel 3167
▲ Doxil Injection (1% to 10%) 2378
Effexor XR Extended-Release Capsules (Rare) 3195
Elitek (Less than or equal to 1%) 2729
Enbrel for Injection (Infrequent) 569
Enjuvia Tablets 1029
Epogen for Injection (Rare) 576
Equetro Extended-Release Capsules 3174
Estratest Tablets 3043
Estratest H.S. Tablets 3043
Femara Tablets (Less than or equal to 2%) 2246
Fluorescite Injection ..... ⊙ 203
Furosemide Tablets 2186
Gabitril Tablets (Infrequent) 973
Geodon Capsules (Rare) 2520
Imitrex Nasal Spray 1470

Imitrex Tablets 1474
Indocin Capsules (Rare) 2024
Indocin I.V. (Less than 1%) 2489
Indocin (Rare) 2024
Invanz for Injection (1.6% to 1.9%) 2029
Kaletra (Less than 2%) 452
Klonopin (Infrequent) 2639
Lunesta Tablets (Rare) 2994
Lybrel Tablets 3204
Megace ES Oral Suspension 2499
Merrem I.V. (0.8%) 684
Miacalcin Nasal Spray (Less than 1%) 2274
Mirapex Tablets 857
Mircette Tablets 1034
Mustargen for Injection 2492
Mycamine for Injection 616
Namenda (Infrequent) 1180
NovoSeven 2367
NovoSeven RT 2370
NuvaRing 2897
Ortho-Cyclen Tablets 2449
Ortho Evra Transdermal System 2437
Ortho Tri-Cyclen Tablets 2449
Ortho Tri-Cyclen Lo Tablets 2458
Paxil (Rare) 1535
Paxil CR Controlled-Release Tablets (Rare) 1544
Premarin Intravenous 3217
Premarin Tablets 3221
Premarin Vaginal Cream 3228
Premphase Tablets 3232
Prempro Tablets 3232
▲ Primaxin I.V. (3.1%) 2083
Procrit for Injection (Rare) 2391
Protonix for Delayed-Release Oral Suspension (Less than 1%) 3254
Protonix Delayed-Release Tablets (Less than 1%) 3254
Protonix I.V. (Less than 1%) 3257
Prozac Weekly Capsules (Rare) 1852
Prozac Pulvules and Liquid (Rare) 1852
ReFacto Vials 3269
Remicade for IV Injection (Greater than or equal to 0.2%) 950
ReoPro Vials (0.1%) 1860
Risperdal Consta Long-Acting Injection (Rare) 1753
▲ Romazicon Injection (1% to 3%) 2646
Sandostatin Injection (Less than 1%) 2300
Seasonique Tablets 1046
Sustiva Capsules (Less than 2%) 930
Sustiva Tablets (Less than 2%) 930
Taxotere Injection Concentrate 2773
Timentin ADD-Vantage 1606
Timentin Injection Galaxy Container 1609
Timentin IV Infusion 1603
Timentin Pharmacy Bulk Package 1613
Torisel Injection (1%) 3272
Trasylol Injection (1% to 2%) 799
Tygacil for Injection (0% to less than 2%) 3276
Venlafaxine Hydrochloride Tablets (Infrequent) 2199
Yaz Tablets 805
Zinacef for Injection (1 in 60 patients) 1678
Zinacef Injection (1 in 60 patients) 1678
Zomig Tablets (Rare) 694
Zomig Nasal Spray (Infrequent) 689
Zomig-ZMT Tablets (Rare) 694
Zonegran Capsules (Infrequent) 1089
Zosyn for Injection (0.2% to 1.3%) 3284

Thrombophlebitis, deep-vein
▲ Avastin IV (6% to 34%) 1192
Azilect Tablets (Infrequent) 3106
Cardene I.V. (Rare) 1093
Effexor XR Extended-Release Capsules 3195
Estratest Tablets 3043
Estratest H.S. Tablets 3043
Evoxac Capsules (Less than 1%) 1013
Exelon Capsules (Infrequent) 2229
Exelon Oral Solution (Infrequent) 2229
▲ Gliadel Wafer (10%) 1076
Ionsys Transdermal System (.1% to less than 1%) 2410
Lamictal (Rare) 1488
Lyrica Capsules (0.1% to 1%) 2527
▲ Prograf Capsules and Injection (3% to 15%) 622
Requip Tablets (Rare) 1561
Venlafaxine Hydrochloride Tablets 2199

Thrombophlebitis, leg
Requip Tablets (Rare) 1561

Thrombophlebitis, peripheral
BeneFIX Vials 3191

Thromboplastin decrease
Avelox (Less than 0.1%) 2803

Thromboplastin time, increase
▲ CellCept Capsules (3% to less than 20%) 2622
▲ CellCept Intravenous (3% to less than 20%) 2622
▲ CellCept Oral Suspension (3% to less than 20%) 2622
▲ CellCept Tablets (3% to less than 20%) 2622
Elspar for Injection 2488
Oncaspar Injection 1138
Panhematin for Injection 2497
Testim 1% Gel (Less than 1%) 701
Zosyn for Injection 3284

Thrombosis
▲ Alimta for Injection (1% to 7%) 1786
AlphaNine SD 1713
Ambien Tablets (Rare) 2692
Ambien CR Tablets (Rare) 2696
▲ Aranesp for Injection (5.6%) 564
▲ Avastin IV (15.1%) 1192
BeneFIX Vials 3191
▲ Busulfex Injection (33%) 2477
Celexa 1160
▲ CellCept Capsules (3% to less than 20%) 2622
▲ CellCept Intravenous (3% to less than 20%) 2622
▲ CellCept Oral Suspension (3% to less than 20%) 2622
▲ CellCept Tablets (3% to less than 20%) 2622
Chantix Tablets (Infrequent) 2511
Doxil Injection (Less than 1%) 2378
Elitek (Less than or equal to 1%) 2729
▲ Eloxatin for Injection (3% to 6%) 2731
Elspar for Injection 2488
Estratest Tablets 3043
Estratest H.S. Tablets 3043
Exelon Capsules (Infrequent) 2229
Exelon Oral Solution (Infrequent) 2229
Follistim AQ Cartridge 2844
Gamunex 3094
Gleevec Tablets (Rare) 2255
Herceptin I.V. 1199
Imitrex Nasal Spray 1470
Imitrex Tablets (Rare) 1474
Ixempra Kit for Injection 915
Leukine 774
Leustatin Injection (2%) 2384
Lexapro Oral Suspension 1174
Lexapro Tablets 1174
Lovenox Injection (Rare) 2756
Mirapex Tablets 857
Mustargen for Injection 2492
NovoSeven (Two patients) 2367
NovoSeven RT 2370
▲ Oncaspar Injection (Greater than or equal to 2% to 3%) 1138
Paxil (Rare) 1535
Paxil CR Controlled-Release Tablets (Rare) 1544
Premarin Intravenous 3217
Premarin Vaginal Cream 3228
Profilnine SD Solvent Detergent 1721
Proleukin for Injection (Less than 1%) 2287
Protonix for Delayed-Release Oral Suspension (Less than 1%) 3254
Protonix Delayed-Release Tablets (Less than 1%) 3254
Protonix I.V. (Less than 1%) 3257
Prozac Weekly Capsules (Rare) 1852
Prozac Pulvules and Liquid (Rare) 1852
Requip Tablets (Infrequent to rare) 1561
Rilutek Tablets (Rare) 2771
Rythmol SR Capsules 1590
Salagen Tablets (Less than 1%) 1082
▲ Simulect for Injection (3% to 10%) 2306
Tasigna Capsules 2316
TNKase 1233
Trasylol Injection (1% to 2%) 799

Thrombosis, arterial
Argatroban Injection (1.8%) 1308
Azilect Tablets (Rare) 3106
▲ CellCept Capsules (3% to less than 20%) 2622
▲ CellCept Intravenous (3% to less than 20%) 2622
▲ CellCept Oral Suspension (3% to less than 20%) 2622
▲ CellCept Tablets (3% to less than 20%) 2622
NovoSeven 2367
NovoSeven RT 2370
Orthoclone OKT3 Sterile Solution 2387
Sandostatin LAR Depot 2302
Trasylol Injection (1% to 2%) 799

Thrombosis, central nervous system
Elspar for Injection 2488

Thrombosis, cerebral
(*see under* Cerebral thrombosis)

Thrombosis, coronary
(*see under* Coronary thrombosis)

Thrombosis, deep-vein
Abilify Injection (Greater than or equal to 1 in 1000 patients and less than 1 in 100 patients) 2466
Abilify Oral Solution (Greater than or equal to 1 in 1000 patients and less than 1 in 100 patients) 2466
Abilify Discmelt Orally Disintegrating Tablets (Greater than or equal to 1 in 1000 patients and less than 1 in 100 patients) 2466
Abilify Tablets (Greater than or equal to 1 in 1000 patients and less than 1 in 100 patients) 2466
Activella Tablets 2347
AndroGel (2 patients) 3159
Angeliq Tablets 751
Aranesp for Injection 564
Arimidex Tablets (2%) 672
BeneFIX Vials 3191
Betaseron for SC Injection 756
Celebrex Capsules (Greater than or equal to 0.1% to less than 1%) 2979
Climara Transdermal System 763
Climara Pro Transdermal System 768
Divigel 3167
Emend Capsules (Greater than 0.5%) 1992
Emend for Injection (Greater than 0.5%) 1999
Enjuvia Tablets 1029
▲ Epogen for Injection (5% to 10%) 576
Evista Tablets 1810
Fenoglide Tablets 2960
Fentora Tablets (Greater than 1%) 968
Mirapex Tablets 857
Mycamine for Injection 616
Namenda 1180
NovoSeven 2367
NovoSeven RT 2370
Premarin Intravenous 3217
Premarin Tablets 3221
Premarin Vaginal Cream 3228
Premphase Tablets 3232
Prempro Tablets 3232
Procrit for Injection 2391
▲ Rapamune (Greater than or equal to 3% to less than 20%) 3260
Rythmol SR Capsules 1590
▲ Sutent Capsules (3%) 2540
Taxotere Injection Concentrate 2773
Torisel Injection (2%) 3272
Tricor Tablets 520
Velcade for Injection 2168
Vivitrol 988

Thrombosis, glomerular capillary
Gengraf Capsules 435
Neoral Oral Solution 2280
Neoral Soft Gelatin Capsules 2280
Sandimmune 2296

Thrombosis, intraabdominal
▲ Avastin IV (3% to 10%) 1192

Thrombosis, leg
▲ Humira Injection (Less than 5%) 442
Zolinza Capsules 2142

Thrombosis, mesenteric
Estratest Tablets 3043
Estratest H.S. Tablets 3043
Lybrel Tablets 3204
Mircette Tablets 1034
NuvaRing 2897
Ortho-Cyclen Tablets 2449
Ortho Evra Transdermal System 2437
Ortho Tri-Cyclen Tablets 2449
Premarin Intravenous 3217
Premarin Vaginal Cream 3228
Seasonique Tablets 1046
Yaz Tablets 805

Thrombosis, mesenteric venous
Avastin IV (Rare) 1192

Thrombosis, mesenteric arterial
Campral Tablets (Rare) 1158

Cosopt Sterile Ophthalmic Solution 1969
Nadolol Tablets 2191
Timoptic-XE Sterile Ophthalmic Gel Forming Solution 2125

Thrombosis, portal vein
Femara Tablets (Less than or equal to 2%) 2246
Mylotarg for Injection 3212
Velcade for Injection 2168

Thrombosis, pulmonary
Divigel 3167
Estratest Tablets 3043
Estratest H.S. Tablets 3043
Trasylol Injection (1% to 2%) 799

Thrombosis, renal artery
Epogen for Injection (Rare) 576
Procrit for Injection (Rare) 2391

Thrombosis, retinal, unspecified
Mircette Tablets 1034
NuvaRing 2897

Thrombosis, retinal artery
Seasonique Tablets 1046
Yaz Tablets 805

Thrombosis, retinal vascular
Activella Tablets 2347
Angeliq Tablets 751
Divigel 3167
Enjuvia Tablets 1029
Epogen for Injection (Rare) 576
Estratest Tablets 3043
Estratest H.S. Tablets 3043
Imitrex Tablets 1474
Intron A for Injection 2859
Lybrel Tablets 3204
Ortho-Cyclen Tablets 2449
Ortho Evra Transdermal System 2437
Ortho Tri-Cyclen Tablets 2449
Ortho Tri-Cyclen Lo Tablets 2458
PegIntron Powder for Injection (Less than or equal to 1%) 2903
Premarin Intravenous 3217
Premarin Tablets 3221
Premarin Vaginal Cream 3228
Premphase Tablets 3232
Prempro Tablets 3232
Procrit for Injection (Rare) 2391
Seasonique Tablets 1046
Yaz Tablets 805

Thrombosis, retinal vein
Sandostatin LAR Depot 2302

Thrombosis, sagittal sinus
Elspar for Injection 2488
Oncaspar Injection 1138

Thrombosis, shunt
Demadex Injection 2630
Demadex Tablets 2630

Thrombosis, subacute
Pletal Tablets 2481

Thrombosis, venous
Actimmune (Rare) 1743
Activase I.V. 1188
Activella Tablets 2347
Alphanate 1709
Angeliq Tablets 751
▲ Aranesp for Injection (5.6%) 564
Aricept Tablets (Infrequent) 1062
Aricept ODT Tablets (Infrequent) 1062
Betaseron for SC Injection 756
Cathflo Activase 1198
Climara Transdermal System 763
Climara Pro Transdermal System 768
Divigel 3167
Enbrel for Injection (Infrequent) 569
Enjuvia Tablets 1029
Epogen for Injection (Rare) 576
Femara Tablets (Less than or equal to 2%) 2246
Kaletra (Less than 2%) 452
Lybrel Tablets 3204
Mircette Tablets 1034
Nimotop Capsules (Less than 1%) 790
NuvaRing 2897
Ortho-Cyclen Tablets 2449
Ortho Evra Transdermal System 2437
Ortho Tri-Cyclen Tablets 2449
Ortho Tri-Cyclen Lo Tablets 2458
Orthoclone OKT3 Sterile Solution 2387
Premarin Intravenous 3217
Premarin Tablets 3221
Premarin Vaginal Cream 3228
Premphase Tablets 3232

Prempro Tablets ... 3232
▲ Procrit for Injection (Up to 10%) ... 2391
Prograf Capsules and Injection ... 622
▲ Taxotere Injection Concentrate (2.3% to 3.6%) ... 2773
▲ Xeloda Tablets (Less than 1% to 8%) ... 2662

Thrombosis at injection site
Mycamine for Injection ... 616

Thrombosis of vascular access
▲ Aranesp for Injection (5.6% to 6%) .. 564
Epogen for Injection (0.25%) ... 576
Furosemide Tablets ... 2186
Procrit for Injection ... 2391

Thrombotic events, cardivascular
Flector Patch ... 561
Vicoprofen Tablets ... 533
Voltaren Tablets ... 2334

Thrombotic events, unspecified
▲ Aranesp for Injection (6.2%) ... 564
BeneFIX Vials ... 3191
Gammagard S/D ... 734
Herceptin I.V. ... 1199
Lybrel Tablets ... 3204
Mobic Oral Suspension ... 863
Mobic Tablets ... 863
▲ Ontak Vials (7%) ... 1079
Procrit for Injection ... 2391

Thrombotic microangiopathy
Rapamune ... 3260
Sutent Capsules (Rare) ... 2540

Thrombotic vascular disease
Accutane Capsules ... 2607
Ortho-Cyclen/Ortho Tri-Cyclen ... 2449
Ortho Tri-Cyclen Lo Tablets ... 2458

Thrombus formation, increased risk of
Angiomax for Injection ... 1933

Thrush, oral
(*see under* Candidiasis, oral)

Thymol turbidity test, positive
Cuprimine Capsules ... 1986

Thymus gland abnormalities, fetal
Accutane Capsules ... 2607

Thyroid binding globulin, increase
(*see under* T4, increase)

Thyroid disease, exacerbation
Proleukin for Injection ... 2287

Thyroid disorder, unspecified
Betaseron for SC Injection ... 756
Chantix Tablets (Infrequent) ... 2511
▲ Rebif Prefilled Syringe for Injection (4% to 6%) ... 1107
Solodyn Extended Release Tablets .. 1938

Thyroid disorders
(*see under* T3, decrease; T4, decrease; T4, increase)

Thyroid function test, abnormal
Crestor Tablets ... 677
Depakote ER Tablets ... 423
Lescol Capsules ... 2268
Lescol XL Tablets ... 2268
Mevacor Tablets ... 2063
Somatuline Depot Injection ... 3102

Thyroid gland discoloration
Solodyn Extended Release Tablets .. 1938

Thyroid hormone, changes
(*see under* T3, decrease; T4, decrease; T4, increase)

Thyroid nodule
Effexor XR Extended-Release Capsules (Rare) ... 3195
Venlafaxine Hydrochloride Tablets (Rare) ... 2199

Thyroid stimulating hormone elevation
Avodart Soft Gelatin Capsules ... 1359
WelChol Tablets (Rare) ... 1015

Thyroiditis
Aldara Cream, 5% ... 1699
Cuprimine Capsules (Rare) ... 1986
Effexor XR Extended-Release Capsules (Rare) ... 3195
▲ Ontak Vials (Less than 5%) ... 1079
Paxil (Rare) ... 1535
Paxil CR Controlled-Release Tablets (Rare) ... 1544
PegIntron Powder for Injection ... 2903
Sular Extended Release Tablets (Less than or equal to 1%) ... 2975
Tasigna Capsules ... 2316
Venlafaxine Hydrochloride Tablets (Rare) ... 2199

Thyrotoxicosis
▲ Ontak Vials (Less than 5%) ... 1079
Synthroid Tablets ... 507

Thyroxin-binding globulin, decrease
AndroGel ... 3159
Testim 1% Gel ... 701

Tics
Abilify Injection (Greater than or equal to 1 in 1000 patients and less than 1 in 100 patients) ... 2466
Abilify Oral Solution (Greater than or equal to 1 in 1000 patients and less than 1 in 100 patients) ... 2466
Abilify Discmelt Orally Disintegrating Tablets (Greater than or equal to 1 in 1000 patients and less than 1 in 100 patients) ... 2466
Abilify Tablets (Greater than or equal to 1 in 1000 patients and less than 1 in 100 patients) ... 2466
Concerta Extended-Release Tablets ... 1925
▲ Daytrana Transdermal Patch (7%) ... 3022
Lamictal ... 1488
Lexapro Oral Suspension (Infrequent) ... 1174
Lexapro Tablets (Infrequent) ... 1174
▲ Vyvanse Capsules (2%) ... 3033

Tightness, feeling of
▲ Imitrex Injection (5%) ... 1465

Tightness, head
Imitrex Injection (2%) ... 1465

Tinea, unspecified
Aceon Tablets (2 mg, 4 mg, 8 mg) (0.3% to 1%) ... 3038

Tinea cruris
Aldara Cream, 5% (More than 1%) ... 1699

Tinea pedis
Xyrem Oral Solution (Infrequent) ... 1766

Tingling
Avelox ... 2803
Bentyl Capsules ... 703
Bentyl Injection ... 703
Bentyl Syrup ... 703
Bentyl Tablets ... 703
Cipro I.V. ... 2817
Cipro ... 2810
Cipro XR Tablets ... 2823
DynaCirc CR Controlled Release Tablets (0.5% to 1%) ... 1407
▲ Elocon Ointment 0.1% (4.8%) ... 2842
Engerix-B Vaccine (Less than 1%) ... 1409
▲ Finacea Gel (4% to 16%) ... 1742
Gengraf Capsules (Rare) ... 435
Humulin 50/50, 100 Units ... 1843
Humulin 70/30 Vial ... 1844
Humulin N Vial ... 1846
Humulin R ... 1849
▲ Imitrex Injection (14%) ... 1465
Imitrex Nasal Spray (Infrequent) ... 1470
▲ Imitrex Tablets (4% to 8%) ... 1474
K-Phos Original (Sodium Free) Tablets (Less frequent) ... 814
K-Phos Neutral Tablets ... 813
Levaquin ... 2416
Levaquin in 5% Dextrose Injection ... 2416
Neoral Oral Solution (Rare) ... 2280
Neoral Soft Gelatin Capsules (Rare) ... 2280
Niaspan Extended-Release Tablets (Among most common) ... 480
Noroxin Tablets ... 2069
▲ Panretin Gel 0.1% (3% to 22%) ... 1081
Profilnine SD Solvent Detergent ... 1721
▲ Protopic Ointment (1% to 8%) ... 628
Reyataz Capsules ... 3299
Sandimmune (Rare) ... 2296
Twinrix Vaccine (Less than 1%) ... 1628

Tingling, ears
Ciprodex Otic Suspension (1 patient) ... 541

Tingling, extremities
Humulin R ... 1849
▲ Indapamide Tablets (Less than 5%) ... 2188

Tingling, feet
Alferon N Injection (1%) ... 1726
Humulin 50/50, 100 Units ... 1843
Humulin 70/30 Vial ... 1844
Humulin N Vial ... 1846
Humulin R ... 1849
Uroqid-Acid No. 2 Tablets ... 814

Tingling, fingers
Noroxin Tablets (0.3% to 1%) ... 2069

Tingling, hands
Adenocard IV Injection (1%) ... 603
Humulin 50/50, 100 Units ... 1843
Humulin 70/30 Vial ... 1844
Humulin N Vial ... 1846
Humulin R ... 1849
Uroqid-Acid No. 2 Tablets ... 814

Tingling, legs
Alferon N Injection (1%) ... 1726

Tingling, lips
Humulin 50/50, 100 Units ... 1843
Humulin 70/30 Vial ... 1844
Humulin N Vial ... 1846
Humulin R ... 1849
K-Phos Original (Sodium Free) Tablets (Less frequent) ... 814
K-Phos Neutral Tablets ... 813
Uroqid-Acid No. 2 Tablets ... 814

Tingling, tongue
Humulin 50/50, 100 Units ... 1843
Humulin 70/30 Vial ... 1844
Humulin N Vial ... 1846
Humulin R ... 1849

Tinnitus
Abelcet Injection ... 1134
Accutane Capsules ... 2607
Aceon Tablets (2 mg, 4 mg, 8 mg) (1.5%) ... 3038
Actiq (1% or greater) ... 959
Aggrenox Capsules (Less than 1%) .. 819
▲ Agrylin Capsules (1% to less than 5%) ... 3017
Alferon N Injection (One patient) ... 1726
Aloxi Injection (Less than 1%) ... 1059
Ambien Tablets (Infrequent) ... 2692
Ambien CR Tablets (1%) ... 2696
Amerge Tablets (Infrequent) ... 1301
▲ Anaprox Tablets (3% to 9%) ... 2632
▲ Anaprox DS Tablets (3% to 9%) ... 2632
Anzemet Injection (Infrequently) ... 2701
Anzemet Tablets (Rare) ... 2704
Aricept Tablets (Infrequent) ... 1062
Aricept ODT Tablets (Infrequent) ... 1062
Asacol Delayed-Release Tablets ... 2579
Atacand HCT (0.5% or greater) ... 642
Atripla Tablets ... 938
Atrovent Nasal Spray 0.06% (Less than 1%) ... 836
Avelox (Less than 0.1%) ... 2803
Axert Tablets (Rare) ... 2431
Bayer Aspirin ... 750
Biaxin/Biaxin XL ... 411
Bicillin C-R Injectable Suspension ... 1775
Bicillin L-A Injection ... 1777
Campral Tablets (Infrequent) ... 1158
Capastat Sulfate for Injection ... 1791
Carbatrol Capsules ... 3019
Cardene I.V. (Rare) ... 1093
Cardizem LA Extended Release Tablets (Less than 2%) ... 421
Celebrex Capsules (0.1% to 1.9%) ... 2979
Celexa (Infrequent) ... 1160
▲ CellCept Capsules (3% to less than 20%) ... 2622
▲ CellCept Intravenous (3% to less than 20%) ... 2622
▲ CellCept Oral Suspension (3% to less than 20%) ... 2622
▲ CellCept Tablets (3% to less than 20%) ... 2622
Chantix Tablets (Infrequent) ... 2511
Cialis Tablets (Less than 2%) ... 1792
Cipro I.V. (1% or less) ... 2817
Cipro (Less than 1%) ... 2810
Cipro XR Tablets ... 2823
Clinoril Tablets (Greater than 1%) ... 1962
Combigan Ophthalmic Solution ... 553
Copaxone for Injection (At least 2%) ... 3110
Coreg Tablets (Greater than 0.1% to 1%) ... 1387
Coreg CR Extended-Release Capsules (0.1% to less than or equal to 1%) ... 1393
Cosopt Sterile Ophthalmic Solution ... 1969
Cozaar Tablets (Less than 1%) ... 1973
Cubicin for Injection (Less than 1%) ... 995
Cuprimine Capsules ... 1986
Cymbalta Delayed-Release Capsules (Infrequent) ... 1801
Dapsone Tablets USP ... 1746
Demadex Injection ... 2630
Demadex Tablets ... 2630
▲ Depakote ER Tablets (Greater than 1% to 7%) ... 423
Diovan HCT Tablets (Greater than 0.2%) ... 2216
Doxil Injection (Less than 1%) ... 2378
▲ EC-Naprosyn Delayed-Release Tablets (3% to 9%) ... 2632
Edecrin ... 698
Effexor XR Extended-Release Capsules (Frequent) ... 3195
Eldepryl Capsules ... 3052
Elmiron Capsules (Less than or equal to 1%) ... 2435
▲ Emend Capsules (3.7%) ... 1992
▲ Emend for Injection (3.7%) ... 1999
Emsam Transdermal System (Frequent) ... 905
Engerix-B Vaccine ... 1409
Equetro Extended-Release Capsules ... 3174
Evoxac Capsules (Less than 1%) ... 1013
Exelon Capsules (Frequent) ... 2229
Exelon Oral Solution (Frequent) ... 2229
Exelon Patch (Infrequent) ... 2233
Exforge Tablets (Greater than 0.1% but less than 1%) ... 2238
▲ Fabrazyme for Intravenous Infusion (8%) ... 1241
Fansidar Tablets ... 2636
Flumadine (0.3% to 1%) ... 1167
Frova Tablets (Frequent) ... 1111
Furosemide Tablets ... 2186
Gabitril Tablets (Frequent) ... 973
Gantrisin Pediatric Suspension ... 2638
Gengraf Capsules (1% to less than 3%) ... 435
Geodon Capsules (Infrequent) ... 2520
Gleevec Tablets (Infrequent) ... 2255
Imitrex Nasal Spray ... 1470
Indocin (Greater than 1%) ... 2024
▲ Intron A for Injection (Less than 5%) ... 2859
Kaletra (Less than 2%) ... 452
Lamictal (Infrequent) ... 1488
Levaquin ... 2416
Levaquin in 5% Dextrose Injection ... 2416
Levitra Tablets (Less than 2%) ... 2876
Lexapro Oral Suspension (Frequent) ... 1174
Lexapro Tablets (Frequent) ... 1174
Lidoderm Patch ... 1114
Lipitor Tablets (Less than 2%) ... 2501
Lunesta Tablets (Infrequent) ... 2994
Lyrica Capsules (Greater than or equal to 1%) ... 2527
Marinol Capsules (Less than 1%) ... 3163
Maxalt Tablets (Infrequent) ... 2056
Maxalt-MLT Orally Disintegrating Tablets (Infrequent) ... 2056
Meridia Capsules ... 475
Miacalcin Nasal Spray (Less than 1%) ... 2274
Micardis Tablets (More than 0.3%) ... 852
Micardis HCT Tablets ... 854
Mirapex Tablets (Greater than or equal to 1%) ... 857
Mobic Oral Suspension (Less than 2%) ... 863
Mobic Tablets (Less than 2%) ... 863
Mustargen for Injection (Infrequent) .. 2492
Nadolol Tablets (1 to 5 of 1000 patients) ... 2191
▲ Nalfon Capsules (4.5%) ... 2508
Namenda (Infrequent) ... 1180
▲ Naprosyn Suspension (3% to 9%) ... 2632
▲ Naprosyn Tablets (3% to 9%) ... 2632
Neoral Oral Solution (1% to less than 3%) ... 2280
Neoral Soft Gelatin Capsules (1% to less than 3%) ... 2280
Neupro Transdermal System ... 3149
Nexavar Tablets (0.1% to less than 1%) ... 784
Nexium Delayed-Release Capsules (Less than 1%) ... 645
Nexium I.V. (Less than 1%) ... 652
Nexium Delayed-Release Oral Suspension (Less than 1%) ... 645

Noroxin Tablets 2069
Norvir (Less than 2%) 489
Orthoclone OKT3 Sterile Solution 2387
OxyContin Tablets (Less than 1%) 2589
Parnate Tablets 1532
Paxil (Frequent) 1535
Paxil CR Controlled-Release Tablets (Frequent) 1544
Pepcid Tablets (Infrequent) 2075
Pepto-Bismol Original Liquid, Maximum Strength Liquid, Original and Cherry Tablets, Chewable Tablets and Easy-To-Swallow Caplets 2564
Percocet Tablets 1127
Percodan Tablets 1130
Pletal Tablets (Less than 2%) 2481
Primaxin I.M. 2080
Primaxin I.V. (Less than 0.2%) 2083
Prinivil Tablets (0.3% to 1%) 2087
Prinzide Tablets (0.3% to 1%) 2092
Pristiq Extended-Release Tablets (1% to 2%) 3247
▲ Prograf Capsules and Injection (3% to 15%) 622
Protonix for Delayed-Release Oral Suspension (Less than 1%) 3254
Protonix Delayed-Release Tablets (Less than 1%) 3254
Protonix I.V. (Less than 1%) 3257
Proventil HFA Inhalation Aerosol (Less than 3%) 2914
Prozac Weekly Capsules (Frequent) 1852
Prozac Pulvules and Liquid (Frequent) 1852
Pylera Capsules 714
Recombivax HB (Less than 1%) 2107
Requip Tablets (Infrequent) 1561
Romazicon Injection (Less than 1%) 2646
Rythmol Tablets (Less than 1% to 2%) 1586
Rythmol SR Capsules 1590
St. Joseph 81 mg Aspirin Chewable and Enteric Coated Tablets 1903
Salagen Tablets (1% to 2%) 1082
Sandimmune (2% or less) 2296
Solodyn Extended Release Tablets (2%) 1938
▲ Soriatane Capsules (Less than 1% to 10%) 3062
Sular Extended Release Tablets (Less than or equal to 1%) 2975
Sustiva Capsules (Less than 2%) 930
Sustiva Tablets (Less than 2%) 930
Symbyax Capsules (Frequent) 1871
Tarka Tablets (Less frequent) 511
Teveten Tablets (Less than 1%) 515
Teveten HCT Tablets (Less than 1%) 517
Timoptic Sterile Ophthalmic Solution 2121
Timoptic in Ocudose 2124
Timoptic-XE Sterile Ophthalmic Gel Forming Solution 2125
Toprol-XL Tablets 666
Treximet Tablets (Infrequent) 1616
Tricor Tablets 520
▲ Trisenox Injection (5%) 986
Twinrix Vaccine 1628
Ultram ER Extended-Release Tablets (0.5% to less than 1%) 2428
Venlafaxine Hydrochloride Tablets (2%) 2199
Vicoprofen Tablets (Less than 3%) 533
▲ Voltaren Tablets (1% to 10%) 2334
▲ Voltaren-XR Tablets (1% to 10%) 2337
Wellbutrin Tablets 1648
▲ Wellbutrin SR Sustained-Release Tablets (5% to 6%) 1653
▲ Wellbutrin XL Extended-Release Tablets (3% to 6%) 1659
Xifaxan Tablets (Less than 2%) 2682
▲ Xyrem Oral Solution (5.9%) 1766
Zomig Tablets (Infrequent) 694
Zomig Nasal Spray (Infrequent) 689
Zomig-ZMT Tablets (Infrequent) 694
Zonegran Capsules (Frequent) 1089
Zosyn for Injection (1% or less) 3284
Zyban Sustained-Release Tablets (1%) 1692
Zyprexa Tablets (Infrequent) 1883
Zyprexa ZYDIS Orally Disintegrating Tablets (Infrequent) 1883
Zyrtec Chewable Tablets (Less than 2%) 1920
Zyrtec Syrup (Less than 2%) 1920
Zyrtec Tablets (Less than 2%) 1920
Zyrtec-D 12 Hour Extended Release Tablets (Less than 2%) 1923

Tiredness
(*see under* Fatigue)

Tobacco misuse
Zyprexa Tablets (Rare) 1883
Zyprexa ZYDIS Orally Disintegrating Tablets (Rare) 1883

Toenails, ingrown
Crixivan Capsules 1979
Prevnar 3241

Tolerance
Adipex-P 1185
Concerta Extended-Release Tablets 1925
Daytrana Transdermal Patch 3022
Duragesic Transdermal System 2405
Lortab 5/500 Tablets 3143
Lortab 7.5/500 Tablets 3144
Lortab 10/500 Tablets 3144
MS Contin Tablets 2585
Nembutal Sodium Solution, USP 2494
Percocet Tablets 1127
Percodan Tablets 1130
Vicodin Tablets 529
Vicodin HP Tablets 531
Vicoprofen Tablets 533
Xyrem Oral Solution 1766
Zemuron Injection 2947

Tolerance, diminished
Symbyax Capsules (Rare) 1871

Tolerance, increased
Ambien Tablets (Rare) 2692
Ambien CR Tablets (Rare) 2696

Tongue, black
Marplan Tablets 3177

Tongue, black "hairy"
(*see under* Glossotrichia)

Tongue, burning
Imitrex Injection 1465
Imitrex Nasal Spray (Infrequent) 1470
Imitrex Tablets 1474
Nalfon Capsules (Less than 1%) 2508
Stalevo Tablets 2309

Tongue, darkening of
Pepto-Bismol Original Liquid, Original and Cherry Chewable Tablets & Caplets ▣ 613
Pepto-Bismol Maximum Strength Liquid ▣ 613

Tongue, dry
Abilify Injection (Greater than or equal to 1 in 1000 patients and less than 1 in 100 patients) 881
Abilify Injection (Greater than or equal to 1 in 1000 patients and less than 1 in 100 patients) 2466
Abilify Oral Solution (Greater than or equal to 1 in 1000 patients and less than 1 in 100 patients) 881
Abilify Oral Solution (Greater than or equal to 1 in 1000 patients and less than 1 in 100 patients) 2466
Abilify Discmelt Orally Disintegrating Tablets (Greater than or equal to 1 in 1000 patients and less than 1 in 100 patients) 881
Abilify Discmelt Orally Disintegrating Tablets (Greater than or equal to 1 in 1000 patients and less than 1 in 100 patients) 2466
Abilify Tablets (Greater than or equal to 1 in 1000 patients and less than 1 in 100 patients) 881
Abilify Tablets (Greater than or equal to 1 in 1000 patients and less than 1 in 100 patients) 2466

Tongue, fine vermicular movements
Moban Tablets 1116
Thioridazine Hydrochloride Tablets 2195
Thiothixene Capsules 2197

Tongue, furry
Pylera Capsules 714

Tongue, geographic
Evoxac Capsules (Less than 1%) 1013

Tongue, protrusion
Geodon 2520
Moban Tablets 1116
Risperdal Consta Long-Acting Injection 1753
Symbyax Capsules 1871
Thioridazine Hydrochloride Tablets 2195
Thiothixene Capsules 2197
Zyprexa Tablets 1883
Zyprexa IntraMuscular 1883
Zyprexa ZYDIS Orally Disintegrating Tablets 1883

Tongue, sore
(*see under* Glossodynia)

Tongue, swelling
(*see under* Glossoncus)

Tongue, thickening of
▲ Kepivance (17%) 583

Tongue discoloration
Avelox (Less than 0.1%) 2803
Biaxin/Biaxin XL 411
Copaxone for Injection (Infrequent) 3110
Effexor XR Extended-Release Capsules (Rare) 3195
Evoxac Capsules (Less than 1%) 1013
▲ Kepivance (17%) 583
Paxil (Rare) 1535
Paxil CR Controlled-Release Tablets (Rare) 1544
Pepto-Bismol Original Liquid, Maximum Strength Liquid, Original and Cherry Tablets, Chewable Tablets and Easy-To-Swallow Caplets 2564
Primaxin I.M. 2080
Primaxin I.V. (Less than 0.2%) 2083
Protonix for Delayed-Release Oral Suspension (Less than 1%) 3254
Protonix Delayed-Release Tablets (Less than 1%) 3254
Protonix I.V. (Less than 1%) 3257
Pylera Capsules 714
Remeron Tablets (Rare) 2924
RemeronSolTab Tablets (Rare) 2927
Rilutek Tablets (Rare) 2771
Venlafaxine Hydrochloride Tablets (Rare) 2199
Zyprexa Tablets (Rare) 1883
Zyprexa ZYDIS Orally Disintegrating Tablets (Rare) 1883
Zyrtec Chewable Tablets (Less than 2%) 1920
Zyrtec Syrup (Less than 2%) 1920
Zyrtec Tablets (Less than 2%) 1920
Zyrtec-D 12 Hour Extended Release Tablets (Less than 2%) 1923
Zyvox (0.2% to 1.1%) 2552

Tongue disorder, unspecified
Emsam Transdermal System (Infrequent) 905
Evoxac Capsules (Less than 1%) 1013
▲ Flovent Diskus 50 mcg (1% to 3%) 1435
Gengraf Capsules (1% to less than 3%) 435
Neoral Oral Solution (1% to less than 3%) 2280
Neoral Soft Gelatin Capsules (1% to less than 3%) 2280
Nexium Delayed-Release Capsules (Less than 1%) 645
Nexium I.V. (Less than 1%) 652
Nexium Delayed-Release Oral Suspension (Less than 1%) 645
Salagen Tablets (Less than 1%) 1082
▲ Soriatane Capsules (1% to 10%) 3062

Tongue numbness
(*see under* Numbness, buccal mucosa)

Tongue sensation, abnormal
Eloxatin for Injection 2731

Tongue spasm
Abilify Injection (Greater than or equal to 1 in 1000 patients and less than 1 in 100 patients) 881
Abilify Injection (Greater than or equal to 1 in 1000 patients and less than 1 in 100 patients) 2466
Abilify Oral Solution (Greater than or equal to 1 in 1000 patients and less than 1 in 100 patients) 881
Abilify Oral Solution (Greater than or equal to 1 in 1000 patients and less than 1 in 100 patients) 2466
Abilify Discmelt Orally Disintegrating Tablets (Greater than or equal to 1 in 1000 patients and less than 1 in 100 patients) 881
Abilify Discmelt Orally Disintegrating Tablets (Greater than or equal to 1 in 1000 patients and less than 1 in 100 patients) 2466
Abilify Tablets (Greater than or equal to 1 in 1000 patients and less than 1 in 100 patients) 881
Abilify Tablets (Greater than or equal to 1 in 1000 patients and less than 1 in 100 patients) 2466

Tonsillitis
Advair HFA 45/21 Inhalation Aerosol 1288
Advair HFA 115/21 Inhalation Aerosol 1288
Advair HFA 230/21 Inhalation Aerosol 1288
▲ Elidel Cream 1% (0.4% to 6.3%) 2221
Exforge Tablets (Greater than or equal to 0.2%) 2238
▲ Flovent Diskus 50 mcg (1% to 3%) 1435
Fluarix Vaccine 1446
Foradil Aerolizer (1.2%) 2849
Gengraf Capsules (1% to less than 3%) 435
Genotropin Lyophilized Powder 2547
Neoral Oral Solution (1% to less than 3%) 2280
Neoral Soft Gelatin Capsules (1% to less than 3%) 2280
Requip Tablets (Infrequent) 1561
Singulair (Greater than or equal to 2%) 2114

Tonsillitis, acute
Elidel Cream 1% (0% to 2.6%) 2221
▲ Exjade Tablets (6.4%) 2244
Mirapex Tablets 857

Tonsils pain/discomfort
▲ Relenza Inhalation Powder (8% to 19%) 1556

Tooth caries, aggravated
Zyrtec Chewable Tablets (Less than 2%) 1920
Zyrtec Syrup (Less than 2%) 1920
Zyrtec Tablets (Less than 2%) 1920

Tooth discoloration
Amoxil Capsules (Rare) 1305
Amoxil Chewable Tablets (Rare) 1305
Amoxil Pediatric Drops for Oral Suspension (Rare) 1305
Amoxil Powder for Oral Suspension (Rare) 1305
Amoxil Tablets (Rare) 1305
Augmentin (Rare) 1323
Augmentin Tablets (Rare) 1327
Augmentin XR Extended Release Tablets (Rare) 1333
Augmentin ES-600 Powder for Oral Suspension (Rare) 1329
Biaxin/Biaxin XL 411
Moxatag Tablets 2165
Solodyn Extended Release Tablets 1938
Zyvox 2552

Tooth disorder
Actiq (Less than 1%) 959
Actonel with Calcium Tablets (2.1%) 2574
▲ ActoPlus Met Tablets (5.3%) 3071
▲ Actos Tablets (5.3%) 3077
▲ Adderall XR Capsules (2% to 4%) 3012
▲ Advair HFA 45/21 Inhalation Aerosol (1% to 3%) 1288
▲ Advair HFA 115/21 Inhalation Aerosol (1% to 3%) 1288
▲ Advair HFA 230/21 Inhalation Aerosol (1% to 3%) 1288
Axid Capsules (1%) 1364
Boniva Injection (3.5%) 2614
Boniva Tablets (3.5%) 2618
Celebrex Capsules (0.1% to 1.9%) 2979
▲ Depakote ER Tablets (Greater than 1% to less than 5%) 423
▲ Duetact Tablets (At least 5%) 3085
▲ Evoxac Capsules (1% to 3%) 1013
Flomax Capsules (1.2% to 2%) 848
▲ Flovent Diskus 50 mcg (1% to 3%) 1435
Forteo for Injection (2%) 1816
Gengraf Capsules (1% to less than 3%) 435
Geodon for Injection (Up to 1%) 2520
▲ Lamictal (3%) 1488

Lescol Capsules (2.1%) 2268
Lescol XL Tablets (1.4%) 2268
Luvox CR Extended-Release Capsules (2%) 1759
Meridia Capsules (Greater than or equal to 1%) 475
Mirapex Tablets (1% or more) 857
Neoral Oral Solution (1% to less than 3%) 2280
Neoral Soft Gelatin Capsules (1% to less than 3%) 2280
Paxil (Rare) 1535
Paxil CR Controlled-Release Tablets (Rare) 1544
Prandin Tablets (Less than 1% to 2%) 2971
Prometrium Capsules (100 mg, 200 mg) 3047
Protopic Ointment (Greater than or equal to 1% to 2%) 628
Provigil Tablets (At least 1%) 977
Rilutek Tablets (Up to 1.2%) 2771
Risperdal Consta Long-Acting Injection (2%) 1753
Salagen Tablets (Less than 1%) 1082
Symbyax Capsules (1% to 2%) 1871
Tricor Tablets 520
Wellbutrin SR Sustained-Release Tablets (At least 1%) 1653
Wellbutrin XL Extended-Release Tablets (At least 1%) 1659
▲ Xenical Capsules (2.9% to 4.3%) 2672
Yaz Tablets (Greater than 1%) 805
Zyprexa Tablets 1883
Zyprexa ZYDIS Orally Disintegrating Tablets 1883

Toothache

▲ Abilify Injection (4%) 2466
▲ Abilify Oral Solution (4%) 881
▲ Abilify Oral Solution (4%) 2466
▲ Abilify Discmelt Orally Disintegrating Tablets (4%) 881
▲ Abilify Discmelt Orally Disintegrating Tablets (4%) 2466
▲ Abilify Tablets (4%) 881
▲ Abilify Tablets (4%) 2466
Aricept Tablets (Infrequent) 1062
Aricept ODT Tablets (Infrequent) 1062
▲ Azmacort Inhalation Aerosol (1% to 3%) 407
Crinone 4% Gel 992
Crinone 8% Gel 992
Elidel Cream 1% (0.4% to 2.6%) 2221
▲ Evoxac Capsules (1% to 3%) 1013
▲ Fabrazyme for Intravenous Infusion (6%) 1241
Frova Tablets (Rare) 1111
Gardasil Injection (1.5%) 2019
Klonopin (Infrequent) 2639
Lamisil Oral Granules (1%) 2264
Lexapro Oral Suspension (2%) 1174
Lexapro Tablets (2%) 1174
Micardis Tablets (More than 0.3%) 852
Micardis HCT Tablets 854
Mirapex Tablets 857
Requip Tablets (Infrequent to frequent) 1561
▲ Risperdal Consta Long-Acting Injection (3%) 1753
Teveten Tablets (Less than 1%) 515
Teveten HCT Tablets (Less than 1%) 517
Ultram ER Extended-Release Tablets (0.5% to less than 1%) 2428
Vivitrol 988
Wellbutrin Tablets (Infrequent) 1648
Xyrem Oral Solution (Frequent) 1766

Torsade de pointes

Adenocard IV Injection 603
Avelox 2803
Biaxin/Biaxin XL (Rare) 411
Celexa 1160
Cipro I.V. 2817
Cipro 2810
Cipro XR Tablets 2823
E.E.S. (Rare) 433
Effexor XR Extended-Release Capsules (Rare) 3195
EryPed (Rare) 431
Geodon (Rare) 2520
Ketek Tablets 2744
Levaquin 2416
Levaquin in 5% Dextrose Injection 2416
Lexapro Oral Suspension 1174
Lexapro Tablets 1174
Luvox CR Extended-Release Capsules 1759
Meridia Capsules 475
Noroxin Tablets (Rare) 2069
Noxafil Oral Suspension 2889
Paxil 1535
Paxil CR Controlled-Release Tablets 1544
Pletal Tablets 2481
Prograf Capsules and Injection 622
Prozac Weekly Capsules 1852
Remeron Tablets (Four cases) 2924
RemeronSolTab Tablets (Four cases) 2927
Risperdal Consta Long-Acting Injection 1753
Rythmol Tablets 1586
Sutent Capsules (Less than 0.1%) 2540
Thioridazine Hydrochloride Tablets 2195
Velcade for Injection 2168
Venlafaxine Hydrochloride Tablets 2199
VESIcare Tablets 636

Torticollis

Aceon Tablets (2 mg, 4 mg, 8 mg) (1.4%) 3038
Actiq (1% or greater) 959
▲ Actonel with Calcium Tablets (1.2% to 5.3%) 2574
Adenocard IV Injection (Less than 1%) 603
▲ Agrylin Capsules (1% to less than 5%) 3017
AmBisome for Injection (Less common) 606
Amerge Tablets (1% to 2%) 1301
▲ Arimidex Tablets (2% to 5%) 672
Asacol Delayed-Release Tablets 2579
Axert Tablets (Infrequent) 2431
▲ Azilect Tablets (2% to 3%) 3106
▲ Bexxar (1% to 6%) 1371
▲ BOTOX Purified Neurotoxin Complex (3 % to 11%) 550
Campral Tablets (Rare) 1158
Cardene I.V. (Rare) 1093
Cipro I.V. (1% or less) 2817
▲ Copaxone for Injection (8%) 3110
Depakote ER Tablets (Greater than or equal to 1%) 423
▲ DepoCyt Injection (14% to 15%) 1136
Doxil Injection (Less than 1%) 2378
DynaCirc CR Controlled Release Tablets (0.5% to 1%) 1407
▲ Effexor XR Extended-Release Capsules (3%) 3195
Emsam Transdermal System (Frequent) 905
Engerix-B Vaccine (Less than 1%) 1409
▲ Fabrazyme for Intravenous Infusion (5%) 1241
Fentora Tablets (Greater than 1%) 968
▲ Flolan for Injection (84%) 1426
▲ Forteo for Injection (3%) 1816
Gabitril Tablets (Frequent) 973
Geodon Capsules (Rare) 2520
Gliadel Wafer (2%) 1076
▲ Imitrex Injection (5%) 1465
▲ Imitrex Tablets (Less than 1% to 3%) 1474
Ionsys Transdermal System (.1% to less than 1%) 2410
Klonopin (Infrequent) 2639
Lamictal (2%) 1488
▲ Lexapro Oral Suspension (3%) 1174
▲ Lexapro Tablets (3%) 1174
Lipitor Tablets (Less than 2%) 2501
Lovaza Capsules 1520
Luvox CR Extended-Release Capsules (Rare) 1759
Lyrica Capsules (Rare) 2527
Meridia Capsules (1.6%) 475
Mirapex Tablets (Greater than or equal to 1%) 857
Norvir (Less than 2%) 489
▲ Orthoclone OKT3 Sterile Solution (14%) 2387
OxyContin Tablets (Less than 1%) 2589
Paxil (Infrequent) 1535
Paxil CR Controlled-Release Tablets (Infrequent) 1544
Prinivil Tablets (0.3% to 1%) 2087
Prinzide Tablets 2092
ProQuad 2099
Protonix for Delayed-Release Oral Suspension (Greater than or equal to 1%) 3254
Protonix Delayed-Release Tablets (Greater than or equal to 1%) 3254
Protonix I.V. (Greater than or equal to 1%) 3257
Protopic Ointment (Greater than or equal to 1%) 628
Provigil Tablets (Greater than or equal to 1%) 977
▲ Pulmicort Flexhaler (Greater than or equal to 1% to 3%) 654
Recombivax HB (Less than 1%) 2107
Remeron Tablets (Infrequent) 2924
RemeronSolTab Tablets (Infrequent) 2927
Requip Tablets (Infrequent to frequent) 1561
Risperdal Consta Long-Acting Injection (Infrequent) 1753
Rythmol SR Capsules 1590
Stromectol Tablets 2120
Symbyax Capsules (Frequent) 1871
Thioridazine Hydrochloride Tablets 2195
▲ Trisenox Injection (13%) 986
▲ Ultram ER Extended-Release Tablets (1% to less than 5%) 2428
Vantas (Less than 2%) 1737
Venlafaxine Hydrochloride Tablets (Rare) 2199
Wellbutrin SR Sustained-Release Tablets (At least 1%) 1653
Wellbutrin XL Extended-Release Tablets (At least 1%) 1659
Xifaxan Tablets (Less than 2%) 2682
Xyrem Oral Solution (Frequent) 1766
Zomig Tablets (Infrequent) 694
Zomig Nasal Spray (Infrequent) 689
Zomig-ZMT Tablets (Infrequent) 694
Zyban Sustained-Release Tablets (2%) 1692
▲ Zyprexa Tablets (2% to 3%) 1883
▲ Zyprexa ZYDIS Orally Disintegrating Tablets (2% to 3%) 1883

Total proteins, decrease

(*see under* Hypoproteinemia)

Tourette's syndrome

Adderall XR Capsules 3012
Concerta Extended-Release Tablets (Rare) 1925
Daytrana Transdermal Patch 3022
Dexedrine 1401
Focalin XR Capsules 2251
Meridia Capsules 475
Metadate CD Capsules (Rare) 3146
Vyvanse Capsules 3033

Toxic shock syndrome

Amevive 611
NuvaRing (Very rare) 2897

Toxicity, cutaneous

▲ Taxotere Injection Concentrate (0.8% to 26.5%) 2773
▲ Vectibix (16% to 90%) 597

Toxicity, drug

Mirapex Tablets 857
Vicodin Tablets 529
Vicodin ES Tablets 530
Vicodin HP Tablets 531

Toxicity, mucosal

Vectibix 597

Toxicity, unspecified

▲ Advair HFA 45/21 Inhalation Aerosol (1% to 3%) 1288
▲ Advair HFA 115/21 Inhalation Aerosol (1% to 3%) 1288
▲ Advair HFA 230/21 Inhalation Aerosol (1% to 3%) 1288

Toxicity, vascular

Gemzar for Injection (Very rare) 1820

Toxoplasmosis

Doxil Injection 2378
Velcade for Injection 2168

Tracheitis

Advair Diskus 100/50 1276
Advair Diskus 250/50 1276
Advair Diskus 500/50 1276
Advair HFA 45/21 Inhalation Aerosol 1288
Advair HFA 115/21 Inhalation Aerosol 1288
Advair HFA 230/21 Inhalation Aerosol 1288
Amerge Tablets (Rare) 1301
Lexapro Oral Suspension (Infrequent) 1174
Lexapro Tablets (Infrequent) 1174
Liquid PedvaxHIB (One case) 2073
▲ Serevent Diskus (7%) 1594

Tracheobronchitis

Avalide Tablets 892
Avalide Tablets 2713
Avapro Tablets (Less than 1%) 897
Avapro Tablets (Less than 1%) 2718

Transaminase, elevation

(*see under* Serum transaminase, elevation)

Transfusion reactions

▲ Clolar for Intravenous Infusion (10%) 1239
▲ Dacogen Injection (7%) 1066

Transfusions, platelet

Treanda for Injection (Less than 1%) 983

Transfusions, red blood cell

▲ Treanda for Injection (20%) 983

Trauma

Ambien CR Tablets (Infrequent) 2696
▲ Cozaar Tablets (4%) 1973
Exelon Capsules (Frequent) 2229
Exelon Oral Solution (Frequent) 2229
▲ Gengraf Capsules (4%) 435
▲ Neoral Oral Solution (4%) 2280
▲ Neoral Soft Gelatin Capsules (4%) 2280
ProQuad 2099
▲ Simulect for Injection (3% to 10%) 2306
Singulair (1%) 2114
Venlafaxine Hydrochloride Tablets (2%) 2199

Trauma, unspecified

Ambien Tablets (Infrequent) 2692
▲ Lescol Capsules (5.1%) 2268
▲ Lescol XL Tablets (4.2%) 2268
▲ Paxil (1.4% to 6%) 1535
Paxil CR Controlled-Release Tablets (1.4%) 1544
Prinzide Tablets (0.3% to 1%) 2092
▲ Zyvox (2.8% to 3.3%) 2552

Trembling

(*see also under* Tremors)

Ultram ER Extended-Release Tablets (0.5% to 4%) 2428

Tremors

▲ Abilify Injection (2% to 9%) 881
▲ Abilify Injection (2% to 11.8%) 2466
▲ Abilify Oral Solution (2% to 9%) 881
▲ Abilify Oral Solution (2% to 11.8%) 2466
▲ Abilify Discmelt Orally Disintegrating Tablets (2% to 9%) 881
▲ Abilify Discmelt Orally Disintegrating Tablets (2% to 11.8%) 2466
▲ Abilify Tablets (2% to 9%) 881
▲ Abilify Tablets (2% to 11.8%) 2466
Adderall XR Capsules 3012
Adenoscan (Less than 1%) 605
Adipex-P 1185
Advicor Tablets 402
▲ Aerobid/Aerobid-M (3% to 9%) 1153
Alferon N Injection (One patient) 1726
Alimta for Injection (Less than 1%) 1786
Alinia for Oral Suspension (Less than 1%) 2677
Alinia Tablets (Less than 1%) 2677
Ambien Tablets (Infrequent) 2692
Ambien CR Tablets (1%) 2696
AmBisome for Injection (Less common) 606
Amerge Tablets (Infrequent) 1301
Amitiza Capsules (Less than 1%) 3082
Amrix Capsules 966
Anaprox Tablets (Less than 1%) 2632
Anaprox DS Tablets (Less than 1%) 2632
Anzemet Injection (Infrequently) 2701
Anzemet Tablets (1.3% to 2.2%) 2704
Aricept Tablets (Frequent) 1062
Aricept ODT Tablets (Frequent) 1062
▲ Arranon Injection (0% to 5%) 1319
Asacol Delayed-Release Tablets 2579
Atripla Tablets 938
Avalide Tablets 892
Avalide Tablets 2713
Avapro Tablets (Less than 1%) 897
Avapro Tablets (Less than 1%) 2718
Avelox (Greater than or equal to 0.1% to less than 2%) 2803
▲ Avinza Capsules (Less than 5%) 1772
Axert Tablets (Infrequent) 2431
Azilect Tablets (Frequent) 3106
▲ BeneFIX Vials (3.1%) 3191
Biaxin/Biaxin XL 411
Bicillin C-R Injectable Suspension 1775
Bicillin L-A Injection 1777
Brovana Inhalation Solution (Less than 2%) 2990
▲ Campath Ampules (3%) 761
Campral Tablets (Frequent) 1158
Cancidas for Injection 1953
Cardizem LA Extended Release Tablets (Less than 2%) 421
▲ Celexa (8%) 1160

▲ CellCept Capsules (24.2% to 33.9%) 2622
▲ CellCept Intravenous (24.2% to 33.9%) 2622
▲ CellCept Oral Suspension (24.2% to 33.9%) 2622
▲ CellCept Tablets (24.2% to 33.9%) 2622
Chantix Tablets (Infrequent) 2511
Cipro I.V. (1% or less) 2817
Cipro (Less than 1%) 2810
Cipro XR Tablets (Less than 1%) 2823
▲ Clolar for Intravenous Infusion (10%) 1239
Combivent Inhalation Aerosol (Less than 2%) 845
Concerta Extended-Release Tablets (2.7%) 1925
▲ Copaxone for Injection (7%) 3110
Cozaar Tablets (Less than 1%) 1973
Crinone 4% Gel 992
Crinone 8% Gel 992
▲ Cymbalta Delayed-Release Capsules (0% to 5%) 1801
▲ Demser Capsules (10%) 1989
▲ Depakote ER Tablets (Greater than 1% to 57%) 423
▲ DepoCyt Injection (9% to 15%) 1136
Dexedrine 1401
Duragesic Transdermal System (1% or greater) 2405
Dyazide Capsules 1405
EC-Naprosyn Delayed-Release Tablets (Less than 1%) 2632
▲ Effexor XR Extended-Release Capsules (4% to 5%) 3195
Eldepryl Capsules 3052
Eligard 7.5 mg (Less than 2%) 2724
Eligard 22.5 mg (Less than 2%) 2724
Eligard 30 mg (Less than 2%) 2724
Eligard 45 mg (Less than 2%) 2724
Elspar for Injection 1990
Emend Capsules (Greater than 0.5%) 1992
Emend for Injection (Greater than 0.5%) 1999
Emsam Transdermal System (Infrequent) 905
EpiPen 1024
Erbitux 912
▲ Evoxac Capsules (1% to 3%) 1013
▲ Exelon Capsules (4% to 10%) 2229
▲ Exelon Oral Solution (4% to 10%) 2229
Exelon Patch (Frequent) 2233
Exforge Tablets (Greater than 0.1% to less than 1%) 2238
Flebogamma 5% 1715
Flebogamma 5% DIF 1718
▲ Flolan for Injection (7% to 21%) 1426
▲ Fluarix Vaccine (3.3% to 6.9%) 1446
Flumadine (Less than 0.3%) 1167
Foradil Aerolizer (1.9%) 2849
Frova Tablets (Infrequent) 1111
▲ Gabitril Tablets (9%) 973
Gammagard Liquid 730
Gammagard S/D 734
Gamunex 3094
▲ Gengraf Capsules (13%) 435
▲ Geodon Capsules (14%) 2520
▲ Gliadel Wafer (5%) 1076
▲ Humira Injection (Less than 5%) 442
Humulin 50/50, 100 Units 1843
Humulin 70/30 Vial 1844
Humulin N Vial 1846
Humulin R 1849
Imitrex Injection (Infrequent) 1465
Imitrex Nasal Spray (Infrequent) 1470
Imitrex Tablets (Rare to infrequent) 1474
Intelence Tablets (Less than 2%) 3119
▲ Intron A for Injection (Less than 5%) 2859
Invanz for Injection (Greater than 0.1%) 2029
▲ Invega Extended-Release Tablets (3% to 4%) 1748
Ionsys Transdermal System (.1% to less than 1%) 2410
Kaletra (Less than 2%) 452
Keppra Oral Solution (1% to greater than or equal to 2%) 3131
Keppra Tablets (1% to greater than or equal to 2%) 3131
Klonopin (Infrequent) 2639
▲ Lamictal (10%) 1488
Lescol Capsules 2268
Lescol XL Tablets 2268
Leukeran Tablets (Rare) 1508
Levaquin 2416
Levaquin in 5% Dextrose Injection 2416
Levothroid Tablets 1170
Levoxyl Tablets 1780
Lexapro Oral Suspension (Infrequent) 1174
Lexapro Tablets (Infrequent) 1174
Lialda Tablets (Infrequent) 3029
Lidoderm Patch 1114
Lunesta Tablets (Rare) 2994
▲ Luvox CR Extended-Release Capsules (1% to 8%) 1759
▲ Lyrica Capsules (1% to 11%) 2527
▲ Marplan Tablets (4%) 3177
▲ Maxair Autohaler (1.3% to 6%) 1705
Maxalt Tablets (Frequent) 2056
Maxalt-MLT Orally Disintegrating Tablets (Frequent) 2056
Meridia Capsules 475
Mevacor Tablets (0.5% to 1%) 2063
Mirapex Tablets (1% or more) 857
Moban Tablets 1116
Mobic Oral Suspension (Less than 2%) 863
Mobic Tablets (Less than 2%) 863
MS Contin Tablets (Less frequent) 2585
▲ Myfortic Tablets (3% to less than 20%) 2276
Nalfon Capsules (2.2%) 2508
Namenda (Infrequent) 1180
Naprosyn Suspension (Less than 1%) 2632
Naprosyn Tablets (Less than 1%) 2632
Natrecor for Injection (Greater than or equal to 1%) 2977
▲ Neoral Oral Solution (12% to 55%) 2280
▲ Neoral Soft Gelatin Capsules (12% to 55%) 2280
Neupro Transdermal System (Greater than or equal to 2%) 3149
Nexium Delayed-Release Capsules (Less than 1%) 645
Nexium I.V. (Less than 1%) 652
Nexium Delayed-Release Oral Suspension (Less than 1%) 645
Noroxin Tablets 2069
Norvir (Less than 2%) 489
Noxafil Oral Suspension (1%) 2889
▲ Orthoclone OKT3 Sterile Solution (13%) 2387
OxyContin Tablets (Less than 1%) 2589
Parnate Tablets 1532
▲ Paxil (1% to 14.7%) 1535
▲ Paxil CR Controlled-Release Tablets (5% to 14.7%) 1544
Percocet Tablets 1127
Perforomist Inhalation Solution 1025
Phenytek Capsules (Rare) 2192
Primaxin I.M. 2080
Primaxin I.V. (Less than 0.2%) 2083
Prinivil Tablets (0.3% to 1%) 2087
Prinzide Tablets 2092
▲ Pristiq Extended-Release Tablets (2% to 9%) 3247
ProAir HFA Inhalation Aerosol (Frequent) 3113
▲ Prograf Capsules and Injection (15% to 56%) 622
ProQuad 2099
Protonix for Delayed-Release Oral Suspension (Less than 1%) 3254
Protonix Delayed-Release Tablets (Less than 1%) 3254
Protonix I.V. (Less than 1%) 3257
▲ Proventil HFA Inhalation Aerosol (7%) 2914
Provigil Tablets (1%) 977
▲ Prozac Weekly Capsules (3% to 13%) 1852
▲ Prozac Pulvules and Liquid (3% to 13%) 1852
Remeron Tablets (2%) 2924
RemeronSolTab Tablets (2%) 2927
Requip Tablets (1% or more) 1561
Retrovir Capsules 1574
Retrovir IV Infusion 1579
Retrovir 1574
Rilutek Tablets (Frequent) 2771
▲ Risperdal Consta Long-Acting Injection (3%) 1753
▲ Romazicon Injection (3% to 9%) 2646
Rythmol Tablets (1% to 2%) 1586
Rythmol SR Capsules (2%) 1590
Salagen Tablets (Less than 1% to 2%) 1082
▲ Sandimmune (12% to 55%) 2296
Sandostatin Injection (Less than 1%) 2300
Seromycin Capsules 1864
▲ Simulect for Injection (Greater than or equal to 10%) 2306
Singulair 2114
Soma Tablets 1931
Stalevo Tablets 2309
▲ Strattera Capsules (1% to 5%) 1864
Stromectol Tablets (0.9%) 2120
Sular Extended Release Tablets (Less than or equal to 1%) 2975
Sustiva Capsules (Less than 2%) 930
Sustiva Tablets (Less than 2%) 930
▲ Symbyax Capsules (Greater than or equal to 5% to 9%) 1871
Tarka Tablets 511
Tasigna Capsules (0.1% to 1%) 2316
Teveten Tablets (Less than 1%) 515
Teveten HCT Tablets (Less than 1%) 517
Thioridazine Hydrochloride Tablets 2195
Treximet Tablets (Infrequent) 1616
▲ Trisenox Injection (13%) 986
▲ Ultane Liquid for Inhalation (6%) 524
▲ Ultram ER Extended-Release Tablets (1% to less than 5%) 2428
▲ Valcyte Tablets (28%) 2654
Valium Tablets (Infrequent) 2658
Vantas (Less than 2%) 1737
▲ Venlafaxine Hydrochloride Tablets (1.1% to 10.2%) 2199
Ventolin HFA Inhalation Aerosol 1638
▲ Vesanoid Capsules (3%) 2660
Viadur Implant (Rare) 802
Vicoprofen Tablets (Less than 1%) 533
Voltaren Tablets (Occasionally) 2334
Voltaren-XR Tablets (Occasionally) 2337
Vyvanse Capsules (2%) 3033
▲ Wellbutrin Tablets (21.1%) 1648
▲ Wellbutrin SR Sustained-Release Tablets (3% to 6%) 1653
▲ Wellbutrin XL Extended-Release Tablets (3% to 6%) 1659
▲ Xeloda Tablets (Less than 5%) 2662
▲ Xopenex Inhalation Solution (6.8%) 3001
▲ Xopenex Inhalation Solution Concentrate (6.8%) 3005
▲ Xopenex HFA Inhalation Aerosol (6.8%) 3009
Xyrem Oral Solution (Less than 1%) 1766
▲ Zofran Injection (7%) 1682
▲ Zofran (5%) 1687
▲ Zofran ODT Orally Disintegrating Tablets (5%) 1687
Zometa for Intravenous Infusion 2341
Zomig Tablets (Infrequent) 694
Zomig Nasal Spray (Infrequent) 689
Zomig-ZMT Tablets (Infrequent) 694
Zonegran Capsules (Frequent) 1089
Zosyn for Injection (1% or less) 3284
Zovirax 1690
Zyban Sustained-Release Tablets (1% to 2%) 1692
▲ Zyprexa Tablets (5% to 23%) 1883
▲ Zyprexa IntraMuscular (1% to 4%) 1883
▲ Zyprexa ZYDIS Orally Disintegrating Tablets (5% to 23%) 1883
Zyrtec Chewable Tablets (Less than 2%) 1920
Zyrtec Syrup (Less than 2%) 1920
Zyrtec Tablets (Less than 2%) 1920
Zyrtec-D 12 Hour Extended Release Tablets (Less than 2%) 1923

Tremulousness
(*see under* Tremors)

Trigeminal neuralgia
(*see under* Neuralgia, trigeminal)

Trigeminy
Lanoxin Injection 1498
Lanoxin Injection Pediatric 1502
Lanoxin Tablets 1505

Triglycerides, increase
(*see under* Hypertriglyceridemia)

Trismus
Ceftin Tablets (0.1% to 1%) 1380
Cymbalta Delayed-Release Capsules 1801
Demser Capsules 1989
Effexor XR Extended-Release Capsules (2%) 3195
Geodon Capsules (Rare) 2520
Invega Extended-Release Tablets 1748
Ixempra Kit for Injection 915
Luvox CR Extended-Release Capsules (Rare) 1759
Lyrica Capsules (Rare) 2527
Paxil (Rare) 1535
Paxil CR Controlled-Release Tablets (Rare) 1544
Rilutek Tablets (Rare) 2771
Stalevo Tablets 2309
Thioridazine Hydrochloride Tablets 2195
Venlafaxine Hydrochloride Tablets (Frequent) 2199

Troponin, increased
Tasigna Capsules 2316

TSH, increase
Aciphex Tablets 1053
Sutent Capsules (2%) 2540

Tuberculosis
CellCept Capsules 2622
CellCept Intravenous 2622
CellCept Oral Suspension 2622
CellCept Tablets 2622
Cimzia 3127
Enbrel for Injection (0.007% to 0.01%) 569
Humira Injection 442
Myfortic Tablets 2276
Rapamune Oral Solution 3260
Remicade for IV Injection 950

Tuberculosis, disseminated
Cimzia 3127

Tuberculosis, reactivation
Enbrel for Injection 569

Tubulopathy
Atripla Tablets 938
Hepsera Tablets 1253
Truvada Tablets 1262
Viread Tablets 1268

Tumor, central nervous system
Nutropin for Injection 1208
Nutropin AQ Injection 1212
Nutropin AQ NuSpin Injection 1212
Nutropin AQ Pen 1212
Nutropin AQ Pen Cartridge 1212

Tumor, gastrointestinal stromal
Requip Tablets (Infrequent) 1561

Tumor, progression time, decreased
Aranesp for Injection 564
Epogen for Injection 576

Tumor flare
▲ Arimidex Tablets (3%) 672
Gengraf Capsules (1% to less than 3%) 435
Neoral Oral Solution (1% to less than 3%) 2280
Neoral Soft Gelatin Capsules (1% to less than 3%) 2280

Tumor lysis syndrome
Campath Ampules 761
Leustatin Injection (Rare) 2384
Mylotarg for Injection 3212
Rituxan I.V. 1223
Treanda for Injection 983
Velcade for Injection 2168

Tumors, intracranial
Norditropin Cartridges 2354

Tumors, solid, non-cutaneous
Raptiva for Injection 1218

Tumors, solid, non-malignant
Nutropin for Injection (0.1%) 1208
Nutropin AQ Injection (0.1%) 1212
Nutropin AQ NuSpin Injection (0.1%) 1212
Nutropin AQ Pen (0.1%) 1212
Nutropin AQ Pen Cartridge (0.1%) 1212
Raptiva for Injection 1218

T-wave, inverted
Risperdal Consta Long-Acting Injection (Rare) 1753
Ultane Liquid for Inhalation (Less than 1%) 524

T-wave flattening
(*see under* EKG changes, T-wave)

Twitching
▲ Adderall XR Capsules (2% to 4%) 3012
Anzemet Injection (Rare) 2701
Anzemet Tablets (Rare) 2704
Campral Tablets (Rare) 1158
Cipro I.V. 2817
Cipro 2810
Cipro XR Tablets 2823
Concerta Extended-Release Tablets (1%) 1925
Depakote ER Tablets (Greater than 1%) 423
Effexor XR Extended-Release Capsules (2%) 3195
Emsam Transdermal System (Infrequent) 905
Exforge Tablets (Less than or equal to 0.1%) 2238
Focalin XR Capsules 2251
Gabitril Tablets (1% or more) 973
▲ Geodon Capsules (14%) 2520

Imitrex Tablets (Rare) 1474
Klonopin (Infrequent) 2639
Lamictal (Infrequent) 1488
Lexapro Oral Suspension (Infrequent) 1174
Lexapro Tablets (Infrequent) 1174
Lidoderm Patch 1114
Lunesta Tablets (Infrequent) 2994
Luvox CR Extended-Release Capsules (Infrequent to 2%) 1759
▲ Lyrica Capsules (4% to 5%) 2527
Marplan Tablets (2%) 3177
Meridia Capsules 475
Mirapex Tablets (Greater than or equal to 1% to 2%) 857
Norvir (Less than 2%) 489
▲ OxyContin Tablets (Between 1% and 5%) 2589
Phenytek Capsules 2192
Remeron Tablets (Frequent) 2924
RemeronSolTab Tablets (Frequent) 2927
Retrovir Capsules 1574
Retrovir IV Infusion 1579
Retrovir 1574
Salagen Tablets (Less than 1%) 1082
▲ Symbyax Capsules (2% to 6%) 1871
Venlafaxine Hydrochloride Tablets (1%) 2199
Wellbutrin SR Sustained-Release Tablets (1% to 2%) 1653
Wellbutrin XL Extended-Release Tablets (1% to 2%) 1659
Zomig Tablets (Rare) 694
Zomig Nasal Spray (Rare) 689
Zomig-ZMT Tablets (Rare) 694
Zonegran Capsules (Infrequent) 1089
Zyban Sustained-Release Tablets (Infrequent) 1692
▲ Zyprexa Tablets (1% to 5%) 1883
▲ Zyprexa IntraMuscular (2% to 4%) 1883
▲ Zyprexa ZYDIS Orally Disintegrating Tablets (1% to 5%) 1883
Zyrtec Chewable Tablets (Less than 2%) 1920
Zyrtec Syrup (Less than 2%) 1920
Zyrtec Tablets (Less than 2%) 1920
Zyrtec-D 12 Hour Extended Release Tablets (Less than 2%) 1923

Tympanic membrane disorder, unspecified
Tamiflu Capsules (1%) 2649
Tamiflu Oral Suspension (1%) 2649

Tympanometry, abnormal
▲ Increlex Injection (Greater than or equal to 5%) 3100

U

Ulceration
▲ Aldara Cream, 5% (0% to 48%) 1699
Eligard 7.5 mg (0.1%) 2724
Eligard 22.5 mg 2724
Eligard 30 mg 2724
Eligard 45 mg 2724
Veramyst Nasal Spray 1643

Ulceration, bucial mucosa
Nalfon Capsules (Less than 1%) 2508

Ulceration, gastrointestinal
▲ Actonel Tablets (39%) 2568
Celebrex Capsules 2979
CellCept Capsules 2622
CellCept Intravenous 2622
CellCept Oral Suspension 2622
CellCept Tablets 2622
Flector Patch 561
▲ Treximet Tablets (1% to 4%) 1616
Vicoprofen Tablets 533

Ulceration, lip
▲ Dacogen Injection (5%) 1066

Ulceration, tongue
▲ Dacogen Injection (7%) 1066
Evoxac Capsules (Less than 1%) 1013
Soriatane Capsules (Less than 1%) 3062

Ulcers
Paxil (Rare) 1535
Paxil CR Controlled-Release Tablets (Rare) 1544
Remeron Tablets (Infrequent) 2924
RemeronSolTab Tablets (Infrequent) 2927
▲ Vesanoid Capsules (3%) 2660
Zomig Tablets (Rare) 694
Zomig-ZMT Tablets (Rare) 694

Ulcers, aphthous
Captopril Tablets (About 0.5% to 2%) 2182
OsmoPrep Tablets 2680

Ulcers, corneal
Copaxone for Injection (Infrequent) 3110
FML Ophthalmic Ointment (Occasional) ⊙223
FML Ophthalmic Suspension (Occasional) ⊙224
FML Forte Ophthalmic Suspension (Occasional) ⊙222
Iquix Ophthalmic Solution (Less than 1%) 3183
Lyrica Capsules (Rare) 2527

Ulcers, cutaneous
Actiq (1% or greater) 959
AmBisome for Injection (Less common) 606
Aricept Tablets (Frequent) 1062
Aricept ODT Tablets (Frequent) 1062
▲ CellCept Capsules (3% to less than 20%) 2622
▲ CellCept Intravenous (3% to less than 20%) 2622
▲ CellCept Oral Suspension (3% to less than 20%) 2622
▲ CellCept Tablets (3% to less than 20%) 2622
Doxil Injection (Less than 1%) 2378
Enbrel for Injection 569
Evoxac Capsules (Less than 1%) 1013
Exelon Capsules (Infrequent) 2229
Exelon Oral Solution (Infrequent) 2229
▲ Flolan for Injection (39%) 1426
Gabitril Tablets (Infrequent) 973
Gengraf Capsules 435
Kaletra (Less than 2%) 452
Lipitor Tablets (Less than 2%) 2501
Miacalcin Nasal Spray (Less than 1%) 2274
Neoral Oral Solution 2280
Neoral Soft Gelatin Capsules 2280
Paxil (Rare) 1535
Paxil CR Controlled-Release Tablets (Rare) 1544
Plavix Tablets (1% to 2.5%) 926
Plavix Tablets (1% to 2.5%) 2767
▲ Prograf Capsules and Injection (3% to 15%) 622
Protonix for Delayed-Release Oral Suspension (Less than 1%) 3254
Protonix Delayed-Release Tablets (Less than 1%) 3254
Protonix I.V. (Less than 1%) 3257
Prozac Weekly Capsules (Infrequent) 1852
Prozac Pulvules and Liquid (Infrequent) 1852
Remeron Tablets (Rare) 2924
RemeronSolTab Tablets (Rare) 2927
Remicade for IV Injection (Greater than or equal to 0.2%) 950
Requip Tablets (Infrequent) 1561
Rilutek Tablets (Infrequent) 2771
▲ Simulect for Injection (3% to 10%) 2306
▲ Soriatane Capsules (1% to 10%) 3062
Sular Extended Release Tablets (Less than or equal to 1%) 2975
Tricor Tablets 520
▲ Xeloda Tablets (Less than 5%) 2662
Zyprexa Tablets (Infrequent) 1883
Zyprexa ZYDIS Orally Disintegrating Tablets (Infrequent) 1883

Ulcers, decubitus
▲ Mycamine for Injection (4.5% to 5.9%) 616

Ulcers, duodenal
Agrylin Capsules 3017
▲ Anaprox Tablets (1% to 10%) 2632
▲ Anaprox DS Tablets (1% to 10%) 2632
Aricept Tablets (Infrequent) 1062
Aricept ODT Tablets (Infrequent) 1062
Campral Tablets (Rare) 1158
Celexa (Rare) 1160
Copaxone for Injection (Infrequent) 3110
▲ EC-Naprosyn Delayed-Release Tablets (1% to 10%) 2632
Exelon Capsules (Infrequent) 2229
Exelon Oral Solution (Infrequent) 2229
Fosamax 2005
Fosamax Plus D Tablets 2013
Indocin Capsules (Less than 1%) 2024
Indocin I.V. (Less than 1%) 2489
Indocin (Less than 1%) 2024
Lipitor Tablets (Less than 2%) 2501
Meridia Capsules 475
Mirapex Tablets 857
Mobic Oral Suspension (Less than 2%) 863
Mobic Tablets (Less than 2%) 863
Myfortic Tablets 2276
▲ Naprosyn Suspension (1% to 10%) 2632
▲ Naprosyn Tablets (1% to 10%) 2632
Pentasa Capsules (Less than 1%) 3030
Plavix Tablets 926
Plavix Tablets 2767
Pletal Tablets (Less than 2%) 2481
Proleukin for Injection 2287
Prozac Weekly Capsules (Rare) 1852
Prozac Pulvules and Liquid (Rare) 1852
Requip Tablets (Infrequent) 1561
Stalevo Tablets 2309
Taxotere Injection Concentrate 2773
Tricor Tablets 520
▲ Voltaren Tablets (1% to 10%) 2334
▲ Voltaren-XR Tablets (1% to 10%) 2337
Zonegran Capsules (Infrequent) 1089
Zosyn for Injection (1.3%) 3284

Ulcers, duodenal, hemorrhagic
Mirapex Tablets 857
Mobic Oral Suspension (Less than 2%) 863
Mobic Tablets (Less than 2%) 863
Percodan Tablets 1130

Ulcers, duodenal, perforated
Mobic Oral Suspension (Less than 2%) 863
Mobic Tablets (Less than 2%) 863

Ulcers, esophageal
Accutane Capsules 2607
Actonel Tablets 2568
Copaxone for Injection (Infrequent) 3110
Doxil Injection (Less than 1%) 2378
Fosamax (0.1% to 1.5%) 2005
Lyrica Capsules (Rare) 2527
Namenda (Infrequent) 1180
Nexium Delayed-Release Capsules (Less than 1%) 645
Nexium I.V. (Less than 1%) 652
Nexium Delayed-Release Oral Suspension (Less than 1%) 645
Pentasa Capsules (Less than 1%) 3030
Prozac Weekly Capsules (Rare) 1852
Prozac Pulvules and Liquid (Rare) 1852
Zyprexa Tablets (Rare) 1883
Zyprexa ZYDIS Orally Disintegrating Tablets (Rare) 1883

Ulcers, gastric
Actonel Tablets 2568
Actonel with Calcium Tablets 2574
Agrylin Capsules 3017
Amerge Tablets (Rare) 1301
▲ Anaprox Tablets (Less than 1% to 10%) 2632
▲ Anaprox DS Tablets (Less than 1% to 10%) 2632
Aricept Tablets (Infrequent) 1062
Aricept ODT Tablets (Infrequent) 1062
Campral Tablets (Rare) 1158
Celexa (Rare) 1160
▲ CellCept Capsules (3% to less than 20%) 2622
▲ CellCept Intravenous (3% to less than 20%) 2622
▲ CellCept Oral Suspension (3% to less than 20%) 2622
▲ CellCept Tablets (3% to less than 20%) 2622
Chantix Tablets (Rare) 2511
Cymbalta Delayed-Release Capsules (Rare) 1801
▲ EC-Naprosyn Delayed-Release Tablets (Less than 1% to 10%) 2632
Evoxac Capsules (Less than 1%) 1013
Exelon Capsules (Infrequent) 2229
Exelon Oral Solution (Infrequent) 2229
Fosamax (Up to 1.1%) 2005
Fosamax Plus D Tablets (0% to 1.1%) 2013
Gengraf Capsules (1% to less than 3%) 435
Lunesta Tablets (Rare) 2994
Meridia Capsules 475
Mirapex Tablets 857
Mobic Oral Suspension (Less than 2%) 863
Mobic Tablets (Less than 2%) 863
Myfortic Tablets 2276
▲ Naprosyn Suspension (Less than 1% to 10%) 2632
▲ Naprosyn Tablets (Less than 1% to 10%) 2632
Neoral Oral Solution (1% to less than 3%) 2280
Neoral Soft Gelatin Capsules (1% to less than 3%) 2280
Nexium Delayed-Release Capsules (Less than 1%) 645
Nexium I.V. (Less than 1%) 652
Nexium Delayed-Release Oral Suspension (Less than 1%) 645
Plavix Tablets (Less than 1%) 926
Plavix Tablets (Less than 1%) 2767
Pletal Tablets (Less than 2%) 2481
Prograf Capsules and Injection 622
Prozac Weekly Capsules (Infrequent) 1852
Prozac Pulvules and Liquid (Infrequent) 1852
Requip Tablets (Infrequent) 1561
Risperdal Consta Long-Acting Injection (Infrequent) 1753
Sandostatin Injection (Less than 1%) 2300
Sandostatin LAR Depot 2302
Tasigna Capsules 2316
Treximet Tablets (Rare) 1616
▲ Voltaren Tablets (1% to 10%) 2334
▲ Voltaren-XR Tablets (1% to 10%) 2337
Wellbutrin SR Sustained-Release Tablets 1653
Wellbutrin XL Extended-Release Tablets 1659
Zonegran Capsules (Infrequent) 1089

Ulcers, gastric, hemorrhage
Mirapex Tablets 857
Prozac Weekly Capsules (Rare) 1852

Ulcers, gastrointestinal
Abilify Injection (Greater than or equal to 1 in 1000 patients and less than 1 in 100 patients) 2466
Abilify Oral Solution (Greater than or equal to 1 in 1000 patients and less than 1 in 100 patients) 2466
Abilify Discmelt Orally Disintegrating Tablets (Greater than or equal to 1 in 1000 patients and less than 1 in 100 patients) 2466
Abilify Tablets (Greater than or equal to 1 in 1000 patients and less than 1 in 100 patients) 2466
Aggrenox Capsules (Less than 1%) 819
▲ Anaprox Tablets (1% to 10%) 2632
▲ Anaprox DS Tablets (1% to 10%) 2632
Bayer Aspirin 750
Clinoril Tablets 1962
Cosmegen for Injection 2485
▲ EC-Naprosyn Delayed-Release Tablets (1% to 10%) 2632
Effexor XR Extended-Release Capsules (Infrequent) 3195
Gleevec Tablets (Infrequent) 2255
Indocin Capsules (Less than 1%) 2024
Indocin I.V. (Less than 1%) 2489
Indocin (Less than 1%) 2024
▲ Intron A for Injection (Less than 5%) 2859
Luvox CR Extended-Release Capsules (Infrequent) 1759
Mobic Oral Suspension 863
Mobic Tablets 863
Nalfon Capsules 2508
▲ Naprosyn Suspension (1% to 10%) 2632
▲ Naprosyn Tablets (1% to 10%) 2632
Paxil (Rare) 1535
Paxil CR Controlled-Release Tablets (Rare) 1544
▲ Photofrin for Injection (Less than 5%) 708
Plavix Tablets (Less than 1%) 926
Plavix Tablets (Less than 1%) 2767
Rilutek Tablets (Infrequent) 2771
St. Joseph 81 mg Aspirin Chewable and Enteric Coated Tablets 1903
Sandostatin Injection (Less than 1%) 2300
Venlafaxine Hydrochloride Tablets (Infrequent) 2199
▲ Voltaren Tablets (1% to 10%) 2334
▲ Voltaren-XR Tablets (1% to 10%) 2337
Wellbutrin Tablets (Rare) 1648

Ulcers, leg
Enbrel for Injection 569

Ulcers, oral mucosal
Actiq (Less than 1%) 959
Asacol Delayed-Release Tablets 2579
Campral Tablets (Rare) 1158
Carbatrol Capsules 3019
Ceftin Tablets (0.1% to 1%) 1380
Cipro I.V. (1% or less) 2817
Cipro XR Tablets 2823
Combivent Inhalation Aerosol 845
Copaxone for Injection (Infrequent) 3110
Cuprimine Capsules 1986
Depakote ER Tablets (Greater than 1%) 423
▲ Doxil Injection (1% to 5%) 2378

Effexor XR Extended-Release Capsules (Infrequent) 3195
Elmiron Capsules (Less than or equal to 1%) 2435
▲ Enbrel for Injection (2% to 6%) 569
▲ Flovent Diskus 50 mcg (1% to 3%) 1435
Gabitril Tablets (1%) 973
Gleevec Tablets (Less common) 2255
▲ Intron A for Injection (Less than 5%) 2859
Invanz for Injection (Greater than 0.1%) 2029
Kaletra (Less than 2%) 452
Lamictal (Infrequent) 1488
Leukeran Tablets (Infrequent) 1508
Lipitor Tablets (Less than 2%) 2501
Lunesta Tablets (Infrequent) 2994
▲ Malarone Pediatric Tablets (2% to 6%) 1521
▲ Malarone Tablets (2% to 6%) 1521
Meridia Capsules 475
Noroxin Tablets (Less frequent) 2069
Norvir (Less than 2%) 489
▲ Ontak Vials (Less than 5%) 1079
Paxil (Infrequent) 1535
Paxil CR Controlled-Release Tablets (Infrequent) 1544
Pentasa Capsules (Less than 1%) 3030
ProAmatine Tablets (Rare) 3032
Protonix for Delayed-Release Oral Suspension (Less than 1%) 3254
Protonix Delayed-Release Tablets (Less than 1%) 3254
Protonix I.V. (Less than 1%) 3257
Provigil Tablets (1%) 977
Prozac Pulvules and Liquid (Infrequent) 1852
Requip Tablets (Infrequent) 1561
Retrovir Capsules 1574
Retrovir IV Infusion 1579
Retrovir 1574
Rythmol SR Capsules 1590
Sular Extended Release Tablets (Less than or equal to 1%) 2975
Trizivir Tablets 1622
Vicoprofen Tablets (Less than 3%) 533
Wellbutrin SR Sustained-Release Tablets (Infrequent) 1653
Wellbutrin XL Extended-Release Tablets (Infrequent) 1659
Ziagen 1673
Zonegran Capsules (Rare) 1089
Zyban Sustained-Release Tablets (2%) 1692
Zyprexa Tablets (Infrequent) 1883
Zyprexa ZYDIS Orally Disintegrating Tablets (Infrequent) 1883

Ulcers, oropharyngeal
Fosamax 2005
Fosamax Plus D Tablets (Rarely) 2013

Ulcers, peptic
Advicor Tablets 402
Aricept Tablets (Infrequent) 1062
Aricept ODT Tablets (Infrequent) 1062
Captopril Tablets (About 0.5% to 2%) 2182
Clinoril Tablets (Less than 1 in 100) 1962
Effexor XR Extended-Release Capsules 3195
Evoxac Capsules (Less than 1%) 1013
Exelon Patch (Infrequent) 2233
Frova Tablets (Rare) 1111
Gengraf Capsules (1% to less than 3%) 435
Imitrex Injection (Rare) 1465
Imitrex Nasal Spray 1470
Imitrex Tablets (Rare) 1474
Indocin Capsules (Less than 1%) 2024
Indocin I.V. (Less than 1%) 2489
Indocin (Less than 1%) 2024
Lamictal (Rare) 1488
Lipitor Tablets (Less than 2%) 2501
▲ Lupron Depot 7.5 mg (Less than 5%) 469
Nalfon Capsules (Less than 1%) 2508
Neoral Oral Solution (1% to less than 3%) 2280
Neoral Soft Gelatin Capsules (1% to less than 3%) 2280
Niaspan Extended-Release Tablets 480
Omnicef Capsules 497
Omnicef for Oral Suspension 497
Paxil (Rare) 1535
Paxil CR Controlled-Release Tablets (Rare) 1544
Percodan Tablets 1130
Plavix Tablets 926
Plavix Tablets 2767
Pletal Tablets (Less than 2%) 2481
Prograf Capsules and Injection 622
Protonix for Delayed-Release Oral Suspension (Less than 1%) 3254
Protonix Delayed-Release Tablets (Less than 1%) 3254
Protonix I.V. (Less than 1%) 3257
Prozac Weekly Capsules (Rare) 1852
Prozac Pulvules and Liquid (Rare) 1852
Requip Tablets (Infrequent) 1561
Rythmol SR Capsules 1590
Sandimmune (2% or less) 2296
Sandostatin Injection (Less than 1%) 2300
Sandostatin LAR Depot 2302
Symbyax Capsules (Infrequent) 1871
Tricor Tablets 520
Urso 250 Tablets (1%) 720
Urso Forte Tablets (1%) 720
Zosyn for Injection (1% or less) 3284
Zyban Sustained-Release Tablets 1692

Ulcers, peptic, aggravation of
Eldepryl Capsules 3052
Niaspan Extended-Release Tablets 480

Ulcers, peptic, hemorrhagic
Mobic Oral Suspension (Less than 2%) 863
Mobic Tablets (Less than 2%) 863
Prozac Pulvules and Liquid (Rare) 1852
Tarceva Tablets 1228

Ulcers, peptic, reactivation of
Cuprimine Capsules 1986
Didronel Tablets (A few patients) 2583

Ulcers, peptic with or without perforation
Asacol Delayed-Release Tablets (Rare) 2579
Didronel Tablets (One report) 2583

Ulcers, peptic with perforation and hemorrhage
▲ Anaprox Tablets (Less than 1% to 4%) 2632
▲ Anaprox DS Tablets (Less than 1% to 4%) 2632
▲ EC-Naprosyn Delayed-Release Tablets (Less than 1% to 4%) 2632
Mobic Oral Suspension (Less than 2%) 863
Mobic Tablets (Less than 2%) 863
▲ Naprosyn Suspension (Less than 1% to 4%) 2632
▲ Naprosyn Tablets (Less than 1% to 4%) 2632

Ulcers, skin
▲ Avastin IV (6%) 1192
Bicillin C-R Injectable Suspension 1775
Bicillin L-A Injection 1777
Exelon Patch (Infrequent) 2233
Lyrica Capsules (0.1% to 1%) 2527
Merrem I.V. (Greater than 0.1% to 1%) 684
Mirapex Tablets 857
Namenda (Infrequent) 1180
Protopic Ointment (0.2% to less than 1%) 628
Salagen Tablets (Less than 1%) 1082
Symbyax Capsules (Rare) 1871
Tasigna Capsules 2316

Unconsciousness
(*see under* Consciousness, loss of)

Underventilation
(*see under* Hypoventilation)

Unresponsiveness, unspecified
Cipro XR Tablets 2823
Synagis Intramuscular Solution 1948

Unsteadiness
Carbatrol Capsules (Among most frequent) 3019
Effexor XR Extended-Release Capsules 3195
Equetro Extended-Release Capsules 3174
Symbyax Capsules 1871

Upper respiratory symptoms
▲ Bactroban Nasal (5%) 1367
▲ Chantix Tablets (5% to 7%) 2511
Engerix-B Vaccine (Less than 1%) 1409
▲ Neoral Oral Solution (13%) 2280
▲ Neoral Soft Gelatin Capsules (13%) 2280
Tarka Tablets (2.4%) 511
Varivax (Greater than or equal to 1%) 2133
▲ Vesanoid Capsules (63%) 2660
▲ Wellbutrin Tablets (5%) 1648

Uremia
(*see under* Azotemia)

Ureteral obstruction
Zolinza Capsules 2142

Ureteral spasm
Lortab 5/500 Tablets 3143
Lortab 7.5/500 Tablets 3144
Lortab 10/500 Tablets 3144
Tussionex Pennkinetic Extended-Release Suspension 3154
Vicodin Tablets 529
Vicodin ES Tablets 530
Vicodin HP Tablets 531
Zydone Tablets 1132

Urethral disorder
Chantix Tablets (Infrequent) 2511
Evoxac Capsules (Less than 1%) 1013
▲ Selzentry Tablets (4.5%) 2534

Urethritis
Copaxone for Injection (Infrequent) 3110
Gabitril Tablets (Infrequent) 973
Imitrex Injection 1465
Imitrex Nasal Spray 1470
Lunesta Tablets (Rare) 2994
Mirapex Tablets 857
Norvir (Less than 2%) 489
Paxil (Rare to infrequent) 1535
Paxil CR Controlled-Release Tablets (Rare to infrequent) 1544
Protonix for Delayed-Release Oral Suspension (Less than 1%) 3254
Protonix Delayed-Release Tablets (Less than 1%) 3254
Protonix I.V. (Less than 1%) 3257
Remeron Tablets (Rare) 2924
RemeronSolTab Tablets (Rare) 2927
Tice BCG (Less than or equal to 1%) 2936
Valstar Sterile Solution for Intravesical Instillation (Less than 1%) 1735

Uric acid, reduction of
Cipro XR Tablets 2823
Timentin ADD-Vantage 1606
Timentin IV Infusion 1603

Uric acid level, changes in
Elitek 2729
▲ Sutent Capsules (8% to 15%) 2540

Uric acid level, increase
(*see under* Hyperuricemia)

Urinary bladder, inflammation of
Amerge Tablets (Infrequent) 1301

Urinary casts
Primaxin I.M. 2080
Primaxin I.V. 2083
Rocephin Injectable Vials, ADD-Vantage, Galaxy, Bulk (Less than 1%) 2642
Rythmol SR Capsules 1590

Urinary cytology, abnormal
Orthoclone OKT3 Sterile Solution 2387

Urinary debris, unspecified
Tice BCG (2%) 2936

Urinary difficulty
(*see under* Micturition, difficulty)

Urinary disorders, unspecified
▲ AndroGel (3.7%) 3159
Ionsys Transdermal System (.1% to less than 1%) 2410
Somatuline Depot Injection 3102

Urinary disturbances
Avapro Tablets (Less than 1%) 897
Avapro Tablets (Less than 1%) 2718
Eldepryl Capsules 3052
▲ Lupron Depot 7.5 mg (12.5%) 469
Lupron Depot–3 Month 11.25 mg 462
▲ Neoral Oral Solution (24.2%) 2280
▲ Neoral Soft Gelatin Capsules (24.2%) 2280
Selzentry Tablets 2534

Urinary findings, abnormal
Capastat Sulfate for Injection 1791

Urinary frequency
(*see under* Polyuria)

Urinary glucose, false-positive
Augmentin 1323
Augmentin Tablets 1327
Augmentin XR Extended Release Tablets 1333
Ceftin 1380
Fortaz 1450
Moxatag Tablets 2165
Rocephin Injectable Vials, ADD-Vantage, Galaxy, Bulk 2642

Urinary hesitancy
AndroGel 3159
Donnatal Extentabs 2507
Eldepryl Capsules 3052
▲ Marplan Tablets (1% to 4%) 3177
MS Contin Tablets (Less frequent) 2585
▲ Paxil (3%) 1535
▲ Paxil CR Controlled-Release Tablets (3%) 1544
Retrovir Capsules 1574
Retrovir IV Infusion 1579
Retrovir 1574
▲ Strattera Capsules (3% to 8%) 1864
Valium Tablets (Infrequent) 2658

Urinary incontinence
Actiq (Less than 1%) 959
Ambien Tablets (Infrequent) 2692
Ambien CR Tablets (Infrequent) 2696
AmBisome for Injection (Less common) 606
Amerge Tablets (Rare) 1301
AndroGel 3159
Aricept Tablets (2%) 1062
Aricept ODT Tablets (2%) 1062
Campral Tablets (Infrequent) 1158
Celebrex Capsules (0.1% to 1.9%) 2979
Celexa (Infrequent) 1160
▲ CellCept Capsules (3% to less than 20%) 2622
▲ CellCept Intravenous (3% to less than 20%) 2622
▲ CellCept Oral Suspension (3% to less than 20%) 2622
▲ CellCept Tablets (3% to less than 20%) 2622
Copaxone for Injection (At least 2%) 3110
Dantrium Capsules (Less frequent) 2580
Depakote ER Tablets (Greater than 1%) 423
DepoCyt Injection (Less than 3%) 1136
▲ Doxil Injection (1% to 10%) 2378
Effexor XR Extended-Release Capsules (Infrequent) 3195
▲ Eloxatin for Injection (2% to less than 5%) 2731
Evoxac Capsules (Less than 1%) 1013
Exelon Capsules (2% or more) 2229
Exelon Oral Solution (2% or more) 2229
Exelon Patch (Frequent) 2233
Gabitril Tablets (Frequent) 973
Gengraf Capsules (1% to less than 3%) 435
Geodon (Rare) 2520
▲ Gliadel Wafer (2% to 8%) 1076
▲ Intron A for Injection (Less than 5%) 2859
Keppra Oral Solution (Greater than or equal to 2%) 3131
Keppra Tablets (Greater than or equal to 2%) 3131
Klonopin (Infrequent) 2639
Lamictal (Infrequent) 1488
Lipitor Tablets (Less than 2%) 2501
Lunesta Tablets (Infrequent) 2994
Lupron Depot-PED 7.5 mg, 11.25 mg and 15 mg (Less than 2%) 471
Luvox CR Extended-Release Capsules (Infrequent) 1759
Lyrica Capsules (1% to 2%) 2527
▲ Megace ES Oral Suspension (1% to 3%) 2499
Merrem I.V. (Greater than 0.1% to 1%) 684
Mirapex Tablets (2%) 857
Neoral Oral Solution (1% to less than 3%) 2280
Neoral Soft Gelatin Capsules (1% to less than 3%) 2280
Neupro Transdermal System 3149
Parnate Tablets 1532
Paxil (Infrequent) 1535
Paxil CR Controlled-Release Tablets (Infrequent) 1544
▲ Prograf Capsules and Injection (3% to 15%) 622
Prozac Weekly Capsules (Infrequent) 1852
Prozac Pulvules and Liquid (Infrequent) 1852
▲ Rebif Prefilled Syringe for Injection (2% to 4%) 1107

Remeron Tablets (Infrequent) **2924**
RemeronSolTab Tablets (Infrequent) **2927**
ReoPro Vials (0.1%) **1860**
Requip Tablets (2%) **1561**
Rilutek Tablets (Infrequent) **2771**
Risperdal Consta Long-Acting Injection (Frequent) **1753**
Rythmol SR Capsules **1590**
Salagen Tablets (1% to 2%) **1082**
Stalevo Tablets **2309**
Stromectol Tablets **2120**
Symbyax Capsules (Frequent) **1871**
Targretin Capsules **1084**
Tasigna Capsules **2316**
▲ Temodar Capsules (2% to 8%) **2931**
Teveten Tablets (Less than 1%) **515**
Teveten HCT Tablets (Less than 1%) **517**
Thioridazine Hydrochloride Tablets ... **2195**
Tice BCG (2%) **2936**
▲ Travatan Z Ophthalmic Solution (1% to 5%) **547**
▲ Trisenox Injection (5%) **986**
▲ Valstar Sterile Solution for Intravesical Instillation (22%) **1735**
Velcade for Injection **2168**
Venlafaxine Hydrochloride Tablets (Infrequent) **2199**
Vicoprofen Tablets (Less than 1%) ... **533**
Wellbutrin Tablets (Rare) **1648**
Wellbutrin SR Sustained-Release Tablets **1653**
Wellbutrin XL Extended-Release Tablets **1659**
▲ Xyrem Oral Solution (Infrequent to 7%) **1766**
Zomig Tablets (Rare) **694**
Zomig Nasal Spray (Rare) **689**
Zomig-ZMT Tablets (Rare) **694**
Zonegran Capsules (Infrequent) **1089**
Zosyn for Injection (1% or less) **3284**
Zyban Sustained-Release Tablets **1692**
Zyprexa Tablets (2%) **1883**
Zyprexa ZYDIS Orally Disintegrating Tablets (2%) **1883**
Zyrtec Chewable Tablets (Less than 2%) **1920**
Zyrtec Syrup (Less than 2%) **1920**
Zyrtec Tablets (Less than 2%) **1920**
Zyrtec-D 12 Hour Extended Release Tablets (Less than 2%) **1923**

Urinary obstruction

Tice BCG (Less than or equal to 1%) **2936**

Urinary retention

Abilify Injection (Greater than or equal to 1 in 1000 patients and less than 1 in 100 patients) **881**
Abilify Injection (Greater than or equal to 1 in 1000 patients and less than 1 in 100 patients) **2466**
Abilify Oral Solution (Greater than or equal to 1 in 1000 patients and less than 1 in 100 patients) **881**
Abilify Oral Solution (Greater than or equal to 1 in 1000 patients and less than 1 in 100 patients) **2466**
Abilify Discmelt Orally Disintegrating Tablets (Greater than or equal to 1 in 1000 patients and less than 1 in 100 patients) **881**
Abilify Discmelt Orally Disintegrating Tablets (Greater than or equal to 1 in 1000 patients and less than 1 in 100 patients) **2466**
Abilify Tablets (Greater than or equal to 1 in 1000 patients and less than 1 in 100 patients) **881**
Abilify Tablets (Greater than or equal to 1 in 1000 patients and less than 1 in 100 patients) **2466**
Aceon Tablets (2 mg, 4 mg, 8 mg) (0.3% to 1%) **3038**
Actiq (Less than 1%) **959**
Aloxi Injection (Less than 1%) **1059**
Ambien Tablets (Rare) **2692**
Ambien CR Tablets (Rare) **2696**
AndroGel **3159**
▲ Angiomax for Injection (4%) **1933**
Anzemet Injection (2%) **2701**
Arixtra Injection (Up to 2.9%) **1313**
Atrovent HFA Inhalation Aerosol **839**
Atrovent Nasal Spray 0.03% **834**
Atrovent Nasal Spray 0.06% **836**
▲ Avinza Capsules (Less than 5%) **1772**
Bentyl Capsules **703**
Bentyl Injection **703**
Bentyl Syrup **703**
Bentyl Tablets **703**
Carbatrol Capsules **3019**
Catapres Tablets (About 1 in 1,000 patients) **841**
Celexa (Infrequent) **1160**
▲ CellCept Capsules (3% to less than 20%) **2622**
▲ CellCept Intravenous (3% to less than 20%) **2622**
▲ CellCept Oral Suspension (3% to less than 20%) **2622**
▲ CellCept Tablets (3% to less than 20%) **2622**
Chantix Tablets (Rare) **2511**
Cipro I.V. (1% or less) **2817**
Cipro (Less than 1%) **2810**
Cipro XR Tablets **2823**
Clorpres Tablets (About 1 in 1,000) **2185**
Combivent Inhalation Aerosol **845**
Copaxone for Injection (At least 2%) **3110**
Cymbalta Delayed-Release Capsules **1801**
Dantrium Capsules (Less frequent) .. **2580**
▲ DepoCyt Injection (5%) **1136**
▲ DepoDur Injection (Greater than 10%) **1095**
Donnatal Extentabs **2507**
▲ Duragesic Transdermal System (3% to 10%) **2405**
Effexor XR Extended-Release Capsules (Frequent) **3195**
Eldepryl Capsules (1 of 49 patients) **3052**
Enablex Extended-Release Tablets ... **2225**
▲ Entereg Capsules (3.2% to 3.5%) ... **3293**
Equetro Extended-Release Capsules **3174**
Evoxac Capsules **1013**
Exelon Capsules (Infrequent) **2229**
Exelon Oral Solution (Infrequent) **2229**
Gabitril Tablets (Infrequent) **973**
Gantrisin Pediatric Suspension **2638**
Geodon Capsules (Infrequent) **2520**
Invanz for Injection (Greater than 0.1%) **2029**
▲ Ionsys Transdermal System (3%) **2410**
Klonopin (Infrequent) **2639**
Lamictal (Rare) **1488**
Lortab 5/500 Tablets **3143**
Lortab 7.5/500 Tablets **3144**
Lortab 10/500 Tablets **3144**
Lyrica Capsules (0.1% to 1%) **2527**
Marplan Tablets **3177**
Mirapex Tablets **857**
Moban Tablets **1116**
Mobic Oral Suspension **863**
Mobic Tablets **863**
MS Contin Tablets (Less frequent) **2585**
▲ Myfortic Tablets (3% to less than 20%) **2276**
Namenda (Infrequent) **1180**
Norvir (Less than 2%) **489**
Opana Tablets (Less than 1%) **1117**
Opana ER Tablets (Less than 1%) **1121**
OxyContin Tablets (Less than 1%) **2589**
Parnate Tablets **1532**
Paxil (Infrequent) **1535**
Paxil CR Controlled-Release Tablets (Infrequent) **1544**
Percocet Tablets **1127**
Percodan Tablets **1130**
ProAmatine Tablets (Among most frequent) **3032**
Provigil Tablets (1%) **977**
Prozac Weekly Capsules (Infrequent) **1852**
Prozac Pulvules and Liquid (Infrequent) **1852**
Remeron Tablets (Infrequent) **2924**
RemeronSolTab Tablets (Infrequent) **2927**
ReoPro Vials (0.4%) **1860**
Requip Tablets (Infrequent) **1561**
Rilutek Tablets (Infrequent) **2771**
Risperdal Consta Long-Acting Injection (Infrequent) **1753**
Rythmol SR Capsules **1590**
Sanctura XR Capsules (Less than 1%) **557**
▲ Simulect for Injection (3% to 10%) ... **2306**
Spiriva HandiHaler (Less than 1%) **870**
Stalevo Tablets **2309**
▲ Strattera Capsules (0.7% to 8%) **1864**
Symbyax Capsules (Infrequent) **1871**
Thioridazine Hydrochloride Tablets ... **2195**
▲ Trasylol Injection (3%) **799**
Tussionex Pennkinetic Extended-Release Suspension **3154**
Ultane Liquid for Inhalation (Less than 1%) **524**
Ultram ER Extended-Release Tablets (0.5% to less than 1%) **2428**
Valium Tablets **2658**
▲ Valstar Sterile Solution for Intravesical Instillation (4%) **1735**
Vantas (Less than 2%) **1737**
Velcade for Injection **2168**
Venlafaxine Hydrochloride Tablets (1%) **2199**
VESIcare Tablets (0% to 1.4%) **636**
Viadur Implant (Less than 2%) **802**
Vicodin Tablets **529**
Vicodin ES Tablets **530**
Vicodin HP Tablets **531**
Vicoprofen Tablets (Less than 1%) **533**
Wellbutrin Tablets (1.9%) **1648**
Wellbutrin SR Sustained-Release Tablets **1653**
Wellbutrin XL Extended-Release Tablets **1659**
▲ Zofran Injection (3%) **1682**
▲ Zofran (5%) **1687**
▲ Zofran ODT Orally Disintegrating Tablets (5%) **1687**
Zolinza Capsules **2142**
Zonegran Capsules (Infrequent) **1089**
Zosyn for Injection (1% or less) **3284**
Zyban Sustained-Release Tablets **1692**
Zydone Tablets **1132**
Zyprexa Tablets (Infrequent) **1883**
Zyprexa ZYDIS Orally Disintegrating Tablets (Infrequent) **1883**
Zyrtec Chewable Tablets (Less than 2%) **1920**
Zyrtec Syrup (Less than 2%) **1920**
Zyrtec Tablets (Less than 2%) **1920**
Zyrtec-D 12 Hour Extended Release Tablets (Less than 2%) **1923**

Urinary sediment, abnormalities

Capastat Sulfate for Injection **1791**
Dyazide Capsules **1405**

Urinary stream, weak

AndroGel **3159**

Urinary tract disorder, unspecified

Brovana Inhalation Solution (Less than 2%) **2990**
▲ CellCept Capsules (3% to less than 20%) **2622**
▲ CellCept Intravenous (3% to less than 20%) **2622**
▲ CellCept Oral Suspension (3% to less than 20%) **2622**
▲ CellCept Tablets (3% to less than 20%) **2622**
Enablex Extended-Release Tablets (Greater than or equal to 1%) **2225**
▲ Leukine (14%) **774**
Lupron Depot 3.75 mg **462**
Protonix for Delayed-Release Oral Suspension (Less than 1%) **3254**
Protonix Delayed-Release Tablets (Less than 1%) **3254**
Protonix I.V. (Less than 1%) **3257**
Selzentry Tablets (2.6%) **2534**
Zomig Tablets (Rare) **694**
Zomig Nasal Spray (Rare) **689**
Zomig-ZMT Tablets (Rare) **694**
Zyban Sustained-Release Tablets **1692**

Urinary urgency

Actiq (1% or greater) **959**
Adenoscan (Less than 1%) **605**
Amerge Tablets (Rare) **1301**
AndroGel **3159**
Aricept Tablets (Infrequent) **1062**
Aricept ODT Tablets (Infrequent) **1062**
Asacol Delayed-Release Tablets **2579**
▲ Avastin IV (3% to 6%) **1192**
▲ Betaseron for SC Injection (11%) **756**
Campral Tablets (Rare) **1158**
▲ Copaxone for Injection (10%) **3110**
Effexor XR Extended-Release Capsules (Infrequent) **3195**
Eligard 7.5 mg (Less than 2%) **2724**
Eligard 22.5 mg (Less than 2%) **2724**
Eligard 30 mg (Less than 2%) **2724**
Eligard 45 mg (Less than 2%) **2724**
Emsam Transdermal System (Infrequent) **905**
Gabitril Tablets (Infrequent) **973**
Ionsys Transdermal System (.1% to less than 1%) **2410**
Lamictal (Rare) **1488**
Lexapro Oral Suspension (Infrequent) **1174**
Lexapro Tablets (Infrequent) **1174**
Lipitor Tablets (Less than 2%) **2501**
Luvox CR Extended-Release Capsules (Infrequent) **1759**
Mirapex Tablets **857**
Paxil (Infrequent) **1535**
Paxil CR Controlled-Release Tablets (Infrequent) **1544**
ProAmatine Tablets (Among most frequent) **3032**
Prozac Weekly Capsules (Infrequent) **1852**
Prozac Pulvules and Liquid (Infrequent) **1852**
Remeron Tablets (Rare) **2924**
RemeronSolTab Tablets (Rare) **2927**
Rilutek Tablets (Infrequent) **2771**
Salagen Tablets (Less than 1%) **1082**
Symbyax Capsules (Infrequent) **1871**
Targretin Capsules **1084**
▲ Tice BCG (6% to 50%) **2936**
▲ Valstar Sterile Solution for Intravesical Instillation (57%) **1735**
Venlafaxine Hydrochloride Tablets (Infrequent) **2199**
Viadur Implant (Less than 2%) **802**
Wellbutrin SR Sustained-Release Tablets (Up to 2%) **1653**
Wellbutrin XL Extended-Release Tablets (2%) **1659**
Zomig Tablets (Infrequent) **694**
Zomig-ZMT Tablets (Infrequent) **694**
Zyban Sustained-Release Tablets (Infrequent) **1692**
Zyprexa Tablets (Infrequent) **1883**

Urination, difficult

(*see under* Micturition, difficulty)

Urination, excessive

▲ Demadex Injection (6.7%) **2630**
▲ Demadex Tablets (6.7%) **2630**

Urination, impaired

Actiq (1% or greater) **959**
AndroGel (Less than 1%) **3159**
Emsam Transdermal System (Infrequent) **905**
Ionsys Transdermal System (.1% to less than 1%) **2410**
Luvox CR Extended-Release Capsules (Infrequent) **1759**
Symbyax Capsules (Infrequent) **1871**
Ultane Liquid for Inhalation (Less than 1%) **524**
Venlafaxine Hydrochloride Tablets (2%) **2199**

Urination, painful

(*see under* Micturition, painful)

Urine, abnormal

Brovana Inhalation Solution (Less than 2%) **2990**
▲ CellCept Capsules (3% to less than 20%) **2622**
▲ CellCept Intravenous (3% to less than 20%) **2622**
▲ CellCept Oral Suspension (3% to less than 20%) **2622**
▲ CellCept Tablets (3% to less than 20%) **2622**
Chantix Tablets (Infrequent) **2511**
Evoxac Capsules (Less than 1%) **1013**
Frova Tablets (Rare) **1111**
Gengraf Capsules (1% to less than 3%) **435**
Kaletra (Less than 2%) **452**
Keppra Oral Solution (2%) **3131**
Keppra Tablets (2%) **3131**
Lamictal (Infrequent) **1488**
Lyrica Capsules (0.1% to 1%) **2527**
Neoral Oral Solution (1% to less than 3%) **2280**
Neoral Soft Gelatin Capsules (1% to less than 3%) **2280**
▲ Novantrone for Injection Concentrate (5% to 11%) **1100**
Provigil Tablets (1%) **977**
Rilutek Tablets (Infrequent) **2771**
Rythmol SR Capsules **1590**
Soriatane Capsules (Less than 1%) .. **3062**
Ultane Liquid for Inhalation (Less than 1%) **524**
Yaz Tablets **805**

Urine, cells in

Accutane Capsules **2607**
Merrem I.V. (Greater than 0.2%) **684**

Urine, color change
Alinia for Oral Suspension (Less than 1%) 2677
Alinia Tablets (Less than 1%) 2677
Clinoril Tablets (Less than 1%) 1962
▲ Comtan Tablets (10%) 2208
Fluorescite Injection ⊙ 203
Klonopin (Infrequent) 2639
Lamisil Tablets 2266
Levaquin 2416
Levaquin in 5% Dextrose Injection 2416
Ortho-Cyclen Tablets 2449
Ortho Evra Transdermal System 2437
Ortho Tri-Cyclen Tablets 2449
Ortho Tri-Cyclen Lo Tablets 2458
Primaxin I.M. 2080
Primaxin I.V. (Less than 0.2%) 2083
▲ Stalevo Tablets (5% to 10%) 2309

Urine, microscopic deposits
Carbatrol Capsules 3019
Equetro Extended-Release Capsules 3174

Urine, output low
(*see under* Hypouresis)

Urine, presence of RBC's
(*see under* Hematuria)

Urine, presence of urobilinogen
Primaxin I.M. 2080
Primaxin I.V. 2083

Urine analysis abnormal
Celebrex Capsules 2979
Chantix Tablets (Infrequent) 2511
Xyrem Oral Solution (Infrequent) 1766

Urine flow decreased
Evoxac Capsules (Less than 1%) 1013
Valstar Sterile Solution for Intravesical Instillation (Less than 1%) 1735

Urine odor, abnormal
Cymbalta Delayed-Release Capsules (Infrequent) 1801

Urolithiasis
Cosopt Sterile Ophthalmic Solution (Less than 1%) 1969
▲ Crixivan Capsules (Approximately 12.4%) 1979
Effexor XR Extended-Release Capsules (Rare) 3195
Paxil (Rare) 1535
Paxil CR Controlled-Release Tablets (Rare) 1544
Tricor Tablets 520
Trusopt Sterile Ophthalmic Solution (Rare) 2128
Venlafaxine Hydrochloride Tablets (Rare) 2199

Urosepsis
Betaseron for SC Injection 756

Urticaria
Abilify Injection (Greater than or equal to 1 in 1000 patients and less than 1 in 100 patients) 881
Abilify Injection (Greater than or equal to 1 in 1000 patients and less than 1 in 100 patients) 2466
Abilify Oral Solution 881
Abilify Oral Solution (Greater than or equal to 1 in 1000 patients and less than 1 in 100 patients) 2466
Abilify Discmelt Orally Disintegrating Tablets 881
Abilify Discmelt Orally Disintegrating Tablets (Greater than or equal to 1 in 1000 patients and less than 1 in 100 patients) 2466
Abilify Tablets 881
Abilify Tablets (Greater than or equal to 1 in 1000 patients and less than 1 in 100 patients) 2466
Accolate Tablets 669
Accutane Capsules 2607
▲ Acetadote Injection (0.2% to 20.8%) 1001
Actiq (Less than 1%) 959
Activase I.V. (Very rare) 1188
Adderall XR Capsules 3012
Adipex-P 1185
Advair Diskus 100/50 1276
Advair Diskus 250/50 1276
Advair Diskus 500/50 1276
Advicor Tablets 402
▲ Aerobid/Aerobid-M (1% to 3%) 1153
Aggrenox Capsules (Less than 1%) 819
▲ Agrylin Capsules (8.3%) 3017
Albenza Tablets (Less than 1%) 1297
Alferon N Injection 1726
Allegra Oral Solution (Less than 1%) 2684
Allegra Tablets (Rare) 2684
Allegra-D 12 Hour Extended-Release Tablets (Rare) 2687
Allegra-D 24 Hour Extended-Release Tablets (Rare) 2690
Alphanate 1709
▲ Alvesco Inhalation Aerosol (Greater than or equal to 3%) 2985
Ambien Tablets (Rare) 2692
Ambien CR Tablets (1%) 2696
AmBisome for Injection (Less common) 606
Amerge Tablets (Infrequent) 1301
Amevive (Less than 1%) 611
Aminohippurate Sodium "PAH" Injection 1950
Amoxil Capsules 1305
Amoxil Chewable Tablets 1305
Amoxil Pediatric Drops for Oral Suspension 1305
Amoxil Powder for Oral Suspension 1305
Amoxil Tablets 1305
Amrix Capsules 966
Anaprox Tablets (Less than 1%) 2632
Anaprox DS Tablets (Less than 1%) 2632
Angeliq Tablets 751
Anzemet Injection (Rare) 2701
Anzemet Tablets (Rare) 2704
Appearex Tablets 2163
Aricept Tablets (Infrequent) 1062
Aricept ODT Tablets (Infrequent) 1062
Arimidex Tablets (Very rare) 672
Asacol Delayed-Release Tablets 2579
Atacand Tablets 639
Atacand HCT 642
▲ Atripla Tablets (Greater than or equal to 5%) 938
Atrovent HFA Inhalation Aerosol 839
Atrovent Nasal Spray 0.03% 834
Atrovent Nasal Spray 0.06% (Rare) 836
Attenuvax (Rare) 1951
▲ Augmentin (3%) 1323
▲ Augmentin Tablets (3%) 1327
Augmentin XR Extended Release Tablets 1333
Augmentin ES-600 Powder for Oral Suspension 1329
Avalide Tablets (Rare) 892
Avalide Tablets (Rare) 2713
Avandamet Tablets 1336
Avandaryl Tablets (Less than 1%) 1344
Avandia Tablets 1351
Avapro Tablets (Rare) 897
Avapro Tablets (Less than 1%) 2718
Avelox (Greater than or equal to 0.1% to less than 2%) 2803
▲ Avinza Capsules (Less than 5%) 1772
Avodart Soft Gelatin Capsules 1359
Axid Capsules (0.5%) 1364
Azmacort Inhalation Aerosol (Rare) 407
Azopt Ophthalmic Suspension (Less than 1%) 540
Azor Tablets 1005
Bactroban Cream (One report) 1366
Bayer Aspirin 750
Beconase AQ Nasal Spray (Rare) 1369
▲ BeneFIX Vials (3.1% to 4.8%) 3191
Benicar Tablets 1009
Benicar HCT Tablets (Rare) 1010
Bentyl Capsules 703
Bentyl Injection 703
Bentyl Syrup 703
Bentyl Tablets 703
Betaseron for SC Injection 756
Betimol Ophthalmic Solution 3181
Biaxin/Biaxin XL 411
Bicillin C-R Injectable Suspension 1775
Bicillin L-A Injection 1777
Boostrix (Rarely) 1377
Brovana Inhalation Solution 2990
Byetta Injection 600
Bystolic Tablets 1155
▲ Campath Ampules (10% to 35%) 761
Campral Tablets (Infrequent) 1158
Cancidas for Injection 1953
Capastat Sulfate for Injection 1791
Carafate Suspension 706
Carafate Tablets 707
Carbatrol Capsules 3019
Catapres Tablets (About 5 in 1,000 patients) 841
Catapres-TTS (2 cases of 3,539 patients) 842
Ceftin (0.1% to 1%) 1380
Celebrex Capsules (0.1% to 1.9%) 2979
Celexa (Infrequent) 1160
▲ Cerezyme for Injection (Approximately 6.6%) 1238
Chantix Tablets (Infrequent) 2511
Cialis Tablets 1792
Cimzia (Rare) 3127
Cipro I.V. (1% or less) 2817
Cipro (Less than 1%) 2810
Cipro XR Tablets 2823
Clarinex Syrup (Rare) 2828
Clarinex Tablets (Rare) 2828
Clarinex Reditabs Tablets (Rare) 2828
Clarinex-D 12-Hour Extended-Release Tablets (Rare) 2831
Clarinex-D 24-Hour Extended-Release Tablets 2834
Climara Transdermal System 763
Climara Pro Transdermal System 768
Clorpres Tablets (About 5 in 1,000) 2185
Combigan Ophthalmic Solution 553
Combivent Inhalation Aerosol (Rare) 845
Combivir Tablets 1384
Comvax 1966
▲ Copaxone for Injection (5%) 3110
Coreg CR Extended-Release Capsules 1393
Cosopt Sterile Ophthalmic Solution 1969
Cozaar Tablets (Less than 1%) 1973
Crestor Tablets 677
Crixivan Capsules (Less than 2%) 1979
Cubicin for Injection 995
Cuprimine Capsules 1986
Cyanokit 5g Antidote 1021
Cymbalta Delayed-Release Capsules 1801
▲ Dacogen Injection (6%) 1066
Dantrium Capsules (Less frequent) 2580
Dantrium Intravenous (Rare) 2582
Daytrana Transdermal Patch 3022
Demser Capsules (Rare) 1989
Denavir Cream 2205
Dexedrine 1401
Didronel Tablets 2583
Diovan HCT Tablets 2216
Divigel 3167
Donnatal Extentabs 2507
▲ Doribax Injection (1% to 5%) 2400
▲ Doxil Injection (1% to 5%) 2378
Duetact Tablets (Less than 1%) 3085
Dyazide Capsules 1405
DynaCirc CR Controlled Release Tablets (0.5% to 1%) 1407
EC-Naprosyn Delayed-Release Tablets (Less than 1%) 2632
E.E.S. 433
Effexor XR Extended-Release Capsules 3195
Elidel Cream 1% (0.3% to 1.1%) 2221
Elitek 2729
Elmiron Capsules (Less than or equal to 1%) 2435
▲ Eloxatin for Injection (2% to less than 5%) 2731
Elspar for Injection 1990
▲ Emend Capsules (Greater than 0.5%) 1992
▲ Emend for Injection (Greater than 0.5%) 1999
Emsam Transdermal System (Infrequent) 905
▲ Emtriva Capsules (17% to 30%) 1246
▲ Emtriva Oral Solution (17% to 30%) 1246
Enbrel for Injection 569
Engerix-B Vaccine (Less than 1%) 1409
Enjuvia Tablets 1029
Epivir 1412
Epivir-HBV 1417
Epogen for Injection (Rare) 576
Epzicom Tablets 1422
Equetro Extended-Release Capsules 3174
Erbitux 912
EryPed 431
Estratest Tablets 3043
Estratest H.S. Tablets 3043
Evoxac Capsules (Less than 1%) 1013
Exelon Capsules (Infrequent) 2229
Exelon Oral Solution (Infrequent) 2229
Exforge Tablets (Less than or equal to 0.1%) 2238
▲ Exjade Tablets (3.7%) 2244
▲ Fabrazyme for Intravenous Infusion (Greater than or equal to 5%) 1241
Fansidar Tablets 2636
Faslodex Injection (Less than 1%) 682
Feiba VH 728
Fleet Phospho-soda (Rare) 1145
Fleet Phospho-soda EZ-PREP (Rare) 1147
Fleet Prep Kits 1149
Flexbumin 25% I.V. (Occasional) 729
▲ Flolan for Injection (25%) 1426
Flomax Capsules 848
Flonase Nasal Spray (Less than 1%) 1431
Flovent Diskus 50 mcg 1435
Flovent HFA (Rare) 1440
Fluarix Vaccine 1446
Flulaval Injection Vaccine 1448
FluMist Vaccine 1945
Fluorescite Injection ⊙ 203
Focalin XR Capsules 2251
Fortaz 1450
Forteo for Injection (Less than 1/1000 patients) 1816
Fosamax 2005
Fosamax Plus D Tablets 2013
Furosemide Tablets 2186
Gabitril Tablets (Infrequent) 973
Gammagard Liquid 730
Gammagard S/D (Occasional) 734
▲ Gamunex (0.5% to 5%) 3094
Gantrisin Pediatric Suspension 2638
Gardasil Injection 2019
Gengraf Capsules (1% to less than 3%) 435
Geodon (Infrequent to rare) 2520
Glucagon for Injection Vials and Emergency Kit 1827
Gris-PEG Tablets 2507
Havrix Injection Vaccine (Less than 1%) 1454
Hemofil M (Extremely rare) 737
Human Albumin Grifols 25% 1706
Hyalgan Solution 2742
▲ Hycamtin for Injection (Less than 1% to 16%) 1459
Imitrex Injection 1465
Imitrex Nasal Spray 1470
Imitrex Tablets 1474
Indocin Capsules (Less than 1%) 2024
Indocin I.V. (Less than 1%) 2489
Indocin (Less than 1%) 2024
Infanrix Vaccine 1479
Intravenous Sodium Diuril 2490
▲ Intron A for Injection (Rare; Less than 5%) 2859
Invanz for Injection (Greater than 0.1%) 2029
Janumet Tablets 2041
Januvia Tablets 2048
Ketek Tablets (Less than 0.2%) 2744
Kinrix Injection Vaccine 1486
Kogenate FS (Rare) 746
Lamictal (Infrequent) 1488
Lamisil Oral Granules (1%) 2264
Lamisil Tablets (1.1%) 2266
Lescol Capsules (Rare) 2268
Lescol XL Tablets 2268
Leukeran Tablets 1508
Leustatin Injection 2384
Levaquin (0.1% to 1%) 2416
Levaquin in 5% Dextrose Injection (0.1% to 1%) 2416
Levothroid Tablets 1170
Levoxyl Tablets 1780
Lialda Tablets (Infrequent) 3029
Lipitor Tablets (Less than 2%) 2501
Lotrisone 2881
Lovenox Injection 2756
Lunesta Tablets (Infrequent) 2994
Lupron Depot 3.75 mg 462
Lupron Depot 7.5 mg 469
Lupron Depot–3 Month 11.25 mg 462
Lupron Depot-PED 7.5 mg, 11.25 mg and 15 mg 471
Luvox CR Extended-Release Capsules (Infrequent) 1759
Lybrel Tablets 3204
Lyrica Capsules (0.1% to 1%) 2527
Malarone Pediatric Tablets 1521
Malarone Tablets 1521
Maxalt Tablets (Infrequent) 2056
Maxalt-MLT Orally Disintegrating Tablets (Infrequent) 2056
Meribin Capsules 2163
Meridia Capsules 475
Merrem I.V. (Greater than 0.1% to 1%) 684
Meruvax II 2061
Metadate CD Capsules 3146
Mevacor Tablets (Rare) 2063
Micardis Tablets 852
Micardis HCT Tablets 854
Mirapex Tablets 857
M-M-R II 2054
Mobic Oral Suspension (Less than 2%) 863
Mobic Tablets (Less than 2%) 863

Motrin IB Tablets and Caplets 1900
Children's Motrin Oral Suspension 1901
Children's Motrin Non-Staining Dye-Free Oral Suspension 1901
Children's Motrin Cold Oral Suspension 1899
Infants' Motrin Concentrated Drops 1901
Infants' Motrin Non-Staining Dye-Free Concentrated Drops 1901
Junior Strength Motrin Caplets and Chewable Tablets 1901
MoviPrep Oral Solution 2679
Moxatag Tablets 2165
MS Contin Tablets (Less frequent) 2585
Mumpsvax (Extremely rare) 2068
Mycamine for Injection 616
Myleran Tablets 1530
Nalfon Capsules (Less than 1%) 2508
Namenda (Infrequent) 1180
Naprosyn Suspension (Less than 1%) 2632
Naprosyn Tablets (Less than 1%) 2632
Neoral Oral Solution (1% to less than 3%) 2280
Neoral Soft Gelatin Capsules (1% to less than 3%) 2280
Neulasta Injection 587
Neupogen for Injection 589
Nexium Delayed-Release Capsules (Less than 1%) 645
Nexium I.V. (Less than 1%) 652
Nexium Delayed-Release Oral Suspension (Less than 1%) 645
Niaspan Extended-Release Tablets ... 480
Noroxin Tablets (Less frequent) 2069
Norvir (Less than 2%) 489
Novantrone for Injection Concentrate 1100
▲ Oncaspar Injection (Greater than 5%) 1138
Opana Tablets (Less than 1%) 1117
Opana ER Tablets (Less than 1%) 1121
Orencia Powder for Intravenous Infusion (Greater than 0.1% and less than or equal to 1%) 921
Ortho-Cyclen Tablets 2449
Ortho Evra Transdermal System 2437
Ortho Tri-Cyclen Tablets 2449
Ortho Tri-Cyclen Lo Tablets 2458
Orthoclone OKT3 Sterile Solution 2387
OsmoPrep Tablets (Rare) 2680
OxyContin Tablets (Less than 1%) 2589
ParaGard T 380A Intrauterine Copper Contraceptive 1041
Parnate Tablets 1532
Paxil (Infrequent) 1535
Paxil CR Controlled-Release Tablets (Infrequent) 1544
Pediarix Vaccine (Rare) 1552
Liquid PedvaxHIB (Two children) 2073
PegIntron Powder for Injection (Less than or equal to 1%) 2903
Pentasa Capsules (Less than 1%) 3030
Pepcid Tablets (Infrequent) 2075
Percocet Tablets 1127
Percodan Tablets 1130
Persantine Tablets (Rare) 869
Plavix Tablets (Less than 1%) 926
Plavix Tablets (Less than 1%) 2767
Pletal Tablets (Less than 2%) 2481
Pneumovax 23 2078
Premarin Intravenous 3217
Premarin Tablets 3221
Premarin Vaginal Cream 3228
Premphase Tablets 3232
Prempro Tablets 3232
Primaxin I.M. 2080
Primaxin I.V. (0.2%) 2083
Prinivil Tablets (0.3% to 1%) 2087
Prinzide Tablets 2092
Procrit for Injection (Rare) 2391
Profilnine SD Solvent Detergent 1721
Proleukin for Injection 2287
Propecia Tablets 2095
Proscar Tablets 2102
Protonix for Delayed-Release Oral Suspension (Less than 1%) 3254
Protonix Delayed-Release Tablets (Less than 1%) 3254
Protonix I.V. (Less than 1%) 3257
▲ Protopic Ointment (3% to 5%) 628
Proventil HFA Inhalation Aerosol (Rare) 2914
Prozac Weekly Capsules 1852
Prozac Pulvules and Liquid 1852
Pulmicort Flexhaler 654
Pulmozyme Inhalation Solution 1217
Pylera Capsules 714
Qvar Inhalation Aerosol (Rare) 3116
Raptiva for Injection (1%) 1218
Recombinate (Extremely rare) 738
Recombivax HB (Less than 1%) 2107
ReFacto Vials 3269
Refludan for Injection (Uncommon) ... 795
Relenza Inhalation Powder (Less than 1.5%) 1556
Remeron Tablets (Rare) 2924
RemeronSolTab Tablets (Rare) 2927
Remicade for IV Injection (Less than 1%) 950
Requip Tablets (Infrequent) 1561
Retrovir Capsules 1574
Retrovir IV Infusion 1579
Retrovir 1574
Rilutek Tablets (Infrequent) 2771
▲ Rituxan I.V. (1% to 8%) 1223
Rocaltrol Capsules 1150
Rocaltrol Oral Solution 1150
Rocephin Injectable Vials, ADD-Vantage, Galaxy, Bulk 2642
RotaTeq 2110
Rythmol SR Capsules 1590
St. Joseph 81 mg Aspirin Chewable and Enteric Coated Tablets 1903
Sandostatin Injection (Less than 1%) 2300
Sandostatin LAR Depot 2302
Seasonique Tablets 1046
▲ Serevent Diskus (3%) 1594
Singulair (Greater than or equal to 2%) 2114
Solodyn Extended Release Tablets (2%) 1938
Soriatane Capsules (Less than 1%) .. 3062
Spiriva HandiHaler 870
Stalevo Tablets 2309
Starlix Tablets 2314
Stromectol Tablets (0.9%) 2120
Sular Extended Release Tablets (Less than or equal to 1%) 2975
Sulfamylon Cream 2194
Sulfamylon for 5% Topical Solution .. 2194
Suprax for Oral Suspension (Less than 2%) 1891
Suprax Tablets (Less than 2%) 1891
Sustiva Capsules (Less than 2%) 930
Sustiva Tablets (Less than 2%) 930
Synagis Intramuscular Solution 1948
Synthroid Tablets 507
Tamiflu Oral Suspension 2649
Tarka Tablets 511
▲ Tasigna Capsules (1% to 10%) 2316
Tekturna HCT Tablets 2324
Teveten HCT Tablets 517
Thioridazine Hydrochloride Tablets (Infrequent) 2195
Thiothixene Capsules 2197
Thyrogen for Injection 1244
Timentin ADD-Vantage 1606
Timentin Injection Galaxy Container 1609
Timentin IV Infusion 1603
Timentin Pharmacy Bulk Package 1613
Timoptic Sterile Ophthalmic Solution (Less frequent) 2121
Timoptic in Ocudose (Less frequent) 2124
Timoptic-XE Sterile Ophthalmic Gel Forming Solution 2125
TNKase (Less than 1%) 1233
Toprol-XL Tablets 666
Treximet Tablets (Infrequent) 1616
Tricor Tablets (1.1%) 520
▲ Trisenox Injection (8%) 986
Trizivir Tablets 1622
Trusopt Sterile Ophthalmic Solution 2128
Twinrix Vaccine (Less than 1%) 1628
Ultane Liquid for Inhalation (Less than 1%) 524
Ultram ER Extended-Release Tablets (0.5% to less than 1%) 2428
Uroxatral Tablets 2786
Valtrex Caplets 1635
Vaqta (Less than 1%) 2130
Varivax (Greater than or equal to 1%) 2133
Velcade for Injection 2168
Venlafaxine Hydrochloride Tablets (Infrequent) 2199
Ventolin HFA Inhalation Aerosol 1638
Vicoprofen Tablets (Less than 1%) 533
Viramune Oral Suspension 873
Viramune Tablets 873
▲ Viread Tablets (5% to 18%) 1268
Visudyne for Injection 2332
Vivitrol 988
▲ Voltaren Ophthalmic Solution (Less than or equal to 3%) 2336
Voltaren Tablets (Rarely) 2334
Voltaren-XR Tablets (Rarely) 2337
Vytorin 10/10 Tablets 2149
Vytorin 10/10 Tablets 2939
Vytorin 10/20 Tablets 2149
Vytorin 10/20 Tablets 2939
Vytorin 10/40 Tablets 2149
Vytorin 10/40 Tablets 2939
Vytorin 10/80 Tablets 2149
Vytorin 10/80 Tablets 2939
Vyvanse Capsules 3033
Wellbutrin Tablets 1648
Wellbutrin SR Sustained-Release Tablets (1% to 2%) 1653
Wellbutrin XL Extended-Release Tablets (1% to 2%) 1659
Xenical Capsules 2672
Xifaxan Tablets 2682
Xolair 1235
Xolair 2339
▲ Xopenex Inhalation Solution (3%) 3001
▲ Xopenex Inhalation Solution Concentrate (3%) 3005
▲ Xopenex HFA Inhalation Aerosol (3%) 3009
Xyrem Oral Solution (Infrequent) 1766
Xyzal Oral Solution 2789
Xyzal Oral Solution 3155
Yaz Tablets 805
Zemplar Injection 538
Zetia Tablets 2157
Zetia Tablets 2951
Zinacef for Injection (Fewer than 1 in 250 patients) 1678
Zinacef Injection (Fewer than 1 in 250 patients) 1678
Zocor Tablets (Rare) 2136
Zofran Injection (Rare) 1682
Zofran 1687
Zofran ODT Orally Disintegrating Tablets 1687
Zomig Tablets (Infrequent) 694
Zomig-ZMT Tablets (Infrequent) 694
Zonegran Capsules (Infrequent) 1089
Zovirax 1690
Zyban Sustained-Release Tablets (1% to 2%) 1692
Zyprexa Tablets (Infrequent) 1883
Zyprexa ZYDIS Orally Disintegrating Tablets (Infrequent) 1883
Zyrtec Chewable Tablets (Less than 2%) 1920
Zyrtec Syrup (Less than 2%) 1920
Zyrtec Tablets (Less than 2%) 1920
Zyrtec-D 12 Hour Extended Release Tablets (Less than 2%) 1923

Urticarial reaction, generalized

Atrovent Nasal Spray 0.03% 834
Xyntha Vials 3280

Uterine contractions, abnormal

Cervidil Vaginal Insert (2% to 4.7%) .. 1165

Uterine disorder, unspecified

Evista Tablets 1810
Zomig Tablets (Rare) 694
Zomig Nasal Spray (Rare) 689
Zomig-ZMT Tablets (Rare) 694

Uterine fibroids

▲ Activella Tablets (0% to 5%) 2347
Zomig Tablets (Rare) 694
Zomig Nasal Spray (Rare) 689
Zomig-ZMT Tablets (Rare) 694

Uterine fibroids, enlarged

Prozac Weekly Capsules (Rare) 1852
Symbyax Capsules (Rare) 1871

Uterine fibromyomata, increase in size

Climara Transdermal System 763
Estratest Tablets 3043
Estratest H.S. Tablets 3043
Premarin Intravenous 3217
Premarin Tablets 3221
Premarin Vaginal Cream 3228
Premphase Tablets 3232
Prempro Tablets 3232
Prozac Pulvules and Liquid (Rare) 1852
Zyprexa Tablets (Infrequent) 1883
Zyprexa ZYDIS Orally Disintegrating Tablets (Infrequent) 1883

Uterine leiomyoma

Requip Tablets (Infrequent) 1561

Uterine leiomyomata, enlargement

Activella Tablets 2347
Angeliq Tablets 751
Climara Transdermal System 763
Climara Pro Transdermal System 768
Divigel 3167
Enjuvia Tablets 1029
Mirapex Tablets 857
Premarin Vaginal Cream 3228

Uterine rupture

Cervidil Vaginal Insert 1165

Uterine spasm

Effexor XR Extended-Release Capsules (Rare) 3195
Paxil (Rare) 1535
Paxil CR Controlled-Release Tablets (Rare) 1544
Venlafaxine Hydrochloride Tablets (Rare) 2199

Uveitis

Actonel Tablets (Rare) 2568
Actonel with Calcium Tablets (Very rare) 2574
▲ Alrex Ophthalmic Suspension 0.2% (Less than 5%) .... ⊙236
Cimzia 3127
Durezol Ophthalmic Emulsion (Less than 1%) .... ⊙275
Effexor XR Extended-Release Capsules (Rare) 3195
FML Ophthalmic Ointment .... ⊙223
FML Ophthalmic Suspension .... ⊙224
FML Forte Ophthalmic Suspension .... ⊙222
Fosamax (Rare) 2005
Fosamax Plus D Tablets (Rarely) 2013
Lamictal (Rare) 1488
▲ Lotemax Ophthalmic Suspension 0.5% (Less than 5%) .... ⊙241
Lyrica Capsules (Rare) 2527
Norvir (Less than 2%) 489
OptiPranolol Metipranolol Ophthalmic Solution 0.3% .... ⊙245
Pred Forte Ophthalmic Suspension .... ⊙227
Pred Mild Ophthalmic Suspension ... ⊙230
Rituxan I.V. 1223
Stromectol Tablets 2120
Venlafaxine Hydrochloride Tablets (Rare) 2199
Zometa for Intravenous Infusion 2341

V

Vagina, dryness

▲ Arimidex Tablets (2% to 5%) 672
▲ Intron A for Injection (Less than 5%) 2859
▲ Prometrium Capsules (100 mg, 200 mg) (Less than 6%) 3047
Pylera Capsules 714

Vaginal bleeding pattern, changes in

Activella Tablets 2347

Vaginal candidiasis

Advair HFA 45/21 Inhalation Aerosol 1288
Advair HFA 115/21 Inhalation Aerosol 1288
Advair HFA 230/21 Inhalation Aerosol 1288
Angeliq Tablets 751
Ceftin (Less frequent) 1380
Cipro I.V. 2817
Climara Transdermal System 763
Climara Pro Transdermal System 768
▲ Copaxone for Injection (8%) 3110
Cubicin for Injection (1.7%) 995
Doxil Injection (Less than 1%) 2378
Estratest Tablets 3043
Estratest H.S. Tablets 3043
Ketek Tablets (Greater than or equal to 0.2% to less than 2%) 2744
Lamictal (Infrequent) 1488
Meridia Capsules (1.2%) 475
Mircette Tablets 1034
Noroxin Tablets 2069
NuvaRing 2897
▲ Omnicef Capsules (5%) 497
Omnicef for Oral Suspension (0.3%) 497
Ortho-Cyclen Tablets 2449
Ortho Evra Transdermal System 2437
Ortho Tri-Cyclen Tablets 2449
Ortho Tri-Cyclen Lo Tablets 2458
Premarin Intravenous 3217
Premarin Tablets 3221
Premarin Vaginal Cream 3228
Premphase Tablets 3232
Prempro Tablets 3232
▲ Prometrium Capsules (100 mg, 200 mg) (Less than 5%) 3047
Protopic Ointment (Greater than or equal to 1%) 628

Soriatane Capsules ... 3062
Tricor Tablets ... 520
Yaz Tablets ... 805
Zinacef for Injection ... 1678
Zinacef Injection ... 1678
Zyvox (1% to 1.6%) ... 2552

Vaginal discharge
▲ Arimidex Tablets (4%) ... 672
Ceftin Tablets (0.1% to 1%) ... 1380
▲ Crinone 4% Gel (11%) ... 992
▲ Crinone 8% Gel (3% to 7%) ... 992
Divigel ... 3167
Lupron Depot-PED 7.5 mg, 11.25 mg and 15 mg (2%) ... 471
Mirapex Tablets ... 857
▲ NuvaRing (5% to 14%) ... 2897
▲ Prometrium Capsules (100 mg, 200 mg) (10%) ... 3047

Vaginal pressure
Adenoscan (Less than 1%) ... 605

Vaginitis
Aceon Tablets (2 mg, 4 mg, 8 mg) (0.3% to 1%) ... 3038
Actiq (1% or greater) ... 959
Activella Tablets ... 2347
Advair HFA 45/21 Inhalation Aerosol ... 1288
Advair HFA 115/21 Inhalation Aerosol ... 1288
Advair HFA 230/21 Inhalation Aerosol ... 1288
Ambien Tablets (Infrequent) ... 2692
Ambien CR Tablets (Infrequent) ... 2696
Amerge Tablets (Rare) ... 1301
Angeliq Tablets ... 751
Aricept Tablets (Infrequent) ... 1062
Aricept ODT Tablets (Infrequent) ... 1062
▲ Arimidex Tablets (4%) ... 672
Augmentin (1%) ... 1323
Augmentin Tablets (1%) ... 1327
Augmentin XR Extended Release Tablets (1%) ... 1333
Avelox (Greater than or equal to 0.1% to less than 2%) ... 2803
Campral Tablets (Infrequent) ... 1158
▲ Ceftin Tablets (0.1% to 5.4%) ... 1380
Celebrex Capsules (0.1% to 1.9%) ... 2979
Cipro I.V. (1% or less) ... 2817
Cipro (Less than 1%) ... 2810
Cipro XR Tablets (Less than 1%) ... 2823
Climara Transdermal System ... 763
Climara Pro Transdermal System (1.9%) ... 768
Copaxone for Injection (At least 2%) ... 3110
▲ Depakote ER Tablets (Greater than 1% to less than 5%) ... 423
Divigel ... 3167
Doxil Injection (Less than 1%) ... 2378
Effexor XR Extended-Release Capsules (Frequent) ... 3195
Elmiron Capsules ... 2435
Emsam Transdermal System (Infrequent) ... 905
Enablex Extended-Release Tablets (Greater than or equal to 1%) ... 2225
▲ Enjuvia Tablets (2% to 7%) ... 1029
▲ Evista Tablets (4.3%) ... 1810
▲ Evoxac Capsules (1% to 3%) ... 1013
Fortaz (Less than 1%) ... 1450
Gabitril Tablets (Frequent) ... 973
▲ Invanz for Injection (1.4% to 3.3%) ... 2029
Ketek Tablets (Greater than or equal to 0.2% to less than 2%) ... 2744
Klonopin (1%) ... 2639
▲ Lamictal (4%) ... 1488
Levaquin (1%) ... 2416
Levaquin in 5% Dextrose Injection (1%) ... 2416
Lunesta Tablets (Infrequent) ... 2994
▲ Lupron Depot 3.75 mg (10%) ... 462
▲ Lupron Depot–3 Month 11.25 mg (10%) ... 462
Lupron Depot-PED 7.5 mg, 11.25 mg and 15 mg (2%) ... 471
Luvox CR Extended-Release Capsules (Infrequent) ... 1759
Lybrel Tablets ... 3204
Mircette Tablets ... 1034
▲ Mirena Intrauterine System (5% or more) ... 779
Nexium Delayed-Release Capsules (Less than 1%) ... 645
Nexium I.V. (Less than 1%) ... 652
Nexium Delayed-Release Oral Suspension (Less than 1%) ... 645
▲ NuvaRing (5% to 14%) ... 2897
Omnicef Capsules (1%) ... 497
Omnicef for Oral Suspension (0.3%) ... 497
Ortho-Cyclen Tablets ... 2449
Ortho Evra Transdermal System ... 2437
Ortho Tri-Cyclen Tablets ... 2449
Ortho Tri-Cyclen Lo Tablets ... 2458
ParaGard T 380A Intrauterine Copper Contraceptive ... 1041
Paxil (Infrequent) ... 1535
Paxil CR Controlled-Release Tablets (Infrequent) ... 1544
Pletal Tablets (Less than 2%) ... 2481
Premarin Intravenous ... 3217
▲ Premarin Tablets (5% to 7%) ... 3221
Premarin Vaginal Cream ... 3228
▲ Premphase Tablets (4% to 7%) ... 3232
▲ Prempro Tablets (4% to 7%) ... 3232
▲ Prograf Capsules and Injection (3% to 15%) ... 622
▲ Prometrium Capsules (100 mg, 200 mg) (Less than 5%) ... 3047
Protonix for Delayed-Release Oral Suspension (Less than 1%) ... 3254
Protonix Delayed-Release Tablets (Less than 1%) ... 3254
Protonix I.V. (Less than 1%) ... 3257
Protopic Ointment (0.2% to less than 1%) ... 628
Remeron Tablets (Infrequent) ... 2924
RemeronSolTab Tablets (Infrequent) ... 2927
Risperdal Consta Long-Acting Injection (Infrequent) ... 1753
Rocephin Injectable Vials, ADD-Vantage, Galaxy, Bulk (Less than 1%) ... 2642
Salagen Tablets (1% to 2%) ... 1082
Sandostatin Injection (Less than 1%) ... 2300
Seasonique Tablets ... 1046
Sular Extended Release Tablets (Less than or equal to 1%) ... 2975
Suprax for Oral Suspension (Less than 2%) ... 1891
Suprax Tablets (Less than 2%) ... 1891
Symbyax Capsules (Infrequent) ... 1871
Tygacil for Injection (0% to less than 2%) ... 3276
▲ Vagifem Tablets (3% to 5%) ... 2375
Venlafaxine Hydrochloride Tablets (Frequent) ... 2199
Wellbutrin Tablets (Infrequent) ... 1648
Wellbutrin SR Sustained-Release Tablets ... 1653
Wellbutrin XL Extended-Release Tablets ... 1659
▲ Xenical Capsules (2.6% to 3.8%) ... 2672
Yaz Tablets (Greater than 1%) ... 805
Zinacef for Injection ... 1678
Zinacef Injection ... 1678
Zomig Tablets (Rare) ... 694
Zomig Nasal Spray (Rare) ... 689
Zomig-ZMT Tablets (Rare) ... 694
Zosyn for Injection (1% or less) ... 3284
Zyban Sustained-Release Tablets ... 1692
Zyprexa Tablets (2%) ... 1883
Zyprexa ZYDIS Orally Disintegrating Tablets (2%) ... 1883
Zyrtec Chewable Tablets (Less than 2%) ... 1920
Zyrtec Syrup (Less than 2%) ... 1920
Zyrtec Tablets (Less than 2%) ... 1920
Zyrtec-D 12 Hour Extended Release Tablets (Less than 2%) ... 1923

Vaginitis, atrophic
Evoxac Capsules (Less than 1%) ... 1013
Exelon Capsules (Infrequent) ... 2229
Exelon Oral Solution (Infrequent) ... 2229
Soriatane Capsules (Less than 1%) ... 3062

Vaginosis, fungal
▲ Augmentin XR Extended Release Tablets (3.3%) ... 1333
Ketek Tablets (Greater than or equal to 0.2% to less than 2%) ... 2744

Varicella
▲ Clarinex Syrup (3.6%) ... 2828
Elidel Cream 1% (0.3% to 2.9%) ... 2221
ProQuad (Greater than or equal to 0.2% to less than 1%) ... 2099
Singulair (Greater than or equal to 2%) ... 2114

Varices, esophageal
Myleran Tablets ... 1530
Nexium Delayed-Release Capsules (Less than 1%) ... 645
Nexium I.V. (Less than 1%) ... 652
Nexium Delayed-Release Oral Suspension (Less than 1%) ... 645
Tabloid Tablets ... 1601

Varicose vein
Mirapex Tablets ... 857

Varicose vein, aggravation of
Lybrel Tablets ... 3204
Seasonique Tablets ... 1046
Yaz Tablets ... 805

Vascular access, clotting
▲ Epogen for Injection (0.25% to 7%) ... 576
▲ Procrit for Injection (0.25 to 7%) ... 2391

Vascular anomaly
Angiomax for Injection (Greater than 0.1% to less than 1%) ... 1933

Vascular collapse
Flebogamma 5% ... 1715
Flebogamma 5% DIF ... 1718
Gammagard Liquid ... 730
Gammagard S/D (Rare) ... 734
Gamunex (Rare) ... 3094

Vascular complications, unspecified
▲ Cozaar Tablets (4%) ... 1973
▲ Flolan for Injection (95%) ... 1426
Follistim AQ Cartridge ... 2844
▲ Humira Injection (Less than 5%) ... 442
Ortho-Cyclen/Ortho Tri-Cyclen ... 2449
Ortho Tri-Cyclen Lo Tablets ... 2458
ReoPro Vials (1.8%) ... 1860
Tricor Tablets ... 520
Zofran (Rare) ... 1687
Zofran ODT Orally Disintegrating Tablets (Rare) ... 1687
Zomig Tablets (Rare) ... 694
Zomig Nasal Spray (Rare) ... 689
Zomig-ZMT Tablets (Rare) ... 694

Vascular disorders, unspecified
▲ Cancidas for Injection (17.5% to 24.6%) ... 1953
▲ Femara Tablets (2.3% to 53.6%) ... 2246
▲ Mycamine for Injection (20.8% to 52.7%) ... 616

Vascular hypertensive disorders
▲ Selzentry Tablets (3.1%) ... 2534

Vascular insufficiency
Zonegran Capsules (Infrequent) ... 1089

Vascular leak syndrome
▲ Ontak Vials (27%) ... 1079

Vascular permeability, increase
Follistim AQ Cartridge ... 2844

Vasculitis
Accutane Capsules ... 2607
Aceon Tablets (2 mg, 4 mg, 8 mg) ... 3038
Advair Diskus 100/50 ... 1276
Advair Diskus 250/50 ... 1276
Advair Diskus 500/50 ... 1276
Advicor Tablets ... 402
Anaprox Tablets (Less than 1%) ... 2632
Anaprox DS Tablets (Less than 1%) ... 2632
Atacand HCT ... 642
Attenuvax ... 1951
Avalide Tablets ... 892
Avalide Tablets ... 2713
Axid Capsules ... 1364
Captopril Tablets ... 2182
Celebrex Capsules (Less than 0.1%) ... 2979
Cimzia ... 3127
Cipro I.V. (1% or less) ... 2817
Cipro ... 2810
Cipro XR Tablets ... 2823
Clorpres Tablets ... 2185
Combivir Tablets ... 1384
Cozaar Tablets ... 1973
Crixivan Capsules ... 1979
Cuprimine Capsules (Rare) ... 1986
Diovan HCT Tablets ... 2216
Dyazide Capsules ... 1405
EC-Naprosyn Delayed-Release Tablets (Less than 1%) ... 2632
Evoxac Capsules (Less than 1%) ... 1013
Exelon Capsules (Infrequent) ... 2229
Exelon Oral Solution (Infrequent) ... 2229
Exforge Tablets (Greater than 0.1% to less than 1%) ... 2238
Fluarix Vaccine ... 1446
Flulaval Injection Vaccine ... 1448
Furosemide Tablets ... 2186
Gantrisin Pediatric Suspension ... 2638
Gemzar for Injection (Very rare) ... 1820
Intravenous Sodium Diuril ... 2490
Intron A for Injection ... 2859
Ixempra Kit for Injection ... 915
Kaletra (Less than 2%) ... 452
Lamictal ... 1488
Lescol Capsules (Rare) ... 2268
Lescol XL Tablets ... 2268
Levaquin ... 2416
Levaquin in 5% Dextrose Injection ... 2416
Luvox CR Extended-Release Capsules ... 1759
Malarone Pediatric Tablets ... 1521
Malarone Tablets ... 1521
Meruvax II ... 2061
Mevacor Tablets (Rare) ... 2063
Micardis HCT Tablets ... 854
M-M-R II ... 2054
Mobic Oral Suspension (Less than 2%) ... 863
Mobic Tablets (Less than 2%) ... 863
Mumpsvax (Rare) ... 2068
Naprosyn Suspension (Less than 1%) ... 2632
Naprosyn Tablets (Less than 1%) ... 2632
Noroxin Tablets ... 2069
Orthoclone OKT3 Sterile Solution ... 2387
Paser Granules ... 1747
PegIntron Powder for Injection (Less than or equal to 1%) ... 2903
Plavix Tablets ... 926
Plavix Tablets ... 2767
Prinivil Tablets (0.3% to 1%) ... 2087
Prinzide Tablets ... 2092
Prozac Weekly Capsules ... 1852
Recombivax HB ... 2107
Remicade for IV Injection ... 950
Retrovir Capsules (Rare) ... 1574
Retrovir IV Infusion (Rare) ... 1579
Retrovir (Rare) ... 1574
Rituxan I.V. ... 1223
Tarka Tablets ... 511
Tekturna HCT Tablets ... 2324
Teveten HCT Tablets ... 517
Trizivir Tablets ... 1622
Vesanoid Capsules ... 2660
Voltaren Tablets (Rarely) ... 2334
Voltaren-XR Tablets (Rarely) ... 2337
Vytorin 10/10 Tablets ... 2149
Vytorin 10/10 Tablets ... 2939
Vytorin 10/20 Tablets ... 2149
Vytorin 10/20 Tablets ... 2939
Vytorin 10/40 Tablets ... 2149
Vytorin 10/40 Tablets ... 2939
Vytorin 10/80 Tablets ... 2149
Vytorin 10/80 Tablets ... 2939
Zantac 25 EFFERdose Tablets (Rare) ... 1670
Zantac Injection (Rare) ... 1666
Zantac Injection Pharmacy Bulk Package (Rare) ... 1668
Zantac Injection Premixed (Rare) ... 1666
Zantac (Rare) ... 1670
Zocor Tablets (Rare) ... 2136
Zolinza Capsules ... 2142

Vasculitis, allergic
Aggrenox Capsules ... 819
Amoxil Capsules ... 1305
Amoxil Chewable Tablets ... 1305
Amoxil Pediatric Drops for Oral Suspension ... 1305
Amoxil Powder for Oral Suspension ... 1305
Amoxil Tablets ... 1305
Avandaryl Tablets ... 1344
Bicillin C-R Injectable Suspension ... 1775
Bicillin L-A Injection ... 1777
Bystolic Tablets ... 1155
Duetact Tablets (Less than 1%) ... 3085
Imitrex Nasal Spray ... 1470
Imitrex Tablets ... 1474
Omnicef Capsules ... 497
Omnicef for Oral Suspension ... 497

Vasculitis, central nervous system
Imitrex Nasal Spray ... 1470
Imitrex Tablets ... 1474

Vasculitis, cutaneous
Atacand HCT ... 642
Avalide Tablets ... 892
Avalide Tablets ... 2713
Clorpres Tablets ... 2185
Depakote ER Tablets ... 423
Diovan HCT Tablets ... 2216
Enbrel for Injection ... 569
Humira Injection ... 442
Intravenous Sodium Diuril ... 2490
Micardis HCT Tablets ... 854
Neupogen for Injection (Infrequent) ... 589
Prinzide Tablets ... 2092
Remicade for IV Injection ... 950
Tekturna HCT Tablets ... 2324
Teveten HCT Tablets ... 517

Vasculitis, eosinophilic
Accolate Tablets (Rare) 669
Advair HFA 45/21 Inhalation Aerosol 1288
Advair HFA 115/21 Inhalation Aerosol 1288
Advair HFA 230/21 Inhalation Aerosol 1288

Vasculitis, hypersensitivity
Augmentin 1323
Augmentin Tablets 1327
Augmentin XR Extended Release Tablets 1333
Augmentin ES-600 Powder for Oral Suspension 1329
Clinoril Tablets (Less than 1 in 100) 1962
Lovenox Injection (Rare) 2756
Moxatag Tablets 2165
Rapamune 3260

Vasculitis, leukocytoclastic
Exjade Tablets 2244
Levaquin 2416
Levaquin in 5% Dextrose Injection 2416
Prozac Weekly Capsules 1852
Valtrex Caplets 1635
Velcade for Injection 2168
Zovirax 1690

Vasculitis, necrotizing
Daytrana Transdermal Patch 3022
Focalin XR Capsules 2251
Metadate CD Capsules 3146

Vasculitis, renal
Cuprimine Capsules (Rare) 1986

Vasodilation
Aceon Tablets (2 mg, 4 mg, 8 mg) (0.3% to 1%) 3038
▲ Acetadote Injection (1.47% to 9.84%) 1001
Actiq (Up to 2%) 959
Actonel with Calcium Tablets (1.4% to 2.3%) 2574
▲ Agrylin Capsules (1% to less than 5%) 3017
Alphagan P Ophthalmic Solution 549
AmBisome for Injection (Less common) 606
Amrix Capsules 966
AndroGel (Less than 1%) 3159
Aralast (0.1%) 726
▲ Argatroban Injection (1% to 10%) 1308
Aricept Tablets (Infrequent) 1062
Aricept ODT Tablets (Infrequent) 1062
▲ Arimidex Tablets (25% to 36%) 672
Asacol Delayed-Release Tablets (2% or greater) 2579
Avelox (Greater than or equal to 0.1% to less than 2%) 2803
▲ Avinza Capsules (Less than 5%) 1772
Axert Tablets (Infrequent) 2431
▲ Betaseron for SC Injection (8%) 756
▲ Bexxar (0% to 5%) 1371
Bicillin C-R Injectable Suspension 1775
Bicillin L-A Injection 1777
▲ Busulfex Injection (25%) 2477
Campral Tablets (Frequent) 1158
Cardene I.V. (0.7%) 1093
▲ CellCept Capsules (3% to less than 20%) 2622
▲ CellCept Intravenous (3% to less than 20%) 2622
▲ CellCept Oral Suspension (3% to less than 20%) 2622
▲ CellCept Tablets (3% to less than 20%) 2622
Cipro I.V. (1% or less) 2817
Combigan Ophthalmic Solution 553
▲ Copaxone for Injection (27%) 3110
Cosopt Sterile Ophthalmic Solution 1969
▲ Doxil Injection (1% to 10%) 2378
▲ Effexor XR Extended-Release Capsules (3% to 5%) 3195
Emsam Transdermal System (Infrequent) 905
Enbrel for Injection 569
▲ Faslodex Injection (17.7%) 682
▲ Flolan for Injection (Most common) 1426
Gabitril Tablets (2%) 973
Geodon for Injection (Up to 1%) 2520
Imitrex Injection (Rare) 1465
Imitrex Nasal Spray 1470
Imitrex Tablets (Rare) 1474
Ionsys Transdermal System (.1% to less than 1%) 2410
Lamictal (Infrequent) 1488
Levaquin 2416
Levaquin in 5% Dextrose Injection 2416
Lexiscan Injection 614
Lipitor Tablets (Less than 2%) 2501
Lovaza Capsules 1520
Lupron Depot-PED 7.5 mg, 11.25 mg and 15 mg (Less than 2%) 471
Luvox CR Extended-Release Capsules (2%) 1759
Marinol Capsules (Greater than 1%) 3163
Meridia Capsules (2.4%) 475
Mirapex Tablets (1% or more) 857
Mycamine for Injection 616
Norvir (1.7%) 489
▲ Ontak Vials (22%) 1079
OxyContin Tablets (Less than 1%) 2589
▲ Paxil (3% to 4%) 1535
▲ Paxil CR Controlled-Release Tablets (3% to 4%) 1544
Pentasa Capsules (Less than 1%) 3030
Pletal Tablets (Less than 2%) 2481
ProAmatine Tablets (Less frequent) 3032
▲ Proleukin for Injection (13%) 2287
Protonix for Delayed-Release Oral Suspension (Less than 1%) 3254
Protonix Delayed-Release Tablets (Less than 1%) 3254
Protonix I.V. (Less than 1%) 3257
Protopic Ointment (Greater than or equal to 1%) 628
Provigil Tablets (2%) 977
▲ Prozac Weekly Capsules (1% to 5%) 1852
▲ Prozac Pulvules and Liquid (1% to 5%) 1852
ReFacto Vials 3269
Remeron Tablets (Frequent) 2924
RemeronSolTab Tablets (Frequent) 2927
Retrovir Capsules 1574
Retrovir IV Infusion 1579
Retrovir 1574
▲ Suboxone Tablets (9.3%) 2601
▲ Subutex Tablets (3.9%) 2601
▲ Sular Extended Release Tablets (4%) 2975
Symbyax Capsules (Frequent) 1871
▲ Taxotere Injection Concentrate (1.1% to 27%) 2773
Timoptic Sterile Ophthalmic Solution 2121
Timoptic in Ocudose 2124
Timoptic-XE Sterile Ophthalmic Gel Forming Solution 2125
Tricor Tablets 520
Tygacil for Injection (0% to less than 2%) 3276
▲ Ultram ER Extended-Release Tablets (1% to less than 5%) 2428
Valstar Sterile Solution for Intravesical Instillation (2%) 1735
▲ Venlafaxine Hydrochloride Tablets (2.3% to 5.6%) 2199
▲ Viadur Implant (67.9%) 802
Vicoprofen Tablets (Less than 3%) 533
Wellbutrin SR Sustained-Release Tablets (Infrequent) 1653
Wellbutrin XL Extended-Release Tablets (Infrequent) 1659
WinRho SDF 741
Zomig Tablets (Rare) 694
Zomig Nasal Spray (Rare) 689
Zomig-ZMT Tablets (Rare) 694
Zyban Sustained-Release Tablets (Infrequent) 1692
Zyprexa Tablets (Infrequent) 1883
Zyprexa ZYDIS Orally Disintegrating Tablets (Infrequent) 1883

Vasodilation, peripheral
Aggrenox Capsules 819
Persantine Tablets 869
Ventolin HFA Inhalation Aerosol 1638

Vasomotor disturbances
Aminohippurate Sodium "PAH" Injection 1950

Vasospasm, coronary artery
Amerge Tablets 1301
Frova Tablets 1111
Imitrex Tablets 1474
Treximet Tablets 1616
Zomig Tablets 694
Zomig Nasal Spray 689
Zomig-ZMT Tablets 694

Vasospasm, rebound
Nimotop Capsules (Less than 1%) 790

Vasospasm, unspecified
Bicillin C-R Injectable Suspension 1775
Bicillin L-A Injection 1777
▲ CellCept Capsules (3% to less than 20%) 2622
▲ CellCept Intravenous (3% to less than 20%) 2622
▲ CellCept Oral Suspension (3% to less than 20%) 2622
▲ CellCept Tablets (3% to less than 20%) 2622
Prozac Weekly Capsules (Rare) 1852
Prozac Pulvules and Liquid (Rare) 1852

Vasospastic reactions
Imitrex Tablets 1474
Treximet Tablets 1616

Vasovagal episode
Alferon N Injection (2%) 1726
Bicillin C-R Injectable Suspension 1775
Bicillin L-A Injection 1777
Exelon Capsules (Infrequent) 2229
Exelon Oral Solution (Infrequent) 2229
Visudyne for Injection (Less than 1%) 2332

Vein, pigmentation of
Aloxi Injection (Less than 1%) 1059

Vein distention
Aloxi Injection (Less than 1%) 1059

Veins, varicosis
Ambien Tablets (Rare) 2692
Ambien CR Tablets (Rare) 2696
Amerge Tablets (Rare) 1301
Campral Tablets (Infrequent) 1158
Copaxone for Injection (Infrequent) .. 3110
Kaletra (Less than 2%) 452
Lexapro Oral Suspension (Infrequent) 1174
Lexapro Tablets (Infrequent) 1174
Paxil (Rare) 1535
Paxil CR Controlled-Release Tablets (Rare) 1544
Pletal Tablets (Less than 2%) 2481
Requip Tablets (Infrequent) 1561
Tricor Tablets 520
▲ Visudyne for Injection (1% to 10%) 2332

Venipuncture site bruise
Abilify Injection (Greater than or equal to 1 in 1000 patients and less than 1 in 100 patients) 881

Veno-occlusive disease, unspecified
▲ Mylotarg for Injection (1% to 20%) 3212

Venous infection at injection site
Primaxin I.V. (0.1%) 2083

Venous pressure, increased
▲ CellCept Capsules (3% to less than 20%) 2622
▲ CellCept Intravenous (3% to less than 20%) 2622
▲ CellCept Oral Suspension (3% to less than 20%) 2622
▲ CellCept Tablets (3% to less than 20%) 2622

Venous thromboembolism
▲ Arimidex Tablets (2% to 5%) 672
Evista Tablets 1810
Prempro Tablets 3232
▲ Rapamune (Greater than or equal to 3% to less than 20%) 3260
Torisel Injection (2%) 3272

Venous thrombophlebitis
Follistim AQ Cartridge 2844
▲ Xeloda Tablets (Less than 5%) 2662

Ventricular contractions
▲ Lexiscan Injection (14%) 614

Ventricular contractions, premature
Adenocard IV Injection 603
Amerge Tablets (Infrequent) 1301
▲ Indapamide Tablets (Less than 5%) 2188
Lanoxin Injection (Less common) 1498
Lanoxin Injection Pediatric (Less common) 1502
Zantac 25 EFFERdose Tablets (Rare) 1670
Zantac Injection (Rare) 1666
Zantac Injection Pharmacy Bulk Package (Rare) 1668
Zantac Injection Premixed (Rare) 1666
Zantac (Rare) 1670
Zofran Injection 1682

Ventricular contractions, premature, multifocal
Lanoxin Injection 1498
Lanoxin Injection Pediatric (Less common) 1502
Lanoxin Tablets (Among most common) 1505

Ventricular contractions, premature, unifocal
Lanoxin Injection 1498
Lanoxin Injection Pediatric (Less common) 1502
Lanoxin Tablets (Among most common) 1505

Ventricular dilation, left-side
Retrovir Capsules (0.8%) 1574
Retrovir IV Infusion (1%) 1579
Retrovir (0.8%) 1574

Ventricular dysfunction
Herceptin I.V. 1199
Prograf Capsules and Injection (Rare) 622
Tasigna Capsules 2316

Ventricular ectopic beats
Cipro I.V. (1% or less) 2817
Digibind for Injection 1403
Imitrex Tablets 1474

Ventricular extrasystoles
Aceon Tablets (2 mg, 4 mg, 8 mg) (0.3% to 1%) 3038
Aricept Tablets (Infrequent) 1062
Aricept ODT Tablets (Infrequent) 1062
Busulfex Injection (2%) 2477
Cardizem LA Extended Release Tablets (Less than 2%) 421
▲ CellCept Capsules (3% to less than 20%) 2622
▲ CellCept Intravenous (3% to less than 20%) 2622
▲ CellCept Oral Suspension (3% to less than 20%) 2622
▲ CellCept Tablets (3% to less than 20%) 2622
Chantix Tablets (Infrequent) 2511
Concerta Extended-Release Tablets 1925
Cyanokit 5g Antidote 1021
Effexor XR Extended-Release Capsules 3195
Lanoxin Injection 1498
Lanoxin Injection Pediatric 1502
Lanoxin Tablets 1505
Meridia Capsules 475
Mirapex Tablets 857
▲ Natrecor for Injection (3% to 4%) 2977
Paxil (Rare) 1535
Paxil CR Controlled-Release Tablets (Rare) 1544
Pletal Tablets (Less than 2%) 2481
Prograf Capsules and Injection 622
Proleukin for Injection (Less than 1%) 2287
Provigil Tablets (At least 1%) 977
Prozac Weekly Capsules (Rare) 1852
Prozac Pulvules and Liquid (Rare) 1852
Remeron Tablets (Infrequent) 2924
RemeronSolTab Tablets (Infrequent) 2927
Rilutek Tablets (Infrequent) 2771
Romazicon Injection (Less than 1%) 2646
Rythmol SR Capsules 1590
Sular Extended Release Tablets (Less than or equal to 1%) 2975
▲ Trasylol Injection (6%) 799
Treximet Tablets (Rare) 1616
Tricor Tablets 520
Ultane Liquid for Inhalation (Less than 1%) 524
Vantas (Less than 2%) 1737
Venlafaxine Hydrochloride Tablets 2199
▲ Xeloda Tablets (Less than 5%) 2662
Zonegran Capsules (Rare) 1089
Zyprexa Tablets (Infrequent) 1883
Zyprexa ZYDIS Orally Disintegrating Tablets (Infrequent) 1883

Ventricular failure
Flolan for Injection 1426

Ventricular gallop
Retrovir Capsules (0.8%) 1574
Retrovir IV Infusion (1%) 1579
Retrovir (0.8%) 1574

Ventricular hypertrophy
Celebrex Capsules (Greater than or equal to 0.1% to less than 1%) 2979
Mirapex Tablets 857
Rythmol SR Capsules 1590

Vyvanse Capsules ... 3033

Ventricular wall thickening

▲ Fabrazyme for Intravenous Infusion (5%) ... 1241

Verruca

Copaxone for Injection (Frequent) ... 3110
Evoxac Capsules (Less than 1%) ... 1013
▲ Prometrium Capsules (100 mg, 200 mg) (Less than 5%) ... 3047
Soriatane Capsules (Less than 1%) ... 3062

Vertebral compression fractures

Fentora Tablets (Greater than 1%) ... 968

Vertical deviation

▲ BOTOX Purified Neurotoxin Complex (2.1% to 16.9%) ... 550

Vertigo

Abelcet Injection ... 1134
Aceon Tablets (2 mg, 4 mg, 8 mg) (0.3% to 1%) ... 3038
Actiq (Up to 1%) ... 959
▲ Actonel with Calcium Tablets (1.6% to 3.3%) ... 2574
Advicor Tablets ... 402
▲ Aerobid/Aerobid-M (1% to 3%) ... 1153
Albenza Tablets (Less than 1% to 1.2%) ... 1297
Ambien Tablets (Frequent) ... 2692
Ambien CR Tablets (2%) ... 2696
Amerge Tablets (Frequent) ... 1301
Anaprox Tablets (Less than 3%) ... 2632
Anaprox DS Tablets (Less than 3%) ... 2632
Anzemet Injection (Infrequently) ... 2701
Anzemet Tablets ... 2704
Aricept Tablets (Infrequent) ... 1062
Aricept ODT Tablets (Infrequent) ... 1062
Asacol Delayed-Release Tablets ... 2579
Atacand Tablets (0.5% or greater) ... 639
Atacand HCT (0.5% or greater) ... 642
Avalide Tablets ... 892
Avalide Tablets ... 2713
Avapro Tablets ... 897
Avapro Tablets ... 2718
Avelox (Greater than or equal to 0.1% to less than 2%) ... 2803
▲ Avinza Capsules (Less than 5%) ... 1772
Axert Tablets (Infrequent) ... 2431
Azilect Tablets (2%) ... 3106
Benicar Tablets (Greater than 0.5%) ... 1009
Benicar HCT Tablets (Greater than 1%) ... 1010
Biaxin/Biaxin XL ... 411
▲ Boniva Injection (3%) ... 2614
▲ Boniva Tablets (3%) ... 2618
Bystolic Tablets ... 1155
Campral Tablets (Infrequent) ... 1158
Capastat Sulfate for Injection ... 1791
Carafate Suspension (Less than 0.5%) ... 706
Carafate Tablets (Less than 0.5%) ... 707
Celebrex Capsules (0.1% to 1.9%) ... 2979
Celexa (Infrequent) ... 1160
▲ CellCept Capsules (3% to less than 20%) ... 2622
▲ CellCept Intravenous (3% to less than 20%) ... 2622
▲ CellCept Oral Suspension (3% to less than 20%) ... 2622
▲ CellCept Tablets (3% to less than 20%) ... 2622
Chantix Tablets (Infrequent) ... 2511
Cialis Tablets (Less than 2%) ... 1792
Cipro XR Tablets (Less than 1%) ... 2823
Clinoril Tablets (Less than 1 in 100) ... 1962
Clorpres Tablets ... 2185
Combigan Ophthalmic Solution ... 553
Concerta Extended-Release Tablets (1.7%) ... 1925
▲ Copaxone for Injection (6%) ... 3110
▲ Coreg Tablets (Greater than 1% to 3%) ... 1387
▲ Coreg CR Extended-Release Capsules (Greater than 1% to less than or equal to 3%) ... 1393
Cosopt Sterile Ophthalmic Solution ... 1969
Cozaar Tablets (Less than 1%) ... 1973
Cubicin for Injection (Less than 1%) ... 995
Cymbalta Delayed-Release Capsules (Frequent) ... 1801
Dapsone Tablets USP ... 1746
▲ Depakote ER Tablets (Greater than 1% to less than 5%) ... 423
Diovan Tablets ... 2212
Diovan HCT Tablets (Greater than 0.2%) ... 2216
▲ Doxil Injection (1% to 10%) ... 2378
Duragesic Transdermal System (Less than 1%) ... 2405
Dyazide Capsules ... 1405
EC-Naprosyn Delayed-Release Tablets (Less than 3%) ... 2632
Edecrin ... 698
Effexor XR Extended-Release Capsules (Frequent) ... 3195
Eldepryl Capsules ... 3052
Eligard 7.5 mg (Less than 2%) ... 2724
Eligard 22.5 mg (Less than 2%) ... 2724
Eligard 30 mg (Less than 2%) ... 2724
Eligard 45 mg (Less than 2%) ... 2724
▲ Eloxatin for Injection (2% to less than 5%) ... 2731
Emsam Transdermal System (Infrequent) ... 905
Engerix-B Vaccine ... 1409
▲ Epzicom Tablets (6%) ... 1422
▲ Evoxac Capsules (1% to 3%) ... 1013
Exelon Capsules (2% or more) ... 2229
Exelon Oral Solution (2% or more) ... 2229
Exelon Patch (0% to 2%) ... 2233
Exforge Tablets (0.2%) ... 2238
Fansidar Tablets ... 2636
Faslodex Injection (Less than 1%) ... 682
Femara Tablets (Less frequent) ... 2246
Flomax Capsules (0.6% to 1%) ... 848
Fluarix Vaccine ... 1446
▲ Forteo for Injection (3.8%) ... 1816
Fosamax ... 2005
Fosamax Plus D Tablets ... 2013
Frova Tablets (Infrequent) ... 1111
Furosemide Tablets ... 2186
Gabitril Tablets (Frequent) ... 973
Gantrisin Pediatric Suspension ... 2638
Gengraf Capsules (1% to less than 3%) ... 435
Geodon Capsules (Frequent) ... 2520
Gleevec Tablets (Infrequent) ... 2255
Havrix Injection Vaccine (Less than 1%) ... 1454
Hexalen Capsules ... 1078
▲ Imitrex Injection (12%) ... 1465
Imitrex Nasal Spray (1% to 1.7%) ... 1470
Imitrex Tablets (Less than 1%) ... 1474
▲ Indapamide Tablets (Less than 5%) ... 2188
Indocin (Greater than 1%) ... 2024
Intelence Tablets (Less than 2%) ... 3119
Intravenous Sodium Diuril ... 2490
▲ Intron A for Injection (Less than 5% to 23%) ... 2859
Invanz for Injection (Greater than 0.1%) ... 2029
Kaletra (Less than 2%) ... 452
▲ Keppra Injection (3% to 5%) ... 3137
▲ Keppra Oral Solution (3% to 5%) ... 3131
▲ Keppra Tablets (3% to 5%) ... 3131
Ketek Tablets (Greater than or equal to 0.2% to less than 2%) ... 2744
Klonopin (Infrequent) ... 2639
Lamictal (2%) ... 1488
Lescol Capsules ... 2268
Lescol XL Tablets ... 2268
Levaquin (0.1% to 1%) ... 2416
Levaquin in 5% Dextrose Injection (0.1% to 1%) ... 2416
Levitra Tablets (Less than 2%) ... 2876
Lexapro Oral Suspension (Infrequent) ... 1174
Lexapro Tablets (Infrequent) ... 1174
Lovaza Capsules ... 1520
Lunesta Tablets (Infrequent) ... 2994
▲ Lupron Depot 3.75 mg (8%) ... 462
▲ Lupron Depot–3 Month 11.25 mg (8%) ... 462
Luvox CR Extended-Release Capsules (Infrequent) ... 1759
▲ Lyrica Capsules (1% to 4%) ... 2527
Mavik Tablets (0.3% to 1%) ... 472
Maxalt Tablets (Infrequent) ... 2056
Maxalt-MLT Orally Disintegrating Tablets (Infrequent) ... 2056
Meridia Capsules ... 475
Mevacor Tablets (0.5% to 1%) ... 2063
Miacalcin Nasal Spray (Less than 1%) ... 2274
Micardis Tablets (More than 0.3%) ... 852
Micardis HCT Tablets ... 854
Mirapex Tablets (1% or more) ... 857
Mobic Oral Suspension (Less than 2%) ... 863
Mobic Tablets (Less than 2%) ... 863
Mustargen for Injection (Infrequent) ... 2492
Namenda (Frequent) ... 1180
Naprosyn Suspension (Less than 3%) ... 2632
Naprosyn Tablets (Less than 3%) ... 2632
Neoral Oral Solution (1% to less than 3%) ... 2280
Neoral Soft Gelatin Capsules (1% to less than 3%) ... 2280
▲ Neupro Transdermal System (3%) ... 3149
Nexium Delayed-Release Capsules (Less than 1%) ... 645
Nexium I.V. (Less than 1%) ... 652
Nexium Delayed-Release Oral Suspension (Less than 1%) ... 645
Norvir (Less than 2%) ... 489
▲ Opana Tablets (6.5%) ... 1117
▲ Opana ER Tablets (0% to 17.8%) ... 1121
Orthoclone OKT3 Sterile Solution ... 2387
OxyContin Tablets (Less than 1%) ... 2589
Paxil (Frequent) ... 1535
Paxil CR Controlled-Release Tablets (Frequent) ... 1544
PegIntron Powder for Injection ... 2903
Plavix Tablets (1% to 2.5%) ... 926
Plavix Tablets (1% to 2.5%) ... 2767
▲ Pletal Tablets (1% to 3%) ... 2481
Primaxin I.M. ... 2080
Primaxin I.V. (Less than 0.2%) ... 2083
Prinivil Tablets (0.2%) ... 2087
Prinzide Tablets (0.3% to 1%) ... 2092
Protonix for Delayed-Release Oral Suspension (Less than 1%) ... 3254
Protonix Delayed-Release Tablets (Less than 1%) ... 3254
Protonix I.V. (Less than 1%) ... 3257
Protopic Ointment (Greater than or equal to 1%) ... 628
Proventil HFA Inhalation Aerosol ... 2914
Provigil Tablets (1%) ... 977
Prozac Weekly Capsules (Infrequent) ... 1852
Prozac Pulvules and Liquid (Infrequent) ... 1852
Rebetol ... 2917
Remeron Tablets (Frequent) ... 2924
RemeronSolTab Tablets (Frequent) ... 2927
Requip Tablets (2%) ... 1561
▲ Requip XL Tablets (4%) ... 1568
Retrovir Capsules ... 1574
Retrovir IV Infusion ... 1579
Retrovir ... 1574
▲ Rilutek Tablets (2.5% to 4.5%) ... 2771
Risperdal Consta Long-Acting Injection (Infrequent) ... 1753
▲ Romazicon Injection (10%) ... 2646
Rythmol Tablets (Less than 1%) ... 1586
Rythmol SR Capsules ... 1590
Seromycin Capsules ... 1864
Solodyn Extended Release Tablets (1%) ... 1938
Soma Tablets ... 1931
Stromectol Tablets (0.9%) ... 2120
Sular Extended Release Tablets (Less than or equal to 1%) ... 2975
Sustiva Capsules (Less than 2%) ... 930
Sustiva Tablets (Less than 2%) ... 930
Symbyax Capsules (Infrequent) ... 1871
Tamiflu Capsules (Less than or equal to 1%) ... 2649
Tamiflu Oral Suspension (Less than or equal to 1%) ... 2649
Tarka Tablets (Less frequent) ... 511
▲ Tasigna Capsules (1% to 10%) ... 2316
Tekturna HCT Tablets (1.2%) ... 2324
Testim 1% Gel ... 701
Teveten Tablets (Less than 1%) ... 515
Teveten HCT Tablets (Less than 1%) ... 517
Timoptic Sterile Ophthalmic Solution ... 2121
Timoptic in Ocudose ... 2124
Timoptic-XE Sterile Ophthalmic Gel Forming Solution ... 2125
Toprol-XL Tablets (1.8%) ... 666
Treximet Tablets (Rare) ... 1616
Tricor Tablets ... 520
Twinrix Vaccine (Less than 1%) ... 1628
Ultram ER Extended-Release Tablets (0.5% to less than 1%) ... 2428
Valium Tablets (Infrequent) ... 2658
Velcade for Injection ... 2168
Venlafaxine Hydrochloride Tablets (Frequent) ... 2199
Vicoprofen Tablets (Less than 1%) ... 533
▲ Visudyne for Injection (1% to 10%) ... 2332
Voltaren Tablets (Occasionally) ... 2334
Voltaren-XR Tablets (Occasionally) ... 2337
Vytorin 10/10 Tablets ... 2149
Vytorin 10/10 Tablets ... 2939
Vytorin 10/20 Tablets ... 2149
Vytorin 10/20 Tablets ... 2939
Vytorin 10/40 Tablets ... 2149
Vytorin 10/40 Tablets ... 2939
Vytorin 10/80 Tablets ... 2149
Vytorin 10/80 Tablets ... 2939
Wellbutrin Tablets (Infrequent) ... 1648
Wellbutrin SR Sustained-Release Tablets (Infrequent) ... 1653
Wellbutrin XL Extended-Release Tablets (Infrequent) ... 1659
▲ Xeloda Tablets (Less than 5%) ... 2662
Xyrem Oral Solution (Less than 1% to frequent) ... 1766
Zantac 25 EFFERdose Tablets (Rare) ... 1670
Zantac Injection ... 1666
Zantac Injection Pharmacy Bulk Package (Rare) ... 1668
Zantac Injection Premixed ... 1666
Zantac (Rare) ... 1670
▲ Zocor Tablets (4.5%) ... 2136
Zomig Tablets (Infrequent) ... 694
Zomig Nasal Spray (Infrequent) ... 689
Zomig-ZMT Tablets (Infrequent) ... 694
Zonegran Capsules (Infrequent) ... 1089
Zosyn for Injection (1.0% or less) ... 3284
Zyban Sustained-Release Tablets (Infrequent) ... 1692
Zyprexa Tablets (Infrequent) ... 1883
Zyprexa ZYDIS Orally Disintegrating Tablets (Infrequent) ... 1883
Zyrtec Chewable Tablets (Less than 2%) ... 1920
Zyrtec Syrup (Less than 2%) ... 1920
Zyrtec Tablets (Less than 2%) ... 1920
Zyrtec-D 12 Hour Extended Release Tablets (Less than 2%) ... 1923
Zyvox (0% to 1.2%) ... 2552

Vesicles

Avelox ... 2803
Cipro I.V. ... 2817
Cipro XR Tablets ... 2823
Daytrana Transdermal Patch ... 3022
Levaquin ... 2416
Levaquin in 5% Dextrose Injection ... 2416
Noroxin Tablets ... 2069

Vesicles at application site

▲ Flector Patch (4%) ... 561
▲ Ionsys Transdermal System (1% to less than 10%) ... 2410
Kinrix Injection Vaccine ... 1486
Lidoderm Patch ... 1114

Vesiculation

▲ Aldara Cream, 5% (0% to 9%) ... 1699
Attenuvax ... 1951
▲ Catapres-TTS (7 of 101 patients) ... 842
Cipro I.V. (1% or less) ... 2817
Diprolene Lotion 0.05% (Less than 1%) ... 2838
Diprolene Ointment 0.05% (Less than 1%) ... 2839
M-M-R II ... 2054

Vesiculobullous reaction

▲ Busulfex Injection (10%) ... 2477

Vestibular disturbances

Lunesta Tablets (Infrequent) ... 2994

Vestibular dysfunction

Gengraf Capsules (1% to less than 3%) ... 435
Neoral Oral Solution (1% to less than 3%) ... 2280
Neoral Soft Gelatin Capsules (1% to less than 3%) ... 2280
Rilutek Tablets (Rare) ... 2771

Viremia

▲ Campath Ampules (55%) ... 761

Virilization

Delatestryl Injection ... 1730
Estratest Tablets (Among most common) ... 3043
Estratest H.S. Tablets (Among most common) ... 3043
▲ Intron A for Injection (Less than 5%) ... 2859

Virilization, female fetus

Delatestryl Injection ... 1730

Vision, blurred

▲ Abilify Injection (3% to 8%) ... 881
▲ Abilify Injection (3% to 8%) ... 2466
▲ Abilify Oral Solution (3% to 8%) ... 881
▲ Abilify Oral Solution (3% to 8%) ... 2466
▲ Abilify Discmelt Orally Disintegrating Tablets (3% to 8%) ... 881
▲ Abilify Discmelt Orally Disintegrating Tablets (3% to 8%) ... 2466
▲ Abilify Tablets (3% to 8%) ... 881
▲ Abilify Tablets (3% to 8%) ... 2466
ActoPlus Met Tablets ... 3071
Adderall XR Capsules ... 3012
Adenocard IV Injection (Less than 1%) ... 603

Adenoscan (Less than 1%) 605
▲ Aerobid/Aerobid-M (1% to 3%) 1153
▲ Alferon N Injection (3% to 6%) 1726
▲ Alphagan P Ophthalmic Solution (1% to 4%) 549
▲ Alrex Ophthalmic Suspension 0.2% (5% to 15%) ⊙236
Ambien CR Tablets (2%) 2696
Amerge Tablets (Infrequent) 1301
Amrix Capsules 966
Anaprox Tablets (Less than 1%) 2632
Anaprox DS Tablets (Less than 1%) 2632
Aricept Tablets (Frequent) 1062
Aricept ODT Tablets (Frequent) 1062
▲ Arranon Injection (4%) 1319
Asacol Delayed-Release Tablets 2579
Atacand HCT 642
Atrovent Nasal Spray 0.03% (Less than 2%) 834
Atrovent Nasal Spray 0.06% (Less than 1%) 836
Avalide Tablets 892
Avalide Tablets 2713
Avandaryl Tablets 1344
▲ Azopt Ophthalmic Suspension (5% to 10%) 540
▲ Bentyl Capsules (27%) 703
▲ Bentyl Injection (27%) 703
▲ Bentyl Syrup (27%) 703
▲ Bentyl Tablets (27%) 703
▲ Betimol Ophthalmic Solution (1% to 5%) 3181
Bicillin C-R Injectable Suspension 1775
Bicillin L-A Injection 1777
Captopril Tablets 2182
Carbatrol Capsules 3019
Catapres Tablets 841
Catapres-TTS (0.5% or less) 842
Celebrex Capsules (0.1% to 1.9%) 2979
Chantix Tablets (Infrequent) 2511
Cialis Tablets (Less than 2%) 1792
Cipro I.V. (1% or less) 2817
Cipro (Less than 1%) 2810
Cipro XR Tablets 2823
Clear Eyes for Dry Eyes ⊙255
Clinoril Tablets (Less than 1 in 100) 1962
Clorpres Tablets 2185
Combigan Ophthalmic Solution (0.1% to 0.2%) 553
Combivent Inhalation Aerosol 845
Concerta Extended-Release Tablets (1.7%) 1925
▲ Coreg Tablets (Greater than 1% to 3%) 1387
▲ Coreg CR Extended-Release Capsules (Greater than 1% to less than or equal to 3%) 1393
▲ Cosopt Sterile Ophthalmic Solution (5% to 15%) 1969
Cozaar Tablets (Less than 1%) 1973
Cubicin for Injection (Less than 1%) 995
Cymbalta Delayed-Release Capsules (Frequent to 2%) 1801
▲ Dacogen Injection (6%) 1066
Dapsone Tablets USP 1746
Daytrana Transdermal Patch 3022
▲ Depakote ER Tablets (4% to 12%) 423
▲ DepoCyt Injection (11% to 12%) 1136
▲ Diclofenac Sodium Ophthalmic Solution (Less than or equal to 5%) ⊙240
Diovan HCT Tablets (Less frequent) 2216
Donnatal Extentabs 2507
Duetact Tablets (Less than 1%) 3085
Duragesic Transdermal System 2405
Dyazide Capsules 1405
EC-Naprosyn Delayed-Release Tablets (Less than 1%) 2632
Edecrin 698
▲ Effexor XR Extended-Release Capsules (4% to 8%) 3195
Eldepryl Capsules 3052
Equetro Extended-Release Capsules 3174
Exelon Capsules (Infrequent) 2229
Exelon Oral Solution (Infrequent) 2229
Exelon Patch (Infrequent) 2233
Femara Tablets (Less than 1%) 2246
Flonase Nasal Spray 1431
FML Ophthalmic Suspension ⊙224
FML Forte Ophthalmic Suspension ⊙222
Focalin XR Capsules 2251
Furosemide Tablets 2186
Gleevec Tablets (Less common) 2255
Humulin 50/50, 100 Units 1843
Humulin 70/30 Vial 1844
Humulin N Vial 1846
Humulin R 1849
Indocin (Less than 1%) 2024
Intelence Tablets (Less than 2%) 3119
Intravenous Sodium Diuril 2490
▲ Intron A for Injection (Less than 5%) 2859
Ionsys Transdermal System (.1% to less than 1%) 2410
Iquix Ophthalmic Solution (1% to 2%) 3183
Ketek Tablets (Greater than or equal to 0.2% to less than 2%) 2744
Klonopin (1%) 2639
Lacrisert Sterile Ophthalmic Insert ⊙233
▲ Lamictal (11% to 25%) 1488
Lanoxin Injection 1498
Lanoxin Injection Pediatric 1502
Lanoxin Tablets 1505
Levaquin 2416
Levaquin in 5% Dextrose Injection 2416
Levitra Tablets (Less than 2%) 2876
Lexapro Oral Suspension (Frequent) 1174
Lexapro Tablets (Frequent) 1174
Lidoderm Patch 1114
▲ Lotemax Ophthalmic Suspension 0.5% (5% to 15%) ⊙241
▲ Lucentis Injection (4% to 17%) 1205
▲ Lyrica Capsules (1% to 12%) 2527
Maxalt Tablets (Infrequent) 2056
Maxalt-MLT Orally Disintegrating Tablets (Infrequent) 2056
Meridia Capsules 475
Metadate CD Capsules 3146
Mevacor Tablets (0.9% to 1.5%) 2063
Miacalcin Nasal Spray (Less than 1%) 2274
Micardis HCT Tablets 854
Mirapex Tablets 857
Moban Tablets (Occasional) 1116
MS Contin Tablets (Less frequent) 2585
▲ Myfortic Tablets (3% to less than 20%) 2276
Nadolol Tablets (1 to 5 of 1000 patients) 2191
Nalfon Capsules (2.2%) 2508
Namenda (Infrequent) 1180
Naprosyn Suspension (Less than 1%) 2632
Naprosyn Tablets (Less than 1%) 2632
Nexium Delayed-Release Capsules 645
Nexium I.V. (Rare) 652
Nexium Delayed-Release Oral Suspension 645
Noroxin Tablets (Less frequent) 2069
Norvir (Less than 2%) 489
▲ Novantrone for Injection Concentrate (3%) 1100
Noxafil Oral Suspension (1%) 2889
Ofloxacin Ophthalmic Solution 0.3% ⊙243
Opana Tablets (Less than 1%) 1117
Opana ER Tablets (Less than 1%) 1121
OptiPranolol Metipranolol Ophthalmic Solution 0.3% (A small number of patients) ⊙245
Orthoclone OKT3 Sterile Solution 2387
Parnate Tablets 1532
▲ Pataday Ophthalmic Solution (Less than or equal to 5%) 543
▲ Patanol Ophthalmic Solution (Less than 5%) 546
▲ Paxil (2% to 7.8%) 1535
▲ Paxil CR Controlled-Release Tablets (2% to 7.8%) 1544
PegIntron Powder for Injection (2%) 2903
Pred Forte Ophthalmic Suspension ⊙227
Prinivil Tablets (0.3% to 1%) 2087
Prinzide Tablets (0.3% to 1%) 2092
▲ Pristiq Extended-Release Tablets (3% to 4%) 3247
Proglycem Capsules (Infrequent) 1185
Proglycem Suspension (Infrequent) 1185
Protonix for Delayed-Release Oral Suspension 3254
Protonix Delayed-Release Tablets 3254
Protonix I.V. 3257
▲ Rebetol (5% to 6%) 2917
Requip Tablets (Infrequent) 1561
▲ Restasis Ophthalmic Emulsion (1% to 5%) 557
▲ Romazicon Injection (1% to 9%) 2646
▲ Rythmol Tablets (2% to 6%) 1586
▲ Rythmol SR Capsules (1% to 6%) 1590
Salagen Tablets (1% to 2%) 1082
Sanctura XR Capsules (Less than 1%) 557
▲ Sandostatin Injection (1% to 4%) 2300
▲ Soriatane Capsules (1% to 10%) 3062
Stalevo Tablets 2309
Tarka Tablets (Less frequent) 511
Tasigna Capsules 2316
Tekturna HCT Tablets 2324
▲ Temodar Capsules (5% to 9%) 2931
Teveten HCT Tablets 517
Thioridazine Hydrochloride Tablets 2195
Thiothixene Capsules (Infrequently) 2197
Timoptic-XE Sterile Ophthalmic Gel Forming Solution 2125
Toprol-XL Tablets 666
Transderm Scōp Transdermal Therapeutic System 2206
▲ Travatan Z Ophthalmic Solution (1% to 4%) 547
▲ Trisenox Injection (10%) 986
▲ Trusopt Sterile Ophthalmic Solution (Approximately 1% to 5%) 2128
▲ Ultram ER Extended-Release Tablets (1% to less than 5%) 2428
Valium Tablets (Infrequent) 2658
Velcade for Injection 2168
▲ Venlafaxine Hydrochloride Tablets (6%) 2199
▲ VESIcare Tablets (3.8% to 4.8%) 636
▲ Visudyne for Injection (10% to 30%) 2332
▲ Voltaren Ophthalmic Solution (Less than or equal to 5%) 2336
Voltaren Tablets (Occasionally) 2334
Voltaren-XR Tablets (Occasionally) 2337
Vyvanse Capsules 3033
▲ Wellbutrin Tablets (14.6%) 1648
▲ Wellbutrin SR Sustained-Release Tablets (2% to 3%) 1653
▲ Xyrem Oral Solution (Less than 1% to 5.9%) 1766
Zantac 25 EFFERdose Tablets (Rare) 1670
Zantac Injection (Rare) 1666
Zantac Injection Pharmacy Bulk Package (Rare) 1668
Zantac Injection Premixed (Rare) 1666
Zantac (Rare) 1670
Zofran Injection 1682
Zolinza Capsules 2142
Zometa for Intravenous Infusion 2341
Zyban Sustained-Release Tablets (Frequent) 1692

Vision, changes
(*see under* Visual disturbances)

Vision, complete loss
Lybrel Tablets 3204
Ortho-Cyclen/Ortho Tri-Cyclen 2449
Ortho Tri-Cyclen Lo Tablets 2458
Premphase Tablets 3232
Prempro Tablets 3232

Vision, decreased
Iquix Ophthalmic Solution (1% to 2%) 3183

Vision, double
(*see under* Diplopia)

Vision, loss of
Imitrex Injection 1465
Imitrex Nasal Spray 1470
Imitrex Tablets 1474
Intron A for Injection 2859
Levitra Tablets (Rare) 2876
Ontak Vials 1079
Ortho Evra Transdermal System 2437
PegIntron Powder for Injection 2903
Prinivil Tablets (0.3% to 1%) 2087
Prinzide Tablets 2092
Sutent Capsules 2540
Thyrogen for Injection 1244
▲ Visudyne for Injection (1% to 10%) 2332
Zyvox 2552

Vision, loss of color
Cipro I.V. (1% or less) 2817
Ontak Vials 1079

Vision, partial loss
Imitrex Tablets 1474
Lybrel Tablets 3204
Ortho-Cyclen/Ortho Tri-Cyclen 2449
Ortho Tri-Cyclen Lo Tablets 2458
Premphase Tablets 3232
Prempro Tablets 3232
Treximet Tablets 1616

Vision, temporary loss of
Eloxatin for Injection 2731
Sular Extended Release Tablets (Less than or equal to 1%) 2975

Vision abnormalities
(*see under* Visual disturbances)

Visual acuity, decreased
ActoPlus Met Tablets 3071
Avandaryl Tablets (Very rare) 1344
Avandia Tablets 1351
Cipro (Less than 1%) 2810
Cipro XR Tablets 2823
Combigan Ophthalmic Solution (0.1% to 0.2%) 553
Duetact Tablets 3085
▲ Durezol Ophthalmic Emulsion (1% to 5%) ⊙275
Eloxatin for Injection 2731
Emend Capsules (Less than or equal to 0.5%) 1992
Emend for Injection (Less than or equal to 0.5%) 1999
Ketek Tablets (Greater than or equal to 0.2% to less than 2%) 2744
Lamisil Oral Granules 2264
Levaquin 2416
Levaquin in 5% Dextrose Injection 2416
Levitra Tablets (Rare) 2876
Mirapex Tablets 857
Namenda (Infrequent) 1180
▲ Nevanac Ophthalmic Suspension 0.1% (5% to 10%) ⊙205
Requip Tablets (Infrequent) 1561
Rythmol SR Capsules 1590
Tasigna Capsules (0.1% to 1%) 2316
▲ Travatan Z Ophthalmic Solution (5% to 10%) 547
Triesence Injectable Suspension (2%) ⊙209
▲ Vigamox Ophthalmic Solution (1% to 6%) 548

Visual acuity, defects
▲ Alphagan P Ophthalmic Solution (1% to 4%) 549
Alrex Ophthalmic Suspension 0.2% ⊙236
Cipro I.V. (1% or less) 2817
Cozaar Tablets (Less than 1%) 1973
FML Ophthalmic Ointment ⊙223
FML Ophthalmic Suspension ⊙224
FML Forte Ophthalmic Suspension ⊙222
Intron A for Injection 2859
Lotemax Ophthalmic Suspension 0.5% ⊙241
PegIntron Powder for Injection (Less than or equal to 1%) 2903
Pred Forte Ophthalmic Suspension ⊙227
Pred Mild Ophthalmic Suspension ⊙230
Pred-G Ophthalmic Ointment ⊙229
Pred-G Ophthalmic Suspension ⊙228
▲ Vesanoid Capsules (6%) 2660
▲ Vigamox Ophthalmic Solution (1% to 6%) ⊙213
▲ Visudyne for Injection (10% to 30%) 2332

Visual depth perception, altered
Ambien CR Tablets (1%) 2696

Visual disturbances
Accutane Capsules 2607
Actiq (1% to 2%) 959
▲ Agrylin Capsules (1% to less than 5%) 3017
Alferon N Injection (1%) 1726
▲ Alphagan P Ophthalmic Solution (Approximately 5% to 9%) 549
▲ Alrex Ophthalmic Suspension 0.2% (5% to 15%) ⊙236
Ambien Tablets (Frequent) 2692
▲ Ambien CR Tablets (3%) 2696
Anaprox Tablets (Less than 3%) 2632
Anaprox DS Tablets (Less than 3%) 2632
Anzemet Injection (Infrequently) 2701
Anzemet Tablets 2704
Aralast (0.1%) 726
Aricept Tablets (Infrequent) 1062
Aricept ODT Tablets (Infrequent) 1062
Asacol Delayed-Release Tablets (2% or greater) 2579
Atripla Tablets 938
Avalide Tablets 892
Avalide Tablets 2713
Avapro Tablets (Less than 1%) 897
Avapro Tablets (Less than 1%) 2718
Avelox (Less than 0.1%) 2803
BeneFIX Vials (1.5%) 3191
▲ Betimol Ophthalmic Solution (More than 5%) 3181
Brovana Inhalation Solution (Less than 2%) 2990
Campral Tablets (Frequent) 1158
Celexa (At least 2%) 1160
▲ CellCept Capsules (3% to less than 20%) 2622
▲ CellCept Intravenous (3% to less than 20%) 2622
▲ CellCept Oral Suspension (3% to less than 20%) 2622

▲ CellCept Tablets (3% to less than 20%) **2622**
Chantix Tablets (Infrequent) **2511**
Cipro I.V. (1% or less) **2817**
Cipro (Less than 1%) **2810**
Cipro XR Tablets **2823**
Clinoril Tablets (Less than 1 in 100) **1962**
▲ Combigan Ophthalmic Solution (1% to 5%) **553**
Comvax **1966**
Concerta Extended-Release Tablets **1925**
Copaxone for Injection (At least 2%) **3110**
▲ Coreg Tablets (5%) **1387**
▲ Coreg CR Extended-Release Capsules (2% to 5%) **1393**
Cosopt Sterile Ophthalmic Solution **1969**
Cuprimine Capsules **1986**
Cymbalta Delayed-Release Capsules (Infrequent) **1801**
Dantrium Capsules (Less frequent) **2580**
Daytrana Transdermal Patch **3022**
▲ Depakote ER Tablets (Greater than 1% to less than 5%) **423**
DepoCyt Injection **1136**
▲ Diclofenac Sodium Ophthalmic Solution (Less than or equal to 5%) ⊙ **240**
Diovan HCT Tablets (Greater than 0.2%) **2216**
Doxil Injection (Less than 1%) **2378**
DynaCirc CR Controlled Release Tablets (0.5% to 1%) **1407**
EC-Naprosyn Delayed-Release Tablets (Less than 3%) **2632**
Edex Injection (1%) **2957**
▲ Effexor XR Extended-Release Capsules (4% to 5%) **3195**
▲ Eloxatin for Injection (1% to 6%) **2731**
Enablex Extended-Release Tablets (Greater than or equal to 1%) **2225**
Engerix-B Vaccine **1409**
Erbitux **912**
Estratest Tablets **3043**
Estratest H.S. Tablets **3043**
▲ Evoxac Capsules (1% to 3%) **1013**
Exforge Tablets (Greater than 0.1 % to less than 1%) **2238**
▲ Flolan for Injection (4%) **1426**
FML Ophthalmic Suspension ⊙ **224**
FML Forte Ophthalmic Suspension ⊙ **222**
Focalin XR Capsules **2251**
Frova Tablets (Frequent) **1111**
Gabitril Tablets (Frequent) **973**
Gengraf Capsules (1% to less than 3%) **435**
Genotropin Lyophilized Powder **2547**
▲ Geodon Capsules (3% to 6%) **2520**
▲ Gliadel Wafer (6%) **1076**
Humatrope Vials and Cartridges **1838**
▲ Hycamtin for Injection (5%) **1459**
Imitrex Injection (Frequent) **1465**
Imitrex Nasal Spray (Infrequent) **1470**
▲ Imitrex Tablets (Up to 3%) **1474**
Increlex Injection **3100**
InnoPran XL Extended Release Capsules **1484**
▲ Intron A for Injection (Less than 5%) **2859**
Ionsys Transdermal System (.1% to less than 1%) **2410**
Kaletra (Less than 2%) **452**
Ketek Tablets **2744**
Klonopin (Infrequent) **2639**
▲ Lamictal (2% to 3%) **1488**
Lamisil Tablets (1.1%) **2266**
Lanoxin Injection **1498**
Lanoxin Injection Pediatric **1502**
Lanoxin Tablets **1505**
Levaquin **2416**
Levaquin in 5% Dextrose Injection **2416**
Levitra Tablets (Rare to less than 2%) **2876**
Lexapro Oral Suspension (Infrequent) **1174**
Lexapro Tablets (Infrequent) **1174**
Lidoderm Patch **1114**
▲ Lotemax Ophthalmic Suspension 0.5% (5% to 15%) ⊙ **241**
▲ Lucentis Injection (0% to 14%) **1205**
▲ Lumigan Ophthalmic Solution (3% to 10%) **556**
▲ Lyrica Capsules (1% to 5%) **2527**
Malarone Pediatric Tablets (2%) **1521**
Malarone Tablets (2%) **1521**
Marinol Capsules (Less than 1%) **3163**
Meridia Capsules **475**
Metadate CD Capsules **3146**
Micardis Tablets (More than 0.3%) **852**
Micardis HCT Tablets **854**
▲ Mirapex Tablets (3%) **857**
Mobic Oral Suspension (Less than 2%) **863**
Mobic Tablets (Less than 2%) **863**
MS Contin Tablets (Less frequent) **2585**
Nadolol Tablets **2191**
Naprosyn Suspension (Less than 3%) **2632**
Naprosyn Tablets (Less than 3%) **2632**
Neoral Oral Solution (1% to less than 3%) **2280**
Neoral Soft Gelatin Capsules (1% to less than 3%) **2280**
▲ Neupro Transdermal System (3%) **3149**
Nexium Delayed-Release Capsules (Less than 1%) **645**
Nexium I.V. (Less than 1%) **652**
Nexium Delayed-Release Oral Suspension (Less than 1%) **645**
Norditropin Cartridges (Small number of patients) **2354**
Noroxin Tablets **2069**
Norvir (Less than 2%) **489**
Nutropin for Injection (A small number of patients) **1208**
Nutropin AQ Injection (A small number of patients) **1212**
Nutropin AQ NuSpin Injection (A small number of patients) **1212**
Nutropin AQ Pen (A small number of patients) **1212**
Nutropin AQ Pen Cartridge (A small number of patients) **1212**
Ontak Vials **1079**
Opana Tablets (Less than 1%) **1117**
Opana ER Tablets (Less than 1%) **1121**
OptiPranolol Metipranolol Ophthalmic Solution 0.3% (A small number of patients) ⊙ **245**
Ortho-Cyclen Tablets **2449**
Ortho Evra Transdermal System **2437**
Ortho Tri-Cyclen Tablets **2449**
Ortho Tri-Cyclen Lo Tablets **2458**
OxyContin Tablets (Less than 1%) **2589**
▲ Paxil (2% to 4%) **1535**
▲ Paxil CR Controlled-Release Tablets (2% to 4%) **1544**
PegIntron Powder for Injection (1%) **2903**
Percocet Tablets **1127**
Percodan Tablets **1130**
Photofrin for Injection **708**
Pred Forte Ophthalmic Suspension ⊙ **227**
Premarin Tablets **3221**
Premphase Tablets **3232**
Prempro Tablets **3232**
▲ Prograf Capsules and Injection (3% to 15%) **622**
▲ Prometrium Capsules (100 mg, 200 mg) (Less than 5%) **3047**
Protonix for Delayed-Release Oral Suspension (Less than 1%) **3254**
Protonix Delayed-Release Tablets (Less than 1%) **3254**
Protonix I.V. (Less than 1%) **3257**
Protopic Ointment (0.2% to less than 1%) **628**
Provigil Tablets (1%) **977**
Prozac Weekly Capsules (2%) **1852**
Prozac Pulvules and Liquid (2%) **1852**
Pylera Capsules **714**
▲ Quixin Ophthalmic Solution (1% to 3%) **3184**
▲ Rebif Prefilled Syringe for Injection (7% to 13%) **1107**
Recombivax HB (Less than 1%) **2107**
ReFacto Vials **3269**
ReoPro Vials (0.7%) **1860**
▲ Requip Tablets (Infrequent to 6%) **1561**
▲ Restasis Ophthalmic Emulsion (1% to 5%) **557**
▲ Risperdal Consta Long-Acting Injection (3%) **1753**
▲ Romazicon Injection (1% to 9%) **2646**
Rythmol Tablets (Less than 1% to 2%) **1586**
Salagen Tablets (Less than 1% to 2%) **1082**
Sanctura XR Capsules **557**
Sandimmune (Rare) **2296**
▲ Sandostatin Injection (1% to 4%) **2300**
▲ Simulect for Injection (3% to 10%) **2306**
▲ Soriatane Capsules (1% to 10%) **3062**
Sular Extended Release Tablets (Less than or equal to 1%) **2975**
Sustiva Capsules **930**
Sustiva Tablets **930**
Symbyax Capsules (Frequent) **1871**
Taxotere Injection Concentrate (Rare) **2773**
▲ Temodar Capsules (5%) **2931**
Teveten Tablets (Less than 1%) **515**
Teveten HCT Tablets (Less than 1%) **517**
Tev-Tropin for Injection (Small number of patients) **1187**
Timoptic Sterile Ophthalmic Solution (Less frequent) **2121**
Timoptic in Ocudose (Less frequent) **2124**
Timoptic-XE Sterile Ophthalmic Gel Forming Solution **2125**
▲ Travatan Z Ophthalmic Solution (1% to 4%) **547**
Treximet Tablets (Rare) **1616**
Tricor Tablets **520**
Twinrix Vaccine **1628**
Valtrex Caplets **1635**
Vantas **1737**
Venlafaxine Hydrochloride Tablets (Frequent) **2199**
▲ Vesanoid Capsules (17%) **2660**
Vicoprofen Tablets (Less than 1%) **533**
▲ Visudyne for Injection (10% to 30%) **2332**
▲ Voltaren Ophthalmic Solution (Less than or equal to 5%) **2336**
Wellbutrin Tablets (Infrequent) **1648**
▲ Xeloda Tablets (5%) **2662**
Xyzal Oral Solution **2789**
Xyzal Oral Solution **3155**
Zovirax **1690**
Zyprexa Tablets (2%) **1883**
Zyprexa ZYDIS Orally Disintegrating Tablets (2%) **1883**

Visual disturbances, flashing lights

Cipro XR Tablets **2823**
Taxotere Injection Concentrate (Rare) **2773**
▲ Visudyne for Injection (10% to 30%) **2332**

Visual field defect

▲ Agrylin Capsules (1% to less than 5%) **3017**
▲ Alphagan P Ophthalmic Solution (1% to 4%) **549**
Alrex Ophthalmic Suspension 0.2% ⊙ **236**
Chantix Tablets (Rare) **2511**
Cialis Tablets **1792**
Combigan Ophthalmic Solution (0.1% to 0.2%) **553**
▲ Cosopt Sterile Ophthalmic Solution (1% to 5%) **1969**
Doxil Injection (Less than 1%) **2378**
Effexor XR Extended-Release Capsules (Rare) **3195**
Eloxatin for Injection **2731**
Emsam Transdermal System (Rare) **905**
FML Ophthalmic Ointment ⊙ **223**
FML Ophthalmic Suspension ⊙ **224**
FML Forte Ophthalmic Suspension ⊙ **222**
Gabitril Tablets (Infrequent) **973**
Geodon Capsules (Rare) **2520**
▲ Gliadel Wafer (2% to 5%) **1076**
Intron A for Injection **2859**
Klonopin (Infrequent) **2639**
Lamictal (Rare) **1488**
Lamisil Oral Granules **2264**
Levitra Tablets (Rare) **2876**
Lotemax Ophthalmic Suspension 0.5% ⊙ **241**
Luvox CR Extended-Release Capsules (Infrequent) **1759**
Lyrica Capsules (Greater than or equal to 2%) **2527**
Nexium Delayed-Release Capsules (Less than 1%) **645**
Nexium I.V. (Less than 1%) **652**
Nexium Delayed-Release Oral Suspension (Less than 1%) **645**
Norvir (Less than 2%) **489**
Paxil (Infrequent) **1535**
Paxil CR Controlled-Release Tablets (Infrequent) **1544**
Pred Forte Ophthalmic Suspension ⊙ **227**
Pred Mild Ophthalmic Suspension ⊙ **230**
Pred-G Ophthalmic Suspension ⊙ **228**
ProAmatine Tablets (Rare) **3032**
Prozac Weekly Capsules (Rare) **1852**
Prozac Pulvules and Liquid (Rare) **1852**
▲ Romazicon Injection (1% to 3%) **2646**
Sandostatin LAR Depot **2302**
Targretin Capsules **1084**
Venlafaxine Hydrochloride Tablets (Infrequent) **2199**
▲ Vesanoid Capsules (3%) **2660**
▲ Visudyne for Injection (10% to 30%) **2332**
Zomig Tablets (Rare) **694**
Zomig Nasal Spray (Rare) **689**
Zomig-ZMT Tablets (Rare) **694**
Zonegran Capsules (Infrequent) **1089**
Zyrtec Chewable Tablets (Less than 2%) **1920**
Zyrtec Syrup (Less than 2%) **1920**
Zyrtec Tablets (Less than 2%) **1920**
Zyrtec-D 12 Hour Extended Release Tablets (Less than 2%) **1923**

Visual impairment

Abelcet Injection **1134**
Ortho-Cyclen/Ortho Tri-Cyclen (Rare) **2449**
Ortho Tri-Cyclen Lo Tablets **2458**
Salagen Tablets **1082**

Vital signs, fluctuations of

Remeron Tablets **2924**
RemeronSolTab Tablets **2927**

Vitamin B12 deficiency

Aricept Tablets (Infrequent) **1062**
Aricept ODT Tablets (Infrequent) **1062**
Nexium Delayed-Release Capsules (Less than 1%) **645**
Nexium I.V. (Less than 1%) **652**
Nexium Delayed-Release Oral Suspension (Less than 1%) **645**

Vitiligo

Finacea Gel (Rare) **1742**
▲ Intron A for Injection (Less than 5%) **2859**
Proleukin for Injection **2287**

Vitreous detachment

▲ Alphagan P Ophthalmic Solution (1% to 4%) **549**
Combigan Ophthalmic Solution (0.1% to 0.2%) **553**
▲ Cosopt Sterile Ophthalmic Solution (1% to 5%) **1969**
Evoxac Capsules (Less than 1%) **1013**
▲ Lucentis Injection (7% to 22%) **1205**
▲ Nevanac Ophthalmic Suspension 0.1% (1% to 5%) ⊙ **205**

Vitreous disorder, unspecified

Combigan Ophthalmic Solution (0.1% to 0.2%) **553**

Vitreous floaters

▲ Alphagan P Ophthalmic Solution (1% to 4%) **549**
Celebrex Capsules (Greater than or equal to 0.1% to less than 1%) **2979**
Chantix Tablets (Rare) **2511**
Combigan Ophthalmic Solution (0.1% to 0.2%) **553**
Iquix Ophthalmic Solution (Less than 1%) **3183**
▲ Lucentis Injection (3% to 32%) **1205**
Miacalcin Nasal Spray (Less than 1%) **2274**
Mirapex Tablets **857**
Sular Extended Release Tablets (Less than or equal to 1%) **2975**
Triesence Injectable Suspension (2%) ⊙ **209**

Voice, deepening of

Delatestryl Injection **1730**
Estratest Tablets **3043**
Estratest H.S. Tablets **3043**

Voice, hoarseness

Estratest Tablets **3043**
Estratest H.S. Tablets **3043**

Voice, loss of

(*see under* Aphonia)

Voice alteration

Accutane Capsules **2607**
Actiq (Less than 1%) **959**
▲ Avastin IV (6% to 9%) **1192**
▲ Avinza Capsules (Less than 5%) **1772**
▲ Azmacort Inhalation Aerosol (1% to 3%) **407**
Brovana Inhalation Solution (Less than 2%) **2990**
▲ CellCept Capsules (3% to less than 20%) **2622**
▲ CellCept Intravenous (3% to less than 20%) **2622**
▲ CellCept Oral Suspension (3% to less than 20%) **2622**
▲ CellCept Tablets (3% to less than 20%) **2622**
Copaxone for Injection (Infrequent) **3110**
Doxil Injection (Less than 1%) **2378**
Effexor XR Extended-Release Capsules (Infrequent) **3195**

Emend Capsules (Greater than 0.5%) **1992**
Emend for Injection (Greater than 0.5%) **1999**
Flonase Nasal Spray **1431**
Gabitril Tablets (Infrequent) **973**
Imitrex Injection **1465**
Imitrex Nasal Spray (Rare) **1470**
Imitrex Tablets (Rare) **1474**
Invanz for Injection (Greater than 0.1%) **2029**
▲ Mirapex Tablets (Greater than or equal to 1%) **857**
OxyContin Tablets (Less than 1%) **2589**
Paxil (Infrequent) **1535**
Paxil CR Controlled-Release Tablets (Infrequent) **1544**
▲ Prograf Capsules and Injection (3% to 15%) **622**
Protonix for Delayed-Release Oral Suspension (Less than 1%) **3254**
Protonix Delayed-Release Tablets (Less than 1%) **3254**
Protonix I.V. (Less than 1%) **3257**
▲ Pulmicort Flexhaler (Greater than or equal to 1% to 3%) **654**
▲ Pulmozyme Inhalation Solution (12% to 18%) **1217**
Salagen Tablets (Less than 1% to 2%) **1082**
Symbyax Capsules (Infrequent) **1871**
Venlafaxine Hydrochloride Tablets (Infrequent) **2199**
Zomig Tablets (Rare) **694**
Zomig Nasal Spray (Infrequent) **689**
Zomig-ZMT Tablets (Rare) **694**
Zyprexa Tablets (Infrequent) **1883**
Zyprexa ZYDIS Orally Disintegrating Tablets (Infrequent) **1883**

Voice disorders

Exubera Inhalation Powder (0.1% to 1.3%) **2515**

Vomiting

▲ Abelcet Injection (3% to 8%) **1134**
▲ Abilify Injection (3% to 11%) **881**
▲ Abilify Injection (4% to 11%) **2466**
▲ Abilify Oral Solution (3% to 11%) **881**
▲ Abilify Oral Solution (4% to 11%) **2466**
▲ Abilify Discmelt Orally Disintegrating Tablets (3% to 11%) **881**
▲ Abilify Discmelt Orally Disintegrating Tablets (4% to 11%) **2466**
▲ Abilify Tablets (3% to 11%) **881**
▲ Abilify Tablets (4% to 11%) **2466**
Accolate Tablets (1.5%) **669**
Accutane Capsules **2607**
Aceon Tablets (2 mg, 4 mg, 8 mg) (1.5%) **3038**
▲ Acetadote Injection (9% to 12%) **1001**
▲ Aciphex Tablets (3.6%) **1053**
▲ Actimmune (13%) **1743**
▲ Actiq (6% to 15%) **959**
Activase I.V. **1188**
Activella Tablets **2347**
Actonel Tablets (0.2% to 1%) **2568**
Actonel with Calcium Tablets (1.9% to 2.5%) **2574**
Aczone Gel 5% **3296**
▲ Adderall XR Capsules (7%) **3012**
Advair Diskus 100/50 **1276**
▲ Advair Diskus 250/50 (Greater than or equal to 3% to 6%) **1276**
▲ Advair Diskus 500/50 (Greater than or equal to 3%) **1276**
▲ Advair HFA 45/21 Inhalation Aerosol (3% to 5%) **1288**
▲ Advair HFA 115/21 Inhalation Aerosol (3% to 5%) **1288**
▲ Advair HFA 230/21 Inhalation Aerosol (3% to 5%) **1288**
▲ Advicor Tablets (3%) **402**
▲ Aerobid/Aerobid-M (25%) **1153**
▲ Aggrenox Capsules (8.4%) **819**
▲ Agrylin Capsules (9.7%) **3017**
▲ Albenza Tablets (3.7% to 6.2%) **1297**
Albutein 5% **1707**
Albutein 25% **1708**
Aldara Cream, 5% (1%) **1699**
▲ Alferon N Injection (3% to 29%) **1726**
▲ Alimta for Injection (Up to 58%) **1786**
Alinia for Oral Suspension (1.1%) **2677**
Alinia Tablets (1.1%) **2677**
▲ Allegra Oral Solution (4.2% to 12%) **2684**
▲ Allegra Tablets (4.2% to 12%) **2684**
Alphanate **1709**
Ambien Tablets (Infrequent) **2692**
Ambien CR Tablets (1%) **2696**
▲ AmBisome for Injection (22.4% to 31.8%) **606**
Amerge Tablets (Frequent) **1301**
Aminohippurate Sodium "PAH" Injection **1950**
▲ Amitiza Capsules (0% to 3%) **3082**
Amoxil Capsules **1305**
Amoxil Chewable Tablets **1305**
Amoxil Pediatric Drops for Oral Suspension **1305**
Amoxil Powder for Oral Suspension **1305**
Amoxil Tablets **1305**
Amrix Capsules **966**
▲ Anaprox Tablets (Less than 1% to 10%) **2632**
▲ Anaprox DS Tablets (Less than 1% to 10%) **2632**
Angeliq Tablets **751**
▲ Angiomax for Injection (6%) **1933**
▲ Aptivus Capsules (5.5% to 5.9%) **823**
▲ Aptivus Oral Solution (5.5% to 5.9%) **823**
▲ Aranesp for Injection (14%) **564**
▲ Argatroban Injection (4.2% to 6.3%) **1308**
▲ Aricept Tablets (8%) **1062**
▲ Aricept ODT Tablets (8%) **1062**
▲ Arimidex Tablets (8% to 13%) **672**
▲ Arixtra Injection (0.6% to 5.9%) **1313**
▲ Arranon Injection (0% to 22%) **1319**
▲ Asacol Delayed-Release Tablets (5%) **2579**
Asmanex Twisthaler (1% to less than 3%) **2797**
Atacand Tablets (More than 1%) **639**
Atacand HCT (0.5% or greater) **642**
Atripla Tablets (2%) **938**
Atrovent HFA Inhalation Aerosol **839**
Atrovent Nasal Spray 0.03% **834**
Atrovent Nasal Spray 0.06% **836**
Attenuvax **1951**
Augmentin (1%) **1323**
Augmentin Tablets (1%) **1327**
Augmentin XR Extended Release Tablets **1333**
Augmentin ES-600 Powder for Oral Suspension (2.2%) **1329**
▲ Avalide Tablets (3%) **892**
▲ Avalide Tablets (3%) **2713**
▲ Avandamet Tablets (16%) **1336**
Avandaryl Tablets (Less than 1%) **1344**
Avandia Tablets **1351**
Avapro Tablets (1% or greater) **897**
Avapro Tablets (1% or greater) **2718**
▲ Avastin IV (5.5% to 52%) **1192**
Avelox (Greater than or equal to 0.1% to less than 2%) **2803**
▲ Avinza Capsules (Greater than 10%) **1772**
Axert Tablets (Infrequent) **2431**
▲ Axid Capsules (1.2% to 3.6%) **1364**
▲ Azilect Tablets (7%) **3106**
▲ Azmacort Inhalation Aerosol (1% to 3%) **407**
Azor Tablets **1005**
Baraclude (Less than 1%) **900**
Bayer Aspirin (2.1%) **750**
BeneFIX Vials (1.5%) **3191**
Benicar Tablets **1009**
Benicar HCT Tablets (Rare) **1010**
Bentyl Capsules **703**
Bentyl Injection **703**
Bentyl Syrup **703**
Bentyl Tablets **703**
Betaseron for SC Injection **756**
▲ Bexxar (1% to 15%) **1371**
▲ Biaxin/Biaxin XL (6%) **411**
Bicillin C-R Injectable Suspension **1775**
Bicillin L-A Injection **1777**
Boniva Injection (2.7%) **2614**
Boniva Tablets (2.7%) **2618**
▲ Boostrix (3% to 26%) **1377**
Brovana Inhalation Solution **2990**
▲ Busulfex Injection (43% to 95%) **2477**
▲ Byetta Injection (13%) **600**
Bystolic Tablets **1155**
Calcijex Injection **419**
Campath Ampules **761**
Campral Tablets **1158**
▲ Cancidas for Injection (7.4% to 16.7%) **1953**
Captopril Tablets (About 0.5% to 2%) **2182**
Carafate Suspension (Less than 0.5%) **706**
Carafate Tablets (Less than 0.5%) **707**
Carbatrol Capsules (Among most frequent) **3019**
▲ Cardene I.V. (4.9%) **1093**
▲ Catapres Tablets (About 5 in 100 patients) **841**
Catapres-TTS (0.5% or less) **842**
Ceftin (2.6%) **1380**
▲ Celebrex Capsules (0.1% to 6%) **2979**
▲ Celexa (1% to 4%) **1160**
▲ CellCept Capsules (3% to 33.9%) **2622**
▲ CellCept Intravenous (3% to 33.9%) **2622**
▲ CellCept Oral Suspension (3% to 33.9%) **2622**
▲ CellCept Tablets (3% to 33.9%) **2622**
▲ Cerezyme for Injection (Approximately 6.5%) **1238**
Cervidil Vaginal Insert (Less than 1%) **1165**
▲ Chantix Tablets (1% to greater than 5%) **2511**
▲ Chemet Capsules (12% to 20.9%) **2484**
Cialis Tablets (Less than 2%) **1792**
▲ Cipro I.V. (1% to 4.8%) **2817**
▲ Cipro (1% to 4.8%) **2810**
Cipro XR Tablets (1% to 2%) **2823**
▲ Clarinex Syrup (6.1%) **2828**
▲ Cleviprex (3.2%) **1936**
Climara Transdermal System **763**
Climara Pro Transdermal System **768**
Clinoril Tablets (Greater than 1%) **1962**
▲ Clolar for Intravenous Infusion (83%) **1239**
▲ Clorpres Tablets (About 5%) **2185**
Combigan Ophthalmic Solution **553**
Combivent Inhalation Aerosol (Less than 2%) **845**
▲ Combivir Tablets (13%) **1384**
▲ Comtan Tablets (4%) **2208**
Comvax (1% to 2.5%) **1966**
Concerta Extended-Release Tablets (1.7% to 2.8%) **1925**
▲ Copaxone for Injection (6%) **3110**
▲ Coreg Tablets (1% to 6%) **1387**
▲ Coreg CR Extended-Release Capsules (1% to 6%) **1393**
Cosmegen for Injection (Common) **2485**
▲ Cosopt Sterile Ophthalmic Solution (1% to 5%) **1969**
Cozaar Tablets (Less than 1%) **1973**
Creon 5 Capsules (Among most frequent) **3041**
Creon 10 Capsules (Among most frequent) **3042**
Creon 20 Capsules (Among most frequent) **3042**
▲ Crinone 8% Gel (5%) **992**
▲ Crixivan Capsules (8.4%) **1979**
▲ Cubicin for Injection (3.2% to 11.7%) **995**
▲ Cuprimine Capsules (17%) **1986**
Cyanokit 5g Antidote **1021**
▲ Cymbalta Delayed-Release Capsules (5% to 6%) **1801**
▲ Dacogen Injection (25%) **1066**
Dantrium Capsules (Rare) **2580**
Dapsone Tablets USP **1746**
Daraprim Tablets **1400**
▲ Daytrana Transdermal Patch (10%) **3022**
Demadex Injection **2630**
Demadex Tablets **2630**
Demser Capsules (Infrequent) **1989**
▲ Depakote ER Tablets (5% to 27%) **423**
▲ DepoCyt Injection (3% to 44%) **1136**
▲ DepoDur Injection (Greater than 10%) **1095**
Diclofenac Sodium Ophthalmic Solution ⊙ **240**
Diovan Tablets (Greater than 0.2%) **2212**
Diovan HCT Tablets (Greater than 0.2%) **2216**
Divigel **3167**
Donnatal Extentabs **2507**
▲ Doxil Injection (7.8% to 32.6%) **2378**
Duetact Tablets (Less than 1%) **3085**
▲ Duragesic Transdermal System (Greater than 10% to 33%) **2405**
Dyazide Capsules **1405**
DynaCirc CR Controlled Release Tablets (0.5% to 1%) **1407**
Dyrenium Capsules (Rare) **3189**
▲ EC-Naprosyn Delayed-Release Tablets (Less than 1% to 10%) **2632**
Edecrin **698**
E.E.S. (Among most frequent) **433**
▲ Effexor XR Extended-Release Capsules (3% to 5%) **3195**
Eldepryl Capsules **3052**
▲ Elidel Cream 1% (0.6% to 6.6%) **2221**
▲ Elitek (50%) **2729**
Elmiron Capsules (Less than or equal to 1%) **2435**
▲ Eloxatin for Injection (4% to 64%) **2731**
Elspar for Injection **1990**
▲ Emend Capsules (7.5%) **1992**
▲ Emend for Injection (7.5%) **1999**
Emsam Transdermal System (Frequent) **905**
▲ Emtriva Capsules (2% to 23%) **1246**
▲ Emtriva Oral Solution (2% to 23%) **1246**
Enablex Extended-Release Tablets (Greater than or equal to 1%) **2225**
▲ Enbrel for Injection (3% to 5%) **569**
Engerix-B Vaccine (Less than 1%) **1409**
Enjuvia Tablets **1029**
EpiPen **1024**
▲ Epivir (13%) **1412**
▲ Epivir-HBV (15%) **1417**
▲ Epogen for Injection (0.26% to 29%) **576**
▲ Equetro Extended-Release Capsules (18%) **3174**
▲ Erbitux (2% to 37%) **912**
EryPed (Among most frequent) **431**
Estratest Tablets **3043**
Estratest H.S. Tablets **3043**
▲ Evista Tablets (3.4% to 4.8%) **1810**
▲ Evoxac Capsules (4.6%) **1013**
▲ Exelon Capsules (17% to 31%) **2229**
▲ Exelon Oral Solution (17% to 31%) **2229**
▲ Exelon Patch (6% to 19%) **2233**
Exforge Tablets (Greater than or equal to 0.2%) **2238**
▲ Exjade Tablets (10.1%) **2244**
▲ Fabrazyme for Intravenous Infusion (24%) **1241**
Fansidar Tablets **2636**
▲ Faslodex Injection (13%) **682**
▲ Femara Tablets (0.2% to 7%) **2246**
▲ Fentora Tablets (0% to 37%) **968**
Ferralet 90 Tablets **2175**
Flebogamma 5% DIF **1718**
▲ Flector Patch (3%) **561**
Fleet Phospho-soda EZ-PREP **1147**
Fleet Prep Kits **1149**
▲ Flolan for Injection (32% to 67%) **1426**
Flomax Capsules (Infrequent) **848**
▲ Flonase Nasal Spray (2.6% to 4.8%) **1431**
▲ Flovent Diskus 50 mcg (4% to 9%) **1435**
Flovent HFA **1440**
Fluarix Vaccine (1.4%) **1446**
Flulaval Injection Vaccine **1448**
Flumadine (1.7%) **1167**
FluMist Vaccine **1945**
Fluorescite Injection ⊙ **203**
Follistim AQ Cartridge **2844**
Fortaz (1 in 500 patients) **1450**
▲ Forteo for Injection (3%) **1816**
Fosamax (0.2% to 1%) **2005**
Fosamax Plus D Tablets (0.2% to 1%) **2013**
▲ Fosrenol Chewable Tablets (9% to 26%) **3027**
Fosteum Capsules **2963**
Frova Tablets (Frequent) **1111**
Furosemide Tablets **2186**
▲ Gabitril Tablets (7%) **973**
▲ Gammagard Liquid (1.21% to 14.8%) **730**
Gammagard S/D (Occasional) **734**
▲ Gamunex (13% to 21%) **3094**
Gantrisin Pediatric Suspension **2638**
Gardasil Injection (2.4%) **2019**
▲ Gemzar for Injection (58% to 71%) **1820**
▲ Gengraf Capsules (2% to 10%) **435**
Genotropin Lyophilized Powder **2547**
▲ Geodon (5%) **2520**
▲ Gleevec Tablets (22.5% to 58%) **2255**
▲ Gliadel Wafer (8% to 21%) **1076**
Glucagon for Injection Vials and Emergency Kit (Occasional) **1827**
Gris-PEG Tablets (Occasional) **2507**
Havrix Injection Vaccine (Less than 1%) **1454**
Hepsera Tablets **1253**
▲ Herceptin I.V. (8% to 23%) **1199**
▲ Hexalen Capsules (33%) **1078**
Human Albumin Grifols 25% **1706**
Humatrope Vials and Cartridges **1838**
▲ Humira Injection (Less than 5%) **442**
Hycamtin Capsules (19% to 21%) **1456**
▲ Hycamtin for Injection (Less than 1% to 58%) **1459**
▲ Imitrex Injection (4%) **1465**
▲ Imitrex Nasal Spray (11% to 13.5%) **1470**
Imitrex Tablets (Greater than 1%) **1474**
▲ Increlex Injection (Greater than or equal to 5%) **3100**
▲ Indapamide Tablets (Less than 5%) **2188**
▲ Indocin I.V. (1% to 3%) **2489**
▲ Infanrix Vaccine (3.3% to 6.6.%) **1479**
InnoPran XL Extended Release Capsules **1484**
Intelence Tablets (2.3%) **3119**
Intravenous Sodium Diuril **2490**
▲ Intron A for Injection (1% to 66%) **2859**
▲ Invanz for Injection (3.7% to 10.2%) **2029**
▲ Ionsys Transdermal System (12%) **2410**
Isentress Tablets (1% to less than 2%) **2036**
▲ Ixempra Kit for Injection (29%) **915**

▲ Janumet Tablets (1.1% to greater than 5%) 2041
▲ Kaletra (2% to 21%) 452
▲ Keppra Oral Solution (1% to 15%) 3131
▲ Keppra Tablets (1% to 15%) 3131
Ketek Tablets (2.4% to 2.9%) 2744
K-Phos Original (Sodium Free) Tablets 814
K-Phos Neutral Tablets 813
Kristalose for Oral Solution 1004
▲ Lamictal (5% to 20%) 1488
▲ Lamisil Oral Granules (5%) 2264
Lamisil Tablets 2266
Lanoxin Injection (Common) 1498
Lanoxin Injection Pediatric 1502
Lanoxin Tablets (Common) 1505
Lescol Capsules 2268
Lescol XL Tablets 2268
Leukeran Tablets (Infrequent) 1508
▲ Leukine (46% to 85%) 774
▲ Leustatin Injection (13%) 2384
Levaquin (2%) 2416
Levaquin in 5% Dextrose Injection (2%) 2416
Levitra Tablets (Less than 2%) 2876
Levothroid Tablets 1170
Levoxyl Tablets 1780
▲ Lexapro Oral Suspension (3%) 1174
▲ Lexapro Tablets (3%) 1174
▲ Lexiva Oral Suspension (Less than or equal to 1% to 8%) 1510
▲ Lexiva Tablets (Less than or equal to 1% to 8%) 1510
Lialda Tablets (Infrequent) 3029
Lidoderm Patch 1114
Lipitor Tablets (Less than 2%) 2501
Lortab 5/500 Tablets (Among most frequent) 3143
Lortab 7.5/500 Tablets (Among most frequent) 3144
Lortab 10/500 Tablets (Among most frequent) 3144
Lovaza Capsules 1520
▲ Lunesta Tablets (0% to 3%) 2994
▲ Lupron Depot 3.75 mg (13%) 462
▲ Lupron Depot–3 Month 11.25 mg (13%) 462
Lupron Depot-PED 7.5 mg, 11.25 mg and 15 mg (Less than 2%) 471
▲ Luvox CR Extended-Release Capsules (6%) 1759
Lybrel Tablets 3204
▲ Lyrica Capsules (1% to 3%) 2527
▲ Malarone Pediatric Tablets (Less than 1% to 19%) 1521
▲ Malarone Tablets (Less than 1% to 19%) 1521
▲ Marinol Capsules (3% to 10%) 3163
Mavik Tablets (0.3% to 1%) 472
Maxair Autohaler 1705
Maxalt Tablets (Frequent) 2056
Maxalt-MLT Orally Disintegrating Tablets (Frequent) 2056
▲ Megace ES Oral Suspension (0% to 6%) 2499
▲ Mepron Suspension (1.3% to 22%) 1526
Meridia Capsules (1.5%) 475
▲ Merrem I.V. (0.8% to 3.6%) 684
Meruvax II 2061
Mevacor Tablets (0.5% to 1%) 2063
▲ Miacalcin Injection (About 10%) 2273
Miacalcin Nasal Spray (Less than 1% to 1.8%) 2274
Micardis Tablets (More than 0.3%) 852
Micardis HCT Tablets (Less than 2%) 854
Mirapex Tablets (2% or more) 857
Mircette Tablets 1034
M-M-R II 2054
Mobic Oral Suspension (0.6% to 2.6%) 863
Mobic Tablets (0.6% to 2.6%) 863
▲ MoviPrep Oral Solution (7.8%) 2679
Moxatag Tablets (0.7%) 2165
MS Contin Tablets (Among most frequent) 2585
Mustargen for Injection 2492
▲ Mycamine for Injection (6.5% to 66.1%) 616
▲ Myfortic Tablets (3% to 23%) 2276
Myleran Tablets 1530
▲ Mylotarg for Injection (53% to 66%) 3212
Nadolol Tablets (1 to 5 of 1000 patients) 2191
Nalfon Capsules (2.6%) 2508
▲ Namenda (3%) 1180
▲ Naprosyn Suspension (Less than 1% to 10%) 2632
▲ Naprosyn Tablets (Less than 1% to 10%) 2632
Nasacort AQ Nasal Spray 2765
▲ Nasonex Nasal Spray (1% to 5%) 2883
▲ Natrecor for Injection (1% to 4%) 2977
Nembutal Sodium Solution, USP (Less than 1%) 2494
▲ Neoral Oral Solution (2% to 10%) 2280
▲ Neoral Soft Gelatin Capsules (2% to 10%) 2280
▲ Neulasta Injection (15% to 72%) 587
▲ Neupogen for Injection (7% to 57%) 589
▲ Neupro Transdermal System (1% to 13%) 3149
▲ Nevanac Ophthalmic Suspension 0.1% (1% to 4%) ⊙ 205
Nexium Delayed-Release Capsules (Less than 1%) 645
Nexium I.V. (Less than 1%) 652
Nexium Delayed-Release Oral Suspension (Less than 1%) 645
Nimotop Capsules (Less than 1%) 790
Nitrolingual Pumpspray (Uncommon) 2965
Norditropin Cartridges (Small number of patients) 2354
Noroxin Tablets (0.3% to 1%) 2069
▲ Norvir (13.7% to 17.4%) 489
▲ Novantrone for Injection Concentrate (9% to 72%) 1100
NovoSeven (1%) 2367
NovoSeven RT (1%) 2370
▲ Noxafil Oral Suspension (4% to 29%) 2889
Nutropin for Injection (A small number of patients) 1208
Nutropin AQ Injection (A small number of patients) 1212
Nutropin AQ NuSpin Injection (A small number of patients) 1212
Nutropin AQ Pen (A small number of patients) 1212
Nutropin AQ Pen Cartridge (A small number of patients) 1212
NuvaRing 2897
Omnicef Capsules (0.7%) 497
Omnicef for Oral Suspension (1%) 497
▲ Ontak Vials (64%) 1079
▲ Opana Tablets (6.8%) 1117
▲ Opana ER Tablets (0% to 15.6%) 1121
Ortho-Cyclen Tablets 2449
Ortho Evra Transdermal System (1% to 2.4%) 2437
Ortho Tri-Cyclen Tablets 2449
Ortho Tri-Cyclen Lo Tablets 2458
▲ Orthoclone OKT3 Sterile Solution (19%) 2387
▲ OsmoPrep Tablets (4% to 10%) 2680
▲ OxyContin Tablets (Less than 1% to 12%) 2589
OxyIR Capsules (Among most frequent) 2593
Paser Granules (Among most common) 1747
▲ Paxil (1% to 3%) 1535
▲ Paxil CR Controlled-Release Tablets (1% to 3%) 1544
Pediarix Vaccine 1552
▲ PegIntron Powder for Injection (7%) 2903
Pentacel 2792
Pentasa Capsules (1.5%) 3030
Pepcid Tablets (Infrequent) 2075
Percocet Tablets (Among most frequent) 1127
Percodan Tablets (Among most frequent) 1130
Perforomist Inhalation Solution (2.4%) 1025
Persantine Tablets 869
Phenytek Capsules 2192
PhosLo GelCaps 1184
▲ Photofrin for Injection (17% to 34%) 708
▲ Plan B Tablets (5.6%) 1044
Plavix Tablets (1% to 2.5%) 926
Plavix Tablets (1% to 2.5%) 2767
Pletal Tablets (2% or greater) 2481
Pneumovax 23 2078
▲ PrandiMet Tablets (Greater than 5%) 2967
▲ Prandin Tablets (2% to 3%) 2971
Premarin Intravenous 3217
Premarin Tablets 3221
Premarin Vaginal Cream 3228
Premphase Tablets 3232
Prempro Tablets 3232
▲ Prevnar (4.9% to 16.8%) 3241
Primaxin I.M. (0.3%) 2080
Primaxin I.V. (Up to 1.5%) 2083
Prinivil Tablets (0.3% to 1%) 2087
Prinzide Tablets (1.4%) 2092
▲ Pristiq Extended-Release Tablets (2% to 9%) 3247
▲ Procrit for Injection (0.26% to 29%) 2391
Profilnine SD Solvent Detergent 1721
Proglycem Capsules (Frequent) 1185
Proglycem Suspension (Frequent) 1185
▲ Prograf Capsules and Injection (14% to 29%) 622
▲ Proleukin for Injection (Less than 1% to 50%) 2287
▲ Prometrium Capsules (100 mg, 200 mg) (5% to 8%) 3047
ProQuad (Greater than or equal to 0.2% to less than 1%) 2099
Protonix for Delayed-Release Oral Suspension (2%) 3254
Protonix Delayed-Release Tablets (2%) 3254
Protonix I.V. (Greater than 1%) 3257
▲ Protopic Ointment (1% to 5%) 628
▲ Proventil HFA Inhalation Aerosol (7%) 2914
Provigil Tablets (Greater than or equal to 1%) 977
▲ Prozac Weekly Capsules (Infrequent to 3%) 1852
▲ Prozac Pulvules and Liquid (3%) 1852
▲ Pulmicort Flexhaler (Greater than or equal to 1% to 3%) 654
Pylera Capsules 714
▲ Rebetol (9% to 42%) 2917
Reclast Injection (2%) 2291
Recombivax HB (Less to greater than 1%) 2107
ReFacto Vials 3269
Relenza Inhalation Powder (1% to 2%) 1556
Remeron Tablets (Frequent) 2924
RemeronSolTab Tablets (Frequent) 2927
▲ ReoPro Vials (11.4%) 1860
▲ Requip Tablets (7% to 12%) 1561
Requip XL Tablets 1568
▲ Retrovir Capsules (4.8% to 25%) 1574
▲ Retrovir IV Infusion (6% to 25%) 1579
▲ Retrovir (4.8% to 25%) 1574
▲ Reyataz Capsules (3% to 8%) 3299
▲ Rilutek Tablets (4.2% to 4.5%) 2771
Risperdal Consta Long-Acting Injection (Frequent) 1753
▲ Rituxan I.V. (1% to 10%) 1223
Rocaltrol Capsules 1150
Rocaltrol Oral Solution 1150
Rocephin Injectable Vials, ADD-Vantage, Galaxy, Bulk (Less than 1%) 2642
▲ Romazicon Injection (11%) 2646
▲ Rotarix Oral Suspension (8% to 13%) 1582
▲ RotaTeq (2.9% to 15.2%) 2110
▲ Rythmol Tablets (3% to 11%) 1586
▲ Rythmol SR Capsules (1% to 6%) 1590
St. Joseph 81 mg Aspirin Chewable and Enteric Coated Tablets 1903
▲ Salagen Tablets (Less than 1% to 4%) 1082
▲ Sandimmune (2% to 10%) 2296
▲ Sandostatin Injection (Less than 10% to 35%) 2300
Sandostatin LAR Depot (6.5% to 21%) 2302
Seasonique Tablets 1046
▲ Sensipar Tablets (27%) 594
▲ Serevent Diskus (3%) 1594
▲ Simulect for Injection (Greater than or equal to 10%) 2306
Singulair 2114
Skelaxin Tablets (Most frequent) 1784
Soma Tablets 1931
▲ Somatuline Depot Injection (Greater than 5% to 7%) 3102
Soriatane Capsules 3062
▲ Spiriva HandiHaler (1% to 4%) 870
▲ Stalevo Tablets (4%) 2309
▲ Strattera Capsules (0.2% to 11%) 1864
Stromectol Tablets (0.9%) 2120
▲ Suboxone Tablets (5% to 7.5%) 2601
▲ Subutex Tablets (5% to 7.8%) 2601
Suprax for Oral Suspension (Less than 2%) 1891
Suprax Tablets (Less than 2%) 1891
▲ Sustiva Capsules (3% to 16%) 930
▲ Sustiva Tablets (3% to 16%) 930
▲ Sutent Capsules (2% to 37%) 2540
Symbicort 80/4.5 Inhalation Aerosol (1.4%) 659
▲ Symbicort 160/4.5 Inhalation Aerosol (3.2%) 659
Symbyax Capsules (Infrequent) 1871
Synagis Intramuscular Solution (More than 1%) 1948
Tabloid Tablets (Less frequent) 1601
▲ Tamiflu Capsules (2% to 15%) 2649
▲ Tamiflu Oral Suspension (2% to 15%) 2649
▲ Tarceva Tablets (Less than 1% to 42%) 1228
▲ Targretin Capsules (3.6% to 13.2%) 1084
▲ Tasigna Capsules (Greater than 10%) 2316
▲ Taxotere Injection Concentrate (0.6% to 56.2%) 2773
▲ Temodar Capsules (3% to 51%) 2931
Teveten Tablets (Less than 1%) 515
Teveten HCT Tablets (Less than 1%) 517
Tev-Tropin for Injection (Small number of patients) 1187
Thioridazine Hydrochloride Tablets 2195
Thiothixene Capsules 2197
Thyrogen for Injection (2.9%) 1244
▲ Tice BCG (3%) 2936
Timentin ADD-Vantage 1606
Timentin Injection Galaxy Container 1609
Timentin IV Infusion 1603
Timentin Pharmacy Bulk Package 1613
Timoptic Sterile Ophthalmic Solution 2121
Timoptic in Ocudose 2124
Timoptic-XE Sterile Ophthalmic Gel Forming Solution 2125
TNKase 1233
Toprol-XL Tablets 666
▲ Torisel Injection (2% to 19%) 3272
Tracleer Tablets 3289
Transderm Scōp Transdermal Therapeutic System (Few patients) 2206
▲ Trasylol Injection (3%) 799
▲ Treanda for Injection (Less than 1% to 16%) 983
Treximet Tablets (Infrequent) 1616
Tricor Tablets 520
▲ Trisenox Injection (58%) 986
▲ Trizivir Tablets (12% to 30%) 1622
Truvada Tablets (2%) 1262
Tussionex Pennkinetic Extended-Release Suspension 3154
Twinrix Vaccine (0% to 1%) 1628
▲ Tygacil for Injection (19.5% to 20%) 3276
▲ Tykerb Tablets (0% to 26%) 1631
Tylenol with Codeine Tablets 2427
▲ Tyzeka Tablets (7%) 2328
▲ Ultane Liquid for Inhalation (18%) 524
▲ Ultram ER Extended-Release Tablets (5% to 9.4%) 2428
Uniphyl Tablets 2595
Urocit-K Tablets (Some patients) 2176
Uroqid-Acid No. 2 Tablets 814
Urso 250 Tablets 720
Urso Forte Tablets 720
▲ Valcyte Tablets (16% to 21%) 2654
Valstar Sterile Solution for Intravesical Instillation (2%) 1735
▲ Valtrex Caplets (Less than 1% to 6%) 1635
Vantas 1737
▲ Vaprisol (5% to 7%) 632
▲ Vaqta (1% to 4%) 2130
Varivax (Greater than or equal to 1%) 2133
▲ Vectibix (2% to 19%) 597
▲ Velcade for Injection (3% to 35%) 2168
▲ Venlafaxine Hydrochloride Tablets (3.4% to 7.9%) 2199
▲ Vesanoid Capsules (57%) 2660
VESIcare Tablets (0.2% to 1.1%) 636
Viadur Implant (Rare) 802
Vicodin Tablets (Among most frequent) 529
Vicodin ES Tablets (Among most frequent) 530
Vicodin HP Tablets (Among most frequent) 531
▲ Vicoprofen Tablets (3% to 9%) 533
Viramune Oral Suspension 873
Viramune Tablets 873
▲ Viread Tablets (2% to 7%) 1268
▲ Vivitrol (10% to 14%) 988
▲ Voltaren Ophthalmic Solution (Less than or equal to 3%) 2336
▲ Voltaren Tablets (1% to 10%) 2334
▲ Voltaren-XR Tablets (1% to 10%) 2337
Vytorin 10/10 Tablets 2149
Vytorin 10/10 Tablets 2939
Vytorin 10/20 Tablets 2149
Vytorin 10/20 Tablets 2939
Vytorin 10/40 Tablets 2149
Vytorin 10/40 Tablets 2939
Vytorin 10/80 Tablets 2149
Vytorin 10/80 Tablets 2939
▲ Vyvanse Capsules (9%) 3033
▲ Wellbutrin Tablets (22.9%) 1648
▲ Wellbutrin SR Sustained-Release Tablets (2% to 4%) 1653
▲ Wellbutrin XL Extended-Release Tablets (2% to 4%) 1659
WinRho SDF 741

▲ Xeloda Tablets (4% to 27%) 2662
▲ Xenical Capsules (3.8%) 2672
Xifaxan Tablets (2.2%) 2682
Xopenex Inhalation Solution 3001
Xopenex Inhalation Solution Concentrate 3005
Xopenex HFA Inhalation Aerosol 3009
▲ Xyntha Vials (5%) 3280
▲ Xyrem Oral Solution (1% to 22.9%) 1766
Yaz Tablets (Greater than 1%) 805
Zantac 25 EFFERdose Tablets 1670
Zantac Injection 1666
Zantac Injection Pharmacy Bulk Package (Frequent) 1668
Zantac Injection Premixed 1666
Zantac 1670
▲ Zemplar Capsules (8%) 536
▲ Zemplar Injection (8%) 538
Zemuron Injection (Less than 1%) 2947
▲ Ziagen (2% to 10%) 1673
Zinacef for Injection 1678
Zinacef Injection 1678
Zocor Tablets 2136
▲ Zolinza Capsules (13% to 15.1%) 2142
▲ Zometa for Intravenous Infusion (14% to 32%) 2341
Zomig Tablets (1% to less than 2%) 694
Zomig Nasal Spray (1% to less than 2%) 689
Zomig-ZMT Tablets (1% to less than 2%) 694
Zonegran Capsules (Frequent) 1089
▲ Zosyn for Injection (2.6% to 3.7%) 3284
Zovirax (2.7%) 1690
Zyban Sustained-Release Tablets (Frequent) 1692
Zydone Tablets (Among most frequent) 1132
▲ Zyprexa Tablets (4%) 1883
▲ Zyprexa ZYDIS Orally Disintegrating Tablets (4%) 1883
Zyrtec Chewable Tablets (2.3% to 2.5%) 1920
Zyrtec Syrup (2.3% to 2.5%) 1920
Zyrtec Tablets (2.3% to 2.5%) 1920
▲ Zyvox (0.9% to 9.4%) 2552

Vulva, dryness
(*see under* Vagina, dryness)

Vulvitis
Zovirax Ointment (0.3%) 819

Vulvovaginitis
Advair HFA 45/21 Inhalation Aerosol 1288
Advair HFA 115/21 Inhalation Aerosol 1288
Advair HFA 230/21 Inhalation Aerosol 1288
▲ Arimidex Tablets (6%) 672
Invanz for Injection (Greater than 0.1%) 2029

W

Walking disorders
Imitrex Nasal Spray (Rare) 1470

Wandering
Aricept Tablets (Frequent) 1062
Aricept ODT Tablets (Frequent) 1062

Warm sensation
Cancidas for Injection 1953
▲ Imitrex Injection (11%) 1465
▲ Imitrex Tablets (2% to 3%) 1474
ProQuad 2099
Zomig Tablets (Common) 694
▲ Zomig-ZMT Tablets (Common) 694

Warm to touch
ProQuad 2099

Warmth
Aceon Tablets (2 mg, 4 mg, 8 mg) (0.3% to 1%) 3038
Bicillin C-R Injectable Suspension 1775
Bicillin L-A Injection 1777
Daytrana Transdermal Patch 3022
Extina Foam, 2% (Less than or equal to 1%) 3057
▲ Imitrex Injection (11%) 1465
Imitrex Nasal Spray (Infrequent) 1470
Miacalcin Injection 2273
Niaspan Extended-Release Tablets (Among most common) 480
Recombivax HB (Less than 1%) 2107
▲ Zomig Tablets (0% to 4%) 694
▲ Zomig Nasal Spray (0% to 4%) 689
▲ Zomig-ZMT Tablets (0% to 4%) 694

Warmth at injection site
Boostrix 1377
Fluarix Vaccine 1446
Hyalgan Solution 2742
Pneumovax 23 (Common) 2078
Rocephin Injectable Vials, ADD-Vantage, Galaxy, Bulk 2642
▲ Vaqta (0.6% to 17.4%) 2130
Xolair 1235
Xolair 2339
Zostavax Injection (1.5%) 2145

Warts
(*see under* Verruca)

Water excretion, impaired
Marplan Tablets 3177

Water intoxication
Carbatrol Capsules 3019
Equetro Extended-Release Capsules 3174
Risperdal Consta Long-Acting Injection 1753
Zyprexa Tablets (Rare) 1883
Zyprexa ZYDIS Orally Disintegrating Tablets (Rare) 1883

Water retention
(*see under* Edema)

WBC, abnormal
Concerta Extended-Release Tablets 1925
Salagen Tablets (Less than 1%) 1082
▲ Targretin Gel 1% (6%) 1088
▲ Temodar Capsules (11%) 2931

WBC, immature
Cipro I.V. (Infrequent) 2817
Cipro XR Tablets 2823
Lupron Depot 3.75 mg 462
Lupron Depot–3 Month 11.25 mg 462

WBC counts, fluctuation
Invanz for Injection (0.8% to 1.5%) 2029
▲ Lupron Depot 3.75 mg (Approximately 5% to 8%) 462
Noroxin Tablets (1.3% to 1.4%) 2069
Primaxin I.M. 2080
▲ Visudyne for Injection (1% to 10%) 2332

WBC counts, increase
Janumet Tablets 2041

Weakness
(*see under* Asthenia)

Weakness, feet
K-Phos Original (Sodium Free) Tablets (Less frequent) 814
K-Phos Neutral Tablets 813
Uroqid-Acid No. 2 Tablets 814

Weakness, hands
K-Phos Original (Sodium Free) Tablets (Less frequent) 814
K-Phos Neutral Tablets 813
Uroqid-Acid No. 2 Tablets 814

Weakness, legs
Dantrium Intravenous 2582
K-Phos Original (Sodium Free) Tablets (Less frequent) 814
K-Phos Neutral Tablets 813
Uroqid-Acid No. 2 Tablets 814
▲ Vesanoid Capsules (3%) 2660

Weakness, local
Amrix Capsules 966
Combigan Ophthalmic Solution 553
Cosopt Sterile Ophthalmic Solution 1969
Timoptic Sterile Ophthalmic Solution 2121
Timoptic in Ocudose (Less frequent) 2124
Timoptic-XE Sterile Ophthalmic Gel Forming Solution 2125

Weakness, muscle
(*see also under* Asthenia)
Ambien Tablets (Rare) 2692
Avalide Tablets 2713
▲ DepoCyt Injection (10% to 15%) 1136
Exforge Tablets (Less than or equal to 0.1%) 2238
Tasigna Capsules (0.1% to 1%) 2316
Zyrtec-D 12 Hour Extended Release Tablets (Less than 2%) 1923

Weeping, skin
▲ Aldara Cream, 5% (0% to 22%) 1699

Weight change, unspecified
Anaprox Tablets (Less than 1%) 2632
Anaprox DS Tablets (Less than 1%) 2632
EC-Naprosyn Delayed-Release Tablets (Less than 1%) 2632
Focalin XR Capsules 2251
▲ Lupron Depot 3.75 mg (6%) 462
▲ Lupron Depot–3 Month 11.25 mg (6%) 462
Naprosyn Suspension (Less than 1%) 2632
Naprosyn Tablets (Less than 1%) 2632
Voltaren Tablets (Occasionally) 2334
Voltaren-XR Tablets (Occasionally) 2337

Weight changes, increase or decrease
▲ Avastin IV (15% to 16%) 1192
Climara Transdermal System 763
▲ Clolar for Intravenous Infusion (15%) 1239
Divigel 3167
Estratest Tablets 3043
Estratest H.S. Tablets 3043
Klonopin (Infrequent) 2639
Lybrel Tablets 3204
Moban Tablets 1116
Ortho-Cyclen Tablets 2449
Ortho Evra Transdermal System 2437
Ortho Tri-Cyclen Tablets 2449
Ortho Tri-Cyclen Lo Tablets 2458
Premphase Tablets 3232
Prempro Tablets 3232
Prometrium Capsules (100 mg, 200 mg) 3047
Seasonique Tablets 1046
Yaz Tablets 805

Weight decrease
(*see under* Weight loss)

Weight gain
▲ Abilify Injection (Less than or equal to 1 in 100 patients to 25%) 881
▲ Abilify Injection (2% to 30%) 2466
▲ Abilify Oral Solution (Less than or equal to 1 in 100 patients to 25%) 881
▲ Abilify Oral Solution (2% to 30%) 2466
▲ Abilify Discmelt Orally Disintegrating Tablets (Less than or equal to 1 in 100 patients to 25%) 881
▲ Abilify Discmelt Orally Disintegrating Tablets (2% to 30%) 2466
▲ Abilify Tablets (Less than or equal to 1 in 100 patients to 25%) 881
▲ Abilify Tablets (2% to 30%) 2466
▲ Activella Tablets (0% to 9%) 2347
▲ ActoPlus Met Tablets (2.9% to 6.7%) 3071
▲ Actos Tablets (0.9% to 3.6%) 3077
Advair Diskus 100/50 1276
Advair Diskus 250/50 1276
Advair Diskus 500/50 1276
▲ Advair HFA 45/21 Inhalation Aerosol (1% to 3%) 1288
▲ Advair HFA 115/21 Inhalation Aerosol (1% to 3%) 1288
▲ Advair HFA 230/21 Inhalation Aerosol (1% to 3%) 1288
▲ Aerobid/Aerobid-M (1% to 3%) 1153
Amitiza Capsules (Less than 1%) 3082
AndroGel 3159
Angeliq Tablets 751
Aricept Tablets (Infrequent) 1062
Aricept ODT Tablets (Infrequent) 1062
▲ Arimidex Tablets (2% to 13%) 672
Avandamet Tablets 1336
Avandaryl Tablets 1344
Avandia Tablets 1351
▲ Azmacort Inhalation Aerosol (1% to 3%) 407
Betaseron for SC Injection 756
▲ Busulfex Injection (8%) 2477
Campral Tablets (Frequent) 1158
Cardizem LA Extended Release Tablets (Less than 2%) 421
Catapres Tablets (About 1 in 100 patients) 841
Catapres-TTS (0.5% or less) 842
Celebrex Capsules (0.1% to 1.9%) 2979
Celexa (Frequent) 1160
▲ CellCept Capsules (3% to less than 20%) 2622
▲ CellCept Intravenous (3% to less than 20%) 2622
▲ CellCept Oral Suspension (3% to less than 20%) 2622
▲ CellCept Tablets (3% to less than 20%) 2622
Chantix Tablets (Frequent) 2511
Climara Pro Transdermal System (2.8%) 768
Clorpres Tablets (About 1%) 2185
▲ Copaxone for Injection (3%) 3110
▲ Coreg Tablets (10% to 12%) 1387
▲ Coreg CR Extended-Release Capsules (10% to 12%) 1393
▲ Cozaar Tablets (4%) 1973
Cymbalta Delayed-Release Capsules (Frequent to 2%) 1801
▲ Depakote ER Tablets (Greater than 1% to 9%) 423
Doxil Injection (Less than 1%) 2378
▲ Duetact Tablets (9.1% to 13.4%) 3085
DynaCirc CR Controlled Release Tablets (0.5% to 1%) 1407
Effexor XR Extended-Release Capsules (Frequent) 3195
Eligard 7.5 mg (Less than 2%) 2724
Eligard 22.5 mg (Less than 2%) 2724
Eligard 30 mg (Less than 2%) 2724
Eligard 45 mg (Less than 2%) 2724
▲ Eloxatin for Injection (10%) 2731
Emsam Transdermal System (2.1%) 905
Enablex Extended-Release Tablets (Greater than or equal to 1%) 2225
Enbrel for Injection 569
Enjuvia Tablets 1029
▲ Evista Tablets (8.8%) 1810
Evoxac Capsules (Less than 1%) 1013
Exforge Tablets (Greater than 0.1% to less than 1%) 2238
Femara Tablets (2%) 2246
▲ Flolan for Injection (6%) 1426
▲ Flovent Diskus 50 mcg (1% to 3%) 1435
Flovent HFA 1440
Follistim AQ Cartridge 2844
Gabitril Tablets (Frequent) 973
Gengraf Capsules (1% to less than 3%) 435
▲ Geodon Capsules (10%) 2520
▲ Gleevec Tablets (5% to 32%) 2255
▲ Hycamtin for Injection (69%) 1459
Imitrex Injection 1465
Imitrex Nasal Spray 1470
Imitrex Tablets (Rare) 1474
Indocin Capsules (Less than 1%) 2024
Indocin I.V. (Less than 1%) 2489
Indocin (Less than 1%) 2024
▲ Intron A for Injection (Less than or equal to 5%) 2859
▲ Invega Extended-Release Tablets (6% to 9%) 1748
Kaletra (Less than 2%) 452
Keppra Oral Solution (1% or more) 3131
Keppra Tablets (1% or more) 3131
K-Phos Neutral Tablets 813
▲ Lamictal (Greater than 1% to less than 5%) 1488
▲ Leukine (8%) 774
Levemir Injection 2352
Lexapro Oral Suspension (Frequent) 1174
Lexapro Tablets (Frequent) 1174
Lipitor Tablets (Less than 2%) 2501
Lunesta Tablets (Infrequent) 2994
Lupron Depot-PED 7.5 mg, 11.25 mg and 15 mg (Less than 2%) 471
Luvox CR Extended-Release Capsules (Frequent) 1759
▲ Lyrica Capsules (4% to 16%) 2527
Maxair Autohaler 1705
Miacalcin Nasal Spray (Less than 1%) 2274
Mirapex Tablets 857
Mircette Tablets 1034
▲ Mirena Intrauterine System (5% or more) 779
Mobic Oral Suspension (Less than 2%) 863
Mobic Tablets (Less than 2%) 863
▲ Myfortic Tablets (3% to less than 20%) 2276
Nadolol Tablets (1 to 5 of 1000 patients) 2191
Neoral Oral Solution (1% to less than 3%) 2280
Neoral Soft Gelatin Capsules (1% to less than 3%) 2280
▲ Neupro Transdermal System (3%) 3149
Nexium Delayed-Release Capsules (Less than 1%) 645
Nexium I.V. (Less than 1%) 652
Nexium Delayed-Release Oral Suspension (Less than 1%) 645
▲ Novantrone for Injection Concentrate (14%) 1100
NovoLog Injection 2359
▲ NuvaRing (5% to 14%) 2897
Ortho Micronor Tablets (Rare) 2446
Patanase Nasal Spray 544
Paxil (Frequent) 1535
Paxil CR Controlled-Release Tablets (Frequent) 1544

Premarin Intravenous 3217
Premarin Tablets 3221
Premarin Vaginal Cream 3228
Prinivil Tablets (0.3% to 1%) 2087
Prinzide Tablets 2092
▲ Prograf Capsules and Injection (3% to 15%) 622
▲ Proleukin for Injection (16%) 2287
Protonix for Delayed-Release Oral Suspension (Less than 1%) 3254
Protonix Delayed-Release Tablets (Less than 1%) 3254
Protonix I.V. (Less than 1%) 3257
Provigil Tablets (At least 1%) 977
Prozac Weekly Capsules (Frequent) 1852
Prozac Pulvules and Liquid (Frequent) 1852
▲ Pulmicort Flexhaler (Greater than or equal to 1% to 3%) 654
Requip Tablets (Infrequent) 1561
Reyataz Capsules 3299
Rilutek Tablets (Infrequent) 2771
▲ Risperdal Consta Long-Acting Injection (4% to 9%) 1753
Rythmol SR Capsules 1590
▲ Simulect for Injection (3% to 10%) 2306
Soriatane Capsules (Less than 1%) 3062
Stalevo Tablets 2309
Sular Extended Release Tablets (Less than or equal to 1%) 2975
Supprelin LA Implant 1731
▲ Symbyax Capsules (Up to 21%) 1871
Targretin Capsules 1084
▲ Tasigna Capsules (1% to 10%) 2316
▲ Taxotere Injection Concentrate (0% to 12.9%) 2773
▲ Temodar Capsules (5%) 2931
Thioridazine Hydrochloride Tablets 2195
Thiothixene Capsules 2197
Tricor Tablets 520
▲ Trisenox Injection (13%) 986
Uroqid-Acid No. 2 Tablets 814
Vantas (2.3%) 1737
Venlafaxine Hydrochloride Tablets (Frequent) 2199
▲ Vesanoid Capsules (23%) 2660
Viadur Implant (2.3%) 802
Vicoprofen Tablets 533
▲ Wellbutrin Tablets (9.4% to 13.6%) 1648
▲ Wellbutrin SR Sustained-Release Tablets (2% to 3%) 1653
▲ Wellbutrin XL Extended-Release Tablets (11%) 1659
Xyzal Oral Solution (0.5%) 2789
Xyzal Oral Solution (0.5%) 3155
Xyzal Tablets (0.5%) 2789
Xyzal Tablets (0.5%) 3155
Yaz Tablets (Greater than 1%) 805
Zometa for Intravenous Infusion 2341
Zomig Tablets (Rare) 694
Zomig Nasal Spray (Rare) 689
Zomig-ZMT Tablets (Rare) 694
Zonegran Capsules (Infrequent) 1089
Zyban Sustained-Release Tablets (Infrequent) 1692
▲ Zyprexa Tablets (5% to 56%) 1883
▲ Zyprexa ZYDIS Orally Disintegrating Tablets (5% to 56%) 1883
Zyrtec Chewable Tablets (Less than 2%) 1920
Zyrtec Syrup (Less than 2%) 1920
Zyrtec Tablets (Less than 2%) 1920
Zyrtec-D 12 Hour Extended Release Tablets (Less than 2%) 1923

Weight gain, delayed

Elocon Cream 0.1% 2840
Elocon Lotion 0.1% 2841
Elocon Ointment 0.1% 2842
▲ Sandostatin Injection (32%) 2300
Verdeso Foam 3069

Weight loss

Abelcet Injection 1134
Abilify Injection (Greater than or equal to 1 in 100 patients) 2466
Abilify Oral Solution (Greater than or equal to 1 in 100 patients) 881
Abilify Oral Solution (Greater than or equal to 1 in 100 patients) 2466
Abilify Discmelt Orally Disintegrating Tablets (Greater than or equal to 1 in 100 patients) 881
Abilify Discmelt Orally Disintegrating Tablets (Greater than or equal to 1 in 100 patients) 2466
Abilify Tablets (Greater than or equal to 1 in 100 patients) 881
Abilify Tablets (Greater than or equal to 1 in 100 patients) 2466
Accutane Capsules 2607
▲ Actimmune (6%) 1743
Actiq (Less than 1%) 959
Activella Tablets 2347
▲ Adderall XR Capsules (1.2% to 11%) 3012
Alferon N Injection (1%) 1726
Ambien Tablets (Rare) 2692
Ambien CR Tablets (Rare) 2696
Angeliq Tablets 751
▲ Aptivus Capsules (3.1%) 823
▲ Aptivus Oral Solution (3.1%) 823
Aricept Tablets (Frequent) 1062
Aricept ODT Tablets (Frequent) 1062
▲ Arimidex Tablets (2% to 5%) 672
▲ Avinza Capsules (Less than 5%) 1772
▲ Azilect Tablets (9%) 3106
Betaseron for SC Injection 756
▲ Bexxar (Less than 1% to 6%) 1371
Calcijex Injection 419
Campral Tablets (Infrequent) 1158
Captopril Tablets 2182
Celexa (Frequent) 1160
▲ CellCept Capsules (3% to less than 20%) 2622
▲ CellCept Intravenous (3% to less than 20%) 2622
▲ CellCept Oral Suspension (3% to less than 20%) 2622
▲ CellCept Tablets (3% to less than 20%) 2622
Climara Pro Transdermal System 768
Combigan Ophthalmic Solution 553
▲ Concerta Extended-Release Tablets (6.5%) 1925
Copaxone for Injection (Infrequent) 3110
▲ Coreg Tablets (Greater than 1% to 3%) 1387
▲ Coreg CR Extended-Release Capsules (Greater than 1% to less than or equal to 3%) 1393
Cosopt Sterile Ophthalmic Solution 1969
Cymbalta Delayed-Release Capsules (2%) 1801
▲ Daytrana Transdermal Patch (9%) 3022
▲ Depakote ER Tablets (6%) 423
Dexedrine 1401
▲ Doxil Injection (1% to 10%) 2378
Duragesic Transdermal System 2405
▲ Effexor XR Extended-Release Capsules (2% to 3%) 3195
Eldepryl Capsules (1 of 49 patients) 3052
Eloxatin for Injection 2731
Elspar for Injection 1990
Emend Capsules (Greater than 0.5%) 1992
Emend for Injection (Greater than 0.5%) 1999
▲ Emsam Transdermal System (5%) 905
Enjuvia Tablets 1029
▲ Erbitux (11% to 84%) 912
Evoxac Capsules (Less than 1%) 1013
▲ Exelon Capsules (3%) 2229
▲ Exelon Oral Solution (3%) 2229
▲ Exelon Patch (3% to 8%) 2233
Exforge Tablets (Greater than 0.1% to less than 1%) 2238
▲ Femara Tablets (7%) 2246
Fentora Tablets (3% to 11%) 968
▲ Flolan for Injection (27% to 45%) 1426
Focalin XR Capsules 2251
Gabitril Tablets (Frequent) 973
Gengraf Capsules (1% to less than 3%) 435
Gleevec Tablets (Infrequent) 2255
▲ Hycamtin for Injection (69%) 1459
Imitrex Injection 1465
Imitrex Nasal Spray (Rare) 1470
Imitrex Tablets (Rare) 1474
▲ Indapamide Tablets (Less than 5%) 2188
▲ Intron A for Injection (Less than 1% to 10%) 2859
Invanz for Injection (Greater than 0.1%) 2029
▲ Ixempra Kit for Injection (6%) 915
▲ Kaletra (Up to 3%) 452
Keppra Injection 3137
Keppra Oral Solution 3131
Keppra Tablets 3131
▲ Lamictal (5%) 1488
Lamisil Tablets 2266
▲ Leukine (37%) 774
Levothroid Tablets 1170
Levoxyl Tablets 1780
Lexapro Oral Suspension (Infrequent) 1174
Lexapro Tablets (Infrequent) 1174
Lunesta Tablets (Infrequent) 2994
Luvox CR Extended-Release Capsules (2%) 1759
Metadate CD Capsules 3146
Mirapex Tablets (2%) 857
Mircette Tablets 1034
Mobic Oral Suspension (Less than 2%) 863
Mobic Tablets (Less than 2%) 863
Myleran Tablets 1530
Namenda (Frequent) 1180
Neoral Oral Solution (1% to less than 3%) 2280
Neoral Soft Gelatin Capsules (1% to less than 3%) 2280
▲ Neupro Transdermal System (2% to 3%) 3149
▲ Nexavar Tablets (10% to 30%) 784
Nexium Delayed-Release Capsules (Less than 1%) 645
Nexium I.V. (Less than 1%) 652
Nexium Delayed-Release Oral Suspension (Less than 1%) 645
Norvir (0% to 2.4%) 489
▲ Novantrone for Injection Concentrate (17%) 1100
▲ Noxafil Oral Suspension (1% to 14%) 2889
▲ Ontak Vials (14%) 1079
Opana Tablets (Less than 1%) 1117
Opana ER Tablets (Less than 1%) 1121
Paxil (Frequent) 1535
Paxil CR Controlled-Release Tablets (Frequent) 1544
▲ PegIntron Powder for Injection (11%) 2903
▲ Photofrin for Injection (6% to 9%) 708
Premarin Intravenous 3217
Premarin Tablets 3221
Premarin Vaginal Cream 3228
Prinivil Tablets (0.3% to 1%) 2087
Prinzide Tablets 2092
Pristiq Extended-Release Tablets (1% to 2%) 3247
Prograf Capsules and Injection 622
Protonix for Delayed-Release Oral Suspension (Less than 1%) 3254
Protonix Delayed-Release Tablets (Less than 1%) 3254
Protonix I.V. (Less than 1%) 3257
Provigil Tablets (Greater than or equal to 1%) 977
Prozac Weekly Capsules (1.4% to 2%) 1852
Prozac Pulvules and Liquid (1.4% to 2%) 1852
Pulmozyme Inhalation Solution 1217
▲ Rebetol (20% to 29%) 2917
Remeron Tablets (Infrequent) 2924
RemeronSolTab Tablets (Infrequent) 2927
Requip Tablets (Infrequent to greater than or equal to 1%) 1561
Retrovir Capsules (0.8%) 1574
Retrovir IV Infusion (1%) 1579
Retrovir (0.8%) 1574
Reyataz Capsules 3299
▲ Rilutek Tablets (3.7% to 4.6%) 2771
Risperdal Consta Long-Acting Injection (1%) 1753
Rocaltrol Capsules 1150
Rocaltrol Oral Solution 1150
Rythmol SR Capsules 1590
Sandimmune (Rare) 2296
Sandostatin Injection (Less than 1%) 2300
▲ Somatuline Depot Injection (5% to 11%) 3102
Stalevo Tablets 2309
▲ Strattera Capsules (2% to 7%) 1864
Sular Extended Release Tablets (Less than or equal to 1%) 2975
▲ Sutent Capsules (12%) 2540
Symbyax Capsules (Frequent) 1871
▲ Tarceva Tablets (0% to 39%) 1228
Targretin Capsules 1084
▲ Tasigna Capsules (1% to 10%) 2316
▲ Taxotere Injection Concentrate (1.6% to 20.7%) 2773
Tice BCG (2%) 2936
Timoptic Sterile Ophthalmic Solution 2121
Timoptic in Ocudose 2124
Timoptic-XE Sterile Ophthalmic Gel Forming Solution 2125
▲ Torisel Injection (1% to 19%) 3272
▲ Treanda for Injection (0% to 7%) 983
Tricor Tablets 520
▲ Trisenox Injection (8%) 986
▲ Ultram ER Extended-Release Tablets (1% to less than 5%) 2428
Vantas (Less than 2%) 1737
▲ Venlafaxine Hydrochloride Tablets (1% to 18%) 2199
▲ Vesanoid Capsules (17%) 2660
Vicoprofen Tablets (Less than 1%) 533
▲ Viread Tablets (2% to 4%) 1268
Vivitrol 988
▲ Vyvanse Capsules (9%) 3033
▲ Wellbutrin Tablets (23.2% to 28%) 1648
▲ Wellbutrin SR Sustained-Release Tablets (14% to 19%) 1653
▲ Wellbutrin XL Extended-Release Tablets (23%) 1659
▲ Xeloda Tablets (Up to 7%) 2662
Xifaxan Tablets (Less than 2%) 2682
Xyrem Oral Solution (Frequent) 1766
▲ Zolinza Capsules (18% to 20.9%) 2142
▲ Zonegran Capsules (3%) 1089
Zyprexa Tablets (Frequent) 1883
Zyprexa ZYDIS Orally Disintegrating Tablets (Frequent) 1883

Wenckebach block

Lanoxin Injection 1498
Lanoxin Injection Pediatric 1502
Lanoxin Tablets 1505

Wenckebach's period

(*see under* A-V conduction, prolongation)

Wheal at injection site

ProQuad 2099

Wheals

Attenuvax (Rare) 1951
Meruvax II 2061
M-M-R II 2054
Mumpsvax (Extremely rare) 2068

Wheezing

Abelcet Injection 1134
Advair Diskus 100/50 1276
Advair Diskus 250/50 1276
Advair Diskus 500/50 1276
Advair HFA 45/21 Inhalation Aerosol 1288
Advair HFA 115/21 Inhalation Aerosol 1288
Advair HFA 230/21 Inhalation Aerosol 1288
▲ Aerobid/Aerobid-M (3% to 9%) 1153
Alferon N Injection 1726
Aricept Tablets (Infrequent) 1062
Aricept ODT Tablets (Infrequent) 1062
▲ Arranon Injection (0% to 5%) 1319
Atrovent Nasal Spray 0.03% 834
Atrovent Nasal Spray 0.06% 836
Avalide Tablets 892
Avalide Tablets 2713
Avapro Tablets (Less than 1%) 897
Avapro Tablets (Less than 1%) 2718
Azmacort Inhalation Aerosol 407
Beconase AQ Nasal Spray (Rare) 1369
BeneFIX Vials 3191
Combivent Inhalation Aerosol 845
Combivir Tablets 1384
Elidel Cream 1% (0% to 1.2%) 2221
Emend Capsules (Less than or equal to 0.5%) 1992
Emend for Injection (Less than or equal to 0.5%) 1999
▲ Epivir (7%) 1412
Epivir-HBV 1417
Epzicom Tablets 1422
▲ Fabrazyme for Intravenous Infusion (6%) 1241
Fentora Tablets (Greater than 1%) 968
▲ Flebogamma 5% (18%) 1715
Flebogamma 5% DIF 1718
Flonase Nasal Spray 1431
Flovent Diskus 50 mcg 1435
Flovent HFA 1440
▲ FluMist Vaccine (2.1% to 5.9%) 1945
Gammagard Liquid 730
Humalog-Pen and KwikPen (Less common) 1829
Humalog Mix 50/50-Pen and KwikPen 1833
Humalog Mix 75/25-Pen and KwikPen (Less common) 1835
Humulin 50/50, 100 Units 1843
Humulin 70/30 Vial (Less common) 1844
Humulin N Vial (Less common) 1846
Humulin R 1849
Humulin R (U-500) 1850
Imitrex Tablets 1474
▲ Intron A for Injection (Less than or equal to 5%) 2859
Invanz for Injection (1%) 2029
Levothroid Tablets 1170
Levoxyl Tablets 1780
Lyrica Capsules 2527
Maxair Autohaler 1705
Maxalt Tablets 2056

Maxalt-MLT Orally Disintegrating Tablets 2056
Mirapex Tablets 857
Motrin IB Tablets and Caplets 1900
Children's Motrin Oral Suspension 1901
Children's Motrin Non-Staining Dye-Free Oral Suspension 1901
Children's Motrin Cold Oral Suspension 1899
Infants' Motrin Concentrated Drops 1901
Infants' Motrin Non-Staining Dye-Free Concentrated Drops 1901
Junior Strength Motrin Caplets and Chewable Tablets 1901
Nasonex Nasal Spray (Greater than or equal to 2%) 2883
Neupogen for Injection 589
Nimotop Capsules (Less than 1%) 790
NovoLog Injection 2359
Omnaris Nasal Spray (Rare) 2998
Orencia Powder for Intravenous Infusion (Greater than 0.1% and less than or equal to 1%) 921
▲ Orthoclone OKT3 Sterile Solution (13%) 2387
Prevnar 3241
Prinivil Tablets (0.3% to 1%) 2087
Prinzide Tablets 2092
ProQuad 2099
Pulmicort Flexhaler 654
Pulmozyme Inhalation Solution 1217
Requip Tablets (Infrequent) 1561
Rythmol SR Capsules (2%) 1590
Sandimmune 2296
Simulect for Injection 2306
Singulair (Greater than or equal to 2%) 2114
Sular Extended Release Tablets (Less than or equal to 1%) 2975
Synagis Intramuscular Solution (More than 1%) 1948
Toprol-XL Tablets (About 1 of 100 patients) 666
▲ Trisenox Injection (13%) 986
Trizivir Tablets 1622
Ultane Liquid for Inhalation (Less than 1%) 524
Vaqta (Less than 1%) 2130
▲ Vesanoid Capsules (14%) 2660
Xopenex Inhalation Solution 3001
Xopenex Inhalation Solution Concentrate 3005
Xopenex HFA Inhalation Aerosol 3009
Xyntha Vials 3280
Zemuron Injection (Less than 1%) 2947

White blood cell count, decreased
▲ Aptivus Capsules (0.3% to 5.4%) 823
▲ Aptivus Oral Solution (0.3% to 5.4%) 823
▲ Betaseron for SC Injection (13%) 756
▲ Cancidas for Injection (12%) 1953
Fenoglide Tablets 2960
▲ Keppra Injection (3.2%) 3137
▲ Keppra Oral Solution (3% to 3.2%) 3131
▲ Keppra Tablets (3% to 3.2%) 3131
Lupron Depot 7.5 mg 469
Lupron Depot-PED 7.5 mg, 11.25 mg and 15 mg 471
Mycamine for Injection 616
▲ Novantrone for Injection Concentrate (87% to 100%) 1100

White blood cell count, increased
Avelox (Greater than or equal to 2%) 2803
Janumet Tablets 2041
Januvia Tablets 2048

Withdrawal bleeding, abnormal
Activella Tablets 2347

Withdrawal reactions
Ambien Tablets (Rare) 2692
Aricept Tablets (Infrequent) 1062
Aricept ODT Tablets (Infrequent) 1062
▲ Avinza Capsules (Less than 5%) 1772
Catapres Tablets 841
Catapres-TTS (0.5% or less) 842
Celexa 1160
Dexedrine 1401
Effexor XR Extended-Release Capsules (Infrequent) 3195
Klonopin 2639
Lortab 5/500 Tablets 3143
Lortab 7.5/500 Tablets 3144
Lortab 10/500 Tablets 3144
Mirapex Tablets 857
MS Contin Tablets 2585
Nembutal Sodium Solution, USP 2494
OxyContin Tablets (Less than 1%) 2589
Paxil (Rare) 1535
Paxil CR Controlled-Release Tablets (Rare) 1544
Remeron Tablets (Rare) 2924
RemeronSolTab Tablets (Rare) 2927
▲ Suboxone Tablets (22% to 25.2%) 2601
▲ Subutex Tablets (18.4% to 22%) 2601
Valium Tablets 2658
Viramune Oral Suspension 873
Viramune Tablets 873
Zyprexa Tablets (Infrequent) 1883
Zyprexa ZYDIS Orally Disintegrating Tablets (Infrequent) 1883

Withdrawal syndrome
Ambien CR Tablets 2696
Campral Tablets (Infrequent) 1158
Daytrana Transdermal Patch 3022
Parnate Tablets 1532
Soma Tablets 1931
Symbyax Capsules (Rare) 1871
Transderm Scōp Transdermal Therapeutic System 2206
Ultram ER Extended-Release Tablets (0.5% to less than 1%) 2428
Venlafaxine Hydrochloride Tablets (Infrequent) 2199
Vivitrol 988

Worsening of underlying illness
Tylenol Chest Congestion Caplets with Cool Burst 1910
Tylenol Chest Congestion Liquid with Cool Burst 1910
Tylenol Cold Severe Congestion Daytime Caplets with Cool Burst 1912

Wound complication
Invanz for Injection (2.9%) 2029

Wound dehiscence
Emend Capsules (Greater than 0.5%) 1992
Emend for Injection (Greater than 0.5%) 1999
▲ Gliadel Wafer (16%) 1076
Invanz for Injection (1.3%) 2029
Rapamune 3260
▲ Valcyte Tablets (Less than 5%) 2654

Wound drainage, increased
▲ Arixtra Injection (0.6% to 4.5%) 1313
▲ Valcyte Tablets (Less than 5%) 2654

Wound effusion
▲ Gliadel Wafer (16%) 1076

Wound healing, impaired
▲ Avastin IV (15%) 1192
FML Ophthalmic Ointment (Infrequent) ⊙ 223
FML Ophthalmic Suspension ⊙ 224
FML Forte Ophthalmic Suspension (Infrequent) ⊙ 222
▲ Gliadel Wafer (16%) 1076
Mirapex Tablets 857
Nexavar Tablets 784
Pred Forte Ophthalmic Suspension ⊙ 227
Pred Mild Ophthalmic Suspension (Infrequent) ⊙ 230
Pred-G Ophthalmic Ointment ⊙ 229
Pred-G Ophthalmic Suspension ⊙ 228
Rapamune 3260
Torisel Injection (1%) 3272
Veramyst Nasal Spray 1643
Voltaren Ophthalmic Solution 2336
▲ Zofran (28%) 1687
▲ Zofran ODT Orally Disintegrating Tablets (28%) 1687

Wound infection
▲ Arixtra Injection (4.9%) 1313
Enbrel for Injection 569
▲ Gengraf Capsules (7%) 435
▲ Invanz for Injection (6.5%) 2029
Mirapex Tablets 857
▲ Myfortic Tablets (3% to less than 20%) 2276
▲ Neoral Oral Solution (7%) 2280
▲ Neoral Soft Gelatin Capsules (7%) 2280
Requip Tablets (Infrequent) 1561
▲ Sandimmune (7% to 10.1%) 2296
Supprelin LA Implant 1731
▲ Valcyte Tablets (Less than 5%) 2654

Wound secretion
Invanz for Injection (1.9%) 2029

Wrist fracture
Arimidex Tablets (2%) 672

Wrist-drop
Azilect Tablets (Rare) 3106
Rilutek Tablets (Rare) 2771

X

Xanthomas, eruptive
Accutane Capsules 2607

Xanthopsia
Atacand HCT 642
Avalide Tablets 892
Avalide Tablets 2713
Clorpres Tablets 2185
Diovan HCT Tablets 2216
Dyazide Capsules 1405
Furosemide Tablets 2186
Indapamide Tablets 2188
Intravenous Sodium Diuril 2490
Lanoxin Injection 1498
Lanoxin Injection Pediatric 1502
Lanoxin Tablets 1505
Micardis HCT Tablets 854
Prinzide Tablets 2092
Tekturna HCT Tablets 2324
Teveten HCT Tablets 517

Xerochilia
Lexapro Oral Suspension (Infrequent) 1174
Lexapro Tablets (Infrequent) 1174
Xifaxan Tablets (Less than 2%) 2682
Zovirax Cream (Less than 1%) 817

Xeroderma
(*see under* Xerosis cutis)

Xeromycteria
Accutane Capsules 2607
▲ Advair HFA 45/21 Inhalation Aerosol (1% to 3%) 1288
▲ Advair HFA 115/21 Inhalation Aerosol (1% to 3%) 1288
▲ Advair HFA 230/21 Inhalation Aerosol (1% to 3%) 1288
Alphagan P Ophthalmic Solution (Less than 1%) 549
AmBisome for Injection (Less common) 606
▲ Atrovent Nasal Spray 0.03% (5.1%) 834
▲ Atrovent Nasal Spray 0.06% (4.8%) 836
Beconase AQ Nasal Spray 1369
Catapres Tablets 841
Clorpres Tablets 2185
Combigan Ophthalmic Solution (0.1% to 0.2%) 553
Flonase Nasal Spray (Less than 1%) 1431
Maxalt Tablets (Infrequent) 2056
Maxalt-MLT Orally Disintegrating Tablets (Infrequent) 2056
▲ Miacalcin Nasal Spray (10.6%) 2274
Mirapex Tablets 857
Protopic Ointment (0.2% to less than 1%) 628
Sanctura XR Capsules (1% to less than 2%) 557

Xerophthalmia
Accutane Capsules 2607
Advair Diskus 100/50 1276
Advair Diskus 250/50 1276
Advair Diskus 500/50 1276
▲ Alamast Ophthalmic Solution (Less than 5%) 3181
▲ Alphagan P Ophthalmic Solution (1% to 4%) 549
▲ Alrex Ophthalmic Suspension 0.2% (5% to 15%) ⊙ 236
AmBisome for Injection (Less common) 606
Amerge Tablets (Rare) 1301
Aricept Tablets (Infrequent) 1062
Aricept ODT Tablets (Infrequent) 1062
Axert Tablets (Rare) 2431
AzaSite Ophthalmic Drops (Less than 1%) 1740
▲ Azopt Ophthalmic Suspension (1% to 5%) 540
▲ Betimol Ophthalmic Solution (More than 5%) 3181
BOTOX Purified Neurotoxin Complex 550
Catapres Tablets 841
Catapres-TTS (0.5% or less) 842
Celexa (Infrequent) 1160
Chantix Tablets (Infrequent) 2511
Clorpres Tablets 2185
▲ Combigan Ophthalmic Solution (1% to 5%) 553
Concerta Extended-Release Tablets 1925
Copaxone for Injection (Infrequent) 3110
▲ Cosopt Sterile Ophthalmic Solution (1% to 5%) 1969
Crinone 4% Gel 992
Crinone 8% Gel 992
Depakote ER Tablets (Greater than 1%) 423
▲ Doxil Injection (1% to 10%) 2378
Effexor XR Extended-Release Capsules (Infrequent) 3195
Emsam Transdermal System (Infrequent) 905
Enablex Extended-Release Tablets (1.5% to 2.1%) 2225
Enbrel for Injection 569
▲ Evoxac Capsules (1% to 3%) 1013
Exforge Tablets (Less than or equal to 0.1%) 2238
Flonase Nasal Spray 1431
Geodon Capsules (Infrequent) 2520
Gleevec Tablets (Infrequent) 2255
InnoPran XL Extended Release Capsules 1484
▲ Intron A for Injection (Less than 5%) 2859
Klonopin (Infrequent) 2639
Lamictal (Infrequent) 1488
Lexapro Oral Suspension (Infrequent) 1174
Lexapro Tablets (Infrequent) 1174
Lipitor Tablets (Less than 2%) 2501
▲ Lotemax Ophthalmic Suspension 0.5% (5% to 15%) ⊙ 241
▲ Lucentis Injection (3% to 14%) 1205
▲ Lumigan Ophthalmic Solution (3% to 10%) 556
Lunesta Tablets (Infrequent) 2994
Lyrica Capsules (0.1% to 1%) 2527
Maxalt Tablets (Infrequent) 2056
Maxalt-MLT Orally Disintegrating Tablets (Infrequent) 2056
Meridia Capsules 475
Mirapex Tablets 857
Nadolol Tablets (1 to 5 of 1000 patients) 2191
Namenda (Infrequent) 1180
▲ Nevanac Ophthalmic Suspension 0.1% (1% to 5%) ⊙ 205
▲ Pataday Ophthalmic Solution (Less than or equal to 5%) 543
▲ Patanol Ophthalmic Solution (Less than 5%) 546
Protopic Ointment (0.2% to less than 1%) 628
Prozac Weekly Capsules (Infrequent) 1852
Prozac Pulvules and Liquid (Infrequent) 1852
Quixin Ophthalmic Solution (Less than 1%) 3184
▲ Rebif Prefilled Syringe for Injection (1% to 3%) 1107
Requip Tablets (2%) 1561
Salagen Tablets (Less than 1%) 1082
Sanctura XR Capsules (1.6% to less than 2%) 557
▲ Soriatane Capsules (10% to 25%) 3062
Symbyax Capsules (Infrequent) 1871
Targretin Capsules 1084
Tasigna Capsules (0.1% to 1%) 2316
Teveten Tablets (Less than 1%) 515
Teveten HCT Tablets (Less than 1%) 517
Timoptic Sterile Ophthalmic Solution 2121
Timoptic in Ocudose 2124
Timoptic-XE Sterile Ophthalmic Gel Forming Solution 2125
Toprol-XL Tablets (Rare) 666
Transderm Scōp Transdermal Therapeutic System (Infrequent) 2206
▲ Travatan Z Ophthalmic Solution (1% to 4%) 547
▲ Trisenox Injection (8%) 986
▲ Trusopt Sterile Ophthalmic Solution (Approximately 1% to 5%) 2128
Venlafaxine Hydrochloride Tablets (Infrequent) 2199
VESIcare Tablets (0.3% to 1.6%) 636
Vicoprofen Tablets (Less than 1%) 533
▲ Vigamox Ophthalmic Solution (1% to 6%) 548
▲ Visudyne for Injection (1% to 10%) 2332
Wellbutrin SR Sustained-Release Tablets (Infrequent) 1653
Wellbutrin XL Extended-Release Tablets (Infrequent) 1659
Zomig Tablets (Infrequent) 694
Zomig Nasal Spray (Rare) 689
Zomig-ZMT Tablets (Infrequent) 694
Zyban Sustained-Release Tablets (Infrequent) 1692
Zyprexa Tablets (Infrequent) 1883

Zyprexa ZYDIS Orally Disintegrating Tablets (Infrequent) 1883
Zyrtec Chewable Tablets (Less than 2%) 1920
Zyrtec Syrup (Less than 2%) 1920
Zyrtec Tablets (Less than 2%) 1920
Zyrtec-D 12 Hour Extended Release Tablets (Less than 2%) 1923

Xerosis cutis

Accutane Capsules 2607
Aceon Tablets (2 mg, 4 mg, 8 mg) (0.3% to 1%) 3038
Advicor Tablets 402
▲ Aldara Cream, 5% (7% to 93%) 1699
AmBisome for Injection (Less common) 606
Amerge Tablets (Rare) 1301
AndroGel (1% to 1.9%) 3159
Aricept Tablets (Infrequent) 1062
Aricept ODT Tablets (Infrequent) 1062
Asacol Delayed-Release Tablets 2579
▲ Avastin IV (7% to 20%) 1192
▲ Avinza Capsules (Less than 5%) 1772
Bactroban Cream (One report) 1366
Bactroban Ointment (Less than 1%) 1368
▲ Benzaclin Topical Gel (3%) *2721
Brovana Inhalation Solution (Less than 2%) 2990
Campral Tablets (Infrequent) 1158
▲ Carac Cream 0.5% (83.4%) 2722
Celebrex Capsules (0.1% to 1.9%) 2979
Celexa (Infrequent) 1160
Chantix Tablets (Infrequent) 2511
Cipro XR Tablets (Less than 1%) 2823
▲ Clolar for Intravenous Infusion (10%) 1239
Copaxone for Injection (Infrequent) 3110
Cozaar Tablets (Less than 1%) 1973
Crixivan Capsules 1979
Depakote ER Tablets (Greater than 1%) 423
Diprolene Lotion 0.05% (Infrequent) 2838
Diprolene Ointment 0.05% 2839
Diprolene AF Cream 0.05% (Infrequent) 2837
▲ Doxil Injection (1% to 10%) 2378
▲ Duac Topical Gel (0% to 15%) 3054
Effexor XR Extended-Release Capsules (Infrequent) 3195
Elocon Cream 0.1% (Infrequent) 2840
Elocon Ointment 0.1% (Infrequent) 2842
▲ Eloxatin for Injection (5% to 6%) 2731
Emsam Transdermal System (Infrequent) 905
Enablex Extended-Release Tablets (Greater than or equal to 1%) 2225
▲ Erbitux (0% to 49%) 912
Evoxac Capsules (Less than 1%) 1013
Exforge Tablets (Less than or equal to 0.1%) 2238
▲ Finacea Gel (1% to 5%) 1742
Follistim AQ Cartridge 2844
Gabitril Tablets (Frequent) 973
Gengraf Capsules (1% to less than 3%) 435
Gleevec Tablets (Less common) 2255
Imitrex Injection 1465
Imitrex Nasal Spray 1470
Imitrex Tablets (Rare) 1474
Intelence Tablets (Less than 2%) 3119
▲ Intron A for Injection (Up to 10%) 2859
Kaletra (Less than 2%) 452
Klonopin (Infrequent) 2639
▲ Lamictal (2% to 5%) 1488
Lescol Capsules 2268
Lescol XL Tablets 2268
Lexapro Oral Suspension (Infrequent) 1174
Lexapro Tablets (Infrequent) 1174
Lipitor Tablets (Less than 2%) 2501
Lotrisone (1.6%) 2881
Lunesta Tablets (Infrequent) 2994
Luvox CR Extended-Release Capsules (Infrequent) 1759
Luxíq Foam 3058
Lyrica Capsules (0.1% to 1%) 2527
Mevacor Tablets 2063
Mirapex Tablets 857
Myleran Tablets (Rare) 1530
Neoral Oral Solution (1% to less than 3%) 2280
Neoral Soft Gelatin Capsules (1% to less than 3%) 2280
▲ Nexavar Tablets (10% to 11%) 784
Niaspan Extended-Release Tablets 480
Norvir (Less than 2%) 489
Olux Foam (One case) 3061
OxyContin Tablets (Less than 1%) 2589
Paxil (Infrequent) 1535
Paxil CR Controlled-Release Tablets (Infrequent) 1544
▲ PegIntron Powder for Injection (11%) 2903
Pentasa Capsules (Less than 1%) 3030
Pepcid Tablets (Infrequent) 2075
Pletal Tablets (Less than 2%) 2481
ProAmatine Tablets (Rare) 3032
Protonix for Delayed-Release Oral Suspension (Less than 1%) 3254
Protonix Delayed-Release Tablets (Less than 1%) 3254
▲ Protopic Ointment (Up to 3%) 628
Provigil Tablets (1%) 977
▲ Rebetol (23% to 24%) 2917
Remeron Tablets (Infrequent) 2924
RemeronSolTab Tablets (Infrequent) 2927
Risperdal Consta Long-Acting Injection (Up to 2%) 1753
Rythmol SR Capsules 1590
Salagen Tablets (Less than 1%) 1082
Sanctura XR Capsules (Less than 1%) 557
▲ Soriatane Capsules (25% to 50%) 3062
Sular Extended Release Tablets (Less than or equal to 1%) 2975
▲ Sutent Capsules (0% to 17%) 2540
Symbyax Capsules (Infrequent) 1871
▲ Tarceva Tablets (0% to 12%) 1228
▲ Targretin Capsules (9.4% to 10.7%) 1084
▲ Tasigna Capsules (1% to 10%) 2316
▲ Taxotere Injection Concentrate (0% to 5.7%) 2773
▲ Temodar Capsules (5%) 2931
▲ Torisel Injection (1% to 11%) 3272
▲ Trisenox Injection (15%) 986
▲ Tykerb Tablets (0% to 10%) 1631
Varivax (Greater than or equal to 1%) 2133
▲ Vectibix (0% to 10%) 597
Venlafaxine Hydrochloride Tablets (Infrequent) 2199
▲ Vesanoid Capsules (77%) 2660
Vytorin 10/10 Tablets 2149
Vytorin 10/10 Tablets 2939
Vytorin 10/20 Tablets 2149
Vytorin 10/20 Tablets 2939
Vytorin 10/40 Tablets 2149
Vytorin 10/40 Tablets 2939
Vytorin 10/80 Tablets 2149
Vytorin 10/80 Tablets 2939
Wellbutrin Tablets (Infrequent) 1648
Xenical Capsules (2.1%) 2672
Ziana Gel (1%) 1942
Zocor Tablets 2136
Zonegran Capsules (Infrequent) 1089
Zovirax Cream (Less than 1%) 817
Zyban Sustained-Release Tablets (2%) 1692
Zyprexa Tablets (Infrequent) 1883
Zyprexa ZYDIS Orally Disintegrating Tablets (Infrequent) 1883
Zyrtec Chewable Tablets (Less than 2%) 1920
Zyrtec Syrup (Less than 2%) 1920
Zyrtec Tablets (Less than 2%) 1920
Zyrtec-D 12 Hour Extended Release Tablets (Less than 2%) 1923

Xerostomia

▲ Abilify Injection (2% to 5%) 881
▲ Abilify Injection (2% to 5%) 2466
▲ Abilify Oral Solution (2% to 5%) 881
▲ Abilify Oral Solution (2% to 5%) 2466
▲ Abilify Discmelt Orally Disintegrating Tablets (2% to 5%) 881
▲ Abilify Discmelt Orally Disintegrating Tablets (2% to 5%) 2466
▲ Abilify Tablets (2% to 5%) 881
▲ Abilify Tablets (2% to 5%) 2466
Accutane Capsules 2607
Aceon Tablets (2 mg, 4 mg, 8 mg) (0.3% to 1%) 3038
Aciphex Tablets 1053
Actiq (1% to 2%) 959
Actonel with Calcium Tablets (1.4% to 2.5%) 2574
▲ Adderall XR Capsules (35%) 3012
Adenoscan (Less than 1%) 605
Adipex-P 1185
Advair Diskus 100/50 1276
Advair Diskus 250/50 1276
Advair Diskus 500/50 1276
Advair HFA 45/21 Inhalation Aerosol 1288
Advair HFA 115/21 Inhalation Aerosol 1288
Advair HFA 230/21 Inhalation Aerosol 1288
Advicor Tablets 402
Alferon N Injection (One patient) 1726
Alimta for Injection (Less than 1%) 1786
Allegra-D 12 Hour Extended-Release Tablets (2.8%) 2687
Allegra-D 24 Hour Extended-Release Tablets (2.8%) 2690
Aloxi Injection (Less than 1%) 1059
▲ Alphagan P Ophthalmic Solution (Approximately 5% to 9%) 549
Alvesco Inhalation Aerosol (Less than 1%) 2985
▲ Ambien Tablets (3%) 2692
AmBisome for Injection (Less common) 606
Amitiza Capsules (0% to 1%) 3082
Amrix Capsules 966
Anaprox Tablets (Less than 1%) 2632
Anaprox DS Tablets (Less than 1%) 2632
Aricept Tablets (Infrequent) 1062
Aricept ODT Tablets (Infrequent) 1062
▲ Arimidex Tablets (4% to 6%) 672
Asacol Delayed-Release Tablets 2579
▲ Atrovent HFA Inhalation Aerosol (1.6% to 4%) 839
Atrovent Nasal Spray 0.03% (Less than 2%) 834
Atrovent Nasal Spray 0.06% (1.4%) 836
Avalide Tablets 892
Avalide Tablets 2713
▲ Avastin IV (4% to 7%) 1192
Avelox (Greater than or equal to 0.1% to less than 2%) 2803
▲ Avinza Capsules (5% to 10%) 1772
Axert Tablets (1%) 2431
Axid Capsules (1.4%) 1364
▲ Azilect Tablets (6%) 3106
▲ Azmacort Inhalation Aerosol (1% to 3%) 407
Azopt Ophthalmic Suspension (Less than 1%) 540
Bactroban Nasal (Less than 1%) 1367
▲ Bentyl Capsules (33%) 703
▲ Bentyl Injection (33%) 703
▲ Bentyl Syrup (33%) 703
▲ Bentyl Tablets (33%) 703
▲ Betimol Ophthalmic Solution (More than 5%) 3181
Brovana Inhalation Solution 2990
▲ Busulfex Injection (26%) 2477
Calcijex Injection 419
▲ Campral Tablets (1% to 3%) 1158
Captopril Tablets (About 0.5% to 2%) 2182
Carafate Suspension (Less than 0.5%) 706
Carafate Tablets (Less than 0.5%) 707
Carbatrol Capsules 3019
Cardizem LA Extended Release Tablets (Less than 2%) 421
▲ Catapres Tablets (40 of 100 patients) 841
▲ Catapres-TTS (25 of 101 patients) 842
Celebrex Capsules (0.1% to 1.9%) 2979
▲ Celexa (1% to 20%) 1160
▲ CellCept Capsules (3% to less than 20%) 2622
▲ CellCept Intravenous (3% to less than 20%) 2622
▲ CellCept Oral Suspension (3% to less than 20%) 2622
▲ CellCept Tablets (3% to less than 20%) 2622
▲ Chantix Tablets (4% to 6%) 2511
Cialis Tablets (Less than 2%) 1792
Cipro I.V. (1% or less) 2817
Cipro XR Tablets (Less than 1%) 2823
▲ Clarinex Tablets (3%) 2828
▲ Clarinex Reditabs Tablets (3%) 2828
▲ Clarinex-D 12-Hour Extended-Release Tablets (8%) 2831
▲ Clarinex-D 24-Hour Extended-Release Tablets (8%) 2834
Clinoril Tablets (Less than 1%) 1962
▲ Clorpres Tablets (40%) 2185
▲ Combigan Ophthalmic Solution (1% to 5%) 553
Combivent Inhalation Aerosol (Less than 2%) 845
▲ Comtan Tablets (3%) 2208
▲ Concerta Extended-Release Tablets (14%) 1925
Copaxone for Injection (At least 2%) 3110
Coreg Tablets (Greater than 0.1% to 1%) 1387
Coreg CR Extended-Release Capsules (0.1% to less than or equal to 1%) 1393
Cosopt Sterile Ophthalmic Solution (Less than 1%) 1969
Cozaar Tablets (Less than 1%) 1973
Crinone 4% Gel 992
Crinone 8% Gel 992
Cubicin for Injection (Less than 1%) 995
▲ Cymbalta Delayed-Release Capsules (5% to 18%) 1801
Demadex Injection 2630
Demadex Tablets 2630
Demser Capsules (Infrequent) 1989
▲ Depakote ER Tablets (Greater than 1% to less than 5%) 423
Dexedrine 1401
Diovan Tablets (Greater than 0.2%) 2212
Diovan HCT Tablets (Greater than 0.2%) 2216
Donnatal Extentabs 2507
▲ Doxil Injection (1% to 10%) 2378
▲ Duragesic Transdermal System (10% or more) 2405
Dyazide Capsules 1405
DynaCirc CR Controlled Release Tablets (0.5% to 1%) 1407
Dyrenium Capsules (Rare) 3189
EC-Naprosyn Delayed-Release Tablets (Less than 1%) 2632
▲ Effexor XR Extended-Release Capsules (5% to 17%) 3195
▲ Eldepryl Capsules (3 of 49 patients) 3052
Elocon Lotion 0.1% (1 in 65 patients) 2841
▲ Eloxatin for Injection (2% to 5%) 2731
Emend Capsules (Greater than 0.5%) 1992
Emend for Injection (Greater than 0.5%) 1999
▲ Emsam Transdermal System (8%) 905
▲ Enablex Extended-Release Tablets (18.7% to 35.3%) 2225
Enbrel for Injection 569
▲ Equetro Extended-Release Capsules (8%) 3174
▲ Erbitux (0% to 11%) 912
▲ Evoxac Capsules (1% to 3%) 1013
Exelon Capsules (Infrequent) 2229
Exelon Oral Solution (Infrequent) 2229
Exforge Tablets (Greater than or equal to 0.2%) 2238
Exubera Inhalation Powder (2.4%) 2515
Fentora Tablets (Greater than 1%) 968
▲ Flector Patch (3%) 561
Flumadine (1.5%) 1167
▲ Focalin XR Capsules (7% to 20%) 2251
Foradil Aerolizer (1.2%) 2849
▲ Frova Tablets (3%) 1111
Furosemide Tablets 2186
Gabitril Tablets (1% or more) 973
Gengraf Capsules (1% to less than 3%) 435
▲ Geodon (4% to 5%) 2520
Imitrex Injection 1465
Imitrex Nasal Spray (Infrequent) 1470
Imitrex Tablets 1474
Intelence Tablets (Less than 2%) 3119
Intravenous Sodium Diuril 2490
▲ Intron A for Injection (Up to 28%) 2859
▲ Invega Extended-Release Tablets (1% to 3%) 1748
Ionsys Transdermal System (.1% to less than 1%) 2410
Kaletra (Less than 2%) 452
Ketek Tablets (Greater than or equal to 0.2% to less than 2%) 2744
Klonopin 2639
▲ Lamictal (6%) 1488
Levitra Tablets (Less than 2%) 2876
▲ Lexapro Oral Suspension (4% to 9%) 1174
▲ Lexapro Tablets (4% to 9%) 1174
Lipitor Tablets (Less than 2%) 2501
Lovaza Capsules 1520
▲ Lunesta Tablets (3% to 7%) 2994
▲ Lupron Depot 3.75 mg (Less than 5%) 462
▲ Lupron Depot–3 Month 11.25 mg (Less than 5%) 462
▲ Luvox CR Extended-Release Capsules (10% to 11%) 1759
▲ Lyrica Capsules (3% to 15%) 2527
▲ Marplan Tablets (6% to 9%) 3177
Maxair Autohaler (1.3%) 1705
▲ Maxalt Tablets (3%) 2056
▲ Maxalt-MLT Orally Disintegrating Tablets (3%) 2056
▲ Megace ES Oral Suspension (1% to 3%) 2499
▲ Meridia Capsules (17.2%) 475
Mevacor Tablets (0.5% to 1%) 2063
Miacalcin Nasal Spray (Less than 1%) 2274
Micardis Tablets (More than 0.3%) 852

Micardis HCT Tablets 854
▲ Mirapex Tablets (Greater than or equal to 1% to 7%) 857
Moban Tablets (Occasional) 1116
Mobic Oral Suspension (Less than 2%) 863
Mobic Tablets (Less than 2%) 863
MS Contin Tablets (Less frequent) 2585
Nadolol Tablets (1 to 5 of 1000 patients) 2191
Nalfon Capsules (Less than 1%) 2508
Naprosyn Suspension (Less than 1%) 2632
Naprosyn Tablets (Less than 1%) 2632
Neoral Oral Solution (1% to less than 3%) 2280
Neoral Soft Gelatin Capsules (1% to less than 3%) 2280
▲ Neupro Transdermal System (3%) 3149
▲ Nexavar Tablets (1% to less than 10%) 784
Nexium Delayed-Release Capsules (Greater than or equal to 1%) 645
Nexium I.V. (Greater than or equal to 1%) 652
Nexium Delayed-Release Oral Suspension (Greater than or equal to 1%) 645
Niaspan Extended-Release Tablets 480
Noroxin Tablets (0.3% to 1%) 2069
Norvir (Less than 2%) 489
Noxafil Oral Suspension (1% to 2%) 2889
Omnicef Capsules (0.3%) 497
▲ Opana Tablets (1% to less than 10%) 1117
▲ Opana ER Tablets (1% to less than 10%) 1121
▲ OxyContin Tablets (6%) 2589
Parnate Tablets 1532
Patanase Nasal Spray (0.9%) 544
▲ Paxil (1% to 20.6%) 1535
▲ Paxil CR Controlled-Release Tablets (1% to 20.6%) 1544
▲ PegIntron Powder for Injection (6%) 2903
Pepcid Tablets (Infrequent) 2075
Percocet Tablets 1127
Percodan Tablets 1130
▲ Perforomist Inhalation Solution (3.3%) 1025
Prinivil Tablets (0.3% to 1%) 2087
Prinzide Tablets (0.3% to 1%) 2092
▲ Pristiq Extended-Release Tablets (11% to 25%) 3247
ProAmatine Tablets (Less frequent) 3032
▲ Prometrium Capsules (100 mg, 200 mg) (Less than 5%) 3047
Protonix for Delayed-Release Oral Suspension (Less than 1%) 3254
Protonix Delayed-Release Tablets (Less than 1%) 3254
Protonix I.V. (Less than 1%) 3257
Protopic Ointment (0.2% to less than 1%) 628
Proventil HFA Inhalation Aerosol (Less than 3%) 2914
▲ Provigil Tablets (4%) 977
▲ Prozac Weekly Capsules (4% to 12%) 1852
▲ Prozac Pulvules and Liquid (4% to 12%) 1852
▲ Pulmicort Flexhaler (Greater than or equal to 1% to 3%) 654
Pylera Capsules 714
▲ Rebetol (8% to 12%) 2917
▲ Rebif Prefilled Syringe for Injection (1% to 5%) 1107
▲ Remeron Tablets (25%) 2924
▲ RemeronSolTab Tablets (25%) 2927
ReoPro Vials (0.1%) 1860
▲ Requip Tablets (3% to 5%) 1561
Requip XL Tablets (2%) 1568
▲ Rilutek Tablets (2% to 3%) 2771
▲ Risperdal Consta Long-Acting Injection (5% to 7%) 1753
Rocaltrol Capsules 1150
Rocaltrol Oral Solution 1150
▲ Romazicon Injection (3% to 9%) 2646
▲ Rythmol Tablets (2% to 6%) 1586
▲ Rythmol SR Capsules (1% to 4%) 1590
Salagen Tablets (Less than 1%) 1082
▲ Sanctura XR Capsules (10.7% to 11.1%) 557
Solodyn Extended Release Tablets (1%) 1938
▲ Spiriva HandiHaler (12% to 16%) 870
▲ Stalevo Tablets (3%) 2309
▲ Strattera Capsules (1% to 21%) 1864
Sular Extended Release Tablets (Less than or equal to 1%) 2975
▲ Sutent Capsules (12%) 2540
▲ Symbyax Capsules (11% to 16%) 1871
Targretin Capsules 1084
Tarka Tablets (0.3% or more) 511
Tasigna Capsules (0.1% to 1%) 2316
Teveten Tablets (Less than 1%) 515
Teveten HCT Tablets (Less than 1%) 517
Thioridazine Hydrochloride Tablets 2195
Thiothixene Capsules (Infrequently) 2197
Timoptic Sterile Ophthalmic Solution (Less frequent) 2121
Timoptic in Ocudose (Less frequent) 2124
Timoptic-XE Sterile Ophthalmic Gel Forming Solution 2125
Toprol-XL Tablets (About 1 of 100 patients) 666
▲ Transderm Scōp Transdermal Therapeutic System (29% to about two-thirds) 2206
Treanda for Injection 983
Treximet Tablets (2%) 1616
Tricor Tablets 520
▲ Trisenox Injection (8%) 986
Trusopt Sterile Ophthalmic Solution 2128
Tygacil for Injection (0% to less than 2%) 3276
Ultane Liquid for Inhalation (Less than 1%) 524
▲ Ultram ER Extended-Release Tablets (5% to 9.8%) 2428
Valium Tablets 2658
▲ Vaprisol (3.8%) 632
▲ Venlafaxine Hydrochloride Tablets (2% to 22%) 2199
▲ VESIcare Tablets (10.9% to 27.6%) 636
Viadur Implant (Less than 2%) 802
▲ Vicoprofen Tablets (3% to 9%) 533
▲ Vivitrol (4% to 24%) 988
Voltaren Tablets (Occasionally) 2334
Voltaren-XR Tablets (Occasionally) 2337
▲ Vyvanse Capsules (5% to 26%) 3033
▲ Wellbutrin Tablets (27.6%) 1648
▲ Wellbutrin SR Sustained-Release Tablets (5% to 24%) 1653
▲ Wellbutrin XL Extended-Release Tablets (5% to 26%) 1659
▲ Xeloda Tablets (Less than 1% to 6%) 2662
Xopenex Inhalation Solution 3001
Xopenex Inhalation Solution Concentrate 3005
Xopenex HFA Inhalation Aerosol 3009
▲ Xyzal Oral Solution (2% to 3%) 2789
▲ Xyzal Oral Solution (2% to 3%) 3155
▲ Xyzal Tablets (2% to 3%) 2789
▲ Xyzal Tablets (2% to 3%) 3155
▲ Zemplar Capsules (3%) 536
▲ Zemplar Injection (3%) 538
Zofran (1% to 2%) 1687
Zofran ODT Orally Disintegrating Tablets (1% to 2%) 1687
▲ Zolinza Capsules (14% to 16.3%) 2142
Zometa for Intravenous Infusion 2341
▲ Zomig Tablets (1% to 3%) 694
▲ Zomig Nasal Spray (1% to 3%) 689
▲ Zomig-ZMT Tablets (1% to 3%) 694
Zonegran Capsules (2%) 1089
▲ Zyban Sustained-Release Tablets (10% to 11%) 1692
▲ Zyprexa Tablets (2% to 32%) 1883
Zyprexa IntraMuscular 1883
▲ Zyprexa ZYDIS Orally Disintegrating Tablets (2% to 32%) 1883
▲ Zyrtec Chewable Tablets (5%) 1920
▲ Zyrtec Syrup (5%) 1920
▲ Zyrtec Tablets (5%) 1920
▲ Zyrtec-D 12 Hour Extended Release Tablets (3.6% to 5%) 1923

Y

Yawning

Ambien Tablets (Rare) 2692
Ambien CR Tablets (Rare) 2696
Celexa (2%) 1160
Cymbalta Delayed-Release Capsules (Frequent to 2%) 1801
▲ Effexor XR Extended-Release Capsules (3% to 5%) 3195
Emsam Transdermal System (Infrequent) 905
Evoxac Capsules 1013
Imitrex Injection (Rare) 1465
Imitrex Nasal Spray 1470
Imitrex Tablets 1474
Klonopin (Infrequent) 2639
Lamictal (Infrequent) 1488
Lexapro Oral Suspension (2%) 1174
Lexapro Tablets (2%) 1174
▲ Luvox CR Extended-Release Capsules (2% to 5%) 1759
Lyrica Capsules (Rare) 2527
Maxalt Tablets (Infrequent) 2056
Maxalt-MLT Orally Disintegrating Tablets (Infrequent) 2056
Meridia Capsules 475
▲ Paxil (4%) 1535
▲ Paxil CR Controlled-Release Tablets (4%) 1544
▲ Pristiq Extended-Release Tablets (1% to 4%) 3247
▲ Prozac Weekly Capsules (1% to 11%) 1852
▲ Prozac Pulvules and Liquid (3%) 1852
▲ Requip Tablets (Infrequent to 3%) 1561
Rilutek Tablets (Infrequent) 2771
Salagen Tablets (Less than 1%) 1082
Symbyax Capsules (Infrequent) 1871
Ultram ER Extended-Release Tablets (0.5% to less than 1%) 2428
▲ Venlafaxine Hydrochloride Tablets (3% to 8%) 2199
Zomig Tablets (Infrequent) 694
Zomig Nasal Spray (Rare) 689
Zomig-ZMT Tablets (Infrequent) 694

Z

Zinc, increased excretion of

Cuprimine Capsules (Rare) 1986
Sandostatin LAR Depot 2302

SECTION 4

INDICATIONS INDEX

This section lists in alphabetical order every indication cited in *PDR®* and its companion volumes, with cross-references to each product entry in which the indication is found. For easy comparison, each listing includes the product's brand name, generic ingredients, and manufacturer. Page numbers refer to the 2009 editions of *PDR®*, *PDR® For Ophthalmic Medicines* and *PDR® For Nonprescription Drugs, Dietary Supplements and Herbs.* A key to the symbols denoting the companion volumes appears in the bottom margin.

Because *PDR®* publishes only official product labeling, only approved indications are cited here. No unapproved uses are listed.

This index is intended to assist you in identifying the extent and nature of your prescribing alternatives as quickly and easily as possible. However, it is by its nature only an extract of the official labeling as it appears in *PDR®*. For more definitive information, always consult the underlying *PDR®* text.

A

A. baumanii infections
Zosyn for Injection (Piperacillin Sodium, Tazobactam Sodium) Wyeth 3284

Abrasions, pain associated with
(*see under* Pain, topical relief of)

Abrasions, skin
(*see under* Infections, skin, bacterial, minor)

Abscess, cutaneous
(*see also under* Infections, skin and skin structure)
Levaquin (Levofloxacin) Ortho-McNeil 2416
Levaquin in 5% Dextrose Injection (Levofloxacin) Ortho-McNeil 2416
Zosyn for Injection (Piperacillin Sodium, Tazobactam Sodium) Wyeth 3284

Abscess, hepatic
(*see under* Infections, intra-abdominal)

Abscess, intra-abdominal
(*see also under* Infections, intra-abdominal)
Cancidas for Injection (Caspofungin acetate) Merck 1953

Abscess, lung
(*see under* Infections, lower respiratory tract)

Abscess, tubo-ovarian
(*see under* Infections, gynecologic)

Acetaminophen overdose, management of
Acetadote Injection (Acetylcysteine) Cumberland 1001

Aches
(*see under* Pain, general)

Aches, muscular
(*see under* Pain, muscular, temporary relief of)

Aches due to common cold
(*see under* Pain associated with upper respiratory infection)

Acid indigestion
(*see under* Hyperacidity, gastric, symptomatic relief of)

Acinetobacter baumannii urinary tract infections
Doribax Injection (Doripenem) Ortho-McNeil 2400

Acinetobacter calcoaceticus infections
Primaxin I.M. (Cilastatin Sodium, Imipenem) Merck 2080
Rocephin Injectable Vials, ADD-Vantage, Galaxy, Bulk (Ceftriaxone Sodium) Roche 2642

Acinetobacter calcoaceticus infections, ocular
Quixin Ophthalmic Solution (Levofloxacin) Vistakon 3184
Zylet Ophthalmic Suspension (Loteprednol Etabonate, Tobramycin) Bausch & Lomb .... ⊙247

Acinetobacter calcoaceticus skin and skin structure infections
Primaxin I.M. (Cilastatin Sodium, Imipenem) Merck 2080

Acinetobacter iwoffi
Vigamox Ophthalmic Solution (Moxifloxacin Hydrochloride) Alcon 548

Acinetobacter species infections
Doribax Injection (Doripenem) Ortho-McNeil 2400
Primaxin I.M. (Cilastatin Sodium, Imipenem) Merck 2080
Primaxin I.V. (Cilastatin Sodium, Imipenem) Merck 2083

Acinetobacter species lower respiratory tract infections
Primaxin I.V. (Cilastatin Sodium, Imipenem) Merck 2083

Acinetobacter species skin and skin structure infections
Primaxin I.M. (Cilastatin Sodium, Imipenem) Merck 2080
Primaxin I.V. (Cilastatin Sodium, Imipenem) Merck 2083
Rocephin Injectable Vials, ADD-Vantage, Galaxy, Bulk (Ceftriaxone Sodium) Roche 2642

Acne, cystic, severe recalcitrant
Accutane Capsules (Isotretinoin) Roche 2607

Acne rosacea
Rosac Wash (Sodium Sulfacetamide) Stiefel 3062

Acne rosacea, ocular
Lotemax Ophthalmic Suspension 0.5% (Loteprednol Etabonate) Bausch & Lomb .... ⊙241
Zylet Ophthalmic Suspension (Loteprednol Etabonate, Tobramycin) Bausch & Lomb .... ⊙247

Acne vulgaris
Aczone Gel 5% (Dapsone) Allergan 3296
Benzaclin Topical Gel (Benzoyl Peroxide, Clindamycin Phosphate) sanofi-aventis 2721
Brevoxyl-4 Creamy Wash (Benzoyl Peroxide) Stiefel 3054
Brevoxyl-4 Gel (Benzoyl Peroxide) Stiefel 3054
Brevoxyl-8 Creamy Wash (Benzoyl Peroxide) Stiefel 3054
Brevoxyl-8 Gel (Benzoyl Peroxide) Stiefel 3054
Duac Topical Gel (Benzoyl Peroxide, Clindamycin) Stiefel 3054
Evoclin Foam, 1% (Clindamycin Phosphate) Stiefel 3056
Ortho Tri-Cyclen Tablets (Ethinyl Estradiol, Norgestimate) Ortho Women's 2449
Rosac Wash (Sodium Sulfacetamide) Stiefel 3062
Solodyn Extended Release Tablets (Minocycline Hydrochloride) Medicis 1938
Yaz Tablets (Ethinyl Estradiol, Drospirenone) Bayer HealthCare Pharmaceuticals 805
Ziana Gel (Clindamycin Phosphate, Tretinoin) Medicis 1942

Acquired immunodeficiency syndrome
(*see under* Infections, human immunodeficiency virus)

Acromegaly
Sandostatin Injection (Octreotide Acetate) Novartis 2300
Sandostatin LAR Depot (Octreotide Acetate) Novartis 2302
Somatuline Depot Injection (Lanreotide) Tercica 3102

Adenocarcinoma, cervical, prevention of
Gardasil Injection (Quadrivalent Human Papillomavirus (Types 6, 11, 16, 18) Recombinant Vaccine) Merck 2019

Adenoma, islet cell, insulin-secreting
Proglycem Capsules (Diazoxide) Gate 1185
Proglycem Suspension (Diazoxide) Gate 1185

Adenomatous polyposis, familial
Celebrex Capsules (Celecoxib) Searle 2979

Adenosine deaminase, enzyme replacement therapy for
Flebogamma 5% (Globulin, Immune (Human)) Grifols 1715
Flebogamma 5% DIF (Immune Globulin Intravenous (Human)) Grifols 1718
Gamunex (Immune Globulin Intravenous (Human)) Talecris 3094

ADHD
(*see under* Attention Deficit Hyperactivity Disorder)

Aerobacter aerogenes infections
(*see under* Enterobacter aerogenes infections)

Agammaglobulinemias, congenital
Gammagard Liquid (Immune Globulin Intravenous (Human)) Baxter Healthcare 730
Gammagard S/D (Immune Globulin Intravenous (Human)) Baxter Healthcare 734
Gamunex (Immune Globulin Intravenous (Human)) Talecris 3094

Agitation associated with bipolar disorder
Abilify Injection (Aripiprazole) Bristol-Myers Squibb 881
Abilify Injection (Aripiprazole) Otsuka 2466
Zyprexa IntraMuscular (Olanzapine) Lilly 1883

Agitation associated with schizophrenia
Abilify Injection (Aripiprazole) Bristol-Myers Squibb 881
Abilify Injection (Aripiprazole) Otsuka 2466
Zyprexa IntraMuscular (Olanzapine) Lilly 1883

AIDS
(*see under* Infections, human immunodeficiency virus)

AIDS related complex
(*see under* Infections, acquired immunodeficiency syndrome-related complex)

Airway obstruction disorders
(*see under* Bronchial asthma; Emphysema)

Alcohol dependence
Vivitrol (Naltrexone) Cephalon 988

Alcohol withdrawal, acute, symptomatic relief of
Valium Tablets (Diazepam) Roche 2658

Alcoholism, chronic, an aid in the management of
Campral Tablets (Acamprosate Calcium) Forest 1158

Allergic reactions, drug-induced
(*see under* Hypersensitivity reactions, drug-induced)

Allergic reactions, general
EpiPen (Epinephrine) Dey 1024

Allergic rhinitis
(*see under* Rhinitis, allergic)

Allergies, respiratory
Actifed Cold & Allergy Tablets (Chlorpheniramine Maleate, Phenylephrine Hydrochloride) McNeil Consumer 1895
Benadryl Severe Allergy & Sinus Headache Caplets (Acetaminophen, Diphenhydramine Hydrochloride, Phenylephrine Hydrochloride) McNeil Consumer 1897
Benadryl Dye-Free Allergy Liqui-gels Softgels (Diphenhydramine Hydrochloride) McNeil Consumer 1897
Benadryl Allergy Kapgels (Diphenhydramine Hydrochloride) McNeil Consumer 1895
Benadryl Allergy Quick Dissolve Strips (Diphenhydramine Hydrochloride) McNeil Consumer 1896
Benadryl Allergy Ultratab Tablets (Diphenhydramine Hydrochloride) McNeil Consumer 1896
Children's Benadryl Dye-Free Allergy Liquid (Diphenhydramine Hydrochloride) McNeil Consumer 1897
Children's Benadryl Allergy Fastmelts (Diphenhydramine Hydrochloride) McNeil Consumer 1897
Children's Benadryl Allergy Liquid (Diphenhydramine Hydrochloride) McNeil Consumer 1898
Children's Benadryl Allergy Perfect Measure (Diphenhydramine Hydrochloride) McNeil Consumer 1896
Children's Benadryl-D Allergy & Sinus Liquid (Diphenhydramine Hydrochloride, Phenylephrine Hydrochloride) McNeil Consumer 1896
Benadryl-D Allergy & Sinus Tablet (Diphenhydramine Hydrochloride, Phenylephrine Hydrochloride) McNeil Consumer 1896
PediaCare Children's Allergy & Cold Liquid (Diphenhydramine Hydrochloride, Phenylephrine Hydrochloride) McNeil Consumer 1902
PediaCare Children's Allergy Liquid (Diphenhydramine Hydrochloride) McNeil Consumer 1902
PediaCare Children's Decongestant Liquid (Phenylephrine Hydrochloride) McNeil Consumer 1902
PediaCare Children's Liquid Multi-Symptom Cold (Dextromethorphan Hydrobromide, Phenylephrine Hydrochloride) McNeil Consumer 1902
Sudafed 12 Hour Nasal Decongestant Non-Drowsy Caplets (Pseudoephedrine Hydrochloride) McNeil Consumer 1909
Sudafed 24 Hour Non-Drowsy Nasal Decongestant Tablets (Pseudoephedrine Hydrochloride) McNeil Consumer 1906
Children's Sudafed Nasal Decongestant Liquid (Pseudoephedrine Hydrochloride) McNeil Consumer 1906
Children's Sudafed PE Cold & Cough Liquid (Dextromethorphan Hydrobromide, Phenylephrine Hydrochloride) McNeil Consumer 1907
Children's Sudafed PE Nasal Decongestant Liquid (Phenylephrine Hydrochloride) McNeil Consumer 1906
Sudafed Nasal Decongestant Tablets (Pseudoephedrine Hydrochloride) McNeil Consumer 1906
Sudafed OM Sinus Cold Moisturizing Nasal Spray (Oxymetazoline Hydrochloride) McNeil Consumer 1906
Sudafed OM Sinus Congestion Moisturizing Nasal Spray (Oxymetazoline Hydrochloride) McNeil Consumer 1906
Sudafed PE Nasal Decongestant Tablets (Phenylephrine Hydrochloride) McNeil Consumer 1907
Sudafed PE Sinus & Allergy Tablets (Chlorpheniramine Maleate, Phenylephrine Hydrochloride) McNeil Consumer 1908
Tussionex Pennkinetic Extended-Release Suspension (Chlorpheniramine Polistirex, Hydrocodone Polistirex) UCB, Inc. 3154
Tylenol Allergy Multi-Symptom Nighttime Caplets with Cool Burst (Acetaminophen, Diphenhydramine Hydrochloride, Phenylephrine Hydrochloride) McNeil Consumer 1916
Children's Tylenol Plus Cold & Allergy Suspension Liquid (Acetaminophen, Diphenhydramine Hydrochloride, Phenylephrine Hydrochloride) McNeil Consumer 1914
Tylenol Sinus Congestion & Pain Severe Caplets with Cool Burst (Acetaminophen, Guaifenesin, Phenylephrine Hydrochloride) McNeil Consumer 1917
Children's Zyrtec Allergy Syrup (Cetirizine Hydrochloride) McNeil Consumer 1920

Alopecia, androgenetic
Propecia Tablets (Finasteride) Merck 2095

Alzheimer's disease
(*see under* Dementia, Alzheimer's type)

Amebiasis, acute intestinal
E.E.S. (Erythromycin Ethylsuccinate) Abbott 433
EryPed (Erythromycin Ethylsuccinate) Abbott 431

Amenorrhea, secondary
Crinone 4% Gel (Progesterone) Columbia 992
Prometrium Capsules (100 mg, 200 mg) (Progesterone) Solvay 3047

Amyotrophic lateral sclerosis
Rilutek Tablets (Riluzole) sanofi-aventis 2771

Analgesia
(*see under* Pain, general)

Anaphylactoid reactions
EpiPen (Epinephrine) Dey 1024

Anaphylaxis, idiopathic
EpiPen (Epinephrine) Dey 1024

Anaphylaxis, treatment of
EpiPen (Epinephrine) Dey 1024

Androgen, absence or deficiency of
AndroGel (Testosterone) Unimed 3159
Delatestryl Injection (Testosterone Enanthate) Indevus 1730
Testim 1% Gel (Testosterone) Auxilium 701

Anemia, AZT-treated HIV-infected patients, treatment of
Epogen for Injection (Epoetin Alfa) Amgen 576
Procrit for Injection (Epoetin Alfa) Ortho Biotech 2391

Anemia, chemotherapy-induced in cancer patients
Aranesp for Injection (Darbepoetin alfa) Amgen 564
Epogen for Injection (Epoetin Alfa) Amgen 576
Procrit for Injection (Epoetin Alfa) Ortho Biotech 2391

Anemia, iron deficiency
Nu-Iron 150 Capsules (Polysaccharide Iron Complex) Merz 2165

Anemia, surgical procedure-induced, to reduce the need for allogeneic blood transfusions
Epogen for Injection (Epoetin Alfa) Amgen 576
Procrit for Injection (Epoetin Alfa) Ortho Biotech 2391

Anemia associated with chronic renal failure
Aranesp for Injection (Darbepoetin alfa) Amgen 564
Epogen for Injection (Epoetin Alfa) Amgen 576
Procrit for Injection (Epoetin Alfa) Ortho Biotech 2391

Anesthesia, general
Ultane Liquid for Inhalation (Sevoflurane) Abbott 524

Anesthesia, general, adjunct in
Nembutal Sodium Solution, USP (Pentobarbital Sodium) Ovation 2494
Nimbex Injection (Cisatracurium Besylate) Abbott 484
Zemuron Injection (Rocuronium Bromide) Schering 2947

Anesthesia, general, supplement to
(*see under* Anesthesia, general, adjunct in)

Anesthesia, local
Hurricaine Topical Anesthetic (Benzocaine) Beutlich 815

Anesthesia, local, oral cavity
Hurricaine Topical Anesthetic (Benzocaine) Beutlich 815

Anesthesia, local, pharyngeal
Hurricaine Topical Anesthetic (Benzocaine) Beutlich 815

Angina
(*see under* Angina pectoris)

Angina, crescendo
(*see under* Angina, unstable)

Angina, pre-infarction
(*see under* Angina, unstable)

Angina, reduce risk of
Advicor Tablets (Lovastatin, Niacin) Abbott 402
Lipitor Tablets (Atorvastatin Calcium) Parke-Davis 2501

Angina, unstable
Bayer Aspirin (Aspirin) Bayer HealthCare Consumer 750
Mevacor Tablets (Lovastatin) Merck 2063

Angina, unstable, adjuvant therapy for
ReoPro Vials (Abciximab) Lilly 1860

Angina, unstable, ischemic complications of, prophylaxis of
Fragmin Injection (Dalteparin Sodium) Eisai 1070
Lovenox Injection (Enoxaparin Sodium) sanofi-aventis 2756

Angina pectoris
Nitro-Dur Transdermal Infusion System (Nitroglycerin) Schering 2887
Nitrolingual Pumpspray (Nitroglycerin) Sciele 2965
Toprol-XL Tablets (Metoprolol Succinate) AstraZeneca LP 666

Angina pectoris, acute, prophylaxis
Nitrolingual Pumpspray (Nitroglycerin) Sciele 2965

Angina pectoris, reduce complications from
Bayer Aspirin (Aspirin) Bayer HealthCare Consumer 750

Angiography, fluorescein, fundus
Fluorescite Injection (Fluorescein Sodium) Alcon .... ⊙203

Angiography, fluorescein, iris vasculature
Fluorescite Injection (Fluorescein Sodium) Alcon .... ⊙203

Ankylosing spondylitis
Anaprox Tablets (Naproxen Sodium) Roche 2632

Anaprox DS Tablets (Naproxen Sodium) Roche ... 2632
Celebrex Capsules (Celecoxib) Searle ... 2979
Clinoril Tablets (Sulindac) Merck ... 1962
EC-Naprosyn Delayed-Release Tablets (Naproxen) Roche ... 2632
Enbrel for Injection (Etanercept) Amgen ... 569
Humira Injection (Adalimumab) Abbott ... 442
Indocin (Indomethacin) Merck ... 2024
Naprosyn Suspension (Naproxen) Roche ... 2632
Naprosyn Tablets (Naproxen) Roche ... 2632
Remicade for IV Injection (Infliximab) Centocor ... 950
Traumeel Injection Solution (Homeopathic Formulations) Heel ... 1725
Voltaren Tablets (Diclofenac Sodium) Novartis ... 2334

Anorexia associated with weight loss, AIDS-induced
Marinol Capsules (Dronabinol) Unimed ... 3163
Megace ES Oral Suspension (Megestrol Acetate) Par ... 2499

Anterior segment inflammation
(*see under* Inflammation, anterior segment)

Anthrax
(*see under* B. anthracis infections)

Anxiety, short-term symptomatic relief of
Hyland's Nerve Tonic Tablets and Caplets (Homeopathic Formulations) Standard Homeopathic ... ▣620
Valium Tablets (Diazepam) Roche ... 2658

Anxiety disorder, generalized
Cymbalta Delayed-Release Capsules (Duloxetine Hydrochloride) Lilly ... 1801
Effexor XR Extended-Release Capsules (Venlafaxine Hydrochloride) Wyeth ... 3195
Lexapro Oral Suspension (Escitalopram Oxalate) Forest ... 1174
Lexapro Tablets (Escitalopram Oxalate) Forest ... 1174
Paxil (Paroxetine Hydrochloride) GlaxoSmithKline ... 1535

Anxiety disorder, social
Effexor XR Extended-Release Capsules (Venlafaxine Hydrochloride) Wyeth ... 3195
Luvox CR Extended-Release Capsules (Fluvoxamine Maleate) Jazz ... 1759
Paxil (Paroxetine Hydrochloride) GlaxoSmithKline ... 1535
Paxil CR Controlled-Release Tablets (Paroxetine Hydrochloride) GlaxoSmithKline ... 1544

Anxiety disorders, management of
Valium Tablets (Diazepam) Roche ... 2658

Aphthous ulcers
(*see under* Stomatitis, recurrent aphthous, symptomatic relief of)

Apnea, sleep
Provigil Tablets (Modafinil) Cephalon ... 977

Appendicitis, gangrenous
Primaxin I.M. (Cilastatin Sodium, Imipenem) Merck ... 2080

Appendicitis, perforated
Primaxin I.M. (Cilastatin Sodium, Imipenem) Merck ... 2080

Appendicitis with peritonitis
Merrem I.V. (Meropenem) AstraZeneca Pharmaceuticals ... 684
Primaxin I.M. (Cilastatin Sodium, Imipenem) Merck ... 2080
Zosyn for Injection (Piperacillin Sodium, Tazobactam Sodium) Wyeth ... 3284

Appetite, suppression of
(*see under* Obesity, exogenous)

Apprehension
(*see under* Anxiety disorders, management of)

ARC
(*see under* Infections, acquired immunodeficiency syndrome-related complex)

Arrhythmias, ventricular
Rythmol Tablets (Propafenone Hydrochloride) GlaxoSmithKline ... 1586

Arterial occlusive disease, peripheral
Plavix Tablets (Clopidogrel Bisulfate) Bristol-Myers Squibb ... 926
Plavix Tablets (Clopidogrel Bisulfate) sanofi-aventis ... 2767

Arteritis, temporal
Triesence Injectable Suspension (Triamcinolone Acetonide) Alcon ... ⊙209

Arthralgia, topical relief of
(*see under* Pain, topical relief of)

Arthritis
(*see also under* Arthritis, rheumatoid; Arthritis, unspecified; Osteoarthritis)
Motrin IB Tablets and Caplets (Ibuprofen) McNeil Consumer ... 1900
ThermaCare Therapeutic Heat Wraps (Device) Procter & Gamble ... 2566

Arthritis, acute, gouty
Clinoril Tablets (Sulindac) Merck ... 1962
Indocin (Indomethacin) Merck ... 2024
Traumeel Injection Solution (Homeopathic Formulations) Heel ... 1725

Arthritis, juvenile
Anaprox Tablets (Naproxen Sodium) Roche ... 2632
Anaprox DS Tablets (Naproxen Sodium) Roche ... 2632
EC-Naprosyn Delayed-Release Tablets (Naproxen) Roche ... 2632
Naprosyn Suspension (Naproxen) Roche ... 2632
Naprosyn Tablets (Naproxen) Roche ... 2632
Orencia Powder for Intravenous Infusion (Abatacept) Bristol-Myers Squibb ... 921

Arthritis, osteo-
(*see under* Osteoarthritis)

Arthritis, psoriatic
Enbrel for Injection (Etanercept) Amgen ... 569
Humira Injection (Adalimumab) Abbott ... 442
Remicade for IV Injection (Infliximab) Centocor ... 950

Arthritis, rheumatoid
Anaprox Tablets (Naproxen Sodium) Roche ... 2632
Anaprox DS Tablets (Naproxen Sodium) Roche ... 2632
Bayer Aspirin (Aspirin) Bayer HealthCare Consumer ... 750
Celebrex Capsules (Celecoxib) Searle ... 2979
Clinoril Tablets (Sulindac) Merck ... 1962
Cuprimine Capsules (Penicillamine) Merck ... 1986
EC-Naprosyn Delayed-Release Tablets (Naproxen) Roche ... 2632
Enbrel for Injection (Etanercept) Amgen ... 569
Gengraf Capsules (Cyclosporine) Abbott ... 435
Humira Injection (Adalimumab) Abbott ... 442
Indocin (Indomethacin) Merck ... 2024
Kineret Injection (Anakinra) Amgen ... 585
Mobic Oral Suspension (Meloxicam) Boehringer Ingelheim ... 863
Mobic Tablets (Meloxicam) Boehringer Ingelheim ... 863
Nalfon Capsules (Fenoprofen Calcium) Pedinol ... 2508
Naprosyn Suspension (Naproxen) Roche ... 2632
Naprosyn Tablets (Naproxen) Roche ... 2632
Neoral Oral Solution (Cyclosporine) Novartis ... 2280
Neoral Soft Gelatin Capsules (Cyclosporine) Novartis ... 2280
Orencia Powder for Intravenous Infusion (Abatacept) Bristol-Myers Squibb ... 921
Remicade for IV Injection (Infliximab) Centocor ... 950
Rituxan I.V. (Rituximab) Genentech ... 1223
Voltaren Tablets (Diclofenac Sodium) Novartis ... 2334
Voltaren-XR Tablets (Diclofenac Sodium) Novartis ... 2337

Arthritis, topical adjunct to
Thera-Gesic Creme (Menthol, Methyl Salicylate) Mission ... ▣610

Arthritis, unspecified
Salonpas Aqua-Patch (Menthol) Hisamitsu ... ▣610
Salonpas Arthritis Pain Patches (Menthol, Methyl Salicylate) Hisamitsu ... ▣608
Salonpas Gel (Menthol, Methyl Salicylate) Hisamitsu ... ▣609
Salonpas Gel-Patch Hot Soothing (Capsicum Extract, Menthol) Hisamitsu ... ▣609
Salonpas Pain Relief Patch (Menthol, Methyl Salicylate) Hisamitsu ... ▣608
Salonpas-Hot Patch (Capsicum Extract) Hisamitsu ... ▣609

Articular inflammation, relief of
Zeel Injection Solution (Homeopathic Formulations) Heel ... 1726

Articular stiffness, relief of
Zeel Injection Solution (Homeopathic Formulations) Heel ... 1726

Aspergillosis
Abelcet Injection (Amphotericin B Lipid Complex) Enzon ... 1134
AmBisome for Injection (Amphotericin B, liposomal) Astellas ... 606
Cancidas for Injection (Caspofungin acetate) Merck ... 1953

Aspergillus fumigatus infections
(*see under* Aspergillosis)

Aspergillus infections, prophylaxis of
Noxafil Oral Suspension (Posaconazole) Schering ... 2889

Asthma, allergen induced
Xolair (Omalizumab) Genentech ... 1235
Xolair (Omalizumab) Novartis ... 2339

Asthma, bronchial
(*see under* Bronchial asthma)

Asthma, nocturnal
Serevent Diskus (Salmeterol Xinafoate) GlaxoSmithKline ... 1594

Astrocytoma, anaplastic
Temodar Capsules (Temozolomide) Schering ... 2931

Athetosis, adjunctive therapy in
Valium Tablets (Diazepam) Roche ... 2658

Athlete's foot
(*see under* Tinea pedis infections)

Atrial fibrillation
Lanoxin Injection (Digoxin) GlaxoSmithKline ... 1498
Lanoxin Injection Pediatric (Digoxin) GlaxoSmithKline ... 1502
Lanoxin Tablets (Digoxin) GlaxoSmithKline ... 1505
Rythmol SR Capsules (Propafenone Hydrochloride) GlaxoSmithKline ... 1590

Atrial fibrillation, paroxysmal
Rythmol Tablets (Propafenone Hydrochloride) GlaxoSmithKline ... 1586

Atrial flutter, paroxysmal
Rythmol Tablets (Propafenone Hydrochloride) GlaxoSmithKline ... 1586

Attention Deficit Hyperactivity Disorder
Adderall XR Capsules (Amphetamine Aspartate, Amphetamine Sulfate, Dextroamphetamine Saccharate, Dextroamphetamine Sulfate) Shire US ... 3012
Concerta Extended-Release Tablets (Methylphenidate Hydrochloride) McNeil Pediatrics ... 1925
Daytrana Transdermal Patch (Methylphenidate) Shire US ... 3022
Dexedrine (Dextroamphetamine Sulfate) GlaxoSmithKline ... 1401
Focalin XR Capsules (Dexmethylphenidate Hydrochloride) Novartis ... 2251
Metadate CD Capsules (Methylphenidate Hydrochloride) UCB, Inc. ... 3146
Strattera Capsules (Atomoxetine Hydrochloride) Lilly ... 1864
Vyvanse Capsules (Lisdexamfetamine Dimesylate) Shire US ... 3033

B

B. anthracis infections
Cipro (Ciprofloxacin) Schering ... 2810
Levaquin (Levofloxacin) Ortho-McNeil ... 2416
Levaquin in 5% Dextrose Injection (Levofloxacin) Ortho-McNeil ... 2416

B. caccae intra-abdominal infections
Doribax Injection (Doripenem) Ortho-McNeil ... 2400

B. distasonis infections
Invanz for Injection (Ertapenem) Merck ... 2029
Primaxin I.M. (Cilastatin Sodium, Imipenem) Merck ... 2080

B. distasonis intra-abdominal infections
Invanz for Injection (Ertapenem) Merck ... 2029
Primaxin I.M. (Cilastatin Sodium, Imipenem) Merck ... 2080

B. fragilis endomyometritis
Invanz for Injection (Ertapenem) Merck ... 2029

B. fragilis gynecologic infections
Primaxin I.V. (Cilastatin Sodium, Imipenem) Merck ... 2083

B. fragilis infections
Avelox (Moxifloxacin Hydrochloride) Schering ... 2803
Cipro I.V. (Ciprofloxacin) Schering ... 2817
Cipro (Ciprofloxacin) Schering ... 2810
Doribax Injection (Doripenem) Ortho-McNeil ... 2400
Invanz for Injection (Ertapenem) Merck ... 2029
Merrem I.V. (Meropenem) AstraZeneca Pharmaceuticals ... 684
Primaxin I.M. (Cilastatin Sodium, Imipenem) Merck ... 2080
Primaxin I.V. (Cilastatin Sodium, Imipenem) Merck ... 2083
Rocephin Injectable Vials, ADD-Vantage, Galaxy, Bulk (Ceftriaxone Sodium) Roche ... 2642
Timentin ADD-Vantage (Clavulanate Potassium, Ticarcillin Disodium) GlaxoSmithKline ... 1606
Timentin Injection Galaxy Container (Clavulanate Potassium, Ticarcillin Disodium) GlaxoSmithKline ... 1609
Timentin IV Infusion (Clavulanate Potassium, Ticarcillin Disodium) GlaxoSmithKline ... 1603
Timentin Pharmacy Bulk Package (Clavulanate Potassium, Ticarcillin Disodium) GlaxoSmithKline ... 1613
Tygacil for Injection (Tigecycline) Wyeth ... 3276
Zosyn for Injection (Piperacillin Sodium, Tazobactam Sodium) Wyeth ... 3284

(▣ Described in PDR® For Nonprescription Drugs) (⊙ Described in PDR® For Ophthalmic Medicines)

B. fragilis intra-abdominal infections
Avelox (Moxifloxacin Hydrochloride) Schering ... 2803
Cipro I.V. (Ciprofloxacin) Schering ... 2817
Cipro (Ciprofloxacin) Schering ... 2810
Doribax Injection (Doripenem) Ortho-McNeil ... 2400
Fortaz (Ceftazidime) GlaxoSmithKline ... 1450
Invanz for Injection (Ertapenem) Merck ... 2029
Merrem I.V. (Meropenem) AstraZeneca Pharmaceuticals ... 684
Primaxin I.M. (Cilastatin Sodium, Imipenem) Merck ... 2080
Primaxin I.V. (Cilastatin Sodium, Imipenem) Merck ... 2083
Rocephin Injectable Vials, ADD-Vantage, Galaxy, Bulk (Ceftriaxone Sodium) Roche ... 2642
Timentin ADD-Vantage (Clavulanate Potassium, Ticarcillin Disodium) GlaxoSmithKline ... 1606
Timentin Injection Galaxy Container (Clavulanate Potassium, Ticarcillin Disodium) GlaxoSmithKline ... 1609
Timentin IV Infusion (Clavulanate Potassium, Ticarcillin Disodium) GlaxoSmithKline ... 1603
Timentin Pharmacy Bulk Package (Clavulanate Potassium, Ticarcillin Disodium) GlaxoSmithKline ... 1613
Tygacil for Injection (Tigecycline) Wyeth ... 3276

B. fragilis peritonitis
Merrem I.V. (Meropenem) AstraZeneca Pharmaceuticals ... 684
Timentin ADD-Vantage (Clavulanate Potassium, Ticarcillin Disodium) GlaxoSmithKline ... 1606
Timentin Injection Galaxy Container (Clavulanate Potassium, Ticarcillin Disodium) GlaxoSmithKline ... 1609
Timentin IV Infusion (Clavulanate Potassium, Ticarcillin Disodium) GlaxoSmithKline ... 1603
Timentin Pharmacy Bulk Package (Clavulanate Potassium, Ticarcillin Disodium) GlaxoSmithKline ... 1613
Zosyn for Injection (Piperacillin Sodium, Tazobactam Sodium) Wyeth ... 3284

B. fragilis septicemia
Primaxin I.V. (Cilastatin Sodium, Imipenem) Merck ... 2083

B. fragilis skin and skin structure infections
Invanz for Injection (Ertapenem) Merck ... 2029
Merrem I.V. (Meropenem) AstraZeneca Pharmaceuticals ... 684
Primaxin I.M. (Cilastatin Sodium, Imipenem) Merck ... 2080
Primaxin I.V. (Cilastatin Sodium, Imipenem) Merck ... 2083
Rocephin Injectable Vials, ADD-Vantage, Galaxy, Bulk (Ceftriaxone Sodium) Roche ... 2642
Tygacil for Injection (Tigecycline) Wyeth ... 3276

B. intermedius infections
Primaxin I.M. (Cilastatin Sodium, Imipenem) Merck ... 2080

B. intermedius intra-abdominal infections
Primaxin I.M. (Cilastatin Sodium, Imipenem) Merck ... 2080

B. melaninogenicus endometritis
Timentin ADD-Vantage (Clavulanate Potassium, Ticarcillin Disodium) GlaxoSmithKline ... 1606
Timentin IV Infusion (Clavulanate Potassium, Ticarcillin Disodium) GlaxoSmithKline ... 1603
Timentin Pharmacy Bulk Package (Clavulanate Potassium, Ticarcillin Disodium) GlaxoSmithKline ... 1613

B. melaninogenicus infections
Timentin ADD-Vantage (Clavulanate Potassium, Ticarcillin Disodium) GlaxoSmithKline ... 1606
Timentin IV Infusion (Clavulanate Potassium, Ticarcillin Disodium) GlaxoSmithKline ... 1603
Timentin Pharmacy Bulk Package (Clavulanate Potassium, Ticarcillin Disodium) GlaxoSmithKline ... 1613

B. ovatus infections
Zosyn for Injection (Piperacillin Sodium, Tazobactam Sodium) Wyeth ... 3284

B. ovatus peritonitis
Zosyn for Injection (Piperacillin Sodium, Tazobactam Sodium) Wyeth ... 3284

B. pertussis infections
E.E.S. (Erythromycin Ethylsuccinate) Abbott ... 433
EryPed (Erythromycin Ethylsuccinate) Abbott ... 431

B. pertussis respiratory tract infections
E.E.S. (Erythromycin Ethylsuccinate) Abbott ... 433
EryPed (Erythromycin Ethylsuccinate) Abbott ... 431

B. thetaiotaomicron infections
Avelox (Moxifloxacin Hydrochloride) Schering ... 2803
Doribax Injection (Doripenem) Ortho-McNeil ... 2400
Merrem I.V. (Meropenem) AstraZeneca Pharmaceuticals ... 684
Primaxin I.M. (Cilastatin Sodium, Imipenem) Merck ... 2080
Tygacil for Injection (Tigecycline) Wyeth ... 3276
Zosyn for Injection (Piperacillin Sodium, Tazobactam Sodium) Wyeth ... 3284

B. thetaiotaomicron intra-abdominal infections
Avelox (Moxifloxacin Hydrochloride) Schering ... 2803
Doribax Injection (Doripenem) Ortho-McNeil ... 2400
Merrem I.V. (Meropenem) AstraZeneca Pharmaceuticals ... 684
Primaxin I.M. (Cilastatin Sodium, Imipenem) Merck ... 2080
Tygacil for Injection (Tigecycline) Wyeth ... 3276

B. thetaiotaomicron peritonitis
Merrem I.V. (Meropenem) AstraZeneca Pharmaceuticals ... 684
Zosyn for Injection (Piperacillin Sodium, Tazobactam Sodium) Wyeth ... 3284

B. uniformis infections
Doribax Injection (Doripenem) Ortho-McNeil ... 2400
Tygacil for Injection (Tigecycline) Wyeth ... 3276

B. uniformis intra-abdominal infections
Doribax Injection (Doripenem) Ortho-McNeil ... 2400
Tygacil for Injection (Tigecycline) Wyeth ... 3276

B. vulgatus infections
Doribax Injection (Doripenem) Ortho-McNeil ... 2400
Tygacil for Injection (Tigecycline) Wyeth ... 3276
Zosyn for Injection (Piperacillin Sodium, Tazobactam Sodium) Wyeth ... 3284

B. vulgatus intra-abdominal infections
Doribax Injection (Doripenem) Ortho-McNeil ... 2400
Tygacil for Injection (Tigecycline) Wyeth ... 3276

B. vulgatus peritonitis
Zosyn for Injection (Piperacillin Sodium, Tazobactam Sodium) Wyeth ... 3284

Backache
Hyland's BackAche with Arnica Caplets (Homeopathic Formulations) Standard Homeopathic ... ■ 618
Motrin IB Tablets and Caplets (Ibuprofen) McNeil Consumer ... 1900
Salonpas Aqua-Patch (Menthol) Hisamitsu ... ■ 610
Salonpas Arthritis Pain Patches (Menthol, Methyl Salicylate) Hisamitsu ... ■ 608
Salonpas Gel (Menthol, Methyl Salicylate) Hisamitsu ... ■ 609
Salonpas Gel-Patch Hot Soothing (Capsicum Extract, Menthol) Hisamitsu ... ■ 609
Salonpas Pain Relief Patch (Menthol, Methyl Salicylate) Hisamitsu ... ■ 608
Salonpas-Hot Patch (Capsicum Extract) Hisamitsu ... ■ 609
Thera-Gesic Creme (Menthol, Methyl Salicylate) Mission ... ■ 610
Extra Strength Tylenol Rapid Release Gels (Acetaminophen) McNeil Consumer ... 1915
Women's Tylenol Menstrual Relief Caplets (Acetaminophen, Pamabrom) McNeil Consumer ... 1919

Backache, systemic, symptomatic relief of
Traumeel Injection Solution (Homeopathic Formulations) Heel ... 1725
Tylenol 8 Hour Extended Release Caplets (Acetaminophen) McNeil Consumer ... 1915

Backache, temporary relief of
(*see under* Pain, topical relief of)

Bacteremia
(*see under* Septicemia, bacterial)

Bacteriuria associated with cystitis, elimination or suppression of
(*see also under* Infections, urinary tract)
Uroqid-Acid No. 2 Tablets (Methenamine Mandelate, Sodium Acid Phosphate) Beach ... 814

Bacteriuria associated with polynephritis, elimination or suppression of
(*see under* Infections, urinary tract)

Bacteroides distasonis infections
(*see under* B. distasonis infections)

Bacteroides fragilis infections
(*see under* B. fragilis infections)

Bacteroides ovatus infections
(*see under* B. ovatus infections)

Bacteroides species gynecologic infections
Primaxin I.M. (Cilastatin Sodium, Imipenem) Merck ... 2080
Primaxin I.V. (Cilastatin Sodium, Imipenem) Merck ... 2083

Bacteroides species infections
(*see also under* B. distasonis infections; B. fragilis infections; B. ovatus infections; B. thetaiotaomicron infections; B. vulgatus infections)
Doribax Injection (Doripenem) Ortho-McNeil ... 2400
Fortaz (Ceftazidime) GlaxoSmithKline ... 1450
Invanz for Injection (Ertapenem) Merck ... 2029
Primaxin I.M. (Cilastatin Sodium, Imipenem) Merck ... 2080
Primaxin I.V. (Cilastatin Sodium, Imipenem) Merck ... 2083
Tygacil for Injection (Tigecycline) Wyeth ... 3276

Bacteroides species intra-abdominal infections
Doribax Injection (Doripenem) Ortho-McNeil ... 2400
Fortaz (Ceftazidime) GlaxoSmithKline ... 1450
Invanz for Injection (Ertapenem) Merck ... 2029
Primaxin I.M. (Cilastatin Sodium, Imipenem) Merck ... 2080
Primaxin I.V. (Cilastatin Sodium, Imipenem) Merck ... 2083

Bacteroides species meningitis
Merrem I.V. (Meropenem) AstraZeneca Pharmaceuticals ... 684

Bacteroides species peritonitis
Primaxin I.M. (Cilastatin Sodium, Imipenem) Merck ... 2080

Bacteroides species septicemia
Primaxin I.V. (Cilastatin Sodium, Imipenem) Merck ... 2083

Bacteroides species skin and skin structure infections
Primaxin I.M. (Cilastatin Sodium, Imipenem) Merck ... 2080
Primaxin I.V. (Cilastatin Sodium, Imipenem) Merck ... 2083

Bacteroides thetaiotaomicron infections
(*see under* B. thetaiotaomicron infections)

Bacteroides vulgatus infections
(*see under* B. vulgatus infections)

Baldness, male pattern of vertex of scalp
Propecia Tablets (Finasteride) Merck ... 2095

Barber's itch
(*see under* Folliculitis barbae)

Barrett's esophagus
Photofrin for Injection (Porfimer Sodium) Axcan Pharma ... 708

Bedsores
(*see under* Ulcers, decubitus, adjunctive therapy in)

Benzodiazepine overdose, management of
Romazicon Injection (Flumazenil) Roche ... 2646

Bifidobacterium species gynecologic infections
Primaxin I.V. (Cilastatin Sodium, Imipenem) Merck ... 2083

Bifidobacterium species infections
Primaxin I.V. (Cilastatin Sodium, Imipenem) Merck ... 2083

Bifidobacterium species intra-abdominal infections
Primaxin I.V. (Cilastatin Sodium, Imipenem) Merck ... 2083

Biotin, deficiency of
Appearex Tablets (Biotin) Merz ... 2163
Meribin Capsules (Biotin) Mericon ... 2163

Bipolar disorder
Lamictal (Lamotrigine) GlaxoSmithKline ... 1488

Bipolar disorder, acute mixed
Abilify Oral Solution (Aripiprazole) Bristol-Myers Squibb ... 881
Abilify Oral Solution (Aripiprazole) Otsuka ... 2466
Abilify Discmelt Orally Disintegrating Tablets (Aripiprazole) Bristol-Myers Squibb ... 881
Abilify Discmelt Orally Disintegrating Tablets (Aripiprazole) Otsuka ... 2466
Abilify Tablets (Aripiprazole) Bristol-Myers Squibb ... 881
Abilify Tablets (Aripiprazole) Otsuka ... 2466
Depakote ER Tablets (Divalproex Sodium) Abbott ... 423
Equetro Extended-Release Capsules (Carbamazepine) Validus ... 3174
Zyprexa Tablets (Olanzapine) Lilly ... 1883
Zyprexa ZYDIS Orally Disintegrating Tablets (Olanzapine) Lilly ... 1883

Bipolar disorder, manic episodes
(*see also under* Manic episodes associated with bipolar disorder)
Abilify Oral Solution (Aripiprazole) Bristol-Myers Squibb ... 881

Abilify Oral Solution (Aripiprazole) Otsuka 2466
Abilify Discmelt Orally Disintegrating Tablets (Aripiprazole) Bristol-Myers Squibb 881
Abilify Discmelt Orally Disintegrating Tablets (Aripiprazole) Otsuka 2466
Abilify Tablets (Aripiprazole) Bristol-Myers Squibb 881
Abilify Tablets (Aripiprazole) Otsuka .. 2466
Depakote ER Tablets (Divalproex Sodium) Abbott 423
Equetro Extended-Release Capsules (Carbamazepine) Validus 3174
Zyprexa Tablets (Olanzapine) Lilly 1883
Zyprexa ZYDIS Orally Disintegrating Tablets (Olanzapine) Lilly 1883

Bites, black widow spider
Antivenin (Black Widow Spider Antivenin) (Black Widow Spider Antivenin (Equine)) Merck 1951

Bites, insect
EpiPen (Epinephrine) Dey 1024

Bleeding associated with acquired hemophilia
NovoSeven RT (Coagulation Factor VIIa, Recombinant) Novo Nordisk .. 2370
NovoSeven (Antihemophilic Factor (Recombinant)) Novo Nordisk 2367

Bleeding associated with congenital hemophiliacs
NovoSeven (Antihemophilic Factor (Recombinant)) Novo Nordisk 2367
NovoSeven RT (Coagulation Factor VIIa, Recombinant) Novo Nordisk .. 2370

Bleeding associated with hemophilia A
Advate (Antihemophilic Factor (Recombinant)) Baxter Healthcare . 721
Alphanate (Antihemophilic Factor (Human), von Willebrand Factor (Human)) Grifols 1709
Feiba VH (Anti-Inhibitor Coagulant Complex) Baxter Healthcare 728
NovoSeven RT (Coagulation Factor VIIa, Recombinant) Novo Nordisk .. 2370
NovoSeven (Antihemophilic Factor (Recombinant)) Novo Nordisk 2367
Xyntha Vials (Antihemophilic Factor (Recombinant), Plasma/Albumin-Free) Wyeth 3280

Bleeding associated with hemophilia B
Feiba VH (Anti-Inhibitor Coagulant Complex) Baxter Healthcare 728
NovoSeven (Antihemophilic Factor (Recombinant)) Novo Nordisk 2367
NovoSeven RT (Coagulation Factor VIIa, Recombinant) Novo Nordisk .. 2370
Profilnine SD Solvent Detergent (Factor IX Complex) Grifols 1721

Blepharitis
Pred Mild Ophthalmic Suspension (Prednisolone Acetate) Allergan .... ⊙230

Blepharitis, fungal
Natacyn Antifungal Ophthalmic Suspension (Natamycin) Alcon ..... ⊙204

Blepharospasm
BOTOX Purified Neurotoxin Complex (Botulinum Toxin Type A) Allergan 550

Blood loss, perioperative, reduction of
Trasylol Injection (Aprotinin) Bayer HealthCare Pharmaceuticals 799

Body aches
(*see under* Pain, general)

Boils, symptomatic relief of
(*see under* Furunculosis, symptomatic relief of)

Bone disease, metabolic, with chronic renal failure
(*see under* Osteodystrophy, renal)

Bone marrow transplantation, allogeneic or autologous, delayed or failed
Leukine (Sargramostim) Bayer HealthCare Pharmaceuticals 774

Bone mass, loss of
(*see under* Osteoporosis)

Bone metastases of solid tumors
Zometa for Intravenous Infusion (Zoledronic acid) Novartis 2341

Bordetella pertussis
(*see under* B. pertussis infections)

Bordetella pertussis, immunization against
(*see also under* Immunization, diphtheria, tetanus and pertussis)
Boostrix (Diphtheria & Tetanus Toxoids and Acellular Pertussis Vaccine Adsorbed) GlaxoSmithKline 1377
Infanrix Vaccine (Diphtheria & Tetanus Toxoids and Acellular Pertussis Vaccine Adsorbed) GlaxoSmithKline 1479
Pediarix Vaccine (Diphtheria & Tetanus Toxoids and Acellular Pertussis Vaccine Adsorbed, Hepatitis B Vaccine, Recombinant, Poliovirus Vaccine Inactivated) GlaxoSmithKline 1552

Borrelia burgdorferi infection
Ceftin Tablets (Cefuroxime Axetil) GlaxoSmithKline 1380

Bowel, evacuation of
Fleet Bisacodyl Laxatives (Bisacodyl) Fleet 1143
Fleet Enema (Sodium Phosphate) Fleet 1143
Fleet Enema Extra (Sodium Phosphate) Fleet 1143
Fleet Enema for Children (Sodium Phosphate) Fleet 1143
Fleet Mineral Oil Enema (Mineral Oil) Fleet 1144
Fleet Pedia-Lax Enema (Sodium Phosphate) Fleet 1143
Fleet Phospho-soda (Sodium Phosphate) Fleet 1145
Fleet Phospho-soda EZ-PREP (Sodium Phosphate) Fleet 1147
Fleet Prep Kits (Bisacodyl, Sodium Phosphate) Fleet 1149
MoviPrep Oral Solution (PEG-3350, Potassium Chloride, Sodium Ascorbate, Sodium Chloride, Sodium Sulfate, Vitamin C) Salix ... 2679
OsmoPrep Tablets (Sodium Phosphate) Salix 2680

Bowel, irritable, syndrome
Amitiza Capsules (Lubiprostone) Takeda 3082
Bentyl Capsules (Dicyclomine Hydrochloride) Axcan Pharma 703
Bentyl Injection (Dicyclomine Hydrochloride) Axcan Pharma 703
Bentyl Syrup (Dicyclomine Hydrochloride) Axcan Pharma 703
Bentyl Tablets (Dicyclomine Hydrochloride) Axcan Pharma 703
Donnatal Extentabs (Atropine Sulfate, Hyoscyamine Sulfate, Phenobarbital, Scopolamine Hydrobromide) PBM 2507
Metamucil Capsules (Psyllium Preparations) Procter & Gamble ... 2563
Metamucil (Psyllium Preparations) Procter & Gamble 2563

Bowel movements, irregular
Dulcolax Stool Softener (Docusate Sodium) Boehringer Ingelheim ..... ▣602
Dulcolax Suppositories (Bisacodyl) Boehringer Ingelheim .... ▣602
Dulcolax Tablets (Bisacodyl) Boehringer Ingelheim .... ▣602

Bowel resection surgery, accelerate time to recovery
Adolor 3293

Branhamella catarrhalis
(*see under* M. catarrhalis infections)

Breast cancer
(*see under* Carcinoma, breast)

Breast carcinoma
(*see under* Carcinoma, breast)

Bromidrosis
Formadon Solution (Formaldehyde) Gordon 1699

Bronchial asthma
Accolate Tablets (Zafirlukast) AstraZeneca Pharmaceuticals 669
Advair Diskus 100/50 (Fluticasone Propionate, Salmeterol Xinafoate) GlaxoSmithKline 1276
Advair Diskus 250/50 (Fluticasone Propionate, Salmeterol Xinafoate) GlaxoSmithKline 1276
Advair Diskus 500/50 (Fluticasone Propionate, Salmeterol Xinafoate) GlaxoSmithKline 1276
Advair HFA 45/21 Inhalation Aerosol (Fluticasone Propionate, Salmeterol Xinafoate) GlaxoSmithKline 1288
Advair HFA 115/21 Inhalation Aerosol (Fluticasone Propionate, Salmeterol Xinafoate) GlaxoSmithKline 1288
Advair HFA 230/21 Inhalation Aerosol (Fluticasone Propionate, Salmeterol Xinafoate) GlaxoSmithKline 1288
Aerobid/Aerobid-M (Flunisolide) Forest 1153
Alvesco Inhalation Aerosol (Ciclesonide) Sepracor 2985
Atrovent HFA Inhalation Aerosol (Ipratropium Bromide) Boehringer Ingelheim 839
Azmacort Inhalation Aerosol (Triamcinolone Acetonide) Abbott 407
Flovent Diskus 50 mcg (Fluticasone Propionate) GlaxoSmithKline 1435
Flovent HFA (Fluticasone Propionate HFA) GlaxoSmithKline 1440
Foradil Aerolizer (Formoterol Fumarate) Schering 2849
Maxair Autohaler (Pirbuterol Acetate) Graceway 1705
Pulmicort Flexhaler (Budesonide) AstraZeneca LP 654
Qvar Inhalation Aerosol (Beclomethasone Dipropionate) Teva Specialty 3116
Serevent Diskus (Salmeterol Xinafoate) GlaxoSmithKline 1594
Singulair (Montelukast Sodium) Merck 2114
Uniphyl Tablets (Theophylline Anhydrous) Purdue Pharmaceutical 2595
Xopenex Inhalation Solution (Levalbuterol Hydrochloride) Sepracor ... 3001
Xopenex Inhalation Solution Concentrate (Levalbuterol Hydrochloride) Sepracor 3005
Xopenex HFA Inhalation Aerosol (Levalbuterol Tartrate) Sepracor 3009

Bronchial asthma, maintenance treatment of
Advair Diskus 100/50 (Fluticasone Propionate, Salmeterol Xinafoate) GlaxoSmithKline 1276
Advair Diskus 250/50 (Fluticasone Propionate, Salmeterol Xinafoate) GlaxoSmithKline 1276
Advair Diskus 500/50 (Fluticasone Propionate, Salmeterol Xinafoate) GlaxoSmithKline 1276
Alvesco Inhalation Aerosol (Ciclesonide) Sepracor 2985
Asmanex Twisthaler (Mometasone Furoate) Schering 2797
Symbicort 80/4.5 Inhalation Aerosol (Budesonide, Formoterol fumarate dihydrate) AstraZeneca LP 659
Symbicort 160/4.5 Inhalation Aerosol (Budesonide, Formoterol fumarate dihydrate) AstraZeneca LP 659

Bronchial asthma, prophylactic therapy
Accolate Tablets (Zafirlukast) AstraZeneca Pharmaceuticals 669
Alvesco Inhalation Aerosol (Ciclesonide) Sepracor 2985

Bronchial congestion
Sinutab Non-Drying Caplets (Guaifenesin, Phenylephrine Hydrochloride) McNeil Consumer .. 1905

Bronchial secretions, thinning of
Sudafed PE Cold & Cough Caplets (Acetaminophen, Dextromethorphan Hydrobromide, Guaifenesin, Phenylephrine Hydrochloride) McNeil Consumer 1907
Sudafed PE Non-Drying Sinus Caplets (Guaifenesin, Phenylephrine Hydrochloride) McNeil Consumer 1908
Tylenol Chest Congestion Caplets with Cool Burst (Acetaminophen, Guaifenesin) McNeil Consumer 1910
Tylenol Chest Congestion Liquid with Cool Burst (Acetaminophen, Guaifenesin) McNeil Consumer 1910
Tylenol Cold Severe Congestion Daytime Caplets with Cool Burst (Acetaminophen, Dextromethorphan Hydrobromide, Guaifenesin, Pseudoephedrine Hydrochloride) McNeil Consumer 1912
Tylenol Cold Head Congestion Severe Daytime Caplets with Cool Burst (Acetaminophen, Dextromethorphan Hydrobromide, Guaifenesin, Phenylephrine Hydrochloride) McNeil Consumer .. 1910
Tylenol Cold Multi-Symptom Severe Caplets with Cool Burst (Acetaminophen, Dextromethorphan Hydrobromide, Guaifenesin, Phenylephrine Hydrochloride) McNeil Consumer 1913
Tylenol Cold Multi-Symptom Severe Daytime Liquid with Citrus Burst (Acetaminophen, Dextromethorphan Hydrobromide, Guaifenesin, Phenylephrine Hydrochloride) McNeil Consumer 1913
Tylenol Sinus Congestion & Pain Severe Caplets with Cool Burst (Acetaminophen, Guaifenesin, Phenylephrine Hydrochloride) McNeil Consumer 1917
Tylenol Sinus Severe Congestion Caplets with Cool Burst (Acetaminophen, Guaifenesin, Pseudoephedrine Hydrochloride) McNeil Consumer 1917

Bronchitis, acute
Omnicef Capsules (Cefdinir) Abbott .. 497
Omnicef for Oral Suspension (Cefdinir) Abbott 497
Suprax for Oral Suspension (Cefixime) Lupin 1891
Suprax Tablets (Cefixime) Lupin 1891

Bronchitis, chronic
Advair Diskus 250/50 (Fluticasone Propionate, Salmeterol Xinafoate) GlaxoSmithKline 1276
Atrovent HFA Inhalation Aerosol (Ipratropium Bromide) Boehringer Ingelheim 839
Brovana Inhalation Solution (Arformoterol Tartrate) Sepracor 2990
Perforomist Inhalation Solution (Formoterol Fumarate) Dey 1025
Serevent Diskus (Salmeterol Xinafoate) GlaxoSmithKline 1594
Spiriva HandiHaler (Tiotropium bromide) Boehringer Ingelheim 870
Uniphyl Tablets (Theophylline Anhydrous) Purdue Pharmaceutical 2595

Bronchitis, chronic, acute exacerbation of
Avelox (Moxifloxacin Hydrochloride) Schering 2803
Biaxin/Biaxin XL (Clarithromycin) Abbott 411
Ceftin Tablets (Cefuroxime Axetil) GlaxoSmithKline 1380
Cipro (Ciprofloxacin) Schering 2810
Levaquin (Levofloxacin) Ortho-McNeil 2416
Levaquin in 5% Dextrose Injection (Levofloxacin) Ortho-McNeil 2416
Omnicef Capsules (Cefdinir) Abbott .. 497
Omnicef for Oral Suspension (Cefdinir) Abbott 497
Primaxin I.M. (Cilastatin Sodium, Imipenem) Merck 2080

Suprax for Oral Suspension (Cefixime) Lupin 1891
Suprax Tablets (Cefixime) Lupin........ 1891

Bronchoconstriction, exercise-induced
Singulair (Montelukast Sodium) Merck 2114

Bronchospasm, exercise-induced
Foradil Aerolizer (Formoterol Fumarate) Schering 2849
ProAir HFA Inhalation Aerosol (Albuterol Sulfate) Teva Specialty... 3113
Proventil HFA Inhalation Aerosol (Albuterol Sulfate) Schering 2914
Serevent Diskus (Salmeterol Xinafoate) GlaxoSmithKline 1594

Bronchospasm, exercise-induced, prevention of
Ventolin HFA Inhalation Aerosol (Albuterol Sulfate) GlaxoSmithKline 1638

Bronchospasm, prevention and relief of
Serevent Diskus (Salmeterol Xinafoate) GlaxoSmithKline 1594
Ventolin HFA Inhalation Aerosol (Albuterol Sulfate) GlaxoSmithKline 1638
Xopenex Inhalation Solution (Levalbuterol Hydrochloride) Sepracor ...3001
Xopenex Inhalation Solution Concentrate (Levalbuterol Hydrochloride) Sepracor 3005
Xopenex HFA Inhalation Aerosol (Levalbuterol Tartrate) Sepracor 3009

Bronchospasm, reversible
(*see also under* Bronchial asthma)
Atrovent HFA Inhalation Aerosol (Ipratropium Bromide) Boehringer Ingelheim 839
Proventil HFA Inhalation Aerosol (Albuterol Sulfate) Schering 2914
Uniphyl Tablets (Theophylline Anhydrous) Purdue Pharmaceutical 2595
Xopenex Inhalation Solution (Levalbuterol Hydrochloride) Sepracor ...3001
Xopenex Inhalation Solution Concentrate (Levalbuterol Hydrochloride) Sepracor 3005
Xopenex HFA Inhalation Aerosol (Levalbuterol Tartrate) Sepracor 3009

Bronchospasm associated with chronic obstructive pulmonary disease
Atrovent HFA Inhalation Aerosol (Ipratropium Bromide) Boehringer Ingelheim 839
Brovana Inhalation Solution (Arformoterol Tartrate) Sepracor 2990
Combivent Inhalation Aerosol (Albuterol Sulfate, Ipratropium Bromide) Boehringer Ingelheim 845
Foradil Aerolizer (Formoterol Fumarate) Schering 2849
Maxair Autohaler (Pirbuterol Acetate) Graceway 1705
Serevent Diskus (Salmeterol Xinafoate) GlaxoSmithKline 1594
Spiriva HandiHaler (Tiotropium bromide) Boehringer Ingelheim 870
Uniphyl Tablets (Theophylline Anhydrous) Purdue Pharmaceutical 2595

Bronchospasm associated with reversible obstructive airways disease
Foradil Aerolizer (Formoterol Fumarate) Schering 2849
ProAir HFA Inhalation Aerosol (Albuterol Sulfate) Teva Specialty ..3113
Serevent Diskus (Salmeterol Xinafoate) GlaxoSmithKline 1594
Xopenex Inhalation Solution (Levalbuterol Hydrochloride) Sepracor ...3001
Xopenex Inhalation Solution Concentrate (Levalbuterol Hydrochloride) Sepracor 3005
Xopenex HFA Inhalation Aerosol (Levalbuterol Tartrate) Sepracor 3009

Bruises
Salonpas Aqua-Patch (Menthol) Hisamitsu ....▣610
Salonpas Arthritis Pain Patches (Menthol, Methyl Salicylate) Hisamitsu...................................▣608
Salonpas Gel (Menthol, Methyl Salicylate) Hisamitsu ....▣609
Salonpas Gel-Patch Hot Soothing (Capsicum Extract, Menthol) Hisamitsu...................................▣609
Salonpas Pain Relief Patch (Menthol, Methyl Salicylate) Hisamitsu...................................▣608
Salonpas-Hot Patch (Capsicum Extract) Hisamitsu ....▣609
Thera-Gesic Creme (Menthol, Methyl Salicylate) Mission............▣610

Bruises, topical relief of
(*see under* Pain, topical relief of)

"Bubble boy" disease
(*see under* Adenosine deaminase, enzyme replacement therapy for)

Bulbar conjunctiva inflammation
Blephamide Ophthalmic Ointment Allergan ....⊙217
Blephamide Ophthalmic Suspension Allergan ....⊙216
FML Ophthalmic Ointment (Fluorometholone) Allergan ....⊙223
FML Ophthalmic Suspension (Fluorometholone) Allergan ....⊙224
FML Forte Ophthalmic Suspension (Fluorometholone) Allergan ....⊙222
Pred Forte Ophthalmic Suspension (Prednisolone Acetate) Allergan ....⊙227
Pred-G Ophthalmic Ointment (Gentamicin Sulfate, Prednisolone Acetate) Allergan ....⊙229
Pred-G Ophthalmic Suspension (Gentamicin Sulfate, Prednisolone Acetate) Allergan ....⊙228
Zylet Ophthalmic Suspension (Loteprednol Etabonate, Tobramycin) Bausch & Lomb ....⊙247

Bulimia nervosa
Prozac Weekly Capsules (Fluoxetine Hydrochloride) Lilly 1852
Prozac Pulvules and Liquid (Fluoxetine Hydrochloride) Lilly 1852

Burn wound infections
(*see under* Infections, burn wound)

Burns, adjunctive therapy in
Accuzyme SE Spray Emulsion (Papain, Urea) Healthpoint 1723
Flexbumin 25% I.V. (Albumin (human)) Baxter Healthcare 729
Panafil Ointment (Chlorophyllin Copper Complex Sodium, Papain, Urea) Healthpoint 1723
Panafil SE Spray Emulsion (Chlorophyllin Copper Complex Sodium, Papain, Urea) Healthpoint 1724

Burns, pain associated with
(*see under* Pain, topical relief of)

Burns, second- and third-degree, adjunctive therapy in
Sulfamylon for 5% Topical Solution (Mafenide Acetate) Mylan 2194

Bursitis
Anaprox Tablets (Naproxen Sodium) Roche 2632
Anaprox DS Tablets (Naproxen Sodium) Roche 2632
Indocin (Indomethacin) Merck 2024
Naprosyn Suspension (Naproxen) Roche 2632
Naprosyn Tablets (Naproxen) Roche 2632
Traumeel Injection Solution (Homeopathic Formulations) Heel 1725

Bursitis, subacromial, acute, symptomatic relief of
Clinoril Tablets (Sulindac) Merck 1962
Indocin (Indomethacin) Merck 2024

C

C. diphtheriae infections
E.E.S. (Erythromycin Ethylsuccinate) Abbott 433
EryPed (Erythromycin Ethylsuccinate) Abbott................................ 431

C. minutissimum infections
E.E.S. (Erythromycin Ethylsuccinate) Abbott.................................. 433
EryPed (Erythromycin Ethylsuccinate) Abbott................................ 431

C. perfringens infections
Avelox (Moxifloxacin Hydrochloride) Schering.. 2803
Tygacil for Injection (Tigecycline) Wyeth... 3276

C. perfringens intra-abdominal infections
Avelox (Moxifloxacin Hydrochloride) Schering... 2803
Tygacil for Injection (Tigecycline) Wyeth... 3276

Cachexia associated with weight loss, AIDS-induced
Megace ES Oral Suspension (Megestrol Acetate) Par 2499

Calcium deficiency
(*see under* Hypocalcemia)

Campylobacter jejuni infectious diarrhea
Cipro (Ciprofloxacin) Schering 2810

Cancer, prostatic
(*see under* Carcinoma, prostate, palliative treatment of)

Candida albicans infections
Nystop Topical Powder USP (Nystatin) Paddock 2498

Candida infections, prophylaxis in hematopoietic stem cell transplantation
Mycamine for Injection (Micafungin Sodium) Astellas 616

Candida infections, prophylaxis of
Noxafil Oral Suspension (Posaconazole) Schering 2889

Candidemia
Cancidas for Injection (Caspofungin acetate) Merck 1953
Mycamine for Injection (Micafungin Sodium) Astellas 616

Candidiasis, cutaneous
Nystop Topical Powder USP (Nystatin) Paddock 2498

Candidiasis, disseminated
Mycamine for Injection (Micafungin Sodium) Astellas 616

Candidiasis, esophageal
Cancidas for Injection (Caspofungin acetate) Merck 1953
Mycamine for Injection (Micafungin Sodium) Astellas 616

Candidiasis, oropharyngeal
Noxafil Oral Suspension (Posaconazole) Schering 2889

Candidiasis, systemic
Abelcet Injection (Amphotericin B Lipid Complex) Enzon 1134
AmBisome for Injection (Amphotericin B, liposomal) Astellas 606

Canker sores
(*see under* Stomatitis, recurrent aphthous, symptomatic relief of)

Carbuncles
(*see under* Furunculosis, symptomatic relief of)

Carbuncles, adjunctive therapy in
Accuzyme SE Spray Emulsion (Papain, Urea) Healthpoint 1723
Panafil Ointment (Chlorophyllin Copper Complex Sodium, Papain, Urea) Healthpoint 1723

Carcinoma, advanced renal cell, treatment of
Nexavar Tablets (Sorafenib) Bayer HealthCare Pharmaceuticals.......... 784
Torisel Injection (Temsirolimus) Wyeth.. 3272

Carcinoma, basal cell
Aldara Cream, 5% (Imiquimod) Graceway 1699

Carcinoma, breast
Arimidex Tablets (Anastrozole) AstraZeneca Pharmaceuticals 672
Faslodex Injection (Fulvestrant) AstraZeneca Pharmaceuticals 682
Femara Tablets (Letrozole) Novartis 2246
Ixempra Kit for Injection (Ixabepilone) Bristol-Myers Squibb............ 915
Taxotere Injection Concentrate (Docetaxel) sanofi-aventis.............. 2773
Tykerb Tablets (Lapatinib) GlaxoSmithKline 1631
Xeloda Tablets (Capecitabine) Roche.. 2662

Carcinoma, breast, adjunctive therapy in
Avastin IV (Bevacizumab) Genentech 1192
Femara Tablets (Letrozole) Novartis 2246
Herceptin I.V. (Trastuzumab) Genentech 1199
Taxotere Injection Concentrate (Docetaxel) sanofi-aventis 2773

Carcinoma, breast, metastatic, resistant, treatment of (Monotherapy)
Ixempra Kit for Injection (Ixabepilone) Bristol-Myers Squibb 915
Xeloda Tablets (Capecitabine) Roche 2662

Carcinoma, breast, metastatic, treatment of
Faslodex Injection (Fulvestrant) AstraZeneca Pharmaceuticals 682
Gemzar for Injection (Gemcitabine Hydrochloride) Lilly 1820
Herceptin I.V. (Trastuzumab) Genentech 1199
Ixempra Kit for Injection (Ixabepilone) Bristol-Myers Squibb 915
Taxotere Injection Concentrate (Docetaxel) sanofi-aventis 2773
Tykerb Tablets (Lapatinib) GlaxoSmithKline 1631
Xeloda Tablets (Capecitabine) Roche 2662

Carcinoma, breast, palliative therapy in
Premarin Tablets (Estrogens, Conjugated) Wyeth 3221

Carcinoma, breast, postmenopausal women
Evista Tablets (Raloxifene Hydrochloride) Lilly 1810

Carcinoma, breast, to reduce the incidence of
Evista Tablets (Raloxifene Hydrochloride) Lilly 1810

Carcinoma, bronchogenic
Mustargen for Injection (Mechlorethamine Hydrochloride) Ovation ...2492

Carcinoma, cervical, prevention of
Gardasil Injection (Quadrivalent Human Papillomavirus (Types 6, 11, 16, 18) Recombinant Vaccine) Merck 2019

Carcinoma, colon, Dukes' stage C, adjunctive treatment in
Xeloda Tablets (Capecitabine) Roche 2662

Carcinoma, colon, metastatic
Vectibix (Panitumumab) Amgen 597
Xeloda Tablets (Capecitabine) Roche 2662

Carcinoma, colorectal
Eloxatin for Injection (Oxaliplatin) sanofi-aventis ... 2731
Erbitux (Cetuximab) Bristol-Myers Squibb ... 912
Xeloda Tablets (Capecitabine) Roche ... 2662

Carcinoma, colorectal, adjunctive therapy in
Avastin IV (Bevacizumab) Genentech ... 1192
Erbitux (Cetuximab) Bristol-Myers Squibb ... 912

Carcinoma, esophageal, obstructing, palliative treatment of
Photofrin for Injection (Porfimer Sodium) Axcan Pharma ... 708

Carcinoma, gastric, adjunctive therapy in
Taxotere Injection Concentrate (Docetaxel) sanofi-aventis ... 2773

Carcinoma, gastroesophageal junction, adjunctive therapy in
Taxotere Injection Concentrate (Docetaxel) sanofi-aventis ... 2773

Carcinoma, head and neck
Erbitux (Cetuximab) Bristol-Myers Squibb ... 912

Carcinoma, head and neck, adjunct in
Erbitux (Cetuximab) Bristol-Myers Squibb ... 912

Carcinoma, lung, non-small cell
Alimta for Injection (Pemetrexed) Lilly ... 1786
Avastin IV (Bevacizumab) Genentech ... 1192
Gemzar for Injection (Gemcitabine Hydrochloride) Lilly ... 1820
Hycamtin Capsules (Topotecan Hydrochloride) GlaxoSmithKline ... 1456
Photofrin for Injection (Porfimer Sodium) Axcan Pharma ... 708
Tarceva Tablets (Erlotinib) Genentech ... 1228
Taxotere Injection Concentrate (Docetaxel) sanofi-aventis ... 2773

Carcinoma, lung, non-small cell, adjunctive therapy in
Taxotere Injection Concentrate (Docetaxel) sanofi-aventis ... 2773

Carcinoma, lung, small cell
Hycamtin for Injection (Topotecan Hydrochloride) GlaxoSmithKline ... 1459

Carcinoma, mammary, metastatic, postmenopausal
Delatestryl Injection (Testosterone Enanthate) Indevus ... 1730

Carcinoma, metastatic, palliative treatment of
Mustargen for Injection (Mechlorethamine Hydrochloride) Ovation ... 2492

Carcinoma, ovary
Doxil Injection (Doxorubicin Hydrochloride Liposome) Ortho Biotech ... 2378
Gemzar for Injection (Gemcitabine Hydrochloride) Lilly ... 1820
Hycamtin Capsules (Topotecan Hydrochloride) GlaxoSmithKline ... 1456
Hycamtin for Injection (Topotecan Hydrochloride) GlaxoSmithKline ... 1459

Carcinoma, ovary, palliative therapy in
Hexalen Capsules (Altretamine) Eisai ... 1078

Carcinoma, pancreas
Gemzar for Injection (Gemcitabine Hydrochloride) Lilly ... 1820
Tarceva Tablets (Erlotinib) Genentech ... 1228

Carcinoma, prostate, adjunctive therapy in
Novantrone for Injection Concentrate (Mitoxantrone Hydrochloride) EMD Serono ... 1100
Taxotere Injection Concentrate (Docetaxel) sanofi-aventis ... 2773

Carcinoma, prostate, palliative treatment of
Eligard 7.5 mg (Leuprolide Acetate) sanofi-aventis ... 2724
Eligard 22.5 mg (Leuprolide Acetate) sanofi-aventis ... 2724
Eligard 30 mg (Leuprolide Acetate) sanofi-aventis ... 2724
Eligard 45 mg (Leuprolide Acetate) sanofi-aventis ... 2724
Lupron Depot 7.5 mg (Leuprolide Acetate) Abbott ... 469
Premarin Tablets (Estrogens, Conjugated) Wyeth ... 3221
Vantas (Histrelin Acetate) Indevus ... 1737
Viadur Implant (Leuprolide Acetate) Bayer HealthCare Pharmaceuticals ... 802

Carcinoma, renal cell
Sutent Capsules (Sunitinib malate) Pfizer ... 2540

Carcinoma, renal cell, metastatic, in adults
Proleukin for Injection (Aldesleukin) Novartis ... 2287

Carcinoma, squamous cell, head and neck, adjunctive therapy in
Taxotere Injection Concentrate (Docetaxel) sanofi-aventis ... 2773

Carcinoma, testis, advanced
Cosmegen for Injection (Dactinomycin) Ovation ... 2485

Carcinoma, thyroid
Cytomel Tablets (Liothyronine Sodium) King ... 1778
Levothroid Tablets (Levothyroxine Sodium) Forest ... 1170
Levoxyl Tablets (Levothyroxine Sodium) King ... 1780
Naturethroid Tablets (Levothyroxine, Liothyronine, Thyroid) RLC ... 2605
Synthroid Tablets (Levothyroxine Sodium) Abbott ... 507

Carcinoma, thyroid, adjunctive diagnostic tool for serum thyroglobulin testing
Thyrogen for Injection (Thyrotropin alfa) Genzyme ... 1244

Carcinoma, unresectable hepatocellular, treatment of
Nexavar Tablets (Sorafenib) Bayer HealthCare Pharmaceuticals ... 784

Carcinoma, urinary bladder, in-situ
Tice BCG (BCG, Live (Intravesical)) Schering ... 2936
Valstar Sterile Solution for Intravesical Instillation (Valrubicin) Indevus ... 1735

Cardiac failure
(*see under* Congestive heart failure, adjunct in)

Cardiac ischemic complications, acute, prevention of, adjunct to PTCA
ReoPro Vials (Abciximab) Lilly ... 1860

Cardiopulmonary bypass surgery, adjunct in
Albutein 5% (Albumin (human)) Grifols ... 1707
Albutein 25% (Albumin (human)) Grifols ... 1708
Flexbumin 25% I.V. (Albumin (human)) Baxter Healthcare ... 729
Human Albumin Grifols 25% (Albumin (human)) Grifols ... 1706

Cardiovascular disease, prevention of
Lipitor Tablets (Atorvastatin Calcium) Parke-Davis ... 2501

Cardiovascular mortality, reduction of, post-MI
Diovan Tablets (Valsartan) Novartis .. 2212

Cataplexy
Xyrem Oral Solution (Sodium Oxybate) Jazz ... 1766

Cataract surgery, treatment adjunct
Diclofenac Sodium Ophthalmic Solution (Diclofenac Sodium) Bausch & Lomb ... ⊙240
Nevanac Ophthalmic Suspension 0.1% (Nepafenac) Alcon ... ⊙205

Cellulitis
Levaquin (Levofloxacin) Ortho-McNeil ... 2416
Levaquin in 5% Dextrose Injection (Levofloxacin) Ortho-McNeil ... 2416

Cellulitis, pelvic
(*see under* Pelvic cellulitis)

Cephalalgia, histaminic
Imitrex Injection (Sumatriptan Succinate) GlaxoSmithKline ... 1465

Cervix, ripening of, in pregnant women at or near term
Cervidil Vaginal Insert (Dinoprostone) Forest ... 1165

Chancroid
Gantrisin Pediatric Suspension (Acetyl Sulfisoxazole) Roche ... 2638

Chickenpox
(*see under* Varicella, acute, treatment of)

Chlamydia pneumoniae infections
Avelox (Moxifloxacin Hydrochloride) Schering ... 2803
Biaxin/Biaxin XL (Clarithromycin) Abbott ... 411
Ketek Tablets (Telithromycin) sanofi-aventis ... 2744
Levaquin (Levofloxacin) Ortho-McNeil ... 2416
Levaquin in 5% Dextrose Injection (Levofloxacin) Ortho-McNeil ... 2416

Chlamydia pneumoniae lower respiratory tract infections
Avelox (Moxifloxacin Hydrochloride) Schering ... 2803
Biaxin/Biaxin XL (Clarithromycin) Abbott ... 411
Ketek Tablets (Telithromycin) sanofi-aventis ... 2744
Levaquin (Levofloxacin) Ortho-McNeil ... 2416
Levaquin in 5% Dextrose Injection (Levofloxacin) Ortho-McNeil ... 2416

Chlamydia trachomatis conjunctivitis of the newborn
E.E.S. (Erythromycin Ethylsuccinate) Abbott ... 433
EryPed (Erythromycin Ethylsuccinate) Abbott ... 431

Chlamydia trachomatis endocervical infections
E.E.S. (Erythromycin Ethylsuccinate) Abbott ... 433
EryPed (Erythromycin Ethylsuccinate) Abbott ... 431

Chlamydia trachomatis infections
E.E.S. (Erythromycin Ethylsuccinate) Abbott ... 433
EryPed (Erythromycin Ethylsuccinate) Abbott ... 431
Vigamox Ophthalmic Solution (Moxifloxacin Hydrochloride) Alcon ... 548

Chlamydia trachomatis infections, ocular
(*see under* Trachoma)

Chlamydia trachomatis pneumonia of infancy
E.E.S. (Erythromycin Ethylsuccinate) Abbott ... 433
EryPed (Erythromycin Ethylsuccinate) Abbott ... 431

Chlamydia trachomatis rectal infections
E.E.S. (Erythromycin Ethylsuccinate) Abbott ... 433
EryPed (Erythromycin Ethylsuccinate) Abbott ... 431

Chlamydia trachomatis urethral infections
E.E.S. (Erythromycin Ethylsuccinate) Abbott ... 433
EryPed (Erythromycin Ethylsuccinate) Abbott ... 431

Chlamydia trachomatis urogenital infections during pregnancy
E.E.S. (Erythromycin Ethylsuccinate) Abbott ... 433
EryPed (Erythromycin Ethylsuccinate) Abbott ... 431

Chloasma
(*see under* Hyperpigmentation, skin, bleaching of)

Cholangitis
(*see under* Infections, intra-abdominal)

Cholecystitis, acute
(*see under* Infections, intra-abdominal)

Cholesterol levels, elevated
(*see under* Hypercholesterolemia, primary, adjunct to diet)

Choroidal neovascularization, secondary to macular degeneration
Visudyne for Injection (Verteporfin) Novartis ... 2332

Christmas disease
(*see under* Hemophilia B)

Cirrhosis, biliary
Urso 250 Tablets (Ursodiol) Axcan Pharma ... 720
Urso Forte Tablets (Ursodiol) Axcan Pharma ... 720

Citrobacter diversus infections
Cipro I.V. (Ciprofloxacin) Schering ... 2817
Cipro (Ciprofloxacin) Schering ... 2810

Citrobacter diversus urinary tract infections
Cipro I.V. (Ciprofloxacin) Schering ... 2817
Cipro (Ciprofloxacin) Schering ... 2810

Citrobacter freundii infections
Cipro I.V. (Ciprofloxacin) Schering ... 2817
Cipro (Ciprofloxacin) Schering ... 2810
Noroxin Tablets (Norfloxacin) Merck . 2069
Tygacil for Injection (Tigecycline) Wyeth ... 3276

Citrobacter freundii intra-abdominal infections
Tygacil for Injection (Tigecycline) Wyeth ... 3276

Citrobacter freundii skin and skin structure infections
Cipro I.V. (Ciprofloxacin) Schering ... 2817
Cipro (Ciprofloxacin) Schering ... 2810

Citrobacter freundii urinary tract infections
Cipro I.V. (Ciprofloxacin) Schering ... 2817
Cipro (Ciprofloxacin) Schering ... 2810
Noroxin Tablets (Norfloxacin) Merck . 2069

Citrobacter species infections
Fortaz (Ceftazidime) GlaxoSmithKline ... 1450
Primaxin I.M. (Cilastatin Sodium, Imipenem) Merck ... 2080
Primaxin I.V. (Cilastatin Sodium, Imipenem) Merck ... 2083
Timentin ADD-Vantage (Clavulanate Potassium, Ticarcillin Disodium) GlaxoSmithKline ... 1606
Timentin Injection Galaxy Container (Clavulanate Potassium, Ticarcillin Disodium) GlaxoSmithKline ... 1609

Timentin IV Infusion (Clavulanate Potassium, Ticarcillin Disodium) GlaxoSmithKline 1603
Timentin Pharmacy Bulk Package (Clavulanate Potassium, Ticarcillin Disodium) GlaxoSmithKline 1613

Citrobacter species intra-abdominal infections
Primaxin I.V. (Cilastatin Sodium, Imipenem) Merck 2083

Citrobacter species lower respiratory tract infections
Fortaz (Ceftazidime) GlaxoSmithKline 1450

Citrobacter species skin and skin structure infections
Primaxin I.M. (Cilastatin Sodium, Imipenem) Merck 2080
Primaxin I.V. (Cilastatin Sodium, Imipenem) Merck 2083

Citrobacter species urinary tract infections
Timentin ADD-Vantage (Clavulanate Potassium, Ticarcillin Disodium) GlaxoSmithKline 1606
Timentin Injection Galaxy Container (Clavulanate Potassium, Ticarcillin Disodium) GlaxoSmithKline 1609
Timentin IV Infusion (Clavulanate Potassium, Ticarcillin Disodium) GlaxoSmithKline 1603
Timentin Pharmacy Bulk Package (Clavulanate Potassium, Ticarcillin Disodium) GlaxoSmithKline 1613

Claudication, intermittent
Pletal Tablets (Cilostazol) Otsuka 2481

Clostridium species infections
Primaxin I.V. (Cilastatin Sodium, Imipenem) Merck 2083
Rocephin Injectable Vials, ADD-Vantage, Galaxy, Bulk (Ceftriaxone Sodium) Roche 2642

Clostridium species intra-abdominal infections
Invanz for Injection (Ertapenem) Merck 2029
Primaxin I.V. (Cilastatin Sodium, Imipenem) Merck 2083
Rocephin Injectable Vials, ADD-Vantage, Galaxy, Bulk (Ceftriaxone Sodium) Roche 2642

Clostridium tetani, immunization against
(*see also under* Immunization, diphtheria, tetanus and pertussis)
Boostrix (Diphtheria & Tetanus Toxoids and Acellular Pertussis Vaccine Adsorbed) GlaxoSmithKline 1377
Infanrix Vaccine (Diphtheria & Tetanus Toxoids and Acellular Pertussis Vaccine Adsorbed) GlaxoSmithKline 1479
Pediarix Vaccine (Diphtheria & Tetanus Toxoids and Acellular Pertussis Vaccine Adsorbed, Hepatitis B Vaccine, Recombinant, Poliovirus Vaccine Inactivated) GlaxoSmithKline 1552

Cold, common, symptomatic relief of
(*see also under* Influenza syndrome, symptomatic relief of)
Actifed Cold & Allergy Tablets (Chlorpheniramine Maleate, Phenylephrine Hydrochloride) McNeil Consumer 1895
Benadryl Allergy & Cold Kapgels (Acetaminophen, Diphenhydramine Hydrochloride, Phenylephrine Hydrochloride) McNeil Consumer 1895
Benadryl Allergy & Sinus Headache Kapgels (Acetaminophen, Diphenhydramine Hydrochloride, Phenylephrine Hydrochloride) McNeil Consumer 1895
Benadryl Severe Allergy & Sinus Headache Caplets (Acetaminophen, Diphenhydramine Hydrochloride, Phenylephrine Hydrochloride) McNeil Consumer 1897
Benadryl Dye-Free Allergy Liqui-gels Softgels (Diphenhydramine Hydrochloride) McNeil Consumer 1897
Benadryl Allergy Kapgels (Diphenhydramine Hydrochloride) McNeil Consumer 1895
Benadryl Allergy Quick Dissolve Strips (Diphenhydramine Hydrochloride) McNeil Consumer 1896
Benadryl Allergy Ultratab Tablets (Diphenhydramine Hydrochloride) McNeil Consumer 1896
Children's Benadryl Allergy Fastmelts (Diphenhydramine Hydrochloride) McNeil Consumer 1897
Children's Benadryl-D Allergy & Sinus Liquid (Diphenhydramine Hydrochloride, Phenylephrine Hydrochloride) McNeil Consumer 1896
Benadryl-D Allergy & Sinus Tablet (Diphenhydramine Hydrochloride, Phenylephrine Hydrochloride) McNeil Consumer 1896
Hyland's Sniffles 'N Sneezes 4 Kids Tablets (Dietary Supplement) Standard Homeopathic .... ■ 621
PediaCare Children's Allergy & Cold Liquid (Diphenhydramine Hydrochloride, Phenylephrine Hydrochloride) McNeil Consumer 1902
PediaCare Children's Decongestant Liquid (Phenylephrine Hydrochloride) McNeil Consumer 1902
PediaCare Children's Liquid Multi-Symptom Cold (Dextromethorphan Hydrobromide, Phenylephrine Hydrochloride) McNeil Consumer 1902
PediaCare Children's Long-Acting Cough (Dextromethorphan Hydrobromide) McNeil Consumer 1902
Sudafed 12 Hour Nasal Decongestant Non-Drowsy Caplets (Pseudoephedrine Hydrochloride) McNeil Consumer 1909
Sudafed 24 Hour Non-Drowsy Nasal Decongestant Tablets (Pseudoephedrine Hydrochloride) McNeil Consumer 1906
Children's Sudafed Nasal Decongestant Liquid (Pseudoephedrine Hydrochloride) McNeil Consumer 1906
Children's Sudafed PE Cold & Cough Liquid (Dextromethorphan Hydrobromide, Phenylephrine Hydrochloride) McNeil Consumer 1907
Children's Sudafed PE Nasal Decongestant Liquid (Phenylephrine Hydrochloride) McNeil Consumer 1906
Sudafed Nasal Decongestant Tablets (Pseudoephedrine Hydrochloride) McNeil Consumer 1906
Sudafed OM Sinus Cold Moisturizing Nasal Spray (Oxymetazoline Hydrochloride) McNeil Consumer 1906
Sudafed OM Sinus Congestion Moisturizing Nasal Spray (Oxymetazoline Hydrochloride) McNeil Consumer 1906
Sudafed PE Cold & Cough Caplets (Acetaminophen, Dextromethorphan Hydrobromide, Guaifenesin, Phenylephrine Hydrochloride) McNeil Consumer 1907
Sudafed PE Nasal Decongestant Tablets (Phenylephrine Hydrochloride) McNeil Consumer 1907
Sudafed PE Nighttime Cold Caplets (Acetaminophen, Diphenhydramine Hydrochloride, Phenylephrine Hydrochloride) McNeil Consumer 1907
Sudafed PE Severe Cold Caplets (Acetaminophen, Diphenhydramine Hydrochloride, Phenylephrine Hydrochloride) McNeil Consumer 1908
Regular Strength Tylenol Tablets (Acetaminophen) McNeil Consumer 1915
Tylenol 8 Hour Extended Release Caplets (Acetaminophen) McNeil Consumer 1915
Extra Strength Tylenol Caplets, Cool Caplets, and EZ Tabs (Acetaminophen) McNeil Consumer 1915
Extra Strength Tylenol Adult Rapid Blast Liquid (Acetaminophen) McNeil Consumer 1915
Extra Strength Tylenol Rapid Release Gels (Acetaminophen) McNeil Consumer 1915
Tylenol Arthritis Pain Extended Release Geltabs/Caplets (Acetaminophen) McNeil Consumer 1915
Tylenol Chest Congestion Caplets with Cool Burst (Acetaminophen, Guaifenesin) McNeil Consumer 1910
Tylenol Chest Congestion Liquid with Cool Burst (Acetaminophen, Guaifenesin) McNeil Consumer 1910
Children's Tylenol Plus Cold Suspension Liquid (Acetaminophen, Chlorpheniramine Maleate, Phenylephrine Hydrochloride) McNeil Consumer 1912
Children's Tylenol Plus Cold & Allergy Suspension Liquid (Acetaminophen, Diphenhydramine Hydrochloride, Phenylephrine Hydrochloride) McNeil Consumer 1914
Children's Tylenol Plus Cough & Runny Nose Suspension Liquid (Acetaminophen, Chlorpheniramine Maleate, Dextromethorphan Hydrobromide) McNeil Consumer 1912
Children's Tylenol Plus Cough & Sore Throat Suspension Liquid (Acetaminophen, Dextromethorphan Hydrobromide) McNeil Consumer 1912
Children's Tylenol Plus Flu Suspension Liquid (Acetaminophen, Chlorpheniramine Maleate, Dextromethorphan Hydrobromide, Phenylephrine Hydrochloride) McNeil Consumer 1914
Children's Tylenol Suspension Liquid (Acetaminophen) McNeil Consumer 1909
Children's Tylenol Meltaways (Acetaminophen) McNeil Consumer 1909
Children's Tylenol Plus Multi-Symptom Cold Suspension Liquid (Acetaminophen, Chlorpheniramine Maleate, Dextromethorphan Hydrobromide, Phenylephrine Hydrochloride) McNeil Consumer 1912
Tylenol Cold Head Congestion Daytime Caplets with Cool Burst (Acetaminophen, Dextromethorphan Hydrobromide, Phenylephrine Hydrochloride) McNeil Consumer 1910
Tylenol Cold Head Congestion Nighttime Caplets with Cool Burst (Acetaminophen, Chlorpheniramine Maleate, Dextromethorphan Hydrobromide, Phenylephrine Hydrochloride) McNeil Consumer 1910
Tylenol Cold Head Congestion Severe Daytime Caplets with Cool Burst (Acetaminophen, Dextromethorphan Hydrobromide, Guaifenesin, Phenylephrine Hydrochloride) McNeil Consumer 1910
Tylenol Cold Multi-Symptom Daytime Caplets with Cool Burst and Rapid Release Gels (Acetaminophen, Dextromethorphan Hydrobromide, Phenylephrine Hydrochloride) McNeil Consumer 1913
Tylenol Cold Multi-Symptom Daytime Liquid with Citrus Burst (Acetaminophen, Dextromethorphan Hydrobromide, Phenylephrine Hydrochloride) McNeil Consumer 1913
Tylenol Cold Multi-Symptom Nighttime Caplets with Cool Burst (Acetaminophen, Chlorpheniramine Maleate, Dextromethorphan Hydrobromide, Phenylephrine Hydrochloride) McNeil Consumer 1913
Tylenol Cold Multi-Symptom Nighttime Liquid with Cool Burst (Acetaminophen, Dextromethorphan Hydrobromide, Doxylamine Succinate, Phenylephrine Hydrochloride) McNeil Consumer 1913
Tylenol Cold Multi-Symptom Severe Caplets with Cool Burst (Acetaminophen, Dextromethorphan Hydrobromide, Guaifenesin, Phenylephrine Hydrochloride) McNeil Consumer 1913
Tylenol Cold Multi-Symptom Severe Daytime Liquid with Citrus Burst (Acetaminophen, Dextromethorphan Hydrobromide, Guaifenesin, Phenylephrine Hydrochloride) McNeil Consumer 1913
Tylenol Cough & Sore Throat Nighttime Liquid with Cool Burst (Acetaminophen, Dextromethorphan Hydrobromide, Doxylamine Succinate) McNeil Consumer 1918
Concentrated Tylenol Infants' Drops (Acetaminophen) McNeil Consumer 1909
Jr. Tylenol Meltaways (Acetaminophen) McNeil Consumer 1909
Tylenol Sinus Congestion & Pain Severe Caplets with Cool Burst (Acetaminophen, Guaifenesin, Phenylephrine Hydrochloride) McNeil Consumer 1917
Tylenol Sore Throat Daytime Liquid with Cool Burst (Acetaminophen) McNeil Consumer 1918
Vicks DayQuil Cold & Flu Multi-Symptom Relief (Acetaminophen, Dextromethorphan Hydrobromide, Phenylephrine Hydrochloride) Procter & Gamble .... ■ 616
Vicks DayQuil LiquiCaps (Acetaminophen, Dextromethorphan Hydrobromide, Phenylephrine Hydrochloride) Procter & Gamble 2567
Vicks DayQuil (Acetaminophen, Dextromethorphan Hydrobromide, Phenylephrine Hydrochloride) Procter & Gamble .... ■ 616
Vicks DayQuil Liquid (Acetaminophen, Dextromethorphan Hydrobromide, Phenylephrine Hydrochloride) Procter & Gamble 2567
Vicks DayQuil Multi-Symptom Cold/Flu Relief (Acetaminophen, Dextromethorphan Hydrobromide, Phenylephrine Hydrochloride) Procter & Gamble 2567
Vicks NyQuil (Acetaminophen, Dextromethorphan Hydrobromide, Doxylamine Succinate) Procter & Gamble .... ■ 617

Cold sores
(*see under* Herpetic manifestations, oral, symptomatic relief of)

Colic, symptomatic relief of
Hyland's Colic Tablets (Chamomilla, Disocorea, Colocynthis, Homeopathic Formulations) Standard Homeopathic .... ■ 619

Colitis, mucous
(*see under* Bowel, irritable, syndrome)

Colitis, ulcerative
Asacol Delayed-Release Tablets (Mesalamine) Procter & Gamble Pharmaceuticals 2579
Lialda Tablets (Mesalamine) Shire US 3029
Pentasa Capsules (Mesalamine) Shire US 3030
Remicade for IV Injection (Infliximab) Centocor 950

Colon, irritable
(*see under* Bowel, irritable, syndrome)

Colon, spastic
(*see under* Bowel, irritable, syndrome)

Colorectal polyps, adenomatous
Celebrex Capsules (Celecoxib) Searle 2979

Condylomata acuminata
Aldara Cream, 5% (Imiquimod) Graceway 1699

Alferon N Injection (Interferon alfa-N3 (Human Leukocyte Derived)) Hemispherx ... 1726
Intron A for Injection (Interferon alfa-2b, Recombinant) Schering ... 2859

Condylomata acuminata, prevention of
Gardasil Injection (Quadrivalent Human Papillomavirus (Types 6, 11, 16, 18) Recombinant Vaccine) Merck ... 2019

Congestive heart failure, adjunct in
(*see also under* Edema, adjunctive therapy in)
Captopril Tablets (Captopril) Mylan ... 2182
Coreg Tablets (Carvedilol) GlaxoSmithKline ... 1387
Coreg CR Extended-Release Capsules (Carvedilol Phosphate) GlaxoSmithKline ... 1393
Demadex Tablets (Torsemide) Roche ... 2630
Dyrenium Capsules (Triamterene) WellSpring ... 3189
Edecrin (Ethacrynic Acid) Aton ... 698
Furosemide Tablets (Furosemide) Mylan ... 2186
Indapamide Tablets (Indapamide) Mylan ... 2188
Intravenous Sodium Diuril (Chlorothiazide Sodium) Ovation ... 2490
Lanoxin Injection (Digoxin) GlaxoSmithKline ... 1498
Lanoxin Injection Pediatric (Digoxin) GlaxoSmithKline ... 1502
Lanoxin Tablets (Digoxin) GlaxoSmithKline ... 1505
Natrecor for Injection (Nesiritide) Scios ... 2977
Prinivil Tablets (Lisinopril) Merck ... 2087

Congestive heart failure, post-myocardial infarction
Mavik Tablets (Trandolapril) Abbott ... 472

Conjunctival hyperemia, reduction of signs and symptoms
(*see under* Ocular redness)

Conjunctival inflammation, bulbar, steroid-responsive
Lotemax Ophthalmic Suspension 0.5% (Loteprednol Etabonate) Bausch & Lomb ... ⊙241

Conjunctival inflammation, palpebral, steroid-responsive
Lotemax Ophthalmic Suspension 0.5% (Loteprednol Etabonate) Bausch & Lomb ... ⊙241

Conjunctivitis, allergic
Alamast Ophthalmic Solution (Pemirolast Potassium) Vistakon ... 3181
Alrex Ophthalmic Suspension 0.2% (Loteprednol Etabonate) Bausch & Lomb ... ⊙236
Elestat Ophthalmic Solution (Epinastine Hydrochloride) Inspire ... 1741
Lotemax Ophthalmic Suspension 0.5% (Loteprednol Etabonate) Bausch & Lomb ... ⊙241
Optivar Ophthalmic Solution (Azelastine Hydrochloride) Meda ... ⊙254
Pataday Ophthalmic Solution (Olopatadine Hydrochloride) Alcon ... 543
Patanol Ophthalmic Solution (Olopatadine Hydrochloride) Alcon ... 546
Zylet Ophthalmic Suspension (Loteprednol Etabonate, Tobramycin) Bausch & Lomb ... ⊙247

Conjunctivitis, bacterial
AzaSite Ophthalmic Drops (Azithromycin) Inspire ... 1740
Ofloxacin Ophthalmic Solution 0.3% (Ofloxacin) Bausch & Lomb ... ⊙243
Quixin Ophthalmic Solution (Levofloxacin) Vistakon ... 3184
Vigamox Ophthalmic Solution (Moxifloxacin Hydrochloride) Alcon ... 548

Conjunctivitis, fungal
Natacyn Antifungal Ophthalmic Suspension (Natamycin) Alcon ... ⊙204

Conjunctivitis, granular
(*see under* Trachoma)

Conjunctivitis, inclusion
Gantrisin Pediatric Suspension (Acetyl Sulfisoxazole) Roche ... 2638

Conjunctivitis, infective
Blephamide Ophthalmic Ointment Allergan ... ⊙217
Blephamide Ophthalmic Suspension Allergan ... ⊙216
Pred-G Ophthalmic Ointment (Gentamicin Sulfate, Prednisolone Acetate) Allergan ... ⊙229
Pred-G Ophthalmic Suspension (Gentamicin Sulfate, Prednisolone Acetate) Allergan ... ⊙228
Zylet Ophthalmic Suspension (Loteprednol Etabonate, Tobramycin) Bausch & Lomb ... ⊙247

Conjunctivitis, unspecified
Bleph-10 Ophthalmic Solution 10% (Sulfacetamide Sodium) Allergan ... ⊙215
Pred Mild Ophthalmic Suspension (Prednisolone Acetate) Allergan ... ⊙230

Constipation
Metamucil Capsules (Psyllium Preparations) Procter & Gamble ... ■611

Constipation, chronic
Kristalose for Oral Solution (Lactulose) Cumberland ... 1004
Metamucil Capsules (Psyllium Preparations) Procter & Gamble ... 2563
Metamucil (Psyllium Preparations) Procter & Gamble ... 2563

Constipation, chronic idiopathic
Amitiza Capsules (Lubiprostone) Takeda ... 3082

Constipation, opioid-induced
Relistor Injection (Methylnaltrexone Bromide) Progenics ... 3310

Constipation, temporary
Ceo-Two Laxative Suppository (Potassium Bitartrate, Sodium Bicarbonate) Beutlich ... 815
Dulcolax Stool Softener (Docusate Sodium) Boehringer Ingelheim ... ■602
Dulcolax Suppositories (Bisacodyl) Boehringer Ingelheim ... ■602
Dulcolax Tablets (Bisacodyl) Boehringer Ingelheim ... ■602
Fleet Babylax Suppositories (Glycerin) Fleet ... 1142
Fleet Bisacodyl Laxatives (Bisacodyl) Fleet ... 1143
Fleet Enema (Sodium Phosphate) Fleet ... 1143
Fleet Enema Extra (Sodium Phosphate) Fleet ... 1143
Fleet Enema for Children (Sodium Phosphate) Fleet ... 1143
Fleet Glycerin Laxatives (Glycerin) Fleet ... 1142
Fleet Glycerin Suppositories (Glycerin) Fleet ... 1142
Fleet Mineral Oil Enema (Mineral Oil) Fleet ... 1144
Fleet Pedia-Lax Chewable Tablets (Magnesium Hydroxide) Fleet ... 1145
Fleet Pedia-Lax Enema (Sodium Phosphate) Fleet ... 1143
Fleet Pedia-Lax Liquid Stool Softener (Docusate Sodium) Fleet ... 1144
Fleet Pedia-Lax Liquid Suppositories (Glycerin) Fleet ... ■605
Fleet Pedia-Lax Senna Quick Dissolve Strips (Sennosides) Fleet ... 1145
Fleet Pedia-Lax Suppositories (Glycerin) Fleet ... 1142
Fleet Phospho-soda (Sodium Phosphate) Fleet ... 1145

Contraception
(*see under* Pregnancy, prevention of)

Contraception, postcoital
Plan B Tablets (Levonorgestrel) Duramed ... 1044

Convulsive disorders, adjunctive therapy in
Valium Tablets (Diazepam) Roche ... 2658

Convulsive episodes, control of
Nembutal Sodium Solution, USP (Pentobarbital Sodium) Ovation ... 2494

Corneal edema
(*see under* Edema, corneal, temporary relief of)

Corneal erosions, recurrent
Lacrisert Sterile Ophthalmic Insert (Hydroxypropyl Cellulose) Aton ... ⊙233

Corneal inflammation, steroid-responsive
Blephamide Ophthalmic Ointment Allergan ... ⊙217
Blephamide Ophthalmic Suspension Allergan ... ⊙216
FML Ophthalmic Ointment (Fluorometholone) Allergan ... ⊙223
FML Ophthalmic Suspension (Fluorometholone) Allergan ... ⊙224
FML Forte Ophthalmic Suspension (Fluorometholone) Allergan ... ⊙222
Lotemax Ophthalmic Suspension 0.5% (Loteprednol Etabonate) Bausch & Lomb ... ⊙241
Pred Forte Ophthalmic Suspension (Prednisolone Acetate) Allergan ... ⊙227
Pred-G Ophthalmic Ointment (Gentamicin Sulfate, Prednisolone Acetate) Allergan ... ⊙229
Pred-G Ophthalmic Suspension (Gentamicin Sulfate, Prednisolone Acetate) Allergan ... ⊙228
Zylet Ophthalmic Suspension (Loteprednol Etabonate, Tobramycin) Bausch & Lomb ... ⊙247

Corneal injury, chemical
Blephamide Ophthalmic Ointment Allergan ... ⊙217
Blephamide Ophthalmic Suspension Allergan ... ⊙216
Pred Mild Ophthalmic Suspension (Prednisolone Acetate) Allergan ... ⊙230
Pred-G Ophthalmic Ointment (Gentamicin Sulfate, Prednisolone Acetate) Allergan ... ⊙229
Pred-G Ophthalmic Suspension (Gentamicin Sulfate, Prednisolone Acetate) Allergan ... ⊙228
Zylet Ophthalmic Suspension (Loteprednol Etabonate, Tobramycin) Bausch & Lomb ... ⊙247

Corneal injury, foreign bodies
Blephamide Ophthalmic Ointment Allergan ... ⊙217
Blephamide Ophthalmic Suspension Allergan ... ⊙216
Pred-G Ophthalmic Ointment (Gentamicin Sulfate, Prednisolone Acetate) Allergan ... ⊙229
Pred-G Ophthalmic Suspension (Gentamicin Sulfate, Prednisolone Acetate) Allergan ... ⊙228
Zylet Ophthalmic Suspension (Loteprednol Etabonate, Tobramycin) Bausch & Lomb ... ⊙247

Corneal injury, radiation
Blephamide Ophthalmic Ointment Allergan ... ⊙217
Blephamide Ophthalmic Suspension Allergan ... ⊙216
Pred-G Ophthalmic Ointment (Gentamicin Sulfate, Prednisolone Acetate) Allergan ... ⊙229
Pred-G Ophthalmic Suspension (Gentamicin Sulfate, Prednisolone Acetate) Allergan ... ⊙228
Zylet Ophthalmic Suspension (Loteprednol Etabonate, Tobramycin) Bausch & Lomb ... ⊙247

Corneal injury, thermal burns
Blephamide Ophthalmic Ointment Allergan ... ⊙217
Blephamide Ophthalmic Suspension Allergan ... ⊙216
Pred Mild Ophthalmic Suspension (Prednisolone Acetate) Allergan ... ⊙230
Pred-G Ophthalmic Ointment (Gentamicin Sulfate, Prednisolone Acetate) Allergan ... ⊙229
Pred-G Ophthalmic Suspension (Gentamicin Sulfate, Prednisolone Acetate) Allergan ... ⊙228
Zylet Ophthalmic Suspension (Loteprednol Etabonate, Tobramycin) Bausch & Lomb ... ⊙247

Corneal refractive surgery, treatment adjunct
Diclofenac Sodium Ophthalmic Solution (Diclofenac Sodium) Bausch & Lomb ... ⊙240

Corneal sensitivity, decreased
Lacrisert Sterile Ophthalmic Insert (Hydroxypropyl Cellulose) Aton ... ⊙233

Corneal ulcers
Bleph-10 Ophthalmic Solution 10% (Sulfacetamide Sodium) Allergan ... ⊙215
Iquix Ophthalmic Solution (Levofloxacin) Vistakon ... 3183
Ofloxacin Ophthalmic Solution 0.3% (Ofloxacin) Bausch & Lomb ... ⊙243

Coronary angioplasty or atherectomy, percutaneous transluminal, adjunct in
Angiomax for Injection (Bivalirudin) The Medicines Company ... 1933

Coronary artery disease, reducing the risk of
Aceon Tablets (2 mg, 4 mg, 8 mg) (Perindopril Erbumine) Solvay ... 3038
Metamucil Dietary Fiber Supplement (Psyllium Preparations) Procter & Gamble ... 2563
Mevacor Tablets (Lovastatin) Merck ... 2063
Zocor Tablets (Simvastatin) Merck ... 2136

Coronary atherosclerosis, to slow the progression of
(*see also under* Coronary artery disease, reducing the risk of)
Advicor Tablets (Lovastatin, Niacin) Abbott ... 402
Lescol Capsules (Fluvastatin Sodium) Novartis ... 2268
Lescol XL Tablets (Fluvastatin Sodium) Novartis ... 2268
Mevacor Tablets (Lovastatin) Merck ... 2063
Niaspan Extended-Release Tablets (Niacin) Abbott ... 480

Coronary syndrome, acute
(*see also under* Cardiac ischemic complications, acute, prevention of, adjunct to PTCA; Coronary angioplasty or atherectomy, percutaneous transluminal, adjunct in)
Integrilin Injection (Eptifibatide) Schering ... 2855
Plavix Tablets (Clopidogrel Bisulfate) Bristol-Myers Squibb ... 926
Plavix Tablets (Clopidogrel Bisulfate) sanofi-aventis ... 2767

Corynebacterium diphtheriae
(*see under* C. diphtheriae infections)

Corynebacterium diphtheriae, immunization against
(*see also under* Immunization, diphtheria, tetanus and pertussis)
Boostrix (Diphtheria & Tetanus Toxoids and Acellular Pertussis Vaccine Adsorbed) GlaxoSmithKline ... 1377
Infanrix Vaccine (Diphtheria & Tetanus Toxoids and Acellular Pertussis Vaccine Adsorbed) GlaxoSmithKline ... 1479
Pediarix Vaccine (Diphtheria & Tetanus Toxoids and Acellular Pertussis Vaccine Adsorbed, Hepatitis B Vaccine, Recombinant, Poliovirus Vaccine Inactivated) GlaxoSmithKline ... 1552

Corynebacterium infections, ocular
Vigamox Ophthalmic Solution (Moxifloxacin Hydrochloride) Alcon ... 548

Corynebacterium infections, unspecified
Vigamox Ophthalmic Solution (Moxifloxacin Hydrochloride) Alcon ... ⊙213

Corynebacterium minutissimum
(*see under* C. minutissimum infections)

Coryza, acute
(*see under* Cold, common, symptomatic relief of)

Cough, symptomatic relief of
Benadryl Allergy & Cold Kapgels (Acetaminophen, Diphenhydramine Hydrochloride, Phenylephrine Hydrochloride) McNeil Consumer ... 1895
Hyland's Cough Syrup with Honey (Homeopathic Formulations) Standard Homeopathic ... ▣619
PediaCare Children's Allergy & Cold Liquid (Diphenhydramine Hydrochloride, Phenylephrine Hydrochloride) McNeil Consumer .. 1902
PediaCare Children's Allergy Liquid (Diphenhydramine Hydrochloride) McNeil Consumer ... 1902
PediaCare Children's Liquid Multi-Symptom Cold (Dextromethorphan Hydrobromide, Phenylephrine Hydrochloride) McNeil Consumer ... 1902
PediaCare Children's Long-Acting Cough (Dextromethorphan Hydrobromide) McNeil Consumer ... 1902
Children's Sudafed PE Cold & Cough Liquid (Dextromethorphan Hydrobromide, Phenylephrine Hydrochloride) McNeil Consumer .. 1907
Sudafed PE Cold & Cough Caplets (Acetaminophen, Dextromethorphan Hydrobromide, Guaifenesin, Phenylephrine Hydrochloride) McNeil Consumer ... 1907
Sudafed PE Severe Cold Caplets (Acetaminophen, Diphenhydramine Hydrochloride, Phenylephrine Hydrochloride) McNeil Consumer ... 1908
Tessalon Capsules (Benzonatate) Forest ... 1183
Tessalon Perles (Benzonatate) Forest ... 1183
Tussionex Pennkinetic Extended-Release Suspension (Chlorpheniramine Polistirex, Hydrocodone Polistirex) UCB, Inc. ... 3154
Tylenol Chest Congestion Caplets with Cool Burst (Acetaminophen, Guaifenesin) McNeil Consumer ... 1910
Tylenol Chest Congestion Liquid with Cool Burst (Acetaminophen, Guaifenesin) McNeil Consumer ... 1910
Children's Tylenol Plus Cough & Runny Nose Suspension Liquid (Acetaminophen, Chlorpheniramine Maleate, Dextromethorphan Hydrobromide) McNeil Consumer .. 1912
Children's Tylenol Plus Cough & Sore Throat Suspension Liquid (Acetaminophen, Dextromethorphan Hydrobromide) McNeil Consumer ... 1912
Children's Tylenol Plus Flu Suspension Liquid (Acetaminophen, Chlorpheniramine Maleate, Dextromethorphan Hydrobromide, Phenylephrine Hydrochloride) McNeil Consumer ... 1914
Children's Tylenol Plus Multi-Symptom Cold Suspension Liquid (Acetaminophen, Chlorpheniramine Maleate, Dextromethorphan Hydrobromide, Phenylephrine Hydrochloride) McNeil Consumer ... 1912
Tylenol Cold Severe Congestion Daytime Caplets with Cool Burst (Acetaminophen, Dextromethorphan Hydrobromide, Guaifenesin, Pseudoephedrine Hydrochloride) McNeil Consumer ... 1912
Tylenol Cold Head Congestion Daytime Caplets with Cool Burst (Acetaminophen, Dextromethorphan Hydrobromide, Phenylephrine Hydrochloride) McNeil Consumer ... 1910
Tylenol Cold Head Congestion Nighttime Caplets with Cool Burst (Acetaminophen, Chlorpheniramine Maleate, Dextromethorphan Hydrobromide, Phenylephrine Hydrochloride) McNeil Consumer ... 1910
Tylenol Cold Head Congestion Severe Daytime Caplets with Cool Burst (Acetaminophen, Dextromethorphan Hydrobromide, Guaifenesin, Phenylephrine Hydrochloride) McNeil Consumer .. 1910
Tylenol Cold Multi-Symptom Daytime Caplets with Cool Burst and Rapid Release Gels (Acetaminophen, Dextromethorphan Hydrobromide, Phenylephrine Hydrochloride) McNeil Consumer .. 1913
Tylenol Cold Multi-Symptom Daytime Liquid with Citrus Burst (Acetaminophen, Dextromethorphan Hydrobromide, Phenylephrine Hydrochloride) McNeil Consumer ... 1913
Tylenol Cold Multi-Symptom Nighttime Caplets with Cool Burst (Acetaminophen, Chlorpheniramine Maleate, Dextromethorphan Hydrobromide, Phenylephrine Hydrochloride) McNeil Consumer ... 1913
Tylenol Cold Multi-Symptom Nighttime Liquid with Cool Burst (Acetaminophen, Dextromethorphan Hydrobromide, Doxylamine Succinate, Phenylephrine Hydrochloride) McNeil Consumer ... 1913
Tylenol Cold Multi-Symptom Severe Caplets with Cool Burst (Acetaminophen, Dextromethorphan Hydrobromide, Guaifenesin, Phenylephrine Hydrochloride) McNeil Consumer ... 1913
Tylenol Cold Multi-Symptom Severe Daytime Liquid with Citrus Burst (Acetaminophen, Dextromethorphan Hydrobromide, Guaifenesin, Phenylephrine Hydrochloride) McNeil Consumer ... 1913
Tylenol Cough & Sore Throat Daytime Liquid with Cool Burst (Acetaminophen, Dextromethorphan Hydrobromide) McNeil Consumer ... 1918
Tylenol Cough & Sore Throat Nighttime Liquid with Cool Burst (Acetaminophen, Dextromethorphan Hydrobromide, Doxylamine Succinate) McNeil Consumer ... 1918
Vicks DayQuil Cold & Flu Multi-Symptom Relief (Acetaminophen, Dextromethorphan Hydrobromide, Phenylephrine Hydrochloride) Procter & Gamble ... ▣616
Vicks DayQuil LiquiCaps (Acetaminophen, Dextromethorphan Hydrobromide, Phenylephrine Hydrochloride) Procter & Gamble .. 2567
Vicks DayQuil Liquid (Acetaminophen, Dextromethorphan Hydrobromide, Phenylephrine Hydrochloride) Procter & Gamble ... 2567
Vicks DayQuil Multi-Symptom Cold/Flu Relief (Acetaminophen, Dextromethorphan Hydrobromide, Phenylephrine Hydrochloride) Procter & Gamble ... 2567
Vicks NyQuil Cold & Flu Multi-Symptom Relief (Acetaminophen, Dextromethorphan Hydrobromide, Doxylamine Succinate) Procter & Gamble ... ▣617
Vicks NyQuil LiquiCaps (Acetaminophen, Dextromethorphan Hydrobromide, Doxylamine Succinate, Pseudoephedrine Hydrochloride) Procter & Gamble ... 2567
Vicks NyQuil Liquid (Acetaminophen, Dextromethorphan Hydrobromide, Doxylamine Succinate, Pseudoephedrine Hydrochloride) Procter & Gamble ... 2567
Vicks NyQuil Multi-Symptom Cold/Flu Relief (Acetaminophen, Dextromethorphan Hydrobromide, Doxylamine Succinate, Pseudoephedrine Hydrochloride) Procter & Gamble ... 2567

Cough, whooping
(*see under* Pertussis)

Cradle cap
(*see under* Dermatitis, seborrheic)

Cramps, leg
(*see under* Leg muscle cramps)

Cretinism
(*see under* Hypothyroidism, replacement or supplemental therapy in)

Crohn's disease
Cimzia (Certolizumab pegol) UCB, Inc. ... 3127
Humira Injection (Adalimumab) Abbott ... 442
Remicade for IV Injection (Infliximab) Centocor ... 950

Cryptococcosis
Abelcet Injection (Amphotericin B Lipid Complex) Enzon ... 1134
AmBisome for Injection (Amphotericin B, liposomal) Astellas ... 606

Cuts, minor, infection from
(*see under* Infections, skin, bacterial, minor)

Cuts, minor, pain associated with
(*see under* Pain, topical relief of)

Cyanide poisoning, treatment of
Cyanokit 5g Antidote (Hydroxocobalamin) Dey ... 1021

Cyclitis
Lotemax Ophthalmic Suspension 0.5% (Loteprednol Etabonate) Bausch & Lomb ... ⊙241
Zylet Ophthalmic Suspension (Loteprednol Etabonate, Tobramycin) Bausch & Lomb ... ⊙247

Cystic fibrosis, adjunctive therapy in
Pulmozyme Inhalation Solution (Dornase Alfa) Genentech ... 1217

Cystinuria
Cuprimine Capsules (Penicillamine) Merck ... 1986

Cystitis
Cipro (Ciprofloxacin) Schering ... 2810
Cipro XR Tablets (Ciprofloxacin) Schering ... 2823
Gantrisin Pediatric Suspension (Acetyl Sulfisoxazole) Roche ... 2638
Noroxin Tablets (Norfloxacin) Merck . 2069
Uroqid-Acid No. 2 Tablets (Methenamine Mandelate, Sodium Acid Phosphate) Beach ... 814

Cystitis, interstitial, symptomatic relief of
Elmiron Capsules (Pentosan Polysulfate Sodium) Ortho Women's ... 2435

D

Dandruff
(*see also under* Dermatitis, seborrheic)
Nizoral A-D Shampoo (Ketoconazole) McNeil Consumer ... 1901

Dementia, Alzheimer's type
Aricept Tablets (Donepezil Hydrochloride) Eisai ... 1062
Aricept ODT Tablets (Donepezil Hydrochloride) Eisai ... 1062
Exelon Capsules (Rivastigmine Tartrate) Novartis ... 2229
Exelon Oral Solution (Rivastigmine Tartrate) Novartis ... 2229
Exelon Patch (Rivastigmine Tartrate) Novartis ... 2233
Namenda (Memantine Hydrochloride) Forest ... 1180

Dementia, Parkinson's disease, associated with
Exelon Capsules (Rivastigmine Tartrate) Novartis ... 2229
Exelon Oral Solution (Rivastigmine Tartrate) Novartis ... 2229
Exelon Patch (Rivastigmine Tartrate) Novartis ... 2233

Dental procedures, adjunct to
Hurricaine Topical Anesthetic (Benzocaine) Beutlich ... 815

Dentures, irritation of
Hurricaine Topical Anesthetic (Benzocaine) Beutlich ... 815

Depression, bipolar
Symbyax Capsules (Fluoxetine Hydrochloride, Olanzapine) Lilly ... 1871

Depression, major, without melancholia
Parnate Tablets (Tranylcypromine Sulfate) GlaxoSmithKline ... 1532

Depression, manic-depressive
(*see under* Mania, bipolar)

Depression, treatment of
Celexa (Citalopram Hydrobromide) Forest ... 1160
Effexor XR Extended-Release Capsules (Venlafaxine Hydrochloride) Wyeth ... 3195
Lexapro Oral Suspension (Escitalopram Oxalate) Forest ... 1174
Lexapro Tablets (Escitalopram Oxalate) Forest ... 1174
Marplan Tablets (Isocarboxazid) Validus ... 3177
Paxil (Paroxetine Hydrochloride) GlaxoSmithKline ... 1535
Paxil CR Controlled-Release Tablets (Paroxetine Hydrochloride) GlaxoSmithKline ... 1544
Wellbutrin Tablets (Bupropion Hydrochloride) GlaxoSmithKline ... 1648
Wellbutrin SR Sustained-Release Tablets (Bupropion Hydrochloride) GlaxoSmithKline ... 1653
Wellbutrin XL Extended-Release Tablets (Bupropion Hydrochloride) GlaxoSmithKline ... 1659

Depressive disorder, major, adjunctive treatment
Abilify Oral Solution (Aripiprazole) Bristol-Myers Squibb ... 881
Abilify Oral Solution (Aripiprazole) Otsuka ... 2466
Abilify Discmelt Orally Disintegrating Tablets (Aripiprazole) Bristol-Myers Squibb ... 881
Abilify Discmelt Orally Disintegrating Tablets (Aripiprazole) Otsuka ... 2466
Abilify Tablets (Aripiprazole) Bristol-Myers Squibb ... 881
Abilify Tablets (Aripiprazole) Otsuka .. 2466

Dermatitis, allergic
MimyX Cream (Glycerin) Stiefel ... 3059

Dermatitis, atopic
Elidel Cream 1% (Pimecrolimus) Novartis ... 2221
MimyX Cream (Glycerin) Stiefel ... 3059
Protopic Ointment (Tacrolimus) Astellas ... 628
Verdeso Foam (Desonide) Stiefel ... 3069

Dermatitis, contact
(*see under* Dermatoses, corticosteroid-responsive)

Dermatitis, corticosteroid-responsive, anal region
Analpram-HC (Hydrocortisone Acetate, Pramoxine Hydrochloride) Ferndale ... 1140

Dermatitis, herpetiformis
Dapsone Tablets USP (Dapsone) Jacobus ... 1746

Dermatitis, radiation
MimyX Cream (Glycerin) Stiefel ... 3059

Dermatitis, seborrheic
Extina Foam, 2% (Ketoconazole) Stiefel ... 3057
Rosac Wash (Sodium Sulfacetamide) Stiefel ... 3062

Dermatofibrosarcoma protuberans
Gleevec Tablets (Imatinib Mesylate) Novartis ... 2255

(▣ Described in PDR® For Nonprescription Drugs) (⊙ Described in PDR® For Ophthalmic Medicines)

Dermatomyositis, possibly effective in
Potaba (Aminobenzoate Potassium) Glenwood ... 1698

Dermatoses, corticosteroid-responsive
(*see also under* Skin, inflammatory conditions)
Diprolene Lotion 0.05% (Betamethasone Dipropionate) Schering ... 2838
Diprolene Ointment 0.05% (Betamethasone Dipropionate) Schering ... 2839
Diprolene AF Cream 0.05% (Betamethasone Dipropionate) Schering ... 2837
Elocon Cream 0.1% (Mometasone Furoate) Schering ... 2840
Elocon Lotion 0.1% (Mometasone Furoate) Schering ... 2841
Elocon Ointment 0.1% (Mometasone Furoate) Schering ... 2842
Luxíq Foam (Betamethasone Valerate) Stiefel ... 3058
Olux Foam (Clobetasol Propionate) Stiefel ... 3061
Olux-E Foam (Clobetasol Propionate) Stiefel ... 3059
Pramosone (Hydrocortisone Acetate, Pramoxine Hydrochloride) Ferndale ... 1141

Diabetes mellitus
(*see under* Hyperglycemia, control of, adjunct to diet)

Diabetes mellitus, insulin-dependent
Apidra Injection (Insulin Glulisine) sanofi-aventis ... 2706
Exubera Inhalation Powder (Insulin, Human (rDNA origin)) Pfizer ... 2515
Humalog-Pen and KwikPen (Insulin Lispro, Human) Lilly ... 1829
Humalog Mix 50/50-Pen and KwikPen (Insulin Lispro, Human, Insulin Lispro Protamine, Human) Lilly ... 1833
Humalog Mix 75/25-Pen and KwikPen (Insulin Lispro, Human, Insulin Lispro Protamine, Human) Lilly ... 1835
Humulin 50/50, 100 Units (Insulin, Human Regular and Human NPH Mixture) Lilly ... 1843
Humulin 70/30 Vial (Insulin, Human Regular and Human NPH Mixture) Lilly ... 1844
Humulin N Vial (Insulin, Human NPH) Lilly ... 1846
Humulin R (Insulin, Human Regular) Lilly ... 1849
Humulin R (U-500) (Insulin, Human Regular) Lilly ... 1850
Lantus Injection (Insulin glargine) sanofi-aventis ... 2749
NovoLog Mix 70/30 (Insulin Aspart, Human, Insulin Aspart Protamine, Human) Novo Nordisk ... 2364
NovoLog Injection (Insulin Aspart, Human Regular) Novo Nordisk ... 2359

Diabetes mellitus, non-insulin-dependent
ActoPlus Met Tablets (Metformin Hydrochloride, Pioglitazone Hydrochloride) Takeda ... 3071
Actos Tablets (Pioglitazone Hydrochloride) Takeda ... 3077
Avandamet Tablets (Rosiglitazone Maleate, Metformin Hydrochloride) GlaxoSmithKline ... 1336
Avandaryl Tablets (Rosiglitazone Maleate, Glimepiride) GlaxoSmithKline ... 1344
Avandia Tablets (Rosiglitazone Maleate) GlaxoSmithKline ... 1351
Byetta Injection (Exenatide) Amylin ... 600
Lantus Injection (Insulin glargine) sanofi-aventis ... 2749
Precose Tablets (Acarbose) Bayer HealthCare Pharmaceuticals ... 792

Diabetes mellitus, type 1
Exubera Inhalation Powder (Insulin, Human (rDNA origin)) Pfizer ... 2515
Lantus Injection (Insulin glargine) sanofi-aventis ... 2749
Levemir Injection (Insulin Detemir (rDNA Origin)) Novo Nordisk ... 2352

Diabetes mellitus, type 2
ActoPlus Met Tablets (Metformin Hydrochloride, Pioglitazone Hydrochloride) Takeda ... 3071
Actos Tablets (Pioglitazone Hydrochloride) Takeda ... 3077
Avandamet Tablets (Rosiglitazone Maleate, Metformin Hydrochloride) GlaxoSmithKline ... 1336
Avandaryl Tablets (Rosiglitazone Maleate, Glimepiride) GlaxoSmithKline ... 1344
Avandia Tablets (Rosiglitazone Maleate) GlaxoSmithKline ... 1351
Byetta Injection (Exenatide) Amylin ... 600
Duetact Tablets (Glimepiride, Pioglitazone Hydrochloride) Takeda ... 3085
Exubera Inhalation Powder (Insulin, Human (rDNA origin)) Pfizer ... 2515
Janumet Tablets (Sitagliptin Phosphate, Metformin Hydrochloride) Merck ... 2041
Januvia Tablets (Sitagliptin Phosphate) Merck ... 2048
Lantus Injection (Insulin glargine) sanofi-aventis ... 2749
Levemir Injection (Insulin Detemir (rDNA Origin)) Novo Nordisk ... 2352
PrandiMet Tablets (Repaglinide, Metformin Hydrochloride) Sciele ... 2967
Prandin Tablets (Repaglinide) Sciele ... 2971
Precose Tablets (Acarbose) Bayer HealthCare Pharmaceuticals ... 792
Starlix Tablets (Nateglinide) Novartis ... 2314
WelChol Tablets (Colesevelam Hydrochloride) Daiichi Sankyo ... 1015

Diabetic nephropathy
(*see under* Nephropathy, diabetic)

Diarrhea, adjunctive therapy in
Imodium Multi-Symptom Relief Caplets and Chewable Tablets (Loperamide Hydrochloride, Simethicone) McNeil Consumer ... 1899

Diarrhea, bacterial
(*see under* Diarrhea, infectious)

Diarrhea, cryptosporidium parvum-induced
Alinia for Oral Suspension (Nitazoxanide) Romark ... 2677
Alinia Tablets (Nitazoxanide) Romark ... 2677

Diarrhea, E. coli-induced
Cipro (Ciprofloxacin) Schering ... 2810

Diarrhea, giardia lamblia-induced
Alinia for Oral Suspension (Nitazoxanide) Romark ... 2677
Alinia Tablets (Nitazoxanide) Romark ... 2677

Diarrhea, infectious
Alinia for Oral Suspension (Nitazoxanide) Romark ... 2677
Alinia Tablets (Nitazoxanide) Romark ... 2677
Cipro (Ciprofloxacin) Schering ... 2810

Diarrhea, protozoal
(*see under* Diarrhea, infectious)

Diarrhea, symptomatic relief of
Imodium A-D Liquid, Caplets, and EZ Chews (Loperamide Hydrochloride) McNeil Consumer ... 1898
Imodium Multi-Symptom Relief Caplets and Chewable Tablets (Loperamide Hydrochloride, Simethicone) McNeil Consumer ... 1899
Pepto-Bismol Original Liquid, Maximum Strength Liquid, Original and Cherry Tablets, Chewable Tablets and Easy-To-Swallow Caplets (Bismuth Subsalicylate) Procter & Gamble ... 2564
Pepto-Bismol Original Liquid, Original and Cherry Chewable Tablets & Caplets (Bismuth Subsalicylate) Procter & Gamble ... ■613
Pepto-Bismol Maximum Strength Liquid (Bismuth Subsalicylate) Procter & Gamble ... ■613

Diarrhea, traveler's
Imodium A-D Liquid, Caplets, and EZ Chews (Loperamide Hydrochloride) McNeil Consumer ... 1898
Xifaxan Tablets (Rifaximin) Salix ... 2682

Diarrhea associated with vasoactive intestinal peptide tumors
Sandostatin Injection (Octreotide Acetate) Novartis ... 2300
Sandostatin LAR Depot (Octreotide Acetate) Novartis ... 2302

Diet, supplementation of
Accelerator Tablets (Amino Acid Preparations, Calcium Carbonate, Calcium Phosphate, Dibasic, Herbals, Multiple) Wellness International ... ■634
Active Calcium Tablets (Calcium Citrate, Vitamin D) Usana ... 3173
Align Daily Probiotic Supplement (Bifidobacteria) Procter & Gamble ... 2563
Andromon Dietary Supplement (Vitex agnus-castus, Dehydroepiandrosterone, Herbal Medicines, unspecified) CPH ... 995
Animi-3 Capsules (Omega-3 Acids, Docosahexaenoic Acid (DHA), Eicosapentaenoic Acid (EPA), Folic Acid, Vitamin B_6, Vitamin B_{12}, Phytosterols) PBM ... 2506
Authia Cream (Thiamine Disulfide, Vitamin B_{12}) Westlake ... 3190
Awareness Clear Capsules (Herbals, Multiple) Awareness Corporation/Awareness Life ... ■624
Bausch & Lomb Ocuvite Adult 50+ Vitamin and Mineral Supplement (Lutein, Copper, Omega-3 Acids, Vitamin C, Vitamin E, Vitamins with Minerals, Zinc Oxide) Bausch & Lomb ... ⊙237
Bausch & Lomb Ocuvite DF Vitamin Supplement (Alpha Lipoic Acid, Genistein, Niacin, Vitamins, Multiple) Bausch & Lomb ... ⊙238
Bausch & Lomb Ocuvite Lutein Vitamin and Mineral Supplement (Lutein, Vitamins with Minerals) Bausch & Lomb ... ⊙238
Bausch & Lomb Ocuvite PreserVision AREDS Tablets (Vitamins with Minerals) Bausch & Lomb ... ⊙238
Beelith Tablets (Magnesium Oxide, Vitamin B_6) Beach ... 813
Bevitamel Tablets (Folic Acid, Melatonin, Vitamin B_{12}) Westlake ... 3190
BioLean Free Tablets (Amino Acid Preparations, Caffeine, Ginkgo biloba, Herbals with Vitamins & Minerals, Green Tea Extract, Niacinamide, Ginseng, Potassium Citrate, Vitamin B_6) Wellness International ... ■635
BioLean II Tablets (Amino Acid Preparations, Caffeine, Calcium Carbonate, Herbals, Multiple) Wellness International ... ■635
Bios Life Drink Mix (Fiber, Vitamins with Minerals, Phytosterols) Unicity ... 3158
Calcet Triple Calcium + Vitamin D Tablets (Calcium Carbonate, Calcium Gluconate, Calcium Lactate, Cholecalciferol) Mission ... ■629
CardioEssentials Capsules (Coenzyme Q-10, Levocarnitine, Taurine) Unicity ... 3159
Catasod-Ocuxtra Mega-30 mg Plus MCT Dietary Supplement (Lutein, Medium-Chain Triglycerides, Vitamins with Minerals, Zeaxanthin) CPH ... 995
Chelated Mineral Tablets (Minerals, Multiple) Usana ... 3173
CitraNatal DHA Capsules (Docosahexaenoic Acid (DHA)) Mission ... 2175
CitraNatal DHA Tablets (Calcium Citrate, Copper, Docusate Sodium, Ferrous Gluconate, Folic Acid, Multivitamins with Minerals, Potassium Iodide, Iron Carbonyl, Zinc Oxide) Mission ... 2175
CitraNatal 90 DHA Capsules (Docosahexaenoic Acid (DHA)) Mission ... 2175
CitraNatal 90 DHA Tablets (Calcium Citrate, Copper, Docusate Sodium, Folic Acid, Multivitamins with Minerals, Potassium Iodide, Iron Carbonyl, Zinc Oxide) Mission ... 2175
Clarity Capsules (Amino Acid Preparations, Bee Pollen, Ginkgo biloba, Herbals with Vitamins & Minerals, Hydroxypropyl Methylcellulose, Lecithin) Wellness International ... ■636
CM Plex Softgels (Fatty Acids, Soy oil, Salmon Oil) Unicity ... 3159
Comax Dietary Supplement (Lutein, Alpha Lipoic Acid, Rutoside, Selenium, Peptidase, Vitamin B_{12}, Vitamin C, Vitamin E, Zinc, Zeaxanthin) CPH ... 995
CoQuinone 30 Capsules (Coenzyme Q-10, Lipoic Acid) Usana ... 3173
CordyMax Cs-4 Capsules (Herbals, Multiple) Pharmanex ... 2560
Daily Complete Liquid (Amino Acid Preparations, Herbals with Vitamins & Minerals, Antioxidants) Awareness Corporation/Awareness Life ... ■624
D-Cal Chewable Caplets (Calcium Carbonate, Vitamin D) A&Z Pharm ... ■624
DHEA Plus Tablets (Dihydroepiandrosterone (DHEA), Ginkgo biloba) Wellness International ... ■636
Dismutax Dietary Supplement (L-Arginine, Coenzyme Q-10, Minerals, Niacin, Superoxide Dismutase) CPH ... 995
Efacor Dietary Supplement (Essential Fatty Acids, Omega-3 Acids, Dietary Supplement, Docosahexaenoic Acid (DHA), Eicosapentaenoic Acid (EPA), Fish Oils) Eniva ... ■626
Elasticity Capsules (Amino Acid Preparations, Herbals with Vitamins & Minerals) Wellness International ... ■636
Eldertonic (Vitamins with Minerals) Merz ... 2163
Elixir Capsules (Amino Acid Preparations, Bee Pollen, Calcium Carbonate, Iron Amino Acid Chelate, Folic Acid, Ginkgo biloba, Herbals with Vitamins & Minerals) Wellness International ... ■636
Essential Capsules (Amino Acid Preparations, Bee Pollen, Herbals with Vitamins & Minerals, Hydroxypropyl Methylcellulose, Soy-containing dietary supplements) Wellness International ... ■637
Experience Capsules (Psyllium Preparations, Herbals, Multiple) Awareness Corporation/Awareness Life ... ■624
Feminine Capsules (Amino Acid Preparations, Hydroxypropyl Methylcellulose, Soy-containing dietary supplements, Minerals, Multiple) Wellness International ... ■637
Ferralet 90 Tablets (Docusate Sodium, Folic Acid, Iron Carbonyl, Vitamin B_{12}, Vitamin C) Mission ... 2175
Fibrinase Dietary Supplement (Vitex agnus-castus, Dehydroepiandrosterone, Herbal Medicines, unspecified) CPH ... 995
Flexibility Capsules (Amino Acid Preparations, Hydroxypropyl Methylcellulose, Vitamins with Minerals) Wellness International ... ■637
Food For Thought Dietary Supplement (Amino Acid Preparations, Vitamins with Minerals) Wellness International ... ■637
Glaucofit Dietary Supplement (Lutein, Alpha Lipoic Acid, Rutoside, Selenium, Peptidase, Vitamin B_{12}, Vitamin C, Vitamin E, Zinc, Zeaxanthin) CPH ... 995
Glauma Dietary Supplement (Lutein, Alpha Lipoic Acid, Rutoside, Selenium, Peptidase, Vitamin B_{12}, Vitamin C, Vitamin E, Zinc, Zeaxanthin) CPH ... 995
Hyland's Earache Drops (Herbals, Multiple) Standard Homeopathic ... ■619

i26 Capsules (Egg product, hyperimmune) Legacy for Life ▣ 629
i26 Chewable Tablets (Egg product, hyperimmune) Legacy for Life ▣ 629
Immune Formulation 200 (Amino Acid Preparations, L-Cysteine, Selenomethionine, L-Glutamic Acid, L-Glutamine, Glycine) ProImmune 2585
Immunocal Powder Sachets (Whey Protein Isolate) Immunotec 1729
Intelectol Tablets (Vinpocetine) Memory Secret ▣ 629
Lifegenes Spray (Thymus polypeptide) America Pharma 564
Lifepak Capsules (Vitamins with Minerals) Pharmanex 2560
LipoTrim Capsules (Herbals with Minerals) Wellness International ▣ 638
L-O-M MUS Softgel Capsules (Carotenoids, Phytofluene, Phytoene, Soy oil, Soy-containing dietary supplements) Panatoz 2499
Lovpil Capsules (Amino Acid Preparations, Herbals with Vitamins & Minerals, Soy-containing dietary supplements) Wellness International ▣ 638
Macutein Mega-30 mg Plus MCT Dietary Supplement (Lutein, Medium-Chain Triglycerides, Vitamins with Minerals, Zeaxanthin) CPH 995
MarineOmega Softgel Capsules (Fatty Acids, Vitamin E) Pharmanex 2560
Marlyn Formula 50 Capsules (Amino Acid Preparations, Vitamin B_6) Marlyn 1894
Masculine Capsules (Amino Acid Preparations, Bee Pollen, Hydroxypropyl Methylcellulose, Herbals with Minerals) Wellness International ▣ 638
Mass Appeal Tablets (Amino Acid Preparations, Dicalcium Phosphate, Minerals) Wellness International ▣ 638
Med Omega Fish Oil 2800 (Omega-3 Acids, Docosahexaenoic Acid (DHA), Eicosapentaenoic Acid (EPA)) Carlson 949
Medizym Tablets (Ananas comosus, Bromelains, Chymotrypsin, Carica papaya, Pancreatin, Papain, Trypsin) Marlyn 1894
Mega Antioxidant Tablets (Dietary Supplement, Vitamins, Multiple) Usana 3174
Metamucil Dietary Fiber Supplement (Psyllium Preparations) Procter & Gamble 2563
Metamucil Smooth Texture Sugar-Free Orange Flavor Powder (Psyllium Preparations) Procter & Gamble 2563
Natural Joint Capsules (Dietary Supplement) Greek Island Labs ▣ 628
Norwegian Cod Liver Oil (Cod Liver Oil, Omega-3 Acids, Docosahexaenoic Acid (DHA), Eicosapentaenoic Acid (EPA), ALA (Alpha-Linolenic Acid), Vitamin A, Vitamin D, Vitamin E) Carlson 949
NT-Kinase Dietary Supplement (L-Arginine, Coenzyme Q-10, Minerals, Niacin, Superoxide Dismutase) CPH 995
Nu-Iron 150 Capsules (Polysaccharide Iron Complex) Merz 2165
Omega 3-10 Softgels (Coenzyme Q-10, Omega-3 Acids) Statacor Biosciences ▣ 632
Optigold Mega-30 mg Plus MCT Dietary Supplement (Lutein, Medium-Chain Triglycerides, Vitamins with Minerals, Zeaxanthin) CPH 995
Phyto-Vite Tablets (Bioflavonoids, Calcium, Phytonutrients, Potassium, Folate, Ginkgo biloba, Herbals with Vitamins & Minerals, Iron, Soy Extract, Antioxidants) Wellness International ▣ 639
Procosa II Tablets (Manganese, Glucosamine Sulfate, Vitamin C) Usana 3174
Proflavanol 90 Tablets (Dietary Supplement, Herbals with Vitamins & Minerals, Vitamin C) Usana 3174
Prostate Olympus Dietary Supplement (Herbals, Multiple) Greek Island Labs ▣ 628
Protector Capsules (Amino Acid Preparations, Bee Pollen, Cellulose, Hydroxypropyl Methylcellulose, Magnesium, Soy-containing dietary supplements, Astragalus, Silicon Dioxide, Stearic Acid, Herbals, Multiple) Wellness International ▣ 639
ProXtreme Protein Supplement (Amino Acid Preparations, Folic Acid, Protein Preparations, Vitamins with Minerals) Wellness International ▣ 639
PureTrim Mediterranean Wellness Shake (Fatty Acids, Rice Protein, Antioxidants) Awareness Corporation/Awareness Life ▣ 624
Reishimax Capsules (Ganoderma lucinum mushroom extract) Pharmanex 2561
Relief Capsules (Amino Acid Preparations, Psyllium Preparations, Herbals with Vitamins) Wellness International ▣ 641
Rolaids Original Peppermint Tablets (Calcium Carbonate, Magnesium Hydroxide) McNeil Consumer 1903
Satieté Tablets (Amino Acid Preparations, Folic Acid, Ginkgo biloba, Herbals with Vitamins & Minerals, Hypericum) Wellness International ▣ 640
Sen-Sei-Ro Liquid (Dietary Supplement) Kyowa 1785
Sen-Sei-Ro Powder Gold (Dietary Supplement) Kyowa 1786
Sleep-Tite Caplets (Herbals with Minerals) Wellness International ▣ 640
SON Formula Tablets (Amino Acid Preparations) International Nutrition Research 1745
Sure2Endure Tablets (Herbals with Vitamins & Minerals, Glucosamine Hydrochloride) Wellness International ▣ 641
SynergyDefense Capsules (Herbals, Multiple) Awareness Corporation/Awareness Life ▣ 625
Tahitian Noni Liquid (Dietary Supplement) Tahitian Noni International ▣ 633
Tēgreen 97 Capsules (Camellia sinensis) Pharmanex 2561
Tofipan Dietary Supplement (Vitex agnus-castus, Dehydroepiandrosterone, Herbal Medicines, unspecified) CPH 995
Tofipan-Z Dietary Supplement (Vitex agnus-castus, Dehydroepiandrosterone, Herbal Medicines, unspecified) CPH 995
Tonox Dietary Supplement (Lutein, Alpha Lipoic Acid, Rutoside, Selenium, Peptidase, Vitamin B_{12}, Vitamin C, Vitamin E, Zinc, Zeaxanthin) CPH 995
Tranquility Capsules (Amino Acid Preparations, Valeriana officinalis, Herbals with Vitamins & Minerals, Soy-containing dietary supplements) Wellness International ▣ 641
4Life Transfer Factor Plus Tri-Factor Formula (Polysaccharides, Transfer factor, Colostrum) 4Life ▣ 628
Vibe Liquid Multi-Nutrient Supplement (Aloe vera, Amino Acid Preparations, Bioflavonoids, Calcium, Dietary Supplement, Phytonutrients, Folic Acid, Potassium, Herbals with Vitamins & Minerals, Minerals, Green Tea Extract, Magnesium, Herbals with Vitamins, Herbals with Minerals, Herbals, Multiple, Minerals, Multiple, Vitamin B_6, Vitamin C, Vitamin E, Vitamins with Minerals, Vitamins, Multiple, Zinc, Antioxidants) Eniva ▣ 626
Visutein Capsules (Lutein, Acetylcysteine, Carotenoids, Vitamin B_2, Zinc) Unicity 3159
WIN CoQ10 Gelcaps (Coenzyme Q-10) Wellness International ▣ 641
WINOmeg3complex Gelcaps (Omega-3-acid ethyl esters, Omega-3 Acids, Docosahexaenoic Acid (DHA), Eicosapentaenoic Acid (EPA), Omega-6 Polyunsaturates) Wellness International ▣ 642
Winrgy Dietary Supplement (Amino Acid Preparations, Caffeine, Vitamins with Minerals) Wellness International ▣ 642
Youthgenes Spray (Placenta factor) America Pharma 564
Zinc-220 Capsules (Zinc Sulfate) Alto 564

Digestive disorders, symptomatic relief of
DDS-Acidophilus Capsules, Tablets, and Powder (Lactobacillus Acidophilus) UAS Labs ▣ 634
Pepto-Bismol Original Liquid, Original and Cherry Chewable Tablets & Caplets (Bismuth Subsalicylate) Procter & Gamble ▣ 613
Pepto-Bismol Maximum Strength Liquid (Bismuth Subsalicylate) Procter & Gamble ▣ 613
Extra Strength Rolaids Freshmint Tablets (Calcium Carbonate, Magnesium Hydroxide) McNeil Consumer 1903

Digestive insufficiencies, symptomatic relief of
Rolaids Original Peppermint Tablets (Calcium Carbonate, Magnesium Hydroxide) McNeil Consumer 1903

Digoxin intoxication, life-threatening
Digibind for Injection (Digoxin Immune Fab (Ovine)) GlaxoSmithKline 1403

Diphtheria
(*see under* C. diphtheriae infections)

Diphtheria, tetanus, pertussis vaccine
(*see also under* Immunization, diphtheria, tetanus and pertussis)
Boostrix (Diphtheria & Tetanus Toxoids and Acellular Pertussis Vaccine Adsorbed) GlaxoSmithKline 1377
Infanrix Vaccine (Diphtheria & Tetanus Toxoids and Acellular Pertussis Vaccine Adsorbed) GlaxoSmithKline 1479
Pediarix Vaccine (Diphtheria & Tetanus Toxoids and Acellular Pertussis Vaccine Adsorbed, Hepatitis B Vaccine, Recombinant, Poliovirus Vaccine Inactivated) GlaxoSmithKline 1552

Diplococcus pneumoniae infections
(*see under* S. pneumoniae infections)

Dizziness
Dramamine Chewable Tablets (Dimenhydrinate) McNeil Consumer 1898
Dramamine Less Drowsy Tablets (Meclizine Hydrochloride) McNeil Consumer 1898
Dramamine Original Tablets (Dimenhydrinate) McNeil Consumer 1898

Dry eye syndrome
Lacrisert Sterile Ophthalmic Insert (Hydroxypropyl Cellulose) Aton ⊙ 233

Dryness, vaginal
Enjuvia Tablets (Estrogens, Conjugated, Synthetic B) Duramed 1029

Ductus arteriosus, patent, palliative maintenance
Indocin I.V. (Indomethacin Sodium Trihydrate) Ovation 2489
NeoProfen Injection (Ibuprofen Lysine) Ovation 2496

Dukes' stage C colon cancer
(*see under* Carcinoma, colon, Dukes' stage C, adjunctive treatment in)

Duodenal ulcer and H. pylori infection, adjunct in
Aciphex Tablets (Rabeprazole Sodium) Eisai 1053
Biaxin/Biaxin XL (Clarithromycin) Abbott 411

Duodenal ulcers, active, short-term treatment of
Aciphex Tablets (Rabeprazole Sodium) Eisai 1053
Axid Capsules (Nizatidine) GlaxoSmithKline 1364
Carafate Suspension (Sucralfate) Axcan Pharma 706
Carafate Tablets (Sucralfate) Axcan Pharma 707
Pepcid Tablets (Famotidine) Merck 2075
Zantac 25 EFFERdose Tablets (Ranitidine Hydrochloride) GlaxoSmithKline 1670
Zantac Injection (Ranitidine Hydrochloride) GlaxoSmithKline 1666
Zantac Injection Pharmacy Bulk Package (Ranitidine Hydrochloride) GlaxoSmithKline 1668
Zantac Injection Premixed (Ranitidine Hydrochloride) GlaxoSmithKline 1666
Zantac (Ranitidine Hydrochloride) GlaxoSmithKline 1670

Duodenal ulcers, adjunctive therapy for
Donnatal Extentabs (Atropine Sulfate, Hyoscyamine Sulfate, Phenobarbital, Scopolamine Hydrobromide) PBM 2507

Duodenal ulcers, maintenance therapy for
Axid Capsules (Nizatidine) GlaxoSmithKline 1364
Carafate Tablets (Sucralfate) Axcan Pharma 707
Pepcid Tablets (Famotidine) Merck 2075
Zantac (Ranitidine Hydrochloride) GlaxoSmithKline 1670

Duodenal ulcers, to reduce the risk of recurrence
Pylera Capsules (Metronidazole, Tetracycline Hydrochloride, Bismuth Subcitrate Potassium) Axcan Pharma 714

Dysbetalipoproteinemia
Lipitor Tablets (Atorvastatin Calcium) Parke-Davis 2501
Simcor Tablets (Niacin, Simvastatin) Abbott 502
Zocor Tablets (Simvastatin) Merck 2136

Dysentery, amoebic
(*see under* Amebiasis, acute intestinal)

Dyslipidemia, mixed, adjunct to diet
Fenoglide Tablets (Fenofibrate) Sciele 2960

Dysmenorrhea, primary
Anaprox Tablets (Naproxen Sodium) Roche 2632
Anaprox DS Tablets (Naproxen Sodium) Roche 2632
Celebrex Capsules (Celecoxib) Searle 2979
Naprosyn Suspension (Naproxen) Roche 2632
Naprosyn Tablets (Naproxen) Roche 2632

Dyspepsia
(*see under* Digestive disorders, symptomatic relief of)

Dysphoric disorder, premenstrual
Paxil CR Controlled-Release Tablets (Paroxetine Hydrochloride) GlaxoSmithKline 1544
Yaz Tablets (Ethinyl Estradiol, Drospirenone) Bayer HealthCare Pharmaceuticals 805

Dyspnea associated with congestive heart failure
Natrecor for Injection (Nesiritide) Scios ... 2977

Dystonia, cervical
BOTOX Purified Neurotoxin Complex (Botulinum Toxin Type A) Allergan ... 550

E

E. cloacae gynecologic infections
Timentin ADD-Vantage (Clavulanate Potassium, Ticarcillin Disodium) GlaxoSmithKline ... 1606
Timentin Injection Galaxy Container (Clavulanate Potassium, Ticarcillin Disodium) GlaxoSmithKline ... 1609
Timentin IV Infusion (Clavulanate Potassium, Ticarcillin Disodium) GlaxoSmithKline ... 1603
Timentin Pharmacy Bulk Package (Clavulanate Potassium, Ticarcillin Disodium) GlaxoSmithKline ... 1613

E. coli bone and joint infections
Rocephin Injectable Vials, ADD-Vantage, Galaxy, Bulk (Ceftriaxone Sodium) Roche ... 2642

E. coli cystitis
Cipro (Ciprofloxacin) Schering ... 2810

E. coli genital infections
Amoxil Capsules (Amoxicillin) GlaxoSmithKline ... 1305
Amoxil Chewable Tablets (Amoxicillin) GlaxoSmithKline ... 1305
Amoxil Pediatric Drops for Oral Suspension (Amoxicillin) GlaxoSmithKline ... 1305
Amoxil Powder for Oral Suspension (Amoxicillin) GlaxoSmithKline ... 1305
Amoxil Tablets (Amoxicillin) GlaxoSmithKline ... 1305

E. coli gynecological infections
Amoxil Capsules (Amoxicillin) GlaxoSmithKline ... 1305
Amoxil Chewable Tablets (Amoxicillin) GlaxoSmithKline ... 1305
Amoxil Pediatric Drops for Oral Suspension (Amoxicillin) GlaxoSmithKline ... 1305
Amoxil Powder for Oral Suspension (Amoxicillin) GlaxoSmithKline ... 1305
Amoxil Tablets (Amoxicillin) GlaxoSmithKline ... 1305
Fortaz (Ceftazidime) GlaxoSmithKline ... 1450
Invanz for Injection (Ertapenem) Merck ... 2029
Primaxin I.M. (Cilastatin Sodium, Imipenem) Merck ... 2080
Primaxin I.V. (Cilastatin Sodium, Imipenem) Merck ... 2083
Timentin ADD-Vantage (Clavulanate Potassium, Ticarcillin Disodium) GlaxoSmithKline ... 1606
Timentin Injection Galaxy Container (Clavulanate Potassium, Ticarcillin Disodium) GlaxoSmithKline ... 1609
Timentin IV Infusion (Clavulanate Potassium, Ticarcillin Disodium) GlaxoSmithKline ... 1603
Timentin Pharmacy Bulk Package (Clavulanate Potassium, Ticarcillin Disodium) GlaxoSmithKline ... 1613
Zosyn for Injection (Piperacillin Sodium, Tazobactam Sodium) Wyeth ... 3284

E. coli infections
Amoxil Capsules (Amoxicillin) GlaxoSmithKline ... 1305
Amoxil Chewable Tablets (Amoxicillin) GlaxoSmithKline ... 1305
Amoxil Pediatric Drops for Oral Suspension (Amoxicillin) GlaxoSmithKline ... 1305
Amoxil Powder for Oral Suspension (Amoxicillin) GlaxoSmithKline ... 1305
Amoxil Tablets (Amoxicillin) GlaxoSmithKline ... 1305
Augmentin (Amoxicillin, Clavulanate Potassium) GlaxoSmithKline ... 1323
Augmentin Tablets (Amoxicillin, Clavulanate Potassium) GlaxoSmithKline ... 1327
Avelox (Moxifloxacin Hydrochloride) Schering ... 2803
Ceftin Tablets (Cefuroxime Axetil) GlaxoSmithKline ... 1380
Cipro I.V. (Ciprofloxacin) Schering ... 2817
Cipro (Ciprofloxacin) Schering ... 2810
Doribax Injection (Doripenem) Ortho-McNeil ... 2400
Fortaz (Ceftazidime) GlaxoSmithKline ... 1450
Invanz for Injection (Ertapenem) Merck ... 2029
Levaquin (Levofloxacin) Ortho-McNeil ... 2416
Levaquin in 5% Dextrose Injection (Levofloxacin) Ortho-McNeil ... 2416
Merrem I.V. (Meropenem) AstraZeneca Pharmaceuticals ... 684
Noroxin Tablets (Norfloxacin) Merck ... 2069
Primaxin I.M. (Cilastatin Sodium, Imipenem) Merck ... 2080
Primaxin I.V. (Cilastatin Sodium, Imipenem) Merck ... 2083
Rocephin Injectable Vials, ADD-Vantage, Galaxy, Bulk (Ceftriaxone Sodium) Roche ... 2642
Seromycin Capsules (Cycloserine) Lilly ... 1864
Suprax for Oral Suspension (Cefixime) Lupin ... 1891
Suprax Tablets (Cefixime) Lupin ... 1891
Timentin ADD-Vantage (Clavulanate Potassium, Ticarcillin Disodium) GlaxoSmithKline ... 1606
Timentin Injection Galaxy Container (Clavulanate Potassium, Ticarcillin Disodium) GlaxoSmithKline ... 1609
Timentin IV Infusion (Clavulanate Potassium, Ticarcillin Disodium) GlaxoSmithKline ... 1603
Timentin Pharmacy Bulk Package (Clavulanate Potassium, Ticarcillin Disodium) GlaxoSmithKline ... 1613
Tygacil for Injection (Tigecycline) Wyeth ... 3276
Zinacef for Injection (Cefuroxime) GlaxoSmithKline ... 1678
Zinacef Injection (Cefuroxime) GlaxoSmithKline ... 1678
Zosyn for Injection (Piperacillin Sodium, Tazobactam Sodium) Wyeth ... 3284

E. coli infections, ocular
Blephamide Ophthalmic Ointment Allergan ... ⊙ 217
Blephamide Ophthalmic Suspension Allergan ... ⊙ 216
Neosporin Ophthalmic Solution Sterile (Gramicidin, Neomycin Sulfate, Polymyxin B Sulfate) King ... ⊙ 252
Pred-G Ophthalmic Ointment (Gentamicin Sulfate, Prednisolone Acetate) Allergan ... ⊙ 229
Pred-G Ophthalmic Suspension (Gentamicin Sulfate, Prednisolone Acetate) Allergan ... ⊙ 228
Zylet Ophthalmic Suspension (Loteprednol Etabonate, Tobramycin) Bausch & Lomb ... ⊙ 247

E. coli intra-abdominal infections
Avelox (Moxifloxacin Hydrochloride) Schering ... 2803
Cipro I.V. (Ciprofloxacin) Schering ... 2817
Cipro (Ciprofloxacin) Schering ... 2810
Doribax Injection (Doripenem) Ortho-McNeil ... 2400
Fortaz (Ceftazidime) GlaxoSmithKline ... 1450
Invanz for Injection (Ertapenem) Merck ... 2029
Merrem I.V. (Meropenem) AstraZeneca Pharmaceuticals ... 684
Primaxin I.M. (Cilastatin Sodium, Imipenem) Merck ... 2080
Primaxin I.V. (Cilastatin Sodium, Imipenem) Merck ... 2083
Rocephin Injectable Vials, ADD-Vantage, Galaxy, Bulk (Ceftriaxone Sodium) Roche ... 2642
Timentin ADD-Vantage (Clavulanate Potassium, Ticarcillin Disodium) GlaxoSmithKline ... 1606
Timentin Injection Galaxy Container (Clavulanate Potassium, Ticarcillin Disodium) GlaxoSmithKline ... 1609
Timentin IV Infusion (Clavulanate Potassium, Ticarcillin Disodium) GlaxoSmithKline ... 1603
Timentin Pharmacy Bulk Package (Clavulanate Potassium, Ticarcillin Disodium) GlaxoSmithKline ... 1613
Tygacil for Injection (Tigecycline) Wyeth ... 3276

E. coli lower respiratory tract infections
Cipro I.V. (Ciprofloxacin) Schering ... 2817
Cipro (Ciprofloxacin) Schering ... 2810
Fortaz (Ceftazidime) GlaxoSmithKline ... 1450
Levaquin (Levofloxacin) Ortho-McNeil ... 2416
Levaquin in 5% Dextrose Injection (Levofloxacin) Ortho-McNeil ... 2416
Primaxin I.V. (Cilastatin Sodium, Imipenem) Merck ... 2083
Rocephin Injectable Vials, ADD-Vantage, Galaxy, Bulk (Ceftriaxone Sodium) Roche ... 2642
Zinacef for Injection (Cefuroxime) GlaxoSmithKline ... 1678
Zinacef Injection (Cefuroxime) GlaxoSmithKline ... 1678

E. coli meningitis
Rocephin Injectable Vials, ADD-Vantage, Galaxy, Bulk (Ceftriaxone Sodium) Roche ... 2642

E. coli peritonitis
Fortaz (Ceftazidime) GlaxoSmithKline ... 1450
Merrem I.V. (Meropenem) AstraZeneca Pharmaceuticals ... 684
Timentin ADD-Vantage (Clavulanate Potassium, Ticarcillin Disodium) GlaxoSmithKline ... 1606
Timentin Injection Galaxy Container (Clavulanate Potassium, Ticarcillin Disodium) GlaxoSmithKline ... 1609
Timentin IV Infusion (Clavulanate Potassium, Ticarcillin Disodium) GlaxoSmithKline ... 1603
Timentin Pharmacy Bulk Package (Clavulanate Potassium, Ticarcillin Disodium) GlaxoSmithKline ... 1613
Zosyn for Injection (Piperacillin Sodium, Tazobactam Sodium) Wyeth ... 3284

E. coli prostatitis
Cipro I.V. (Ciprofloxacin) Schering ... 2817
Cipro (Ciprofloxacin) Schering ... 2810
Levaquin (Levofloxacin) Ortho-McNeil ... 2416
Levaquin in 5% Dextrose Injection (Levofloxacin) Ortho-McNeil ... 2416
Noroxin Tablets (Norfloxacin) Merck ... 2069

E. coli pyelonephritis
Levaquin (Levofloxacin) Ortho-McNeil ... 2416
Levaquin in 5% Dextrose Injection (Levofloxacin) Ortho-McNeil ... 2416

E. coli septicemia
Cipro I.V. (Ciprofloxacin) Schering ... 2817
Fortaz (Ceftazidime) GlaxoSmithKline ... 1450
Primaxin I.V. (Cilastatin Sodium, Imipenem) Merck ... 2083
Rocephin Injectable Vials, ADD-Vantage, Galaxy, Bulk (Ceftriaxone Sodium) Roche ... 2642
Timentin ADD-Vantage (Clavulanate Potassium, Ticarcillin Disodium) GlaxoSmithKline ... 1606
Timentin Injection Galaxy Container (Clavulanate Potassium, Ticarcillin Disodium) GlaxoSmithKline ... 1609
Timentin IV Infusion (Clavulanate Potassium, Ticarcillin Disodium) GlaxoSmithKline ... 1603
Timentin Pharmacy Bulk Package (Clavulanate Potassium, Ticarcillin Disodium) GlaxoSmithKline ... 1613
Zinacef for Injection (Cefuroxime) GlaxoSmithKline ... 1678
Zinacef Injection (Cefuroxime) GlaxoSmithKline ... 1678

E. coli skin and skin structure infections
Amoxil Capsules (Amoxicillin) GlaxoSmithKline ... 1305
Amoxil Chewable Tablets (Amoxicillin) GlaxoSmithKline ... 1305
Amoxil Pediatric Drops for Oral Suspension (Amoxicillin) GlaxoSmithKline ... 1305
Amoxil Powder for Oral Suspension (Amoxicillin) GlaxoSmithKline ... 1305
Amoxil Tablets (Amoxicillin) GlaxoSmithKline ... 1305
Augmentin (Amoxicillin, Clavulanate Potassium) GlaxoSmithKline ... 1323
Augmentin Tablets (Amoxicillin, Clavulanate Potassium) GlaxoSmithKline ... 1327
Cipro I.V. (Ciprofloxacin) Schering ... 2817
Cipro (Ciprofloxacin) Schering ... 2810
Fortaz (Ceftazidime) GlaxoSmithKline ... 1450
Invanz for Injection (Ertapenem) Merck ... 2029
Merrem I.V. (Meropenem) AstraZeneca Pharmaceuticals ... 684
Primaxin I.M. (Cilastatin Sodium, Imipenem) Merck ... 2080
Primaxin I.V. (Cilastatin Sodium, Imipenem) Merck ... 2083
Rocephin Injectable Vials, ADD-Vantage, Galaxy, Bulk (Ceftriaxone Sodium) Roche ... 2642
Timentin ADD-Vantage (Clavulanate Potassium, Ticarcillin Disodium) GlaxoSmithKline ... 1606
Timentin Injection Galaxy Container (Clavulanate Potassium, Ticarcillin Disodium) GlaxoSmithKline ... 1609
Timentin IV Infusion (Clavulanate Potassium, Ticarcillin Disodium) GlaxoSmithKline ... 1603
Timentin Pharmacy Bulk Package (Clavulanate Potassium, Ticarcillin Disodium) GlaxoSmithKline ... 1613
Tygacil for Injection (Tigecycline) Wyeth ... 3276
Zinacef for Injection (Cefuroxime) GlaxoSmithKline ... 1678
Zinacef Injection (Cefuroxime) GlaxoSmithKline ... 1678

E. coli urinary tract infections
Amoxil Capsules (Amoxicillin) GlaxoSmithKline ... 1305
Amoxil Chewable Tablets (Amoxicillin) GlaxoSmithKline ... 1305
Amoxil Pediatric Drops for Oral Suspension (Amoxicillin) GlaxoSmithKline ... 1305
Amoxil Powder for Oral Suspension (Amoxicillin) GlaxoSmithKline ... 1305
Amoxil Tablets (Amoxicillin) GlaxoSmithKline ... 1305
Augmentin (Amoxicillin, Clavulanate Potassium) GlaxoSmithKline ... 1323
Augmentin Tablets (Amoxicillin, Clavulanate Potassium) GlaxoSmithKline ... 1327
Ceftin Tablets (Cefuroxime Axetil) GlaxoSmithKline ... 1380
Cipro I.V. (Ciprofloxacin) Schering ... 2817
Cipro (Ciprofloxacin) Schering ... 2810
Cipro XR Tablets (Ciprofloxacin) Schering ... 2823
Doribax Injection (Doripenem) Ortho-McNeil ... 2400
Fortaz (Ceftazidime) GlaxoSmithKline ... 1450
Gantrisin Pediatric Suspension (Acetyl Sulfisoxazole) Roche ... 2638
Invanz for Injection (Ertapenem) Merck ... 2029
Levaquin (Levofloxacin) Ortho-McNeil ... 2416
Levaquin in 5% Dextrose Injection (Levofloxacin) Ortho-McNeil ... 2416
Noroxin Tablets (Norfloxacin) Merck ... 2069
Primaxin I.V. (Cilastatin Sodium, Imipenem) Merck ... 2083
Rocephin Injectable Vials, ADD-Vantage, Galaxy, Bulk (Ceftriaxone Sodium) Roche ... 2642
Seromycin Capsules (Cycloserine) Lilly ... 1864
Suprax for Oral Suspension (Cefixime) Lupin ... 1891
Suprax Tablets (Cefixime) Lupin ... 1891
Timentin ADD-Vantage (Clavulanate Potassium, Ticarcillin Disodium) GlaxoSmithKline ... 1606

Timentin Injection Galaxy Container (Clavulanate Potassium, Ticarcillin Disodium) GlaxoSmithKline 1609
Timentin IV Infusion (Clavulanate Potassium, Ticarcillin Disodium) GlaxoSmithKline 1603
Timentin Pharmacy Bulk Package (Clavulanate Potassium, Ticarcillin Disodium) GlaxoSmithKline 1613
Zinacef for Injection (Cefuroxime) GlaxoSmithKline 1678
Zinacef Injection (Cefuroxime) GlaxoSmithKline 1678

E. coli-induced diarrhea
(*see under* Diarrhea, E. coli-induced)

E. faecalis (vancomycin susceptible strains) skin and skin structure infections
Cubicin for Injection (Daptomycin) Cubist 995
Tygacil for Injection (Tigecycline) Wyeth 3276

E. faecalis (vancomycin-susceptible strains) intra-abdominal infections
Tygacil for Injection (Tigecycline) Wyeth 3276

E. faecalis infections
Amoxil Capsules (Amoxicillin) GlaxoSmithKline 1305
Amoxil Chewable Tablets (Amoxicillin) GlaxoSmithKline 1305
Amoxil Pediatric Drops for Oral Suspension (Amoxicillin) GlaxoSmithKline 1305
Amoxil Powder for Oral Suspension (Amoxicillin) GlaxoSmithKline 1305
Amoxil Tablets (Amoxicillin) GlaxoSmithKline 1305
Avelox (Moxifloxacin Hydrochloride) Schering 2803
Levaquin (Levofloxacin) Ortho-McNeil 2416
Levaquin in 5% Dextrose Injection (Levofloxacin) Ortho-McNeil 2416
Merrem I.V. (Meropenem) AstraZeneca Pharmaceuticals 684
Tygacil for Injection (Tigecycline) Wyeth 3276

E. faecalis intra-abdominal infections
Avelox (Moxifloxacin Hydrochloride) Schering 2803

E. faecalis prostatitis
Amoxil Capsules (Amoxicillin) GlaxoSmithKline 1305
Amoxil Chewable Tablets (Amoxicillin) GlaxoSmithKline 1305
Amoxil Pediatric Drops for Oral Suspension (Amoxicillin) GlaxoSmithKline 1305
Amoxil Powder for Oral Suspension (Amoxicillin) GlaxoSmithKline 1305
Amoxil Tablets (Amoxicillin) GlaxoSmithKline 1305
Levaquin (Levofloxacin) Ortho-McNeil 2416
Levaquin in 5% Dextrose Injection (Levofloxacin) Ortho-McNeil 2416

E. faecalis skin and skin structure infections
Levaquin (Levofloxacin) Ortho-McNeil 2416
Levaquin in 5% Dextrose Injection (Levofloxacin) Ortho-McNeil 2416
Merrem I.V. (Meropenem) AstraZeneca Pharmaceuticals 684

E. faecalis urinary tract infections
Amoxil Capsules (Amoxicillin) GlaxoSmithKline 1305
Amoxil Chewable Tablets (Amoxicillin) GlaxoSmithKline 1305
Amoxil Pediatric Drops for Oral Suspension (Amoxicillin) GlaxoSmithKline 1305
Amoxil Powder for Oral Suspension (Amoxicillin) GlaxoSmithKline 1305
Amoxil Tablets (Amoxicillin) GlaxoSmithKline 1305
Cipro XR Tablets (Ciprofloxacin) Schering 2823
Levaquin (Levofloxacin) Ortho-McNeil 2416
Levaquin in 5% Dextrose Injection (Levofloxacin) Ortho-McNeil 2416

Ear, infection
(*see under* Otitis media, acute)

Echinococcus granulosus infections
Albenza Tablets (Albendazole) GlaxoSmithKline 1297

Eczema, unspecified
(*see under* Skin, inflammatory conditions)

Edema, adjunctive therapy in
Demadex Tablets (Torsemide) Roche 2630
Dyazide Capsules (Hydrochlorothiazide, Triamterene) GlaxoSmithKline 1405
Dyrenium Capsules (Triamterene) WellSpring 3189
Edecrin (Ethacrynic Acid) Aton 698
Furosemide Tablets (Furosemide) Mylan 2186
Indapamide Tablets (Indapamide) Mylan 2188
Intravenous Sodium Diuril (Chlorothiazide Sodium) Ovation 2490

Edema, congestive heart failure-induced, treatment of
Demadex Injection (Torsemide) Roche 2630

Edema, corneal, temporary relief of
Muro 128 Ophthalmic Ointment (Sodium Chloride) Bausch & Lomb ....⊙243
Muro 128 Ophthalmic Solution 2% and 5% (Sodium Chloride) Bausch & Lomb ....⊙242

Edema, hepatic disease-induced, treatment of
Demadex Injection (Torsemide) Roche 2630

Edema, renal disease-induced, treatment of
Demadex Injection (Torsemide) Roche 2630

Embolism, pulmonary
Activase I.V. (Alteplase) Genentech ..1188
Arixtra Injection (Fondaparinux Sodium) GlaxoSmithKline 1313

Embolism, pulmonary, acute, lysis of
Activase I.V. (Alteplase) Genentech ..1188

Emotionalism
Hyland's Calms Forté 4 Kids Tablets (Homeopathic Formulations, Sulfur) Standard Homeopathic ....▣619

Emphysema
Atrovent HFA Inhalation Aerosol (Ipratropium Bromide) Boehringer Ingelheim 839
Brovana Inhalation Solution (Arformoterol Tartrate) Sepracor 2990
Perforomist Inhalation Solution (Formoterol Fumarate) Dey 1025
Serevent Diskus (Salmeterol Xinafoate) GlaxoSmithKline 1594
Spiriva HandiHaler (Tiotropium bromide) Boehringer Ingelheim 870
Uniphyl Tablets (Theophylline Anhydrous) Purdue Pharmaceutical 2595

Emphysema, panacinar, due to congenital Alpha1-antitrypsin deficiency
Aralast (Alpha$_1$-Proteinase Inhibitor (Human)) Baxter Healthcare 726
Prolastin (Alpha$_1$-Proteinase Inhibitor (Human)) Talecris 3099

Empyema
Bicillin C-R Injectable Suspension (Penicillin G Benzathine, Penicillin G Procaine) King 1775
Bicillin L-A Injection (Penicillin G Benzathine, Penicillin G Procaine) King 1777

Endocarditis, bacterial
Primaxin I.V. (Cilastatin Sodium, Imipenem) Merck 2083

Endocrine adenomas, multiple
(*see also under* Hypersecretory conditions, pathological)
Pepcid Tablets (Famotidine) Merck ... 2075

Endometrial hyperplasia, prevention of
Prometrium Capsules (100 mg, 200 mg) (Progesterone) Solvay 3047

Endometriosis
Lupron Depot 3.75 mg (Leuprolide Acetate) Abbott............................ 462
Lupron Depot–3 Month 11.25 mg (Leuprolide Acetate) Abbott........... 462

Endometritis
(*see also under* Infections, gynecologic)
Fortaz (Ceftazidime) GlaxoSmithKline........................... 1450
Timentin ADD-Vantage (Clavulanate Potassium, Ticarcillin Disodium) GlaxoSmithKline 1606
Timentin Injection Galaxy Container (Clavulanate Potassium, Ticarcillin Disodium) GlaxoSmithKline 1609
Timentin IV Infusion (Clavulanate Potassium, Ticarcillin Disodium) GlaxoSmithKline 1603
Timentin Pharmacy Bulk Package (Clavulanate Potassium, Ticarcillin Disodium) GlaxoSmithKline 1613
Zosyn for Injection (Piperacillin Sodium, Tazobactam Sodium) Wyeth 3284

Endomyometritis
Invanz for Injection (Ertapenem) Merck 2029
Primaxin I.M. (Cilastatin Sodium, Imipenem) Merck 2080

Entamoeba histolytica
(*see under* Amebiasis, acute intestinal)

Enterobacter aerogenes infections
Noroxin Tablets (Norfloxacin) Merck .2069
Rocephin Injectable Vials, ADD-Vantage, Galaxy, Bulk (Ceftriaxone Sodium) Roche 2642

Enterobacter aerogenes infections, ocular
Pred-G Ophthalmic Ointment (Gentamicin Sulfate, Prednisolone Acetate) Allergan ....⊙229
Pred-G Ophthalmic Suspension (Gentamicin Sulfate, Prednisolone Acetate) Allergan ....⊙228
Zylet Ophthalmic Suspension (Loteprednol Etabonate, Tobramycin) Bausch & Lomb ....⊙247

Enterobacter aerogenes lower respiratory tract infections
Rocephin Injectable Vials, ADD-Vantage, Galaxy, Bulk (Ceftriaxone Sodium) Roche 2642

Enterobacter aerogenes urinary tract infections
Noroxin Tablets (Norfloxacin) Merck .2069

Enterobacter cloacae bone and joint infections
Cipro I.V. (Ciprofloxacin) Schering 2817
Cipro (Ciprofloxacin) Schering 2810

Enterobacter cloacae infections
Avelox (Moxifloxacin Hydrochloride) Schering 2803
Cipro I.V. (Ciprofloxacin) Schering 2817
Cipro (Ciprofloxacin) Schering 2810
Levaquin (Levofloxacin) Ortho-McNeil 2416
Levaquin in 5% Dextrose Injection (Levofloxacin) Ortho-McNeil 2416
Noroxin Tablets (Norfloxacin) Merck .2069
Primaxin I.M. (Cilastatin Sodium, Imipenem) Merck 2080
Rocephin Injectable Vials, ADD-Vantage, Galaxy, Bulk (Ceftriaxone Sodium) Roche 2642

Timentin ADD-Vantage (Clavulanate Potassium, Ticarcillin Disodium) GlaxoSmithKline 1606
Timentin Injection Galaxy Container (Clavulanate Potassium, Ticarcillin Disodium) GlaxoSmithKline 1609
Timentin IV Infusion (Clavulanate Potassium, Ticarcillin Disodium) GlaxoSmithKline 1603
Timentin Pharmacy Bulk Package (Clavulanate Potassium, Ticarcillin Disodium) GlaxoSmithKline 1613
Tygacil for Injection (Tigecycline) Wyeth... 3276

Enterobacter cloacae infections, ocular
Neosporin Ophthalmic Solution Sterile (Gramicidin, Neomycin Sulfate, Polymyxin B Sulfate) King ....⊙252
Ofloxacin Ophthalmic Solution 0.3% (Ofloxacin) Bausch & Lomb ....⊙243

Enterobacter cloacae intra-abdominal infections
Tygacil for Injection (Tigecycline) Wyeth 3276

Enterobacter cloacae lower respiratory tract infections
Cipro I.V. (Ciprofloxacin) Schering 2817
Cipro (Ciprofloxacin) Schering 2810

Enterobacter cloacae skin and skin structure infections
Cipro I.V. (Ciprofloxacin) Schering 2817
Cipro (Ciprofloxacin) Schering 2810
Primaxin I.M. (Cilastatin Sodium, Imipenem) Merck 2080
Rocephin Injectable Vials, ADD-Vantage, Galaxy, Bulk (Ceftriaxone Sodium) Roche 2642

Enterobacter cloacae urinary tract infections
Cipro I.V. (Ciprofloxacin) Schering 2817
Cipro (Ciprofloxacin) Schering 2810
Levaquin (Levofloxacin) Ortho-McNeil 2416
Levaquin in 5% Dextrose Injection (Levofloxacin) Ortho-McNeil 2416
Noroxin Tablets (Norfloxacin) Merck .2069
Timentin ADD-Vantage (Clavulanate Potassium, Ticarcillin Disodium) GlaxoSmithKline 1606
Timentin Injection Galaxy Container (Clavulanate Potassium, Ticarcillin Disodium) GlaxoSmithKline 1609
Timentin IV Infusion (Clavulanate Potassium, Ticarcillin Disodium) GlaxoSmithKline 1603
Timentin Pharmacy Bulk Package (Clavulanate Potassium, Ticarcillin Disodium) GlaxoSmithKline 1613

Enterobacter species bone and joint infections
Fortaz (Ceftazidime) GlaxoSmithKline 1450
Primaxin I.V. (Cilastatin Sodium, Imipenem) Merck 2083
Rocephin Injectable Vials, ADD-Vantage, Galaxy, Bulk (Ceftriaxone Sodium) Roche 2642

Enterobacter species gynecologic infections
Primaxin I.V. (Cilastatin Sodium, Imipenem) Merck 2083
Timentin ADD-Vantage (Clavulanate Potassium, Ticarcillin Disodium) GlaxoSmithKline 1606
Timentin Injection Galaxy Container (Clavulanate Potassium, Ticarcillin Disodium) GlaxoSmithKline 1609
Timentin IV Infusion (Clavulanate Potassium, Ticarcillin Disodium) GlaxoSmithKline 1603
Timentin Pharmacy Bulk Package (Clavulanate Potassium, Ticarcillin Disodium) GlaxoSmithKline 1613

Enterobacter species infections
Augmentin (Amoxicillin, Clavulanate Potassium) GlaxoSmithKline 1323
Augmentin Tablets (Amoxicillin, Clavulanate Potassium) GlaxoSmithKline 1327

Fortaz (Ceftazidime) GlaxoSmithKline ... 1450
Primaxin I.V. (Cilastatin Sodium, Imipenem) Merck ... 2083
Rocephin Injectable Vials, ADD-Vantage, Galaxy, Bulk (Ceftriaxone Sodium) Roche ... 2642
Seromycin Capsules (Cycloserine) Lilly ... 1864
Timentin ADD-Vantage (Clavulanate Potassium, Ticarcillin Disodium) GlaxoSmithKline ... 1606
Timentin Injection Galaxy Container (Clavulanate Potassium, Ticarcillin Disodium) GlaxoSmithKline ... 1609
Timentin IV Infusion (Clavulanate Potassium, Ticarcillin Disodium) GlaxoSmithKline ... 1603
Timentin Pharmacy Bulk Package (Clavulanate Potassium, Ticarcillin Disodium) GlaxoSmithKline ... 1613
Zinacef for Injection (Cefuroxime) GlaxoSmithKline ... 1678
Zinacef Injection (Cefuroxime) GlaxoSmithKline ... 1678

Enterobacter species infections, ocular
Pred-G Ophthalmic Ointment (Gentamicin Sulfate, Prednisolone Acetate) Allergan ... ⊙229

Enterobacter species intra-abdominal infections
Primaxin I.V. (Cilastatin Sodium, Imipenem) Merck ... 2083

Enterobacter species lower respiratory tract infections
Fortaz (Ceftazidime) GlaxoSmithKline ... 1450
Primaxin I.V. (Cilastatin Sodium, Imipenem) Merck ... 2083

Enterobacter species septicemia
Primaxin I.V. (Cilastatin Sodium, Imipenem) Merck ... 2083

Enterobacter species skin and skin structure infections
Fortaz (Ceftazidime) GlaxoSmithKline ... 1450
Primaxin I.V. (Cilastatin Sodium, Imipenem) Merck ... 2083
Zinacef for Injection (Cefuroxime) GlaxoSmithKline ... 1678
Zinacef Injection (Cefuroxime) GlaxoSmithKline ... 1678

Enterobacter species urinary tract infections
Augmentin (Amoxicillin, Clavulanate Potassium) GlaxoSmithKline ... 1323
Augmentin Tablets (Amoxicillin, Clavulanate Potassium) GlaxoSmithKline ... 1327
Fortaz (Ceftazidime) GlaxoSmithKline ... 1450
Primaxin I.V. (Cilastatin Sodium, Imipenem) Merck ... 2083
Seromycin Capsules (Cycloserine) Lilly ... 1864

Enterobiasis
Reese's Pinworm Treatments (Pyrantel Pamoate) Reese ... ▣618

Enterobius vermicularis infestation
(*see under* Enterobiasis)

Enterococci faecalis infections
Amoxil Capsules (Amoxicillin) GlaxoSmithKline ... 1305
Amoxil Chewable Tablets (Amoxicillin) GlaxoSmithKline ... 1305
Amoxil Pediatric Drops for Oral Suspension (Amoxicillin) GlaxoSmithKline ... 1305
Amoxil Powder for Oral Suspension (Amoxicillin) GlaxoSmithKline ... 1305
Amoxil Tablets (Amoxicillin) GlaxoSmithKline ... 1305

Enterococci faecalis urinary tract infections
Cipro (Ciprofloxacin) Schering ... 2810
Cipro XR Tablets (Ciprofloxacin) Schering ... 2823

Enterococci infections
(*see under* Streptococci group D infections)

Enterococcus faecium, vancomycin-resistant bacteremia
Zyvox (Linezolid) Pharmacia & Upjohn ... 2552

Enterococcus faecium, vancomycin-resistant infections
Zyvox (Linezolid) Pharmacia & Upjohn ... 2552

Enterocolitis, acute
Donnatal Extentabs (Atropine Sulfate, Hyoscyamine Sulfate, Phenobarbital, Scopolamine Hydrobromide) PBM ... 2507

Epicondylitis
Traumeel Injection Solution (Homeopathic Formulations) Heel ... 1725

Epidermophyton floccosum infections
Gris-PEG Tablets (Griseofulvin) Pedinol ... 2507
Lotrisone (Betamethasone Dipropionate, Clotrimazole) Schering ... 2881
Naftin Cream (Naftifine Hydrochloride) Merz ... 2164
Naftin Gel (Naftifine Hydrochloride) Merz ... 2164

Epilepsy
Lamictal (Lamotrigine) GlaxoSmithKline ... 1488

Epilepsy, generalized
(*see under* Seizures, generalized, tonic-clonic)

Epilepsy, grand mal
(*see under* Seizures, generalized, tonic-clonic)

Epilepsy, petit mal
(*see under* Seizures, generalized, absence)

Epilepticus, status
Nembutal Sodium Solution, USP (Pentobarbital Sodium) Ovation ... 2494

Episiotomy, topical debriding in
(*see under* Wounds, debridement of)

Erectile dysfunction
Cialis Tablets (Tadalafil) Lilly ... 1792
Edex Injection (Alprostadil) Schwarz ... 2957
Levitra Tablets (Vardenafil Hydrochloride) Schering ... 2876

Erysipelas
Bicillin C-R Injectable Suspension (Penicillin G Benzathine, Penicillin G Procaine) King ... 1775
Bicillin L-A Injection (Penicillin G Benzathine, Penicillin G Procaine) King ... 1777

Erythrasma
E.E.S. (Erythromycin Ethylsuccinate) Abbott ... 433
EryPed (Erythromycin Ethylsuccinate) Abbott ... 431

Escherichia coli
(*see under* E. coli infections)

Esophagitis, erosive
(*see also under* Gastroesophageal reflux disease)
Axid Capsules (Nizatidine) GlaxoSmithKline ... 1364
Nexium Delayed-Release Capsules (Esomeprazole Magnesium) AstraZeneca LP ... 645
Nexium I.V. (Esomeprazole Sodium) AstraZeneca LP ... 652
Nexium Delayed-Release Oral Suspension (Esomeprazole Magnesium) AstraZeneca LP ... 645
Protonix for Delayed-Release Oral Suspension (Pantoprazole Sodium) Wyeth ... 3254
Protonix Delayed-Release Tablets (Pantoprazole Sodium) Wyeth ... 3254
Protonix I.V. (Pantoprazole Sodium) Wyeth ... 3257
Zantac (Ranitidine Hydrochloride) GlaxoSmithKline ... 1670

Esophagitis, ulcerative
Axid Capsules (Nizatidine) GlaxoSmithKline ... 1364

Estrogen, deficiency
(*see under* Hypoestrogenism)

Eubacterium species infections
Invanz for Injection (Ertapenem) Merck ... 2029
Primaxin I.V. (Cilastatin Sodium, Imipenem) Merck ... 2083

Eubacterium species intra-abdominal infections
Invanz for Injection (Ertapenem) Merck ... 2029
Primaxin I.V. (Cilastatin Sodium, Imipenem) Merck ... 2083

Ewing's sarcoma, palliative treatment of
Cosmegen for Injection (Dactinomycin) Ovation ... 2485

Eye, anterior segment inflammation
(*see under* Inflammation, anterior segment)

Eyes, burning, reduction of
Clear Eyes for Dry Eyes (Carboxymethylcellulose Sodium, Glycerin) Medtech ... ⊙255
Clear Eyes Itchy Eye Relief (Glycerin, Naphazoline Hydrochloride, Zinc Sulfate) Medtech ... ⊙255
Clear Eyes Triple Action Relief (Polyvinyl Alcohol, Povidone, Tetrahydrozoline Hydrochloride) Medtech ... ⊙255
Optive Lubricant Eye Drops (Carboxymethylcellulose Sodium, Glycerin) Allergan ... ⊙227
Optive Sensitive Lubricant Eye Drops (Carboxymethylcellulose Sodium, Glycerin) Allergan ... ⊙227
Refresh Celluvisc Lubricant Eye Drops (Carboxymethylcellulose Sodium) Allergan ... ⊙231
Refresh Plus Lubricant Eye Drops (Carboxymethylcellulose Sodium) Allergan ... ⊙232
Refresh Tears Lubricant Eye Drops (Carboxymethylcellulose Sodium) Allergan ... ⊙232
Soothe XP Eye Drops (Mineral Oil) Bausch & Lomb ... ⊙246
Systane Ultra Lubricating Eye Drops (Polyethylene Glycol, Propylene Glycol) Alcon ... 547

Eyes, dry
(*see under* Keratoconjunctivitis sicca)

Eyes, inflammation
(*see under* Ocular inflammation)

Eyes, irrigation of
Betadine 5% Ophthalmic Solution (Povidone Iodine) Alcon ... ⊙202

Eyes, irritation, symptomatic relief of
Clear Eyes for Dry Eyes (Carboxymethylcellulose Sodium, Glycerin) Medtech ... ⊙255
Clear Eyes Itchy Eye Relief (Glycerin, Naphazoline Hydrochloride, Zinc Sulfate) Medtech ... ⊙255
Clear Eyes Triple Action Relief (Polyvinyl Alcohol, Povidone, Tetrahydrozoline Hydrochloride) Medtech ... ⊙255
Optive Lubricant Eye Drops (Carboxymethylcellulose Sodium, Glycerin) Allergan ... ⊙227
Optive Sensitive Lubricant Eye Drops (Carboxymethylcellulose Sodium, Glycerin) Allergan ... ⊙227
Refresh Celluvisc Lubricant Eye Drops (Carboxymethylcellulose Sodium) Allergan ... ⊙231
Refresh Plus Lubricant Eye Drops (Carboxymethylcellulose Sodium) Allergan ... ⊙232
Refresh Tears Lubricant Eye Drops (Carboxymethylcellulose Sodium) Allergan ... ⊙232
Soothe XP Eye Drops (Mineral Oil) Bausch & Lomb ... ⊙246
Systane Ultra Lubricating Eye Drops (Polyethylene Glycol, Propylene Glycol) Alcon ... 547
Visine Pure Tears Dry Eye Relief Lubricant Eye Drops (Hypromellose, Glycerin, Polyethylene Glycol) Johnson & Johnson ... ⊙251

Eyes, lubrication of
(*see also under* Keratoconjunctivitis sicca)
Restasis Ophthalmic Emulsion (Cyclosporine) Allergan ... 557

Eyes, red
(*see under* Ocular redness)

Eyes, watery
(*see also under* Lacrimation, symptomatic relief of)
PediaCare Children's Allergy & Cold Liquid (Diphenhydramine Hydrochloride, Phenylephrine Hydrochloride) McNeil Consumer ... 1902
PediaCare Children's Allergy Liquid (Diphenhydramine Hydrochloride) McNeil Consumer ... 1902
Sudafed PE Sinus & Allergy Tablets (Chlorpheniramine Maleate, Phenylephrine Hydrochloride) McNeil Consumer ... 1908
Zyrtec-D Allergy & Congestion Extended-Release Tablets (Cetirizine Hydrochloride, Pseudoephedrine Hydrochloride) McNeil Consumer ... 1923

Eyes, dryness, symptomatic relief of
Clear Eyes Itchy Eye Relief (Glycerin, Naphazoline Hydrochloride, Zinc Sulfate) Medtech ... ⊙255

F

Fabry disease
Fabrazyme for Intravenous Infusion (Agalsidase beta) Genzyme ... 1241

Factor IX, deficiency of, hemophilia B caused
AlphaNine SD (Factor IX (Human)) Grifols ... 1713
Profilnine SD Solvent Detergent (Factor IX Complex) Grifols ... 1721

Female castration
(*see under* Ovaries, castration of)

Fever, reduction of
Benadryl Allergy & Cold Kapgels (Acetaminophen, Diphenhydramine Hydrochloride, Phenylephrine Hydrochloride) McNeil Consumer ... 1895
Motrin IB Tablets and Caplets (Ibuprofen) McNeil Consumer ... 1900
Children's Motrin Oral Suspension (Ibuprofen) McNeil Consumer ... 1901
Children's Motrin Non-Staining Dye-Free Oral Suspension (Ibuprofen) McNeil Consumer ... 1901
Infants' Motrin Concentrated Drops (Ibuprofen) McNeil Consumer ... 1901
Infants' Motrin Non-Staining Dye-Free Concentrated Drops (Ibuprofen) McNeil Consumer ... 1901
Junior Strength Motrin Caplets and Chewable Tablets (Ibuprofen) McNeil Consumer ... 1901
Sudafed PE Cold & Cough Caplets (Acetaminophen, Dextromethorphan Hydrobromide, Guaifenesin, Phenylephrine Hydrochloride) McNeil Consumer ... 1907
Sudafed PE Nighttime Cold Caplets (Acetaminophen, Diphenhydramine Hydrochloride, Phenylephrine Hydrochloride) McNeil Consumer ... 1907
Regular Strength Tylenol Tablets (Acetaminophen) McNeil Consumer ... 1915
Tylenol 8 Hour Extended Release Caplets (Acetaminophen) McNeil Consumer ... 1915

Extra Strength Tylenol Caplets, Cool Caplets, and EZ Tabs (Acetaminophen) McNeil Consumer 1915
Extra Strength Tylenol Adult Rapid Blast Liquid (Acetaminophen) McNeil Consumer 1915
Extra Strength Tylenol Rapid Release Gels (Acetaminophen) McNeil Consumer 1915
Tylenol Chest Congestion Caplets with Cool Burst (Acetaminophen, Guaifenesin) McNeil Consumer 1910
Tylenol Chest Congestion Liquid with Cool Burst (Acetaminophen, Guaifenesin) McNeil Consumer 1910
Children's Tylenol Plus Cold Suspension Liquid (Acetaminophen, Chlorpheniramine Maleate, Phenylephrine Hydrochloride) McNeil Consumer 1912
Children's Tylenol Plus Cold & Allergy Suspension Liquid (Acetaminophen, Diphenhydramine Hydrochloride, Phenylephrine Hydrochloride) McNeil Consumer .. 1914
Children's Tylenol Plus Cough & Runny Nose Suspension Liquid (Acetaminophen, Chlorpheniramine Maleate, Dextromethorphan Hydrobromide) McNeil Consumer .. 1912
Children's Tylenol Plus Cough & Sore Throat Suspension Liquid (Acetaminophen, Dextromethorphan Hydrobromide) McNeil Consumer 1912
Children's Tylenol Plus Flu Suspension Liquid (Acetaminophen, Chlorpheniramine Maleate, Dextromethorphan Hydrobromide, Phenylephrine Hydrochloride) McNeil Consumer 1914
Children's Tylenol Plus Multi-Symptom Cold Suspension Liquid (Acetaminophen, Chlorpheniramine Maleate, Dextromethorphan Hydrobromide, Phenylephrine Hydrochloride) McNeil Consumer 1912
Tylenol Cold Severe Congestion Daytime Caplets with Cool Burst (Acetaminophen, Dextromethorphan Hydrobromide, Guaifenesin, Pseudoephedrine Hydrochloride) McNeil Consumer 1912
Tylenol Cold Head Congestion Severe Daytime Caplets with Cool Burst (Acetaminophen, Dextromethorphan Hydrobromide, Guaifenesin, Phenylephrine Hydrochloride) McNeil Consumer .. 1910
Tylenol Cold Multi-Symptom Daytime Caplets with Cool Burst and Rapid Release Gels (Acetaminophen, Dextromethorphan Hydrobromide, Phenylephrine Hydrochloride) McNeil Consumer .. 1913
Tylenol Cold Multi-Symptom Daytime Liquid with Citrus Burst (Acetaminophen, Dextromethorphan Hydrobromide, Phenylephrine Hydrochloride) McNeil Consumer 1913
Tylenol Cold Multi-Symptom Nighttime Caplets with Cool Burst (Acetaminophen, Chlorpheniramine Maleate, Dextromethorphan Hydrobromide, Phenylephrine Hydrochloride) McNeil Consumer 1913
Tylenol Cold Multi-Symptom Nighttime Liquid with Cool Burst (Acetaminophen, Dextromethorphan Hydrobromide, Doxylamine Succinate, Phenylephrine Hydrochloride) McNeil Consumer 1913
Tylenol Cold Multi-Symptom Severe Caplets with Cool Burst (Acetaminophen, Dextromethorphan Hydrobromide, Guaifenesin, Phenylephrine Hydrochloride) McNeil Consumer 1913
Tylenol Cold Multi-Symptom Severe Daytime Liquid with Citrus Burst (Acetaminophen, Dextromethorphan Hydrobromide, Guaifenesin, Phenylephrine Hydrochloride) McNeil Consumer 1913
Concentrated Tylenol Infants' Drops (Acetaminophen) McNeil Consumer 1909
Jr. Tylenol Meltaways (Acetaminophen) McNeil Consumer 1909
Tylenol Sore Throat Daytime Liquid with Cool Burst (Acetaminophen) McNeil Consumer 1918
Tylenol Sore Throat Nighttime Liquid with Cool Burst (Acetaminophen, Diphenhydramine Hydrochloride) McNeil Consumer 1918
Vicks DayQuil Cold & Flu Multi-Symptom Relief (Acetaminophen, Dextromethorphan Hydrobromide, Phenylephrine Hydrochloride) Procter & Gamble .... ■616
Vicks DayQuil LiquiCaps (Acetaminophen, Dextromethorphan Hydrobromide, Phenylephrine Hydrochloride) Procter & Gamble .. 2567
Vicks DayQuil Liquid (Acetaminophen, Dextromethorphan Hydrobromide, Phenylephrine Hydrochloride) Procter & Gamble 2567
Vicks DayQuil Multi-Symptom Cold/Flu Relief (Acetaminophen, Dextromethorphan Hydrobromide, Phenylephrine Hydrochloride) Procter & Gamble 2567

Fever, unspecified
Vicks NyQuil LiquiCaps (Acetaminophen, Dextromethorphan Hydrobromide, Doxylamine Succinate, Pseudoephedrine Hydrochloride) Procter & Gamble 2567
Vicks NyQuil Liquid (Acetaminophen, Dextromethorphan Hydrobromide, Doxylamine Succinate, Pseudoephedrine Hydrochloride) Procter & Gamble 2567
Vicks NyQuil Multi-Symptom Cold/Flu Relief (Acetaminophen, Dextromethorphan Hydrobromide, Doxylamine Succinate, Pseudoephedrine Hydrochloride) Procter & Gamble 2567

Fever associated with common cold
Children's Motrin Cold Oral Suspension (Ibuprofen, Pseudoephedrine Hydrochloride) McNeil Consumer 1899
Children's Tylenol Plus Cold Suspension Liquid (Acetaminophen, Chlorpheniramine Maleate, Phenylephrine Hydrochloride) McNeil Consumer 1912
Tylenol Cold Multi-Symptom Daytime Caplets with Cool Burst and Rapid Release Gels (Acetaminophen, Dextromethorphan Hydrobromide, Phenylephrine Hydrochloride) McNeil Consumer .. 1913
Tylenol Cold Multi-Symptom Daytime Liquid with Citrus Burst (Acetaminophen, Dextromethorphan Hydrobromide, Phenylephrine Hydrochloride) McNeil Consumer 1913
Tylenol Cold Multi-Symptom Nighttime Liquid with Cool Burst (Acetaminophen, Dextromethorphan Hydrobromide, Doxylamine Succinate, Phenylephrine Hydrochloride) McNeil Consumer 1913
Tylenol Cold Multi-Symptom Severe Caplets with Cool Burst (Acetaminophen, Dextromethorphan Hydrobromide, Guaifenesin, Phenylephrine Hydrochloride) McNeil Consumer 1913
Tylenol Cold Multi-Symptom Severe Daytime Liquid with Citrus Burst (Acetaminophen, Dextromethorphan Hydrobromide, Guaifenesin, Phenylephrine Hydrochloride) McNeil Consumer 1913
Vicks NyQuil Cold & Flu Multi-Symptom Relief (Acetaminophen, Dextromethorphan Hydrobromide, Doxylamine Succinate) Procter & Gamble .... ■617
Vicks NyQuil LiquiCaps (Acetaminophen, Dextromethorphan Hydrobromide, Doxylamine Succinate) Procter & Gamble .... ■617

Fever blisters
(*see under* Herpetic manifestations, oral, symptomatic relief of)

Fiber, deficiency of
Metamucil Dietary Fiber Supplement (Psyllium Preparations) Procter & Gamble 2563

Fibromyalgia
Cymbalta Delayed-Release Capsules (Duloxetine Hydrochloride) Lilly 1801
Lyrica Capsules (Pregabalin) Pfizer ... 2527

Flu symptoms
(*see under* Influenza syndrome, symptomatic relief of)

Folliculitis barbae
Gris-PEG Tablets (Griseofulvin) Pedinol 2507

Fungal infections, skin
(*see under* Infections, mycotic, cutaneous)

Furunculosis
Levaquin (Levofloxacin) Ortho-McNeil 2416
Levaquin in 5% Dextrose Injection (Levofloxacin) Ortho-McNeil 2416

Furunculosis, symptomatic relief of
Panafil Ointment (Chlorophyllin Copper Complex Sodium, Papain, Urea) Healthpoint 1723
Panafil SE Spray Emulsion (Chlorophyllin Copper Complex Sodium, Papain, Urea) Healthpoint 1724

Fusobacterium species infections
Primaxin I.M. (Cilastatin Sodium, Imipenem) Merck 2080
Primaxin I.V. (Cilastatin Sodium, Imipenem) Merck 2083

Fusobacterium species intra-abdominal infections
Primaxin I.M. (Cilastatin Sodium, Imipenem) Merck 2080
Primaxin I.V. (Cilastatin Sodium, Imipenem) Merck 2083

Fusobacterium species skin and skin structure infections
Primaxin I.V. (Cilastatin Sodium, Imipenem) Merck 2083

G

Gardnerella vaginalis infections
Primaxin I.V. (Cilastatin Sodium, Imipenem) Merck 2083

Gas
Extra Strength Rolaids Plus Gas Relief Tropical Fruit Softchews (Calcium Carbonate, Simethicone) McNeil Consumer 1903
Rolaids Multi-Symptom Berry Tablets (Calcium Carbonate, Magnesium Hydroxide, Simethicone) McNeil Consumer 1903

Gastric hyperacidity
(*see under* Hyperacidity, gastric)

Gastric ulcer, NSAID-associated, risk reductions
Nexium Delayed-Release Capsules (Esomeprazole Magnesium) AstraZeneca LP 645
Nexium Delayed-Release Oral Suspension (Esomeprazole Magnesium) AstraZeneca LP 645

Gastric ulcers, active, benign, short-term treatment of
Axid Capsules (Nizatidine) GlaxoSmithKline 1364
Pepcid Tablets (Famotidine) Merck ... 2075
Zantac (Ranitidine Hydrochloride) GlaxoSmithKline 1670

Gastroenteritis, rotavirus, prevention of
Rotarix Oral Suspension (Rotavirus Vaccine, Live, Oral) GlaxoSmithKline 1582
RotaTeq (Rotavirus vaccine, live, oral, pentavalent) Merck 2110

Gastroesophageal reflux disease
Aciphex Tablets (Rabeprazole Sodium) Eisai 1053
Nexium Delayed-Release Capsules (Esomeprazole Magnesium) AstraZeneca LP 645
Nexium I.V. (Esomeprazole Sodium) AstraZeneca LP 652
Nexium Delayed-Release Oral Suspension (Esomeprazole Magnesium) AstraZeneca LP 645
Pepcid Tablets (Famotidine) Merck ... 2075
Protonix for Delayed-Release Oral Suspension (Pantoprazole Sodium) Wyeth 3254
Protonix Delayed-Release Tablets (Pantoprazole Sodium) Wyeth 3254
Protonix I.V. (Pantoprazole Sodium) Wyeth 3257
Zantac (Ranitidine Hydrochloride) GlaxoSmithKline 1670

Gastrointestinal stromal tumors
(*see under* Tumors, gastrointestinal stromal)

Gaucher disease, Type 1
Cerezyme for Injection (Imiglucerase) Genzyme 1238

Gelineau's syndrome
(*see under* Narcolepsy)

Genital warts
(*see under* Condylomata acuminata)

GERD
(*see under* Gastroesophageal reflux disease)

German measles
(*see under* Rubella, prophylaxis)

Gestational trophoblastic neoplasia
Cosmegen for Injection (Dactinomycin) Ovation 2485

GIST
(*see under* Tumors, gastrointestinal stromal)

Glaucoma, chronic open-angle
OptiPranolol Metipranolol Ophthalmic Solution 0.3% (Metipranolol) Bausch & Lomb ..... ⊙245
Timoptic Sterile Ophthalmic Solution (Timolol Maleate) Merck ... 2121
Timoptic in Ocudose (Timolol Maleate) Merck 2124
Timoptic-XE Sterile Ophthalmic Gel Forming Solution (Timolol Maleate) Merck 2125

Glaucoma, open-angle
Alphagan P Ophthalmic Solution (Brimonidine Tartrate) Allergan 549
Azopt Ophthalmic Suspension (Brinzolamide) Alcon 540
Cosopt Sterile Ophthalmic Solution (Dorzolamide Hydrochloride, Timolol Maleate) Merck 1969
Lumigan Ophthalmic Solution (Bimatoprost) Allergan 556
Trusopt Sterile Ophthalmic Solution (Dorzolamide Hydrochloride) Merck 2128
Xalatan Ophthalmic Solution (Latanoprost) Pharmacia & Upjohn .... ⊙273

Glaucoma, unspecified
Combigan Ophthalmic Solution (Brimonidine Tartrate, Timolol Maleate) Allergan 553

Glioblastoma multiforme
Temodar Capsules (Temozolomide) Schering 2931

Glioblastoma multiforme, recurrent, adjunctive therapy in
Gliadel Wafer (Polifeprosan 20 with Carmustine) Eisai 1076

Gliomas, cerebral
Gliadel Wafer (Polifeprosan 20 with Carmustine) Eisai ... 1076

Goiter, euthyroid, treatment or prevention of
Naturethroid Tablets (Levothyroxine, Liothyronine, Thyroid) RLC ... 2605
Synthroid Tablets (Levothyroxine Sodium) Abbott ... 507

Goiter, suppression of pituitary TSH in
Cytomel Tablets (Liothyronine Sodium) King ... 1778
Levothroid Tablets (Levothyroxine Sodium) Forest ... 1170
Levoxyl Tablets (Levothyroxine Sodium) King ... 1780
Naturethroid Tablets (Levothyroxine, Liothyronine, Thyroid) RLC ... 2605
Synthroid Tablets (Levothyroxine Sodium) Abbott ... 507

Gonococcal infections, uncomplicated
Rocephin Injectable Vials, ADD-Vantage, Galaxy, Bulk (Ceftriaxone Sodium) Roche ... 2642
Zinacef for Injection (Cefuroxime) GlaxoSmithKline ... 1678
Zinacef Injection (Cefuroxime) GlaxoSmithKline ... 1678

Gonorrhea
(*see also under* N. gonorrhoeae infections)
Amoxil Capsules (Amoxicillin) GlaxoSmithKline ... 1305
Amoxil Chewable Tablets (Amoxicillin) GlaxoSmithKline ... 1305
Amoxil Pediatric Drops for Oral Suspension (Amoxicillin) GlaxoSmithKline ... 1305
Amoxil Powder for Oral Suspension (Amoxicillin) GlaxoSmithKline ... 1305
Amoxil Tablets (Amoxicillin) GlaxoSmithKline ... 1305
Rocephin Injectable Vials, ADD-Vantage, Galaxy, Bulk (Ceftriaxone Sodium) Roche ... 2642
Zinacef for Injection (Cefuroxime) GlaxoSmithKline ... 1678
Zinacef Injection (Cefuroxime) GlaxoSmithKline ... 1678

Gonorrhea, cervical/urethral
Amoxil Capsules (Amoxicillin) GlaxoSmithKline ... 1305
Amoxil Chewable Tablets (Amoxicillin) GlaxoSmithKline ... 1305
Amoxil Pediatric Drops for Oral Suspension (Amoxicillin) GlaxoSmithKline ... 1305
Amoxil Powder for Oral Suspension (Amoxicillin) GlaxoSmithKline ... 1305
Amoxil Tablets (Amoxicillin) GlaxoSmithKline ... 1305
Cipro (Ciprofloxacin) Schering ... 2810
Noroxin Tablets (Norfloxacin) Merck ... 2069
Rocephin Injectable Vials, ADD-Vantage, Galaxy, Bulk (Ceftriaxone Sodium) Roche ... 2642

Gonorrhea, pharyngeal
Rocephin Injectable Vials, ADD-Vantage, Galaxy, Bulk (Ceftriaxone Sodium) Roche ... 2642

Gonorrhea, rectal
Amoxil Capsules (Amoxicillin) GlaxoSmithKline ... 1305
Amoxil Chewable Tablets (Amoxicillin) GlaxoSmithKline ... 1305
Amoxil Pediatric Drops for Oral Suspension (Amoxicillin) GlaxoSmithKline ... 1305
Amoxil Powder for Oral Suspension (Amoxicillin) GlaxoSmithKline ... 1305
Amoxil Tablets (Amoxicillin) GlaxoSmithKline ... 1305
Rocephin Injectable Vials, ADD-Vantage, Galaxy, Bulk (Ceftriaxone Sodium) Roche ... 2642

Gonorrhea, uncomplicated
Amoxil Capsules (Amoxicillin) GlaxoSmithKline ... 1305
Amoxil Chewable Tablets (Amoxicillin) GlaxoSmithKline ... 1305
Amoxil Pediatric Drops for Oral Suspension (Amoxicillin) GlaxoSmithKline ... 1305
Amoxil Powder for Oral Suspension (Amoxicillin) GlaxoSmithKline ... 1305
Amoxil Tablets (Amoxicillin) GlaxoSmithKline ... 1305
Ceftin Tablets (Cefuroxime Axetil) GlaxoSmithKline ... 1380
Cipro (Ciprofloxacin) Schering ... 2810
Noroxin Tablets (Norfloxacin) Merck ... 2069
Rocephin Injectable Vials, ADD-Vantage, Galaxy, Bulk (Ceftriaxone Sodium) Roche ... 2642

Gout, acute
Anaprox Tablets (Naproxen Sodium) Roche ... 2632
Anaprox DS Tablets (Naproxen Sodium) Roche ... 2632
Naprosyn Suspension (Naproxen) Roche ... 2632
Naprosyn Tablets (Naproxen) Roche ... 2632

Grand mal epilepsy
(*see under* Seizures, generalized, tonic-clonic)

Granulomatous disease, chronic
Actimmune (Interferon Gamma-1B) InterMune ... 1743

Growth, in children, stimulation of
Increlex Injection (Mecasermin [rDNA origin]) Tercica ... 3100

Growth failure, children
Humatrope Vials and Cartridges (Somatropin) Lilly ... 1838

Growth failure, chronic renal insufficiency-induced in children
Nutropin for Injection (Somatropin) Genentech ... 1208
Nutropin AQ Injection (Somatropin) Genentech ... 1212
Nutropin AQ NuSpin Injection (Somatropin) Genentech ... 1212
Nutropin AQ Pen (Somatropin) Genentech ... 1212
Nutropin AQ Pen Cartridge (Somatropin) Genentech ... 1212

Growth hormone secretion, inadequate
Genotropin Lyophilized Powder (Somatropin) Pharmacia & Upjohn ... 2547
Humatrope Vials and Cartridges (Somatropin) Lilly ... 1838
Norditropin Cartridges (Somatropin (rDNA Origin)) Novo Nordisk ... 2354
Nutropin for Injection (Somatropin) Genentech ... 1208
Nutropin AQ Injection (Somatropin) Genentech ... 1212
Nutropin AQ NuSpin Injection (Somatropin) Genentech ... 1212
Nutropin AQ Pen (Somatropin) Genentech ... 1212
Nutropin AQ Pen Cartridge (Somatropin) Genentech ... 1212
Tev-Tropin for Injection (Somatropin (rDNA Origin)) Gate ... 1187

Gums, irritation of
Hurricaine Topical Anesthetic (Benzocaine) Beutlich ... 815

Gums, sore
(*see under* Pain, dental)

H

H. aegypticus infections, ocular
Zylet Ophthalmic Suspension (Loteprednol Etabonate, Tobramycin) Bausch & Lomb ... ⊙247

H. influenzae, central nervous system infections
Fortaz (Ceftazidime) GlaxoSmithKline ... 1450

H. influenzae bronchitis
Amoxil Capsules (Amoxicillin) GlaxoSmithKline ... 1305
Amoxil Chewable Tablets (Amoxicillin) GlaxoSmithKline ... 1305
Amoxil Pediatric Drops for Oral Suspension (Amoxicillin) GlaxoSmithKline ... 1305
Amoxil Powder for Oral Suspension (Amoxicillin) GlaxoSmithKline ... 1305
Amoxil Tablets (Amoxicillin) GlaxoSmithKline ... 1305
Avelox (Moxifloxacin Hydrochloride) Schering ... 2803
Biaxin/Biaxin XL (Clarithromycin) Abbott ... 411
Ceftin Tablets (Cefuroxime Axetil) GlaxoSmithKline ... 1380
Levaquin (Levofloxacin) Ortho-McNeil ... 2416
Levaquin in 5% Dextrose Injection (Levofloxacin) Ortho-McNeil ... 2416
Omnicef Capsules (Cefdinir) Abbott ... 497
Omnicef for Oral Suspension (Cefdinir) Abbott ... 497
Suprax for Oral Suspension (Cefixime) Lupin ... 1891
Suprax Tablets (Cefixime) Lupin ... 1891

H. influenzae infections
Amoxil Capsules (Amoxicillin) GlaxoSmithKline ... 1305
Amoxil Chewable Tablets (Amoxicillin) GlaxoSmithKline ... 1305
Amoxil Pediatric Drops for Oral Suspension (Amoxicillin) GlaxoSmithKline ... 1305
Amoxil Powder for Oral Suspension (Amoxicillin) GlaxoSmithKline ... 1305
Amoxil Tablets (Amoxicillin) GlaxoSmithKline ... 1305
Augmentin (Amoxicillin, Clavulanate Potassium) GlaxoSmithKline ... 1323
Augmentin Tablets (Amoxicillin, Clavulanate Potassium) GlaxoSmithKline ... 1327
Augmentin XR Extended Release Tablets (Amoxicillin, Clavulanate Potassium) GlaxoSmithKline ... 1333
Augmentin ES-600 Powder for Oral Suspension (Amoxicillin, Clavulanate Potassium) GlaxoSmithKline ... 1329
Avelox (Moxifloxacin Hydrochloride) Schering ... 2803
Biaxin/Biaxin XL (Clarithromycin) Abbott ... 411
Ceftin (Cefuroxime Axetil) GlaxoSmithKline ... 1380
Cipro I.V. (Ciprofloxacin) Schering ... 2817
Cipro (Ciprofloxacin) Schering ... 2810
E.E.S. (Erythromycin Ethylsuccinate) Abbott ... 433
EryPed (Erythromycin Ethylsuccinate) Abbott ... 431
Fortaz (Ceftazidime) GlaxoSmithKline ... 1450
Invanz for Injection (Ertapenem) Merck ... 2029
Ketek Tablets (Telithromycin) sanofi-aventis ... 2744
Levaquin (Levofloxacin) Ortho-McNeil ... 2416
Levaquin in 5% Dextrose Injection (Levofloxacin) Ortho-McNeil ... 2416
Merrem I.V. (Meropenem) AstraZeneca Pharmaceuticals ... 684
Omnicef Capsules (Cefdinir) Abbott ... 497
Omnicef for Oral Suspension (Cefdinir) Abbott ... 497
Primaxin I.M. (Cilastatin Sodium, Imipenem) Merck ... 2080
Primaxin I.V. (Cilastatin Sodium, Imipenem) Merck ... 2083
Rocephin Injectable Vials, ADD-Vantage, Galaxy, Bulk (Ceftriaxone Sodium) Roche ... 2642
Suprax for Oral Suspension (Cefixime) Lupin ... 1891
Suprax Tablets (Cefixime) Lupin ... 1891
Timentin ADD-Vantage (Clavulanate Potassium, Ticarcillin Disodium) GlaxoSmithKline ... 1606
Timentin Injection Galaxy Container (Clavulanate Potassium, Ticarcillin Disodium) GlaxoSmithKline ... 1609
Timentin IV Infusion (Clavulanate Potassium, Ticarcillin Disodium) GlaxoSmithKline ... 1603
Timentin Pharmacy Bulk Package (Clavulanate Potassium, Ticarcillin Disodium) GlaxoSmithKline ... 1613
Vigamox Ophthalmic Solution (Moxifloxacin Hydrochloride) Alcon ... ⊙213
Zinacef for Injection (Cefuroxime) GlaxoSmithKline ... 1678
Zinacef Injection (Cefuroxime) GlaxoSmithKline ... 1678
Zosyn for Injection (Piperacillin Sodium, Tazobactam Sodium) Wyeth ... 3284

H. influenzae infections, ocular
Blephamide Ophthalmic Ointment Allergan ... ⊙217
Blephamide Ophthalmic Suspension Allergan ... ⊙216
Neosporin Ophthalmic Solution Sterile (Gramicidin, Neomycin Sulfate, Polymyxin B Sulfate) King ... ⊙252
Ofloxacin Ophthalmic Solution 0.3% (Ofloxacin) Bausch & Lomb ... ⊙243
Pred-G Ophthalmic Ointment (Gentamicin Sulfate, Prednisolone Acetate) Allergan ... ⊙229
Pred-G Ophthalmic Suspension (Gentamicin Sulfate, Prednisolone Acetate) Allergan ... ⊙228
Quixin Ophthalmic Solution (Levofloxacin) Vistakon ... 3184
Vigamox Ophthalmic Solution (Moxifloxacin Hydrochloride) Alcon ... 548
Zylet Ophthalmic Suspension (Loteprednol Etabonate, Tobramycin) Bausch & Lomb ... ⊙247

H. influenzae lower respiratory tract infections
Amoxil Capsules (Amoxicillin) GlaxoSmithKline ... 1305
Amoxil Chewable Tablets (Amoxicillin) GlaxoSmithKline ... 1305
Amoxil Pediatric Drops for Oral Suspension (Amoxicillin) GlaxoSmithKline ... 1305
Amoxil Powder for Oral Suspension (Amoxicillin) GlaxoSmithKline ... 1305
Amoxil Tablets (Amoxicillin) GlaxoSmithKline ... 1305
Augmentin (Amoxicillin, Clavulanate Potassium) GlaxoSmithKline ... 1323
Augmentin Tablets (Amoxicillin, Clavulanate Potassium) GlaxoSmithKline ... 1327
Augmentin XR Extended Release Tablets (Amoxicillin, Clavulanate Potassium) GlaxoSmithKline ... 1333
Biaxin/Biaxin XL (Clarithromycin) Abbott ... 411
Cipro I.V. (Ciprofloxacin) Schering ... 2817
Cipro (Ciprofloxacin) Schering ... 2810
Fortaz (Ceftazidime) GlaxoSmithKline ... 1450
Invanz for Injection (Ertapenem) Merck ... 2029
Ketek Tablets (Telithromycin) sanofi-aventis ... 2744
Levaquin (Levofloxacin) Ortho-McNeil ... 2416
Levaquin in 5% Dextrose Injection (Levofloxacin) Ortho-McNeil ... 2416
Primaxin I.M. (Cilastatin Sodium, Imipenem) Merck ... 2080
Primaxin I.V. (Cilastatin Sodium, Imipenem) Merck ... 2083
Rocephin Injectable Vials, ADD-Vantage, Galaxy, Bulk (Ceftriaxone Sodium) Roche ... 2642
Timentin ADD-Vantage (Clavulanate Potassium, Ticarcillin Disodium) GlaxoSmithKline ... 1606
Timentin Injection Galaxy Container (Clavulanate Potassium, Ticarcillin Disodium) GlaxoSmithKline ... 1609
Timentin IV Infusion (Clavulanate Potassium, Ticarcillin Disodium) GlaxoSmithKline ... 1603
Timentin Pharmacy Bulk Package (Clavulanate Potassium, Ticarcillin Disodium) GlaxoSmithKline ... 1613
Zinacef for Injection (Cefuroxime) GlaxoSmithKline ... 1678
Zinacef Injection (Cefuroxime) GlaxoSmithKline ... 1678
Zosyn for Injection (Piperacillin Sodium, Tazobactam Sodium) Wyeth ... 3284

H. influenzae meningitis
Fortaz (Ceftazidime) GlaxoSmithKline 1450
Gantrisin Pediatric Suspension (Acetyl Sulfisoxazole) Roche 2638
Merrem I.V. (Meropenem) AstraZeneca Pharmaceuticals 684
Rocephin Injectable Vials, ADD-Vantage, Galaxy, Bulk (Ceftriaxone Sodium) Roche 2642
Zinacef for Injection (Cefuroxime) GlaxoSmithKline 1678
Zinacef Injection (Cefuroxime) GlaxoSmithKline 1678

H. influenzae otitis externa
Amoxil Capsules (Amoxicillin) GlaxoSmithKline 1305
Amoxil Chewable Tablets (Amoxicillin) GlaxoSmithKline 1305
Amoxil Pediatric Drops for Oral Suspension (Amoxicillin) GlaxoSmithKline 1305
Amoxil Powder for Oral Suspension (Amoxicillin) GlaxoSmithKline 1305
Amoxil Tablets (Amoxicillin) GlaxoSmithKline 1305

H. influenzae otitis media
Amoxil Capsules (Amoxicillin) GlaxoSmithKline 1305
Amoxil Chewable Tablets (Amoxicillin) GlaxoSmithKline 1305
Amoxil Pediatric Drops for Oral Suspension (Amoxicillin) GlaxoSmithKline 1305
Amoxil Powder for Oral Suspension (Amoxicillin) GlaxoSmithKline 1305
Amoxil Tablets (Amoxicillin) GlaxoSmithKline 1305
Augmentin (Amoxicillin, Clavulanate Potassium) GlaxoSmithKline 1323
Augmentin Tablets (Amoxicillin, Clavulanate Potassium) GlaxoSmithKline 1327
Augmentin ES-600 Powder for Oral Suspension (Amoxicillin, Clavulanate Potassium) GlaxoSmithKline 1329
Biaxin/Biaxin XL (Clarithromycin) Abbott 411
Ceftin (Cefuroxime Axetil) GlaxoSmithKline 1380
Omnicef Capsules (Cefdinir) Abbott 497
Omnicef for Oral Suspension (Cefdinir) Abbott 497
Rocephin Injectable Vials, ADD-Vantage, Galaxy, Bulk (Ceftriaxone Sodium) Roche 2642
Suprax for Oral Suspension (Cefixime) Lupin 1891
Suprax Tablets (Cefixime) Lupin 1891

H. influenzae otitis media, adjunctive therapy in
Gantrisin Pediatric Suspension (Acetyl Sulfisoxazole) Roche 2638

H. influenzae pneumonia
Avelox (Moxifloxacin Hydrochloride) Schering 2803
Biaxin/Biaxin XL (Clarithromycin) Abbott 411
Invanz for Injection (Ertapenem) Merck 2029
Ketek Tablets (Telithromycin) sanofi-aventis 2744
Omnicef Capsules (Cefdinir) Abbott 497
Omnicef for Oral Suspension (Cefdinir) Abbott 497

H. influenzae septicemia
Fortaz (Ceftazidime) GlaxoSmithKline 1450
Rocephin Injectable Vials, ADD-Vantage, Galaxy, Bulk (Ceftriaxone Sodium) Roche 2642
Zinacef for Injection (Cefuroxime) GlaxoSmithKline 1678
Zinacef Injection (Cefuroxime) GlaxoSmithKline 1678

H. influenzae sinusitis
Amoxil Capsules (Amoxicillin) GlaxoSmithKline 1305
Amoxil Chewable Tablets (Amoxicillin) GlaxoSmithKline 1305
Amoxil Pediatric Drops for Oral Suspension (Amoxicillin) GlaxoSmithKline 1305
Amoxil Powder for Oral Suspension (Amoxicillin) GlaxoSmithKline 1305
Amoxil Tablets (Amoxicillin) GlaxoSmithKline 1305
Augmentin (Amoxicillin, Clavulanate Potassium) GlaxoSmithKline 1323
Augmentin Tablets (Amoxicillin, Clavulanate Potassium) GlaxoSmithKline 1327
Augmentin XR Extended Release Tablets (Amoxicillin, Clavulanate Potassium) GlaxoSmithKline 1333
Avelox (Moxifloxacin Hydrochloride) Schering 2803
Biaxin/Biaxin XL (Clarithromycin) Abbott 411
Ceftin Tablets (Cefuroxime Axetil) GlaxoSmithKline 1380
Cipro I.V. (Ciprofloxacin) Schering 2817
Cipro (Ciprofloxacin) Schering 2810
Levaquin (Levofloxacin) Ortho-McNeil 2416
Levaquin in 5% Dextrose Injection (Levofloxacin) Ortho-McNeil 2416
Omnicef Capsules (Cefdinir) Abbott 497
Omnicef for Oral Suspension (Cefdinir) Abbott 497

H. influenzae upper respiratory tract infections
Amoxil Capsules (Amoxicillin) GlaxoSmithKline 1305
Amoxil Chewable Tablets (Amoxicillin) GlaxoSmithKline 1305
Amoxil Pediatric Drops for Oral Suspension (Amoxicillin) GlaxoSmithKline 1305
Amoxil Powder for Oral Suspension (Amoxicillin) GlaxoSmithKline 1305
Amoxil Tablets (Amoxicillin) GlaxoSmithKline 1305
E.E.S. (Erythromycin Ethylsuccinate) Abbott 433
EryPed (Erythromycin Ethylsuccinate) Abbott 431

H. parainfluenzae bronchitis
Avelox (Moxifloxacin Hydrochloride) Schering 2803
Ceftin Tablets (Cefuroxime Axetil) GlaxoSmithKline 1380
Levaquin (Levofloxacin) Ortho-McNeil 2416
Levaquin in 5% Dextrose Injection (Levofloxacin) Ortho-McNeil 2416

H. parainfluenzae infections
Augmentin XR Extended Release Tablets (Amoxicillin, Clavulanate Potassium) GlaxoSmithKline 1333
Avelox (Moxifloxacin Hydrochloride) Schering 2803
Biaxin/Biaxin XL (Clarithromycin) Abbott 411
Ceftin Tablets (Cefuroxime Axetil) GlaxoSmithKline 1380
Cipro (Ciprofloxacin) Schering 2810
Levaquin (Levofloxacin) Ortho-McNeil 2416
Levaquin in 5% Dextrose Injection (Levofloxacin) Ortho-McNeil 2416
Primaxin I.V. (Cilastatin Sodium, Imipenem) Merck 2083
Rocephin Injectable Vials, ADD-Vantage, Galaxy, Bulk (Ceftriaxone Sodium) Roche 2642
Vigamox Ophthalmic Solution (Moxifloxacin Hydrochloride) Alcon ⊙213

H. parainfluenzae infections, ocular
Vigamox Ophthalmic Solution (Moxifloxacin Hydrochloride) Alcon 548

H. parainfluenzae lower respiratory tract infections
Augmentin XR Extended Release Tablets (Amoxicillin, Clavulanate Potassium) GlaxoSmithKline 1333
Biaxin/Biaxin XL (Clarithromycin) Abbott 411
Cipro I.V. (Ciprofloxacin) Schering 2817
Cipro (Ciprofloxacin) Schering 2810
Levaquin (Levofloxacin) Ortho-McNeil 2416
Levaquin in 5% Dextrose Injection (Levofloxacin) Ortho-McNeil 2416
Primaxin I.V. (Cilastatin Sodium, Imipenem) Merck 2083
Rocephin Injectable Vials, ADD-Vantage, Galaxy, Bulk (Ceftriaxone Sodium) Roche 2642

H. parainfluenzae pneumonia
Augmentin XR Extended Release Tablets (Amoxicillin, Clavulanate Potassium) GlaxoSmithKline 1333
Biaxin/Biaxin XL (Clarithromycin) Abbott 411
Omnicef Capsules (Cefdinir) Abbott 497
Omnicef for Oral Suspension (Cefdinir) Abbott 497

H. parainfluenzae sinusitis
Levaquin (Levofloxacin) Ortho-McNeil 2416
Levaquin in 5% Dextrose Injection (Levofloxacin) Ortho-McNeil 2416

H. pylori infection and duodenal ulcer
Amoxil Capsules (Amoxicillin) GlaxoSmithKline 1305
Amoxil Chewable Tablets (Amoxicillin) GlaxoSmithKline 1305
Amoxil Pediatric Drops for Oral Suspension (Amoxicillin) GlaxoSmithKline 1305
Amoxil Powder for Oral Suspension (Amoxicillin) GlaxoSmithKline 1305
Amoxil Tablets (Amoxicillin) GlaxoSmithKline 1305
Pylera Capsules (Metronidazole, Tetracycline Hydrochloride, Bismuth Subcitrate Potassium) Axcan Pharma 714

H. pylori infection and duodenal ulcer, adjunct in
Aciphex Tablets (Rabeprazole Sodium) Eisai 1053
Amoxil Capsules (Amoxicillin) GlaxoSmithKline 1305
Amoxil Chewable Tablets (Amoxicillin) GlaxoSmithKline 1305
Amoxil Pediatric Drops for Oral Suspension (Amoxicillin) GlaxoSmithKline 1305
Amoxil Powder for Oral Suspension (Amoxicillin) GlaxoSmithKline 1305
Amoxil Tablets (Amoxicillin) GlaxoSmithKline 1305
Biaxin/Biaxin XL (Clarithromycin) Abbott 411
Nexium Delayed-Release Capsules (Esomeprazole Magnesium) AstraZeneca LP 645
Nexium Delayed-Release Oral Suspension (Esomeprazole Magnesium) AstraZeneca LP 645

Haemophilus influenzae
(*see under* H. influenzae infections)

Haemophilus influenzae type b, immunization against
(*see also under* Immunization, haemophilus influenzae type b)
Comvax (Haemophilus B Conjugate Vaccine, Hepatitis B Vaccine, Recombinant) Merck 1966
Liquid PedvaxHIB (Haemophilus B Conjugate Vaccine) Merck 2073

Haemophilus influenzae type b vaccine
(*see also under* Immunization, haemophilus influenzae type b; Immunization, haemophilus influenzae type B and hepatitis B virus)
Comvax (Haemophilus B Conjugate Vaccine, Hepatitis B Vaccine, Recombinant) Merck 1966
Liquid PedvaxHIB (Haemophilus B Conjugate Vaccine) Merck 2073

Hairy cell leukemias
(*see under* Leukemia, hairy cell)

Hansen's disease
(*see under* Leprosy)

Hashimoto's thyroiditis
Naturethroid Tablets (Levothyroxine, Liothyronine, Thyroid) RLC 2605
Synthroid Tablets (Levothyroxine Sodium) Abbott 507

Hay fever
(*see under* Pollinosis)

Headache
Benadryl Allergy & Cold Kapgels (Acetaminophen, Diphenhydramine Hydrochloride, Phenylephrine Hydrochloride) McNeil Consumer 1895
Benadryl Allergy & Sinus Headache Kapgels (Acetaminophen, Diphenhydramine Hydrochloride, Phenylephrine Hydrochloride) McNeil Consumer 1895
Benadryl Severe Allergy & Sinus Headache Caplets (Acetaminophen, Diphenhydramine Hydrochloride, Phenylephrine Hydrochloride) McNeil Consumer 1897
Motrin IB Tablets and Caplets (Ibuprofen) McNeil Consumer 1900
Children's Motrin Oral Suspension (Ibuprofen) McNeil Consumer 1901
Children's Motrin Non-Staining Dye-Free Oral Suspension (Ibuprofen) McNeil Consumer 1901
Infants' Motrin Concentrated Drops (Ibuprofen) McNeil Consumer 1901
Infants' Motrin Non-Staining Dye-Free Concentrated Drops (Ibuprofen) McNeil Consumer 1901
Junior Strength Motrin Caplets and Chewable Tablets (Ibuprofen) McNeil Consumer 1901
Sinutab Sinus Caplets (Acetaminophen, Phenylephrine Hydrochloride) McNeil Consumer 1905
Sudafed PE Cold & Cough Caplets (Acetaminophen, Dextromethorphan Hydrobromide, Guaifenesin, Phenylephrine Hydrochloride) McNeil Consumer 1907
Sudafed PE Nighttime Cold Caplets (Acetaminophen, Diphenhydramine Hydrochloride, Phenylephrine Hydrochloride) McNeil Consumer 1907
Sudafed PE Severe Cold Caplets (Acetaminophen, Diphenhydramine Hydrochloride, Phenylephrine Hydrochloride) McNeil Consumer 1908
Sudafed PE Sinus Headache Caplets (Acetaminophen, Phenylephrine Hydrochloride) McNeil Consumer 1908
Regular Strength Tylenol Tablets (Acetaminophen) McNeil Consumer 1915
Tylenol 8 Hour Extended Release Caplets (Acetaminophen) McNeil Consumer 1915
Extra Strength Tylenol Caplets, Cool Caplets, and EZ Tabs (Acetaminophen) McNeil Consumer 1915
Extra Strength Tylenol Adult Rapid Blast Liquid (Acetaminophen) McNeil Consumer 1915
Extra Strength Tylenol PM Caplets, Geltabs, Liquid, and Rapid Release Gels (Acetaminophen, Diphenhydramine Hydrochloride) McNeil Consumer 1915
Extra Strength Tylenol Rapid Release Gels (Acetaminophen) McNeil Consumer 1915
Tylenol Allergy Multi-Symptom Caplets with Cool Burst and Rapid Release Gelcaps (Acetaminophen, Chlorpheniramine Maleate, Phenylephrine Hydrochloride) McNeil Consumer 1916
Tylenol Allergy Multi-Symptom Nighttime Caplets with Cool Burst (Acetaminophen, Diphenhydramine Hydrochloride, Phenylephrine Hydrochloride) McNeil Consumer 1916
Tylenol Severe Allergy Caplets (Acetaminophen, Diphenhydramine Hydrochloride) McNeil Consumer 1916
Tylenol Arthritis Pain Extended Release Geltabs/Caplets (Acetaminophen) McNeil Consumer 1915
Tylenol Chest Congestion Caplets with Cool Burst (Acetaminophen, Guaifenesin) McNeil Consumer 1910
Tylenol Chest Congestion Liquid with Cool Burst (Acetaminophen, Guaifenesin) McNeil Consumer 1910

Children's Tylenol Plus Cold Suspension Liquid (Acetaminophen, Chlorpheniramine Maleate, Phenylephrine Hydrochloride) McNeil Consumer 1912
Children's Tylenol Plus Cold & Allergy Suspension Liquid (Acetaminophen, Diphenhydramine Hydrochloride, Phenylephrine Hydrochloride) McNeil Consumer .. 1914
Children's Tylenol Plus Cough & Runny Nose Suspension Liquid (Acetaminophen, Chlorpheniramine Maleate, Dextromethorphan Hydrobromide) McNeil Consumer .. 1912
Children's Tylenol Plus Cough & Sore Throat Suspension Liquid (Acetaminophen, Dextromethorphan Hydrobromide) McNeil Consumer 1912
Children's Tylenol Plus Flu Suspension Liquid (Acetaminophen, Chlorpheniramine Maleate, Dextromethorphan Hydrobromide, Phenylephrine Hydrochloride) McNeil Consumer 1914
Children's Tylenol Suspension Liquid (Acetaminophen) McNeil Consumer 1909
Children's Tylenol Meltaways (Acetaminophen) McNeil Consumer 1909
Children's Tylenol Plus Multi-Symptom Cold Suspension Liquid (Acetaminophen, Chlorpheniramine Maleate, Dextromethorphan Hydrobromide, Phenylephrine Hydrochloride) McNeil Consumer 1912
Tylenol Cold Severe Congestion Daytime Caplets with Cool Burst (Acetaminophen, Dextromethorphan Hydrobromide, Guaifenesin, Pseudoephedrine Hydrochloride) McNeil Consumer 1912
Tylenol Cold Head Congestion Daytime Caplets with Cool Burst (Acetaminophen, Dextromethorphan Hydrobromide, Phenylephrine Hydrochloride) McNeil Consumer 1910
Tylenol Cold Head Congestion Nighttime Caplets with Cool Burst (Acetaminophen, Chlorpheniramine Maleate, Dextromethorphan Hydrobromide, Phenylephrine Hydrochloride) McNeil Consumer 1910
Tylenol Cold Head Congestion Severe Daytime Caplets with Cool Burst (Acetaminophen, Dextromethorphan Hydrobromide, Guaifenesin, Phenylephrine Hydrochloride) McNeil Consumer .. 1910
Tylenol Cough & Sore Throat Daytime Liquid with Cool Burst (Acetaminophen, Dextromethorphan Hydrobromide) McNeil Consumer 1918
Tylenol Cough & Sore Throat Nighttime Liquid with Cool Burst (Acetaminophen, Dextromethorphan Hydrobromide, Doxylamine Succinate) McNeil Consumer 1918
Concentrated Tylenol Infants' Drops (Acetaminophen) McNeil Consumer 1909
Jr. Tylenol Meltaways (Acetaminophen) McNeil Consumer 1909
Tylenol Sinus Congestion & Pain Daytime Caplets with Cool Burst and Gelcaps (Acetaminophen, Phenylephrine Hydrochloride) McNeil Consumer 1917
Tylenol Sinus Congestion & Pain Nighttime Caplets with Cool Burst (Acetaminophen, Chlorpheniramine Maleate, Phenylephrine Hydrochloride) McNeil Consumer 1917
Tylenol Sinus Congestion & Pain Severe Caplets with Cool Burst (Acetaminophen, Guaifenesin, Phenylephrine Hydrochloride) McNeil Consumer 1917
Tylenol Sinus Severe Congestion Caplets with Cool Burst (Acetaminophen, Guaifenesin, Pseudoephedrine Hydrochloride) McNeil Consumer 1917
Tylenol Sore Throat Daytime Liquid with Cool Burst (Acetaminophen) McNeil Consumer 1918
Tylenol Sore Throat Nighttime Liquid with Cool Burst (Acetaminophen, Diphenhydramine Hydrochloride) McNeil Consumer 1918
Women's Tylenol Menstrual Relief Caplets (Acetaminophen, Pamabrom) McNeil Consumer 1919
Vicks NyQuil Cold & Flu Multi-Symptom Relief (Acetaminophen, Dextromethorphan Hydrobromide, Doxylamine Succinate) Procter & Gamble .... ▣ 617
Vicks NyQuil LiquiCaps (Acetaminophen, Dextromethorphan Hydrobromide, Doxylamine Succinate, Pseudoephedrine Hydrochloride) Procter & Gamble 2567
Vicks NyQuil Liquid (Acetaminophen, Dextromethorphan Hydrobromide, Doxylamine Succinate, Pseudoephedrine Hydrochloride) Procter & Gamble 2567
Vicks NyQuil Multi-Symptom Cold/Flu Relief (Acetaminophen, Dextromethorphan Hydrobromide, Doxylamine Succinate, Pseudoephedrine Hydrochloride) Procter & Gamble 2567

Headache, cluster
(*see under* Cephalalgia, histaminic)

Headache, migraine
Amerge Tablets (Naratriptan Hydrochloride) GlaxoSmithKline 1301
Axert Tablets (Almotriptan Malate) Ortho-McNeil Neurologics 2431
Frova Tablets (Frovatriptan Succinate) Endo 1111
Imitrex Injection (Sumatriptan Succinate) GlaxoSmithKline 1465
Imitrex Nasal Spray (Sumatriptan) GlaxoSmithKline 1470
Imitrex Tablets (Sumatriptan Succinate) GlaxoSmithKline 1474
Maxalt Tablets (Rizatriptan Benzoate) Merck 2056
Maxalt-MLT Orally Disintegrating Tablets (Rizatriptan Benzoate) Merck 2056
Treximet Tablets (Naproxen Sodium, Sumatriptan Succinate) GlaxoSmithKline 1616
Zomig Tablets (Zolmitriptan) AstraZeneca Pharmaceuticals 694
Zomig Nasal Spray (Zolmitriptan) AstraZeneca Pharmaceuticals 689
Zomig-ZMT Tablets (Zolmitriptan) AstraZeneca Pharmaceuticals 694

Headache, migraine, prophylaxis of
Depakote ER Tablets (Divalproex Sodium) Abbott 423

Headache, sinus, symptomatic relief of
(*see under* Sinus headache)

Headache, vascular
(*see under* Headache, migraine)

Headache accompanied by insomnia
Extra Strength Tylenol PM Caplets, Geltabs, Liquid, and Rapid Release Gels (Acetaminophen, Diphenhydramine Hydrochloride) McNeil Consumer 1915

Headache associated with common cold
(*see also under* Sinus headache)
Children's Motrin Cold Oral Suspension (Ibuprofen, Pseudoephedrine Hydrochloride) McNeil Consumer 1899
Tylenol Chest Congestion Caplets with Cool Burst (Acetaminophen, Guaifenesin) McNeil Consumer 1910
Tylenol Chest Congestion Liquid with Cool Burst (Acetaminophen, Guaifenesin) McNeil Consumer 1910
Children's Tylenol Plus Cold Suspension Liquid (Acetaminophen, Chlorpheniramine Maleate, Phenylephrine Hydrochloride) McNeil Consumer 1912
Children's Tylenol Plus Cough & Runny Nose Suspension Liquid (Acetaminophen, Chlorpheniramine Maleate, Dextromethorphan Hydrobromide) McNeil Consumer .. 1912
Children's Tylenol Plus Cough & Sore Throat Suspension Liquid (Acetaminophen, Dextromethorphan Hydrobromide) McNeil Consumer 1912
Children's Tylenol Plus Multi-Symptom Cold Suspension Liquid (Acetaminophen, Chlorpheniramine Maleate, Dextromethorphan Hydrobromide, Phenylephrine Hydrochloride) McNeil Consumer 1912
Tylenol Cold Head Congestion Daytime Caplets with Cool Burst (Acetaminophen, Dextromethorphan Hydrobromide, Phenylephrine Hydrochloride) McNeil Consumer 1910
Tylenol Cold Head Congestion Nighttime Caplets with Cool Burst (Acetaminophen, Chlorpheniramine Maleate, Dextromethorphan Hydrobromide, Phenylephrine Hydrochloride) McNeil Consumer 1910
Tylenol Cold Head Congestion Severe Daytime Caplets with Cool Burst (Acetaminophen, Dextromethorphan Hydrobromide, Guaifenesin, Phenylephrine Hydrochloride) McNeil Consumer .. 1910
Tylenol Cold Multi-Symptom Daytime Caplets with Cool Burst and Rapid Release Gels (Acetaminophen, Dextromethorphan Hydrobromide, Phenylephrine Hydrochloride) McNeil Consumer .. 1913
Tylenol Cold Multi-Symptom Daytime Liquid with Citrus Burst (Acetaminophen, Dextromethorphan Hydrobromide, Phenylephrine Hydrochloride) McNeil Consumer 1913
Tylenol Cold Multi-Symptom Nighttime Caplets with Cool Burst (Acetaminophen, Chlorpheniramine Maleate, Dextromethorphan Hydrobromide, Phenylephrine Hydrochloride) McNeil Consumer 1913
Tylenol Cold Multi-Symptom Nighttime Liquid with Cool Burst (Acetaminophen, Dextromethorphan Hydrobromide, Doxylamine Succinate, Phenylephrine Hydrochloride) McNeil Consumer 1913
Tylenol Cold Multi-Symptom Severe Caplets with Cool Burst (Acetaminophen, Dextromethorphan Hydrobromide, Guaifenesin, Phenylephrine Hydrochloride) McNeil Consumer 1913
Tylenol Cold Multi-Symptom Severe Daytime Liquid with Citrus Burst (Acetaminophen, Dextromethorphan Hydrobromide, Guaifenesin, Phenylephrine Hydrochloride) McNeil Consumer 1913
Vicks DayQuil Cold & Flu Multi-Symptom Relief (Acetaminophen, Dextromethorphan Hydrobromide, Phenylephrine Hydrochloride) Procter & Gamble .... ▣ 616
Vicks DayQuil LiquiCaps (Acetaminophen, Dextromethorphan Hydrobromide, Phenylephrine Hydrochloride) Procter & Gamble .. 2567
Vicks DayQuil (Acetaminophen, Dextromethorphan Hydrobromide, Phenylephrine Hydrochloride) Procter & Gamble .... ▣ 616
Vicks DayQuil Liquid (Acetaminophen, Dextromethorphan Hydrobromide, Phenylephrine Hydrochloride) Procter & Gamble 2567
Vicks DayQuil Multi-Symptom Cold/Flu Relief (Acetaminophen, Dextromethorphan Hydrobromide, Phenylephrine Hydrochloride) Procter & Gamble 2567

Heart, allogeneic transplants, prophylaxis of organ rejection in
CellCept Capsules (Mycophenolate Mofetil) Roche 2622
CellCept Intravenous (Mycophenolate Mofetil Hydrochloride) Roche .. 2622
CellCept Oral Suspension (Mycophenolate Mofetil) Roche 2622
CellCept Tablets (Mycophenolate Mofetil) Roche 2622
Gengraf Capsules (Cyclosporine) Abbott 435
Neoral Oral Solution (Cyclosporine) Novartis 2280
Neoral Soft Gelatin Capsules (Cyclosporine) Novartis 2280
Orthoclone OKT3 Sterile Solution (Muromonab-CD3) Ortho Biotech ... 2387
Prograf Capsules and Injection (Tacrolimus) Astellas 622
Sandimmune (Cyclosporine) Novartis 2296

Heart failure
(*see under* Congestive heart failure, adjunct in)

Heart failure, congestive
(*see under* Congestive heart failure, adjunct in)

Heart failure, NYHA Class II - IV
Atacand Tablets (Candesartan Cilexetil) AstraZeneca LP 639
Diovan Tablets (Valsartan) Novartis .. 2212
Toprol-XL Tablets (Metoprolol Succinate) AstraZeneca LP 666

Heartburn
(*see under* Hyperacidity, gastric, symptomatic relief of)

Heartburn, frequent
Prilosec OTC Tablets (Omeprazole Magnesium) Procter & Gamble...... 2565

Hematopoietic progenitor cells, mobilization of
Neupogen for Injection (Filgrastim) Amgen 589

Hemodialysis, adjunct in
Albutein 5% (Albumin (human)) Grifols 1707
Albutein 25% (Albumin (human)) Grifols 1708

Hemolytic disease, newborn
Flexbumin 25% I.V. (Albumin (human)) Baxter Healthcare 729

Hemophilia A
Advate (Antihemophilic Factor (Recombinant)) Baxter Healthcare . 721
Hemofil M (Antihemophilic Factor (Human)) Baxter Healthcare 737
Kogenate FS (Antihemophilic Factor (Recombinant)) Bayer Healthcare 746
Kogenate FS with Bio-Set (Antihemophilic Factor (Recombinant)) Bayer Healthcare 748
Recombinate (Antihemophilic Factor (Recombinant)) Baxter Healthcare 738
ReFacto Vials (Antihemophilic Factor (Recombinant)) Wyeth 3269

Hemophilia A, perioperative management of
Advate (Antihemophilic Factor (Recombinant)) Baxter Healthcare . 721
Xyntha Vials (Antihemophilic Factor (Recombinant), Plasma/Albumin-Free) Wyeth 3280

Hemophilia A with Factor VIII inhibitors
Alphanate (Antihemophilic Factor (Human), von Willebrand Factor (Human)) Grifols 1709

Hemophilia B
BeneFIX Vials (Antihemophilic Factor (Recombinant)) Wyeth 3191

Hemorrhage, subarachnoid, resulting in neurological deficits
Nimotop Capsules (Nimodipine) Bayer HealthCare Pharmaceuticals 790

Hemostasis, an aid in
Trasylol Injection (Aprotinin) Bayer HealthCare Pharmaceuticals 799

Hepatitis A virus, immunization against
(*see also under* Hepatitis A virus vaccine; Immunization, hepatitis A and B virus; Immunization, hepatitis A virus)
Havrix Injection Vaccine (Hepatitis A Vaccine, Inactivated) GlaxoSmithKline 1454
Twinrix Vaccine (Hepatitis A Vaccine, Inactivated, Hepatitis B Vaccine, Recombinant) GlaxoSmithKline 1628
Vaqta (Hepatitis A Vaccine, Inactivated) Merck 2130

Hepatitis A virus vaccine
(*see also under* Hepatitis A virus, immunization against; Immunization, hepatitis A and B virus; Immunization, hepatitis A virus)
Havrix Injection Vaccine (Hepatitis A Vaccine, Inactivated) GlaxoSmithKline 1454
Twinrix Vaccine (Hepatitis A Vaccine, Inactivated, Hepatitis B Vaccine, Recombinant) GlaxoSmithKline 1628
Vaqta (Hepatitis A Vaccine, Inactivated) Merck 2130

Hepatitis B, chronic
Baraclude (Entecavir) Bristol-Myers Squibb 900
Epivir-HBV (Lamivudine) GlaxoSmithKline 1417
Hepsera Tablets (Adefovir dipivoxil) Gilead 1253
Intron A for Injection (Interferon alfa-2b, Recombinant) Schering 2859
Tyzeka Tablets (Telbivudine) Novartis 2328

Hepatitis B virus, immunization against
(*see also under* Immunization, haemophilus influenzae type B and hepatitis B virus; Immunization, hepatitis A and B virus)
Comvax (Haemophilus B Conjugate Vaccine, Hepatitis B Vaccine, Recombinant) Merck 1966
Engerix-B Vaccine (Hepatitis B Vaccine, Recombinant) GlaxoSmithKline 1409
Pediarix Vaccine (Diphtheria & Tetanus Toxoids and Acellular Pertussis Vaccine Adsorbed, Hepatitis B Vaccine, Recombinant, Poliovirus Vaccine Inactivated) GlaxoSmithKline 1552
Recombivax HB (Hepatitis B Vaccine, Recombinant) Merck 2107
Twinrix Vaccine (Hepatitis A Vaccine, Inactivated, Hepatitis B Vaccine, Recombinant) GlaxoSmithKline 1628

Hepatitis B virus, postexposure prophylaxis
Nabi-HB (Hepatitis B Immune Globulin (Human)) Biotest 815

Hepatitis B virus vaccine
(*see also under* Haemophilus influenzae type b, immunization against; Haemophilus influenzae type b vaccine; Hepatitis B virus, immunization against; Immunization, haemophilus influenzae type B and hepatitis B virus; Immunization, hepatitis A and B virus; Immunization, hepatitis B virus)
Comvax (Haemophilus B Conjugate Vaccine, Hepatitis B Vaccine, Recombinant) Merck 1966
Engerix-B Vaccine (Hepatitis B Vaccine, Recombinant) GlaxoSmithKline 1409
Pediarix Vaccine (Diphtheria & Tetanus Toxoids and Acellular Pertussis Vaccine Adsorbed, Hepatitis B Vaccine, Recombinant, Poliovirus Vaccine Inactivated) GlaxoSmithKline 1552
Recombivax HB (Hepatitis B Vaccine, Recombinant) Merck 2107
Twinrix Vaccine (Hepatitis A Vaccine, Inactivated, Hepatitis B Vaccine, Recombinant) GlaxoSmithKline 1628

Hepatitis C, chronic
Intron A for Injection (Interferon alfa-2b, Recombinant) Schering 2859
PegIntron Powder for Injection (Peginterferon Alfa-2b) Schering 2903
Rebetol (Ribavirin) Schering 2917

Herellea vaginicola
(*see under* Acinetobacter calcoaceticus infections, ocular)

Herpes, genital, initial and recurrent episodes
Zovirax (Acyclovir) GlaxoSmithKline 1690

Herpes genitalis
Valtrex Caplets (Valacyclovir Hydrochloride) GlaxoSmithKline 1635
Zovirax Capsules (Acyclovir) GlaxoSmithKline 1690
Zovirax Cream (Acyclovir) Biovail 817
Zovirax Ointment (Acyclovir) Biovail 819
Zovirax (Acyclovir) GlaxoSmithKline 1690

Herpes labialis
Valtrex Caplets (Valacyclovir Hydrochloride) GlaxoSmithKline 1635

Herpes labialis, recurrent
Zovirax Cream (Acyclovir) Biovail 817

Herpes simplex keratitis
Viroptic Ophthalmic Solution (Trifluridine) King .... ⊙253

Herpes simplex virus infections
Denavir Cream (Penciclovir) Novartis Consumer 2205
Zovirax Cream (Acyclovir) Biovail 817
Zovirax Ointment (Acyclovir) Biovail 819

Herpes simplex virus mucocutaneous infection
Zovirax Cream (Acyclovir) Biovail 817
Zovirax Ointment (Acyclovir) Biovail 819

Herpes zoster, prevention of
Zostavax Injection (Zoster Vaccine Live) Merck 2145

Herpes zoster infections
Valtrex Caplets (Valacyclovir Hydrochloride) GlaxoSmithKline 1635
Zovirax (Acyclovir) GlaxoSmithKline 1690

Herpetic manifestations, oral, symptomatic relief of
(*see also under* Herpes simplex virus infections)
Denavir Cream (Penciclovir) Novartis Consumer 2205
Valtrex Caplets (Valacyclovir Hydrochloride) GlaxoSmithKline 1635

HIV Infection
(*see under* Infections, human immunodeficiency virus)

Hodgkin's disease
Leukeran Tablets (Chlorambucil) GlaxoSmithKline 1508

Hodgkin's disease, adjunctive therapy in
Leukine (Sargramostim) Bayer HealthCare Pharmaceuticals 774

Hodgkin's disease, stages III and IV, palliative treatment of
Mustargen for Injection (Mechlorethamine Hydrochloride) Ovation 2492

Horton's headache
(*see under* Cephalalgia, histaminic)

Human papillomavirus vaccine
Gardasil Injection (Quadrivalent Human Papillomavirus (Types 6, 11, 16, 18) Recombinant Vaccine) Merck 2019

Hydatid disease, cystic
Albenza Tablets (Albendazole) GlaxoSmithKline 1297

Hyperacidity, gastric
Maximum Strength Zantac 150 Tablets (Ranitidine Hydrochloride) Boehringer Ingelheim .... ■603
Maximum Strength Zantac 150 Cool Mint Tablets (Ranitidine Hydrochloride) Boehringer Ingelheim .... ■603

Hyperacidity, gastric, symptomatic relief of
Axid Capsules (Nizatidine) GlaxoSmithKline 1364
Nexium Delayed-Release Capsules (Esomeprazole Magnesium) AstraZeneca LP 645
Nexium Delayed-Release Oral Suspension (Esomeprazole Magnesium) AstraZeneca LP 645
Original Strength Pepcid AC Gelcaps (Famotidine) J&J – Merck 1771
Original Strength Pepcid AC Tablets (Famotidine) J&J – Merck 1771
Maximum Strength Pepcid AC Tablets (Famotidine) J&J – Merck 1771
Pepcid Complete Chewable Tablets (Calcium Carbonate, Famotidine, Magnesium Hydroxide) J&J – Merck 1771
Pepto-Bismol Original Liquid, Original and Cherry Chewable Tablets & Caplets (Bismuth Subsalicylate) Procter & Gamble .... ■613
Pepto-Bismol Maximum Strength Liquid (Bismuth Subsalicylate) Procter & Gamble .... ■613
Prilosec OTC Tablets (Omeprazole Magnesium) Procter & Gamble 2565
Extra Strength Rolaids Plus Gas Relief Tropical Fruit Softchews (Calcium Carbonate, Simethicone) McNeil Consumer 1903
Extra Strength Rolaids Softchews Vanilla Creme (Calcium Carbonate) McNeil Consumer 1903
Extra Strength Rolaids Freshmint Tablets (Calcium Carbonate, Magnesium Hydroxide) McNeil Consumer 1903
Rolaids Multi-Symptom Berry Tablets (Calcium Carbonate, Magnesium Hydroxide, Simethicone) McNeil Consumer 1903
Rolaids Original Peppermint Tablets (Calcium Carbonate, Magnesium Hydroxide) McNeil Consumer 1903
Zantac 75 Tablets (Ranitidine Hydrochloride) Boehringer Ingelheim .... ■603

Hyperbetalipoproteinemia
(*see under* Hyperlipoproteinemia, types IIa and IIb, adjunct to diet)

Hyperbilirubinemia, neonatal
Albutein 25% (Albumin (human)) Grifols 1708
Human Albumin Grifols 25% (Albumin (human)) Grifols 1706

Hypercalcemia associated with cancer
Sensipar Tablets (Cinacalcet Hydrochloride) Amgen 594
Zometa for Intravenous Infusion (Zoledronic acid) Novartis 2341

Hypercalcemic emergencies, adjunct in
Miacalcin Injection (Calcitonin-Salmon) Novartis 2273

Hypercapnia, acute, with COPD
(*see under* Respiratory insufficiency, acute, with chronic obstructive pulmonary disease)

Hypercholesterolemia
Niaspan Extended-Release Tablets (Niacin) Abbott 480
Simcor Tablets (Niacin, Simvastatin) Abbott 502
Zetia Tablets (Ezetimibe) Merck/Schering Plough 2157

Hypercholesterolemia, homozygous, familial, adjunct to other agents
Crestor Tablets (Rosuvastatin Calcium) AstraZeneca Pharmaceuticals 677
Vytorin 10/10 Tablets (Ezetimibe, Simvastatin) Merck/Schering Plough 2149
Vytorin 10/10 Tablets (Ezetimibe, Simvastatin) Schering 2939
Vytorin 10/20 Tablets (Ezetimibe, Simvastatin) Merck/Schering Plough 2149
Vytorin 10/20 Tablets (Ezetimibe, Simvastatin) Schering 2939
Vytorin 10/40 Tablets (Ezetimibe, Simvastatin) Merck/Schering Plough 2149
Vytorin 10/40 Tablets (Ezetimibe, Simvastatin) Schering 2939
Vytorin 10/80 Tablets (Ezetimibe, Simvastatin) Merck/Schering Plough 2149
Vytorin 10/80 Tablets (Ezetimibe, Simvastatin) Schering 2939
Zetia Tablets (Ezetimibe) Merck/Schering Plough 2157
Zetia Tablets (Ezetimibe) Schering 2951

Hypercholesterolemia, primary, adjunct to diet
Advicor Tablets (Lovastatin, Niacin) Abbott 402
Crestor Tablets (Rosuvastatin Calcium) AstraZeneca Pharmaceuticals 677
Lescol Capsules (Fluvastatin Sodium) Novartis 2268
Lescol XL Tablets (Fluvastatin Sodium) Novartis 2268
Lipitor Tablets (Atorvastatin Calcium) Parke-Davis 2501
Mevacor Tablets (Lovastatin) Merck 2063
Niaspan Extended-Release Tablets (Niacin) Abbott 480
Simcor Tablets (Niacin, Simvastatin) Abbott 502
Tricor Tablets (Fenofibrate) Abbott 520
Vytorin 10/10 Tablets (Ezetimibe, Simvastatin) Merck/Schering Plough 2149
Vytorin 10/10 Tablets (Ezetimibe, Simvastatin) Schering 2939
Vytorin 10/20 Tablets (Ezetimibe, Simvastatin) Merck/Schering Plough 2149
Vytorin 10/20 Tablets (Ezetimibe, Simvastatin) Schering 2939
Vytorin 10/40 Tablets (Ezetimibe, Simvastatin) Merck/Schering Plough 2149
Vytorin 10/40 Tablets (Ezetimibe, Simvastatin) Schering 2939
Vytorin 10/80 Tablets (Ezetimibe, Simvastatin) Merck/Schering Plough 2149
Vytorin 10/80 Tablets (Ezetimibe, Simvastatin) Schering 2939
WelChol Tablets (Colesevelam Hydrochloride) Daiichi Sankyo 1015
Zetia Tablets (Ezetimibe) Merck/Schering Plough 2157
Zetia Tablets (Ezetimibe) Schering 2951
Zocor Tablets (Simvastatin) Merck 2136

Hypereosinophilic syndrome
Gleevec Tablets (Imatinib Mesylate) Novartis 2255

Hyperglycemia, control of, adjunct to diet
(*see also under* Diabetes mellitus, insulin-dependent; Diabetes mellitus, non-insulin-dependent)
ActoPlus Met Tablets (Metformin Hydrochloride, Pioglitazone Hydrochloride) Takeda 3071
Actos Tablets (Pioglitazone Hydrochloride) Takeda 3077
Apidra Injection (Insulin Glulisine) sanofi-aventis 2706
Avandamet Tablets (Rosiglitazone Maleate, Metformin Hydrochloride) GlaxoSmithKline 1336
Avandaryl Tablets (Rosiglitazone Maleate, Glimepiride) GlaxoSmithKline 1344
Avandia Tablets (Rosiglitazone Maleate) GlaxoSmithKline 1351

Byetta Injection (Exenatide) Amylin ... 600
Exubera Inhalation Powder (Insulin, Human (rDNA origin)) Pfizer 2515
Janumet Tablets (Sitagliptin Phosphate, Metformin Hydrochloride) Merck 2041
Januvia Tablets (Sitagliptin Phosphate) Merck 2048
Precose Tablets (Acarbose) Bayer HealthCare Pharmaceuticals.......... 792

Hyperhidrosis
BOTOX Purified Neurotoxin Complex (Botulinum Toxin Type A) Allergan 550
Formadon Solution (Formaldehyde) Gordon 1699

Hyperlipidemia
Crestor Tablets (Rosuvastatin Calcium) AstraZeneca Pharmaceuticals 677
Zetia Tablets (Ezetimibe) Schering.... 2951

Hyperlipidemia, adjunct to diet
Fenoglide Tablets (Fenofibrate) Sciele 2960

Hyperlipoproteinemia, type III, adjunct to diet
Zocor Tablets (Simvastatin) Merck ... 2136

Hyperlipoproteinemia, types IIa and IIb, adjunct to diet
Advicor Tablets (Lovastatin, Niacin) Abbott 402
Crestor Tablets (Rosuvastatin Calcium) AstraZeneca Pharmaceuticals 677
Lescol Capsules (Fluvastatin Sodium) Novartis 2268
Lescol XL Tablets (Fluvastatin Sodium) Novartis 2268
Lipitor Tablets (Atorvastatin Calcium) Parke-Davis 2501
Mevacor Tablets (Lovastatin) Merck . 2063
Niaspan Extended-Release Tablets (Niacin) Abbott 480
Zocor Tablets (Simvastatin) Merck ... 2136

Hyperlipoproteinemia, types IV and V, adjunct to diet
Advicor Tablets (Lovastatin, Niacin) Abbott 402
Niaspan Extended-Release Tablets (Niacin) Abbott 480
Tricor Tablets (Fenofibrate) Abbott ... 520

Hyperparathyroidism, secondary
Rocaltrol Capsules (Calcitriol) Fontus 1150
Rocaltrol Oral Solution (Calcitriol) Fontus 1150
Sensipar Tablets (Cinacalcet Hydrochloride) Amgen 594
Zemplar Capsules (Paricalcitol) Abbott 536
Zemplar Injection (Paricalcitol) Abbott 538

Hyperphosphatemia
Fosrenol Chewable Tablets (Lanthanum Carbonate) Shire US 3027
PhosLo GelCaps (Calcium Acetate) Fresenius 1184

Hyperpigmentation, skin, bleaching of
Pure Gardens Cream (Herbals with Vitamins) Awareness Corporation/Awareness Life .... ▣ 624

Hypersecretory conditions, pathological
Aciphex Tablets (Rabeprazole Sodium) Eisai 1053
Nexium Delayed-Release Capsules (Esomeprazole Magnesium) AstraZeneca LP 645
Nexium Delayed-Release Oral Suspension (Esomeprazole Magnesium) AstraZeneca LP 645
Pepcid Tablets (Famotidine) Merck ... 2075
Protonix for Delayed-Release Oral Suspension (Pantoprazole Sodium) Wyeth 3254
Protonix Delayed-Release Tablets (Pantoprazole Sodium) Wyeth 3254
Protonix I.V. (Pantoprazole Sodium) Wyeth 3257

Zantac 25 EFFERdose Tablets (Ranitidine Hydrochloride) GlaxoSmithKline 1670
Zantac Injection (Ranitidine Hydrochloride) GlaxoSmithKline 1666
Zantac Injection Pharmacy Bulk Package (Ranitidine Hydrochloride) GlaxoSmithKline 1668
Zantac Injection Premixed (Ranitidine Hydrochloride) GlaxoSmithKline 1666
Zantac (Ranitidine Hydrochloride) GlaxoSmithKline 1670

Hypersensitivity reactions, drug-induced
EpiPen (Epinephrine) Dey 1024

Hypertension
Aceon Tablets (2 mg, 4 mg, 8 mg) (Perindopril Erbumine) Solvay........ 3038
Atacand Tablets (Candesartan Cilexetil) AstraZeneca LP 639
Atacand HCT (Hydrochlorothiazide, Candesartan Cilexetil) AstraZeneca LP 642
Avalide Tablets (Irbesartan, Hydrochlorothiazide) Bristol-Myers Squibb 892
Avalide Tablets (Irbesartan, Hydrochlorothiazide) sanofi-aventis........ 2713
Avapro Tablets (Irbesartan) Bristol-Myers Squibb 897
Avapro Tablets (Irbesartan) sanofi-aventis 2718
Azor Tablets (Olmesartan Medoxomil, Amlodipine Besylate) Daiichi Sankyo 1005
Benicar Tablets (Olmesartan Medoxomil) Daiichi Sankyo........ 1009
Benicar HCT Tablets (Olmesartan Medoxomil, Hydrochlorothiazide) Daiichi Sankyo 1010
Bystolic Tablets (Nebivolol) Forest.... 1155
Captopril Tablets (Captopril) Mylan ... 2182
Cardene I.V. (Nicardipine Hydrochloride) EKR........ 1093
Cardizem LA Extended Release Tablets (Diltiazem Hydrochloride) Abbott 421
Catapres Tablets (Clonidine Hydrochloride) Boehringer Ingelheim 841
Catapres-TTS (Clonidine) Boehringer Ingelheim 842
Cleviprex (Clevidipine Butyrate) The Medicines Company........ 1936
Clorpres Tablets (Chlorthalidone, Clonidine Hydrochloride) Mylan...... 2185
Coreg Tablets (Carvedilol) GlaxoSmithKline 1387
Coreg CR Extended-Release Capsules (Carvedilol Phosphate) GlaxoSmithKline 1393
Cozaar Tablets (Losartan Potassium) Merck 1973
Demadex Injection (Torsemide) Roche 2630
Demadex Tablets (Torsemide) Roche 2630
Diovan Tablets (Valsartan) Novartis .. 2212
Diovan HCT Tablets (Hydrochlorothiazide, Valsartan) Novartis........ 2216
Dyazide Capsules (Hydrochlorothiazide, Triamterene) GlaxoSmithKline 1405
DynaCirc CR Controlled Release Tablets (Isradipine) GlaxoSmithKline 1407
Exforge Tablets (Amlodipine Besylate, Valsartan) Novartis........ 2238
Furosemide Tablets (Furosemide) Mylan 2186
Indapamide Tablets (Indapamide) Mylan 2188
InnoPran XL Extended Release Capsules (Propranolol Hydrochloride) GlaxoSmithKline 1484
Mavik Tablets (Trandolapril) Abbott ... 472
Micardis Tablets (Telmisartan) Boehringer Ingelheim 852
Micardis HCT Tablets (Hydrochlorothiazide, Telmisartan) Boehringer Ingelheim 854
Nadolol Tablets (Nadolol) Mylan........ 2191
Prinivil Tablets (Lisinopril) Merck....... 2087
Prinzide Tablets (Hydrochlorothiazide, Lisinopril) Merck........ 2092
Sular Extended Release Tablets (Nisoldipine) Sciele........ 2975
Tarka Tablets (Trandolapril, Verapamil Hydrochloride) Abbott........ 511

Tekturna Tablets (Aliskiren) Novartis 2321
Tekturna HCT Tablets (Aliskiren, Hydrochlorothiazide) Novartis........ 2324
Teveten Tablets (Eprosartan Mesylate) Abbott 515
Teveten HCT Tablets (Eprosartan Mesylate, Hydrochlorothiazide) Abbott 517
Toprol-XL Tablets (Metoprolol Succinate) AstraZeneca LP 666

Hypertension, adjunctive treatment
Micardis Tablets (Telmisartan) Boehringer Ingelheim 852

Hypertension, essential
(*see under* Hypertension)

Hypertension, ocular
(*see also under* Glaucoma, chronic open-angle)
Alphagan P Ophthalmic Solution (Brimonidine Tartrate) Allergan 549
Azopt Ophthalmic Suspension (Brinzolamide) Alcon 540
Betimol Ophthalmic Solution (Timolol Hemihydrate) Vistakon 3181
Combigan Ophthalmic Solution (Brimonidine Tartrate, Timolol Maleate) Allergan 553
Cosopt Sterile Ophthalmic Solution (Dorzolamide Hydrochloride, Timolol Maleate) Merck 1969
Lumigan Ophthalmic Solution (Bimatoprost) Allergan 556
OptiPranolol Metipranolol Ophthalmic Solution 0.3% (Metipranolol) Bausch & Lomb ..... ⊙ 245
Timoptic Sterile Ophthalmic Solution (Timolol Maleate) Merck ... 2121
Timoptic in Ocudose (Timolol Maleate) Merck 2124
Timoptic-XE Sterile Ophthalmic Gel Forming Solution (Timolol Maleate) Merck 2125
Travatan Z Ophthalmic Solution (Travoprost) Alcon 547
Trusopt Sterile Ophthalmic Solution (Dorzolamide Hydrochloride) Merck 2128
Xalatan Ophthalmic Solution (Latanoprost) Pharmacia & Upjohn .... ⊙ 273

Hypertension, pulmonary
Flolan for Injection (Epoprostenol Sodium) GlaxoSmithKline 1426
Tracleer Tablets (Bosentan) Actelion 3289

Hypertension, pulmonary arterial
Letairis Tablets (Ambrisentan) Gilead 1258

Hypertensive crises
(*see under* Hypertension)

Hypertensive episodes, control of, in pheochromocytoma
Dibenzyline Capsules (Phenoxybenzamine Hydrochloride) WellSpring . 3188

Hyperthermia, malignant, prophylaxis
Dantrium Capsules (Dantrolene Sodium) Procter & Gamble Pharmaceuticals 2580
Dantrium Intravenous (Dantrolene Sodium) Procter & Gamble Pharmaceuticals 2582

Hyperthermia, malignant, treatment adjunct
Dantrium Intravenous (Dantrolene Sodium) Procter & Gamble Pharmaceuticals 2582

Hypertriglyceridemia, adjunct to diet
(*see also under* Dysbetalipoproteinemia)
Crestor Tablets (Rosuvastatin Calcium) AstraZeneca Pharmaceuticals 677
Fenoglide Tablets (Fenofibrate) Sciele 2960
Lescol Capsules (Fluvastatin Sodium) Novartis 2268

Lescol XL Tablets (Fluvastatin Sodium) Novartis........ 2268
Lipitor Tablets (Atorvastatin Calcium) Parke-Davis 2501
Lovaza Capsules (Omega-3-acid ethyl esters) GlaxoSmithKline 1520
Simcor Tablets (Niacin, Simvastatin) Abbott 502
Tricor Tablets (Fenofibrate) Abbott.... 520
Zocor Tablets (Simvastatin) Merck.... 2136

Hypertriglyceridemia, primary, adjunct to diet
Advicor Tablets (Lovastatin, Niacin) Abbott 402
Simcor Tablets (Niacin, Simvastatin) Abbott 502

Hyperuricemia
Elitek (Rasburicase) sanofi-aventis 2729

Hypnotic
(*see under* Sleep, induction of)

Hypoalbuminemia
Albutein 5% (Albumin (human)) Grifols 1707
Flexbumin 25% I.V. (Albumin (human)) Baxter Healthcare 729

Hypocalcemia
Rocaltrol Capsules (Calcitriol) Fontus 1150
Rocaltrol Oral Solution (Calcitriol) Fontus 1150

Hypocalcemia associated with chronic renal failure
Calcijex Injection (Calcitriol) Abbott... 419
Rocaltrol Capsules (Calcitriol) Fontus 1150
Rocaltrol Oral Solution (Calcitriol) Fontus 1150

Hypocalcemia associated with idiopathic hypoparathyroidism
Rocaltrol Capsules (Calcitriol) Fontus 1150
Rocaltrol Oral Solution (Calcitriol) Fontus 1150

Hypocalcemia associated with postsurgical hypoparathyroidism
Rocaltrol Capsules (Calcitriol) Fontus 1150
Rocaltrol Oral Solution (Calcitriol) Fontus 1150

Hypocalcemia associated with pseudohypoparathyroidism
Rocaltrol Capsules (Calcitriol) Fontus 1150
Rocaltrol Oral Solution (Calcitriol) Fontus 1150

Hypoestrogenism
Climara Transdermal System (Estradiol) Bayer HealthCare Pharmaceuticals 763
Premarin Intravenous (Estrogens, Conjugated) Wyeth........ 3217
Premarin Tablets (Estrogens, Conjugated) Wyeth........ 3221

Hypoglycemia
Glucagon for Injection Vials and Emergency Kit (Glucagon) Lilly...... 1827

Hypoglycemia, hyperinsulinemic
Proglycem Capsules (Diazoxide) Gate 1185
Proglycem Suspension (Diazoxide) Gate 1185

Hypogonadism, hypogonadotropic, in males
AndroGel (Testosterone) Unimed 3159
Delatestryl Injection (Testosterone Enanthate) Indevus........ 1730
Testim 1% Gel (Testosterone) Auxilium 701

Hypogonadism, male, primary
AndroGel (Testosterone) Unimed 3159
Testim 1% Gel (Testosterone) Auxilium 701

Hypogonadism, male, secondary to pituitary failure
AndroGel (Testosterone) Unimed 3159

Hyponatremia, euvolemic
Vaprisol (Conivaptan Hydrochloride) Astellas ... 632

Hypophosphatemia
K-Phos Neutral Tablets (Potassium Phosphate, Sodium Phosphate) Beach ... 813

Hypoprothrombinemia, drug-induced
Mephyton Tablets (Vitamin K_1) Aton.. 700

Hypoprothrombinemia, salicylate-induced
Mephyton Tablets (Vitamin K_1) Aton.. 700

Hypoprothrombinemia, secondary factors-induced
Mephyton Tablets (Vitamin K_1) Aton.. 700

Hypotension, orthostatic
ProAmatine Tablets (Midodrine Hydrochloride) Shire US ... 3032

Hypothyroidism, ordinary
(*see under* Hypothyroidism, replacement or supplemental therapy in)

Hypothyroidism, primary
(*see under* Hypothyroidism, replacement or supplemental therapy in)

Hypothyroidism, replacement or supplemental therapy in
Cytomel Tablets (Liothyronine Sodium) King ... 1778
Levothroid Tablets (Levothyroxine Sodium) Forest ... 1170
Levoxyl Tablets (Levothyroxine Sodium) King ... 1780
Naturethroid Tablets (Levothyroxine, Liothyronine, Thyroid) RLC ... 2605
Synthroid Tablets (Levothyroxine Sodium) Abbott ... 507

Hypothyroidism, secondary
(*see under* Hypothyroidism, replacement or supplemental therapy in)

Hypothyroidism, tertiary
(*see under* Hypothyroidism, replacement or supplemental therapy in)

Hypovolemia
Flexbumin 25% I.V. (Albumin (human)) Baxter Healthcare ... 729

Hypovolemic shock
Albutein 5% (Albumin (human)) Grifols ... 1707
Albutein 25% (Albumin (human)) Grifols ... 1708
Human Albumin Grifols 25% (Albumin (human)) Grifols ... 1706

I

Idiopathic thrombocytopenic purpura
(*see under* Purpura, idiopathic thrombocytopenic)

Immunization, diphtheria, tetanus, pertussis, and haemophilus influenzae type B
Pentacel (Diphtheria and Tetanus Toxoids and Acellular Pertussis Adsorbed, Inactivated Poliovirus and Haemophilus b Conjugate (Tetanus Toxoid Conjugate) Vaccine) Sanofi Pasteur ... 2792

Immunization, diphtheria, tetanus and pertussis
Boostrix (Diphtheria & Tetanus Toxoids and Acellular Pertussis Vaccine Adsorbed) GlaxoSmithKline ... 1377
Infanrix Vaccine (Diphtheria & Tetanus Toxoids and Acellular Pertussis Vaccine Adsorbed) GlaxoSmithKline ... 1479
Kinrix Injection Vaccine (Diphtheria and Tetanus Toxoids and Acellular Pertussis Adsorbed and Inactivated Poliovirus Vaccine) GlaxoSmithKline ... 1486
Pediarix Vaccine (Diphtheria & Tetanus Toxoids and Acellular Pertussis Vaccine Adsorbed, Hepatitis B Vaccine, Recombinant, Poliovirus Vaccine Inactivated) GlaxoSmithKline ... 1552

Immunization, haemophilus influenzae type b
Liquid PedvaxHIB (Haemophilus B Conjugate Vaccine) Merck ... 2073

Immunization, haemophilus influenzae type B and hepatitis B virus
Comvax (Haemophilus B Conjugate Vaccine, Hepatitis B Vaccine, Recombinant) Merck ... 1966

Immunization, hepatitis A and B virus
Twinrix Vaccine (Hepatitis A Vaccine, Inactivated, Hepatitis B Vaccine, Recombinant) GlaxoSmithKline ... 1628

Immunization, hepatitis A virus
Havrix Injection Vaccine (Hepatitis A Vaccine, Inactivated) GlaxoSmithKline ... 1454
Vaqta (Hepatitis A Vaccine, Inactivated) Merck ... 2130

Immunization, hepatitis B virus
Engerix-B Vaccine (Hepatitis B Vaccine, Recombinant) GlaxoSmithKline ... 1409
Pediarix Vaccine (Diphtheria & Tetanus Toxoids and Acellular Pertussis Vaccine Adsorbed, Hepatitis B Vaccine, Recombinant, Poliovirus Vaccine Inactivated) GlaxoSmithKline ... 1552
Recombivax HB (Hepatitis B Vaccine, Recombinant) Merck ... 2107

Immunization, human papillomavirus
Gardasil Injection (Quadrivalent Human Papillomavirus (Types 6, 11, 16, 18) Recombinant Vaccine) Merck ... 2019

Immunization, influenza virus, types A and B
Fluarix Vaccine (Influenza Virus Vaccine) GlaxoSmithKline ... 1446
Flulaval Injection Vaccine (Influenza Virus Vaccine) GlaxoSmithKline ... 1448
FluMist Vaccine (Influenza Virus Vaccine Live, Intranasal) MedImmune ... 1945

Immunization, pneumococcal disease
(*see also under* Pneumococcal disease, immunization against)
Pneumovax 23 (Pneumococcal Vaccine, Polyvalent) Merck ... 2078
Prevnar (Pneumococcal vaccine, diphtheria conjugate) Wyeth ... 3241

Immunization, poliovirus 1, 2, and 3
Kinrix Injection Vaccine (Diphtheria and Tetanus Toxoids and Acellular Pertussis Adsorbed and Inactivated Poliovirus Vaccine) GlaxoSmithKline ... 1486
Pediarix Vaccine (Diphtheria & Tetanus Toxoids and Acellular Pertussis Vaccine Adsorbed, Hepatitis B Vaccine, Recombinant, Poliovirus Vaccine Inactivated) GlaxoSmithKline ... 1552
Pentacel (Diphtheria and Tetanus Toxoids and Acellular Pertussis Adsorbed, Inactivated Poliovirus and Haemophilus b Conjugate (Tetanus Toxoid Conjugate) Vaccine) Sanofi Pasteur ... 2792

Immunization, varicella
Varivax (Varicella Virus Vaccine Live) Merck ... 2133

Immunodeficiencies
Flebogamma 5% DIF (Immune Globulin Intravenous (Human)) Grifols ... 1718
Gammagard Liquid (Immune Globulin Intravenous (Human)) Baxter Healthcare ... 730
Gammagard S/D (Immune Globulin Intravenous (Human)) Baxter Healthcare ... 734
Gamunex (Immune Globulin Intravenous (Human)) Talecris ... 3094

Immunodeficiency, common variable
Flebogamma 5% (Globulin, Immune (Human)) Grifols ... 1715
Flebogamma 5% DIF (Immune Globulin Intravenous (Human)) Grifols ... 1718
Gammagard S/D (Immune Globulin Intravenous (Human)) Baxter Healthcare ... 734
Gamunex (Immune Globulin Intravenous (Human)) Talecris ... 3094

Immunodeficiency disease, severe combined
(*see under* Adenosine deaminase, enzyme replacement therapy for)

Impetigo contagiosa
Altabax Ointment (Retapamulin) GlaxoSmithKline ... 1299
Bactroban Ointment (Mupirocin) GlaxoSmithKline ... 1368
Ceftin for Oral Suspension (Cefuroxime Axetil) GlaxoSmithKline ... 1380
Levaquin (Levofloxacin) Ortho-McNeil ... 2416
Levaquin in 5% Dextrose Injection (Levofloxacin) Ortho-McNeil ... 2416

Impotence, male
(*see under* Erectile dysfunction)

Indigestion
(*see under* Digestive disorders, symptomatic relief of)

Infection, pleural space
Cancidas for Injection (Caspofungin acetate) Merck ... 1953

Infections, acquired immunodeficiency syndrome-related complex
AmBisome for Injection (Amphotericin B, liposomal) Astellas ... 606
Biaxin/Biaxin XL (Clarithromycin) Abbott ... 411
Intron A for Injection (Interferon alfa-2b, Recombinant) Schering ... 2859
Marinol Capsules (Dronabinol) Unimed ... 3163
Retrovir IV Infusion (Zidovudine) GlaxoSmithKline ... 1579
Valcyte Tablets (Valganciclovir Hydrochloride) Roche ... 2654
WinRho SDF (Rh_o (D) Immune Globulin (Human)) Baxter Healthcare ... 741

Infections, aerobic organisms
Fortaz (Ceftazidime) GlaxoSmithKline ... 1450

Infections, anaerobic organisms
Fortaz (Ceftazidime) GlaxoSmithKline ... 1450
Primaxin I.V. (Cilastatin Sodium, Imipenem) Merck ... 2083

Infections, bacterial, various types
Merrem I.V. (Meropenem) AstraZeneca Pharmaceuticals ... 684

Infections, beta-lactamase producing organisms
Augmentin (Amoxicillin, Clavulanate Potassium) GlaxoSmithKline ... 1323
Augmentin Tablets (Amoxicillin, Clavulanate Potassium) GlaxoSmithKline ... 1327
Augmentin XR Extended Release Tablets (Amoxicillin, Clavulanate Potassium) GlaxoSmithKline ... 1333
Ceftin (Cefuroxime Axetil) GlaxoSmithKline ... 1380
Merrem I.V. (Meropenem) AstraZeneca Pharmaceuticals ... 684
Suprax for Oral Suspension (Cefixime) Lupin ... 1891
Suprax Tablets (Cefixime) Lupin ... 1891
Zosyn for Injection (Piperacillin Sodium, Tazobactam Sodium) Wyeth ... 3284

Infections, bone and joint
Cipro I.V. (Ciprofloxacin) Schering ... 2817
Cipro (Ciprofloxacin) Schering ... 2810
Fortaz (Ceftazidime) GlaxoSmithKline ... 1450
Primaxin I.V. (Cilastatin Sodium, Imipenem) Merck ... 2083
Rocephin Injectable Vials, ADD-Vantage, Galaxy, Bulk (Ceftriaxone Sodium) Roche ... 2642
Timentin ADD-Vantage (Clavulanate Potassium, Ticarcillin Disodium) GlaxoSmithKline ... 1606
Timentin Injection Galaxy Container (Clavulanate Potassium, Ticarcillin Disodium) GlaxoSmithKline ... 1609
Timentin IV Infusion (Clavulanate Potassium, Ticarcillin Disodium) GlaxoSmithKline ... 1603
Timentin Pharmacy Bulk Package (Clavulanate Potassium, Ticarcillin Disodium) GlaxoSmithKline ... 1613
Zinacef for Injection (Cefuroxime) GlaxoSmithKline ... 1678
Zinacef Injection (Cefuroxime) GlaxoSmithKline ... 1678

Infections, burn wound
(*see also under* Infections, skin, bacterial, minor)
Sulfamylon Cream (Mafenide Acetate) Mylan ... 2194

Infections, central nervous system
Fortaz (Ceftazidime) GlaxoSmithKline ... 1450

Infections, diabetic foot
Zosyn for Injection (Piperacillin Sodium, Tazobactam Sodium) Wyeth ... 3284
Zyvox (Linezolid) Pharmacia & Upjohn ... 2552

Infections, ear, nose and throat
Amoxil Capsules (Amoxicillin) GlaxoSmithKline ... 1305
Amoxil Chewable Tablets (Amoxicillin) GlaxoSmithKline ... 1305
Amoxil Pediatric Drops for Oral Suspension (Amoxicillin) GlaxoSmithKline ... 1305
Amoxil Powder for Oral Suspension (Amoxicillin) GlaxoSmithKline ... 1305
Amoxil Tablets (Amoxicillin) GlaxoSmithKline ... 1305

Infections, fungal, empirical therapy for febrile, neutropenic patients
Cancidas for Injection (Caspofungin acetate) Merck ... 1953

Infections, fungal, systemic
Abelcet Injection (Amphotericin B Lipid Complex) Enzon ... 1134

Infections, genitourinary tract
Amoxil Capsules (Amoxicillin) GlaxoSmithKline ... 1305
Amoxil Chewable Tablets (Amoxicillin) GlaxoSmithKline ... 1305
Amoxil Pediatric Drops for Oral Suspension (Amoxicillin) GlaxoSmithKline ... 1305
Amoxil Powder for Oral Suspension (Amoxicillin) GlaxoSmithKline ... 1305
Amoxil Tablets (Amoxicillin) GlaxoSmithKline ... 1305

Infections, gram-negative bacteria
Primaxin I.V. (Cilastatin Sodium, Imipenem) Merck ... 2083
Seromycin Capsules (Cycloserine) Lilly ... 1864
Suprax for Oral Suspension (Cefixime) Lupin ... 1891
Suprax Tablets (Cefixime) Lupin ... 1891

Infections, gram-positive bacteria
Primaxin I.V. (Cilastatin Sodium, Imipenem) Merck 2083
Seromycin Capsules (Cycloserine) Lilly 1864
Suprax for Oral Suspension (Cefixime) Lupin 1891
Suprax Tablets (Cefixime) Lupin........ 1891

Infections, gynecologic
Fortaz (Ceftazidime) GlaxoSmithKline 1450
Primaxin I.M. (Cilastatin Sodium, Imipenem) Merck 2080
Primaxin I.V. (Cilastatin Sodium, Imipenem) Merck 2083
Timentin ADD-Vantage (Clavulanate Potassium, Ticarcillin Disodium) GlaxoSmithKline 1606
Timentin Injection Galaxy Container (Clavulanate Potassium, Ticarcillin Disodium) GlaxoSmithKline 1609
Timentin IV Infusion (Clavulanate Potassium, Ticarcillin Disodium) GlaxoSmithKline 1603
Timentin Pharmacy Bulk Package (Clavulanate Potassium, Ticarcillin Disodium) GlaxoSmithKline 1613
Zosyn for Injection (Piperacillin Sodium, Tazobactam Sodium) Wyeth 3284

Infections, human immunodeficiency virus
Atripla Tablets (Tenofovir Disoproxil Fumarate, Efavirenz, Emtricitabine) Bristol-Myers Squibb & Gilead Sciences 938
Combivir Tablets (Lamivudine, Zidovudine) GlaxoSmithKline 1384
Crixivan Capsules (Indinavir Sulfate) Merck 1979
Emtriva Capsules (Emtricitabine) Gilead 1246
Emtriva Oral Solution (Emtricitabine) Gilead 1246
Epivir (Lamivudine) GlaxoSmithKline . 1412
Epzicom Tablets (Lamivudine, Abacavir Sulfate) GlaxoSmithKline 1422
Intelence Tablets (Etravirine) Tibotec 3119
Isentress Tablets (Raltegravir) Merck 2036
Kaletra (Lopinavir, Ritonavir) Abbott .. 452
Lexiva Oral Suspension (Fosamprenavir Calcium) GlaxoSmithKline 1510
Lexiva Tablets (Fosamprenavir Calcium) GlaxoSmithKline 1510
Retrovir Capsules (Zidovudine) GlaxoSmithKline 1574
Retrovir IV Infusion (Zidovudine) GlaxoSmithKline 1579
Retrovir (Zidovudine) GlaxoSmithKline 1574
Reyataz Capsules (Atazanavir Sulfate) Bristol-Myers Squibb 3299
Selzentry Tablets (Maraviroc) Pfizer . 2534
Sustiva Capsules (Efavirenz) Bristol-Myers Squibb 930
Sustiva Tablets (Efavirenz) Bristol-Myers Squibb 930
Trizivir Tablets (Lamivudine, Abacavir Sulfate, Zidovudine) GlaxoSmithKline 1622
Truvada Tablets (Tenofovir Disoproxil Fumarate, Emtricitabine) Gilead 1262
Viramune Oral Suspension (Nevirapine) Boehringer Ingelheim 873
Viramune Tablets (Nevirapine) Boehringer Ingelheim 873
Viread Tablets (Tenofovir Disoproxil Fumarate) Gilead 1268
Ziagen (Abacavir Sulfate) GlaxoSmithKline 1673

Infections, human immunodeficiency virus, adjunct
Norvir (Ritonavir) Abbott 489

Infections, human immunodeficiency virus, in combination with ritonavir
Aptivus Capsules (Tipranavir) Boehringer Ingelheim 823
Aptivus Oral Solution (Tipranavir) Boehringer Ingelheim 823

Infections, intra-abdominal
Avelox (Moxifloxacin Hydrochloride) Schering 2803
Cipro I.V. (Ciprofloxacin) Schering 2817
Cipro (Ciprofloxacin) Schering 2810
Doribax Injection (Doripenem) Ortho-McNeil 2400
Fortaz (Ceftazidime) GlaxoSmithKline 1450
Invanz for Injection (Ertapenem) Merck 2029
Merrem I.V. (Meropenem) AstraZeneca Pharmaceuticals 684
Primaxin I.M. (Cilastatin Sodium, Imipenem) Merck 2080
Primaxin I.V. (Cilastatin Sodium, Imipenem) Merck 2083
Rocephin Injectable Vials, ADD-Vantage, Galaxy, Bulk (Ceftriaxone Sodium) Roche 2642
Timentin ADD-Vantage (Clavulanate Potassium, Ticarcillin Disodium) GlaxoSmithKline 1606
Timentin Injection Galaxy Container (Clavulanate Potassium, Ticarcillin Disodium) GlaxoSmithKline 1609
Timentin IV Infusion (Clavulanate Potassium, Ticarcillin Disodium) GlaxoSmithKline 1603
Timentin Pharmacy Bulk Package (Clavulanate Potassium, Ticarcillin Disodium) GlaxoSmithKline 1613

Infections, lower respiratory tract
Amoxil Capsules (Amoxicillin) GlaxoSmithKline 1305
Amoxil Chewable Tablets (Amoxicillin) GlaxoSmithKline 1305
Amoxil Pediatric Drops for Oral Suspension (Amoxicillin) GlaxoSmithKline 1305
Amoxil Powder for Oral Suspension (Amoxicillin) GlaxoSmithKline 1305
Amoxil Tablets (Amoxicillin) GlaxoSmithKline 1305
Augmentin (Amoxicillin, Clavulanate Potassium) GlaxoSmithKline 1323
Augmentin Tablets (Amoxicillin, Clavulanate Potassium) GlaxoSmithKline 1327
Augmentin XR Extended Release Tablets (Amoxicillin, Clavulanate Potassium) GlaxoSmithKline 1333
Avelox (Moxifloxacin Hydrochloride) Schering 2803
Biaxin/Biaxin XL (Clarithromycin) Abbott 411
Cipro I.V. (Ciprofloxacin) Schering 2817
Cipro (Ciprofloxacin) Schering 2810
E.E.S. (Erythromycin Ethylsuccinate) Abbott 433
EryPed (Erythromycin Ethylsuccinate) Abbott 431
Fortaz (Ceftazidime) GlaxoSmithKline 1450
Invanz for Injection (Ertapenem) Merck 2029
Levaquin (Levofloxacin) Ortho-McNeil 2416
Levaquin in 5% Dextrose Injection (Levofloxacin) Ortho-McNeil 2416
Omnicef Capsules (Cefdinir) Abbott .. 497
Omnicef for Oral Suspension (Cefdinir) Abbott 497
Primaxin I.M. (Cilastatin Sodium, Imipenem) Merck 2080
Primaxin I.V. (Cilastatin Sodium, Imipenem) Merck 2083
Rocephin Injectable Vials, ADD-Vantage, Galaxy, Bulk (Ceftriaxone Sodium) Roche 2642
Suprax for Oral Suspension (Cefixime) Lupin 1891
Suprax Tablets (Cefixime) Lupin 1891
Timentin ADD-Vantage (Clavulanate Potassium, Ticarcillin Disodium) GlaxoSmithKline 1606
Timentin Injection Galaxy Container (Clavulanate Potassium, Ticarcillin Disodium) GlaxoSmithKline 1609
Timentin IV Infusion (Clavulanate Potassium, Ticarcillin Disodium) GlaxoSmithKline 1603
Timentin Pharmacy Bulk Package (Clavulanate Potassium, Ticarcillin Disodium) GlaxoSmithKline 1613
Zinacef for Injection (Cefuroxime) GlaxoSmithKline 1678
Zinacef Injection (Cefuroxime) GlaxoSmithKline 1678
Zosyn for Injection (Piperacillin Sodium, Tazobactam Sodium) Wyeth 3284

Infections, lower respiratory tract, RSV-induced, prevention of
Synagis Intramuscular Solution (Palivizumab) MedImmune 1948

Infections, mycotic, cutaneous
Nystop Topical Powder USP (Nystatin) Paddock 2498

Infections, mycotic, mucocutaneous
Nystop Topical Powder USP (Nystatin) Paddock 2498

Infections, ocular, bacterial
Bleph-10 Ophthalmic Solution 10% (Sulfacetamide Sodium) Allergan .. ⊙215
Ofloxacin Ophthalmic Solution 0.3% (Ofloxacin) Bausch & Lomb .... ⊙243
Quixin Ophthalmic Solution (Levofloxacin) Vistakon 3184

Infections, perioperative, reduction of the incidence of
Rocephin Injectable Vials, ADD-Vantage, Galaxy, Bulk (Ceftriaxone Sodium) Roche 2642
Zinacef for Injection (Cefuroxime) GlaxoSmithKline 1678
Zinacef Injection (Cefuroxime) GlaxoSmithKline 1678

Infections, polymicrobic
Fortaz (Ceftazidime) GlaxoSmithKline 1450
Primaxin I.V. (Cilastatin Sodium, Imipenem) Merck 2083

Infections, respiratory tract, unspecified
E.E.S. (Erythromycin Ethylsuccinate) Abbott 433
EryPed (Erythromycin Ethylsuccinate) Abbott 431
Omnicef Capsules (Cefdinir) Abbott .. 497
Omnicef for Oral Suspension (Cefdinir) Abbott 497

Infections, skin, bacterial, minor
Bactroban Ointment (Mupirocin) GlaxoSmithKline 1368
Clorpactin WCS-90 (Sodium Oxychlorosene) Guardian 1722

Infections, skin and skin structure
Amoxil Capsules (Amoxicillin) GlaxoSmithKline 1305
Amoxil Chewable Tablets (Amoxicillin) GlaxoSmithKline 1305
Amoxil Pediatric Drops for Oral Suspension (Amoxicillin) GlaxoSmithKline 1305
Amoxil Powder for Oral Suspension (Amoxicillin) GlaxoSmithKline 1305
Amoxil Tablets (Amoxicillin) GlaxoSmithKline 1305
Augmentin (Amoxicillin, Clavulanate Potassium) GlaxoSmithKline 1323
Augmentin Tablets (Amoxicillin, Clavulanate Potassium) GlaxoSmithKline 1327
Avelox (Moxifloxacin Hydrochloride) Schering 2803
Bactroban Cream (Mupirocin Calcium) GlaxoSmithKline 1366
Biaxin/Biaxin XL (Clarithromycin) Abbott 411
Ceftin Tablets (Cefuroxime Axetil) GlaxoSmithKline 1380
Cipro I.V. (Ciprofloxacin) Schering 2817
Cipro (Ciprofloxacin) Schering 2810
E.E.S. (Erythromycin Ethylsuccinate) Abbott 433
EryPed (Erythromycin Ethylsuccinate) Abbott 431
Fortaz (Ceftazidime) GlaxoSmithKline 1450
Invanz for Injection (Ertapenem) Merck 2029
Levaquin (Levofloxacin) Ortho-McNeil 2416
Levaquin in 5% Dextrose Injection (Levofloxacin) Ortho-McNeil 2416
Merrem I.V. (Meropenem) AstraZeneca Pharmaceuticals 684
Omnicef Capsules (Cefdinir) Abbott .. 497
Omnicef for Oral Suspension (Cefdinir) Abbott 497
Primaxin I.M. (Cilastatin Sodium, Imipenem) Merck 2080
Primaxin I.V. (Cilastatin Sodium, Imipenem) Merck 2083
Rocephin Injectable Vials, ADD-Vantage, Galaxy, Bulk (Ceftriaxone Sodium) Roche 2642
Timentin ADD-Vantage (Clavulanate Potassium, Ticarcillin Disodium) GlaxoSmithKline 1606
Timentin Injection Galaxy Container (Clavulanate Potassium, Ticarcillin Disodium) GlaxoSmithKline 1609
Timentin IV Infusion (Clavulanate Potassium, Ticarcillin Disodium) GlaxoSmithKline 1603
Timentin Pharmacy Bulk Package (Clavulanate Potassium, Ticarcillin Disodium) GlaxoSmithKline 1613
Zinacef for Injection (Cefuroxime) GlaxoSmithKline 1678
Zinacef Injection (Cefuroxime) GlaxoSmithKline 1678
Zosyn for Injection (Piperacillin Sodium, Tazobactam Sodium) Wyeth 3284
Zyvox (Linezolid) Pharmacia & Upjohn 2552

Infections, soft tissues
(*see under* Infections, skin and skin structure)

Infections, surgical, colorectal, prevention of
Invanz for Injection (Ertapenem) Merck 2029

Infections, surgical, ophthalmic, prevention of
Betadine 5% Ophthalmic Solution (Povidone Iodine) Alcon .... ⊙202

Infections, tapeworm
Albenza Tablets (Albendazole) GlaxoSmithKline 1297

Infections, upper respiratory tract
Avelox (Moxifloxacin Hydrochloride) Schering 2803
Biaxin/Biaxin XL (Clarithromycin) Abbott 411
Bicillin C-R Injectable Suspension (Penicillin G Benzathine, Penicillin G Procaine) King 1775
Bicillin L-A Injection (Penicillin G Benzathine, Penicillin G Procaine) King 1777
E.E.S. (Erythromycin Ethylsuccinate) Abbott 433
EryPed (Erythromycin Ethylsuccinate) Abbott 431
Omnicef Capsules (Cefdinir) Abbott .. 497
Omnicef for Oral Suspension (Cefdinir) Abbott 497
Suprax for Oral Suspension (Cefixime) Lupin 1891
Suprax Tablets (Cefixime) Lupin 1891

Infections, urinary tract
Augmentin (Amoxicillin, Clavulanate Potassium) GlaxoSmithKline 1323
Augmentin Tablets (Amoxicillin, Clavulanate Potassium) GlaxoSmithKline 1327
Ceftin Tablets (Cefuroxime Axetil) GlaxoSmithKline 1380
Cipro I.V. (Ciprofloxacin) Schering 2817
Cipro (Ciprofloxacin) Schering 2810
Cipro XR Tablets (Ciprofloxacin) Schering 2823
Doribax Injection (Doripenem) Ortho-McNeil 2400
E.E.S. (Erythromycin Ethylsuccinate) Abbott 433
EryPed (Erythromycin Ethylsuccinate) Abbott 431
Fortaz (Ceftazidime) GlaxoSmithKline 1450
Gantrisin Pediatric Suspension (Acetyl Sulfisoxazole) Roche 2638
Invanz for Injection (Ertapenem) Merck 2029
Levaquin (Levofloxacin) Ortho-McNeil 2416

(▣ Described in PDR® For Nonprescription Drugs) (⊙ Described in PDR® For Ophthalmic Medicines)

Levaquin in 5% Dextrose Injection (Levofloxacin) Ortho-McNeil ... 2416
Noroxin Tablets (Norfloxacin) Merck . 2069
Primaxin I.V. (Cilastatin Sodium, Imipenem) Merck ... 2083
Rocephin Injectable Vials, ADD-Vantage, Galaxy, Bulk (Ceftriaxone Sodium) Roche ... 2642
Seromycin Capsules (Cycloserine) Lilly ... 1864
Suprax for Oral Suspension (Cefixime) Lupin ... 1891
Suprax Tablets (Cefixime) Lupin ... 1891
Timentin ADD-Vantage (Clavulanate Potassium, Ticarcillin Disodium) GlaxoSmithKline ... 1606
Timentin Injection Galaxy Container (Clavulanate Potassium, Ticarcillin Disodium) GlaxoSmithKline ... 1609
Timentin IV Infusion (Clavulanate Potassium, Ticarcillin Disodium) GlaxoSmithKline ... 1603
Timentin Pharmacy Bulk Package (Clavulanate Potassium, Ticarcillin Disodium) GlaxoSmithKline ... 1613
Uroqid-Acid No. 2 Tablets (Methenamine Mandelate, Sodium Acid Phosphate) Beach ... 814
Zinacef for Injection (Cefuroxime) GlaxoSmithKline ... 1678
Zinacef Injection (Cefuroxime) GlaxoSmithKline ... 1678

Infections, venereal
(*see under* Gonorrhea)

Infectious diarrhea
(*see under* Diarrhea, infectious)

Infertility, progesterone deficiency-induced
Crinone 8% Gel (Progesterone) Columbia ... 992

Inflammation, anorectal
Analpram-HC (Hydrocortisone Acetate, Pramoxine Hydrochloride) Ferndale ... 1140

Inflammation, anterior segment
Blephamide Ophthalmic Ointment Allergan ... ⊙217
Blephamide Ophthalmic Suspension Allergan ... ⊙216
FML Ophthalmic Ointment (Fluorometholone) Allergan ... ⊙223
FML Ophthalmic Suspension (Fluorometholone) Allergan ... ⊙224
FML Forte Ophthalmic Suspension (Fluorometholone) Allergan ... ⊙222
Lotemax Ophthalmic Suspension 0.5% (Loteprednol Etabonate) Bausch & Lomb ... ⊙241
Pred Forte Ophthalmic Suspension (Prednisolone Acetate) Allergan ... ⊙227
Pred-G Ophthalmic Ointment (Gentamicin Sulfate, Prednisolone Acetate) Allergan ... ⊙229
Pred-G Ophthalmic Suspension (Gentamicin Sulfate, Prednisolone Acetate) Allergan ... ⊙228
Zylet Ophthalmic Suspension (Loteprednol Etabonate, Tobramycin) Bausch & Lomb ... ⊙247

Inflammation, postoperative
Durezol Ophthalmic Emulsion (Difluprednate) Sirion ... ⊙275

Inflammation due to trauma
Traumeel Injection Solution (Homeopathic Formulations) Heel ... 1725

Influenza, prophylaxis of
Relenza Inhalation Powder (Zanamivir) GlaxoSmithKline ... 1556
Tamiflu Capsules (Oseltamivir Phosphate) Roche ... 2649
Tamiflu Oral Suspension (Oseltamivir Phosphate) Roche ... 2649

Influenza, symptomatic relief of
Oscillococcinum (Anas Barbariae Hepatis et Cordis Extractum) Boiron ... ▣604
Children's Tylenol Plus Cold Suspension Liquid (Acetaminophen, Chlorpheniramine Maleate, Phenylephrine Hydrochloride) McNeil Consumer ... 1912
Children's Tylenol Plus Cough & Runny Nose Suspension Liquid (Acetaminophen, Chlorpheniramine Maleate, Dextromethorphan Hydrobromide) McNeil Consumer .. 1912
Children's Tylenol Plus Cough & Sore Throat Suspension Liquid (Acetaminophen, Dextromethorphan Hydrobromide) McNeil Consumer ... 1912
Children's Tylenol Plus Multi-Symptom Cold Suspension Liquid (Acetaminophen, Chlorpheniramine Maleate, Dextromethorphan Hydrobromide, Phenylephrine Hydrochloride) McNeil Consumer ... 1912
Tylenol Cold Head Congestion Severe Daytime Caplets with Cool Burst (Acetaminophen, Dextromethorphan Hydrobromide, Guaifenesin, Phenylephrine Hydrochloride) McNeil Consumer .. 1910
Vicks NyQuil Liquid (Acetaminophen, Dextromethorphan Hydrobromide, Doxylamine Succinate) Procter & Gamble ... ▣617

Influenza, treatment of
Tamiflu Capsules (Oseltamivir Phosphate) Roche ... 2649
Tamiflu Oral Suspension (Oseltamivir Phosphate) Roche ... 2649

Influenza A virus, acute illness, treatment of
Relenza Inhalation Powder (Zanamivir) GlaxoSmithKline ... 1556

Influenza A virus, respiratory tract illness, chemoprophylaxis of
Flumadine (Rimantadine Hydrochloride) Forest ... 1167

Influenza A virus, respiratory tract illness, treatment of
Flumadine (Rimantadine Hydrochloride) Forest ... 1167

Influenza B virus, acute illness, treatment of
Relenza Inhalation Powder (Zanamivir) GlaxoSmithKline ... 1556

Influenza syndrome, symptomatic relief of
Children's Motrin Cold Oral Suspension (Ibuprofen, Pseudoephedrine Hydrochloride) McNeil Consumer ... 1899
Tussionex Pennkinetic Extended-Release Suspension (Chlorpheniramine Polistirex, Hydrocodone Polistirex) UCB, Inc. ... 3154
Children's Tylenol Suspension Liquid (Acetaminophen) McNeil Consumer ... 1909
Children's Tylenol Meltaways (Acetaminophen) McNeil Consumer ... 1909
Concentrated Tylenol Infants' Drops (Acetaminophen) McNeil Consumer ... 1909
Jr. Tylenol Meltaways (Acetaminophen) McNeil Consumer ... 1909
Vicks NyQuil Cold & Flu Multi-Symptom Relief (Acetaminophen, Dextromethorphan Hydrobromide, Doxylamine Succinate) Procter & Gamble ... ▣617
Vicks NyQuil LiquiCaps (Acetaminophen, Dextromethorphan Hydrobromide, Doxylamine Succinate, Pseudoephedrine Hydrochloride) Procter & Gamble ... 2567
Vicks NyQuil Liquid (Acetaminophen, Dextromethorphan Hydrobromide, Doxylamine Succinate, Pseudoephedrine Hydrochloride) Procter & Gamble ... 2567
Vicks NyQuil Multi-Symptom Cold/Flu Relief (Acetaminophen, Dextromethorphan Hydrobromide, Doxylamine Succinate, Pseudoephedrine Hydrochloride) Procter & Gamble ... 2567

Influenza virus type A and B, immunization against
(*see also under* Immunization, influenza virus, types A and B)
Fluarix Vaccine (Influenza Virus Vaccine) GlaxoSmithKline ... 1446
FluMist Vaccine (Influenza Virus Vaccine Live, Intranasal) MedImmune ... 1945

Influenza virus type A and B vaccine
(*see also under* Immunization, influenza virus, types A and B)
Fluarix Vaccine (Influenza Virus Vaccine) GlaxoSmithKline ... 1446
FluMist Vaccine (Influenza Virus Vaccine Live, Intranasal) MedImmune ... 1945

Injury, gums
Hurricaine Topical Anesthetic (Benzocaine) Beutlich ... 815

Injury, mouth
Hurricaine Topical Anesthetic (Benzocaine) Beutlich ... 815

Insect bites, pain due to
(*see under* Pain, topical relief of)

Insomnia
(*see also under* Sleep, induction of)
Hyland's Calms Forté 4 Kids Tablets (Homeopathic Formulations, Sulfur) Standard Homeopathic ... ▣619

Intermittent claudication
(*see under* Claudication, intermittent)

Intertrigo
(*see under* Skin, inflammatory conditions)

Intraocular pressure, elevation
(*see under* Hypertension, ocular)

Intravascular device, maintenance of patency
Cathflo Activase (Alteplase) Genentech ... 1198

Intubation, endotracheal
Nimbex Injection (Cisatracurium Besylate) Abbott ... 484
Zemuron Injection (Rocuronium Bromide) Schering ... 2947

Iritis
Lotemax Ophthalmic Suspension 0.5% (Loteprednol Etabonate) Bausch & Lomb ... ⊙241
Zylet Ophthalmic Suspension (Loteprednol Etabonate, Tobramycin) Bausch & Lomb ... ⊙247

Iron overload, chronic
Exjade Tablets (Deferasirox) Novartis ... 2244

Irritable bowel syndrome
(*see under* Bowel, irritable, syndrome)

Ischemic attacks, transient
Bayer Aspirin (Aspirin) Bayer HealthCare Consumer ... 750

Ischemic attacks, transient, reduce risk of
Bayer Aspirin (Aspirin) Bayer HealthCare Consumer ... 750

Itching, eyes
Actifed Cold & Allergy Tablets (Chlorpheniramine Maleate, Phenylephrine Hydrochloride) McNeil Consumer ... 1895
Bausch & Lomb Alaway Eye Drops (Ketotifen Fumarate) Bausch & Lomb ... ⊙237
Benadryl Allergy & Sinus Headache Kapgels (Acetaminophen, Diphenhydramine Hydrochloride, Phenylephrine Hydrochloride) McNeil Consumer ... 1895
Benadryl Severe Allergy & Sinus Headache Caplets (Acetaminophen, Diphenhydramine Hydrochloride, Phenylephrine Hydrochloride) McNeil Consumer ... 1897
Benadryl Dye-Free Allergy Liqui-gels Softgels (Diphenhydramine Hydrochloride) McNeil Consumer .. 1897
Benadryl Allergy Kapgels (Diphenhydramine Hydrochloride) McNeil Consumer ... 1895
Benadryl Allergy Quick Dissolve Strips (Diphenhydramine Hydrochloride) McNeil Consumer ... 1896
Benadryl Allergy Ultratab Tablets (Diphenhydramine Hydrochloride) McNeil Consumer ... 1896
Children's Benadryl Dye-Free Allergy Liquid (Diphenhydramine Hydrochloride) McNeil Consumer .. 1897
Children's Benadryl Allergy Fastmelts (Diphenhydramine Hydrochloride) McNeil Consumer .. 1897
Children's Benadryl Allergy Liquid (Diphenhydramine Hydrochloride) McNeil Consumer ... 1898
Children's Benadryl Allergy Perfect Measure (Diphenhydramine Hydrochloride) McNeil Consumer .. 1896
Children's Benadryl-D Allergy & Sinus Liquid (Diphenhydramine Hydrochloride, Phenylephrine Hydrochloride) McNeil Consumer .. 1896
Benadryl-D Allergy & Sinus Tablet (Diphenhydramine Hydrochloride, Phenylephrine Hydrochloride) McNeil Consumer ... 1896
Pataday Ophthalmic Solution (Olopatadine Hydrochloride) Alcon ... 543
PediaCare Children's Allergy & Cold Liquid (Diphenhydramine Hydrochloride, Phenylephrine Hydrochloride) McNeil Consumer .. 1902
PediaCare Children's Allergy Liquid (Diphenhydramine Hydrochloride) McNeil Consumer ... 1902
Refresh Eye Itch Relief (Ketotifen Fumarate) Allergan ... ⊙231
Sudafed PE Nighttime Cold Caplets (Acetaminophen, Diphenhydramine Hydrochloride, Phenylephrine Hydrochloride) McNeil Consumer ... 1907
Sudafed PE Sinus & Allergy Tablets (Chlorpheniramine Maleate, Phenylephrine Hydrochloride) McNeil Consumer ... 1908
Tylenol Allergy Multi-Symptom Caplets with Cool Burst and Rapid Release Gelcaps (Acetaminophen, Chlorpheniramine Maleate, Phenylephrine Hydrochloride) McNeil Consumer ... 1916
Tylenol Allergy Multi-Symptom Nighttime Caplets with Cool Burst (Acetaminophen, Diphenhydramine Hydrochloride, Phenylephrine Hydrochloride) McNeil Consumer ... 1916
Tylenol Severe Allergy Caplets (Acetaminophen, Diphenhydramine Hydrochloride) McNeil Consumer ... 1916
Children's Tylenol Plus Cold & Allergy Suspension Liquid (Acetaminophen, Diphenhydramine Hydrochloride, Phenylephrine Hydrochloride) McNeil Consumer .. 1914
Zyrtec Allergy Tablets (Cetirizine Hydrochloride) McNeil Consumer .. 1919
Children's Zyrtec Allergy Syrup (Cetirizine Hydrochloride) McNeil Consumer ... 1920
Zyrtec-D Allergy & Congestion Extended-Release Tablets (Cetirizine Hydrochloride, Pseudoephedrine Hydrochloride) McNeil Consumer ... 1923

Itching, skin
(*see under* Pruritus, topical relief of)

Itching, sunburn
(*see under* Pruritus, topical relief of)

J

Jock itch
(*see under* Tinea cruris infections)

Joint disease, degenerative, unspecified
Traumeel Injection Solution (Homeopathic Formulations) Heel ... 1725

Joint pain
(*see under* Pain, arthritic, minor)

Juvenile arthritis, idiopathic
Humira Injection (Adalimumab) Abbott ... 442

K

K. pneumoniae bacteremia
Rocephin Injectable Vials, ADD-Vantage, Galaxy, Bulk (Ceftriaxone Sodium) Roche ... 2642

K. pneumoniae bone and joint infections
Rocephin Injectable Vials, ADD-Vantage, Galaxy, Bulk (Ceftriaxone Sodium) Roche ... 2642

K. pneumoniae gynecologic infections
Primaxin I.M. (Cilastatin Sodium, Imipenem) Merck ... 2080
Timentin ADD-Vantage (Clavulanate Potassium, Ticarcillin Disodium) GlaxoSmithKline ... 1606
Timentin Injection Galaxy Container (Clavulanate Potassium, Ticarcillin Disodium) GlaxoSmithKline ... 1609
Timentin IV Infusion (Clavulanate Potassium, Ticarcillin Disodium) GlaxoSmithKline ... 1603
Timentin Pharmacy Bulk Package (Clavulanate Potassium, Ticarcillin Disodium) GlaxoSmithKline ... 1613

K. pneumoniae infections
Augmentin XR Extended Release Tablets (Amoxicillin, Clavulanate Potassium) GlaxoSmithKline ... 1333
Avelox (Moxifloxacin Hydrochloride) Schering ... 2803
Ceftin Tablets (Cefuroxime Axetil) GlaxoSmithKline ... 1380
Cipro I.V. (Ciprofloxacin) Schering ... 2817
Cipro (Ciprofloxacin) Schering ... 2810
Invanz for Injection (Ertapenem) Merck ... 2029
Levaquin (Levofloxacin) Ortho-McNeil ... 2416
Levaquin in 5% Dextrose Injection (Levofloxacin) Ortho-McNeil ... 2416
Merrem I.V. (Meropenem) AstraZeneca Pharmaceuticals ... 684
Noroxin Tablets (Norfloxacin) Merck ... 2069
Primaxin I.M. (Cilastatin Sodium, Imipenem) Merck ... 2080
Rocephin Injectable Vials, ADD-Vantage, Galaxy, Bulk (Ceftriaxone Sodium) Roche ... 2642
Timentin ADD-Vantage (Clavulanate Potassium, Ticarcillin Disodium) GlaxoSmithKline ... 1606
Timentin Injection Galaxy Container (Clavulanate Potassium, Ticarcillin Disodium) GlaxoSmithKline ... 1609
Timentin IV Infusion (Clavulanate Potassium, Ticarcillin Disodium) GlaxoSmithKline ... 1603
Timentin Pharmacy Bulk Package (Clavulanate Potassium, Ticarcillin Disodium) GlaxoSmithKline ... 1613
Tygacil for Injection (Tigecycline) Wyeth ... 3276
Zosyn for Injection (Piperacillin Sodium, Tazobactam Sodium) Wyeth ... 3284

K. pneumoniae infections, ocular
Pred-G Ophthalmic Ointment (Gentamicin Sulfate, Prednisolone Acetate) Allergan ... ⊙229

K. pneumoniae intra-abdominal infections
Cipro I.V. (Ciprofloxacin) Schering ... 2817
Cipro (Ciprofloxacin) Schering ... 2810
Doribax Injection (Doripenem) Ortho-McNeil ... 2400
Merrem I.V. (Meropenem) AstraZeneca Pharmaceuticals ... 684
Primaxin I.M. (Cilastatin Sodium, Imipenem) Merck ... 2080
Rocephin Injectable Vials, ADD-Vantage, Galaxy, Bulk (Ceftriaxone Sodium) Roche ... 2642
Timentin ADD-Vantage (Clavulanate Potassium, Ticarcillin Disodium) GlaxoSmithKline ... 1606
Timentin Injection Galaxy Container (Clavulanate Potassium, Ticarcillin Disodium) GlaxoSmithKline ... 1609
Timentin IV Infusion (Clavulanate Potassium, Ticarcillin Disodium) GlaxoSmithKline ... 1603
Timentin Pharmacy Bulk Package (Clavulanate Potassium, Ticarcillin Disodium) GlaxoSmithKline ... 1613

K. pneumoniae lower respiratory tract infections
Augmentin XR Extended Release Tablets (Amoxicillin, Clavulanate Potassium) GlaxoSmithKline ... 1333
Cipro I.V. (Ciprofloxacin) Schering ... 2817
Cipro (Ciprofloxacin) Schering ... 2810
Invanz for Injection (Ertapenem) Merck ... 2029
Levaquin (Levofloxacin) Ortho-McNeil ... 2416
Levaquin in 5% Dextrose Injection (Levofloxacin) Ortho-McNeil ... 2416
Rocephin Injectable Vials, ADD-Vantage, Galaxy, Bulk (Ceftriaxone Sodium) Roche ... 2642

K. pneumoniae respiratory tract infections
Avelox (Moxifloxacin Hydrochloride) Schering ... 2803

K. pneumoniae septicemia
Rocephin Injectable Vials, ADD-Vantage, Galaxy, Bulk (Ceftriaxone Sodium) Roche ... 2642

K. pneumoniae skin and skin structure infections
Cipro I.V. (Ciprofloxacin) Schering ... 2817
Cipro (Ciprofloxacin) Schering ... 2810
Invanz for Injection (Ertapenem) Merck ... 2029
Primaxin I.M. (Cilastatin Sodium, Imipenem) Merck ... 2080
Rocephin Injectable Vials, ADD-Vantage, Galaxy, Bulk (Ceftriaxone Sodium) Roche ... 2642

K. pneumoniae urinary tract infections
Ceftin Tablets (Cefuroxime Axetil) GlaxoSmithKline ... 1380
Cipro I.V. (Ciprofloxacin) Schering ... 2817
Cipro (Ciprofloxacin) Schering ... 2810
Cipro XR Tablets (Ciprofloxacin) Schering ... 2823
Doribax Injection (Doripenem) Ortho-McNeil ... 2400
Levaquin (Levofloxacin) Ortho-McNeil ... 2416
Levaquin in 5% Dextrose Injection (Levofloxacin) Ortho-McNeil ... 2416
Noroxin Tablets (Norfloxacin) Merck ... 2069
Rocephin Injectable Vials, ADD-Vantage, Galaxy, Bulk (Ceftriaxone Sodium) Roche ... 2642

Kaposi's sarcoma, AIDS-related
Doxil Injection (Doxorubicin Hydrochloride Liposome) Ortho Biotech ... 2378
Intron A for Injection (Interferon alfa-2b, Recombinant) Schering ... 2859
Panretin Gel 0.1% (Alitretinoin) Eisai ... 1081

Kawasaki syndrome
Gammagard S/D (Immune Globulin Intravenous (Human)) Baxter Healthcare ... 734

Keratitis, exposure
Lacrisert Sterile Ophthalmic Insert (Hydroxypropyl Cellulose) Aton ... ⊙233

Keratitis, fungal
Natacyn Antifungal Ophthalmic Suspension (Natamycin) Alcon ... ⊙204

Keratitis, Fusarium solani
Natacyn Antifungal Ophthalmic Suspension (Natamycin) Alcon ... ⊙204

Keratitis, herpes zoster
Zylet Ophthalmic Suspension (Loteprednol Etabonate, Tobramycin) Bausch & Lomb ... ⊙247

Keratitis, punctate, superficial
Lotemax Ophthalmic Suspension 0.5% (Loteprednol Etabonate) Bausch & Lomb ... ⊙241
Zylet Ophthalmic Suspension (Loteprednol Etabonate, Tobramycin) Bausch & Lomb ... ⊙247

Keratitis, recurrent epithelial
Viroptic Ophthalmic Solution (Trifluridine) King ... ⊙253

Keratitis sicca
(*see under* Keratoconjunctivitis sicca)

Keratoconjunctivitis, primary
Viroptic Ophthalmic Solution (Trifluridine) King ... ⊙253

Keratoconjunctivitis sicca
Clear Eyes for Dry Eyes (Carboxymethylcellulose Sodium, Glycerin) Medtech ... ⊙255
Clear Eyes Triple Action Relief (Polyvinyl Alcohol, Povidone, Tetrahydrozoline Hydrochloride) Medtech ... ⊙255
Freshkote Sterile Ophthalmic Solution (Polyvinyl Alcohol, Povidone) Focus ... ⊙248
Lacrisert Sterile Ophthalmic Insert (Hydroxypropyl Cellulose) Aton ... ⊙233
Optive Lubricant Eye Drops (Carboxymethylcellulose Sodium, Glycerin) Allergan ... ⊙227
Optive Sensitive Lubricant Eye Drops (Carboxymethylcellulose Sodium, Glycerin) Allergan ... ⊙227
Refresh Celluvisc Lubricant Eye Drops (Carboxymethylcellulose Sodium) Allergan ... ⊙231
Refresh Plus Lubricant Eye Drops (Carboxymethylcellulose Sodium) Allergan ... ⊙232
Refresh Tears Lubricant Eye Drops (Carboxymethylcellulose Sodium) Allergan ... ⊙232
Restasis Ophthalmic Emulsion (Cyclosporine) Allergan ... 557
Soothe Lubricant Eye Drops (Glycerin, Propylene Glycol) Bausch & Lomb ... ⊙246
Soothe XP Eye Drops (Mineral Oil) Bausch & Lomb ... ⊙246
Systane Ultra Lubricating Eye Drops (Polyethylene Glycol, Propylene Glycol) Alcon ... 547

Keratosis, actinic
Aldara Cream, 5% (Imiquimod) Graceway ... 1699
Carac Cream 0.5% (Fluorouracil) sanofi-aventis ... 2722

Keratosis, solar
Carac Cream 0.5% (Fluorouracil) sanofi-aventis ... 2722

Klebsiella oxytoca infections
Rocephin Injectable Vials, ADD-Vantage, Galaxy, Bulk (Ceftriaxone Sodium) Roche ... 2642
Tygacil for Injection (Tigecycline) Wyeth ... 3276

Klebsiella oxytoca intra-abdominal infections
Tygacil for Injection (Tigecycline) Wyeth ... 3276

Klebsiella oxytoca skin and structure infections
Rocephin Injectable Vials, ADD-Vantage, Galaxy, Bulk (Ceftriaxone Sodium) Roche ... 2642

Klebsiella pneumonia intra-abdominal infections
Tygacil for Injection (Tigecycline) Wyeth ... 3276

Klebsiella pneumoniae infections
(*see under* K. pneumoniae infections)

Klebsiella species bone and joint infections
Fortaz (Ceftazidime) GlaxoSmithKline ... 1450

Klebsiella species gynecologic infections
Primaxin I.V. (Cilastatin Sodium, Imipenem) Merck ... 2083

Klebsiella species infections
Augmentin (Amoxicillin, Clavulanate Potassium) GlaxoSmithKline ... 1323
Augmentin Tablets (Amoxicillin, Clavulanate Potassium) GlaxoSmithKline ... 1327
Doribax Injection (Doripenem) Ortho-McNeil ... 2400
Fortaz (Ceftazidime) GlaxoSmithKline ... 1450
Primaxin I.V. (Cilastatin Sodium, Imipenem) Merck ... 2083
Timentin ADD-Vantage (Clavulanate Potassium, Ticarcillin Disodium) GlaxoSmithKline ... 1606
Timentin Injection Galaxy Container (Clavulanate Potassium, Ticarcillin Disodium) GlaxoSmithKline ... 1609
Timentin IV Infusion (Clavulanate Potassium, Ticarcillin Disodium) GlaxoSmithKline ... 1603
Timentin Pharmacy Bulk Package (Clavulanate Potassium, Ticarcillin Disodium) GlaxoSmithKline ... 1613
Zinacef for Injection (Cefuroxime) GlaxoSmithKline ... 1678
Zinacef Injection (Cefuroxime) GlaxoSmithKline ... 1678

Klebsiella species infections, ocular
Neosporin Ophthalmic Solution Sterile (Gramicidin, Neomycin Sulfate, Polymyxin B Sulfate) King ... ⊙252

Klebsiella species intra-abdominal infections
Doribax Injection (Doripenem) Ortho-McNeil ... 2400
Fortaz (Ceftazidime) GlaxoSmithKline ... 1450
Primaxin I.V. (Cilastatin Sodium, Imipenem) Merck ... 2083
Tygacil for Injection (Tigecycline) Wyeth ... 3276

Klebsiella species lower respiratory tract infections
Fortaz (Ceftazidime) GlaxoSmithKline ... 1450
Primaxin I.V. (Cilastatin Sodium, Imipenem) Merck ... 2083
Timentin ADD-Vantage (Clavulanate Potassium, Ticarcillin Disodium) GlaxoSmithKline ... 1606
Timentin Injection Galaxy Container (Clavulanate Potassium, Ticarcillin Disodium) GlaxoSmithKline ... 1609
Timentin IV Infusion (Clavulanate Potassium, Ticarcillin Disodium) GlaxoSmithKline ... 1603
Timentin Pharmacy Bulk Package (Clavulanate Potassium, Ticarcillin Disodium) GlaxoSmithKline ... 1613
Zinacef for Injection (Cefuroxime) GlaxoSmithKline ... 1678
Zinacef Injection (Cefuroxime) GlaxoSmithKline ... 1678

Klebsiella species septicemia
Fortaz (Ceftazidime) GlaxoSmithKline ... 1450
Primaxin I.V. (Cilastatin Sodium, Imipenem) Merck ... 2083
Timentin ADD-Vantage (Clavulanate Potassium, Ticarcillin Disodium) GlaxoSmithKline ... 1606
Timentin Injection Galaxy Container (Clavulanate Potassium, Ticarcillin Disodium) GlaxoSmithKline ... 1609
Timentin IV Infusion (Clavulanate Potassium, Ticarcillin Disodium) GlaxoSmithKline ... 1603
Timentin Pharmacy Bulk Package (Clavulanate Potassium, Ticarcillin Disodium) GlaxoSmithKline ... 1613
Zinacef for Injection (Cefuroxime) GlaxoSmithKline ... 1678
Zinacef Injection (Cefuroxime) GlaxoSmithKline ... 1678

Klebsiella species skin and skin structure infections
Augmentin (Amoxicillin, Clavulanate Potassium) GlaxoSmithKline ... 1323

Augmentin Tablets (Amoxicillin, Clavulanate Potassium) GlaxoSmithKline ... 1327
Fortaz (Ceftazidime) GlaxoSmithKline ... 1450
Primaxin I.V. (Cilastatin Sodium, Imipenem) Merck ... 2083
Timentin ADD-Vantage (Clavulanate Potassium, Ticarcillin Disodium) GlaxoSmithKline ... 1606
Timentin Injection Galaxy Container (Clavulanate Potassium, Ticarcillin Disodium) GlaxoSmithKline ... 1609
Timentin IV Infusion (Clavulanate Potassium, Ticarcillin Disodium) GlaxoSmithKline ... 1603
Timentin Pharmacy Bulk Package (Clavulanate Potassium, Ticarcillin Disodium) GlaxoSmithKline ... 1613
Zinacef for Injection (Cefuroxime) GlaxoSmithKline ... 1678
Zinacef Injection (Cefuroxime) GlaxoSmithKline ... 1678

Klebsiella species urinary tract infections
Augmentin (Amoxicillin, Clavulanate Potassium) GlaxoSmithKline ... 1323
Augmentin Tablets (Amoxicillin, Clavulanate Potassium) GlaxoSmithKline ... 1327
Doribax Injection (Doripenem) Ortho-McNeil ... 2400
Fortaz (Ceftazidime) GlaxoSmithKline ... 1450
Primaxin I.V. (Cilastatin Sodium, Imipenem) Merck ... 2083
Timentin ADD-Vantage (Clavulanate Potassium, Ticarcillin Disodium) GlaxoSmithKline ... 1606
Timentin Injection Galaxy Container (Clavulanate Potassium, Ticarcillin Disodium) GlaxoSmithKline ... 1609
Timentin IV Infusion (Clavulanate Potassium, Ticarcillin Disodium) GlaxoSmithKline ... 1603
Timentin Pharmacy Bulk Package (Clavulanate Potassium, Ticarcillin Disodium) GlaxoSmithKline ... 1613
Zinacef for Injection (Cefuroxime) GlaxoSmithKline ... 1678
Zinacef Injection (Cefuroxime) GlaxoSmithKline ... 1678

Klebsiella-Enterobacter species infections, ocular
Blephamide Ophthalmic Ointment Allergan ... ⊙217
Blephamide Ophthalmic Suspension Allergan ... ⊙216
Pred-G Ophthalmic Suspension (Gentamicin Sulfate, Prednisolone Acetate) Allergan ... ⊙228
Zylet Ophthalmic Suspension (Loteprednol Etabonate, Tobramycin) Bausch & Lomb ... ⊙247

Koch-Weeks bacillus infections, ocular
(*see under* H. aegypticus infections, ocular)

L

Lacrimation, symptomatic relief of
Actifed Cold & Allergy Tablets (Chlorpheniramine Maleate, Phenylephrine Hydrochloride) McNeil Consumer ... 1895
Allegra-D 12 Hour Extended-Release Tablets (Fexofenadine Hydrochloride, Pseudoephedrine Hydrochloride) sanofi-aventis ... 2687
Benadryl Allergy & Sinus Headache Kapgels (Acetaminophen, Diphenhydramine Hydrochloride, Phenylephrine Hydrochloride) McNeil Consumer ... 1895
Benadryl Severe Allergy & Sinus Headache Caplets (Acetaminophen, Diphenhydramine Hydrochloride, Phenylephrine Hydrochloride) McNeil Consumer ... 1897
Benadryl Dye-Free Allergy Liqui-gels Softgels (Diphenhydramine Hydrochloride) McNeil Consumer ... 1897
Benadryl Allergy Kapgels (Diphenhydramine Hydrochloride) McNeil Consumer ... 1895
Benadryl Allergy Quick Dissolve Strips (Diphenhydramine Hydrochloride) McNeil Consumer ... 1896
Benadryl Allergy Ultratab Tablets (Diphenhydramine Hydrochloride) McNeil Consumer ... 1896
Children's Benadryl Dye-Free Allergy Liquid (Diphenhydramine Hydrochloride) McNeil Consumer ... 1897
Children's Benadryl Allergy Fastmelts (Diphenhydramine Hydrochloride) McNeil Consumer ... 1897
Children's Benadryl Allergy Liquid (Diphenhydramine Hydrochloride) McNeil Consumer ... 1898
Children's Benadryl Allergy Perfect Measure (Diphenhydramine Hydrochloride) McNeil Consumer ... 1896
Children's Benadryl-D Allergy & Sinus Liquid (Diphenhydramine Hydrochloride, Phenylephrine Hydrochloride) McNeil Consumer ... 1896
Benadryl-D Allergy & Sinus Tablet (Diphenhydramine Hydrochloride, Phenylephrine Hydrochloride) McNeil Consumer ... 1896
Sudafed PE Nighttime Cold Caplets (Acetaminophen, Diphenhydramine Hydrochloride, Phenylephrine Hydrochloride) McNeil Consumer ... 1907
Tylenol Allergy Multi-Symptom Caplets with Cool Burst and Rapid Release Gelcaps (Acetaminophen, Chlorpheniramine Maleate, Phenylephrine Hydrochloride) McNeil Consumer ... 1916
Tylenol Allergy Multi-Symptom Nighttime Caplets with Cool Burst (Acetaminophen, Diphenhydramine Hydrochloride, Phenylephrine Hydrochloride) McNeil Consumer ... 1916
Tylenol Severe Allergy Caplets (Acetaminophen, Diphenhydramine Hydrochloride) McNeil Consumer ... 1916
Children's Tylenol Plus Cold & Allergy Suspension Liquid (Acetaminophen, Diphenhydramine Hydrochloride, Phenylephrine Hydrochloride) McNeil Consumer ... 1914
Zyrtec Allergy Tablets (Cetirizine Hydrochloride) McNeil Consumer ... 1919
Children's Zyrtec Allergy Syrup (Cetirizine Hydrochloride) McNeil Consumer ... 1920
Children's Zyrtec Allergy Chewable Tablets (Cetirizine Hydrochloride) McNeil Consumer ... 1922

Lactobacillus acidophilus, deficiency of
DDS-Acidophilus Capsules, Tablets, and Powder (Lactobacillus Acidophilus) UAS Labs ... ▣634

LDL cholesterol, elevation
(*see under* Hyperlipoproteinemia, types IIa and IIb, adjunct to diet)

Lead poisoning
Chemet Capsules (Succimer) Ovation ... 2484

Leg muscle cramps
Hyland's Leg Cramps with Quinine Tablets and Caplets (Homeopathic Formulations) Standard Homeopathic ... ▣620

Legionella pneumophila infections
(*see under* Legionnaires' disease)

Legionnaires' disease
E.E.S. (Erythromycin Ethylsuccinate) Abbott ... 433
EryPed (Erythromycin Ethylsuccinate) Abbott ... 431
Levaquin (Levofloxacin) Ortho-McNeil ... 2416
Levaquin in 5% Dextrose Injection (Levofloxacin) Ortho-McNeil ... 2416

Lennox-Gastaut syndrome
Klonopin (Clonazepam) Roche ... 2639
Lamictal (Lamotrigine) GlaxoSmithKline ... 1488

Leprosy
Dapsone Tablets USP (Dapsone) Jacobus ... 1746

Leukemia, acute, nonlymphocytic, adjunctive therapy
Novantrone for Injection Concentrate (Mitoxantrone Hydrochloride) EMD Serono ... 1100

Leukemia, acute, promyelocytic
Trisenox Injection (Arsenic Trioxide) Cephalon ... 986
Vesanoid Capsules (Tretinoin) Roche ... 2660

Leukemia, acute lymphoblastic
Arranon Injection (Nelarabine) GlaxoSmithKline ... 1319
Clolar for Intravenous Infusion (Clofarabine) Genzyme ... 1239
Gleevec Tablets (Imatinib Mesylate) Novartis ... 2255
Oncaspar Injection (Pegaspargase) Enzon ... 1138

Leukemia, acute lymphocytic
Elspar for Injection (Asparaginase) Merck ... 1990
Elspar for Injection (Asparaginase) Ovation ... 2488

Leukemia, acute myelogenous
Leukine (Sargramostim) Bayer HealthCare Pharmaceuticals ... 774

Leukemia, acute myeloid, adjunctive therapy in
Neupogen for Injection (Filgrastim) Amgen ... 589

Leukemia, acute myeloid, CD33 positive
Mylotarg for Injection (Gemtuzumab Ozogamicin) Wyeth ... 3212

Leukemia, acute nonlymphocytic
Tabloid Tablets (Thioguanine) GlaxoSmithKline ... 1601

Leukemia, adjunctive therapy in
Elitek (Rasburicase) sanofi-aventis ... 2729

Leukemia, chronic eosinophic
Gleevec Tablets (Imatinib Mesylate) Novartis ... 2255

Leukemia, chronic lymphocytic
Leukeran Tablets (Chlorambucil) GlaxoSmithKline ... 1508
Mustargen for Injection (Mechlorethamine Hydrochloride) Ovation ... 2492
Treanda for Injection (Bendamustine Hydrochloride) Cephalon ... 983

Leukemia, chronic lymphocytic, B-cell
Campath Ampules (Alemtuzumab) Bayer HealthCare Pharmaceuticals ... 761

Leukemia, chronic lymphocytic, B-cell, prevention of bacterial infection in
Gammagard S/D (Immune Globulin Intravenous (Human)) Baxter Healthcare ... 734

Leukemia, chronic myeloid
Busulfex Injection (Busulfan) Otsuka ... 2477
Gleevec Tablets (Imatinib Mesylate) Novartis ... 2255
Mustargen for Injection (Mechlorethamine Hydrochloride) Ovation ... 2492
Myleran Tablets (Busulfan) GlaxoSmithKline ... 1530

Leukemia, hairy cell
Intron A for Injection (Interferon alfa-2b, Recombinant) Schering ... 2859
Leustatin Injection (Cladribine) Ortho Biotech ... 2384

Leukemia, lymphoblastic, adjunctive therapy in
Leukine (Sargramostim) Bayer HealthCare Pharmaceuticals ... 774

Listeria monocytogenes infections
E.E.S. (Erythromycin Ethylsuccinate) Abbott ... 433
EryPed (Erythromycin Ethylsuccinate) Abbott ... 431

Listeriosis
E.E.S. (Erythromycin Ethylsuccinate) Abbott ... 433
EryPed (Erythromycin Ethylsuccinate) Abbott ... 431

Liver, allogeneic transplants, prophylaxis of organ rejection in
CellCept Capsules (Mycophenolate Mofetil) Roche ... 2622
CellCept Intravenous (Mycophenolate Mofetil Hydrochloride) Roche ... 2622
CellCept Oral Suspension (Mycophenolate Mofetil) Roche ... 2622
CellCept Tablets (Mycophenolate Mofetil) Roche ... 2622
Gengraf Capsules (Cyclosporine) Abbott ... 435
Neoral Oral Solution (Cyclosporine) Novartis ... 2280
Neoral Soft Gelatin Capsules (Cyclosporine) Novartis ... 2280
Orthoclone OKT3 Sterile Solution (Muromonab-CD3) Ortho Biotech ... 2387
Prograf Capsules and Injection (Tacrolimus) Astellas ... 622
Sandimmune (Cyclosporine) Novartis ... 2296

Locoregional solid malignancies
Cosmegen for Injection (Dactinomycin) Ovation ... 2485

Lou Gehrig's disease
(*see under* Amyotrophic lateral sclerosis)

Lupus erythematosus, systemic
Bayer Aspirin (Aspirin) Bayer HealthCare Consumer ... 750

Lyme disease
(*see under* Borrelia burgdorferi infection)

Lymphoma, cutaneous T-cell
Ontak Vials (Denileukin Diftitox) Eisai ... 1079
Targretin Capsules (Bexarotene) Eisai ... 1084
Targretin Gel 1% (Bexarotene) Eisai ... 1088
Zolinza Capsules (Vorinostat) Merck ... 2142

Lymphoma, lymphoblastic
Arranon Injection (Nelarabine) GlaxoSmithKline ... 1319

Lymphoma, mantle cell
Velcade for Injection (Bortezomib) Millennium ... 2168

Lymphoma, non-Hodgkin's, follicular
Bexxar (Iodine I 131 Tositumomab, Tositumomab) GlaxoSmithKline ... 1371
Intron A for Injection (Interferon alfa-2b, Recombinant) Schering ... 2859

Lymphoma, unspecified, adjunctive therapy in
Elitek (Rasburicase) sanofi-aventis ... 2729

Lymphomas, giant follicular
Leukeran Tablets (Chlorambucil) GlaxoSmithKline ... 1508

Lymphomas, Hodgkin's
(*see under* Hodgkin's disease)

Lymphomas, malignant
Leukeran Tablets (Chlorambucil) GlaxoSmithKline ... 1508

Lymphomas, non-Hodgkin's
Bexxar (Iodine I 131 Tositumomab, Tositumomab) GlaxoSmithKline ... 1371
Leukeran Tablets (Chlorambucil) GlaxoSmithKline ... 1508
Rituxan I.V. (Rituximab) Genentech ... 1223

Lymphomas, non-Hodgkin's, adjunctive therapy in
Leukine (Sargramostim) Bayer HealthCare Pharmaceuticals 774

Lymphomas, non-Hodgkin's, refractory
Bexxar (Iodine I 131 Tositumomab, Tositumomab) GlaxoSmithKline 1371

Lymphomatous meningitis
DepoCyt Injection (Cytarabine Liposome) Enzon 1136

Lymphosarcoma
(*see under* Lymphomas, non-Hodgkin's)

M

M. catarrhalis, otitis media
Augmentin (Amoxicillin, Clavulanate Potassium) GlaxoSmithKline 1323
Augmentin Tablets (Amoxicillin, Clavulanate Potassium) GlaxoSmithKline 1327
Augmentin ES-600 Powder for Oral Suspension (Amoxicillin, Clavulanate Potassium) GlaxoSmithKline 1329
Biaxin/Biaxin XL (Clarithromycin) Abbott 411
Ceftin (Cefuroxime Axetil) GlaxoSmithKline 1380
Omnicef Capsules (Cefdinir) Abbott .. 497
Omnicef for Oral Suspension (Cefdinir) Abbott 497
Rocephin Injectable Vials, ADD-Vantage, Galaxy, Bulk (Ceftriaxone Sodium) Roche 2642
Suprax for Oral Suspension (Cefixime) Lupin 1891
Suprax Tablets (Cefixime) Lupin 1891

M. catarrhalis bronchitis
Avelox (Moxifloxacin Hydrochloride) Schering 2803
Levaquin (Levofloxacin) Ortho-McNeil 2416
Levaquin in 5% Dextrose Injection (Levofloxacin) Ortho-McNeil 2416

M. catarrhalis infections
Augmentin (Amoxicillin, Clavulanate Potassium) GlaxoSmithKline 1323
Augmentin Tablets (Amoxicillin, Clavulanate Potassium) GlaxoSmithKline 1327
Augmentin XR Extended Release Tablets (Amoxicillin, Clavulanate Potassium) GlaxoSmithKline 1333
Augmentin ES-600 Powder for Oral Suspension (Amoxicillin, Clavulanate Potassium) GlaxoSmithKline 1329
Avelox (Moxifloxacin Hydrochloride) Schering 2803
Biaxin/Biaxin XL (Clarithromycin) Abbott 411
Ceftin (Cefuroxime Axetil) GlaxoSmithKline 1380
Cipro (Ciprofloxacin) Schering 2810
Invanz for Injection (Ertapenem) Merck 2029
Ketek Tablets (Telithromycin) sanofi-aventis 2744
Levaquin (Levofloxacin) Ortho-McNeil 2416
Levaquin in 5% Dextrose Injection (Levofloxacin) Ortho-McNeil 2416
Omnicef Capsules (Cefdinir) Abbott .. 497
Omnicef for Oral Suspension (Cefdinir) Abbott 497
Suprax for Oral Suspension (Cefixime) Lupin 1891

M. catarrhalis lower respiratory tract infections
Augmentin (Amoxicillin, Clavulanate Potassium) GlaxoSmithKline 1323
Augmentin Tablets (Amoxicillin, Clavulanate Potassium) GlaxoSmithKline 1327
Augmentin XR Extended Release Tablets (Amoxicillin, Clavulanate Potassium) GlaxoSmithKline 1333
Avelox (Moxifloxacin Hydrochloride) Schering 2803
Biaxin/Biaxin XL (Clarithromycin) Abbott 411
Cipro (Ciprofloxacin) Schering 2810
Invanz for Injection (Ertapenem) Merck 2029
Ketek Tablets (Telithromycin) sanofi-aventis 2744
Levaquin (Levofloxacin) Ortho-McNeil 2416
Levaquin in 5% Dextrose Injection (Levofloxacin) Ortho-McNeil 2416
Omnicef Capsules (Cefdinir) Abbott .. 497
Omnicef for Oral Suspension (Cefdinir) Abbott 497

M. catarrhalis pneumonia
Avelox (Moxifloxacin Hydrochloride) Schering 2803
Invanz for Injection (Ertapenem) Merck 2029
Ketek Tablets (Telithromycin) sanofi-aventis 2744
Omnicef Capsules (Cefdinir) Abbott .. 497
Omnicef for Oral Suspension (Cefdinir) Abbott 497

M. catarrhalis sinusitis
Augmentin (Amoxicillin, Clavulanate Potassium) GlaxoSmithKline 1323
Augmentin Tablets (Amoxicillin, Clavulanate Potassium) GlaxoSmithKline 1327
Augmentin XR Extended Release Tablets (Amoxicillin, Clavulanate Potassium) GlaxoSmithKline 1333
Avelox (Moxifloxacin Hydrochloride) Schering 2803
Biaxin/Biaxin XL (Clarithromycin) Abbott 411
Cipro I.V. (Ciprofloxacin) Schering 2817
Cipro (Ciprofloxacin) Schering 2810
Levaquin (Levofloxacin) Ortho-McNeil 2416
Levaquin in 5% Dextrose Injection (Levofloxacin) Ortho-McNeil 2416

Macular degeneration
Lucentis Injection (Ranibizumab) Genentech 1205

Major depression disorder, treatment of
Remeron Tablets (Mirtazapine) Schering 2924
RemeronSolTab Tablets (Mirtazapine) Schering 2927

Major depressive disorder
Cymbalta Delayed-Release Capsules (Duloxetine Hydrochloride) Lilly 1801
Emsam Transdermal System (Selegiline) Bristol-Myers Squibb 905
Pristiq Extended-Release Tablets (Desvenlafaxine Succinate) Wyeth . 3247
Prozac Weekly Capsules (Fluoxetine Hydrochloride) Lilly 1852
Prozac Pulvules and Liquid (Fluoxetine Hydrochloride) Lilly 1852
Venlafaxine Hydrochloride Tablets (Venlafaxine Hydrochloride) Mylan . 2199

Malaria
(*see under* P. falciparum infections; P. malariae infections; P. ovale infections; P. vivax infections)

Malaria, prophylaxis of
Daraprim Tablets (Pyrimethamine) GlaxoSmithKline 1400
Malarone Pediatric Tablets (Atovaquone, Proguanil Hydrochloride) GlaxoSmithKline 1521
Malarone Tablets (Atovaquone, Proguanil Hydrochloride) GlaxoSmithKline 1521

Malaria, treatment or prophylaxis of
Fansidar Tablets (Pyrimethamine, Sulfadoxine) Roche 2636

Malassezia furfur
(*see under* Pityrosporon orbiculare infections)

Mania, bipolar
Abilify Oral Solution (Aripiprazole) Bristol-Myers Squibb 881
Abilify Oral Solution (Aripiprazole) Otsuka 2466
Abilify Discmelt Orally Disintegrating Tablets (Aripiprazole) Bristol-Myers Squibb 881
Abilify Discmelt Orally Disintegrating Tablets (Aripiprazole) Otsuka 2466
Abilify Tablets (Aripiprazole) Bristol-Myers Squibb 881
Abilify Tablets (Aripiprazole) Otsuka .. 2466
Geodon (Ziprasidone Hydrochloride) Pfizer 2520
Zyprexa Tablets (Olanzapine) Lilly 1883
Zyprexa ZYDIS Orally Disintegrating Tablets (Olanzapine) Lilly 1883

Mastocytosis, systemic
Gleevec Tablets (Imatinib Mesylate) Novartis 2255
Zantac (Ranitidine Hydrochloride) GlaxoSmithKline 1670

Measles, prophylaxis
Attenuvax (Measles Virus Vaccine Live) Merck 1951
M-M-R II (Measles, Mumps & Rubella Virus Vaccine, Live) Merck 2054
ProQuad (Measles, Mumps, Rubella and Varicella Virus Vaccine Live) Merck 2099

Melanin hyperpigmentation
(*see under* Hyperpigmentation, skin, bleaching of)

Melanoma
Intron A for Injection (Interferon alfa-2b, Recombinant) Schering 2859
Proleukin for Injection (Aldesleukin) Novartis 2287

Melasma
(*see under* Hyperpigmentation, skin, bleaching of)

Meningitis
Bicillin C-R Injectable Suspension (Penicillin G Benzathine, Penicillin G Procaine) King 1775
Bicillin L-A Injection (Penicillin G Benzathine, Penicillin G Procaine) King 1777
Fortaz (Ceftazidime) GlaxoSmithKline 1450
Merrem I.V. (Meropenem) AstraZeneca Pharmaceuticals 684
Rocephin Injectable Vials, ADD-Vantage, Galaxy, Bulk (Ceftriaxone Sodium) Roche 2642
Zinacef for Injection (Cefuroxime) GlaxoSmithKline 1678
Zinacef Injection (Cefuroxime) GlaxoSmithKline 1678

Meningitis, meningococcal, prophylaxis of
Gantrisin Pediatric Suspension (Acetyl Sulfisoxazole) Roche 2638

Meningitis, meningococcal, treatment of
Gantrisin Pediatric Suspension (Acetyl Sulfisoxazole) Roche 2638

Menopause, vasomotor symptoms of
Activella Tablets (Estradiol, Norethindrone Acetate) Novo Nordisk 2347
Angeliq Tablets (Estradiol, Drospirenone) Bayer HealthCare Pharmaceuticals 751
Climara Transdermal System (Estradiol) Bayer HealthCare Pharmaceuticals 763
Climara Pro Transdermal System (Estradiol, Levonorgestrel) Bayer HealthCare Pharmaceuticals 768
Divigel (Estradiol) Upsher-Smith 3167
Enjuvia Tablets (Estrogens, Conjugated, Synthetic B) Duramed 1029
Estratest Tablets (Estrogens, Esterified, Methyltestosterone) Solvay ... 3043
Estratest H.S. Tablets (Estrogens, Esterified, Methyltestosterone) Solvay 3043
Premarin Tablets (Estrogens, Conjugated) Wyeth 3221
Premphase Tablets (Estrogens, Conjugated, Medroxyprogesterone Acetate) Wyeth 3232
Prempro Tablets (Estrogens, Conjugated, Medroxyprogesterone Acetate) Wyeth 3232

Menstrual, signs and symptoms, temporary relief of
Women's Tylenol Menstrual Relief Caplets (Acetaminophen, Pamabrom) McNeil Consumer 1919

Menstrual cramps
(*see under* Pain, menstrual)

Micrococcus luteus
Vigamox Ophthalmic Solution (Moxifloxacin Hydrochloride) Alcon 548

Microsporum audouinii infections
Gris-PEG Tablets (Griseofulvin) Pedinol 2507

Microsporum canis infections
Gris-PEG Tablets (Griseofulvin) Pedinol 2507

Microsporum gypseum infections
Gris-PEG Tablets (Griseofulvin) Pedinol 2507

Migraine headache
(*see under* Headache, migraine; Headache, migraine, prophylaxis of)

Mima-Herellea species infections
(*see under* Acinetobacter species infections)

Moraxella catarrhalis
(*see under* M. catarrhalis infections)

Moraxella lacunata infections, ocular
Zylet Ophthalmic Suspension (Loteprednol Etabonate, Tobramycin) Bausch & Lomb .... ⊙ 247

Morganella morganii infections
Cipro I.V. (Ciprofloxacin) Schering 2817
Cipro (Ciprofloxacin) Schering 2810
Fortaz (Ceftazidime) GlaxoSmithKline 1450
Primaxin I.V. (Cilastatin Sodium, Imipenem) Merck 2083
Rocephin Injectable Vials, ADD-Vantage, Galaxy, Bulk (Ceftriaxone Sodium) Roche 2642

Morganella morganii infections, ocular
Zylet Ophthalmic Suspension (Loteprednol Etabonate, Tobramycin) Bausch & Lomb .... ⊙ 247

Morganella morganii skin and skin structure infections
Cipro I.V. (Ciprofloxacin) Schering 2817
Cipro (Ciprofloxacin) Schering 2810
Primaxin I.V. (Cilastatin Sodium, Imipenem) Merck 2083
Rocephin Injectable Vials, ADD-Vantage, Galaxy, Bulk (Ceftriaxone Sodium) Roche 2642

Morganella morganii urinary tract infections
Cipro I.V. (Ciprofloxacin) Schering 2817
Cipro (Ciprofloxacin) Schering 2810
Primaxin I.V. (Cilastatin Sodium, Imipenem) Merck 2083
Rocephin Injectable Vials, ADD-Vantage, Galaxy, Bulk (Ceftriaxone Sodium) Roche 2642

Morphea, possibly effective in
Potaba (Aminobenzoate Potassium) Glenwood 1698

Motion sickness
Dramamine Chewable Tablets (Dimenhydrinate) McNeil Consumer 1898
Dramamine Less Drowsy Tablets (Meclizine Hydrochloride) McNeil Consumer 1898
Dramamine Original Tablets (Dimenhydrinate) McNeil Consumer 1898
Transderm Scōp Transdermal Therapeutic System (Scopolamine) Novartis Consumer 2206

Mouth, irritation of
Hurricaine Topical Anesthetic (Benzocaine) Beutlich 815

Mouth, sore, pain
Hurricaine Topical Anesthetic (Benzocaine) Beutlich 815

Mucormycosis
(*see under* Zygomycosis)

Mucositis
Kepivance (Palifermin) Amgen 583

Multiple follicles, development of in an ART program
Follistim AQ Cartridge (Follitropin Beta) Schering 2844

Multiple sclerosis, acute exacerbations
Copaxone for Injection (Glatiramer Acetate) Teva Neuroscience 3110

Multiple sclerosis, alleviation of signs and symptoms
Dantrium Capsules (Dantrolene Sodium) Procter & Gamble Pharmaceuticals 2580

Multiple sclerosis, chronic progressive
Novantrone for Injection Concentrate (Mitoxantrone Hydrochloride) EMD Serono 1100

Multiple sclerosis, relapsing-remitting
Betaseron for SC Injection (Interferon Beta-1b) Bayer HealthCare Pharmaceuticals 756
Copaxone for Injection (Glatiramer Acetate) Teva Neuroscience 3110
Novantrone for Injection Concentrate (Mitoxantrone Hydrochloride) EMD Serono 1100
Rebif Prefilled Syringe for Injection (Interferon Beta-1a) EMD Serono 1107

Mumps, prophylaxis
M-M-R II (Measles, Mumps & Rubella Virus Vaccine, Live) Merck 2054
Mumpsvax (Mumps Virus Vaccine, Live) Merck 2068
ProQuad (Measles, Mumps, Rubella and Varicella Virus Vaccine Live) Merck 2099

Muscle spasm
(*see under* Spasticity, muscle, symptomatic alleviation of)

Muscles, skeletal, relaxation, preoperative
Nimbex Injection (Cisatracurium Besylate) Abbott 484
Zemuron Injection (Rocuronium Bromide) Schering 2947

Musculo-skeletal discomfort, adjunct in
Skelaxin Tablets (Metaxalone) King 1784

Myalgia
(*see under* Pain, muscular, temporary relief of)

Myalgia, topical relief of
(*see under* Pain, topical relief of)

Mycobacterium avium complex (MAC) disease, disseminated
Biaxin/Biaxin XL (Clarithromycin) Abbott 411

Mycobacterium avium complex (MAC) disease, disseminated, prophylaxis of
Biaxin/Biaxin XL (Clarithromycin) Abbott 411

Mycobacterium intracellulare infections
Biaxin/Biaxin XL (Clarithromycin) Abbott 411

Mycobacterium leprae infections
(*see under* Leprosy)

Mycobacterium tuberculosis infection, pulmonary
Capastat Sulfate for Injection (Capreomycin Sulfate) Lilly 1791

Mycoplasma pneumoniae infection
Avelox (Moxifloxacin Hydrochloride) Schering 2803
Biaxin/Biaxin XL (Clarithromycin) Abbott 411
E.E.S. (Erythromycin Ethylsuccinate) Abbott 433
EryPed (Erythromycin Ethylsuccinate) Abbott 431
Ketek Tablets (Telithromycin) sanofi-aventis 2744
Levaquin (Levofloxacin) Ortho-McNeil 2416
Levaquin in 5% Dextrose Injection (Levofloxacin) Ortho-McNeil 2416

Mycoplasma pneumoniae respiratory tract infections
Biaxin/Biaxin XL (Clarithromycin) Abbott 411
E.E.S. (Erythromycin Ethylsuccinate) Abbott 433
EryPed (Erythromycin Ethylsuccinate) Abbott 431
Ketek Tablets (Telithromycin) sanofi-aventis 2744
Levaquin (Levofloxacin) Ortho-McNeil 2416
Levaquin in 5% Dextrose Injection (Levofloxacin) Ortho-McNeil 2416

Mycosis fungoides
Mustargen for Injection (Mechlorethamine Hydrochloride) Ovation 2492

Myelodysplastic diseases associated with PDGFR gene rearrangements
Gleevec Tablets (Imatinib Mesylate) Novartis 2255

Myelodysplastic syndrome
Dacogen Injection (Decitabine) Eisai 1066

Myeloid recovery, acceleration of
Leukine (Sargramostim) Bayer HealthCare Pharmaceuticals 774

Myeloma, multiple
Doxil Injection (Doxorubicin Hydrochloride Liposome) Ortho Biotech 2378
Velcade for Injection (Bortezomib) Millennium 2168

Myeloma, multiple, adjunct in
Zometa for Intravenous Infusion (Zoledronic acid) Novartis 2341

Myeloprolifertive diseases associated with PDGFR gene rearrangements
Gleevec Tablets (Imatinib Mesylate) Novartis 2255

Myocardial infarction, acute
Activase I.V. (Alteplase) Genentech 1188
Bayer Aspirin (Aspirin) Bayer HealthCare Consumer 750
Integrilin Injection (Eptifibatide) Schering 2855
Plavix Tablets (Clopidogrel Bisulfate) Bristol-Myers Squibb 926
Plavix Tablets (Clopidogrel Bisulfate) sanofi-aventis 2767
TNKase (Tenecteplase) Genentech 1233

Myocardial infarction, acute ST-segment elevation
Lovenox Injection (Enoxaparin Sodium) sanofi-aventis 2756

Myocardial infarction, non-Q-wave
Fragmin Injection (Dalteparin Sodium) Eisai 1070
Integrilin Injection (Eptifibatide) Schering 2855
Lovenox Injection (Enoxaparin Sodium) sanofi-aventis 2756

Myocardial infarction, post, left ventricular dysfunction
Captopril Tablets (Captopril) Mylan 2182
Coreg Tablets (Carvedilol) GlaxoSmithKline 1387
Coreg CR Extended-Release Capsules (Carvedilol Phosphate) GlaxoSmithKline 1393
Mavik Tablets (Trandolapril) Abbott 472

Myocardial infarction, prophylaxis, adjunct in
Mevacor Tablets (Lovastatin) Merck 2063

Myocardial infarction, to reduce the risk of
Advicor Tablets (Lovastatin, Niacin) Abbott 402
Bayer Aspirin (Aspirin) Bayer HealthCare Consumer 750
Lipitor Tablets (Atorvastatin Calcium) Parke-Davis 2501
Niaspan Extended-Release Tablets (Niacin) Abbott 480
Zocor Tablets (Simvastatin) Merck 2136

Myocardial infarction, treatment adjunct
Mavik Tablets (Trandolapril) Abbott 472
Prinivil Tablets (Lisinopril) Merck 2087

Myocardial perfusion imaging, radionuclide
Lexiscan Injection (Regadenoson) Astellas 614

Myocardial perfusion imaging, thallium, adjunct in
Adenoscan (Adenosine) Astellas 605

Myocardial reinfarction, prophylaxis
Bayer Aspirin (Aspirin) Bayer HealthCare Consumer 750
Plavix Tablets (Clopidogrel Bisulfate) Bristol-Myers Squibb 926
Plavix Tablets (Clopidogrel Bisulfate) sanofi-aventis 2767

Myocardial revascularization procedures, to reduce the risk of
Advicor Tablets (Lovastatin, Niacin) Abbott 402
Bayer Aspirin (Aspirin) Bayer HealthCare Consumer 750
Lescol Capsules (Fluvastatin Sodium) Novartis 2268
Lescol XL Tablets (Fluvastatin Sodium) Novartis 2268
Lipitor Tablets (Atorvastatin Calcium) Parke-Davis 2501
Mevacor Tablets (Lovastatin) Merck 2063
Zocor Tablets (Simvastatin) Merck 2136

Myxedema
(*see under* Hypothyroidism, replacement or supplemental therapy in)

Myxedema coma/precoma
(*see under* Hypothyroidism, replacement or supplemental therapy in)

N

N. gonorrhoeae endocervical infections
Ceftin Tablets (Cefuroxime Axetil) GlaxoSmithKline 1380
Cipro (Ciprofloxacin) Schering 2810
Noroxin Tablets (Norfloxacin) Merck 2069
Rocephin Injectable Vials, ADD-Vantage, Galaxy, Bulk (Ceftriaxone Sodium) Roche 2642

N. gonorrhoeae gynecologic infections
Noroxin Tablets (Norfloxacin) Merck 2069

N. gonorrhoeae infections
Amoxil Capsules (Amoxicillin) GlaxoSmithKline 1305
Amoxil Chewable Tablets (Amoxicillin) GlaxoSmithKline 1305
Amoxil Pediatric Drops for Oral Suspension (Amoxicillin) GlaxoSmithKline 1305
Amoxil Powder for Oral Suspension (Amoxicillin) GlaxoSmithKline 1305
Amoxil Tablets (Amoxicillin) GlaxoSmithKline 1305
Ceftin Tablets (Cefuroxime Axetil) GlaxoSmithKline 1380
Cipro (Ciprofloxacin) Schering 2810
E.E.S. (Erythromycin Ethylsuccinate) Abbott 433
EryPed (Erythromycin Ethylsuccinate) Abbott 431
Fortaz (Ceftazidime) GlaxoSmithKline 1450
Noroxin Tablets (Norfloxacin) Merck 2069
Rocephin Injectable Vials, ADD-Vantage, Galaxy, Bulk (Ceftriaxone Sodium) Roche 2642
Suprax for Oral Suspension (Cefixime) Lupin 1891
Suprax Tablets (Cefixime) Lupin 1891
Zinacef for Injection (Cefuroxime) GlaxoSmithKline 1678
Zinacef Injection (Cefuroxime) GlaxoSmithKline 1678

N. gonorrhoeae infections, ocular
Pred-G Ophthalmic Ointment (Gentamicin Sulfate, Prednisolone Acetate) Allergan .... ⊙229
Pred-G Ophthalmic Suspension (Gentamicin Sulfate, Prednisolone Acetate) Allergan .... ⊙228

N. gonorrhoeae pelvic inflammatory disease
E.E.S. (Erythromycin Ethylsuccinate) Abbott 433
EryPed (Erythromycin Ethylsuccinate) Abbott 431
Rocephin Injectable Vials, ADD-Vantage, Galaxy, Bulk (Ceftriaxone Sodium) Roche 2642

N. gonorrhoeae pharyngeal infections
Rocephin Injectable Vials, ADD-Vantage, Galaxy, Bulk (Ceftriaxone Sodium) Roche 2642

N. gonorrhoeae rectal infections
Amoxil Capsules (Amoxicillin) GlaxoSmithKline 1305
Amoxil Chewable Tablets (Amoxicillin) GlaxoSmithKline 1305
Amoxil Pediatric Drops for Oral Suspension (Amoxicillin) GlaxoSmithKline 1305
Amoxil Powder for Oral Suspension (Amoxicillin) GlaxoSmithKline 1305
Amoxil Tablets (Amoxicillin) GlaxoSmithKline 1305
Ceftin Tablets (Cefuroxime Axetil) GlaxoSmithKline 1380
Rocephin Injectable Vials, ADD-Vantage, Galaxy, Bulk (Ceftriaxone Sodium) Roche 2642

N. gonorrhoeae urethral infections
Amoxil Capsules (Amoxicillin) GlaxoSmithKline 1305
Amoxil Chewable Tablets (Amoxicillin) GlaxoSmithKline 1305
Amoxil Pediatric Drops for Oral Suspension (Amoxicillin) GlaxoSmithKline 1305
Amoxil Powder for Oral Suspension (Amoxicillin) GlaxoSmithKline 1305
Amoxil Tablets (Amoxicillin) GlaxoSmithKline 1305
Ceftin Tablets (Cefuroxime Axetil) GlaxoSmithKline 1380
Cipro (Ciprofloxacin) Schering 2810
Noroxin Tablets (Norfloxacin) Merck 2069
Rocephin Injectable Vials, ADD-Vantage, Galaxy, Bulk (Ceftriaxone Sodium) Roche 2642

N. gonorrhoeae urinary tract infections
Suprax for Oral Suspension (Cefixime) Lupin 1891
Suprax Tablets (Cefixime) Lupin 1891

N. meningitidis infections
Fortaz (Ceftazidime) GlaxoSmithKline 1450
Merrem I.V. (Meropenem) AstraZeneca Pharmaceuticals 684
Rocephin Injectable Vials, ADD-Vantage, Galaxy, Bulk (Ceftriaxone Sodium) Roche 2642
Zinacef for Injection (Cefuroxime) GlaxoSmithKline 1678

Zinacef Injection (Cefuroxime) GlaxoSmithKline 1678

N. meningitidis meningitis

Fortaz (Ceftazidime) GlaxoSmithKline 1450
Merrem I.V. (Meropenem) AstraZeneca Pharmaceuticals 684
Rocephin Injectable Vials, ADD-Vantage, Galaxy, Bulk (Ceftriaxone Sodium) Roche 2642
Zinacef for Injection (Cefuroxime) GlaxoSmithKline 1678
Zinacef Injection (Cefuroxime) GlaxoSmithKline 1678

Nail, dry brittle

Appearex Tablets (Biotin) Merz 2163

Narcolepsy

Dexedrine (Dextroamphetamine Sulfate) GlaxoSmithKline 1401
Provigil Tablets (Modafinil) Cephalon 977

Nasal congestion, symptomatic relief of

Actifed Cold & Allergy Tablets (Chlorpheniramine Maleate, Phenylephrine Hydrochloride) McNeil Consumer 1895
Allegra-D 12 Hour Extended-Release Tablets (Fexofenadine Hydrochloride, Pseudoephedrine Hydrochloride) sanofi-aventis 2687
Allegra-D 24 Hour Extended-Release Tablets (Fexofenadine Hydrochloride, Pseudoephedrine Hydrochloride) sanofi-aventis 2690
Benadryl Allergy & Cold Kapgels (Acetaminophen, Diphenhydramine Hydrochloride, Phenylephrine Hydrochloride) McNeil Consumer 1895
Benadryl Allergy & Sinus Headache Kapgels (Acetaminophen, Diphenhydramine Hydrochloride, Phenylephrine Hydrochloride) McNeil Consumer 1895
Benadryl Severe Allergy & Sinus Headache Caplets (Acetaminophen, Diphenhydramine Hydrochloride, Phenylephrine Hydrochloride) McNeil Consumer 1897
Children's Benadryl-D Allergy & Sinus Liquid (Diphenhydramine Hydrochloride, Phenylephrine Hydrochloride) McNeil Consumer 1896
Benadryl-D Allergy & Sinus Tablet (Diphenhydramine Hydrochloride, Phenylephrine Hydrochloride) McNeil Consumer 1896
Clarinex-D 12-Hour Extended-Release Tablets (Desloratadine, Pseudoephedrine Sulfate) Schering 2831
Clarinex-D 24-Hour Extended-Release Tablets (Desloratadine, Pseudoephedrine Sulfate) Schering 2834
PediaCare Children's Allergy & Cold Liquid (Diphenhydramine Hydrochloride, Phenylephrine Hydrochloride) McNeil Consumer 1902
PediaCare Children's Decongestant Liquid (Phenylephrine Hydrochloride) McNeil Consumer 1902
PediaCare Children's Liquid Multi-Symptom Cold (Dextromethorphan Hydrobromide, Phenylephrine Hydrochloride) McNeil Consumer 1902
Simply Soothing (Sodium Chloride) McNeil Consumer 1905
Sinutab Non-Drying Caplets (Guaifenesin, Phenylephrine Hydrochloride) McNeil Consumer 1905
Sinutab Sinus Caplets (Acetaminophen, Phenylephrine Hydrochloride) McNeil Consumer 1905
Sudafed 12 Hour Nasal Decongestant Non-Drowsy Caplets (Pseudoephedrine Hydrochloride) McNeil Consumer 1909
Sudafed 24 Hour Non-Drowsy Nasal Decongestant Tablets (Pseudoephedrine Hydrochloride) McNeil Consumer 1906
Children's Sudafed Nasal Decongestant Liquid (Pseudoephedrine Hydrochloride) McNeil Consumer 1906
Children's Sudafed PE Cold & Cough Liquid (Dextromethorphan Hydrobromide, Phenylephrine Hydrochloride) McNeil Consumer 1907
Children's Sudafed PE Nasal Decongestant Liquid (Phenylephrine Hydrochloride) McNeil Consumer 1906
Sudafed Nasal Decongestant Tablets (Pseudoephedrine Hydrochloride) McNeil Consumer 1906
Sudafed OM Sinus Cold Moisturizing Nasal Spray (Oxymetazoline Hydrochloride) McNeil Consumer 1906
Sudafed OM Sinus Congestion Moisturizing Nasal Spray (Oxymetazoline Hydrochloride) McNeil Consumer 1906
Sudafed PE Cold & Cough Caplets (Acetaminophen, Dextromethorphan Hydrobromide, Guaifenesin, Phenylephrine Hydrochloride) McNeil Consumer 1907
Sudafed PE Nasal Decongestant Tablets (Phenylephrine Hydrochloride) McNeil Consumer 1907
Sudafed PE Nighttime Cold Caplets (Acetaminophen, Diphenhydramine Hydrochloride, Phenylephrine Hydrochloride) McNeil Consumer 1907
Sudafed PE Non-Drying Sinus Caplets (Guaifenesin, Phenylephrine Hydrochloride) McNeil Consumer 1908
Sudafed PE Severe Cold Caplets (Acetaminophen, Diphenhydramine Hydrochloride, Phenylephrine Hydrochloride) McNeil Consumer 1908
Sudafed PE Sinus & Allergy Tablets (Chlorpheniramine Maleate, Phenylephrine Hydrochloride) McNeil Consumer 1908
Sudafed PE Sinus Headache Caplets (Acetaminophen, Phenylephrine Hydrochloride) McNeil Consumer 1908
Tylenol Allergy Multi-Symptom Caplets with Cool Burst and Rapid Release Gelcaps (Acetaminophen, Chlorpheniramine Maleate, Phenylephrine Hydrochloride) McNeil Consumer 1916
Tylenol Allergy Multi-Symptom Nighttime Caplets with Cool Burst (Acetaminophen, Diphenhydramine Hydrochloride, Phenylephrine Hydrochloride) McNeil Consumer 1916
Tylenol Chest Congestion Caplets with Cool Burst (Acetaminophen, Guaifenesin) McNeil Consumer 1910
Tylenol Chest Congestion Liquid with Cool Burst (Acetaminophen, Guaifenesin) McNeil Consumer 1910
Children's Tylenol Plus Cold Suspension Liquid (Acetaminophen, Chlorpheniramine Maleate, Phenylephrine Hydrochloride) McNeil Consumer 1912
Children's Tylenol Plus Cold & Allergy Suspension Liquid (Acetaminophen, Diphenhydramine Hydrochloride, Phenylephrine Hydrochloride) McNeil Consumer 1914
Children's Tylenol Plus Flu Suspension Liquid (Acetaminophen, Chlorpheniramine Maleate, Dextromethorphan Hydrobromide, Phenylephrine Hydrochloride) McNeil Consumer 1914
Children's Tylenol Plus Multi-Symptom Cold Suspension Liquid (Acetaminophen, Chlorpheniramine Maleate, Dextromethorphan Hydrobromide, Phenylephrine Hydrochloride) McNeil Consumer 1912
Tylenol Cold Severe Congestion Daytime Caplets with Cool Burst (Acetaminophen, Dextromethorphan Hydrobromide, Guaifenesin, Pseudoephedrine Hydrochloride) McNeil Consumer 1912
Tylenol Cold Head Congestion Daytime Caplets with Cool Burst (Acetaminophen, Dextromethorphan Hydrobromide, Phenylephrine Hydrochloride) McNeil Consumer 1910
Tylenol Cold Head Congestion Nighttime Caplets with Cool Burst (Acetaminophen, Chlorpheniramine Maleate, Dextromethorphan Hydrobromide, Phenylephrine Hydrochloride) McNeil Consumer 1910
Tylenol Cold Head Congestion Severe Daytime Caplets with Cool Burst (Acetaminophen, Dextromethorphan Hydrobromide, Guaifenesin, Phenylephrine Hydrochloride) McNeil Consumer 1910
Tylenol Cold Multi-Symptom Daytime Caplets with Cool Burst and Rapid Release Gels (Acetaminophen, Dextromethorphan Hydrobromide, Phenylephrine Hydrochloride) McNeil Consumer 1913
Tylenol Cold Multi-Symptom Daytime Liquid with Citrus Burst (Acetaminophen, Dextromethorphan Hydrobromide, Phenylephrine Hydrochloride) McNeil Consumer 1913
Tylenol Cold Multi-Symptom Nighttime Caplets with Cool Burst (Acetaminophen, Chlorpheniramine Maleate, Dextromethorphan Hydrobromide, Phenylephrine Hydrochloride) McNeil Consumer 1913
Tylenol Cold Multi-Symptom Nighttime Liquid with Cool Burst (Acetaminophen, Dextromethorphan Hydrobromide, Doxylamine Succinate, Phenylephrine Hydrochloride) McNeil Consumer 1913
Tylenol Cold Multi-Symptom Severe Caplets with Cool Burst (Acetaminophen, Dextromethorphan Hydrobromide, Guaifenesin, Phenylephrine Hydrochloride) McNeil Consumer 1913
Tylenol Cold Multi-Symptom Severe Daytime Liquid with Citrus Burst (Acetaminophen, Dextromethorphan Hydrobromide, Guaifenesin, Phenylephrine Hydrochloride) McNeil Consumer 1913
Tylenol Sinus Congestion & Pain Daytime Caplets with Cool Burst and Gelcaps (Acetaminophen, Phenylephrine Hydrochloride) McNeil Consumer 1917
Tylenol Sinus Congestion & Pain Nighttime Caplets with Cool Burst (Acetaminophen, Chlorpheniramine Maleate, Phenylephrine Hydrochloride) McNeil Consumer 1917
Tylenol Sinus Congestion & Pain Severe Caplets with Cool Burst (Acetaminophen, Guaifenesin, Phenylephrine Hydrochloride) McNeil Consumer 1917
Vicks DayQuil Cold & Flu Multi-Symptom Relief (Acetaminophen, Dextromethorphan Hydrobromide, Phenylephrine Hydrochloride) Procter & Gamble .... ▣616
Vicks DayQuil LiquiCaps (Acetaminophen, Dextromethorphan Hydrobromide, Phenylephrine Hydrochloride) Procter & Gamble 2567
Vicks DayQuil (Acetaminophen, Dextromethorphan Hydrobromide, Phenylephrine Hydrochloride) Procter & Gamble .... ▣616
Vicks DayQuil Liquid (Acetaminophen, Dextromethorphan Hydrobromide, Phenylephrine Hydrochloride) Procter & Gamble 2567
Vicks DayQuil Multi-Symptom Cold/Flu Relief (Acetaminophen, Dextromethorphan Hydrobromide, Phenylephrine Hydrochloride) Procter & Gamble 2567
Vicks NyQuil LiquiCaps (Acetaminophen, Dextromethorphan Hydrobromide, Doxylamine Succinate, Pseudoephedrine Hydrochloride) Procter & Gamble 2567
Vicks NyQuil Liquid (Acetaminophen, Dextromethorphan Hydrobromide, Doxylamine Succinate, Pseudoephedrine Hydrochloride) Procter & Gamble 2567
Vicks NyQuil Multi-Symptom Cold/Flu Relief (Acetaminophen, Dextromethorphan Hydrobromide, Doxylamine Succinate, Pseudoephedrine Hydrochloride) Procter & Gamble 2567
Zyrtec-D Allergy & Congestion Extended-Release Tablets (Cetirizine Hydrochloride, Pseudoephedrine Hydrochloride) McNeil Consumer 1923

Nasal dryness

Simply Soothing (Sodium Chloride) McNeil Consumer 1905

Nausea

(*see also under* Motion sickness)
Dramamine Chewable Tablets (Dimenhydrinate) McNeil Consumer 1898
Dramamine Less Drowsy Tablets (Meclizine Hydrochloride) McNeil Consumer 1898
Dramamine Original Tablets (Dimenhydrinate) McNeil Consumer 1898

Nausea, emetogenic, cancer chemotherapy-induced

Aloxi Injection (Palonosetron Hydrochloride) Eisai 1059
Anzemet Injection (Dolasetron Mesylate) sanofi-aventis 2701
Anzemet Tablets (Dolasetron Mesylate) sanofi-aventis 2704
Emend Capsules (Aprepitant) Merck 1992
Emend for Injection (Fosaprepitant Dimeglumine) Merck 1999
Marinol Capsules (Dronabinol) Unimed 3163
Zofran Injection (Ondansetron Hydrochloride) GlaxoSmithKline 1682
Zofran (Ondansetron Hydrochloride) GlaxoSmithKline 1687
Zofran ODT Orally Disintegrating Tablets (Ondansetron) GlaxoSmithKline 1687

Nausea, emetogenic, radiation therapy-induced

Zofran (Ondansetron Hydrochloride) GlaxoSmithKline 1687
Zofran ODT Orally Disintegrating Tablets (Ondansetron) GlaxoSmithKline 1687

Nausea, postoperative

Aloxi Injection (Palonosetron Hydrochloride) Eisai 1059
Anzemet Injection (Dolasetron Mesylate) sanofi-aventis 2701
Anzemet Tablets (Dolasetron Mesylate) sanofi-aventis 2704
Emend Capsules (Aprepitant) Merck 1992
Zofran Injection (Ondansetron Hydrochloride) GlaxoSmithKline 1682
Zofran (Ondansetron Hydrochloride) GlaxoSmithKline 1687
Zofran ODT Orally Disintegrating Tablets (Ondansetron) GlaxoSmithKline 1687

Necrotic tissue, debridement of

Accuzyme SE Spray Emulsion (Papain, Urea) Healthpoint 1723
Panafil Ointment (Chlorophyllin Copper Complex Sodium, Papain, Urea) Healthpoint 1723
Panafil SE Spray Emulsion (Chlorophyllin Copper Complex Sodium, Papain, Urea) Healthpoint 1724
Santyl Collagenase Ointment (Collagenase) Healthpoint 1724

Neisseria gonorrhoeae

(*see under* N. gonorrhoeae infections)

Neisseria meningitidis

(*see under* N. gonorrhoeae infections)

Neisseria species infections, ocular
Neosporin Ophthalmic Solution Sterile (Gramicidin, Neomycin Sulfate, Polymyxin B Sulfate) King ..... ⊙252
Pred-G Ophthalmic Suspension (Gentamicin Sulfate, Prednisolone Acetate) Allergan ..... ⊙228
Zylet Ophthalmic Suspension (Loteprednol Etabonate, Tobramycin) Bausch & Lomb ..... ⊙247

Neoplasia, cervical intraepithelial, prevention of
Gardasil Injection (Quadrivalent Human Papillomavirus (Types 6, 11, 16, 18) Recombinant Vaccine) Merck 2019

Neoplasia, vaginal intraepithelial, prevention of
Gardasil Injection (Quadrivalent Human Papillomavirus (Types 6, 11, 16, 18) Recombinant Vaccine) Merck 2019

Neoplasia, vulvar intraepithelial, prevention of
Gardasil Injection (Quadrivalent Human Papillomavirus (Types 6, 11, 16, 18) Recombinant Vaccine) Merck 2019

Nephroblastoma
(*see under* Wilms' tumor)

Nephrolithiasis, calcium
Urocit-K Tablets (Potassium Citrate) Mission 2176

Nephropathy, diabetic
Avapro Tablets (Irbesartan) Bristol-Myers Squibb 897
Avapro Tablets (Irbesartan) sanofi-aventis 2718
Cozaar Tablets (Losartan Potassium) Merck 1973

Nephrosis, acute, adjunctive therapy
Flexbumin 25% I.V. (Albumin (human)) Baxter Healthcare 729
Human Albumin Grifols 25% (Albumin (human)) Grifols 1706

Neuralgia, glossopharyngeal
Carbatrol Capsules (Carbamazepine) Shire US 3019

Neuralgia, postherpetic
Lidoderm Patch (Lidocaine) Endo 1114
Lyrica Capsules (Pregabalin) Pfizer 2527

Neuralgia, trigeminal
Carbatrol Capsules (Carbamazepine) Shire US 3019

Neurocysticercosis
Albenza Tablets (Albendazole) GlaxoSmithKline 1297

Neurological deficits, post-SAH, improvement of
Nimotop Capsules (Nimodipine) Bayer HealthCare Pharmaceuticals 790

Neutropenia, chemotherapy-induced
Neulasta Injection (Pegfilgrastim) Amgen 587
Neupogen for Injection (Filgrastim) Amgen 589

Neutropenia, febrile, to decrease the incidence of infection
AmBisome for Injection (Amphotericin B, liposomal) Astellas 606
Cipro I.V. (Ciprofloxacin) Schering 2817
Neulasta Injection (Pegfilgrastim) Amgen 587
Neupogen for Injection (Filgrastim) Amgen 589

Neutropenia, post-bone marrow transplant
Neupogen for Injection (Filgrastim) Amgen 589

Neutropenia, severe, chronic
Neupogen for Injection (Filgrastim) Amgen 589

Neutropenia-related clinical sequelae, post-bone marrow transplant
Neupogen for Injection (Filgrastim) Amgen 589

Night-terrors
Hyland's Calms Forté 4 Kids Tablets (Homeopathic Formulations, Sulfur) Standard Homeopathic ..... ▣619

Nocardia asteroides infections
(*see under* Nocardiosis)

Nocardiosis
Gantrisin Pediatric Suspension (Acetyl Sulfisoxazole) Roche 2638

Noonan's syndrome, growth failure associated with
Norditropin Cartridges (Somatropin (rDNA Origin)) Novo Nordisk 2354

Nose, itchy
(*see under* Pruritus, rhinopharyngeal, symptomatic relief of)

Nose, runny
(*see under* Rhinorrhea)

Nutrients, deficiency of
ProNutra Protein Supplement (Vitamins with Minerals, Whey Protein Isolate) Immunotec Medical 1730

Nutrients, deficiency of, stress-induced
(*see under* Nutrients, deficiency of)

Nutrients, deficiency of, surgery-induced
(*see under* Nutrients, deficiency of)

O

Obesity, exogenous
Adipex-P (Phentermine Hydrochloride) Gate 1185
Meridia Capsules (Sibutramine Hydrochloride Monohydrate) Abbott 475
Xenical Capsules (Orlistat) Roche 2672

Obsessive compulsive disorder
Luvox CR Extended-Release Capsules (Fluvoxamine Maleate) Jazz 1759
Paxil (Paroxetine Hydrochloride) GlaxoSmithKline 1535
Prozac Weekly Capsules (Fluoxetine Hydrochloride) Lilly 1852
Prozac Pulvules and Liquid (Fluoxetine Hydrochloride) Lilly 1852

Ocular health, maintenance
Bausch & Lomb PreserVision AREDS Softgels (Vitamins with Minerals) Bausch & Lomb ..... ⊙239
Bausch & Lomb PreserVision Lutein Softgels (Lutein, Vitamins with Minerals) Bausch & Lomb ..... ⊙239

Ocular inflammation
Durezol Ophthalmic Emulsion (Difluprednate) Sirion ..... ⊙275
Pred Mild Ophthalmic Suspension (Prednisolone Acetate) Allergan ..... ⊙230
Triesence Injectable Suspension (Triamcinolone Acetonide) Alcon ..... ⊙209

Ocular inflammation, postoperative
Voltaren Ophthalmic Solution (Diclofenac Sodium) Novartis 2336

Ocular inflammation, steroid-responsive
FML Ophthalmic Suspension (Fluorometholone) Allergan ..... ⊙224
Lotemax Ophthalmic Suspension 0.5% (Loteprednol Etabonate) Bausch & Lomb ..... ⊙241
Pred Forte Ophthalmic Suspension (Prednisolone Acetate) Allergan ..... ⊙227

Ocular inflammation with bacterial infection, steroid-responsive
Blephamide Ophthalmic Ointment Allergan ..... ⊙217
Blephamide Ophthalmic Suspension Allergan ..... ⊙216
Pred-G Ophthalmic Ointment (Gentamicin Sulfate, Prednisolone Acetate) Allergan ..... ⊙229
Pred-G Ophthalmic Suspension (Gentamicin Sulfate, Prednisolone Acetate) Allergan ..... ⊙228
Zylet Ophthalmic Suspension (Loteprednol Etabonate, Tobramycin) Bausch & Lomb ..... ⊙247

Ocular redness
Clear Eyes Itchy Eye Relief (Glycerin, Naphazoline Hydrochloride, Zinc Sulfate) Medtech ..... ⊙255
Clear Eyes Triple Action Relief (Polyvinyl Alcohol, Povidone, Tetrahydrozoline Hydrochloride) Medtech ..... ⊙255

Onchocerciasis
Stromectol Tablets (Ivermectin) Merck 2120

Onychomycosis
(*see under* Tinea unguium infections)

Ophthalmia, Egyptian
(*see under* Trachoma)

Ophthalmia, sympathetic
Triesence Injectable Suspension (Triamcinolone Acetonide) Alcon ..... ⊙209

Opioid dependence, treatment of
Suboxone Tablets (Buprenorphine Hydrochloride, Naloxone Hydrochloride) Reckitt Benckiser 2601
Subutex Tablets (Buprenorphine Hydrochloride) Reckitt Benckiser 2601

Orthodontic appliances, irritation
Hurricaine Topical Anesthetic (Benzocaine) Beutlich 815

Ossification, heterotopic
Didronel Tablets (Etidronate Disodium) Procter & Gamble Pharmaceuticals 2583

Osteitis deformans
(*see under* Paget's disease of bone)

Osteoarthritis
Anaprox Tablets (Naproxen Sodium) Roche 2632
Anaprox DS Tablets (Naproxen Sodium) Roche 2632
Bayer Aspirin (Aspirin) Bayer HealthCare Consumer 750
Celebrex Capsules (Celecoxib) Searle 2979
Clinoril Tablets (Sulindac) Merck 1962
CM Plex Cream (Fatty Acids, Olive Oil) Unicity 3159
EC-Naprosyn Delayed-Release Tablets (Naproxen) Roche 2632
Hyalgan Solution (Sodium Hyaluronate) sanofi-aventis 2742
Indocin (Indomethacin) Merck 2024
Limbrel Capsules (Flavocoxid) Primus 2561
Mobic Oral Suspension (Meloxicam) Boehringer Ingelheim 863
Mobic Tablets (Meloxicam) Boehringer Ingelheim 863
Nalfon Capsules (Fenoprofen Calcium) Pedinol 2508
Naprosyn Suspension (Naproxen) Roche 2632
Naprosyn Tablets (Naproxen) Roche 2632
Traumeel Injection Solution (Homeopathic Formulations) Heel 1725
Voltaren Tablets (Diclofenac Sodium) Novartis 2334
Voltaren-XR Tablets (Diclofenac Sodium) Novartis 2337

Osteoarthritis, symptoms of
Zeel Injection Solution (Homeopathic Formulations) Heel 1726

Osteodystrophy, renal
Calcijex Injection (Calcitriol) Abbott 419

Osteopenia
Fosteum Capsules (Genistein Aglycone, Zinc Bisglycinate, Cholecalciferol) Sciele 2963

Osteoporosis
Activella Tablets (Estradiol, Norethindrone Acetate) Novo Nordisk 2347
Boniva Injection (Ibandronate Sodium) Roche 2614
Boniva Tablets (Ibandronate Sodium) Roche 2618
Evista Tablets (Raloxifene Hydrochloride) Lilly 1810
Forteo for Injection (Teriparatide) Lilly 1816
Fosamax (Alendronate Sodium) Merck 2005
Fosamax Plus D Tablets (Alendronate Sodium, Cholecalciferol) Merck 2013
Fosteum Capsules (Genistein Aglycone, Zinc Bisglycinate, Cholecalciferol) Sciele 2963
Premphase Tablets (Estrogens, Conjugated, Medroxyprogesterone Acetate) Wyeth 3232
Prempro Tablets (Estrogens, Conjugated, Medroxyprogesterone Acetate) Wyeth 3232

Osteoporosis, corticosteroid-induced
Fosamax (Alendronate Sodium) Merck 2005

Osteoporosis, glucocorticoid-induced, prevention of
Actonel Tablets (Risedronate Sodium) Procter & Gamble Pharmaceuticals 2568

Osteoporosis, glucocorticoid-induced, treatment of
Actonel Tablets (Risedronate Sodium) Procter & Gamble Pharmaceuticals 2568

Osteoporosis, postmenopausal, prevention of
Activella Tablets (Estradiol, Norethindrone Acetate) Novo Nordisk 2347
Actonel Tablets (Risedronate Sodium) Procter & Gamble Pharmaceuticals 2568
Actonel with Calcium Tablets (Risedronate Sodium, Calcium Carbonate) Procter & Gamble Pharmaceuticals 2574
Boniva Injection (Ibandronate Sodium) Roche 2614
Boniva Tablets (Ibandronate Sodium) Roche 2618
Climara Transdermal System (Estradiol) Bayer HealthCare Pharmaceuticals 763
Climara Pro Transdermal System (Estradiol, Levonorgestrel) Bayer HealthCare Pharmaceuticals 768
Premphase Tablets (Estrogens, Conjugated, Medroxyprogesterone Acetate) Wyeth 3232
Prempro Tablets (Estrogens, Conjugated, Medroxyprogesterone Acetate) Wyeth 3232

Osteoporosis, postmenopausal, treatment adjunct
Miacalcin Injection (Calcitonin-Salmon) Novartis 2273
Miacalcin Nasal Spray (Calcitonin-Salmon) Novartis 2274
Premarin Tablets (Estrogens, Conjugated) Wyeth 3221

Osteoporosis, postmenopausal, treatment of
Actonel Tablets (Risedronate Sodium) Procter & Gamble Pharmaceuticals 2568
Actonel with Calcium Tablets (Risedronate Sodium, Calcium Carbonate) Procter & Gamble Pharmaceuticals 2574
Evista Tablets (Raloxifene Hydrochloride) Lilly 1810

Miacalcin Nasal Spray (Calcitonin-Salmon) Novartis 2274
Reclast Injection (Zoledronic acid) Novartis 2291

Osteoporosis in men
Actonel Tablets (Risedronate Sodium) Procter & Gamble Pharmaceuticals 2568

Otitis externa, acute
Ciprodex Otic Suspension (Ciprofloxacin, Dexamethasone) Alcon 541

Otitis media
Bicillin C-R Injectable Suspension (Penicillin G Benzathine, Penicillin G Procaine) King 1775
Bicillin L-A Injection (Penicillin G Benzathine, Penicillin G Procaine) King 1777
Suprax Tablets (Cefixime) Lupin 1891

Otitis media, acute
Augmentin (Amoxicillin, Clavulanate Potassium) GlaxoSmithKline 1323
Augmentin Tablets (Amoxicillin, Clavulanate Potassium) GlaxoSmithKline 1327
Augmentin ES-600 Powder for Oral Suspension (Amoxicillin, Clavulanate Potassium) GlaxoSmithKline 1329
Biaxin/Biaxin XL (Clarithromycin) Abbott 411
Ceftin (Cefuroxime Axetil) GlaxoSmithKline 1380
Ciprodex Otic Suspension (Ciprofloxacin, Dexamethasone) Alcon 541
Omnicef Capsules (Cefdinir) Abbott 497
Omnicef for Oral Suspension (Cefdinir) Abbott 497
Rocephin Injectable Vials, ADD-Vantage, Galaxy, Bulk (Ceftriaxone Sodium) Roche 2642
Suprax for Oral Suspension (Cefixime) Lupin 1891

Otitis media, adjunctive therapy
Hyland's Earache Tablets (Homeopathic Formulations) Standard Homeopathic .... ▣620

Otitis media, H. influenzae-induced
(*see under* H. influenzae otitis media)

Otitis media, S. pneumoniae-induced
(*see under* S. pneumoniae otitis media)

Otitis media, S. pyogenes-induced
(*see under* S. pyogenes otitis media)

Otitis media, Staphylococci-induced
(*see under* Staphylococci otitis media)

Ovarian failure, primary
Premarin Tablets (Estrogens, Conjugated) Wyeth 3221

Ovaries, castration of
Premarin Tablets (Estrogens, Conjugated) Wyeth 3221

Ovary, adenocarcinoma
(*see under* Carcinoma, ovary)

Ovulation, induction of
Follistim AQ Cartridge (Follitropin Beta) Schering 2844

Oxyuriasis
(*see under* Enterobiasis)

P

P. aeruginosa bone and joint infections
Cipro I.V. (Ciprofloxacin) Schering 2817
Cipro (Ciprofloxacin) Schering 2810
Fortaz (Ceftazidime) GlaxoSmithKline 1450
Primaxin I.V. (Cilastatin Sodium, Imipenem) Merck 2083

P. aeruginosa infections
Cipro I.V. (Ciprofloxacin) Schering 2817
Cipro (Ciprofloxacin) Schering 2810
Doribax Injection (Doripenem) Ortho-McNeil 2400
Fortaz (Ceftazidime) GlaxoSmithKline 1450
Levaquin (Levofloxacin) Ortho-McNeil 2416
Levaquin in 5% Dextrose Injection (Levofloxacin) Ortho-McNeil 2416
Merrem I.V. (Meropenem) AstraZeneca Pharmaceuticals 684
Noroxin Tablets (Norfloxacin) Merck 2069
Primaxin I.M. (Cilastatin Sodium, Imipenem) Merck 2080
Primaxin I.V. (Cilastatin Sodium, Imipenem) Merck 2083
Rocephin Injectable Vials, ADD-Vantage, Galaxy, Bulk (Ceftriaxone Sodium) Roche 2642
Timentin ADD-Vantage (Clavulanate Potassium, Ticarcillin Disodium) GlaxoSmithKline 1606
Timentin Injection Galaxy Container (Clavulanate Potassium, Ticarcillin Disodium) GlaxoSmithKline 1609
Timentin IV Infusion (Clavulanate Potassium, Ticarcillin Disodium) GlaxoSmithKline 1603
Timentin Pharmacy Bulk Package (Clavulanate Potassium, Ticarcillin Disodium) GlaxoSmithKline 1613
Zosyn for Injection (Piperacillin Sodium, Tazobactam Sodium) Wyeth 3284

P. aeruginosa infections, ocular
Ofloxacin Ophthalmic Solution 0.3% (Ofloxacin) Bausch & Lomb .... ⊙243
Pred-G Ophthalmic Ointment (Gentamicin Sulfate, Prednisolone Acetate) Allergan .... ⊙229
Pred-G Ophthalmic Suspension (Gentamicin Sulfate, Prednisolone Acetate) Allergan .... ⊙228
Zylet Ophthalmic Suspension (Loteprednol Etabonate, Tobramycin) Bausch & Lomb .... ⊙247

P. aeruginosa intra-abdominal infections
Cipro I.V. (Ciprofloxacin) Schering 2817
Cipro (Ciprofloxacin) Schering 2810
Doribax Injection (Doripenem) Ortho-McNeil 2400
Merrem I.V. (Meropenem) AstraZeneca Pharmaceuticals 684
Primaxin I.M. (Cilastatin Sodium, Imipenem) Merck 2080
Primaxin I.V. (Cilastatin Sodium, Imipenem) Merck 2083

P. aeruginosa lower respiratory tract infections
Cipro I.V. (Ciprofloxacin) Schering 2817
Cipro (Ciprofloxacin) Schering 2810
Fortaz (Ceftazidime) GlaxoSmithKline 1450
Levaquin (Levofloxacin) Ortho-McNeil 2416
Levaquin in 5% Dextrose Injection (Levofloxacin) Ortho-McNeil 2416

P. aeruginosa meningitis
Fortaz (Ceftazidime) GlaxoSmithKline 1450

P. aeruginosa septicemia
Fortaz (Ceftazidime) GlaxoSmithKline 1450
Primaxin I.V. (Cilastatin Sodium, Imipenem) Merck 2083
Timentin ADD-Vantage (Clavulanate Potassium, Ticarcillin Disodium) GlaxoSmithKline 1606
Timentin Injection Galaxy Container (Clavulanate Potassium, Ticarcillin Disodium) GlaxoSmithKline 1609
Timentin IV Infusion (Clavulanate Potassium, Ticarcillin Disodium) GlaxoSmithKline 1603
Timentin Pharmacy Bulk Package (Clavulanate Potassium, Ticarcillin Disodium) GlaxoSmithKline 1613

P. aeruginosa skin and skin structure infections
Cipro I.V. (Ciprofloxacin) Schering 2817
Cipro (Ciprofloxacin) Schering 2810
Fortaz (Ceftazidime) GlaxoSmithKline 1450
Merrem I.V. (Meropenem) AstraZeneca Pharmaceuticals 684
Primaxin I.M. (Cilastatin Sodium, Imipenem) Merck 2080
Primaxin I.V. (Cilastatin Sodium, Imipenem) Merck 2083
Rocephin Injectable Vials, ADD-Vantage, Galaxy, Bulk (Ceftriaxone Sodium) Roche 2642

P. aeruginosa urinary tract infections
Cipro I.V. (Ciprofloxacin) Schering 2817
Cipro (Ciprofloxacin) Schering 2810
Cipro XR Tablets (Ciprofloxacin) Schering 2823
Doribax Injection (Doripenem) Ortho-McNeil 2400
Fortaz (Ceftazidime) GlaxoSmithKline 1450
Levaquin (Levofloxacin) Ortho-McNeil 2416
Levaquin in 5% Dextrose Injection (Levofloxacin) Ortho-McNeil 2416
Noroxin Tablets (Norfloxacin) Merck 2069
Primaxin I.V. (Cilastatin Sodium, Imipenem) Merck 2083
Timentin ADD-Vantage (Clavulanate Potassium, Ticarcillin Disodium) GlaxoSmithKline 1606
Timentin Injection Galaxy Container (Clavulanate Potassium, Ticarcillin Disodium) GlaxoSmithKline 1609
Timentin IV Infusion (Clavulanate Potassium, Ticarcillin Disodium) GlaxoSmithKline 1603
Timentin Pharmacy Bulk Package (Clavulanate Potassium, Ticarcillin Disodium) GlaxoSmithKline 1613

P. falciparum infections
Daraprim Tablets (Pyrimethamine) GlaxoSmithKline 1400
Fansidar Tablets (Pyrimethamine, Sulfadoxine) Roche 2636
Malarone Pediatric Tablets (Atovaquone, Proguanil Hydrochloride) GlaxoSmithKline 1521
Malarone Tablets (Atovaquone, Proguanil Hydrochloride) GlaxoSmithKline 1521

P. falciparum infections, adjunct in
Gantrisin Pediatric Suspension (Acetyl Sulfisoxazole) Roche 2638

P. malariae infections
Daraprim Tablets (Pyrimethamine) GlaxoSmithKline 1400

P. melaninogenicus, endometritis
Timentin ADD-Vantage (Clavulanate Potassium, Ticarcillin Disodium) GlaxoSmithKline 1606
Timentin Injection Galaxy Container (Clavulanate Potassium, Ticarcillin Disodium) GlaxoSmithKline 1609
Timentin IV Infusion (Clavulanate Potassium, Ticarcillin Disodium) GlaxoSmithKline 1603

P. melaninogenicus, infections
Timentin ADD-Vantage (Clavulanate Potassium, Ticarcillin Disodium) GlaxoSmithKline 1606
Timentin Injection Galaxy Container (Clavulanate Potassium, Ticarcillin Disodium) GlaxoSmithKline 1609
Timentin IV Infusion (Clavulanate Potassium, Ticarcillin Disodium) GlaxoSmithKline 1603

P. mirabilis bone and joint infections
Rocephin Injectable Vials, ADD-Vantage, Galaxy, Bulk (Ceftriaxone Sodium) Roche 2642

P. mirabilis genitourinary tract infections
Amoxil Capsules (Amoxicillin) GlaxoSmithKline 1305
Amoxil Chewable Tablets (Amoxicillin) GlaxoSmithKline 1305
Amoxil Pediatric Drops for Oral Suspension (Amoxicillin) GlaxoSmithKline 1305
Amoxil Powder for Oral Suspension (Amoxicillin) GlaxoSmithKline 1305
Amoxil Tablets (Amoxicillin) GlaxoSmithKline 1305

P. mirabilis gynecologic infections
Amoxil Capsules (Amoxicillin) GlaxoSmithKline 1305
Amoxil Chewable Tablets (Amoxicillin) GlaxoSmithKline 1305
Amoxil Pediatric Drops for Oral Suspension (Amoxicillin) GlaxoSmithKline 1305
Amoxil Powder for Oral Suspension (Amoxicillin) GlaxoSmithKline 1305
Amoxil Tablets (Amoxicillin) GlaxoSmithKline 1305

P. mirabilis infections
Amoxil Capsules (Amoxicillin) GlaxoSmithKline 1305
Amoxil Chewable Tablets (Amoxicillin) GlaxoSmithKline 1305
Amoxil Pediatric Drops for Oral Suspension (Amoxicillin) GlaxoSmithKline 1305
Amoxil Powder for Oral Suspension (Amoxicillin) GlaxoSmithKline 1305
Amoxil Tablets (Amoxicillin) GlaxoSmithKline 1305
Avelox (Moxifloxacin Hydrochloride) Schering 2803
Cipro I.V. (Ciprofloxacin) Schering 2817
Cipro (Ciprofloxacin) Schering 2810
Fortaz (Ceftazidime) GlaxoSmithKline 1450
Levaquin (Levofloxacin) Ortho-McNeil 2416
Levaquin in 5% Dextrose Injection (Levofloxacin) Ortho-McNeil 2416
Merrem I.V. (Meropenem) AstraZeneca Pharmaceuticals 684
Noroxin Tablets (Norfloxacin) Merck 2069
Rocephin Injectable Vials, ADD-Vantage, Galaxy, Bulk (Ceftriaxone Sodium) Roche 2642
Suprax for Oral Suspension (Cefixime) Lupin 1891
Suprax Tablets (Cefixime) Lupin 1891

P. mirabilis infections, ocular
Ofloxacin Ophthalmic Solution 0.3% (Ofloxacin) Bausch & Lomb .... ⊙243
Zylet Ophthalmic Suspension (Loteprednol Etabonate, Tobramycin) Bausch & Lomb .... ⊙247

P. mirabilis intra-abdominal infections
Avelox (Moxifloxacin Hydrochloride) Schering 2803
Cipro I.V. (Ciprofloxacin) Schering 2817
Cipro (Ciprofloxacin) Schering 2810

P. mirabilis lower respiratory tract infections
Cipro I.V. (Ciprofloxacin) Schering 2817
Cipro (Ciprofloxacin) Schering 2810
Fortaz (Ceftazidime) GlaxoSmithKline 1450
Rocephin Injectable Vials, ADD-Vantage, Galaxy, Bulk (Ceftriaxone Sodium) Roche 2642

P. mirabilis prostatitis
Amoxil Capsules (Amoxicillin) GlaxoSmithKline 1305
Amoxil Chewable Tablets (Amoxicillin) GlaxoSmithKline 1305
Amoxil Pediatric Drops for Oral Suspension (Amoxicillin) GlaxoSmithKline 1305
Amoxil Powder for Oral Suspension (Amoxicillin) GlaxoSmithKline 1305
Amoxil Tablets (Amoxicillin) GlaxoSmithKline 1305
Cipro I.V. (Ciprofloxacin) Schering 2817
Cipro (Ciprofloxacin) Schering 2810

P. mirabilis skin and skin structure infections
Cipro I.V. (Ciprofloxacin) Schering 2817
Cipro (Ciprofloxacin) Schering 2810
Fortaz (Ceftazidime) GlaxoSmithKline 1450
Invanz for Injection (Ertapenem) Merck 2029
Levaquin (Levofloxacin) Ortho-McNeil 2416
Levaquin in 5% Dextrose Injection (Levofloxacin) Ortho-McNeil 2416
Merrem I.V. (Meropenem) AstraZeneca Pharmaceuticals 684

(▣ Described in PDR® For Nonprescription Drugs)

(⊙ Described in PDR® For Ophthalmic Medicines)

Rocephin Injectable Vials, ADD-Vantage, Galaxy, Bulk (Ceftriaxone Sodium) Roche 2642

P. mirabilis urinary tract infections
Amoxil Capsules (Amoxicillin) GlaxoSmithKline 1305
Amoxil Chewable Tablets (Amoxicillin) GlaxoSmithKline 1305
Amoxil Pediatric Drops for Oral Suspension (Amoxicillin) GlaxoSmithKline 1305
Amoxil Powder for Oral Suspension (Amoxicillin) GlaxoSmithKline 1305
Amoxil Tablets (Amoxicillin) GlaxoSmithKline 1305
Cipro I.V. (Ciprofloxacin) Schering 2817
Cipro (Ciprofloxacin) Schering 2810
Cipro XR Tablets (Ciprofloxacin) Schering 2823
Doribax Injection (Doripenem) Ortho-McNeil 2400
Fortaz (Ceftazidime) GlaxoSmithKline 1450
Levaquin (Levofloxacin) Ortho-McNeil 2416
Levaquin in 5% Dextrose Injection (Levofloxacin) Ortho-McNeil 2416
Noroxin Tablets (Norfloxacin) Merck . 2069
Rocephin Injectable Vials, ADD-Vantage, Galaxy, Bulk (Ceftriaxone Sodium) Roche 2642
Suprax for Oral Suspension (Cefixime) Lupin 1891
Suprax Tablets (Cefixime) Lupin 1891

P. ovale infections
Daraprim Tablets (Pyrimethamine) GlaxoSmithKline 1400

P. vivax infections
Daraprim Tablets (Pyrimethamine) GlaxoSmithKline 1400

P. vulgaris infections
Cipro I.V. (Ciprofloxacin) Schering 2817
Cipro (Ciprofloxacin) Schering 2810
Noroxin Tablets (Norfloxacin) Merck . 2069
Primaxin I.V. (Cilastatin Sodium, Imipenem) Merck 2083
Rocephin Injectable Vials, ADD-Vantage, Galaxy, Bulk (Ceftriaxone Sodium) Roche 2642

P. vulgaris infections, ocular
Zylet Ophthalmic Suspension (Loteprednol Etabonate, Tobramycin) Bausch & Lomb .... ⊙247

P. vulgaris skin and skin structure infections
Cipro I.V. (Ciprofloxacin) Schering 2817
Cipro (Ciprofloxacin) Schering 2810
Primaxin I.V. (Cilastatin Sodium, Imipenem) Merck 2083

P. vulgaris urinary tract infections
Gantrisin Pediatric Suspension (Acetyl Sulfisoxazole) Roche 2638
Noroxin Tablets (Norfloxacin) Merck . 2069
Primaxin I.V. (Cilastatin Sodium, Imipenem) Merck 2083
Rocephin Injectable Vials, ADD-Vantage, Galaxy, Bulk (Ceftriaxone Sodium) Roche 2642

Paget's disease of bone
Actonel Tablets (Risedronate Sodium) Procter & Gamble Pharmaceuticals 2568
Didronel Tablets (Etidronate Disodium) Procter & Gamble Pharmaceuticals 2583
Fosamax (Alendronate Sodium) Merck 2005
Miacalcin Injection (Calcitonin-Salmon) Novartis 2273
Reclast Injection (Zoledronic acid) Novartis 2291

Pain, acute
Flector Patch (Diclofenac Epolamine) Alpharma 561

Pain, arthritic, minor
Motrin IB Tablets and Caplets (Ibuprofen) McNeil Consumer 1900
ThermaCare Therapeutic Heat Wraps (Device) Procter & Gamble 2566
Traumeel Injection Solution (Homeopathic Formulations) Heel 1725
Regular Strength Tylenol Tablets (Acetaminophen) McNeil Consumer 1915
Tylenol 8 Hour Extended Release Caplets (Acetaminophen) McNeil Consumer 1915
Extra Strength Tylenol Caplets, Cool Caplets, and EZ Tabs (Acetaminophen) McNeil Consumer 1915
Extra Strength Tylenol Adult Rapid Blast Liquid (Acetaminophen) McNeil Consumer 1915
Extra Strength Tylenol Rapid Release Gels (Acetaminophen) McNeil Consumer 1915
Tylenol Arthritis Pain Extended Release Geltabs/Caplets (Acetaminophen) McNeil Consumer 1915

Pain, arthritic, relief of
Zeel Injection Solution (Homeopathic Formulations) Heel 1726

Pain, breakthrough
Fentora Tablets (Fentanyl Citrate) Cephalon 968

Pain, cancer
Fentora Tablets (Fentanyl Citrate) Cephalon 968

Pain, cancer, opioid-tolerant patients
Actiq (Fentanyl Citrate) Cephalon 959

Pain, chronic, moderate to moderately severe
Ultram ER Extended-Release Tablets (Tramadol Hydrochloride) Ortho-McNeil 2428

Pain, dental
Celebrex Capsules (Celecoxib) Searle 2979
Hurricaine Topical Anesthetic (Benzocaine) Beutlich 815
Hyland's Teething Gel (Homeopathic Formulations) Standard Homeopathic .... ▣621
Hyland's Teething Tablets (Belladonna Alkaloids, Homeopathic Formulations) Standard Homeopathic .... ▣621
Children's Motrin Oral Suspension (Ibuprofen) McNeil Consumer 1901
Children's Motrin Non-Staining Dye-Free Oral Suspension (Ibuprofen) McNeil Consumer 1901
Infants' Motrin Concentrated Drops (Ibuprofen) McNeil Consumer 1901
Infants' Motrin Non-Staining Dye-Free Concentrated Drops (Ibuprofen) McNeil Consumer 1901
Junior Strength Motrin Caplets and Chewable Tablets (Ibuprofen) McNeil Consumer 1901
Regular Strength Tylenol Tablets (Acetaminophen) McNeil Consumer 1915
Tylenol 8 Hour Extended Release Caplets (Acetaminophen) McNeil Consumer 1915
Extra Strength Tylenol Caplets, Cool Caplets, and EZ Tabs (Acetaminophen) McNeil Consumer 1915
Extra Strength Tylenol Adult Rapid Blast Liquid (Acetaminophen) McNeil Consumer 1915
Extra Strength Tylenol Rapid Release Gels (Acetaminophen) McNeil Consumer 1915
Tylenol Arthritis Pain Extended Release Geltabs/Caplets (Acetaminophen) McNeil Consumer 1915

Pain, general
Benadryl Allergy & Cold Kapgels (Acetaminophen, Diphenhydramine Hydrochloride, Phenylephrine Hydrochloride) McNeil Consumer 1895
Benadryl Allergy & Sinus Headache Kapgels (Acetaminophen, Diphenhydramine Hydrochloride, Phenylephrine Hydrochloride) McNeil Consumer 1895
Benadryl Severe Allergy & Sinus Headache Caplets (Acetaminophen, Diphenhydramine Hydrochloride, Phenylephrine Hydrochloride) McNeil Consumer 1897
Motrin IB Tablets and Caplets (Ibuprofen) McNeil Consumer 1900
Children's Motrin Oral Suspension (Ibuprofen) McNeil Consumer 1901
Children's Motrin Non-Staining Dye-Free Oral Suspension (Ibuprofen) McNeil Consumer 1901
Infants' Motrin Concentrated Drops (Ibuprofen) McNeil Consumer 1901
Infants' Motrin Non-Staining Dye-Free Concentrated Drops (Ibuprofen) McNeil Consumer 1901
St. Joseph 81 mg Aspirin Chewable and Enteric Coated Tablets (Aspirin) McNeil Consumer 1903
Sinutab Sinus Caplets (Acetaminophen, Phenylephrine Hydrochloride) McNeil Consumer 1905
Sudafed PE Nighttime Cold Caplets (Acetaminophen, Diphenhydramine Hydrochloride, Phenylephrine Hydrochloride) McNeil Consumer 1907
Sudafed PE Severe Cold Caplets (Acetaminophen, Diphenhydramine Hydrochloride, Phenylephrine Hydrochloride) McNeil Consumer 1908
Sudafed PE Sinus Headache Caplets (Acetaminophen, Phenylephrine Hydrochloride) McNeil Consumer 1908
ThermaCare Therapeutic Heat Wraps (Device) Procter & Gamble 2566
Traumeel Injection Solution (Homeopathic Formulations) Heel 1725
Regular Strength Tylenol Tablets (Acetaminophen) McNeil Consumer 1915
Tylenol 8 Hour Extended Release Caplets (Acetaminophen) McNeil Consumer 1915
Extra Strength Tylenol Caplets, Cool Caplets, and EZ Tabs (Acetaminophen) McNeil Consumer 1915
Extra Strength Tylenol Adult Rapid Blast Liquid (Acetaminophen) McNeil Consumer 1915
Extra Strength Tylenol PM Caplets, Geltabs, Liquid, and Rapid Release Gels (Acetaminophen, Diphenhydramine Hydrochloride) McNeil Consumer 1915
Extra Strength Tylenol Rapid Release Gels (Acetaminophen) McNeil Consumer 1915
Tylenol Allergy Multi-Symptom Caplets with Cool Burst and Rapid Release Gelcaps (Acetaminophen, Chlorpheniramine Maleate, Phenylephrine Hydrochloride) McNeil Consumer 1916
Tylenol Allergy Multi-Symptom Nighttime Caplets with Cool Burst (Acetaminophen, Diphenhydramine Hydrochloride, Phenylephrine Hydrochloride) McNeil Consumer 1916
Tylenol Severe Allergy Caplets (Acetaminophen, Diphenhydramine Hydrochloride) McNeil Consumer 1916
Tylenol Chest Congestion Caplets with Cool Burst (Acetaminophen, Guaifenesin) McNeil Consumer 1910
Tylenol Chest Congestion Liquid with Cool Burst (Acetaminophen, Guaifenesin) McNeil Consumer 1910
Children's Tylenol Plus Cold Suspension Liquid (Acetaminophen, Chlorpheniramine Maleate, Phenylephrine Hydrochloride) McNeil Consumer 1912
Children's Tylenol Plus Cold & Allergy Suspension Liquid (Acetaminophen, Diphenhydramine Hydrochloride, Phenylephrine Hydrochloride) McNeil Consumer .. 1914
Children's Tylenol Plus Cough & Runny Nose Suspension Liquid (Acetaminophen, Chlorpheniramine Maleate, Dextromethorphan Hydrobromide) McNeil Consumer .. 1912
Children's Tylenol Plus Cough & Sore Throat Suspension Liquid (Acetaminophen, Dextromethorphan Hydrobromide) McNeil Consumer 1912
Children's Tylenol Plus Flu Suspension Liquid (Acetaminophen, Chlorpheniramine Maleate, Dextromethorphan Hydrobromide, Phenylephrine Hydrochloride) McNeil Consumer 1914
Children's Tylenol Plus Multi-Symptom Cold Suspension Liquid (Acetaminophen, Chlorpheniramine Maleate, Dextromethorphan Hydrobromide, Phenylephrine Hydrochloride) McNeil Consumer 1912
Tylenol Cold Severe Congestion Daytime Caplets with Cool Burst (Acetaminophen, Dextromethorphan Hydrobromide, Guaifenesin, Pseudoephedrine Hydrochloride) McNeil Consumer 1912
Tylenol Cold Head Congestion Daytime Caplets with Cool Burst (Acetaminophen, Dextromethorphan Hydrobromide, Phenylephrine Hydrochloride) McNeil Consumer 1910
Tylenol Cold Head Congestion Nighttime Caplets with Cool Burst (Acetaminophen, Chlorpheniramine Maleate, Dextromethorphan Hydrobromide, Phenylephrine Hydrochloride) McNeil Consumer 1910
Tylenol Cold Head Congestion Severe Daytime Caplets with Cool Burst (Acetaminophen, Dextromethorphan Hydrobromide, Guaifenesin, Phenylephrine Hydrochloride) McNeil Consumer .. 1910
Tylenol Sinus Congestion & Pain Daytime Caplets with Cool Burst and Gelcaps (Acetaminophen, Phenylephrine Hydrochloride) McNeil Consumer 1917
Tylenol Sinus Congestion & Pain Nighttime Caplets with Cool Burst (Acetaminophen, Chlorpheniramine Maleate, Phenylephrine Hydrochloride) McNeil Consumer 1917
Tylenol Sinus Congestion & Pain Severe Caplets with Cool Burst (Acetaminophen, Guaifenesin, Phenylephrine Hydrochloride) McNeil Consumer 1917
Tylenol Sinus Severe Congestion Caplets with Cool Burst (Acetaminophen, Guaifenesin, Pseudoephedrine Hydrochloride) McNeil Consumer 1917
Women's Tylenol Menstrual Relief Caplets (Acetaminophen, Pamabrom) McNeil Consumer 1919

Pain, intractable chronic
(*see under* Pain, severe)

Pain, joint
Salonpas Aqua-Patch (Menthol) Hisamitsu .... ▣610
Salonpas Arthritis Pain Patches (Menthol, Methyl Salicylate) Hisamitsu .... ▣608
Salonpas Gel (Menthol, Methyl Salicylate) Hisamitsu .... ▣609
Salonpas Gel-Patch Hot Soothing (Capsicum Extract, Menthol) Hisamitsu .... ▣609
Salonpas Pain Relief Patch (Menthol, Methyl Salicylate) Hisamitsu .... ▣608
Salonpas-Hot Patch (Capsicum Extract) Hisamitsu .... ▣609
ThermaCare Therapeutic Heat Wraps (Device) Procter & Gamble 2566

Pain, major surgical
DepoDur Injection (Morphine Sulfate) EKR 1095

Pain, menstrual
Motrin IB Tablets and Caplets (Ibuprofen) McNeil Consumer 1900
ThermaCare Therapeutic Heat Wraps (Device) Procter & Gamble 2566

Regular Strength Tylenol Tablets (Acetaminophen) McNeil Consumer 1915
Tylenol 8 Hour Extended Release Caplets (Acetaminophen) McNeil Consumer 1915
Extra Strength Tylenol Caplets, Cool Caplets, and EZ Tabs (Acetaminophen) McNeil Consumer 1915
Extra Strength Tylenol Adult Rapid Blast Liquid (Acetaminophen) McNeil Consumer 1915
Extra Strength Tylenol Rapid Release Gels (Acetaminophen) McNeil Consumer 1915
Tylenol Arthritis Pain Extended Release Geltabs/Caplets (Acetaminophen) McNeil Consumer 1915
Women's Tylenol Menstrual Relief Caplets (Acetaminophen, Pamabrom) McNeil Consumer 1919

Pain, mild
Junior Strength Motrin Caplets and Chewable Tablets (Ibuprofen) McNeil Consumer 1901
Regular Strength Tylenol Tablets (Acetaminophen) McNeil Consumer 1915
Tylenol 8 Hour Extended Release Caplets (Acetaminophen) McNeil Consumer 1915
Extra Strength Tylenol Caplets, Cool Caplets, and EZ Tabs (Acetaminophen) McNeil Consumer 1915
Extra Strength Tylenol Adult Rapid Blast Liquid (Acetaminophen) McNeil Consumer 1915
Extra Strength Tylenol Rapid Release Gels (Acetaminophen) McNeil Consumer 1915
Tylenol Cough & Sore Throat Daytime Liquid with Cool Burst (Acetaminophen, Dextromethorphan Hydrobromide) McNeil Consumer 1918
Tylenol Sore Throat Nighttime Liquid with Cool Burst (Acetaminophen, Diphenhydramine Hydrochloride) McNeil Consumer 1918

Pain, mild to moderate
Anaprox Tablets (Naproxen Sodium) Roche 2632
Anaprox DS Tablets (Naproxen Sodium) Roche 2632
Nalfon Capsules (Fenoprofen Calcium) Pedinol 2508
Naprosyn Suspension (Naproxen) Roche 2632
Naprosyn Tablets (Naproxen) Roche 2632

Pain, mild to moderate, acute musculo-skeletal
Amrix Capsules (Cyclobenzaprine Hydrochloride) Cephalon 966
Soma Tablets (Carisoprodol) Meda 1931

Pain, mild to moderately severe
Tylenol with Codeine Tablets (Acetaminophen, Codeine Phosphate) Ortho-McNeil 2427

Pain, moderate
Opana Tablets (Oxymorphone Hydrochloride) Endo 1117
Opana ER Tablets (Oxymorphone Hydrochloride) Endo 1121

Pain, moderate to moderately severe
Lortab 5/500 Tablets (Acetaminophen, Hydrocodone Bitartrate) UCB, Inc. 3143
Lortab 7.5/500 Tablets (Acetaminophen, Hydrocodone Bitartrate) UCB, Inc. 3144
Lortab 10/500 Tablets (Acetaminophen, Hydrocodone Bitartrate) UCB, Inc. 3144
OxyIR Capsules (Oxycodone Hydrochloride) Purdue Pharma 2593
Percocet Tablets (Acetaminophen, Oxycodone Hydrochloride) Endo 1127
Percodan Tablets (Aspirin, Oxycodone Hydrochloride) Endo 1130
Vicodin Tablets (Acetaminophen, Hydrocodone Bitartrate) Abbott 529
Vicodin ES Tablets (Acetaminophen, Hydrocodone Bitartrate) Abbott 530
Vicodin HP Tablets (Acetaminophen, Hydrocodone Bitartrate) Abbott 531
Zydone Tablets (Acetaminophen, Hydrocodone Bitartrate) Endo 1132

Pain, moderate to severe
Avinza Capsules (Morphine Sulfate) King 1772
Celebrex Capsules (Celecoxib) Searle 2979
Duragesic Transdermal System (Fentanyl) Ortho-McNeil 2405
MS Contin Tablets (Morphine Sulfate) Purdue Pharma 2585
Opana Tablets (Oxymorphone Hydrochloride) Endo 1117
Opana ER Tablets (Oxymorphone Hydrochloride) Endo 1121
OxyContin Tablets (Oxycodone Hydrochloride) Purdue Pharma 2589
Vicoprofen Tablets (Hydrocodone Bitartrate, Ibuprofen) Abbott 533

Pain, muscular, temporary relief of
Motrin IB Tablets and Caplets (Ibuprofen) McNeil Consumer 1900
Thera-Gesic Creme (Menthol, Methyl Salicylate) Mission .... ▣610
ThermaCare Therapeutic Heat Wraps (Device) Procter & Gamble 2566
Traumeel Injection Solution (Homeopathic Formulations) Heel 1725
Regular Strength Tylenol Tablets (Acetaminophen) McNeil Consumer 1915
Tylenol 8 Hour Extended Release Caplets (Acetaminophen) McNeil Consumer 1915
Extra Strength Tylenol Caplets, Cool Caplets, and EZ Tabs (Acetaminophen) McNeil Consumer 1915
Extra Strength Tylenol Adult Rapid Blast Liquid (Acetaminophen) McNeil Consumer 1915
Extra Strength Tylenol Rapid Release Gels (Acetaminophen) McNeil Consumer 1915
Tylenol Arthritis Pain Extended Release Geltabs/Caplets (Acetaminophen) McNeil Consumer 1915
Tylenol Sore Throat Daytime Liquid with Cool Burst (Acetaminophen) McNeil Consumer 1918

Pain, neuropathic, associated with diabetic peripheral neuropathy
Cymbalta Delayed-Release Capsules (Duloxetine Hydrochloride) Lilly 1801
Lyrica Capsules (Pregabalin) Pfizer 2527

Pain, ocular
Durezol Ophthalmic Emulsion (Difluprednate) Sirion .... ⊙275

Pain, oral
Hurricaine Topical Anesthetic (Benzocaine) Beutlich 815

Pain, postoperative, relief of
Celebrex Capsules (Celecoxib) Searle 2979
Durezol Ophthalmic Emulsion (Difluprednate) Sirion .... ⊙275
Ionsys Transdermal System (Fentanyl) Ortho-McNeil 2410
Voltaren Ophthalmic Solution (Diclofenac Sodium) Novartis 2336

Pain, rheumatic
Traumeel Injection Solution (Homeopathic Formulations) Heel 1725

Pain, severe
Opana Tablets (Oxymorphone Hydrochloride) Endo 1117
Opana ER Tablets (Oxymorphone Hydrochloride) Endo 1121

Pain, teething
(*see under* Pain, dental)

Pain, tooth
Motrin IB Tablets and Caplets (Ibuprofen) McNeil Consumer 1900
Regular Strength Tylenol Tablets (Acetaminophen) McNeil Consumer 1915
Tylenol 8 Hour Extended Release Caplets (Acetaminophen) McNeil Consumer 1915
Extra Strength Tylenol Caplets, Cool Caplets, and EZ Tabs (Acetaminophen) McNeil Consumer 1915
Extra Strength Tylenol Adult Rapid Blast Liquid (Acetaminophen) McNeil Consumer 1915
Extra Strength Tylenol Rapid Release Gels (Acetaminophen) McNeil Consumer 1915
Tylenol Arthritis Pain Extended Release Geltabs/Caplets (Acetaminophen) McNeil Consumer 1915
Children's Tylenol Suspension Liquid (Acetaminophen) McNeil Consumer 1909
Children's Tylenol Meltaways (Acetaminophen) McNeil Consumer 1909
Concentrated Tylenol Infants' Drops (Acetaminophen) McNeil Consumer 1909

Pain, topical relief of
Salonpas Aqua-Patch (Menthol) Hisamitsu .... ▣610
Salonpas Arthritis Pain Patches (Menthol, Methyl Salicylate) Hisamitsu .... ▣608
Salonpas Gel (Menthol, Methyl Salicylate) Hisamitsu .... ▣609
Salonpas Gel-Patch Hot Soothing (Capsicum Extract, Menthol) Hisamitsu .... ▣609
Salonpas Pain Relief Patch (Menthol, Methyl Salicylate) Hisamitsu .... ▣608
Salonpas-Hot Patch (Capsicum Extract) Hisamitsu .... ▣609
Smile's Prid Salve (Homeopathic Formulations) Standard Homeopathic .... ▣620
Tahitian Noni Leaf Serum Soothing Gel (Herbal Medicines, unspecified) Tahitian Noni International .... ▣632
Thera-Gesic Creme (Menthol, Methyl Salicylate) Mission .... ▣610
ThermaCare Therapeutic Heat Wraps (Device) Procter & Gamble 2566
Topricin Pain Relief and Healing Cream (Homeopathic Formulations) Topical BioMedics .... ▣621
Regular Strength Tylenol Tablets (Acetaminophen) McNeil Consumer 1915
Tylenol 8 Hour Extended Release Caplets (Acetaminophen) McNeil Consumer 1915
Extra Strength Tylenol Caplets, Cool Caplets, and EZ Tabs (Acetaminophen) McNeil Consumer 1915
Extra Strength Tylenol Adult Rapid Blast Liquid (Acetaminophen) McNeil Consumer 1915
Extra Strength Tylenol Rapid Release Gels (Acetaminophen) McNeil Consumer 1915
Tylenol Arthritis Pain Extended Release Geltabs/Caplets (Acetaminophen) McNeil Consumer 1915

Pain associated with arthritis, topical
(*see under* Pain, topical relief of)

Pain associated with sports injuries
(*see under* Pain, topical relief of)

Pain associated with upper respiratory infection
Motrin IB Tablets and Caplets (Ibuprofen) McNeil Consumer 1900
Children's Motrin Oral Suspension (Ibuprofen) McNeil Consumer 1901
Children's Motrin Non-Staining Dye-Free Oral Suspension (Ibuprofen) McNeil Consumer 1901
Children's Motrin Cold Oral Suspension (Ibuprofen, Pseudoephedrine Hydrochloride) McNeil Consumer 1899
Infants' Motrin Concentrated Drops (Ibuprofen) McNeil Consumer 1901
Infants' Motrin Non-Staining Dye-Free Concentrated Drops (Ibuprofen) McNeil Consumer 1901
Junior Strength Motrin Caplets and Chewable Tablets (Ibuprofen) McNeil Consumer 1901
Sudafed PE Cold & Cough Caplets (Acetaminophen, Dextromethorphan Hydrobromide, Guaifenesin, Phenylephrine Hydrochloride) McNeil Consumer 1907
Regular Strength Tylenol Tablets (Acetaminophen) McNeil Consumer 1915
Tylenol 8 Hour Extended Release Caplets (Acetaminophen) McNeil Consumer 1915
Extra Strength Tylenol Caplets, Cool Caplets, and EZ Tabs (Acetaminophen) McNeil Consumer 1915
Extra Strength Tylenol Adult Rapid Blast Liquid (Acetaminophen) McNeil Consumer 1915
Extra Strength Tylenol Rapid Release Gels (Acetaminophen) McNeil Consumer 1915
Tylenol Arthritis Pain Extended Release Geltabs/Caplets (Acetaminophen) McNeil Consumer 1915
Tylenol Chest Congestion Caplets with Cool Burst (Acetaminophen, Guaifenesin) McNeil Consumer 1910
Tylenol Chest Congestion Liquid with Cool Burst (Acetaminophen, Guaifenesin) McNeil Consumer 1910
Children's Tylenol Plus Cold Suspension Liquid (Acetaminophen, Chlorpheniramine Maleate, Phenylephrine Hydrochloride) McNeil Consumer 1912
Children's Tylenol Plus Cough & Runny Nose Suspension Liquid (Acetaminophen, Chlorpheniramine Maleate, Dextromethorphan Hydrobromide) McNeil Consumer 1912
Children's Tylenol Plus Cough & Sore Throat Suspension Liquid (Acetaminophen, Dextromethorphan Hydrobromide) McNeil Consumer 1912
Children's Tylenol Suspension Liquid (Acetaminophen) McNeil Consumer 1909
Children's Tylenol Meltaways (Acetaminophen) McNeil Consumer 1909
Children's Tylenol Plus Multi-Symptom Cold Suspension Liquid (Acetaminophen, Chlorpheniramine Maleate, Dextromethorphan Hydrobromide, Phenylephrine Hydrochloride) McNeil Consumer 1912
Tylenol Cold Head Congestion Daytime Caplets with Cool Burst (Acetaminophen, Dextromethorphan Hydrobromide, Phenylephrine Hydrochloride) McNeil Consumer 1910
Tylenol Cold Head Congestion Nighttime Caplets with Cool Burst (Acetaminophen, Chlorpheniramine Maleate, Dextromethorphan Hydrobromide, Phenylephrine Hydrochloride) McNeil Consumer 1910
Tylenol Cold Head Congestion Severe Daytime Caplets with Cool Burst (Acetaminophen, Dextromethorphan Hydrobromide, Guaifenesin, Phenylephrine Hydrochloride) McNeil Consumer 1910
Tylenol Cold Multi-Symptom Daytime Caplets with Cool Burst and Rapid Release Gels (Acetaminophen, Dextromethorphan Hydrobromide, Phenylephrine Hydrochloride) McNeil Consumer 1913
Tylenol Cold Multi-Symptom Daytime Liquid with Citrus Burst (Acetaminophen, Dextromethorphan Hydrobromide, Phenylephrine Hydrochloride) McNeil Consumer 1913
Tylenol Cold Multi-Symptom Nighttime Caplets with Cool Burst (Acetaminophen, Chlorpheniramine Maleate, Dextromethorphan Hydrobromide, Phenylephrine Hydrochloride) McNeil Consumer 1913

(▣ Described in PDR® For Nonprescription Drugs) (⊙ Described in PDR® For Ophthalmic Medicines)

Tylenol Cold Multi-Symptom Nighttime Liquid with Cool Burst (Acetaminophen, Dextromethorphan Hydrobromide, Doxylamine Succinate, Phenylephrine Hydrochloride) McNeil Consumer **1913**
Tylenol Cold Multi-Symptom Severe Caplets with Cool Burst (Acetaminophen, Dextromethorphan Hydrobromide, Guaifenesin, Phenylephrine Hydrochloride) McNeil Consumer **1913**
Tylenol Cold Multi-Symptom Severe Daytime Liquid with Citrus Burst (Acetaminophen, Dextromethorphan Hydrobromide, Guaifenesin, Phenylephrine Hydrochloride) McNeil Consumer **1913**
Tylenol Cough & Sore Throat Nighttime Liquid with Cool Burst (Acetaminophen, Dextromethorphan Hydrobromide, Doxylamine Succinate) McNeil Consumer **1918**
Concentrated Tylenol Infants' Drops (Acetaminophen) McNeil Consumer **1909**
Jr. Tylenol Meltaways (Acetaminophen) McNeil Consumer **1909**
Vicks DayQuil Cold & Flu Multi-Symptom Relief (Acetaminophen, Dextromethorphan Hydrobromide, Phenylephrine Hydrochloride) Procter & Gamble .... ▣**616**
Vicks DayQuil LiquiCaps (Acetaminophen, Dextromethorphan Hydrobromide, Phenylephrine Hydrochloride) Procter & Gamble .. **2567**
Vicks DayQuil Liquid (Acetaminophen, Dextromethorphan Hydrobromide, Phenylephrine Hydrochloride) Procter & Gamble **2567**
Vicks DayQuil Multi-Symptom Cold/Flu Relief (Acetaminophen, Dextromethorphan Hydrobromide, Phenylephrine Hydrochloride) Procter & Gamble **2567**
Vicks NyQuil Cold & Flu Multi-Symptom Relief (Acetaminophen, Dextromethorphan Hydrobromide, Doxylamine Succinate) Procter & Gamble .... ▣**617**
Vicks NyQuil LiquiCaps (Acetaminophen, Dextromethorphan Hydrobromide, Doxylamine Succinate, Pseudoephedrine Hydrochloride) Procter & Gamble **2567**
Vicks NyQuil Liquid (Acetaminophen, Dextromethorphan Hydrobromide, Doxylamine Succinate, Pseudoephedrine Hydrochloride) Procter & Gamble **2567**
Vicks NyQuil Multi-Symptom Cold/Flu Relief (Acetaminophen, Dextromethorphan Hydrobromide, Doxylamine Succinate, Pseudoephedrine Hydrochloride) Procter & Gamble **2567**

Pain due to common cold
(*see under* Pain associated with upper respiratory infection)

Palpebral conjunctiva inflammation
Blephamide Ophthalmic Ointment Allergan .... ⊙**217**
Blephamide Ophthalmic Suspension Allergan .... ⊙**216**
FML Ophthalmic Ointment (Fluorometholone) Allergan .... ⊙**223**
FML Ophthalmic Suspension (Fluorometholone) Allergan .... ⊙**224**
FML Forte Ophthalmic Suspension (Fluorometholone) Allergan .... ⊙**222**
Pred Forte Ophthalmic Suspension (Prednisolone Acetate) Allergan .... ⊙**227**
Pred-G Ophthalmic Ointment (Gentamicin Sulfate, Prednisolone Acetate) Allergan .... ⊙**229**
Pred-G Ophthalmic Suspension (Gentamicin Sulfate, Prednisolone Acetate) Allergan .... ⊙**228**
Zylet Ophthalmic Suspension (Loteprednol Etabonate, Tobramycin) Bausch & Lomb .... ⊙**247**

Pancreas, disseminated adenocarcinoma
(*see under* Carcinoma, pancreas)

Pancreatic cystic fibrosis
Viokase (Pancrelipase) Axcan Pharma **721**

Pancreatic insufficiency
Creon 5 Capsules (Pancrelipase) Solvay **3041**
Creon 10 Capsules (Pancrelipase) Solvay **3042**
Creon 20 Capsules (Pancrelipase) Solvay **3042**
Ultrase Capsules (Pancrelipase) Axcan Pharma **718**
Ultrase MT Capsules (Pancrelipase) Axcan Pharma **719**
Viokase (Pancrelipase) Axcan Pharma **721**

Panic disorder
Effexor XR Extended-Release Capsules (Venlafaxine Hydrochloride) Wyeth **3195**
Klonopin (Clonazepam) Roche **2639**
Paxil (Paroxetine Hydrochloride) GlaxoSmithKline **1535**
Paxil CR Controlled-Release Tablets (Paroxetine Hydrochloride) GlaxoSmithKline **1544**
Prozac Weekly Capsules (Fluoxetine Hydrochloride) Lilly **1852**
Prozac Pulvules and Liquid (Fluoxetine Hydrochloride) Lilly **1852**

Paralysis agitans
(*see under* Parkinson's disease)

Parkinson's disease
Azilect Tablets (Rasagiline Mesylate) Teva Neuroscience **3106**
Comtan Tablets (Entacapone) Novartis **2208**
Eldepryl Capsules (Selegiline Hydrochloride) Somerset **3052**
Mirapex Tablets (Pramipexole Dihydrochloride) Boehringer Ingelheim **857**
Requip Tablets (Ropinirole Hydrochloride) GlaxoSmithKline **1561**
Requip XL Tablets (Ropinirole Hydrochloride) GlaxoSmithKline **1568**
Stalevo Tablets (Carbidopa, Levodopa, Entacapone) Novartis ... **2309**

Parkinson's disease, adjunct to levodopa/carbidopa therapy in the management of
Azilect Tablets (Rasagiline Mesylate) Teva Neuroscience **3106**

Parkinson's disease, idiopathic
Azilect Tablets (Rasagiline Mesylate) Teva Neuroscience **3106**
Neupro Transdermal System (Rotigotine) UCB, Inc. **3149**

PCP
(*see under* Pneumocystis carinii pneumonia)

Pelvic cellulitis
(*see also under* Infections, gynecologic)
Fortaz (Ceftazidime) GlaxoSmithKline **1450**

Pelvic inflammatory disease
(*see also under* Infections, gynecologic)
E.E.S. (Erythromycin Ethylsuccinate) Abbott **433**
EryPed (Erythromycin Ethylsuccinate) Abbott **431**
Rocephin Injectable Vials, ADD-Vantage, Galaxy, Bulk (Ceftriaxone Sodium) Roche **2642**
Zosyn for Injection (Piperacillin Sodium, Tazobactam Sodium) Wyeth **3284**

Pemphigus, possibly effective in
Potaba (Aminobenzoate Potassium) Glenwood **1698**

Penicillin therapy, an adjuvant to
E.E.S. (Erythromycin Ethylsuccinate) Abbott **433**

Peptococcus species gynecologic infections
Primaxin I.V. (Cilastatin Sodium, Imipenem) Merck **2083**

Peptococcus species infections
Doribax Injection (Doripenem) Ortho-McNeil **2400**
Primaxin I.V. (Cilastatin Sodium, Imipenem) Merck **2083**

Peptococcus species intra-abdominal infections
Primaxin I.M. (Cilastatin Sodium, Imipenem) Merck **2080**
Primaxin I.V. (Cilastatin Sodium, Imipenem) Merck **2083**

Peptococcus species skin and skin structure infections
Primaxin I.V. (Cilastatin Sodium, Imipenem) Merck **2083**

Peptostreptococcus species endomyometritis
Invanz for Injection (Ertapenem) Merck **2029**

Peptostreptococcus species gynecologic infections
Primaxin I.M. (Cilastatin Sodium, Imipenem) Merck **2080**
Primaxin I.V. (Cilastatin Sodium, Imipenem) Merck **2083**

Peptostreptococcus species infections
Avelox (Moxifloxacin Hydrochloride) Schering **2803**
Invanz for Injection (Ertapenem) Merck **2029**
Merrem I.V. (Meropenem) AstraZeneca Pharmaceuticals **684**
Primaxin I.M. (Cilastatin Sodium, Imipenem) Merck **2080**
Primaxin I.V. (Cilastatin Sodium, Imipenem) Merck **2083**
Rocephin Injectable Vials, ADD-Vantage, Galaxy, Bulk (Ceftriaxone Sodium) Roche **2642**
Tygacil for Injection (Tigecycline) Wyeth **3276**

Peptostreptococcus species intra-abdominal infections
Avelox (Moxifloxacin Hydrochloride) Schering **2803**
Doribax Injection (Doripenem) Ortho-McNeil **2400**
Invanz for Injection (Ertapenem) Merck **2029**
Merrem I.V. (Meropenem) AstraZeneca Pharmaceuticals **684**
Primaxin I.M. (Cilastatin Sodium, Imipenem) Merck **2080**
Primaxin I.V. (Cilastatin Sodium, Imipenem) Merck **2083**
Rocephin Injectable Vials, ADD-Vantage, Galaxy, Bulk (Ceftriaxone Sodium) Roche **2642**
Tygacil for Injection (Tigecycline) Wyeth **3276**

Peptostreptococcus species peritonitis
Merrem I.V. (Meropenem) AstraZeneca Pharmaceuticals **684**

Peptostreptococcus species skin and skin structure infections
Invanz for Injection (Ertapenem) Merck **2029**
Merrem I.V. (Meropenem) AstraZeneca Pharmaceuticals **684**
Primaxin I.V. (Cilastatin Sodium, Imipenem) Merck **2083**
Rocephin Injectable Vials, ADD-Vantage, Galaxy, Bulk (Ceftriaxone Sodium) Roche **2642**

Percutaneous coronary intervention, adjunct in
Angiomax for Injection (Bivalirudin) The Medicines Company **1933**
ReoPro Vials (Abciximab) Lilly **1860**

Pericarditis, bacterial
Bicillin C-R Injectable Suspension (Penicillin G Benzathine, Penicillin G Procaine) King **1775**
Bicillin L-A Injection (Penicillin G Benzathine, Penicillin G Procaine) King **1777**

Periodontitis
Merrem I.V. (Meropenem) AstraZeneca Pharmaceuticals **684**

Peripheral blood progenitor cell transplantation
(*see under* Hematopoietic progenitor cells, mobilization of)

Peritonitis
(*see also under* Infections, intra-abdominal)
Bicillin C-R Injectable Suspension (Penicillin G Benzathine, Penicillin G Procaine) King **1775**
Bicillin L-A Injection (Penicillin G Benzathine, Penicillin G Procaine) King **1777**
Fortaz (Ceftazidime) GlaxoSmithKline **1450**
Timentin ADD-Vantage (Clavulanate Potassium, Ticarcillin Disodium) GlaxoSmithKline **1606**
Timentin Injection Galaxy Container (Clavulanate Potassium, Ticarcillin Disodium) GlaxoSmithKline **1609**
Timentin IV Infusion (Clavulanate Potassium, Ticarcillin Disodium) GlaxoSmithKline **1603**
Timentin Pharmacy Bulk Package (Clavulanate Potassium, Ticarcillin Disodium) GlaxoSmithKline **1613**

Peritonitis, candidal
Cancidas for Injection (Caspofungin acetate) Merck **1953**
Mycamine for Injection (Micafungin Sodium) Astellas **616**

Pertussis
E.E.S. (Erythromycin Ethylsuccinate) Abbott **433**
EryPed (Erythromycin Ethylsuccinate) Abbott **431**

Petit mal epilepsy
(*see under* Seizures, generalized, absence)

Peyronie's disease, possibly effective in
Potaba (Aminobenzoate Potassium) Glenwood **1698**

Pharyngitis, symptomatic relief of
Hurricaine Topical Anesthetic (Benzocaine) Beutlich **815**
Junior Strength Motrin Caplets and Chewable Tablets (Ibuprofen) McNeil Consumer **1901**

Pharyngitis, treatment of
Biaxin/Biaxin XL (Clarithromycin) Abbott **411**
Ceftin (Cefuroxime Axetil) GlaxoSmithKline **1380**
E.E.S. (Erythromycin Ethylsuccinate) Abbott **433**
EryPed (Erythromycin Ethylsuccinate) Abbott **431**
Omnicef Capsules (Cefdinir) Abbott .. **497**
Omnicef for Oral Suspension (Cefdinir) Abbott **497**
Suprax for Oral Suspension (Cefixime) Lupin **1891**
Suprax Tablets (Cefixime) Lupin **1891**

Pheochromocytoma
Demser Capsules (Metyrosine) Merck **1989**
Dibenzyline Capsules (Phenoxybenzamine Hydrochloride) WellSpring . **3188**

Philadelphia chromosome positive chronic myelogenous leukemia, acute phase
Tasigna Capsules (Nilotinib) Novartis **2316**

Philadelphia chromosome positive chronic myelogenous leukemia, chronic phase
Tasigna Capsules (Nilotinib) Novartis ... 2316

Phlegm, loosen
Sinutab Non-Drying Caplets (Guaifenesin, Phenylephrine Hydrochloride) McNeil Consumer .. 1905
Sudafed PE Cold & Cough Caplets (Acetaminophen, Dextromethorphan Hydrobromide, Guaifenesin, Phenylephrine Hydrochloride) McNeil Consumer ... 1907
Sudafed PE Non-Drying Sinus Caplets (Guaifenesin, Phenylephrine Hydrochloride) McNeil Consumer ... 1908
Tylenol Chest Congestion Caplets with Cool Burst (Acetaminophen, Guaifenesin) McNeil Consumer ... 1910
Tylenol Chest Congestion Liquid with Cool Burst (Acetaminophen, Guaifenesin) McNeil Consumer ... 1910
Tylenol Cold Severe Congestion Daytime Caplets with Cool Burst (Acetaminophen, Dextromethorphan Hydrobromide, Guaifenesin, Pseudoephedrine Hydrochloride) McNeil Consumer ... 1912
Tylenol Cold Head Congestion Severe Daytime Caplets with Cool Burst (Acetaminophen, Dextromethorphan Hydrobromide, Guaifenesin, Phenylephrine Hydrochloride) McNeil Consumer .. 1910
Tylenol Cold Multi-Symptom Severe Caplets with Cool Burst (Acetaminophen, Dextromethorphan Hydrobromide, Guaifenesin, Phenylephrine Hydrochloride) McNeil Consumer ... 1913
Tylenol Cold Multi-Symptom Severe Daytime Liquid with Citrus Burst (Acetaminophen, Dextromethorphan Hydrobromide, Guaifenesin, Phenylephrine Hydrochloride) McNeil Consumer ... 1913
Tylenol Sinus Congestion & Pain Severe Caplets with Cool Burst (Acetaminophen, Guaifenesin, Phenylephrine Hydrochloride) McNeil Consumer ... 1917
Tylenol Sinus Severe Congestion Caplets with Cool Burst (Acetaminophen, Guaifenesin, Pseudoephedrine Hydrochloride) McNeil Consumer ... 1917

Phosphorus deficiency
(*see under* Hypophosphatemia)

Photophobia
Voltaren Ophthalmic Solution (Diclofenac Sodium) Novartis ... 2336

Phycomycosis
(*see under* Zygomycosis)

Pinworm infestation
(*see under* Enterobiasis)

Pityrosporon orbiculare infections
Mentax Cream (Butenafine Hydrochloride) Mylan ... 2190

Plasmodium infection
(*see under* P. falciparum infections; P. malariae infections; P. ovale infections; P. vivax infections)

Pleural effusion, malignant
Alimta for Injection (Pemetrexed) Lilly ... 1786

PMDD
(*see under* Dysphoric disorder, premenstrual)

PMS
(*see under* Premenstrual syndrome, management of)

Pneumococcal disease, immunization against
Pneumovax 23 (Pneumococcal Vaccine, Polyvalent) Merck ... 2078
Prevnar (Pneumococcal vaccine, diphtheria conjugate) Wyeth ... 3241

Pneumocystis carinii pneumonia
Mepron Suspension (Atovaquone) GlaxoSmithKline ... 1526

Pneumonia
(*see also under* Infections, lower respiratory tract)
Avelox (Moxifloxacin Hydrochloride) Schering ... 2803
Biaxin/Biaxin XL (Clarithromycin) Abbott ... 411
Bicillin C-R Injectable Suspension (Penicillin G Benzathine, Penicillin G Procaine) King ... 1775
Bicillin L-A Injection (Penicillin G Benzathine, Penicillin G Procaine) King ... 1777
Fortaz (Ceftazidime) GlaxoSmithKline ... 1450
Invanz for Injection (Ertapenem) Merck ... 2029
Ketek Tablets (Telithromycin) sanofi-aventis ... 2744
Levaquin (Levofloxacin) Ortho-McNeil ... 2416
Levaquin in 5% Dextrose Injection (Levofloxacin) Ortho-McNeil ... 2416
Omnicef Capsules (Cefdinir) Abbott .. 497
Omnicef for Oral Suspension (Cefdinir) Abbott ... 497
Zinacef for Injection (Cefuroxime) GlaxoSmithKline ... 1678
Zinacef Injection (Cefuroxime) GlaxoSmithKline ... 1678
Zyvox (Linezolid) Pharmacia & Upjohn ... 2552

Pneumonia, community-acquired
Augmentin XR Extended Release Tablets (Amoxicillin, Clavulanate Potassium) GlaxoSmithKline ... 1333
Avelox (Moxifloxacin Hydrochloride) Schering ... 2803
Invanz for Injection (Ertapenem) Merck ... 2029
Ketek Tablets (Telithromycin) sanofi-aventis ... 2744
Levaquin (Levofloxacin) Ortho-McNeil ... 2416
Levaquin in 5% Dextrose Injection (Levofloxacin) Ortho-McNeil ... 2416
Zosyn for Injection (Piperacillin Sodium, Tazobactam Sodium) Wyeth ... 3284
Zyvox (Linezolid) Pharmacia & Upjohn ... 2552

Pneumonia, nosocomial
(*see also under* Infections, lower respiratory tract)
Cipro I.V. (Ciprofloxacin) Schering ... 2817
Levaquin (Levofloxacin) Ortho-McNeil ... 2416
Levaquin in 5% Dextrose Injection (Levofloxacin) Ortho-McNeil ... 2416
Zosyn for Injection (Piperacillin Sodium, Tazobactam Sodium) Wyeth ... 3284
Zyvox (Linezolid) Pharmacia & Upjohn ... 2552

Pneumonia, pneumocystis carinii
(*see under* Pneumocystis carinii pneumonia)

Pneumonococcal septic arthritis, acute
Bicillin C-R Injectable Suspension (Penicillin G Benzathine, Penicillin G Procaine) King ... 1775
Bicillin L-A Injection (Penicillin G Benzathine, Penicillin G Procaine) King ... 1777

Poliomyelitis, prevention of
(*see under* Immunization, poliovirus 1, 2, and 3)

Poliovirus types 1, 2, and 3, immunization against
(*see also under* Immunization, poliovirus 1, 2, and 3)
Pediarix Vaccine (Diphtheria & Tetanus Toxoids and Acellular Pertussis Vaccine Adsorbed, Hepatitis B Vaccine, Recombinant, Poliovirus Vaccine Inactivated) GlaxoSmithKline ... 1552

Poliovirus types 1, 2, and 3 vaccine
(*see also under* Immunization, poliovirus 1, 2, and 3)
Pediarix Vaccine (Diphtheria & Tetanus Toxoids and Acellular Pertussis Vaccine Adsorbed, Hepatitis B Vaccine, Recombinant, Poliovirus Vaccine Inactivated) GlaxoSmithKline ... 1552

Pollinosis
(*see also under* Rhinitis, seasonal allergic)
Benadryl Allergy & Sinus Headache Kapgels (Acetaminophen, Diphenhydramine Hydrochloride, Phenylephrine Hydrochloride) McNeil Consumer ... 1895
Benadryl Severe Allergy & Sinus Headache Caplets (Acetaminophen, Diphenhydramine Hydrochloride, Phenylephrine Hydrochloride) McNeil Consumer ... 1897
Benadryl Dye-Free Allergy Liqui-gels Softgels (Diphenhydramine Hydrochloride) McNeil Consumer .. 1897
Benadryl Allergy Kapgels (Diphenhydramine Hydrochloride) McNeil Consumer ... 1895
Benadryl Allergy Quick Dissolve Strips (Diphenhydramine Hydrochloride) McNeil Consumer ... 1896
Benadryl Allergy Ultratab Tablets (Diphenhydramine Hydrochloride) McNeil Consumer ... 1896
Children's Benadryl Dye-Free Allergy Liquid (Diphenhydramine Hydrochloride) McNeil Consumer .. 1897
Children's Benadryl Allergy Fastmelts (Diphenhydramine Hydrochloride) McNeil Consumer .. 1897
Children's Benadryl Allergy Liquid (Diphenhydramine Hydrochloride) McNeil Consumer ... 1898
Children's Benadryl Allergy Perfect Measure (Diphenhydramine Hydrochloride) McNeil Consumer .. 1896
Children's Benadryl-D Allergy & Sinus Liquid (Diphenhydramine Hydrochloride, Phenylephrine Hydrochloride) McNeil Consumer .. 1896
Benadryl-D Allergy & Sinus Tablet (Diphenhydramine Hydrochloride, Phenylephrine Hydrochloride) McNeil Consumer ... 1896
PediaCare Children's Allergy & Cold Liquid (Diphenhydramine Hydrochloride, Phenylephrine Hydrochloride) McNeil Consumer .. 1902
PediaCare Children's Allergy Liquid (Diphenhydramine Hydrochloride) McNeil Consumer ... 1902
PediaCare Children's Decongestant Liquid (Phenylephrine Hydrochloride) McNeil Consumer ... 1902
PediaCare Children's Liquid Multi-Symptom Cold (Dextromethorphan Hydrobromide, Phenylephrine Hydrochloride) McNeil Consumer ... 1902
Sudafed 12 Hour Nasal Decongestant Non-Drowsy Caplets (Pseudoephedrine Hydrochloride) McNeil Consumer ... 1909
Sudafed 24 Hour Non-Drowsy Nasal Decongestant Tablets (Pseudoephedrine Hydrochloride) McNeil Consumer ... 1906
Children's Sudafed Nasal Decongestant Liquid (Pseudoephedrine Hydrochloride) McNeil Consumer ... 1906
Children's Sudafed PE Cold & Cough Liquid (Dextromethorphan Hydrobromide, Phenylephrine Hydrochloride) McNeil Consumer .. 1907
Children's Sudafed PE Nasal Decongestant Liquid (Phenylephrine Hydrochloride) McNeil Consumer ... 1906
Sudafed Nasal Decongestant Tablets (Pseudoephedrine Hydrochloride) McNeil Consumer ... 1906
Sudafed OM Sinus Cold Moisturizing Nasal Spray (Oxymetazoline Hydrochloride) McNeil Consumer ... 1906
Sudafed OM Sinus Congestion Moisturizing Nasal Spray (Oxymetazoline Hydrochloride) McNeil Consumer ... 1906
Sudafed PE Nasal Decongestant Tablets (Phenylephrine Hydrochloride) McNeil Consumer ... 1907
Sudafed PE Nighttime Cold Caplets (Acetaminophen, Diphenhydramine Hydrochloride, Phenylephrine Hydrochloride) McNeil Consumer ... 1907
Sudafed PE Severe Cold Caplets (Acetaminophen, Diphenhydramine Hydrochloride, Phenylephrine Hydrochloride) McNeil Consumer ... 1908
Sudafed PE Sinus & Allergy Tablets (Chlorpheniramine Maleate, Phenylephrine Hydrochloride) McNeil Consumer ... 1908
Tylenol Allergy Multi-Symptom Caplets with Cool Burst and Rapid Release Gelcaps (Acetaminophen, Chlorpheniramine Maleate, Phenylephrine Hydrochloride) McNeil Consumer ... 1916
Tylenol Allergy Multi-Symptom Nighttime Caplets with Cool Burst (Acetaminophen, Diphenhydramine Hydrochloride, Phenylephrine Hydrochloride) McNeil Consumer ... 1916
Tylenol Severe Allergy Caplets (Acetaminophen, Diphenhydramine Hydrochloride) McNeil Consumer ... 1916
Tylenol Sinus Congestion & Pain Severe Caplets with Cool Burst (Acetaminophen, Guaifenesin, Phenylephrine Hydrochloride) McNeil Consumer ... 1917
Children's Zyrtec Allergy Syrup (Cetirizine Hydrochloride) McNeil Consumer ... 1920
Zyrtec-D Allergy & Congestion Extended-Release Tablets (Cetirizine Hydrochloride, Pseudoephedrine Hydrochloride) McNeil Consumer ... 1923

Polycythemia vera
Mustargen for Injection (Mechlorethamine Hydrochloride) Ovation ... 2492

Polyps, nasal, prevention of recurrence
Beconase AQ Nasal Spray (Beclomethasone Dipropionate Monohydrate) GlaxoSmithKline ... 1369

Polyps, nasal, treatment of
Nasonex Nasal Spray (Mometasone Furoate Monohydrate) Schering ... 2883

Porphyria, acute intermittent, amelioration of recurrent attacks of
Panhematin for Injection (Hemin) Ovation ... 2497

Porphyria variegata
Panhematin for Injection (Hemin) Ovation ... 2497

Porphyromonas asaccharolytica endomyometritis
Invanz for Injection (Ertapenem) Merck ... 2029

Porphyromonas asaccharolytica skin and structure infections
Invanz for Injection (Ertapenem) Merck ... 2029

Postnasal drip
(*see under* Cold, common, symptomatic relief of)

Post-traumatic stress disorder
(*see under* Stress disorder, post-traumatic)

Prader-Willi syndrome, growth failure due to
Genotropin Lyophilized Powder (Somatropin) Pharmacia & Upjohn 2547

Pregnancy, prevention of
Lybrel Tablets (Ethinyl Estradiol, Levonorgestrel) Wyeth 3204
Mircette Tablets (Desogestrel, Ethinyl Estradiol) Duramed 1034
Mirena Intrauterine System (Levonorgestrel) Bayer HealthCare Pharmaceuticals 779
NuvaRing (Etonogestrel, Ethinyl Estradiol) Schering 2897
Ortho-Cyclen Tablets (Ethinyl Estradiol, Norgestimate) Ortho Women's 2449
Ortho Evra Transdermal System (Norelgestromin, Ethinyl Estradiol) Ortho Women's 2437
Ortho Micronor Tablets (Norethindrone) Ortho Women's 2446
Ortho Tri-Cyclen Tablets (Ethinyl Estradiol, Norgestimate) Ortho Women's 2449
Ortho Tri-Cyclen Lo Tablets (Ethinyl Estradiol, Norgestimate) Ortho Women's 2458
ParaGard T 380A Intrauterine Copper Contraceptive (Copper, Intrauterine) Duramed 1041
Seasonique Tablets (Ethinyl Estradiol, Levonorgestrel) Duramed 1046
Yaz Tablets (Ethinyl Estradiol, Drospirenone) Bayer HealthCare Pharmaceuticals 805

Pregnancy, vitamin supplement for
(*see under* Vitamin deficiency, postpartum; Vitamin deficiency, prenatal)

Premenstrual, signs and symptoms, temporary relief of
Women's Tylenol Menstrual Relief Caplets (Acetaminophen, Pamabrom) McNeil Consumer 1919

Premenstrual dysphoric disorder
(*see under* Dysphoric disorder, premenstrual)

Premenstrual syndrome
(*see under* Premenstrual syndrome, management of)

Premenstrual syndrome, management of
(*see also under* Dysphoric disorder, premenstrual)
Awareness Female Balance (Herbals, Multiple) Awareness Corporation/Awareness Life .... ■ 624

Prevotella bivia endomyometritis
Invanz for Injection (Ertapenem) Merck 2029

Prevotella bivia skin and skin structure infections
Invanz for Injection (Ertapenem) Merck 2029

Proctitis, ulcerative
Canasa Rectal Suppositories (Mesalamine) Axcan Pharma 705

Promote the natural immune system of the body
SynergyDefense Capsules (Herbals, Multiple) Awareness Corporation/Awareness Life .... ■ 625

Propionibacterium acnes infections
Ofloxacin Ophthalmic Solution 0.3% (Ofloxacin) Bausch & Lomb .... ⊙ 243

Propionibacterium species gynecologic infections
Primaxin I.V. (Cilastatin Sodium, Imipenem) Merck 2083

Propionibacterium species infections
Primaxin I.V. (Cilastatin Sodium, Imipenem) Merck 2083

Propionibacterium species intra-abdominal infections
Primaxin I.V. (Cilastatin Sodium, Imipenem) Merck 2083

Prostatic cancer, palliative treatment of
(*see under* Carcinoma, prostate, palliative treatment of)

Prostatic hyperplasia, benign, symptomatic treatment
Avodart Soft Gelatin Capsules (Dutasteride) GlaxoSmithKline 1359
Flomax Capsules (Tamsulosin Hydrochloride) Boehringer Ingelheim 848
Proscar Tablets (Finasteride) Merck.. 2102
Uroxatral Tablets (Alfuzosin Hydrochloride) sanofi-aventis 2786

Prostatic hyperplasia, benign, symptomatic treatment, adjunctive therapy
Avodart Soft Gelatin Capsules (Dutasteride) GlaxoSmithKline 1359

Prostatitis
Cipro I.V. (Ciprofloxacin) Schering 2817
Cipro (Ciprofloxacin) Schering 2810
Levaquin (Levofloxacin) Ortho-McNeil 2416
Levaquin in 5% Dextrose Injection (Levofloxacin) Ortho-McNeil 2416
Noroxin Tablets (Norfloxacin) Merck . 2069

Proteus, indole-positive, infections
(*see under* Morganella morganii infections)

Proteus mirabilis
(*see under* P. mirabilis infections)

Proteus species gynecologic infections
Primaxin I.V. (Cilastatin Sodium, Imipenem) Merck 2083

Proteus species infections
Fortaz (Ceftazidime) GlaxoSmithKline 1450
Primaxin I.V. (Cilastatin Sodium, Imipenem) Merck 2083

Proteus species infections, ocular, indole-negative
Pred-G Ophthalmic Suspension (Gentamicin Sulfate, Prednisolone Acetate) Allergan .... ⊙ 228

Proteus species intra-abdominal infections
Primaxin I.V. (Cilastatin Sodium, Imipenem) Merck 2083

Proteus species skin and skin structure infections
Fortaz (Ceftazidime) GlaxoSmithKline 1450

Proteus species urinary tract infections
Doribax Injection (Doripenem) Ortho-McNeil 2400
Fortaz (Ceftazidime) GlaxoSmithKline 1450
Gantrisin Pediatric Suspension (Acetyl Sulfisoxazole) Roche 2638

Proteus vulgaris
(*see under* P. vulgaris infections)

Prothrombin deficiency, anticoagulant-induced
Mephyton Tablets (Vitamin K_1) Aton .. 700

Providencia rettgeri infections
Cipro I.V. (Ciprofloxacin) Schering 2817
Cipro (Ciprofloxacin) Schering 2810
Primaxin I.V. (Cilastatin Sodium, Imipenem) Merck 2083

Providencia rettgeri skin and skin structure infections
Primaxin I.V. (Cilastatin Sodium, Imipenem) Merck 2083

Providencia rettgeri urinary tract infections
Cipro I.V. (Ciprofloxacin) Schering 2817
Cipro (Ciprofloxacin) Schering 2810
Primaxin I.V. (Cilastatin Sodium, Imipenem) Merck 2083

Providencia stuartii infections
Cipro I.V. (Ciprofloxacin) Schering 2817
Cipro (Ciprofloxacin) Schering 2810

Providencia stuartii skin and skin structure infections
Cipro I.V. (Ciprofloxacin) Schering 2817
Cipro (Ciprofloxacin) Schering 2810

Pruritus
Hyland's Restful Legs Tablets (Homeopathic Formulations) Standard Homeopathic .... ■ 620

Pruritus, anogenital
Analpram-HC (Hydrocortisone Acetate, Pramoxine Hydrochloride) Ferndale 1140

Pruritus, pharyngeal
Actifed Cold & Allergy Tablets (Chlorpheniramine Maleate, Phenylephrine Hydrochloride) McNeil Consumer 1895
PediaCare Children's Allergy & Cold Liquid (Diphenhydramine Hydrochloride, Phenylephrine Hydrochloride) McNeil Consumer .. 1902
Sudafed PE Sinus & Allergy Tablets (Chlorpheniramine Maleate, Phenylephrine Hydrochloride) McNeil Consumer 1908

Pruritus, rhinal
Actifed Cold & Allergy Tablets (Chlorpheniramine Maleate, Phenylephrine Hydrochloride) McNeil Consumer 1895
PediaCare Children's Allergy & Cold Liquid (Diphenhydramine Hydrochloride, Phenylephrine Hydrochloride) McNeil Consumer .. 1902
Sudafed PE Sinus & Allergy Tablets (Chlorpheniramine Maleate, Phenylephrine Hydrochloride) McNeil Consumer 1908

Pruritus, rhinopharyngeal, symptomatic relief of
Allegra-D 12 Hour Extended-Release Tablets (Fexofenadine Hydrochloride, Pseudoephedrine Hydrochloride) sanofi-aventis 2687
Benadryl Allergy & Sinus Headache Kapgels (Acetaminophen, Diphenhydramine Hydrochloride, Phenylephrine Hydrochloride) McNeil Consumer 1895
Benadryl Severe Allergy & Sinus Headache Caplets (Acetaminophen, Diphenhydramine Hydrochloride, Phenylephrine Hydrochloride) McNeil Consumer 1897
Benadryl Dye-Free Allergy Liqui-gels Softgels (Diphenhydramine Hydrochloride) McNeil Consumer .. 1897
Benadryl Allergy Kapgels (Diphenhydramine Hydrochloride) McNeil Consumer 1895
Benadryl Allergy Quick Dissolve Strips (Diphenhydramine Hydrochloride) McNeil Consumer 1896
Benadryl Allergy Ultratab Tablets (Diphenhydramine Hydrochloride) McNeil Consumer 1896
Children's Benadryl Dye-Free Allergy Liquid (Diphenhydramine Hydrochloride) McNeil Consumer .. 1897
Children's Benadryl Allergy Fastmelts (Diphenhydramine Hydrochloride) McNeil Consumer .. 1897
Children's Benadryl Allergy Liquid (Diphenhydramine Hydrochloride) McNeil Consumer 1898
Children's Benadryl Allergy Perfect Measure (Diphenhydramine Hydrochloride) McNeil Consumer .. 1896
Children's Benadryl-D Allergy & Sinus Liquid (Diphenhydramine Hydrochloride, Phenylephrine Hydrochloride) McNeil Consumer .. 1896
Benadryl-D Allergy & Sinus Tablet (Diphenhydramine Hydrochloride, Phenylephrine Hydrochloride) McNeil Consumer 1896
Sudafed PE Nighttime Cold Caplets (Acetaminophen, Diphenhydramine Hydrochloride, Phenylephrine Hydrochloride) McNeil Consumer 1907
Tylenol Allergy Multi-Symptom Caplets with Cool Burst and Rapid Release Gelcaps (Acetaminophen, Chlorpheniramine Maleate, Phenylephrine Hydrochloride) McNeil Consumer 1916
Tylenol Allergy Multi-Symptom Nighttime Caplets with Cool Burst (Acetaminophen, Diphenhydramine Hydrochloride, Phenylephrine Hydrochloride) McNeil Consumer 1916
Tylenol Severe Allergy Caplets (Acetaminophen, Diphenhydramine Hydrochloride) McNeil Consumer 1916
Zyrtec Allergy Tablets (Cetirizine Hydrochloride) McNeil Consumer .. 1919
Children's Zyrtec Allergy Syrup (Cetirizine Hydrochloride) McNeil Consumer 1920
Children's Zyrtec Allergy Chewable Tablets (Cetirizine Hydrochloride) McNeil Consumer 1922
Zyrtec-D Allergy & Congestion Extended-Release Tablets (Cetirizine Hydrochloride, Pseudoephedrine Hydrochloride) McNeil Consumer 1923

Pruritus, topical relief of
Diprolene Lotion 0.05% (Betamethasone Dipropionate) Schering 2838
Diprolene Ointment 0.05% (Betamethasone Dipropionate) Schering 2839
Diprolene AF Cream 0.05% (Betamethasone Dipropionate) Schering 2837
Elocon Cream 0.1% (Mometasone Furoate) Schering 2840
Elocon Lotion 0.1% (Mometasone Furoate) Schering 2841
Elocon Ointment 0.1% (Mometasone Furoate) Schering 2842
Luxiq Foam (Betamethasone Valerate) Stiefel 3058
Olux Foam (Clobetasol Propionate) Stiefel 3061
Olux-E Foam (Clobetasol Propionate) Stiefel 3059
Pramosone (Hydrocortisone Acetate, Pramoxine Hydrochloride) Ferndale 1141

Pruritus ani
(*see under* Pruritus, anogenital)

Pseudomonas aeruginosa infections
(*see under* P. aeruginosa infections)

Pseudomonas species infections
Doribax Injection (Doripenem) Ortho-McNeil 2400
Fortaz (Ceftazidime) GlaxoSmithKline 1450

Pseudomonas species infections, ocular
Blephamide Ophthalmic Ointment Allergan .... ⊙ 217
Blephamide Ophthalmic Suspension Allergan .... ⊙ 216
Neosporin Ophthalmic Solution Sterile (Gramicidin, Neomycin Sulfate, Polymyxin B Sulfate) King .... ⊙ 252
Ofloxacin Ophthalmic Solution 0.3% (Ofloxacin) Bausch & Lomb .... ⊙ 243

Pseudomonas species septicemia
Timentin ADD-Vantage (Clavulanate Potassium, Ticarcillin Disodium) GlaxoSmithKline 1606
Timentin Injection Galaxy Container (Clavulanate Potassium, Ticarcillin Disodium) GlaxoSmithKline 1609

Timentin IV Infusion (Clavulanate Potassium, Ticarcillin Disodium) GlaxoSmithKline 1603
Timentin Pharmacy Bulk Package (Clavulanate Potassium, Ticarcillin Disodium) GlaxoSmithKline 1613

Pseudomonas species urinary tract infections
Doribax Injection (Doripenem) Ortho-McNeil 2400
Timentin ADD-Vantage (Clavulanate Potassium, Ticarcillin Disodium) GlaxoSmithKline 1606
Timentin Injection Galaxy Container (Clavulanate Potassium, Ticarcillin Disodium) GlaxoSmithKline 1609
Timentin IV Infusion (Clavulanate Potassium, Ticarcillin Disodium) GlaxoSmithKline 1603
Timentin Pharmacy Bulk Package (Clavulanate Potassium, Ticarcillin Disodium) GlaxoSmithKline 1613

Psoriasis
Amevive (Alefacept) Astellas 611
Olux Foam (Clobetasol Propionate) Stiefel 3061
Raptiva for Injection (Efalizumab) Genentech 1218

Psoriasis, erythrodermic
Soriatane Capsules (Acitretin) Stiefel 3062

Psoriasis, generalized pustular
Soriatane Capsules (Acitretin) Stiefel 3062

Psoriasis, plaque-type
Enbrel for Injection (Etanercept) Amgen 569
Humira Injection (Adalimumab) Abbott 442
Remicade for IV Injection (Infliximab) Centocor 950
Vanos Cream (Fluocinonide) Medicis 1941

Psoriasis, pustular
Soriatane Capsules (Acitretin) Stiefel 3062

Psoriasis, severe
Enbrel for Injection (Etanercept) Amgen 569

Psoriasis, severe recalcitrant
Gengraf Capsules (Cyclosporine) Abbott 435
Neoral Oral Solution (Cyclosporine) Novartis 2280
Neoral Soft Gelatin Capsules (Cyclosporine) Novartis 2280

Psoriatic arthritis
(*see under* Arthritis, psoriatic)

Psoriatic plaques
Amevive (Alefacept) Astellas 611
Enbrel for Injection (Etanercept) Amgen 569
Gengraf Capsules (Cyclosporine) Abbott 435
Neoral Oral Solution (Cyclosporine) Novartis 2280
Neoral Soft Gelatin Capsules (Cyclosporine) Novartis 2280
Raptiva for Injection (Efalizumab) Genentech 1218

Psychotic disorders, management of the manifestations of
(*see under* Schizophrenia)

Puberty, central precocious
Lupron Depot-PED 7.5 mg, 11.25 mg and 15 mg (Leuprolide Acetate) Abbott 471
Supprelin LA Implant (Histrelin Acetate) Indevus 1731

Puberty, delayed, in male
Delatestryl Injection (Testosterone Enanthate) Indevus 1730

Pulmonary disease, obstruction, exacerbation of
Advair Diskus 100/50 (Fluticasone Propionate, Salmeterol Xinafoate) GlaxoSmithKline 1276
Advair Diskus 250/50 (Fluticasone Propionate, Salmeterol Xinafoate) GlaxoSmithKline 1276
Advair Diskus 500/50 (Fluticasone Propionate, Salmeterol Xinafoate) GlaxoSmithKline 1276

Pulmonary emphysema
(*see under* Emphysema)

Purpura, idiopathic thrombocytopenic
Gammagard S/D (Immune Globulin Intravenous (Human)) Baxter Healthcare 734
Gamunex (Immune Globulin Intravenous (Human)) Talecris 3094
WinRho SDF (Rh_0 (D) Immune Globulin (Human)) Baxter Healthcare 741

Pyelitis
Gantrisin Pediatric Suspension (Acetyl Sulfisoxazole) Roche 2638
Uroqid-Acid No. 2 Tablets (Methenamine Mandelate, Sodium Acid Phosphate) Beach 814

Pyelonephritis
Cipro I.V. (Ciprofloxacin) Schering 2817
Cipro (Ciprofloxacin) Schering 2810
Cipro XR Tablets (Ciprofloxacin) Schering 2823
Doribax Injection (Doripenem) Ortho-McNeil 2400
Gantrisin Pediatric Suspension (Acetyl Sulfisoxazole) Roche 2638
Invanz for Injection (Ertapenem) Merck 2029
Levaquin (Levofloxacin) Ortho-McNeil 2416
Levaquin in 5% Dextrose Injection (Levofloxacin) Ortho-McNeil 2416
Uroqid-Acid No. 2 Tablets (Methenamine Mandelate, Sodium Acid Phosphate) Beach 814

Pyoderma gangrenosum
Levaquin (Levofloxacin) Ortho-McNeil 2416
Levaquin in 5% Dextrose Injection (Levofloxacin) Ortho-McNeil 2416

R

Radiography, gastrointestinal tract, adjunct in
Glucagon for Injection Vials and Emergency Kit (Glucagon) Lilly 1827

Rash, drug
(*see under* Hypersensitivity reactions, drug-induced)

Rash, protection of
Ivy Block (Bentoquatam) Standard Homeopathic .... ▣ 621

Rash, unspecified
(*see under* Skin, inflammatory conditions)

RDS
(*see under* Respiratory distress syndrome)

Renal, allogeneic transplants, prophylaxis of organ rejection in
CellCept Oral Suspension (Mycophenolate Mofetil) Roche 2622

Renal allogeneic transplants, prophylaxis of organ rejection in
CellCept Capsules (Mycophenolate Mofetil) Roche 2622
CellCept Intravenous (Mycophenolate Mofetil Hydrochloride) Roche 2622
CellCept Tablets (Mycophenolate Mofetil) Roche 2622

Renal allograft transplants, acute rejection in
Orthoclone OKT3 Sterile Solution (Muromonab-CD3) Ortho Biotech 2387

Renal allograft transplants, prophylaxis of organ rejection
Myfortic Tablets (Mycophenolic Acid) Novartis 2276

Renal plasma flow, estimation of
Aminohippurate Sodium "PAH" Injection (Aminohippurate Sodium) Merck 1950

Renal transplantation, prevention of rejection in
Gengraf Capsules (Cyclosporine) Abbott 435
Neoral Oral Solution (Cyclosporine) Novartis 2280
Neoral Soft Gelatin Capsules (Cyclosporine) Novartis 2280
Prograf Capsules and Injection (Tacrolimus) Astellas 622
Rapamune (Sirolimus) Wyeth 3260
Sandimmune (Cyclosporine) Novartis 2296
Simulect for Injection (Basiliximab) Novartis 2306

Renal tubular acidosis, management of
Urocit-K Tablets (Potassium Citrate) Mission 2176

Renal tubular secretory mechanism, measurement of the functional capacity of
Aminohippurate Sodium "PAH" Injection (Aminohippurate Sodium) Merck 1950

Respiratory distress syndrome
Flexbumin 25% I.V. (Albumin (human)) Baxter Healthcare 729
Infasurf Intratracheal Suspension (Calfactant) Forest 1168

Respiratory insufficiency, acute, with chronic obstructive pulmonary disease
Combivent Inhalation Aerosol (Albuterol Sulfate, Ipratropium Bromide) Boehringer Ingelheim 845
Perforomist Inhalation Solution (Formoterol Fumarate) Dey 1025

Respiratory symptoms, upper, relief of
(*see under* Influenza syndrome, symptomatic relief of)

Restless legs syndrome
Hyland's Restful Legs Tablets (Homeopathic Formulations) Standard Homeopathic .... ▣ 620
Mirapex Tablets (Pramipexole Dihydrochloride) Boehringer Ingelheim 857
Requip Tablets (Ropinirole Hydrochloride) GlaxoSmithKline 1561

Retinitis, cytomegalovirus
Valcyte Tablets (Valganciclovir Hydrochloride) Roche 2654

Rhabdomyosarcoma
Cosmegen for Injection (Dactinomycin) Ovation 2485

Rheumatic fever, prophylaxis of
E.E.S. (Erythromycin Ethylsuccinate) Abbott 433
EryPed (Erythromycin Ethylsuccinate) Abbott 431

Rheumatoid arthritis, juvenile
Bayer Aspirin (Aspirin) Bayer HealthCare Consumer 750
Celebrex Capsules (Celecoxib) Searle 2979
Enbrel for Injection (Etanercept) Amgen 569
Mobic Oral Suspension (Meloxicam) Boehringer Ingelheim 863
Mobic Tablets (Meloxicam) Boehringer Ingelheim 863

Rhinitis, allergic
Actifed Cold & Allergy Tablets (Chlorpheniramine Maleate, Phenylephrine Hydrochloride) McNeil Consumer 1895
Atrovent Nasal Spray 0.03% (Ipratropium Bromide) Boehringer Ingelheim 834
Sudafed PE Sinus & Allergy Tablets (Chlorpheniramine Maleate, Phenylephrine Hydrochloride) McNeil Consumer 1908
Xyzal Oral Solution (Levocetirizine Dihydrochloride) sanofi-aventis 2789
Xyzal Oral Solution (Levocetirizine Dihydrochloride) UCB, Inc. 3155
Xyzal Tablets (Levocetirizine Dihydrochloride) sanofi-aventis 2789
Xyzal Tablets (Levocetirizine Dihydrochloride) UCB, Inc. 3155

Rhinitis, perennial allergic
Atrovent Nasal Spray 0.03% (Ipratropium Bromide) Boehringer Ingelheim 834
Beconase AQ Nasal Spray (Beclomethasone Dipropionate Monohydrate) GlaxoSmithKline 1369
Clarinex Syrup (Desloratadine) Schering 2828
Clarinex Tablets (Desloratadine) Schering 2828
Clarinex Reditabs Tablets (Desloratadine) Schering 2828
Flonase Nasal Spray (Fluticasone Propionate) GlaxoSmithKline 1431
Nasacort AQ Nasal Spray (Triamcinolone Acetonide) sanofi-aventis 2765
Nasonex Nasal Spray (Mometasone Furoate Monohydrate) Schering 2883
Omnaris Nasal Spray (Ciclesonide) Sepracor 2998
Singulair (Montelukast Sodium) Merck 2114
Veramyst Nasal Spray (Fluticasone Furoate) GlaxoSmithKline 1643
Zyrtec Chewable Tablets (Cetirizine Hydrochloride) McNeil Consumer 1920
Zyrtec Syrup (Cetirizine Hydrochloride) McNeil Consumer 1920
Zyrtec Tablets (Cetirizine Hydrochloride) McNeil Consumer 1920
Zyrtec-D 12 Hour Extended Release Tablets (Cetirizine Hydrochloride, Pseudoephedrine Hydrochloride) McNeil Consumer 1923

Rhinitis, seasonal allergic
Allegra Oral Solution (Fexofenadine Hydrochloride) sanofi-aventis 2684
Allegra Tablets (Fexofenadine Hydrochloride) sanofi-aventis 2684
Allegra-D 12 Hour Extended-Release Tablets (Fexofenadine Hydrochloride, Pseudoephedrine Hydrochloride) sanofi-aventis 2687
Allegra-D 24 Hour Extended-Release Tablets (Fexofenadine Hydrochloride, Pseudoephedrine Hydrochloride) sanofi-aventis 2690
Beconase AQ Nasal Spray (Beclomethasone Dipropionate Monohydrate) GlaxoSmithKline 1369
Clarinex Syrup (Desloratadine) Schering 2828
Clarinex Tablets (Desloratadine) Schering 2828
Clarinex Reditabs Tablets (Desloratadine) Schering 2828
Clarinex-D 12-Hour Extended-Release Tablets (Desloratadine, Pseudoephedrine Sulfate) Schering 2831
Clarinex-D 24-Hour Extended-Release Tablets (Desloratadine, Pseudoephedrine Sulfate) Schering 2834
Flonase Nasal Spray (Fluticasone Propionate) GlaxoSmithKline 1431
Nasacort AQ Nasal Spray (Triamcinolone Acetonide) sanofi-aventis 2765
Nasonex Nasal Spray (Mometasone Furoate Monohydrate) Schering 2883
Omnaris Nasal Spray (Ciclesonide) Sepracor 2998
Patanase Nasal Spray (Olopatadine Hydrochloride) Alcon 544
Singulair (Montelukast Sodium) Merck 2114
Veramyst Nasal Spray (Fluticasone Furoate) GlaxoSmithKline 1643

Zyrtec Chewable Tablets (Cetirizine Hydrochloride) McNeil Consumer .. 1920
Zyrtec Syrup (Cetirizine Hydrochloride) McNeil Consumer 1920
Zyrtec Tablets (Cetirizine Hydrochloride) McNeil Consumer 1920
Zyrtec-D 12 Hour Extended Release Tablets (Cetirizine Hydrochloride, Pseudoephedrine Hydrochloride) McNeil Consumer .. 1923

Rhinitis, vasomotor
Beconase AQ Nasal Spray (Beclomethasone Dipropionate Monohydrate) GlaxoSmithKline 1369

Rhinorrhea
Actifed Cold & Allergy Tablets (Chlorpheniramine Maleate, Phenylephrine Hydrochloride) McNeil Consumer 1895
Allegra-D 12 Hour Extended-Release Tablets (Fexofenadine Hydrochloride, Pseudoephedrine Hydrochloride) sanofi-aventis 2687
Allegra-D 24 Hour Extended-Release Tablets (Fexofenadine Hydrochloride, Pseudoephedrine Hydrochloride) sanofi-aventis 2690
Atrovent Nasal Spray 0.03% (Ipratropium Bromide) Boehringer Ingelheim 834
Atrovent Nasal Spray 0.06% (Ipratropium Bromide) Boehringer Ingelheim 836
Benadryl Allergy & Cold Kapgels (Acetaminophen, Diphenhydramine Hydrochloride, Phenylephrine Hydrochloride) McNeil Consumer 1895
Benadryl Allergy & Sinus Headache Kapgels (Acetaminophen, Diphenhydramine Hydrochloride, Phenylephrine Hydrochloride) McNeil Consumer 1895
Benadryl Severe Allergy & Sinus Headache Caplets (Acetaminophen, Diphenhydramine Hydrochloride, Phenylephrine Hydrochloride) McNeil Consumer 1897
Benadryl Dye-Free Allergy Liqui-gels Softgels (Diphenhydramine Hydrochloride) McNeil Consumer .. 1897
Benadryl Allergy Kapgels (Diphenhydramine Hydrochloride) McNeil Consumer 1895
Benadryl Allergy Quick Dissolve Strips (Diphenhydramine Hydrochloride) McNeil Consumer 1896
Benadryl Allergy Ultratab Tablets (Diphenhydramine Hydrochloride) McNeil Consumer 1896
Children's Benadryl Dye-Free Allergy Liquid (Diphenhydramine Hydrochloride) McNeil Consumer .. 1897
Children's Benadryl Allergy Fastmelts (Diphenhydramine Hydrochloride) McNeil Consumer .. 1897
Children's Benadryl Allergy Liquid (Diphenhydramine Hydrochloride) McNeil Consumer 1898
Children's Benadryl Allergy Perfect Measure (Diphenhydramine Hydrochloride) McNeil Consumer .. 1896
Children's Benadryl-D Allergy & Sinus Liquid (Diphenhydramine Hydrochloride, Phenylephrine Hydrochloride) McNeil Consumer .. 1896
Benadryl-D Allergy & Sinus Tablet (Diphenhydramine Hydrochloride, Phenylephrine Hydrochloride) McNeil Consumer 1896
PediaCare Children's Allergy & Cold Liquid (Diphenhydramine Hydrochloride, Phenylephrine Hydrochloride) McNeil Consumer .. 1902
PediaCare Children's Allergy Liquid (Diphenhydramine Hydrochloride) McNeil Consumer 1902
Sudafed PE Nighttime Cold Caplets (Acetaminophen, Diphenhydramine Hydrochloride, Phenylephrine Hydrochloride) McNeil Consumer 1907
Sudafed PE Severe Cold Caplets (Acetaminophen, Diphenhydramine Hydrochloride, Phenylephrine Hydrochloride) McNeil Consumer 1908
Sudafed PE Sinus & Allergy Tablets (Chlorpheniramine Maleate, Phenylephrine Hydrochloride) McNeil Consumer 1908
Tylenol Allergy Multi-Symptom Caplets with Cool Burst and Rapid Release Gelcaps (Acetaminophen, Chlorpheniramine Maleate, Phenylephrine Hydrochloride) McNeil Consumer 1916
Tylenol Allergy Multi-Symptom Nighttime Caplets with Cool Burst (Acetaminophen, Diphenhydramine Hydrochloride, Phenylephrine Hydrochloride) McNeil Consumer 1916
Tylenol Severe Allergy Caplets (Acetaminophen, Diphenhydramine Hydrochloride) McNeil Consumer 1916
Children's Tylenol Plus Cold Suspension Liquid (Acetaminophen, Chlorpheniramine Maleate, Phenylephrine Hydrochloride) McNeil Consumer 1912
Children's Tylenol Plus Cold & Allergy Suspension Liquid (Acetaminophen, Diphenhydramine Hydrochloride, Phenylephrine Hydrochloride) McNeil Consumer .. 1914
Children's Tylenol Plus Cough & Runny Nose Suspension Liquid (Acetaminophen, Chlorpheniramine Maleate, Dextromethorphan Hydrobromide) McNeil Consumer .. 1912
Children's Tylenol Plus Flu Suspension Liquid (Acetaminophen, Chlorpheniramine Maleate, Dextromethorphan Hydrobromide, Phenylephrine Hydrochloride) McNeil Consumer 1914
Children's Tylenol Plus Multi-Symptom Cold Suspension Liquid (Acetaminophen, Chlorpheniramine Maleate, Dextromethorphan Hydrobromide, Phenylephrine Hydrochloride) McNeil Consumer 1912
Tylenol Cold Head Congestion Nighttime Caplets with Cool Burst (Acetaminophen, Chlorpheniramine Maleate, Dextromethorphan Hydrobromide, Phenylephrine Hydrochloride) McNeil Consumer 1910
Tylenol Cold Multi-Symptom Nighttime Caplets with Cool Burst (Acetaminophen, Chlorpheniramine Maleate, Dextromethorphan Hydrobromide, Phenylephrine Hydrochloride) McNeil Consumer 1913
Tylenol Cold Multi-Symptom Nighttime Liquid with Cool Burst (Acetaminophen, Dextromethorphan Hydrobromide, Doxylamine Succinate, Phenylephrine Hydrochloride) McNeil Consumer 1913
Tylenol Cough & Sore Throat Nighttime Liquid with Cool Burst (Acetaminophen, Dextromethorphan Hydrobromide, Doxylamine Succinate) McNeil Consumer 1918
Tylenol Sinus Congestion & Pain Nighttime Caplets with Cool Burst (Acetaminophen, Chlorpheniramine Maleate, Phenylephrine Hydrochloride) McNeil Consumer 1917
Tylenol Sore Throat Nighttime Liquid with Cool Burst (Acetaminophen, Diphenhydramine Hydrochloride) McNeil Consumer 1918
Vicks NyQuil Cold & Flu Multi-Symptom Relief (Acetaminophen, Dextromethorphan Hydrobromide, Doxylamine Succinate) Procter & Gamble .... ▣617
Vicks NyQuil LiquiCaps (Acetaminophen, Dextromethorphan Hydrobromide, Doxylamine Succinate, Pseudoephedrine Hydrochloride) Procter & Gamble 2567
Vicks NyQuil Liquid (Acetaminophen, Dextromethorphan Hydrobromide, Doxylamine Succinate, Pseudoephedrine Hydrochloride) Procter & Gamble 2567
Vicks NyQuil Multi-Symptom Cold/Flu Relief (Acetaminophen, Dextromethorphan Hydrobromide, Doxylamine Succinate, Pseudoephedrine Hydrochloride) Procter & Gamble 2567
Zyrtec Allergy Tablets (Cetirizine Hydrochloride) McNeil Consumer .. 1919
Children's Zyrtec Allergy Chewable Tablets (Cetirizine Hydrochloride) McNeil Consumer 1922
Zyrtec-D Allergy & Congestion Extended-Release Tablets (Cetirizine Hydrochloride, Pseudoephedrine Hydrochloride) McNeil Consumer 1923

Ringworm infections of the body
(*see under* Tinea corporis infections)

Ringworm infections of the feet
(*see under* Tinea pedis infections)

Ringworm infections of the groin
(*see under* Tinea cruris infections)

Ringworm infections of the nails
(*see under* Tinea unguium infections)

Ringworm infections of the scalp
(*see under* Tinea capitis infections)

Rosacea
Finacea Gel (Azelaic Acid) Intendis ... 1742

Rubella, prophylaxis
Meruvax II (Rubella Virus Vaccine Live) Merck 2061
M-M-R II (Measles, Mumps & Rubella Virus Vaccine, Live) Merck 2054
ProQuad (Measles, Mumps, Rubella and Varicella Virus Vaccine Live) Merck 2099

S

S. agalactiae infections
Invanz for Injection (Ertapenem) Merck 2029
Merrem I.V. (Meropenem) AstraZeneca Pharmaceuticals 684
Noroxin Tablets (Norfloxacin) Merck . 2069
Tygacil for Injection (Tigecycline) Wyeth 3276
Zyvox (Linezolid) Pharmacia & Upjohn 2552

S. agalactiae pelvic inflammatory disease
Invanz for Injection (Ertapenem) Merck 2029

S. agalactiae skin and skin structure infections
Cubicin for Injection (Daptomycin) Cubist 995
Invanz for Injection (Ertapenem) Merck 2029
Merrem I.V. (Meropenem) AstraZeneca Pharmaceuticals 684
Tygacil for Injection (Tigecycline) Wyeth 3276
Zyvox (Linezolid) Pharmacia & Upjohn 2552

S. agalactiae urinary tract infections
Noroxin Tablets (Norfloxacin) Merck . 2069

S. anginosus infections
Avelox (Moxifloxacin Hydrochloride) Schering 2803
Tygacil for Injection (Tigecycline) Wyeth 3276

S. anginosus intra-abdominal infections
Avelox (Moxifloxacin Hydrochloride) Schering 2803
Tygacil for Injection (Tigecycline) Wyeth 3276

S. anginosus skin and skin structure infections
Tygacil for Injection (Tigecycline) Wyeth 3276

S. aureus (methicillin-susceptible strains) intra-abdominal infections
Tygacil for Injection (Tigecycline) Wyeth 3276

S. aureus (non-penicillinase producing) infections
Primaxin I.V. (Cilastatin Sodium, Imipenem) Merck 2083

S. aureus (penicillinase producing) infections
Primaxin I.M. (Cilastatin Sodium, Imipenem) Merck 2080
Primaxin I.V. (Cilastatin Sodium, Imipenem) Merck 2083

S. aureus (penicillinase and non-penicillinase producing strains) skin and skin structure infections
Tygacil for Injection (Tigecycline) Wyeth 3276
Zinacef for Injection (Cefuroxime) GlaxoSmithKline 1678
Zinacef Injection (Cefuroxime) GlaxoSmithKline 1678

S. aureus bone and joint infections
Fortaz (Ceftazidime) GlaxoSmithKline 1450
Primaxin I.V. (Cilastatin Sodium, Imipenem) Merck 2083
Rocephin Injectable Vials, ADD-Vantage, Galaxy, Bulk (Ceftriaxone Sodium) Roche 2642
Timentin ADD-Vantage (Clavulanate Potassium, Ticarcillin Disodium) GlaxoSmithKline 1606
Timentin Injection Galaxy Container (Clavulanate Potassium, Ticarcillin Disodium) GlaxoSmithKline 1609
Timentin IV Infusion (Clavulanate Potassium, Ticarcillin Disodium) GlaxoSmithKline 1603
Timentin Pharmacy Bulk Package (Clavulanate Potassium, Ticarcillin Disodium) GlaxoSmithKline 1613
Zinacef for Injection (Cefuroxime) GlaxoSmithKline 1678
Zinacef Injection (Cefuroxime) GlaxoSmithKline 1678

S. aureus bronchitis
Levaquin (Levofloxacin) Ortho-McNeil 2416
Levaquin in 5% Dextrose Injection (Levofloxacin) Ortho-McNeil 2416

S. aureus endocarditis
Cubicin for Injection (Daptomycin) Cubist 995
Primaxin I.V. (Cilastatin Sodium, Imipenem) Merck 2083

S. aureus gynecologic infections
Primaxin I.V. (Cilastatin Sodium, Imipenem) Merck 2083
Timentin ADD-Vantage (Clavulanate Potassium, Ticarcillin Disodium) GlaxoSmithKline 1606
Timentin Injection Galaxy Container (Clavulanate Potassium, Ticarcillin Disodium) GlaxoSmithKline 1609
Timentin IV Infusion (Clavulanate Potassium, Ticarcillin Disodium) GlaxoSmithKline 1603
Timentin Pharmacy Bulk Package (Clavulanate Potassium, Ticarcillin Disodium) GlaxoSmithKline 1613

S. aureus infection, eradication of nasal colonization of
Bactroban Nasal (Mupirocin Calcium) GlaxoSmithKline 1367

S. aureus infections
Augmentin (Amoxicillin, Clavulanate Potassium) GlaxoSmithKline 1323
Augmentin Tablets (Amoxicillin, Clavulanate Potassium) GlaxoSmithKline 1327
Augmentin XR Extended Release Tablets (Amoxicillin, Clavulanate Potassium) GlaxoSmithKline 1333
Avelox (Moxifloxacin Hydrochloride) Schering 2803
Bactroban Ointment (Mupirocin) GlaxoSmithKline 1368
Biaxin/Biaxin XL (Clarithromycin) Abbott 411

Ceftin (Cefuroxime Axetil) GlaxoSmithKline ... 1380
Cipro I.V. (Ciprofloxacin) Schering ... 2817
Cipro (Ciprofloxacin) Schering ... 2810
E.E.S. (Erythromycin Ethylsuccinate) Abbott ... 433
EryPed (Erythromycin Ethylsuccinate) Abbott ... 431
Fortaz (Ceftazidime) GlaxoSmithKline ... 1450
Invanz for Injection (Ertapenem) Merck ... 2029
Levaquin (Levofloxacin) Ortho-McNeil ... 2416
Levaquin in 5% Dextrose Injection (Levofloxacin) Ortho-McNeil ... 2416
Merrem I.V. (Meropenem) AstraZeneca Pharmaceuticals ... 684
Noroxin Tablets (Norfloxacin) Merck ... 2069
Primaxin I.M. (Cilastatin Sodium, Imipenem) Merck ... 2080
Primaxin I.V. (Cilastatin Sodium, Imipenem) Merck ... 2083
Rocephin Injectable Vials, ADD-Vantage, Galaxy, Bulk (Ceftriaxone Sodium) Roche ... 2642
Timentin ADD-Vantage (Clavulanate Potassium, Ticarcillin Disodium) GlaxoSmithKline ... 1606
Timentin Injection Galaxy Container (Clavulanate Potassium, Ticarcillin Disodium) GlaxoSmithKline ... 1609
Timentin IV Infusion (Clavulanate Potassium, Ticarcillin Disodium) GlaxoSmithKline ... 1603
Timentin Pharmacy Bulk Package (Clavulanate Potassium, Ticarcillin Disodium) GlaxoSmithKline ... 1613
Tygacil for Injection (Tigecycline) Wyeth ... 3276
Zinacef for Injection (Cefuroxime) GlaxoSmithKline ... 1678
Zinacef Injection (Cefuroxime) GlaxoSmithKline ... 1678
Zosyn for Injection (Piperacillin Sodium, Tazobactam Sodium) Wyeth ... 3284
Zyvox (Linezolid) Pharmacia & Upjohn ... 2552

S. aureus infections (erythromycin susceptible strains)
Ketek Tablets (Telithromycin) sanofi-aventis ... 2744

S. aureus infections (methicillin-susceptible strains)
Avelox (Moxifloxacin Hydrochloride) Schering ... 2803
Ketek Tablets (Telithromycin) sanofi-aventis ... 2744
Levaquin (Levofloxacin) Ortho-McNeil ... 2416
Levaquin in 5% Dextrose Injection (Levofloxacin) Ortho-McNeil ... 2416
Merrem I.V. (Meropenem) AstraZeneca Pharmaceuticals ... 684

S. aureus infections, ocular
Blephamide Ophthalmic Ointment Allergan ... ⊙217
Blephamide Ophthalmic Suspension Allergan ... ⊙216
Neosporin Ophthalmic Solution Sterile (Gramicidin, Neomycin Sulfate, Polymyxin B Sulfate) King ... ⊙252
Ofloxacin Ophthalmic Solution 0.3% (Ofloxacin) Bausch & Lomb ... ⊙243
Pred-G Ophthalmic Ointment (Gentamicin Sulfate, Prednisolone Acetate) Allergan ... ⊙229
Pred-G Ophthalmic Suspension (Gentamicin Sulfate, Prednisolone Acetate) Allergan ... ⊙228
Quixin Ophthalmic Solution (Levofloxacin) Vistakon ... 3184
Vigamox Ophthalmic Solution (Moxifloxacin Hydrochloride) Alcon ... 548
Zylet Ophthalmic Suspension (Loteprednol Etabonate, Tobramycin) Bausch & Lomb ... ⊙247

S. aureus intra-abdominal infections
Fortaz (Ceftazidime) GlaxoSmithKline ... 1450
Primaxin I.V. (Cilastatin Sodium, Imipenem) Merck ... 2083

S. aureus lower respiratory tract infections
Augmentin XR Extended Release Tablets (Amoxicillin, Clavulanate Potassium) GlaxoSmithKline ... 1333
Fortaz (Ceftazidime) GlaxoSmithKline ... 1450
Levaquin (Levofloxacin) Ortho-McNeil ... 2416
Levaquin in 5% Dextrose Injection (Levofloxacin) Ortho-McNeil ... 2416
Primaxin I.V. (Cilastatin Sodium, Imipenem) Merck ... 2083
Rocephin Injectable Vials, ADD-Vantage, Galaxy, Bulk (Ceftriaxone Sodium) Roche ... 2642
Timentin ADD-Vantage (Clavulanate Potassium, Ticarcillin Disodium) GlaxoSmithKline ... 1606
Timentin Injection Galaxy Container (Clavulanate Potassium, Ticarcillin Disodium) GlaxoSmithKline ... 1609
Timentin IV Infusion (Clavulanate Potassium, Ticarcillin Disodium) GlaxoSmithKline ... 1603
Timentin Pharmacy Bulk Package (Clavulanate Potassium, Ticarcillin Disodium) GlaxoSmithKline ... 1613
Zinacef for Injection (Cefuroxime) GlaxoSmithKline ... 1678
Zinacef Injection (Cefuroxime) GlaxoSmithKline ... 1678
Zosyn for Injection (Piperacillin Sodium, Tazobactam Sodium) Wyeth ... 3284
Zyvox (Linezolid) Pharmacia & Upjohn ... 2552

S. aureus meningitis
Zinacef for Injection (Cefuroxime) GlaxoSmithKline ... 1678
Zinacef Injection (Cefuroxime) GlaxoSmithKline ... 1678

S. aureus respiratory tract infections
Avelox (Moxifloxacin Hydrochloride) Schering ... 2803

S. aureus septicemia
Cubicin for Injection (Daptomycin) Cubist ... 995
Fortaz (Ceftazidime) GlaxoSmithKline ... 1450
Primaxin I.V. (Cilastatin Sodium, Imipenem) Merck ... 2083
Rocephin Injectable Vials, ADD-Vantage, Galaxy, Bulk (Ceftriaxone Sodium) Roche ... 2642
Timentin ADD-Vantage (Clavulanate Potassium, Ticarcillin Disodium) GlaxoSmithKline ... 1606
Timentin Injection Galaxy Container (Clavulanate Potassium, Ticarcillin Disodium) GlaxoSmithKline ... 1609
Timentin IV Infusion (Clavulanate Potassium, Ticarcillin Disodium) GlaxoSmithKline ... 1603
Timentin Pharmacy Bulk Package (Clavulanate Potassium, Ticarcillin Disodium) GlaxoSmithKline ... 1613
Zinacef for Injection (Cefuroxime) GlaxoSmithKline ... 1678
Zinacef Injection (Cefuroxime) GlaxoSmithKline ... 1678

S. aureus skin and skin structure infections
Augmentin (Amoxicillin, Clavulanate Potassium) GlaxoSmithKline ... 1323
Augmentin Tablets (Amoxicillin, Clavulanate Potassium) GlaxoSmithKline ... 1327
Avelox (Moxifloxacin Hydrochloride) Schering ... 2803
Bactroban Cream (Mupirocin Calcium) GlaxoSmithKline ... 1366
Bactroban Ointment (Mupirocin) GlaxoSmithKline ... 1368
Biaxin/Biaxin XL (Clarithromycin) Abbott ... 411
Ceftin Tablets (Cefuroxime Axetil) GlaxoSmithKline ... 1380
Cipro I.V. (Ciprofloxacin) Schering ... 2817
Cipro (Ciprofloxacin) Schering ... 2810
Cubicin for Injection (Daptomycin) Cubist ... 995
E.E.S. (Erythromycin Ethylsuccinate) Abbott ... 433
EryPed (Erythromycin Ethylsuccinate) Abbott ... 431
Fortaz (Ceftazidime) GlaxoSmithKline ... 1450
Invanz for Injection (Ertapenem) Merck ... 2029
Levaquin (Levofloxacin) Ortho-McNeil ... 2416
Levaquin in 5% Dextrose Injection (Levofloxacin) Ortho-McNeil ... 2416
Merrem I.V. (Meropenem) AstraZeneca Pharmaceuticals ... 684
Omnicef Capsules (Cefdinir) Abbott ... 497
Omnicef for Oral Suspension (Cefdinir) Abbott ... 497
Primaxin I.M. (Cilastatin Sodium, Imipenem) Merck ... 2080
Primaxin I.V. (Cilastatin Sodium, Imipenem) Merck ... 2083
Rocephin Injectable Vials, ADD-Vantage, Galaxy, Bulk (Ceftriaxone Sodium) Roche ... 2642
Timentin ADD-Vantage (Clavulanate Potassium, Ticarcillin Disodium) GlaxoSmithKline ... 1606
Timentin Injection Galaxy Container (Clavulanate Potassium, Ticarcillin Disodium) GlaxoSmithKline ... 1609
Timentin IV Infusion (Clavulanate Potassium, Ticarcillin Disodium) GlaxoSmithKline ... 1603
Timentin Pharmacy Bulk Package (Clavulanate Potassium, Ticarcillin Disodium) GlaxoSmithKline ... 1613
Zinacef for Injection (Cefuroxime) GlaxoSmithKline ... 1678
Zinacef Injection (Cefuroxime) GlaxoSmithKline ... 1678
Zosyn for Injection (Piperacillin Sodium, Tazobactam Sodium) Wyeth ... 3284
Zyvox (Linezolid) Pharmacia & Upjohn ... 2552

S. aureus urinary tract infections
Noroxin Tablets (Norfloxacin) Merck ... 2069
Primaxin I.V. (Cilastatin Sodium, Imipenem) Merck ... 2083
Timentin ADD-Vantage (Clavulanate Potassium, Ticarcillin Disodium) GlaxoSmithKline ... 1606
Timentin Injection Galaxy Container (Clavulanate Potassium, Ticarcillin Disodium) GlaxoSmithKline ... 1609
Timentin IV Infusion (Clavulanate Potassium, Ticarcillin Disodium) GlaxoSmithKline ... 1603
Timentin Pharmacy Bulk Package (Clavulanate Potassium, Ticarcillin Disodium) GlaxoSmithKline ... 1613

S. constellatus infections
Avelox (Moxifloxacin Hydrochloride) Schering ... 2803

S. constellatus intra-abdominal infections
Avelox (Moxifloxacin Hydrochloride) Schering ... 2803
Doribax Injection (Doripenem) Ortho-McNeil ... 2400

S. dysgalactiae (subspecies equisimilis) skin and skin structure infections
Cubicin for Injection (Daptomycin) Cubist ... 995

S. epidermis bone and joint infections
Primaxin I.V. (Cilastatin Sodium, Imipenem) Merck ... 2083

S. epidermis gynecologic infections
Primaxin I.V. (Cilastatin Sodium, Imipenem) Merck ... 2083
Timentin ADD-Vantage (Clavulanate Potassium, Ticarcillin Disodium) GlaxoSmithKline ... 1606
Timentin Injection Galaxy Container (Clavulanate Potassium, Ticarcillin Disodium) GlaxoSmithKline ... 1609
Timentin IV Infusion (Clavulanate Potassium, Ticarcillin Disodium) GlaxoSmithKline ... 1603
Timentin Pharmacy Bulk Package (Clavulanate Potassium, Ticarcillin Disodium) GlaxoSmithKline ... 1613

S. epidermis infections
Cipro I.V. (Ciprofloxacin) Schering ... 2817
Cipro (Ciprofloxacin) Schering ... 2810
Noroxin Tablets (Norfloxacin) Merck ... 2069
Primaxin I.V. (Cilastatin Sodium, Imipenem) Merck ... 2083
Rocephin Injectable Vials, ADD-Vantage, Galaxy, Bulk (Ceftriaxone Sodium) Roche ... 2642
Timentin ADD-Vantage (Clavulanate Potassium, Ticarcillin Disodium) GlaxoSmithKline ... 1606
Timentin Injection Galaxy Container (Clavulanate Potassium, Ticarcillin Disodium) GlaxoSmithKline ... 1609
Timentin IV Infusion (Clavulanate Potassium, Ticarcillin Disodium) GlaxoSmithKline ... 1603
Timentin Pharmacy Bulk Package (Clavulanate Potassium, Ticarcillin Disodium) GlaxoSmithKline ... 1613

S. epidermis infections, ocular
Ofloxacin Ophthalmic Solution 0.3% (Ofloxacin) Bausch & Lomb ... ⊙243
Quixin Ophthalmic Solution (Levofloxacin) Vistakon ... 3184
Vigamox Ophthalmic Solution (Moxifloxacin Hydrochloride) Alcon ... 548
Zylet Ophthalmic Suspension (Loteprednol Etabonate, Tobramycin) Bausch & Lomb ... ⊙247

S. epidermis intra-abdominal infections
Primaxin I.V. (Cilastatin Sodium, Imipenem) Merck ... 2083

S. epidermis meningitis
Rocephin Injectable Vials, ADD-Vantage, Galaxy, Bulk (Ceftriaxone Sodium) Roche ... 2642

S. epidermis prostatitis
Levaquin (Levofloxacin) Ortho-McNeil ... 2416
Levaquin in 5% Dextrose Injection (Levofloxacin) Ortho-McNeil ... 2416

S. epidermis skin and skin structure infections
Cipro I.V. (Ciprofloxacin) Schering ... 2817
Cipro (Ciprofloxacin) Schering ... 2810
Primaxin I.V. (Cilastatin Sodium, Imipenem) Merck ... 2083
Rocephin Injectable Vials, ADD-Vantage, Galaxy, Bulk (Ceftriaxone Sodium) Roche ... 2642

S. epidermis urinary tract infections
Cipro I.V. (Ciprofloxacin) Schering ... 2817
Cipro (Ciprofloxacin) Schering ... 2810
Noroxin Tablets (Norfloxacin) Merck ... 2069

S. faecalis infections
Amoxil Pediatric Drops for Oral Suspension (Amoxicillin) GlaxoSmithKline ... 1305
Cipro I.V. (Ciprofloxacin) Schering ... 2817
Noroxin Tablets (Norfloxacin) Merck ... 2069

S. faecalis urinary tract infections
Cipro I.V. (Ciprofloxacin) Schering ... 2817
Noroxin Tablets (Norfloxacin) Merck ... 2069

S. haemolyticus
Vigamox Ophthalmic Solution (Moxifloxacin Hydrochloride) Alcon ... 548

S. hominis
Vigamox Ophthalmic Solution (Moxifloxacin Hydrochloride) Alcon ... 548

S. intermedius intra-abdominal infections
Doribax Injection (Doripenem) Ortho-McNeil ... 2400

S. pneumoniae bone and joint infections
Rocephin Injectable Vials, ADD-Vantage, Galaxy, Bulk (Ceftriaxone Sodium) Roche ... 2642

S. pneumoniae bronchitis
Amoxil Capsules (Amoxicillin) GlaxoSmithKline ... 1305

Amoxil Chewable Tablets (Amoxicillin) GlaxoSmithKline ... 1305
Amoxil Pediatric Drops for Oral Suspension (Amoxicillin) GlaxoSmithKline ... 1305
Amoxil Powder for Oral Suspension (Amoxicillin) GlaxoSmithKline ... 1305
Amoxil Tablets (Amoxicillin) GlaxoSmithKline ... 1305
Avelox (Moxifloxacin Hydrochloride) Schering ... 2803
Biaxin/Biaxin XL (Clarithromycin) Abbott ... 411
Ceftin Tablets (Cefuroxime Axetil) GlaxoSmithKline ... 1380
Levaquin (Levofloxacin) Ortho-McNeil ... 2416
Levaquin in 5% Dextrose Injection (Levofloxacin) Ortho-McNeil ... 2416
Omnicef Capsules (Cefdinir) Abbott ... 497
Omnicef for Oral Suspension (Cefdinir) Abbott ... 497
Suprax for Oral Suspension (Cefixime) Lupin ... 1891
Suprax Tablets (Cefixime) Lupin ... 1891

S. pneumoniae central nervous system infections

Fortaz (Ceftazidime) GlaxoSmithKline ... 1450

S. pneumoniae infections

Amoxil Capsules (Amoxicillin) GlaxoSmithKline ... 1305
Amoxil Chewable Tablets (Amoxicillin) GlaxoSmithKline ... 1305
Amoxil Pediatric Drops for Oral Suspension (Amoxicillin) GlaxoSmithKline ... 1305
Amoxil Powder for Oral Suspension (Amoxicillin) GlaxoSmithKline ... 1305
Amoxil Tablets (Amoxicillin) GlaxoSmithKline ... 1305
Augmentin Tablets (Amoxicillin, Clavulanate Potassium) GlaxoSmithKline ... 1327
Augmentin XR Extended Release Tablets (Amoxicillin, Clavulanate Potassium) GlaxoSmithKline ... 1333
Augmentin ES-600 Powder for Oral Suspension (Amoxicillin, Clavulanate Potassium) GlaxoSmithKline ... 1329
Avelox (Moxifloxacin Hydrochloride) Schering ... 2803
Biaxin/Biaxin XL (Clarithromycin) Abbott ... 411
Ceftin (Cefuroxime Axetil) GlaxoSmithKline ... 1380
Cipro I.V. (Ciprofloxacin) Schering ... 2817
Cipro (Ciprofloxacin) Schering ... 2810
E.E.S. (Erythromycin Ethylsuccinate) Abbott ... 433
EryPed (Erythromycin Ethylsuccinate) Abbott ... 431
Fortaz (Ceftazidime) GlaxoSmithKline ... 1450
Invanz for Injection (Ertapenem) Merck ... 2029
Ketek Tablets (Telithromycin) sanofi-aventis ... 2744
Levaquin (Levofloxacin) Ortho-McNeil ... 2416
Levaquin in 5% Dextrose Injection (Levofloxacin) Ortho-McNeil ... 2416
Merrem I.V. (Meropenem) AstraZeneca Pharmaceuticals ... 684
Omnicef Capsules (Cefdinir) Abbott ... 497
Omnicef for Oral Suspension (Cefdinir) Abbott ... 497
Primaxin I.M. (Cilastatin Sodium, Imipenem) Merck ... 2080
Primaxin I.V. (Cilastatin Sodium, Imipenem) Merck ... 2083
Rocephin Injectable Vials, ADD-Vantage, Galaxy, Bulk (Ceftriaxone Sodium) Roche ... 2642
Suprax for Oral Suspension (Cefixime) Lupin ... 1891
Suprax Tablets (Cefixime) Lupin ... 1891
Zinacef for Injection (Cefuroxime) GlaxoSmithKline ... 1678
Zinacef Injection (Cefuroxime) GlaxoSmithKline ... 1678
Zyvox (Linezolid) Pharmacia & Upjohn ... 2552

S. pneumoniae infections, ocular

Blephamide Ophthalmic Ointment Allergan ... ⊙217
Blephamide Ophthalmic Suspension Allergan ... ⊙216
Ofloxacin Ophthalmic Solution 0.3% (Ofloxacin) Bausch & Lomb ... ⊙243
Pred-G Ophthalmic Ointment (Gentamicin Sulfate, Prednisolone Acetate) Allergan ... ⊙229
Pred-G Ophthalmic Suspension (Gentamicin Sulfate, Prednisolone Acetate) Allergan ... ⊙228
Quixin Ophthalmic Solution (Levofloxacin) Vistakon ... 3184
Vigamox Ophthalmic Solution (Moxifloxacin Hydrochloride) Alcon ... 548
Zylet Ophthalmic Suspension (Loteprednol Etabonate, Tobramycin) Bausch & Lomb ... ⊙247

S. pneumoniae lower respiratory tract infections

Amoxil Capsules (Amoxicillin) GlaxoSmithKline ... 1305
Amoxil Chewable Tablets (Amoxicillin) GlaxoSmithKline ... 1305
Amoxil Pediatric Drops for Oral Suspension (Amoxicillin) GlaxoSmithKline ... 1305
Amoxil Powder for Oral Suspension (Amoxicillin) GlaxoSmithKline ... 1305
Amoxil Tablets (Amoxicillin) GlaxoSmithKline ... 1305
Augmentin XR Extended Release Tablets (Amoxicillin, Clavulanate Potassium) GlaxoSmithKline ... 1333
Avelox (Moxifloxacin Hydrochloride) Schering ... 2803
Biaxin/Biaxin XL (Clarithromycin) Abbott ... 411
Cipro I.V. (Ciprofloxacin) Schering ... 2817
Cipro (Ciprofloxacin) Schering ... 2810
E.E.S. (Erythromycin Ethylsuccinate) Abbott ... 433
EryPed (Erythromycin Ethylsuccinate) Abbott ... 431
Fortaz (Ceftazidime) GlaxoSmithKline ... 1450
Invanz for Injection (Ertapenem) Merck ... 2029
Ketek Tablets (Telithromycin) sanofi-aventis ... 2744
Levaquin (Levofloxacin) Ortho-McNeil ... 2416
Levaquin in 5% Dextrose Injection (Levofloxacin) Ortho-McNeil ... 2416
Omnicef Capsules (Cefdinir) Abbott ... 497
Omnicef for Oral Suspension (Cefdinir) Abbott ... 497
Primaxin I.M. (Cilastatin Sodium, Imipenem) Merck ... 2080
Rocephin Injectable Vials, ADD-Vantage, Galaxy, Bulk (Ceftriaxone Sodium) Roche ... 2642
Zinacef for Injection (Cefuroxime) GlaxoSmithKline ... 1678
Zinacef Injection (Cefuroxime) GlaxoSmithKline ... 1678
Zyvox (Linezolid) Pharmacia & Upjohn ... 2552

S. pneumoniae meningitis

Fortaz (Ceftazidime) GlaxoSmithKline ... 1450
Merrem I.V. (Meropenem) AstraZeneca Pharmaceuticals ... 684
Rocephin Injectable Vials, ADD-Vantage, Galaxy, Bulk (Ceftriaxone Sodium) Roche ... 2642
Zinacef for Injection (Cefuroxime) GlaxoSmithKline ... 1678
Zinacef Injection (Cefuroxime) GlaxoSmithKline ... 1678

S. pneumoniae otitis media

Amoxil Capsules (Amoxicillin) GlaxoSmithKline ... 1305
Amoxil Chewable Tablets (Amoxicillin) GlaxoSmithKline ... 1305
Amoxil Pediatric Drops for Oral Suspension (Amoxicillin) GlaxoSmithKline ... 1305
Amoxil Powder for Oral Suspension (Amoxicillin) GlaxoSmithKline ... 1305
Amoxil Tablets (Amoxicillin) GlaxoSmithKline ... 1305
Augmentin Tablets (Amoxicillin, Clavulanate Potassium) GlaxoSmithKline ... 1327
Augmentin ES-600 Powder for Oral Suspension (Amoxicillin, Clavulanate Potassium) GlaxoSmithKline ... 1329
Biaxin/Biaxin XL (Clarithromycin) Abbott ... 411
Ceftin (Cefuroxime Axetil) GlaxoSmithKline ... 1380
Omnicef Capsules (Cefdinir) Abbott ... 497
Omnicef for Oral Suspension (Cefdinir) Abbott ... 497
Prevnar (Pneumococcal vaccine, diphtheria conjugate) Wyeth ... 3241
Rocephin Injectable Vials, ADD-Vantage, Galaxy, Bulk (Ceftriaxone Sodium) Roche ... 2642
Suprax for Oral Suspension (Cefixime) Lupin ... 1891

S. pneumoniae pharyngitis

Amoxil Capsules (Amoxicillin) GlaxoSmithKline ... 1305
Amoxil Chewable Tablets (Amoxicillin) GlaxoSmithKline ... 1305
Amoxil Pediatric Drops for Oral Suspension (Amoxicillin) GlaxoSmithKline ... 1305
Amoxil Powder for Oral Suspension (Amoxicillin) GlaxoSmithKline ... 1305
Amoxil Tablets (Amoxicillin) GlaxoSmithKline ... 1305
EryPed (Erythromycin Ethylsuccinate) Abbott ... 431

S. pneumoniae respiratory tract infections

Amoxil Capsules (Amoxicillin) GlaxoSmithKline ... 1305
Amoxil Chewable Tablets (Amoxicillin) GlaxoSmithKline ... 1305
Amoxil Pediatric Drops for Oral Suspension (Amoxicillin) GlaxoSmithKline ... 1305
Amoxil Powder for Oral Suspension (Amoxicillin) GlaxoSmithKline ... 1305
Amoxil Tablets (Amoxicillin) GlaxoSmithKline ... 1305

S. pneumoniae septicemia

Fortaz (Ceftazidime) GlaxoSmithKline ... 1450
Rocephin Injectable Vials, ADD-Vantage, Galaxy, Bulk (Ceftriaxone Sodium) Roche ... 2642
Zinacef for Injection (Cefuroxime) GlaxoSmithKline ... 1678
Zinacef Injection (Cefuroxime) GlaxoSmithKline ... 1678

S. pneumoniae sinusitis

Amoxil Capsules (Amoxicillin) GlaxoSmithKline ... 1305
Amoxil Chewable Tablets (Amoxicillin) GlaxoSmithKline ... 1305
Amoxil Pediatric Drops for Oral Suspension (Amoxicillin) GlaxoSmithKline ... 1305
Amoxil Powder for Oral Suspension (Amoxicillin) GlaxoSmithKline ... 1305
Amoxil Tablets (Amoxicillin) GlaxoSmithKline ... 1305
Augmentin XR Extended Release Tablets (Amoxicillin, Clavulanate Potassium) GlaxoSmithKline ... 1333
Avelox (Moxifloxacin Hydrochloride) Schering ... 2803
Biaxin/Biaxin XL (Clarithromycin) Abbott ... 411
Ceftin Tablets (Cefuroxime Axetil) GlaxoSmithKline ... 1380
Cipro I.V. (Ciprofloxacin) Schering ... 2817
Cipro (Ciprofloxacin) Schering ... 2810
Levaquin (Levofloxacin) Ortho-McNeil ... 2416
Levaquin in 5% Dextrose Injection (Levofloxacin) Ortho-McNeil ... 2416

S. pneumoniae upper respiratory tract infections

Amoxil Capsules (Amoxicillin) GlaxoSmithKline ... 1305
Amoxil Chewable Tablets (Amoxicillin) GlaxoSmithKline ... 1305
Amoxil Pediatric Drops for Oral Suspension (Amoxicillin) GlaxoSmithKline ... 1305
Amoxil Powder for Oral Suspension (Amoxicillin) GlaxoSmithKline ... 1305
Amoxil Tablets (Amoxicillin) GlaxoSmithKline ... 1305
Biaxin/Biaxin XL (Clarithromycin) Abbott ... 411
E.E.S. (Erythromycin Ethylsuccinate) Abbott ... 433
EryPed (Erythromycin Ethylsuccinate) Abbott ... 431

S. pyogenes infections

Avelox (Moxifloxacin Hydrochloride) Schering ... 2803
Bactroban Ointment (Mupirocin) GlaxoSmithKline ... 1368
Biaxin/Biaxin XL (Clarithromycin) Abbott ... 411
Ceftin (Cefuroxime Axetil) GlaxoSmithKline ... 1380
Cipro I.V. (Ciprofloxacin) Schering ... 2817
Cipro (Ciprofloxacin) Schering ... 2810
E.E.S. (Erythromycin Ethylsuccinate) Abbott ... 433
EryPed (Erythromycin Ethylsuccinate) Abbott ... 431
Fortaz (Ceftazidime) GlaxoSmithKline ... 1450
Invanz for Injection (Ertapenem) Merck ... 2029
Levaquin (Levofloxacin) Ortho-McNeil ... 2416
Levaquin in 5% Dextrose Injection (Levofloxacin) Ortho-McNeil ... 2416
Merrem I.V. (Meropenem) AstraZeneca Pharmaceuticals ... 684
Omnicef Capsules (Cefdinir) Abbott ... 497
Omnicef for Oral Suspension (Cefdinir) Abbott ... 497
Primaxin I.M. (Cilastatin Sodium, Imipenem) Merck ... 2080
Primaxin I.V. (Cilastatin Sodium, Imipenem) Merck ... 2083
Rocephin Injectable Vials, ADD-Vantage, Galaxy, Bulk (Ceftriaxone Sodium) Roche ... 2642
Suprax for Oral Suspension (Cefixime) Lupin ... 1891
Suprax Tablets (Cefixime) Lupin ... 1891
Tygacil for Injection (Tigecycline) Wyeth ... 3276
Zinacef for Injection (Cefuroxime) GlaxoSmithKline ... 1678
Zinacef Injection (Cefuroxime) GlaxoSmithKline ... 1678
Zyvox (Linezolid) Pharmacia & Upjohn ... 2552

S. pyogenes infections, ocular

Pred-G Ophthalmic Ointment (Gentamicin Sulfate, Prednisolone Acetate) Allergan ... ⊙229

S. pyogenes lower respiratory tract infections

E.E.S. (Erythromycin Ethylsuccinate) Abbott ... 433
EryPed (Erythromycin Ethylsuccinate) Abbott ... 431
Zinacef for Injection (Cefuroxime) GlaxoSmithKline ... 1678
Zinacef Injection (Cefuroxime) GlaxoSmithKline ... 1678

S. pyogenes otitis media

Ceftin (Cefuroxime Axetil) GlaxoSmithKline ... 1380
Suprax for Oral Suspension (Cefixime) Lupin ... 1891
Suprax Tablets (Cefixime) Lupin ... 1891

S. pyogenes pharyngitis

Biaxin/Biaxin XL (Clarithromycin) Abbott ... 411
Ceftin (Cefuroxime Axetil) GlaxoSmithKline ... 1380
Moxatag Tablets (Amoxicillin) MiddleBrook ... 2165
Omnicef Capsules (Cefdinir) Abbott ... 497
Omnicef for Oral Suspension (Cefdinir) Abbott ... 497
Suprax for Oral Suspension (Cefixime) Lupin ... 1891
Suprax Tablets (Cefixime) Lupin ... 1891

S. pyogenes skin and skin structure infections

Avelox (Moxifloxacin Hydrochloride) Schering ... 2803
Bactroban Cream (Mupirocin Calcium) GlaxoSmithKline ... 1366
Biaxin/Biaxin XL (Clarithromycin) Abbott ... 411
Ceftin Tablets (Cefuroxime Axetil) GlaxoSmithKline ... 1380
Cipro I.V. (Ciprofloxacin) Schering ... 2817
Cipro (Ciprofloxacin) Schering ... 2810
Cubicin for Injection (Daptomycin) Cubist ... 995
E.E.S. (Erythromycin Ethylsuccinate) Abbott ... 433
EryPed (Erythromycin Ethylsuccinate) Abbott ... 431

Fortaz (Ceftazidime) GlaxoSmithKline ... 1450
Invanz for Injection (Ertapenem) Merck ... 2029
Levaquin (Levofloxacin) Ortho-McNeil ... 2416
Levaquin in 5% Dextrose Injection (Levofloxacin) Ortho-McNeil ... 2416
Merrem I.V. (Meropenem) AstraZeneca Pharmaceuticals ... 684
Omnicef Capsules (Cefdinir) Abbott .. 497
Omnicef for Oral Suspension (Cefdinir) Abbott ... 497
Primaxin I.M. (Cilastatin Sodium, Imipenem) Merck ... 2080
Primaxin I.V. (Cilastatin Sodium, Imipenem) Merck ... 2083
Rocephin Injectable Vials, ADD-Vantage, Galaxy, Bulk (Ceftriaxone Sodium) Roche ... 2642
Tygacil for Injection (Tigecycline) Wyeth ... 3276
Zinacef for Injection (Cefuroxime) GlaxoSmithKline ... 1678
Zinacef Injection (Cefuroxime) GlaxoSmithKline ... 1678
Zyvox (Linezolid) Pharmacia & Upjohn ... 2552

S. pyogenes tonsillitis
Biaxin/Biaxin XL (Clarithromycin) Abbott ... 411
Ceftin (Cefuroxime Axetil) GlaxoSmithKline ... 1380
Moxatag Tablets (Amoxicillin) MiddleBrook ... 2165
Omnicef Capsules (Cefdinir) Abbott .. 497
Omnicef for Oral Suspension (Cefdinir) Abbott ... 497
Suprax for Oral Suspension (Cefixime) Lupin ... 1891
Suprax Tablets (Cefixime) Lupin ... 1891

S. pyogenes upper respiratory tract infections
Biaxin/Biaxin XL (Clarithromycin) Abbott ... 411
E.E.S. (Erythromycin Ethylsuccinate) Abbott ... 433
EryPed (Erythromycin Ethylsuccinate) Abbott ... 431
Omnicef Capsules (Cefdinir) Abbott .. 497
Omnicef for Oral Suspension (Cefdinir) Abbott ... 497
Suprax for Oral Suspension (Cefixime) Lupin ... 1891
Suprax Tablets (Cefixime) Lupin ... 1891

S. saprophyticus cystitis
Cipro (Ciprofloxacin) Schering ... 2810

S. saprophyticus urinary tract infections
Cipro (Ciprofloxacin) Schering ... 2810
Cipro XR Tablets (Ciprofloxacin) Schering ... 2823
Levaquin (Levofloxacin) Ortho-McNeil ... 2416
Levaquin in 5% Dextrose Injection (Levofloxacin) Ortho-McNeil ... 2416
Noroxin Tablets (Norfloxacin) Merck . 2069

S. viridans skin and skin structure infections
Merrem I.V. (Meropenem) AstraZeneca Pharmaceuticals ... 684

S. warnerii infections, ocular
Vigamox Ophthalmic Solution (Moxifloxacin Hydrochloride) Alcon ... 548

SAH
(*see under* Hemorrhage, subarachnoid, resulting in neurological deficits)

Salmonella typhi infections
Cipro (Ciprofloxacin) Schering ... 2810

Sarcoma botryoides
Cosmegen for Injection (Dactinomycin) Ovation ... 2485

Scar tissue
Mederma Topical Gel (Allantoin, Allium cepa) Merz ... 2163
Mederma Cream Plus SPF 30 (Octocrylene, Avobenzone, Oxybenzone) Merz ... 2163
Mederma for Kids Topical Gel (Allantoin, Allium cepa) Merz ... 2164

Scarlatina
Bicillin C-R Injectable Suspension (Penicillin G Benzathine, Penicillin G Procaine) King ... 1775
Bicillin L-A Injection (Penicillin G Benzathine, Penicillin G Procaine) King ... 1777

Scarlet fever
(*see under* Scarlatina)

Schizophrenia
Abilify Oral Solution (Aripiprazole) Bristol-Myers Squibb ... 881
Abilify Oral Solution (Aripiprazole) Otsuka ... 2466
Abilify Discmelt Orally Disintegrating Tablets (Aripiprazole) Bristol-Myers Squibb ... 881
Abilify Discmelt Orally Disintegrating Tablets (Aripiprazole) Otsuka ... 2466
Abilify Tablets (Aripiprazole) Bristol-Myers Squibb ... 881
Abilify Tablets (Aripiprazole) Otsuka .. 2466
Geodon (Ziprasidone Hydrochloride) Pfizer ... 2520
Invega Extended-Release Tablets (Paliperidone) Janssen ... 1748
Moban Tablets (Molindone Hydrochloride) Endo ... 1116
Risperdal Consta Long-Acting Injection (Risperidone) Janssen ... 1753
Thioridazine Hydrochloride Tablets (Thioridazine Hydrochloride) Mylan ... 2195
Thiothixene Capsules (Thiothixene) Mylan ... 2197
Zyprexa Tablets (Olanzapine) Lilly ... 1883
Zyprexa ZYDIS Orally Disintegrating Tablets (Olanzapine) Lilly ... 1883

Scleroderma, linear, possibly effective in
Potaba (Aminobenzoate Potassium) Glenwood ... 1698

Scleroderma, possibly effective in
Potaba (Aminobenzoate Potassium) Glenwood ... 1698

Seasonal Affective Disorder
Wellbutrin XL Extended-Release Tablets (Bupropion Hydrochloride) GlaxoSmithKline ... 1659

Seborrhea
(*see under* Dandruff)

Sedation
(*see also under* Sleep, induction of)
Nembutal Sodium Solution, USP (Pentobarbital Sodium) Ovation ... 2494

Sedation, benzodiazepine-induced, complete or partial reversal of
Romazicon Injection (Flumazenil) Roche ... 2646

Sedation, daytime
Xyrem Oral Solution (Sodium Oxybate) Jazz ... 1766

Seizures, absence, adjunctive therapy in
Depakote ER Tablets (Divalproex Sodium) Abbott ... 423

Seizures, akinetic
Klonopin (Clonazepam) Roche ... 2639

Seizures, centrencephalic
(*see under* Seizures, generalized, absence; Seizures, generalized, tonic-clonic)

Seizures, focal
Carbatrol Capsules (Carbamazepine) Shire US ... 3019
Lyrica Capsules (Pregabalin) Pfizer ... 2527
Phenytek Capsules (Phenytoin Sodium) Mylan ... 2192

Seizures, generalized, absence
Depakote ER Tablets (Divalproex Sodium) Abbott ... 423
Klonopin (Clonazepam) Roche ... 2639

Seizures, generalized, tonic-clonic
Carbatrol Capsules (Carbamazepine) Shire US ... 3019
Phenytek Capsules (Phenytoin Sodium) Mylan ... 2192

Seizures, generalized, tonic-clonic, adjunctive therapy in
Keppra Injection (Levetiracetam) UCB, Inc. ... 3137
Keppra Oral Solution (Levetiracetam) UCB, Inc. ... 3131
Keppra Tablets (Levetiracetam) UCB, Inc. ... 3131
Lamictal (Lamotrigine) GlaxoSmithKline ... 1488

Seizures, multiple, adjunctive therapy in
Depakote ER Tablets (Divalproex Sodium) Abbott ... 423

Seizures, myoclonic
Klonopin (Clonazepam) Roche ... 2639

Seizures, myoclonic, adjunctive therapy in
Keppra Injection (Levetiracetam) UCB, Inc. ... 3137
Keppra Oral Solution (Levetiracetam) UCB, Inc. ... 3131
Keppra Tablets (Levetiracetam) UCB, Inc. ... 3131

Seizures, neurosurgery-induced
Phenytek Capsules (Phenytoin Sodium) Mylan ... 2192

Seizures, neurosurgery-induced, prophylaxis of
Phenytek Capsules (Phenytoin Sodium) Mylan ... 2192

Seizures, partial
(*see under* Seizures, focal)

Seizures, partial, adjunctive therapy in
Depakote ER Tablets (Divalproex Sodium) Abbott ... 423
Gabitril Tablets (Tiagabine Hydrochloride) Cephalon ... 973
Keppra Injection (Levetiracetam) UCB, Inc. ... 3137
Keppra Oral Solution (Levetiracetam) UCB, Inc. ... 3131
Keppra Tablets (Levetiracetam) UCB, Inc. ... 3131
Lamictal (Lamotrigine) GlaxoSmithKline ... 1488
Zonegran Capsules (Zonisamide) Eisai ... 1089

Seizures, partial, complex
Depakote ER Tablets (Divalproex Sodium) Abbott ... 423

Seizures, psychomotor
Carbatrol Capsules (Carbamazepine) Shire US ... 3019
Phenytek Capsules (Phenytoin Sodium) Mylan ... 2192

Senile lentigines
(*see under* Hyperpigmentation, skin, bleaching of)

Sepsis
Zinacef for Injection (Cefuroxime) GlaxoSmithKline ... 1678
Zinacef Injection (Cefuroxime) GlaxoSmithKline ... 1678

Sepsis, severe
Xigris Powder for Intravenous Infusion (Drotrecogin alfa (activated)) Lilly ... 1880

Septicemia, bacterial
Bicillin C-R Injectable Suspension (Penicillin G Benzathine, Penicillin G Procaine) King ... 1775
Bicillin L-A Injection (Penicillin G Benzathine, Penicillin G Procaine) King ... 1777
Cipro I.V. (Ciprofloxacin) Schering ... 2817
Fortaz (Ceftazidime) GlaxoSmithKline ... 1450
Invanz for Injection (Ertapenem) Merck ... 2029
Primaxin I.V. (Cilastatin Sodium, Imipenem) Merck ... 2083
Rocephin Injectable Vials, ADD-Vantage, Galaxy, Bulk (Ceftriaxone Sodium) Roche ... 2642
Timentin ADD-Vantage (Clavulanate Potassium, Ticarcillin Disodium) GlaxoSmithKline ... 1606
Timentin Injection Galaxy Container (Clavulanate Potassium, Ticarcillin Disodium) GlaxoSmithKline ... 1609
Timentin IV Infusion (Clavulanate Potassium, Ticarcillin Disodium) GlaxoSmithKline ... 1603
Timentin Pharmacy Bulk Package (Clavulanate Potassium, Ticarcillin Disodium) GlaxoSmithKline ... 1613
Zinacef for Injection (Cefuroxime) GlaxoSmithKline ... 1678
Zinacef Injection (Cefuroxime) GlaxoSmithKline ... 1678
Zyvox (Linezolid) Pharmacia & Upjohn ... 2552

Serratia marcescens bone and joint infections
Cipro I.V. (Ciprofloxacin) Schering ... 2817
Cipro (Ciprofloxacin) Schering ... 2810

Serratia marcescens infections
Cipro I.V. (Ciprofloxacin) Schering ... 2817
Cipro (Ciprofloxacin) Schering ... 2810
Levaquin (Levofloxacin) Ortho-McNeil ... 2416
Levaquin in 5% Dextrose Injection (Levofloxacin) Ortho-McNeil ... 2416
Noroxin Tablets (Norfloxacin) Merck . 2069
Primaxin I.V. (Cilastatin Sodium, Imipenem) Merck ... 2083
Rocephin Injectable Vials, ADD-Vantage, Galaxy, Bulk (Ceftriaxone Sodium) Roche ... 2642
Timentin ADD-Vantage (Clavulanate Potassium, Ticarcillin Disodium) GlaxoSmithKline ... 1606
Timentin Injection Galaxy Container (Clavulanate Potassium, Ticarcillin Disodium) GlaxoSmithKline ... 1609
Timentin IV Infusion (Clavulanate Potassium, Ticarcillin Disodium) GlaxoSmithKline ... 1603
Timentin Pharmacy Bulk Package (Clavulanate Potassium, Ticarcillin Disodium) GlaxoSmithKline ... 1613

Serratia marcescens infections, ocular
Ofloxacin Ophthalmic Solution 0.3% (Ofloxacin) Bausch & Lomb ... ⊙243
Pred-G Ophthalmic Ointment (Gentamicin Sulfate, Prednisolone Acetate) Allergan ... ⊙229
Pred-G Ophthalmic Suspension (Gentamicin Sulfate, Prednisolone Acetate) Allergan ... ⊙228
Quixin Ophthalmic Solution (Levofloxacin) Vistakon ... 3184

Serratia marcescens lower respiratory tract infections
Levaquin (Levofloxacin) Ortho-McNeil ... 2416
Levaquin in 5% Dextrose Injection (Levofloxacin) Ortho-McNeil ... 2416
Primaxin I.V. (Cilastatin Sodium, Imipenem) Merck ... 2083
Rocephin Injectable Vials, ADD-Vantage, Galaxy, Bulk (Ceftriaxone Sodium) Roche ... 2642

Serratia marcescens skin and skin structure infections
Rocephin Injectable Vials, ADD-Vantage, Galaxy, Bulk (Ceftriaxone Sodium) Roche ... 2642

Serratia marcescens urinary tract infections
Cipro I.V. (Ciprofloxacin) Schering ... 2817
Cipro (Ciprofloxacin) Schering ... 2810
Noroxin Tablets (Norfloxacin) Merck . 2069
Timentin ADD-Vantage (Clavulanate Potassium, Ticarcillin Disodium) GlaxoSmithKline ... 1606

Timentin Injection Galaxy Container (Clavulanate Potassium, Ticarcillin Disodium) GlaxoSmithKline 1609
Timentin IV Infusion (Clavulanate Potassium, Ticarcillin Disodium) GlaxoSmithKline 1603
Timentin Pharmacy Bulk Package (Clavulanate Potassium, Ticarcillin Disodium) GlaxoSmithKline 1613

Serratia species infections
Fortaz (Ceftazidime) GlaxoSmithKline 1450
Primaxin I.V. (Cilastatin Sodium, Imipenem) Merck 2083

Serratia species lower respiratory tract infections
Fortaz (Ceftazidime) GlaxoSmithKline 1450

Serratia species septicemia
Fortaz (Ceftazidime) GlaxoSmithKline 1450
Primaxin I.V. (Cilastatin Sodium, Imipenem) Merck 2083

Serratia species skin and skin structure infections
Fortaz (Ceftazidime) GlaxoSmithKline 1450
Primaxin I.V. (Cilastatin Sodium, Imipenem) Merck 2083

Shigella boydii infectious diarrhea
Cipro (Ciprofloxacin) Schering 2810

Shigella dysenteriae infectious diarrhea
Cipro (Ciprofloxacin) Schering 2810

Shigella flexneri infectious diarrhea
Cipro (Ciprofloxacin) Schering 2810

Shigella sonnei infectious diarrhea
Cipro (Ciprofloxacin) Schering 2810

Shingles
(*see under* Herpes zoster infections)

Short stature, children
Humatrope Vials and Cartridges (Somatropin) Lilly 1838
Norditropin Cartridges (Somatropin (rDNA Origin)) Novo Nordisk 2354
Nutropin for Injection (Somatropin) Genentech 1208
Nutropin AQ Injection (Somatropin) Genentech 1212
Nutropin AQ NuSpin Injection (Somatropin) Genentech 1212
Nutropin AQ Pen (Somatropin) Genentech 1212
Nutropin AQ Pen Cartridge (Somatropin) Genentech 1212

Short stature, idiopathic
Genotropin Lyophilized Powder (Somatropin) Pharmacia & Upjohn 2547
Humatrope Vials and Cartridges (Somatropin) Lilly 1838
Nutropin for Injection (Somatropin) Genentech 1208
Nutropin AQ Injection (Somatropin) Genentech 1212
Nutropin AQ NuSpin Injection (Somatropin) Genentech 1212
Nutropin AQ Pen (Somatropin) Genentech 1212
Nutropin AQ Pen Cartridge (Somatropin) Genentech 1212

Shoulder, acute painful
(*see under* Bursitis, subacromial, acute, symptomatic relief of)

Sinus congestion, symptomatic relief of
Benadryl Severe Allergy & Sinus Headache Caplets (Acetaminophen, Diphenhydramine Hydrochloride, Phenylephrine Hydrochloride) McNeil Consumer 1897
Sinutab Non-Drying Caplets (Guaifenesin, Phenylephrine Hydrochloride) McNeil Consumer 1905
Sinutab Sinus Caplets (Acetaminophen, Phenylephrine Hydrochloride) McNeil Consumer 1905
Sudafed 12 Hour Nasal Decongestant Non-Drowsy Caplets (Pseudoephedrine Hydrochloride) McNeil Consumer 1909
Sudafed 24 Hour Non-Drowsy Nasal Decongestant Tablets (Pseudoephedrine Hydrochloride) McNeil Consumer 1906
Children's Sudafed Nasal Decongestant Liquid (Pseudoephedrine Hydrochloride) McNeil Consumer 1906
Sudafed Nasal Decongestant Tablets (Pseudoephedrine Hydrochloride) McNeil Consumer 1906
Sudafed OM Sinus Cold Moisturizing Nasal Spray (Oxymetazoline Hydrochloride) McNeil Consumer 1906
Sudafed OM Sinus Congestion Moisturizing Nasal Spray (Oxymetazoline Hydrochloride) McNeil Consumer 1906
Sudafed PE Nasal Decongestant Tablets (Phenylephrine Hydrochloride) McNeil Consumer 1907
Sudafed PE Non-Drying Sinus Caplets (Guaifenesin, Phenylephrine Hydrochloride) McNeil Consumer 1908
Tylenol Allergy Multi-Symptom Caplets with Cool Burst and Rapid Release Gelcaps (Acetaminophen, Chlorpheniramine Maleate, Phenylephrine Hydrochloride) McNeil Consumer 1916
Tylenol Allergy Multi-Symptom Nighttime Caplets with Cool Burst (Acetaminophen, Diphenhydramine Hydrochloride, Phenylephrine Hydrochloride) McNeil Consumer 1916
Tylenol Chest Congestion Caplets with Cool Burst (Acetaminophen, Guaifenesin) McNeil Consumer 1910
Tylenol Chest Congestion Liquid with Cool Burst (Acetaminophen, Guaifenesin) McNeil Consumer 1910
Tylenol Cold Head Congestion Daytime Caplets with Cool Burst (Acetaminophen, Dextromethorphan Hydrobromide, Phenylephrine Hydrochloride) McNeil Consumer 1910
Tylenol Cold Head Congestion Nighttime Caplets with Cool Burst (Acetaminophen, Chlorpheniramine Maleate, Dextromethorphan Hydrobromide, Phenylephrine Hydrochloride) McNeil Consumer 1910
Tylenol Cold Multi-Symptom Daytime Caplets with Cool Burst and Rapid Release Gels (Acetaminophen, Dextromethorphan Hydrobromide, Phenylephrine Hydrochloride) McNeil Consumer 1913
Tylenol Cold Multi-Symptom Daytime Liquid with Citrus Burst (Acetaminophen, Dextromethorphan Hydrobromide, Phenylephrine Hydrochloride) McNeil Consumer 1913
Tylenol Sinus Congestion & Pain Daytime Caplets with Cool Burst and Gelcaps (Acetaminophen, Phenylephrine Hydrochloride) McNeil Consumer 1917
Tylenol Sinus Congestion & Pain Nighttime Caplets with Cool Burst (Acetaminophen, Chlorpheniramine Maleate, Phenylephrine Hydrochloride) McNeil Consumer 1917
Tylenol Sinus Congestion & Pain Severe Caplets with Cool Burst (Acetaminophen, Guaifenesin, Phenylephrine Hydrochloride) McNeil Consumer 1917
Tylenol Sinus Severe Congestion Caplets with Cool Burst (Acetaminophen, Guaifenesin, Pseudoephedrine Hydrochloride) McNeil Consumer 1917
Zyrtec-D Allergy & Congestion Extended-Release Tablets (Cetirizine Hydrochloride, Pseudoephedrine Hydrochloride) McNeil Consumer 1923

Sinus headache
Vicks NyQuil LiquiCaps (Acetaminophen, Dextromethorphan Hydrobromide, Doxylamine Succinate) Procter & Gamble .... ■617

Sinus pressure, relief of
Benadryl Severe Allergy & Sinus Headache Caplets (Acetaminophen, Diphenhydramine Hydrochloride, Phenylephrine Hydrochloride) McNeil Consumer 1897
Sinutab Non-Drying Caplets (Guaifenesin, Phenylephrine Hydrochloride) McNeil Consumer 1905
Sinutab Sinus Caplets (Acetaminophen, Phenylephrine Hydrochloride) McNeil Consumer 1905
Sudafed 12 Hour Nasal Decongestant Non-Drowsy Caplets (Pseudoephedrine Hydrochloride) McNeil Consumer 1909
Children's Sudafed Nasal Decongestant Liquid (Pseudoephedrine Hydrochloride) McNeil Consumer 1906
Sudafed OM Sinus Cold Moisturizing Nasal Spray (Oxymetazoline Hydrochloride) McNeil Consumer 1906
Sudafed OM Sinus Congestion Moisturizing Nasal Spray (Oxymetazoline Hydrochloride) McNeil Consumer 1906
Sudafed PE Nasal Decongestant Tablets (Phenylephrine Hydrochloride) McNeil Consumer 1907
Sudafed PE Non-Drying Sinus Caplets (Guaifenesin, Phenylephrine Hydrochloride) McNeil Consumer 1908
Tylenol Allergy Multi-Symptom Caplets with Cool Burst and Rapid Release Gelcaps (Acetaminophen, Chlorpheniramine Maleate, Phenylephrine Hydrochloride) McNeil Consumer 1916
Tylenol Allergy Multi-Symptom Nighttime Caplets with Cool Burst (Acetaminophen, Diphenhydramine Hydrochloride, Phenylephrine Hydrochloride) McNeil Consumer 1916
Tylenol Sinus Congestion & Pain Daytime Caplets with Cool Burst and Gelcaps (Acetaminophen, Phenylephrine Hydrochloride) McNeil Consumer 1917
Tylenol Sinus Congestion & Pain Nighttime Caplets with Cool Burst (Acetaminophen, Chlorpheniramine Maleate, Phenylephrine Hydrochloride) McNeil Consumer 1917
Tylenol Sinus Congestion & Pain Severe Caplets with Cool Burst (Acetaminophen, Guaifenesin, Phenylephrine Hydrochloride) McNeil Consumer 1917
Tylenol Sinus Severe Congestion Caplets with Cool Burst (Acetaminophen, Guaifenesin, Pseudoephedrine Hydrochloride) McNeil Consumer 1917
Zyrtec-D Allergy & Congestion Extended-Release Tablets (Cetirizine Hydrochloride, Pseudoephedrine Hydrochloride) McNeil Consumer 1923

Sinusitis, adjunctive therapy
Children's Motrin Cold Oral Suspension (Ibuprofen, Pseudoephedrine Hydrochloride) McNeil Consumer 1899

Sinusitis, treatment of
Augmentin (Amoxicillin, Clavulanate Potassium) GlaxoSmithKline 1323
Augmentin Tablets (Amoxicillin, Clavulanate Potassium) GlaxoSmithKline 1327
Augmentin XR Extended Release Tablets (Amoxicillin, Clavulanate Potassium) GlaxoSmithKline 1333
Avelox (Moxifloxacin Hydrochloride) Schering 2803
Biaxin/Biaxin XL (Clarithromycin) Abbott 411
Ceftin Tablets (Cefuroxime Axetil) GlaxoSmithKline 1380
Cipro I.V. (Ciprofloxacin) Schering 2817
Cipro (Ciprofloxacin) Schering 2810
E.E.S. (Erythromycin Ethylsuccinate) Abbott 433
EryPed (Erythromycin Ethylsuccinate) Abbott 431
Levaquin (Levofloxacin) Ortho-McNeil 2416
Levaquin in 5% Dextrose Injection (Levofloxacin) Ortho-McNeil 2416
Omnicef Capsules (Cefdinir) Abbott 497
Omnicef for Oral Suspension (Cefdinir) Abbott 497

Sitosterolemia
Zetia Tablets (Ezetimibe) Merck/Schering Plough 2157
Zetia Tablets (Ezetimibe) Schering 2951

Sjogren's syndrome
Evoxac Capsules (Cevimeline Hydrochloride) Daiichi Sankyo 1013
Salagen Tablets (Pilocarpine Hydrochloride) Eisai 1082

Skin, dry, moisturization of
MimyX Cream (Glycerin) Stiefel 3059
Pure Gardens Cream (Herbals with Vitamins) Awareness Corporation/Awareness Life .... ■624
Tahitian Noni Seed Oil (Herbal Medicines, unspecified) Tahitian Noni International .... ■634

Skin, fine wrinkles, mitigation of
Pure Gardens Cream (Herbals with Vitamins) Awareness Corporation/Awareness Life .... ■624

Skin, hyperpigmentation
(*see under* Hyperpigmentation, skin, bleaching of)

Skin, inflammatory conditions
(*see also under* Dermatoses, corticosteroid-responsive)
Diprolene Lotion 0.05% (Betamethasone Dipropionate) Schering 2838

Skin, irritation, minor, pain associated with
(*see under* Pain, topical relief of)

Skin, irritation, minor, temporary relief of
Smile's Prid Salve (Homeopathic Formulations) Standard Homeopathic .... ■620

Skin abscesses
(*see under* Infections, skin and skin structure)

Skin and skin structure disorders
Levaquin (Levofloxacin) Ortho-McNeil 2416
Levaquin in 5% Dextrose Injection (Levofloxacin) Ortho-McNeil 2416

Skin infections, bacterial, minor
(*see under* Infections, skin, bacterial, minor)

Skin lacerations, infected
(*see under* Infections, skin and skin structure)

Skin ulcers, venous insufficiency-induced, non-infected
ProNutra Protein Supplement (Vitamins with Minerals, Whey Protein Isolate) Immunotec Medical 1730

Sleep, induction of
(*see also under* Sedation)
Ambien Tablets (Zolpidem Tartrate) sanofi-aventis 2692
Ambien CR Tablets (Zolpidem Tartrate) sanofi-aventis 2696

Hyland's Calms Forté Tablets and Caplets (Homeopathic Formulations) Standard Homeopathic ...... ▣618
Lunesta Tablets (Eszopiclone) Sepracor **2994**
Nembutal Sodium Solution, USP (Pentobarbital Sodium) Ovation **2494**
Rozerem Tablets (Ramelteon) Takeda **3091**
Simply Sleep Caplets (Diphenhydramine Hydrochloride) McNeil Consumer **1905**

Sleep disorders
Provigil Tablets (Modafinil) Cephalon **977**

Slough, liquefaction of
Accuzyme SE Spray Emulsion (Papain, Urea) Healthpoint **1723**

Smoking cessation, temporary aid to
Chantix Tablets (Varenicline Tartrate) Pfizer **2511**
NoSmo[King] Stop Smoking Aid (Herbals, Multiple) NOSMO .... ▣630
Zyban Sustained-Release Tablets (Bupropion Hydrochloride) GlaxoSmithKline **1692**

Sneezing
Actifed Cold & Allergy Tablets (Chlorpheniramine Maleate, Phenylephrine Hydrochloride) McNeil Consumer **1895**
Allegra-D 12 Hour Extended-Release Tablets (Fexofenadine Hydrochloride, Pseudoephedrine Hydrochloride) sanofi-aventis **2687**
Benadryl Allergy & Cold Kapgels (Acetaminophen, Diphenhydramine Hydrochloride, Phenylephrine Hydrochloride) McNeil Consumer **1895**
Benadryl Allergy & Sinus Headache Kapgels (Acetaminophen, Diphenhydramine Hydrochloride, Phenylephrine Hydrochloride) McNeil Consumer **1895**
Benadryl Severe Allergy & Sinus Headache Caplets (Acetaminophen, Diphenhydramine Hydrochloride, Phenylephrine Hydrochloride) McNeil Consumer **1897**
Benadryl Dye-Free Allergy Liqui-gels Softgels (Diphenhydramine Hydrochloride) McNeil Consumer .. **1897**
Benadryl Allergy Kapgels (Diphenhydramine Hydrochloride) McNeil Consumer **1895**
Benadryl Allergy Quick Dissolve Strips (Diphenhydramine Hydrochloride) McNeil Consumer **1896**
Benadryl Allergy Ultratab Tablets (Diphenhydramine Hydrochloride) McNeil Consumer **1896**
Children's Benadryl Dye-Free Allergy Liquid (Diphenhydramine Hydrochloride) McNeil Consumer .. **1897**
Children's Benadryl Allergy Fastmelts (Diphenhydramine Hydrochloride) McNeil Consumer .. **1897**
Children's Benadryl Allergy Liquid (Diphenhydramine Hydrochloride) McNeil Consumer **1898**
Children's Benadryl Allergy Perfect Measure (Diphenhydramine Hydrochloride) McNeil Consumer .. **1896**
Children's Benadryl-D Allergy & Sinus Liquid (Diphenhydramine Hydrochloride, Phenylephrine Hydrochloride) McNeil Consumer .. **1896**
Benadryl-D Allergy & Sinus Tablet (Diphenhydramine Hydrochloride, Phenylephrine Hydrochloride) McNeil Consumer **1896**
PediaCare Children's Allergy & Cold Liquid (Diphenhydramine Hydrochloride, Phenylephrine Hydrochloride) McNeil Consumer .. **1902**
PediaCare Children's Allergy Liquid (Diphenhydramine Hydrochloride) McNeil Consumer **1902**
Sudafed PE Nighttime Cold Caplets (Acetaminophen, Diphenhydramine Hydrochloride, Phenylephrine Hydrochloride) McNeil Consumer **1907**
Sudafed PE Severe Cold Caplets (Acetaminophen, Diphenhydramine Hydrochloride, Phenylephrine Hydrochloride) McNeil Consumer **1908**
Sudafed PE Sinus & Allergy Tablets (Chlorpheniramine Maleate, Phenylephrine Hydrochloride) McNeil Consumer **1908**
Tylenol Allergy Multi-Symptom Caplets with Cool Burst and Rapid Release Gelcaps (Acetaminophen, Chlorpheniramine Maleate, Phenylephrine Hydrochloride) McNeil Consumer **1916**
Tylenol Allergy Multi-Symptom Nighttime Caplets with Cool Burst (Acetaminophen, Diphenhydramine Hydrochloride, Phenylephrine Hydrochloride) McNeil Consumer **1916**
Tylenol Severe Allergy Caplets (Acetaminophen, Diphenhydramine Hydrochloride) McNeil Consumer **1916**
Children's Tylenol Plus Cold Suspension Liquid (Acetaminophen, Chlorpheniramine Maleate, Phenylephrine Hydrochloride) McNeil Consumer **1912**
Children's Tylenol Plus Cold & Allergy Suspension Liquid (Acetaminophen, Diphenhydramine Hydrochloride, Phenylephrine Hydrochloride) McNeil Consumer .. **1914**
Children's Tylenol Plus Cough & Runny Nose Suspension Liquid (Acetaminophen, Chlorpheniramine Maleate, Dextromethorphan Hydrobromide) McNeil Consumer .. **1912**
Children's Tylenol Plus Flu Suspension Liquid (Acetaminophen, Chlorpheniramine Maleate, Dextromethorphan Hydrobromide, Phenylephrine Hydrochloride) McNeil Consumer **1914**
Children's Tylenol Plus Multi-Symptom Cold Suspension Liquid (Acetaminophen, Chlorpheniramine Maleate, Dextromethorphan Hydrobromide, Phenylephrine Hydrochloride) McNeil Consumer **1912**
Tylenol Cold Head Congestion Nighttime Caplets with Cool Burst (Acetaminophen, Chlorpheniramine Maleate, Dextromethorphan Hydrobromide, Phenylephrine Hydrochloride) McNeil Consumer **1910**
Tylenol Cold Multi-Symptom Nighttime Caplets with Cool Burst (Acetaminophen, Chlorpheniramine Maleate, Dextromethorphan Hydrobromide, Phenylephrine Hydrochloride) McNeil Consumer **1913**
Tylenol Cold Multi-Symptom Nighttime Liquid with Cool Burst (Acetaminophen, Dextromethorphan Hydrobromide, Doxylamine Succinate, Phenylephrine Hydrochloride) McNeil Consumer **1913**
Tylenol Cough & Sore Throat Nighttime Liquid with Cool Burst (Acetaminophen, Dextromethorphan Hydrobromide, Doxylamine Succinate) McNeil Consumer **1918**
Tylenol Sinus Congestion & Pain Nighttime Caplets with Cool Burst (Acetaminophen, Chlorpheniramine Maleate, Phenylephrine Hydrochloride) McNeil Consumer **1917**
Tylenol Sore Throat Nighttime Liquid with Cool Burst (Acetaminophen, Diphenhydramine Hydrochloride) McNeil Consumer **1918**
Vicks NyQuil Cold & Flu Multi-Symptom Relief (Acetaminophen, Dextromethorphan Hydrobromide, Doxylamine Succinate) Procter & Gamble .... ▣617
Vicks NyQuil LiquiCaps (Acetaminophen, Dextromethorphan Hydrobromide, Doxylamine Succinate, Pseudoephedrine Hydrochloride) Procter & Gamble **2567**
Vicks NyQuil Liquid (Acetaminophen, Dextromethorphan Hydrobromide, Doxylamine Succinate, Pseudoephedrine Hydrochloride) Procter & Gamble **2567**
Vicks NyQuil Multi-Symptom Cold/Flu Relief (Acetaminophen, Dextromethorphan Hydrobromide, Doxylamine Succinate, Pseudoephedrine Hydrochloride) Procter & Gamble **2567**
Zyrtec Allergy Tablets (Cetirizine Hydrochloride) McNeil Consumer .. **1919**
Children's Zyrtec Allergy Syrup (Cetirizine Hydrochloride) McNeil Consumer **1920**
Children's Zyrtec Allergy Chewable Tablets (Cetirizine Hydrochloride) McNeil Consumer **1922**
Zyrtec-D Allergy & Congestion Extended-Release Tablets (Cetirizine Hydrochloride, Pseudoephedrine Hydrochloride) McNeil Consumer **1923**

Snoring
SnoreStop Extinguisher 120 Oral Spray (Homeopathic Formulations) Green .... ▣607
SnoreStop Maximum Strength Chewable Tablets (Homeopathic Formulations) Green .... ▣607

Social phobia
(*see under* Anxiety disorder, social)

Solar lentigines
(*see under* Hyperpigmentation, skin, bleaching of)

Somatotropin deficiency syndrome
Humatrope Vials and Cartridges (Somatropin) Lilly **1838**

Sour stomach
(*see under* Hyperacidity, gastric, symptomatic relief of)

Spasm, skeletal muscle
Valium Tablets (Diazepam) Roche **2658**

Spasticity, cerebral palsy-induced
(*see under* Spasticity, upper motor neuron disorder-induced)

Spasticity, multiple sclerosis-induced
(*see under* Spasticity, upper motor neuron disorder-induced)

Spasticity, muscle, symptomatic alleviation of
Amrix Capsules (Cyclobenzaprine Hydrochloride) Cephalon **966**

Spasticity, spinal cord injury-induced
(*see under* Spasticity, upper motor neuron disorder-induced)

Spasticity, stroke-induced
(*see under* Spasticity, upper motor neuron disorder-induced)

Spasticity, upper motor neuron disorder-induced
Dantrium Capsules (Dantrolene Sodium) Procter & Gamble Pharmaceuticals **2580**
Valium Tablets (Diazepam) Roche **2658**

Spondyloarthropathy
Bayer Aspirin (Aspirin) Bayer HealthCare Consumer **750**

Sprains, topical relief of
(*see under* Pain, topical relief of)

Staphylococci, coagulase-negative, infections, ocular
Pred-G Ophthalmic Suspension (Gentamicin Sulfate, Prednisolone Acetate) Allergan .... ⊙228
Zylet Ophthalmic Suspension (Loteprednol Etabonate, Tobramycin) Bausch & Lomb .... ⊙247

Staphylococci, coagulase-positive, infections, ocular
Pred-G Ophthalmic Suspension (Gentamicin Sulfate, Prednisolone Acetate) Allergan .... ⊙228
Zylet Ophthalmic Suspension (Loteprednol Etabonate, Tobramycin) Bausch & Lomb .... ⊙247

Staphylococci, nonpenicillinase-producing, infections
Amoxil Capsules (Amoxicillin) GlaxoSmithKline **1305**
Amoxil Chewable Tablets (Amoxicillin) GlaxoSmithKline **1305**
Amoxil Pediatric Drops for Oral Suspension (Amoxicillin) GlaxoSmithKline **1305**
Amoxil Powder for Oral Suspension (Amoxicillin) GlaxoSmithKline **1305**
Amoxil Tablets (Amoxicillin) GlaxoSmithKline **1305**

Staphylococci, urinary tract infections
Gantrisin Pediatric Suspension (Acetyl Sulfisoxazole) Roche **2638**

Staphylococci lower respiratory tract infections
Amoxil Capsules (Amoxicillin) GlaxoSmithKline **1305**
Amoxil Chewable Tablets (Amoxicillin) GlaxoSmithKline **1305**
Amoxil Pediatric Drops for Oral Suspension (Amoxicillin) GlaxoSmithKline **1305**
Amoxil Powder for Oral Suspension (Amoxicillin) GlaxoSmithKline **1305**
Amoxil Tablets (Amoxicillin) GlaxoSmithKline **1305**

Staphylococci otitis media
Amoxil Capsules (Amoxicillin) GlaxoSmithKline **1305**
Amoxil Chewable Tablets (Amoxicillin) GlaxoSmithKline **1305**
Amoxil Pediatric Drops for Oral Suspension (Amoxicillin) GlaxoSmithKline **1305**
Amoxil Powder for Oral Suspension (Amoxicillin) GlaxoSmithKline **1305**
Amoxil Tablets (Amoxicillin) GlaxoSmithKline **1305**

Staphylococci skin and skin structure infections
Amoxil Capsules (Amoxicillin) GlaxoSmithKline **1305**
Amoxil Chewable Tablets (Amoxicillin) GlaxoSmithKline **1305**
Amoxil Pediatric Drops for Oral Suspension (Amoxicillin) GlaxoSmithKline **1305**
Amoxil Powder for Oral Suspension (Amoxicillin) GlaxoSmithKline **1305**
Amoxil Tablets (Amoxicillin) GlaxoSmithKline **1305**

Staphylococcus aureus
(*see under* S. aureus infections)

Staphylococcus epidermidis
(*see under* S. epidermis infections)

Staphylococcus species infections
Amoxil Capsules (Amoxicillin) GlaxoSmithKline **1305**
Amoxil Chewable Tablets (Amoxicillin) GlaxoSmithKline **1305**
Amoxil Pediatric Drops for Oral Suspension (Amoxicillin) GlaxoSmithKline **1305**
Amoxil Powder for Oral Suspension (Amoxicillin) GlaxoSmithKline **1305**
Amoxil Tablets (Amoxicillin) GlaxoSmithKline **1305**

Status epilepticus
(*see under* Epilepticus, status)

Steatorrhea, adjunctive therapy in
Ultrase MT Capsules (Pancrelipase) Axcan Pharma **719**

Stiff-man syndrome, adjunctive therapy in
Valium Tablets (Diazepam) Roche 2658

Stomach, sour
(*see under* Hyperacidity, gastric, symptomatic relief of)

Stomach, upset
(*see under* Digestive disorders, symptomatic relief of)

Stomatitis, recurrent aphthous, symptomatic relief of
Hurricaine Topical Anesthetic (Benzocaine) Beutlich 815

Strabismus
BOTOX Purified Neurotoxin Complex (Botulinum Toxin Type A) Allergan 550

Strep throat
(*see under* Streptococci species upper respiratory tract infections)

Streptococcal pharyngitis
E.E.S. (Erythromycin Ethylsuccinate) Abbott 433
Omnicef Capsules (Cefdinir) Abbott 497
Omnicef for Oral Suspension (Cefdinir) Abbott 497
Suprax for Oral Suspension (Cefixime) Lupin 1891
Suprax Tablets (Cefixime) Lupin 1891

Streptococci, alpha-hemolytic (viridans group), infections
Amoxil Capsules (Amoxicillin) GlaxoSmithKline 1305
Amoxil Chewable Tablets (Amoxicillin) GlaxoSmithKline 1305
Amoxil Pediatric Drops for Oral Suspension (Amoxicillin) GlaxoSmithKline 1305
Amoxil Powder for Oral Suspension (Amoxicillin) GlaxoSmithKline 1305
Amoxil Tablets (Amoxicillin) GlaxoSmithKline 1305

Streptococci (viridans group) infections, ocular
Blephamide Ophthalmic Ointment Allergan ..... ⊙217
Blephamide Ophthalmic Suspension Allergan ..... ⊙216
Quixin Ophthalmic Solution (Levofloxacin) Vistakon 3184

Streptococci group A beta-hemolytic infections
(*see also under* Erysipelas)
Amoxil Capsules (Amoxicillin) GlaxoSmithKline 1305
Amoxil Chewable Tablets (Amoxicillin) GlaxoSmithKline 1305
Amoxil Pediatric Drops for Oral Suspension (Amoxicillin) GlaxoSmithKline 1305
Amoxil Powder for Oral Suspension (Amoxicillin) GlaxoSmithKline 1305
Amoxil Tablets (Amoxicillin) GlaxoSmithKline 1305
Primaxin I.V. (Cilastatin Sodium, Imipenem) Merck 2083

Streptococci group A beta-hemolytic otitis media
Amoxil Capsules (Amoxicillin) GlaxoSmithKline 1305
Amoxil Chewable Tablets (Amoxicillin) GlaxoSmithKline 1305
Amoxil Pediatric Drops for Oral Suspension (Amoxicillin) GlaxoSmithKline 1305
Amoxil Powder for Oral Suspension (Amoxicillin) GlaxoSmithKline 1305
Amoxil Tablets (Amoxicillin) GlaxoSmithKline 1305

Streptococci group A beta-hemolytic skin and skin structure infections
Amoxil Capsules (Amoxicillin) GlaxoSmithKline 1305
Amoxil Chewable Tablets (Amoxicillin) GlaxoSmithKline 1305
Amoxil Pediatric Drops for Oral Suspension (Amoxicillin) GlaxoSmithKline 1305
Amoxil Powder for Oral Suspension (Amoxicillin) GlaxoSmithKline 1305
Amoxil Tablets (Amoxicillin) GlaxoSmithKline 1305
Fortaz (Ceftazidime) GlaxoSmithKline 1450
Primaxin I.V. (Cilastatin Sodium, Imipenem) Merck 2083

Streptococci group A beta-hemolytic species infections, ocular
Pred-G Ophthalmic Ointment (Gentamicin Sulfate, Prednisolone Acetate) Allergan ..... ⊙229
Pred-G Ophthalmic Suspension (Gentamicin Sulfate, Prednisolone Acetate) Allergan ..... ⊙228
Zylet Ophthalmic Suspension (Loteprednol Etabonate, Tobramycin) Bausch & Lomb ..... ⊙247

Streptococci group B infections
Primaxin I.V. (Cilastatin Sodium, Imipenem) Merck 2083

Streptococci group D bone and joint infections
Primaxin I.V. (Cilastatin Sodium, Imipenem) Merck 2083

Streptococci group D genitourinary tract infections
Primaxin I.V. (Cilastatin Sodium, Imipenem) Merck 2083

Streptococci group D gynecologic infections
Primaxin I.M. (Cilastatin Sodium, Imipenem) Merck 2080

Streptococci group D infections
Primaxin I.V. (Cilastatin Sodium, Imipenem) Merck 2083

Streptococci group D intra-abdominal infections
Primaxin I.M. (Cilastatin Sodium, Imipenem) Merck 2080
Primaxin I.V. (Cilastatin Sodium, Imipenem) Merck 2083

Streptococci group D septicemia
Primaxin I.V. (Cilastatin Sodium, Imipenem) Merck 2083

Streptococci group D skin and skin structure infections
Primaxin I.M. (Cilastatin Sodium, Imipenem) Merck 2080
Primaxin I.V. (Cilastatin Sodium, Imipenem) Merck 2083

Streptococci infections, ocular
Neosporin Ophthalmic Solution Sterile (Gramicidin, Neomycin Sulfate, Polymyxin B Sulfate) King ..... ⊙252
Quixin Ophthalmic Solution (Levofloxacin) Vistakon 3184
Zylet Ophthalmic Suspension (Loteprednol Etabonate, Tobramycin) Bausch & Lomb ..... ⊙247

Streptococci non-hemolytic species infections, ocular
Pred-G Ophthalmic Suspension (Gentamicin Sulfate, Prednisolone Acetate) Allergan ..... ⊙228
Zylet Ophthalmic Suspension (Loteprednol Etabonate, Tobramycin) Bausch & Lomb ..... ⊙247

Streptococci skin and skin structure infections
Amoxil Capsules (Amoxicillin) GlaxoSmithKline 1305
Amoxil Chewable Tablets (Amoxicillin) GlaxoSmithKline 1305
Amoxil Pediatric Drops for Oral Suspension (Amoxicillin) GlaxoSmithKline 1305
Amoxil Powder for Oral Suspension (Amoxicillin) GlaxoSmithKline 1305
Amoxil Tablets (Amoxicillin) GlaxoSmithKline 1305
Bicillin C-R Injectable Suspension (Penicillin G Benzathine, Penicillin G Procaine) King 1775
Bicillin L-A Injection (Penicillin G Benzathine, Penicillin G Procaine) King 1777

Streptococci species infections
Bicillin C-R Injectable Suspension (Penicillin G Benzathine, Penicillin G Procaine) King 1775
Bicillin L-A Injection (Penicillin G Benzathine, Penicillin G Procaine) King 1777

Streptococci species upper respiratory tract infections
Amoxil Capsules (Amoxicillin) GlaxoSmithKline 1305
Amoxil Chewable Tablets (Amoxicillin) GlaxoSmithKline 1305
Amoxil Pediatric Drops for Oral Suspension (Amoxicillin) GlaxoSmithKline 1305
Amoxil Powder for Oral Suspension (Amoxicillin) GlaxoSmithKline 1305
Amoxil Tablets (Amoxicillin) GlaxoSmithKline 1305
Ceftin (Cefuroxime Axetil) GlaxoSmithKline 1380
Omnicef Capsules (Cefdinir) Abbott 497
Omnicef for Oral Suspension (Cefdinir) Abbott 497
Suprax for Oral Suspension (Cefixime) Lupin 1891
Suprax Tablets (Cefixime) Lupin 1891

Streptococcus agalactiae infections
(*see under* S. agalactiae infections)

Streptococcus faecalis
(*see under* S. faecalis infections)

Streptococcus pneumoniae
(*see under* S. pneumoniae infections)

Streptococcus pneumoniae, immunization against
(*see also under* Pneumococcal disease, immunization against)
Pneumovax 23 (Pneumococcal Vaccine, Polyvalent) Merck 2078
Prevnar (Pneumococcal vaccine, diphtheria conjugate) Wyeth 3241

Streptococcus pneumoniae infections, ocular
Neosporin Ophthalmic Solution Sterile (Gramicidin, Neomycin Sulfate, Polymyxin B Sulfate) King ..... ⊙252

Streptococcus pyogenes
(*see under* S. pyogenes infections)

Streptococcus species infections
Amoxil Capsules (Amoxicillin) GlaxoSmithKline 1305
Amoxil Chewable Tablets (Amoxicillin) GlaxoSmithKline 1305
Amoxil Pediatric Drops for Oral Suspension (Amoxicillin) GlaxoSmithKline 1305
Amoxil Powder for Oral Suspension (Amoxicillin) GlaxoSmithKline 1305
Amoxil Tablets (Amoxicillin) GlaxoSmithKline 1305
Bactroban Ointment (Mupirocin) GlaxoSmithKline 1368
Doribax Injection (Doripenem) Ortho-McNeil 2400
Omnicef Capsules (Cefdinir) Abbott 497
Omnicef for Oral Suspension (Cefdinir) Abbott 497
Suprax for Oral Suspension (Cefixime) Lupin 1891
Suprax Tablets (Cefixime) Lupin 1891

Streptococcus species intra-abdominal infections
Doribax Injection (Doripenem) Ortho-McNeil 2400

Streptococcus tonsillitis
(*see under* Streptococci species upper respiratory tract infections)

Streptococcus viridans group infections
Merrem I.V. (Meropenem) AstraZeneca Pharmaceuticals 684
Primaxin I.M. (Cilastatin Sodium, Imipenem) Merck 2080
Rocephin Injectable Vials, ADD-Vantage, Galaxy, Bulk (Ceftriaxone Sodium) Roche 2642
Vigamox Ophthalmic Solution (Moxifloxacin Hydrochloride) Alcon 548

Stress disorder, post-traumatic
Paxil (Paroxetine Hydrochloride) GlaxoSmithKline 1535

Stroke, ischemic
Activase I.V. (Alteplase) Genentech 1188

Stroke, to reduce the risk of
Aggrenox Capsules (Aspirin, Dipyridamole) Boehringer Ingelheim 819
Bayer Aspirin (Aspirin) Bayer HealthCare Consumer 750
Cozaar Tablets (Losartan Potassium) Merck 1973
Lipitor Tablets (Atorvastatin Calcium) Parke-Davis 2501
Plavix Tablets (Clopidogrel Bisulfate) Bristol-Myers Squibb 926
Plavix Tablets (Clopidogrel Bisulfate) sanofi-aventis 2767
Zocor Tablets (Simvastatin) Merck 2136

Strongyloidiasis
Stromectol Tablets (Ivermectin) Merck 2120

Sunburn, pain associated with
(*see under* Pain, topical relief of)

Swelling, nasal passages
Sudafed 24 Hour Non-Drowsy Nasal Decongestant Tablets (Pseudoephedrine Hydrochloride) McNeil Consumer 1906
Sudafed OM Sinus Cold Moisturizing Nasal Spray (Oxymetazoline Hydrochloride) McNeil Consumer 1906
Sudafed OM Sinus Congestion Moisturizing Nasal Spray (Oxymetazoline Hydrochloride) McNeil Consumer 1906
Tylenol Sinus Congestion & Pain Nighttime Caplets with Cool Burst (Acetaminophen, Chlorpheniramine Maleate, Phenylephrine Hydrochloride) McNeil Consumer 1917
Zyrtec-D Allergy & Congestion Extended-Release Tablets (Cetirizine Hydrochloride, Pseudoephedrine Hydrochloride) McNeil Consumer 1923

Sympathetic ophthalmia
(*see under* Ophthalmia, sympathetic)

T

T. pallidum infections
E.E.S. (Erythromycin Ethylsuccinate) Abbott 433
EryPed (Erythromycin Ethylsuccinate) Abbott 431

Tachycardia, paroxysmal supraventricular
Adenocard IV Injection (Adenosine) Astellas 603
Rythmol Tablets (Propafenone Hydrochloride) GlaxoSmithKline 1586

Tachycardia, paroxysmal supraventricular associated with Wolff-Parkinson-White syndrome
(*see under* Wolff-Parkinson-White syndrome)

Tachycardia, ventricular, sustained
Rythmol Tablets (Propafenone Hydrochloride) GlaxoSmithKline 1586

Tachycardias, paroxysmal atrial
(*see under* Tachycardia, paroxysmal supraventricular)

Taenia solium infections
Albenza Tablets (Albendazole) GlaxoSmithKline 1297

Tapeworm infections
(*see under* Infections, tapeworm)

Tendonitis
Anaprox Tablets (Naproxen Sodium) Roche 2632
Anaprox DS Tablets (Naproxen Sodium) Roche 2632
Clinoril Tablets (Sulindac) Merck 1962
Indocin (Indomethacin) Merck 2024
Naprosyn Suspension (Naproxen) Roche 2632
Naprosyn Tablets (Naproxen) Roche 2632
Traumeel Injection Solution (Homeopathic Formulations) Heel 1725

Testis, advanced carcinoma of
(*see under* Carcinoma, testis, advanced)

Testosterone, deficiency of
(*see under* Androgen, absence or deficiency of)

Threadworm infestations
(*see under* Strongyloidiasis)

Throat, itchy
(*see under* Pruritus, rhinopharyngeal, symptomatic relief of)

Throat, sore
(*see also under* Pharyngitis, symptomatic relief of)
Benadryl Allergy & Cold Kapgels (Acetaminophen, Diphenhydramine Hydrochloride, Phenylephrine Hydrochloride) McNeil Consumer 1895
Hurricaine Topical Anesthetic (Benzocaine) Beutlich 815
Children's Motrin Oral Suspension (Ibuprofen) McNeil Consumer 1901
Children's Motrin Non-Staining Dye-Free Oral Suspension (Ibuprofen) McNeil Consumer 1901
Infants' Motrin Concentrated Drops (Ibuprofen) McNeil Consumer 1901
Infants' Motrin Non-Staining Dye-Free Concentrated Drops (Ibuprofen) McNeil Consumer 1901
Junior Strength Motrin Caplets and Chewable Tablets (Ibuprofen) McNeil Consumer 1901
Sudafed PE Cold & Cough Caplets (Acetaminophen, Dextromethorphan Hydrobromide, Guaifenesin, Phenylephrine Hydrochloride) McNeil Consumer 1907
Sudafed PE Nighttime Cold Caplets (Acetaminophen, Diphenhydramine Hydrochloride, Phenylephrine Hydrochloride) McNeil Consumer 1907
Sudafed PE Severe Cold Caplets (Acetaminophen, Diphenhydramine Hydrochloride, Phenylephrine Hydrochloride) McNeil Consumer 1908
Tylenol Allergy Multi-Symptom Nighttime Caplets with Cool Burst (Acetaminophen, Diphenhydramine Hydrochloride, Phenylephrine Hydrochloride) McNeil Consumer 1916
Tylenol Chest Congestion Caplets with Cool Burst (Acetaminophen, Guaifenesin) McNeil Consumer 1910
Tylenol Chest Congestion Liquid with Cool Burst (Acetaminophen, Guaifenesin) McNeil Consumer 1910
Children's Tylenol Plus Cold Suspension Liquid (Acetaminophen, Chlorpheniramine Maleate, Phenylephrine Hydrochloride) McNeil Consumer 1912
Children's Tylenol Plus Cold & Allergy Suspension Liquid (Acetaminophen, Diphenhydramine Hydrochloride, Phenylephrine Hydrochloride) McNeil Consumer 1914
Children's Tylenol Plus Cough & Runny Nose Suspension Liquid (Acetaminophen, Chlorpheniramine Maleate, Dextromethorphan Hydrobromide) McNeil Consumer 1912
Children's Tylenol Plus Cough & Sore Throat Suspension Liquid (Acetaminophen, Dextromethorphan Hydrobromide) McNeil Consumer 1912
Children's Tylenol Plus Flu Suspension Liquid (Acetaminophen, Chlorpheniramine Maleate, Dextromethorphan Hydrobromide, Phenylephrine Hydrochloride) McNeil Consumer 1914
Children's Tylenol Suspension Liquid (Acetaminophen) McNeil Consumer 1909
Children's Tylenol Meltaways (Acetaminophen) McNeil Consumer 1909
Children's Tylenol Plus Multi-Symptom Cold Suspension Liquid (Acetaminophen, Chlorpheniramine Maleate, Dextromethorphan Hydrobromide, Phenylephrine Hydrochloride) McNeil Consumer 1912
Tylenol Cold Severe Congestion Daytime Caplets with Cool Burst (Acetaminophen, Dextromethorphan Hydrobromide, Guaifenesin, Pseudoephedrine Hydrochloride) McNeil Consumer 1912
Tylenol Cold Head Congestion Daytime Caplets with Cool Burst (Acetaminophen, Dextromethorphan Hydrobromide, Phenylephrine Hydrochloride) McNeil Consumer 1910
Tylenol Cold Head Congestion Nighttime Caplets with Cool Burst (Acetaminophen, Chlorpheniramine Maleate, Dextromethorphan Hydrobromide, Phenylephrine Hydrochloride) McNeil Consumer 1910
Tylenol Cold Head Congestion Severe Daytime Caplets with Cool Burst (Acetaminophen, Dextromethorphan Hydrobromide, Guaifenesin, Phenylephrine Hydrochloride) McNeil Consumer 1910
Tylenol Cold Multi-Symptom Daytime Caplets with Cool Burst and Rapid Release Gels (Acetaminophen, Dextromethorphan Hydrobromide, Phenylephrine Hydrochloride) McNeil Consumer 1913
Tylenol Cold Multi-Symptom Daytime Liquid with Citrus Burst (Acetaminophen, Dextromethorphan Hydrobromide, Phenylephrine Hydrochloride) McNeil Consumer 1913
Tylenol Cold Multi-Symptom Nighttime Caplets with Cool Burst (Acetaminophen, Chlorpheniramine Maleate, Dextromethorphan Hydrobromide, Phenylephrine Hydrochloride) McNeil Consumer 1913
Tylenol Cold Multi-Symptom Nighttime Liquid with Cool Burst (Acetaminophen, Dextromethorphan Hydrobromide, Doxylamine Succinate, Phenylephrine Hydrochloride) McNeil Consumer 1913
Tylenol Cold Multi-Symptom Severe Caplets with Cool Burst (Acetaminophen, Dextromethorphan Hydrobromide, Guaifenesin, Phenylephrine Hydrochloride) McNeil Consumer 1913
Tylenol Cold Multi-Symptom Severe Daytime Liquid with Citrus Burst (Acetaminophen, Dextromethorphan Hydrobromide, Guaifenesin, Phenylephrine Hydrochloride) McNeil Consumer 1913
Tylenol Cough & Sore Throat Daytime Liquid with Cool Burst (Acetaminophen, Dextromethorphan Hydrobromide) McNeil Consumer 1918
Tylenol Cough & Sore Throat Nighttime Liquid with Cool Burst (Acetaminophen, Dextromethorphan Hydrobromide, Doxylamine Succinate) McNeil Consumer 1918
Concentrated Tylenol Infants' Drops (Acetaminophen) McNeil Consumer 1909
Tylenol Sore Throat Daytime Liquid with Cool Burst (Acetaminophen) McNeil Consumer 1918
Tylenol Sore Throat Nighttime Liquid with Cool Burst (Acetaminophen, Diphenhydramine Hydrochloride) McNeil Consumer 1918
Vicks DayQuil Cold & Flu Multi-Symptom Relief (Acetaminophen, Dextromethorphan Hydrobromide, Phenylephrine Hydrochloride) Procter & Gamble .... ▣616
Vicks DayQuil LiquiCaps (Acetaminophen, Dextromethorphan Hydrobromide, Phenylephrine Hydrochloride) Procter & Gamble 2567
Vicks DayQuil (Acetaminophen, Dextromethorphan Hydrobromide, Phenylephrine Hydrochloride) Procter & Gamble .... ▣616
Vicks DayQuil Liquid (Acetaminophen, Dextromethorphan Hydrobromide, Phenylephrine Hydrochloride) Procter & Gamble 2567
Vicks DayQuil Multi-Symptom Cold/Flu Relief (Acetaminophen, Dextromethorphan Hydrobromide, Phenylephrine Hydrochloride) Procter & Gamble 2567
Vicks NyQuil Cold & Flu Multi-Symptom Relief (Acetaminophen, Dextromethorphan Hydrobromide, Doxylamine Succinate) Procter & Gamble .... ▣617
Vicks NyQuil LiquiCaps (Acetaminophen, Dextromethorphan Hydrobromide, Doxylamine Succinate, Pseudoephedrine Hydrochloride) Procter & Gamble 2567
Vicks NyQuil Liquid (Acetaminophen, Dextromethorphan Hydrobromide, Doxylamine Succinate, Pseudoephedrine Hydrochloride) Procter & Gamble 2567
Vicks NyQuil Multi-Symptom Cold/Flu Relief (Acetaminophen, Dextromethorphan Hydrobromide, Doxylamine Succinate, Pseudoephedrine Hydrochloride) Procter & Gamble 2567

Thrombocythemia
Agrylin Capsules (Anagrelide Hydrochloride) Shire US 3017

Thrombocytopenia, heparin-induced
Argatroban Injection (Argatroban) GlaxoSmithKline 1308
Refludan for Injection (Lepirudin) Bayer HealthCare Pharmaceuticals 795

Thromboembolic complications
Fragmin Injection (Dalteparin Sodium) Eisai 1070
Refludan for Injection (Lepirudin) Bayer HealthCare Pharmaceuticals 795

Thromboembolism, postoperative, adjunct in
Persantine Tablets (Dipyridamole) Boehringer Ingelheim 869

Thrombosis, deep venous, prophylaxis of
Arixtra Injection (Fondaparinux Sodium) GlaxoSmithKline 1313
Fragmin Injection (Dalteparin Sodium) Eisai 1070
Lovenox Injection (Enoxaparin Sodium) sanofi-aventis 2756

Thrombosis, deep venous, treatment of
Arixtra Injection (Fondaparinux Sodium) GlaxoSmithKline 1313
Lovenox Injection (Enoxaparin Sodium) sanofi-aventis 2756

Thrush
(*see under* Candidiasis, oropharyngeal)

Thyroid function, aid in the diagnosis of
Cytomel Tablets (Liothyronine Sodium) King 1778
Levothroid Tablets (Levothyroxine Sodium) Forest 1170
Levoxyl Tablets (Levothyroxine Sodium) King 1780
Naturethroid Tablets (Levothyroxine, Liothyronine, Thyroid) RLC 2605
Synthroid Tablets (Levothyroxine Sodium) Abbott 507

Thyroiditis, chronic lymphocytic
(*see under* Hashimoto's thyroiditis)

Tinea barbae
(*see under* Folliculitis barbae)

Tinea capitis infections
Gris-PEG Tablets (Griseofulvin) Pedinol 2507
Lamisil Oral Granules (Terbinafine Hydrochloride) Novartis 2264

Tinea corporis infections
Gris-PEG Tablets (Griseofulvin) Pedinol 2507
Lotrisone (Betamethasone Dipropionate, Clotrimazole) Schering 2881
Naftin Cream (Naftifine Hydrochloride) Merz 2164
Naftin Gel (Naftifine Hydrochloride) Merz 2164

Tinea cruris infections
Gris-PEG Tablets (Griseofulvin) Pedinol 2507
Lotrisone (Betamethasone Dipropionate, Clotrimazole) Schering 2881
Naftin Cream (Naftifine Hydrochloride) Merz 2164
Naftin Gel (Naftifine Hydrochloride) Merz 2164

Tinea pedis infections
Gordochom Solution (Chloroxylenol, Undecylenic Acid) Gordon 1699
Gris-PEG Tablets (Griseofulvin) Pedinol 2507
Lotrisone (Betamethasone Dipropionate, Clotrimazole) Schering 2881
Naftin Cream (Naftifine Hydrochloride) Merz 2164
Naftin Gel (Naftifine Hydrochloride) Merz 2164

Tinea unguium infections
Gris-PEG Tablets (Griseofulvin) Pedinol 2507
Lamisil Tablets (Terbinafine Hydrochloride) Novartis 2266

Tinea versicolor infections
(*see under* Pityrosporon orbiculare infections)

Tonsillitis
Biaxin/Biaxin XL (Clarithromycin) Abbott 411
Ceftin (Cefuroxime Axetil) GlaxoSmithKline 1380
E.E.S. (Erythromycin Ethylsuccinate) Abbott 433
Omnicef Capsules (Cefdinir) Abbott 497
Omnicef for Oral Suspension (Cefdinir) Abbott 497
Suprax for Oral Suspension (Cefixime) Lupin 1891
Suprax Tablets (Cefixime) Lupin 1891

Torulosis
(*see under* Cryptococcosis)

Toxoplasmosis, adjunctive therapy in
Daraprim Tablets (Pyrimethamine) GlaxoSmithKline 1400
Gantrisin Pediatric Suspension (Acetyl Sulfisoxazole) Roche 2638

Trachoma
Gantrisin Pediatric Suspension (Acetyl Sulfisoxazole) Roche 2638

Trachoma, adjunct in
Bleph-10 Ophthalmic Solution 10% (Sulfacetamide Sodium) Allergan .... ⊙215

Treponema pallidum
(*see under* T. pallidum infections)

Trichophyton crateriform infections
Gris-PEG Tablets (Griseofulvin) Pedinol 2507

Trichophyton gallinae infections
Gris-PEG Tablets (Griseofulvin) Pedinol 2507

Trichophyton interdigitalis infections
Gris-PEG Tablets (Griseofulvin) Pedinol 2507

Trichophyton megnini infections
Gris-PEG Tablets (Griseofulvin) Pedinol 2507

Trichophyton mentagrophytes infections
Gris-PEG Tablets (Griseofulvin) Pedinol 2507
Lotrisone (Betamethasone Dipropionate, Clotrimazole) Schering 2881
Naftin Cream (Naftifine Hydrochloride) Merz 2164
Naftin Gel (Naftifine Hydrochloride) Merz 2164

Trichophyton rubrum infections
Gris-PEG Tablets (Griseofulvin) Pedinol 2507
Lotrisone (Betamethasone Dipropionate, Clotrimazole) Schering 2881
Naftin Cream (Naftifine Hydrochloride) Merz 2164
Naftin Gel (Naftifine Hydrochloride) Merz 2164

Trichophyton schoenleini infections
Gris-PEG Tablets (Griseofulvin) Pedinol 2507

Trichophyton sulfureum infections
Gris-PEG Tablets (Griseofulvin) Pedinol 2507

Trichophyton tonsurans infections
Gris-PEG Tablets (Griseofulvin) Pedinol 2507
Naftin Gel (Naftifine Hydrochloride) Merz 2164

Trichophyton verrucosum infections
Gris-PEG Tablets (Griseofulvin) Pedinol 2507

Triglyceride levels, elevated
(*see under* Hypertriglyceridemia, adjunct to diet)

Tuberculosis, pulmonary
Seromycin Capsules (Cycloserine) Lilly 1864

Tuberculosis, treatment
Seromycin Capsules (Cycloserine) Lilly 1864

Tuberculosis, treatment adjunct
Capastat Sulfate for Injection (Capreomycin Sulfate) Lilly 1791
Paser Granules (Aminosalicylic Acid) Jacobus 1747

Tumor, papillary, prophylaxis of
Tice BCG (BCG, Live (Intravesical)) Schering 2936

Tumor therapy adjuntive
Elitek (Rasburicase) sanofi-aventis 2729

Tumors, benign epithelial
(*see under* Warts, common, removal of)

Tumors, carcinoid, symptomatic relief of
Sandostatin Injection (Octreotide Acetate) Novartis 2300
Sandostatin LAR Depot (Octreotide Acetate) Novartis 2302

Tumors, gastrointestinal stromal
Gleevec Tablets (Imatinib Mesylate) Novartis 2255
Sutent Capsules (Sunitinib malate) Pfizer 2540

Turner's syndrome
Humatrope Vials and Cartridges (Somatropin) Lilly 1838

Turner's syndrome, growth failure associated with
Genotropin Lyophilized Powder (Somatropin) Pharmacia & Upjohn 2547
Norditropin Cartridges (Somatropin (rDNA Origin)) Novo Nordisk 2354

Typhoid fever
Cipro (Ciprofloxacin) Schering 2810

U

Ulcerative colitis
(*see under* Colitis, ulcerative)

Ulcers, decubitus, adjunctive therapy in
Panafil Ointment (Chlorophyllin Copper Complex Sodium, Papain, Urea) Healthpoint 1723
Panafil SE Spray Emulsion (Chlorophyllin Copper Complex Sodium, Papain, Urea) Healthpoint 1724

Ulcers, dermal
Accuzyme SE Spray Emulsion (Papain, Urea) Healthpoint 1723
Primaxin I.M. (Cilastatin Sodium, Imipenem) Merck 2080

Ulcers, diabetic, adjunctive therapy in
Accuzyme Debriding Ointment (Papain, Urea) Healthpoint 1723
Accuzyme SE Spray Emulsion (Papain, Urea) Healthpoint 1723
Panafil Ointment (Chlorophyllin Copper Complex Sodium, Papain, Urea) Healthpoint 1723
Panafil SE Spray Emulsion (Chlorophyllin Copper Complex Sodium, Papain, Urea) Healthpoint 1724

Ulcers, varicose, adjunctive therapy in
Accuzyme Debriding Ointment (Papain, Urea) Healthpoint 1723
Accuzyme SE Spray Emulsion (Papain, Urea) Healthpoint 1723
Panafil Ointment (Chlorophyllin Copper Complex Sodium, Papain, Urea) Healthpoint 1723
Panafil SE Spray Emulsion (Chlorophyllin Copper Complex Sodium, Papain, Urea) Healthpoint 1724

Ureaplasma urealyticum infections
E.E.S. (Erythromycin Ethylsuccinate) Abbott 433
EryPed (Erythromycin Ethylsuccinate) Abbott 431

Ureaplasma urealyticum urethritis
E.E.S. Granules (Erythromycin Ethylsuccinate) Abbott 433
EryPed (Erythromycin Ethylsuccinate) Abbott 431

Ureaplasma urealyticum urethritis, nongonococcal
E.E.S. (Erythromycin Ethylsuccinate) Abbott 433
EryPed (Erythromycin Ethylsuccinate) Abbott 431

Urethritis
E.E.S. (Erythromycin Ethylsuccinate) Abbott 433
EryPed (Erythromycin Ethylsuccinate) Abbott 431

Urethritis, nongonococcal
E.E.S. (Erythromycin Ethylsuccinate) Abbott 433

Uric acid lithiasis
(*see under* Urolithiasis, management of)

Urinary bladder, overactive
Enablex Extended-Release Tablets (Darifenacin) Novartis 2225
Sanctura XR Capsules (Trospium Chloride) Allergan 557
VESIcare Tablets (Solifenacin Succinate) Astellas 636

Urine, acidification of
K-Phos Original (Sodium Free) Tablets (Potassium Acid Phosphate) Beach 814

Urolithiasis, management of
Urocit-K Tablets (Potassium Citrate) Mission 2176

Urticaria, chronic
Allegra Oral Solution (Fexofenadine Hydrochloride) sanofi-aventis 2684
Allegra Tablets (Fexofenadine Hydrochloride) sanofi-aventis 2684
Clarinex Syrup (Desloratadine) Schering 2828
Clarinex Tablets (Desloratadine) Schering 2828
Clarinex Reditabs Tablets (Desloratadine) Schering 2828
Xyzal Oral Solution (Levocetirizine Dihydrochloride) sanofi-aventis 2789
Xyzal Oral Solution (Levocetirizine Dihydrochloride) UCB, Inc. 3155
Xyzal Tablets (Levocetirizine Dihydrochloride) sanofi-aventis 2789
Xyzal Tablets (Levocetirizine Dihydrochloride) UCB, Inc. 3155
Zyrtec Chewable Tablets (Cetirizine Hydrochloride) McNeil Consumer 1920
Children's Zyrtec Hives Relief Syrup (Cetirizine Hydrochloride) McNeil Consumer 1920
Zyrtec Syrup (Cetirizine Hydrochloride) McNeil Consumer 1920
Zyrtec Tablets (Cetirizine Hydrochloride) McNeil Consumer 1920

Urticarial manifestations, relief of
(*see under* Urticaria, chronic)

Uterine bleeding, abnormal
Premarin Intravenous (Estrogens, Conjugated) Wyeth 3217

Uterine leiomyomata
Lupron Depot 3.75 mg (Leuprolide Acetate) Abbott 462
Lupron Depot–3 Month 11.25 mg (Leuprolide Acetate) Abbott 462

Uveitis
Triesence Injectable Suspension (Triamcinolone Acetonide) Alcon .... ⊙ 209

Uveitis, chronic anterior, steroid-responsive
Blephamide Ophthalmic Ointment Allergan .... ⊙ 217
Blephamide Ophthalmic Suspension Allergan .... ⊙ 216
Pred-G Ophthalmic Ointment (Gentamicin Sulfate, Prednisolone Acetate) Allergan .... ⊙ 229
Pred-G Ophthalmic Suspension (Gentamicin Sulfate, Prednisolone Acetate) Allergan .... ⊙ 228
Zylet Ophthalmic Suspension (Loteprednol Etabonate, Tobramycin) Bausch & Lomb .... ⊙ 247

V

Vaginal atrophy
Activella Tablets (Estradiol, Norethindrone Acetate) Novo Nordisk 2347
Angeliq Tablets (Estradiol, Drospirenone) Bayer HealthCare Pharmaceuticals 751
Climara Transdermal System (Estradiol) Bayer HealthCare Pharmaceuticals 763
Premarin Tablets (Estrogens, Conjugated) Wyeth 3221
Premphase Tablets (Estrogens, Conjugated, Medroxyprogesterone Acetate) Wyeth 3232
Prempro Tablets (Estrogens, Conjugated, Medroxyprogesterone Acetate) Wyeth 3232

Vaginal atrophy, postmenopausal
Enjuvia Tablets (Estrogens, Conjugated, Synthetic B) Duramed 1029

Vaginitis, atrophic
Premarin Vaginal Cream (Estrogens, Conjugated) Wyeth 3228
Vagifem Tablets (Estradiol) Novo Nordisk 2375

Varicella, acute, treatment of
Zovirax (Acyclovir) GlaxoSmithKline 1690

Varicella vaccine
(*see also under* Immunization, varicella)
ProQuad (Measles, Mumps, Rubella and Varicella Virus Vaccine Live) Merck 2099
Varivax (Varicella Virus Vaccine Live) Merck 2133

Varicella virus, immunization against
(*see also under* Immunization, varicella)
Varivax (Varicella Virus Vaccine Live) Merck 2133

Ventilation, mechanical, facilitation of
Nimbex Injection (Cisatracurium Besylate) Abbott 484
Zemuron Injection (Rocuronium Bromide) Schering 2947

Ventricular arrhythmias
(*see under* Arrhythmias, ventricular)

Ventricular dysfunction, left, asymptomatic
(*see under* Myocardial infarction, post, left ventricular dysfunction)

Ventricular tachycardia, sustained
(*see under* Tachycardia, ventricular, sustained)

Ventriculitis
(*see under* Infections, central nervous system)

Verrucae vulgaris infection
(*see under* Warts, common, removal of)

VIPomas diarrhea
(*see under* Diarrhea associated with vasoactive intestinal peptide tumors)

Vitamin, multiple, deficiency of
Hep-Forte Capsules (Vitamins with Minerals) Marlyn 1894
Mega Antioxidant Tablets (Dietary Supplement, Vitamins, Multiple) Usana 3174

Vitamin B complex, deficiency of
Eldertonic (Vitamins with Minerals) Merz 2163

Vitamin deficiency, postpartum
CitraNatal DHA Capsules (Docosahexaenoic Acid (DHA)) Mission 2175
CitraNatal DHA Tablets (Calcium Citrate, Copper, Docusate Sodium, Ferrous Gluconate, Folic Acid, Multivitamins with Minerals, Potassium Iodide, Iron Carbonyl, Zinc Oxide) Mission 2175
CitraNatal 90 DHA Capsules (Docosahexaenoic Acid (DHA)) Mission 2175
CitraNatal 90 DHA Tablets (Calcium Citrate, Copper, Docusate Sodium, Folic Acid, Multivitamins with Minerals, Potassium Iodide, Iron Carbonyl, Zinc Oxide) Mission 2175

Vitamin deficiency, prenatal
Animi-3 Capsules (Omega-3 Acids, Docosahexaenoic Acid (DHA), Eicosapentaenoic Acid (EPA), Folic Acid, Vitamin B_6, Vitamin B_{12}, Phytosterols) PBM 2506
CitraNatal DHA Capsules (Docosahexaenoic Acid (DHA)) Mission 2175

CitraNatal DHA Tablets (Calcium Citrate, Copper, Docusate Sodium, Ferrous Gluconate, Folic Acid, Multivitamins with Minerals, Potassium Iodide, Iron Carbonyl, Zinc Oxide) Mission **2175**
CitraNatal 90 DHA Capsules (Docosahexaenoic Acid (DHA)) Mission **2175**
CitraNatal 90 DHA Tablets (Calcium Citrate, Copper, Docusate Sodium, Folic Acid, Multivitamins with Minerals, Potassium Iodide, Iron Carbonyl, Zinc Oxide) Mission **2175**

Vomiting
(*see also under* Motion sickness)
Dramamine Chewable Tablets (Dimenhydrinate) McNeil Consumer **1898**
Dramamine Less Drowsy Tablets (Meclizine Hydrochloride) McNeil Consumer **1898**
Dramamine Original Tablets (Dimenhydrinate) McNeil Consumer **1898**

Vomiting, emetogenic, cancer chemotherapy-induced
Aloxi Injection (Palonosetron Hydrochloride) Eisai **1059**
Anzemet Injection (Dolasetron Mesylate) sanofi-aventis **2701**
Anzemet Tablets (Dolasetron Mesylate) sanofi-aventis **2704**
Emend Capsules (Aprepitant) Merck **1992**
Emend for Injection (Fosaprepitant Dimeglumine) Merck **1999**
Marinol Capsules (Dronabinol) Unimed **3163**
Zofran Injection (Ondansetron Hydrochloride) GlaxoSmithKline **1682**
Zofran (Ondansetron Hydrochloride) GlaxoSmithKline **1687**
Zofran ODT Orally Disintegrating Tablets (Ondansetron) GlaxoSmithKline **1687**

Vomiting, emetogenic, radiation therapy-induced
Zofran (Ondansetron Hydrochloride) GlaxoSmithKline **1687**
Zofran ODT Orally Disintegrating Tablets (Ondansetron) GlaxoSmithKline **1687**

Vomiting, postoperative
Aloxi Injection (Palonosetron Hydrochloride) Eisai **1059**
Anzemet Injection (Dolasetron Mesylate) sanofi-aventis **2701**
Anzemet Tablets (Dolasetron Mesylate) sanofi-aventis **2704**
Emend Capsules (Aprepitant) Merck **1992**
Zofran Injection (Ondansetron Hydrochloride) GlaxoSmithKline **1682**
Zofran (Ondansetron Hydrochloride) GlaxoSmithKline **1687**
Zofran ODT Orally Disintegrating Tablets (Ondansetron) GlaxoSmithKline **1687**

von Willebrand's disease
Alphanate (Antihemophilic Factor (Human), von Willebrand Factor (Human)) Grifols **1709**

Vulvae, kraurosis
Premarin Vaginal Cream (Estrogens, Conjugated) Wyeth **3228**

Vulvar atrophy
Activella Tablets (Estradiol, Norethindrone Acetate) Novo Nordisk **2347**
Angeliq Tablets (Estradiol, Drospirenone) Bayer HealthCare Pharmaceuticals **751**
Climara Transdermal System (Estradiol) Bayer HealthCare Pharmaceuticals **763**
Enjuvia Tablets (Estrogens, Conjugated, Synthetic B) Duramed **1029**
Premarin Tablets (Estrogens, Conjugated) Wyeth **3221**
Premphase Tablets (Estrogens, Conjugated, Medroxyprogesterone Acetate) Wyeth **3232**
Prempro Tablets (Estrogens, Conjugated, Medroxyprogesterone Acetate) Wyeth **3232**

W

Warts, common, removal of
Formadon Solution (Formaldehyde) Gordon **1699**

Warts, genital
(*see under* Condylomata acuminata)

Wheezing, symptomatic relief of
(*see under* Bronchial asthma)

Whooping cough
(*see under* Pertussis)

Wilms' tumor
Cosmegen for Injection (Dactinomycin) Ovation **2485**

Wilson's disease
Cuprimine Capsules (Penicillamine) Merck **1986**

Wiskott-Aldrich syndrome
Flebogamma 5% (Globulin, Immune (Human)) Grifols **1715**
Flebogamma 5% DIF (Immune Globulin Intravenous (Human)) Grifols **1718**
Gammagard Liquid (Immune Globulin Intravenous (Human)) Baxter Healthcare **730**
Gammagard S/D (Immune Globulin Intravenous (Human)) Baxter Healthcare **734**
Gamunex (Immune Globulin Intravenous (Human)) Talecris **3094**

Wolff-Parkinson-White syndrome
Adenocard IV Injection (Adenosine) Astellas **603**

Wound care, adjunctive therapy in
Panafil Ointment (Chlorophyllin Copper Complex Sodium, Papain, Urea) Healthpoint **1723**
Xenaderm Ointment (Balsam Peru, Castor Oil, Trypsin) Healthpoint **1725**

Wounds, debridement of
Accuzyme Debriding Ointment (Papain, Urea) Healthpoint **1723**
Accuzyme SE Spray Emulsion (Papain, Urea) Healthpoint **1723**
Panafil Ointment (Chlorophyllin Copper Complex Sodium, Papain, Urea) Healthpoint **1723**
Panafil SE Spray Emulsion (Chlorophyllin Copper Complex Sodium, Papain, Urea) Healthpoint **1724**
Santyl Collagenase Ointment (Collagenase) Healthpoint **1724**

Wounds, infected, adjunctive therapy in
Accuzyme SE Spray Emulsion (Papain, Urea) Healthpoint **1723**
Panafil Ointment (Chlorophyllin Copper Complex Sodium, Papain, Urea) Healthpoint **1723**
Panafil SE Spray Emulsion (Chlorophyllin Copper Complex Sodium, Papain, Urea) Healthpoint **1724**

Wounds, pilonidal cyst, adjunctive therapy in
Accuzyme SE Spray Emulsion (Papain, Urea) Healthpoint **1723**
Panafil Ointment (Chlorophyllin Copper Complex Sodium, Papain, Urea) Healthpoint **1723**
Panafil SE Spray Emulsion (Chlorophyllin Copper Complex Sodium, Papain, Urea) Healthpoint **1724**

Wounds, postoperative, adjunctive therapy in
Accuzyme SE Spray Emulsion (Papain, Urea) Healthpoint **1723**
Panafil Ointment (Chlorophyllin Copper Complex Sodium, Papain, Urea) Healthpoint **1723**
Panafil SE Spray Emulsion (Chlorophyllin Copper Complex Sodium, Papain, Urea) Healthpoint **1724**

Wounds, removal of exudates, aids in
Panafil Ointment (Chlorophyllin Copper Complex Sodium, Papain, Urea) Healthpoint **1723**

Wounds, superficial
Levaquin (Levofloxacin) Ortho-McNeil **2416**
Levaquin in 5% Dextrose Injection (Levofloxacin) Ortho-McNeil **2416**

Wounds, traumatic, adjunctive therapy in
Accuzyme SE Spray Emulsion (Papain, Urea) Healthpoint **1723**
Panafil Ointment (Chlorophyllin Copper Complex Sodium, Papain, Urea) Healthpoint **1723**
Panafil SE Spray Emulsion (Chlorophyllin Copper Complex Sodium, Papain, Urea) Healthpoint **1724**

Wrinkles, fine
(*see under* Skin, fine wrinkles, mitigation of)

X

Xerostomia, radiotherapy-induced
Salagen Tablets (Pilocarpine Hydrochloride) Eisai **1082**

X-linked agammaglobulinemia
Flebogamma 5% (Globulin, Immune (Human)) Grifols **1715**
Flebogamma 5% DIF (Immune Globulin Intravenous (Human)) Grifols **1718**

X-linked immunodeficiency with hyper IgM
Gamunex (Immune Globulin Intravenous (Human)) Talecris **3094**

XO syndrome
(*see under* Turner's syndrome)

Z

Zollinger-Ellison syndrome
Aciphex Tablets (Rabeprazole Sodium) Eisai **1053**
Nexium Delayed-Release Capsules (Esomeprazole Magnesium) AstraZeneca LP **645**
Nexium Delayed-Release Oral Suspension (Esomeprazole Magnesium) AstraZeneca LP **645**
Pepcid Tablets (Famotidine) Merck ... **2075**
Protonix for Delayed-Release Oral Suspension (Pantoprazole Sodium) Wyeth **3254**
Protonix Delayed-Release Tablets (Pantoprazole Sodium) Wyeth **3254**
Protonix I.V. (Pantoprazole Sodium) Wyeth **3257**
Zantac (Ranitidine Hydrochloride) GlaxoSmithKline **1670**

Zygomycosis
Abelcet Injection (Amphotericin B Lipid Complex) Enzon **1134**

SECTION 5

CONTRAINDICATIONS INDEX

This section lists in alphabetical order every medical condition cited as a contraindication in *PDR*® and its companion volumes, with cross-references to all product entries in which the contraindication is found. Page numbers refer to the 2009 editions of *PDR*®, *PDR*® *For Ophthalmic Medicines* and *PDR*® *For Nonprescription Drugs, Dietary Supplements and Herbs*. A key to the symbols denoting the companion volumes appears in the bottom margin.

These listings will enable you to quickly identify drugs that generally threaten to be inappropriate in the presence of a given complication. However, a drug's suitability is sometimes affected by the severity of the complicating condition, the age or gender of the patient, and the drug's route of administration. In ambiguous situations, a quick review of the underlying *PDR*® text may therefore prove helpful.

Note, too, that the index does not list other drugs and dietary items whose use would present a contraindication. Contraindicated combinations can be found in the Interactions Index and the Food Interactions Cross-Reference. Hypersensitivity to the product's ingredients—an almost universal contraindication—also has not been indexed here. If the clinical picture includes the risk of allergic reaction, be sure to check individual product labeling for additional information.

A

Abortion, infected
Mirena Intrauterine System 779

Abortion, missed
Crinone 4% Gel............ 992
Crinone 8% Gel............ 992
Prometrium Capsules (100 mg, 200 mg) 3047

Achalasia, esophageal
Fosamax............ 2005
Fosamax Plus D Tablets 2013

Acid base imbalance, uncorrected
(*see under* Acidosis, metabolic, unspecified; Ketoacidosis, diabetic)

Acidosis, metabolic, unspecified
(*see also under* Ketoacidosis, diabetic)
ActoPlus Met Tablets 3071
Avandamet Tablets 1336
Janumet Tablets 2041
PrandiMet Tablets 2967

Acquired immune deficiency syndrome
(*see also under* Human immunodeficiency virus)
Attenuvax 1951
Meruvax II 2061
M-M-R II 2054
Mumpsvax 2068
Tice BCG 2936
Varivax 2133
Zostavax Injection 2145

Actinomycosis, genital
Mirena Intrauterine System 779

Adenoma, hepatic
Lybrel Tablets 3204
Mircette Tablets 1034
NuvaRing 2897
Ortho-Cyclen Tablets 2449
Ortho Evra Transdermal System 2437
Ortho Tri-Cyclen Tablets 2449
Ortho Tri-Cyclen Lo Tablets 2458

Adrenal cortical insufficiency
(*see under* Adrenal insufficiency, uncorrected; Adrenal insufficiency, unspecified)

Adrenal cortical insufficiency, uncorrected
Naturethroid Tablets 2605

Adrenal dysfunction, uncontrolled
Follistim AQ Cartridge 2844

Adrenal dysfunction, uncorrected
(*see under* Adrenal insufficiency, uncorrected)

Adrenal gland failure
(*see under* Adrenal insufficiency, unspecified)

Adrenal insufficiency, uncorrected
Cytomel Tablets 1778
Levothroid Tablets 1170
Levoxyl Tablets 1780
Synthroid Tablets 507

Adrenal insufficiency, unspecified
Angeliq Tablets 751
Urocit-K Tablets 2176
Yaz Tablets 805

Adrenocortical insufficiency
(*see under* Adrenal insufficiency, uncorrected; Adrenal insufficiency, unspecified)

Agitated states
(*see also under* Agitation)
Vyvanse Capsules 3033

Agitation
Adderall XR Capsules 3012
Adipex-P 1185
Concerta Extended-Release Tablets 1925
Daytrana Transdermal Patch 3022
Dexedrine 1401
Focalin XR Capsules 2251
Metadate CD Capsules 3146
Vyvanse Capsules 3033

Agranulocytosis, penicillamine-related
Cuprimine Capsules 1986

AIDS
(*see under* Acquired immune deficiency syndrome)

Alcohol discontinuation, abrupt
Zyban Sustained-Release Tablets 1692

Alcoholism
Seromycin Capsules 1864

Allergic reaction to aspirin
Aggrenox Capsules 819
Anaprox Tablets 2632
Anaprox DS Tablets 2632
Clinoril Tablets 1962
EC-Naprosyn Delayed-Release Tablets 2632
Flector Patch 561
Naprosyn Suspension 2632
Naprosyn Tablets 2632
Salonpas Arthritis Pain Patches .... ▣ 608
Salonpas Gel .... ▣ 609
Salonpas Pain Relief Patch .... ▣ 608
Voltaren Tablets 2334

Allergic reaction to non-steroidal anti-inflammatory drugs
Aggrenox Capsules 819
Anaprox Tablets 2632
Anaprox DS Tablets 2632
Celebrex Capsules 2979
Clinoril Tablets 1962
EC-Naprosyn Delayed-Release Tablets 2632
Flector Patch 561
Naprosyn Suspension 2632
Naprosyn Tablets 2632
Salonpas Arthritis Pain Patches .... ▣ 608
Salonpas Gel .... ▣ 609
Salonpas Pain Relief Patch .... ▣ 608
Voltaren Tablets 2334

Allergic reaction to sulfonamides
Avalide Tablets 2713
Celebrex Capsules 2979
Micardis HCT Tablets 854
Tekturna HCT Tablets 2324

Allograft
(*see under* Organ allograft)

ALT greater than or equal to 2.5x ULN, in combination with capecitabine
Ixempra Kit for Injection 915

Amino acid metabolism disorders
(*see under* Electrolyte imbalance, uncorrected)

Anastomosis, unspecified
(*see under* Ileocolostomy)

Anemia, aplastic, penicillamine-related
Cuprimine Capsules 1986

Anemia, hemolytic, history of
Elitek 2729
Skelaxin Tablets 1784

Anemia, megaloblastic, unspecified
Daraprim Tablets 1400
Fansidar Tablets 2636

Anemia, sickle cell
Edex Injection 2957
Rebetol 2917

Anemia, unspecified
Albutein 5% 1707
Albutein 25% 1708
Flexbumin 25% I.V. 729
Human Albumin Grifols 25% 1706

Anemia, unspecified, history of
Skelaxin Tablets 1784

Anesthesia, general
Metadate CD Capsules 3146
Parnate Tablets 1532

Anesthesia, local
Parnate Tablets 1532

Aneurysm
(*see also under* Cerebrovascular accident)
Activase I.V. 1188
ReoPro Vials 1860
TNKase 1233

Angina, Prinzmetal's
Amerge Tablets 1301
Axert Tablets 2431
Frova Tablets 1111
Imitrex Injection 1465
Imitrex Nasal Spray 1470
Imitrex Tablets 1474
Maxalt Tablets 2056
Maxalt-MLT Orally Disintegrating Tablets 2056
Treximet Tablets 1616
Zomig Tablets 694
Zomig Nasal Spray 689
Zomig-ZMT Tablets 694

Angina, unspecified, history of
Proleukin for Injection 2287

Angina, vasospastic, unspecified
Treximet Tablets 1616

Angina pectoris
Amerge Tablets 1301
Axert Tablets 2431
Frova Tablets 1111
Imitrex Injection 1465
Imitrex Nasal Spray 1470
Imitrex Tablets 1474
Maxalt Tablets 2056
Maxalt-MLT Orally Disintegrating Tablets 2056
Treximet Tablets 1616
Zomig Tablets 694
Zomig Nasal Spray 689
Zomig-ZMT Tablets 694

Angioedema, hereditary
Prinivil Tablets 2087
Prinzide Tablets 2092

Angioedema, idiopathic
Prinivil Tablets 2087
Prinzide Tablets 2092

Angulation, penile
Edex Injection 2957

Anorexia nervosa
Meridia Capsules 475
Wellbutrin Tablets 1648
Wellbutrin SR Sustained-Release Tablets 1653
Wellbutrin XL Extended-Release Tablets 1659
Zyban Sustained-Release Tablets 1692

Anuria
Atacand HCT 642
Avalide Tablets 892
Avalide Tablets 2713
Benicar HCT Tablets 1010
Clorpres Tablets 2185
Demadex Injection 2630
Demadex Tablets 2630
Diovan HCT Tablets 2216
Dyazide Capsules 1405
Dyrenium Capsules 3189
Edecrin 698
Furosemide Tablets 2186
Indapamide Tablets 2188
Intravenous Sodium Diuril 2490
Micardis HCT Tablets 854
Prinzide Tablets 2092
Tekturna HCT Tablets 2324
Teveten HCT Tablets 517

Anxiety
Concerta Extended-Release Tablets 1925
Daytrana Transdermal Patch 3022
Focalin XR Capsules 2251
Metadate CD Capsules 3146
Seromycin Capsules 1864

Aortic coarctation
(*see under* Stenosis, aortic)

Aortic stenosis
(*see under* Stenosis, aortic)

Apoplexy, cerebral
(*see under* Cerebrovascular accident)

Aprotinin exposure within last 12 months
Trasylol Injection 799

Arrhythmia, cardiac, history of
Proleukin for Injection 2287
Thioridazine Hydrochloride Tablets 2195

Arrhythmia, cardiac, unspecified
(*see also under* Bradycardia, sinus; Bradycardia, unspecified; Fibrillation, ventricular; Heart block, first degree; Heart block, greater than first degree; Heart block, sinoatrial; Heart block, unspecified; Lown-Ganong-Levine syndrome; Q-T interval prolongation; Sick sinus syndrome; Sinus node dysfunction, unspecified; Tachycardia, ventricular; Tachycardia, ventricular, history of; Wolff-Parkinson-White syndrome)
Amrix Capsules 966
Rythmol SR Capsules 1590

Arrhythmia, ventricular
Rythmol Tablets 1586

Arrhythmia, ventricular, unspecified
(*see under* Fibrillation, ventricular; Tachycardia, ventricular; Tachycardia, ventricular, history of; Ventricular dysfunction, left)

Arterial disease, unspecified
(*see under* Angina, Prinzmetal's; Angina pectoris; Arteriosclerosis, unspecified; Arteriovenous malformation; Coronary artery disease; Coronary artery disease, history of; Coronary artery vasospasm; Stenosis, aortic)

Arteriosclerosis, advanced
Adderall XR Capsules 3012
Vyvanse Capsules 3033

Arteriosclerosis, unspecified
(*see also under* Coronary artery disease; Stenosis, aortic)
Adderall XR Capsules 3012
Adipex-P 1185
Dexedrine 1401

Arteriovenous malformation
Activase I.V. 1188
ReoPro Vials 1860
TNKase 1233

As primary therapy in patients with cardiogenic shock
Natrecor for Injection 2977

Ascites
Fleet Enema 1143
Fleet Enema Extra 1143
Fleet Enema for Children 1143
Fleet Pedia-Lax Enema 1143
Fleet Phospho-soda 1145
Fleet Phospho-soda EZ-PREP 1147
Fleet Prep Kits 1149

AST greater than or equal to 2.5x ULN, in combination with capecitabine
Ixempra Kit for Injection 915

Asthma, acute
(*see also under* Status asthmaticus)
Advair Diskus 100/50 1276
Advair Diskus 250/50 1276
Advair Diskus 500/50 1276
Advair HFA 45/21 Inhalation Aerosol 1288
Advair HFA 115/21 Inhalation Aerosol 1288
Advair HFA 230/21 Inhalation Aerosol 1288
Asmanex Twisthaler 2797
Avinza Capsules 1772
Azmacort Inhalation Aerosol 407
Combigan Ophthalmic Solution 553
DepoDur Injection 1095
Duragesic Transdermal System 2405
Flovent Diskus 50 mcg 1435
InnoPran XL Extended Release Capsules 1484
MS Contin Tablets 2585
OxyContin Tablets 2589
OxyIR Capsules 2593
Pulmicort Flexhaler 654
Qvar Inhalation Aerosol 3116
Symbicort 80/4.5 Inhalation Aerosol 659
Symbicort 160/4.5 Inhalation Aerosol 659

Asthma, history of
Betimol Ophthalmic Solution 3181
Combigan Ophthalmic Solution 553
Cosopt Sterile Ophthalmic Solution 1969
DepoDur Injection 1095
Duragesic Transdermal System 2405
InnoPran XL Extended Release Capsules 1484
OptiPranolol Metipranolol Ophthalmic Solution 0.3% .... ⊙245
Timoptic Sterile Ophthalmic Solution 2121
Timoptic in Ocudose 2124
Timoptic-XE Sterile Ophthalmic Gel Forming Solution 2125

Asthma, uncontrolled
Salagen Tablets 1082

Asthma, unspecified
Adenoscan 605
Avinza Capsules 1772
Betimol Ophthalmic Solution 3181
Coreg Tablets 1387
Coreg CR Extended-Release Capsules 1393
Cosopt Sterile Ophthalmic Solution 1969
DepoDur Injection 1095
InnoPran XL Extended Release Capsules 1484
MS Contin Tablets 2585
Nadolol Tablets 2191
Opana ER Tablets 1121
OptiPranolol Metipranolol Ophthalmic Solution 0.3% .... ⊙245
OxyContin Tablets 2589
OxyIR Capsules 2593
Timoptic Sterile Ophthalmic Solution 2121
Timoptic in Ocudose 2124
Timoptic-XE Sterile Ophthalmic Gel Forming Solution 2125

Asthmatic attack
(*see under* Asthma, acute)

Atony, intestinal
Donnatal Extentabs 2507

Atresia, pulmonary
Indocin I.V. 2489
NeoProfen Injection 2496

Atrioventricular block
(*see under* Heart block, first degree; Heart block, greater than first degree; Heart block, unspecified)

Atrioventricular block, Second degree
Combigan Ophthalmic Solution 553
Lexiscan Injection 614
Rythmol Tablets 1586

Atrioventricular block, third degree
Combigan Ophthalmic Solution 553
Lexiscan Injection 614
Rythmol Tablets 1586

AV block
(*see under* Heart block, first degree; Heart block, greater than first degree; Heart block, unspecified)

Azotemia
Edecrin 698

B

Bacterial endocarditis
(*see under* Endocarditis, bacterial)

Bilirubin greater than 1x ULN, in combination with capecitabine
Ixempra Kit for Injection 915

Bleeding, abnormal, unspecified
(*see also under* Hematuria)
Indocin I.V. 2489

Bleeding, active major
Angiomax for Injection 1933

Bleeding, arterial
Advicor Tablets 402
Niaspan Extended-Release Tablets 480
Simcor Tablets 502

Bleeding, cerebrovascular
(*see under* Bleeding, intracranial; Cerebrovascular accident)

Bleeding, gastrointestinal
Indocin I.V. 2489
NeoProfen Injection 2496
Plavix Tablets 926
Plavix Tablets 2767
ReoPro Vials 1860

Bleeding, gastrointestinal, history of
Proleukin for Injection 2287

Bleeding, genital, abnormal
(*see also under* Bleeding, genitourinary)
Activella Tablets 2347
Angeliq Tablets 751
Cervidil Vaginal Insert 1165
Climara Transdermal System 763
Climara Pro Transdermal System 768
Enjuvia Tablets 1029
Estratest Tablets 3043
Estratest H.S. Tablets 3043
Follistim AQ Cartridge 2844
Lupron Depot 3.75 mg 462
Lupron Depot–3 Month 11.25 mg 462
Lybrel Tablets 3204
Mircette Tablets 1034

Mirena Intrauterine System 779
NuvaRing 2897
Ortho-Cyclen Tablets 2449
Ortho Evra Transdermal System 2437
Ortho Micronor Tablets 2446
Ortho Tri-Cyclen Tablets 2449
Ortho Tri-Cyclen Lo Tablets 2458
ParaGard T 380A Intrauterine Copper Contraceptive 1041
Plan B Tablets 1044
Premarin Intravenous 3217
Premarin Tablets 3221
Premarin Vaginal Cream 3228
Premphase Tablets 3232
Prempro Tablets 3232
Prometrium Capsules (100 mg, 200 mg) 3047
Vagifem Tablets 2375

Bleeding, genitourinary
(*see also under* Bleeding, genital, abnormal)
ReoPro Vials 1860

Bleeding, history of
Integrilin Injection 2855
Oncaspar Injection 1138

Bleeding, internal, unspecified
(*see also under* Hematuria)
Activase I.V. 1188
NeoProfen Injection 2496
ReoPro Vials 1860
TNKase 1233
Xigris Powder for Intravenous Infusion 1880

Bleeding, intracranial
(*see also under* Cerebrovascular accident)
Activase I.V. 1188
Indocin I.V. 2489
NeoProfen Injection 2496
Plavix Tablets 926
Plavix Tablets 2767
Pletal Tablets 2481

Bleeding, pathological, active
Plavix Tablets 926
Plavix Tablets 2767
Pletal Tablets 2481

Bleeding, rectal
Indocin Suppositories 2024

Bleeding, ulcer, peptic
Pletal Tablets 2481

Bleeding, unspecified
(*see also under* Bleeding, internal, unspecified; Hematuria)
Argatroban Injection 1308
Arixtra Injection 1313
Lovenox Injection 2756

Bleeding, uterine
(*see under* Bleeding, genital, abnormal)

Bleeding, vaginal, abnormal
(*see under* Bleeding, genital, abnormal)

Bleeding, vaginal, undiagnosed
Crinone 4% Gel 992
Crinone 8% Gel 992
Divigel 3167
Follistim AQ Cartridge 2844
Seasonique Tablets 1046
Yaz Tablets 805

Bleeding disorders, unspecified
(*see also under* Bleeding tendencies; Hemophilia; Thrombocytopenia, unspecified)
Elspar for Injection 2488
Indocin I.V. 2489
Pletal Tablets 2481

Bleeding tendencies
Activase I.V. 1188
Elspar for Injection 2488
Fragmin Injection 1070
ReoPro Vials 1860
TNKase 1233

Blood disorders, unspecified
NeoProfen Injection 2496

Blood dyscrasias, unspecified
(*see also under* Anemia, hemolytic, history of; Anemia, megaloblastic, unspecified; Anemia, sickle cell; Anemia, unspecified; Anemia, unspecified, history of; Bleeding disorders, unspecified; Hemophilia; Neutropenia; Thrombocytopenia, unspecified)
Attenuvax 1951
Fansidar Tablets 2636
Meruvax II 2061
M-M-R II 2054
Mumpsvax 2068
ProQuad 2099
Thiothixene Capsules 2197
Varivax 2133

Blood vessel, major, tumors eroding into
Photofrin for Injection 708

Body weight less than 50 kg
Arixtra Injection 1313

Bone marrow aplasia
(*see under* Bone marrow depression)

Bone marrow damage
(*see under* Bone marrow depression)

Bone marrow depression
Hycamtin for Injection 1459

Bone marrow depression, history of
Carbatrol Capsules 3019
Equetro Extended-Release Capsules 3174
Hexalen Capsules 1078

Bone marrow function impairment
(*see under* Bone marrow depression)

Bone marrow hypoplasia
(*see under* Bone marrow depression)

Bowel disease, inflammatory
(*see under* Inflammation, gastrointestinal tract)

Bowel ischemia, history of
Amerge Tablets 1301
Frova Tablets 1111
Imitrex Nasal Spray 1470
Imitrex Tablets 1474
Proleukin for Injection 2287
Treximet Tablets 1616

Bowel obstruction
(*see under* Bowel ischemia, history of; Obstruction, gastrointestinal tract)

Bowel perforation
(*see under* Perforation, gastrointestinal tract)

Bowel perforation, history of
(*see under* Perforation, gastrointestinal tract, history of)

Bradycardia, severe
Bystolic Tablets 1155

Bradycardia, sinus
Adenocard IV Injection 603
Adenoscan 605
Betimol Ophthalmic Solution 3181
Combigan Ophthalmic Solution 553
InnoPran XL Extended Release Capsules 1484
Nadolol Tablets 2191
OptiPranolol Metipranolol Ophthalmic Solution 0.3% ⊙245
Timoptic Sterile Ophthalmic Solution 2121
Timoptic in Ocudose 2124
Timoptic-XE Sterile Ophthalmic Gel Forming Solution 2125
Toprol-XL Tablets 666

Bradycardia, unspecified
Coreg Tablets 1387
Coreg CR Extended-Release Capsules 1393
Rythmol Tablets 1586
Rythmol SR Capsules 1590

Brain tumor
(*see under* Tumor, pituitary, unspecified)

Breast cancer
(*see also under* Carcinoma, breast, history of; Carcinoma, breast, male; Carcinoma, breast, unspecified)
Fosteum Capsules 2963
Lybrel Tablets 3204
NuvaRing 2897
Seasonique Tablets 1046
Yaz Tablets 805

Breastfeeding
Advicor Tablets 402
AndroGel 3159
Bentyl Capsules 703
Bentyl Injection 703
Bentyl Syrup 703
Bentyl Tablets 703
Crestor Tablets 677
Cuprimine Capsules 1986
Doxil Injection 2378
Estratest Tablets 3043
Estratest H.S. Tablets 3043
Evista Tablets 1810
Fansidar Tablets 2636
Fenoglide Tablets 2960
Gantrisin Pediatric Suspension 2638
Hycamtin for Injection 1459
Lescol Capsules 2268
Lescol XL Tablets 2268
Lipitor Tablets 2501
Lupron Depot 3.75 mg 462
Lupron Depot–3 Month 11.25 mg 462
Mevacor Tablets 2063
Mylotarg for Injection 3212
Orthoclone OKT3 Sterile Solution 2387
Pylera Capsules 714
Simcor Tablets 502
Testim 1% Gel 701
Vytorin 10/10 Tablets 2149
Vytorin 10/10 Tablets 2939
Vytorin 10/20 Tablets 2149
Vytorin 10/20 Tablets 2939
Vytorin 10/40 Tablets 2149
Vytorin 10/40 Tablets 2939
Vytorin 10/80 Tablets 2149
Vytorin 10/80 Tablets 2939
Zetia Tablets 2157
Zetia Tablets 2951
Zocor Tablets 2136

Breathing problems, unspecified
(*see under* Pulmonary disorders, unspecified; Respiratory illness, febrile)

Bronchial asthma
(*see under* Asthma, acute; Asthma, history of; Asthma, unspecified)

Bronchoesophageal, fistula, existence of
Photofrin for Injection 708

Bronchospastic disorders, unspecified
(*see also under* Asthma, acute; Asthma, history of; Asthma, unspecified)
Adenoscan 605
Coreg Tablets 1387
Coreg CR Extended-Release Capsules 1393
Rythmol Tablets 1586
Rythmol SR Capsules 1590

Bulimia
Meridia Capsules 475
Wellbutrin Tablets 1648
Wellbutrin SR Sustained-Release Tablets 1653
Wellbutrin XL Extended-Release Tablets 1659
Zyban Sustained-Release Tablets 1692

Bundle branch block
(*see under* Heart block, unspecified)

C

CAD
(*see under* Coronary artery disease)

Cancer
(*see under* Carcinoma, breast, history of; Carcinoma, breast, male; Carcinoma, breast, unspecified; Carcinoma, cervical; Carcinoma, endometrium; Carcinoma, genital, unspecified; Carcinoma, hepatic; Carcinoma, prostate; Carcinoma, uterine; Neoplasm, bone marrow system, malignant; Neoplasm, lymphatic system, malignant)

Carcinoma, breast, history of
Activella Tablets 2347
Angeliq Tablets 751
Crinone 4% Gel 992
Crinone 8% Gel 992
Divigel 3167
Mircette Tablets 1034
NuvaRing 2897
Premphase Tablets 3232
Prempro Tablets 3232

Carcinoma, breast, male
(*see also under* Carcinoma, breast, unspecified)
AndroGel 3159
Delatestryl Injection 1730
Testim 1% Gel 701

Carcinoma, breast, unspecified
(*see also under* Carcinoma, breast, history of; Carcinoma, breast, male; Neoplasm, estrogen dependent)
Activella Tablets 2347
Climara Transdermal System 763
Climara Pro Transdermal System 768
Divigel 3167
Enjuvia Tablets 1029
Estratest Tablets 3043
Estratest H.S. Tablets 3043
Fosteum Capsules 2963
Lybrel Tablets 3204
Mirena Intrauterine System 779
Ortho-Cyclen Tablets 2449
Ortho Evra Transdermal System 2437
Ortho Micronor Tablets 2446
Ortho Tri-Cyclen Tablets 2449
Ortho Tri-Cyclen Lo Tablets 2458
Premarin Intravenous 3217
Premarin Tablets 3221
Premarin Vaginal Cream 3228
Premphase Tablets 3232
Prempro Tablets 3232
Prometrium Capsules (100 mg, 200 mg) 3047
Vagifem Tablets 2375

Carcinoma, cervical
(*see also under* Carcinoma, genital, unspecified)
Mirena Intrauterine System 779

Carcinoma, endometrium
(*see also under* Carcinoma, uterine)
Lybrel Tablets 3204
Mircette Tablets 1034
NuvaRing 2897
Ortho-Cyclen Tablets 2449
Ortho Evra Transdermal System 2437
Ortho Tri-Cyclen Tablets 2449
Ortho Tri-Cyclen Lo Tablets 2458
Seasonique Tablets 1046
Yaz Tablets 805

Carcinoma, female reproductive organs
(*see under* Carcinoma, cervical; Carcinoma, endometrium; Carcinoma, genital, unspecified; Carcinoma, uterine)

Carcinoma, genital, unspecified
(*see also under* Carcinoma, cervical; Carcinoma, prostate)
Crinone 4% Gel 992
Crinone 8% Gel 992

Carcinoma, hepatic
Lybrel Tablets 3204
Mircette Tablets 1034
Mirena Intrauterine System 779
NuvaRing 2897
Ortho-Cyclen Tablets 2449
Ortho Evra Transdermal System 2437
Ortho Micronor Tablets 2446
Ortho Tri-Cyclen Tablets 2449
Ortho Tri-Cyclen Lo Tablets 2458
Seasonique Tablets 1046
Yaz Tablets 805

Carcinoma, prostate
(*see also under* Carcinoma, genital, unspecified)
AndroGel 3159
Delatestryl Injection 1730
Testim 1% Gel 701

Carcinoma, reproductive organs
Fosteum Capsules 2963

Carcinoma, skin, unspecified
(*see under* Melanoma, history of)

Carcinoma, uterine
(*see also under* Carcinoma, endometrium)
Mirena Intrauterine System 779

Cardiac arrhythmia
(*see under* Arrhythmia, cardiac, unspecified)

Cardiac decompensation
(*see under* Heart failure, unspecified)

Cardiac disease
(*see under* Cardiovascular disorders, unspecified)

Cardiac dysfunction
(*see under* Cardiovascular disorders, unspecified)

Cardiac failure
(*see under* Heart failure, unspecified)

Cardiac failure, NYHA class III
Avandamet Tablets 1336
Avandaryl Tablets 1344

Cardiac failure, NYHA class IV
Avandamet Tablets 1336
Avandaryl Tablets 1344

Cardiac failure, NYHA class IV decompensated
Coreg Tablets 1387
Coreg CR Extended-Release Capsules 1393
Toprol-XL Tablets 666

Cardiac insufficiency
(*see under* Cardiovascular disorders, unspecified)

Cardiac rhythm disturbances, unspecified
(*see under* Arrhythmia, cardiac, unspecified)

Cardiogenic shock
Betimol Ophthalmic Solution 3181
Bystolic Tablets 1155
Combigan Ophthalmic Solution 553
Coreg Tablets 1387
Coreg CR Extended-Release Capsules 1393
Cosopt Sterile Ophthalmic Solution 1969
InnoPran XL Extended Release Capsules 1484
Nadolol Tablets 2191
OptiPranolol Metipranolol Ophthalmic Solution 0.3% .... ⊙245
Rythmol Tablets 1586
Rythmol SR Capsules 1590
Tarka Tablets 511
Timoptic Sterile Ophthalmic Solution 2121
Timoptic in Ocudose 2124
Timoptic-XE Sterile Ophthalmic Gel Forming Solution 2125
Toprol-XL Tablets 666

Cardiovascular collapse
(*see under* Shock, unspecified)

Cardiovascular disease, symptomatic
Vyvanse Capsules 3033

Cardiovascular disorders, unspecified
(*see also under* Angina, Prinzmetal's; Angina, vasospastic, unspecified; Angina pectoris; Arrhythmia, cardiac, unspecified; Cardiogenic shock; Congestive heart failure, uncontrolled; Congestive heart failure, unspecified; Coronary artery disease; Coronary artery disease, history of; ECG changes, history of; Endocarditis, bacterial; Heart disease, ischemic; Heart failure, unspecified; Hypertension, unspecified; Myocardial infarction; Myocardial infarction, history of)
Adderall XR Capsules 3012
Adipex-P 1185
Amerge Tablets 1301
Dexedrine 1401
Imitrex Injection 1465
Indocin I.V. 2489
Marplan Tablets 3177
Parnate Tablets 1532
Zomig Tablets 694
Zomig Nasal Spray 689
Zomig-ZMT Tablets 694

Cardiovascular status, unstable in acute hemorrhage
Bentyl Capsules 703
Bentyl Injection 703
Bentyl Syrup 703
Bentyl Tablets 703
Donnatal Extentabs 2507

Cavernosal fibrosis
(*see under* Fibrosis, cavernosal)

Cellular immune deficiency
(*see under* Immunodeficiency, unspecified)

Central nervous system depression
Moban Tablets 1116
Thioridazine Hydrochloride Tablets 2195
Thiothixene Capsules 2197

Cephalopelvic disproportion
Cervidil Vaginal Insert 1165

Cerebral apoplexy
(*see under* Cerebrovascular accident)

Cerebral herniation
Xigris Powder for Intravenous Infusion 1880

Cerebral vascular accident
(*see under* Cerebrovascular accident)

Cerebral vascular disease
(*see also under* Bleeding, intracranial; Cerebrovascular accident)
Lybrel Tablets 3204
Marplan Tablets 3177
Mircette Tablets 1034
NuvaRing 2897
Ortho-Cyclen Tablets 2449
Ortho Evra Transdermal System 2437
Ortho Tri-Cyclen Tablets 2449
Ortho Tri-Cyclen Lo Tablets 2458
Parnate Tablets 1532
Seasonique Tablets 1046
Yaz Tablets 805

Cerebral vascular disease, history of
(*see also under* Cerebrovascular accident, history of)
NuvaRing 2897
Seasonique Tablets 1046
Yaz Tablets 805

Cerebrovascular accident
(*see also under* Bleeding, intracranial)
Activella Tablets 2347
Amerge Tablets 1301
Divigel 3167
Estratest H.S. Tablets 3043
Frova Tablets 1111
Imitrex Injection 1465
Imitrex Nasal Spray 1470
Imitrex Tablets 1474
Premarin Vaginal Cream 3228
Premphase Tablets 3232
Prempro Tablets 3232
Prometrium Capsules (100 mg, 200 mg) 3047
ReoPro Vials 1860
Treximet Tablets 1616

Cerebrovascular accident, history of
Activase I.V. 1188
Activella Tablets 2347
Estratest H.S. Tablets 3043
Integrilin Injection 2855
Prempro Tablets 3232
Prometrium Capsules (100 mg, 200 mg) 3047
ReoPro Vials 1860
TNKase 1233

Cerebrovascular defects
(*see under* Cerebral vascular disease)

Cerebrovascular disorders, unspecified
(*see under* Cerebral vascular disease; Neurological disorders, unspecified)

Cerebrovascular hemorrhage
(*see under* Bleeding, intracranial; Cerebrovascular accident)

Cerebrovascular syndrome
Amerge Tablets 1301
Imitrex Nasal Spray 1470
Imitrex Tablets 1474
Treximet Tablets 1616

Cervicitis, mucopurulent
ParaGard T 380A Intrauterine Copper Contraceptive 1041

Cervicitis, untreated
Mirena Intrauterine System 779

Cesarean section, history of
Cervidil Vaginal Insert 1165

Chest pain, unspecified, history of
(*see also under* Angina, unspecified, history of)
Proleukin for Injection 2287

CHF
(*see under* Congestive heart failure, uncontrolled; Congestive heart failure, unspecified)

Chicken pox
(*see under* Varicella)

Children
Avodart Soft Gelatin Capsules 1359
Edex Injection 2957
Eligard 22.5 mg 2724
Eligard 30 mg 2724
Vantas 1737

Cholestasis
Xenical Capsules 2672

Chronic obstructive pulmonary disease
(*see also under* Asthma, history of; Asthma, uncontrolled; Asthma, unspecified)
Betimol Ophthalmic Solution 3181
Combigan Ophthalmic Solution 553
Cosopt Sterile Ophthalmic Solution 1969
OptiPranolol Metipranolol Ophthalmic Solution 0.3% .... ⊙245
Timoptic Sterile Ophthalmic Solution 2121
Timoptic in Ocudose 2124
Timoptic-XE Sterile Ophthalmic Gel Forming Solution 2125

Chronic obstructive pulmonary disease, acute
Advair Diskus 100/50 1276
Advair Diskus 250/50 1276
Advair Diskus 500/50 1276

Circulatory collapse
(*see under* Shock, unspecified)

Cirrhosis, primary biliary
Fenoglide Tablets 2960
Tricor Tablets 520

Cirrhosis, unspecified
Dantrium Capsules 2580
Precose Tablets 792

Coagulation disorders
(*see under* Bleeding disorders, unspecified; Hemophilia)

Colitis, antibiotic-associated
Duac Topical Gel 3054
Evoclin Foam, 1% 3056
Ziana Gel 1942

Colitis, pseudomembranous
Duac Topical Gel 3054

Colitis, ulcerative
Bentyl Capsules 703
Bentyl Injection 703
Bentyl Syrup 703
Bentyl Tablets 703
Donnatal Extentabs 2507
Evoclin Foam, 1% 3056
Fleet Phospho-soda 1145
Fleet Phospho-soda EZ-PREP 1147
Precose Tablets 792
Ziana Gel 1942

Colitis, ulcerative, history of
Benzaclin Topical Gel 2721
Duac Topical Gel 3054

Colitis, unspecified
(*see under* Colitis, ulcerative; Enterocolitis, necrotizing)

Colitis, unspecified, history of
Benzaclin Topical Gel 2721

Colonic ulceration
(*see under* Colitis, ulcerative)

Coma, diabetic
Avandamet Tablets 1336
Thiothixene Capsules 2197

Coma, hepatic
Thiothixene Capsules 2197

Coma, unspecified
Infanrix Vaccine 1479
Moban Tablets 1116
Thioridazine Hydrochloride Tablets 2195
Thiothixene Capsules 2197

Coma, unspecified, history of
Proleukin for Injection 2287

Comatose states
(*see under* Coma, diabetic; Coma, hepatic; Coma, unspecified)

Conduction disorders, cardiac
(*see under* Arrhythmia, cardiac, unspecified)

Conduction disturbances
(*see under* Arrhythmia, cardiac, unspecified)

Congestive heart failure, uncontrolled
Rythmol Tablets ... 1586
Rythmol SR Capsules ... 1590

Congestive heart failure, unspecified
Amrix Capsules ... 966
Fleet Enema ... 1143
Fleet Enema Extra ... 1143
Fleet Enema for Children ... 1143
Fleet Pedia-Lax Enema ... 1143
Fleet Phospho-soda ... 1145
Fleet Phospho-soda EZ-PREP ... 1147
Fleet Prep Kits ... 1149
Flolan for Injection ... 1426
Pletal Tablets ... 2481
Remicade for IV Injection ... 950

Convulsions, history of
(*see under* Seizure disorders, history of)

Convulsive disorders
(*see under* Seizure disorders, unspecified)

Convulsive disorders, history of
(*see under* Seizure disorders, history of)

COPD
(*see under* Chronic obstructive pulmonary disease)

Coronary artery disease
(*see also under* Coronary artery vasospasm; Stenosis, aortic)
Lybrel Tablets ... 3204
Mircette Tablets ... 1034
NuvaRing ... 2897
Ortho-Cyclen Tablets ... 2449
Ortho Evra Transdermal System ... 2437
Ortho Tri-Cyclen Tablets ... 2449
Ortho Tri-Cyclen Lo Tablets ... 2458
Seasonique Tablets ... 1046
Yaz Tablets ... 805

Coronary artery disease, history of
NuvaRing ... 2897
Seasonique Tablets ... 1046
Yaz Tablets ... 805

Coronary artery disease, severe
Allegra-D 12 Hour Extended-Release Tablets ... 2687
Allegra-D 24 Hour Extended-Release Tablets ... 2690
Clarinex-D 12-Hour Extended-Release Tablets ... 2831
Clarinex-D 24-Hour Extended-Release Tablets ... 2834
Zyrtec-D 12 Hour Extended Release Tablets ... 1923

Coronary artery vasospasm
(*see also under* Angina, Prinzmetal's; Angina pectoris)
Axert Tablets ... 2431
Frova Tablets ... 1111
Imitrex Injection ... 1465
Maxalt Tablets ... 2056
Maxalt-MLT Orally Disintegrating Tablets ... 2056
Zomig Tablets ... 694
Zomig Nasal Spray ... 689
Zomig-ZMT Tablets ... 694

Coronary heart disease
(*see under* Cardiovascular disorders, unspecified)

Coronary insufficiency
(*see under* Cardiovascular disorders, unspecified)

Coronary occlusion
(*see under* Myocardial infarction)

Creatinine clearance, abnormal
(*see under* Renal dysfunction)

Cremophor EL, history of hypersensitivity
Ixempra Kit for Injection ... 915

Critical illness, acute
Genotropin Lyophilized Powder ... 2547
Humatrope Vials and Cartridges ... 1838
Norditropin Cartridges ... 2354
Nutropin for Injection ... 1208
Nutropin AQ Injection ... 1212
Nutropin AQ NuSpin Injection ... 1212
Nutropin AQ Pen ... 1212
Nutropin AQ Pen Cartridge ... 1212
Tev-Tropin for Injection ... 1187

Crohn's disease
Fleet Phospho-soda ... 1145
Fleet Phospho-soda EZ-PREP ... 1147
Fleet Prep Kits ... 1149

Cysts, ovarian
Follistim AQ Cartridge ... 2844

D

Deep vein thrombophlebitis, history of
(*see under* Thrombophlebitis, history of)

Deep vein thrombosis
Activella Tablets ... 2347
Climara Transdermal System ... 763
Climara Pro Transdermal System ... 768
Divigel ... 3167
Enjuvia Tablets ... 1029
Estratest Tablets ... 3043
Estratest H.S. Tablets ... 3043
Premarin Intravenous ... 3217
Premarin Tablets ... 3221
Premarin Vaginal Cream ... 3228
Prempro Tablets ... 3232
Prometrium Capsules (100 mg, 200 mg) ... 3047

Deep vein thrombosis, history of
Activella Tablets ... 2347
Climara Transdermal System ... 763
Climara Pro Transdermal System ... 768
Divigel ... 3167
Enjuvia Tablets ... 1029
Estratest Tablets ... 3043
Estratest H.S. Tablets ... 3043
Premarin Intravenous ... 3217
Premarin Tablets ... 3221
Premarin Vaginal Cream ... 3228
Premphase Tablets ... 3232
Prempro Tablets ... 3232
Prometrium Capsules (100 mg, 200 mg) ... 3047

Dehydration, unspecified
Fleet Enema ... 1143
Fleet Enema Extra ... 1143
Fleet Pedia-Lax Enema ... 1143
Urocit-K Tablets ... 2176
Uroqid-Acid No. 2 Tablets ... 814

Dendritic keratitis
(*see under* Herpes simplex keratitis)

Depression, mental
Seromycin Capsules ... 1864

Diabetes mellitus
Urocit-K Tablets ... 2176

Diabetes mellitus, type 1, sole therapy
Prandin Tablets ... 2971
Starlix Tablets ... 2314

Diabetes with vascular involvement
Lybrel Tablets ... 3204
NuvaRing ... 2897
Ortho-Cyclen Tablets ... 2449
Ortho Evra Transdermal System ... 2437
Ortho Tri-Cyclen Tablets ... 2449
Ortho Tri-Cyclen Lo Tablets ... 2458
Seasonique Tablets ... 1046
Yaz Tablets ... 805

Diabetic ketoacidosis
(*see under* Ketoacidosis, diabetic)

Diarrhea, severe
Edecrin ... 698

Dihydropyrimidine Dehydrogenase (DPD) Deficiency
Carac Cream 0.5% ... 2722
Xeloda Tablets ... 2662

Disease, infectious, unspecified
Mustargen for Injection ... 2492

Drug abuse, history of
Adderall XR Capsules ... 3012
Adipex-P ... 1185
Dexedrine ... 1401
Vyvanse Capsules ... 3033

Dysgammaglobulinemia
Attenuvax ... 1951
Meruvax II ... 2061
M-M-R II ... 2054
Mumpsvax ... 2068
ProQuad ... 2099
Varivax ... 2133

E

ECG, QT syndrome, long
Tasigna Capsules ... 2316
Thioridazine Hydrochloride Tablets ... 2195

ECG changes, history of
Proleukin for Injection ... 2287

Electrocardiogram changes
(*see under* ECG changes, history of)

Electrolyte depletion
(*see under* Electrolyte imbalance, uncorrected)

Electrolyte disturbances
(*see under* Electrolyte imbalance, uncorrected)

Electrolyte imbalance, uncorrected
(*see also under* Hypercalcemia; Hyperkalemia; Hyperphosphatemia; Hypocalcemia; Hypokalemia)
Edecrin ... 698
Rythmol Tablets ... 1586
Rythmol SR Capsules ... 1590

Encephalopathy, history of
Boostrix ... 1377
Infanrix Vaccine ... 1479
Kinrix Injection Vaccine ... 1486
Pediarix Vaccine ... 1552
Pentacel ... 2792

Endocarditis, bacterial
Arixtra Injection ... 1313

Endometrial cancer
(*see under* Carcinoma, endometrium)

Endometritis, postpartum
Mirena Intrauterine System ... 779
ParaGard T 380A Intrauterine Copper Contraceptive ... 1041

Enteritis, history of
Benzaclin Topical Gel ... 2721
Duac Topical Gel ... 3054
Evoclin Foam, 1% ... 3056

Enteritis, regional
Ziana Gel ... 1942

Enterocolitis, necrotizing
Indocin I.V. ... 2489
NeoProfen Injection ... 2496

Epidural catheter, presence of
Xigris Powder for Intravenous Infusion ... 1880

Epilepsy
Seromycin Capsules ... 1864

Epilepsy, uncontrolled
(*see also under* Status epilepticus)
Boostrix ... 1377
Infanrix Vaccine ... 1479
Kinrix Injection Vaccine ... 1486
Pediarix Vaccine ... 1552

Epiphyses, closed
Genotropin Lyophilized Powder ... 2547
Humatrope Vials and Cartridges ... 1838
Increlex Injection ... 3100
Norditropin Cartridges ... 2354
Nutropin for Injection ... 1208
Nutropin AQ Injection ... 1212
Nutropin AQ NuSpin Injection ... 1212
Nutropin AQ Pen ... 1212
Nutropin AQ Pen Cartridge ... 1212
Tev-Tropin for Injection ... 1187

Epiphyses, fused
(*see under* Epiphyses, closed)

Epithelial herpes simplex keratitis
(*see under* Herpes simplex keratitis)

Esophageal abnormalities, unspecified
(*see also under* Achalasia, esophageal; Esophagitis, reflux; Stricture, esophageal)
Fosamax ... 2005
Fosamax Plus D Tablets ... 2013

Esophageal achalasia
(*see under* Achalasia, esophageal)

Esophageal stricture
(*see under* Stricture, esophageal)

Esophageal ulcers less than 1 cm
Photofrin for Injection ... 708

Esophageal varices
Photofrin for Injection ... 708

Esophagitis, reflux
Bentyl Capsules ... 703
Bentyl Injection ... 703
Bentyl Syrup ... 703
Bentyl Tablets ... 703

Exercise, strenuous physical
Urocit-K Tablets ... 2176

Eye infection
(*see under* Infection, ophthalmic, fungal; Infection, ophthalmic, mycobacterial; Infection, ophthalmic, viral; Iritis, acute)

F

Fallot's tetralogy
(*see under* Tetralogy of Fallot)

Febrile illness
(*see under* Fever; Infection, febrile; Respiratory illness, febrile)

Fetal distress, non-imminent delivery
Cervidil Vaginal Insert ... 1165

Fever
(*see also under* Infection, febrile; Respiratory illness, febrile)
ProQuad ... 2099
Tice BCG ... 2936

Fibrillation, ventricular
Lanoxin Injection ... 1498
Lanoxin Injection Pediatric ... 1502
Lanoxin Tablets ... 1505
Rythmol Tablets ... 1586

Fibrosis, cavernosal
Edex Injection ... 2957

Fibrosis, unspecified
(*see under* Fibrosis, cavernosal)

Fibrotic processes
(*see under* Fibrosis, cavernosal)

Fluid overload
Orthoclone OKT3 Sterile Solution 2387

Fructose intolerance
Metadate CD Capsules 3146

FSH, high levels of
Follistim AQ Cartridge 2844

Fungal disease, ophthalmic
Durezol Ophthalmic Emulsion ..... ⊙ 275
Triesence Injectable Suspension ..... ⊙ 209

Fungal infections
(*see under* Actinomycosis, genital; Infection, ophthalmic, fungal)

G

Galactose malabsorption
Metadate CD Capsules 3146

Gallbladder disease, unspecified
Fenoglide Tablets 2960
Tricor Tablets 520

Gastric retention
Enablex Extended-Release Tablets 2225
Sanctura XR Capsules 557
VESIcare Tablets 636

Gastric varices
Photofrin for Injection 708

Gastrointestinal disorders
(*see under* Bleeding, gastrointestinal; Esophageal abnormalities, unspecified; Gastric retention; Hernia, hiatal; Inflammation, gastrointestinal tract; Intestinal disorders, unspecified; Obstruction, gastrointestinal tract; Perforation, gastrointestinal tract)

Gastrointestinal obstruction
(*see under* Obstruction, gastrointestinal tract)

Gastrointestinal perforation
(*see under* Perforation, gastrointestinal tract)

Gastrointestinal tract malformation, congenital
Rotarix Oral Suspension 1582

General anesthesia
(*see under* Anesthesia, general)

Genital bleeding
(*see under* Bleeding, genital, abnormal)

Glaucoma, angle closure
Allegra-D 12 Hour Extended-Release Tablets 2687
Allegra-D 24 Hour Extended-Release Tablets 2690
Clarinex-D 12-Hour Extended-Release Tablets 2831
Clarinex-D 24-Hour Extended-Release Tablets 2834
Evoxac Capsules 1013
Klonopin 2639
Salagen Tablets 1082
Stalevo Tablets 2309
Strattera Capsules 1864
Transderm Scōp Transdermal Therapeutic System 2206
Valium Tablets 2658
Zyrtec-D 12 Hour Extended Release Tablets 1923

Glaucoma, narrow angle
(*see under* Glaucoma, angle closure)

Glaucoma, narrow-angle, uncontrolled
Cymbalta Delayed-Release Capsules 1801
Enablex Extended-Release Tablets 2225
Sanctura XR Capsules 557
VESIcare Tablets 636

Glaucoma, open angle, untreated
Klonopin 2639
Valium Tablets 2658

Glaucoma, unspecified
Adderall XR Capsules 3012
Adipex-P 1185
Bentyl Capsules 703
Bentyl Injection 703
Bentyl Syrup 703
Bentyl Tablets 703
Concerta Extended-Release Tablets 1925
Daytrana Transdermal Patch 3022
Dexedrine 1401
Donnatal Extentabs 2507
Focalin XR Capsules 2251
Metadate CD Capsules 3146
Vyvanse Capsules 3033

Glucose malabsorption
Metadate CD Capsules 3146

Glucose-6-phosphate dehydrogenase
Elitek 2729

H

Head injury
(*see also under* Trauma, intracranial)
DepoDur Injection 1095

Headache
(*see under* Headache, history of; Migraine, basilar; Migraine, hemiplegic)

Headache, history of
Marplan Tablets 3177
Parnate Tablets 1532

Headaches with focal neurological symptoms
Lybrel Tablets 3204
NuvaRing 2897
Ortho-Cyclen Tablets 2449
Ortho Evra Transdermal System 2437
Ortho Tri-Cyclen Tablets 2449
Ortho Tri-Cyclen Lo Tablets 2458
Seasonique Tablets 1046
Yaz Tablets 805

Heart attack
(*see under* Myocardial infarction)

Heart block, first degree
Rythmol Tablets 1586

Heart block, greater than first degree
Adenocard IV Injection 603
Adenoscan 605
Betimol Ophthalmic Solution 3181
Bystolic Tablets 1155
Cardizem LA Extended Release Tablets 421
Coreg Tablets 1387
Coreg CR Extended-Release Capsules 1393
InnoPran XL Extended Release Capsules 1484
Nadolol Tablets 2191
OptiPranolol Metipranolol Ophthalmic Solution 0.3% ..... ⊙ 245
Tarka Tablets 511
Timoptic Sterile Ophthalmic Solution 2121
Timoptic in Ocudose 2124
Timoptic-XE Sterile Ophthalmic Gel Forming Solution 2125
Toprol-XL Tablets 666

Heart block, sinoatrial
Rythmol Tablets 1586

Heart block, unspecified
Amrix Capsules 966
Primaxin I.M. 2080

Heart damage
(*see under* Cardiovascular disorders, unspecified)

Heart disease, ischemic
(*see also under* Angina pectoris; Ischemia, silent; Myocardial infarction)
Amerge Tablets 1301
Axert Tablets 2431
Frova Tablets 1111
Imitrex Injection 1465
Imitrex Nasal Spray 1470
Imitrex Tablets 1474
Maxalt Tablets 2056
Maxalt-MLT Orally Disintegrating Tablets 2056
Treximet Tablets 1616
Zomig Tablets 694
Zomig Nasal Spray 689
Zomig-ZMT Tablets 694

Heart disease, severe organic
ProAmatine Tablets 3032

Heart disease, unspecified
(*see under* Cardiovascular disorders, unspecified)

Heart disease, valvular
Lybrel Tablets 3204
NuvaRing 2897
Ortho-Cyclen/Ortho Tri-Cyclen 2449

Heart failure, intravascular volume, increased
Albutein 5% 1707
Albutein 25% 1708

Heart failure, unspecified
(*see also under* Congestive heart failure, unspecified)
ActoPlus Met Tablets 3071
Actos Tablets 3077
Albutein 5% 1707
Albutein 25% 1708
Betimol Ophthalmic Solution 3181
Bystolic Tablets 1155
Combigan Ophthalmic Solution 553
Cosopt Sterile Ophthalmic Solution 1969
Duetact Tablets 3085
Flexbumin 25% I.V. 729
Geodon 2520
Human Albumin Grifols 25% 1706
Nadolol Tablets 2191
OptiPranolol Metipranolol Ophthalmic Solution 0.3% ..... ⊙ 245
Orthoclone OKT3 Sterile Solution 2387
Timoptic Sterile Ophthalmic Solution 2121
Timoptic in Ocudose 2124
Timoptic-XE Sterile Ophthalmic Gel Forming Solution 2125
Toprol-XL Tablets 666

Hematologic disorders
(*see under* Bleeding disorders, unspecified; Blood dyscrasias, unspecified)

Hematopoietic disorders
(*see under* Blood dyscrasias, unspecified; Bone marrow depression)

Hematuria
Tice BCG 2936

Hemochromatosis
Ferralet 90 Tablets 2175
Nu-Iron 150 Capsules 2165

Hemoglobinopathies
Rebetol 2917

Hemolytic anemia
Ferralet 90 Tablets 2175

Hemophilia
Percodan Tablets 1130

Hemorrhage
(*see under* Bleeding, abnormal, unspecified; Bleeding, gastrointestinal; Bleeding, gastrointestinal, history of; Bleeding, genital, abnormal; Bleeding, genitourinary; Bleeding, history of; Bleeding, internal, unspecified; Bleeding, intracranial; Bleeding, rectal; Bleeding, unspecified; Bleeding disorders, unspecified; Bleeding tendencies; Cardiovascular status, unstable in acute hemorrhage)

Hemorrhagic diathesis
(*see under* Bleeding tendencies)

Hemorrhagic stroke
(*see under* Stroke, hemorrhagic)

Hemosiderosis
Ferralet 90 Tablets 2175
Nu-Iron 150 Capsules 2165

Hemostatic disorders
(*see under* Bleeding disorders, unspecified)

Hepatic adenoma
(*see under* Adenoma, hepatic)

Hepatic cancer
(*see under* Carcinoma, hepatic)

Hepatic coma
(*see under* Coma, hepatic)

Hepatic damage
(*see under* Liver dysfunction)

Hepatic decompensation
PegIntron Powder for Injection 2903

Hepatic disease
(*see under* Liver disease, unspecified)

Hepatic dysfunction
(*see also under* Liver dysfunction)
Yaz Tablets 805

Hepatic failure
(*see under* Liver failure)

Hepatic impairment
(*see under* Liver dysfunction)

Hepatic impairment, moderate
Aptivus Capsules 823
Aptivus Oral Solution 823
Opana Tablets 1117
Uroxatral Tablets 2786
Viramune Oral Suspension 873
Viramune Tablets 873

Hepatic impairment, severe
Agrylin Capsules 3017
Amerge Tablets 1301
Aptivus Capsules 823
Aptivus Oral Solution 823
Bystolic Tablets 1155
Coreg Tablets 1387
Imitrex Injection 1465
Imitrex Nasal Spray 1470
Imitrex Tablets 1474
Opana Tablets 1117
Uroxatral Tablets 2786
Viramune Oral Suspension 873
Viramune Tablets 873

Hepatic injury
(*see under* Liver dysfunction)

Hepatic insufficiency
(*see under* Liver dysfunction)

Hepatitis
Dantrium Capsules 2580

Hepatitis, autoimmune
Intron A for Injection 2859
PegIntron Powder for Injection 2903

Hepatitis, history of
Ketek Tablets 2744

Hepatocellular failure
(*see under* Liver failure)

Hereditary or acquired thrombophilias
Lybrel Tablets ... 3204

Hernia, hiatal
Donnatal Extentabs ... 2507

Herpes simplex keratitis
Alrex Ophthalmic Suspension 0.2% ... ⊙ 236
Durezol Ophthalmic Emulsion ... ⊙ 275
FML Ophthalmic Ointment ... ⊙ 223
FML Ophthalmic Suspension ... ⊙ 224
FML Forte Ophthalmic Suspension ... ⊙ 222
Lotemax Ophthalmic Suspension 0.5% ... ⊙ 241
Pred Forte Ophthalmic Suspension ... ⊙ 227
Pred Mild Ophthalmic Suspension ... ⊙ 230
Pred-G Ophthalmic Ointment ... ⊙ 229
Pred-G Ophthalmic Suspension ... ⊙ 228

Herpes zoster
Cosmegen for Injection ... 2485

Hiatal hernia
(*see under* Hernia, hiatal)

HIV
(*see under* Human immunodeficiency virus)

Human Immunodeficiency Syndrome
Zostavax Injection ... 2145

Human immunodeficiency virus
(*see also under* Acquired immune deficiency syndrome)
Amevive ... 611
Attenuvax ... 1951
Mumpsvax ... 2068
Pediarix Vaccine ... 1552
ProQuad ... 2099
Tice BCG ... 2936
Varivax ... 2133

Hypercalcemia
Actonel with Calcium Tablets ... 2574
Calcijex Injection ... 419
PhosLo GelCaps ... 1184
Rocaltrol Capsules ... 1150
Rocaltrol Oral Solution ... 1150
Zemplar Capsules ... 536
Zemplar Injection ... 538

Hypercarbia
MS Contin Tablets ... 2585
Opana ER Tablets ... 1121
OxyContin Tablets ... 2589
OxyIR Capsules ... 2593
Percodan Tablets ... 1130

Hyperkalemia
Dyazide Capsules ... 1405
Dyrenium Capsules ... 3189
K-Phos Original (Sodium Free) Tablets ... 814
Urocit-K Tablets ... 2176

Hyperlipemia
Cleviprex ... 1936

Hyperparathyroidism
Fleet Enema ... 1143
Fleet Enema Extra ... 1143
Fleet Enema for Children ... 1143
Fleet Pedia-Lax Enema ... 1143
Fleet Phospho-soda ... 1145
Fleet Phospho-soda EZ-PREP ... 1147
Fleet Prep Kits ... 1149

Hyperphosphatemia
K-Phos Original (Sodium Free) Tablets ... 814
K-Phos Neutral Tablets ... 813
Uroqid-Acid No. 2 Tablets ... 814

Hypersensitivity to benzyl alcohol
Lovenox Injection ... 2756
Nutropin for Injection ... 1208

Hypersensitivity to pork products
Lovenox Injection ... 2756

Hypertension, excessive supine
ProAmatine Tablets ... 3032

Hypertension, moderate
Adderall XR Capsules ... 3012
Vyvanse Capsules ... 3033

Hypertension, severe
Adderall XR Capsules ... 3012
Allegra-D 12 Hour Extended-Release Tablets ... 2687
Allegra-D 24 Hour Extended-Release Tablets ... 2690
Clarinex-D 12-Hour Extended-Release Tablets ... 2831
Clarinex-D 24-Hour Extended-Release Tablets ... 2834
NuvaRing ... 2897
Ortho-Cyclen/Ortho Tri-Cyclen ... 2449
Seasonique Tablets ... 1046
Vyvanse Capsules ... 3033
Yaz Tablets ... 805
Zyrtec-D 12 Hour Extended Release Tablets ... 1923

Hypertension, uncontrolled
Activase I.V. ... 1188
Amerge Tablets ... 1301
Aranesp for Injection ... 564
Axert Tablets ... 2431
Epogen for Injection ... 576
Frova Tablets ... 1111
Gengraf Capsules ... 435
Imitrex Nasal Spray ... 1470
Imitrex Tablets ... 1474
Integrilin Injection ... 2855
Lybrel Tablets ... 3204
Maxalt Tablets ... 2056
Maxalt-MLT Orally Disintegrating Tablets ... 2056
Neoral Oral Solution ... 2280
Neoral Soft Gelatin Capsules ... 2280
Orthoclone OKT3 Sterile Solution ... 2387
Procrit for Injection ... 2391
ReoPro Vials ... 1860
TNKase ... 1233
Treximet Tablets ... 1616
Zomig Tablets ... 694
Zomig Nasal Spray ... 689
Zomig-ZMT Tablets ... 694

Hypertension, unspecified
Adipex-P ... 1185
Dexedrine ... 1401
Imitrex Injection ... 1465
Marplan Tablets ... 3177
Ortho Evra Transdermal System ... 2437
Ortho Tri-Cyclen Lo Tablets ... 2458
Parnate Tablets ... 1532

Hyperthermia, malignant, susceptibility to
Ultane Liquid for Inhalation ... 524

Hyperthyroidism
(*see also under* Thyrotoxicosis; Thyrotoxicosis, untreated)
Adderall XR Capsules ... 3012
Adipex-P ... 1185
Amrix Capsules ... 966
Dexedrine ... 1401
Vyvanse Capsules ... 3033

Hypervitaminosis D
(*see under* Toxicity, vitamin D)

Hypocalcemia
Actonel Tablets ... 2568
Actonel with Calcium Tablets ... 2574
Boniva Injection ... 2614
Boniva Tablets ... 2618
Fosamax ... 2005
Fosamax Plus D Tablets ... 2013
Reclast Injection ... 2291

Hypogammaglobulinemia
(*see also under* Immunodeficiency, unspecified)
Attenuvax ... 1951
Meruvax II ... 2061
M-M-R II ... 2054
Mumpsvax ... 2068
ProQuad ... 2099
Varivax ... 2133

Hypoglycemia, functional
Proglycem Capsules ... 1185
Proglycem Suspension ... 1185

Hypoglycemia, unspecified
Apidra Injection ... 2706
Humalog-Pen and KwikPen ... 1829
Humalog Mix 50/50-Pen and KwikPen ... 1833
Humulin R ... 1849
Humulin R (U-500) ... 1850
NovoLog Mix 70/30 ... 2364
NovoLog Injection ... 2359

Hypokalemia
Tasigna Capsules ... 2316

Hypomagnesemia
Tasigna Capsules ... 2316

Hyponatremia, hypovolemic
Vaprisol ... 632

Hypotension, unspecified
Cardizem LA Extended Release Tablets ... 421
Rythmol Tablets ... 1586
Rythmol SR Capsules ... 1590
Tarka Tablets ... 511

Hypovolemia
(*see under* Shock, unspecified)

I

IgA deficiencies, selective
(*see under* Immunoglobulin A deficiency)

Ileocolostomy
Activase I.V. ... 1188

Ileus, paralytic
Avinza Capsules ... 1772
DepoDur Injection ... 1095
Donnatal Extentabs ... 2507
Duragesic Transdermal System ... 2405
MS Contin Tablets ... 2585
Opana Tablets ... 1117
Opana ER Tablets ... 1121
OxyContin Tablets ... 2589
OxyIR Capsules ... 2593
Percodan Tablets ... 1130

Ileus, unspecified
(*see also under* Ileus, paralytic)
Fleet Phospho-soda ... 1145
Fleet Phospho-soda EZ-PREP ... 1147
Fleet Prep Kits ... 1149

Immunodeficiency, family history of
Meruvax II ... 2061
M-M-R II ... 2054
Mumpsvax ... 2068
ProQuad ... 2099

Immunodeficiency, history of
Attenuvax ... 1951
ProQuad ... 2099
Varivax ... 2133
Zostavax Injection ... 2145

Immunodeficiency, unspecified
(*see also under* Acquired immune deficiency syndrome; Dysgammaglobulinemia; Human immunodeficiency virus; Hypogammaglobulinemia; Immunodeficiency, family history of; Immunodeficiency, history of; Immunoglobulin A deficiency; Immunosuppression)
Attenuvax ... 1951
Meruvax II ... 2061
M-M-R II ... 2054
Mumpsvax ... 2068
ProQuad ... 2099
Tice BCG ... 2936
Varivax ... 2133

Immunodeficient state
(*see under* Immunodeficiency, unspecified)

Immunoglobulin A deficiency
Aralast ... 726
Flebogamma 5% ... 1715
Flebogamma 5% DIF ... 1718
Gammagard S/D ... 734
Prolastin ... 3099

Immunosuppression
Attenuvax ... 1951
Meruvax II ... 2061
M-M-R II ... 2054
Mumpsvax ... 2068
ProQuad ... 2099
Tice BCG ... 2936
Varivax ... 2133

Imperforate anus
Fleet Enema ... 1143
Fleet Enema Extra ... 1143
Fleet Enema for Children ... 1143
Fleet Pedia-Lax Enema ... 1143

Impulse generation disorders
(*see under* Arrhythmia, cardiac, unspecified)

Inability to stand or sit upright for at least 30 minutes
Actonel Tablets ... 2568
Actonel with Calcium Tablets ... 2574
Fosamax ... 2005
Fosamax Plus D Tablets ... 2013

Inability to stand or sit upright for at least 60 minutes
Boniva Tablets ... 2618

Increased intracranial pressure
(*see under* Intracranial pressure, increased)

Infants
Bentyl Capsules ... 703
Bentyl Injection ... 703
Bentyl Syrup ... 703
Bentyl Tablets ... 703
Fansidar Tablets ... 2636
Gantrisin Pediatric Suspension ... 2638
WinRho SDF ... 741

Infection, bacterial, unspecified
(*see under* Endocarditis, bacterial)

Infection, febrile
Attenuvax ... 1951
Meruvax II ... 2061
M-M-R II ... 2054
Mumpsvax ... 2068
ProQuad ... 2099
Varivax ... 2133

Infection, fungal
(*see under* Actinomycosis, genital; Infection, ophthalmic, fungal)

Infection, fungal, unspecified
(*see under* Actinomycosis, genital)

Infection, injection site
BOTOX Purified Neurotoxin Complex ... 550
Hyalgan Solution ... 2742

Infection, mycobacterial
(*see under* Infection, ophthalmic, mycobacterial)

Infection, ocular
Lucentis Injection ... 1205

Infection, ophthalmic, active
Restasis Ophthalmic Emulsion ... 557

Infection, ophthalmic, fungal
Alrex Ophthalmic Suspension 0.2% ... ⊙ 236
FML Ophthalmic Ointment ... ⊙ 223
FML Ophthalmic Suspension ... ⊙ 224
FML Forte Ophthalmic Suspension ... ⊙ 222
Lotemax Ophthalmic Suspension 0.5% ... ⊙ 241
Pred Forte Ophthalmic Suspension ... ⊙ 227
Pred Mild Ophthalmic Suspension ... ⊙ 230
Pred-G Ophthalmic Ointment ... ⊙ 229
Pred-G Ophthalmic Suspension ... ⊙ 228

Infection, ophthalmic, mycobacterial
Alrex Ophthalmic Suspension 0.2% ... ⊙ 236
FML Ophthalmic Ointment ... ⊙ 223
FML Ophthalmic Suspension ... ⊙ 224
FML Forte Ophthalmic Suspension ... ⊙ 222
Lotemax Ophthalmic Suspension 0.5% ... ⊙ 241

Pred Forte Ophthalmic Suspension ⊙ 227
Pred Mild Ophthalmic Suspension ⊙ 230
Pred-G Ophthalmic Ointment ⊙ 229
Pred-G Ophthalmic Suspension ⊙ 228

Infection, ophthalmic, unspecified
(*see under* Iritis, acute)

Infection, ophthalmic, untreated
Pred Forte Ophthalmic Suspension ⊙ 227
Pred Mild Ophthalmic Suspension ⊙ 230

Infection, ophthalmic, viral
(*see also under* Herpes simplex keratitis)
FML Ophthalmic Ointment ⊙ 223
FML Ophthalmic Suspension ⊙ 224
FML Forte Ophthalmic Suspension ⊙ 222
Lotemax Ophthalmic Suspension 0.5% ⊙ 241
Pred Forte Ophthalmic Suspension ⊙ 227
Pred Mild Ophthalmic Suspension ⊙ 230
Pred-G Ophthalmic Ointment ⊙ 229
Pred-G Ophthalmic Suspension ⊙ 228

Infection, periocular
Lucentis Injection 1205

Infection, respiratory
(*see under* Respiratory illness, febrile)

Infection, untreated
(*see also under* Infection, ophthalmic, untreated)
Indocin I.V. 2489
NeoProfen Injection 2496

Infection, urinary tract
Tice BCG 2936

Infection, vaginal
(*see under* Cervicitis, untreated; Vaginitis, untreated; Vaginosis, bacterial, untreated)

Infection, viral
(*see also under* Herpes simplex keratitis; Herpes zoster; Human immunodeficiency virus; Infection, ophthalmic, viral; Varicella)
Bayer Aspirin 750
Percodan Tablets 1130

Infection, viral, external canal
Ciprodex Otic Suspension 541

Infertility, treatment of
Synthroid Tablets 507

Inflammation, gastrointestinal tract
(*see also under* Colitis, ulcerative; Colitis, ulcerative, history of; Colitis, unspecified, history of; Enteritis, history of; Enterocolitis, necrotizing; Esophagitis, reflux)
Fleet Enema 1143
Fleet Enema Extra 1143
Fleet Enema for Children 1143
Fleet Pedia-Lax Enema 1143
Fleet Phospho-soda 1145
Fleet Phospho-soda EZ-PREP 1147
Fleet Prep Kits 1149
Precose Tablets 792

Inflammatory bowel disease
(*see under* Inflammation, gastrointestinal tract)

Intestinal atony
(*see under* Atony, intestinal)

Intestinal disorders, unspecified
(*see also under* Atony, intestinal; Bowel ischemia, history of; Inflammation, gastrointestinal tract; Megacolon, unspecified; Obstruction, gastrointestinal tract; Perforation, gastrointestinal tract)
Precose Tablets 792

Intestinal obstruction
(*see under* Obstruction, gastrointestinal tract)

Intoxication, unspecified
Ultram ER Extended-Release Tablets 2428

Intracranial pressure, increased
DepoDur Injection 1095
Romazicon Injection 2646

Intracranial trauma
(*see under* Trauma, intracranial)

Intravenous administration
Increlex Injection 3100

Intubation, history of
Proleukin for Injection 2287

Iritis, acute
Evoxac Capsules 1013
Salagen Tablets 1082

Ischemia, silent
Amerge Tablets 1301
Axert Tablets 2431
Frova Tablets 1111
Imitrex Injection 1465
Imitrex Nasal Spray 1470
Imitrex Tablets 1474
Maxalt Tablets 2056
Maxalt-MLT Orally Disintegrating Tablets 2056
Zomig Tablets 694
Zomig Nasal Spray 689
Zomig-ZMT Tablets 694

Ischemia, unspecified
Imitrex Injection 1465

Ischemic attacks, transient
Amerge Tablets 1301
Frova Tablets 1111
Imitrex Injection 1465
Imitrex Nasal Spray 1470
Imitrex Tablets 1474
Treximet Tablets 1616

Ischemic heart disease
(*see under* Heart disease, ischemic)

Ischemic myocardial disease
(*see under* Heart disease, ischemic)

Isomaltase insuffiency
Metadate CD Capsules 3146

J

Jaundice, cholestatic of pregnancy, history of
Lybrel Tablets 3204
Mircette Tablets 1034
NuvaRing 2897
Ortho-Cyclen Tablets 2449
Ortho Evra Transdermal System 2437
Ortho Tri-Cyclen Tablets 2449
Ortho Tri-Cyclen Lo Tablets 2458
Seasonique Tablets 1046
Yaz Tablets 805

Jaundice, history of
Augmentin 1323
Augmentin Tablets 1327
Augmentin XR Extended Release Tablets 1333
Augmentin ES-600 Powder for Oral Suspension 1329
Ketek Tablets 2744
Mircette Tablets 1034
Ortho-Cyclen Tablets 2449
Ortho Evra Transdermal System 2437
Ortho Tri-Cyclen Tablets 2449
Ortho Tri-Cyclen Lo Tablets 2458
Seasonique Tablets 1046
Yaz Tablets 805

K

Keratitis, dendritic
(*see under* Herpes simplex keratitis)

Ketoacidosis, diabetic
ActoPlus Met Tablets 3071
Avandamet Tablets 1336
Avandaryl Tablets 1344
Duetact Tablets 3085
Janumet Tablets 2041
PrandiMet Tablets 2967
Prandin Tablets 2971
Precose Tablets 792
Starlix Tablets 2314

Kidney damage
(*see under* Renal dysfunction)

Kidney disease
(*see under* Renal disease, unspecified)

Kidney failure
(*see under* Renal failure)

L

Lactation
(*see under* Breastfeeding)

Left ventricular dysfunction
(*see under* Ventricular dysfunction, left)

Lesions, gastrointestinal, unspecified
(*see under* Colitis, ulcerative; Colitis, ulcerative, history of)

Lesions, intracranial, unspecified
(*see also under* Tumor, intracranial, unspecified; Tumor, pituitary, unspecified)
Tev-Tropin for Injection 1187

Lesions, malignant, unspecified
(*see under* Carcinoma, breast, history of; Carcinoma, breast, male; Carcinoma, breast, unspecified; Carcinoma, cervical; Carcinoma, endometrium; Carcinoma, genital, unspecified; Carcinoma, hepatic; Carcinoma, prostate; Melanoma, history of; Neoplasm, bone marrow system, malignant; Neoplasm, lymphatic system, malignant)

Lesions, skin, unspecified
Stalevo Tablets 2309

Lesions, skin, viral
(*see under* Herpes zoster; Varicella)

Leukemia, acute
Zostavax Injection 2145

Leukemia, chronic myelogenous, without definitive diagnosis
Myleran Tablets 1530

Leukemia, unspecified
Attenuvax 1951
Edex Injection 2957
Meruvax II 2061
M-M-R II 2054
Mumpsvax 2068
ProQuad 2099
Tice BCG 2936
Varivax 2133

Lipid metabolism, defect
Cleviprex 1936

Liver adenoma
(*see under* Adenoma, hepatic)

Liver cancer
(*see under* Carcinoma, hepatic)

Liver damage
(*see under* Liver dysfunction)

Liver disease, active
Fenoglide Tablets 2960
Lipitor Tablets 2501
Lybrel Tablets 3204
NuvaRing 2897
Seasonique Tablets 1046
Simcor Tablets 502
Vytorin 10/10 Tablets 2149
Vytorin 10/20 Tablets 2149
Vytorin 10/40 Tablets 2149
Vytorin 10/80 Tablets 2149
Yaz Tablets 805

Liver disease, decompensated
Intron A for Injection 2859
PegIntron Powder for Injection 2903

Liver disease, history of
(*see also under* Hepatitis, history of; Liver dysfunction, history of)
Marplan Tablets 3177
Parnate Tablets 1532

Liver disease, unspecified
(*see also under* Cirrhosis, primary biliary; Cirrhosis, unspecified; Hepatitis; Liver dysfunction)
Activella Tablets 2347
Advicor Tablets 402
Climara Transdermal System 763
Climara Pro Transdermal System 768
Crestor Tablets 677
Crinone 4% Gel 992
Crinone 8% Gel 992
Dantrium Capsules 2580
Depakote ER Tablets 423
Dyrenium Capsules 3189
Enjuvia Tablets 1029
Estratest Tablets 3043
Estratest H.S. Tablets 3043
Klonopin 2639
Lescol Capsules 2268
Lescol XL Tablets 2268
Mevacor Tablets 2063
Mirena Intrauterine System 779
Ortho Micronor Tablets 2446
Premarin Intravenous 3217
Premarin Tablets 3221
Premarin Vaginal Cream 3228
Premphase Tablets 3232
Prempro Tablets 3232
Prometrium Capsules (100 mg, 200 mg) 3047
Uroqid-Acid No. 2 Tablets 814
Vytorin 10/10 Tablets 2939
Vytorin 10/20 Tablets 2939
Vytorin 10/40 Tablets 2939
Vytorin 10/80 Tablets 2939
Ziagen Tablets 1673
Zocor Tablets 2136

Liver disorders, history of
Augmentin 1323
Augmentin ES-600 Powder for Oral Suspension 1329

Liver disorders, unspecified
(*see under* Liver dysfunction)

Liver dysfunction
(*see also under* Jaundice, cholestatic of pregnancy, history of; Jaundice, history of; Liver disease, unspecified; Liver failure; Serum transaminase elevation)
Activella Tablets 2347
Advicor Tablets 402
Angeliq Tablets 751
Climara Transdermal System 763
Climara Pro Transdermal System 768
Coreg CR Extended-Release Capsules 1393
Divigel 3167

Enjuvia Tablets 1029
Epzicom Tablets 1422
Estratest Tablets 3043
Estratest H.S. Tablets 3043
Fenoglide Tablets 2960
Niaspan Extended-Release Tablets 480
Opana ER Tablets 1121
Ortho-Cyclen/Ortho Tri-Cyclen 2449
Premarin Intravenous 3217
Premarin Tablets 3221
Premarin Vaginal Cream 3228
Premphase Tablets 3232
Prempro Tablets 3232
Prometrium Capsules (100 mg, 200 mg) 3047
Seasonique Tablets 1046
Skelaxin Tablets 1784
Treximet Tablets 1616
Tricor Tablets 520
Trizivir Tablets 1622
Yaz Tablets 805
Ziagen 1673

Liver dysfunction, history of
(*see also under* Liver disease, history of)
Augmentin Tablets 1327
Augmentin XR Extended Release Tablets 1333

Liver dysfunction, severe
(*see under* Hepatic impairment, severe)

Liver failure
(*see also under* Coma, hepatic; Liver dysfunction)
Fansidar Tablets 2636
Gris-PEG Tablets 2507
Ortho-Cyclen/Ortho Tri-Cyclen 2449
Soriatane Capsules 3062

Liver function tests, abnormal
(*see under* Serum transaminase elevation)

Liver insufficiency
(*see under* Liver dysfunction)

Liver tumor
(*see under* Adenoma, hepatic; Carcinoma, hepatic; Tumor, liver, benign)

Local anesthesia
(*see under* Anesthesia, local)

Lown-Ganong-Levine syndrome
Tarka Tablets 511

Lung disease, unspecified
(*see under* Pulmonary disorders, unspecified)

Lymphoma
(*see also under* Neoplasm, lymphatic system, malignant)
Attenuvax 1951
Meruvax II 2061
M-M-R II 2054
Mumpsvax 2068
ProQuad 2099
Tice BCG 2936
Varivax 2133
Zostavax Injection 2145

M

Malabsorption syndrome
Xenical Capsules 2672

Malignancies, unspecified
Gengraf Capsules 435
Humatrope Vials and Cartridges 1838
Neoral Oral Solution 2280
Neoral Soft Gelatin Capsules 2280
Nutropin for Injection 1208
Nutropin AQ Injection 1212
Nutropin AQ NuSpin Injection 1212
Nutropin AQ Pen 1212
Nutropin AQ Pen Cartridge 1212
Tev-Tropin for Injection 1187

Malignancy
(*see under* Carcinoma, breast, history of; Carcinoma, breast, male; Carcinoma, breast, unspecified; Carcinoma, endometrium; Carcinoma, hepatic; Carcinoma, prostate; Leukemia, unspecified; Lymphoma; Melanoma, history of; Neoplasm, bone marrow system, malignant; Neoplasm, lymphatic system, malignant)

Malignancy, active
Genotropin Lyophilized Powder 2547
Norditropin Cartridges 2354

Malignancy, breast
Crinone 4% Gel 992
Crinone 8% Gel 992

Malignancy, cervical
ParaGard T 380A Intrauterine Copper Contraceptive 1041

Malignancy, uterine
ParaGard T 380A Intrauterine Copper Contraceptive 1041

Mechanical disorders of ventilation
(*see under* Asthma, acute; Asthma, history of; Asthma, unspecified; Obstruction, respiratory tract)

Megacolon, unspecified
Fleet Enema 1143
Fleet Enema Extra 1143
Fleet Enema for Children 1143
Fleet Pedia-Lax Enema 1143
Fleet Phospho-soda 1145
Fleet Phospho-soda EZ-PREP 1147
Fleet Prep Kits 1149

Megaloblastic anemia
(*see under* Anemia, megaloblastic, unspecified)

Melanoma, history of
Stalevo Tablets 2309

Mental depression
(*see under* Depression, mental)

Metabolic acidosis
(*see under* Acidosis, metabolic, unspecified; Ketoacidosis, diabetic)

Migraine, basilar
Amerge Tablets 1301
Axert Tablets 2431
Frova Tablets 1111
Imitrex Injection 1465
Imitrex Nasal Spray 1470
Imitrex Tablets 1474
Maxalt Tablets 2056
Maxalt-MLT Orally Disintegrating Tablets 2056
Treximet Tablets 1616
Zomig Tablets 694
Zomig Nasal Spray 689
Zomig-ZMT Tablets 694

Migraine, hemiplegic
Amerge Tablets 1301
Axert Tablets 2431
Frova Tablets 1111
Imitrex Injection 1465
Imitrex Nasal Spray 1470
Imitrex Tablets 1474
Maxalt Tablets 2056
Maxalt-MLT Orally Disintegrating Tablets 2056
Treximet Tablets 1616
Zomig Tablets 694
Zomig Nasal Spray 689
Zomig-ZMT Tablets 694

Multipara, unspecified
Cervidil Vaginal Insert 1165

Myasthenia gravis
Bentyl Capsules 703
Bentyl Injection 703
Bentyl Syrup 703
Bentyl Tablets 703
Donnatal Extentabs 2507
Ketek Tablets 2744

Mycobacterial infection
(*see under* Infection, ophthalmic, mycobacterial)

Mycobacterial infections, ophthalmic
Durezol Ophthalmic Emulsion ....⊙275

Myeloid blasts, leukemic
Leukine 774

Myeloma, multiple
Edex Injection 2957

Myeloproliferative disorders
(*see under* Leukemia, acute; Leukemia, unspecified; Myeloma, multiple)

Myelosuppression
(*see under* Bone marrow depression)

Myocardial damage
(*see under* Cardiovascular disorders, unspecified)

Myocardial disease
(*see under* Cardiovascular disorders, unspecified)

Myocardial infarction
Activella Tablets 2347
Cardizem LA Extended Release Tablets 421
Cytomel Tablets 1778
Divigel 3167
Estratest Tablets 3043
Estratest H.S. Tablets 3043
Geodon 2520
Levothroid Tablets 1170
Levoxyl Tablets 1780
Premarin Vaginal Cream 3228
Premphase Tablets 3232
Prempro Tablets 3232
Prometrium Capsules (100 mg, 200 mg) 3047
Zomig-ZMT Tablets 694

Myocardial Infarction, acute, recovery phase
Amrix Capsules 966

Myocardial infarction, history of
Amerge Tablets 1301
Axert Tablets 2431
Estratest Tablets 3043
Estratest H.S. Tablets 3043
Frova Tablets 1111
Imitrex Injection 1465
Imitrex Nasal Spray 1470
Imitrex Tablets 1474
Maxalt Tablets 2056
Maxalt-MLT Orally Disintegrating Tablets 2056
Proleukin for Injection 2287
Prometrium Capsules (100 mg, 200 mg) 3047
Treximet Tablets 1616
Zomig Tablets 694
Zomig Nasal Spray 689

N

Naloxone challenge test, failed
Vivitrol 988

Narcotic dependence
Vivitrol 988

Narcotic withdrawal, acute
Vivitrol 988

Narrow angle glaucoma
(*see under* Glaucoma, angle closure)

Nausea
Fleet Prep Kits 1149

Necrosis
(*see also under* Enterocolitis, necrotizing)
Urocit-K Tablets 2176

Neonates
(*see under* Infants)

Neoplasia, estrogen dependent
(*see under* Neoplasm, estrogen dependent)

Neoplasia, hepatic
(*see under* Adenoma, hepatic; Carcinoma, hepatic; Tumor, liver, benign)

Neoplasia, unspecified
(*see also under* Neoplasm, unspecified)
Divigel 3167
Increlex Injection 3100

Neoplasm, androgen dependent
(*see under* Carcinoma, prostate)

Neoplasm, bone marrow system, malignant
(*see also under* Myeloid blasts, leukemic; Myeloma, multiple)
Attenuvax 1951
Meruvax II 2061
M-M-R II 2054
Mumpsvax 2068
ProQuad 2099
Varivax 2133
Zostavax Injection 2145

Neoplasm, estrogen dependent
(*see also under* Carcinoma, breast, male; Carcinoma, breast, unspecified)
Activella Tablets 2347
Angeliq Tablets 751
Climara Transdermal System 763
Climara Pro Transdermal System 768
Enjuvia Tablets 1029
Estratest Tablets 3043
Estratest H.S. Tablets 3043
Lybrel Tablets 3204
Mircette Tablets 1034
NuvaRing 2897
Ortho-Cyclen Tablets 2449
Ortho Evra Transdermal System 2437
Ortho Tri-Cyclen Tablets 2449
Ortho Tri-Cyclen Lo Tablets 2458
Premarin Intravenous 3217
Premarin Tablets 3221
Premarin Vaginal Cream 3228
Premphase Tablets 3232
Prempro Tablets 3232
Seasonique Tablets 1046
Vagifem Tablets 2375
Yaz Tablets 805

Neoplasm, estrogen dependent, history of
(*see under* Carcinoma, breast, history of)

Neoplasm, hepatic, unspecified
(*see under* Adenoma, hepatic; Carcinoma, hepatic; Tumor, liver, benign)

Neoplasm, intracranial
(*see under* Tumor, intracranial, unspecified)

Neoplasm, lymphatic system, malignant
(*see also under* Lymphoma)
Attenuvax 1951
Meruvax II 2061
M-M-R II 2054
Mumpsvax 2068
ProQuad 2099
Varivax 2133

Neoplasm, ovarian
(*see under* Cysts, ovarian)

Neoplasm, unspecified
Nutropin for Injection 1208
Nutropin AQ Injection 1212
Nutropin AQ NuSpin Injection 1212
Nutropin AQ Pen 1212
Nutropin AQ Pen Cartridge 1212

Neoplastic activity, unspecified
(*see under* Neoplasm, unspecified; Tumor activity, unspecified)

Nephrosis, lipoid
Cleviprex 1936

Neurologic toxicity
(*see under* Toxicity, neurologic)

Neurological disorders, unspecified
(*see also under* Central nervous system depression; Cerebral vascular disease; Cerebral vascular disease, history of; Cerebrovascular accident; Cerebrovascular accident, history of; Depression, mental; Encephalopathy, history of; Epilepsy; Epilepsy, uncontrolled; Intracranial pressure, increased; Myasthenia gravis; Psychosis; Psychosis, toxic, history of; Seizure disorders, history of; Seizure disorders, unspecified; Tourette's syndrome; Toxicity, neurologic)
Boostrix 1377
Fluarix Vaccine 1446
Flulaval Injection Vaccine 1448
Infanrix Vaccine 1479
Kinrix Injection Vaccine 1486
Pediarix Vaccine 1552
Pentacel 2792

Neutropenia
Taxotere Injection Concentrate 2773

Neutrophil count, baseline, less than 1500 cells/mm3
Ixempra Kit for Injection 915

Nursing mothers
(*see under* Breastfeeding)

O

Obesity
Humatrope Vials and Cartridges 1838

Obesity, therapy of
Synthroid Tablets 507

Obstruction, biliary tract
(*see under* Jaundice, cholestatic of pregnancy, history of; Jaundice, history of)

Obstruction, bladder neck
(*see under* Obstruction, urinary tract)

Obstruction, gastrointestinal tract
(*see also under* Achalasia, esophageal; Bowel ischemia, history of; Ileus, paralytic; Ileus, unspecified; Stricture, esophageal)
Amitiza Capsules 3082
Bentyl Capsules 703
Bentyl Injection 703
Bentyl Syrup 703
Bentyl Tablets 703
Donnatal Extentabs 2507
Fleet Enema 1143
Fleet Enema Extra 1143
Fleet Enema for Children 1143
Fleet Pedia-Lax Enema 1143
Fleet Phospho-soda 1145
Fleet Phospho-soda EZ-PREP 1147
Fleet Prep Kits 1149
Precose Tablets 792
WelChol Tablets 1015

Obstruction, respiratory tract
DepoDur Injection 1095

Obstruction, urinary tract
(*see also under* Urinary retention)
Bentyl Capsules 703
Bentyl Injection 703
Bentyl Syrup 703
Bentyl Tablets 703
Donnatal Extentabs 2507

Obstruction, urogenital tract
(*see under* Obstruction, urinary tract)

Obstructive uropathy
(*see under* Obstruction, urinary tract)

Ocular herpes simplex
(*see under* Herpes simplex keratitis)

Oliguria
Edecrin 698

Opioid dependence
(*see under* Narcotic dependence)

Opioid intolerance
Duragesic Transdermal System 2405

Opioid non-tolerant patients
Actiq 959

Opioid urine screen, positive
Vivitrol 988

Opioid use, more than 7 consecutive days immediately prior to therapy
Entereg Capsules 3293

Opioid withdrawal
(*see under* Narcotic withdrawal, acute)

Organ allograft
Proleukin for Injection 2287

Organic heart disease
(*see under* Cardiovascular disorders, unspecified; Heart disease, ischemic)

Ovarian enlargement, unspecified
Follistim AQ Cartridge 2844

Ovarian failure, primary
Follistim AQ Cartridge 2844

Overt cardiac failure
(*see under* Heart failure, unspecified)

P

Pain, abdominal
Fleet Prep Kits 1149

Pain, acute
Actiq 959
Duragesic Transdermal System 2405
Fentora Tablets 968

Pain, intermittent
Duragesic Transdermal System 2405

Pain, mild
Duragesic Transdermal System 2405
Opana ER Tablets 1121

Pain, peri-operative, coronary artery bypass graft surgery
Anaprox Tablets 2632
Anaprox DS Tablets 2632
Celebrex Capsules 2979
Clinoril Tablets 1962
EC-Naprosyn Delayed-Release Tablets 2632
Flector Patch 561
Indocin 2024
Mobic Oral Suspension 863
Mobic Tablets 863
Naprosyn Suspension 2632
Naprosyn Tablets 2632
Vicoprofen Tablets 533
Voltaren Tablets 2334
Voltaren-XR Tablets 2337

Pain, post operative
Actiq 959
Duragesic Transdermal System 2405
Fentora Tablets 968
Opana ER Tablets 1121

Pancreatic diseases, unspecified
Ultrase Capsules 718
Ultrase MT Capsules 719

Pancreatitis
Cleviprex 1936
Creon 5 Capsules 3041
Creon 10 Capsules 3042
Creon 20 Capsules 3042
Elspar for Injection 1990
Elspar for Injection 2488
Ultrase Capsules 718
Ultrase MT Capsules 719

Pancreatitis, history of
Elspar for Injection 1990
Elspar for Injection 2488
Oncaspar Injection 1138

Pancreatitis, history of hypertriglyceridemia-induced
WelChol Tablets 1015

Paralytic ileus
(*see under* Ileus, paralytic)

Pediatric patients 18 years of age and younger
Anzemet Injection 2701
Pylera Capsules 714

Pediatric patients under 6 years of age
Tussionex Pennkinetic Extended-Release Suspension 3154

Pediatric patients under 18 years of age
Fleet Prep Kits 1149

Pelvic inflammatory disease
Mirena Intrauterine System 779
ParaGard T 380A Intrauterine Copper Contraceptive 1041

Pelvic inflammatory disease, history of
ParaGard T 380A Intrauterine Copper Contraceptive 1041

Penile deformation
(*see under* Angulation, penile; Fibrosis, cavernosal; Peyronie's disease)

Penile implants
Edex Injection 2957

Peptic ulcer
(*see under* Ulcer, peptic)

Perforation, gastrointestinal tract
Fleet Enema 1143
Fleet Enema Extra 1143
Fleet Enema for Children 1143
Fleet Pedia-Lax Enema 1143
Fleet Phospho-soda 1145
Fleet Phospho-soda EZ-PREP 1147
Fleet Prep Kits 1149

Perforation, gastrointestinal tract, history of
Proleukin for Injection 2287

Perforation, intestinal
(*see under* Perforation, gastrointestinal tract)

Pericardial tamponade, history of
Proleukin for Injection 2287

Peripheral arterial disease
(*see under* Peripheral vascular disease)

Peripheral vascular disease
(*see also under* Arteriosclerosis, unspecified; Thrombophlebitis)
Amerge Tablets 1301
Frova Tablets 1111
Imitrex Injection 1465
Imitrex Nasal Spray 1470
Imitrex Tablets 1474
Treximet Tablets 1616

Peripheral vascular insufficiency
(*see under* Peripheral vascular disease)

Peyronie's disease
Edex Injection 2957

Pheochromocytoma
Azilect Tablets 3106
Emsam Transdermal System 905
Glucagon for Injection Vials and Emergency Kit 1827
Marplan Tablets 3177
Parnate Tablets 1532
ProAmatine Tablets 3032

Phlebitis
(*see under* Thrombophlebitis)

Phosphate stones, infected
K-Phos Original (Sodium Free) Tablets 814
K-Phos Neutral Tablets 813

Photosensitivity diseases, unspecified
(*see under* Porphyria, acute; Porphyria, unspecified)

Platelet count less than 100,000 cells/mm3
Ixempra Kit for Injection 915

Poor nutritional state
(*see under* Electrolyte imbalance, uncorrected)

Porphyria, acute
Donnatal Extentabs 2507
Soma Tablets 1931

Porphyria, unspecified
Gris-PEG Tablets 2507
Nembutal Sodium Solution, USP 2494
Photofrin for Injection 708
Vagifem Tablets 2375
Visudyne for Injection 2332

Prader-Willi Syndrome
Humatrope Vials and Cartridges 1838
Nutropin for Injection 1208
Nutropin AQ Injection 1212
Nutropin AQ NuSpin Injection 1212
Nutropin AQ Pen 1212
Nutropin AQ Pen Cartridge 1212
Tev-Tropin for Injection 1187

Prader-Willi syndrome and severe obesity
Genotropin Lyophilized Powder 2547
Norditropin Cartridges 2354

Prader-Willi syndrome and severe respiratory impairment
Genotropin Lyophilized Powder 2547
Norditropin Cartridges 2354

Prader-Willi syndrome and sleep apnea
Norditropin Cartridges 2354

Prader-Willi syndrome and upper airway obstruction
Norditropin Cartridges 2354

Pregnancy
Accutane Capsules 2607
Aceon Tablets (2 mg, 4 mg, 8 mg) 3038
Activella Tablets 2347
Advicor Tablets 402
AndroGel 3159
Attenuvax 1951
Carac Cream 0.5% 2722
Climara Transdermal System 763
Climara Pro Transdermal System 768
Crestor Tablets 677
Cuprimine Capsules 1986
Delatestryl Injection 1730
Divigel 3167
Eligard 7.5 mg 2724
Eligard 22.5 mg 2724
Eligard 30 mg 2724
Eligard 45 mg 2724
Enjuvia Tablets 1029
Estratest Tablets 3043
Estratest H.S. Tablets 3043

Evista Tablets 1810
Fansidar Tablets 2636
Faslodex Injection 682
Follistim AQ Cartridge 2844
Fosteum Capsules 2963
Gantrisin Pediatric Suspension 2638
Gris-PEG Tablets 2507
Hycamtin for Injection 1459
Lescol Capsules 2268
Lescol XL Tablets 2268
Letairis Tablets 1258
Lipitor Tablets 2501
Lupron Depot 3.75 mg 462
Lupron Depot 7.5 mg 469
Lupron Depot–3 Month 11.25 mg 462
Lupron Depot-PED 7.5 mg, 11.25 mg and 15 mg 471
Lybrel Tablets 3204
Meruvax II 2061
Mevacor Tablets 2063
Mircette Tablets 1034
Mirena Intrauterine System 779
M-M-R II 2054
Mumpsvax 2068
NuvaRing 2897
Ortho-Cyclen Tablets 2449
Ortho Evra Transdermal System 2437
Ortho Micronor Tablets 2446
Ortho Tri-Cyclen Tablets 2449
Ortho Tri-Cyclen Lo Tablets 2458
Orthoclone OKT3 Sterile Solution 2387
ParaGard T 380A Intrauterine Copper Contraceptive 1041
Plan B Tablets 1044
Premarin Intravenous 3217
Premarin Tablets 3221
Premarin Vaginal Cream 3228
Premphase Tablets 3232
Prempro Tablets 3232
Prometrium Capsules (100 mg, 200 mg) 3047
Propecia Tablets 2095
ProQuad 2099
Proscar Tablets 2102
Pylera Capsules 714
Rebetol 2917
Seasonique Tablets 1046
Simcor Tablets 502
Soriatane Capsules 3062
Supprelin LA Implant 1731
Targretin Capsules 1084
Targretin Gel 1% 1088
Testim 1% Gel 701
Tracleer Tablets 3289
Vagifem Tablets 2375
Varivax 2133
Viadur Implant 802
Vytorin 10/10 Tablets 2149
Vytorin 10/10 Tablets 2939
Vytorin 10/20 Tablets 2149
Vytorin 10/20 Tablets 2939
Vytorin 10/40 Tablets 2149
Vytorin 10/40 Tablets 2939
Vytorin 10/80 Tablets 2149
Vytorin 10/80 Tablets 2939
Yaz Tablets 805
Zetia Tablets 2157
Zetia Tablets 2951
Zocor Tablets 2136
Zostavax Injection 2145

Pregnancy, diagnostic test for
Prometrium Capsules (100 mg, 200 mg) 3047

Priapism, predisposition to
Edex Injection 2957

Proctitis, history of
Indocin Suppositories 2024

Prolactinoma, pituitary
(*see under* Tumor, intracranial, unspecified)

Psychic disturbances
(*see under* Psychosis)

Psychosis
Seromycin Capsules 1864

Psychosis, toxic, history of
Proleukin for Injection 2287

Pulmonary atresia
(*see under* Atresia, pulmonary)

Pulmonary congestion
Cardizem LA Extended Release Tablets 421

Pulmonary disorders, unspecified
(*see also under* Asthma, acute; Asthma, unspecified; Atresia, pulmonary; Chronic obstructive pulmonary disease; Pulmonary congestion; Pulmonary function test, abnormal)
Exubera Inhalation Powder 2515

Pulmonary embolism
Activella Tablets 2347
Angeliq Tablets 751
Climara Transdermal System 763
Climara Pro Transdermal System 768
Divigel 3167
Enjuvia Tablets 1029
Estratest Tablets 3043
Estratest H.S. Tablets 3043
Evista Tablets 1810
Premarin Intravenous 3217
Premarin Tablets 3221
Premarin Vaginal Cream 3228
Premphase Tablets 3232
Prempro Tablets 3232
Prometrium Capsules (100 mg, 200 mg) 3047

Pulmonary embolism, history of
Activella Tablets 2347
Climara Transdermal System 763
Climara Pro Transdermal System 768
Divigel 3167
Enjuvia Tablets 1029
Estratest Tablets 3043
Estratest H.S. Tablets 3043
Premarin Intravenous 3217
Premarin Tablets 3221
Premarin Vaginal Cream 3228
Premphase Tablets 3232
Prempro Tablets 3232
Prometrium Capsules (100 mg, 200 mg) 3047

Pulmonary function test, abnormal
Proleukin for Injection 2287

Q

Q-T interval prolongation
Geodon 2520

R

Radiation therapy
Gengraf Capsules 435
Leukine 774
Neoral Oral Solution 2280
Neoral Soft Gelatin Capsules 2280
Tice BCG 2936

Radiotherapy
(*see under* Radiation therapy)

Rectal bleeding
(*see under* Bleeding, rectal)

Renal decompensation
(*see under* Renal failure)

Renal dialysis
Augmentin XR Extended Release Tablets 1333
Integrilin Injection 2855

Renal disease, unspecified
(*see also under* Renal dysfunction)
ActoPlus Met Tablets 3071
Avandamet Tablets 1336
Dyrenium Capsules 3189
Janumet Tablets 2041
Paser Granules 1747
ProAmatine Tablets 3032
Rosac Wash 3062
Xyzal Tablets 2789
Xyzal Tablets 3155

Renal dysfunction
(*see also under* Anuria; Oliguria; Renal disease, unspecified; Renal failure)
ActoPlus Met Tablets 3071
Angeliq Tablets 751
Augmentin XR Extended Release Tablets 1333
Augmentin ES-600 Powder for Oral Suspension 1329
Avandamet Tablets 1336
Dyazide Capsules 1405
Dyrenium Capsules 3189
Fleet Prep Kits 1149
Gengraf Capsules 435
Indocin I.V. 2489
Integrilin Injection 2855
Janumet Tablets 2041
K-Phos Original (Sodium Free) Tablets 814
K-Phos Neutral Tablets 813
Nalfon Capsules 2508
NeoProfen Injection 2496
Neoral Oral Solution 2280
Neoral Soft Gelatin Capsules 2280
PrandiMet Tablets 2967
Pylera Capsules 714
Seromycin Capsules 1864
Skelaxin Tablets 1784
Uroqid-Acid No. 2 Tablets 814
Xeloda Tablets 2662
Xyzal Tablets 2789
Xyzal Tablets 3155
Yaz Tablets 805

Renal dysfunction, history of
Marplan Tablets 3177
Proleukin for Injection 2287

Renal dysfunction, pedatric
Xyzal Oral Solution 2789
Xyzal Oral Solution 3155

Renal dysfunction, rheumatoid arthritis patients with
Cuprimine Capsules 1986

Renal dysfunction, severe
Amerge Tablets 1301
Fenoglide Tablets 2960
Malarone Pediatric Tablets 1521
Malarone Tablets 1521
Marplan Tablets 3177
Tricor Tablets 520
Xyzal Oral Solution 2789
Xyzal Oral Solution 3155

Renal excretory function impairment
(*see under* Renal dysfunction)

Renal failure
(*see also under* Renal dysfunction)
Fansidar Tablets 2636
Fleet Phospho-soda 1145
Fleet Phospho-soda EZ-PREP 1147
Soriatane Capsules 3062
Urocit-K Tablets 2176

Renal failure, dialysis-dependent
Fleet Enema 1143
Fleet Enema Extra 1143
Fleet Enema for Children 1143
Fleet Pedia-Lax Enema 1143
Xyzal Oral Solution 2789
Xyzal Oral Solution 3155

Renal impairment
(*see under* Renal dysfunction)

Renal insufficiency
(*see under* Renal dysfunction)

Respiratory depression
Avinza Capsules 1772
DepoDur Injection 1095
Duragesic Transdermal System 2405
MS Contin Tablets 2585
Opana Tablets 1117
Opana ER Tablets 1121
OxyContin Tablets 2589
OxyIR Capsules 2593

Respiratory depression, in absence of resuscitative equipment
Percodan Tablets 1130

Respiratory disease, unspecified
(*see under* Respiratory illness, febrile)

Respiratory disorders
(*see under* Bronchospastic disorders, unspecified; Obstruction, respiratory tract; Pulmonary disorders, unspecified; Respiratory depression)

Respiratory distress
(*see under* Asthma, acute; Respiratory depression)

Respiratory distress, acute, caused by obstructing endobronchial lesion
Photofrin for Injection 708

Respiratory failure
Humatrope Vials and Cartridges 1838

Respiratory illness, febrile
Attenuvax 1951
Meruvax II 2061
M-M-R II 2054
Mumpsvax 2068
Varivax 2133

Respiratory illness, unspecified
(*see under* Pulmonary disorders, unspecified; Respiratory illness, febrile)

Respiratory insufficiency, unspecified
(*see also under* Obstruction, respiratory tract; Pulmonary disorders, unspecified; Respiratory illness, febrile)
Humatrope Vials and Cartridges 1838

Respiratory obstruction
(*see under* Obstruction, respiratory tract)

Respiratory tract conditions, lower
(*see under* Pulmonary disorders, unspecified)

Retinopathy, diabetic
Humatrope Vials and Cartridges 1838
Norditropin Cartridges 2354
Nutropin for Injection 1208
Nutropin AQ Injection 1212
Nutropin AQ NuSpin Injection 1212
Nutropin AQ Pen 1212
Nutropin AQ Pen Cartridge 1212
Tev-Tropin for Injection 1187

Retinopathy, diabetic, active proliferative
Genotropin Lyophilized Powder 2547

Retinopathy, diabetic, severe non-profilerative
Genotropin Lyophilized Powder 2547

S

SA block
(*see under* Heart block, sinoatrial)

Seizure disorders, history of
Orthoclone OKT3 Sterile Solution 2387
Proleukin for Injection 2287

Seizure disorders, unspecified
(*see also under* Epilepsy; Epilepsy, uncontrolled; Status epilepticus)
Wellbutrin Tablets 1648
Wellbutrin SR Sustained-Release Tablets 1653
Wellbutrin XL Extended-Release Tablets 1659
Zyban Sustained-Release Tablets 1692

Seizure disorders, untreated
(*see under* Epilepsy, uncontrolled)

Seizures, history of
(*see under* Seizure disorders, history of)

Sepsis
Enbrel for Injection 569

Septicemia
(*see under* Sepsis)

Serum transaminase elevation
(*see also under* Liver dysfunction)
Advicor Tablets 402
Crestor Tablets 677
Lescol Capsules 2268
Lescol XL Tablets 2268
Lipitor Tablets 2501
Marplan Tablets 3177
Mevacor Tablets 2063
Parnate Tablets 1532
Vytorin 10/10 Tablets 2149
Vytorin 10/10 Tablets 2939
Vytorin 10/20 Tablets 2149
Vytorin 10/20 Tablets 2939
Vytorin 10/40 Tablets 2149
Vytorin 10/40 Tablets 2939
Vytorin 10/80 Tablets 2149
Vytorin 10/80 Tablets 2939
Zocor Tablets 2136

Serum triglyceride concentration greater than 500 mg/dL
WelChol Tablets 1015

Severe left ventricular dysfunction
(*see under* Ventricular dysfunction, left)

Sexual activity inadvisable, males
Edex Injection 2957

Shingles
(*see under* Herpes zoster)

Shock, cardiogenic
(*see under* Cardiogenic shock)

Shock, unspecified
(*see also under* Cardiogenic shock)
Primaxin I.M. 2080
Thiothixene Capsules 2197

Sick sinus node syndrome
(*see under* Sick sinus syndrome)

Sick sinus syndrome
Adenocard IV Injection 603
Adenoscan 605
Bystolic Tablets 1155
Cardizem LA Extended Release Tablets 421
Coreg Tablets 1387
Coreg CR Extended-Release Capsules 1393
Rythmol Tablets 1586
Rythmol SR Capsules 1590
Tarka Tablets 511
Toprol-XL Tablets 666

Sickle cell anemia
(*see under* Anemia, sickle cell)

Sino-atrial block
(*see under* Heart block, first degree; Heart block, greater than first degree; Heart block, unspecified)

Sinus node disease
(*see under* Bradycardia, sinus; Sick sinus syndrome; Sinus node dysfunction, unspecified)

Sinus node dysfunction, unspecified
Adenocard IV Injection 603
Adenoscan 605
Lexiscan Injection 614

Skin, damaged
Flector Patch 561

Skin, non-intact
Flector Patch 561

Skin disorders, unspecified
(*see under* Lesions, skin, unspecified; Melanoma, history of)

Skin lesions
(*see under* Lesions, skin, unspecified)

Smoking
Exubera Inhalation Powder 2515

Smoking, heavy
NuvaRing 2897
Yaz Tablets 805

Spasms, infantile, history of
Infanrix Vaccine 1479
Kinrix Injection Vaccine 1486
Pediarix Vaccine 1552

Status asthmaticus
Advair Diskus 100/50 1276
Advair Diskus 250/50 1276
Advair Diskus 500/50 1276
Advair HFA 45/21 Inhalation Aerosol 1288
Advair HFA 115/21 Inhalation Aerosol 1288
Advair HFA 230/21 Inhalation Aerosol 1288
Aerobid/Aerobid-M 1153
Alvesco Inhalation Aerosol 2985
Asmanex Twisthaler 2797
Azmacort Inhalation Aerosol 407
Flovent HFA 1440
Pulmicort Flexhaler 654
Qvar Inhalation Aerosol 3116
Symbicort 80/4.5 Inhalation Aerosol 659
Symbicort 160/4.5 Inhalation Aerosol 659

Status epilepticus
Romazicon Injection 2646

Stenosis, aortic
Cardene I.V. 1093
Cleviprex 1936
Indocin I.V. 2489
NeoProfen Injection 2496

Stress test, abnormal
Proleukin for Injection 2287

Stricture, esophageal
Fosamax 2005
Fosamax Plus D Tablets 2013

Stroke
(*see under* Cerebrovascular accident)

Stroke, hemorrhagic
Xigris Powder for Intravenous Infusion 1880

Stroke, history of
(*see under* Cerebrovascular accident, history of)

Succinic semialdehyde dehydrogenase deficiency
Xyrem Oral Solution 1766

Sucrase insuffiency
Metadate CD Capsules 3146

Superficial herpes simplex keratitis
(*see under* Herpes simplex keratitis)

Surgery, central nervous system
(*see under* Surgery, intracranial; Surgery, intraspinal)

Surgery, elective
Parnate Tablets 1532

Surgery, intracranial
Activase I.V. 1188
TNKase 1233
Xigris Powder for Intravenous Infusion 1880

Surgery, intraspinal
Activase I.V. 1188
Xigris Powder for Intravenous Infusion 1880

Surgery, major, with prolonged immobilization
Lybrel Tablets 3204
NuvaRing 2897
Ortho-Cyclen Tablets 2449
Ortho Evra Transdermal System 2437
Ortho Tri-Cyclen Tablets 2449
Ortho Tri-Cyclen Lo Tablets 2458
Seasonique Tablets 1046
Yaz Tablets 805

Surgery, unspecified
Integrilin Injection 2855
Metadate CD Capsules 3146
ReoPro Vials 1860

Surgery, uterine, history of
(*see also under* Cesarean section, history of)
Cervidil Vaginal Insert 1165

Systolic blood pressure less than 90 mm Hg
Natrecor for Injection 2977

T

Tachyarrhythmia
(*see under* Arrhythmia, cardiac, unspecified)

Tachycardia, ventricular
Rythmol Tablets 1586

Tachycardia, ventricular, history of
Proleukin for Injection 2287

Tendinitis, history of
Noroxin Tablets 2069

Tendon rupture, history of
Noroxin Tablets 2069

Tension
Concerta Extended-Release Tablets 1925
Daytrana Transdermal Patch 3022
Focalin XR Capsules 2251
Metadate CD Capsules 3146

Tetralogy of Fallot
Indocin I.V. 2489
NeoProfen Injection 2496

Thallium stress test, abnormal
(*see under* Stress test, abnormal)

Thrombocytopathy, unspecified
(*see under* Thrombocytopenia, unspecified)

Thrombocytopenia, unspecified
Arixtra Injection 1313
Fragmin Injection 1070
Indocin I.V. 2489
Integrilin Injection 2855
Lovenox Injection 2756
NeoProfen Injection 2496
ReoPro Vials 1860

Thromboembolic disorders
(*see also under* Cerebrovascular accident)
Activella Tablets 2347
Climara Transdermal System 763
Climara Pro Transdermal System 768
Crinone 4% Gel 992
Crinone 8% Gel 992
Enjuvia Tablets 1029
Estratest Tablets 3043
Estratest H.S. Tablets 3043
Lybrel Tablets 3204
Mircette Tablets 1034
NuvaRing 2897
Ortho-Cyclen Tablets 2449
Ortho Evra Transdermal System 2437
Ortho Tri-Cyclen Tablets 2449
Ortho Tri-Cyclen Lo Tablets 2458
Premarin Intravenous 3217
Premarin Tablets 3221
Premarin Vaginal Cream 3228
Premphase Tablets 3232
Prempro Tablets 3232
Prometrium Capsules (100 mg, 200 mg) 3047
Seasonique Tablets 1046
Yaz Tablets 805

Thromboembolic disorders, arterial
Angeliq Tablets 751
Divigel 3167

Thromboembolic disorders, history of
(*see also under* Cerebrovascular accident, history of)
Activella Tablets 2347
Estratest Tablets 3043
Estratest H.S. Tablets 3043
Evista Tablets 1810
Mircette Tablets 1034
NuvaRing 2897
Ortho-Cyclen Tablets 2449
Ortho Evra Transdermal System 2437
Ortho Tri-Cyclen Tablets 2449
Ortho Tri-Cyclen Lo Tablets 2458
Premarin Intravenous 3217
Premarin Vaginal Cream 3228
Premphase Tablets 3232
Prempro Tablets 3232
Prometrium Capsules (100 mg, 200 mg) 3047
Seasonique Tablets 1046
Vagifem Tablets 2375
Yaz Tablets 805

Thrombogenic rhythm disorders
Lybrel Tablets 3204

Thrombogenic valvulopathies
Lybrel Tablets 3204
Seasonique Tablets 1046
Yaz Tablets 805

Thrombophlebitis
Crinone 4% Gel 992
Crinone 8% Gel 992
Lybrel Tablets 3204
Mircette Tablets 1034
NuvaRing 2897
Ortho-Cyclen Tablets 2449
Ortho Evra Transdermal System 2437
Ortho Tri-Cyclen Tablets 2449
Ortho Tri-Cyclen Lo Tablets 2458
Seasonique Tablets 1046
Vagifem Tablets 2375
Yaz Tablets 805

Thrombophlebitis, history of
Crinone 4% Gel 992
Crinone 8% Gel 992
Lybrel Tablets 3204
Mircette Tablets 1034
NuvaRing 2897
Ortho-Cyclen Tablets 2449
Ortho Evra Transdermal System 2437
Ortho Tri-Cyclen Tablets 2449
Ortho Tri-Cyclen Lo Tablets 2458
Seasonique Tablets 1046
Yaz Tablets 805

Thrombosis
Elspar for Injection 2488

Thrombosis, deep vein
Angeliq Tablets 751
Premphase Tablets 3232

Thrombosis, history of
Angeliq Tablets 751
Elspar for Injection 2488
Estratest Tablets 3043
Estratest H.S. Tablets 3043
Evista Tablets 1810
Oncaspar Injection 1138
Premarin Intravenous 3217
Premarin Vaginal Cream 3228

Thyroid dysfunction, uncontrolled
Follistim AQ Cartridge 2844

Thyrotoxicosis
ProAmatine Tablets 3032

Thyrotoxicosis, untreated
Cytomel Tablets 1778
Levothroid Tablets 1170
Levoxyl Tablets 1780
Naturethroid Tablets 2605
Synthroid Tablets 507

Tics, motor
Concerta Extended-Release Tablets 1925
Daytrana Transdermal Patch 3022
Focalin XR Capsules 2251
Metadate CD Capsules 3146

Tissue breakdown
(*see under* Necrosis)

Tourette's syndrome
Concerta Extended-Release Tablets 1925
Daytrana Transdermal Patch 3022
Focalin XR Capsules 2251
Metadate CD Capsules 3146

Tourette's syndrome, history of
Concerta Extended-Release Tablets 1925
Daytrana Transdermal Patch 3022
Focalin XR Capsules 2251
Metadate CD Capsules 3146

Toxicity, neurologic
Hexalen Capsules 1078

Toxicity, vitamin D
Calcijex Injection 419
Rocaltrol Capsules 1150
Rocaltrol Oral Solution 1150
Zemplar Capsules 536
Zemplar Injection 538

Tracheoesophageal fistula, existence of
Photofrin for Injection 708

Transaminases elevation, serum
(*see under* Serum transaminase elevation)

Transplant
(*see under* Organ allograft)

Trauma, intracranial
(*see also under* Cerebrovascular accident; Head injury)
Activase I.V. 1188
TNKase 1233

Trauma, intracranial, unspecified
TNKase 1233
Xigris Powder for Intravenous Infusion 1880

Trauma, intraspinal
Activase I.V. 1188
TNKase 1233

Trauma, unspecified
ReoPro Vials 1860

Tuberculosis, active
Tice BCG 2936

Tuberculosis, unspecified
(*see under* Infection, ophthalmic, mycobacterial)

Tuberculosis, untreated
Attenuvax 1951
Meruvax II 2061
M-M-R II 2054
Mumpsvax 2068
ProQuad 2099
Varivax 2133

Tumor, adrenal
(*see under* Pheochromocytoma)

Tumor, breast
Follistim AQ Cartridge 2844

Tumor, breast, malignant
(*see under* Carcinoma, breast, history of; Carcinoma, breast, male; Carcinoma, breast, unspecified)

Tumor, hepatic
(*see under* Adenoma, hepatic; Carcinoma, hepatic; Tumor, liver, benign)

Tumor, hormone dependent
(*see under* Neoplasm, estrogen dependent)

Tumor, hypothalamus
Follistim AQ Cartridge 2844

Tumor, intracranial, progression of
Norditropin Cartridges 2354

Tumor, intracranial, recurrence of
Norditropin Cartridges 2354

Tumor, intracranial, unspecified
(*see also under* Lesions, intracranial, unspecified; Tumor, pituitary, unspecified)
Activase I.V. 1188
Humatrope Vials and Cartridges 1838
Nutropin for Injection 1208
Nutropin AQ Injection 1212
Nutropin AQ NuSpin Injection 1212
Nutropin AQ Pen 1212
Nutropin AQ Pen Cartridge 1212
ReoPro Vials 1860
TNKase 1233
Xigris Powder for Intravenous Infusion 1880

Tumor, liver, benign
Mirena Intrauterine System 779
Seasonique Tablets 1046
Yaz Tablets 805

Tumor, liver, malignant
(*see under* Carcinoma, hepatic)

Tumor, ovarian
Follistim AQ Cartridge 2844

Tumor, pituitary, unspecified
(*see also under* Tumor, intracranial, unspecified)
Follistim AQ Cartridge 2844

Tumor, unspecified
(*see under* Neoplasm, unspecified)

Tumor, uterine
Follistim AQ Cartridge 2844

Tumor activity, unspecified
Genotropin Lyophilized Powder 2547
Humatrope Vials and Cartridges 1838

Tumors, intracranial, in hypopituitary children
Norditropin Cartridges 2354

U

Ulcer, gastrointestinal
(*see under* Perforation, gastrointestinal tract; Ulcer, peptic)

Ulcer, peptic
Advicor Tablets 402
Niaspan Extended-Release Tablets 480
Plavix Tablets 926
Simcor Tablets 502

Ulcerative colitis
(*see under* Colitis, ulcerative)

Unstable cardiovascular status in acute hemorrhage
(*see under* Cardiovascular status, unstable in acute hemorrhage)

Urea cycle disorders
Depakote ER Tablets 423

Uremia
(*see under* Azotemia)

Urinary obstruction
(*see under* Obstruction, urinary tract)

Urinary retention
(*see also under* Obstruction, urinary tract)
Allegra-D 12 Hour Extended-Release Tablets 2687
Allegra-D 24 Hour Extended-Release Tablets 2690
Clarinex-D 12-Hour Extended-Release Tablets 2831
Clarinex-D 24-Hour Extended-Release Tablets 2834
Enablex Extended-Release Tablets 2225
ProAmatine Tablets 3032
Sanctura XR Capsules 557
VESIcare Tablets 636
Zyrtec-D 12 Hour Extended Release Tablets 1923

Urinary tract disorders
(*see under* Infection, urinary tract; Obstruction, urinary tract; Renal disease, unspecified; Renal dysfunction)

Uropathy, obstructive
(*see under* Obstruction, urinary tract)

Uterine abnormalities, unspecified
Mirena Intrauterine System 779

Uterine cavity distortion
ParaGard T 380A Intrauterine Copper Contraceptive 1041

V

Vaccinia
Alrex Ophthalmic Suspension 0.2% ⊙ 236
Durezol Ophthalmic Emulsion ⊙ 275
FML Ophthalmic Ointment ⊙ 223
FML Ophthalmic Suspension ⊙ 224
FML Forte Ophthalmic Suspension ⊙ 222
Lotemax Ophthalmic Suspension 0.5% ⊙ 241
Pred Forte Ophthalmic Suspension ⊙ 227
Pred Mild Ophthalmic Suspension ⊙ 230
Pred-G Ophthalmic Ointment ⊙ 229
Pred-G Ophthalmic Suspension ⊙ 228

Vaginal bleeding, abnormal
(*see under* Bleeding, genital, abnormal)

Vaginitis, untreated
Mirena Intrauterine System 779

Vaginosis, bacterial, untreated
Mirena Intrauterine System 779

Varicella
Alrex Ophthalmic Suspension 0.2% ⊙ 236
Cosmegen for Injection 2485
Durezol Ophthalmic Emulsion ⊙ 275
FML Ophthalmic Ointment ⊙ 223
FML Ophthalmic Suspension ⊙ 224
FML Forte Ophthalmic Suspension ⊙ 222
Lotemax Ophthalmic Suspension 0.5% ⊙ 241
Pred Forte Ophthalmic Suspension ⊙ 227
Pred Mild Ophthalmic Suspension ⊙ 230
Pred-G Ophthalmic Ointment ⊙ 229
Pred-G Ophthalmic Suspension ⊙ 228

Vascular impairment of extremities
(*see under* Peripheral vascular disease)

Vasculitis, history of
ReoPro Vials 1860

Vasospasm, coronary artery
(*see under* Coronary artery vasospasm)

Ventilatory function depression
(*see under* Respiratory depression)

Ventricular dysfunction, left
Flolan for Injection 1426
Tarka Tablets 511

Ventricular fibrillation
(*see under* Fibrillation, ventricular)

Viral disease, conjunctiva
Durezol Ophthalmic Emulsion ⊙ 275

Viral disease, cornea
Durezol Ophthalmic Emulsion ⊙ 275

Viral infections
(*see under* Herpes simplex keratitis; Herpes zoster; Human immunodeficiency virus; Infection, ophthalmic, viral; Varicella)

Vitamin D toxicity
(*see under* Toxicity, vitamin D)

Vomiting
Fleet Prep Kits 1149

W

Wilson's disease
ParaGard T 380A Intrauterine Copper Contraceptive 1041

Wolff-Parkinson-White syndrome
Tarka Tablets 511

Women
Avodart Soft Gelatin Capsules 1359
Edex Injection 2957
Eligard 22.5 mg 2724
Eligard 30 mg 2724
Eligard 45 mg 2724
Vantas 1737

Women of childbearing potential
Avodart Soft Gelatin Capsules 1359

Women of Premenopausal Endocrine Status
Femara Tablets 2246

SECTION 6

INTERNATIONAL DRUG NAME INDEX

This section names the *PDR®* equivalents of over 33,000 foreign pharmaceutical products. Organized alphabetically by overseas trade name, it shows the country (or countries) in which the name is used, gives the product's closest U.S. generic equivalent, and lists the associated brand-name prescription drugs described by *PDR®*, together with the page on which they are found.

Products from the following nations are included:

Argentina	France	Malaysia	Spain
Australia	Germany	Mexico	Sweden
Austria	Greece	Monaco	Switzerland
Belgium	Hong Kong	New Zealand	Thailand
Brazil	Hungary	Norway	The Netherlands
Canada	India	Poland	The Philippines
Chile	Irish Republic	Portugal	Turkey
Czech Republic	Israel	Russia	United Arab Emirates
Denmark	Italy	Singapore	United Kingdom
Finland	Japan	South Africa	Venezuela

Page numbers refer to the 2009 editions of *PDR®* and *PDR® For Ophthalmic Medicines*. The symbol denoting an entry in *PDR® For Ophthalmic Medicines* appears in the bottom margin.

These entries are intended only as an aid in approximating the contents of a foreign prescription. For proper dosing guidelines, indications, contraindications, warnings, and precautions of its U.S. equivalents, always consult the underlying *PDR®* text. Foreign trade names are courtesy of *PDR's* affiliate, MICROMEDEX, Inc.

3A OFTENO (Chile, Mexico, Venezuela)
DICLOFENAC SODIUM
Voltaren Tablets **2334**
Voltaren-XR Tablets **2337**

3TC (Argentina, Australia, Canada, Hong Kong, Malaysia, Mexico, New Zealand, South Africa, Switzerland)
LAMIVUDINE
Epivir Oral Solution **1412**
Epivir Tablets **1412**
Epivir-HBV Oral Solution **1417**
Epivir-HBV Tablets **1417**

3TC COMPLEX (Argentina)
LAMIVUDINE
Epivir Oral Solution **1412**
Epivir Tablets **1412**
Epivir-HBV Oral Solution **1417**
Epivir-HBV Tablets **1417**

3TC/AZT (Argentina)
LAMIVUDINE
Epivir Oral Solution **1412**
Epivir Tablets **1412**
Epivir-HBV Oral Solution **1417**
Epivir-HBV Tablets **1417**

3TC/EPIVIR (Chile)
LAMIVUDINE
Epivir Oral Solution **1412**
Epivir Tablets **1412**
Epivir-HBV Oral Solution **1417**
Epivir-HBV Tablets **1417**

9PM (India)
LATANOPROST
Xalatan Ophthalmic Solution . . . . ⊙**273**

A ACIDO (Argentina)
TRETINOIN
Vesanoid Capsules. **2660**

ABAMUNE (India)
ABACAVIR SULFATE
Ziagen Oral Solution. **1673**
Ziagen Tablets **1673**

ABBOCALCIJEX (Greece)
CALCITRIOL
Calcijex Injection **419**
Rocaltrol Capsules. **1150**
Rocaltrol Oral Solution **1150**

ABENTEL (Thailand)
ALBENDAZOLE
Albenza Tablets. **1297**

ABEREL (France)
TRETINOIN
Vesanoid Capsules. **2660**

ABERELA (Norway, Sweden)
TRETINOIN
Vesanoid Capsules. **2660**

ABERTEN (Greece)
THEOPHYLLINE
Uniphyl Tablets **2595**

ABIOLEX (Chile)
AMOXICILLIN
Amoxil Pediatric Drops for Oral Suspension. **1305**
Amoxil Tablets **1305**

ABIOTYL (Argentina)
AMOXICILLIN
Amoxil Pediatric Drops for Oral Suspension. **1305**
Amoxil Tablets **1305**

ABITREN (Hong Kong, Israel, Thailand)
DICLOFENAC SODIUM
Voltaren Tablets **2334**
Voltaren-XR Tablets **2337**

ABRILAR (Argentina)
SALMETEROL XINAFOATE
Serevent Diskus **1594**

ABSORLENT (Spain)
ESTRADIOL
Climara Transdermal System. **763**

ABUTIROI (Mexico)
LEVOTHYROXINE SODIUM
Levothroid Tablets **1170**
Levoxyl Tablets. **1780**
Synthroid Tablets. **507**

AC VASCULAR (Argentina)
NIMODIPINE
Nimotop Capsules **790**

ACALIX (Argentina, Venezuela)
DILTIAZEM HYDROCHLORIDE
Cardizem LA Extended Release Tablets. . . . **421**

ACALKA (Brazil, Chile, Portugal, Spain, Thailand, The Philippines)
POTASSIUM CITRATE
Urocit-K Tablets. **2176**

ACANTEX (Chile)
CEFTRIAXONE SODIUM
Rocephin Injectable Vials, ADD-Vantage, Galaxy, Bulk **2642**

ACARBAY (India)
ACARBOSE
Precose Tablets **792**

ACASMUL (Chile)
DILTIAZEM HYDROCHLORIDE
Cardizem LA Extended Release Tablets. . . . **421**

ACCOLATE (Argentina, Australia, Belgium, Brazil, Canada, Chile, Czech Republic, Finland, Hong Kong, Hungary, Irish Republic, Israel, Mexico, Poland, Portugal, Russia, Singapore, South Africa, Spain, Switzerland, Thailand, The Philippines, Turkey, United Kingdom, Venezuela)
ZAFIRLUKAST
Accolate Tablets **669**

ACCOLEIT (Italy)
ZAFIRLUKAST
Accolate Tablets **669**

ACCURAN (Greece)
ISOTRETINOIN
Accutane Capsules **2607**

ACCURE (Australia)
ISOTRETINOIN
Accutane Capsules **2607**

ACCUTANE (Canada)
ISOTRETINOIN
Accutane Capsules **2607**

ACCUTIN (Denmark)
ISOTRETINOIN
Accutane Capsules **2607**

ACECOMB (Austria)
HYDROCHLOROTHIAZIDE/LISINOPRIL
Prinzide Tablets **2092**

ACE-HEMMER COMP (Germany)
CAPTOPRIL
Captopril Tablets. **2182**

ACELISINO COMP (Austria)
LISINOPRIL
Prinivil Tablets **2087**

ACEMIN (Austria)
LISINOPRIL
Prinivil Tablets **2087**

ACENORM (Australia, Germany)
CAPTOPRIL
Captopril Tablets. **2182**

ACENORM HCT (Germany)
CAPTOPRIL
Captopril Tablets. **2182**

ACEOMEL (Hungary, Irish Republic)
CAPTOPRIL
Captopril Tablets. **2182**

ACEOTO (Spain)
CIPROFLOXACIN
Cipro Oral Suspension **2810**

ACEPRAN (Chile)
CLONAZEPAM
Klonopin Tablets **2639**

ACEPRESS (Italy)
CAPTOPRIL
Captopril Tablets **2182**

ACEPRIL (Denmark, Hong Kong, United Kingdom)
LISINOPRIL
Prinivil Tablets **2087**

ACEPRILEX (Italy)
CAPTOPRIL
Captopril Tablets **2182**

ACEPTIN (The Philippines)
RANITIDINE HYDROCHLORIDE
Zantac 25 EFFERdose Tablets **1670**
Zantac 150 Tablets **1670**
Zantac 300 Tablets **1670**
Zantac Injection **1666**
Zantac Injection Premixed **1666**
Zantac Syrup **1670**

ACER (Poland)
CETIRIZINE HYDROCHLORIDE
Zyrtec Syrup **1920**
Zyrtec Tablets **1920**

ACERCOMP (Finland)
HYDROCHLOROTHIAZIDE/LISINOPRIL
Prinzide Tablets **2092**

ACERDIL (Chile)
LISINOPRIL
Prinivil Tablets **2087**

ACERDIL-D (Chile)
HYDROCHLOROTHIAZIDE/LISINOPRIL
Prinzide Tablets **2092**

ACERIL (Israel)
CAPTOPRIL
Captopril Tablets **2182**

ACERILIN (Turkey)
LISINOPRIL
Prinivil Tablets **2087**

ACETAN (Austria)
LISINOPRIL
Prinivil Tablets **2087**

ACETEN (India, Russia, South Africa)
CAPTOPRIL
Captopril Tablets **2182**

ACETOXYL (Canada, United Kingdom)
BENZOYL PEROXIDE
Brevoxyl-4 Creamy Wash **3054**
Brevoxyl-4 Gel **3054**
Brevoxyl-8 Creamy Wash **3054**
Brevoxyl-8 Gel **3054**

ACID A VIT (Belgium, The Netherlands)
TRETINOIN
Vesanoid Capsules **2660**

ACID HALT (Canada)
FAMOTIDINE
Pepcid for Oral Suspension **2075**
Pepcid Tablets **2075**

ACIDEX (Argentina)
RANITIDINE HYDROCHLORIDE
Zantac 25 EFFERdose Tablets **1670**
Zantac 150 Tablets **1670**
Zantac 300 Tablets **1670**
Zantac Injection **1666**
Zantac Injection Premixed **1666**
Zantac Syrup **1670**

ACIDINE (Malaysia)
FAMOTIDINE
Pepcid for Oral Suspension **2075**
Pepcid Tablets **2075**

ACIFLUX (Chile)
RANITIDINE HYDROCHLORIDE
Zantac 25 EFFERdose Tablets **1670**
Zantac 150 Tablets **1670**
Zantac 300 Tablets **1670**
Zantac Injection **1666**
Zantac Injection Premixed **1666**
Zantac Syrup **1670**

ACILAC (Canada)
LACTULOSE
Kristalose for Oral Solution **1004**

ACILOC (India, Thailand, The Philippines)
RANITIDINE HYDROCHLORIDE
Zantac 150 Tablets **1670**
Zantac 25 EFFERdose Tablets **1670**
Zantac 300 Tablets **1670**
Zantac Injection **1666**
Zantac Injection Premixed **1666**
Zantac Syrup **1670**

ACILOC RD (India)
RANITIDINE HYDROCHLORIDE
Zantac 25 EFFERdose Tablets **1670**
Zantac 150 Tablets **1670**
Zantac 300 Tablets **1670**
Zantac Injection **1666**
Zantac Injection Premixed **1666**
Zantac Syrup **1670**

ACIVAL (Argentina)
NIMODIPINE
Nimotop Capsules **790**

ACLAREX (Greece)
CELECOXIB
Celebrex Capsules **2979**

ACLAV (Argentina)
AMOXICILLIN
Amoxil Pediatric Drops for Oral Suspension **1305**
Amoxil Tablets **1305**

ACLIN (Australia, Hong Kong)
SULINDAC
Clinoril Tablets **1962**

ACLORAL (Mexico)
RANITIDINE HYDROCHLORIDE
Zantac 25 EFFERdose Tablets **1670**
Zantac 150 Tablets **1670**
Zantac 300 Tablets **1670**
Zantac Injection **1666**
Zantac Injection Premixed **1666**
Zantac Syrup **1670**

ACLOSAN (Argentina)
TAMSULOSIN HYDROCHLORIDE
Flomax Capsules **848**

ACNACYL (Australia, Hong Kong, Singapore)
BENZOYL PEROXIDE
Brevoxyl-4 Creamy Wash **3054**
Brevoxyl-4 Gel **3054**
Brevoxyl-8 Creamy Wash **3054**
Brevoxyl-8 Gel **3054**

ACNE DERM (Israel)
BENZOYL PEROXIDE
Brevoxyl-4 Creamy Wash **3054**
Brevoxyl-4 Gel **3054**
Brevoxyl-8 Creamy Wash **3054**
Brevoxyl-8 Gel **3054**

ACNE MASK (Israel)
BENZOYL PEROXIDE
Brevoxyl-4 Creamy Wash **3054**
Brevoxyl-4 Gel **3054**
Brevoxyl-8 Creamy Wash **3054**
Brevoxyl-8 Gel **3054**

ACNE-AID (Spain)
BENZOYL PEROXIDE
Brevoxyl-4 Creamy Wash **3054**
Brevoxyl-4 Gel **3054**
Brevoxyl-8 Creamy Wash **3054**
Brevoxyl-8 Gel **3054**

ACNECARE (The Netherlands)
BENZOYL PEROXIDE
Brevoxyl-4 Creamy Wash **3054**
Brevoxyl-4 Gel **3054**
Brevoxyl-8 Creamy Wash **3054**
Brevoxyl-8 Gel **3054**

ACNECIDE (Irish Republic, United Kingdom)
BENZOYL PEROXIDE
Brevoxyl-4 Creamy Wash **3054**
Brevoxyl-4 Gel **3054**
Brevoxyl-8 Creamy Wash **3054**
Brevoxyl-8 Gel **3054**

ACNECLEAR (Hong Kong)
BENZOYL PEROXIDE
Brevoxyl-4 Creamy Wash **3054**
Brevoxyl-4 Gel **3054**
Brevoxyl-8 Creamy Wash **3054**
Brevoxyl-8 Gel **3054**

ACNEFUGE (Switzerland)
BENZOYL PEROXIDE
Brevoxyl-4 Creamy Wash **3054**
Brevoxyl-4 Gel **3054**
Brevoxyl-8 Creamy Wash **3054**
Brevoxyl-8 Gel **3054**

ACNEGEL (United Kingdom)
BENZOYL PEROXIDE
Brevoxyl-4 Creamy Wash **3054**
Brevoxyl-4 Gel **3054**
Brevoxyl-8 Creamy Wash **3054**
Brevoxyl-8 Gel **3054**

ACNELYSE (Turkey)
TRETINOIN
Vesanoid Capsules **2660**

ACNE-MED (Hungary)
BENZOYL PEROXIDE
Brevoxyl-4 Creamy Wash **3054**
Brevoxyl-4 Gel **3054**
Brevoxyl-8 Creamy Wash **3054**
Brevoxyl-8 Gel **3054**

ACNEMIN (Spain)
ISOTRETINOIN
Accutane Capsules **2607**

ACNEOUT (Argentina)
TRETINOIN
Vesanoid Capsules **2660**

ACNEPAS (Argentina)
BENZOYL PEROXIDE
Brevoxyl-4 Creamy Wash **3054**
Brevoxyl-4 Gel **3054**
Brevoxyl-8 Creamy Wash **3054**
Brevoxyl-8 Gel **3054**

ACNEPAS E (Argentina)
BENZOYL PEROXIDE
Brevoxyl-4 Creamy Wash **3054**
Brevoxyl-4 Gel **3054**
Brevoxyl-8 Creamy Wash **3054**
Brevoxyl-8 Gel **3054**

ACNEPLUS (Belgium)
BENZOYL PEROXIDE
Brevoxyl-4 Creamy Wash **3054**
Brevoxyl-4 Gel **3054**
Brevoxyl-8 Creamy Wash **3054**
Brevoxyl-8 Gel **3054**

ACNESAN (Argentina, Brazil)
BENZOYL PEROXIDE
Brevoxyl-4 Creamy Wash **3054**
Brevoxyl-4 Gel **3054**
Brevoxyl-8 Creamy Wash **3054**
Brevoxyl-8 Gel **3054**

ACNETANE (South Africa)
ISOTRETINOIN
Accutane Capsules **2607**

ACNETREX (The Philippines)
ISOTRETINOIN
Accutane Capsules **2607**

ACNEX (Venezuela)
BENZOYL PEROXIDE
Brevoxyl-4 Creamy Wash **3054**
Brevoxyl-4 Gel **3054**
Brevoxyl-8 Creamy Wash **3054**
Brevoxyl-8 Gel **3054**

ACNEXYL (Thailand)
BENZOYL PEROXIDE
Brevoxyl-4 Creamy Wash **3054**
Brevoxyl-4 Gel **3054**
Brevoxyl-8 Creamy Wash **3054**
Brevoxyl-8 Gel **3054**

ACNIL (Mexico)
TRETINOIN
Vesanoid Capsules **2660**

ACNOTIN (Chile, Hong Kong, Thailand)
ISOTRETINOIN
Accutane Capsules **2607**

A-CNOTREN (Greece)
ISOTRETINOIN
Accutane Capsules **2607**

ACOFLAM (United Kingdom)
DICLOFENAC SODIUM
Voltaren Tablets **2334**
Voltaren-XR Tablets **2337**

ACREL (Spain)
RISEDRONATE SODIUM
Actonel Tablets **2568**

ACREXON (The Philippines)
CEFTRIAXONE SODIUM
Rocephin Injectable Vials, ADD-Vantage, Galaxy, Bulk **2642**

ACRIDILOLE (Russia)
CARVEDILOL
Coreg Tablets **1387**

ACTA (Hong Kong, Singapore)
TRETINOIN
Vesanoid Capsules **2660**

ACTICIN (United Kingdom)
TRETINOIN
Vesanoid Capsules **2660**

ACTIDINE (Hong Kong)
FAMOTIDINE
Pepcid for Oral Suspension **2075**
Pepcid Tablets **2075**

ACTILAX (Australia)
LACTULOSE
Kristalose for Oral Solution **1004**

ACTIMAX (Argentina)
ALENDRONATE SODIUM
Fosamax Tablets **2005**

ACTIMOL (India)
DICLOFENAC SODIUM
Voltaren Tablets **2334**
Voltaren-XR Tablets **2337**

ACTINERVAL (Argentina)
CARBAMAZEPINE
Carbatrol Capsules **3019**

ACTINOMA (Turkey)
DICLOFENAC SODIUM
Voltaren Tablets **2334**
Voltaren-XR Tablets **2337**

ACTIPRAM (Chile)
CITALOPRAM HYDROBROMIDE
Celexa Tablets **1160**

ACTIQ (Australia, Denmark, Finland, France, Germany, Greece, Irish Republic, Italy, Norway, Spain, Sweden, Switzerland, The Netherlands, United Kingdom)
FENTANYL CITRATE
Actiq **959**

ACTIQUIM (Mexico)
NAPROXEN
EC-Naprosyn Delayed-Release Tablets **2632**
Naprosyn Suspension **2632**
Naprosyn Tablets **2632**

ACTISKENAN (France)
MORPHINE SULFATE
MS Contin Tablets **2585**

ACTIVELLE (Argentina, Brazil, Czech Republic, France, Hong Kong, Hungary, Irish Republic, Israel, Malaysia, Poland, Portugal, South Africa, Spain, Thailand, The Netherlands, Turkey)
ESTRADIOL
Climara Transdermal System **763**

ACTONEL (Argentina, Australia, Austria, Belgium, Brazil, Canada, Chile, Czech Republic, France, Greece, Hong Kong, Hungary, India, Israel, Italy, Mexico, Poland, Portugal, Singapore, South Africa, Spain, Switzerland, Thailand, The Netherlands, The Philippines, Turkey, Venezuela)
RISEDRONATE SODIUM
Actonel Tablets **2568**

ACTOPRIL (Irish Republic)
CAPTOPRIL
Captopril Tablets **2182**

ACTOS (Argentina, Australia, Austria, Belgium, Brazil, Canada, Chile, Czech Republic, Denmark, Finland, France, Germany, Greece, Hong Kong, Italy, Japan, New Zealand, Norway, Portugal, Russia, South Africa, Spain, Sweden, Switzerland, Thailand, The Netherlands, The Philippines, United Kingdom, Venezuela)
PIOGLITAZONE HYDROCHLORIDE
Actos Tablets **3077**

ACUGESIC (Hong Kong)
TRAMADOL HYDROCHLORIDE
Ultram ER Tablets **2428**

ACURA (Norway, Sweden)
CETIRIZINE HYDROCHLORIDE
Zyrtec Syrup **1920**
Zyrtec Tablets **1920**

ACUSPRAIN (South Africa)
NAPROXEN
EC-Naprosyn Delayed-Release Tablets **2632**

Naprosyn Suspension 2632
Naprosyn Tablets 2632

ACUTRET (India)
ISOTRETINOIN
Accutane Capsules 2607

ADAMON (Argentina, Austria, Hungary, Italy)
TRAMADOL HYDROCHLORIDE
Ultram ER Tablets 2428

ADANA (Argentina)
IRBESARTAN
Avapro Tablets 897

ADANA PLUS (Argentina)
IRBESARTAN
Avapro Tablets 897

ADANT (France, Israel, Thailand, Turkey)
SODIUM HYALURONATE
Hyalgan Solution 2742

ADARTREL (Switzerland)
ROPINIROLE HYDROCHLORIDE
Requip Tablets 1561

ADCO-CIPRIN (South Africa)
CIPROFLOXACIN HYDROCHLORIDE
Cipro Tablets 2810

ADCO-LIQUILAX (South Africa)
LACTULOSE
Kristalose for Oral Solution 1004

ADCORTYL (Irish Republic, Israel, United Kingdom)
TRIAMCINOLONE ACETONIDE
Azmacort Inhalation Aerosol 407
Nasacort AQ Nasal Spray 2765

ADCORTYL IN ORABASE (Irish Republic, United Kingdom)
TRIAMCINOLONE ACETONIDE
Azmacort Inhalation Aerosol 407
Nasacort AQ Nasal Spray 2765

ADCO-TALOMIL (South Africa)
CITALOPRAM HYDROBROMIDE
Celexa Tablets 1160

ADEL (Mexico)
CLARITHROMYCIN
Biaxin Filmtab Tablets 411
Biaxin Granules 411

ADENOCARD (Brazil, Canada)
ADENOSINE
Adenocard IV Injection 603
Adenoscan 605

ADENOCOR (Australia, Belgium, Czech Republic, Denmark, Finland, Greece, Hungary, Irish Republic, Israel, Malaysia, New Zealand, Norway, Poland, Portugal, Singapore, South Africa, Spain, Sweden, Thailand, The Netherlands, United Kingdom, Venezuela)
ADENOSINE
Adenocard IV Injection 603
Adenoscan 605

ADENOJECT (India)
ADENOSINE
Adenocard IV Injection 603
Adenoscan 605

ADENOSCAN (Australia, Austria, Czech Republic, Finland, France, Germany, Hong Kong, Italy, Japan, Spain, The Netherlands, United Kingdom)
ADENOSINE
Adenocard IV Injection 603
Adenoscan 605

ADEPRIL (Mexico)
CARBAMAZEPINE
Carbatrol Capsules 3019

ADERAN (Argentina)
SIBUTRAMINE HYDROCHLORIDE
Meridia Capsules 475

ADESIPRESS-TTS (Italy)
CLONIDINE
Catapres-TTS 842

ADEZAN (Greece)
DIPYRIDAMOLE
Persantine Tablets 869

ADEZIO (Hong Kong, Malaysia, Singapore)
CETIRIZINE HYDROCHLORIDE
Zyrtec Syrup 1920
Zyrtec Tablets 1920

ADGYN ESTRO (United Kingdom)
ESTRADIOL
Climara Transdermal System 763

ADIATIN (Mexico)
FAMOTIDINE
Pepcid for Oral Suspension 2075
Pepcid Tablets 2075

ADICANIL (Greece)
LISINOPRIL
Prinivil Tablets 2087

ADICLAIR (Germany)
NYSTATIN
Nystop Topical Powder USP 2498

ADIPUR (Switzerland)
SIMVASTATIN
Zocor Tablets 2136

ADISAR (Chile)
SIBUTRAMINE HYDROCHLORIDE
Meridia Capsules 475

ADIZEM (Irish Republic, Israel, United Kingdom)
DILTIAZEM HYDROCHLORIDE
Cardizem LA Extended Release Tablets 421

ADMON (Spain)
NIMODIPINE
Nimotop Capsules 790

ADOCOMP (Germany)
CAPTOPRIL
Captopril Tablets 2182

ADOCOR (Germany)
CAPTOPRIL
Captopril Tablets 2182

ADOLONTA (Spain)
TRAMADOL HYDROCHLORIDE
Ultram ER Tablets 2428

ADREKAR (Austria, Germany)
ADENOSINE
Adenocard IV Injection 603
Adenoscan 605

ADRONAT (Italy, Portugal)
ALENDRONATE SODIUM
Fosamax Tablets 2005

ADUCIN (Denmark)
RANITIDINE HYDROCHLORIDE
Zantac 25 EFFERdose Tablets 1670
Zantac 150 Tablets 1670
Zantac 300 Tablets 1670
Zantac Injection 1666
Zantac Injection Premixed 1666
Zantac Syrup 1670

ADVAGRAF (United Kingdom)
TACROLIMUS
Prograf Capsules and Injection 622

AERFLU (Italy)
FLUNISOLIDE
Aerobid Inhaler System 1153
Aerobid-M Inhaler System 1153

AERODIOL (Argentina, Australia, Austria, Belgium, Brazil, Denmark, France, Germany, Greece, Hong Kong, Irish Republic, Italy, New Zealand, Switzerland, The Netherlands, Turkey, United Kingdom, Venezuela)
ESTRADIOL
Climara Transdermal System 763

AEROLID (Italy)
FLUNISOLIDE
Aerobid Inhaler System 1153
Aerobid-M Inhaler System 1153

AEROMAX (Germany)
SALMETEROL XINAFOATE
Serevent Diskus 1594

AEROMETROL PLUS (Chile)
SALMETEROL XINAFOATE
Serevent Diskus 1594

AERONIX (Spain)
ZAFIRLUKAST
Accolate Tablets 669

AEROTROP (Argentina)
IPRATROPIUM BROMIDE
Atrovent Nasal Spray 0.03% 834
Atrovent Nasal Spray 0.06% 836

AEROVENT (Israel)
IPRATROPIUM BROMIDE
Atrovent Nasal Spray 0.03% 834
Atrovent Nasal Spray 0.06% 836

AEROXINA (Argentina)
CLARITHROMYCIN
Biaxin Filmtab Tablets 411
Biaxin Granules 411

AERUGINOX (The Philippines)
CEFUROXIME SODIUM
Zinacef Injection 1678

AFENEXIL (Argentina)
PAROXETINE HYDROCHLORIDE
Paxil Oral Suspension 1535
Paxil Tablets 1535

AFENIL (Greece)
TRANDOLAPRIL
Mavik Tablets 472

AFENOXIN (Greece)
CIPROFLOXACIN HYDROCHLORIDE
Cipro Tablets 2810

AFLODAC (Italy)
SULINDAC
Clinoril Tablets 1962

AFONILUM (Austria, Czech Republic, Germany, Poland)
THEOPHYLLINE
Uniphyl Tablets 2595

AFPRED-THEO (Germany)
THEOPHYLLINE
Uniphyl Tablets 2595

AFTAB (Finland, Germany, Italy)
TRIAMCINOLONE ACETONIDE
Azmacort Inhalation Aerosol 407
Nasacort AQ Nasal Spray 2765

AFTACH (Hong Kong, Japan, Portugal)
TRIAMCINOLONE ACETONIDE
Azmacort Inhalation Aerosol 407
Nasacort AQ Nasal Spray 2765

AFTER BURN (Israel)
LIDOCAINE
Lidoderm Patch 1114

AFUGIN (Poland)
TERBINAFINE HYDROCHLORIDE
Lamisil Tablets 2266

AFUNGINAL (The Philippines)
NYSTATIN
Nystop Topical Powder USP 2498

AGELAN (Hong Kong, Irish Republic)
INDAPAMIDE
Indapamide Tablets 2188

AGELMIN (Greece, Singapore)
CETIRIZINE HYDROCHLORIDE
Zyrtec Syrup 1920
Zyrtec Tablets 1920

AGGRENOX (Belgium, Canada, Czech Republic, Germany, Hong Kong, Portugal, Thailand, The Philippines)
DIPYRIDAMOLE
Persantine Tablets 869

AGILOMED (Austria)
DICLOFENAC SODIUM
Voltaren Tablets 2334
Voltaren-XR Tablets 2337

AGOFENAC (Switzerland)
DICLOFENAC SODIUM
Voltaren Tablets 2334
Voltaren-XR Tablets 2337

AGREDAMOL (Belgium)
DIPYRIDAMOLE
Persantine Tablets 869

AGRELID (Argentina)
ANAGRELIDE HYDROCHLORIDE
Agrylin Capsules 3017

AGREMOL (Thailand)
DIPYRIDAMOLE
Persantine Tablets 869

AGRENOX (Argentina)
DIPYRIDAMOLE
Persantine Tablets 869

AGRYLIN (Australia, Brazil, Canada, Greece, Hong Kong, Israel, South Africa, The Philippines)
ANAGRELIDE HYDROCHLORIDE
Agrylin Capsules 3017

AGUFAM (Thailand)
FAMOTIDINE
Pepcid for Oral Suspension 2075
Pepcid Tablets 2075

AGYR (Austria)
CIPROFLOXACIN HYDROCHLORIDE
Cipro Tablets 2810

AIRBRONAL (Argentina)
THEOPHYLLINE
Uniphyl Tablets 2595

AIRCLIN (Brazil)
TRIAMCINOLONE ACETONIDE
Azmacort Inhalation Aerosol 407
Nasacort AQ Nasal Spray 2765

AIROL (Australia, Austria, Czech Republic, Germany, Greece, Israel, Italy, Mexico, Norway, South Africa, Switzerland, The Philippines)
TRETINOIN
Vesanoid Capsules 2660

AIRON (Venezuela)
MONTELUKAST SODIUM
Singulair Chewable Tablets 2114
Singulair Tablets 2114

AISOSKIN (Italy)
ISOTRETINOIN
Accutane Capsules 2607

AK-CIDE (Canada)
PREDNISOLONE ACETATE/SULFACETAMIDE SODIUM
Blephamide Ophthalmic Ointment . . . . ⊙217
Blephamide Ophthalmic Suspension . . . . ⊙216

AK-FLUOR (Canada)
FLUORESCEIN SODIUM
Fluorescite Injection . . . . ⊙203

AKNE-AID-LOTION MILD (Germany)
BENZOYL PEROXIDE
Brevoxyl-4 Creamy Wash 3054
Brevoxyl-4 Gel 3054
Brevoxyl-8 Creamy Wash 3054
Brevoxyl-8 Gel 3054

AKNECIDE (Czech Republic)
BENZOYL PEROXIDE
Brevoxyl-4 Creamy Wash 3054
Brevoxyl-4 Gel 3054
Brevoxyl-8 Creamy Wash 3054
Brevoxyl-8 Gel 3054

AKNEDERM OXID (Germany)
BENZOYL PEROXIDE
Brevoxyl-4 Creamy Wash 3054
Brevoxyl-4 Gel 3054
Brevoxyl-8 Creamy Wash 3054
Brevoxyl-8 Gel 3054

AKNEFUG (Czech Republic)
ESTRADIOL
Climara Transdermal System 763

AKNEFUG BP (Turkey)
BENZOYL PEROXIDE
Brevoxyl-4 Creamy Wash 3054
Brevoxyl-4 Gel 3054
Brevoxyl-8 Creamy Wash 3054
Brevoxyl-8 Gel 3054

AKNEFUG ISO (Germany)
ISOTRETINOIN
Accutane Capsules 2607

AKNEFUG-OXID (Czech Republic, Germany, Hungary)
BENZOYL PEROXIDE
Brevoxyl-4 Creamy Wash 3054
Brevoxyl-4 Gel 3054
Brevoxyl-8 Creamy Wash 3054
Brevoxyl-8 Gel 3054

AKNENORMIN (Germany, Poland)
ISOTRETINOIN
Accutane Capsules 2607

AKNEROXID (Austria, Belgium, Czech Republic, Germany, Hungary, Malaysia, Poland, Singapore, Switzerland, The Netherlands)
BENZOYL PEROXIDE
Brevoxyl-4 Creamy Wash . . . 3054
Brevoxyl-4 Gel . . . 3054
Brevoxyl-8 Creamy Wash . . . 3054
Brevoxyl-8 Gel . . . 3054

AKNESIL (Greece)
ISOTRETINOIN
Accutane Capsules . . . 2607

AKNEX (Switzerland)
BENZOYL PEROXIDE
Brevoxyl-4 Creamy Wash . . . 3054
Brevoxyl-4 Gel . . . 3054
Brevoxyl-8 Creamy Wash . . . 3054
Brevoxyl-8 Gel . . . 3054

AKRIPAMIDE (Russia)
INDAPAMIDE
Indapamide Tablets . . . 2188

AKSEF (Turkey)
CEFUROXIME AXETIL
Ceftin for Oral Suspension . . . 1380
Ceftin Tablets . . . 1380

AKSIL (Turkey)
BENZOYL PEROXIDE
Brevoxyl-4 Creamy Wash . . . 3054
Brevoxyl-4 Gel . . . 3054
Brevoxyl-8 Creamy Wash . . . 3054
Brevoxyl-8 Gel . . . 3054

AKTIOSAN (Argentina)
DICLOFENAC SODIUM
Voltaren Tablets . . . 2334
Voltaren-XR Tablets . . . 2337

AKUDOL (Italy)
NAPROXEN SODIUM
Anaprox DS Tablets . . . 2632
Anaprox Tablets . . . 2632

ALACETAN NNA (Germany)
NAPROXEN SODIUM
Anaprox DS Tablets . . . 2632
Anaprox Tablets . . . 2632

ALAMIL (Brazil)
TERBINAFINE HYDROCHLORIDE
Lamisil Tablets . . . 2266

ALANDIEM (Portugal)
DILTIAZEM HYDROCHLORIDE
Cardizem LA Extended Release Tablets . . . 421

ALAPRIL (Italy)
LISINOPRIL
Prinivil Tablets . . . 2087

ALBA-3 (Brazil)
ALBENDAZOLE
Albenza Tablets . . . 1297

ALBATEL (Thailand)
ALBENDAZOLE
Albenza Tablets . . . 1297

ALBEN (Brazil, Thailand)
ALBENDAZOLE
Albenza Tablets . . . 1297

ALBENDA (Thailand, United Arab Emirates)
ALBENDAZOLE
Albenza Tablets . . . 1297

ALBENDOL (Malaysia)
ALBENDAZOLE
Albenza Tablets . . . 1297

ALBENDROX (Brazil)
ALBENDAZOLE
Albenza Tablets . . . 1297

ALBENDY (Brazil)
ALBENDAZOLE
Albenza Tablets . . . 1297

ALBENIX (Brazil)
ALBENDAZOLE
Albenza Tablets . . . 1297

ALBENSIL (Mexico)
ALBENDAZOLE
Albenza Tablets . . . 1297

ALBENTEL (Brazil)
ALBENDAZOLE
Albenza Tablets . . . 1297

ALBENZONIL (Brazil)
ALBENDAZOLE
Albenza Tablets . . . 1297

ALBEOLER (Chile)
FLUTICASONE PROPIONATE
Flonase Nasal Spray . . . 1431

ALBESINE BIOTIC (Argentina)
AMOXICILLIN
Amoxil Pediatric Drops for Oral Suspension . . . 1305
Amoxil Tablets . . . 1305

ALBEZIN (Brazil)
ALBENDAZOLE
Albenza Tablets . . . 1297

ALBEZOL (Venezuela)
ALBENDAZOLE
Albenza Tablets . . . 1297

ALBEZOLE (India)
ALBENDAZOLE
Albenza Tablets . . . 1297

ALBICAR (Venezuela)
ALBENDAZOLE
Albenza Tablets . . . 1297

ALBICORT (Belgium, The Netherlands)
TRIAMCINOLONE ACETONIDE
Azmacort Inhalation Aerosol . . . 407
Nasacort AQ Nasal Spray . . . 2765

ALBISTIN (Brazil)
NYSTATIN
Nystop Topical Powder USP . . . 2498

ALBORAL (Mexico)
DIAZEPAM
Valium Tablets . . . 2658

ALCIS (Spain)
ESTRADIOL
Climara Transdermal System . . . 763

ALCOPHYLLIN (South Africa)
THEOPHYLLINE
Uniphyl Tablets . . . 2595

ALDA (Thailand)
ALBENDAZOLE
Albenza Tablets . . . 1297

ALDARA (Argentina, Australia, Belgium, Brazil, Canada, Chile, Czech Republic, Denmark, Finland, France, Germany, Greece, Hong Kong, Irish Republic, Israel, Italy, Malaysia, Mexico, New Zealand, Norway, Poland, Singapore, South Africa, Spain, Sweden, Switzerland, Thailand, The Netherlands, The Philippines, United Kingdom)
IMIQUIMOD
Aldara Cream, 5% . . . 1699

ALDAZINE (Australia, New Zealand)
THIORIDAZINE HYDROCHLORIDE
Thioridazine Hydrochloride Tablets . . . 2195

ALDIC (Thailand)
FUROSEMIDE
Furosemide Tablets . . . 2186

ALDIZEM (Czech Republic)
DILTIAZEM HYDROCHLORIDE
Cardizem LA Extended Release Tablets . . . 421

ALDOACNE (Spain)
BENZOYL PEROXIDE
Brevoxyl-4 Creamy Wash . . . 3054
Brevoxyl-4 Gel . . . 3054
Brevoxyl-8 Creamy Wash . . . 3054
Brevoxyl-8 Gel . . . 3054

ALDORON NF (Argentina)
DICLOFENAC SODIUM
Voltaren Tablets . . . 2334
Voltaren-XR Tablets . . . 2337

ALDRONAC (Venezuela)
ALENDRONATE SODIUM
Fosamax Tablets . . . 2005

ALDROX (Chile)
ALENDRONATE SODIUM
Fosamax Tablets . . . 2005

ALENAT (Sweden)
ALENDRONATE SODIUM
Fosamax Tablets . . . 2005

ALENATO (Argentina, Poland)
ALENDRONATE SODIUM
Fosamax Tablets . . . 2005

ALENBIT (Greece)
NORFLOXACIN
Noroxin Tablets . . . 2069

ALENDIL (Brazil)
ALENDRONATE SODIUM
Fosamax Tablets . . . 2005

ALENDROS (Italy)
ALENDRONATE SODIUM
Fosamax Tablets . . . 2005

ALENSTRAN (Greece)
CETIRIZINE HYDROCHLORIDE
Zyrtec Syrup . . . 1920
Zyrtec Tablets . . . 1920

ALERCINA (Spain)
CETIRIZINE HYDROCHLORIDE
Zyrtec Syrup . . . 1920
Zyrtec Tablets . . . 1920

ALERID (Austria, Czech Republic, Germany, India, Sweden)
CETIRIZINE HYDROCHLORIDE
Zyrtec Syrup . . . 1920
Zyrtec Tablets . . . 1920

ALERION (Argentina)
CLONAZEPAM
Klonopin Tablets . . . 2639

ALERLISIN (Spain)
CETIRIZINE HYDROCHLORIDE
Zyrtec Syrup . . . 1920
Zyrtec Tablets . . . 1920

ALERMED (Poland)
CETIRIZINE HYDROCHLORIDE
Zyrtec Syrup . . . 1920
Zyrtec Tablets . . . 1920

ALERTEC (Canada)
MODAFINIL
Provigil Tablets . . . 977

ALERTOP (Chile)
CETIRIZINE HYDROCHLORIDE
Zyrtec Syrup . . . 1920
Zyrtec Tablets . . . 1920

ALERTOP-D (Chile)
CETIRIZINE HYDROCHLORIDE
Zyrtec Syrup . . . 1920
Zyrtec Tablets . . . 1920

ALERZINA (Poland)
CETIRIZINE HYDROCHLORIDE
Zyrtec Syrup . . . 1920
Zyrtec Tablets . . . 1920

ALETIR (Brazil)
CETIRIZINE HYDROCHLORIDE
Zyrtec Syrup . . . 1920
Zyrtec Tablets . . . 1920

ALEVE (Argentina, Australia, Austria, Czech Republic, France, Germany, Hungary, Italy, Poland, South Africa, Spain, Switzerland, The Netherlands, Turkey)
NAPROXEN SODIUM
Anaprox DS Tablets . . . 2632
Anaprox Tablets . . . 2632

ALFAKEN (Mexico)
LISINOPRIL
Prinivil Tablets . . . 2087

ALFASIN (Brazil)
FINASTERIDE
Propecia Tablets . . . 2095
Proscar Tablets . . . 2102

ALFATE (India)
SUCRALFATE
Carafate Suspension . . . 706
Carafate Tablets . . . 707

ALFAZOL (Mexico)
ALBENDAZOLE
Albenza Tablets . . . 1297

ALFOXIL (Turkey)
AMOXICILLIN
Amoxil Pediatric Drops for Oral Suspension . . . 1305
Amoxil Tablets . . . 1305

ALFUCA (Thailand)
ALBENDAZOLE
Albenza Tablets . . . 1297

ALGEDOL (Argentina)
MORPHINE SULFATE
MS Contin Tablets . . . 2585

ALGEFIT (Austria)
DICLOFENAC SODIUM
Voltaren Tablets . . . 2334
Voltaren-XR Tablets . . . 2337

ALGIOPRUX (Argentina)
NAPROXEN
EC-Naprosyn Delayed-Release Tablets . . . 2632
Naprosyn Suspension . . . 2632
Naprosyn Tablets . . . 2632

ALGIOXIB (Argentina)
DICLOFENAC SODIUM
Voltaren Tablets . . . 2334
Voltaren-XR Tablets . . . 2337

ALGIREM (Russia)
RIMANTADINE HYDROCHLORIDE
Flumadine Syrup . . . 1167
Flumadine Tablets . . . 1167

ALGOCETIL (Italy)
SULINDAC
Clinoril Tablets . . . 1962

ALGONAPRIL (Italy)
NAPROXEN
EC-Naprosyn Delayed-Release Tablets . . . 2632
Naprosyn Suspension . . . 2632
Naprosyn Tablets . . . 2632

ALGOSENAC (Italy)
DICLOFENAC SODIUM
Voltaren Tablets . . . 2334
Voltaren-XR Tablets . . . 2337

ALGYBREX (Argentina)
CELECOXIB
Celebrex Capsules . . . 2979

ALIB (Brazil)
ALBENDAZOLE
Albenza Tablets . . . 1297

ALIDASE (Argentina)
NAPROXEN
EC-Naprosyn Delayed-Release Tablets . . . 2632
Naprosyn Suspension . . . 2632
Naprosyn Tablets . . . 2632

ALIFLUS (Italy)
SALMETEROL XINAFOATE
Serevent Diskus . . . 1594

ALIN (Brazil)
ALBENDAZOLE
Albenza Tablets . . . 1297

ALIOT (Venezuela)
ALENDRONATE SODIUM
Fosamax Tablets . . . 2005

ALIPASE (France)
PANCRELIPASE
Ultrase Capsules . . . 718
Ultrase MT Capsules . . . 719

ALISEUM (Italy)
DIAZEPAM
Valium Tablets . . . 2658

ALIVIOMAS (Spain)
NAPROXEN
EC-Naprosyn Delayed-Release Tablets . . . 2632
Naprosyn Suspension . . . 2632
Naprosyn Tablets . . . 2632

ALKADIL (Czech Republic)
CAPTOPRIL
Captopril Tablets . . . 2182

ALKALIT (Czech Republic)
POTASSIUM CITRATE
Urocit-K Tablets . . . 2176

ALLECET (South Africa)
CETIRIZINE HYDROCHLORIDE
Zyrtec Syrup . . . 1920
Zyrtec Tablets . . . 1920

ALLEGRA-D (Canada, Chile, Venezuela)
FEXOFENADINE HYDROCHLORIDE/ PSEUDOEPHEDRINE HYDROCHLORIDE
Allegra-D 12 Hour Extended-Release Tablets . . . 2687

ALLEGRO (Israel)
FLUTICASONE PROPIONATE
Flonase Nasal Spray . . . 1431

ALLENOPAR (Austria)
PAROXETINE HYDROCHLORIDE
Paxil Oral Suspension . . . 1535

Paxil Tablets 1535

ALLERCET (Thailand)
CETIRIZINE HYDROCHLORIDE
Zyrtec Syrup 1920
Zyrtec Tablets 1920

ALLERGY RELIEF (Canada)
CETIRIZINE HYDROCHLORIDE
Zyrtec Syrup 1920
Zyrtec Tablets 1920

ALLERMAX (Australia)
MOMETASONE FUROATE
Elocon Cream 0.1% 2840
Elocon Lotion 0.1% 2841
Elocon Ointment 0.1% 2842
Nasonex Nasal Spray 2883

ALLERMINE (South Africa)
CETIRIZINE HYDROCHLORIDE
Zyrtec Syrup 1920
Zyrtec Tablets 1920

ALLERSET (Turkey)
CETIRIZINE HYDROCHLORIDE
Zyrtec Syrup 1920
Zyrtec Tablets 1920

ALLERTEC (Poland, Russia, Singapore)
CETIRIZINE HYDROCHLORIDE
Zyrtec Syrup 1920
Zyrtec Tablets 1920

ALLURENE (Austria, The Netherlands)
ESTRADIOL
Climara Transdermal System 763

ALLVORAN (Germany)
DICLOFENAC SODIUM
Voltaren Tablets 2334
Voltaren-XR Tablets 2337

ALMARION (Thailand)
THEOPHYLLINE
Uniphyl Tablets 2595

ALMIRAL (Hong Kong, Russia)
DICLOFENAC SODIUM
Voltaren Tablets 2334
Voltaren-XR Tablets 2337

ALMODAN (United Kingdom)
AMOXICILLIN
Amoxil Pediatric Drops for Oral Suspension 1305
Amoxil Tablets 1305

ALNA (Austria, Germany)
TAMSULOSIN HYDROCHLORIDE
Flomax Capsules 848

ALNOK (Denmark)
CETIRIZINE HYDROCHLORIDE
Zyrtec Syrup 1920
Zyrtec Tablets 1920

ALOPRESIN (Spain)
CAPTOPRIL
Captopril Tablets 2182

ALOVENT (Venezuela)
IPRATROPIUM BROMIDE
Atrovent Nasal Spray 0.03% 834
Atrovent Nasal Spray 0.06% 836

ALPERTAN (Argentina)
VALSARTAN
Diovan Tablets 2212

ALPHADINE (Greece)
RANITIDINE HYDROCHLORIDE
Zantac 25 EFFERdose Tablets 1670
Zantac 150 Tablets 1670
Zantac 300 Tablets 1670
Zantac Injection 1666
Zantac Injection Premixed 1666
Zantac Syrup 1670

ALPHA-LAC (Canada)
LACTULOSE
Kristalose for Oral Solution 1004

ALPOXEN (Denmark, Finland, Norway, Sweden)
NAPROXEN
EC-Naprosyn Delayed-Release Tablets 2632
Naprosyn Suspension 2632
Naprosyn Tablets 2632

ALPROFEN (Spain)
NAPROXEN
EC-Naprosyn Delayed-Release Tablets 2632
Naprosyn Suspension 2632
Naprosyn Tablets 2632

ALPRON (The Philippines)
NAPROXEN
EC-Naprosyn Delayed-Release Tablets 2632
Naprosyn Suspension 2632
Naprosyn Tablets 2632

ALQUEN (Spain)
RANITIDINE HYDROCHLORIDE
Zantac 25 EFFERdose Tablets 1670
Zantac 150 Tablets 1670
Zantac 300 Tablets 1670
Zantac Injection 1666
Zantac Injection Premixed 1666
Zantac Syrup 1670

ALSART (Venezuela)
VALSARTAN
Diovan Tablets 2212

ALSARTAN (India)
LOSARTAN POTASSIUM
Cozaar Tablets 1973

ALSARTAN-AM (India)
LOSARTAN POTASSIUM
Cozaar Tablets 1973

ALSARTAN-H (India)
LOSARTAN POTASSIUM
Cozaar Tablets 1973

ALSIDEXTEN (Mexico)
DICLOFENAC SODIUM
Voltaren Tablets 2334
Voltaren-XR Tablets 2337

ALSUCRAL (Finland, Malaysia, Singapore)
SUCRALFATE
Carafate Suspension 706
Carafate Tablets 707

ALTACEF (India)
CEFUROXIME AXETIL
Ceftin for Oral Suspension 1380
Ceftin Tablets 1380

ALTEMOL (Mexico)
INTERFERON ALFA-N3
Alferon N Injection 1726

ALTEN (Hong Kong, Malaysia, Singapore)
TRETINOIN
Vesanoid Capsules 2660

ALTERCOR (The Netherlands)
SIMVASTATIN
Zocor Tablets 2136

ALTERGEN (Italy)
SODIUM HYALURONATE
Hyalgan Solution 2742

ALTER-H2 (Mexico)
RANITIDINE HYDROCHLORIDE
Zantac 25 EFFERdose Tablets 1670
Zantac 150 Tablets 1670
Zantac 300 Tablets 1670
Zantac Injection 1666
Zantac Injection Premixed 1666
Zantac Syrup 1670

ALTIAZEM (Hong Kong, Italy, Russia, Singapore, Thailand)
DILTIAZEM HYDROCHLORIDE
Cardizem LA Extended Release Tablets 421

ALTIVER (Mexico)
CAPTOPRIL
Captopril Tablets 2182

ALTIZEM (Turkey)
DILTIAZEM HYDROCHLORIDE
Cardizem LA Extended Release Tablets 421

ALTOSONE (Italy)
MOMETASONE FUROATE
Elocon Cream 0.1% 2840
Elocon Lotion 0.1% 2841
Elocon Ointment 0.1% 2842
Nasonex Nasal Spray 2883

ALTRAZ (India)
ANASTROZOLE
Arimidex Tablets 672

ALTRICAL (Mexico)
CALCITRIOL
Calcijex Injection 419
Rocaltrol Capsules 1150
Rocaltrol Oral Solution 1150

ALTROL (Mexico)
CALCITRIOL
Calcijex Injection 419
Rocaltrol Capsules 1150
Rocaltrol Oral Solution 1150

ALUDROX AC (Argentina)
RANITIDINE HYDROCHLORIDE
Zantac 25 EFFERdose Tablets 1670
Zantac 150 Tablets 1670
Zantac 300 Tablets 1670
Zantac Injection 1666
Zantac Injection Premixed 1666
Zantac Syrup 1670

ALUPRAM (United Kingdom)
DIAZEPAM
Valium Tablets 2658

ALUSULIN (Hungary)
SUCRALFATE
Carafate Suspension 706
Carafate Tablets 707

ALUTAN (Switzerland)
CITALOPRAM HYDROBROMIDE
Celexa Tablets 1160

ALUZINE (United Kingdom)
FUROSEMIDE
Furosemide Tablets 2186

ALVENT (Brazil)
IPRATROPIUM BROMIDE
Atrovent Nasal Spray 0.03% 834
Atrovent Nasal Spray 0.06% 836

ALVIDINA (Mexico)
RANITIDINE HYDROCHLORIDE
Zantac 25 EFFERdose Tablets 1670
Zantac 150 Tablets 1670
Zantac 300 Tablets 1670
Zantac Injection 1666
Zantac Injection Premixed 1666
Zantac Syrup 1670

ALVI-TEC (Mexico)
AMOXICILLIN
Amoxil Pediatric Drops for Oral Suspension 1305
Amoxil Tablets 1305

ALXEN (Mexico)
NAPROXEN
EC-Naprosyn Delayed-Release Tablets 2632
Naprosyn Suspension 2632
Naprosyn Tablets 2632

ALZAIMAX (Argentina)
DONEPEZIL HYDROCHLORIDE
Aricept Tablets 1062

ALZENTAL (Singapore)
ALBENDAZOLE
Albenza Tablets 1297

ALZOBEN (Brazil)
ALBENDAZOLE
Albenza Tablets 1297

ALZOL (Thailand)
ALBENDAZOLE
Albenza Tablets 1297

ALZOMED-F (Mexico)
BENZONATATE
Tessalon Perles 1183

ALZYR (Finland)
CETIRIZINE HYDROCHLORIDE
Zyrtec Syrup 1920
Zyrtec Tablets 1920

ALZYTEC (Singapore)
CETIRIZINE HYDROCHLORIDE
Zyrtec Syrup 1920
Zyrtec Tablets 1920

AMANDA (Thailand)
TRAMADOL HYDROCHLORIDE
Ultram ER Tablets 2428

AMATINE (Canada)
MIDODRINE HYDROCHLORIDE
ProAmatine Tablets 3032

AMBONEURAL (Austria)
SELEGILINE HYDROCHLORIDE
Eldepryl Capsules 3052

AMBULASE (Poland)
FINASTERIDE
Propecia Tablets 2095
Proscar Tablets 2102

AMCEF (Mexico)
CEFTRIAXONE SODIUM
Rocephin Injectable Vials, ADD-Vantage, Galaxy, Bulk 2642

AMCOLD (India)
CETIRIZINE HYDROCHLORIDE
Zyrtec Syrup 1920
Zyrtec Tablets 1920

AMEKET (The Philippines)
RANITIDINE HYDROCHLORIDE
Zantac 25 EFFERdose Tablets 1670
Zantac 150 Tablets 1670
Zantac 300 Tablets 1670
Zantac Injection 1666
Zantac Injection Premixed 1666
Zantac Syrup 1670

AMERGE (Canada)
NARATRIPTAN HYDROCHLORIDE
Amerge Tablets 1301

AMERTIL (Poland)
CETIRIZINE HYDROCHLORIDE
Zyrtec Syrup 1920
Zyrtec Tablets 1920

AMFAMOX (Australia)
FAMOTIDINE
Pepcid for Oral Suspension 2075
Pepcid Tablets 2075

AMIADA (Germany)
TERBINAFINE HYDROCHLORIDE
Lamisil Tablets 2266

AMIAS (The Netherlands, United Kingdom)
CANDESARTAN CILEXETIL
Atacand Tablets 639

AMICROBIN (Spain)
NORFLOXACIN
Noroxin Tablets 2069

AMIGRENIN (Russia)
SUMATRIPTAN SUCCINATE
Imitrex Injection 1465
Imitrex Tablets 1474

AMILENE (Chile)
ONDANSETRON
Zofran ODT Orally Disintegrating Tablets 1687

AMILITRAP (Argentina)
LAMIVUDINE
Epivir Oral Solution 1412
Epivir Tablets 1412
Epivir-HBV Oral Solution 1417
Epivir-HBV Tablets 1417

AMIMOX (Norway)
AMOXICILLIN
Amoxil Pediatric Drops for Oral Suspension 1305
Amoxil Tablets 1305

AMINDAN (Germany)
SELEGILINE HYDROCHLORIDE
Eldepryl Capsules 3052

AMINOFILIN (Argentina)
THEOPHYLLINE
Uniphyl Tablets 2595

AMINOMAL (Italy)
THEOPHYLLINE
Uniphyl Tablets 2595

AMIXEN (Argentina)
AMOXICILLIN
Amoxil Pediatric Drops for Oral Suspension 1305
Amoxil Tablets 1305

AMIZEPIN (Poland)
CARBAMAZEPINE
Carbatrol Capsules 3019

AMMINAC (Thailand)
DICLOFENAC SODIUM
Voltaren Tablets 2334
Voltaren-XR Tablets 2337

AMMITRAM (Thailand)
TRAMADOL HYDROCHLORIDE
Ultram ER Tablets 2428

AMMI-VOTARA (Thailand)
DICLOFENAC SODIUM
Voltaren Tablets 2334
Voltaren-XR Tablets 2337

AMO VITRAX (Australia, New Zealand, Singapore, South Africa, Sweden, Switzerland, Thailand)
SODIUM HYALURONATE
Hyalgan Solution 2742

AMOBIOTIC (Chile)
AMOXICILLIN
Amoxil Pediatric Drops for Oral Suspension 1305
Amoxil Tablets 1305

AMOCLANE (Belgium)
AMOXICILLIN
Amoxil Pediatric Drops for Oral Suspension 1305
Amoxil Tablets 1305

AMOCLAV (The Philippines)
AMOXICILLIN
Amoxil Pediatric Drops for Oral Suspension 1305
Amoxil Tablets 1305

AMOFAT (Mexico)
FAMOTIDINE
Pepcid for Oral Suspension 2075
Pepcid Tablets 2075

AMOKSILIN (Turkey)
AMOXICILLIN
Amoxil Pediatric Drops for Oral Suspension 1305
Amoxil Tablets 1305

AMOKSINA (Turkey)
AMOXICILLIN
Amoxil Pediatric Drops for Oral Suspension 1305
Amoxil Tablets 1305

AMOPEN (United Kingdom)
AMOXICILLIN
Amoxil Pediatric Drops for Oral Suspension 1305
Amoxil Tablets 1305

AMOSPES (Greece)
AMOXICILLIN
Amoxil Pediatric Drops for Oral Suspension 1305
Amoxil Tablets 1305

AMOVAL (Chile)
AMOXICILLIN
Amoxil Pediatric Drops for Oral Suspension 1305
Amoxil Tablets 1305

AMOVAL DUO (Chile)
AMOXICILLIN
Amoxil Pediatric Drops for Oral Suspension 1305
Amoxil Tablets 1305

AMOX (Brazil)
AMOXICILLIN
Amoxil Pediatric Drops for Oral Suspension 1305
Amoxil Tablets 1305

AMOXAL (Venezuela)
AMOXICILLIN
Amoxil Pediatric Drops for Oral Suspension 1305
Amoxil Tablets 1305

AMOXAPEN (Hong Kong, Singapore)
AMOXICILLIN
Amoxil Pediatric Drops for Oral Suspension 1305
Amoxil Tablets 1305

AMOXCILLIN (Thailand)
AMOXICILLIN
Amoxil Pediatric Drops for Oral Suspension 1305
Amoxil Tablets 1305

AMOX-G (Argentina)
AMOXICILLIN
Amoxil Pediatric Drops for Oral Suspension 1305
Amoxil Tablets 1305

AMOX-G BRONQUIAL (Argentina)
AMOXICILLIN
Amoxil Pediatric Drops for Oral Suspension 1305
Amoxil Tablets 1305

AMOXI (Argentina)
AMOXICILLIN
Amoxil Pediatric Drops for Oral Suspension 1305
Amoxil Tablets 1305

AMOXI PLUS (Argentina)
AMOXICILLIN
Amoxil Pediatric Drops for Oral Suspension 1305
Amoxil Tablets 1305

AMOXI RESPIRATORIO (Argentina)
AMOXICILLIN
Amoxil Pediatric Drops for Oral Suspension 1305
Amoxil Tablets 1305

AMOXI-BASAN (Switzerland)
AMOXICILLIN
Amoxil Pediatric Drops for Oral Suspension 1305
Amoxil Tablets 1305

AMOXIBIOCIN (Germany)
AMOXICILLIN
Amoxil Pediatric Drops for Oral Suspension 1305
Amoxil Tablets 1305

AMOXIBIOT (Argentina)
AMOXICILLIN
Amoxil Pediatric Drops for Oral Suspension 1305
Amoxil Tablets 1305

AMOXIBRON (Brazil)
AMOXICILLIN
Amoxil Pediatric Drops for Oral Suspension 1305
Amoxil Tablets 1305

AMOXICAP (Brazil)
AMOXICILLIN
Amoxil Pediatric Drops for Oral Suspension 1305
Amoxil Tablets 1305

AMOXICINA (Argentina)
AMOXICILLIN
Amoxil Pediatric Drops for Oral Suspension 1305
Amoxil Tablets 1305

AMOXICOM (Brazil)
AMOXICILLIN
Amoxil Pediatric Drops for Oral Suspension 1305
Amoxil Tablets 1305

AMOXIDAL (Argentina)
AMOXICILLIN
Amoxil Pediatric Drops for Oral Suspension 1305
Amoxil Tablets 1305

AMOXIDENT (United Kingdom)
AMOXICILLIN
Amoxil Pediatric Drops for Oral Suspension 1305
Amoxil Tablets 1305

AMOXIFAR BALSAMICO (Brazil)
AMOXICILLIN
Amoxil Pediatric Drops for Oral Suspension 1305
Amoxil Tablets 1305

AMOXIGA (Venezuela)
AMOXICILLIN
Amoxil Pediatric Drops for Oral Suspension 1305
Amoxil Tablets 1305

AMOXIGRAND (Argentina)
AMOXICILLIN
Amoxil Pediatric Drops for Oral Suspension 1305
Amoxil Tablets 1305

AMOXIGRAND BRONQUIAL (Argentina)
AMOXICILLIN
Amoxil Pediatric Drops for Oral Suspension 1305
Amoxil Tablets 1305

AMOXIGRAND COMPUESTO (Argentina)
AMOXICILLIN
Amoxil Pediatric Drops for Oral Suspension 1305
Amoxil Tablets 1305

AMOXIL (Hong Kong, Singapore)
AMOXICILLIN
Amoxil Pediatric Drops for Oral Suspension 1305
Amoxil Tablets 1305

AMOXIMED (Brazil)
AMOXICILLIN
Amoxil Pediatric Drops for Oral Suspension 1305
Amoxil Tablets 1305

AMOXINA (Brazil)
AMOXICILLIN
Amoxil Pediatric Drops for Oral Suspension 1305
Amoxil Tablets 1305

AMOXI-PED (Brazil)
AMOXICILLIN
Amoxil Pediatric Drops for Oral Suspension 1305
Amoxil Tablets 1305

AMOXIPOTEN (Argentina)
AMOXICILLIN
Amoxil Pediatric Drops for Oral Suspension 1305
Amoxil Tablets 1305

AMOXITAN (Brazil)
AMOXICILLIN
Amoxil Pediatric Drops for Oral Suspension 1305
Amoxil Tablets 1305

AMOXITENK RESPIRATORIO (Argentina)
AMOXICILLIN
Amoxil Pediatric Drops for Oral Suspension 1305
Amoxil Tablets 1305

AMOXIVAN (India)
AMOXICILLIN
Amoxil Pediatric Drops for Oral Suspension 1305
Amoxil Tablets 1305

AMOXOL (Argentina)
AMOXICILLIN
Amoxil Pediatric Drops for Oral Suspension 1305
Amoxil Tablets 1305

AMPINA (Argentina)
NIMODIPINE
Nimotop Capsules 790

AMPLAL (Brazil)
AMOXICILLIN
Amoxil Pediatric Drops for Oral Suspension 1305
Amoxil Tablets 1305

AMPLIAR (Argentina)
ATORVASTATIN CALCIUM
Lipitor Tablets 2501

AMPLOSPEC (Brazil)
CEFTRIAXONE SODIUM
Rocephin Injectable Vials, ADD-Vantage, Galaxy, Bulk 2642

AMPLOZOL (Brazil)
ALBENDAZOLE
Albenza Tablets 1297

AMUSA (The Philippines)
AMOXICILLIN
Amoxil Pediatric Drops for Oral Suspension 1305
Amoxil Tablets 1305

AMVISC (Austria, Canada, Israel, Norway, South Africa, Sweden, Turkey)
SODIUM HYALURONATE
Hyalgan Solution 2742

AMX (Mexico)
AMOXICILLIN
Amoxil Pediatric Drops for Oral Suspension 1305
Amoxil Tablets 1305

ANABET (Portugal)
NADOLOL
Nadolol Tablets 2191

ANADOL (Thailand)
TRAMADOL HYDROCHLORIDE
Ultram ER Tablets 2428

ANA-FLEX (Brazil)
DICLOFENAC SODIUM
Voltaren Tablets 2334
Voltaren-XR Tablets 2337

ANAFLIN (Mexico)
NAPROXEN
EC-Naprosyn Delayed-Release Tablets 2632
Naprosyn Suspension 2632
Naprosyn Tablets 2632

ANALAB (Malaysia, Thailand)
TRAMADOL HYDROCHLORIDE
Ultram ER Tablets 2428

ANALERGIN (Russia)
CETIRIZINE HYDROCHLORIDE
Zyrtec Syrup 1920
Zyrtec Tablets 1920

ANALFIN (Mexico)
MORPHINE SULFATE
MS Contin Tablets 2585

ANALPAN (Hong Kong)
DICLOFENAC SODIUM
Voltaren Tablets 2334
Voltaren-XR Tablets 2337

ANAMORPH (Australia)
MORPHINE SULFATE
MS Contin Tablets 2585

ANANGOR (Brazil)
TRAMADOL HYDROCHLORIDE
Ultram ER Tablets 2428

ANAPRAN (Poland)
NAPROXEN SODIUM
Anaprox DS Tablets 2632
Anaprox Tablets 2632

ANAPROTAB (Turkey)
NAPROXEN SODIUM
Anaprox DS Tablets 2632
Anaprox Tablets 2632

ANAPROX (Australia, Canada, Greece, Spain)
NAPROXEN SODIUM
Anaprox DS Tablets 2632
Anaprox Tablets 2632

ANAPSYL (Mexico)
NAPROXEN SODIUM
Anaprox DS Tablets 2632
Anaprox Tablets 2632

ANAPTIVAN (Greece)
CEFUROXIME SODIUM
Zinacef Injection 1678

ANASKEBIR (Argentina)
ANASTROZOLE
Arimidex Tablets 672

ANASTRAZE (Argentina)
ANASTROZOLE
Arimidex Tablets 672

ANATINE (Argentina)
FINASTERIDE
Propecia Tablets 2095
Proscar Tablets 2102

ANAX (Singapore)
NAPROXEN SODIUM
Anaprox DS Tablets 2632
Anaprox Tablets 2632

ANDAPSIN (Sweden)
SUCRALFATE
Carafate Suspension 706
Carafate Tablets 707

ANDAZOL (Turkey)
ALBENDAZOLE
Albenza Tablets 1297

ANDROFLOXIN (Brazil)
NORFLOXACIN
Noroxin Tablets 2069

ANDROLIP (Brazil)
SIMVASTATIN
Zocor Tablets 2136

ANDROPEL (Argentina)
FINASTERIDE
Propecia Tablets 2095
Proscar Tablets 2102

ANDROTIN (Mexico)
FAMOTIDINE
Pepcid for Oral Suspension 2075
Pepcid Tablets 2075

ANEBOL (Argentina)
ANASTROZOLE
Arimidex Tablets 672

ANESTOL (Turkey)
LIDOCAINE
Lidoderm Patch 1114

ANEUROL (Spain)
DIAZEPAM
Valium Tablets 2658

ANEXATE (Australia, Austria, Belgium, Canada, Czech Republic, France, Germany, Greece, Hong Kong, Hungary, Irish Republic, Israel, Italy, New Zealand, Norway, Poland, Portugal, Singapore, South Africa, Spain, Switzerland, Thailand, The Netherlands, The Philippines, Turkey, United Kingdom)
FLUMAZENIL
Romazicon Injection 2646

ANFENAX (New Zealand, South Africa)
DICLOFENAC SODIUM
Voltaren Tablets 2334
Voltaren-XR Tablets 2337

ANFOZAN (Greece)
ETIDRONATE DISODIUM
Didronel Tablets 2583

ANGELIQ (Argentina, Australia, Austria, Belgium, Chile, Finland, Germany, Greece, Hong Kong, Irish Republic, Israel, Italy, Poland, South Africa, Spain, Thailand, The Netherlands, The Philippines, United Kingdom)
ESTRADIOL
Climara Transdermal System 763

ANGEMIN (Sweden)
ESTRADIOL
Climara Transdermal System 763

ANGIACT (Denmark)
DILTIAZEM HYDROCHLORIDE
Cardizem LA Extended Release Tablets 421

ANGICONTIN (Denmark)
DILTIAZEM HYDROCHLORIDE
Cardizem LA Extended Release Tablets 421

ANGIDIL (Italy)
DILTIAZEM HYDROCHLORIDE
Cardizem LA Extended Release Tablets 421

ANGIODROX (Spain)
DILTIAZEM HYDROCHLORIDE
Cardizem LA Extended Release Tablets 421

ANGIOFLUOR (Argentina)
FLUORESCEIN SODIUM
Fluorescite Injection . . . . . ⊙203

ANGIOLONG (Brazil)
DILTIAZEM HYDROCHLORIDE
Cardizem LA Extended Release Tablets 421

ANGIOSAN (Austria)
VALSARTAN
Diovan Tablets 2212

ANGIOTROFIN (Mexico)
DILTIAZEM HYDROCHLORIDE
Cardizem LA Extended Release Tablets 421

ANGIOZEM (The Philippines, United Kingdom)
DILTIAZEM HYDROCHLORIDE
Cardizem LA Extended Release Tablets 421

ANGIPRESS (Italy)
DILTIAZEM HYDROCHLORIDE
Cardizem LA Extended Release Tablets 421

ANGITIL (United Kingdom)
DILTIAZEM HYDROCHLORIDE
Cardizem LA Extended Release Tablets 421

ANGIZEM (Italy, Singapore, Thailand)
DILTIAZEM HYDROCHLORIDE
Cardizem LA Extended Release Tablets 421

ANIDUV (Argentina)
NIMODIPINE
Nimotop Capsules 790

ANISTAL (Mexico)
RANITIDINE HYDROCHLORIDE
Zantac 25 EFFERdose Tablets 1670
Zantac 150 Tablets 1670
Zantac 300 Tablets 1670
Zantac Injection 1666
Zantac Injection Premixed 1666
Zantac Syrup 1670

ANLOSTIN (Poland)
LOVASTATIN
Mevacor Tablets 2063

ANNOXEN (Thailand)
NAPROXEN SODIUM
Anaprox DS Tablets 2632
Anaprox Tablets 2632

A-NOX (Turkey)
NAPROXEN SODIUM
Anaprox DS Tablets 2632
Anaprox Tablets 2632

ANSENTRON (Brazil)
ONDANSETRON HYDROCHLORIDE
Zofran Injection 1682
Zofran Injection Premixed 1682
Zofran Oral Solution 1687
Zofran Tablets 1687

ANSILAN (Greece)
FAMOTIDINE
Pepcid for Oral Suspension 2075
Pepcid Tablets 2075

ANSILIVE (Brazil)
DIAZEPAM
Valium Tablets 2658

ANSIOLIN (Italy)
DIAZEPAM
Valium Tablets 2658

ANSIUM (Spain)
DIAZEPAM
Valium Tablets 2658

ANTAFIT (Thailand)
CARBAMAZEPINE
Carbatrol Capsules 3019

ANTAGON (Brazil)
RANITIDINE HYDROCHLORIDE
Zantac 25 EFFERdose Tablets 1670
Zantac 150 Tablets 1670
Zantac 300 Tablets 1670
Zantac Injection 1666
Zantac Injection Premixed 1666
Zantac Syrup 1670

ANTAGOSAN (France, Germany, Italy)
APROTININ
Trasylol Injection 799

ANTAK (Brazil)
RANITIDINE HYDROCHLORIDE
Zantac 25 EFFERdose Tablets 1670
Zantac 150 Tablets 1670
Zantac 300 Tablets 1670
Zantac Injection 1666
Zantac Injection Premixed 1666
Zantac Syrup 1670

ANTALGIN (Spain)
NAPROXEN SODIUM
Anaprox DS Tablets 2632
Anaprox Tablets 2632

ANTASTEN (Argentina)
CAPTOPRIL
Captopril Tablets 2182

ANTELEPSIN (Czech Republic, Germany)
CLONAZEPAM
Klonopin Tablets 2639

ANTENEX (Australia)
DIAZEPAM
Valium Tablets 2658

ANTEPSIN (Argentina, Brazil, Denmark, Finland, Irish Republic, Italy, Norway, Turkey)
SUCRALFATE
Carafate Suspension 706
Carafate Tablets 707

ANTHEL (Thailand)
ALBENDAZOLE
Albenza Tablets 1297

ANTHRAXITON (Greece)
DICLOFENAC SODIUM
Voltaren Tablets 2334
Voltaren-XR Tablets 2337

ANTI CD3 (Brazil)
MUROMONAB-CD3
Orthoclone OKT3 Sterile Solution 2387

ANTIBACIN (Greece)
CEFTRIAXONE SODIUM
Rocephin Injectable Vials, ADD-Vantage, Galaxy, Bulk 2642

ANTIBIOCILINA (Argentina)
AMOXICILLIN
Amoxil Pediatric Drops for Oral Suspension 1305
Amoxil Tablets 1305

ANTIBIOTREX (France)
ISOTRETINOIN
Accutane Capsules 2607

ANTIBLOC (Argentina)
CARVEDILOL
Coreg Tablets 1387

ANTICHOL (Greece)
SIMVASTATIN
Zocor Tablets 2136

ANTIDIN (Brazil)
RANITIDINE HYDROCHLORIDE
Zantac 25 EFFERdose Tablets 1670
Zantac 150 Tablets 1670
Zantac 300 Tablets 1670
Zantac Injection 1666
Zantac Injection Premixed 1666
Zantac Syrup 1670

ANTI-FOSFAT CA (Turkey)
CALCIUM ACETATE
PhosLo GelCaps 1184

ANTILYSIN (Czech Republic)
APROTININ
Trasylol Injection 799

ANTIMED (Mexico)
CIPROFLOXACIN
Cipro Oral Suspension 2810

ANTIMIGRIN (Austria)
NARATRIPTAN HYDROCHLORIDE
Amerge Tablets 1301

ANTIOBIOCILINA (Argentina)
AMOXICILLIN
Amoxil Pediatric Drops for Oral Suspension 1305
Amoxil Tablets 1305

ANTIPARKIN (Germany)
SELEGILINE HYDROCHLORIDE
Eldepryl Capsules 3052

ANTIPLAQ (Argentina)
CLOPIDOGREL BISULFATE
Plavix Tablets 926, 2767

ANTOPAR (Czech Republic, Hong Kong)
BENZOYL PEROXIDE
Brevoxyl-4 Creamy Wash 3054
Brevoxyl-4 Gel 3054
Brevoxyl-8 Creamy Wash 3054
Brevoxyl-8 Gel 3054

ANTORIL (Argentina)
GEMCITABINE HYDROCHLORIDE
Gemzar for Injection 1820

ANULBET (Chile)
FAMOTIDINE
Pepcid for Oral Suspension 2075
Pepcid Tablets 2075

ANXICALM (Irish Republic)
DIAZEPAM
Valium Tablets 2658

ANXOL (India)
DIAZEPAM
Valium Tablets 2658

ANZEM (South Africa)
DILTIAZEM HYDROCHLORIDE
Cardizem LA Extended Release Tablets 421

AORTEN (Brazil)
CAPTOPRIL
Captopril Tablets 2182

AOVA (Greece)
RANITIDINE HYDROCHLORIDE
Zantac 25 EFFERdose Tablets 1670
Zantac 150 Tablets 1670
Zantac 300 Tablets 1670
Zantac Injection 1666
Zantac Injection Premixed 1666
Zantac Syrup 1670

APARO (Austria)
PAROXETINE HYDROCHLORIDE
Paxil Oral Suspension 1535
Paxil Tablets 1535

APAURIN (Czech Republic, Russia)
DIAZEPAM
Valium Tablets 2658

APECITAB (Argentina)
CAPECITABINE
Xeloda Tablets 2662

APEPLUS (Chile)
FINASTERIDE
Propecia Tablets 2095
Proscar Tablets 2102

APIROL (Israel)
NORFLOXACIN
Noroxin Tablets 2069

A-PLEX (Mexico)
TRETINOIN
Vesanoid Capsules 2660

APLOM (Venezuela)
RANITIDINE HYDROCHLORIDE
Zantac 25 EFFERdose Tablets 1670
Zantac 150 Tablets 1670
Zantac 300 Tablets 1670
Zantac Injection 1666
Zantac Injection Premixed 1666
Zantac Syrup 1670

APO-AMOXI (Hong Kong)
AMOXICILLIN
Amoxil Pediatric Drops for Oral Suspension 1305
Amoxil Tablets 1305

APOBACE (Mexico)
CARBAMAZEPINE
Carbatrol Capsules 3019

APOCAPEN (Israel)
CAPTOPRIL
Captopril Tablets 2182

APO-CAPTO (Canada, Czech Republic, Hong Kong, Malaysia, Russia, Singapore)
CAPTOPRIL
Captopril Tablets 2182

APO-CARVE (Czech Republic)
CARVEDILOL
Coreg Tablets 1387

APO-DICLO (Czech Republic, Malaysia, New Zealand, Russia)
DICLOFENAC SODIUM
Voltaren Tablets 2334
Voltaren-XR Tablets 2337

APO-DILTIAZ (Canada, Hong Kong)
DILTIAZEM HYDROCHLORIDE
Cardizem LA Extended Release Tablets 421

APO-FENO (Canada, Czech Republic, Poland)
FENOFIBRATE
Tricor Tablets 520

APO-FENO-MICRO (Hong Kong, Malaysia)
FENOFIBRATE
Tricor Tablets 520

APOFLOX (Mexico)
CIPROFLOXACIN
Cipro Oral Suspension 2810

APOGASTINE (Israel)
FAMOTIDINE
Pepcid for Oral Suspension 2075
Pepcid Tablets 2075

APO-INDAP (Poland)
INDAPAMIDE
Indapamide Tablets 2188

APO-IPRAVENT (Canada, New Zealand)
IPRATROPIUM BROMIDE
Atrovent Nasal Spray 0.03% 834
Atrovent Nasal Spray 0.06% 836

APOLLONSET (Greece)
DIAZEPAM
Valium Tablets 2658

APO-LOVA (Poland)
LOVASTATIN
Mevacor Tablets 2063

APOMEX (Israel)
SELEGILINE HYDROCHLORIDE
Eldepryl Capsules 3052

(⊙ Described in PDR® For Ophthalmic Medicines)

APOMOXYN (Israel)
AMOXICILLIN
Amoxil Pediatric Drops for Oral Suspension.... 1305
Amoxil Tablets 1305

APONACIN (Israel)
NAPROXEN
EC-Naprosyn Delayed-Release Tablets.... 2632
Naprosyn Suspension.... 2632
Naprosyn Tablets 2632

APO-NADOL (Canada, Hong Kong)
NADOLOL
Nadolol Tablets.... 2191

APO-NAPRO-NA (Canada, Hong Kong, Malaysia, Singapore)
NAPROXEN SODIUM
Anaprox DS Tablets 2632
Anaprox Tablets 2632

APONISTAN V (Mexico)
NYSTATIN
Nystop Topical Powder USP.... 2498

APO-NORFLOX (Canada)
NORFLOXACIN
Noroxin Tablets.... 2069

APO-PAROX (Czech Republic)
PAROXETINE HYDROCHLORIDE
Paxil Oral Suspension.... 1535
Paxil Tablets.... 1535

APO-SELEG (Czech Republic)
SELEGILINE HYDROCHLORIDE
Eldepryl Capsules 3052

APO-SELIN (Poland)
SELEGILINE HYDROCHLORIDE
Eldepryl Capsules 3052

APO-SIMVA (Czech Republic)
SIMVASTATIN
Zocor Tablets.... 2136

APO-SULIN (Canada, Malaysia)
SULINDAC
Clinoril Tablets 1962

APOTEOPROL (Mexico)
THEOPHYLLINE
Uniphyl Tablets 2595

APO-THEO (Canada, Hong Kong, Malaysia, Singapore)
THEOPHYLLINE
Uniphyl Tablets 2595

APOTIL (Israel)
TIMOLOL MALEATE
Timoptic in Ocudose 2124
Timoptic Sterile Ophthalmic Solution 2121
Timoptic-XE Sterile Ophthalmic Gel Forming Solution 2125

APO-TIMOL (Canada, New Zealand)
TIMOLOL MALEATE
Timoptic in Ocudose 2124
Timoptic Sterile Ophthalmic Solution 2121
Timoptic-XE Sterile Ophthalmic Gel Forming Solution 2125

APO-TIMOP (Canada, Hong Kong, New Zealand)
TIMOLOL MALEATE
Timoptic in Ocudose 2124
Timoptic Sterile Ophthalmic Solution 2121
Timoptic-XE Sterile Ophthalmic Gel Forming Solution 2125

APO-TRIAZIDE (Hong Kong, Russia, Singapore)
HYDROCHLOROTHIAZIDE/TRIAMTERENE
Dyazide Capsules 1405

APOVEN (Australia)
IPRATROPIUM BROMIDE
Atrovent Nasal Spray 0.03%.... 834
Atrovent Nasal Spray 0.06%.... 836

APOVENT (Israel)
IPRATROPIUM BROMIDE
Atrovent Nasal Spray 0.03%.... 834
Atrovent Nasal Spray 0.06%.... 836

APOZAN (Israel)
RANITIDINE HYDROCHLORIDE
Zantac 25 EFFERdose Tablets 1670
Zantac 150 Tablets 1670
Zantac 300 Tablets 1670
Zantac Injection 1666
Zantac Injection Premixed 1666
Zantac Syrup 1670

APOZEPAM (Denmark, Sweden)
DIAZEPAM
Valium Tablets 2658

APRACUR BIOTIC (Argentina)
AMOXICILLIN
Amoxil Pediatric Drops for Oral Suspension.... 1305
Amoxil Tablets 1305

APRA-GEL (Belgium)
NAPROXEN
EC-Naprosyn Delayed-Release Tablets.... 2632
Naprosyn Suspension.... 2632
Naprosyn Tablets 2632

APRALJIN (Turkey)
NAPROXEN SODIUM
Anaprox DS Tablets 2632
Anaprox Tablets 2632

APRANAX (Belgium, France, Hungary, Switzerland, Turkey, Venezuela)
NAPROXEN SODIUM
Anaprox DS Tablets 2632
Anaprox Tablets 2632

APROL (Turkey)
NAPROXEN SODIUM
Anaprox DS Tablets 2632
Anaprox Tablets 2632

APROMED (Turkey)
NAPROXEN SODIUM
Anaprox DS Tablets 2632
Anaprox Tablets 2632

APROTEX (Russia)
APROTININ
Trasylol Injection 799

APROVEL (Argentina, Belgium, Brazil, Chile, Czech Republic, Denmark, Finland, France, Germany, Greece, Hong Kong, Hungary, Italy, Malaysia, Mexico, Norway, Russia, Singapore, South Africa, Spain, Thailand, The Philippines, Venezuela)
IRBESARTAN
Avapro Tablets 897

APROVEL HCT (Hong Kong, Thailand)
IRBESARTAN
Avapro Tablets 897

APROWELL (Turkey)
NAPROXEN SODIUM
Anaprox DS Tablets 2632
Anaprox Tablets 2632

APROZIDE (Brazil)
IRBESARTAN
Avapro Tablets 897

APUZIN (Malaysia)
CAPTOPRIL
Captopril Tablets.... 2182

AQUANIL (Denmark, Finland, Norway, Sweden)
TIMOLOL MALEATE
Timoptic in Ocudose 2124
Timoptic Sterile Ophthalmic Solution 2121
Timoptic-XE Sterile Ophthalmic Gel Forming Solution 2125

AQUARID (South Africa)
FUROSEMIDE
Furosemide Tablets 2186

AQUEDUX (Portugal)
FUROSEMIDE
Furosemide Tablets 2186

AQUIFY (Argentina)
SODIUM HYALURONATE
Hyalgan Solution.... 2742

ARADOIS (Brazil)
LOSARTAN POTASSIUM
Cozaar Tablets 1973

ARADOIS H (Brazil)
LOSARTAN POTASSIUM
Cozaar Tablets 1973

ARATAN (Chile)
LOSARTAN POTASSIUM
Cozaar Tablets 1973

ARBIL (United Kingdom)
CARBAMAZEPINE
Carbatrol Capsules 3019

ARCANAFENAC (South Africa)
DICLOFENAC SODIUM
Voltaren Tablets 2334
Voltaren-XR Tablets 2337

ARCANAMIDE (South Africa)
FUROSEMIDE
Furosemide Tablets 2186

ARCID (Spain)
RANITIDINE HYDROCHLORIDE
Zantac 25 EFFERdose Tablets 1670
Zantac 150 Tablets 1670
Zantac 300 Tablets 1670
Zantac Injection 1666
Zantac Injection Premixed 1666
Zantac Syrup 1670

ARCLONAC (Thailand)
DICLOFENAC SODIUM
Voltaren Tablets 2334
Voltaren-XR Tablets 2337

ARCOIRAN (Spain)
SUMATRIPTAN SUCCINATE
Imitrex Injection 1465
Imitrex Tablets 1474

ARDORAL (Spain)
RANITIDINE HYDROCHLORIDE
Zantac 25 EFFERdose Tablets 1670
Zantac 150 Tablets 1670
Zantac 300 Tablets 1670
Zantac Injection 1666
Zantac Injection Premixed 1666
Zantac Syrup 1670

ARENDAL (Argentina, Chile)
ALENDRONATE SODIUM
Fosamax Tablets 2005

AREPLEX (Poland)
CLOPIDOGREL BISULFATE
Plavix Tablets 926, 2767

ARFLOXINA (Mexico)
CIPROFLOXACIN
Cipro Oral Suspension 2810

ARGEFLOX (Argentina)
CIPROFLOXACIN HYDROCHLORIDE
Cipro Tablets 2810

ARIAL (Italy)
SALMETEROL XINAFOATE
Serevent Diskus 1594

ARICEPT (Australia, Austria, Belgium, Canada, Czech Republic, Denmark, Finland, France, Greece, Hong Kong, Hungary, Irish Republic, Israel, Italy, Japan, Malaysia, New Zealand, Norway, Poland, Portugal, Singapore, South Africa, Spain, Sweden, Switzerland, Thailand, The Philippines, Turkey, United Kingdom)
DONEPEZIL HYDROCHLORIDE
Aricept Tablets 1062

ARIDIL (United Kingdom)
FUROSEMIDE
Furosemide Tablets 2186

ARIFON (Russia)
INDAPAMIDE
Indapamide Tablets 2188

ARIMIDEX (Argentina, Australia, Austria, Belgium, Brazil, Canada, Chile, Czech Republic, Denmark, Finland, France, Greece, Hong Kong, Hungary, Irish Republic, Israel, Italy, Malaysia, Mexico, New Zealand, Norway, Poland, Portugal, Russia, Singapore, South Africa, Spain, Sweden, Switzerland, Thailand, The Netherlands, The Philippines, Turkey, United Kingdom, Venezuela)
ANASTROZOLE
Arimidex Tablets 672

ARISTIN-C (Greece)
CIPROFLOXACIN
Cipro Oral Suspension 2810

ARISTO (Hong Kong)
TRIAMCINOLONE ACETONIDE
Azmacort Inhalation Aerosol.... 407
Nasacort AQ Nasal Spray 2765

ARISTOCORT (Australia, Hong Kong, New Zealand, Thailand)
TRIAMCINOLONE ACETONIDE
Azmacort Inhalation Aerosol.... 407
Nasacort AQ Nasal Spray 2765

ARISTROL (India)
CALCITRIOL
Calcijex Injection 419
Rocaltrol Capsules.... 1150
Rocaltrol Oral Solution 1150

ARISTROL FORTE (India)
CALCITRIOL
Calcijex Injection 419
Rocaltrol Capsules.... 1150
Rocaltrol Oral Solution 1150

ARKAMIN (India)
CLONIDINE HYDROCHLORIDE
Catapres Tablets 841

ARKAMIN-H (India)
CLONIDINE HYDROCHLORIDE
Catapres Tablets 841

ARMISTOR (Mexico)
ESTRADIOL
Climara Transdermal System 763

ARMONIL (Italy)
ESTRADIOL
Climara Transdermal System 763

ARMOPHYLLINE (France)
THEOPHYLLINE
Uniphyl Tablets 2595

ARMOTRAZ (India)
ANASTROZOLE
Arimidex Tablets 672

ARMOXIN (Mexico)
AMOXICILLIN
Amoxil Pediatric Drops for Oral Suspension.... 1305
Amoxil Tablets 1305

ARNETIN (Czech Republic, Malaysia)
RANITIDINE HYDROCHLORIDE
Zantac 150 Tablets 1670
Zantac 25 EFFERdose Tablets 1670
Zantac 300 Tablets 1670
Zantac Injection 1666
Zantac Injection Premixed 1666
Zantac Syrup 1670

AROMENAL (Argentina)
ANASTROZOLE
Arimidex Tablets 672

AROPAX (Argentina, Australia, Belgium, Brazil, Mexico, New Zealand, South Africa, Spain)
PAROXETINE HYDROCHLORIDE
Paxil Oral Suspension.... 1535
Paxil Tablets.... 1535

AROXAT (Chile)
PAROXETINE HYDROCHLORIDE
Paxil Oral Suspension.... 1535
Paxil Tablets.... 1535

ARRETIN (Mexico, Poland)
TRETINOIN
Vesanoid Capsules.... 2660

ARSENAL (Mexico)
NAPROXEN
EC-Naprosyn Delayed-Release Tablets.... 2632
Naprosyn Suspension.... 2632
Naprosyn Tablets 2632

ARSENAL COMPUESTO (Mexico)
NAPROXEN SODIUM
Anaprox DS Tablets 2632
Anaprox Tablets 2632

ARTAGEN (India, Thailand)
NAPROXEN
EC-Naprosyn Delayed-Release Tablets.... 2632
Naprosyn Suspension.... 2632
Naprosyn Tablets 2632

ARTEROSAN (Chile)
SIMVASTATIN
Zocor Tablets.... 2136

ARTESOL (Chile)
CILOSTAZOL
Pletal Tablets 2481

ARTFLEX (Argentina)
SODIUM HYALURONATE
Hyalgan Solution.... 2742

ARTHOTEC (Germany)
DICLOFENAC SODIUM
Voltaren Tablets 2334

Voltaren-XR Tablets 2337

ARTHREASE (Germany, Israel, United Kingdom)
SODIUM HYALURONATE
Hyalgan Solution 2742

ARTHREX (Germany)
DICLOFENAC SODIUM
Voltaren Tablets 2334
Voltaren-XR Tablets 2337

ARTHREX DUO (Germany)
DICLOFENAC SODIUM
Voltaren Tablets 2334
Voltaren-XR Tablets 2337

ARTHROCINE (France)
SULINDAC
Clinoril Tablets 1962

ARTHROSIN (United Kingdom)
NAPROXEN
EC-Naprosyn Delayed-Release Tablets 2632
Naprosyn Suspension 2632
Naprosyn Tablets 2632

ARTHROTEC (Australia, Austria, Belgium, Canada, Czech Republic, Denmark, Finland, Greece, Hong Kong, Irish Republic, Israel, Norway, Poland, Portugal, Russia, Singapore, South Africa, Sweden, Switzerland, Thailand, The Netherlands, United Kingdom, Venezuela)
DICLOFENAC SODIUM
Voltaren Tablets 2334
Voltaren-XR Tablets 2337

ARTHROXEN (United Kingdom)
NAPROXEN
EC-Naprosyn Delayed-Release Tablets 2632
Naprosyn Suspension 2632
Naprosyn Tablets 2632

ARTHRU-DERM (South Africa)
DICLOFENAC SODIUM
Voltaren Tablets 2334
Voltaren-XR Tablets 2337

ARTHRUM H (France)
SODIUM HYALURONATE
Hyalgan Solution 2742

ARTILOG (Italy)
CELECOXIB
Celebrex Capsules 2979

ARTONIL (Sweden)
RANITIDINE HYDROCHLORIDE
Zantac 25 EFFERdose Tablets 1670
Zantac 150 Tablets 1670
Zantac 300 Tablets 1670
Zantac Injection 1666
Zantac Injection Premixed 1666
Zantac Syrup 1670

ARTOTEC (France)
DICLOFENAC SODIUM
Voltaren Tablets 2334
Voltaren-XR Tablets 2337

ARTREN (Brazil, Venezuela)
DICLOFENAC SODIUM
Voltaren Tablets 2334
Voltaren-XR Tablets 2337

ARTRENAC (Mexico)
DICLOFENAC SODIUM
Voltaren Tablets 2334
Voltaren-XR Tablets 2337

ARTRENAC PRO (Mexico)
DICLOFENAC SODIUM
Voltaren Tablets 2334
Voltaren-XR Tablets 2337

ARTRENE (Mexico)
DICLOFENAC SODIUM
Voltaren Tablets 2334
Voltaren-XR Tablets 2337

ARTRIBID (Portugal)
SULINDAC
Clinoril Tablets 1962

ARTROFENAC (Italy)
DICLOFENAC SODIUM
Voltaren Tablets 2334
Voltaren-XR Tablets 2337

ARTRON (Mexico)
NAPROXEN
EC-Naprosyn Delayed-Release Tablets 2632
Naprosyn Suspension 2632
Naprosyn Tablets 2632

ARTROTEC (Italy, Mexico, Spain, The Netherlands)
DICLOFENAC SODIUM
Voltaren Tablets 2334
Voltaren-XR Tablets 2337

ARTROXEN (Italy)
NAPROXEN
EC-Naprosyn Delayed-Release Tablets 2632
Naprosyn Suspension 2632
Naprosyn Tablets 2632

ARTZ (Denmark, Italy)
SODIUM HYALURONATE
Hyalgan Solution 2742

ARTZAL (Austria, Finland, Sweden)
SODIUM HYALURONATE
Hyalgan Solution 2742

ARUCLONIN (Czech Republic, Germany, Hungary)
CLONIDINE HYDROCHLORIDE
Catapres Tablets 841

ARUDEL (Spain)
SIMVASTATIN
Zocor Tablets 2136

ARUTIMOL (Czech Republic, Hungary, Russia)
TIMOLOL MALEATE
Timoptic in Ocudose 2124
Timoptic Sterile Ophthalmic Solution 2121
Timoptic-XE Sterile Ophthalmic Gel Forming Solution 2125

ARUTRIN (Germany)
TRIAMCINOLONE ACETONIDE
Azmacort Inhalation Aerosol 407
Nasacort AQ Nasal Spray 2765

ARUTROPID (Germany)
IPRATROPIUM BROMIDE
Atrovent Nasal Spray 0.03% 834
Atrovent Nasal Spray 0.06% 836

ARXEN (Mexico)
NAPROXEN
EC-Naprosyn Delayed-Release Tablets 2632
Naprosyn Suspension 2632
Naprosyn Tablets 2632

ARXEN COMPOSITUM (Mexico)
NAPROXEN
EC-Naprosyn Delayed-Release Tablets 2632
Naprosyn Suspension 2632
Naprosyn Tablets 2632

ARYTHMOL (Irish Republic, United Kingdom)
PROPAFENONE HYDROCHLORIDE
Rythmol SR Capsules 1590

ARZEDYN (Greece)
CETIRIZINE HYDROCHLORIDE
Zyrtec Syrup 1920
Zyrtec Tablets 1920

ARZEPAM (Mexico)
DIAZEPAM
Valium Tablets 2658

ASASANTIN (Australia, Austria, Denmark, Finland, Hungary, Mexico, Sweden, The Netherlands)
DIPYRIDAMOLE
Persantine Tablets 869

ASASANTINE (France)
DIPYRIDAMOLE
Persantine Tablets 869

ASAX (Chile)
FUROSEMIDE
Furosemide Tablets 2186

ASENTA (Israel)
DONEPEZIL HYDROCHLORIDE
Aricept Tablets 1062

ASIOLEX (Argentina)
ANASTROZOLE
Arimidex Tablets 672

ASMABIOL (Argentina)
THEOPHYLLINE
Uniphyl Tablets 2595

ASMAFLU (Italy)
FLUNISOLIDE
Aerobid Inhaler System 1153
Aerobid-M Inhaler System 1153

ASMANEX (Austria, Brazil, Czech Republic, Denmark, Finland, Germany, Greece, Irish Republic, New Zealand, Spain, Sweden, Switzerland, The Netherlands, United Kingdom, Venezuela)
MOMETASONE FUROATE
Elocon Cream 0.1% 2840
Elocon Lotion 0.1% 2841
Elocon Ointment 0.1% 2842
Nasonex Nasal Spray 2883

ASMASOLON (The Philippines)
THEOPHYLLINE
Uniphyl Tablets 2595

ASMATIL (Portugal)
FLUTICASONE PROPIONATE
Flonase Nasal Spray 1431

ASMO (Spain)
THEOPHYLLINE
Uniphyl Tablets 2595

ASMO-LAVI (Portugal)
FLUTICASONE PROPIONATE
Flonase Nasal Spray 1431

ASODOCEL (Argentina)
DOCETAXEL
Taxotere Injection Concentrate 2773

ASONACOR (Austria)
PROPAFENONE HYDROCHLORIDE
Rythmol SR Capsules 1590

ASPASERINE B6 TRANQ (Spain)
DIAZEPAM
Valium Tablets 2658

ASPENIL (Italy)
AMOXICILLIN
Amoxil Pediatric Drops for Oral Suspension 1305
Amoxil Tablets 1305

ASSIVAL (Israel)
DIAZEPAM
Valium Tablets 2658

ASSOLID (Italy)
FLUNISOLIDE
Aerobid Inhaler System 1153
Aerobid-M Inhaler System 1153

ASTHMA T (Israel)
THEOPHYLLINE
Uniphyl Tablets 2595

ASTMEROLE (Turkey)
SALMETEROL XINAFOATE
Serevent Diskus 1594

ASTRAMORPH (Brazil)
MORPHINE SULFATE
MS Contin Tablets 2585

ASUCROSE (India)
ACARBOSE
Precose Tablets 792

ASYTEC (Denmark)
CETIRIZINE HYDROCHLORIDE
Zyrtec Syrup 1920
Zyrtec Tablets 1920

ATAC (Chile)
NAPROXEN SODIUM
Anaprox DS Tablets 2632
Anaprox Tablets 2632

ATACAND (Argentina, Australia, Austria, Belgium, Brazil, Canada, Chile, Czech Republic, Denmark, Finland, France, Greece, Hungary, Irish Republic, Israel, Malaysia, Mexico, New Zealand, Norway, Poland, Portugal, Russia, Singapore, South Africa, Spain, Sweden, Switzerland, The Netherlands, Turkey, Venezuela)
CANDESARTAN CILEXETIL
Atacand Tablets 639

ATACAND PLUS (Australia, Belgium, Canada, Czech Republic, Hungary, Israel, Malaysia, Mexico, Norway, Singapore, South Africa, Spain, Switzerland, The Netherlands, Turkey, Venezuela)
CANDESARTAN CILEXETIL
Atacand Tablets 639

ATACAND-D (Argentina)
CANDESARTAN CILEXETIL
Atacand Tablets 639

ATACANDZID (Denmark)
CANDESARTAN CILEXETIL
Atacand Tablets 639

ATARVA (Argentina)
ATORVASTATIN CALCIUM
Lipitor Tablets 2501

ATARVITON (Greece)
DIAZEPAM
Valium Tablets 2658

ATAZID (Denmark)
CANDESARTAN CILEXETIL
Atacand Tablets 639

ATEM (Italy)
IPRATROPIUM BROMIDE
Atrovent Nasal Spray 0.03% 834
Atrovent Nasal Spray 0.06% 836

ATEMUR (Germany)
FLUTICASONE PROPIONATE
Flonase Nasal Spray 1431

ATENFAR (Chile)
ATORVASTATIN CALCIUM
Lipitor Tablets 2501

ATENIX (Chile)
SIBUTRAMINE HYDROCHLORIDE
Meridia Capsules 475

ATENSINA (Brazil)
CLONIDINE HYDROCHLORIDE
Catapres Tablets 841

ATENSINE (Irish Republic, United Kingdom)
DIAZEPAM
Valium Tablets 2658

ATERKEY (Spain)
LOVASTATIN
Mevacor Tablets 2063

ATEROCLAR (Argentina)
ATORVASTATIN CALCIUM
Lipitor Tablets 2501

ATHROFEN (Switzerland)
DICLOFENAC SODIUM
Voltaren Tablets 2334
Voltaren-XR Tablets 2337

ATIBAX C (Argentina)
CIPROFLOXACIN
Cipro Oral Suspension 2810

ATIFLAN (Mexico)
NAPROXEN
EC-Naprosyn Delayed-Release Tablets 2632
Naprosyn Suspension 2632
Naprosyn Tablets 2632

A-TINIC (Thailand)
TRETINOIN
Vesanoid Capsules 2660

ATLACNE (Argentina)
ISOTRETINOIN
Accutane Capsules 2607

ATORLIP (Chile, India)
ATORVASTATIN CALCIUM
Lipitor Tablets 2501

ATORVA (India)
ATORVASTATIN CALCIUM
Lipitor Tablets 2501

ATRAM (Poland)
CARVEDILOL
Coreg Tablets 1387

ATREDERM (Poland)
TRETINOIN
Vesanoid Capsules 2660

ATRISER (Mexico)
SULINDAC
Clinoril Tablets 1962

ATRISOL (Mexico)
CAPTOPRIL
Captopril Tablets 2182

ATRIVAL (Argentina)
AMOXICILLIN
Amoxil Pediatric Drops for Oral Suspension 1305

Amoxil Tablets 1305

ATROMBIN (Finland)
DIPYRIDAMOLE
Persantine Tablets 869

ATRONASE (Austria, Belgium, South Africa)
IPRATROPIUM BROMIDE
Atrovent Nasal Spray 0.03% 834
Atrovent Nasal Spray 0.06% 836

ATROVENT (Argentina, Australia, Austria, Belgium, Brazil, Canada, Chile, Czech Republic, Denmark, Finland, France, Germany, Greece, Hong Kong, Hungary, Irish Republic, Israel, Italy, Japan, Malaysia, Mexico, New Zealand, Norway, Poland, Portugal, Russia, Singapore, South Africa, Spain, Sweden, Switzerland, Thailand, The Netherlands, The Philippines, Turkey, United Kingdom)
IPRATROPIUM BROMIDE
Atrovent Nasal Spray 0.03% 834
Atrovent Nasal Spray 0.06% 836

ATROX (Poland)
ATORVASTATIN CALCIUM
Lipitor Tablets 2501

ATROZOL (Poland)
ANASTROZOLE
Arimidex Tablets 672

ATTOR (India)
ATORVASTATIN CALCIUM
Lipitor Tablets 2501

AT-V (Mexico)
DIAZEPAM
Valium Tablets 2658

AUDOCAINA (Venezuela)
LIDOCAINE
Lidoderm Patch 1114

AUGELIT (Brazil)
DICLOFENAC SODIUM
Voltaren Tablets 2334
Voltaren-XR Tablets 2337

AUGMENTIN (Turkey)
AMOXICILLIN
Amoxil Pediatric Drops for Oral Suspension 1305
Amoxil Tablets 1305

AUGMENTIN BID (Venezuela)
AMOXICILLIN
Amoxil Pediatric Drops for Oral Suspension 1305
Amoxil Tablets 1305

AUGMEX (Singapore)
AMOXICILLIN
Amoxil Pediatric Drops for Oral Suspension 1305
Amoxil Tablets 1305

AUGURCIN (The Philippines)
AMOXICILLIN
Amoxil Pediatric Drops for Oral Suspension 1305
Amoxil Tablets 1305

AUREX (Poland)
CITALOPRAM HYDROBROMIDE
Celexa Tablets 1160

AURODIPINE (Greece)
NIMODIPINE
Nimotop Capsules 790

AUROFOX (Mexico)
CEFTRIAXONE SODIUM
Rocephin Injectable Vials, ADD-Vantage, Galaxy, Bulk 2642

AUROSTATIN (Greece)
LOVASTATIN
Mevacor Tablets 2063

AUSCARD (Australia)
DILTIAZEM HYDROCHLORIDE
Cardizem LA Extended Release Tablets 421

AUSFAM (Australia, Hong Kong)
FAMOTIDINE
Pepcid for Oral Suspension 2075
Pepcid Tablets 2075

AUSRAN (Australia)
RANITIDINE HYDROCHLORIDE
Zantac 25 EFFERdose Tablets 1670
Zantac 150 Tablets 1670
Zantac 300 Tablets 1670
Zantac Injection 1666
Zantac Injection Premixed 1666
Zantac Syrup 1670

AUSTYN (Australia, Singapore)
THEOPHYLLINE
Uniphyl Tablets 2595

AUTDOL (Chile)
DICLOFENAC SODIUM
Voltaren Tablets 2334
Voltaren-XR Tablets 2337

AUXXIL (Chile)
LEVOFLOXACIN
Levaquin Injection 2416
Levaquin Tablets 2416

AVALIDE (Mexico)
IRBESARTAN
Avapro Tablets 897

AVANDAMET (Argentina, Australia, Belgium, Canada, Chile, Denmark, Finland, France, Germany, Greece, Irish Republic, Italy, Malaysia, Mexico, Norway, Poland, Singapore, Sweden, Switzerland, The Netherlands, The Philippines, United Kingdom, Venezuela)
ROSIGLITAZONE MALEATE
Avandia Tablets 1351

AVANDIA (Argentina, Australia, Belgium, Brazil, Canada, Chile, Czech Republic, Denmark, Finland, France, Germany, Greece, Hong Kong, Hungary, Irish Republic, Israel, Italy, Malaysia, Mexico, New Zealand, Norway, Poland, Portugal, Singapore, South Africa, Spain, Sweden, Switzerland, Thailand, The Netherlands, The Philippines, Turkey, United Kingdom, Venezuela)
ROSIGLITAZONE MALEATE
Avandia Tablets 1351

AVAPRO (Argentina, Australia, Brazil, Mexico)
IRBESARTAN
Avapro Tablets 897

AVAPRO HCT (Argentina, Australia)
IRBESARTAN
Avapro Tablets 897

AVASTINEE (Hong Kong)
SIMVASTATIN
Zocor Tablets 2136

AVERTEX (Argentina)
FINASTERIDE
Propecia Tablets 2095
Proscar Tablets 2102

AVICIS (Brazil)
ESTRADIOL
Climara Transdermal System 763

AVILAC (Israel)
LACTULOSE
Kristalose for Oral Solution 1004

AVITCID (Finland)
TRETINOIN
Vesanoid Capsules 2660

AVLOSULFON (Canada, Israel)
DAPSONE
Dapsone Tablets USP 1746

AVUXILAN (Mexico)
AMOXICILLIN
Amoxil Pediatric Drops for Oral Suspension 1305
Amoxil Tablets 1305

AXACEF (Denmark, Sweden)
CEFUROXIME SODIUM
Zinacef Injection 1678

AXANT (Chile)
LACTULOSE
Kristalose for Oral Solution 1004

AXCIL (Mexico)
AMOXICILLIN
Amoxil Pediatric Drops for Oral Suspension 1305
Amoxil Tablets 1305

AXELVIN (Greece)
LISINOPRIL
Prinivil Tablets 2087

AXER (Italy)
NAPROXEN SODIUM
Anaprox DS Tablets 2632
Anaprox Tablets 2632

AXETINE (Belgium, Czech Republic, Hong Kong, Russia, Thailand)
CEFUROXIME AXETIL
Ceftin for Oral Suspension 1380
Ceftin Tablets 1380

AXOBAT (Italy)
CEFTRIAXONE SODIUM
Rocephin Injectable Vials, ADD-Vantage, Galaxy, Bulk 2642

AXONE (India)
CEFTRIAXONE SODIUM
Rocephin Injectable Vials, ADD-Vantage, Galaxy, Bulk 2642

AXOTIDE (Switzerland)
FLUTICASONE PROPIONATE
Flonase Nasal Spray 1431

AXTAR (Mexico)
CEFTRIAXONE SODIUM
Rocephin Injectable Vials, ADD-Vantage, Galaxy, Bulk 2642

AXUROCEF (Thailand)
CEFUROXIME AXETIL
Ceftin for Oral Suspension 1380
Ceftin Tablets 1380

AYRA (Turkey)
CANDESARTAN CILEXETIL
Atacand Tablets 639

AZANTAC (France, Mexico, The Netherlands)
RANITIDINE HYDROCHLORIDE
Zantac 150 Tablets 1670
Zantac 25 EFFERdose Tablets 1670
Zantac 300 Tablets 1670
Zantac Injection 1666
Zantac Injection Premixed 1666
Zantac Syrup 1670

AZATYL (Greece)
CEFTRIAXONE SODIUM
Rocephin Injectable Vials, ADD-Vantage, Galaxy, Bulk 2642

AZEPAL (Hungary)
CARBAMAZEPINE
Carbatrol Capsules 3019

AZEPAM (Thailand)
DIAZEPAM
Valium Tablets 2658

AZETAVIR (Mexico)
ZIDOVUDINE
Retrovir Capsules 1574
Retrovir IV Infusion 1579
Retrovir Syrup 1574
Retrovir Tablets 1574

AZILIV (Brazil)
RANITIDINE HYDROCHLORIDE
Zantac 25 EFFERdose Tablets 1670
Zantac 150 Tablets 1670
Zantac 300 Tablets 1670
Zantac Injection 1666
Zantac Injection Premixed 1666
Zantac Syrup 1670

AZIMAX (Spain)
ZAFIRLUKAST
Accolate Tablets 669

AZMACORT (Brazil, Canada, Czech Republic)
TRIAMCINOLONE ACETONIDE
Azmacort Inhalation Aerosol 407
Nasacort AQ Nasal Spray 2765

AZOAZOL (Argentina)
ZIDOVUDINE
Retrovir Capsules 1574
Retrovir IV Infusion 1579
Retrovir Syrup 1574
Retrovir Tablets 1574

AZOPT (Argentina, Australia, Austria, Belgium, Brazil, Canada, Chile, Czech Republic, Denmark, Finland, France, Germany, Greece, Hong Kong, Hungary, Irish Republic, Israel, Italy, Malaysia, Mexico, New Zealand, Norway, Poland, Portugal, Russia, Singapore, Spain, Sweden, Switzerland, Thailand, The Netherlands, The Philippines, Turkey, United Kingdom, Venezuela)
BRINZOLAMIDE
Azopt Ophthalmic Suspension 540

AZOPTIC (South Africa)
BRINZOLAMIDE
Azopt Ophthalmic Suspension 540

AZOTINE (Argentina)
ZIDOVUDINE
Retrovir Capsules 1574
Retrovir IV Infusion 1579
Retrovir Syrup 1574
Retrovir Tablets 1574

AZOVIR (Poland)
ZIDOVUDINE
Retrovir Capsules 1574
Retrovir IV Infusion 1579
Retrovir Syrup 1574
Retrovir Tablets 1574

AZURANIT (Germany)
RANITIDINE HYDROCHLORIDE
Zantac 25 EFFERdose Tablets 1670
Zantac 150 Tablets 1670
Zantac 300 Tablets 1670
Zantac Injection 1666
Zantac Injection Premixed 1666
Zantac Syrup 1670

BACCIDAL (Japan, Spain)
NORFLOXACIN
Noroxin Tablets 2069

BACIGYL (India)
NORFLOXACIN
Noroxin Tablets 2069

BACIGYL-N (India)
NORFLOXACIN
Noroxin Tablets 2069

BACIPRO (Venezuela)
CIPROFLOXACIN
Cipro Oral Suspension 2810

BACPROIN (Mexico)
CIPROFLOXACIN HYDROCHLORIDE
Cipro Tablets 2810

BACROCIN (Brazil)
MUPIROCIN
Bactroban Ointment 1368

BACTEX (Thailand)
MUPIROCIN
Bactroban Ointment 1368

BACTIFLOX (Malaysia)
CIPROFLOXACIN HYDROCHLORIDE
Cipro Tablets 2810

BACTIFREE (The Philippines)
MUPIROCIN
Bactroban Ointment 1368

BACTIMED (Belgium)
AMOXICILLIN
Amoxil Pediatric Drops for Oral Suspension 1305
Amoxil Tablets 1305

BACTODERM (Israel)
MUPIROCIN
Bactroban Ointment 1368

BACTOQUIN (India)
CIPROFLOXACIN HYDROCHLORIDE
Cipro Tablets 2810

BACTRACID (Germany)
NORFLOXACIN
Noroxin Tablets 2069

BACTROBAN (Argentina, Australia, Belgium, Brazil, Chile, Czech Republic, France, Greece, Hong Kong, Hungary, India, Japan, Malaysia, Mexico, New Zealand, Poland, Portugal, Russia, Singapore, South Africa, Spain, Thailand, The Philippines, Turkey, United Kingdom, Venezuela)
MUPIROCIN CALCIUM
Bactroban Cream 2% 1366

Bactroban Nasal 2% ... 1367

BACTROBANDOS (Venezuela)
MUPIROCIN CALCIUM
Bactroban Cream 2% ... 1366
Bactroban Nasal 2% ... 1367

BACTRONEO (Brazil)
MUPIROCIN
Bactroban Ointment ... 1368

BAC-ZIDIM (Mexico)
CEFTAZIDIME
Fortaz for Injection ... 1450

BAFLOX (Venezuela)
CIPROFLOXACIN
Cipro Oral Suspension ... 2810

BAJATEN (Argentina)
INDAPAMIDE
Indapamide Tablets ... 2188

B-ALCERIN (Greece)
RANITIDINE HYDROCHLORIDE
Zantac 25 EFFERdose Tablets ... 1670
Zantac 150 Tablets ... 1670
Zantac 300 Tablets ... 1670
Zantac Injection ... 1666
Zantac Injection Premixed ... 1666
Zantac Syrup ... 1670

BALCOR (Brazil, Portugal)
DILTIAZEM HYDROCHLORIDE
Cardizem LA Extended Release Tablets ... 421

BALEPTON (Greece)
CIPROFLOXACIN HYDROCHLORIDE
Cipro Tablets ... 2810

BANATIN (Greece)
FAMOTIDINE
Pepcid for Oral Suspension ... 2075
Pepcid Tablets ... 2075

BANTIX (Chile)
MUPIROCIN CALCIUM
Bactroban Cream 2% ... 1366
Bactroban Nasal 2% ... 1367

BARAZAN (Germany)
NORFLOXACIN
Noroxin Tablets ... 2069

BARCLYD (France)
CLONIDINE HYDROCHLORIDE
Catapres Tablets ... 841

BAROXAL (Greece)
RANITIDINE HYDROCHLORIDE
Zantac 25 EFFERdose Tablets ... 1670
Zantac 150 Tablets ... 1670
Zantac 300 Tablets ... 1670
Zantac Injection ... 1666
Zantac Injection Premixed ... 1666
Zantac Syrup ... 1670

BASIRON (Denmark, Finland, Norway, Russia, Sweden, Switzerland, The Netherlands)
BENZOYL PEROXIDE
Brevoxyl-4 Creamy Wash ... 3054
Brevoxyl-4 Gel ... 3054
Brevoxyl-8 Creamy Wash ... 3054
Brevoxyl-8 Gel ... 3054

BAXAMED (Mexico)
NORFLOXACIN
Noroxin Tablets ... 2069

BAXIDYME (The Philippines)
CEFTAZIDIME
Fortaz for Injection ... 1450

BAZETHAM (Poland)
TAMSULOSIN HYDROCHLORIDE
Flomax Capsules ... 848

BEATIZEM (Singapore)
DILTIAZEM HYDROCHLORIDE
Cardizem LA Extended Release Tablets ... 421

BECABIL (Spain)
AMOXICILLIN
Amoxil Pediatric Drops for Oral Suspension ... 1305
Amoxil Tablets ... 1305

BECENUN (Brazil, Denmark, Norway, Sweden)
CARMUSTINE
Gliadel Wafer ... 1076

BECONASE ALLERGY (Australia)
FLUTICASONE PROPIONATE
Flonase Nasal Spray ... 1431

BECTAM (Chile)
PAROXETINE HYDROCHLORIDE
Paxil Oral Suspension ... 1535
Paxil Tablets ... 1535

BEDOL (United Kingdom)
ESTRADIOL
Climara Transdermal System ... 763

BEFIMAT (Greece)
NIMODIPINE
Nimotop Capsules ... 790

BEGLAN (Spain)
SALMETEROL XINAFOATE
Serevent Diskus ... 1594

BEILANDE (Hong Kong)
FAMOTIDINE
Pepcid for Oral Suspension ... 2075
Pepcid Tablets ... 2075

BEKNOL (Mexico)
BENZONATATE
Tessalon Perles ... 1183

BEL (Germany)
SIMVASTATIN
Zocor Tablets ... 2136

BELMACINA (Spain)
CIPROFLOXACIN HYDROCHLORIDE
Cipro Tablets ... 2810

BELMALAX (Spain)
LACTULOSE
Kristalose for Oral Solution ... 1004

BELMALIP (Spain)
SIMVASTATIN
Zocor Tablets ... 2136

BELOC (Turkey)
METOPROLOL SUCCINATE
Toprol-XL Tablets ... 666

BELOC-ZOK (Switzerland)
METOPROLOL SUCCINATE
Toprol-XL Tablets ... 666

BELOKEN (Spain)
METOPROLOL SUCCINATE
Toprol-XL Tablets ... 666

BELOZOK (Argentina)
METOPROLOL SUCCINATE
Toprol-XL Tablets ... 666

BEMPLAS (Argentina)
CLONIDINE HYDROCHLORIDE
Catapres Tablets ... 841

BENACNE (Portugal)
BENZOYL PEROXIDE
Brevoxyl-4 Creamy Wash ... 3054
Brevoxyl-4 Gel ... 3054
Brevoxyl-8 Creamy Wash ... 3054
Brevoxyl-8 Gel ... 3054

BENADAY (Denmark)
CETIRIZINE HYDROCHLORIDE
Zyrtec Syrup ... 1920
Zyrtec Tablets ... 1920

BENADRYL ALLERGY ORAL SOLUTION (United Kingdom)
CETIRIZINE HYDROCHLORIDE
Zyrtec Syrup ... 1920
Zyrtec Tablets ... 1920

BENADRYL ONE A DAY (United Kingdom)
CETIRIZINE HYDROCHLORIDE
Zyrtec Syrup ... 1920
Zyrtec Tablets ... 1920

BENAXONA (Mexico)
CEFTRIAXONE SODIUM
Rocephin Injectable Vials, ADD-Vantage, Galaxy, Bulk ... 2642

BENDAPAR (Mexico)
ALBENDAZOLE
Albenza Tablets ... 1297

BENDEX (India, South Africa)
ALBENDAZOLE
Albenza Tablets ... 1297

BENECUT (Austria)
NAFTIFINE HYDROCHLORIDE
Naftin Cream ... 2164
Naftin Gel ... 2164

BENET (Japan)
RISEDRONATE SODIUM
Actonel Tablets ... 2568

BENFOFEN (Germany)
DICLOFENAC SODIUM
Voltaren Tablets ... 2334
Voltaren-XR Tablets ... 2337

BENOXID (Italy)
BENZOYL PEROXIDE
Brevoxyl-4 Creamy Wash ... 3054
Brevoxyl-4 Gel ... 3054
Brevoxyl-8 Creamy Wash ... 3054
Brevoxyl-8 Gel ... 3054

BENOXYGEL (Portugal, Spain)
BENZOYL PEROXIDE
Brevoxyl-4 Creamy Wash ... 3054
Brevoxyl-4 Gel ... 3054
Brevoxyl-8 Creamy Wash ... 3054
Brevoxyl-8 Gel ... 3054

BENOXYL (Australia, Canada, Irish Republic, Mexico, New Zealand, South Africa, The Philippines, United Kingdom, Venezuela)
BENZOYL PEROXIDE
Brevoxyl-4 Creamy Wash ... 3054
Brevoxyl-4 Gel ... 3054
Brevoxyl-8 Creamy Wash ... 3054
Brevoxyl-8 Gel ... 3054

BENTIAMIN (Brazil)
ALBENDAZOLE
Albenza Tablets ... 1297

BENZAC (Australia, Belgium, Brazil, Canada, Italy, New Zealand, Portugal, Singapore, Switzerland, Thailand, The Netherlands)
BENZOYL PEROXIDE
Brevoxyl-4 Creamy Wash ... 3054
Brevoxyl-4 Gel ... 3054
Brevoxyl-8 Creamy Wash ... 3054
Brevoxyl-8 Gel ... 3054

BENZAC AC (Brazil, Hong Kong, India, Malaysia, Mexico, South Africa, The Philippines, Turkey, Venezuela)
BENZOYL PEROXIDE
Brevoxyl-4 Creamy Wash ... 3054
Brevoxyl-4 Gel ... 3054
Brevoxyl-8 Creamy Wash ... 3054
Brevoxyl-8 Gel ... 3054

BENZAC PLUS (Chile, Mexico)
BENZOYL PEROXIDE
Brevoxyl-4 Creamy Wash ... 3054
Brevoxyl-4 Gel ... 3054
Brevoxyl-8 Creamy Wash ... 3054
Brevoxyl-8 Gel ... 3054

BENZAC-AC (Israel)
BENZOYL PEROXIDE
Brevoxyl-4 Creamy Wash ... 3054
Brevoxyl-4 Gel ... 3054
Brevoxyl-8 Creamy Wash ... 3054
Brevoxyl-8 Gel ... 3054

BENZACNE (Poland)
BENZOYL PEROXIDE
Brevoxyl-4 Creamy Wash ... 3054
Brevoxyl-4 Gel ... 3054
Brevoxyl-8 Creamy Wash ... 3054
Brevoxyl-8 Gel ... 3054

BENZAC-W (Greece)
BENZOYL PEROXIDE
Brevoxyl-4 Creamy Wash ... 3054
Brevoxyl-4 Gel ... 3054
Brevoxyl-8 Creamy Wash ... 3054
Brevoxyl-8 Gel ... 3054

BENZADERM (Mexico)
BENZOYL PEROXIDE
Brevoxyl-4 Creamy Wash ... 3054
Brevoxyl-4 Gel ... 3054
Brevoxyl-8 Creamy Wash ... 3054
Brevoxyl-8 Gel ... 3054

BENZAGEL (Brazil, France, United Kingdom)
BENZOYL PEROXIDE
Brevoxyl-4 Creamy Wash ... 3054
Brevoxyl-4 Gel ... 3054
Brevoxyl-8 Creamy Wash ... 3054
Brevoxyl-8 Gel ... 3054

BENZAKNEN (Austria, Germany)
BENZOYL PEROXIDE
Brevoxyl-4 Creamy Wash ... 3054
Brevoxyl-4 Gel ... 3054
Brevoxyl-8 Creamy Wash ... 3054
Brevoxyl-8 Gel ... 3054

BENZAMYCIN (Argentina, Belgium, Canada, Chile, Hong Kong, Israel, Mexico, Turkey, United Kingdom)
BENZOYL PEROXIDE
Brevoxyl-4 Creamy Wash ... 3054
Brevoxyl-4 Gel ... 3054
Brevoxyl-8 Creamy Wash ... 3054
Brevoxyl-8 Gel ... 3054

BENZAMYCINE (South Africa)
BENZOYL PEROXIDE
Brevoxyl-4 Creamy Wash ... 3054
Brevoxyl-4 Gel ... 3054
Brevoxyl-8 Creamy Wash ... 3054
Brevoxyl-8 Gel ... 3054

BENZAPUR (Poland)
BENZOYL PEROXIDE
Brevoxyl-4 Creamy Wash ... 3054
Brevoxyl-4 Gel ... 3054
Brevoxyl-8 Creamy Wash ... 3054
Brevoxyl-8 Gel ... 3054

BENZEVIT (Brazil)
NYSTATIN
Nystop Topical Powder USP ... 2498

BENZIHEX (Argentina)
BENZOYL PEROXIDE
Brevoxyl-4 Creamy Wash ... 3054
Brevoxyl-4 Gel ... 3054
Brevoxyl-8 Creamy Wash ... 3054
Brevoxyl-8 Gel ... 3054

BENZOL (Brazil)
ALBENDAZOLE
Albenza Tablets ... 1297

BENZOMIX (Italy)
BENZOYL PEROXIDE
Brevoxyl-4 Creamy Wash ... 3054
Brevoxyl-4 Gel ... 3054
Brevoxyl-8 Creamy Wash ... 3054
Brevoxyl-8 Gel ... 3054

BENZONAL (Mexico)
BENZONATATE
Tessalon Perles ... 1183

BENZOPIN (South Africa)
DIAZEPAM
Valium Tablets ... 2658

BENZOYT (Germany)
BENZOYL PEROXIDE
Brevoxyl-4 Creamy Wash ... 3054
Brevoxyl-4 Gel ... 3054
Brevoxyl-8 Creamy Wash ... 3054
Brevoxyl-8 Gel ... 3054

BENZPEROX (Germany)
BENZOYL PEROXIDE
Brevoxyl-4 Creamy Wash ... 3054
Brevoxyl-4 Gel ... 3054
Brevoxyl-8 Creamy Wash ... 3054
Brevoxyl-8 Gel ... 3054

BENZYME (Mexico)
DIAZEPAM
Valium Tablets ... 2658

BEPSAR (The Philippines)
LOSARTAN POTASSIUM
Cozaar Tablets ... 1973

BERLEX (Argentina)
ALENDRONATE SODIUM
Fosamax Tablets ... 2005

BERLTHYROX (Germany)
LEVOTHYROXINE SODIUM
Levothroid Tablets ... 1170
Levoxyl Tablets ... 1780
Synthroid Tablets ... 507

BERMACIA (Brazil)
THEOPHYLLINE
Uniphyl Tablets ... 2595

BESTATIN (Thailand)
SIMVASTATIN
Zocor Tablets ... 2136

BETABIOT (Mexico)
AMOXICILLIN
Amoxil Pediatric Drops for Oral Suspension ... 1305
Amoxil Tablets ... 1305

BETACAINE (Canada, Mexico)
LIDOCAINE
Lidoderm Patch ... 1114

BETACLAV (Brazil)
AMOXICILLIN
Amoxil Pediatric Drops for Oral Suspension ... 1305
Amoxil Tablets ... 1305

BETAFERON (Argentina, Australia, Austria, Belgium, Brazil, Chile, Czech Republic, Denmark, Finland, France, Germany, Hong Kong, Hungary, India, Irish Republic, Israel, Italy, Malaysia, Mexico, New Zealand, Norway, Poland, Portugal, Russia, Singapore, South Africa, Spain, Sweden, Switzerland, Thailand, The Netherlands, The Philippines, Turkey, United Kingdom)
INTERFERON BETA-1B
Betaseron for SC Injection ... 756

BETALOC (Czech Republic, Hungary, New Zealand, Poland)
METOPROLOL SUCCINATE
Toprol-XL Tablets ... 666

BETALOC ZOK (Russia)
METOPROLOL SUCCINATE
Toprol-XL Tablets ... 666

BETAMICAN (Spain)
SALMETEROL XINAFOATE
Serevent Diskus ... 1594

BETAPAM (South Africa)
DIAZEPAM
Valium Tablets ... 2658

BETAPLEX (Chile)
CARVEDILOL
Coreg Tablets ... 1387

BETAREN (Israel)
DICLOFENAC SODIUM
Voltaren Tablets ... 2334
Voltaren-XR Tablets ... 2337

BETARRETIN (Venezuela)
TRETINOIN
Vesanoid Capsules ... 2660

BETASERON (Canada)
INTERFERON BETA-1B
Betaseron for SC Injection ... 756

BETA-TIM (Canada)
TIMOLOL MALEATE
Timoptic in Ocudose ... 2124
Timoptic Sterile Ophthalmic Solution ... 2121
Timoptic-XE Sterile Ophthalmic Gel Forming Solution ... 2125

BETAZIDIM (Venezuela)
CEFTAZIDIME
Fortaz for Injection ... 1450

BETAZOK (Irish Republic, The Philippines)
METOPROLOL SUCCINATE
Toprol-XL Tablets ... 666

BETIM (Irish Republic, Norway, United Kingdom)
TIMOLOL MALEATE
Timoptic in Ocudose ... 2124
Timoptic Sterile Ophthalmic Solution ... 2121
Timoptic-XE Sterile Ophthalmic Gel Forming Solution ... 2125

BETO (Poland)
METOPROLOL SUCCINATE
Toprol-XL Tablets ... 666

BETULAC (Sweden)
LACTULOSE
Kristalose for Oral Solution ... 1004

BEURISES (South Africa)
FUROSEMIDE
Furosemide Tablets ... 2186

BEVINDAZOL (Venezuela)
ALBENDAZOLE
Albenza Tablets ... 1297

BEXID (Sweden)
BENZOYL PEROXIDE
Brevoxyl-4 Creamy Wash ... 3054
Brevoxyl-4 Gel ... 3054
Brevoxyl-8 Creamy Wash ... 3054
Brevoxyl-8 Gel ... 3054

BEXINOR (Singapore)
NORFLOXACIN
Noroxin Tablets ... 2069

BGB NORFLOX (Thailand)
NORFLOXACIN
Noroxin Tablets ... 2069

BI PRETERAX (Belgium)
PERINDOPRIL ERBUMINE
Aceon Tablets (2 mg, 4 mg, 8 mg) ... 3038

BIALZEPAM (Portugal)
DIAZEPAM
Valium Tablets ... 2658

BIAMOTIL (Brazil)
CIPROFLOXACIN HYDROCHLORIDE
Cipro Tablets ... 2810

BIAXIN (Canada, Germany)
CLARITHROMYCIN
Biaxin Filmtab Tablets ... 411
Biaxin Granules ... 411

BICLAR (Belgium)
CLARITHROMYCIN
Biaxin Filmtab Tablets ... 411
Biaxin Granules ... 411

BICLOPAN (Singapore)
DICLOFENAC SODIUM
Voltaren Tablets ... 2334
Voltaren-XR Tablets ... 2337

BICNU (Argentina, Australia, Canada, Chile, Czech Republic, France, Hong Kong, Hungary, Irish Republic, Israel, Malaysia, Mexico, New Zealand, Singapore, South Africa, Thailand, The Philippines, United Kingdom)
CARMUSTINE
Gliadel Wafer ... 1076

BIDECAR (Argentina)
CARVEDILOL
Coreg Tablets ... 1387

BIFARDOL (Mexico)
NAPROXEN SODIUM
Anaprox DS Tablets ... 2632
Anaprox Tablets ... 2632

BIFINORMA (Germany)
LACTULOSE
Kristalose for Oral Solution ... 1004

BIFITERAL (Austria, Belgium, Germany)
LACTULOSE
Kristalose for Oral Solution ... 1004

BIFOSA (India)
ALENDRONATE SODIUM
Fosamax Tablets ... 2005

BILATEN (Chile)
CANDESARTAN CILEXETIL
Atacand Tablets ... 639

BILATEN-D (Chile)
CANDESARTAN CILEXETIL
Atacand Tablets ... 639

BILORDYL (Germany)
THEOPHYLLINE
Uniphyl Tablets ... 2595

BIMOXIN (Brazil)
AMOXICILLIN
Amoxil Pediatric Drops for Oral Suspension ... 1305
Amoxil Tablets ... 1305

BINANIDDA (The Netherlands)
TERBINAFINE HYDROCHLORIDE
Lamisil Tablets ... 2266

BINDAZAC (Greece)
RANITIDINE HYDROCHLORIDE
Zantac 25 EFFERdose Tablets ... 1670
Zantac 150 Tablets ... 1670
Zantac 300 Tablets ... 1670
Zantac Injection ... 1666
Zantac Injection Premixed ... 1666
Zantac Syrup ... 1670

BINOCLAR (Hong Kong, Venezuela)
CLARITHROMYCIN
Biaxin Filmtab Tablets ... 411
Biaxin Granules ... 411

BIO TARBUN (Argentina)
NORFLOXACIN
Noroxin Tablets ... 2069

BIO-AMOKSICLAV (South Africa)
AMOXICILLIN
Amoxil Pediatric Drops for Oral Suspension ... 1305
Amoxil Tablets ... 1305

BIOCARD (Irish Republic)
CARVEDILOL
Coreg Tablets ... 1387

BIOCICLIN (Italy)
CEFUROXIME SODIUM
Zinacef Injection ... 1678

BIOCIP (India, South Africa)
CIPROFLOXACIN
Cipro Oral Suspension ... 2810

BIOCIPRO (Greece)
CIPROFLOXACIN
Cipro Oral Suspension ... 2810

BIOCIP-TZ (India)
CIPROFLOXACIN
Cipro Oral Suspension ... 2810

BIOCLAR (India)
CLARITHROMYCIN
Biaxin Filmtab Tablets ... 411
Biaxin Granules ... 411

BIO-DAC (Mexico)
SULINDAC
Clinoril Tablets ... 1962

BIODALGIC (France)
TRAMADOL HYDROCHLORIDE
Ultram ER Tablets ... 2428

BIODEZIL (Mexico)
CAPTOPRIL
Captopril Tablets ... 2182

BIODOL (Irish Republic)
TRAMADOL HYDROCHLORIDE
Ultram ER Tablets ... 2428

BIODRIBIN (Poland)
CLADRIBINE
Leustatin Injection ... 2384

BIODROP (Argentina)
DORZOLAMIDE HYDROCHLORIDE
Trusopt Sterile Ophthalmic Solution ... 2128

BIOFANAL (Germany)
NYSTATIN
Nystop Topical Powder USP ... 2498

BIOFERON (Thailand)
INTERFERON ALFA-2B
Intron A for Injection ... 2859

BIOFLOX (Mexico)
CIPROFLOXACIN
Cipro Oral Suspension ... 2810

BIOFLOXCIN (Irish Republic)
CIPROFLOXACIN
Cipro Oral Suspension ... 2810

BIOFLOXIN (India)
NORFLOXACIN
Noroxin Tablets ... 2069

BIOFLOX-TZ (India)
NORFLOXACIN
Noroxin Tablets ... 2069

BIOFUREX (Italy)
CEFUROXIME SODIUM
Zinacef Injection ... 1678

BIOFUROKSYM (Poland)
CEFUROXIME SODIUM
Zinacef Injection ... 1678

BIOLAC (Italy)
LACTULOSE
Kristalose for Oral Solution ... 1004

BIOLAN (Germany)
SODIUM HYALURONATE
Hyalgan Solution ... 2742

BIOLON (Brazil, Canada, Chile, Germany, Israel, Italy, Mexico, South Africa, Switzerland, Turkey)
SODIUM HYALURONATE
Hyalgan Solution ... 2742

BIOLONE (South Africa)
SODIUM HYALURONATE
Hyalgan Solution ... 2742

BIOMENT (Turkey)
AMOXICILLIN
Amoxil Pediatric Drops for Oral Suspension ... 1305
Amoxil Tablets ... 1305

BIOMISEN (Mexico)
FUROSEMIDE
Furosemide Tablets ... 2186

BIOMOX (Thailand)
AMOXICILLIN
Amoxil Pediatric Drops for Oral Suspension ... 1305
Amoxil Tablets ... 1305

BIOMOXIL (India)
AMOXICILLIN
Amoxil Pediatric Drops for Oral Suspension ... 1305
Amoxil Tablets ... 1305

BIOMOXIL-LB (India)
AMOXICILLIN
Amoxil Pediatric Drops for Oral Suspension ... 1305
Amoxil Tablets ... 1305

BIONEURYL (Mexico)
CARBAMAZEPINE
Carbatrol Capsules ... 3019

BIOPHYLLIN (South Africa)
THEOPHYLLINE
Uniphyl Tablets ... 2595

BIOPRIL (India)
LISINOPRIL
Prinivil Tablets ... 2087

BIOPRIL-AM (India)
LISINOPRIL
Prinivil Tablets ... 2087

BIORACEF (Poland)
CEFUROXIME AXETIL
Ceftin for Oral Suspension ... 1380
Ceftin Tablets ... 1380

BIOREUNIL (Mexico)
CARBAMAZEPINE
Carbatrol Capsules ... 3019

BIORTAN (Venezuela)
LOSARTAN POTASSIUM
Cozaar Tablets ... 1973

BIOSEMIDA (Venezuela)
FUROSEMIDE
Furosemide Tablets ... 2186

BIOSETRON (Greece)
ONDANSETRON
Zofran ODT Orally Disintegrating Tablets ... 1687

BIOSIM (India)
SIMVASTATIN
Zocor Tablets ... 2136

BIOTIC (Argentina)
CIPROFLOXACIN HYDROCHLORIDE
Cipro Tablets ... 2810

BIOTRAKSON (Poland)
CEFTRIAXONE SODIUM
Rocephin Injectable Vials, ADD-Vantage, Galaxy, Bulk ... 2642

BIOTREDINE (Greece)
ETIDRONATE DISODIUM
Didronel Tablets ... 2583

BIOTUM (Poland)
CEFTAZIDIME
Fortaz for Injection ... 1450

BIOVIR (Brazil)
LAMIVUDINE
Epivir Oral Solution ... 1412
Epivir Tablets ... 1412
Epivir-HBV Oral Solution ... 1417
Epivir-HBV Tablets ... 1417

BIOXAN (Mexico)
NAPROXEN
EC-Naprosyn Delayed-Release Tablets ... 2632
Naprosyn Suspension ... 2632
Naprosyn Tablets ... 2632

BIOXILINA (Argentina)
AMOXICILLIN
Amoxil Pediatric Drops for Oral Suspension ... 1305
Amoxil Tablets ... 1305

BIOXILINA PLUS (Argentina)
AMOXICILLIN
Amoxil Pediatric Drops for Oral Suspension 1305
Amoxil Tablets 1305

BIOXIMA (Italy)
CEFUROXIME SODIUM
Zinacef Injection 1678

BIOZIDIMA (Venezuela)
CEFTAZIDIME
Fortaz for Injection 1450

BIPOLAM (Austria)
LAMOTRIGINE
Lamictal Chewable Dispersible Tablets 1488
Lamictal Tablets 1488

BIPREDONIUM (Spain)
INDAPAMIDE
Indapamide Tablets 2188

BIPRETERAX (Argentina, Irish Republic, South Africa, Venezuela)
PERINDOPRIL ERBUMINE
Aceon Tablets (2 mg, 4 mg, 8 mg) 3038

BI-PRETERAX (The Philippines)
PERINDOPRIL ERBUMINE
Aceon Tablets (2 mg, 4 mg, 8 mg) 3038

BIPRONYL (Singapore)
NAPROXEN
EC-Naprosyn Delayed-Release Tablets 2632
Naprosyn Suspension 2632
Naprosyn Tablets 2632

BIRVAC (Argentina)
LAMIVUDINE
Epivir Oral Solution 1412
Epivir Tablets 1412
Epivir-HBV Oral Solution 1417
Epivir-HBV Tablets 1417

BISTATIN V (Mexico)
NYSTATIN
Nystop Topical Powder USP 2498

BISTON (Czech Republic)
CARBAMAZEPINE
Carbatrol Capsules 3019

BI-TILDIEM (France)
DILTIAZEM HYDROCHLORIDE
Cardizem LA Extended Release Tablets 421

BITIRON (Turkey)
LEVOTHYROXINE SODIUM
Levothroid Tablets 1170
Levoxyl Tablets 1780
Synthroid Tablets 507

BIVORILAN (Greece)
CIPROFLOXACIN HYDROCHLORIDE
Cipro Tablets 2810

BIXON (Italy)
CEFTRIAXONE SODIUM
Rocephin Injectable Vials, ADD-Vantage, Galaxy, Bulk 2642

BLADER (Argentina)
CIPROFLOXACIN
Cipro Oral Suspension 2810

BLEFAMIDE (Chile)
PREDNISOLONE ACETATE/SULFACETAMIDE SODIUM
Blephamide Ophthalmic Ointment ⊙217
Blephamide Ophthalmic Suspension ⊙216

BLENOX (Spain)
AMOXICILLIN
Amoxil Pediatric Drops for Oral Suspension 1305
Amoxil Tablets 1305

BLEPHAMIDE (Switzerland)
PREDNISOLONE ACETATE/SULFACETAMIDE SODIUM
Blephamide Ophthalmic Ointment ⊙217
Blephamide Ophthalmic Suspension ⊙216

BLEZAMONT (Greece)
CETIRIZINE HYDROCHLORIDE
Zyrtec Syrup 1920
Zyrtec Tablets 1920

BLOCACID (India, Mexico, Singapore)
NAPROXEN
EC-Naprosyn Delayed-Release Tablets 2632
Naprosyn Suspension 2632
Naprosyn Tablets 2632

BLOCADREN (Australia, Austria, Belgium, Canada, Hong Kong, Irish Republic, Italy, Mexico, Norway, Portugal, South Africa, Spain, Sweden, Switzerland, The Netherlands, United Kingdom)
TIMOLOL MALEATE
Timoptic in Ocudose 2124
Timoptic Sterile Ophthalmic Solution 2121
Timoptic-XE Sterile Ophthalmic Gel Forming Solution 2125

BLOCALCIN (Czech Republic, Hungary, Poland, Russia)
DILTIAZEM HYDROCHLORIDE
Cardizem LA Extended Release Tablets 421

BLOCANOL (Finland)
TIMOLOL MALEATE
Timoptic in Ocudose 2124
Timoptic Sterile Ophthalmic Solution 2121
Timoptic-XE Sterile Ophthalmic Gel Forming Solution 2125

BLOCAR (Chile)
CARVEDILOL
Coreg Tablets 1387

BLOKIUM FLEX (Argentina)
DICLOFENAC SODIUM
Voltaren Tablets 2334
Voltaren-XR Tablets 2337

BLOKTUS (Mexico)
BENZONATATE
Tessalon Perles 1183

BLOPRESID (Italy, The Netherlands)
CANDESARTAN CILEXETIL
Atacand Tablets 639

BLOPRESS (Austria, Brazil, Chile, Czech Republic, Germany, Hong Kong, Italy, Japan, Malaysia, Mexico, Portugal, Spain, Switzerland, Thailand, The Netherlands, The Philippines, Venezuela)
CANDESARTAN CILEXETIL
Atacand Tablets 639

BLOPRESS 16 MG + 12,5 MG (Portugal)
CANDESARTAN CILEXETIL
Atacand Tablets 639

BLOPRESS PLUS (Germany, Mexico, Switzerland, The Philippines, Venezuela)
CANDESARTAN CILEXETIL
Atacand Tablets 639

B-LOVATIN (Greece)
LOVASTATIN
Mevacor Tablets 2063

BLOX (Chile)
CANDESARTAN CILEXETIL
Atacand Tablets 639

BLUMOL (Greece)
RANITIDINE HYDROCHLORIDE
Zantac 25 EFFERdose Tablets 1670
Zantac 150 Tablets 1670
Zantac 300 Tablets 1670
Zantac Injection 1666
Zantac Injection Premixed 1666
Zantac Syrup 1670

BOCATRIOL (Austria, Denmark, Germany, Switzerland)
CALCITRIOL
Calcijex Injection 419
Rocaltrol Capsules 1150
Rocaltrol Oral Solution 1150

BOLBAMOX (Mexico)
AMOXICILLIN
Amoxil Pediatric Drops for Oral Suspension 1305
Amoxil Tablets 1305

BOLOXEN (Poland)
NAPROXEN SODIUM
Anaprox DS Tablets 2632
Anaprox Tablets 2632

BONALEN (Brazil)
ALENDRONATE SODIUM
Fosamax Tablets 2005

BONEMASS (Brazil)
ETIDRONATE DISODIUM
Didronel Tablets 2583

BONEMAX (Turkey)
ALENDRONATE SODIUM
Fosamax Tablets 2005

BONJELA TEETHING GEL (United Kingdom)
LIDOCAINE
Lidoderm Patch 1114

BONMAX (India)
RALOXIFENE HYDROCHLORIDE
Evista Tablets 1810

BONMIN (Turkey)
NAPROXEN SODIUM
Anaprox DS Tablets 2632
Anaprox Tablets 2632

BONYL (Denmark)
NAPROXEN
EC-Naprosyn Delayed-Release Tablets 2632
Naprosyn Suspension 2632
Naprosyn Tablets 2632

BRADELMIN (Mexico)
ALBENDAZOLE
Albenza Tablets 1297

BRAINAL (Chile, Czech Republic, Russia, Spain)
NIMODIPINE
Nimotop Capsules 790

BREK (Argentina)
ALENDRONATE SODIUM
Fosamax Tablets 2005

BRELCIP (The Philippines)
CIPROFLOXACIN HYDROCHLORIDE
Cipro Tablets 2810

BRELLERCET (The Philippines)
CETIRIZINE HYDROCHLORIDE
Zyrtec Syrup 1920
Zyrtec Tablets 1920

BREMON (Spain)
CLARITHROMYCIN
Biaxin Filmtab Tablets 411
Biaxin Granules 411

BRENOXIL (Mexico)
AMOXICILLIN
Amoxil Pediatric Drops for Oral Suspension 1305
Amoxil Tablets 1305

BRESEC (Greece)
CEFTRIAXONE SODIUM
Rocephin Injectable Vials, ADD-Vantage, Galaxy, Bulk 2642

BRETHAL (Turkey)
FLUTICASONE PROPIONATE
Flonase Nasal Spray 1431

BREVOXYL (Australia, Austria, Belgium, Finland, France, Germany, Greece, Hong Kong, Irish Republic, Malaysia, New Zealand, Norway, Poland, Singapore, South Africa, Sweden, Thailand, The Philippines, United Kingdom)
BENZOYL PEROXIDE
Brevoxyl-4 Creamy Wash 3054
Brevoxyl-4 Gel 3054
Brevoxyl-8 Creamy Wash 3054
Brevoxyl-8 Gel 3054

BREXONASE (Chile)
FLUTICASONE PROPIONATE
Flonase Nasal Spray 1431

BREXOVENT (Chile)
FLUTICASONE PROPIONATE
Flonase Nasal Spray 1431

BRINAF (Czech Republic)
TERBINAFINE HYDROCHLORIDE
Lamisil Tablets 2266

BRINTENAL (Argentina)
SELEGILINE HYDROCHLORIDE
Eldepryl Capsules 3052

BRISOVENT (Portugal)
FLUTICASONE PROPIONATE
Flonase Nasal Spray 1431

BRISTAMOX (Sweden)
AMOXICILLIN
Amoxil Pediatric Drops for Oral Suspension 1305
Amoxil Tablets 1305

BRITIAZIM (United Kingdom)
DILTIAZEM HYDROCHLORIDE
Cardizem LA Extended Release Tablets 421

BRIXORAL (Greece)
RANITIDINE HYDROCHLORIDE
Zantac 25 EFFERdose Tablets 1670
Zantac 150 Tablets 1670
Zantac 300 Tablets 1670
Zantac Injection 1666
Zantac Injection Premixed 1666
Zantac Syrup 1670

BROLIN (Spain)
FAMOTIDINE
Pepcid for Oral Suspension 2075
Pepcid Tablets 2075

BRONALIDE (Canada, Germany, Greece)
FLUNISOLIDE
Aerobid Inhaler System 1153
Aerobid-M Inhaler System 1153

BRONCHOPHEN (South Africa)
THEOPHYLLINE
Uniphyl Tablets 2595

BRONCHOPHYLLINE (Israel)
THEOPHYLLINE
Uniphyl Tablets 2595

BRONCHORETARD (Germany)
THEOPHYLLINE
Uniphyl Tablets 2595

BRONCOFOL (India)
THEOPHYLLINE
Uniphyl Tablets 2595

BRONCOFOL-P (India)
THEOPHYLLINE
Uniphyl Tablets 2595

BRONCONEX (New Zealand)
MOMETASONE FUROATE
Elocon Cream 0.1% 2840
Elocon Lotion 0.1% 2841
Elocon Ointment 0.1% 2842
Nasonex Nasal Spray 2883

BRONCORT (Belgium, Switzerland)
FLUNISOLIDE
Aerobid Inhaler System 1153
Aerobid-M Inhaler System 1153

BRONDIL (REFORMULATED) (The Philippines)
THEOPHYLLINE
Uniphyl Tablets 2595

BRONILIDE (Czech Republic, France, Switzerland)
FLUNISOLIDE
Aerobid Inhaler System 1153
Aerobid-M Inhaler System 1153

BRONKASMA (Argentina)
THEOPHYLLINE
Uniphyl Tablets 2595

BRONKOLIN (Turkey)
THEOPHYLLINE
Uniphyl Tablets 2595

BRONPAX (Mexico)
BENZONATATE
Tessalon Perles 1183

BRONQUIASMA (Brazil)
THEOPHYLLINE
Uniphyl Tablets 2595

BROVAFLAMP (South Africa)
DICLOFENAC SODIUM
Voltaren Tablets 2334
Voltaren-XR Tablets 2337

BROXOLIM-AM (Mexico)
AMOXICILLIN
Amoxil Pediatric Drops for Oral Suspension 1305
Amoxil Tablets 1305

BRUCAP (Mexico)
CAPTOPRIL
Captopril Tablets 2182

BUGAZON (Mexico)
CAPTOPRIL
Captopril Tablets 2182

BUMAFLEX N (Argentina)
NAPROXEN
EC-Naprosyn Delayed-Release Tablets 2632

(⊙ Described in PDR® For Ophthalmic Medicines)

Naprosyn Suspension . . . 2632
Naprosyn Tablets . . . 2632

BUROFIX (Hungary)
CALCIUM ACETATE
PhosLo GelCaps . . . 1184

BUSILVEX (Denmark, Germany, Greece, Italy, Norway, Poland, Spain, Sweden, Switzerland, The Netherlands, United Kingdom)
BUSULFAN
Myleran Tablets . . . 1530

BUSULFEX (Canada, Hong Kong, Israel, Turkey)
BUSULFAN
Myleran Tablets . . . 1530

BUTOP (India)
BUTENAFINE HYDROCHLORIDE
Mentax Cream . . . 2190

BUTOSALI (Mexico)
FUROSEMIDE
Furosemide Tablets . . . 2186

BUXON (Chile)
BUPROPION HYDROCHLORIDE
Wellbutrin SR Sustained-Release Tablets . . 1653
Wellbutrin Tablets . . . 1648
Zyban Sustained-Release Tablets . . . 1692

BY-MADOL (Irish Republic)
TRAMADOL HYDROCHLORIDE
Ultram ER Tablets . . . 2428

BYSCLAS (The Philippines)
CLARITHROMYCIN
Biaxin Filmtab Tablets . . . 411
Biaxin Granules . . . 411

BYZESTRA (Irish Republic)
LISINOPRIL
Prinivil Tablets . . . 2087

CABAL (Argentina)
CETIRIZINE HYDROCHLORIDE
Zyrtec Syrup . . . 1920
Zyrtec Tablets . . . 1920

CABIOTEN (Brazil)
CAPTOPRIL
Captopril Tablets . . . 2182

CAL-ANTAGON (Portugal)
DILTIAZEM HYDROCHLORIDE
Cardizem LA Extended Release Tablets . . . 421

CALAZEM (United Kingdom)
DILTIAZEM HYDROCHLORIDE
Cardizem LA Extended Release Tablets . . . 421

CALCETAT (Italy)
CALCIUM ACETATE
PhosLo GelCaps . . . 1184

CALCICARD (United Kingdom)
DILTIAZEM HYDROCHLORIDE
Cardizem LA Extended Release Tablets . . . 421

CALCIJEX (Australia, Austria, Brazil, Canada, Czech Republic, Finland, Hong Kong, Hungary, Irish Republic, Israel, Italy, Malaysia, Mexico, Norway, Poland, Singapore, Spain, Sweden, Switzerland, The Netherlands, Turkey, United Kingdom)
CALCITRIOL
Calcijex Injection . . . 419
Rocaltrol Capsules . . . 1150
Rocaltrol Oral Solution . . . 1150

CALCIT (Thailand)
CALCITRIOL
Calcijex Injection . . . 419
Rocaltrol Capsules . . . 1150
Rocaltrol Oral Solution . . . 1150

CALFATE (Portugal)
SUCRALFATE
Carafate Suspension . . . 706
Carafate Tablets . . . 707

CALIDIOL (Hungary, Poland)
ESTRADIOL
Climara Transdermal System . . . 763

CALMADOR (Argentina)
TRAMADOL HYDROCHLORIDE
Ultram ER Tablets . . . 2428

CALMANTE DE DENTICION (Chile)
LIDOCAINE
Lidoderm Patch . . . 1114

CALMARIL (Thailand)
THIORIDAZINE HYDROCHLORIDE
Thioridazine Hydrochloride Tablets . . . 2195

CALMAVEN (Spain)
DIAZEPAM
Valium Tablets . . . 2658

CALMIDAN (Spain)
SUCRALFATE
Carafate Suspension . . . 706
Carafate Tablets . . . 707

CALMIGEN (Irish Republic)
DIAZEPAM
Valium Tablets . . . 2658

CALMOCITENO (Brazil)
DIAZEPAM
Valium Tablets . . . 2658

CALMOFLEX (Argentina)
DICLOFENAC SODIUM
Voltaren Tablets . . . 2334
Voltaren-XR Tablets . . . 2337

CALMOSERPIN (Germany)
HYDROCHLOROTHIAZIDE/TRIAMTERENE
Dyazide Capsules . . . 1405

CALMPOSE (India, South Africa)
DIAZEPAM
Valium Tablets . . . 2658

CALNIT (Spain)
NIMODIPINE
Nimotop Capsules . . . 790

CALZEM (Brazil)
DILTIAZEM HYDROCHLORIDE
Cardizem LA Extended Release Tablets . . . 421

CAMOXIN (Brazil)
AMOXICILLIN
Amoxil Pediatric Drops for Oral Suspension . . . 1305
Amoxil Tablets . . . 1305

CAMPAL (Venezuela)
DICLOFENAC SODIUM
Voltaren Tablets . . . 2334
Voltaren-XR Tablets . . . 2337

CANDACIDE (South Africa)
NYSTATIN
Nystop Topical Powder USP . . . 2498

CANDERMIL (Argentina)
NYSTATIN
Nystop Topical Powder USP . . . 2498

CANDIDA-LOKALICID (Germany)
NYSTATIN
Nystop Topical Powder USP . . . 2498

CANDIDIAS (Argentina)
NYSTATIN
Nystop Topical Powder USP . . . 2498

CANDIO (Austria, Germany, Switzerland)
NYSTATIN
Nystop Topical Powder USP . . . 2498

CANDISTATIN (Brazil, Canada)
NYSTATIN
Nystop Topical Powder USP . . . 2498

CANEF (Denmark, Finland, Mexico, Norway, Portugal, Sweden, The Netherlands)
FLUVASTATIN SODIUM
Lescol Capsules . . . 2268

CANSTAT (South Africa)
NYSTATIN
Nystop Topical Powder USP . . . 2498

CANTANIDIN (Austria)
CLONIDINE HYDROCHLORIDE
Catapres Tablets . . . 841

CAPACE (Australia, Austria, India, South Africa)
CAPTOPRIL
Captopril Tablets . . . 2182

CAPIN (Hungary)
CAPTOPRIL
Captopril Tablets . . . 2182

CAPOCARD (Hong Kong)
CAPTOPRIL
Captopril Tablets . . . 2182

CAPOMED (The Philippines)
CAPTOPRIL
Captopril Tablets . . . 2182

CAPOSTAD (Austria)
CAPTOPRIL
Captopril Tablets . . . 2182

CAPOTEN (Australia, Belgium, Brazil, Canada, Chile, Czech Republic, Denmark, Finland, Greece, Hong Kong, Irish Republic, Italy, Malaysia, New Zealand, Norway, Portugal, Singapore, South Africa, Spain, Sweden, Thailand, The Netherlands, The Philippines, United Kingdom, Venezuela)
CAPTOPRIL
Captopril Tablets . . . 2182

CAPOTENA (Mexico)
CAPTOPRIL
Captopril Tablets . . . 2182

CAPOTRIL (Brazil)
CAPTOPRIL
Captopril Tablets . . . 2182

CAPOX (Brazil)
CAPTOPRIL
Captopril Tablets . . . 2182

CAPOX H (Brazil)
CAPTOPRIL
Captopril Tablets . . . 2182

CAPOZID (Denmark)
CAPTOPRIL
Captopril Tablets . . . 2182

CAPOZIDE (Germany, Mexico, New Zealand, South Africa, United Kingdom, Venezuela)
CAPTOPRIL
Captopril Tablets . . . 2182

CAPRIL (Brazil, Hong Kong)
CAPTOPRIL
Captopril Tablets . . . 2182

CAPRILL (Irish Republic)
CAPTOPRIL
Captopril Tablets . . . 2182

CAPRILTOP (Belgium)
CAPTOPRIL
Captopril Tablets . . . 2182

CAPROS (Germany)
MORPHINE SULFATE
MS Contin Tablets . . . 2585

CAPRYSIN (Finland)
CLONIDINE HYDROCHLORIDE
Catapres Tablets . . . 841

CAPSICOF (Mexico)
BENZONATATE
Tessalon Perles . . . 1183

CAPTI (Israel)
CAPTOPRIL
Captopril Tablets . . . 2182

CAPTIL (Brazil)
CAPTOPRIL
Captopril Tablets . . . 2182

CAPTIREX (France)
CAPTOPRIL
Captopril Tablets . . . 2182

CAPTO PLUS (Germany)
CAPTOPRIL
Captopril Tablets . . . 2182

CAPTO-BASAN (Switzerland)
CAPTOPRIL
Captopril Tablets . . . 2182

CAPTOBEL (Brazil)
CAPTOPRIL
Captopril Tablets . . . 2182

CAPTOBETA (Germany)
CAPTOPRIL
Captopril Tablets . . . 2182

CAPTOBETA COMP (Germany)
CAPTOPRIL
Captopril Tablets . . . 2182

CAPTO-CO (United Kingdom)
CAPTOPRIL
Captopril Tablets . . . 2182

CAPTOCORD (Brazil)
CAPTOPRIL
Captopril Tablets . . . 2182

CAPTODAN (Denmark)
CAPTOPRIL
Captopril Tablets . . . 2182

CAPTODOC (Germany)
CAPTOPRIL
Captopril Tablets . . . 2182

CAPTODOC COMP (Germany)
CAPTOPRIL
Captopril Tablets . . . 2182

CAPTO-DURA COR (Germany)
CAPTOPRIL
Captopril Tablets . . . 2182

CAPTO-DURA M (Germany)
CAPTOPRIL
Captopril Tablets . . . 2182

CAPTOFLUX (Germany)
CAPTOPRIL
Captopril Tablets . . . 2182

CAPTOGAMMA (Germany, Hungary)
CAPTOPRIL
Captopril Tablets . . . 2182

CAPTOGAMMA HCT (Germany)
CAPTOPRIL
Captopril Tablets . . . 2182

CAPTOHEXAL (Australia, Germany, New Zealand, South Africa)
CAPTOPRIL
Captopril Tablets . . . 2182

CAPTOHEXAL COMP (Austria, Czech Republic, Germany)
CAPTOPRIL
Captopril Tablets . . . 2182

CAPTOL (Denmark)
CAPTOPRIL
Captopril Tablets . . . 2182

CAPTOLAB (Brazil)
CAPTOPRIL
Captopril Tablets . . . 2182

CAPTOLANE (France)
CAPTOPRIL
Captopril Tablets . . . 2182

CAPTOLIN (Brazil)
CAPTOPRIL
Captopril Tablets . . . 2182

CAPTOMAX (South Africa)
CAPTOPRIL
Captopril Tablets . . . 2182

CAPTOMED (Austria, Brazil)
CAPTOPRIL
Captopril Tablets . . . 2182

CAPTOMERCK (Germany)
CAPTOPRIL
Captopril Tablets . . . 2182

CAPTOMIN (Finland)
CAPTOPRIL
Captopril Tablets . . . 2182

CAPTON (Brazil)
CAPTOPRIL
Captopril Tablets . . . 2182

CAPTOPHAR (United Arab Emirates)
CAPTOPRIL
Captopril Tablets . . . 2182

CAPTOPIRIL (Brazil)
CAPTOPRIL
Captopril Tablets . . . 2182

CAPTOPLUS (Austria)
CAPTOPRIL
Captopril Tablets . . . 2182

CAPTOPRESS (Germany)
CAPTOPRIL
Captopril Tablets . . . 2182

CAPTOPRIL PLUS (Germany)
CAPTOPRIL
Captopril Tablets . . . 2182

CAPTOPRIL-HCT (Austria)
CAPTOPRIL
Captopril Tablets . . . 2182

CAPTOPRIMED (Belgium)
CAPTOPRIL
Captopril Tablets . . . 2182

CAPTOPRON (Brazil)
CAPTOPRIL
Captopril Tablets . . . 2182

CAPTOR (Austria, Irish Republic)
CAPTOPRIL
Captopril Tablets . . . 2182

CAPTOREAL (Germany)
CAPTOPRIL
Captopril Tablets . . . 2182

CAPTORETIC (South Africa)
CAPTOPRIL
Captopril Tablets . . . 2182

CAPTOR-HCT (Irish Republic)
CAPTOPRIL
Captopril Tablets . . . 2182

CAPTOSEN (Brazil)
CAPTOPRIL
Captopril Tablets . . . 2182

CAPTOSER (Mexico)
CAPTOPRIL
Captopril Tablets . . . 2182

CAPTOSIF (Brazil)
CAPTOPRIL
Captopril Tablets . . . 2182

CAPTOSINA (Spain)
CAPTOPRIL
Captopril Tablets . . . 2182

CAPTOSOL (Switzerland)
CAPTOPRIL
Captopril Tablets . . . 2182

CAPTOSOL COMP (Switzerland)
CAPTOPRIL
Captopril Tablets . . . 2182

CAPTOSTAD (Finland)
CAPTOPRIL
Captopril Tablets . . . 2182

CAPTOTEC (Brazil)
CAPTOPRIL
Captopril Tablets . . . 2182

CAPTOTEC + HCT (Brazil)
CAPTOPRIL
Captopril Tablets . . . 2182

CAPTOTYROL (Austria)
CAPTOPRIL
Captopril Tablets . . . 2182

CAPTOZEN (Brazil)
CAPTOPRIL
Captopril Tablets . . . 2182

CAPTRAL (Mexico)
CAPTOPRIL
Captopril Tablets . . . 2182

CAPTRIL (Canada)
CAPTOPRIL
Captopril Tablets . . . 2182

CAPTRIZIN (Brazil)
CAPTOPRIL
Captopril Tablets . . . 2182

CARACE (Irish Republic, United Kingdom)
LISINOPRIL
Prinivil Tablets . . . 2087

CARACE PLUS (Irish Republic, United Kingdom)
HYDROCHLOROTHIAZIDE/LISINOPRIL
Prinzide Tablets . . . 2092

CARAFATE (Australia, New Zealand)
SUCRALFATE
Carafate Suspension . . . 706
Carafate Tablets . . . 707

CARALPHA (United Kingdom)
LISINOPRIL
Prinivil Tablets . . . 2087

CARBA (Germany)
CARBAMAZEPINE
Carbatrol Capsules . . . 3019

CARBABETA (Germany)
CARBAMAZEPINE
Carbatrol Capsules . . . 3019

CARBACONTIN (India)
CARBAMAZEPINE
Carbatrol Capsules . . . 3019

CARBACTOL RETARD (Chile)
CARBAMAZEPINE
Carbatrol Capsules . . . 3019

CARBADURA (Germany)
CARBAMAZEPINE
Carbatrol Capsules . . . 3019

CARBAFLUX (Germany)
CARBAMAZEPINE
Carbatrol Capsules . . . 3019

CARBAGAMMA (Germany)
CARBAMAZEPINE
Carbatrol Capsules . . . 3019

CARBAGEN (United Kingdom)
CARBAMAZEPINE
Carbatrol Capsules . . . 3019

CARBAGRAMON (Argentina)
CARBAMAZEPINE
Carbatrol Capsules . . . 3019

CARBALAN (Mexico)
CARBAMAZEPINE
Carbatrol Capsules . . . 3019

CARBAMAT (Argentina)
CARBAMAZEPINE
Carbatrol Capsules . . . 3019

CARBAPIN (Russia)
CARBAMAZEPINE
Carbatrol Capsules . . . 3019

CARBASAL (Mexico)
CARBAMAZEPINE
Carbatrol Capsules . . . 3019

CARBATIL (Venezuela)
CARVEDILOL
Coreg Tablets . . . 1387

CARBATOL (Thailand)
CARBAMAZEPINE
Carbatrol Capsules . . . 3019

CARBAVAL (Mexico)
CARBAMAZEPINE
Carbatrol Capsules . . . 3019

CARBAZENE (Thailand)
CARBAMAZEPINE
Carbatrol Capsules . . . 3019

CARBAZEP (Mexico)
CARBAMAZEPINE
Carbatrol Capsules . . . 3019

CARBAZINA (Mexico)
CARBAMAZEPINE
Carbatrol Capsules . . . 3019

CARBI (Israel)
CARBAMAZEPINE
Carbatrol Capsules . . . 3019

CARBILEPP (The Philippines)
CARBAMAZEPINE
Carbatrol Capsules . . . 3019

CARBIUM (Australia, Germany)
CARBAMAZEPINE
Carbatrol Capsules . . . 3019

CARBRITAL (Australia)
PENTOBARBITAL SODIUM
Nembutal Sodium Solution, USP . . . 2494

CARDCAL (Australia)
DILTIAZEM HYDROCHLORIDE
Cardizem LA Extended Release Tablets . . . 421

CARDCOR (Brazil)
DIGOXIN
Lanoxin Injection . . . 1498
Lanoxin Injection Pediatric . . . 1502
Lanoxin Tablets . . . 1505

CARDIACE (South Africa)
CAPTOPRIL
Captopril Tablets . . . 2182

CARDIACTON (Austria)
DILTIAZEM HYDROCHLORIDE
Cardizem LA Extended Release Tablets . . . 421

CARDIAGEN (Germany)
CAPTOPRIL
Captopril Tablets . . . 2182

CARDIAGEN HCT (Germany)
CAPTOPRIL
Captopril Tablets . . . 2182

CARDIL (Denmark, Greece, Malaysia, Russia, Singapore, Thailand)
DILTIAZEM HYDROCHLORIDE
Cardizem LA Extended Release Tablets . . . 421

CARDILOL (Brazil)
CARVEDILOL
Coreg Tablets . . . 1387

CARDILOM (Brazil)
CAPTOPRIL
Captopril Tablets . . . 2182

CARDIN (Poland)
SIMVASTATIN
Zocor Tablets . . . 2136

CARDIOFENONE (Italy)
PROPAFENONE HYDROCHLORIDE
Rythmol SR Capsules . . . 1590

CARDIOGOXIN (Argentina)
DIGOXIN
Lanoxin Injection . . . 1498
Lanoxin Injection Pediatric . . . 1502
Lanoxin Tablets . . . 1505

CARDIOL (Finland, Portugal)
CARVEDILOL
Coreg Tablets . . . 1387

CARDIOREG (Italy)
DIGOXIN
Lanoxin Injection . . . 1498
Lanoxin Injection Pediatric . . . 1502
Lanoxin Tablets . . . 1505

CARDIOSTATIN (Russia)
LOVASTATIN
Mevacor Tablets . . . 2063

CARDIOVERT (The Philippines)
ADENOSINE
Adenocard IV Injection . . . 603
Adenoscan . . . 605

CARDIOXIN (India)
DIGOXIN
Lanoxin Injection . . . 1498
Lanoxin Injection Pediatric . . . 1502
Lanoxin Tablets . . . 1505

CARDIPRIL (Mexico)
CAPTOPRIL
Captopril Tablets . . . 2182

CARDISER (Spain)
DILTIAZEM HYDROCHLORIDE
Cardizem LA Extended Release Tablets . . . 421

CARDITRIL (Brazil)
CAPTOPRIL
Captopril Tablets . . . 2182

CARDIUM (Hong Kong, Singapore)
DILTIAZEM HYDROCHLORIDE
Cardizem LA Extended Release Tablets . . . 421

CARDIVAS (Russia)
CARVEDILOL
Coreg Tablets . . . 1387

CARDIZEM (Australia, Brazil, Canada, Denmark, Finland, New Zealand, Norway, Sweden)
DILTIAZEM HYDROCHLORIDE
Cardizem LA Extended Release Tablets . . . 421

CARDOXIN (Israel)
DIPYRIDAMOLE
Persantine Tablets . . . 869

CARDYL (Spain, The Netherlands)
ATORVASTATIN CALCIUM
Lipitor Tablets . . . 2501

CAREFLU (Italy)
FLUNISOLIDE
Aerobid Inhaler System . . . 1153
Aerobid-M Inhaler System . . . 1153

CARENCIL (Portugal)
CAPTOPRIL
Captopril Tablets . . . 2182

CARLICH (Germany)
CARVEDILOL
Coreg Tablets . . . 1387

CARLOC (India, South Africa)
CARVEDILOL
Coreg Tablets . . . 1387

CARMAPINE (Thailand)
CARBAMAZEPINE
Carbatrol Capsules . . . 3019

CARMAZIN (Brazil)
CARBAMAZEPINE
Carbatrol Capsules . . . 3019

CARMICINA (Portugal)
CIPROFLOXACIN HYDROCHLORIDE
Cipro Tablets . . . 2810

CARMUBRIS (Austria, Germany)
CARMUSTINE
Gliadel Wafer . . . 1076

CARPAZ (South Africa)
CARBAMAZEPINE
Carbatrol Capsules . . . 3019

CARPIN (Mexico)
CARBAMAZEPINE
Carbatrol Capsules . . . 3019

CARPINE (Thailand)
CARBAMAZEPINE
Carbatrol Capsules . . . 3019

CARRELDON (Spain)
DILTIAZEM HYDROCHLORIDE
Cardizem LA Extended Release Tablets . . . 421

CARSOL (Switzerland)
CARBAMAZEPINE
Carbatrol Capsules . . . 3019

CARTAZID (Venezuela)
CAPTOPRIL
Captopril Tablets . . . 2182

CARVE (Germany)
CARVEDILOL
Coreg Tablets . . . 1387

CARVECARD (Germany)
CARVEDILOL
Coreg Tablets . . . 1387

CARVEDEXXON (Israel)
CARVEDILOL
Coreg Tablets . . . 1387

CARVEDIGAMMA (Germany, Poland)
CARVEDILOL
Coreg Tablets . . . 1387

CARVEDIL (Argentina, Venezuela)
CARVEDILOL
Coreg Tablets . . . 1387

CARVEDIL D (Argentina)
CARVEDILOL
Coreg Tablets . . . 1387

CARVEL (Argentina)
CARVEDILOL
Coreg Tablets . . . 1387

CARVETONE (Denmark)
CARVEDILOL
Coreg Tablets . . . 1387

CARVETREND (Poland, South Africa)
CARVEDILOL
Coreg Tablets . . . 1387

CARVIL (India)
CARVEDILOL
Coreg Tablets . . . 1387

CARVIPRESS (Italy)
CARVEDILOL
Coreg Tablets . . . 1387

CARZEM (Italy, Thailand)
DILTIAZEM HYDROCHLORIDE
Cardizem LA Extended Release Tablets . . . 421

CARZEPIN (Hong Kong)
CARBAMAZEPINE
Carbatrol Capsules . . . 3019

CARZEPINE (Thailand)
CARBAMAZEPINE
Carbatrol Capsules . . . 3019

CASBAME (Mexico)
LOVASTATIN
Mevacor Tablets . . . 2063

CASBOL (Spain)
PAROXETINE HYDROCHLORIDE
Paxil Oral Suspension . . . 1535
Paxil Tablets . . . 1535

CASCOR (Malaysia, Thailand)
DILTIAZEM HYDROCHLORIDE
Cardizem LA Extended Release Tablets . . . 421

CATALIP (Portugal)
FENOFIBRATE
Tricor Tablets 520

CATAPRES (Australia, Canada, Hong Kong, India, Irish Republic, Japan, New Zealand, South Africa, Thailand, The Philippines, United Kingdom)
CLONIDINE HYDROCHLORIDE
Catapres Tablets 841

CATAPRES DIU (India)
CLONIDINE HYDROCHLORIDE
Catapres Tablets 841

CATAPRESAN (Austria, Chile, Czech Republic, Denmark, Finland, Germany, Greece, Mexico, Norway, Portugal, Spain, Sweden, Switzerland, The Netherlands, Venezuela)
CLONIDINE HYDROCHLORIDE
Catapres Tablets 841

CATAPRESSAN (Belgium, France)
CLONIDINE HYDROCHLORIDE
Catapres Tablets 841

CATEGOR (Argentina)
CAPECITABINE
Xeloda Tablets 2662

CATEX (Spain)
CIPROFLOXACIN HYDROCHLORIDE
Cipro Tablets 2810

CATEXAN (South Africa)
INDAPAMIDE
Indapamide Tablets 2188

CATONA (Mexico)
CAPTOPRIL
Captopril Tablets 2182

CATONET (Denmark)
CAPTOPRIL
Captopril Tablets 2182

CATOPLIN (Singapore)
CAPTOPRIL
Captopril Tablets 2182

CATOPROL (Brazil)
CAPTOPRIL
Captopril Tablets 2182

CAUSALON PRO (Argentina)
NAPROXEN
EC-Naprosyn Delayed-Release Tablets 2632
Naprosyn Suspension 2632
Naprosyn Tablets 2632

C-BILDZ (Austria)
CIPROFLOXACIN HYDROCHLORIDE
Cipro Tablets 2810

CEBRALAT (Brazil)
CILOSTAZOL
Pletal Tablets 2481

CEBRILIN (Brazil)
PAROXETINE HYDROCHLORIDE
Paxil Oral Suspension 1535
Paxil Tablets 1535

CEBROCAL (Argentina)
DONEPEZIL HYDROCHLORIDE
Aricept Tablets 1062

CEBROFORT (Argentina)
NIMODIPINE
Nimotop Capsules 790

CECNOIN (Brazil)
ISOTRETINOIN
Accutane Capsules 2607

CECURAL (Greece)
LOVASTATIN
Mevacor Tablets 2063

CEDETRIN-T (Czech Republic)
MUROMONAB-CD3
Orthoclone OKT3 Sterile Solution 2387

CEDIZIM (Italy)
CEFTAZIDIME
Fortaz for Injection 1450

CEF-3 (Thailand, The Philippines)
CEFTRIAXONE SODIUM
Rocephin Injectable Vials, ADD-Vantage, Galaxy, Bulk 2642

CEF-4 (Thailand)
CEFTAZIDIME
Fortaz for Injection 1450

CEFADAY (Turkey)
CEFTRIAXONE SODIUM
Rocephin Injectable Vials, ADD-Vantage, Galaxy, Bulk 2642

CEFAMAR (Italy, Thailand)
CEFUROXIME SODIUM
Zinacef Injection 1678

CEFASYN (India, South Africa)
CEFUROXIME AXETIL
Ceftin for Oral Suspension 1380
Ceftin Tablets 1380

CEFATIN (Turkey)
CEFUROXIME AXETIL
Ceftin for Oral Suspension 1380
Ceftin Tablets 1380

CEFAXONA (Mexico)
CEFTRIAXONE SODIUM
Rocephin Injectable Vials, ADD-Vantage, Galaxy, Bulk 2642

CEFAXONE (Czech Republic, Malaysia, Singapore)
CEFTRIAXONE SODIUM
Rocephin Injectable Vials, ADD-Vantage, Galaxy, Bulk 2642

CEFAZID (India)
CEFTAZIDIME
Fortaz for Injection 1450

CEFAZIMA (Brazil)
CEFTAZIDIME
Fortaz for Injection 1450

CEFAZIME (Singapore)
CEFTAZIDIME
Fortaz for Injection 1450

CEF-DIME (Thailand)
CEFTAZIDIME
Fortaz for Injection 1450

CEFGRAM (Venezuela)
CEFTAZIDIME
Fortaz for Injection 1450

CEFIN (Singapore, Venezuela)
CEFTRIAXONE SODIUM
Rocephin Injectable Vials, ADD-Vantage, Galaxy, Bulk 2642

CEFINE (Thailand)
CEFTRIAXONE SODIUM
Rocephin Injectable Vials, ADD-Vantage, Galaxy, Bulk 2642

CEFIX (Venezuela)
CEFTRIAXONE SODIUM
Rocephin Injectable Vials, ADD-Vantage, Galaxy, Bulk 2642

CEFLOUR (Malaysia)
CEFUROXIME SODIUM
Zinacef Injection 1678

CEFOCEF (India)
CEFTRIAXONE SODIUM
Rocephin Injectable Vials, ADD-Vantage, Galaxy, Bulk 2642

CEFODIME (Thailand)
CEFTAZIDIME
Fortaz for Injection 1450

CEFOFIX (Portugal, The Netherlands)
CEFUROXIME SODIUM
Zinacef Injection 1678

CEFOGEN (India, Thailand)
CEFUROXIME SODIUM
Zinacef Injection 1678

CEFOMAX (Argentina)
CEFTRIAXONE SODIUM
Rocephin Injectable Vials, ADD-Vantage, Galaxy, Bulk 2642

CEFOPRIM (Greece, Italy)
CEFUROXIME SODIUM
Zinacef Injection 1678

CEFORTAM (Portugal)
CEFTAZIDIME SODIUM
Fortaz for Injection 1450

CEFOTRIX (Denmark, Germany, Hungary)
CEFTRIAXONE SODIUM
Rocephin Injectable Vials, ADD-Vantage, Galaxy, Bulk 2642

CEFOXIM (India)
CEFUROXIME AXETIL
Ceftin for Oral Suspension 1380
Ceftin Tablets 1380

CEFRADEN (Mexico)
CEFTRIAXONE SODIUM
Rocephin Injectable Vials, ADD-Vantage, Galaxy, Bulk 2642

CEFT (Brazil)
CEFTRIAXONE SODIUM
Rocephin Injectable Vials, ADD-Vantage, Galaxy, Bulk 2642

CEFTAL (Irish Republic)
CEFUROXIME AXETIL
Ceftin for Oral Suspension 1380
Ceftin Tablets 1380

CEFTANORTH (Brazil)
CEFTAZIDIME
Fortaz for Injection 1450

CEFTARIDEM (Greece)
CEFTAZIDIME
Fortaz for Injection 1450

CEFTAZ (India)
CEFTAZIDIME
Fortaz for Injection 1450

CEFTAZIDON (Brazil)
CEFTAZIDIME
Fortaz for Injection 1450

CEFTEN (Brazil)
CEFTAZIDIME
Fortaz for Injection 1450

CEFTIDIN (India)
CEFTAZIDIME
Fortaz for Injection 1450

CEFTIM (Italy)
CEFTAZIDIME
Fortaz for Injection 1450

CEFTIN (Canada)
CEFUROXIME AXETIL
Ceftin for Oral Suspension 1380
Ceftin Tablets 1380

CEFTREX (Malaysia, Mexico, Thailand)
CEFTRIAXONE SODIUM
Rocephin Injectable Vials, ADD-Vantage, Galaxy, Bulk 2642

CEFTRILEM (Mexico)
CEFTRIAXONE SODIUM
Rocephin Injectable Vials, ADD-Vantage, Galaxy, Bulk 2642

CEFTRINAL (Greece)
RANITIDINE HYDROCHLORIDE
Zantac 25 EFFERdose Tablets 1670
Zantac 150 Tablets 1670
Zantac 300 Tablets 1670
Zantac Injection 1666
Zantac Injection Premixed 1666
Zantac Syrup 1670

CEFTRIPHIN (Thailand)
CEFTRIAXONE SODIUM
Rocephin Injectable Vials, ADD-Vantage, Galaxy, Bulk 2642

CEFU (Germany)
CEFUROXIME AXETIL
Ceftin for Oral Suspension 1380
Ceftin Tablets 1380

CEFUDURA (Germany)
CEFUROXIME AXETIL
Ceftin for Oral Suspension 1380
Ceftin Tablets 1380

CEFUHEXAL (Germany)
CEFUROXIME AXETIL
Ceftin for Oral Suspension 1380
Ceftin Tablets 1380

CEFU-HEXAL (South Africa)
CEFUROXIME AXETIL
Ceftin for Oral Suspension 1380
Ceftin Tablets 1380

CEFUMAX (Italy)
CEFUROXIME SODIUM
Zinacef Injection 1678

CEFUR (Italy)
CEFUROXIME SODIUM
Zinacef Injection 1678

CEFURACET (Mexico)
CEFUROXIME AXETIL
Ceftin for Oral Suspension 1380
Ceftin Tablets 1380

CEFURAX (Germany, Israel)
CEFUROXIME AXETIL
Ceftin for Oral Suspension 1380
Ceftin Tablets 1380

CEFUREX (Italy)
CEFUROXIME SODIUM
Zinacef Injection 1678

CEFURIM (Switzerland)
CEFUROXIME AXETIL
Ceftin for Oral Suspension 1380
Ceftin Tablets 1380

CEFURIN (Italy)
CEFUROXIME SODIUM
Zinacef Injection 1678

CEFURO-PUREN (Germany)
CEFUROXIME AXETIL
Ceftin for Oral Suspension 1380
Ceftin Tablets 1380

CEFUROX (Argentina)
CEFUROXIME AXETIL
Ceftin for Oral Suspension 1380
Ceftin Tablets 1380

CEFUROX-REU (Germany)
CEFUROXIME SODIUM
Zinacef Injection 1678

CEFUROX-WOLFF (Germany)
CEFUROXIME AXETIL
Ceftin for Oral Suspension 1380
Ceftin Tablets 1380

CEFUZIME (United Arab Emirates)
CEFUROXIME AXETIL
Ceftin for Oral Suspension 1380
Ceftin Tablets 1380

CEFZON (Japan)
CEFDINIR
Omnicef Capsules 497
Omnicef for Oral Suspension 497

CEF-ZONE (Thailand)
CEFTRIAXONE SODIUM
Rocephin Injectable Vials, ADD-Vantage, Galaxy, Bulk 2642

CELAPRAM (Australia, New Zealand)
CITALOPRAM HYDROBROMIDE
Celexa Tablets 1160

CELAY (Venezuela)
CETIRIZINE HYDROCHLORIDE
Zyrtec Syrup 1920
Zyrtec Tablets 1920

CELCOX (Israel)
CELECOXIB
Celebrex Capsules 2979

CELEBRA (Brazil, Chile, Denmark, Finland, Israel, Sweden)
CELECOXIB
Celebrex Capsules 2979

CELEBREX (Argentina, Australia, Austria, Belgium, Canada, Czech Republic, France, Germany, Greece, Hong Kong, Hungary, Irish Republic, Italy, Malaysia, Mexico, New Zealand, Poland, Portugal, Russia, Singapore, South Africa, Spain, Switzerland, Thailand, The Netherlands, The Philippines, United Kingdom, Venezuela)
CELECOXIB
Celebrex Capsules 2979

CELEDOL (India)
CELECOXIB
Celebrex Capsules 2979

CELEFER (Spain)
MUPIROCIN
Bactroban Ointment 1368

CELEMAX (Argentina)
CELECOXIB
Celebrex Capsules 2979

CELEXA (Canada)
CITALOPRAM HYDROBROMIDE
Celexa Tablets 1160

CELIB (India)
CELECOXIB
Celebrex Capsules 2979

CELVISTA (Thailand)
RALOXIFENE HYDROCHLORIDE
Evista Tablets **1810**

CENCENAG (Thailand)
DICLOFENAC SODIUM
Voltaren Tablets **2334**
Voltaren-XR Tablets **2337**

CENLIDAC (Thailand)
SULINDAC
Clinoril Tablets **1962**

CENTOCORT (Thailand)
TRIAMCINOLONE ACETONIDE
Azmacort Inhalation Aerosol **407**
Nasacort AQ Nasal Spray **2765**

CENTRAPRYL (United Kingdom)
SELEGILINE HYDROCHLORIDE
Eldepryl Capsules **3052**

CENTROMICINA (Argentina)
CLARITHROMYCIN
Biaxin Filmtab Tablets **411**
Biaxin Granules **411**

CEPAL (Greece)
FAMOTIDINE
Pepcid for Oral Suspension **2075**
Pepcid Tablets **2075**

CEPARIDIN (Spain)
TRAMADOL HYDROCHLORIDE
Ultram ER Tablets **2428**

CEPAZINE (France)
CEFUROXIME AXETIL
Ceftin for Oral Suspension **1380**
Ceftin Tablets **1380**

CEPHULAC (Canada)
LACTULOSE
Kristalose for Oral Solution **1004**

CEPLON (Venezuela)
CAPTOPRIL
Captopril Tablets **2182**

CEPRAZOL (Chile)
ALBENDAZOLE
Albenza Tablets **1297**

CEPRIMAX (Spain)
CIPROFLOXACIN HYDROCHLORIDE
Cipro Tablets **2810**

CEPTAZ (Canada)
CEFTAZIDIME
Fortaz for Injection **1450**

CERANID (The Philippines)
RANITIDINE HYDROCHLORIDE
Zantac 25 EFFERdose Tablets **1670**
Zantac 150 Tablets **1670**
Zantac 300 Tablets **1670**
Zantac Injection **1666**
Zantac Injection Premixed **1666**
Zantac Syrup **1670**

CERATIO (Poland)
CETIRIZINE HYDROCHLORIDE
Zyrtec Syrup **1920**
Zyrtec Tablets **1920**

CEREBROVASE (United Kingdom)
DIPYRIDAMOLE
Persantine Tablets **869**

CERELLA (Germany)
ESTRADIOL
Climara Transdermal System **763**

CERELUC (Argentina)
PIOGLITAZONE HYDROCHLORIDE
Actos Tablets **3077**

CEREX (Czech Republic)
CETIRIZINE HYDROCHLORIDE
Zyrtec Syrup **1920**
Zyrtec Tablets **1920**

CEREZYME (Australia, Austria, Belgium, Canada, Czech Republic, Denmark, Finland, France, Germany, Hong Kong, Israel, Italy, Japan, New Zealand, Norway, Poland, Portugal, South Africa, Spain, Sweden, Switzerland, The Netherlands, United Kingdom)
IMIGLUCERASE
Cerezyme for Injection **1238**

CERINA (Switzerland)
ESTRADIOL
Climara Transdermal System **763**

CEROFENE (Greece)
CEFUROXIME SODIUM
Zinacef Injection **1678**

CEROXIM (Hungary, Poland, South Africa)
CEFUROXIME AXETIL
Ceftin for Oral Suspension **1380**
Ceftin Tablets **1380**

CERTALAC (Belgium)
LACTULOSE
Kristalose for Oral Solution **1004**

CERUXIM (Greece)
CEFUROXIME SODIUM
Zinacef Injection **1678**

CERVIDIL (Australia, Canada, New Zealand)
DINOPROSTONE
Cervidil Vaginal Insert **1165**

CERVIN (The Philippines)
CEFUROXIME SODIUM
Zinacef Injection **1678**

CERVIPRIME (India)
DINOPROSTONE
Cervidil Vaginal Insert **1165**

CERVIPROST (Austria, Germany, Norway, Sweden, Switzerland, The Netherlands)
DINOPROSTONE
Cervidil Vaginal Insert **1165**

CERZINE (Switzerland)
CETIRIZINE HYDROCHLORIDE
Zyrtec Syrup **1920**
Zyrtec Tablets **1920**

CESPLON (Spain)
CAPTOPRIL
Captopril Tablets **2182**

CET ECO (Switzerland)
CETIRIZINE HYDROCHLORIDE
Zyrtec Syrup **1920**
Zyrtec Tablets **1920**

CETALERG (Germany)
CETIRIZINE HYDROCHLORIDE
Zyrtec Syrup **1920**
Zyrtec Tablets **1920**

CETALERGIN (Poland)
CETIRIZINE HYDROCHLORIDE
Zyrtec Syrup **1920**
Zyrtec Tablets **1920**

CETALLERG (Switzerland)
CETIRIZINE HYDROCHLORIDE
Zyrtec Syrup **1920**
Zyrtec Tablets **1920**

CETAPRED (Belgium)
PREDNISOLONE ACETATE/SULFACETAMIDE SODIUM
Blephamide Ophthalmic Ointment . . . . . . ⊙**217**
Blephamide Ophthalmic Suspension . . . . ⊙**216**

CETAZ (Brazil)
CEFTAZIDIME
Fortaz for Injection **1450**

CETAZIME (Hungary)
CEFTAZIDIME
Fortaz for Injection **1450**

CETCIP (India)
CETIRIZINE HYDROCHLORIDE
Zyrtec Syrup **1920**
Zyrtec Tablets **1920**

CETERIFUG (Germany)
CETIRIZINE HYDROCHLORIDE
Zyrtec Syrup **1920**
Zyrtec Tablets **1920**

CETI (Germany)
CETIRIZINE HYDROCHLORIDE
Zyrtec Syrup **1920**
Zyrtec Tablets **1920**

CETICAD (India)
CETIRIZINE HYDROCHLORIDE
Zyrtec Syrup **1920**
Zyrtec Tablets **1920**

CETIDAC (Argentina)
CETIRIZINE HYDROCHLORIDE
Zyrtec Syrup **1920**
Zyrtec Tablets **1920**

CETIDERM (Austria, Germany)
CETIRIZINE HYDROCHLORIDE
Zyrtec Syrup **1920**
Zyrtec Tablets **1920**

CETIDURA (Germany)
CETIRIZINE HYDROCHLORIDE
Zyrtec Syrup **1920**
Zyrtec Tablets **1920**

CETIHEXAL (Brazil)
CETIRIZINE HYDROCHLORIDE
Zyrtec Syrup **1920**
Zyrtec Tablets **1920**

CETIHIS (Hong Kong, Thailand)
CETIRIZINE HYDROCHLORIDE
Zyrtec Syrup **1920**
Zyrtec Tablets **1920**

CETIL (Germany)
CETIRIZINE HYDROCHLORIDE
Zyrtec Syrup **1920**
Zyrtec Tablets **1920**

CETILICH (Germany)
CETIRIZINE HYDROCHLORIDE
Zyrtec Syrup **1920**
Zyrtec Tablets **1920**

CETIMIN (The Philippines)
CETIRIZINE HYDROCHLORIDE
Zyrtec Syrup **1920**
Zyrtec Tablets **1920**

CETI-PUREN (Germany)
CETIRIZINE HYDROCHLORIDE
Zyrtec Syrup **1920**
Zyrtec Tablets **1920**

CETIRAM (Greece)
CETIRIZINE HYDROCHLORIDE
Zyrtec Syrup **1920**
Zyrtec Tablets **1920**

CETIRHEXAL (Austria)
CETIRIZINE HYDROCHLORIDE
Zyrtec Syrup **1920**
Zyrtec Tablets **1920**

CETIRIGAMMA (Germany)
CETIRIZINE HYDROCHLORIDE
Zyrtec Syrup **1920**
Zyrtec Tablets **1920**

CETIRIN (Hong Kong)
CETIRIZINE HYDROCHLORIDE
Zyrtec Syrup **1920**
Zyrtec Tablets **1920**

CETIRISTAD (Austria)
CETIRIZINE HYDROCHLORIDE
Zyrtec Syrup **1920**
Zyrtec Tablets **1920**

CETIRIVAX (Venezuela)
CETIRIZINE HYDROCHLORIDE
Zyrtec Syrup **1920**
Zyrtec Tablets **1920**

CETIRIVAX D (Venezuela)
CETIRIZINE HYDROCHLORIDE
Zyrtec Syrup **1920**
Zyrtec Tablets **1920**

CETIRLAN (Germany)
CETIRIZINE HYDROCHLORIDE
Zyrtec Syrup **1920**
Zyrtec Tablets **1920**

CETIROCOL (United Kingdom)
CETIRIZINE HYDROCHLORIDE
Zyrtec Syrup **1920**
Zyrtec Tablets **1920**

CETIZINE (Argentina)
CETIRIZINE HYDROCHLORIDE
Zyrtec Syrup **1920**
Zyrtec Tablets **1920**

CETRALON (United Arab Emirates)
CETIRIZINE HYDROCHLORIDE
Zyrtec Syrup **1920**
Zyrtec Tablets **1920**

CETRAPHYLLINE (France)
THEOPHYLLINE
Uniphyl Tablets **2595**

CETRAXAL PLUS (Spain)
CIPROFLOXACIN
Cipro Oral Suspension **2810**

CETRILER (Argentina)
CETIRIZINE HYDROCHLORIDE
Zyrtec Syrup **1920**
Zyrtec Tablets **1920**

CETRIMED (Thailand)
CETIRIZINE HYDROCHLORIDE
Zyrtec Syrup **1920**
Zyrtec Tablets **1920**

CETRINE (Irish Republic, Russia, Singapore, Switzerland, Thailand, Venezuela)
CETIRIZINE HYDROCHLORIDE
Zyrtec Syrup **1920**
Zyrtec Tablets **1920**

CETRIVAX (Poland)
CETIRIZINE HYDROCHLORIDE
Zyrtec Syrup **1920**
Zyrtec Tablets **1920**

CETRIWAL (India)
CETIRIZINE HYDROCHLORIDE
Zyrtec Syrup **1920**
Zyrtec Tablets **1920**

CETRIZEN (Poland)
CETIRIZINE HYDROCHLORIDE
Zyrtec Syrup **1920**
Zyrtec Tablets **1920**

CETRIZET (India, Thailand)
CETIRIZINE HYDROCHLORIDE
Zyrtec Syrup **1920**
Zyrtec Tablets **1920**

CETRIZIN (Brazil, Thailand)
CETIRIZINE HYDROCHLORIDE
Zyrtec Syrup **1920**
Zyrtec Tablets **1920**

CETRON (Argentina)
ONDANSETRON
Zofran ODT Orally Disintegrating Tablets . . **1687**

CETRYN (Turkey)
CETIRIZINE HYDROCHLORIDE
Zyrtec Syrup **1920**
Zyrtec Tablets **1920**

CETY (Hong Kong)
CETIRIZINE HYDROCHLORIDE
Zyrtec Syrup **1920**
Zyrtec Tablets **1920**

CETYROL (Austria)
CETIRIZINE HYDROCHLORIDE
Zyrtec Syrup **1920**
Zyrtec Tablets **1920**

CETYRYZYNA (Poland)
CETIRIZINE HYDROCHLORIDE
Zyrtec Syrup **1920**
Zyrtec Tablets **1920**

CEVAS (India)
CARVEDILOL
Coreg Tablets **1387**

CEXB (Venezuela)
CELECOXIB
Celebrex Capsules **2979**

CEXIDAL OTICO (Spain)
CIPROFLOXACIN
Cipro Oral Suspension **2810**

CEXIM (Hungary)
CEFUROXIME SODIUM
Zinacef Injection **1678**

CEZA (Thailand)
CETIRIZINE HYDROCHLORIDE
Zyrtec Syrup **1920**
Zyrtec Tablets **1920**

C-FLOX (Australia)
CIPROFLOXACIN HYDROCHLORIDE
Cipro Tablets **2810**

C-FLOXACIN (Thailand)
CIPROFLOXACIN HYDROCHLORIDE
Cipro Tablets **2810**

CHAMPS D-WORMS (Malaysia)
ALBENDAZOLE
Albenza Tablets **1297**

CHANTALINE (Spain)
THEOPHYLLINE
Uniphyl Tablets **2595**

CHARLYN (Italy)
FLUNISOLIDE
Aerobid Inhaler System **1153**
Aerobid-M Inhaler System **1153**

CHEMISTS OWN PERIOD PAIN TABLETS (Australia)
NAPROXEN SODIUM
Anaprox DS Tablets **2632**

Anaprox Tablets 2632

CHIBRO-PROSCAR (France)
FINASTERIDE
Propecia Tablets 2095
Proscar Tablets 2102

CHIBRO-TIMOPTOL (Germany)
TIMOLOL MALEATE
Timoptic in Ocudose 2124
Timoptic Sterile Ophthalmic Solution 2121
Timoptic-XE Sterile Ophthalmic Gel Forming Solution 2125

CHIBROXIN (Argentina, Brazil, Chile, Germany, Hong Kong, Israel, Malaysia, Poland, Singapore, Spain, Venezuela)
NORFLOXACIN
Noroxin Tablets 2069

CHIBROXINE (France)
NORFLOXACIN
Noroxin Tablets 2069

CHIBROXOL (Belgium, Portugal, Switzerland, The Netherlands)
NORFLOXACIN
Noroxin Tablets 2069

CHLORAMINOPHENE (Monaco)
CHLORAMBUCIL
Leukeran Tablets 1508

CHOLEMED (Belgium)
SIMVASTATIN
Zocor Tablets 2136

CHOLESTAD (The Philippines)
SIMVASTATIN
Zocor Tablets 2136

CHRISTATIN (Greece)
SIMVASTATIN
Zocor Tablets 2136

CHRONOPHYLLIN (South Africa)
THEOPHYLLINE
Uniphyl Tablets 2595

CHRONULAC (Canada)
LACTULOSE
Kristalose for Oral Solution 1004

CIAZIL (Australia)
CITALOPRAM HYDROBROMIDE
Celexa Tablets 1160

CIBRAMICINA (Brazil)
AMOXICILLIN
Amoxil Pediatric Drops for Oral Suspension 1305
Amoxil Tablets 1305

CIBROGAN (Argentina)
CILOSTAZOL
Pletal Tablets 2481

CICLODIN (The Philippines)
CIPROFLOXACIN HYDROCHLORIDE
Cipro Tablets 2810

CICLOTRAN (Argentina)
RALOXIFENE HYDROCHLORIDE
Evista Tablets 1810

CICLOX (Argentina)
CLONAZEPAM
Klonopin Tablets 2639

CIDANAMOX (Spain)
AMOXICILLIN
Amoxil Pediatric Drops for Oral Suspension 1305
Amoxil Tablets 1305

CIDRON (Denmark, Finland, Sweden)
CETIRIZINE HYDROCHLORIDE
Zyrtec Syrup 1920
Zyrtec Tablets 1920

CIDROPS (Greece)
CIPROFLOXACIN
Cipro Oral Suspension 2810

CIDROXAL (The Philippines)
CIPROFLOXACIN HYDROCHLORIDE
Cipro Tablets 2810

CIFIN (Denmark)
CIPROFLOXACIN HYDROCHLORIDE
Cipro Tablets 2810

CIFLAN (Portugal)
CIPROFLOXACIN HYDROCHLORIDE
Cipro Tablets 2810

CIFLO (Thailand)
CIPROFLOXACIN HYDROCHLORIDE
Cipro Tablets 2810

CIFLOC (South Africa)
CIPROFLOXACIN HYDROCHLORIDE
Cipro Tablets 2810

CIFLOCINA (Brazil)
CIPROFLOXACIN
Cipro Oral Suspension 2810

CIFLOLAN (Thailand)
CIPROFLOXACIN
Cipro Oral Suspension 2810

CIFLOSIN (Turkey)
CIPROFLOXACIN
Cipro Oral Suspension 2810

CIFLOX (Austria, Brazil, Italy, Venezuela)
CIPROFLOXACIN HYDROCHLORIDE
Cipro Tablets 2810

CIFLOXAGER (Irish Republic)
CIPROFLOXACIN HYDROCHLORIDE
Cipro Tablets 2810

CIFLOXAN (Brazil)
CIPROFLOXACIN
Cipro Oral Suspension 2810

CIFLOXIN (Chile, Hong Kong)
CIPROFLOXACIN
Cipro Oral Suspension 2810

CIFLOXINAL (Czech Republic, Russia)
CIPROFLOXACIN HYDROCHLORIDE
Cipro Tablets 2810

CIFLOXTRON (Brazil)
CIPROFLOXACIN HYDROCHLORIDE
Cipro Tablets 2810

CIFLURON (Turkey)
CIPROFLOXACIN
Cipro Oral Suspension 2810

CIFRAN (Czech Republic, Hungary, Malaysia, Poland, South Africa)
CIPROFLOXACIN
Cipro Oral Suspension 2810

CIL (Germany)
FENOFIBRATE
Tricor Tablets 520

CILAB (Thailand)
CIPROFLOXACIN
Cipro Oral Suspension 2810

CILETIN (The Philippines)
CILOSTAZOL
Pletal Tablets 2481

CILEX (Germany)
CITALOPRAM HYDROBROMIDE
Celexa Tablets 1160

CILIFT (South Africa)
CITALOPRAM HYDROBROMIDE
Celexa Tablets 1160

CILODAC (India)
CILOSTAZOL
Pletal Tablets 2481

CILODEX (Chile, Mexico)
CIPROFLOXACIN HYDROCHLORIDE
Cipro Tablets 2810

CILON (Poland)
CITALOPRAM HYDROBROMIDE
Celexa Tablets 1160

CILOQUIN (Australia)
CIPROFLOXACIN HYDROCHLORIDE
Cipro Tablets 2810

CILOSTAL (Argentina)
CILOSTAZOL
Pletal Tablets 2481

CILOVAS (Argentina)
CILOSTAZOL
Pletal Tablets 2481

CILOX (Norway)
CIPROFLOXACIN HYDROCHLORIDE
Cipro Tablets 2810

CILOXACIN (Chile)
CIPROFLOXACIN HYDROCHLORIDE
Cipro Tablets 2810

CILOXADEX (Argentina)
CIPROFLOXACIN HYDROCHLORIDE
Cipro Tablets 2810

CILOXAN (Argentina, Australia, Austria, Belgium, Brazil, Canada, Czech Republic, Denmark, France, Germany, Greece, Hong Kong, Hungary, Israel, Malaysia, Mexico, New Zealand, Poland, Russia, Singapore, South Africa, Sweden, Switzerland, Thailand, The Netherlands, The Philippines, Turkey, United Kingdom, Venezuela)
CIPROFLOXACIN HYDROCHLORIDE
Cipro Tablets 2810

CIMAL (Chile)
CITALOPRAM HYDROBROMIDE
Celexa Tablets 1160

CIMECARD (Brazil)
DIGOXIN
Lanoxin Injection 1498
Lanoxin Injection Pediatric 1502
Lanoxin Tablets 1505

CIMOGAL (Mexico)
CIPROFLOXACIN HYDROCHLORIDE
Cipro Tablets 2810

CINFLOXINE (Thailand)
CIPROFLOXACIN HYDROCHLORIDE
Cipro Tablets 2810

CINIE (Poland)
SUMATRIPTAN SUCCINATE
Imitrex Injection 1465
Imitrex Tablets 1474

CINOFLAX (Brazil)
CIPROFLOXACIN HYDROCHLORIDE
Cipro Tablets 2810

CIP ECO (Switzerland)
CIPROFLOXACIN HYDROCHLORIDE
Cipro Tablets 2810

CIPFLOCIN (Thailand)
CIPROFLOXACIN
Cipro Oral Suspension 2810

CIPFLOX (New Zealand)
CIPROFLOXACIN
Cipro Oral Suspension 2810

CIPGEN (India)
CIPROFLOXACIN
Cipro Oral Suspension 2810

CIPGEN TZ (India)
CIPROFLOXACIN
Cipro Oral Suspension 2810

CIPHIN (Czech Republic)
CIPROFLOXACIN
Cipro Oral Suspension 2810

CIPIDE (Hong Kong)
CIPROFLOXACIN HYDROCHLORIDE
Cipro Tablets 2810

CIPLACEF (India, Venezuela)
CEFTRIAXONE SODIUM
Rocephin Injectable Vials, ADD-Vantage, Galaxy, Bulk 2642

CIPLOX (Hong Kong, Israel, Portugal)
CIPROFLOXACIN
Cipro Oral Suspension 2810

CIPLOX D (India)
CIPROFLOXACIN
Cipro Oral Suspension 2810

CIPLOX TZ (India)
CIPROFLOXACIN
Cipro Oral Suspension 2810

CIPLOXX (South Africa)
CIPROFLOXACIN HYDROCHLORIDE
Cipro Tablets 2810

CIPOBACTER (Spain)
CIPROFLOXACIN HYDROCHLORIDE
Cipro Tablets 2810

CIPOFIX (South Africa)
CEFUROXIME SODIUM
Zinacef Injection 1678

CIPON (Thailand)
CIPROFLOXACIN
Cipro Oral Suspension 2810

CIPRAGER (Irish Republic)
CITALOPRAM HYDROBROMIDE
Celexa Tablets 1160

CIPRAIN (Mexico)
CIPROFLOXACIN
Cipro Oral Suspension 2810

CIPRAM (Hong Kong, Malaysia, Singapore, Thailand, Turkey)
CITALOPRAM HYDROBROMIDE
Celexa Tablets 1160

CIPRAMIL (Australia, Chile, Germany, Israel, New Zealand, Norway, Poland, Russia, South Africa)
CITALOPRAM HYDROBROMIDE
Celexa Tablets 1160

CIPRAPINE (Irish Republic, The Netherlands)
CITALOPRAM HYDROBROMIDE
Celexa Tablets 1160

CIPRASID (Turkey)
CIPROFLOXACIN
Cipro Oral Suspension 2810

CIPRENIT OTICO (Spain)
CIPROFLOXACIN HYDROCHLORIDE
Cipro Tablets 2810

CIPREX (Brazil)
CIPROFLOXACIN HYDROCHLORIDE
Cipro Tablets 2810

CIPRIL (Hong Kong, India)
LISINOPRIL
Prinivil Tablets 2087

CIPRIL-H (India)
LISINOPRIL
Prinivil Tablets 2087

CIPRINOL (The Netherlands)
CIPROFLOXACIN HYDROCHLORIDE
Cipro Tablets 2810

CIPRIVAX (Venezuela)
CIPROFLOXACIN
Cipro Oral Suspension 2810

CIPRO (Argentina, Turkey)
CIPROFLOXACIN
Cipro Oral Suspension 2810

CIPRO HC (Argentina, Brazil, Hong Kong)
CIPROFLOXACIN HYDROCHLORIDE
Cipro Tablets 2810

CIPROANT (Brazil)
CIPROFLOXACIN
Cipro Oral Suspension 2810

CIPROBAY (Czech Republic, Greece, Hungary, Poland)
CIPROFLOXACIN
Cipro Oral Suspension 2810

CIPROBAY HC (Singapore, South Africa)
CIPROFLOXACIN
Cipro Oral Suspension 2810

CIPROBAY HC OTIC (Czech Republic)
CIPROFLOXACIN HYDROCHLORIDE
Cipro Tablets 2810

CIPROBEL (Belgium)
CIPROFLOXACIN
Cipro Oral Suspension 2810

CIPROBETA (Germany)
CIPROFLOXACIN HYDROCHLORIDE
Cipro Tablets 2810

CIPROBID (Czech Republic, Thailand)
CIPROFLOXACIN
Cipro Oral Suspension 2810

CIPROBIOT (Brazil)
CIPROFLOXACIN HYDROCHLORIDE
Cipro Tablets 2810

CIPROBIOTIC (Mexico)
CIPROFLOXACIN HYDROCHLORIDE
Cipro Tablets 2810

CIPRO-CENT (India)
CIPROFLOXACIN HYDROCHLORIDE
Cipro Tablets 2810

CIPROCEP (Thailand)
CIPROFLOXACIN
Cipro Oral Suspension 2810

CIPROCIN (Brazil)
CIPROFLOXACIN
Cipro Oral Suspension 2810

CIPROCINA (Brazil)
CIPROFLOXACIN
Cipro Oral Suspension 2810

CIPROCTAL (Spain)
CIPROFLOXACIN HYDROCHLORIDE
Cipro Tablets 2810

CIPRODEX (Israel)
CIPROFLOXACIN HYDROCHLORIDE
Cipro Tablets 2810

CIPRODINE (Brazil)
CIPROFLOXACIN HYDROCHLORIDE
Cipro Tablets 2810

CIPRODOC (Germany)
CIPROFLOXACIN HYDROCHLORIDE
Cipro Tablets 2810

CIPRODURA (Germany)
CIPROFLOXACIN HYDROCHLORIDE
Cipro Tablets 2810

CIPROFAL (Greece)
CIPROFLOXACIN
Cipro Oral Suspension 2810

CIPROFAR (Brazil)
CIPROFLOXACIN HYDROCHLORIDE
Cipro Tablets 2810

CIPROFAT (Germany)
CIPROFLOXACIN HYDROCHLORIDE
Cipro Tablets 2810

CIPROFIN (Thailand)
CIPROFLOXACIN
Cipro Oral Suspension 2810

CIPROFLONAX (Brazil)
CIPROFLOXACIN
Cipro Oral Suspension 2810

CIPROFLOX (Brazil, Germany, Switzerland, Venezuela)
CIPROFLOXACIN
Cipro Oral Suspension 2810

CIPROFLOXIL (Brazil)
CIPROFLOXACIN
Cipro Oral Suspension 2810

CIPROFLOX-OTIC (Argentina)
CIPROFLOXACIN HYDROCHLORIDE
Cipro Tablets 2810

CIPROFLOX-PUREN (Germany)
CIPROFLOXACIN HYDROCHLORIDE
Cipro Tablets 2810

CIPROFUR (Mexico)
CIPROFLOXACIN HYDROCHLORIDE
Cipro Tablets 2810

CIPROGAMMA (Germany)
CIPROFLOXACIN HYDROCHLORIDE
Cipro Tablets 2810

CIPROGEN (South Africa, Thailand)
CIPROFLOXACIN
Cipro Oral Suspension 2810

CIPROGIS (Israel)
CIPROFLOXACIN
Cipro Oral Suspension 2810

CIPROGLEN (Thailand)
CIPROFLOXACIN
Cipro Oral Suspension 2810

CIPROHEXAL (Mexico)
CIPROFLOXACIN HYDROCHLORIDE
Cipro Tablets 2810

CIPRO-HEXAL (South Africa)
CIPROFLOXACIN
Cipro Oral Suspension 2810

CIPROK (Spain)
CIPROFLOXACIN HYDROCHLORIDE
Cipro Tablets 2810

CIPROKTAN (Turkey)
CIPROFLOXACIN HYDROCHLORIDE
Cipro Tablets 2810

CIPROL (Australia, Hong Kong)
CIPROFLOXACIN HYDROCHLORIDE
Cipro Tablets 2810

CIPROLET (Russia, Singapore, Venezuela)
CIPROFLOXACIN
Cipro Oral Suspension 2810

CIPRO-LICH (Germany)
CIPROFLOXACIN HYDROCHLORIDE
Cipro Tablets 2810

CIPROLONE (Russia)
CIPROFLOXACIN HYDROCHLORIDE
Cipro Tablets 2810

CIPROMAX (The Philippines)
CIPROFLOXACIN HYDROCHLORIDE
Cipro Tablets 2810

CIPROMED (Austria, Finland, Russia)
CIPROFLOXACIN HYDROCHLORIDE
Cipro Tablets 2810

CIPRO-MED (Switzerland)
CIPROFLOXACIN HYDROCHLORIDE
Cipro Tablets 2810

CIPROMET (The Philippines)
CIPROFLOXACIN HYDROCHLORIDE
Cipro Tablets 2810

CIPROMIZIN (Brazil)
CIPROFLOXACIN
Cipro Oral Suspension 2810

CIPROMYCIN (Greece)
CIPROFLOXACIN HYDROCHLORIDE
Cipro Tablets 2810

CIPRONAL (Brazil)
CIPROFLOXACIN HYDROCHLORIDE
Cipro Tablets 2810

CIPRONAX (Venezuela)
CIPROFLOXACIN HYDROCHLORIDE
Cipro Tablets 2810

CIPRONEX (Poland)
CIPROFLOXACIN HYDROCHLORIDE
Cipro Tablets 2810

CIPRONOM (Brazil)
CIPROFLOXACIN
Cipro Oral Suspension 2810

CIPRO-OTICO (Argentina)
CIPROFLOXACIN HYDROCHLORIDE
Cipro Tablets 2810

CIPROPOL (Poland)
CIPROFLOXACIN HYDROCHLORIDE
Cipro Tablets 2810

CIPROQUINOL (Portugal)
CIPROFLOXACIN
Cipro Oral Suspension 2810

CIPRO-SAAR (Germany)
CIPROFLOXACIN HYDROCHLORIDE
Cipro Tablets 2810

CIPROSER (Mexico)
CIPROFLOXACIN
Cipro Oral Suspension 2810

CIPROSPES (Greece)
CIPROFLOXACIN HYDROCHLORIDE
Cipro Tablets 2810

CIPROSTAD (Austria)
CIPROFLOXACIN HYDROCHLORIDE
Cipro Tablets 2810

CIPROSUN (Russia, Thailand)
CIPROFLOXACIN
Cipro Oral Suspension 2810

CIPROTAN (Irish Republic)
CITALOPRAM HYDROBROMIDE
Celexa Tablets 1160

CIPROTENK (Argentina)
CIPROFLOXACIN HYDROCHLORIDE
Cipro Tablets 2810

CIPROTOR (The Philippines)
CIPROFLOXACIN HYDROCHLORIDE
Cipro Tablets 2810

CIPROVAL (Chile)
CIPROFLOXACIN
Cipro Oral Suspension 2810

CIPROWIN (India)
CIPROFLOXACIN
Cipro Oral Suspension 2810

CIPRO-WOLFF (Germany)
CIPROFLOXACIN HYDROCHLORIDE
Cipro Tablets 2810

CIPROX (Germany)
CIPROFLOXACIN HYDROCHLORIDE
Cipro Tablets 2810

CIPROXAN (Brazil, Thailand)
CIPROFLOXACIN
Cipro Oral Suspension 2810

CIPROXEN (Brazil)
CIPROFLOXACIN
Cipro Oral Suspension 2810

CIPROXIL (Brazil)
CIPROFLOXACIN HYDROCHLORIDE
Cipro Tablets 2810

CIPROXIN (Israel, Turkey)
CIPROFLOXACIN
Cipro Oral Suspension 2810

CIPROXIN HC (Australia, Israel, New Zealand, Switzerland)
CIPROFLOXACIN HYDROCHLORIDE
Cipro Tablets 2810

CIPROXINA (Portugal, Venezuela)
CIPROFLOXACIN
Cipro Oral Suspension 2810

CIPROXINA HC (Mexico)
CIPROFLOXACIN
Cipro Oral Suspension 2810

CIPROXINA SIMPLE (Spain)
CIPROFLOXACIN HYDROCHLORIDE
Cipro Tablets 2810

CIPROXINE (Belgium)
CIPROFLOXACIN
Cipro Oral Suspension 2810

CIPROXINO (Chile)
CIPROFLOXACIN
Cipro Oral Suspension 2810

CIPROXYL (Hong Kong, Thailand)
CIPROFLOXACIN
Cipro Oral Suspension 2810

CIPTINI (India)
CIPROFLOXACIN
Cipro Oral Suspension 2810

CIQFADIN (Mexico)
CIPROFLOXACIN
Cipro Oral Suspension 2810

CIRFLOX-G (Argentina)
CIPROFLOXACIN
Cipro Oral Suspension 2810

CIRIAX (Argentina)
CIPROFLOXACIN
Cipro Oral Suspension 2810

CIRIAX OTIC (Argentina)
CIPROFLOXACIN HYDROCHLORIDE
Cipro Tablets 2810

CIRIZINE (Greece)
CETIRIZINE HYDROCHLORIDE
Zyrtec Syrup 1920
Zyrtec Tablets 1920

CIROK (Singapore, The Philippines, Venezuela)
CIPROFLOXACIN
Cipro Oral Suspension 2810

CIROXIN (Singapore)
CIPROFLOXACIN HYDROCHLORIDE
Cipro Tablets 2810

CISCUTAN (Austria)
ISOTRETINOIN
Accutane Capsules 2607

CI-SONS (Mexico)
CIPROFLOXACIN HYDROCHLORIDE
Cipro Tablets 2810

CISTAMINE (Thailand)
CETIRIZINE HYDROCHLORIDE
Zyrtec Syrup 1920
Zyrtec Tablets 1920

CITADEP (India)
CITALOPRAM HYDROBROMIDE
Celexa Tablets 1160

CITADUR (Denmark)
CITALOPRAM HYDROBROMIDE
Celexa Tablets 1160

CITADURA (Germany)
CITALOPRAM HYDROBROMIDE
Celexa Tablets 1160

CITAHAM (Denmark)
CITALOPRAM HYDROBROMIDE
Celexa Tablets 1160

CITAL (Hong Kong, Poland)
CITALOPRAM HYDROBROMIDE
Celexa Tablets 1160

CITALEC (Czech Republic)
CITALOPRAM HYDROBROMIDE
Celexa Tablets 1160

CITALHEXAL (Austria)
CITALOPRAM HYDROBROMIDE
Celexa Tablets 1160

CITALICH (Germany)
CITALOPRAM HYDROBROMIDE
Celexa Tablets 1160

CITALOHEXAL (South Africa)
CITALOPRAM HYDROBROMIDE
Celexa Tablets 1160

CITALON (Austria, Germany)
CITALOPRAM HYDROBROMIDE
Celexa Tablets 1160

CITALOSTAD (Austria)
CITALOPRAM HYDROBROMIDE
Celexa Tablets 1160

CITALVIR (Spain)
CITALOPRAM HYDROBROMIDE
Celexa Tablets 1160

CITARA (Turkey)
CITALOPRAM HYDROBROMIDE
Celexa Tablets 1160

CITARATIO (Poland)
CITALOPRAM HYDROBROMIDE
Celexa Tablets 1160

CITARCANA (Austria)
CITALOPRAM HYDROBROMIDE
Celexa Tablets 1160

CITAVIE (Sweden)
CITALOPRAM HYDROBROMIDE
Celexa Tablets 1160

CITAXIN (Poland)
CITALOPRAM HYDROBROMIDE
Celexa Tablets 1160

CITIFLUX (Italy)
FLUNISOLIDE
Aerobid Inhaler System 1153
Aerobid-M Inhaler System 1153

CITIREUMA (Italy)
SULINDAC
Clinoril Tablets 1962

CITIZEM (Italy)
DILTIAZEM HYDROCHLORIDE
Cardizem LA Extended Release Tablets 421

CITIZOL (India)
CIPROFLOXACIN
Cipro Oral Suspension 2810

CITOGEL (Austria, Italy)
SUCRALFATE
Carafate Suspension 706
Carafate Tablets 707

CITOL (Turkey)
CITALOPRAM HYDROBROMIDE
Celexa Tablets 1160

CITOLAP (Turkey)
CITALOPRAM HYDROBROMIDE
Celexa Tablets 1160

CITOR (Austria)
CITALOPRAM HYDROBROMIDE
Celexa Tablets 1160

CITRIHEXAL (Australia)
CALCITRIOL
Calcijex Injection 419
Rocaltrol Capsules 1150
Rocaltrol Oral Solution 1150

CITROL (Irish Republic)
CITALOPRAM HYDROBROMIDE
Celexa Tablets 1160

CITROVENOT (Greece)
CIPROFLOXACIN HYDROCHLORIDE
Cipro Tablets 2810

CIZETOL (India)
CARBAMAZEPINE
Carbatrol Capsules 3019

CLACEE (South Africa)
CLARITHROMYCIN
Biaxin Filmtab Tablets 411
Biaxin Granules 411

CLACIN (Hong Kong)
CLARITHROMYCIN
Biaxin Filmtab Tablets 411
Biaxin Granules 411

CLACINA (Portugal)
CLARITHROMYCIN
Biaxin Filmtab Tablets 411
Biaxin Granules 411

CLAMICIN (Brazil)
CLARITHROMYCIN
Biaxin Filmtab Tablets 411
Biaxin Granules 411

CLAMYCIN (United Arab Emirates)
CLARITHROMYCIN
Biaxin Filmtab Tablets 411
Biaxin Granules 411

CLANEKSI (The Philippines)
AMOXICILLIN
Amoxil Pediatric Drops for Oral Suspension 1305
Amoxil Tablets 1305

CLARAC (Australia)
CLARITHROMYCIN
Biaxin Filmtab Tablets 411
Biaxin Granules 411

CLARANTA (The Philippines, Venezuela)
CLARITHROMYCIN
Biaxin Filmtab Tablets 411
Biaxin Granules 411

CLARARCANA (Austria)
CLARITHROMYCIN
Biaxin Filmtab Tablets 411
Biaxin Granules 411

CLARBACT (India)
CLARITHROMYCIN
Biaxin Filmtab Tablets 411
Biaxin Granules 411

CLARIBID (India)
CLARITHROMYCIN
Biaxin Filmtab Tablets 411
Biaxin Granules 411

CLARIBIOTIC (Argentina)
CLARITHROMYCIN
Biaxin Filmtab Tablets 411
Biaxin Granules 411

CLARICIDE (Turkey)
CLARITHROMYCIN
Biaxin Filmtab Tablets 411
Biaxin Granules 411

CLARICINA (Argentina, Brazil)
CLARITHROMYCIN
Biaxin Filmtab Tablets 411
Biaxin Granules 411

CLARICIP (India)
CLARITHROMYCIN
Biaxin Filmtab Tablets 411
Biaxin Granules 411

CLARIGET (The Philippines)
CLARITHROMYCIN
Biaxin Filmtab Tablets 411
Biaxin Granules 411

CLARIHEXAL (South Africa)
CLARITHROMYCIN
Biaxin Filmtab Tablets 411
Biaxin Granules 411

CLARIMAC (India)
CLARITHROMYCIN
Biaxin Filmtab Tablets 411
Biaxin Granules 411

CLARIMAX (Argentina, Brazil, Chile)
CLARITHROMYCIN
Biaxin Filmtab Tablets 411
Biaxin Granules 411

CLARIMID (Argentina)
CLARITHROMYCIN
Biaxin Filmtab Tablets 411
Biaxin Granules 411

CLARINEO (Brazil)
CLARITHROMYCIN
Biaxin Filmtab Tablets 411
Biaxin Granules 411

CLARIPEN (Greece, Singapore)
CLARITHROMYCIN
Biaxin Filmtab Tablets 411
Biaxin Granules 411

CLARITAB (Brazil)
CLARITHROMYCIN
Biaxin Filmtab Tablets 411
Biaxin Granules 411

CLARITH (Japan, Thailand)
CLARITHROMYCIN
Biaxin Filmtab Tablets 411
Biaxin Granules 411

CLARITHROBETA (Germany)
CLARITHROMYCIN
Biaxin Filmtab Tablets 411
Biaxin Granules 411

CLARITIC (Venezuela)
CLARITHROMYCIN
Biaxin Filmtab Tablets 411
Biaxin Granules 411

CLARITROMAX (Brazil)
CLARITHROMYCIN
Biaxin Filmtab Tablets 411
Biaxin Granules 411

CLARITRON (Brazil, Venezuela)
CLARITHROMYCIN
Biaxin Filmtab Tablets 411
Biaxin Granules 411

CLARITUR (Spain)
CLARITHROMYCIN
Biaxin Filmtab Tablets 411
Biaxin Granules 411

CLARIVAX (Venezuela)
CLARITHROMYCIN
Biaxin Filmtab Tablets 411
Biaxin Granules 411

CLAROMYCIN (Greece)
CLARITHROMYCIN
Biaxin Filmtab Tablets 411
Biaxin Granules 411

CLAROMYCINE (Switzerland)
CLARITHROMYCIN
Biaxin Filmtab Tablets 411
Biaxin Granules 411

CLARON (Thailand)
CLARITHROMYCIN
Biaxin Filmtab Tablets 411
Biaxin Granules 411

CLAROPRAM (Switzerland)
CITALOPRAM HYDROBROMIDE
Celexa Tablets 1160

CLAROSIP (Chile, Irish Republic, The Netherlands, United Kingdom)
CLARITHROMYCIN
Biaxin Filmtab Tablets 411
Biaxin Granules 411

CLAROVIL (Argentina)
CLARITHROMYCIN
Biaxin Filmtab Tablets 411
Biaxin Granules 411

CLATIC (Chile)
CLARITHROMYCIN
Biaxin Filmtab Tablets 411
Biaxin Granules 411

CLATORIN (Brazil)
CLARITHROMYCIN
Biaxin Filmtab Tablets 411
Biaxin Granules 411

CLATROCIN (Mexico)
CLARITHROMYCIN
Biaxin Filmtab Tablets 411
Biaxin Granules 411

CLATROMICIN (Argentina)
CLARITHROMYCIN
Biaxin Filmtab Tablets 411
Biaxin Granules 411

CLAV-AIR (Brazil)
AMOXICILLIN
Amoxil Pediatric Drops for Oral Suspension 1305
Amoxil Tablets 1305

CLEAN & CLEAR CONTINUOUS CONTROL (Canada)
BENZOYL PEROXIDE
Brevoxyl-4 Creamy Wash 3054
Brevoxyl-4 Gel 3054
Brevoxyl-8 Creamy Wash 3054
Brevoxyl-8 Gel 3054

CLEAN & CLEAR PERSA GEL (Canada)
BENZOYL PEROXIDE
Brevoxyl-4 Creamy Wash 3054
Brevoxyl-4 Gel 3054
Brevoxyl-8 Creamy Wash 3054
Brevoxyl-8 Gel 3054

CLEARAMED (Spain, Sweden, The Netherlands)
BENZOYL PEROXIDE
Brevoxyl-4 Creamy Wash 3054
Brevoxyl-4 Gel 3054
Brevoxyl-8 Creamy Wash 3054
Brevoxyl-8 Gel 3054

CLEARASIL B.P. PLUS (Canada)
BENZOYL PEROXIDE
Brevoxyl-4 Creamy Wash 3054
Brevoxyl-4 Gel 3054
Brevoxyl-8 Creamy Wash 3054
Brevoxyl-8 Gel 3054

CLEARASIL BENZOYL P (South Africa)
BENZOYL PEROXIDE
Brevoxyl-4 Creamy Wash 3054
Brevoxyl-4 Gel 3054
Brevoxyl-8 Creamy Wash 3054
Brevoxyl-8 Gel 3054

CLEARASIL EXTRA STRENGTH (Australia)
BENZOYL PEROXIDE
Brevoxyl-4 Creamy Wash 3054
Brevoxyl-4 Gel 3054
Brevoxyl-8 Creamy Wash 3054
Brevoxyl-8 Gel 3054

CLEARASIL MAX 10 (United Kingdom)
BENZOYL PEROXIDE
Brevoxyl-4 Creamy Wash 3054
Brevoxyl-4 Gel 3054
Brevoxyl-8 Creamy Wash 3054
Brevoxyl-8 Gel 3054

CLEARASIL PLUS (Mexico)
BENZOYL PEROXIDE
Brevoxyl-4 Creamy Wash 3054
Brevoxyl-4 Gel 3054
Brevoxyl-8 Creamy Wash 3054
Brevoxyl-8 Gel 3054

CLEARASIL ULTRA (Australia, Italy, New Zealand, Poland)
BENZOYL PEROXIDE
Brevoxyl-4 Creamy Wash 3054
Brevoxyl-4 Gel 3054
Brevoxyl-8 Creamy Wash 3054
Brevoxyl-8 Gel 3054

CLEAREX COVER UP (Israel)
BENZOYL PEROXIDE
Brevoxyl-4 Creamy Wash 3054
Brevoxyl-4 Gel 3054
Brevoxyl-8 Creamy Wash 3054
Brevoxyl-8 Gel 3054

CLERIDIUM (France)
DIPYRIDAMOLE
Persantine Tablets 869

CLERON (Hong Kong)
CLARITHROMYCIN
Biaxin Filmtab Tablets 411
Biaxin Granules 411

CLETONOL (Argentina)
NIMODIPINE
Nimotop Capsules 790

CLEVERON (Brazil)
ALENDRONATE SODIUM
Fosamax Tablets 2005

CLEXANE (Argentina, Australia, Belgium, Brazil, Chile, Czech Republic, Germany, Greece, Hong Kong, Hungary, India, Irish Republic, Israel, Italy, Malaysia, Mexico, New Zealand, Poland, Russia, Singapore, South Africa, Spain, Switzerland, Thailand, The Netherlands, The Philippines, Turkey, United Kingdom, Venezuela)
ENOXAPARIN SODIUM
Lovenox Injection 2756

CLIANE (Brazil, New Zealand, Venezuela)
ESTRADIOL
Climara Transdermal System 763

CLIARVAS (Argentina)
LOSARTAN POTASSIUM
Cozaar Tablets 1973

CLIDAN B (Argentina)
BENZOYL PEROXIDE
Brevoxyl-4 Creamy Wash 3054
Brevoxyl-4 Gel 3054
Brevoxyl-8 Creamy Wash 3054
Brevoxyl-8 Gel 3054

CLIMADERM (Argentina, Brazil, Chile, Mexico, Venezuela)
ESTRADIOL
Climara Transdermal System 763

CLIMARA (Australia, Austria, Belgium, Canada, Czech Republic, Denmark, Finland, France, Irish Republic, Israel, Italy, New Zealand, Norway, Poland, Portugal, Russia, South Africa, Sweden, Switzerland, Thailand, The Netherlands, The Philippines, Turkey)
ESTRADIOL
Climara Transdermal System 763

CLIMASTON (France)
ESTRADIOL
Climara Transdermal System 763

CLIMASTON CONTINU (The Netherlands)
ESTRADIOL
Climara Transdermal System 763

CLINDOXYL (Argentina, Austria)
BENZOYL PEROXIDE
Brevoxyl-4 Creamy Wash 3054
Brevoxyl-4 Gel 3054
Brevoxyl-8 Creamy Wash 3054
Brevoxyl-8 Gel 3054

CLINFAR (Brazil)
SIMVASTATIN
Zocor Tablets 2136

CLINIFLAM (South Africa)
DICLOFENAC SODIUM
Voltaren Tablets 2334
Voltaren-XR Tablets 2337

CLINORIL (Australia, Austria, Belgium, Canada, Czech Republic, Denmark, Hong Kong, Irish Republic, Italy, Malaysia, Mexico, New Zealand, Norway, South Africa, Sweden, Switzerland, Thailand, The Netherlands, United Kingdom, Venezuela)
SULINDAC
Clinoril Tablets 1962

CLINOSYN (South Africa)
NAPROXEN
EC-Naprosyn Delayed-Release Tablets 2632
Naprosyn Suspension 2632
Naprosyn Tablets 2632

CLIOGAN (Spain)
ESTRADIOL
Climara Transdermal System 763

CLISON (Mexico)
SULINDAC
Clinoril Tablets 1962

CLISUNDAC (Italy)
SULINDAC
Clinoril Tablets 1962

CLIVOTEN (Italy)
ISRADIPINE
DynaCirc CR Tablets 1407

CLOBENDIAN (Spain)
DILTIAZEM HYDROCHLORIDE
Cardizem LA Extended Release Tablets 421

CLODIAN (Argentina)
CLOPIDOGREL BISULFATE
Plavix Tablets 926, 2767

CLODREL (Argentina)
CLOPIDOGREL BISULFATE
Plavix Tablets 926, 2767

CLOFAMOX (Argentina)
AMOXICILLIN
Amoxil Pediatric Drops for Oral Suspension 1305
Amoxil Tablets 1305

CLOFEC (Hong Kong, Malaysia, Singapore, Thailand)
DICLOFENAC SODIUM
Voltaren Tablets . . . 2334
Voltaren-XR Tablets . . . 2337

CLOFENAC (Hong Kong, Malaysia, Singapore, Venezuela)
DICLOFENAC SODIUM
Voltaren Tablets . . . 2334
Voltaren-XR Tablets . . . 2337

CLOFENID (Brazil)
DICLOFENAC SODIUM
Voltaren Tablets . . . 2334
Voltaren-XR Tablets . . . 2337

CLOFENIX (The Philippines)
DICLOFENAC SODIUM
Voltaren Tablets . . . 2334
Voltaren-XR Tablets . . . 2337

CLOFIL (The Philippines)
DICLOFENAC SODIUM
Voltaren Tablets . . . 2334
Voltaren-XR Tablets . . . 2337

CLOFLOW (India)
CLOPIDOGREL BISULFATE
Plavix Tablets . . . 926, 2767

CLOFLOW PLUS (India)
CLOPIDOGREL BISULFATE
Plavix Tablets . . . 926, 2767

CLOFON (Thailand)
DICLOFENAC SODIUM
Voltaren Tablets . . . 2334
Voltaren-XR Tablets . . . 2337

CLONABAY (Argentina)
CLONAZEPAM
Klonopin Tablets . . . 2639

CLONAC (Australia, Greece)
DICLOFENAC SODIUM
Voltaren Tablets . . . 2334
Voltaren-XR Tablets . . . 2337

CLONAGIN (Argentina)
CLONAZEPAM
Klonopin Tablets . . . 2639

CLONAPAM (Canada, Chile, Hungary)
CLONAZEPAM
Klonopin Tablets . . . 2639

CLONAREN (The Philippines)
DICLOFENAC SODIUM
Voltaren Tablets . . . 2334
Voltaren-XR Tablets . . . 2337

CLONAX (Argentina)
CLONAZEPAM
Klonopin Tablets . . . 2639

CLONAZEN 2 (Argentina)
CLONAZEPAM
Klonopin Tablets . . . 2639

CLONDEPRYL (Irish Republic)
SELEGILINE HYDROCHLORIDE
Eldepryl Capsules . . . 3052

CLONER (Argentina)
CLONAZEPAM
Klonopin Tablets . . . 2639

CLONESINA (Brazil)
CLONIDINE HYDROCHLORIDE
Catapres Tablets . . . 841

CLONEX (Chile, Israel)
CLONAZEPAM
Klonopin Tablets . . . 2639

CLONID-OPHTAL (Germany)
CLONIDINE HYDROCHLORIDE
Catapres Tablets . . . 841

CLONIDURAL (Argentina)
CLONIDINE
Catapres-TTS . . . 842

CLONILIX (Irish Republic)
INDAPAMIDE
Indapamide Tablets . . . 2188

CLONIPRES (Venezuela)
CLONIDINE HYDROCHLORIDE
Catapres Tablets . . . 841

CLONISTADA (Germany)
CLONIDINE HYDROCHLORIDE
Catapres Tablets . . . 841

CLONNIRIT (Israel)
CLONIDINE HYDROCHLORIDE
Catapres Tablets . . . 841

CLONOCID (Irish Republic)
CLARITHROMYCIN
Biaxin Filmtab Tablets . . . 411
Biaxin Granules . . . 411

CLONODIFEN (Mexico)
DICLOFENAC SODIUM
Voltaren Tablets . . . 2334
Voltaren-XR Tablets . . . 2337

CLONOGAL (Hungary)
CLONAZEPAM
Klonopin Tablets . . . 2639

CLONOTRIL (Brazil)
CLONAZEPAM
Klonopin Tablets . . . 2639

CLOPACT (India)
CLOPIDOGREL BISULFATE
Plavix Tablets . . . 926, 2767

CLOPACT A (India)
CLOPIDOGREL BISULFATE
Plavix Tablets . . . 926, 2767

CLOPIVAS (India)
CLOPIDOGREL BISULFATE
Plavix Tablets . . . 926, 2767

CLOPIVAS AP (India)
CLOPIDOGREL BISULFATE
Plavix Tablets . . . 926, 2767

CLOPOD (India)
CLOPIDOGREL BISULFATE
Plavix Tablets . . . 926, 2767

CLOPOD-A (India)
CLOPIDOGREL BISULFATE
Plavix Tablets . . . 926, 2767

CLOROM (Irish Republic)
CLARITHROMYCIN
Biaxin Filmtab Tablets . . . 411
Biaxin Granules . . . 411

CLORPAX (Australia)
BUPROPION HYDROCHLORIDE
Wellbutrin SR Sustained-Release Tablets . . 1653
Wellbutrin Tablets . . . 1648
Zyban Sustained-Release Tablets . . . 1692

CLOSINA (Australia)
CYCLOSERINE
Seromycin Capsules . . . 1864

CLOSTEDAL (Mexico)
CARBAMAZEPINE
Carbatrol Capsules . . . 3019

CLOVIXIME (The Philippines)
CEFUROXIME SODIUM
Zinacef Injection . . . 1678

CLOXIB (Argentina)
CELECOXIB
Celebrex Capsules . . . 2979

CLOZANIL (Chile)
CLONAZEPAM
Klonopin Tablets . . . 2639

CLUSINOL (Australia)
SULINDAC
Clinoril Tablets . . . 1962

CMP (Argentina)
CARBAMAZEPINE
Carbatrol Capsules . . . 3019

CO-ACETAN (Austria)
HYDROCHLOROTHIAZIDE/LISINOPRIL
Prinzide Tablets . . . 2092

CO-AMOXI (Belgium)
AMOXICILLIN
Amoxil Pediatric Drops for Oral Suspension . . . 1305
Amoxil Tablets . . . 1305

CO-AMOXYCLAV (South Africa)
AMOXICILLIN
Amoxil Pediatric Drops for Oral Suspension . . . 1305
Amoxil Tablets . . . 1305

CO-ANGIOSAN (Austria)
VALSARTAN
Diovan Tablets . . . 2212

COAPROVEL (Argentina, Belgium, Chile, Czech Republic, Denmark, Germany, Hong Kong, Hungary, Irish Republic, Italy, Malaysia, Mexico, Norway, Singapore, South Africa, Spain, Thailand, The Philippines, Venezuela)
HYDROCHLOROTHIAZIDE/IRBESARTAN
Avalide Tablets . . . 892

COBAY (Thailand)
CIPROFLOXACIN HYDROCHLORIDE
Cipro Tablets . . . 2810

COBIX (India)
CELECOXIB
Celebrex Capsules . . . 2979

CO-CAPTOPRIL (Austria)
CAPTOPRIL
Captopril Tablets . . . 2182

CO-CAPTOTYROL (Austria)
CAPTOPRIL
Captopril Tablets . . . 2182

CO-CAPTRAL (Mexico)
CAPTOPRIL
Captopril Tablets . . . 2182

CO-DIOVAN (Austria, Czech Republic, Germany, Hong Kong, Irish Republic, Israel, Malaysia, Mexico, Poland, Portugal, Russia, Singapore, South Africa, Spain, Switzerland, Thailand, The Netherlands, The Philippines, Turkey, United Kingdom)
HYDROCHLOROTHIAZIDE/VALSARTAN
Diovan HCT Tablets . . . 2216

CO-DIOVANE (Belgium)
HYDROCHLOROTHIAZIDE/VALSARTAN
Diovan HCT Tablets . . . 2216

CODRINAN (Brazil)
THEOPHYLLINE
Uniphyl Tablets . . . 2595

COFENAC (India)
DICLOFENAC SODIUM
Voltaren Tablets . . . 2334
Voltaren-XR Tablets . . . 2337

COGITON (Poland)
DONEPEZIL HYDROCHLORIDE
Aricept Tablets . . . 1062

COGNITIV (Austria, Czech Republic, Russia)
SELEGILINE HYDROCHLORIDE
Eldepryl Capsules . . . 3052

CO-HYPOMED (Austria)
LISINOPRIL
Prinivil Tablets . . . 2087

COLATAN (Spain)
NARATRIPTAN HYDROCHLORIDE
Amerge Tablets . . . 1301

COLEDIS (Argentina)
SIMVASTATIN
Zocor Tablets . . . 2136

COLEMIN (Spain)
SIMVASTATIN
Zocor Tablets . . . 2136

COLESTERMINOL (Argentina)
SIMVASTATIN
Zocor Tablets . . . 2136

COLESVIR (Spain)
LOVASTATIN
Mevacor Tablets . . . 2063

COLEVIX (Chile)
LOVASTATIN
Mevacor Tablets . . . 2063

COLIFOSSIM (Italy)
CEFUROXIME SODIUM
Zinacef Injection . . . 1678

CO-LISINOPRIL (Switzerland)
LISINOPRIL
Prinivil Tablets . . . 2087

CO-LISINOSTAD (Austria)
LISINOPRIL
Prinivil Tablets . . . 2087

COLPROSTERONE (Spain)
PROGESTERONE
Crinone 4% Gel . . . 992
Prometrium Capsules (100 mg, 200 mg) . 3047

COLSANAC (Portugal)
LACTULOSE
Kristalose for Oral Solution . . . 1004

COLVER (Italy)
CARVEDILOL
Coreg Tablets . . . 1387

COMALOSE-R (Canada)
LACTULOSE
Kristalose for Oral Solution . . . 1004

COMBANTRIN-A (India)
ALBENDAZOLE
Albenza Tablets . . . 1297

COMBAREN (Venezuela)
DICLOFENAC SODIUM
Voltaren Tablets . . . 2334
Voltaren-XR Tablets . . . 2337

COMBID (Thailand)
LAMIVUDINE
Epivir Oral Solution . . . 1412
Epivir Tablets . . . 1412
Epivir-HBV Oral Solution . . . 1417
Epivir-HBV Tablets . . . 1417

COMBINED (Argentina)
OLANZAPINE
Zyprexa Tablets . . . 1883

COMBIPUL (The Philippines)
IPRATROPIUM BROMIDE
Atrovent Nasal Spray 0.03% . . . 834
Atrovent Nasal Spray 0.06% . . . 836

COMBIREX (India)
LAMIVUDINE
Epivir Oral Solution . . . 1412
Epivir Tablets . . . 1412
Epivir-HBV Oral Solution . . . 1417
Epivir-HBV Tablets . . . 1417

COMBISARTAN (Italy)
HYDROCHLOROTHIAZIDE/VALSARTAN
Diovan HCT Tablets . . . 2216

COMBIVENT (Argentina, Australia, Brazil, Malaysia, The Philippines, Turkey, Venezuela)
IPRATROPIUM BROMIDE
Atrovent Nasal Spray 0.03% . . . 834
Atrovent Nasal Spray 0.06% . . . 836

COMBIVIR (Australia, Austria, Belgium, Brazil, Canada, Chile, Czech Republic, Denmark, Finland, France, Germany, Greece, Hong Kong, Irish Republic, Israel, Italy, Malaysia, Mexico, New Zealand, Norway, Poland, Portugal, Russia, Singapore, South Africa, Spain, Sweden, Switzerland, The Netherlands, The Philippines, United Kingdom, Venezuela)
LAMIVUDINE/ZIDOVUDINE
Combivir Tablets . . . 1384

COMBIZAR (The Philippines)
LOSARTAN POTASSIUM
Cozaar Tablets . . . 1973

CO-MICARDIS (South Africa)
TELMISARTAN
Micardis Tablets . . . 852

COMPAZ (Brazil)
DIAZEPAM
Valium Tablets . . . 2658

COMPLUTINE (Spain)
DIAZEPAM
Valium Tablets . . . 2658

CONDROTEC (United Kingdom)
NAPROXEN
EC-Naprosyn Delayed-Release Tablets . . . 2632
Naprosyn Suspension . . . 2632
Naprosyn Tablets . . . 2632

CONEF (Argentina)
FINASTERIDE
Propecia Tablets . . . 2095
Proscar Tablets . . . 2102

CONFOBOS (Spain)
FAMOTIDINE
Pepcid for Oral Suspension . . . 2075
Pepcid Tablets . . . 2075

CONFORMAL (Argentina)
CARBAMAZEPINE
Carbatrol Capsules . . . 3019

CONGEX (Argentina)
NAPROXEN
EC-Naprosyn Delayed-Release Tablets 2632
Naprosyn Suspension 2632
Naprosyn Tablets 2632

CONNETTIVINA (Austria, Hong Kong, Italy, Thailand)
SODIUM HYALURONATE
Hyalgan Solution 2742

CONPRES (Hungary)
LISINOPRIL
Prinivil Tablets 2087

CONSEC (India)
RANITIDINE HYDROCHLORIDE
Zantac 25 EFFERdose Tablets 1670
Zantac 150 Tablets 1670
Zantac 300 Tablets 1670
Zantac Injection 1666
Zantac Injection Premixed 1666
Zantac Syrup 1670

CONSTILAX (Greece)
NORFLOXACIN
Noroxin Tablets 2069

CONTALGIN (Denmark)
MORPHINE SULFATE
MS Contin Tablets 2585

CONTIFLO (United Kingdom)
TAMSULOSIN HYDROCHLORIDE
Flomax Capsules 848

CONTIPHYLLIN (Germany)
THEOPHYLLINE
Uniphyl Tablets 2595

CONTRACNE (France)
ISOTRETINOIN
Accutane Capsules 2607

CONTRAMAL (Austria, Belgium, France, India, Italy, Turkey)
TRAMADOL HYDROCHLORIDE
Ultram ER Tablets 2428

CONTROLIP (Mexico)
FENOFIBRATE
Tricor Tablets 520

CONTROLPROS (Argentina)
TAMSULOSIN HYDROCHLORIDE
Flomax Capsules 848

CONTRYKAL (Russia)
APROTININ
Trasylol Injection 799

CONVADEN (Czech Republic)
ESTRADIOL
Climara Transdermal System 763

CONVECTAL (Spain)
DILTIAZEM HYDROCHLORIDE
Cardizem LA Extended Release Tablets 421

CONVERTAL (Portugal)
CAPTOPRIL
Captopril Tablets 2182

CONVULEX (Venezuela)
CARBAMAZEPINE
Carbatrol Capsules 3019

CONVULSAN (Brazil)
CARBAMAZEPINE
Carbatrol Capsules 3019

COOLIPS (Chile)
CETIRIZINE HYDROCHLORIDE
Zyrtec Syrup 1920
Zyrtec Tablets 1920

COPAL (Mexico)
SULINDAC
Clinoril Tablets 1962

COPAXONE (Argentina, Australia, Austria, Belgium, Brazil, Canada, Czech Republic, Denmark, Finland, France, Greece, Hungary, Irish Republic, Israel, Italy, New Zealand, Norway, Poland, Portugal, Russia, Spain, Sweden, Switzerland, The Netherlands, Turkey)
GLATIRAMER ACETATE
Copaxone for Injection 3110

COR TENSOBON (Germany)
CAPTOPRIL
Captopril Tablets 2182

CORAFEN (Argentina)
CARVEDILOL
Coreg Tablets 1387

CORAGOXINE (France)
DIGOXIN
Lanoxin Injection 1498
Lanoxin Injection Pediatric 1502
Lanoxin Tablets 1505

CORAL (Mexico)
DICLOFENAC SODIUM
Voltaren Tablets 2334
Voltaren-XR Tablets 2337

CORALEN (Spain)
RANITIDINE HYDROCHLORIDE
Zantac 25 EFFERdose Tablets 1670
Zantac 150 Tablets 1670
Zantac 300 Tablets 1670
Zantac Injection 1666
Zantac Injection Premixed 1666
Zantac Syrup 1670

CORAMIL (Sweden)
DILTIAZEM HYDROCHLORIDE
Cardizem LA Extended Release Tablets 421

CORAS (Australia)
DILTIAZEM HYDROCHLORIDE
Cardizem LA Extended Release Tablets 421

CORAZEM (Austria, Venezuela)
DILTIAZEM HYDROCHLORIDE
Cardizem LA Extended Release Tablets 421

CORAZET (Germany)
DILTIAZEM HYDROCHLORIDE
Cardizem LA Extended Release Tablets 421

CORDES BPO (Germany)
BENZOYL PEROXIDE
Brevoxyl-4 Creamy Wash 3054
Brevoxyl-4 Gel 3054
Brevoxyl-8 Creamy Wash 3054
Brevoxyl-8 Gel 3054

CORDES NYSTATIN SOFT (Germany)
NYSTATIN
Nystop Topical Powder USP 2498

CORDES VAS (Germany)
TRETINOIN
Vesanoid Capsules 2660

CORDINATE (Germany)
VALSARTAN
Diovan Tablets 2212

CORDINATE PLUS (Germany)
VALSARTAN
Diovan Tablets 2212

CORDIRON (Brazil)
SIMVASTATIN
Zocor Tablets 2136

CORDISIL (Venezuela)
DILTIAZEM HYDROCHLORIDE
Cardizem LA Extended Release Tablets 421

COREG (Brazil, Canada)
CARVEDILOL
Coreg Tablets 1387

CORGARD (Argentina, Belgium, Brazil, Canada, Chile, France, Hong Kong, Irish Republic, Italy, Malaysia, Mexico, New Zealand, South Africa, Spain, Switzerland, United Kingdom, Venezuela)
NADOLOL
Nadolol Tablets 2191

CORGARETIC (Irish Republic, Mexico, South Africa, Switzerland, United Kingdom)
BENDROFLUMETHIAZIDE/NADOLOL
Corzide Tablets

CORIBON (Italy)
DIPYRIDAMOLE
Persantine Tablets 869

CORIC (Germany)
LISINOPRIL
Prinivil Tablets 2087

CORIC PLUS (Germany)
HYDROCHLOROTHIAZIDE/LISINOPRIL
Prinzide Tablets 2092

CORIDIL (Switzerland)
DILTIAZEM HYDROCHLORIDE
Cardizem LA Extended Release Tablets 421

CORITENSIL (Argentina)
CARVEDILOL
Coreg Tablets 1387

CORIXA (Argentina)
CLARITHROMYCIN
Biaxin Filmtab Tablets 411
Biaxin Granules 411

CORIXIL (Italy)
VALSARTAN
Diovan Tablets 2212

CORMAC (Venezuela)
LOSARTAN POTASSIUM
Cozaar Tablets 1973

CORMATIC (Venezuela)
LOSARTAN POTASSIUM
Cozaar Tablets 1973

CORODIN (Chile)
LOSARTAN POTASSIUM
Cozaar Tablets 1973

COROLATER (Spain)
DILTIAZEM HYDROCHLORIDE
Cardizem LA Extended Release Tablets 421

COROLIN (Finland)
SIMVASTATIN
Zocor Tablets 2136

CORONAIR (Belgium)
DIPYRIDAMOLE
Persantine Tablets 869

CORONARINE (France)
DIPYRIDAMOLE
Persantine Tablets 869

CORONORM (Germany)
CAPTOPRIL
Captopril Tablets 2182

COROPRES (Spain)
CARVEDILOL
Coreg Tablets 1387

COROSAN (Italy)
DIPYRIDAMOLE
Persantine Tablets 869

COROXIN (Italy)
DIPYRIDAMOLE
Persantine Tablets 869

CORPRILIN (Switzerland)
LISINOPRIL
Prinivil Tablets 2087

CORPRIRETIC (Switzerland)
LISINOPRIL
Prinivil Tablets 2087

CORSTAT (Hong Kong)
SIMVASTATIN
Zocor Tablets 2136

CORTICOSAN (Argentina)
LOSARTAN POTASSIUM
Cozaar Tablets 1973

CORTICOTHERAPIQUE (Switzerland)
TRIAMCINOLONE ACETONIDE
Azmacort Inhalation Aerosol 407
Nasacort AQ Nasal Spray 2765

CORTRAN (Chile)
CITALOPRAM HYDROBROMIDE
Celexa Tablets 1160

CORTYNASE (Venezuela)
MOMETASONE FUROATE
Elocon Cream 0.1% 2840
Elocon Lotion 0.1% 2841
Elocon Ointment 0.1% 2842
Nasonex Nasal Spray 2883

CORUBIN (Argentina)
CARVEDILOL
Coreg Tablets 1387

CORUS (Brazil)
LOSARTAN POTASSIUM
Cozaar Tablets 1973

CORUS H (Brazil)
LOSARTAN POTASSIUM
Cozaar Tablets 1973

CORYOL (Poland)
CARVEDILOL
Coreg Tablets 1387

CORZIDE (Canada)
NADOLOL
Nadolol Tablets 2191

COSAAR (Austria, Switzerland)
LOSARTAN POTASSIUM
Cozaar Tablets 1973

COSMOPRIL (Greece)
SELEGILINE HYDROCHLORIDE
Eldepryl Capsules 3052

COSOPT (Argentina, Australia, Brazil, Chile, Czech Republic, Greece, Hong Kong, Hungary, Irish Republic, New Zealand, Poland, Portugal, Singapore, Thailand, The Netherlands, Turkey, Venezuela)
DORZOLAMIDE HYDROCHLORIDE/TIMOLOL MALEATE
Cosopt Sterile Ophthalmic Solution 1969

COTAREG (Brazil, France, Italy, The Netherlands)
HYDROCHLOROTHIAZIDE/VALSARTAN
Diovan HCT Tablets 2216

CO-TAREG (Portugal)
VALSARTAN
Diovan Tablets 2212

COTAZYM (Canada, New Zealand)
PANCRELIPASE
Ultrase Capsules 718
Ultrase MT Capsules 719

COTAZYM S FORTE (Australia)
PANCRELIPASE
Ultrase Capsules 718
Ultrase MT Capsules 719

COTAZYM-S (The Netherlands)
PANCRELIPASE
Ultrase Capsules 718
Ultrase MT Capsules 719

COTENSIL (Venezuela)
LISINOPRIL
Prinivil Tablets 2087

COULERGIN (Spain)
CETIRIZINE HYDROCHLORIDE
Zyrtec Syrup 1920
Zyrtec Tablets 1920

CO-VALS (Spain)
HYDROCHLOROTHIAZIDE/VALSARTAN
Diovan HCT Tablets 2216

COVANCE (India)
LOSARTAN POTASSIUM
Cozaar Tablets 1973

COVASTIN (Hong Kong, Malaysia, Singapore)
SIMVASTATIN
Zocor Tablets 2136

COVENTROL (Venezuela)
CARVEDILOL
Coreg Tablets 1387

COVERENE (Argentina)
PERINDOPRIL ERBUMINE
Aceon Tablets (2 mg, 4 mg, 8 mg) 3038

COVEREX (Hungary, Poland, The Netherlands)
PERINDOPRIL ERBUMINE
Aceon Tablets (2 mg, 4 mg, 8 mg) 3038

COVEREX KOMB (Hungary)
PERINDOPRIL ERBUMINE
Aceon Tablets (2 mg, 4 mg, 8 mg) 3038

COVERSUM (Austria, Germany, Switzerland)
PERINDOPRIL ERBUMINE
Aceon Tablets (2 mg, 4 mg, 8 mg) 3038

COVERSUM COMBI (Germany, Switzerland)
PERINDOPRIL ERBUMINE
Aceon Tablets (2 mg, 4 mg, 8 mg) 3038

COVERSYL (Australia, Belgium, Brazil, Canada, Chile, Denmark, Finland, France, Greece, India, Irish Republic, Italy, Japan, Malaysia, Mexico, New Zealand, Portugal, Singapore, South Africa, Spain, Thailand, The Netherlands, The Philippines, Turkey, United Kingdom, Venezuela)
PERINDOPRIL ERBUMINE
Aceon Tablets (2 mg, 4 mg, 8 mg) 3038

COVERSYL COMP (Denmark, Finland)
PERINDOPRIL ERBUMINE
Aceon Tablets (2 mg, 4 mg, 8 mg) **3038**

COVERSYL PLUS (Australia, Belgium, Canada, India, Irish Republic, Malaysia, New Zealand, South Africa, The Netherlands, Turkey, United Kingdom)
PERINDOPRIL ERBUMINE
Aceon Tablets (2 mg, 4 mg, 8 mg) **3038**

COXEL (Argentina)
CELECOXIB
Celebrex Capsules **2979**

COXTENK (Argentina)
CELECOXIB
Celebrex Capsules **2979**

COZAAR (Australia, Belgium, Brazil, Canada, Chile, Czech Republic, Denmark, Finland, France, Greece, Hong Kong, Hungary, Irish Republic, Malaysia, Mexico, New Zealand, Norway, Poland, Portugal, Russia, Singapore, South Africa, Spain, Sweden, Thailand, The Netherlands, The Philippines, Turkey, United Kingdom, Venezuela)
LOSARTAN POTASSIUM
Cozaar Tablets **1973**

COZAAR PLUS (The Netherlands)
LOSARTAN POTASSIUM
Cozaar Tablets **1973**

COZAAREX (Argentina)
LOSARTAN POTASSIUM
Cozaar Tablets **1973**

COZAAREX D (Argentina)
LOSARTAN POTASSIUM
Cozaar Tablets **1973**

CP-CARBA (Hong Kong)
CARBAMAZEPINE
Carbatrol Capsules **3019**

CP-FURO (Hong Kong)
FUROSEMIDE
Furosemide Tablets **2186**

CP-THEO (Hong Kong)
THEOPHYLLINE
Uniphyl Tablets **2595**

CRAFILM (Italy)
SUCRALFATE
Carafate Suspension **706**
Carafate Tablets **707**

CRALSANIC (South Africa)
SUCRALFATE
Carafate Suspension **706**
Carafate Tablets **707**

CRANOC (Germany)
FLUVASTATIN SODIUM
Lescol Capsules **2268**

CRASNITIN (Germany, Italy, The Netherlands)
ASPARAGINASE
Elspar for Injection **2488**

CRASNITINE (Switzerland)
ASPARAGINASE
Elspar for Injection **2488**

CRAVERIL (Argentina)
FENOFIBRATE
Tricor Tablets **520**

CRAVIT (Japan, Malaysia, Singapore, Turkey)
LEVOFLOXACIN
Levaquin Injection **2416**
Levaquin Tablets **2416**

CREDAXOL (Mexico)
RANITIDINE HYDROCHLORIDE
Zantac 25 EFFERdose Tablets **1670**
Zantac 150 Tablets **1670**
Zantac 300 Tablets **1670**
Zantac Injection **1666**
Zantac Injection Premixed **1666**
Zantac Syrup **1670**

CRIMA (Argentina)
CEFTAZIDIME
Fortaz for Injection **1450**

CRINONE (Argentina, Belgium, Brazil, Canada, Chile, Denmark, Finland, Germany, Greece, Hong Kong, India, Irish Republic, Israel, Italy, Malaysia, Mexico, New Zealand, Norway, Portugal, Singapore, South Africa, Spain, Sweden, Switzerland, Thailand, The Philippines, United Kingdom, Venezuela)
PROGESTERONE
Crinone 4% Gel **992**
Prometrium Capsules (100 mg, 200 mg) . **3047**

CRISACIDE (Argentina)
CIPROFLOXACIN
Cipro Oral Suspension **2810**

CRISASMA (Argentina)
THEOPHYLLINE
Uniphyl Tablets **2595**

CRISAZET (Argentina)
ZIDOVUDINE
Retrovir Capsules **1574**
Retrovir IV Infusion **1579**
Retrovir Syrup **1574**
Retrovir Tablets **1574**

CRISMOL (Chile)
CLONAZEPAM
Klonopin Tablets **2639**

CRISOMET (Spain)
LAMOTRIGINE
Lamictal Chewable Dispersible Tablets . . . **1488**
Lamictal Tablets **1488**

CRISPLUS (Argentina)
ORLISTAT
Xenical Capsules **2672**

CRISTACLAR (Argentina)
DONEPEZIL HYDROCHLORIDE
Aricept Tablets **1062**

CRISTERONA (Argentina)
ESTRADIOL
Climara Transdermal System **763**

CRIXAN (Malaysia, Singapore, Thailand)
CLARITHROMYCIN
Biaxin Filmtab Tablets **411**
Biaxin Granules **411**

CRIXIVAN (Argentina, Australia, Austria, Belgium, Brazil, Canada, Chile, Czech Republic, Denmark, Finland, France, Germany, Greece, Hong Kong, Irish Republic, Israel, Italy, Malaysia, Mexico, New Zealand, Norway, Poland, Portugal, Russia, Singapore, South Africa, Spain, Sweden, Switzerland, Thailand, The Netherlands, The Philippines, Turkey, United Kingdom, Venezuela)
INDINAVIR SULFATE
Crixivan Capsules **1979**

CROMATODOL (Austria)
TRAMADOL HYDROCHLORIDE
Ultram ER Tablets **2428**

CROMIDIN (Chile)
TACROLIMUS
Prograf Capsules and Injection **622**

CRONASMA (Germany)
THEOPHYLLINE
Uniphyl Tablets **2595**

CRONODINE (Spain)
DILTIAZEM HYDROCHLORIDE
Cardizem LA Extended Release Tablets **421**

CRONOL (Spain)
FAMOTIDINE
Pepcid for Oral Suspension **2075**
Pepcid Tablets **2075**

CRYAXON (The Philippines)
CEFTRIAXONE SODIUM
Rocephin Injectable Vials, ADD-Vantage, Galaxy, Bulk **2642**

CRYOPRIL (Mexico)
CAPTOPRIL
Captopril Tablets **2182**

CRYSANAL (Australia)
NAPROXEN SODIUM
Anaprox DS Tablets **2632**
Anaprox Tablets **2632**

CRYSTACIT (South Africa)
POTASSIUM CITRATE
Urocit-K Tablets **2176**

CTZ (India)
CETIRIZINE HYDROCHLORIDE
Zyrtec Syrup **1920**
Zyrtec Tablets **1920**

CUADEL (Argentina)
DIAZEPAM
Valium Tablets **2658**

CUANTIN (Spain)
FAMOTIDINE
Pepcid for Oral Suspension **2075**
Pepcid Tablets **2075**

CUERPO AMARILLO FUERTE (Mexico)
PROGESTERONE
Crinone 4% Gel **992**
Prometrium Capsules (100 mg, 200 mg) . **3047**

CUNESIN (Spain)
CIPROFLOXACIN HYDROCHLORIDE
Cipro Tablets **2810**

CUPAX (Greece)
CEFUROXIME AXETIL
Ceftin for Oral Suspension **1380**
Ceftin Tablets **1380**

CURACNE (Argentina, France, Poland)
ISOTRETINOIN
Accutane Capsules **2607**

CURAKNE (Switzerland)
ISOTRETINOIN
Accutane Capsules **2607**

CURAM (Hong Kong, Malaysia, South Africa)
AMOXICILLIN
Amoxil Pediatric Drops for Oral Suspension **1305**
Amoxil Tablets **1305**

CURANTYL (Russia)
DIPYRIDAMOLE
Persantine Tablets **869**

CURANTYL N (Czech Republic, Germany)
DIPYRIDAMOLE
Persantine Tablets **869**

CURATANE (Israel)
ISOTRETINOIN
Accutane Capsules **2607**

CURAVISC (Israel)
SODIUM HYALURONATE
Hyalgan Solution **2742**

CURBAN (Greece)
NIMODIPINE
Nimotop Capsules **790**

CURIOSIN (Czech Republic)
SODIUM HYALURONATE
Hyalgan Solution **2742**

CUROCEF (Austria, Chile)
CEFUROXIME AXETIL
Ceftin for Oral Suspension **1380**
Ceftin Tablets **1380**

CUROXIM (Italy)
CEFUROXIME SODIUM
Zinacef Injection **1678**

CUROXIMA (Spain)
CEFUROXIME SODIUM
Zinacef Injection **1678**

CUROXIME (Portugal)
CEFUROXIME SODIUM
Zinacef Injection **1678**

CUSIMOLOL (Hong Kong, Hungary, Italy, Mexico, Poland, Portugal, Spain, Turkey)
TIMOLOL MALEATE
Timoptic in Ocudose **2124**
Timoptic Sterile Ophthalmic Solution **2121**
Timoptic-XE Sterile Ophthalmic Gel Forming Solution **2125**

CUTACNYL (France)
BENZOYL PEROXIDE
Brevoxyl-4 Creamy Wash **3054**
Brevoxyl-4 Gel **3054**
Brevoxyl-8 Creamy Wash **3054**
Brevoxyl-8 Gel **3054**

CUTANUM (Germany)
ESTRADIOL
Climara Transdermal System **763**

CUTENOX (Brazil)
ENOXAPARIN SODIUM
Lovenox Injection **2756**

CUTICLIN (Venezuela)
ISOTRETINOIN
Accutane Capsules **2607**

CUTIFITOL (Spain)
PROGESTERONE
Crinone 4% Gel **992**
Prometrium Capsules (100 mg, 200 mg) . **3047**

CUTIVAT (Denmark)
FLUTICASONE PROPIONATE
Flonase Nasal Spray **1431**

CUTIVATE (Argentina, Austria, Belgium, Czech Republic, Hong Kong, Hungary, Israel, Malaysia, Mexico, Poland, Portugal, Russia, Singapore, South Africa, Spain, Switzerland, The Netherlands, The Philippines, Turkey, United Kingdom, Venezuela)
FLUTICASONE PROPIONATE
Flonase Nasal Spray **1431**

CUXAFENON (Germany)
PROPAFENONE HYDROCHLORIDE
Rythmol SR Capsules **1590**

CYCIN (Singapore)
CIPROFLOXACIN HYDROCHLORIDE
Cipro Tablets **2810**

CYCLOBIOL (Chile)
ESTRADIOL
Climara Transdermal System **763**

CYCLODERM (Austria)
ESTRADIOL
Climara Transdermal System **763**

CYCLOGEST (Malaysia, Singapore, South Africa, Thailand, Turkey, United Kingdom)
PROGESTERONE
Crinone 4% Gel **992**
Prometrium Capsules (100 mg, 200 mg) . **3047**

CYCLORINE (India)
CYCLOSERINE
Seromycin Capsules **1864**

CYCLOSERINE (TM) (United Kingdom)
CYCLOSERINE
Seromycin Capsules **1864**

CYFLOX (Thailand)
CIPROFLOXACIN
Cipro Oral Suspension **2810**

CYFLOXIN (Hong Kong)
CIPROFLOXACIN HYDROCHLORIDE
Cipro Tablets **2810**

CYLLIND (Germany)
CLARITHROMYCIN
Biaxin Filmtab Tablets **411**
Biaxin Granules **411**

CYLOCORT (Brazil)
CIPROFLOXACIN HYDROCHLORIDE
Cipro Tablets **2810**

CYMALON CRANBERRY (United Kingdom)
POTASSIUM CITRATE
Urocit-K Tablets **2176**

CYNOMEL (Brazil, France, Greece, Mexico)
LIOTHYRONINE SODIUM
Cytomel Tablets **1778**

CYNT (Venezuela)
SIMVASTATIN
Zocor Tablets **2136**

CYPRAL (Venezuela)
CIPROFLOXACIN
Cipro Oral Suspension **2810**

CYSTISTAT (Canada, United Kingdom)
SODIUM HYALURONATE
Hyalgan Solution **2742**

CYSTOPURIN (United Kingdom)
POTASSIUM CITRATE
Urocit-K Tablets 2176

CYTOMEL (Belgium, Canada, The Netherlands)
LIOTHYRONINE SODIUM
Cytomel Tablets 1778

CYZINE (Thailand)
CETIRIZINE HYDROCHLORIDE
Zyrtec Syrup 1920
Zyrtec Tablets 1920

DABENZOL (Mexico)
ALBENDAZOLE
Albenza Tablets 1297

DACALA (Spain)
AMOXICILLIN
Amoxil Pediatric Drops for Oral Suspension 1305
Amoxil Tablets 1305

DACLIN (New Zealand)
SULINDAC
Clinoril Tablets 1962

DACTEN (Argentina)
CANDESARTAN CILEXETIL
Atacand Tablets 639

DACTEN D (Argentina)
CANDESARTAN CILEXETIL
Atacand Tablets 639

DAFEX (Argentina)
LAMOTRIGINE
Lamictal Chewable Dispersible Tablets 1488
Lamictal Tablets 1488

DAFLOXEN (Mexico)
NAPROXEN SODIUM
Anaprox DS Tablets 2632
Anaprox Tablets 2632

DAFLOXEN-F (Mexico)
NAPROXEN SODIUM
Anaprox DS Tablets 2632
Anaprox Tablets 2632

DAIV (Argentina)
DIAZEPAM
Valium Tablets 2658

DAKSOL (Chile)
LAMOTRIGINE
Lamictal Chewable Dispersible Tablets 1488
Lamictal Tablets 1488

DALTAZEN (Venezuela)
DILTIAZEM HYDROCHLORIDE
Cardizem LA Extended Release Tablets 421

DALTROID (Mexico)
LEVOTHYROXINE SODIUM
Levothroid Tablets 1170
Levoxyl Tablets 1780
Synthroid Tablets 507

DALYCRID (The Philippines)
RANITIDINE HYDROCHLORIDE
Zantac 25 EFFERdose Tablets 1670
Zantac 150 Tablets 1670
Zantac 300 Tablets 1670
Zantac Injection 1666
Zantac Injection Premixed 1666
Zantac Syrup 1670

DALZAD (Greece)
VALSARTAN
Diovan Tablets 2212

DAMIDE (Italy)
INDAPAMIDE
Indapamide Tablets 2188

DAMOSAL (Mexico)
DIPYRIDAMOLE
Persantine Tablets 869

DANILAX (Denmark, Hong Kong)
LACTULOSE
Kristalose for Oral Solution 1004

DANILON (Venezuela)
NORFLOXACIN
Noroxin Tablets 2069

DANLENE (Italy)
DANTROLENE SODIUM
Dantrium Capsules 2580
Dantrium Intravenous 2582

DANOPTIN (Poland)
LAMOTRIGINE
Lamictal Chewable Dispersible Tablets 1488
Lamictal Tablets 1488

DANTAMACRIN (Austria, Germany, Switzerland)
DANTROLENE SODIUM
Dantrium Capsules 2580
Dantrium Intravenous 2582

DANTENK (Argentina)
ONDANSETRON HYDROCHLORIDE
Zofran Injection 1682
Zofran Injection Premixed 1682
Zofran Oral Solution 1687
Zofran Tablets 1687

DANTRALEN (Spain)
DANTROLENE SODIUM
Dantrium Capsules 2580
Dantrium Intravenous 2582

DANTRIUM (Australia, Belgium, Canada, Chile, Denmark, France, Greece, Hong Kong, Irish Republic, Israel, Italy, New Zealand, Portugal, South Africa, The Netherlands, United Kingdom)
DANTROLENE SODIUM
Dantrium Capsules 2580
Dantrium Intravenous 2582

DANTROLEN (Brazil, Greece)
DANTROLENE SODIUM
Dantrium Capsules 2580
Dantrium Intravenous 2582

DANTRON (PREPARATION) (South Africa, Thailand)
ONDANSETRON HYDROCHLORIDE
Zofran Injection 1682
Zofran Injection Premixed 1682
Zofran Oral Solution 1687
Zofran Tablets 1687

DAPAMAX (South Africa)
INDAPAMIDE
Indapamide Tablets 2188

DAPA-TABS (Australia, Hong Kong)
INDAPAMIDE
Indapamide Tablets 2188

DAPRIL (Czech Republic, Russia, Singapore)
LISINOPRIL
Prinivil Tablets 2087

DAPROX (Denmark)
NAPROXEN
EC-Naprosyn Delayed-Release Tablets 2632
Naprosyn Suspension 2632
Naprosyn Tablets 2632

DAPS (Argentina)
DAPSONE
Dapsone Tablets USP 1746

DAPSODERM-X (Mexico)
DAPSONE
Dapsone Tablets USP 1746

DAPTRIL (South Africa)
INDAPAMIDE
Indapamide Tablets 2188

DARAPRIM (Argentina, Australia, Austria, Belgium, Brazil, Canada, Chile, Germany, Irish Republic, Israel, Mexico, Poland, South Africa, Spain, Sweden, Switzerland, Thailand, The Netherlands, United Kingdom)
PYRIMETHAMINE
Daraprim Tablets 1400

DARAPRIN (Brazil)
PYRIMETHAMINE
Daraprim Tablets 1400

DARDEX (Spain)
CAPTOPRIL
Captopril Tablets 2182

DARIC (Argentina)
FINASTERIDE
Propecia Tablets 2095
Proscar Tablets 2102

DARMOL LACTULOSE (Austria)
LACTULOSE
Kristalose for Oral Solution 1004

DARSTIN (Spain)
PROGESTERONE
Crinone 4% Gel 992
Prometrium Capsules (100 mg, 200 mg) 3047

DARTROX (Mexico)
NAPROXEN
EC-Naprosyn Delayed-Release Tablets 2632
Naprosyn Suspension 2632
Naprosyn Tablets 2632

DASKIL (Austria, Italy)
TERBINAFINE HYDROCHLORIDE
Lamisil Tablets 2266

DASKYL (Portugal)
TERBINAFINE HYDROCHLORIDE
Lamisil Tablets 2266

DATEVAN (Argentina)
PAROXETINE HYDROCHLORIDE
Paxil Oral Suspension 1535
Paxil Tablets 1535

DATRON (Spain)
ONDANSETRON HYDROCHLORIDE
Zofran Injection 1682
Zofran Injection Premixed 1682
Zofran Oral Solution 1687
Zofran Tablets 1687

DAVIXON (Italy)
CEFTRIAXONE SODIUM
Rocephin Injectable Vials, ADD-Vantage, Galaxy, Bulk 2642

DAXOTEL (India, Thailand, Venezuela)
DOCETAXEL
Taxotere Injection Concentrate 2773

DAYTRIX (Italy)
CEFTRIAXONE SODIUM
Rocephin Injectable Vials, ADD-Vantage, Galaxy, Bulk 2642

DAZID (Thailand)
TRIAMTERENE
Dyrenium Capsules 3189

DAZINE (Thailand)
THIORIDAZINE HYDROCHLORIDE
Thioridazine Hydrochloride Tablets 2195

DAZOCAN (Mexico)
ALBENDAZOLE
Albenza Tablets 1297

DAZOL (Brazil)
ALBENDAZOLE
Albenza Tablets 1297

DAZOLIN (Chile, Mexico)
ALBENDAZOLE
Albenza Tablets 1297

D-CYCLOSERIN (Greece)
CYCLOSERINE
Seromycin Capsules 1864

DEALGIC (Italy)
DICLOFENAC SODIUM
Voltaren Tablets 2334
Voltaren-XR Tablets 2337

DEBAX (Austria)
CAPTOPRIL
Captopril Tablets 2182

DEBRIL (Argentina)
NAPROXEN
EC-Naprosyn Delayed-Release Tablets 2632
Naprosyn Suspension 2632
Naprosyn Tablets 2632

DECIPAR (Spain)
ENOXAPARIN SODIUM
Lovenox Injection 2756

DECLOFON (Greece)
DICLOFENAC SODIUM
Voltaren Tablets 2334
Voltaren-XR Tablets 2337

DECOSIL (Mexico)
NAPROXEN SODIUM
Anaprox DS Tablets 2632
Anaprox Tablets 2632

DECOSTRIOL (Germany, Hong Kong, Thailand)
CALCITRIOL
Calcijex Injection 419
Rocaltrol Capsules 1150
Rocaltrol Oral Solution 1150

DEDOLOR (Austria)
DICLOFENAC SODIUM
Voltaren Tablets 2334
Voltaren-XR Tablets 2337

DEFANAC (United Kingdom)
DICLOFENAC SODIUM
Voltaren Tablets 2334
Voltaren-XR Tablets 2337

DEFIXAL (Venezuela)
ALENDRONATE SODIUM
Fosamax Tablets 2005

DEFLAMAT (Austria, Italy, Switzerland, Turkey)
DICLOFENAC SODIUM
Voltaren Tablets 2334
Voltaren-XR Tablets 2337

DEFLAMM (Austria)
DICLOFENAC SODIUM
Voltaren Tablets 2334
Voltaren-XR Tablets 2337

DEFLAMOX (Mexico)
NAPROXEN SODIUM
Anaprox DS Tablets 2632
Anaprox Tablets 2632

DEGRANOL (South Africa)
CARBAMAZEPINE
Carbatrol Capsules 3019

DEIXIM (Italy)
CEFTRIAXONE SODIUM
Rocephin Injectable Vials, ADD-Vantage, Galaxy, Bulk 2642

DELEPTIN (Austria)
CARBAMAZEPINE
Carbatrol Capsules 3019

DELIDOSE (France)
ESTRADIOL
Climara Transdermal System 763

DELIMON (Greece)
DICLOFENAC SODIUM
Voltaren Tablets 2334
Voltaren-XR Tablets 2337

DELOS OTIC (Argentina)
CIPROFLOXACIN
Cipro Oral Suspension 2810

DELPHI (Belgium, The Netherlands)
TRIAMCINOLONE ACETONIDE
Azmacort Inhalation Aerosol 407
Nasacort AQ Nasal Spray 2765

DELPHIMIX 1 (Germany)
DICLOFENAC SODIUM
Voltaren Tablets 2334
Voltaren-XR Tablets 2337

DELPHINAC (Germany)
DICLOFENAC SODIUM
Voltaren Tablets 2334
Voltaren-XR Tablets 2337

DELTA 80 (Italy)
BENZOYL PEROXIDE
Brevoxyl-4 Creamy Wash 3054
Brevoxyl-4 Gel 3054
Brevoxyl-8 Creamy Wash 3054
Brevoxyl-8 Gel 3054

DELTACEF (Italy)
CEFUROXIME SODIUM
Zinacef Injection 1678

DELTAZEN (France)
DILTIAZEM HYDROCHLORIDE
Cardizem LA Extended Release Tablets 421

DEMSIL (Greece)
TERBINAFINE HYDROCHLORIDE
Lamisil Tablets 2266

DENACLOF (Greece)
DICLOFENAC SODIUM
Voltaren Tablets 2334
Voltaren-XR Tablets 2337

DENAN (Germany)
SIMVASTATIN
Zocor Tablets 2136

DENAXPREN (Spain)
NAPROXEN
EC-Naprosyn Delayed-Release Tablets 2632
Naprosyn Suspension 2632
Naprosyn Tablets 2632

DENAZOX (Thailand)
DILTIAZEM HYDROCHLORIDE
Cardizem LA Extended Release Tablets 421

DENCORUB ANTI-INFLAMMATORY (Australia)
DICLOFENAC SODIUM
Voltaren Tablets . . . **2334**
Voltaren-XR Tablets . . . **2337**

DENERVAL (Portugal)
PAROXETINE HYDROCHLORIDE
Paxil Oral Suspension . . . **1535**
Paxil Tablets . . . **1535**

DENIREN (Mexico)
AMOXICILLIN
Amoxil Pediatric Drops for Oral Suspension . . . **1305**
Amoxil Tablets . . . **1305**

DENKACORT (Hong Kong)
TRIAMCINOLONE ACETONIDE
Azmacort Inhalation Aerosol . . . **407**
Nasacort AQ Nasal Spray . . . **2765**

DENULCER (Spain)
RANITIDINE HYDROCHLORIDE
Zantac 25 EFFERdose Tablets . . . **1670**
Zantac 150 Tablets . . . **1670**
Zantac 300 Tablets . . . **1670**
Zantac Injection . . . **1666**
Zantac Injection Premixed . . . **1666**
Zantac Syrup . . . **1670**

DEPALGOS (Italy)
OXYCODONE HYDROCHLORIDE
OxyContin Tablets . . . **2589**
OxyIR Capsules . . . **2593**

DEPAROC (South Africa)
PAROXETINE HYDROCHLORIDE
Paxil Oral Suspension . . . **1535**
Paxil Tablets . . . **1535**

DEPRAMIL (South Africa)
CITALOPRAM HYDROBROMIDE
Celexa Tablets . . . **1160**

DEPRENYL (France, Germany)
SELEGILINE HYDROCHLORIDE
Eldepryl Capsules . . . **3052**

DEPRILAN (Brazil)
SELEGILINE HYDROCHLORIDE
Eldepryl Capsules . . . **3052**

DEPUROL (Chile)
VENLAFAXINE HYDROCHLORIDE
Effexor XR Capsules . . . **3195**

DERCOME (Germany)
BENZOYL PEROXIDE
Brevoxyl-4 Creamy Wash . . . **3054**
Brevoxyl-4 Gel . . . **3054**
Brevoxyl-8 Creamy Wash . . . **3054**
Brevoxyl-8 Gel . . . **3054**

DERCUTANE (Spain)
ISOTRETINOIN
Accutane Capsules . . . **2607**

DERGENTIL (Venezuela)
MOMETASONE FUROATE
Elocon Cream 0.1% . . . **2840**
Elocon Lotion 0.1% . . . **2841**
Elocon Ointment 0.1% . . . **2842**
Nasonex Nasal Spray . . . **2883**

DERICIP (India)
THEOPHYLLINE
Uniphyl Tablets . . . **2595**

DERICIP PLUS (India)
THEOPHYLLINE
Uniphyl Tablets . . . **2595**

DERM A (The Philippines)
TRETINOIN
Vesanoid Capsules . . . **2660**

DERMABAZ (Hong Kong)
TRETINOIN
Vesanoid Capsules . . . **2660**

DERMACLEAN (Argentina)
BENZOYL PEROXIDE
Brevoxyl-4 Creamy Wash . . . **3054**
Brevoxyl-4 Gel . . . **3054**
Brevoxyl-8 Creamy Wash . . . **3054**
Brevoxyl-8 Gel . . . **3054**

DERMACNE (Canada)
BENZOYL PEROXIDE
Brevoxyl-4 Creamy Wash . . . **3054**
Brevoxyl-4 Gel . . . **3054**
Brevoxyl-8 Creamy Wash . . . **3054**
Brevoxyl-8 Gel . . . **3054**

DERMACOM (Chile)
BUTENAFINE HYDROCHLORIDE
Mentax Cream . . . **2190**

DERMACORT (Hong Kong, Malaysia, Singapore)
TRIAMCINOLONE ACETONIDE
Azmacort Inhalation Aerosol . . . **407**
Nasacort AQ Nasal Spray . . . **2765**

DERMAIROL (Sweden)
TRETINOIN
Vesanoid Capsules . . . **2660**

DERMANCE (Canada)
BENZOYL PEROXIDE
Brevoxyl-4 Creamy Wash . . . **3054**
Brevoxyl-4 Gel . . . **3054**
Brevoxyl-8 Creamy Wash . . . **3054**
Brevoxyl-8 Gel . . . **3054**

DERMAORAL (Denmark)
ISOTRETINOIN
Accutane Capsules . . . **2607**

DERMATIN (Germany)
TERBINAFINE HYDROCHLORIDE
Lamisil Tablets . . . **2266**

DERMATRANS (Chile)
ESTRADIOL
Climara Transdermal System . . . **763**

DERMAX (South Africa)
TERBINAFINE HYDROCHLORIDE
Lamisil Tablets . . . **2266**

DERMENET (Chile)
MOMETASONE FUROATE
Elocon Cream 0.1% . . . **2840**
Elocon Lotion 0.1% . . . **2841**
Elocon Ointment 0.1% . . . **2842**
Nasonex Nasal Spray . . . **2883**

DERMESTRIL (Australia, Austria, Belgium, Czech Republic, Finland, France, Germany, Greece, Hong Kong, Hungary, Irish Republic, Italy, Portugal, Spain, Switzerland, The Netherlands, United Kingdom)
ESTRADIOL
Climara Transdermal System . . . **763**

DERMINOIN (Greece)
ISOTRETINOIN
Accutane Capsules . . . **2607**

DERMODAN (Chile)
TRETINOIN
Vesanoid Capsules . . . **2660**

DERMOJUVENTUS (Spain)
TRETINOIN
Vesanoid Capsules . . . **2660**

DERMOPERO (Argentina)
IVERMECTIN
Stromectol Tablets . . . **2120**

DERMORETIN (Brazil)
TRETINOIN
Vesanoid Capsules . . . **2660**

DERMOSONA (Chile)
MOMETASONE FUROATE
Elocon Cream 0.1% . . . **2840**
Elocon Lotion 0.1% . . . **2841**
Elocon Ointment 0.1% . . . **2842**
Nasonex Nasal Spray . . . **2883**

DERMOVAGISIL (Spain)
LIDOCAINE
Lidoderm Patch . . . **1114**

DERMOXYL (Canada, Chile)
BENZOYL PEROXIDE
Brevoxyl-4 Creamy Wash . . . **3054**
Brevoxyl-4 Gel . . . **3054**
Brevoxyl-8 Creamy Wash . . . **3054**
Brevoxyl-8 Gel . . . **3054**

DERONGA HEILPASTE (Germany)
NATAMYCIN
Natacyn Antifungal Ophthalmic Suspension . . . ⊙**204**

DEROXAT (France, Switzerland)
PAROXETINE HYDROCHLORIDE
Paxil Oral Suspension . . . **1535**
Paxil Tablets . . . **1535**

DESAFLU (Italy)
FLUNISOLIDE
Aerobid Inhaler System . . . **1153**
Aerobid-M Inhaler System . . . **1153**

DESAL (Turkey)
FUROSEMIDE
Furosemide Tablets . . . **2186**

DESANDEN (Switzerland)
BENZOYL PEROXIDE
Brevoxyl-4 Creamy Wash . . . **3054**
Brevoxyl-4 Gel . . . **3054**
Brevoxyl-8 Creamy Wash . . . **3054**
Brevoxyl-8 Gel . . . **3054**

DESINFLAM (Argentina)
DICLOFENAC SODIUM
Voltaren Tablets . . . **2334**
Voltaren-XR Tablets . . . **2337**

DESITAL (Norway)
CITALOPRAM HYDROBROMIDE
Celexa Tablets . . . **1160**

DESQUAM-X (Canada)
BENZOYL PEROXIDE
Brevoxyl-4 Creamy Wash . . . **3054**
Brevoxyl-4 Gel . . . **3054**
Brevoxyl-8 Creamy Wash . . . **3054**
Brevoxyl-8 Gel . . . **3054**

DETIDRON (Austria)
ETIDRONATE DISODIUM
Didronel Tablets . . . **2583**

DEUCOVAL (Chile)
NAPROXEN SODIUM
Anaprox DS Tablets . . . **2632**
Anaprox Tablets . . . **2632**

DEXA AMINOFILIN (Argentina)
THEOPHYLLINE
Uniphyl Tablets . . . **2595**

DEXA TEOSONA (Argentina)
THEOPHYLLINE
Uniphyl Tablets . . . **2595**

DEXACAP (Hong Kong)
CAPTOPRIL
Captopril Tablets . . . **2182**

DEXANTOL (Switzerland)
PAROXETINE HYDROCHLORIDE
Paxil Oral Suspension . . . **1535**
Paxil Tablets . . . **1535**

DEXIVEN (Argentina)
CALCITRIOL
Calcijex Injection . . . **419**
Rocaltrol Capsules . . . **1150**
Rocaltrol Oral Solution . . . **1150**

DEXNON (Spain)
LEVOTHYROXINE SODIUM
Levothroid Tablets . . . **1170**
Levoxyl Tablets . . . **1780**
Synthroid Tablets . . . **507**

DEXOMON (United Kingdom)
DICLOFENAC SODIUM
Voltaren Tablets . . . **2334**
Voltaren-XR Tablets . . . **2337**

DEZABIL (Mexico)
ALBENDAZOLE
Albenza Tablets . . . **1297**

DEZEPAN (Argentina)
DIAZEPAM
Valium Tablets . . . **2658**

DHACTULOSE (Singapore)
LACTULOSE
Kristalose for Oral Solution . . . **1004**

DI RETARD (Spain)
DICLOFENAC SODIUM
Voltaren Tablets . . . **2334**
Voltaren-XR Tablets . . . **2337**

DIABEN (Argentina)
ROSIGLITAZONE MALEATE
Avandia Tablets . . . **1351**

DIABESTAT (Chile)
PIOGLITAZONE HYDROCHLORIDE
Actos Tablets . . . **3077**

DIACARDIN (Italy)
DILTIAZEM HYDROCHLORIDE
Cardizem LA Extended Release Tablets . . . **421**

DIACEPAM (Mexico)
DIAZEPAM
Valium Tablets . . . **2658**

DIACEPLEX (Spain)
DIAZEPAM
Valium Tablets . . . **2658**

DIACEPLEX SIMPLE (Spain)
DIAZEPAM
Valium Tablets . . . **2658**

DIA-COLON (Italy)
LACTULOSE
Kristalose for Oral Solution . . . **1004**

DIACOR (France)
DILTIAZEM HYDROCHLORIDE
Cardizem LA Extended Release Tablets . . . **421**

DIACORDIN (Czech Republic, Poland)
DILTIAZEM HYDROCHLORIDE
Cardizem LA Extended Release Tablets . . . **421**

DIACTAL (Argentina)
DIAZEPAM
Valium Tablets . . . **2658**

DIAGLIT (India)
PIOGLITAZONE HYDROCHLORIDE
Actos Tablets . . . **3077**

DIALAR (United Kingdom)
DIAZEPAM
Valium Tablets . . . **2658**

DIANO (Thailand)
DIAZEPAM
Valium Tablets . . . **2658**

DIAPAM (Finland, Thailand, Turkey)
DIAZEPAM
Valium Tablets . . . **2658**

DIAPANIL (Mexico)
DIAZEPAM
Valium Tablets . . . **2658**

DIAPINE (Malaysia, Singapore, Thailand)
DIAZEPAM
Valium Tablets . . . **2658**

DIAPO (Malaysia)
DIAZEPAM
Valium Tablets . . . **2658**

DIAQUEL (South Africa)
DIAZEPAM
Valium Tablets . . . **2658**

DIASTAT (Canada)
DIAZEPAM
Valium Tablets . . . **2658**

DIASTONE (Argentina)
DICLOFENAC SODIUM
Voltaren Tablets . . . **2334**
Voltaren-XR Tablets . . . **2337**

DIATEX (Mexico)
DIAZEPAM
Valium Tablets . . . **2658**

DIATIL (South Africa)
DILTIAZEM HYDROCHLORIDE
Cardizem LA Extended Release Tablets . . . **421**

DIAXONE (Italy)
CEFTRIAXONE SODIUM
Rocephin Injectable Vials, ADD-Vantage, Galaxy, Bulk . . . **2642**

DIAZ (Israel)
DIAZEPAM
Valium Tablets . . . **2658**

DIAZEFAST (Brazil)
DIAZEPAM
Valium Tablets . . . **2658**

DIAZELONG (Brazil)
DIAZEPAM
Valium Tablets . . . **2658**

DIAZEM (Russia, Turkey)
DILTIAZEM HYDROCHLORIDE
Cardizem LA Extended Release Tablets . . . **421**

DIAZEMULS (Australia, Canada, Germany, Hong Kong, Irish Republic, Italy, The Netherlands, United Kingdom)
DIAZEPAM
Valium Tablets . . . **2658**

DIAZEPAN (Brazil)
DIAZEPAM
Valium Tablets . . . **2658**

DICEPIN B6 (Spain)
DIAZEPAM
Valium Tablets . . . **2658**

DICIL (Chile)
TERBINAFINE HYDROCHLORIDE
Lamisil Tablets 2266

DICLAC (Australia, Austria, Brazil, Germany, Hungary, Republic, Mexico, Poland, Switzerland)
DICLOFENAC SODIUM
Voltaren Tablets 2334
Voltaren-XR Tablets 2337

DICLAX (New Zealand)
DICLOFENAC SODIUM
Voltaren Tablets 2334
Voltaren-XR Tablets 2337

DICLAXOL (Austria)
DICLOFENAC SODIUM
Voltaren Tablets 2334
Voltaren-XR Tablets 2337

DICLO (Irish Republic, Switzerland)
DICLOFENAC SODIUM
Voltaren Tablets 2334
Voltaren-XR Tablets 2337

DICLO-ATTRITIN (Germany)
DICLOFENAC SODIUM
Voltaren Tablets 2334
Voltaren-XR Tablets 2337

DICLO-BASAN (Switzerland)
DICLOFENAC SODIUM
Voltaren Tablets 2334
Voltaren-XR Tablets 2337

DICLOBENE (Russia)
DICLOFENAC SODIUM
Voltaren Tablets 2334
Voltaren-XR Tablets 2337

DICLOBERL (Germany, Russia)
DICLOFENAC SODIUM
Voltaren Tablets 2334
Voltaren-XR Tablets 2337

DICLOCULAR (Italy)
DICLOFENAC SODIUM
Voltaren Tablets 2334
Voltaren-XR Tablets 2337

DICLO-DENK (Hong Kong, Singapore)
DICLOFENAC SODIUM
Voltaren Tablets 2334
Voltaren-XR Tablets 2337

DICLO-DIVIDO (Germany)
DICLOFENAC SODIUM
Voltaren Tablets 2334
Voltaren-XR Tablets 2337

DICLODOC (Germany)
DICLOFENAC SODIUM
Voltaren Tablets 2334
Voltaren-XR Tablets 2337

DICLODOL (Italy)
DICLOFENAC SODIUM
Voltaren Tablets 2334
Voltaren-XR Tablets 2337

DICLODUO (Poland)
DICLOFENAC SODIUM
Voltaren Tablets 2334
Voltaren-XR Tablets 2337

DICLO-F (Russia)
DICLOFENAC SODIUM
Voltaren Tablets 2334
Voltaren-XR Tablets 2337

DICLOFAN (Italy)
DICLOFENAC SODIUM
Voltaren Tablets 2334
Voltaren-XR Tablets 2337

DICLOFEMED (Belgium)
DICLOFENAC SODIUM
Voltaren Tablets 2334
Voltaren-XR Tablets 2337

DICLOFEN (Czech Republic, Thailand)
DICLOFENAC SODIUM
Voltaren Tablets 2334
Voltaren-XR Tablets 2337

DICLOFENBETA (Germany)
DICLOFENAC SODIUM
Voltaren Tablets 2334
Voltaren-XR Tablets 2337

DICLOFLAM (South Africa)
DICLOFENAC SODIUM
Voltaren Tablets 2334
Voltaren-XR Tablets 2337

DICLOFLEX (United Kingdom)
DICLOFENAC SODIUM
Voltaren Tablets 2334
Voltaren-XR Tablets 2337

DICLOFTAL (Portugal)
DICLOFENAC SODIUM
Voltaren Tablets 2334
Voltaren-XR Tablets 2337

DICLOFTIL (Italy)
DICLOFENAC SODIUM
Voltaren Tablets 2334
Voltaren-XR Tablets 2337

DICLOGEA (Denmark)
DICLOFENAC SODIUM
Voltaren Tablets 2334
Voltaren-XR Tablets 2337

DICLO-GEL (Germany)
DICLOFENAC SODIUM
Voltaren Tablets 2334
Voltaren-XR Tablets 2337

DICLOGENOM (Brazil)
DICLOFENAC SODIUM
Voltaren Tablets 2334
Voltaren-XR Tablets 2337

DICLOGENTA (India)
DICLOFENAC SODIUM
Voltaren Tablets 2334
Voltaren-XR Tablets 2337

DICLOGESIC (Hong Kong)
DICLOFENAC SODIUM
Voltaren Tablets 2334
Voltaren-XR Tablets 2337

DICLOGESIC RELAX (Argentina)
DICLOFENAC SODIUM
Voltaren Tablets 2334
Voltaren-XR Tablets 2337

DICLOGRUN (Germany)
DICLOFENAC SODIUM
Voltaren Tablets 2334
Voltaren-XR Tablets 2337

DICLOHEXAL (Australia, New Zealand)
DICLOFENAC SODIUM
Voltaren Tablets 2334
Voltaren-XR Tablets 2337

DICLOLAN (Thailand)
DICLOFENAC SODIUM
Voltaren Tablets 2334
Voltaren-XR Tablets 2337

DICLOMAX (Irish Republic, United Kingdom)
DICLOFENAC SODIUM
Voltaren Tablets 2334
Voltaren-XR Tablets 2337

DICLOMEC (Turkey)
DICLOFENAC SODIUM
Voltaren Tablets 2334
Voltaren-XR Tablets 2337

DICLOMEL (Hungary, Irish Republic)
DICLOFENAC SODIUM
Voltaren Tablets 2334
Voltaren-XR Tablets 2337

DICLOMELAN (Austria)
DICLOFENAC SODIUM
Voltaren Tablets 2334
Voltaren-XR Tablets 2337

DICLOMERCK (Germany)
DICLOFENAC SODIUM
Voltaren Tablets 2334
Voltaren-XR Tablets 2337

DICLOMETIN (Finland)
DICLOFENAC SODIUM
Voltaren Tablets 2334
Voltaren-XR Tablets 2337

DICLOMOL (India, Thailand)
DICLOFENAC SODIUM
Voltaren Tablets 2334
Voltaren-XR Tablets 2337

DICLONAC (India)
DICLOFENAC SODIUM
Voltaren Tablets 2334
Voltaren-XR Tablets 2337

DICLONACO (Brazil)
DICLOFENAC SODIUM
Voltaren Tablets 2334
Voltaren-XR Tablets 2337

DICLONAT (Russia)
DICLOFENAC SODIUM
Voltaren Tablets 2334
Voltaren-XR Tablets 2337

DICLONATRIUM (Brazil)
DICLOFENAC SODIUM
Voltaren Tablets 2334
Voltaren-XR Tablets 2337

DICLONEX RELAX (Argentina)
DICLOFENAC SODIUM
Voltaren Tablets 2334
Voltaren-XR Tablets 2337

DICLO-OPT (Germany)
DICLOFENAC SODIUM
Voltaren Tablets 2334
Voltaren-XR Tablets 2337

DICLOPHLOGONT (Germany, Greece)
DICLOFENAC SODIUM
Voltaren Tablets 2334
Voltaren-XR Tablets 2337

DICLO-PUREN (Germany)
DICLOFENAC SODIUM
Voltaren Tablets 2334
Voltaren-XR Tablets 2337

DICLORAN (Mexico)
DICLOFENAC SODIUM
Voltaren Tablets 2334
Voltaren-XR Tablets 2337

DICLORAN-A (India)
DICLOFENAC SODIUM
Voltaren Tablets 2334
Voltaren-XR Tablets 2337

DICLOREKTAL (Germany)
DICLOFENAC SODIUM
Voltaren Tablets 2334
Voltaren-XR Tablets 2337

DICLORENGEL (Israel)
DICLOFENAC SODIUM
Voltaren Tablets 2334
Voltaren-XR Tablets 2337

DICLOREUM (Czech Republic)
DICLOFENAC SODIUM
Voltaren Tablets 2334
Voltaren-XR Tablets 2337

DICLO-SAAR (Germany)
DICLOFENAC SODIUM
Voltaren Tablets 2334
Voltaren-XR Tablets 2337

DICLOSAL (Venezuela)
DICLOFENAC SODIUM
Voltaren Tablets 2334
Voltaren-XR Tablets 2337

DICLOSIAN (Thailand)
DICLOFENAC SODIUM
Voltaren Tablets 2334
Voltaren-XR Tablets 2337

DICLOSIFAR (Switzerland)
DICLOFENAC SODIUM
Voltaren Tablets 2334
Voltaren-XR Tablets 2337

DICLOSOD (Brazil)
DICLOFENAC SODIUM
Voltaren Tablets 2334
Voltaren-XR Tablets 2337

DICLOSODICO (Brazil)
DICLOFENAC SODIUM
Voltaren Tablets 2334
Voltaren-XR Tablets 2337

DICLO-SPONDYRIL (Germany)
DICLOFENAC SODIUM
Voltaren Tablets 2334
Voltaren-XR Tablets 2337

DICLOSTAD (Austria)
DICLOFENAC SODIUM
Voltaren Tablets 2334
Voltaren-XR Tablets 2337

DICLOSTAN (Venezuela)
DICLOFENAC SODIUM
Voltaren Tablets 2334
Voltaren-XR Tablets 2337

DICLOSYL (Austria)
DICLOFENAC SODIUM
Voltaren Tablets 2334
Voltaren-XR Tablets 2337

DICLO-TABLINEN (Germany)
DICLOFENAC SODIUM
Voltaren Tablets 2334
Voltaren-XR Tablets 2337

DICLOTARD (United Kingdom)
DICLOFENAC SODIUM
Voltaren Tablets 2334
Voltaren-XR Tablets 2337

DICLOTEARS (Italy)
DICLOFENAC SODIUM
Voltaren Tablets 2334
Voltaren-XR Tablets 2337

DICLOTEC (Canada, Portugal)
DICLOFENAC SODIUM
Voltaren Tablets 2334
Voltaren-XR Tablets 2337

DICLOTOP (Belgium)
DICLOFENAC SODIUM
Voltaren Tablets 2334
Voltaren-XR Tablets 2337

DICLOVIT (Russia)
DICLOFENAC SODIUM
Voltaren Tablets 2334
Voltaren-XR Tablets 2337

DICLOVOL (United Kingdom)
DICLOFENAC SODIUM
Voltaren Tablets 2334
Voltaren-XR Tablets 2337

DICLOWAL (Hong Kong, Singapore)
DICLOFENAC SODIUM
Voltaren Tablets 2334
Voltaren-XR Tablets 2337

DICLOZIP (United Kingdom)
DICLOFENAC SODIUM
Voltaren Tablets 2334
Voltaren-XR Tablets 2337

DIDAMOL (Belgium)
DIPYRIDAMOLE
Persantine Tablets 869

DIDRONAT (Turkey)
ETIDRONATE DISODIUM
Didronel Tablets 2583

DIDRONATE (Denmark, Finland, Norway, Sweden)
ETIDRONATE DISODIUM
Didronel Tablets 2583

DIDRONEL (Australia, Austria, Belgium, Canada, France, Germany, Hong Kong, Irish Republic, Israel, Italy, Japan, New Zealand, Portugal, South Africa, Switzerland, The Netherlands, United Kingdom)
ETIDRONATE DISODIUM
Didronel Tablets 2583

DIENPAX (Brazil)
DIAZEPAM
Valium Tablets 2658

DIFEN (Germany, Thailand)
DICLOFENAC SODIUM
Voltaren Tablets 2334
Voltaren-XR Tablets 2337

DIFENA (Hong Kong)
DICLOFENAC SODIUM
Voltaren Tablets 2334
Voltaren-XR Tablets 2337

DIFENAC (Argentina, Hong Kong, Singapore, South Africa, Thailand)
DICLOFENAC SODIUM
Voltaren Tablets 2334
Voltaren-XR Tablets 2337

DIFENAK (Turkey)
DICLOFENAC SODIUM
Voltaren Tablets 2334
Voltaren-XR Tablets 2337

DIFENAN (Brazil)
DICLOFENAC SODIUM
Voltaren Tablets 2334
Voltaren-XR Tablets 2337

DIFENAX (The Philippines)
DICLOFENAC SODIUM
Voltaren Tablets 2334
Voltaren-XR Tablets 2337

DIFEND (Greece)
DICLOFENAC SODIUM
Voltaren Tablets 2334

Voltaren-XR Tablets **2337**

DIFENE (Austria, Irish Republic)
DICLOFENAC SODIUM
Voltaren Tablets **2334**
Voltaren-XR Tablets **2337**

DIFENET (Denmark)
DICLOFENAC SODIUM
Voltaren Tablets **2334**
Voltaren-XR Tablets **2337**

DIFENO (Thailand)
DICLOFENAC SODIUM
Voltaren Tablets **2334**
Voltaren-XR Tablets **2337**

DIFENOL (Hong Kong)
DICLOFENAC SODIUM
Voltaren Tablets **2334**
Voltaren-XR Tablets **2337**

DIFERBEST (Mexico)
NAPROXEN SODIUM
Anaprox DS Tablets **2632**
Anaprox Tablets **2632**

DIFFUMAL (Italy)
THEOPHYLLINE
Uniphyl Tablets **2595**

DIFIX (Italy)
CALCITRIOL
Calcijex Injection **419**
Rocaltrol Capsules **1150**
Rocaltrol Oral Solution **1150**

DIFLAPANE (The Philippines)
DICLOFENAC SODIUM
Voltaren Tablets **2334**
Voltaren-XR Tablets **2337**

DIFLERIX (Hong Kong, Malaysia)
INDAPAMIDE
Indapamide Tablets **2188**

DIFNAL (Singapore)
DICLOFENAC SODIUM
Voltaren Tablets **2334**
Voltaren-XR Tablets **2337**

DIFOSFEN (Argentina, Singapore, Spain)
ETIDRONATE DISODIUM
Didronel Tablets **2583**

DIFOXACIL (Mexico)
NORFLOXACIN
Noroxin Tablets **2069**

DIGACIN (Germany)
DIGOXIN
Lanoxin Injection **1498**
Lanoxin Injection Pediatric **1502**
Lanoxin Tablets **1505**

DIGAOL (France)
TIMOLOL MALEATE
Timoptic in Ocudose **2124**
Timoptic Sterile Ophthalmic Solution **2121**
Timoptic-XE Sterile Ophthalmic Gel Forming Solution **2125**

DIGARIL (Spain)
FLUVASTATIN SODIUM
Lescol Capsules **2268**

DIGENAC (United Kingdom)
DICLOFENAC SODIUM
Voltaren Tablets **2334**
Voltaren-XR Tablets **2337**

DIGERVIN (Spain)
FAMOTIDINE
Pepcid for Oral Suspension **2075**
Pepcid Tablets **2075**

DIGESS (Canada)
PANCRELIPASE
Ultrase Capsules **718**
Ultrase MT Capsules **719**

DIGESTOSAN (Austria)
RANITIDINE HYDROCHLORIDE
Zantac 25 EFFERdose Tablets **1670**
Zantac 150 Tablets **1670**
Zantac 300 Tablets **1670**
Zantac Injection **1666**
Zantac Injection Premixed **1666**
Zantac Syrup **1670**

DIGEZANOL (Mexico)
ALBENDAZOLE
Albenza Tablets **1297**

DIGITAX (Brazil)
DIGOXIN
Lanoxin Injection **1498**
Lanoxin Injection Pediatric **1502**
Lanoxin Tablets **1505**

DIGIXINA (Brazil)
DIGOXIN
Lanoxin Injection **1498**
Lanoxin Injection Pediatric **1502**
Lanoxin Tablets **1505**

DIGNOFENAC (Chile, Germany)
DICLOFENAC SODIUM
Voltaren Tablets **2334**
Voltaren-XR Tablets **2337**

DIGOCARD-G (Argentina)
DIGOXIN
Lanoxin Injection **1498**
Lanoxin Injection Pediatric **1502**
Lanoxin Tablets **1505**

DIGOMAL (Italy)
DIGOXIN
Lanoxin Injection **1498**
Lanoxin Injection Pediatric **1502**
Lanoxin Tablets **1505**

DIGOREGEN (Germany)
DIGOXIN
Lanoxin Injection **1498**
Lanoxin Injection Pediatric **1502**
Lanoxin Tablets **1505**

DIGOSIN (Japan)
DIGOXIN
Lanoxin Injection **1498**
Lanoxin Injection Pediatric **1502**
Lanoxin Tablets **1505**

DIGOX (Brazil)
DIGOXIN
Lanoxin Injection **1498**
Lanoxin Injection Pediatric **1502**
Lanoxin Tablets **1505**

DIGOXAN (Brazil)
DIGOXIN
Lanoxin Injection **1498**
Lanoxin Injection Pediatric **1502**
Lanoxin Tablets **1505**

DIGOXEN (Brazil)
DIGOXIN
Lanoxin Injection **1498**
Lanoxin Injection Pediatric **1502**
Lanoxin Tablets **1505**

DIGOXIL (Brazil)
DIGOXIN
Lanoxin Injection **1498**
Lanoxin Injection Pediatric **1502**
Lanoxin Tablets **1505**

DIKLONAT P (Poland)
DICLOFENAC SODIUM
Voltaren Tablets **2334**
Voltaren-XR Tablets **2337**

DILABAR (Spain)
CAPTOPRIL
Captopril Tablets **2182**

DILACLAN (Spain)
DILTIAZEM HYDROCHLORIDE
Cardizem LA Extended Release Tablets **421**

DILADEL (Italy)
DILTIAZEM HYDROCHLORIDE
Cardizem LA Extended Release Tablets **421**

DILAHIM (Argentina)
DILTIAZEM HYDROCHLORIDE
Cardizem LA Extended Release Tablets **421**

DILAMAX (Portugal)
SALMETEROL XINAFOATE
Serevent Diskus **1594**

DILANACIN (Germany)
DIGOXIN
Lanoxin Injection **1498**
Lanoxin Injection Pediatric **1502**
Lanoxin Tablets **1505**

DILAPLUS (Austria)
CARVEDILOL
Coreg Tablets **1387**

DILAPROST (Turkey)
FINASTERIDE
Propecia Tablets **2095**
Proscar Tablets **2102**

DILATAM (Israel, South Africa, Thailand)
DILTIAZEM HYDROCHLORIDE
Cardizem LA Extended Release Tablets **421**

DILATAME (Austria)
DILTIAZEM HYDROCHLORIDE
Cardizem LA Extended Release Tablets **421**

DILATOL (Portugal)
ISRADIPINE
DynaCirc CR Tablets **1407**

DILATREND (Argentina, Australia, Austria, Brazil, Chile, Czech Republic, Germany, Greece, Hong Kong, Hungary, Italy, Mexico, New Zealand, Norway, Poland, Singapore, South Africa, Switzerland, Thailand, The Philippines, Turkey, Venezuela)
CARVEDILOL
Coreg Tablets **1387**

DILBLOC (Portugal)
CARVEDILOL
Coreg Tablets **1387**

DILCARD (New Zealand)
DILTIAZEM HYDROCHLORIDE
Cardizem LA Extended Release Tablets **421**

DILCARDIA (India, Russia, The Philippines, United Kingdom)
DILTIAZEM HYDROCHLORIDE
Cardizem LA Extended Release Tablets **421**

DILCEREN (Czech Republic)
NIMODIPINE
Nimotop Capsules **790**

DILCONTIN (India)
DILTIAZEM HYDROCHLORIDE
Cardizem LA Extended Release Tablets **421**

DILCOR (Denmark)
DILTIAZEM HYDROCHLORIDE
Cardizem LA Extended Release Tablets **421**

DILEM (Hong Kong, Italy, Malaysia)
DILTIAZEM HYDROCHLORIDE
Cardizem LA Extended Release Tablets **421**

DILETAN (Portugal)
SUMATRIPTAN SUCCINATE
Imitrex Injection **1465**
Imitrex Tablets **1474**

DILFAR (Portugal)
DILTIAZEM HYDROCHLORIDE
Cardizem LA Extended Release Tablets **421**

DILGARD (India)
DILTIAZEM HYDROCHLORIDE
Cardizem LA Extended Release Tablets **421**

DILITER (Italy)
DILTIAZEM HYDROCHLORIDE
Cardizem LA Extended Release Tablets **421**

DILIZEM (Singapore, Thailand)
DILTIAZEM HYDROCHLORIDE
Cardizem LA Extended Release Tablets **421**

DILMIN (Finland)
DILTIAZEM HYDROCHLORIDE
Cardizem LA Extended Release Tablets **421**

DILOC (The Netherlands)
DILTIAZEM HYDROCHLORIDE
Cardizem LA Extended Release Tablets **421**

DILOCAR (Italy)
CARVEDILOL
Coreg Tablets **1387**

DILOCARD (Poland)
DILTIAZEM HYDROCHLORIDE
Cardizem LA Extended Release Tablets **421**

DILONGO (Portugal)
DILTIAZEM HYDROCHLORIDE
Cardizem LA Extended Release Tablets **421**

DILPRAL (Finland)
DILTIAZEM HYDROCHLORIDE
Cardizem LA Extended Release Tablets **421**

DILRENE (France, Hungary)
DILTIAZEM HYDROCHLORIDE
Cardizem LA Extended Release Tablets **421**

DILSAL (Germany)
DILTIAZEM HYDROCHLORIDE
Cardizem LA Extended Release Tablets **421**

DIL-SANORANIA (Germany)
DILTIAZEM HYDROCHLORIDE
Cardizem LA Extended Release Tablets **421**

DILTA (Germany)
DILTIAZEM HYDROCHLORIDE
Cardizem LA Extended Release Tablets **421**

DILTABETA (Germany)
DILTIAZEM HYDROCHLORIDE
Cardizem LA Extended Release Tablets **421**

DILTAHEXAL (Australia, Austria, Germany, New Zealand)
DILTIAZEM HYDROCHLORIDE
Cardizem LA Extended Release Tablets **421**

DILTAM (Irish Republic)
DILTIAZEM HYDROCHLORIDE
Cardizem LA Extended Release Tablets **421**

DILTAN (Hong Kong, Hungary, Thailand)
DILTIAZEM HYDROCHLORIDE
Cardizem LA Extended Release Tablets **421**

DILTAPHAM (Germany)
DILTIAZEM HYDROCHLORIDE
Cardizem LA Extended Release Tablets **421**

DILTARETARD (Germany)
DILTIAZEM HYDROCHLORIDE
Cardizem LA Extended Release Tablets **421**

DILTEC (Thailand)
DILTIAZEM HYDROCHLORIDE
Cardizem LA Extended Release Tablets **421**

DILTELAN (The Philippines)
DILTIAZEM HYDROCHLORIDE
Cardizem LA Extended Release Tablets **421**

DILTEM (Greece)
DILTIAZEM HYDROCHLORIDE
Cardizem LA Extended Release Tablets **421**

DILTI (Germany)
DILTIAZEM HYDROCHLORIDE
Cardizem LA Extended Release Tablets **421**

DILTIACOR (Argentina, Brazil)
DILTIAZEM HYDROCHLORIDE
Cardizem LA Extended Release Tablets **421**

DILTIAGAMMA (Germany)
DILTIAZEM HYDROCHLORIDE
Cardizem LA Extended Release Tablets **421**

DILTIAMAX (Australia)
DILTIAZEM HYDROCHLORIDE
Cardizem LA Extended Release Tablets **421**

DILTIAMERCK (Germany)
DILTIAZEM HYDROCHLORIDE
Cardizem LA Extended Release Tablets **421**

DILTIANGINA (Portugal)
DILTIAZEM HYDROCHLORIDE
Cardizem LA Extended Release Tablets **421**

DILTIASTAD (Austria)
DILTIAZEM HYDROCHLORIDE
Cardizem LA Extended Release Tablets **421**

DILTICARD (Turkey)
DILTIAZEM HYDROCHLORIDE
Cardizem LA Extended Release Tablets **421**

DILTIEM (Portugal)
DILTIAZEM HYDROCHLORIDE
Cardizem LA Extended Release Tablets **421**

DILTI-ESSEX (Germany)
DILTIAZEM HYDROCHLORIDE
Cardizem LA Extended Release Tablets **421**

DILTIKARD (Norway)
DILTIAZEM HYDROCHLORIDE
Cardizem LA Extended Release Tablets **421**

DILTIME (The Philippines)
DILTIAZEM HYDROCHLORIDE
Cardizem LA Extended Release Tablets **421**

DILTIPRESS (Brazil)
DILTIAZEM HYDROCHLORIDE
Cardizem LA Extended Release Tablets **421**

DILTIUC (Germany)
DILTIAZEM HYDROCHLORIDE
Cardizem LA Extended Release Tablets **421**

DILTIWAS (Spain)
DILTIAZEM HYDROCHLORIDE
Cardizem LA Extended Release Tablets **421**

DILTIZEM (Brazil, Turkey)
DILTIAZEM HYDROCHLORIDE
Cardizem LA Extended Release Tablets **421**

DILTOR (Brazil)
DILTIAZEM HYDROCHLORIDE
Cardizem LA Extended Release Tablets **421**

DILUCID (Mexico)
LOVASTATIN
Mevacor Tablets . . . 2063

DILUTOL (Argentina)
ENOXAPARIN SODIUM
Lovenox Injection . . . 2756

DILZATYROL (Austria)
DILTIAZEM HYDROCHLORIDE
Cardizem LA Extended Release Tablets . . . 421

DILZEM (Australia, Austria, Czech Republic, Finland, Germany, Hong Kong, Hungary, India, Irish Republic, New Zealand, Switzerland, Thailand, The Philippines, United Kingdom)
DILTIAZEM HYDROCHLORIDE
Cardizem LA Extended Release Tablets . . . 421

DILZENE (Italy)
DILTIAZEM HYDROCHLORIDE
Cardizem LA Extended Release Tablets . . . 421

DILZEREAL (Germany)
DILTIAZEM HYDROCHLORIDE
Cardizem LA Extended Release Tablets . . . 421

DILZICARDIN (Germany)
DILTIAZEM HYDROCHLORIDE
Cardizem LA Extended Release Tablets . . . 421

DIMALOSIO (Italy)
LACTULOSE
Kristalose for Oral Solution . . . 1004

DIMASE (Thailand)
CEFTAZIDIME
Fortaz for Injection . . . 1450

DIMENFORMON (The Netherlands)
ESTRADIOL
Climara Transdermal System . . . 763

DIMETIL (Germany)
CARVEDILOL
Coreg Tablets . . . 1387

DIMITONE (Belgium, Denmark, Israel)
CARVEDILOL
Coreg Tablets . . . 1387

DIMORF (Brazil)
MORPHINE SULFATE
MS Contin Tablets . . . 2585

DINAC (Australia, Thailand)
DICLOFENAC SODIUM
Voltaren Tablets . . . 2334
Voltaren-XR Tablets . . . 2337

DINACLON (Greece)
DICLOFENAC SODIUM
Voltaren Tablets . . . 2334
Voltaren-XR Tablets . . . 2337

DINAFLOX (Mexico)
CIPROFLOXACIN HYDROCHLORIDE
Cipro Tablets . . . 2810

DINAMOT (Venezuela)
FAMOTIDINE
Pepcid for Oral Suspension . . . 2075
Pepcid Tablets . . . 2075

DINAVIR (Brazil)
INDINAVIR SULFATE
Crixivan Capsules . . . 1979

DINAXIN (Mexico)
RANITIDINE HYDROCHLORIDE
Zantac 25 EFFERdose Tablets . . . 1670
Zantac 150 Tablets . . . 1670
Zantac 300 Tablets . . . 1670
Zantac Injection . . . 1666
Zantac Injection Premixed . . . 1666
Zantac Syrup . . . 1670

DINAZIDE (Thailand)
HYDROCHLOROTHIAZIDE/TRIAMTERENE
Dyazide Capsules . . . 1405

DINILL-D (Mexico)
CIPROFLOXACIN HYDROCHLORIDE
Cipro Tablets . . . 2810

DINISOR (Spain)
DILTIAZEM HYDROCHLORIDE
Cardizem LA Extended Release Tablets . . . 421

DINUL (Portugal)
FAMOTIDINE
Pepcid for Oral Suspension . . . 2075
Pepcid Tablets . . . 2075

DIOCAM (Argentina)
CLONAZEPAM
Klonopin Tablets . . . 2639

DIOFLUOR (Canada)
FLUORESCEIN SODIUM
Fluorescite Injection . . . ⊙203

DIOVAN (Argentina, Austria, Brazil, Canada, Czech Republic, Denmark, Finland, Germany, Greece, Hong Kong, Hungary, India, Irish Republic, Israel, Malaysia, Mexico, New Zealand, Norway, Poland, Portugal, Russia, Singapore, South Africa, Spain, Sweden, Switzerland, Thailand, The Netherlands, The Philippines, Turkey, United Kingdom, Venezuela)
VALSARTAN
Diovan Tablets . . . 2212

DIOVAN A (Argentina)
VALSARTAN
Diovan Tablets . . . 2212

DIOVAN COMP (Denmark, Finland, Norway, Sweden)
HYDROCHLOROTHIAZIDE/VALSARTAN
Diovan HCT Tablets . . . 2216

DIOVAN D (Argentina)
VALSARTAN
Diovan Tablets . . . 2212

DIOVAN HCT (Brazil, Canada, Hungary, Mexico, Venezuela)
HYDROCHLOROTHIAZIDE/VALSARTAN
Diovan HCT Tablets . . . 2216

DIOVANE (Belgium)
VALSARTAN
Diovan Tablets . . . 2212

DIOXAFLEX (Brazil)
DICLOFENAC SODIUM
Voltaren Tablets . . . 2334
Voltaren-XR Tablets . . . 2337

DIOXAFLEX FORTE (Argentina)
DICLOFENAC SODIUM
Voltaren Tablets . . . 2334
Voltaren-XR Tablets . . . 2337

DIOXAFLEX PLUS (Argentina)
DICLOFENAC SODIUM
Voltaren Tablets . . . 2334
Voltaren-XR Tablets . . . 2337

DIP (Venezuela)
SUCRALFATE
Carafate Suspension . . . 706
Carafate Tablets . . . 707

DIPARENE (Belgium)
NAPROXEN
EC-Naprosyn Delayed-Release Tablets . . . 2632
Naprosyn Suspension . . . 2632
Naprosyn Tablets . . . 2632

DIPEDYNE (Mexico)
ZIDOVUDINE
Retrovir Capsules . . . 1574
Retrovir IV Infusion . . . 1579
Retrovir Syrup . . . 1574
Retrovir Tablets . . . 1574

DIPEZONA (Argentina)
DIAZEPAM
Valium Tablets . . . 2658

DIPHAR (France)
DIPYRIDAMOLE
Persantine Tablets . . . 869

DIPHOS (Germany)
ETIDRONATE DISODIUM
Didronel Tablets . . . 2583

DIPNI (Argentina)
NYSTATIN
Nystop Topical Powder USP . . . 2498

DIPRES (Mexico)
DIPYRIDAMOLE
Persantine Tablets . . . 869

DI-PROMAL (Austria)
IPRATROPIUM BROMIDE
Atrovent Nasal Spray 0.03% . . . 834
Atrovent Nasal Spray 0.06% . . . 836

DIPSIN (Portugal)
FAMOTIDINE
Pepcid for Oral Suspension . . . 2075
Pepcid Tablets . . . 2075

DIPYRIDAN (Belgium)
DIPYRIDAMOLE
Persantine Tablets . . . 869

DIPYRIN (Finland)
DIPYRIDAMOLE
Persantine Tablets . . . 869

DIPYROL (South Africa)
DIPYRIDAMOLE
Persantine Tablets . . . 869

DIRALON (Venezuela)
DICLOFENAC SODIUM
Voltaren Tablets . . . 2334
Voltaren-XR Tablets . . . 2337

DIRINE (Malaysia, Singapore, Thailand)
FUROSEMIDE
Furosemide Tablets . . . 2186

DIRINOL (Mexico)
DIPYRIDAMOLE
Persantine Tablets . . . 869

DIROTON (Czech Republic, Poland, Russia)
LISINOPRIL
Prinivil Tablets . . . 2087

DIRRET (Mexico)
DICLOFENAC SODIUM
Voltaren Tablets . . . 2334
Voltaren-XR Tablets . . . 2337

DIRUNEZ (Greece)
NORFLOXACIN
Noroxin Tablets . . . 2069

DISCOID (Germany)
FUROSEMIDE
Furosemide Tablets . . . 2186

DISEQUENS (Argentina)
ESTRADIOL
Climara Transdermal System . . . 763

DISIPAN (Argentina)
DICLOFENAC SODIUM
Voltaren Tablets . . . 2334
Voltaren-XR Tablets . . . 2337

DISLIPIN (Venezuela)
LOVASTATIN
Mevacor Tablets . . . 2063

DISLIPINA (Portugal)
SIMVASTATIN
Zocor Tablets . . . 2136

DISLIPOR (Chile)
ATORVASTATIN CALCIUM
Lipitor Tablets . . . 2501

DISMAM (Chile)
LACTULOSE
Kristalose for Oral Solution . . . 1004

DISMOLAN (Argentina, Venezuela)
ONDANSETRON HYDROCHLORIDE
Zofran Injection . . . 1682
Zofran Injection Premixed . . . 1682
Zofran Oral Solution . . . 1687
Zofran Tablets . . . 1687

DISNE ASMOL (Spain)
IPRATROPIUM BROMIDE
Atrovent Nasal Spray 0.03% . . . 834
Atrovent Nasal Spray 0.06% . . . 836

DISOGRAM (United Kingdom)
DILTIAZEM HYDROCHLORIDE
Cardizem LA Extended Release Tablets . . . 421

DISOPAM (Israel)
DIAZEPAM
Valium Tablets . . . 2658

DISPACLONIDIN (Germany)
CLONIDINE HYDROCHLORIDE
Catapres Tablets . . . 841

DISPASAN (Germany)
SODIUM HYALURONATE
Hyalgan Solution . . . 2742

DISPATIM (Austria, Germany)
TIMOLOL MALEATE
Timoptic in Ocudose . . . 2124
Timoptic Sterile Ophthalmic Solution . . . 2121
Timoptic-XE Sterile Ophthalmic Gel Forming Solution . . . 2125

DISPROMIL (Spain)
FAMOTIDINE
Pepcid for Oral Suspension . . . 2075
Pepcid Tablets . . . 2075

DISTALENE (Argentina)
ANASTROZOLE
Arimidex Tablets . . . 672

DITENATE N (Germany)
THEOPHYLLINE
Uniphyl Tablets . . . 2595

DITIZEM (Thailand)
DILTIAZEM HYDROCHLORIDE
Cardizem LA Extended Release Tablets . . . 421

DIUMIDE-K CONTINUS (United Kingdom)
FUROSEMIDE
Furosemide Tablets . . . 2186

DIURAL (Denmark, Norway, Sweden)
FUROSEMIDE
Furosemide Tablets . . . 2186

DIURAPID (Germany)
FUROSEMIDE
Furosemide Tablets . . . 2186

DIUREMIDA (Brazil)
FUROSEMIDE
Furosemide Tablets . . . 2186

DIURESAL (Switzerland)
FUROSEMIDE
Furosemide Tablets . . . 2186

DIURESIN (Poland)
INDAPAMIDE
Indapamide Tablets . . . 2188

DIURET (Brazil)
FUROSEMIDE
Furosemide Tablets . . . 2186

DIURETIKUM VERLA (Germany)
HYDROCHLOROTHIAZIDE/TRIAMTERENE
Dyazide Capsules . . . 1405

DIUREX (Brazil)
FUROSEMIDE
Furosemide Tablets . . . 2186

DIURID (Austria)
HYDROCHLOROTHIAZIDE/TRIAMTERENE
Dyazide Capsules . . . 1405

DIURIL (The Philippines)
FUROSEMIDE
Furosemide Tablets . . . 2186

DIURIN (New Zealand)
FUROSEMIDE
Furosemide Tablets . . . 2186

DIURIT (Brazil)
FUROSEMIDE
Furosemide Tablets . . . 2186

DIURIX (Brazil, Switzerland)
FUROSEMIDE
Furosemide Tablets . . . 2186

DIUROLAN (Mexico)
FUROSEMIDE
Furosemide Tablets . . . 2186

DIUROLASA (Spain)
FUROSEMIDE
Furosemide Tablets . . . 2186

DIUTENSAT (Germany)
HYDROCHLOROTHIAZIDE/TRIAMTERENE
Dyazide Capsules . . . 1405

DIU-TONOLYTRIL (Germany)
HYDROCHLOROTHIAZIDE/TRIAMTERENE
Dyazide Capsules . . . 1405

DIVAL (Venezuela)
DICLOFENAC SODIUM
Voltaren Tablets . . . 2334
Voltaren-XR Tablets . . . 2337

DIVELOL (Brazil)
CARVEDILOL
Coreg Tablets . . . 1387

DIVIGEL (Czech Republic, Denmark, Finland, Hungary, India, Irish Republic, Malaysia, Poland, Singapore, Sweden, Switzerland, Thailand)
ESTRADIOL
Climara Transdermal System . . . 763

DIXAMID (Greece)
INDAPAMIDE
Indapamide Tablets ... 2188

DIXARIT (Australia, Belgium, Canada, Germany, Hong Kong, Irish Republic, Malaysia, New Zealand, Singapore, South Africa, The Netherlands, United Kingdom)
CLONIDINE HYDROCHLORIDE
Catapres Tablets ... 841

DIZAN (Thailand)
DIAZEPAM
Valium Tablets ... 2658

DIZATEC (Italy)
CEFTAZIDIME
Fortaz for Injection ... 1450

DIZEPAM (Thailand)
DIAZEPAM
Valium Tablets ... 2658

DNAREN (Brazil)
DICLOFENAC SODIUM
Voltaren Tablets ... 2334
Voltaren-XR Tablets ... 2337

DOBET (Venezuela)
DORZOLAMIDE HYDROCHLORIDE
Trusopt Sterile Ophthalmic Solution ... 2128

DOBUPAL (Spain)
VENLAFAXINE HYDROCHLORIDE
Effexor XR Capsules ... 3195

DOCAMOCLAF (Belgium)
AMOXICILLIN
Amoxil Pediatric Drops for Oral Suspension ... 1305
Amoxil Tablets ... 1305

DOCAMOXICI (Belgium)
AMOXICILLIN
Amoxil Pediatric Drops for Oral Suspension ... 1305
Amoxil Tablets ... 1305

DOCCAPTOPRI (Belgium)
CAPTOPRIL
Captopril Tablets ... 2182

DOCCIPROFLO (Belgium)
CIPROFLOXACIN
Cipro Oral Suspension ... 2810

DOCDICLOFE (Belgium)
DICLOFENAC SODIUM
Voltaren Tablets ... 2334
Voltaren-XR Tablets ... 2337

DOCDIPYRI (Belgium)
DIPYRIDAMOLE
Persantine Tablets ... 869

DOCEKEBIR (Argentina)
DOCETAXEL
Taxotere Injection Concentrate ... 2773

DOCETAX (India)
DOCETAXEL
Taxotere Injection Concentrate ... 2773

DOCFENOFI (Belgium)
FENOFIBRATE
Tricor Tablets ... 520

DOCFUROSE (Belgium)
FUROSEMIDE
Furosemide Tablets ... 2186

DOCINDAPA (Belgium)
INDAPAMIDE
Indapamide Tablets ... 2188

DOCLIS (Spain)
DILTIAZEM HYDROCHLORIDE
Cardizem LA Extended Release Tablets ... 421

DOCSIMVASTA (Belgium)
SIMVASTATIN
Zocor Tablets ... 2136

DOCTRAMADO (Belgium)
TRAMADOL HYDROCHLORIDE
Ultram ER Tablets ... 2428

DOFEN (Mexico)
DICLOFENAC SODIUM
Voltaren Tablets ... 2334
Voltaren-XR Tablets ... 2337

DOFLEX (India)
DICLOFENAC SODIUM
Voltaren Tablets ... 2334
Voltaren-XR Tablets ... 2337

DOFLEX PLUS (India)
DICLOFENAC SODIUM
Voltaren Tablets ... 2334
Voltaren-XR Tablets ... 2337

DOGOXINE (Mexico)
DIGOXIN
Lanoxin Injection ... 1498
Lanoxin Injection Pediatric ... 1502
Lanoxin Tablets ... 1505

DOLAUT (Italy)
DICLOFENAC SODIUM
Voltaren Tablets ... 2334
Voltaren-XR Tablets ... 2337

DOLCET (The Philippines)
TRAMADOL HYDROCHLORIDE
Ultram ER Tablets ... 2428

DOLCONTIN (Finland, Norway, Sweden)
MORPHINE SULFATE
MS Contin Tablets ... 2585

DOLECTRAN (Argentina)
DOCETAXEL
Taxotere Injection Concentrate ... 2773

DOLFLAM (Mexico)
DICLOFENAC SODIUM
Voltaren Tablets ... 2334
Voltaren-XR Tablets ... 2337

DOLGIT-DICLO (Germany)
DICLOFENAC SODIUM
Voltaren Tablets ... 2334
Voltaren-XR Tablets ... 2337

DOLILUX (Italy)
RANITIDINE HYDROCHLORIDE
Zantac 25 EFFERdose Tablets ... 1670
Zantac 150 Tablets ... 1670
Zantac 300 Tablets ... 1670
Zantac Injection ... 1666
Zantac Injection Premixed ... 1666
Zantac Syrup ... 1670

DOLMAL (The Philippines)
TRAMADOL HYDROCHLORIDE
Ultram ER Tablets ... 2428

DOLMIGRAL (Spain)
SUMATRIPTAN SUCCINATE
Imitrex Injection ... 1465
Imitrex Tablets ... 1474

DOLMINA (Czech Republic)
DICLOFENAC SODIUM
Voltaren Tablets ... 2334
Voltaren-XR Tablets ... 2337

DOLNAXEN (Mexico)
NAPROXEN
EC-Naprosyn Delayed-Release Tablets ... 2632
Naprosyn Suspension ... 2632
Naprosyn Tablets ... 2632

DOLO NERVOBION (Spain)
DICLOFENAC SODIUM
Voltaren Tablets ... 2334
Voltaren-XR Tablets ... 2337

DOLOATRIXEN (Mexico)
NAPROXEN
EC-Naprosyn Delayed-Release Tablets ... 2632
Naprosyn Suspension ... 2632
Naprosyn Tablets ... 2632

DOLOBASAN (Germany)
DICLOFENAC SODIUM
Voltaren Tablets ... 2334
Voltaren-XR Tablets ... 2337

DOLODOL (Spain)
TRAMADOL HYDROCHLORIDE
Ultram ER Tablets ... 2428

DOLOFENAC (Argentina)
DICLOFENAC SODIUM
Voltaren Tablets ... 2334
Voltaren-XR Tablets ... 2337

DOLOFLAM (The Philippines)
DICLOFENAC SODIUM
Voltaren Tablets ... 2334
Voltaren-XR Tablets ... 2337

DOLOL (Austria, Denmark)
TRAMADOL HYDROCHLORIDE
Ultram ER Tablets ... 2428

DOLORMIN MIT NAPROXEN (Germany)
NAPROXEN
EC-Naprosyn Delayed-Release Tablets ... 2632
Naprosyn Suspension ... 2632
Naprosyn Tablets ... 2632

DOLOTANDAX (Mexico)
NAPROXEN SODIUM
Anaprox DS Tablets ... 2632
Anaprox Tablets ... 2632

DOLOTRAL (The Philippines)
TRAMADOL HYDROCHLORIDE
Ultram ER Tablets ... 2428

DOLOTRAM (South Africa)
TRAMADOL HYDROCHLORIDE
Ultram ER Tablets ... 2428

DOLOTRAMINE (Switzerland)
TRAMADOL HYDROCHLORIDE
Ultram ER Tablets ... 2428

DOLOVISANO DICLO (Germany)
DICLOFENAC SODIUM
Voltaren Tablets ... 2334
Voltaren-XR Tablets ... 2337

DOLO-VOLTAREN (Spain)
DICLOFENAC SODIUM
Voltaren Tablets ... 2334
Voltaren-XR Tablets ... 2337

DOLPASSE (Austria)
DICLOFENAC SODIUM
Voltaren Tablets ... 2334
Voltaren-XR Tablets ... 2337

DOLPAZ (The Philippines)
TRAMADOL HYDROCHLORIDE
Ultram ER Tablets ... 2428

DOLTARD (Czech Republic, Denmark, Poland, The Netherlands)
MORPHINE SULFATE
MS Contin Tablets ... 2585

DOLVAN (Argentina)
DICLOFENAC SODIUM
Voltaren Tablets ... 2334
Voltaren-XR Tablets ... 2337

DOLVAN FLEX (Argentina)
DICLOFENAC SODIUM
Voltaren Tablets ... 2334
Voltaren-XR Tablets ... 2337

DOLXEN (Mexico)
NAPROXEN
EC-Naprosyn Delayed-Release Tablets ... 2632
Naprosyn Suspension ... 2632
Naprosyn Tablets ... 2632

DOLZAM (Belgium)
TRAMADOL HYDROCHLORIDE
Ultram ER Tablets ... 2428

DONAPROX (Mexico)
NAPROXEN
EC-Naprosyn Delayed-Release Tablets ... 2632
Naprosyn Suspension ... 2632
Naprosyn Tablets ... 2632

DONATAXEL (Argentina)
DOCETAXEL
Taxotere Injection Concentrate ... 2773

DONAZ (India)
DONEPEZIL HYDROCHLORIDE
Aricept Tablets ... 1062

DONECEPT (India)
DONEPEZIL HYDROCHLORIDE
Aricept Tablets ... 1062

DONEKA (Spain)
LISINOPRIL
Prinivil Tablets ... 2087

DONEKA PLUS (Spain)
HYDROCHLOROTHIAZIDE/LISINOPRIL
Prinzide Tablets ... 2092

DONEPES (Argentina)
DONEPEZIL HYDROCHLORIDE
Aricept Tablets ... 1062

DONEPEX (Poland)
DONEPEZIL HYDROCHLORIDE
Aricept Tablets ... 1062

DOPSAN (Thailand)
DAPSONE
Dapsone Tablets USP ... 1746

DORCALOR (Portugal)
DICLOFENAC SODIUM
Voltaren Tablets ... 2334
Voltaren-XR Tablets ... 2337

DORGEN (Brazil)
DICLOFENAC SODIUM
Voltaren Tablets ... 2334
Voltaren-XR Tablets ... 2337

DORICOFLU (Italy)
FLUNISOLIDE
Aerobid Inhaler System ... 1153
Aerobid-M Inhaler System ... 1153

DORIMAN (Spain)
CIPROFLOXACIN HYDROCHLORIDE
Cipro Tablets ... 2810

DORLAMIDA (Argentina)
DORZOLAMIDE HYDROCHLORIDE
Trusopt Sterile Ophthalmic Solution ... 2128

DORLAMIDA T (Argentina)
DORZOLAMIDE HYDROCHLORIDE
Trusopt Sterile Ophthalmic Solution ... 2128

DOROXAN (Italy)
DICLOFENAC SODIUM
Voltaren Tablets ... 2334
Voltaren-XR Tablets ... 2337

DORPIEL (Argentina)
TRETINOIN
Vesanoid Capsules ... 2660

DORSOF T (Chile)
DORZOLAMIDE HYDROCHLORIDE/TIMOLOL MALEATE
Cosopt Sterile Ophthalmic Solution ... 1969

DORZOFLAX (Argentina)
DORZOLAMIDE HYDROCHLORIDE
Trusopt Sterile Ophthalmic Solution ... 2128

DORZOL (Venezuela)
DORZOLAMIDE HYDROCHLORIDE
Trusopt Sterile Ophthalmic Solution ... 2128

DORZOX (India)
DORZOLAMIDE HYDROCHLORIDE
Trusopt Sterile Ophthalmic Solution ... 2128

DOSAVASTATIN (Argentina)
SIMVASTATIN
Zocor Tablets ... 2136

DOSIER (Chile)
BUPROPION HYDROCHLORIDE
Wellbutrin SR Sustained-Release Tablets ... 1653
Wellbutrin Tablets ... 1648
Zyban Sustained-Release Tablets ... 1692

DOVAL (South Africa)
DIAZEPAM
Valium Tablets ... 2658

DOXAPRIL (Argentina)
LISINOPRIL
Prinivil Tablets ... 2087

DOXETAL (Argentina)
DOCETAXEL
Taxotere Injection Concentrate ... 2773

DOXMIL (Argentina)
DOCETAXEL
Taxotere Injection Concentrate ... 2773

DOXTRAN FLEX (Argentina)
DICLOFENAC SODIUM
Voltaren Tablets ... 2334
Voltaren-XR Tablets ... 2337

DP GESIC (India)
DICLOFENAC SODIUM
Voltaren Tablets ... 2334
Voltaren-XR Tablets ... 2337

D-PAM (New Zealand)
DIAZEPAM
Valium Tablets ... 2658

DRALEN (Greece)
ETIDRONATE DISODIUM
Didronel Tablets ... 2583

DRENIAN (Spain)
DIAZEPAM
Valium Tablets ... 2658

DRILYNA (Argentina)
THEOPHYLLINE
Uniphyl Tablets ... 2595

DRISENTIN (Turkey)
DIPYRIDAMOLE
Persantine Tablets ... 869

DROLASONA (Spain)
FLUTICASONE PROPIONATE
Flonase Nasal Spray 1431

DROMADOL (United Kingdom)
TRAMADOL HYDROCHLORIDE
Ultram ER Tablets 2428

DRONAL (Italy)
ALENDRONATE SODIUM
Fosamax Tablets 2005

DRONATE-OS (India)
ETIDRONATE DISODIUM
Didronel Tablets 2583

DROPAXIN (Italy)
PAROXETINE HYDROCHLORIDE
Paxil Oral Suspension 1535
Paxil Tablets 1535

DROPFLAM (Italy)
DICLOFENAC SODIUM
Voltaren Tablets 2334
Voltaren-XR Tablets 2337

DROPSTAR (Argentina, Italy)
SODIUM HYALURONATE
Hyalgan Solution 2742

DROPTIMOL (Italy)
TIMOLOL MALEATE
Timoptic in Ocudose 2124
Timoptic Sterile Ophthalmic Solution 2121
Timoptic-XE Sterile Ophthalmic Gel Forming Solution 2125

DRY & CLEAR (South Africa)
BENZOYL PEROXIDE
Brevoxyl-4 Creamy Wash 3054
Brevoxyl-4 Gel 3054
Brevoxyl-8 Creamy Wash 3054
Brevoxyl-8 Gel 3054

DRYPTAL (Czech Republic, Hong Kong, Irish Republic, United Kingdom)
FUROSEMIDE
Furosemide Tablets 2186

D-TATO (Mexico)
BENZONATATE
Tessalon Perles 1183

D-TRIOL (Greece)
CALCITRIOL
Calcijex Injection 419
Rocaltrol Capsules 1150
Rocaltrol Oral Solution 1150

DUAC (Australia, Hong Kong, Irish Republic, Poland, Spain, Sweden, The Netherlands)
BENZOYL PEROXIDE
Brevoxyl-4 Creamy Wash 3054
Brevoxyl-4 Gel 3054
Brevoxyl-8 Creamy Wash 3054
Brevoxyl-8 Gel 3054

DUAC ONCE DAILY (United Kingdom)
BENZOYL PEROXIDE
Brevoxyl-4 Creamy Wash 3054
Brevoxyl-4 Gel 3054
Brevoxyl-8 Creamy Wash 3054
Brevoxyl-8 Gel 3054

DUALTEN (Chile)
CARVEDILOL
Coreg Tablets 1387

DUAVENT (The Philippines)
IPRATROPIUM BROMIDE
Atrovent Nasal Spray 0.03% 834
Atrovent Nasal Spray 0.06% 836

DUBAGEST (India)
PROGESTERONE
Crinone 4% Gel 992
Prometrium Capsules (100 mg, 200 mg) . 3047

DUBE (Singapore)
LIDOCAINE
Lidoderm Patch 1114

DUCENE (Australia)
DIAZEPAM
Valium Tablets 2658

DUCTOCINA (Brazil)
CIPROFLOXACIN
Cipro Oral Suspension 2810

DUCTONAR (Argentina)
RISEDRONATE SODIUM
Actonel Tablets 2568

DUCTOPRIL (Brazil)
CAPTOPRIL
Captopril Tablets 2182

DULAX (Irish Republic)
LACTULOSE
Kristalose for Oral Solution 1004

DUNOX (Argentina)
AMOXICILLIN
Amoxil Pediatric Drops for Oral Suspension 1305
Amoxil Tablets 1305

DUOBLOC (Argentina)
CARVEDILOL
Coreg Tablets 1387

DUOFLEX (Mexico)
DICLOFENAC SODIUM
Voltaren Tablets 2334
Voltaren-XR Tablets 2337

DUOKLIMAN (Austria)
ESTRADIOL
Climara Transdermal System 763

DUOLAX (Spain)
LACTULOSE
Kristalose for Oral Solution 1004

DUOLIN (India, New Zealand, South Africa, Venezuela)
IPRATROPIUM BROMIDE
Atrovent Nasal Spray 0.03% 834
Atrovent Nasal Spray 0.06% 836

DUORAN (Italy)
RANITIDINE HYDROCHLORIDE
Zantac 25 EFFERdose Tablets 1670
Zantac 150 Tablets 1670
Zantac 300 Tablets 1670
Zantac Injection 1666
Zantac Injection Premixed 1666
Zantac Syrup 1670

DUOVEL (Turkey)
FAMOTIDINE
Pepcid for Oral Suspension 2075
Pepcid Tablets 2075

DUOVIR (Brazil, India, South Africa, Venezuela)
LAMIVUDINE
Epivir Oral Solution 1412
Epivir Tablets 1412
Epivir-HBV Oral Solution 1417
Epivir-HBV Tablets 1417

DUOVIR N (India)
LAMIVUDINE
Epivir Oral Solution 1412
Epivir Tablets 1412
Epivir-HBV Oral Solution 1417
Epivir-HBV Tablets 1417

DUPHALAC (Australia, Austria, Belgium, Canada, Chile, Czech Republic, Finland, France, Greece, Hong Kong, Hungary, India, Irish Republic, Italy, Malaysia, New Zealand, Norway, Poland, Portugal, Russia, Singapore, South Africa, Spain, Sweden, Switzerland, Thailand, The Netherlands, The Philippines, Turkey, United Kingdom)
LACTULOSE
Kristalose for Oral Solution 1004

DURACRALFAT (Germany)
SUCRALFATE
Carafate Suspension 706
Carafate Tablets 707

DURADIAZEPAM (Germany)
DIAZEPAM
Valium Tablets 2658

DURADIURET (Germany)
HYDROCHLOROTHIAZIDE/TRIAMTERENE
Dyazide Capsules 1405

DURAFENAT (Germany)
FENOFIBRATE
Tricor Tablets 520

DURAFURID (Germany)
FUROSEMIDE
Furosemide Tablets 2186

DURAGESIC (Canada)
FENTANYL
Duragesic Transdermal System 2405

DURALGIN (Denmark)
MORPHINE SULFATE
MS Contin Tablets 2585

DURALMOR (Mexico)
MORPHINE SULFATE
MS Contin Tablets 2585

DURAMORPH (Argentina)
MORPHINE SULFATE
MS Contin Tablets 2585

DURAPHYLLIN (Germany)
THEOPHYLLINE
Uniphyl Tablets 2595

DURATER (Mexico)
FAMOTIDINE
Pepcid for Oral Suspension 2075
Pepcid Tablets 2075

DURATIMOL (Germany)
TIMOLOL MALEATE
Timoptic in Ocudose 2124
Timoptic Sterile Ophthalmic Solution 2121
Timoptic-XE Sterile Ophthalmic Gel Forming Solution 2125

DURAVOLTEN (Germany)
DICLOFENAC SODIUM
Voltaren Tablets 2334
Voltaren-XR Tablets 2337

DURA-ZOK (Denmark)
METOPROLOL SUCCINATE
Toprol-XL Tablets 666

DUREMID (Argentina)
INDAPAMIDE
Indapamide Tablets 2188

DUROGESIC (Argentina, Australia, Austria, Belgium, Brazil, Chile, Czech Republic, Denmark, Finland, France, Germany, Greece, Hong Kong, Hungary, India, Irish Republic, Israel, Italy, Malaysia, Mexico, New Zealand, Norway, Poland, Portugal, Russia, Singapore, South Africa, Spain, Sweden, Switzerland, Thailand, The Netherlands, The Philippines, Turkey, United Kingdom, Venezuela)
FENTANYL
Duragesic Transdermal System 2405

DUXIMA (Italy)
CEFUROXIME SODIUM
Zinacef Injection 1678

DUZIMICIN (Brazil)
AMOXICILLIN
Amoxil Pediatric Drops for Oral Suspension 1305
Amoxil Tablets 1305

DYALAC (The Philippines)
DILTIAZEM HYDROCHLORIDE
Cardizem LA Extended Release Tablets 421

DYAZIDE (Canada, Hong Kong, Irish Republic, Mexico, New Zealand, Portugal, Singapore, South Africa, Switzerland)
HYDROCHLOROTHIAZIDE/TRIAMTERENE
Dyazide Capsules 1405

DYCON (The Philippines)
DICLOFENAC SODIUM
Voltaren Tablets 2334
Voltaren-XR Tablets 2337

DYNACIRC (Argentina, Canada, Chile, Hong Kong, Malaysia, Mexico, New Zealand, Singapore, South Africa, Thailand, Turkey, Venezuela)
ISRADIPINE
DynaCirc CR Tablets 1407

DYNAFLOC (South Africa)
CIPROFLOXACIN
Cipro Oral Suspension 2810

DYNAPAM (South Africa)
DIAZEPAM
Valium Tablets 2658

DYRENIUM (Canada, Switzerland)
TRIAMTERENE
Dyrenium Capsules 3189

DYSMENALGIT (Germany)
NAPROXEN
EC-Naprosyn Delayed-Release Tablets 2632
Naprosyn Suspension 2632
Naprosyn Tablets 2632

DYTAC (Australia, Belgium, Irish Republic, The Netherlands, United Kingdom)
TRIAMTERENE
Dyrenium Capsules 3189

DYTA-URESE (Belgium, The Netherlands)
TRIAMTERENE
Dyrenium Capsules 3189

DYTENZIDE (Belgium, The Netherlands)
HYDROCHLOROTHIAZIDE/TRIAMTERENE
Dyazide Capsules 1405

DYTERENE (Thailand)
HYDROCHLOROTHIAZIDE/TRIAMTERENE
Dyazide Capsules 1405

DYTIDE H (Austria, Germany)
HYDROCHLOROTHIAZIDE/TRIAMTERENE
Dyazide Capsules 1405

EASY DAYZ (India)
NAPROXEN SODIUM
Anaprox DS Tablets 2632
Anaprox Tablets 2632

ECAMAIS (Portugal)
LISINOPRIL
Prinivil Tablets 2087

ECAPRESAN (Mexico)
CAPTOPRIL
Captopril Tablets 2182

ECAPRIL (Mexico, Portugal)
CAPTOPRIL
Captopril Tablets 2182

ECATEN (Mexico)
CAPTOPRIL
Captopril Tablets 2182

ECLARAN (Argentina, Czech Republic, France, Portugal)
BENZOYL PEROXIDE
Brevoxyl-4 Creamy Wash 3054
Brevoxyl-4 Gel 3054
Brevoxyl-8 Creamy Wash 3054
Brevoxyl-8 Gel 3054

ECNAGEL PB (Argentina)
BENZOYL PEROXIDE
Brevoxyl-4 Creamy Wash 3054
Brevoxyl-4 Gel 3054
Brevoxyl-8 Creamy Wash 3054
Brevoxyl-8 Gel 3054

ECODOLOR (Switzerland)
TRAMADOL HYDROCHLORIDE
Ultram ER Tablets 2428

ECOFENAC (Switzerland)
DICLOFENAC SODIUM
Voltaren Tablets 2334
Voltaren-XR Tablets 2337

ECOLINE (Greece)
CEFUROXIME AXETIL
Ceftin for Oral Suspension 1380
Ceftin Tablets 1380

ECONAC (United Kingdom)
DICLOFENAC SODIUM
Voltaren Tablets 2334
Voltaren-XR Tablets 2337

ECOPACE (United Kingdom)
CAPTOPRIL
Captopril Tablets 2182

ECTIVA (Italy, Mexico)
SIBUTRAMINE HYDROCHLORIDE
Meridia Capsules 475

ECUADERM (Venezuela)
BENZOYL PEROXIDE
Brevoxyl-4 Creamy Wash 3054
Brevoxyl-4 Gel 3054
Brevoxyl-8 Creamy Wash 3054
Brevoxyl-8 Gel 3054

ECURAL (Germany)
MOMETASONE FUROATE
Elocon Cream 0.1% 2840
Elocon Lotion 0.1% 2841
Elocon Ointment 0.1% 2842
Nasonex Nasal Spray 2883

EDEM (Mexico)
NAPROXEN SODIUM
Anaprox DS Tablets 2632

Anaprox Tablets . . . 2632

EDEMANN (The Philippines)
FUROSEMIDE
Furosemide Tablets . . . 2186

EDEMID (Venezuela)
FUROSEMIDE
Furosemide Tablets . . . 2186

EDENOL (Mexico)
FUROSEMIDE
Furosemide Tablets . . . 2186

EDICTUM (Argentina)
CLONAZEPAM
Klonopin Tablets . . . 2639

EDOLGLAU (Portugal)
CLONIDINE HYDROCHLORIDE
Catapres Tablets . . . 841

EEZE (Finland)
DICLOFENAC SODIUM
Voltaren Tablets . . . 2334
Voltaren-XR Tablets . . . 2337

EFAVILEA (Argentina)
EFAVIRENZ
Sustiva Capsules . . . 930

EFAVIR (India, Venezuela)
EFAVIRENZ
Sustiva Capsules . . . 930

EFECTIN (Austria, Czech Republic, Hungary, Poland)
VENLAFAXINE HYDROCHLORIDE
Effexor XR Capsules . . . 3195

EFEMOLINA (Argentina)
FLUOROMETHOLONE
FML Ophthalmic Ointment . . . ⊙223

EFEMOLINE (The Philippines, Turkey)
FLUOROMETHOLONE
FML Ophthalmic Ointment . . . ⊙223

EFEROX (Germany, Poland)
LEVOTHYROXINE SODIUM
Levothroid Tablets . . . 1170
Levoxyl Tablets . . . 1780
Synthroid Tablets . . . 507

EFEROX JOD (Germany)
LEVOTHYROXINE SODIUM
Levothroid Tablets . . . 1170
Levoxyl Tablets . . . 1780
Synthroid Tablets . . . 507

EFEXOR (Argentina, Australia, Austria, Belgium, Brazil, Chile, Denmark, Finland, Greece, Hong Kong, Irish Republic, Israel, Italy, Malaysia, Mexico, New Zealand, Norway, Portugal, Singapore, South Africa, Sweden, Switzerland, Thailand, The Netherlands, The Philippines, Turkey, United Kingdom, Venezuela)
VENLAFAXINE HYDROCHLORIDE
Effexor XR Capsules . . . 3195

EFFACNE (France, Switzerland)
BENZOYL PEROXIDE
Brevoxyl-4 Creamy Wash . . . 3054
Brevoxyl-4 Gel . . . 3054
Brevoxyl-8 Creamy Wash . . . 3054
Brevoxyl-8 Gel . . . 3054

EFFECTSAL (Singapore)
NORFLOXACIN
Noroxin Tablets . . . 2069

EFFEDERM (France)
TRETINOIN
Vesanoid Capsules . . . 2660

EFFEKTON (Germany)
DICLOFENAC SODIUM
Voltaren Tablets . . . 2334
Voltaren-XR Tablets . . . 2337

EFFEXOR (Canada)
VENLAFAXINE HYDROCHLORIDE
Effexor XR Capsules . . . 3195

EFFLUMIDEX (Czech Republic, Germany, Hungary)
FLUOROMETHOLONE
FML Ophthalmic Ointment . . . ⊙223

EFTRIVAL (Venezuela)
CEFTRIAXONE SODIUM
Rocephin Injectable Vials, ADD-Vantage, Galaxy, Bulk . . . 2642

EFTRY (Italy)
CEFTRIAXONE SODIUM
Rocephin Injectable Vials, ADD-Vantage, Galaxy, Bulk . . . 2642

EGIBREN (Italy)
SELEGILINE HYDROCHLORIDE
Eldepryl Capsules . . . 3052

EGIFILIN (Hungary)
THEOPHYLLINE
Uniphyl Tablets . . . 2595

EHLIXACIN (Mexico)
CIPROFLOXACIN
Cipro Oral Suspension . . . 2810

EISMYCIN (Germany)
MUPIROCIN
Bactroban Ointment . . . 1368

EKLIPS (Turkey)
LOSARTAN POTASSIUM
Cozaar Tablets . . . 1973

EKLIPS PLUS (Turkey)
LOSARTAN POTASSIUM
Cozaar Tablets . . . 1973

ELAFAX (Argentina)
VENLAFAXINE HYDROCHLORIDE
Effexor XR Capsules . . . 3195

ELANDUR (Argentina)
ALENDRONATE SODIUM
Fosamax Tablets . . . 2005

ELCION (India)
DIAZEPAM
Valium Tablets . . . 2658

ELDEPRINE (France)
SELEGILINE HYDROCHLORIDE
Eldepryl Capsules . . . 3052

ELDEPRYL (Australia, Belgium, Canada, Denmark, Finland, Irish Republic, New Zealand, Norway, South Africa, Sweden, The Netherlands, United Kingdom)
SELEGILINE HYDROCHLORIDE
Eldepryl Capsules . . . 3052

ELEBE (Argentina)
CARBAMAZEPINE
Carbatrol Capsules . . . 3019

ELEGELIN (Singapore, Thailand)
SELEGILINE HYDROCHLORIDE
Eldepryl Capsules . . . 3052

ELEOMOX (The Philippines)
AMOXICILLIN
Amoxil Pediatric Drops for Oral Suspension . . . 1305
Amoxil Tablets . . . 1305

ELEQUINE (Mexico)
LEVOFLOXACIN
Levaquin Injection . . . 2416
Levaquin Tablets . . . 2416

ELEVAT (South Africa)
DRONABINOL
Marinol Capsules . . . 3163

ELEVEX (The Philippines)
TIMOLOL MALEATE
Timoptic in Ocudose . . . 2124
Timoptic Sterile Ophthalmic Solution . . . 2121
Timoptic-XE Sterile Ophthalmic Gel Forming Solution . . . 2125

ELFAXONE (The Netherlands)
CEFTRIAXONE SODIUM
Rocephin Injectable Vials, ADD-Vantage, Galaxy, Bulk . . . 2642

ELICA (Mexico, South Africa, Spain, The Philippines)
MOMETASONE FUROATE
Elocon Cream 0.1% . . . 2840
Elocon Lotion 0.1% . . . 2841
Elocon Ointment 0.1% . . . 2842
Nasonex Nasal Spray . . . 2883

ELIOSID (Italy)
FLUNISOLIDE
Aerobid Inhaler System . . . 1153
Aerobid-M Inhaler System . . . 1153

ELIUR (Argentina)
FUROSEMIDE
Furosemide Tablets . . . 2186

ELIXIFILIN (Spain)
THEOPHYLLINE
Uniphyl Tablets . . . 2595

ELIXINE (Chile)
THEOPHYLLINE
Uniphyl Tablets . . . 2595

ELIXOFILINA (Mexico)
THEOPHYLLINE
Uniphyl Tablets . . . 2595

ELIXOPHYLLIN (Australia, Canada)
THEOPHYLLINE
Uniphyl Tablets . . . 2595

ELLANCO (Hong Kong)
LOVASTATIN
Mevacor Tablets . . . 2063

ELLESTE (Czech Republic)
ESTRADIOL
Climara Transdermal System . . . 763

ELLESTE-SOLO (United Kingdom)
ESTRADIOL
Climara Transdermal System . . . 763

ELMENDOS (Australia, Germany)
LAMOTRIGINE
Lamictal Chewable Dispersible Tablets . . . 1488
Lamictal Tablets . . . 1488

ELMIRON (Argentina, Australia, Canada, Hong Kong)
PENTOSAN POLYSULFATE SODIUM
Elmiron Capsules . . . 2435

ELOBACT (Germany)
CEFUROXIME AXETIL
Ceftin for Oral Suspension . . . 1380
Ceftin Tablets . . . 1380

ELOCOM (Belgium, Brazil, Canada, Chile, Czech Republic, Hungary, Israel, Poland, Portugal, Russia, Spain, Switzerland)
MOMETASONE FUROATE
Elocon Cream 0.1% . . . 2840
Elocon Lotion 0.1% . . . 2841
Elocon Ointment 0.1% . . . 2842
Nasonex Nasal Spray . . . 2883

ELOCON (Argentina, Australia, Austria, Denmark, Finland, Greece, India, Irish Republic, Italy, New Zealand, Norway, South Africa, Sweden, The Netherlands, The Philippines, Turkey, United Kingdom, Venezuela)
MOMETASONE FUROATE
Elocon Cream 0.1% . . . 2840
Elocon Lotion 0.1% . . . 2841
Elocon Ointment 0.1% . . . 2842
Nasonex Nasal Spray . . . 2883

ELOCONEX (Venezuela)
MOMETASONE FUROATE
Elocon Cream 0.1% . . . 2840
Elocon Lotion 0.1% . . . 2841
Elocon Ointment 0.1% . . . 2842
Nasonex Nasal Spray . . . 2883

ELOMET (Hong Kong, Malaysia, Mexico, Singapore, Thailand, Venezuela)
MOMETASONE FUROATE
Elocon Cream 0.1% . . . 2840
Elocon Lotion 0.1% . . . 2841
Elocon Ointment 0.1% . . . 2842
Nasonex Nasal Spray . . . 2883

ELONGAL (Chile)
DIAZEPAM
Valium Tablets . . . 2658

ELOSALIC (Argentina, Austria, Brazil, Germany, Hong Kong, Poland, South Africa, Sweden, Thailand, Turkey, Venezuela)
MOMETASONE FUROATE
Elocon Cream 0.1% . . . 2840
Elocon Lotion 0.1% . . . 2841
Elocon Ointment 0.1% . . . 2842
Nasonex Nasal Spray . . . 2883

ELOSONE (Poland)
MOMETASONE FUROATE
Elocon Cream 0.1% . . . 2840
Elocon Lotion 0.1% . . . 2841
Elocon Ointment 0.1% . . . 2842
Nasonex Nasal Spray . . . 2883

ELOVENT (Austria, Greece, The Netherlands)
MOMETASONE FUROATE
Elocon Cream 0.1% . . . 2840
Elocon Lotion 0.1% . . . 2841
Elocon Ointment 0.1% . . . 2842
Nasonex Nasal Spray . . . 2883

ELSPAR (Brazil, Hong Kong)
ASPARAGINASE
Elspar for Injection . . . 2488

ELSTATIN (Singapore)
LOVASTATIN
Mevacor Tablets . . . 2063

ELTHYRO (Thailand)
LEVOTHYROXINE SODIUM
Levothroid Tablets . . . 1170
Levoxyl Tablets . . . 1780
Synthroid Tablets . . . 507

ELTHYRONE (Belgium)
LEVOTHYROXINE SODIUM
Levothroid Tablets . . . 1170
Levoxyl Tablets . . . 1780
Synthroid Tablets . . . 507

ELTROXIN (Canada, Czech Republic, Denmark, Hong Kong, India, Irish Republic, Israel, New Zealand, Poland, Singapore, South Africa, Thailand, The Netherlands, The Philippines, United Kingdom)
LEVOTHYROXINE SODIUM
Levothroid Tablets . . . 1170
Levoxyl Tablets . . . 1780
Synthroid Tablets . . . 507

ELTROXINE (Switzerland)
LEVOTHYROXINE SODIUM
Levothroid Tablets . . . 1170
Levoxyl Tablets . . . 1780
Synthroid Tablets . . . 507

ELVENAVIR (Argentina)
INDINAVIR SULFATE
Crixivan Capsules . . . 1979

EMANTHAL (India)
ALBENDAZOLE
Albenza Tablets . . . 1297

EMESET (Czech Republic, India, Thailand, Venezuela)
ONDANSETRON HYDROCHLORIDE
Zofran Injection . . . 1682
Zofran Injection Premixed . . . 1682
Zofran Oral Solution . . . 1687
Zofran Tablets . . . 1687

EMETRON (Czech Republic, Hungary, Poland, Russia)
ONDANSETRON HYDROCHLORIDE
Zofran Injection . . . 1682
Zofran Injection Premixed . . . 1682
Zofran Oral Solution . . . 1687
Zofran Tablets . . . 1687

EMITAL (Irish Republic)
ONDANSETRON HYDROCHLORIDE
Zofran Injection . . . 1682
Zofran Injection Premixed . . . 1682
Zofran Oral Solution . . . 1687
Zofran Tablets . . . 1687

EMIVOX (Argentina)
ONDANSETRON
Zofran ODT Orally Disintegrating Tablets . . . 1687

EMLA (Czech Republic, Finland, Poland, The Philippines, Turkey, United Kingdom)
LIDOCAINE
Lidoderm Patch . . . 1114

EMOCAL (Finland)
CITALOPRAM HYDROBROMIDE
Celexa Tablets . . . 1160

EMOCHOL (Poland)
NAPROXEN
EC-Naprosyn Delayed-Release Tablets . . . 2632
Naprosyn Suspension . . . 2632
Naprosyn Tablets . . . 2632

EMODAN (The Philippines)
ONDANSETRON HYDROCHLORIDE
Zofran Injection . . . 1682

Zofran Injection Premixed 1682
Zofran Oral Solution 1687
Zofran Tablets 1687

EMOFORM (France, United Kingdom)
FORMALDEHYDE
Formadon Solution 1699

ENADIOL NETA (Chile)
ESTRADIOL
Climara Transdermal System 763

ENBREL (Argentina, Australia, Belgium, Brazil, Canada, Chile, Czech Republic, Denmark, Finland, France, Germany, Greece, Hong Kong, Hungary, India, Irish Republic, Israel, Italy, Mexico, New Zealand, Norway, Poland, Portugal, South Africa, Spain, Sweden, Switzerland, Thailand, The Netherlands, The Philippines, Turkey, United Kingdom, Venezuela)
ETANERCEPT
Enbrel for Injection 569

ENDOCLAR (Argentina)
DONEPEZIL HYDROCHLORIDE
Aricept Tablets 1062

ENDOGEL (Germany)
SODIUM HYALURONATE
Hyalgan Solution 2742

ENDOMETRIN (Hong Kong, Israel)
PROGESTERONE
Crinone 4% Gel 992
Prometrium Capsules (100 mg, 200 mg) . 3047

ENDOMINA (Spain)
ESTRADIOL
Climara Transdermal System 763

ENDONE (Australia)
OXYCODONE HYDROCHLORIDE
OxyContin Tablets 2589
OxyIR Capsules 2593

ENDRONAX (Brazil)
ALENDRONATE SODIUM
Fosamax Tablets 2005

ENFEXIA (Turkey)
CEFUROXIME AXETIL
Ceftin for Oral Suspension 1380
Ceftin Tablets 1380

ENI (Mexico)
CIPROFLOXACIN HYDROCHLORIDE
Cipro Tablets 2810

ENLACE (Mexico)
CAPTOPRIL
Captopril Tablets 2182

ENOPARIN (Venezuela)
ENOXAPARIN SODIUM
Lovenox Injection 2756

ENOXIN (Hong Kong, Malaysia)
CIPROFLOXACIN HYDROCHLORIDE
Cipro Tablets 2810

ENPER (Argentina)
ZIDOVUDINE
Retrovir Capsules 1574
Retrovir IV Infusion 1579
Retrovir Syrup 1574
Retrovir Tablets 1574

ENROMIC (Argentina)
LOSARTAN POTASSIUM
Cozaar Tablets 1973

ENTERAL (Venezuela)
RANITIDINE HYDROCHLORIDE
Zantac 25 EFFERdose Tablets 1670
Zantac 150 Tablets 1670
Zantac 300 Tablets 1670
Zantac Injection 1666
Zantac Injection Premixed 1666
Zantac Syrup 1670

ENTOPLUS (Mexico)
ALBENDAZOLE
Albenza Tablets 1297

ENTRYDIL (Irish Republic)
DILTIAZEM HYDROCHLORIDE
Cardizem LA Extended Release Tablets 421

ENZACE (Australia)
CAPTOPRIL
Captopril Tablets 2182

ENZIPAN (Italy)
PANCRELIPASE
Ultrase Capsules 718
Ultrase MT Capsules 719

EOSTAR (Austria)
CITALOPRAM HYDROBROMIDE
Celexa Tablets 1160

EPADOREN (Greece)
RANITIDINE HYDROCHLORIDE
Zantac 25 EFFERdose Tablets 1670
Zantac 150 Tablets 1670
Zantac 300 Tablets 1670
Zantac Injection 1666
Zantac Injection Premixed 1666
Zantac Syrup 1670

EPALAT EPS (Italy)
LACTULOSE
Kristalose for Oral Solution 1004

EPALFEN (Italy, The Netherlands)
LACTULOSE
Kristalose for Oral Solution 1004

EPAZIN (The Philippines)
CARBAMAZEPINE
Carbatrol Capsules 3019

EPHELIA (Germany, Italy)
ESTRADIOL
Climara Transdermal System 763

EPI-ABEREL (Germany)
TRETINOIN
Vesanoid Capsules 2660

EPICLODINA (Mexico)
CLONIDINE
Catapres-TTS 842

EPICORDIN (Germany)
CAPTOPRIL
Captopril Tablets 2182

EPIESTROL (Chile, Irish Republic, Italy, Switzerland)
ESTRADIOL
Climara Transdermal System 763

EPIFON (Venezuela)
LAMOTRIGINE
Lamictal Chewable Dispersible Tablets . . . 1488
Lamictal Tablets 1488

EPIKOR (The Philippines)
CARBAMAZEPINE
Carbatrol Capsules 3019

EPILACTAL (Poland)
LAMOTRIGINE
Lamictal Chewable Dispersible Tablets . . . 1488
Lamictal Tablets 1488

EPILEPAX (Argentina)
LAMOTRIGINE
Lamictal Chewable Dispersible Tablets . . . 1488
Lamictal Tablets 1488

EPIMAZ (United Kingdom)
CARBAMAZEPINE
Carbatrol Capsules 3019

EPIMORPH (Canada)
MORPHINE SULFATE
MS Contin Tablets 2585

EPITEC (South Africa)
LAMOTRIGINE
Lamictal Chewable Dispersible Tablets . . . 1488
Lamictal Tablets 1488

EPITREL (Mexico)
TRETINOIN
Vesanoid Capsules 2660

EPITRIAM (The Netherlands)
TRIAMTERENE
Dyrenium Capsules 3189

EPITRIL (India)
CLONAZEPAM
Klonopin Tablets 2639

EPIVIR (Austria, Belgium, Brazil, Czech Republic, Denmark, Finland, France, Germany, Greece, Irish Republic, Israel, Italy, Japan, Norway, Poland, Portugal, Russia, Singapore, Spain, Sweden, Thailand, The Netherlands, Turkey, United Kingdom, Venezuela)
LAMIVUDINE
Epivir Oral Solution 1412
Epivir Tablets 1412
Epivir-HBV Oral Solution 1417
Epivir-HBV Tablets 1417

EPIZAM (India)
CLONAZEPAM
Klonopin Tablets 2639

EPOALLEN (Austria)
EPOPROSTENOL SODIUM
Flolan for Injection 1426

EPOGEN (Argentina)
EPOETIN ALFA
Epogen for Injection 576
Procrit for Injection 2391

EPOKINE (Thailand)
EPOETIN ALFA
Epogen for Injection 576
Procrit for Injection 2391

EPOPEN (Spain)
EPOETIN ALFA
Epogen for Injection 576
Procrit for Injection 2391

EPOSAL (Chile)
CARBAMAZEPINE
Carbatrol Capsules 3019

EPOSINO (The Philippines)
EPOETIN ALFA
Epogen for Injection 576
Procrit for Injection 2391

EPOXITIN (Italy)
EPOETIN ALFA
Epogen for Injection 576
Procrit for Injection 2391

EPREX (Argentina, Australia, Belgium, Brazil, Canada, Chile, Czech Republic, Denmark, Finland, France, Germany, Greece, Hong Kong, Hungary, Irish Republic, Israel, Italy, Malaysia, Mexico, New Zealand, Norway, Poland, Russia, Singapore, South Africa, Spain, Sweden, Switzerland, Thailand, The Netherlands, The Philippines, Turkey, United Kingdom, Venezuela)
EPOETIN ALFA
Epogen for Injection 576
Procrit for Injection 2391

EPSITRON (Hong Kong, Thailand)
CAPTOPRIL
Captopril Tablets 2182

ERADIX (Austria)
FAMOTIDINE
Pepcid for Oral Suspension 2075
Pepcid Tablets 2075

ERANZ (Argentina, Brazil, Chile, Mexico, Venezuela)
DONEPEZIL HYDROCHLORIDE
Aricept Tablets 1062

ERDON (Hong Kong)
DICLOFENAC SODIUM
Voltaren Tablets 2334
Voltaren-XR Tablets 2337

ERIDAN (Italy)
DIAZEPAM
Valium Tablets 2658

ERIMICIN (Argentina, Chile)
BENZOYL PEROXIDE
Brevoxyl-4 Creamy Wash 3054
Brevoxyl-4 Gel 3054
Brevoxyl-8 Creamy Wash 3054
Brevoxyl-8 Gel 3054

ERIOX (Argentina)
DOCETAXEL
Taxotere Injection Concentrate 2773

ERITINA (Brazil)
EPOETIN ALFA
Epogen for Injection 576
Procrit for Injection 2391

ERROLON (Argentina)
FUROSEMIDE
Furosemide Tablets 2186

ERWINASE (Greece)
ASPARAGINASE
Elspar for Injection 2488

ERYPO (Austria, Germany)
EPOETIN ALFA
Epogen for Injection 576
Procrit for Injection 2391

ESALDOX (Chile)
LEVOTHYROXINE SODIUM
Levothroid Tablets 1170
Levoxyl Tablets 1780
Synthroid Tablets 507

ESCLEBIN (Spain)
NORFLOXACIN
Noroxin Tablets 2069

ESCLIMA (Italy)
ESTRADIOL
Climara Transdermal System 763

ESCOZEM (Switzerland)
DILTIAZEM HYDROCHLORIDE
Cardizem LA Extended Release Tablets 421

ESCUDO (Italy)
SUCRALFATE
Carafate Suspension 706
Carafate Tablets 707

ESGIPYRIN (India)
DICLOFFNAC SODIUM
Voltaren Tablets 2334
Voltaren-XR Tablets 2337

ESGIPYRIN DS (India)
DICLOFENAC SODIUM
Voltaren Tablets 2334
Voltaren-XR Tablets 2337

ESITEREN (Germany)
HYDROCHLOROTHIAZIDE/TRIAMTERENE
Dyazide Capsules 1405

ESKAZOLE (Australia, Austria, France, Germany, Greece, Israel, Mexico, Spain, The Netherlands, United Kingdom)
ALBENDAZOLE
Albenza Tablets 1297

ESLOFEN (The Philippines)
DICLOFENAC SODIUM
Voltaren Tablets 2334
Voltaren-XR Tablets 2337

ESOFEX (Finland)
RANITIDINE HYDROCHLORIDE
Zantac 25 EFFERdose Tablets 1670
Zantac 150 Tablets 1670
Zantac 300 Tablets 1670
Zantac Injection 1666
Zantac Injection Premixed 1666
Zantac Syrup 1670

ESOLUT (Italy)
PROGESTERONE
Crinone 4% Gel 992
Prometrium Capsules (100 mg, 200 mg) . 3047

ESOTRAN (Spain)
ESTRADIOL
Climara Transdermal System 763

ESPA-LEPSIN (Germany)
CARBAMAZEPINE
Carbatrol Capsules 3019

ESPARIL (Germany)
CAPTOPRIL
Captopril Tablets 2182

ESPASEVIT (Argentina)
ONDANSETRON
Zofran ODT Orally Disintegrating Tablets . . 1687

ESPEDEN (Spain)
NORFLOXACIN
Noroxin Tablets 2069

ESPO (Japan)
EPOETIN ALFA
Epogen for Injection 576
Procrit for Injection 2391

ESPOGEN (Thailand)
EPOETIN ALFA
Epogen for Injection 576
Procrit for Injection 2391

ESPONTAL (Argentina)
TAMSULOSIN HYDROCHLORIDE
Flomax Capsules 848

ESPRASONE (Spain)
ESTRADIOL
Climara Transdermal System 763

ESRADIN (Italy)
ISRADIPINE
DynaCirc CR Tablets 1407

ESSELDON (Greece)
FAMOTIDINE
Pepcid for Oral Suspension 2075
Pepcid Tablets 2075

ESSVENTIA (Mexico)
ESTRADIOL
Climara Transdermal System 763

ESTALIS (Argentina, Austria, Belgium, Brazil, Canada, Czech Republic, Irish Republic, Norway, Poland, Portugal, Spain, Switzerland, The Netherlands)
ESTRADIOL
Climara Transdermal System 763

ESTALIS CONTINUOUS (Australia)
ESTRADIOL
Climara Transdermal System 763

ESTIMA (France)
PROGESTERONE
Crinone 4% Gel. 992
Prometrium Capsules (100 mg, 200 mg) . 3047

ESTRABETA (Germany)
ESTRADIOL
Climara Transdermal System 763

ESTRACE (Canada, Czech Republic)
ESTRADIOL
Climara Transdermal System 763

ESTRACE-C (Czech Republic)
ESTRADIOL
Climara Transdermal System 763

ESTRACUTAN (Austria)
ESTRADIOL
Climara Transdermal System 763

ESTRADELLE (Brazil)
ESTRADIOL
Climara Transdermal System 763

ESTRADERM (Argentina, Australia, Austria, Belgium, Brazil, Canada, Czech Republic, Denmark, Finland, France, Germany, Hong Kong, Hungary, India, Irish Republic, Israel, Italy, Mexico, New Zealand, Norway, Poland, Portugal, Singapore, South Africa, Spain, Sweden, Switzerland, The Netherlands, Turkey, United Kingdom, Venezuela)
ESTRADIOL
Climara Transdermal System 763

ESTRADERM TTS (Greece)
ESTRADIOL
Climara Transdermal System 763

ESTRADOT (Argentina, Australia, Austria, Brazil, Canada, Finland, Germany, Greece, Hungary, Irish Republic, Norway, Poland, Portugal, South Africa, Spain, Sweden, Switzerland, The Netherlands, United Kingdom, Venezuela)
ESTRADIOL
Climara Transdermal System 763

ESTRAGEST (Argentina, Brazil, Czech Republic, Hungary, Venezuela)
ESTRADIOL
Climara Transdermal System 763

ESTRAHEXAL (Czech Republic)
ESTRADIOL
Climara Transdermal System 763

ESTRAMON (Austria, Germany, Greece, Hungary, Irish Republic, Mexico, Switzerland, Turkey)
ESTRADIOL
Climara Transdermal System 763

ESTRAPATCH (France, Poland)
ESTRADIOL
Climara Transdermal System 763

ESTRENA (Finland)
ESTRADIOL
Climara Transdermal System 763

ESTREVA (Argentina, Belgium, Brazil, Chile, Czech Republic, Germany, Hong Kong, Mexico, Monaco, Poland, Singapore, Switzerland, The Netherlands, Turkey)
ESTRADIOL
Climara Transdermal System 763

ESTRIFAM (Germany)
ESTRADIOL
Climara Transdermal System 763

ESTRIMAX (Czech Republic, Hungary, Russia)
ESTRADIOL
Climara Transdermal System 763

ESTRING (Argentina, Australia, Austria, Canada, Czech Republic, Denmark, Finland, Germany, Greece, New Zealand, Norway, South Africa, Switzerland, The Netherlands, United Kingdom)
ESTRADIOL
Climara Transdermal System 763

ESTROACT (India)
RALOXIFENE HYDROCHLORIDE
Evista Tablets. 1810

ESTROCLIM (Italy)
ESTRADIOL
Climara Transdermal System 763

ESTRODOSE (Italy)
ESTRADIOL
Climara Transdermal System 763

ESTROFEM (Argentina, Australia, Austria, Belgium, Brazil, Czech Republic, Denmark, Finland, France, Greece, Hong Kong, Hungary, Irish Republic, Israel, Italy, Malaysia, New Zealand, Poland, Portugal, Russia, Singapore, South Africa, Thailand, The Netherlands, The Philippines)
ESTRADIOL
Climara Transdermal System 763

ESTROFEM N (Switzerland)
ESTRADIOL
Climara Transdermal System 763

ESTROFFIK (Spain)
ESTRADIOL
Climara Transdermal System 763

ESTROGEL (Austria, Canada, Denmark, Finland, Greece, Venezuela)
ESTRADIOL
Climara Transdermal System 763

ESTRONAR (Portugal)
ESTRADIOL
Climara Transdermal System 763

ESTRONORM (Germany)
ESTRADIOL
Climara Transdermal System 763

ESTROPLAST (Poland)
ESTRADIOL
Climara Transdermal System 763

ETAMUCIN (Austria)
SODIUM HYALURONATE
Hyalgan Solution 2742

ETAZIM (Italy)
CEFTAZIDIME
Fortaz for Injection 1450

ETHEOPHYL (Germany)
THEOPHYLLINE
Uniphyl Tablets 2595

ETHIPAM (South Africa)
DIAZEPAM
Valium Tablets 2658

ETIDRATE (New Zealand)
ETIDRONATE DISODIUM
Didronel Tablets 2583

ETIDREL (Sweden)
ETIDRONATE DISODIUM
Didronel Tablets 2583

ETIDRON (Germany, Greece, Italy)
ETIDRONATE DISODIUM
Didronel Tablets 2583

ETIPLUS (Greece)
ETIDRONATE DISODIUM
Didronel Tablets 2583

ETIZEM (Czech Republic, Portugal)
DILTIAZEM HYDROCHLORIDE
Cardizem LA Extended Release Tablets. . . . 421

ETYOFIL (India)
THEOPHYLLINE
Uniphyl Tablets 2595

ETYZEM (Italy)
DILTIAZEM HYDROCHLORIDE
Cardizem LA Extended Release Tablets. . . . 421

EU 2000 (Thailand)
TERBINAFINE HYDROCHLORIDE
Lamisil Tablets 2266

EUBINE (France)
OXYCODONE HYDROCHLORIDE
OxyContin Tablets 2589
OxyIR Capsules. 2593

EUCARDIC (Irish Republic, Sweden, The Netherlands, United Kingdom)
CARVEDILOL
Coreg Tablets. 1387

EUCOPROST (Spain)
FINASTERIDE
Propecia Tablets 2095
Proscar Tablets. 2102

EUCOR (Thailand)
SIMVASTATIN
Zocor Tablets. 2136

EUDIGOX (Italy)
DIGOXIN
Lanoxin Injection 1498
Lanoxin Injection Pediatric 1502
Lanoxin Tablets. 1505

EUDYNA (Austria, Germany, Hong Kong, India, Mexico, Singapore)
TRETINOIN
Vesanoid Capsules. 2660

EUFATIN (Mexico)
FAMOTIDINE
Pepcid for Oral Suspension 2075
Pepcid Tablets 2075

EUFILINA (Portugal, Spain)
THEOPHYLLINE
Uniphyl Tablets 2595

EUFLEXXA (United Kingdom)
SODIUM HYALURONATE
Hyalgan Solution 2742

EUFLOXIN (Mexico)
CIPROFLOXACIN
Cipro Oral Suspension 2810

EUGALAC (Austria, Germany)
LACTULOSE
Kristalose for Oral Solution 1004

EUGERIAL (Argentina, Brazil)
NIMODIPINE
Nimotop Capsules 790

EUKODAL (Germany)
OXYCODONE HYDROCHLORIDE
OxyContin Tablets 2589
OxyIR Capsules. 2593

EUPEN (Chile)
TAMSULOSIN HYDROCHLORIDE
Flomax Capsules. 848

EUPHYLLIN (Belgium, Czech Republic, Finland, Germany, Norway, Poland, South Africa, Switzerland)
THEOPHYLLINE
Uniphyl Tablets 2595

EUPHYLLIN 200 (Germany)
THEOPHYLLINE
Uniphyl Tablets 2595

EUPHYLLINA (Italy)
THEOPHYLLINE
Uniphyl Tablets 2595

EUPHYLLINE (France)
THEOPHYLLINE
Uniphyl Tablets 2595

EUPHYLONG (Czech Republic, Germany, Hong Kong, Hungary, Sweden, Switzerland, The Netherlands)
THEOPHYLLINE
Uniphyl Tablets 2595

EURALBEN (Mexico)
ALBENDAZOLE
Albenza Tablets. 1297

EU-RAN (The Philippines)
RANITIDINE HYDROCHLORIDE
Zantac 25 EFFERdose Tablets 1670
Zantac 150 Tablets 1670
Zantac 300 Tablets 1670
Zantac Injection 1666
Zantac Injection Premixed 1666
Zantac Syrup 1670

EURITSIN (Argentina)
ADENOSINE
Adenocard IV Injection 603
Adenoscan. 605

EUROCOR (The Philippines)
SIMVASTATIN
Zocor Tablets. 2136

EUROFENAC (Hong Kong)
DICLOFENAC SODIUM
Voltaren Tablets 2334
Voltaren-XR Tablets 2337

EUROFLOX (The Philippines)
NORFLOXACIN
Noroxin Tablets. 2069

EUROFLU (Italy)
FLUNISOLIDE
Aerobid Inhaler System. 1153
Aerobid-M Inhaler System 1153

EUROGESIC (Chile)
NAPROXEN
EC-Naprosyn Delayed-Release Tablets. . . . 2632
Naprosyn Suspension. 2632
Naprosyn Tablets 2632

EUROMICINA (Chile)
CLARITHROMYCIN
Biaxin Filmtab Tablets. 411
Biaxin Granules 411

EUROSEF (The Philippines)
CEFTRIAXONE SODIUM
Rocephin Injectable Vials, ADD-Vantage, Galaxy, Bulk 2642

EUROTRETIN (Argentina)
TRETINOIN
Vesanoid Capsules. 2660

EUSTIDIL (Portugal)
FLUTICASONE PROPIONATE
Flonase Nasal Spray 1431

EUTHYROX (Argentina, Austria, Belgium, Brazil, Czech Republic, Germany, Hungary, Poland, Russia, Singapore, Sweden, Switzerland, Thailand, The Netherlands, The Philippines, Venezuela)
LEVOTHYROXINE SODIUM
Levothroid Tablets. 1170
Levoxyl Tablets. 1780
Synthroid Tablets. 507

EUTIMIL (Italy)
PAROXETINE HYDROCHLORIDE
Paxil Oral Suspension. 1535
Paxil Tablets. 1535

EUTIROX (Chile, Italy, Mexico, Spain)
LEVOTHYROXINE SODIUM
Levothroid Tablets. 1170
Levoxyl Tablets. 1780
Synthroid Tablets. 507

EUTIZ (Argentina)
FINASTERIDE
Propecia Tablets 2095
Proscar Tablets. 2102

EUTROXSIG (Australia)
LEVOTHYROXINE SODIUM
Levothroid Tablets. 1170
Levoxyl Tablets. 1780
Synthroid Tablets. 507

EUVASTEN (The Philippines)
SIMVASTATIN
Zocor Tablets. 2136

EVACALM (United Kingdom)
DIAZEPAM
Valium Tablets 2658

EVADOL (Mexico)
DICLOFENAC SODIUM
Voltaren Tablets 2334
Voltaren-XR Tablets 2337

EVAFILM (France)
ESTRADIOL
Climara Transdermal System 763

EVAPAUSE (France)
PROGESTERONE
Crinone 4% Gel. 992

Prometrium Capsules (100 mg, 200 mg) . 3047

EVIANTRINA (Spain)
FAMOTIDINE
Pepcid for Oral Suspension 2075
Pepcid Tablets 2075

EVIMAL (Chile)
DONEPEZIL HYDROCHLORIDE
Aricept Tablets 1062

EVINOPON (Greece)
DICLOFENAC SODIUM
Voltaren Tablets 2334
Voltaren-XR Tablets 2337

EVISTA (Argentina, Australia, Austria, Belgium, Brazil, Canada, Chile, Czech Republic, Denmark, Finland, France, Germany, Greece, Hong Kong, Hungary, Irish Republic, Israel, Italy, Malaysia, Mexico, New Zealand, Norway, Poland, Portugal, Singapore, South Africa, Spain, Sweden, Switzerland, The Netherlands, The Philippines, Turkey, United Kingdom, Venezuela)
RALOXIFENE HYDROCHLORIDE
Evista Tablets 1810

EVOPAD (Spain)
ESTRADIOL
Climara Transdermal System 763

EVOREL (Argentina, Denmark, Finland, Germany, Irish Republic, Israel, Mexico, Norway, South Africa, Sweden, United Kingdom)
ESTRADIOL
Climara Transdermal System 763

EVOREL CONTI (Argentina, Irish Republic, Israel, Mexico, United Kingdom)
ESTRADIOL
Climara Transdermal System 763

EVOTROX (United Kingdom)
LEVOTHYROXINE SODIUM
Levothroid Tablets 1170
Levoxyl Tablets 1780
Synthroid Tablets 507

EXERTIAL (Argentina)
CIPROFLOXACIN HYDROCHLORIDE
Cipro Tablets 2810

EXFOLIUM (Argentina)
TRIAMCINOLONE ACETONIDE
Azmacort Inhalation Aerosol 407
Nasacort AQ Nasal Spray 2765

EXIFINE (India, Malaysia, Russia)
TERBINAFINE HYDROCHLORIDE
Lamisil Tablets 2266

EXINOL (Venezuela)
SUCRALFATE
Carafate Suspension 706
Carafate Tablets 707

EXIREL (Austria)
PIRBUTEROL ACETATE
Maxair Autohaler 1705

EXODERIL (Austria, Czech Republic, Germany, Hong Kong, Hungary, Israel, Malaysia, Poland, Singapore, Switzerland, Turkey)
NAFTIFINE HYDROCHLORIDE
Naftin Cream 2164
Naftin Gel 2164

EXOGRAN (Austria, The Netherlands)
CEFTRIAXONE SODIUM
Rocephin Injectable Vials, ADD-Vantage, Galaxy, Bulk 2642

EXOVIR (Argentina)
ZIDOVUDINE
Retrovir Capsules 1574
Retrovir IV Infusion 1579
Retrovir Syrup 1574
Retrovir Tablets 1574

EXPLANER (Argentina)
NIMODIPINE
Nimotop Capsules 790

EXPROS (Finland)
TAMSULOSIN HYDROCHLORIDE
Flomax Capsules 848

EXTRACORT (Germany)
TRIAMCINOLONE ACETONIDE
Azmacort Inhalation Aerosol 407
Nasacort AQ Nasal Spray 2765

EXTUR (Spain)
INDAPAMIDE
Indapamide Tablets 2188

EYECLOF (Greece)
DICLOFENAC SODIUM
Voltaren Tablets 2334
Voltaren-XR Tablets 2337

EYECON (Israel)
SODIUM HYALURONATE
Hyalgan Solution 2742

EYESTIL (Canada)
SODIUM HYALURONATE
Hyalgan Solution 2742

EZOPTA (Greece)
RANITIDINE HYDROCHLORIDE
Zantac 25 EFFERdose Tablets 1670
Zantac 150 Tablets 1670
Zantac 300 Tablets 1670
Zantac Injection 1666
Zantac Injection Premixed 1666
Zantac Syrup 1670

EZUMYCIN (Greece)
CLARITHROMYCIN
Biaxin Filmtab Tablets 411
Biaxin Granules 411

FABAMOX (Argentina)
AMOXICILLIN
Amoxil Pediatric Drops for Oral Suspension 1305
Amoxil Tablets 1305

FABOFUROX (Argentina)
FUROSEMIDE
Furosemide Tablets 2186

FABOTRANIL (Argentina)
DIAZEPAM
Valium Tablets 2658

FABRALGINA (Argentina)
NAPROXEN
EC-Naprosyn Delayed-Release Tablets 2632
Naprosyn Suspension 2632
Naprosyn Tablets 2632

FABUTIN (Mexico)
FAMOTIDINE
Pepcid for Oral Suspension 2075
Pepcid Tablets 2075

FACORT (Thailand)
TRIAMCINOLONE ACETONIDE
Azmacort Inhalation Aerosol 407
Nasacort AQ Nasal Spray 2765

FADAFLUMAZ (Argentina)
FLUMAZENIL
Romazicon Injection 2646

FADALIVIO (Argentina)
NAPROXEN
EC-Naprosyn Delayed-Release Tablets 2632
Naprosyn Suspension 2632
Naprosyn Tablets 2632

FADINE (Hong Kong, India, Malaysia, Thailand)
FAMOTIDINE
Pepcid for Oral Suspension 2075
Pepcid Tablets 2075

FADIPINA (Venezuela)
FAMOTIDINE
Pepcid for Oral Suspension 2075
Pepcid Tablets 2075

FADUL (Germany)
FAMOTIDINE
Pepcid for Oral Suspension 2075
Pepcid Tablets 2075

FAGASTRIL (Spain)
FAMOTIDINE
Pepcid for Oral Suspension 2075
Pepcid Tablets 2075

FAGATRIM (Mexico)
FAMOTIDINE
Pepcid for Oral Suspension 2075
Pepcid Tablets 2075

FAGUS (Spain)
RANITIDINE HYDROCHLORIDE
Zantac 25 EFFERdose Tablets 1670
Zantac 150 Tablets 1670
Zantac 300 Tablets 1670
Zantac Injection 1666
Zantac Injection Premixed 1666
Zantac Syrup 1670

FAMEC (Turkey)
FAMOTIDINE
Pepcid for Oral Suspension 2075
Pepcid Tablets 2075

FAMIDYNA (Poland)
FAMOTIDINE
Pepcid for Oral Suspension 2075
Pepcid Tablets 2075

FAMILY MEDICATED SUNBURN RELIEF (Canada)
LIDOCAINE
Lidoderm Patch 1114

FAMINE (Hong Kong)
FAMOTIDINE
Pepcid for Oral Suspension 2075
Pepcid Tablets 2075

FAMO (Germany, Israel, Turkey)
FAMOTIDINE
Pepcid for Oral Suspension 2075
Pepcid Tablets 2075

FAMOBETA (Germany)
FAMOTIDINE
Pepcid for Oral Suspension 2075
Pepcid Tablets 2075

FAMOC (Singapore, Thailand)
FAMOTIDINE
Pepcid for Oral Suspension 2075
Pepcid Tablets 2075

FAMOCID (Hong Kong, Russia, Singapore, Thailand)
FAMOTIDINE
Pepcid for Oral Suspension 2075
Pepcid Tablets 2075

FAMODIL (Italy)
FAMOTIDINE
Pepcid for Oral Suspension 2075
Pepcid Tablets 2075

FAMODIN (India, Turkey)
FAMOTIDINE
Pepcid for Oral Suspension 2075
Pepcid Tablets 2075

FAMODINE (Brazil, Hong Kong)
FAMOTIDINE
Pepcid for Oral Suspension 2075
Pepcid Tablets 2075

FAMOGAST (Poland, Turkey)
FAMOTIDINE
Pepcid for Oral Suspension 2075
Pepcid Tablets 2075

FAMOGEL (Venezuela)
FAMOTIDINE
Pepcid for Oral Suspension 2075
Pepcid Tablets 2075

FAMOHEXAL (Australia, Austria)
FAMOTIDINE
Pepcid for Oral Suspension 2075
Pepcid Tablets 2075

FAMOKEY (Spain)
FAMOTIDINE
Pepcid for Oral Suspension 2075
Pepcid Tablets 2075

FAMOLTA (Hong Kong)
FAMOTIDINE
Pepcid for Oral Suspension 2075
Pepcid Tablets 2075

FAMONERTON (Germany)
FAMOTIDINE
Pepcid for Oral Suspension 2075
Pepcid Tablets 2075

FAMONIT (Russia)
FAMOTIDINE
Pepcid for Oral Suspension 2075
Pepcid Tablets 2075

FAMONITE (India)
FAMOTIDINE
Pepcid for Oral Suspension 2075
Pepcid Tablets 2075

FAMONOX (Thailand)
FAMOTIDINE
Pepcid for Oral Suspension 2075
Pepcid Tablets 2075

FAMOPRIL (Singapore)
FAMOTIDINE
Pepcid for Oral Suspension 2075
Pepcid Tablets 2075

FAMOPSIN (Hong Kong, Malaysia, Thailand)
FAMOTIDINE
Pepcid for Oral Suspension 2075
Pepcid Tablets 2075

FAMORILA (The Philippines)
FAMOTIDINE
Pepcid for Oral Suspension 2075
Pepcid Tablets 2075

FAMOSAN (Czech Republic, Russia)
FAMOTIDINE
Pepcid for Oral Suspension 2075
Pepcid Tablets 2075

FAMOSER (Turkey)
FAMOTIDINE
Pepcid for Oral Suspension 2075
Pepcid Tablets 2075

FAMOSET (Brazil)
FAMOTIDINE
Pepcid for Oral Suspension 2075
Pepcid Tablets 2075

FAMOSIA (Thailand)
FAMOTIDINE
Pepcid for Oral Suspension 2075
Pepcid Tablets 2075

FAMOSIN (Austria)
FAMOTIDINE
Pepcid for Oral Suspension 2075
Pepcid Tablets 2075

FAMOTAB (Thailand)
FAMOTIDINE
Pepcid for Oral Suspension 2075
Pepcid Tablets 2075

FAMOTAL (Norway)
FAMOTIDINE
Pepcid for Oral Suspension 2075
Pepcid Tablets 2075

FAMOTEC (United Arab Emirates)
FAMOTIDINE
Pepcid for Oral Suspension 2075
Pepcid Tablets 2075

FAMOTEP (Turkey)
FAMOTIDINE
Pepcid for Oral Suspension 2075
Pepcid Tablets 2075

FAMOTID (Brazil)
FAMOTIDINE
Pepcid for Oral Suspension 2075
Pepcid Tablets 2075

FAMOTIL (Brazil)
FAMOTIDINE
Pepcid for Oral Suspension 2075
Pepcid Tablets 2075

FAMOTIN (Hong Kong, Singapore, Thailand)
FAMOTIDINE
Pepcid for Oral Suspension 2075
Pepcid Tablets 2075

FAMOTSAN (Turkey)
FAMOTIDINE
Pepcid for Oral Suspension 2075
Pepcid Tablets 2075

FAMOWAL (India)
FAMOTIDINE
Pepcid for Oral Suspension 2075
Pepcid Tablets 2075

FAMOX (Brazil, Hong Kong, New Zealand)
FAMOTIDINE
Pepcid for Oral Suspension 2075
Pepcid Tablets 2075

FAMOXAL (Mexico)
FAMOTIDINE
Pepcid for Oral Suspension 2075
Pepcid Tablets 2075

FAMOXIL (Brazil)
FAMOTIDINE
Pepcid for Oral Suspension 2075
Pepcid Tablets 2075

FAMTAC (India)
FAMOTIDINE
Pepcid for Oral Suspension 2075

Pepcid Tablets . . . 2075

FAMTINE (The Philippines)
FAMOTIDINE
Pepcid for Oral Suspension . . . 2075
Pepcid Tablets . . . 2075

FAMULCER (Spain, Venezuela)
FAMOTIDINE
Pepcid for Oral Suspension . . . 2075
Pepcid Tablets . . . 2075

FANOSIN (Spain)
FAMOTIDINE
Pepcid for Oral Suspension . . . 2075
Pepcid Tablets . . . 2075

FANOX (Spain)
FAMOTIDINE
Pepcid for Oral Suspension . . . 2075
Pepcid Tablets . . . 2075

FARAXEN (Mexico)
NAPROXEN
EC-Naprosyn Delayed-Release Tablets . . . 2632
Naprosyn Suspension . . . 2632
Naprosyn Tablets . . . 2632

FARCEF (Greece)
CEFTRIAXONE SODIUM
Rocephin Injectable Vials, ADD-Vantage, Galaxy, Bulk . . . 2642

FARGO (Australia)
LIDOCAINE
Lidoderm Patch . . . 1114

FARLAC (Brazil)
LACTULOSE
Kristalose for Oral Solution . . . 1004

FARMACEF (Thailand)
CEFUROXIME AXETIL
Ceftin for Oral Suspension . . . 1380
Ceftin Tablets . . . 1380

FARMACNE (Spain)
ISOTRETINOIN
Accutane Capsules . . . 2607

FARMIN (Mexico)
DIAZEPAM
Valium Tablets . . . 2658

FARMOTEX (Mexico)
FAMOTIDINE
Pepcid for Oral Suspension . . . 2075
Pepcid Tablets . . . 2075

FARPRESSE (Portugal)
LISINOPRIL
Prinivil Tablets . . . 2087

FARXEN (Mexico)
NAPROXEN
EC-Naprosyn Delayed-Release Tablets . . . 2632
Naprosyn Suspension . . . 2632
Naprosyn Tablets . . . 2632

FASCAR (Thailand)
CLARITHROMYCIN
Biaxin Filmtab Tablets . . . 411
Biaxin Granules . . . 411

FASE (Italy)
APROTININ
Trasylol Injection . . . 799

FASELUT (Argentina)
PROGESTERONE
Crinone 4% Gel . . . 992
Prometrium Capsules (100 mg, 200 mg) . 3047

FASIDINE (Thailand)
FAMOTIDINE
Pepcid for Oral Suspension . . . 2075
Pepcid Tablets . . . 2075

FASTIN (Canada)
PHENTERMINE HYDROCHLORIDE
Adipex-P Capsules . . . 1185
Adipex-P Tablets . . . 1185

FATEC (Thailand)
CETIRIZINE HYDROCHLORIDE
Zyrtec Syrup . . . 1920
Zyrtec Tablets . . . 1920

FATIDIN (Portugal)
FAMOTIDINE
Pepcid for Oral Suspension . . . 2075
Pepcid Tablets . . . 2075

FATORIL (Mexico)
FAMOTIDINE
Pepcid for Oral Suspension . . . 2075
Pepcid Tablets . . . 2075

FAUSTAN (Germany)
DIAZEPAM
Valium Tablets . . . 2658

FAWODIN (Mexico)
FAMOTIDINE
Pepcid for Oral Suspension . . . 2075
Pepcid Tablets . . . 2075

FAXINE (Italy)
VENLAFAXINE HYDROCHLORIDE
Effexor XR Capsules . . . 3195

FEACEF (Greece)
CEFUROXIME AXETIL
Ceftin for Oral Suspension . . . 1380
Ceftin Tablets . . . 1380

FEBRAX (Mexico)
NAPROXEN SODIUM
Anaprox DS Tablets . . . 2632
Anaprox Tablets . . . 2632

FEGENOR (France, Hong Kong)
FENOFIBRATE
Tricor Tablets . . . 520

FELANOR (Argentina)
CLONAZEPAM
Klonopin Tablets . . . 2639

FELIPRAM (Italy)
CITALOPRAM HYDROBROMIDE
Celexa Tablets . . . 1160

FELISELIN (Greece)
SELEGILINE HYDROCHLORIDE
Eldepryl Capsules . . . 3052

FELIXENE (Spain)
CIPROFLOXACIN HYDROCHLORIDE
Cipro Tablets . . . 2810

FELIXIMIR (Italy)
CITALOPRAM HYDROBROMIDE
Celexa Tablets . . . 1160

FELORAN (Czech Republic)
DICLOFENAC SODIUM
Voltaren Tablets . . . 2334
Voltaren-XR Tablets . . . 2337

FEM 7 (Argentina, Brazil, Chile, Czech Republic, Germany, Hong Kong, Mexico, Poland, Singapore, Switzerland, The Netherlands)
ESTRADIOL
Climara Transdermal System . . . 763

FEMALON (Chile)
ESTRADIOL
Climara Transdermal System . . . 763

FEMANEST (Denmark, Sweden)
ESTRADIOL
Climara Transdermal System . . . 763

FEMATAB (Irish Republic)
ESTRADIOL
Climara Transdermal System . . . 763

FEMATRIX (Irish Republic, United Kingdom)
ESTRADIOL
Climara Transdermal System . . . 763

FEMEX (The Netherlands)
NAPROXEN SODIUM
Anaprox DS Tablets . . . 2632
Anaprox Tablets . . . 2632

FEMIDERM (Chile)
ESTRADIOL
Climara Transdermal System . . . 763

FEMIDOT (Chile)
ESTRADIOL
Climara Transdermal System . . . 763

FEMIGEL (South Africa)
ESTRADIOL
Climara Transdermal System . . . 763

FEMINOFLEX (Greece)
ETIDRONATE DISODIUM
Didronel Tablets . . . 2583

FEMINOVA (Belgium)
ESTRADIOL
Climara Transdermal System . . . 763

FEMITY (Italy)
ESTRADIOL
Climara Transdermal System . . . 763

FEMME FREE (Australia)
NAPROXEN
EC-Naprosyn Delayed-Release Tablets . . . 2632
Naprosyn Suspension . . . 2632
Naprosyn Tablets . . . 2632

FEMOSTON 1/5 (Portugal)
ESTRADIOL
Climara Transdermal System . . . 763

FEMOSTON CONTI (Austria, Belgium, Brazil, Chile, Finland, Germany, Italy, Poland, South Africa, Switzerland, Thailand, United Kingdom, Venezuela)
ESTRADIOL
Climara Transdermal System . . . 763

FEMOSTON CONTINU (The Netherlands)
ESTRADIOL
Climara Transdermal System . . . 763

FEMOSTON MONO (Germany)
ESTRADIOL
Climara Transdermal System . . . 763

FEMPHASCYL CONTI (Austria)
ESTRADIOL
Climara Transdermal System . . . 763

FEMPHASCYL CONTINU (The Netherlands)
ESTRADIOL
Climara Transdermal System . . . 763

FEMSEPT (France)
ESTRADIOL
Climara Transdermal System . . . 763

FEMSEVEN (Austria, Denmark, Finland, Italy, Sweden, Switzerland, United Kingdom, Venezuela)
ESTRADIOL
Climara Transdermal System . . . 763

FEMSEVEN CONTI (United Kingdom)
ESTRADIOL
Climara Transdermal System . . . 763

FEMSIEBEN (Austria)
ESTRADIOL
Climara Transdermal System . . . 763

FEMTAB CONTINUOUS (United Kingdom)
ESTRADIOL
Climara Transdermal System . . . 763

FEMTRAN (Australia, New Zealand)
ESTRADIOL
Climara Transdermal System . . . 763

FENAC (Australia, Thailand)
DICLOFENAC SODIUM
Voltaren Tablets . . . 2334
Voltaren-XR Tablets . . . 2337

FENACTOL (United Kingdom)
DICLOFENAC SODIUM
Voltaren Tablets . . . 2334
Voltaren-XR Tablets . . . 2337

FENADIUM (Malaysia)
DICLOFENAC SODIUM
Voltaren Tablets . . . 2334
Voltaren-XR Tablets . . . 2337

FENADOL (Italy)
DICLOFENAC SODIUM
Voltaren Tablets . . . 2334
Voltaren-XR Tablets . . . 2337

FENAPLUS (India)
DICLOFENAC SODIUM
Voltaren Tablets . . . 2334
Voltaren-XR Tablets . . . 2337

FENARDIN (Poland)
FENOFIBRATE
Tricor Tablets . . . 520

FENAREN (Austria)
DICLOFENAC SODIUM
Voltaren Tablets . . . 2334
Voltaren-XR Tablets . . . 2337

FENASPEC (The Philippines)
DICLOFENAC SODIUM
Voltaren Tablets . . . 2334
Voltaren-XR Tablets . . . 2337

FENBURIL (Brazil)
DICLOFENAC SODIUM
Voltaren Tablets . . . 2334
Voltaren-XR Tablets . . . 2337

FENDER (Italy)
DICLOFENAC SODIUM
Voltaren Tablets . . . 2334
Voltaren-XR Tablets . . . 2337

FENIL-V (Portugal)
DICLOFENAC SODIUM
Voltaren Tablets . . . 2334
Voltaren-XR Tablets . . . 2337

FENISONA (Argentina)
MOMETASONE FUROATE
Elocon Cream 0.1% . . . 2840
Elocon Lotion 0.1% . . . 2841
Elocon Ointment 0.1% . . . 2842
Nasonex Nasal Spray . . . 2883

FENOBETA (Germany)
FENOFIBRATE
Tricor Tablets . . . 520

FENOBRAT (Hungary)
FENOFIBRATE
Tricor Tablets . . . 520

FENOBRATE (Argentina)
FENOFIBRATE
Tricor Tablets . . . 520

FENOCLOF (Greece)
DICLOFENAC SODIUM
Voltaren Tablets . . . 2334
Voltaren-XR Tablets . . . 2337

FENODID (Mexico)
FENTANYL CITRATE
Actiq . . . 959

FENOFITOP (Belgium)
FENOFIBRATE
Tricor Tablets . . . 520

FENOGAL (Belgium, United Kingdom)
FENOFIBRATE
Tricor Tablets . . . 520

FENOGAL LIDOSE (Singapore)
FENOFIBRATE
Tricor Tablets . . . 520

FENOLIP (Argentina, Austria, India)
FENOFIBRATE
Tricor Tablets . . . 520

FENORATIO (Poland)
FENOFIBRATE
Tricor Tablets . . . 520

FENORIT (Italy)
PROPAFENONE HYDROCHLORIDE
Rythmol SR Capsules . . . 1590

FENOX (Thailand)
FENOFIBRATE
Tricor Tablets . . . 520

FENSAIDE (India)
DICLOFENAC SODIUM
Voltaren Tablets . . . 2334
Voltaren-XR Tablets . . . 2337

FENSAIDE-P (India)
DICLOFENAC SODIUM
Voltaren Tablets . . . 2334
Voltaren-XR Tablets . . . 2337

FENSARTAN (Argentina)
LOSARTAN POTASSIUM
Cozaar Tablets . . . 1973

FENSARTAN D (Argentina)
LOSARTAN POTASSIUM
Cozaar Tablets . . . 1973

FENTABBOTT (Brazil)
FENTANYL CITRATE
Actiq . . . 959

FENTAHEXAL (Poland)
FENTANYL
Duragesic Transdermal System . . . 2405

FENTAL (Irish Republic)
FENTANYL
Duragesic Transdermal System . . . 2405

FENTANEST (Brazil, Italy, Mexico, Spain)
FENTANYL CITRATE
Actiq . . . 959

FENTATIL (Brazil)
FENTANYL
Duragesic Transdermal System . . . 2405

FENTAX (Argentina)
FENTANYL CITRATE
Actiq 959

FERLEX (Mexico)
AMOXICILLIN
Amoxil Pediatric Drops for Oral Suspension 1305
Amoxil Tablets 1305

FERMATHRON (Australia, Germany, United Kingdom)
SODIUM HYALURONATE
Hyalgan Solution 2742

FERMAVISC (Switzerland)
SODIUM HYALURONATE
Hyalgan Solution 2742

FERVEX (Mexico)
DICLOFENAC SODIUM
Voltaren Tablets 2334
Voltaren-XR Tablets 2337

FESTAL REFORMULADO (Venezuela)
AMYLASE/LIPASE/PROTEASE
Creon 5 Capsules 3041
Creon 10 Capsules 3042
Creon 20 Capsules 3042
Ultrase Capsules 718
Ultrase MT Capsules 719
Viokase Powder 721
Viokase Tablets 721

FIBONEL (Chile, Spain)
FAMOTIDINE
Pepcid for Oral Suspension 2075
Pepcid Tablets 2075

FIBRAFEN (The Philippines)
FENOFIBRATE
Tricor Tablets 520

FIBRAMOX (Venezuela)
AMOXICILLIN
Amoxil Pediatric Drops for Oral Suspension 1305
Amoxil Tablets 1305

FIBRASE (Italy)
PENTOSAN POLYSULFATE SODIUM
Elmiron Capsules 2435

FIBREZYM (Germany)
PENTOSAN POLYSULFATE SODIUM
Elmiron Capsules 2435

FIBROCID (Spain)
PENTOSAN POLYSULFATE SODIUM
Elmiron Capsules 2435

FIBROCIDE (Portugal)
PENTOSAN POLYSULFATE SODIUM
Elmiron Capsules 2435

FIBROLAN (Thailand)
FENOFIBRATE
Tricor Tablets 520

FIBROXYN (South Africa)
NAPROXEN
EC-Naprosyn Delayed-Release Tablets 2632
Naprosyn Suspension 2632
Naprosyn Tablets 2632

FIBSOL (Australia)
LISINOPRIL
Prinivil Tablets 2087

FIDATO (Italy)
CEFTRIAXONE SODIUM
Rocephin Injectable Vials, ADD-Vantage, Galaxy, Bulk 2642

FIDECAINA (Argentina)
LIDOCAINE
Lidoderm Patch 1114

FIGOZANT (Greece)
NIMODIPINE
Nimotop Capsules 790

FIGREL (Greece)
DICLOFENAC SODIUM
Voltaren Tablets 2334
Voltaren-XR Tablets 2337

FILAZEM (The Philippines)
DILTIAZEM HYDROCHLORIDE
Cardizem LA Extended Release Tablets 421

FILGINASE (Argentina)
EFAVIRENZ
Sustiva Capsules 930

FILTEN (Argentina)
CARVEDILOL
Coreg Tablets 1387

FILXINE (Argentina)
ALENDRONATE SODIUM
Fosamax Tablets 2005

FINABER (Argentina)
ONDANSETRON
Zofran ODT Orally Disintegrating Tablets 1687

FINABURG (The Netherlands)
FINASTERIDE
Propecia Tablets 2095
Proscar Tablets 2102

FINACILEN (Argentina)
NIMODIPINE
Nimotop Capsules 790

FINALOP (Brazil)
FINASTERIDE
Propecia Tablets 2095
Proscar Tablets 2102

FINANIDDA (The Netherlands)
TERBINAFINE HYDROCHLORIDE
Lamisil Tablets 2266

FINAP (Chile)
CITALOPRAM HYDROBROMIDE
Celexa Tablets 1160

FINARID (Turkey)
FINASTERIDE
Propecia Tablets 2095
Proscar Tablets 2102

FINARIDE (Poland)
FINASTERIDE
Propecia Tablets 2095
Proscar Tablets 2102

FINASEPT (Argentina)
CLARITHROMYCIN
Biaxin Filmtab Tablets 411
Biaxin Granules 411

FINAST (Russia, Venezuela)
FINASTERIDE
Propecia Tablets 2095
Proscar Tablets 2102

FINASTEC (Brazil)
FINASTERIDE
Propecia Tablets 2095
Proscar Tablets 2102

FINASTER (Poland)
FINASTERIDE
Propecia Tablets 2095
Proscar Tablets 2102

FINASTERIN (Argentina)
FINASTERIDE
Propecia Tablets 2095
Proscar Tablets 2102

FINASTID (Italy)
FINASTERIDE
Propecia Tablets 2095
Proscar Tablets 2102

FINASTIL (Brazil)
FINASTERIDE
Propecia Tablets 2095
Proscar Tablets 2102

FINAVITA (The Netherlands)
TERBINAFINE HYDROCHLORIDE
Lamisil Tablets 2266

FINCAR (India)
FINASTERIDE
Propecia Tablets 2095
Proscar Tablets 2102

FINDALER (Chile)
CETIRIZINE HYDROCHLORIDE
Zyrtec Syrup 1920
Zyrtec Tablets 1920

FINDECLIN (Argentina)
ALENDRONATE SODIUM
Fosamax Tablets 2005

FINEX (Brazil, Czech Republic)
TERBINAFINE HYDROCHLORIDE
Lamisil Tablets 2266

FINGRAS (Argentina)
ORLISTAT
Xenical Capsules 2672

FINLEPSIN (Germany, Hungary, Poland, Russia)
CARBAMAZEPINE
Carbatrol Capsules 3019

FINLIPOL (Argentina)
ATORVASTATIN CALCIUM
Lipitor Tablets 2501

FINOXI (Argentina)
ONDANSETRON
Zofran ODT Orally Disintegrating Tablets 1687

FINPECIA (India)
FINASTERIDE
Propecia Tablets 2095
Proscar Tablets 2102

FINPROSTAT (Argentina)
FINASTERIDE
Propecia Tablets 2095
Proscar Tablets 2102

FINTOP (India)
BUTENAFINE HYDROCHLORIDE
Mentax Cream 2190

FIRIDE (Thailand)
FINASTERIDE
Propecia Tablets 2095
Proscar Tablets 2102

FIRIN (Germany)
NORFLOXACIN
Noroxin Tablets 2069

FITAXAL (France)
LACTULOSE
Kristalose for Oral Solution 1004

FITZECALM (United Arab Emirates)
CARBAMAZEPINE
Carbatrol Capsules 3019

FIXCA (Spain)
ONDANSETRON HYDROCHLORIDE
Zofran Injection 1682
Zofran Injection Premixed 1682
Zofran Oral Solution 1687
Zofran Tablets 1687

FIXOPAN (Venezuela)
ALENDRONATE SODIUM
Fosamax Tablets 2005

FLADON (Brazil)
DICLOFENAC SODIUM
Voltaren Tablets 2334
Voltaren-XR Tablets 2337

FLAMALGEN (Brazil)
DICLOFENAC SODIUM
Voltaren Tablets 2334
Voltaren-XR Tablets 2337

FLAMAR (The Philippines)
CELECOXIB
Celebrex Capsules 2979

FLAMATAK (United Kingdom)
DICLOFENAC SODIUM
Voltaren Tablets 2334
Voltaren-XR Tablets 2337

FLAMRASE (United Kingdom)
DICLOFENAC SODIUM
Voltaren Tablets 2334
Voltaren-XR Tablets 2337

FLANAREN (Brazil)
DICLOFENAC SODIUM
Voltaren Tablets 2334
Voltaren-XR Tablets 2337

FLANAX (Brazil, Mexico, The Philippines)
NAPROXEN SODIUM
Anaprox DS Tablets 2632
Anaprox Tablets 2632

FLANKOL (Mexico)
DICLOFENAC SODIUM
Voltaren Tablets 2334
Voltaren-XR Tablets 2337

FLATEZOL (Mexico)
ALBENDAZOLE
Albenza Tablets 1297

FLAVIX (India)
VENLAFAXINE HYDROCHLORIDE
Effexor XR Capsules 3195

FLAVOXEN (Mexico)
NAPROXEN
EC-Naprosyn Delayed-Release Tablets 2632
Naprosyn Suspension 2632
Naprosyn Tablets 2632

FLAXENDOL (Mexico)
NAPROXEN SODIUM
Anaprox DS Tablets 2632
Anaprox Tablets 2632

FLAXIN (Brazil)
FINASTERIDE
Propecia Tablets 2095
Proscar Tablets 2102

FLAXVAN (Argentina)
NAPROXEN
EC-Naprosyn Delayed-Release Tablets 2632
Naprosyn Suspension 2632
Naprosyn Tablets 2632

FLEMING (Hong Kong)
AMOXICILLIN
Amoxil Pediatric Drops for Oral Suspension 1305
Amoxil Tablets 1305

FLEMOXIN (Greece, New Zealand, Russia, Switzerland)
AMOXICILLIN
Amoxil Pediatric Drops for Oral Suspension 1305
Amoxil Tablets 1305

FLEXAGEN (South Africa)
DICLOFENAC SODIUM
Voltaren Tablets 2334
Voltaren-XR Tablets 2337

FLEXAMINA (Brazil)
DICLOFENAC SODIUM
Voltaren Tablets 2334
Voltaren-XR Tablets 2337

FLEXEN (Mexico)
NAPROXEN
EC-Naprosyn Delayed-Release Tablets 2632
Naprosyn Suspension 2632
Naprosyn Tablets 2632

FLEXIN (Argentina)
DICLOFENAC SODIUM
Voltaren Tablets 2334
Voltaren-XR Tablets 2337

FLEXOTARD (United Kingdom)
DICLOFENAC SODIUM
Voltaren Tablets 2334
Voltaren-XR Tablets 2337

FLEXRESAN (Spain)
ISOTRETINOIN
Accutane Capsules 2607

FLIXODERM (Italy)
FLUTICASONE PROPIONATE
Flonase Nasal Spray 1431

FLIXONASE (Argentina, Australia, Austria, Belgium, Brazil, Chile, Czech Republic, Denmark, Finland, France, Greece, Hong Kong, Hungary, Israel, Italy, Malaysia, Mexico, New Zealand, Poland, Russia, Singapore, South Africa, Spain, Thailand, The Netherlands, Turkey, United Kingdom, Venezuela)
FLUTICASONE PROPIONATE
Flonase Nasal Spray 1431

FLIXOTAIDE (Portugal)
FLUTICASONE PROPIONATE
Flonase Nasal Spray 1431

FLIXOTIDE (Argentina, Australia, Austria, Belgium, Brazil, Chile, Czech Republic, Denmark, Finland, France, Greece, Hong Kong, Hungary, Irish Republic, Israel, Italy, Malaysia, Mexico, New Zealand, Poland, Russia, Singapore, South Africa, Spain, Thailand, The Netherlands, The Philippines, Turkey, United Kingdom, Venezuela)
FLUTICASONE PROPIONATE
Flonase Nasal Spray 1431

FLIXOVATE (France)
FLUTICASONE PROPIONATE
Flonase Nasal Spray 1431

FLOBAC (Brazil)
CIPROFLOXACIN
Cipro Oral Suspension 2810

FLOCIPRIN (Greece)
CIPROFLOXACIN HYDROCHLORIDE
Cipro Tablets 2810

FLOGAREN (Venezuela)
DICLOFENAC SODIUM
Voltaren Tablets 2334

Voltaren-XR Tablets ... 2337

FLOGEN (Mexico)
NAPROXEN SODIUM
Anaprox DS Tablets ... 2632
Anaprox Tablets ... 2632

FLOGENAC (Argentina)
DICLOFENAC SODIUM
Voltaren Tablets ... 2334
Voltaren-XR Tablets ... 2337

FLOGESIC (Brazil)
DICLOFENAC SODIUM
Voltaren Tablets ... 2334
Voltaren-XR Tablets ... 2337

FLOGINAX (Italy)
NAPROXEN
EC-Naprosyn Delayed-Release Tablets ... 2632
Naprosyn Suspension ... 2632
Naprosyn Tablets ... 2632

FLOGOCEFAL (Argentina)
NAPROXEN
EC-Naprosyn Delayed-Release Tablets ... 2632
Naprosyn Suspension ... 2632
Naprosyn Tablets ... 2632

FLOGOCORT (Chile)
MOMETASONE FUROATE
Elocon Cream 0.1% ... 2840
Elocon Lotion 0.1% ... 2841
Elocon Ointment 0.1% ... 2842
Nasonex Nasal Spray ... 2883

FLOGOGIN (Italy)
NAPROXEN SODIUM
Anaprox DS Tablets ... 2632
Anaprox Tablets ... 2632

FLOGOLISIN (Argentina)
DICLOFENAC SODIUM
Voltaren Tablets ... 2334
Voltaren-XR Tablets ... 2337

FLOHALE (India)
FLUTICASONE PROPIONATE
Flonase Nasal Spray ... 1431

FLOHALE DP (South Africa)
FLUTICASONE PROPIONATE
Flonase Nasal Spray ... 1431

FLOLAN (Australia, Austria, Belgium, Canada, Czech Republic, Denmark, France, Irish Republic, Israel, Italy, Norway, Singapore, Spain, Switzerland, The Netherlands, United Kingdom)
EPOPROSTENOL SODIUM
Flolan for Injection ... 1426

FLOMAX (Australia, Canada, New Zealand, South Africa, Turkey, United Kingdom)
TAMSULOSIN HYDROCHLORIDE
Flomax Capsules ... 848

FLOMAXTRA (United Kingdom)
TAMSULOSIN HYDROCHLORIDE
Flomax Capsules ... 848

FLOMEX (India)
FLUOROMETHOLONE
FML Ophthalmic Ointment ... ⊙223

FLOMEX N (India)
FLUOROMETHOLONE
FML Ophthalmic Ointment ... ⊙223

FLOMIST (India, South Africa)
FLUTICASONE PROPIONATE
Flonase Nasal Spray ... 1431

FLONASE (Canada)
FLUTICASONE PROPIONATE
Flonase Nasal Spray ... 1431

FLORALAC (Austria)
LACTULOSE
Kristalose for Oral Solution ... 1004

FLORAXINA (Argentina)
CIPROFLOXACIN HYDROCHLORIDE
Cipro Tablets ... 2810

FLOROC (The Philippines)
CIPROFLOXACIN HYDROCHLORIDE
Cipro Tablets ... 2810

FLOSEF (India)
FLUOROMETHOLONE
FML Ophthalmic Ointment ... ⊙223

FLOSSAC (Italy)
NORFLOXACIN
Noroxin Tablets ... 2069

FLOVENT (Canada)
FLUTICASONE PROPIONATE
Flonase Nasal Spray ... 1431

FLOX (Brazil)
NORFLOXACIN
Noroxin Tablets ... 2069

FLOXACIN (Austria, Brazil, Mexico)
NORFLOXACIN
Noroxin Tablets ... 2069

FLOXACIPRON (Portugal)
CIPROFLOXACIN
Cipro Oral Suspension ... 2810

FLOXAGER (Mexico)
CIPROFLOXACIN HYDROCHLORIDE
Cipro Tablets ... 2810

FLOXAKIN (Mexico)
CIPROFLOXACIN
Cipro Oral Suspension ... 2810

FLOXALIN (Italy)
NAPROXEN SODIUM
Anaprox DS Tablets ... 2632
Anaprox Tablets ... 2632

FLOXAMICIN (Argentina)
NORFLOXACIN
Noroxin Tablets ... 2069

FLOXAN (Brazil)
CIPROFLOXACIN
Cipro Oral Suspension ... 2810

FLOXANOR (Brazil)
NORFLOXACIN
Noroxin Tablets ... 2069

FLOXANTINA (Mexico)
CIPROFLOXACIN HYDROCHLORIDE
Cipro Tablets ... 2810

FLOXATOM (Brazil)
NORFLOXACIN
Noroxin Tablets ... 2069

FLOXATRAL (Argentina)
NORFLOXACIN
Noroxin Tablets ... 2069

FLOXATRAT (Brazil)
NORFLOXACIN
Noroxin Tablets ... 2069

FLOXEL (The Philippines)
LEVOFLOXACIN
Levaquin Injection ... 2416
Levaquin Tablets ... 2416

FLOXELENA (Mexico)
CIPROFLOXACIN
Cipro Oral Suspension ... 2810

FLOXEN (Hong Kong)
NORFLOXACIN
Noroxin Tablets ... 2069

FLOXENOR (Thailand)
NORFLOXACIN
Noroxin Tablets ... 2069

FLOXILIN (Brazil)
NORFLOXACIN
Noroxin Tablets ... 2069

FLOXIN (South Africa)
NORFLOXACIN
Noroxin Tablets ... 2069

FLOXINOL (Brazil)
NORFLOXACIN
Noroxin Tablets ... 2069

FLOXLEVO (Argentina)
LEVOFLOXACIN
Levaquin Injection ... 2416
Levaquin Tablets ... 2416

FLOZEPAN (Argentina)
CLONAZEPAM
Klonopin Tablets ... 2639

FLU OPH (Thailand)
FLUOROMETHOLONE
FML Ophthalmic Ointment ... ⊙223

FLUACORT (Belgium)
FLUOROMETHOLONE
FML Ophthalmic Ointment ... ⊙223

FLUATON (Italy)
FLUOROMETHOLONE
FML Ophthalmic Ointment ... ⊙223

FLUBEST (Turkey)
INDAPAMIDE
Indapamide Tablets ... 2188

FLUCOL (Mexico)
NAPROXEN
EC-Naprosyn Delayed-Release Tablets ... 2632
Naprosyn Suspension ... 2632
Naprosyn Tablets ... 2632

FLUCON (Australia, Belgium, Czech Republic, France, Greece, Hong Kong, Hungary, New Zealand, Poland, South Africa, Switzerland, Thailand, The Netherlands)
FLUOROMETHOLONE
FML Ophthalmic Ointment ... ⊙223

FLUDAPAMIDE (Switzerland)
INDAPAMIDE
Indapamide Tablets ... 2188

FLUDEX (Austria, Belgium, Denmark, France, Greece, Portugal, Switzerland, The Netherlands, Turkey)
INDAPAMIDE
Indapamide Tablets ... 2188

FLUDIN (Turkey)
INDAPAMIDE
Indapamide Tablets ... 2188

FLUFORTE (Chile, Mexico)
FLUOROMETHOLONE
FML Ophthalmic Ointment ... ⊙223

FLUFORTE N (Mexico)
FLUOROMETHOLONE
FML Ophthalmic Ointment ... ⊙223

FLUGEN (Spain)
FLUOROMETHOLONE
FML Ophthalmic Ointment ... ⊙223

FLUIDEMA (Portugal)
INDAPAMIDE
Indapamide Tablets ... 2188

FLUINOL (Spain)
FLUTICASONE PROPIONATE
Flonase Nasal Spray ... 1431

FLUI-THEOPHYLLINE (Germany)
THEOPHYLLINE
Uniphyl Tablets ... 2595

FLULON (The Philippines)
FLUOROMETHOLONE
FML Ophthalmic Ointment ... ⊙223

FLUMADINE (Israel)
RIMANTADINE HYDROCHLORIDE
Flumadine Syrup ... 1167
Flumadine Tablets ... 1167

FLUMAGE (Argentina)
FLUMAZENIL
Romazicon Injection ... 2646

FLUMANOVAG (Argentina)
FLUMAZENIL
Romazicon Injection ... 2646

FLUMAZEN (Argentina)
FLUMAZENIL
Romazicon Injection ... 2646

FLUMAZIL (Brazil)
FLUMAZENIL
Romazicon Injection ... 2646

FLUMETHOLON (Hong Kong)
FLUOROMETHOLONE
FML Ophthalmic Ointment ... ⊙223

FLUMETOL (Greece, Italy, Turkey)
TIMOLOL MALEATE
Timoptic in Ocudose ... 2124
Timoptic Sterile Ophthalmic Solution ... 2121
Timoptic-XE Sterile Ophthalmic Gel Forming Solution ... 2125

FLUMETOL S (Czech Republic)
FLUOROMETHOLONE
FML Ophthalmic Ointment ... ⊙223

FLUMETOL SEMPLICE (Italy)
FLUOROMETHOLONE
FML Ophthalmic Ointment ... ⊙223

FLUMEX (Brazil)
FLUOROMETHOLONE
FML Ophthalmic Ointment ... ⊙223

FLUMEZINA (Italy)
FLUOROMETHOLONE
FML Ophthalmic Ointment ... ⊙223

FLUMINEX (Italy)
FLUNISOLIDE
Aerobid Inhaler System ... 1153
Aerobid-M Inhaler System ... 1153

FLUMOX (South Africa)
AMOXICILLIN
Amoxil Pediatric Drops for Oral Suspension ... 1305
Amoxil Tablets ... 1305

FLUNASE (Israel)
FLUNISOLIDE
Aerobid Inhaler System ... 1153
Aerobid-M Inhaler System ... 1153

FLUNIGAR (Italy)
FLUNISOLIDE
Aerobid Inhaler System ... 1153
Aerobid-M Inhaler System ... 1153

FLUNITEC (Argentina, Brazil, Denmark, Norway)
FLUNISOLIDE
Aerobid Inhaler System ... 1153
Aerobid-M Inhaler System ... 1153

FLUNITOP (Italy)
FLUNISOLIDE
Aerobid Inhaler System ... 1153
Aerobid-M Inhaler System ... 1153

FLUOFTAL (Austria)
FLUORESCEIN SODIUM
Fluorescite Injection ... ⊙203

FLUORALFA (Italy)
FLUORESCEIN SODIUM
Fluorescite Injection ... ⊙203

FLUOR-AMPS (United Kingdom)
FLUORESCEIN SODIUM
Fluorescite Injection ... ⊙203

FLUORE STAIN STRIPS (India)
FLUORESCEIN SODIUM
Fluorescite Injection ... ⊙203

FLUORES (South Africa)
FLUORESCEIN SODIUM
Fluorescite Injection ... ⊙203

FLUORESCITE (Argentina, Australia, Canada, Czech Republic, Hong Kong, Malaysia, New Zealand, Poland, Singapore, South Africa, Thailand, Turkey)
FLUORESCEIN SODIUM
Fluorescite Injection ... ⊙203

FLUORETS (Australia, Canada, Irish Republic, New Zealand, Singapore, South Africa)
FLUORESCEIN SODIUM
Fluorescite Injection ... ⊙203

FLUOR-I-STRIP AT (Canada)
FLUORESCEIN SODIUM
Fluorescite Injection ... ⊙203

FLUOROMETIL (Mexico)
FLUOROMETHOLONE
FML Ophthalmic Ointment ... ⊙223

FLUORO-OPHTAL (Germany)
FLUOROMETHOLONE
FML Ophthalmic Ointment ... ⊙223

FLUOROPOS (Czech Republic, Germany)
FLUOROMETHOLONE
FML Ophthalmic Ointment ... ⊙223

FLUPAMID (Turkey)
INDAPAMIDE
Indapamide Tablets ... 2188

FLURESS (Australia)
FLUORESCEIN SODIUM
Fluorescite Injection ... ⊙203

FLUROLON (Denmark)
FLUOROMETHOLONE
FML Ophthalmic Ointment ... ⊙223

FLUROP (Portugal)
FLUOROMETHOLONE
FML Ophthalmic Ointment ... ⊙223

FLUSEMINAL (Greece)
NORFLOXACIN
Noroxin Tablets ... 2069

FLUSONAL (Spain)
FLUTICASONE PROPIONATE
Flonase Nasal Spray . . . 1431

FLUSPIRAL (Italy)
FLUTICASONE PROPIONATE
Flonase Nasal Spray . . . 1431

FLUTAIDE (Portugal)
FLUTICASONE PROPIONATE
Flonase Nasal Spray . . . 1431

FLUTANS (Turkey)
INDAPAMIDE
Indapamide Tablets . . . 2188

FLUTIAMIK (Argentina)
FINASTERIDE
Propecia Tablets . . . 2095
Proscar Tablets . . . 2102

FLUTICAPS (Brazil)
FLUTICASONE PROPIONATE
Flonase Nasal Spray . . . 1431

FLUTICORT (Argentina, Venezuela)
FLUTICASONE PROPIONATE
Flonase Nasal Spray . . . 1431

FLUTIDE (Germany, Norway, Sweden, The Netherlands)
FLUTICASONE PROPIONATE
Flonase Nasal Spray . . . 1431

FLUTI-K (Argentina)
FLUTICASONE PROPIONATE
Flonase Nasal Spray . . . 1431

FLUTINASE (Switzerland)
FLUTICASONE PROPIONATE
Flonase Nasal Spray . . . 1431

FLUTIVATE (Brazil, Chile, Germany, Norway, Sweden)
FLUTICASONE PROPIONATE
Flonase Nasal Spray . . . 1431

FLUTIVENT (Argentina)
FLUTICASONE PROPIONATE
Flonase Nasal Spray . . . 1431

FLUXIFARM (Argentina)
FLUMAZENIL
Romazicon Injection . . . 2646

FLUXIL (Brazil)
FUROSEMIDE
Furosemide Tablets . . . 2186

FLUXINAM (Greece)
FLUOROMETHOLONE
FML Ophthalmic Ointment . . . ⊙223

FLUXOCOR (Brazil)
DIPYRIDAMOLE
Persantine Tablets . . . 869

FLUXPIREN (Argentina)
DICLOFENAC SODIUM
Voltaren Tablets . . . 2334
Voltaren-XR Tablets . . . 2337

FML (Argentina, Australia, Belgium, Canada, Finland, Greece, Hong Kong, Irish Republic, Israel, Malaysia, Mexico, New Zealand, Portugal, Singapore, South Africa, Spain, Switzerland, Thailand, The Netherlands, The Philippines, Turkey, United Kingdom)
FLUOROMETHOLONE
FML Ophthalmic Ointment . . . ⊙223

FML NEO (Argentina)
FLUOROMETHOLONE
FML Ophthalmic Ointment . . . ⊙223

FOKALEPSIN (Germany)
CARBAMAZEPINE
Carbatrol Capsules . . . 3019

FOKUSIN (Poland)
TAMSULOSIN HYDROCHLORIDE
Flomax Capsules . . . 848

FOLCRES (Argentina)
FINASTERIDE
Propecia Tablets . . . 2095
Proscar Tablets . . . 2102

FOLITABS (Spain)
FINASTERIDE
Propecia Tablets . . . 2095
Proscar Tablets . . . 2102

FORCAD (The Philippines)
SIMVASTATIN
Zocor Tablets . . . 2136

FORCEF (India)
CEFUROXIME AXETIL
Ceftin for Oral Suspension . . . 1380
Ceftin Tablets . . . 1380

FORCILIN (Argentina)
MODAFINIL
Provigil Tablets . . . 977

FOREXIN (Thailand)
CIPROFLOXACIN
Cipro Oral Suspension . . . 2810

FORGRAM (The Philippines)
CEFTRIAXONE SODIUM
Rocephin Injectable Vials, ADD-Vantage, Galaxy, Bulk . . . 2642

FORMISTIN (Italy)
CETIRIZINE HYDROCHLORIDE
Zyrtec Syrup . . . 1920
Zyrtec Tablets . . . 1920

FORMOL (Argentina)
FORMALDEHYDE
Formadon Solution . . . 1699

FORSEF (Turkey)
CEFTRIAXONE SODIUM
Rocephin Injectable Vials, ADD-Vantage, Galaxy, Bulk . . . 2642

FORTADIM (Thailand)
CEFTAZIDIME
Fortaz for Injection . . . 1450

FORTAM (Spain, Switzerland)
CEFTAZIDIME
Fortaz for Injection . . . 1450

FORTAZ (Brazil, Canada)
CEFTAZIDIME
Fortaz for Injection . . . 1450

FORTENAC (Switzerland)
DICLOFENAC SODIUM
Voltaren Tablets . . . 2334
Voltaren-XR Tablets . . . 2337

FORTERRA (Greece)
CIPROFLOXACIN HYDROCHLORIDE
Cipro Tablets . . . 2810

FORTFEN (South Africa)
DICLOFENAC SODIUM
Voltaren Tablets . . . 2334
Voltaren-XR Tablets . . . 2337

FORTIMAX (Spain)
NORFLOXACIN
Noroxin Tablets . . . 2069

FORTRADOL (Italy)
TRAMADOL HYDROCHLORIDE
Ultram ER Tablets . . . 2428

FORTUM (Argentina, Australia, Austria, Chile, Czech Republic, Denmark, France, Germany, Hong Kong, Hungary, India, Irish Republic, Israel, Malaysia, Mexico, New Zealand, Norway, Poland, Russia, Singapore, South Africa, Sweden, Thailand, The Netherlands, The Philippines, Turkey, United Kingdom, Venezuela)
CEFTAZIDIME
Fortaz for Injection . . . 1450

FORTUMSET (France)
CEFTAZIDIME
Fortaz for Injection . . . 1450

FORTZAAR (Denmark, Germany, Malaysia, Portugal, South Africa, Spain, Thailand, The Netherlands)
LOSARTAN POTASSIUM
Cozaar Tablets . . . 1973

FORZAAR (Italy)
LOSARTAN POTASSIUM
Cozaar Tablets . . . 1973

FORZID (Thailand, The Philippines)
CEFTAZIDIME
Fortaz for Injection . . . 1450

FOSALAN (Israel)
ALENDRONATE SODIUM
Fosamax Tablets . . . 2005

FOSALEN (Greece)
ALENDRONATE SODIUM
Fosamax Tablets . . . 2005

FOSAMAX (Argentina, Australia, Austria, Belgium, Brazil, Canada, Chile, Czech Republic, Denmark, Finland, France, Germany, Greece, Hong Kong, Hungary, Irish Republic, Italy, Malaysia, Mexico, New Zealand, Norway, Poland, Portugal, Russia, Singapore, South Africa, Spain, Sweden, Switzerland, Thailand, The Netherlands, The Philippines, Turkey, United Kingdom, Venezuela)
ALENDRONATE SODIUM
Fosamax Tablets . . . 2005

FOSAMAX PLUS (Argentina, Australia, Hong Kong)
ALENDRONATE SODIUM
Fosamax Tablets . . . 2005

FOSAVANCE (Belgium, Finland, Germany, Irish Republic, Italy, Spain, The Philippines)
ALENDRONATE SODIUM
Fosamax Tablets . . . 2005

FOSKINA (The Philippines)
MUPIROCIN
Bactroban Ointment . . . 1368

FOSVAL (Chile)
ALENDRONATE SODIUM
Fosamax Tablets . . . 2005

FOUCACILLIN (Greece)
CEFUROXIME AXETIL
Ceftin for Oral Suspension . . . 1380
Ceftin Tablets . . . 1380

FOURNOX (Thailand)
CEFTAZIDIME
Fortaz for Injection . . . 1450

FOXIN (Thailand)
NORFLOXACIN
Noroxin Tablets . . . 2069

FOXINON (Thailand)
NORFLOXACIN
Noroxin Tablets . . . 2069

FP TAB (Japan)
SELEGILINE HYDROCHLORIDE
Eldepryl Capsules . . . 3052

FRACTAL (France)
FLUVASTATIN SODIUM
Lescol Capsules . . . 2268

FRANOL (Thailand)
THEOPHYLLINE
Uniphyl Tablets . . . 2595

FRAXIDOL (Italy)
TRAMADOL HYDROCHLORIDE
Ultram ER Tablets . . . 2428

FRECUENTAL (Argentina)
FUROSEMIDE
Furosemide Tablets . . . 2186

FREDYR (Greece)
CEFUROXIME SODIUM
Zinacef Injection . . . 1678

FREMID (The Philippines)
FUROSEMIDE
Furosemide Tablets . . . 2186

FRETIC (The Philippines)
FUROSEMIDE
Furosemide Tablets . . . 2186

FREUDAL (Mexico)
DIAZEPAM
Valium Tablets . . . 2658

FRIBAT (Italy)
CEFTAZIDIME
Fortaz for Injection . . . 1450

FRIMAIND (Italy)
CITALOPRAM HYDROBROMIDE
Celexa Tablets . . . 1160

FRINEG (Italy)
CEFTRIAXONE SODIUM
Rocephin Injectable Vials, ADD-Vantage, Galaxy, Bulk . . . 2642

FRIVENT (Italy)
THEOPHYLLINE
Uniphyl Tablets . . . 2595

FROLICIN (Greece)
AMOXICILLIN
Amoxil Pediatric Drops for Oral Suspension . . . 1305
Amoxil Tablets . . . 1305

FROMIL (Venezuela)
FUROSEMIDE
Furosemide Tablets . . . 2186

FROMILID (Czech Republic, Hungary, Poland, Russia)
CLARITHROMYCIN
Biaxin Filmtab Tablets . . . 411
Biaxin Granules . . . 411

FROOP (United Kingdom)
FUROSEMIDE
Furosemide Tablets . . . 2186

FROSINOR (Spain)
PAROXETINE HYDROCHLORIDE
Paxil Oral Suspension . . . 1535
Paxil Tablets . . . 1535

FROXAL (Mexico)
CEFUROXIME SODIUM
Zinacef Injection . . . 1678

FRUDEMISAN (Mexico)
FUROSEMIDE
Furosemide Tablets . . . 2186

FRUMAX (United Kingdom)
FUROSEMIDE
Furosemide Tablets . . . 2186

FRUMERON (Hong Kong, Thailand)
INDAPAMIDE
Indapamide Tablets . . . 2188

FRUMIL (Greece)
FUROSEMIDE
Furosemide Tablets . . . 2186

FRUSEHEXAL (Australia)
FUROSEMIDE
Furosemide Tablets . . . 2186

FRUSEMA (The Philippines)
FUROSEMIDE
Furosemide Tablets . . . 2186

FRUSEMIX (India)
FUROSEMIDE
Furosemide Tablets . . . 2186

FRUSENE (Irish Republic, United Kingdom)
FUROSEMIDE
Furosemide Tablets . . . 2186

FRUSENEX (India)
FUROSEMIDE
Furosemide Tablets . . . 2186

FRUSETIC (United Kingdom)
FUROSEMIDE
Furosemide Tablets . . . 2186

FRUSID (Australia, Hong Kong, New Zealand, Singapore, United Kingdom)
FUROSEMIDE
Furosemide Tablets . . . 2186

FRUSIDE (Irish Republic)
FUROSEMIDE
Furosemide Tablets . . . 2186

FRUSIX (India)
FUROSEMIDE
Furosemide Tablets . . . 2186

FRUSOL (United Kingdom)
FUROSEMIDE
Furosemide Tablets . . . 2186

FTAZIDIME (Greece)
CEFTAZIDIME
Fortaz for Injection . . . 1450

FTONAVIL (Greece)
CAPTOPRIL
Captopril Tablets . . . 2182

FTOROCORT (Hungary, Russia, Thailand)
TRIAMCINOLONE ACETONIDE
Azmacort Inhalation Aerosol . . . 407
Nasacort AQ Nasal Spray . . . 2765

FUBAXYN (The Philippines)
CEFUROXIME AXETIL
Ceftin for Oral Suspension . . . 1380
Ceftin Tablets . . . 1380

FUCEROX (Mexico)
CEFUROXIME SODIUM
Zinacef Injection 1678

FUDIRINE (Thailand)
FUROSEMIDE
Furosemide Tablets 2186

FUDONE (India)
FAMOTIDINE
Pepcid for Oral Suspension 2075
Pepcid Tablets 2075

FULCRO (Italy)
FENOFIBRATE
Tricor Tablets 520

FUL-GLO (Australia, New Zealand)
FLUORESCEIN SODIUM
Fluorescite Injection . . . . . ⊙203

FULGRAM (Chile, Italy, Venezuela)
NORFLOXACIN
Noroxin Tablets 2069

FUMARENID (Germany)
FUROSEMIDE
Furosemide Tablets 2186

FUNCID (The Philippines)
BUTENAFINE HYDROCHLORIDE
Mentax Cream 2190

FUNDUSCEIN (Canada)
FLUORESCEIN SODIUM
Fluorescite Injection . . . . . ⊙203

FUNGAFINE (Irish Republic)
TERBINAFINE HYDROCHLORIDE
Lamisil Tablets 2266

FUNGASIL (Irish Republic)
TERBINAFINE HYDROCHLORIDE
Lamisil Tablets 2266

FUNGICIDIN (Czech Republic)
NYSTATIN
Nystop Topical Powder USP 2498

FUNGIREDUCT (Germany)
NYSTATIN
Nystop Topical Powder USP 2498

FUNGITIF (The Netherlands)
TERBINAFINE HYDROCHLORIDE
Lamisil Tablets 2266

FUNGOSTATIN (Turkey)
NYSTATIN
Nystop Topical Powder USP 2498

FUNGOTERBINE (Russia)
TERBINAFINE HYDROCHLORIDE
Lamisil Tablets 2266

FUNGUEAL (Argentina)
TERBINAFINE HYDROCHLORIDE
Lamisil Tablets 2266

FUNTOPIC (Venezuela)
TERBINAFINE HYDROCHLORIDE
Lamisil Tablets 2266

FUNTYL (Brazil)
TERBINAFINE HYDROCHLORIDE
Lamisil Tablets 2266

FURAGRAND (Argentina)
FUROSEMIDE
Furosemide Tablets 2186

FURAL (Austria)
FUROSEMIDE
Furosemide Tablets 2186

FURANTHRIL (Czech Republic, Germany)
FUROSEMIDE
Furosemide Tablets 2186

FURAXIL (Greece)
CEFUROXIME AXETIL
Ceftin for Oral Suspension 1380
Ceftin Tablets 1380

FURDIUREN (Venezuela)
FUROSEMIDE
Furosemide Tablets 2186

FURESE (Denmark)
FUROSEMIDE
Furosemide Tablets 2186

FURESIN (Brazil)
FUROSEMIDE
Furosemide Tablets 2186

FURESIS (Finland)
FUROSEMIDE
Furosemide Tablets 2186

FURESIS COMP (Finland)
FUROSEMIDE
Furosemide Tablets 2186

FURETIC (Thailand)
FUROSEMIDE
Furosemide Tablets 2186

FURIDE (Thailand)
FUROSEMIDE
Furosemide Tablets 2186

FURINE (Thailand)
FUROSEMIDE
Furosemide Tablets 2186

FURITAL (Argentina)
FUROSEMIDE
Furosemide Tablets 2186

FURIX (Argentina, Denmark, Norway, Sweden)
FUROSEMIDE
Furosemide Tablets 2186

FURMIDAL (Mexico)
FUROSEMIDE
Furosemide Tablets 2186

FURMIDE (Malaysia)
FUROSEMIDE
Furosemide Tablets 2186

FURO-BASAN (Switzerland)
FUROSEMIDE
Furosemide Tablets 2186

FURO-BASF (Germany)
FUROSEMIDE
Furosemide Tablets 2186

FUROBETA (Germany)
FUROSEMIDE
Furosemide Tablets 2186

FUROCEF (The Philippines)
CEFUROXIME SODIUM
Zinacef Injection 1678

FUROCEM (The Philippines)
CEFUROXIME SODIUM
Zinacef Injection 1678

FUROGAMMA (Germany)
FUROSEMIDE
Furosemide Tablets 2186

FUROHEXAL (Austria)
FUROSEMIDE
Furosemide Tablets 2186

FUROMED (Germany)
FUROSEMIDE
Furosemide Tablets 2186

FUROMID (Turkey)
FUROSEMIDE
Furosemide Tablets 2186

FUROMIL (Mexico)
FUROSEMIDE
Furosemide Tablets 2186

FUROMIN (Finland)
FUROSEMIDE
Furosemide Tablets 2186

FURON (Czech Republic, Hungary)
FUROSEMIDE
Furosemide Tablets 2186

FURONET (Denmark)
FUROSEMIDE
Furosemide Tablets 2186

FURONEX (Mexico)
FUROSEMIDE
Furosemide Tablets 2186

FURO-PUREN (Germany)
FUROSEMIDE
Furosemide Tablets 2186

FURORESE (Czech Republic)
FUROSEMIDE
Furosemide Tablets 2186

FUROSAL (Germany)
FUROSEMIDE
Furosemide Tablets 2186

FUROSAN (Brazil, Mexico)
FUROSEMIDE
Furosemide Tablets 2186

FUROSCAN (The Philippines)
FUROSEMIDE
Furosemide Tablets 2186

FUROSCAND (Sweden)
FUROSEMIDE
Furosemide Tablets 2186

FUROSECORD (Brazil)
FUROSEMIDE
Furosemide Tablets 2186

FUROSEM (Brazil)
FUROSEMIDE
Furosemide Tablets 2186

FUROSEMIX (France)
FUROSEMIDE
Furosemide Tablets 2186

FUROSEN (Brazil)
FUROSEMIDE
Furosemide Tablets 2186

FUROSETRON (Brazil)
FUROSEMIDE
Furosemide Tablets 2186

FUROSIFAR (Switzerland)
FUROSEMIDE
Furosemide Tablets 2186

FUROSIX (Brazil)
FUROSEMIDE
Furosemide Tablets 2186

FUROSTAD (Austria)
FUROSEMIDE
Furosemide Tablets 2186

FUROTER (Mexico)
FUROSEMIDE
Furosemide Tablets 2186

FUROTOP (Belgium)
FUROSEMIDE
Furosemide Tablets 2186

FUROTYROL (Austria)
FUROSEMIDE
Furosemide Tablets 2186

FUROVITE (Israel)
FUROSEMIDE
Furosemide Tablets 2186

FUROXIM (Austria)
CEFUROXIME AXETIL
Ceftin for Oral Suspension 1380
Ceftin Tablets 1380

FUROXY (The Philippines)
CEFUROXIME SODIUM
Zinacef Injection 1678

FUROZIX (Brazil)
FUROSEMIDE
Furosemide Tablets 2186

FURSEMIDA (Brazil)
FUROSEMIDE
Furosemide Tablets 2186

FURSOL (Switzerland)
FUROSEMIDE
Furosemide Tablets 2186

FURTENK (Argentina)
FUROSEMIDE
Furosemide Tablets 2186

FUSERIDE (Thailand)
FUROSEMIDE
Furosemide Tablets 2186

FUSID (Germany, Israel, The Netherlands)
FUROSEMIDE
Furosemide Tablets 2186

FUSIMEX (The Philippines)
FUROSEMIDE
Furosemide Tablets 2186

FUSTAREN (Mexico)
DICLOFENAC SODIUM
Voltaren Tablets 2334
Voltaren-XR Tablets 2337

FUXEN (Mexico)
NAPROXEN
EC-Naprosyn Delayed-Release Tablets 2632
Naprosyn Suspension 2632
Naprosyn Tablets 2632

GAAP OFTENO (Venezuela)
LATANOPROST
Xalatan Ophthalmic Solution . . . . . ⊙273

GAAX (Chile)
LATANOPROST
Xalatan Ophthalmic Solution . . . . . ⊙273

GAAX T (Chile)
LATANOPROST
Xalatan Ophthalmic Solution . . . . . ⊙273

GABATRIL (Mexico)
TIAGABINE HYDROCHLORIDE
Gabitril Tablets 973

GABIROL (Mexico)
RIMANTADINE HYDROCHLORIDE
Flumadine Syrup 1167
Flumadine Tablets 1167

GABITRIL (Australia, Austria, Belgium, Brazil, Czech Republic, Denmark, Finland, France, Germany, Greece, Hungary, Irish Republic, Italy, Poland, Portugal, Spain, Switzerland, United Kingdom)
TIAGABINE HYDROCHLORIDE
Gabitril Tablets 973

GABOX (Venezuela)
CARBAMAZEPINE
Carbatrol Capsules 3019

GALEBIRON (Greece)
RANITIDINE HYDROCHLORIDE
Zantac 25 EFFERdose Tablets 1670
Zantac 150 Tablets 1670
Zantac 300 Tablets 1670
Zantac Injection 1666
Zantac Injection Premixed 1666
Zantac Syrup 1670

GALEDOL (Mexico)
DICLOFENAC SODIUM
Voltaren Tablets 2334
Voltaren-XR Tablets 2337

GALEMIN (Greece)
CEFUROXIME SODIUM
Zinacef Injection 1678

GALIDRIN (Mexico)
RANITIDINE HYDROCHLORIDE
Zantac 25 EFFERdose Tablets 1670
Zantac 150 Tablets 1670
Zantac 300 Tablets 1670
Zantac Injection 1666
Zantac Injection Premixed 1666
Zantac Syrup 1670

GAMMAKINE (Italy)
INTERFERON GAMMA-1B
Actimmune 1743

GANAVAX (Argentina)
VENLAFAXINE HYDROCHLORIDE
Effexor XR Capsules 3195

GANOR (Germany)
FAMOTIDINE
Pepcid for Oral Suspension 2075
Pepcid Tablets 2075

GANVIREL (Argentina)
LAMIVUDINE
Epivir Oral Solution 1412
Epivir Tablets 1412
Epivir-HBV Oral Solution 1417
Epivir-HBV Tablets 1417

GANVIREL DUO (Argentina)
LAMIVUDINE
Epivir Oral Solution 1412
Epivir Tablets 1412
Epivir-HBV Oral Solution 1417
Epivir-HBV Tablets 1417

GAOPTOL (Monaco)
TIMOLOL MALEATE
Timoptic in Ocudose 2124
Timoptic Sterile Ophthalmic Solution 2121
Timoptic-XE Sterile Ophthalmic Gel Forming Solution 2125

GAPROXEN (Greece)
RANITIDINE HYDROCHLORIDE
Zantac 25 EFFERdose Tablets 1670
Zantac 150 Tablets 1670
Zantac 300 Tablets 1670
Zantac Injection 1666
Zantac Injection Premixed 1666
Zantac Syrup 1670

GARANIL (Spain)
CAPTOPRIL
Captopril Tablets 2182

GARDEX (Denmark, Finland)
CETIRIZINE HYDROCHLORIDE
Zyrtec Syrup 1920

Zyrtec Tablets 1920

GARDOTON (Chile)
ONDANSETRON
Zofran ODT Orally Disintegrating Tablets .. 1687

GARRANIL (Spain)
CAPTOPRIL
Captopril Tablets 2182

GASCOP (Mexico)
ALBENDAZOLE
Albenza Tablets 1297

GASTAC (Venezuela)
RANITIDINE HYDROCHLORIDE
Zantac 25 EFFERdose Tablets 1670
Zantac 150 Tablets 1670
Zantac 300 Tablets 1670
Zantac Injection 1666
Zantac Injection Premixed 1666
Zantac Syrup 1670

GASTENIN (Spain)
FAMOTIDINE
Pepcid for Oral Suspension 2075
Pepcid Tablets 2075

GASTER (Japan)
FAMOTIDINE
Pepcid for Oral Suspension 2075
Pepcid Tablets 2075

GASTEROGEN (Greece)
FAMOTIDINE
Pepcid for Oral Suspension 2075
Pepcid Tablets 2075

GASTEROL (Turkey)
FAMOTIDINE
Pepcid for Oral Suspension 2075
Pepcid Tablets 2075

GASTIFAM (Turkey)
FAMOTIDINE
Pepcid for Oral Suspension 2075
Pepcid Tablets 2075

GASTOPRIDE (Portugal)
FAMOTIDINE
Pepcid for Oral Suspension 2075
Pepcid Tablets 2075

GASTRAL (Spain)
SUCRALFATE
Carafate Suspension 706
Carafate Tablets 707

GASTRIDIN (Italy, Mexico)
FAMOTIDINE
Pepcid for Oral Suspension 2075
Pepcid Tablets 2075

GASTRIDINA (Portugal)
RANITIDINE HYDROCHLORIDE
Zantac 25 EFFERdose Tablets 1670
Zantac 150 Tablets 1670
Zantac 300 Tablets 1670
Zantac Injection 1666
Zantac Injection Premixed 1666
Zantac Syrup 1670

GASTRIFAM (Portugal)
FAMOTIDINE
Pepcid for Oral Suspension 2075
Pepcid Tablets 2075

GASTRIL (Hong Kong)
RANITIDINE HYDROCHLORIDE
Zantac 25 EFFERdose Tablets 1670
Zantac 150 Tablets 1670
Zantac 300 Tablets 1670
Zantac Injection 1666
Zantac Injection Premixed 1666
Zantac Syrup 1670

GASTRION (Spain)
FAMOTIDINE
Pepcid for Oral Suspension 2075
Pepcid Tablets 2075

GASTRIUM (Chile)
FAMOTIDINE
Pepcid for Oral Suspension 2075
Pepcid Tablets 2075

GASTRO (Israel)
FAMOTIDINE
Pepcid for Oral Suspension 2075
Pepcid Tablets 2075

GASTROCOL (Chile)
SUCRALFATE
Carafate Suspension 706
Carafate Tablets 707

GASTRODOMINA (Hong Kong, Spain)
FAMOTIDINE
Pepcid for Oral Suspension 2075
Pepcid Tablets 2075

GASTROFAM (Turkey)
FAMOTIDINE
Pepcid for Oral Suspension 2075
Pepcid Tablets 2075

GASTROGEL (Italy, Switzerland)
SUCRALFATE
Carafate Suspension 706
Carafate Tablets 707

GASTROLAV (Portugal)
RANITIDINE HYDROCHLORIDE
Zantac 25 EFFERdose Tablets 1670
Zantac 150 Tablets 1670
Zantac 300 Tablets 1670
Zantac Injection 1666
Zantac Injection Premixed 1666
Zantac Syrup 1670

GASTROLETS (Argentina)
RANITIDINE HYDROCHLORIDE
Zantac 25 EFFERdose Tablets 1670
Zantac 150 Tablets 1670
Zantac 300 Tablets 1670
Zantac Injection 1666
Zantac Injection Premixed 1666
Zantac Syrup 1670

GASTROPEN (Spain)
FAMOTIDINE
Pepcid for Oral Suspension 2075
Pepcid Tablets 2075

GASTROSEDOL (Argentina)
RANITIDINE HYDROCHLORIDE
Zantac 25 EFFERdose Tablets 1670
Zantac 150 Tablets 1670
Zantac 300 Tablets 1670
Zantac Injection 1666
Zantac Injection Premixed 1666
Zantac Syrup 1670

GASTROSIDIN (Russia, Turkey)
FAMOTIDINE
Pepcid for Oral Suspension 2075
Pepcid Tablets 2075

GASTRULCER (Portugal)
RANITIDINE HYDROCHLORIDE
Zantac 25 EFFERdose Tablets 1670
Zantac 150 Tablets 1670
Zantac 300 Tablets 1670
Zantac Injection 1666
Zantac Injection Premixed 1666
Zantac Syrup 1670

GATINAR (Spain, Switzerland)
LACTULOSE
Kristalose for Oral Solution 1004

GAVILAST (United Kingdom)
RANITIDINE HYDROCHLORIDE
Zantac 25 EFFERdose Tablets 1670
Zantac 150 Tablets 1670
Zantac 300 Tablets 1670
Zantac Injection 1666
Zantac Injection Premixed 1666
Zantac Syrup 1670

GEFINA (Finland)
FINASTERIDE
Propecia Tablets 2095
Proscar Tablets 2102

GELBAG (Germany)
SODIUM HYALURONATE
Hyalgan Solution 2742

GELCAIN (Chile)
LIDOCAINE
Lidoderm Patch 1114

GELESTRA (Italy)
ESTRADIOL
Climara Transdermal System 763

GEL-LIDO (Brazil)
LIDOCAINE
Lidoderm Patch 1114

GEL-OSE (Canada)
LACTULOSE
Kristalose for Oral Solution 1004

GEMCITE (India)
GEMCITABINE HYDROCHLORIDE
Gemzar for Injection 1820

GEMISTATIN (Argentina)
SIMVASTATIN
Zocor Tablets 2136

GEMTRO (Argentina)
GEMCITABINE HYDROCHLORIDE
Gemzar for Injection 1820

GEMZAR (Australia, Austria, Belgium, Brazil, Canada, Chile, Czech Republic, Denmark, Finland, France, Germany, Greece, Hong Kong, Hungary, Irish Republic, Israel, Italy, Malaysia, Mexico, New Zealand, Norway, Poland, Portugal, Russia, Singapore, South Africa, Spain, Sweden, Switzerland, Thailand, The Netherlands, The Philippines, Turkey, United Kingdom, Venezuela)
GEMCITABINE HYDROCHLORIDE
Gemzar for Injection 1820

GEMZIL (Thailand)
CAPTOPRIL
Captopril Tablets 2182

GENALEN (Italy)
ALENDRONATE SODIUM
Fosamax Tablets 2005

GENALGEN (Mexico)
NAPROXEN
EC-Naprosyn Delayed-Release Tablets 2632
Naprosyn Suspension 2632
Naprosyn Tablets 2632

GENAPROST (Italy)
FINASTERIDE
Propecia Tablets 2095
Proscar Tablets 2102

GENDAZEL (Thailand)
ALBENDAZOLE
Albenza Tablets 1297

GENEPHOXAL (Greece)
CEFUROXIME AXETIL
Ceftin for Oral Suspension 1380
Ceftin Tablets 1380

GENERLOG (Thailand)
TRIAMCINOLONE ACETONIDE
Azmacort Inhalation Aerosol 407
Nasacort AQ Nasal Spray 2765

GENGIGEL (Portugal)
SODIUM HYALURONATE
Hyalgan Solution 2742

GENITOFLOX (Brazil)
NORFLOXACIN
Noroxin Tablets 2069

GENLAC (Australia)
LACTULOSE
Kristalose for Oral Solution 1004

GEN-LAC (Canada)
LACTULOSE
Kristalose for Oral Solution 1004

GENMOX (India)
AMOXICILLIN
Amoxil Pediatric Drops for Oral Suspension 1305
Amoxil Tablets 1305

GENOCOLAN (Argentina)
LACTULOSE
Kristalose for Oral Solution 1004

GENOVOX (Greece)
NIMODIPINE
Nimotop Capsules 790

GENOXEN (Hong Kong, Irish Republic)
NAPROXEN
EC-Naprosyn Delayed-Release Tablets 2632
Naprosyn Suspension 2632
Naprosyn Tablets 2632

GENPROL (Spain)
CITALOPRAM HYDROBROMIDE
Celexa Tablets 1160

GEN-TIMOLOL (New Zealand)
TIMOLOL MALEATE
Timoptic in Ocudose 2124
Timoptic Sterile Ophthalmic Solution 2121
Timoptic-XE Sterile Ophthalmic Gel Forming Solution 2125

GENTIRAN (Greece)
CETIRIZINE HYDROCHLORIDE
Zyrtec Syrup 1920
Zyrtec Tablets 1920

GEPROMI (Mexico)
PROGESTERONE
Crinone 4% Gel 992
Prometrium Capsules (100 mg, 200 mg) . 3047

GERELAX (Irish Republic, Israel)
LACTULOSE
Kristalose for Oral Solution 1004

GERICARB (Irish Republic)
CARBAMAZEPINE
Carbatrol Capsules 3019

GERINAP (Irish Republic)
NAPROXEN
EC-Naprosyn Delayed-Release Tablets 2632
Naprosyn Suspension 2632
Naprosyn Tablets 2632

GEROLAMIC (Austria)
LAMOTRIGINE
Lamictal Chewable Dispersible Tablets 1488
Lamictal Tablets 1488

GEROSIM (Austria)
SIMVASTATIN
Zocor Tablets 2136

GEROTEN (Irish Republic)
CAPTOPRIL
Captopril Tablets 2182

GERTAC (Irish Republic)
RANITIDINE HYDROCHLORIDE
Zantac 25 EFFERdose Tablets 1670
Zantac 150 Tablets 1670
Zantac 300 Tablets 1670
Zantac Injection 1666
Zantac Injection Premixed 1666
Zantac Syrup 1670

GERTOCALM (Greece)
RANITIDINE HYDROCHLORIDE
Zantac 25 EFFERdose Tablets 1670
Zantac 150 Tablets 1670
Zantac 300 Tablets 1670
Zantac Injection 1666
Zantac Injection Premixed 1666
Zantac Syrup 1670

GERVAKEN (Mexico)
CLARITHROMYCIN
Biaxin Filmtab Tablets 411
Biaxin Granules 411

GERXIDIN (Venezuela)
CIPROFLOXACIN
Cipro Oral Suspension 2810

GESICAIN (India)
LIDOCAINE
Lidoderm Patch 1114

GESIPROX (Singapore)
NAPROXEN SODIUM
Anaprox DS Tablets 2632
Anaprox Tablets 2632

GESLUTIN (Mexico)
PROGESTERONE
Crinone 4% Gel 992
Prometrium Capsules (100 mg, 200 mg) . 3047

GESTER (Argentina)
PROGESTERONE
Crinone 4% Gel 992
Prometrium Capsules (100 mg, 200 mg) . 3047

GESTEROL (Canada)
PROGESTERONE
Crinone 4% Gel 992
Prometrium Capsules (100 mg, 200 mg) . 3047

GESTONE (Israel, New Zealand, Thailand, United Kingdom)
PROGESTERONE
Crinone 4% Gel 992
Prometrium Capsules (100 mg, 200 mg) . 3047

GEWACALM (Austria)
DIAZEPAM
Valium Tablets 2658

GEWAZEM (Austria)
DILTIAZEM HYDROCHLORIDE
Cardizem LA Extended Release Tablets 421

GEZT (Argentina)
GEMCITABINE HYDROCHLORIDE
Gemzar for Injection 1820

GIBAC (Mexico)
CIPROFLOXACIN
Cipro Oral Suspension 2810

GIBICEF (Italy)
CEFUROXIME SODIUM
Zinacef Injection 1678

GIBIFLU (Italy)
FLUNISOLIDE
Aerobid Inhaler System 1153
Aerobid-M Inhaler System 1153

GIBINAP (Italy)
NAPROXEN SODIUM
Anaprox DS Tablets 2632
Anaprox Tablets 2632

GIBIXEN (Italy)
NAPROXEN
EC-Naprosyn Delayed-Release Tablets 2632
Naprosyn Suspension 2632
Naprosyn Tablets 2632

GIMABROL (Mexico)
AMOXICILLIN
Amoxil Pediatric Drops for Oral Suspension 1305
Amoxil Tablets 1305

GINAIKOS (Italy)
ESTRADIOL
Climara Transdermal System 763

GINATEX (Argentina)
ESTRADIOL
Climara Transdermal System 763

GINECOSID (Venezuela)
PROGESTERONE
Crinone 4% Gel 992
Prometrium Capsules (100 mg, 200 mg) . 3047

GINECOSIDE (Brazil)
PROGESTERONE
Crinone 4% Gel 992
Prometrium Capsules (100 mg, 200 mg) . 3047

GINEDISC (Brazil, Mexico)
ESTRADIOL
Climara Transdermal System 763

GINEFOLIN (Chile)
ESTRADIOL
Climara Transdermal System 763

GINO CIRIAX (Argentina)
CIPROFLOXACIN HYDROCHLORIDE
Cipro Tablets 2810

GINODERM (Chile)
ESTRADIOL
Climara Transdermal System 763

GINORECTOL (Greece, Singapore)
CIPROFLOXACIN HYDROCHLORIDE
Cipro Tablets 2810

GIROFLOX (Portugal, Spain)
CIPROFLOXACIN
Cipro Oral Suspension 2810

GI-TAK (South Africa)
RANITIDINE HYDROCHLORIDE
Zantac 25 EFFERdose Tablets 1670
Zantac 150 Tablets 1670
Zantac 300 Tablets 1670
Zantac Injection 1666
Zantac Injection Premixed 1666
Zantac Syrup 1670

GIVAIR (Italy)
FLUNISOLIDE
Aerobid Inhaler System 1153
Aerobid-M Inhaler System 1153

GLADIUS (Greece)
CEFTRIAXONE SODIUM
Rocephin Injectable Vials, ADD-Vantage, Galaxy, Bulk 2642

GLAFEMAK (Greece)
TIMOLOL MALEATE
Timoptic in Ocudose 2124
Timoptic Sterile Ophthalmic Solution 2121
Timoptic-XE Sterile Ophthalmic Gel Forming Solution 2125

GLATIM (Argentina)
TIMOLOL MALEATE
Timoptic in Ocudose 2124
Timoptic Sterile Ophthalmic Solution 2121
Timoptic-XE Sterile Ophthalmic Gel Forming Solution 2125

GLAUCOL (United Kingdom)
TIMOLOL MALEATE
Timoptic in Ocudose 2124
Timoptic Sterile Ophthalmic Solution 2121
Timoptic-XE Sterile Ophthalmic Gel Forming Solution 2125

GLAUCO-OPH (Hong Kong, Thailand)
TIMOLOL MALEATE
Timoptic in Ocudose 2124
Timoptic Sterile Ophthalmic Solution 2121
Timoptic-XE Sterile Ophthalmic Gel Forming Solution 2125

GLAUCOSAN (South Africa)
TIMOLOL MALEATE
Timoptic in Ocudose 2124
Timoptic Sterile Ophthalmic Solution 2121
Timoptic-XE Sterile Ophthalmic Gel Forming Solution 2125

GLAUCOSTAT (Argentina)
LATANOPROST
Xalatan Ophthalmic Solution . . . . . ⊙273

GLAUCOTENSIL (Chile)
DORZOLAMIDE HYDROCHLORIDE
Trusopt Sterile Ophthalmic Solution 2128

GLAUCOTENSIL D (Venezuela)
DORZOLAMIDE HYDROCHLORIDE
Trusopt Sterile Ophthalmic Solution 2128

GLAUCOTENSIL T (Chile, Venezuela)
DORZOLAMIDE HYDROCHLORIDE/ TIMOLOL MALEATE
Cosopt Sterile Ophthalmic Solution 1969

GLAUSINE (Austria)
CLONIDINE HYDROCHLORIDE
Catapres Tablets 841

GLAUSOLETS (Chile)
TIMOLOL MALEATE
Timoptic in Ocudose 2124
Timoptic Sterile Ophthalmic Solution 2121
Timoptic-XE Sterile Ophthalmic Gel Forming Solution 2125

GLAUSOLETS PLUS (Chile)
DORZOLAMIDE HYDROCHLORIDE
Trusopt Sterile Ophthalmic Solution 2128

GLAUTIMOL (Brazil)
TIMOLOL MALEATE
Timoptic in Ocudose 2124
Timoptic Sterile Ophthalmic Solution 2121
Timoptic-XE Sterile Ophthalmic Gel Forming Solution 2125

GLAXOPROST (Austria)
EPOPROSTENOL SODIUM
Flolan for Injection 1426

GLAXOSETRON (Austria)
ONDANSETRON
Zofran ODT Orally Disintegrating Tablets . . 1687

GLAXOTRIPTAN (Austria)
SUMATRIPTAN SUCCINATE
Imitrex Injection 1465
Imitrex Tablets 1474

GLAZIDIM (Belgium, Finland, Italy)
CEFTAZIDIME
Fortaz for Injection 1450

GLEVO (India)
LEVOFLOXACIN
Levaquin Injection 2416
Levaquin Tablets 2416

GLIADEL (Australia, Brazil, Canada, Chile, France, Greece, Israel, Italy, New Zealand, Portugal, Singapore, South Africa, Spain, The Netherlands, United Kingdom)
CARMUSTINE
Gliadel Wafer 1076

GLICOBASE (Italy)
ACARBOSE
Precose Tablets 792

GLIFAPEN (Argentina)
AMOXICILLIN
Amoxil Pediatric Drops for Oral Suspension 1305
Amoxil Tablets 1305

GLIMIDE (Argentina)
ROSIGLITAZONE MALEATE
Avandia Tablets 1351

GLIOSARTAN (Argentina)
TELMISARTAN
Micardis Tablets 852

GLIOSARTAN PLUS (Argentina)
TELMISARTAN
Micardis Tablets 852

GLITA (India)
PIOGLITAZONE HYDROCHLORIDE
Actos Tablets 3077

GLOBITAN (Venezuela)
TIMOLOL MALEATE
Timoptic in Ocudose 2124
Timoptic Sterile Ophthalmic Solution 2121
Timoptic-XE Sterile Ophthalmic Gel Forming Solution 2125

GLOBUCE (Spain)
CIPROFLOXACIN HYDROCHLORIDE
Cipro Tablets 2810

GLOBUREN (Italy)
EPOETIN ALFA
Epogen for Injection 576
Procrit for Injection 2391

GLOCURE-OPTA (The Philippines)
TIMOLOL MALEATE
Timoptic in Ocudose 2124
Timoptic Sterile Ophthalmic Solution 2121
Timoptic-XE Sterile Ophthalmic Gel Forming Solution 2125

GLORIXONE (Greece)
CEFTRIAXONE SODIUM
Rocephin Injectable Vials, ADD-Vantage, Galaxy, Bulk 2642

GLOSSYFIN (Greece)
CIPROFLOXACIN HYDROCHLORIDE
Cipro Tablets 2810

GLUBOSE (India)
ACARBOSE
Precose Tablets 792

GLUCAGEN (Argentina, Australia, Austria, Belgium, Czech Republic, Denmark, Finland, France, Germany, Greece, Hong Kong, Hungary, India, Irish Republic, Israel, Italy, Malaysia, New Zealand, Poland, Portugal, Russia, Singapore, South Africa, Spain, Switzerland, Thailand, The Netherlands, Turkey, United Kingdom)
GLUCAGON HYDROCHLORIDE
Glucagon for Injection Vials and Emergency Kit 1827

GLUCAR (India)
ACARBOSE
Precose Tablets 792

GLUCOBAY (Argentina, Australia, Austria, Belgium, Brazil, Chile, Czech Republic, Denmark, Finland, Greece, Hong Kong, Hungary, India, Irish Republic, Italy, Malaysia, Mexico, New Zealand, Norway, Poland, Portugal, Russia, Singapore, South Africa, Spain, Sweden, Switzerland, Thailand, The Netherlands, The Philippines, Turkey, United Kingdom, Venezuela)
ACARBOSE
Precose Tablets 792

GLUCOMOL (India)
TIMOLOL MALEATE
Timoptic in Ocudose 2124
Timoptic Sterile Ophthalmic Solution 2121
Timoptic-XE Sterile Ophthalmic Gel Forming Solution 2125

GLUCONASE (The Philippines)
ACARBOSE
Precose Tablets 792

GLUCOR (France)
ACARBOSE
Precose Tablets 792

GLUCOTIM (India)
TIMOLOL MALEATE
Timoptic in Ocudose 2124
Timoptic Sterile Ophthalmic Solution 2121
Timoptic-XE Sterile Ophthalmic Gel Forming Solution 2125

GLUDEX (Argentina)
ROSIGLITAZONE MALEATE
Avandia Tablets 1351

GLUDEX PLUS (Argentina)
ROSIGLITAZONE MALEATE
Avandia Tablets 1351

GLUMIDA (Spain)
ACARBOSE
Precose Tablets 792

GLUSTAR (Venezuela)
ATORVASTATIN CALCIUM
Lipitor Tablets 2501

GLUSTIN (The Netherlands)
PIOGLITAZONE HYDROCHLORIDE
Actos Tablets 3077

GLUTASEDAN (Argentina)
DIAZEPAM
Valium Tablets 2658

GLUTASEY (Spain)
SIMVASTATIN
Zocor Tablets 2136

GLYMOL (Russia)
TIMOLOL MALEATE
Timoptic in Ocudose 2124
Timoptic Sterile Ophthalmic Solution 2121
Timoptic-XE Sterile Ophthalmic Gel Forming Solution 2125

GLYNOSE (Turkey)
ACARBOSE
Precose Tablets 792

GLYTOP (Argentina)
TRIAMCINOLONE ACETONIDE
Azmacort Inhalation Aerosol 407
Nasacort AQ Nasal Spray 2765

GNOSTOVAL (Greece)
LISINOPRIL
Prinivil Tablets 2087

GOBANAL (Spain)
DIAZEPAM
Valium Tablets 2658

GOBBICAINA (Argentina)
LIDOCAINE
Lidoderm Patch 1114

GODAFILIN (Spain)
THEOPHYLLINE
Uniphyl Tablets 2595

GOLAN (Mexico)
FUROSEMIDE
Furosemide Tablets 2186

GOLDASTATIN (Greece)
SIMVASTATIN
Zocor Tablets 2136

GOLYSINE (Argentina)
CIPROFLOXACIN
Cipro Oral Suspension 2810

GONDONAR (Argentina)
ANASTROZOLE
Arimidex Tablets 672

GONIF (Greece)
CEFUROXIME SODIUM
Zinacef Injection 1678

GONNING (Hong Kong)
CIPROFLOXACIN
Cipro Oral Suspension 2810

GONORCIN (Thailand)
NORFLOXACIN
Noroxin Tablets 2069

GO-ON (Germany, Hong Kong, Italy, Malaysia)
SODIUM HYALURONATE
Hyalgan Solution 2742

GOPTEN (Australia, Austria, Brazil, Denmark, Finland, France, Germany, Hungary, Irish Republic, Italy, Mexico, New Zealand, Norway, Poland, Portugal, South Africa, Spain, Sweden, Switzerland, The Netherlands, Turkey, United Kingdom)
TRANDOLAPRIL
Mavik Tablets 472

GORDOX (Czech Republic, Hungary, Russia)
APROTININ
Trasylol Injection 799

GOTAS OTOLOGICAS (Chile)
LIDOCAINE
Lidoderm Patch 1114

GOTELY (Chile)
TAMSULOSIN HYDROCHLORIDE
Flomax Capsules 848

GRAMAGEN (Argentina)
GEMCITABINE HYDROCHLORIDE
Gemzar for Injection 1820

GRATEN (Mexico)
MORPHINE SULFATE
MS Contin Tablets 2585

(⊙ Described in PDR® For Ophthalmic Medicines)

GRAVIDEX (Spain)
DINOPROSTONE
Cervidil Vaginal Insert 1165

GRAY-F (Argentina)
FENTANYL CITRATE
Actiq 959

GRENIS (Greece)
NORFLOXACIN
Noroxin Tablets 2069

GRENIS-CIPRO (Greece)
CIPROFLOXACIN HYDROCHLORIDE
Cipro Tablets 2810

GREPIFLOX (Argentina)
LEVOFLOXACIN
Levaquin Injection 2416
Levaquin Tablets 2416

GREXIN (Thailand)
DIGOXIN
Lanoxin Injection 1498
Lanoxin Injection Pediatric 1502
Lanoxin Tablets 1505

GRIFOCIPROX (Chile)
CIPROFLOXACIN
Cipro Oral Suspension 2810

GRIFODILZEM (Chile)
DILTIAZEM HYDROCHLORIDE
Cardizem LA Extended Release Tablets 421

GRIFONIMOD (Chile)
NIMODIPINE
Nimotop Capsules 790

GRIFOTRIAXONA (Chile)
CEFTRIAXONE SODIUM
Rocephin Injectable Vials, ADD-Vantage, Galaxy, Bulk 2642

GROFENAC (Hong Kong, Switzerland)
DICLOFENAC SODIUM
Voltaren Tablets 2334
Voltaren-XR Tablets 2337

GROFIBRAT (Czech Republic, Poland)
FENOFIBRATE
Tricor Tablets 520

GUTRON (Austria, Chile, Czech Republic, France, Germany, Hong Kong, Hungary, Israel, Italy, Mexico, New Zealand, Poland, Portugal, Russia, Singapore, Switzerland, Thailand, The Netherlands)
MIDODRINE HYDROCHLORIDE
ProAmatine Tablets 3032

GYNESTREL (Italy)
NAPROXEN SODIUM
Anaprox DS Tablets 2632
Anaprox Tablets 2632

GYNPOLAR (Germany)
ESTRADIOL
Climara Transdermal System 763

GYRABLOCK (Czech Republic, Russia, Singapore, Thailand)
NORFLOXACIN
Noroxin Tablets 2069

GYRACIP (Germany)
CIPROFLOXACIN
Cipro Oral Suspension 2810

H2 BLOC (The Philippines)
FAMOTIDINE
Pepcid for Oral Suspension 2075
Pepcid Tablets 2075

H2OXYL (Canada, Germany, Switzerland)
BENZOYL PEROXIDE
Brevoxyl-4 Creamy Wash 3054
Brevoxyl-4 Gel 3054
Brevoxyl-8 Creamy Wash 3054
Brevoxyl-8 Gel 3054

HAEMITON (Germany, Russia)
CLONIDINE HYDROCHLORIDE
Catapres Tablets 841

HAEMITON-AUGENTROPFEN (Germany)
CLONIDINE HYDROCHLORIDE
Catapres Tablets 841

HALDID (Denmark)
FENTANYL CITRATE
Actiq 959

HALF CAPOZIDE (Irish Republic)
CAPTOPRIL
Captopril Tablets 2182

HALONIX (India)
SODIUM HYALURONATE
Hyalgan Solution 2742

HAMOXILLIN (Hong Kong)
AMOXICILLIN
Amoxil Pediatric Drops for Oral Suspension 1305
Amoxil Tablets 1305

HARIFIN (Thailand)
FINASTERIDE
Propecia Tablets 2095
Proscar Tablets 2102

HARNAL (Hong Kong, Japan, Thailand, The Philippines)
TAMSULOSIN HYDROCHLORIDE
Flomax Capsules 848

HART (Argentina)
DILTIAZEM HYDROCHLORIDE
Cardizem LA Extended Release Tablets 421

HARTYLOX (The Philippines)
CAPTOPRIL
Captopril Tablets 2182

HAWKMIDE (Thailand)
FUROSEMIDE
Furosemide Tablets 2186

HAYFEVER & ALLERGY RELIEF (United Kingdom)
CETIRIZINE HYDROCHLORIDE
Zyrtec Syrup 1920
Zyrtec Tablets 1920

HAYFEVER RELIEF (United Kingdom)
CETIRIZINE HYDROCHLORIDE
Zyrtec Syrup 1920
Zyrtec Tablets 1920

HEALON (Australia, Belgium, Brazil, Canada, Chile, Czech Republic, Finland, France, Germany, Hong Kong, Hungary, Israel, Italy, Malaysia, New Zealand, Norway, Russia, Singapore, South Africa, Sweden, Switzerland, Thailand, The Netherlands, Turkey, Venezuela)
SODIUM HYALURONATE
Hyalgan Solution 2742

HEALONID (Austria, France, Irish Republic, United Kingdom)
SODIUM HYALURONATE
Hyalgan Solution 2742

HEARTBURN RELIEF (Australia)
RANITIDINE HYDROCHLORIDE
Zantac 25 EFFERdose Tablets 1670
Zantac 150 Tablets 1670
Zantac 300 Tablets 1670
Zantac Injection 1666
Zantac Injection Premixed 1666
Zantac Syrup 1670

HEINIX (Finland)
CETIRIZINE HYDROCHLORIDE
Zyrtec Syrup 1920
Zyrtec Tablets 1920

HEKTULOSE (Germany)
LACTULOSE
Kristalose for Oral Solution 1004

HELAL (Venezuela)
ALBENDAZOLE
Albenza Tablets 1297

HELICLAR (Belgium)
CLARITHROMYCIN
Biaxin Filmtab Tablets 411
Biaxin Granules 411

HELICODID (Brazil)
CLARITHROMYCIN
Biaxin Filmtab Tablets 411
Biaxin Granules 411

HELIMOX (Italy)
AMOXICILLIN
Amoxil Pediatric Drops for Oral Suspension 1305
Amoxil Tablets 1305

HELIPAC (India)
AMOXICILLIN
Amoxil Pediatric Drops for Oral Suspension 1305
Amoxil Tablets 1305

HELMINE (Spain)
ONDANSETRON HYDROCHLORIDE
Zofran Injection 1682
Zofran Injection Premixed 1682
Zofran Oral Solution 1687
Zofran Tablets 1687

HELMINTAL (Brazil)
ALBENDAZOLE
Albenza Tablets 1297

HELMISONS (Mexico)
ALBENDAZOLE
Albenza Tablets 1297

HEMAX (Thailand)
EPOETIN ALFA
Epogen for Injection 576
Procrit for Injection 2391

HEMIGOXINE NATIVELLE (France)
DIGOXIN
Lanoxin Injection 1498
Lanoxin Injection Pediatric 1502
Lanoxin Tablets 1505

HENEXAL (Mexico)
FUROSEMIDE
Furosemide Tablets 2186

HEPALAC (Thailand)
LACTULOSE
Kristalose for Oral Solution 1004

HEPA-MERZ LACT (Germany)
LACTULOSE
Kristalose for Oral Solution 1004

HEPATICUM-LAC-MEDICE (Germany)
LACTULOSE
Kristalose for Oral Solution 1004

HEPRONE (Spain)
SUCRALFATE
Carafate Suspension 706
Carafate Tablets 707

HEPTODINE (Argentina, Venezuela)
LAMIVUDINE
Epivir Oral Solution 1412
Epivir Tablets 1412
Epivir-HBV Oral Solution 1417
Epivir-HBV Tablets 1417

HEPTOVIR (Canada)
LAMIVUDINE
Epivir Oral Solution 1412
Epivir Tablets 1412
Epivir-HBV Oral Solution 1417
Epivir-HBV Tablets 1417

HERBESSER (Hong Kong, Japan, Malaysia, Portugal, Singapore, Thailand)
DILTIAZEM HYDROCHLORIDE
Cardizem LA Extended Release Tablets 421

HERCEPTIN (Argentina, Australia, Belgium, Brazil, Canada, Chile, Czech Republic, Denmark, Finland, France, Germany, Greece, Hong Kong, Hungary, Irish Republic, Israel, Italy, Mexico, New Zealand, Norway, Poland, Portugal, Singapore, South Africa, Spain, Sweden, Switzerland, Thailand, The Netherlands, The Philippines, Turkey, United Kingdom, Venezuela)
TRASTUZUMAB
Herceptin I.V. 1199

HERMOLEPSIN (Sweden)
CARBAMAZEPINE
Carbatrol Capsules 3019

HEVRONAZ (Greece)
MUPIROCIN
Bactroban Ointment 1368

HEXAGASTRON (Denmark)
SUCRALFATE
Carafate Suspension 706
Carafate Tablets 707

HEXALID (Denmark)
DIAZEPAM
Valium Tablets 2658

HEXATRON (Denmark)
ONDANSETRON HYDROCHLORIDE
Zofran Injection 1682
Zofran Injection Premixed 1682
Zofran Oral Solution 1687
Zofran Tablets 1687

HIALID (Hong Kong, Singapore, Thailand, The Philippines)
SODIUM HYALURONATE
Hyalgan Solution 2742

HIALUDORF (Argentina)
SODIUM HYALURONATE
Hyalgan Solution 2742

HICONCIL (The Netherlands)
AMOXICILLIN
Amoxil Pediatric Drops for Oral Suspension 1305
Amoxil Tablets 1305

HIDRASAL (Mexico)
FUROSEMIDE
Furosemide Tablets 2186

HIDROPRIL (Brazil)
CAPTOPRIL
Captopril Tablets 2182

HIDRORONOL T (Chile)
HYDROCHLOROTHIAZIDE/TRIAMTERENE
Dyazide Capsules 1405

HIDROTIAZIDA (Brazil)
NYSTATIN
Nystop Topical Powder USP 2498

HIGLUCEM (Argentina)
PIOGLITAZONE HYDROCHLORIDE
Actos Tablets 3077

HINCOMOX (Brazil)
AMOXICILLIN
Amoxil Pediatric Drops for Oral Suspension 1305
Amoxil Tablets 1305

HIPEN (India)
AMOXICILLIN
Amoxil Pediatric Drops for Oral Suspension 1305
Amoxil Tablets 1305

HIPERTEX (Mexico)
CAPTOPRIL
Captopril Tablets 2182

HIPERTIL (Portugal)
CAPTOPRIL
Captopril Tablets 2182

HIPOCATRIL (Brazil)
CAPTOPRIL
Captopril Tablets 2182

HIPOSTEROL (Chile)
LOVASTATIN
Mevacor Tablets 2063

HIPOTEN (Argentina, Brazil)
CAPTOPRIL
Captopril Tablets 2182

HIPOTENSIL (Portugal)
CAPTOPRIL
Captopril Tablets 2182

HIPOVASTIN (Argentina)
LOVASTATIN
Mevacor Tablets 2063

HIPRESS (Brazil)
LOSARTAN POTASSIUM
Cozaar Tablets 1973

HISPLENIL (Venezuela)
SIMVASTATIN
Zocor Tablets 2136

HISTAC (Czech Republic, Hungary, India, Malaysia, Russia, Singapore, Thailand)
RANITIDINE HYDROCHLORIDE
Zantac 150 Tablets 1670
Zantac 25 EFFERdose Tablets 1670
Zantac 300 Tablets 1670
Zantac Injection 1666
Zantac Injection Premixed 1666

Zantac Syrup 1670

HISTACET (Hong Kong)
CETIRIZINE HYDROCHLORIDE
Zyrtec Syrup 1920
Zyrtec Tablets 1920

HISTAFILIN (Spain)
THEOPHYLLINE
Uniphyl Tablets 2595

HISTAFREN (Greece)
CETIRIZINE HYDROCHLORIDE
Zyrtec Syrup 1920
Zyrtec Tablets 1920

HISTAK (South Africa)
RANITIDINE HYDROCHLORIDE
Zantac 25 EFFERdose Tablets 1670
Zantac 150 Tablets 1670
Zantac 300 Tablets 1670
Zantac Injection 1666
Zantac Injection Premixed 1666
Zantac Syrup 1670

HISTALEN D (Chile)
CETIRIZINE HYDROCHLORIDE
Zyrtec Syrup 1920
Zyrtec Tablets 1920

HISTATEC (Switzerland)
CETIRIZINE HYDROCHLORIDE
Zyrtec Syrup 1920
Zyrtec Tablets 1920

HISTAX (Chile)
CETIRIZINE HYDROCHLORIDE
Zyrtec Syrup 1920
Zyrtec Tablets 1920

HISTAZINE (Hong Kong)
CETIRIZINE HYDROCHLORIDE
Zyrtec Syrup 1920
Zyrtec Tablets 1920

HISTEC (Finland)
CETIRIZINE HYDROCHLORIDE
Zyrtec Syrup 1920
Zyrtec Tablets 1920

HISTEK (Irish Republic)
CETIRIZINE HYDROCHLORIDE
Zyrtec Syrup 1920
Zyrtec Tablets 1920

HISTICA (Thailand)
CETIRIZINE HYDROCHLORIDE
Zyrtec Syrup 1920
Zyrtec Tablets 1920

HISTIMED (Belgium)
CETIRIZINE HYDROCHLORIDE
Zyrtec Syrup 1920
Zyrtec Tablets 1920

HISTOP (Spain)
SIMVASTATIN
Zocor Tablets 2136

HITRIZIN (Turkey)
CETIRIZINE HYDROCHLORIDE
Zyrtec Syrup 1920
Zyrtec Tablets 1920

HIVIRUX (Argentina)
LAMIVUDINE
Epivir Oral Solution 1412
Epivir Tablets 1412
Epivir-HBV Oral Solution 1417
Epivir-HBV Tablets 1417

HIVIRUX COMPLEX (Argentina)
LAMIVUDINE
Epivir Oral Solution 1412
Epivir Tablets 1412
Epivir-HBV Oral Solution 1417
Epivir-HBV Tablets 1417

H-MIDE (Thailand)
FUROSEMIDE
Furosemide Tablets 2186

HOLADREN (Chile)
ALENDRONATE SODIUM
Fosamax Tablets 2005

HOLETAR (Czech Republic, Russia)
LOVASTATIN
Mevacor Tablets 2063

HOREX (Mexico)
TIMOLOL MALEATE
Timoptic in Ocudose 2124
Timoptic Sterile Ophthalmic Solution 2121
Timoptic-XE Sterile Ophthalmic Gel Forming Solution 2125

HORIZEM (United Kingdom)
DILTIAZEM HYDROCHLORIDE
Cardizem LA Extended Release Tablets 421

HORMODIOL (Argentina)
ESTRADIOL
Climara Transdermal System 763

HORMODOSE (Brazil)
ESTRADIOL
Climara Transdermal System 763

HORMORAL (Chile)
PROGESTERONE
Crinone 4% Gel 992
Prometrium Capsules (100 mg, 200 mg) . 3047

HOSBOCIN (Spain)
CEFTRIAXONE SODIUM
Rocephin Injectable Vials, ADD-Vantage, Galaxy, Bulk 2642

HPB (Argentina)
FINASTERIDE
Propecia Tablets 2095
Proscar Tablets 2102

HUBERDINA (Spain)
FAMOTIDINE
Pepcid for Oral Suspension 2075
Pepcid Tablets 2075

HUMA-CAPTORIL (Hungary)
CAPTOPRIL
Captopril Tablets 2182

HUMA-DIFENAC (Hungary)
DICLOFENAC SODIUM
Voltaren Tablets 2334
Voltaren-XR Tablets 2337

HUMA-RANIDINE (Hungary)
RANITIDINE HYDROCHLORIDE
Zantac 25 EFFERdose Tablets 1670
Zantac 150 Tablets 1670
Zantac 300 Tablets 1670
Zantac Injection 1666
Zantac Injection Premixed 1666
Zantac Syrup 1670

HUMA-SEMIDE (Hungary)
FUROSEMIDE
Furosemide Tablets 2186

HUMORAP (Argentina)
CITALOPRAM HYDROBROMIDE
Celexa Tablets 1160

HYABAK (Italy)
SODIUM HYALURONATE
Hyalgan Solution 2742

HYA-JECT (Germany)
SODIUM HYALURONATE
Hyalgan Solution 2742

HYAL (Malaysia)
SODIUM HYALURONATE
Hyalgan Solution 2742

HYALART (Argentina, Germany, Greece, Italy, Portugal, Spain)
SODIUM HYALURONATE
Hyalgan Solution 2742

HYAL-DROP (France, Switzerland)
SODIUM HYALURONATE
Hyalgan Solution 2742

HYALEIN (Japan)
SODIUM HYALURONATE
Hyalgan Solution 2742

HYALGAN (Austria, Canada, Chile, Czech Republic, Denmark, Finland, France, Hong Kong, Hungary, Irish Republic, Italy, Poland, Singapore, Spain, Sweden, Turkey, United Kingdom, Venezuela)
SODIUM HYALURONATE
Hyalgan Solution 2742

HYALISTIL (Italy)
SODIUM HYALURONATE
Hyalgan Solution 2742

HYAL-SYSTEM (Germany)
SODIUM HYALURONATE
Hyalgan Solution 2742

HYALUBRIX (Germany)
SODIUM HYALURONATE
Hyalgan Solution 2742

HYALUDERMIN (Brazil)
SODIUM HYALURONATE
Hyalgan Solution 2742

HYANAC (Argentina)
DICLOFENAC SODIUM
Voltaren Tablets 2334
Voltaren-XR Tablets 2337

HYA-OPHTAL (Germany)
SODIUM HYALURONATE
Hyalgan Solution 2742

HYASOL (Argentina, Mexico)
SODIUM HYALURONATE
Hyalgan Solution 2742

HYBRIDIL (Austria)
CARVEDILOL
Coreg Tablets 1387

HYCAMPTIN (Turkey)
TOPOTECAN HYDROCHLORIDE
Hycamtin for Injection 1459

HYCAMTIN (Argentina, Australia, Austria, Belgium, Brazil, Canada, Chile, Czech Republic, Denmark, Finland, France, Germany, Greece, Hong Kong, Hungary, Irish Republic, Israel, Italy, Norway, Poland, Portugal, Russia, Singapore, South Africa, Spain, Sweden, Switzerland, Thailand, The Netherlands, United Kingdom, Venezuela)
TOPOTECAN HYDROCHLORIDE
Hycamtin for Injection 1459

HYCOSAN5 (Switzerland)
SODIUM HYALURONATE
Hyalgan Solution 2742

HYDRENE (Australia)
TRIAMTERENE
Dyrenium Capsules 3189

HYDREX (South Africa)
FUROSEMIDE
Furosemide Tablets 2186

HYDROFLUX (Greece)
FUROSEMIDE
Furosemide Tablets 2186

HYDRO-LESS (South Africa)
INDAPAMIDE
Indapamide Tablets 2188

HY-DROP (Italy)
SODIUM HYALURONATE
Hyalgan Solution 2742

HYDRO-RAPID (Germany)
FUROSEMIDE
Furosemide Tablets 2186

HYDRO-RAPID-TABLINEN (Switzerland)
FUROSEMIDE
Furosemide Tablets 2186

HY-GAG (Germany)
SODIUM HYALURONATE
Hyalgan Solution 2742

HYLAN (Germany)
SODIUM HYALURONATE
Hyalgan Solution 2742

HYLO-CARE (Germany)
SODIUM HYALURONATE
Hyalgan Solution 2742

HYLO-COMOD (France, Germany, Israel, Italy, Portugal, Switzerland)
SODIUM HYALURONATE
Hyalgan Solution 2742

HYLO-VISION (Germany)
SODIUM HYALURONATE
Hyalgan Solution 2742

HYLUPROTECT (France, Italy)
SODIUM HYALURONATE
Hyalgan Solution 2742

HYPERMOL (New Zealand)
TIMOLOL MALEATE
Timoptic in Ocudose 2124
Timoptic Sterile Ophthalmic Solution 2121
Timoptic-XE Sterile Ophthalmic Gel Forming Solution 2125

HYPERTORR (Germany)
HYDROCHLOROTHIAZIDE/TRIAMTERENE
Dyazide Capsules 1405

HYPODINE (Thailand)
CLONIDINE HYDROCHLORIDE
Catapres Tablets 841

HYPOLIP (Czech Republic)
FENOFIBRATE
Tricor Tablets 520

HYPOMED (Austria)
LISINOPRIL
Prinivil Tablets 2087

HYPOTENSOR (Greece)
CAPTOPRIL
Captopril Tablets 2182

HYRUAN (Hong Kong, Thailand)
SODIUM HYALURONATE
Hyalgan Solution 2742

HYSAN (Germany, Israel, Switzerland)
SODIUM HYALURONATE
Hyalgan Solution 2742

HYTACAND (Portugal)
CANDESARTAN CILEXETIL
Atacand Tablets 639

HYTENEZE (United Kingdom)
CAPTOPRIL
Captopril Tablets 2182

HYZAAR (Brazil, Czech Republic, Hungary, Malaysia, New Zealand, Poland, The Philippines, Turkey, Venezuela)
LOSARTAN POTASSIUM
Cozaar Tablets 1973

HYZAAR PLUS (Venezuela)
LOSARTAN POTASSIUM
Cozaar Tablets 1973

HYZAN (Hong Kong, Malaysia, Singapore)
RANITIDINE HYDROCHLORIDE
Zantac 150 Tablets 1670
Zantac 25 EFFERdose Tablets 1670
Zantac 300 Tablets 1670
Zantac Injection 1666
Zantac Injection Premixed 1666
Zantac Syrup 1670

IAL (Hong Kong, Hungary, Italy, Switzerland, Turkey)
SODIUM HYALURONATE
Hyalgan Solution 2742

IALECT (Italy)
SODIUM HYALURONATE
Hyalgan Solution 2742

IALUGEN (Switzerland)
SODIUM HYALURONATE
Hyalgan Solution 2742

IALUGEN PLUS (Czech Republic, Hungary)
SODIUM HYALURONATE
Hyalgan Solution 2742

IALUM (Italy)
SODIUM HYALURONATE
Hyalgan Solution 2742

IALUREX (Italy)
SODIUM HYALURONATE
Hyalgan Solution 2742

IALUSET (France)
SODIUM HYALURONATE
Hyalgan Solution 2742

IALUTIM (Italy)
TIMOLOL MALEATE
Timoptic in Ocudose 2124
Timoptic Sterile Ophthalmic Solution 2121
Timoptic-XE Sterile Ophthalmic Gel Forming Solution 2125

IBAMOXIL (Brazil)
AMOXICILLIN
Amoxil Pediatric Drops for Oral Suspension 1305
Amoxil Tablets 1305

IBIAMOX (Thailand)
AMOXICILLIN
Amoxil Pediatric Drops for Oral Suspension 1305
Amoxil Tablets 1305

ICAZ (France, The Philippines)
ISRADIPINE
DynaCirc CR Tablets 1407

ICORAN (Greece)
LISINOPRIL
Prinivil Tablets ... **2087**

ICTUS (Brazil)
CARVEDILOL
Coreg Tablets ... **1387**

IDROLAC (Italy)
LACTULOSE
Kristalose for Oral Solution ... **1004**

IDUVO (Argentina)
ZIDOVUDINE
Retrovir Capsules ... **1574**
Retrovir IV Infusion ... **1579**
Retrovir Syrup ... **1574**
Retrovir Tablets ... **1574**

IESEF (Turkey)
CEFTRIAXONE SODIUM
Rocephin Injectable Vials, ADD-Vantage, Galaxy, Bulk ... **2642**

IESETUM (Turkey)
CEFTAZIDIME
Fortaz for Injection ... **1450**

IFA REDUCCING (Mexico)
PHENTERMINE HYDROCHLORIDE
Adipex-P Capsules ... **1185**
Adipex-P Tablets ... **1185**

IFADA (Spain)
FAMOTIDINE
Pepcid for Oral Suspension ... **2075**
Pepcid Tablets ... **2075**

IFICIPRO (Russia)
CIPROFLOXACIN
Cipro Oral Suspension ... **2810**

IFISTATIN (Singapore)
SIMVASTATIN
Zocor Tablets ... **2136**

I-GESIC (India)
DICLOFENAC SODIUM
Voltaren Tablets ... **2334**
Voltaren-XR Tablets ... **2337**

IGLODINE FLEX (Argentina)
DICLOFENAC SODIUM
Voltaren Tablets ... **2334**
Voltaren-XR Tablets ... **2337**

IGUASSINA (Brazil)
HYDROCHLOROTHIAZIDE/TRIAMTERENE
Dyazide Capsules ... **1405**

IKTORIVIL (Sweden)
CLONAZEPAM
Klonopin Tablets ... **2639**

ILAGANE (Spain)
NAPROXEN
EC-Naprosyn Delayed-Release Tablets ... **2632**
Naprosyn Suspension ... **2632**
Naprosyn Tablets ... **2632**

ILIAXONE (Italy)
CEFTRIAXONE SODIUM
Rocephin Injectable Vials, ADD-Vantage, Galaxy, Bulk ... **2642**

ILOPAR (Greece)
LOVASTATIN
Mevacor Tablets ... **2063**

ILOSTAL (Chile)
CILOSTAZOL
Pletal Tablets ... **2481**

ILOTYCIN-A (South Africa)
TRETINOIN
Vesanoid Capsules ... **2660**

IMACILLIN (Denmark)
AMOXICILLIN
Amoxil Pediatric Drops for Oral Suspension ... **1305**
Amoxil Tablets ... **1305**

IMAVERMIL (Brazil)
ALBENDAZOLE
Albenza Tablets ... **1297**

IMBISTAD (Mexico)
SIMVASTATIN
Zocor Tablets ... **2136**

IMEPAS (Mexico)
DIAZEPAM
Valium Tablets ... **2658**

IMFLAC (Australia)
DICLOFENAC SODIUM
Voltaren Tablets ... **2334**
Voltaren-XR Tablets ... **2337**

IMIGRAN (Argentina, Australia, Brazil, Chile, Czech Republic, Germany, Greece, Hong Kong, Hungary, Irish Republic, Malaysia, New Zealand, Norway, Poland, Portugal, Russia, Singapore, South Africa, Spain, Thailand, The Philippines, Turkey, United Kingdom, Venezuela)
SUMATRIPTAN SUCCINATE
Imitrex Injection ... **1465**
Imitrex Tablets ... **1474**

IMIJECT (France)
SUMATRIPTAN SUCCINATE
Imitrex Injection ... **1465**
Imitrex Tablets ... **1474**

IMIMOR (Chile)
IMIQUIMOD
Aldara Cream, 5% ... **1699**

IMIMORE (Argentina)
IMIQUIMOD
Aldara Cream, 5% ... **1699**

IMIPEM (Italy)
CILASTATIN SODIUM/IMIPENEM
Primaxin I.M. ... **2080**
Primaxin I.V. ... **2083**

IMITREX (Argentina, Israel)
SUMATRIPTAN SUCCINATE
Imitrex Injection ... **1465**
Imitrex Tablets ... **1474**

IMMUKIN (Irish Republic)
INTERFERON GAMMA-1B
Actimmune ... **1743**

IMMUKINE (The Netherlands)
INTERFERON GAMMA-1B
Actimmune ... **1743**

IMOT (Mexico, Venezuela)
TIMOLOL MALEATE
Timoptic in Ocudose ... **2124**
Timoptic Sterile Ophthalmic Solution ... **2121**
Timoptic-XE Sterile Ophthalmic Gel Forming Solution ... **2125**

IMPOSERGON (Greece)
FAMOTIDINE
Pepcid for Oral Suspension ... **2075**
Pepcid Tablets ... **2075**

IMPUGAN (Denmark, Sweden, Switzerland, Thailand)
FUROSEMIDE
Furosemide Tablets ... **2186**

IMUFOR (Argentina, Austria)
INTERFERON GAMMA-1B
Actimmune ... **1743**

IMUKIN (Austria, Denmark, Finland, France, Germany, Italy, Norway, Portugal, Spain, Sweden)
INTERFERON GAMMA-1B
Actimmune ... **1743**

IMUNOXA (Argentina)
LAMIVUDINE
Epivir Oral Solution ... **1412**
Epivir Tablets ... **1412**
Epivir-HBV Oral Solution ... **1417**
Epivir-HBV Tablets ... **1417**

IMUNOXA COMPLEX (Argentina)
LAMIVUDINE
Epivir Oral Solution ... **1412**
Epivir Tablets ... **1412**
Epivir-HBV Oral Solution ... **1417**
Epivir-HBV Tablets ... **1417**

INAC (Singapore)
DICLOFENAC SODIUM
Voltaren Tablets ... **2334**
Voltaren-XR Tablets ... **2337**

INALACOR (Spain)
FLUTICASONE PROPIONATE
Flonase Nasal Spray ... **1431**

INALCORT (Italy)
FLUNISOLIDE
Aerobid Inhaler System ... **1153**
Aerobid-M Inhaler System ... **1153**

INAMIDE (Irish Republic)
INDAPAMIDE
Indapamide Tablets ... **2188**

INASPIR (Spain)
SALMETEROL XINAFOATE
Serevent Diskus ... **1594**

INASTMOL (Argentina)
THEOPHYLLINE
Uniphyl Tablets ... **2595**

INCID (The Philippines)
RANITIDINE HYDROCHLORIDE
Zantac 25 EFFERdose Tablets ... **1670**
Zantac 150 Tablets ... **1670**
Zantac 300 Tablets ... **1670**
Zantac Injection ... **1666**
Zantac Injection Premixed ... **1666**
Zantac Syrup ... **1670**

INCIDAL-OD (Thailand)
CETIRIZINE HYDROCHLORIDE
Zyrtec Syrup ... **1920**
Zyrtec Tablets ... **1920**

INCLENS (Venezuela)
FUROSEMIDE
Furosemide Tablets ... **2186**

INCORIL (Argentina, Brazil, Chile)
DILTIAZEM HYDROCHLORIDE
Cardizem LA Extended Release Tablets ... **421**

INDACAR (Denmark)
INDAPAMIDE
Indapamide Tablets ... **2188**

INDAFLEX (Italy)
INDAPAMIDE
Indapamide Tablets ... **2188**

INDAHEXAL (Australia)
INDAPAMIDE
Indapamide Tablets ... **2188**

INDALIX (South Africa)
INDAPAMIDE
Indapamide Tablets ... **2188**

INDAMID (Turkey)
INDAPAMIDE
Indapamide Tablets ... **2188**

INDAMOL (Italy)
INDAPAMIDE
Indapamide Tablets ... **2188**

INDANORM (United Arab Emirates)
INDAPAMIDE
Indapamide Tablets ... **2188**

INDAP (Czech Republic, Russia)
INDAPAMIDE
Indapamide Tablets ... **2188**

INDAPEN (Brazil, Poland, Turkey)
INDAPAMIDE
Indapamide Tablets ... **2188**

INDAPRES (Poland)
INDAPAMIDE
Indapamide Tablets ... **2188**

INDAPRESS (Chile)
INDAPAMIDE
Indapamide Tablets ... **2188**

INDAPSAN (Poland)
INDAPAMIDE
Indapamide Tablets ... **2188**

INDA-PUREN (Germany)
INDAPAMIDE
Indapamide Tablets ... **2188**

INDICONTIN (India)
INDAPAMIDE
Indapamide Tablets ... **2188**

INDITOR (India)
INDAPAMIDE
Indapamide Tablets ... **2188**

INDIVAN (India, Venezuela)
INDINAVIR SULFATE
Crixivan Capsules ... **1979**

INDIX (Poland)
INDAPAMIDE
Indapamide Tablets ... **2188**

INDOLIN (Italy)
INDAPAMIDE
Indapamide Tablets ... **2188**

INDURIN (Turkey)
INDAPAMIDE
Indapamide Tablets ... **2188**

INDUZEPAM (Argentina)
CLONAZEPAM
Klonopin Tablets ... **2639**

INF (Argentina)
INTERFERON ALFA-2B
Intron A for Injection ... **2859**

INFASURF (Israel)
CALFACTANT
Infasurf Intratracheal Suspension ... **1168**

INFECTOFLAM (Belgium, Brazil, Czech Republic, Malaysia, The Philippines)
FLUOROMETHOLONE
FML Ophthalmic Ointment ... **⊙223**

INFECTOMOX (Germany)
AMOXICILLIN
Amoxil Pediatric Drops for Oral Suspension ... **1305**
Amoxil Tablets ... **1305**

INFECTOPYODERM (Germany)
MUPIROCIN
Bactroban Ointment ... **1368**

INFECTOZIDIM (Germany)
CEFTAZIDIME
Fortaz for Injection ... **1450**

INFEKOR (The Philippines)
CEFUROXIME SODIUM
Zinacef Injection ... **1678**

INFESTAT (United Kingdom)
NYSTATIN
Nystop Topical Powder USP ... **2498**

INFLA-BAN (South Africa)
DICLOFENAC SODIUM
Voltaren Tablets ... **2334**
Voltaren-XR Tablets ... **2337**

INFLAMAX (Brazil)
DICLOFENAC SODIUM
Voltaren Tablets ... **2334**
Voltaren-XR Tablets ... **2337**

INFLANAC (Hong Kong, Singapore, Thailand)
DICLOFENAC SODIUM
Voltaren Tablets ... **2334**
Voltaren-XR Tablets ... **2337**

INFLANOX (Mexico)
NAPROXEN
EC-Naprosyn Delayed-Release Tablets ... **2632**
Naprosyn Suspension ... **2632**
Naprosyn Tablets ... **2632**

INFLASED (Turkey)
DICLOFENAC SODIUM
Voltaren Tablets ... **2334**
Voltaren-XR Tablets ... **2337**

INFLOXA (Mexico)
CIPROFLOXACIN
Cipro Oral Suspension ... **2810**

INGASTRI (Spain)
FAMOTIDINE
Pepcid for Oral Suspension ... **2075**
Pepcid Tablets ... **2075**

INGECLOF (Argentina)
DICLOFENAC SODIUM
Voltaren Tablets ... **2334**
Voltaren-XR Tablets ... **2337**

INGETIM (Argentina)
TIMOLOL MALEATE
Timoptic in Ocudose ... **2124**
Timoptic Sterile Ophthalmic Solution ... **2121**
Timoptic-XE Sterile Ophthalmic Gel Forming Solution ... **2125**

INHACORT (Germany)
FLUNISOLIDE
Aerobid Inhaler System ... **1153**
Aerobid-M Inhaler System ... **1153**

INHALEX (Thailand)
IPRATROPIUM BROMIDE
Atrovent Nasal Spray 0.03% ... **834**
Atrovent Nasal Spray 0.06% ... **836**

INHIBACE (Israel)
CAPTOPRIL
Captopril Tablets ... **2182**

INIBIL (Italy)
APROTININ
Trasylol Injection ... **799**

INIPROL (Belgium, France, Italy)
APROTININ
Trasylol Injection 799

INKAMIL (Spain)
CIPROFLOXACIN HYDROCHLORIDE
Cipro Tablets 2810

INOFUNGIN (Brazil)
NYSTATIN
Nystop Topical Powder USP 2498

INOTRIN (Greece)
ISOTRETINOIN
Accutane Capsules 2607

INOVAL (Brazil)
FENTANYL CITRATE
Actiq 959

INPAMIDE (Thailand)
INDAPAMIDE
Indapamide Tablets 2188

INSENSYE (Australia)
NORFLOXACIN
Noroxin Tablets 2069

INSIDE (Sweden)
RANITIDINE HYDROCHLORIDE
Zantac 25 EFFERdose Tablets 1670
Zantac 150 Tablets 1670
Zantac 300 Tablets 1670
Zantac Injection 1666
Zantac Injection Premixed 1666
Zantac Syrup 1670

INSIDE BRUS (Finland, Norway)
RANITIDINE HYDROCHLORIDE
Zantac 25 EFFERdose Tablets 1670
Zantac 150 Tablets 1670
Zantac 300 Tablets 1670
Zantac Injection 1666
Zantac Injection Premixed 1666
Zantac Syrup 1670

INSIG (Australia)
INDAPAMIDE
Indapamide Tablets 2188

INTEGRILIN (Australia, Belgium, Brazil, Canada, Chile, Czech Republic, Denmark, Finland, France, Germany, Greece, Hong Kong, Hungary, Irish Republic, Israel, Italy, Malaysia, New Zealand, Norway, Poland, Portugal, Russia, Singapore, South Africa, Spain, Sweden, Switzerland, Thailand, The Netherlands, The Philippines, United Kingdom)
EPTIFIBATIDE
Integrilin Injection 2855

INTER 2-B (Argentina)
INTERFERON ALFA-2B
Intron A for Injection 2859

INTERBERIN (Austria)
SARGRAMOSTIM
Leukine 774

INTERBION (Greece)
CEFUROXIME AXETIL
Ceftin for Oral Suspension 1380
Ceftin Tablets 1380

INTOCEL (Argentina)
CLADRIBINE
Leustatin Injection 2384

INTRACEF (Brazil, South Africa)
CEFTAZIDIME
Fortaz for Injection 1450

INTRON (Venezuela)
INTERFERON ALFA-2B
Intron A for Injection 2859

INTRON A (Canada, Czech Republic, Hong Kong, Hungary, Israel, Malaysia, Mexico, Poland, Portugal, Singapore, South Africa, Spain, Switzerland, Thailand, The Philippines, Turkey, Venezuela)
INTERFERON ALFA-2B
Intron A for Injection 2859

INTRONA (Austria, Denmark, Finland, France, Irish Republic, Norway, Sweden, The Netherlands)
INTERFERON ALFA-2B
Intron A for Injection 2859

INVEOXEL (Chile)
NAPROXEN
EC-Naprosyn Delayed-Release Tablets 2632
Naprosyn Suspension 2632
Naprosyn Tablets 2632

INVIGAN (Spain)
FAMOTIDINE
Pepcid for Oral Suspension 2075
Pepcid Tablets 2075

INZA (Australia, Hong Kong)
NAPROXEN
EC-Naprosyn Delayed-Release Tablets 2632
Naprosyn Suspension 2632
Naprosyn Tablets 2632

IOR T3 (Chile, Mexico)
MUROMONAB-CD3
Orthoclone OKT3 Sterile Solution 2387

IPACEF (Italy)
CEFUROXIME SODIUM
Zinacef Injection 1678

IPAGASTRIL (Italy)
SUCRALFATE
Carafate Suspension 706
Carafate Tablets 707

IPAMIX (Italy)
INDAPAMIDE
Indapamide Tablets 2188

IPOMEX (Argentina)
SIBUTRAMINE HYDROCHLORIDE
Meridia Capsules 475

IPOREL (Poland)
CLONIDINE HYDROCHLORIDE
Catapres Tablets 841

IPOTENSIUM (Italy)
CLONIDINE HYDROCHLORIDE
Catapres Tablets 841

IPRA (New Zealand)
IPRATROPIUM BROMIDE
Atrovent Nasal Spray 0.03% 834
Atrovent Nasal Spray 0.06% 836

IPRABON (Brazil)
IPRATROPIUM BROMIDE
Atrovent Nasal Spray 0.03% 834
Atrovent Nasal Spray 0.06% 836

IPRABRON (Argentina)
IPRATROPIUM BROMIDE
Atrovent Nasal Spray 0.03% 834
Atrovent Nasal Spray 0.06% 836

IPRADUAL (Argentina)
IPRATROPIUM BROMIDE
Atrovent Nasal Spray 0.03% 834
Atrovent Nasal Spray 0.06% 836

IPRALIN (Venezuela)
IPRATROPIUM BROMIDE
Atrovent Nasal Spray 0.03% 834
Atrovent Nasal Spray 0.06% 836

IPRAMID (Greece)
SIMVASTATIN
Zocor Tablets 2136

IPRAMOL (Irish Republic, United Kingdom)
IPRATROPIUM BROMIDE
Atrovent Nasal Spray 0.03% 834
Atrovent Nasal Spray 0.06% 836

IPRANASE (India)
IPRATROPIUM BROMIDE
Atrovent Nasal Spray 0.03% 834
Atrovent Nasal Spray 0.06% 836

IPRANEO (Brazil)
IPRATROPIUM BROMIDE
Atrovent Nasal Spray 0.03% 834
Atrovent Nasal Spray 0.06% 836

IPRASALB (Argentina)
IPRATROPIUM BROMIDE
Atrovent Nasal Spray 0.03% 834
Atrovent Nasal Spray 0.06% 836

IPRATRIN (Australia)
IPRATROPIUM BROMIDE
Atrovent Nasal Spray 0.03% 834
Atrovent Nasal Spray 0.06% 836

IPRAVENT (Australia, Hong Kong, India)
IPRATROPIUM BROMIDE
Atrovent Nasal Spray 0.03% 834
Atrovent Nasal Spray 0.06% 836

IPRAXA (The Netherlands)
IPRATROPIUM BROMIDE
Atrovent Nasal Spray 0.03% 834
Atrovent Nasal Spray 0.06% 836

IPRES (Poland)
INDAPAMIDE
Indapamide Tablets 2188

IPROLAN (The Philippines)
CIPROFLOXACIN HYDROCHLORIDE
Cipro Tablets 2810

IPROXIN (Venezuela)
CIPROFLOXACIN
Cipro Oral Suspension 2810

IPVENT (South Africa)
IPRATROPIUM BROMIDE
Atrovent Nasal Spray 0.03% 834
Atrovent Nasal Spray 0.06% 836

IQFADINA (Mexico)
RANITIDINE HYDROCHLORIDE
Zantac 25 EFFERdose Tablets 1670
Zantac 150 Tablets 1670
Zantac 300 Tablets 1670
Zantac Injection 1666
Zantac Injection Premixed 1666
Zantac Syrup 1670

IQFASOL (Mexico)
NAPROXEN
EC-Naprosyn Delayed-Release Tablets 2632
Naprosyn Suspension 2632
Naprosyn Tablets 2632

IRA (Argentina)
CLARITHROMYCIN
Biaxin Filmtab Tablets 411
Biaxin Granules 411

IRBAN (Israel)
IRBESARTAN
Avapro Tablets 897

IRBAN PLUS (Israel)
IRBESARTAN
Avapro Tablets 897

IRICIL (Spain)
LISINOPRIL
Prinivil Tablets 2087

IRICIL PLUS (Spain)
LISINOPRIL
Prinivil Tablets 2087

IRILENS (Italy)
SODIUM HYALURONATE
Hyalgan Solution 2742

IROVEL (India)
IRBESARTAN
Avapro Tablets 897

IRPAX (Poland)
PERINDOPRIL ERBUMINE
Aceon Tablets (2 mg, 4 mg, 8 mg) 3038

IRUMED (Czech Republic)
LISINOPRIL
Prinivil Tablets 2087

IRUXOL (Argentina, Brazil, Finland)
COLLAGENASE
Santyl Collagenase Ointment 1724

IRUXOL MONO (Belgium, Brazil, Greece, Hong Kong, Switzerland)
COLLAGENASE
Santyl Collagenase Ointment 1724

IRUXOL SIMPLEX (Venezuela)
COLLAGENASE
Santyl Collagenase Ointment 1724

ISADOL (Mexico)
ZIDOVUDINE
Retrovir Capsules 1574
Retrovir IV Infusion 1579
Retrovir Syrup 1574
Retrovir Tablets 1574

ISCLOFEN (United Kingdom)
DICLOFENAC SODIUM
Voltaren Tablets 2334
Voltaren-XR Tablets 2337

ISCOVER (Argentina, Australia, Brazil, Germany, Greece, Italy, Mexico, Portugal, Spain, Switzerland, The Netherlands)
CLOPIDOGREL BISULFATE
Plavix Tablets 926, 2767

ISDIBEN (Spain)
ISOTRETINOIN
Accutane Capsules 2607

ISELPIN (The Philippines)
SUCRALFATE
Carafate Suspension 706
Carafate Tablets 707

ISET (Argentina)
CLARITHROMYCIN
Biaxin Filmtab Tablets 411
Biaxin Granules 411

ISIMOXIN (Italy)
AMOXICILLIN
Amoxil Pediatric Drops for Oral Suspension 1305
Amoxil Tablets 1305

ISO ESTEDI (Spain)
ISOTRETINOIN
Accutane Capsules 2607

ISOACNE (Brazil)
ISOTRETINOIN
Accutane Capsules 2607

ISOBLOC (Argentina)
CARVEDILOL
Coreg Tablets 1387

ISOCUTAN (Austria)
ISOTRETINOIN
Accutane Capsules 2607

ISODERM (Germany)
ISOTRETINOIN
Accutane Capsules 2607

ISODERMAL (Greece)
ISOTRETINOIN
Accutane Capsules 2607

ISOFACE (Mexico, Venezuela)
ISOTRETINOIN
Accutane Capsules 2607

ISOGERIL (Greece)
ISOTRETINOIN
Accutane Capsules 2607

ISOGLAUCON (Austria, Germany, Italy, Spain)
CLONIDINE HYDROCHLORIDE
Catapres Tablets 841

ISOHEXAL (Australia)
ISOTRETINOIN
Accutane Capsules 2607

ISOMINA (Venezuela)
FAMOTIDINE
Pepcid for Oral Suspension 2075
Pepcid Tablets 2075

ISOPTO CETAPRED (Belgium, Canada, Greece)
PREDNISOLONE ACETATE/SULFACETAMIDE SODIUM
Blephamide Ophthalmic Ointment . . . . ⊙217
Blephamide Ophthalmic Suspension . . . . ⊙216

ISOPTO FLUCON (Germany, Spain)
FLUOROMETHOLONE
FML Ophthalmic Ointment . . . . ⊙223

ISOSKIN (Greece)
ISOTRETINOIN
Accutane Capsules 2607

ISOSOL (Austria)
ISOTRETINOIN
Accutane Capsules 2607

ISOSUPRA LIDOSE (Belgium)
ISOTRETINOIN
Accutane Capsules 2607

ISOTANE (New Zealand, Thailand)
ISOTRETINOIN
Accutane Capsules 2607

ISOTRET (Germany)
ISOTRETINOIN
Accutane Capsules 2607

ISOTREX (Argentina, Australia, Austria, Brazil, Canada, Chile, Czech Republic, Denmark, France, Germany, Hong Kong, Hungary, Irish Republic, Israel, Italy, Malaysia, Mexico, New Zealand, Poland, Portugal, Singapore, South Africa, Spain, Thailand, The Philippines, United Kingdom, Venezuela)
ISOTRETINOIN
Accutane Capsules 2607

ISOTREX ERITROMICINA (Spain)
ISOTRETINOIN
Accutane Capsules 2607

ISOTREXIN (Austria, Brazil, Germany, Irish Republic, Italy, Poland, Portugal, Singapore, Thailand, United Kingdom)
ISOTRETINOIN
Accutane Capsules 2607

ISOTROIN (Greece, India)
ISOTRETINOIN
Accutane Capsules 2607

ITALNIK (Mexico)
CIPROFLOXACIN
Cipro Oral Suspension 2810

ITAMI (Italy)
DICLOFENAC SODIUM
Voltaren Tablets 2334
Voltaren-XR Tablets 2337

ITOREX (Italy)
CEFUROXIME SODIUM
Zinacef Injection 1678

ITROP (Austria, Czech Republic, Germany, Switzerland)
IPRATROPIUM BROMIDE
Atrovent Nasal Spray 0.03% 834
Atrovent Nasal Spray 0.06% 836

IURONICO BIOTIC (Argentina)
SODIUM HYALURONATE
Hyalgan Solution 2742

IVERMEC (Brazil)
IVERMECTIN
Stromectol Tablets 2120

IVEXTERM (Mexico)
IVERMECTIN
Stromectol Tablets 2120

IZADIMA (Mexico)
CEFTAZIDIME
Fortaz for Injection 1450

IZOTEK (Poland)
ISOTRETINOIN
Accutane Capsules 2607

JABASTATINA (Portugal)
SIMVASTATIN
Zocor Tablets 2136

JALVASE (The Netherlands)
LOSARTAN POTASSIUM
Cozaar Tablets 1973

JANACIN (Hong Kong, Malaysia, Thailand)
NORFLOXACIN
Noroxin Tablets 2069

JATROPUR (Germany)
TRIAMTERENE
Dyrenium Capsules 3189

JATROSOM N (Germany)
TRANYLCYPROMINE SULFATE
Parnate Tablets 1532

JENAFENAC (Germany)
DICLOFENAC SODIUM
Voltaren Tablets 2334
Voltaren-XR Tablets 2337

JENATEREN COMP (Germany)
HYDROCHLOROTHIAZIDE/TRIAMTERENE
Dyazide Capsules 1405

JENOQUINE (United Arab Emirates)
LEVOFLOXACIN
Levaquin Injection 2416
Levaquin Tablets 2416

JODTHYROX (Czech Republic, Poland)
LEVOTHYROXINE SODIUM
Levothroid Tablets 1170
Levoxyl Tablets 1780
Synthroid Tablets 507

JOHNSONS CLEAN & CLEAR PERSA GEL (Canada)
BENZOYL PEROXIDE
Brevoxyl-4 Creamy Wash 3054
Brevoxyl-4 Gel 3054
Brevoxyl-8 Creamy Wash 3054
Brevoxyl-8 Gel 3054

JOSIR (France)
TAMSULOSIN HYDROCHLORIDE
Flomax Capsules 848

JOSKEN (Mexico)
SIMVASTATIN
Zocor Tablets 2136

JOSSALIND (Germany)
SODIUM HYALURONATE
Hyalgan Solution 2742

JOYZOL (India)
OLANZAPINE
Zyprexa Tablets 1883

JULAB (Hong Kong, Thailand)
SELEGILINE HYDROCHLORIDE
Eldepryl Capsules 3052

JUMEX (Argentina, Austria, Czech Republic, Hong Kong, Hungary, Israel, Italy, Malaysia, Poland, Portugal, Singapore, Thailand, The Philippines, Venezuela)
SELEGILINE HYDROCHLORIDE
Eldepryl Capsules 3052

JUMEXAL (Switzerland)
SELEGILINE HYDROCHLORIDE
Eldepryl Capsules 3052

JUMEXIL (Brazil)
SELEGILINE HYDROCHLORIDE
Eldepryl Capsules 3052

JUNO (Argentina)
LEVOTHYROXINE SODIUM
Levothroid Tablets 1170
Levoxyl Tablets 1780
Synthroid Tablets 507

KADIAN (Canada)
MORPHINE SULFATE
MS Contin Tablets 2585

KAILASA (Argentina)
CLARITHROMYCIN
Biaxin Filmtab Tablets 411
Biaxin Granules 411

KAIMIL (Italy)
FLUNISOLIDE
Aerobid Inhaler System 1153
Aerobid-M Inhaler System 1153

KAIZEM (India)
DILTIAZEM HYDROCHLORIDE
Cardizem LA Extended Release Tablets 421

KAJOS (Norway, Sweden)
POTASSIUM CITRATE
Urocit-K Tablets 2176

KALCYTRIOL (Poland)
CALCITRIOL
Calcijex Injection 419
Rocaltrol Capsules 1150
Rocaltrol Oral Solution 1150

KALINOR (Turkey)
POTASSIUM CITRATE
Urocit-K Tablets 2176

KALIUM (Germany)
POTASSIUM CITRATE
Urocit-K Tablets 2176

KALIXOCIN (Australia)
CLARITHROMYCIN
Biaxin Filmtab Tablets 411
Biaxin Granules 411

KALPRESS (Spain)
VALSARTAN
Diovan Tablets 2212

KALPRESS PLUS (Spain)
VALSARTAN
Diovan Tablets 2212

KALTIAZEM (Argentina)
DILTIAZEM HYDROCHLORIDE
Cardizem LA Extended Release Tablets 421

KANDISTAT (Brazil)
NYSTATIN
Nystop Topical Powder USP 2498

KANOLONE (Thailand)
TRIAMCINOLONE ACETONIDE
Azmacort Inhalation Aerosol 407
Nasacort AQ Nasal Spray 2765

KAPABLOC (Austria)
MORPHINE SULFATE
MS Contin Tablets 2585

KAPANOL (Australia, Austria, Belgium, Denmark, France, Germany, Israel, Mexico, New Zealand, Norway, Switzerland, The Netherlands)
MORPHINE SULFATE
MS Contin Tablets 2585

KAPLON (United Kingdom)
CAPTOPRIL
Captopril Tablets 2182

KAPNAX (Turkey)
NAPROXEN SODIUM
Anaprox DS Tablets 2632
Anaprox Tablets 2632

KAPPACEF (Italy)
CEFTRIAXONE SODIUM
Rocephin Injectable Vials, ADD-Vantage, Galaxy, Bulk 2642

KAPRIL (Turkey)
CAPTOPRIL
Captopril Tablets 2182

KAPTORIL (Turkey)
CAPTOPRIL
Captopril Tablets 2182

KARAZEPIN (Turkey)
CARBAMAZEPINE
Carbatrol Capsules 3019

KARBAC (Brazil)
CARBAMAZEPINE
Carbatrol Capsules 3019

KARBALEX (Turkey)
CARBAMAZEPINE
Carbatrol Capsules 3019

KARBASIF (Turkey)
CARBAMAZEPINE
Carbatrol Capsules 3019

KARBEROL (Turkey)
CARBAMAZEPINE
Carbatrol Capsules 3019

KARDIL (Norway, Turkey)
DILTIAZEM HYDROCHLORIDE
Cardizem LA Extended Release Tablets 421

KARDISENTIN (Turkey)
DIPYRIDAMOLE
Persantine Tablets 869

KARIN (Israel)
CLARITHROMYCIN
Biaxin Filmtab Tablets 411
Biaxin Granules 411

KAROKSEN (Turkey)
NAPROXEN SODIUM
Anaprox DS Tablets 2632
Anaprox Tablets 2632

KARVEA (Australia, Germany, Greece, Italy, Spain, The Netherlands, Turkey)
IRBESARTAN
Avapro Tablets 897

KARVEZIDE (Australia, Germany, Italy, Spain, The Netherlands, Turkey)
HYDROCHLOROTHIAZIDE/IRBESARTAN
Avalide Tablets 892

KATION (Italy)
POTASSIUM CITRATE
Urocit-K Tablets 2176

KATOPIL (Czech Republic)
CAPTOPRIL
Captopril Tablets 2182

KATOPRIL (Singapore)
CAPTOPRIL
Captopril Tablets 2182

KATTWILACT (Germany)
LACTULOSE
Kristalose for Oral Solution 1004

KAVELOR (Venezuela)
SIMVASTATIN
Zocor Tablets 2136

KAZEPIN (Turkey)
CARBAMAZEPINE
Carbatrol Capsules 3019

K-CITRA (Canada)
POTASSIUM CITRATE
Urocit-K Tablets 2176

KEAL (France)
SUCRALFATE
Carafate Suspension 706
Carafate Tablets 707

KECIFLOX (Germany)
CIPROFLOXACIN HYDROCHLORIDE
Cipro Tablets 2810

KEEFLOXIN (Portugal)
CIPROFLOXACIN HYDROCHLORIDE
Cipro Tablets 2810

KEFADIM (Belgium, Brazil, Czech Republic, Thailand, United Kingdom)
CEFTAZIDIME
Fortaz for Injection 1450

KEFAMIN (Spain)
CEFTAZIDIME
Fortaz for Injection 1450

KEFAZIM (Austria)
CEFTAZIDIME
Fortaz for Injection 1450

KEFNIR (India)
CEFDINIR
Omnicef Capsules 497
Omnicef for Oral Suspension 497

KEFOX (Italy, The Philippines)
CEFUROXIME SODIUM
Zinacef Injection 1678

KEFTRAGARD (India)
CEFTRIAXONE SODIUM
Rocephin Injectable Vials, ADD-Vantage, Galaxy, Bulk 2642

KEFTRIAXON (Israel)
CEFTRIAXONE SODIUM
Rocephin Injectable Vials, ADD-Vantage, Galaxy, Bulk 2642

KEFURIM (Israel)
CEFUROXIME SODIUM
Zinacef Injection 1678

KEFURION (Finland)
CEFUROXIME SODIUM
Zinacef Injection 1678

KEFUROX (Belgium, Canada)
CEFUROXIME SODIUM
Zinacef Injection 1678

KEFZIM (Chile, South Africa)
CEFTAZIDIME
Fortaz for Injection 1450

KELA (Thailand)
TRIAMCINOLONE ACETONIDE
Azmacort Inhalation Aerosol 407
Nasacort AQ Nasal Spray 2765

KEMZID (Hong Kong, Singapore, Thailand)
TRIAMCINOLONE ACETONIDE
Azmacort Inhalation Aerosol 407
Nasacort AQ Nasal Spray 2765

KENACORT (Belgium, France, India, Italy, Thailand, The Philippines)
TRIAMCINOLONE ACETONIDE
Azmacort Inhalation Aerosol 407
Nasacort AQ Nasal Spray 2765

KENACORT-A (Argentina, Australia, Belgium, Chile, Greece, Hong Kong, Irish Republic, Malaysia, New Zealand, Singapore, Switzerland, The Netherlands, The Philippines, Turkey)
TRIAMCINOLONE ACETONIDE
Azmacort Inhalation Aerosol 407
Nasacort AQ Nasal Spray 2765

KENACORT-T (Finland, Norway, Sweden)
TRIAMCINOLONE ACETONIDE
Azmacort Inhalation Aerosol 407
Nasacort AQ Nasal Spray 2765

KENALIN (Mexico)
SULINDAC
Clinoril Tablets 1962

KENA-LITE (Thailand)
TRIAMCINOLONE ACETONIDE
Azmacort Inhalation Aerosol 407
Nasacort AQ Nasal Spray 2765

KENALOG (Canada, Czech Republic, Denmark, Germany, Hungary, Irish Republic, Israel, United Kingdom, Venezuela)
TRIAMCINOLONE ACETONIDE
Azmacort Inhalation Aerosol 407
Nasacort AQ Nasal Spray 2765

KENALOG IN ORABASE (Australia, Canada, Hong Kong, Israel, Malaysia, New Zealand, Singapore, South Africa, Spain, Thailand)
TRIAMCINOLONE ACETONIDE
Azmacort Inhalation Aerosol 407

Nasacort AQ Nasal Spray 2765

KENALONE (Australia)
TRIAMCINOLONE ACETONIDE
Azmacort Inhalation Aerosol 407
Nasacort AQ Nasal Spray 2765

KENAPRIL (Mexico)
CAPTOPRIL
Captopril Tablets 2182

KENAPROX (Mexico)
NAPROXEN
EC-Naprosyn Delayed-Release Tablets 2632
Naprosyn Suspension 2632
Naprosyn Tablets 2632

KENERGON (Switzerland)
LIDOCAINE
Lidoderm Patch 1114

KENESIL (Spain)
NIMODIPINE
Nimotop Capsules 790

KENICET (Mexico)
CETIRIZINE HYDROCHLORIDE
Zyrtec Syrup 1920
Zyrtec Tablets 1920

KENO (Thailand)
TRIAMCINOLONE ACETONIDE
Azmacort Inhalation Aerosol 407
Nasacort AQ Nasal Spray 2765

KENOIDAL (Belgium)
TRIAMCINOLONE ACETONIDE
Azmacort Inhalation Aerosol 407
Nasacort AQ Nasal Spray 2765

KENOKET (Mexico)
CLONAZEPAM
Klonopin Tablets 2639

KENOLAN (Mexico)
CAPTOPRIL
Captopril Tablets 2182

KENSEDAL (Mexico)
NAPROXEN
EC-Naprosyn Delayed-Release Tablets 2632
Naprosyn Suspension 2632
Naprosyn Tablets 2632

KENZEN (France)
CANDESARTAN CILEXETIL
Atacand Tablets 639

KENZOFLEX (Mexico)
CIPROFLOXACIN HYDROCHLORIDE
Cipro Tablets 2810

KENZOLOL (Mexico)
NIMODIPINE
Nimotop Capsules 790

KEPTRIX (The Philippines)
CEFTRIAXONE SODIUM
Rocephin Injectable Vials, ADD-Vantage, Galaxy, Bulk 2642

KERLOCAL (France)
TRETINOIN
Vesanoid Capsules 2660

KESINT (Italy)
CEFUROXIME SODIUM
Zinacef Injection 1678

KESS (Argentina)
LAMIVUDINE
Epivir Oral Solution 1412
Epivir Tablets 1412
Epivir-HBV Oral Solution 1417
Epivir-HBV Tablets 1417

KESS COMPLEX (Argentina)
LAMIVUDINE
Epivir Oral Solution 1412
Epivir Tablets 1412
Epivir-HBV Oral Solution 1417
Epivir-HBV Tablets 1417

KESTERINA (Venezuela)
CEFTAZIDIME
Fortaz for Injection 1450

KETANINE (Singapore)
CAPTOPRIL
Captopril Tablets 2182

KETIDIN (Argentina)
RALOXIFENE HYDROCHLORIDE
Evista Tablets 1810

KETOCEF (Russia)
CEFUROXIME SODIUM
Zinacef Injection 1678

KETREL (France, Portugal)
TRETINOIN
Vesanoid Capsules 2660

KEYERPRIL (Mexico)
CAPTOPRIL
Captopril Tablets 2182

KEZEPIN (Mexico)
CARBAMAZEPINE
Carbatrol Capsules 3019

KIATRIUM (Brazil)
DIAZEPAM
Valium Tablets 2658

KIDROLASE (Argentina, Canada, Czech Republic, France, Israel)
ASPARAGINASE
Elspar for Injection 2488

KIMAFAN (Hong Kong)
CAPTOPRIL
Captopril Tablets 2182

KINABIDE (Argentina)
SELEGILINE HYDROCHLORIDE
Eldepryl Capsules 3052

KINDAREN (Brazil)
DICLOFENAC SODIUM
Voltaren Tablets 2334
Voltaren-XR Tablets 2337

KINLINE (Thailand)
SELEGILINE HYDROCHLORIDE
Eldepryl Capsules 3052

KINZAL (Switzerland)
TELMISARTAN
Micardis Tablets 852

KINZALKOMB (Belgium, Denmark, Finland, Germany, Sweden, The Netherlands)
TELMISARTAN
Micardis Tablets 852

KINZALMONO (Belgium, Denmark, Finland, Germany, Sweden, The Netherlands)
TELMISARTAN
Micardis Tablets 852

KINZALPLUS (Switzerland)
TELMISARTAN
Micardis Tablets 852

KIPRES (Japan)
MONTELUKAST SODIUM
Singulair Chewable Tablets 2114
Singulair Tablets 2114

KIR RICHTER (Italy)
APROTININ
Trasylol Injection 799

KIVEXA (Argentina, Denmark, Finland, Germany, Irish Republic, Italy, Norway, Poland, Spain, Sweden, The Netherlands)
ABACAVIR SULFATE
Ziagen Oral Solution 1673
Ziagen Tablets 1673

KLABAX (Poland, Russia)
CLARITHROMYCIN
Biaxin Filmtab Tablets 411
Biaxin Granules 411

KLABET (Mexico)
CLARITHROMYCIN
Biaxin Filmtab Tablets 411
Biaxin Granules 411

KLABION (Poland)
CLARITHROMYCIN
Biaxin Filmtab Tablets 411
Biaxin Granules 411

KLACID (Australia, Czech Republic, Denmark, Finland, Germany, Hong Kong, Hungary, Irish Republic, Israel, Italy, Malaysia, New Zealand, Norway, Poland, Portugal, Russia, Singapore, South Africa, Spain, Sweden, Thailand, The Netherlands, Turkey)
CLARITHROMYCIN
Biaxin Filmtab Tablets 411
Biaxin Granules 411

KLACIPED (Switzerland)
CLARITHROMYCIN
Biaxin Filmtab Tablets 411
Biaxin Granules 411

KLAMIRAN (Hungary)
CLARITHROMYCIN
Biaxin Filmtab Tablets 411
Biaxin Granules 411

KLARI (Hungary)
CLARITHROMYCIN
Biaxin Filmtab Tablets 411
Biaxin Granules 411

KLARICID (Argentina, Brazil, Chile, Greece, The Netherlands, The Philippines, United Kingdom, Venezuela)
CLARITHROMYCIN
Biaxin Filmtab Tablets 411
Biaxin Granules 411

KLARIDEX (Israel)
CLARITHROMYCIN
Biaxin Filmtab Tablets 411
Biaxin Granules 411

KLARIFAR (Greece)
CLARITHROMYCIN
Biaxin Filmtab Tablets 411
Biaxin Granules 411

KLARITHRAN (South Africa)
CLARITHROMYCIN
Biaxin Filmtab Tablets 411
Biaxin Granules 411

KLARITHRIN (Greece)
CLARITHROMYCIN
Biaxin Filmtab Tablets 411
Biaxin Granules 411

KLARITRIL (Brazil)
CLARITHROMYCIN
Biaxin Filmtab Tablets 411
Biaxin Granules 411

KLARIX (Mexico)
CLARITHROMYCIN
Biaxin Filmtab Tablets 411
Biaxin Granules 411

KLARMIN (Poland)
CLARITHROMYCIN
Biaxin Filmtab Tablets 411
Biaxin Granules 411

KLARMYN (Mexico, The Philippines)
CLARITHROMYCIN
Biaxin Filmtab Tablets 411
Biaxin Granules 411

KLAROLID (Turkey)
CLARITHROMYCIN
Biaxin Filmtab Tablets 411
Biaxin Granules 411

KLAROMIN (Turkey)
CLARITHROMYCIN
Biaxin Filmtab Tablets 411
Biaxin Granules 411

KLARPHARMA (Mexico)
CLARITHROMYCIN
Biaxin Filmtab Tablets 411
Biaxin Granules 411

KLAX (Turkey)
CLARITHROMYCIN
Biaxin Filmtab Tablets 411
Biaxin Granules 411

KLAZ (The Philippines)
CLARITHROMYCIN
Biaxin Filmtab Tablets 411
Biaxin Granules 411

KLEREN (Venezuela)
NIMODIPINE
Nimotop Capsules 790

KLERIMED (Hong Kong, Russia, Singapore)
CLARITHROMYCIN
Biaxin Filmtab Tablets 411
Biaxin Granules 411

KLEXANE (Denmark, Finland, Norway, Sweden)
ENOXAPARIN SODIUM
Lovenox Injection 2756

KLIANE (Czech Republic)
ESTRADIOL
Climara Transdermal System 763

KLICINA (Venezuela)
CIPROFLOXACIN
Cipro Oral Suspension 2810

KLIMAPUR (Austria)
ESTRADIOL
Climara Transdermal System 763

KLIMAREDUCT (Austria)
ESTRADIOL
Climara Transdermal System 763

KLINOTAL (Venezuela)
FAMOTIDINE
Pepcid for Oral Suspension 2075
Pepcid Tablets 2075

KLINOXID (Germany)
BENZOYL PEROXIDE
Brevoxyl-4 Creamy Wash 3054
Brevoxyl-4 Gel 3054
Brevoxyl-8 Creamy Wash 3054
Brevoxyl-8 Gel 3054

KLIOFEM (United Kingdom)
ESTRADIOL
Climara Transdermal System 763

KLIOGEST (Argentina, Australia, Belgium, Brazil, Czech Republic, Hungary, Malaysia, New Zealand, Poland, The Philippines, Turkey)
ESTRADIOL
Climara Transdermal System 763

KLIOVANCE (Australia, New Zealand)
ESTRADIOL
Climara Transdermal System 763

KLONACID (Argentina)
CLARITHROMYCIN
Biaxin Filmtab Tablets 411
Biaxin Granules 411

KLONALMOX (Argentina)
AMOXICILLIN
Amoxil Pediatric Drops for Oral Suspension 1305
Amoxil Tablets 1305

KLONAPROST (Argentina)
LATANOPROST
Xalatan Ophthalmic Solution .... ⊙273

KLONASTIN (Argentina)
SIMVASTATIN
Zocor Tablets 2136

KLOSARTAN D (Argentina)
LOSARTAN POTASSIUM
Cozaar Tablets 1973

K-LYTE (Canada)
POTASSIUM CITRATE
Urocit-K Tablets 2176

KOCEFAN (Italy)
CEFTRIAXONE SODIUM
Rocephin Injectable Vials, ADD-Vantage, Galaxy, Bulk 2642

KOFRON (Spain)
CLARITHROMYCIN
Biaxin Filmtab Tablets 411
Biaxin Granules 411

KOLKIN (Argentina)
FUROSEMIDE
Furosemide Tablets 2186

KOLLAGENASE (Brazil)
COLLAGENASE
Santyl Collagenase Ointment 1724

KOLLAGENASE COM CLORANFENICOL (Brazil)
COLLAGENASE
Santyl Collagenase Ointment 1724

KOLLOSTERIL (Argentina)
CARVEDILOL
Coreg Tablets 1387

KOLPAZOL (Brazil)
NYSTATIN
Nystop Topical Powder USP 2498

KOLPOVENT (Chile)
SALMETEROL XINAFOATE
Serevent Diskus 1594

KORTIKOID-RATIOPHARM (Germany)
TRIAMCINOLONE ACETONIDE
Azmacort Inhalation Aerosol 407
Nasacort AQ Nasal Spray 2765

KOSTAL (Chile)
CILOSTAZOL
Pletal Tablets 2481

KOSTEO (Australia)
CALCITRIOL
Calcijex Injection . . . 419
Rocaltrol Capsules . . . 1150
Rocaltrol Oral Solution . . . 1150

KRATIUM (Hong Kong)
DIAZEPAM
Valium Tablets . . . 2658

KRAUTIN (Greece)
SELEGILINE HYDROCHLORIDE
Eldepryl Capsules . . . 3052

KREBSILASI (Italy)
PANCRELIPASE
Ultrase Capsules . . . 718
Ultrase MT Capsules . . . 719

KREDEX (Australia, Belgium, France, Italy, Norway, Portugal, Spain, Sweden)
CARVEDILOL
Coreg Tablets . . . 1387

KRENOSIN (France, Italy, Mexico)
ADENOSINE
Adenocard IV Injection . . . 603
Adenoscan . . . 605

KRENOSINE (Switzerland)
ADENOSINE
Adenocard IV Injection . . . 603
Adenoscan . . . 605

KRIADEX (Mexico)
CLONAZEPAM
Klonopin Tablets . . . 2639

KROBICIN (Mexico)
CLARITHROMYCIN
Biaxin Filmtab Tablets . . . 411
Biaxin Granules . . . 411

KSILIDIN (Turkey)
LIDOCAINE
Lidoderm Patch . . . 1114

KURACID (Denmark)
RANITIDINE HYDROCHLORIDE
Zantac 25 EFFERdose Tablets . . . 1670
Zantac 150 Tablets . . . 1670
Zantac 300 Tablets . . . 1670
Zantac Injection . . . 1666
Zantac Injection Premixed . . . 1666
Zantac Syrup . . . 1670

KYMAZOL (Greece)
SIMVASTATIN
Zocor Tablets . . . 2136

LA MORPH (New Zealand)
MORPHINE SULFATE
MS Contin Tablets . . . 2585

LABEL (Brazil)
RANITIDINE HYDROCHLORIDE
Zantac 25 EFFERdose Tablets . . . 1670
Zantac 150 Tablets . . . 1670
Zantac 300 Tablets . . . 1670
Zantac Injection . . . 1666
Zantac Injection Premixed . . . 1666
Zantac Syrup . . . 1670

LABENDA (Thailand)
ALBENDAZOLE
Albenza Tablets . . . 1297

LABENTROL (Greece)
CIPROFLOXACIN HYDROCHLORIDE
Cipro Tablets . . . 2810

LABILENO (Spain)
LAMOTRIGINE
Lamictal Chewable Dispersible Tablets . . . 1488
Lamictal Tablets . . . 1488

LABILEX (Greece)
CEFTRIAXONE SODIUM
Rocephin Injectable Vials, ADD-Vantage, Galaxy, Bulk . . . 2642

LABIMIQ (Chile)
IMIQUIMOD
Aldara Cream, 5% . . . 1699

LABISTATIN (Argentina)
SIMVASTATIN
Zocor Tablets . . . 2136

LABISTATIN DUO (Argentina)
SIMVASTATIN
Zocor Tablets . . . 2136

LAC-DOL (Australia)
LACTULOSE
Kristalose for Oral Solution . . . 1004

LACEROL (Spain)
DILTIAZEM HYDROCHLORIDE
Cardizem LA Extended Release Tablets . . . 421

LACRIPHARMA (Argentina)
SODIUM HYALURONATE
Hyalgan Solution . . . 2742

LACSON (South Africa)
LACTULOSE
Kristalose for Oral Solution . . . 1004

LACTOCUR (Australia, Germany)
LACTULOSE
Kristalose for Oral Solution . . . 1004

LACTOFALK (Germany)
LACTULOSE
Kristalose for Oral Solution . . . 1004

LACTOGER (Italy)
LACTULOSE
Kristalose for Oral Solution . . . 1004

LACTUFLOR (Germany)
LACTULOSE
Kristalose for Oral Solution . . . 1004

LACTUGAL (United Kingdom)
LACTULOSE
Kristalose for Oral Solution . . . 1004

LACTUL (Malaysia)
LACTULOSE
Kristalose for Oral Solution . . . 1004

LACTULAC (Turkey)
LACTULOSE
Kristalose for Oral Solution . . . 1004

LACTULAX (Canada, Israel, Mexico)
LACTULOSE
Kristalose for Oral Solution . . . 1004

LACTULOL (Poland)
LACTULOSE
Kristalose for Oral Solution . . . 1004

LACTULON (Argentina)
LACTULOSE
Kristalose for Oral Solution . . . 1004

LACTULONA (Brazil, Venezuela)
LACTULOSE
Kristalose for Oral Solution . . . 1004

LACTUMED (Malaysia)
LACTULOSE
Kristalose for Oral Solution . . . 1004

LACTUS (Singapore)
LACTULOSE
Kristalose for Oral Solution . . . 1004

LACTUVERLAN (Germany)
LACTULOSE
Kristalose for Oral Solution . . . 1004

LACTYL (Italy)
LACTULOSE
Kristalose for Oral Solution . . . 1004

LADIWIN (India)
LAMIVUDINE
Epivir Oral Solution . . . 1412
Epivir Tablets . . . 1412
Epivir-HBV Oral Solution . . . 1417
Epivir-HBV Tablets . . . 1417

LAEVILAC S (Germany)
LACTULOSE
Kristalose for Oral Solution . . . 1004

LAEVOLAC (Austria, Czech Republic, Hong Kong, Hungary, Israel, Italy, New Zealand, Portugal, South Africa, Switzerland, Thailand, Turkey)
LACTULOSE
Kristalose for Oral Solution . . . 1004

LAFAMO (Hong Kong)
FAMOTIDINE
Pepcid for Oral Suspension . . . 2075
Pepcid Tablets . . . 2075

LAFEDAM (Argentina)
ALENDRONATE SODIUM
Fosamax Tablets . . . 2005

LAFELAX (Argentina)
LACTULOSE
Kristalose for Oral Solution . . . 1004

LAFUREX (Italy)
CEFUROXIME SODIUM
Zinacef Injection . . . 1678

LAGOTRAN (Argentina)
LAMOTRIGINE
Lamictal Chewable Dispersible Tablets . . . 1488
Lamictal Tablets . . . 1488

LAGRICEL (Mexico)
SODIUM HYALURONATE
Hyalgan Solution . . . 2742

LAGRICEL OFTENO (Chile, Venezuela)
SODIUM HYALURONATE
Hyalgan Solution . . . 2742

LAGUR (Brazil)
CLARITHROMYCIN
Biaxin Filmtab Tablets . . . 411
Biaxin Granules . . . 411

LAITUN (The Philippines)
CIPROFLOXACIN HYDROCHLORIDE
Cipro Tablets . . . 2810

LAKE (Spain)
RANITIDINE HYDROCHLORIDE
Zantac 25 EFFERdose Tablets . . . 1670
Zantac 150 Tablets . . . 1670
Zantac 300 Tablets . . . 1670
Zantac Injection . . . 1666
Zantac Injection Premixed . . . 1666
Zantac Syrup . . . 1670

LAKEA (Poland)
LOSARTAN POTASSIUM
Cozaar Tablets . . . 1973

LAKTIPEX (Sweden)
LACTULOSE
Kristalose for Oral Solution . . . 1004

LAKTOL (Turkey)
LACTULOSE
Kristalose for Oral Solution . . . 1004

LAKTULAX (Austria)
LACTULOSE
Kristalose for Oral Solution . . . 1004

LAMBIPOL (Belgium)
LAMOTRIGINE
Lamictal Chewable Dispersible Tablets . . . 1488
Lamictal Tablets . . . 1488

LAMDA (India)
LAMIVUDINE
Epivir Oral Solution . . . 1412
Epivir Tablets . . . 1412
Epivir-HBV Oral Solution . . . 1417
Epivir-HBV Tablets . . . 1417

LAMDA-Z (India)
LAMIVUDINE
Epivir Oral Solution . . . 1412
Epivir Tablets . . . 1412
Epivir-HBV Oral Solution . . . 1417
Epivir-HBV Tablets . . . 1417

LAMEPIL (India)
LAMOTRIGINE
Lamictal Chewable Dispersible Tablets . . . 1488
Lamictal Tablets . . . 1488

LAMETEC (India)
LAMOTRIGINE
Lamictal Chewable Dispersible Tablets . . . 1488
Lamictal Tablets . . . 1488

LAMI (Brazil)
LAMIVUDINE
Epivir Oral Solution . . . 1412
Epivir Tablets . . . 1412
Epivir-HBV Oral Solution . . . 1417
Epivir-HBV Tablets . . . 1417

LAMIA (Poland)
LAMOTRIGINE
Lamictal Chewable Dispersible Tablets . . . 1488
Lamictal Tablets . . . 1488

LAMIBERGEN (Argentina)
LAMIVUDINE
Epivir Oral Solution . . . 1412
Epivir Tablets . . . 1412
Epivir-HBV Oral Solution . . . 1417
Epivir-HBV Tablets . . . 1417

LAMICOSIL (Spain)
TERBINAFINE HYDROCHLORIDE
Lamisil Tablets . . . 2266

LAMICSTART (France)
LAMOTRIGINE
Lamictal Chewable Dispersible Tablets . . . 1488
Lamictal Tablets . . . 1488

LAMICTAL (Argentina, Australia, Austria, Belgium, Brazil, Canada, Chile, Czech Republic, Denmark, Finland, France, Germany, Greece, Hong Kong, Hungary, Irish Republic, Israel, Italy, Malaysia, Mexico, New Zealand, Norway, Portugal, Russia, Singapore, Spain, Sweden, Switzerland, Thailand, The Netherlands, The Philippines, Turkey, United Kingdom, Venezuela)
LAMOTRIGINE
Lamictal Chewable Dispersible Tablets . . . 1488
Lamictal Tablets . . . 1488

LAMICTIN (South Africa)
LAMOTRIGINE
Lamictal Chewable Dispersible Tablets . . . 1488
Lamictal Tablets . . . 1488

LAMIDAC (India)
LAMIVUDINE
Epivir Oral Solution . . . 1412
Epivir Tablets . . . 1412
Epivir-HBV Oral Solution . . . 1417
Epivir-HBV Tablets . . . 1417

LAMIDEN (Brazil)
LAMIVUDINE
Epivir Oral Solution . . . 1412
Epivir Tablets . . . 1412
Epivir-HBV Oral Solution . . . 1417
Epivir-HBV Tablets . . . 1417

LAMIDUS (Australia)
LAMOTRIGINE
Lamictal Chewable Dispersible Tablets . . . 1488
Lamictal Tablets . . . 1488

LAMIFEN (The Philippines)
TERBINAFINE HYDROCHLORIDE
Lamisil Tablets . . . 2266

LAMILEA (Argentina)
LAMIVUDINE
Epivir Oral Solution . . . 1412
Epivir Tablets . . . 1412
Epivir-HBV Oral Solution . . . 1417
Epivir-HBV Tablets . . . 1417

LAMILEPT (Poland)
LAMOTRIGINE
Lamictal Chewable Dispersible Tablets . . . 1488
Lamictal Tablets . . . 1488

LAMIRAX (Argentina)
LAMOTRIGINE
Lamictal Chewable Dispersible Tablets . . . 1488
Lamictal Tablets . . . 1488

LAMIREX (India)
LAMIVUDINE
Epivir Oral Solution . . . 1412
Epivir Tablets . . . 1412
Epivir-HBV Oral Solution . . . 1417
Epivir-HBV Tablets . . . 1417

LAMISIL (Argentina, Belgium, Canada, Czech Republic, Denmark, Finland, France, Hong Kong, India, Irish Republic, Israel, Italy, Mexico, New Zealand, Poland, Portugal, Singapore, South Africa, Spain, Thailand, The Philippines, Turkey, United Kingdom)
TERBINAFINE HYDROCHLORIDE
Lamisil Tablets . . . 2266

LAMISILATE (France)
TERBINAFINE HYDROCHLORIDE
Lamisil Tablets . . . 2266

LAMISILATT (Poland)
TERBINAFINE HYDROCHLORIDE
Lamisil Tablets . . . 2266

LAMITOR (Brazil, South Africa, The Netherlands)
LAMOTRIGINE
Lamictal Chewable Dispersible Tablets . . . 1488
Lamictal Tablets . . . 1488

LAMITRIN (Australia, Poland)
LAMOTRIGINE
Lamictal Chewable Dispersible Tablets . . . 1488
Lamictal Tablets . . . 1488

LAMIVIR (India, Venezuela)
LAMIVUDINE
Epivir Oral Solution . . . 1412
Epivir Tablets . . . 1412
Epivir-HBV Oral Solution . . . 1417
Epivir-HBV Tablets . . . 1417

LAMIVIR S (India)
LAMIVUDINE
Epivir Oral Solution . . . 1412

Epivir Tablets 1412
Epivir-HBV Oral Solution 1417
Epivir-HBV Tablets 1417

LAMO (Germany)
LAMOTRIGINE
Lamictal Chewable Dispersible Tablets . . . 1488
Lamictal Tablets 1488

LAMOCHEM (The Netherlands)
LAMOTRIGINE
Lamictal Chewable Dispersible Tablets . . . 1488
Lamictal Tablets 1488

LAMODEX (Israel)
LAMOTRIGINE
Lamictal Chewable Dispersible Tablets . . . 1488
Lamictal Tablets 1488

LAMOGINE (Israel)
LAMOTRIGINE
Lamictal Chewable Dispersible Tablets . . . 1488
Lamictal Tablets 1488

LAMOMONT (The Netherlands)
LAMOTRIGINE
Lamictal Chewable Dispersible Tablets . . . 1488
Lamictal Tablets 1488

LAMOTIFI (The Netherlands)
LAMOTRIGINE
Lamictal Chewable Dispersible Tablets . . . 1488
Lamictal Tablets 1488

LAMOTRIAX (Germany)
LAMOTRIGINE
Lamictal Chewable Dispersible Tablets . . . 1488
Lamictal Tablets 1488

LAMOTRIG (Germany)
LAMOTRIGINE
Lamictal Chewable Dispersible Tablets . . . 1488
Lamictal Tablets 1488

LAMOTRIGLAX (Austria)
LAMOTRIGINE
Lamictal Chewable Dispersible Tablets . . . 1488
Lamictal Tablets 1488

LAMOTRIHEXAL (Poland)
LAMOTRIGINE
Lamictal Chewable Dispersible Tablets . . . 1488
Lamictal Tablets 1488

LAMOTRIL (Argentina)
LAMOTRIGINE
Lamictal Chewable Dispersible Tablets . . . 1488
Lamictal Tablets 1488

LAMOTRIX (Poland)
LAMOTRIGINE
Lamictal Chewable Dispersible Tablets . . . 1488
Lamictal Tablets 1488

LAMPOSPORIN (Italy)
CEFUROXIME SODIUM
Zinacef Injection 1678

LAMRA (Germany)
DIAZEPAM
Valium Tablets 2658

LAMUZID (India)
LAMIVUDINE
Epivir Oral Solution 1412
Epivir Tablets 1412
Epivir-HBV Oral Solution 1417
Epivir-HBV Tablets 1417

LAMZID (South Africa)
ZIDOVUDINE
Retrovir Capsules 1574
Retrovir IV Infusion. 1579
Retrovir Syrup 1574
Retrovir Tablets. 1574

LANACARD (Germany)
DIGOXIN
Lanoxin Injection 1498
Lanoxin Injection Pediatric 1502
Lanoxin Tablets. 1505

LANACORDIN (Spain)
DIGOXIN
Lanoxin Injection 1498
Lanoxin Injection Pediatric 1502
Lanoxin Tablets. 1505

LANACRIST (Sweden)
DIGOXIN
Lanoxin Injection 1498
Lanoxin Injection Pediatric 1502
Lanoxin Tablets. 1505

LANAFINE (Irish Republic)
TERBINAFINE HYDROCHLORIDE
Lamisil Tablets 2266

LANALGET (Austria)
TRAMADOL HYDROCHLORIDE
Ultram ER Tablets 2428

LANATIN (Denmark)
LISINOPRIL
Prinivil Tablets 2087

LANDOLAXIN (Greece)
LISINOPRIL
Prinivil Tablets 2087

LANDROLEN (Mexico)
ALENDRONATE SODIUM
Fosamax Tablets 2005

LANEXAT (Argentina, Brazil, Chile, Denmark, Finland, Mexico, Sweden, Venezuela)
FLUMAZENIL
Romazicon Injection. 2646

LANICOR (Argentina, Austria, Germany, Italy, The Netherlands, Venezuela)
DIGOXIN
Lanoxin Injection 1498
Lanoxin Injection Pediatric 1502
Lanoxin Tablets. 1505

LANOXICAPS (The Netherlands)
DIGOXIN
Lanoxin Injection 1498
Lanoxin Injection Pediatric 1502
Lanoxin Tablets. 1505

LANOXIN (Argentina, Australia, Belgium, Brazil, Canada, Hong Kong, India, Irish Republic, Israel, Italy, Malaysia, Mexico, New Zealand, Norway, Portugal, Singapore, South Africa, Sweden, Switzerland, Thailand, The Netherlands, The Philippines, United Kingdom)
DIGOXIN
Lanoxin Injection 1498
Lanoxin Injection Pediatric 1502
Lanoxin Tablets. 1505

LAPROST (Venezuela)
LATANOPROST
Xalatan Ophthalmic Solution . . . . . . ⊙273

LARA (India)
LOSARTAN POTASSIUM
Cozaar Tablets 1973

LARAFLEX (United Kingdom)
NAPROXEN
EC-Naprosyn Delayed-Release Tablets. . . . 2632
Naprosyn Suspension. 2632
Naprosyn Tablets 2632

LARGOPEN (Turkey)
AMOXICILLIN
Amoxil Pediatric Drops for Oral Suspension. 1305
Amoxil Tablets 1305

LARICID (Turkey)
CLARITHROMYCIN
Biaxin Filmtab Tablets. 411
Biaxin Granules 411

LARIG (Irish Republic)
LAMOTRIGINE
Lamictal Chewable Dispersible Tablets . . . 1488
Lamictal Tablets 1488

LARJANCAINA (Argentina)
LIDOCAINE
Lidoderm Patch 1114

LARSIMAL (Argentina)
FLUOROMETHOLONE
FML Ophthalmic Ointment. . . . . ⊙223

LASER (Italy)
NAPROXEN
EC-Naprosyn Delayed-Release Tablets. . . . 2632
Naprosyn Suspension. 2632
Naprosyn Tablets 2632

LASERVIS (Germany, Malaysia, Switzerland)
SODIUM HYALURONATE
Hyalgan Solution. 2742

LASIKAL (United Kingdom)
FUROSEMIDE
Furosemide Tablets 2186

LASILACTON (Mexico)
FUROSEMIDE
Furosemide Tablets 2186

LASILACTONE (United Kingdom)
FUROSEMIDE
Furosemide Tablets 2186

LASILETTEN (The Netherlands)
FUROSEMIDE
Furosemide Tablets 2186

LASILIX (France)
FUROSEMIDE
Furosemide Tablets 2186

LASIPRESSIN (United Kingdom)
FUROSEMIDE
Furosemide Tablets 2186

LASIVEN (Thailand)
FUROSEMIDE
Furosemide Tablets 2186

LASIX (Argentina, Australia, Belgium, Brazil, Canada, Czech Republic, Denmark, Finland, Hong Kong, India, Irish Republic, Israel, Malaysia, Mexico, New Zealand, Norway, Portugal, Russia, Singapore, South Africa, Sweden, Thailand, The Netherlands, The Philippines, Turkey, United Kingdom, Venezuela)
FUROSEMIDE
Furosemide Tablets 2186

LASMA (Irish Republic, United Kingdom)
THEOPHYLLINE
Uniphyl Tablets 2595

LASORIDE (United Kingdom)
FUROSEMIDE
Furosemide Tablets 2186

L-ASP (Argentina)
ASPARAGINASE
Elspar for Injection 2488

LASPAR (South Africa)
ASPARAGINASE
Elspar for Injection 2488

LASSIFAR (Italy)
LACTULOSE
Kristalose for Oral Solution 1004

LATAC (Hong Kong)
RANITIDINE HYDROCHLORIDE
Zantac 25 EFFERdose Tablets 1670
Zantac 150 Tablets 1670
Zantac 300 Tablets 1670
Zantac Injection 1666
Zantac Injection Premixed 1666
Zantac Syrup 1670

LATANOFLAX (Argentina)
LATANOPROST
Xalatan Ophthalmic Solution . . . . . . ⊙273

LATANOPRESS (Venezuela)
LATANOPROST
Xalatan Ophthalmic Solution . . . . . . ⊙273

LATOF (Chile)
LATANOPROST
Xalatan Ophthalmic Solution . . . . . . ⊙273

LATRIGIN (Argentina)
LAMOTRIGINE
Lamictal Chewable Dispersible Tablets . . . 1488
Lamictal Tablets 1488

LATTUBIO (Italy)
LACTULOSE
Kristalose for Oral Solution 1004

LATTULAC (Italy)
LACTULOSE
Kristalose for Oral Solution 1004

LAVER (Thailand)
TRIAMCINOLONE ACETONIDE
Azmacort Inhalation Aerosol. 407
Nasacort AQ Nasal Spray 2765

LAXARON (France)
LACTULOSE
Kristalose for Oral Solution 1004

LAXEERSIROOP (The Netherlands)
LACTULOSE
Kristalose for Oral Solution 1004

LAXETTE (South Africa)
LACTULOSE
Kristalose for Oral Solution 1004

LAXILOSE (Canada)
LACTULOSE
Kristalose for Oral Solution 1004

LAXINAT (The Philippines)
CEFUROXIME SODIUM
Zinacef Injection 1678

LAXOMUNDIN (Germany)
LACTULOSE
Kristalose for Oral Solution 1004

LAXOSE (Irish Republic, United Kingdom)
LACTULOSE
Kristalose for Oral Solution 1004

LAXULAC (Italy)
LACTULOSE
Kristalose for Oral Solution 1004

LAXYL (Mexico)
DIAZEPAM
Valium Tablets 2658

LEDERCORT (Argentina, Sweden)
TRIAMCINOLONE ACETONIDE
Azmacort Inhalation Aerosol. 407
Nasacort AQ Nasal Spray 2765

LEDERCORT CON NEOMICINA (Argentina)
TRIAMCINOLONE ACETONIDE
Azmacort Inhalation Aerosol. 407
Nasacort AQ Nasal Spray 2765

LEDERCORT-N (India)
TRIAMCINOLONE ACETONIDE
Azmacort Inhalation Aerosol. 407
Nasacort AQ Nasal Spray 2765

LEDERLIND (Germany)
NYSTATIN
Nystop Topical Powder USP. 2498

LEDOX (Norway)
NAPROXEN
EC-Naprosyn Delayed-Release Tablets. . . . 2632
Naprosyn Suspension. 2632
Naprosyn Tablets 2632

LEDOXID ACNE (Switzerland)
BENZOYL PEROXIDE
Brevoxyl-4 Creamy Wash. 3054
Brevoxyl-4 Gel 3054
Brevoxyl-8 Creamy Wash. 3054
Brevoxyl-8 Gel 3054

LEEFLOX (India)
LEVOFLOXACIN
Levaquin Injection 2416
Levaquin Tablets. 2416

LEFLOXIN (Thailand)
LEVOFLOXACIN
Levaquin Injection 2416
Levaquin Tablets. 2416

LEFLUMAX (Argentina)
LEVOFLOXACIN
Levaquin Injection 2416
Levaquin Tablets. 2416

LEGENDAL (Switzerland, The Netherlands)
LACTULOSE
Kristalose for Oral Solution 1004

LEGIL (Greece)
SELEGILINE HYDROCHLORIDE
Eldepryl Capsules 3052

LEGIS (Spain)
IPRATROPIUM BROMIDE
Atrovent Nasal Spray 0.03%. 834
Atrovent Nasal Spray 0.06%. 836

LEKOKLAR (Czech Republic, Poland)
CLARITHROMYCIN
Biaxin Filmtab Tablets. 411
Biaxin Granules 411

LELONG CONTUSIONS (France)
PENTOSAN POLYSULFATE SODIUM
Elmiron Capsules 2435

LEMBROL (Argentina)
DIAZEPAM
Valium Tablets 2658

LEMERON (Mexico)
INTERFERON ALFA-2B
Intron A for Injection. 2859

LEMLAX (United Kingdom)
LACTULOSE
Kristalose for Oral Solution 1004

LEMORCAN (Greece)
NORFLOXACIN
Noroxin Tablets . . . 2069

LEMOXOL (Greece)
CEFTAZIDIME
Fortaz for Injection . . . 1450

LEMTOSID (Mexico)
BENZONATATE
Tessalon Perles . . . 1183

LEMYTRIOL (Mexico)
CALCITRIOL
Calcijex Injection . . . 419
Rocaltrol Capsules . . . 1150
Rocaltrol Oral Solution . . . 1150

LENDACIN (Czech Republic, Hungary, Poland, Russia)
CEFTRIAXONE SODIUM
Rocephin Injectable Vials, ADD-Vantage, Galaxy, Bulk . . . 2642

LENDRONAL (Argentina)
ALENDRONATE SODIUM
Fosamax Tablets . . . 2005

LENIARTRIL (Italy)
NAPROXEN
EC-Naprosyn Delayed-Release Tablets . . . 2632
Naprosyn Suspension . . . 2632
Naprosyn Tablets . . . 2632

LENITIL (Argentina)
DICLOFENAC SODIUM
Voltaren Tablets . . . 2334
Voltaren-XR Tablets . . . 2337

LENOXICAPS (Germany)
DIGOXIN
Lanoxin Injection . . . 1498
Lanoxin Injection Pediatric . . . 1502
Lanoxin Tablets . . . 1505

LENOXIN (Germany)
DIGOXIN
Lanoxin Injection . . . 1498
Lanoxin Injection Pediatric . . . 1502
Lanoxin Tablets . . . 1505

LENPRYL (Mexico)
CAPTOPRIL
Captopril Tablets . . . 2182

LEO-400 (Thailand)
ALBENDAZOLE
Albenza Tablets . . . 1297

LEODRIN (Chile)
ALENDRONATE SODIUM
Fosamax Tablets . . . 2005

LEPHIN (Thailand)
CEFTRIAXONE SODIUM
Rocephin Injectable Vials, ADD-Vantage, Galaxy, Bulk . . . 2642

LEPOBRON (Portugal)
THEOPHYLLINE
Uniphyl Tablets . . . 2595

LEPRAVIR (The Philippines)
DAPSONE
Dapsone Tablets USP . . . 1746

LEPROFEN (Argentina)
ANASTROZOLE
Arimidex Tablets . . . 672

LEPTANAL (Norway, Sweden)
FENTANYL CITRATE
Actiq . . . 959

LEPTANAL COMP (Sweden)
FENTANYL CITRATE
Actiq . . . 959

LEPTIC (Argentina)
CLONAZEPAM
Klonopin Tablets . . . 2639

LEPUR (Greece)
SIMVASTATIN
Zocor Tablets . . . 2136

LERTUS CD (Mexico)
DICLOFENAC SODIUM
Voltaren Tablets . . . 2334
Voltaren-XR Tablets . . . 2337

LERUZE (Greece)
LISINOPRIL
Prinivil Tablets . . . 2087

LESCOL (Argentina, Australia, Austria, Belgium, Brazil, Canada, Czech Republic, Denmark, Finland, France, Greece, Hong Kong, Hungary, Irish Republic, Israel, Italy, Malaysia, Mexico, New Zealand, Norway, Poland, Portugal, Russia, Singapore, South Africa, Spain, Sweden, Switzerland, Thailand, The Netherlands, The Philippines, Turkey, United Kingdom, Venezuela)
FLUVASTATIN SODIUM
Lescol Capsules . . . 2268

LESTRIC (Malaysia)
LOVASTATIN
Mevacor Tablets . . . 2063

LETANSIL (Brazil)
DIAZEPAM
Valium Tablets . . . 2658

LETEQUATRO (Portugal)
LEVOTHYROXINE SODIUM
Levothroid Tablets . . . 1170
Levoxyl Tablets . . . 1780
Synthroid Tablets . . . 507

LETIZEN (Czech Republic, Poland, Russia)
CETIRIZINE HYDROCHLORIDE
Zyrtec Syrup . . . 1920
Zyrtec Tablets . . . 1920

LETROX (Czech Republic, Hungary, Poland)
LEVOTHYROXINE SODIUM
Levothroid Tablets . . . 1170
Levoxyl Tablets . . . 1780
Synthroid Tablets . . . 507

LETTER (Portugal)
LEVOTHYROXINE SODIUM
Levothroid Tablets . . . 1170
Levoxyl Tablets . . . 1780
Synthroid Tablets . . . 507

LEUCOGEN (Spain)
ASPARAGINASE
Elspar for Injection . . . 2488

LEUKAST (Chile)
MONTELUKAST SODIUM
Singulair Chewable Tablets . . . 2114
Singulair Tablets . . . 2114

LEUKERAN (Argentina, Australia, Austria, Belgium, Brazil, Canada, Chile, Czech Republic, Denmark, Finland, Germany, Greece, Hong Kong, India, Irish Republic, Israel, Italy, Malaysia, Mexico, New Zealand, Norway, Poland, Portugal, Russia, Singapore, South Africa, Spain, Sweden, Switzerland, Thailand, The Netherlands, The Philippines, Turkey, United Kingdom)
CHLORAMBUCIL
Leukeran Tablets . . . 1508

LEUNASE (Hong Kong, India, Japan, Malaysia, Mexico, Singapore, Thailand, The Philippines, Turkey)
ASPARAGINASE
Elspar for Injection . . . 2488

LEUSTAT (Argentina, United Kingdom)
CLADRIBINE
Leustatin Injection . . . 2384

LEUSTATIN (Australia, Austria, Belgium, Brazil, Canada, Czech Republic, Denmark, Finland, Germany, Greece, Hong Kong, Israel, Italy, New Zealand, Norway, South Africa, Spain, Sweden, Switzerland, Thailand, The Netherlands, The Philippines, Venezuela)
CLADRIBINE
Leustatin Injection . . . 2384

LEUSTATINE (France)
CLADRIBINE
Leustatin Injection . . . 2384

LEVAQUIN (Argentina, Brazil, Canada, Venezuela)
LEVOFLOXACIN
Levaquin Injection . . . 2416
Levaquin Tablets . . . 2416

LEVAXIN (Norway, Sweden)
LEVOTHYROXINE SODIUM
Levothroid Tablets . . . 1170
Levoxyl Tablets . . . 1780
Synthroid Tablets . . . 507

LEVEDAD (Argentina)
DICLOFENAC SODIUM
Voltaren Tablets . . . 2334
Voltaren-XR Tablets . . . 2337

LEVIOGEL (Italy)
DICLOFENAC SODIUM
Voltaren Tablets . . . 2334
Voltaren-XR Tablets . . . 2337

LEVISTAN (Venezuela)
LOVASTATIN
Mevacor Tablets . . . 2063

LEVO (Israel)
LEVOFLOXACIN
Levaquin Injection . . . 2416
Levaquin Tablets . . . 2416

LEVOCIDE (India)
LEVOFLOXACIN
Levaquin Injection . . . 2416
Levaquin Tablets . . . 2416

LEVODEX (Israel)
DILTIAZEM HYDROCHLORIDE
Cardizem LA Extended Release Tablets . . . 421

LEVOFF (India)
LEVOFLOXACIN
Levaquin Injection . . . 2416
Levaquin Tablets . . . 2416

LEVOFLOX (India)
LEVOFLOXACIN
Levaquin Injection . . . 2416
Levaquin Tablets . . . 2416

LEVOFLOX OZ KIT (India)
LEVOFLOXACIN
Levaquin Injection . . . 2416
Levaquin Tablets . . . 2416

LEVOLAC (Finland, Norway)
LACTULOSE
Kristalose for Oral Solution . . . 1004

LEVONIS (Italy)
FLUNISOLIDE
Aerobid Inhaler System . . . 1153
Aerobid-M Inhaler System . . . 1153

LEVO-T (Canada)
LEVOTHYROXINE SODIUM
Levothroid Tablets . . . 1170
Levoxyl Tablets . . . 1780
Synthroid Tablets . . . 507

LEVOTAC (Brazil)
LEVOFLOXACIN
Levaquin Injection . . . 2416
Levaquin Tablets . . . 2416

LEVOTEC (Canada)
LEVOTHYROXINE SODIUM
Levothroid Tablets . . . 1170
Levoxyl Tablets . . . 1780
Synthroid Tablets . . . 507

LEVOTHROID (Greece, Spain)
LEVOTHYROXINE SODIUM
Levothroid Tablets . . . 1170
Levoxyl Tablets . . . 1780
Synthroid Tablets . . . 507

LEVOTHYROX (France)
LEVOTHYROXINE SODIUM
Levothroid Tablets . . . 1170
Levoxyl Tablets . . . 1780
Synthroid Tablets . . . 507

LEVOTIRON (Turkey)
LEVOTHYROXINE SODIUM
Levothroid Tablets . . . 1170
Levoxyl Tablets . . . 1780
Synthroid Tablets . . . 507

LEVOTIROX (Italy)
LEVOTHYROXINE SODIUM
Levothroid Tablets . . . 1170
Levoxyl Tablets . . . 1780
Synthroid Tablets . . . 507

LEVOTRIN (Argentina)
LIOTHYRONINE SODIUM
Cytomel Tablets . . . 1778

LEVOX (The Philippines)
LEVOFLOXACIN
Levaquin Injection . . . 2416
Levaquin Tablets . . . 2416

LEVOXACIN (Italy)
LEVOFLOXACIN
Levaquin Injection . . . 2416
Levaquin Tablets . . . 2416

LEVOXIN (Brazil)
LEVOFLOXACIN
Levaquin Injection . . . 2416
Levaquin Tablets . . . 2416

LEWIXIN (The Philippines)
AMOXICILLIN
Amoxil Pediatric Drops for Oral Suspension . . . 1305
Amoxil Tablets . . . 1305

LEXEMIN (Hong Kong, Singapore, Thailand)
FENOFIBRATE
Tricor Tablets . . . 520

LEXFOR (Thailand)
NORFLOXACIN
Noroxin Tablets . . . 2069

LEXIFLOX (Hong Kong)
NORFLOXACIN
Noroxin Tablets . . . 2069

LEXINOR (Finland, Hong Kong, Malaysia, Singapore, Sweden, Thailand, The Philippines)
NORFLOXACIN
Noroxin Tablets . . . 2069

LEXOBENE (Germany)
DICLOFENAC SODIUM
Voltaren Tablets . . . 2334
Voltaren-XR Tablets . . . 2337

LEZIDIM (Mexico)
CEFTAZIDIME
Fortaz for Injection . . . 1450

LEZOLE (Argentina)
ANASTROZOLE
Arimidex Tablets . . . 672

LGHYAL (India)
SODIUM HYALURONATE
Hyalgan Solution . . . 2742

LIBERALGIUM (Spain)
DICLOFENAC SODIUM
Voltaren Tablets . . . 2334
Voltaren-XR Tablets . . . 2337

LICUAGEN (Argentina)
CILOSTAZOL
Pletal Tablets . . . 2481

LIDERMA (Switzerland)
ISOTRETINOIN
Accutane Capsules . . . 2607

LIDIAL (Brazil)
LIDOCAINE
Lidoderm Patch . . . 1114

LIDIL CORT (Argentina)
FLUTICASONE PROPIONATE
Flonase Nasal Spray . . . 1431

LIDOCAINA SPRAY (Italy)
LIDOCAINE
Lidoderm Patch . . . 1114

LIDONOSTRUM (Portugal)
LIDOCAINE
Lidoderm Patch . . . 1114

LIDOPOSTERIN (Poland)
LIDOCAINE
Lidoderm Patch . . . 1114

LIDOPOSTERINE (Germany)
LIDOCAINE
Lidoderm Patch . . . 1114

LIDOSPRAY (Brazil)
LIDOCAINE
Lidoderm Patch . . . 1114

LIDOSTON (Brazil)
LIDOCAINE
Lidoderm Patch . . . 1114

LIFAMOX (Brazil)
AMOXICILLIN
Amoxil Pediatric Drops for Oral Suspension . . . 1305
Amoxil Tablets . . . 1305

LIFENAC (Mexico)
DICLOFENAC SODIUM
Voltaren Tablets . . . 2334

Voltaren-XR Tablets 2337

LIFERXINA (Mexico)
CIPROFLOXACIN
Cipro Oral Suspension 2810

LIFERZIT (Greece)
LOVASTATIN
Mevacor Tablets 2063

LIFEZAR (The Philippines)
LOSARTAN POTASSIUM
Cozaar Tablets 1973

LIFIN (Poland)
FINASTERIDE
Propecia Tablets 2095
Proscar Tablets 2102

LIFUROM (South Africa)
CEFUROXIME SODIUM
Zinacef Injection 1678

LIFUROX (Czech Republic, Denmark, Finland, Norway, Spain, Sweden, Venezuela)
CEFUROXIME SODIUM
Zinacef Injection 1678

LIGNOSPAN SPECIAL (South Africa)
LIDOCAINE
Lidoderm Patch 1114

LIKENIL (Spain)
LISINOPRIL
Prinivil Tablets 2087

LILAC (The Philippines)
LACTULOSE
Kristalose for Oral Solution 1004

LIMOX (Greece)
CIPROFLOXACIN
Cipro Oral Suspension 2810

LIMOXIN (Mexico)
AMOXICILLIN
Amoxil Pediatric Drops for Oral Suspension 1305
Amoxil Tablets 1305

LINDISC (Argentina, Brazil)
ESTRADIOL
Climara Transdermal System 763

LINDRON (Poland)
ALENDRONATE SODIUM
Fosamax Tablets 2005

LINFOLYSIN (Italy)
CHLORAMBUCIL
Leukeran Tablets 1508

LINOLA CORT TRIAM (Germany)
TRIAMCINOLONE ACETONIDE
Azmacort Inhalation Aerosol 407
Nasacort AQ Nasal Spray 2765

LINOLADIOL (Austria)
ESTRADIOL
Climara Transdermal System 763

LINOLADIOL N (Czech Republic, Germany, Hungary)
ESTRADIOL
Climara Transdermal System 763

LINOLADIOL-H N (Czech Republic, Germany, Hungary)
ESTRADIOL
Climara Transdermal System 763

LINOPRIL (Brazil)
LISINOPRIL
Prinivil Tablets 2087

LINORIL (India)
LISINOPRIL
Prinivil Tablets 2087

LINVAS (India)
LISINOPRIL
Prinivil Tablets 2087

LIOTIXIL (Italy)
CEFTAZIDIME
Fortaz for Injection 1450

LIOTREX (Chile)
SUMATRIPTAN SUCCINATE
Imitrex Injection 1465
Imitrex Tablets 1474

LIPANON (Brazil)
FENOFIBRATE
Tricor Tablets 520

LIPANTHYL (Belgium, Finland, France, Germany, Greece, Hong Kong, Hungary, Italy, Malaysia, Poland, Portugal, Russia, Singapore, Sweden, Switzerland, Thailand, The Philippines, Turkey)
FENOFIBRATE
Tricor Tablets 520

LIPANTIL (Irish Republic, United Kingdom)
FENOFIBRATE
Tricor Tablets 520

LIPAREX (Argentina)
ATORVASTATIN CALCIUM
Lipitor Tablets 2501

LIPARISON (Spain)
FENOFIBRATE
Tricor Tablets 520

LIPAXAN (Italy)
FLUVASTATIN SODIUM
Lescol Capsules 2268

LIPAZ (Portugal)
SIMVASTATIN
Zocor Tablets 2136

LIPCOR (Austria)
FENOFIBRATE
Tricor Tablets 520

LIPCUT (Finland)
SIMVASTATIN
Zocor Tablets 2136

LIPDAUNE (Portugal)
LOVASTATIN
Mevacor Tablets 2063

LIPEROL (Mexico)
LOVASTATIN
Mevacor Tablets 2063

LIPEX (Australia, New Zealand)
SIMVASTATIN
Zocor Tablets 2136

LIPIBEC (Argentina)
ATORVASTATIN CALCIUM
Lipitor Tablets 2501

LIPICARD (India)
FENOFIBRATE
Tricor Tablets 520

LIPIDAX (Italy)
FENOFIBRATE
Tricor Tablets 520

LIPIDEX (South Africa)
SIMVASTATIN
Zocor Tablets 2136

LIPIDIL (Argentina, Australia, Brazil, Canada, Chile, Germany, Greece, Hungary, Mexico)
FENOFIBRATE
Tricor Tablets 520

LIPIDLESS (Greece)
LOVASTATIN
Mevacor Tablets 2063

LIPIFEN (Argentina)
ATORVASTATIN CALCIUM
Lipitor Tablets 2501

LIPIL (Italy)
FENOFIBRATE
Tricor Tablets 520

LIPIMIBE (Argentina)
SIMVASTATIN
Zocor Tablets 2136

LIPIREX (Czech Republic, France)
FENOFIBRATE
Tricor Tablets 520

LIPITOR (Argentina, Australia, Belgium, Brazil, Canada, Chile, Finland, Greece, Hong Kong, Irish Republic, Israel, Italy, Japan, Malaysia, Mexico, New Zealand, Norway, Singapore, South Africa, Sweden, Thailand, The Netherlands, The Philippines, Turkey, United Kingdom, Venezuela)
ATORVASTATIN CALCIUM
Lipitor Tablets 2501

LIPIVAS (Denmark, The Philippines)
LOVASTATIN
Mevacor Tablets 2063

LIPO RED (Spain)
FENOFIBRATE
Tricor Tablets 520

LIPOCAMBI (Argentina)
ATORVASTATIN CALCIUM
Lipitor Tablets 2501

LIPOCIDEN (Spain)
SIMVASTATIN
Zocor Tablets 2136

LIPOCLAR (Italy)
FENOFIBRATE
Tricor Tablets 520

LIPOFEN (Portugal, Turkey)
FENOFIBRATE
Tricor Tablets 520

LIPOFENE (Italy)
FENOFIBRATE
Tricor Tablets 520

LIPOFIN (Argentina)
ATORVASTATIN CALCIUM
Lipitor Tablets 2501

LIPOFREN (Spain)
LOVASTATIN
Mevacor Tablets 2063

LIPONORM (Argentina, Italy)
ATORVASTATIN CALCIUM
Lipitor Tablets 2501

LIPOPLASMIN (Argentina)
FENOFIBRATE
Tricor Tablets 520

LIPOREST (India)
ATORVASTATIN CALCIUM
Lipitor Tablets 2501

LIPOREX (Greece)
SIMVASTATIN
Zocor Tablets 2136

LIPOSCLER (Spain)
LOVASTATIN
Mevacor Tablets 2063

LIPOSIT (Italy, Spain)
FENOFIBRATE
Tricor Tablets 520

LIPOVAS (Spain, Turkey)
FENOFIBRATE
Tricor Tablets 520

LIPRACE (Australia)
LISINOPRIL
Prinivil Tablets 2087

LIPREREN (Chile)
LISINOPRIL
Prinivil Tablets 2087

LIPRIL (India, Portugal)
LISINOPRIL
Prinivil Tablets 2087

LIPRIMAR (Hungary, Russia)
ATORVASTATIN CALCIUM
Lipitor Tablets 2501

LIPROX (Poland)
LOVASTATIN
Mevacor Tablets 2063

LIPSIN (Austria, France, Italy, South Africa)
FENOFIBRATE
Tricor Tablets 520

LIPUS (Portugal)
LOVASTATIN
Mevacor Tablets 2063

LIPWAY (The Philippines)
FENOFIBRATE
Tricor Tablets 520

LIROKEN (Mexico)
DICLOFENAC SODIUM
Voltaren Tablets 2334
Voltaren-XR Tablets 2337

LIS (Italy)
LACTULOSE
Kristalose for Oral Solution 1004

LISAC (Argentina)
SIMVASTATIN
Zocor Tablets 2136

LISACNE (Chile)
ISOTRETINOIN
Accutane Capsules 2607

LISDENE (Poland, Singapore, Thailand)
LISINOPRIL
Prinivil Tablets 2087

LISI LICH (Germany)
LISINOPRIL
Prinivil Tablets 2087

LISIBETA (Germany)
LISINOPRIL
Prinivil Tablets 2087

LISIBETA COMP (Germany)
LISINOPRIL
Prinivil Tablets 2087

LISICOSTAD (United Kingdom)
LISINOPRIL
Prinivil Tablets 2087

LISIDOC (Germany)
LISINOPRIL
Prinivil Tablets 2087

LISIFLEN (Italy)
DICLOFENAC SODIUM
Voltaren Tablets 2334
Voltaren-XR Tablets 2337

LISIGAMMA (Germany)
LISINOPRIL
Prinivil Tablets 2087

LISIGAMMA HCT (Germany)
LISINOPRIL
Prinivil Tablets 2087

LISIHEXAL (Austria, Germany, Poland)
LISINOPRIL
Prinivil Tablets 2087

LISIHEXAL COMB (Austria)
LISINOPRIL
Prinivil Tablets 2087

LISILET (Venezuela)
LISINOPRIL
Prinivil Tablets 2087

LISILETIC (Venezuela)
LISINOPRIL
Prinivil Tablets 2087

LISILICH COMP (Germany)
LISINOPRIL
Prinivil Tablets 2087

LISINAL (Argentina)
LISINOPRIL
Prinivil Tablets 2087

LISINOBELL (Australia)
LISINOPRIL
Prinivil Tablets 2087

LISINOCOMP (Austria)
LISINOPRIL
Prinivil Tablets 2087

LISINOGEN (Denmark)
LISINOPRIL
Prinivil Tablets 2087

LISINOPLUS (Denmark)
LISINOPRIL
Prinivil Tablets 2087

LISINOPRIL COMP (Austria)
LISINOPRIL
Prinivil Tablets 2087

LISINORATIO (Poland)
LISINOPRIL
Prinivil Tablets 2087

LISINORETIC (Brazil)
LISINOPRIL
Prinivil Tablets 2087

LISINOSPES (Greece)
LISINOPRIL
Prinivil Tablets 2087

LISINOSTAD (Austria)
LISINOPRIL
Prinivil Tablets 2087

LISINOTYROL (Austria)
LISINOPRIL
Prinivil Tablets 2087

LISIPIN (Venezuela)
CIPROFLOXACIN HYDROCHLORIDE
Cipro Tablets ... **2810**

LISIPRIL (Finland)
LISINOPRIL
Prinivil Tablets ... **2087**

LISIPRIL COMP (Finland)
HYDROCHLOROTHIAZIDE/LISINOPRIL
Prinzide Tablets ... **2092**

LISIPROL (Poland)
LISINOPRIL
Prinivil Tablets ... **2087**

LISI-PUREN (Germany)
LISINOPRIL
Prinivil Tablets ... **2087**

LISI-PUREN COMP (Germany)
LISINOPRIL
Prinivil Tablets ... **2087**

LISITRIL (Switzerland)
LISINOPRIL
Prinivil Tablets ... **2087**

LISITRIL COMP (Switzerland)
LISINOPRIL
Prinivil Tablets ... **2087**

LISOCLOR (Brazil)
LISINOPRIL
Prinivil Tablets ... **2087**

LISODER (Chile)
MOMETASONE FUROATE
Elocon Cream 0.1% ... **2840**
Elocon Lotion 0.1% ... **2841**
Elocon Ointment 0.1% ... **2842**
Nasonex Nasal Spray ... **2883**

LISODUR (Australia)
LISINOPRIL
Prinivil Tablets ... **2087**

LISODURA (Germany)
LISINOPRIL
Prinivil Tablets ... **2087**

LISODURA PLUS (Germany)
LISINOPRIL
Prinivil Tablets ... **2087**

LISONOTEC (Brazil)
LISINOPRIL
Prinivil Tablets ... **2087**

LISOPRESS (Hungary, Irish Republic)
LISINOPRIL
Prinivil Tablets ... **2087**

LISOPRIL (Switzerland)
LISINOPRIL
Prinivil Tablets ... **2087**

LISOPRIL PLUS (Switzerland)
LISINOPRIL
Prinivil Tablets ... **2087**

LISORETIC (South Africa)
LISINOPRIL
Prinivil Tablets ... **2087**

LISORIL (India, Russia, Singapore)
LISINOPRIL
Prinivil Tablets ... **2087**

LISORIL-5HT (India)
LISINOPRIL
Prinivil Tablets ... **2087**

LISPOR (Chile)
LOVASTATIN
Mevacor Tablets ... **2063**

LISPRIL (Irish Republic, Thailand)
LISINOPRIL
Prinivil Tablets ... **2087**

LISPRIL-HYDROCHLOROTHIAZIDE (Irish Republic)
LISINOPRIL
Prinivil Tablets ... **2087**

LISTRIL (Brazil, Czech Republic)
LISINOPRIL
Prinivil Tablets ... **2087**

LITAK (Australia, Denmark, Finland, France, Germany, Israel, Switzerland, The Netherlands, United Kingdom)
CLADRIBINE
Leustatin Injection ... **2384**

LITHIMOLE (Greece)
TIMOLOL MALEATE
Timoptic in Ocudose ... **2124**
Timoptic Sterile Ophthalmic Solution ... **2121**
Timoptic-XE Sterile Ophthalmic Gel Forming Solution ... **2125**

LITOCID (Poland)
POTASSIUM CITRATE
Urocit-K Tablets ... **2176**

LITOCIT (Brazil)
POTASSIUM CITRATE
Urocit-K Tablets ... **2176**

LIVESAN (France)
FENOFIBRATE
Tricor Tablets ... **520**

LIVOLUK (India)
LACTULOSE
Kristalose for Oral Solution ... **1004**

LIXAMIDE (South Africa)
INDAPAMIDE
Indapamide Tablets ... **2188**

LIXOGAN (Mexico)
NAPROXEN
EC-Naprosyn Delayed-Release Tablets ... **2632**
Naprosyn Suspension ... **2632**
Naprosyn Tablets ... **2632**

LIZAN (Turkey)
DIAZEPAM
Valium Tablets ... **2658**

LIZIK (Turkey)
FUROSEMIDE
Furosemide Tablets ... **2186**

LOBAFEN (The Philippines)
DICLOFENAC SODIUM
Voltaren Tablets ... **2334**
Voltaren-XR Tablets ... **2337**

LOCACID (Argentina, Czech Republic, France, Hong Kong, Israel, Poland, Portugal)
TRETINOIN
Vesanoid Capsules ... **2660**

LOCASYN (Denmark)
FLUNISOLIDE
Aerobid Inhaler System ... **1153**
Aerobid-M Inhaler System ... **1153**

LOCEPTIN (Sweden)
MORPHINE SULFATE
MS Contin Tablets ... **2585**

LOCHOL (Hungary, Thailand)
FLUVASTATIN SODIUM
Lescol Capsules ... **2268**

LOCOL (Germany)
FLUVASTATIN SODIUM
Lescol Capsules ... **2268**

LOCTENK (Argentina)
LOSARTAN POTASSIUM
Cozaar Tablets ... **1973**

LOCTENK D (Argentina)
LOSARTAN POTASSIUM
Cozaar Tablets ... **1973**

LODALES (France)
SIMVASTATIN
Zocor Tablets ... **2136**

LODIMOL (Mexico)
DIPYRIDAMOLE
Persantine Tablets ... **869**

LODIPRES (Chile)
CARVEDILOL
Coreg Tablets ... **1387**

LODYFEN (Mexico)
DICLOFENAC SODIUM
Voltaren Tablets ... **2334**
Voltaren-XR Tablets ... **2337**

LOFACOL (Hong Kong)
LOVASTATIN
Mevacor Tablets ... **2063**

LOFENAX (The Philippines)
DICLOFENAC SODIUM
Voltaren Tablets ... **2334**
Voltaren-XR Tablets ... **2337**

LOFENSAID (United Kingdom)
DICLOFENAC SODIUM
Voltaren Tablets ... **2334**
Voltaren-XR Tablets ... **2337**

LOGAT (Brazil)
RANITIDINE HYDROCHLORIDE
Zantac 25 EFFERdose Tablets ... **1670**
Zantac 150 Tablets ... **1670**
Zantac 300 Tablets ... **1670**
Zantac Injection ... **1666**
Zantac Injection Premixed ... **1666**
Zantac Syrup ... **1670**

LOGESIC (Mexico)
DICLOFENAC SODIUM
Voltaren Tablets ... **2334**
Voltaren-XR Tablets ... **2337**

LOGOMED AKNE-GEL (Germany)
BENZOYL PEROXIDE
Brevoxyl-4 Creamy Wash ... **3054**
Brevoxyl-4 Gel ... **3054**
Brevoxyl-8 Creamy Wash ... **3054**
Brevoxyl-8 Gel ... **3054**

LOKALEN (Turkey)
LIDOCAINE
Lidoderm Patch ... **1114**

LOKILAN (Norway)
FLUNISOLIDE
Aerobid Inhaler System ... **1153**
Aerobid-M Inhaler System ... **1153**

LOKILAN NASAL (Sweden)
FLUNISOLIDE
Aerobid Inhaler System ... **1153**
Aerobid-M Inhaler System ... **1153**

LOMADRYL (Greece)
RANITIDINE HYDROCHLORIDE
Zantac 25 EFFERdose Tablets ... **1670**
Zantac 150 Tablets ... **1670**
Zantac 300 Tablets ... **1670**
Zantac Injection ... **1666**
Zantac Injection Premixed ... **1666**
Zantac Syrup ... **1670**

LOMAR (Hong Kong)
LOVASTATIN
Mevacor Tablets ... **2063**

LOMARIN (Chile)
LAMOTRIGINE
Lamictal Chewable Dispersible Tablets ... **1488**
Lamictal Tablets ... **1488**

LOMIR (Austria, Belgium, Brazil, Czech Republic, Denmark, Finland, Germany, Greece, Hungary, Italy, Norway, Poland, Portugal, Russia, Spain, Sweden, Switzerland, The Netherlands)
ISRADIPINE
DynaCirc CR Tablets ... **1407**

LONGACEPH (Czech Republic)
CEFTRIAXONE SODIUM
Rocephin Injectable Vials, ADD-Vantage, Galaxy, Bulk ... **2642**

LONGAZEM (Italy)
DILTIAZEM HYDROCHLORIDE
Cardizem LA Extended Release Tablets ... **421**

LONTAX (The Netherlands)
CITALOPRAM HYDROBROMIDE
Celexa Tablets ... **1160**

LOORTAN (Belgium)
LOSARTAN POTASSIUM
Cozaar Tablets ... **1973**

LO-P-CAPS (Thailand)
CALCIUM ACETATE
PhosLo GelCaps ... **1184**

LOPIRETIC (Portugal)
CAPTOPRIL
Captopril Tablets ... **2182**

LOPIRIN (Austria, Germany, Switzerland)
CAPTOPRIL
Captopril Tablets ... **2182**

LOPLAC (Argentina)
LOSARTAN POTASSIUM
Cozaar Tablets ... **1973**

LOPLAC-D (Argentina)
LOSARTAN POTASSIUM
Cozaar Tablets ... **1973**

LOPRATIN (The Netherlands)
CEFTRIAXONE SODIUM
Rocephin Injectable Vials, ADD-Vantage, Galaxy, Bulk ... **2642**

LOPRIL (Brazil, Finland, France)
CAPTOPRIL
Captopril Tablets ... **2182**

LOPTOMIT (The Netherlands)
TIMOLOL MALEATE
Timoptic in Ocudose ... **2124**
Timoptic Sterile Ophthalmic Solution ... **2121**
Timoptic-XE Sterile Ophthalmic Gel Forming Solution ... **2125**

LORAGA (Finland, Sweden)
LACTULOSE
Kristalose for Oral Solution ... **1004**

LORBIFENAC (Argentina)
DICLOFENAC SODIUM
Voltaren Tablets ... **2334**
Voltaren-XR Tablets ... **2337**

LORBIFLOXACINA (Argentina)
CIPROFLOXACIN
Cipro Oral Suspension ... **2810**

LORCAMIN (Greece)
NORFLOXACIN
Noroxin Tablets ... **2069**

LORETIC (South Africa)
HYDROCHLOROTHIAZIDE/TRIAMTERENE
Dyazide Capsules ... **1405**

LOREXEN (Mexico)
NAPROXEN
EC-Naprosyn Delayed-Release Tablets ... **2632**
Naprosyn Suspension ... **2632**
Naprosyn Tablets ... **2632**

LOREXIL M (Mexico)
AMOXICILLIN
Amoxil Pediatric Drops for Oral Suspension ... **1305**
Amoxil Tablets ... **1305**

LORISTA (Czech Republic, Poland)
LOSARTAN POTASSIUM
Cozaar Tablets ... **1973**

LORISTA H (Poland)
LOSARTAN POTASSIUM
Cozaar Tablets ... **1973**

LORITER (Argentina)
LOVASTATIN
Mevacor Tablets ... **2063**

LOROXIDE (Canada)
BENZOYL PEROXIDE
Brevoxyl-4 Creamy Wash ... **3054**
Brevoxyl-4 Gel ... **3054**
Brevoxyl-8 Creamy Wash ... **3054**
Brevoxyl-8 Gel ... **3054**

LORSACOR (Brazil)
LOSARTAN POTASSIUM
Cozaar Tablets ... **1973**

LORSAR + HCT (Brazil)
LOSARTAN POTASSIUM
Cozaar Tablets ... **1973**

LORTAAN (Italy, Portugal)
LOSARTAN POTASSIUM
Cozaar Tablets ... **1973**

LORVAS (India, Thailand)
INDAPAMIDE
Indapamide Tablets ... **2188**

LORZAAR (Germany)
LOSARTAN POTASSIUM
Cozaar Tablets ... **1973**

LOSACAR (India)
LOSARTAN POTASSIUM
Cozaar Tablets ... **1973**

LOSACAR-H (India)
LOSARTAN POTASSIUM
Cozaar Tablets ... **1973**

LOSACOR (Argentina, Poland)
LOSARTAN POTASSIUM
Cozaar Tablets ... **1973**

LOSACOR D (Argentina)
LOSARTAN POTASSIUM
Cozaar Tablets ... **1973**

LOSANORM (India)
LOSARTAN POTASSIUM
Cozaar Tablets ... **1973**

LOSAPRES (Chile)
LOSARTAN POTASSIUM
Cozaar Tablets **1973**

LOSAPREX (Italy)
LOSARTAN POTASSIUM
Cozaar Tablets **1973**

LOSARTEC (Brazil)
LOSARTAN POTASSIUM
Cozaar Tablets **1973**

LOSATAL (Brazil)
LOSARTAN POTASSIUM
Cozaar Tablets **1973**

LOSAZID (The Netherlands)
LOSARTAN POTASSIUM
Cozaar Tablets **1973**

LOSE.LAX (Austria)
LACTULOSE
Kristalose for Oral Solution **1004**

LOSIL-T (Mexico)
TERBINAFINE HYDROCHLORIDE
Lamisil Tablets **2266**

LOSIUM (India)
LOSARTAN POTASSIUM
Cozaar Tablets **1973**

LOSTAM (Argentina)
TAMSULOSIN HYDROCHLORIDE
Flomax Capsules **848**

LOSTATIN (Malaysia, Singapore, Venezuela)
LOVASTATIN
Mevacor Tablets **2063**

LOTIOBLANC (Argentina)
TRETINOIN
Vesanoid Capsules **2660**

LOUTEN (Argentina, Chile)
LATANOPROST
Xalatan Ophthalmic Solution . . . . ⊙**273**

LOUTEN T (Argentina)
LATANOPROST
Xalatan Ophthalmic Solution . . . . ⊙**273**

LOVA (Germany)
LOVASTATIN
Mevacor Tablets **2063**

LOVABETA (Germany)
LOVASTATIN
Mevacor Tablets **2063**

LOVACARD (Czech Republic, India)
LOVASTATIN
Mevacor Tablets **2063**

LOVACHOL (South Africa)
LOVASTATIN
Mevacor Tablets **2063**

LOVACODAN (Denmark)
LOVASTATIN
Mevacor Tablets **2063**

LOVACOL (Chile, Finland)
LOVASTATIN
Mevacor Tablets **2063**

LOVACOR (Brazil)
SIMVASTATIN
Zocor Tablets **2136**

LOVADRUG (Greece)
LOVASTATIN
Mevacor Tablets **2063**

LOVADURA (Germany)
LOVASTATIN
Mevacor Tablets **2063**

LOVAGAMMA (Germany)
LOVASTATIN
Mevacor Tablets **2063**

LOVAHEXAL (Germany)
LOVASTATIN
Mevacor Tablets **2063**

LOVALIP (Israel)
LOVASTATIN
Mevacor Tablets **2063**

LOVANIL (Venezuela)
LOVASTATIN
Mevacor Tablets **2063**

LOVAPEN (Greece)
LOVASTATIN
Mevacor Tablets **2063**

LOVAS (Venezuela)
LOVASTATIN
Mevacor Tablets **2063**

LOVASC (Brazil)
LOVASTATIN
Mevacor Tablets **2063**

LOVAST (Brazil)
LOVASTATIN
Mevacor Tablets **2063**

LOVASTEN (Greece)
LOVASTATIN
Mevacor Tablets **2063**

LOVASTEROL (Poland, Russia)
LOVASTATIN
Mevacor Tablets **2063**

LOVASTIN (Malaysia, Poland)
LOVASTATIN
Mevacor Tablets **2063**

LOVATEX (Greece)
LOVASTATIN
Mevacor Tablets **2063**

LOVATON (Brazil)
LOVASTATIN
Mevacor Tablets **2063**

LOVATOP (Greece)
LOVASTATIN
Mevacor Tablets **2063**

LOVAX (Brazil)
LOVASTATIN
Mevacor Tablets **2063**

LOVENOX (Austria, Canada, France, Portugal, Switzerland)
ENOXAPARIN SODIUM
Lovenox Injection **2756**

LOVERAL (Mexico)
ALBENDAZOLE
Albenza Tablets **1297**

LOVINACOR (Italy)
LOVASTATIN
Mevacor Tablets **2063**

LOWCHOLID (Greece)
SIMVASTATIN
Zocor Tablets **2136**

LOWLIPID (Greece)
LOVASTATIN
Mevacor Tablets **2063**

LOWPRE (Mexico)
CAPTOPRIL
Captopril Tablets **2182**

LOWPRES (Venezuela)
CLONIDINE HYDROCHLORIDE
Catapres Tablets **841**

LOXASID (Turkey)
CIPROFLOXACIN HYDROCHLORIDE
Cipro Tablets **2810**

LOXIFEN (Argentina)
RALOXIFENE HYDROCHLORIDE
Evista Tablets **1810**

LOXONE (Thailand)
NORFLOXACIN
Noroxin Tablets **2069**

LOZAP (Czech Republic, Poland)
LOSARTAN POTASSIUM
Cozaar Tablets **1973**

LOZIDE (Canada)
INDAPAMIDE
Indapamide Tablets **2188**

LOZITAN (India)
LOSARTAN POTASSIUM
Cozaar Tablets **1973**

L-THYROX (Germany)
LEVOTHYROXINE SODIUM
Levothroid Tablets **1170**
Levoxyl Tablets **1780**
Synthroid Tablets **507**

L-THYROX JOD (Germany)
LEVOTHYROXINE SODIUM
Levothroid Tablets **1170**
Levoxyl Tablets **1780**
Synthroid Tablets **507**

LTK250 (Argentina)
POTASSIUM CITRATE
Urocit-K Tablets **2176**

LUASE (Spain)
DICLOFENAC SODIUM
Voltaren Tablets **2334**
Voltaren-XR Tablets **2337**

LUBEXYL (Hungary, Poland, Switzerland)
BENZOYL PEROXIDE
Brevoxyl-4 Creamy Wash **3054**
Brevoxyl-4 Gel **3054**
Brevoxyl-8 Creamy Wash **3054**
Brevoxyl-8 Gel **3054**

LUFAC-Z (Mexico)
DICLOFENAC SODIUM
Voltaren Tablets **2334**
Voltaren-XR Tablets **2337**

LUFI (India)
LEVOFLOXACIN
Levaquin Injection **2416**
Levaquin Tablets **2416**

LUGESTERON (Finland)
PROGESTERONE
Crinone 4% Gel **992**
Prometrium Capsules (100 mg, 200 mg) . **3047**

LUITASE (Italy)
PANCRELIPASE
Ultrase Capsules **718**
Ultrase MT Capsules **719**

LUKAIR (Argentina)
MONTELUKAST SODIUM
Singulair Chewable Tablets **2114**
Singulair Tablets **2114**

LUKASM (Italy)
MONTELUKAST SODIUM
Singulair Chewable Tablets **2114**
Singulair Tablets **2114**

LUMAREN (Greece, Singapore)
RANITIDINE HYDROCHLORIDE
Zantac 150 Tablets **1670**
Zantac 25 EFFERdose Tablets **1670**
Zantac 300 Tablets **1670**
Zantac Injection **1666**
Zantac Injection Premixed **1666**
Zantac Syrup **1670**

LUMERAN (Hong Kong)
RANITIDINE HYDROCHLORIDE
Zantac 25 EFFERdose Tablets **1670**
Zantac 150 Tablets **1670**
Zantac 300 Tablets **1670**
Zantac Injection **1666**
Zantac Injection Premixed **1666**
Zantac Syrup **1670**

LUMOX (Mexico)
AMOXICILLIN
Amoxil Pediatric Drops for Oral Suspension **1305**
Amoxil Tablets **1305**

LUMOXBRON S (Mexico)
AMOXICILLIN
Amoxil Pediatric Drops for Oral Suspension **1305**
Amoxil Tablets **1305**

LUNDIRAN (Spain)
NAPROXEN
EC-Naprosyn Delayed-Release Tablets **2632**
Naprosyn Suspension **2632**
Naprosyn Tablets **2632**

LUNIBRON (Italy)
FLUNISOLIDE
Aerobid Inhaler System **1153**
Aerobid-M Inhaler System **1153**

LUNIS (Italy)
FLUNISOLIDE
Aerobid Inhaler System **1153**
Aerobid-M Inhaler System **1153**

LUPAREN (Brazil)
DICLOFENAC SODIUM
Voltaren Tablets **2334**
Voltaren-XR Tablets **2337**

LURANTAL (Austria)
ISOTRETINOIN
Accutane Capsules **2607**

LURDEX (Mexico)
ALBENDAZOLE
Albenza Tablets **1297**

LUTEINA (Poland)
PROGESTERONE
Crinone 4% Gel **992**
Prometrium Capsules (100 mg, 200 mg) . **3047**

LUTOGIN (Italy)
PROGESTERONE
Crinone 4% Gel **992**
Prometrium Capsules (100 mg, 200 mg) . **3047**

LYCEFT (India)
CEFTRIAXONE SODIUM
Rocephin Injectable Vials, ADD-Vantage, Galaxy, Bulk **2642**

LYMETEL (Spain)
FLUVASTATIN SODIUM
Lescol Capsules **2268**

LYNDAK (Italy)
SULINDAC
Clinoril Tablets **1962**

LYOTRET (Greece)
ISOTRETINOIN
Accutane Capsules **2607**

LYSOFORM (Germany, Spain)
FORMALDEHYDE
Formadon Solution **1699**

LYSOFORMIN (Germany)
FORMALDEHYDE
Formadon Solution **1699**

LYSTIN (Hong Kong, Thailand)
NYSTATIN
Nystop Topical Powder USP **2498**

MAALOX H2 ACID CONTROLLER (Canada)
FAMOTIDINE
Pepcid for Oral Suspension **2075**
Pepcid Tablets **2075**

MABICROL (Mexico)
CLARITHROMYCIN
Biaxin Filmtab Tablets **411**
Biaxin Granules **411**

MABRON (Czech Republic, Hong Kong, Malaysia, Russia, Singapore, Thailand, United Kingdom)
TRAMADOL HYDROCHLORIDE
Ultram ER Tablets **2428**

MABTHERA (Argentina, Australia, Austria, Belgium, Brazil, Chile, Czech Republic, Denmark, Finland, France, Germany, Greece, Hong Kong, Hungary, Irish Republic, Israel, Italy, Mexico, New Zealand, Norway, Poland, Portugal, Singapore, South Africa, Spain, Sweden, Switzerland, Thailand, The Netherlands, The Philippines, Turkey, United Kingdom, Venezuela)
RITUXIMAB
Rituxan I.V. **1223**

MACLADIN (Italy)
CLARITHROMYCIN
Biaxin Filmtab Tablets **411**
Biaxin Granules **411**

MACLAR (Austria, Belgium, India, Portugal)
CLARITHROMYCIN
Biaxin Filmtab Tablets **411**
Biaxin Granules **411**

MACOBAL (Argentina)
NIMODIPINE
Nimotop Capsules **790**

MACROL (Turkey)
CLARITHROMYCIN
Biaxin Filmtab Tablets **411**
Biaxin Granules **411**

MACROMICINA (Argentina)
CLARITHROMYCIN
Biaxin Filmtab Tablets **411**
Biaxin Granules **411**

MADAPROX (Spain)
NAPROXEN
EC-Naprosyn Delayed-Release Tablets **2632**
Naprosyn Suspension **2632**
Naprosyn Tablets **2632**

MADOL (Thailand)
TRAMADOL HYDROCHLORIDE
Ultram ER Tablets **2428**

MADOLA (Thailand)
TRAMADOL HYDROCHLORIDE
Ultram ER Tablets **2428**

(⊙ Described in PDR® For Ophthalmic Medicines)

MAFEL (Argentina)
PROGESTERONE
Crinone 4% Gel ... 992
Prometrium Capsules (100 mg, 200 mg) ... 3047

MAFENA (Mexico)
DICLOFENAC SODIUM
Voltaren Tablets ... 2334
Voltaren-XR Tablets ... 2337

MAGLUPHEN (Austria)
DICLOFENAC SODIUM
Voltaren Tablets ... 2334
Voltaren-XR Tablets ... 2337

MAGNASPOR (Thailand)
CEFUROXIME AXETIL
Ceftin for Oral Suspension ... 1380
Ceftin Tablets ... 1380

MAGNITON-R (Greece)
INDAPAMIDE
Indapamide Tablets ... 2188

MALANIL (South Africa)
ATOVAQUONE
Mepron Suspension ... 1526

MALARONE (Australia, Brazil, Irish Republic, Israel, Italy, New Zealand, Norway, Poland, Spain, The Netherlands, United Kingdom)
ATOVAQUONE
Mepron Suspension ... 1526

MALASTOP (Belgium)
PYRIMETHAMINE
Daraprim Tablets ... 1400

MALEXIN (Germany)
NAPROXEN
EC-Naprosyn Delayed-Release Tablets ... 2632
Naprosyn Suspension ... 2632
Naprosyn Tablets ... 2632

MALFIN (Denmark)
MORPHINE SULFATE
MS Contin Tablets ... 2585

MALOCEF (Greece)
CEFTAZIDIME
Fortaz for Injection ... 1450

MALOCIDE (France)
PYRIMETHAMINE
Daraprim Tablets ... 1400

MALOPRIM (Belgium, Irish Republic)
PYRIMETHAMINE
Daraprim Tablets ... 1400

MANDOLGIN (Denmark)
TRAMADOL HYDROCHLORIDE
Ultram ER Tablets ... 2428

MANDROLAX LACTU (Germany)
LACTULOSE
Kristalose for Oral Solution ... 1004

MANDRO-ZEP (Germany)
DIAZEPAM
Valium Tablets ... 2658

MANOFLOX (Thailand)
NORFLOXACIN
Noroxin Tablets ... 2069

MANOL (Chile)
TRAMADOL HYDROCHLORIDE
Ultram ER Tablets ... 2428

MANOLONE (Thailand)
TRIAMCINOLONE ACETONIDE
Azmacort Inhalation Aerosol ... 407
Nasacort AQ Nasal Spray ... 2765

MANOVERM (Thailand)
ALBENDAZOLE
Albenza Tablets ... 1297

MAOTIL (Germany)
SELEGILINE HYDROCHLORIDE
Eldepryl Capsules ... 3052

MAPELOR (The Netherlands)
TAMSULOSIN HYDROCHLORIDE
Flomax Capsules ... 848

MAPEZINE (Thailand)
CARBAMAZEPINE
Carbatrol Capsules ... 3019

MAPLUXIN (Mexico)
DIGOXIN
Lanoxin Injection ... 1498
Lanoxin Injection Pediatric ... 1502
Lanoxin Tablets ... 1505

MARDUK (Germany)
BENZOYL PEROXIDE
Brevoxyl-4 Creamy Wash ... 3054
Brevoxyl-4 Gel ... 3054
Brevoxyl-8 Creamy Wash ... 3054
Brevoxyl-8 Gel ... 3054

MARINOL (Canada)
DRONABINOL
Marinol Capsules ... 3163

MARIZINE (Hong Kong)
CETIRIZINE HYDROCHLORIDE
Zyrtec Syrup ... 1920
Zyrtec Tablets ... 1920

MARMODINE (Hong Kong)
FAMOTIDINE
Pepcid for Oral Suspension ... 2075
Pepcid Tablets ... 2075

MARTULOSE (Hong Kong)
LACTULOSE
Kristalose for Oral Solution ... 1004

MARVIL (Argentina)
ALENDRONATE SODIUM
Fosamax Tablets ... 2005

MASAWORM (Thailand)
ALBENDAZOLE
Albenza Tablets ... 1297

MASDIL (Spain)
DILTIAZEM HYDROCHLORIDE
Cardizem LA Extended Release Tablets ... 421

MATIGEL (Venezuela)
TIMOLOL MALEATE
Timoptic in Ocudose ... 2124
Timoptic Sterile Ophthalmic Solution ... 2121
Timoptic-XE Sterile Ophthalmic Gel Forming Solution ... 2125

MATILOL (Venezuela)
TIMOLOL MALEATE
Timoptic in Ocudose ... 2124
Timoptic Sterile Ophthalmic Solution ... 2121
Timoptic-XE Sterile Ophthalmic Gel Forming Solution ... 2125

MATRIFEN (Sweden, United Kingdom)
FENTANYL
Duragesic Transdermal System ... 2405

MAURAN (Italy)
RANITIDINE HYDROCHLORIDE
Zantac 25 EFFERdose Tablets ... 1670
Zantac 150 Tablets ... 1670
Zantac 300 Tablets ... 1670
Zantac Injection ... 1666
Zantac Injection Premixed ... 1666
Zantac Syrup ... 1670

MAVID (Germany)
CLARITHROMYCIN
Biaxin Filmtab Tablets ... 411
Biaxin Granules ... 411

MAVIFLOX (Mexico)
CIPROFLOXACIN
Cipro Oral Suspension ... 2810

MAVIK (Canada, South Africa)
TRANDOLAPRIL
Mavik Tablets ... 472

MAXAIR (France, Switzerland)
PIRBUTEROL ACETATE
Maxair Autohaler ... 1705

MAXALT (Argentina, Austria, Belgium, Brazil, Canada, Chile, Czech Republic, Denmark, Finland, Germany, Greece, Hungary, Italy, Mexico, New Zealand, Norway, Poland, Portugal, South Africa, Spain, Sweden, Switzerland, The Netherlands, United Kingdom, Venezuela)
RIZATRIPTAN BENZOATE
Maxalt Tablets ... 2056
Maxalt-MLT Orally Disintegrating Tablets ... 2056

MAXIBONE (Israel)
ALENDRONATE SODIUM
Fosamax Tablets ... 2005

MAXIBRAL (Greece)
ETIDRONATE DISODIUM
Didronel Tablets ... 2583

MAXICARDIL (Argentina)
DIPYRIDAMOLE
Persantine Tablets ... 869

MAXIDON (Sweden)
MORPHINE SULFATE
MS Contin Tablets ... 2585

MAXIFLOX (Brazil)
CIPROFLOXACIN HYDROCHLORIDE
Cipro Tablets ... 2810

MAXIFLOX D (Brazil)
CIPROFLOXACIN HYDROCHLORIDE
Cipro Tablets ... 2810

MAXILERG (Brazil)
DICLOFENAC SODIUM
Voltaren Tablets ... 2334
Voltaren-XR Tablets ... 2337

MAXINT (Mexico)
AMOXICILLIN
Amoxil Pediatric Drops for Oral Suspension ... 1305
Amoxil Tablets ... 1305

MAXIOSTENIL (Argentina)
SODIUM HYALURONATE
Hyalgan Solution ... 2742

MAXIPRIL (Italy)
CAPTOPRIL
Captopril Tablets ... 2182

MAXTRAL (Argentina)
ALENDRONATE SODIUM
Fosamax Tablets ... 2005

MAXULID (The Philippines)
CLARITHROMYCIN
Biaxin Filmtab Tablets ... 411
Biaxin Granules ... 411

MAXZIDE (Belgium)
TRIAMTERENE
Dyrenium Capsules ... 3189

MAZEPINE (Canada)
CARBAMAZEPINE
Carbatrol Capsules ... 3019

MAZETOL (India)
CARBAMAZEPINE
Carbatrol Capsules ... 3019

M-BETA (Germany)
MORPHINE SULFATE
MS Contin Tablets ... 2585

MCR (Israel)
MORPHINE SULFATE
MS Contin Tablets ... 2585

MDILTIWAS (Spain)
DILTIAZEM HYDROCHLORIDE
Cardizem LA Extended Release Tablets ... 421

M-DOLOR (Austria, Germany)
MORPHINE SULFATE
MS Contin Tablets ... 2585

MEBENIX (Brazil)
ALBENDAZOLE
Albenza Tablets ... 1297

MEBUMAL (Denmark)
PENTOBARBITAL SODIUM
Nembutal Sodium Solution, USP ... 2494

MECTIZAN (France)
IVERMECTIN
Stromectol Tablets ... 2120

MEDAFLOX (Argentina)
CIPROFLOXACIN
Cipro Oral Suspension ... 2810

MEDALIN (Venezuela)
FAMOTIDINE
Pepcid for Oral Suspension ... 2075
Pepcid Tablets ... 2075

MEDAREN (Thailand)
DICLOFENAC SODIUM
Voltaren Tablets ... 2334
Voltaren-XR Tablets ... 2337

MEDAXIME (South Africa)
CEFUROXIME SODIUM
Zinacef Injection ... 1678

MEDAXONE (Russia)
CEFTRIAXONE SODIUM
Rocephin Injectable Vials, ADD-Vantage, Galaxy, Bulk ... 2642

MEDAXONUM (Hong Kong)
CEFTRIAXONE SODIUM
Rocephin Injectable Vials, ADD-Vantage, Galaxy, Bulk ... 2642

MEDIBIOX (Chile)
LEVOFLOXACIN
Levaquin Injection ... 2416
Levaquin Tablets ... 2416

MEDICLEAR (United Kingdom)
BENZOYL PEROXIDE
Brevoxyl-4 Creamy Wash ... 3054
Brevoxyl-4 Gel ... 3054
Brevoxyl-8 Creamy Wash ... 3054
Brevoxyl-8 Gel ... 3054

MEDILAX (Denmark)
LACTULOSE
Kristalose for Oral Solution ... 1004

MEDILET (Austria, Germany)
LACTULOSE
Kristalose for Oral Solution ... 1004

MEDINOX MONO (Germany)
PENTOBARBITAL SODIUM
Nembutal Sodium Solution, USP ... 2494

MEDIPAM (Finland)
DIAZEPAM
Valium Tablets ... 2658

MEDIPHYLLIN CHRONO (Greece)
THEOPHYLLINE
Uniphyl Tablets ... 2595

MEDIPO (Italy)
SIMVASTATIN
Zocor Tablets ... 2136

MEDITROL (Thailand)
CALCITRIOL
Calcijex Injection ... 419
Rocaltrol Capsules ... 1150
Rocaltrol Oral Solution ... 1150

MEDIURESIX (Thailand)
FUROSEMIDE
Furosemide Tablets ... 2186

MEDIXIL (Chile)
SIBUTRAMINE HYDROCHLORIDE
Meridia Capsules ... 475

MEDIXIN (Argentina)
LACTULOSE
Kristalose for Oral Solution ... 1004

MEDOCIPRIN (Hong Kong, Russia, Thailand)
CIPROFLOXACIN
Cipro Oral Suspension ... 2810

MEDOSTATIN (Czech Republic, Hong Kong, Malaysia, Russia, Singapore)
LOVASTATIN
Mevacor Tablets ... 2063

MEDOVASCIN (Greece)
LOVASTATIN
Mevacor Tablets ... 2063

MEDOXEM (Greece)
CEFUROXIME SODIUM
Zinacef Injection ... 1678

MEDOXIM (Italy)
CEFUROXIME SODIUM
Zinacef Injection ... 1678

MEDOZEM (Thailand)
DILTIAZEM HYDROCHLORIDE
Cardizem LA Extended Release Tablets ... 421

MED-PHYLLINE (Thailand)
THEOPHYLLINE
Uniphyl Tablets ... 2595

MEGACID (Turkey)
CLARITHROMYCIN
Biaxin Filmtab Tablets ... 411
Biaxin Granules ... 411

MEGAFLOX (Portugal)
CIPROFLOXACIN HYDROCHLORIDE
Cipro Tablets ... 2810

MEGALEX (Argentina)
RANITIDINE HYDROCHLORIDE
Zantac 25 EFFERdose Tablets ... 1670

Zantac 150 Tablets . . . 1670
Zantac 300 Tablets . . . 1670
Zantac Injection . . . 1666
Zantac Injection Premixed . . . 1666
Zantac Syrup . . . 1670

MEGALIS (Venezuela)
DIPYRIDAMOLE
Persantine Tablets . . . 869

MEGANOX (Chile)
LAMOTRIGINE
Lamictal Chewable Dispersible Tablets . . . 1488
Lamictal Tablets . . . 1488

MEGION (Hungary, Mexico, The Philippines, Venezuela)
CEFTRIAXONE SODIUM
Rocephin Injectable Vials, ADD-Vantage, Galaxy, Bulk . . . 2642

MELAXOSE (France)
LACTULOSE
Kristalose for Oral Solution . . . 1004

MELERIL (Spain, Venezuela)
THIORIDAZINE HYDROCHLORIDE
Thioridazine Hydrochloride Tablets . . . 2195

MELGAR (Argentina)
NAPROXEN
EC-Naprosyn Delayed-Release Tablets . . . 2632
Naprosyn Suspension . . . 2632
Naprosyn Tablets . . . 2632

MELLERETTEN (Germany, The Netherlands)
THIORIDAZINE HYDROCHLORIDE
Thioridazine Hydrochloride Tablets . . . 2195

MELLERETTES (Switzerland, Turkey)
THIORIDAZINE HYDROCHLORIDE
Thioridazine Hydrochloride Tablets . . . 2195

MELLERIL (Austria, Belgium, Brazil, Denmark, Finland, Greece, Hong Kong, Hungary, Irish Republic, Israel, Italy, Malaysia, New Zealand, Norway, Portugal, South Africa, Switzerland, The Netherlands, Turkey)
THIORIDAZINE HYDROCHLORIDE
Thioridazine Hydrochloride Tablets . . . 2195

MELZINE (Irish Republic)
THIORIDAZINE HYDROCHLORIDE
Thioridazine Hydrochloride Tablets . . . 2195

MEMAC (Italy)
DONEPEZIL HYDROCHLORIDE
Aricept Tablets . . . 1062

MEMENTO NF (Argentina)
NORFLOXACIN
Noroxin Tablets . . . 2069

MENAELLE (Monaco)
PROGESTERONE
Crinone 4% Gel . . . 992
Prometrium Capsules (100 mg, 200 mg) . 3047

MENOGRAINE (South Africa)
CLONIDINE HYDROCHLORIDE
Catapres Tablets . . . 841

MENO-IMPLANT (Belgium, The Netherlands)
ESTRADIOL
Climara Transdermal System . . . 763

MENO-PATCH (Israel)
ESTRADIOL
Climara Transdermal System . . . 763

MENOREST (Australia, Austria, Brazil, Czech Republic, Denmark, Finland, France, Germany, Greece, Irish Republic, Italy, Norway, Portugal, South Africa, Spain, Sweden, Switzerland, The Netherlands, United Kingdom)
ESTRADIOL
Climara Transdermal System . . . 763

MENSOMA (Portugal)
FAMOTIDINE
Pepcid for Oral Suspension . . . 2075
Pepcid Tablets . . . 2075

MENTAX (Brazil, Israel, Japan)
BUTENAFINE HYDROCHLORIDE
Mentax Cream . . . 2190

MENTIX (Chile)
MODAFINIL
Provigil Tablets . . . 977

MEPLAR (Argentina)
PAROXETINE HYDROCHLORIDE
Paxil Oral Suspension . . . 1535
Paxil Tablets . . . 1535

MEPRON (Canada)
ATOVAQUONE
Mepron Suspension . . . 1526

MERANOL (Venezuela)
DIPYRIDAMOLE
Persantine Tablets . . . 869

MERAPRIL (Italy)
CAPTOPRIL
Captopril Tablets . . . 2182

MERCK-CO-LISINOPRIL (Belgium)
LISINOPRIL
Prinivil Tablets . . . 2087

MEREPRINE (Portugal)
CAPTOPRIL
Captopril Tablets . . . 2182

MERIDIA (Austria, Canada, Poland, Russia)
SIBUTRAMINE HYDROCHLORIDE
Meridia Capsules . . . 475

MEROEFECTIL (Argentina)
MEROPENEM
Merrem I.V. . . . 684

MERONEM (Belgium, Brazil, Chile, Czech Republic, Denmark, Finland, Germany, Greece, Hong Kong, Hungary, India, Irish Republic, Israel, Malaysia, Norway, Poland, Portugal, Russia, Singapore, South Africa, Spain, Sweden, Switzerland, Thailand, The Netherlands, The Philippines, Turkey, United Kingdom, Venezuela)
MEROPENEM
Merrem I.V. . . . 684

MEROPEN (Japan)
MEROPENEM
Merrem I.V. . . . 684

MEROTENK (Argentina)
MEROPENEM
Merrem I.V. . . . 684

MEROXIL (Brazil)
MEROPENEM
Merrem I.V. . . . 684

MEROZEN (Argentina)
MEROPENEM
Merrem I.V. . . . 684

MERPEM (Argentina)
MEROPENEM
Merrem I.V. . . . 684

MERREM (Australia, Canada, Italy, Mexico, New Zealand)
MEROPENEM
Merrem I.V. . . . 684

MERXIL (Mexico)
DICLOFENAC SODIUM
Voltaren Tablets . . . 2334
Voltaren-XR Tablets . . . 2337

MESIN (Thailand)
ALBENDAZOLE
Albenza Tablets . . . 1297

M-ESLON (Canada, Chile, Czech Republic, Hong Kong, Hungary, New Zealand, Turkey)
MORPHINE SULFATE
MS Contin Tablets . . . 2585

MESPORIN (Hong Kong, Portugal)
CEFTRIAXONE SODIUM
Rocephin Injectable Vials, ADD-Vantage, Galaxy, Bulk . . . 2642

METAFLEX PLUS NF (Argentina)
DICLOFENAC SODIUM
Voltaren Tablets . . . 2334
Voltaren-XR Tablets . . . 2337

METAMIDOL (Portugal)
DIAZEPAM
Valium Tablets . . . 2658

METASON (Argentina)
MOMETASONE FUROATE
Elocon Cream 0.1% . . . 2840
Elocon Lotion 0.1% . . . 2841
Elocon Ointment 0.1% . . . 2842
Nasonex Nasal Spray . . . 2883

METASPRAY (India)
MOMETASONE FUROATE
Elocon Cream 0.1% . . . 2840
Elocon Lotion 0.1% . . . 2841
Elocon Ointment 0.1% . . . 2842
Nasonex Nasal Spray . . . 2883

METAZEM (Hong Kong, Singapore, Thailand, United Kingdom)
DILTIAZEM HYDROCHLORIDE
Cardizem LA Extended Release Tablets . . . 421

METICEL (Spain)
RANITIDINE HYDROCHLORIDE
Zantac 25 EFFERdose Tablets . . . 1670
Zantac 150 Tablets . . . 1670
Zantac 300 Tablets . . . 1670
Zantac Injection . . . 1666
Zantac Injection Premixed . . . 1666
Zantac Syrup . . . 1670

METIMYD (Canada, Sweden)
PREDNISOLONE ACETATE/SULFACETAMIDE SODIUM
Blephamide Ophthalmic Ointment . . . ⊙217
Blephamide Ophthalmic Suspension . . . ⊙216

METLIGINE (Japan)
MIDODRINE HYDROCHLORIDE
ProAmatine Tablets . . . 3032

METOHEXAL (Germany, Poland)
METOPROLOL SUCCINATE
Toprol-XL Tablets . . . 666

METORAL (Thailand)
TRIAMCINOLONE ACETONIDE
Azmacort Inhalation Aerosol . . . 407
Nasacort AQ Nasal Spray . . . 2765

METO-SUCCINAT (Germany)
METOPROLOL SUCCINATE
Toprol-XL Tablets . . . 666

METRACIN (Mexico)
DICLOFENAC SODIUM
Voltaren Tablets . . . 2334
Voltaren-XR Tablets . . . 2337

METRONOM (Austria)
PROPAFENONE HYDROCHLORIDE
Rythmol SR Capsules . . . 1590

MEVACOR (Austria, Brazil, Canada, Chile, Czech Republic, Denmark, Finland, Greece, Hong Kong, Hungary, Malaysia, Mexico, Norway, Spain, Venezuela)
LOVASTATIN
Mevacor Tablets . . . 2063

MEVAL (Canada)
DIAZEPAM
Valium Tablets . . . 2658

MEVASTEROL (Spain)
LOVASTATIN
Mevacor Tablets . . . 2063

MEVASTIN (Greece)
LOVASTATIN
Mevacor Tablets . . . 2063

MEVECAN (Greece)
CEFUROXIME AXETIL
Ceftin for Oral Suspension . . . 1380
Ceftin Tablets . . . 1380

MEVINACOR (Germany, Portugal)
LOVASTATIN
Mevacor Tablets . . . 2063

MEVINOL (Greece)
LOVASTATIN
Mevacor Tablets . . . 2063

MEVLOR (Argentina, Portugal)
LOVASTATIN
Mevacor Tablets . . . 2063

M-FLOX (Thailand)
NORFLOXACIN
Noroxin Tablets . . . 2069

M-FURO (Turkey)
MOMETASONE FUROATE
Elocon Cream 0.1% . . . 2840
Elocon Lotion 0.1% . . . 2841
Elocon Ointment 0.1% . . . 2842
Nasonex Nasal Spray . . . 2883

MIBESAN-S (Mexico)
NYSTATIN
Nystop Topical Powder USP . . . 2498

MICARDIS (Argentina, Australia, Austria, Belgium, Brazil, Canada, Chile, Czech Republic, Denmark, Finland, France, Germany, Greece, Hong Kong, Hungary, Irish Republic, Italy, Japan, Malaysia, Mexico, Norway, Poland, Portugal, Russia, Singapore, South Africa, Spain, Sweden, Switzerland, Thailand, The Netherlands, The Philippines, Turkey, United Kingdom, Venezuela)
TELMISARTAN
Micardis Tablets . . . 852

MICARDIS HCT (Brazil)
TELMISARTAN
Micardis Tablets . . . 852

MICARDIS PLUS (Argentina, Australia, Belgium, Canada, Greece, Hong Kong, Italy, Malaysia, Mexico, Poland, Portugal, Singapore, Spain, Sweden, The Netherlands, The Philippines, Turkey, Venezuela)
TELMISARTAN
Micardis Tablets . . . 852

MICARDISPLUS (Austria, Denmark, Finland, France, Germany, Irish Republic, Norway, Switzerland, United Kingdom)
TELMISARTAN
Micardis Tablets . . . 852

MICOBAN (Greece)
MUPIROCIN
Bactroban Ointment . . . 1368

MICONACINA (Mexico)
NATAMYCIN
Natacyn Antifungal Ophthalmic Suspension . . . ⊙204

MICOSET (Chile)
TERBINAFINE HYDROCHLORIDE
Lamisil Tablets . . . 2266

MICOSIL (Brazil)
TERBINAFINE HYDROCHLORIDE
Lamisil Tablets . . . 2266

MICOSONA (Spain)
NAFTIFINE HYDROCHLORIDE
Naftin Cream . . . 2164
Naftin Gel . . . 2164

MICOSTAL (Brazil)
NYSTATIN
Nystop Topical Powder USP . . . 2498

MICOSTALAB (Brazil)
NYSTATIN
Nystop Topical Powder USP . . . 2498

MICOSTATIN (Argentina, Brazil, Chile, Mexico, Venezuela)
NYSTATIN
Nystop Topical Powder USP . . . 2498

MICOSTATIN BABY (Mexico)
NYSTATIN
Nystop Topical Powder USP . . . 2498

MICOSTOP (Chile)
TERBINAFINE HYDROCHLORIDE
Lamisil Tablets . . . 2266

MICRANIL (Argentina)
SUMATRIPTAN SUCCINATE
Imitrex Injection . . . 1465
Imitrex Tablets . . . 1474

MICRODIT (Mexico)
RANITIDINE HYDROCHLORIDE
Zantac 25 EFFERdose Tablets . . . 1670
Zantac 150 Tablets . . . 1670
Zantac 300 Tablets . . . 1670
Zantac Injection . . . 1666
Zantac Injection Premixed . . . 1666
Zantac Syrup . . . 1670

MICROFLOX (Thailand)
CIPROFLOXACIN HYDROCHLORIDE
Cipro Tablets . . . 2810

MICRONOAN (Italy)
DIAZEPAM
Valium Tablets . . . 2658

MICROPHYLLIN (South Africa)
THEOPHYLLINE
Uniphyl Tablets 2595

MICRORGAN (Mexico)
CIPROFLOXACIN HYDROCHLORIDE
Cipro Tablets 2810

MICROSULF (Argentina)
CIPROFLOXACIN HYDROCHLORIDE
Cipro Tablets 2810

MICROXIN (Mexico)
NORFLOXACIN
Noroxin Tablets 2069

MICTASOL (Mexico)
NORFLOXACIN
Noroxin Tablets 2069

MIDAVEN (Mexico)
RANITIDINE HYDROCHLORIDE
Zantac 25 EFFERdose Tablets 1670
Zantac 150 Tablets 1670
Zantac 300 Tablets 1670
Zantac Injection 1666
Zantac Injection Premixed 1666
Zantac Syrup 1670

MIDAX (Argentina)
OLANZAPINE
Zyprexa Tablets 1883

MIDON (Irish Republic)
MIDODRINE HYDROCHLORIDE
ProAmatine Tablets 3032

MIDRAN (Italy, South Africa)
APROTININ
Trasylol Injection 799

MIDRAT (Mexico)
CAPTOPRIL
Captopril Tablets 2182

MIELUCIN (Brazil)
BUSULFAN
Myleran Tablets 1530

MIGRANEITOR (Argentina)
SUMATRIPTAN
Imitrex Nasal Spray 1470

MIGRAVAL (Venezuela)
SUMATRIPTAN SUCCINATE
Imitrex Injection 1465
Imitrex Tablets 1474

MIGRIL (Brazil)
SUMATRIPTAN SUCCINATE
Imitrex Injection 1465
Imitrex Tablets 1474

MIKOSTAT (United Arab Emirates)
NYSTATIN
Nystop Topical Powder USP 2498

MIKOSTAT BABY OINTMENT (United Arab Emirates)
NYSTATIN
Nystop Topical Powder USP 2498

MIKOSTATIN (Turkey)
NYSTATIN
Nystop Topical Powder USP 2498

MILADOR (The Philippines)
TRAMADOL HYDROCHLORIDE
Ultram ER Tablets 2428

MILANOLONE (Thailand)
TRIAMCINOLONE ACETONIDE
Azmacort Inhalation Aerosol 407
Nasacort AQ Nasal Spray 2765

MILICAL (Chile, Venezuela)
SIBUTRAMINE HYDROCHLORIDE
Meridia Capsules 475

MILLIBAR (Hong Kong, Italy, Singapore)
INDAPAMIDE
Indapamide Tablets 2188

MILLIDOL (Thailand)
TRAMADOL HYDROCHLORIDE
Ultram ER Tablets 2428

MINIDOL (Chile)
TRAMADOL HYDROCHLORIDE
Ultram ER Tablets 2428

MINIDOL PLUS (Chile)
TRAMADOL HYDROCHLORIDE
Ultram ER Tablets 2428

MINIOSTENIL (Argentina)
SODIUM HYALURONATE
Hyalgan Solution 2742

MINOBESE (South Africa)
PHENTERMINE HYDROCHLORIDE
Adipex-P Capsules 1185
Adipex-P Tablets 1185

MINOR (Brazil)
LOVASTATIN
Mevacor Tablets 2063

MINPROSTIN (Denmark, Finland, Greece, Norway, Sweden)
DINOPROSTONE
Cervidil Vaginal Insert 1165

MINPROSTIN E2 (Germany)
DINOPROSTONE
Cervidil Vaginal Insert 1165

MINTAGRAS (Chile)
SIBUTRAMINE HYDROCHLORIDE
Meridia Capsules 475

MINUSLIP (Argentina)
FENOFIBRATE
Tricor Tablets 520

MINUSORB (Brazil)
ALENDRONATE SODIUM
Fosamax Tablets 2005

MIO ALDORON NF (Argentina)
DICLOFENAC SODIUM
Voltaren Tablets 2334
Voltaren-XR Tablets 2337

MIOCALM (Argentina)
DICLOFENAC SODIUM
Voltaren Tablets 2334
Voltaren-XR Tablets 2337

MIOCAP (Mexico)
CAPTOPRIL
Captopril Tablets 2182

MIOSEN (Spain)
DIPYRIDAMOLE
Persantine Tablets 869

MIO-VIROBRON NF (Argentina)
DICLOFENAC SODIUM
Voltaren Tablets 2334
Voltaren-XR Tablets 2337

MIOZEPAM (Argentina)
CLONAZEPAM
Klonopin Tablets 2639

MIPHAR (Israel)
FUROSEMIDE
Furosemide Tablets 2186

MIQUIMOD (Argentina)
IMIQUIMOD
Aldara Cream, 5% 1699

MIR (Israel)
MORPHINE SULFATE
MS Contin Tablets 2585

MIRAGRAN (Chile)
NARATRIPTAN HYDROCHLORIDE
Amerge Tablets 1301

MIRANAX (Austria, Denmark, Finland, Sweden)
NAPROXEN SODIUM
Anaprox DS Tablets 2632
Anaprox Tablets 2632

MIRFAT (Germany)
CLONIDINE HYDROCHLORIDE
Catapres Tablets 841

MIROCEF (Poland)
CEFTAZIDIME SODIUM
Fortaz for Injection 1450

MIRUBAL (Venezuela)
PHENTERMINE HYDROCHLORIDE
Adipex-P Capsules 1185
Adipex-P Tablets 1185

MISODOMIN (Greece)
LOVASTATIN
Mevacor Tablets 2063

MISOFENAC (Italy, The Netherlands)
DICLOFENAC SODIUM
Voltaren Tablets 2334
Voltaren-XR Tablets 2337

MISULBAN (Italy, Monaco)
BUSULFAN
Myleran Tablets 1530

MITATONIN (Hong Kong)
NORFLOXACIN
Noroxin Tablets 2069

MITEN (Spain)
VALSARTAN
Diovan Tablets 2212

MITEN PLUS (Spain)
VALSARTAN
Diovan Tablets 2212

MITROKEN (Mexico)
CIPROFLOXACIN HYDROCHLORIDE
Cipro Tablets 2810

MIVALEN (Brazil)
SIMVASTATIN
Zocor Tablets 2136

MIXCILIN (Argentina)
AMOXICILLIN
Amoxil Pediatric Drops for Oral Suspension 1305
Amoxil Tablets 1305

MIYADREN (Turkey)
DICLOFENAC SODIUM
Voltaren Tablets 2334
Voltaren-XR Tablets 2337

M-LONG (Austria, Germany)
MORPHINE SULFATE
MS Contin Tablets 2585

MOBAN (Hong Kong)
MOLINDONE HYDROCHLORIDE
Moban Tablets 1116

MOCIMED (Mexico)
AMOXICILLIN
Amoxil Pediatric Drops for Oral Suspension 1305
Amoxil Tablets 1305

MODAPLATE (United Kingdom)
DIPYRIDAMOLE
Persantine Tablets 869

MODASOMIL (Austria, Switzerland)
MODAFINIL
Provigil Tablets 977

MODAVIGIL (Australia, New Zealand)
MODAFINIL
Provigil Tablets 977

MODERAN (Venezuela)
LACTULOSE
Kristalose for Oral Solution 1004

MODIFENAC (Denmark, Norway, Sweden)
DICLOFENAC SODIUM
Voltaren Tablets 2334
Voltaren-XR Tablets 2337

MODIFICAL (Brazil)
ONDANSETRON HYDROCHLORIDE
Zofran Injection 1682
Zofran Injection Premixed 1682
Zofran Oral Solution 1687
Zofran Tablets 1687

MODINA (Portugal)
NIMODIPINE
Nimotop Capsules 790

MODINOL (Greece)
RIZATRIPTAN BENZOATE
Maxalt Tablets 2056
Maxalt-MLT Orally Disintegrating Tablets .. 2056

MODIODAL (Denmark, France, Greece, Mexico, Norway, Portugal, Spain, Sweden, The Netherlands, Turkey)
MODAFINIL
Provigil Tablets 977

MODUS (Spain)
NIMODIPINE
Nimotop Capsules 790

MOGETIC (Germany)
MORPHINE SULFATE
MS Contin Tablets 2585

MOKCAN (India)
AMOXICILLIN
Amoxil Pediatric Drops for Oral Suspension 1305
Amoxil Tablets 1305

MOMATE (India, The Philippines)
MOMETASONE FUROATE
Elocon Cream 0.1% 2840
Elocon Lotion 0.1% 2841
Elocon Ointment 0.1% 2842
Nasonex Nasal Spray 2883

MOMATE-S (India)
MOMETASONE FUROATE
Elocon Cream 0.1% 2840
Elocon Lotion 0.1% 2841
Elocon Ointment 0.1% 2842
Nasonex Nasal Spray 2883

MOMELAB (Chile)
MOMETASONE FUROATE
Elocon Cream 0.1% 2840
Elocon Lotion 0.1% 2841
Elocon Ointment 0.1% 2842
Nasonex Nasal Spray 2883

MOMEN (Spain)
NAPROXEN
EC-Naprosyn Delayed-Release Tablets 2632
Naprosyn Suspension 2632
Naprosyn Tablets 2632

MOMENDOL (Italy, Portugal, The Netherlands)
NAPROXEN SODIUM
Anaprox DS Tablets 2632
Anaprox Tablets 2632

MONARIT (Argentina)
NAPROXEN SODIUM
Anaprox DS Tablets 2632
Anaprox Tablets 2632

MONAXIN (Belgium)
CLARITHROMYCIN
Biaxin Filmtab Tablets 411
Biaxin Granules 411

MONDRIAN (Chile)
BUPROPION HYDROCHLORIDE
Wellbutrin SR Sustained-Release Tablets .. 1653
Wellbutrin Tablets 1648
Zyban Sustained-Release Tablets 1692

MONILAC (Japan)
LACTULOSE
Kristalose for Oral Solution 1004

MONOCEF (India)
CEFTRIAXONE SODIUM
Rocephin Injectable Vials, ADD-Vantage, Galaxy, Bulk 2642

MONOCID (Austria)
CLARITHROMYCIN
Biaxin Filmtab Tablets 411
Biaxin Granules 411

MONOCRIN (The Philippines)
CEFTRIAXONE SODIUM
Rocephin Injectable Vials, ADD-Vantage, Galaxy, Bulk 2642

MONOCRIXO (France)
TRAMADOL HYDROCHLORIDE
Ultram ER Tablets 2428

MONOFLAM (Germany)
DICLOFENAC SODIUM
Voltaren Tablets 2334
Voltaren-XR Tablets 2337

MONONAXY (France)
CLARITHROMYCIN
Biaxin Filmtab Tablets 411
Biaxin Granules 411

MONOTAX (India)
CEFTRIAXONE SODIUM
Rocephin Injectable Vials, ADD-Vantage, Galaxy, Bulk 2642

MONO-TILDIEM (France, Malaysia, Singapore, Thailand, The Philippines)
DILTIAZEM HYDROCHLORIDE
Cardizem LA Extended Release Tablets 421

MONOXAR (Italy)
CEFTRIAXONE SODIUM
Rocephin Injectable Vials, ADD-Vantage, Galaxy, Bulk 2642

MONOZECLAR (France)
CLARITHROMYCIN
Biaxin Filmtab Tablets 411
Biaxin Granules 411

MONOZOL (Brazil)
ALBENDAZOLE
Albenza Tablets 1297

MONSALIC (Czech Republic)
MOMETASONE FUROATE
Elocon Cream 0.1% 2840

Elocon Lotion 0.1% 2841
Elocon Ointment 0.1% 2842
Nasonex Nasal Spray 2883

MONTAIR (India)
MONTELUKAST SODIUM
Singulair Chewable Tablets 2114
Singulair Tablets 2114

MONTAIR PLUS (India)
MONTELUKAST SODIUM
Singulair Chewable Tablets 2114
Singulair Tablets 2114

MONTEGEN (Italy)
MONTELUKAST SODIUM
Singulair Chewable Tablets 2114
Singulair Tablets 2114

MORAPID (Austria)
MORPHINE SULFATE
MS Contin Tablets 2585

MORAXEN (United Kingdom)
MORPHINE SULFATE
MS Contin Tablets 2585

MORCAP (United Kingdom)
MORPHINE SULFATE
MS Contin Tablets 2585

MORCONTIN (India)
MORPHINE SULFATE
MS Contin Tablets 2585

MORETAL (Hungary)
MORPHINE SULFATE
MS Contin Tablets 2585

MORONAL (Germany)
NYSTATIN
Nystop Topical Powder USP 2498

MORPH (Germany)
MORPHINE SULFATE
MS Contin Tablets 2585

MORPHGESIC (United Kingdom)
MORPHINE SULFATE
MS Contin Tablets 2585

MORSTEL (Irish Republic)
MORPHINE SULFATE
MS Contin Tablets 2585

MOSALAN (Greece)
CEFUROXIME AXETIL
Ceftin for Oral Suspension 1380
Ceftin Tablets 1380

MOSCONTIN (France)
MORPHINE SULFATE
MS Contin Tablets 2585

MOSTRELAN (Greece)
FAMOTIDINE
Pepcid for Oral Suspension 2075
Pepcid Tablets 2075

MOTIAX (Italy)
FAMOTIDINE
Pepcid for Oral Suspension 2075
Pepcid Tablets 2075

MOTID (The Philippines)
FAMOTIDINE
Pepcid for Oral Suspension 2075
Pepcid Tablets 2075

MOTIDIN (Hungary)
FAMOTIDINE
Pepcid for Oral Suspension 2075
Pepcid Tablets 2075

MOTIDINE (Hong Kong, Singapore, Thailand)
FAMOTIDINE
Pepcid for Oral Suspension 2075
Pepcid Tablets 2075

MOTIFENE (Belgium, Finland, United Kingdom)
DICLOFENAC SODIUM
Voltaren Tablets 2334
Voltaren-XR Tablets 2337

MOTIVAN (Spain)
PAROXETINE HYDROCHLORIDE
Paxil Oral Suspension 1535
Paxil Tablets 1535

MOVERDIN (Turkey)
SELEGILINE HYDROCHLORIDE
Eldepryl Capsules 3052

MOVERGAN (Germany)
SELEGILINE HYDROCHLORIDE
Eldepryl Capsules 3052

MOVESAN (Greece)
MOMETASONE FUROATE
Elocon Cream 0.1% 2840
Elocon Lotion 0.1% 2841
Elocon Ointment 0.1% 2842
Nasonex Nasal Spray 2883

MOVEX (Mexico)
NAPROXEN
EC-Naprosyn Delayed-Release Tablets 2632
Naprosyn Suspension 2632
Naprosyn Tablets 2632

MOX (India)
AMOXICILLIN
Amoxil Pediatric Drops for Oral Suspension 1305
Amoxil Tablets 1305

MOXADENT (Portugal)
AMOXICILLIN
Amoxil Pediatric Drops for Oral Suspension 1305
Amoxil Tablets 1305

MOXICEL (Mexico)
AMOXICILLIN
Amoxil Pediatric Drops for Oral Suspension 1305
Amoxil Tablets 1305

MOXICLINA (Mexico)
AMOXICILLIN
Amoxil Pediatric Drops for Oral Suspension 1305
Amoxil Tablets 1305

MOXIPEN (Portugal, Singapore)
AMOXICILLIN
Amoxil Pediatric Drops for Oral Suspension 1305
Amoxil Tablets 1305

MOXITOP (Belgium)
AMOXICILLIN
Amoxil Pediatric Drops for Oral Suspension 1305
Amoxil Tablets 1305

MOXITRAL (Argentina)
AMOXICILLIN
Amoxil Pediatric Drops for Oral Suspension 1305
Amoxil Tablets 1305

MOXLIN CLV (Mexico)
AMOXICILLIN
Amoxil Pediatric Drops for Oral Suspension 1305
Amoxil Tablets 1305

MOXYCARB (India)
AMOXICILLIN
Amoxil Pediatric Drops for Oral Suspension 1305
Amoxil Tablets 1305

MOXYCARB-DT (India)
AMOXICILLIN
Amoxil Pediatric Drops for Oral Suspension 1305
Amoxil Tablets 1305

MOXYCLAV (South Africa)
AMOXICILLIN
Amoxil Pediatric Drops for Oral Suspension 1305
Amoxil Tablets 1305

MOXYMAX (South Africa)
AMOXICILLIN
Amoxil Pediatric Drops for Oral Suspension 1305
Amoxil Tablets 1305

MS CONTIN (Australia, Belgium, Canada, Italy, The Netherlands, Venezuela)
MORPHINE SULFATE
MS Contin Tablets 2585

MS DIRECT (Belgium)
MORPHINE SULFATE
MS Contin Tablets 2585

MS MONO (Australia)
MORPHINE SULFATE
MS Contin Tablets 2585

MSI (Germany)
MORPHINE SULFATE
MS Contin Tablets 2585

MSIR (Canada)
MORPHINE SULFATE
MS Contin Tablets 2585

MS-LONG (Brazil)
MORPHINE SULFATE
MS Contin Tablets 2585

MSP (Israel)
MORPHINE SULFATE
MS Contin Tablets 2585

MSR (Germany)
MORPHINE SULFATE
MS Contin Tablets 2585

MST (Portugal)
MORPHINE SULFATE
MS Contin Tablets 2585

MST CONTINUS (Argentina, Brazil, Hong Kong, Irish Republic, Mexico, New Zealand, Poland, Singapore, South Africa, Spain, Switzerland, The Philippines, United Kingdom)
MORPHINE SULFATE
MS Contin Tablets 2585

MST MONO (New Zealand)
MORPHINE SULFATE
MS Contin Tablets 2585

MST UNICONTINUS (Spain)
MORPHINE SULFATE
MS Contin Tablets 2585

MST UNO (Czech Republic)
MORPHINE SULFATE
MS Contin Tablets 2585

MUCLOX (Spain)
FAMOTIDINE
Pepcid for Oral Suspension 2075
Pepcid Tablets 2075

MULCATEL (Chile)
SUCRALFATE
Carafate Suspension 706
Carafate Tablets 707

MULTILIND (Germany, United Kingdom)
NYSTATIN
Nystop Topical Powder USP 2498

MULTISEF (Turkey)
CEFUROXIME SODIUM
Zinacef Injection 1678

MUNDIDOL (Austria)
MORPHINE SULFATE
MS Contin Tablets 2585

MUNDIL (Germany)
CAPTOPRIL
Captopril Tablets 2182

MUPAX (Argentina)
MUPIROCIN
Bactroban Ointment 1368

MUPIDERM (France)
MUPIROCIN
Bactroban Ointment 1368

MUPIRAN (Greece)
MUPIROCIN
Bactroban Ointment 1368

MUPIROX (Argentina, Poland)
MUPIROCIN
Bactroban Ointment 1368

MUPISKIN (Italy)
MUPIROCIN
Bactroban Ointment 1368

MUPORIN (Thailand)
MUPIROCIN
Bactroban Ointment 1368

MUS (Chile)
CLARITHROMYCIN
Biaxin Filmtab Tablets 411
Biaxin Granules 411

MUSTOPIC (India)
TACROLIMUS
Prograf Capsules and Injection 622

MUVIDINA (Argentina)
ZIDOVUDINE
Retrovir Capsules 1574
Retrovir IV Infusion 1579
Retrovir Syrup 1574
Retrovir Tablets 1574

MXL (Irish Republic, Portugal, United Kingdom)
MORPHINE SULFATE
MS Contin Tablets 2585

MYCARZEM (Greece)
DILTIAZEM HYDROCHLORIDE
Cardizem LA Extended Release Tablets 421

MYCOCUR (Turkey)
TERBINAFINE HYDROCHLORIDE
Lamisil Tablets 2266

MYCO-INTRADERMI (Germany)
NYSTATIN
Nystop Topical Powder USP 2498

MYCONAFINE (Poland)
TERBINAFINE HYDROCHLORIDE
Lamisil Tablets 2266

MYCONORMIN (Germany, Switzerland)
TERBINAFINE HYDROCHLORIDE
Lamisil Tablets 2266

MYCOSTATIN (Australia, Austria, Denmark, Finland, Greece, Hong Kong, India, Irish Republic, Italy, Malaysia, New Zealand, Norway, Portugal, Singapore, South Africa, Spain, Sweden, Thailand, The Philippines)
NYSTATIN
Nystop Topical Powder USP 2498

MYCOSTATINE (France, Switzerland)
NYSTATIN
Nystop Topical Powder USP 2498

MYCOTEL (Thailand)
ALBENDAZOLE
Albenza Tablets 1297

MYFLOXIN (Thailand)
NORFLOXACIN
Noroxin Tablets 2069

MYKODERM HEILSALBE (Germany)
NYSTATIN
Nystop Topical Powder USP 2498

MYKOPOSTERINE N (Germany)
NYSTATIN
Nystop Topical Powder USP 2498

MYKUNDEX (Germany)
NYSTATIN
Nystop Topical Powder USP 2498

MYKUNDEX HEILSALBE (Germany)
NYSTATIN
Nystop Topical Powder USP 2498

MYKUNDEX MONO (Germany)
NYSTATIN
Nystop Topical Powder USP 2498

MYKUNDEX OVULA (Germany)
NYSTATIN
Nystop Topical Powder USP 2498

MYLERAN (Argentina, Australia, Austria, Belgium, Brazil, Canada, Chile, Czech Republic, France, Germany, Greece, Hong Kong, India, Irish Republic, Israel, Italy, Malaysia, Mexico, New Zealand, Norway, Poland, Portugal, Russia, Singapore, South Africa, Sweden, Switzerland, Thailand, The Netherlands, Turkey, United Kingdom)
BUSULFAN
Myleran Tablets 1530

MYOCARDON N (Germany)
THEOPHYLLINE
Uniphyl Tablets 2595

MYODIPINE (Greece)
NIMODIPINE
Nimotop Capsules 790

MYOGIT (Czech Republic, Germany)
DICLOFENAC SODIUM
Voltaren Tablets 2334
Voltaren-XR Tablets 2337

MYONIL (Denmark)
DILTIAZEM HYDROCHLORIDE
Cardizem LA Extended Release Tablets 421

MYTOLAC (Sweden)
BENZOYL PEROXIDE
Brevoxyl-4 Creamy Wash 3054

Brevoxyl-4 Gel . . . 3054
Brevoxyl-8 Creamy Wash . . . 3054
Brevoxyl-8 Gel . . . 3054

NABICORTIN (Greece)
LOVASTATIN
Mevacor Tablets . . . 2063

NABOREL (Greece)
NIMODIPINE
Nimotop Capsules . . . 790

NABRATIN (Argentina)
CLOPIDOGREL BISULFATE
Plavix Tablets . . . 926, 2767

NAC (India)
DICLOFENAC SODIUM
Voltaren Tablets . . . 2334
Voltaren-XR Tablets . . . 2337

NACLODIN (Venezuela)
CLONIDINE HYDROCHLORIDE
Catapres Tablets . . . 841

NACLOF (Austria, Czech Republic, Norway, Poland, Russia, South Africa, Sweden, Thailand, The Netherlands)
DICLOFENAC SODIUM
Voltaren Tablets . . . 2334
Voltaren-XR Tablets . . . 2337

NACTOL (Mexico)
BENZONATATE
Tessalon Perles . . . 1183

NACUA (Venezuela)
FUROSEMIDE
Furosemide Tablets . . . 2186

NADOSTINE (Canada, Hong Kong)
NYSTATIN
Nystop Topical Powder USP . . . 2498

NAFASOL (South Africa)
NAPROXEN
EC-Naprosyn Delayed-Release Tablets . . . 2632
Naprosyn Suspension . . . 2632
Naprosyn Tablets . . . 2632

NAFINA (Venezuela)
TERBINAFINE HYDROCHLORIDE
Lamisil Tablets . . . 2266

NAFLAPEN (Mexico)
NAPROXEN
EC-Naprosyn Delayed-Release Tablets . . . 2632
Naprosyn Suspension . . . 2632
Naprosyn Tablets . . . 2632

NAFLUVENT (Argentina)
FENTANYL
Duragesic Transdermal System . . . 2405

NAFORDYL (Greece)
LISINOPRIL
Prinivil Tablets . . . 2087

NAFTIN (Canada)
NAFTIFINE HYDROCHLORIDE
Naftin Cream . . . 2164
Naftin Gel . . . 2164

NAILDERM (Irish Republic)
TERBINAFINE HYDROCHLORIDE
Lamisil Tablets . . . 2266

NAKLOFEN (Czech Republic, Russia)
DICLOFENAC SODIUM
Voltaren Tablets . . . 2334
Voltaren-XR Tablets . . . 2337

NAKLOFEN DUO (Russia)
DICLOFENAC SODIUM
Voltaren Tablets . . . 2334
Voltaren-XR Tablets . . . 2337

NALAPRES (Italy)
HYDROCHLOROTHIAZIDE/LISINOPRIL
Prinzide Tablets . . . 2092

NALGESIN (Czech Republic, Russia)
NAPROXEN SODIUM
Anaprox DS Tablets . . . 2632
Anaprox Tablets . . . 2632

NALGIFLEX RELAX (Argentina)
DICLOFENAC SODIUM
Voltaren Tablets . . . 2334
Voltaren-XR Tablets . . . 2337

NALION (Spain)
NORFLOXACIN
Noroxin Tablets . . . 2069

NAPAMIDE (Australia, Hong Kong, Malaysia, New Zealand, Singapore)
INDAPAMIDE
Indapamide Tablets . . . 2188

NAPFLAM (South Africa)
NAPROXEN
EC-Naprosyn Delayed-Release Tablets . . . 2632
Naprosyn Suspension . . . 2632
Naprosyn Tablets . . . 2632

NAPLIN (New Zealand)
INDAPAMIDE
Indapamide Tablets . . . 2188

NAPMEL (Hungary, Irish Republic)
NAPROXEN
EC-Naprosyn Delayed-Release Tablets . . . 2632
Naprosyn Suspension . . . 2632
Naprosyn Tablets . . . 2632

NAPONAL (Turkey)
NAPROXEN
EC-Naprosyn Delayed-Release Tablets . . . 2632
Naprosyn Suspension . . . 2632
Naprosyn Tablets . . . 2632

NAPRADOL (Turkey)
NAPROXEN SODIUM
Anaprox DS Tablets . . . 2632
Anaprox Tablets . . . 2632

NAPRATEC (United Kingdom)
NAPROXEN
EC-Naprosyn Delayed-Release Tablets . . . 2632
Naprosyn Suspension . . . 2632
Naprosyn Tablets . . . 2632

NAPREL (South Africa)
NAPROXEN
EC-Naprosyn Delayed-Release Tablets . . . 2632
Naprosyn Suspension . . . 2632
Naprosyn Tablets . . . 2632

NAPRELAN (Sweden, The Netherlands, The Philippines)
NAPROXEN SODIUM
Anaprox DS Tablets . . . 2632
Anaprox Tablets . . . 2632

NAPREN (Norway, Turkey)
NAPROXEN SODIUM
Anaprox DS Tablets . . . 2632
Anaprox Tablets . . . 2632

NAPREX (Irish Republic, Israel)
NAPROXEN SODIUM
Anaprox DS Tablets . . . 2632
Anaprox Tablets . . . 2632

NAPRIUM (Italy)
NAPROXEN
EC-Naprosyn Delayed-Release Tablets . . . 2632
Naprosyn Suspension . . . 2632
Naprosyn Tablets . . . 2632

NAPRIUS (Italy)
NAPROXEN
EC-Naprosyn Delayed-Release Tablets . . . 2632
Naprosyn Suspension . . . 2632
Naprosyn Tablets . . . 2632

NAPROBENE (Austria, Czech Republic)
NAPROXEN
EC-Naprosyn Delayed-Release Tablets . . . 2632
Naprosyn Suspension . . . 2632
Naprosyn Tablets . . . 2632

NAPROCOAT (The Netherlands)
NAPROXEN
EC-Naprosyn Delayed-Release Tablets . . . 2632
Naprosyn Suspension . . . 2632
Naprosyn Tablets . . . 2632

NAPRODEVA (Turkey)
NAPROXEN
EC-Naprosyn Delayed-Release Tablets . . . 2632
Naprosyn Suspension . . . 2632
Naprosyn Tablets . . . 2632

NAPRODIL (Mexico)
NAPROXEN
EC-Naprosyn Delayed-Release Tablets . . . 2632
Naprosyn Suspension . . . 2632
Naprosyn Tablets . . . 2632

NAPRODIL PLUS (Mexico)
NAPROXEN SODIUM
Anaprox DS Tablets . . . 2632
Anaprox Tablets . . . 2632

NAPRODOL (Italy)
NAPROXEN SODIUM
Anaprox DS Tablets . . . 2632
Anaprox Tablets . . . 2632

NAPRO-DORSCH (Germany)
NAPROXEN
EC-Naprosyn Delayed-Release Tablets . . . 2632
Naprosyn Suspension . . . 2632
Naprosyn Tablets . . . 2632

NAPROFIDEX (Argentina)
NAPROXEN
EC-Naprosyn Delayed-Release Tablets . . . 2632
Naprosyn Suspension . . . 2632
Naprosyn Tablets . . . 2632

NAPROFLAM (Belgium)
NAPROXEN
EC-Naprosyn Delayed-Release Tablets . . . 2632
Naprosyn Suspension . . . 2632
Naprosyn Tablets . . . 2632

NAPROFLEX (Thailand)
NAPROXEN SODIUM
Anaprox DS Tablets . . . 2632
Anaprox Tablets . . . 2632

NAPROGEN (Argentina)
NAPROXEN
EC-Naprosyn Delayed-Release Tablets . . . 2632
Naprosyn Suspension . . . 2632
Naprosyn Tablets . . . 2632

NAPROGESIC (Australia, Chile, New Zealand)
NAPROXEN SODIUM
Anaprox DS Tablets . . . 2632
Anaprox Tablets . . . 2632

NAPROKES (Spain)
NAPROXEN
EC-Naprosyn Delayed-Release Tablets . . . 2632
Naprosyn Suspension . . . 2632
Naprosyn Tablets . . . 2632

NAPROLAG (Switzerland)
NAPROXEN
EC-Naprosyn Delayed-Release Tablets . . . 2632
Naprosyn Suspension . . . 2632
Naprosyn Tablets . . . 2632

NAPROMETIN (Finland)
NAPROXEN
EC-Naprosyn Delayed-Release Tablets . . . 2632
Naprosyn Suspension . . . 2632
Naprosyn Tablets . . . 2632

NAPROMEX (Finland)
NAPROXEN
EC-Naprosyn Delayed-Release Tablets . . . 2632
Naprosyn Suspension . . . 2632
Naprosyn Tablets . . . 2632

NAPRONAX (Brazil)
NAPROXEN SODIUM
Anaprox DS Tablets . . . 2632
Anaprox Tablets . . . 2632

NAPRONET (Denmark)
NAPROXEN
EC-Naprosyn Delayed-Release Tablets . . . 2632
Naprosyn Suspension . . . 2632
Naprosyn Tablets . . . 2632

NAPRONTAG (Argentina)
NAPROXEN
EC-Naprosyn Delayed-Release Tablets . . . 2632
Naprosyn Suspension . . . 2632
Naprosyn Tablets . . . 2632

NAPRONTAG FLEX (Argentina)
NAPROXEN
EC-Naprosyn Delayed-Release Tablets . . . 2632
Naprosyn Suspension . . . 2632
Naprosyn Tablets . . . 2632

NAPROREX (Hong Kong, Italy)
NAPROXEN SODIUM
Anaprox DS Tablets . . . 2632
Anaprox Tablets . . . 2632

NAPROSCRIPT (South Africa)
NAPROXEN
EC-Naprosyn Delayed-Release Tablets . . . 2632
Naprosyn Suspension . . . 2632
Naprosyn Tablets . . . 2632

NAPROSIAN (Thailand)
NAPROXEN
EC-Naprosyn Delayed-Release Tablets . . . 2632
Naprosyn Suspension . . . 2632
Naprosyn Tablets . . . 2632

NAPROSO (Thailand)
NAPROXEN SODIUM
Anaprox DS Tablets . . . 2632
Anaprox Tablets . . . 2632

NAPROSYN (Australia, Brazil, Canada, Czech Republic, Denmark, Finland, Greece, Hong Kong, Hungary, India, Irish Republic, Italy, New Zealand, Norway, Portugal, Singapore, South Africa, Spain, Sweden, Switzerland, Thailand, The Philippines, Turkey, United Kingdom)
NAPROXEN SODIUM
Anaprox DS Tablets . . . 2632
Anaprox Tablets . . . 2632

NAPROSYNE (Belgium, France, The Netherlands)
NAPROXEN
EC-Naprosyn Delayed-Release Tablets . . . 2632
Naprosyn Suspension . . . 2632
Naprosyn Tablets . . . 2632

NAPROTAB (Turkey)
NAPROXEN
EC-Naprosyn Delayed-Release Tablets . . . 2632
Naprosyn Suspension . . . 2632
Naprosyn Tablets . . . 2632

NAPROVAL (Spain)
NAPROXEN
EC-Naprosyn Delayed-Release Tablets . . . 2632
Naprosyn Suspension . . . 2632
Naprosyn Tablets . . . 2632

NAPROVITE (The Netherlands)
NAPROXEN SODIUM
Anaprox DS Tablets . . . 2632
Anaprox Tablets . . . 2632

NAPROX (Brazil)
NAPROXEN
EC-Naprosyn Delayed-Release Tablets . . . 2632
Naprosyn Suspension . . . 2632
Naprosyn Tablets . . . 2632

NAPROXI (Israel)
NAPROXEN
EC-Naprosyn Delayed-Release Tablets . . . 2632
Naprosyn Suspension . . . 2632
Naprosyn Tablets . . . 2632

NAPRUX (Argentina)
NAPROXEN
EC-Naprosyn Delayed-Release Tablets . . . 2632
Naprosyn Suspension . . . 2632
Naprosyn Tablets . . . 2632

NAPSEN (Thailand)
NAPROXEN
EC-Naprosyn Delayed-Release Tablets . . . 2632
Naprosyn Suspension . . . 2632
Naprosyn Tablets . . . 2632

NAPSYN (Czech Republic)
NAPROXEN
EC-Naprosyn Delayed-Release Tablets . . . 2632
Naprosyn Suspension . . . 2632
Naprosyn Tablets . . . 2632

NAPXEN (Hong Kong, Thailand)
NAPROXEN
EC-Naprosyn Delayed-Release Tablets . . . 2632
Naprosyn Suspension . . . 2632
Naprosyn Tablets . . . 2632

NAQUA (Hong Kong, Portugal)
FUROSEMIDE
Furosemide Tablets . . . 2186

NARAGRAN (Denmark)
NARATRIPTAN HYDROCHLORIDE
Amerge Tablets . . . 1301

NARAMIG (Argentina, Australia, Austria, Belgium, Brazil, Chile, Czech Republic, Finland, France, Greece, Hungary, Israel, Mexico, New Zealand, Norway, Portugal, Russia, Singapore, South Africa, Spain, Sweden, Switzerland, Thailand, The Netherlands, Turkey, United Kingdom)
NARATRIPTAN HYDROCHLORIDE
Amerge Tablets . . . 1301

NARIDE (Australia)
INDAPAMIDE
Indapamide Tablets . . . 2188

NARIGEN (Greece)
RANITIDINE HYDROCHLORIDE
Zantac 25 EFFERdose Tablets . . . 1670
Zantac 150 Tablets . . . 1670
Zantac 300 Tablets . . . 1670
Zantac Injection . . . 1666
Zantac Injection Premixed . . . 1666

Zantac Syrup 1670

NARILET (Spain)
IPRATROPIUM BROMIDE
Atrovent Nasal Spray 0.03% 834
Atrovent Nasal Spray 0.06% 836

NAROCIN (Israel)
NAPROXEN SODIUM
Anaprox DS Tablets 2632
Anaprox Tablets 2632

NARZEN (Thailand)
NAPROXEN
EC-Naprosyn Delayed-Release Tablets 2632
Naprosyn Suspension 2632
Naprosyn Tablets 2632

NASACOR (South Africa)
TRIAMCINOLONE ACETONIDE
Azmacort Inhalation Aerosol 407
Nasacort AQ Nasal Spray 2765

NASACORT (Argentina, Austria, Brazil, Canada, Chile, Czech Republic, Denmark, Finland, France, Germany, Greece, Hong Kong, Irish Republic, Italy, Mexico, New Zealand, Norway, Singapore, Spain, Sweden, Switzerland, Thailand, The Netherlands, Turkey, United Kingdom, Venezuela)
TRIAMCINOLONE ACETONIDE
Azmacort Inhalation Aerosol 407
Nasacort AQ Nasal Spray 2765

NASACORT AQ (Australia, Malaysia)
TRIAMCINOLONE ACETONIDE
Azmacort Inhalation Aerosol 407
Nasacort AQ Nasal Spray 2765

NASALIDE (France)
FLUNISOLIDE
Aerobid Inhaler System 1153
Aerobid-M Inhaler System 1153

NASOCAN (Mexico)
NAPROXEN SODIUM
Anaprox DS Tablets 2632
Anaprox Tablets 2632

NASOFAN (Irish Republic, United Kingdom)
FLUTICASONE PROPIONATE
Flonase Nasal Spray 1431

NASOMET (Portugal)
MOMETASONE FUROATE
Elocon Cream 0.1% 2840
Elocon Lotion 0.1% 2841
Elocon Ointment 0.1% 2842
Nasonex Nasal Spray 2883

NASONEX (Argentina, Australia, Austria, Belgium, Brazil, Canada, Chile, Czech Republic, Denmark, Finland, France, Germany, Greece, Hong Kong, Hungary, Irish Republic, Israel, Italy, Malaysia, Norway, Poland, Russia, Singapore, South Africa, Spain, Sweden, Switzerland, Thailand, The Netherlands, The Philippines, Turkey, United Kingdom, Venezuela)
MOMETASONE FUROATE
Elocon Cream 0.1% 2840
Elocon Lotion 0.1% 2841
Elocon Ointment 0.1% 2842
Nasonex Nasal Spray 2883

NASTERID (Brazil)
FINASTERIDE
Propecia Tablets 2095
Proscar Tablets 2102

NASTERID A (Brazil)
FINASTERIDE
Propecia Tablets 2095
Proscar Tablets 2102

NASTERIL (Argentina)
FINASTERIDE
Propecia Tablets 2095
Proscar Tablets 2102

NASTEROL (Venezuela)
FINASTERIDE
Propecia Tablets 2095
Proscar Tablets 2102

NATACYN (Argentina, Singapore, South Africa, Thailand)
NATAMYCIN
Natacyn Antifungal Ophthalmic Suspension . . . . . ⊙204

NATADROPS (India)
NATAMYCIN
Natacyn Antifungal Ophthalmic Suspension . . . . . ⊙204

NATAFUCIN (Italy)
NATAMYCIN
Natacyn Antifungal Ophthalmic Suspension . . . . . ⊙204

NATIFA (Brazil)
ESTRADIOL
Climara Transdermal System 763

NATIFA PRO (Brazil)
ESTRADIOL
Climara Transdermal System 763

NATRAMID (United Kingdom)
INDAPAMIDE
Indapamide Tablets 2188

NATRAX (Poland)
NAPROXEN
EC-Naprosyn Delayed-Release Tablets 2632
Naprosyn Suspension 2632
Naprosyn Tablets 2632

NATRILIX (Argentina, Australia, Brazil, Chile, Denmark, Finland, Germany, Hong Kong, India, Irish Republic, Italy, Malaysia, Mexico, New Zealand, Singapore, South Africa, Thailand, The Philippines, United Kingdom, Venezuela)
INDAPAMIDE
Indapamide Tablets 2188

NATRIOXEN (Italy)
NAPROXEN SODIUM
Anaprox DS Tablets 2632
Anaprox Tablets 2632

NATULAX (Germany)
LACTULOSE
Kristalose for Oral Solution 1004

NATURA FENAC (Argentina)
DICLOFENAC SODIUM
Voltaren Tablets 2334
Voltaren-XR Tablets 2337

NATUROGEST (India)
PROGESTERONE
Crinone 4% Gel 992
Prometrium Capsules (100 mg, 200 mg) . 3047

NATYL (Switzerland)
DIPYRIDAMOLE
Persantine Tablets 869

NAUSEDRON (Brazil)
ONDANSETRON HYDROCHLORIDE
Zofran Injection 1682
Zofran Injection Premixed 1682
Zofran Oral Solution 1687
Zofran Tablets 1687

NAUSETRON (South Africa)
ONDANSETRON HYDROCHLORIDE
Zofran Injection 1682
Zofran Injection Premixed 1682
Zofran Oral Solution 1687
Zofran Tablets 1687

NAVIXEN (Mexico)
NAPROXEN
EC-Naprosyn Delayed-Release Tablets 2632
Naprosyn Suspension 2632
Naprosyn Tablets 2632

NAXELAN (Chile)
MODAFINIL
Provigil Tablets 977

NAXEN (Australia, Canada, Mexico, New Zealand, South Africa)
NAPROXEN
EC-Naprosyn Delayed-Release Tablets 2632
Naprosyn Suspension 2632
Naprosyn Tablets 2632

NAXIL (Mexico)
NAPROXEN
EC-Naprosyn Delayed-Release Tablets 2632
Naprosyn Suspension 2632
Naprosyn Tablets 2632

NAXODOL (Mexico)
NAPROXEN
EC-Naprosyn Delayed-Release Tablets 2632
Naprosyn Suspension 2632
Naprosyn Tablets 2632

NAXOPAAR (Mexico)
NAPROXEN
EC-Naprosyn Delayed-Release Tablets 2632
Naprosyn Suspension 2632
Naprosyn Tablets 2632

NAXOPREN (Finland)
NAPROXEN
EC-Naprosyn Delayed-Release Tablets 2632
Naprosyn Suspension 2632
Naprosyn Tablets 2632

NAXY (France)
CLARITHROMYCIN
Biaxin Filmtab Tablets 411
Biaxin Granules 411

NAXYN (Israel)
NAPROXEN
EC-Naprosyn Delayed-Release Tablets 2632
Naprosyn Suspension 2632
Naprosyn Tablets 2632

NEBULCORT (Italy)
FLUNISOLIDE
Aerobid Inhaler System 1153
Aerobid-M Inhaler System 1153

NEBULEX (Chile)
FLUTICASONE PROPIONATE
Flonase Nasal Spray 1431

NEDICLON (Mexico)
DICLOFENAC SODIUM
Voltaren Tablets 2334
Voltaren-XR Tablets 2337

NEDOXAL (Mexico)
NAPROXEN SODIUM
Anaprox DS Tablets 2632
Anaprox Tablets 2632

NEFAZAN (Argentina)
CLOPIDOGREL BISULFATE
Plavix Tablets 926, 2767

NEFLOX (Argentina)
CIPROFLOXACIN
Cipro Oral Suspension 2810

NEFOBEN (Argentina)
THEOPHYLLINE
Uniphyl Tablets 2595

NEFROTAL (Venezuela)
LOSARTAN POTASSIUM
Cozaar Tablets 1973

NEFROTAL H (Venezuela)
LOSARTAN POTASSIUM
Cozaar Tablets 1973

NEGACEF (United Arab Emirates)
CEFTAZIDIME
Fortaz for Injection 1450

NEGAFLOX (Russia)
NORFLOXACIN
Noroxin Tablets 2069

NELABOCIN (Greece)
CEFUROXIME AXETIL
Ceftin for Oral Suspension 1380
Ceftin Tablets 1380

NELBINEX (Greece)
NIMODIPINE
Nimotop Capsules 790

NEMBUTAL (Australia, Canada, Hong Kong, Thailand)
PENTOBARBITAL SODIUM
Nembutal Sodium Solution, USP 2494

NEMODINE (Venezuela)
NIMODIPINE
Nimotop Capsules 790

NEMOTAN (Russia)
NIMODIPINE
Nimotop Capsules 790

NEMOXIL (Brazil)
AMOXICILLIN
Amoxil Pediatric Drops for Oral Suspension 1305
Amoxil Tablets 1305

NEMOZOLE (India, Russia)
ALBENDAZOLE
Albenza Tablets 1297

NEO BENDAZOL (Brazil)
ALBENDAZOLE
Albenza Tablets 1297

NEO CLODIL (Brazil)
CLONIDINE HYDROCHLORIDE
Catapres Tablets 841

NEO EBLIMON (Italy)
NAPROXEN
EC-Naprosyn Delayed-Release Tablets 2632
Naprosyn Suspension 2632
Naprosyn Tablets 2632

NEO ELIXIFILIN (Spain)
THEOPHYLLINE
Uniphyl Tablets 2595

NEO MISTATIN (Brazil)
NYSTATIN
Nystop Topical Powder USP 2498

NEO STRATA ASTRINGENT ACNE TREATMENT (Canada)
BENZOYL PEROXIDE
Brevoxyl-4 Creamy Wash 3054
Brevoxyl-4 Gel 3054
Brevoxyl-8 Creamy Wash 3054
Brevoxyl-8 Gel 3054

NEO STRATA BLEMISH SPOT (Canada)
BENZOYL PEROXIDE
Brevoxyl-4 Creamy Wash 3054
Brevoxyl-4 Gel 3054
Brevoxyl-8 Creamy Wash 3054
Brevoxyl-8 Gel 3054

NEOCEFTRIONA (Brazil)
CEFTRIAXONE SODIUM
Rocephin Injectable Vials, ADD-Vantage, Galaxy, Bulk 2642

NEOCEL (Argentina)
DOCETAXEL
Taxotere Injection Concentrate 2773

NEOCIP (India)
CIPROFLOXACIN
Cipro Oral Suspension 2810

NEOCIP M (India)
CIPROFLOXACIN
Cipro Oral Suspension 2810

NEO-DISTERIN (Greece)
FENOFIBRATE
Tricor Tablets 520

NEODOLPASSE (Czech Republic, Hungary)
DICLOFENAC SODIUM
Voltaren Tablets 2334
Voltaren-XR Tablets 2337

NEOFLOXIN (Brazil, Singapore)
CIPROFLOXACIN
Cipro Oral Suspension 2810

NEO-IPERTAS (Greece)
CAPTOPRIL
Captopril Tablets 2182

NEOLIPID (Brazil)
LOVASTATIN
Mevacor Tablets 2063

NEO-LOTAN (Italy)
LOSARTAN POTASSIUM
Cozaar Tablets 1973

NEONAXIL (Mexico)
NAPROXEN
EC-Naprosyn Delayed-Release Tablets 2632
Naprosyn Suspension 2632
Naprosyn Tablets 2632

NEO-PREOCIL (Portugal)
FLUOROMETHOLONE
FML Ophthalmic Ointment . . . . . ⊙223

NEOPRESS (Brazil)
LOSARTAN POTASSIUM
Cozaar Tablets 1973

NEO-PYRAZON (Malaysia, Singapore, The Philippines)
DICLOFENAC SODIUM
Voltaren Tablets 2334
Voltaren-XR Tablets 2337

NEORINOL (Chile)
IPRATROPIUM BROMIDE
Atrovent Nasal Spray 0.03% 834

Atrovent Nasal Spray 0.06% ... 836

NEORPAN PLUS (Mexico)
NAPROXEN SODIUM
Anaprox DS Tablets ... 2632
Anaprox Tablets ... 2632

NEOSAC (Brazil)
RANITIDINE HYDROCHLORIDE
Zantac 25 EFFERdose Tablets ... 1670
Zantac 150 Tablets ... 1670
Zantac 300 Tablets ... 1670
Zantac Injection ... 1666
Zantac Injection Premixed ... 1666
Zantac Syrup ... 1670

NEOSEMID (Brazil)
FUROSEMIDE
Furosemide Tablets ... 2186

NEOSTATIN (Argentina, Brazil)
NYSTATIN
Nystop Topical Powder USP ... 2498

NEOTAB (Turkey)
FAMOTIDINE
Pepcid for Oral Suspension ... 2075
Pepcid Tablets ... 2075

NEOTAREN (Brazil)
DICLOFENAC SODIUM
Voltaren Tablets ... 2334
Voltaren-XR Tablets ... 2337

NEOTHYRON (Austria)
LEVOTHYROXINE SODIUM
Levothroid Tablets ... 1170
Levoxyl Tablets ... 1780
Synthroid Tablets ... 507

NEOTIGASON (Argentina, Australia, Austria, Belgium, Brazil, Chile, Czech Republic, Denmark, Finland, Germany, Greece, Hong Kong, Hungary, Irish Republic, Israel, Italy, Mexico, New Zealand, Norway, Poland, Portugal, Singapore, South Africa, Spain, Sweden, Switzerland, Thailand, The Netherlands, The Philippines, Turkey, United Kingdom, Venezuela)
ACITRETIN
Soriatane Capsules ... 3062

NEO-TIROIMADE (Portugal)
LIOTHYRONINE SODIUM
Cytomel Tablets ... 1778

NEOTRETIN (Argentina)
TRETINOIN
Vesanoid Capsules ... 2660

NEOTREX (Mexico)
ISOTRETINOIN
Accutane Capsules ... 2607

NEOTUL (Spain)
FAMOTIDINE
Pepcid for Oral Suspension ... 2075
Pepcid Tablets ... 2075

NEOVISC (Canada)
SODIUM HYALURONATE
Hyalgan Solution ... 2742

NEPENTHE (The Philippines)
DICLOFENAC SODIUM
Voltaren Tablets ... 2334
Voltaren-XR Tablets ... 2337

NEPHRAL (Germany)
HYDROCHLOROTHIAZIDE/TRIAMTERENE
Dyazide Capsules ... 1405

NEPHREX (Australia, Hong Kong)
CALCIUM ACETATE
PhosLo GelCaps ... 1184

NEREFLUN (Italy)
FLUNISOLIDE
Aerobid Inhaler System ... 1153
Aerobid-M Inhaler System ... 1153

NERGADAN (Spain)
LOVASTATIN
Mevacor Tablets ... 2063

NERICUR (United Kingdom)
BENZOYL PEROXIDE
Brevoxyl-4 Creamy Wash ... 3054
Brevoxyl-4 Gel ... 3054
Brevoxyl-8 Creamy Wash ... 3054
Brevoxyl-8 Gel ... 3054

NEROLID (Mexico)
DIAZEPAM
Valium Tablets ... 2658

NERVIUM (Turkey)
DIAZEPAM
Valium Tablets ... 2658

NERVIX (Chile)
VENLAFAXINE HYDROCHLORIDE
Effexor XR Capsules ... 3195

NESBILER (Argentina)
FLUOROMETHOLONE
FML Ophthalmic Ointment ... ⊙223

NETUNAL (Argentina)
SUCRALFATE
Carafate Suspension ... 706
Carafate Tablets ... 707

NEUGAL (Mexico)
RANITIDINE HYDROCHLORIDE
Zantac 25 EFFERdose Tablets ... 1670
Zantac 150 Tablets ... 1670
Zantac 300 Tablets ... 1670
Zantac Injection ... 1666
Zantac Injection Premixed ... 1666
Zantac Syrup ... 1670

NEUGERON (Mexico)
CARBAMAZEPINE
Carbatrol Capsules ... 3019

NEUMOTIDE (Argentina)
SALMETEROL XINAFOATE
Serevent Diskus ... 1594

NEURAL (Brazil)
LAMOTRIGINE
Lamictal Chewable Dispersible Tablets ... 1488
Lamictal Tablets ... 1488

NEURALPRONA (Argentina)
NAPROXEN
EC-Naprosyn Delayed-Release Tablets ... 2632
Naprosyn Suspension ... 2632
Naprosyn Tablets ... 2632

NEURIUM (Brazil)
LAMOTRIGINE
Lamictal Chewable Dispersible Tablets ... 1488
Lamictal Tablets ... 1488

NEUROCEFAL TRANQUI (Spain)
DIAZEPAM
Valium Tablets ... 2658

NEURODOL TISSUGEL (Switzerland)
LIDOCAINE
Lidoderm Patch ... 1114

NEUROGERON (Chile)
NIMODIPINE
Nimotop Capsules ... 790

NEUROLEP (Mexico)
CARBAMAZEPINE
Carbatrol Capsules ... 3019

NEUROLYTRIL (Germany)
DIAZEPAM
Valium Tablets ... 2658

NEURON (Brazil)
NIMODIPINE
Nimotop Capsules ... 790

NEUROTOL (Finland)
CARBAMAZEPINE
Carbatrol Capsules ... 3019

NEUROTOP (Austria, Czech Republic, Hungary, Poland, Singapore, Switzerland)
CARBAMAZEPINE
Carbatrol Capsules ... 3019

NEURYL (Argentina, Chile)
CLONAZEPAM
Klonopin Tablets ... 2639

NEUTRACID (Venezuela)
FAMOTIDINE
Pepcid for Oral Suspension ... 2075
Pepcid Tablets ... 2075

NEUTROGENA ACNE MASK (Australia, Canada)
BENZOYL PEROXIDE
Brevoxyl-4 Creamy Wash ... 3054
Brevoxyl-4 Gel ... 3054
Brevoxyl-8 Creamy Wash ... 3054
Brevoxyl-8 Gel ... 3054

NEUTROGENA ON THE SPOT ACNE TREATMENT (Canada)
BENZOYL PEROXIDE
Brevoxyl-4 Creamy Wash ... 3054
Brevoxyl-4 Gel ... 3054
Brevoxyl-8 Creamy Wash ... 3054
Brevoxyl-8 Gel ... 3054

NEVOFAM (Turkey)
FAMOTIDINE
Pepcid for Oral Suspension ... 2075
Pepcid Tablets ... 2075

NEXPROXYN (The Philippines)
CIPROFLOXACIN HYDROCHLORIDE
Cipro Tablets ... 2810

NIAR (Brazil, Mexico)
SELEGILINE HYDROCHLORIDE
Eldepryl Capsules ... 3052

NICOSTAT (Brazil)
NYSTATIN
Nystop Topical Powder USP ... 2498

NICOTEX (India)
BUPROPION HYDROCHLORIDE
Wellbutrin SR Sustained-Release Tablets ... 1653
Wellbutrin Tablets ... 1648
Zyban Sustained-Release Tablets ... 1692

NIDAZOLIN (Brazil)
NYSTATIN
Nystop Topical Powder USP ... 2498

NIDDAFIN (The Netherlands)
TERBINAFINE HYDROCHLORIDE
Lamisil Tablets ... 2266

NIDDAVITA (The Netherlands)
TERBINAFINE HYDROCHLORIDE
Lamisil Tablets ... 2266

NIFATIN (Brazil)
NYSTATIN
Nystop Topical Powder USP ... 2498

NIFLAM (Argentina)
CELECOXIB
Celebrex Capsules ... 2979

NIJ-TEROL (Chile)
LOVASTATIN
Mevacor Tablets ... 2063

NILPERIDOL (Brazil)
FENTANYL CITRATE
Actiq ... 959

NILSON (Italy)
CEFTRIAXONE SODIUM
Rocephin Injectable Vials, ADD-Vantage, Galaxy, Bulk ... 2642

NILSTAT (Australia, Belgium, Canada, New Zealand)
NYSTATIN
Nystop Topical Powder USP ... 2498

NIM (Germany)
NIMODIPINE
Nimotop Capsules ... 790

NIMEGEN (Singapore)
ISOTRETINOIN
Accutane Capsules ... 2607

NIMICOR (Chile)
SIMVASTATIN
Zocor Tablets ... 2136

NIMODIL (Greece)
NIMODIPINE
Nimotop Capsules ... 790

NIMODILAT (Argentina)
NIMODIPINE
Nimotop Capsules ... 790

NIMODILAT PLUS (Argentina)
NIMODIPINE
Nimotop Capsules ... 790

NIMOPAX (Brazil)
NIMODIPINE
Nimotop Capsules ... 790

NIMOREAGIN (Argentina)
NIMODIPINE
Nimotop Capsules ... 790

NIMOTOP (Argentina, Australia, Austria, Belgium, Brazil, Canada, Chile, Czech Republic, Denmark, Finland, France, Germany, Greece, Hong Kong, Hungary, Irish Republic, Israel, Italy, Malaysia, Mexico, New Zealand, Norway, Poland, Portugal, Russia, Singapore, South Africa, Spain, Sweden, Switzerland, Thailand, The Netherlands, The Philippines, Turkey, United Kingdom, Venezuela)
NIMODIPINE
Nimotop Capsules ... 790

NIMOVAS (Brazil)
NIMODIPINE
Nimotop Capsules ... 790

NINDAXA (United Kingdom)
INDAPAMIDE
Indapamide Tablets ... 2188

NIPODUR (Greece)
RANITIDINE HYDROCHLORIDE
Zantac 25 EFFERdose Tablets ... 1670
Zantac 150 Tablets ... 1670
Zantac 300 Tablets ... 1670
Zantac Injection ... 1666
Zantac Injection Premixed ... 1666
Zantac Syrup ... 1670

NIPOGALIN (Greece)
CEFUROXIME SODIUM
Zinacef Injection ... 1678

NISIS (France)
VALSARTAN
Diovan Tablets ... 2212

NISISCO (France)
HYDROCHLOROTHIAZIDE/VALSARTAN
Diovan HCT Tablets ... 2216

NISOLID (Italy)
FLUNISOLIDE
Aerobid Inhaler System ... 1153
Aerobid-M Inhaler System ... 1153

NISORAN (Italy)
FLUNISOLIDE
Aerobid Inhaler System ... 1153
Aerobid-M Inhaler System ... 1153

NISTAFESA (Venezuela)
NYSTATIN
Nystop Topical Powder USP ... 2498

NISTAGEN (Brazil)
NYSTATIN
Nystop Topical Powder USP ... 2498

NISTAGRAND (Argentina)
NYSTATIN
Nystop Topical Powder USP ... 2498

NISTAGYN (Brazil)
NYSTATIN
Nystop Topical Powder USP ... 2498

NISTAKEN (Mexico)
PROPAFENONE HYDROCHLORIDE
Rythmol SR Capsules ... 1590

NISTAMED (Argentina)
NYSTATIN
Nystop Topical Powder USP ... 2498

NISTAN (Mexico)
NYSTATIN
Nystop Topical Powder USP ... 2498

NISTANIL (Brazil)
NYSTATIN
Nystop Topical Powder USP ... 2498

NISTAQUIM (Mexico)
NYSTATIN
Nystop Topical Powder USP ... 2498

NISTAT (Argentina)
NYSTATIN
Nystop Topical Powder USP ... 2498

NISTATIN (Brazil)
NYSTATIN
Nystop Topical Powder USP ... 2498

NISTAVAL (Brazil)
NYSTATIN
Nystop Topical Powder USP ... 2498

NISTAX (Brazil)
NYSTATIN
Nystop Topical Powder USP ... 2498

NISTINOL (Argentina)
NYSTATIN
Nystop Topical Powder USP ... 2498

NISTORAL (Chile)
NYSTATIN
Nystop Topical Powder USP ... 2498

NITASTIN (Greece)
SIMVASTATIN
Zocor Tablets ... 2136

NITEN (Argentina)
LOSARTAN POTASSIUM
Cozaar Tablets ... 1973

NITEN D (Argentina)
LOSARTAN POTASSIUM
Cozaar Tablets 1973

NITEREY (Argentina)
TRETINOIN
Vesanoid Capsules 2660

NITISED (Greece)
RANITIDINE HYDROCHLORIDE
Zantac 25 EFFERdose Tablets 1670
Zantac 150 Tablets 1670
Zantac 300 Tablets 1670
Zantac Injection 1666
Zantac Injection Premixed 1666
Zantac Syrup 1670

NITROCIT (South Africa)
POTASSIUM CITRATE
Urocit-K Tablets 2176

NITROUREAN (Spain)
CARMUSTINE
Gliadel Wafer 1076

NITRUMON (Belgium, Greece, Italy, Turkey)
CARMUSTINE
Gliadel Wafer 1076

NIVADOR (Spain)
CEFUROXIME AXETIL
Ceftin for Oral Suspension 1380
Ceftin Tablets 1380

NIVAS (Argentina)
NIMODIPINE
Nimotop Capsules 790

NIVAS PLUS (Argentina)
NIMODIPINE
Nimotop Capsules 790

NIVELIPOL (Argentina)
SIMVASTATIN
Zocor Tablets 2136

NIVOFLOX (Mexico)
CIPROFLOXACIN HYDROCHLORIDE
Cipro Tablets 2810

NIXAL (Mexico)
NAPROXEN SODIUM
Anaprox DS Tablets 2632
Anaprox Tablets 2632

NIXIN (Brazil, Portugal)
CIPROFLOXACIN HYDROCHLORIDE
Cipro Tablets 2810

NIXTENSYN (The Philippines)
DIAZEPAM
Valium Tablets 2658

NIZIN-V (Mexico)
NYSTATIN
Nystop Topical Powder USP 2498

NM POWDER (India)
NORFLOXACIN
Noroxin Tablets 2069

NOAN (Brazil, Italy)
DIAZEPAM
Valium Tablets 2658

NOAX UNO (Czech Republic)
TRAMADOL HYDROCHLORIDE
Ultram ER Tablets 2428

NOBLIGAN (Argentina, Austria, Denmark, Mexico, Norway, Sweden)
TRAMADOL HYDROCHLORIDE
Ultram ER Tablets 2428

NOCEPTIN (The Netherlands)
MORPHINE SULFATE
MS Contin Tablets 2585

NODOL (Italy)
RANITIDINE HYDROCHLORIDE
Zantac 25 EFFERdose Tablets 1670
Zantac 150 Tablets 1670
Zantac 300 Tablets 1670
Zantac Injection 1666
Zantac Injection Premixed 1666
Zantac Syrup 1670

NOFLAM (New Zealand)
NAPROXEN
EC-Naprosyn Delayed-Release Tablets 2632
Naprosyn Suspension 2632
Naprosyn Tablets 2632

NOFLAM-N (Hong Kong)
NAPROXEN SODIUM
Anaprox DS Tablets 2632
Anaprox Tablets 2632

NOFLOROX (Mexico)
NORFLOXACIN
Noroxin Tablets 2069

NOITRON (Greece)
ISOTRETINOIN
Accutane Capsules 2607

NOKLOT (India)
CLOPIDOGREL BISULFATE
Plavix Tablets 926, 2767

NOKTONE (Norway)
RANITIDINE HYDROCHLORIDE
Zantac 25 EFFERdose Tablets 1670
Zantac 150 Tablets 1670
Zantac 300 Tablets 1670
Zantac Injection 1666
Zantac Injection Premixed 1666
Zantac Syrup 1670

NOLICIN (Czech Republic, Hungary, Poland, Russia)
NORFLOXACIN
Noroxin Tablets 2069

NOLIPAX (Italy)
FENOFIBRATE
Tricor Tablets 520

NOLIPREL (Czech Republic, Hungary)
PERINDOPRIL ERBUMINE
Aceon Tablets (2 mg, 4 mg, 8 mg) 3038

NOODIPINA (Brazil)
NIMODIPINE
Nimotop Capsules 790

NOR 2 (Argentina)
NORFLOXACIN
Noroxin Tablets 2069

NOR T (India)
NORFLOXACIN
Noroxin Tablets 2069

NORACIN (Brazil, Thailand)
NORFLOXACIN
Noroxin Tablets 2069

NORANAT (Argentina)
INDAPAMIDE
Indapamide Tablets 2188

NORAXIN (Thailand)
NORFLOXACIN
Noroxin Tablets 2069

NORBACTIN (India, Malaysia, Russia, Singapore, Thailand, The Philippines)
NORFLOXACIN
Noroxin Tablets 2069

NORDOTOL (Denmark)
CARBAMAZEPINE
Carbatrol Capsules 3019

NORFCIN (Thailand)
NORFLOXACIN
Noroxin Tablets 2069

NORFENON (Mexico)
PROPAFENONE HYDROCHLORIDE
Rythmol SR Capsules 1590

NORFLAMIN (Brazil)
NORFLOXACIN
Noroxin Tablets 2069

NORFLO (Thailand)
NORFLOXACIN
Noroxin Tablets 2069

NORFLOCIN (Thailand)
NORFLOXACIN
Noroxin Tablets 2069

NORFLOCINE (Switzerland)
NORFLOXACIN
Noroxin Tablets 2069

NORFLOHEXAL (Australia, Germany)
NORFLOXACIN
Noroxin Tablets 2069

NORFLOK (Spain)
NORFLOXACIN
Noroxin Tablets 2069

NORFLOL (Argentina)
NORFLOXACIN
Noroxin Tablets 2069

NORFLOSAL (Germany)
NORFLOXACIN
Noroxin Tablets 2069

NORFLOSAN (Venezuela)
NORFLOXACIN
Noroxin Tablets 2069

NORFLOSTAD (Austria)
NORFLOXACIN
Noroxin Tablets 2069

NORFLOVAL (Venezuela)
NORFLOXACIN
Noroxin Tablets 2069

NORFLOX (Brazil, India)
NORFLOXACIN
Noroxin Tablets 2069

NORFLOX TZ (India)
NORFLOXACIN
Noroxin Tablets 2069

NORFLOXASAN (Brazil)
NORFLOXACIN
Noroxin Tablets 2069

NORFLOX-AZU (Germany)
NORFLOXACIN
Noroxin Tablets 2069

NORFLOXBETA (Germany)
NORFLOXACIN
Noroxin Tablets 2069

NORFLOXIL (Brazil)
NORFLOXACIN
Noroxin Tablets 2069

NORFLOXIN (Thailand)
NORFLOXACIN
Noroxin Tablets 2069

NORFLOXINOR (Malaysia)
NORFLOXACIN
Noroxin Tablets 2069

NORFLOXMED (Brazil)
NORFLOXACIN
Noroxin Tablets 2069

NORFLOX-PUREN (Germany)
NORFLOXACIN
Noroxin Tablets 2069

NORFLOXYL (Thailand)
NORFLOXACIN
Noroxin Tablets 2069

NORFLUXX (Germany)
NORFLOXACIN
Noroxin Tablets 2069

NORILET (Russia, Venezuela)
NORFLOXACIN
Noroxin Tablets 2069

NORIMOX (South Africa)
AMOXICILLIN
Amoxil Pediatric Drops for Oral Suspension 1305
Amoxil Tablets 1305

NORIPLEX (Hungary)
INDAPAMIDE
Indapamide Tablets 2188

NORMAFENAC (Greece)
CEFUROXIME SODIUM
Zinacef Injection 1678

NORMALAC (Poland)
LACTULOSE
Kristalose for Oral Solution 1004

NORMALIP PRO (Germany)
FENOFIBRATE
Tricor Tablets 520

NORMAPRIL (Brazil)
CAPTOPRIL
Captopril Tablets 2182

NORMASE (Italy, Poland)
LACTULOSE
Kristalose for Oral Solution 1004

NORMASTIN (The Philippines)
SIMVASTATIN
Zocor Tablets 2136

NORMAX (India, Russia)
NORFLOXACIN
Noroxin Tablets 2069

NORMAX TZ (India)
NORFLOXACIN
Noroxin Tablets 2069

NORMIL (The Philippines)
CAPTOPRIL
Captopril Tablets 2182

NORMOLOSE (Greece)
CAPTOPRIL
Captopril Tablets 2182

NORMOLOSE-H (Greece)
CAPTOPRIL
Captopril Tablets 2182

NORMOMENSIL (Brazil)
PROGESTERONE
Crinone 4% Gel 992
Prometrium Capsules (100 mg, 200 mg) 3047

NORMOPRESAN (Israel)
CLONIDINE HYDROCHLORIDE
Catapres Tablets 841

NORMOPRIL (India)
LISINOPRIL
Prinivil Tablets 2087

NORMORYTMIN (Argentina, Irish Republic)
PROPAFENONE HYDROCHLORIDE
Rythmol SR Capsules 1590

NORMOTEN (The Philippines)
LOSARTAN POTASSIUM
Cozaar Tablets 1973

NORMOTENSOR (Brazil)
FUROSEMIDE
Furosemide Tablets 2186

NORMOTHERIN (Greece)
SIMVASTATIN
Zocor Tablets 2136

NORMOTIL (Portugal)
CAPTOPRIL
Captopril Tablets 2182

NORMULEN (Spain, The Netherlands)
DICLOFENAC SODIUM
Voltaren Tablets 2334
Voltaren-XR Tablets 2337

NOROCIN (Greece)
NORFLOXACIN
Noroxin Tablets 2069

NOROXIN (Argentina, Australia, Canada, Chile, Finland, Italy, Mexico, New Zealand, Portugal, South Africa, Spain, Switzerland, The Netherlands, Turkey, United Kingdom, Venezuela)
NORFLOXACIN
Noroxin Tablets 2069

NOROXINE (France)
NORFLOXACIN
Noroxin Tablets 2069

NORQUINOL (Mexico)
NORFLOXACIN
Noroxin Tablets 2069

NORSA (Thailand)
NORFLOXACIN
Noroxin Tablets 2069

NORSOL (Argentina, Switzerland)
NORFLOXACIN
Noroxin Tablets 2069

NORTENSIN (Argentina)
TRANDOLAPRIL
Mavik Tablets 472

NORTOLAN (Greece)
NIMODIPINE
Nimotop Capsules 790

NORTON (Brazil)
NIMODIPINE
Nimotop Capsules 790

NORTRAM (The Philippines)
NORFLOXACIN
Noroxin Tablets 2069

NORUXOL (Italy)
COLLAGENASE
Santyl Collagenase Ointment 1724

NORVIR (Australia, Belgium, Canada, Chile, Czech Republic, Denmark, Finland, France, Germany, Greece, Hong Kong, Hungary, Irish Republic, Israel, Italy, Japan, Malaysia, Mexico, New Zealand, Norway, Poland, Portugal, Russia, South Africa, Spain, Sweden, Switzerland, Thailand, The Netherlands, Turkey, United Kingdom, Venezuela)
RITONAVIR
Norvir Oral Solution . . . 489
Norvir Soft Gelatin Capsules . . . 489

NORXACIN (Brazil, Thailand)
NORFLOXACIN
Noroxin Tablets . . . 2069

NORXIA (Thailand)
NORFLOXACIN
Noroxin Tablets . . . 2069

NORXIN (Brazil)
NORFLOXACIN
Noroxin Tablets . . . 2069

NOS (Spain)
FAMOTIDINE
Pepcid for Oral Suspension . . . 2075
Pepcid Tablets . . . 2075

NOSTEROL (Argentina)
SIMVASTATIN
Zocor Tablets . . . 2136

NOTIDIN (Turkey)
FAMOTIDINE
Pepcid for Oral Suspension . . . 2075
Pepcid Tablets . . . 2075

NOVA (Canada)
PENTOBARBITAL SODIUM
Nembutal Sodium Solution, USP . . . 2494

NOVA RECTAL (Canada)
PENTOBARBITAL SODIUM
Nembutal Sodium Solution, USP . . . 2494

NOVACIL (Brazil)
AMOXICILLIN
Amoxil Pediatric Drops for Oral Suspension . . . 1305
Amoxil Tablets . . . 1305

NOVACILINA (Chile)
LEVOFLOXACIN
Levaquin Injection . . . 2416
Levaquin Tablets . . . 2416

NOVACLAV (India)
AMOXICILLIN
Amoxil Pediatric Drops for Oral Suspension . . . 1305
Amoxil Tablets . . . 1305

NOVACLOX LB (India)
AMOXICILLIN
Amoxil Pediatric Drops for Oral Suspension . . . 1305
Amoxil Tablets . . . 1305

NOVADEX (Mexico)
NAPROXEN
EC-Naprosyn Delayed-Release Tablets . . . 2632
Naprosyn Suspension . . . 2632
Naprosyn Tablets . . . 2632

NOVAL (Greece)
TIMOLOL MALEATE
Timoptic in Ocudose . . . 2124
Timoptic Sterile Ophthalmic Solution . . . 2121
Timoptic-XE Sterile Ophthalmic Gel Forming Solution . . . 2125

NOVAMOX (India, The Philippines)
AMOXICILLIN
Amoxil Pediatric Drops for Oral Suspension . . . 1305
Amoxil Tablets . . . 1305

NOVAMOX AX (India)
AMOXICILLIN
Amoxil Pediatric Drops for Oral Suspension . . . 1305
Amoxil Tablets . . . 1305

NOVAMOX LB (India)
AMOXICILLIN
Amoxil Pediatric Drops for Oral Suspension . . . 1305
Amoxil Tablets . . . 1305

NOVAPHYLLINE (Greece)
THEOPHYLLINE
Uniphyl Tablets . . . 2595

NOVAPIRINA (Italy)
DICLOFENAC SODIUM
Voltaren Tablets . . . 2334
Voltaren-XR Tablets . . . 2337

NOVAPRES (Mexico)
CAPTOPRIL
Captopril Tablets . . . 2182

NOVAPSYL (Mexico)
BENZONATATE
Tessalon Perles . . . 1183

NOVASONE (Argentina, Australia)
MOMETASONE FUROATE
Elocon Cream 0.1% . . . 2840
Elocon Lotion 0.1% . . . 2841
Elocon Ointment 0.1% . . . 2842
Nasonex Nasal Spray . . . 2883

NOVASULFON (Mexico)
DAPSONE
Dapsone Tablets USP . . . 1746

NOVATEC (Belgium, The Netherlands)
LISINOPRIL
Prinivil Tablets . . . 2087

NOVAVIR (Mexico)
ZIDOVUDINE
Retrovir Capsules . . . 1574
Retrovir IV Infusion . . . 1579
Retrovir Syrup . . . 1574
Retrovir Tablets . . . 1574

NOVAXEN (Mexico)
NAPROXEN
EC-Naprosyn Delayed-Release Tablets . . . 2632
Naprosyn Suspension . . . 2632
Naprosyn Tablets . . . 2632

NOVAZAM (France)
DIAZEPAM
Valium Tablets . . . 2658

NOVAZYD (Belgium, The Netherlands)
LISINOPRIL
Prinivil Tablets . . . 2087

NOVELIAN (Spain)
SUMATRIPTAN SUCCINATE
Imitrex Injection . . . 1465
Imitrex Tablets . . . 1474

NOVIDAT (Argentina)
CIPROFLOXACIN HYDROCHLORIDE
Cipro Tablets . . . 2810

NOVO-AZT (Canada)
ZIDOVUDINE
Retrovir Capsules . . . 1574
Retrovir IV Infusion . . . 1579
Retrovir Syrup . . . 1574
Retrovir Tablets . . . 1574

NOVO-CAPTORIL (Canada, Hong Kong)
CAPTOPRIL
Captopril Tablets . . . 2182

NOVOCAR (Chile)
CARVEDILOL
Coreg Tablets . . . 1387

NOVO-CARBAMAZ (Canada)
CARBAMAZEPINE
Carbatrol Capsules . . . 3019

NOVOCEF (Poland)
CEFUROXIME AXETIL
Ceftin for Oral Suspension . . . 1380
Ceftin Tablets . . . 1380

NOVOCRAL (Greece)
CEFTAZIDIME
Fortaz for Injection . . . 1450

NOVO-DIFENAC (Hong Kong)
DICLOFENAC SODIUM
Voltaren Tablets . . . 2334
Voltaren-XR Tablets . . . 2337

NOVODIL (Italy)
DIPYRIDAMOLE
Persantine Tablets . . . 869

NOVO-DILTAZEM (Canada)
DILTIAZEM HYDROCHLORIDE
Cardizem LA Extended Release Tablets . . . 421

NOVO-DIPAM (Canada)
DIAZEPAM
Valium Tablets . . . 2658

NOVO-DIPIRADOL (Canada)
DIPYRIDAMOLE
Persantine Tablets . . . 869

NOVO-IPRAMIDE (Canada)
IPRATROPIUM BROMIDE
Atrovent Nasal Spray 0.03% . . . 834
Atrovent Nasal Spray 0.06% . . . 836

NOVO-NAPROX (Canada)
NAPROXEN
EC-Naprosyn Delayed-Release Tablets . . . 2632
Naprosyn Suspension . . . 2632
Naprosyn Tablets . . . 2632

NOVOQUIN (Mexico)
CIPROFLOXACIN HYDROCHLORIDE
Cipro Tablets . . . 2810

NOVO-RANIDINE (Canada, Hong Kong, Poland)
RANITIDINE HYDROCHLORIDE
Zantac 150 Tablets . . . 1670
Zantac 25 EFFERdose Tablets . . . 1670
Zantac 300 Tablets . . . 1670
Zantac Injection . . . 1666
Zantac Injection Premixed . . . 1666
Zantac Syrup . . . 1670

NOVO-RIDAZINE (Canada)
THIORIDAZINE HYDROCHLORIDE
Thioridazine Hydrochloride Tablets . . . 2195

NOVOSEF (Czech Republic, Turkey)
CEFTRIAXONE SODIUM
Rocephin Injectable Vials, ADD-Vantage, Galaxy, Bulk . . . 2642

NOVO-SEMIDE (Canada)
FUROSEMIDE
Furosemide Tablets . . . 2186

NOVO-SUCRALATE (Canada)
SUCRALFATE
Carafate Suspension . . . 706
Carafate Tablets . . . 707

NOVO-SUNDAC (Canada)
SULINDAC
Clinoril Tablets . . . 1962

NOVO-THEOPHYL (Canada, Hong Kong)
THEOPHYLLINE
Uniphyl Tablets . . . 2595

NOVOTHYRAL (Czech Republic, Poland)
LIOTHYRONINE SODIUM
Cytomel Tablets . . . 1778

NOVO-TIMOL (Canada)
TIMOLOL MALEATE
Timoptic in Ocudose . . . 2124
Timoptic Sterile Ophthalmic Solution . . . 2121
Timoptic-XE Sterile Ophthalmic Gel Forming Solution . . . 2125

NOVO-TRIAMZIDE (Canada)
HYDROCHLOROTHIAZIDE/TRIAMTERENE
Dyazide Capsules . . . 1405

NOVOXIL (Brazil)
AMOXICILLIN
Amoxil Pediatric Drops for Oral Suspension . . . 1305
Amoxil Tablets . . . 1305

NOVRAL (Brazil)
LISINOPRIL
Prinivil Tablets . . . 2087

NOVUXOL (The Netherlands, Turkey)
COLLAGENASE
Santyl Collagenase Ointment . . . 1724

NOXINE (Thailand)
NORFLOXACIN
Noroxin Tablets . . . 2069

NOXINOR (Thailand)
NORFLOXACIN
Noroxin Tablets . . . 2069

NOXORAM (The Philippines)
CEFTRIAXONE SODIUM
Rocephin Injectable Vials, ADD-Vantage, Galaxy, Bulk . . . 2642

NOXUFEN (Switzerland)
NORFLOXACIN
Noroxin Tablets . . . 2069

N-STATIN (Australia)
NYSTATIN
Nystop Topical Powder USP . . . 2498

NUBREX (The Philippines)
FENOFIBRATE
Tricor Tablets . . . 520

NU-CAPTO (Canada)
CAPTOPRIL
Captopril Tablets . . . 2182

NU-DICLO (Canada)
DICLOFENAC SODIUM
Voltaren Tablets . . . 2334
Voltaren-XR Tablets . . . 2337

NU-DILTIAZ (Canada)
DILTIAZEM HYDROCHLORIDE
Cardizem LA Extended Release Tablets . . . 421

NUELIN (Australia, Denmark, Finland, Hong Kong, Irish Republic, Malaysia, New Zealand, Norway, Singapore, South Africa, Thailand, The Philippines, United Kingdom, Venezuela)
THEOPHYLLINE
Uniphyl Tablets . . . 2595

NUFLOXIB (Australia)
NORFLOXACIN
Noroxin Tablets . . . 2069

NULCERIN (Spain)
FAMOTIDINE
Pepcid for Oral Suspension . . . 2075
Pepcid Tablets . . . 2075

NU-LOTAN (Japan)
LOSARTAN POTASSIUM
Cozaar Tablets . . . 1973

NUMEN (Spain)
CIPROFLOXACIN HYDROCHLORIDE
Cipro Tablets . . . 2810

NU-NAPROX (Canada)
NAPROXEN
EC-Naprosyn Delayed-Release Tablets . . . 2632
Naprosyn Suspension . . . 2632
Naprosyn Tablets . . . 2632

NUPRAFEN (Singapore)
NAPROXEN
EC-Naprosyn Delayed-Release Tablets . . . 2632
Naprosyn Suspension . . . 2632
Naprosyn Tablets . . . 2632

NU-RANIT (Canada)
RANITIDINE HYDROCHLORIDE
Zantac 25 EFFERdose Tablets . . . 1670
Zantac 150 Tablets . . . 1670
Zantac 300 Tablets . . . 1670
Zantac Injection . . . 1666
Zantac Injection Premixed . . . 1666
Zantac Syrup . . . 1670

NUROCAIN (New Zealand)
LIDOCAINE
Lidoderm Patch . . . 1114

NUROLASTS (Australia)
NAPROXEN SODIUM
Anaprox DS Tablets . . . 2632
Anaprox Tablets . . . 2632

NU-ROX (Chile)
ENOXAPARIN SODIUM
Lovenox Injection . . . 2756

NU-TRIAZIDE (Canada)
HYDROCHLOROTHIAZIDE/TRIAMTERENE
Dyazide Capsules . . . 1405

NYADERM (Canada)
NYSTATIN
Nystop Topical Powder USP . . . 2498

NYCODOL (Austria)
TRAMADOL HYDROCHLORIDE
Ultram ER Tablets . . . 2428

NYCOPREN (Austria, Belgium, Denmark, Finland, Greece, Switzerland, The Netherlands, United Kingdom)
NAPROXEN
EC-Naprosyn Delayed-Release Tablets . . . 2632
Naprosyn Suspension . . . 2632
Naprosyn Tablets . . . 2632

NYOGEL (Australia, Belgium, France, Germany, Greece, Irish Republic, Italy, New Zealand, Portugal, South Africa, The Netherlands, United Kingdom)
TIMOLOL MALEATE
Timoptic in Ocudose . . . 2124

Timoptic Sterile Ophthalmic Solution 2121
Timoptic-XE Sterile Ophthalmic Gel Forming Solution 2125

NYOLOL (Belgium, Brazil, Chile, France, Greece, Hong Kong, Israel, Malaysia, Mexico, Poland, Portugal, Singapore, Spain, Switzerland, Thailand, The Philippines, Turkey, Venezuela)
TIMOLOL MALEATE
Timoptic in Ocudose 2124
Timoptic Sterile Ophthalmic Solution 2121
Timoptic-XE Sterile Ophthalmic Gel Forming Solution 2125

NYSPES (United Kingdom)
NYSTATIN
Nystop Topical Powder USP 2498

NYSTACID (South Africa)
NYSTATIN
Nystop Topical Powder USP 2498

NYSTADERM (Austria, Germany)
NYSTATIN
Nystop Topical Powder USP 2498

NYSTADERMAL (United Kingdom)
NYSTATIN
Nystop Topical Powder USP 2498

NYSTAFORM (United Kingdom)
NYSTATIN
Nystop Topical Powder USP 2498

NYSTAMONT (Greece, United Kingdom)
NYSTATIN
Nystop Topical Powder USP 2498

NYSTAN (United Kingdom)
NYSTATIN
Nystop Topical Powder USP 2498

NYSTASAN (Mexico)
NYSTATIN
Nystop Topical Powder USP 2498

NYSTATIN-DOME (United Kingdom)
NYSTATIN
Nystop Topical Powder USP 2498

NYSTAVESCENT (United Kingdom)
NYSTATIN
Nystop Topical Powder USP 2498

NYZOC (Austria)
SIMVASTATIN
Zocor Tablets 2136

OAC HP7 (The Philippines)
CLARITHROMYCIN
Biaxin Filmtab Tablets 411
Biaxin Granules 411

OBESTAT (India)
SIBUTRAMINE HYDROCHLORIDE
Meridia Capsules 475

OBLIOSER (Italy, Spain)
MORPHINE SULFATE
MS Contin Tablets 2585

OCEFAX (Argentina)
CIPROFLOXACIN
Cipro Oral Suspension 2810

OCLOVIR (Argentina)
RIMANTADINE HYDROCHLORIDE
Flumadine Syrup 1167
Flumadine Tablets 1167

OCSAAR (Israel)
LOSARTAN POTASSIUM
Cozaar Tablets 1973

OCTIL (Israel)
TIMOLOL MALEATE
Timoptic in Ocudose 2124
Timoptic Sterile Ophthalmic Solution 2121
Timoptic-XE Sterile Ophthalmic Gel Forming Solution 2125

OCTODIOL (Czech Republic)
ESTRADIOL
Climara Transdermal System 763

OCUBRAX (Belgium, Hungary, Spain, Turkey)
DICLOFENAC SODIUM
Voltaren Tablets 2334
Voltaren-XR Tablets 2337

OCUMED (Russia)
TIMOLOL MALEATE
Timoptic in Ocudose 2124
Timoptic Sterile Ophthalmic Solution 2121
Timoptic-XE Sterile Ophthalmic Gel Forming Solution 2125

OCUPROST (Argentina)
LATANOPROST
Xalatan Ophthalmic Solution .... ⊙273

OCUPROSTIM (Argentina)
LATANOPROST
Xalatan Ophthalmic Solution .... ⊙273

OCUSTIL (Italy)
SODIUM HYALURONATE
Hyalgan Solution 2742

OCUTIM (India)
TIMOLOL MALEATE
Timoptic in Ocudose 2124
Timoptic Sterile Ophthalmic Solution 2121
Timoptic-XE Sterile Ophthalmic Gel Forming Solution 2125

ODANET (Greece)
RANITIDINE HYDROCHLORIDE
Zantac 25 EFFERdose Tablets 1670
Zantac 150 Tablets 1670
Zantac 300 Tablets 1670
Zantac Injection 1666
Zantac Injection Premixed 1666
Zantac Syrup 1670

ODANEX (Chile)
ONDANSETRON
Zofran ODT Orally Disintegrating Tablets 1687

ODEMASE (Germany)
FUROSEMIDE
Furosemide Tablets 2186

ODIVIR KIT (India)
EFAVIRENZ
Sustiva Capsules 930

ODRIC (Japan)
TRANDOLAPRIL
Mavik Tablets 472

ODRIK (Australia, Brazil, Denmark, France, Greece, Irish Republic, New Zealand, Portugal, Spain, The Netherlands, United Kingdom)
TRANDOLAPRIL
Mavik Tablets 472

ODUPRIL (Greece)
CAPTOPRIL
Captopril Tablets 2182

OEDEMEX (Switzerland)
FUROSEMIDE
Furosemide Tablets 2186

OESCLIM (Austria, Brazil, Canada, Chile, Czech Republic, France, Greece, Hungary, Poland, Sweden)
ESTRADIOL
Climara Transdermal System 763

OESTRACLIN (Spain)
ESTRADIOL
Climara Transdermal System 763

OESTRING (Sweden)
ESTRADIOL
Climara Transdermal System 763

OESTRO GEL (Argentina)
ESTRADIOL
Climara Transdermal System 763

OESTRODOSE (France, Israel, Spain)
ESTRADIOL
Climara Transdermal System 763

OESTROGEL (Belgium, Brazil, Czech Republic, France, Greece, Hong Kong, Hungary, Irish Republic, Israel, Malaysia, Mexico, Russia, Singapore, Switzerland, Thailand, United Kingdom)
ESTRADIOL
Climara Transdermal System 763

OFAL (Argentina)
TIMOLOL MALEATE
Timoptic in Ocudose 2124
Timoptic Sterile Ophthalmic Solution 2121
Timoptic-XE Sterile Ophthalmic Gel Forming Solution 2125

OFAL P (Argentina)
TIMOLOL MALEATE
Timoptic in Ocudose 2124
Timoptic Sterile Ophthalmic Solution 2121
Timoptic-XE Sterile Ophthalmic Gel Forming Solution 2125

OFAMIX (Venezuela)
AMOXICILLIN
Amoxil Pediatric Drops for Oral Suspension 1305
Amoxil Tablets 1305

OFF-TEN (Chile)
CARVEDILOL
Coreg Tablets 1387

OFLOCIN (Greece)
ETIDRONATE DISODIUM
Didronel Tablets 2583

OFLONO (Chile)
CIPROFLOXACIN HYDROCHLORIDE
Cipro Tablets 2810

OFLONO-D (Chile)
CIPROFLOXACIN HYDROCHLORIDE
Cipro Tablets 2810

OFOXIN (Brazil)
CIPROFLOXACIN HYDROCHLORIDE
Cipro Tablets 2810

OFRAMAX (Czech Republic, India, Poland, Russia, Singapore, South Africa, Thailand)
CEFTRIAXONE SODIUM
Rocephin Injectable Vials, ADD-Vantage, Galaxy, Bulk 2642

OFTACILOX (Italy, Portugal, Spain)
CIPROFLOXACIN
Cipro Oral Suspension 2810

OFTACIPROX (Chile)
CIPROFLOXACIN HYDROCHLORIDE
Cipro Tablets 2810

OFTAMOLOL (Denmark, Norway)
TIMOLOL MALEATE
Timoptic in Ocudose 2124
Timoptic Sterile Ophthalmic Solution 2121
Timoptic-XE Sterile Ophthalmic Gel Forming Solution 2125

OFTAN (Hong Kong, Israel, Norway, Poland, Switzerland, Thailand, The Philippines)
TIMOLOL MALEATE
Timoptic in Ocudose 2124
Timoptic Sterile Ophthalmic Solution 2121
Timoptic-XE Sterile Ophthalmic Gel Forming Solution 2125

OFTAN TIMOLOL (Russia)
TIMOLOL MALEATE
Timoptic in Ocudose 2124
Timoptic Sterile Ophthalmic Solution 2121
Timoptic-XE Sterile Ophthalmic Gel Forming Solution 2125

OFTAQUIN (Mexico)
CIPROFLOXACIN
Cipro Oral Suspension 2810

OFTAQUIX (Denmark, Finland, Germany, Italy, Poland, Sweden, The Netherlands, The Philippines, United Kingdom)
LEVOFLOXACIN
Levaquin Injection 2416
Levaquin Tablets 2416

OFTENSIN (Czech Republic, Poland)
TIMOLOL MALEATE
Timoptic in Ocudose 2124
Timoptic Sterile Ophthalmic Solution 2121
Timoptic-XE Sterile Ophthalmic Gel Forming Solution 2125

OFTIC (Chile)
DICLOFENAC SODIUM
Voltaren Tablets 2334
Voltaren-XR Tablets 2337

OFTIMOLO (Italy)
TIMOLOL MALEATE
Timoptic in Ocudose 2124
Timoptic Sterile Ophthalmic Solution 2121
Timoptic-XE Sterile Ophthalmic Gel Forming Solution 2125

OKLARICID (Greece)
CLARITHROMYCIN
Biaxin Filmtab Tablets 411
Biaxin Granules 411

OLBENDITAL (Mexico)
ALBENDAZOLE
Albenza Tablets 1297

OLDINOT (Argentina)
DONEPEZIL HYDROCHLORIDE
Aricept Tablets 1062

OLEXAR (India)
OLANZAPINE
Zyprexa Tablets 1883

OLFEN (Brazil, Czech Republic, Hong Kong, Hungary, Israel, Malaysia, Portugal, Singapore, Thailand)
DICLOFENAC SODIUM
Voltaren Tablets 2334
Voltaren-XR Tablets 2337

OLIMER (Argentina)
CLONAZEPAM
Klonopin Tablets 2639

OLIVIN (Chile)
OLANZAPINE
Zyprexa Tablets 1883

OLMORAN (Spain)
ZAFIRLUKAST
Accolate Tablets 669

OLTENS (France)
CAPTOPRIL
Captopril Tablets 2182

OLWORM (India)
ALBENDAZOLE
Albenza Tablets 1297

OLZAPIN (Poland)
OLANZAPINE
Zyprexa Tablets 1883

OMAFLAXINA (Argentina)
CIPROFLOXACIN
Cipro Oral Suspension 2810

OMCILON A ORABASE (Brazil)
TRIAMCINOLONE ACETONIDE
Azmacort Inhalation Aerosol 407
Nasacort AQ Nasal Spray 2765

OMIC (Belgium)
TAMSULOSIN HYDROCHLORIDE
Flomax Capsules 848

OMINOL (Mexico)
PROGESTERONE
Crinone 4% Gel 992
Prometrium Capsules (100 mg, 200 mg) 3047

OMIX (Austria, France, Switzerland)
TAMSULOSIN HYDROCHLORIDE
Flomax Capsules 848

OMNEXEL (Irish Republic)
TAMSULOSIN HYDROCHLORIDE
Flomax Capsules 848

OMNIC (Argentina, Brazil, Chile, Czech Republic, Denmark, Finland, Germany, Greece, Hungary, Irish Republic, Israel, Italy, Norway, Poland, Portugal, Russia, Spain, The Netherlands)
TAMSULOSIN HYDROCHLORIDE
Flomax Capsules 848

OMNICEF (Austria, Thailand)
CEFDINIR
Omnicef Capsules 497
Omnicef for Oral Suspension 497

OMSAL (Poland)
TAMSULOSIN HYDROCHLORIDE
Flomax Capsules 848

OMSIL (Irish Republic)
TAMSULOSIN HYDROCHLORIDE
Flomax Capsules 848

ONAPAN (Mexico)
DIAZEPAM
Valium Tablets 2658

ONCASPAR (Argentina, Canada, Germany, Poland, Russia)
PEGASPARGASE
Oncaspar Injection 1138

ONCLAST (Japan)
ALENDRONATE SODIUM
Fosamax Tablets 2005

ONCOEMET (Chile)
ONDANSETRON HYDROCHLORIDE
Zofran Injection . . . 1682
Zofran Injection Premixed . . . 1682
Zofran Oral Solution . . . 1687
Zofran Tablets . . . 1687

ONCOGEM (India)
GEMCITABINE HYDROCHLORIDE
Gemzar for Injection . . . 1820

ONDANOGLAX (Austria)
ONDANSETRON
Zofran ODT Orally Disintegrating Tablets . . 1687

ONDAREN (Greece)
ONDANSETRON
Zofran ODT Orally Disintegrating Tablets . . 1687

ONDAZ (Australia)
ONDANSETRON
Zofran ODT Orally Disintegrating Tablets . . 1687

ONDEMET (Czech Republic, United Kingdom)
ONDANSETRON HYDROCHLORIDE
Zofran Injection . . . 1682
Zofran Injection Premixed . . . 1682
Zofran Oral Solution . . . 1687
Zofran Tablets . . . 1687

ONDENSAN (Austria)
ONDANSETRON HYDROCHLORIDE
Zofran Injection . . . 1682
Zofran Injection Premixed . . . 1682
Zofran Oral Solution . . . 1687
Zofran Tablets . . . 1687

ONEXID (The Philippines)
CLARITHROMYCIN
Biaxin Filmtab Tablets . . . 411
Biaxin Granules . . . 411

ONEXMOL (Mexico)
NAPROXEN SODIUM
Anaprox DS Tablets . . . 2632
Anaprox Tablets . . . 2632

ONKOMORPHIN (Germany)
MORPHINE SULFATE
MS Contin Tablets . . . 2585

ONSENAL (France, Norway, Spain, Sweden, The Netherlands)
CELECOXIB
Celebrex Capsules . . . 2979

ONSIA (Thailand)
ONDANSETRON HYDROCHLORIDE
Zofran Injection . . . 1682
Zofran Injection Premixed . . . 1682
Zofran Oral Solution . . . 1687
Zofran Tablets . . . 1687

ONTRAX (Brazil)
ONDANSETRON HYDROCHLORIDE
Zofran Injection . . . 1682
Zofran Injection Premixed . . . 1682
Zofran Oral Solution . . . 1687
Zofran Tablets . . . 1687

ONYCHON (Czech Republic)
TERBINAFINE HYDROCHLORIDE
Lamisil Tablets . . . 2266

ONYMAX (Poland, Switzerland)
TERBINAFINE HYDROCHLORIDE
Lamisil Tablets . . . 2266

OPATANOL (Belgium, Denmark, Finland, France, Germany, Greece, Hungary, Irish Republic, Italy, Norway, Portugal, Spain, Sweden, Switzerland, The Netherlands, United Kingdom)
OLOPATADINE HYDROCHLORIDE
Patanol Ophthalmic Solution . . . 546

OPHTALIN (Italy)
SODIUM HYALURONATE
Hyalgan Solution . . . 2742

OPHTALIN PLUS (Turkey)
SODIUM HYALURONATE
Hyalgan Solution . . . 2742

OPHTHALIN (Australia, Hong Kong, Hungary, Irish Republic, Israel, New Zealand, Singapore, Thailand, United Kingdom)
SODIUM HYALURONATE
Hyalgan Solution . . . 2742

OPHTILAN (Austria)
TIMOLOL MALEATE
Timoptic in Ocudose . . . 2124
Timoptic Sterile Ophthalmic Solution . . . 2121
Timoptic-XE Sterile Ophthalmic Gel Forming Solution . . . 2125

OPHTIM (France)
TIMOLOL MALEATE
Timoptic in Ocudose . . . 2124
Timoptic Sterile Ophthalmic Solution . . . 2121
Timoptic-XE Sterile Ophthalmic Gel Forming Solution . . . 2125

OPRAKS (Turkey)
NAPROXEN SODIUM
Anaprox DS Tablets . . . 2632
Anaprox Tablets . . . 2632

OPRIDAN (Greece)
ISOTRETINOIN
Accutane Capsules . . . 2607

OPTAMAX (Brazil)
DICLOFENAC SODIUM
Voltaren Tablets . . . 2334
Voltaren-XR Tablets . . . 2337

OPTHAFLOX (Mexico)
CIPROFLOXACIN HYDROCHLORIDE
Cipro Tablets . . . 2810

OPTIFLUOR (Mexico)
FLUORESCEIN SODIUM
Fluorescite Injection . . . ⊙203

OPTIL (United Kingdom)
DILTIAZEM HYDROCHLORIDE
Cardizem LA Extended Release Tablets . . . 421

OPTIMOL (Australia, Denmark, Hong Kong, Russia, Sweden)
TIMOLOL MALEATE
Timoptic in Ocudose . . . 2124
Timoptic Sterile Ophthalmic Solution . . . 2121
Timoptic-XE Sterile Ophthalmic Gel Forming Solution . . . 2125

OPTINATE (Finland, Italy, Norway, Sweden)
RISEDRONATE SODIUM
Actonel Tablets . . . 2568

OPTINATE SEPTIMUM (Sweden)
RISEDRONATE SODIUM
Actonel Tablets . . . 2568

OPTINEM (Austria)
MEROPENEM
Merrem I.V. . . . 684

OPTIPAR (Finland)
PAROXETINE HYDROCHLORIDE
Paxil Oral Suspension . . . 1535
Paxil Tablets . . . 1535

OPTOBET (Greece)
DICLOFENAC SODIUM
Voltaren Tablets . . . 2334
Voltaren-XR Tablets . . . 2337

OPTREX CONTACT LENS FRIENDLY EYE DROPS (United Kingdom)
SODIUM HYALURONATE
Hyalgan Solution . . . 2742

OPTROL (Australia)
SALMETEROL XINAFOATE
Serevent Diskus . . . 1594

OPTRUMA (Austria, Finland, France, Germany, Italy, Portugal, Spain, The Netherlands)
RALOXIFENE HYDROCHLORIDE
Evista Tablets . . . 1810

OPUMIDE (United Kingdom)
INDAPAMIDE
Indapamide Tablets . . . 2188

ORABIOT UD (Argentina)
CLARITHROMYCIN
Biaxin Filmtab Tablets . . . 411
Biaxin Granules . . . 411

ORACORT (Canada, Israel, New Zealand, Thailand)
TRIAMCINOLONE ACETONIDE
Azmacort Inhalation Aerosol . . . 407
Nasacort AQ Nasal Spray . . . 2765

ORALMUV (Argentina)
LAMIVUDINE
Epivir Oral Solution . . . 1412
Epivir Tablets . . . 1412
Epivir-HBV Oral Solution . . . 1417
Epivir-HBV Tablets . . . 1417

ORALOG (Thailand)
TRIAMCINOLONE ACETONIDE
Azmacort Inhalation Aerosol . . . 407
Nasacort AQ Nasal Spray . . . 2765

ORAL-T (Thailand)
TRIAMCINOLONE ACETONIDE
Azmacort Inhalation Aerosol . . . 407
Nasacort AQ Nasal Spray . . . 2765

ORAMEDY (Singapore)
TRIAMCINOLONE ACETONIDE
Azmacort Inhalation Aerosol . . . 407
Nasacort AQ Nasal Spray . . . 2765

ORAMINAX (Portugal)
AMOXICILLIN
Amoxil Pediatric Drops for Oral Suspension . . . 1305
Amoxil Tablets . . . 1305

ORAMORPH (Austria, Belgium, Canada, Czech Republic, France, Germany, Irish Republic, Italy, Spain, Sweden, The Netherlands, United Kingdom)
MORPHINE SULFATE
MS Contin Tablets . . . 2585

ORANOR (Mexico)
NORFLOXACIN
Noroxin Tablets . . . 2069

ORAQIX (Denmark, Finland, Norway, Sweden, The Netherlands, United Kingdom)
LIDOCAINE
Lidoderm Patch . . . 1114

ORA-SED LOTION (Australia)
LIDOCAINE
Lidoderm Patch . . . 1114

ORATANE (Australia, Hong Kong, Malaysia, Mexico, New Zealand, Singapore, South Africa)
ISOTRETINOIN
Accutane Capsules . . . 2607

ORAXIM (Italy)
CEFUROXIME AXETIL
Ceftin for Oral Suspension . . . 1380
Ceftin Tablets . . . 1380

ORCILONE (Thailand)
TRIAMCINOLONE ACETONIDE
Azmacort Inhalation Aerosol . . . 407
Nasacort AQ Nasal Spray . . . 2765

OROMONE (France)
ESTRADIOL
Climara Transdermal System . . . 763

OROTREX (Portugal)
ISOTRETINOIN
Accutane Capsules . . . 2607

OROVAS (The Philippines)
SIMVASTATIN
Zocor Tablets . . . 2136

OROXINE (Australia, Malaysia, Singapore)
LEVOTHYROXINE SODIUM
Levothroid Tablets . . . 1170
Levoxyl Tablets . . . 1780
Synthroid Tablets . . . 507

ORPIC (South Africa)
CIPROFLOXACIN HYDROCHLORIDE
Cipro Tablets . . . 2810

ORREPASTE (Malaysia, Singapore)
TRIAMCINOLONE ACETONIDE
Azmacort Inhalation Aerosol . . . 407
Nasacort AQ Nasal Spray . . . 2765

ORTHOCEL (India)
CELECOXIB
Celebrex Capsules . . . 2979

ORTHOCLONE (Greece, South Africa)
MUROMONAB-CD3
Orthoclone OKT3 Sterile Solution . . . 2387

ORTHOCLONE OKT3 (Australia, Belgium, Brazil, Canada, Czech Republic, Finland, France, Germany, Hong Kong, Israel, Italy, Malaysia, Mexico, New Zealand, Norway, Sweden, Switzerland, Thailand, The Netherlands, Turkey)
MUROMONAB-CD3
Orthoclone OKT3 Sterile Solution . . . 2387

ORTHOVISC (Canada, Germany, Israel, United Kingdom)
SODIUM HYALURONATE
Hyalgan Solution . . . 2742

ORTOFLAN (Brazil)
DICLOFENAC SODIUM
Voltaren Tablets . . . 2334
Voltaren-XR Tablets . . . 2337

ORTOPSIQUE (Mexico)
DIAZEPAM
Valium Tablets . . . 2658

OSALEN (Poland)
ALENDRONATE SODIUM
Fosamax Tablets . . . 2005

OSDRON (Brazil)
ALENDRONATE SODIUM
Fosamax Tablets . . . 2005

OSEMIN (Mexico)
FUROSEMIDE
Furosemide Tablets . . . 2186

OSEOFEM (Argentina)
RALOXIFENE HYDROCHLORIDE
Evista Tablets . . . 1810

OSEOTENK (Argentina)
ALENDRONATE SODIUM
Fosamax Tablets . . . 2005

OSFO (Greece)
ETIDRONATE DISODIUM
Didronel Tablets . . . 2583

OSMOLAC (Italy)
LACTULOSE
Kristalose for Oral Solution . . . 1004

OSMOLAK (Turkey)
LACTULOSE
Kristalose for Oral Solution . . . 1004

OSPAMOX (Greece, Hungary, Poland, Portugal, Venezuela)
AMOXICILLIN
Amoxil Pediatric Drops for Oral Suspension . . . 1305
Amoxil Tablets . . . 1305

OSSOMAX (Brazil)
ALENDRONATE SODIUM
Fosamax Tablets . . . 2005

OSTALERT (Greece)
ALENDRONATE SODIUM
Fosamax Tablets . . . 2005

OSTAREN (Thailand)
DICLOFENAC SODIUM
Voltaren Tablets . . . 2334
Voltaren-XR Tablets . . . 2337

OSTEDRON (Greece, Poland)
ETIDRONATE DISODIUM
Didronel Tablets . . . 2583

OSTEMAX (Poland)
ALENDRONATE SODIUM
Fosamax Tablets . . . 2005

OSTENAN (Brazil)
ALENDRONATE SODIUM
Fosamax Tablets . . . 2005

OSTENIL (France, Germany, Poland, Switzerland, Turkey, United Kingdom)
ALENDRONATE SODIUM
Fosamax Tablets . . . 2005

OSTEO D (Israel)
CALCITRIOL
Calcijex Injection . . . 419
Rocaltrol Capsules . . . 1150
Rocaltrol Oral Solution . . . 1150

OSTEOBON (South Africa)
ALENDRONATE SODIUM
Fosamax Tablets . . . 2005

OSTEOD (Thailand)
CALCITRIOL
Calcijex Injection . . . 419
Rocaltrol Capsules . . . 1150
Rocaltrol Oral Solution . . . 1150

OSTEO-D (Turkey)
CALCITRIOL
Calcijex Injection . . . 419
Rocaltrol Capsules . . . 1150
Rocaltrol Oral Solution . . . 1150

OSTEODIDRONEL (Belgium)
ETIDRONATE DISODIUM
Didronel Tablets . . . 2583

(⊙ Described in PDR® For Ophthalmic Medicines)

OSTEODRUG (Greece)
ETIDRONATE DISODIUM
Didronel Tablets 2583

OSTEODUR (Venezuela)
ALENDRONATE SODIUM
Fosamax Tablets 2005

OSTEOFAR (Brazil)
ALENDRONATE SODIUM
Fosamax Tablets 2005

OSTEOFEM (Chile)
ALENDRONATE SODIUM
Fosamax Tablets 2005

OSTEOFENE (Argentina)
ALENDRONATE SODIUM
Fosamax Tablets 2005

OSTEOFORM (Brazil)
ALENDRONATE SODIUM
Fosamax Tablets 2005

OSTEOFOS (Hong Kong, India)
ALENDRONATE SODIUM
Fosamax Tablets 2005

OSTEOMAX (Turkey, Venezuela)
ALENDRONATE SODIUM
Fosamax Tablets 2005

OSTEOMEG (The Philippines)
CALCITRIOL
Calcijex Injection 419
Rocaltrol Capsules 1150
Rocaltrol Oral Solution 1150

OSTEOMEL (Irish Republic)
ALENDRONATE SODIUM
Fosamax Tablets 2005

OSTEONATE (Argentina)
ALENDRONATE SODIUM
Fosamax Tablets 2005

OSTEORAL (Brazil)
ALENDRONATE SODIUM
Fosamax Tablets 2005

OSTEOSAN (Chile)
ALENDRONATE SODIUM
Fosamax Tablets 2005

OSTEOTON (Greece)
ETIDRONATE DISODIUM
Didronel Tablets 2583

OSTEOTOP (Chile)
ETIDRONATE DISODIUM
Didronel Tablets 2583

OSTEOTRAT (Brazil)
ALENDRONATE SODIUM
Fosamax Tablets 2005

OSTEOTRIOL (Germany, Russia)
CALCITRIOL
Calcijex Injection 419
Rocaltrol Capsules 1150
Rocaltrol Oral Solution 1150

OSTEUM (Spain)
ETIDRONATE DISODIUM
Didronel Tablets 2583

OSTOGENE (Greece)
ETIDRONATE DISODIUM
Didronel Tablets 2583

OSTOLEK (Poland)
ALENDRONATE SODIUM
Fosamax Tablets 2005

OSTOPOR (Greece)
ETIDRONATE DISODIUM
Didronel Tablets 2583

OSTRIOL (Brazil)
CALCITRIOL
Calcijex Injection 419
Rocaltrol Capsules 1150
Rocaltrol Oral Solution 1150

OTALEX (Venezuela)
CIPROFLOXACIN
Cipro Oral Suspension 2810

OTARI (Greece)
CALCITRIOL
Calcijex Injection 419
Rocaltrol Capsules 1150
Rocaltrol Oral Solution 1150

OTEX HC (Argentina, Chile)
CIPROFLOXACIN HYDROCHLORIDE
Cipro Tablets 2810

OTO BIOTAER (Argentina)
CIPROFLOXACIN
Cipro Oral Suspension 2810

OTOBIOTIC (Argentina)
CIPROFLOXACIN
Cipro Oral Suspension 2810

OTOCIPRIN (Spain)
CIPROFLOXACIN HYDROCHLORIDE
Cipro Tablets 2810

OTODON (Venezuela)
LIDOCAINE
Lidoderm Patch 1114

OTOIAL (Italy)
SODIUM HYALURONATE
Hyalgan Solution 2742

OTOSAT (Spain)
CIPROFLOXACIN HYDROCHLORIDE
Cipro Tablets 2810

OTOSPORIN C (Argentina)
CIPROFLOXACIN HYDROCHLORIDE
Cipro Tablets 2810

OTRASEL (France)
SELEGILINE HYDROCHLORIDE
Eldepryl Capsules 3052

OVESTAL (The Netherlands)
ESTRADIOL
Climara Transdermal System 763

OVINOL (Greece)
NORFLOXACIN
Noroxin Tablets 2069

OXA FORTE (Argentina)
DICLOFENAC SODIUM
Voltaren Tablets 2334
Voltaren-XR Tablets 2337

OXAL (Mexico)
ALBENDAZOLE
Albenza Tablets 1297

OXALGIN (India)
DICLOFENAC SODIUM
Voltaren Tablets 2334
Voltaren-XR Tablets 2337

OXALGIN-D (India)
DICLOFENAC SODIUM
Voltaren Tablets 2334
Voltaren-XR Tablets 2337

OXALGIN-DP (India)
DICLOFENAC SODIUM
Voltaren Tablets 2334
Voltaren-XR Tablets 2337

OXALGIN-SR (India)
DICLOFENAC SODIUM
Voltaren Tablets 2334
Voltaren-XR Tablets 2337

OXANEST (Finland)
OXYCODONE HYDROCHLORIDE
OxyContin Tablets 2589
OxyIR Capsules 2593

OXAPROST (Argentina)
DICLOFENAC SODIUM
Voltaren Tablets 2334
Voltaren-XR Tablets 2337

OXEPAR (Portugal)
PAROXETINE HYDROCHLORIDE
Paxil Oral Suspension 1535
Paxil Tablets 1535

OXET (Germany)
PAROXETINE HYDROCHLORIDE
Paxil Oral Suspension 1535
Paxil Tablets 1535

OXETINE (Australia, Denmark)
PAROXETINE HYDROCHLORIDE
Paxil Oral Suspension 1535
Paxil Tablets 1535

OXICALMANS (Argentina)
OXYCODONE HYDROCHLORIDE
OxyContin Tablets 2589
OxyIR Capsules 2593

OXIDERMA (Spain)
BENZOYL PEROXIDE
Brevoxyl-4 Creamy Wash 3054
Brevoxyl-4 Gel 3054
Brevoxyl-8 Creamy Wash 3054
Brevoxyl-8 Gel 3054

OXIGEN (Brazil)
NIMODIPINE
Nimotop Capsules 790

OXINOVAG (Argentina)
OXYCODONE HYDROCHLORIDE
OxyContin Tablets 2589
OxyIR Capsules 2593

OXINOVAG COMPLEX (Argentina)
OXYCODONE HYDROCHLORIDE
OxyContin Tablets 2589
OxyIR Capsules 2593

OXTIN (Venezuela)
CIPROFLOXACIN HYDROCHLORIDE
Cipro Tablets 2810

OXY (Australia, Canada, Czech Republic, Germany, Hong Kong, Israel, Mexico, The Netherlands, United Kingdom)
BENZOYL PEROXIDE
Brevoxyl-4 Creamy Wash 3054
Brevoxyl-4 Gel 3054
Brevoxyl-8 Creamy Wash 3054
Brevoxyl-8 Gel 3054

OXY IR (Canada)
OXYCODONE HYDROCHLORIDE
OxyContin Tablets 2589
OxyIR Capsules 2593

OXY SENSITIVE (Israel)
BENZOYL PEROXIDE
Brevoxyl-4 Creamy Wash 3054
Brevoxyl-4 Gel 3054
Brevoxyl-8 Creamy Wash 3054
Brevoxyl-8 Gel 3054

OXYAL (Germany, Italy)
SODIUM HYALURONATE
Hyalgan Solution 2742

OXYCARDIL (Poland)
DILTIAZEM HYDROCHLORIDE
Cardizem LA Extended Release Tablets 421

OXYCOD (Israel)
OXYCODONE HYDROCHLORIDE
OxyContin Tablets 2589
OxyIR Capsules 2593

OXYCONTIN (Argentina, Australia, Austria, Belgium, Brazil, Canada, Chile, Czech Republic, Denmark, Finland, France, Irish Republic, Israel, Italy, Mexico, New Zealand, Norway, Spain, Sweden, Switzerland, The Netherlands, The Philippines, United Kingdom, Venezuela)
OXYCODONE HYDROCHLORIDE
OxyContin Tablets 2589
OxyIR Capsules 2593

OXYDERM (Canada)
BENZOYL PEROXIDE
Brevoxyl-4 Creamy Wash 3054
Brevoxyl-4 Gel 3054
Brevoxyl-8 Creamy Wash 3054
Brevoxyl-8 Gel 3054

OXYGESIC (Germany)
OXYCODONE HYDROCHLORIDE
OxyContin Tablets 2589
OxyIR Capsules 2593

OXYNORM (Australia, Austria, Denmark, Finland, France, Irish Republic, New Zealand, Norway, Spain, Sweden, Switzerland, The Netherlands, United Kingdom)
OXYCODONE HYDROCHLORIDE
OxyContin Tablets 2589
OxyIR Capsules 2593

OXYTOKO (Spain)
BENZOYL PEROXIDE
Brevoxyl-4 Creamy Wash 3054
Brevoxyl-4 Gel 3054
Brevoxyl-8 Creamy Wash 3054
Brevoxyl-8 Gel 3054

OZAPIN (India)
OLANZAPINE
Zyprexa Tablets 1883

OZEPAM (India)
CLONAZEPAM
Klonopin Tablets 2639

PACEUM (Switzerland)
DIAZEPAM
Valium Tablets 2658

PACINAX (Chile)
DIAZEPAM
Valium Tablets 2658

PACIUM (Spain)
DIAZEPAM
Valium Tablets 2658

PACTENS (Mexico)
NAPROXEN SODIUM
Anaprox DS Tablets 2632
Anaprox Tablets 2632

PAFTEC (Portugal)
FLUNISOLIDE
Aerobid Inhaler System 1153
Aerobid-M Inhaler System 1153

PAINBREAK (Germany)
MORPHINE SULFATE
MS Contin Tablets 2585

PAINDOL (Thailand)
TRAMADOL HYDROCHLORIDE
Ultram ER Tablets 2428

PAINEX (Portugal)
DICLOFENAC SODIUM
Voltaren Tablets 2334
Voltaren-XR Tablets 2337

PAINFORT (Venezuela)
DICLOFENAC SODIUM
Voltaren Tablets 2334
Voltaren-XR Tablets 2337

PALDAR (Argentina)
MUPIROCIN
Bactroban Ointment 1368

PALUXETIL (Austria)
PAROXETINE HYDROCHLORIDE
Paxil Oral Suspension 1535
Paxil Tablets 1535

PAMID (Israel)
INDAPAMIDE
Indapamide Tablets 2188

PANALBA (Greece)
FAMOTIDINE
Pepcid for Oral Suspension 2075
Pepcid Tablets 2075

PANAMOR (South Africa)
DICLOFENAC SODIUM
Voltaren Tablets 2334
Voltaren-XR Tablets 2337

PANATRIX (Italy)
CEFTRIAXONE SODIUM
Rocephin Injectable Vials, ADD-Vantage, Galaxy, Bulk 2642

PANAXIM (The Philippines)
CEFUROXIME SODIUM
Zinacef Injection 1678

PANBESY (Belgium, Hong Kong, Singapore, Thailand)
PHENTERMINE HYDROCHLORIDE
Adipex-P Capsules 1185
Adipex-P Tablets 1185

PANCLOFLEX (Argentina)
DICLOFENAC SODIUM
Voltaren Tablets 2334
Voltaren-XR Tablets 2337

PANCREASE (Australia, Belgium, Brazil, Canada, Denmark, Finland, Israel, Italy, Mexico, New Zealand, Norway, Spain, Sweden, The Netherlands, United Kingdom, Venezuela)
PANCRELIPASE
Ultrase Capsules 718
Ultrase MT Capsules 719

PANDERMIN CICATRIZANTE (Spain)
SODIUM HYALURONATE
Hyalgan Solution 2742

PANGEL (Belgium)
BENZOYL PEROXIDE
Brevoxyl-4 Creamy Wash 3054
Brevoxyl-4 Gel 3054
Brevoxyl-8 Creamy Wash 3054
Brevoxyl-8 Gel 3054

PANGRAF (India)
TACROLIMUS
Prograf Capsules and Injection 622

PANITOL (Thailand)
CARBAMAZEPINE
Carbatrol Capsules ... **3019**

PANKREADEN (Italy)
PANCRELIPASE
Ultrase Capsules ... **718**
Ultrase MT Capsules ... **719**

PANKREASE (South Africa)
PANCRELIPASE
Ultrase Capsules ... **718**
Ultrase MT Capsules ... **719**

PANNOGEL (France)
BENZOYL PEROXIDE
Brevoxyl-4 Creamy Wash ... **3054**
Brevoxyl-4 Gel ... **3054**
Brevoxyl-8 Creamy Wash ... **3054**
Brevoxyl-8 Gel ... **3054**

PANOTILE CIPRO (Germany)
CIPROFLOXACIN HYDROCHLORIDE
Cipro Tablets ... **2810**

PANOXYL (Australia, Austria, Brazil, Canada, Finland, France, Germany, Hong Kong, Irish Republic, Israel, Italy, Malaysia, Mexico, New Zealand, Norway, Portugal, Singapore, South Africa, Spain, Switzerland, Thailand, The Philippines, United Kingdom, Venezuela)
BENZOYL PEROXIDE
Brevoxyl-4 Creamy Wash ... **3054**
Brevoxyl-4 Gel ... **3054**
Brevoxyl-8 Creamy Wash ... **3054**
Brevoxyl-8 Gel ... **3054**

PANSULFOX (Chile)
BENZOYL PEROXIDE
Brevoxyl-4 Creamy Wash ... **3054**
Brevoxyl-4 Gel ... **3054**
Brevoxyl-8 Creamy Wash ... **3054**
Brevoxyl-8 Gel ... **3054**

PANTASOL (Italy)
FLUNISOLIDE
Aerobid Inhaler System ... **1153**
Aerobid-M Inhaler System ... **1153**

PANTESTONE (Argentina)
ANASTROZOLE
Arimidex Tablets ... **672**

PANTINOL (Austria)
APROTININ
Trasylol Injection ... **799**

PANTOK (Spain)
SIMVASTATIN
Zocor Tablets ... **2136**

PANTOXON (Italy)
CEFTRIAXONE SODIUM
Rocephin Injectable Vials, ADD-Vantage, Galaxy, Bulk ... **2642**

PANTRIXON (The Philippines)
CEFTRIAXONE SODIUM
Rocephin Injectable Vials, ADD-Vantage, Galaxy, Bulk ... **2642**

PANZID (Italy)
CEFTAZIDIME
Fortaz for Injection ... **1450**

PANZYTRAT (Australia, New Zealand)
PANCRELIPASE
Ultrase Capsules ... **718**
Ultrase MT Capsules ... **719**

PAPASINE (Argentina)
NAPROXEN
EC-Naprosyn Delayed-Release Tablets ... **2632**
Naprosyn Suspension ... **2632**
Naprosyn Tablets ... **2632**

PARABACT (India)
NORFLOXACIN
Noroxin Tablets ... **2069**

PARACEFAN (Belgium)
CLONIDINE HYDROCHLORIDE
Catapres Tablets ... **841**

PARACNE (Argentina)
BENZOYL PEROXIDE
Brevoxyl-4 Creamy Wash ... **3054**
Brevoxyl-4 Gel ... **3054**
Brevoxyl-8 Creamy Wash ... **3054**
Brevoxyl-8 Gel ... **3054**

PARAFORTAN (The Philippines)
DICLOFENAC SODIUM
Voltaren Tablets ... **2334**
Voltaren-XR Tablets ... **2337**

PARAIOP (Argentina)
LATANOPROST
Xalatan Ophthalmic Solution ... **⊙273**

PARANTHIL (South Africa)
ALBENDAZOLE
Albenza Tablets ... **1297**

PARAPRES (Spain)
CANDESARTAN CILEXETIL
Atacand Tablets ... **639**

PARAPRES PLUS (Spain)
CANDESARTAN CILEXETIL
Atacand Tablets ... **639**

PARASIN (Brazil)
ALBENDAZOLE
Albenza Tablets ... **1297**

PARASTHMAN (Germany)
THEOPHYLLINE
Uniphyl Tablets ... **2595**

PARATONINA (Spain)
PAROXETINE HYDROCHLORIDE
Paxil Oral Suspension ... **1535**
Paxil Tablets ... **1535**

PARCETIN (Argentina)
NORFLOXACIN
Noroxin Tablets ... **2069**

PAREXAT (Switzerland)
PAROXETINE HYDROCHLORIDE
Paxil Oral Suspension ... **1535**
Paxil Tablets ... **1535**

PARI (India)
PAROXETINE HYDROCHLORIDE
Paxil Oral Suspension ... **1535**
Paxil Tablets ... **1535**

PARKEXIN (Brazil)
SELEGILINE HYDROCHLORIDE
Eldepryl Capsules ... **3052**

PARKILYNE (South Africa)
SELEGILINE HYDROCHLORIDE
Eldepryl Capsules ... **3052**

PARLAZIN (Hungary)
CETIRIZINE HYDROCHLORIDE
Zyrtec Syrup ... **1920**
Zyrtec Tablets ... **1920**

PARNATE (Argentina, Australia, Brazil, Canada, Czech Republic, Germany, Irish Republic, New Zealand, South Africa, Spain)
TRANYLCYPROMINE SULFATE
Parnate Tablets ... **1532**

PAROCETAN (Austria)
PAROXETINE HYDROCHLORIDE
Paxil Oral Suspension ... **1535**
Paxil Tablets ... **1535**

PAROLICH (Germany)
PAROXETINE HYDROCHLORIDE
Paxil Oral Suspension ... **1535**
Paxil Tablets ... **1535**

PAROMERCK (Poland)
PAROXETINE HYDROCHLORIDE
Paxil Oral Suspension ... **1535**
Paxil Tablets ... **1535**

PARONAL (Belgium, The Netherlands)
ASPARAGINASE
Elspar for Injection ... **2488**

PARONEX (Switzerland)
PAROXETINE HYDROCHLORIDE
Paxil Oral Suspension ... **1535**
Paxil Tablets ... **1535**

PAROSER (Irish Republic)
PAROXETINE HYDROCHLORIDE
Paxil Oral Suspension ... **1535**
Paxil Tablets ... **1535**

PAROTIN (India)
PAROXETINE HYDROCHLORIDE
Paxil Oral Suspension ... **1535**
Paxil Tablets ... **1535**

PAROTUR (Spain)
PAROXETINE HYDROCHLORIDE
Paxil Oral Suspension ... **1535**
Paxil Tablets ... **1535**

PAROX (Irish Republic)
PAROXETINE HYDROCHLORIDE
Paxil Oral Suspension ... **1535**
Paxil Tablets ... **1535**

PAROXAT (Austria, Germany, Hungary)
PAROXETINE HYDROCHLORIDE
Paxil Oral Suspension ... **1535**
Paxil Tablets ... **1535**

PAROXEDURA (Germany)
PAROXETINE HYDROCHLORIDE
Paxil Oral Suspension ... **1535**
Paxil Tablets ... **1535**

PAROXETOP (Switzerland)
PAROXETINE HYDROCHLORIDE
Paxil Oral Suspension ... **1535**
Paxil Tablets ... **1535**

PAROXIFLEX (Sweden)
PAROXETINE HYDROCHLORIDE
Paxil Oral Suspension ... **1535**
Paxil Tablets ... **1535**

PARVEN (Mexico)
BENZONATATE
Tessalon Perles ... **1183**

PASODRON (Chile)
ALENDRONATE SODIUM
Fosamax Tablets ... **2005**

PATANOL (Argentina, Australia, Brazil, Canada, Chile, Hong Kong, Israel, Malaysia, Mexico, New Zealand, Singapore, South Africa, Thailand, The Philippines, Turkey, Venezuela)
OLOPATADINE HYDROCHLORIDE
Patanol Ophthalmic Solution ... **546**

PATOX (Mexico)
CIPROFLOXACIN HYDROCHLORIDE
Cipro Tablets ... **2810**

PATXEN (Mexico)
NAPROXEN
EC-Naprosyn Delayed-Release Tablets ... **2632**
Naprosyn Suspension ... **2632**
Naprosyn Tablets ... **2632**

PAUSOGEST (Czech Republic, Hungary)
ESTRADIOL
Climara Transdermal System ... **763**

PAX (South Africa)
DIAZEPAM
Valium Tablets ... **2658**

PAXAM (Australia, New Zealand)
CLONAZEPAM
Klonopin Tablets ... **2639**

PAXATE (Mexico)
DIAZEPAM
Valium Tablets ... **2658**

PAXERATIO (Poland)
PAROXETINE HYDROCHLORIDE
Paxil Oral Suspension ... **1535**
Paxil Tablets ... **1535**

PAXETIL (Portugal)
PAROXETINE HYDROCHLORIDE
Paxil Oral Suspension ... **1535**
Paxil Tablets ... **1535**

PAXIL (Argentina, Canada, Mexico, Russia, South Africa, Turkey, Venezuela)
PAROXETINE HYDROCHLORIDE
Paxil Oral Suspension ... **1535**
Paxil Tablets ... **1535**

PAXILFAR (Portugal)
TRAMADOL HYDROCHLORIDE
Ultram ER Tablets ... **2428**

PAXON (Argentina)
LOSARTAN POTASSIUM
Cozaar Tablets ... **1973**

PAXON-D (Argentina)
LOSARTAN POTASSIUM
Cozaar Tablets ... **1973**

PAXT (Irish Republic)
PAROXETINE HYDROCHLORIDE
Paxil Oral Suspension ... **1535**
Paxil Tablets ... **1535**

PAXTIN (Poland)
PAROXETINE HYDROCHLORIDE
Paxil Oral Suspension ... **1535**
Paxil Tablets ... **1535**

PAXTINE (Australia)
PAROXETINE HYDROCHLORIDE
Paxil Oral Suspension ... **1535**
Paxil Tablets ... **1535**

PAXUM (India)
DIAZEPAM
Valium Tablets ... **2658**

PAXXET (Israel)
PAROXETINE HYDROCHLORIDE
Paxil Oral Suspension ... **1535**
Paxil Tablets ... **1535**

PAZITAL (Spain)
TRAMADOL HYDROCHLORIDE
Ultram ER Tablets ... **2428**

PAZOLINI (Brazil)
DIAZEPAM
Valium Tablets ... **2658**

PB GEL (Argentina)
BENZOYL PEROXIDE
Brevoxyl-4 Creamy Wash ... **3054**
Brevoxyl-4 Gel ... **3054**
Brevoxyl-8 Creamy Wash ... **3054**
Brevoxyl-8 Gel ... **3054**

PEAULINE (The Netherlands)
BENZOYL PEROXIDE
Brevoxyl-4 Creamy Wash ... **3054**
Brevoxyl-4 Gel ... **3054**
Brevoxyl-8 Creamy Wash ... **3054**
Brevoxyl-8 Gel ... **3054**

PEBEGAL (Mexico)
BENZONATATE
Tessalon Perles ... **1183**

PEDIAPHYLLIN PL (The Netherlands)
THEOPHYLLINE
Uniphyl Tablets ... **2595**

PELICREP (Argentina)
FINASTERIDE
Propecia Tablets ... **2095**
Proscar Tablets ... **2102**

PENCLA (Thailand)
AMOXICILLIN
Amoxil Pediatric Drops for Oral Suspension ... **1305**
Amoxil Tablets ... **1305**

PENESTER (Czech Republic, Poland)
FINASTERIDE
Propecia Tablets ... **2095**
Proscar Tablets ... **2102**

PENGESIC (Malaysia, Singapore, The Philippines)
TRAMADOL HYDROCHLORIDE
Ultram ER Tablets ... **2428**

PENGON (Greece)
DICLOFENAC SODIUM
Voltaren Tablets ... **2334**
Voltaren-XR Tablets ... **2337**

PENLES (Japan)
LIDOCAINE
Lidoderm Patch ... **1114**

PENMOX (South Africa)
AMOXICILLIN
Amoxil Pediatric Drops for Oral Suspension ... **1305**
Amoxil Tablets ... **1305**

PENNSAID (Canada, Italy, Portugal, United Kingdom)
DICLOFENAC SODIUM
Voltaren Tablets ... **2334**
Voltaren-XR Tablets ... **2337**

PENSODIL (Mexico)
NAPROXEN SODIUM
Anaprox DS Tablets ... **2632**
Anaprox Tablets ... **2632**

PENTALAC (Brazil)
LACTULOSE
Kristalose for Oral Solution ... **1004**

PENTICLOX (Mexico)
AMOXICILLIN
Amoxil Pediatric Drops for Oral Suspension 1305
Amoxil Tablets 1305

PENTILZENO (Portugal)
DILTIAZEM HYDROCHLORIDE
Cardizem LA Extended Release Tablets 421

PENVICILIN (Brazil)
AMOXICILLIN
Amoxil Pediatric Drops for Oral Suspension 1305
Amoxil Tablets 1305

PEPAR (India)
PIOGLITAZONE HYDROCHLORIDE
Actos Tablets 3077

PEP-BLOC (The Philippines)
RANITIDINE HYDROCHLORIDE
Zantac 25 EFFERdose Tablets 1670
Zantac 150 Tablets 1670
Zantac 300 Tablets 1670
Zantac Injection 1666
Zantac Injection Premixed 1666
Zantac Syrup 1670

PEPCID (Australia, Austria, Finland, Germany, Hong Kong, Irish Republic, New Zealand, Norway, South Africa, Spain, Sweden, Switzerland, The Netherlands)
FAMOTIDINE
Pepcid for Oral Suspension 2075
Pepcid Tablets 2075

PEPCIDAC (France)
FAMOTIDINE
Pepcid for Oral Suspension 2075
Pepcid Tablets 2075

PEPCIDIN (Denmark, Finland, Norway, Sweden, The Netherlands)
FAMOTIDINE
Pepcid for Oral Suspension 2075
Pepcid Tablets 2075

PEPCIDINA (Portugal)
FAMOTIDINE
Pepcid for Oral Suspension 2075
Pepcid Tablets 2075

PEPCIDINE (Australia, Austria, Belgium, Hong Kong, Malaysia, Mexico, New Zealand, Singapore, Switzerland, Thailand, The Philippines, Venezuela)
FAMOTIDINE
Pepcid for Oral Suspension 2075
Pepcid Tablets 2075

PEPCINE (Thailand)
FAMOTIDINE
Pepcid for Oral Suspension 2075
Pepcid Tablets 2075

PEPDENAL (Thailand)
FAMOTIDINE
Pepcid for Oral Suspension 2075
Pepcid Tablets 2075

PEPDIF (Turkey)
FAMOTIDINE
Pepcid for Oral Suspension 2075
Pepcid Tablets 2075

PEPDINE (France)
FAMOTIDINE
Pepcid for Oral Suspension 2075
Pepcid Tablets 2075

PEPDUL (Germany)
FAMOTIDINE
Pepcid for Oral Suspension 2075
Pepcid Tablets 2075

PEPFAMIN (Thailand)
FAMOTIDINE
Pepcid for Oral Suspension 2075
Pepcid Tablets 2075

PEP-RANI (Portugal)
RANITIDINE HYDROCHLORIDE
Zantac 25 EFFERdose Tablets 1670
Zantac 150 Tablets 1670
Zantac 300 Tablets 1670
Zantac Injection 1666
Zantac Injection Premixed 1666
Zantac Syrup 1670

PEPTAB (Portugal)
RANITIDINE HYDROCHLORIDE
Zantac 25 EFFERdose Tablets 1670
Zantac 150 Tablets 1670
Zantac 300 Tablets 1670
Zantac Injection 1666
Zantac Injection Premixed 1666
Zantac Syrup 1670

PEPTAN (Greece)
FAMOTIDINE
Pepcid for Oral Suspension 2075
Pepcid Tablets 2075

PEPTIC GUARD (Canada)
FAMOTIDINE
Pepcid for Oral Suspension 2075
Pepcid Tablets 2075

PEPTIC RELIEF (Canada)
RANITIDINE HYDROCHLORIDE
Zantac 25 EFFERdose Tablets 1670
Zantac 150 Tablets 1670
Zantac 300 Tablets 1670
Zantac Injection 1666
Zantac Injection Premixed 1666
Zantac Syrup 1670

PEPTIFAR (Portugal)
RANITIDINE HYDROCHLORIDE
Zantac 25 EFFERdose Tablets 1670
Zantac 150 Tablets 1670
Zantac 300 Tablets 1670
Zantac Injection 1666
Zantac Injection Premixed 1666
Zantac Syrup 1670

PEPTIGAL (Hungary)
FAMOTIDINE
Pepcid for Oral Suspension 2075
Pepcid Tablets 2075

PEPTOCI (Thailand)
FAMOTIDINE
Pepcid for Oral Suspension 2075
Pepcid Tablets 2075

PEPTONORM (Greece)
SUCRALFATE
Carafate Suspension 706
Carafate Tablets 707

PEPTRAD (The Philippines)
TRAMADOL HYDROCHLORIDE
Ultram ER Tablets 2428

PEPZAN (Australia, Hong Kong, Malaysia, New Zealand, Singapore)
FAMOTIDINE
Pepcid for Oral Suspension 2075
Pepcid Tablets 2075

PERASTHMAN N (Germany)
THEOPHYLLINE
Uniphyl Tablets 2595

PERCLODIN (Irish Republic)
DIPYRIDAMOLE
Persantine Tablets 869

PERENAL (Greece)
LISINOPRIL
Prinivil Tablets 2087

PERICHOL (Denmark)
SIMVASTATIN
Zocor Tablets 2136

PERIPLUM (Italy)
NIMODIPINE
Nimotop Capsules 790

PERISET (India)
ONDANSETRON HYDROCHLORIDE
Zofran Injection 1682
Zofran Injection Premixed 1682
Zofran Oral Solution 1687
Zofran Tablets 1687

PERKOD (France)
DIPYRIDAMOLE
Persantine Tablets 869

PEROXACNE (Spain)
BENZOYL PEROXIDE
Brevoxyl-4 Creamy Wash 3054
Brevoxyl-4 Gel 3054
Brevoxyl-8 Creamy Wash 3054
Brevoxyl-8 Gel 3054

PEROXIBEN (Spain)
BENZOYL PEROXIDE
Brevoxyl-4 Creamy Wash 3054
Brevoxyl-4 Gel 3054
Brevoxyl-8 Creamy Wash 3054
Brevoxyl-8 Gel 3054

PEROXIBEN PLUS (Chile)
BENZOYL PEROXIDE
Brevoxyl-4 Creamy Wash 3054
Brevoxyl-4 Gel 3054
Brevoxyl-8 Creamy Wash 3054
Brevoxyl-8 Gel 3054

PEROXIMICINA (Argentina)
BENZOYL PEROXIDE
Brevoxyl-4 Creamy Wash 3054
Brevoxyl-4 Gel 3054
Brevoxyl-8 Creamy Wash 3054
Brevoxyl-8 Gel 3054

PERSA-GEL W (Australia)
BENZOYL PEROXIDE
Brevoxyl-4 Creamy Wash 3054
Brevoxyl-4 Gel 3054
Brevoxyl-8 Creamy Wash 3054
Brevoxyl-8 Gel 3054

PERSANTIN (Argentina, Australia, Austria, Brazil, Chile, Czech Republic, Denmark, Finland, Germany, Hong Kong, India, Irish Republic, Italy, Japan, Malaysia, Mexico, New Zealand, Norway, Portugal, Russia, Singapore, South Africa, Sweden, Thailand, The Netherlands, The Philippines, United Kingdom, Venezuela)
DIPYRIDAMOLE
Persantine Tablets 869

PERSANTIN PLUS (Hong Kong)
DIPYRIDAMOLE
Persantine Tablets 869

PERSANTIN S (Brazil)
DIPYRIDAMOLE
Persantine Tablets 869

PERSANTINE (Belgium, Canada, France, Switzerland)
DIPYRIDAMOLE
Persantine Tablets 869

PERSOL (India)
BENZOYL PEROXIDE
Brevoxyl-4 Creamy Wash 3054
Brevoxyl-4 Gel 3054
Brevoxyl-8 Creamy Wash 3054
Brevoxyl-8 Gel 3054

PERSOL FORTE (India)
BENZOYL PEROXIDE
Brevoxyl-4 Creamy Wash 3054
Brevoxyl-4 Gel 3054
Brevoxyl-8 Creamy Wash 3054
Brevoxyl-8 Gel 3054

PERTACILON (Greece, Singapore)
CAPTOPRIL
Captopril Tablets 2182

PERTENSO (Argentina)
CLONIDINE
Catapres-TTS 842

PETSIX (India)
FUROSEMIDE
Furosemide Tablets 2186

P-GLITZ (India)
PIOGLITAZONE HYDROCHLORIDE
Actos Tablets 3077

PHAMOPRIL (Germany)
CAPTOPRIL
Captopril Tablets 2182

PHAMORANIT (Germany)
RANITIDINE HYDROCHLORIDE
Zantac 25 EFFERdose Tablets 1670
Zantac 150 Tablets 1670
Zantac 300 Tablets 1670
Zantac Injection 1666
Zantac Injection Premixed 1666
Zantac Syrup 1670

PHARCINA (Mexico)
CIPROFLOXACIN HYDROCHLORIDE
Cipro Tablets 2810

PHARMADOL (Thailand)
TRAMADOL HYDROCHLORIDE
Ultram ER Tablets 2428

PHARMAFIL (Mexico)
THEOPHYLLINE
Uniphyl Tablets 2595

PHARMAFLAM (South Africa)
DICLOFENAC SODIUM
Voltaren Tablets 2334
Voltaren-XR Tablets 2337

PHARMALOSE (Canada)
LACTULOSE
Kristalose for Oral Solution 1004

PHARMAMOX (Switzerland)
AMOXICILLIN
Amoxil Pediatric Drops for Oral Suspension 1305
Amoxil Tablets 1305

PHARMOTIDINE (Thailand)
FAMOTIDINE
Pepcid for Oral Suspension 2075
Pepcid Tablets 2075

PHARMOX (Brazil)
AMOXICILLIN
Amoxil Pediatric Drops for Oral Suspension 1305
Amoxil Tablets 1305

PHARPHYLLINE (The Netherlands)
THEOPHYLLINE
Uniphyl Tablets 2595

PHENEDRINE (Hong Kong, The Philippines)
THEOPHYLLINE
Uniphyl Tablets 2595

PHOS-EX (Austria, Denmark, Finland, Germany, Norway, Sweden, The Netherlands, Turkey, United Kingdom)
CALCIUM ACETATE
PhosLo GelCaps 1184

PHOSFORID (India)
CALCIUM ACETATE
PhosLo GelCaps 1184

PHOSLO (Chile)
CALCIUM ACETATE
PhosLo GelCaps 1184

PHOSTARAC (Argentina)
ALENDRONATE SODIUM
Fosamax Tablets 2005

PHYLOBID (India)
THEOPHYLLINE
Uniphyl Tablets 2595

PHYLODAY (India)
THEOPHYLLINE
Uniphyl Tablets 2595

PHYZIDINE (Hong Kong)
FAMOTIDINE
Pepcid for Oral Suspension 2075
Pepcid Tablets 2075

PIAMFUCIN (Russia)
NATAMYCIN
Natacyn Antifungal Ophthalmic Suspension . . . . ⊙204

PIECIDEX NF (Argentina)
TERBINAFINE HYDROCHLORIDE
Lamisil Tablets 2266

PILOTIM (Argentina)
TIMOLOL MALEATE
Timoptic in Ocudose 2124
Timoptic Sterile Ophthalmic Solution 2121
Timoptic-XE Sterile Ophthalmic Gel Forming Solution 2125

PIMA BICIRON N (Germany)
NATAMYCIN
Natacyn Antifungal Ophthalmic Suspension . . . . ⊙204

PIMAFUCIN (Belgium, Czech Republic, Finland, Germany, Hungary, Poland, Russia, The Netherlands, Turkey, United Kingdom)
NATAMYCIN
Natacyn Antifungal Ophthalmic Suspension . . . . ⊙204

PIMAFUCORT (Poland)
NATAMYCIN
Natacyn Antifungal Ophthalmic Suspension . . . . ⊙204

PINAMOX (Irish Republic)
AMOXICILLIN
Amoxil Pediatric Drops for Oral Suspension 1305
Amoxil Tablets 1305

PIOGLIT (Argentina)
PIOGLITAZONE HYDROCHLORIDE
Actos Tablets 3077

PIOMED (India)
PIOGLITAZONE HYDROCHLORIDE
Actos Tablets 3077

PIOSAFE (India)
PIOGLITAZONE HYDROCHLORIDE
Actos Tablets . . . 3077

PIOZULIN (India)
PIOGLITAZONE HYDROCHLORIDE
Actos Tablets . . . 3077

PIPLEX (Chile)
ISOTRETINOIN
Accutane Capsules . . . 2607

PIPROL (Spain)
CIPROFLOXACIN HYDROCHLORIDE
Cipro Tablets . . . 2810

PIRASMIN (Turkey)
THEOPHYLLINE
Uniphyl Tablets . . . 2595

PIREXYL (Chile)
DICLOFENAC SODIUM
Voltaren Tablets . . . 2334
Voltaren-XR Tablets . . . 2337

PIRIDASMIN (Spain)
THEOPHYLLINE
Uniphyl Tablets . . . 2595

PIRIMECIDAN (Spain)
PYRIMETHAMINE
Daraprim Tablets . . . 1400

PIRITEZE (United Kingdom)
CETIRIZINE HYDROCHLORIDE
Zyrtec Syrup . . . 1920
Zyrtec Tablets . . . 1920

PIROBAC (Chile)
BENZOYL PEROXIDE
Brevoxyl-4 Creamy Wash . . . 3054
Brevoxyl-4 Gel . . . 3054
Brevoxyl-8 Creamy Wash . . . 3054
Brevoxyl-8 Gel . . . 3054

PISTOFIL (Greece)
NORFLOXACIN
Noroxin Tablets . . . 2069

PLACIDIAX (Argentina)
CLONAZEPAM
Klonopin Tablets . . . 2639

PLACIDOX (India)
DIAZEPAM
Valium Tablets . . . 2658

PLAMOX (Argentina)
AMOXICILLIN
Amoxil Pediatric Drops for Oral Suspension . . . 1305
Amoxil Tablets . . . 1305

PLAN (Argentina)
ATORVASTATIN CALCIUM
Lipitor Tablets . . . 2501

PLANITRIX (Greece)
FENOFIBRATE
Tricor Tablets . . . 520

PLASIMINE (Spain)
MUPIROCIN
Bactroban Ointment . . . 1368

PLATELET (Italy)
DIPYRIDAMOLE
Persantine Tablets . . . 869

PLATO (South Africa)
DIPYRIDAMOLE
Persantine Tablets . . . 869

PLAUCINA (Spain)
ENOXAPARIN SODIUM
Lovenox Injection . . . 2756

PLAUDIT (Italy)
FLUNISOLIDE
Aerobid Inhaler System . . . 1153
Aerobid-M Inhaler System . . . 1153

PLAVIX (Argentina, Australia, Austria, Belgium, Brazil, Chile, Czech Republic, Denmark, Germany, Greece, Hungary, India, Israel, Italy, Mexico, New Zealand, Norway, Portugal, Russia, South Africa, Spain, Thailand, The Philippines, Turkey, Venezuela)
CLOPIDOGREL BISULFATE
Plavix Tablets . . . 926, 2767

PLENOLYT (Spain)
CIPROFLOXACIN HYDROCHLORIDE
Cipro Tablets . . . 2810

PLENTY (Brazil)
SIBUTRAMINE HYDROCHLORIDE
Meridia Capsules . . . 475

PLETAAL (Argentina, Hong Kong, Japan, Thailand, The Philippines)
CILOSTAZOL
Pletal Tablets . . . 2481

PLETAL (United Kingdom)
CILOSTAZOL
Pletal Tablets . . . 2481

PLETOZ (India)
CILOSTAZOL
Pletal Tablets . . . 2481

PLEXXO (Poland, The Netherlands)
LAMOTRIGINE
Lamictal Chewable Dispersible Tablets . . . 1488
Lamictal Tablets . . . 1488

PLEYAR (Argentina)
CLOPIDOGREL BISULFATE
Plavix Tablets . . . 926, 2767

PLIDAN (Argentina)
DIAZEPAM
Valium Tablets . . . 2658

PLIDEX (Argentina)
DIAZEPAM
Valium Tablets . . . 2658

PLIDEX T (Argentina)
DIAZEPAM
Valium Tablets . . . 2658

PLIXYM (Poland)
CEFUROXIME SODIUM
Zinacef Injection . . . 1678

PLOSTIM (Argentina)
TIMOLOL MALEATE
Timoptic in Ocudose . . . 2124
Timoptic Sterile Ophthalmic Solution . . . 2121
Timoptic-XE Sterile Ophthalmic Gel Forming Solution . . . 2125

PLURAIR (Brazil)
FLUTICASONE PROPIONATE
Flonase Nasal Spray . . . 1431

PLURIMEN (Spain)
SELEGILINE HYDROCHLORIDE
Eldepryl Capsules . . . 3052

PLUSEPTIC (Argentina)
CEFTAZIDIME
Fortaz for Injection . . . 1450

PLUSGIN (Argentina)
CIPROFLOXACIN
Cipro Oral Suspension . . . 2810

PLUSTAXANO (Argentina)
DOCETAXEL
Taxotere Injection Concentrate . . . 2773

PODIUM (Spain)
DIAZEPAM
Valium Tablets . . . 2658

POENTIMOL (Argentina)
TIMOLOL MALEATE
Timoptic in Ocudose . . . 2124
Timoptic Sterile Ophthalmic Solution . . . 2121
Timoptic-XE Sterile Ophthalmic Gel Forming Solution . . . 2125

POINT (Israel)
NAPROXEN SODIUM
Anaprox DS Tablets . . . 2632
Anaprox Tablets . . . 2632

POLCORTOLON TC (Poland)
TRIAMCINOLONE ACETONIDE
Azmacort Inhalation Aerosol . . . 407
Nasacort AQ Nasal Spray . . . 2765

POLET (Mexico)
NAPROXEN
EC-Naprosyn Delayed-Release Tablets . . . 2632
Naprosyn Suspension . . . 2632
Naprosyn Tablets . . . 2632

POLFENON (Poland)
PROPAFENONE HYDROCHLORIDE
Rythmol SR Capsules . . . 1590

POLIBAC (Brazil)
AMOXICILLIN
Amoxil Pediatric Drops for Oral Suspension . . . 1305
Amoxil Tablets . . . 1305

POLICANO (Greece)
ISOTRETINOIN
Accutane Capsules . . . 2607

POLI-CIFLOXIN (Thailand)
CIPROFLOXACIN
Cipro Oral Suspension . . . 2810

POLICOR (Argentina)
CILOSTAZOL
Pletal Tablets . . . 2481

POLIREUMIN (Brazil)
SODIUM HYALURONATE
Hyalgan Solution . . . 2742

POLIXIMA (Italy)
CEFUROXIME SODIUM
Zinacef Injection . . . 1678

POLLENSHIELD (United Kingdom)
CETIRIZINE HYDROCHLORIDE
Zyrtec Syrup . . . 1920
Zyrtec Tablets . . . 1920

POLTAX (Brazil)
DICLOFENAC SODIUM
Voltaren Tablets . . . 2334
Voltaren-XR Tablets . . . 2337

POLTRAM (Poland)
TRAMADOL HYDROCHLORIDE
Ultram ER Tablets . . . 2428

POLYANION (Austria)
PENTOSAN POLYSULFATE SODIUM
Elmiron Capsules . . . 2435

POLYCITRA-K (Canada)
POTASSIUM CITRATE
Urocit-K Tablets . . . 2176

POLYFLAM (Belgium)
DICLOFENAC SODIUM
Voltaren Tablets . . . 2334
Voltaren-XR Tablets . . . 2337

POLYXEN (Thailand)
NAPROXEN
EC-Naprosyn Delayed-Release Tablets . . . 2632
Naprosyn Suspension . . . 2632
Naprosyn Tablets . . . 2632

PONDERA (Brazil)
PAROXETINE HYDROCHLORIDE
Paxil Oral Suspension . . . 1535
Paxil Tablets . . . 1535

PONDTROXIN (Thailand)
LEVOTHYROXINE SODIUM
Levothroid Tablets . . . 1170
Levoxyl Tablets . . . 1780
Synthroid Tablets . . . 507

PONTALSIC (Spain)
TRAMADOL HYDROCHLORIDE
Ultram ER Tablets . . . 2428

POROSAL (Venezuela)
ALENDRONATE SODIUM
Fosamax Tablets . . . 2005

PORUXIN (Greece)
FINASTERIDE
Propecia Tablets . . . 2095
Proscar Tablets . . . 2102

POSANIN (Thailand)
DIPYRIDAMOLE
Persantine Tablets . . . 869

POSIVYL (Chile)
PAROXETINE HYDROCHLORIDE
Paxil Oral Suspension . . . 1535
Paxil Tablets . . . 1535

POSNAC (Thailand)
DICLOFENAC SODIUM
Voltaren Tablets . . . 2334
Voltaren-XR Tablets . . . 2337

POTCIT (Malaysia)
POTASSIUM CITRATE
Urocit-K Tablets . . . 2176

POTENCORT (United Arab Emirates)
FLUTICASONE PROPIONATE
Flonase Nasal Spray . . . 1431

POTENDAL (Spain)
CEFTAZIDIME
Fortaz for Injection . . . 1450

POVANIL (Thailand)
CLONAZEPAM
Klonopin Tablets . . . 2639

POWERCEF (India)
CEFTRIAXONE SODIUM
Rocephin Injectable Vials, ADD-Vantage, Galaxy, Bulk . . . 2642

POWERGYL (India)
NORFLOXACIN
Noroxin Tablets . . . 2069

PRACAP (Brazil)
FINASTERIDE
Propecia Tablets . . . 2095
Proscar Tablets . . . 2102

PRACEM (Mexico)
DIPYRIDAMOLE
Persantine Tablets . . . 869

PRADIF (Greece, Italy, Portugal, Switzerland)
TAMSULOSIN HYDROCHLORIDE
Flomax Capsules . . . 848

PRAM (Austria)
CITALOPRAM HYDROBROMIDE
Celexa Tablets . . . 1160

PRAMCIL (Chile)
CITALOPRAM HYDROBROMIDE
Celexa Tablets . . . 1160

PRAMEXYL (Italy)
CITALOPRAM HYDROBROMIDE
Celexa Tablets . . . 1160

PRANADOX (Mexico)
ZIDOVUDINE
Retrovir Capsules . . . 1574
Retrovir IV Infusion . . . 1579
Retrovir Syrup . . . 1574
Retrovir Tablets . . . 1574

PRANDASE (Canada, Israel)
ACARBOSE
Precose Tablets . . . 792

PRANDIN E2 (South Africa)
DINOPROSTONE
Cervidil Vaginal Insert . . . 1165

PRANDIOL (France)
DIPYRIDAMOLE
Persantine Tablets . . . 869

PRANOXEN (South Africa)
NAPROXEN
EC-Naprosyn Delayed-Release Tablets . . . 2632
Naprosyn Suspension . . . 2632
Naprosyn Tablets . . . 2632

PRANOXEN CONTINUS (United Kingdom)
NAPROXEN
EC-Naprosyn Delayed-Release Tablets . . . 2632
Naprosyn Suspension . . . 2632
Naprosyn Tablets . . . 2632

PRAXEDOL (Mexico)
NAPROXEN
EC-Naprosyn Delayed-Release Tablets . . . 2632
Naprosyn Suspension . . . 2632
Naprosyn Tablets . . . 2632

PRECAPTIL (Mexico)
CAPTOPRIL
Captopril Tablets . . . 2182

PRECAR (Venezuela)
DIPYRIDAMOLE
Persantine Tablets . . . 869

PRE-CLAR (Chile)
CLARITHROMYCIN
Biaxin Filmtab Tablets . . . 411
Biaxin Granules . . . 411

PREDALGIC (France)
TRAMADOL HYDROCHLORIDE
Ultram ER Tablets . . . 2428

PREDONIUM (Austria, Hong Kong, New Zealand, Portugal, The Netherlands)
PERINDOPRIL ERBUMINE
Aceon Tablets (2 mg, 4 mg, 8 mg) . . . 3038

PREDXAL (Mexico)
TELMISARTAN
Micardis Tablets . . . 852

PREDXAL PLUS (Mexico)
TELMISARTAN
Micardis Tablets . . . 852

PREFEST (Brazil)
ESTRADIOL
Climara Transdermal System . . . 763

PRELAT (The Philippines)
CAPTOPRIL
Captopril Tablets . . . 2182

PRELECTAL (Italy)
PERINDOPRIL ERBUMINE
Aceon Tablets (2 mg, 4 mg, 8 mg) . . . 3038

PREMASTAN (Mexico)
PROGESTERONE
Crinone 4% Gel . . . 992
Prometrium Capsules (100 mg, 200 mg) . 3047

PREMJACT (United Kingdom)
LIDOCAINE
Lidoderm Patch . . . 1114

PRENESSA (Poland)
PERINDOPRIL ERBUMINE
Aceon Tablets (2 mg, 4 mg, 8 mg) . . . 3038

PREPIDIL (Austria, Belgium, Canada, Czech Republic, France, Germany, Hong Kong, Hungary, Irish Republic, Israel, Italy, Mexico, New Zealand, Poland, Russia, South Africa, Spain, Switzerland, The Netherlands, United Kingdom)
DINOPROSTONE
Cervidil Vaginal Insert . . . 1165

PRERAN (Japan)
TRANDOLAPRIL
Mavik Tablets . . . 472

PRESAR (Spain)
CITALOPRAM HYDROBROMIDE
Celexa Tablets . . . 1160

PRESARTAN (Venezuela)
LOSARTAN POTASSIUM
Cozaar Tablets . . . 1973

PRESCAL (Irish Republic, United Kingdom)
ISRADIPINE
DynaCirc CR Tablets . . . 1407

PRESINOR (Argentina)
LOSARTAN POTASSIUM
Cozaar Tablets . . . 1973

PRESINOR D (Argentina)
LOSARTAN POTASSIUM
Cozaar Tablets . . . 1973

PRESOKIN (Chile)
LISINOPRIL
Prinivil Tablets . . . 2087

PRESOQUIN (Venezuela)
DILTIAZEM HYDROCHLORIDE
Cardizem LA Extended Release Tablets . . . 421

PRESS-12 (Greece)
LISINOPRIL
Prinivil Tablets . . . 2087

PRESSOMAX (Brazil)
CAPTOPRIL
Captopril Tablets . . . 2182

PRESSURAL (Italy)
INDAPAMIDE
Indapamide Tablets . . . 2188

PRESSURIL (Greece)
LISINOPRIL
Prinivil Tablets . . . 2087

PRESTARIUM (Czech Republic)
PERINDOPRIL ERBUMINE
Aceon Tablets (2 mg, 4 mg, 8 mg) . . . 3038

PRESTARIUM PLUS (Poland)
PERINDOPRIL ERBUMINE
Aceon Tablets (2 mg, 4 mg, 8 mg) . . . 3038

PRESTOLE (France)
HYDROCHLOROTHIAZIDE/TRIAMTERENE
Dyazide Capsules . . . 1405

PRETANIX (Hungary)
INDAPAMIDE
Indapamide Tablets . . . 2188

PRETERAX (Argentina, Austria, Belgium, Brazil, Canada, Germany, Greece, Irish Republic, Italy, Mexico, Portugal, Singapore, South Africa, Spain, Switzerland, The Netherlands, The Philippines, Turkey, Venezuela)
PERINDOPRIL ERBUMINE
Aceon Tablets (2 mg, 4 mg, 8 mg) . . . 3038

PREVENCOR (Spain)
ATORVASTATIN CALCIUM
Lipitor Tablets . . . 2501

PREXAN (Italy)
NAPROXEN
EC-Naprosyn Delayed-Release Tablets . . . 2632
Naprosyn Suspension . . . 2632
Naprosyn Tablets . . . 2632

PREXUM (South Africa)
PERINDOPRIL ERBUMINE
Aceon Tablets (2 mg, 4 mg, 8 mg) . . . 3038

PREXUM PLUS (South Africa)
PERINDOPRIL ERBUMINE
Aceon Tablets (2 mg, 4 mg, 8 mg) . . . 3038

PRIALTA (The Philippines)
PIOGLITAZONE HYDROCHLORIDE
Actos Tablets . . . 3077

PRILOSIN (South Africa)
LISINOPRIL
Prinivil Tablets . . . 2087

PRILOVASE (Portugal)
CAPTOPRIL
Captopril Tablets . . . 2182

PRILPRESSIN (Brazil)
CAPTOPRIL
Captopril Tablets . . . 2182

PRIMAQUIN (Chile)
ESTRADIOL
Climara Transdermal System . . . 763

PRIMAXIN (Canada, Greece, United Kingdom)
CILASTATIN SODIUM/IMIPENEM
Primaxin I.M. . . . 2080
Primaxin I.V. . . . 2083

PRIMERAL (Italy)
NAPROXEN SODIUM
Anaprox DS Tablets . . . 2632
Anaprox Tablets . . . 2632

PRIMESIN (Italy, Switzerland)
FLUVASTATIN SODIUM
Lescol Capsules . . . 2268

PRIMIPROST (India)
DINOPROSTONE
Cervidil Vaginal Insert . . . 1165

PRIMOCID (Greece)
CLARITHROMYCIN
Biaxin Filmtab Tablets . . . 411
Biaxin Granules . . . 411

PRIMOFENAC (Switzerland)
DICLOFENAC SODIUM
Voltaren Tablets . . . 2334
Voltaren-XR Tablets . . . 2337

PRIMOSON-F (Mexico)
PROGESTERONE
Crinone 4% Gel . . . 992
Prometrium Capsules (100 mg, 200 mg) . 3047

PRIMULEX (Hungary)
SELEGILINE HYDROCHLORIDE
Eldepryl Capsules . . . 3052

PRINARTEN (Mexico)
CAPTOPRIL
Captopril Tablets . . . 2182

PRINCESS PROLIB (Spain)
FLUVASTATIN SODIUM
Lescol Capsules . . . 2268

PRINCIPROX (Switzerland)
CIPROFLOXACIN HYDROCHLORIDE
Cipro Tablets . . . 2810

PRINIL (Switzerland)
LISINOPRIL
Prinivil Tablets . . . 2087

PRINISER (Mexico)
LISINOPRIL
Prinivil Tablets . . . 2087

PRINIVIL (Australia, Austria, Brazil, Canada, Czech Republic, France, Greece, Hong Kong, Italy, Malaysia, Mexico, New Zealand, Poland, Portugal, Singapore, South Africa, Spain, Venezuela)
LISINOPRIL
Prinivil Tablets . . . 2087

PRINIVIL PLUS (Spain)
HYDROCHLOROTHIAZIDE/LISINOPRIL
Prinzide Tablets . . . 2092

PRINZIDE (Austria, Brazil, Canada, France, Italy, Mexico, New Zealand, Portugal, Switzerland)
HYDROCHLOROTHIAZIDE/LISINOPRIL
Prinzide Tablets . . . 2092

PRISDAL (Spain)
CITALOPRAM HYDROBROMIDE
Celexa Tablets . . . 1160

PRISMA (Chile)
CITALOPRAM HYDROBROMIDE
Celexa Tablets . . . 1160

PRITOR (Argentina, Australia, Brazil, Czech Republic, France, Greece, Hungary, Italy, Poland, Portugal, Russia, Spain, The Netherlands, The Philippines, Turkey, Venezuela)
TELMISARTAN
Micardis Tablets . . . 852

PRITOR HCT (Brazil)
TELMISARTAN
Micardis Tablets . . . 852

PRITOR PLUS (Greece, Poland, Portugal, Spain, Turkey, Venezuela)
TELMISARTAN
Micardis Tablets . . . 852

PRITORAL (Chile)
TELMISARTAN
Micardis Tablets . . . 852

PRITORPLUS (France, Hungary, Italy, The Netherlands, The Philippines)
TELMISARTAN
Micardis Tablets . . . 852

PRIXAR (Italy, The Netherlands)
LEVOFLOXACIN
Levaquin Injection . . . 2416
Levaquin Tablets . . . 2416

PRIXLAE (The Philippines)
CETIRIZINE HYDROCHLORIDE
Zyrtec Syrup . . . 1920
Zyrtec Tablets . . . 1920

PRIZEM (Mexico)
DIAZEPAM
Valium Tablets . . . 2658

PROACNE (Thailand)
ISOTRETINOIN
Accutane Capsules . . . 2607

PROAIR (Argentina)
FLUTICASONE PROPIONATE
Flonase Nasal Spray . . . 1431

PROCAPTAN (Italy)
PERINDOPRIL ERBUMINE
Aceon Tablets (2 mg, 4 mg, 8 mg) . . . 3038

PROCARDIN (Hong Kong, Singapore)
DIPYRIDAMOLE
Persantine Tablets . . . 869

PROCETOKEN (Argentina)
FENOFIBRATE
Tricor Tablets . . . 520

PROCIN (Brazil)
CIPROFLOXACIN
Cipro Oral Suspension . . . 2810

PROCIP (India)
CIPROFLOXACIN
Cipro Oral Suspension . . . 2810

PROCOR (Brazil)
DIPYRIDAMOLE
Persantine Tablets . . . 869

PROCOR S (Brazil)
DIPYRIDAMOLE
Persantine Tablets . . . 869

PROCTOCREM (Argentina)
LIDOCAINE
Lidoderm Patch . . . 1114

PRO-CURE (Israel)
FINASTERIDE
Propecia Tablets . . . 2095
Proscar Tablets . . . 2102

PROCUTA (France)
ISOTRETINOIN
Accutane Capsules . . . 2607

PROCYTHOL (Greece)
SELEGILINE HYDROCHLORIDE
Eldepryl Capsules . . . 3052

PRODOLOR (Germany)
NAPROXEN
EC-Naprosyn Delayed-Release Tablets . . . 2632
Naprosyn Suspension . . . 2632
Naprosyn Tablets . . . 2632

PRODOXIN (Brazil)
CEFTRIAXONE SODIUM
Rocephin Injectable Vials, ADD-Vantage, Galaxy, Bulk . . . 2642

PRODUVIR (Brazil)
ZIDOVUDINE
Retrovir Capsules . . . 1574
Retrovir IV Infusion . . . 1579
Retrovir Syrup . . . 1574
Retrovir Tablets . . . 1574

PROFENAC (India)
DICLOFENAC SODIUM
Voltaren Tablets . . . 2334
Voltaren-XR Tablets . . . 2337

PROFEX (Israel)
PROPAFENONE HYDROCHLORIDE
Rythmol SR Capsules . . . 1590

PROFINE (India)
PROGESTERONE
Crinone 4% Gel . . . 992
Prometrium Capsules (100 mg, 200 mg) . 3047

PROFLAX (Argentina)
TIMOLOL MALEATE
Timoptic in Ocudose . . . 2124
Timoptic Sterile Ophthalmic Solution . . . 2121
Timoptic-XE Sterile Ophthalmic Gel Forming Solution . . . 2125

PROFLOX (Brazil, Thailand)
CIPROFLOXACIN
Cipro Oral Suspension . . . 2810

PROFLOXIN (Australia, Irish Republic)
CIPROFLOXACIN HYDROCHLORIDE
Cipro Tablets . . . 2810

PROFUREX (The Philippines)
CEFUROXIME SODIUM
Zinacef Injection . . . 1678

PROGEFFIK (Italy, Spain)
PROGESTERONE
Crinone 4% Gel . . . 992
Prometrium Capsules (100 mg, 200 mg) . 3047

PROGENAR (Portugal)
PROGESTERONE
Crinone 4% Gel . . . 992
Prometrium Capsules (100 mg, 200 mg) . 3047

PROGENDO (Chile, Venezuela)
PROGESTERONE
Crinone 4% Gel . . . 992
Prometrium Capsules (100 mg, 200 mg) . 3047

PROGERING (Chile)
PROGESTERONE
Crinone 4% Gel . . . 992
Prometrium Capsules (100 mg, 200 mg) . 3047

PROGEST (Argentina, India)
PROGESTERONE
Crinone 4% Gel . . . 992
Prometrium Capsules (100 mg, 200 mg) . 3047

PROGESTAN (The Netherlands, Turkey)
PROGESTERONE
Crinone 4% Gel . . . 992
Prometrium Capsules (100 mg, 200 mg) . 3047

PROGESTASERT (Canada, France)
PROGESTERONE
Crinone 4% Gel . . . 992
Prometrium Capsules (100 mg, 200 mg) . 3047

PROGESTERONE IMPLANTS (United Kingdom)
PROGESTERONE
Crinone 4% Gel . . . 992
Prometrium Capsules (100 mg, 200 mg) . 3047

PROGESTOGEL (Belgium, France, Hong Kong, Italy, Portugal, Russia, Spain, Switzerland, Thailand, Venezuela)
PROGESTERONE
Crinone 4% Gel . . . 992

Prometrium Capsules (100 mg, 200 mg) . 3047

PROGESTOL (Italy)
PROGESTERONE
Crinone 4% Gel . . . 992
Prometrium Capsules (100 mg, 200 mg) . 3047

PROGESTOSOL (France, Spain, Switzerland)
PROGESTERONE
Crinone 4% Gel . . . 992
Prometrium Capsules (100 mg, 200 mg) . 3047

PROGOR (Belgium, Thailand)
DILTIAZEM HYDROCHLORIDE
Cardizem LA Extended Release Tablets . . . 421

PROGRAF (Argentina, Australia, Austria, Brazil, Canada, Chile, Czech Republic, Denmark, Finland, France, Germany, Greece, Hong Kong, Hungary, Irish Republic, Israel, Italy, Japan, Malaysia, Mexico, New Zealand, Norway, Poland, Portugal, Singapore, South Africa, Spain, Sweden, Switzerland, Thailand, The Philippines, Turkey, United Kingdom, Venezuela)
TACROLIMUS
Prograf Capsules and Injection . . . 622

PROGRAFT (Belgium, The Netherlands)
TACROLIMUS
Prograf Capsules and Injection . . . 622

PROGYNOVA (United Kingdom)
ESTRADIOL
Climara Transdermal System . . . 763

PROHAIR (Brazil, Chile)
FINASTERIDE
Propecia Tablets . . . 2095
Proscar Tablets . . . 2102

PRO-HDL (India)
LOVASTATIN
Mevacor Tablets . . . 2063

PROLDIN (Mexico)
CAPTOPRIL
Captopril Tablets . . . 2182

PROLEKOFEN (Czech Republic)
PROPAFENONE HYDROCHLORIDE
Rythmol SR Capsules . . . 1590

PROLIDON (Mexico)
PROGESTERONE
Crinone 4% Gel . . . 992
Prometrium Capsules (100 mg, 200 mg) . 3047

PROLIPASE (Argentina, Austria, Switzerland)
PANCRELIPASE
Ultrase Capsules . . . 718
Ultrase MT Capsules . . . 719

PROLISINA E2 (Argentina)
DINOPROSTONE
Cervidil Vaginal Insert . . . 1165

PROLONG (Chile)
LIDOCAINE
Lidoderm Patch . . . 1114

PROLUTON (Argentina, Australia, Italy, Thailand)
PROGESTERONE
Crinone 4% Gel . . . 992
Prometrium Capsules (100 mg, 200 mg) . 3047

PROMAL (Austria)
ATOVAQUONE
Mepron Suspension . . . 1526

PROMETRIUM (Canada, Italy)
PROGESTERONE
Crinone 4% Gel . . . 992
Prometrium Capsules (100 mg, 200 mg) . 3047

PRONASTERON (Brazil)
FINASTERIDE
Propecia Tablets . . . 2095
Proscar Tablets . . . 2102

PRONAT (Mexico)
NAPROXEN
EC-Naprosyn Delayed-Release Tablets . . . 2632
Naprosyn Suspension . . . 2632
Naprosyn Tablets . . . 2632

PRONAXEN (Finland, Sweden)
NAPROXEN
EC-Naprosyn Delayed-Release Tablets . . . 2632
Naprosyn Suspension . . . 2632
Naprosyn Tablets . . . 2632

PRONAXIL (Mexico)
NAPROXEN
EC-Naprosyn Delayed-Release Tablets . . . 2632
Naprosyn Suspension . . . 2632
Naprosyn Tablets . . . 2632

PRONAX-P (Mexico)
NAPROXEN SODIUM
Anaprox DS Tablets . . . 2632
Anaprox Tablets . . . 2632

PRONIX (Argentina)
DICLOFENAC SODIUM
Voltaren Tablets . . . 2334
Voltaren-XR Tablets . . . 2337

PRONOXEN (Mexico)
NAPROXEN
EC-Naprosyn Delayed-Release Tablets . . . 2632
Naprosyn Suspension . . . 2632
Naprosyn Tablets . . . 2632

PRONTALGIN (Italy)
TRAMADOL HYDROCHLORIDE
Ultram ER Tablets . . . 2428

PRONTOCID N (Germany)
FORMALDEHYDE
Formadon Solution . . . 1699

PRONTOFORT (Mexico)
TRAMADOL HYDROCHLORIDE
Ultram ER Tablets . . . 2428

PRONTOGEST (Italy)
PROGESTERONE
Crinone 4% Gel . . . 992
Prometrium Capsules (100 mg, 200 mg) . 3047

PROOTOCIPRO (Argentina)
CIPROFLOXACIN
Cipro Oral Suspension . . . 2810

PROPAFEN (Germany)
PROPAFENONE HYDROCHLORIDE
Rythmol SR Capsules . . . 1590

PROPAM (New Zealand)
DIAZEPAM
Valium Tablets . . . 2658

PRO-PAM (Australia)
DIAZEPAM
Valium Tablets . . . 2658

PROPAMERCK (Germany)
PROPAFENONE HYDROCHLORIDE
Rythmol SR Capsules . . . 1590

PROPANORM (Czech Republic, Russia)
PROPAFENONE HYDROCHLORIDE
Rythmol SR Capsules . . . 1590

PROPA-ORAMON (Germany)
PROPAFENONE HYDROCHLORIDE
Rythmol SR Capsules . . . 1590

PROPASTAD (Germany)
PROPAFENONE HYDROCHLORIDE
Rythmol SR Capsules . . . 1590

PROPA-TABLETTEN (Czech Republic)
PROPAFENONE HYDROCHLORIDE
Rythmol SR Capsules . . . 1590

PROPECIA (Argentina, Australia, Austria, Brazil, Canada, Czech Republic, Denmark, Finland, France, Germany, Greece, Hong Kong, Israel, Italy, Malaysia, New Zealand, Poland, Portugal, Singapore, South Africa, Spain, Sweden, Switzerland, Thailand, The Netherlands, The Philippines, Turkey, United Kingdom, Venezuela)
FINASTERIDE
Propecia Tablets . . . 2095
Proscar Tablets . . . 2102

PROPERIL (Chile)
CAPTOPRIL
Captopril Tablets . . . 2182

PROPESHIA (Mexico)
FINASTERIDE
Propecia Tablets . . . 2095
Proscar Tablets . . . 2102

PROPESS (Argentina, Austria, Czech Republic, Denmark, Finland, France, Germany, Greece, Hong Kong, Hungary, Irish Republic, Israel, Italy, Mexico, Poland, Portugal, South Africa, Spain, Sweden, Switzerland, The Netherlands, United Kingdom)
DINOPROSTONE
Cervidil Vaginal Insert . . . 1165

PROPIONAL (Mexico)
NAPROXEN
EC-Naprosyn Delayed-Release Tablets . . . 2632
Naprosyn Suspension . . . 2632
Naprosyn Tablets . . . 2632

PROQUIN (Australia)
CIPROFLOXACIN HYDROCHLORIDE
Cipro Tablets . . . 2810

PRORYNORM (Germany)
PROPAFENONE HYDROCHLORIDE
Rythmol SR Capsules . . . 1590

PROSAID (United Kingdom)
NAPROXEN
EC-Naprosyn Delayed-Release Tablets . . . 2632
Naprosyn Suspension . . . 2632
Naprosyn Tablets . . . 2632

PROSCAR (Argentina, Australia, Austria, Belgium, Brazil, Canada, Chile, Czech Republic, Denmark, Finland, Germany, Greece, Hong Kong, Hungary, Irish Republic, Italy, Malaysia, Mexico, New Zealand, Norway, Poland, Portugal, Russia, Singapore, South Africa, Spain, Sweden, Switzerland, Thailand, The Netherlands, The Philippines, Turkey, United Kingdom, Venezuela)
FINASTERIDE
Propecia Tablets . . . 2095
Proscar Tablets . . . 2102

PROSDINA (Venezuela)
FINASTERIDE
Propecia Tablets . . . 2095
Proscar Tablets . . . 2102

PROSERINE (Thailand)
CYCLOSERINE
Seromycin Capsules . . . 1864

PROSMIN (Argentina)
FINASTERIDE
Propecia Tablets . . . 2095
Proscar Tablets . . . 2102

PROSTALL (Chile)
TAMSULOSIN HYDROCHLORIDE
Flomax Capsules . . . 848

PROSTAMNIC (Poland)
TAMSULOSIN HYDROCHLORIDE
Flomax Capsules . . . 848

PROSTANIL (Argentina)
FINASTERIDE
Propecia Tablets . . . 2095
Proscar Tablets . . . 2102

PROSTANOVAG (Argentina)
FINASTERIDE
Propecia Tablets . . . 2095
Proscar Tablets . . . 2102

PROSTENE (Argentina)
FINASTERIDE
Propecia Tablets . . . 2095
Proscar Tablets . . . 2102

PROSTERID (Hungary)
FINASTERIDE
Propecia Tablets . . . 2095
Proscar Tablets . . . 2102

PROSTERIT (Turkey)
FINASTERIDE
Propecia Tablets . . . 2095
Proscar Tablets . . . 2102

PROSTIDE (Brazil, Italy)
FINASTERIDE
Propecia Tablets . . . 2095
Proscar Tablets . . . 2102

PROSTIN E2 (Australia, Austria, Belgium, Canada, Czech Republic, Greece, Hong Kong, Hungary, Irish Republic, Israel, Italy, Malaysia, New Zealand, Portugal, Russia, Singapore, South Africa, Switzerland, Thailand, The Netherlands, United Kingdom)
DINOPROSTONE
Cervidil Vaginal Insert . . . 1165

PROSTINE E2 (France)
DINOPROSTONE
Cervidil Vaginal Insert . . . 1165

PROTANGIX (France)
DIPYRIDAMOLE
Persantine Tablets . . . 869

PROTEVIS (Argentina)
TIMOLOL MALEATE
Timoptic in Ocudose . . . 2124
Timoptic Sterile Ophthalmic Solution . . . 2121
Timoptic-XE Sterile Ophthalmic Gel Forming Solution . . . 2125

PROTININ (Mexico)
APROTININ
Trasylol Injection . . . 799

PROTOPIC (Argentina, Austria, Belgium, Canada, Chile, Denmark, Finland, France, Germany, Greece, Hong Kong, Irish Republic, Israel, Italy, Japan, Norway, Poland, Portugal, Spain, Sweden, Switzerland, Thailand, The Netherlands, United Kingdom)
TACROLIMUS
Prograf Capsules and Injection . . . 622

PROTOPY (The Netherlands)
TACROLIMUS
Prograf Capsules and Injection . . . 622

PROTOSOL (Israel)
APROTININ
Trasylol Injection . . . 799

PROTRADON (Czech Republic)
TRAMADOL HYDROCHLORIDE
Ultram ER Tablets . . . 2428

PROVAMES (France)
ESTRADIOL
Climara Transdermal System . . . 763

PROVAS (Switzerland)
VALSARTAN
Diovan Tablets . . . 2212

PROVAS COMP (Switzerland)
VALSARTAN
Diovan Tablets . . . 2212

PROVAS MAXX (Switzerland)
VALSARTAN
Diovan Tablets . . . 2212

PRO-VENT (Irish Republic, United Kingdom)
THEOPHYLLINE
Uniphyl Tablets . . . 2595

PROVIGIL (Belgium, Irish Republic, Israel, Italy, South Africa, United Kingdom)
MODAFINIL
Provigil Tablets . . . 977

PROVISC (Argentina, Australia, Austria, Belgium, France, Germany, Hong Kong, Hungary, Irish Republic, Italy, Malaysia, New Zealand, Norway, Singapore, South Africa, Thailand, The Philippines, Turkey, United Kingdom, Venezuela)
SODIUM HYALURONATE
Hyalgan Solution . . . 2742

PROXACIN (Brazil, Hong Kong, Turkey)
CIPROFLOXACIN
Cipro Oral Suspension . . . 2810

PROXALIN (Mexico)
NAPROXEN
EC-Naprosyn Delayed-Release Tablets . . . 2632
Naprosyn Suspension . . . 2632
Naprosyn Tablets . . . 2632

PROXALIN PLUS (Mexico)
NAPROXEN
EC-Naprosyn Delayed-Release Tablets . . . 2632

Naprosyn Suspension . . . 2632
Naprosyn Tablets . . . 2632

PROXEM (Mexico)
NAPROXEN
EC-Naprosyn Delayed-Release Tablets . . . 2632
Naprosyn Suspension . . . 2632
Naprosyn Tablets . . . 2632

PROXEN (Australia, Austria, Germany, Hong Kong, South Africa, Switzerland, Thailand)
NAPROXEN
EC-Naprosyn Delayed-Release Tablets . . . 2632
Naprosyn Suspension . . . 2632
Naprosyn Tablets . . . 2632

PROXIME (Venezuela)
LEVOFLOXACIN
Levaquin Injection . . . 2416
Levaquin Tablets . . . 2416

PROXINE (Italy)
NAPROXEN
EC-Naprosyn Delayed-Release Tablets . . . 2632
Naprosyn Suspension . . . 2632
Naprosyn Tablets . . . 2632

PROXINOR (Thailand)
NORFLOXACIN
Noroxin Tablets . . . 2069

PROXITEC (Mexico)
CIPROFLOXACIN
Cipro Oral Suspension . . . 2810

PROZINE (South Africa)
CARBAMAZEPINE
Carbatrol Capsules . . . 3019

PSICOASTEN (Argentina)
PAROXETINE HYDROCHLORIDE
Paxil Oral Suspension . . . 1535
Paxil Tablets . . . 1535

PSICONOR (Argentina)
CITALOPRAM HYDROBROMIDE
Celexa Tablets . . . 1160

PSYCHOLANZ (India)
OLANZAPINE
Zyprexa Tablets . . . 1883

PSYCHOPAX (Austria, Switzerland)
DIAZEPAM
Valium Tablets . . . 2658

PTINOLIN (Greece)
RANITIDINE HYDROCHLORIDE
Zantac 25 EFFERdose Tablets . . . 1670
Zantac 150 Tablets . . . 1670
Zantac 300 Tablets . . . 1670
Zantac Injection . . . 1666
Zantac Injection Premixed . . . 1666
Zantac Syrup . . . 1670

PULMENO (Spain)
THEOPHYLLINE
Uniphyl Tablets . . . 2595

PULMIDUR (Austria)
THEOPHYLLINE
Uniphyl Tablets . . . 2595

PULMILIDE (Austria)
FLUNISOLIDE
Aerobid Inhaler System . . . 1153
Aerobid-M Inhaler System . . . 1153

PULMIST (Italy)
FLUNISOLIDE
Aerobid Inhaler System . . . 1153
Aerobid-M Inhaler System . . . 1153

PULMOPHYLLIN (South Africa)
THEOPHYLLINE
Uniphyl Tablets . . . 2595

PULMOPHYLLINE (Canada)
THEOPHYLLINE
Uniphyl Tablets . . . 2595

PULMO-TIMELETS (Denmark, Germany)
THEOPHYLLINE
Uniphyl Tablets . . . 2595

PURAN T4 (Brazil)
LEVOTHYROXINE SODIUM
Levothroid Tablets . . . 1170
Levoxyl Tablets . . . 1780
Synthroid Tablets . . . 507

PURESIS (South Africa)
FUROSEMIDE
Furosemide Tablets . . . 2186

PURGOLAC (Greece)
LACTULOSE
Kristalose for Oral Solution . . . 1004

PURGOXIN (South Africa)
DIGOXIN
Lanoxin Injection . . . 1498
Lanoxin Injection Pediatric . . . 1502
Lanoxin Tablets . . . 1505

PURICAP (Argentina)
ANASTROZOLE
Arimidex Tablets . . . 672

PUTAREN (Thailand)
DICLOFENAC SODIUM
Voltaren Tablets . . . 2334
Voltaren-XR Tablets . . . 2337

PYRALFIN (India)
PYRIMETHAMINE
Daraprim Tablets . . . 1400

PYRAMET (India)
PYRIMETHAMINE
Daraprim Tablets . . . 1400

PYRIDAMEL (Irish Republic)
DIPYRIDAMOLE
Persantine Tablets . . . 869

PYTAZEN (New Zealand)
DIPYRIDAMOLE
Persantine Tablets . . . 869

QINOSYN (The Philippines)
CIPROFLOXACIN HYDROCHLORIDE
Cipro Tablets . . . 2810

QUAGU-TEST (Argentina)
APROTININ
Trasylol Injection . . . 799

QUALECON (Argentina)
FENOFIBRATE
Tricor Tablets . . . 520

QUALI-A (Hong Kong)
TRETINOIN
Vesanoid Capsules . . . 2660

QUALICOR (Hong Kong)
SIMVASTATIN
Zocor Tablets . . . 2136

QUALI-MENTIN (Hong Kong)
AMOXICILLIN
Amoxil Pediatric Drops for Oral Suspension . . . 1305
Amoxil Tablets . . . 1305

QUALIPANTYL (Hong Kong)
FENOFIBRATE
Tricor Tablets . . . 520

QUAMATEL (Czech Republic, Hong Kong, Hungary, Poland, Russia)
FAMOTIDINE
Pepcid for Oral Suspension . . . 2075
Pepcid Tablets . . . 2075

QUANTOR (Spain)
RANITIDINE HYDROCHLORIDE
Zantac 25 EFFERdose Tablets . . . 1670
Zantac 150 Tablets . . . 1670
Zantac 300 Tablets . . . 1670
Zantac Injection . . . 1666
Zantac Injection Premixed . . . 1666
Zantac Syrup . . . 1670

QUARDIN (Portugal)
RANITIDINE HYDROCHLORIDE
Zantac 25 EFFERdose Tablets . . . 1670
Zantac 150 Tablets . . . 1670
Zantac 300 Tablets . . . 1670
Zantac Injection . . . 1666
Zantac Injection Premixed . . . 1666
Zantac Syrup . . . 1670

QUEDOX (Mexico)
CLARITHROMYCIN
Biaxin Filmtab Tablets . . . 411
Biaxin Granules . . . 411

QUERATAL (Mexico)
TRETINOIN
Vesanoid Capsules . . . 2660

QUER-OUT (Argentina)
DICLOFENAC SODIUM
Voltaren Tablets . . . 2334
Voltaren-XR Tablets . . . 2337

QUERTO (Germany)
CARVEDILOL
Coreg Tablets . . . 1387

QUIBRON (Thailand)
THEOPHYLLINE
Uniphyl Tablets . . . 2595

QUIBRON-T (Canada)
THEOPHYLLINE
Uniphyl Tablets . . . 2595

QUIDEX (Argentina)
CIPROFLOXACIN
Cipro Oral Suspension . . . 2810

QUIFLOX (Brazil)
CIPROFLOXACIN HYDROCHLORIDE
Cipro Tablets . . . 2810

QUIFLOXONA (Mexico)
CIPROFLOXACIN
Cipro Oral Suspension . . . 2810

QUILAREX (Argentina)
VENLAFAXINE HYDROCHLORIDE
Effexor XR Capsules . . . 3195

QUILOX (The Philippines)
CIPROFLOXACIN
Cipro Oral Suspension . . . 2810

QUINOBIOT (Chile)
LEVOFLOXACIN
Levaquin Injection . . . 2416
Levaquin Tablets . . . 2416

QUINOCIN (Hong Kong)
CIPROFLOXACIN
Cipro Oral Suspension . . . 2810

QUINOCORT (Venezuela)
CIPROFLOXACIN HYDROCHLORIDE
Cipro Tablets . . . 2810

QUINOFLEX (Portugal)
NORFLOXACIN
Noroxin Tablets . . . 2069

QUINOFLOX (Mexico)
CIPROFLOXACIN HYDROCHLORIDE
Cipro Tablets . . . 2810

QUINOFORM (Brazil)
NORFLOXACIN
Noroxin Tablets . . . 2069

QUINOFTAL (Venezuela)
CIPROFLOXACIN
Cipro Oral Suspension . . . 2810

QUINORYL (The Philippines)
CIPROFLOXACIN HYDROCHLORIDE
Cipro Tablets . . . 2810

QUINOTIC (Venezuela)
CIPROFLOXACIN HYDROCHLORIDE
Cipro Tablets . . . 2810

QUINOTIC HC (Venezuela)
CIPROFLOXACIN HYDROCHLORIDE
Cipro Tablets . . . 2810

QUINOX (Portugal)
CIPROFLOXACIN
Cipro Oral Suspension . . . 2810

QUINTOR (Czech Republic)
CIPROFLOXACIN HYDROCHLORIDE
Cipro Tablets . . . 2810

QUIPRIME (The Philippines)
CIPROFLOXACIN HYDROCHLORIDE
Cipro Tablets . . . 2810

QUIPRO (Czech Republic, Spain)
CIPROFLOXACIN HYDROCHLORIDE
Cipro Tablets . . . 2810

QUISEGEN (Argentina)
CIPROFLOXACIN HYDROCHLORIDE
Cipro Tablets . . . 2810

QUOMEM (Austria, Italy, Spain, Thailand, The Netherlands)
BUPROPION HYDROCHLORIDE
Wellbutrin SR Sustained-Release Tablets . . . 1653
Wellbutrin Tablets . . . 1648
Zyban Sustained-Release Tablets . . . 1692

RABIODINA (Brazil)
RANITIDINE HYDROCHLORIDE
Zantac 25 EFFERdose Tablets . . . 1670
Zantac 150 Tablets . . . 1670
Zantac 300 Tablets . . . 1670
Zantac Injection . . . 1666
Zantac Injection Premixed . . . 1666
Zantac Syrup . . . 1670

RADAN (Brazil)
RANITIDINE HYDROCHLORIDE
Zantac 25 EFFERdose Tablets . . . 1670
Zantac 150 Tablets . . . 1670
Zantac 300 Tablets . . . 1670
Zantac Injection . . . 1666
Zantac Injection Premixed . . . 1666
Zantac Syrup . . . 1670

RADICACINE (Argentina)
CELECOXIB
Celebrex Capsules . . . 2979

RADIN (Hong Kong)
RANITIDINE HYDROCHLORIDE
Zantac 25 EFFERdose Tablets . . . 1670
Zantac 150 Tablets . . . 1670
Zantac 300 Tablets . . . 1670
Zantac Injection . . . 1666
Zantac Injection Premixed . . . 1666
Zantac Syrup . . . 1670

RADINE (Thailand)
RANITIDINE HYDROCHLORIDE
Zantac 25 EFFERdose Tablets . . . 1670
Zantac 150 Tablets . . . 1670
Zantac 300 Tablets . . . 1670
Zantac Injection . . . 1666
Zantac Injection Premixed . . . 1666
Zantac Syrup . . . 1670

RADUCTIL (Argentina, Mexico)
SIBUTRAMINE HYDROCHLORIDE
Meridia Capsules . . . 475

RAFFONIN (Chile)
FLUTICASONE PROPIONATE
Flonase Nasal Spray . . . 1431

RAGEX (Italy)
CEFTRIAXONE SODIUM
Rocephin Injectable Vials, ADD-Vantage, Galaxy, Bulk . . . 2642

RALISTA (India)
RALOXIFENE HYDROCHLORIDE
Evista Tablets . . . 1810

RALIZON (Greece)
CETIRIZINE HYDROCHLORIDE
Zyrtec Syrup . . . 1920
Zyrtec Tablets . . . 1920

RAN (Portugal)
RANITIDINE HYDROCHLORIDE
Zantac 25 EFFERdose Tablets . . . 1670
Zantac 150 Tablets . . . 1670
Zantac 300 Tablets . . . 1670
Zantac Injection . . . 1666
Zantac Injection Premixed . . . 1666
Zantac Syrup . . . 1670

RAN H2 (Spain)
RANITIDINE HYDROCHLORIDE
Zantac 25 EFFERdose Tablets . . . 1670
Zantac 150 Tablets . . . 1670
Zantac 300 Tablets . . . 1670
Zantac Injection . . . 1666
Zantac Injection Premixed . . . 1666
Zantac Syrup . . . 1670

RAN LICH (Germany)
RANITIDINE HYDROCHLORIDE
Zantac 25 EFFERdose Tablets . . . 1670
Zantac 150 Tablets . . . 1670
Zantac 300 Tablets . . . 1670
Zantac Injection . . . 1666
Zantac Injection Premixed . . . 1666
Zantac Syrup . . . 1670

RANACID (Norway)
RANITIDINE HYDROCHLORIDE
Zantac 25 EFFERdose Tablets . . . 1670
Zantac 150 Tablets . . . 1670
Zantac 300 Tablets . . . 1670
Zantac Injection . . . 1666
Zantac Injection Premixed . . . 1666
Zantac Syrup . . . 1670

RANAPS (United Kingdom)
RANITIDINE HYDROCHLORIDE
Zantac 25 EFFERdose Tablets . . . 1670
Zantac 150 Tablets . . . 1670
Zantac 300 Tablets . . . 1670
Zantac Injection . . . 1666
Zantac Injection Premixed . . . 1666
Zantac Syrup . . . 1670

RANI (Singapore)
RANITIDINE HYDROCHLORIDE
Zantac 25 EFFERdose Tablets . . . 1670
Zantac 150 Tablets . . . 1670
Zantac 300 Tablets . . . 1670
Zantac Injection . . . 1666
Zantac Injection Premixed . . . 1666
Zantac Syrup . . . 1670

RANI 2 (Australia)
RANITIDINE HYDROCHLORIDE
Zantac 25 EFFERdose Tablets . . . 1670

Zantac 150 Tablets 1670
Zantac 300 Tablets 1670
Zantac Injection 1666
Zantac Injection Premixed 1666
Zantac Syrup 1670

RANIBEN (Italy)
RANITIDINE HYDROCHLORIDE
Zantac 25 EFFERdose Tablets 1670
Zantac 150 Tablets 1670
Zantac 300 Tablets 1670
Zantac Injection 1666
Zantac Injection Premixed 1666
Zantac Syrup 1670

RANIBERL (Czech Republic, Germany, Poland)
RANITIDINE HYDROCHLORIDE
Zantac 150 Tablets 1670
Zantac 25 EFFERdose Tablets 1670
Zantac 300 Tablets 1670
Zantac Injection 1666
Zantac Injection Premixed 1666
Zantac Syrup 1670

RANIBETA (Germany)
RANITIDINE HYDROCHLORIDE
Zantac 25 EFFERdose Tablets 1670
Zantac 150 Tablets 1670
Zantac 300 Tablets 1670
Zantac Injection 1666
Zantac Injection Premixed 1666
Zantac Syrup 1670

RANIBLOC (Germany, Italy, Venezuela)
RANITIDINE HYDROCHLORIDE
Zantac 150 Tablets 1670
Zantac 25 EFFERdose Tablets 1670
Zantac 300 Tablets 1670
Zantac Injection 1666
Zantac Injection Premixed 1666
Zantac Syrup 1670

RANIC (Austria, Belgium, Poland)
RANITIDINE HYDROCHLORIDE
Zantac 150 Tablets 1670
Zantac 25 EFFERdose Tablets 1670
Zantac 300 Tablets 1670
Zantac Injection 1666
Zantac Injection Premixed 1666
Zantac Syrup 1670

RANICEL (Chile)
RANITIDINE HYDROCHLORIDE
Zantac 25 EFFERdose Tablets 1670
Zantac 150 Tablets 1670
Zantac 300 Tablets 1670
Zantac Injection 1666
Zantac Injection Premixed 1666
Zantac Syrup 1670

RANICID (Thailand)
RANITIDINE HYDROCHLORIDE
Zantac 25 EFFERdose Tablets 1670
Zantac 150 Tablets 1670
Zantac 300 Tablets 1670
Zantac Injection 1666
Zantac Injection Premixed 1666
Zantac Syrup 1670

RANICLON (Greece)
RANITIDINE HYDROCHLORIDE
Zantac 25 EFFERdose Tablets 1670
Zantac 150 Tablets 1670
Zantac 300 Tablets 1670
Zantac Injection 1666
Zantac Injection Premixed 1666
Zantac Syrup 1670

RANICLOR (Brazil)
RANITIDINE HYDROCHLORIDE
Zantac 25 EFFERdose Tablets 1670
Zantac 150 Tablets 1670
Zantac 300 Tablets 1670
Zantac Injection 1666
Zantac Injection Premixed 1666
Zantac Syrup 1670

RANICODAN (Denmark)
RANITIDINE HYDROCHLORIDE
Zantac 25 EFFERdose Tablets 1670
Zantac 150 Tablets 1670
Zantac 300 Tablets 1670
Zantac Injection 1666
Zantac Injection Premixed 1666
Zantac Syrup 1670

RANICUR (Finland)
RANITIDINE HYDROCHLORIDE
Zantac 25 EFFERdose Tablets 1670
Zantac 150 Tablets 1670
Zantac 300 Tablets 1670
Zantac Injection 1666
Zantac Injection Premixed 1666
Zantac Syrup 1670

RANICUX (Germany)
RANITIDINE HYDROCHLORIDE
Zantac 25 EFFERdose Tablets 1670
Zantac 150 Tablets 1670
Zantac 300 Tablets 1670
Zantac Injection 1666
Zantac Injection Premixed 1666
Zantac Syrup 1670

RANIDEX (Italy)
RANITIDINE HYDROCHLORIDE
Zantac 25 EFFERdose Tablets 1670
Zantac 150 Tablets 1670
Zantac 300 Tablets 1670
Zantac Injection 1666
Zantac Injection Premixed 1666
Zantac Syrup 1670

RANIDIL (Italy)
RANITIDINE HYDROCHLORIDE
Zantac 25 EFFERdose Tablets 1670
Zantac 150 Tablets 1670
Zantac 300 Tablets 1670
Zantac Injection 1666
Zantac Injection Premixed 1666
Zantac Syrup 1670

RANIDIN (Brazil, Spain)
RANITIDINE HYDROCHLORIDE
Zantac 25 EFFERdose Tablets 1670
Zantac 150 Tablets 1670
Zantac 300 Tablets 1670
Zantac Injection 1666
Zantac Injection Premixed 1666
Zantac Syrup 1670

RANIDINA (Brazil)
RANITIDINE HYDROCHLORIDE
Zantac 25 EFFERdose Tablets 1670
Zantac 150 Tablets 1670
Zantac 300 Tablets 1670
Zantac Injection 1666
Zantac Injection Premixed 1666
Zantac Syrup 1670

RANIDINE (Thailand)
RANITIDINE HYDROCHLORIDE
Zantac 25 EFFERdose Tablets 1670
Zantac 150 Tablets 1670
Zantac 300 Tablets 1670
Zantac Injection 1666
Zantac Injection Premixed 1666
Zantac Syrup 1670

RANIDURA T (Germany)
RANITIDINE HYDROCHLORIDE
Zantac 25 EFFERdose Tablets 1670
Zantac 150 Tablets 1670
Zantac 300 Tablets 1670
Zantac Injection 1666
Zantac Injection Premixed 1666
Zantac Syrup 1670

RANIFESA (Venezuela)
RANITIDINE HYDROCHLORIDE
Zantac 25 EFFERdose Tablets 1670
Zantac 150 Tablets 1670
Zantac 300 Tablets 1670
Zantac Injection 1666
Zantac Injection Premixed 1666
Zantac Syrup 1670

RANIFLEX (Brazil)
RANITIDINE HYDROCHLORIDE
Zantac 25 EFFERdose Tablets 1670
Zantac 150 Tablets 1670
Zantac 300 Tablets 1670
Zantac Injection 1666
Zantac Injection Premixed 1666
Zantac Syrup 1670

RANIGAST (Poland, Russia)
RANITIDINE HYDROCHLORIDE
Zantac 25 EFFERdose Tablets 1670
Zantac 150 Tablets 1670
Zantac 300 Tablets 1670
Zantac Injection 1666
Zantac Injection Premixed 1666
Zantac Syrup 1670

RANIHEXAL (Australia, South Africa)
RANITIDINE HYDROCHLORIDE
Zantac 150 Tablets 1670
Zantac 25 EFFERdose Tablets 1670
Zantac 300 Tablets 1670
Zantac Injection 1666
Zantac Injection Premixed 1666
Zantac Syrup 1670

RANIL (Finland)
RANITIDINE HYDROCHLORIDE
Zantac 25 EFFERdose Tablets 1670
Zantac 150 Tablets 1670
Zantac 300 Tablets 1670
Zantac Injection 1666
Zantac Injection Premixed 1666
Zantac Syrup 1670

RANILONGA (Spain)
RANITIDINE HYDROCHLORIDE
Zantac 25 EFFERdose Tablets 1670
Zantac 150 Tablets 1670
Zantac 300 Tablets 1670
Zantac Injection 1666
Zantac Injection Premixed 1666
Zantac Syrup 1670

RANIMED (Argentina, Switzerland)
RANITIDINE HYDROCHLORIDE
Zantac 150 Tablets 1670
Zantac 25 EFFERdose Tablets 1670
Zantac 300 Tablets 1670
Zantac Injection 1666
Zantac Injection Premixed 1666
Zantac Syrup 1670

RANIMERCK (Germany)
RANITIDINE HYDROCHLORIDE
Zantac 25 EFFERdose Tablets 1670
Zantac 150 Tablets 1670
Zantac 300 Tablets 1670
Zantac Injection 1666
Zantac Injection Premixed 1666
Zantac Syrup 1670

RANIMEX (Finland)
RANITIDINE HYDROCHLORIDE
Zantac 25 EFFERdose Tablets 1670
Zantac 150 Tablets 1670
Zantac 300 Tablets 1670
Zantac Injection 1666
Zantac Injection Premixed 1666
Zantac Syrup 1670

RANI-NERTON (Germany)
RANITIDINE HYDROCHLORIDE
Zantac 25 EFFERdose Tablets 1670
Zantac 150 Tablets 1670
Zantac 300 Tablets 1670
Zantac Injection 1666
Zantac Injection Premixed 1666
Zantac Syrup 1670

RANINORM (Austria)
RANITIDINE HYDROCHLORIDE
Zantac 25 EFFERdose Tablets 1670
Zantac 150 Tablets 1670
Zantac 300 Tablets 1670
Zantac Injection 1666
Zantac Injection Premixed 1666
Zantac Syrup 1670

RANIPLEX (France)
RANITIDINE HYDROCHLORIDE
Zantac 25 EFFERdose Tablets 1670
Zantac 150 Tablets 1670
Zantac 300 Tablets 1670
Zantac Injection 1666
Zantac Injection Premixed 1666
Zantac Syrup 1670

RANIPROTECT (Germany)
RANITIDINE HYDROCHLORIDE
Zantac 25 EFFERdose Tablets 1670
Zantac 150 Tablets 1670
Zantac 300 Tablets 1670
Zantac Injection 1666
Zantac Injection Premixed 1666
Zantac Syrup 1670

RANI-Q (Sweden)
RANITIDINE HYDROCHLORIDE
Zantac 25 EFFERdose Tablets 1670
Zantac 150 Tablets 1670
Zantac 300 Tablets 1670
Zantac Injection 1666
Zantac Injection Premixed 1666
Zantac Syrup 1670

RANISAN (Czech Republic, Poland, Russia)
RANITIDINE HYDROCHLORIDE
Zantac 150 Tablets 1670
Zantac 25 EFFERdose Tablets 1670
Zantac 300 Tablets 1670
Zantac Injection 1666
Zantac Injection Premixed 1666
Zantac Syrup 1670

RANISEN (Mexico)
RANITIDINE HYDROCHLORIDE
Zantac 25 EFFERdose Tablets 1670
Zantac 150 Tablets 1670
Zantac 300 Tablets 1670
Zantac Injection 1666
Zantac Injection Premixed 1666
Zantac Syrup 1670

RANISIFAR (Switzerland)
RANITIDINE HYDROCHLORIDE
Zantac 25 EFFERdose Tablets 1670
Zantac 150 Tablets 1670
Zantac 300 Tablets 1670
Zantac Injection 1666
Zantac Injection Premixed 1666
Zantac Syrup 1670

RANITAB (Germany, The Philippines, Turkey)
RANITIDINE HYDROCHLORIDE
Zantac 150 Tablets 1670
Zantac 25 EFFERdose Tablets 1670
Zantac 300 Tablets 1670
Zantac Injection 1666
Zantac Injection Premixed 1666
Zantac Syrup 1670

RANITAK (Brazil)
RANITIDINE HYDROCHLORIDE
Zantac 25 EFFERdose Tablets 1670
Zantac 150 Tablets 1670
Zantac 300 Tablets 1670
Zantac Injection 1666
Zantac Injection Premixed 1666
Zantac Syrup 1670

RANITAL (Czech Republic)
RANITIDINE HYDROCHLORIDE
Zantac 25 EFFERdose Tablets 1670
Zantac 150 Tablets 1670
Zantac 300 Tablets 1670
Zantac Injection 1666
Zantac Injection Premixed 1666
Zantac Syrup 1670

RANITIC (Argentina, Australia, Germany, Hungary, Irish Republic, United Kingdom)
RANITIDINE HYDROCHLORIDE
Zantac 150 Tablets 1670
Zantac 25 EFFERdose Tablets 1670
Zantac 300 Tablets 1670
Zantac Injection 1666
Zantac Injection Premixed 1666
Zantac Syrup 1670

RANITIDOC (Germany)
RANITIDINE HYDROCHLORIDE
Zantac 25 EFFERdose Tablets 1670
Zantac 150 Tablets 1670
Zantac 300 Tablets 1670
Zantac Injection 1666
Zantac Injection Premixed 1666
Zantac Syrup 1670

RANITIL (Brazil, United Kingdom)
RANITIDINE HYDROCHLORIDE
Zantac 150 Tablets 1670
Zantac 25 EFFERdose Tablets 1670
Zantac 300 Tablets 1670
Zantac Injection 1666
Zantac Injection Premixed 1666
Zantac Syrup 1670

RANITIN (Brazil, Czech Republic, Poland)
RANITIDINE HYDROCHLORIDE
Zantac 150 Tablets 1670
Zantac 25 EFFERdose Tablets 1670
Zantac 300 Tablets 1670
Zantac Injection 1666
Zantac Injection Premixed 1666
Zantac Syrup 1670

RANITINE (Portugal, Turkey)
RANITIDINE HYDROCHLORIDE
Zantac 150 Tablets 1670
Zantac 25 EFFERdose Tablets 1670
Zantac 300 Tablets 1670
Zantac Injection 1666
Zantac Injection Premixed 1666
Zantac Syrup 1670

RANITINOL (Brazil)
RANITIDINE HYDROCHLORIDE
Zantac 25 EFFERdose Tablets 1670
Zantac 150 Tablets 1670
Zantac 300 Tablets 1670
Zantac Injection 1666
Zantac Injection Premixed 1666
Zantac Syrup 1670

RANITION (Brazil)
RANITIDINE HYDROCHLORIDE
Zantac 25 EFFERdose Tablets 1670
Zantac 150 Tablets 1670
Zantac 300 Tablets 1670
Zantac Injection 1666
Zantac Injection Premixed 1666

Zantac Syrup . . . 1670

RANITRAL (Argentina)
RANITIDINE HYDROCHLORIDE
Zantac 25 EFFERdose Tablets . . . 1670
Zantac 150 Tablets . . . 1670
Zantac 300 Tablets . . . 1670
Zantac Injection . . . 1666
Zantac Injection Premixed . . . 1666
Zantac Syrup . . . 1670

RANITRAT (Brazil)
RANITIDINE HYDROCHLORIDE
Zantac 25 EFFERdose Tablets . . . 1670
Zantac 150 Tablets . . . 1670
Zantac 300 Tablets . . . 1670
Zantac Injection . . . 1666
Zantac Injection Premixed . . . 1666
Zantac Syrup . . . 1670

RANITYROL (Austria)
RANITIDINE HYDROCHLORIDE
Zantac 25 EFFERdose Tablets . . . 1670
Zantac 150 Tablets . . . 1670
Zantac 300 Tablets . . . 1670
Zantac Injection . . . 1666
Zantac Injection Premixed . . . 1666
Zantac Syrup . . . 1670

RANIVEL (Spain)
RANITIDINE HYDROCHLORIDE
Zantac 25 EFFERdose Tablets . . . 1670
Zantac 150 Tablets . . . 1670
Zantac 300 Tablets . . . 1670
Zantac Injection . . . 1666
Zantac Injection Premixed . . . 1666
Zantac Syrup . . . 1670

RANIX (Spain, Venezuela)
RANITIDINE HYDROCHLORIDE
Zantac 150 Tablets . . . 1670
Zantac 25 EFFERdose Tablets . . . 1670
Zantac 300 Tablets . . . 1670
Zantac Injection . . . 1666
Zantac Injection Premixed . . . 1666
Zantac Syrup . . . 1670

RANIXAL (Finland)
RANITIDINE HYDROCHLORIDE
Zantac 25 EFFERdose Tablets . . . 1670
Zantac 150 Tablets . . . 1670
Zantac 300 Tablets . . . 1670
Zantac Injection . . . 1666
Zantac Injection Premixed . . . 1666
Zantac Syrup . . . 1670

RANIZAC (Greece)
RANITIDINE HYDROCHLORIDE
Zantac 25 EFFERdose Tablets . . . 1670
Zantac 150 Tablets . . . 1670
Zantac 300 Tablets . . . 1670
Zantac Injection . . . 1666
Zantac Injection Premixed . . . 1666
Zantac Syrup . . . 1670

RANIZAN (Venezuela)
RANITIDINE HYDROCHLORIDE
Zantac 25 EFFERdose Tablets . . . 1670
Zantac 150 Tablets . . . 1670
Zantac 300 Tablets . . . 1670
Zantac Injection . . . 1666
Zantac Injection Premixed . . . 1666
Zantac Syrup . . . 1670

RANOBEL (Turkey)
RANITIDINE HYDROCHLORIDE
Zantac 25 EFFERdose Tablets . . . 1670
Zantac 150 Tablets . . . 1670
Zantac 300 Tablets . . . 1670
Zantac Injection . . . 1666
Zantac Injection Premixed . . . 1666
Zantac Syrup . . . 1670

RANOLTA (Hong Kong)
RANITIDINE HYDROCHLORIDE
Zantac 25 EFFERdose Tablets . . . 1670
Zantac 150 Tablets . . . 1670
Zantac 300 Tablets . . . 1670
Zantac Injection . . . 1666
Zantac Injection Premixed . . . 1666
Zantac Syrup . . . 1670

RANOPINE (Irish Republic)
RANITIDINE HYDROCHLORIDE
Zantac 25 EFFERdose Tablets . . . 1670
Zantac 150 Tablets . . . 1670
Zantac 300 Tablets . . . 1670
Zantac Injection . . . 1666
Zantac Injection Premixed . . . 1666
Zantac Syrup . . . 1670

RANOPRIL (Malaysia)
LISINOPRIL
Prinivil Tablets . . . 2087

RANOXYL (Australia)
RANITIDINE HYDROCHLORIDE
Zantac 25 EFFERdose Tablets . . . 1670
Zantac 150 Tablets . . . 1670
Zantac 300 Tablets . . . 1670
Zantac Injection . . . 1666
Zantac Injection Premixed . . . 1666
Zantac Syrup . . . 1670

RANSIM (Australia)
SIMVASTATIN
Zocor Tablets . . . 2136

RANTAC (India, Russia, Thailand)
RANITIDINE HYDROCHLORIDE
Zantac 150 Tablets . . . 1670
Zantac 25 EFFERdose Tablets . . . 1670
Zantac 300 Tablets . . . 1670
Zantac Injection . . . 1666
Zantac Injection Premixed . . . 1666
Zantac Syrup . . . 1670

RANTAG (United Arab Emirates)
RANITIDINE HYDROCHLORIDE
Zantac 25 EFFERdose Tablets . . . 1670
Zantac 150 Tablets . . . 1670
Zantac 300 Tablets . . . 1670
Zantac Injection . . . 1666
Zantac Injection Premixed . . . 1666
Zantac Syrup . . . 1670

RANTEC (United Kingdom)
RANITIDINE HYDROCHLORIDE
Zantac 25 EFFERdose Tablets . . . 1670
Zantac 150 Tablets . . . 1670
Zantac 300 Tablets . . . 1670
Zantac Injection . . . 1666
Zantac Injection Premixed . . . 1666
Zantac Syrup . . . 1670

RANTEEN (South Africa)
RANITIDINE HYDROCHLORIDE
Zantac 25 EFFERdose Tablets . . . 1670
Zantac 150 Tablets . . . 1670
Zantac 300 Tablets . . . 1670
Zantac Injection . . . 1666
Zantac Injection Premixed . . . 1666
Zantac Syrup . . . 1670

RANTEX (Venezuela)
LISINOPRIL
Prinivil Tablets . . . 2087

RANUBER (Spain)
RANITIDINE HYDROCHLORIDE
Zantac 25 EFFERdose Tablets . . . 1670
Zantac 150 Tablets . . . 1670
Zantac 300 Tablets . . . 1670
Zantac Injection . . . 1666
Zantac Injection Premixed . . . 1666
Zantac Syrup . . . 1670

RANZAC (United Kingdom)
RANITIDINE HYDROCHLORIDE
Zantac 25 EFFERdose Tablets . . . 1670
Zantac 150 Tablets . . . 1670
Zantac 300 Tablets . . . 1670
Zantac Injection . . . 1666
Zantac Injection Premixed . . . 1666
Zantac Syrup . . . 1670

RAPICLAV (India)
AMOXICILLIN
Amoxil Pediatric Drops for Oral Suspension . . . 1305
Amoxil Tablets . . . 1305

RAPIDIN (The Philippines)
RANITIDINE HYDROCHLORIDE
Zantac 25 EFFERdose Tablets . . . 1670
Zantac 150 Tablets . . . 1670
Zantac 300 Tablets . . . 1670
Zantac Injection . . . 1666
Zantac Injection Premixed . . . 1666
Zantac Syrup . . . 1670

RAPIQURE (The Philippines)
CIPROFLOXACIN
Cipro Oral Suspension . . . 2810

RASITOL (Malaysia)
FUROSEMIDE
Furosemide Tablets . . . 2186

RATACAND (Italy, The Netherlands)
CANDESARTAN CILEXETIL
Atacand Tablets . . . 639

RATACAND PLUS (Italy)
CANDESARTAN CILEXETIL
Atacand Tablets . . . 639

RATIC (Singapore, Thailand)
RANITIDINE HYDROCHLORIDE
Zantac 150 Tablets . . . 1670
Zantac 25 EFFERdose Tablets . . . 1670
Zantac 300 Tablets . . . 1670
Zantac Injection . . . 1666
Zantac Injection Premixed . . . 1666
Zantac Syrup . . . 1670

RATICINA (Argentina)
RANITIDINE HYDROCHLORIDE
Zantac 25 EFFERdose Tablets . . . 1670
Zantac 150 Tablets . . . 1670
Zantac 300 Tablets . . . 1670
Zantac Injection . . . 1666
Zantac Injection Premixed . . . 1666
Zantac Syrup . . . 1670

RATIOALLERG (Austria)
CETIRIZINE HYDROCHLORIDE
Zyrtec Syrup . . . 1920
Zyrtec Tablets . . . 1920

RATIOGEL (Poland)
DICLOFENAC SODIUM
Voltaren Tablets . . . 2334
Voltaren-XR Tablets . . . 2337

RATIO-IPRA SAL UDV (Canada)
IPRATROPIUM BROMIDE
Atrovent Nasal Spray 0.03% . . . 834
Atrovent Nasal Spray 0.06% . . . 836

RAUDIL (Mexico)
RANITIDINE HYDROCHLORIDE
Zantac 25 EFFERdose Tablets . . . 1670
Zantac 150 Tablets . . . 1670
Zantac 300 Tablets . . . 1670
Zantac Injection . . . 1666
Zantac Injection Premixed . . . 1666
Zantac Syrup . . . 1670

RAVALTON (Greece)
CIPROFLOXACIN HYDROCHLORIDE
Cipro Tablets . . . 2810

RAVOTAF (Mexico)
AMOXICILLIN
Amoxil Pediatric Drops for Oral Suspension . . . 1305
Amoxil Tablets . . . 1305

RAVOTRIL (Chile)
CLONAZEPAM
Klonopin Tablets . . . 2639

RAWEL (Poland)
INDAPAMIDE
Indapamide Tablets . . . 2188

RAXENOL (Mexico)
NAPROXEN
EC-Naprosyn Delayed-Release Tablets . . . 2632
Naprosyn Suspension . . . 2632
Naprosyn Tablets . . . 2632

RAXIDE (The Philippines)
RANITIDINE HYDROCHLORIDE
Zantac 25 EFFERdose Tablets . . . 1670
Zantac 150 Tablets . . . 1670
Zantac 300 Tablets . . . 1670
Zantac Injection . . . 1666
Zantac Injection Premixed . . . 1666
Zantac Syrup . . . 1670

RAYNE (Mexico)
DIAZEPAM
Valium Tablets . . . 2658

RAZENE (New Zealand)
CETIRIZINE HYDROCHLORIDE
Zyrtec Syrup . . . 1920
Zyrtec Tablets . . . 1920

REACEL-A (Mexico)
TRETINOIN
Vesanoid Capsules . . . 2660

REACTINE (Austria, Belgium, Canada, France, Germany, Norway, Spain, Sweden, The Netherlands)
CETIRIZINE HYDROCHLORIDE
Zyrtec Syrup . . . 1920
Zyrtec Tablets . . . 1920

REALDIRON (Russia)
INTERFERON ALFA-2B
Intron A for Injection . . . 2859

REBETRON (South Africa)
INTERFERON ALFA-2B
Intron A for Injection . . . 2859

RECAMICINA (Chile)
LEVOFLOXACIN
Levaquin Injection . . . 2416
Levaquin Tablets . . . 2416

REC-DZ (India)
DIAZEPAM
Valium Tablets . . . 2658

RECEANT (Greece)
CEFUROXIME SODIUM
Zinacef Injection . . . 1678

RECITAL (Israel)
CITALOPRAM HYDROBROMIDE
Celexa Tablets . . . 1160

RECO (Argentina)
RANITIDINE HYDROCHLORIDE
Zantac 25 EFFERdose Tablets . . . 1670
Zantac 150 Tablets . . . 1670
Zantac 300 Tablets . . . 1670
Zantac Injection . . . 1666
Zantac Injection Premixed . . . 1666
Zantac Syrup . . . 1670

REDUCOL (Brazil)
LOVASTATIN
Mevacor Tablets . . . 2063

REDUCTEL (Mexico)
CAPTOPRIL
Captopril Tablets . . . 2182

REDUCTIL (Australia, Austria, Belgium, Brazil, Chile, Denmark, Finland, Germany, Greece, Hong Kong, Hungary, Irish Republic, Italy, Malaysia, New Zealand, Norway, Portugal, Singapore, South Africa, Spain, Sweden, Switzerland, Thailand, The Netherlands, The Philippines, Turkey, United Kingdom, Venezuela)
SIBUTRAMINE HYDROCHLORIDE
Meridia Capsules . . . 475

REDUPRESS (Brazil)
LOSARTAN POTASSIUM
Cozaar Tablets . . . 1973

REDUSA (Hong Kong)
PHENTERMINE HYDROCHLORIDE
Adipex-P Capsules . . . 1185
Adipex-P Tablets . . . 1185

REDUSCAR (Brazil)
FINASTERIDE
Propecia Tablets . . . 2095
Proscar Tablets . . . 2102

REDUSTEROL (Argentina)
SIMVASTATIN
Zocor Tablets . . . 2136

REDUSTEROL DUO (Argentina)
SIMVASTATIN
Zocor Tablets . . . 2136

REDUTEN (Chile)
SIBUTRAMINE HYDROCHLORIDE
Meridia Capsules . . . 475

REDUTENSIL (Argentina)
VALSARTAN
Diovan Tablets . . . 2212

REDUXADE (Italy)
SIBUTRAMINE HYDROCHLORIDE
Meridia Capsules . . . 475

REGENESIS (Argentina)
ALENDRONATE SODIUM
Fosamax Tablets . . . 2005

REGENTAL (Chile)
NIMODIPINE
Nimotop Capsules . . . 790

REGEPAR (Austria, Switzerland)
SELEGILINE HYDROCHLORIDE
Eldepryl Capsules . . . 3052

REGIOCAINA (Argentina)
LIDOCAINE
Lidoderm Patch . . . 1114

REGULACT (Mexico)
LACTULOSE
Kristalose for Oral Solution . . . 1004

REGULOSE (United Kingdom)
LACTULOSE
Kristalose for Oral Solution . . . 1004

REICHAMOX (Hong Kong)
AMOXICILLIN
Amoxil Pediatric Drops for Oral Suspension . . . 1305
Amoxil Tablets . . . 1305

REJUVA-A (Canada)
TRETINOIN
Vesanoid Capsules. 2660

REKOSTIN (Poland)
ALENDRONATE SODIUM
Fosamax Tablets 2005

RELANIUM (Russia)
DIAZEPAM
Valium Tablets 2658

RELAPAZ (Spain)
CITALOPRAM HYDROBROMIDE
Celexa Tablets 1160

RELASAN (Mexico)
DIAZEPAM
Valium Tablets 2658

RELASTEF (Italy)
TRETINOIN
Vesanoid Capsules. 2660

RELAXYL (India)
DICLOFENAC SODIUM
Voltaren Tablets 2334
Voltaren-XR Tablets 2337

RELAXYL PLUS (India)
DICLOFENAC SODIUM
Voltaren Tablets 2334
Voltaren-XR Tablets 2337

RELAZEPAM (Mexico)
DIAZEPAM
Valium Tablets 2658

RELIMAL (The Philippines)
MORPHINE SULFATE
MS Contin Tablets 2585

RELIPAIN (Greece, Italy)
MORPHINE SULFATE
MS Contin Tablets 2585

RELIUM (Russia)
DIAZEPAM
Valium Tablets 2658

RELOKAP (Turkey)
NAPROXEN SODIUM
Anaprox DS Tablets 2632
Anaprox Tablets 2632

RELOVA (Switzerland)
DICLOFENAC SODIUM
Voltaren Tablets 2334
Voltaren-XR Tablets 2337

RELOXYL (Italy)
BENZOYL PEROXIDE
Brevoxyl-4 Creamy Wash. 3054
Brevoxyl-4 Gel 3054
Brevoxyl-8 Creamy Wash. 3054
Brevoxyl-8 Gel 3054

RELSED (Poland)
DIAZEPAM
Valium Tablets 2658

REMAFEN (Hong Kong, Malaysia, Singapore)
DICLOFENAC SODIUM
Voltaren Tablets 2334
Voltaren-XR Tablets 2337

REMENA (Greece)
CIPROFLOXACIN HYDROCHLORIDE
Cipro Tablets 2810

REMENS (India)
PROGESTERONE
Crinone 4% Gel. 992
Prometrium Capsules (100 mg, 200 mg) . 3047

REMETHAN (Hong Kong, Malaysia)
DICLOFENAC SODIUM
Voltaren Tablets 2334
Voltaren-XR Tablets 2337

REMICADE (Argentina, Australia, Belgium, Brazil, Canada, Chile, Czech Republic, Denmark, Finland, France, Germany, Greece, Hong Kong, Hungary, Irish Republic, Israel, Italy, Japan, Mexico, New Zealand, Norway, Poland, Portugal, Russia, Singapore, Spain, Sweden, Switzerland, Thailand, The Netherlands, The Philippines, Turkey, United Kingdom, Venezuela)
INFLIXIMAB
Remicade for IV Injection. 950

REMITEX (Chile)
CETIRIZINE HYDROCHLORIDE
Zyrtec Syrup 1920
Zyrtec Tablets 1920

REMONTAL (Spain)
NIMODIPINE
Nimotop Capsules 790

REN (Hong Kong)
DICLOFENAC SODIUM
Voltaren Tablets 2334
Voltaren-XR Tablets 2337

RENACIDIN (Argentina)
FINASTERIDE
Propecia Tablets 2095
Proscar Tablets. 2102

RENCEF (Chile)
LACTULOSE
Kristalose for Oral Solution 1004

RENEZIDE (South Africa)
HYDROCHLOROTHIAZIDE/TRIAMTERENE
Dyazide Capsules 1405

RENFORT (The Philippines)
RANITIDINE HYDROCHLORIDE
Zantac 25 EFFERdose Tablets 1670
Zantac 150 Tablets 1670
Zantac 300 Tablets 1670
Zantac Injection 1666
Zantac Injection Premixed 1666
Zantac Syrup 1670

RENIDAC (Mexico)
SULINDAC
Clinoril Tablets 1962

RENOGEN (The Philippines)
EPOETIN ALFA
Epogen for Injection. 576
Procrit for Injection 2391

RENOTENS (South Africa)
LISINOPRIL
Prinivil Tablets 2087

RENOVA (Canada, Malaysia, South Africa, Thailand)
TRETINOIN
Vesanoid Capsules. 2660

RENOXACIN (Italy)
NORFLOXACIN
Noroxin Tablets. 2069

RENTOP (Argentina)
RISEDRONATE SODIUM
Actonel Tablets. 2568

RENTREX (Thailand)
CETIRIZINE HYDROCHLORIDE
Zyrtec Syrup 1920
Zyrtec Tablets 1920

REOPRO (Argentina, Australia, Austria, Belgium, Brazil, Canada, Chile, Czech Republic, Denmark, Finland, France, Germany, Greece, Hong Kong, India, Irish Republic, Israel, Italy, Malaysia, Mexico, New Zealand, Norway, Poland, Russia, Singapore, South Africa, Spain, Sweden, Switzerland, Thailand, The Netherlands, United Kingdom)
ABCIXIMAB
ReoPro Vials 1860

REPENTIL (Venezuela)
SIBUTRAMINE HYDROCHLORIDE
Meridia Capsules. 475

REPLASYN (Argentina)
ESTRADIOL
Climara Transdermal System 763

REPRIADOL (Denmark)
MORPHINE SULFATE
MS Contin Tablets 2585

REPROST (Chile)
NAPROXEN
EC-Naprosyn Delayed-Release Tablets. . . . 2632
Naprosyn Suspension. 2632
Naprosyn Tablets 2632

REQUIP (Argentina, Austria, Belgium, Canada, Chile, Czech Republic, Denmark, Finland, France, Germany, Greece, Hong Kong, Hungary, Irish Republic, Israel, Italy, Malaysia, New Zealand, Norway, Poland, Portugal, Singapore, South Africa, Spain, Sweden, Switzerland, The Netherlands, Turkey, United Kingdom)
ROPINIROLE HYDROCHLORIDE
Requip Tablets 1561

RESIMIDA (Venezuela)
FUROSEMIDE
Furosemide Tablets 2186

RESMA (Belgium)
ZAFIRLUKAST
Accolate Tablets 669

RESOSTYL (Greece)
SELEGILINE HYDROCHLORIDE
Eldepryl Capsules 3052

RESOTYL (Chile)
MODAFINIL
Provigil Tablets 977

RESPEXIL (Brazil)
NORFLOXACIN
Noroxin Tablets. 2069

RESPICORT (Switzerland)
TRIAMCINOLONE ACETONIDE
Azmacort Inhalation Aerosol 407
Nasacort AQ Nasal Spray 2765

RESPICUR (Austria, Italy)
THEOPHYLLINE
Uniphyl Tablets 2595

RESPIDUAL (Venezuela)
IPRATROPIUM BROMIDE
Atrovent Nasal Spray 0.03%. 834
Atrovent Nasal Spray 0.06%. 836

RESPONTIN (Norway, United Kingdom)
IPRATROPIUM BROMIDE
Atrovent Nasal Spray 0.03%. 834
Atrovent Nasal Spray 0.06%. 836

RESSITAL (Turkey)
CETIRIZINE HYDROCHLORIDE
Zyrtec Syrup 1920
Zyrtec Tablets 1920

RESTOPON (Greece)
RANITIDINE HYDROCHLORIDE
Zantac 25 EFFERdose Tablets 1670
Zantac 150 Tablets 1670
Zantac 300 Tablets 1670
Zantac Injection 1666
Zantac Injection Premixed 1666
Zantac Syrup 1670

RETACNYL (Argentina, Brazil, Chile, France, Hong Kong, Malaysia, Mexico, Singapore, South Africa, Thailand, The Philippines, Venezuela)
TRETINOIN
Vesanoid Capsules. 2660

RETAFYLLIN (Finland, Hungary, Malaysia, Singapore, Thailand)
THEOPHYLLINE
Uniphyl Tablets 2595

RETALZEM (Hong Kong)
DILTIAZEM HYDROCHLORIDE
Cardizem LA Extended Release Tablets. . . . 421

RETAMIN (Venezuela)
RANITIDINE HYDROCHLORIDE
Zantac 25 EFFERdose Tablets 1670
Zantac 150 Tablets 1670
Zantac 300 Tablets 1670
Zantac Injection 1666
Zantac Injection Premixed 1666
Zantac Syrup 1670

RET-A-PRES (Mexico)
TRETINOIN
Vesanoid Capsules. 2660

RETAVIT (Israel)
TRETINOIN
Vesanoid Capsules. 2660

RETENSIN (The Philippines)
CAPTOPRIL
Captopril Tablets. 2182

RETEP (Argentina)
FUROSEMIDE
Furosemide Tablets 2186

RETICNE (Argentina)
TRETINOIN
Vesanoid Capsules. 2660

RETIN-A (Argentina, Australia, Austria, Brazil, Canada, Chile, Czech Republic, France, Hong Kong, Irish Republic, Israel, Italy, Malaysia, Mexico, New Zealand, Poland, Portugal, Singapore, South Africa, Switzerland, Thailand, The Philippines, United Kingdom)
TRETINOIN
Vesanoid Capsules. 2660

RETINEI (Venezuela)
TRETINOIN
Vesanoid Capsules. 2660

RETINIDE (Argentina)
ISOTRETINOIN
Accutane Capsules 2607

RETINO (Turkey)
TRETINOIN
Vesanoid Capsules. 2660

RETINOVA (Belgium, Brazil, Denmark, France, New Zealand, Singapore, Spain, Sweden, United Kingdom)
TRETINOIN
Vesanoid Capsules. 2660

RETIRIDES (Spain)
TRETINOIN
Vesanoid Capsules. 2660

RETISOL-A (Canada)
TRETINOIN
Vesanoid Capsules. 2660

RETITOP (France)
TRETINOIN
Vesanoid Capsules. 2660

RETRIEVE (Australia, Hong Kong)
TRETINOIN
Vesanoid Capsules. 2660

RETROKOR (The Philippines)
CEFTRIAXONE SODIUM
Rocephin Injectable Vials, ADD-Vantage, Galaxy, Bulk 2642

RETROVIR (Argentina, Australia, Austria, Belgium, Brazil, Canada, Chile, Czech Republic, Denmark, Finland, France, Germany, Greece, Hong Kong, India, Irish Republic, Israel, Italy, Malaysia, Mexico, New Zealand, Norway, Poland, Portugal, Russia, Singapore, South Africa, Spain, Sweden, Switzerland, Thailand, The Netherlands, The Philippines, Turkey, United Kingdom, Venezuela)
ZIDOVUDINE
Retrovir Capsules 1574
Retrovir IV Infusion. 1579
Retrovir Syrup 1574
Retrovir Tablets. 1574

REUCORTIL (Mexico)
NAPROXEN
EC-Naprosyn Delayed-Release Tablets. . . . 2632
Naprosyn Suspension. 2632
Naprosyn Tablets 2632

REUMAREN (Brazil)
DICLOFENAC SODIUM
Voltaren Tablets 2334
Voltaren-XR Tablets 2337

REUMYL (Italy)
SULINDAC
Clinoril Tablets 1962

REUXEN (Portugal)
NAPROXEN
EC-Naprosyn Delayed-Release Tablets. . . . 2632
Naprosyn Suspension. 2632
Naprosyn Tablets 2632

REVALINTABS (The Netherlands)
CETIRIZINE HYDROCHLORIDE
Zyrtec Syrup 1920
Zyrtec Tablets 1920

REVASTIN (Brazil)
SIMVASTATIN
Zocor Tablets. 2136

REVECTINA (Brazil)
IVERMECTIN
Stromectol Tablets **2120**

REVELLEX (Argentina, South Africa)
INFLIXIMAB
Remicade for IV Injection **950**

REVELOL (India)
METOPROLOL SUCCINATE
Toprol-XL Tablets **666**

REVION (Greece)
CIPROFLOXACIN HYDROCHLORIDE
Cipro Tablets **2810**

REVIRAX (Brazil)
ZIDOVUDINE
Retrovir Capsules **1574**
Retrovir IV Infusion **1579**
Retrovir Syrup **1574**
Retrovir Tablets **1574**

REWODINA (Czech Republic, Germany)
DICLOFENAC SODIUM
Voltaren Tablets **2334**
Voltaren-XR Tablets **2337**

REXACIN (Hong Kong, Thailand)
NORFLOXACIN
Noroxin Tablets **2069**

REXAMAT (Argentina)
CALCITRIOL
Calcijex Injection **419**
Rocaltrol Capsules **1150**
Rocaltrol Oral Solution **1150**

REXETIN (Poland, Russia)
PAROXETINE HYDROCHLORIDE
Paxil Oral Suspension **1535**
Paxil Tablets **1535**

REXNER (Argentina)
CIPROFLOXACIN HYDROCHLORIDE
Cipro Tablets **2810**

REXTAT (Italy)
LOVASTATIN
Mevacor Tablets **2063**

REZAMID (Argentina)
TRIAMCINOLONE ACETONIDE
Azmacort Inhalation Aerosol **407**
Nasacort AQ Nasal Spray **2765**

REZAMID D, REZAMID F, REZAMID M (Argentina)
TRIAMCINOLONE ACETONIDE
Azmacort Inhalation Aerosol **407**
Nasacort AQ Nasal Spray **2765**

REZULT (India)
ROSIGLITAZONE MALEATE
Avandia Tablets **1351**

RFG-KIT (Argentina)
FLUORESCEIN SODIUM
Fluorescite Injection .... ⊙**203**

R-FLEX (South Africa)
SULINDAC
Clinoril Tablets **1962**

RHEMOFENAX (Hong Kong)
DICLOFENAC SODIUM
Voltaren Tablets **2334**
Voltaren-XR Tablets **2337**

RHEUFENAC (Switzerland)
DICLOFENAC SODIUM
Voltaren Tablets **2334**
Voltaren-XR Tablets **2337**

RHEUFLAM (The Philippines)
DICLOFENAC SODIUM
Voltaren Tablets **2334**
Voltaren-XR Tablets **2337**

RHEUFLEX (United Kingdom)
NAPROXEN
EC-Naprosyn Delayed-Release Tablets **2632**
Naprosyn Suspension **2632**
Naprosyn Tablets **2632**

RHEUMABENE (Austria)
DICLOFENAC SODIUM
Voltaren Tablets **2334**
Voltaren-XR Tablets **2337**

RHEUMASAN D (Germany)
DICLOFENAC SODIUM
Voltaren Tablets **2334**
Voltaren-XR Tablets **2337**

RHEUMATAC (United Kingdom)
DICLOFENAC SODIUM
Voltaren Tablets **2334**
Voltaren-XR Tablets **2337**

RHEUMAVEK (Greece)
DICLOFENAC SODIUM
Voltaren Tablets **2334**
Voltaren-XR Tablets **2337**

RHEWLIN (Malaysia)
DICLOFENAC SODIUM
Voltaren Tablets **2334**
Voltaren-XR Tablets **2337**

RHINALAR (Australia, Canada, Hong Kong)
FLUNISOLIDE
Aerobid Inhaler System **1153**
Aerobid-M Inhaler System **1153**

RHINARIS-F (Canada)
FLUNISOLIDE
Aerobid Inhaler System **1153**
Aerobid-M Inhaler System **1153**

RHINIL (Hong Kong)
CETIRIZINE HYDROCHLORIDE
Zyrtec Syrup **1920**
Zyrtec Tablets **1920**

RHINISAN (Germany)
TRIAMCINOLONE ACETONIDE
Azmacort Inhalation Aerosol **407**
Nasacort AQ Nasal Spray **2765**

RHINOGEN (Switzerland)
SODIUM HYALURONATE
Hyalgan Solution **2742**

RHINOVENT (Switzerland)
IPRATROPIUM BROMIDE
Atrovent Nasal Spray 0.03% **834**
Atrovent Nasal Spray 0.06% **836**

RHIZIN (Singapore)
CETIRIZINE HYDROCHLORIDE
Zyrtec Syrup **1920**
Zyrtec Tablets **1920**

RHODIALAX (Canada)
LACTULOSE
Kristalose for Oral Solution **1004**

RHODIALOSE (Canada)
LACTULOSE
Kristalose for Oral Solution **1004**

RHODIAPROX (Canada)
NAPROXEN
EC-Naprosyn Delayed-Release Tablets **2632**
Naprosyn Suspension **2632**
Naprosyn Tablets **2632**

RHOTARD (United Kingdom)
MORPHINE SULFATE
MS Contin Tablets **2585**

RHUMALGAN (Switzerland, United Kingdom)
DICLOFENAC SODIUM
Voltaren Tablets **2334**
Voltaren-XR Tablets **2337**

RHYTHMOCOR (Austria)
PROPAFENONE HYDROCHLORIDE
Rythmol SR Capsules **1590**

RIBASTAMIN (Argentina)
RISEDRONATE SODIUM
Actonel Tablets **2568**

RIBEX FLU (Italy)
DICLOFENAC SODIUM
Voltaren Tablets **2334**
Voltaren-XR Tablets **2337**

RIBOLIN (Greece)
RANITIDINE HYDROCHLORIDE
Zantac 25 EFFERdose Tablets **1670**
Zantac 150 Tablets **1670**
Zantac 300 Tablets **1670**
Zantac Injection **1666**
Zantac Injection Premixed **1666**
Zantac Syrup **1670**

RIDAZIN (Israel)
THIORIDAZINE HYDROCHLORIDE
Thioridazine Hydrochloride Tablets **2195**

RIDAZINE (South Africa, Thailand)
THIORIDAZINE HYDROCHLORIDE
Thioridazine Hydrochloride Tablets **2195**

RIDRON (Argentina)
RISEDRONATE SODIUM
Actonel Tablets **2568**

RIDRON PACK (Argentina)
RISEDRONATE SODIUM
Actonel Tablets **2568**

RIFAXI (Argentina)
RITONAVIR
Norvir Oral Solution **489**
Norvir Soft Gelatin Capsules **489**

RIFLUX (Poland)
RANITIDINE HYDROCHLORIDE
Zantac 25 EFFERdose Tablets **1670**
Zantac 150 Tablets **1670**
Zantac 300 Tablets **1670**
Zantac Injection **1666**
Zantac Injection Premixed **1666**
Zantac Syrup **1670**

RIGIX (Austria)
CETIRIZINE HYDROCHLORIDE
Zyrtec Syrup **1920**
Zyrtec Tablets **1920**

RILACE (Turkey)
LISINOPRIL
Prinivil Tablets **2087**

RILACE PLUS (Turkey)
LISINOPRIL
Prinivil Tablets **2087**

RILASAT (Argentina)
RILUZOLE
Rilutek Tablets **2771**

RILCAPTON (Hong Kong, Russia, Singapore)
CAPTOPRIL
Captopril Tablets **2182**

RILUTEK (Argentina, Australia, Austria, Belgium, Brazil, Canada, Chile, Czech Republic, Denmark, Finland, France, Germany, Greece, Hong Kong, Hungary, Irish Republic, Israel, Italy, Japan, Mexico, Norway, Poland, Portugal, Singapore, South Africa, Spain, Sweden, Switzerland, Thailand, The Netherlands, Turkey, United Kingdom, Venezuela)
RILUZOLE
Rilutek Tablets **2771**

RIMAPAM (United Kingdom)
DIAZEPAM
Valium Tablets **2658**

RIMOXYN (United Kingdom)
NAPROXEN
EC-Naprosyn Delayed-Release Tablets **2632**
Naprosyn Suspension **2632**
Naprosyn Tablets **2632**

RINALIX (Malaysia, Singapore)
INDAPAMIDE
Indapamide Tablets **2188**

RINATEC (Irish Republic, United Kingdom)
IPRATROPIUM BROMIDE
Atrovent Nasal Spray 0.03% **834**
Atrovent Nasal Spray 0.06% **836**

RINELON (Italy, Mexico, South Africa, Spain, Thailand, The Philippines)
MOMETASONE FUROATE
Elocon Cream 0.1% **2840**
Elocon Lotion 0.1% **2841**
Elocon Ointment 0.1% **2842**
Nasonex Nasal Spray **2883**

RINISONA (Argentina)
FLUTICASONE PROPIONATE
Flonase Nasal Spray **1431**

RINITRIN (India)
CETIRIZINE HYDROCHLORIDE
Zyrtec Syrup **1920**
Zyrtec Tablets **1920**

RINOBEREN (Spain)
IPRATROPIUM BROMIDE
Atrovent Nasal Spray 0.03% **834**
Atrovent Nasal Spray 0.06% **836**

RINOLAST D (Venezuela)
FEXOFENADINE HYDROCHLORIDE/PSEUDOEPHEDRINE HYDROCHLORIDE
Allegra-D 12 Hour Extended-Release Tablets **2687**

RINOSONE (Spain)
FLUTICASONE PROPIONATE
Flonase Nasal Spray **1431**

RINOVAGOS (Italy)
IPRATROPIUM BROMIDE
Atrovent Nasal Spray 0.03% **834**
Atrovent Nasal Spray 0.06% **836**

RINOVAL (Chile)
MOMETASONE FUROATE
Elocon Cream 0.1% **2840**
Elocon Lotion 0.1% **2841**
Elocon Ointment 0.1% **2842**
Nasonex Nasal Spray **2883**

RINSTEAD TEETHING GEL (United Kingdom)
LIDOCAINE
Lidoderm Patch **1114**

RINXOFAY (Thailand)
CEFTRIAXONE SODIUM
Rocephin Injectable Vials, ADD-Vantage, Galaxy, Bulk **2642**

RISEDON (Argentina)
RISEDRONATE SODIUM
Actonel Tablets **2568**

RISELLE (Brazil, Czech Republic)
ESTRADIOL
Climara Transdermal System **763**

RISOFOS (India)
RISEDRONATE SODIUM
Actonel Tablets **2568**

RISTO (Thailand)
TRIAMCINOLONE ACETONIDE
Azmacort Inhalation Aerosol **407**
Nasacort AQ Nasal Spray **2765**

RITECHOL (Irish Republic)
SIMVASTATIN
Zocor Tablets **2136**

RITHROPROL (Greece)
CLARITHROMYCIN
Biaxin Filmtab Tablets **411**
Biaxin Granules **411**

RITMOCOR (Chile)
PROPAFENONE HYDROCHLORIDE
Rythmol SR Capsules **1590**

RITMONORM (Brazil)
PROPAFENONE HYDROCHLORIDE
Rythmol SR Capsules **1590**

RITOMUNE (India)
RITONAVIR
Norvir Oral Solution **489**
Norvir Soft Gelatin Capsules **489**

RITOVIR (Brazil)
RITONAVIR
Norvir Oral Solution **489**
Norvir Soft Gelatin Capsules **489**

RITROMINE (Argentina)
NORFLOXACIN
Noroxin Tablets **2069**

RITUXAN (Canada, Japan)
RITUXIMAB
Rituxan I.V. **1223**

RIUCLONAZ (Argentina)
CLONAZEPAM
Klonopin Tablets **2639**

RIVATRIL (Finland)
CLONAZEPAM
Klonopin Tablets **2639**

RIVAZOL (Mexico)
ALBENDAZOLE
Albenza Tablets **1297**

RIVILINA (Argentina)
APROTININ
Trasylol Injection **799**

RIVOSTATIN (Switzerland)
NYSTATIN
Nystop Topical Powder USP **2498**

RIVOTRIL (Argentina, Australia, Austria, Belgium, Brazil, Canada, Czech Republic, Denmark, France, Germany, Hong Kong, Hungary, Irish Republic, Israel, Italy, Mexico, New Zealand, Norway, Poland, Portugal, Singapore, South Africa, Spain, Switzerland, Thailand, The Netherlands, The Philippines, Turkey, United Kingdom, Venezuela)
CLONAZEPAM
Klonopin Tablets **2639**

RIVOXICILLIN (Switzerland)
AMOXICILLIN
Amoxil Pediatric Drops for Oral Suspension **1305**
Amoxil Tablets **1305**

RIXIL (Italy)
VALSARTAN
Diovan Tablets **2212**

RIZACT (India)
RIZATRIPTAN BENZOATE
Maxalt Tablets **2056**
Maxalt-MLT Orally Disintegrating Tablets .. **2056**

RIZALIEF (Austria)
RIZATRIPTAN BENZOATE
Maxalt Tablets **2056**
Maxalt-MLT Orally Disintegrating Tablets .. **2056**

RIZALIV (Italy)
RIZATRIPTAN BENZOATE
Maxalt Tablets **2056**
Maxalt-MLT Orally Disintegrating Tablets .. **2056**

RIZATAN (The Netherlands)
RIZATRIPTAN BENZOATE
Maxalt Tablets **2056**
Maxalt-MLT Orally Disintegrating Tablets .. **2056**

RMS (New Zealand)
MORPHINE SULFATE
MS Contin Tablets **2585**

ROACCUTAN (Argentina, Austria, Denmark, Finland, Germany, Hungary, Italy, Mexico, Portugal, Venezuela)
ISOTRETINOIN
Accutane Capsules **2607**

ROACCUTANE (Australia, Belgium, Czech Republic, France, Greece, Hong Kong, Irish Republic, Israel, New Zealand, Poland, Singapore, South Africa, Switzerland, Thailand, The Netherlands, The Philippines, Turkey, United Kingdom)
ISOTRETINOIN
Accutane Capsules **2607**

ROACNETAN (Chile)
ISOTRETINOIN
Accutane Capsules **2607**

ROACUTAN (Brazil, Spain)
ISOTRETINOIN
Accutane Capsules **2607**

ROCALTROL (Australia, Austria, Belgium, Brazil, Canada, Chile, Czech Republic, Denmark, France, Germany, Hong Kong, Hungary, Irish Republic, Italy, Japan, Mexico, New Zealand, Norway, Poland, Portugal, Singapore, South Africa, Spain, Sweden, Switzerland, Thailand, The Netherlands, The Philippines, Turkey, United Kingdom, Venezuela)
CALCITRIOL
Calcijex Injection **419**
Rocaltrol Capsules **1150**
Rocaltrol Oral Solution **1150**

ROCEFALIN (Spain)
CEFTRIAXONE SODIUM
Rocephin Injectable Vials, ADD-Vantage, Galaxy, Bulk **2642**

ROCEFIN (Brazil, Italy)
CEFTRIAXONE SODIUM
Rocephin Injectable Vials, ADD-Vantage, Galaxy, Bulk **2642**

ROCEPHALIN (Denmark, Finland, Norway, Sweden)
CEFTRIAXONE SODIUM
Rocephin Injectable Vials, ADD-Vantage, Galaxy, Bulk **2642**

ROCEPHIN (Australia, Austria, Canada, Czech Republic, Germany, Greece, Hong Kong, Hungary, Irish Republic, Israel, Japan, Mexico, New Zealand, Poland, Portugal, Singapore, South Africa, Thailand, The Netherlands, The Philippines, Turkey, United Kingdom, Venezuela)
CEFTRIAXONE SODIUM
Rocephin Injectable Vials, ADD-Vantage, Galaxy, Bulk **2642**

ROCEPHINE (Belgium, France, Switzerland)
CEFTRIAXONE SODIUM
Rocephin Injectable Vials, ADD-Vantage, Galaxy, Bulk **2642**

ROCHE (Canada)
NAPROXEN SODIUM
Anaprox DS Tablets **2632**
Anaprox Tablets **2632**

RODIPAL (Argentina)
CARVEDILOL
Coreg Tablets **1387**

ROFANTEN (Spain)
NAPROXEN
EC-Naprosyn Delayed-Release Tablets **2632**
Naprosyn Suspension **2632**
Naprosyn Tablets **2632**

ROFLAZIN (Turkey)
CIPROFLOXACIN HYDROCHLORIDE
Cipro Tablets **2810**

ROFLUAL (France)
RIMANTADINE HYDROCHLORIDE
Flumadine Syrup **1167**
Flumadine Tablets **1167**

ROFOXIN (Brazil)
CEFTRIAXONE SODIUM
Rocephin Injectable Vials, ADD-Vantage, Galaxy, Bulk **2642**

ROFUNIL (The Philippines)
FUROSEMIDE
Furosemide Tablets **2186**

ROFY (Thailand)
TRAMADOL HYDROCHLORIDE
Ultram ER Tablets **2428**

ROGASTI (Israel)
FAMOTIDINE
Pepcid for Oral Suspension **2075**
Pepcid Tablets **2075**

ROGLIN (India)
ROSIGLITAZONE MALEATE
Avandia Tablets **1351**

ROGLIN-M (India)
ROSIGLITAZONE MALEATE
Avandia Tablets **1351**

ROICAL (Malaysia, Singapore)
CALCITRIOL
Calcijex Injection **419**
Rocaltrol Capsules **1150**
Rocaltrol Oral Solution **1150**

ROLAB-AMOCLAV (South Africa)
AMOXICILLIN
Amoxil Pediatric Drops for Oral Suspension **1305**
Amoxil Tablets **1305**

ROLICYTIN (Mexico)
CLARITHROMYCIN
Biaxin Filmtab Tablets **411**
Biaxin Granules **411**

ROLSICAL (India)
CALCITRIOL
Calcijex Injection **419**
Rocaltrol Capsules **1150**
Rocaltrol Oral Solution **1150**

ROMAKSEN (Turkey)
NAPROXEN SODIUM
Anaprox DS Tablets **2632**
Anaprox Tablets **2632**

ROMALINA (Venezuela)
NYSTATIN
Nystop Topical Powder USP **2498**

ROMATIM (Turkey)
NAPROXEN
EC-Naprosyn Delayed-Release Tablets **2632**
Naprosyn Suspension **2632**
Naprosyn Tablets **2632**

ROMICEF (The Philippines)
CEFUROXIME SODIUM
Zinacef Injection **1678**

ROMIR (Mexico)
CAPTOPRIL
Captopril Tablets **2182**

RONABIN (Israel)
DRONABINOL
Marinol Capsules **3163**

RONTAGEL (Argentina)
ESTRADIOL
Climara Transdermal System **763**

RONTILONA (Portugal, Spain)
FLUTICASONE PROPIONATE
Flonase Nasal Spray **1431**

ROPRIL (Hong Kong)
CAPTOPRIL
Captopril Tablets **2182**

ROPSIL (Chile)
CLONAZEPAM
Klonopin Tablets **2639**

ROSAGENUS (Greece)
FAMOTIDINE
Pepcid for Oral Suspension **2075**
Pepcid Tablets **2075**

ROSICON (India)
ROSIGLITAZONE MALEATE
Avandia Tablets **1351**

ROSICON MF (India)
ROSIGLITAZONE MALEATE
Avandia Tablets **1351**

ROSIGLIT (Argentina)
ROSIGLITAZONE MALEATE
Avandia Tablets **1351**

ROSIGLIT-MET (Argentina)
ROSIGLITAZONE MALEATE
Avandia Tablets **1351**

ROSITAL (Greece)
NIMODIPINE
Nimotop Capsules **790**

ROTHONAL (Greece)
RANITIDINE HYDROCHLORIDE
Zantac 25 EFFERdose Tablets **1670**
Zantac 150 Tablets **1670**
Zantac 300 Tablets **1670**
Zantac Injection **1666**
Zantac Injection Premixed **1666**
Zantac Syrup **1670**

ROVACOR (India, Russia, Singapore)
LOVASTATIN
Mevacor Tablets **2063**

ROWESTIN (Venezuela)
SIMVASTATIN
Zocor Tablets **2136**

ROXATINE (Australia)
PAROXETINE HYDROCHLORIDE
Paxil Oral Suspension **1535**
Paxil Tablets **1535**

ROXEN (Thailand)
NAPROXEN
EC-Naprosyn Delayed-Release Tablets **2632**
Naprosyn Suspension **2632**
Naprosyn Tablets **2632**

ROXIN (Australia, Turkey)
CIPROFLOXACIN HYDROCHLORIDE
Cipro Tablets **2810**

ROXON (The Philippines)
CEFTRIAXONE SODIUM
Rocephin Injectable Vials, ADD-Vantage, Galaxy, Bulk **2642**

ROYCEFAX (Brazil)
CEFTAZIDIME
Fortaz for Injection **1450**

ROYEN (Argentina, Spain)
CALCIUM ACETATE
PhosLo GelCaps **1184**

ROZON (Turkey)
RANITIDINE HYDROCHLORIDE
Zantac 25 EFFERdose Tablets **1670**
Zantac 150 Tablets **1670**
Zantac 300 Tablets **1670**
Zantac Injection **1666**
Zantac Injection Premixed **1666**
Zantac Syrup **1670**

RUBACINA (Spain)
FAMOTIDINE
Pepcid for Oral Suspension **2075**
Pepcid Tablets **2075**

RUBIULCER (Spain)
RANITIDINE HYDROCHLORIDE
Zantac 25 EFFERdose Tablets **1670**
Zantac 150 Tablets **1670**
Zantac 300 Tablets **1670**
Zantac Injection **1666**
Zantac Injection Premixed **1666**
Zantac Syrup **1670**

RUCAINA (Mexico)
LIDOCAINE
Lidoderm Patch **1114**

RUDOLAC (Switzerland)
LACTULOSE
Kristalose for Oral Solution **1004**

RUDOPRAM (Switzerland)
CITALOPRAM HYDROBROMIDE
Celexa Tablets **1160**

RUDOXIL (Argentina)
CARVEDILOL
Coreg Tablets **1387**

RUMATAB (Thailand)
DICLOFENAC SODIUM
Voltaren Tablets **2334**
Voltaren-XR Tablets **2337**

RUMAZOLIDIN (Turkey)
NAPROXEN
EC-Naprosyn Delayed-Release Tablets **2632**
Naprosyn Suspension **2632**
Naprosyn Tablets **2632**

RUPEDIZ (Argentina)
DIAZEPAM
Valium Tablets **2658**

RUSYDE (United Kingdom)
FUROSEMIDE
Furosemide Tablets **2186**

RUVOMINOX (Greece)
DICLOFENAC SODIUM
Voltaren Tablets **2334**
Voltaren-XR Tablets **2337**

RUXIM (The Philippines)
CEFUROXIME SODIUM
Zinacef Injection **1678**

RYTHMEX (Israel)
PROPAFENONE HYDROCHLORIDE
Rythmol SR Capsules **1590**

RYTHMOL (Canada, France, South Africa)
PROPAFENONE HYDROCHLORIDE
Rythmol SR Capsules **1590**

RYTHMONORM (Greece)
PROPAFENONE HYDROCHLORIDE
Rythmol SR Capsules **1590**

RYTMOCARD (The Philippines)
PROPAFENONE HYDROCHLORIDE
Rythmol SR Capsules **1590**

RYTMOGENAT (Germany)
PROPAFENONE HYDROCHLORIDE
Rythmol SR Capsules **1590**

RYTMONORM (Belgium, Chile, Denmark, Finland, Germany, Hong Kong, Hungary, Italy, Malaysia, New Zealand, Poland, Portugal, Russia, Singapore, Spain, Sweden, Switzerland, Thailand, The Netherlands, Turkey, Venezuela)
PROPAFENONE HYDROCHLORIDE
Rythmol SR Capsules **1590**

RYTMONORMA (Austria)
PROPAFENONE HYDROCHLORIDE
Rythmol SR Capsules **1590**

RYTMO-PUREN (Germany)
PROPAFENONE HYDROCHLORIDE
Rythmol SR Capsules **1590**

RYVEL (Hong Kong)
CETIRIZINE HYDROCHLORIDE
Zyrtec Syrup **1920**
Zyrtec Tablets **1920**

SABAX COMBINEB (South Africa)
IPRATROPIUM BROMIDE
Atrovent Nasal Spray 0.03% **834**
Atrovent Nasal Spray 0.06% **836**

SABIDAL RECTIOL (Italy)
THEOPHYLLINE
Uniphyl Tablets **2595**

SALCA (Venezuela)
FUROSEMIDE
Furosemide Tablets **2186**

SALDAC (Australia, New Zealand)
SULINDAC
Clinoril Tablets . . . 1962

SALI-PUREN (Germany)
HYDROCHLOROTHIAZIDE/TRIAMTERENE
Dyazide Capsules . . . 1405

SALMETEDUR (Italy)
SALMETEROL XINAFOATE
Serevent Diskus . . . 1594

SALMETER (Venezuela)
SALMETEROL XINAFOATE
Serevent Diskus . . . 1594

SALODIUR (Austria)
HYDROCHLOROTHIAZIDE/TRIAMTERENE
Dyazide Capsules . . . 1405

SALSPRAY (Venezuela)
SALMETEROL XINAFOATE
Serevent Diskus . . . 1594

SALTERMOX (South Africa)
AMOXICILLIN
Amoxil Pediatric Drops for Oral Suspension . . . 1305
Amoxil Tablets . . . 1305

SALUPRAN (Mexico)
NAPROXEN
EC-Naprosyn Delayed-Release Tablets . . . 2632
Naprosyn Suspension . . . 2632
Naprosyn Tablets . . . 2632

SALURIN (United Arab Emirates)
FUROSEMIDE
Furosemide Tablets . . . 2186

SALVALERG (Argentina)
CETIRIZINE HYDROCHLORIDE
Zyrtec Syrup . . . 1920
Zyrtec Tablets . . . 1920

SAMERTAN (Chile)
TELMISARTAN
Micardis Tablets . . . 852

SAMIL-O2 (Italy)
BENZOYL PEROXIDE
Brevoxyl-4 Creamy Wash . . . 3054
Brevoxyl-4 Gel . . . 3054
Brevoxyl-8 Creamy Wash . . . 3054
Brevoxyl-8 Gel . . . 3054

SAMOX (Thailand)
AMOXICILLIN
Amoxil Pediatric Drops for Oral Suspension . . . 1305
Amoxil Tablets . . . 1305

SAMOXIN (Thailand)
AMOXICILLIN
Amoxil Pediatric Drops for Oral Suspension . . . 1305
Amoxil Tablets . . . 1305

SANALER (Chile)
CETIRIZINE HYDROCHLORIDE
Zyrtec Syrup . . . 1920
Zyrtec Tablets . . . 1920

SANCAP (Greece)
CAPTOPRIL
Captopril Tablets . . . 2182

SANCIPRO (Denmark)
CIPROFLOXACIN HYDROCHLORIDE
Cipro Tablets . . . 2810

SANDOSTATIN (Canada, Finland, Germany, Irish Republic, Singapore, The Philippines, United Kingdom)
OCTREOTIDE ACETATE
Sandostatin LAR Depot . . . 2302

SANDOSTATINE (France, Switzerland, The Netherlands)
OCTREOTIDE ACETATE
Sandostatin LAR Depot . . . 2302

SANDRENA (Australia, Austria, Brazil, Chile, Denmark, Germany, Italy, Mexico, New Zealand, Switzerland, The Netherlands, United Kingdom)
ESTRADIOL
Climara Transdermal System . . . 763

SANELOR (Chile)
LOVASTATIN
Mevacor Tablets . . . 2063

SANIPRESIN (Chile)
LOSARTAN POTASSIUM
Cozaar Tablets . . . 1973

SANIPROSTOL (Chile)
FINASTERIDE
Propecia Tablets . . . 2095
Proscar Tablets . . . 2102

SANOMED (The Philippines)
NAPROXEN SODIUM
Anaprox DS Tablets . . . 2632
Anaprox Tablets . . . 2632

SANOXIT (Germany)
BENZOYL PEROXIDE
Brevoxyl-4 Creamy Wash . . . 3054
Brevoxyl-4 Gel . . . 3054
Brevoxyl-8 Creamy Wash . . . 3054
Brevoxyl-8 Gel . . . 3054

SANSANAL (Germany)
CAPTOPRIL
Captopril Tablets . . . 2182

SANSET (Turkey)
CIPROFLOXACIN
Cipro Oral Suspension . . . 2810

SANTANOL (Turkey)
RANITIDINE HYDROCHLORIDE
Zantac 25 EFFERdose Tablets . . . 1670
Zantac 150 Tablets . . . 1670
Zantac 300 Tablets . . . 1670
Zantac Injection . . . 1666
Zantac Injection Premixed . . . 1666
Zantac Syrup . . . 1670

SANTYL (Canada)
COLLAGENASE
Santyl Collagenase Ointment . . . 1724

SARF (United Arab Emirates)
CIPROFLOXACIN HYDROCHLORIDE
Cipro Tablets . . . 2810

SAROMET (Argentina)
DIAZEPAM
Valium Tablets . . . 2658

SARTON (Czech Republic)
VALSARTAN
Diovan Tablets . . . 2212

SARVAL (Argentina)
VALSARTAN
Diovan Tablets . . . 2212

SAUBASIN (Greece)
DILTIAZEM HYDROCHLORIDE
Cardizem LA Extended Release Tablets . . . 421

SCF (Australia)
SUCRALFATE
Carafate Suspension . . . 706
Carafate Tablets . . . 707

SCHEINPHARM TRIAMCINE-A (Canada)
TRIAMCINOLONE ACETONIDE
Azmacort Inhalation Aerosol . . . 407
Nasacort AQ Nasal Spray . . . 2765

SCHERITONIN (Argentina)
ISOTRETINOIN
Accutane Capsules . . . 2607

SCHEROGEL (Austria, Belgium, Germany, Italy, Spain)
BENZOYL PEROXIDE
Brevoxyl-4 Creamy Wash . . . 3054
Brevoxyl-4 Gel . . . 3054
Brevoxyl-8 Creamy Wash . . . 3054
Brevoxyl-8 Gel . . . 3054

SCHOLL ATHLETE'S FOOT (Canada)
BUTENAFINE HYDROCHLORIDE
Mentax Cream . . . 2190

SCLERIL (Italy)
FENOFIBRATE
Tricor Tablets . . . 520

SCLEROFIN (Argentina)
FENOFIBRATE
Tricor Tablets . . . 520

SCRIPTOPAM (South Africa)
DIAZEPAM
Valium Tablets . . . 2658

SEBERCIM (Italy)
NORFLOXACIN
Noroxin Tablets . . . 2069

SECALIP (France, Spain)
FENOFIBRATE
Tricor Tablets . . . 520

SECOTEX (Argentina, Brazil, Chile, Mexico, Venezuela)
TAMSULOSIN HYDROCHLORIDE
Flomax Capsules . . . 848

SECUBAR (Spain)
LISINOPRIL
Prinivil Tablets . . . 2087

SECUBAR DIU (Spain)
HYDROCHLOROTHIAZIDE/LISINOPRIL
Prinzide Tablets . . . 2092

SECURO (Argentina)
IVERMECTIN
Stromectol Tablets . . . 2120

SEDACRIS (Argentina)
THEOPHYLLINE
Uniphyl Tablets . . . 2595

SEDALIN (Thailand)
CEFTRIAXONE SODIUM
Rocephin Injectable Vials, ADD-Vantage, Galaxy, Bulk . . . 2642

SEDANGOR (Argentina)
DIPYRIDAMOLE
Persantine Tablets . . . 869

SEDANIUM-R (Greece)
FAMOTIDINE
Pepcid for Oral Suspension . . . 2075
Pepcid Tablets . . . 2075

SEDIVER (Mexico)
DIAZEPAM
Valium Tablets . . . 2658

SEDONERVIL COMPLEX (Spain)
DIAZEPAM
Valium Tablets . . . 2658

SEDOPAN (Greece)
CEFUROXIME AXETIL
Ceftin for Oral Suspension . . . 1380
Ceftin Tablets . . . 1380

SEDOTENSIL (Argentina)
LISINOPRIL
Prinivil Tablets . . . 2087

SEDOVANON (Argentina)
CLONAZEPAM
Klonopin Tablets . . . 2639

SEDUXEN (Czech Republic, Hungary, Russia)
DIAZEPAM
Valium Tablets . . . 2658

SEDUXEN RG (Czech Republic)
DIAZEPAM
Valium Tablets . . . 2658

SEFAKTIL (Turkey)
CEFUROXIME AXETIL
Ceftin for Oral Suspension . . . 1380
Ceftin Tablets . . . 1380

SEFDIN (India)
CEFDINIR
Omnicef Capsules . . . 497
Omnicef for Oral Suspension . . . 497

SEFMAL (Hong Kong, Singapore, Thailand)
TRAMADOL HYDROCHLORIDE
Ultram ER Tablets . . . 2428

SEFMEX (Hong Kong, Thailand)
SELEGILINE HYDROCHLORIDE
Eldepryl Capsules . . . 3052

SEFNAC (Thailand)
DICLOFENAC SODIUM
Voltaren Tablets . . . 2334
Voltaren-XR Tablets . . . 2337

SEFNOR (Singapore, Thailand)
NORFLOXACIN
Noroxin Tablets . . . 2069

SEGALIN (Czech Republic)
SELEGILINE HYDROCHLORIDE
Eldepryl Capsules . . . 3052

SEGAN (Poland, Russia)
SELEGILINE HYDROCHLORIDE
Eldepryl Capsules . . . 3052

SEGURIL (Spain)
FUROSEMIDE
Furosemide Tablets . . . 2186

SEKUSEPT FORTE S (Germany)
FORMALDEHYDE
Formadon Solution . . . 1699

SELADIN (Malaysia, Singapore)
NAPROXEN
EC-Naprosyn Delayed-Release Tablets . . . 2632
Naprosyn Suspension . . . 2632
Naprosyn Tablets . . . 2632

SELAN (Spain)
CEFUROXIME AXETIL
Ceftin for Oral Suspension . . . 1380
Ceftin Tablets . . . 1380

SELDEPAR (Turkey)
SELEGILINE HYDROCHLORIDE
Eldepryl Capsules . . . 3052

SELECIM (Switzerland)
SELEGILINE HYDROCHLORIDE
Eldepryl Capsules . . . 3052

SELECOM (Italy)
SELEGILINE HYDROCHLORIDE
Eldepryl Capsules . . . 3052

SELECTOFEN (Mexico)
DICLOFENAC SODIUM
Voltaren Tablets . . . 2334
Voltaren-XR Tablets . . . 2337

SELECTOFUR (Mexico)
FUROSEMIDE
Furosemide Tablets . . . 2186

SELEDAT (Italy)
SELEGILINE HYDROCHLORIDE
Eldepryl Capsules . . . 3052

SELEGAM (Germany)
SELEGILINE HYDROCHLORIDE
Eldepryl Capsules . . . 3052

SELEGOS (Hong Kong, Malaysia, Russia, Singapore)
SELEGILINE HYDROCHLORIDE
Eldepryl Capsules . . . 3052

SELEMERCK (Germany)
SELEGILINE HYDROCHLORIDE
Eldepryl Capsules . . . 3052

SELEPARK (Germany)
SELEGILINE HYDROCHLORIDE
Eldepryl Capsules . . . 3052

SELERIN (India, Poland)
SELEGILINE HYDROCHLORIDE
Eldepryl Capsules . . . 3052

SELGENE (Australia, New Zealand, Thailand)
SELEGILINE HYDROCHLORIDE
Eldepryl Capsules . . . 3052

SELGIMED (Germany)
SELEGILINE HYDROCHLORIDE
Eldepryl Capsules . . . 3052

SELGIN (India, Poland)
SELEGILINE HYDROCHLORIDE
Eldepryl Capsules . . . 3052

SELGINA (Chile)
SELEGILINE HYDROCHLORIDE
Eldepryl Capsules . . . 3052

SELINE (Thailand)
SELEGILINE HYDROCHLORIDE
Eldepryl Capsules . . . 3052

SELOKEN (Austria, Mexico, Spain)
METOPROLOL SUCCINATE
Toprol-XL Tablets . . . 666

SELOKEN ZOC (Finland, Sweden)
METOPROLOL SUCCINATE
Toprol-XL Tablets . . . 666

SELOZOK (France)
METOPROLOL SUCCINATE
Toprol-XL Tablets . . . 666

SELO-ZOK (Belgium, Brazil, Denmark, Norway)
METOPROLOL SUCCINATE
Toprol-XL Tablets . . . 666

SELPAR (Italy)
SELEGILINE HYDROCHLORIDE
Eldepryl Capsules . . . 3052

SEMUELE (Greece)
RANITIDINE HYDROCHLORIDE
Zantac 25 EFFERdose Tablets . . . 1670
Zantac 150 Tablets . . . 1670
Zantac 300 Tablets . . . 1670
Zantac Injection . . . 1666

Zantac Injection Premixed **1666**
Zantac Syrup **1670**

SENIREX (Finland)
CETIRIZINE HYDROCHLORIDE
Zyrtec Syrup **1920**
Zyrtec Tablets **1920**

SENRO (Spain)
NORFLOXACIN
Noroxin Tablets **2069**

SENSATON (Argentina)
CLONAZEPAM
Klonopin Tablets **2639**

SENSIGARD (Italy)
RANITIDINE HYDROCHLORIDE
Zantac 25 EFFERdose Tablets **1670**
Zantac 150 Tablets **1670**
Zantac 300 Tablets **1670**
Zantac Injection **1666**
Zantac Injection Premixed **1666**
Zantac Syrup **1670**

SENSIPHARMA (Mexico)
LIDOCAINE
Lidoderm Patch **1114**

SENSITRAM (Brazil)
TRAMADOL HYDROCHLORIDE
Ultram ER Tablets **2428**

SEPATREM (Czech Republic)
SELEGILINE HYDROCHLORIDE
Eldepryl Capsules **3052**

SEPCEN (Spain)
CIPROFLOXACIN HYDROCHLORIDE
Cipro Tablets **2810**

SEPIBEST (Mexico)
CARBAMAZEPINE
Carbatrol Capsules **3019**

SEPRAFILM (United Kingdom)
SODIUM HYALURONATE
Hyalgan Solution **2742**

SEPRAM (Finland, Germany)
CITALOPRAM HYDROBROMIDE
Celexa Tablets **1160**

SEPTIBIOTIC (Argentina)
LEVOFLOXACIN
Levaquin Injection **2416**
Levaquin Tablets **2416**

SEPTICIDE (Argentina)
CIPROFLOXACIN HYDROCHLORIDE
Cipro Tablets **2810**

SEPTINOR (The Philippines)
NORFLOXACIN
Noroxin Tablets **2069**

SEPTOCIPRO (Spain)
CIPROFLOXACIN HYDROCHLORIDE
Cipro Tablets **2810**

SERALGAN (Austria)
CITALOPRAM HYDROBROMIDE
Celexa Tablets **1160**

SERASA (Mexico)
ASPARAGINASE
Elspar for Injection **2488**

SERBENDAZOL (Mexico)
ALBENDAZOLE
Albenza Tablets **1297**

SEREDYN (Mexico)
DIAZEPAM
Valium Tablets **2658**

SERESTILL (Italy)
PAROXETINE HYDROCHLORIDE
Paxil Oral Suspension **1535**
Paxil Tablets **1535**

SERETIDE (Argentina, Australia, Belgium, Czech Republic, Hong Kong, Hungary, India, Malaysia, New Zealand, Poland, Russia, Turkey, Venezuela)
SALMETEROL XINAFOATE
Serevent Diskus **1594**

SERETRAN (Chile)
PAROXETINE HYDROCHLORIDE
Paxil Oral Suspension **1535**
Paxil Tablets **1535**

SEREUPIN (Italy)
PAROXETINE HYDROCHLORIDE
Paxil Oral Suspension **1535**
Paxil Tablets **1535**

SEREVENT (Argentina, Australia, Austria, Belgium, Brazil, Canada, Chile, Czech Republic, Denmark, Finland, France, Germany, Greece, Hong Kong, Hungary, Irish Republic, Israel, Italy, Malaysia, Mexico, New Zealand, Norway, Poland, Portugal, Russia, Singapore, South Africa, Spain, Sweden, Switzerland, Thailand, The Netherlands, The Philippines, Turkey, United Kingdom, Venezuela)
SALMETEROL XINAFOATE
Serevent Diskus **1594**

SERGIMAX (The Philippines)
CEFTRIAXONE SODIUM
Rocephin Injectable Vials, ADD-Vantage, Galaxy, Bulk **2642**

SERITAL (Germany)
CITALOPRAM HYDROBROMIDE
Celexa Tablets **1160**

SERMOXOL (Mexico)
AMOXICILLIN
Amoxil Pediatric Drops for Oral Suspension **1305**
Amoxil Tablets **1305**

SEROBID (India)
SALMETEROL XINAFOATE
Serevent Diskus **1594**

SERODUR (Denmark)
PAROXETINE HYDROCHLORIDE
Paxil Oral Suspension **1535**
Paxil Tablets **1535**

SEROMYCIN (Canada, Hong Kong)
CYCLOSERINE
Seromycin Capsules **1864**

SEROPRAM (Argentina, Hungary, Mexico, Spain)
CITALOPRAM HYDROBROMIDE
Celexa Tablets **1160**

SEROVIDINA (Mexico)
ZIDOVUDINE
Retrovir Capsules **1574**
Retrovir IV Infusion **1579**
Retrovir Syrup **1574**
Retrovir Tablets **1574**

SEROXAT (Austria, Belgium, Czech Republic, Denmark, Finland, Germany, Greece, Hong Kong, Hungary, Irish Republic, Israel, Italy, Malaysia, Norway, Poland, Portugal, Singapore, Spain, Sweden, Thailand, The Netherlands, The Philippines, Turkey, United Kingdom)
PAROXETINE HYDROCHLORIDE
Paxil Oral Suspension **1535**
Paxil Tablets **1535**

SERTIDINE (Mexico)
FAMOTIDINE
Pepcid for Oral Suspension **2075**
Pepcid Tablets **2075**

SERTINAL (Argentina)
SIBUTRAMINE HYDROCHLORIDE
Meridia Capsules **475**

SERTRIXEN (Mexico)
NAPROXEN
EC-Naprosyn Delayed-Release Tablets **2632**
Naprosyn Suspension **2632**
Naprosyn Tablets **2632**

SERVAMOX (Thailand)
AMOXICILLIN
Amoxil Pediatric Drops for Oral Suspension **1305**
Amoxil Tablets **1305**

SERVIFLOX (Singapore, Thailand, Venezuela)
CIPROFLOXACIN
Cipro Oral Suspension **2810**

SERVINAPROX (Switzerland)
NAPROXEN
EC-Naprosyn Delayed-Release Tablets **2632**
Naprosyn Suspension **2632**
Naprosyn Tablets **2632**

SERVIPEP (Hong Kong, Hungary, Singapore)
FAMOTIDINE
Pepcid for Oral Suspension **2075**
Pepcid Tablets **2075**

SERVIPROXAN (Thailand)
NAPROXEN SODIUM
Anaprox DS Tablets **2632**
Anaprox Tablets **2632**

SERVIRADINE (Mexico)
RANITIDINE HYDROCHLORIDE
Zantac 25 EFFERdose Tablets **1670**
Zantac 150 Tablets **1670**
Zantac 300 Tablets **1670**
Zantac Injection **1666**
Zantac Injection Premixed **1666**
Zantac Syrup **1670**

SESAREN (Argentina, Chile, Venezuela)
VENLAFAXINE HYDROCHLORIDE
Effexor XR Capsules **3195**

SETANOL (Greece)
NORFLOXACIN
Noroxin Tablets **2069**

SETIN (Thailand)
CETIRIZINE HYDROCHLORIDE
Zyrtec Syrup **1920**
Zyrtec Tablets **1920**

SETIRAL (Turkey)
CETIRIZINE HYDROCHLORIDE
Zyrtec Syrup **1920**
Zyrtec Tablets **1920**

SETRIOX (Italy)
CEFTRIAXONE SODIUM
Rocephin Injectable Vials, ADD-Vantage, Galaxy, Bulk **2642**

SETRON (Czech Republic)
ONDANSETRON HYDROCHLORIDE
Zofran Injection **1682**
Zofran Injection Premixed **1682**
Zofran Oral Solution **1687**
Zofran Tablets **1687**

SETRONIL (Chile)
CITALOPRAM HYDROBROMIDE
Celexa Tablets **1160**

SETRONON (Poland)
ONDANSETRON HYDROCHLORIDE
Zofran Injection **1682**
Zofran Injection Premixed **1682**
Zofran Oral Solution **1687**
Zofran Tablets **1687**

SEVACOL (Argentina)
SIMVASTATIN
Zocor Tablets **2136**

SEVERAL (Argentina)
SIMVASTATIN
Zocor Tablets **2136**

SEVREDOL (Czech Republic, France, Germany, Irish Republic, New Zealand, Poland, Portugal, Spain, Switzerland, The Netherlands, United Kingdom)
MORPHINE SULFATE
MS Contin Tablets **2585**

SEVRE-LONG (Switzerland)
MORPHINE SULFATE
MS Contin Tablets **2585**

SFINAC (Greece)
DICLOFENAC SODIUM
Voltaren Tablets **2334**
Voltaren-XR Tablets **2337**

SHAROX (The Philippines)
CEFUROXIME AXETIL
Ceftin for Oral Suspension **1380**
Ceftin Tablets **1380**

SHEMOL (Mexico)
TIMOLOL MALEATE
Timoptic in Ocudose **2124**
Timoptic Sterile Ophthalmic Solution **2121**
Timoptic-XE Sterile Ophthalmic Gel Forming Solution **2125**

SHINCEF (Singapore)
CEFUROXIME SODIUM
Zinacef Injection **1678**

SHINCORT (Malaysia, Singapore, Thailand)
TRIAMCINOLONE ACETONIDE
Azmacort Inhalation Aerosol **407**
Nasacort AQ Nasal Spray **2765**

SIBUNAR (Denmark)
CIPROFLOXACIN HYDROCHLORIDE
Cipro Tablets **2810**

SIBUTRAL (France)
SIBUTRAMINE HYDROCHLORIDE
Meridia Capsules **475**

SIBU-TRATOBES (Argentina)
SIBUTRAMINE HYDROCHLORIDE
Meridia Capsules **475**

SICADENTOL PLUS (Argentina)
NAPROXEN
EC-Naprosyn Delayed-Release Tablets **2632**
Naprosyn Suspension **2632**
Naprosyn Tablets **2632**

SICCO (Germany)
INDAPAMIDE
Indapamide Tablets **2188**

SICO RELAX (Spain)
DIAZEPAM
Valium Tablets **2658**

SICOR (Hungary)
SIMVASTATIN
Zocor Tablets **2136**

SICOTRAL (Argentina)
PAROXETINE HYDROCHLORIDE
Paxil Oral Suspension **1535**
Paxil Tablets **1535**

SIFLOKS (Russia, Turkey)
CIPROFLOXACIN
Cipro Oral Suspension **2810**

SIFLOXAN (Brazil)
CIPROFLOXACIN
Cipro Oral Suspension **2810**

SIGACAP COR (Germany)
CAPTOPRIL
Captopril Tablets **2182**

SIGAFAM (Mexico)
FAMOTIDINE
Pepcid for Oral Suspension **2075**
Pepcid Tablets **2075**

SIGAFENAC (Germany)
DICLOFENAC SODIUM
Voltaren Tablets **2334**
Voltaren-XR Tablets **2337**

SIGAMOPEN (Switzerland)
AMOXICILLIN
Amoxil Pediatric Drops for Oral Suspension **1305**
Amoxil Tablets **1305**

SIGASALUR (Germany)
FUROSEMIDE
Furosemide Tablets **2186**

SIGMA CLAV (Brazil)
AMOXICILLIN
Amoxil Pediatric Drops for Oral Suspension **1305**
Amoxil Tablets **1305**

SIGMATRIOL (Brazil)
CALCITRIOL
Calcijex Injection **419**
Rocaltrol Capsules **1150**
Rocaltrol Oral Solution **1150**

SIGMAXIN (Australia)
DIGOXIN
Lanoxin Injection **1498**
Lanoxin Injection Pediatric **1502**
Lanoxin Tablets **1505**

SIKLOCAP (Turkey)
CYCLOSERINE
Seromycin Capsules **1864**

SILCOR (Argentina)
CALCITRIOL
Calcijex Injection **419**
Rocaltrol Capsules **1150**
Rocaltrol Oral Solution **1150**

SILFOX (Argentina)
DICLOFENAC SODIUM
Voltaren Tablets **2334**
Voltaren-XR Tablets **2337**

SILFOX FLEX (Argentina)
DICLOFENAC SODIUM
Voltaren Tablets **2334**
Voltaren-XR Tablets **2337**

SILIDRAL (Argentina)
ALENDRONATE SODIUM
Fosamax Tablets **2005**

SILINO (Germany)
DICLOFENAC SODIUM
Voltaren Tablets 2334
Voltaren-XR Tablets 2337

SILKIS (Austria, Belgium, Brazil, Chile, Finland, France, Germany, Greece, Hong Kong, Irish Republic, Italy, Mexico, Norway, Poland, Portugal, Singapore, Spain, Switzerland, The Netherlands, The Philippines, United Kingdom, Venezuela)
CALCITRIOL
Calcijex Injection 419
Rocaltrol Capsules 1150
Rocaltrol Oral Solution 1150

SIMASPEN (South Africa)
SIMVASTATIN
Zocor Tablets 2136

SIMATOR (Irish Republic)
SIMVASTATIN
Zocor Tablets 2136

SIMCARD (Hong Kong, India, South Africa)
SIMVASTATIN
Zocor Tablets 2136

SIMCHOL (India)
SIMVASTATIN
Zocor Tablets 2136

SIMCORA (Switzerland)
SIMVASTATIN
Zocor Tablets 2136

SIMCORHEXAL (Austria)
SIMVASTATIN
Zocor Tablets 2136

SIMETAC (Hong Kong)
RANITIDINE HYDROCHLORIDE
Zantac 25 EFFERdose Tablets 1670
Zantac 150 Tablets 1670
Zantac 300 Tablets 1670
Zantac Injection 1666
Zantac Injection Premixed 1666
Zantac Syrup 1670

SIMGAL (Poland, Russia)
SIMVASTATIN
Zocor Tablets 2136

SIMIREX (Czech Republic)
SIMVASTATIN
Zocor Tablets 2136

SIMLO (India, Russia)
SIMVASTATIN
Zocor Tablets 2136

SIMOVIL (Israel)
SIMVASTATIN
Zocor Tablets 2136

SIMPERTEN (Chile)
LOSARTAN POTASSIUM
Cozaar Tablets 1973

SIMPLAQOR (Mexico, Venezuela)
SIMVASTATIN
Zocor Tablets 2136

SIMRATIO (Poland)
SIMVASTATIN
Zocor Tablets 2136

SIMREDIN (Poland)
SIMVASTATIN
Zocor Tablets 2136

SIMSTIN (Austria)
SIMVASTATIN
Zocor Tablets 2136

SIMTAN (Irish Republic)
SIMVASTATIN
Zocor Tablets 2136

SIMTEC (Hong Kong, Malaysia)
CETIRIZINE HYDROCHLORIDE
Zyrtec Syrup 1920
Zyrtec Tablets 1920

SIMTIN (Hong Kong, Singapore, The Philippines)
SIMVASTATIN
Zocor Tablets 2136

SIMULECT (Argentina, Australia, Belgium, Brazil, Canada, Chile, Czech Republic, Denmark, Finland, France, Germany, Greece, Hong Kong, Irish Republic, Israel, Italy, Malaysia, Mexico, New Zealand, Norway, Poland, Portugal, Russia, Singapore, South Africa, Spain, Sweden, Switzerland, Thailand, The Netherlands, The Philippines, Turkey, United Kingdom)
BASILIXIMAB
Simulect for Injection 2306

SIMULTAN (Argentina, Chile)
VALSARTAN
Diovan Tablets 2212

SIMULTAN D (Argentina)
VALSARTAN
Diovan Tablets 2212

SIMULTEC (Venezuela)
BASILIXIMAB
Simulect for Injection 2306

SIMVA (The Netherlands)
SIMVASTATIN
Zocor Tablets 2136

SIMVAAPS (Germany)
SIMVASTATIN
Zocor Tablets 2136

SIMVABELL (Australia)
SIMVASTATIN
Zocor Tablets 2136

SIMVABETA (Germany)
SIMVASTATIN
Zocor Tablets 2136

SIMVACARD (Czech Republic, Germany, Poland, Russia)
SIMVASTATIN
Zocor Tablets 2136

SIMVACHOL (Greece, Poland)
SIMVASTATIN
Zocor Tablets 2136

SIMVACOL (Hungary, Portugal)
SIMVASTATIN
Zocor Tablets 2136

SIMVACOR (Germany, Greece, Israel, Malaysia, Poland, Singapore, South Africa)
SIMVASTATIN
Zocor Tablets 2136

SIMVADOC (Germany)
SIMVASTATIN
Zocor Tablets 2136

SIMVADOR (United Kingdom)
SIMVASTATIN
Zocor Tablets 2136

SIMVADURA (Germany)
SIMVASTATIN
Zocor Tablets 2136

SIMVAFOUR (Belgium)
SIMVASTATIN
Zocor Tablets 2136

SIMVAGAMMA (Germany)
SIMVASTATIN
Zocor Tablets 2136

SIMVAHEXAL (Australia, Poland)
SIMVASTATIN
Zocor Tablets 2136

SIMVAKOL (Turkey)
SIMVASTATIN
Zocor Tablets 2136

SIMVALIP (Germany)
SIMVASTATIN
Zocor Tablets 2136

SIMVAPROL (Greece)
SIMVASTATIN
Zocor Tablets 2136

SIMVAR (Australia)
SIMVASTATIN
Zocor Tablets 2136

SIMVARCANA (Austria)
SIMVASTATIN
Zocor Tablets 2136

SIMVASINE (Switzerland)
SIMVASTATIN
Zocor Tablets 2136

SIMVASS (Chile)
SIMVASTATIN
Zocor Tablets 2136

SIMVAST (Switzerland)
SIMVASTATIN
Zocor Tablets 2136

SIMVASTAD (Austria)
SIMVASTATIN
Zocor Tablets 2136

SIMVASTAMED (Belgium)
SIMVASTATIN
Zocor Tablets 2136

SIMVASTEN (Spain)
SIMVASTATIN
Zocor Tablets 2136

SIMVASTEROL (Poland)
SIMVASTATIN
Zocor Tablets 2136

SIMVASTIN (Switzerland)
SIMVASTATIN
Zocor Tablets 2136

SIMVASTOL (Russia)
SIMVASTATIN
Zocor Tablets 2136

SIMVASTUR (Spain)
SIMVASTATIN
Zocor Tablets 2136

SIMVATIN (Austria, Greece)
SIMVASTATIN
Zocor Tablets 2136

SIMVAX (Czech Republic)
SIMVASTATIN
Zocor Tablets 2136

SIMVAXON (Israel)
SIMVASTATIN
Zocor Tablets 2136

SIMVOR (Czech Republic, Hungary, Malaysia, Russia, Singapore, Thailand)
SIMVASTATIN
Zocor Tablets 2136

SIMVOTIN (India, South Africa)
SIMVASTATIN
Zocor Tablets 2136

SIMZOR (Irish Republic)
SIMVASTATIN
Zocor Tablets 2136

SINAKORT-A (Turkey)
TRIAMCINOLONE ACETONIDE
Azmacort Inhalation Aerosol 407
Nasacort AQ Nasal Spray 2765

SINCROSA (Mexico)
ACARBOSE
Precose Tablets 792

SINFEXINA (Mexico)
CIPROFLOXACIN
Cipro Oral Suspension 2810

SINFRACT (Mexico)
ALENDRONATE SODIUM
Fosamax Tablets 2005

SINGULAIR (Argentina, Australia, Austria, Belgium, Brazil, Canada, Chile, Czech Republic, Denmark, Finland, France, Germany, Greece, Hong Kong, Hungary, Irish Republic, Israel, Italy, Malaysia, Mexico, New Zealand, Norway, Poland, Portugal, Singapore, South Africa, Spain, Sweden, Switzerland, Thailand, The Netherlands, The Philippines, Turkey, United Kingdom, Venezuela)
MONTELUKAST SODIUM
Singulair Chewable Tablets 2114
Singulair Tablets 2114

SINOBID (Greece)
NORFLOXACIN
Noroxin Tablets 2069

SINOLIP (The Philippines)
LISINOPRIL
Prinivil Tablets 2087

SINOPREN (South Africa)
LISINOPRIL
Prinivil Tablets 2087

SINOPRIL (Russia)
LISINOPRIL
Prinivil Tablets 2087

SINOPRYL (Turkey)
LISINOPRIL
Prinivil Tablets 2087

SINORETIK (Turkey)
LISINOPRIL
Prinivil Tablets 2087

SINOVIAL (France)
SODIUM HYALURONATE
Hyalgan Solution 2742

SINPEBAC (Mexico)
MUPIROCIN
Bactroban Ointment 1368

SINPET (Mexico)
PHENTERMINE HYDROCHLORIDE
Adipex-P Capsules 1185
Adipex-P Tablets 1185

SINPOR (Portugal)
SIMVASTATIN
Zocor Tablets 2136

SINTENYL (Switzerland)
FENTANYL CITRATE
Actiq 959

SINTOFENAC (Brazil)
DICLOFENAC SODIUM
Voltaren Tablets 2334
Voltaren-XR Tablets 2337

SINTOLATT (Italy)
LACTULOSE
Kristalose for Oral Solution 1004

SINVACOR (Italy)
SIMVASTATIN
Zocor Tablets 2136

SINVALIP (Brazil)
SIMVASTATIN
Zocor Tablets 2136

SINVASCOR (Brazil)
SIMVASTATIN
Zocor Tablets 2136

SINVASTACOR (Brazil)
SIMVASTATIN
Zocor Tablets 2136

SINVASTAMED (Brazil)
SIMVASTATIN
Zocor Tablets 2136

SINVASTIL (Portugal)
SIMVASTATIN
Zocor Tablets 2136

SINVASTIN (Brazil)
SIMVASTATIN
Zocor Tablets 2136

SINVATROX (Brazil)
SIMVASTATIN
Zocor Tablets 2136

SINVAX (Brazil)
SIMVASTATIN
Zocor Tablets 2136

SINVAZ (Brazil, Venezuela)
SIMVASTATIN
Zocor Tablets 2136

SIPAM (Thailand)
DIAZEPAM
Valium Tablets 2658

SIPRION (Finland)
CIPROFLOXACIN HYDROCHLORIDE
Cipro Tablets 2810

SIPROBEL (Turkey)
CIPROFLOXACIN HYDROCHLORIDE
Cipro Tablets 2810

SIPROGUT (Turkey)
CIPROFLOXACIN
Cipro Oral Suspension 2810

SIPROSAN (Turkey)
CIPROFLOXACIN HYDROCHLORIDE
Cipro Tablets 2810

SIROLAX (Israel)
LACTULOSE
Kristalose for Oral Solution . . . 1004

SIRTAL (Austria, Germany)
CARBAMAZEPINE
Carbatrol Capsules . . . 3019

SIRTAP (Italy)
CEFTRIAXONE SODIUM
Rocephin Injectable Vials, ADD-Vantage, Galaxy, Bulk . . . 2642

SISARE MONO (Germany)
ESTRADIOL
Climara Transdermal System . . . 763

SISPRES (Turkey)
CIPROFLOXACIN
Cipro Oral Suspension . . . 2810

SITERIN (Finland)
CETIRIZINE HYDROCHLORIDE
Zyrtec Syrup . . . 1920
Zyrtec Tablets . . . 1920

SITRIOL (Australia)
CALCITRIOL
Calcijex Injection . . . 419
Rocaltrol Capsules . . . 1150
Rocaltrol Oral Solution . . . 1150

SIVASTIN (Brazil, Italy)
SIMVASTATIN
Zocor Tablets . . . 2136

SIVATIN (Irish Republic)
SIMVASTATIN
Zocor Tablets . . . 2136

SIVEROL (The Philippines)
TRAMADOL HYDROCHLORIDE
Ultram ER Tablets . . . 2428

SIVLOR (Argentina)
LOVASTATIN
Mevacor Tablets . . . 2063

SIXACINA (Chile)
CETIRIZINE HYDROCHLORIDE
Zyrtec Syrup . . . 1920
Zyrtec Tablets . . . 1920

SKENAN (Belgium, Czech Republic, France, Italy, Portugal, Spain, The Netherlands)
MORPHINE SULFATE
MS Contin Tablets . . . 2585

SKEZIDE (Thailand)
HYDROCHLOROTHIAZIDE/TRIAMTERENE
Dyazide Capsules . . . 1405

SKITZ (Australia)
BENZOYL PEROXIDE
Brevoxyl-4 Creamy Wash . . . 3054
Brevoxyl-4 Gel . . . 3054
Brevoxyl-8 Creamy Wash . . . 3054
Brevoxyl-8 Gel . . . 3054

SLIMIN (Germany)
HYDROCHLOROTHIAZIDE/TRIAMTERENE
Dyazide Capsules . . . 1405

SLO-BID (Australia, Canada, Hong Kong, Mexico)
THEOPHYLLINE
Uniphyl Tablets . . . 2595

SLOFENAC (United Kingdom)
DICLOFENAC SODIUM
Voltaren Tablets . . . 2334
Voltaren-XR Tablets . . . 2337

SLO-MORPH (Irish Republic)
MORPHINE SULFATE
MS Contin Tablets . . . 2585

SLO-PHYLLIN (Irish Republic, Italy, United Kingdom)
THEOPHYLLINE
Uniphyl Tablets . . . 2595

SLO-THEO (Hong Kong)
THEOPHYLLINE
Uniphyl Tablets . . . 2595

SLOVALGIN (Czech Republic)
MORPHINE SULFATE
MS Contin Tablets . . . 2585

SLOZEM (United Kingdom)
DILTIAZEM HYDROCHLORIDE
Cardizem LA Extended Release Tablets . . . 421

SMARIL (Greece)
RANITIDINE HYDROCHLORIDE
Zantac 25 EFFERdose Tablets . . . 1670
Zantac 150 Tablets . . . 1670
Zantac 300 Tablets . . . 1670
Zantac Injection . . . 1666
Zantac Injection Premixed . . . 1666
Zantac Syrup . . . 1670

SNOFFOCIN (Thailand)
NORFLOXACIN
Noroxin Tablets . . . 2069

SOBREPINA (Portugal)
NIMODIPINE
Nimotop Capsules . . . 790

SOBRONIL (Spain)
NAPROXEN
EC-Naprosyn Delayed-Release Tablets . . . 2632
Naprosyn Suspension . . . 2632
Naprosyn Tablets . . . 2632

SODEN (Hong Kong, Singapore)
NAPROXEN SODIUM
Anaprox DS Tablets . . . 2632
Anaprox Tablets . . . 2632

SODEXX FAMOTIDINE (Austria)
FAMOTIDINE
Pepcid for Oral Suspension . . . 2075
Pepcid Tablets . . . 2075

SODICLO (South Africa)
DICLOFENAC SODIUM
Voltaren Tablets . . . 2334
Voltaren-XR Tablets . . . 2337

SODIP-PHYLLINE (Switzerland)
THEOPHYLLINE
Uniphyl Tablets . . . 2595

SODIXEN (Mexico)
NAPROXEN SODIUM
Anaprox DS Tablets . . . 2632
Anaprox Tablets . . . 2632

SOFASIN (Greece)
NORFLOXACIN
Noroxin Tablets . . . 2069

SOFLAX (United Arab Emirates)
LACTULOSE
Kristalose for Oral Solution . . . 1004

SOLARAZE (Denmark, Finland, France, Germany, Irish Republic, Italy, Norway, Sweden, United Kingdom)
DICLOFENAC SODIUM
Voltaren Tablets . . . 2334
Voltaren-XR Tablets . . . 2337

SOLARCAINE (Switzerland)
LIDOCAINE
Lidoderm Patch . . . 1114

SOLEXA (Austria, Italy, Portugal, The Netherlands)
CELECOXIB
Celebrex Capsules . . . 2979

SOLFIDIN (Argentina)
CLONAZEPAM
Klonopin Tablets . . . 2639

SOLGERETIK Austria, Germany
BENDROFLUMETHIAZIDE/NADOLOL
Corzide Tablets

SOLGOL (Austria, Germany, Spain)
NADOLOL
Nadolol Tablets . . . 2191

SOLIS (United Kingdom)
DIAZEPAM
Valium Tablets . . . 2658

SOLOSIN (Germany)
THEOPHYLLINE
Uniphyl Tablets . . . 2595

SOLUCEL (Spain)
BENZOYL PEROXIDE
Brevoxyl-4 Creamy Wash . . . 3054
Brevoxyl-4 Gel . . . 3054
Brevoxyl-8 Creamy Wash . . . 3054
Brevoxyl-8 Gel . . . 3054

SOLUGEL (Argentina, Brazil, Canada, Chile, Mexico, Venezuela)
BENZOYL PEROXIDE
Brevoxyl-4 Creamy Wash . . . 3054
Brevoxyl-4 Gel . . . 3054
Brevoxyl-8 Creamy Wash . . . 3054
Brevoxyl-8 Gel . . . 3054

SOLVEASY (Australia)
TERBINAFINE HYDROCHLORIDE
Lamisil Tablets . . . 2266

SOLVETAN (Greece)
CEFTAZIDIME
Fortaz for Injection . . . 1450

SOMAC (Spain)
CITALOPRAM HYDROBROMIDE
Celexa Tablets . . . 1160

SOMAFLEX (Greece)
ETIDRONATE DISODIUM
Didronel Tablets . . . 2583

SOMALGESIC (Mexico)
NAPROXEN
EC-Naprosyn Delayed-Release Tablets . . . 2632
Naprosyn Suspension . . . 2632
Naprosyn Tablets . . . 2632

SOMAPLUS (Brazil)
DIAZEPAM
Valium Tablets . . . 2658

SOMATRAN (Chile)
SUMATRIPTAN
Imitrex Nasal Spray . . . 1470

SOMOFILLINA (Italy)
THEOPHYLLINE
Uniphyl Tablets . . . 2595

SOMOPHYLLIN (Canada, South Africa)
THEOPHYLLINE
Uniphyl Tablets . . . 2595

SONAP (Thailand)
NAPROXEN SODIUM
Anaprox DS Tablets . . . 2632
Anaprox Tablets . . . 2632

SOPENTAL (South Africa)
PENTOBARBITAL SODIUM
Nembutal Sodium Solution, USP . . . 2494

SOPHIXIN (Mexico, Venezuela)
CIPROFLOXACIN HYDROCHLORIDE
Cipro Tablets . . . 2810

SOPROXEN (Singapore, Thailand)
NAPROXEN SODIUM
Anaprox DS Tablets . . . 2632
Anaprox Tablets . . . 2632

SOREDINE (Greece)
RANITIDINE HYDROCHLORIDE
Zantac 25 EFFERdose Tablets . . . 1670
Zantac 150 Tablets . . . 1670
Zantac 300 Tablets . . . 1670
Zantac Injection . . . 1666
Zantac Injection Premixed . . . 1666
Zantac Syrup . . . 1670

SOREN (Hong Kong)
NAPROXEN SODIUM
Anaprox DS Tablets . . . 2632
Anaprox Tablets . . . 2632

SORIATANE (Canada, France)
ACITRETIN
Soriatane Capsules . . . 3062

SORTAL (Venezuela)
LOSARTAN POTASSIUM
Cozaar Tablets . . . 1973

SORTIS (Austria, Czech Republic, Hungary, Poland, Switzerland)
ATORVASTATIN CALCIUM
Lipitor Tablets . . . 2501

SOSTRIL (Germany, Venezuela)
ALBENDAZOLE
Albenza Tablets . . . 1297

SOTAZIDEN N (Germany)
NADOLOL
Nadolol Tablets . . . 2191

SOTOVASTIN (Greece)
SIMVASTATIN
Zocor Tablets . . . 2136

SOTRET (Thailand)
ISOTRETINOIN
Accutane Capsules . . . 2607

SP 54 (Hong Kong, Hungary)
PENTOSAN POLYSULFATE SODIUM
Elmiron Capsules . . . 2435

SPATANIL (Greece)
CETIRIZINE HYDROCHLORIDE
Zyrtec Syrup . . . 1920
Zyrtec Tablets . . . 1920

SPAZMO-VALIBRIN (Turkey)
DIAZEPAM
Valium Tablets . . . 2658

SPECINOR (Greece)
RANITIDINE HYDROCHLORIDE
Zantac 25 EFFERdose Tablets . . . 1670
Zantac 150 Tablets . . . 1670
Zantac 300 Tablets . . . 1670
Zantac Injection . . . 1666
Zantac Injection Premixed . . . 1666
Zantac Syrup . . . 1670

SPECTROFLEX (Mexico)
CIPROFLOXACIN
Cipro Oral Suspension . . . 2810

SPECTROXYL (Switzerland)
AMOXICILLIN
Amoxil Pediatric Drops for Oral Suspension . . . 1305
Amoxil Tablets . . . 1305

SPECTRUM (Italy)
CEFTAZIDIME
Fortaz for Injection . . . 1450

SPIROLAIR (Belgium)
PIRBUTEROL ACETATE
Maxair Autohaler . . . 1705

SPOPHYLLIN (Czech Republic)
THEOPHYLLINE
Uniphyl Tablets . . . 2595

SPREDIOL (Italy)
ESTRADIOL
Climara Transdermal System . . . 763

SRM-RHOTARD (Singapore, South Africa)
MORPHINE SULFATE
MS Contin Tablets . . . 2585

STACER (Portugal)
RANITIDINE HYDROCHLORIDE
Zantac 25 EFFERdose Tablets . . . 1670
Zantac 150 Tablets . . . 1670
Zantac 300 Tablets . . . 1670
Zantac Injection . . . 1666
Zantac Injection Premixed . . . 1666
Zantac Syrup . . . 1670

STACORT-A (Hong Kong)
TRIAMCINOLONE ACETONIDE
Azmacort Inhalation Aerosol . . . 407
Nasacort AQ Nasal Spray . . . 2765

STARCEF (Italy)
CEFTAZIDIME
Fortaz for Injection . . . 1450

STAREZIN (Greece)
SIMVASTATIN
Zocor Tablets . . . 2136

STARVAL (India)
VALSARTAN
Diovan Tablets . . . 2212

STASIVA (Greece)
SIMVASTATIN
Zocor Tablets . . . 2136

STATEX (Canada, Singapore)
MORPHINE SULFATE
MS Contin Tablets . . . 2585

STATINAL (Greece)
SIMVASTATIN
Zocor Tablets . . . 2136

STATIVER (Greece)
SIMVASTATIN
Zocor Tablets . . . 2136

STAZEPINE (Hungary)
CARBAMAZEPINE
Carbatrol Capsules . . . 3019

STEDON (Greece)
DIAZEPAM
Valium Tablets . . . 2658

STEINACLOX (Greece)
NORFLOXACIN
Noroxin Tablets . . . 2069

STENOCOR (Italy)
DIPYRIDAMOLE
Persantine Tablets . . . 869

STERICEF (India, Russia)
CEFTRIAXONE SODIUM
Rocephin Injectable Vials, ADD-Vantage, Galaxy, Bulk . . . 2642

STERIGIN (Austria)
ESTRADIOL
Climara Transdermal System . . . 763

STERODOME (Greece)
ETIDRONATE DISODIUM
Didronel Tablets . . . 2583

STERONASE AQ (Israel)
TRIAMCINOLONE ACETONIDE
Azmacort Inhalation Aerosol . . . 407
Nasacort AQ Nasal Spray . . . 2765

STEROSTATINE (Belgium)
NYSTATIN
Nystop Topical Powder USP . . . 2498

STESOLID (Austria, Czech Republic, Denmark, Finland, Germany, Greece, Hong Kong, Hungary, Irish Republic, Israel, Norway, Portugal, Singapore, Spain, Sweden, Switzerland, Thailand, The Netherlands, United Kingdom)
DIAZEPAM
Valium Tablets . . . 2658

STEVENCILLIN (Greece)
AMOXICILLIN
Amoxil Pediatric Drops for Oral Suspension . . . 1305
Amoxil Tablets . . . 1305

STIEFOTREX (Greece)
ISOTRETINOIN
Accutane Capsules . . . 2607

STIEVA-A (Australia, Canada, Chile, Hong Kong, Malaysia, Mexico, Singapore, Thailand, The Philippines)
TRETINOIN
Vesanoid Capsules . . . 2660

STIEVAMYCIN (Argentina, Canada, Mexico)
TRETINOIN
Vesanoid Capsules . . . 2660

STIGMICARPIN (Greece)
NIMODIPINE
Nimotop Capsules . . . 790

STILIDEN (Italy)
PAROXETINE HYDROCHLORIDE
Paxil Oral Suspension . . . 1535
Paxil Tablets . . . 1535

STILL (Brazil, Mexico)
DICLOFENAC SODIUM
Voltaren Tablets . . . 2334
Voltaren-XR Tablets . . . 2337

STILLINE (United Kingdom)
SELEGILINE HYDROCHLORIDE
Eldepryl Capsules . . . 3052

STILOZ (India)
CILOSTAZOL
Pletal Tablets . . . 2481

STIMOLCARDIO (Italy)
DIPYRIDAMOLE
Persantine Tablets . . . 869

STIOXYL (Sweden)
BENZOYL PEROXIDE
Brevoxyl-4 Creamy Wash . . . 3054
Brevoxyl-4 Gel . . . 3054
Brevoxyl-8 Creamy Wash . . . 3054
Brevoxyl-8 Gel . . . 3054

STOCRIN (Argentina, Australia, Austria, Belgium, Brazil, Chile, Czech Republic, Denmark, Finland, Greece, Hong Kong, Israel, Malaysia, Mexico, New Zealand, Norway, Poland, Portugal, Russia, Singapore, South Africa, Sweden, Switzerland, Thailand, The Netherlands, Venezuela)
EFAVIRENZ
Sustiva Capsules . . . 930

STOP ESPINILLA NORMADERM (Spain)
BENZOYL PEROXIDE
Brevoxyl-4 Creamy Wash . . . 3054
Brevoxyl-4 Gel . . . 3054
Brevoxyl-8 Creamy Wash . . . 3054
Brevoxyl-8 Gel . . . 3054

STRIMOX (Venezuela)
AMOXICILLIN
Amoxil Pediatric Drops for Oral Suspension . . . 1305
Amoxil Tablets . . . 1305

STROMECTOL (Australia, France, Japan, The Netherlands)
IVERMECTIN
Stromectol Tablets . . . 2120

STRONAZON (United Kingdom)
TAMSULOSIN HYDROCHLORIDE
Flomax Capsules . . . 848

STROX (India)
CIPROFLOXACIN HYDROCHLORIDE
Cipro Tablets . . . 2810

STUD (United Kingdom)
LIDOCAINE
Lidoderm Patch . . . 1114

STUD 100 (Australia, Israel)
LIDOCAINE
Lidoderm Patch . . . 1114

SUADIAN (Italy)
NAFTIFINE HYDROCHLORIDE
Naftin Cream . . . 2164
Naftin Gel . . . 2164

SUBELAN (Chile)
VENLAFAXINE HYDROCHLORIDE
Effexor XR Capsules . . . 3195

SUBLIMAZE (Argentina, Australia, Canada, Irish Republic, New Zealand, South Africa, The Philippines, United Kingdom)
FENTANYL CITRATE
Actiq . . . 959

SUBSTITOL (Austria)
ESTRADIOL
Climara Transdermal System . . . 763
MORPHINE SULFATE
MS Contin Tablets . . . 2585

SUBSYDE (Thailand)
DICLOFENAC SODIUM
Voltaren Tablets . . . 2334
Voltaren-XR Tablets . . . 2337

SUCARI (Hong Kong)
SUCRALFATE
Carafate Suspension . . . 706
Carafate Tablets . . . 707

SUCCOSA (Sweden)
SUCRALFATE
Carafate Suspension . . . 706
Carafate Tablets . . . 707

SUCRABEST (Germany)
SUCRALFATE
Carafate Suspension . . . 706
Carafate Tablets . . . 707

SUCRAFEN (Thailand)
SUCRALFATE
Carafate Suspension . . . 706
Carafate Tablets . . . 707

SUCRAFILM (Brazil)
SUCRALFATE
Carafate Suspension . . . 706
Carafate Tablets . . . 707

SUCRAGER (Italy)
SUCRALFATE
Carafate Suspension . . . 706
Carafate Tablets . . . 707

SUCRAL (Italy, Thailand)
SUCRALFATE
Carafate Suspension . . . 706
Carafate Tablets . . . 707

SUCRALAN (Austria, Czech Republic)
SUCRALFATE
Carafate Suspension . . . 706
Carafate Tablets . . . 707

SUCRALBENE (Austria)
SUCRALFATE
Carafate Suspension . . . 706
Carafate Tablets . . . 707

SUCRALFIN (Italy)
SUCRALFATE
Carafate Suspension . . . 706
Carafate Tablets . . . 707

SUCRALMAX (Argentina)
SUCRALFATE
Carafate Suspension . . . 706
Carafate Tablets . . . 707

SUCRALOSE (PREPARATION) (United Arab Emirates)
SUCRALFATE
Carafate Suspension . . . 706
Carafate Tablets . . . 707

SUCRALSTAD (Austria)
SUCRALFATE
Carafate Suspension . . . 706
Carafate Tablets . . . 707

SUCRALUM (Portugal)
SUCRALFATE
Carafate Suspension . . . 706
Carafate Tablets . . . 707

SUCRAMAL (Italy)
SUCRALFATE
Carafate Suspension . . . 706
Carafate Tablets . . . 707

SUCRAMED (Austria)
SUCRALFATE
Carafate Suspension . . . 706
Carafate Tablets . . . 707

SUCRAPHIL (Germany)
SUCRALFATE
Carafate Suspension . . . 706
Carafate Tablets . . . 707

SUCRASE (India)
SUCRALFATE
Carafate Suspension . . . 706
Carafate Tablets . . . 707

SUCRATE (Greece, Italy, Thailand)
SUCRALFATE
Carafate Suspension . . . 706
Carafate Tablets . . . 707

SUCRATYROL (Austria)
SUCRALFATE
Carafate Suspension . . . 706
Carafate Tablets . . . 707

SUCRORIL (Italy)
SUCRALFATE
Carafate Suspension . . . 706
Carafate Tablets . . . 707

SUDAC (Italy)
SULINDAC
Clinoril Tablets . . . 1962

SUGAR (Italy)
SUCRALFATE
Carafate Suspension . . . 706
Carafate Tablets . . . 707

SUGAST (Italy)
SUCRALFATE
Carafate Suspension . . . 706
Carafate Tablets . . . 707

SUIFLOX (Mexico)
CIPROFLOXACIN HYDROCHLORIDE
Cipro Tablets . . . 2810

SULARTRENE (Italy)
SULINDAC
Clinoril Tablets . . . 1962

SULCRAN (Chile)
SUCRALFATE
Carafate Suspension . . . 706
Carafate Tablets . . . 707

SULCRATE (Canada)
SUCRALFATE
Carafate Suspension . . . 706
Carafate Tablets . . . 707

SULEN (Italy)
SULINDAC
Clinoril Tablets . . . 1962

SULEXON (Spain)
DICLOFENAC SODIUM
Voltaren Tablets . . . 2334
Voltaren-XR Tablets . . . 2337

SULFAMYLON (Canada, United Kingdom)
MAFENIDE ACETATE
Sulfamylon Cream . . . 2194
Sulfamylon for 5% Topical Solution . . . 2194

SULFINAV (Argentina)
EFAVIRENZ
Sustiva Capsules . . . 930

SULFONA (Portugal, Spain)
DAPSONE
Dapsone Tablets USP . . . 1746

SULFOXYL (Canada)
BENZOYL PEROXIDE
Brevoxyl-4 Creamy Wash . . . 3054
Brevoxyl-4 Gel . . . 3054
Brevoxyl-8 Creamy Wash . . . 3054
Brevoxyl-8 Gel . . . 3054

SULIFUR (Mexico)
SULINDAC
Clinoril Tablets . . . 1962

SULINDAL (Spain)
SULINDAC
Clinoril Tablets . . . 1962

SULINOL (Italy)
SULINDAC
Clinoril Tablets . . . 1962

SULIX (Chile)
TAMSULOSIN HYDROCHLORIDE
Flomax Capsules . . . 848

SULREUMA (Italy)
SULINDAC
Clinoril Tablets . . . 1962

SUMACLINA (Portugal)
SIMVASTATIN
Zocor Tablets . . . 2136

SUMADOL (Italy)
SUMATRIPTAN SUCCINATE
Imitrex Injection . . . 1465
Imitrex Tablets . . . 1474

SUMAMIGREN (Poland)
SUMATRIPTAN SUCCINATE
Imitrex Injection . . . 1465
Imitrex Tablets . . . 1474

SUMATRAN (Turkey)
SUMATRIPTAN
Imitrex Nasal Spray . . . 1470

SUMAX (Brazil)
SUMATRIPTAN SUCCINATE
Imitrex Injection . . . 1465
Imitrex Tablets . . . 1474

SUMIGRA (Poland)
SUMATRIPTAN
Imitrex Nasal Spray . . . 1470

SUMIGRENE (Italy)
SUMATRIPTAN SUCCINATE
Imitrex Injection . . . 1465
Imitrex Tablets . . . 1474

SUMINAT (India)
SUMATRIPTAN SUCCINATE
Imitrex Injection . . . 1465
Imitrex Tablets . . . 1474

SUMITREX (Mexico)
SUMATRIPTAN
Imitrex Nasal Spray . . . 1470

SUNPROX (Malaysia, Singapore)
NAPROXEN SODIUM
Anaprox DS Tablets . . . 2632
Anaprox Tablets . . . 2632

SUPARTZ (United Kingdom)
SODIUM HYALURONATE
Hyalgan Solution . . . 2742

SUPERO (Italy)
CEFUROXIME SODIUM
Zinacef Injection . . . 1678

SUPEUDOL (Canada)
OXYCODONE HYDROCHLORIDE
OxyContin Tablets . . . 2589
OxyIR Capsules . . . 2593

SUPIROCIN (India)
MUPIROCIN
Bactroban Ointment . . . 1368

SUPIROCIN-B (India)
MUPIROCIN
Bactroban Ointment . . . 1368

SUPLASYN (Canada, France, Germany, Irish Republic, Israel, Switzerland, United Kingdom)
SODIUM HYALURONATE
Hyalgan Solution . . . 2742

SUPRACOF (Mexico)
BENZONATATE
Tessalon Perles . . . 1183

SUPRAHYAL (Chile, Mexico, Venezuela)
SODIUM HYALURONATE
Hyalgan Solution . . . 2742

SUPRALIP (Thailand, United Kingdom)
FENOFIBRATE
Tricor Tablets . . . 520

SUPRAMOX (Switzerland)
AMOXICILLIN
Amoxil Pediatric Drops for Oral Suspension . . . 1305
Amoxil Tablets . . . 1305

SUPRIMOX (India)
AMOXICILLIN
Amoxil Pediatric Drops for Oral Suspension . . . 1305
Amoxil Tablets . . . 1305

SURAZEM (The Netherlands)
DILTIAZEM HYDROCHLORIDE
Cardizem LA Extended Release Tablets . . . 421

SURIL (Italy)
SUCRALFATE
Carafate Suspension . . . 706
Carafate Tablets . . . 707

SUSTAC (Argentina)
RANITIDINE HYDROCHLORIDE
Zantac 25 EFFERdose Tablets . . . 1670
Zantac 150 Tablets . . . 1670
Zantac 300 Tablets . . . 1670
Zantac Injection . . . 1666
Zantac Injection Premixed . . . 1666
Zantac Syrup . . . 1670

SUSTIVA (Canada, France, Germany, Irish Republic, Italy, Spain, The Netherlands, United Kingdom)
EFAVIRENZ
Sustiva Capsules . . . 930

SUTAC (Thailand)
CETIRIZINE HYDROCHLORIDE
Zyrtec Syrup . . . 1920
Zyrtec Tablets . . . 1920

SUTRICO (Argentina)
FINASTERIDE
Propecia Tablets . . . 2095
Proscar Tablets . . . 2102

SUVALAN (Australia)
SUMATRIPTAN SUCCINATE
Imitrex Injection . . . 1465
Imitrex Tablets . . . 1474

SVELTANET (Greece)
RANITIDINE HYDROCHLORIDE
Zantac 25 EFFERdose Tablets . . . 1670
Zantac 150 Tablets . . . 1670
Zantac 300 Tablets . . . 1670
Zantac Injection . . . 1666
Zantac Injection Premixed . . . 1666
Zantac Syrup . . . 1670

SVIROXIT (Greece)
ETIDRONATE DISODIUM
Didronel Tablets . . . 2583

SYLADOR (Brazil)
TRAMADOL HYDROCHLORIDE
Ultram ER Tablets . . . 2428

SYMBYAX (Argentina, Chile, Mexico)
OLANZAPINE
Zyprexa Tablets . . . 1883

SYMLA (The Netherlands)
LAMOTRIGINE
Lamictal Chewable Dispersible Tablets . . . 1488
Lamictal Tablets . . . 1488

SYMOXYL (India)
AMOXICILLIN
Amoxil Pediatric Drops for Oral Suspension . . . 1305
Amoxil Tablets . . . 1305

SYNAPROSYN (Venezuela)
NAPROXEN
EC-Naprosyn Delayed-Release Tablets . . . 2632
Naprosyn Suspension . . . 2632
Naprosyn Tablets . . . 2632

SYNAX (Turkey)
NAPROXEN SODIUM
Anaprox DS Tablets . . . 2632
Anaprox Tablets . . . 2632

SYNCLAR (Hong Kong, India)
CLARITHROMYCIN
Biaxin Filmtab Tablets . . . 411
Biaxin Granules . . . 411

SYNDOL (Turkey)
NAPROXEN SODIUM
Anaprox DS Tablets . . . 2632
Anaprox Tablets . . . 2632

SYNERGON (Turkey)
PROGESTERONE
Crinone 4% Gel . . . 992
Prometrium Capsules (100 mg, 200 mg) . 3047

SYNFLEX (Australia, Canada, Hong Kong, Irish Republic, Italy, New Zealand, Singapore, South Africa, Thailand, United Kingdom)
NAPROXEN SODIUM
Anaprox DS Tablets . . . 2632
Anaprox Tablets . . . 2632

SYNITIDINE (Hong Kong)
RANITIDINE HYDROCHLORIDE
Zantac 25 EFFERdose Tablets . . . 1670
Zantac 150 Tablets . . . 1670
Zantac 300 Tablets . . . 1670
Zantac Injection . . . 1666
Zantac Injection Premixed . . . 1666
Zantac Syrup . . . 1670

SYNOCROM (Italy)
SODIUM HYALURONATE
Hyalgan Solution . . . 2742

SYNOGIL (Germany)
NATAMYCIN
Natacyn Antifungal Ophthalmic Suspension . . . ⊙204

SYNOGIN (Thailand)
NAPROXEN
EC-Naprosyn Delayed-Release Tablets . . . 2632
Naprosyn Suspension . . . 2632
Naprosyn Tablets . . . 2632

SYNTARIS (Austria, Belgium, Czech Republic, Germany, Irish Republic, Italy, South Africa, Switzerland, The Netherlands, United Kingdom)
FLUNISOLIDE
Aerobid Inhaler System . . . 1153
Aerobid-M Inhaler System . . . 1153

SYNTHOMANET (Greece)
RANITIDINE HYDROCHLORIDE
Zantac 25 EFFERdose Tablets . . . 1670
Zantac 150 Tablets . . . 1670
Zantac 300 Tablets . . . 1670
Zantac Injection . . . 1666
Zantac Injection Premixed . . . 1666
Zantac Syrup . . . 1670

SYNTHROID (Brazil, Canada)
LEVOTHYROXINE SODIUM
Levothroid Tablets . . . 1170
Levoxyl Tablets . . . 1780
Synthroid Tablets . . . 507

SYSTEN (Austria, Belgium, Brazil, Czech Republic, France, Hungary, Italy, Mexico, Poland, Switzerland, The Netherlands)
ESTRADIOL
Climara Transdermal System . . . 763

SYSTEN CONTI (Brazil, Czech Republic, Poland)
ESTRADIOL
Climara Transdermal System . . . 763

T.O.VIR (Thailand)
ZIDOVUDINE
Retrovir Capsules . . . 1574
Retrovir IV Infusion . . . 1579
Retrovir Syrup . . . 1574
Retrovir Tablets . . . 1574

T/H-BASAN (Switzerland)
HYDROCHLOROTHIAZIDE/TRIAMTERENE
Dyazide Capsules . . . 1405

T-1 (Thailand)
TRIAMCINOLONE ACETONIDE
Azmacort Inhalation Aerosol . . . 407
Nasacort AQ Nasal Spray . . . 2765

T3 (Greece)
LIOTHYRONINE SODIUM
Cytomel Tablets . . . 1778

T4 (Argentina, Greece)
LEVOTHYROXINE SODIUM
Levothroid Tablets . . . 1170
Levoxyl Tablets . . . 1780
Synthroid Tablets . . . 507

TA OSOTH (Thailand)
TRIAMCINOLONE ACETONIDE
Azmacort Inhalation Aerosol . . . 407
Nasacort AQ Nasal Spray . . . 2765

TABPHYN (United Kingdom)
TAMSULOSIN HYDROCHLORIDE
Flomax Capsules . . . 848

TABULAN (Venezuela)
CAPTOPRIL
Captopril Tablets . . . 2182

TACEX (Mexico)
CEFTRIAXONE SODIUM
Rocephin Injectable Vials, ADD-Vantage, Galaxy, Bulk . . . 2642

TACHYFENON (Germany)
PROPAFENONE HYDROCHLORIDE
Rythmol SR Capsules . . . 1590

TACICUL (Argentina)
LOSARTAN POTASSIUM
Cozaar Tablets . . . 1973

TACINES (Argentina)
CIPROFLOXACIN
Cipro Oral Suspension . . . 2810

TACINOL (Thailand)
TRIAMCINOLONE ACETONIDE
Azmacort Inhalation Aerosol . . . 407
Nasacort AQ Nasal Spray . . . 2765

TACLAR (Poland)
CLARITHROMYCIN
Biaxin Filmtab Tablets . . . 411
Biaxin Granules . . . 411

TACRAF (Argentina)
TACROLIMUS
Prograf Capsules and Injection . . . 622

TACROINMUN (Argentina)
TACROLIMUS
Prograf Capsules and Injection . . . 622

TACRON (Spain)
NAPROXEN
EC-Naprosyn Delayed-Release Tablets . . . 2632
Naprosyn Suspension . . . 2632
Naprosyn Tablets . . . 2632

TACRO-TIC (Argentina)
TACROLIMUS
Prograf Capsules and Injection . . . 622

TACROZ (India)
TACROLIMUS
Prograf Capsules and Injection . . . 622

TADOL (Denmark)
TRAMADOL HYDROCHLORIDE
Ultram ER Tablets . . . 2428

TAFLOX (Portugal)
NORFLOXACIN
Noroxin Tablets . . . 2069

TAGAL (Mexico)
CEFTAZIDIME
Fortaz for Injection . . . 1450

TAGONIS (Germany)
PAROXETINE HYDROCHLORIDE
Paxil Oral Suspension . . . 1535
Paxil Tablets . . . 1535

TAHOR (France)
ATORVASTATIN CALCIUM
Lipitor Tablets . . . 2501

TAIRAL (Spain)
FAMOTIDINE
Pepcid for Oral Suspension . . . 2075
Pepcid Tablets . . . 2075

TAKADOL (France)
TRAMADOL HYDROCHLORIDE
Ultram ER Tablets . . . 2428

TAKS (Malaysia, Thailand)
DICLOFENAC SODIUM
Voltaren Tablets . . . 2334
Voltaren-XR Tablets . . . 2337

TALAM (Australia)
CITALOPRAM HYDROBROMIDE
Celexa Tablets . . . 1160

TALEMA (Venezuela)
DIAZEPAM
Valium Tablets . . . 2658

TALGESIL (Malaysia)
FENTANYL
Duragesic Transdermal System . . . 2405

TALICIX (Spain)
CLARITHROMYCIN
Biaxin Filmtab Tablets . . . 411
Biaxin Granules . . . 411

TALIRAX (Greece)
FLUOROMETHOLONE
FML Ophthalmic Ointment . . . ⊙223

TALLITON (Hungary, Russia)
CARVEDILOL
Coreg Tablets . . . 1387

TALNUR (Argentina)
FENTANYL
Duragesic Transdermal System . . . 2405

TALOFILINA (Brazil)
THEOPHYLLINE
Uniphyl Tablets . . . 2595

TALOHEXAL (Australia)
CITALOPRAM HYDROBROMIDE
Celexa Tablets . . . 1160

TALOKEN (Mexico)
CEFTAZIDIME
Fortaz for Injection . . . 1450

TALOMIL (South Africa)
CITALOPRAM HYDROBROMIDE
Celexa Tablets . . . 1160

TALOTREN (Turkey)
THEOPHYLLINE
Uniphyl Tablets . . . 2595

TALZIC (Venezuela)
CETIRIZINE HYDROCHLORIDE
Zyrtec Syrup . . . 1920
Zyrtec Tablets . . . 1920

TAM (Spain)
CIPROFLOXACIN HYDROCHLORIDE
Cipro Tablets . . . 2810

TAMERAN (Spain)
FAMOTIDINE
Pepcid for Oral Suspension . . . 2075
Pepcid Tablets . . . 2075

TAMICTOR (Finland)
TAMSULOSIN HYDROCHLORIDE
Flomax Capsules . . . 848

TAMIN (Spain)
FAMOTIDINE
Pepcid for Oral Suspension . . . 2075
Pepcid Tablets . . . 2075

TAMIRAM (Brazil)
LEVOFLOXACIN
Levaquin Injection . . . 2416
Levaquin Tablets . . . 2416

TAMOLAN (Thailand)
TRAMADOL HYDROCHLORIDE
Ultram ER Tablets . . . 2428

TAMSU (Irish Republic)
TAMSULOSIN HYDROCHLORIDE
Flomax Capsules . . . 848

TAMSUDIL (Poland)
TAMSULOSIN HYDROCHLORIDE
Flomax Capsules . . . 848

TAMSULEK (Poland)
TAMSULOSIN HYDROCHLORIDE
Flomax Capsules . . . 848

TAMSULON (Venezuela)
TAMSULOSIN HYDROCHLORIDE
Flomax Capsules . . . 848

TAMSUMIN (Finland)
TAMSULOSIN HYDROCHLORIDE
Flomax Capsules . . . 848

TAMSUNA (Argentina)
TAMSULOSIN HYDROCHLORIDE
Flomax Capsules . . . 848

TANAMOF (Argentina)
LATANOPROST
Xalatan Ophthalmic Solution . . . ⊙273

TANAVAT (Argentina)
SIMVASTATIN
Zocor Tablets . . . 2136

TANDAX (Mexico)
NAPROXEN SODIUM
Anaprox DS Tablets . . . 2632

Anaprox Tablets 2632

TANDIAL (Mexico)
DIAZEPAM
Valium Tablets 2658

TANDIX (Portugal)
INDAPAMIDE
Indapamide Tablets 2188

TANFEDIN (Venezuela)
CARBAMAZEPINE
Carbatrol Capsules 3019

TANIDINA (Spain)
RANITIDINE HYDROCHLORIDE
Zantac 25 EFFERdose Tablets 1670
Zantac 150 Tablets 1670
Zantac 300 Tablets 1670
Zantac Injection 1666
Zantac Injection Premixed 1666
Zantac Syrup 1670

TANIZONA (Mexico)
NAPROXEN
EC-Naprosyn Delayed-Release Tablets 2632
Naprosyn Suspension 2632
Naprosyn Tablets 2632

TANSILOPROST (Argentina)
TAMSULOSIN HYDROCHLORIDE
Flomax Capsules 848

TANYL (Israel, South Africa)
FENTANYL CITRATE
Actiq 959

TANYZ (Poland)
TAMSULOSIN HYDROCHLORIDE
Flomax Capsules 848

TARDOTOL (Denmark)
CARBAMAZEPINE
Carbatrol Capsules 3019

TAREG (Brazil, Chile, France, Italy, Portugal, South Africa)
VALSARTAN
Diovan Tablets 2212

TAREG-D (Chile)
HYDROCHLOROTHIAZIDE/VALSARTAN
Diovan HCT Tablets 2216

TARIMYL (Venezuela)
ATORVASTATIN CALCIUM
Lipitor Tablets 2501

TARJEN (Thailand)
DICLOFENAC SODIUM
Voltaren Tablets 2334
Voltaren-XR Tablets 2337

TARJENA (Thailand)
DICLOFENAC SODIUM
Voltaren Tablets 2334
Voltaren-XR Tablets 2337

TARKA (Denmark, Finland, France, Germany, Greece, Italy, Mexico, Poland, South Africa, Spain, Sweden, Switzerland, The Netherlands)
TRANDOLAPRIL
Mavik Tablets 472

TARON (Venezuela)
ALBENDAZOLE
Albenza Tablets 1297

TARSIME (Poland)
CEFUROXIME SODIUM
Zinacef Injection 1678

TARTRIAKSON (Poland)
CEFTRIAXONE SODIUM
Rocephin Injectable Vials, ADD-Vantage, Galaxy, Bulk 2642

TAUCOR (Spain)
LOVASTATIN
Mevacor Tablets 2063

TAVACOR (Italy)
LOVASTATIN
Mevacor Tablets 2063

TAVANIC (Argentina, Austria, Belgium, Brazil, Chile, Czech Republic, Finland, France, Germany, Greece, Hungary, India, Irish Republic, Israel, Italy, Mexico, Portugal, Russia, South Africa, Spain, Sweden, Switzerland, The Netherlands, Turkey, United Kingdom, Venezuela)
LEVOFLOXACIN
Levaquin Injection 2416
Levaquin Tablets 2416

TAVAN-SP 54 (South Africa)
PENTOSAN POLYSULFATE SODIUM
Elmiron Capsules 2435

TAVER (Malaysia, Thailand)
CARBAMAZEPINE
Carbatrol Capsules 3019

TAVOR (Venezuela)
SIMVASTATIN
Zocor Tablets 2136

TAXENAN (Mexico)
NAPROXEN
EC-Naprosyn Delayed-Release Tablets 2632
Naprosyn Suspension 2632
Naprosyn Tablets 2632

TAXIFUR (Mexico)
CEFTAZIDIME
Fortaz for Injection 1450

TAXOTERE (Argentina, Australia, Austria, Belgium, Brazil, Canada, Chile, Czech Republic, Denmark, Finland, France, Germany, Greece, Hong Kong, Hungary, Irish Republic, Israel, Italy, Japan, Malaysia, Mexico, New Zealand, Norway, Poland, Portugal, Russia, Singapore, South Africa, Spain, Sweden, Switzerland, Thailand, The Netherlands, The Philippines, Turkey, United Kingdom, Venezuela)
DOCETAXEL
Taxotere Injection Concentrate 2773

TAZALUX (The Netherlands)
CEFTAZIDIME
Fortaz for Injection 1450

TAZEPIN (Brazil)
RANITIDINE HYDROCHLORIDE
Zantac 25 EFFERdose Tablets 1670
Zantac 150 Tablets 1670
Zantac 300 Tablets 1670
Zantac Injection 1666
Zantac Injection Premixed 1666
Zantac Syrup 1670

TAZICEF (The Philippines)
CEFTAZIDIME
Fortaz for Injection 1450

TAZIDAN (The Philippines)
CEFTAZIDIME
Fortaz for Injection 1450

TAZIDEM (Brazil, The Philippines)
CEFTAZIDIME
Fortaz for Injection 1450

TAZIDIF (Italy)
CEFTAZIDIME
Fortaz for Injection 1450

TAZIDIME (Canada)
CEFTAZIDIME
Fortaz for Injection 1450

TAZIJECT (South Africa)
CEFTAZIDIME
Fortaz for Injection 1450

TAZOBAC (Germany, Italy, Portugal, Switzerland)
PIPERACILLIN SODIUM/TAZOBACTAM SODIUM
Zosyn for Injection 3284

TAZOCILLINE (France)
PIPERACILLIN SODIUM/TAZOBACTAM SODIUM
Zosyn for Injection 3284

TAZOCIN (Belgium, Denmark, Finland, Greece, Hong Kong, Irish Republic, Israel, Italy, Mexico, New Zealand, Singapore, South Africa, Sweden, Thailand, The Netherlands)
PIPERACILLIN SODIUM/TAZOBACTAM SODIUM
Zosyn for Injection 3284

TAZONAM (Austria, Chile)
PIPERACILLIN SODIUM/TAZOBACTAM SODIUM
Zosyn for Injection 3284

TDL (The Philippines)
TRAMADOL HYDROCHLORIDE
Ultram ER Tablets 2428

TEALEP (Argentina)
FINASTERIDE
Propecia Tablets 2095
Proscar Tablets 2102

TEBEGRAN (Mexico)
SUMATRIPTAN SUCCINATE
Imitrex Injection 1465
Imitrex Tablets 1474

TECHNIPHYLLINE (Monaco)
THEOPHYLLINE
Uniphyl Tablets 2595

TECNOLIP (Portugal)
LOVASTATIN
Mevacor Tablets 2063

TEDRAL (United Kingdom)
THEOPHYLLINE
Uniphyl Tablets 2595

TEDRALAN (Monaco)
THEOPHYLLINE
Uniphyl Tablets 2595

TEFOR (Turkey)
LEVOTHYROXINE SODIUM
Levothroid Tablets 1170
Levoxyl Tablets 1780
Synthroid Tablets 507

TEGRETAL (Chile, Germany)
CARBAMAZEPINE
Carbatrol Capsules 3019

TEGRETARD (Brazil)
CARBAMAZEPINE
Carbatrol Capsules 3019

TEGRETOL (Argentina, Australia, Austria, Belgium, Brazil, Canada, Czech Republic, Denmark, Finland, France, Greece, Hong Kong, Hungary, Irish Republic, Israel, Italy, Malaysia, Mexico, New Zealand, Norway, Poland, Portugal, Russia, Singapore, South Africa, Spain, Sweden, Switzerland, Thailand, The Netherlands, The Philippines, Turkey, United Kingdom, Venezuela)
CARBAMAZEPINE
Carbatrol Capsules 3019

TEGREX (Brazil)
CARBAMAZEPINE
Carbatrol Capsules 3019

TEGREZIN (Brazil)
CARBAMAZEPINE
Carbatrol Capsules 3019

TEGRITAL (India)
CARBAMAZEPINE
Carbatrol Capsules 3019

TELARIX (Greece)
CETIRIZINE HYDROCHLORIDE
Zyrtec Syrup 1920
Zyrtec Tablets 1920

TELFAST DECONGESTANT (New Zealand)
FEXOFENADINE HYDROCHLORIDE/ PSEUDOEPHEDRINE HYDROCHLORIDE
Allegra-D 12 Hour Extended-Release Tablets 2687

TELFAST-D (Malaysia, Singapore)
FEXOFENADINE HYDROCHLORIDE/ PSEUDOEPHEDRINE HYDROCHLORIDE
Allegra-D 12 Hour Extended-Release Tablets 2687

TELMA (India)
TELMISARTAN
Micardis Tablets 852

TELMOX (Argentina)
AMOXICILLIN
Amoxil Pediatric Drops for Oral Suspension 1305
Amoxil Tablets 1305

TELNASE (Australia, New Zealand)
TRIAMCINOLONE ACETONIDE
Azmacort Inhalation Aerosol 407
Nasacort AQ Nasal Spray 2765

TELPRES (India)
TELMISARTAN
Micardis Tablets 852

TELSOMET (Venezuela)
DIAZEPAM
Valium Tablets 2658

TEMACO (Thailand)
THEOPHYLLINE
Uniphyl Tablets 2595

TEMISARTAN (Argentina)
LOSARTAN POTASSIUM
Cozaar Tablets 1973

TEMPERAX (Chile)
CITALOPRAM HYDROBROMIDE
Celexa Tablets 1160

TEMPOROL (Irish Republic, South Africa)
CARBAMAZEPINE
Carbatrol Capsules 3019

TEMSERIN (Germany, Greece)
TIMOLOL MALEATE
Timoptic in Ocudose 2124
Timoptic Sterile Ophthalmic Solution 2121
Timoptic-XE Sterile Ophthalmic Gel Forming Solution 2125

TENACID (Italy)
CILASTATIN SODIUM/IMIPENEM
Primaxin I.M. 2080
Primaxin I.V. 2083

TENASIL (Poland)
TERBINAFINE HYDROCHLORIDE
Lamisil Tablets 2266

TENDOX (The Netherlands)
BENZOYL PEROXIDE
Brevoxyl-4 Creamy Wash 3054
Brevoxyl-4 Gel 3054
Brevoxyl-8 Creamy Wash 3054
Brevoxyl-8 Gel 3054

TENIBEX (Mexico)
ALBENDAZOLE
Albenza Tablets 1297

TENKAFRUSE (United Kingdom)
FUROSEMIDE
Furosemide Tablets 2186

TENOCARD (Argentina)
NIMODIPINE
Nimotop Capsules 790

TENOPRES (Argentina)
LOSARTAN POTASSIUM
Cozaar Tablets 1973

TENOPRES D (Argentina)
LOSARTAN POTASSIUM
Cozaar Tablets 1973

TENOPT (Australia)
TIMOLOL MALEATE
Timoptic in Ocudose 2124
Timoptic Sterile Ophthalmic Solution 2121
Timoptic-XE Sterile Ophthalmic Gel Forming Solution 2125

TENPRIL (Italy)
CAPTOPRIL
Captopril Tablets 2182

TENSERPIL (Venezuela)
LOSARTAN POTASSIUM
Cozaar Tablets 1973

TENSIKEY (Spain)
LISINOPRIL
Prinivil Tablets 2087

TENSIKEY COMPLEX (Spain)
LISINOPRIL
Prinivil Tablets 2087

TENSIL (Mexico)
CAPTOPRIL
Captopril Tablets 2182

TENSIOMIN (Czech Republic, Germany, Hong Kong, Hungary, Thailand)
CAPTOPRIL
Captopril Tablets 2182

TENSIOMIN-COR (Germany)
CAPTOPRIL
Captopril Tablets 2182

TENSIUM (United Kingdom)
DIAZEPAM
Valium Tablets 2658

TENSOBON (Germany, Switzerland)
CAPTOPRIL
Captopril Tablets 2182

TENSOBON COMP (Germany)
CAPTOPRIL
Captopril Tablets 2182

TENSOPREL (Singapore, Spain)
CAPTOPRIL
Captopril Tablets . . . 2182

TENSOPRIL (Argentina, Irish Republic, Israel, Portugal, United Kingdom)
CAPTOPRIL
Captopril Tablets . . . 2182

TENSOPRIL D (Argentina)
LISINOPRIL
Prinivil Tablets . . . 2087

TENSOSTAD (Germany)
CAPTOPRIL
Captopril Tablets . . . 2182

TENSO-TIMELETS (Germany)
CLONIDINE HYDROCHLORIDE
Catapres Tablets . . . 841

TENUALAX (Argentina)
LACTULOSE
Kristalose for Oral Solution . . . 1004

TEOBAG (Turkey)
THEOPHYLLINE
Uniphyl Tablets . . . 2595

TEOBID (Italy, Venezuela)
THEOPHYLLINE
Uniphyl Tablets . . . 2595

TEODELIN (Spain)
THEOPHYLLINE
Uniphyl Tablets . . . 2595

TEODOSIS (Argentina)
THEOPHYLLINE
Uniphyl Tablets . . . 2595

TEOFILAB (Brazil)
THEOPHYLLINE
Uniphyl Tablets . . . 2595

TEOGEL (Spain)
THEOPHYLLINE
Uniphyl Tablets . . . 2595

TEOKAP (Turkey)
THEOPHYLLINE
Uniphyl Tablets . . . 2595

TEOLIXIR (Spain)
THEOPHYLLINE
Uniphyl Tablets . . . 2595

TEOLONG (Brazil, Mexico)
THEOPHYLLINE
Uniphyl Tablets . . . 2595

TEONIBSA (Portugal)
THEOPHYLLINE
Uniphyl Tablets . . . 2595

TEONOVA (Italy)
THEOPHYLLINE
Uniphyl Tablets . . . 2595

TEOPHYL (Brazil)
THEOPHYLLINE
Uniphyl Tablets . . . 2595

TEOPLUS (Italy)
THEOPHYLLINE
Uniphyl Tablets . . . 2595

TEOSEL (Turkey)
THEOPHYLLINE
Uniphyl Tablets . . . 2595

TEOSONA (Argentina)
THEOPHYLLINE
Uniphyl Tablets . . . 2595

TEOSONA SOL (Argentina)
THEOPHYLLINE
Uniphyl Tablets . . . 2595

TEOSTON (Brazil)
THEOPHYLLINE
Uniphyl Tablets . . . 2595

TEOTARD (Czech Republic, Russia)
THEOPHYLLINE
Uniphyl Tablets . . . 2595

TEOVAL/R (Italy)
THEOPHYLLINE
Uniphyl Tablets . . . 2595

TEOVENT (Portugal)
THEOPHYLLINE
Uniphyl Tablets . . . 2595

TERAFIN (Turkey)
TERBINAFINE HYDROCHLORIDE
Lamisil Tablets . . . 2266

TERAQUIN (Argentina)
LEVOFLOXACIN
Levaquin Injection . . . 2416
Levaquin Tablets . . . 2416

TERBAC (Mexico)
CEFTRIAXONE SODIUM
Rocephin Injectable Vials, ADD-Vantage, Galaxy, Bulk . . . 2642

TERBAFIN (New Zealand)
TERBINAFINE HYDROCHLORIDE
Lamisil Tablets . . . 2266

TERBICIL (South Africa)
TERBINAFINE HYDROCHLORIDE
Lamisil Tablets . . . 2266

TERBIDERM (Germany, Poland, The Netherlands)
TERBINAFINE HYDROCHLORIDE
Lamisil Tablets . . . 2266

TERBIFIL (Switzerland)
TERBINAFINE HYDROCHLORIDE
Lamisil Tablets . . . 2266

TERBIFIN (Hong Kong, India)
TERBINAFINE HYDROCHLORIDE
Lamisil Tablets . . . 2266

TERBIGALEN (Germany)
TERBINAFINE HYDROCHLORIDE
Lamisil Tablets . . . 2266

TERBIGEN (Poland)
TERBINAFINE HYDROCHLORIDE
Lamisil Tablets . . . 2266

TERBIGRAM (Greece)
TERBINAFINE HYDROCHLORIDE
Lamisil Tablets . . . 2266

TERBINAVITA (The Netherlands)
TERBINAFINE HYDROCHLORIDE
Lamisil Tablets . . . 2266

TERBISIL (Czech Republic, Hungary, Poland, Turkey)
TERBINAFINE HYDROCHLORIDE
Lamisil Tablets . . . 2266

TEREKOL (Argentina)
TERBINAFINE HYDROCHLORIDE
Lamisil Tablets . . . 2266

TERFEX (Chile, Venezuela)
TERBINAFINE HYDROCHLORIDE
Lamisil Tablets . . . 2266

TERFIN (Argentina)
TERBINAFINE HYDROCHLORIDE
Lamisil Tablets . . . 2266

TERFUNGIN (The Netherlands)
TERBINAFINE HYDROCHLORIDE
Lamisil Tablets . . . 2266

TERIAM (France)
TRIAMTERENE
Dyrenium Capsules . . . 3189

TERIL (Australia, Hong Kong, Israel, New Zealand, United Kingdom)
CARBAMAZEPINE
Carbatrol Capsules . . . 3019

TERNAF (Irish Republic)
TERBINAFINE HYDROCHLORIDE
Lamisil Tablets . . . 2266

TERODUL (Mexico)
RANITIDINE HYDROCHLORIDE
Zantac 25 EFFERdose Tablets . . . 1670
Zantac 150 Tablets . . . 1670
Zantac 300 Tablets . . . 1670
Zantac Injection . . . 1666
Zantac Injection Premixed . . . 1666
Zantac Syrup . . . 1670

TEROLINAL (Greece)
LISINOPRIL
Prinivil Tablets . . . 2087

TEROMOL (Spain)
THEOPHYLLINE
Uniphyl Tablets . . . 2595

TEROST (Brazil)
ALENDRONATE SODIUM
Fosamax Tablets . . . 2005

TERPOSEN (Spain)
RANITIDINE HYDROCHLORIDE
Zantac 25 EFFERdose Tablets . . . 1670
Zantac 150 Tablets . . . 1670
Zantac 300 Tablets . . . 1670
Zantac Injection . . . 1666
Zantac Injection Premixed . . . 1666
Zantac Syrup . . . 1670

TERSIF (Argentina)
LISINOPRIL
Prinivil Tablets . . . 2087

TERTENSIF (Czech Republic, Poland, Spain)
INDAPAMIDE
Indapamide Tablets . . . 2188

TERTROXIN (Australia, Czech Republic, Irish Republic, New Zealand, South Africa, Thailand, United Kingdom, Venezuela)
LIOTHYRONINE SODIUM
Cytomel Tablets . . . 1778

TERVESON (Greece)
LOVASTATIN
Mevacor Tablets . . . 2063

TERYSOL (Venezuela)
FUROSEMIDE
Furosemide Tablets . . . 2186

TERZINE (Thailand)
CETIRIZINE HYDROCHLORIDE
Zyrtec Syrup . . . 1920
Zyrtec Tablets . . . 1920

TESALON (Mexico)
BENZONATATE
Tessalon Perles . . . 1183

TESOPEN (Mexico)
BENZONATATE
Tessalon Perles . . . 1183

TESS (India)
TRIAMCINOLONE ACETONIDE
Azmacort Inhalation Aerosol . . . 407
Nasacort AQ Nasal Spray . . . 2765

TESSALON (Canada)
BENZONATATE
Tessalon Perles . . . 1183

TETACID (Austria)
FAMOTIDINE
Pepcid for Oral Suspension . . . 2075
Pepcid Tablets . . . 2075

TETROID (Brazil)
LEVOTHYROXINE SODIUM
Levothroid Tablets . . . 1170
Levoxyl Tablets . . . 1780
Synthroid Tablets . . . 507

TEVANATE (Germany)
ALENDRONATE SODIUM
Fosamax Tablets . . . 2005

TEXA (South Africa)
CETIRIZINE HYDROCHLORIDE
Zyrtec Syrup . . . 1920
Zyrtec Tablets . . . 1920

TEXOT (Argentina)
DOCETAXEL
Taxotere Injection Concentrate . . . 2773

TEXOVEN (Mexico)
BENZONATATE
Tessalon Perles . . . 1183

TEYLOR (Spain)
SIMVASTATIN
Zocor Tablets . . . 2136

THAIS (France)
ESTRADIOL
Climara Transdermal System . . . 763

THEANORF (Italy)
NORFLOXACIN
Noroxin Tablets . . . 2069

THELBAN (Malaysia)
ALBENDAZOLE
Albenza Tablets . . . 1297

THEO (Germany)
THEOPHYLLINE
Uniphyl Tablets . . . 2595

THEO MAX (Spain)
THEOPHYLLINE
Uniphyl Tablets . . . 2595

THEO PA (India)
THEOPHYLLINE
Uniphyl Tablets . . . 2595

THEO2 (The Netherlands)
THEOPHYLLINE
Uniphyl Tablets . . . 2595

THEO-2 (Belgium)
THEOPHYLLINE
Uniphyl Tablets . . . 2595

THEO-24 (Italy)
THEOPHYLLINE
Uniphyl Tablets . . . 2595

THEOBID (India)
THEOPHYLLINE
Uniphyl Tablets . . . 2595

THEO-BROS (Greece)
THEOPHYLLINE
Uniphyl Tablets . . . 2595

THEOCHRON (Canada)
THEOPHYLLINE
Uniphyl Tablets . . . 2595

THEODAY (India)
THEOPHYLLINE
Uniphyl Tablets . . . 2595

THEODUR (Japan)
THEOPHYLLINE
Uniphyl Tablets . . . 2595

THEO-DUR (Argentina, Australia, Belgium, Canada, Czech Republic, Denmark, Finland, Greece, Hong Kong, Irish Republic, Italy, New Zealand, Norway, Singapore, South Africa, Spain, Sweden, Thailand, The Philippines, Turkey, United Kingdom)
THEOPHYLLINE
Uniphyl Tablets . . . 2595

THEOFOL (Finland)
THEOPHYLLINE
Uniphyl Tablets . . . 2595

THEOFOL COMP (Finland)
THEOPHYLLINE
Uniphyl Tablets . . . 2595

THEOHEXAL (Austria)
THEOPHYLLINE
Uniphyl Tablets . . . 2595

THEOLAIR (Belgium, Canada, France, Germany, Italy, Spain, Switzerland, The Netherlands)
THEOPHYLLINE
Uniphyl Tablets . . . 2595

THEOLAN (Irish Republic)
THEOPHYLLINE
Uniphyl Tablets . . . 2595

THEOLIN (Malaysia, Singapore, The Netherlands)
THEOPHYLLINE
Uniphyl Tablets . . . 2595

THEOLONG (Japan)
THEOPHYLLINE
Uniphyl Tablets . . . 2595

THEON (Switzerland)
THEOPHYLLINE
Uniphyl Tablets . . . 2595

THEOPED (India)
THEOPHYLLINE
Uniphyl Tablets . . . 2595

THEOPEXINE (France)
THEOPHYLLINE
Uniphyl Tablets . . . 2595

THEOPHAR (United Arab Emirates)
THEOPHYLLINE
Uniphyl Tablets . . . 2595

THEOPHTARD (Hungary)
THEOPHYLLINE
Uniphyl Tablets . . . 2595

THEOPHYLLARD (Belgium, Czech Republic, Germany)
THEOPHYLLINE
Uniphyl Tablets . . . 2595

THEOPHYLLINE SEDATIVE BRUNEAU (Belgium)
THEOPHYLLINE
Uniphyl Tablets . . . 2595

TIMODROP (Thailand)
TIMOLOL MALEATE
Timoptic in Ocudose 2124
Timoptic Sterile Ophthalmic Solution 2121
Timoptic-XE Sterile Ophthalmic Gel Forming Solution 2125

TIMOEDO (Germany)
TIMOLOL MALEATE
Timoptic in Ocudose 2124
Timoptic Sterile Ophthalmic Solution 2121
Timoptic-XE Sterile Ophthalmic Gel Forming Solution 2125

TIMOFTAL (Austria, Turkey)
TIMOLOL MALEATE
Timoptic in Ocudose 2124
Timoptic Sterile Ophthalmic Solution 2121
Timoptic-XE Sterile Ophthalmic Gel Forming Solution 2125

TIMOFTOL (Spain)
TIMOLOL MALEATE
Timoptic in Ocudose 2124
Timoptic Sterile Ophthalmic Solution 2121
Timoptic-XE Sterile Ophthalmic Gel Forming Solution 2125

TIMOGAL (Czech Republic)
TIMOLOL MALEATE
Timoptic in Ocudose 2124
Timoptic Sterile Ophthalmic Solution 2121
Timoptic-XE Sterile Ophthalmic Gel Forming Solution 2125

TIMOGEL (Spain)
TIMOLOL MALEATE
Timoptic in Ocudose 2124
Timoptic Sterile Ophthalmic Solution 2121
Timoptic-XE Sterile Ophthalmic Gel Forming Solution 2125

TIMOGLAU (Portugal)
TIMOLOL MALEATE
Timoptic in Ocudose 2124
Timoptic Sterile Ophthalmic Solution 2121
Timoptic-XE Sterile Ophthalmic Gel Forming Solution 2125

TIMOHEXAL (Austria, Czech Republic, Germany, Poland, Russia)
TIMOLOL MALEATE
Timoptic in Ocudose 2124
Timoptic Sterile Ophthalmic Solution 2121
Timoptic-XE Sterile Ophthalmic Gel Forming Solution 2125

TIMOLABAK (Italy)
TIMOLOL MALEATE
Timoptic in Ocudose 2124
Timoptic Sterile Ophthalmic Solution 2121
Timoptic-XE Sterile Ophthalmic Gel Forming Solution 2125

TIMOLEN (Portugal)
TIMOLOL MALEATE
Timoptic in Ocudose 2124
Timoptic Sterile Ophthalmic Solution 2121
Timoptic-XE Sterile Ophthalmic Gel Forming Solution 2125

TIMOLER (Argentina)
TIMOLOL MALEATE
Timoptic in Ocudose 2124
Timoptic Sterile Ophthalmic Solution 2121
Timoptic-XE Sterile Ophthalmic Gel Forming Solution 2125

TIMOLO (India)
TIMOLOL MALEATE
Timoptic in Ocudose 2124
Timoptic Sterile Ophthalmic Solution 2121
Timoptic-XE Sterile Ophthalmic Gel Forming Solution 2125

TIMOLUX (Italy)
TIMOLOL MALEATE
Timoptic in Ocudose 2124
Timoptic Sterile Ophthalmic Solution 2121
Timoptic-XE Sterile Ophthalmic Gel Forming Solution 2125

TIMOMANN (Germany)
TIMOLOL MALEATE
Timoptic in Ocudose 2124
Timoptic Sterile Ophthalmic Solution 2121
Timoptic-XE Sterile Ophthalmic Gel Forming Solution 2125

TIMONIL (Czech Republic, Germany, Hong Kong, Hungary, Israel, Poland, Switzerland, United Kingdom)
CARBAMAZEPINE
Carbatrol Capsules 3019

TIMO-OPTAL (Thailand)
TIMOLOL MALEATE
Timoptic in Ocudose 2124
Timoptic Sterile Ophthalmic Solution 2121
Timoptic-XE Sterile Ophthalmic Gel Forming Solution 2125

TIMOP (Chile)
TIMOLOL MALEATE
Timoptic in Ocudose 2124
Timoptic Sterile Ophthalmic Solution 2121
Timoptic-XE Sterile Ophthalmic Gel Forming Solution 2125

TIM-OPHTAL (Austria, Germany)
TIMOLOL MALEATE
Timoptic in Ocudose 2124
Timoptic Sterile Ophthalmic Solution 2121
Timoptic-XE Sterile Ophthalmic Gel Forming Solution 2125

TIMO-POS (Belgium)
TIMOLOL MALEATE
Timoptic in Ocudose 2124
Timoptic Sterile Ophthalmic Solution 2121
Timoptic-XE Sterile Ophthalmic Gel Forming Solution 2125

TIMOPOS COMOD (Germany)
TIMOLOL MALEATE
Timoptic in Ocudose 2124
Timoptic Sterile Ophthalmic Solution 2121
Timoptic-XE Sterile Ophthalmic Gel Forming Solution 2125

TIMOPTIC (Argentina, Austria, Canada, Poland, Switzerland, Turkey)
TIMOLOL MALEATE
Timoptic in Ocudose 2124
Timoptic Sterile Ophthalmic Solution 2121
Timoptic-XE Sterile Ophthalmic Gel Forming Solution 2125

TIMOPTOL (Australia, Belgium, Brazil, Czech Republic, France, Hong Kong, Irish Republic, Italy, Japan, Malaysia, Mexico, New Zealand, Portugal, Singapore, South Africa, Thailand, The Netherlands, United Kingdom, Venezuela)
TIMOLOL MALEATE
Timoptic in Ocudose 2124
Timoptic Sterile Ophthalmic Solution 2121
Timoptic-XE Sterile Ophthalmic Gel Forming Solution 2125

TIMOPTOLGEL (Belgium)
TIMOLOL MALEATE
Timoptic in Ocudose 2124
Timoptic Sterile Ophthalmic Solution 2121
Timoptic-XE Sterile Ophthalmic Gel Forming Solution 2125

TIMOPTOL-XE (Australia, Chile)
TIMOLOL MALEATE
Timoptic in Ocudose 2124
Timoptic Sterile Ophthalmic Solution 2121
Timoptic-XE Sterile Ophthalmic Gel Forming Solution 2125

TIMOSAN (Denmark, Finland, Norway, Sweden)
TIMOLOL MALEATE
Timoptic in Ocudose 2124
Timoptic Sterile Ophthalmic Solution 2121
Timoptic-XE Sterile Ophthalmic Gel Forming Solution 2125

TIMOSIL (Thailand)
TIMOLOL MALEATE
Timoptic in Ocudose 2124
Timoptic Sterile Ophthalmic Solution 2121
Timoptic-XE Sterile Ophthalmic Gel Forming Solution 2125

TIMOSINE (Germany)
TIMOLOL MALEATE
Timoptic in Ocudose 2124
Timoptic Sterile Ophthalmic Solution 2121
Timoptic-XE Sterile Ophthalmic Gel Forming Solution 2125

TIMOSOFT (Italy)
TIMOLOL MALEATE
Timoptic in Ocudose 2124
Timoptic Sterile Ophthalmic Solution 2121
Timoptic-XE Sterile Ophthalmic Gel Forming Solution 2125

TIMOSOL (Turkey)
TIMOLOL MALEATE
Timoptic in Ocudose 2124
Timoptic Sterile Ophthalmic Solution 2121
Timoptic-XE Sterile Ophthalmic Gel Forming Solution 2125

TIMO-STULLN (Germany)
TIMOLOL MALEATE
Timoptic in Ocudose 2124
Timoptic Sterile Ophthalmic Solution 2121
Timoptic-XE Sterile Ophthalmic Gel Forming Solution 2125

TIMOZZARD (Mexico)
TIMOLOL MALEATE
Timoptic in Ocudose 2124
Timoptic Sterile Ophthalmic Solution 2121
Timoptic-XE Sterile Ophthalmic Gel Forming Solution 2125

TIMPILO (Argentina, Australia, Czech Republic, Malaysia)
TIMOLOL MALEATE
Timoptic in Ocudose 2124
Timoptic Sterile Ophthalmic Solution 2121
Timoptic-XE Sterile Ophthalmic Gel Forming Solution 2125

TIMPRON (United Kingdom)
NAPROXEN
EC-Naprosyn Delayed-Release Tablets 2632
Naprosyn Suspension 2632
Naprosyn Tablets 2632

TIMSOPT (Austria)
DORZOLAMIDE HYDROCHLORIDE/ TIMOLOL MALEATE
Cosopt Sterile Ophthalmic Solution 1969

TINACEF (Argentina)
CEFTAZIDIME
Fortaz for Injection 1450

TINAGEL (Belgium, The Netherlands)
BENZOYL PEROXIDE
Brevoxyl-4 Creamy Wash 3054
Brevoxyl-4 Gel 3054
Brevoxyl-8 Creamy Wash 3054
Brevoxyl-8 Gel 3054

TINASIN (Venezuela)
SIMVASTATIN
Zocor Tablets 2136

TINEAFINE (Switzerland)
TERBINAFINE HYDROCHLORIDE
Lamisil Tablets 2266

T-INMUN (Chile)
TACROLIMUS
Prograf Capsules and Injection 622

TIOF (Chile, Mexico)
TIMOLOL MALEATE
Timoptic in Ocudose 2124
Timoptic Sterile Ophthalmic Solution 2121
Timoptic-XE Sterile Ophthalmic Gel Forming Solution 2125

TIOF PLUS (Chile)
DORZOLAMIDE HYDROCHLORIDE
Trusopt Sterile Ophthalmic Solution 2128

TIONER (Spain)
TRAMADOL HYDROCHLORIDE
Ultram ER Tablets 2428

TIOSALIS (Argentina)
ONDANSETRON HYDROCHLORIDE
Zofran Injection 1682
Zofran Injection Premixed 1682
Zofran Oral Solution 1687
Zofran Tablets 1687

TIPAC (Chile)
RANITIDINE HYDROCHLORIDE
Zantac 25 EFFERdose Tablets 1670
Zantac 150 Tablets 1670
Zantac 300 Tablets 1670
Zantac Injection 1666
Zantac Injection Premixed 1666
Zantac Syrup 1670

TIPAROL (Sweden)
TRAMADOL HYDROCHLORIDE
Ultram ER Tablets 2428

TIPODEX (Spain)
FAMOTIDINE
Pepcid for Oral Suspension 2075
Pepcid Tablets 2075

TIRACRIN (Italy)
LEVOTHYROXINE SODIUM
Levothroid Tablets 1170
Levoxyl Tablets 1780
Synthroid Tablets 507

TIRIZIN (Austria)
CETIRIZINE HYDROCHLORIDE
Zyrtec Syrup 1920
Zyrtec Tablets 1920

TIROCAL (Mexico)
CALCITRIOL
Calcijex Injection 419
Rocaltrol Capsules 1150
Rocaltrol Oral Solution 1150

TIROIDIN (Brazil)
LEVOTHYROXINE SODIUM
Levothroid Tablets 1170
Levoxyl Tablets 1780
Synthroid Tablets 507

TIROIDINE (Mexico)
LEVOTHYROXINE SODIUM
Levothroid Tablets 1170
Levoxyl Tablets 1780
Synthroid Tablets 507

TIROMEL (Turkey)
LIOTHYRONINE SODIUM
Cytomel Tablets 1778

TIROSINT (Italy)
LEVOTHYROXINE SODIUM
Levothroid Tablets 1170
Levoxyl Tablets 1780
Synthroid Tablets 507

TISOGEN (Argentina)
TOPOTECAN HYDROCHLORIDE
Hycamtin for Injection 1459

TISOREK (Argentina)
CELECOXIB
Celebrex Capsules 2979

TI-TRE (Italy)
LIOTHYRONINE SODIUM
Cytomel Tablets 1778

TIVIRLON (Greece)
LISINOPRIL
Prinivil Tablets 2087

TIZINE (Thailand)
CETIRIZINE HYDROCHLORIDE
Zyrtec Syrup 1920
Zyrtec Tablets 1920

T-LONG (Germany)
TRAMADOL HYDROCHLORIDE
Ultram ER Tablets 2428

TOBICOR (Switzerland)
LISINOPRIL
Prinivil Tablets 2087

TOBICOR PLUS (Switzerland)
LISINOPRIL
Prinivil Tablets 2087

TOBIN (Switzerland)
CETIRIZINE HYDROCHLORIDE
Zyrtec Syrup 1920
Zyrtec Tablets 1920

TOBRAFEN (Switzerland)
DICLOFENAC SODIUM
Voltaren Tablets 2334
Voltaren-XR Tablets 2337

TOBRATLAS (Argentina)
DICLOFENAC SODIUM
Voltaren Tablets 2334
Voltaren-XR Tablets 2337

TOCASOL (Chile)
IMIQUIMOD
Aldara Cream, 5% 1699

TOCODERM (Mexico)
TRETINOIN
Vesanoid Capsules 2660

TOLMA (The Philippines)
TRAMADOL HYDROCHLORIDE
Ultram ER Tablets 2428

TOLOXIN (Thailand)
DIGOXIN
Lanoxin Injection 1498
Lanoxin Injection Pediatric 1502
Lanoxin Tablets 1505

TOLYDOL (India)
TRAMADOL HYDROCHLORIDE
Ultram ER Tablets 2428

TOMAG (Argentina)
RANITIDINE HYDROCHLORIDE
Zantac 25 EFFERdose Tablets 1670

Zantac 150 Tablets . . . 1670
Zantac 300 Tablets . . . 1670
Zantac Injection . . . 1666
Zantac Injection Premixed . . . 1666
Zantac Syrup . . . 1670

TOMANIL FLEX (Argentina)
DICLOFENAC SODIUM
Voltaren Tablets . . . 2334
Voltaren-XR Tablets . . . 2337

TOMPRIL (Brazil)
CAPTOPRIL
Captopril Tablets . . . 2182

TONOFTAL-N (Germany)
NYSTATIN
Nystop Topical Powder USP . . . 2498

TONOTEN (Venezuela)
LISINOPRIL
Prinivil Tablets . . . 2087

TONOTENSIL (Chile)
LISINOPRIL
Prinivil Tablets . . . 2087

TONOTENSIL D (Chile)
HYDROCHLOROTHIAZIDE/LISINOPRIL
Prinzide Tablets . . . 2092

TOPACE (Australia)
CAPTOPRIL
Captopril Tablets . . . 2182

TOPALGIC (France)
TRAMADOL HYDROCHLORIDE
Ultram ER Tablets . . . 2428

TOPCORT (Hong Kong, India)
MOMETASONE FUROATE
Elocon Cream 0.1% . . . 2840
Elocon Lotion 0.1% . . . 2841
Elocon Ointment 0.1% . . . 2842
Nasonex Nasal Spray . . . 2883

TOPESTIN (Argentina)
TOPOTECAN HYDROCHLORIDE
Hycamtin for Injection . . . 1459

TOPEX (Australia)
BENZOYL PEROXIDE
Brevoxyl-4 Creamy Wash . . . 3054
Brevoxyl-4 Gel . . . 3054
Brevoxyl-8 Creamy Wash . . . 3054
Brevoxyl-8 Gel . . . 3054

TOPFANS (Italy)
DICLOFENAC SODIUM
Voltaren Tablets . . . 2334
Voltaren-XR Tablets . . . 2337

TOPILONE (Thailand)
TRIAMCINOLONE ACETONIDE
Azmacort Inhalation Aerosol . . . 407
Nasacort AQ Nasal Spray . . . 2765

TOPISTIN (Greece)
CIPROFLOXACIN
Cipro Oral Suspension . . . 2810

TOPLA (South Africa)
LIDOCAINE
Lidoderm Patch . . . 1114

TOPOKEBIR (Argentina)
TOPOTECAN HYDROCHLORIDE
Hycamtin for Injection . . . 1459

TOPOTAG (Argentina)
TOPOTECAN HYDROCHLORIDE
Hycamtin for Injection . . . 1459

TOPOTEL (India, Thailand)
TOPOTECAN HYDROCHLORIDE
Hycamtin for Injection . . . 1459

TOPRILEM (Mexico)
CAPTOPRIL
Captopril Tablets . . . 2182

TOPROL (Australia)
METOPROLOL SUCCINATE
Toprol-XL Tablets . . . 666

TOPTEAR (Chile, Venezuela)
SODIUM HYALURONATE
Hyalgan Solution . . . 2742

TORIO (Thailand)
SIMVASTATIN
Zocor Tablets . . . 2136

TORIOL (Spain)
RANITIDINE HYDROCHLORIDE
Zantac 25 EFFERdose Tablets . . . 1670
Zantac 150 Tablets . . . 1670
Zantac 300 Tablets . . . 1670
Zantac Injection . . . 1666
Zantac Injection Premixed . . . 1666
Zantac Syrup . . . 1670

TORIVAS (Argentina)
ATORVASTATIN CALCIUM
Lipitor Tablets . . . 2501

TORLOS (Brazil)
LOSARTAN POTASSIUM
Cozaar Tablets . . . 1973

TORLOS H (Brazil)
LOSARTAN POTASSIUM
Cozaar Tablets . . . 1973

TORVACARD (Poland)
ATORVASTATIN CALCIUM
Lipitor Tablets . . . 2501

TORVAST (Italy)
ATORVASTATIN CALCIUM
Lipitor Tablets . . . 2501

TORVIC (Mexico)
CLARITHROMYCIN
Biaxin Filmtab Tablets . . . 411
Biaxin Granules . . . 411

TORYXIL (Germany)
DICLOFENAC SODIUM
Voltaren Tablets . . . 2334
Voltaren-XR Tablets . . . 2337

TOTALIP (Italy)
ATORVASTATIN CALCIUM
Lipitor Tablets . . . 2501

TOTELLE (Sweden)
ESTRADIOL
Climara Transdermal System . . . 763

TOTELLE CONTINUO (Argentina, Chile, Mexico, Venezuela)
ESTRADIOL
Climara Transdermal System . . . 763

TOTELMIN (Brazil)
ALBENDAZOLE
Albenza Tablets . . . 1297

TOTTIZIM (Italy)
CEFTAZIDIME
Fortaz for Injection . . . 1450

TRABAR (Czech Republic, Israel)
TRAMADOL HYDROCHLORIDE
Ultram ER Tablets . . . 2428

TRABILIN (Brazil)
TRAMADOL HYDROCHLORIDE
Ultram ER Tablets . . . 2428

TRACINE (Thailand)
TRAMADOL HYDROCHLORIDE
Ultram ER Tablets . . . 2428

TRACIX (Spain)
CILASTATIN SODIUM/IMIPENEM
Primaxin I.M. . . . 2080
Primaxin I.V. . . . 2083

TRADELIA (Germany)
ESTRADIOL
Climara Transdermal System . . . 763

TRADOL (Germany, Irish Republic, Mexico, Singapore)
TRAMADOL HYDROCHLORIDE
Ultram ER Tablets . . . 2428

TRADOLAN (Austria, Denmark, Finland, Norway, Sweden)
TRAMADOL HYDROCHLORIDE
Ultram ER Tablets . . . 2428

TRADOLGESIC (Thailand)
TRAMADOL HYDROCHLORIDE
Ultram ER Tablets . . . 2428

TRADONAL (Belgium, Hong Kong, Italy, Spain, The Netherlands, The Philippines)
TRAMADOL HYDROCHLORIDE
Ultram ER Tablets . . . 2428

TRADOX (Chile)
LAMOTRIGINE
Lamictal Chewable Dispersible Tablets . . . 1488
Lamictal Tablets . . . 1488

TRAFLASH (Italy)
TRAMADOL HYDROCHLORIDE
Ultram ER Tablets . . . 2428

TRALGIOL (Spain)
TRAMADOL HYDROCHLORIDE
Ultram ER Tablets . . . 2428

TRALGIT (Czech Republic)
TRAMADOL HYDROCHLORIDE
Ultram ER Tablets . . . 2428

TRALIC (Mexico)
TRAMADOL HYDROCHLORIDE
Ultram ER Tablets . . . 2428

TRALODIE (Italy)
TRAMADOL HYDROCHLORIDE
Ultram ER Tablets . . . 2428

TRAMA (Germany)
TRAMADOL HYDROCHLORIDE
Ultram ER Tablets . . . 2428

TRAMABENE (Austria, Czech Republic)
TRAMADOL HYDROCHLORIDE
Ultram ER Tablets . . . 2428

TRAMABETA (Germany)
TRAMADOL HYDROCHLORIDE
Ultram ER Tablets . . . 2428

TRAMACET (Argentina, Canada, Mexico, South Africa, United Kingdom)
TRAMADOL HYDROCHLORIDE
Ultram ER Tablets . . . 2428

TRAMACIP (India)
TRAMADOL HYDROCHLORIDE
Ultram ER Tablets . . . 2428

TRAMACIP PLUS (India)
TRAMADOL HYDROCHLORIDE
Ultram ER Tablets . . . 2428

TRAMADA (Malaysia)
TRAMADOL HYDROCHLORIDE
Ultram ER Tablets . . . 2428

TRAMADEX (Israel)
TRAMADOL HYDROCHLORIDE
Ultram ER Tablets . . . 2428

TRAMADIL (Thailand)
TRAMADOL HYDROCHLORIDE
Ultram ER Tablets . . . 2428

TRAMADIN (Finland)
TRAMADOL HYDROCHLORIDE
Ultram ER Tablets . . . 2428

TRAMADOC (Germany)
TRAMADOL HYDROCHLORIDE
Ultram ER Tablets . . . 2428

TRAMADOLOR (Austria, Germany, Hungary, Switzerland, Turkey)
TRAMADOL HYDROCHLORIDE
Ultram ER Tablets . . . 2428

TRAMADON (Brazil)
TRAMADOL HYDROCHLORIDE
Ultram ER Tablets . . . 2428

TRAMA-DORSCH (Germany)
TRAMADOL HYDROCHLORIDE
Ultram ER Tablets . . . 2428

TRAMADURA (Germany)
TRAMADOL HYDROCHLORIDE
Ultram ER Tablets . . . 2428

TRAMAGETIC (Finland, Germany, Norway, The Netherlands)
TRAMADOL HYDROCHLORIDE
Ultram ER Tablets . . . 2428

TRAMAGIT (Czech Republic, Germany)
TRAMADOL HYDROCHLORIDE
Ultram ER Tablets . . . 2428

TRAMAHEXAL (Australia, Poland, South Africa)
TRAMADOL HYDROCHLORIDE
Ultram ER Tablets . . . 2428

TRAMAKE (Irish Republic, United Kingdom)
TRAMADOL HYDROCHLORIDE
Ultram ER Tablets . . . 2428

TRAMA-KLOSIDOL (Argentina)
TRAMADOL HYDROCHLORIDE
Ultram ER Tablets . . . 2428

TRAMAL (Argentina, Australia, Austria, Brazil, Chile, Finland, Germany, Hong Kong, Israel, Malaysia, New Zealand, Poland, Portugal, Russia, Singapore, South Africa, Switzerland, Thailand, The Netherlands, Venezuela)
TRAMADOL HYDROCHLORIDE
Ultram ER Tablets . . . 2428

TRAMALAN (Argentina, Thailand)
TRAMADOL HYDROCHLORIDE
Ultram ER Tablets . . . 2428

TRAMALGIC (Hungary)
TRAMADOL HYDROCHLORIDE
Ultram ER Tablets . . . 2428

TRAMALIN (Italy)
TRAMADOL HYDROCHLORIDE
Ultram ER Tablets . . . 2428

TRAMAMED (Austria, Thailand)
TRAMADOL HYDROCHLORIDE
Ultram ER Tablets . . . 2428

TRAMAMERCK (Germany)
TRAMADOL HYDROCHLORIDE
Ultram ER Tablets . . . 2428

TRAMAPINE (Irish Republic)
TRAMADOL HYDROCHLORIDE
Ultram ER Tablets . . . 2428

TRAMASTAD (Austria)
TRAMADOL HYDROCHLORIDE
Ultram ER Tablets . . . 2428

TRAMATYROL (Austria)
TRAMADOL HYDROCHLORIDE
Ultram ER Tablets . . . 2428

TRAMAX (Thailand)
TRAMADOL HYDROCHLORIDE
Ultram ER Tablets . . . 2428

TRAMAZAC (India, South Africa)
TRAMADOL HYDROCHLORIDE
Ultram ER Tablets . . . 2428

TRAMBO (Finland)
TRAMADOL HYDROCHLORIDE
Ultram ER Tablets . . . 2428

TRAMCOD (Poland)
TRAMADOL HYDROCHLORIDE
Ultram ER Tablets . . . 2428

TRAMEDPHANO (Germany)
TRAMADOL HYDROCHLORIDE
Ultram ER Tablets . . . 2428

TRAMELENE (The Netherlands)
TRAMADOL HYDROCHLORIDE
Ultram ER Tablets . . . 2428

TRAMEX (Irish Republic)
TRAMADOL HYDROCHLORIDE
Ultram ER Tablets . . . 2428

TRAMIUM (Belgium)
TRAMADOL HYDROCHLORIDE
Ultram ER Tablets . . . 2428

TRAMO (Hong Kong)
TRAMADOL HYDROCHLORIDE
Ultram ER Tablets . . . 2428

TRAMODA (Thailand)
TRAMADOL HYDROCHLORIDE
Ultram ER Tablets . . . 2428

TRAMSILONE (Thailand)
TRIAMCINOLONE ACETONIDE
Azmacort Inhalation Aerosol . . . 407
Nasacort AQ Nasal Spray . . . 2765

TRAMUNDAL (Austria)
TRAMADOL HYDROCHLORIDE
Ultram ER Tablets . . . 2428

TRAMUNDIN (Austria, Czech Republic, Germany, Poland, Switzerland, The Philippines)
TRAMADOL HYDROCHLORIDE
Ultram ER Tablets . . . 2428

TRANCOCARD (Italy)
DIPYRIDAMOLE
Persantine Tablets . . . 869

TRANJECT (South Africa)
DIAZEPAM
Valium Tablets . . . 2658

TRANKIL (The Philippines)
DIAZEPAM
Valium Tablets 2658

TRANQUASE (Germany)
DIAZEPAM
Valium Tablets 2658

TRANQUIRIT (Italy)
DIAZEPAM
Valium Tablets 2658

TRANQUO (Germany)
DIAZEPAM
Valium Tablets 2658

TRANSDIOL (Argentina)
ESTRADIOL
Climara Transdermal System 763

TRANSIPEN (Greece)
INDAPAMIDE
Indapamide Tablets 2188

TRANSVITAL (Chile)
ESTRADIOL
Climara Transdermal System 763

TRANTIL (Mexico)
CARBAMAZEPINE
Carbatrol Capsules 3019

TRASEDAL (France)
TRAMADOL HYDROCHLORIDE
Ultram ER Tablets 2428

TRASKOLAN (Poland)
APROTININ
Trasylol Injection 799

TRASTOCIR (Argentina)
CILOSTAZOL
Pletal Tablets 2481

TRASYLOL (Australia, Austria, Belgium, Brazil, Canada, Chile, Czech Republic, Denmark, Finland, France, Germany, Greece, Hong Kong, Hungary, Irish Republic, Italy, Malaysia, Mexico, New Zealand, Poland, Russia, Singapore, South Africa, Spain, Sweden, Switzerland, Thailand, The Netherlands, Turkey, United Kingdom, Venezuela)
APROTININ
Trasylol Injection 799

TRATACNE (Argentina)
TRETINOIN
Vesanoid Capsules 2660

TRAUMOX (South Africa)
NAPROXEN
EC-Naprosyn Delayed-Release Tablets 2632
Naprosyn Suspension 2632
Naprosyn Tablets 2632

TRAVEX (Portugal)
TRAMADOL HYDROCHLORIDE
Ultram ER Tablets 2428

TRAVIATA (Chile)
PAROXETINE HYDROCHLORIDE
Paxil Oral Suspension 1535
Paxil Tablets 1535

TRAVILAN (Greece)
CEFTRIAXONE SODIUM
Rocephin Injectable Vials, ADD-Vantage, Galaxy, Bulk 2642

TRAZINAC (Venezuela)
DICLOFENAC SODIUM
Voltaren Tablets 2334
Voltaren-XR Tablets 2337

TRAZOTEVA (Argentina)
DOCETAXEL
Taxotere Injection Concentrate 2773

TRD-CONTIN (India)
TRAMADOL HYDROCHLORIDE
Ultram ER Tablets 2428

TRECIFAN (Greece)
ISOTRETINOIN
Accutane Capsules 2607

TREMOREX (Denmark)
SELEGILINE HYDROCHLORIDE
Eldepryl Capsules 3052

TREPINA (Mexico)
CARBAMAZEPINE
Carbatrol Capsules 3019

TREPOL (Mexico)
DIPYRIDAMOLE
Persantine Tablets 869

TRETIN (Greece)
ISOTRETINOIN
Accutane Capsules 2607

TRETINAC (Switzerland)
ISOTRETINOIN
Accutane Capsules 2607

TRETINAX (Venezuela)
TRETINOIN
Vesanoid Capsules 2660

TRETINEX (Poland)
ISOTRETINOIN
Accutane Capsules 2607

TRETINODERM (Argentina)
TRETINOIN
Vesanoid Capsules 2660

TRETINOINE KEFRANE (France)
TRETINOIN
Vesanoid Capsules 2660

TRETINON (Malaysia, Mexico)
TRETINOIN
Vesanoid Capsules 2660

TREVILOR (Germany)
VENLAFAXINE HYDROCHLORIDE
Effexor XR Capsules 3195

TREWILOR (Austria)
VENLAFAXINE HYDROCHLORIDE
Effexor XR Capsules 3195

TREXOFIN (Singapore)
CEFTRIAXONE SODIUM
Rocephin Injectable Vials, ADD-Vantage, Galaxy, Bulk 2642

TREXOL (Mexico)
TRAMADOL HYDROCHLORIDE
Ultram ER Tablets 2428

TRIACORT (Italy, Russia)
TRIAMCINOLONE ACETONIDE
Azmacort Inhalation Aerosol 407
Nasacort AQ Nasal Spray 2765

TRIADERM (Canada)
TRIAMCINOLONE ACETONIDE
Azmacort Inhalation Aerosol 407
Nasacort AQ Nasal Spray 2765

TRIAKEN (Mexico)
CEFTRIAXONE SODIUM
Rocephin Injectable Vials, ADD-Vantage, Galaxy, Bulk 2642

TRIAKLIM (Hungary)
ESTRADIOL
Climara Transdermal System 763

TRIAL GEL (Argentina)
ESTRADIOL
Climara Transdermal System 763

TRIAL GEST (Argentina)
ESTRADIOL
Climara Transdermal System 763

TRIAL SAT (Argentina)
ESTRADIOL
Climara Transdermal System 763

TRIALONA (Spain)
FLUTICASONE PROPIONATE
Flonase Nasal Spray 1431

TRIAM (Hong Kong, Singapore)
TRIAMCINOLONE ACETONIDE
Azmacort Inhalation Aerosol 407
Nasacort AQ Nasal Spray 2765

TRIAMA (Thailand)
TRIAMCINOLONE ACETONIDE
Azmacort Inhalation Aerosol 407
Nasacort AQ Nasal Spray 2765

TRIAMAXCO (United Kingdom)
HYDROCHLOROTHIAZIDE/TRIAMTERENE
Dyazide Capsules 1405

TRIAMCINOLON COMPOSITUM (Czech Republic)
TRIAMCINOLONE ACETONIDE
Azmacort Inhalation Aerosol 407
Nasacort AQ Nasal Spray 2765

TRIAMCINOLON E (Czech Republic)
TRIAMCINOLONE ACETONIDE
Azmacort Inhalation Aerosol 407
Nasacort AQ Nasal Spray 2765

TRIAMCINOLON S (Czech Republic)
TRIAMCINOLONE ACETONIDE
Azmacort Inhalation Aerosol 407
Nasacort AQ Nasal Spray 2765

TRIAMCO (United Kingdom)
HYDROCHLOROTHIAZIDE/TRIAMTERENE
Dyazide Capsules 1405

TRIAM-CO (Hong Kong, Russia)
HYDROCHLOROTHIAZIDE/TRIAMTERENE
Dyazide Capsules 1405

TRIAMCORT (Switzerland)
TRIAMCINOLONE ACETONIDE
Azmacort Inhalation Aerosol 407
Nasacort AQ Nasal Spray 2765

TRIAMCREME (Germany)
TRIAMCINOLONE ACETONIDE
Azmacort Inhalation Aerosol 407
Nasacort AQ Nasal Spray 2765

TRIAMGALEN (Germany)
TRIAMCINOLONE ACETONIDE
Azmacort Inhalation Aerosol 407
Nasacort AQ Nasal Spray 2765

TRIAMHEXAL (Austria, Germany)
TRIAMCINOLONE ACETONIDE
Azmacort Inhalation Aerosol 407
Nasacort AQ Nasal Spray 2765

TRIAMIZIDE (New Zealand)
HYDROCHLOROTHIAZIDE/TRIAMTERENE
Dyazide Capsules 1405

TRIAMPUR COMPOSITUM (Germany, Russia)
HYDROCHLOROTHIAZIDE/TRIAMTERENE
Dyazide Capsules 1405

TRIAMSALBE (Germany)
TRIAMCINOLONE ACETONIDE
Azmacort Inhalation Aerosol 407
Nasacort AQ Nasal Spray 2765

TRIAMTEREN COMP (Austria)
HYDROCHLOROTHIAZIDE/TRIAMTERENE
Dyazide Capsules 1405

TRIAMTEREN/HCT (Austria)
TRIAMTERENE
Dyrenium Capsules 3189

TRIAMTEREN-H (Germany)
HYDROCHLOROTHIAZIDE/TRIAMTERENE
Dyazide Capsules 1405

TRIAMTERIL (Turkey)
TRIAMTERENE
Dyrenium Capsules 3189

TRIAMTERIL COMPLEX (Italy)
HYDROCHLOROTHIAZIDE/TRIAMTERENE
Dyazide Capsules 1405

TRIAMTHIAZID (Germany)
HYDROCHLOROTHIAZIDE/TRIAMTERENE
Dyazide Capsules 1405

TRIAM-TIAZIDA R (Portugal)
HYDROCHLOROTHIAZIDE/TRIAMTERENE
Dyazide Capsules 1405

TRIAMVIRGI (Italy)
TRIAMCINOLONE ACETONIDE
Azmacort Inhalation Aerosol 407
Nasacort AQ Nasal Spray 2765

TRIANCIL (Brazil)
TRIAMCINOLONE ACETONIDE
Azmacort Inhalation Aerosol 407
Nasacort AQ Nasal Spray 2765

TRI-ANEMUL (Germany)
TRIAMCINOLONE ACETONIDE
Azmacort Inhalation Aerosol 407
Nasacort AQ Nasal Spray 2765

TRIARESE (Germany)
HYDROCHLOROTHIAZIDE/TRIAMTERENE
Dyazide Capsules 1405

TRIASTAD HCT (Austria)
HYDROCHLOROTHIAZIDE/TRIAMTERENE
Dyazide Capsules 1405

TRIAX (Israel)
CEFTRIAXONE SODIUM
Rocephin Injectable Vials, ADD-Vantage, Galaxy, Bulk 2642

TRIAXON (Brazil)
CEFTRIAXONE SODIUM
Rocephin Injectable Vials, ADD-Vantage, Galaxy, Bulk 2642

TRIAXONE (United Arab Emirates)
CEFTRIAXONE SODIUM
Rocephin Injectable Vials, ADD-Vantage, Galaxy, Bulk 2642

TRIAXTON (Brazil)
CEFTRIAXONE SODIUM
Rocephin Injectable Vials, ADD-Vantage, Galaxy, Bulk 2642

TRIAZID (Germany)
HYDROCHLOROTHIAZIDE/TRIAMTERENE
Dyazide Capsules 1405

TRICEFIN (Singapore)
CEFTRIAXONE SODIUM
Rocephin Injectable Vials, ADD-Vantage, Galaxy, Bulk 2642

TRICEN (Spain)
TRANDOLAPRIL/VERAPAMIL HYDROCHLORIDE
Tarka Tablets 511

TRICEPHIN (Thailand)
CEFTRIAXONE SODIUM
Rocephin Injectable Vials, ADD-Vantage, Galaxy, Bulk 2642

TRICOCET (Brazil)
NYSTATIN
Nystop Topical Powder USP 2498

TRICOFARMA (Argentina)
FINASTERIDE
Propecia Tablets 2095
Proscar Tablets 2102

TRICOR (Chile)
ADENOSINE
Adenocard IV Injection 603
Adenoscan 605

TRICORTONE (Australia)
TRIAMCINOLONE ACETONIDE
Azmacort Inhalation Aerosol 407
Nasacort AQ Nasal Spray 2765

TRIFAMOX (Argentina)
AMOXICILLIN
Amoxil Pediatric Drops for Oral Suspension 1305
Amoxil Tablets 1305

TRIGEN (Mexico)
CIPROFLOXACIN HYDROCHLORIDE
Cipro Tablets 2810

TRIGGER (Italy)
RANITIDINE HYDROCHLORIDE
Zantac 25 EFFERdose Tablets 1670
Zantac 150 Tablets 1670
Zantac 300 Tablets 1670
Zantac Injection 1666
Zantac Injection Premixed 1666
Zantac Syrup 1670

TRIGINET (Poland)
LAMOTRIGINE
Lamictal Chewable Dispersible Tablets . . . 1488
Lamictal Tablets 1488

TRIGON DEPOT (Spain)
TRIAMCINOLONE ACETONIDE
Azmacort Inhalation Aerosol 407
Nasacort AQ Nasal Spray 2765

TRIIODOTHYRONINE INJECTION (United Kingdom)
LIOTHYRONINE SODIUM
Cytomel Tablets 1778

TRIKAL (Italy)
CALCITRIOL
Calcijex Injection 419
Rocaltrol Capsules 1150
Rocaltrol Oral Solution 1150

TRILOSIL (Thailand)
TRIAMCINOLONE ACETONIDE
Azmacort Inhalation Aerosol 407
Nasacort AQ Nasal Spray 2765

TRIM (Malaysia, Thailand)
TRIAMCINOLONE ACETONIDE
Azmacort Inhalation Aerosol 407
Nasacort AQ Nasal Spray 2765

TRIMASONE (Thailand)
TRIAMCINOLONE ACETONIDE
Azmacort Inhalation Aerosol 407

Nasacort AQ Nasal Spray 2765

TRIMEBA (Mexico)
CLARITHROMYCIN
Biaxin Filmtab Tablets 411
Biaxin Granules 411

TRIMONIL (Denmark, Finland, Norway, Sweden)
CARBAMAZEPINE
Carbatrol Capsules 3019

TRIMOX (Brazil)
AMOXICILLIN
Amoxil Pediatric Drops for Oral Suspension 1305
Amoxil Tablets 1305

TRINALION (Portugal)
NIMODIPINE
Nimotop Capsules 790

TRINOLONE (Singapore)
TRIAMCINOLONE ACETONIDE
Azmacort Inhalation Aerosol 407
Nasacort AQ Nasal Spray 2765

TRIOMUNE (India, South Africa, Venezuela)
LAMIVUDINE
Epivir Oral Solution 1412
Epivir Tablets 1412
Epivir-HBV Oral Solution 1417
Epivir-HBV Tablets 1417

TRIORAL/HCT (Austria)
TRIAMTERENE
Dyrenium Capsules 3189

TRIOX (Mexico)
CEFTRIAXONE SODIUM
Rocephin Injectable Vials, ADD-Vantage, Galaxy, Bulk 2642

TRIOX NF (Chile)
NAPROXEN SODIUM
Anaprox DS Tablets 2632
Anaprox Tablets 2632

TRI-THIAZID (Germany)
HYDROCHLOROTHIAZIDE/TRIAMTERENE
Dyazide Capsules 1405

TRI-THIAZID RESERPIN (Germany)
HYDROCHLOROTHIAZIDE/TRIAMTERENE
Dyazide Capsules 1405

TRIVUDIN (Argentina)
LAMIVUDINE
Epivir Oral Solution 1412
Epivir Tablets 1412
Epivir-HBV Oral Solution 1417
Epivir-HBV Tablets 1417

TRIXONE (Thailand)
CEFTRIAXONE SODIUM
Rocephin Injectable Vials, ADD-Vantage, Galaxy, Bulk 2642

TRIXOPHIN (The Philippines)
CEFTRIAXONE SODIUM
Rocephin Injectable Vials, ADD-Vantage, Galaxy, Bulk 2642

TRIXOTENE (Argentina)
DOCETAXEL
Taxotere Injection Concentrate 2773

TRIYOTEX (Mexico)
LIOTHYRONINE SODIUM
Cytomel Tablets 1778

TRIZ (Thailand)
CETIRIZINE HYDROCHLORIDE
Zyrtec Syrup 1920
Zyrtec Tablets 1920

TRIZID (Hong Kong, New Zealand)
HYDROCHLOROTHIAZIDE/TRIAMTERENE
Dyazide Capsules 1405

TRIZOL (Chile)
LAMOTRIGINE
Lamictal Chewable Dispersible Tablets . . . 1488
Lamictal Tablets 1488

TRIZOLIN (Malaysia, Singapore, Thailand)
NORFLOXACIN
Noroxin Tablets 2069

TROFENTYL (India)
FENTANYL CITRATE
Actiq 959

TROKEN (Argentina)
CLOPIDOGREL BISULFATE
Plavix Tablets 926, 2767

TROLIP (Hong Kong, The Philippines)
FENOFIBRATE
Tricor Tablets 520

TROMAGESIC (India)
DICLOFENAC SODIUM
Voltaren Tablets 2334
Voltaren-XR Tablets 2337

TROMAX (India)
DICLOFENAC SODIUM
Voltaren Tablets 2334
Voltaren-XR Tablets 2337

TROMBENOX (Italy)
ENOXAPARIN SODIUM
Lovenox Injection 2756

TROMBOLIZ (Turkey)
DIPYRIDAMOLE
Persantine Tablets 869

TROMBONOT (Argentina)
CILOSTAZOL
Pletal Tablets 2481

TROMBOXANIL (Brazil)
DIPYRIDAMOLE
Persantine Tablets 869

TROMPERSANTIN (Mexico)
DIPYRIDAMOLE
Persantine Tablets 869

TROMPHYLLIN (Germany)
THEOPHYLLINE
Uniphyl Tablets 2595

TROPIOVENT (United Kingdom)
IPRATROPIUM BROMIDE
Atrovent Nasal Spray 0.03% 834
Atrovent Nasal Spray 0.06% 836

TROPISOL (Mexico)
CAPTOPRIL
Captopril Tablets 2182

TROPIX-HC (Mexico)
CAPTOPRIL
Captopril Tablets 2182

TROPOCER (Venezuela)
NIMODIPINE
Nimotop Capsules 790

TRORIX (Chile)
ONDANSETRON
Zofran ODT Orally Disintegrating Tablets . . 1687

TROSIC (Thailand)
TRAMADOL HYDROCHLORIDE
Ultram ER Tablets 2428

TROZOLET (Chile, Venezuela)
ANASTROZOLE
Arimidex Tablets 672

TROZOLITE (Argentina)
ANASTROZOLE
Arimidex Tablets 672

TRUCTUM (Venezuela)
ONDANSETRON
Zofran ODT Orally Disintegrating Tablets . . 1687

TRUMSAL (Spain)
DILTIAZEM HYDROCHLORIDE
Cardizem LA Extended Release Tablets 421

TRUOXIN (Irish Republic)
CIPROFLOXACIN HYDROCHLORIDE
Cipro Tablets 2810

TRUSOPT (Argentina, Australia, Austria, Belgium, Brazil, Canada, Chile, Czech Republic, Denmark, Finland, France, Germany, Greece, Hong Kong, Hungary, Irish Republic, Israel, Italy, Malaysia, Mexico, New Zealand, Norway, Poland, Portugal, Russia, Singapore, South Africa, Spain, Sweden, Switzerland, Thailand, The Netherlands, The Philippines, Turkey, United Kingdom, Venezuela)
DORZOLAMIDE HYDROCHLORIDE
Trusopt Sterile Ophthalmic Solution 2128

TULIP (Mexico, Poland, Russia)
ATORVASTATIN CALCIUM
Lipitor Tablets 2501

TULOTRACT (Germany)
LACTULOSE
Kristalose for Oral Solution 1004

TUNDRA (Argentina)
NAPROXEN
EC-Naprosyn Delayed-Release Tablets 2632
Naprosyn Suspension 2632
Naprosyn Tablets 2632

TUPAST (Greece)
RANITIDINE HYDROCHLORIDE
Zantac 25 EFFERdose Tablets 1670
Zantac 150 Tablets 1670
Zantac 300 Tablets 1670
Zantac Injection 1666
Zantac Injection Premixed 1666
Zantac Syrup 1670

TURFA (Germany)
HYDROCHLOROTHIAZIDE/TRIAMTERENE
Dyazide Capsules 1405

TURIXIN (Germany)
MUPIROCIN CALCIUM
Bactroban Cream 2% 1366
Bactroban Nasal 2% 1367

TURM (Italy)
FLUNISOLIDE
Aerobid Inhaler System 1153
Aerobid-M Inhaler System 1153

TUSEHLI (Mexico)
BENZONATATE
Tessalon Perles 1183

TUSICAL (Mexico)
BENZONATATE
Tessalon Perles 1183

TUSITATO (Mexico)
BENZONATATE
Tessalon Perles 1183

TUZZIL (Mexico)
BENZONATATE
Tessalon Perles 1183

TWICE (Italy)
MORPHINE SULFATE
MS Contin Tablets 2585

TWINVISC (Germany)
SODIUM HYALURONATE
Hyalgan Solution 2742

TYMASIL (United Kingdom)
NATAMYCIN
Natacyn Antifungal Ophthalmic Suspension . . . . ⊙204

T-ZA (Thailand)
ZIDOVUDINE
Retrovir Capsules 1574
Retrovir IV Infusion 1579
Retrovir Syrup 1574
Retrovir Tablets 1574

UBICOR (Switzerland)
DILTIAZEM HYDROCHLORIDE
Cardizem LA Extended Release Tablets 421

UBIZOL (Portugal)
FLUTICASONE PROPIONATE
Flonase Nasal Spray 1431

UDRAMIL (Germany)
TRANDOLAPRIL/VERAPAMIL HYDROCHLORIDE
Tarka Tablets 511

UDRIK (Germany)
TRANDOLAPRIL
Mavik Tablets 472

UGOTREX (Greece)
CEFTRIAXONE SODIUM
Rocephin Injectable Vials, ADD-Vantage, Galaxy, Bulk 2642

ULCAID (South Africa)
RANITIDINE HYDROCHLORIDE
Zantac 25 EFFERdose Tablets 1670
Zantac 150 Tablets 1670
Zantac 300 Tablets 1670
Zantac Injection 1666
Zantac Injection Premixed 1666
Zantac Syrup 1670

ULCAR (France)
SUCRALFATE
Carafate Suspension 706
Carafate Tablets 707

ULCECUR (Portugal)
RANITIDINE HYDROCHLORIDE
Zantac 25 EFFERdose Tablets 1670
Zantac 150 Tablets 1670
Zantac 300 Tablets 1670
Zantac Injection 1666
Zantac Injection Premixed 1666
Zantac Syrup 1670

ULCEDIN (Mexico)
RANITIDINE HYDROCHLORIDE
Zantac 25 EFFERdose Tablets 1670
Zantac 150 Tablets 1670
Zantac 300 Tablets 1670
Zantac Injection 1666
Zantac Injection Premixed 1666
Zantac Syrup 1670

ULCEFAM (The Philippines)
FAMOTIDINE
Pepcid for Oral Suspension 2075
Pepcid Tablets 2075

ULCEFATE (South Africa, Thailand)
SUCRALFATE
Carafate Suspension 706
Carafate Tablets 707

ULCEKON (India)
SUCRALFATE
Carafate Suspension 706
Carafate Tablets 707

ULCELAC (Argentina)
FAMOTIDINE
Pepcid for Oral Suspension 2075
Pepcid Tablets 2075

ULCENOL (Venezuela)
FAMOTIDINE
Pepcid for Oral Suspension 2075
Pepcid Tablets 2075

ULCERAGON (The Philippines)
RANITIDINE HYDROCHLORIDE
Zantac 25 EFFERdose Tablets 1670
Zantac 150 Tablets 1670
Zantac 300 Tablets 1670
Zantac Injection 1666
Zantac Injection Premixed 1666
Zantac Syrup 1670

ULCERAL (Austria, The Philippines)
SUCRALFATE
Carafate Suspension 706
Carafate Tablets 707

ULCERAN (Czech Republic, Hong Kong, Hungary, Malaysia, Russia, Singapore, Thailand)
FAMOTIDINE
Pepcid for Oral Suspension 2075
Pepcid Tablets 2075

ULCERASE (Portugal)
COLLAGENASE
Santyl Collagenase Ointment 1724

ULCERGO (The Philippines)
RANITIDINE HYDROCHLORIDE
Zantac 25 EFFERdose Tablets 1670
Zantac 150 Tablets 1670
Zantac 300 Tablets 1670
Zantac Injection 1666
Zantac Injection Premixed 1666
Zantac Syrup 1670

ULCERIT (Brazil)
RANITIDINE HYDROCHLORIDE
Zantac 25 EFFERdose Tablets 1670
Zantac 150 Tablets 1670
Zantac 300 Tablets 1670
Zantac Injection 1666
Zantac Injection Premixed 1666
Zantac Syrup 1670

ULCERIX (The Philippines)
RANITIDINE HYDROCHLORIDE
Zantac 25 EFFERdose Tablets 1670
Zantac 150 Tablets 1670
Zantac 300 Tablets 1670
Zantac Injection 1666
Zantac Injection Premixed 1666
Zantac Syrup 1670

ULCERLMIN (Japan)
SUCRALFATE
Carafate Suspension 706
Carafate Tablets 707

ULCERMIN (Portugal, Spain)
SUCRALFATE
Carafate Suspension 706
Carafate Tablets 707

ULCEROL (Portugal)
RANITIDINE HYDROCHLORIDE
Zantac 25 EFFERdose Tablets 1670

Zantac 150 Tablets **1670**
Zantac 300 Tablets **1670**
Zantac Injection **1666**
Zantac Injection Premixed **1666**
Zantac Syrup **1670**

ULCERTEC (Malaysia, Singapore)
SUCRALFATE
Carafate Suspension **706**
Carafate Tablets **707**

ULCETAB (South Africa)
SUCRALFATE
Carafate Suspension **706**
Carafate Tablets **707**

ULCETIC (South Africa)
SUCRALFATE
Carafate Suspension **706**
Carafate Tablets **707**

ULCETRAX (Spain)
FAMOTIDINE
Pepcid for Oral Suspension **2075**
Pepcid Tablets **2075**

ULCEVIT (Mexico)
RANITIDINE HYDROCHLORIDE
Zantac 25 EFFERdose Tablets **1670**
Zantac 150 Tablets **1670**
Zantac 300 Tablets **1670**
Zantac Injection **1666**
Zantac Injection Premixed **1666**
Zantac Syrup **1670**

ULCEX (Italy)
RANITIDINE HYDROCHLORIDE
Zantac 25 EFFERdose Tablets **1670**
Zantac 150 Tablets **1670**
Zantac 300 Tablets **1670**
Zantac Injection **1666**
Zantac Injection Premixed **1666**
Zantac Syrup **1670**

ULCIDINE (Canada, Switzerland)
FAMOTIDINE
Pepcid for Oral Suspension **2075**
Pepcid Tablets **2075**

ULCIMAX (India)
FAMOTIDINE
Pepcid for Oral Suspension **2075**
Pepcid Tablets **2075**

ULCIN (The Philippines)
RANITIDINE HYDROCHLORIDE
Zantac 25 EFFERdose Tablets **1670**
Zantac 150 Tablets **1670**
Zantac 300 Tablets **1670**
Zantac Injection **1666**
Zantac Injection Premixed **1666**
Zantac Syrup **1670**

ULCIRAM (Venezuela)
SUCRALFATE
Carafate Suspension **706**
Carafate Tablets **707**

ULCIREX (France)
RANITIDINE HYDROCHLORIDE
Zantac 25 EFFERdose Tablets **1670**
Zantac 150 Tablets **1670**
Zantac 300 Tablets **1670**
Zantac Injection **1666**
Zantac Injection Premixed **1666**
Zantac Syrup **1670**

ULCODERMA (Mexico)
COLLAGENASE
Santyl Collagenase Ointment **1724**

ULCOFAM (Thailand)
FAMOTIDINE
Pepcid for Oral Suspension **2075**
Pepcid Tablets **2075**

ULCOGANT (Austria, Belgium, Czech Republic, Germany, Hungary, Switzerland, The Netherlands)
SUCRALFATE
Carafate Suspension **706**
Carafate Tablets **707**

ULCOLIND RANI (Germany)
RANITIDINE HYDROCHLORIDE
Zantac 25 EFFERdose Tablets **1670**
Zantac 150 Tablets **1670**
Zantac 300 Tablets **1670**
Zantac Injection **1666**
Zantac Injection Premixed **1666**
Zantac Syrup **1670**

ULCON (Venezuela)
SUCRALFATE
Carafate Suspension **706**
Carafate Tablets **707**

ULCONA (Spain)
SUCRALFATE
Carafate Suspension **706**
Carafate Tablets **707**

ULCOREN (Brazil)
RANITIDINE HYDROCHLORIDE
Zantac 25 EFFERdose Tablets **1670**
Zantac 150 Tablets **1670**
Zantac 300 Tablets **1670**
Zantac Injection **1666**
Zantac Injection Premixed **1666**
Zantac Syrup **1670**

ULCOSIN (Hungary)
RANITIDINE HYDROCHLORIDE
Zantac 25 EFFERdose Tablets **1670**
Zantac 150 Tablets **1670**
Zantac 300 Tablets **1670**
Zantac Injection **1666**
Zantac Injection Premixed **1666**
Zantac Syrup **1670**

ULCOTENK (Argentina)
RANITIDINE HYDROCHLORIDE
Zantac 25 EFFERdose Tablets **1670**
Zantac 150 Tablets **1670**
Zantac 300 Tablets **1670**
Zantac Injection **1666**
Zantac Injection Premixed **1666**
Zantac Syrup **1670**

ULCRAFATE (Thailand)
SUCRALFATE
Carafate Suspension **706**
Carafate Tablets **707**

ULCRAST (Italy)
SUCRALFATE
Carafate Suspension **706**
Carafate Tablets **707**

ULCUFATO (Spain)
SUCRALFATE
Carafate Suspension **706**
Carafate Tablets **707**

ULCURAN (Turkey)
RANITIDINE HYDROCHLORIDE
Zantac 25 EFFERdose Tablets **1670**
Zantac 150 Tablets **1670**
Zantac 300 Tablets **1670**
Zantac Injection **1666**
Zantac Injection Premixed **1666**
Zantac Syrup **1670**

ULCUSAN (Austria)
FAMOTIDINE
Pepcid for Oral Suspension **2075**
Pepcid Tablets **2075**

ULCYTE (Australia)
SUCRALFATE
Carafate Suspension **706**
Carafate Tablets **707**

ULFAMET (Thailand)
FAMOTIDINE
Pepcid for Oral Suspension **2075**
Pepcid Tablets **2075**

ULFAMID (Czech Republic, Poland, Russia)
FAMOTIDINE
Pepcid for Oral Suspension **2075**
Pepcid Tablets **2075**

ULGARINE (Spain)
FAMOTIDINE
Pepcid for Oral Suspension **2075**
Pepcid Tablets **2075**

ULGASTRAN (Poland)
SUCRALFATE
Carafate Suspension **706**
Carafate Tablets **707**

ULKOBRIN (Italy)
RANITIDINE HYDROCHLORIDE
Zantac 25 EFFERdose Tablets **1670**
Zantac 150 Tablets **1670**
Zantac 300 Tablets **1670**
Zantac Injection **1666**
Zantac Injection Premixed **1666**
Zantac Syrup **1670**

ULKODIN (Mexico)
RANITIDINE HYDROCHLORIDE
Zantac 25 EFFERdose Tablets **1670**
Zantac 150 Tablets **1670**
Zantac 300 Tablets **1670**
Zantac Injection **1666**
Zantac Injection Premixed **1666**
Zantac Syrup **1670**

ULRAN (Czech Republic, Russia, The Philippines)
RANITIDINE HYDROCHLORIDE
Zantac 150 Tablets **1670**
Zantac 25 EFFERdose Tablets **1670**
Zantac 300 Tablets **1670**
Zantac Injection **1666**
Zantac Injection Premixed **1666**
Zantac Syrup **1670**

ULSAL (Austria)
RANITIDINE HYDROCHLORIDE
Zantac 25 EFFERdose Tablets **1670**
Zantac 150 Tablets **1670**
Zantac 300 Tablets **1670**
Zantac Injection **1666**
Zantac Injection Premixed **1666**
Zantac Syrup **1670**

ULSANIC (Hong Kong, Israel, South Africa, Thailand)
SUCRALFATE
Carafate Suspension **706**
Carafate Tablets **707**

ULSAVEN (Mexico)
RANITIDINE HYDROCHLORIDE
Zantac 25 EFFERdose Tablets **1670**
Zantac 150 Tablets **1670**
Zantac 300 Tablets **1670**
Zantac Injection **1666**
Zantac Injection Premixed **1666**
Zantac Syrup **1670**

ULTAK (South Africa)
RANITIDINE HYDROCHLORIDE
Zantac 25 EFFERdose Tablets **1670**
Zantac 150 Tablets **1670**
Zantac 300 Tablets **1670**
Zantac Injection **1666**
Zantac Injection Premixed **1666**
Zantac Syrup **1670**

ULTICER (Hong Kong)
RANITIDINE HYDROCHLORIDE
Zantac 25 EFFERdose Tablets **1670**
Zantac 150 Tablets **1670**
Zantac 300 Tablets **1670**
Zantac Injection **1666**
Zantac Injection Premixed **1666**
Zantac Syrup **1670**

ULTIDIN (Mexico)
FAMOTIDINE
Pepcid for Oral Suspension **2075**
Pepcid Tablets **2075**

ULTRA CLEARASIL (The Philippines, United Kingdom)
BENZOYL PEROXIDE
Brevoxyl-4 Creamy Wash **3054**
Brevoxyl-4 Gel **3054**
Brevoxyl-8 Creamy Wash **3054**
Brevoxyl-8 Gel **3054**

ULTRA HEARTBURN RELIEF (United Kingdom)
FAMOTIDINE
Pepcid for Oral Suspension **2075**
Pepcid Tablets **2075**

ULTRABETA (Portugal)
SALMETEROL XINAFOATE
Serevent Diskus **1594**

ULTRABIOTIC (Chile)
MUPIROCIN
Bactroban Ointment **1368**

ULTRACELE (India)
CELECOXIB
Celebrex Capsules **2979**

ULTRACET (Thailand, Venezuela)
TRAMADOL HYDROCHLORIDE
Ultram ER Tablets **2428**

ULTRA-CLEAR-A-MED (Austria)
BENZOYL PEROXIDE
Brevoxyl-4 Creamy Wash **3054**
Brevoxyl-4 Gel **3054**
Brevoxyl-8 Creamy Wash **3054**
Brevoxyl-8 Gel **3054**

ULTRAFINA (India)
FINASTERIDE
Propecia Tablets **2095**
Proscar Tablets **2102**

ULTRAFLOX (Thailand)
CIPROFLOXACIN HYDROCHLORIDE
Cipro Tablets **2810**

ULTRAMICINA (Argentina, Spain)
CIPROFLOXACIN
Cipro Oral Suspension **2810**

ULTRAMICINA PLUS (Spain)
CIPROFLOXACIN
Cipro Oral Suspension **2810**

ULTRAMOX (Brazil)
AMOXICILLIN
Amoxil Pediatric Drops for Oral Suspension **1305**
Amoxil Tablets **1305**

ULTRAQUIN (Argentina)
LEVOFLOXACIN
Levaquin Injection **2416**
Levaquin Tablets **2416**

ULTRASE (Brazil, Canada)
PANCRELIPASE
Ultrase Capsules **718**
Ultrase MT Capsules **719**

ULTRAVIRAL (Argentina)
LAMIVUDINE
Epivir Oral Solution **1412**
Epivir Tablets **1412**
Epivir-HBV Oral Solution **1417**
Epivir-HBV Tablets **1417**

ULTRAVIRAL DUO (Argentina)
LAMIVUDINE
Epivir Oral Solution **1412**
Epivir Tablets **1412**
Epivir-HBV Oral Solution **1417**
Epivir-HBV Tablets **1417**

ULTRAZAC (India)
TRAMADOL HYDROCHLORIDE
Ultram ER Tablets **2428**

ULTROXIM (Italy)
CEFUROXIME SODIUM
Zinacef Injection **1678**

UMAREN (Hungary)
RANITIDINE HYDROCHLORIDE
Zantac 25 EFFERdose Tablets **1670**
Zantac 150 Tablets **1670**
Zantac 300 Tablets **1670**
Zantac Injection **1666**
Zantac Injection Premixed **1666**
Zantac Syrup **1670**

UMBRIUM (Austria)
DIAZEPAM
Valium Tablets **2658**

UMINE (New Zealand, Singapore)
PHENTERMINE HYDROCHLORIDE
Adipex-P Capsules **1185**
Adipex-P Tablets **1185**

UNDERACID (Spain)
RANITIDINE HYDROCHLORIDE
Zantac 25 EFFERdose Tablets **1670**
Zantac 150 Tablets **1670**
Zantac 300 Tablets **1670**
Zantac Injection **1666**
Zantac Injection Premixed **1666**
Zantac Syrup **1670**

UNDERAN (Chile)
MUPIROCIN
Bactroban Ointment **1368**

UNI CARBAMAZ (Brazil)
CARBAMAZEPINE
Carbatrol Capsules **3019**

UNI DIAZEPAX (Brazil)
DIAZEPAM
Valium Tablets **2658**

UNI MASDIL (Spain)
DILTIAZEM HYDROCHLORIDE
Cardizem LA Extended Release Tablets **421**

UNI MIST (Spain)
MORPHINE SULFATE
MS Contin Tablets **2585**

UNICET (Thailand)
CETIRIZINE HYDROCHLORIDE
Zyrtec Syrup **1920**
Zyrtec Tablets **1920**

UNICLAR (Argentina, Chile, Italy, Mexico, Venezuela)
MOMETASONE FUROATE
Elocon Cream 0.1% **2840**
Elocon Lotion 0.1% **2841**
Elocon Ointment 0.1% **2842**

Nasonex Nasal Spray . . . 2883

UNICLONAX (The Philippines)
DICLOFENAC SODIUM
Voltaren Tablets . . . 2334
Voltaren-XR Tablets . . . 2337

UNICLOPHEN (Czech Republic)
DICLOFENAC SODIUM
Voltaren Tablets . . . 2334
Voltaren-XR Tablets . . . 2337

UNICONTIN (India, Portugal)
THEOPHYLLINE
Uniphyl Tablets . . . 2595

UNI-DUR (Czech Republic, Italy, Mexico, South Africa)
THEOPHYLLINE
Uniphyl Tablets . . . 2595

UNIF (Thailand)
TRIAMCINOLONE ACETONIDE
Azmacort Inhalation Aerosol . . . 407
Nasacort AQ Nasal Spray . . . 2765

UNIFLOX (Argentina, France)
CIPROFLOXACIN HYDROCHLORIDE
Cipro Tablets . . . 2810

UNIFYL (Austria, Switzerland)
THEOPHYLLINE
Uniphyl Tablets . . . 2595

UNIGET (Germany)
TIMOLOL MALEATE
Timoptic in Ocudose . . . 2124
Timoptic Sterile Ophthalmic Solution . . . 2121
Timoptic-XE Sterile Ophthalmic Gel Forming Solution . . . 2125

UNIKLAR (Turkey)
CLARITHROMYCIN
Biaxin Filmtab Tablets . . . 411
Biaxin Granules . . . 411

UNILAIR (Czech Republic, Germany)
THEOPHYLLINE
Uniphyl Tablets . . . 2595

UNILONG (Spain)
THEOPHYLLINE
Uniphyl Tablets . . . 2595

UNIMOX (South Africa)
AMOXICILLIN
Amoxil Pediatric Drops for Oral Suspension . . . 1305
Amoxil Tablets . . . 1305

UNINAPRO (Italy)
NAPROXEN SODIUM
Anaprox DS Tablets . . . 2632
Anaprox Tablets . . . 2632

UNIPHYL (Canada, Hong Kong, South Africa)
THEOPHYLLINE
Uniphyl Tablets . . . 2595

UNIPHYLLIN (Germany, Greece)
THEOPHYLLINE
Uniphyl Tablets . . . 2595

UNIPHYLLIN CONTINUS (Irish Republic, United Kingdom)
THEOPHYLLINE
Uniphyl Tablets . . . 2595

UNIRELAXED (Mexico)
NAPROXEN
EC-Naprosyn Delayed-Release Tablets . . . 2632
Naprosyn Suspension . . . 2632
Naprosyn Tablets . . . 2632

UNIREN (Hong Kong)
DICLOFENAC SODIUM
Voltaren Tablets . . . 2334
Voltaren-XR Tablets . . . 2337

UNISEDIL (Portugal)
DIAZEPAM
Valium Tablets . . . 2658

UNITIMOFTOL (Spain)
TIMOLOL MALEATE
Timoptic in Ocudose . . . 2124
Timoptic Sterile Ophthalmic Solution . . . 2121
Timoptic-XE Sterile Ophthalmic Gel Forming Solution . . . 2125

UNITRAL (The Philippines)
TRAMADOL HYDROCHLORIDE
Ultram ER Tablets . . . 2428

UNIVAL (Mexico)
SUCRALFATE
Carafate Suspension . . . 706
Carafate Tablets . . . 707

UNIXAN (Denmark)
THEOPHYLLINE
Uniphyl Tablets . . . 2595

UNO (Czech Republic)
DICLOFENAC SODIUM
Voltaren Tablets . . . 2334
Voltaren-XR Tablets . . . 2337

UNOCARDIL (Denmark)
DILTIAZEM HYDROCHLORIDE
Cardizem LA Extended Release Tablets . . . 421

UNOXIMED (The Philippines)
CEFUROXIME SODIUM
Zinacef Injection . . . 1678

UPHASTATIN (Malaysia)
NYSTATIN
Nystop Topical Powder USP . . . 2498

UPROX (Poland)
TAMSULOSIN HYDROCHLORIDE
Flomax Capsules . . . 848

U-PROXYN (Thailand)
NAPROXEN
EC-Naprosyn Delayed-Release Tablets . . . 2632
Naprosyn Suspension . . . 2632
Naprosyn Tablets . . . 2632

URASIN (Thailand)
FUROSEMIDE
Furosemide Tablets . . . 2186

URASIX (Brazil)
FUROSEMIDE
Furosemide Tablets . . . 2186

URBAL (Spain)
SUCRALFATE
Carafate Suspension . . . 706
Carafate Tablets . . . 707

UREKOLIN (Chile)
NORFLOXACIN
Noroxin Tablets . . . 2069

UREMIDE (Australia, South Africa)
FUROSEMIDE
Furosemide Tablets . . . 2186

UREN (Chile)
HYDROCHLOROTHIAZIDE/TRIAMTERENE
Dyazide Capsules . . . 1405

URETIC (South Africa)
FUROSEMIDE
Furosemide Tablets . . . 2186

UREX (Australia, Hong Kong, Turkey)
FUROSEMIDE
Furosemide Tablets . . . 2186

URGENDOL (India)
TRAMADOL HYDROCHLORIDE
Ultram ER Tablets . . . 2428

URIBETA (Mexico)
INTERFERON BETA-1B
Betaseron for SC Injection . . . 756

URIFRON (Mexico)
INTERFERON ALFA-2B
Intron A for Injection . . . 2859

URIGON (Greece)
DICLOFENAC SODIUM
Voltaren Tablets . . . 2334
Voltaren-XR Tablets . . . 2337

URIMAX (India)
TAMSULOSIN HYDROCHLORIDE
Flomax Capsules . . . 848

URIMAX F (India)
TAMSULOSIN HYDROCHLORIDE
Flomax Capsules . . . 848

URINOX (Malaysia, Thailand)
NORFLOXACIN
Noroxin Tablets . . . 2069

URITOL (Canada)
FUROSEMIDE
Furosemide Tablets . . . 2186

URITRACIN (The Philippines)
NORFLOXACIN
Noroxin Tablets . . . 2069

URITRAT (Brazil)
NORFLOXACIN
Noroxin Tablets . . . 2069

URIZIDE (South Africa)
HYDROCHLOROTHIAZIDE/TRIAMTERENE
Dyazide Capsules . . . 1405

UROBACID (Austria, Greece, Malaysia, Singapore, The Philippines)
NORFLOXACIN
Noroxin Tablets . . . 2069

UROCAUDAL (Spain)
TRIAMTERENE
Dyrenium Capsules . . . 3189

UROCAUDAL TIAZIDA (Spain)
HYDROCHLOROTHIAZIDE/TRIAMTERENE
Dyazide Capsules . . . 1405

UROCID-K (Turkey)
POTASSIUM CITRATE
Urocit-K Tablets . . . 2176

UROCIPROXIN (Turkey)
CIPROFLOXACIN
Cipro Oral Suspension . . . 2810

UROCIT-K (Australia, Hong Kong, Malaysia, Singapore)
POTASSIUM CITRATE
Urocit-K Tablets . . . 2176

UROCTAL (Hong Kong, Spain)
NORFLOXACIN
Noroxin Tablets . . . 2069

URODIXIN (Greece)
CIPROFLOXACIN
Cipro Oral Suspension . . . 2810

UROFIN (Argentina)
FINASTERIDE
Propecia Tablets . . . 2095
Proscar Tablets . . . 2102

UROFLOX (Brazil, Portugal)
NORFLOXACIN
Noroxin Tablets . . . 2069

UROFOS (Argentina)
NORFLOXACIN
Noroxin Tablets . . . 2069

UROKIT (Argentina)
POTASSIUM CITRATE
Urocit-K Tablets . . . 2176

URO-LINFOL (Argentina)
NORFLOXACIN
Noroxin Tablets . . . 2069

UROLOSIN (Spain)
TAMSULOSIN HYDROCHLORIDE
Flomax Capsules . . . 848

URONOVAG (Argentina)
NORFLOXACIN
Noroxin Tablets . . . 2069

UROPLEX (Brazil)
NORFLOXACIN
Noroxin Tablets . . . 2069

UROSEPTAL (Argentina, Brazil)
NORFLOXACIN
Noroxin Tablets . . . 2069

UROSPES-N (Greece)
NORFLOXACIN
Noroxin Tablets . . . 2069

UROSTAD (Poland)
TAMSULOSIN HYDROCHLORIDE
Flomax Capsules . . . 848

UROTEM (Argentina)
NORFLOXACIN
Noroxin Tablets . . . 2069

UROTOTAL (Argentina)
FINASTERIDE
Propecia Tablets . . . 2095
Proscar Tablets . . . 2102

UROXACIN (Argentina)
NORFLOXACIN
Noroxin Tablets . . . 2069

UROXAZOL-N (Brazil)
NORFLOXACIN
Noroxin Tablets . . . 2069

UROXIN (Hong Kong, Singapore, Thailand, United Arab Emirates)
CIPROFLOXACIN
Cipro Oral Suspension . . . 2810

URPROSAN (Spain)
FINASTERIDE
Propecia Tablets . . . 2095
Proscar Tablets . . . 2102

UTAC (Thailand)
RANITIDINE HYDROCHLORIDE
Zantac 25 EFFERdose Tablets . . . 1670
Zantac 150 Tablets . . . 1670
Zantac 300 Tablets . . . 1670
Zantac Injection . . . 1666
Zantac Injection Premixed . . . 1666
Zantac Syrup . . . 1670

UTAHZONE (Hong Kong)
CIPROFLOXACIN HYDROCHLORIDE
Cipro Tablets . . . 2810

UTERONE (India)
PROGESTERONE
Crinone 4% Gel . . . 992
Prometrium Capsules (100 mg, 200 mg) . 3047

UTICINA (Italy)
NORFLOXACIN
Noroxin Tablets . . . 2069

UTIFLOX (The Philippines)
NORFLOXACIN
Noroxin Tablets . . . 2069

UTIN (South Africa)
NORFLOXACIN
Noroxin Tablets . . . 2069

UTINOR (Italy, The Philippines, United Kingdom)
NORFLOXACIN
Noroxin Tablets . . . 2069

UTROGESTAN (Argentina, Austria, Belgium, Brazil, Czech Republic, France, Greece, Hong Kong, Hungary, Irish Republic, Israel, Malaysia, Mexico, Portugal, Russia, Singapore, South Africa, Spain, Switzerland, Thailand, Venezuela)
PROGESTERONE
Crinone 4% Gel . . . 992
Prometrium Capsules (100 mg, 200 mg) . 3047

UV IX (Mexico)
CIPROFLOXACIN
Cipro Oral Suspension . . . 2810

V DAY ZEPAM (Thailand)
DIAZEPAM
Valium Tablets . . . 2658

VACINOLONE (Thailand)
TRIAMCINOLONE ACETONIDE
Azmacort Inhalation Aerosol . . . 407
Nasacort AQ Nasal Spray . . . 2765

VADINAR (Mexico)
DIPYRIDAMOLE
Persantine Tablets . . . 869

VADITON (Spain, The Netherlands)
FLUVASTATIN SODIUM
Lescol Capsules . . . 2268

VAGIFEM (Australia, Austria, Belgium, Canada, Chile, Czech Republic, Denmark, Finland, Germany, Greece, Hong Kong, Hungary, Irish Republic, Israel, Italy, New Zealand, Norway, Poland, Portugal, Singapore, South Africa, Spain, Sweden, Switzerland, Thailand, The Netherlands, The Philippines, Turkey, United Kingdom)
ESTRADIOL
Climara Transdermal System . . . 763

VAGISIL (United Kingdom)
LIDOCAINE
Lidoderm Patch . . . 1114

VAGOSTAL (Spain)
FAMOTIDINE
Pepcid for Oral Suspension . . . 2075
Pepcid Tablets . . . 2075

VALAPLEX (Chile)
VALSARTAN
Diovan Tablets . . . 2212

VALAPLEX-D (Chile)
VALSARTAN
Diovan Tablets . . . 2212

VALAXONA (Denmark, Germany)
DIAZEPAM
Valium Tablets . . . 2658

VALCLAIR (United Kingdom)
DIAZEPAM
Valium Tablets . . . 2658

VALDERMA ACTIVE (United Kingdom)
BENZOYL PEROXIDE
Brevoxyl-4 Creamy Wash **3054**
Brevoxyl-4 Gel **3054**
Brevoxyl-8 Creamy Wash **3054**
Brevoxyl-8 Gel **3054**

VALENAC (United Kingdom)
DICLOFENAC SODIUM
Voltaren Tablets **2334**
Voltaren-XR Tablets **2337**

VALENIUM (Thailand)
DIAZEPAM
Valium Tablets **2658**

VALEXIME (Italy)
CEFTRIAXONE SODIUM
Rocephin Injectable Vials, ADD-Vantage, Galaxy, Bulk **2642**

VALIFLOX (Argentina)
LEVOFLOXACIN
Levaquin Injection **2416**
Levaquin Tablets **2416**

VALIQUID (Germany)
DIAZEPAM
Valium Tablets **2658**

VALITRAN (Italy)
DIAZEPAM
Valium Tablets **2658**

VALIUM (Argentina, Australia, Austria, Belgium, Brazil, Canada, Denmark, France, Germany, India, Irish Republic, Israel, Italy, Mexico, Norway, Portugal, Singapore, South Africa, Spain, Sweden, Switzerland, Thailand, The Netherlands, The Philippines, United Kingdom, Venezuela)
DIAZEPAM
Valium Tablets **2658**

VALIX (Brazil)
DIAZEPAM
Valium Tablets **2658**

VALMETOL-3 (Mexico)
CALCITRIOL
Calcijex Injection **419**
Rocaltrol Capsules. **1150**
Rocaltrol Oral Solution **1150**

VALOCORDIN-DIAZEPAM (Germany)
DIAZEPAM
Valium Tablets **2658**

VALOXIN (Brazil)
DIGOXIN
Lanoxin Injection **1498**
Lanoxin Injection Pediatric **1502**
Lanoxin Tablets. **1505**

VALPAM (Australia, Hong Kong)
DIAZEPAM
Valium Tablets **2658**

VALPAX (Chile)
CLONAZEPAM
Klonopin Tablets **2639**

VALPEX (Argentina)
DONEPEZIL HYDROCHLORIDE
Aricept Tablets **1062**

VALPRESSION (Italy)
VALSARTAN
Diovan Tablets **2212**

VALROX (United Kingdom)
NAPROXEN
EC-Naprosyn Delayed-Release Tablets. . . . **2632**
Naprosyn Suspension. **2632**
Naprosyn Tablets **2632**

VALS (Spain)
VALSARTAN
Diovan Tablets **2212**

VALSARTAN/HCTZ (Austria)
VALSARTAN
Diovan Tablets **2212**

VALSTAR (Israel)
VALRUBICIN
Valstar Sterile Solution for Intravesical Instillation. **1735**

VALTAXIN (Canada)
VALRUBICIN
Valstar Sterile Solution for Intravesical Instillation. **1735**

VANDRAL (Spain)
VENLAFAXINE HYDROCHLORIDE
Effexor XR Capsules **3195**

VANTICON (Argentina)
ZAFIRLUKAST
Accolate Tablets **669**

VANTIN (Mexico)
NAPROXEN
EC-Naprosyn Delayed-Release Tablets. . . . **2632**
Naprosyn Suspension. **2632**
Naprosyn Tablets **2632**

VANZOR (Mexico)
DIAZEPAM
Valium Tablets **2658**

VARAXIL (Mexico)
CAPTOPRIL
Captopril Tablets **2182**

VARILISIN (Belgium)
COLLAGENASE
Santyl Collagenase Ointment **1724**

VARTALAN (Chile)
VALSARTAN
Diovan Tablets **2212**

VARTALAN D (Chile)
HYDROCHLOROTHIAZIDE/VALSARTAN
Diovan HCT Tablets **2216**

VARTELON (Hong Kong)
DICLOFENAC SODIUM
Voltaren Tablets **2334**
Voltaren-XR Tablets **2337**

VASALEN (Thailand)
DICLOFENAC SODIUM
Voltaren Tablets **2334**
Voltaren-XR Tablets **2337**

VASATEN (Venezuela)
VALSARTAN
Diovan Tablets **2212**

VASATEN HCT (Venezuela)
VALSARTAN
Diovan Tablets **2212**

VASCAL (Germany)
ISRADIPINE
DynaCirc CR Tablets. **1407**

VASCOR (Malaysia, Singapore, Thailand)
SIMVASTATIN
Zocor Tablets. **2136**

VASCORIM (Portugal)
SIMVASTATIN
Zocor Tablets. **2136**

VASILIP (Czech Republic, Hong Kong, Poland, Russia)
SIMVASTATIN
Zocor Tablets. **2136**

VASLAN (Spain)
ISRADIPINE
DynaCirc CR Tablets. **1407**

VASLIP (Brazil)
SIMVASTATIN
Zocor Tablets. **2136**

VASMULAX (The Philippines)
DILTIAZEM HYDROCHLORIDE
Cardizem LA Extended Release Tablets. . . . **421**

VASOCARDOL (Australia)
DILTIAZEM HYDROCHLORIDE
Cardizem LA Extended Release Tablets. . . . **421**

VASODIPINA (Brazil)
NIMODIPINE
Nimotop Capsules **790**

VASOFLEX (Chile)
NIMODIPINE
Nimotop Capsules **790**

VASOGARD (Brazil)
CILOSTAZOL
Pletal Tablets **2481**

VASOJET (Brazil)
LISINOPRIL
Prinivil Tablets **2087**

VASOMED (Chile)
SIMVASTATIN
Zocor Tablets. **2136**

VASOSTAD (The Philippines)
CAPTOPRIL
Captopril Tablets **2182**

VASOTENAL (Argentina, Chile, Venezuela)
SIMVASTATIN
Zocor Tablets. **2136**

VASOTENAL EZ (Argentina)
SIMVASTATIN
Zocor Tablets. **2136**

VASOTOP (India)
NIMODIPINE
Nimotop Capsules **790**

VASTAN (Poland, Venezuela)
SIMVASTATIN
Zocor Tablets. **2136**

VASTATIL (Brazil)
SIMVASTATIN
Zocor Tablets. **2136**

VASTATIN (Greece)
SIMVASTATIN
Zocor Tablets. **2136**

VASTILAN (The Philippines)
SIMVASTATIN
Zocor Tablets. **2136**

VASTIN (Australia, New Zealand)
FLUVASTATIN SODIUM
Lescol Capsules **2268**

VASTRIPINE (Greece)
NIMODIPINE
Nimotop Capsules **790**

VASTUS (Argentina, Chile)
ALBENDAZOLE
Albenza Tablets. **1297**

VASYROL (United Kingdom)
DIPYRIDAMOLE
Persantine Tablets **869**

VATRAN (Italy)
DIAZEPAM
Valium Tablets **2658**

VAXMAN (The Philippines)
AMOXICILLIN
Amoxil Pediatric Drops for Oral Suspension. **1305**
Amoxil Tablets **1305**

VECLAM (Italy)
CLARITHROMYCIN
Biaxin Filmtab Tablets **411**
Biaxin Granules **411**

VEENAC (Thailand)
DICLOFENAC SODIUM
Voltaren Tablets **2334**
Voltaren-XR Tablets **2337**

VEFRON (Greece)
ONDANSETRON
Zofran ODT Orally Disintegrating Tablets . . **1687**

VEKFAZOLIN (Greece)
CEFUROXIME SODIUM
Zinacef Injection **1678**

VELAFAX (Poland)
VENLAFAXINE HYDROCHLORIDE
Effexor XR Capsules **3195**

VELAMOX (Brazil)
AMOXICILLIN
Amoxil Pediatric Drops for Oral Suspension. **1305**
Amoxil Tablets **1305**

VELARIL (Venezuela)
CLONIDINE HYDROCHLORIDE
Catapres Tablets **841**

VELAXIN (Poland)
VENLAFAXINE HYDROCHLORIDE
Effexor XR Capsules **3195**

VELDROL (Mexico)
TRAMADOL HYDROCHLORIDE
Ultram ER Tablets **2428**

VELKALOV (Greece)
LOVASTATIN
Mevacor Tablets **2063**

VELMONIT (Spain)
CIPROFLOXACIN HYDROCHLORIDE
Cipro Tablets **2810**

VELPRO (Mexico)
BENZONATATE
Tessalon Perles **1183**

VELSAY (Mexico)
NAPROXEN
EC-Naprosyn Delayed-Release Tablets. . . . **2632**
Naprosyn Suspension. **2632**
Naprosyn Tablets **2632**

VELSAY-S COMPUESTO (Mexico)
NAPROXEN
EC-Naprosyn Delayed-Release Tablets. . . . **2632**
Naprosyn Suspension. **2632**
Naprosyn Tablets **2632**

VELTEX (South Africa)
DICLOFENAC SODIUM
Voltaren Tablets **2334**
Voltaren-XR Tablets **2337**

VELTION (Greece)
MUPIROCIN
Bactroban Ointment. **1368**

VEMIZOL (Malaysia)
ALBENDAZOLE
Albenza Tablets. **1297**

VENDAZOL (Venezuela)
ALBENDAZOLE
Albenza Tablets. **1297**

VENDREX (Brazil)
DICLOFENAC SODIUM
Voltaren Tablets **2334**
Voltaren-XR Tablets **2337**

VENLA (Israel)
VENLAFAXINE HYDROCHLORIDE
Effexor XR Capsules **3195**

VENLIFT (Brazil)
VENLAFAXINE HYDROCHLORIDE
Effexor XR Capsules **3195**

VENLOR (India, South Africa)
VENLAFAXINE HYDROCHLORIDE
Effexor XR Capsules **3195**

VENOPRIL (Brazil)
CAPTOPRIL
Captopril Tablets **2182**

VENOZEL (Poland)
DICLOFENAC SODIUM
Voltaren Tablets **2334**
Voltaren-XR Tablets **2337**

VENT RETARD (Spain)
THEOPHYLLINE
Uniphyl Tablets **2595**

VENTARONE (Thailand)
DICLOFENAC SODIUM
Voltaren Tablets **2334**
Voltaren-XR Tablets **2337**

VENTER (Czech Republic, Hungary, Poland, Russia)
SUCRALFATE
Carafate Suspension **706**
Carafate Tablets **707**

VENTOFLU (Italy)
FLUNISOLIDE
Aerobid Inhaler System. **1153**
Aerobid-M Inhaler System **1153**

VERACOL (Greece)
CEFTRIAXONE SODIUM
Rocephin Injectable Vials, ADD-Vantage, Galaxy, Bulk **2642**

VERACUR (United Kingdom)
FORMALDEHYDE
Formadon Solution. **1699**

VERADOL (Argentina)
NAPROXEN
EC-Naprosyn Delayed-Release Tablets. . . . **2632**
Naprosyn Suspension. **2632**
Naprosyn Tablets **2632**

VERAL (Czech Republic, Hungary)
DICLOFENAC SODIUM
Voltaren Tablets **2334**
Voltaren-XR Tablets **2337**

VERANZOL (Mexico)
ALBENDAZOLE
Albenza Tablets. **1297**

VERASPIR (Portugal)
SALMETEROL XINAFOATE
Serevent Diskus 1594

VERATEN (Argentina)
CARVEDILOL
Coreg Tablets. 1387

VERCOL (Greece)
LISINOPRIL
Prinivil Tablets 2087

VERDAZOL (Brazil)
ALBENDAZOLE
Albenza Tablets. 1297

VERELAIT (Italy)
LACTULOSE
Kristalose for Oral Solution 1004

VERLOST (Greece)
RANITIDINE HYDROCHLORIDE
Zantac 25 EFFERdose Tablets 1670
Zantac 150 Tablets 1670
Zantac 300 Tablets 1670
Zantac Injection 1666
Zantac Injection Premixed 1666
Zantac Syrup 1670

VERMECTIL (Brazil)
IVERMECTIN
Stromectol Tablets. 2120

VERMICLASE (Brazil)
ALBENDAZOLE
Albenza Tablets. 1297

VERMILAN (Mexico)
ALBENDAZOLE
Albenza Tablets. 1297

VERMIN PLUS (Mexico)
ALBENDAZOLE
Albenza Tablets. 1297

VERMISEN (Mexico)
ALBENDAZOLE
Albenza Tablets. 1297

VERMITAL (Brazil)
ALBENDAZOLE
Albenza Tablets. 1297

VERMIXIDE (Thailand)
ALBENDAZOLE
Albenza Tablets. 1297

VERMOIL (Chile)
ALBENDAZOLE
Albenza Tablets. 1297

VERNTHOL (South Africa)
THEOPHYLLINE
Uniphyl Tablets 2595

VEROXIL (Greece, Italy)
INDAPAMIDE
Indapamide Tablets 2188

VERSATIS (United Kingdom)
LIDOCAINE
Lidoderm Patch 1114

VESALION FLEX (Argentina)
DICLOFENAC SODIUM
Voltaren Tablets 2334
Voltaren-XR Tablets 2337

VESANOID (Argentina, Australia, Austria, Belgium, Brazil, Canada, Chile, Czech Republic, Finland, France, Germany, Greece, Hong Kong, Hungary, Irish Republic, Israel, Italy, Mexico, New Zealand, Norway, Poland, Portugal, Singapore, South Africa, Spain, Sweden, Switzerland, Thailand, The Netherlands, The Philippines, Turkey, United Kingdom, Venezuela)
TRETINOIN
Vesanoid Capsules. 2660

VESIX (Finland, The Netherlands)
FUROSEMIDE
Furosemide Tablets 2186

VESPROCIN (Thailand)
CIPROFLOXACIN
Cipro Oral Suspension 2810

VESTACLAV (Malaysia)
AMOXICILLIN
Amoxil Pediatric Drops for Oral Suspension. 1305
Amoxil Tablets 1305

VESXACIN (Thailand)
NORFLOXACIN
Noroxin Tablets. 2069

VETAMOL (Greece)
NORFLOXACIN
Noroxin Tablets. 2069

VETANSIL (Brazil)
DIAZEPAM
Valium Tablets 2658

VETIPROST (Argentina)
FINASTERIDE
Propecia Tablets 2095
Proscar Tablets. 2102

VEXURAT (Greece)
FAMOTIDINE
Pepcid for Oral Suspension 2075
Pepcid Tablets 2075

VIAFUROX (Argentina)
FUROSEMIDE
Furosemide Tablets 2186

VIANI (The Netherlands)
SALMETEROL XINAFOATE
Serevent Diskus 1594

VIARTRIL FLEX (Argentina)
DICLOFENAC SODIUM
Voltaren Tablets 2334
Voltaren-XR Tablets 2337

VIARTRIL NF (Argentina)
DICLOFENAC SODIUM
Voltaren Tablets 2334
Voltaren-XR Tablets 2337

VIATOPIN (Hungary)
TOPOTECAN HYDROCHLORIDE
Hycamtin for Injection. 1459

VIAVOX (Venezuela)
DICLOFENAC SODIUM
Voltaren Tablets 2334
Voltaren-XR Tablets 2337

VIAZEM (Denmark, Sweden, United Kingdom)
DILTIAZEM HYDROCHLORIDE
Cardizem LA Extended Release Tablets. . . . 421

VICARDOL (Argentina)
CARVEDILOL
Coreg Tablets. 1387

VICK-ZYRT (Hong Kong)
CETIRIZINE HYDROCHLORIDE
Zyrtec Syrup 1920
Zyrtec Tablets 1920

VICNAS (Spain)
NORFLOXACIN
Noroxin Tablets. 2069

VIDA FAMODINE (Hong Kong)
FAMOTIDINE
Pepcid for Oral Suspension 2075
Pepcid Tablets 2075

VIDAPRIL (Portugal)
CAPTOPRIL
Captopril Tablets. 2182

VIDASTAT (Hong Kong, The Philippines)
SIMVASTATIN
Zocor Tablets. 2136

VIDOX (Argentina)
MUPIROCIN
Bactroban Ointment. 1368

VIEPAX (Israel)
VENLAFAXINE HYDROCHLORIDE
Effexor XR Capsules 3195

VIFLOXINA (Mexico)
CIPROFLOXACIN
Cipro Oral Suspension 2810

VIGICER (Argentina)
MODAFINIL
Provigil Tablets 977

VIGIL (Czech Republic, Germany, Poland)
MODAFINIL
Provigil Tablets 977

VIKING (Greece)
LOVASTATIN
Mevacor Tablets 2063

VIKROL (Mexico)
CLARITHROMYCIN
Biaxin Filmtab Tablets 411
Biaxin Granules. 411

VILACRIL (Greece)
DICLOFENAC SODIUM
Voltaren Tablets 2334
Voltaren-XR Tablets 2337

VILONIT (Greece)
DICLOFENAC SODIUM
Voltaren Tablets 2334
Voltaren-XR Tablets 2337

VINCOSEDAN (Spain)
DIAZEPAM
Valium Tablets 2658

VINDACIN (Mexico)
SULINDAC
Clinoril Tablets 1962

VINGIONAL (Argentina)
RANITIDINE HYDROCHLORIDE
Zantac 25 EFFERdose Tablets 1670
Zantac 150 Tablets 1670
Zantac 300 Tablets 1670
Zantac Injection 1666
Zantac Injection Premixed 1666
Zantac Syrup 1670

VINSEN (Thailand)
NAPROXEN
EC-Naprosyn Delayed-Release Tablets. . . . 2632
Naprosyn Suspension. 2632
Naprosyn Tablets 2632

VINTIX (Venezuela)
SIBUTRAMINE HYDROCHLORIDE
Meridia Capsules. 475

VIOKASE (Belgium, Canada)
PANCRELIPASE
Ultrase Capsules. 718
Ultrase MT Capsules 719

VIPLENA (Chile)
ORLISTAT
Xenical Capsules. 2672

VIPLUS (Mexico)
NAPROXEN SODIUM
Anaprox DS Tablets 2632
Anaprox Tablets 2632

VIRAFERON (France, Mexico, Spain, The Netherlands)
INTERFERON ALFA-2B
Intron A for Injection. 2859

VIR-COMPLEX (Brazil)
LAMIVUDINE
Epivir Oral Solution 1412
Epivir Tablets 1412
Epivir-HBV Oral Solution 1417
Epivir-HBV Tablets 1417

VIRDOX (Spain)
CETIRIZINE HYDROCHLORIDE
Zyrtec Syrup 1920
Zyrtec Tablets 1920

VIRLIX (Austria, Czech Republic, Denmark, France, Italy, Mexico, Norway, Poland, Portugal, Spain, The Philippines, Turkey, Venezuela)
CETIRIZINE HYDROCHLORIDE
Zyrtec Syrup 1920
Zyrtec Tablets 1920

VIROBRON NF (Argentina)
DICLOFENAC SODIUM
Voltaren Tablets 2334
Voltaren-XR Tablets 2337

VIRORREVER (Argentina)
EFAVIRENZ
Sustiva Capsules. 930

VIROZID (Brazil)
ZIDOVUDINE
Retrovir Capsules 1574
Retrovir IV Infusion. 1579
Retrovir Syrup 1574
Retrovir Tablets. 1574

VIRUSTAT (Brazil)
ZIDOVUDINE
Retrovir Capsules 1574
Retrovir IV Infusion. 1579
Retrovir Syrup 1574
Retrovir Tablets. 1574

VISCOR (Italy)
DIPYRIDAMOLE
Persantine Tablets 869

VISCOSEAL (Germany, Malaysia, Switzerland, United Kingdom)
SODIUM HYALURONATE
Hyalgan Solution 2742

VISIAL (India)
SODIUM HYALURONATE
Hyalgan Solution 2742

VISIOL (Germany, Malaysia, Switzerland)
SODIUM HYALURONATE
Hyalgan Solution 2742

VISLUBE (Germany, Malaysia, Switzerland)
SODIUM HYALURONATE
Hyalgan Solution 2742

VISMED (Australia, France, Germany, Hong Kong, Italy, Switzerland)
SODIUM HYALURONATE
Hyalgan Solution 2742

VISTHESIA (Germany)
SODIUM HYALURONATE
Hyalgan Solution 2742

VITABIN (The Netherlands)
TERBINAFINE HYDROCHLORIDE
Lamisil Tablets 2266

VITACID (Portugal)
TRETINOIN
Vesanoid Capsules. 2660

VITAMIN A ACID (Hong Kong)
TRETINOIN
Vesanoid Capsules. 2660

VITANOL (Spain)
TRETINOIN
Vesanoid Capsules. 2660

VITANOL-A (Argentina, Brazil)
TRETINOIN
Vesanoid Capsules. 2660

VITINOIN (Canada)
TRETINOIN
Vesanoid Capsules. 2660

VITRAX (France)
SODIUM HYALURONATE
Hyalgan Solution 2742

VI-URIL (Chile)
TAMSULOSIN HYDROCHLORIDE
Flomax Capsules 848

VIVACOR (Poland)
CARVEDILOL
Coreg Tablets. 1387

VIVAL (Norway)
DIAZEPAM
Valium Tablets 2658

VIVAPRYL (United Kingdom)
SELEGILINE HYDROCHLORIDE
Eldepryl Capsules 3052

VIVATEC (Denmark, Finland, Norway, Sweden)
LISINOPRIL
Prinivil Tablets 2087

VIVATEC COMP (Finland, Norway)
HYDROCHLOROTHIAZIDE/LISINOPRIL
Prinzide Tablets 2092

VIVAZID (Denmark)
HYDROCHLOROTHIAZIDE/LISINOPRIL
Prinzide Tablets 2092

VIVELLE (Belgium, Canada)
ESTRADIOL
Climara Transdermal System 763

VIVELLE DOT (Denmark)
ESTRADIOL
Climara Transdermal System 763

VIVELLEDOT (France)
ESTRADIOL
Climara Transdermal System 763

VIVOL (Canada)
DIAZEPAM
Valium Tablets 2658

VIXIDERM E (Argentina)
BENZOYL PEROXIDE
Brevoxyl-4 Creamy Wash. 3054
Brevoxyl-4 Gel 3054

Brevoxyl-8 Creamy Wash . . . 3054
Brevoxyl-8 Gel . . . 3054

VIZERUL (Argentina, Venezuela)
RANITIDINE HYDROCHLORIDE
Zantac 150 Tablets . . . 1670
Zantac 25 EFFERdose Tablets . . . 1670
Zantac 300 Tablets . . . 1670
Zantac Injection . . . 1666
Zantac Injection Premixed . . . 1666
Zantac Syrup . . . 1670

V-NOLONE (Thailand)
TRIAMCINOLONE ACETONIDE
Azmacort Inhalation Aerosol . . . 407
Nasacort AQ Nasal Spray . . . 2765

VOFENAL (Canada)
DICLOFENAC SODIUM
Voltaren Tablets . . . 2334
Voltaren-XR Tablets . . . 2337

VOKER (Malaysia)
FAMOTIDINE
Pepcid for Oral Suspension . . . 2075
Pepcid Tablets . . . 2075

VOLCIDOL-S (Thailand)
TRAMADOL HYDROCHLORIDE
Ultram ER Tablets . . . 2428

VOLDAL (France)
DICLOFENAC SODIUM
Voltaren Tablets . . . 2334
Voltaren-XR Tablets . . . 2337

VOLFENAC (Thailand)
DICLOFENAC SODIUM
Voltaren Tablets . . . 2334
Voltaren-XR Tablets . . . 2337

VOLFENN (The Philippines)
DICLOFENAC SODIUM
Voltaren Tablets . . . 2334
Voltaren-XR Tablets . . . 2337

VOLNAC (Thailand)
DICLOFENAC SODIUM
Voltaren Tablets . . . 2334
Voltaren-XR Tablets . . . 2337

VOLOGEN (Irish Republic)
DICLOFENAC SODIUM
Voltaren Tablets . . . 2334
Voltaren-XR Tablets . . . 2337

VOLON A (Austria)
TRIAMCINOLONE ACETONIDE
Azmacort Inhalation Aerosol . . . 407
Nasacort AQ Nasal Spray . . . 2765

VOLONIMAT (Germany)
TRIAMCINOLONE ACETONIDE
Azmacort Inhalation Aerosol . . . 407
Nasacort AQ Nasal Spray . . . 2765

VOLONIMAT N (Germany)
TRIAMCINOLONE ACETONIDE
Azmacort Inhalation Aerosol . . . 407
Nasacort AQ Nasal Spray . . . 2765

VOLRAMAN (United Kingdom)
DICLOFENAC SODIUM
Voltaren Tablets . . . 2334
Voltaren-XR Tablets . . . 2337

VOLSAID (United Kingdom)
DICLOFENAC SODIUM
Voltaren Tablets . . . 2334
Voltaren-XR Tablets . . . 2337

VOLTA (Thailand)
DICLOFENAC SODIUM
Voltaren Tablets . . . 2334
Voltaren-XR Tablets . . . 2337

VOLTADOL (Italy)
DICLOFENAC SODIUM
Voltaren Tablets . . . 2334
Voltaren-XR Tablets . . . 2337

VOLTAFLEX (Brazil)
DICLOFENAC SODIUM
Voltaren Tablets . . . 2334
Voltaren-XR Tablets . . . 2337

VOLTAMICIN (Austria, Brazil, Czech Republic, Hungary, Singapore)
DICLOFENAC SODIUM
Voltaren Tablets . . . 2334
Voltaren-XR Tablets . . . 2337

VOLTAPATCH (Belgium)
DICLOFENAC SODIUM
Voltaren Tablets . . . 2334
Voltaren-XR Tablets . . . 2337

VOLTAREN (Brazil, Greece, Norway, Sweden, Turkey, Venezuela)
DICLOFENAC SODIUM
Voltaren Tablets . . . 2334
Voltaren-XR Tablets . . . 2337

VOLTAREN COLIRIO (Argentina, Brazil)
DICLOFENAC SODIUM
Voltaren Tablets . . . 2334
Voltaren-XR Tablets . . . 2337

VOLTAREN FLEX (Argentina)
DICLOFENAC SODIUM
Voltaren Tablets . . . 2334
Voltaren-XR Tablets . . . 2337

VOLTAREN FORTE (Argentina, Mexico)
DICLOFENAC SODIUM
Voltaren Tablets . . . 2334
Voltaren-XR Tablets . . . 2337

VOLTAREN OPHTA (Hungary, Switzerland, Turkey)
DICLOFENAC SODIUM
Voltaren Tablets . . . 2334
Voltaren-XR Tablets . . . 2337

VOLTAREN OPHTHA (Australia, Canada, Germany, Hong Kong, Israel, New Zealand, Norway, Singapore, South Africa, Sweden)
DICLOFENAC SODIUM
Voltaren Tablets . . . 2334
Voltaren-XR Tablets . . . 2337

VOLTAREN PLUS (Germany)
DICLOFENAC SODIUM
Voltaren Tablets . . . 2334
Voltaren-XR Tablets . . . 2337

VOLTARENE (France)
DICLOFENAC SODIUM
Voltaren Tablets . . . 2334
Voltaren-XR Tablets . . . 2337

VOLTAROL OPHTHA (Irish Republic, United Kingdom)
DICLOFENAC SODIUM
Voltaren Tablets . . . 2334
Voltaren-XR Tablets . . . 2337

VOLTEN (Venezuela)
DICLOFENAC SODIUM
Voltaren Tablets . . . 2334
Voltaren-XR Tablets . . . 2337

VOLTENAC (Poland)
DICLOFENAC SODIUM
Voltaren Tablets . . . 2334
Voltaren-XR Tablets . . . 2337

VOLTRIC (Spain)
CETIRIZINE HYDROCHLORIDE
Zyrtec Syrup . . . 1920
Zyrtec Tablets . . . 1920

VOLUTINE (Italy)
FENOFIBRATE
Tricor Tablets . . . 520

VOLUTOL (Mexico)
CARBAMAZEPINE
Carbatrol Capsules . . . 3019

VOLVERAC (Thailand)
DICLOFENAC SODIUM
Voltaren Tablets . . . 2334
Voltaren-XR Tablets . . . 2337

VOMIOF (India)
ONDANSETRON HYDROCHLORIDE
Zofran Injection . . . 1682
Zofran Injection Premixed . . . 1682
Zofran Oral Solution . . . 1687
Zofran Tablets . . . 1687

VOMITRON (Thailand)
ONDANSETRON HYDROCHLORIDE
Zofran Injection . . . 1682
Zofran Injection Premixed . . . 1682
Zofran Oral Solution . . . 1687
Zofran Tablets . . . 1687

VONAU (Brazil)
ONDANSETRON HYDROCHLORIDE
Zofran Injection . . . 1682
Zofran Injection Premixed . . . 1682
Zofran Oral Solution . . . 1687
Zofran Tablets . . . 1687

V-OPTIC (Israel)
TIMOLOL MALEATE
Timoptic in Ocudose . . . 2124
Timoptic Sterile Ophthalmic Solution . . . 2121
Timoptic-XE Sterile Ophthalmic Gel Forming Solution . . . 2125

VOREN (Malaysia, Thailand, The Philippines)
DICLOFENAC SODIUM
Voltaren Tablets . . . 2334
Voltaren-XR Tablets . . . 2337

VOREN PLUS (Malaysia)
DICLOFENAC SODIUM
Voltaren Tablets . . . 2334
Voltaren-XR Tablets . . . 2337

VOSTAR (Denmark)
DICLOFENAC SODIUM
Voltaren Tablets . . . 2334
Voltaren-XR Tablets . . . 2337

VOTAMED (Thailand)
DICLOFENAC SODIUM
Voltaren Tablets . . . 2334
Voltaren-XR Tablets . . . 2337

VOTAXIL (Venezuela)
DICLOFENAC SODIUM
Voltaren Tablets . . . 2334
Voltaren-XR Tablets . . . 2337

VUCLODIR (Argentina)
LAMIVUDINE
Epivir Oral Solution . . . 1412
Epivir Tablets . . . 1412
Epivir-HBV Oral Solution . . . 1417
Epivir-HBV Tablets . . . 1417

VUDIRAX (Brazil)
LAMIVUDINE
Epivir Oral Solution . . . 1412
Epivir Tablets . . . 1412
Epivir-HBV Oral Solution . . . 1417
Epivir-HBV Tablets . . . 1417

VURDON (Greece)
DICLOFENAC SODIUM
Voltaren Tablets . . . 2334
Voltaren-XR Tablets . . . 2337

WARI-DICLOWAL (Malaysia)
DICLOFENAC SODIUM
Voltaren Tablets . . . 2334
Voltaren-XR Tablets . . . 2337

WAUCOSIN (Greece)
TIMOLOL MALEATE
Timoptic in Ocudose . . . 2124
Timoptic Sterile Ophthalmic Solution . . . 2121
Timoptic-XE Sterile Ophthalmic Gel Forming Solution . . . 2125

WAYTRAX (Mexico)
CEFTAZIDIME
Fortaz for Injection . . . 1450

WELLBUTRIN (Argentina, Brazil, Canada, Chile, Czech Republic, Hong Kong, Hungary, Mexico, South Africa, Venezuela)
BUPROPION HYDROCHLORIDE
Wellbutrin SR Sustained-Release Tablets . . . 1653
Wellbutrin Tablets . . . 1648
Zyban Sustained-Release Tablets . . . 1692

WELLVONE (Australia, Austria, Belgium, Denmark, France, Germany, Greece, Italy, South Africa, Spain, Sweden, Switzerland, The Netherlands, United Kingdom)
ATOVAQUONE
Mepron Suspension . . . 1526

WENFLOX (Argentina)
NORFLOXACIN
Noroxin Tablets . . . 2069

WEPOX (India)
EPOETIN ALFA
Epogen for Injection . . . 576
Procrit for Injection . . . 2391

WILSIM (The Philippines)
SIMVASTATIN
Zocor Tablets . . . 2136

WINAFLOX (The Philippines)
NORFLOXACIN
Noroxin Tablets . . . 2069

WONTIZEM (Hong Kong)
DILTIAZEM HYDROCHLORIDE
Cardizem LA Extended Release Tablets . . . 421

XACIN (Thailand)
NORFLOXACIN
Noroxin Tablets . . . 2069

XAGRID (Belgium, Denmark, Finland, France, Germany, Irish Republic, Italy, Norway, Spain, Sweden, Switzerland, The Netherlands, United Kingdom)
ANAGRELIDE HYDROCHLORIDE
Agrylin Capsules . . . 3017

XALACOM (Argentina, Australia, Austria, Belgium, Brazil, Canada, Czech Republic, France, Germany, Greece, Hong Kong, Hungary, Irish Republic, Israel, Italy, Malaysia, Mexico, New Zealand, Poland, Portugal, Singapore, South Africa, Spain, Switzerland, Thailand, The Netherlands, The Philippines, United Kingdom, Venezuela)
LATANOPROST
Xalatan Ophthalmic Solution . . . ⊙273

XALATAN (Argentina, Australia, Austria, Belgium, Brazil, Canada, Chile, Czech Republic, Denmark, Finland, France, Germany, Greece, Hong Kong, Hungary, Irish Republic, Israel, Italy, Malaysia, Mexico, New Zealand, Norway, Poland, Portugal, Russia, Singapore, South Africa, Spain, Sweden, Switzerland, Thailand, The Netherlands, The Philippines, Turkey, United Kingdom, Venezuela)
LATANOPROST
Xalatan Ophthalmic Solution . . . ⊙273

XALCOM (Denmark, Finland, Norway, Sweden)
LATANOPROST
Xalatan Ophthalmic Solution . . . ⊙273

XALOTINA (Argentina)
AMOXICILLIN
Amoxil Pediatric Drops for Oral Suspension . . . 1305
Amoxil Tablets . . . 1305

XANIDINE (Thailand)
RANITIDINE HYDROCHLORIDE
Zantac 25 EFFERdose Tablets . . . 1670
Zantac 150 Tablets . . . 1670
Zantac 300 Tablets . . . 1670
Zantac Injection . . . 1666
Zantac Injection Premixed . . . 1666
Zantac Syrup . . . 1670

XANOMEL (Hungary, Irish Republic)
RANITIDINE HYDROCHLORIDE
Zantac 150 Tablets . . . 1670
Zantac 25 EFFERdose Tablets . . . 1670
Zantac 300 Tablets . . . 1670
Zantac Injection . . . 1666
Zantac Injection Premixed . . . 1666
Zantac Syrup . . . 1670

XANTHIUM (France, Thailand, Turkey)
THEOPHYLLINE
Uniphyl Tablets . . . 2595

XANTIVENT (Switzerland)
THEOPHYLLINE
Uniphyl Tablets . . . 2595

XARATOR (Italy)
ATORVASTATIN CALCIUM
Lipitor Tablets . . . 2501

XARB (India)
IRBESARTAN
Avapro Tablets . . . 897

XARB-H (India)
HYDROCHLOROTHIAZIDE/IRBESARTAN
Avalide Tablets . . . 892

XARTAN (Poland)
LOSARTAN POTASSIUM
Cozaar Tablets . . . 1973

XASMUN (Spain)
NORFLOXACIN
Noroxin Tablets . . . 2069

XEDENOL (Argentina)
DICLOFENAC SODIUM
Voltaren Tablets . . . 2334
Voltaren-XR Tablets . . . 2337

XEDENOL FLEX (Argentina)
DICLOFENAC SODIUM
Voltaren Tablets . . . 2334
Voltaren-XR Tablets . . . 2337

XELODA (Argentina, Australia, Austria, Belgium, Brazil, Canada, Chile, Czech Republic, Denmark, Finland, France, Germany, Greece, Hong Kong, Hungary, Irish Republic, Israel, Italy, Mexico, New Zealand, Norway, Poland, Portugal, Singapore, South Africa, Spain, Sweden, Switzerland, Thailand, The Netherlands, The Philippines, Turkey, United Kingdom, Venezuela)
CAPECITABINE
Xeloda Tablets . . . 2662

XENAR (Italy)
NAPROXEN
EC-Naprosyn Delayed-Release Tablets . . . 2632
Naprosyn Suspension . . . 2632
Naprosyn Tablets . . . 2632

XENICAL (Argentina, Australia, Austria, Belgium, Brazil, Canada, Chile, Czech Republic, Denmark, Finland, France, Germany, Greece, Hong Kong, Hungary, Irish Republic, Israel, Italy, Mexico, New Zealand, Norway, Poland, Portugal, Singapore, South Africa, Spain, Sweden, Switzerland, Thailand, The Netherlands, The Philippines, Turkey, United Kingdom, Venezuela)
ORLISTAT
Xenical Capsules . . . 2672

XENIPLUS (Argentina)
ORLISTAT
Xenical Capsules . . . 2672

XENOBID (India)
NAPROXEN
EC-Naprosyn Delayed-Release Tablets . . . 2632
Naprosyn Suspension . . . 2632
Naprosyn Tablets . . . 2632

XENOPAN (Austria)
NAPROXEN
EC-Naprosyn Delayed-Release Tablets . . . 2632
Naprosyn Suspension . . . 2632
Naprosyn Tablets . . . 2632

XEROTIL (Italy)
MIDODRINE HYDROCHLORIDE
ProAmatine Tablets . . . 3032

XETANOR (Poland)
PAROXETINE HYDROCHLORIDE
Paxil Oral Suspension . . . 1535
Paxil Tablets . . . 1535

XETIN (Spain)
PAROXETINE HYDROCHLORIDE
Paxil Oral Suspension . . . 1535
Paxil Tablets . . . 1535

XICANE (Argentina)
NAPROXEN
EC-Naprosyn Delayed-Release Tablets . . . 2632
Naprosyn Suspension . . . 2632
Naprosyn Tablets . . . 2632

XIDAN EDO (Germany)
SODIUM HYALURONATE
Hyalgan Solution . . . 2742

XILANIC (Argentina)
PAROXETINE HYDROCHLORIDE
Paxil Oral Suspension . . . 1535
Paxil Tablets . . . 1535

XILOCLER (Argentina)
LIDOCAINE
Lidoderm Patch . . . 1114

XILONIBSA (Portugal)
LIDOCAINE
Lidoderm Patch . . . 1114

XILOPAR (Austria, Germany, Italy, Portugal)
SELEGILINE HYDROCHLORIDE
Eldepryl Capsules . . . 3052

XIMAKEN (Mexico)
CEFUROXIME SODIUM
Zinacef Injection . . . 1678

XIMVE (Poland)
SIMVASTATIN
Zocor Tablets . . . 2136

XINA (Argentina)
DICLOFENAC SODIUM
Voltaren Tablets . . . 2334
Voltaren-XR Tablets . . . 2337

XINPLEX (Argentina)
ORLISTAT
Xenical Capsules . . . 2672

XIPRO (The Philippines)
CIPROFLOXACIN HYDROCHLORIDE
Cipro Tablets . . . 2810

XIPROCAN (Mexico)
AMOXICILLIN
Amoxil Pediatric Drops for Oral Suspension . . . 1305
Amoxil Tablets . . . 1305

XONATIL (Mexico)
CEFTRIAXONE SODIUM
Rocephin Injectable Vials, ADD-Vantage, Galaxy, Bulk . . . 2642

XORIM (Hungary, Poland, Venezuela)
CEFUROXIME SODIUM
Zinacef Injection . . . 1678

XORIMAX (Poland, The Philippines)
CEFUROXIME AXETIL
Ceftin for Oral Suspension . . . 1380
Ceftin Tablets . . . 1380

X'TAC (Malaysia)
RANITIDINE HYDROCHLORIDE
Zantac 25 EFFERdose Tablets . . . 1670
Zantac 150 Tablets . . . 1670
Zantac 300 Tablets . . . 1670
Zantac Injection . . . 1666
Zantac Injection Premixed . . . 1666
Zantac Syrup . . . 1670

XTENDA (The Philippines)
CEFTRIAXONE SODIUM
Rocephin Injectable Vials, ADD-Vantage, Galaxy, Bulk . . . 2642

X'TOR (India)
ATORVASTATIN CALCIUM
Lipitor Tablets . . . 2501

XYLESTESIN (Czech Republic)
LIDOCAINE
Lidoderm Patch . . . 1114

XYLOCAINA (Chile, Venezuela)
LIDOCAINE
Lidoderm Patch . . . 1114

XYLOCAINE (Czech Republic, Greece, India, Israel, Malaysia, South Africa, United Kingdom)
LIDOCAINE
Lidoderm Patch . . . 1114

XYLODASE (United Kingdom)
LIDOCAINE
Lidoderm Patch . . . 1114

XYLOPROCT (Hong Kong)
LIDOCAINE
Lidoderm Patch . . . 1114

XYMEL (Irish Republic)
TRAMADOL HYDROCHLORIDE
Ultram ER Tablets . . . 2428

YANURAX (Argentina)
NORFLOXACIN
Noroxin Tablets . . . 2069

YARA (Greece)
RANITIDINE HYDROCHLORIDE
Zantac 25 EFFERdose Tablets . . . 1670
Zantac 150 Tablets . . . 1670
Zantac 300 Tablets . . . 1670
Zantac Injection . . . 1666
Zantac Injection Premixed . . . 1666
Zantac Syrup . . . 1670

YASNAL (Poland)
DONEPEZIL HYDROCHLORIDE
Aricept Tablets . . . 1062

YATROX (Spain)
ONDANSETRON HYDROCHLORIDE
Zofran Injection . . . 1682
Zofran Injection Premixed . . . 1682
Zofran Oral Solution . . . 1687
Zofran Tablets . . . 1687

YENIZIN (Turkey)
CETIRIZINE HYDROCHLORIDE
Zyrtec Syrup . . . 1920
Zyrtec Tablets . . . 1920

YEPOTIN (Mexico)
EPOETIN ALFA
Epogen for Injection . . . 576
Procrit for Injection . . . 2391

YESAN (Greece)
TIMOLOL MALEATE
Timoptic in Ocudose . . . 2124
Timoptic Sterile Ophthalmic Solution . . . 2121
Timoptic-XE Sterile Ophthalmic Gel Forming Solution . . . 2125

YOKEL (Greece)
CEFUROXIME SODIUM
Zinacef Injection . . . 1678

YUREMID (Mexico)
FUROSEMIDE
Furosemide Tablets . . . 2186

ZAARPRESS (Brazil)
LOSARTAN POTASSIUM
Cozaar Tablets . . . 1973

ZAART (India)
LOSARTAN POTASSIUM
Cozaar Tablets . . . 1973

ZAART-H (India)
LOSARTAN POTASSIUM
Cozaar Tablets . . . 1973

ZADIM (The Philippines)
CEFTAZIDIME
Fortaz for Injection . . . 1450

ZADINE (Brazil)
RANITIDINE HYDROCHLORIDE
Zantac 25 EFFERdose Tablets . . . 1670
Zantac 150 Tablets . . . 1670
Zantac 300 Tablets . . . 1670
Zantac Injection . . . 1666
Zantac Injection Premixed . . . 1666
Zantac Syrup . . . 1670

ZADOLINA (Mexico)
CEFTAZIDIME
Fortaz for Injection . . . 1450

ZAEDOC (United Kingdom)
RANITIDINE HYDROCHLORIDE
Zantac 25 EFFERdose Tablets . . . 1670
Zantac 150 Tablets . . . 1670
Zantac 300 Tablets . . . 1670
Zantac Injection . . . 1666
Zantac Injection Premixed . . . 1666
Zantac Syrup . . . 1670

ZAFIMIDA (Mexico)
FUROSEMIDE
Furosemide Tablets . . . 2186

ZAFIRASMAL (Argentina)
ZAFIRLUKAST
Accolate Tablets . . . 669

ZAFIRST (Italy)
ZAFIRLUKAST
Accolate Tablets . . . 669

ZAGORINE (Greece)
CEFUROXIME AXETIL
Ceftin for Oral Suspension . . . 1380
Ceftin Tablets . . . 1380

ZALASTA (Poland)
OLANZAPINE
Zyprexa Tablets . . . 1883

ZALDIAR (Austria, Mexico, Poland, Spain, Switzerland, The Netherlands, Venezuela)
TRAMADOL HYDROCHLORIDE
Ultram ER Tablets . . . 2428

ZAMACORT (Mexico)
TRIAMCINOLONE ACETONIDE
Azmacort Inhalation Aerosol . . . 407
Nasacort AQ Nasal Spray . . . 2765

ZAMADOL (Irish Republic, United Kingdom)
TRAMADOL HYDROCHLORIDE
Ultram ER Tablets . . . 2428

ZAMOCILLINE (France)
AMOXICILLIN
Amoxil Pediatric Drops for Oral Suspension . . . 1305
Amoxil Tablets . . . 1305

ZAMUDOL (France)
TRAMADOL HYDROCHLORIDE
Ultram ER Tablets . . . 2428

ZAMUR (Poland)
CEFUROXIME AXETIL
Ceftin for Oral Suspension . . . 1380
Ceftin Tablets . . . 1380

ZANDID (Turkey)
RANITIDINE HYDROCHLORIDE
Zantac 25 EFFERdose Tablets . . . 1670
Zantac 150 Tablets . . . 1670
Zantac 300 Tablets . . . 1670
Zantac Injection . . . 1666
Zantac Injection Premixed . . . 1666
Zantac Syrup . . . 1670

ZANDIL (The Philippines)
DILTIAZEM HYDROCHLORIDE
Cardizem LA Extended Release Tablets . . . 421

ZANDINE (Irish Republic)
RANITIDINE HYDROCHLORIDE
Zantac 25 EFFERdose Tablets . . . 1670
Zantac 150 Tablets . . . 1670
Zantac 300 Tablets . . . 1670
Zantac Injection . . . 1666
Zantac Injection Premixed . . . 1666
Zantac Syrup . . . 1670

ZANIDEX (Israel)
RANITIDINE HYDROCHLORIDE
Zantac 25 EFFERdose Tablets . . . 1670
Zantac 150 Tablets . . . 1670
Zantac 300 Tablets . . . 1670
Zantac Injection . . . 1666
Zantac Injection Premixed . . . 1666
Zantac Syrup . . . 1670

ZANIDIN (New Zealand)
RANITIDINE HYDROCHLORIDE
Zantac 25 EFFERdose Tablets . . . 1670
Zantac 150 Tablets . . . 1670
Zantac 300 Tablets . . . 1670
Zantac Injection . . . 1666
Zantac Injection Premixed . . . 1666
Zantac Syrup . . . 1670

ZANTAB (Israel)
RANITIDINE HYDROCHLORIDE
Zantac 25 EFFERdose Tablets . . . 1670
Zantac 150 Tablets . . . 1670
Zantac 300 Tablets . . . 1670
Zantac Injection . . . 1666
Zantac Injection Premixed . . . 1666
Zantac Syrup . . . 1670

ZANTAC (Australia, Austria, Belgium, Chile, Czech Republic, Denmark, Finland, Greece, Hong Kong, Hungary, Irish Republic, Israel, Italy, Malaysia, New Zealand, Norway, Poland, Portugal, Russia, Singapore, South Africa, Spain, Sweden, Thailand, The Netherlands, The Philippines, Turkey, United Kingdom, Venezuela)
RANITIDINE HYDROCHLORIDE
Zantac 25 EFFERdose Tablets . . . 1670
Zantac 150 Tablets . . . 1670
Zantac 300 Tablets . . . 1670
Zantac Injection . . . 1666
Zantac Injection Premixed . . . 1666
Zantac Syrup . . . 1670

ZANTARAC (Austria)
RANITIDINE HYDROCHLORIDE
Zantac 25 EFFERdose Tablets . . . 1670
Zantac 150 Tablets . . . 1670
Zantac 300 Tablets . . . 1670
Zantac Injection . . . 1666
Zantac Injection Premixed . . . 1666
Zantac Syrup . . . 1670

ZANTIC (Germany, Switzerland)
RANITIDINE HYDROCHLORIDE
Zantac 150 Tablets . . . 1670
Zantac 25 EFFERdose Tablets . . . 1670
Zantac 300 Tablets . . . 1670
Zantac Injection . . . 1666
Zantac Injection Premixed . . . 1666
Zantac Syrup . . . 1670

ZAPTO (South Africa)
CAPTOPRIL
Captopril Tablets . . . 2182

ZAPTO CO (South Africa)
CAPTOPRIL
Captopril Tablets . . . 2182

ZARATOR (Argentina, Chile, Denmark, Greece, Portugal, Spain, The Netherlands)
ATORVASTATIN CALCIUM
Lipitor Tablets . . . 2501

ZAREX (Israel)
FAMOTIDINE
Pepcid for Oral Suspension . . . 2075

Pepcid Tablets **2075**

ZASTERID (Poland)
FINASTERIDE
Propecia Tablets **2095**
Proscar Tablets **2102**

ZAXEM (Austria)
BUTENAFINE HYDROCHLORIDE
Mentax Cream **2190**

Z-BEC (Greece)
LISINOPRIL
Prinivil Tablets **2087**

ZEBEN (Thailand)
ALBENDAZOLE
Albenza Tablets **1297**

ZECLAR (Czech Republic, Finland, France)
CLARITHROMYCIN
Biaxin Filmtab Tablets **411**
Biaxin Granules **411**

ZECLAREN (Greece)
CLARITHROMYCIN
Biaxin Filmtab Tablets **411**
Biaxin Granules **411**

ZEDDAN (Italy)
TRANDOLAPRIL
Mavik Tablets **472**

ZEFAXONE (Thailand)
CEFTRIAXONE SODIUM
Rocephin Injectable Vials, ADD-Vantage, Galaxy, Bulk **2642**

ZEFFIX (Argentina, Australia, Austria, Belgium, Brazil, Czech Republic, Denmark, Finland, France, Germany, Greece, Hong Kong, Hungary, Irish Republic, Israel, Italy, Malaysia, New Zealand, Norway, Poland, Portugal, Russia, Singapore, Spain, Sweden, Switzerland, Thailand, The Philippines, Turkey, United Kingdom)
LAMIVUDINE
Epivir Oral Solution **1412**
Epivir Tablets **1412**
Epivir-HBV Oral Solution **1417**
Epivir-HBV Tablets **1417**

ZEFROXE (South Africa)
CEFUROXIME AXETIL
Ceftin for Oral Suspension **1380**
Ceftin Tablets **1380**

ZEFTAM (Thailand)
CEFTAZIDIME
Fortaz for Injection **1450**

ZEGEN (The Philippines)
CEFUROXIME AXETIL
Ceftin for Oral Suspension **1380**
Ceftin Tablets **1380**

ZEID (Mexico)
SIMVASTATIN
Zocor Tablets **2136**

ZEISIN (Germany)
PIRBUTEROL ACETATE
Maxair Autohaler **1705**

ZELA (Thailand)
ALBENDAZOLE
Albenza Tablets **1297**

ZELAPAR (Argentina, United Kingdom)
SELEGILINE HYDROCHLORIDE
Eldepryl Capsules **3052**

ZELFIN (Mexico)
ALBENDAZOLE
Albenza Tablets **1297**

ZELIXA (Poland)
SIBUTRAMINE HYDROCHLORIDE
Meridia Capsules **475**

ZEM (Greece)
DILTIAZEM HYDROCHLORIDE
Cardizem LA Extended Release Tablets **421**

ZEMAX (South Africa)
LISINOPRIL
Prinivil Tablets **2087**

ZEMOX (Germany)
SIMVASTATIN
Zocor Tablets **2136**

ZEMPLAR (Austria, Finland, Germany, Greece, Hong Kong, Irish Republic, Italy, Norway, Portugal, Spain, Sweden, Switzerland, The Netherlands, United Kingdom, Venezuela)
PARICALCITOL
Zemplar Injection **538**

ZEMTARD (United Kingdom)
DILTIAZEM HYDROCHLORIDE
Cardizem LA Extended Release Tablets **421**

ZEMTRIAL (The Philippines)
DILTIAZEM HYDROCHLORIDE
Cardizem LA Extended Release Tablets **421**

ZENAXIN (Mexico)
ALBENDAZOLE
Albenza Tablets **1297**

ZENCEF (Venezuela)
CEFUROXIME SODIUM
Zinacef Injection **1678**

ZENDHIN (Hong Kong, Malaysia, Singapore)
RANITIDINE HYDROCHLORIDE
Zantac 150 Tablets **1670**
Zantac 25 EFFERdose Tablets **1670**
Zantac 300 Tablets **1670**
Zantac Injection **1666**
Zantac Injection Premixed **1666**
Zantac Syrup **1670**

ZENODIAN (Italy)
SUCRALFATE
Carafate Suspension **706**
Carafate Tablets **707**

ZENSIL (Thailand)
CETIRIZINE HYDROCHLORIDE
Zyrtec Syrup **1920**
Zyrtec Tablets **1920**

ZENTEL (Australia, Brazil, Chile, Czech Republic, France, India, Italy, Malaysia, Mexico, Poland, Portugal, Singapore, South Africa, Switzerland, Thailand, The Philippines, Venezuela)
ALBENDAZOLE
Albenza Tablets **1297**

ZENTIUS (Argentina, Chile)
CITALOPRAM HYDROBROMIDE
Celexa Tablets **1160**

ZENZERA (Thailand)
ALBENDAZOLE
Albenza Tablets **1297**

ZEPAN (Mexico)
DIAZEPAM
Valium Tablets **2658**

ZEPHOLIN (Greece, Irish Republic)
THEOPHYLLINE
Uniphyl Tablets **2595**

ZEPIKEN (Mexico)
CARBAMAZEPINE
Carbatrol Capsules **3019**

ZEPOSE (India)
DIAZEPAM
Valium Tablets **2658**

ZEPRAT (Mexico)
DIAZEPAM
Valium Tablets **2658**

ZEPROSIL (South Africa)
LISINOPRIL
Prinivil Tablets **2087**

ZEPTAG (The Philippines)
RANITIDINE HYDROCHLORIDE
Zantac 25 EFFERdose Tablets **1670**
Zantac 150 Tablets **1670**
Zantac 300 Tablets **1670**
Zantac Injection **1666**
Zantac Injection Premixed **1666**
Zantac Syrup **1670**

ZEPTOL (Russia, Thailand)
CARBAMAZEPINE
Carbatrol Capsules **3019**

ZEPTRIGEN (The Philippines)
CEFTAZIDIME
Fortaz for Injection **1450**

ZERA (Portugal)
SIMVASTATIN
Zocor Tablets **2136**

ZERELLA (Austria, Italy)
ESTRADIOL
Climara Transdermal System **763**

ZERLUBRON (Greece)
FENOFIBRATE
Tricor Tablets **520**

ZERMED (Thailand)
CETIRIZINE HYDROCHLORIDE
Zyrtec Syrup **1920**
Zyrtec Tablets **1920**

ZEROPENEM (Argentina)
MEROPENEM
Merrem I.V. **684**

ZERTINE (Hong Kong, Thailand)
CETIRIZINE HYDROCHLORIDE
Zyrtec Syrup **1920**
Zyrtec Tablets **1920**

ZESGER (Irish Republic)
LISINOPRIL
Prinivil Tablets **2087**

ZESGER PLUS (Irish Republic)
LISINOPRIL
Prinivil Tablets **2087**

ZESTAN (Irish Republic)
LISINOPRIL
Prinivil Tablets **2087**

ZESTOMAX (South Africa)
LISINOPRIL
Prinivil Tablets **2087**

ZESTORETIC (Argentina, Austria, Belgium, Brazil, Canada, Chile, Denmark, France, Hong Kong, Irish Republic, Italy, Mexico, New Zealand, Norway, Portugal, South Africa, Spain, Sweden, Switzerland, The Netherlands, The Philippines, Turkey, United Kingdom)
LISINOPRIL
Prinivil Tablets **2087**

ZESTRIL (Argentina, Australia, Belgium, Brazil, Canada, Chile, Denmark, Finland, France, Greece, Hong Kong, Irish Republic, Italy, Malaysia, Mexico, New Zealand, Norway, Portugal, Singapore, South Africa, Spain, Sweden, Switzerland, Thailand, The Netherlands, The Philippines, Turkey, United Kingdom)
LISINOPRIL
Prinivil Tablets **2087**

ZETAGAL (Greece)
CEFUROXIME SODIUM
Zinacef Injection **1678**

ZETALERG (Brazil)
CETIRIZINE HYDROCHLORIDE
Zyrtec Syrup **1920**
Zyrtec Tablets **1920**

ZETAVUDIN (Argentina)
ZIDOVUDINE
Retrovir Capsules **1574**
Retrovir IV Infusion **1579**
Retrovir Syrup **1574**
Retrovir Tablets **1574**

ZETIR (Brazil, Germany)
CETIRIZINE HYDROCHLORIDE
Zyrtec Syrup **1920**
Zyrtec Tablets **1920**

ZETOMAX (South Africa)
LISINOPRIL
Prinivil Tablets **2087**

ZETOMAX CO (South Africa)
LISINOPRIL
Prinivil Tablets **2087**

ZETOP (South Africa)
CETIRIZINE HYDROCHLORIDE
Zyrtec Syrup **1920**
Zyrtec Tablets **1920**

ZETRON (Thailand)
ONDANSETRON HYDROCHLORIDE
Zofran Injection **1682**
Zofran Injection Premixed **1682**
Zofran Oral Solution **1687**
Zofran Tablets **1687**

ZETROTAX (Argentina)
ZIDOVUDINE
Retrovir Capsules **1574**
Retrovir IV Infusion **1579**
Retrovir Syrup **1574**
Retrovir Tablets **1574**

ZIAGEN (Australia, Austria, Belgium, Canada, Chile, Czech Republic, Denmark, Finland, France, Germany, Greece, Hong Kong, Irish Republic, Israel, Italy, New Zealand, Norway, Poland, Portugal, Russia, Singapore, South Africa, Spain, Sweden, Switzerland, The Netherlands, Turkey, United Kingdom)
ABACAVIR SULFATE
Ziagen Oral Solution **1673**
Ziagen Tablets **1673**

ZIAGENAVIR (Argentina, Brazil, Mexico, Thailand)
ABACAVIR SULFATE
Ziagen Oral Solution **1673**
Ziagen Tablets **1673**

ZIAXEL (Greece)
TRANDOLAPRIL/VERAPAMIL HYDROCHLORIDE
Tarka Tablets **511**

ZICET (Hong Kong)
CETIRIZINE HYDROCHLORIDE
Zyrtec Syrup **1920**
Zyrtec Tablets **1920**

ZIDAC (France)
RANITIDINE HYDROCHLORIDE
Zantac 25 EFFERdose Tablets **1670**
Zantac 150 Tablets **1670**
Zantac 300 Tablets **1670**
Zantac Injection **1666**
Zantac Injection Premixed **1666**
Zantac Syrup **1670**

ZIDEPRIL (Greece)
CAPTOPRIL
Captopril Tablets **2182**

ZIDIC-C (Mexico)
ZIDOVUDINE
Retrovir Capsules **1574**
Retrovir IV Infusion **1579**
Retrovir Syrup **1574**
Retrovir Tablets **1574**

ZIDICEF (Mexico)
CEFTAZIDIME
Fortaz for Injection **1450**

ZIDIMA (Argentina)
CEFTAZIDIME
Fortaz for Injection **1450**

ZIDIS (Thailand)
ZIDOVUDINE
Retrovir Capsules **1574**
Retrovir IV Infusion **1579**
Retrovir Syrup **1574**
Retrovir Tablets **1574**

ZIDIX (Brazil)
ZIDOVUDINE
Retrovir Capsules **1574**
Retrovir IV Infusion **1579**
Retrovir Syrup **1574**
Retrovir Tablets **1574**

ZIDOLAM (Brazil)
LAMIVUDINE
Epivir Oral Solution **1412**
Epivir Tablets **1412**
Epivir-HBV Oral Solution **1417**
Epivir-HBV Tablets **1417**

ZIDOREX (India)
ZIDOVUDINE
Retrovir Capsules **1574**
Retrovir IV Infusion **1579**
Retrovir Syrup **1574**
Retrovir Tablets **1574**

ZIDOVIR (Brazil, India, Mexico, Venezuela)
ZIDOVUDINE
Retrovir Capsules **1574**
Retrovir IV Infusion **1579**
Retrovir Syrup **1574**
Retrovir Tablets **1574**

ZIDOVUSAN (Brazil)
ZIDOVUDINE
Retrovir Capsules **1574**
Retrovir IV Infusion **1579**
Retrovir Syrup **1574**
Retrovir Tablets **1574**

ZIENAM (Austria)
CILASTATIN SODIUM/IMIPENEM
Primaxin I.M. . . . 2080
Primaxin I.V. . . . 2083

ZILACTIN-L (Canada)
LIDOCAINE
Lidoderm Patch . . . 1114

ZILAK (Brazil)
RANITIDINE HYDROCHLORIDE
Zantac 25 EFFERdose Tablets . . . 1670
Zantac 150 Tablets . . . 1670
Zantac 300 Tablets . . . 1670
Zantac Injection . . . 1666
Zantac Injection Premixed . . . 1666
Zantac Syrup . . . 1670

ZILAST (India)
CILOSTAZOL
Pletal Tablets . . . 2481

ZILDEM (South Africa)
DILTIAZEM HYDROCHLORIDE
Cardizem LA Extended Release Tablets . . . 421

ZILDEN (Greece, Italy)
DILTIAZEM HYDROCHLORIDE
Cardizem LA Extended Release Tablets . . . 421

ZILION (India)
ZIDOVUDINE
Retrovir Capsules . . . 1574
Retrovir IV Infusion . . . 1579
Retrovir Syrup . . . 1574
Retrovir Tablets . . . 1574

ZILISTEN (Greece)
CEFUROXIME SODIUM
Zinacef Injection . . . 1678

ZIMMEX (Thailand)
SIMVASTATIN
Zocor Tablets . . . 2136

ZIMSTAT (Australia)
SIMVASTATIN
Zocor Tablets . . . 2136

ZINACEF (Belgium, Brazil, Canada, Czech Republic, Denmark, Finland, Germany, Greece, Hong Kong, Hungary, Irish Republic, Israel, Malaysia, New Zealand, Norway, Poland, Russia, Singapore, South Africa, Sweden, Switzerland, Thailand, The Netherlands, The Philippines, United Kingdom, Venezuela)
CEFUROXIME AXETIL
Ceftin for Oral Suspension . . . 1380
Ceftin Tablets . . . 1380

ZINADOL (Greece)
CEFUROXIME AXETIL
Ceftin for Oral Suspension . . . 1380
Ceftin Tablets . . . 1380

ZINAT (Switzerland)
CEFUROXIME AXETIL
Ceftin for Oral Suspension . . . 1380
Ceftin Tablets . . . 1380

ZINETAC (India)
RANITIDINE HYDROCHLORIDE
Zantac 25 EFFERdose Tablets . . . 1670
Zantac 150 Tablets . . . 1670
Zantac 300 Tablets . . . 1670
Zantac Injection . . . 1666
Zantac Injection Premixed . . . 1666
Zantac Syrup . . . 1670

ZINEX (The Philippines)
CETIRIZINE HYDROCHLORIDE
Zyrtec Syrup . . . 1920
Zyrtec Tablets . . . 1920

ZINNAT (Australia, Austria, Belgium, Brazil, Chile, Czech Republic, Denmark, Finland, Germany, Hong Kong, Hungary, Irish Republic, Israel, Italy, Malaysia, New Zealand, Poland, Russia, Singapore, South Africa, Spain, Sweden, Thailand, The Netherlands, The Philippines, Turkey, United Kingdom, Venezuela)
CEFUROXIME AXETIL
Ceftin for Oral Suspension . . . 1380
Ceftin Tablets . . . 1380

ZINOCEP (Italy)
CEFUROXIME SODIUM
Zinacef Injection . . . 1678

ZINOPRIL (Brazil)
LISINOPRIL
Prinivil Tablets . . . 2087

ZIPOS (Portugal)
CEFUROXIME AXETIL
Ceftin for Oral Suspension . . . 1380
Ceftin Tablets . . . 1380

ZIPRA (Mexico)
CIPROFLOXACIN HYDROCHLORIDE
Cipro Tablets . . . 2810

ZIPTEK (Greece)
CETIRIZINE HYDROCHLORIDE
Zyrtec Syrup . . . 1920
Zyrtec Tablets . . . 1920

ZIREMEX (Greece)
NIMODIPINE
Nimotop Capsules . . . 790

ZIRPINE (Irish Republic)
CETIRIZINE HYDROCHLORIDE
Zyrtec Syrup . . . 1920
Zyrtec Tablets . . . 1920

ZIRTEC (Italy)
CETIRIZINE HYDROCHLORIDE
Zyrtec Syrup . . . 1920
Zyrtec Tablets . . . 1920

ZIRTEK (Austria, Greece, Irish Republic, United Kingdom)
CETIRIZINE HYDROCHLORIDE
Zyrtec Syrup . . . 1920
Zyrtec Tablets . . . 1920

ZITTEC (Thailand)
CETIRIZINE HYDROCHLORIDE
Zyrtec Syrup . . . 1920
Zyrtec Tablets . . . 1920

ZIVAS (The Philippines)
SIMVASTATIN
Zocor Tablets . . . 2136

ZNUPRIL (Greece)
CETIRIZINE HYDROCHLORIDE
Zyrtec Syrup . . . 1920
Zyrtec Tablets . . . 1920

ZOBEN (Malaysia)
ALBENDAZOLE
Albenza Tablets . . . 1297

ZOBID (The Philippines)
DICLOFENAC SODIUM
Voltaren Tablets . . . 2334
Voltaren-XR Tablets . . . 2337

ZOCOLIP (Denmark)
SIMVASTATIN
Zocor Tablets . . . 2136

ZOCOR (Argentina, Australia, Belgium, Brazil, Canada, Chile, Czech Republic, Denmark, Finland, France, Germany, Greece, Hong Kong, Hungary, Irish Republic, Italy, Malaysia, Mexico, New Zealand, Norway, Poland, Portugal, Russia, Singapore, South Africa, Spain, Switzerland, Thailand, The Netherlands, The Philippines, Turkey, United Kingdom, Venezuela)
SIMVASTATIN
Zocor Tablets . . . 2136

ZOCORD (Austria, Sweden)
SIMVASTATIN
Zocor Tablets . . . 2136

ZODAC (Czech Republic)
CETIRIZINE HYDROCHLORIDE
Zyrtec Syrup . . . 1920
Zyrtec Tablets . . . 1920

ZODOL (Chile)
TRAMADOL HYDROCHLORIDE
Ultram ER Tablets . . . 2428

ZOFER (Turkey)
ONDANSETRON
Zofran ODT Orally Disintegrating Tablets . . 1687

ZOFLUT (India)
FLUTICASONE PROPIONATE
Flonase Nasal Spray . . . 1431

ZOFRAN (Argentina, Australia, Belgium, Brazil, Czech Republic, Germany, Hong Kong, Hungary, Irish Republic, Israel, Italy, Malaysia, Mexico, New Zealand, Norway, Poland, Portugal, Russia, Singapore, South Africa, Spain, Sweden, Switzerland, The Netherlands, The Philippines, Turkey, United Kingdom, Venezuela)
ONDANSETRON HYDROCHLORIDE
Zofran Injection . . . 1682
Zofran Injection Premixed . . . 1682
Zofran Oral Solution . . . 1687
Zofran Tablets . . . 1687

ZOFRON (Greece)
ONDANSETRON HYDROCHLORIDE
Zofran Injection . . . 1682
Zofran Injection Premixed . . . 1682
Zofran Oral Solution . . . 1687
Zofran Tablets . . . 1687

ZOLAFREN (Poland)
OLANZAPINE
Zyprexa Tablets . . . 1883

ZOLBEN (Brazil)
ALBENDAZOLE
Albenza Tablets . . . 1297

ZOLDAN (Brazil)
ALBENDAZOLE
Albenza Tablets . . . 1297

ZOLIDEN (Greece)
RANITIDINE HYDROCHLORIDE
Zantac 25 EFFERdose Tablets . . . 1670
Zantac 150 Tablets . . . 1670
Zantac 300 Tablets . . . 1670
Zantac Injection . . . 1666
Zantac Injection Premixed . . . 1666
Zantac Syrup . . . 1670

ZOLINA (Venezuela)
CIPROFLOXACIN
Cipro Oral Suspension . . . 2810

ZOLTEM (Turkey)
ONDANSETRON HYDROCHLORIDE
Zofran Injection . . . 1682
Zofran Injection Premixed . . . 1682
Zofran Oral Solution . . . 1687
Zofran Tablets . . . 1687

ZOLTEROL (Hong Kong, Malaysia, Singapore)
DICLOFENAC SODIUM
Voltaren Tablets . . . 2334
Voltaren-XR Tablets . . . 2337

ZOLVASTIN (The Philippines)
SIMVASTATIN
Zocor Tablets . . . 2136

ZOMORPH (United Kingdom)
MORPHINE SULFATE
MS Contin Tablets . . . 2585

ZONAKER (Mexico)
SODIUM HYALURONATE
Hyalgan Solution . . . 2742

ZONATIAN (Argentina)
ISOTRETINOIN
Accutane Capsules . . . 2607

ZOPAM (Thailand)
DIAZEPAM
Valium Tablets . . . 2658

ZOPIROL (Argentina)
TIMOLOL MALEATE
Timoptic in Ocudose . . . 2124
Timoptic Sterile Ophthalmic Solution . . . 2121
Timoptic-XE Sterile Ophthalmic Gel Forming Solution . . . 2125

ZORAN (Russia, Singapore, Venezuela)
RANITIDINE HYDROCHLORIDE
Zantac 150 Tablets . . . 1670
Zantac 25 EFFERdose Tablets . . . 1670
Zantac 300 Tablets . . . 1670
Zantac Injection . . . 1666
Zantac Injection Premixed . . . 1666
Zantac Syrup . . . 1670

ZORCED (Mexico)
SIMVASTATIN
Zocor Tablets . . . 2136

ZOREF (Italy, Portugal)
CEFUROXIME AXETIL
Ceftin for Oral Suspension . . . 1380
Ceftin Tablets . . . 1380

ZOROXIN (Austria, Belgium, Denmark)
NORFLOXACIN
Noroxin Tablets . . . 2069

ZOVAST (The Philippines)
SIMVASTATIN
Zocor Tablets . . . 2136

ZOVATIN (Turkey)
SIMVASTATIN
Zocor Tablets . . . 2136

ZOXAN (India)
CIPROFLOXACIN
Cipro Oral Suspension . . . 2810

ZUMALGIC (France)
TRAMADOL HYDROCHLORIDE
Ultram ER Tablets . . . 2428

ZUMENON (Australia, Austria, Belgium, Finland, Portugal, Switzerland, The Netherlands, United Kingdom)
ESTRADIOL
Climara Transdermal System . . . 763

ZURFIX (Greece)
RANITIDINE HYDROCHLORIDE
Zantac 25 EFFERdose Tablets . . . 1670
Zantac 150 Tablets . . . 1670
Zantac 300 Tablets . . . 1670
Zantac Injection . . . 1666
Zantac Injection Premixed . . . 1666
Zantac Syrup . . . 1670

ZUROCID (Greece)
SIMVASTATIN
Zocor Tablets . . . 2136

ZUVAIR (India)
ZAFIRLUKAST
Accolate Tablets . . . 669

ZYBAN (Australia, Austria, Belgium, Brazil, Canada, Czech Republic, Denmark, Finland, France, Germany, Greece, Hong Kong, Hungary, India, Irish Republic, Israel, Italy, New Zealand, Norway, Poland, Portugal, Singapore, South Africa, Sweden, Switzerland, The Netherlands, Turkey, United Kingdom, Venezuela)
BUPROPION HYDROCHLORIDE
Wellbutrin SR Sustained-Release Tablets . . 1653
Wellbutrin Tablets . . . 1648
Zyban Sustained-Release Tablets . . . 1692

ZYCEL (India)
CELECOXIB
Celebrex Capsules . . . 2979

ZYDOL (Australia, Irish Republic, United Kingdom)
TRAMADOL HYDROCHLORIDE
Ultram ER Tablets . . . 2428

ZYDOWIN (India)
ZIDOVUDINE
Retrovir Capsules . . . 1574
Retrovir IV Infusion . . . 1579
Retrovir Syrup . . . 1574
Retrovir Tablets . . . 1574

ZYFLOX (The Philippines)
CIPROFLOXACIN HYDROCHLORIDE
Cipro Tablets . . . 2810

ZYGIUM (Mexico)
CALCITRIOL
Calcijex Injection **419**
Rocaltrol Capsules **1150**
Rocaltrol Oral Solution **1150**

ZYLIUM (Brazil)
RANITIDINE HYDROCHLORIDE
Zantac 25 EFFERdose Tablets **1670**
Zantac 150 Tablets **1670**
Zantac 300 Tablets **1670**
Zantac Injection **1666**
Zantac Injection Premixed **1666**
Zantac Syrup **1670**

ZYLLERGY (Israel)
CETIRIZINE HYDROCHLORIDE
Zyrtec Syrup **1920**
Zyrtec Tablets **1920**

ZYLLT (Poland)
CLOPIDOGREL BISULFATE
Plavix Tablets **926, 2767**

ZYMED (Thailand)
CETIRIZINE HYDROCHLORIDE
Zyrtec Syrup **1920**
Zyrtec Tablets **1920**

ZYNAL (Singapore)
NAPROXEN SODIUM
Anaprox DS Tablets **2632**
Anaprox Tablets **2632**

ZYNO (Thailand)
TRIAMCINOLONE ACETONIDE
Azmacort Inhalation Aerosol **407**
Nasacort AQ Nasal Spray **2765**

ZYNOR (Irish Republic)
CETIRIZINE HYDROCHLORIDE
Zyrtec Syrup **1920**
Zyrtec Tablets **1920**

ZYNTABAC (Spain, The Netherlands)
BUPROPION HYDROCHLORIDE
Wellbutrin SR Sustained-Release Tablets . . **1653**
Wellbutrin Tablets **1648**
Zyban Sustained-Release Tablets **1692**

ZYPI (The Philippines)
PIOGLITAZONE HYDROCHLORIDE
Actos Tablets **3077**

ZYPREXA (Argentina, Australia, Austria, Belgium, Brazil, Canada, Chile, Czech Republic, Denmark, Finland, France, Germany, Greece, Hong Kong, Hungary, Irish Republic, Israel, Italy, Malaysia, Mexico, New Zealand, Norway, Poland, Portugal, Russia, Singapore, South Africa, Spain, Sweden, Switzerland, Thailand, The Netherlands, The Philippines, Turkey, United Kingdom, Venezuela)
OLANZAPINE
Zyprexa Tablets **1883**

ZYRAC (Thailand)
CETIRIZINE HYDROCHLORIDE
Zyrtec Syrup **1920**
Zyrtec Tablets **1920**

ZYRAZINE (Thailand)
CETIRIZINE HYDROCHLORIDE
Zyrtec Syrup **1920**
Zyrtec Tablets **1920**

ZYRCON (Thailand)
CETIRIZINE HYDROCHLORIDE
Zyrtec Syrup **1920**
Zyrtec Tablets **1920**

ZYREX (Thailand)
CETIRIZINE HYDROCHLORIDE
Zyrtec Syrup **1920**
Zyrtec Tablets **1920**

ZYRLEX (Sweden)
CETIRIZINE HYDROCHLORIDE
Zyrtec Syrup **1920**
Zyrtec Tablets **1920**

ZYRRIGIN (The Philippines)
CETIRIZINE HYDROCHLORIDE
Zyrtec Syrup **1920**
Zyrtec Tablets **1920**

ZYRTEC (Argentina, Austria, Belgium, Brazil, Canada, Chile, Czech Republic, Denmark, Finland, France, Germany, Hong Kong, Hungary, India, Israel, Japan, Malaysia, Mexico, New Zealand, Norway, Poland, Portugal, Russia, Singapore, South Africa, Spain, Switzerland, Thailand, The Netherlands, The Philippines, Turkey, Venezuela)
CETIRIZINE HYDROCHLORIDE
Zyrtec Syrup **1920**
Zyrtec Tablets **1920**

ZYRZINE (Thailand)
CETIRIZINE HYDROCHLORIDE
Zyrtec Syrup **1920**
Zyrtec Tablets **1920**

ZYTAZ (India)
CEFTAZIDIME
Fortaz for Injection **1450**

ZYTINE (Thailand)
CETIRIZINE HYDROCHLORIDE
Zyrtec Syrup **1920**
Zyrtec Tablets **1920**

ZYTRAM (New Zealand, Spain)
TRAMADOL HYDROCHLORIDE
Ultram ER Tablets **2428**

SECTION 7

GENERIC AVAILABILITY GUIDE

This section allows you to quickly determine which forms and strengths of a brand-name drug are also available generically. The entries are organized alphabetically by brand name and dosage form, with strengths in ascending order. Please note all active ingredients are not listed, please refer to the FDA prescribing label for more details. Generic availability is indicated by a mark in the "Yes" column. Included are all prescription products described in *PDR®* and *PDR® For Ophthalmic Medicines*. Generic availability information is drawn from the *Red Book® Drug Database* maintained by *PDR*'s parent organization, Thomson Reuters.

STRENGTH	GENERIC YES	GENERIC NO
Abelcet Injection		
5 mg/ml		■
Abilify Tablets		
2 mg		■
5 mg		■
10 mg		■
15 mg		■
20 mg		■
30 mg		■
Accolate Tablets		
10 mg		■
20 mg		■
Accutane Capsules		
10 mg	■	
20 mg	■	
40 mg	■	
Accuzyme Debriding Ointment		
830000 u/gm-10%	■	
Accuzyme SE Spray Emulsion		
830000 u/gm-10%		■
Aceon Tablets (2 mg, 4 mg, 8 mg)		
2 mg		■
4 mg		■
8 mg		■
Acetadote Injection		
200 mg/ml		■
Actimmune		
2 million iu/0.5 ml		■
Actiq		
0.2 mg	■	
0.4 mg	■	
0.6 mg	■	
0.8 mg	■	
1.2 mg	■	
1.6 mg	■	
Activase I.V.		
50 mg		■
100 mg		■
Active Calcium Tablets		
200 mg-100 iu	■	
Activella Tablets		
0.5 mg-0.1 mg		■
1 mg-0.5 mg	■	
Actonel Tablets		
5 mg		■
30 mg		■
35 mg		■
75 mg		■
150 mg		■
Actos Tablets		
15 mg		■
30 mg		■
45 mg		■
Adderall XR Capsules		
5 mg		■
10 mg		■
15 mg		■
20 mg		■
25 mg		■
30 mg		■
Adenocard IV Injection		
3 mg/ml	■	
Adenoscan		
3 mg/ml	■	
Adipex-P Capsules		
37.5 mg	■	
Adipex-P Tablets		
37.5 mg	■	
Advair Diskus 100/50		
0.1 mg/actuation-0.05 mg		■
Advair Diskus 250/50		
0.25 mg/actuation-0.05 mg		■
Advair Diskus 500/50		
0.5 mg/actuation-0.05 mg		■
Advair HFA Inhalation Aerosol		
45 mcg/21 mcg		■
115 mcg/21 mcg		■
230 mcg/21 mcg		■
Advate		
250 iu		■
500 iu		■
1000 iu		■
1500 iu		■
2000 iu		■
3000 iu		■
Advicor Tablets		
500 mg-20 mg		■
750 mg-20 mg		■
1000 mg-20 mg		■
1000 mg-40 mg		■
Aerobid Inhaler System		
0.25 mg/actuation		■
Aerobid-M Inhaler System		
0.25 mg/actuation		■
Aggrenox Capsules		
25 mg-200 mg		■
Agrylin Capsules		
0.5 mg	■	
1 mg	■	
Alamast Ophthalmic Solution		
0.1%		■
Albenza Tablets		
200 mg		■
Albutein 5%		
5%	■	
Albutein 25%		
25%	■	
Aldara Cream, 5%		
5%		■
Alimta for Injection		
100 mg		■
500 mg		■
Alinia for Oral Suspension		
100 mg/5 ml		■
Alinia Tablets		
500 mg		■
Allegra Oral Solution		
30 mg/5 ml		■
Allegra Tablets		
30 mg	■	
60 mg	■	
180 mg	■	
Allegra-D 24 Hour Extended-Release Tablets		
180 mg-240 mg		■
Aloxi Injection		
0.05 mg/ml		■
Alphagan P Ophthalmic Solution		
0.1%		■
0.15%		■
Alphanate		
250 iu/5 ml		■
500 iu/5 ml		■
1000 iu/10 ml		■
1500 iu/10 ml		■

STRENGTH	GENERIC YES	GENERIC NO
AlphaNine SD		
150 iu/mg	■	
Alrex Ophthalmic Suspension 0.2%		
0.2%		■
Altabax Ointment		
1%		■
Alvesco Inhalation Aerosol		
80 mcg/actuation		■
160 mcg/actuation		■
Ambien Tablets		
5 mg	■	
10 mg	■	
Ambien CR Tablets		
6.25 mg		■
12.5 mg		■
AmBisome for Injection		
50 mg		■
Amerge Tablets		
1 mg		■
2.5 mg		■
Aminohippurate Sodium "PAH" Injection		
20%		■
Amitiza Capsules		
8 mcg		■
24 mcg		■
Amoxil Capsules		
250 mg	■	
500 mg	■	
Amoxil Chewable Tablets		
125 mg	■	
200 mg	■	
250 mg	■	
400 mg	■	
Amoxil Pediatric Drops for Oral Suspension		
50 mg/ml	■	
Amoxil Powder for Oral Suspension		
250 mg/5 ml	■	
400 mg/5 ml	■	
Amoxil Tablets		
500 mg	■	
875 mg	■	
Analpram HC Cream, 1% and 2.5%		
1%-1%		■
2.5%-1%		■
Analpram HC Lotion, 2.5%		
2.5%-1%		■
Anaprox Tablets		
275 mg	■	
Anaprox DS Tablets		
550 mg	■	
AndroGel		
1%		■
Angiomax for Injection		
250 mg		■
Antivenin (Black Widow Spider Antivenin)		
6000 u		■
Anzemet Injection		
20 mg/ml	■	
Anzemet Tablets		
50 mg		■
100 mg		■
Apidra Injection		
100 u/ml		■
Appearex Tablets		
2.5 mg		■
Aptivus Capsules		
250 mg		■
Aralast		
1 mg		■
0.5 g/25 ml		■
1 g/50 ml		■
Aranesp for Injection		
0.025 mg/0.42 ml		■
0.04 mg/0.4 ml		■
0.06 mg/0.3 ml		■
0.1 mg/0.5 ml		■
0.15 mg/0.3 ml		■
0.2 mg/0.4 ml		■
0.3 mg/0.6 ml		■
0.5 mg/1 ml		■
Argatroban Injection		
100 mg/ml		■
Aricept ODT Tablets		
5 mg		■
10 mg		■
Arimidex Tablets		
1 mg		■
Arranon Injection		
5 mg/ml		■
Asacol Delayed-Release Tablets		
400 mg		■
Atacand Tablets		
4 mg		■
8 mg		■
16 mg		■
32 mg		■
Atacand HCT Tablets		
16 mg-12.5 mg		■
32 mg-12.5 mg		■
32 mg-25 mg		■
Atripla Tablets		
600 mg-200 mg-300 mg		■
Atrovent HFA Inhalation Aerosol		
0.017 mg/actuation		■
Atrovent Nasal Spray 0.03%		
0.03%	■	
Atrovent Nasal Spray 0.06%		
0.06%	■	
Attenuvax		
1000 tcid50		■
Augmentin Chewable Tablets		
125 mg-31.25 mg		■
200 mg-28.5 mg	■	
250 mg-62.5 mg		■
400 mg-57 mg	■	
Augmentin Powder for Oral Suspension		
125 mg/5 ml-31.25 mg/5 ml		■
200 mg/5 ml-28.5 mg/5 ml	■	
250 mg/5 ml-62.5 mg/5 ml		■
400 mg/5 ml-57 mg/5 ml	■	
Augmentin Tablets		
250 mg-125 mg	■	
500 mg-125 mg	■	
875 mg-125 mg	■	
Augmentin XR Extended Release Tablets		
1000 mg-62.5 mg		■
Augmentin ES-600 Powder for Oral Suspension		
600 mg/5 ml-42.9 mg/5 ml	■	
Avalide Tablets		
150 mg-12.5 mg		■
300 mg-12.5 mg		■
300 mg-25 mg		■
Avandamet Tablets		
500 mg-2 mg		■
500 mg-4 mg		■
1000 mg-2 mg		■
1000 mg-4 mg		■
Avandaryl Tablets		
4 mg-1 mg		■
4 mg-2 mg		■
4 mg-4 mg		■
8 mg-2 mg		■
8 mg-4 mg		■
Avandia Tablets		
2 mg		■
4 mg		■
8 mg		■
Avapro Tablets		
75 mg		■
150 mg		■
300 mg		■
Avastin IV		
25 mg/ml		■
Avelox Tablets		
400 mg		■
Avinza Capsules		
30 mg		■
60 mg		■
90 mg		■
120 mg		■
Avodart Soft Gelatin Capsules		
0.5 mg		■
Axert Tablets		
6.25 mg		■
12.5 mg		■
Azilect Tablets		
0.5 mg		■
1 mg		■
Azopt Ophthalmic Suspension		
1%		■
Azor Tablets		
5 mg-20 mg		■
5 mg-40 mg		■
10 mg-20 mg		■
10 mg-40 mg		■
Bactroban Cream		
2%		■
Bactroban Nasal		
2%		■
Bactroban Ointment		
2%	■	
Baraclude Tablets		
0.5 mg		■
1 mg		■
Bausch & Lomb Ocuvite Lutein Vitamin and Mineral Supplement 1		
60 mg-30 iu-15 mg-2 mg-6 mg		■
Beconase AQ Nasal Spray		
0.042 mg/actuation		■
Beelith Tablets		
600 mg-25 mg		■
BeneFIX Vials		
250 iu		■
500 iu		■
1000 iu		■
2000 iu		■
Benicar Tablets		
5 mg		■
20 mg		■
40 mg		■
Benicar HCT Tablets		
12.5 mg-20 mg		■
12.5 mg-40 mg		■
25 mg-40 mg		■
Benzaclin Topical Gel		
5%-1%		■
Betadine 5% Ophthalmic Solution		
5%		■
Betaseron for SC Injection		
0.3 mg		■
Betimol Ophthalmic Solution		
0.25%		■
0.5%		■
Bevitamel Tablets		
1 mg-0.4 mg-3 mg		■
Biaxin Filmtab Tablets		
250 mg	■	
500 mg	■	
Biaxin Granules		
125 mg/5 ml	■	
250 mg/5 ml	■	
Biaxin XL Filmtab Tablets		
500 mg	■	
Bleph-10 Ophthalmic Solution 10%		
10%	■	
Blephamide Ophthalmic Ointment		
0.2%-10%		■
Blephamide Ophthalmic Suspension		
0.2%-10%		■
Boniva Tablets		
2.5 mg		■
150 mg		■
Boostrix		
2.5 lf/5 lf/2.5 mcg/8 mcg/8 mcg		■
BOTOX Purified Neurotoxin Complex		
100 u		■
Brevoxyl-4 Creamy Wash		
4%	■	
Brevoxyl-4 Gel		
4%		■
Brevoxyl-8 Creamy Wash		
8%	■	
Brevoxyl-8 Gel		
8%		■
Brovana Inhalation Solution		
15 mcg/2 ml		■
Busulfex Injection		
6 mg/ml		■
Byetta Injection		
250 mcg/ml		■
Bystolic Tablets		
2.5 mg		■
5 mg		■
10 mg		■
Calcijex Injection		
1 mcg/ml	■	
2 mcg/ml	■	
Campath Ampules		
30 mg/ml		■
Canasa Rectal Suppositories		
1000 mg		■
Cancidas for Injection		
50 mg		■
70 mg		■
Captopril Tablets		
12.5 mg	■	
25 mg	■	
50 mg	■	
100 mg	■	
Carac Cream 0.5%		
0.5%		■
Carafate Suspension		
1 gm/10 ml	■	
Carafate Tablets		
1 gm	■	
Carbatrol Capsules		
100 mg		■
200 mg		■
300 mg		■
Cardene I.V.		
2.5 mg/ml	■	
Cardizem LA Extended Release Tablets		
120 mg		■
180 mg		■
240 mg		■
300 mg		■
360 mg		■
420 mg		■

STRENGTH	GENERIC YES	GENERIC NO
Catapres Tablets		
0.1 mg	■	
0.2 mg	■	
0.3 mg	■	
Catapres-TTS		
0.1 mg/24 hr		■
0.2 mg/24 hr		■
0.3 mg/24 hr		■
Cathflo Activase		
2 mg		■
Ceftin for Oral Suspension		
125 mg/5 ml	■	
250 mg/5 ml	■	
Ceftin Tablets		
125 mg	■	
250 mg	■	
500 mg	■	
Celebrex Capsules		
50 mg		■
100 mg		■
200 mg		■
400 mg		■
Celexa Oral Solution		
10 mg/5 ml	■	
Celexa Tablets		
10 mg	■	
20 mg	■	
40 mg	■	
CellCept Capsules		
250 mg	■	
CellCept Intravenous		
500 mg		■
CellCept Oral Suspension		
200 mg/ml		■
CellCept Tablets		
500 mg		■
Cerezyme for Injection		
200 u		■
400 u		■
Cervidil Vaginal Insert		
0.3 mg/hr		■
Chantix Tablets		
0.5 mg		■
1 mg		■
Chemet Capsules		
100 mg		■
Cialis Tablets		
2.5 mg		■
5 mg		■
10 mg		■
20 mg		■
Cimzia		
200 mg		■
Cipro Oral Suspension		
250 mg/5 ml		■
500 mg/5 ml		■
Cipro Tablets		
100 mg	■	
250 mg	■	
500 mg	■	
750 mg	■	
Cipro XR Tablets		
500 mg		■
1000 mg		■
CitraNatal DHA Tablets		
120 mg-125 mg-27 mg-400 iu-30 iu-3 mg-3.4 mg-20 mg-20 mg-1 mg-0.15 mg-25 mg-2 mg-50 mg-250 mg		■
CitraNatal 90 DHA Capsules		
120 mg-200 mg-90 mg-400 iu-30 iu-3 mg-3.4 mg-20 mg-20 mg-1 mg-0.15 mg-25 mg-2 mg-50 mg-250 mg	■	
Clarinex Syrup		
.5 mg/ml		■
Clarinex Tablets		
5 mg		■
Clarinex Reditabs Tablets		
2.5 mg		■
5 mg		■

STRENGTH	GENERIC YES	GENERIC NO
Clarinex-D 12-Hour Extended-Release Tablets		
2.5 mg-120 mg		■
Clarinex-D 24-Hour Extended-Release Tablets		
5 mg-240 mg		■
Cleviprex		
0.5 mg/ml		■
Climara Transdermal System		
0.025 mg/24 hr	■	
0.0375 mg/24 hr	■	
0.05 mg/24 hr	■	
0.06 mg/24 hr		■
0.075 mg/24 hr	■	
0.1 mg/24 hr	■	
Clinoril Tablets		
200 mg	■	
Clolar for Intravenous Infusion		
1 mg/ml		■
Clorpres Tablets		
15 mg-0.1 mg	■	
15 mg-0.2 mg	■	
15 mg-0.3 mg	■	
Combigan Ophthalmic Solution		
0.2%-0.5%		■
Combivent Inhalation Aerosol		
0.09 mg-0.018 mg/actuation		■
Combivir Tablets		
150 mg-300 mg		■
Comtan Tablets		
200 mg		■
Comvax		
7.5 mcg-125 mcg-5 mcg		■
Concerta Extended-Release Tablets		
18 mg		■
27 mg		■
36 mg		■
54 mg		■
Copaxone for Injection		
20 mg/ml		■
CordyMax Cs-4 Capsules		
525 mg	■	
Coreg Tablets		
3.125 mg	■	
6.25 mg	■	
12.5 mg	■	
25 mg	■	
Cosopt Sterile Ophthalmic Solution		
2%-0.5%		■
Cozaar Tablets		
25 mg		■
50 mg		■
100 mg		■
Creon 5 Capsules		
16600 u-5000 u-18750 u		■
Creon 10 Capsules		
33200 u-10000 u-37500 u	■	
Creon 20 Capsules		
66400 u-20000 u-75000 u	■	
Crestor Tablets		
5 mg		■
10 mg		■
20 mg		■
40 mg		■
Crinone 8% Gel		
8%		■
Crixivan Capsules		
100 mg		■
200 mg		■
333 mg		■
400 mg		■
Cubicin for Injection		
500 mg		■
Cuprimine Capsules		
250 mg		■

STRENGTH	GENERIC YES	GENERIC NO
Cyanokit 5g Antidote		
2.5 gm		■
Cytomel Tablets		
0.005 mg		■
0.025 mg		■
0.05 mg		■
Dacogen Injection		
50 mg		■
Dantrium Capsules		
25 mg	■	
50 mg	■	
100 mg	■	
Dapsone Tablets USP		
25 mg	■	
100 mg	■	
Daraprim Tablets		
25 mg		■
Daytrana Transdermal Patch		
10 mg/9 hr		■
15 mg/9 hr		■
20 mg/9 hr		■
30 mg/9 hr		■
Delatestryl Injection		
200 mg/ml	■	
Demadex Injection		
10 mg/ml		■
Demadex Tablets		
5 mg	■	
10 mg	■	
20 mg	■	
100 mg	■	
Denavir Cream		
1%		■
Depakote ER Tablets		
250 mg		■
500 mg		■
DepoCyt Injection		
10 mg/ml		■
DepoDur Injection		
10 mg/ml		■
15 mg/1.5 ml		■
Dexedrine Spansule Sustained-Release Capsules		
5 mg	■	
10 mg	■	
15 mg	■	
Dexedrine Tablets		
5 mg	■	
Dibenzyline Capsules		
10 mg		■
Didronel Tablets		
200 mg	■	
400 mg	■	
Digibind for Injection		
38 mg		■
Diovan Tablets		
40 mg		■
80 mg		■
160 mg		■
320 mg		■
Diovan HCT Tablets		
80 mg-12.5 mg		■
160 mg-12.5 mg		■
160 mg-25 mg		■
320 mg-12.5 mg		■
320 mg-25 mg		■
Diprolene Lotion 0.05%		
0.05%	■	
Diprolene Ointment 0.05%		
0.05%	■	
Diprolene AF Cream 0.05%		
0.05%	■	
Divigel		
0.25 mg/packet		■
0.5 mg/packet		■
1 mg/packet		■

STRENGTH	GENERIC YES	GENERIC NO
Donnatal Extentabs		
0.0582 mg-0.3111 mg-48.6 mg-0.0195 mg		■
Doribax Injection		
500 mg		■
Doxil Injection		
2 mg/ml		■
Duac Topical Gel		
5%-1%		■
Duragesic Transdermal System		
12.5 mcg/hr	■	
25 mcg/hr	■	
50 mcg/hr	■	
75 mcg/hr	■	
100 mcg/hr	■	
Dyazide Capsules		
25 mg-37.5 mg	■	
25 mg-50 mg	■	
DynaCirc CR Controlled Release Tablets		
5 mg		■
10 mg		■
Dyrenium Capsules		
50 mg		■
100 mg		■
EC-Naprosyn Delayed-Release Tablets		
375 mg	■	
500 mg	■	
Edecrin Tablets		
25 mg		■
Edecrin Sodium Intravenous		
25 mg		■
Edex Injection		
10 mcg	■	
20 mcg	■	
40 mcg	■	
E.E.S. 200 Liquid		
200 mg/5 ml	■	
E.E.S. 400 Liquid		
400 mg/5 ml	■	
E.E.S. 400 Filmtab Tablets		
400 mg	■	
E.E.S. Granules		
200 mg/5 ml	■	
Effexor XR Extended-Release Capsules		
37.5 mg		■
75 mg		■
150 mg		■
Eldepryl Capsules		
5 mg		■
Elidel Cream 1%		
1%		■
Eligard 7.5 mg		
7.5 mg		■
Eligard 22.5 mg		
22.5 mg		■
Eligard 45 mg		
45 mg		■
Elitek		
1.5 mg		■
7.5 mg		■
Elmiron Capsules		
100 mg		■
Elocon Cream 0.1%		
0.1%	■	
Elocon Lotion 0.1%		
0.1%	■	
Elocon Ointment 0.1%		
0.1%	■	
Eloxatin for Injection		
5 mg/ml		■

STRENGTH	GENERIC YES	GENERIC NO
Elspar for Injection		
10000 iu		■
Emend Capsules		
40 mg		■
80 mg		■
125 mg		■
Emend for Injection		
115 mg		■
Emsam Transdermal System		
6 mg/24 hr		■
9 mg/24 hr		■
12 mg/24 hr		■
Emtriva Capsules		
200 mg		■
Enbrel for Injection		
25 mg/vial		■
50 mg/ml		■
Engerix-B Vaccine		
20 mcg/ml		■
Enjuvia Tablets		
0.3 mg		■
0.45 mg		■
0.625 mg		■
0.9 mg		■
1.25 mg		■
EpiPen Auto-Injector		
0.3 mg/0.3 ml		■
EpiPen Jr. Auto-Injector		
0.15 mg/0.3 ml		■
Epivir Oral Solution		
10 mg/ml		■
Epivir Tablets		
150 mg		■
300 mg		■
Epivir-HBV Oral Solution		
5 mg/ml		■
Epivir-HBV Tablets		
100 mg		■
Epogen for Injection		
2000 u/ml		■
3000 u/ml		■
4000 u/ml		■
10000 u/ml		■
20000 u/ml		■
40000 u/ml		■
Equetro Extended-Release Capsules		
100 mg		■
200 mg		■
300 mg		■
Erbitux		
2 mg/ml		■
EryPed 200 & EryPed 400 Oral Suspension		
200 mg/5 ml	■	
400 mg/5 ml	■	
EryPed Drops		
100 mg/2.5 ml		■
Estratest Tablets		
1.25 mg-2.5 mg	■	
Estratest H.S. Tablets		
0.625 mg-1.25 mg	■	
Evista Tablets		
60 mg		■
Evoclin Foam, 1%		
1%		■
Evoxac Capsules		
30 mg		■
Exelon Capsules		
1.5 mg	■	
3 mg	■	
4.5 mg	■	
6 mg	■	
Exelon Patch		
4.6 mg/24 hr		■
9.5 mg/24 hr		■
Exforge Tablets		
5 mg-160 mg		■
5 mg-320 mg		■
10 mg-160 mg		■
10 mg-320 mg		■
Exjade Tablets		
125 mg		■
250 mg		■
500 mg		■
Extina Foam, 2%		
2%		■
Fabrazyme for Intravenous Infusion		
5 mg		■
35 mg		■
Fansidar Tablets		
25 mg-500 mg		■
Faslodex Injection		
50 mg/ml		■
Feiba VH		
500 u		■
1000 u		■
2500 u		■
Femara Tablets		
2.5 mg		■
Fentora Tablets		
100 mcg		■
200 mcg		■
300 mcg		■
400 mcg		■
600 mcg		■
800 mcg		■
Finacea Gel		
15%		■
Flebogamma 5% DIF		
50 mg/ml		■
Flector Patch		
1.3%		■
Flexbumin 25% I.V.		
25%	■	
Flolan for Injection		
0.5 mg	■	
1.5 mg	■	
Flomax Capsules		
0.4 mg		■
Flonase Nasal Spray		
0.05 mg/actuation	■	
Flovent HFA 44 mcg Inhalation Aerosol		
0.044 mg/actuation		■
Flovent HFA 110 mcg Inhalation Aerosol		
0.11 mg/actuation		■
Flovent HFA 220 mcg Inhalation Aerosol		
0.22 mg/actuation		■
Fluarix Vaccine		
45 mcg/0.5 ml	■	
Flumadine Syrup		
50 mg/5 ml		■
Flumadine Tablets		
100 mg	■	
Fluorescite Injection		
10%		■
FML Ophthalmic Ointment		
0.1%		■
FML Ophthalmic Suspension		
0.1%	■	
FML Forte Ophthalmic Suspension		
0.25%		■
Follistim AQ Cartridge		
75 iu/0.5 ml		■
150 iu/0.5 ml		■
300 iu/0.36 ml		■
600 iu/0.72 ml		■
900 iu/1.08 ml		■
Foradil Aerolizer		
0.012 mg		■
Fortaz Injection		
1 gm	■	
2 gm	■	
6 gm	■	
500 mg	■	
Fortaz for Injection		
1 gm/50 ml-2.2 gm/50 ml		■
2 gm/50 ml-1.6 gm/50 ml		■
Forteo for Injection		
250 mcg/ml		■
Fosamax Oral Solution		
70 mg/75 ml		■
Fosamax Tablets		
5 mg	■	
10 mg	■	
35 mg	■	
40 mg	■	
70 mg	■	
Fosamax Plus D Tablets		
70 mg-2800 iu		■
Fosrenol Chewable Tablets		
250 mg		■
500 mg		■
1000 mg		■
Furosemide Tablets		
20 mg	■	
40 mg	■	
80 mg	■	
Gabitril Tablets		
2 mg		■
4 mg		■
12 mg		■
16 mg		■
20 mg		■
Gammagard Liquid		
100 mg/ml		■
Gammagard S/D		
0.5 gm	■	
2.5 gm	■	
5 gm	■	
10 gm	■	
Gantrisin Pediatric Suspension		
500 mg/5 ml		■
Gemzar for Injection		
1 gm		■
200 mg		■
Gengraf Capsules		
25 mg	■	
100 mg	■	
Genotropin Lyophilized Powder		
5.8 mg		■
13.8 mg		■
Geodon Capsules		
20 mg		■
40 mg		■
60 mg		■
80 mg		■
Geodon for Injection		
20 mg/ml		■
Gleevec Tablets		
100 mg		■
400 mg		■
Gliadel Wafer		
7.7 mg		■
Glucagon for Injection Vials and Emergency Kit		
1 mg		■
Gris-PEG Tablets		
125 mg		■
250 mg		■
Havrix Injection Vaccine		
1440 el u/1 ml		■
Hepsera Tablets		
10 mg		■
Herceptin I.V.		
21 mg/ml		■
Hexalen Capsules		
50 mg		■
Humalog-Pen and KwikPen		
100 u/ml		■
Humalog Mix 50/50-Pen and KwikPen		
50 u/ml-50 u/ml		■
Humalog Mix 75/25-Pen and KwikPen		
75 u/ml-25 u/ml		■
Humatrope Vials and Cartridges		
5 mg		■
6 mg		■
12 mg		■
24 mg		■
Humira Injection		
40 mg/0.8 ml		■
Humulin R (U-500)		
500 u/ml		■
Hyalgan Solution		
10 mg/ml	■	
Hycamtin Capsules		
0.25 mg		■
1 mg		■
Hycamtin for Injection		
4 mg		■
Imitrex Injection		
4 mg/0.5 ml		■
6 mg/0.5 ml		■
Imitrex Nasal Spray		
5 mg		■
20 mg		■
Imitrex Tablets		
25 mg		■
50 mg		■
100 mg		■
Indapamide Tablets		
1.25 mg	■	
2.5 mg	■	
Indocin Capsules		
25 mg	■	
50 mg	■	
Indocin I.V.		
1 mg		■
Indocin Oral Suspension		
25 mg/5 ml		■
Indocin Suppositories		
50 mg	■	
Infanrix Vaccine		
0.5 ml		■
Infasurf Intratracheal Suspension		
35 mg/ml		■
Integrilin Injection		
0.75 mg/ml		■
2 mg/ml		■
Intravenous Sodium Diuril		
0.5 g		■
Intron A for Injection		
10 million iu/ml		■
18 million iu/ml		■
22.5 million iu/1.5 ml		■
22.8 million iu/3.8 ml		■
32 million iu/3.2 ml		■
37.5 million iu/1.5 ml		■
50 million iu/ml		■
75 million iu/1.5 ml		■

STRENGTH	GENERIC YES	GENERIC NO
Invanz for Injection		
1 gm		■
Invega Extended-Release Tablets		
3 mg		■
6 mg		■
9 mg		■
Iquix Ophthalmic Solution		
1.5%		■
Isentress Tablets		
400 mg		■
Ixempra Kit for Injection		
15 mg		■
45 mg		■
Janumet Tablets		
50 mg-500 mg		■
50 mg-1000 mg		■
Januvia Tablets		
25 mg		■
50 mg		■
100 mg		■
Kaletra Oral Solution		
80 mg/20 mg/1 ml		■
Kaletra Tablets		
100 mg/25 mg		■
200 mg/50 mg		■
Kepivance		
6.25 mg		■
Keppra Oral Solution		
100 mg/ml		■
Keppra Tablets		
250 mg		■
500 mg		■
750 mg		■
Ketek Tablets		
300 mg		■
400 mg		■
Kineret Injection		
100 mg/0.67 ml		■
Kinrix Injection Vaccine		
0.5 ml		■
Klonopin Tablets		
0.5 mg	■	
1 mg	■	
2 mg	■	
Klonopin Wafers		
0.125 mg	■	
0.25 mg	■	
0.5 mg	■	
1 mg	■	
2 mg	■	
Kogenate FS		
250 iu/2.5 ml		■
500 iu/2.5 ml		■
1000 iu/2.5 ml		■
2000 iu/5 ml		■
K-Phos Original (Sodium Free) Tablets		
500 mg		■
K-Phos Neutral Tablets		
155 mg-852 mg-130 mg	■	
Kristalose for Oral Solution		
10 gm/packet		■
20 gm/packet		■
Lacrisert Sterile Ophthalmic Insert		
5 mg		■
Lamictal Chewable Dispersible Tablets		
2 mg		■
5 mg	■	
25 mg	■	
Lamictal Tablets		
25 mg	■	
100 mg	■	
150 mg	■	
200 mg	■	
Lamisil Oral Granules		
125 mg/packet		■
187.5 mg/packet		■
Lamisil Tablets		
250 mg	■	
Lanoxin Injection		
0.25 mg/ml	■	
Lanoxin Injection Pediatric		
0.1 mg/ml		■
Lanoxin Tablets		
0.125 mg	■	
0.25 mg	■	
Lantus Injection		
100 u/ml		■
Lescol Capsules		
20 mg		■
40 mg		■
Lescol XL Tablets		
80 mg		■
Letairis Tablets		
5 mg		■
10 mg		■
Leukeran Tablets		
2 mg		■
Leukine		
250 mcg		■
500 mcg/ml		■
Leustatin Injection		
1 mg/ml	■	
Levaquin Injection		
5 mg/ml		■
25 mg/ml		■
Levaquin Oral Solution		
25 mg/ml		■
Levaquin Tablets		
250 mg		■
500 mg		■
750 mg		■
Levaquin in 5% Dextrose Injection		
5 mg/ml		■
Levemir Injection		
100 u/ml		■
Levitra Tablets		
2.5 mg		■
5 mg		■
10 mg		■
20 mg		■
Levothroid Tablets		
0.025 mg	■	
0.05 mg	■	
0.075 mg	■	
0.088 mg	■	
0.1 mg	■	
0.112 mg	■	
0.125 mg	■	
0.137 mg	■	
0.15 mg	■	
0.175 mg	■	
0.2 mg	■	
0.3 mg	■	
Levoxyl Tablets		
0.025 mg	■	
0.05 mg	■	
0.075 mg	■	
0.088 mg	■	
0.1 mg	■	
0.112 mg	■	
0.125 mg	■	
0.137 mg	■	
0.15 mg	■	
0.175 mg	■	
0.2 mg	■	
Lexapro Oral Suspension		
5 mg/5 ml		■
Lexapro Tablets		
5 mg	■	
10 mg	■	
20 mg	■	
Lexiscan Injection		
0.08 mg/ml		■
Lexiva Tablets		
700 mg		■
Lialda Tablets		
1.2 gm		■
Lidoderm Patch		
5%		■
Limbrel Capsules		
250 mg		■
500 mg		■
Lipitor Tablets		
10 mg		■
20 mg		■
40 mg		■
80 mg		■
Lortab Tablets		
500 mg-2.5 mg	■	
500 mg-5 mg	■	
500 mg-7.5 mg	■	
500 mg-10 mg	■	
Lotemax Ophthalmic Suspension 0.5%		
0.5%		■
Lotrisone Cream		
0.05%-1%	■	
Lovaza Capsules		
1 gm		■
Lovenox Injection		
30 mg/0.3 ml		■
40 mg/0.4 ml		■
60 mg/0.6 ml		■
80 mg/0.8 ml		■
100 mg/ml		■
120 mg/0.8 ml		■
150 mg/ml		■
Lucentis Injection		
0.5 mg/0.05 ml		■
Lumigan Ophthalmic Solution		
0.03%		■
Lunesta Tablets		
1 mg		■
2 mg		■
3 mg		■
Lupron Depot 3.75 mg		
3.75 mg		■
Lupron Depot 7.5 mg		
7.5 mg		■
Lupron Depot--3 Month 11.25 mg		
11.25 mg		■
Lupron Depot-PED 7.5 mg, 11.25 mg and 15 mg		
7.5 mg		■
11.25 mg		■
15 mg		■
Luvox CR Extended-Release Capsules		
100 mg		■
150 mg		■
Luxiq Foam		
0.12%		■
Lybrel Tablets		
20 mcg-90 mcg		■
Lyrica Capsules		
25 mg		■
50 mg		■
75 mg		■
100 mg		■
150 mg		■
200 mg		■
225 mg		■
300 mg		■
Malarone Pediatric Tablets		
62.5 mg-25 mg		■
Malarone Tablets		
250 mg-100 mg		■
Marinol Capsules		
2.5 mg	■	
5 mg	■	
10 mg	■	
Marlyn Formula 50 Capsules		
252 mg-1 mg-320 mg	■	
Mavik Tablets		
1 mg	■	
2 mg	■	
4 mg	■	
Maxair Autohaler		
0.2 mg/actuation		■
Maxalt Tablets		
5 mg		■
10 mg		■
Maxalt-MLT Orally Disintegrating Tablets		
5 mg		■
10 mg		■
Megace ES Oral Suspension		
625 mg/5 ml		■
Mentax Cream		
1%		■
Mephyton Tablets		
5 mg		■
Mepron Suspension		
750 mg/5 ml		■
Meridia Capsules		
5 mg		■
10 mg		■
15 mg		■
Merrem I.V.		
1 gm		■
500 mg		■
Meruvax II		
1000 tcid50		■
Metadate CD Capsules		
10 mg		■
20 mg		■
30 mg		■
40 mg		■
50 mg		■
60 mg		■
Mevacor Tablets		
20 mg	■	
40 mg	■	
Miacalcin Injection		
200 iu/ml		■
Miacalcin Nasal Spray		
200 iu/0.09 ml		■
Micardis Tablets		
20 mg		■
40 mg		■
80 mg		■
Micardis HCT Tablets		
40 mg-12.5 mg		■
80 mg-12.5 mg		■
80 mg-25 mg		■
Mirapex Tablets		
0.125 mg		■
0.25 mg		■
0.5 mg		■
0.75 mg		■
1 mg		■
1.5 mg		■
Mirena Intrauterine System		
52 mg		■
Moban Tablets		
5 mg		■
10 mg		■
25 mg		■
50 mg		■
Mobic Tablets		
7.5 mg	■	
15 mg	■	
MS Contin Tablets		
15 mg	■	
30 mg	■	
60 mg	■	
100 mg	■	
200 mg	■	
Mumpsvax		
20000 tcid50		■
Mustargen for Injection		
10 mg		■

STRENGTH	GENERIC YES	GENERIC NO
Mycamine for Injection		
50 mg		■
100 mg		■
Myfortic Tablets		
180 mg		■
360 mg		■
Mylotarg for Injection		
5 mg		■
Nadolol Tablets		
20 mg	■	
40 mg	■	
80 mg	■	
160 mg	■	
Naftin Cream		
1%		■
Naftin Gel		
1%		■
Naprosyn Suspension		
25 mg/ml	■	
Naprosyn Tablets		
250 mg	■	
375 mg	■	
500 mg	■	
Nasacort AQ Nasal Spray		
55 mcg/actuation		■
Nasonex Nasal Spray		
0.05 mg/actuation		■
Natacyn Antifungal Ophthalmic Suspension		
5%		■
Natrecor for Injection		
1.5 mg		■
Naturethroid Tablets		
16.25 mg		■
32.5 mg		■
65 mg		■
130 mg		■
195 mg		■
Nembutal Sodium Solution, USP		
50 mg/ml		■
NeoProfen Injection		
10 mg/ml		■
Neoral Oral Solution		
100 mg/ml	■	
Neoral Soft Gelatin Capsules		
25 mg	■	
100 mg	■	
Neulasta Injection		
6 mg/0.6 ml		■
Neupogen for Injection		
300 mcg/0.5 ml		■
300 mcg/ml		■
480 mcg/0.8 ml		■
480 mcg/1.6 ml		■
Nevanac Ophthalmic Suspension 0.1%		
0.1%		■
Nexavar Tablets		
200 mg		■
Nexium Delayed-Release Capsules		
20 mg		■
40 mg		■
Nexium I.V.		
20 mg		■
40 mg		■
Nexium Delayed-Release Oral Suspension		
10 mg		■
20 mg		■
40 mg		■
Niaspan Extended-Release Tablets		
500 mg		■
750 mg		■
1000 mg		■
Nimotop Capsules		
30 mg	■	
Nitro-Dur Transdermal Infusion System		
0.1 mg/hr	■	
0.2 mg/hr	■	
0.3 mg/hr		■
0.4 mg/hr	■	
0.6 mg/hr	■	
0.8 mg/hr		■
Nitrolingual Pumpspray		
0.4 mg/actuation		■
Norditropin Cartridges		
5 mg/1.5 ml		■
15 mg/1.5 ml		■
Noroxin Tablets		
400 mg		■
Norvir Oral Solution		
80 mg/ml		■
Norvir Soft Gelatin Capsules		
100 mg		■
Novantrone for Injection Concentrate		
2 mg/ml	■	
NovoLog Mix 70/30		
70 u/ml-30 u/ml		■
NovoLog Injection		
100 u/ml		■
NovoSeven		
1 mcg		■
Noxafil Oral Suspension		
40 mg/ml		■
Nu-Iron 150 Capsules		
150 mg	■	
Nutropin for Injection		
5 mg		■
10 mg		■
Nutropin AQ Injection		
5 mg/ml		■
Nutropin AQ Pen Cartridge		
5 mg/ml		■
10 mg/ml		■
NuvaRing		
0.015 mg/0.12 mg/24 hr		■
Nystop Topical Powder USP		
100000 u/gm	■	
Olux Foam		
0.05%	■	
Olux-E Foam		
0.05%		■
Omnicef Capsules		
300 mg	■	
Omnicef for Oral Suspension		
125 mg/5 ml	■	
250 mg/5 ml	■	
Ontak Vials		
150 mcg/ml		■
Opana Tablets		
5 mg		■
10 mg		■
OptiPranolol Metipranolol Ophthalmic Solution 0.3%		
0.3%	■	
Orencia Powder for Intravenous Infusion		
250 mg		■
Ortho-Cyclen Tablets		
35 mcg-0.25 mg	■	
Ortho Evra Transdermal System		
0.75 mg-6 mg		■
Ortho Micronor Tablets		
0.35 mg	■	
Orthoclone OKT3 Sterile Solution		
1 mg/ml		■
OsmoPrep Tablets		
0.398 gm-1.102 gm		■
OxyContin Tablets		
10 mg	■	
15 mg		■
20 mg	■	
30 mg		■
40 mg	■	
60 mg		■
80 mg	■	
OxyIR Capsules		
5 mg	■	
Panafil Ointment		
0.5%-10%-10%		■
Panafil SE Spray Emulsion		
0.5%-10%-10%	■	
Parnate Tablets		
10 mg	■	
Paser Granules		
4 gm/packet		■
Pataday Ophthalmic Solution		
0.2%		■
Patanase Nasal Spray		
0.6%		■
Patanol Ophthalmic Solution		
0.1%		■
Paxil Oral Suspension		
10 mg/5 ml	■	
Paxil Tablets		
10 mg	■	
20 mg	■	
30 mg	■	
40 mg	■	
Paxil CR Controlled-Release Tablets		
12.5 mg	■	
25 mg	■	
37.5 mg	■	
Liquid PedvaxHIB		
7.5 mcg/0.5 ml		■
Pentacel		
0.5 ml	■	
Pentasa Capsules		
250 mg		■
500 mg		■
Pepcid Tablets		
20 mg	■	
40 mg	■	
Percocet Tablets		
325 mg-2.5 mg		■
325 mg-5 mg	■	
325 mg-7.5 mg	■	
325 mg-10 mg	■	
500 mg-7.5 mg	■	
650 mg-10 mg	■	
Percodan Tablets		
325 mg-4.5 mg-0.38 mg	■	
Perforomist Inhalation Solution		
20 mcg/2 ml		■
Persantine Tablets		
25 mg	■	
50 mg	■	
75 mg	■	
Phenytek Capsules		
200 mg		■
300 mg		■
PhosLo GelCaps		
667 mg		■
Photofrin for Injection		
75 mg		■
Plavix Tablets		
75 mg	■	
300 mg		■
Pletal Tablets		
50 mg	■	
100 mg	■	
Pneumovax 23		
25 mcg/0.5 ml		■
Potaba Envules		
2 gm/packet	■	
Potaba Tablets		
0.5 gm		■
Pramosone Cream 1% and 2.5%		
1%-1%		■
2.5%-1%		■
Pramosone Lotion 1% and 2.5%		
1%-1%		■
2.5%-1%		■
Pramosone Ointment 1% and 2.5%		
1%-1%		■
2.5%-1%		■
Prandin Tablets		
0.5 mg		■
1 mg		■
2 mg		■
Precose Tablets		
25 mg	■	
50 mg	■	
100 mg	■	
Pred Forte Ophthalmic Suspension		
1%	■	
Pred Mild Ophthalmic Suspension		
0.12%		■
Pred-G Ophthalmic Ointment		
0.12%	■	
Pred-G Ophthalmic Suspension		
0.3%-1%		■
Premarin Intravenous		
25 mg		■
Premarin Tablets		
0.3 mg		■
0.45 mg		■
0.625 mg		■
0.9 mg		■
1.25 mg		■
Premarin Vaginal Cream		
0.625 mg/gm		■
Premphase Tablets		
0.625 mg-5 mg		■
Prempro Tablets		
0.3 mg-1.5 mg		■
0.45 mg-1.5 mg		■
0.625 mg-2.5 mg		■
0.625 mg-5 mg		■
Prevnar		
16 mcg/0.5 ml		■
Primaxin I.M.		
500 mg-500 mg		■
Primaxin I.V.		
250 mg-250 mg		■
500 mg-500 mg		■
Prinivil Tablets		
5 mg	■	
10 mg	■	
20 mg	■	
Prinzide Tablets		
12.5 mg-10 mg	■	
12.5 mg-20 mg	■	
Pristiq Extended-Release Tablets		
50 mg		■
100 mg		■
ProAmatine Tablets		
2.5 mg	■	
5 mg	■	
10 mg	■	

STRENGTH	GENERIC YES	GENERIC NO
Procrit for Injection		
2000 u/ml		■
3000 u/ml		■
4000 u/ml		■
10000 u/ml		■
20000 u/ml		■
40000 u/ml		■
Profilnine SD Solvent Detergent		
1 iu	■	
Prograf Capsules and Injection		
0.5 mg		■
1 mg		■
5 mg		■
5 mg/ml		■
Prolastin		
500 mg/20 ml		■
1000 mg/40 ml		■
Proleukin for Injection		
22 million iu		■
Prometrium Capsules (100 mg, 200 mg)		
100 mg		■
200 mg		■
Propecia Tablets		
1 mg	■	
Proscar Tablets		
5 mg	■	
Protonix Delayed-Release Tablets		
20 mg	■	
40 mg	■	
Protonix I.V.		
40 mg		■
Protopic Ointment		
0.03%		■
0.1%		■
Proventil HFA Inhalation Aerosol		
0.09 mg/actuation		■
Provigil Tablets		
100 mg		■
200 mg		■
Prozac Weekly Capsules		
90 mg		■
Prozac Pulvules and Liquid		
10 mg	■	
20 mg	■	
20 mg/5 ml	■	
40 mg	■	
Pulmicort Flexhaler		
90 mcg/dose		■
180 mcg/dose		■
Pulmozyme Inhalation Solution		
2.5 mg/2.5 ml		■
Pylera Capsules		
140 mg-125 mg-125 mg		■
Quixin Ophthalmic Solution		
0.5%		■
Qvar Inhalation Aerosol		
0.04 mg/actuation		■
0.08 mg/actuation		■
Rapamune Tablets		
1 mg		■
2 mg		■
Raptiva for Injection		
125 mg		■
Rebetol Capsules		
200 mg	■	
Rebif Prefilled Syringe for Injection		
22 mcg/0.5 ml		■
44 mcg/0.5 ml		■
Reclast Injection		
5 mg/100 ml		■
Recombinate		
1 iu		■
Recombivax HB		
10 mcg/ml		■
40 mcg/ml		■
ReFacto Vials		
250 iu		■
500 iu		■
1000 iu		■
2000 iu		■
Refludan for Injection		
50 mg		■
Relenza Inhalation Powder		
5 mg/actuation		■
Remeron Tablets		
15 mg	■	
30 mg	■	
45 mg	■	
RemeronSolTab Tablets		
15 mg	■	
30 mg	■	
45 mg	■	
Remicade for IV Injection		
100 mg		■
ReoPro Vials		
2 mg/ml		■
Requip Tablets		
0.25 mg	■	
0.5 mg	■	
1 mg	■	
2 mg	■	
3 mg	■	
4 mg	■	
5 mg	■	
Requip XL Tablets		
2 mg		■
4 mg		■
8 mg		■
12 mg		■
Restasis Ophthalmic Emulsion		
0.05%		■
Retrovir Capsules		
100 mg	■	
Retrovir IV Infusion		
10 mg/ml		■
Retrovir Syrup		
50 mg/5 ml	■	
Retrovir Tablets		
300 mg	■	
Reyataz Capsules		
100 mg		■
150 mg		■
200 mg		■
300 mg		■
Rilutek Tablets		
50 mg		■
Risperdal Consta Long-Acting Injection		
12.5 mg		■
25 mg		■
37.5 mg		■
50 mg		■
Rituxan I.V.		
10 mg/ml		■
Rocaltrol Capsules		
0.25 mcg	■	
0.5 mcg	■	
Rocaltrol Oral Solution		
1 mcg/ml	■	
Rocephin Injectable Vials, ADD-Vantage, Galaxy, Bulk		
1 gm	■	
1 gm/50 ml	■	
2 gm	■	
2 gm/50 ml	■	
10 gm	■	
250 mg	■	
500 mg	■	
Romazicon Injection		
0.1 mg/ml	■	
Rosac Wash		
10%-1%		■
Rozerem Tablets		
8 mg		■
Rythmol Tablets		
150 mg	■	
225 mg	■	
300 mg	■	
Rythmol SR Capsules		
225 mg		■
325 mg		■
425 mg		■
Salagen Tablets		
5 mg	■	
7.5 mg	■	
Sanctura XR Capsules		
60 mg		■
Sandimmune Oral Solution		
100 mg/ml	■	
Sandimmune I.V. Ampuls for Infusion		
50 mg/ml	■	
Sandimmune Soft Gelatin Capsules		
25 mg	■	
100 mg/ml	■	
Sandostatin Injection		
50 mcg/ml	■	
100 mcg/ml	■	
200 mcg/ml	■	
500 mcg/ml	■	
1000 mcg/ml	■	
Sandostatin LAR Depot		
10 mg		■
20 mg		■
30 mg		■
Santyl Collagenase Ointment		
250 u/gm		■
Selzentry Tablets		
150 mg		■
300 mg		■
Sensipar Tablets		
30 mg		■
60 mg		■
90 mg		■
Serevent Diskus		
0.046 mg/actuation		■
Simcor Tablets		
500 mg-20 mg		■
750 mg-20 mg		■
1000 mg-20 mg		■
Simulect for Injection		
10 mg		■
20 mg		■
Singulair Tablets		
10 mg		■
Singulair Chewable Tablets		
4 mg		■
5 mg		■
Singulair Oral Granules		
4 mg/packet		■
Skelaxin Tablets		
800 mg		■
Solodyn Extended Release Tablets		
45 mg		■
90 mg		■
135 mg		■
Soma Tablets		
250 mg		■
350 mg	■	
Somatuline Depot Injection		
60 mg		■
90 mg		■
120 mg		■
Soriatane Capsules		
10 mg		■
25 mg		■
Spiriva HandiHaler		
18 mcg		■
Stalevo Tablets		
12.5 mg-50 mg-200 mg		■
18.75 mg-75 mg-200 mg		■
25 mg-100 mg-200 mg		■
31.25 mg-125 mg-200 mg		■
37.5 mg-150 mg-200 mg		■
50 mg-200 mg-200 mg		■
Strattera Capsules		
10 mg		■
18 mg		■
25 mg		■
40 mg		■
60 mg		■
80 mg		■
100 mg		■
Stromectol Tablets		
3 mg		■
Suboxone Tablets		
2 mg-0.5 mg		■
8 mg-2 mg		■
Subutex Tablets		
2 mg		■
8 mg		■
Sular Extended Release Tablets		
8.5 mg		■
17 mg		■
25.5 mg		■
34 mg		■
Sulfamylon Cream		
85 mg/gm		■
Sulfamylon for 5% Topical Solution		
50 gm/packet		■
Supprelin LA Implant		
50 mg		■
Suprax for Oral Suspension		
100 mg/5 ml		■
200 mg/5 ml		■
Suprax Tablets		
400 mg		■
Sustiva Capsules		
50 mg		■
100 mg		■
200 mg		■
Sutent Capsules		
12.5 mg		■
25 mg		■
50 mg		■
Symbyax Capsules		
3 mg-25 mg		■
6 mg-25 mg		■
6 mg-50 mg		■
12 mg-25 mg		■
12 mg-50 mg		■
Synthroid Tablets		
0.025 mg	■	
0.05 mg	■	
0.075 mg	■	
0.088 mg	■	
0.1 mg	■	
0.112 mg	■	
0.125 mg	■	
0.137 mg	■	
0.15 mg	■	
0.175 mg	■	
0.2 mg	■	
0.3 mg	■	
Tabloid Tablets		
40 mg		■
Tamiflu Capsules		
30 mg		■
45 mg		■
75 mg		■
Tamiflu Oral Suspension		
12 mg/ml		■
Tarceva Tablets		
25 mg		■
100 mg		■
150 mg		■
Targretin Capsules		
75 mg		■
Targretin Gel 1%		
1%		■

STRENGTH	GENERIC YES	GENERIC NO
Tarka Tablets		
1 mg-240 mg		■
2 mg-180 mg		■
2 mg-240 mg		■
4 mg-240 mg		■
Taxotere Injection Concentrate		
20 mg/0.5 ml		■
Tegreen 97 Capsules		
250 mg	■	
Tekturna Tablets		
150 mg		■
300 mg		■
Tekturna HCT Tablets		
150 mg-12.5 mg		■
150 mg-25 mg		■
300 mg-12.5 mg		■
300 mg-25 mg		■
Temodar Capsules		
5 mg		■
20 mg		■
100 mg		■
140 mg		■
180 mg		■
250 mg		■
Tessalon Capsules		
200 mg	■	
Tessalon Perles		
100 mg	■	
Testim 1% Gel		
1%		■
Teveten Tablets		
400 mg		■
600 mg		■
Tev-Tropin for Injection		
5 mg		■
Thioridazine Hydrochloride Tablets		
10 mg	■	
25 mg	■	
50 mg	■	
100 mg	■	
Thiothixene Capsules		
1 mg	■	
2 mg	■	
5 mg	■	
10 mg	■	
Thyrogen for Injection		
1.1 mg		■
Tice BCG		
800 million cfu		■
Timentin ADD-Vantage		
3 g-0.1g		■
Timentin IV Infusion		
3 g-0.1g		■
Timentin Pharmacy Bulk Package		
30 g-1g		■
Timoptic Sterile Ophthalmic Solution		
0.25%	■	
0.5%	■	
Timoptic in Ocudose		
0.25%		■
0.5%		■
Timoptic-XE Sterile Ophthalmic Gel Forming Solution		
0.25%	■	
0.5%	■	
TNKase		
50 mg		■
Toprol-XL Tablets		
25 mg	■	
50 mg	■	
100 mg	■	
200 mg	■	
Torisel Injection		
25 mg/ml		■
Tracleer Tablets		
62.5 mg		■
125 mg		■
Transderm Scop Transdermal Therapeutic System		
1 mg/72 hrs		■
Trasylol Injection		
10000 kiu/ml		■
Travatan Z Ophthalmic Solution		
0.004%		■
Treximet Tablets		
500 mg-85 mg		■
Tricor Tablets		
48 mg		■
145 mg		■
Trisenox Injection		
1 mg/ml		■
Trizivir Tablets		
300 mg-150 mg-300 mg		■
Trusopt Sterile Ophthalmic Solution		
2%	■	
Truvada Tablets		
200 mg-300 mg		■
Tussionex Pennkinetic Extended-Release Suspension		
8 mg/5 ml-10 mg/5 ml		■
Twinrix Vaccine		
720 el u/ml-20 mcg/ml		■
Tygacil for Injection		
50 mg		■
Tykerb Tablets		
250 mg		■
Tylenol with Codeine Tablets		
300 mg-30 mg	■	
300 mg-60 mg	■	
Tyzeka Tablets		
600 mg		■
Ultane Liquid for Inhalation		
100%	■	
Ultrase Capsules		
20000 u-4500 u-25000 u	■	
Ultrase MT Capsules		
39000 u-12000 u-39000 u	■	
58500 u-18000 u-58500 u	■	
65000 u-20000 u-65000 u	■	
Uniphyl Tablets		
400 mg	■	
600 mg	■	
Urocit-K Tablets		
5 meq	■	
10 meq	■	
Uroqid-Acid No. 2 Tablets		
500 mg-500 mg		■
Uroxatral Tablets		
10 mg		■
Vagifem Tablets		
25 mcg		■
Valcyte Tablets		
450 mg		■
Valium Tablets		
2 mg	■	
5 mg	■	
10 mg	■	
Valstar Sterile Solution for Intravesical Instillation		
40 mg/ml		■
Valtrex Caplets		
1 gm	■	
500 mg	■	
Vanos Cream		
0.1%		■
Vantas		
50 mg		■
Vaprisol		
20 mg/4 ml		■
Vaqta		
50 u/ml		■
Varivax		
1350 pfu		■
Velcade for Injection		
3.5 mg		■
Venlafaxine Hydrochloride Tablets		
25 mg	■	
37.5 mg	■	
50 mg	■	
100 mg	■	
Ventolin HFA Inhalation Aerosol		
0.09 mg/actuation		■
Veramyst Nasal Spray		
27.5 mcg/actuation		■
Verdeso Foam		
0.05%		■
Vesanoid Capsules		
10 mg	■	
Viadur Implant		
65 mg		■
Vicodin Tablets		
500 mg-5 mg	■	
Vicodin ES Tablets		
750 mg-7.5 mg	■	
Vicodin HP Tablets		
660 mg-10 mg	■	
Vicoprofen Tablets		
7.5 mg-200 mg	■	
Vigamox Ophthalmic Solution		
0.5%		■
Viokase Powder		
70000 u-16800 u-70000 u/0.7 g		■
Viokase Tablets		
30000 u-8000 u-30000 u	■	
60000 u-16000 u-60000 u	■	
Viramune Oral Suspension		
50 mg/5 ml		■
Viramune Tablets		
200 mg		■
Viread Tablets		
300 mg		■
Viroptic Ophthalmic Solution		
1%	■	
Visudyne for Injection		
15 mg		■
Vivitrol		
380 mg		■
Voltaren Ophthalmic Solution		
0.1%	■	
Voltaren Tablets		
75 mg	■	
Voltaren-XR Tablets		
100 mg	■	
Vyvanse Capsules		
20 mg		■
30 mg		■
40 mg		■
50 mg		■
60 mg		■
70 mg		■
WelChol Tablets		
625 mg		■
Wellbutrin Tablets		
75 mg	■	
100 mg	■	
Wellbutrin SR Sustained-Release Tablets		
100 mg	■	
150 mg	■	
200 mg	■	
Wellbutrin XL Extended-Release Tablets		
150 mg	■	
300 mg	■	
WinRho SDF		
600 iu		■
1500 iu		■
2500 iu		■
5000 iu		■
15000 iu		■
Xalatan Ophthalmic Solution		
0.005%		■
Xeloda Tablets		
150 mg		■
500 mg		■
Xenaderm Ointment		
90 u/87 mg/788 mg/1g		■
Xenical Capsules		
120 mg		■
Xifaxan Tablets		
200 mg		■
Xigris Powder for Intravenous Infusion		
5 mg		■
20 mg		■
Xolair		
150 mg		■
Xopenex Inhalation Solution		
0.31 mg/3 ml		■
0.63 mg/3 ml		■
1.25 mg/3 ml		■
Xopenex Inhalation Solution Concentrate		
1.25 mg/0.5 ml		■
Xyntha Vials		
250 iu		■
500 iu		■
1000 iu		■
2000 iu		■
Xyrem Oral Solution		
500 mg/ml		■
Xyzal Tablets		
5 mg		■
Yaz Tablets		
3 mg-0.02 mg		■
Zantac 25 EFFERdose Tablets		
25 mg		■
Zantac Injection		
25 mg/ml	■	
Zantac Injection Premixed		
1 mg/ml		■
Zantac Syrup		
15 mg/ml	■	
Zantac 150 Tablets		
150 mg	■	
Zantac 300 Tablets		
300 mg	■	
Zemplar Injection		
0.002 mg/ml		■
0.005 mg/ml		■
Zemuron Injection		
10 mg/ml		■
Zetia Tablets		
10 mg		■
Ziagen Oral Solution		
20 mg/ml		■
Ziagen Tablets		
300 mg		■
Ziana Gel		
1.2%-0.025%		■

STRENGTH	GENERIC YES	GENERIC NO
Zinacef Injection		
1.5 gm	■	
1.5 gm/50 ml	■	
7.5 gm	■	
750 mg	■	
750 mg/50 ml	■	
Zinc-220 Capsules		
220 mg	■	
Zocor Tablets		
5 mg	■	
10 mg	■	
20 mg	■	
40 mg	■	
80 mg	■	
Zofran Injection		
2 mg/ml	■	
Zofran Injection Premixed		
32 mg/50 ml	■	
Zofran Oral Solution		
4 mg/5 ml	■	
Zofran Tablets		
4 mg	■	
8 mg	■	
Zofran ODT Orally Disintegrating Tablets		
4 mg	■	
8 mg	■	
Zolinza Capsules		
100 mg		■
Zometa for Intravenous Infusion		
4 mg/5 ml		■
Zomig Tablets		
2.5 mg		■
5 mg		■
Zomig Nasal Spray		
5 mg		■
Zomig-ZMT Tablets		
2.5 mg		■
5 mg		■
Zostavax Injection		
19400 pfu/0.65 ml		■
Zosyn for Injection		
2 gm-0.25 gm		■
2 gm/50 ml-0.25 gm/50 ml		■
3 gm-0.375 gm		■
3 gm/50 ml-0.375 gm/50 ml		■
4 gm-0.5 gm		■
4 gm/100 ml-0.5 gm/100 m		■
36 gm-4.5 gm		■
Zovirax Capsules		
200 mg	■	
Zovirax Cream		
5%		■
Zovirax Ointment		
5%		■
Zovirax Suspension		
200 mg/5 ml	■	
Zovirax Tablets		
400 mg	■	
800 mg	■	
Zyban Sustained-Release Tablets		
150 mg	■	
Zydone Tablets		
400 mg-5 mg		■
400 mg-7.5 mg		■
400 mg-10 mg		■
Zylet Ophthalmic Suspension		
0.5%-0.3%		■
Zyprexa Tablets		
2.5 mg		■
5 mg		■
7.5 mg		■
10 mg		■
15 mg		■
20 mg		■
Zyprexa IntraMuscular		
10 mg		■
Zyprexa ZYDIS Orally Disintegrating Tablets		
5 mg		■
10 mg		■
15 mg		■
20 mg		■
Zyvox for Oral Suspension		
100 mg/5 ml		■
Zyvox Injection		
2 mg/ml		■
Zyvox Tablets		
600 mg		■

SECTION 8

IMPRINT IDENTIFICATION GUIDE

Too often, patients on multiple medications have no idea what they're taking; and a "brown-bag inventory" may not help if it confronts you with a collection of unfamiliar tablets and capsules. This section of the *PDR® Guide to Drug Interactions, Side Effects, and Indications* provides you with a handy solution.

The convenient table below allows you to identify thousands of solid oral medications by imprint alone. Imprints beginning with a number are listed first, in ascending order. All numbers with leading zeros, as in "053", are listed before numbers without leading zeros. Imprints beginning with a letter follow in alphabetical order. Most commonly prescribed drugs are represented.

Each entry includes the full imprint code, the product's brand or generic name, and, to confirm identification, its strength, color, form, and shape. The name of the product's manufacturer completes each listing. The information is extracted, with permission, from the Identidex System produced by Micromedex, Inc.

IMPRINT	BRAND/GENERIC NAME	STRENGTH	COLOR	FORM	SHAPE	MANUFACTURER
0.1; RPR ;	Ddavp	0.1 mg	White	Tablet	Oval	Sanofi-Aventis U.S.
0.25 ; SP 321	Niravam	0.25 mg	Yellow	Tablet, Disintegrating	Circle	UCB Pharma
0.25 MG ; HYCAMTIN	Hycamtin	0.25 mg	Opaque White	Capsule		Glaxosmithkline
0.5 ; B 491	Alprazolam	0.5 mg	White	Tablet, Extended Release	Circle	Barr Laboratories
0.5 ; LOGO 4232 ;	Bumetanide	0.5 mg	Light Green	Tablet	Circle	Teva Pharmaceuticals
0.5 ; SP 322	Niravam	0.5 mg	Yellow	Tablet, Disintegrating	Circle	UCB Pharma
006 ; ADAMS	Allerx-D	2.5 mg ; 120 mg	Yellow	Tablet, Extended Release		Adams Laboratories
008 ; ACG	Atacand	8 mg	Light Pink	Tablet	Circle	Astrazeneca
0013 ; 10	Pravastatin Sodium	10 mg	Pink to Peach	Tablet	Ovoid-Rectangular	Watson Laboratories
0014 ; 20	Pravastatin Sodium	20 mg	Yellow	Tablet	Ovoid-Rectangular	Watson Laboratories
0016 ; 40	Pravastatin Sodium	40 mg	Green	Tablet	Ovoid-Rectangular	Watson Laboratories
0019 ; 80	Pravastatin Sodium	80 mg	Yellow	Tablet	Oval	Watson Laboratories
0038; G	Etodolac	200 mg	Light Gray	Capsule		Par Pharmaceutical
0039; G	Etodolac	300 mg	Gray	Capsule		Par Pharmaceutical
0040; G	Etodolac	400 mg	Orange	Tablet	Oval	Par Pharmaceutical
0093; HY-PAM 25 MG	HY-Pam	25 mg	Black or Lavender	Capsule		Teva Pharmaceuticals
0093; HY-PAM 50 MG	HY-Pam 50	50 mg	Dark Green and White Opaque	Capsule		Teva Pharmaceuticals
01 ; CBP	Allerx - AM Dose	120 mg ; 2.5 mg	Yellow	Tablet, Extended Release	Oblong	Adams Laboratories
01 45 ; P400	Pacerone	400 mg	Light Yellow	Tablet	Oval	Upsher-Smith Laboratories
02 ; CBP	Allerx - Pm Dose	8 mg ; 2.5 mg	Blue	Tablet, Extended Release	Oblong	Adams Laboratories
03 ; E ;	Allegra	30 mg	Peach	Tablet		Sanofi-Aventis U.S.
06 ; E ;	Allegra	60 mg	Peach	Tablet		Sanofi-Aventis U.S.
016 ; ACH	Atacand	16 mg	Pink	Tablet	Circle	Astrazeneca
018 ; E ;	Allegra	180 mg	Peach	Tablet		Sanofi-Aventis U.S.
019; DMSP	Cimetidine	200 mg	White	Tablet	Oval	Bristol-Myers Squibb
021 ; KOS	Simcor	500 mg ; 20 mg	Blue	Tablet, Extended Release		Abbott Laboratories
022 ; KOS	Simcor	750 mg ; 20 mg	Blue	Tablet, Extended Release		Abbott Laboratories
023 ; KOS	Simcor	1000 mg ; 20 mg	Blue	Tablet, Extended Release		Abbott Laboratories
026; G	Piroxicam	10 mg	Opaque Olive and Dark Green	Capsule		Par Pharmaceutical
027; G	Piroxicam	20 mg	Opaque Dark Green	Capsule		Par Pharmaceutical
032 ; ACL	Atacand	32 mg	Pink	Tablet	Circle	Astrazeneca
050; DMSP	Cimetidine	300 mg	White	Tablet	Oval	Bristol-Myers Squibb
057; DMSP	Cimetidine	400 mg	White	Tablet	Oval	Bristol-Myers Squibb
058; DMSP	Cimetidine	800 mg	White	Tablet	Oval	Bristol-Myers Squibb
066 100 ; B	Isoniazid	100 mg	White to Off-White	Tablet	Circle	Barr Laboratories
070 ; USL	Potassium Citrate	5 meq	Tan to Yellowish	Tablet	Circle	Upsher-Smith Laboratories
071 ; USL	Potassium Citrate	10 meq	Tan to Yellowish	Tablet	Oval	Upsher-Smith Laboratories

IMPRINT	BRAND/GENERIC NAME	STRENGTH	COLOR	FORM	SHAPE	MANUFACTURER
071 300 ; B	Isoniazid	300 mg	White to Off-White	Tablet	Oval	Barr Laboratories
081 IMPAX/10	Omeprazole Delayed-Release	10 mg	Lavender, Light Brown	Capsule, Delayed Release		Teva Pharmaceuticals
082 IMPAX 20 ;	Omeprazole Delayed-Release	20 mg	Lavender	Capsule, Delayed Release		Teva Pharmaceuticals
091 ; PAR	Doxycycline	50 mg	Yellow	Tablet	Circle	Par Pharmaceutical
092 ; PAR	Doxycycline	75 mg	Light Orange	Tablet	Circle	Par Pharmaceutical
093 ; PAR	Doxycycline	100 mg	Yellow	Tablet	Circle	Par Pharmaceutical
0321; US	Magsal	600 mg ; 25 mg	Light Green	Tablet	Oval	U.S. Pharmaceutical
0430; WALLACE	Felbatol	400 mg	Yellow	Tablet	Capsule-Shape	Meda Pharmaceuticals
0431; WALLACE	Felbatol	600 mg	Peach	Tablet	Capsule-Shape	Meda Pharmaceuticals
0665; 4001	Medroxyprogesterone	10 mg	White	Tablet	Circle, Scored	Novartis Generics
0665; 4001	Medroxyprogesterone	10 mg	White	Tablet	Circle, Scored, Compressed	Warner Chilcott
0665; 4120 ;	Valproic Acid	250 mg	Orange	Capsule, Liquid Filled	Oval	Novartis Generics
0665; 4160	Lithium Carbonate	300 mg	White	Capsule		Novartis Generics
0842 ; V	Phrenilin	50 mg ; 325 mg	Pale Violet	Tablet		Valeant Pharmaceuticals
0863 ; 93	Ciprofloxacin	250 mg	White to Off White	Tablet	Circle	Teva Pharmaceuticals
0865 ; 93	Ciprofloxacin	750 mg	White to Off White	Tablet	Capsule-Shape	Teva Pharmaceuticals
0924 ; 9 3	Oxaprozin	600 mg	White to Off-White	Tablet	Capsule-Shape	Teva Pharmaceuticals
1	Amphedex Tdc Paracotes	15 mg		Capsule		Paddock Labs
1	Lo-Ten	0.1 mg ; 25 mg ; 15 mg		Tablet		Teva Pharmaceuticals
1	Nitrogard	1 mg	Off-White	Sustained-Release Tablet	Circle, Standard Convex	Forest Pharmaceuticals
1 ; B 492	Alprazolam	1 mg	Yellow	Tablet, Extended Release	Circle	Barr Laboratories
1 ; LOGO	Fentora	100 mcg	White	Tablet	Circle	Cephalon
1 ; LOGO 4233 ;	Bumetanide	1 mg	Yellow	Tablet	Circle	Teva Pharmaceuticals
1 ; SP 323	Niravam	1 mg	White	Tablet, Disintegrating	Circle	UCB Pharma
1 7 ; M	Quinapril	5 mg	Orange	Tablet	Circle	Mylan Pharmaceuticals
1 MG ; HYCAMTIN	Hycamtin	1 mg	Opaque Pink	Capsule		Glaxosmithkline
1/90; JC; E2/N; OM	Prefest Estradiol/norgestimate	1 mg ; 0.09 mg	White	Tablet		Monarch Pharmaceuticals
1; 4036 ;	Estazolam	1 mg	White	Tablet	Square, Flat-Faced, Beveled-Edge, Scored	Ivax Pharmaceuticals
1; JC; E2; OM	Prefest Estradiol	1 mg	Pink	Tablet		Monarch Pharmaceuticals
2	Amphedex Tdc Paracotes	10 mg		Capsule		Paddock Labs
2	Detrol LA	2 mg	Blue-Green	Capsule, Extended Release		Pharmacia & Upjohn
2	Nitrogard	2 mg	Off-White	Sustained-Release Tablet	Circle, Standard Convex	Forest Pharmaceuticals
2 ; B 493	Alprazolam	2 mg	Blue	Tablet, Extended Release	Circle	Barr Laboratories
2 ; LOGO	Fentora	200 mcg	White	Tablet	Circle	Cephalon
2 ; LOGO 4234 ;	Bumetanide	2 mg	Peach	Tablet	Circle	Teva Pharmaceuticals
2 ; SB	Avandia	2 mg	Pink	Tablet	Five-Sided	Glaxosmithkline
2 ; SP 324	Niravam	2 mg	White	Tablet, Disintegrating	Circle	UCB Pharma
2 1/2; U; 121	Loniten	2.5 mg	White	Tablet	Circle, Scored	Pharmacia & Upjohn
2 RP ; TENEX	Tenex	2 mg	Yellow	Tablet	Diamond	A.H. Robins
2.5 ; FL	Bystolic	2.5 mg	Light Blue	Tablet	Triangle	Forest Pharmaceuticals
2/500 ; GSK	Avandamet	2 mg ; 500 mg	Pale Pink	Tablet	Oval	Glaxosmithkline
2/1000 ; GSK	Avandamet	1000 mg ; 2 mg	Yellow	Tablet	Oval	Glaxosmithkline
2; 93; 50	Acetaminophen and Codeine No. 2	300 mg ; 15 mg	White	Tablet	Circle, Flat, Beveled Edge	Teva Pharmaceuticals
2; 4037 ;	Estazolam	2 mg	Salmon	Tablet	Square, Flat-Faced, Beveled-Edge, Scored	Ivax Pharmaceuticals
2; VALIUM; R; ROCHE	Valium	2 mg	White	Tablet	Circle, Scored	Roche Products
3	Nitrogard	3 mg	Off-White	Sustained-Release Tablet	Circle, Standard Convex	Forest Pharmaceuticals
3 ; B 494	Alprazolam	3 mg	Green	Tablet, Extended Release	Circle	Barr Laboratories
3 ; LOGO	Fentora	300 mcg	White	Tablet	Circle	Cephalon
3 ; RX 562	Acetaminophen and Codeine Phosphate	300 mg ; 30 mg	White	Tablet	Circle	Ranbaxy Pharmaceuticals
3; 93; 150	Acetaminophen and Codeine Phosphate	300 mg ; 30 mg	White	Tablet	Circle	Teva Pharmaceuticals
3M; 221	Orphenadrine Citrate ER	100 mg	White	Extended-Release Tablet	Circle	Mylan Pharmaceuticals
3M; 342	Theolair	125 mg	White	Tablet	Circle, Scored	3M Pharmaceuticals
3M; SR; 200	Theolair-SR	200 mg	White	Sustained-Release Tablet	Circle, Scored	3M Pharmaceuticals
3M; SR; 250 ;	Theolair-SR	250 mg	White	Sustained-Release Tablet	Circle, Scored	3M Pharmaceuticals
3M; SR; 300 ;	Theolair-SR	300 mg	White	Sustained-Release Tablet	Oval, Scored	3M Pharmaceuticals
3M; SR; 500 ;	Theolair-SR	500 mg	White	Sustained-Release Tablet	Capsule-Shape, Scored	3M Pharmaceuticals
3M; THEOLAIR; 250	Theolair	250 mg	White	Tablet	Capsule-Shape, Scored	3M Pharmaceuticals
3M; TR; 50	Tambocor	50 mg	White	Tablet	Circle	Graceway Pharmaceuticals
3M; TR; 150	Tambocor	150 mg	White	Tablet	Oval	Graceway Pharmaceuticals
3M; UREX	Urex	1 G	White	Tablet	Capsule-Shape, Scored	3M Pharmaceuticals
3RP ; 200	Ribavirin	200 mg	Light Blue	Tablet	Capsule-Shape	Par Pharmaceutical
3RP ; 400	Ribatab	400 mg	Medium Blue	Tablet	Capsule-Shape	Par Pharmaceutical
3RP ; 600	Ribatab	600 mg	Dark Blue	Tablet	Capsule-Shape	Par Pharmaceutical
4	Detrol LA	4 mg	Blue	Capsule, Extended Release		Pharmacia & Upjohn
4 ; LOGO	Fentora	400 mcg	White	Tablet	Circle	Cephalon
4 ; RX 561	Acetaminophen and Codeine Phosphate	300 mg ; 60 mg	White	Tablet	Circle	Ranbaxy Pharmaceuticals
4 ; SB	Avandia	4 mg	Orange	Tablet	Five-Sided	Glaxosmithkline

IMPRINT	BRAND/GENERIC NAME	STRENGTH	COLOR	FORM	SHAPE	MANUFACTURER
4/500 ; GSK	Avandamet	4 mg ; 500 mg	Orange	Tablet	Oval	Glaxosmithkline
4/1000 ; GSK	Avandamet	1000 mg ; 4 mg	Pink	Tablet	Oval	Glaxosmithkline
4; 93; 350	Acetaminophen and Codeine Phosphate	300 mg ; 60 mg	White	Tablet	Circle	Teva Pharmaceuticals
5	Buspirone Hydrochloride	5 mg	White	Tablet	Circle	Actavis Totowa
5	Opana ER	5 mg	Pink	Tablet, Extended Release	Eight-Sided	Endo Pharmaceuticals
5	Rhinspec	300 mg ; 100 mg ; 5 mg	Pink	Tablet		Teva Pharmaceuticals
5	Zyprexa Zydis	5 mg	Yellow	Tablet, Disintegrating	Circle	Eli Lilly
5 ; FL	Bystolic	5 mg	Beige	Tablet	Triangle	Forest Pharmaceuticals
5 ; FL ;	Lexapro	5 mg	White to Off White	Tablet	Circle	Forest Pharmaceuticals
5 ; FL ;	Namenda	5 mg	Tan	Tablet	Capsule-Shape	Forest Pharmaceuticals
5 ; GSI	Letairis	5 mg	Pale Pink	Tablet	Square	Gilead Sciences
5 MG ; RSN	Actonel	5 mg	Yellow	Tablet	Oval	Procter & Gamble Pharmaceuticals
5 MG 3512 5 MG SB	Dexedrine Spansule	5 mg	Brown, Clear	Capsule, Extended Release		Glaxosmithkline
5 MG SONATA	Sonata	5 mg	Green, Light Green	Capsule		Wyeth Pharmaceuticals
5 XL	Ditropan XL	5 mg	Pale Yellow	Tablet, Extended Release	Circle	Ortho-Mcneil Pharmaceutical
5/500 ; LOGO 5712	Glyburide and Metformin Hydrochloride	5 mg ; 500 mg	Yellow	Tablet	Oval	Teva Pharmaceuticals
5; ARICEPT	Aricept Odt	5 mg	White	Disintegrating Tablet		Pfizer
5; R	Sotret	10 mg	Light Pink	Capsule		Ranbaxy Pharmaceuticals
5; VALIUM; R; ROCHE	Valium	5 mg	Yellow	Tablet	Circle, Scored	Roche Products
6	Bevitone	20 mg ; 3 mcg ; 150 mg ; 5 mg ; 20 mg	Pink	Tablet		Teva Pharmaceuticals
6 ; LOGO	Fentora	600 mcg	White	Tablet	Circle	Cephalon
6; R	Sotret	20 mg	Maroon	Capsule		Ranbaxy Pharmaceuticals
7	Luride	1 mg		Tablet, Chewable		Colgate Oral Pharmaceuticals
7; R	Sotret	40 mg	Yellow	Capsule		Ranbaxy Pharmaceuticals
7.5	Opana ER	7.5 mg	Gray	Tablet, Extended Release	Eight-Sided	Endo Pharmaceuticals
7.5 ; G	Meloxicam	7.5 mg	Peach	Tablet	Circle	Mylan Pharmaceuticals
7.5; DF	Enablex	7.5 mg	White	Tablet, Extended Release	Circle	Novartis Pharmaceuticals
8 ; LOGO	Fentora	800 mcg	White	Tablet	Circle	Cephalon
8 ; NO	Ondansetron Hydrochloride	8 mg	Yellow	Tablet	Oval	Actavis Totowa
8 ; SB	Avandia	8 mg	Red-Brown	Tablet	Five-Sided	Glaxosmithkline
8/4 ; GSK	Avandaryl	8 mg ; 4 mg	Red	Tablet	Triangle	Glaxosmithkline
9 3 ; 72 83	Oxcarbazepine	600 mg	Brown to Dark Brown	Tablet	Capsule-Shape	Teva Pharmaceuticals
9 3 ; 2238 ;	Cephalexin	250 mg	White	Tablet	Capsule-Shape	Teva Pharmaceuticals
9 3 ; 2240 ;	Cephalexin	500 mg	White	Tablet	Capsule-Shape	Teva Pharmaceuticals
9 3 ; 4741	Citalopram Hydrobromide	20 mg	Light Pink	Tablet	Capsule-Shape	Teva Pharmaceuticals
9 3 ; 4742	Citalopram Hydrobromide	40 mg	White to Off-White	Tablet	Capsule-Shape	Teva Pharmaceuticals
9 3 ; 7188	Fluoxetine Hydrochloride	10 mg	Blue	Tablet	Oval	Teva Pharmaceuticals
9; 3; 27	Torsemide	5 mg	White to Off-White	Tablet	Oval, Scored	Teva Pharmaceuticals
9; 3; 28	Torsemide	10 mg	White to Off-White	Tablet	Oval, Scored	Teva Pharmaceuticals
9; 3; 29	Torsemide	20 mg	White to Off-White	Tablet	Oval, Scored	Teva Pharmaceuticals
9; 3; 30	Torsemide	100 mg	White to Off-White	Tablet	Oval	Teva Pharmaceuticals
9; 3; 72; 22	Fosinopril Sodium	10 mg	White to Off-White	Tablet	Capsule-Shape	Teva Pharmaceuticals
9; 3; 7127	Torsemide	5 mg	White to Off-White	Tablet	Oval, Scored	Teva Pharmaceuticals
9; 3; 7128	Torsemide	10 mg	White to Off-White	Tablet	Oval, Scored	Teva Pharmaceuticals
9; 3; 7129	Torsemide	20 mg	White to Off-White	Tablet	Oval, Scored	Teva Pharmaceuticals
9; 3; 7130	Torsemide	100 mg	White to Off-White	Tablet	Oval, Scored	Teva Pharmaceuticals
9; 3; 7159	Pergolide Mesylate	0.25 mg	Mottled Green	Tablet	Capsule-Shape, Scored	Teva Pharmaceuticals
9; 3; 7160	Pergolide Mesylate	0.05 mg	Ivory	Tablet	Capsule-Shape, Scored	Teva Pharmaceuticals
9; 3; 7161	Pergolide Mesylate	1 mg	Mottled Pink	Tablet	Capsule-Shape, Scored	Teva Pharmaceuticals
10	Buspirone Hydrochloride	10 mg	White	Tablet	Circle	Actavis Totowa
10	Opana ER	10 mg	Light Orange	Tablet, Extended Release	Eight-Sided	Endo Pharmaceuticals
10	Zyprexa Zydis	10 mg	Yellow	Tablet, Disintegrating	Circle	Eli Lilly
10 ;	Ceenu	10 mg	Two-Tone White	Capsule		Bristol-Myers Oncology
10 ; A 640	Abilify Discmelt	10 mg	Pink	Tablet, Disintegrating	Circle	Otsuka America Pharmaceutical
10 ; ABG	Oxycodone Hydrochloride	10 mg	White	Controlled-Release Tablet	Circle	Ivax Pharmaceuticals
10 ; ABG	Oxycodone Hydrochloride Controlled-Release	10 mg	White	Controlled Release Tablet	Circle	Ivax Pharmaceuticals
10 ; E702	Oxycodone Hydrochloride	10 mg	White	Tablet, Extended Release	Circle	Endo Generics
10 ; FL	Bystolic	10 mg	Pink-Purple	Tablet	Triangle	Forest Pharmaceuticals
10 ; FL ;	Lexapro	10 mg	White to Off White	Tablet	Circle	Forest Pharmaceuticals
10 ; FL ;	Namenda	10 mg	Gray	Tablet	Capsule-Shape	Forest Pharmaceuticals
10 ; OC	Oxycontin	10 mg	White	Tablet, Extended Release	Circle	Purdue Pharmaceutical Products
10 ; ORA	Orapred Odt	10 mg	White	Tablet, Disintegrating		Sciele Pharma
10 ; PD 155	Lipitor	10 mg	White	Coated Tablet	Circle	Parke-Davis
10 10 10 ; A2 80	Buspirone Hydrochloride	30 mg	White to Off-White	Tablet	Capsule-Shape	Actavis Totowa
10 MG ; LILLY 3227	Strattera	10 mg	White	Capsule		Eli Lilly
10 MG 93 810	Nortriptyline Hydrochloride	10 mg	Orange, White	Capsule		Teva Pharmaceuticals
10 MG SONATA	Sonata	10 mg	Green, Light Green	Capsule		Wyeth Pharmaceuticals
10 XL	Ditropan XL	10 mg	Pink	Tablet, Extended Release		Ortho-Mcneil Pharmaceutical
10/100; SP; 341	Parcopa	10 mg ; 100 mg	Blue	Tablet, Disintegrating	Circle	UCB Pharma
10; ARICEPT	Aricept Odt	10 mg	Yellow	Disintegrating Tablet		Pfizer

IMPRINT	BRAND/GENERIC NAME	STRENGTH	COLOR	FORM	SHAPE	MANUFACTURER
10; GILEAD; LIVER SYMBOL	Hepsera	10 mg	White	Tablet		Gilead Sciences
10; VALIUM; R; ROCHE	Valium	10 mg	Blue	Tablet		Roche Products
10MG ; GSK COREG CR	Coreg Cr	10 mg	White, Green	Capsule, Extended Release		Glaxosmithkline
10MG 3513 10MG SB	Dexedrine Spansule	10 mg	Brown, Clear	Capsule, Extended Release		Glaxosmithkline
11	Akineton	2 mg	White	Tablet	Circle	Par Pharmaceutical
11 ; OX	Oxandrolone	2.5 mg	White	Tablet	Oval	Watson Laboratories
11 ; RX	Fosinopril Sodium	10 mg	White to Off White	Tablet	Capsule-Shape	Ranbaxy Pharmaceuticals
12.5 MG 4870 ; LOGO	Hydrochlorothiazide	12.5 mg	White Opaque	Capsule	Capsule-Shape	Teva Pharmaceuticals
14 ; B	Kelnor 1/35 - Light Yellow Tablet	1 mg ; 35 mcg	Light Yellow	Tablet	Circle	Barr Laboratories
15	Opana ER	15 mg	White	Tablet, Extended Release	Eight-Sided	Endo Pharmaceuticals
15	Prevacid Solutab	15 mg	White to Yellowish White with Orange to Dark Brown Speckles	Tablet, Disintegrating		Tap Pharmaceuticals
15	Zyprexa Zydis	15 mg	Yellow	Tablet, Disintegrating	Circle	Eli Lilly
15 ; 93	Nabumetone	500 mg	White	Tablet	Oval	Teva Pharmaceuticals
15 ; A 641	Abilify Discmelt	15 mg	Yellow	Tablet, Disintegrating	Circle	Otsuka America Pharmaceutical
15 ; G	Meloxicam	15 mg	Peach	Tablet	Oblong	Mylan Pharmaceuticals
15 ; OC	Oxycontin	15 mg	Gray	Tablet, Extended Release	Circle	Purdue Pharmaceutical Products
15 ; ORA	Orapred Odt	15 mg	White	Tablet, Disintegrating		Sciele Pharma
15 XL	Ditropan XL	15 mg	Gray	Tablet, Extended Release	Circle	Ortho-Mcneil Pharmaceutical
15/500 ; 4833M	Actoplus Met	15 mg ; 500 mg	White to Off-White	Tablet	Oblong	Takeda Pharmaceuticals
15/850 ; 4833M	Actoplus Met	850 mg ; 15 mg	White to Off-White	Tablet	Oblong	Takeda Pharmaceuticals
15; DF	Enablex	15 mg	Light Peach	Tablet, Extended Release	Circle	Novartis Pharmaceuticals
15MG 3514 15MG SB	Dexedrine Spansule	15 mg	Brown, Clear	Capsule, Extended Release		Glaxosmithkline
16 ; 93	Nabumetone	750 mg	Beige	Tablet	Oval	Par Pharmaceutical
17	Moexipril Hydrochloride	7.5 mg	Pink	Tablet	Oval	Teva Pharmaceuticals
18	Quinapril	5 mg	White to Off-White	Tablet	Circle	Ranbaxy Pharmaceuticals
18 MG ; LILLY 3238	Strattera	18 mg	Gold, White	Capsule		Eli Lilly
19 ; RE	Atenolol	25 mg	White to Off-White	Tablet	Circle	Ranbaxy Pharmaceuticals
20	Neospect	100 mg ; 25 mg ; 15 mg ; 100 mg	Green	Tablet		Teva Pharmaceuticals
20	Opana ER	20 mg	Light Green	Tablet, Extended Release	Eight-Sided	Endo Pharmaceuticals
20	Zegerid	20 mg ; 1100 mg	Light Blue, White	Capsule		Santarus
20	Zyprexa Zydis	20 mg	Yellow	Tablet, Disintegrating	Circle	Eli Lilly
20 ; A 642	Abilify Discmelt	20 mg	White	Tablet, Disintegrating	Circle	Otsuka America Pharmaceutical
20 ; ABG	Oxycodone Hydrochloride	20 mg	Pink	Controlled-Release Tablet	Circle	Ivax Pharmaceuticals
20 ; ABG	Oxycodone Hydrochloride Controlled-Release	20 mg	Pink	Controlled Release Tablet	Circle	Ivax Pharmaceuticals
20 ; E703	Oxycodone Hydrochloride	20 mg	Pink	Tablet, Extended Release	Circle	Endo Generics
20 ; FL ;	Lexapro	20 mg	White to Off White	Tablet	Circle	Forest Pharmaceuticals
20 ; OC	Oxycontin	20 mg	Pink	Tablet, Extended Release	Circle	Purdue Pharmaceutical Products
20 ; P	Hydrochlorothiazide	12.5 mg	Peach	Tablet	Circle	Actavis Elizabeth
20 ; PD 156	Lipitor	20 mg	White	Coated Tablet	Oval	Parke-Davis
20 600 ; DOCS	Mydocs	20 mg ; 600 mg	White	Tablet, Extended Release	Oval	Centurion Labs
20 MG	Nexium	20 mg	Amethyst with Two Yellow Bars	Capsule, Delayed Release		Astrazeneca
20 MG ; GSK COREG CR	Coreg Cr	20 mg	White, Yellow	Capsule, Extended Release		Glaxosmithkline
20 MG; LILLY; 3235	Cymbalta	20 mg	Opaque Green	Delayed-Release Capsule		Eli Lilly
22	Rhinex	150 mg ; 1.25 mg ; 2.5 mg	Pink and White	Tablet		Teva Pharmaceuticals
22 ; M	Albuterol Sulfate	4 mg	White	Tablet, Extended Release	Circle	Mylan Pharmaceuticals
24 ; D	Clarinex-D 24 Hour	5 mg ; 240 mg	Light Blue	Tablet, Extended Release	Oval	Schering
24 ; M	Albuterol Sulfate	8 mg	Blue	Tablet, Extended Release	Circle	Mylan Pharmaceuticals
25	Levoxyl	25 mcg	Orange	Tablet	Oval	King Pharmaceuticals
25 ; TOP	Topamax	25 mg	White	Tablet	Circle	Ortho-Mcneil Pharmaceutical
25 MG ; LILLY 3228	Strattera	25 mg	Blue, White	Capsule		Eli Lilly
25 MG ; WATSON 800	Hydroxyzine Pamoate	25 mg	Dark Green Opaque, Light Green Opaque	Capsule		Watson Laboratories
25 MG 93 811	Nortriptyline Hydrochloride	25 mg	Orange, White	Capsule		Teva Pharmaceuticals
25/100; SP; 342	Parcopa	25 mg ; 100 mg	Yellow	Tablet, Disintegrating	Circle	UCB Pharma
25/250; SP; 343	Parcopa	25 mg ; 250 mg	Blue	Tablet, Disintegrating	Circle	UCB Pharma
25; LL; A; 13	Asendin	25 mg	Off-White	Tablet	Seven-Sided	Lederle Laboratories
25; T4	Levothroid	25 mcg	Orange	Tablet	Capsule-Shape	Forest Pharmaceuticals
30	Opana ER	30 mg	Red	Tablet, Extended Release	Eight-Sided	Endo Pharmaceuticals

IMPRINT	BRAND/GENERIC NAME	STRENGTH	COLOR	FORM	SHAPE	MANUFACTURER
30	Prevacid	30 mg	White to Yellowish White with Orange to Dark Brown Speckles	Tablet, Disintegrating		Takeda Pharmaceuticals
30 ; A 643	Abilify Discmelt	30 mg	Pink	Tablet, Disintegrating	Circle	Otsuka America Pharmaceutical
30 ; B ;	Nifediac CC	30 mg	Mustard Yellow	Tablet, Extended Release	Circle	Teva Pharmaceuticals
30 ; OC	Oxycontin	30 mg	Brown	Tablet, Extended Release	Circle	Purdue Pharmaceutical Products
30 ; ORA	Orapred Odt	30 mg	White	Tablet, Disintegrating		Sciele Pharma
30 MG ; RSN	Actonel	30 mg	White	Tablet	Oval	Procter & Gamble Pharmaceuticals
30 MG; LILLY; 3240	Cymbalta	30 mg	Opaque White and Opaque Blue	Delayed-Release Capsule		Eli Lilly
30/2 ; 4833G ;	Duetact	30 mg ; 2 mg	Off-White to White	Tablet	Circle	Takeda Pharmaceuticals
30/4 ; 4833G ;	Duetact	30 mg ; 4 mg	Off-White to White	Tablet	Circle	Takeda Pharmaceuticals
31	Alendronate Sodium	70 mg	White	Tablet	Oval	Watson Pharma
31; BONE IMAGE	Fosamax	70 mg	White	Tablet	Oval	Merck
32 38 ; WPI	Sertraline Hydrochloride	25 mg	Green	Tablet	Capsule-Shape	Watson Laboratories
32 39 ; WPI	Sertraline Hydrochloride	50 mg	Blue	Tablet	Capsule-Shape	Watson Laboratories
32 40 ; WPI	Sertraline Hydrochloride	100 mg	Yellow	Tablet	Capsule-Shape	Watson Laboratories
35 MG ; RSN	Actonel	35 mg	Orange	Tablet	Oval	Procter & Gamble Pharmaceuticals
35 MG ; RSN	Actonel with Calcium (Risedronate Sodium Tablets)	35 mg	Orange	Tablet	Oval	Procter & Gamble
37; 4401	Depen	250 mg	White	Tablet		Meda Pharmaceuticals
37.5 ; PL PCR	Paroxetine Hydrochloride	37.5 mg	Blue	Tablet, Extended Release	Circle	Mylan Pharmaceuticals
38AV	Ketek	300 mg	Light Orange	Tablet	Oval	Sanofi-Aventis U.S.
39 ; 9 3	Lamotrigine	25 mg	White to Off-White	Tablet	Diamond	Teva Pharmaceuticals
40	Opana ER	40 mg	Yellow	Tablet, Extended Release	Eight-Sided	Endo Pharmaceuticals
40	Zegerid	40 mg ; 1100 mg	Dark Blue, White	Capsule		Santarus
40 ;	Ceenu	40 mg	White and Green	Capsule		Bristol-Myers Oncology
40 ; ABG	Oxycodone Hydrochloride	40 mg	Yellow	Controlled-Release Tablet	Circle	Ivax Pharmaceuticals
40 ; ABG	Oxycodone Hydrochloride Controlled-Release	40 mg	Yellow	Controlled Release Tablet	Circle	Ivax Pharmaceuticals
40 ; CRESTOR	Crestor	40 mg	Pink	Tablet	Oval	Astrazeneca
40 ; E705	Oxycodone Hydrochloride	40 mg	Yellow	Tablet, Extended Release	Circle	Endo Generics
40 ; MYLAN 216	Furosemide	40 mg	White	Tablet	Circle	Mylan Pharmaceuticals
40 ; OC	Oxycontin	40 mg	Yellow	Tablet, Extended Release	Circle	Purdue Pharmaceutical Products
40 ; PD 157	Lipitor	40 mg	White	Tablet	Circle	Pfizer
40 MG	Nexium	40 mg	Opaque, Amethyst with 3 Yellow Bars	Capsule, Delayed Release		Astrazeneca
40 MG ; LILLY 3229	Strattera	40 mg	Blue	Capsule		Eli Lilly
40MG ; GSK COREG CR	Coreg Cr	40 mg	Green, Yellow	Capsule, Extended Release		Glaxosmithkline
42	Neosorb Plus	300 mg ; 150 mg	Green and White	Tablet		Teva Pharmaceuticals
44	Vicks 44 Liquicaps Non-Drowsy Cough & Cold Relief	30 mg ; 60 mg	Transparent Red	Gel/jelly		Procter & Gamble
44	Vicks 44 Liquidaps Cough, Cold & Flu Relief	30 mg ; 10 mg ; 250 mg ; 2 mg	Transparent Blue	Gel/jelly		Procter & Gamble
48 ; RB ;	Glimepiride	1 mg	Blue	Tablet	Hourglass-Shape	Ranbaxy Pharmaceuticals
49 ; RB ;	Glimepiride	2 mg	Blue	Tablet	Hourglass-Shape	Ranbaxy Pharmaceuticals
50	Levoxyl	50 mcg	White	Tablet	Oval	King Pharmaceuticals
50 ; LOGO 4404	Clozapine	50 mg	Pale Yellow	Tablet	Circle	Teva Pharmaceuticals
50 ; RB ;	Glimepiride	4 mg	Blue	Tablet	Hourglass-Shape	Ranbaxy Pharmaceuticals
50 ; TOPAMAX	Topamax	50 mg	White	Tablet	Circle	Ortho-Mcneil Pharmaceutical
50 MG ; WATSON 801	Hydroxyzine Pamoate	50 mg	Dark Green Opaque, White Opaque	Capsule		Watson Laboratories
50 MG 93 812	Nortriptyline Hydrochloride	50 mg	White	Capsule		Teva Pharmaceuticals
50; LL; A; 15	Asendin	50 mg	Orange	Tablet	Seven-Sided	Lederle Laboratories
50; T4	Levothroid	50 mcg	White	Tablet	Capsule-Shape	Forest Pharmaceuticals
50H ; LOGO	Micardis	20 mg	White or Off-White	Tablet	Circle	Boehringer Ingelheim Pharmaceuticals
51 ; 93	Carvedilol	3.125 mg	White	Tablet	Oval	Teva Pharmaceuticals
51 51 ; GEIGY	Lopressor	50 mg	Pink	Tablet	Capsule-Shape	Novartis
51H ; LOGO	Micardis	40 mg	White or Off-White	Tablet	Oblong	Boehringer Ingelheim Pharmaceuticals
52H ; LOGO	Micardis	80 mg	White or Off-White	Tablet	Oblong	Boehringer Ingelheim Pharmaceuticals
54 005	Anagrelide Hydrochloride	0.5 mg	White	Capsule		Roxane Laboratories
54 015	Torsemide	5 mg	White to Off-White	Tablet	Circle	Roxane Laboratories
54 016	Torsemide	10 mg	White to Off-White	Tablet	Circle	Roxane Laboratories
54 017	Torsemide	20 mg	White to Off-White	Tablet	Circle	Roxane Laboratories
54 104	Fluconazole	100 mg	Pink	Tablet	Circle	Roxane Laboratories
54 107	Lithium Carbonate	300 mg	Beige	Tablet, Extended Release	Circle	Roxane Laboratories
54 111	Mefloquine Hydrochloride	250 mg	Off-White to Yellow	Tablet	Circle	Roxane Laboratories
54 145	Ramipril	5 mg	Red Opaque	Capsule		Roxane Laboratories
54 163	Meperidine Hydrochloride	100 mg	White	Tablet		Roxane Laboratories
54 200	Fluconazole	150 mg	Pink	Tablet	Circle	Roxane Laboratories
54 213	Lithium Carbonate	150 mg	White Opaque	Capsule		Roxane Laboratories
54 231	Ropinirole Hydrochloride	2 mg	Orange	Tablet	Circle	Roxane Laboratories
54 262	Morphine Sulfate	30 mg	White	Tablet		Roxane Laboratories
54 271	Clarithromycin	250 mg	White	Tablet	Circle	Roxane Laboratories

IMPRINT	BRAND/GENERIC NAME	STRENGTH	COLOR	FORM	SHAPE	MANUFACTURER
54 273	Ropinirole Hydrochloride	4 mg	Brown	Tablet	Circle	Roxane Laboratories
54 299	Dexamethasone	0.5 mg	Yellow	Tablet		Roxane Laboratories
54 312	Clarithromycin	500 mg	White	Tablet	Capsule-Shape	Roxane Laboratories
54 328	Ramipril	1.25 mg	Yellow Opaque	Capsule		Roxane Laboratories
54 334	Fluconazole	200 mg	Pink	Tablet	Circle	Roxane Laboratories
54 337	Ropinirole Hydrochloride	0.5 mg	Yellow	Tablet	Circle	Roxane Laboratories
54 371	Zolpidem Tartrate	5 mg	Pink	Tablet	Circle	Roxane Laboratories
54 409 ;	Oramorph SR	30 mg	White	Sustained-Release Tablet	Circle	Roxane Laboratories
54 409 30	Oramorph SR	30 mg	White	Tablet, Extended Release		Xanodyne Pharmaceuticals
54 420	Mercaptopurine	50 mg	Pale Yellow	Tablet	Biconvex	Roxane Laboratories
54 452	Lithium Carbonate	300 mg	White	Tablet		Roxane Laboratories
54 463	Lithium Carbonate	300 mg	Flesh	Capsule		Roxane Laboratories
54 489	Dexamethasone	1 mg	Yellow	Tablet		Roxane Laboratories
54 511	Ropinirole Hydrochloride	0.25 mg	White	Tablet	Circle	Roxane Laboratories
54 521	Cilostazol	50 mg	White	Tablet	Triangle	Roxane Laboratories
54 543	Roxicet	5 mg ; 325 mg	White	Tablet		Roxane Laboratories
54 552	Clotrimazole Troche	10 mg	White	Lozenge/troche		Roxane Laboratories
54 553	Zolpidem Tartrate	10 mg	White	Tablet	Circle	Roxane Laboratories
54 575	Ropinirole Hydrochloride	3 mg	Red	Tablet	Circle	Roxane Laboratories
54 582	Roxicodone	5 mg	White	Tablet		Xanodyne Pharmaceuticals
54 602	Ramipril	10 mg	Blue Opaque	Capsule		Roxane Laboratories
54 609 ;	Hydromorphone Hydrochloride	4 mg	White	Tablet	Circle	Roxane Laboratories
54 647	Pilocarpine Hydrochloride	5 mg	White	Tablet	Biconvex	Roxane Laboratories
54 662	Dexamethasone	2 mg	White	Tablet		Roxane Laboratories
54 702	Lithium Carbonate	600 mg	Flesh, White Opaque	Capsule		Roxane Laboratories
54 722	Ropinirole Hydrochloride	5 mg	Blue	Tablet	Circle	Roxane Laboratories
54 733	Morphine Sulfate	15 mg	White	Tablet		Roxane Laboratories
54 743 ;	Hydromorphone Hydrochloride	2 mg	White	Tablet	Circle	Roxane Laboratories
54 744	Terbinafine Hydrochloride	250 mg	White	Tablet	Circle	Roxane Laboratories
54 751	Ropinirole Hydrochloride	1 mg	Green	Tablet	Circle	Roxane Laboratories
54 757	Cilostazol	100 mg	White	Tablet	Circle	Roxane Laboratories
54 769	Dexamethasone	6 mg	Aqua	Tablet		Roxane Laboratories
54 777	Zidovudine	300 mg	White	Tablet	Circle	Roxane Laboratories
54 782 ;	Oramorph SR	15 mg	White	Sustained-Release Tablet	Circle	Roxane Laboratories
54 782 15	Oramorph SR	15 mg	White	Tablet, Extended Release		Xanodyne Pharmaceuticals
54 794	Ramipril	2.5 mg	Orange Opaque	Capsule		Roxane Laboratories
54 840	Furosemide	20 mg	White	Tablet		Roxane Laboratories
54 862 ;	Oramorph SR	100 mg	White	Tablet, Extended Release	Circle	Roxane Laboratories
54 862 100	Oramorph SR	100 mg	White	Tablet, Extended Release		Xanodyne Pharmaceuticals
54 878	Pilocarpine Hydrochloride	7.5 mg	Blue	Tablet	Biconvex	Roxane Laboratories
54 879	Meperidine Hydrochloride	50 mg	White	Tablet		Roxane Laboratories
54 892	Dexamethasone	4 mg	Green	Tablet		Roxane Laboratories
54 922	Granisetron Hydrochloride	1 mg	White	Tablet	Circle	Roxane Laboratories
54 923	Acyclovir	200 mg		Capsule		Roxane Laboratories
54 933 60	Oramorph SR	60 mg	White	Tablet, Extended Release		Xanodyne Pharmaceuticals
54 943	Dexamethasone	1.5 mg	Pink	Tablet		Roxane Laboratories
54 960	Dexamethasone	0.75 mg	Pale Blue	Tablet		Roxane Laboratories
54 996	Fluconazole	50 mg	Pink	Tablet	Circle	Roxane Laboratories
54 998	Anagrelide Hydrochloride	1 mg	Gray	Capsule		Roxane Laboratories
54/943	Dexpak 13 Day Taperpak	1.5 mg	Pink	Tablet	Circle	Ecr Pharmaceuticals
54/943	Dexpak JR. 10 Day Taperpak	1.5 mg	Pink	Tablet	Circle	Ecr Pharmaceuticals
54; 007	Mirtazapine	45 mg	White	Tablet	Circle	Roxane Laboratories
54; 009	Propranolol Hydrochloride	20 mg	White	Tablet	Circle	Roxane Laboratories
54; 010	Diflunisal	250 mg	Orange	Coated Tablet	Capsule-Shape, Biconvex	Roxane Laboratories
54; 012	Amitriptyline Hydrochloride	25 mg	White	Tablet		Roxane Laboratories
54; 013	Leucovorin Calcium	25 mg	Yellow	Tablet	Circle, Scored	Roxane Laboratories
54; 019	Chlorpheniramine Maleate	4 mg	Yellow	Tablet		Roxane Laboratories
54; 024	Flecainide Acetate	50 mg	White	Tablet	Circle	Roxane Laboratories
54; 039	Naproxen	500 mg	Beige	Tablet	Capsule-Shape	Roxane Laboratories
54; 042	Nefazodone Hydrochloride	100 mg	White	Tablet	Oval	Roxane Laboratories
54; 042	Nefazodone Hydrochloride	100 mg	White	Tablet	Oval, Scored	Roxane Laboratories
54; 043	Azathioprine	50 mg	Yellow	Tablet	Circle, Scored	Roxane Laboratories
54; 050	Haloperidol	1 mg		Tablet		Roxane Laboratories
54; 053	Quinidine Sulfate	300 mg	White	Tablet		Roxane Laboratories
54; 062	Propranolol Hydrochloride	60 mg	White	Tablet	Circle	Roxane Laboratories
54; 063	Acetaminophen	325 mg	White	Tablet		Roxane Laboratories
54; 070	Flecainide Acetate	100 mg	White	Tablet	Circle	Roxane Laboratories
54; 072	Hydroxyurea	500 mg	Dark Green and Light Pink	Capsule		Roxane Laboratories
54; 080	Prednisone	25 mg		Tablet		Roxane Laboratories
54; 090	Roxanol SR	30 mg	White	Sustained-Release Tablet		Roxane Laboratories
54; 092	Prednisone	1 mg	White	Tablet		Roxane Laboratories
54; 093	Diflunisal	500 mg	Orange	Coated Tablet	Capsule-Shape, Biconvex	Roxane Laboratories
54; 099	Amitriptyline Hydrochloride	50 mg	White	Tablet		Roxane Laboratories
54; 103	Bisacodyl	5 mg	Orange	Tablet		Roxane Laboratories
54; 133	Calcium Carbonate	1250 mg	Off-White	Tablet, Chewable	Circle	Roxane Laboratories
54; 142	Methadone Hydrochloride	10 mg	White	Tablet		Roxane Laboratories
54; 143	Amitriptyline Hydrochloride	100 mg	White	Tablet		Roxane Laboratories
54; 150	Flecainide Acetate	150 mg	White	Tablet	Capsule-Shape	Roxane Laboratories
54; 162	Dolophine Hydrochloride	5 mg	White	Tablet	Circle	Roxane Laboratories
54; 169	Haloperidol	0.5 mg		Tablet		Roxane Laboratories

IMPRINT	BRAND/GENERIC NAME	STRENGTH	COLOR	FORM	SHAPE	MANUFACTURER
54; 172	Isoxsuprine Hydrochloride	10 mg	White	Tablet		Roxane Laboratories
54; 179	Chloral Hydrate	500 mg	Red	Capsule		Roxane Laboratories
54; 180	Naproxen Sodium Film-Coated	275 mg	Light Blue	Tablet	Oval	Roxane Laboratories
54; 183	Prednisolone	5 mg	White	Tablet		Roxane Laboratories
54; 193	Viramune	200 mg	White	Tablet	Oval, Biconvex, Bisected Scored	Roxane Laboratories
54; 199	Roxicodone	30 mg	Blue	Tablet		Roxane Laboratories
54; 201	Mirtazapine	15 mg	Yellow	Tablet	Circle	Roxane Laboratories
54; 210	Methadone Hydrochloride	5 mg	White	Tablet		Roxane Laboratories
54; 212	Neomycin Sulfate	500 mg	Off-White	Tablet		Roxane Laboratories
54; 223	Diphenhydramine Hydrochloride	50 mg	Pink	Capsule		Roxane Laboratories
54; 249	Propranolol Hydrochloride	80 mg	White	Tablet	Circle	Roxane Laboratories
54; 252	Acetaminophen	500 mg		Tablet		Roxane Laboratories
54; 253	Sulfamethoxazole and Trimethoprim	400 mg ; 80 mg	White	Tablet	Capsule-Shape, Scored	Roxane Laboratories
54; 259	Ferrous Sulfate	300 mg	Red	Tablet		Roxane Laboratories
54; 262	Morphine Sulfate	30 mg	White	Tablet		Roxane Laboratories
54; 263	Phenobarbital	100 mg	White	Tablet		Roxane Laboratories
54; 280	Dht	0.125 mg	White	Tablet		Roxane Laboratories
54; 293	Leucovorin Calcium	5 mg	Off-White	Tablet	Circle, Scored	Roxane Laboratories
54; 302	Calcium Carbonate	1250 mg	White	Tablet	Capsule-Shape	Roxane Laboratories
54; 303	Propantheline Bromide	15 mg	White	Tablet		Roxane Laboratories
54; 310	Nefazodone Hydrochloride	200 mg	Speckled Yellow	Tablet	Oval	Roxane Laboratories
54; 310	Nefazodone Hydrochloride	200 mg	Yellow	Tablet	Oval	Roxane Laboratories
54; 323	Methotrexate	2.5 mg	Yellow	Tablet	Circle, Scored	Roxane Laboratories
54; 329	Indomethacin	50 mg	Light Green	Capsule		Roxane Laboratories
54; 333	Propranolol Hydrochloride	40 mg	White	Tablet	Circle	Roxane Laboratories
54; 339	Prednisone	2.5 mg	White	Tablet		Roxane Laboratories
54; 343	Prednisone	50 mg	White	Tablet		Roxane Laboratories
54; 346	Lithium Carbonate	450 mg	Off-White to Yellow	Extended-Release Tablet		Roxane Laboratories
54; 352	Megestrol Acetate	40 mg	White	Tablet	Circle, Scored	Roxane Laboratories
54; 353	Mirtazapine	30 mg	Biege	Tablet	Circle	Roxane Laboratories
54; 360	Amitriptyline Hydrochloride	75 mg	White	Tablet		Roxane Laboratories
54; 363	Mirtazapine	30 mg	Beige	Tablet	Circle	Roxane Laboratories
54; 369	Loperamide Hydrochloride	2 mg	Light Green	Capsule		Roxane Laboratories
54; 372	Calcium Gluconate	500 mg	White	Tablet		Roxane Laboratories
54; 382	Haloperidol	10 mg		Tablet		Roxane Laboratories
54; 383	Methyldopa	500 mg		Tablet		Roxane Laboratories
54; 392	Oxycodone and Acetaminophen	500 mg ; 5 mg		Capsule		Roxane Laboratories
54; 392	Roxilox	5 mg ; 500 mg		Capsule		Roxane Laboratories
54; 403	Hydromorphone Hydrochloride	8 mg	White	Tablet	Circle, Scored	Roxane Laboratories
54; 409; 30	Morphine Sulfate SR	30 mg	White	Sustained-Release Tablet	Circle, Scored	Roxane Laboratories
54; 410	Levorphanol Tartrate	2 mg	White	Tablet	Circle, Scored	Roxane Laboratories
54; 412	Codeine Sulfate	60 mg	White	Tablet		Roxane Laboratories
54; 422	Indomethacin	25 mg	Light Green	Capsule		Roxane Laboratories
54; 460	Cimetidine	800 mg		Tablet		Roxane Laboratories
54; 472	Piroxicam	10 mg		Capsule		Roxane Laboratories
54; 479	Piroxicam	20 mg	Dark Blue	Capsule		Roxane Laboratories
54; 482	Tamoxifen	20 mg	White	Tablet	Circle	Roxane Laboratories
54; 492	Amitriptyline Hydrochloride	150 mg	White	Tablet		Roxane Laboratories
54; 499	Hydrochlorothiazide	50 mg	Peach	Tablet		Roxane Laboratories
54; 503	Phenobarbital	15 mg	White	Tablet		Roxane Laboratories
54; 512	Alprazolam	0.25 mg	White	Tablet	Oval, Scored	Roxane Laboratories
54; 519	Triazolam	0.125 mg	White	Tablet	Oval	Roxane Laboratories
54; 523	Mexiletine Hydrochloride	150 mg		Capsule		Roxane Laboratories
54; 529	Torecan	10 mg	Yellow	Tablet		Roxane Laboratories
54; 532	Pseudoephedrine Hydrochloride	60 mg	White	Tablet		Roxane Laboratories
54; 533	Furosemide	80 mg	White	Tablet	Circle	Roxane Laboratories
54; 539	Ascorbic Acid	250 mg	White	Tablet		Roxane Laboratories
54; 549	Dolophine Hydrochloride	10 mg	White	Tablet	Circle	Roxane Laboratories
54; 570	Haloperidol	2 mg		Tablet		Roxane Laboratories
54; 572	Phenobarbital	30 mg	White	Tablet		Roxane Laboratories
54; 579	Isoxsuprine Hydrochloride	20 mg	White	Tablet		Roxane Laboratories
54; 583	Furosemide	40 mg	White	Tablet		Roxane Laboratories
54; 592	Diclofenac Sodium	50 mg	White	Timed-Release Tablet	Circle	Roxane Laboratories
54; 599	Alprazolam	0.5 mg	White	Tablet	Oval, Scored	Roxane Laboratories
54; 603	Naproxen Sodium Film-Coated	550 mg	Dark Blue	Tablet	Capsule-Shape	Roxane Laboratories
54; 612	Prednisone	5 mg	White	Tablet		Roxane Laboratories
54; 613	Codeine Sulfate	15 mg		Tablet		Roxane Laboratories
54; 620	Triazolam	0.25 mg	Light Blue	Tablet	Oval, Scored	Roxane Laboratories
54; 622	Methyldopa	250 mg		Tablet		Roxane Laboratories
54; 623	Acetaminophen and Codeine Phosphate	300 mg ; 30 mg	White	Tablet		Roxane Laboratories
54; 632	Mexiletine Hydrochloride	200 mg		Capsule		Roxane Laboratories
54; 639	Cyclophosphamide	25 mg	Light Blue	Tablet	Circle	Roxane Laboratories
54; 643	Naproxen	250 mg	Beige	Tablet	Circle	Roxane Laboratories
54; 650	Leucovorin Calcium	15 mg	Yellow	Tablet	Circle, Scored	Roxane Laboratories
54; 659	Pseudoephedrine Hydrochloride and Triprolidine Hydrochloride	60 mg ; 2.5 mg	White	Tablet		Roxane Laboratories
54; 659	Triprolidine with Pseudoephedrine Hydrochloride	60 mg ; 2.5 mg		Tablet		Roxane Laboratories
54; 680	Ascorbic Acid	500 mg	White	Tablet		Roxane Laboratories
54; 690	Haloperidol	20 mg		Tablet		Roxane Laboratories
54; 699	Niacin	50 mg	White	Tablet		Roxane Laboratories
54; 703	Imipramine Hydrochloride	50 mg	Coral	Tablet		Roxane Laboratories
54; 710	Roxicodone	15 mg	Green	Tablet		Roxane Laboratories
54; 713	Nefazodone Hydrochloride	50 mg	Peach	Tablet	Oval	Roxane Laboratories
54; 713	Nefazodone Hydrochloride	50 mg	Speckled Peach	Tablet	Oval	Roxane Laboratories
54; 730	Roxicet	5 mg ; 500 mg	White	Tablet	Capsule-Shape	Roxane Laboratories

IMPRINT	BRAND/GENERIC NAME	STRENGTH	COLOR	FORM	SHAPE	MANUFACTURER
54; 732	Diphenoxylate Hydrochloride and Atropine Sulfate	2.5 mg ; 0.025 mg	White	Tablet		Roxane Laboratories
54; 733	Morphine Sulfate	15 mg	White	Tablet		Roxane Laboratories
54; 749	Nefazodone Hydrochloride	150 mg	Peach	Tablet	Oval	Roxane Laboratories
54; 749	Nefazodone Hydrochloride	150 mg	Speckled Peach	Tablet	Oval, Scored	Roxane Laboratories
54; 760	Prednisone	20 mg	White	Tablet		Roxane Laboratories
54; 763	Megestrol Acetate	20 mg	White	Tablet	Circle, Scored	Roxane Laboratories
54; 772	Dht	0.4 mg		Tablet		Roxane Laboratories
54; 773	Haloperidol	5 mg	White	Tablet	Six-Sided, Scored	Roxane Laboratories
54; 779	Phenobarbital	60 mg	White	Tablet		Roxane Laboratories
54; 780	Tamoxifen	10 mg	White	Tablet	Circle	Roxane Laboratories
54; 783	Codeine Sulfate	30 mg	White	Tablet		Roxane Laboratories
54; 799	Cimetidine	400 mg		Tablet		Roxane Laboratories
54; 810	Propranolol Hydrochloride	90 mg	White	Tablet	Circle	Roxane Laboratories
54; 812	Hydrochlorothiazide	25 mg	Peach	Tablet		Roxane Laboratories
54; 819	Acetaminophen	650 mg	White	Tablet		Roxane Laboratories
54; 822	Sulfamethoxazole and Trimethoprim Double Strength	800 mg ; 160 mg	White	Tablet	Capsule-Shape, Scored	Roxane Laboratories
54; 823	Pseudoephedrine Hydrochloride	30 mg	White	Tablet		Roxane Laboratories
54; 833	Nefazodone Hydrochloride	250 mg	White	Tablet	Oval	Roxane Laboratories
54; 839	Diclofenac Sodium	75 mg	White	Timed-Release Tablet	Circle	Roxane Laboratories
54; 843	Methadone Hydrochloride	40 mg	White	Tablet	Square with Rounded Corners; Cross-Scored	Roxane Laboratories
54; 853	Methyldopa	125 mg		Tablet		Roxane Laboratories
54; 859	Aminophylline	100 mg	White	Tablet		Roxane Laboratories
54; 860	Alprazolam	1 mg	White	Tablet	Scored, Oval	Roxane Laboratories
54; 880	Imipramine Hydrochloride	25 mg	Coral	Tablet		Roxane Laboratories
54; 883	Methadone Hydrochloride	40 mg	Peach	Tablet		Roxane Laboratories
54; 899	Prednisone	10 mg	White	Tablet		Roxane Laboratories
54; 902	Roxiprin	4.5 mg ; 0.38 mg ; 325 mg	White	Tablet	Circle	Roxane Laboratories
54; 903	Dht	0.2 mg	Pink	Tablet		Roxane Laboratories
54; 912	Cimetidine	300 mg		Tablet		Roxane Laboratories
54; 930	Aminophylline	200 mg	White	Tablet		Roxane Laboratories
54; 932	Acetaminophen and Codeine No. 4	300 mg ; 60 mg	White	Tablet		Roxane Laboratories
54; 939	Imipramine Hydrochloride	10 mg	Coral	Tablet		Roxane Laboratories
54; 942	Leucovorin Calcium	10 mg	Off-White	Tablet	Scored, Circle	Roxane Laboratories
54; 959	Mexiletine Hydrochloride	250 mg		Tablet		Roxane Laboratories
54; 969	Diazepam	2 mg	Peach	Tablet	Scored, Circle	Roxane Laboratories
54; 970	Propranolol Hydrochloride	10 mg	White	Tablet	Circle	Roxane Laboratories
54; 972	Propoxyphene Hydrochloride	65 mg	Pink	Capsule		Roxane Laboratories
54; 973	Diazepam	5 mg	Peach	Tablet	Circle, Scored	Roxane Laboratories
54; 979	Quinidine Sulfate	200 mg	White	Tablet		Roxane Laboratories
54; 980	Cyclophosphamide	50 mg	Light Blue	Tablet	Circle	Roxane Laboratories
54; 982	Diazepam	10 mg	Peach	Tablet	Circle, Scored	Roxane Laboratories
54; 983	Amitriptyline Hydrochloride	10 mg	White	Tablet		Roxane Laboratories
54; 992	Naproxen	375 mg	Pink	Tablet	Capsule-Shape	Roxane Laboratories
54; 997	Mirtazapine	45 mg	White	Tablet	Circle	Roxane Laboratories
56 ; 9 3	Fluvoxamine Maleate	50 mg	Yellow	Tablet	Capsule-Shape	Teva Pharmaceuticals
57	Zorprin	800 mg	White	Extended-Release Tablet	Oblong	Par Pharmaceutical
57 ; 9 3	Fluvoxamine Maleate	100 mg	Pink to Light Brick	Tablet	Capsule-Shape	Teva Pharmaceuticals
60	Terazosin Hydrochloride	1 mg	Grey	Capsule		Teva Pharmaceuticals
60 ; B	Nifediac CC	60 mg	Mustard Yellow	Tablet, Extended Release	Circle	Teva Pharmaceuticals
60 ; OC	Oxycontin	60 mg	Red	Tablet, Extended Release	Circle	Purdue Pharmaceutical Products
60 MG; LILLY; 3237	Cymbalta	60 mg	Opaque Green and Opaque Blue	Capsule, Delayed Release		Eli Lilly
61	Terazosin Hydrochloride	2 mg	Yellow	Capsule		Teva Pharmaceuticals
62	Terazosin Hydrochloride	5 mg	Red	Capsule		Teva Pharmaceuticals
62.5	Tracleer	62.5 mg	Orange-White	Coated Tablet	Circle, Biconvex	Genentech
63	Terazosin Hydrochloride	10 mg	Blue	Capsule		Teva Pharmaceuticals
68; 7	Norpramin	10 mg	Blue	Tablet		Sanofi-Aventis U.S.
70	Adipex 8	8 mg	Blue and White	Tablet		Teva Pharmaceuticals
71 71 ; GEIGY	Lopressor	100 mg	Light Blue	Tablet	Capsule-Shape	Novartis
72 ; 93	Fluvoxamine Maleate	25 mg	White	Tablet	Capsule-Shape	Teva Pharmaceuticals
72 81 ; 9 3	Oxcarbazepine	150 mg	Brown to Dark Brown	Tablet	Capsule-Shape	Teva Pharmaceuticals
72 82 ; 9 3	Oxcarbazepine	300 mg	Brown to Dark Brown	Tablet	Capsule-Shape	Teva Pharmaceuticals
73 ; 93	Zolpidem Tartrate	5 mg	Pink	Tablet	Circle	Teva Pharmaceuticals
74 ; 93	Zolpidem Tartrate	10 mg	White to Off-White	Tablet	Circle	Teva Pharmaceuticals
74; XX	Potassium Chloride	750 mg	Light Brown	Tablet	Oval	Abbott Laboratories
75	Levoxyl	75 mcg	Purple	Tablet	Oval	King Pharmaceuticals
75	Slo-Bid Gyrocaps	75 mg	White and Clear	Extended-Release Capsule		Aventis Pharmaceuticals
75 MG ; RSN	Actonel	75 mg	Pink	Tablet	Oval	Procter & Gamble Pharmaceuticals
75 MG 93 813	Nortriptyline Hydrochloride	75 mg	Orange	Capsule		Teva Pharmaceuticals
75; T4	Levothroid	75 mcg	Violet	Tablet	Capsule-Shape	Forest Pharmaceuticals
77	Alendronate Sodium	35 mg	White	Tablet	Oval	Watson Pharma
77; BONE IMAGE	Fosamax	35 mg	White	Tablet	Oval	Merck
78/27	Belladenal-S	0.25 mg ; 50 mg	Multi-Colored	Tablet	Cross-Scored	Novartis Pharmaceuticals
78/212; 10 ;	Metaprel	10 mg	White	Tablet	Circle, Compressed	Novartis Pharmaceuticals
78/213; 20	Metaprel	20 mg	White	Tablet	Circle, Compressed	Novartis Pharmaceuticals
78; 28 ;	Belladenal	0.25 mg ; 50 mg	White	Tablet	Cross-Scored	Novartis Pharmaceuticals
78; 31	Bellergal-S	40 mg ; 0.6 mg ; 0.2 mg	Dark Green, Orange, Yellow	Tablet	Circle, Compressed	Novartis
78; 52; SANDOZ S ;	Mesantoin	100 mg	Pink	Tablet		Novartis Pharmaceuticals

IMPRINT	BRAND/GENERIC NAME	STRENGTH	COLOR	FORM	SHAPE	MANUFACTURER
80 ; ABG	Oxycodone Hydrochloride	80 mg	Green	Controlled-Release Tablet	Circle	Ivax Pharmaceuticals
80 ; ABG	Oxycodone Hydrochloride Controlled-Release	80 mg	Green	Controlled Release Tablet	Circle	Ivax Pharmaceuticals
80 ; E710	Oxycodone Hydrochloride	80 mg	Green	Tablet, Extended Release	Circle	Endo Generics
80 ; MYLAN 232	Furosemide	80 mg	White	Tablet	Circle	Mylan Pharmaceuticals
80 ; OC	Oxycontin	80 mg	Green	Tablet, Extended Release	Circle	Purdue Pharmaceutical Products
80 ; PD 158	Lipitor	80 mg	White	Tablet	Circle	Pfizer
80 INNOPRANXL LOGO	Innopran XL	80 mg	Gray, White	Capsule, Extended Release		Glaxosmithkline
80MG ; GSK COREG CR	Coreg Cr	80 mg	White	Capsule, Extended Release		Glaxosmithkline
83 ; BI	Mirapex	0.125 mg	White	Tablet	Circle	Boehringer Ingelheim Pharmaceuticals
83 ; STUARTNATAL LOGO	Duet Chewable by Stuartnatal	3000 IU ; 120 mg ; 400 IU ; 30 mg ; 1.8 mg ; 4 mg ; 20 mg ; 25 mg ; 1 mg ; 12 mcg ; 100 mg ; 29 mg ; 25 mg ; 25 mg ; 2 mg	Mottled Orange	Tablet, Chewable	Heart-Shape	Xanodyne Pharmaceuticals
84 ; R	Alprazolam	1 mg	Yellow	Tablet, Extended Release	Circle	Actavis Elizabeth
84 84 ; BI BI	Mirapex	0.25 mg	White	Tablet	Oval	Boehringer Ingelheim Pharmaceuticals
85 85 ; BI BI	Mirapex	0.5 mg	White	Tablet	Oval	Boehringer Ingelheim Pharmaceuticals
85; 05; M	Flecainide Acetate	50 mg	Round	Tablet	Circle, White	Mylan Pharmaceuticals
85; 10; M	Flecainide Acetate	100 mg	White	Tablet	Circle	Mylan Pharmaceuticals
85; 15; M	Flecainide Acetate	150 mg	White	Tablet	Capsule-Shape	Mylan Pharmaceuticals
86 ; R	Alprazolam	3 mg	Light Green	Tablet, Extended Release	Circle	Actavis Elizabeth
86; 62; C ;	Skelaxin	400 mg	Pale Rose	Tablet	Circle, Scored	King Pharmaceuticals
86; 67; S ;	Skelaxin	800 mg	Pink	Tablet	Oval, Scored	King Pharmaceuticals
87	Terramycin with Polymyxin B Sulfate	100 mg ; 100000 U	Yellow	Tablet		Pfizer
87 ; R	Alprazolam	2 mg	Peach	Tablet, Extended Release	Circle	Actavis Elizabeth
88	Levoxyl	88 mcg	Olive	Tablet	Oval	King Pharmaceuticals
88; T4	Levothroid	88 mcg	Mint Green	Tablet	Capsule-Shape	Forest Pharmaceuticals
90 ; B	Nifediac CC	90 mg	Yellow	Tablet, Extended Release	Circle	Teva Pharmaceuticals
90 90 ; BI BI	Mirapex	1 mg	White	Tablet	Circle	Boehringer Ingelheim Pharmaceuticals
91 91 ; BI BI	Mirapex	1.5 mg	White	Tablet	Circle	Boehringer Ingelheim Pharmaceuticals
93	Actihist	2.5 mg ; 60 mg	White	Tablet		Paddock Labs
93 42	Fluoxetine Hydrochloride	10 mg	Powder Blue	Capsule		Teva Pharmaceuticals
93 ; 24 ;	Oxycodone Hydrochloride Extended Release	10 mg	White	Tablet, Extended Release	Oval	Teva Pharmaceuticals
93 ; 31 ;	Oxycodone Hydrochloride Extended Release	20 mg	Pink	Tablet, Extended Release	Oval	Teva Pharmaceuticals
93 ; 32 ;	Oxycodone Hydrochloride Extended Release	40 mg	Yellow	Tablet, Extended Release	Oval	Teva Pharmaceuticals
93 ; 33 ;	Oxycodone Hydrochloride Extended Release	80 mg	Green	Tablet, Extended Release	Oval	Teva Pharmaceuticals
93 ; 83	Amlodipine Besylate	2.5 mg	White to Off-White	Tablet	Circle	Teva Pharmaceuticals
93 ; 688	Lamotrigine	5 mg	White to Off-White	Tablet, Chewable	Circle	Teva Pharmaceuticals
93 ; 1077	Cefprozil	250 mg	Light Orange	Tablet	Circle	Teva Pharmaceuticals
93 ; 1078	Cefprozil	500 mg	White	Tablet	Capsule-Shape	Teva Pharmaceuticals
93 ; 4740	Citalopram Hydrobromide	10 mg	Light Beige	Tablet	Capsule-Shape	Teva Pharmaceuticals
93 ; 5150	Moexipril Hydrochloride	15 mg	Pink	Tablet	Oval	Teva Pharmaceuticals
93 ; 5510 ;	Mercaptopurine	50 mg	Pale Yellow to Buff	Tablet	Circle	Teva Pharmaceuticals
93 ; 7152	Simvastatin	5 mg	Light Yellow	Tablet	Circle	Teva Pharmaceuticals
93 ; 7153	Simvastatin	10 mg	Light Pink	Tablet	Circle	Teva Pharmaceuticals
93 ; 7154	Simvastatin	20 mg	Tan	Tablet	Circle	Teva Pharmaceuticals
93 ; 7155	Simvastatin	40 mg	Red	Tablet	Circle	Teva Pharmaceuticals
93 ; 7156	Simvastatin	80 mg	Brick Red	Tablet	Capsule-Shape	Teva Pharmaceuticals
93 ; 7168	Amlodipine Besylate	10 mg	White to Off-White	Tablet	Circle	Teva Pharmaceuticals
93 ; 7254 ;	Glimepiride	1 mg	Mottled Pink	Tablet	Circle	Teva Pharmaceuticals
93 ; 7255 ;	Glimepiride	2 mg	Mottled Green	Tablet	Circle	Teva Pharmaceuticals
93 ; 7256 ;	Glimepiride	4 mg	Mottled Light Blue	Tablet	Circle	Teva Pharmaceuticals
93 ; 7296	Carvedilol	25 mg	White	Tablet	Oval	Teva Pharmaceuticals
93 ; 8117	Famciclovir	125 mg	White	Tablet	Circle	Teva Pharmaceuticals
93 ; 8118	Famciclovir	250 mg	White	Tablet	Circle	Teva Pharmaceuticals
93 ; 8119	Famciclovir	500 mg	White	Tablet	Capsule-Shape	Teva Pharmaceuticals
93 068	Meprobamate	200 mg		Tablet		Teva Pharmaceuticals
93 069	Meprobamate	400 mg		Tablet		Teva Pharmaceuticals
93 11; 2	Aspirin and Codeine No. 2	325 mg ; 15 mg	White	Tablet	Circle, Convex	Teva Pharmaceuticals
93 39	Gabapentin	300 mg	Orange	Capsule		Teva Pharmaceuticals
93 40	Gabapentin	400 mg	Caramel	Capsule		Teva Pharmaceuticals
93 43	Fluoxetine Hydrochloride	20 mg	Powder Blue	Capsule		Teva Pharmaceuticals
93 76	Isosorbide Mononitrate	20 mg	Yellow	Tablet	Circle	Teva Pharmaceuticals
93 93 852	Metronidazole	500 mg	White	Tablet	Oblong	Teva Pharmaceuticals
93 129	Estazolam	1 mg	White	Tablet	Oval	Teva Pharmaceuticals
93 130	Estazolam	2 mg	Coral	Tablet	Oval	Teva Pharmaceuticals
93 208	Galzin	50 mg	Opaque Orange	Capsule, Liquid Filled		Gate Pharmaceuticals

IMPRINT	BRAND/GENERIC NAME	STRENGTH	COLOR	FORM	SHAPE	MANUFACTURER
93 215	Galzin	25 mg	Opaque Aqua Blue	Capsule, Liquid Filled		Gate Pharmaceuticals
93 294 ;	Carbidopa and Levodopa	25 mg ; 250 mg	Blue, Mottled Blue	Tablet	Circle	Teva Pharmaceuticals
93 490	Propoxyphene Napsylate and Acetaminophen - White Tablets	100 mg ; 650 mg	White	Tablet	Oblong	Teva Pharmaceuticals
93 752	Atenolol	50 mg	White	Tablet	Circle	Teva Pharmaceuticals
93 753	Atenolol	100 mg	White	Tablet	Circle	Teva Pharmaceuticals
93 778	Carbamazepine	100 mg	Pink, Red	Tablet, Chewable	Circle	Teva Pharmaceuticals
93 782	Tamoxifen Citrate	20 mg	White to Off-White	Tablet	Circle	Teva Pharmaceuticals
93 784	Tamoxifen Citrate	10 mg	White	Tablet	Circle	Teva Pharmaceuticals
93 851	Metronidazole	250 mg	White	Tablet	Circle	Teva Pharmaceuticals
93 890	Propoxyphene Napsylate and Acetaminophen - Pink Tablets	100 mg ; 650 mg	Pink	Tablet	Oblong	Teva Pharmaceuticals
93 1036	Hydrochlorothiazide and Lisinopril	12.5 mg ; 20 mg	White	Tablet	Circle	Teva Pharmaceuticals
93 1037	Hydrochlorothiazide and Lisinopril	25 mg ; 20 mg	Peach	Tablet	Circle	Teva Pharmaceuticals
93 3145	Cephalexin	250 mg	Gray, Swedish Orange	Capsule		Teva Pharmaceuticals
93 3147	Cephalexin	500 mg	Swedish Orange	Capsule		Teva Pharmaceuticals
93 3160	Cefdinir	300 mg	Lavender-Opaque, Light Green -Opaque	Capsule		Teva Pharmaceuticals
93 3196	Cefadroxil	500 mg	Orange Opaque, White Opaque	Capsule	Capsule-Shape	Teva Pharmaceuticals
93 4067	Prazosin Hydrochloride	1 mg	Ivory Opaque	Capsule		Teva Pharmaceuticals
93 4068	Prazosin Hydrochloride	2 mg	Pink Opaque	Capsule		Teva Pharmaceuticals
93 4069	Prazosin Hydrochloride	5 mg	Blue	Capsule		Teva Pharmaceuticals
93 5268	Zaleplon	5 mg	Opaque Blue Green, Opaque White	Capsule		Teva Pharmaceuticals
93 5269	Zaleplon	10 mg	Opaque Aqua Blue, Opaque Blue Green	Capsule		Teva Pharmaceuticals
93 7162	Zonisamide	100 mg	Flesh Colored Opaque, Pink Opaque	Capsule		Teva Pharmaceuticals
93 7198	Fluoxetine Hydrochloride	40 mg	Blue, Orange	Capsule		Teva Pharmaceuticals
93 7225	Selfemra	10 mg	Purple	Capsule		Teva Pharmaceuticals
93 7226	Selfemra	20 mg	Flesh, Purple	Capsule		Teva Pharmaceuticals
93 7435	Ramipril	1.25 mg	Rich Yellow Opaque	Capsule		Teva Pharmaceuticals
93 7436	Ramipril	2.5 mg	Light Orange Opaque	Capsule		Teva Pharmaceuticals
93 7437	Ramipril	5 mg	Pink Opaque	Capsule		Teva Pharmaceuticals
93 7438	Ramipril	10 mg	Powder Blue Opaque	Capsule		Teva Pharmaceuticals
93 7439	Divalproex Sodium	125 mg	Reddish-Brown	Tablet, Delayed Release	Oval	Teva Pharmaceuticals
93 7440	Divalproex Sodium	250 mg	Beige	Tablet, Delayed Release	Oval	Teva Pharmaceuticals
93 7441	Divalproex Sodium	500 mg	Dark Pink	Tablet, Delayed Release	Oval	Teva Pharmaceuticals
93 7508	Zonisamide	25 mg	White Opaque	Capsule		Teva Pharmaceuticals
93 7509	Zonisamide	50 mg	Iron Gray Opaque	Capsule		Teva Pharmaceuticals
93 9133	Amiodarone Hydrochloride	200 mg	Pink	Tablet	Circle	Teva Pharmaceuticals
93 9380	Ursodiol	300 mg	Red Opaque, White Opaque	Capsule		Teva Pharmaceuticals
93/11	Pantoprazole Sodium	20 mg	Yellow	Tablet, Delayed Release	Oval	Teva Pharmaceuticals
93/12	Pantoprazole Sodium	40 mg	Yellow	Tablet, Delayed Release	Oval	Teva Pharmaceuticals
93; 027	Dipyridamole	25 mg		Tablet		Teva Pharmaceuticals
93; 088	Sulfamethoxazole and Trimethoprim	400 mg ; 80 mg	White	Tablet	Circle, Convex, Scored	Teva Pharmaceuticals
93; 089	Sulfamethoxazole and Trimethoprim Double Strength	800 mg ; 160 mg	White	Tablet	Oval, Convex, Scored	Teva Pharmaceuticals
93; 5	Naproxen Delayed-Release	375 mg	White	Enteric-Coated Tablet	Capsule-Shape	Teva Pharmaceuticals
93; 6	Naproxen Delayed-Release	500 mg	White	Enteric-Coated Tablet	Capsule-Shape	Teva Pharmaceuticals
93; 7	Chlorpropamide	250 mg	Blue	Tablet	Circle, Convex, Scored	Teva Pharmaceuticals
93; 8	Indapamide	2.5 mg	White	Coated Tablet	Circle	Teva Pharmaceuticals
93; 10	Chlorpropamide	100 mg	Blue	Tablet	Circle, Convex, Scored	Teva Pharmaceuticals
93; 12; 3	Aspirin and Codeine No. 3	325 mg ; 30 mg	White	Tablet	Convex, Circle	Teva Pharmaceuticals
93; 13; 4	Aspirin and Codeine No. 4	325 mg ; 60 mg	White	Tablet	Circle, Convex	Teva Pharmaceuticals
93; 16	Nabumetone	750 mg	Beige	Tablet	Oval	Teva Pharmaceuticals
93; 21	Diltiazem ER	60 mg	Pink and White	Extended-Release Capsule		Teva Pharmaceuticals
93; 22	Diltiazem ER	90 mg	Pink and Yellow	Extended-Release Capsule		Teva Pharmaceuticals
93; 23	Diltiazem ER	120 mg	Pink and Orange	Extended-Release Capsule		Teva Pharmaceuticals
93; 26	Enalapril Maleate	2.5 mg	Yellow	Tablet	Oval, Scored	Teva Pharmaceuticals
93; 27	Enalapril Maleate	5 mg	White	Tablet	Oval, Scored	Teva Pharmaceuticals
93; 28	Enalapril Maleate	10 mg		Tablet		Teva Pharmaceuticals
93; 29	Enalapril Maleate	20 mg	Orange	Tablet	Oblong	Teva Pharmaceuticals
93; 41	Clomiphene Citrate	50 mg	White	Tablet	Circle, Flat, Beveled Edge, Scored	Teva Pharmaceuticals
93; 53	Buspirone Hydrochloride	5 mg		Tablet		Teva Pharmaceuticals
93; 54	Buspirone Hydrochloride	10 mg		Tablet		Teva Pharmaceuticals
93; 58	Tramadol Hydrochloride	50 mg	White	Tablet	Oval	Teva Pharmaceuticals
93; 61	Sotalol Hydrochloride	80 mg	Light Blue	Tablet	Oblong	Teva Pharmaceuticals
93; 62	Sotalol Hydrochloride	160 mg	Light Blue	Tablet	Oval, Scored	Teva Pharmaceuticals
93; 63	Sotalol Hydrochloride	240 mg	Light Blue	Tablet	Oval, Scored	Teva Pharmaceuticals
93; 91	Captopril	12.5 mg	White	Tablet	Oval, Scored	Teva Pharmaceuticals
93; 92	Captopril	25 mg	White	Tablet	Round, Quadrisected Scored	Teva Pharmaceuticals
93; 97	Captopril	50 mg	White	Tablet	Circle, Scored	Teva Pharmaceuticals
93; 98	Captopril	100 mg	White	Tablet	Circle, Scored	Teva Pharmaceuticals
93; 100	Labetalol Hydrochloride	100 mg		Tablet		Teva Pharmaceuticals
93; 102	Labetalol Hydrochloride	200 mg		Tablet		Teva Pharmaceuticals
93; 106	Labetalol Hydrochloride	300 mg		Tablet		Teva Pharmaceuticals
93; 111	Cimetidine	200 mg	White	Coated Tablet	Circle	Teva Pharmaceuticals
93; 112	Cimetidine	300 mg	White	Coated Tablet	Circle	Teva Pharmaceuticals
93; 113	Cimetidine	400 mg	White	Coated Tablet	Oblong, Scored	Teva Pharmaceuticals
93; 115	Haloperidol	0.5 mg	White	Tablet	Circle	Teva Pharmaceuticals
93; 116	Haloperidol	1 mg	Yellow	Tablet	Circle	Teva Pharmaceuticals

IMPRINT	BRAND/GENERIC NAME	STRENGTH	COLOR	FORM	SHAPE	MANUFACTURER
93; 117	Haloperidol	2 mg	Pink	Tablet	Circle	Teva Pharmaceuticals
93; 118	Haloperidol	5 mg	Green	Tablet	Circle	Teva Pharmaceuticals
93; 122	Cimetidine	800 mg	White	Coated Tablet	Oblong, Scored	Teva Pharmaceuticals
93; 132	Acetaminophen and Codeine No. 2	300 mg ; 15 mg	Carmel Opaque and White	Capsule		Teva Pharmaceuticals
93; 138	Diphenhydramine Hydrochloride	25 mg	Pink Transparent and Clear	Capsule		Teva Pharmaceuticals
93; 139	Diphenhydramine Hydrochloride	50 mg	Pink Transparent	Capsule		Teva Pharmaceuticals
93; 147	Naproxen	250 mg	Mottled Light Brick Red	Tablet	Circle, Biconvex	Teva Pharmaceuticals
93; 148	Naproxen	375 mg	Mottled Peach	Tablet	Oval	Teva Pharmaceuticals
93; 149	Naproxen	500 mg	Mottled Light Brick Red	Tablet	Oval	Teva Pharmaceuticals
93; 152	Acetaminophen and Codeine No. 3	300 mg ; 30 mg	Coral and Scarlet, Opaque	Capsule		Teva Pharmaceuticals
93; 153	Phendimetrazine Tartrate	35 mg	Pink	Tablet	Oblong	Teva Pharmaceuticals
93; 154	Ticlopidine Hydrochloride	250 mg	White	Tablet	Oval	Teva Pharmaceuticals
93; 157	Diethylpropion Hydrochloride	25 mg	White	Tablet	Circle, Flat Beveled Edge	Teva Pharmaceuticals
93; 172	Acetaminophen and Codeine No. 4	300 mg ; 60 mg	Brown and Iron Gray, Opaque	Capsule		Teva Pharmaceuticals
93; 176	Captopril and Hydrochlorothiazide	25 mg ; 15 mg	White	Tablet	Round, Quadrisected Scored	Teva Pharmaceuticals
93; 177	Captopril and Hydrochlorothiazide	25 mg ; 25 mg	Tan	Tablet	Round, Quadrisected Scored	Teva Pharmaceuticals
93; 181	Captopril and Hydrochlorothiazide	50 mg ; 15 mg	White	Tablet	Oval, Scored	Teva Pharmaceuticals
93; 182	Captopril and Hydrochlorothiazide	50 mg ; 25 mg	Tan	Tablet	Oval, Scored	Teva Pharmaceuticals
93; 205; LEMMON	Donphen	0.02 mg ; 0.1 mg ; 15 mg ; 6 mcg	Pink	Tablet	Circle, Convex, Scored	Teva Pharmaceuticals
93; 214	Tolmetin Sodium	600 mg	Orange	Tablet	Oblong	Teva Pharmaceuticals
93; 280	Bupropion Hydrochloride	75 mg	Yellow	Coated Tablet	Circle	Teva Pharmaceuticals
93; 290	Bupropion Hydrochloride	100 mg		Coated Tablet		Teva Pharmaceuticals
93; 292	Carbidopa and Levodopa	10 mg ; 100 mg	Mottled Blue	Tablet	Circle	Teva Pharmaceuticals
93; 293	Carbidopa and Levodopa	25 mg ; 100 mg	Mottled Yellow	Tablet	Scored, Circle	Teva Pharmaceuticals
93; 307	Clemastine Fumarate	1.34 mg	White	Tablet	Circle, Convex, Scored	Teva Pharmaceuticals
93; 308	Clemastine Fumarate	2.68 mg	White	Tablet	Circle, Convex, Scored	Teva Pharmaceuticals
93; 318	Diltiazem Hydrochloride	30 mg	Faint Orange	Coated Tablet	Circle, Biconvex	Teva Pharmaceuticals
93; 319	Diltiazem Hydrochloride	60 mg	Orange	Coated Tablet	Circle, Biconvex, Scored	Teva Pharmaceuticals
93; 320	Diltiazem Hydrochloride	90 mg	Faint Orange	Coated Tablet	Oblong, Scored	Teva Pharmaceuticals
93; 321	Diltiazem Hydrochloride	120 mg	Orange	Coated Tablet	Oblong, Scored	Teva Pharmaceuticals
93; 431	Chlorthalidone	50 mg	Blue	Tablet	Circle, Flat, Beveled Edge	Teva Pharmaceuticals
93; 433	Chlorthalidone	100 mg	White	Tablet	Circle, Flat Beveled Edge, Scored	Teva Pharmaceuticals
93; 494	Clonidine Hydrochloride	0.1 mg	Green	Tablet	Circle	Teva Pharmaceuticals
93; 495	Clonidine Hydrochloride	0.2 mg	Yellow	Tablet		Teva Pharmaceuticals
93; 496	Clonidine Hydrochloride	0.3 mg	Peach	Tablet	Circle	Teva Pharmaceuticals
93; 525	Amitriptyline Hydrochloride	10 mg	Pink	Coated Tablet	Circle, Biconvex	Teva Pharmaceuticals
93; 527	Amitriptyline Hydrochloride	25 mg	Green	Coated Tablet	Circle, Biconvex	Teva Pharmaceuticals
93; 529	Amitriptyline Hydrochloride	50 mg	Brown	Coated Tablet	Circle, Biconvex	Teva Pharmaceuticals
93; 531	Amitriptyline Hydrochloride	75 mg	Purple	Coated Tablet	Circle, Biconvex	Teva Pharmaceuticals
93; 533	Amitriptyline Hydrochloride	100 mg	Orange	Coated Tablet	Circle, Biconvex	Teva Pharmaceuticals
93; 535	Amitriptyline Hydrochloride	150 mg	Peach	Coated Tablet	Circle, Biconvex	Teva Pharmaceuticals
93; 536	Naproxen Sodium	275 mg	White to Off-White	Coated Tablet	Oval	Teva Pharmaceuticals
93; 537	Naproxen Sodium	550 mg	White to Off-White	Coated Tablet	Oval	Teva Pharmaceuticals
93; 539	Mepro Compound	150 mg ; 250 mg ; 75 mg		Tablet	Three-Layered	Teva Pharmaceuticals
93; 542	Chlorzoxazone	500 mg	White	Tablet	Oblong, Scored, Convex	Teva Pharmaceuticals
93; 545	Chlorzoxazone and Acetaminophen	300 mg ; 250 mg	Light Green	Tablet	Circle, Flat, Beveled Edge, Scored	Teva Pharmaceuticals
93; 576	Lovastatin	20 mg	Blue	Tablet	Circle	Teva Pharmaceuticals
93; 585	Indo-Lemmon	25 mg	Light Green Opaque	Capsule		Teva Pharmaceuticals
93; 587	Indo-Lemmon	50 mg	Light Green Opaque	Capsule		Teva Pharmaceuticals
93; 613	Amoxicillin	250 mg	Carmel and Ivory, Opaque	Capsule		Teva Pharmaceuticals
93; 615	Amoxicillin	500 mg	Ivory Opaque	Capsule		Teva Pharmaceuticals
93; 617	Chlordinum Sealets	5 mg ; 2.5 mg	White Opaque	Capsule		Teva Pharmaceuticals
93; 620	Propranolol Hydrochloride	20 mg	Blue	Tablet	Circle, Scored	Teva Pharmaceuticals
93; 637	Trazodone Hydrochloride	50 mg	White to Off-White	Tablet	Circle	Teva Pharmaceuticals
93; 638	Trazodone Hydrochloride	100 mg	White to Off-White	Tablet	Circle	Teva Pharmaceuticals
93; 640	Propranolol Hydrochloride	40 mg	Green	Tablet	Scored, Circle	Teva Pharmaceuticals
93; 653	Doxycycline Hyclate	100 mg	Aqua Blue Opaque	Capsule		Teva Pharmaceuticals
93; 657	Calcitriol	0.25 mcg	Red-Brown, Yellow-Brown	Capsule, Liquid Filled	Oval	Teva Pharmaceuticals
93; 658	Calcitriol	0.5 mcg	Brown and Pink	Capsule, Liquid Filled	Oval	Teva Pharmaceuticals
93; 665	Albuterol Sulfate	2 mg	White	Tablet	Circle, Scored	Teva Pharmaceuticals
93; 666	Albuterol	4 mg	White	Tablet	Circle, Scored	Teva Pharmaceuticals
93; 670	Gemcor	600 mg	White to Off-White	Coated Tablet	Oval, Scored	Upsher-Smith Laboratories
93; 670	Gemfibrozil	600 mg	White	Tablet	Oval	Teva Pharmaceuticals
93; 686	Propoxyphene Compound	389 mg ; 32.4 mg ; 65 mg	Gray and Red	Capsule		Teva Pharmaceuticals
93; 711	Flurbiprofen	100 mg	Deep Sky Blue	Coated Tablet	Circle, Convex	Teva Pharmaceuticals
93; 727	Papaverine Hydrochloride	150 mg	Brown and Clear	Timed-Release Capsule		Teva Pharmaceuticals
93; 728	Sulindac	150 mg	Yellow	Tablet	Circle, Convex	Teva Pharmaceuticals
93; 729	Sulindac	200 mg	Yellow	Tablet	Circle, Convex, Scored	Teva Pharmaceuticals
93; 741; 93; 741	Propoxyphene Hydrochloride	65 mg	Opaque Pink	Capsule		Teva Pharmaceuticals
93; 742	Doxy-Lemmon	50 mg	White and Aqua Blue, Opaque	Capsule		Teva Pharmaceuticals
93; 742	Doxycycline Hyclate	50 mg	White and Aqua Blue, Opaque	Capsule		Teva Pharmaceuticals

IMPRINT	BRAND/GENERIC NAME	STRENGTH	COLOR	FORM	SHAPE	MANUFACTURER
93; 743	Doxy-Lemmon	50 mg	Aqua Blue Opaque	Capsule		Teva Pharmaceuticals
93; 754	Diflunisal	250 mg	Blue/lavender	Tablet	Capsule-Shape	Teva Pharmaceuticals
93; 755	Diflunisal	500 mg	Blue	Coated Tablet	Oblong	Teva Pharmaceuticals
93; 756	Piroxicam	10 mg	Dark Green and Olive	Capsule		Teva Pharmaceuticals
93; 757	Piroxicam	20 mg	Dark Green	Capsule		Teva Pharmaceuticals
93; 777	Hydrochlorothiazide	25 mg	Peach	Tablet	Circle, Flat, Beveled Edge, Scored	Teva Pharmaceuticals
93; 779	Hydrochlorothiazide	50 mg	Peach	Tablet	Circle, Flat, Beveled Edge, Scored	Teva Pharmaceuticals
93; 788	Selegiline Hydrochloride	5 mg	White to Off-White	Tablet	Circle, Flat, Beveled Edge	Teva Pharmaceuticals
93; 793	Nicardipine	20 mg	Opaque White and Aqua Blue	Capsule, Liquid Filled		Teva Pharmaceuticals
93; 794	Nicardipine	30 mg	Opaque White and Light Blue	Capsule, Liquid Filled		Teva Pharmaceuticals
93; 798	Indomethacin	25 mg	Light Green Opaque	Capsule		Teva Pharmaceuticals
93; 799	Indomethacin	50 mg	Light Green Opaque	Capsule		Teva Pharmaceuticals
93; 802	Antispasmodic	16.2 mg ; 0.1037 mg ; 0.0194 mg ; 0.0065 mg	Transparent Green and Clear	Capsule		Teva Pharmaceuticals
93; 804	Phentermine Hydrochloride Black and Scarlet	30 mg	Black and Scarlet, Opaque	Capsule		Teva Pharmaceuticals
93; 808	Phentermine Hydrochloride	8 mg	Green	Tablet	Circle	Teva Pharmaceuticals
93; 809	Phentermine Hydrochloride	8 mg	Peach	Tablet	Circle	Teva Pharmaceuticals
93; 816	Belladonna Alkaloids with Phenobarbital	0.1037 mg ; 0.0194 mg ; 0.0065 mg ; 16.2 mg	White	Tablet	Circle, Convex, Scored	Teva Pharmaceuticals
93; 821	Reserpine	0.25 mg	White	Tablet	Circle, Flat, Beveled Edge, Scored	Teva Pharmaceuticals
93; 823	Uridon	0.03 mg ; 50 mg ; 5.5 mg ; 20 mg ; 5 mg ; 0.03 mg	Blue	Coated Tablet		Teva Pharmaceuticals
93; 824	Pseudoephedrine Hydrochloride	60 mg	White	Tablet	Circle, Convex	Teva Pharmaceuticals
93; 827	Reserpine	0.1 mg	White	Tablet	Circle, Flat, Beveled Edge, Scored	Teva Pharmaceuticals
93; 828	Urinary Anteseptic No. 3	7.5 mg ; 0.06 mg ; 0.03 mg ; 120 mg ; 6 mg ; 30 mg	Blue	Coated Tablet	Circle	Teva Pharmaceuticals
93; 828	Uritin	7.5 mg ; 0.06 mg ; 0.03 mg ; 120 mg ; 30 mg ; 6 mg		Tablet		Teva Pharmaceuticals
93; 832	Clonazepam	0.5 mg	Yellow	Tablet	Circle, Single-Scored	Teva Pharmaceuticals
93; 833	Clonazepam	1 mg	Mottled Green	Tablet	Circle, Single-Scored	Teva Pharmaceuticals
93; 834	Clonazepam	2 mg	White to Off-White	Tablet	Circle, Single-Scored	Teva Pharmaceuticals
93; 838	Dicyclomine Hydrochloride with Phenobarbital	10 mg ; 15 mg	Blue and Clear	Capsule		Teva Pharmaceuticals
93; 841	Dicyclomine Hydrochloride	10 mg	Blue Transparent	Capsule		Teva Pharmaceuticals
93; 845	Atrosept	18.1 mg ; 4.5 mg ; 5.4 mg ; 0.03 mg ; 0.03 mg ; 40.8 mg	Dark Blue	Coated Tablet	Circle	Teva Pharmaceuticals
93; 845	Urinary Antiseptic No. 2	0.03 mg ; 0.03 mg ; 40.8 mg ; 5.4 mg ; 18.1 mg ; 4.5 mg	Purple	Coated Tablet	Circle	Teva Pharmaceuticals
93; 845	Uroblue	4.5 mg ; 0.03 mg ; 0.03 mg ; 40.8 mg ; 5.4 mg ; 18.1 mg	Purple	Tablet		Teva Pharmaceuticals
93; 846	Belladonna Extract and Phenobarbital	0.25 Gr ; 0.167 Gr	Green	Tablet	Circle	Teva Pharmaceuticals
93; 848	Triphed	60 mg ; 2.5 mg	White	Tablet	Circle, Convex, Scored	Teva Pharmaceuticals
93; 853	Phentermine Hydrochloride	30 mg	Blue and Clear with Blue and White Pellets	Capsule		Teva Pharmaceuticals
93; 858	VI-Forte	80 mg ; 70 mg ; 25 mg ; 10 mg ; 10 mg ; 5 mg ; 4 mg ; 2 mg ; 12500 IU ; 50 IU ; 150 mg	Black and Orange	Capsule		Teva Pharmaceuticals
93; 859	Phentermine Hydrochloride	30 mg	Brown and Clear with Orange and White Pellets	Capsule		Teva Pharmaceuticals
93; 860	Phentermine Hydrochloride Yellow	30 mg	Yellow Opaque	Capsule		Teva Pharmaceuticals
93; 861	Phentermine Hydrochloride	8 mg	Yellow	Capsule		Teva Pharmaceuticals
93; 862	Phentermine Hydrochloride	8 mg	Black	Capsule		Teva Pharmaceuticals
93; 866	Phendimetrazine Tartrate	35 mg	Black	Capsule		Teva Pharmaceuticals
93; 867	Phendimetrazine Tartrate	35 mg	Brown and Clear	Capsule		Teva Pharmaceuticals
93; 868	Phendimetrazine Tartrate	30 mg	Red and Yellow	Capsule		Teva Pharmaceuticals
93; 869	Phendimetrazine Tartrate	35 mg	Green and Clear	Capsule		Teva Pharmaceuticals
93; 872	Butabarbital Sodium	15 mg	Purple	Tablet	Circle, Convex, Scored	Teva Pharmaceuticals
93; 873	Butabarbital Sodium	30 mg	Green	Tablet	Circle, Convex, Scored	Teva Pharmaceuticals
93; 882	Phentermine Hydrochloride	15 mg	Gray and Yellow	Capsule		Teva Pharmaceuticals
93; 886	Drummergal	20 mg ; 0.3 mg ; 0.1 mg	Tan	Coated Tablet	Circle	Teva Pharmaceuticals
93; 886	Ergobel	0.3 mg ; 0.1 mg ; 20 mg		Tablet		Teva Pharmaceuticals
93; 888	Phentermine Hydrochloride Black	30 mg	Black Opaque	Capsule		Teva Pharmaceuticals
93; 891	Dicyclomine Hydrochloride	20 mg	Blue	Tablet	Circle, Flat Beveled Edge	Teva Pharmaceuticals
93; 892	Etodolac	400 mg	Pink	Tablet	Capsule-Shape	Teva Pharmaceuticals
93; 896	Famotidine	20 mg	Beige	Tablet	Circle	Teva Pharmaceuticals
93; 897	Famotidine	40 mg	Tan	Tablet	Circle	Teva Pharmaceuticals
93; 899	Phentermine Hydrochloride	30 mg	Red and Yellow	Capsule		Teva Pharmaceuticals
93; 900	Ketoconazole	200 mg	White	Tablet	Circle	Teva Pharmaceuticals
93; 911; 10	Isoxsuprine Hydrochloride	10 mg	White	Tablet	Convex, Circle	Teva Pharmaceuticals
93; 913; 20	Isoxsuprine Hydrochloride	20 mg	White	Tablet	Circle, Convex, Scored	Teva Pharmaceuticals

IMPRINT	BRAND/GENERIC NAME	STRENGTH	COLOR	FORM	SHAPE	MANUFACTURER
93; 926	Lovastatin	10 mg		Tablet		Teva Pharmaceuticals
93; 928	Lovastatin	40 mg		Tablet		Teva Pharmaceuticals
93; 943	Nystatin	100,000 units	Light Yellow	Tablet	Diamond	Teva Pharmaceuticals
93; 948	Diclofenac Potassium	50 mg	Orange	Tablet	Circle	Teva Pharmaceuticals
93; 956	Clomipramine Hydrochloride	25 mg	White and Orange	Capsule		Teva Pharmaceuticals
93; 957	Chlordiazepoxide Hydrochloride	5 mg	Light Green and Yellow, Opaque	Capsule		Teva Pharmaceuticals
93; 958	Clomipramine Hydrochloride	50 mg	White and Light Blue	Capsule		Teva Pharmaceuticals
93; 959	Chlordiazepoxide Hydrochloride	10 mg	Black and Light Green, Opaque	Capsule		Teva Pharmaceuticals
93; 960	Clomipramine Hydrochloride	75 mg	White and Tan	Capsule		Teva Pharmaceuticals
93; 961	Chlordiazepoxide Hydrochloride	25 mg	Light Green and White, Opaque	Capsule		Teva Pharmaceuticals
93; 983	Nystatin	500,000 units	Brown	Coated Tablet	Circle, Convex	Teva Pharmaceuticals
93; 1003; 5	Buspirone Hydrochloride	15 mg		Tablet		Teva Pharmaceuticals
93; 1024	Nefazodone Hydrochloride	100 mg	White	Tablet	Capsule-Shape, Scored	Teva Pharmaceuticals
93; 1025	Nefazodone Hydrochloride	200 mg	Yellow	Tablet	Capsule-Shape, Scored	Teva Pharmaceuticals
93; 1026	Nefazodone Hydrochloride	250 mg	White	Tablet	Capsule-Shape, Scored	Teva Pharmaceuticals
93; 1035	Hydrochlorothiazide and Lisinopril	12.5 mg ; 10 mg	Peach	Tablet	Circle	Teva Pharmaceuticals
93; 1041	Diclofenac Sodium	100 mg	Pink	Extended-Release Tablet	Circle	Teva Pharmaceuticals
93; 1044	Enalapril and Hydrochlorothiazide	5 mg ; 12.5 mg	White	Tablet	Capsule-Shape	Teva Pharmaceuticals
93; 1052	Enalapril and Hydrochlorothiazide	10 mg ; 25 mg	Rust	Tablet	Capsule-Shape	Teva Pharmaceuticals
93; 1060	Sotalol Hydrochloride	120 mg	Light Blue	Tablet	Oval, Scored	Teva Pharmaceuticals
93; 1087	Cefaclor	500 mg	Blue	Tablet	Oval	Teva Pharmaceuticals
93; 1111	Lisinopril	2.5 mg	White	Tablet	Circle	Teva Pharmaceuticals
93; 1112	Lisinopril	5 mg	Red	Tablet	Circle, Scored	Teva Pharmaceuticals
93; 1113	Lisinopril	10 mg	Red	Tablet	Circle	Teva Pharmaceuticals
93; 1114	Lisinopril	20 mg	Red	Tablet	Capsule-Shape	Teva Pharmaceuticals
93; 1115	Lisinopril	40 mg	Yellow	Tablet	Capsule-Shape	Teva Pharmaceuticals
93; 1118	Etodolac	600 mg	Light Blue	Extended-Release Tablet	Oval	Teva Pharmaceuticals
93; 1122	Etodolac ER	400 mg	Orange	Extended-Release Tablet	Oval	Teva Pharmaceuticals
93; 1177	Neomycin Sulfate	500 mg	Off-White	Tablet	Circle	Teva Pharmaceuticals
93; 1215	Cefaclor	375 mg	Blue	Tablet	Oval	Teva Pharmaceuticals
93; 1893	Etodolac	500 mg	Blue	Tablet	Oval	Teva Pharmaceuticals
93; 2264	Amoxicillin	875 mg	Off White	Tablet	Capsule-Shape, Scored	Teva Pharmaceuticals
93; 2268	Amoxicillin	250 mg	Off White	Tablet, Chewable	Capsule-Shape	Teva Pharmaceuticals
93; 2274	Amoxicillin and Clavulanate Potassium	500 mg ; 125 mg	White	Tablet	Oblong	Teva Pharmaceuticals
93; 2275 ;	Amoxicillin and Clavulanate Potassium	875 mg ; 125 mg	White	Tablet	Oblong	Teva Pharmaceuticals
93; 3107 ;	Amoxicillin	250 mg	Caramel and Buff	Capsule		Teva Pharmaceuticals
93; 3109	Amoxicillin	500 mg	Buff	Capsule		Teva Pharmaceuticals
93; 3111 ;	Ampicillin	250 mg	Scarlet and Grey	Capsule		Teva Pharmaceuticals
93; 3113 ;	Ampicillin	500 mg	Scarlet and Gray	Capsule		Teva Pharmaceuticals
93; 3115 ;	Oxacillin Sodium	250 mg	Blue Opaque	Capsule		Teva Pharmaceuticals
93; 3117 ;	Oxacillin Sodium	500 mg	Blue Opaque	Capsule		Teva Pharmaceuticals
93; 3119 ;	Cloxacillin	250 mg	Dark Green and Scarlet	Capsule		Teva Pharmaceuticals
93; 3121 ;	Cloxacillin	500 mg	Dark Green and Scarlet	Capsule		Teva Pharmaceuticals
93; 3123 ;	Dicloxacillin Sodium	250 mg	Green and Light Green	Capsule		Teva Pharmaceuticals
93; 3125 ;	Dicloxacillin Sodium	500 mg	Green and Light Green	Capsule		Teva Pharmaceuticals
93; 3127 ;	Disopyramide Phosphate	100 mg	Blue and Scarlet	Capsule		Teva Pharmaceuticals
93; 3129	Disopyramide Phosphate	150 mg	Buff and Scarlet	Capsule		Teva Pharmaceuticals
93; 3153 ;	Cephradine	250 mg	Light Green and Pink	Capsule		Teva Pharmaceuticals
93; 3155 ;	Cephradine	500 mg	Light Green	Capsule		Teva Pharmaceuticals
93; 3165 ;	Minocycline Hydrochloride	50 mg	Pink	Capsule		Teva Pharmaceuticals
93; 3167 ;	Minocycline Hydrochloride	100 mg	Pink and Maroon	Capsule		Teva Pharmaceuticals
93; 3171	Clindamycin Hydrochloride	150 mg	Blue, Red	Capsule		Teva Pharmaceuticals
93; 3193 ;	Ketoprofen	50 mg	Blue and Light Blue	Capsule		Teva Pharmaceuticals
93; 3195 ;	Ketoprofen	75 mg	Blue and White	Capsule		Teva Pharmaceuticals
93; 5157	Lisinopril	30 mg	White	Tablet	Circle	Teva Pharmaceuticals
93; 7113	Nefazodone Hydrochloride	150 mg	Peach	Tablet	Capsule-Shape, Scored	Teva Pharmaceuticals
93; 7120	Flutamide	125 mg	Beige	Capsule		Teva Pharmaceuticals
93; 7172	Etodolac	500 mg	Gray	Extended-Release Tablet	Oval	Teva Pharmaceuticals
93; 7178	Nefazodone Hydrochloride	50 mg	Light Pink	Tablet	Scored, Capsule-Shape	Teva Pharmaceuticals
93; 7180	Ofloxacin	200 mg	Light Yellow	Tablet	Oval	Teva Pharmaceuticals
93; 7181	Ofloxacin	300 mg	White to Off-White	Tablet	Oval	Teva Pharmaceuticals
93; 7182	Ofloxacin	400 mg	Pale Gold	Tablet	Oval	Teva Pharmaceuticals
93; 7223	Fosinopril Sodium	20 mg	White to Off-White	Tablet	Rectangle	Teva Pharmaceuticals
93; 7224	Fosinopril Sodium	40 mg	White to Off-White	Tablet	Circle	Teva Pharmaceuticals
93; 7267	Metformin Hydrochloride	500 mg	White to Off-White	Extended-Release Tablet	Oval	Teva Pharmaceuticals
93; 9411	Methazolamide	25 mg	White	Tablet	Square	Teva Pharmaceuticals
93; 9643	Prochlorperazine Maleate	5 mg	Yellow	Tablet	Circle	Teva Pharmaceuticals
93; 9652	Prochlorperazine Maleate	10 mg	Yellow	Tablet	Circle	Teva Pharmaceuticals
93; DOXY	Doxy-Lemmon	100 mg	Orange	Coated Tablet	Circle	Teva Pharmaceuticals
93; DOXY	Doxycycline Hyclate	100 mg	Orange	Coated Tablet	Circle	Teva Pharmaceuticals
93; SOFARIN; 2 ;	Sofarin	2 mg	Lavender	Tablet	Circle, Scored	Teva Pharmaceuticals
93; SOFARIN; 2 1/2 ;	Sofarin	2.5 mg	Orange	Tablet	Circle, Scored	Teva Pharmaceuticals
93; SOFARIN; 5	Sofarin	5 mg	Pink	Tablet	Circle, Scored	Teva Pharmaceuticals
93-741	Propoxyphene Hydrochloride	65 mg	Pink	Capsule		Par Pharmaceutical
99	Adipex 8	8 mg	Blue and White	Capsule		Teva Pharmaceuticals
99	Vibra-Tabs	100 mg	Peach	Coated Tablet	Circle	Pfizer Laboratories
100	Dicumarol	100 mg		Tablet		Abbott Laboratories
100	Levoxyl	100 mcg	Yellow	Tablet	Oval	King Pharmaceuticals
100 ;	Ceenu	100 mg	Two-Tone Green	Capsule		Bristol-Myers Oncology
100 ; FPI	Endometrin	100 mg	White to Off-White	Tablet	Oblong	Ferring Pharmaceuticals

IMPRINT	BRAND/GENERIC NAME	STRENGTH	COLOR	FORM	SHAPE	MANUFACTURER
100 ; TMC125	Intelence	100 mg	White to Off-White	Tablet	Oval	Tibotec Therapeutics
100 ; TOPAMAX	Topamax	100 mg	Yellow	Tablet	Circle	Ortho-Mcneil Pharmaceutical
100 ; VOLTAREN XR	Voltaren-Xr	100 mg	Light Pink	Tablet, Extended Release	Circle	Novartis Pharmaceuticals
100 ; WELLCOME Y9C	Retrovir	100 mg	Dark Blue Band, White, Opaque	Capsule		Glaxosmithkline
100 DS	Norvir	100 mg	White	Capsule, Liquid Filled		Abbott Laboratories
100 MG ; T	Tegretol-Xr	100 mg	Yellow	Tablet, Extended Release	Circle	Novartis
100; LARODOPA; ROCHE	Larodopa	100 mg	Pink	Tablet	Oval, Scored	Roche Pharmaceuticals
100; LL; A; 17	Asendin	100 mg	Blue	Tablet	Seven-Sided	Lederle Laboratories
100; T4	Levothroid	100 mcg	Yellow	Tablet	Capsule-Shape	Forest Pharmaceuticals
101	Azulfidine	500 mg	Yellow	Tablet	Circle	Pharmacia & Upjohn
101 ; BI	Mirapex	0.75 mg	White	Tablet	Oval	Boehringer Ingelheim Pharmaceuticals
101 ; LOGO	Terbinafine Hydrochloride	250 mg	Light Pink	Tablet	Circle	Actavis Elizabeth
103	Docusate Sodium with Casanthranol	100 mg ; 30 mg	Maroon	Capsule		Paddock Labs
103	Oxoids	20 mg ; 0.3 mg ; 8 mg	Blue	Tablet		Teva Pharmaceuticals
107	Nu'leven	100 mg ; 10 mg ; 150 mg	Aqua	Tablet	Circle, Concave	Teva Pharmaceuticals
108	Lemidyne with Codeine	30 mg ; 230 mg ; 150 mg ; 30 mg	White	Tablet		Teva Pharmaceuticals
110	Amnesteem	10 mg	Reddish Brown	Capsule		Mylan Bertek Pharmaceuticals
110	Moexipril Hydrochloride	7.5 mg	Light Beige	Tablet	Circle	Paddock Laboratories
110	Rhinex DM	2 mg ; 10 mg ; 5 mg	White	Tablet		Teva Pharmaceuticals
112	Januvia	50 mg	Light Beige	Tablet	Circle	Merck & Company
112	Levoxyl	112 mcg	Rose	Tablet	Oval	King Pharmaceuticals
112; T4	Levothroid	112 mcg	Rose	Tablet	Capsule-Shape	Forest Pharmaceuticals
120	Amnesteem	20 mg	Reddish Brown and Cream	Capsule		Mylan Bertek Pharmaceuticals
120 ; B	Cardizem LA	120 mg	White	Tablet, Extended Release	Capsule-Shape	Abbott Laboratories
120 ; IMDUR	Imdur	120 mg	White	Tablet, Extended Release	Capsule-Shape	Schering
120 INNOPRANXL LOGO	Innopran XL	120 mg	Gray, Off-White	Capsule, Extended Release		Glaxosmithkline
123	Atripla	600 mg ; 200 mg ; 300 mg	Pink	Tablet	Capsule-Shape	Bristol-Myers Squibb & Gilead Sciences
125	Levoxyl	125 mcg	Brown	Tablet	Oval	King Pharmaceuticals
125	Slo-Bid Gyrocaps	125 mg	White	Extended-Release Capsule		Aventis Pharmaceuticals
125	Tracleer	125 mg	Orange-White	Coated Tablet	Biconvex, Oval	Genentech
125 ; FAMVIR	Famvir	125 mg	White	Tablet	Circle	Novartis
125; T4	Levothroid	125 mcg	Brown	Tablet	Capsule-Shape	Forest Pharmaceuticals
131; 07	Prednicen-M	5 mg	Red	Coated Tablet	Capsule-Shaped, Bisected Scored	Century Pharmaceuticals
131; 07	Prednicen-M Tablet 5 mg	5 mg	Red	Coated Tablet	Capsule-Shape	Schwarz Pharma
132 ; 93	Lamotrigine	25 mg	White to Off-White	Tablet, Chewable	Oval	Teva Pharmaceuticals
133	Extendryl Chewable	10 mg ; 2 mg ; 1.25 mg	Tan	Tablet, Chewable		Fleming
135 ; 93	Carvedilol	6.25 mg	White	Tablet	Oval	Teva Pharmaceuticals
137	Levoxyl	137 mcg	Dark Blue	Tablet	Oval	King Pharmaceuticals
138 ; B 4	Galantamine	4 mg	Yellow	Tablet	Circle	Barr Laboratories
139 ; B 8	Galantamine	8 mg	Dark Pink	Tablet	Circle	Barr Laboratories
140	Amnesteem	40 mg	Orange and Brown	Capsule		Mylan Bertek Pharmaceuticals
140 ; B 12	Galantamine	12 mg	Red	Tablet	Circle	Barr Laboratories
141 ;	Trilafon Repetab	8 mg	Gray	Timed-Release Tablet		Schering
142	Bupropion Hydrochloride XL	300 mg	Off-White	Tablet, Extended Release, 24 Hr	Oval	Actavis South Atlantic
145	Prinzide	10 mg ; 12.5 mg	Blue	Tablet	Six-Sided	Merck & Company
147 ; THER-RX	Encora - AM	400 mg ; 200 IU ; 25 mg ; 2 mg ; 25 mg	Light Pink	Tablet	Oval	Ther-RX
150	Acetaminophen and Codeine	325 mg ; 30 mg	White	Tablet		Paddock Labs
150	Levoxyl	150 mcg	Blue	Tablet	Oval	King Pharmaceuticals
150 ; BNVA	Boniva	150 mg	White	Tablet	Oblong	Roche Laboratories
150 ; LOGO 701	Demeclocycline Hydrochloride	150 mg	Pink	Tablet	Circle	Barr Laboratories
150 ; LOGO 4357	Ranitidine	150 mg	Beige	Tablet	Circle	Teva Pharmaceuticals
150 ; RELIANT ; AXID	Axid	150 mg	Opaque Dark Yellow, Opaque Pale Yellow	Capsule		Glaxosmithkline
150 MG ; RSN	Actonel	150 mg	Blue	Tablet	Oval	Procter & Gamble Pharmaceuticals
150; LL; A; 18	Asendin	150 mg	Peach	Tablet	Seven-Sided	Lederle Laboratories
150; T4	Levothroid	150 mcg	Blue	Tablet	Capsule-Shape	Forest Pharmaceuticals
151 ; M	Finasteride	5 mg	White	Tablet	Circle	Mylan Pharmaceuticals
155	Lemidyne with Codeine	230 mg ; 150 mg ; 30 mg ; 15 mg	White	Tablet		Teva Pharmaceuticals
155 ; THER-RX	Repliva 21/7	151 mg ; 150 mg ; 140 mg ; 60 mg ; 0.8 mg ; 1 mg ; 10 mcg	Red	Tablet	Oval	Ther-RX
160 ; OC	Oxycontin	160 mg	Blue	Tablet, Extended Release	Capsule-Shape	Purdue Pharmaceutical Products
161 ; THER-RX	Encora - Pm	0.5 mg ; 12.5 mg ; 600 mg ; 600 IU ; 25 mg	Purple	Tablet	Oval	Ther-RX
162 ; THER-RX	Niferex Gold	10 mg ; 50 mg ; 200 mg ; 50 mg ; 60.8 mg ; 1 mg ; 25 mcg	Orange	Tablet	Oval	Ther-RX

IMPRINT	BRAND/GENERIC NAME	STRENGTH	COLOR	FORM	SHAPE	MANUFACTURER
166	Mandelamine	500 mg	Brown	Coated Tablet	Capsule-Shape	Warner Chilcott
167	Mandelamine	1000 mg	Purple	Coated Tablet		Warner Chilcott
172 ;	Meticorten	5 mg	White	Tablet		Schering
175	Levoxyl	175 mcg	Turquoise	Tablet	Oval	King Pharmaceuticals
175 ; LOGO	Carvedilol	3.125 mg	White	Tablet	Oval	Actavis Elizabeth
175; T4	Levothroid	175 mcg	Lilac	Tablet	Capsule-Shape	Forest Pharmaceuticals
176 ; LOGO	Carvedilol	6.25 mg	White	Tablet	Oval	Actavis Elizabeth
177	Kuvan	100 mg	Off-White to Light Yellow	Tablet, Disintegrating	Circle	Biomarin Pharmaceuticals
177 ; LOGO	Carvedilol	12.5 mg	White	Tablet	Oval	Actavis Elizabeth
178 ; LOGO	Carvedilol	25 mg	White	Tablet	Oval	Actavis Elizabeth
180 ; B	Cardizem LA	180 mg	White	Tablet, Extended Release	Capsule-Shape	Abbott Laboratories
191 ; US	Folgard RX	2.2 mg ; 25 mg ; 1	Yellow	Tablet	Oval	Upsher-Smith Laboratories
196 ; THER-RX	Primacare Advantage - Pm Dose	230 IU ; 90 mcg ; 3 mg ; 3.4 mg ; 20 mg ; 50 mg ; 1 mg ; 12 mcg ; 35 mcg ; 7 mg ; 250 mg ; 30 mg ; 11 mg ; 75 mcg ; 1.3 mg ; 45 mcg ; 50 mcg ; 50 mg ; 35 mg ; 100 mg	Pink	Tablet	Oval	Ther-RX
197 ; THER-RX	Chromagen Forte	50 mg ; 101 mg ; 50 mg ; 60 mg ; 0.8 mg ; 1 mg ; 10 mcg	Maroon	Tablet		Ther-RX
198 ; THER-RX	Chromagen	70 mg ; 75 mg ; 150 mg ; 2 mg ; 10 mcg ; 50 mg	Maroon	Tablet		Ther-RX
199 ; 9 3	Venlafaxine Hydrochloride	25 mg	Mottled Peach	Tablet	Circle	Teva Pharmaceuticals
199 ; THER-RX	Chromagen FA	1 mg ; 10 mcg ; 70 mg ; 75 mg ; 150 mg ; 2 mg	Green	Tablet		Ther-RX
200	Hydrochlorothiazide	50 mg	Peach	Tablet		Paddock Labs
200	Levoxyl	200 mcg	Pink	Tablet	Oval	King Pharmaceuticals
200 ; 7111 ;	Cimetidine	200 mg	White to Off-White	Tablet	Circle	Teva Pharmaceuticals
200 ; BAYER CROSS	Nexavar	200 mg	Red	Tablet	Circle	Bayer Pharmaceutical Division
200 ; K	Oxandrolone	2.5 mg	White	Tablet	Circle	Par Pharmaceutical
200 ; LOGO 4405	Clozapine	200 mg	Pale Yellow	Tablet	Oval	Teva Pharmaceuticals
200 ; TOPAMAX	Topamax	200 mg	Salmon	Tablet	Circle	Ortho-Mcneil Pharmaceutical
200 MG ; T	Tegretol-Xr	200 mg	Pink	Tablet, Extended Release	Circle	Novartis
200; T4	Levothroid	200 mcg	Pink	Tablet	Capsule-Shape	Forest Pharmaceuticals
201 ; THER-RX	Repliva 21/7 - Red Tablet	151 mg ; 150 mg ; 140 mg ; 60 mg ; 0.8 mg ; 1 mg ; 10 mcg	Red	Tablet	Oval	Ther-RX
204	Amobarbital D-Lay	60 mg	Orange and White	Tablet		Teva Pharmaceuticals
205 ; C	Nuvigil	50 mg	White	Tablet	Circle	Cephalon
206 ; THER-RX	Repliva 21/7 - Purple Tablet	150 mg	Purple	Tablet	Oval	Ther-RX
207	Corgard	40 mg		Tablet		Monarch Pharmaceuticals
207; LEMMON; 207	Mepriam	400 mg	Yellow	Tablet	Scored, Oblong	Teva Pharmaceuticals
208	Corgard	120 mg		Tablet		Monarch Pharmaceuticals
215 ; C	Nuvigil	150 mg	White	Tablet	Oval	Cephalon
220 ; K	Leflunomide	10 mg	White	Tablet	Circle	Par Pharmaceutical
221	Januvia	25 mg	Pink	Tablet	Circle	Merck & Company
221 ; 93	Risperidone	0.25 mg	Dark Yellow	Tablet	Circle	Teva Pharmaceuticals
221 ; K	Leflunomide	20 mg	White	Tablet	Triangle	Par Pharmaceutical
225 ; 93	Risperidone	0.5 mg	Red-Brown	Tablet	Circle	Teva Pharmaceuticals
225 ; C	Nuvigil	250 mg	White	Tablet	Oval	Cephalon
226 ; M	Quinapril	10 mg	Orange	Tablet	Circle	Mylan Pharmaceuticals
227	Isentress	400 mg	Pink	Tablet	Oval	Merck & Company
227; 555	Erythromycin Estolate	250 mg	Orange	Capsule		Teva Pharmaceuticals
231	Ferrocol	150 mg	Blue	Capsule		Teva Pharmaceuticals
232	Corgard	20 mg		Tablet		Monarch Pharmaceuticals
234 ; M	Metformin Hydrochloride	500 mg	White	Tablet	Circle	Mylan Pharmaceuticals
235	Thyrocrine	2.5 Gr	Tan	Tablet		Teva Pharmaceuticals
235	Thyroid	2.5 Gr	Tan	Tablet		Teva Pharmaceuticals
236 ; PAR	Doxycycline	150 mg	Peach	Tablet	Circle	Par Pharmaceutical
240 ; B	Cardizem LA	240 mg	White	Tablet, Extended Release	Capsule-Shape	Abbott Laboratories
240 ; M	Metformin Hydrochloride	850 mg	White	Tablet	Circle	Mylan Pharmaceuticals
241	Corgard	80 mg		Tablet		Monarch Pharmaceuticals
243 ; WATSON	Leena - Light Blue Tablet	0.5 mg ; 0.035 mg	Light Blue	Tablet	Circle	Watson Laboratories
244 ; MYLAN	Verapamil Hydrochloride	120 mg	Blue	Tablet, Extended Release	Oval	Mylan Pharmaceuticals
244 ; WATSON	Leena - Light Yellow-Green Tablet	1 mg ; 0.035 mg	Light Yellow-Green	Tablet	Circle	Watson Laboratories
245 ; WATSON	Necon 1/50 - White Tablet	1 mg ; 0.05 mg	White	Tablet	Circle	Watson Pharma
246 ;	Corgard	160 mg	Blue	Tablet	Oblong, Scored	Monarch Pharmaceuticals
247 ; B	Junel Fe 1/20 - Brown Tablet	75 mg	Brown	Tablet	Circle	Barr Laboratories
247 ; B	Junel Fe 1.5/30 - Brown Tablet	75 mg	Brown	Tablet	Circle	Barr Laboratories
250	Bendopa	0.25 GM	Clear	Capsule		Valeant Pharmaceuticals
250 ; FAMVIR	Famvir	250 mg	White	Tablet	Circle	Novartis
250 ; LAMISIL	Lamisil	250 mg	White to Yellow-Tinged	Tablet	Circle	Novartis
250 ; LOGO 5311	Ciprofloxacin	250 mg	White to Off-White	Tablet	Oval	Teva Pharmaceuticals
250 ; TM	Tindamax	250 mg	Pink	Tablet	Circle	Mission Pharmacal
250 ; VIRACEPT	Viracept	250 mg	Light Blue	Coated Tablet	Capsule-Shape	Agouron Pharmaceuticals

IMPRINT	BRAND/GENERIC NAME	STRENGTH	COLOR	FORM	SHAPE	MANUFACTURER
250/125 ; AUGMENTIN	Augmentin	125 mg ; 250 mg	White	Tablet	Oval	Glaxosmithkline
250; LARODOPA; ROCHE	Larodopa	250 mg	Pink	Tablet	Circle, Scored	Roche Pharmaceuticals
251; DMSP	Carbidopa and Levodopa	25 mg ; 250 mg	Light Dapple-Blue	Tablet	Oval, Scored	Bristol-Myers Squibb
254 ; M	Quinapril	20 mg	Orange	Tablet	Circle	Mylan Pharmaceuticals
261	Codone	5 mg	White	Tablet		Teva Pharmaceuticals
266 ; MRK	Maxalt	5 mg	Pale Pink	Tablet	Capsule-Shape	Merck & Company
271; DMSP	Carbidopa and Levodopa	10 mg ; 100 mg	Dark Dapple-Blue	Tablet	Oval, Scored	Bristol-Myers Squibb
272 ; M	Quinapril	40 mg	Orange	Tablet	Circle	Mylan Pharmaceuticals
272; DMSP	Carbidopa and Levodopa	25 mg ; 100 mg	Yellow	Tablet	Oval, Scored	Bristol-Myers Squibb
277	Januvia	100 mg	Beige	Tablet	Circle	Merck & Company
283; 200 MCG	Baycol	0.2 mg	Light Yellow	Tablet		Bayer Pharmaceutical
284; 300 MCG	Baycol	0.3 mg	Yellow-Brown	Tablet		Bayer Pharmaceutical
285; 400 MCG	Baycol	0.4 mg	Ocher	Tablet		Bayer Pharmaceutical
286; 800 MCG	Baycol	0.8 mg	Brown-Orange	Tablet		Bayer Pharmaceutical
296	Phyldrox	100 mg ; 25 mg ; 15 mg	White	Tablet		Teva Pharmaceuticals
300 ; 7117	Cimetidine	300 mg	White to Off-White	Tablet	Circle	Teva Pharmaceuticals
300 ; B	Cardizem LA	300 mg	White	Tablet, Extended Release	Capsule-Shape	Abbott Laboratories
300 ; GX CW3	Retrovir	300 mg	White	Tablet	Circle	Glaxosmithkline
300 ; LOGO 702	Demeclocycline Hydrochloride	300 mg	Pink	Tablet	Circle	Barr Laboratories
300 ; RELIANT ; AXID	Axid	300 mg	Opaque Brown, Opaque Pale Yellow	Capsule		Glaxosmithkline
300 ; SEROQUEL	Seroquel	300 mg	White	Tablet	Capsule-Shape	Astrazeneca
300; M30; MOVA	Cimetidine	300 mg	White	Coated Tablet	Round, Bisected Scored	Par Pharmaceutical
300; T4	Levothroid	300 mcg	Green	Tablet	Capsule-Shape	Forest Pharmaceuticals
304	Pyradyne	15 mg ; 210 mg ; 30 mg ; 150 mg	Red	Tablet		Teva Pharmaceuticals
306	Pyradyne Compound	0.12 mg ; 8 mg ; 15 mg ; 120 mg ; 100 mg ; 8 mg ; 10 mg	Yellow	Tablet		Teva Pharmaceuticals
308AV	Allegra-D 24 Hour	180 mg ; 240 mg	White	Tablet, Extended Release	Circle	Sanofi-Aventis U.S.
311	Vytorin 10/10	10 mg ; 10 mg	White to Off-White	Tablet	Capsule-Shape	Merck/schering-Plough Pharmaceuticals
311AV ; E	Allegra Odt	30 mg	White	Tablet, Disintegrating	Circle	Sanofi-Aventis U.S.
312	Vytorin 10/20	10 mg ; 20 mg	White to Off-White	Tablet	Capsule-Shape	Merck/schering-Plough Pharmaceuticals
313	Vytorin 10/40	10 mg ; 40 mg	White to Off-White	Tablet	Capsule-Shape	Merck/schering-Plough Pharmaceuticals
315	Vytorin 10/80	10 mg ; 80 mg	White to Off-White	Tablet	Capsule-Shape	Merck/schering-Plough Pharmaceuticals
321 ; M	Lorazepam	0.5 mg	White to Off-White	Tablet	Circle	Mylan Pharmaceuticals
322	Lemivite	0.4 IU ; 1666 IU ; 1.7 mg ; 8 mg ; 1 mg ; 66 IU ; 0.33 mg ; 16 mg ; 71 mg ; 1.6 mg ; 1 mcg ; 3.33 mg ; 0.33 mg ; 55 mg ; 0.166 mg ; 1 mg ; 1 mg ; 0.4 mg	Red	Tablet		Teva Pharmaceuticals
332 ; B	Velivet - Orange Tablet	0.125 mg ; 0.025 mg	Orange	Tablet	Circle	Barr Laboratories
333	Campral	333 mg	White	Enteric-Coated Tablet	Circle	Forest Pharmaceuticals
335 ; B	Velivet - Pink Tablet	0.15 mg ; 0.025 mg	Pink	Tablet	Circle	Barr Laboratories
336	Diagnex Blue Test Sodium Benzoate and Caffeine	250 mg ;		Tablet		Bristol-Myers Squibb
351; RPR	Slo-Phyllin	100 mg	White	Tablet	Circle	Aventis Pharmaceuticals
355	Aluprin	300 mg ;	Green and White	Tablet		Teva Pharmaceuticals
360 ; B	Cardizem LA	360 mg	White	Tablet, Extended Release	Capsule-Shape	Abbott Laboratories
386; ORGANON	Cotazym	30000 U ; 25 mg ; 8000 U ; 30000 U	Red	Capsule		Organon
393	Diabinese	100 mg	Blue	Tablet	D-Shape	Pfizer Laboratories
394	Diabinese	250 mg	Blue	Tablet	D-Shape	Pfizer Laboratories
400 ; H3647	Ketek	400 mg	Light Orange	Tablet	Oval	Sanofi-Aventis U.S.
400 ; IP 131	Ibuprofen	400 mg	White	Tablet	Circle	Watson Laboratories
400 ; N 943	Acyclovir	400 mg	Blue	Tablet	Capsule-Shape	Teva Pharmaceuticals
400 ; SEROQUEL	Seroquel	400 mg	Yellow	Tablet	Capsule-Shape	Astrazeneca
400 MG ; T	Tegretol-Xr	400 mg	Brown	Tablet, Extended Release	Circle	Novartis
400; M40; MOVA	Cimetidine	400 mg	White	Coated Tablet	Capsule-Shaped, Bisected Scored	Par Pharmaceutical
414	Zetia	10 mg	Off-White	Tablet	Capsule-Shape	Schering
420 ; B	Cardizem LA	420 mg	White	Tablet, Extended Release	Capsule-Shape	Abbott Laboratories
446	Tamoxifen	10 mg	White	Tablet	Circle	Astrazeneca
461 ; ETH	Dazidox	10 mg	Pink	Tablet	Circle	Ther-RX
461; 80 MG	Emend	80 mg	White	Capsule		Merck & Company
462 ; ETH	Dazidox	20 mg	Gray	Tablet	Circle	Ther-RX
462; 125 MG	Emend	125 mg	Pink, White	Capsule		Merck & Company
463 ; 9 3	Lamotrigine	100 mg	Peach	Tablet	Diamond	Teva Pharmaceuticals
464 40MG ;	Emend	40 mg	Opaque Mustard Yellow, Opaque White	Capsule	Capsule-Shape	Merck & Company
496	Adphen-G	35 mg	Green Speckled	Tablet	Oblong, Scored	Ferndale Laboratories
499; SCHERING	Oreton Methyl	25 mg	Peach	Tablet		Schering
500 ; ALINIA	Alinia	500 mg	Yellow	Tablet	Circle	Romark Laboratories
500 ; ANDRX 674	Metformin Hydrochloride	500 mg	White	Tablet	Circle	Watson Pharma

IMPRINT	BRAND/GENERIC NAME	STRENGTH	COLOR	FORM	SHAPE	MANUFACTURER
500 ; FAMVIR	Famvir	500 mg	White	Tablet	Oval	Novartis
500 ; GMZ	Glumetza	500 mg	Blue	Tablet, Extended Release	Oval	Depomed
500 ; HOURGLASS 4331	Metformin Hydrochloride	500 mg	White	Tablet	Oval	Teva Pharmaceuticals
500 ; HOURGLASS 4335	Metformin Hydrochloride ER	500 mg	White to Off White	Tablet, Extended Release	Oval	Ivax Pharmaceuticals
500 ; HOURGLASS 5312	Ciprofloxacin	500 mg	White to Off-White	Tablet	Oval	Teva Pharmaceuticals
500 ; KOS	Niaspan	500 mg	Medium Orange	Tablet, Extended Release	Capsule-Shape	Kos Pharmaceuticals
500 ; LOGO 571	Metformin Hydrochloride	500 mg	White to Off White	Tablet, Extended Release	Capsule-Shape	Watson Pharma
500 ; TM	Tindamax	500 mg	Pink	Tablet	Oval	Mission Pharmacal
500 MG; A5; LEDERLE	Achromycin V	500 mg	Yellow and Blue	Capsule		Lederle Laboratories
500/125 ; AUGMENTIN	Augmentin	125 mg ; 500 mg	White	Tablet	Oval	Glaxosmithkline
500; LARODOPA; ROCHE	Larodopa	500 mg	Pink	Tablet	Oblong, Scored	Roche Pharmaceuticals
500; MG	Mono-Gesic	500 mg	Pink	Coated Tablet	Circle	Schwarz Pharma
502 ; KOS	Advicor	500 mg ; 20 mg	Light Yellow	Tablet, Extended Release	Capsule-Shape	Kos Pharmaceuticals
511 ; PAR	Minocycline Hydrochloride	50 mg	White	Tablet	Capsule-Shape	Par Pharmaceutical
511; 1 MG	Lorazepam	1 mg	White	Tablet	Five-Sided	Wyeth Pharmaceuticals
511; 2 MG	Lorazepam	2 mg	White	Tablet	Five-Sided	Wyeth Pharmaceuticals
512 ; PAR	Minocycline Hydrochloride	75 mg	White	Tablet	Capsule-Shape	Par Pharmaceutical
513 ; PAR	Minocycline Hydrochloride	100 mg	White	Tablet	Capsule-Shape	Par Pharmaceutical
521 SINEMET CR ;	Sinemet Cr 50-200	50 mg ; 200 mg	Peach	Tablet, Extended Release	Oval	Bristol-Myers Squibb
523 ; M	Bisoprolol Fumarate	5 mg	Purple	Tablet	Circle	Mylan Pharmaceuticals
524 ; BMS	Sprycel	70 mg	White to Off-White	Tablet	Circle	Bristol-Myers Squibb
527 ; BMS	Sprycel	20 mg	White to Off-White	Tablet	Circle	Bristol-Myers Squibb
528 ; BMS	Sprycel	50 mg	White to Off-White	Tablet	Oval	Bristol-Myers Squibb
540 ; R	Carbidopa and Levodopa	250 mg ; 25 mg	Mottled Light Blue	Tablet	Circle	Actavis Elizabeth
543; 80 ;	Zocor	80 mg	Brick Red	Coated Tablet	Capsule-Shape	Merck & Company
544 ; B	Terbinafine Hydrochloride	250 mg	White or Almost White	Tablet	Circle	Barr Laboratories
547	Wigrettes	2 mg	White	Tablet		Organon
555; 030	Colchicine	0.65 mg	White	Tablet		Barr Laboratories
555; 19	Hydrochlorothiazide Hydrochloride	25 mg	Peach	Tablet	Circle, Scored	Barr Laboratories
555; 20	Hydrochlorothiazide Hydrochloride	50 mg	Peach	Tablet	Circle, Scored	Barr Laboratories
555; 126	Dicyclomine Hydrochloride	20 mg	Blue	Tablet	Circle	Barr Laboratories
555; 429	Trimethoprim	100 mg	White	Tablet	Circle, Scored	Barr Laboratories
555; 430	Trimethoprim	200 mg		Tablet		Barr Laboratories
562; W615	Westhroid	129.6 mg	Various Colors	Tablet	Circle	Western Research Laboratories
568 100 MG	Zolinza	100 mg	White, Opaque	Capsule		Merck & Company
575	Janumet	50 mg ; 500 mg	Light Pink	Tablet	Capsule-Shape	Merck & Company
576 ; B	Granisetron Hydrochloride	1 mg	White	Tablet	Circle	Barr Laboratories
577	Janumet	50 mg ; 1000 mg	Red	Tablet	Capsule-Shape	Merck & Company
580 ; WC	Ovcon-35 28 Day - Light Peach Tablet	0.4 mg ; 0.035 mg	Light Peach	Tablet	Circle	Warner Chilcott
580 ; WC	Zenchent 0.4/35 28-Day - Light Peach Tablet	0.4 mg ; 0.035 mg	Light Peach	Tablet	Circle	Watson Pharma
581 ; W C	Femcon Fe - White Tablet	0.4 mg ; 0.035 mg	White	Tablet, Chewable	Circle	Warner Chilcott
591; A	Meprobamate	400 mg	White	Tablet	Circle, Scored	Watson Laboratories
591; B	Meprobamate	200 mg	White	Tablet	Circle	Watson Laboratories
600 ; IP 132	Ibuprofen	600 mg	White	Tablet	Oval	Watson Laboratories
600; 4141 ;	Fenoprofen Calcium	600 mg	Peach	Coated Tablet	Oval, Bisected Scored	Ivax Pharmaceuticals
601 SINEMET CR	Sinemet Cr 25-100	25 mg ; 100 mg	Pink	Tablet, Extended Release	Oval	Bristol-Myers Squibb
603	Sumycin	500 mg	Pink	Tablet	Capsule-Shape	Par Pharmaceutical
603	Sumycin 500	500 mg	Pink	Tablet	Capsule-Shape	Par Pharmaceutical
607; 0.5 MG	Prograf	0.5 mg	Light Yellow	Capsule		Fujisawa
617; 1 MG	Prograf	1 mg	White	Capsule		Fujisawa
625 ; V	Viracept	625 mg	White	Coated Tablet	Oval	Agouron Pharmaceuticals
627	Belap Se	10.8 mg	Green	Tablet		Teva Pharmaceuticals
633 ; M	Nifedipine	90 mg	Brown	Tablet, Extended Release	Circle	Andrx Pharmaceuticals
633 ; R	Lovastatin	10 mg	White	Tablet	Circle	Actavis Elizabeth
634 ; R	Lovastatin	20 mg	Pink	Tablet	Circle	Actavis Elizabeth
635 ; R	Lovastatin	40 mg	Yellow	Tablet	Circle	Actavis Elizabeth
643; 2 1/2	Metolazone	2.5 mg	Pink	Tablet	Circle	Celltech
644	Prednisolone	5 mg	Orange	Tablet		Teva Pharmaceuticals
644; 5	Metolazone	5 mg	Blue	Tablet	Circle	Celltech
645	Prednisone	5 mg	White	Tablet		Teva Pharmaceuticals
645; 10	Metolazone	10 mg	Yellow	Tablet	Circle	Celltech
647 SINEMET ;	Sinemet 10-100	10 mg ; 100 mg	Dark Dapple-Blue	Tablet	Oval	Bristol-Myers Squibb
650 SINEMET ;	Sinemet 25-100	25 mg ; 100 mg	Yellow	Tablet	Oval	Bristol-Myers Squibb
654 SINEMET ;	Sinemet 25-250	25 mg ; 250 mg	Light Dapple-Blue	Tablet	Oval	Bristol-Myers Squibb
657; 5 MG	Prograf	5 mg	Gray and Red	Capsule		Fujisawa
663	Sumycin	250 mg	Pink	Tablet	Capsule-Shape	Par Pharmaceutical
663	Sumycin 250	250 mg	Light Pink	Tablet	Capsule-Shape	Par Pharmaceutical
682	Budeprion XL	300 mg	Yellow	Tablet, Extended Release	Oval	Teva Pharmaceuticals
688 ; 93	Lamotrigine	5 mg	White to Off White	Tablet, Chewable	Circle	Teva Pharmaceuticals
701 ; GILEAD	Truvada	200 mg ; 300 mg	Blue	Tablet	Capsule-Shape	Gilead Sciences

IMPRINT	BRAND/GENERIC NAME	STRENGTH	COLOR	FORM	SHAPE	MANUFACTURER
707	Rynatan	9 mg ; 25 mg	Buff	Tablet	Capsule-Shape	Meda Pharmaceuticals
707; SP; 7.5	Univasc	7.5 mg	Pink	Tablet	Circle	UCB Pharma
715; SP; 15	Univasc	15 mg	Salmon	Tablet	Circle	UCB Pharma
719 ; B 35	Alendronate Sodium	35 mg	White	Tablet	Oval	Barr Laboratories
720 ; B 70	Alendronate Sodium	70 mg	White	Tablet	Oval	Barr Laboratories
731	Tamoxifen	20 mg	White	Tablet	Circle, Biconvex	Astrazeneca
732 ; M	Ondansetron	4 mg	White to Off-White	Tablet, Disintegrating	Circle	Mylan Pharmaceuticals
733; 54	Morphine Sulfate	15 mg	White	Tablet		Roxane Laboratories
734 ; M	Ondansetron	8 mg	White to Off-White	Tablet, Disintegrating	Circle	Mylan Pharmaceuticals
745	Hyzaar 100-12.5	12.5 mg ; 100 mg	White	Tablet	Oval	Merck
746 ; LOGO	Tri-Previfem - White Tablet	0.18 mg ; 0.035 mg	White	Tablet	Circle	Teva Pharmaceuticals
747 ; LOGO	Tri-Previfem - Light Blue Tablet	0.215 mg ; 0.035 mg	Light Blue	Tablet	Circle	Teva Pharmaceuticals
748 ; LOGO	Previfem - Blue Tablet	0.25 mg ; 0.035 mg	Blue	Tablet	Circle	Teva Pharmaceuticals
750 ; KOS	Niaspan	750 mg	Medium Orange	Tablet, Extended Release	Capsule-Shape	Kos Pharmaceuticals
750 ; LOGO 577	Metformin Hydrochloride	750 mg	Light Yellow	Tablet, Extended Release	Capsule-Shape	Watson Pharma
750 ; LOGO 5313	Ciprofloxacin	750 mg	White to Off-White	Tablet	Oval	Teva Pharmaceuticals
751 ; M ;	Cyclobenzaprine Hydrochloride	10 mg	Butterscotch Yellow	Tablet	Circle	Mylan Pharmaceuticals
752 ; KOS	Advicor	750 mg ; 20 mg	Light Orange	Tablet, Extended Release	Capsule-Shape	Kos Pharmaceuticals
752 ; M	Fexofenadine Hydrochloride	30 mg	Blue	Tablet	Circle	Mylan Pharmaceuticals
755 ; R	Citalopram Hydrobromide	10 mg	Beige	Tablet	Capsule-Shape	Actavis Elizabeth
770 ; RG	Finasteride	5 mg	White to Off-White	Tablet	Triangle	Barr Laboratories
771 ; M ;	Cyclobenzaprine Hydrochloride	5 mg	Blue	Tablet	Circle	Mylan Pharmaceuticals
787 ; 93	Atenolol	25 mg	White to Off-White	Tablet	Circle	Teva Pharmaceuticals
800 ; 7711 ;	Cimetidine	800 mg	White to Off-White	Tablet	Oval	Teva Pharmaceuticals
800 ; IP 137	Ibuprofen	800 mg	White	Tablet	Capsule-Shape	Watson Laboratories
800 ; N 947	Acyclovir	800 mg	White to Off-White	Tablet	Capsule-Shape	Teva Pharmaceuticals
800; M80; MOVA	Cimetidine	800 mg	White	Coated Tablet	Capsule-Shaped, Bisected Scored	Par Pharmaceutical
803 ; LOGO	Spironolactone	25 mg	White to Off-White	Tablet	Circle	Actavis Elizabeth
810	Thyroid Green	5 Gr	Green	Tablet		Teva Pharmaceuticals
812	Thyroid	3 Gr	Blue	Tablet		Teva Pharmaceuticals
830 ;	Proglycem	100 mg	Orange	Capsule		Schering
832 ; ALP 2 1/2	Amlodipine Besylate	2.5 mg	White	Tablet	Circle	Upsher-Smith Laboratories
832 ; ALP 5	Amlodipine Besylate	5 mg	White	Tablet	Circle	Upsher-Smith Laboratories
832 ; ALP 10	Amlodipine Besylate	10 mg	White	Tablet	Circle	Upsher-Smith Laboratories
832 86	Androxy	10 mg	Green	Tablet	Circle	Upsher-Smith Laboratories
844	Thyroid	2 Gr	Red	Tablet		Teva Pharmaceuticals
848 ; STUARTNATAL LOGO	Duet	25 mg ; 2 mg ; 3000 IU ; 120 mg ; 400 IU ; 30 mg ; 1.8 mg ; 4 mg ; 20 mg ; 25 mg ; 1 mg ; 12 mcg ; 200 mg ; 29 mg ; 25 mg	Yellow	Tablet	Oval	Xanodyne Pharmaceuticals
848 ; STUARTNATAL LOGO	Duet Dha - Duet Tablet	3000 IU ; 120 mg ; 400 IU ; 30 mg ; 1.8 mg ; 4 mg ; 20 mg ; 25 mg ; 1 mg ; 12 mcg ; 200 mg ; 29 mg ; 25 mg ; 25 mg ; 2 mg	Yellow	Tablet	Oval	Xanodyne Pharmaceuticals
850 ; ANDRX 675	Metformin Hydrochloride	850 mg	White	Tablet	Circle	Watson Pharma
850 ; HOURGLASS 4330	Metformin Hydrochloride	850 mg	White	Tablet	Oval	Ivax Pharmaceuticals
850 ; PAR	Meloxicam	7.5 mg	Off-White to Yellow	Tablet	Circle	Par Pharmaceutical
851 ; PAR	Meloxicam	15 mg	Off-White to Yellow	Tablet	Oval	Par Pharmaceutical
852 ; BMS 100	Sprycel	100 mg	White to Off-White	Tablet	Oval	Bristol-Myers Squibb
854	Thyroid Tan	5 Gr	Tan	Tablet		Teva Pharmaceuticals
879; 525	Doxycycline Hyclate	50 mg	Blue and White	Capsule		Novartis Generics
879; 526	Doxycycline Hyclate	100 mg	Blue	Capsule		Novartis Generics
935 ; ANDRX LOGO	Fosinopril Sodium	10 mg	White	Tablet	Capsule-Shape	Watson Pharma
936 ; ANDRX LOGO	Fosinopril Sodium	20 mg	White	Tablet	Oval	Watson Pharma
937 ; ANDRX LOGO	Fosinopril Sodium	40 mg	White	Tablet	Circle	Watson Pharma
949 ; WATSON	Lutera - White Tablet	0.1 mg ; 0.02 mg	White	Tablet	Circle	Watson Laboratories
955	Famotidine	20 mg	White	Tablet	Circle	Watson Pharma
958 ; PAR	Chlordiazepoxide Hydrochloride	5 mg	Opaque Green, Opaque Yellow	Capsule		Par Pharmaceutical
959 ; PAR	Chlordiazepoxide Hydrochloride	10 mg	Opaque Black, Opaque Green	Capsule		Par Pharmaceutical
960 ; PAR	Chlordiazepoxide Hydrochloride	25 mg	Opaque Green, Opaque White	Capsule		Par Pharmaceutical
962 ; PAR	Chlordiazepoxide and Amitriptyline Hydrochloride - Double Strength	10 mg ; 25 mg	White	Tablet		Par Pharmaceutical
966 ; WATSON	Quasense - White Tablet	0.15 mg ; 0.03 mg	White	Tablet	Circle	Watson Pharma
967 ; WATSON	Sronyx - White Tablet	0.1 mg ; 0.02 mg	White	Tablet	Circle	Watson Laboratories
968 ;	Tindal	20 mg	Salmon	Tablet		Schering
977 ; B	Junel 1/20 - Light Yellow Tablet	1 mg ; 20 mcg	Light Yellow	Tablet	Circle	Barr Laboratories
977 ; B	Junel Fe 1/20 - Light Yellow Tablet	1 mg ; 20 mcg	Light Yellow	Tablet	Circle	Barr Laboratories
978 ; B	Junel 1.5/30 - Pink Tablet	1.5 mg ; 30 mcg	Pink	Tablet	Circle	Barr Laboratories
978 ; B	Junel Fe 1.5/30 - Pink Tablet	1.5 mg ; 30 mcg	Pink	Tablet	Circle	Barr Laboratories
992 ; B	Jolessa - Pink Tablet	0.15 mg ; 0.03 mg	Pink	Tablet	Circle	Barr Laboratories
1000 ; ANDRX 676	Metformin Hydrochloride	1000 mg	White	Tablet	Oval	Watson Pharma
1000 ; HOURGLASS 4432	Metformin Hydrochloride	1000 mg	White	Tablet	Oval	Ivax Pharmaceuticals
1000 ; KOS	Niaspan	1000 mg	Medium Orange	Tablet, Extended Release	Capsule-Shape	Abbott Laboratories

IMPRINT	BRAND/GENERIC NAME	STRENGTH	COLOR	FORM	SHAPE	MANUFACTURER
1002 ; KOS	Advicor	1000 mg ; 20 mg	Light Purple/dark Pink	Tablet, Extended Release	Capsule-Shape	Kos Pharmaceuticals
1004 ; KOS	Advicor	1000 mg ; 40 mg	Reddish Brown	Tablet, Extended Release	Capsule-Shape	Abbott Laboratories
1024	Christodyne-Dhc	5 mg ; 150 mg ; 230 mg ; 30 mg	Green and White Speckled	Tablet		Paddock Labs
1045 ; 93	Quinapril	20 mg	Brown	Tablet	Capsule-Shape	Teva Pharmaceuticals
1050 ; 93	Quinapril	5 mg	Brown	Tablet	Circle	Teva Pharmaceuticals
1051 ; 93	Quinapril	10 mg	Brown	Tablet	Oval	Teva Pharmaceuticals
1053 ; 93	Quinapril	40 mg	Brown	Tablet	Capsule-Shape	Teva Pharmaceuticals
1117 ; W	Lybrel	90 mcg ; 20 mcg	Yellow	Tablet	Circle	Wyeth Pharmaceuticals
1171 ; 75	Plavix	75 mg	Pink	Tablet	Circle	Bristol-Myers Squibb
1172 ; 93	Penicillin-VK	250 mg	Mottled White to Off-White	Tablet	Oval	Teva Pharmaceuticals
1174 ; 93	Penicillin-VK	500 mg	Mottled White to Off-White	Tablet	Oval	Teva Pharmaceuticals
1221	Fluvoxamine Maleate	100 mg	Beige	Tablet	Oval	Baypharma
1222	Fluvoxamine Maleate	25 mg	White	Tablet	Oval	Baypharma
1225	Fluvoxamine Maleate	50 mg	Yellow	Tablet	Oval	Baypharma
1332 ; 300	Plavix	300 mg	Pink	Tablet	Oblong	Bristol-Myers Squibb
1492	Monopril HCT	10 mg ; 12.5 mg	Peach	Tablet	Circle	Bristol-Myers Squibb
1493	Monopril HCT	20 mg ; 12.5 mg	Peach	Tablet	Circle, Scored	Bristol-Myers Squibb
1611 ; BMS	Baraclude	0.5 mg	White to Off-White	Tablet	Triangle	Bristol-Myers Squibb
1612 ; BMS	Baraclude	1 mg	Pink	Tablet	Triangle	Bristol-Myers Squibb
1740 40MG	Omeprazole	40 mg	Amethyst, Apricot	Capsule, Delayed Release		Ranbaxy Pharmaceuticals
2080	Axert	6.25 mg	White with Red Ink	Tablet	Circle, Compressed, Biconvex	Pharmacia & Upjohn
2112	Pentetra-Tdc	80 mg	Clear and Green	Capsule		Paddock Labs
2131 Z ZENITH 100 MG	Nitrofurantoin Macrocrystals	100 mg	Pink Opaque	Capsule		Teva Pharmaceuticals
2442 ; G ;	Budeprion SR	100 mg	Yellow	Tablet, Extended Release	Circle	Teva Pharmaceuticals
2444 ; G	Buproban	150 mg	Light Yellow	Tablet, Extended Release	Circle	Teva Pharmaceuticals
2771; HEART SHAPE	Avapro	75 mg	White	Tablet	Oval, Biconvex	Sanofi Pharmaceuticals
2772; HEART SHAPE	Avapro	150 mg	White	Tablet	Oval, Biconvex	Sanofi Pharmaceuticals
2773; HEART SHAPE	Avapro	300 mg	White	Tablet	Oval, Biconvex	Sanofi Pharmaceuticals
2775; HEART	Avalide	150 mg ; 12.5 mg	Peach	Tablet	Oval, Biconvex	Bristol-Myers Squibb
2776 ; HEART	Avalide	300 mg ; 12.5 mg	Peach	Tablet	Oval	Bristol-Myers Squibb
3000	Quinidine Gluconate	324 mg		Sustained-Release Tablet		Roxane Laboratories
3125 VANCOCIN HCL 125 MG	Vancocin	125 mg	Blue, Brown	Capsule		Eli Lilly
3126 VANCOCIN HCL 125 MG	Vancocin	250 mg	Blue, Lavender	Capsule		Eli Lilly
3169 ; WPI	Alendronate Sodium	5 mg	White	Tablet	Circle	Watson Laboratories
3170 ; WPI	Alendronate Sodium	10 mg	White	Tablet	Oval	Watson Laboratories
3171 ; WPI	Alendronate Sodium	35 mg	White	Tablet	Capsule-Shape	Watson Laboratories
3172 ; WPI	Alendronate Sodium	40 mg	White	Tablet	Circle	Watson Laboratories
3173 ; WPI	Alendronate Sodium	70 mg	White	Tablet	Capsule-Shape	Watson Laboratories
3176 ; WPI	Citalopram Hydrobromide	10 mg	White	Tablet	Circle	Watson Laboratories
3220 ; WATSON	Butalbital, Acetaminophen, Caffeine, and Codeine Phosphate	325 mg ; 40 mg ; 30 mg ; 50 mg	Opaque Dark Blue, Opaque White	Capsule		Watson Laboratories
3230 WPI	Meloxicam	7.5 mg	Yellow	Tablet	Circle	Watson Laboratories
3231 WPI	Meloxicam	15 mg	Yellow	Tablet	Circle	Watson Laboratories
3250 ; WATSON	Nitrofurantoin Monohydrate/ macrocrystals	25 mg ; 75 mg	Opaque Black, Yellow	Capsule		Watson Laboratories
3253 ; WATSON	Nitrofurantoin Macrocrystals	50 mg	White, Yellow	Capsule		Watson Laboratories
3254 ; WATSON	Nitrofurantoin Macrocrystals	100 mg	Yellow	Capsule		Watson Laboratories
3322 ; WPI	Terbinafine Hydrochloride	250 mg	White	Tablet	Circle	Watson Laboratories
3344; SB; 10 MG	Compazine Spansule	10 mg	Black and Natural	Sustained-Release Capsule		Glaxosmithkline
3346; SB; 15 MG	Compazine Spansule	15 mg	Black and Natural	Sustained-Release Capsule		Glaxosmithkline
3366 ; WPI	Zolpidem Tartrate	5 mg	Pink	Tablet	Capsule-Shape	Watson Laboratories
3367 ; WPI	Zolpidem Tartrate	10 mg	White	Tablet	Capsule-Shape	Watson Laboratories
3369 ; WATSON	Butalbital, Acetaminophen, and Caffeine	50 mg ; 325 mg ; 40 mg	White	Tablet	Circle	Watson Laboratories
3461 ; WPI	Sertraline Hydrochloride	150 mg	White	Tablet	Capsule-Shape	Watson Laboratories
3757 ; LOGO	Lisinopril	2.5 mg	White	Tablet	Circle	Ivax Pharmaceuticals
3758 ; LOGO	Lisinopril	5 mg	White	Tablet	Square	Ivax Pharmaceuticals
3759 ; I	Lisinopril	10 mg	White	Tablet	Triangle	Teva Pharmaceuticals
3760 ; LOGO	Lisinopril	20 mg	White	Tablet	Five-Sided	Ivax Pharmaceuticals
3761 ; LOGO	Lisinopril	40 mg	White	Tablet	Circle	Ivax Pharmaceuticals
3762 ; LOGO	Lisinopril	30 mg	White	Tablet	Oval	Ivax Pharmaceuticals
3984; 3 ;	Aspirin and Codeine Phosphate	325 mg ; 30 mg	White	Tablet	Circle	Ivax Pharmaceuticals
3985; 4 ;	Aspirin and Codeine Phosphate	325 mg ; 60 mg	White	Tablet	Circle	Ivax Pharmaceuticals
4059 ; 9 3	Cefadroxil	1000 mg	White to Off-White	Tablet	Oval	Teva Pharmaceuticals
4117 ; W	Trecator	250 mg	Orange	Tablet		Wyeth Pharmaceuticals
4266; 200	Acyclovir	200 mg	White	Capsule		Watson Laboratories
4364; 100	Labetalol	100 mg	Yellow	Tablet	Circle, Bisected	Ivax Pharmaceuticals
4365; 200	Labetalol	200 mg	White	Tablet	Circle, Bisected	Ivax Pharmaceuticals
4366; 300	Labetalol	300 mg	Green	Tablet	Circle	Ivax Pharmaceuticals
4440 ; 100 ;	Gabapentin	100 mg	White	Tablet	Circle	Ivax Pharmaceuticals
4441 ; 300 ;	Gabapentin	300 mg	White	Tablet	Circle	Ivax Pharmaceuticals
4442 ; 400 ;	Gabapentin	400 mg	White	Tablet	Oval	Ivax Pharmaceuticals
4443 ; 600 ;	Gabapentin	600 mg	White	Tablet	Oval	Teva Pharmaceuticals
4444 ; 800 ;	Gabapentin	800 mg	White	Tablet	Oval	Teva Pharmaceuticals
4821 ; I 1	Lorazepam	1 mg	White	Tablet	Circle	Teva Pharmaceuticals

IMPRINT	BRAND/GENERIC NAME	STRENGTH	COLOR	FORM	SHAPE	MANUFACTURER
4822 ; I 2	Lorazepam	2 mg	White	Tablet	Circle	Teva Pharmaceuticals
5044 ; SOLVAY	Teveten	400 mg	Pink	Tablet	Oval	Abbott Laboratories
5046 ; SOLVAY	Teveten	600 mg	White	Tablet	Capsule-Shape	Abbott Laboratories
5052 ; DAN	Prednisone	5 mg	White	Tablet	Circle	Watson Laboratories
5124 ; 93	Benazepril Hydrochloride	5 mg	Light Yellow	Tablet	Triangle	Teva Pharmaceuticals
5125 ; 93	Benazepril Hydrochloride	10 mg	Mustard Yellow	Tablet	Triangle	Teva Pharmaceuticals
5126 ; 93	Benazepril Hydrochloride	20 mg	Pink	Tablet	Triangle	Teva Pharmaceuticals
5127 ; 93	Benazepril Hydrochloride	40 mg	Pink to Light Red	Tablet	Triangle	Teva Pharmaceuticals
5140 ; 93	Alendronate Sodium	5 mg	White to Off-White	Tablet	Circle	Teva Pharmaceuticals
5141 ; 93	Alendronate Sodium	10 mg	White to Off-White	Tablet	Circle	Teva Pharmaceuticals
5142 ; 93	Alendronate Sodium	40 mg	White to Off-White	Tablet	Oval	Teva Pharmaceuticals
5147 ; SOLVAY	Teveten HCT	600 mg ; 12.5 mg	Butterscotch	Tablet	Capsule-Shape	Abbott Laboratories
5150 ; SOLVAY	Teveten HCT	600 mg ; 25 mg	Brick Red	Tablet	Capsule-Shape	Abbott Laboratories
5161	Hydrocodone Bitartrate and Ibuprofen	7.5 mg ; 200 mg	White	Tablet	Circle	Teva Pharmaceuticals
5171 ; 93	Alendronate Sodium	70 mg	White to Off-White	Tablet	Rectangle	Teva Pharmaceuticals
5172 ; 93	Alendronate Sodium	35 mg	White to Off-White	Tablet	Rectangle	Teva Pharmaceuticals
5213 ; 9 3	Moexipril Hydrochloride and Hydrochlorothiazide	7.5 mg ; 12.5 mg	Yellow	Tablet	Capsule-Shape	Teva Pharmaceuticals
5214 ; 9 3	Moexipril Hydrochloride and Hydrochlorothiazide	12.5 mg ; 15 mg	White	Tablet	Capsule-Shape	Teva Pharmaceuticals
5215 ; 9 3	Moexipril Hydrochloride and Hydrochlorothiazide	15 mg ; 25 mg	Yellow	Tablet	Capsule-Shape	Teva Pharmaceuticals
5270 93	Bisoprolol Fumarate	5 mg	Pink	Tablet	Circle	Teva Pharmaceuticals
5271 93	Bisoprolol Fumarate	10 mg	White	Tablet	Circle	Teva Pharmaceuticals
5275 ; 93	Dexmethylphenidate Hydrochloride	2.5 mg	Blue	Tablet	Circle	Teva Pharmaceuticals
5276 ; 93	Dexmethylphenidate Hydrochloride	5 mg	Yellow	Tablet	Circle	Teva Pharmaceuticals
5277 ; 93	Dexmethylphenidate Hydrochloride	10 mg	White to Off-White	Tablet	Circle	Teva Pharmaceuticals
5282 ; 93	Ropinirole Hydrochloride	0.25 mg	White	Tablet	Circle	Teva Pharmaceuticals
5283 ; 93	Ropinirole Hydrochloride	0.5 mg	Yellow	Tablet	Circle	Teva Pharmaceuticals
5284 ; 93	Ropinirole Hydrochloride	1 mg	Green	Tablet	Circle	Teva Pharmaceuticals
5285 ; 93	Ropinirole Hydrochloride	2 mg	Pink	Tablet	Circle	Teva Pharmaceuticals
5286 ; 93	Ropinirole Hydrochloride	3 mg	Purple	Tablet	Circle	Teva Pharmaceuticals
5287 ; 93	Ropinirole Hydrochloride	4 mg	Beige	Tablet	Circle	Teva Pharmaceuticals
5288 ; 93	Ropinirole Hydrochloride	5 mg	Blue	Tablet	Circle	Teva Pharmaceuticals
5400 ; FP	Combunox	5 mg ; 400 mg	Off White, White	Tablet	Capsule-Shape	Forest Pharmaceuticals
5401 ; AMB 5	Ambien	5 mg	Pink	Tablet	Capsule-Shape	Sanofi-Aventis U.S.
5410 ; LOGO 50 ;	Fluconazole	50 mg	Pink	Tablet	Oval	Teva Pharmaceuticals
5411 ; LOGO 100 ;	Fluconazole	100 mg	Pink	Tablet	Oval	Teva Pharmaceuticals
5412 ; LOGO 150 ;	Fluconazole	150 mg	Pink	Tablet	Oval	Teva Pharmaceuticals
5413 ; LOGO 200 ;	Fluconazole	200 mg	Pink	Tablet	Oval	Teva Pharmaceuticals
5420 ; LOGO 0.5	Cabergoline	0.5 mg	White	Tablet	Oval	Teva Pharmaceuticals
5421 ; AMB 10	Ambien	10 mg	White	Tablet	Capsule-Shape	Sanofi-Aventis U.S.
5442 ; DAN	Prednisone	10 mg	White	Tablet	Circle	Watson Laboratories
5443 ; DAN	Prednisone	20 mg	Peach	Tablet	Circle	Watson Laboratories
5450 ; 93	Alprazolam	0.5 mg	White	Tablet, Extended Release	Circle	Teva Pharmaceuticals
5451 ; 93	Alprazolam	1 mg	Yellow	Tablet, Extended Release	Circle	Teva Pharmaceuticals
5452 ; 93	Alprazolam	2 mg	Blue	Tablet, Extended Release	Oval	Teva Pharmaceuticals
5453 ; 93	Alprazolam	3 mg	Green	Tablet, Extended Release	Circle	Teva Pharmaceuticals
5623; 150 MG ;	Nizatidine	150 mg	Yellow and White	Capsule		Ivax Pharmaceuticals
5636; DAN	Meclofenamate Sodium	50 mg	Pink	Capsule		Watson Laboratories
5656; 10; HOURGLASS	Tamoxifen	10 mg	White	Tablet	Circle	Ivax Pharmaceuticals
5657; 20; HOURGLASS	Tamoxifen	20 mg	White	Tablet	Circle	Ivax Pharmaceuticals
5672 ; 25	Sertraline Hydrochloride	25 mg	Light Blue	Tablet	Circle	Teva Pharmaceuticals
5673 ; 50	Sertraline Hydrochloride	50 mg	Light Blue	Tablet	Oval	Teva Pharmaceuticals
5674 ; 100	Sertraline Hydrochloride	100 mg	Light Blue	Tablet	Capsule-Shape	Teva Pharmaceuticals
5752; SCS	Piroxicam	10 mg	Opaque Light Blue and Orange	Capsule		Scs Pharmaceuticals
5777; DAN; 50	Atenolol	50 mg	White	Tablet	Circle, Scored	Watson Laboratories
5778; DAN; 100	Atenolol	100 mg	White	Tablet	Circle	Watson Laboratories
6057	Glyburide and Metformin Hydrochloride	1.25 mg ; 250 mg	Pale Yellow	Coated Tablet	Capsule-Shape	Par Pharmaceutical
6058	Glyburide and Metformin Hydrochloride	2.5 mg ; 500 mg	Pale Orange	Coated Tablet	Capsule-Shape	Par Pharmaceutical
6059	Glyburide and Metformin Hydrochloride	5 mg ; 500 mg	Yellow	Coated Tablet	Capsule-Shape	Par Pharmaceutical
7114 ; 93	Paroxetine	10 mg	Yellow	Tablet	Circle	Teva Pharmaceuticals
7115 ; 93	Paroxetine	20 mg	Pink	Tablet	Circle	Teva Pharmaceuticals
7116 ; 93	Paroxetine	30 mg	Blue	Tablet	Circle	Teva Pharmaceuticals
7121 ; 93	Paroxetine	40 mg	Green	Tablet	Circle	Teva Pharmaceuticals
7146 ; 93	Azithromycin	250 mg	Mottled Pink	Tablet	Oval	Teva Pharmaceuticals
7147 ; 93	Azithromycin	600 mg	White to Off-White	Tablet	Capsule-Shape	Teva Pharmaceuticals
7157 ; 93	Clarithromycin	250 mg	Yellow	Tablet	Oval	Teva Pharmaceuticals
7158 ; 93	Clarithromycin	500 mg	Light Yellow	Tablet	Oval	Teva Pharmaceuticals
7167 ; 93	Amlodipine Besylate	5 mg	White to Off-White	Tablet	Circle	Teva Pharmaceuticals
7169 ; 93	Azithromycin	500 mg	Mottled Pink	Tablet	Oval	Teva Pharmaceuticals
7171 ; 400	Cimetidine	400 mg	White to Off-White	Tablet	Capsule-Shape	Teva Pharmaceuticals
7175 ; 93	Sertraline Hydrochloride	25 mg	Light Green	Tablet	Oval	Teva Pharmaceuticals
7176 ; 93	Sertraline Hydrochloride	50 mg	Light Blue	Tablet	Oval	Teva Pharmaceuticals
7177 ; 93	Sertraline Hydrochloride	100 mg	Light Yellow	Tablet	Oval	Teva Pharmaceuticals

IMPRINT	BRAND/GENERIC NAME	STRENGTH	COLOR	FORM	SHAPE	MANUFACTURER
7206 ; 9 3	Mirtazapine	15 mg	Yellow	Tablet	Circle	Teva Pharmaceuticals
7207 ; 9 3	Mirtazapine	30 mg	Red-Brown	Tablet	Circle	Teva Pharmaceuticals
7208 ; 93	Mirtazapine	45 mg	White to Off-White	Tablet	Circle	Teva Pharmaceuticals
7230 ; 93	Cilostazol	50 mg	White to Off White	Tablet	Rectangle	Teva Pharmaceuticals
7231 ; 93	Cilostazol	100 mg	White to Off White	Tablet	Circle	Teva Pharmaceuticals
7232 ; 93	Ribavirin	200 mg	Light Pink to Pink	Tablet	Circle	Teva Pharmaceuticals
7234 ; 93	Meloxicam	7.5 mg	Mottled Yellow	Tablet	Capsule-Shape	Teva Pharmaceuticals
7240 ; 93	Risperidone	1 mg	White to Off-White	Tablet	Circle	Teva Pharmaceuticals
7241 ; 93	Risperidone	2 mg	Orange	Tablet	Circle	Teva Pharmaceuticals
7242 ; 93	Risperidone	3 mg	Yellow	Tablet	Circle	Teva Pharmaceuticals
7243 ; 93	Risperidone	4 mg	Green	Tablet	Circle	Teva Pharmaceuticals
7244 ; 93	Clarithromycin	500 mg	Yellow	Tablet, Extended Release	Oval	Teva Pharmaceuticals
7247 ; 9 3	Lamotrigine	150 mg	Cream	Tablet	Diamond	Teva Pharmaceuticals
7248 ; 9 3	Lamotrigine	200 mg	Blue	Tablet	Diamond	Teva Pharmaceuticals
7251 ; 93	Fexofenadine Hydrochloride	30 mg	Peach	Tablet	Capsule-Shape	Teva Pharmaceuticals
7252 ; 93	Fexofenadine Hydrochloride	60 mg	Peach	Tablet	Circle	Teva Pharmaceuticals
7253 ; 93	Fexofenadine Hydrochloride	180 mg	Peach	Tablet	Circle	Teva Pharmaceuticals
7294 ; 93	Terbinafine Hydrochloride	250 mg	White to Off White	Tablet	Circle	Teva Pharmaceuticals
7295 ; 93	Carvedilol	12.5 mg	White	Tablet	Oval	Teva Pharmaceuticals
7299 ; 93	Meloxicam	15 mg	Mottled Yellow	Tablet	Rectangle	Teva Pharmaceuticals
7301 ; 93	Ondansetron	4 mg	White to Off White	Tablet, Disintegrating	Circle	Teva Pharmaceuticals
7302 ; 93	Ondansetron	8 mg	White to Off White	Tablet, Disintegrating	Circle	Teva Pharmaceuticals
7325 ; 9 3	Trandolapril	1 mg	Mottled Salmon	Tablet	Capsule-Shape	Teva Pharmaceuticals
7326 ; 93	Trandolapril	2 mg	Mottled Yellow	Tablet	Capsule-Shape	Teva Pharmaceuticals
7327 ; 93	Trandolapril	4 mg	Mottled Rose	Tablet	Capsule-Shape	Teva Pharmaceuticals
7330 ; 93	Lofibra	54 mg	Yellow	Tablet	Circle	Gate Pharmaceuticals
7331 ; 93	Lofibra	160 mg	White to Off-White	Tablet	Oval	Gate Pharmaceuticals
7355 ; 93	Finasteride	5 mg	Blue	Tablet	Capsule-Shape	Teva Pharmaceuticals
7380 ; 9 3	Venlafaxine Hydrochloride	37.5 mg	Mottled Peach	Tablet	Circle	Teva Pharmaceuticals
7381 ; 9 3	Venlafaxine Hydrochloride	50 mg	Mottled Peach	Tablet	Circle	Teva Pharmaceuticals
7382 ; 9 3	Venlafaxine Hydrochloride	75 mg	Mottled Peach	Tablet	Circle	Teva Pharmaceuticals
7383 ; 9 3	Venlafaxine Hydrochloride	100 mg	Mottled Peach	Tablet	Circle	Teva Pharmaceuticals
7455 ; 93	Glipizide and Metformin Hydrochloride	2.5 mg ; 250 mg	Pink	Tablet	Capsule-Shape	Barr Laboratories
7456 ; 93	Glipizide and Metformin Hydrochloride	2.5 mg ; 500 mg	White	Tablet	Capsule-Shape	Barr Laboratories
7457 ; 93	Glipizide and Metformin Hydrochloride	5 mg ; 500 mg	Pink	Tablet	Capsule-Shape	Barr Laboratories
7485 ; 93	Granisetron Hydrochloride	1 mg	White to Off-White	Tablet	Capsule-Shape	Teva Pharmaceuticals
7489	Ampicillin	250 mg	Brown and White	Capsule		Bristol-Myers Squibb
7499	Ampicillin	500 mg	Brown and White	Capsule		Bristol-Myers Squibb
7663	Aromasin	25 mg	Off-White to Slightly Gray	Tablet	Circle	Pharmacia & Upjohn
7720; 250 ;	Cefzil	250 mg	Light Orange	Coated Tablet		Bristol-Myers Squibb
7721; 500 ;	Cefzil	500 mg	White	Coated Tablet		Bristol-Myers Squibb
7767 50	Celebrex	50 mg	White with Red Band	Capsule		Pfizer
7767 100	Celebrex	100 mg	White with Blue Band	Capsule		Pfizer
7767 200	Celebrex	200 mg	White with Gold Band	Capsule		Pfizer
7767 400	Celebrex	400 mg	White with Green Band	Capsule		Pfizer
9338	Gabapentin	100 mg	Gray	Capsule		Teva Pharmaceuticals
9550	Mudrane	111 mg ; 16 mg ; 195 mg ; 8 mg	Yellow	Tablet		Ecr Pharmaceuticals
59010; 240	Bupap	50 mg ; 650 mg	Light Blue	Tablet		Ecr Pharmaceuticals
60274; 120MG	Verapamil Hydrochloride	120 mg	Yellow Opaque	Capsule		Watson Laboratories
60274; 180MG	Verapamil Hydrochloride	180 mg	Light Gray Yellow Opaque	Capsule		Watson Laboratories
60274; 240MG	Verapamil Hydrochloride	240 mg	Dark Blue and Yellow Opaque	Capsule		Watson Laboratories
60274; 360MG	Verapamil Hydrochloride	360 mg	Lavender and Yellow Opaque	Capsule		Watson Laboratories
937370 ; 93 7370	Amlodipine Besylate and Benazepril Hydrochloride	10 mg ; 2.5 mg	White Opaque	Capsule	Capsule-Shape	Teva Pharmaceuticals
937371 ; 93 7371	Amlodipine Besylate and Benazepril Hydrochloride	5 mg ; 10 mg	Orange Opaque, White Opaque	Capsule	Capsule-Shape	Teva Pharmaceuticals
937372 ; 93 7372	Amlodipine Besylate and Benazepril Hydrochloride	5 mg ; 20 mg	Pink Opaque, White Opaque	Capsule	Capsule-Shape	Teva Pharmaceuticals
937373 ; 93 7373	Amlodipine Besylate and Benazepril Hydrochloride	10 mg ; 20 mg	Blue Violet Opaque	Capsule	Capsule-Shape	Teva Pharmaceuticals
A	Axert	12.5 mg	White with Blue Ink	Tablet	Circle, Compressed, Biconvex	Ortho-Mcneil Pharmaceutical
A	Cefol	750 mg ; 100 mg ; 20 mg ; 15 mg ; 10 mg ; 5 mg ; 0.5 mg ; 6 mcg ; 30 IU	Green	Coated Tablet	Oval	Abbott Laboratories
A	Children's Aspirin	75 mg	Bright Pink	Tablet, Chewable		Abbott Laboratories
A	Ephedrine and Nembutal 25	25 mg ; 25 mg	Black	Capsule		Abbott Laboratories
A	Fero-Gradumet	525 mg	Red	Tablet		Abbott Laboratories
A	Gerilets	5000 IU ; 400 IU ; 45 IU ; 0.4 mg ; 2.25 mg ; 2.6 mg ; 30 mg ; 0.45 mg ; 15 mg ; 90 mg ; 3 mg ; 9 mcg ; 27 mg	Green	Tablet		Abbott Laboratories
A	Iberet-500	525 mg ; 500 mg ; 25 mcg ; 6 mg ; 6 mg ; 30 mg ; 5 mg ; 10 mg	Red	Coated Tablet	Oblong	Abbott Laboratories
A	Lidone	5 mg	Cream and Blue	Capsule		Abbott Laboratories

IMPRINT	BRAND/GENERIC NAME	STRENGTH	COLOR	FORM	SHAPE	MANUFACTURER
A	Lidone	10 mg	Cream and Red	Capsule		Abbott Laboratories
A	Lidone	25 mg	Cream and Brown	Capsule		Abbott Laboratories
A	Surbex T	15 mg ; 10 mg ; 100 mg ; 5 mg ; 10 mcg ; 20 mg ; 500 mg	Orange	Tablet	Oblong	Abbott Laboratories
A	Tral with Phenobarbital Gradumet	30 mg ; 50 mg	Blue	Tablet		Abbott Laboratories
A ;	Clarinex Reditabs	5 mg	Light Red	Tablet, Disintegrating	Circle	Schering-Plough
A 024	Permax	0.05 mg	Ivory	Tablet		Valeant Pharmaceuticals
A 025	Permax	0.25 mg	Green	Tablet		Valeant Pharmaceuticals
A 026	Permax	1 mg	Pink	Tablet	Oblong	Valeant Pharmaceuticals
A 15	Buspirone Hydrochloride	15 mg	White	Tablet	Rectangle	Actavis Totowa
A 115	Bellamine S	0.2 mg ; 0.6 mg ; 40 mg	Green	Tablet		Actavis Totowa
A 117	Bupropion Hydrochloride	150 mg	Pale Yellow	Tablet, Extended Release, 12 Hr	Circle	Actavis South Atlantic
A 133	Bupropion Hydrochloride	150 mg	Pale Yellow	Tablet, Extended Release, 12 Hr	Circle	Actavis South Atlantic
A 151	Nifedipine	60 mg	Yellow	Tablet, Extended Release	Circle	Actavis South Atlantic
A 153	Nifedipine	30 mg	Yellow	Tablet, Extended Release	Circle	Actavis South Atlantic
A 191	Loxapine	5 mg	Dark Green	Capsule		Actavis Totowa
A 192	Loxapine	10 mg	Dark Green, Yellow	Capsule		Actavis Totowa
A 193	Loxapine	25 mg	Dark Green, Light Green	Capsule		Actavis Totowa
A 194	Loxapine	50 mg	Dark Green, Light Blue	Capsule		Actavis Totowa
A 211	Naloxone and Pentazocine	0.5 mg ; 50 mg	Light Yellow	Tablet	Capsule-Shape	Actavis Totowa
A 219	Dantrolene Sodium	25 mg	Medium Orange Opaque, Yellow Opaque	Capsule		Actavis Totowa
A 220	Dantrolene Sodium	50 mg	Medium Orange Opaque, Yellow Opaque	Capsule		Actavis Totowa
A 221	Dantrolene Sodium	100 mg	Medium Orange Opaque, Yellow Opaque	Capsule		Actavis Totowa
A 234	Tizanidine Hydrochloride	4 mg	White	Tablet		Actavis Totowa
A 236	Tizanidine Hydrochloride	2 mg	White	Tablet	Circle	Actavis Totowa
A 268	Bethanechol Chloride	5 mg	White	Tablet	Circle	Actavis Totowa
A 269	Bethanechol Chloride	10 mg	White	Tablet	Circle	Actavis Totowa
A 270	Bethanechol Chloride	25 mg	Orange-Yellow	Tablet	Circle	Actavis Totowa
A 285	Meloxicam	7.5 mg	Yellow	Tablet	Circle	Actavis Totowa
A 286	Meloxicam	15 mg	Yellow	Tablet	Oval	Actavis Totowa
A 293	Trimipramine Maleate	25 mg	Light Blue Opaque, Yellow Opaque	Capsule		Actavis Totowa
A 294	Trimipramine Maleate	50 mg	Light Blue Opaque, Medium Orange Opaque	Capsule		Actavis Totowa
A 295	Trimipramine Maleate	100 mg	Light Blue Opaque, White Opaque	Capsule		Actavis Totowa
A 301 ;	Cyclobenzaprine Hydrochloride	5 mg	Orange	Tablet	Circle	Actavis Totowa
A 312	Hydroxyzine Hydrochloride	25 mg	Green	Tablet	Circle	Actavis Totowa
A 313	Hydroxyzine Hydrochloride	50 mg	Yellow	Tablet	Circle	Actavis Totowa
A 325 ; LOGO 325	Rythmol SR	325 mg	White	Capsule		Glaxosmithkline
A 327	Phendimetrazine Tartrate	35 mg	Yellow	Tablet	Circle	Actavis Totowa
A 425 ; LOGO 425	Rythmol SR	425 mg	White	Capsule		Glaxosmithkline
A IH	Dutoprol	12.5 mg ; 25 mg	Yellow	Tablet, Extended Release	Circle	Astrazeneca
A IK	Dutoprol	50 mg ; 12.5 mg	Light Orange	Tablet, Extended Release	Circle	Astrazeneca
A IL	Dutoprol	100 mg ; 12.5 mg	Yellow	Tablet, Extended Release	Circle	Astrazeneca
A; 002	Aquatab DM	1200 mg ; 60 mg	Light Blue	Coated Tablet	Circle, Scored	Adams Laboratories
A; 003 ;	Phenazopyridine Hydrochloride	100 mg	Maroon	Tablet	Circle	Actavis Totowa
A; 004 ;	Phenazopyridine Hydrochloride	200 mg	Maroon	Tablet	Circle	Actavis Totowa
A; 018	Chlordiazepoxide Hydrochloride with Clidinium Bromide	5 mg ; 2.5 mg	Green	Capsule		Watson Laboratories
A; 019 ;	Amigesic	500 mg	Yellow	Tablet	Circle	Actavis Totowa
A; 020 ;	Amigesic	750 mg	Yellow	Tablet		Actavis Totowa
A; 031 ;	Multivitamin W/fluoride	2500 IU ; 400 IU ; 15 IU ; 60 mg ; 0.3 mg ; 1.05 mg ; 1.2 mg ; 13.5 mg ; 1.05 mg ; 4.5 mcg ; 0.5 mg	Orange, Pink or Purple	Tablet, Chewable		Actavis Totowa
A; 039 ;	Amidrine	325 mg ; 65 mg ; 100 mg	Maroon or Red and White	Capsule		Actavis Totowa
A; 041	Acetaminophen/oxycodone	500 mg ; 5 mg	White	Capsule		Actavis Totowa
A; 047	Bontril Slow-Release	105 mg	Green and Yellow	Extended-Release Capsule		Amarin Pharmaceuticals
A; 060	Ursodiol	300 mg	Pink and White	Capsule		Actavis Totowa
A; 2	Dilaudid	2 mg	Orange	Tablet	Circle	Purdue Pharma
A; 4	Dilaudid	4 mg	Yellow	Tablet	Circle	Purdue Pharma
A; 5	Oxycodone Hydrochloride	5 mg	White	Tablet	Circle	Actavis Totowa
A; 21	Acetaminophen	325 mg	White	Tablet		Lederle Laboratories
A; 50; G	Atenolol	50 mg	White	Tablet	Circle, Flat; Bevelled Edge; Scored	Par Pharmaceutical
A; 75	Acetaminophen/oxycodone	325 mg ; 5 mg	White	Tablet	Circle	Actavis Totowa
A; 100; G	Atenolol	100 mg	White	Tablet	Circle, Flat; Bevelled Edge	Par Pharmaceutical
A; 105	Naltrexone Hydrochloride	50 mg	Yellow	Tablet	Capsule-Shape	Actavis Totowa

IMPRINT	BRAND/GENERIC NAME	STRENGTH	COLOR	FORM	SHAPE	MANUFACTURER
A; 106	Amibid LA	600 mg	Green	Tablet, Extended Release	Capsule-Shape	Actavis Totowa
A; 106	New Ami-Tex LA	600 mg ; 30 mg	Green	Tablet, Extended Release		Actavis Totowa
A; 111	Methenamine Mandelate	0.5 GM	Brown	Tablet	Oval	Actavis Totowa
A; 127	Sodium Fluoride	0.5 mg	Purple	Tablet, Chewable	Circle	Actavis Totowa
A; 128	Sodium Fluoride	1 mg	Assorted	Tablet, Chewable	Circle	Actavis Totowa
A; 133	Glyburide Micronized	1.5 mg	White	Tablet	Oval	Actavis Totowa
A; 134	Glyburide Micronized	3 mg	Blue	Tablet	Oval	Actavis Totowa
A; 135	Glyburide Micronized	6 mg	Yellow	Tablet	Oval	Actavis Totowa
A; 136	Carisoprodol	350 mg	White	Tablet	Circle	Actavis Totowa
A; 137	Aspirin/carisoprodol	200 mg ; 325 mg	Red and White	Tablet	Circle	Actavis Totowa
A; 138	Aspirin/carisoprodol/codeine	200 mg ; 325 mg ; 16 mg	White and Yellow	Tablet	Circle	Actavis Totowa
A; 139	Amibid DM	30 mg ; 600 mg	Green	Tablet, Extended Release	Capsule-Shape	Actavis Totowa
A; 143	Hyoscyamine Sulfate	0.125 mg	White	Tablet	Circle	Actavis Totowa
A; 155	Hyoscyamine Sulfate	0.125 mg	Blue	Tablet	Circle	Actavis Totowa
A; 156	Hyoscyamine Sulfate	0.375 mg	Orange	Tablet, Extended Release	Capsule-Shape	Actavis Totowa
A; 157	Meperidine Hydrochloride	100 mg	White	Tablet	Circle	Actavis Totowa
A; 158	Meperidine Hydrochloride	50 mg	White	Tablet	Circle	Actavis Totowa
A; 159	Phentermine Hydrochloride	37.5 mg	White with Blue Speckles	Tablet	Capsule-Shape	Actavis Totowa
A; 160	Phentermine Hydrochloride	30 mg	Yellow	Capsule		Actavis Totowa
A; 161	Pemoline	37.5 mg	Peach	Tablet	Circle	Actavis Totowa
A; 162	Pemoline	75 mg	Peach	Tablet	Circle	Actavis Totowa
A; 163	Hyoscyamine Sulfate	0.375 mg	Clear with White and Orange Beads	Capsule, Extended Release		Actavis Totowa
A; 166	Trimethobenzamide Hydrochloride	250 mg	Aqua and Light Blue	Capsule		Actavis Totowa
A; 167	Phentermine Hydrochloride	37.5 mg	White and Blue	Capsule		Actavis Totowa
A; 170	Phentermine Hydrochloride	15 mg	Gray, Orange, Yellow	Capsule		Actavis Totowa
A; 171	Prenatal RX	1.5 mg ; 0.5 mg ; 27 mg ; 50 mg ; 8.5 mg ; 2000 IU ; 0.75 mg ; 0.8 mg ; 2 mg ; 0.00125 mg ; 40 mg ; 200 IU ; 7.5 IU ; 12.5 mg ; 0.015 mg ; 100 mg ; 3.5 mg	White	Tablet	Oblong	Actavis Totowa
A; 172	Codeine Phosphate/guaifenesin	10 mg ; 300 mg	Red	Tablet		Actavis Totowa
A; 173	Phentermine Hydrochloride	30 mg	Clear and Blue	Capsule		Actavis Totowa
A; 179	Betaxolol Hydrochloride	10 mg	White	Tablet	Circle	Actavis Totowa
A; 180	Betaxolol Hydrochloride	20 mg	White	Tablet	Circle	Actavis Totowa
A; 185	Trimethobenzamide Hydrochloride	300 mg	Lavender	Capsule		Actavis Totowa
A; 186	Pemoline	37.5 mg	Peach	Tablet, Chewable	Square	Actavis Totowa
A; 187	Oxycodone Hydrochloride	5 mg	Peach and Brown	Capsule		Actavis Totowa
A; 190	Meperidine Hydrochloride/ promethazine Hydrochloride	50 mg ; 25 mg	Red	Capsule		Actavis Totowa
A; 197	Pemoline	18.75 mg	White	Tablet	Circle	Actavis Totowa
A; 213	Acetaminophen/pentazocine Hydrochloride	650 mg ; 25 mg	Light Blue	Tablet	Capsule-Shape	Actavis Totowa
A; 214	Oxycodone Hydrochloride	15 mg	Green	Tablet	Circle	Actavis Totowa
A; 215	Oxycodone Hydrochloride	30 mg	Blue	Tablet	Circle	Actavis Totowa
A; 216	Carbetapentane Tannate and Chlorpheniramine Tannate	60 mg ; 5 mg	Dark Purple	Tablet	Circle	Actavis Totowa
A; 226	Mirtazapine	15 mg	Yellow	Tablet	Oval	Actavis Totowa
A; 227	Mirtazapine	30 mg	Tan	Tablet	Oval	Actavis Totowa
A; 228	Mirtazapine	45 mg	White	Tablet	Oval	Actavis Totowa
A; 245	Guaifenesin ER	1200 mg	White	Tablet, Extended Release	Capsule-Shape	Actavis Totowa
A; 246	Dextromethorphan/guaifenesin	60 mg ; 1200 mg	Blue	Tablet, Extended Release	Capsule-Shape	Actavis Totowa
A; 247	Guaifenesin/pseudoephedrine	1200 mg ; 120 mg	White	Tablet, Extended Release	Capsule-Shape	Actavis Totowa
A; 273	Tramadol Hydrochloride	50 mg	White to Off-White	Tablet	Circle	Ivax Pharmaceuticals
A; 554	Carbamazepine	200 mg	White	Tablet	Circle, Flat, Scored	Teva Pharmaceuticals
A; 585	Atamet	25 mg ; 100 mg	Mottled Yellow	Tablet	Circle, Scored	Athena Neurosciences
A; 585	Carbidopa and Levodopa	100 mg ; 25 mg	Mottled Yellow	Tablet	Circle	Teva Pharmaceuticals
A; 587	Atamet	25 mg ; 250 mg	Mottled Blue	Tablet	Circle, Scored	Athena Neurosciences
A; 750	Salsalate	750 mg	Blue or Yellow	Tablet		Novartis Generics
A; A; 8	Dilaudid	8 mg	White	Tablet	Triangle	Purdue Pharma
A; AA	Chlorthalidone	25 mg		Tablet		Abbott Laboratories
A; AB	Chlorthalidone	50 mg		Tablet		Abbott Laboratories
A; AD ;	Peganone	250 mg	White	Tablet	Circle, Scored	Abbott Laboratories
A; AE ;	Peganone	500 mg	White	Tablet	Circle, Scored	Abbott Laboratories
A; AF	Colchicine	0.6 mg		Tablet		Abbott Laboratories
A; AM	Tridione	300 mg		Capsule		Abbott Laboratories
A; AN	Dicumarol	25 mg		Tablet		Abbott Laboratories
A; ANTABUSE; 250	Antabuse	250 mg	White to Off-White	Tablet	Eight-Sided, Scored, Compressed	Wyeth Pharmaceuticals
A; ANTABUSE; 500	Antabuse	500 mg	White to Off-White	Tablet	Eight-Sided, Scored, Compressed	Wyeth Pharmaceuticals
A; AO	Dicumarol	50 mg		Tablet		Abbott Laboratories
A; B	Toprol XL	25 mg		Extended-Release Tablet		Astrazeneca
A; CE	Nembutal Sodium	30 mg	Yellow	Capsule		Abbott Laboratories
A; CP	A-Poxide	5 mg	Yellow and Green	Capsule		Abbott Laboratories
A; CS	A-Poxide	10 mg	Green and Evergreen	Capsule		Abbott Laboratories
A; CT	A-Poxide	25 mg		Capsule		Abbott Laboratories
A; EC	Ery-Tab	250 mg	White	Enteric-Coated Tablet	Oval	Abbott Laboratories
A; EE	E.E.S.-400 Filmtab	400 mg	Pink	Coated Tablet	Oblong	Abbott Laboratories

IMPRINT	BRAND/GENERIC NAME	STRENGTH	COLOR	FORM	SHAPE	MANUFACTURER
A; EH	Ery-Tab	333 mg	White	Enteric-Coated Tablet		Abbott Laboratories
A; FI	Tricor	48 mg	Yellow	Tablet		Abbott Laboratories
A; FO	Tricor	145 mg	White	Tablet		Abbott Laboratories
A; FT ;	Mavik	1 mg	Salmon	Tablet	Circle, Scored	Abbott Laboratories
A; FX ;	Mavik	2 mg	Yellow	Tablet	Circle, Compressed	Abbott Laboratories
A; FZ ;	Mavik	4 mg	Rose	Tablet	Circle, Compressed	Abbott Laboratories
A; IA	Cartrol	2.5 mg	Gray	Tablet	Oval	Abbott Laboratories
A; II	Phenurone	500 mg	White	Tablet		Abbott Laboratories
A; KJ	Biaxin XL	500 mg	Yellow	Extended-Release Tablet	Capsule-Shape	Abbott Laboratories
A; KL	Biaxin	500 mg	Yellow	Coated Tablet	Oval	Abbott Laboratories
A; KT	Biaxin	250 mg	Yellow	Coated Tablet	Oval	Abbott Laboratories
A; LE	Tridione Dulcet	150 mg		Tablet, Chewable		Abbott Laboratories
A; LF ;	Panwarfin	10 mg	White	Tablet		Abbott Laboratories
A; LJ ;	Harmonyl	0.1 mg	Light Yellow	Tablet		Abbott Laboratories
A; LK ;	Harmonyl	0.25 mg	Salmon	Tablet		Abbott Laboratories
A; LM ;	Panwarfin	2 mg	Purple	Tablet		Abbott Laboratories
A; LN ;	Panwarfin	2.5 mg	Orange	Tablet		Abbott Laboratories
A; LO ;	Panwarfin	5 mg	Salmon	Tablet		Abbott Laboratories
A; LR ;	Panwarfin	7.5 mg	Yellow	Tablet		Abbott Laboratories
A; MC	Desoxyn Gradumet	5 mg	White	Tablet		Abbott Laboratories
A; ME	Desoxyn Gradumet	10 mg	Light Orange	Tablet		Abbott Laboratories
A; MF	Desoxyn Gradumet	15 mg	Yellow	Tablet		Abbott Laboratories
A; MO	Toprol XL	50 mg	White	Sustained-Release Tablet	Circle, Biconvex, Scored	Astrazeneca
A; MS	Toprol XL	100 mg	White	Sustained-Release Tablet	Biconvex, Scored, Circle	Astrazeneca
A; MY	Toprol XL	200 mg	White	Sustained-Release Tablet	Oval, Biconvex, Scored	Astrazeneca
A; NC	Nicobid	125 mg	Black and Clear	Capsule		Aventis Behring
A; ND	Nicobid	250 mg	Green and Clear	Capsule		Aventis Behring
A; NE	Nicolar	500 mg	Yellow	Tablet		Aventis Behring
A; NJ	Cefol	6 mcg ; 30 IU ; 750 mg ; 100 mg ; 20 mg ; 15 mg ; 10 mg ; 5 mg ; 50 mcg	Green	Coated Tablet	Oval	Abbott Laboratories
A; NR	Depakote	250 mg	Peach	Tablet, Delayed Release		Abbott Laboratories
A; NS ;	Depakote	500 mg	Lavender	Tablet, Delayed Release		Abbott Laboratories
A; NT ;	Depakote	125 mg	Salmon Pink	Tablet, Delayed Release		Abbott Laboratories
A; TC	Armour Thyroid 1/4 grain	15 mg	Light Tan	Tablet	Circle, Convex	Forest Pharmaceuticals
A; TC	Desoxyn	2.5 mg	White	Tablet		Abbott Laboratories
A; TD	Armour Thyroid 1/2 grain	30 mg	Light Tan	Tablet	Circle	Forest Pharmaceuticals
A; TE	Armour Thyroid 1 grain	60 mg	Light Tan	Tablet	Circle	Forest Pharmaceuticals
A; TE	Desoxyn	5 mg	White	Tablet		Abbott Laboratories
A; TF	Armour Thyroid 2 grains	120 mg	Light Tan	Tablet	Circle	Forest Pharmaceuticals
A; TG	Armour Thyroid 3 grains	180 mg	Light Tan	Tablet		Forest Pharmaceuticals
A; TH	Armour Thyroid 4 grains	240 mg	Light Tan	Tablet	Circle, Convex	Forest Pharmaceuticals
A; TI	Armour Thyroid 5 grains	300 mg	Light Tan	Tablet	Round, Bisected Scored	Forest Pharmaceuticals
A; TJ	Armour Thyroid 1-1/2 grains	90 mg	Light Tan	Tablet	Circle, Convex	Forest Pharmaceuticals
A; TL	Tranxene T-Tab	3.75 mg	Blue	Tablet	T-Shaped, Scored	Abbott Laboratories
A; TM	Tranxene T-Tab	7.5 mg	Peach	Tablet	T-Shaped, Scored	Abbott Laboratories
A; TN	Tranxene T-Tab	15 mg	Lavender	Tablet	T-Shaped, Scored	Abbott Laboratories
A; TX	Tranxene-Sd Half Strength	11.25 mg	Blue	Tablet	Circle	Abbott Laboratories
A; YC	Thyrolar-1/4	3.1 mcg ; 12.5 mcg	Violet and White	Tablet		Forest Pharmaceuticals
A; YD	Thyrolar-1/2	6.25 mcg ; 25 mcg	Peach and White	Tablet		Forest Pharmaceuticals
A; YE	Thyrolar-1	12.5 mcg ; 50 mcg	Pink and White	Tablet		Forest Pharmaceuticals
A; YF	Thyrolar-2	25 mcg ; 100 mcg	Green and White	Tablet		Forest Pharmaceuticals
A; YH	Thyrolar-3	37.5 mcg ; 150 mcg	Yellow and White	Tablet		Forest Pharmaceuticals
A; Z	Azathioprine	50 mg	Yellow	Tablet	Circle, Scored	Mylan Pharmaceuticals
A~	Ambien Cr	6.25 mg	Pink	Tablet, Extended Release	Circle	Sanofi-Aventis U.S.
A~	Ambien Cr	12.5 mg	Blue	Tablet, Extended Release	Circle	Sanofi-Aventis U.S.
A-006 2	Abilify	2 mg	Green	Tablet	Rectangle	Bristol-Myers Squibb
A-007 5	Abilify	5 mg	Blue	Tablet	Rectangle	Bristol-Myers Squibb
A-008 10	Abilify	10 mg	Pink	Tablet	Rectangle	Bristol-Myers Squibb
A-009 15	Abilify	15 mg	Yellow	Tablet	Circle	Bristol-Myers Squibb
A-010 20	Abilify	20 mg	White	Tablet	Circle	Bristol-Myers Squibb
A-011 30	Abilify	30 mg	Pink	Tablet	Circle	Bristol-Myers Squibb
A-263	Isradipine	2.5 mg	White Opaque	Capsule		Actavis Totowa
A-264	Isradipine	5 mg	Flesh Opaque	Capsule		Actavis Totowa
A-309	Amantadine Hydrochloride	100 mg	Swedish Orange Opaque	Capsule, Liquid Filled		Actavis Totowa
A2C	Lanoxicaps	0.05 mg	Red	Capsule, Liquid Filled	Oblong, Small	Glaxosmithkline
A8 ; M	Amlodipine Besylate	2.5 mg	Blue	Tablet	Circle	Mylan Pharmaceuticals
A9 ; M	Amlodipine Besylate	5 mg	Blue	Tablet	Circle	Mylan Pharmaceuticals
A9L; RD	Artane Sequels	5 mg	Clear Blue	Sustained-Release Capsule	Oval	Lederle Laboratories
A10 ; M	Amlodipine Besylate	10 mg	Blue	Tablet	Circle	Mylan Pharmaceuticals
A21 ; M	Alprazolam	0.5 mg	White	Tablet, Extended Release	Circle	Mylan Pharmaceuticals
A22 ; M	Alprazolam	1 mg	Light Orange	Tablet, Extended Release	Circle	Mylan Pharmaceuticals
A23 ; M	Alprazolam	2 mg	Light Lavender	Tablet, Extended Release	Circle	Mylan Pharmaceuticals
A24 ; M	Alprazolam	3 mg	Light Pink	Tablet, Extended Release	Circle	Mylan Pharmaceuticals
A77 ; W	Aralen	500 mg	White	Film-Coated, Discoid Tablet	Circle	Sanofi-Aventis U.S.

IMPRINT	BRAND/GENERIC NAME	STRENGTH	COLOR	FORM	SHAPE	MANUFACTURER
A101	Budeprion XL	150 mg	White to Off-White	Tablet, Extended Release	Circle	Teva Pharmaceuticals
A250	Cilostazol	100 mg	White	Tablet	Circle	Actavis Totowa
A254	Mirtazapine	15 mg	White	Tablet, Disintegrating	Circle	Actavis Totowa
A255	Mirtazapine	30 mg	White	Tablet, Disintegrating	Circle	Actavis Totowa
A256	Mirtazapine	45 mg	White	Tablet, Disintegrating	Circle	Actavis Totowa
A265	Dipyridamole	25 mg	Yellow	Tablet	Circle	Actavis Totowa
A266	Dipyridamole	50 mg	Yellow	Tablet	Circle	Actavis Totowa
A267	Dipyridamole	75 mg	Yellow	Tablet	Circle	Actavis Totowa
A311	Hydroxyzine Hydrochloride	10 mg	Orange	Tablet	Circle	Actavis Totowa
A500 ; A500	Darvocet A500	100 mg ; 500 mg	Dark Orange	Tablet	Oval	Xanodyne Pharmaceuticals
AB2 5 ; LOGO	Amlodipine Besylate	2.5 mg	White	Tablet	Circle	Actavis Totowa
AB5 ; LOGO	Amlodipine Besylate	5 mg	White	Tablet	Circle	Actavis Totowa
AB10 ; LOGO	Amlodipine Besylate	10 mg	White	Tablet	Circle	Actavis Totowa
ABBOTT LOGO; 25 MG; OR	Gengraf	25 mg	White with Blue Ink	Capsule		Abbott Laboratories
ABBOTT LOGO; 100 MG; OT	Gengraf	100 mg	White, 2 Blue Stripes, Blue Ink	Capsule		Abbott Laboratories
ABBOTT LOGO; AR	Tricor, Micronized	134 mg	White	Capsule		Abbott Laboratories
ABBOTT LOGO; FR	Tricor, Micronized	67 mg	Yellow	Capsule		Abbott Laboratories
ABBOTT LOGO; HC	Depakote ER	500 mg	Gray	Extended-Release Tablet		Abbott Laboratories
ABBOTT LOGO; HF	Depakote ER	250 mg	White	Extended-Release Tablet	Oval	Abbott Laboratories
ABBOTT LOGO; HH	Hytrin	1 mg	Grey	Capsule		Abbott Laboratories
ABBOTT LOGO; HK	Hytrin	5 mg	Red	Capsule		Abbott Laboratories
ABBOTT LOGO; HN	Hytrin	10 mg	Blue	Capsule		Abbott Laboratories
ABBOTT LOGO; HY	Hytrin	2 mg	Yellow	Capsule		Abbott Laboratories
ABBOTT LOGO; SR	Tricor, Micronized	200 mg	Orange	Capsule		Abbott Laboratories
ABG 15	Morphine Sulfate	15 mg	Blue	Tablet, Extended Release	Circle	Watson Laboratories
ABG 30	Morphine Sulfate	30 mg	Lavender	Tablet, Extended Release	Circle	Watson Laboratories
ABG 60	Morphine Sulfate	60 mg	Orange	Tablet, Extended Release	Circle	Watson Laboratories
ABG 100	Morphine Sulfate	100 mg	Gray	Tablet, Extended Release	Circle	Watson Laboratories
ABG 200	Morphine Sulfate	200 mg	Green	Tablet, Extended Release	Circle	Watson Laboratories
AC; 200; G	Acebutolol Hydrochloride	200 mg	Lavender and Orange	Capsule		Par Pharmaceutical
AC; 200; G	Acebutolol Hydrochloride	200 mg	Orange and Purple	Capsule		Alpharma
AC; 400; G	Acebutolol Hydrochloride	400 mg	Lavender and Orange	Capsule		Par Pharmaceutical
ACCUTANE; 10; ROCHE	Accutane	10 mg	Light Pink	Capsule	Oval	Roche Laboratories
ACCUTANE; 20; ROCHE	Accutane	20 mg	Maroon	Capsule	Oval	Roche Laboratories
ACCUTANE; 40; ROCHE	Accutane	40 mg	Yellow	Capsule	Oval	Roche Laboratories
ACF ; 004	Atacand	4 mg	White to Off-White	Tablet	Circle	Astrazeneca
ACIPHEX; 20 ;	Aciphex	20 mg	Light Yellow	Delayed-Release Tablet		Eisai
ACJ	Atacand HCT	32 mg ; 12.5 mg	Yellow	Tablet	Oval	Astrazeneca
ACJ; 322	Atacand HCT	32 mg ; 12.5 mg	Yellow	Tablet	Oval	Astrazeneca
ACS	Atacand HCT	16 mg ; 12.5 mg	Peach	Tablet	Oval	Astrazeneca
ACS; 162	Atacand HCT	16 mg ; 12.5 mg	Peach	Tablet	Oval	Astrazeneca
ACTIGALL; 300 MG ;	Actigall	300 mg	Pink and White	Capsule		Watson Laboratories
ACTOS 15	Actos	15 mg	White to Off White	Tablet	Circle	Takeda Pharmaceuticals
ACTOS 30	Actos	30 mg	White to Off White	Tablet	Circle	Takeda Pharmaceuticals
ACTOS 45	Actos	45 mg	White to Off White	Tablet	Circle	Takeda Pharmaceuticals
ACY; 200	Acyclovir	200 mg		Tablet		Mylan Pharmaceuticals
ACY; 400	Acyclovir	400 mg	White	Tablet	Oval	Mylan Pharmaceuticals
ACY; 800	Acyclovir	800 mg		Tablet		Mylan Pharmaceuticals
AD; 5	Adderall 5 mg Tablet	1.25 mg ; 1.25 mg ; 1.25 mg ; 1.25 mg	Blue	Tablet	Double-Scored	Shire Pharmaceuticals
AD; 7.5	Adderall 7.5 mg Tablet	1.875 mg ; 1.875 mg ; 1.875 mg ; 1.875 mg	Blue	Tablet	Circle, Double-Scored	Shire Pharmaceuticals
AD; 10	Adderall 10 mg Tablet	2.5 mg ; 2.5 mg ; 2.5 mg ; 2.5 mg	Blue	Tablet	Double-Scored	Shire Pharmaceuticals
AD; 12.5	Adderall 12.5 mg Tablet	3.125 mg ; 3.125 mg ; 3.125 mg ; 3.125 mg	Orange	Tablet	Circle, Double-Scored	Shire Pharmaceuticals
AD; 15	Adderall 15 mg Tablet	3.75 mg ; 3.75 mg ; 3.75 mg ; 3.75 mg	Orange	Tablet	Oval, Double-Scored	Shire Pharmaceuticals
AD; 20	Adderall 20 mg Tablet	5 mg ; 5 mg ; 5 mg ; 5 mg	Orange	Tablet	Double-Scored	Shire Pharmaceuticals
AD; 30	Adderall 30 mg Tablet	7.5 mg ; 7.5 mg ; 7.5 mg ; 7.5 mg	Orange	Tablet	Double-Scored	Shire Pharmaceuticals
ADALAT CC; 30	Adalat CC	30 mg	Pink	Tablet, Extended Release	Circle	Schering
ADALAT CC; 60	Adalat CC	60 mg	Salmon	Tablet, Extended Release	Circle	Schering
ADALAT CC; 90	Adalat CC	90 mg	Dark Red	Tablet, Extended Release	Circle	Schering
ADALAT; 10	Adalat	20 mg	Orange and Light Brown	Capsule, Liquid Filled		Bayer Pharmaceutical
ADALAT; 20	Adalat	10 mg	Orange	Capsule, Liquid Filled		Bayer Pharmaceutical
ADAMS; 063	Aquatab C	120 mg ; 60 mg ; 1200 mg	Light Yellow	Extended-Release Tablet	Oval, Scored	Adams Laboratories
ADAMS; 068	Aquatab D	1200 mg ; 75 mg	Light Green	Extended-Release Tablet	Oval, Scored	Adams Laboratories
ADDERALL XR 10 MG ;	Adderall Xr - 10 mg Capsule	2.5 mg ; 2.5 mg ; 2.5 mg ; 2.5 mg	Blue	Capsule, Extended Release		Shire Pharmaceuticals
ADDERALL XR 15 MG	Adderall Xr - 15 mg Capsule	3.75 mg ; 3.75 mg ; 3.75 mg ; 3.75 mg	White/blue	Capsule, Extended Release		Shire Pharmaceuticals

IMPRINT	BRAND/GENERIC NAME	STRENGTH	COLOR	FORM	SHAPE	MANUFACTURER
ADDERALL XR 20 MG ;	Adderall Xr - 20 mg Capsule	5 mg ; 5 mg ; 5 mg ; 5 mg	Orange	Capsule, Extended Release		Shire Pharmaceuticals
ADDERALL XR 25 MG	Adderall Xr - 25 mg Capsule	6.25 mg ; 6.25 mg ; 6.25 mg ; 6.25 mg	Orange/white	Capsule, Extended Release		Shire Pharmaceuticals
ADDERALL XR 30 MG ;	Adderall Xr - 30 mg Capsule	7.5 mg ; 7.5 mg ; 7.5 mg ; 7.5 mg	Natural/orange	Capsule, Extended Release		Shire Pharmaceuticals
ADDERALL XR; 5 MG	Adderall Xr - 5 mg Capsule	1.25 mg ; 1.25 mg ; 1.25 mg ; 1.25 mg	Clear/blue	Capsule, Extended Release		Shire Pharmaceuticals
ADEFLOR; CHEWABLE; 0.5	Adeflor	5 mg ; 2 mcg ; 18 mg ; 2 mg ; 0.5 mg ; 4000 IU ; 400 IU ; 2 mg ; 75 mg ; 1 mg	Light Brown	Tablet, Chewable	Circle	Pharmacia & Upjohn
ADEFLOR; CHEWABLE; 1.0	Adeflor	5 mg ; 2 mcg ; 18 mg ; 2 mg ; 1 mg ; 4000 IU ; 400 IU ; 2 mg ; 75 mg ; 1 mg	Brown	Tablet, Chewable	Circle	Pharmacia & Upjohn
ADEFLOR; M	Adeflor M	2.5 mg ; 400 IU ; 6000 IU ; 1.5 mg ; 10 mg ; 30 mg ; 0.1 mg ; 250 mg ; 10 mg ; 2 mcg ; 20 mg ; 1 mg ; 100 mg ;	Pink	Tablet	Oval	Pharmacia & Upjohn
ADIPEX-P 9-9	Adipex-P	37.5 mg	Blue and White	Tablet	Oblong	Gate Pharmaceuticals
ADIPEX-P 37.5	Adipex-P	37.5 mg	White and Bright Blue	Capsule		Gate Pharmaceuticals
ADL2698	Entereg	12 mg	Blue	Capsule		Glaxosmithkline
ADX 1 ; A	Arimidex	1 mg	White	Tablet	Biconvex	Astrazeneca LP
AEY; 420	Deronil	0.75 mg	Amber-Yellow	Tablet		Schering
AF ANACIN	Anacin Maximum Strength, Aspirin Free	500 mg	Blue or White	Capsule, Liquid Filled	Capsule-Shape	A.H. Robins
AHR	Cough Calmers	52.5 mg ; 7.5 mg	Red	Lozenge/troche	Square	Wyeth Consumer Healthcare
AHR	Dimacol	30 mg ; 10 mg ; 100 mg	Orange	Tablet	Oval	Wyeth Consumer Healthcare
AHR	Robalate	500 mg	White	Tablet, Chewable		Wyeth Pharmaceuticals
AHR ;	Z-Bec	6 mcg ; 25 mg ; 22.5 mg ; 45 IU ; 600 mg ; 15 mg ; 10.2 mg ; 100 mg ; 10 mg	Green	Coated Tablet	Capsule-Shape	Wyeth Consumer Healthcare
AHR; 0677	Allbee C-800	45 IU ; 800 mg ; 15 mg ; 17 mg ; 100 mg ; 25 mg ; 12 mcg ; 25 mg	Orange	Coated Tablet	Oblong	A.H. Robins
AHR; 0678	Allbee C-800 Plus Iron	27 mg ; 45 IU ; 800 mg ; 0.4 mg ; 15 mg ; 17 mg ; 100 mg ; 25 mg ; 12 mcg ; 25 mg	Dark Red	Coated Tablet	Oblong	A.H. Robins
AHR; 160 ;	Rela	350 mg	Pink	Coated Tablet	Circle	Schering-Plough
AHR; 1650	Dimacol	100 mg ; 30 mg ; 15 mg	Orange and Green	Capsule		Wyeth Consumer Healthcare
AHR; 2117	Dimetane Decongestant	10 mg ; 4 mg	Light Blue	Tablet		A.H. Robins
AHR; 5049	Entozyme	300 mg ; 250 mg ; 150 mg	White	Coated Tablet	Circle	A.H. Robins
AHR; 5449	Exna	50 mg	Yellow	Tablet	Circle, Scored	Wyeth Pharmaceuticals
AHR; 5650	Imavate	50 mg	Pink	Tablet	Circle	Wyeth Consumer Healthcare
AHR; 6207	Phenaphen	325 mg	Dark Brown, Black and Clear	Capsule		A.H. Robins
AHR; 6209	Phenaphen	325 mg	White	Coated Tablet	Capsule-Shape	A.H. Robins
AHR; 6242	Phenaphen with Codeine No. 2	15 mg ; 325 mg	Black and Yellow	Capsule		A.H. Robins
AHR; 6251	Phenaphen-650 with Codeine	30 mg ; 650 mg	White	Tablet	Capsule-Shape	A.H. Robins
AHR; 6257	Phenaphen with Codeine No. 3	30 mg ; 325 mg	Black and Green	Capsule		A.H. Robins
AHR; 6274	Phenaphen with Codeine No. 4	60 mg ; 325 mg	Green and White	Capsule		A.H. Robins
AHR; ROBAXISAL	Robaxisal	325 mg ; 400 mg	Pink and White Layered	Tablet		A.H. Robins
AHR; ROBICAP; 8417	Robitet-250 Robicaps	250 mg	Pink and Brown	Capsule		Wyeth Pharmaceuticals
AHR; ROBICAP; 8427	Robitet-500 Robicaps	500 mg	Cream and Brown	Capsule		Wyeth Pharmaceuticals
AKH; 892 ;	Tremin	2 mg	White	Tablet		Schering
AKJ; 596 ;	Tremin	5 mg	Gray	Tablet		Schering
AL	Clorazepate Dipotassium	3.75 mg	Blue	Tablet	Circle, Scored, Compressed	Novartis Generics
AL 0.5; G	Alprazolam	0.5 mg	Dark Yellow	Tablet	Oval, Scored	Par Pharmaceutical
AL; 1.0; G ;	Alprazolam	1 mg	White	Tablet	Oval, Scored	Par Pharmaceutical
ALBAMYCIN	Albamycin	250 mg	White and Maroon	Capsule		Pharmacia & Upjohn
ALLBEE C; AHR	Allbee with C	10.2 mg ; 50 mg ; 5 mg ; 10 mg ; 300 mg ; 15 mg	Yellow	Tablet	Capsule-Shape	A.H. Robins
ALLEGRA; 60 MG	Allegra	60 mg	White and Pink	Capsule		Aventis Pharmaceuticals
ALLEGRA-D	Allegra-D 12 Hour	60 mg ; 120 mg	White and Tan	Tablet, Extended Release	Oblong	Sanofi-Aventis U.S.
ALLFEN JR	Allfen JR	400 mg		Tablet		Mcr American Pharmaceuticals
ALPHA; 028	Guaifenesin	1200 mg	White	Tablet	Oblong, Scored	Eli Lilly
ALTACE; 1.25; HOECHST	Altace	1.25 mg	Yellow	Capsule		Monarch Pharmaceuticals
ALTACE; 2.5 MG; HOECHST	Altace	2.5 mg	Orange	Capsule		Monarch Pharmaceuticals
ALTACE; 5 MG; HOECHST	Altace	5 mg	Red	Capsule		Monarch Pharmaceuticals
ALTACE; 10 MG; HOECHST	Altace	10 mg	Blue	Capsule		Monarch Pharmaceuticals

IMPRINT	BRAND/GENERIC NAME	STRENGTH	COLOR	FORM	SHAPE	MANUFACTURER
AM	Tridione	300 mg	White	Capsule		Abbott Laboratories
AM; 1	Methenamine Mandelate	1 GM	Purple	Tablet	Oval	Actavis Totowa
AM; 200; G	Amiodarone Hydrochloride	200 mg	White	Tablet	Circle, Scored	Par Pharmaceutical
AMARYL	Amaryl	1 mg	Pink	Tablet	Oblong	Sanofi-Aventis U.S.
AMARYL	Amaryl	2 mg	Green	Tablet	Oblong	Sanofi-Aventis U.S.
AMARYL	Amaryl	4 mg	Blue	Tablet	Oblong	Sanofi-Aventis U.S.
AMBI; G; AMBIFED; G	Ambifed-G	60 mg ; 1000 mg	White	Tablet	Capsule-Shape	Mcr American Pharmaceuticals
AMBI; G; DM; AMBIFED; G	Ambifed-G DM	60 mg ; 1000 mg ; 30 mg	White	Tablet	Capsule-Shape	Mcr American Pharmaceuticals
AMGEN; 30	Sensipar	30 mg	Light Green	Tablet	Oval	Amgen
AMGEN; 60	Sensipar	60 mg	Light Green	Tablet	Oval	Amgen
AMGEN; 90	Sensipar	90 mg	Light Green	Tablet	Oval	Amgen
AMIDE; 009; 10	Isoxsuprine Hydrochloride	10 mg	White	Tablet	Circle	Actavis Totowa
AMIDE; 010; 20	Isoxsuprine Hydrochloride	20 mg	White	Tablet	Circle	Actavis Totowa
AMIDE; 014	Dexchlorpheniramine Maleate	4 mg	Yellow	Tablet	Oval	Watson Laboratories
AMIDE; 015	Dexchlorpheniramine Maleate	6 mg	White	Tablet	Oval	Watson Laboratories
AMIDE; 024	Amidal	20 mg ; 300 mg	White	Tablet, Extended Release	Capsule-Shape	Actavis Totowa
AMIDE; 025	Chlorzoxazone	500 mg	Green	Tablet	Capsule-Shape	Actavis Totowa
AMIDE; 053 ;	Chlorzoxazone	250 mg	Peach	Tablet	Circle	Actavis Totowa
AMIDE; 084	Choline Magnesium Trisalicylate	500 mg	Peach	Tablet	Capsule-Shape	Actavis Totowa
AMIDE; 085	Choline Magnesium Trisalicylate	750 mg	White	Tablet	Capsule-Shape	Actavis Totowa
AMOXIL; 125	Amoxil	125 mg	Pink	Tablet, Chewable	Oval	Glaxosmithkline
AMOXIL; 200	Amoxil	200 mg	Pale Pink	Tablet, Chewable	Circle	Glaxosmithkline
AMOXIL; 250	Amoxil	250 mg	Pink	Tablet, Chewable	Oval	Glaxosmithkline
AMOXIL; 250	Amoxil	250 mg	Royal Blue and Pink	Capsule		Glaxosmithkline
AMOXIL; 400	Amoxil	400 mg	Pale Pink	Tablet, Chewable	Circle	Glaxosmithkline
AMOXIL; 500	Amoxil	500 mg	Pink	Tablet	Capsule-Shape	Glaxosmithkline
AMOXIL; 500	Amoxil	500 mg	Royal Blue and Pink	Capsule		Glaxosmithkline
AMP; 500	Ampicillin	500 mg	Blue and White	Capsule		Teva Pharmaceuticals
AMT; 832	Amantadine Hydrochloride	100 mg	Peach	Tablet	Circle	Upsher-Smith Laboratories
AMX; 500	Amoxicillin	500 mg	Orange and White	Capsule		Par Pharmaceutical
ANAPROX DS; ROCHE ;	Anaprox DS	550 mg	Dark Blue	Coated Tablet	Oblong	Roche Laboratories
ANCOBON; 250 ROCHE	Ancobon	250 mg	Green and Gray	Capsule		Valeant Pharmaceuticals
ANCOBON; 500 ROCHE	Ancobon	500 mg	Gray and White	Capsule		Valeant Pharmaceuticals
ANDRX 610 10 MG	Omeprazole	10 mg	Light Green, White	Capsule, Delayed Release		Watson Pharma
ANDRX 620 20 MG	Omeprazole	20 mg	Dark Green, White	Capsule, Delayed Release		Watson Pharma
ANDRX 640 40 MG	Omeprazole	40 mg	Dark Green, Light Green	Capsule		Watson Pharma
ANDRX 696 120 MG	Taztia Xt	120 mg	Opaque Pink, Pink	Capsule, Extended Release, 24 Hr		Watson Pharma
ANDRX 697 180 MG	Taztia Xt	180 mg	Light Blue, Opaque Buff	Capsule, Extended Release, 24 Hr		Watson Pharma
ANDRX 698 240 MG	Taztia Xt	240 mg	Light Blue, Pink	Capsule, Extended Release, 24 Hr		Watson Pharma
ANDRX 699 300 MG	Taztia Xt	300 mg	Opaque Buff, Pink	Capsule, Extended Release, 24 Hr		Watson Pharma
ANDRX 700 360 MG	Taztia Xt	360 mg	Light Blue, Light Blue Opaque	Capsule, Extended Release, 24 Hr		Watson Pharma
ANDRX 710	Potassium Chloride	10 meq	Off-White	Tablet, Extended Release	Capsule-Shape	Watson Pharma
ANDRX 720	Potassium Chloride	20 meq	Off-White	Tablet, Extended Release	Capsule-Shape	Watson Pharma
ANDRX LOGO 5 ; 531 ;	Quinapril Hydrochloride	5 mg	Pink	Tablet	Oval	Andrx Pharmaceuticals
ANDRX LOGO 10	Altoprev	10 mg	Dark Orange	Tablet, Extended Release	Circle	Watson Pharma
ANDRX LOGO 10 ; 532 ;	Quinapril Hydrochloride	10 mg	Pink	Tablet	Circle	Andrx Pharmaceuticals
ANDRX LOGO 20	Altoprev	20 mg	Orange	Tablet, Extended Release	Circle	Andrx Pharmaceuticals
ANDRX LOGO 20 ; 533 ;	Quinapril Hydrochloride	20 mg	Pink	Tablet	Circle	Andrx Pharmaceuticals
ANDRX LOGO 40	Altoprev	40 mg	Peach	Tablet, Extended Release	Circle	Andrx Pharmaceuticals
ANDRX LOGO 40 ; 534 ;	Quinapril Hydrochloride	40 mg	Pink	Tablet	Circle	Andrx Pharmaceuticals
ANDRX LOGO 60	Altoprev	60 mg	Light Peach	Tablet, Extended Release	Circle	Andrx Pharmaceuticals
ANDRX LOGO 574	Fortamet	500 mg	White	Tablet, Extended Release		Andrx Pharmaceuticals
ANDRX LOGO 575	Fortamet	1000 mg	White	Tablet, Extended Release		Andrx Pharmaceuticals
ANDRX LOGO; 524	Hydrocodone Bitartrate and Ibuprofen	7.5 mg ; 200 mg	White	Tablet		Watson Pharma
ANDRX; 510; 100 MG	Ketoprofen	100 mg	White	Extended-Release Capsule		Andrx Pharmaceuticals
ANDRX; 515; 150 MG	Ketoprofen	150 mg	Light Turquoise Blue and White	Extended-Release Capsule		Andrx Pharmaceuticals
ANDRX; 520; 200 MG	Ketoprofen	200 mg	Light Turquoise Blue	Capsule, Extended Release		Watson Pharma
ANDRX; 548	Diltia Xt	120 mg	White	Capsule, Extended Release, 24 Hr		Watson Pharma

IMPRINT	BRAND/GENERIC NAME	STRENGTH	COLOR	FORM	SHAPE	MANUFACTURER
ANDRX; 549	Diltia Xt	180 mg	Gray and White	Capsule, Extended Release, 24 Hr		Watson Pharma
ANDRX; 550	Diltia Xt	240 mg	Gray	Capsule, Extended Release, 24 Hr		Watson Pharma
ANDRX; 597	Cartia Xt	120 mg	Orange and White	Capsule, Extended Release, 24 Hr		Watson Pharma
ANDRX; 598	Cartia Xt	180 mg	Orange and Yellow	Capsule, Extended Release, 24 Hr		Watson Pharma
ANDRX; 599	Cartia Xt	240 mg	Orange and Brown	Capsule, Extended Release, 24 Hr		Watson Pharma
ANDRX; 600	Cartia Xt	300 mg	Orange	Capsule, Extended Release, 24 Hr		Watson Pharma
ANDRX; 827	Generic Entex LA	400 mg ; 30 mg	Opaque Orange	Capsule, Extended Release		Andrx Pharmaceuticals
ANK; SP ;	Miradon	50 mg	Pink	Tablet	Oval, Scored	Schering
ANOLOR; 300; 51674; 0009	Anolor 300	325 mg ; 50 mg ; 40 mg	White	Capsule		Blansett Pharmacal
ANSAID; 50 MG	Ansaid	50 mg	White	Coated Tablet	Oval	Pharmacia & Upjohn
ANSAID; 100 MG	Ansaid	100 mg	Blue	Tablet	Oval	Pharmacia & Upjohn
ANSPOR; 250; SKF	Anspor	250 mg	Red and White	Capsule		Glaxosmithkline
ANSPOR; 500; SKF	Anspor	500 mg	Red	Capsule		Glaxosmithkline
ANZEMET; 50	Anzemet	50 mg	Light Pink	Tablet	Circle	Sanofi-Aventis U.S.
ANZEMET; 100	Anzemet	100 mg	Pink	Tablet	Oval	Sanofi-Aventis U.S.
AP; 015	Pseudoephedrine Hcl and Triprolidine Hcl	60 mg ; 2.5 mg	White	Tablet	Circle, Scored	Advance Pharmaceutical
AP; 017	Pseudoephedrine Hydrochloride	30 mg	Red	Tablet	Circle	Advance Pharmaceutical
AP; 026	Acetaminophen and Phenyltoloxamine	325 mg ; 30 mg	Peach	Tablet	Circle	Advance Pharmaceutical
AP; 026	Estradiol	1 mg	Lavender	Tablet	Circle	Bristol-Myers Squibb
AP; 027	Estradiol	2 mg	Green	Tablet	Circle	Bristol-Myers Squibb
AP; 1	Phenazopyridine Hydrochloride	100 mg	Dark Maroon	Coated Tablet	Circle, Scored	Novartis Generics
AP; 2	Phenazopyridine Hydrochloride	200 mg	Dark Maroon	Coated Tablet	Circle, Scored	Novartis Generics
AP; 20	Diphenhydramine Hydrochloride	25 mg	Pink and White	Capsule		Advance Pharmaceutical
AP; 21	Diphenhydramine Hydrochloride	50 mg	Bright Pink	Capsule	Small	Advance Pharmaceutical
AP; 35	Docusate Sodium	250 mg	Red and Yellow	Capsule		Advance Pharmaceutical
AP; 37	Acetaminophen	500 mg	Red and Clear with White Powder	Capsule		Advance Pharmaceutical
AP; 5160	Captopril and Hydrochlorothiazide	25 mg ; 15 mg	White and Orange Mottled	Tablet	Rounded Square, Quadrisected Scored	Bristol-Myers Squibb
AP; 5161	Captopril and Hydrochlorothiazide	25 mg ; 25 mg	Peach	Tablet	Rounded Square, Quadrisected Scored	Bristol-Myers Squibb
AP; 5162	Captopril and Hydrochlorothiazide	50 mg ; 15 mg	White and Orange Mottled	Tablet	Oval, Scored	Bristol-Myers Squibb
AP; 5163	Captopril and Hydrochlorothiazide	50 mg ; 25 mg	Peach	Tablet	Oval, Scored	Bristol-Myers Squibb
APSE	Ami-Tex Pse	600 mg ; 120 mg	Yellow	Tablet, Extended Release	Capsule-Shape	Actavis Totowa
ARICEPT ; 5	Aricept	5 mg	White	Tablet	Circle	Pfizer
ARICEPT ; 5	Aricept Odt	5 mg	White	Tablet, Disintegrating		Pfizer
ARICEPT ; 10	Aricept	10 mg	Yellow	Tablet	Circle	Pfizer
ARICEPT ; 10	Aricept Odt	10 mg	Yellow	Tablet, Disintegrating		Pfizer
ASACOL; NE	Asacol	400 mg	Red-Brown	Timed-Release Tablet	Capsule-Shape	Procter & Gamble Pharmaceuticals
ASBRON; G; 78/202 ;	Asbron G	100 mg ; 300 mg	Green with White Inlay	Tablet		Novartis Pharmaceuticals
ASPIRIN	Aspirin	325 mg	White	Coated Tablet	Circle	Pfeiffer Pharmaceuticals
ASPIRIN	Aspirin	325 mg	White	Tablet	Circle	Baxter Healthcare
ATARAX; 10	Atarax	10 mg	Orange	Tablet	Triangle	Pfizer
ATARAX; 25	Atarax	25 mg	Green	Tablet	Triangle	Pfizer Laboratories
ATARAX; 50	Atarax	50 mg	Yellow	Tablet	Triangle	Pfizer Laboratories
ATARAX; 100	Atarax	100 mg	Red	Tablet	Triangle	Pfizer Laboratories
ATHENA LOGO	Carbatrol	200 mg	Light Gray and Blue-Green	Extended-Release Capsule		Shire Pharmaceuticals
ATHENA LOGO	Carbatrol	300 mg	Black and Blue-Green	Extended-Release Capsule		Shire Pharmaceuticals
ATROMID-S; 500	Atromid-S	500 mg	Orange	Capsule, Liquid Filled	Oblong	Wyeth Pharmaceuticals
AUGMENTIN 200	Augmentin	200 mg ; 28.5 mg	Pink	Tablet, Chewable	Circle	Glaxosmithkline
AUGMENTIN 400	Augmentin	400 mg ; 57 mg	Pink	Tablet, Chewable	Circle	Glaxosmithkline
AUGMENTIN 875	Augmentin	125 mg ; 875 mg	White	Tablet	Capsule-Shape	Glaxosmithkline
AUGMENTIN XR	Augmentin Xr	1000 mg ; 62.5 mg	White	Tablet, Extended Release	Oval	Glaxosmithkline
AVINZA 30 MG 505	Avinza	30 mg	White Opaque, Yellow	Capsule, Extended Release, 24 Hr		King Pharmaceuticals
AVINZA 60 MG 506	Avinza	60 mg	Bluish-Green, White Opaque	Capsule, Extended Release, 24 Hr		King Pharmaceuticals
AVINZA 90 MG 507	Avinza	90 mg	Red, White Opaque	Capsule, Extended Release, 24 Hr		King Pharmaceuticals
AVINZA 120 MG 508	Avinza	120 mg	Blue-Violet, White Opaque	Capsule, Extended Release, 24 Hr		King Pharmaceuticals
AXCAN PHARMA BMT	Pylera	125 mg ; 140 mg ; 125 mg	White Opaque	Capsule		Axcan Scandipharm
AXID; 150; RELIANT ;	Axid	150 mg	Opaque Dark Yellow and Opaque Pale Yellow	Capsule		Eli Lilly
AXID; 300; RELIANT ;	Axid	300 mg	Opaque Brown and Opaque Pale Yellow	Capsule		Eli Lilly
AYERST; 878	Premarin with Methyltestosterone	0.625 mg ; 5 mg	White	Tablet	Circle	Wyeth Pharmaceuticals
AYERST; 879	Premarin with Methyltestosterone	1.25 mg ; 10 mg	Yellow	Tablet	Circle	Wyeth Pharmaceuticals
AYERST; 880	Pmb-200	200 mg ; 0.45 mg	Green	Tablet	Oblong	Wyeth Pharmaceuticals

IMPRINT	BRAND/GENERIC NAME	STRENGTH	COLOR	FORM	SHAPE	MANUFACTURER
AYERST; 881	Pmb-400	0.45 mg ; 400 mg	Pink	Tablet	Oblong	Wyeth Pharmaceuticals
AYGESTIN; 5	Aygestin	5 mg	White	Tablet	Oval, Scored	Barr Laboratories
B	Anolor Dh	5 mg ; 325 mg ; 50 mg ; 40 mg	Orange	Capsule		Blansett Pharmacal
B / 778	Oxycodone Hydochloride and Ibuprofen	5 mg ; 400 mg	White to Off-White	Tablet	Capsule-Shape	Barr Laboratories
B ; 333	Velivet - Beige Tablet	0.025 mg ; 0.1 mg	Beige	Tablet	Circle	Barr Laboratories
B ; 735	Balziva - Light Peach Tablet	0.4 mg ; 0.035 mg	Light Peach	Tablet	Circle	Barr Laboratories
B 145	Digitek	0.125 mg	Yellow	Tablet	Circle	Mylan Bertek Pharmaceuticals
B 146	Digitek	0.25 mg	White	Tablet	Circle	Mylan Bertek Pharmaceuticals
B 980	Nimodipine	30 mg	Orange Opaque	Capsule, Liquid Filled	Oblong	Barr Laboratories
B/B	Anolor Dh5	5 mg ; 500 mg	Opaque White	Capsule		Blansett Pharmacal
B; 11 ;	Zagam	200 mg	White	Coated Tablet	Circle, Biconvex	Mylan Bertek Pharmaceuticals
B; 21	Levlen 21	0.15 mg ; 30 mcg	Orange	21-Day Tablet Pack	Circle	Berlex Laboratories
B; 21	Levlen 28 - Orange Tablet	0.15 mg ; 30 mcg	Orange	Tablet	Circle	Bayer Healthcare Pharmaceuticals
B; 30	Nifedical XL	30 mg	Reddish Brown	Extended-Release Tablet	Circle	Teva Pharmaceuticals
B; 50; 902	Naltrexone Hydrochloride	50 mg	Beige	Tablet	Circle, Scored	Barr Laboratories
B; 60	Nifedical XL	60 mg	Reddish Brown	Extended-Release Tablet	Circle	Teva Pharmaceuticals
B; 60	Nifedipine	60 mg	Yellow	Extended-Release Tablet	Circle	Teva Pharmaceuticals
B; 95	Tri-Levlen 21 Brown Tablet	0.05 mg ; 0.03 mg	Brown	21-Day Tablet Pack	Circle	Berlex Laboratories
B; 95	Tri-Levlen 28 Brown Tablet	0.05 mg ; 0.03 mg	Brown	28-Day Tablet Pack	Circle	Berlex Laboratories
B; 96	Tri-Levlen 21 White Tablet	0.075 mg ; 0.04 mg	White	21-Day Tablet Pack	Circle	Berlex Laboratories
B; 96	Tri-Levlen 28 White Tablet	0.075 mg ; 0.04 mg	White	28-Day Tablet Pack	Circle	Berlex Laboratories
B; 97	Tri-Levlen 21 Light Yellow Tablet	0.125 mg ; 0.03 mg	Light Yellow	21-Day Tablet Pack	Circle	Berlex Laboratories
B; 97	Tri-Levlen 28 Light Yellow Tablet	0.125 mg ; 0.03 mg	Light Yellow	28-Day Tablet Pack	Circle	Berlex Laboratories
B; 133	Pyridostigmine Bromide	60 mg	White	Tablet	Round, Quadrisected Scored	Barr Laboratories
B; 171	Mefloquine Hydrochloride	250 mg	White	Tablet	Oval	Barr Laboratories
B; 201; 10	Fluoxetine Hydrochloride	10 mg	Beige	Tablet	Scored, Oval	Barr Laboratories
B; 211; 5	Norethindrone Acetate	5 mg	White	Tablet	Oval	Barr Laboratories
B; 241	Mirtazapine	15 mg	White	Disintegrating Tablet	Circle	Barr Laboratories
B; 241	Mirtazapine	15 mg	White to Off White	Disintegrating Tablet	Circle	Barr Laboratories
B; 242	Mirtazapine	30 mg	White	Disintegrating Tablet	Circle	Barr Laboratories
B; 242	Mirtazapine	30 mg	White to Off White	Disintegrating Tablet	Circle	Barr Laboratories
B; 252	Dipyridamole	25 mg	White	Tablet	Circle	Barr Laboratories
B; 275; REVIA	Revia	50 mg	Beige	Tablet	Circle, Scored	Barr Laboratories
B; 285	Dipyridamole	50 mg	White	Tablet	Circle	Barr Laboratories
B; 298	Hydroxyzine Hydrochloride	25 mg	Orange	Tablet	Circle	Barr Laboratories
B; 301	Hydroxyzine Hydrochloride	10 mg	Yellow	Tablet	Circle	Barr Laboratories
B; 302; 2 ;	Acetaminophen and Codeine	300 mg ; 15 mg	White	Tablet	Circle, Scored	Barr Laboratories
B; 303; 3 ;	Acetaminophen and Codeine	300 mg ; 30 mg	White	Tablet	Circle, Scored	Barr Laboratories
B; 304; 4 ;	Acetaminophen and Codeine	300 mg ; 60 mg	White	Tablet	Circle, Scored	Barr Laboratories
B; 344	Errin	0.35 mg	Yellow	Tablet	Circle	Barr Laboratories
B; 345	Lithium Carbonate	300 mg	Off-White	Extended-Release Tablet	Circle	Barr Laboratories
B; 357	Methyldopa	125 mg	White	Coated Tablet	Circle	Barr Laboratories
B; 381 ;	Meperidine Hydrochloride	50 mg	White	Tablet	Circle	Barr Laboratories
B; 385; 500	Metformin Hydrochloride	500 mg	White	Tablet	Oval	Barr Laboratories
B; 386; 850	Metformin Hydrochloride	850 mg	White	Tablet	Oval	Barr Laboratories
B; 387; 10; 00	Metformin Hydrochloride	1000 mg	White	Tablet	Oval	Barr Laboratories
B; 484	Leucovorin Calcium	5 mg	White	Tablet	Circle	Barr Laboratories
B; 485	Leucovorin Calcium	25 mg	Green	Tablet	Circle	Barr Laboratories
B; 555; 424	Metoclopramide	10 mg	White	Tablet	Circle, Scored, Convex	Barr Laboratories
B; 555; 606	Megestrolacetate	20 mg	White	Tablet		Barr Laboratories
B; 555; 779	Medroxyprogesterone Acetate	10 mg	White	Tablet	Circle, Biconvex, Scored	Barr Laboratories
B; 555; 872	Medroxyprogesterone Acetate	2.5 mg	White	Tablet	Circle, Biconvex, Scored	Barr Laboratories
B; 555; 873	Medroxyprogesterone Acetate	5 mg	White	Tablet	Circle, Biconvex, Scored	Barr Laboratories
B; 572	Methotrexate	2.5 mg	Yellow	Tablet	Oval, Scored	Barr Laboratories
B; 715	Camila	0.35 mg	Light Pink	Tablet	Circle	Barr Laboratories
B; 728	Doxycycline	50 mg	Yellow	Tablet	Circle	Bioglan Pharma
B; 729	Doxycycline	100 mg	Yellow	Tablet	Circle	Bioglan Pharma
B; 730	Doxycycline	75 mg	Light Orange	Tablet	Circle	Bioglan Pharma
B; 775; 7; 1/2	Dextroamphetamine Saccharate, Amphetamine Aspartate, Dextroamphetamine Sulfate, Amphetamine Sulfate 7.5 mg Tablet	1.875 mg ; 1.875 mg ; 1.875 mg ; 1.875 mg	Blue	Tablet	Oval	Barr Laboratories
B; 776; 12; 1/2	Dextroamphetamine Saccharate, Amphetamine Aspartate, Dextroamphetamine Sulfate, Amphetamine Sulfate 12.5 mg Tablet	3.125 mg ; 3.125 mg ; 3.125 mg ; 3.125 mg	Peach	Tablet	Oval	Barr Laboratories
B; 777; 1; 5	Dextroamphetamine Saccharate, Amphetamine Aspartate, Dextroamphetamine Sulfate, Amphetamine Sulfate 15 mg Tablet	3.75 mg ; 3.75 mg ; 3.75 mg ; 3.75 mg	Peach	Tablet	Circle	Barr Laboratories
B; 814; 250	Ciprofloxacin	250 mg	Yellow	Tablet	Circle	Barr Laboratories
B; 815; 500	Ciprofloxacin	500 mg	Yellow	Tablet	Capsule-Shape	Barr Laboratories
B; 816; 750	Ciprofloxacin	750 mg	Yellow	Tablet	Capsule-Shape	Barr Laboratories
B; 859	Flecainide Acetate	50 mg	White to Off White	Tablet	Circle	Barr Laboratories
B; 860; 100	Flecainide Acetate	100 mg	White to Off White	Tablet	Oval, Scored	Barr Laboratories
B; 861; 150	Flecainide Acetate	150 mg	White to Off White	Tablet	Oval, Scored	Barr Laboratories
B; 886; 1	Estradiol	1 mg		Tablet		Barr Laboratories
B; 887; 2	Estradiol	2 mg	Green	Tablet	Oval	Barr Laboratories
B; 899; 1/2	Estradiol	0.5 mg		Tablet		Barr Laboratories
B; 917; 200	Amiodarone Hydrochloride	200 mg	White	Tablet	Circle, Scored	Barr Laboratories
B; 923; 400	Ethambutol Hydrochloride	400 mg	White	Tablet	Oval, Scored	Barr Laboratories
B; 927; 5	Trexall	5 mg	Green	Tablet	Oval	Barr Laboratories
B; 928; 7 1/2	Trexall	7.5 mg	Blue	Tablet	Oval, Scored	Barr Laboratories

IMPRINT	BRAND/GENERIC NAME	STRENGTH	COLOR	FORM	SHAPE	MANUFACTURER
B; 929; 10	Trexall	10 mg	Pink	Tablet	Oval, Scored	Barr Laboratories
B; 941	Nortrel .5/35	35 mcg ; 0.5 mg	Light Yellow	Tablet	Circle	Barr Laboratories
B; 942	Nortrel 7/7/7 Blue Tablet	0.75 mg ; 0.035 mg	Blue	28-Day Tablet Pack	Circle	Barr Laboratories
B; 943	Nortrel 7/7/7 Peach Tablet	1 mg ; 0.035 mg	Peach	28-Day Tablet Pack	Circle	Barr Laboratories
B; 945; 15	Trexall	15 mg	Purple	Tablet	Oval	Barr Laboratories
B; 949	Nortrel 1/35	1 mg ; 35 mcg	Yellow	Tablet	Circle	Barr Laboratories
B; 951	Nortrel 7/7/7 Light Yellow Tablet	0.5 mg ; 0.035 mg	Light Yellow	28-Day Tablet Pack	Circle	Barr Laboratories
B; 952; 5	Dextroamphetamine Sulfate	5 mg	Peach	Tablet	Circle	Barr Laboratories
B; 953; 10	Dextroamphetamine Sulfate	10 mg	Pink	Tablet	Circle, Scored	Barr Laboratories
B; 965	Lessina 28 Pink Tablet	0.1 mg ; 0.02 mg	Pink	Tablet	Circle	Barr Laboratories
B; 967	Fluvoxamine Maleate	25 mg	Off-White	Tablet	Oval	Barr Laboratories
B; 968; 50	Fluvoxamine Maleate	50 mg	Yellow	Tablet	Oval, Scored	Barr Laboratories
B; 969; 100	Fluvoxamine Maleate	100 mg	Brown	Tablet	Oval, Scored	Barr Laboratories
B; 971; 5	Dextroamphetamine Saccharate, Amphetamine Aspartate, Dextroamphetamine Sulfate, Amphetamine Sulfate 5 mg Tablet	1.25 mg ; 1.25 mg ; 1.25 mg ; 1.25 mg	Blue	Tablet	Oval	Barr Laboratories
B; 972; 1; 0	Dextroamphetamine Saccharate, Amphetamine Aspartate, Dextroamphetamine Sulfate, Amphetamine Sulfate 10 mg Tablet	2.5 mg ; 2.5 mg ; 2.5 mg ; 2.5 mg	Blue	Tablet	Oval, Scored, with Partial Bisects	Barr Laboratories
B; 973; 2; 0	Dextroamphetamine Saccharate, Amphetamine Aspartate, Dextroamphetamine Sulfate, Amphetamine Sulfate 20 mg Tablet	5 mg ; 5 mg ; 5 mg ; 5 mg	Peach	Tablet	Oval	Barr Laboratories
B; 974; 3; 0	Dextroamphetamine Saccharate, Amphetamine Aspartate, Dextroamphetamine Sulfate, Amphetamine Sulfate 30 mg Tablet	7.5 mg ; 7.5 mg ; 7.5 mg ; 7.5 mg	Peach	Tablet	Oval	Barr Laboratories
B; 987	Sprintec	35 mcg ; 0.25 mg	Blue	Tablet	Circle	Barr Laboratories
B; 992	Portia 28 Pink Tablet	30 mcg ; 0.15 mg	Pink	28-Day Tablet Pack	Circle	Barr Laboratories
B; 997; 1/10	Fludrocortisone Acetate	0.1 mg	Yellow	Tablet	Oval	Barr Laboratories
B2C	Lanoxicaps	0.1 mg	Yellow	Capsule, Liquid Filled	Oval, Small	Glaxosmithkline
B3; LL	Zebeta	10 mg	White	Coated Tablet	Heart-Shape, Biconvex	Lederle Laboratories
BACTRIM; ROCHE	Bactrim	400 mg ; 80 mg	Light Green	Tablet	Capsule-Shape, Scored	Roche Laboratories
BACTRIM-DS; ROCHE	Bactrim DS	160 mg ; 800 mg	White	Tablet	Capsule-Shape	Roche Laboratories
BARR 302 50 ;	Hydroxyzine Pamoate	50 mg	Light Yellow Opaque, Maroon Opaque	Capsule		Barr Laboratories
BARR 323 25 ;	Hydroxyzine Pamoate	25 mg	Light Yellow Opaque, Pink Opaque	Capsule		Barr Laboratories
BARR 808	Tretinoin	10 mg	Brown Opaque, Dark Yellow Opaque	Capsule, Liquid Filled		Barr Laboratories
BARR 827 25 MG	Zonisamide	25 mg	White Opaque	Capsule		Barr Laboratories
BARR 828 50 MG	Zonisamide	50 mg	Grey Opaque	Capsule		Barr Laboratories
BARR 829 100 MG	Zonisamide	100 mg	Orange Opaque	Capsule		Barr Laboratories
BARR/454 ;	Claravis	30 mg	Orange Opaque	Capsule, Liquid Filled		Barr Laboratories
BARR/934 ;	Claravis	10 mg	Light Gray, Light Gray Opaque	Capsule, Liquid Filled		Barr Laboratories
BARR/935 ;	Claravis	20 mg	Brown Opaque, Brown Orange Opaque	Capsule, Liquid Filled		Barr Laboratories
BARR/936 ;	Claravis	40 mg	Light Orange	Capsule, Liquid Filled		Barr Laboratories
BARR; 010	Tetracycline Hydrochloride	500 mg	Black and Yellow	Capsule		Barr Laboratories
BARR; 011	Tetracycline Hydrochloride	250 mg	Orange and Yellow	Capsule		Barr Laboratories
BARR; 033	Chlordiazepoxide Hydrochloride	10 mg	Black and Green	Capsule		Barr Laboratories
BARR; 059 ;	Diphenhydramine Hydrochloride	50 mg	Pink	Capsule		Barr Laboratories
BARR; 10 MG; 876	Fluoxetine Hydrochloride	10 mg	Blue and Yellow	Capsule		Barr Laboratories
BARR; 20 MG; 877	Fluoxetine Hydrochloride	20 mg	Blue and White	Capsule		Barr Laboratories
BARR; 128	Dicyclomine Hydrochloride	10 mg	Blue	Capsule		Barr Laboratories
BARR; 158	Chlordiazepoxide Hydrochloride	5 mg	Green and Yellow	Capsule		Barr Laboratories
BARR; 159	Chlordiazepoxide Hydrochloride	25 mg	Green and White	Capsule		Barr Laboratories
BARR; 281	Aminophylline	200 mg	White	Tablet	Circle	Barr Laboratories
BARR; 282	Aminophylline	100 mg	White	Tablet	Circle	Barr Laboratories
BARR; 286 ;	Dipyridamole	75 mg	White	Tablet	Circle	Barr Laboratories
BARR; 299	Hydroxyzine Hydrochloride	50 mg	Orange	Tablet	Circle	Barr Laboratories
BARR; 300	Hydroxyzine Hydrochloride	100 mg	Orange	Tablet	Circle	Barr Laboratories
BARR; 324; 100	Hydroxyzine Pamoate	100 mg	Opaque Yellow and Opaque Pink Filled with Yellow Powder	Capsule, Liquid Filled		Barr Laboratories
BARR; 325	Hydrocodone Bitartrate and Acetaminophen	5 mg ; 500 mg	White	Tablet	Capsule-Shape, Scored	Barr Laboratories
BARR; 382 ;	Meperidine Hydrochloride	100 mg	White	Tablet	Circle, Biconvex	Barr Laboratories
BARR; 407	Doxepin Hydrochloride	100 mg	White and Green	Capsule		Barr Laboratories
BARR; 442	Acetohexamide	250 mg	White	Tablet	Oval, Biconvex, Scored	Barr Laboratories
BARR; 443	Acetohexamide	500 mg	White	Tablet	Capsule-Shape, Biconvex, Scored	Barr Laboratories
BARR; 446	Tamoxifen Citrate	10 mg	White	Tablet	Circle, Biconvex	Barr Laboratories
BARR; 555; 163	Diazepam	2 mg	White	Tablet	Round, Flat-Faced, Beveled-Edge, Scored	Barr Laboratories
BARR; 555; 164	Diazepam	10 mg	Blue	Tablet	Round, Flat-Faced, Beveled-Edge, Scored	Barr Laboratories
BARR; 555; 192	Hydrochlorothiazide Hydrochloride	100 mg	Peach	Tablet	Circle, Scored	Barr Laboratories
BARR; 555; 271	Sulfinpyrazone	100 mg	White	Tablet	Round, Flat-Faced, Beveled-Edge, Scored	Barr Laboratories

IMPRINT	BRAND/GENERIC NAME	STRENGTH	COLOR	FORM	SHAPE	MANUFACTURER
BARR; 555; 293	Oxycodone with Aspirin	4.5 mg ; 0.38 mg ; 325 mg	Yellow	Tablet	Circle, Scored	Barr Laboratories
BARR; 555; 363	Diazepam	5 mg	Yellow	Tablet	Round, Flat-Faced, Beveled-Edge, Scored	Barr Laboratories
BARR; 555; 444	Hydrochlorothiazide and Triamterene	50 mg ; 75 mg	Yellow	Tablet	Oval	Barr Laboratories
BARR; 555; 444	Triamterene and Hydrochlorothiazide	50 mg ; 75 mg	Yellow	Tablet	Biconvex, Scored, Oval	Barr Laboratories
BARR; 555; 483 ;	Amiloride Hydrochloride and Hydrochlorothiazide	5 mg ; 50 mg	Light Yellow	Tablet	Circle, Biconvex, Scored	Barr Laboratories
BARR; 555; 489	Trazodone Hydrochloride	50 mg	White	Tablet	Circle	Barr Laboratories
BARR; 555; 490	Trazodone Hydrochloride	100 mg	White	Tablet	Circle	Barr Laboratories
BARR; 555; 585	Chlorzoxazone	500 mg	Light Green	Tablet	Circle	Barr Laboratories
BARR; 555; 607 ;	Megestrol Acetate	40 mg	White	Tablet		Barr Laboratories
BARR; 555; 643	Hydrochlorothiazide and Triamterene	25 mg ; 37.5 mg	Green	Tablet	Oval	Barr Laboratories
BARR; 555; 643	Triamterene and Hydrochlorothiazide	37.5 mg ; 25 mg	Green	Tablet	Scored, Oval	Barr Laboratories
BARR; 555; 727	Estropipate	0.75 mg	Yellow	Tablet	Circle, Scored	Barr Laboratories
BARR; 555; 728	Estropipate	1.5 mg	Peach	Tablet	Circle	Barr Laboratories
BARR; 555; 729	Estropipate	3 mg	Blue	Tablet	Circle, Scored	Barr Laboratories
BARR; 633	Danazol	50 mg	Yellow and White	Capsule		Barr Laboratories
BARR; 634	Danazol	100 mg	Yellow	Capsule		Barr Laboratories
BARR; 635	Danazol	200 mg	Opaque Orange and Transparent Orange	Capsule, Liquid Filled		Barr Laboratories
BARR; 658	Oxycodone and Acetaminophen	500 mg ; 5 mg	Red and White	Capsule		Barr Laboratories
BARR; 732; 50 50 50	Trazodone Hydrochloride	150 mg	White	Tablet	Oblong	Barr Laboratories
BARR; 733; 100 100 100	Trazodone Hydrochloride	300 mg	White	Tablet	Oval	Barr Laboratories
BARR; 831; 1 ;	Warfarin Sodium	1 mg	Pink	Tablet	Oval, Flat-Faced, Beveled-Edge, Scored	Barr Laboratories
BARR; 832; 2 1/2 ;	Warfarin Sodium	2.5 mg	Green	Tablet	Oval, Flat-Faced, Beveled-Edge, Scored	Barr Laboratories
BARR; 833; 5	Warfarin Sodium	5 mg	Peach	Tablet	Oval, Flat-Faced, Beveled-Edge, Scored	Barr Laboratories
BARR; 834; 7 1/2 ;	Warfarin Sodium	7.5 mg	Yellow	Tablet	Oval, Flat-Faced, Beveled-Edge, Scored	Barr Laboratories
BARR; 835; 10 ;	Warfarin Sodium	10 mg	White	Tablet	Oval, Flat-Faced, Beveled-Edge, Scored	Barr Laboratories
BARR; 869; 2 ;	Warfarin Sodium	2 mg	Lavender	Tablet	Oval, Flat-Faced, Beveled-Edge, Scored	Barr Laboratories
BARR; 870	Flutamide	125 mg	Brown and White	Capsule		Barr Laboratories
BARR; 874; 4 ;	Warfarin Sodium	4 mg	Blue	Tablet	Oval, Flat-Faced, Beveled-Edge, Scored	Barr Laboratories
BARR; 882	Hydroxyurea	500 mg	Pink and Purple	Capsule		Barr Laboratories
BARR; 904	Tamoxifen Citrate	20 mg	White	Tablet	Circle, Biconvex	Barr Laboratories
BARR; 925; 3	Warfarin Sodium	3 mg	Tan	Tablet	Oval	Barr Laboratories
BARR; 926; 6	Warfarin Sodium	6 mg	Teal	Tablet	Oval	Barr Laboratories
BARR; 954	Dextroamphetamine Sulfate	5 mg	Beige	Extended-Release Capsule		Barr Laboratories
BARR; 955	Dextroamphetamine Sulfate	10 mg	Brown and Clear	Extended-Release Capsule		Barr Laboratories
BARR; 956	Dextroamphetamine Sulfate	15 mg	Brown and Clear	Extended-Release Capsule		Barr Laboratories
BAYER C500 QD	Cipro Xr	500 mg	White to Light Yellow	Tablet, Extended Release	Oblong	Schering
BAYER; 2.5	Levitra	2.5 mg	Orange	Tablet	Circle	Schering
BAYER; 5	Levitra	5 mg	Orange	Tablet	Circle	Schering
BAYER; 10	Levitra	10 mg	Orange	Tablet	Circle	Schering
BAYER; 20	Levitra	20 mg	Orange	Tablet	Circle	Schering
BAYER; C1000; QD	Cipro Xr	1000 mg	White to Light Yellow	Extended-Release Tablet	Oblong	Bayer Pharmaceutical
BAYER; LG ;	Biltricide	600 mg	White to Orange Tinged	Coated Tablet	Oblong, Triscored	Bayer Pharmaceutical
BAYER; M400	Avelox	400 mg	Red	Tablet	Oblong	Schering-Plough
BCI	Hectorol	0.5 mcg	Citrus Orange	Capsule, Liquid Filled	Oval	Genzyme
BCI	Hectorol	2.5 mcg	Sunshine Yellow	Capsule, Liquid Filled	Oval	Genzyme
BEACH; 1111	K-Phos	500 mg	White	Tablet	Circle	Beach Pharmaceuticals
BEACH; 1112	Uroqid-Acid	350 mg ; 200 mg	Yellow	Tablet	Circle	Beach Pharmaceuticals
BEACH; 1114	Uroqid-Acid No. 2	500 mg ; 500 mg	Yellow	Coated Tablet	Capsule-Shape	Beach Pharmaceuticals
BEACH; 1115	Thiacide	500 mg ; 250 mg ;	Green	Tablet	Capsule-Shape	Beach Pharmaceuticals
BEACH; 1125	K-Phos Neutral	155 mg ; 852 mg ; 130 mg	White	Tablet	Capsule-Shape	Beach Pharmaceuticals
BEACH; 1134	K-Phos No. 2	305 mg ; 700 mg ; 250 mg	Brown	Tablet	Capsule-Shape	Beach Pharmaceuticals
BEACH; 1135	K-Phos M.F.	155 mg ; 250 mg	White	Tablet	Circle	Beach Pharmaceuticals
BEACH; 1136	Citrolith	950 mg ; 50 mg		Tablet		Beach Pharmaceuticals
BEECHAM; 185	Beepen - VK	250 mg	White	Tablet	Oval	Glaxosmithkline
BEECHAM; 186	Beepen - VK	500 mg	White	Tablet	Oval	Glaxosmithkline
BENTYL 10	Bentyl	10 mg	Blue	Capsule		Axcan Scandipharm
BENTYL 20 ;	Bentyl	20 mg	Light Blue	Tablet	Circle	Axcan Scandipharm
BENTYL; 10 ;	Bentyl	10 mg	Blue	Capsule		Aventis Pharmaceuticals
BERLEX	Elixophyllin SR	250 mg	Clear	Extended-Release Capsule		Forest Pharmaceuticals
BERLEX; 80 MG	Betapace Af	80 mg	White	Tablet	Capsule-Shape	Berlex Laboratories
BERLEX; 100	Elixophyllin	100 mg	White	Capsule		Forest Pharmaceuticals
BERLEX; 120 MG	Betapace Af	120 mg	White	Tablet	Capsule-Shape	Berlex Laboratories
BERLEX; 129	Elixophyllin SR	125 mg	White	Extended-Release Capsule		Forest Pharmaceuticals
BERLEX; 131	Aminodur Dura-Tabs	300 mg	White to Off-White	Tablet		Berlex Laboratories

IMPRINT	BRAND/GENERIC NAME	STRENGTH	COLOR	FORM	SHAPE	MANUFACTURER
BERLEX; 160 MG	Betapace Af	160 mg	White	Tablet	Capsule-Shape	Berlex Laboratories
BERLEX; 162	Bilivist	500 mg	Yellow-Tan	Capsule, Liquid Filled		Berlex Laboratories
BERLEX; 200	Elixophyllin	200 mg	White	Capsule		Forest Pharmaceuticals
BEROCCA; PLUS; ROCHE	Berocca Plus	0.15 mg ; 25 mg ; 0.8 mg ; 27 mg ; 0.1 mg ; 50 mg ; 5 mg ; 3 mg ; 22.5 mg ; 500 mg ; 20 ; 20 mg ; 25 mg ; 50 mg ; 5000 IU ; 30 IU ; 100 mg	Yellow-Gold	Tablet	Oblong	Roche Pharmaceuticals
BEROCCA; ROCHE	Berocca	15 mg ; 4 mg ; 5 mcg ; 100 mg ; 18 mg ; 0.5 mg ; 500 mg ; 15 mg	Light Green	Tablet	Capsule-Shape	Roche Pharmaceuticals
BERTEK; 560	Phenytoin	100 mg		Capsule		Mylan Bertek Pharmaceuticals
BERTEK; 670	Phenytek	200 mg	Dark Blue Cap, Blue Body	Extended-Release Capsule		Mylan Bertek Pharmaceuticals
BERTEK; 750	Phenytek	300 mg	Blue Cap and Body	Extended-Release Capsule		Mylan Bertek Pharmaceuticals
BETAPACE; 80 MG	Betapace	80 mg	Light Blue	Tablet	Capsule-Shape	Berlex Laboratories
BETAPACE; 120 MG	Betapace	120 mg	Light Blue	Tablet	Capsule-Shape	Berlex Laboratories
BETAPACE; 160 MG	Betapace	160 mg	Light Blue	Tablet	Capsule-Shape	Berlex Laboratories
BETAPACE; 240 MG	Betapace	240 mg	Light Blue	Tablet	Capsule-Shape	Berlex Laboratories
BI 58 ; FLOMAX 0.4 MG	Flomax	0.4 mg	Olive Green Opaque Cap and Orange Opaque Body	Capsule		Boehringer Ingelheim Pharmaceuticals
BI; 6	Catapres	0.1 mg	Tan	Tablet	Oval, Scored	Boehringer Ingelheim Pharmaceuticals
BI; 7	Catapres	0.2 mg	Orange	Tablet	Oval, Scored	Boehringer Ingelheim Pharmaceuticals
BI; 8	Combipres	0.1 mg ; 15 mg	Pink	Tablet	Oval, Scored	Boehringer Ingelheim Pharmaceuticals
BI; 9	Combipres	0.2 mg ; 15 mg	Blue	Tablet	Oval, Scored	Boehringer Ingelheim Pharmaceuticals
BI; 10	Combipres	15 mg ; 0.3 mg	White	Tablet	Oval, Scored	Boehringer Ingelheim Pharmaceuticals
BI; 11	Catapres	0.3 mg	Orange	Tablet	Oval, Scored	Boehringer Ingelheim Pharmaceuticals
BI; 17	Persantine	25 mg	Orange	Coated Tablet	Circle	Boehringer Ingelheim Pharmaceuticals
BI; 18	Persantine	50 mg	Orange	Tablet	Circle	Boehringer Ingelheim Pharmaceuticals
BI; 19	Persantine	75 mg	Orange	Coated Tablet	Circle	Boehringer Ingelheim Pharmaceuticals
BI; 20	Serentil	10 mg	Red	Coated Tablet		Boehringer Ingelheim Pharmaceuticals
BI; 28	Torecan	10 mg	Yellow	Tablet	Circle	Boehringer Ingelheim Pharmaceuticals
BI; 48	Respbid	250 mg	White	Extended-Release Tablet		Boehringer Ingelheim Pharmaceuticals
BI; 49	Respbid	500 mg	White	Extended-Release Tablet		Boehringer Ingelheim Pharmaceuticals
BI; 49	Respid	500 mg	White	Tablet	Capsule-Shape	3M Pharmaceuticals
BI; 62	Preludin	75 mg	Pink	Tablet		Boehringer Ingelheim Pharmaceuticals
BI; 64	Prelu-2	105 mg	Light and Dark Green	Extended-Release Capsule		Boehringer Ingelheim Pharmaceuticals
BI; 66	Mexitil	150 mg	Red and Tan	Capsule		Boehringer Ingelheim Pharmaceuticals
BI; 67	Mexitil	200 mg	Red	Capsule		Boehringer Ingelheim Pharmaceuticals
BI; 68	Mexitil	250 mg	Red and Aqua Green	Capsule		Boehringer Ingelheim Pharmaceuticals
BI; 79	Preludin	50 mg	White	Tablet	Circle	Boehringer Ingelheim Pharmaceuticals
BI; 100	Serentil	100 mg	Red	Coated Tablet		Boehringer Ingelheim Pharmaceuticals
BIOCAL	Biocal Calcium Supplement	625 mg	White	Tablet, Chewable		Bayer Consumer Care
BIOCAL	Biocal Calcium Supplement	1250 mg	White	Tablet		Bayer Consumer Care
BIOCRAFT; 16	Penicillin VK	250 mg	White	Tablet	Oval	Teva Pharmaceuticals
BIOCRAFT; 32	Sulfamethoxazole and Trimethoprim Single Strength	400 mg ; 80 mg	White	Tablet	Circle, Scored	Teva Pharmaceuticals
BIOCRAFT; 33	Smz-Tmp DS	800 mg ; 160 mg	White	Tablet	Oval, Scored	Teva Pharmaceuticals
BIOCRAFT; 34	Trimethoprim	100 mg	White	Tablet	Circle	Teva Pharmaceuticals
BIOCRAFT; 49	Penicillin-VK	500 mg	White	Tablet	Oval, Scored	Teva Pharmaceuticals
BIOCRAFT; 94	Cyclacillin	250 mg	White	Tablet	Capsule-Shape	Teva Pharmaceuticals
BIOCRAFT; 95	Cyclacillin	500 mg	White	Tablet	Capsule-Shape	Teva Pharmaceuticals
BIOCRAFT; 105 105	Sucralfate	1 G	White	Tablet	Capsule-Shape, Scored	Teva Pharmaceuticals
BIOCRAFT; 148	Clindamycin Hydrochloride	75 mg	Red	Capsule		Teva Pharmaceuticals
BIOCRAFT; 163	Cinoxacin	250 mg	Blue and Yellow	Capsule		Teva Pharmaceuticals
BIOCRAFT; 164	Cinoxacin	500 mg	Blue and Yellow	Capsule		Teva Pharmaceuticals
BIOCRAFT; 177	Potassium Chloride	600 mg	Opaque Blue and White	Extended-Release Capsule		Teva Pharmaceuticals
BIOCRAFT; 178	Potassium Chloride	750 mg	Opaque Blue	Extended-Release Capsule		Teva Pharmaceuticals
BIOCRAFT; 185	Ketoprofen	25 mg	White	Capsule		Teva Pharmaceuticals
BIOCRAFT; 223	Cefaclor	250 mg	Opaque White and Gray	Capsule		Teva Pharmaceuticals

IMPRINT	BRAND/GENERIC NAME	STRENGTH	COLOR	FORM	SHAPE	MANUFACTURER
BIOCRAFT; 224	Cefaclor	500 mg	Opaque Red and White	Capsule		Teva Pharmaceuticals
BJ; 675	Oreton Propionate	10 mg	Pink	Tablet		Schering
BL; 07	Penicillin G Potassium	200,000 units	White	Tablet	Circle	Teva Pharmaceuticals
BL; 09	Penicillin G Potassium	250,000 units	White	Tablet	Circle	Teva Pharmaceuticals
BL; 10	Penicillin G Potassium	400,000 units	White	Tablet	Circle	Teva Pharmaceuticals
BL; 15	Penicillin-VK	250 mg	White	Tablet	Circle, Scored	Teva Pharmaceuticals
BL; 17	Penicillin-VK	500 mg	White	Tablet	Circle, Scored	Teva Pharmaceuticals
BL; 19	Imipramine Hydrochloride	10 mg	Yellow	Tablet	Circle	Teva Pharmaceuticals
BL; 20	Imipramine Hydrochloride	25 mg	Salmon	Tablet	Circle	Teva Pharmaceuticals
BL; 21	Imipramine Hydrochloride	50 mg	Green	Tablet	Circle	Teva Pharmaceuticals
BL; 22	Amitriptyline Hydrochloride	10 mg	Pink	Tablet	Circle	Teva Pharmaceuticals
BL; 23	Amitriptyline Hydrochloride	25 mg	Light Green	Tablet	Circle	Teva Pharmaceuticals
BL; 24	Amitriptyline Hydrochloride	50 mg	Brown	Tablet	Circle	Teva Pharmaceuticals
BL; 25	Amitriptyline Hydrochloride	75 mg	Lavender	Tablet	Circle	Teva Pharmaceuticals
BL; 26	Amitriptyline Hydrochloride	100 mg	Orange	Tablet	Circle	Teva Pharmaceuticals
BL; 32	Smz-Tmp	400 mg ; 80 mg	White	Tablet	Circle	Teva Pharmaceuticals
BL; 35	Trimethoprim	200 mg	White	Tablet	Circle	Teva Pharmaceuticals
BL; 42	Thioridazine Hydrochloride	10 mg	Green	Tablet	Oval	Teva Pharmaceuticals
BL; 46	Thioridazine Hydrochloride	100 mg	Light-Green	Tablet	Oval	Teva Pharmaceuticals
BL; 52	Amiloride Hydrochloride and Hydrochlorothiazide	5 mg ; 50 mg	Yellow	Tablet	Circle, Scored	Warner Chilcott
BL; 82 ;	Saluron	50 mg	White	Tablet	Circle, Scored	Bristol-Myers Squibb
BL; 92	Metoclopramide	5 mg	White	Tablet	Circle	Teva Pharmaceuticals
BL; 93	Metoclopramide	10 mg	White	Tablet	Circle, Scored	Teva Pharmaceuticals
BL; 130	Albuterol Sulfate	2 mg	White	Tablet	Circle	Teva Pharmaceuticals
BL; 131	Albuterol	4 mg	White	Tablet	Round, Bisected Scored	Teva Pharmaceuticals
BL; 132	Metaproterenol	10 mg	White	Tablet	Circle, Scored	Teva Pharmaceuticals
BL; 133	Metaproterenol	20 mg	White	Tablet	Circle	Teva Pharmaceuticals
BL; 141	Baclofen	10 mg	White	Tablet	Circle, Scored	Teva Pharmaceuticals
BL; 142	Baclofen	20 mg	White	Tablet	Circle, Scored	Teva Pharmaceuticals
BL; 207 ;	Corgard	40 mg	Blue	Tablet	Circle, Scored	Bristol Laboratories
BL; 208 ;	Corgard	120 mg	Blue	Tablet	Scored, Oblong	Bristol-Myers Squibb
BL; 221	Amoxicillin	125 mg	White to Off-White	Tablet, Chewable	Capsule-Shape	Teva Pharmaceuticals
BL; 222	Amoxicillin	250 mg	White	Tablet, Chewable	Capsule-Shape	Teva Pharmaceuticals
BL; 232 ;	Corgard	20 mg	Blue	Tablet	Circle, Scored	Bristol-Myers Squibb
BL; 241	Corgard	80 mg	Blue	Tablet	Circle, Scored	Bristol-Myers Squibb
BL; C1	Ultracef	1 GM	White or Yellow	Tablet	Capsule-Shape	Bristol-Myers Squibb
BL; E1 ;	Bristamycin	250 mg	Orange	Tablet	Circle	Bristol-Myers Squibb
BL; L1	Lysodren	500 mg	White	Tablet	Circle, Scored	Bristol-Myers Squibb
BL; N2	Naldagesic	325 mg ; 15 mg	Blue	Tablet	Capsule-Shape	Bristol-Myers Squibb
BL; V1 ;	Betapen-VK	250 mg	White	Coated Tablet		Bristol-Myers Squibb
BLAINE	Mag-Ox 400	400 mg	White	Tablet	Circle	Blaine Pharmaceuticals
BLAINE 0054	Uro-Mag	140 mg	White	Capsule		Blaine Pharmaceuticals
BLANSETT; 3; 08	Nalex-A	4 mg ; 40 mg ; 20 mg	Light Tan	Extended-Release Tablet	Capsule-Shape, Scored	Blansett Pharmacal
BLANSETT; 30	Nalex	120 mg ; 250 mg	Clear and White	Extended-Release Capsule		Blansett Pharmacal
BMP 189	Augmentin	125 mg ; 31.25 mg	Yellow	Tablet, Chewable	Circle	Glaxosmithkline
BMP 190	Augmentin	250 mg ; 62.5 mg	Yellow	Tablet, Chewable	Circle	Glaxosmithkline
BMP; 108	Cotrol-D	60 mg ; 4 mg	Green	Tablet		Glaxosmithkline
BMP; 109	Dasikon	195 mg ; 130 mg ; 0.065 mg ; 2 mg ; 32 mg	Natural and Blue	Capsule		Glaxosmithkline
BMP; 119	Hybephen	0.0094 mg ; 15 mg ; 0.1277 mg ; 0.0233 mg	Green	Tablet		Glaxosmithkline
BMP; 121	Livitamin	3 mg ; 5 mcg ; 0.66 mg ; 2 mg ; 150 mg ; 100 mg ; 3 mg ; 3 mg ; 10 mg ; 100 mg	Pink	Capsule		Glaxosmithkline
BMP; 122	Livitamin-If	0.66 mg ; 2 mg ; 150 mg ; 0.33 Nf U ; 100 mg ; 3 mg ; 3 mg ; 10 mg ; 100 mg ; 3 mg ; 5 mcg	Green	Capsule		Glaxosmithkline
BMP; 123	Livitamin	50 mg ; 3 mg ; 3 mg ; 3 mg ; 10 mg ; 5 mcg ; 100 mg ; 2 mg ; 0.33 mg	Orange	Tablet, Chewable		Glaxosmithkline
BMP; 124	Livitamin Prenatal	20 mg ; 10 mg ; 5 mg ; 3 Mgg ; 3 mg ; 0.5 mg ; 5 mcg ; 350 mg ; 50 mg ; 6000 U.S.P. units ; 400 U.S.P. units ; 100 mg	Yellow	Tablet		Glaxosmithkline
BMP; 135	Semets	3 mg	Red	Troche		Glaxosmithkline
BMP; 139	Thalfed	8 mg ; 0.12 G ; 25 mg	White	Tablet		Glaxosmithkline
BMP; 140	Totacillin	250 mg	Brown and Orange	Capsule		Glaxosmithkline
BMP; 141	Totacillin	500 mg	Brown and Orange	Capsule		Glaxosmithkline
BMP; 143	Bactocill	250 mg	Brown and Yellow	Capsule		Glaxosmithkline
BMP; 144	Bactocill	500 mg	Brown and Yellow	Capsule		Glaxosmithkline
BMP; 145	Daricon	10 mg	White	Tablet	Circle, Grooved	Glaxosmithkline
BMP; 146	Daricon PB	15 mg ; 5 mg	Pink	Tablet		Glaxosmithkline
BMP; 150	Obedrin-LA	10 mg		Tablet		Glaxosmithkline
BMP; 165	Dycill	250 mg	Light Blue and Creme	Capsule		Glaxosmithkline
BMP; 166	Dycill	500 mg	Light Blue and Creme	Capsule		Glaxosmithkline
BMP; 167	Actol Expectorant Tablet	30 mg ; 200 mg	Red	Coated Tablet		Glaxosmithkline
BMP; 169	Cloxapen	250 mg	Lime and Beige	Capsule		Glaxosmithkline

IMPRINT	BRAND/GENERIC NAME	STRENGTH	COLOR	FORM	SHAPE	MANUFACTURER
BMP; 170	Cloxapen	500 mg	Lime and Beige	Capsule		Glaxosmithkline
BMP; 192	Maxolon	10 mg	Blue	Tablet	Scored, Circle	Glaxosmithkline
BMP; 194	Enarax White	5 mg ; 25 mg	White	Tablet		Glaxosmithkline
BMP; 195	Enarax Black and White	10 mg ; 25 mg	Black and White	Tablet		Glaxosmithkline
BMP; 211	Larotid	250 mg	Caramel and Buff	Capsule		Glaxosmithkline
BMS 80	Pravachol	80 mg	Yellow	Tablet	Oval	Bristol-Myers Squibb
BMS 100 MG 3623	Reyataz	100 mg	Blue, White	Capsule		Bristol-Myers Squibb
BMS 150 MG 3624	Reyataz	150 mg	Blue, Powder Blue	Capsule		Bristol-Myers Squibb
BMS 200 MG 3631	Reyataz	200 mg	Blue	Capsule		Bristol-Myers Squibb
BMS 300 MG 3622	Reyataz	300 mg	Blue, Red	Capsule		Bristol-Myers Squibb
BMS 1964; 15	Zerit	15 mg	Light Yellow and Dark Red	Capsule		Bristol-Myers Squibb
BMS 1965; 20	Zerit	20 mg	Light Brown	Capsule		Bristol-Myers Squibb
BMS 1966; 30	Zerit	30 mg	Light Orange and Dark Orange	Capsule		Bristol-Myers Squibb
BMS 1967; 40	Zerit	40 mg	Dark Orange	Capsule		Bristol-Myers Squibb
BMS; 37.5 MG; 1555	Zerit Xr	37.5 mg	Red and Yellow	Extended-Release Capsule		Bristol-Myers Squibb
BMS; 50 MG; 1656	Zerit Xr	50 mg	Orange	Extended-Release Capsule		Bristol-Myers Squibb
BMS; 50; 31	Serzone	50 mg	Light Pink	Tablet	Six-Sided	Bristol-Myers Squibb
BMS; 75 MG; 1557	Zerit Xr	75 mg	Red	Extended-Release Capsule		Bristol-Myers Squibb
BMS; 80 ;	Pravigard Pac	81 mg ; 80 mg	Yellow Oval Tablet and White Tablet	Tablet		Bristol-Myers Squibb
BMS; 80 ;	Pravigard Pac	325 mg ; 80 mg	Yellow Oval Tablet and White Tablet	Tablet		Bristol-Myers Squibb
BMS; 100 MG; 1558	Zerit Xr	100 mg	Yellow	Extended-Release Capsule		Bristol-Myers Squibb
BMS; 100; 32	Serzone	100 mg	White	Tablet	Hexagonal, Bisected, Scored Scored	Bristol-Myers Squibb
BMS; 125 MG; 6671	Videx Ec	125 mg	White with Tan Ink	Capsule, Delayed Release		Bristol-Myers Squibb
BMS; 150; 39	Serzone	150 mg	Peach	Tablet	Six-Sided, Bisect Scored	Bristol-Myers Squibb
BMS; 200 MG; 6672	Videx Ec	200 mg	White with Green Ink	Capsule, Delayed Release		Bristol-Myers Squibb
BMS; 200; 33	Serzone	200 mg	Light Yellow	Tablet	Six-Sided	Bristol-Myers Squibb
BMS; 250 MG; 6673	Videx Ec	250 mg	White with Blue Ink	Capsule, Delayed Release		Bristol-Myers Squibb
BMS; 250; 41	Serzone	250 mg	White	Tablet	Six-Sided	Bristol-Myers Squibb
BMS; 400 MG; 6674	Videx Ec	400 mg	White with Red Ink	Capsule, Delayed Release		Bristol-Myers Squibb
BMS; 6060; 500	Glucophage	500 mg	White	Coated Tablet		Bristol-Myers Squibb
BMS; 6063; 500	Glucophage Xr	500 mg	White	Extended-Release Tablet	Biconvex, Capsule-Shape	Bristol-Myers Squibb
BMS; 6070; 850	Glucophage	850 mg	White	Coated Tablet		Bristol-Myers Squibb
BMS; 6071; 1000	Glucophage	1000 mg	White	Tablet	Oblong, Scored	Bristol-Myers Squibb
BMS; 6072	Glucovance	1.25 mg ; 250 mg	Pale Yellow	Coated Tablet	Capsule-Shape, Bevel-Edged, Biconvex	Bristol-Myers Squibb
BMS; 6073	Glucovance	2.5 mg ; 500 mg	Pale Orange	Coated Tablet	Capsule-Shape, Bevel-Edged, Biconvex	Bristol-Myers Squibb
BMS; 6074	Glucovance	5 mg ; 500 mg	Yellow	Coated Tablet	Capsule-Shape, Bevel-Edged, Biconvex	Bristol-Myers Squibb
BMS; 6077	Metaglip	2.5 mg ; 500 mg	White	Tablet	Oval	Bristol-Myers Squibb
BMS; 6078	Metaglip	5 mg ; 500 mg	Pink	Tablet	Oval	Bristol-Myers Squibb
BMS; 6081	Metaglip	250 mg ; 2.5 mg	Pink	Tablet	Oval	Bristol-Myers Squibb
BMS; MONOPRIL; 10 ;	Monopril	10 mg	White to Off-White	Tablet	Diamond	Bristol-Myers Squibb
BMS; MONOPRIL; 20 ;	Monopril	20 mg	White to Off-White	Tablet	Oval, Compressed	Bristol-Myers Squibb
BMS; MONOPRIL; 40 ;	Monopril	40 mg	White to Off-White	Tablet	Six-Sided, Biconvex Hexagonal Shaped, Compressed	Bristol-Myers Squibb
BMS; TEQUIN; 200	Tequin	200 mg	White	Tablet	Oval	Bristol-Myers Squibb
BMS; TEQUIN; 400	Tequin	400 mg	White	Tablet	Oval	Bristol-Myers Squibb
BNP7600	Elmiron	100 mg	White Opaque	Capsule		Ortho-Mcneil Pharmaceutical
BOCK; 460	Zephrex	400 mg ; 60 mg	White	Coated Tablet	Oval; Bisected Scored	Sanofi Pharmaceuticals
BOCK; HS 33	Hemaspan	110 mg ; 20 mg ; 200 mg	Tan	Tablet	Oblong	Sanofi Pharmaceuticals
BOCK; P; N	Prenate Ultra Prenatal Vitamins	90 mg ; 1 mg ; 2700 I.U. ; 30 I.U. ; 400 IU	White	Tablet	Oval, Scored	Sanofi Pharmaceuticals
BOEHRINGER INGELHEIM LOGO; 01A	Aggrenox	200 mg ; 25 mg	Red and Ivory with Yellow Pellets	Capsule		Boehringer Ingelheim Pharmaceuticals
BOEHRINGER MANNHEIM LOGO; 102; 5	Demadex	5 mg	White	Tablet	Oval, Scored	Roche Laboratories
BOEHRINGER MANNHEIM LOGO; 103; 10	Demadex	10 mg	White	Tablet	Oval, Scored	Roche Laboratories
BOEHRINGER MANNHEIM LOGO; 104; 20	Demadex	20 mg	White	Tablet	Oval, Scored	Roche Laboratories
BOEHRINGER MANNHEIM LOGO; 105; 100	Demadex	100 mg	White	Tablet	Capsule-Shape, Scored	Roche Laboratories
BRA	Halflytely & Bisacodyl Tablets Bowel Prep Kit - Bisacodyl Tablets	5 mg	Pink	Tablet, Delayed Release	Circle	Braintree Laboratories
BRA; 200	Phoslo	667 mg	White	Tablet	Circle	Braintree Laboratories
BRICANYL; 2 1/2 ;	Bricanyl	2.5 mg	White	Tablet	Circle	Aventis Pharmaceuticals

IMPRINT	BRAND/GENERIC NAME	STRENGTH	COLOR	FORM	SHAPE	MANUFACTURER
BRICANYL; 5 ;	Bricanyl	5 mg	White	Tablet	Square, Scored	Aventis Pharmaceuticals
BRISTOL	Bristacycline	250 mg	Green and Yellow	Capsule		Bristol-Myers Squibb
BRISTOL	Tetrex	100 mg	Yellow and Orange	Capsule		Bristol-Myers Squibb
BRISTOL	Tetrex-F	250 mg ; 250000 U		Capsule		Bristol-Myers Squibb
BRISTOL; 500	Bristacycline	500 mg	Green and Yellow	Capsule		Bristol-Myers Squibb
BRISTOL; 518 ;	Quibron Plus	150 mg ; 100 mg ; 25 mg ; 20 mg		Capsule		Bristol-Myers Squibb
BRISTOL; 732	Enkaid	25 mg	Green and Yellow	Capsule		Bristol-Myers Squibb
BRISTOL; 734	Enkaid	35 mg	Green and Orange	Capsule		Bristol-Myers Squibb
BRISTOL; 735	Enkaid	50 mg	Green and Brown	Capsule		Bristol-Myers Squibb
BRISTOL; 3091	Vepesid	50 mg	Pink	Capsule, Liquid Filled		Bristol-Myers Squibb
BRISTOL; 7278	Trimox	250 mg	Maroon and Pink	Capsule		Bristol-Myers Squibb
BRISTOL; 7279	Trimox	500 mg	Maroon and Pink	Capsule		Bristol-Myers Squibb
BRISTOL-MYERS; DATRIL; 500MG	Datril Extra Strength	500 mg	Green and White	Capsule		Bristol-Myers Squibb
BUCET; UAD; 307	Bucet	650 mg ; 50 mg	White	Capsule		Uad Laboratories
BUTISOL; 37-114	Butisol Sodium	50 mg		Tablet		Meda Pharmaceuticals
BVF; 0117	Pentoxifylline	400 mg		Extended-Release Tablet	Oblong, Compressed	Teva Pharmaceuticals
BVF; 120	Diltiazem Hydrochloride	120 mg	Clear Light Green	Extended-Release Capsule		Teva Pharmaceuticals
BVF; 180	Diltiazem Hydrochloride	180 mg	Dark Green and Light Green	Extended-Release Capsule		Teva Pharmaceuticals
BVF; 240	Diltiazem Hydrochloride	240 mg	Clear Dark Green	Extended-Release Capsule		Teva Pharmaceuticals
BVF; 300	Diltiazem Hydrochloride	300 mg	Ivory and Dark Green	Extended-Release Capsule		Teva Pharmaceuticals
C	Comtrex Multi-Symptom Cold Reliever	325 mg ; 30 mg ; 2 mg ; 10 mg	Yellow	Tablet		Bristol-Myers Squibb
C	Myfortic	180 mg ;	Lime Green	Enteric-Coated Tablet	Circle	Novartis
C	Prempro White Tablet	2.5 mg	White	Tablet	Oval, Scored	Wyeth-Ayerst Laboratories
C 2 1/2	Cialis	2.5 mg	Yellow	Tablet	Oval	Eli Lilly
C 5	Cialis	5 mg	Yellow	Tablet	Teardrop-Shape	Eli Lilly
C 10	Cialis	10 mg	Yellow	Tablet	Teardrop-Shape	Eli Lilly
C 20	Cialis	20 mg	Yellow	Tablet	Teardrop-Shape	Eli Lilly
C 21 ; M	Citalopram Hydrobromide	10 mg	Yellow	Tablet	Circle	Mylan Pharmaceuticals
C 22 ; M	Citalopram Hydrobromide	20 mg	Yellow	Tablet	Circle	Mylan Pharmaceuticals
C 24 ; M	Citalopram Hydrobromide	40 mg	Yellow	Tablet	Circle	Mylan Pharmaceuticals
C 402	Gabitril	2 mg	Orange-Peach	Tablet	Circle	Cephalon
C 404	Gabitril	4 mg	Yellow	Tablet	Circle	Cephalon
C 412	Gabitril	12 mg	Green	Tablet	Oval	Cephalon
C 416	Gabitril	16 mg	Blue	Tablet	Oval	Cephalon
C G ; T D	Trileptal	150 mg	Pale Grey-Green	Tablet	Oval	Novartis
C; 1	Choline Magnesium Trisalicylate	1000 mg	Pink	Tablet	Capsule-Shape	Actavis Totowa
C; 83; LL	Centrum Singles	500 mg	White	Coated Tablet	Oval, Convex	Wyeth Consumer Healthcare
C; 86; 72	Salflex	750 mg	White	Coated Tablet	Oblong, Scored	Amarin Pharmaceuticals
C; 119	Famotidine	20 mg	Pale Yellow	Tablet	Circle	Par Pharmaceutical
C; 120	Famotidine	40 mg	Yellow	Tablet	Circle	Par Pharmaceutical
C; 151	Buspirone Hydrochloride	5 mg	White	Tablet	Circle	Ranbaxy Pharmaceuticals
C; 152	Buspirone Hydrochloride	10 mg	White	Tablet	Circle	Ranbaxy Pharmaceuticals
C; 582	Cefadroxil	500 mg	Brown and White	Capsule		Ranbaxy Pharmaceuticals
C; 600; LL	Caltrate 600	600 mg	White	Coated Tablet	Oblong	Wyeth Consumer Healthcare
C; 3227	Nifedipine	10 mg	Tan	Capsule		Warner Chilcott
C; 3453	Nifedipine	20 mg	White	Capsule	Oval	Warner Chilcott
C; 8648	Bontril Pdm	35 mg	Green and Yellow	Tablet	Circle, BI-Layered, Scored	Amarin Pharmaceuticals
C; 8650	Phrenilin	325 mg ; 50 mg		Tablet		Amarin Pharmaceuticals
C; 8657	Hydrocet	5 mg ; 500 mg	Blue and White	Capsule		Amarin Pharmaceuticals
C; 8671	Salflex	500 mg	White	Coated Tablet	Circle	Amarin Pharmaceuticals
C; 8674	Motofen	0.025 mg ; 1 mg	White	Tablet	Five-Sided, Scored	Amarin Pharmaceuticals
C; CLOCK DESIGN	Quinaglute Dura-Tabs	324 mg	White	Extended-Release Tablet	Circle	Berlex Laboratories
C2C	Lanoxicaps	0.2 mg	Green	Capsule, Liquid Filled	Oblong	Glaxosmithkline
C5	Clarinex	5 mg	Light Blue	Tablet	Circle	Schering-Plough
C31 ; M	Carvedilol	3.125 mg	Blue	Tablet	Circle	Mylan Pharmaceuticals
C32 ; M	Carvedilol	6.25 mg	White	Tablet	Circle	Mylan Pharmaceuticals
C33 ; M	Carvedilol	12.5 mg	White	Tablet	Circle	Mylan Pharmaceuticals
C34 ; M	Carvedilol	25 mg	White	Tablet	Circle	Mylan Pharmaceuticals
C73 ;	Azor	5 mg ; 20 mg	White	Tablet		Daiichi Sankyo
C74	Azor	20 mg ; 10 mg	Gray-Orange	Tablet		Daiichi Sankyo
C75 ;	Azor	5 mg ; 40 mg	Cream	Tablet		Daiichi Sankyo
C77 ;	Azor	10 mg ; 40 mg	Brown-Red	Tablet		Daiichi Sankyo
C500 ; G	Clarithromycin	500 mg	White to Off-White	Tablet	Oval	Mylan Pharmaceuticals
CALAN; SR; 120	Calan SR	120 mg	Light Violet	Tablet, Extended Release	Oval	Pfizer Us Pharmaceuticals Group
CALTRATE; M; 600	Caltrate Plus Calcium	600 mg ; 200 IU ; 40 mg ; 7.5 mg ; 1 mg ; 1.8 mg ;	Dusty Rose	Coated Tablet	Oval, Scored	Wyeth Consumer Healthcare
CAPOTEN; 12.5 MG	Capoten	12.5 mg	White	Tablet	Oval, Biconvex, Partially Bisected Scored	Bristol-Myers Squibb
CAPOTEN; 25 MG ;	Capoten	25 mg	White	Tablet	Oval, Biconvex with a Quadrisect Bar Scored	Bristol-Myers Squibb
CAPOTEN; 50 MG ;	Capoten	50 mg	White	Tablet	Oval, Biconvex, Scored	Bristol-Myers Squibb
CAPOTEN; 100 MG ;	Capoten	100 mg	White	Tablet	Oval, Biconvex, Scored	Bristol-Myers Squibb
CAPOZIDE 25/15	Capozide 25/15	15 mg ; 25 mg	White with Orange Mottling	Tablet	Square	Par Pharmaceutical
CAPOZIDE 25/25	Capozide 25/25	25 mg ; 25 mg	Peach	Tablet	Square	Par Pharmaceutical
CAPOZIDE 50/15	Capozide 50/15	50 mg ; 15 mg	White with Orange Mottling	Tablet	Oval	Par Pharmaceutical
CAPOZIDE 50/25	Capozide 50/25	50 mg ; 25 mg	Peach	Tablet	Oval	Par Pharmaceutical
CARAFATE; 1712 ;	Carafate	1 GM	Light Pink	Tablet	Capsule-Shape	Axcan Scandipharm

IMPRINT	BRAND/GENERIC NAME	STRENGTH	COLOR	FORM	SHAPE	MANUFACTURER
CARDENE SR 30MG PDL BIOPHARMA	Cardene SR	30 mg	Opaque Pink	Capsule, Extended Release	Capsule-Shape	Pdl Biopharma
CARDENE SR 45 MG PDL BIOPHARMA	Cardene SR	45 mg	Opaque Powder Blue	Capsule, Extended Release	Capsule-Shape	Ekr Therapeutics
CARDENE SR 60 MG PDL BIOPHARMA	Cardene SR	60 mg	Opaque Light Blue, White	Capsule, Extended Release		Pdl Biopharma
CARDENE SR; 30 MG; SYNTEX; 2440	Cardene SR	30 mg	Pink	Capsule, Extended Release		Roche Laboratories
CARDENE SR; 60 MG; SYNTEX; 2442	Cardene SR	60 mg	Light Blue and White	Capsule, Extended Release		Roche Laboratories
CARDILATE; X7A	Cardilate	10 mg	White	Tablet	Square	Glaxosmithkline
CARDURA; 1 MG	Cardura	1 mg	White	Tablet	Oblong, Scored	Pfizer Laboratories
CARDURA; 2 MG	Cardura	2 mg	Light Orange	Tablet	Oblong, Scored	Pfizer Laboratories
CARDURA; 4 MG	Cardura	4 mg	Orange	Tablet	Oblong, Scored	Pfizer Laboratories
CARDURA; 8 MG	Cardura	8 mg	Green	Tablet	Oblong, Scored	Pfizer Laboratories
CARNITOR ST	Carnitor	330 mg		Tablet		Sigma-Tau Pharmaceuticals
CATAFLAM; 25	Cataflam	25 mg	Light Pink	Tablet	Circle, Biconvex	Novartis Pharmaceuticals
CB; 300	Cimetidine	300 mg	Light Yellow	Coated Tablet	Circle	Lederle Laboratories
CB; 400	Cimetidine	400 mg	Light Yellow	Coated Tablet	Oval	Lederle Laboratories
CB; 800	Cimetidine	800 mg	Light Yellow	Coated Tablet	Oval	Lederle Laboratories
CC	Cycrin	2.5 mg	White	Tablet	Oval, Scored	Esi Pharma
CC; 108	Hydrochlorothiazide	50 mg	Peach	Tablet	Circle	Novartis Generics
CC; 116	Hydrochlorothiazide	25 mg	Peach	Tablet	Circle	Novartis Generics
CC; CYCRIN	Cycrin	10 mg	Peach	Tablet	Oval, Scored	Esi Pharma
CD 129	Ranitidine Hydrochloride	150 mg	Opaque Light Brown	Capsule		Par Pharmaceutical
CD 130	Ranitidine Hydrochloride	300 mg	Opaque Light Brown	Capsule		Par Pharmaceutical
CDX50	Casodex	50 mg	White	Coated Tablet		Astrazeneca
CELGENE / 50 MG LOGO	Thalomid	50 mg	White Opaque	Capsule		Celgene
CELGENE / 100 MG LOGO	Thalomid	100 mg	Tan	Capsule		Celgene
CELGENE / 150 MG LOGO	Thalomid	150 mg	Blue, Tan	Capsule		Celgene
CELGENE / 200 MG LOGO	Thalomid	200 mg	Blue	Capsule		Celgene
CELGENE; DO NOT GET PREGNANT LOGO	Thalomid	50 mg	White	Capsule		Celgene
CELLCEPT; 250; ROCHE	Cellcept	250 mg	Blue and Brown	Capsule, Liquid Filled		Roche
CELLCEPT; 500; ROCHE	Cellcept	500 mg	Lavender	Coated Tablet	Capsule-Shape	Roche Laboratories
CELLTECH; 575; 20 MG	Metadate Cd	20 mg	Blue and White	Extended-Release Capsule		Celltech
CELLTECH; 575; 20 MG ;	Metadate Cd	20 mg	Blue and White	Extended-Release Capsule		Celltech
CELLTECH; 576; 30 MG	Metadate Cd	30 mg	Reddish Brown and White	Extended-Release Capsule		Celltech
CENTRAL; 40	Codimal-L.A.	120 mg ; 8 mg	Clear and Red with Blue Beads	Extended-Release Capsule		Schwarz Pharma
CENTRAL; 130 MG	Theoclear LA	130 mg	Clear	Timed-Release Capsule		Schwarz Pharma
CENTRAL; 260 MG	Theoclear LA	260 mg	Clear	Timed-Release Capsule		Schwarz Pharma
CENTRUM; C;1	Centrum Advanced Formula	6 mcg ; 25 mcg ; 18 mg ; 5000 IU ; 30 IU ; 400 mcg ; 20 mg ; 400 IU ; 30 mcg ; 10 mg ; 162 mg ; 125 mg ; 150 mcg ; 100 mg ; 2 mg ; 15 mg ; 2.5 mg ; 40 mg ; 25 mcg ; 25 mcg ; 25 mcg ; 5 mcg ; 10 mcg ; 60 mg ; 1.5 mg ; 1.7 mg ; 2 mg	Peach	Coated Tablet	Oblong, Scored	Wyeth Consumer Healthcare
CF; 512	Cefadroxil	500 mg	White	Coated Tablet	Oblong, Biconvex, Scored	Ranbaxy Pharmaceuticals
CF; A	Nembutal Sodium	50 mg	Orange and White	Capsule		Abbott Laboratories
CG ; FV	Femara	2.5 mg	Dark Yellow	Tablet	Circle	Novartis
CG CG ; TE TE	Trileptal	300 mg	Yellow	Tablet	Oval	Novartis
CG CG ; TF TF	Trileptal	600 mg	Light Pink	Tablet	Oval	Novartis Pharmaceuticals
CG; FXF	Foradil Aerolizer	12 mcg	Clear	Capsule		Novartis
CGPI 40	Oracea	40 mg	Beige Opaque	Capsule		Galderma
CH; A	Nembutal Sodium	100 mg	Yellow	Capsule		Abbott Laboratories
CHEW; EZ	Eryped	200 mg	White	Tablet, Chewable	Circle, Scored	Abbott Laboratories
CHX 0.5 ; PFIZER	Chantix	0.5 mg	Off-White to White	Tablet	Capsule-Shape	Pfizer
CHX 1.0 ; PFIZER	Chantix	1 mg	Light Blue	Tablet	Capsule-Shape	Pfizer
CIBA	Pyribenzamine Lontabs	50 mg	Light Green	Tablet		Novartis
CIBA 24	Cytadren	250 mg	White	Tablet	Circle	Novartis
CIBA; 3	Ritalin	10 mg	Pale Green	Tablet	Circle, Scored	Novartis Pharmaceuticals
CIBA; 7	Ritalin	5 mg	Yellow	Tablet	Circle	Novartis Pharmaceuticals
CIBA; 13	Serpasil-Esidrix No. 1	0.1 mg ; 25 mg	Light Orange	Tablet	Circle	Novartis
CIBA; 16	Ritalin SR	20 mg	White	Sustained-Release Tablet	Circle, Coated	Novartis Pharmaceuticals
CIBA; 22	Esidrix	25 mg	Pink	Tablet	Circle, Scored	Novartis
CIBA; 26	Ludiomil	50 mg	Dark Orange	Tablet	Circle, Scored	Novartis
CIBA; 31 (ORANGE) ;	Forhistal	1 mg	Orange or Green	Tablet		Novartis

IMPRINT	BRAND/GENERIC NAME	STRENGTH	COLOR	FORM	SHAPE	MANUFACTURER
CIBA; 32	Metandren	25 mg	Yellow	Tablet	Circle, Scored	Novartis
CIBA; 33 ;	Pyribenzamine	50 mg	Light Blue	Tablet		Novartis
CIBA; 34	Ritalin	20 mg	Pale Yellow	Tablet	Circle, Scored	Novartis Pharmaceuticals
CIBA; 35	Serpasil	0.1 mg	White	Tablet	Circle	Novartis
CIBA; 36	Serpasil	0.25 mg	White	Tablet	Circle, Scored	Novartis
CIBA; 40	Serpasil-Apresoline No. 1	25 mg ; 0.1 mg	Yellow	Tablet	Circle	Novartis
CIBA; 45	Forhistal Lontabs	2.5 mg	Orange	Tablet	Oblong	Novartis
CIBA; 47	Esimil	10 mg ; 25 mg	White	Tablet	Circle, Scored	Novartis
CIBA; 49	Ismelin	10 mg	Yellow	Tablet	Circle, Scored	Novartis
CIBA; 64	Metandren Linguets	10 mg	Yellow	Tablet	Capsule-Shape	Novartis
CIBA; 65	Lithobid	300 mg	Peach	Sustained-Release Tablet		Novartis
CIBA; 71	Ser-AP-Es	25 mg ; 15 mg ; 0.1 mg	Pink	Tablet	Circle	Novartis
CIBA; 92	Gammacorten	0.75 mg		Tablet		Novartis
CIBA; 95	Pyribenzamine	25 mg	Green	Tablet		Novartis
CIBA; 96	Ultandren	5 mg	Lavender	Tablet		Novartis
CIBA; 103	Ismelin	25 mg	White	Tablet	Circle, Scored	Novartis
CIBA; 104	Serpasil-Apresoline No. 2	50 mg ; 0.2 mg	Yellow	Tablet	Circle	Novartis
CIBA; 105	Dialog	300 mg ; 15 mg	White	Tablet	Circle, Scored	Novartis
CIBA; 110	Ludiomil	25 mg	Dark Orange	Tablet	Oval, Scored	Novartis
CIBA; 110	Ludiomil	25 mg	Orange	Tablet	Oval, Scored	Novartis
CIBA; 130	Metopirone	250 mg	White	Tablet	Circle, Scored	Novartis
CIBA; 134	Pyribenzamine with Ephedrine	12 mg ; 25 mg	White	Tablet		Novartis
CIBA; 135	Ludiomil	75 mg	White	Coated Tablet	Oval	Novartis
CIBA; 135	Ludiomil	75 mg	White	Tablet	Oval, Scored	Novartis
CIBA; 152	Regitine	50 mg	White	Tablet		Novartis
CIBA; 192	Esidrex	100 mg	Blue	Tablet	Circle, Scored	Novartis
CIBA; 192	Esidrix	100 mg	Blue	Tablet	Circle, Scored	Novartis
CIPRO 250	Cipro	250 mg	White to Slightly Yellow	Tablet	Circle	Schering
CIPRO 500	Cipro	500 mg	White to Slightly Yellow	Tablet	Capsule-Shape	Schering
CIPRO 750	Cipro	750 mg	White to Slightly Yellow	Tablet	Capsule-Shape	Schering
CIR; 3 MG	Entocort Ec	3 mg	Light Grey and Pink	Capsule		Astrazeneca
CITRACAL ; MPC	Citracal Petites	200 IU ; 200 mg	White	Tablet	Oval	Mission Pharmacal
CK	Angeliq	0.5 mg ; 1 mg	Pink	Tablet	Circle	Bayer Healthcare Pharmaceuticals
CL; 101	Methocarbamol	750 mg		Tablet		Roxane Laboratories
CL; 190	Methocarbamol	500 mg		Tablet		Roxane Laboratories
CL; 400	Ercaf	100 mg ; 1 mg	Beige	Coated Tablet	Circle, Scored	Novartis Generics
CL; 418	Phenylbutazone	100 mg	Red	Coated Tablet		Novartis Generics
CL; 503	Papaverine Hydrochloride	150 mg	Brown and Clear	Extended-Release Capsule		Roxane Laboratories
CL; 751	Methyldopa	250 mg		Tablet		Novartis Generics
CL; 752	Methyldopa	500 mg		Tablet		Novartis Generics
CL; 753	Methyldopa and Hydrochlorothiazide	250 mg ; 15 mg		Tablet		Novartis Generics
CL; 754	Methyldopa and Hydrochlorothiazide	25 mg ; 250 mg		Tablet		Novartis Generics
CLARITIN 10 458	Claritin	10 mg	White to Off-White	Tablet	Circle	Schering-Plough Healthcare Products
CLARITIN-D	Claritin-D 12 Hour	5 mg ; 120 mg	White	Tablet, Extended Release		Schering-Plough Healthcare Products
CLARITIN-D 24 HOUR	Claritin-D 24 Hour	240 mg ; 10 mg	White to Off-White	Tablet, Extended Release		Schering-Plough Healthcare Products
CLEOCIN; 75 MG	Cleocin	75 mg	Green	Capsule		Pharmacia & Upjohn
CLEOCIN; 150 MG	Cleocin	150 mg	Blue and Green	Capsule		Pharmacia & Upjohn
CLEOCIN; 300 MG	Cleocin	300 mg	Blue	Capsule		Pharmacia & Upjohn
CLISTIN; MCNEIL	Clistin	4 mg	Pink	Tablet	Scored, Circle	Mcneil Pharmaceutical
CLL ; NVR	Tekturna HCT	150 mg ; 25 mg	Pale Yellow	Tablet	Oval	Novartis
CLOMID; 50 ;	Clomid	50 mg	White to Pale Yellow	Tablet	Circle	Sanofi-Aventis U.S.
CLOZARIL; 25	Clozaril	25 mg	Pale Yellow	Tablet	Circle, Compressed, Embossed	Novartis Pharmaceuticals
CLOZARIL; 100	Clozaril	100 mg	Pale Yellow	Tablet	Circle, Compressed	Novartis Pharmaceuticals
CN 90	Citranatal 90 Dha - Vitamin Tablet	2 mg ; 50 mg ; 120 mg ; 200 mg ; 90 mg ; 400 IU ; 30 IU ; 3 mg ; 3.4 mg ; 20 mg ; 20 mg ; 1 mg ; 150 mcg ; 25 mg	White	Tablet	Oval	Mission Pharmacal
CN RX	Citranatal Dha - Prenatal Tablet	3 mg ; 3.4 mg ; 20 mg ; 20 mg ; 1 mg ; 150 mcg ; 25 mg ; 2 mg ; 50 mg ; 120 mg ; 125 mg ; 27 mg ; 400 IU ; 30 IU	White	Tablet	Oval	Mission Pharmacal
CN RX	Citranatal RX	3 mg ; 3.4 mg ; 20 mg ; 20 mg ; 1 mg ; 150 mcg ; 25 mg ; 2 mg ; 50 mg ; 120 mg ; 125 mg ; 27 mg ; 400 IU ; 30 IU	White	Tablet	Oval	Mission Pharmacal
CN; 0.5; G	Clonazepam	0.5 mg	Light Yellow	Tablet	Circle, Scored	Par Pharmaceutical
CN; 1; G	Clonazepam	1 mg	Dark Yellow	Tablet	Circle, Scored	Par Pharmaceutical
CN; 2; G	Clonazepam	2 mg	White	Tablet	Circle, Scored	Par Pharmaceutical
COGNEX; 10	Cognex	10 mg	Yellow and Dark Green	Capsule		Sciele Pharma
COGNEX; 20	Cognex	20 mg	Yellow and Light Blue	Capsule		Sciele Pharma

IMPRINT	BRAND/GENERIC NAME	STRENGTH	COLOR	FORM	SHAPE	MANUFACTURER
COGNEX; 30	Cognex	30 mg	Yellow and Orange	Capsule		Sciele Pharma
COGNEX; 40	Cognex	40 mg	Yellow and Lavender	Capsule		Sciele Pharma
COMBID; SKF	Combid	5 mg ; 10 mg	Yellow and Clear	Capsule		Glaxosmithkline
COMHIST LA; 01490466	Comhist LA	20 mg ; 4 mg ; 50 mg	Yellow and Clear	Capsule		Procter & Gamble Pharmaceuticals
COMPOZ	Compoz Maximum Strength Nighttime Sleep Aid	50 mg	Blue	Capsule, Liquid Filled	Circle	Medtech
COMPOZ	Compoz Maximum Strength Nighttime Sleep Aid	50 mg	White	Tablet	Oblong	Medtech
COMTAN	Comtan	200 mg	Brown-Orange	Coated Tablet	Oval	Novartis
COP; 014	Luride	0.5 mg		Tablet, Chewable		Colgate Oral Pharmaceuticals
COP; 186	Luride	0.25 mg		Tablet, Chewable		Colgate Oral Pharmaceuticals
COPLEY 158 ;	Multivitamins with Fluoride	1.05 mg ; 4.5 mcg ; 2500 IU ; 400 IU ; 15 IU ; 0.3 mg ; 1.05 mg ; 1.2 mg ; 13.5 mg ; 0.5 mg ; 60 mg	Multi-Colored	Tablet, Chewable	Square	Novartis Generics
COPLEY; 0519	Vitamins with Fluoride	2500 IU ; 400 IU ; 15 IU ; 0.3 mg ; 13.5 mg ; 1 mg ; 60 mg ; 1.05 mg ; 1.2 mg ; 1.05 mg ; 4.5 mcg	Multi-Colored	Tablet, Chewable	Square	Novartis Generics
COPLEY; 107	Mebendazole	100 mg	Light Peach	Tablet, Chewable	Circle	Teva Pharmaceuticals
COPLEY; 111	Prenatal 1+1	65 mg ; 4000 IU ; 400 IU ; 11 mg ; 1 mg ; 1.5 mg ; 3 mg ; 20 mg ; 200 mg ; 2 mg ; 25 mg ; 120 mg ; 10 mg ; 12 mcg	Yellow	Coated Tablet	Capsule-Shape	Novartis Generics
COPLEY; 114	Procainamide Hydrochloride	750 mg	Tan	Tablet, Extended Release	Capsule-Shape	Teva Pharmaceuticals
COPLEY; 131	Sodium Fluoride	2.2 mg	Pink	Tablet, Chewable	Circle	Novartis Generics
COPLEY; 188	Procainamide Hydrochloride	500 mg	Pink	Tablet, Extended Release	Capsule-Shape	Teva Pharmaceuticals
COPLEY; 225	Potassium Chloride	8 meq	Orange	Tablet, Extended Release	Circle	Teva Pharmaceuticals
COPLEY; 225	Potassium Chloride	600 mg	Peach	Extended-Release Tablet	Circle	Teva Pharmaceuticals
COR 130	Dextroamphetamine Saccharate, Amphetamine Aspartate Monohydrate, Dextroamphetamine Sulfate, and Amphetamine Sulfate	1.25 mg ; 1.25 mg ; 1.25 mg ; 1.25 mg	Blue	Tablet	Circle	Ranbaxy Pharmaceuticals
COR 132	Dextroamphetamine Saccharate, Amphetamine Aspartate, Dextroamphetamine Sulfate, and Amphetamine Sulfate	2.5 mg ; 2.5 mg ; 2.5 mg ; 2.5 mg	Blue	Tablet	Circle	Ranbaxy Pharmaceuticals
COR 135	Dextroamphetamine Saccharate, Amphetamine Aspartate, Dextroamphetamine Sulfate, and Amphetamine Sulfate	5 mg ; 5 mg ; 5 mg ; 5 mg	Pink	Tablet	Circle	Ranbaxy Pharmaceuticals
COR 136	Dextroamphetamine Saccharate, Amphetamine Aspartate, Dextroamphetamine Sulfate, and Amphetamine Sulfate	7.5 mg ; 7.5 mg ; 7.5 mg ; 7.5 mg	Pink	Tablet	Circle	Ranbaxy Pharmaceuticals
COR; 103	Carisoprodol	350 mg	White	Tablet	Circle	Ranbaxy Pharmaceuticals
CORTEF; 5	Cortef	5 mg	White	Tablet	Circle, Scored	Pharmacia & Upjohn
CORTEF; 10	Cortef	10 mg	White	Tablet	Scored, Circle	Pharmacia & Upjohn
CORTEF; 20	Cortef	20 mg	White	Tablet	Circle, Scored	Pharmacia & Upjohn
COTRIM DS; 93 93	Cotrim DS	800 mg ; 160 mg	White	Tablet	Oval, Convex, Scored	Teva Pharmaceuticals
COTRIM; 93 93	Cotrim	400 mg ; 80 mg	White	Tablet	Circle, Convex, Scored	Teva Pharmaceuticals
COTYLENOL	Cotylenol Cold Medication	2 mg ; 30 mg ; 15 mg ; 325 mg	Yellow	Tablet	Oblong	Mcneil Consumer Healthcare Division of Mcneil
COUMADIN 2 ;	Coumadin	2 mg	Lavender	Tablet	Circle	Bristol-Myers Squibb
COUMADIN 2 1/2 ;	Coumadin	2.5 mg	Green	Tablet	Circle	Bristol-Myers Squibb
COUMADIN 3 ;	Coumadin	3 mg	Tan	Tablet	Circle	Bristol-Myers Squibb
COUMADIN 4 ;	Coumadin	4 mg	Blue	Tablet	Circle	Bristol-Myers Squibb
COUMADIN 5 ;	Coumadin	5 mg	Peach	Tablet	Circle	Bristol-Myers Squibb
COUMADIN 6 ;	Coumadin	6 mg	Teal	Tablet	Circle	Bristol-Myers Squibb
COUMADIN 7 1/2 ;	Coumadin	7.5 mg	Yellow	Tablet	Circle	Bristol-Myers Squibb
COUMADIN 10 ;	Coumadin	10 mg	White	Tablet	Circle	Bristol-Myers Squibb
CR 250	Ciprofloxacin	250 mg	White to Off-White	Tablet	Circle	Actavis South Atlantic
CR 500	Ciprofloxacin	500 mg	White to Off-White	Tablet	Capsule-Shape	Actavis South Atlantic
CR 750	Ciprofloxacin	750 mg	White to Off-White	Tablet	Capsule-Shape	Actavis South Atlantic
CRESTOR 5	Crestor	5 mg	Yellow	Tablet	Circle	Astrazeneca
CRESTOR 10	Crestor	10 mg	Pink	Tablet	Circle	Astrazeneca
CRESTOR 20	Crestor	20 mg	Pink	Tablet	Circle	Astrazeneca
CRIXIVAN; 100 MG	Crixivan	100 mg	White Semi-Translucent	Capsule		Merck
CRIXIVAN; 200 MG	Crixivan	200 mg	White Semi-Translucent	Capsule		Merck & Company
CRIXIVAN; 333 MG	Crixivan	333 mg	White with a Red Band	Capsule		Merck & Company
CRIXIVAN; 400 MG	Crixivan	400 mg	White Semi-Translucent	Capsule		Merck
CSF ; NVR	Exforge	5 mg ; 320 mg	Very Dark Yellow	Tablet	Oval	Novartis
CT	Myfortic	360 mg	Pale Orange-Red	Enteric-Coated Tablet	Oval	Novartis
CT 1	Zyflo	600 mg	White	Tablet	Oval	Critical Therapeutics
CT2	Zyflo Cr	600 mg	Red, White	Tablet, Extended Release	Oblong	Critical Therapeutics

IMPRINT	BRAND/GENERIC NAME	STRENGTH	COLOR	FORM	SHAPE	MANUFACTURER
CTI ; NVR	Diovan HCT	25 mg ; 320 mg	Yellow	Tablet	Oval	Novartis Pharmaceuticals
CUPRIMINE MSD 602	Cuprimine	250 mg	Ivory	Capsule		Aton Pharma
CUPRIMINE MSD 672	Cuprimine	125 mg	Opaque Gray, Opaque Ivory	Capsule		Aton Pharma
CVI ; NVR	Tekturna HCT	300 mg ; 12.5 mg	Violet White	Tablet	Oval	Novartis
CVT500	Ranexa	500 mg	Light Orange	Tablet, Extended Release	Oblong	Cv Therapeutics
CVT1000	Ranexa	1000 mg	Pale Yellow	Tablet, Extended Release	Oblong	Cv Therapeutics
CVV ; NVR	Tekturna HCT	300 mg ; 25 mg	Light Yellow	Tablet	Oval	Novartis
CXL 4	Cardura XL	4 mg	White	Tablet, Extended Release		Pfizer
CXL 8	Cardura XL	8 mg	White	Tablet, Extended Release		Pfizer
CY	Cyklokapron	500 mg	White	Tablet	Circle, Flat, with Beveled Edges	Pharmacia & Upjohn
CYCRIN; C	Premphase Medroxyprogesterone	5 mg	Light Purple	Tablet	Oval	Wyeth Pharmaceuticals
CYSTA; 50; MYLAN	Cystagon	50 mg	White, Opaque	Capsule		Mylan Pharmaceuticals
CYSTAGON; 150; MYLAN	Cystagon	150 mg	White, Opaque	Capsule		Mylan Pharmaceuticals
CZ	Balsalazide Disodium	750 mg	Beige	Capsule		Watson Laboratories
CZ	Colazal	750 mg	Beige	Capsule		Salix Pharmaceuticals
D	Doan's Ibuprofen Backache Pills	200 mg	White	Tablet		Novartis Consumer
D 24 ; M	Doxycycline	150 mg	Orange	Tablet	Circle	Mylan Pharmaceuticals
D; 2.5 MG	Focalin	2.5 mg	Blue	Tablet	D-Shape	Novartis
D; 5 MG	Focalin	5 mg	Yellow	Tablet	D-Shape	Novartis
D; 10 MG	Focalin	10 mg	White	Tablet	D-Shape	Novartis
D; 92	Drisdol	50000 IU	Green	Capsule, Liquid Filled		Sanofi-Aventis U.S.
D12	Clarinex-D 12 Hour	120 mg ; 2.5 mg	Blue, White	Tablet, Extended Release	Oval	Schering
D21 ; M	Doxycycline	50 mg	Light Yellow	Tablet	Circle	Mylan Pharmaceuticals
D22 ; M	Doxycycline	75 mg	Orange	Tablet	Circle	Mylan Pharmaceuticals
D23 ; M	Doxycycline	100 mg	Light Yellow	Tablet	Circle	Mylan Pharmaceuticals
D35 W	Demerol Hydrochloride	50 mg	White	Tablet	Circle	Sanofi-Aventis U.S.
D37 W	Demerol Hydrochloride	100 mg	White	Tablet	Circle	Sanofi-Aventis U.S.
D75	Doryx	75 mg	White	Tablet, Delayed Release	Oval	Warner Chilcott
D100	Doryx	100 mg	White	Tablet, Delayed Release	Oval	Warner Chilcott
DALMANE; 15; ICN ;	Dalmane	15 mg	Orange and Ivory	Capsule		Valeant Pharmaceuticals
DALMANE; 30; ICN ;	Dalmane	30 mg	Red and Ivory	Capsule		Valeant Pharmaceuticals
DAN ; 5538	Quinidine Gluconate	324 mg	Off White	Tablet, Extended Release	Circle	Watson Laboratories
DAN 5440 DAN 5440	Doxycycline Hyclate	100 mg	Blue	Capsule		Watson Laboratories
DAN 5658	Cyclobenzaprine Hydrochloride	10 mg	White	Tablet	Circle	Watson Laboratories
DAN 5726	Hydroxyzine Pamoate	25 mg	Dark Green, Light Green	Capsule		Watson Laboratories
DAN DAN 5325	Probenecid and Colchicine	500 mg ; 0.5 mg	White	Tablet	Capsule-Shape	Watson Laboratories
DAN DAN; 5600 ;	Trazodone Hydrochloride	50 mg	White	Tablet	Circle	Watson Laboratories
DAN; 2; 5621	Diazepam	2 mg	White	Tablet	Circle, Scored	Watson Laboratories
DAN; 5; 5619	Diazepam	5 mg	Yellow	Tablet	Circle, Scored	Watson Laboratories
DAN; 5; 5882	Methylphenidate Hydrochloride	5 mg	Light Purple	Tablet	Circle	Watson Laboratories
DAN; 5; 5882	Methylphenidate Hydrochloride	5 mg	Purple	Tablet	Circle	Watson Laboratories
DAN; 59; 12	Captopril and Hydrochlorothiazide	50 mg ; 25 mg	Blue	Tablet	Oval, Scored	Danbury Pharmacal
DAN; 10; 5554	Propranolol Hydrochloride	10 mg	Orange	Tablet	Circle, Scored	Watson Laboratories
DAN; 10; 5620	Diazepam	10 mg	Light Blue	Tablet	Circle, Scored	Watson Laboratories
DAN; 10; 5883	Methylphenidate Hydrochloride	10 mg	Green	Tablet	Circle	Watson Laboratories
DAN; 10; 5883	Methylphenidate Hydrochloride	10 mg	Light Green	Tablet	Circle, Scored	Watson Laboratories
DAN; 20; 5884	Methylphenidate Hydrochloride	20 mg	Peach	Tablet	Circle	Watson Laboratories
DAN; 20; 5884	Methylphenidate Hydrochloride	20 mg	Peach	Tablet	Circle, Scored	Watson Laboratories
DAN; 50; 5777	Atenolol	50 mg	White	Tablet	Circle	Watson Laboratories
DAN; 944	Colchicine	0.6 mg	White	Tablet	Circle	Watson Laboratories
DAN; 3120	Clindamycin Hydrochloride	300 mg	Pink	Capsule		Watson Laboratories
DAN; 5059 DAN	Prednisolone	5 mg	Peach	Tablet	Circle	Watson Laboratories
DAN; 5216; DAN	Folic Acid	1 mg	Yellow	Tablet	Circle, Scored	Watson Laboratories
DAN; 5307; DAN	Promethazine Hydrochloride	25 mg	White	Tablet	Circle	Watson Laboratories
DAN; 5319	Promethazine Hydrochloride	50 mg	White	Tablet	Circle	Watson Laboratories
DAN; 5321; DAN	Primidone	250 mg	White	Tablet	Circle, Scored	Watson Laboratories
DAN; 5335; DAN	Trihexyphenidyl Hydrochloride	2 mg	White	Tablet	Circle, Scored	Watson Laboratories
DAN; 5337; DAN	Trihexyphenidyl Hydrochloride	5 mg	White	Tablet	Circle, Scored	Watson Laboratories
DAN; 5347; DAN	Probenecid	500 mg	Yellow	Coated Tablet	Capsule-Shape, Scored	Watson Laboratories
DAN; 5368; DAN	Disulfiram	500 mg	Off-White	Tablet	Circle, Scored	Danbury Pharmacal
DAN; 5376; DAN	Disulfiram	250 mg	Off-White	Tablet	Circle, Scored	Danbury Pharmacal
DAN; 5379	Erythromycin Estolate	250 mg	Orange and White	Capsule		Danbury Pharmacal
DAN; 5381; DAN	Methocarbamol	500 mg	White	Tablet	Circle, Scored	Danbury Pharmacal
DAN; 5428	Hydralazine Complex	15 mg ; 25 mg ; 0.1 mg	Pink	Tablet		Danbury Pharmacal
DAN; 5428	Reserpine, Hydralazine Hydrochloride and Hydrochlorothiazide	25 mg ; 15 mg ; 0.1 mg	Yellow	Tablet	Circle	Danbury Pharmacal
DAN; 5430; DAN	Acetazolamide	250 mg	White	Tablet	Circle, Scored	Watson Laboratories
DAN; 5438 DAN	Quinidine Sulfate	200 mg	White	Tablet	Scored, Circle	Watson Laboratories
DAN; 5440	Doxycycline Hyclate	100 mg	Light Blue	Capsule		Watson Laboratories
DAN; 5453	Quinidine Sulfate	100 mg		Tablet		Danbury Pharmacal
DAN; 5454; DAN	Quinidine Sulfate	300 mg	White	Tablet	Circle, Scored	Watson Laboratories
DAN; 5455; DAN	Chlorpropamide	250 mg	Blue	Tablet	Circle, Scored	Danbury Pharmacal
DAN; 5507	Chlorthalidone	25 mg	Yellow or Orange	Tablet	Circle	Danbury Pharmacal
DAN; 5513	Carisoprodol	350 mg	White	Tablet	Circle	Watson Laboratories
DAN; 5518	Chlorthalidone	50 mg	Light Green or Light Blue	Tablet	Circle	Danbury Pharmacal

IMPRINT	BRAND/GENERIC NAME	STRENGTH	COLOR	FORM	SHAPE	MANUFACTURER
DAN; 5522 ;	Hydroxyzine Hydrochloride	10 mg	Orange	Coated Tablet	Circle	Watson Laboratories
DAN; 5523	Hydroxyzine Hydrochloride	25 mg	Green	Coated Tablet	Circle	Watson Laboratories
DAN; 5535 ;	Doxycycline Hyclate	50 mg	LT. Blue and White	Capsule		Watson Laboratories
DAN; 5540	Metronidazole	250 mg	White to Off-White	Tablet	Circle	Watson Laboratories
DAN; 5543; DAN	Allopurinol	100 mg	White	Tablet	Scored, Circle	Watson Laboratories
DAN; 5544; DAN	Allopurinol	300 mg	Orange	Tablet	Scored, Circle	Watson Laboratories
DAN; 5552; DAN	Metronidazole	500 mg	White to Off-White	Tablet	Circle	Watson Laboratories
DAN; 5553	Doxycycline Hyclate	100 mg	Orange	Coated Tablet	Circle	Watson Laboratories
DAN; 5555; 20	Propranolol Hydrochloride	20 mg	Light Blue	Tablet	Circle, Scored	Watson Laboratories
DAN; 5556; 40	Propranolol Hydrochloride	40 mg	Light Green	Tablet	Circle, Scored	Watson Laboratories
DAN; 5557; 80	Propranolol Hydrochloride	80 mg	Yellow	Tablet	Circle, Scored	Watson Laboratories
DAN; 5560	Disopyramide Phosphate	100 mg	Opaque Orange	Capsule		Watson Laboratories
DAN; 5561	Disopyramide Phosphate	150 mg	Opaque Brown	Capsule		Watson Laboratories
DAN; 5579; DAN	Chlorpropamide	100 mg	Blue	Tablet	Circle, Scored	Danbury Pharmacal
DAN; 5582; DAN	Tolazamide	250 mg	White	Tablet	Circle, Scored	Danbury Pharmacal
DAN; 5584	Ibuprofen	400 mg	White	Coated Tablet	Circle	Danbury Pharmacal
DAN; 5586	Ibuprofen	600 mg	White	Coated Tablet	Oval	Danbury Pharmacal
DAN; 5590; DAN	Tolazamide	500 mg	White	Tablet	Circle, Scored	Danbury Pharmacal
DAN; 5591; DAN	Tolazamide	100 mg	White	Tablet	Circle, Scored	Danbury Pharmacal
DAN; 5599; DAN	Trazodone Hcl	100 mg	White	Coated Tablet	Circle, Scored	Watson Laboratories
DAN; 5629	Doxepin Hydrochloride	10 mg	Buff	Capsule		Watson Laboratories
DAN; 5630	Doxepin Hydrochloride	25 mg	White and Ivory	Capsule		Watson Laboratories
DAN; 5631	Doxepin Hydrochloride	50 mg	Ivory	Capsule		Watson Laboratories
DAN; 5632	Doxepin Hydrochloride	75 mg	Light Green	Capsule		Watson Laboratories
DAN; 5642; 2.5	Minoxidil	2.5 mg	White	Tablet	Circle, Scored	Watson Laboratories
DAN; 5643; 10	Minoxidil	10 mg	White	Tablet	Circle, Scored	Watson Laboratories
DAN; 5644	Ibuprofen	800 mg	White	Coated Tablet	Oval	Danbury Pharmacal
DAN; 5660; DAN	Sulindac	200 mg	Yellow	Tablet	Circle, Scored	Watson Laboratories
DAN; 5661	Sulindac	150 mg	Yellow	Tablet	Circle	Watson Laboratories
DAN; 5682	Triamterene and Hydrochlorothiazide	75 mg ; 50 mg	Yellow	Tablet	Circle, Scored	Danbury Pharmacal
DAN; 5708	Clindamycin Hydrochloride	150 mg	Gray and Pink	Capsule		Danbury Pharmacal
DAN; 5730; 10	Baclofen	10 mg	White	Tablet	Circle, Scored	Watson Laboratories
DAN; 5731; 20	Baclofen	20 mg	White	Tablet	Circle, Scored	Watson Laboratories
DAN; 5778; 100	Atenolol	100 mg	White	Tablet	Circle	Watson Laboratories
DAN; 5782	Atenolol and Chlorthalidone	50 mg ; 25 mg	White	Tablet	Circle, Scored	Watson Laboratories
DAN; 5783	Atenolol and Chlorthalidone	100 mg ; 25 mg	White	Tablet	Circle	Watson Laboratories
DAN; DAN; 5382	Methocarbamol	750 mg	White	Tablet	Oval, Scored	Watson Laboratories
DAN; DAN; 5543	Allopurinol	100 mg	White	Tablet	Circle, Scored	Watson Laboratories
DAN; DAN; 5544	Allopurinol	300 mg	Orange	Tablet	Circle, Scored	Watson Laboratories
DANTRIUM 25 MG; 0149 0030	Dantrium	25 mg	Opaque, Orange and Tan	Capsule		Procter & Gamble Pharmaceuticals
DANTRIUM 50 MG; 0149 0031	Dantrium	50 mg	Opaque, Orange and Tan	Capsule		Procter & Gamble Pharmaceuticals
DANTRIUM 100 MG; 0149 0033	Dantrium	100 mg	Opaque, Orange and Tan	Capsule		Procter & Gamble Pharmaceuticals
DARAPRIM; A3A	Daraprim	25 mg	White	Tablet		Glaxosmithkline
DARVOCET N 50	Darvocet-N 50	50 mg ; 325 mg	Dark Orange	Tablet	Capsule-Shape	Xanodyne Pharmaceuticals
DARVOCET N 100	Darvocet-N 100	100 mg ; 650 mg	Dark Orange	Tablet	Capsule-Shape	Xanodyne Pharmaceuticals
DARVON	Darvon Pulvules	65 mg	Opaque Pink	Capsule		Xanodyne Pharmaceuticals
DARVON COMP	Darvon Compound	32 mg ; 389 mg ; 32.4 mg	Pink	Capsule		Eli Lilly
DARVON-N 100	Darvon-N	100 mg	Buff	Tablet	Oval	Xanodyne Pharmaceuticals
DAYQUIL; SINUS PAIN	Dayquil Sinus Pressure and Pain Relief with Ibuprofen	30 mg ; 200 mg	White	Tablet		Procter & Gamble
DDAVP; 0.2; RPR ;	Ddavp	0.2 mg	White	Tablet	Circle	Sanofi-Aventis U.S.
DEFEN	Defen-LA	60 mg ; 600 mg	White	Sustained-Release Tablet		First Horizon Pharmaceutical
DELTASONE; 2.5	Deltasone	2.5 mg	Pink	Tablet	Circle, Scored	Pharmacia & Upjohn
DELTASONE; 5	Deltasone	5 mg	White	Tablet	Circle, Scored	Pharmacia & Upjohn
DELTASONE; 10	Deltasone	10 mg	White	Tablet	Circle, Scored	Pharmacia & Upjohn
DELTASONE; 20	Deltasone	20 mg	Peach	Tablet	Circle, Scored	Pharmacia & Upjohn
DELTASONE; 50 ;	Deltasone	50 mg	White	Tablet	Circle, Scored	Pharmacia & Upjohn
DEPAKENE	Depakene	250 mg	Orange	Capsule, Liquid Filled		Abbott Laboratories
DEPAKOTE SPRINKLE 125 MG; THIS END UP	Depakote Sprinkle	125 mg	White Opaque/blue	Capsule		Abbott Laboratories
DERMIK; 044	Durrax	10 mg	Lavender	Tablet	Circle	Dermik Laboratories
DERMIK; 045	Durrax	25 mg	Lavender	Tablet	Circle	Dermik Laboratories
DHA 250 ;	Optinate - L-Vcaps	250 mg	Clear with Light Yellow to Dark Orange Mixture	Capsule		Sciele Pharma
DIA; B	Diabeta	1.25 mg	Peach	Tablet	Oblong	Sanofi-Aventis U.S.
DIA; B	Diabeta	2.5 mg	Peach	Tablet	Oblong	Sanofi-Aventis U.S.
DIA; B	Diabeta	5 mg	Light Green	Tablet	Oblong	Sanofi-Aventis U.S.
DIASORB	Diasorb	750 mg	Pink	Tablet	Circle	Columbia Laboratories
DICLOFENAC EPOLAMINE PATCH 1.3%	Flector 1.3%	13 mg/GM		Patch, Extended Release		Alpharma
DIFLUCAN; 50; ROERIG	Diflucan	50 mg	Pink	Tablet	Four-Sided	Pfizer Roerig
DIFLUCAN; 100; ROERIG	Diflucan	100 mg	Pink	Tablet	Four-Sided	Pfizer Roerig
DIFLUCAN; 150; ROERIG	Diflucan	150 mg	Pink	Tablet	Oval	Pfizer Roerig
DIFLUCAN; 200; ROERIG	Diflucan	200 mg	Pink	Tablet	Four-Sided	Pfizer Roerig
DIPENTUM 250 MG	Dipentum	250 mg	Beige	Capsule		UCB Pharma

IMPRINT	BRAND/GENERIC NAME	STRENGTH	COLOR	FORM	SHAPE	MANUFACTURER
DISALCID; 3M	Disalcid	500 mg	Aqua	Coated Tablet	Round, Bisected Scored	3M Pharmaceuticals
DISALCID; 3M	Disalcid	500 mg	Aqua and White	Capsule		3M Pharmaceuticals
DISALCID; 750; 3M	Disalcid	750 mg	Aqua	Coated Tablet	Capsule-Shaped, Bisected Scored	3M Pharmaceuticals
DIUCARDIN; 50	Diucardin	50 mg	White	Tablet	Oval, Scored	Wyeth Pharmaceuticals
DMI ; 500	Proquin Xr	500 mg	Blue	Tablet, Extended Release	Oval	Depomed
DO ; NVR	Diovan	40 mg	Yellow	Tablet	Oval	Novartis
DORAL; 7.5	Doral	7.5 mg	Light Orange with White Speckles	Tablet	Capsule-Shape	Meda Pharmaceuticals
DORMALIN; 722	Dormalin	15 mg	Light Orange	Tablet	Capsule-Shape	Schering
DORSEY	Rautensin	2 mg	Orange	Tablet	Circle, Scored	Novartis Pharmaceuticals
DORSEY	Wilpo	8 mg	Green	Tablet		Novartis Pharmaceuticals
DOW; 11	Novahistine Fortis	10 mg ; 2 mg	Green and White	Capsule		Glaxosmithkline Consumer
DOW; 71	Novahistine Sinus	325 mg ; 30 mg ; 2 mg	White	Tablet	Circle	Glaxosmithkline Consumer
DOW; 603	Phenoxene	50 mg	Beige	Tablet	Circle	Aventis Pharmaceuticals
DP; 016	Aviane 28 Orange Tablet	0.1 mg ; 0.02 mg	Orange	28-Day Tablet Pack	Circle	Barr Laboratories
DP; 021	Kariva White	0.15 mg ; 0.02 mg	White	Tablet	Circle	Barr Laboratories
DP; 022	Kariva Light Blue	0.01 mg	Light Blue	Tablet	Circle	Barr Laboratories
DP; 25	Levoxyl	25 mcg	Orange	Tablet	Oval, Notched	Monarch Pharmaceuticals
DP; 41	Cenestin	0.3 mg	Green	Tablet	Circle	Barr Laboratories
DP; 42	Cenestin	0.625 mg	Red	Tablet	Circle	Barr Laboratories
DP; 43	Cenestin	0.9 mg	White	Tablet	Circle	Barr Laboratories
DP; 44	Cenestin	1.25 mg	Blue	Tablet	Circle	Barr Laboratories
DP; 50 ;	Levoxyl	50 mcg	White	Tablet	Oval	Monarch Pharmaceuticals
DP; 75	Levoxyl	75 mcg	Purple	Tablet	Oval	Monarch Pharmaceuticals
DP; 88	Levoxyl	88 mcg	Olive	Tablet	Oval	Monarch Pharmaceuticals
DP; 100	Levoxyl	100 mcg	Yellow	Tablet	Oval	Monarch Pharmaceuticals
DP; 112	Levoxyl	112 mcg	Rose	Tablet	Oval	Monarch Pharmaceuticals
DP; 125	Levoxyl	125 mcg	Brown	Tablet	Oval	Monarch Pharmaceuticals
DP; 137	Levoxyl	137 mcg	Dark Blue	Tablet	Oval	Monarch Pharmaceuticals
DP; 150	Levoxyl	150 mcg	Blue	Tablet	Oval	Monarch Pharmaceuticals
DP; 175	Levoxyl	175 mcg	Turquoise	Tablet	Oval	Monarch Pharmaceuticals
DP; 200	Levoxyl	200 mcg	Pink	Tablet	Oval, Notched	Monarch Pharmaceuticals
DP; 300	Levoxyl	300 mcg	Green	Tablet	Oval	Monarch Pharmaceuticals
DP; 301	Methylprednisolone	4 mg	White	Tablet	Oval, Scored	Barr Laboratories
DP; 510	Enpresse 28 Pink Tablets	0.05 mg ; 0.03 mg	Pink	Tablet	Circle	Barr Laboratories
DP; 511	Enpresse 28 White Tablets	0.075 mg ; 0.04 mg	White	28-Day Tablet Pack	Circle	Barr Laboratories
DP; 512	Enpresse 28 Orange Tablets	0.03 mg ; 0.125 mg	Orange	28-Day Tablet Pack	Circle	Barr Laboratories
DP; 521	Prochlorperazine Maleate	5 mg	Orange	Tablet	Circle	Barr Laboratories
DP; 522	Prochlorperazine Maleate	10 mg	Yellow	Tablet	Circle	Barr Laboratories
DP; 543	Cryselle 28 White Tablet	0.3 mg ; 0.03 mg	White	Tablet	Circle	Barr Laboratories
DP; 575	Apri 28 Pink Tablets	0.03 mg ; 0.15 mg	Pink	Tablet		Barr Laboratories
DPI; 288	Triamterene and Hydrochlorothiazide	37.5 mg ; 25 mg	White	Capsule		Barr Laboratories
DPI; 364	Duradrin	325 mg ; 65 mg ; 100 mg	White and Scarlet	Capsule		Barr Laboratories
DPI; 488	Hydrochlorothiazide and Triamterene	25 mg ; 37.5 mg	White	Capsule		Barr Laboratories
DRIXORAL C+F	Drixoral Cold & Flu	60 mg ; 3 mg ; 500 mg	Green	Sustained-Release Tablet	Oval	Schering-Plough Healthcare Products
DRL; 50; 1	Nefazodone Hydrochloride	50 mg	White	Tablet	Oval	Par Pharmaceutical
DRL; 100; 2	Nefazodone Hydrochloride	100 mg	White	Tablet	Oval	Par Pharmaceutical
DRL; 150; 3	Nefazodone Hydrochloride	150 mg	White	Tablet	Oval	Par Pharmaceutical
DRL; 200; 4	Nefazodone Hydrochloride	200 mg	White	Tablet	Oval	Par Pharmaceutical
DRL; 250; 5	Nefazodone Hydrochloride	250 mg	White	Tablet	Oval	Par Pharmaceutical
DROXIA; 6335	Droxia	200 mg	Blue-Green	Capsule		Bristol-Myers Squibb
DROXIA; 6336	Droxia	300 mg	Purple	Capsule		Bristol-Myers Squibb
DROXIA; 6337	Droxia	400 mg	Red-Orange	Capsule		Bristol-Myers Squibb
DS	Yaz - Pink Tablet	0.02 mg ; 3 mg	Light Pink	Tablet	Circle	Bayer Healthcare Pharmaceuticals
DT	Detrol	2 mg	White	Tablet	Circle	Pharmacia & Upjohn
DT; I	Pec-Dec	60 mg	Light Brown	Tablet	Circle	Glaxosmithkline
DUPONT; 1 1 ;	Revia	50 mg	Pale Yellow	Coated Tablet	Capsule-Shape, Scored	Bristol-Myers Squibb
DUPONT; TREXAN	Trexan	50 mg	White	Tablet	Circle, Scored	Bristol-Myers Squibb
DUPONT; VALPIN	Valpin 50	50 mg	Beige	Tablet		Bristol-Myers Squibb
DURACT	Duract	25 mg	Opaque Light Yellow Body and Opaque Red Cap with 2 Blue Bands	Capsule		Wyeth-Ayerst Laboratories
DUVOID 10 ; WPC 004	Bethanechol Chloride	10 mg	White	Tablet	Circle	Actavis South Atlantic
DUVOID 25 ; WPC 005	Bethanechol Chloride	25 mg	White	Tablet	Circle	Actavis South Atlantic
DUVOID 50 ; WPC 006	Bethanechol Chloride	50 mg	Tan	Tablet	Circle	Actavis South Atlantic
DV ; NVR	Diovan	80 mg	Pale Red	Tablet	Teardrop-Shape	Novartis
DX ; NVR	Diovan	160 mg	Grey-Orange	Tablet	Teardrop-Shape	Novartis
DX 41	Diclofenac Sodium	100 mg	Pink	Tablet, Extended Release	Circle	Watson Laboratories
DX; 2; G	Doxazosin Mesylate	2 mg	White	Tablet	Capsule-Shape, Scored	Par Pharmaceutical
DX; 4; G	Doxazosin Mesylate	4 mg	White	Tablet	Capsule-Shape, Scored	Par Pharmaceutical
DX; 8; G	Doxazosin Mesylate	8 mg	White	Tablet	Capsule-Shape, Scored	Par Pharmaceutical
DX1; G	Doxazosin Mesylate	1 mg	White	Tablet	Circle	Par Pharmaceutical
DXL ; NVR	Diovan	320 mg	Dark Grey-Violet	Tablet	Teardrop-Shape	Novartis
DYAZIDE; SB	Dyazide	25 mg ; 37.5 mg	Red and White	Capsule		Glaxosmithkline
DYFLEX; 400	Dyflex	400 mg	White	Tablet	Circle, Concave, Scored	Teva Pharmaceuticals
DYN 045	Solodyn	45 mg	Gray	Tablet, Extended Release		Medicis Pharmaceutical

IMPRINT	BRAND/GENERIC NAME	STRENGTH	COLOR	FORM	SHAPE	MANUFACTURER
DYN 090	Solodyn	90 mg	Yellow	Tablet, Extended Release		Medicis Pharmaceutical
DYN 135	Solodyn	135 mg	(Pink) Orange-Brown	Tablet, Extended Release		Medicis Pharmaceutical
DYN-50; 747	Dynacin	50 mg	White	Tablet	Capsule-Shape	Medicis Pharmaceutical
DYN-75; 748	Dynacin	75 mg	Gray	Tablet	Capsule-Shape	Medicis Pharmaceutical
DYN-100; 749	Dynacin	100 mg	Dark Gray	Tablet	Capsule-Shape	Medicis Pharmaceutical
DYNABAC; UC; 5364	Dynabac	250 mg	White	Enteric-Coated Tablet	Circle	Muro Pharmaceutical
DYNACIN 50MG ; 0487	Dynacin	50 mg	Opaque White	Capsule		Medicis Pharmaceutical
DYNACIN 75MG ; 0489	Dynacin	75 mg	Light Gray	Capsule		Medicis Pharmaceutical
DYNACIN 100MG ; 0488	Dynacin	100 mg	Dark Gray, White	Capsule		Medicis Pharmaceutical
DYNACIRC; 2.5; S	Dynacirc	2.5 mg	White	Capsule		Novartis Pharmaceuticals
DYNACIRC; 5; S	Dynacirc	5 mg	Light Pink	Capsule		Novartis Pharmaceuticals
DYNACIRCCR 5	Dynacirc Cr	5 mg	Light Pink	Tablet	Circle	Glaxosmithkline
DYNACIRCCR 10	Dynacirc Cr	10 mg	Beige	Tablet	Circle	Glaxosmithkline
DYRENIUM; SKF; 50	Dyrenium	50 mg	Opaque Red	Capsule		Glaxosmithkline
DYRENIUM; SKF; 100	Dyrenium	100 mg	Opaque Red	Capsule		Glaxosmithkline
E; 121	Captopril	12.5 mg	White	Tablet	Circle, Scored	Par Pharmaceutical
E; 122	Captopril	25 mg	White	Tablet	Round, Quadrisected Scored	Par Pharmaceutical
E; 123	Captopril	50 mg	White	Tablet	Circle, Scored	Par Pharmaceutical
E; 124	Captopril	100 mg	White	Tablet	Circle, Scored	Par Pharmaceutical
E; 5000 ;	Phentermine Hydrochloride Blue/clear	30 mg	Blue and Clear	Capsule		Novartis Generics
E; 5380 ;	Contrin	0.5 mg ; 110 mg ; 240 mg ; 15 mcg ; 75 mg	Maroon and Red	Capsule		Novartis Generics
E50	Etoposide	50 mg	Dark Pink with Black Ink	Capsule	Oblong	Mylan Pharmaceuticals
E612 5	Opana	5 mg	Blue	Tablet	Circle	Endo Pharmaceuticals
E613 10	Opana	10 mg	Red	Tablet	Circle	Endo Pharmaceuticals
EA	Erythromycin	500 mg	Pink	Coated Tablet	Capsule-Shape	Abbott Laboratories
EATON; 036	Furadantin	50 mg	Yellow	Tablet		Procter & Gamble Pharmaceuticals
EB; ABBOTT LOGO	Erythromycin	250 mg	Pink	Tablet	Capsule-Shape	Abbott Laboratories
EC-NAPROSYN; 375	Ec-Naprosyn	375 mg	White	Delayed-Release Tablet	Capsule-Shape	Roche Laboratories
EC-NAPROSYN; 500	Ec-Naprosyn	500 mg	White	Delayed-Release Tablet	Capsule-Shape	Roche Laboratories
ECE ; NVR	Exforge	5 mg ; 160 mg	Dark Yellow	Tablet	Oval	Novartis
ECR 15	Amrix	15 mg	Orange	Capsule, Extended Release		Ecr Pharmaceuticals
ECR 24 D	Lodrane 24d	12 mg ; 90 mg	Blue	Capsule, Extended Release, 24 Hr		Ecr Pharmaceuticals
ECR 30	Amrix	30 mg	Blue, Orange	Capsule, Extended Release		Ecr Pharmaceuticals
ECR; 6006	Lodrane Ld	6 mg ; 60 mg	Clear	Capsule		Ecr Pharmaceuticals
ED; A	Ery-Tab	500 mg	Pink	Enteric-Coated Tablet		Abbott Laboratories
EDECRIN ; MSD 65	Edecrin	25 mg	White	Tablet	Capsule-Shape	Aton Pharma
EF	E.E.S.	200 mg	White	Tablet, Chewable	Circle, Scored	Abbott Laboratories
EK; ABBOTT LOGO	Pce Dispertab	500 mg	White	Tablet	Oval	Abbott Laboratories
ELAVIL; 40	Elavil	10 mg	Blue	Coated Tablet	Circle	Astrazeneca
ELAVIL; 41	Elavil	50 mg	Beige	Coated Tablet	Circle	Astrazeneca
ELAVIL; 42	Elavil	75 mg	Orange	Coated Tablet	Circle	Astrazeneca
ELAVIL; 43	Elavil	100 mg	Mauve	Coated Tablet	Circle	Astrazeneca
ELAVIL; 45	Elavil	25 mg	Yellow	Coated Tablet	Circle	Astrazeneca
ELAVIL; 47	Elavil	150 mg	Blue	Coated Tablet	Capsule-Shape	Astrazeneca
ELN 30	Afeditab Cr	30 mg	Brick Red	Tablet, Extended Release	Circle	Watson Laboratories
ELN 60	Afeditab Cr	60 mg	Brick Red	Tablet, Extended Release	Circle	Watson Laboratories
ELN; 30	Nifedipine	30 mg	Red-Brown	Extended-Release Tablet	Circle	Watson Laboratories
ELN; 60	Nifedipine ER	60 mg	Red-Brown	Extended-Release Tablet	Circle	Watson Laboratories
EM	Dyflex 200	200 mg	White	Tablet	Circle, Concave, Scored	Teva Pharmaceuticals
EM; SP	Estinyl	0.05 mg	Pink	Coated Tablet		Schering
EMCYT; PHARMACIA; 132	Emcyt	140 mg	White	Capsule		Pharmacia & Upjohn
EMPIRIN; 3	Empirin with Codeine No. 3	325 mg ; 30 mg	White	Tablet		Glaxosmithkline
EMPIRIN; 4	Empirin with Codeine No. 4	60 mg ; 325 mg	White	Tablet		Glaxosmithkline
E-MYCIN; 250 MG	E-Mycin	250 mg	Orange	Timed-Release Tablet	Circle	Pharmacia & Upjohn
E-MYCIN; 333 MG	E-Mycin	333 mg	White	Timed-Release Tablet	Circle	Pharmacia & Upjohn
EN; 2.5; G	Enalapril Maleate	2.5 mg	White	Tablet	Circle	Par Pharmaceutical
EN; 5; G; G	Enalapril Maleate	5 mg	White	Tablet	Oval	Par Pharmaceutical
EN; 10; G	Enalapril Maleate	10 mg	Rusty Red	Tablet	Oval	Par Pharmaceutical
EN; 20; G	Enalapril Maleate	20 mg	Peach	Tablet	Oval	Par Pharmaceutical
ENDEP; 50; ROCHE	Endep	50 mg	Orange	Coated Tablet	Circle, Scored	Roche Laboratories
ENDEP; 75; ROCHE	Endep	75 mg	Yellow	Coated Tablet	Circle, Scored	Roche Laboratories
ENDO 610	Endodan	4.8355 mg ; 325 mg	Yellow	Tablet	Circle	Endo Pharmaceuticals
ENDO; 744	Etodolac	400 mg	Pale Yellow	Tablet	Oval	Bristol-Myers Squibb
ENDURON	Enduron	2.5 mg	Orange	Tablet	Square, Scored	Abbott Laboratories
ENDURON	Enduron	5 mg	Salmon	Tablet	Square, Scored	Abbott Laboratories
ENTEX PSE; 032 032	Entex Pse	600 mg ; 120 mg	Yellow	Sustained-Release Tablet	Oval, Elongated, Scored	Andrx Pharmaceuticals
ENTOLASE; AHR	Entolase	20,000 USP units ; 4000 USP units ; 25,000 USP units		Capsule		Wyeth Pharmaceuticals
ENTOLASE-HP; AHR	Entolase-Hp	40,000 USP units ; 8000 USP units ; 50,000 USP units		Capsule		Wyeth Pharmaceuticals

IMPRINT	BRAND/GENERIC NAME	STRENGTH	COLOR	FORM	SHAPE	MANUFACTURER
EPITOL; 93; 93	Epitol	200 mg	White	Tablet	Circle, Scored, Flat	Teva Pharmaceuticals
EPITOL; 93; 758	Epitol	100 mg	Pink with Red Speckles	Tablet, Chewable	Circle, Flat, Beveled Edge, Scored	Teva Pharmaceuticals
ER; ABBOTT LOGO	Erythromycin Delayed-Release	250 mg	Clear and Maroon with Pink and Yellow Particles	Capsule		Abbott Laboratories
ER; SP	Estinyl	0.02 mg	Beige	Coated Tablet		Schering
ES	Erythrocin Stearate Filmtab	250 mg	Pink	Coated Tablet	Circle	Abbott Laboratories
ESKALITH; SB	Eskalith	300 mg	Gray, Yellow	Capsule		Glaxosmithkline
ESR; 1174; MARION	Gaviscon	160 mg ; 105 mg	White	Tablet, Chewable	Circle	Glaxosmithkline Consumer
ESTRADIOL 0.025 MG/DAY (ONCE WEEKLY)	Estradiol	0.025 mg/24 Hr	Peach	Patch, Extended Release	Circle	Mylan Pharmaceuticals
ESTRADIOL 0.0375 MG/DAY (ONCE WEEKLY)	Estradiol	0.0375 mg/24 Hr	Peach	Patch, Extended Release	Circle	Mylan Pharmaceuticals
ESTRADIOL 0.05 MG/DAY (ONCE WEEKLY)	Estradiol	0.05 mg/24 Hr	Peach	Patch, Extended Release	Circle	Mylan Pharmaceuticals
ESTRADIOL 0.06 MG/DAY (ONCE WEEKLY)	Estradiol	0.06 mg/24 Hr	Peach	Patch, Extended Release	Circle	Mylan Pharmaceuticals
ESTRADIOL 0.075 MG/DAY (ONCE WEEKLY)	Estradiol	0.075 mg/24 Hr	Peach	Patch, Extended Release	Circle	Mylan Pharmaceuticals
ESTRADIOL 0.1 MG/DAY (ONCE WEEKLY)	Estradiol	0.1 mg/24 Hr	Peach	Patch, Extended Release	Circle	Mylan Pharmaceuticals
ET	Erythrocin Stearate Filmtab	500 mg	Pink	Coated Tablet	Oblong	Abbott Laboratories
EVOXAC; 30 MG	Evoxac	30 mg	White	Capsule		Daiichi Sankyo
EXELON 1.5 MG	Exelon	1.5 mg	Yellow	Capsule		Novartis
EXELON 3 MG	Exelon	3 mg	Orange	Capsule		Novartis
EXELON 4.5 MG	Exelon	4.5 mg	Red	Capsule		Novartis
EXELON 6 MG	Exelon	6 mg	Orange, Red	Capsule		Novartis
EZFE 200	Ezfe 200	200 mg	Brown Opaque, Orange Opaque	Capsule		Mcneil, R.A.
F JR F JR	Extendryl JR.	10 mg ; 4 mg ; 1.25 mg	Green, Red	Capsule, Extended Release		Fleming
F SR SR	Extendryl SR.	2.5 mg ; 20 mg ; 8 mg	Green, Red	Capsule, Extended Release		Fleming
F; III	Aerolate III	65 mg	Clear, Red	Capsule, Extended Release, 12 Hr		Fleming
F; JR	Aerolate JR.	130 mg	Clear, Red	Capsule, Extended Release, 12 Hr		Fleming
F; SR	Aerolate SR.	260 mg	Clear, Red	Capsule, Extended Release, 12 Hr		Fleming
F5 ;	Ferralet 90	90 mg ; 1 mg ; 12 mcg ; 120 mg ; 50 mg	Green	Tablet	Rectangle	Mission Pharmacal
F11 ; M	Felodipine	2.5 mg	White	Tablet, Extended Release	Circle	Mylan Pharmaceuticals
F12 ; M	Felodipine	5 mg	Yellow	Tablet, Extended Release	Circle	Mylan Pharmaceuticals
F13 ; M	Felodipine	10 mg	Blue	Tablet, Extended Release	Circle	Mylan Pharmaceuticals
FANSIDAR; ROCHE	Fansidar	25 mg ; 500 mg	White	Tablet	Circle, Scored	Roche Laboratories
FASTIN; BEECHAM	Fastin	30 mg	Blue and Clear with Blue and White Beads	Capsule		Glaxosmithkline
FC; 50; G	Flecainide Acetate	50 mg	White	Tablet	Circle	Par Pharmaceutical
FC; 100; G	Flecainide Acetate	100 mg	White	Tablet	Circle, Scored	Par Pharmaceutical
FC; 150; G	Flecainide Acetate	150 mg	White	Tablet	Oval, Scored	Par Pharmaceutical
FELDENE; PFIZER 322	Feldene	10 mg	Maroon and Blue	Capsule		Pfizer Laboratories
FELDENE; PFIZER 323	Feldene	20 mg	Maroon	Capsule		Pfizer Laboratories
FENTANYL 12MCG/HR	Fentanyl Transdermal System	12 mcg/hr	Translucent	Patch, Extended Release	Rectangle	Mylan Pharmaceuticals
FENTANYL 25MCG/HR	Fentanyl Transdermal System	25 mcg/hr	Translucent	Patch, Extended Release	Rectangle	Mylan Pharmaceuticals
FENTANYL 50MCG/HR	Fentanyl Transdermal System	50 mcg/hr	Translucent	Patch, Extended Release	Rectangle	Mylan Pharmaceuticals
FENTANYL 75MCG/HR	Fentanyl Transdermal System	75 mcg/hr	Translucent	Patch, Extended Release	Rectangle	Mylan Pharmaceuticals
FENTANYL 100MCG/HR	Fentanyl Transdermal System	100 mcg/hr	Translucent	Patch, Extended Release	Rectangle	Mylan Pharmaceuticals
FENTANYL TS 25 MCG/H	Fentanyl Transdermal System	25 mcg/hr	Clear	Patch, Extended Release	Rectangle	Watson Laboratories
FENTANYL TS 50 MCG/HR	Fentanyl Transdermal System	50 mcg/hr	Clear	Patch, Extended Release	Triangle	Watson Laboratories
FENTANYL TS 75 MCG/H	Fentanyl Transdermal System	75 mcg/hr	Clear	Patch, Extended Release	Rectangle	Watson Laboratories
FENTANYL TS 100 MCG/H	Fentanyl Transdermal System	100 mcg/hr	Clear	Patch, Extended Release	Rectangle	Watson Laboratories
FEOSOL	Feosol	159 mg		Extended-Release Capsule		Glaxosmithkline Consumer
FH 10 ; 440	Sular	10 mg	Oyster	Tablet, Extended Release	Circle	Sciele Pharma

IMPRINT	BRAND/GENERIC NAME	STRENGTH	COLOR	FORM	SHAPE	MANUFACTURER
FH 20 ; 441	Sular	20 mg	Yellow Cream	Tablet, Extended Release	Circle	Sciele Pharma
FH 30 ; 442	Sular	30 mg	Mustard	Tablet, Extended Release	Circle	Sciele Pharma
FH 40 ; 443	Sular	40 mg	Burnt Orange	Tablet, Extended Release	Circle	Sciele Pharma
FH 50	Triglide	50 mg	Off White	Tablet	Circle	Sciele Pharma
FH 160	Triglide	160 mg	Off White	Tablet	Circle	Sciele Pharma
FHF	Pentone	100 mg	White	Capsule		Faulding Laboratories
FHI	Fenoglide	120 mg	White to Off-White	Tablet	Oval	Sciele Pharma
FIORICET CODEINE LOGO	Fioricet with Codeine	30 mg ; 50 mg ; 40 mg ; 325 mg	Opaque Dark Blue, Opaque Light Grey	Capsule	Circle	Watson Pharma
FIORICET WATSON ;	Fioricet	40 mg ; 325 mg ; 50 mg	Light Blue	Tablet	Circle	Watson Laboratories
FIORINAL CODEINE; WATSON 956	Fiorinal with Codeine	40 mg ; 325 mg ; 30 mg ; 50 mg	Blue, Yellow	Capsule		Watson Laboratories
FIORINAL; 78; 103	Fiorinal	325 mg ; 50 mg ; 40 mg	Kelly Green and Lime Green	Capsule		Watson Laboratories
FL	Adphen	35 mg	Peach	Tablet	Circle, Scored	Ferndale Laboratories
FL	Phendimetrazine Tartrate	35 mg	Yellow or Pink	Tablet	Circle	Ferndale Laboratories
FL	Strifon Forte Dsc	500 mg	Light Green	Tablet	Scored, Circle	Ferndale Laboratories
FL 50 ; G	Fluconazole	50 mg	Pink	Tablet	Rectangle	Par Pharmaceutical
FL 100 ; G	Fluconazole	100 mg	Pink	Tablet	Rectangle	Par Pharmaceutical
FL 150 ; G	Fluconazole	150 mg	Pink	Tablet	Oval	Par Pharmaceutical
FL 200 ; G ;	Fluconazole	200 mg	Pink	Tablet	Rectangle	Par Pharmaceutical
FL; 10; G	Fluoxetine Hydrochloride	10 mg	White	Tablet	Oval	Par Pharmaceutical
FL; 20; G	Fluoxetine Hydrochloride	20 mg	White	Tablet	Oval	Par Pharmaceutical
FL; 1033	Spastrin	40 mg ; 0.6 mg ; 0.2 mg	Blue	Tablet	Circle, Scored	Novartis Generics
FL; DOUBLE HEART	Kronofed-A	120 mg ; 8 mg	White, Clear	Sustained-Release Capsule		Ferndale Laboratories
FL; DOUBLE HEART	Kronofed-A JR	60 mg ; 4 mg	White and Clear	Sustained-Release Capsule		Ferndale Laboratories
FL; DOUBLE HEART	Obestin	30 mg	Blue and Clear with Blue and White Beads	Capsule		Ferndale Laboratories
FL; DOUBLE.HEART	Dapex	37.5 mg	Opaque Blue and Clear	Capsule		Ferndale Laboratories
FLO	Fenoglide	40 mg	White to Off-White	Tablet	Oval	Sciele Pharma
FLOXIN; 200 MG	Floxin	200 mg	Pale Yellow	Coated Tablet		Ortho-Mcneil Pharmaceutical
FLOXIN; 300 MG	Floxin	300 mg	White	Coated Tablet		Ortho-Mcneil Pharmaceutical
FLOXIN; 400 MG	Floxin	400 mg	Pale Gold	Coated Tablet		Ortho-Mcneil Pharmaceutical
FLUMADINE 100; FOREST	Flumadine	100 mg	Orange	Coated Tablet	Oval	Forest Pharmaceuticals
FLUOXETINE; R; 149	Fluoxetine Hydrochloride	40 mg	White	Capsule		Par Pharmaceutical
FOREST; 0372; ESGIC PLUS	Esgic-Plus	500 mg ; 50 mg ; 40 mg	Red	Capsule		Forest Pharmaceuticals
FOREST; 372 ;	Feostat	100 mg	Brown	Tablet, Chewable	Circle	Forest Pharmaceuticals
FOREST; 610A	Bancap Hc	500 mg ; 5 mg	Yellow and Orange	Capsule		Forest Pharmaceuticals
FOREST; 610A	Hydrocodone Bitartrate and Acetaminophen	5 mg ; 500 mg	Orange and Yellow	Capsule		Forest Pharmaceuticals
FOREST; 642	Elixophyllin Df 100	100 mg	White	Gel/jelly		Forest Pharmaceuticals
FOREST; 643	Elixophyllin Df 200	200 mg	White	Capsule, Liquid Filled		Forest Pharmaceuticals
FOREST; 678	Esgic-Plus	50 mg ; 500 mg ; 40 mg	White	Tablet	Capsule-Shape, Scored	Forest Pharmaceuticals
FP; 10 MG	Celexa	10 mg	Beige	Coated Tablet	Oval	Forest Pharmaceuticals
FP; 20 MG	Celexa	20 mg	Pink	Tablet	Oval	Forest Pharmaceuticals
FP; 40 MG	Celexa	40 mg	White	Tablet	Oval	Forest Pharmaceuticals
FULVICIN; P/G; 352	Fulvicin P/g	330 mg	White	Tablet	Oval, Compressed, Scored	Schering
FULVICIN; P/G; 654	Fulvicin P/g	165 mg	White	Tablet	Oval, Compressed, Scored	Schering
G ; BN/10	Baclofen	10 mg	White	Tablet	Circle	Mylan Pharmaceuticals
G ; BN/20	Baclofen	20 mg	White	Tablet	Circle	Mylan Pharmaceuticals
G ; C250	Clarithromycin	250 mg	White to Off-White	Tablet	Oval	Mylan Pharmaceuticals
G ; CF 250	Ciprofloxacin	250 mg	White to Off-White	Tablet	Circle	Par Pharmaceutical
G ; CF 500	Ciprofloxacin	500 mg	White to Off-White	Tablet	Capsule-Shape	Par Pharmaceutical
G ; CF 750	Ciprofloxacin	750 mg	White to Off-White	Tablet	Capsule-Shape	Par Pharmaceutical
G ; ED 200	Etidronate Disodium	200 mg	White	Tablet	Rectangle	Mylan Pharmaceuticals
G ; ED 400	Etidronate Disodium	400 mg	White	Tablet	Capsule-Shape	Mylan Pharmaceuticals
G ; GT 4	Galantamine Hydrobromide	4 mg	White	Tablet	Circle	Mylan Pharmaceuticals
G ; GT 8	Galantamine Hydrobromide	8 mg	White	Tablet	Circle	Mylan Pharmaceuticals
G ; GT 12	Galantamine Hydrobromide	12 mg	White	Tablet	Circle	Mylan Pharmaceuticals
G ; P1 ;	Paroxetine Hydrochloride	10 mg	White	Tablet	Circle	Watson Pharma
G ; P2	Paroxetine Hydrochloride	20 mg	White	Tablet	Circle	Andrx Pharmaceuticals
G ; P3	Paroxetine Hydrochloride	30 mg	White	Tablet	Circle	Andrx Pharmaceuticals
G ; P4 ;	Paroxetine Hydrochloride	40 mg	White	Tablet	Circle	Watson Pharma
G ; TL 50	Tramadol Hydrochloride	50 mg	White	Tablet		Par Pharmaceutical
G 11 ; MYLAN ;	Glimepiride	1 mg	White	Tablet	Oval	Mylan Pharmaceuticals
G 12 ; MYLAN ;	Glimepiride	2 mg	Yellow	Tablet	Oval	Mylan Pharmaceuticals
G 13 ; MYLAN ;	Glimepiride	4 mg	Peach	Tablet	Oval	Mylan Pharmaceuticals
G 341	Oxybutynin Chloride	5 mg	Purple	Tablet, Extended Release	Circle	Teva Pharmaceuticals
G 342	Oxybutynin Chloride	10 mg	Pink	Tablet, Extended Release	Circle	Teva Pharmaceuticals
G 343	Oxybutynin Chloride	15 mg	Off-White	Tablet, Extended Release	Circle	Teva Pharmaceuticals
G ZA5	Zaleplon	5 mg	Opaque Peach	Capsule		Mylan Pharmaceuticals
G ZA10	Zaleplon	10 mg	Opaque White	Capsule		Mylan Pharmaceuticals
G; 00; 30	Ranitidine Hydrochloride	150 mg	White	Tablet	Circle	Mylan Pharmaceuticals
G; 00; 53	Oxaprozin	600 mg	White	Tablet	Oval	Par Pharmaceutical

IMPRINT	BRAND/GENERIC NAME	STRENGTH	COLOR	FORM	SHAPE	MANUFACTURER
G; 0031	Ranitidine Hydrochloride	300 mg	White	Tablet	Capsule-Shape	Mylan Pharmaceuticals
G; 0034	Acyclovir	200 mg	Blue, Opaque	Capsule		Par Pharmaceutical
G; 0036	Acyclovir	400 mg	White	Tablet	Five-Sided	Par Pharmaceutical
G; 0037	Acyclovir	800 mg	Blue	Tablet	Oval	Par Pharmaceutical
G; 25	Atenolol	25 mg	White	Tablet	Circle, Flat; Bevelled Edge; Scored	Par Pharmaceutical
G; 50; BAYER LOGO	Glucobay	50 mg	White to Brown Tinged	Tablet	Circle, Convex	Bayer Pharmaceutical
G; 100; BAYER LOGO	Glucobay	100 mg	White to Brown Tinged	Tablet	Circle, Convex, Scored	Bayer Pharmaceutical
G; 2444	Budeprion SR	150 mg	Light Yellow	Extended-Release Tablet	Circle	Teva Pharmaceuticals
G; 3327; 4	Methylprednisolone Acetate	4 mg	White	Tablet	Oval	Pharmacia & Upjohn
G; ET; 500	Etodolac	500 mg	Light Blue	Tablet	Oval	Par Pharmaceutical
G; FL; 10	Fluoxetine Hydrochloride	10 mg	Purple and Green	Capsule		Par Pharmaceutical
G; FL; 20	Fluoxetine Hydrochloride	20 mg	Purple and Green	Capsule		Par Pharmaceutical
G; GU; 1	Guanfacine Hydrochloride	1 mg	White	Tablet	Oval	Par Pharmaceutical
G; GU; 2	Guanfacine Hydrochloride	2 mg	White	Tablet	Oval	Par Pharmaceutical
G; S; 80	Sotalol Hydrochloride	80 mg	White	Tablet	Capsule-Shape	Par Pharmaceutical
G; S; 120	Sotalol Hydrochloride	120 mg	White	Tablet	Capsule-Shape	Par Pharmaceutical
G; S; 160	Sotalol Hydrochloride	160 mg	White	Tablet	Capsule-Shape	Par Pharmaceutical
G; S; 240	Sotalol Hydrochloride	240 mg	White	Tablet	Capsule-Shape	Par Pharmaceutical
G; SE; 5	Selegiline Hydrochloride	5 mg	White	Tablet	Circle	Par Pharmaceutical
G; T250	Ticlopidine Hydrochloride	250 mg	White to Off-White	Tablet	Oval	Par Pharmaceutical
G3 ; M	Granisetron Hydrochloride	1 mg	White	Tablet	Circle	Mylan Pharmaceuticals
G31 ; M	Glipizide and Metformin Hydrochloride	2.5 mg ; 250 mg	White	Tablet	Circle	Mylan Pharmaceuticals
G32 ; M	Glipizide and Metformin Hydrochloride	500 mg ; 2.5 mg	White	Tablet	Oval	Mylan Pharmaceuticals
G33 ; M	Glipizide and Metformin Hydrochloride	5 mg ; 500 mg	Peach	Tablet	Capsule-Shape	Mylan Pharmaceuticals
GAL 8	Razadyne ER	8 mg	White Opaque	Capsule, Extended Release		Ortho-Mcneil Neurologics
GAL 16	Razadyne ER	16 mg	Pink Opaque	Capsule, Extended Release		Ortho-Mcneil Neurologics
GAL 24	Razadyne ER	24 mg	Caramel Opaque	Capsule, Extended Release		Ortho-Mcneil Neurologics
GANTANOL; ROCHE	Gantanol	0.5 G	Pale Green	Tablet	Circle, Scored	Roche Laboratories
GANTANOL-DS; ROCHE	Gantanol-DS	1 G	Light Orange	Tablet	Capsule-Shape, Scored	Roche Laboratories
GEIGY GM	Lamprene	50 mg	Brown	Capsule	Oblong	Novartis
GEIGY; 14	Butazolidin	100 mg	Red	Coated Tablet	Circle	Novartis
GEIGY; 35 35	Lopressor HCT	25 mg ; 50 mg	White and Blue	Tablet		Novartis
GEIGY; 44; BUTAZOLIDIN; 100 MG	Butazolidin	100 mg	Orange and White	Capsule		Novartis
GEIGY; 48	Pbz-SR	100 mg	Lavender	Extended-Release Tablet	Circle	Novartis
GEIGY; 111	Pbz	25 mg	White	Tablet	Circle, Scored	Novartis
GEIGY; 117	Pbz	50 mg	White	Tablet	Circle, Scored	Novartis
GEIGY; GM	Lamprene	100 mg	Brown	Capsule	Oblong	Novartis
GG ; 157 157	Benazepril Hydrochloride and Hydrochlorothiazide	5 mg ; 6.25 mg	White	Tablet	Oval	Par Pharmaceutical
GG ; 158 158	Benazepril Hydrochloride and Hydrochlorothiazide	10 mg ; 12.5 mg	White	Tablet	Oval	Par Pharmaceutical
GG ; 159 159	Benazepril Hydrochloride and Hydrochlorothiazide	20 mg ; 12.5 mg	White	Tablet	Oval	Par Pharmaceutical
GG ; 160 160	Benazepril Hydrochloride and Hydrochlorothiazide	20 mg ; 25 mg	White	Tablet	Oval	Par Pharmaceutical
GG 517	Indomethacin	25 mg	Light Green	Capsule		Novartis Generics
GG 518	Indomethacin	50 mg	Light Green	Capsule		Novartis Generics
GG; 9 ;	Dexamethasone	0.75 mg	Blue	Tablet	Five-Sided	Novartis Generics
GG; 11 ;	Chlorthalidone	25 mg	Yellow	Tablet	Circle	Novartis Generics
GG; 12	Medroxyprogesterone	10 mg	White	Tablet	Circle, Scored	Novartis Generics
GG; 13 ;	Chlorthalidone	50 mg	Green	Tablet	Circle, Scored	Novartis Generics
GG; 14 ;	Prednisolone	5 mg	Peach	Tablet	Circle, Scored	Novartis Generics
GG; 17	Chlorthalidone and Reserpine	50 mg ; 0.25 mg		Tablet		Novartis Generics
GG; 23	T.E.P.	130 mg ; 24.3 mg ; 8.1 mg	White	Tablet	Circle	Novartis Generics
GG; 24 ;	T.E.H.	25 mg ; 10 mg ; 130 mg	White	Tablet	Circle, Scored; Compressed	Novartis Generics
GG; 27 ;	Hydrochlorothiazide	50 mg	Peach	Tablet	Circle, Scored	Novartis Generics
GG; 28 ;	Hydrochlorothiazide	25 mg	Peach	Tablet	Circle, Scored	Novartis Generics
GG; 29 ;	Triamcinolone	4 mg	White	Tablet	Capsule-Shape	Novartis Generics
GG; 37	Hydroxyzine Hydrochloride	10 mg	Lavender	Coated Tablet		Novartis Generics
GG; 38	Hydroxyzine Hydrochloride	25 mg	Lavender	Coated Tablet	Circle	Novartis Generics
GG; 39	Hydroxyzine Hydrochloride	50 mg	Purple	Coated Tablet		Novartis Generics
GG; 45 ;	Dipyridamole	50 mg	White	Coated Tablet	Circle	Novartis Generics
GG; 49 ;	Dipyridamole	25 mg	White	Coated Tablet	Circle	Novartis Generics
GG; 56	Disopyramide Phosphate	100 mg	Opaque Orange	Capsule		Novartis Generics
GG; 57	Disopyramide Phosphate	150 mg		Capsule		Novartis Generics
GG; 61	Chlorpropamide	100 mg	White	Tablet	Circle, Scored	Novartis Generics
GG; 62	Sodium Fluoride	2.2 mg	Pink	Tablet	Circle	Novartis Generics
GG; 66	Diazepam	2 mg	White	Tablet	Circle, Scored	Novartis Generics
GG; 67	Diazepam	5 mg	Orange	Tablet	Circle, Scored	Novartis Generics
GG; 68	Diazepam	10 mg	Green	Tablet	Circle, Scored	Novartis Generics
GG; 70	Propranolol Hydrochloride	90 mg		Tablet		Novartis Generics
GG; 71	Propranolol Hydrochloride	10 mg	Peach Colored	Tablet	Circle, Scored	Novartis Generics
GG; 72	Propranolol Hydrochloride	20 mg	Blue	Tablet	Circle, Scored	Novartis Generics
GG; 73	Propranolol Hydrochloride	40 mg	Green	Tablet	Circle, Scored	Novartis Generics
GG; 74	Propranolol Hydrochloride	60 mg	Salmon Colored	Tablet	Circle, Scored	Novartis Generics
GG; 75	Propranolol Hydrochloride	80 mg	Yellow	Tablet	Circle, Scored	Novartis Generics

IMPRINT	BRAND/GENERIC NAME	STRENGTH	COLOR	FORM	SHAPE	MANUFACTURER
GG; 79	Prednisone	5 mg	White	Tablet	Circle, Scored	Novartis Generics
GG; 81	Clonidine Hydrochloride	0.1 mg	Light Green	Tablet	Circle, Scored	Novartis Generics
GG; 82	Clonidine Hydrochloride	0.2 mg	Yellow	Tablet	Circle, Scored	Novartis Generics
GG; 83	Clonidine Hydrochloride	0.3 mg	Blue	Tablet	Circle, Scored	Novartis Generics
GG; 84	Timolol Maleate	5 mg	White	Tablet	Circle	Novartis Generics
GG; 86	Clonidine Hydrochloride and Chlorthalidone	0.1 mg ; 15 mg		Tablet		Novartis Generics
GG; 87	Clonidine Hydrochloride and Chlorthalidone	15 mg ; 0.2 mg		Tablet		Novartis Generics
GG; 88	Clonidine Hydrochloride and Chlorthalidone	15 mg ; 0.3 mg		Tablet		Novartis Generics
GG; 96	Clorazepate Dipotassium	3.75 mg	Blue	Tablet	Circle, Scored, Compressed	Novartis Generics
GG; 98	Clorazepate Dipotassium	7.5 mg	Peach	Tablet	Circle, Scored, Compressed	Novartis Generics
GG; 99	Clorazepate Dipotassium	15 mg	White	Tablet	Circle, Scored, Compressed	Novartis Generics
GG; 101 ;	Methocarbamol	750 mg	White	Tablet	Oblong	Novartis Generics
GG; 103 ;	Metronidazole	250 mg	White	Coated Tablet	Circle, Scored	Novartis Generics
GG; 104	Methyldopa	125 mg	White	Coated Tablet	Circle	Novartis Generics
GG; 111	Methyldopa	250 mg	White	Coated Tablet	Circle	Novartis Generics
GG; 113	Metoclopramide Hydrochloride	10 mg	White	Tablet	Circle, Scored	Novartis Generics
GG; 119 ;	Butal Compound	40 mg ; 50 mg ; 325 mg	White	Tablet	Circle	Novartis Generics
GG; 122	Sulfasalazine	500 mg	Butterscotch	Tablet	Circle	Novartis Generics
GG; 127	Quiphile	260 mg	White	Tablet	Circle	Novartis Generics
GG; 135	Clorazepate Dipotassium	11.25 mg		Sustained-Release Tablet		Novartis Generics
GG; 136	Clorazepate Dipotassium	22.5 mg		Sustained-Release Tablet		Novartis Generics
GG; 138 ;	Sulfamethoxazole	500 mg	Green	Tablet	Circle, Scored	Novartis Generics
GG; 139	Buspirone Hydrochloride	5 mg		Tablet		Novartis Generics
GG; 140	Buspirone Hydrochloride	10 mg		Tablet		Novartis Generics
GG; 144	Chlorpropamide	250 mg	White	Tablet	Circle, Scored	Novartis Generics
GG; 145 ;	Dimenhydrinate	50 mg	Yellow	Tablet	Circle, Scored	Novartis Generics
GG; 146	Hydrochlorothiazide and Reserpine	50 mg ; 0.125 mg		Tablet		Novartis Generics
GG; 150 ;	Meprobamate	400 mg	White	Tablet	Circle, Scored	Novartis Generics
GG; 153	Propranolol Hydrochloride and Hydrochlorothiazide	25 mg ; 40 mg	White	Tablet	Circle, Scored	Novartis Generics
GG; 154	Propranolol Hydrochloride and Hydrochlorothiazide	80 mg ; 25 mg	White	Tablet	Circle, Scored	Novartis Generics
GG; 155 ;	Prednisone	20 mg	Peach-Colored	Tablet	Circle, Scored	Novartis Generics
GG; 156	Prednisone	10 mg	White	Tablet	Circle	Novartis Generics
GG; 157	Prednisone	50 mg	White	Tablet	Circle, Scored	Novartis Generics
GG; 158 ;	Sulfisoxazole	500 mg	White	Tablet	Circle	Novartis Generics
GG; 173	Methotrexate	2.5 mg		Tablet		Novartis Generics
GG; 177	Captopril	25 mg		Tablet		Novartis Generics
GG; 178	Captopril	50 mg		Tablet		Novartis Generics
GG; 179	Captopril	100 mg		Tablet		Novartis Generics
GG; 182	Timolol Maleate	10 mg	White	Tablet	Circle, Scored	Novartis Generics
GG; 183	Timolol Maleate	20 mg	Blue	Tablet	Circle, Scored	Novartis Generics
GG; 184	Oxybutynin Chloride	5 mg	Light Blue	Tablet	Round, Convex, Bisected Scored	Novartis Generics
GG; 186	Metaproterenol Sulfate	10 mg		Tablet		Novartis Generics
GG; 187	Metaproterenol Sulfate	20 mg		Tablet		Novartis Generics
GG; 188	Guanabenz Acetate	4 mg		Tablet		Novartis Generics
GG; 189	Guanabenz Acetate	8 mg		Tablet		Novartis Generics
GG; 190 ;	Methocarbamol	500 mg	White	Tablet	Circle, Scored	Novartis Generics
GG; 193	Naloxone and Pentazocine	0.5 mg ; 50 mg		Tablet		Novartis Generics
GG; 194	Indapamide	2.5 mg		Tablet		Novartis Generics
GG; 195 ;	Metronidazole	500 mg	White	Coated Tablet	Oblong	Novartis Generics
GG; 204	Tolmetin Sodium	200 mg		Tablet		Novartis Generics
GG; 206	Captopril and Hydrochlorothiazide	25 mg ; 15 mg		Tablet		Novartis Generics
GG; 207	Captopril and Hydrochlorothiazide	25 mg ; 25 mg		Tablet		Novartis Generics
GG; 208	Captopril and Hydrochlorothiazide	50 mg ; 15 mg		Tablet		Novartis Generics
GG; 209	Captopril and Hydrochlorothiazide	50 mg ; 25 mg		Tablet		Novartis Generics
GG; 219	Methyldopa and Hydrochlorothiazide	15 mg ; 250 mg	Light Green	Coated Tablet	Circle	Novartis Generics
GG; 221	Theophylline	100 mg		Tablet		Novartis Generics
GG; 222	Theophylline	200 mg		Tablet		Novartis Generics
GG; 223	Theophylline	300 mg		Tablet		Novartis Generics
GG; 234	Methylprednisolone	4 mg	White	Tablet	Oval, Scored	Novartis Generics
GG; 238	Glyburide	1.25 mg	White	Tablet	Circle, Scored	Novartis Generics
GG; 240	Glyburide	5 mg	Blue	Tablet	Circle, Scored	Novartis Generics
GG; 242	Methyclothiazide	5 mg	Salmon-Colored	Tablet	Circle, Scored	Novartis Generics
GG; 243	Methyldopa and Hydrochlorothiazide	30 mg ; 500 mg	Light Green	Coated Tablet	Circle	Novartis Generics
GG; 244	Methyclothiazide	2.5 mg	Orange	Tablet	Circle, Scored	Novartis Generics
GG; 246	Bumetanide	0.5 mg		Tablet		Novartis Generics
GG; 247	Bumetanide	1 mg		Tablet		Novartis Generics
GG; 248	Bumetanide	2 mg		Tablet		Novartis Generics
GG; 250	Quinidine Gluconate	324 mg	White	Sustained-Release Tablet	Circle	Novartis Generics
GG; 251	Carbidopa and Levodopa	10 mg ; 100 mg	Blue	Tablet	Circle, Scored	Novartis Generics
GG; 252	Carbidopa and Levodopa	25 mg ; 100 mg	Yellow	Tablet	Circle, Scored	Novartis Generics
GG; 253	Carbidopa and Levodopa	25 mg ; 250 mg	Light Blue	Tablet	Circle, Scored	Novartis Generics
GG; 254	Fenoprofen Calcium	600 mg	White	Coated Tablet	Oval, Scored, Embossed	Novartis Generics
GG; 255	Disobrom	120 mg ; 6 mg	White	Timed-Release Tablet	Circle	Novartis Generics

IMPRINT	BRAND/GENERIC NAME	STRENGTH	COLOR	FORM	SHAPE	MANUFACTURER
GG; 265	Methyldopa and Hydrochlorothiazide	25 mg ; 250 mg	White	Coated Tablet	Circle	Novartis Generics
GG; 270	Tolazamide	100 mg	White	Tablet	Circle, Scored	Novartis Generics
GG; 271	Tolazamide	250 mg	White	Tablet	Circle, Scored	Novartis Generics
GG; 272	Tolazamide	500 mg	White	Tablet	Circle, Scored	Novartis Generics
GG; 273	Quinidine Sulfate	300 mg		Sustained-Release Tablet		Novartis Generics
GG; 277	Sucralfate	1 GM		Tablet		Novartis Generics
GG; 280	Minocycline	50 mg		Tablet		Novartis Generics
GG; 281	Minocycline	100 mg		Tablet		Novartis Generics
GG; 285 ;	Quinidine Sulfate	200 mg	White	Tablet	Circle, Scored	Novartis Generics
GG; 286	Quinidine Sulfate	300 mg	White	Tablet	Circle, Scored	Novartis Generics
GG; 289	Methyldopa and Hydrochlorothiazide	50 mg ; 500 mg	White	Coated Tablet	Circle	Novartis Generics
GG; 297	Doxycycline Hyclate	100 mg		Tablet		Novartis Generics
GG; 406	Probucol	250 mg		Tablet		Novartis Generics
GG; 407 ;	Chlorpromazine Hydrochloride	50 mg	Off-White	Coated Tablet	Circle	Novartis Generics
GG; 409	Leucovorin Calcium	5 mg		Tablet		Novartis Generics
GG; 410	Leucovorin Calcium	25 mg		Tablet		Novartis Generics
GG; 412	Carisoprodol Compound	325 mg ; 200 mg		Tablet		Novartis Generics
GG; 414	Probenecid	500 mg	Yellow	Coated Tablet	Capsule-Shape	Novartis Generics
GG; 421	Chlorzoxazone	250 mg	Orange	Tablet	Circle, Scored	Novartis Generics
GG; 422	Chlorzoxazone	500 mg	Orange	Tablet	Circle, Scored	Novartis Generics
GG; 425	Erythromycin Ethylsuccinate	400 mg		Coated Tablet		Novartis Generics
GG; 436	Nystatin	500,000 units	Brown	Coated Tablet	Circle	Novartis Generics
GG; 437 ;	Chlorpromazine Hydrochloride	100 mg	Off-White	Coated Tablet	Circle	Novartis Generics
GG; 447	Pentoxifylline	400 mg		Sustained-Release Tablet		Novartis Generics
GG; 452	Orphenadrine Citrate, Aspirin and Caffeine	385 mg ; 30 mg ; 25 mg		Tablet		Novartis Generics
GG; 453	Orphenadrine Citrate, Aspirin and Caffeine	60 mg ; 50 mg ; 770 mg		Tablet		Novartis Generics
GG; 454	Diflunisal	250 mg		Tablet		Novartis Generics
GG; 455 ;	Chlorpromazine Hydrochloride	10 mg	Off-White	Coated Tablet	Circle	Novartis Generics
GG; 456	Diflunisal	500 mg		Tablet		Novartis Generics
GG; 457 ;	Chlorpromazine Hydrochloride	200 mg	Off-White	Coated Tablet	Circle	Novartis Generics
GG; 462	Tocainide	400 mg		Tablet		Novartis Generics
GG; 463	Tocainide	600 mg		Tablet		Novartis Generics
GG; 464 ;	Dipyridamole	75 mg	White	Coated Tablet	Circle	Novartis Generics
GG; 465	Nadolol	20 mg		Tablet		Novartis Generics
GG; 466	Nadolol	40 mg		Tablet		Novartis Generics
GG; 467	Nadolol	80 mg		Tablet		Novartis Generics
GG; 468	Nadolol	120 mg		Tablet		Novartis Generics
GG; 469	Nadolol	160 mg		Tablet		Novartis Generics
GG; 471	Methyldopa	500 mg	White	Coated Tablet	Circle	Novartis Generics
GG; 472	Procainamide Hydrochloride	250 mg	White	Sustained-Release Tablet	Oblong	Novartis Generics
GG; 473	Procainamide Hydrochloride	500 mg	White	Sustained-Release Tablet	Oblong, Scored	Novartis Generics
GG; 476 ;	Chlorpromazine Hydrochloride	25 mg	Off-White	Coated Tablet	Circle	Novartis Generics
GG; 487	Probenecid and Colchicine	0.5 mg ; 500 mg	White	Tablet	Oblong	Novartis Generics
GG; 492	Divalproex Sodium	125 mg		Tablet		Novartis Generics
GG; 493	Divalproex Sodium	250 mg		Tablet		Novartis Generics
GG; 494	Divalproex Sodium	500 mg		Tablet		Novartis Generics
GG; 501 ;	Nitroglycerin	6.5 mg	Blue and Dark Yellow	Sustained-Release Capsule		Novartis Generics
GG; 504	Tolmetin Sodium	400 mg		Capsule		Novartis Generics
GG; 509 ;	Cyclandelate	400 mg	Blue and Red	Capsule		Novartis Generics
GG; 510	Sulfinpyrazone	200 mg		Capsule		Novartis Generics
GG; 511 ;	Nitroglycerin	2.5 mg	Lavender and Clear	Sustained-Release Capsule		Novartis Generics
GG; 512 ;	Nitroglycerin SR	9 mg	Clear Yellow and Green	Sustained-Release Capsule		Novartis Generics
GG; 513	Gemfibrozil	300 mg		Capsule		Novartis Generics
GG; 514 ;	Phenylbutazone	100 mg	Light Blue	Capsule		Novartis Generics
GG; 515	Quinidine Sulfate	325 mg		Tablet		Novartis Generics
GG; 516 ;	Phendimetrazine	105 mg	Blue and Clear with Blue Beads	Sustained-Release Capsule		Novartis Generics
GG; 519	Indomethacin	75 mg		Extended-Release Capsule		Novartis Generics
GG; 520 ;	Butal Compound	50 mg ; 325 mg ; 40 mg		Capsule		Novartis Generics
GG; 522	Flurazepam	15 mg	Powder Blue and White	Capsule		Novartis Generics
GG; 523	Flurazepam	30 mg	Powder Blue	Capsule		Novartis Generics
GG; 524	Meclofenamate Sodium	50 mg	Maroon and Pink	Capsule		Novartis Generics
GG; 525	Meclofenamate Sodium	100 mg	Maroon and White	Capsule		Novartis Generics
GG; 526	Clorazepate Dipotassium	3.75 mg	Opaque White with Bands	Capsule		Novartis Generics
GG; 527	Clorazepate	7.5 mg	Opaque White with Bands	Capsule		Novartis Generics
GG; 528	Clorazepate	15 mg	Opaque White with Bands	Capsule		Novartis Generics
GG; 529 ;	Cyclandelate	200 mg	Powder Blue	Capsule		Novartis Generics
GG; 533 ;	Diphenhydramine Hydrochloride	25 mg	Pink and Clear with White Powder	Capsule		Novartis Generics
GG; 534	Clofibrate	500 mg		Capsule		Novartis Generics
GG; 541 ;	Diphenhydramine Hydrochloride	50 mg	Pink	Capsule		Novartis Generics
GG; 542	Prazepam	5 mg		Capsule		Novartis Generics

IMPRINT	BRAND/GENERIC NAME	STRENGTH	COLOR	FORM	SHAPE	MANUFACTURER
GG; 543	Prazepam	10 mg		Capsule		Novartis Generics
GG; 544	Prazepam	20 mg		Capsule		Novartis Generics
GG; 545	Cephalexin	250 mg	Opaque Orange and Gray	Capsule		Novartis Generics
GG; 546	Cephalexin	500 mg	Opaque Orange and Gray	Capsule		Novartis Generics
GG; 555	Cephalexin	500 mg	Swedish Orange	Capsule		Novartis Generics
GG; 556	Cephalexin	250 mg	Swedish Orange and Gray	Capsule		Novartis Generics
GG; 558	Fenoprofen Calcium	200 mg	White with Gold and Black Bands	Capsule		Novartis Generics
GG; 559	Fenoprofen Calcium	300 mg	White with Gold Bands	Capsule		Novartis Generics
GG; 560	Ferrous Sulfate	250 mg		Sustained-Release Capsule		Novartis Generics
GG; 560 ;	Ferrous Sulfate	250 mg	Red and Clear with Brown and White Beads	Sustained-Release Capsule		Novartis Generics
GG; 561	Danazol	50 mg		Capsule		Novartis Generics
GG; 571	Clinoxide	5 mg ; 2.5 mg	Opaque White	Capsule		Novartis Generics
GG; 572	Doxepin Hydrochloride	25 mg	Opaque White with Pink and Gold Bands	Capsule		Novartis Generics
GG; 573	Doxepin Hydrochloride	50 mg	Opaque White with Pink and Green Bands	Capsule		Novartis Generics
GG; 574	Doxepin Hydrochloride	75 mg	Opaque White with Black and Gold Bands	Capsule		Novartis Generics
GG; 576	Doxepin Hydrochloride	10 mg	White with Red and Gold Band	Capsule		Novartis Generics
GG; 577	Doxepin Hydrochloride	100 mg	White with Blue and Green Bands	Capsule		Novartis Generics
GG; 578	Doxepin Hydrochloride	150 mg		Capsule		Novartis Generics
GG; 582	Hydroxyzine Pamoate	25 mg	Two-Toned Green	Capsule		Novartis Generics
GG; 583	Hydroxyzine Pamoate	50 mg	Opaque White and Green	Capsule		Novartis Generics
GG; 584	Hydroxyzine Pamoate	100 mg		Capsule		Novartis Generics
GG; 585	Loxapine Succinate	5 mg		Capsule		Novartis Generics
GG; 586	Loxapine Succinate	10 mg		Capsule		Novartis Generics
GG; 587	Loxapine Succinate	25 mg		Capsule		Novartis Generics
GG; 588	Loxapine Succinate	50 mg		Capsule		Novartis Generics
GG; 591 ;	Propoxyphene Hydrochloride	65 mg	Opaque Pale Pink	Capsule		Novartis Generics
GG; 592	Prazosin Hydrochloride	1 mg	White with Black Ink Bands	Capsule		Novartis Generics
GG; 593	Prazosin Hydrochloride	2 mg	White with Pink and Black Ink Bands	Capsule		Novartis Generics
GG; 594	Prazosin Hydrochloride	5 mg	White with Blue and Black Ink Bands	Capsule		Novartis Generics
GG; 601	Isotretinoin	10 mg		Capsule		Novartis Generics
GG; 602	Isotretinoin	20 mg		Capsule		Novartis Generics
GG; 603	Isotretinoin	40 mg		Capsule		Novartis Generics
GG; 604	Cyclosporine	25 mg		Capsule		Novartis Generics
GG; 605	Cyclosporine	100 mg		Capsule		Novartis Generics
GG; 625	Flutamide	125 mg		Capsule		Novartis Generics
GG; 702	Isosorbide Mononitrate	20 mg		Tablet		Novartis Generics
GG; 704	Tolmetin Sodium	600 mg		Tablet		Novartis Generics
GG; 714	Erythromycin Stearate	250 mg		Tablet		Novartis Generics
GG; 715	Erythromycin Stearate	500 mg		Tablet		Novartis Generics
GG; 730	Pseudoephedrine and Terfenadine	60 mg ; 120 mg		Sustained-Release Tablet		Novartis Generics
GG; 733	Salsalate	500 mg	Light Green	Coated Tablet	Circle	Novartis Generics
GG; 734	Salsalate	750 mg		Coated Tablet	Capsule-Shape, Scored	Novartis Generics
GG; 755	Doxazosin	1 mg		Tablet		Novartis Generics
GG; 756	Doxazosin	2 mg		Tablet		Novartis Generics
GG; 757	Doxazosin	4 mg		Tablet		Novartis Generics
GG; 758	Doxazosin	8 mg		Tablet		Novartis Generics
GG; 774	Etodolac	400 mg		Tablet		Novartis Generics
GG; 801	Ketoprofen	75 mg		Capsule		Novartis Generics
GG; 802	Ketoprofen	50 mg		Capsule		Novartis Generics
GG; 805	Piroxicam	10 mg		Capsule		Novartis Generics
GG; 806	Piroxicam	20 mg		Capsule		Novartis Generics
GG; 808	Tetracycline Hydrochloride	250 mg	Yellow and Orange	Capsule		Novartis Generics
GG; 809	Tetracycline Hydrochloride	500 mg	Yellow and Black	Capsule		Novartis Generics
GG; 810	Oxytetracycline	250 mg		Capsule		Novartis Generics
GG; 811	Erythromycin Estolate	250 mg	Orange and Buff	Capsule		Novartis Generics
GG; 812	Minocycline	50 mg		Capsule		Novartis Generics
GG; 813	Minocycline	100 mg		Capsule		Novartis Generics
GG; 814	Doxycycline	50 mg	Blue and White	Capsule		Novartis Generics
GG; 815	Doxycycline	100 mg	Blue	Capsule		Novartis Generics
GG; 816	Nizatidine	150 mg		Capsule		Novartis Generics
GG; 817	Nizatidine	300 mg		Capsule		Novartis Generics
GG; 818	Propranolol	60 mg		Sustained-Release Capsule		Novartis Generics
GG; 819	Propranolol	80 mg		Sustained-Release Capsule		Novartis Generics
GG; 820	Propranolol	120 mg		Sustained-Release Capsule		Novartis Generics
GG; 821	Propranolol	160 mg		Sustained-Release Capsule		Novartis Generics

IMPRINT	BRAND/GENERIC NAME	STRENGTH	COLOR	FORM	SHAPE	MANUFACTURER
GG; 832	Etodolac	200 mg		Capsule		Novartis Generics
GG; 833	Etodolac	300 mg		Capsule		Novartis Generics
GG; 835	Erythromycin	250 mg		Capsule		Novartis Generics
GG; 842	Nicardipine Hydrochloride	20 mg		Capsule		Novartis Generics
GG; 843	Nicardipine Hydrochloride	30 mg		Capsule		Novartis Generics
GG; 958 ;	Metoclopramide	5 mg	White	Tablet	Circle	Novartis Generics
GG; 9533	Mudrane GG-2	111 mg ; 100 mg	Green Mottled	Tablet		Ecr Pharmaceuticals
GG; 9551	Mudrane GG	111 mg ; 16 mg ; 100 mg ; 8 mg	Yellow Mottled	Tablet		Ecr Pharmaceuticals
GG; D5	Selegiline Hydrochloride	5 mg		Tablet		Novartis Generics
GG; M1	Metoclopramide Hydrochloride	1 mg		Tablet		Novartis Generics
GIL 0.5	Azilect	0.5 mg	White to Off-White	Tablet	Circle	Teva Pharmaceuticals
GIL 1	Azilect	1 mg	White to Off-White	Tablet	Circle	Teva Pharmaceuticals
GILEAD; 200 MG	Emtriva	200 mg	Blue and White	Capsule		Gilead Sciences
GILEAD; 4331; 300	Viread	300 mg	Light Blue	Coated Tablet	Teardrop-Shape	Gilead Sciences
GL; 81	Renoquid	250 mg	White	Tablet	Circle, Scored	Glenwood
GLAXO	Vicon-C	100 mg ; 80 mg ; 70 mg ; 20 mg ; 20 mg ; 10 mg ; 5 mg ; 300 mg	Orange and Yellow	Capsule		Glaxosmithkline
GLAXO	Vicon Plus	10 mg ; 5 mg ; 4 mg ; 2 mg ; 4000 IU ; 50 IU ; 150 mg ; 80 mg ; 70 mg ; 25 mg ; 10 mg	Red and Beige	Capsule		Glaxosmithkline
GLAXO ; ZANTAC 300	Zantac 300	300 mg	Yellow	Tablet	Capsule-Shape	Glaxosmithkline
GLAXO; 268	Theobid Duracap	260 mg	Blue and Clear	Sustained-Release Capsule		Glaxosmithkline
GLAXO; 316	Vicon Forte	10 mg ; 5 mg ; 4 mg ; 2 mg ; 1 mg ; 10 mg ; 8000 IU ; 50 IU ; 150 mg ; 80 mg ; 70 mg ; 25 mg ; 10 mg	Orange and Black	Capsule		Glaxosmithkline
GLAXO; 371	Trandate HCT	100 mg ; 25 mg	Pale Peach	Coated Tablet	Oval	Glaxosmithkline
GLAXO; 372	Trandate HCT	25 mg ; 200 mg	White	Coated Tablet	Oval	Glaxosmithkline
GLAXO; 373	Trandate HCT	25 mg ; 300 mg	Medium Peach	Coated Tablet	Oval	Glaxosmithkline
GLAXO; AMESEC	Amesec	130 mg ; 25 mg	Orange and Blue	Capsule		Glaxosmithkline
GLAXO; TRINSICON	Trinsicon	110 mg ; 240 mg ; 15 mcg ; 0.5 mg ; 75 mg	Dark Pink and Dark Red	Capsule		Glaxosmithkline
GLAXO; VENTOLIN; 2	Ventolin	2 mg	White	Tablet	Circle, Compressed	Glaxosmithkline
GLUCOTROL XL; 2.5	Glucotrol XL	2.5 mg	Blue	Extended-Release Tablet		Pfizer Laboratories
GLUCOTROL XL; 5	Glucotrol XL	5 mg	White	Extended-Release Tablet	Circle, Biconvex	Pfizer Laboratories
GLUCOTROL XL; 10	Glucotrol XL	10 mg	White	Extended-Release Tablet	Biconvex, Circle	Pfizer Laboratories
GLYBUR 364; 364	Glyburide	5 mg	Blue	Tablet	Oblong	Teva Pharmaceuticals
GLYBUR 433; 433	Glyburide	2.5 mg	Pink	Tablet	Oblong, Scored	Teva Pharmaceuticals
GLYNASE 1.5; PT; PT	Glynase Prestab	1.5 mg	White	Tablet	Egg-Shape, Contour, Scored	Pharmacia & Upjohn
GLYNASE 3; PT; PT	Glynase Prestab	3 mg	Blue	Tablet	Egg-Shape	Pharmacia & Upjohn
GLYNASE 6; PT; PT	Glynase Prestab	6 mg	Yellow	Tablet	Egg-Shape, Contour, Scored	Pharmacia & Upjohn
GLYSET; 25	Glyset	25 mg	White	Tablet	Circle	Pharmacia & Upjohn
GLYSET; 50	Glyset	50 mg	White	Tablet	Circle	Pharmacia & Upjohn
GLYSET; 100	Glyset	100 mg	White	Tablet	Circle	Pharmacia & Upjohn
GP 5; G	Glipizide	5 mg	White	Tablet	Oval, Convex	Par Pharmaceutical
GP 10; G	Glipizide	10 mg	White	Tablet	Oval, Convex	Par Pharmaceutical
GRISACTIN ULTRA; 125	Grisactin Ultra	125 mg	White	Tablet		Wyeth Pharmaceuticals
GRISACTIN ULTRA; 250	Grisactin Ultra	250 mg	White	Tablet		Wyeth Pharmaceuticals
GRISACTIN ULTRA; 330	Grisactin Ultra	330 mg	White	Tablet		Wyeth Pharmaceuticals
GRISACTIN; 125	Grisactin	125 mg	Orange	Capsule, Liquid Filled		Wyeth Pharmaceuticals
GRISACTIN; 250	Grisactin	250 mg	Yellow	Capsule, Liquid Filled		Wyeth Pharmaceuticals
GRISACTIN; 500	Grisactin	500 mg	Pink	Tablet	Circle	Wyeth Pharmaceuticals
GRIS-PEG; 125	Gris-Peg	125 mg	White	Coated Tablet	Circle, Scored	Pedinol
GRIS-PEG; 250	Gris-Peg	250 mg	White	Coated Tablet	Capsule-Shape, Scored	Pedinol
GS ; 25C	Zantac 25 Efferdose	25 mg	White to Pale Yellow	Tablet, Effervescent	Circle	Glaxosmithkline
GS 3V2	Requip XL	2 mg	Pink	Tablet, Extended Release	Capsule-Shape	Glaxosmithkline
GS 5CC	Requip XL	8 mg	Red	Tablet, Extended Release	Capsule-Shape	Glaxosmithkline
GS WXG	Requip XL	4 mg	Light Brown	Tablet, Extended Release	Capsule-Shape	Glaxosmithkline
GS XJG	Tykerb	250 mg	Orange	Tablet	Oval	Glaxosmithkline
GS YYG	Treximet	85 mg ; 500 mg	Blue	Tablet		Glaxosmithkline
GS; FC2	Epzicom	600 mg ; 300 mg	Orange	Tablet	Modified, Capsule-Shape	Glaxosmithkline
GSI ; 10	Letairis	10 mg	Deep Pink	Tablet	Oval	Gilead Sciences
GSK ; 4/1 ;	Avandaryl	4 mg ; 1 mg	Yellow	Tablet	Triangle	Glaxosmithkline
GSK ; 4/2 ;	Avandaryl	4 mg ; 2 mg	Orange	Tablet	Triangle	Glaxosmithkline
GSK ; 4/4 ;	Avandaryl	4 mg ; 4 mg	Pink	Tablet	Triangle	Glaxosmithkline
GSK ; 8/2 ;	Avandaryl	8 mg ; 2 mg	Pale Pink	Tablet	Triangle	Glaxosmithkline
GUAIFED; MURO 120-250	Guaifed	120 mg ; 250 mg	White and Clear	Extended-Release Capsule		Muro Pharmaceutical
GUAIFED-PD	Guaifed-PD	60 mg ; 300 mg	Blue and Clear	Extended-Release Capsule		Muro Pharmaceutical
GUAIMAX-D; SP; 2055	Guaimax-D	600 mg ; 120 mg	White	Tablet, Extended Release	Capsule-Shape	UCB Pharma
GX CC1	Agenerase	50 mg	Off White to Cream	Capsule, Liquid Filled		Glaxosmithkline

IMPRINT	BRAND/GENERIC NAME	STRENGTH	COLOR	FORM	SHAPE	MANUFACTURER
GX CE2	Avodart	0.5 mg	Dull Yellow	Capsule, Liquid Filled		Glaxosmithkline
GX CF7 24	Zofran	24 mg	Pink	Tablet	Oval	Glaxosmithkline
GX CL2	Lamictal	5 mg	White to Off White	Tablet, Chewable	Capsule-Shape	Glaxosmithkline
GX CL5	Lamictal	25 mg	White	Tablet, Chewable	Oval	Glaxosmithkline
GX LL7	Lexiva	700 mg	Pink	Tablet	Capsule-Shape	Glaxosmithkline
GX; 623	Ziagen	300 mg	Yellow	Coated Tablet	Biconvex, Capsule-Shape	Glaxosmithkline
GX; CE3	Amerge	1 mg	White	Coated Tablet	D-Shape	Glaxosmithkline
GX; CE5	Amerge	2.5 mg	Green	Coated Tablet	D-Shape	Glaxosmithkline
GX; CG5	Epivir-Hbv	100 mg	Butterscotch	Coated Tablet	Capsule-Shape, Biconvex	Glaxosmithkline
GX; CG7	Malarone Pediatric	62.5 mg ; 25 mg	Pink	Coated Tablet	Circle, Biconvex	Glaxosmithkline
GX; CJ7; 150 ;	Epivir	150 mg	White	Coated Tablet	Diamond, Modified	Glaxosmithkline
GX; CK3	Raxar	200 mg	White to Pale Yellow	Coated Tablet	Circle, Biconvex, Bevel-Edged	Glaxosmithkline
GX; CM3	Malarone	250 mg ; 100 mg	Pink	Coated Tablet	Circle, Biconvex	Glaxosmithkline
GX; CT1	Lotronex	1 mg	Blue	Coated Tablet	Oval	Glaxosmithkline
GX; EG2	Ceftin	500 mg	White	Tablet	Capsule-Shape	Glaxosmithkline
GX; EG3; L	Leukeran	2 mg	Brown	Tablet	Circle, Biconvex	Glaxosmithkline
GX; EH3; A	Alkeran	2 mg	White	Coated Tablet	Circle, Biconvex	Glaxosmithkline
GX; EJ7	Epivir	300 mg	Gray	Coated Tablet	Diamond, Modified	Glaxosmithkline
GX; ES7	Ceftin	250 mg	White	Tablet	Capsule-Shape	Glaxosmithkline
GX; LL1	Trizivir	300 mg ; 150 mg ; 300 mg	Blue-Green	Coated Tablet	Capsule-Shape	Glaxosmithkline
GXFC3	Combivir	150 mg ; 300 mg	White	Coated Tablet	Capsule-Shape	Glaxosmithkline
H; 1; LL	Hydromox	50 mg	White	Tablet	Circle, Flat, Scored, Beveled	Lederle Laboratories
H3 ; M	Hydrochlorothiazide	12.5 mg	White to Off-White	Tablet	Circle	Mylan Pharmaceuticals
H4	Micardis HCT	40 mg ; 12.5 mg	White and Red	Tablet	Oblong	Boehringer Ingelheim Pharmaceuticals
H8	Micardis HCT	12.5 mg ; 80 mg	White and Red	Tablet	Oblong	Boehringer Ingelheim Pharmaceuticals
H9	Micardis HCT	25 mg ; 80 mg	White and Yellow	Tablet	Oblong	Boehringer Ingelheim Pharmaceuticals
HALCION; 0.25 ;	Halcion	0.25 mg	Powder-Blue	Tablet	Oval	Pharmacia & Upjohn
HALCION; 0.5	Halcion	0.5 mg	White	Tablet	Oval, Scored	Pharmacia & Upjohn
HALDOL; 1; MCNEIL	Haldol	1 mg	Yellow	Tablet	U-Shape, with "H" Cut Out in Center, Scored	Ortho-Mcneil Pharmaceutical
HALDOL; 2; MCNEIL	Haldol	2 mg	Pink	Tablet	U-Shape, with "H" Cut Out in Center, Scored	Ortho-Mcneil Pharmaceutical
HALDOL; 5; MCNEIL	Haldol	5 mg	Green	Tablet	with "H" Cut Out in Center, Scored, U-Shape	Ortho-Mcneil Pharmaceutical
HALDOL; 10; MCNEIL	Haldol	10 mg	Aqua	Tablet	U-Shape, with "H" Cut Out in Center, Scored	Ortho-Mcneil Pharmaceutical
HALDOL; 20; MCNEIL	Haldol	20 mg	Salmon	Tablet	U-Shape, with "H" Cut Out in Center, Scored	Ortho-Mcneil Pharmaceutical
HALFAN	Halfan	250 mg	White	Tablet	Capsule-Shape	Glaxosmithkline
HALOTESTIN; 2 ;	Halotestin	2 mg	Peach	Tablet	Circle, Scored	Pharmacia & Upjohn
HALOTESTIN; 5 ;	Halotestin	5 mg	Light Green	Tablet	Scored, Circle	Pharmacia & Upjohn
HALOTESTIN; 10 ;	Halotestin	10 mg	Green	Tablet	Circle, Scored	Pharmacia & Upjohn
HB; 93; 614	Belap	10.8 mg ; 16.2 mg	Green	Tablet	Circle, Convex	Teva Pharmaceuticals
HCQS	Hydroxychloroquine Sulfate	200 mg	White to Off-White	Tablet	Capsule-Shape	Ranbaxy Pharmaceuticals
HD 567	Butalbital, Acetaminophen and Caffeine	50 mg ; 325 mg ; 40 mg	White	Tablet	Circle	Watson Laboratories
HD; 532	Roxilox	5 mg ; 500 mg	Scarlet Red and Buff White	Capsule		Roxane Laboratories
HD; 544	Diazepam	5 mg	Yellow	Tablet	Circle, Scored	Warner Chilcott
HD; 546	Diazepam	2 mg	White	Tablet	Circle, Scored	Warner Chilcott
HD; 549	Diazepam	10 mg	Blue	Tablet	Circle, Scored	Warner Chilcott
HD; 725	Doxycycline Hyclate	100 mg	Beige	Coated Tablet	Circle	Novartis Generics
HGH ; CG	Diovan HCT	12.5 mg ; 80 mg	Light Orange	Tablet	Oval	Novartis Pharmaceuticals
HHH ; CG	Diovan HCT	12.5 mg ; 160 mg	Dark Red	Tablet	Oval	Novartis Pharmaceuticals
HIL ; NVR	Diovan HCT	12.5 mg ; 320 mg	Pink	Tablet	Oval	Novartis Pharmaceuticals
HIVID; 0.375; ROCHE	Hivid	0.375 mg	Beige	Tablet	Oval	Roche Pharmaceuticals
HIVID; 0.750; ROCHE	Hivid	0.75 mg	Gray	Tablet	Oval	Roche Pharmaceuticals
HOECHST; 73	Festalan	30,000 units ; 6000 units ; 20,000 units ; 1 mg	Orange	Tablet	Circle	Aventis Pharmaceuticals
HOECHST; LASIX	Lasix	20 mg	White	Tablet	Oval	Sanofi-Aventis U.S.
HORIZON; 205	Robinul Forte	2 mg	White	Tablet	Circle, Compressed, Scored	Sciele Pharma
HOURGLASS 4346 40 MG	Fluoxetine Hydrochloride	40 mg	Light Blue Opaque	Capsule		Ivax Pharmaceuticals
HOURGLASS 4356 20 MG ;	Fluoxetine Hydrochloride	20 mg	Aqua Blue	Capsule		Ivax Pharmaceuticals
HOURGLASS 4358 ; 300 ;	Ranitidine	300 mg	Beige	Tablet	Oval	Teva Pharmaceuticals
HOURGLASS 4363 10 MG ;	Fluoxetine Hydrochloride	10 mg	Aqua Blue, Opaque White	Capsule		Ivax Pharmaceuticals
HOURGLASS 4382 300MG ;	Gabapentin	300 mg	White, Opaque, Yellow, Opaque	Capsule		Teva Pharmaceuticals
HOURGLASS 4383 400MG ;	Gabapentin	400 mg	Orange, Opaque, White, Opaque	Capsule		Teva Pharmaceuticals
HOURGLASS 4980 ;	Propoxyphene Napsylate and Acetaminophen	100 mg ; 650 mg	Pink	Tablet	Capsule-Shape	Ivax Pharmaceuticals
HOURGLASS; 56; 65; 5; 5; 5	Buspirone Hydrochloride	15 mg	White	Tablet	Capsule-Shape	Ivax Pharmaceuticals
HOURGLASS; 120	Verapamil Hydrochloride	120 mg	Ivory	Extended-Release Tablet	Circle	Ivax Pharmaceuticals
HOURGLASS; 3667	Perphenazine	2 mg	White	Coated Tablet	Circle	Ivax Pharmaceuticals
HOURGLASS; 3668	Perphenazine	4 mg	White	Coated Tablet	Oval	Ivax Pharmaceuticals
HOURGLASS; 3669	Perphenazine	8 mg	White	Coated Tablet	Circle	Ivax Pharmaceuticals
HOURGLASS; 3670	Perphenazine	16 mg	White	Coated Tablet	Oval	Ivax Pharmaceuticals
HOURGLASS; 3685; 1	Doxazosin Mesylate	1 mg	White	Tablet	Circle	Ivax Pharmaceuticals

IMPRINT	BRAND/GENERIC NAME	STRENGTH	COLOR	FORM	SHAPE	MANUFACTURER
HOURGLASS; 3686; 2	Doxazosin Mesylate	2 mg	White	Tablet	Circle	Ivax Pharmaceuticals
HOURGLASS; 3687; 4	Doxazosin Mesylate	4 mg	Orange	Tablet	Circle	Ivax Pharmaceuticals
HOURGLASS; 3688; 8	Doxazosin Mesylate	8 mg	Green	Tablet	Circle	Ivax Pharmaceuticals
HOURGLASS; 3966	Diphenoxylate Hydrochloride and Atropine Sulfate	2.5 mg ; 0.025 mg	White	Tablet	Circle	Ivax Pharmaceuticals
HOURGLASS; 4058	Cefadroxil	500 mg	Clear and White	Capsule		Ivax Pharmaceuticals
HOURGLASS; 4059 ;	Cefadroxil	1000 mg	White	Tablet		Ivax Pharmaceuticals
HOURGLASS; 4194; 500	Cefaclor Extended-Release	500 mg	Blue	Extended-Release Tablet	Oval	Ivax Pharmaceuticals
HOURGLASS; 4195; 2.5	Enalapril Maleate	2.5 mg	Yellow	Tablet	Circle, Scored	Ivax Pharmaceuticals
HOURGLASS; 4196; 5	Enalapril Maleate	5 mg	White	Tablet	Circle, Scored	Ivax Pharmaceuticals
HOURGLASS; 4197; 10	Enalapril Maleate	10 mg	Salmon	Tablet	Circle	Ivax Pharmaceuticals
HOURGLASS; 4198; 20	Enalapril Maleate	20 mg	Peach	Tablet	Circle	Ivax Pharmaceuticals
HOURGLASS; 4303	Clozapine	12.5 mg	Pale Yellow	Tablet	Oval	Ivax Pharmaceuticals
HOURGLASS; 4332; 100	Nefazodone Hydrochloride	100 mg	Peach	Tablet	Oval	Ivax Pharmaceuticals
HOURGLASS; 4333; 150	Nefazodone Hydrochloride	150 mg	Peach	Tablet	Circle	Ivax Pharmaceuticals
HOURGLASS; 4334; 200	Nefazodone Hydrochloride	200 mg	Peach	Tablet	Oval	Ivax Pharmaceuticals
HOURGLASS; 4335; 250	Nefazodone Hydrochloride	250 mg	Peach	Tablet	Circle	Ivax Pharmaceuticals
HOURGLASS; 4343; 50	Nefazodone Hydrochloride	50 mg	Peach	Tablet	Oval	Ivax Pharmaceuticals
HOURGLASS; 4392	Fluvoxamine Maleate	100 mg	Beige	Tablet	Circle	Ivax Pharmaceuticals
HOURGLASS; 4430; 100	Misoprostol	100 mcg		Tablet		Ivax Pharmaceuticals
HOURGLASS; 4431; 200	Misoprostol	200 mcg	White	Tablet	Circle, Scored	Ivax Pharmaceuticals
HOURGLASS; 4510	Fluoxetine Hydrochloride	10 mg	Light Green	Tablet	Oval	Ivax Pharmaceuticals
HOURGLASS; 4960	Flutamide	125 mg	Light Brown Opaque	Capsule		Ivax Pharmaceuticals
HOURGLASS; 5032; 20/25	Lisinopril and Hydrochlorothiazide	20 mg ; 25 mg	Peach	Tablet	Circle	Ivax Pharmaceuticals
HOURGLASS; 5033; 10/12.5	Lisinopril and Hydrochlorothiazide	10 mg ; 12.5 mg	Blue	Tablet	Circle	Ivax Pharmaceuticals
HOURGLASS; 5034; 20/12.5	Lisinopril and Hydrochlorothiazide	12.5 mg ; 20 mg	Yellow	Tablet	Circle	Ivax Pharmaceuticals
HOURGLASS; 5663; 5	Buspirone Hydrochloride	5 mg	White	Tablet	Oval	Ivax Pharmaceuticals
HOURGLASS; 5664; 10	Buspirone Hydrochloride	10 mg	White	Tablet	Oval	Ivax Pharmaceuticals
HOURGLASS; 5675; 15	Mirtazapine	15 mg	Yellow	Tablet	Circle	Ivax Pharmaceuticals
HOURGLASS; 5676; 30	Mirtazapine	30 mg	Tan	Tablet	Circle	Ivax Pharmaceuticals
HOURGLASS; 5695; 45	Mirtazapine	45 mg	White	Tablet	Circle	Ivax Pharmaceuticals
HOURGLASS; 7300 ;	Verapamil Hydrochloride	240 mg	Ivory	Extended-Release Tablet	Oblong	Ivax Pharmaceuticals
HOURGLASS; 9200	Glipizide	10 mg	White	Tablet	Circle, Scored	Ivax Pharmaceuticals
HOURGLASS; 9201	Glipizide	5 mg	White	Tablet	Circle	Ivax Pharmaceuticals
HOURLASS; 7301 ;	Verapamil Hydrochloride	180 mg	Orange	Extended-Release Tablet	Oblong, Scored	Ivax Pharmaceuticals
HP; 15	Mescolor	8 mg ; 120 mg ; 2.5 mg	White	Sustained-Release Tablet	Film-Coated, Scored	First Horizon Pharmaceutical
HPC; 170; HORIZON LOGO	Zebutal	500 mg ; 50 mg ; 40 mg	Pink and Red	Capsule		First Horizon Pharmaceutical
HPC; 200	Robinul	1 mg	White	Tablet	Circle, Compressed, Scored	Sciele Pharma
HTI; 77 ;	Thalitone	15 mg	White	Tablet	Kidney-Shape, Compressed	Monarch Pharmaceuticals
HXH ; NVR	Diovan HCT	25 mg ; 160 mg	Brown Orange	Tablet	Oval	Novartis Pharmaceuticals
HYDERGINE; 0.5; S ;	Hydergine	0.167 mg ; 0.167 mg ; 0.167 mg	White	Tablet	Circle	Novartis
HYDREA; 830	Hydrea	500 mg	Pink and Green	Capsule		Bristol-Myers Squibb
HYZAAR ; MRK 717	Hyzaar 50-12.5	12.5 mg ; 50 mg	Yellow	Tablet	Teardrop-Shape	Merck
HYZAAR ; MRK 747	Hyzaar 100-25	25 mg ; 100 mg	Light Yellow	Tablet	Teardrop-Shape	Merck
I	Visicol	1.102 GM ; 0.398 GM	White to Off-White	Tablet	Circle	Salix Pharmaceuticals
I; 25	Imitrex	25 mg	White	Coated Tablet	Triangle	Glaxosmithkline
IBU 400	Ibu	400 mg	White	Tablet	Oval	Par Pharmaceutical
IBU 400	Ibuprofen	400 mg	White	Tablet	Oval	Watson Laboratories
IBU 600	Ibu	600 mg	White	Tablet		Par Pharmaceutical
IBU 600	Ibuprofen	600 mg	White	Tablet		Watson Laboratories
IBU 800	Ibu	800 mg	White	Tablet		Par Pharmaceutical
IBU 800	Ibuprofen	800 mg	White	Tablet		Watson Laboratories
IBU; 400	Ibuprofen	400 mg	White	Tablet		Warner Chilcott
IBU; 600	Ibuprofen	600 mg	White	Coated Tablet		Warner Chilcott
IBU; 800	Ibuprofen	800 mg	White	Tablet		Warner Chilcott
IC	Cartrol	5 mg	White	Tablet	Oval	Abbott Laboratories
ICN; 0901	Testred	10 mg	Red	Capsule		Valeant Pharmaceuticals
ICN; 311	Android-10	10 mg	White	Capsule		Valeant Pharmaceuticals
ICN; 600	8-Mop	10 mg	Pink	Capsule	Oblong	Valeant Pharmaceuticals
ICN; 600 ;	Oxsoralen	10 mg		Capsule		Valeant Pharmaceuticals
ICN; 650	Oxsoralen-Ultra	10 mg		Capsule		Valeant Pharmaceuticals
ICN; M180 ;	Mestinon Timespan	180 mg		Sustained-Release Tablet	Capsule-Shape, Scored	Valeant Pharmaceuticals

IMPRINT	BRAND/GENERIC NAME	STRENGTH	COLOR	FORM	SHAPE	MANUFACTURER
IE; 1.25; G	Indapamide	1.25 mg	Orange	Tablet	Circle	Par Pharmaceutical
IE; 2.5; G	Indapamide	2.5 mg	White	Tablet	Circle	Par Pharmaceutical
IG226 ; 25 MG	Zonisamide	25 mg	White Opaque	Capsule		Ranbaxy Pharmaceuticals
IG227 ; 50 MG	Zonisamide	50 mg	Blue Opaque, White Opaque	Capsule		Ranbaxy Pharmaceuticals
IG228 ; 100 MG	Zonisamide	100 mg	Brown Opaque, White Opaque	Capsule		Ranbaxy Pharmaceuticals
IKA	Serophene	50 mg	White	Tablet		Serono
IL ; NVR	Tekturna	150 mg	Light Pink	Tablet	Circle	Novartis Pharmaceuticals
IL; 3581	Theochron	300 mg	White	Tablet, Extended Release	Capsule-Shape	Forest Pharmaceuticals
IL; 3584	Theochron	100 mg	White	Extended-Release Tablet	Circle, Convex, Scored	Forest Pharmaceuticals
IL; 3609	Propranolol Hydrochloride	60 mg	Brown and Clear	Extended-Release Capsule		Novartis Generics
IL; 3610	Propranolol Hydrochloride	80 mg	Opaque Blue and Clear	Extended-Release Capsule		Novartis Generics
IL; 3611	Propranolol Hydrochloride	120 mg	Opaque Blue and Clear	Extended-Release Capsule		Novartis Generics
IL; 3612	Propranolol Hydrochloride	160 mg	Opaque Blue and Clear	Extended-Release Capsule		Novartis Generics
IL; 3613	Isochron	40 mg	Peach	Capsule, Extended Release	Circle	Forest Pharmaceuticals
IL; 3625	Theocap	300 mg	Clear with Off-White Beads	Capsule, Extended Release, 12 Hr		Forest Pharmaceuticals
IL; 3634	Theocap	200 mg	Clear and White with Off-White Beads	Capsule, Extended Release, 12 Hr		Forest Pharmaceuticals
IL; 3638	Theocap	125 mg	Clear with Off-White Beads	Capsule, Extended Release, 12 Hr		Forest Pharmaceuticals
IMDUR	Imdur	30 mg	White	Tablet, Extended Release	Capsule-Shape	Schering
IMDUR ; 60-60	Imdur	60 mg	White	Tablet, Extended Release	Capsule-Shape	Schering
IMITREX 50 LOGO	Imitrex	50 mg	White	Tablet	Triangle	Glaxosmithkline
IMITREX 100 LOGO	Imitrex	100 mg	Pink	Tablet	Triangle	Glaxosmithkline
INDERAL; 40 ;	Inderal	40 mg	Green	Tablet	Six-Sided	Wyeth Pharmaceuticals
INDERAL; 60; I	Inderal	60 mg	Pink	Tablet	Six-Sided	Wyeth Pharmaceuticals
INDERAL; 80; I	Inderal	80 mg	Yellow	Tablet	Six-Sided	Wyeth Pharmaceuticals
INDERAL; 90; I	Inderal	90 mg	Lavender	Tablet	Six-Sided, Scored	Wyeth Pharmaceuticals
INDERIDE LA; 80/50	Inderide LA	80 mg ; 50 mg	Beige with 4 Gold Bands	Extended-Release Capsule		Wyeth Pharmaceuticals
INDERIDE LA; 120/ 50	Inderide LA	120 mg ; 50 mg	Beige and Brown with 4 Gold Bands	Extended-Release Capsule		Wyeth Pharmaceuticals
INDERIDE LA; 160/ 50	Inderide LA	160 mg ; 50 mg	Brown with 4 Gold Bands	Extended-Release Capsule		Wyeth Pharmaceuticals
INDERIDE; 40/25; I	Inderide	25 mg ; 40 mg	Off-White	Tablet	Six-Sided	Wyeth Pharmaceuticals
INDERIDE; 80/25; I	Inderide	80 mg ; 25 mg	Off-White	Tablet	Six-Sided, Scored	Wyeth Pharmaceuticals
INDOCIN MSD 25	Indocin	25 mg	Opaque Blue and White	Capsule		Merck & Company
INDOCIN MSD 50	Indocin	50 mg	Opaque Blue and White	Capsule		Merck & Company
IP 146	Reprexain	5 mg ; 200 mg	White	Tablet	Oval	Watson Laboratories
ISMO 20	Ismo	20 mg	Orange	Tablet	Circle	Wyeth Pharmaceuticals
IU ; NVR	Tekturna	300 mg	Light Red	Tablet	Oval	Novartis Pharmaceuticals
J; 19	Potassium Permanganate	300 mg		Tablet		Eli Lilly
J; 37	Phenobarbital	60 mg	White	Tablet	Circle	Eli Lilly
J; 94	Tapazole	5 mg	White	Tablet	Circle, Scored	Jones Pharma
J; 95	Tapazole	10 mg	White	Tablet	Scored, Circle	Jones Pharma
J05	Caffeine, Citrated	65 mg		Tablet		Eli Lilly
JANSSEN ; G4 ;	Razadyne	4 mg	Off-White	Tablet		Ortho-Mcneil Neurologics
JANSSEN ; G8	Razadyne	8 mg	Pink	Tablet		Ortho-Mcneil Neurologics
JANSSEN ; G12 ;	Razadyne	12 mg	Orange-Brown	Tablet		Ortho-Mcneil Neurologics
JANSSEN R 1	Risperdal	1 mg	White	Tablet		Janssen Pharmaceutica Products
JANSSEN R 2	Risperdal	2 mg	Orange	Tablet		Janssen Pharmaceutica Products
JANSSEN R 3	Risperdal	3 mg	Yellow	Tablet		Janssen Pharmaceutica Products
JANSSEN R 4	Risperdal	4 mg	Green	Tablet		Janssen Pharmaceutica Products
JANSSEN RIS 0.25	Risperdal	0.25 mg	Dark Yellow	Tablet		Janssen Pharmaceutica Products
JANSSEN RIS 0.5	Risperdal	0.5 mg	Red-Brown	Tablet		Janssen Pharmaceutica Products
JANSSEN; AST; 10	Hismanal	10 mg	White	Tablet		Janssen Pharmaceutica Products
JANSSEN; CIS; 10	Prepulsid	10 mg		Tablet		Janssen Pharmaceutica Products
JANSSEN; IMODIUM	Imodium	2 mg	Light Green and Dark Green	Capsule		Mcneil Consumer Healthcare Division of Mcneil
JANSSEN; L; 50	Ergamisol	50 mg	White	Coated Tablet		Janssen Pharmaceutica Products
JANSSEN; NIZORAL	Nizoral	200 mg	White	Tablet		Janssen Pharmaceutica Products
JANSSEN; P; 10	Propulsid	10 mg	White	Tablet	Circle, Small, Scored	Janssen Pharmaceutica Products
JANSSEN; P; 20	Propulsid	20 mg	Blue	Tablet	Oval	Janssen Pharmaceutica Products
JANSSEN; R; 2	Risperdal	2 mg	Orange	Tablet		Janssen Pharmaceutica Products

IMPRINT	BRAND/GENERIC NAME	STRENGTH	COLOR	FORM	SHAPE	MANUFACTURER
JANSSEN; R; 3	Risperdal	3 mg	Yellow	Tablet		Janssen Pharmaceutica Products
JANSSEN; R; 4	Risperdal	4 mg	Green	Tablet		Janssen Pharmaceutica Products
JANSSEN; SPORANOX; 100	Sporanox	100 mg	Blue and Pink	Capsule		Janssen Pharmaceutica Products
JDS	Stavzor	125 mg	Orange	Capsule, Delayed Release	Oval	Jds Pharmaceuticals
JDS1	Stavzor	250 mg	Orange	Capsule, Delayed Release	Oval	Jds Pharmaceuticals
JDS2	Stavzor	500 mg	Orange	Capsule, Delayed Release	Oval	Jds Pharmaceuticals
JMI; 626	Thyroid Strong 0.5 grain	0.75 Gr	Orange or Reddish Brown	Coated Tablet		Western Research Laboratories
JMI; 627	Thyroid Strong 1 grain	1.5 Gr	Orange or Reddish Brown	Coated Tablet		Western Research Laboratories
JMI; 628	Thyroid Strong 2 grains	3 Gr	Red or Reddish Brown	Coated Tablet		Western Research Laboratories
JMI; 629	Thyroid Strong 3 grains	4.5 Gr	Red or Reddish Brown	Coated Tablet		Western Research Laboratories
JMI; 674	Thyroid Strong 1 grain Natural	1.5 Gr	Tan	Tablet	Compressed	Western Research Laboratories
JMI; 675	Thyroid Strong 2 grains Natural	3 Gr	Tan	Tablet	Compressed	Western Research Laboratories
JMI; 686	Thyroid Strong 0.5 grain Natural	0.75 Gr	Tan	Tablet	Compressed	Western Research Laboratories
JMI; APT	Thyroid with Pituitary	194.4 mg ;	Lemon Yellow	Coated Tablet	Circle	Western Research Laboratories
JMI; D16	Cytomel	25 mcg	White	Tablet	Circle	Jones Pharma
JSP; 513	Unithroid	25 mcg	Peach	Tablet	Round, Partially Bisected Scored	Watson Laboratories
JSP; 514	Unithroid	50 mcg	White	Tablet	Round, Partially Bisected Scored	Watson Laboratories
JSP; 515	Unithroid	75 mcg	Purple	Tablet	Round, Partially Bisected Scored	Watson Laboratories
JSP; 516	Unithroid	100 mcg	Yellow	Tablet	Round, Partially Bisected Scored	Watson Laboratories
JSP; 519	Unithroid	125 mcg	Tan	Tablet	Round, Partially Bisected Scored	Watson Laboratories
JSP; 520	Unithroid	150 mcg	Blue	Tablet	Round, Partially Bisected Scored	Watson Laboratories
JSP; 522	Unithroid	200 mcg	Pink	Tablet	Round, Partially Bisected Scored	Watson Laboratories
JSP; 523	Unithroid	300 mcg	Green	Tablet	Round, Partially Bisected Scored	Watson Laboratories
JSP; 561	Unithroid	88 mcg	Olive	Tablet	Round, Partially Bisected Scored	Watson Laboratories
JSP; 562	Unithroid	112 mcg	Rose	Tablet	Round, Partially Bisected Scored	Watson Laboratories
JSP; 563	Unithroid	175 mcg	Lilac	Tablet	Round, Partially Bisected Scored	Watson Laboratories
JSP; 873	Thyrox	25 mcg	Peach	Tablet		Watson Laboratories
JSP; 874	Thyrox	50 mcg	White	Tablet		Watson Laboratories
JSP; 875	Thyrox	75 mcg	Purple	Tablet		Watson Laboratories
JSP; 876	Thyrox	88 mcg	Olive	Tablet		Watson Laboratories
JSP; 877	Thyrox	100 mcg	Yellow	Tablet		Watson Laboratories
JSP; 878	Thyrox	112 mcg	Rose	Tablet		Watson Laboratories
JSP; 879	Thyrox	125 mcg	Tan	Tablet		Watson Laboratories
JSP; 880	Thyrox	150 mcg	Blue	Tablet		Watson Laboratories
JSP; 881	Thyrox	175 mcg	Lilac	Tablet		Watson Laboratories
JSP; 882	Thyrox	200 mcg	Pink	Tablet		Watson Laboratories
JSP; 883	Thyrox	300 mcg	Green	Tablet		Watson Laboratories
K	Clarinex Reditabs	2.5 mg	Light Red	Tablet, Disintegrating		Schering-Plough
K ; 201	Oxandrolone	10 mg	White	Tablet	Capsule-Shape	Par Pharmaceutical
K ; 250	Tranylcypromine Sulfate	10 mg	Red	Tablet	Circle	Par Pharmaceutical
K 400 ;	Glycopyrrolate	1 mg	White	Tablet	Circle	Par Pharmaceutical
K 401 ;	Glycopyrrolate	2 mg	White	Tablet	Circle	Par Pharmaceutical
K; U	Levsin Forte	0.25 mg	White	Tablet		Schwarz Pharma
K1	Kytril	1 mg	White	Tablet	Triangle	Roche Laboratories
K5	Clonazepam Odt	0.125 mg	White	Tablet, Disintegrating	Circle	Par Pharmaceutical
K6	Clonazepam Odt	0.25 mg	White	Tablet, Disintegrating	Circle	Par Pharmaceutical
K7	Clonazepam Odt	0.5 mg	White	Tablet, Disintegrating	Circle	Par Pharmaceutical
K8	Clonazepam Odt	1 mg	White	Tablet, Disintegrating	Circle	Par Pharmaceutical
K9	Clonazepam Odt	2 mg	White	Tablet, Disintegrating	Circle	Par Pharmaceutical
KADIAN 10 MG	Kadian	10 mg	Light Blue Opaque	Capsule, Extended Release		Alpharma Branded Products Division
KADIAN 20 MG	Kadian	20 mg	Yellow Opaque	Capsule, Extended Release		Alpharma Branded Products Division
KADIAN 30 MG	Kadian	30 mg	Blue Violet Opaque	Capsule, Extended Release		Alpharma Branded Products Division
KADIAN 50 MG	Kadian	50 mg	Blue Opaque	Capsule, Extended Release		Alpharma Branded Products Division
KADIAN 60 MG	Kadian	60 mg	Pink Opaque	Capsule, Extended Release		Alpharma Branded Products Division
KADIAN 80 MG	Kadian	80 mg	Light Orange Opaque	Capsule, Extended Release		Alpharma Branded Products Division
KADIAN 100 MG	Kadian	100 mg	Green Opaque	Capsule, Extended Release		Alpharma Branded Products Division
KADIAN 200 MG	Kadian	200 mg	Light Brown Opaque	Capsule, Extended Release		Alpharma Branded Products Division
KALI ; 083	Tramadol Hydrochloride and Acetaminophen	325 mg ; 37.5 mg	Orange	Tablet	Capsule-Shape	Par Pharmaceutical
KC; M10	Klor-Con M10	10 meq	White	Extended-Release Tablet	Oblong	Upsher-Smith Laboratories
KC; M20	Klor-Con M20	20 meq	White	Extended-Release Tablet	Oblong, Scored	Upsher-Smith Laboratories
KC; M20	Klor-Con M20	1500 mg	White	Tablet	Oblong	Upsher-Smith Laboratories
KEFLEX 333 MG	Keflex	333 mg	Opaque Light Green	Capsule		Advancis Pharmaceutical
KEMADRIN; S3A	Kemadrin	5 mg	White	Tablet		Glaxosmithkline
KERLONE; 10	Kerlone	10 mg	White	Tablet	Circle	Sanofi-Aventis U.S.
KERLONE; 20; B	Kerlone	20 mg	White	Tablet	Circle	Sanofi-Aventis U.S.
KLOR-CON 10	Klor-Con 10	750 mg	Yellow	Coated Tablet	Circle	Upsher-Smith Laboratories
KLOR-CON; 8	Klor-Con 8	600 mg	Blue	Coated Tablet	Circle, Bevel-Edged	Upsher-Smith Laboratories
KLOTRIX; BL; 10MEQ; 770	Klotrix	750 mg	Orange	Timed-Release Tablet	Circle	Bristol-Myers Squibb
KPH; 102	Azulfidine En-Tabs	500 mg	Gold	Enteric-Coated Tablet	Oval	Pharmacia & Upjohn

IMPRINT	BRAND/GENERIC NAME	STRENGTH	COLOR	FORM	SHAPE	MANUFACTURER
KPI/283 ; CORZIDE 40/5 ;	Corzide 40/5	40 mg ; 5 mg	White to Bluish White with Dark Blue Specks	Tablet	Circle	King Pharmaceuticals
KPI/284 ; CORZIDE 80/5 ;	Corzide 80/5	80 mg ; 5 mg	White to Bluish White with Dark Blue Specks	Tablet	Circle	King Pharmaceuticals
KPI; 1	Acetaminophen and Hydrocodone Bitartrate	500 mg ; 5 mg		Tablet		King Pharmaceuticals
KPI; 2	Acetaminophen and Hydrocodone Bitartrate	7.5 mg ; 750 mg	Light Blue	Tablet	Circle	King Pharmaceuticals
KPI115 ; KPI 115	Cytomel	5 mcg	White to Off-White	Tablet	Circle	King Pharmaceuticals
KPI116 ; KPI 116	Cytomel	25 mcg	White to Off-White	Tablet	Circle	King Pharmaceuticals
KPI117 ; KPI 117	Cytomel	50 mcg	White to Off-White	Tablet	Circle	King Pharmaceuticals
KREMERS URBAN; 320	Nitrocine Timecaps	2.5 mg	Violet and Clear	Sustained-Release Capsule		Schwarz Pharma
KREMERS URBAN; 330	Nitrocine Timecaps	6.5 mg	Blue and Orange	Sustained-Release Capsule		Schwarz Pharma
KREMERS URBAN; 340	Nitrocine Timecaps	9 mg	Clear	Sustained-Release Capsule		Schwarz Pharma
KU; 114	Omeprazole	10 mg	White	Delayed-Release Capsule		Schwarz Pharma
KU; 118	Omeprazole	20 mg	White and Gold	Delayed-Release Capsule		Schwarz Pharma
L ; I	Lorazepam	0.5 mg	White	Tablet	Circle	Teva Pharmaceuticals
L 4 ; M	Levothyroxine Sodium	25 mcg	Orange	Tablet	Capsule-Shape	Mylan Pharmaceuticals
L 5 ; M	Levothyroxine Sodium	50 mcg	White	Tablet	Capsule-Shape	Mylan Pharmaceuticals
L 6 ; M	Levothyroxine Sodium	75 mcg	Violet	Tablet	Capsule-Shape	Mylan Pharmaceuticals
L 7 ; M	Levothyroxine Sodium	88 mcg	Olive	Tablet	Capsule-Shape	Mylan Pharmaceuticals
L 8 ; M	Levothyroxine Sodium	100 mcg	Yellow	Tablet	Capsule-Shape	Mylan Pharmaceuticals
L 9 ; M	Levothyroxine Sodium	112 mcg	Rose	Tablet	Capsule-Shape	Mylan Pharmaceuticals
L 10 ; M	Levothyroxine Sodium	125 mcg	Gray	Tablet	Capsule-Shape	Mylan Pharmaceuticals
L 11 ; M	Levothyroxine Sodium	150 mcg	Blue	Tablet	Capsule-Shape	Mylan Pharmaceuticals
L 12 ; M	Levothyroxine Sodium	175 mcg	Lilac	Tablet	Capsule-Shape	Mylan Pharmaceuticals
L 13 ; M	Levothyroxine Sodium	200 mcg	Pink	Tablet	Capsule-Shape	Mylan Pharmaceuticals
L 14 ; M	Levothyroxine Sodium	300 mcg	Green	Tablet	Capsule-Shape	Mylan Pharmaceuticals
L 15 ; M	Levothyroxine Sodium	137 mcg	Turquoise	Tablet	Capsule-Shape	Mylan Pharmaceuticals
L; 9; LL	Ledercillin VK	500 mg	White	Tablet	Round, Convex, Bisected Scored	Lederle Laboratories
L; 10; LL	Ledercillin VK	250 mg	White	Tablet	Round, Convex, Bisected Scored	Lederle Laboratories
L3 ; IT	Boniva	2.5 mg	White	Tablet	Oblong	Roche Laboratories
LAMICTAL; 25	Lamictal	25 mg	White	Tablet	Shield-Shape	Glaxosmithkline
LAMICTAL; 100	Lamictal	100 mg	Peach	Tablet	Shield-Shape	Glaxosmithkline
LAMICTAL; 150	Lamictal	150 mg	Cream	Tablet	Shield-Shape	Glaxosmithkline
LAMICTAL; 200	Lamictal	200 mg	Blue	Tablet	Shield-Shape	Glaxosmithkline
LANOXIN; T9A	Lanoxin	0.5 mg	Green	Tablet	Circle, Scored	Glaxosmithkline
LANOXIN; X3A	Lanoxin	0.25 mg	White	Tablet	Circle, Scored	Glaxosmithkline
LANOXIN; Y3B	Lanoxin	0.125 mg	Yellow	Tablet	Circle, Scored	Glaxosmithkline
LARIAM; 250; ROCHE	Lariam	250 mg	White	Tablet	Circle, Scored	Roche Pharmaceuticals
LAROBEC; ROCHE	Larobec	100 mg ; 18 mg ; 0.5 mg ; 500 mg ; 15 mg ; 15 mg ; 5 mcg	Orange	Coated Tablet	Oblong	Roche Pharmaceuticals
LARODOPA; ROCHE; 100	Larodopa	100 mg	Pink and Scarlet	Capsule		Roche Pharmaceuticals
LARODOPA; ROCHE; 250	Larodopa	250 mg	Pink and Beige	Capsule		Roche Pharmaceuticals
LARODOPA; ROCHE; 500	Larodopa	500 mg	Pink	Capsule		Roche Pharmaceuticals
LAROTID; 500; BMP; 212	Larotid	500 mg	Buff	Capsule		Glaxosmithkline
LASIX; 40; HOECHST	Lasix	40 mg	White	Tablet	Circle	Sanofi-Aventis U.S.
LASIX; 80; HOECHST	Lasix	80 mg	White	Tablet	Circle	Sanofi-Aventis U.S.
LBS01	Inversine	2.5 mg	Yellow	Tablet	Circle	Targacept
LCE 50	Stalevo 50	12.5 mg ; 50 mg ; 200 mg	Brownish or Greyish-Red	Tablet	Circle	Novartis Pharmaceuticals
LCE 100	Stalevo 100	25 mg ; 100 mg ; 200 mg	Brownish or Greyish-Red	Tablet	Oval	Novartis Pharmaceuticals
LCE 150	Stalevo 150	150 mg ; 200 mg ; 37.5 mg	Brownish or Greyish-Red	Tablet	Oblong	Novartis Pharmaceuticals
LCE 200	Stalevo 200	50 mg ; 200 mg ; 200 mg	Dark Brownish Red	Tablet	Oval	Novartis Pharmaceuticals
LCI ; NVR	Tekturna HCT	150 mg ; 12.5 mg	White	Tablet	Oval	Novartis
LDT	Tyzeka	600 mg	White to Slightly Yellow	Tablet	Oval	Novartis Pharmaceuticals
LE	Tridione	150 mg	White	Tablet, Chewable		Abbott Laboratories
LEDERLE; A; 20	Acetaminophen	500 mg	Blue	Capsule		Lederle Laboratories
LEDERLE; A3; 250 MG	Achromycin V	250 mg	Yellow and Blue	Capsule		Lederle Laboratories
LEDERLE; A31	Ampicillin Trihydrate	250 mg	Green and White	Capsule		Lederle Laboratories
LEDERLE; A32	Ampicillin Trihydrate	500 mg	Green and White	Capsule		Lederle Laboratories
LEDERLE; A33	Amoxicillin	250 mg	Grey and Green	Capsule		Lederle Laboratories
LEDERLE; A34	Amoxicillin	500 mg	Gray and Green	Capsule		Lederle Laboratories
LEDERLE; C; 61	Cephradine	250 mg	Green and Light Pink	Capsule		Lederle Laboratories
LEDERLE; C; 62	Cephradine	500 mg	Light Green	Capsule		Lederle Laboratories
LEDERLE; C54; CEFACLOR; 250MG	Cefaclor	250 mg	Opaque Pink and Blue	Capsule		Lederle Laboratories
LEDERLE; C55	Clorazepate Dipotassium	3.75 mg	White and Lavender	Capsule		Lederle Laboratories
LEDERLE; C56	Clorazepate Dipotassium	7.5 mg	Lavender and Maroon	Capsule		Lederle Laboratories
LEDERLE; C57	Clorazepate Dipotassium	15 mg	Lavender	Capsule		Lederle Laboratories

IMPRINT	BRAND/GENERIC NAME	STRENGTH	COLOR	FORM	SHAPE	MANUFACTURER
LEDERLE; C58; CEFACLOR; 500MG	Cefaclor	500 mg	Opaque Lavender and Blue	Capsule		Lederle Laboratories
LEDERLE; D16	Dicloxacillin Sodium	250 mg	Green	Capsule		Lederle Laboratories
LEDERLE; D17	Dicloxacillin Sodium	500 mg	Light Green	Capsule		Lederle Laboratories
LEDERLE; D25	Doxycycline Hyclate	100 mg	Blue	Capsule		Lederle Laboratories
LEDERLE; D36	Dolene	65 mg	Pink	Capsule		Lederle Laboratories
LEDERLE; D47	Doxepin Hydrochloride	25 mg	Ivory and Yellow	Capsule		Lederle Laboratories
LEDERLE; D48	Doxepin Hydrochloride	50 mg	Lavendar and Dark Red	Capsule		Lederle Laboratories
LEDERLE; D49	Doxepin Hydrochloride	75 mg	Purple and Dark Pink	Capsule		Lederle Laboratories
LEDERLE; D50	Doxepin Hydrochloride	10 mg	Buff or Blue	Capsule		Lederle Laboratories
LEDERLE; D54	Doxepin Hydrochloride	100 mg	Green and White	Capsule		Lederle Laboratories
LEDERLE; D55	Doxepin Hydrochloride	150 mg	Gray and Orange	Capsule		Lederle Laboratories
LEDERLE; D62	Disopyramide	100 mg	Dark Red and Blue	Capsule		Lederle Laboratories
LEDERLE; I19	Indomethacin	25 mg	Pink and White	Capsule		Lederle Laboratories
LEDERLE; I20 ;	Indomethacin	50 mg	Opaque Pink and Opaque White	Capsule		Lederle Laboratories
LEDERLE; K1	Ketoprofen	25 mg	Dark Green	Capsule		Lederle Laboratories
LEDERLE; K2	Ketoprofen	50 mg	Light Green	Capsule		Lederle Laboratories
LEDERLE; K3	Ketoprofen	75 mg	White	Capsule		Lederle Laboratories
LEDERLE; O; P69	Prazosin Hydrochloride	1 mg	Flesh	Capsule		Lederle Laboratories
LEDERLE; O; P70	Prazosin Hydrochloride	2 mg	Pink	Capsule		Lederle Laboratories
LEDERLE; O; P71	Prazosin Hydrochloride	5 mg	Blue	Capsule		Lederle Laboratories
LEDERLE;C2; CENTRUM JR	Centrum JR. Plus Iron	10 mg ; 10 mcg ; 50 mg ; 108 mg ; 18 mg ; 5000 IU ; 400 IU ; 30 IU ; 60 mg ; 400 mcg ; 1.5 mg ; 1.7 mg ; 20 mg ; 2 mg ; 6 mcg ; 40 mg ; 2 mg ; 15 mg ; 1 mg ; 45 mcg ; 150 mg ; 20 mcg ; 20 mcg	Various	Tablet, Chewable	Oval	Wyeth Consumer Healthcare
LEMMON	Dralserp	25 mg ; 0.1 mg	Orange	Tablet		Teva Pharmaceuticals
LEMMON	Promethazine Hydrochloride	25 mg	Blue	Tablet	Circle, Convex, Scored	Teva Pharmaceuticals
LEMMON; 30	Neothylline	200 mg	White	Tablet	Circle, Convex, Scored	Teva Pharmaceuticals
LEMMON; 37	Neothylline	400 mg	White	Tablet	Oblong, Scored	Teva Pharmaceuticals
LEMMON; 52	Uristat	50 mg ; 0.03 mg ; 5 mg ; 0.03 mg ; 5.5 mg ; 20 mg	Blue	Tablet		Teva Pharmaceuticals
LEMMON; 71; 71	Statobex	35 mg	Green and White	Tablet	Oblong, Convex; Scored	Teva Pharmaceuticals
LEMMON; 77	Statobex-G	35 mg	Green	Tablet	Oblong, Scored	Teva Pharmaceuticals
LEMMON; 86; 86	S.B.P.	50 mg ; 30 mg ; 15 mg	White	Tablet	Circle, Flat, Beveled Edge, Scored	Teva Pharmaceuticals
LEMMON; 93-10; GLUCAMIDE; 100	Glucamide	100 mg	Blue	Tablet	Circle, Convex, Scored	Teva Pharmaceuticals
LEMMON; 93-7; GLUCAMIDE; 250	Glucamide	250 mg	Blue	Tablet	Circle, Convex, Scored	Teva Pharmaceuticals
LEMMON; 105	Dralzine	25 mg	Yellow	Tablet	Oblong	Teva Pharmaceuticals
LEMMON; 123	Sed-Tens S.E.	10 mg	Red and White Speckled	Tablet	Oblong	Teva Pharmaceuticals
LEMMON; 128 128	Neothylline GG	200 mg ; 200 mg	White	Tablet	Circle, Flat, Beveled Edge, Scored	Teva Pharmaceuticals
LEMMON; 133	Dexampex	15 mg	Green Transparent and Clear	Capsule		Teva Pharmaceuticals
LEMMON; 137	Dipav	150 mg	Brown and Clear	Capsule		Teva Pharmaceuticals
LEMMON; 169	B.P.P.	1.2 mg ; 120 mg ; 15 mg ; 120 mg ; 15 mg	Yellow	Tablet	Circle, Convex	Teva Pharmaceuticals
LEMMON; 178 178	Methampex	10 mg	Pink	Tablet	Oblong, Scored	Teva Pharmaceuticals
LEMMON; 179	Dexampex	15 mg	Blue	Tablet	Oblong	Teva Pharmaceuticals
LEMMON; 180	Dexampex	10 mg	Pink	Tablet	Oblong	Teva Pharmaceuticals
LEMMON; 211	Lexor	50 mg	Peach	Tablet		Teva Pharmaceuticals
LEMMON; 238	Diacin	200 mg	Red and Clear with Red and White Pellets Inside	Capsule		Teva Pharmaceuticals
LEMMON; 277	Statobex	35 mg	Green and White, Opaque	Capsule		Teva Pharmaceuticals
LEMMON; 341	Ruhexatal with Reserpine	30 mg ; 10 mg ; 0.1 mg ; 20 mg		Tablet		Teva Pharmaceuticals
LESCOL XL; 80	Lescol XL	80 mg	Yellow	Extended-Release Tablet	Circle	Novartis
LEVAQUIN; 250	Levaquin	250 mg	Terra Cotta Pink	Coated Tablet		Ortho-Mcneil Pharmaceutical
LEVAQUIN; 500	Levaquin	500 mg	Peach	Coated Tablet		Ortho-Mcneil Pharmaceutical
LEVAQUIN; 750	Levaquin	750 mg	White	Coated Tablet	Rectangle, Modified	Ortho-Mcneil Pharmaceutical
LEVO-DROMORAN; ROCHE ;	Levo-Dromoran	2 mg	White	Tablet	Circle, Scored, Beveled	Valeant Pharmaceuticals
LEXXEL 2; 5-2.5	Lexxel	5 mg ; 2.5 mg	White	Extended-Release Tablet	Circle, Biconvex, Film-Coated	Astrazeneca
LEXXEL; 1; 5-5	Lexxel	5 mg ; 5 mg	White	Extended-Release Tablet	Circle	Astrazeneca
LIBRAX; ICN ;	Librax	5 mg ; 2.5 mg	Blue-Green	Capsule, Liquid Filled		Valeant Pharmaceuticals
LIBRITABS; 5; ROCHE	Libritabs	5 mg	Green	Coated Tablet	Circle, Scored	Roche Products
LIBRITABS; 10; ROCHE	Libritabs	10 mg	Green	Coated Tablet	Scored, Circle	Roche Products
LIBRITABS; 25; ROCHE	Libritabs	25 mg	Green	Coated Tablet	Circle, Scored	Roche Products
LIBRIUM 5; ROCHE	Librium	5 mg	Green and Yellow	Capsule		Valeant Pharmaceuticals
LIBRIUM 10; ROCHE	Librium	10 mg	Green and Black	Capsule		Valeant Pharmaceuticals
LIBRIUM 25; ROCHE	Librium	25 mg	Green and White	Capsule		Valeant Pharmaceuticals
LILLY 3230 3/25	Symbyax	3 mg ; 25 mg	Light Yellow, Peach	Capsule		Eli Lilly

IMPRINT	BRAND/GENERIC NAME	STRENGTH	COLOR	FORM	SHAPE	MANUFACTURER
LILLY 3231 6/25	Symbyax	6 mg ; 25 mg	Light Yellow, Mustard Yellow	Capsule		Eli Lilly
LILLY 3232 12/25	Symbyax	12 mg ; 25 mg	Light Yellow, Red	Capsule		Eli Lilly
LILLY 3233 6/50	Symbyax	50 mg ; 6 mg	Light Grey, Mustard Yellow	Capsule		Eli Lilly
LILLY 3234 12/50	Symbyax	12 mg ; 50 mg	Light Grey, Red	Capsule		Eli Lilly
LILLY 3239 ; 60 MG	Strattera	60 mg	Blue, Gold	Capsule		Eli Lilly
LILLY F04 ; LILLY F04	Seromycin	250 mg	Opaque Gray, Opaque Red	Capsule		Eli Lilly
LILLY F40	Seconal	100 mg	Orange or Red	Capsule		Eli Lilly
LILLY T03	Novacebrin with Fluoride	2.5 mg ; 1 mg ; 1.2 mg ; 10 mcg ; 60 mg ; 1.5 mg ; 2 mg ; 1 mg ; 3 mcg ; 12 mg	Orange	Tablet, Chewable		Eli Lilly
LILLY; 3004; 90 MG	Prozac Weekly	90 mg	Green and Clear with White Enteric-Coated Pellets	Timed-Release Capsule		Eli Lilly
LILLY; 3061	Ceclor	250 mg	White and Purple	Capsule		Eli Lilly
LILLY; 3062	Ceclor	500 mg	Gray and Purple	Capsule		Eli Lilly
LILLY; 3110; DARVON COMP	Darvon Compound	389 mg ; 32.4 mg ; 32 mg	Pink and Gray	Capsule		Eli Lilly
LILLY; 3111; DARVON COMP 65	Darvon Compound 65	32.4 mg ; 65 mg ; 389 mg	Red and Grey	Capsule		Eli Lilly
LILLY; 3132; PINDAC; 12.5	Pindac	12.5 mg	Blue and Clear with Orange Beads	Capsule		Eli Lilly
LILLY; 3133; PINDAC; 25	Pindac	25 mg	Blue and Clear with White Beads	Capsule		Eli Lilly
LILLY; 3170	Lorabid Pulvules	200 mg	Blue and Gray	Capsule		Monarch Pharmaceuticals
LILLY; 3210; 10 MG	Sarafem	10 mg	Lavender	Capsule		Warner Chilcott
LILLY; 3220; 20 MG	Sarafem	20 mg	Lavender, Pink	Capsule		Warner Chilcott
LILLY; 4112	Zyprexa	2.5 mg	White	Tablet	Circle	Eli Lilly
LILLY; 4115	Zyprexa	5 mg	White	Tablet	Circle	Eli Lilly
LILLY; 4116	Zyprexa	7.5 mg	White	Tablet	Circle	Eli Lilly
LILLY; 4117	Zyprexa	10 mg	White	Tablet	Circle	Eli Lilly
LILLY; 4165	Evista	60 mg	White with Blue Ink	Tablet	Circle	Eli Lilly
LILLY; 4415	Zyprexa	15 mg	Blue	Tablet	Egg-Shape	Eli Lilly
LILLY; 4420	Zyprexa	20 mg	Pink	Tablet	Egg-Shape	Eli Lilly
LILLY; A01	Ammonium Chloride	500 mg		Sustained-Release Tablet		Eli Lilly
LILLY; A02	Ferrous Sulfate	325 mg	Red	Sustained-Release Tablet		Eli Lilly
LILLY; A04	Pancreatin, Triple Strength	1 G		Sustained-Release Tablet		Eli Lilly
LILLY; A05	Potassium Chloride	300 mg		Tablet		Eli Lilly
LILLY; A06	Potassium Iodide	300 mg		Enteric-Coated Tablet		Eli Lilly
LILLY; A09	Sodium Chloride	1 GM		Enteric-Coated Tablet		Eli Lilly
LILLY; A10	Sodium Salicylate	325 mg		Coated Tablet		Eli Lilly
LILLY; A11	Sodium Salicylate	650 mg		Enteric-Coated Tablet		Eli Lilly
LILLY; A12	Ammonium Chloride	15 Gr		Sustained-Release Tablet		Eli Lilly
LILLY; A14	Thyroid	30 mg		Enteric-Coated Tablet		Eli Lilly
LILLY; A15	Thyroid	60 mg		Enteric-Coated Tablet		Eli Lilly
LILLY; A16	Thyroid	120 mg		Enteric-Coated Tablet		Eli Lilly
LILLY; A17	Thyroid	200 mg		Enteric-Coated Tablet		Eli Lilly
LILLY; A25	A.S.A.	325 mg		Enteric-Coated Tablet		Eli Lilly
LILLY; A27	Amesec	25 mg ; 130 mg ; 25 mg		Sustained-Release Tablet		Eli Lilly
LILLY; A30	Aminosalicylic Acid	500 mg		Sustained-Release Tablet		Eli Lilly
LILLY; A31	Potassium Chloride	1 GM		Enteric-Coated Tablet		Eli Lilly
LILLY; A32	A.S.A.	650 mg		Enteric-Coated Tablet		Eli Lilly
LILLY; A36	Ferrous Sulfate	325 mg	Green	Sustained-Release Tablet		Eli Lilly
LILLY; A39	Quinidine Sulfate	200 mg		Enteric-Coated Tablet		Eli Lilly
LILLY; B51	Alphalin	7.5 mg		Capsule		Eli Lilly
LILLY; B52	Alphalin	15 mg		Capsule		Eli Lilly
LILLY; B60	Deltalin	1.25 mg		Capsule, Liquid Filled		Eli Lilly
LILLY; C06	Cascara	325 mg	Chocolate	Coated Tablet		Eli Lilly
LILLY; C07	Cascara Compound	10 mg ; 8 mg ; 4 mg ; 16 mg ; 16 mg	Pink	Coated Tablet		Eli Lilly
LILLY; C11	Rhinitis, Full Strength	32.5 mg ; 32.5 mg ; 5.8 mg	Chocolate	Coated Tablet		Eli Lilly
LILLY; C13	Ferrous Sulfate	325 mg	Chocolate	Coated Tablet		Eli Lilly
LILLY; C27	V-Cillin K	125 mg	White	Tablet		Eli Lilly
LILLY; C29	V-Cillin K	250 mg	White	Tablet		Eli Lilly
LILLY; C31	Anhydron K	2 mg ; 500 mg		Coated Tablet		Eli Lilly
LILLY; C32	Anhydron Kr	2 mg ; 500 mg ; 0.25 mg		Coated Tablet		Eli Lilly
LILLY; C36	Quinine Sulfate	325 mg	Chocolate	Coated Tablet		Eli Lilly
LILLY; C46	V-Cillin K	500 mg	White	Tablet		Eli Lilly
LILLY; C47	Hepicebrin	1.5 mg ; 10 mcg ; 20 mg ; 75 mg ; 2 mg ; 3 mg		Coated Tablet		Eli Lilly
LILLY; C71	Multi-Cebrin	3 mg ; 25 mcg ; 3 mg ; 3 mg ; 1.2 mg ; 3 mcg ; 75 mg ; 5 mg ; 25 mg ; 6 mg	Dark Red	Tablet		Eli Lilly

IMPRINT	BRAND/GENERIC NAME	STRENGTH	COLOR	FORM	SHAPE	MANUFACTURER
LILLY; DARVOCET-N 50	Darvocet-N 50	325 mg ; 50 mg	Dark Orange	Coated Tablet	Capsule-Shape	Eli Lilly
LILLY; DARVOCET-N 100	Darvocet-N 100	650 mg ; 100 mg	Dark Orange	Coated Tablet	Capsule-Shape	Eli Lilly
LILLY; DARVON-N; 100 ;	Darvon-N	100 mg	Buff	Tablet	Oblong	Eli Lilly
LILLY; DARVON-N; ASA	Darvon-N with A.S.A.	100 mg ; 325 mg	Orange	Tablet	Circle	Eli Lilly
LILLY; F09	Seromycin with Isoniazid	150 mg ; 250 mg		Capsule		Eli Lilly
LILLY; F11 ;	A.S.A.	325 mg	Clear or Pink	Capsule		Eli Lilly
LILLY; F13	A.S.A. Compound	227 mg ; 32.5 mg ; 160 mg	White Opaque	Capsule		Eli Lilly
LILLY; F14	Ephedrine and Amytal	25 mg ; 50 mg	Yellow	Capsule		Eli Lilly
LILLY; F20	Ephedrine and Seconal Sodium	25 mg ; 50 mg	Scarlet	Capsule		Eli Lilly
LILLY; F23	Amytal Sodium No. 4	65 mg	Blue	Capsule		Eli Lilly
LILLY; F24	Ephedrine Sulfate	25 mg	Pink	Capsule		Eli Lilly
LILLY; F25	Ephedrine Sulfate	50 mg	Pink	Capsule		Eli Lilly
LILLY; F26	Quinine Sulfate	130 mg	White Opaque	Capsule		Eli Lilly
LILLY; F27	Quinine Sulfate	200 mg	White Opaque	Capsule		Eli Lilly
LILLY; F29	Quinine Sulfate	325 mg	White Opaque	Capsule		Eli Lilly
LILLY; F30	A.S.A. Compound	227 mg ; 160 mg ; 32.5 mg	Pink	Capsule		Eli Lilly
LILLY; F33	Amytal Sodium No. 2	200 mg	Blue	Capsule		Eli Lilly
LILLY; F36	Copavin	15 mg ; 15 mg	Clear	Capsule		Eli Lilly
LILLY; F39	Quinidine Sulfate	200 mg		Capsule		Eli Lilly
LILLY; F41	Bilron	300 mg	Green	Capsule		Eli Lilly
LILLY; F42	Seconal Sodium	50 mg	Red	Capsule		Eli Lilly
LILLY; F45	Epragen	227 mg ; 50 mg ; 22 mg ; 130 mg	Yellow and Brown	Capsule		Eli Lilly
LILLY; F47	Amesec	130 mg ; 25 mg ; 25 mg	Blue and Orange	Capsule		Eli Lilly
LILLY; F50	A.S.A. and Codeine, No. 2	230 mg ; 30 mg ; 15 mg ; 150 mg	White and Light Gray	Capsule		Eli Lilly
LILLY; F51	A.S.A. and Codeine, No. 3	230 mg ; 30 mg ; 30 mg ; 150 mg	White and Dark Gray	Capsule		Eli Lilly
LILLY; F52	Dibasic Calcium Phosphate with Vitamin D	500 mg ; 0.825 mg	Clear	Capsule		Eli Lilly
LILLY; F53	Trisogel	4 1/2 grains	Pink	Capsule		Eli Lilly
LILLY; F56	Calcium Gluconate with Vitamin D	325 mg ; 0.825 mcg	Opaque White	Capsule		Eli Lilly
LILLY; F57	Dicalcium Phosphate and Calcium Gluconate with Vitamin D	200 mg ; 8.25 mcg ; 290 mg	White Opaque	Capsule		Eli Lilly
LILLY; F61	Bilron	150 mg	Green	Capsule		Eli Lilly
LILLY; F63	Dicalcium Phosphate with Vitamin D and Iron	500 mg ; 33 IU ; 10 mg	Pink	Capsule		Eli Lilly
LILLY; F64	Tuinal	25 mg ; 25 mg	Blue and Orange	Capsule		Eli Lilly
LILLY; F67	A.S.A. and Codeine, No. 4	230 mg ; 30 mg ; 60 mg ; 150 mg	Dark Gray	Capsule		Eli Lilly
LILLY; F76	Prenalac	16.6 mg ; 2.5 mg ; 0.3 mg ; 1.7 mcg ; 2.5 mg ; 0.8 mg ; 1 mg ; 0.25 mg ; 0.5 mg ; 1.25 mcg	Pink and Light Blue	Capsule		Eli Lilly
LILLY; F97	CO-Elorine	8 mg	Yellow and Turquoise	Capsule		Eli Lilly
LILLY; G01	Alphalin	3 mg		Capsule		Eli Lilly
LILLY; H03; DARVON	Darvon	65 mg	Pink	Capsule	Capsule-Shape	Eli Lilly
LILLY; H04; DARVON; C; ASA	Darvon with Asa	65 mg ; 325 mg	Red and Light Pink	Capsule		Eli Lilly
LILLY; H10	En-Cebrin F	2 mg ; 1 mg ; 5 mcg ; 5 mg ; 50 mg ; 10 mcg ; 250 mg ; 30 mg ; 0.15 mg ; 1 mg ; 5 mg ; 1 mg ; 1.5 mg ; 1.2 mg ; 3 mg ; 2 mg ; 10 mg	Pink and Blue	Capsule		Eli Lilly
LILLY; H12	En-Cebrin	3 mg ; 2 mg ; 1.7 mg ; 5 mcg ; 50 mg ; 1.2 mg ; 10 mg ; 5 mg ; 10 mcg ; 250 mg ; 30 mg ; 0.15 mg ; 1 mg ; 5 mg ; 1 mg ; 1.5 mg	Pink and Blue	Capsule		Eli Lilly
LILLY; H13	Novrad	50 mg	Ivory and Light Brown	Capsule		Eli Lilly
LILLY; H14	Novrad	100 mg	Ivory and Light Brown	Capsule		Eli Lilly
LILLY; H15	Novrad with A.S.A.	50 mg ; 300 mg	Ivory and Dark Brown	Capsule		Eli Lilly
LILLY; H17	Aventyl	10 mg	White and Yellow	Capsule		Eli Lilly
LILLY; H19	Aventyl	25 mg	White and Yellow	Capsule		Eli Lilly
LILLY; H72	Theracebrin	150 mg ; 12.5 mg ; 7.5 mg ; 37.5 mcg ; 15 mg ; 10 mg ; 2.5 mg ; 10 mcg ; 150 mg ; 20 mg	Black	Capsule		Eli Lilly
LILLY; H91	Doloxene Compound	375 mg ; 30 mg ; 100 mg	Red and Gray	Capsule		Eli Lilly
LILLY; HO2	Darvon	32 mg	Light Pink	Capsule		Eli Lilly
LILLY; J01	Ammonium Chloride	325 mg		Tablet	Compressed	Eli Lilly
LILLY; J02	Atropine Sulfate	0.4 mg		Tablet		Eli Lilly

IMPRINT	BRAND/GENERIC NAME	STRENGTH	COLOR	FORM	SHAPE	MANUFACTURER
LILLY; J03	Belladonna Extract	15 mg		Tablet	Compressed	Eli Lilly
LILLY; J05	Caffeine, Citrated	65 mg		Tablet	Compressed	Eli Lilly
LILLY; J09	Codeine Sulfate	15 mg		Tablet		Eli Lilly
LILLY; J11	Codeine Sulfate	60 mg		Tablet		Eli Lilly
LILLY; J13	Colchicine	0.6 mg		Tablet	Compressed	Eli Lilly
LILLY; J20	Quinidine Sulfate	200 mg		Tablet	Compressed	Eli Lilly
LILLY; J23	Soda Mint	5 Gr		Tablet	Compressed	Eli Lilly
LILLY; J24	Sodium Bicarbonate	325 mg		Tablet		Eli Lilly
LILLY; J25	Thyroid	60 mg		Tablet	Compressed	Eli Lilly
LILLY; J26	Thyroid	120 mg		Tablet	Compressed	Eli Lilly
LILLY; J29	Thyroid	30 mg		Tablet	Compressed	Eli Lilly
LILLY; J30	Thyroid	15 mg		Tablet	Compressed	Eli Lilly
LILLY; J31	Phenobarbital	15 mg		Tablet		Eli Lilly
LILLY; J32	Phenobarbital	30 mg		Tablet		Eli Lilly
LILLY; J33	Phenobarbital	100 mg	White	Tablet	Circle, Scored	Eli Lilly
LILLY; J36	Ergotrate Maleate	0.2 mg		Tablet		Eli Lilly
LILLY; J41	Niacin	20 mg		Tablet	Compressed	Eli Lilly
LILLY; J43	Niacin	50 mg		Tablet	Compressed, Scored	Eli Lilly
LILLY; J45	Hexa-Betalin	25 mg ; 0.5%		Tablet	Compressed	Eli Lilly
LILLY; J46	Niacinamide	50 mg		Tablet	Compressed	Eli Lilly
LILLY; J47	Riboflavin	5 mg		Tablet	Compressed	Eli Lilly
LILLY; J49	Diethylstilbestrol	0.1 mg		Tablet		Eli Lilly
LILLY; J53	Pantholin	10 mg		Tablet	Compressed	Eli Lilly
LILLY; J55	Phenobarbital and Belladonna, No. 1	30 mg ; 8 mg		Tablet	Compressed, Scored	Eli Lilly
LILLY; J56	Hexa-Betalin	10 mg		Tablet	Compressed	Eli Lilly
LILLY; J57	Crystodigin	0.2 mg	White	Tablet		Eli Lilly
LILLY; J59	Phenobarbital and Belladonna, No. 2	15 mg ; 4 mg		Tablet	Compressed	Eli Lilly
LILLY; J60	Crystodigin	0.1 mg	Pink	Tablet		Eli Lilly
LILLY; J61	Papaverine Hydrochloride	30 mg		Tablet	Compressed	Eli Lilly
LILLY; J62	Papaverine Hydrochloride	60 mg		Tablet		Eli Lilly
LILLY; J63	Riboflavin	10 mg		Tablet		Eli Lilly
LILLY; J64	Dolophine Hydrochloride	5 mg		Tablet		Eli Lilly
LILLY; J66	Folic Acid	5 mg		Tablet	Compressed	Eli Lilly
LILLY; J69	Propylthiouracil	50 mg		Tablet	Compressed, Scored	Eli Lilly
LILLY; J70	Phenobarbital and Belladonna, No. 3	8 mg ; 15 mg		Tablet	Compressed	Eli Lilly
LILLY; J72	Dolophine Hydrochloride	10 mg		Tablet		Eli Lilly
LILLY; J73	Methyltestosterone	10 mg		Tablet	Compressed, Scored	Eli Lilly
LILLY; J74	Methyltestosterone	25 mg		Tablet		Eli Lilly
LILLY; J75	Crystodigin	0.05 mg	Orange	Tablet		Eli Lilly
LILLY; J76	Crystodigin	0.15 mg	Yellow	Tablet		Eli Lilly
LILLY; J99	Sandril	0.1 mg	Orange	Tablet	Compressed	Eli Lilly
LILLY; L01	Sandril	0.25 mg	Green	Tablet	Compressed, Scored	Eli Lilly
LILLY; L02	Tylandril	0.25 mg ; 5 mg ; 0.1 mg		Tablet	Compressed	Eli Lilly
LILLY; S04	Metycaine Hydrochloride and Zinc Oxide Compound	125 mg ; 250 mg ; 12.5 mg		Suppository		Eli Lilly
LILLY; S05	Seconal Sodium Suppositories	120 mg		Suppository		Eli Lilly
LILLY; S06	Amytal Sodium	200 mg		Suppository		Eli Lilly
LILLY; S11	Seconal Sodium Suppositories	200 mg		Suppository		Eli Lilly
LILLY; S14	Seconal Sodium Suppositories	60 mg		Suppository		Eli Lilly
LILLY; S17	Seconal Sodium Suppositories	30 mg		Suppository		Eli Lilly
LILLY; T02	Novacebrin	4000 IU ; 400 IU ; 60 mg ; 1.5 mg ; 2 mg ; 0.8 mg ; 3 mcg ; 12 mg ; 2.5 mg	Yellow	Tablet, Chewable	Compressed	Eli Lilly
LILLY; T05	A.S.A.	325 mg		Tablet	Compressed	Eli Lilly
LILLY; T06	A.S.A.	325 mg	Pink	Tablet	Compressed	Eli Lilly
LILLY; T07	A.S.A. Compound	227 mg ; 160 mg ; 32.5 mg	White	Tablet	Compressed	Eli Lilly
LILLY; T13	Calcium Lactate	325 mg		Tablet	Compressed	Eli Lilly
LILLY; T14	Calcium Lactate	650 mg		Tablet	Compressed	Eli Lilly
LILLY; T19	Methenamine	325 mg		Tablet	Compressed	Eli Lilly
LILLY; T20	Methenamine	500 mg		Tablet	Compressed	Eli Lilly
LILLY; T21	Methenamine and Sodium Biphosphate	325 mg ; 325 mg		Tablet	Compressed	Eli Lilly
LILLY; T23	Sodium Chloride	2.25 GM		Tablet	Compressed	Eli Lilly
LILLY; T24	Sodium Chloride	1 GM		Tablet	Compressed	Eli Lilly
LILLY; T26	Pancreatin	325 mg		Tablet	Compressed	Eli Lilly
LILLY; T32	Amytal	100 mg	Pink	Tablet		Eli Lilly
LILLY; T35	Calcium Carbonate, Aromatic	650 mg		Tablet	Compressed	Eli Lilly
LILLY; T36	Calcium Gluconate	1 GM		Tablet	Compressed	Eli Lilly
LILLY; T37	Amytal	50 mg	Orange	Tablet		Eli Lilly
LILLY; T39	Calcium Gluconate	500 mg		Tablet	Compressed	Eli Lilly
LILLY; T40	Amytal	15 mg	Green	Tablet	Capsule-Shape	Eli Lilly
LILLY; T42	A.S.A. and Codeine, N0. 2	150 mg ; 230 mg ; 30 mg ; 15 mg		Tablet	Compressed	Eli Lilly
LILLY; T44	Calcium Gluconate with Vitamin D	1.65 mcg ; 1 GM		Tablet	Compressed	Eli Lilly
LILLY; T46	Sulfapyridine	0.5 GM		Tablet	Compressed	Eli Lilly
LILLY; T49	A.S.A. and Codeine, No. 3	230 mg ; 30 mg ; 30 mg ; 150 mg		Tablet	Compressed	Eli Lilly
LILLY; T50	A.S.A. Compound	227 mg ; 160 mg ; 32.5 mg	Pink	Tablet	Compressed	Eli Lilly
LILLY; T52	Betalin S	10 mg		Tablet	Compressed	Eli Lilly
LILLY; T55	Papaverine Hydrochloride	100 mg		Tablet	Compressed	Eli Lilly
LILLY; T56	Amytal	30 mg	Yellow	Tablet		Eli Lilly

IMPRINT	BRAND/GENERIC NAME	STRENGTH	COLOR	FORM	SHAPE	MANUFACTURER
LILLY; T59	Betalin S	25 mg		Tablet	Compressed	Eli Lilly
LILLY; T61	Dicalcium Phosphate	500 mg		Tablet	Compressed	Eli Lilly
LILLY; T62	Betalin S	50 mg		Tablet	Compressed	Eli Lilly
LILLY; T63	Betalin S	100 mg		Tablet	Compressed	Eli Lilly
LILLY; T71	Sulfonamides Triplex	0.167 GM ; 0.167 GM ; 0.167 GM		Tablet	Compressed	Eli Lilly
LILLY; T72	Hexa-Betalin	50 mg		Tablet	Compressed	Eli Lilly
LILLY; T73	Papaverine Hydrochloride	200 mg		Tablet	Compressed	Eli Lilly
LILLY; T75	Neotrizine	167 mg ; 167 mg ; 167 mg		Tablet	Compressed, Scored	Eli Lilly
LILLY; T77	Neopenzine 150	167 mg ; 167 mg ; 167 mg ; 150,000 units		Tablet	Compressed	Eli Lilly
LILLY; T92	Neopenzine 300	167 mg ; 167 mg ; 167 mg ; 300,000 units		Tablet		Eli Lilly
LILLY; T95	V-Cillin Sulfa	125 mg ; 167 mg ; 167 mg ; 167 mg		Tablet		Eli Lilly
LILLY; T96	Neomycin Sulfate	500 mg		Tablet		Eli Lilly
LILLY; U; 29	Sandril	0.25 mg		Tablet		Eli Lilly
LILLY; U02	Sandril	1 mg		Tablet		Eli Lilly
LILLY; U03	Dymelor	250 mg	White	Tablet	Capsule-Shape, Scored	Eli Lilly
LILLY; U04	V-Cillin K Sulfa	0.167 GM ; 0.167 GM ; 0.167 GM ; 125 mg		Tablet		Eli Lilly
LILLY; U07	Dymelor	500 mg	Yellow	Tablet	Scored, Capsule-Shape	Eli Lilly
LILLY; U09	Anhydron	2 mg	Pink	Tablet		Eli Lilly
LILLY; U30	Tylandril	0.25 mg ; 5 mg ; 0.1 mg	Green	Tablet		Eli Lilly
LILLY; U56	Folic Acid	1 mg		Tablet		Eli Lilly
LILLY; Y18	Penicillin G Potassium Solvets	100,000 units		Tablet		Eli Lilly
LILLY; Y23	Castor Oil	0.62 ml		Capsule		Eli Lilly
LILLY; Y40	Apomorphine Hydrochloride	6 mg		Tablet		Eli Lilly
LILLY; Y41	Atropine Sulfate Hypodermic Tablet	0.3 mg		Tablet		Eli Lilly
LILLY; Y42	Atropine Sulfate Hypodermic Tablet	0.4 mg		Tablet		Eli Lilly
LILLY; Y43	Atropine Sulfate Hypodermic Tablet	0.6 mg		Tablet		Eli Lilly
LILLY; Y52	Morphine and Atropine Hypodermic	15 mg ; 0.4 mg		Tablet		Eli Lilly
LILLY; Y53	Scopolamine Hydrobromide Hypodermic	0.6 mg		Tablet		Eli Lilly
LILLY; Y54	Scopolamine Hydrobromide Hypodermic	0.4 mg		Tablet		Eli Lilly
LILLY; Y56	Codeine Phosphate Hypodermic Tablet	15 mg		Tablet		Eli Lilly
LILLY; Y57	Codeine Phosphate	30 mg		Tablet		Eli Lilly
LIMBITROL	Limbitrol	5 mg ; 12.5 mg	Blue	Coated Tablet	Circle	Valeant Pharmaceuticals
LIMBITROL DS	Limbitrol DS	10 mg ; 25 mg	White	Coated Tablet		Valeant Pharmaceuticals
LIMBREL 52001	Limbrel	250 mg	Teal	Capsule		Primus Pharmaceutical
LINCOCIN; 250 MG ;	Lincocin Pediatric	250 mg	Light Blue	Capsule		Pharmacia & Upjohn
LINCOCIN; 500 MG ;	Lincocin	500 mg	Light Blue and Dark Blue	Capsule		Pharmacia & Upjohn
LIORESAL; 10/10	Lioresal	10 mg	White	Tablet	Oval, Scored	Novartis
LIORESAL; 20/20	Lioresal	20 mg	White	Tablet	Capsule-Shape, Scored	Novartis
LL A4	Aristocort	4 mg	White	Tablet	Oblong	Lederle Laboratories
LL; 5; C; 33	Leucovorin Calcium	5 mg	Yellow-White	Tablet	Circle, Convex, Scored	Xanodyne Pharmaceuticals
LL; 10; C; 12	Leucovorin Calcium	10 mg	Light Yellow	Tablet	Square with Rounded Corners, Convex, Bisected Scored	Lederle Laboratories
LL; 15; C; 35	Leucovorin Calcium	15 mg	Yellow-White	Tablet	Convex, Scored, Oval	Xanodyne Pharmaceuticals
LL; A 24	Amitriptyline Hydrochloride	10 mg	Pink	Coated Tablet	Circle	Lederle Laboratories
LL; A 25	Amitriptyline Hydrochloride	25 mg	Green	Coated Tablet	Circle	Lederle Laboratories
LL; A 26	Amitriptyline Hydrochloride	50 mg	Brown	Coated Tablet	Circle	Lederle Laboratories
LL; A; 7	Atenolol	25 mg	White	Tablet	Circle	Lederle Laboratories
LL; A; 27	Amitriptyline Hydrochloride	75 mg	Light Purple	Coated Tablet	Circle	Lederle Laboratories
LL; A; 28	Amitriptyline Hydrochloride	100 mg	Red-Orange	Coated Tablet	Circle	Lederle Laboratories
LL; A; 45	Albuterol Sulfate	2 mg	White	Tablet	Round, Flat, Bisected Scored	Lederle Laboratories
LL; A; 46	Albuterol Sulfate	4 mg	White	Tablet	Round, Flat, Bisected Scored	Lederle Laboratories
LL; A; 49	Atenolol	50 mg	White	Tablet	Circle, Scored	Lederle Laboratories
LL; A; 51	Alprazolam	0.25 mg	White	Tablet	Oval, Convex, Scored	Lederle Laboratories
LL; A; 52	Alprazolam	0.5 mg	Yellow	Tablet	Oval, Convex, Scored	Lederle Laboratories
LL; A; 53	Alprazolam	1 mg	Green	Tablet	Oval, Convex, Scored	Lederle Laboratories
LL; A; 54	Alprazolam	2 mg	Green	Tablet	Oblong, Convex	Lederle Laboratories
LL; A1 ;	Aristocort	1 mg	Yellow	Tablet	Oblong, Flat; Scored	Lederle Laboratories
LL; A2 ;	Triamcinolone	2 mg	Pink	Tablet	Oblong, Flat, Scored	Lederle Laboratories
LL; A8 ;	Aristocort	8 mg	Yellow	Tablet	Oblong, Flat, Scored	Lederle Laboratories
LL; A11; ARTANE; 2	Artane	2 mg	White	Tablet	Circle, Flat, Scored	Lederle Laboratories
LL; A12; ARTANE; 5	Artane	5 mg	White	Tablet	Circle, Flat, Scored	Lederle Laboratories
LL; B; 10	Benztropine Mesylate	1 mg	White	Tablet	Oval, Scored	Lederle Laboratories
LL; B; 11	Benztropine Mesylate	2 mg	White	Tablet	Circle, Scored	Lederle Laboratories
LL; B1	Zebeta	5 mg	Pink	Coated Tablet	Heart-Shape	Lederle Laboratories
LL; C; 15	Chlorthalidone	50 mg	Dark Blue	Tablet	Circle, Scored	Lederle Laboratories
LL; C; 40	Caltrate 600 Plus Vitamin D	125 IU ; 600 mg	Light Brown	Coated Tablet	Oblong, Scored	Wyeth Consumer Healthcare
LL; C; 42	Clonidine Hydrochloride	0.1 mg	Blue	Tablet	Circle, Convex	Lederle Laboratories
LL; C; 43	Clonidine Hydrochloride	0.2 mg	Light Yellow	Tablet	Circle, Convex	Lederle Laboratories
LL; C; 44	Clonidine Hydrochloride	0.3 mg	Light Green	Tablet	Circle, Convex	Lederle Laboratories
LL; C; 67	Chlordiazepoxide and Amitriptyline Hydrochloride	12.5 mg ; 5 mg	Green	Coated Tablet	Circle	Lederle Laboratories

IMPRINT	BRAND/GENERIC NAME	STRENGTH	COLOR	FORM	SHAPE	MANUFACTURER
LL; C; 68	Chlordiazepoxide and Amitriptyline Hydrochloride	10 mg ; 25 mg	White	Coated Tablet	Circle	Lederle Laboratories
LL; C; 69	Clorazepate Dipotassium	3.75 mg	Blue	Tablet	Circle, Scored	Lederle Laboratories
LL; C; 70	Clorazepate Dipotassium	7.5 mg	Peach	Tablet	Circle, Scored	Lederle Laboratories
LL; C; 71	Clorazepate Dipotassium	15 mg	White	Tablet	Circle, Scored	Lederle Laboratories
LL; C; 81	Cephalexin	250 mg	White	Coated Tablet	Oblong	Lederle Laboratories
LL; C; 82	Cephalexin	500 mg	White	Coated Tablet	Oblong	Lederle Laboratories
LL; C;7	Chlorthalidone	25 mg	Dark Orange	Tablet	Circle, Scored	Lederle Laboratories
LL; C37	Chlorpropamide	100 mg	White	Tablet	Circle, Scored	Lederle Laboratories
LL; C38	Chlorpropamide	250 mg	White	Tablet	Circle, Scored	Lederle Laboratories
LL; C60; CENTRUM JR	Centrum JR. with Extra Calcium	15 mg ; 1 mg ; 20 mcg ; 20 mcg ; 60 mg ; 2 mg ; 6 mcg ; 10 mcg ; 18 mg ; 5000 IU ; 400 IU ; 30 IU ; 400 mcg ; 45 mcg ; 1.5 mg ; 10 mg ; 1.7 mg ; 20 mg ; 40 mg ; 150 mcg ; 2 mg ; 50 mg ; 160 mg	Red	Tablet	Oblong, Scored	Wyeth Consumer Healthcare
LL; D; 31	Diphenoxylate Hydrochloride and Atropine Sulfate	2.5 mg ; 0.025 mg	White	Tablet	Circle	Lederle Laboratories
LL; D; 41	Doxycycline Hyclate	100 mg	Green	Coated Tablet	Circle	Lederle Laboratories
LL; D; 44	Dipyridamole	25 mg	Purple or White	Coated Tablet	Circle	Lederle Laboratories
LL; D; 45	Dipyridamole	50 mg	Purple or White	Coated Tablet	Circle	Lederle Laboratories
LL; D; 46	Dipyridamole	75 mg	Purple or White	Coated Tablet	Circle	Lederle Laboratories
LL; D; 51	Diazepam	2 mg	White	Tablet	Scored, Circle	Lederle Laboratories
LL; D; 72	Diltiazem	60 mg	Blue	Coated Tablet	Round, Convex, Bisected Scored	Lederle Laboratories
LL; D; 75	Diltiazem	90 mg	Blue	Coated Tablet	Oblong, Convex, Bisected Scored	Lederle Laboratories
LL; D; 77	Diltiazem	120 mg	Blue	Coated Tablet	Oblong, Convex, Bisected Scored	Lederle Laboratories
LL; D11	Declomycin	150 mg	Red	Coated Tablet	Circle, Convex	Lederle Laboratories
LL; D12	Declomycin	300 mg	Red	Coated Tablet	Circle, Convex	Lederle Laboratories
LL; D52	Diazepam	5 mg	Light Brown	Tablet	Circle, Scored	Lederle Laboratories
LL; D53	Diazepam	10 mg	Light Green	Tablet	Circle, Scored	Lederle Laboratories
LL; D71	Diltiazem	30 mg	Blue	Coated Tablet	Circle, Convex	Lederle Laboratories
LL; E2	Erythromycin Stearate	250 mg	Yellow	Coated Tablet	Circle	Lederle Laboratories
LL; E5 ;	Erythromycin Stearate	500 mg	Yellow	Coated Tablet	Oval	Lederle Laboratories
LL; E10	Erythromycin Ethylsuccinate	400 mg	Beige	Tablet	Oval	Lederle Laboratories
LL; EXTRA C; C39; CENTRUM JR	Centrum JR. Plus Extra C, Advanced Formula	10 mg ; 1.7 mg ; 20 mg ; 40 mg ; 150 mcg ; 2 mg ; 50 mg ; 108 mg ; 15 mg ; 1 mg ; 20 mcg ; 20 mcg ; 300 mg ; 2 mg ; 6 mcg ; 10 mcg ; 18 mg ; 5000 IU ; 400 IU ; 30 IU ; 400 mcg ; 45 mcg ; 1.5 mg		Tablet, Chewable	Oblong, Scored	Wyeth Consumer Healthcare
LL; F; 12	Furosemide	40 mg	White to Off-White	Tablet	Circle, Scored	Lederle Laboratories
LL; F; 13	Furosemide	80 mg	White to Off-White	Tablet	Circle, Scored	Lederle Laboratories
LL; F; 22	Fenoprofen Calcium	600 mg	White	Coated Tablet	Capsule-Shape, Scored	Lederle Laboratories
LL; F11	Furosemide	20 mg	White to Off-White	Tablet	Circle	Lederle Laboratories
LL; F21	Ferrous Gluconate	300 mg	Green	Coated Tablet	Circle	Lederle Laboratories
LL; G2	Gevral T	2.25 mg ; 2.6 mg ; 30 mg ; 3 mg ; 9 mcg ; 162 mg ; 225 mcg ; 100 mg ; 1.5 mg ; 22.5 mg ; 27 mg ; 5000 IU ; 400 IU ; 45 IU ; 90 mg ; 0.4 mg	Maroon	Coated Tablet	Oblong	Lederle Laboratories
LL; G17	Gemfibrozil	600 mg	White to Off-White	Coated Tablet	Oval, Scored	Lederle Laboratories
LL; H; 2	Hydromox R	50 mg ; 0.125 mg	Yellow	Tablet	Circle, Scored	Lederle Laboratories
LL; H; 14	Hydrochlorothiazide	25 mg	Peach	Tablet	Circle, Scored	Lederle Laboratories
LL; H11	Hydralazine Hydrochloride	25 mg	Red	Coated Tablet	Circle, Convex	Lederle Laboratories
LL; H12	Hydralazine Hydrochloride	50 mg	Red	Coated Tablet	Circle, Convex	Lederle Laboratories
LL; HEART; B; 12	Ziac	2.5 mg ; 6.25 mg	Yellow	Coated Tablet	Circle, Convex	Wyeth Pharmaceuticals
LL; HEART; B; 13	Ziac	5 mg ; 6.25 mg	Pink	Coated Tablet	Circle, Convex	Wyeth Pharmaceuticals
LL; HEART; B; 14	Ziac	6.25 mg ; 10 mg	White	Coated Tablet	Circle, Convex	Wyeth Pharmaceuticals
LL; I11	Imipramine Hydrochloride	10 mg	Yellow	Tablet	Circle	Lederle Laboratories
LL; I12	Imipramine Hydrochloride	25 mg	Rust	Tablet	Circle	Lederle Laboratories
LL; I13	Imipramine Hydrochloride	50 mg	Green	Tablet	Circle	Lederle Laboratories
LL; J1	Methazolamide	25 mg	White	Tablet	Square, Convex	Lederle Laboratories
LL; J2	Methazolamide	50 mg	White	Tablet	Circle, Convex	Lederle Laboratories
LL; M; 1	Methotrexate	2.5 mg	Yellow	Tablet	Round, Convex, Bisected Scored	Lederle Laboratories
LL; M; 7	Myambutol	400 mg	White	Coated Tablet	Circle, Convex, Scored	Lederle Laboratories
LL; M; 19	Methocarbamol	500 mg	White	Tablet	Circle, Scored	Lederle Laboratories
LL; M; 20	Methocarbamol	750 mg	White	Tablet	Capsule-Shape, Scored	Lederle Laboratories
LL; M; 36	Methyldopa and Hydrochlorothiazide	250 mg ; 15 mg	Yellow	Coated Tablet	Circle	Lederle Laboratories
LL; M; 37	Methyldopa and Hydrochlorothiazide	250 mg ; 25 mg	Pink	Coated Tablet	Circle	Lederle Laboratories
LL; M1	Rheumatrex	2.5 mg	Yellow	Tablet	Circle, Convex, Scored	Lederle Laboratories
LL; M3	Minocin	50 mg	Orange	Coated Tablet	Circle, Convex	Lederle Laboratories
LL; M5	Minocin	100 mg	Orange	Coated Tablet	Circle, Convex, Scored	Lederle Laboratories
LL; M6	Myambutol	100 mg	White	Coated Tablet	Circle, Convex	Lederle Laboratories
LL; M8; MAXZIDE	Maxzide	50 mg ; 75 mg	Yellow	Tablet	Bowtie	Lederle Laboratories
LL; M22	Methyldopa	250 mg	Peach	Coated Tablet	Circle	Lederle Laboratories
LL; M23	Methyldopa	500 mg	Peach	Coated Tablet	Circle	Lederle Laboratories
LL; M28	Metoclopramide Hydrochloride	10 mg	White		Circle, Scored	Lederle Laboratories

IMPRINT	BRAND/GENERIC NAME	STRENGTH	COLOR	FORM	SHAPE	MANUFACTURER
LL; N; 11	Naproxen	250 mg	Light Green	Tablet	Circle	Lederle Laboratories
LL; N; 17	Naproxen	375 mg	White	Tablet	Capsule-Shape	Lederle Laboratories
LL; N; 77	Naproxen	500 mg	Light Green	Tablet	Capsule-Shape	Lederle Laboratories
LL; N6	Nilstat	100,000 units	Yellow	Tablet	Oval, Convex	Lederle Laboratories
LL; P; 33	Propylthiouracil	50 mg	White	Tablet	Circle, Scored	Lederle Laboratories
LL; P; 36	Pyrazinamide	500 mg	White	Tablet	Circle, Scored, Convex	Lederle Laboratories
LL; P; 44	Propranolol Hydrochloride	10 mg	Gray	Tablet	Circle, Scored	Lederle Laboratories
LL; P; 45	Propranolol Hydrochloride	20 mg	Purple	Tablet	Circle, Scored	Lederle Laboratories
LL; P; 46	Propranolol Hydrochloride	40 mg	Light Brown	Tablet	Circle	Lederle Laboratories
LL; P; 47	Propranolol Hydrochloride	80 mg	Light Blue	Tablet	Circle, Scored	Lederle Laboratories
LL; P; 48	Procainamide Hydrochloride SR	250 mg	Light Blue	Coated Tablet	Oval, Scored	Lederle Laboratories
LL; P; 65	Propranolol Hydrochloride	60 mg	White	Tablet	Circle	Lederle Laboratories
LL; P; 76	Perphenazine and Amitriptyline Hydrochloride	4 mg ; 50 mg	Orange	Coated Tablet	Circle	Lederle Laboratories
LL; P9	Pronemia	75 mg ; 115 mg ; 150 mg ; 1 mg ; 15 mcg	Red	Capsule		Lederle Laboratories
LL; P72	Perphenazine and Amitriptyline Hydrochloride	2 mg ; 10 mg	Blue	Coated Tablet	Circle	Lederle Laboratories
LL; P73	Perphenazine with Amitriptyline Hydrochloride	2 mg ; 25 mg	Orange	Coated Tablet	Circle	Lederle Laboratories
LL; P74	Perphenazine and Amitriptyline Hydrochloride	4 mg ; 10 mg	Light Peach	Coated Tablet	Circle	Lederle Laboratories
LL; P75	Perphenazine and Amitriptyline Hydrochloride	4 mg ; 25 mg	Yellow	Coated Tablet	Circle	Lederle Laboratories
LL; Q; 11	Quinidine Sulfate	200 mg	White	Tablet	Circle, Convex, Scored	Lederle Laboratories
LL; S; 1	Advanced Formula Stresstabs 600	45 mcg ; 400 mcg ; 100 mg ; 30 IU ; 20 mg ; 15 mg ; 5 mg ; 500 mg ; 15 mg ; 12 mcg	Orange	Tablet	Oblong	Lederle Laboratories
LL; S; 3	Stresstabs 600 Plus Zinc	30 IU ; 600 mg ; 400 mcg ; 20 mg ; 10 mg ; 100 mg ; 5 mg ; 12 mcg ; 45 mcg ; 25 mg ; 3 mg ; 23.9 mg	Peach	Tablet	Oblong, Scored	Lederle Laboratories
LL; S; 3	Stresstabs Plus Zinc	20 mg ; 3 mg ; 23.9 mg ; 30 IU ; 500 mg ; 400 mcg ; 10 mg ; 10 mg ; 100 mg ; 5 mg ; 12 mcg ; 45 mcg	Peach	Tablet	Oblong, Scored	Lederle Laboratories
LL; S; 14	Sulfasalazine	500 mg	Brown	Tablet	Circle, Scored	Lederle Laboratories
LL; S; 16	Sulindac	150 mg	Yellow	Tablet	Circle, Scored	Lederle Laboratories
LL; S; 17	Sulindac	200 mg	Yellow	Tablet	Circle, Scored	Lederle Laboratories
LL; T; 29	Trazodone Hydrochloride	50 mg	White	Tablet	Circle, Scored	Lederle Laboratories
LL; T; 30	Trazodone Hydrochloride	100 mg	White	Tablet	Circle, Scored	Lederle Laboratories
LL; T; 34	Theophylline C.R.	100 mg	White	Timed-Release Tablet	Circle, Convex	Lederle Laboratories
LL; T1	Tri-Hemic 600	30 IU ; 75 mg ; 1 mg ; 115 mg ; 50 mg ; 600 mg ; 25 mcg	Red	Coated Tablet	Oblong	Lederle Laboratories
LL; T13	Sulfamethoxazole and Trimethoprim	400 mg ; 80 mg	White	Tablet	Circle, Scored	Lederle Laboratories
LL; T16	Sulfamethoxazole and Trimethoprim	800 mg ; 160 mg	White	Tablet	Oblong	Lederle Laboratories
LL; T31; 50; 100	Trazodone Hydrochloride	150 mg	White	Tablet	Scored, Four-Sided	Lederle Laboratories
LL; V; 5	Verapamil Hydrochloride	120 mg	White	Coated Tablet	Circle, Scored	Lederle Laboratories
LL;A 14	Amiloride and Hydrochlorothiazide	50 mg ; 5 mg	Yellow	Tablet	Circle	Lederle Laboratories
LODINE XL; 400	Lodine XL	400 mg	Orange-Red	Extended-Release Tablet	Capsule-Shape	Wyeth Pharmaceuticals
LODINE XL; 500	Lodine XL	500 mg	Grey-Green	Extended-Release Tablet	Capsule-Shape, Biconvex	Wyeth Pharmaceuticals
LODINE XL; 600	Lodine XL	600 mg	Light Grey	Extended-Release Tablet	Capsule-Shape, Biconvex	Wyeth Pharmaceuticals
LODINE; 200	Lodine	200 mg	Light Gray with a Wide Red Band	Capsule		Wyeth Pharmaceuticals
LODINE; 300	Lodine	300 mg	Light Gray with a Wide Red Band, Light Gray with 2 Narrow Red Bands	Capsule		Wyeth Pharmaceuticals
LODINE; 400	Lodine	400 mg	Yellow-Orange	Coated Tablet	Oval	Wyeth Pharmaceuticals
LODINE; 500	Lodine	500 mg	Blue	Coated Tablet	Oval	Wyeth Pharmaceuticals
LOFIBRA 67MG GATE 322	Lofibra	67 mg	Opaque Pink	Capsule		Gate Pharmaceuticals
LOFIBRA 134MG GATE 323	Lofibra	134 mg	Opaque Light Blue	Capsule		Gate Pharmaceuticals
LOFIBRA 200MG GATE 324	Lofibra	200 mg	Opaque Orange	Capsule		Gate Pharmaceuticals
LOGO	Maxalt-Mlt	5 mg	White to Off-White	Tablet, Disintegrating	Circle	Merck & Company
LOGO ;	Maxalt-Mlt	10 mg	White to Off-White	Tablet, Disintegrating	Circle	Merck & Company
LOGO ; 1MG/500MG ;	Prandimet	1 mg ; 500 mg	Yellow	Tablet		Novo Nordisk
LOGO ; 2MG/500MG ;	Prandimet	2 mg ; 500 mg	Pink	Tablet		Novo Nordisk
LOGO ; 270	Fosamax Plus D	5600 IU ; 70 mg	White to Off-White	Tablet	Rectangle	Merck & Company
LOGO ; 600	Prezista	600 mg	Orange	Tablet	Oval	Tibotec Therapeutics
LOGO ; 710	Fosamax Plus D	70 mg ; 2800 IU	White to Off-White	Tablet	Capsule-Shape	Merck & Company
LOGO ; 748	Tri-Previfem - Blue Tablet	0.25 mg ; 0.035 mg	Blue	Tablet	Circle	Teva Pharmaceuticals
LOGO ; B8	Subutex	8 mg	White	Tablet	Oval	Reckitt Benckiser
LOGO ; F5	Finasteride	5 mg	Blue	Tablet	Circle	Actavis Totowa
LOGO ; NOVO 288	Activella	1 mg ; 0.5 mg	White	Tablet	Circle	Pharmacia & Upjohn
LOGO ; NOVO 291	Activella	0.5 mg ; 0.1 mg	White	Tablet	Circle	Novo Nordisk
LOGO 0400 5MG	Zaleplon	5 mg	Opaque White	Capsule		Upsher-Smith Laboratories

IMPRINT	BRAND/GENERIC NAME	STRENGTH	COLOR	FORM	SHAPE	MANUFACTURER
LOGO 0401 10MG	Zaleplon	10 mg	Green	Capsule		Upsher-Smith Laboratories
LOGO 20 ; 5728 ;	Famotidine	20 mg	Beige	Tablet	Circle	Ivax Pharmaceuticals
LOGO 29	Oxycodone Hydrochloride and Ibuprofen	5 mg ; 400 mg	Yellow	Tablet	Capsule-Shape	Actavis Elizabeth
LOGO 40 ; 5729	Famotidine	40 mg	Tan	Tablet	Circle	Teva Pharmaceuticals
LOGO 100 MG 2131	Nitrofurantoin Macrocrystals	100 mg	Pink Opaque	Capsule		Teva Pharmaceuticals
LOGO 225	Rythmol SR	225 mg	White	Capsule		Glaxosmithkline
LOGO 559 ;	Potassium Chloride	8 meq	Opaque White	Capsule, Extended Release		Watson Pharma
LOGO 560 ;	Potassium Chloride	10 meq	Opaque Dark Blue	Capsule, Extended Release		Watson Pharma
LOGO 567 ; TRIANGLE; 567	Hydrocodone Bitartrate and Acetaminophen	660 mg ; 10 mg	White	Tablet	Capsule-Shape	Watson Pharma
LOGO 721	Sertraline Hydrochloride	25 mg	White to Off White	Tablet	Capsule-Shape	Actavis Elizabeth
LOGO 722	Sertraline Hydrochloride	50 mg	Orange	Tablet	Capsule-Shape	Actavis Elizabeth
LOGO 723	Sertraline Hydrochloride	100 mg	Pink	Tablet	Capsule-Shape	Actavis Elizabeth
LOGO 777	Clarithromycin	500 mg	Orange	Tablet, Extended Release	Oval	Watson Pharma
LOGO 2898	Glipizide	2.5 mg	Blue	Tablet, Extended Release	Circle	Actavis Elizabeth
LOGO 2899	Glipizide	5 mg	White	Tablet, Extended Release	Circle	Actavis Elizabeth
LOGO 2900	Glipizide	10 mg	White	Tablet, Extended Release	Circle	Actavis Elizabeth
LOGO 4359 ; 25 ;	Clozapine	25 mg	Pale Yellow	Tablet	Circle	Teva Pharmaceuticals
LOGO 4360 ; 100 ;	Clozapine	100 mg	Pale Yellow	Tablet	Circle	Teva Pharmaceuticals
LOGO 5710 ; 1.25/ 250 ;	Glyburide and Metformin Hydrochloride	1.25 mg ; 250 mg	Light Yellow	Tablet	Oval	Teva Pharmaceuticals
LOGO 5711 ; 2.5/500 ;	Glyburide and Metformin Hydrochloride	2.5 mg ; 500 mg	Light Orange	Tablet	Oval	Teva Pharmaceuticals
LOGO JC	Rythmol	150 mg		Tablet	Circle	Glaxosmithkline
LOGO JI	Rythmol	225 mg		Tablet	Circle	Glaxosmithkline
LOGO JN	Rythmol	300 mg		Tablet	Circle	Glaxosmithkline
LOGO KA ;	Kaletra	200 mg ; 50 mg	Yellow	Tablet	Oval	Abbott Laboratories
LOGO KC ;	Kaletra	100 mg ; 25 mg	Pale Yellow	Tablet	Oval	Abbott Laboratories
LOGO LCR 100	Luvox Cr	100 mg	Opaque Dark Blue, Opaque White	Capsule, Extended Release		Jazz Pharmaceuticals
LOGO LCR 150	Luvox Cr	150 mg	Opaque Dark Blue, Opaque Powder Blue	Capsule, Extended Release		Jazz Pharmaceuticals
LOGO ZA	Zemplar	1 mcg	Gray	Capsule, Liquid Filled	Oval	Abbott Laboratories
LOGO ZF	Zemplar	2 mcg	Orange-Brown	Capsule, Liquid Filled	Oval	Abbott Laboratories
LOGO ZK	Zemplar	4 mcg	Gold	Capsule, Liquid Filled	Oval	Abbott Laboratories
LONITEN; 10 ;	Loniten	10 mg	White	Tablet	Circle, Scored	Pharmacia & Upjohn
LORTREL 2265	Lotrel	5 mg ; 20 mg	Pink, White	Capsule		Novartis
LOTENSIN HCT; 57 ;	Lotensin HCT	5 mg ; 6.25 mg	White	Tablet	Oblong, Scored	Novartis Pharmaceuticals
LOTENSIN HCT; 72	Lotensin HCT	10 mg ; 12.5 mg	Light Pink	Tablet	Oblong, Scored	Novartis Pharmaceuticals
LOTENSIN HCT; 74 ;	Lotensin HCT	20 mg ; 12.5 mg	Grayish-Violet	Tablet	Oblong, Scored	Novartis Pharmaceuticals
LOTENSIN HCT; 75 ;	Lotensin HCT	25 mg ; 20 mg	Red	Tablet	Scored, Oblong	Novartis Pharmaceuticals
LOTENSIN; 5 ;	Lotensin	5 mg	Light Yellow	Tablet	Circle	Novartis Pharmaceuticals
LOTENSIN; 10 ;	Lotensin	10 mg	Dark Yellow	Tablet	Circle	Novartis Pharmaceuticals
LOTENSIN; 20 ;	Lotensin	20 mg	Tan	Tablet	Circle	Novartis Pharmaceuticals
LOTENSIN; 40 ;	Lotensin	40 mg	Dark Rose	Tablet	Circle	Novartis Pharmaceuticals
LOTREL 0364	Lotrel	10 mg ; 20 mg	Purple, White	Capsule		Novartis
LOTREL 0379	Lotrel	10 mg ; 40 mg	Dark Blue, White	Capsule		Novartis
LOTREL 0384	Lotrel	5 mg ; 40 mg	Light Blue, White	Capsule		Novartis
LOTREL 2255	Lotrel	10 mg ; 2.5 mg	Gold, White	Capsule		Novartis
LOTREL 2260	Lotrel	10 mg ; 5 mg	Light Brown, White	Capsule		Novartis
LTG; 2	Lamictal	2 mg	White to Off White	Tablet, Chewable	Circle	Glaxosmithkline
LUF ; NVR	Exforge	10 mg ; 320 mg	Dark Yellow	Tablet	Oval	Novartis
LUPIN; 302	Cefuroxime Axetil	250 mg	White to Off-White	Tablet	Capsule-Shape	Watson Laboratories
LV; 10; G	Lovastatin	10 mg	Peach	Tablet	Circle	Par Pharmaceutical
LV; 20; G	Lovastatin	20 mg	Light Blue	Tablet	Circle	Par Pharmaceutical
LV; 40; G	Lovastatin	40 mg	Green	Tablet	Circle	Par Pharmaceutical
M ; 15	Meloxicam	15 mg	Pastel Yellow	Tablet	Oblong	Roxane Laboratories
M ; 15	Mobic	15 mg	Pastel Yellow	Tablet	Oblong	Boehringer Ingelheim Pharmaceuticals
M ; 315	Ondansetron Hydrochloride	4 mg	White	Tablet	Circle	Mylan Pharmaceuticals
M ; 322	Ciprofloxacin	250 mg	Orange	Tablet	Circle	Mylan Pharmaceuticals
M ; 344	Ondansetron Hydrochloride	8 mg	Orange	Tablet	Circle	Mylan Pharmaceuticals
M ; 354	Ondansetron Hydrochloride	16 mg	Orange	Tablet	Circle	Mylan Pharmaceuticals
M ; 374	Ondansetron Hydrochloride	24 mg	Orange	Tablet	Circle	Mylan Pharmaceuticals
M ; 524	Bisoprolol Fumarate	10 mg	White	Tablet	Circle	Mylan Pharmaceuticals
M ; A6	Alendronate Sodium	5 mg	White	Tablet	Circle	Mylan Pharmaceuticals
M ; A7	Alendronate Sodium	10 mg	White	Tablet	Circle	Mylan Pharmaceuticals
M ; GX EF3	Myleran	2 mg	White	Tablet	Circle	Glaxosmithkline
M ; "H" 1 ;	Hydrochlorothiazide	25 mg	White to Off-White	Tablet	Circle	Mylan Pharmaceuticals
M ; "H" 2 ;	Hydrochlorothiazide	50 mg	White to Off-White	Tablet	Circle	Mylan Pharmaceuticals
M ; L 24	Lisinopril	10 mg	White	Tablet	Circle	Mylan Pharmaceuticals
M ; L 25	Lisinopril	20 mg	Yellow	Tablet	Circle	Mylan Pharmaceuticals
M ; L 26	Lisinopril	40 mg	Green	Tablet	Circle	Mylan Pharmaceuticals
M ; LOGO	Meloxicam	7.5 mg	Pastel Yellow	Tablet	Circle	Roxane Laboratories
M ; LOGO	Mobic	7.5 mg	Pastel Yellow	Tablet	Circle	Boehringer Ingelheim Pharmaceuticals
M ; V 1	Venlafaxine Hydrochloride	25 mg	Yellow	Tablet	Circle	Mylan Pharmaceuticals
M ; V 2	Venlafaxine Hydrochloride	37.5 mg	Yellow	Tablet	Circle	Mylan Pharmaceuticals
M ; V 3	Venlafaxine Hydrochloride	50 mg	Yellow	Tablet	Circle	Mylan Pharmaceuticals
M 18	Metoprolol Tartrate	25 mg	White	Tablet	Circle	Mylan Pharmaceuticals
M 32	Metoprolol Tartrate	50 mg	Pink	Tablet	Circle	Mylan Pharmaceuticals
M 44	Cyproheptadine Hydrochloride	4 mg	White	Tablet	Circle, Scored, Flat Beveled Edge	Mylan Pharmaceuticals

IMPRINT	BRAND/GENERIC NAME	STRENGTH	COLOR	FORM	SHAPE	MANUFACTURER
M 47	Metoprolol Tartrate	100 mg	Light Blue	Tablet	Circle	Mylan Pharmaceuticals
M 50	Metoprolol Succinate	50 mg	White	Tablet, Extended Release	Circle	Par Pharmaceutical
M 54; 10	Thioridazine Hydrochloride	10 mg		Tablet		Roxane Laboratories
M 66	Meloxicam	7.5 mg	Yellow	Tablet	Circle	Mylan Pharmaceuticals
M 89	Meloxicam	15 mg	Yellow	Tablet	Circle	Mylan Pharmaceuticals
M 96 ;	Nadolol and Bendroflumethiazide	40 mg ; 5 mg	Yellow	Tablet	Circle	Mylan Pharmaceuticals
M 99 ;	Nadolol and Bendroflumethiazide	80 mg ; 5 mg	Yellow	Tablet	Circle	Mylan Pharmaceuticals
M 100	Metoprolol Succinate	100 mg	White	Tablet, Extended Release	Circle	Par Pharmaceutical
M 200	Metoprolol Succinate	200 mg	White	Tablet, Extended Release	Oval	Par Pharmaceutical
M 244	Metformin Hydrochloride	1000 mg	White	Tablet	Oval	Mylan Pharmaceuticals
M 350	Metformin Hydrochloride	750 mg	Tan	Tablet, Extended Release	Oval	Mylan Pharmaceuticals
M 352	Metformin Hydrochloride	500 mg	Tan	Tablet, Extended Release	Oval	Mylan Pharmaceuticals
M 515	Mirtazapine	15 mg	Beige	Tablet	Circle	Mylan Pharmaceuticals
M 530	Mirtazapine	30 mg	Beige	Tablet	Circle	Mylan Pharmaceuticals
M 533	Azithromycin	250 mg	Blue	Tablet	Circle	Mylan Pharmaceuticals
M 534	Azithromycin	500 mg	Blue	Tablet	Capsule-Shape	Mylan Pharmaceuticals
M 535	Azithromycin	600 mg	Blue	Tablet	Oval	Mylan Pharmaceuticals
M 542 ;	Quinapril Hydrochloride and Hydrochlorothiazide	10 mg ; 12.5 mg	Pink	Tablet	Circle	Mylan Pharmaceuticals
M 543 ;	Quinapril Hydrochloride and Hydrochlorothiazide	20 mg ; 12.5 mg	Yellow	Tablet	Circle	Mylan Pharmaceuticals
M 544 ;	Quinapril Hydrochloride and Hydrochlorothiazide	20 mg ; 25 mg	Pink	Tablet	Circle	Mylan Pharmaceuticals
M 545	Mirtazapine	45 mg	Beige	Tablet	Circle	Mylan Pharmaceuticals
M 571	Terbinafine Hydrochloride	250 mg	White to Off-White	Tablet	Capsule-Shape	Mylan Pharmaceuticals
M 724	Tizanidine Hydrochloride	4 mg	White to Off-White	Tablet		Mylan Pharmaceuticals
M 753 ;	Fexofenadine Hydrochloride	60 mg	Blue	Tablet	Circle	Mylan Pharmaceuticals
M 755	Fexofenadine Hydrochloride	180 mg	Blue	Tablet	Capsule-Shape	Mylan Pharmaceuticals
M 1743 ;	Ciprofloxacin	500 mg	Orange	Tablet, Extended Release	Capsule-Shape	Mylan Pharmaceuticals
M 1745 ;	Ciprofloxacin	1000 mg	Orange	Tablet, Extended Release	Capsule-Shape	Mylan Pharmaceuticals
M A11	Alendronate Sodium	35 mg	White	Tablet	Capsule-Shape	Mylan Pharmaceuticals
M A12	Alendronate Sodium	70 mg	White	Tablet	Capsule-Shape	Mylan Pharmaceuticals
M B	Metoprolol Succinate	25 mg	White	Tablet, Extended Release	Oval	Par Pharmaceutical
M C41	Cilostazol	50 mg	White to Off-White	Tablet	Circle	Mylan Pharmaceuticals
M C42	Cilostazol	100 mg	White to Off-White	Tablet	Circle	Mylan Pharmaceuticals
M C51 ;	Carbidopa and Levodopa	10 mg ; 100 mg	Green	Tablet, Disintegrating	Circle	Mylan Pharmaceuticals
M C52 ;	Carbidopa and Levodopa	25 mg ; 100 mg	Blue	Tablet, Disintegrating	Circle	Mylan Pharmaceuticals
M C53 ;	Carbidopa and Levodopa	25 mg ; 250 mg	Green	Tablet, Disintegrating	Circle	Mylan Pharmaceuticals
M L23	Lisinopril	5 mg	Peach	Tablet	Circle	Mylan Pharmaceuticals
M N3	Paroxetine	30 mg	Blue	Tablet	Circle	Mylan Pharmaceuticals
M N4	Paroxetine	40 mg	Blue	Tablet	Circle	Mylan Pharmaceuticals
M O 5	Oxybutynin Chloride	5 mg	Light Green	Tablet, Extended Release	Circle	Mylan Pharmaceuticals
M O 10	Oxybutynin Chloride	10 mg	Peach	Tablet, Extended Release	Circle	Mylan Pharmaceuticals
M O 17	Oxybutynin Chloride	15 mg	Gray	Tablet, Extended Release	Circle	Mylan Pharmaceuticals
M P3	Paroxetine Hydrochloride	12.5 mg	White	Tablet, Extended Release	Circle	Mylan Pharmaceuticals
M P4	Paroxetine Hydrochloride	25 mg	Lavender	Tablet, Extended Release	Circle	Mylan Pharmaceuticals
M S1 ;	Sertraline Hydrochloride	25 mg	Light Green	Tablet	Circle	Mylan Pharmaceuticals
M S2	Sertraline Hydrochloride	50 mg	Light Green	Tablet	Circle	Mylan Pharmaceuticals
M S3	Sertraline Hydrochloride	100 mg	Light Green	Tablet	Oval	Mylan Pharmaceuticals
M S23 ;	Sotalol Hydrochloride	80 mg	Light Orange	Tablet	Circle	Mylan Pharmaceuticals
M S24 ;	Sotalol Hydrochloride	120 mg	Light Orange	Tablet	Circle	Mylan Pharmaceuticals
M S25 ;	Sotalol Hydrochloride	160 mg	Light Orange	Tablet	Circle	Mylan Pharmaceuticals
M V4 ;	Venlafaxine Hydrochloride	75 mg	Yellow	Tablet	Circle	Mylan Pharmaceuticals
M V5 ;	Venlafaxine Hydrochloride	100 mg	Yellow	Tablet	Circle	Mylan Pharmaceuticals
M Z1	Zolpidem Tartrate	5 mg	Lavender	Tablet	Circle	Mylan Pharmaceuticals
M Z2	Zolpidem Tartrate	10 mg	Lavender	Tablet	Circle	Mylan Pharmaceuticals
M; 018	Nucofed	20 mg ; 60 mg	Green and Clear	Capsule		Monarch Pharmaceuticals
M; 019 ;	Quibron-T/SR	300 mg	White	Sustained-Release Tablet	Accudose (Triple-Scored)	Monarch Pharmaceuticals
M; 020	Quibron-T	300 mg	Ivory	Tablet	Accudose (Triple-Scored)	Monarch Pharmaceuticals
M; 022 ;	Quibron	150 mg ; 90 mg	Clear Yellow	Capsule, Liquid Filled		Monarch Pharmaceuticals
M; 052 ;	Septra	400 mg ; 80 mg	Pink	Tablet	Circle, Scored	Monarch Pharmaceuticals
M; 053 ;	Septra DS	160 mg ; 800 mg	Pink	Tablet	Oval, Scored	Monarch Pharmaceuticals
M; 1	Clonidine Hydrochloride and Chlorthalidone	0.1 mg ; 15 mg	Yellow	Tablet	Circle, Scored, Biconvex	Mylan Pharmaceuticals
M; 1	Clorpres	15 mg ; 0.1 mg	Yellow	Tablet	Circle, Scored	Mylan Bertek Pharmaceuticals
M; 4	Fluphenazine Hydrochloride	1 mg	White	Tablet	Triangle	Mylan Pharmaceuticals
M; 9	Fluphenazine Hydrochloride	2.5 mg	Yellow	Tablet	Triangle	Mylan Pharmaceuticals
M; 11	Penicillin V Potassium	250 mg	White	Tablet	Oval	Mylan Pharmaceuticals
M; 12	Penicillin V Potassium	500 mg	White	Tablet	Circle, Scored	Mylan Pharmaceuticals
M; 12	Penicillin VK	500 mg		Tablet		Teva Pharmaceuticals
M; 13	Tolbutamide	500 mg	White	Tablet	Circle	Mylan Pharmaceuticals
M; 14	Methotrexate Sodium	2.5 mg	Orange	Tablet	Circle	Mylan Pharmaceuticals
M; 15	Atropine Sulfate and Diphenoxylate Hydrochloride	0.025 mg ; 2.5 mg	White	Tablet	Circle	Mylan Pharmaceuticals
M; 15	Klor-Con M15	1125 mg	White	Tablet	Oblong	Upsher-Smith Laboratories

IMPRINT	BRAND/GENERIC NAME	STRENGTH	COLOR	FORM	SHAPE	MANUFACTURER
M; 23	Diltiazem Hydrochloride	30 mg	White	Tablet	Circle	Mylan Pharmaceuticals
M; 25	L-Thyroxine	0.025 mg	Blue	Tablet	Circle, Scored	Warner Chilcott
M; 27	Clonidine Hydrochloride and Chlorthalidone	0.2 mg ; 15 mg	Yellow	Tablet	Scored, Biconvex, Circle	Mylan Pharmaceuticals
M; 27	Clorpres	15 mg ; 0.2 mg	Yellow	Tablet	Circle, Scored	Mylan Bertek Pharmaceuticals
M; 28	Nadolol	20 mg	Yellow	Tablet	Circle	Mylan Pharmaceuticals
M; 29	Methyclothiazide	5 mg	Blue	Tablet	Circle, Scored	Mylan Pharmaceuticals
M; 31	Allopurinol	100 mg	White	Tablet	Circle	Mylan Pharmaceuticals
M; 33	Chlorothiazide and Reserpine	0.125 mg ; 250 mg	Light Orange	Tablet	Circle, Scored, Flat Beveled Edge	Mylan Pharmaceuticals
M; 33; 56	Orphenadrine Citrate, Aspirin and Caffeine Double Strength	50 mg ; 770 mg ; 60 mg	White and Yellow Layered	Tablet	Capsule-Shape	Mylan Pharmaceuticals
M; 35	Chlorthalidone	25 mg	Yellow	Tablet	Circle	Mylan Pharmaceuticals
M; 36	Amitriptyline Hydrochloride	50 mg	Brown	Tablet	Circle	Mylan Pharmaceuticals
M; 37	Amitriptyline Hydrochloride	75 mg	Blue	Tablet	Circle	Mylan Pharmaceuticals
M; 38	Amitriptyline Hydrochloride	100 mg	Orange	Tablet	Circle	Mylan Pharmaceuticals
M; 39	Amitriptyline Hydrochloride	150 mg	Flesh	Coated Tablet	Capsule-Shape	Mylan Pharmaceuticals
M; 40	Clorazepate Dipotassium	7.5 mg	Peach	Tablet	Circle, Scored, Flat Beveled Edge	Mylan Pharmaceuticals
M; 40; MATERNA	Materna Prenatal Vitamin and Mineral	5000 IU ; 10 mg ; 25 mg ; 30 IU ; 400 IU ; 3.4 mg ; 10 mg ; 12 mcg ; 3 mg ; 25 mcg ; 25 mg ; 150 mcg ; 2 mg ; 250 mg ; 100 mg ; 30 mcg ; 25 mcg ; 1 mg ; 60 mg ; 5 mg ; 20 mg	Off-White	Coated Tablet	Oval, Scored	Wyeth-Ayerst Laboratories
M; 41	Spironolactone and Hydrochlorothiazide	25 mg ; 25 mg	Ivory	Tablet	Circle	Mylan Pharmaceuticals
M; 43	Chlorothiazide and Reserpine	0.125 mg ; 500 mg	Light Orange	Tablet	Circle, Scored, Flat Beveled Edge	Mylan Pharmaceuticals
M; 45	Diltiazem Hydrochloride	60 mg	White	Tablet	Circle	Mylan Pharmaceuticals
M; 46	Spironolactone	25 mg	Orange	Tablet		Mylan Pharmaceuticals
M; 50	Chlorothiazide	250 mg	White	Tablet	Circle, Scored	Mylan Pharmaceuticals
M; 50	L-Thyroxine	0.05 mg	Blue	Tablet	Circle, Scored	Warner Chilcott
M; 51	Amitriptyline Hydrochloride	25 mg	Light Green	Tablet	Circle	Mylan Pharmaceuticals
M; 52	Pindolol	5 mg	White	Tablet	Circle, Scored, Biconvex	Mylan Pharmaceuticals
M; 53	Cimetidine	200 mg	Green	Coated Tablet	Five-Sided, House Shaped, Biconvex, Beveled Edge	Mylan Pharmaceuticals
M; 54; 10	Thioridazine Hydrochloride	10 mg	Orange	Tablet	Circle	Mylan Pharmaceuticals
M; 55	Timolol Maleate	5 mg	Green	Tablet	Circle, Flat Beveled Edge	Mylan Pharmaceuticals
M; 58; 25	Thioridazine Hydrochloride	25 mg		Tablet		Roxane Laboratories
M; 58; 25	Thioridazine Hydrochloride	25 mg	Orange	Tablet	Circle	Mylan Pharmaceuticals
M; 59; 50	Thioridazine Hydrochloride	50 mg		Tablet		Roxane Laboratories
M; 59; 50	Thioridazine Hydrochloride	50 mg	Orange	Tablet	Circle	Mylan Pharmaceuticals
M; 60	Maprotiline Hydrochloride	25 mg	White	Coated Tablet	Circle, Scored, Biconvex, Beveled Edge	Mylan Pharmaceuticals
M; 61; 100	Thioridazine Hydrochloride	100 mg		Tablet		Roxane Laboratories
M; 61; 100	Thioridazine Hydrochloride	100 mg	Orange	Tablet	Circle	Mylan Pharmaceuticals
M; 63	Atenolol and Chlorthalidone	50 mg ; 25 mg	White	Tablet	Circle, Scored, Biconvex	Mylan Pharmaceuticals
M; 64	Atenolol and Chlorthalidone	100 mg ; 25 mg	White	Tablet	Circle, Biconvex	Mylan Pharmaceuticals
M; 65	Acetaminophen and Propoxyphene Hydrochloride	65 mg ; 650 mg	Orange	Capsule		Mylan Pharmaceuticals
M; 69	Indapamide	1.25 mg		Tablet		Mylan Pharmaceuticals
M; 70	Clorazepate Dipotassium	15 mg	White	Tablet	Circle, Scored, Flat Beveled Edge	Mylan Pharmaceuticals
M; 71	Allopurinol	300 mg	White	Tablet	Circle	Mylan Pharmaceuticals
M; 72	Clonidine Hydrochloride and Chlorthalidone	0.3 mg ; 15 mg	Yellow	Tablet	Circle, Scored, Biconvex	Mylan Pharmaceuticals
M; 72	Clorpres	0.3 mg ; 15 mg	Yellow	Tablet	Circle, Scored	Mylan Bertek Pharmaceuticals
M; 72	Menest	0.3 mg	Yellow	Coated Tablet	Oblong	Monarch Pharmaceuticals
M; 73	Menest	0.625 mg	Orange	Coated Tablet	Oblong	Monarch Pharmaceuticals
M; 74	Fluphenazine Hydrochloride	5 mg	Green	Tablet	Triangle	Mylan Pharmaceuticals
M; 74	Menest	1.25 mg	Green	Coated Tablet	Oblong	Monarch Pharmaceuticals
M; 75	Chlorthalidone	50 mg	Green	Tablet	Circle	Mylan Pharmaceuticals
M; 75	L-Thyroxine	0.075 mg	Blue	Tablet	Circle, Scored	Warner Chilcott
M; 75	Menest	2.5 mg	Pink	Coated Tablet	Oblong	Monarch Pharmaceuticals
M; 76	Flurbiprofen	50 mg	Beige	Coated Tablet	Circle	Mylan Pharmaceuticals
M; 77	Amitriptyline Hydrochloride	10 mg	White	Tablet	Circle	Mylan Pharmaceuticals
M; 80	Indapamide	2.5 mg	White	Tablet	Circle	Mylan Pharmaceuticals
M; 81	Captopril and Hydrochlorothiazide	25 mg ; 15 mg	White	Tablet	Circle, Scored	Mylan Pharmaceuticals
M; 83	Captopril and Hydrochlorothiazide	25 mg ; 25 mg	Peach	Tablet	Circle, Scored	Mylan Pharmaceuticals
M; 84	Captopril and Hydrochlorothiazide	15 mg ; 50 mg	White	Tablet	Capsule-Shape, Scored	Mylan Pharmaceuticals
M; 86	Captopril and Hydrochlorothiazide	50 mg ; 25 mg	Peach	Tablet	Capsule-Shape, Scored	Mylan Pharmaceuticals
M; 87	Maprotiline Hydrochloride	50 mg	Blue	Coated Tablet	Circle, Scored, Biconvex, Beveled Edge	Mylan Pharmaceuticals
M; 92	Maprotiline Hydrochloride	75 mg	White	Coated Tablet	Scored, Biconvex, Beveled Edge, Circle	Mylan Pharmaceuticals
M; 93	Flurbiprofen	100 mg	Beige	Coated Tablet	Circle	Mylan Pharmaceuticals
M; 95	Penicillin V Potassium	250 mg	White	Tablet	Circle, Scored	Mylan Pharmaceuticals
M; 97	Fluphenazine Hydrochloride	10 mg	Orange	Tablet	Triangle	Mylan Pharmaceuticals
M; 98	Penicillin V Potassium	500 mg	White	Tablet	Oval	Mylan Pharmaceuticals
M; 100	L-Thyroxine	0.1 mg	Blue	Tablet	Circle, Scored	Warner Chilcott
M; 100	Motrin	100 mg	White	Tablet	Capsule-Shape, Scored	Mcneil Consumer Healthcare Division of Mcneil
M; 100; LEVO; T	L-Thyroxine	0.1 mg	Yellow	Tablet	Circle, Scored	Novartis Generics
M; 113	Glyburide, Micronized	1.5 mg	White	Tablet	Oval, Scored	Mylan Pharmaceuticals
M; 125	Glyburide, Micronized	3 mg	Light Yellow	Tablet	Oval, Scored	Mylan Pharmaceuticals

IMPRINT	BRAND/GENERIC NAME	STRENGTH	COLOR	FORM	SHAPE	MANUFACTURER
M; 125	L-Thyroxine	0.125 mg	Blue	Tablet	Circle, Scored	Warner Chilcott
M; 127	Pindolol	10 mg	White	Tablet	Circle, Scored, Biconvex	Mylan Pharmaceuticals
M; 132	Nadolol	80 mg	Yellow	Tablet	Circle	Mylan Pharmaceuticals
M; 134	Ketorolac Tromethamine	10 mg	White	Tablet	Circle	Mylan Pharmaceuticals
M; 135	Diltiazem Hydrochloride	90 mg	White	Tablet	Capsule-Shape	Mylan Pharmaceuticals
M; 142	Glyburide	6 mg	Green	Tablet	Scored, Oval	Mylan Pharmaceuticals
M; 144	Tamoxifen Citrate	10 mg	White	Tablet	Circle	Mylan Pharmaceuticals
M; 146	Spironolactone	25 mg	White	Tablet	Circle	Mylan Pharmaceuticals
M; 150	L-Thyroxine	0.15 mg	Blue	Tablet	Circle, Scored	Warner Chilcott
M; 150; LEVO; T	L-Thyroxine	0.15 mg	Blue	Tablet	Circle, Scored	Novartis Generics
M; 171	Nadolol	40 mg	Yellow	Tablet	Circle	Mylan Pharmaceuticals
M; 172	Metolazone	2.5 mg	Peach	Tablet	Circle	Mylan Pharmaceuticals
M; 200	L-Thyroxine	0.2 mg	Blue	Tablet	Circle, Scored	Warner Chilcott
M; 200; LEVO; T	L-Thyroxine	0.2 mg	Pink	Tablet	Circle, Scored	Novartis Generics
M; 221	Timolol Maleate	10 mg	Green	Tablet	Circle, Scored, Flat Beveled Edge	Mylan Pharmaceuticals
M; 231	Atenolol	50 mg	White	Tablet	Circle	Mylan Pharmaceuticals
M; 243	Spironolactone	50 mg	White	Coated Tablet	Circle, Biconvex, Bevel-Edged, Scored	Mylan Pharmaceuticals
M; 253	Acyclovir	400 mg	White	Tablet	Circle	Mylan Pharmaceuticals
M; 255	Albuterol	2 mg	White	Tablet	Circle	Mylan Pharmaceuticals
M; 261	Ketoconazole	200 mg	White	Tablet	Circle	Mylan Pharmaceuticals
M; 273	Penicillin V Potassium	250 mg	White	Coated Tablet	Circle, Biconvex, Scored	Mylan Pharmaceuticals
M; 274	Tamoxifen Citrate	20 mg	White to Off-White	Tablet	Circle	Mylan Pharmaceuticals
M; 275	Penicillin V Potassium	500 mg	White	Coated Tablet	Oblong, Biconvex, Scored on Both Sides	Mylan Pharmaceuticals
M; 300	L-Thyroxine	0.3 mg	Blue	Tablet	Circle, Scored	Warner Chilcott
M; 300; LEVO; T	L-Thyroxine	0.3 mg	Green	Tablet	Circle, Scored	Novartis Generics
M; 302	Acyclovir	800 mg	White	Tablet	Oval	Mylan Pharmaceuticals
M; 305	Sotalol Hydrochloride	80 mg	Orange	Tablet	Circle, Scored	Mylan Pharmaceuticals
M; 310	Sotalol Hydrochloride	120 mg	Orange	Tablet	Circle, Scored	Mylan Pharmaceuticals
M; 313	Tolmetin Sodium	600 mg	Beige	Coated Tablet	Oval	Mylan Pharmaceuticals
M; 314	Sotalol Hydrochloride	160 mg	Orange	Tablet	Circle, Scored	Mylan Pharmaceuticals
M; 316	Sotalol Hydrochloride	240 mg	Orange	Tablet	Circle, Scored	Mylan Pharmaceuticals
M; 317	Cimetidine	300 mg	Green	Tablet	Five-Sided	Mylan Pharmaceuticals
M; 355	Diclofenac Sodium	100 mg	Yellow	Extended-Release Tablet	Circle, Biconvex, Bevel-Edged	Mylan Pharmaceuticals
M; 365	Procet	5 mg ; 325 mg	White	Tablet	Capsule-Shape, Scored	Andrx Pharmaceuticals
M; 366	Procet	7.5 mg ; 325 mg	White	Tablet	Oval, Scored	Andrx Pharmaceuticals
M; 372	Cimetidine	400 mg	Green	Coated Tablet	Five-Sided, House Shaped	Mylan Pharmaceuticals
M; 373	Hydroxychloroquine Sulfate	200 mg	White	Tablet	Circle	Mylan Pharmaceuticals
M; 400	Erythromycin Ethylsuccinate	400 mg	Beige	Coated Tablet	Capsule-Shape, Biconvex, Beveled Edge	Mylan Pharmaceuticals
M; 407	Fluvoxamine Maleate	25 mg	Off-White to Yellow	Tablet	Oval	Mylan Pharmaceuticals
M; 407	Fluvoxamine Maleate	25 mg	Orange	Tablet	Oval	Mylan Pharmaceuticals
M; 412	Fluvoxamine Maleate	50 mg	Off-White to Yellow	Tablet	Oval, Scored	Mylan Pharmaceuticals
M; 412	Fluvoxamine Maleate	50 mg	Orange	Tablet	Oval, Scored	Mylan Pharmaceuticals
M; 414	Fluvoxamine Maleate	100 mg	Off-White to Yellow	Tablet	Oval, Scored	Mylan Pharmaceuticals
M; 414	Fluvoxamine Maleate	100 mg	Orange	Tablet	Oval, Scored	Mylan Pharmaceuticals
M; 433	Bupropion Hydrochloride	75 mg	Peach	Tablet	Circle	Mylan Pharmaceuticals
M; 435	Bupropion Hydrochloride	100 mg	Light Blue	Tablet	Circle	Mylan Pharmaceuticals
M; 437	Spironolactone	100 mg	White	Coated Tablet	Circle, Biconvex, Bevel-Edged, Scored	Mylan Pharmaceuticals
M; 441	Benazepril Hydrochloride	5 mg	White	Tablet	Circle	Mylan Pharmaceuticals
M; 443	Benazepril Hydrochloride	10 mg	White	Tablet	Circle	Mylan Pharmaceuticals
M; 444	Benazepril Hydrochloride	20 mg	White	Tablet	Circle	Mylan Pharmaceuticals
M; 447	Benazepril Hydrochloride	40 mg	White	Tablet	Oval	Mylan Pharmaceuticals
M; 471	Fenoprofen Calcium	600 mg	Orange	Coated Tablet	Capsule-Shape, Scored	Mylan Pharmaceuticals
M; 475	Nifedipine ER	30 mg	Rose-Pink	Extended-Release Tablet	Circle	Mylan Pharmaceuticals
M; 482	Nifedipine ER	60 mg	Rose-Pink	Extended-Release Tablet	Circle	Mylan Pharmaceuticals
M; 495	Nifedipine ER	90 mg	Rose-Pink	Extended-Release Tablet	Circle	Mylan Pharmaceuticals
M; 501	Bisoprolol Fumarate and Hydrochlorothiazide	2.5 mg ; 6.25 mg	Orange	Tablet	Circle	Mylan Pharmaceuticals
M; 503	Bisoprolol Fumarate and Hydrochlorothiazide	5 mg ; 6.25 mg	Blue	Tablet	Circle	Mylan Pharmaceuticals
M; 505	Bisoprolol Fumarate and Hydrochlorothiazide	10 mg ; 6.25 mg	White	Tablet	Circle	Mylan Pharmaceuticals
M; 525	Diltiazem Hydrochloride	120 mg	White with Clear Film Coat	Coated Tablet	Capsule-Shape, Scored	Mylan Pharmaceuticals
M; 537	Naproxen Sodium	275 mg	Light Blue	Coated Tablet	Circle	Mylan Pharmaceuticals
M; 541	Cimetidine	800 mg	Green	Coated Tablet	Oval, Scored	Mylan Pharmaceuticals
M; 572	Albuterol	4 mg	White	Tablet	Circle	Mylan Pharmaceuticals
M; 577	Amiloride Hydrochloride and Hydrochlorothiazide	5 mg ; 50 mg	Orange	Tablet	Circle, Scored	Mylan Pharmaceuticals
M; 712	Enalapril and Hydrochlorothiazide	5 mg ; 12.5 mg	White	Tablet	Circle, Biconvex	Mylan Pharmaceuticals
M; 715	Timolol Maleate	20 mg	Green	Tablet	Capsule-Shape, Scored, Biconvex, Beveled Edge	Mylan Pharmaceuticals
M; 723	Enalapril and Hydrochlorothiazide	10 mg ; 25 mg	White	Tablet	Circle, Biconvex	Mylan Pharmaceuticals
M; 725	Benazepril Hydrochloride and Hydrochlorothiazide	6.25 mg ; 5 mg	Beige	Tablet	Scored, Oval	Mylan Pharmaceuticals
M; 735	Benazepril Hydrochloride and Hydrochlorothiazide	12.5 mg ; 10 mg	Beige	Tablet	Circle, Scored	Mylan Pharmaceuticals
M; 745	Benazepril Hydrochloride and Hydrochlorothiazide	20 mg ; 12.5 mg	Beige	Tablet	Capsule-Shape, Scored	Mylan Pharmaceuticals
M; 757	Atenolol	100 mg	White	Tablet	Circle	Mylan Pharmaceuticals
M; 775	Benazepril Hydrochloride and Hydrochlorothiazide	20 mg ; 25 mg	Beige	Tablet	Oval, Scored	Mylan Pharmaceuticals
M; 3354	Orphenadrine Citrate, Aspirin and Caffeine	385 mg ; 30 mg ; 25 mg	White and Yellow Layered	Tablet	Circle	Mylan Pharmaceuticals
M; 3358	Orphenadrine Citrate	100 mg	White	Extended-Release Tablet	Circle	Mylan Pharmaceuticals
M; A2	Atenolol	25 mg	White	Tablet	Circle	Mylan Pharmaceuticals

IMPRINT	BRAND/GENERIC NAME	STRENGTH	COLOR	FORM	SHAPE	MANUFACTURER
M; B1	Buspirone Hydrochloride	5 mg	White	Tablet	Oval, Biconvex, Scored	Mylan Pharmaceuticals
M; B2	Buspirone Hydrochloride	10 mg	White	Tablet	Oval, Biconvex, Scored	Mylan Pharmaceuticals
M; B3; 5 5 5	Buspirone Hydrochloride	15 mg	White	Tablet	Capsule-Shape	Mylan Pharmaceuticals
M; B4; 10 10 10	Buspirone Hydrochloride	30 mg	White	Tablet	Capsule-Shape, Bevel-Edged, trisected	Mylan Pharmaceuticals
M; C; 7	Clozapine	25 mg	Peach	Tablet	Circle	Mylan Pharmaceuticals
M; C; 11	Clozapine	100 mg	Green	Tablet	Circle	Mylan Pharmaceuticals
M; C; 13	Clonazepam	0.5 mg	Yellow	Tablet	Circle	Mylan Pharmaceuticals
M; C; 14	Clonazepam	1 mg	Green	Tablet	Circle	Mylan Pharmaceuticals
M; C; 15	Clonazepam	2 mg	White	Tablet	Circle	Mylan Pharmaceuticals
M; C1	Captopril	12.5 mg	White	Tablet	Oval	Mylan Pharmaceuticals
M; C2	Captopril	25 mg	White	Tablet	Circle	Mylan Pharmaceuticals
M; C3	Captopril	50 mg	White	Tablet	Circle, Scored	Mylan Pharmaceuticals
M; C4	Captopril	100 mg	White	Tablet	Circle, Scored	Mylan Pharmaceuticals
M; D5	Diclofenac Potassium	50 mg	White	Coated Tablet	Circle, Biconvex	Mylan Pharmaceuticals
M; D6	Dicyclomine Hydrochloride	20 mg	Blue	Tablet	Circle	Mylan Pharmaceuticals
M; D9	Doxazosin Mesylate	1 mg	White	Tablet	Circle	Mylan Pharmaceuticals
M; D10	Doxazosin Mesylate	2 mg	Pink	Tablet	Circle	Mylan Pharmaceuticals
M; D11	Doxazosin Mesylate	4 mg	Blue	Tablet	Circle	Mylan Pharmaceuticals
M; D12	Doxazosin Mesylate	8 mg	Purple	Tablet	Circle, Scored	Mylan Pharmaceuticals
M; E3	Estradiol	0.5 mg	White	Tablet	Circle	Mylan Pharmaceuticals
M; E4	Estradiol	1 mg	Pink	Tablet	Circle	Mylan Pharmaceuticals
M; E5	Estradiol	2 mg	Blue	Tablet	Circle	Mylan Pharmaceuticals
M; E7	Estropipate	0.75 mg	Yellow	Tablet	Circle	Mylan Pharmaceuticals
M; E8	Estropipate	1.5 mg	Peach	Tablet	Circle	Mylan Pharmaceuticals
M; E9	Estropipate	3 mg	Blue	Tablet	Circle	Mylan Pharmaceuticals
M; E15	Enalapril Maleate	2.5 mg	White	Tablet	Circle	Mylan Pharmaceuticals
M; E16	Enalapril Maleate	5 mg	White	Tablet	Circle	Mylan Pharmaceuticals
M; E17	Enalapril Maleate	10 mg	Light Blue	Tablet	Circle	Mylan Pharmaceuticals
M; E18	Enalapril Maleate	20 mg	Blue	Tablet	Circle	Mylan Pharmaceuticals
M; F1	Famotidine	20 mg	Yellow	Tablet	Circle	Mylan Pharmaceuticals
M; F2	Famotidine	40 mg	Green	Coated Tablet	Circle, Biconvex, Bevel-Edged	Mylan Pharmaceuticals
M; G4	Guanfacine	1 mg	White	Tablet	Circle	Mylan Pharmaceuticals
M; G5	Guanfacine	2 mg	Blue	Tablet	Circle	Mylan Pharmaceuticals
M; L19	Lovastatin	10 mg	White to Off-White	Tablet	Circle, Flat-Faced, Bevel-Edged	Mylan Pharmaceuticals
M; L20	Lovastatin	20 mg	Yellow	Tablet	Circle, Flat-Faced, Bevel-Edged	Mylan Pharmaceuticals
M; L21	Lovastatin	40 mg	Pink	Tablet	Circle, Flat-Faced, Bevel-Edged	Mylan Pharmaceuticals
M; L22	Lisinopril	2.5 mg	Light Blue	Tablet	Circle	Mylan Pharmaceuticals
M; L27	Lisinopril	30 mg	Light Blue	Tablet	Circle	Mylan Pharmaceuticals
M; LH1	Hydrochlorothiazide and Lisinopril	12.5 mg ; 10 mg		Tablet		Mylan Pharmaceuticals
M; LH2	Hydrochlorothiazide and Lisinopril	12.5 mg ; 20 mg		Tablet		Mylan Pharmaceuticals
M; LH3	Hydrochlorothiazide and Lisinopril	25 mg ; 20 mg		Tablet		Mylan Pharmaceuticals
M; N; 52	Nefazodone Hydrochloride	100 mg	White	Tablet	Circle	Mylan Pharmaceuticals
M; N; 53	Nefazodone Hydrochloride	150 mg	White	Tablet	Circle	Mylan Pharmaceuticals
M; N; 54	Nefazodone Hydrochloride	200 mg	White	Tablet	Circle	Mylan Pharmaceuticals
M; N; 55	Nefazodone Hydrochloride	250 mg	White	Tablet	Circle	Mylan Pharmaceuticals
M; P1	Prochlorperazine Maleate	5 mg	Maroon	Tablet	Circle	Mylan Pharmaceuticals
M; P2	Prochlorperazine Maleate	10 mg	Maroon	Tablet	Circle	Mylan Pharmaceuticals
M; R	Nu-Iron-V	3 mg ; 2 mg ; 10 mg ; 312 mg ; 60 mg ; 1 mg ; 50 mg ; 3 mcg ; 4000 IU ; 400 IU ; 3 mg	Red	Tablet	Oblong, Scored	Merz
M; T3	Trifluoperazine Hydrochloride	1 mg	White	Tablet	Circle	Mylan Pharmaceuticals
M; T4	Trifluoperazine Hydrochloride	2 mg	White	Tablet	Circle	Mylan Pharmaceuticals
M; T5	Trifluoperazine Hydrochloride	5 mg	Lavender	Tablet	Circle	Mylan Pharmaceuticals
M; T6	Trifluoperazine Hydrochloride	10 mg	Lavender	Tablet	Circle	Mylan Pharmaceuticals
M03; 1.5; MOVA	Glyburide Micronized	1.5 mg	White	Tablet	Oval, Bisected Scored	Watson Laboratories
M04; 3.0; MOVA	Glyburide Micronized	3 mg	Blue	Tablet	Oval, Bisected Scored	Watson Laboratories
M07; 6.0; MOVA	Glyburide Micronized	6 mg	Light Yellow	Tablet	Oval, Bisected Scored	Watson Laboratories
M2	Furosemide	20 mg	White	Tablet	Circle	Mylan Pharmaceuticals
M4	Mesnex	400 mg	White	Tablet	Oblong	Baxter Healthcare
M30 ;	Clorazepate Dipotassium	3.75 mg	Blue	Tablet	Circle	Mylan Pharmaceuticals
M118	Pentazocine and Naloxone Hydrochloride	50 mg ; 0.5 mg	Light Yellow	Tablet	Capsule-Shape, Scored	Ranbaxy Pharmaceuticals
M312 ;	Verapamil Hydrochloride	180 mg	Blue	Tablet, Extended Release	Oval	Mylan Pharmaceuticals
M411 ;	Verapamil Hydrochloride	240 mg	Blue	Tablet, Extended Release	Capsule-Shape	Mylan Pharmaceuticals
M1000	Glumetza	1000 mg	White	Tablet, Extended Release	Oval	Depomed
MACROBID; NORWICH EATON	Macrobid	100 mg	Opaque, Black and Yellow	Capsule		Procter & Gamble Pharmaceuticals
MACRODANTIN; 25 MG; 0149; 0007	Macrodantin	25 mg	Opaque, White	Capsule		Procter & Gamble Pharmaceuticals
MACRODANTIN; 50 MG; 0149-0008	Macrodantin	50 mg	Opaque, Yellow and White	Capsule		Procter & Gamble Pharmaceuticals
MACRODANTIN; 100 MG; 0149; 0009	Macrodantin	100 mg	Opaque, Yellow	Capsule		Procter & Gamble Pharmaceuticals
MAOLATE	Maolate	400 mg	Tan	Tablet	Circle, Scored	Upjohn
MARION; 1525	Duotrate	30 mg	Black and Clear with White Pellets	Capsule		Aventis Pharmaceuticals
MARION; 1530	Duotrate	45 mg	Black and Light Blue with White Pellets	Capsule		Aventis Pharmaceuticals
MARION; 1555	Pavabid	150 mg		Extended-Release Capsule		Aventis Pharmaceuticals
MARION; 1555	Pavabid Plateau	150 mg		Timed-Release Capsule		Aventis Pharmaceuticals
MARION; 1555; PAVABID	Pavabid	150 mg	Black and White	Capsule		Aventis Pharmaceuticals

IMPRINT	BRAND/GENERIC NAME	STRENGTH	COLOR	FORM	SHAPE	MANUFACTURER
MARION; 1656	Os-Cal-Gesic	400 mg ; 100 mg ; 50 U	Blue-Green	Tablet	Oblong	Aventis Pharmaceuticals
MARION; PAVABID HP	Pavabid Hp Capsulets	300 mg	Light Orange	Tablet		Aventis Pharmaceuticals
MARION; PAVABID: HP	Pavabid Hp	300 mg	Light Orange	Capsule		Aventis Pharmaceuticals
MARION; PRETTS; 1177	Pretts Diet Aid	200 mg ; 100 mg ; 70 mg	Yellow	Tablet	Circle	Aventis Pharmaceuticals
MATULANE; O; SIGMA-TAU ;	Matulane	50 mg	Ivory	Capsule		Sigma-Tau Pharmaceuticals
MAXIDONE; 634	Maxidone	750 mg ; 10 mg	Yellow	Tablet	Capsule-Shape, Scored	Watson Laboratories
MAXZIDE; B; M8	Maxzide	75 mg ; 50 mg	Yellow	Tablet	Bowtie	Mylan Bertek Pharmaceuticals
MAXZIDE; B; M9	Maxzide	37.5 mg ; 25 mg	Green	Tablet	Bowtie	Mylan Bertek Pharmaceuticals
MAYRAND	Eldercaps	110 mg ; 70 mg ; 5 mg ; 1 mg ; 400 IU ; 4000 IU ; 25 IU ; 200 mg ; 10 mg ; 5 mg ; 2 mg ; 25 mg ; 10 mg	Opaque Red	Capsule		Merz
MAYRAND	Trimcaps	105 mg	Lavender and White	Sustained-Release Capsule		Merz
MC	Desoxyn	5 mg	White	Sustained-Release Tablet		Abbott Laboratories
MCNEIL; 058 ;	Butibel-Zyme	15 mg ; 15 mg	Pink	Tablet		Mcneil Pharmaceutical
MCNEIL; 1/2; HALDOL	Haldol	0.5 mg	White	Tablet	U-Shape, with "H" Cut Out in Center, Scored	Ortho-Mcneil Pharmaceutical
MCNEIL; 151	Clistin-Ra	8 mg	Orange	Coated Tablet		Mcneil Pharmaceutical
MCNEIL; 153	Clistin-Ra	12 mg	Yellow	Coated Tablet		Mcneil Pharmaceutical
MCNEIL; 659 ;	Ultram	50 mg	White	Coated Tablet	Capsule-Shape, Scored	Ortho-Mcneil Pharmaceutical
MCNEIL; BUTIBEL ;	Butibel	15 mg ; 15 mg	Red	Tablet		Mcneil Pharmaceutical
MCNEIL; BUTICAPS ;	Buticaps	15 mg	Lavender and White	Capsule		Mcneil Pharmaceutical
MCNEIL; BUTICAPS ;	Buticaps	30 mg	Aqua-Green and White	Capsule		Mcneil Pharmaceutical
MCNEIL; BUTICAPS ;	Buticaps	50 mg	Orange and White	Capsule		Mcneil Pharmaceutical
MCNEIL; BUTICAPS ;	Buticaps	100 mg	Pink and White	Capsule		Mcneil Pharmaceutical
MCNEIL; BUTISOL SODIUM ;	Butisol Sodium	30 mg	Green	Tablet	Circle, Scored	Mcneil Pharmaceutical
MCNEIL; BUTISOL SODIUM ;	Butisol Sodium	50 mg	Orange	Tablet	Circle, Scored	Mcneil Pharmaceutical
MCNEIL; BUTISOL SODIUM ;	Butisol Sodium	100 mg	Pink	Tablet		Mcneil Pharmaceutical
MCNEIL; PANCREASE	Pancrease	4500 U ; 20000 U ; 25000 U	White	Capsule		Ortho-Mcneil Pharmaceutical
MCNEIL; PANCREASE; MT 4	Pancrease Mt 4	12,000 USP units ; 12,000 USP units ; 4000 USP units	Yellow and Clear	Capsule		Mcneil Pharmaceutical
MCNEIL; PANCREASE; MT 10	Pancrease Mt 10	30,000 USP units ; 10,000 USP units ; 30,000 USP units	Pink and Clear	Capsule		Mcneil Pharmaceutical
MCNEIL; PANCREASE; MT 16	Pancrease Mt 16	16,000 USP units ; 48,000 USP units ; 48,000 USP units	Salmon and Clear	Capsule		Mcneil Pharmaceutical
MCNEIL; PANCREASE; MT 25	Pancrease Mt 25	25000 U ; 75000 U ; 75000 U	White	Capsule		Mcneil Pharmaceutical
MCNEIL; PANCREASE; MT 32	Pancrease Mt 32	32000 U ; 90000 U ; 70000 U	White	Capsule		Mcneil Pharmaceutical
MCNEIL; TYLENOL CODEINE 2 ;	Tylenol with Codeine No. 2	15 mg ; 300 mg	White	Tablet		Mcneil Pharmaceutical
MCNEIL; TYLENOL; CODEINE 1	Tylenol with Codeine No. 1	7.5 mg ; 300 mg	White	Tablet	Circle	Mcneil Pharmaceutical
MD; 518	Diethylpropion Hydrochloride	25 mg	Medium Blue		Circle	Novartis Generics
ME	Desoxyn	10 mg	Orange	Sustained-Release Tablet		Abbott Laboratories
MEDACID	Medacid Antacid	223 mg ; 127 mg ; 59 mg	Blue	Tablet		Bristol-Myers Squibb
MEDROL 4 ;	Medrol	4 mg	White	Tablet	Oval	Pharmacia & Upjohn
MEDROL; 2	Medrol	2 mg	Pink	Tablet	Oval, Scored	Pharmacia & Upjohn
MEDROL; 8 ;	Medrol	8 mg	Peach	Tablet	Oval, Scored	Pharmacia & Upjohn
MEDROL; 16	Medrol	16 mg	White	Tablet	Oval, Scored	Pharmacia & Upjohn
MEDROL; 24 ;	Medrol	24 mg	Yellow	Tablet	Oval, Scored	Pharmacia & Upjohn
MEDROL; 32 ;	Medrol	32 mg	Peach	Tablet	Oval, Scored	Pharmacia & Upjohn
MERIDIA; 5	Meridia	5 mg	Blue and Yellow	Capsule		Abbott Laboratories
MERIDIA; 10	Meridia	10 mg	Blue and White	Capsule		Abbott Laboratories
MERIDIA; 15	Meridia	15 mg	Yellow and White	Capsule		Abbott Laboratories
MERRELL; 37	Cantil	25 mg	Yellow	Tablet		Sanofi-Aventis U.S.
MERRELL; 62	Metahydrin	2 mg	Pink	Tablet	Circle, Debossed	Aventis Pharmaceuticals
MERRELL; 63	Metahydrin	4 mg	Aqua Blue	Tablet	Circle, Debossed	Aventis Pharmaceuticals
MERRELL; 64	Metatensin	2 mg ; 0.1 mg	Yellow	Tablet		Aventis Pharmaceuticals
MERRELL; 65	Metatensin	4 mg ; 0.1 mg	Lavender	Tablet		Aventis Pharmaceuticals
MERRELL; 277	Hiprex	1 GM	Yellow	Tablet	Capsule-Shape	Sanofi-Aventis U.S.
MESTINON; 60; ICN	Mestinon	60 mg		Tablet		Valeant Pharmaceuticals
METRYL; 93	Metryl	250 mg	White	Tablet	Circle, Convex	Teva Pharmaceuticals
METRYL; 500; 93; 93	Metryl	500 mg	White	Tablet	Oblong, Scored	Teva Pharmaceuticals
MF	Desoxyn	15 mg	Yellow	Sustained-Release Tablet		Abbott Laboratories

IMPRINT	BRAND/GENERIC NAME	STRENGTH	COLOR	FORM	SHAPE	MANUFACTURER
MF; 1; G	Metformin Hydrochloride	500 mg	White	Tablet	Circle	Par Pharmaceutical
MF; 2; G	Metformin Hydrochloride	850 mg	White	Tablet	Circle	Par Pharmaceutical
MF; 3; G	Metformin Hydrochloride	1000 mg	White	Tablet	Oblong	Par Pharmaceutical
MH; 1; M	Midodrine Hydrochloride	2.5 mg	White to Off White	Tablet	Circle, Scored	Mylan Pharmaceuticals
MH; 2; M	Midodrine Hydrochloride	5 mg	White to Off White	Tablet	Scored, Circle	Mylan Pharmaceuticals
MH; 3; M	Midodrine Hydrochloride	10 mg	White to Off White	Tablet	Circle, Scored	Mylan Pharmaceuticals
MIA; 110	Butalbital, Acetaminophen and Caffeine	325 mg ; 50 mg ; 40 mg	White	Tablet	Capsule-Shape, Scored	Novartis Generics
MICRO-K 10; THER-RX 009	Micro-K 10	10 meq	Light Orange and White	Extended-Release Capsule		Ther-RX
MICRO-K; THER-RX 010	Micro-K	8 meq	Light Orange	Extended-Release Capsule		Ther-RX
MICRONASE; 1.25	Micronase	1.25 mg	White	Tablet	Circle, Scored	Pharmacia & Upjohn
MICRONASE; 2.5	Micronase	2.5 mg	Dark Pink	Tablet	Circle, Scored	Pharmacia & Upjohn
MICRONASE; 5	Micronase	5 mg	Blue	Tablet	Circle	Pharmacia & Upjohn
MICROZIDE; 12.5	Microzide	12.5 mg	Opaque Teal	Capsule, Liquid Filled		Watson Laboratories
MILES; 721	Niclocide	500 mg		Tablet		Bayer Pharmaceutical
MILES; 951	Lithane	300 mg	Green	Tablet	Circle, Scocred(Scored)	Bayer Pharmaceutical
MINOCYCLINE 50 DAN 5694 ;	Minocycline Hydrochloride	50 mg	Opaque Yellow	Capsule		Watson Laboratories
MINOCYCLINE 75 WPI ;	Minocycline Hydrochloride	75 mg	Opaque White, Opaque Yellow	Capsule		Watson Laboratories
MINOCYCLINE 100 DAN 5695 ;	Minocycline Hydrochloride	100 mg	Opaque Yelllow, Opaque Dark Gray	Capsule		Watson Laboratories
MINOXIDIL 2 1/2 ; PAR 256	Minoxidil	2.5 mg	White	Tablet	Circle	Par Pharmaceutical
MINOXIDIL 10 ; PAR 257	Minoxidil	10 mg	White	Tablet	Circle	Par Pharmaceutical
MJ 503 50	Cytoxan	50 mg	White with Blue Speckles	Tablet		Bristol-Myers Squibb
MJ; 021	Estrace	0.5 mg		Tablet		Warner Chilcott
MJ; 5 MG ;	Buspar	5 mg	White	Tablet	Ovoid-Rectangular, Scored	Mead Johnson
MJ; 10 MG ;	Buspar	10 mg	White	Tablet	Ovoid-Rectangular, Scored	Mead Johnson
MJ; 468	Poly-VI-Flor	0.3 mg ; 1.05 mg ; 1.2 mg ; 13.5 mg ; 60 mg ; 1.05 mg ; 4.5 mcg ; 0.5 mg ; 2500 IU ; 400 IU ; 15 IU	Purple, Orange, or Pink	Tablet, Chewable	Rectangle	Mead Johnson
MJ; 474	Poly-VI-Flor	15 IU ; 0.3 mg ; 1.05 mg ; 1.2 mg ; 4.5 mcg ; 1 mg ; 2500 U ; 13.5 mg ; 1.05 mg ; 60 mg ; 400 U	Pink, Purple, or Orange	Tablet, Chewable	Square	Mead Johnson
MJ; 487	Poly-VI-Flor	13.5 mg ; 1.2 mg ; 1.05 mg ; 45 mcg ; 60 mg ; 0.3 mg ; 0.25 mg ; 15 IU ; 400 IU ; 1.05 mg ; 2500 IU	Light Purple	Tablet, Chewable	Circle	Mead Johnson
MJ; 504; 25	Cytoxan	25 mg	White with Blue Speckles	Tablet		Bristol-Myers Squibb
MJ; 543	Vasodilan	10 mg	White	Tablet		Bristol-Myers Squibb
MJ; 555	Deapril-ST	1 mg		Tablet		Mead Johnson
MJ; 583	Ovcon-35-21	0.4 mg ; 35 mcg	Peach	21-Day Tablet Pack	Circle	Warner Chilcott
MJ; 584	Ovcon-50 Yellow Tablet	1 mg ; 50 mcg	Yellow	28-Day Tablet Pack	Circle	Warner Chilcott
MJ; 595	Megace	20 mg	Light Blue	Tablet		Mead Johnson Oncology
MJ; 596	Megace	40 mg	Light Blue	Tablet		Mead Johnson Oncology
MJ; 702	Enfamil Natalins RX	25 mg ; 3 mg ; 4000 IU ; 80 mg ; 400 IU ; 15 IU ; 1.5 mg ; 1.6 mg ; 17 mg ; 4 mg ; 1 mg ; 2.5 mcg ; 30 mcg ; 7 mg ; 200 mg ; 54 mg ; 100 mg	White Speckled	Tablet	Oval	Mead Johnson
MJ; 702	Natalins RX	4 mg ; 25 mg ; 15 IU ; 400 IU ; 4000 IU ; 1.6 mg ; 17 mg ; 60 mg ; 3 mg ; 0.03 mg ; 200 mg ; 1 mg ; 100 mg ; 7 mg ; 1.5 mg ; 2.5 mcg ; 80 mg	White	Tablet	Oval	Mead Johnson
MJ; 755	Estrace	1 mg	Lavender	Tablet		Warner Chilcott
MJ; 784; DURICEF; 500MG ;	Duricef	500 mg	Maroon and White	Capsule		Bristol-Myers Squibb
MJ; 785	Duricef	1 G	White	Tablet		Bristol-Myers Squibb
MJ; 822; 5	Buspar Dividose	15 mg	White	Tablet		Bristol-Myers Squibb
ML; 674	Thyroid Strong	65 mg	Light Tan	Tablet		Western Research Laboratories
ML; 824; 10	Buspar Dividose	30 mg	Pink	Tablet	Trisected	Bristol-Myers Squibb
MOTRIN 600MG	Motrin	600 mg	Peach	Tablet	Oval	Pharmacia & Upjohn
MOTRIN; 50	Motrin	50 mg	Orange	Tablet, Chewable	Circle, Scored	Mcneil Consumer Healthcare Division of Mcneil
MOTRIN; 100	Motrin	100 mg	Orange	Tablet, Chewable	Circle, Scored	Mcneil Consumer Healthcare Division of Mcneil
MOTRIN; 300 MG	Motrin	300 mg	White	Coated Tablet	Circle	Pharmacia & Upjohn
MOTRIN; 400 MG	Motrin	400 mg	Orange	Coated Tablet	Circle	Pharmacia & Upjohn
MOTRIN; 800 MG	Motrin	800 mg	Apricot	Tablet	Oblong	Pharmacia & Upjohn
MPC; 100	Tussend	5 mg ; 60 mg ; 4 mg	Yellow	Tablet	Capsule-Shape, Scored	Monarch Pharmaceuticals
MR	Hydro-Z-50	50 mg	Peach	Tablet	Circle, Scored	Merz
MR	Sterapred	5 mg	Blue	Tablet	Circle	Merz
MR	Trimtabs	35 mg	Lavender	Tablet		Merz

IMPRINT	BRAND/GENERIC NAME	STRENGTH	COLOR	FORM	SHAPE	MANUFACTURER
MR; 15; G	Mirtazapine	15 mg	Yellow	Tablet	Circle	Par Pharmaceutical
MR; 30; G	Mirtazapine	30 mg	Buff	Tablet	Circle	Par Pharmaceutical
MR; 45; G	Mirtazapine	45 mg	White	Tablet	Circle	Par Pharmaceutical
MRK 267 ; MAXALT	Maxalt	10 mg	Pale Pink	Tablet	Capsule-Shape	Merck & Company
MRK; 212; FOSAMAX	Fosamax	40 mg	White	Tablet	Triangle	Merck & Company
MRK; 925	Fosamax	5 mg	White	Tablet	Circle	Merck & Company
MRK; 936	Fosamax	10 mg	White	Tablet	Oval	Merck & Company
MRK; 951	Cozaar	25 mg	Light Green	Coated Tablet	Teardrop-Shape	Merck
MRK; 952; COZAAR	Cozaar	50 mg	Green	Coated Tablet	Teardrop-Shape	Merck
MRK; 960	Cozaar	100 mg	Dark Green	Coated Tablet	Teardrop-Shape	Merck
MSAP	Arthritis Pain Formula	500 mg ; 27 mg ; 100 mg	Light Brown or White	Tablet		Wyeth Consumer Healthcare
MSD 19	Prinivil	5 mg	White	Tablet	Oval	Merck & Company
MSD 106	Prinivil	10 mg	Light Yellow	Tablet	Oval	Merck & Company
MSD 207	Prinivil	20 mg	Peach	Tablet	Oval	Merck & Company
MSD 661 ; SYPRINE	Syprine	250 mg	Light Brown Opaque	Capsule		Aton Pharma
MSD 690 DEMSER	Demser	250 mg	Opaque Blue	Capsule	Capsule-Shape	Aton Pharma
MSD/140	Prinzide	20 mg ; 12.5 mg	Yellow	Tablet	Six-Sided	Merck & Company
MSD; 14; VASOTEC	Vasotec	2.5 mg	Yellow	Tablet	Barrel, Biconvex, Scored, Compressed	Merck & Company
MSD; 15	Prinivil	2.5 mg	White	Tablet	Circle, Small	Merck Sharp & Dohme
MSD; 20	Decadron	0.25 mg	Orange	Tablet	Five-Sided, Compressed, Scored	Merck & Company
MSD; 21	Cogentin	0.5 mg	White	Tablet	Circle, Scored	Merck & Company
MSD; 41	Decadron	0.5 mg	Yellow	Tablet	Five-Sided, Compressed, Score	Merck & Company
MSD; 42	Hydrodiuril	25 mg	Peach	Tablet	Circle, Scored, Compressed	Merck & Company
MSD; 53	Hydropres-25	25 mg ; 0.125 mg	Green	Tablet	Circle, Scored	Merck & Company
MSD; 59; BLOCADREN	Blocadren	5 mg	Light Blue	Tablet	Circle, Compressed	Merck & Company
MSD; 60	Cogentin	2 mg	White	Tablet	Circle, Scored, Compressed	Merck & Company
MSD; 62	Periactin	4 mg	White	Tablet	Circle, Compressed, Scored	Merck & Company
MSD; 63	Decadron	0.75 mg	Bluish-Green	Tablet	Five-Sided, Compressed, Scored	Merck & Company
MSD; 67	Timolide	10 mg ; 25 mg	Light Blue	Tablet		Merck & Company
MSD; 72; PROSCAR	Proscar	5 mg	Blue	Coated Tablet	Character-Shape, Modified Apple	Merck & Company
MSD; 92	Midamor	5 mg	Yellow	Tablet	Diamond-Shaped, Compressed	Merck & Company
MSD; 95	Decadron	1.5 mg	Pink	Tablet	Five-Sided, Compressed, Scored	Merck & Company
MSD; 97	Decadron	4 mg	White	Tablet	Five-Sided, Compressed, Scored	Merck & Company
MSD; 105	Hydrodiuril	50 mg	Peach	Tablet	Circle, Scored, Compressed	Merck & Company
MSD; 127	Hydropres-50	50 mg ; 0.125 mg	Green	Tablet	Circle, Scored	Merck & Company
MSD; 135	Aldomet	125 mg	Yellow	Coated Tablet	Circle	Merck & Company
MSD; 136; BLOCADREN	Blocadren	10 mg	Light Blue	Tablet	Circle, Scored, Compressed	Merck & Company
MSD; 139	Stromectol	6 mg	White	Tablet	Scored, Beveled-Edge	Merck & Company
MSD; 147	Decadron	6 mg	Green	Tablet	Five-Sided, Compressed, Scored	Merck & Company
MSD; 173	Vaseretic	5 mg ; 12.5 mg	Green	Tablet	Capsule-Shape, Squared, Compressed	Merck & Company
MSD; 214	Diuril	250 mg	White	Tablet	Circle, Scored, Compressed	Merck & Company
MSD; 219	Cortone Acetate	25 mg	White	Tablet	Circle, Scored, Compressed	Merck & Company
MSD; 230	Diupres-250	250 mg ; 0.125 mg	Pink	Tablet	Circle, Scored	Merck & Company
MSD; 237; PRINIVIL	Prinivil	40 mg	Rose-Red	Tablet	Shield-Shape, Compressed	Merck & Company
MSD; 401	Aldomet	250 mg	Yellow	Coated Tablet	Circle	Merck & Company
MSD; 403	Urecholine	5 mg	White	Tablet	Circle, Scored, Compressed	Merck & Company
MSD; 405	Diupres-500	500 mg ; 0.125 mg	Pink	Tablet	Circle, Scored	Merck & Company
MSD; 410	Hydrodiuril	100 mg	Peach	Tablet	Circle, Scored, Compressed	Merck & Company
MSD; 412	Urecholine	10 mg	Pink	Tablet	Circle, Compressed, Scored	Merck & Company
MSD; 423	Aldoril-15	250 mg ; 15 mg	Salmon	Coated Tablet	Circle	Merck & Company
MSD; 432	Diuril	500 mg	White	Tablet	Circle, Scored, Compressed	Merck & Company
MSD; 437; BLOCADREN	Blocadren	20 mg	Light Blue	Tablet	Capsule-Shape, Scored, Compressed	Merck & Company
MSD; 456	Aldoril-25	250 mg ; 25 mg	White	Coated Tablet	Circle	Merck & Company
MSD; 457	Urecholine	25 mg	Yellow	Tablet	Circle, Compressed, Scored	Merck & Company
MSD; 460	Urecholine	50 mg	Yellow	Tablet	Circle, Compressed, Scored	Merck & Company
MSD; 501	Benemid	500 mg	Yellow	Coated Tablet	Capsule-Shape, Scored	Merck & Company
MSD; 516	Aldomet	500 mg	Yellow	Coated Tablet	Circle	Merck & Company
MSD; 517	Triavil 4-50	4 mg ; 50 mg	Orange	Coated Tablet	Diamond	Merck & Company
MSD; 612	Aldoclor 150	250 mg ; 150 mg	Beige	Coated Tablet	Oval	Merck & Company
MSD; 614	Colbenemid	0.5 GM ; 0.5 mg	White to Off-White	Tablet	Capsule-Shape, Scored	Merck & Company
MSD; 619	Hydrocortone	10 mg	White	Tablet	Oval, Compressed, Scored	Merck & Company
MSD; 634	Aldoclor 250	250 mg ; 250 mg	Green	Coated Tablet	Oval	Merck & Company
MSD; 635	Cogentin	1 mg	White	Tablet	Oval, Scored, Compressed	Merck & Company
MSD; 675	Dolobid	250 mg	Peach	Coated Tablet	Capsule-Shape	Merck & Company
MSD; 693	Indocin SR	75 mg	Blue and Clear with White Pellets	Extended-Release Capsule		Merck & Company
MSD; 694	Aldoril D30	500 mg ; 30 mg	Salmon	Coated Tablet	Oval	Merck & Company
MSD; 697	Dolobid	500 mg	Orange	Coated Tablet	Capsule-Shape	Merck & Company
MSD; 705; NOROXIN	Noroxin	400 mg	Dark Pink	Coated Tablet	Oval	Merck Sharp & Dohme
MSD; 712; VASOTEC	Vasotec	5 mg	White	Tablet	Barrel, Scored, Compressed	Merck & Company
MSD; 713; VASOTEC	Vasotec	10 mg	Salmon	Tablet	Barrel, Compressed	Merck & Company
MSD; 714; VASOTEC	Vasotec	20 mg	Peach	Tablet	Barrel, Compressed	Merck & Company
MSD; 720; VASERETIC	Vaseretic	25 mg ; 10 mg	Rust	Tablet	Squared, Compressed, Capsule-Shape	Merck & Company
MSD; 726; ZOCOR	Zocor	5 mg	Buff	Coated Tablet	Shield-Shape	Merck & Company
MSD; 730; MEVACOR	Mevacor	10 mg	Peach	Tablet	Eight-Sided	Merck & Company
MSD; 731; MEVACOR	Mevacor	20 mg	Light Blue	Tablet	Eight-Sided	Merck & Company
MSD; 732; MEVACOR	Mevacor	40 mg	Green	Tablet	Eight-Sided	Merck & Company
MSD; 735; ZOCOR	Zocor	10 mg	Peach	Coated Tablet	Shield-Shape	Merck & Company

IMPRINT	BRAND/GENERIC NAME	STRENGTH	COLOR	FORM	SHAPE	MANUFACTURER
MSD; 740; ZOCOR	Zocor	20 mg	Tan	Coated Tablet	Shield-Shape	Merck & Company
MSD; 749; ZOCOR	Zocor	40 mg	Brick Red	Coated Tablet	Shield-Shape	Merck & Company
MSD; 907	Mintezol	500 mg	White	Tablet, Chewable	Circle, Scored	Merck & Company
MSD; 914	Triavil 2-10	2 mg ; 10 mg	Blue	Coated Tablet	Triangle	Merck & Company
MSD; 917	Moduretic	5 mg ; 50 mg	Peach	Tablet	Diamond	Merck & Company
MSD; 921	Triavil 2-25	2 mg ; 25 mg	Orange	Coated Tablet	Triangle	Merck & Company
MSD; 934	Triavil 4-10	4 mg ; 10 mg	Salmon	Coated Tablet	Triangle	Merck & Company
MSD; 935	Aldoril D50	500 mg ; 50 mg	White	Coated Tablet	Oval	Merck & Company
MSD; 941	Clinoril	150 mg	Yellow	Tablet	Six-Sided, Compressed	Merck & Company
MSD; 942	Clinoril	200 mg	Yellow	Tablet	Six-Sided, Scored, Compressed	Merck & Company
MSD; 946	Triavil 4-25	4 mg ; 25 mg	Yellow	Coated Tablet	Triangle	Merck & Company
MSD; 964	Pepcid	40 mg	Light Brownish-Orange	Coated Tablet	U-Shape	Merck & Company
MSM	Momentum Extra Strength	580 mg	White	Tablet	Oblong	Medtech
MURO; 6-60 ;	Bromfed-PD	6 mg ; 60 mg	Dark-Green and Clear with White Beads	Timed-Release Capsule		Muro Pharmaceutical
MURO; 12-120 ;	Bromfed	12 mg ; 120 mg	Light Green and Clear	Timed-Release Capsule		Muro Pharmaceutical
MURO; 60/40	Guaitab	60 mg ; 400 mg	Purple	Tablet	Layered, Scored	Muro Pharmaceutical
MURO; 4060	Bromfed	4 mg ; 60 mg	White	Tablet		Muro Pharmaceutical
MVC 150 ; PFIZER	Selzentry	150 mg	Blue	Tablet	Oval	Pfizer
MX31	Citalopram	10 mg	Beige	Tablet	Circle	Mylan Pharmaceuticals
MX32	Citalopram	20 mg	Pink	Tablet	Circle	Mylan Pharmaceuticals
MX33	Citalopram	40 mg	White	Tablet	Circle	Mylan Pharmaceuticals
MYCOBUTIN; PHARMACIA	Mycobutin	150 mg	Red-Brown	Capsule		Pharmacia & Upjohn
MYLAN ; 323	Ciprofloxacin	500 mg	Orange	Tablet	Capsule-Shape	Mylan Pharmaceuticals
MYLAN ; 324	Ciprofloxacin	750 mg	Orange	Tablet	Capsule-Shape	Mylan Pharmaceuticals
MYLAN 143	Indomethacin	25 mg	Light Green Opaque	Capsule		Mylan Pharmaceuticals
MYLAN 147	Indomethacin	50 mg	Light Green Opaque	Capsule		Mylan Pharmaceuticals
MYLAN 152	Clonidine Hydrochloride	0.1 mg	White	Tablet	Circle	Mylan Pharmaceuticals
MYLAN 186	Clonidine Hydrochloride	0.2 mg	White	Tablet	Circle	Mylan Pharmaceuticals
MYLAN 199	Clonidine Hydrochloride	0.3 mg	White	Tablet	Circle	Mylan Pharmaceuticals
MYLAN 214	Haloperidol	2 mg	Orange	Tablet	Circle	Mylan Pharmaceuticals
MYLAN 257	Haloperidol	1 mg	Orange	Tablet	Circle	Mylan Pharmaceuticals
MYLAN 327	Haloperidol	5 mg	Orange	Tablet	Circle	Mylan Pharmaceuticals
MYLAN 351	Haloperidol	0.5 mg	Orange	Tablet	Circle	Mylan Pharmaceuticals
MYLAN 457	Lorazepam	1 mg	White to Off-White, White	Tablet	Circle	Mylan Pharmaceuticals
MYLAN 777	Lorazepam	2 mg	White to Off-White	Tablet	Circle	Mylan Pharmaceuticals
MYLAN 1410	Nortriptyline Hydrochloride	10 mg	Opaque Swedish Orange	Capsule		Mylan Pharmaceuticals
MYLAN 1560 ;	Extended Phenytoin Sodium	100 mg	Lavender, White	Capsule, Extended Release		Mylan Pharmaceuticals
MYLAN 1650	Nitrofurantoin Macrocrystals	50 mg	Light Brown Opaque	Capsule		Mylan Pharmaceuticals
MYLAN 1700	Nitrofurantoin Macrocrystals	100 mg	Gray Opaque	Capsule		Mylan Pharmaceuticals
MYLAN 2325	Nortriptyline Hydrochloride	25 mg	Opaque Orange and Opaque Swedish Orange	Capsule		Mylan Pharmaceuticals
MYLAN 3250	Nortriptyline Hydrochloride	50 mg	Opaque Swedish Orange, Opaque Yellow	Capsule		Mylan Pharmaceuticals
MYLAN 4210	Fluoxetine	10 mg	Flesh Opaque, White Opaque	Capsule		Mylan Pharmaceuticals
MYLAN 4220	Fluoxetine	20 mg	Flesh Opaque, Light Turquoise Blue Opaque	Capsule		Mylan Pharmaceuticals
MYLAN 4350	Fluoxetine	40 mg	Light Blue Opaque, White Opaque	Capsule		Mylan Pharmaceuticals
MYLAN 6160	Propranolol Hydrochloride	60 mg	Blue-Violet Opaque, Pink Opaque	Capsule, Extended Release		Mylan Pharmaceuticals
MYLAN 6180	Propranolol Hydrochloride	80 mg	Orange Opaque, Pink Opaque	Capsule, Extended Release		Mylan Pharmaceuticals
MYLAN 6201	Verapamil Hydrochloride	100 mg	Red Opaque, White Opaque	Capsule, Extended Release		Mylan Pharmaceuticals
MYLAN 6202	Verapamil Hydrochloride	200 mg	Light Orange Opaque, Red Opaque	Capsule, Extended Release		Mylan Pharmaceuticals
MYLAN 6203	Verapamil Hydrochloride	300 mg	Red Opaque	Capsule, Extended Release		Mylan Pharmaceuticals
MYLAN 6220	Propranolol Hydrochloride	120 mg	Blue-Violet Opaque	Capsule, Extended Release		Mylan Pharmaceuticals
MYLAN 6260	Propranolol Hydrochloride	160 mg	Pink Opaque	Capsule, Extended Release		Mylan Pharmaceuticals
MYLAN 6750	Balsalazide Disodium	750 mg	Orange Opaque	Capsule		Mylan Pharmaceuticals
MYLAN 7005	Loxapine	5 mg	Olive	Capsule		Mylan Pharmaceuticals
MYLAN 7010	Loxapine	10 mg	Olive, Yellow	Capsule		Mylan Pharmaceuticals
MYLAN 7025	Loxapine	25 mg	Light Green, Olive	Capsule		Mylan Pharmaceuticals
MYLAN 7050	Loxapine	50 mg	Light Blue, Olive	Capsule		Mylan Pharmaceuticals
MYLAN 7065	Propoxyphene Hydrochloride	65 mg	Rose	Capsule		Mylan Pharmaceuticals
MYLAN; 9; 4	Carbidopa and Levodopa	50 mg ; 200 mg	Purple	Tablet, Extended Release	Oval	Mylan Pharmaceuticals
MYLAN; 11; 77	Oxaprozin	600 mg	White	Coated Tablet	Oval, Biconvex, Bevel-Edged, Scored	Mylan Pharmaceuticals
MYLAN; 43	Reserpine and Chlorothiazide	0.125 mg ; 500 mg	Peach	Tablet	Circle, Scored	Mylan Pharmaceuticals
MYLAN; 73	Perphenazine and Amitriptyline Hydrochloride	50 mg ; 4 mg	Purple	Coated Tablet	Circle, Biconvex, Beveled Edge	Mylan Pharmaceuticals
MYLAN; 88	Carbidopa and Levodopa	25 mg ; 100 mg	Purple	Extended-Release Tablet	Oval	Mylan Pharmaceuticals
MYLAN; 101	Tetracycline Hydrochloride	250 mg	Orange and Yellow	Capsule		Mylan Pharmaceuticals
MYLAN; 102	Tetracycline Hydrochloride	500 mg	Black and Yellow	Capsule		Mylan Pharmaceuticals

IMPRINT	BRAND/GENERIC NAME	STRENGTH	COLOR	FORM	SHAPE	MANUFACTURER
MYLAN; 106; 250	Erythromycin Stearate	250 mg	Yellow	Coated Tablet	Biconvex, Circle	Mylan Pharmaceuticals
MYLAN; 107; 500	Erythromycin Stearate	500 mg	Yellow	Coated Tablet	Oval, Biconvex	Mylan Pharmaceuticals
MYLAN; 115	Ampicillin Trihydrate	250 mg	Scarlet and Light Gray	Capsule		Mylan Pharmaceuticals
MYLAN; 116	Ampicillin Trihydrate	500 mg	Scarlet and Light Gray	Capsule		Mylan Pharmaceuticals
MYLAN; 131	Propoxyphene Compound	65 mg ; 389 mg ; 32.4 mg	Red and Grey	Capsule		Mylan Pharmaceuticals
MYLAN; 145	Doxycycline Hyclate	50 mg	Aqua Blue and White	Capsule		Mylan Pharmaceuticals
MYLAN; 148	Doxycycline Hyclate	100 mg	Aqua Blue	Capsule		Mylan Pharmaceuticals
MYLAN; 155	Acetaminophen and Propoxyphene Napsylate	650 mg ; 100 mg	Pink	Coated Tablet	Capsule-Shape	Mylan Pharmaceuticals
MYLAN; 156; 500	Probenecid	500 mg	Yellow	Coated Tablet	Capsule-Shape	Mylan Pharmaceuticals
MYLAN; 162	Chlorothiazide	500 mg	White	Tablet	Circle, Scored, Flat Beveled Edge	Mylan Pharmaceuticals
MYLAN; 167; 100	Doxycycline Hyclate	100 mg	Beige	Coated Tablet	Circle, Biconvex, Beveled Edge	Mylan Pharmaceuticals
MYLAN; 182; 10	Propranolol Hydrochloride	10 mg	Orange	Tablet	Circle	Mylan Pharmaceuticals
MYLAN; 183; 20	Propranolol Hydrochloride	20 mg	Blue	Tablet	Circle	Mylan Pharmaceuticals
MYLAN; 184; 40	Propranolol Hydrochloride	40 mg	Green	Tablet	Circle	Mylan Pharmaceuticals
MYLAN; 185; 80	Propranolol Hydrochloride	80 mg	Yellow	Tablet	Circle	Mylan Pharmaceuticals
MYLAN; 197; 100	Chlorpropamide	100 mg	Green	Tablet	Circle	Mylan Pharmaceuticals
MYLAN; 204	Amoxicillin Trihydrate	250 mg	Caramel and Buff	Capsule		Mylan Pharmaceuticals
MYLAN; 205	Amoxicillin Trihydrate	500 mg	Buff	Capsule		Mylan Pharmaceuticals
MYLAN; 210; 250	Chlorpropamide	250 mg	Green	Tablet	Circle, Scored	Mylan Pharmaceuticals
MYLAN; 211	Chlordiazepoxide and Amitriptyline Hydrochloride	12.5 mg ; 5 mg	Green	Coated Tablet	Circle, Biconvex	Mylan Pharmaceuticals
MYLAN; 217; 250	Tolazamide	250 mg	White	Tablet	Circle, Scored, Biconvex	Mylan Pharmaceuticals
MYLAN; 237	Etodolac	400 mg	White	Tablet	Oval	Mylan Pharmaceuticals
MYLAN; 242	Etodolac	500 mg	Pink	Tablet	Oval	Mylan Pharmaceuticals
MYLAN; 245	Bumetanide	0.5 mg	Light Green	Tablet	Oval, Scored	Mylan Pharmaceuticals
MYLAN; 251	Trazodone Hydrochloride	50 mg	Clear	Coated Tablet	Circle, Scored, Biconvex, Beveled Edge	Mylan Pharmaceuticals
MYLAN; 252	Trazodone Hydrochloride	100 mg	Clear	Coated Tablet	Circle, Scored, Biconvex, Beveled Edge	Mylan Pharmaceuticals
MYLAN; 271	Diazepam	2 mg	White	Tablet	Circle	Mylan Pharmaceuticals
MYLAN; 277	Chlordiazepoxide and Amitriptyline Hydrochloride	25 mg ; 10 mg	White	Coated Tablet	Circle, Biconvex	Mylan Pharmaceuticals
MYLAN; 330	Perphenazine and Amitriptyline Hydrochloride	2 mg ; 10 mg	White	Coated Tablet	Circle, Biconvex, Beveled Edge	Mylan Pharmaceuticals
MYLAN; 345	Diazepam	5 mg	Orange	Tablet	Circle	Mylan Pharmaceuticals
MYLAN; 347	Propranolol Hydrochloride and Hydrochlorothiazide	25 mg ; 80 mg	White	Tablet	Circle, Scored, Biconvex	Mylan Pharmaceuticals
MYLAN; 357	Pentoxifylline	400 mg	Lavender	Tablet, Extended Release	Capsule-Shape	Mylan Pharmaceuticals
MYLAN; 370	Bumetanide	1 mg	Yellow	Tablet	Oval, Scored	Mylan Pharmaceuticals
MYLAN; 377	Naproxen	250 mg	White	Tablet	Circle	Mylan Pharmaceuticals
MYLAN; 417	Bumetanide	2 mg	Peach	Tablet	Scored, Oval	Mylan Pharmaceuticals
MYLAN; 421	Methyldopa	500 mg	Beige	Tablet	Capsule-Shape	Mylan Pharmaceuticals
MYLAN; 427	Sulindac	150 mg	Yellow-Orange	Tablet	Circle	Mylan Pharmaceuticals
MYLAN; 442	Perphenazine and Amitriptyline Hydrochloride	25 mg ; 2 mg	Purple	Coated Tablet	Circle, Biconvex, Beveled Edge	Mylan Pharmaceuticals
MYLAN; 451	Naproxen	500 mg	White	Tablet	Capsule-Shape	Mylan Pharmaceuticals
MYLAN; 477	Diazepam	10 mg	Green	Tablet	Circle, Scored	Mylan Pharmaceuticals
MYLAN; 507	Methyldopa and Hydrochlorothiazide	250 mg ; 15 mg	Green	Coated Tablet	Circle, Biconvex, Beveled Edge	Mylan Pharmaceuticals
MYLAN; 512	Verapamil Hydrochloride	80 mg	White	Tablet	Circle	Mylan Pharmaceuticals
MYLAN; 517	Gemfibrozil	600 mg	White	Coated Tablet	Oval, Partially Scored	Mylan Pharmaceuticals
MYLAN; 521	Acetaminophen and Propoxyphene Napsylate	100 mg ; 650 mg	White	Coated Tablet	Capsule-Shape, Biconvex, Beveled Edge	Mylan Pharmaceuticals
MYLAN; 531	Sulindac	200 mg	Yellow-Orange	Tablet	Circle	Mylan Pharmaceuticals
MYLAN; 551	Tolazamide	500 mg	White	Tablet	Circle, Scored, Biconvex	Mylan Pharmaceuticals
MYLAN; 555	Naproxen	375 mg	White	Tablet	Capsule-Shape	Mylan Pharmaceuticals
MYLAN; 574	Perphenazine and Amitriptyline Hydrochloride	25 mg ; 4 mg	Orange	Coated Tablet	Circle, Biconvex, Beveled Edge	Mylan Pharmaceuticals
MYLAN; 611	Methyldopa	250 mg	Beige	Tablet	Circle	Mylan Pharmaceuticals
MYLAN; 711	Methyldopa and Hydrochlorothiazide	250 mg ; 25 mg	Green	Coated Tablet	Capsule-Shape, Biconvex	Mylan Pharmaceuticals
MYLAN; 727	Perphenazine and Amitriptyline Hydrochloride	4 mg ; 10 mg	Blue	Coated Tablet	Circle, Biconvex, Beveled Edge	Mylan Pharmaceuticals
MYLAN; 731	Propranolol Hydrochloride and Hydrochlorothiazide	40 mg ; 25 mg	White	Tablet	Circle, Scored, Biconvex	Mylan Pharmaceuticals
MYLAN; 733	Naproxen Sodium	550 mg	Light Blue	Coated Tablet	Oval, Modified	Mylan Pharmaceuticals
MYLAN; 772	Verapamil Hydrochloride	120 mg	White	Tablet	Circle	Mylan Pharmaceuticals
MYLAN; 810	Hydrochlorothiazide	12.5 mg	White	Capsule		Mylan Pharmaceuticals
MYLAN; 1001	Thiothixene	1 mg	Tan and Blue	Capsule		Mylan Pharmaceuticals
MYLAN; 1010	Piroxicam	10 mg	Green and Olive	Capsule		Mylan Pharmaceuticals
MYLAN; 1020	Nicardipine Hydrochloride	20 mg	Opaque Blue-Green and Yellow	Capsule		Mylan Pharmaceuticals
MYLAN; 1049	Doxepin Hydrochloride	10 mg	Buff	Capsule		Mylan Pharmaceuticals
MYLAN; 1101	Prazosin Hydrochloride	1 mg	Green and Brown	Capsule		Mylan Pharmaceuticals
MYLAN; 1155	Acetaminophen and Propoxyphene Napsylate	650 mg ; 100 mg	White	Tablet	Capsule-Shape, Biconvex, Beveled Edge	Mylan Pharmaceuticals
MYLAN; 1155	Acetaminophen and Propoxyphene Napsylate	650 mg ; 100 mg	White	Tablet	Capsule-Shape	Mylan Pharmaceuticals
MYLAN; 1200	Acebutolol Hydrochloride	200 mg	Medium Orange Opaque	Capsule		Mylan Pharmaceuticals
MYLAN; 1204	Amoxicillin	250 mg	Yellow	Capsule		Mylan Pharmaceuticals
MYLAN; 1205	Amoxicillin	500 mg	Yellow	Capsule		Mylan Pharmaceuticals
MYLAN; 1400	Acebutolol Hydrochloride	400 mg	Medium Orange Opaque	Capsule		Mylan Pharmaceuticals

IMPRINT	BRAND/GENERIC NAME	STRENGTH	COLOR	FORM	SHAPE	MANUFACTURER
MYLAN; 1401	Ibuprofen	400 mg	White	Coated Tablet	Circle	Mylan Pharmaceuticals
MYLAN; 1401 ;	Ibuprofen	400 mg	White	Coated Tablet	Circle, Biconvex, Beveled Edge	Mylan Pharmaceuticals
MYLAN; 1430	Nicardipine Hydrochloride	30 mg	Opaque Blue-Green and Yellow	Capsule		Mylan Pharmaceuticals
MYLAN; 1570	Terazosin Hydrochloride	10 mg	Lavender	Capsule		Mylan Pharmaceuticals
MYLAN; 1601	Ibuprofen	600 mg	White	Coated Tablet	Oval	Mylan Pharmaceuticals
MYLAN; 1601 ;	Ibuprofen	600 mg	White	Coated Tablet	Capsule-Shape, Biconvex, Beveled Edge	Mylan Pharmaceuticals
MYLAN; 1610	Dicyclomine Hydrochloride	10 mg	Light Turquoise Blue	Capsule		Mylan Pharmaceuticals
MYLAN; 1801	Ibuprofen	800 mg	White	Coated Tablet	Capsule-Shape	Mylan Pharmaceuticals
MYLAN; 1801 ;	Ibuprofen	800 mg	White	Coated Tablet	Oval, Biconvex, Beveled Edge	Mylan Pharmaceuticals
MYLAN; 2002	Thiothixene	2 mg	Tan and Yellow	Capsule		Mylan Pharmaceuticals
MYLAN; 2020	Piroxicam	20 mg	Green	Capsule		Mylan Pharmaceuticals
MYLAN; 2100	Loperamide Hydrochloride	2 mg	Brown	Capsule		Mylan Pharmaceuticals
MYLAN; 2115	Ampicillin	250 mg	White Opaque	Capsule		Mylan Pharmaceuticals
MYLAN; 2116	Ampicillin	500 mg	White	Capsule		Mylan Pharmaceuticals
MYLAN; 2150	Meclofenamate Sodium	50 mg	Coral	Capsule		Mylan Pharmaceuticals
MYLAN; 2200	Acyclovir	200 mg	Purple	Capsule		Mylan Pharmaceuticals
MYLAN; 2252	Selegiline Hydrochloride	5 mg	Light Blue Opaque and Aqua Blue	Capsule		Mylan Pharmaceuticals
MYLAN; 2260	Terazosin Hydrochloride	1 mg	Rich Yellow and Light Lavender	Capsule		Mylan Pharmaceuticals
MYLAN; 2264	Terazosin Hydrochloride	2 mg	Black and Light Lavender	Capsule		Mylan Pharmaceuticals
MYLAN; 2268	Terazosin Hydrochloride	5 mg	Gray and Lavender	Capsule		Mylan Pharmaceuticals
MYLAN; 2302	Prazosin Hydrochloride	2 mg	Brown	Capsule		Mylan Pharmaceuticals
MYLAN; 2537	Triamterene and Hydrochlorothiazide	25 mg ; 37.5 mg	Olive and Yellow	Capsule		Mylan Pharmaceuticals
MYLAN; 3000	Meclofenamate Sodium	100 mg	Coral and White	Capsule		Mylan Pharmaceuticals
MYLAN; 3005	Thiothixene	5 mg	Tan and White	Capsule		Mylan Pharmaceuticals
MYLAN; 3025	Clomipramine Hydrochloride	25 mg	Orange and Flesh	Capsule		Mylan Pharmaceuticals
MYLAN; 3050	Clomipramine Hydrochloride	50 mg	Yellow and Flesh	Capsule		Mylan Pharmaceuticals
MYLAN; 3075	Clomipramine Hydrochloride	75 mg	Orange and Flesh	Capsule		Mylan Pharmaceuticals
MYLAN; 3125	Doxepin Hydrochloride	25 mg	Ivory and White	Capsule		Mylan Pharmaceuticals
MYLAN; 3205	Prazosin Hydrochloride	5 mg	Blue and Brown	Capsule		Mylan Pharmaceuticals
MYLAN; 3422	Nitrofurantoin Monohydrate/ macrocrystals	25 mg ; 75 mg	Light Gray and Light Brown	Capsule		Mylan Pharmaceuticals
MYLAN; 4010	Temazepam	15 mg	Peach	Capsule		Mylan Pharmaceuticals
MYLAN; 4070	Ketoprofen	50 mg	Light Green	Capsule		Mylan Pharmaceuticals
MYLAN; 4175	Nortriptyline Hydrochloride	75 mg	Brown and Orange	Capsule		Mylan Pharmaceuticals
MYLAN; 4250	Doxepin Hydrochloride	50 mg	Ivory	Capsule		Mylan Pharmaceuticals
MYLAN; 4415	Flurazepam Hydrochloride	15 mg	White and Blue	Capsule		Mylan Pharmaceuticals
MYLAN; 4430	Flurazepam Hydrochloride	30 mg	Blue	Capsule		Mylan Pharmaceuticals
MYLAN; 4700	Gemfibrozil	300 mg	Swedish Orange and White	Capsule		Mylan Pharmaceuticals
MYLAN; 5010	Thiothixene	10 mg	Tan and Peach	Capsule		Mylan Pharmaceuticals
MYLAN; 5050	Temazepam	30 mg	Yellow	Capsule		Mylan Pharmaceuticals
MYLAN; 5200	Tolmetin Sodium	400 mg	Light Blue	Capsule		Mylan Pharmaceuticals
MYLAN; 5211	Omeprazole	10 mg	Dark Green	Delayed-Release Capsule		Mylan Pharmaceuticals
MYLAN; 5220	Diltiazem Hydrochloride	120 mg	Light Pink and Flesh	Capsule, Extended Release		Mylan Pharmaceuticals
MYLAN; 5280	Diltiazem Hydrochloride	180 mg	Lavender and Flesh	Capsule, Extended Release		Mylan Pharmaceuticals
MYLAN; 5340	Diltiazem Hydrochloride	240 mg	Light Blue and Flesh	Capsule, Extended Release		Mylan Pharmaceuticals
MYLAN; 5375	Doxepin Hydrochloride	75 mg	Brite Light Green	Capsule		Mylan Pharmaceuticals
MYLAN; 5750	Ketoprofen	75 mg		Capsule		Mylan Pharmaceuticals
MYLAN; 6025	Cephalexin	250 mg	Dark Blue and Opaque White	Capsule		Mylan Pharmaceuticals
MYLAN; 6050	Cephalexin	500 mg	Dark Blue and Light Blue	Capsule		Mylan Pharmaceuticals
MYLAN; 6060	Diltiazem Hydrochloride	60 mg	Coral and White	Capsule, Extended Release		Mylan Pharmaceuticals
MYLAN; 6090	Diltiazem Hydrochloride	90 mg	Coral and Ivory	Capsule, Extended Release		Mylan Pharmaceuticals
MYLAN; 6120	Diltiazem Hydrochloride	120 mg	Coral	Capsule, Extended Release		Mylan Pharmaceuticals
MYLAN; 6150	Omeprazole	20 mg	Dark Green and Blue Green	Delayed-Release Capsule		Mylan Pharmaceuticals
MYLAN; 6320	Verapamil Hydrochloride	120 mg	Blue-Green and White	Capsule, Extended Release		Mylan Pharmaceuticals
MYLAN; 6380	Verapamil Hydrochloride	180 mg	Blue-Green and Light Green	Capsule, Extended Release		Mylan Pharmaceuticals
MYLAN; 6410	Doxepin Hydrochloride	100 mg	Bbright Light Green and White	Capsule		Mylan Pharmaceuticals
MYLAN; 6440	Verapamil Hydrochloride	240 mg	Blue-Green	Capsule, Extended Release		Mylan Pharmaceuticals
MYLAN; 7200	Etodolac	200 mg	Brown Opaque	Capsule		Mylan Pharmaceuticals
MYLAN; 7233	Etodolac	300 mg	Light Brown Opaque	Capsule		Mylan Pharmaceuticals
MYLAN; 7250	Cefaclor	250 mg	Pink and White	Capsule		Mylan Pharmaceuticals
MYLAN; 7500	Cefaclor	500 mg	Pink and Grey	Capsule		Mylan Pharmaceuticals
MYLAN; A	Alprazolam	0.25 mg	White	Tablet	Circle	Mylan Pharmaceuticals
MYLAN; A1	Alprazolam	1 mg	Blue	Tablet	Circle	Mylan Pharmaceuticals
MYLAN; A3	Alprazolam	0.5 mg	Peach	Tablet	Circle	Mylan Pharmaceuticals
MYLAN; A4	Alprazolam	2 mg	White	Tablet	Circle	Mylan Pharmaceuticals
MYLAN; G1	Glipizide	5 mg	White	Tablet	Circle	Mylan Pharmaceuticals
MYLAN; G2	Glipizide	10 mg	White	Tablet	Circle	Mylan Pharmaceuticals

IMPRINT	BRAND/GENERIC NAME	STRENGTH	COLOR	FORM	SHAPE	MANUFACTURER
MYLAN; TH: 2	Triamterene and Hydrochlorothiazide	75 mg ; 50 mg	Yellow	Tablet	Circle	Mylan Pharmaceuticals
N	Nephrocaps	100 mg ; 1 mg ; 20 mg ; 1.5 mg ; 1.7 mg ; 10 mg ; 5 mg ; 150 mcg ; 6 mcg	Black	Capsule, Liquid Filled	Oval	Fleming
N 1 ; M	Paroxetine	10 mg	Blue	Tablet	Capsule-Shape	Mylan Pharmaceuticals
N 2 ; M	Paroxetine	20 mg	Blue	Tablet	Capsule-Shape	Mylan Pharmaceuticals
N 5 ; M	Ropinirole Hydrochloride	0.5 mg	Yellow	Tablet	Circle	Mylan Pharmaceuticals
N 10 ; M	Ropinirole Hydrochloride	1 mg	Green	Tablet	Circle	Mylan Pharmaceuticals
N 20 ; M	Ropinirole Hydrochloride	2 mg	Orange	Tablet	Circle	Mylan Pharmaceuticals
N 22 ; M	Nisoldipine	20 mg	Beige	Tablet, Extended Release	Circle	Mylan Pharmaceuticals
N 23 ; M	Nisoldipine	30 mg	Orange	Tablet, Extended Release	Circle	Mylan Pharmaceuticals
N 24 ; M	Nisoldipine	40 mg	Yellow	Tablet, Extended Release	Circle	Mylan Pharmaceuticals
N 25 ; M	Ropinirole Hydrochloride	0.25 mg	White	Tablet	Circle	Mylan Pharmaceuticals
N 30 ; M	Ropinirole Hydrochloride	3 mg	Lavender	Tablet	Circle	Mylan Pharmaceuticals
N 40 ; M	Ropinirole Hydrochloride	4 mg	Grayish Beige	Tablet	Circle	Mylan Pharmaceuticals
N 50 ; M	Ropinirole Hydrochloride	5 mg	Blue	Tablet	Circle	Mylan Pharmaceuticals
N 894 150	Nizatidine	150 mg	Opaque White, Opaque Light Tan	Capsule		Teva Pharmaceuticals
N 899 300	Nizatidine	300 mg	Opaque Light Tan	Capsule		Teva Pharmaceuticals
N 940 200	Acyclovir	200 mg	Opaque Blue	Capsule		Teva Pharmaceuticals
N; 1.5; 034	Glyburide	1.5 mg		Tablet		Teva Pharmaceuticals
N; 3	Nitrostat	0.3 mg	White	Tablet	Circle, Flat-Faced	Parke-Davis
N; 3; 035	Glyburide	3 mg	Pale Blue	Tablet	Oval, Scored	Teva Pharmaceuticals
N; 4	Nitrostat	0.4 mg	White	Tablet	Circle, Flat-Faced	Parke-Davis
N; 6	Nitrostat	0.6 mg	White	Tablet	Circle, Flat-Faced	Parke-Davis
N; 126; 0.25	Alprazolam	0.25 mg	White	Tablet	Circle, Scored	Warner Chilcott
N; 127; 0.5	Alprazolam	0.5 mg	Orange	Tablet	Circle, Scored	Warner Chilcott
N; 131; 1.0	Alprazolam	1 mg	Blue	Tablet	Circle, Scored	Warner Chilcott
N; 132; 12.5	Captopril	12.5 mg	White	Tablet	Oval, Scored	Teva Pharmaceuticals
N; 134; 50	Captopril	50 mg	White	Tablet	Oval, Scored	Teva Pharmaceuticals
N; 135; 100	Captopril	100 mg	White	Tablet	Oval, Scored	Teva Pharmaceuticals
N; 171; 10	Nifedipine	10 mg	Brown	Capsule		Teva Pharmaceuticals
N; 240; 67	Fenofibrate	67 mg	Pink	Capsule		Teva Pharmaceuticals
N; 342; 1.25	Glyburide	1.25 mg	White	Tablet	Circle, Scored	Teva Pharmaceuticals
N; 343; 2.5	Glyburide	2.5 mg	Peach	Tablet	Circle, Scored	Teva Pharmaceuticals
N; 344; 5	Glyburide	5 mg	Light Green	Tablet	Circle, Scored	Teva Pharmaceuticals
N; 397; 300	Etodolac	300 mg	Red	Capsule		Teva Pharmaceuticals
N; 411; 134	Fenofibrate	134 mg	Light Blue	Capsule		Teva Pharmaceuticals
N; 412; 200	Fenofibrate	200 mg	Orange	Capsule		Teva Pharmaceuticals
N; 590; 1	Doxazosin Mesylate	1 mg	White to Off-White	Tablet	Circle, Scored	Teva Pharmaceuticals
N; 593; 2	Doxazosin Mesylate	2 mg	White to Off-White	Tablet	Capsule-Shape	Teva Pharmaceuticals
N; 596; 4	Doxazosin Mesylate	4 mg	White to Off-White	Tablet	Diamond, Scored	Teva Pharmaceuticals
N; 598; 8	Doxazosin Mesylate	8 mg	White to Off-White	Tablet	Circle	Teva Pharmaceuticals
N; 739; 150	Mexiletine Hydrochloride	150 mg	Light Orange and Tan	Capsule		Teva Pharmaceuticals
N; 740; 200	Mexiletine Hydrochloride	200 mg	Light Orange	Capsule		Teva Pharmaceuticals
N; 741; 250	Mexiletine Hydrochloride	250 mg	Light Orange and Dark Green	Capsule		Teva Pharmaceuticals
N; 815; 400	Tolmetin Sodium	400 mg	Red	Capsule		Teva Pharmaceuticals
N2; SWORD LOGO	Suboxone	2 mg ; 0.5 mg	Orange	Tablet	Six-Sided	Reckitt Benckiser
N5; LL	Nilstat	500,000 units	Pink	Coated Tablet	Circle, Convex	Lederle Laboratories
N8; SWORD LOGO	Suboxone	8 mg ; 2 mg	Orange	Tablet	Six-Sided	Reckitt Benckiser
NAPROSYN; 250; ROCHE ;	Naprosyn	250 mg	Yellow	Tablet	Circle, Biconvex	Roche Laboratories
NAPROSYN; 375 ;	Naprosyn	375 mg	Peach	Tablet	Capsule-Shape	Roche Laboratories
NAPROSYN; 500 ;	Naprosyn	500 mg	Yellow	Tablet	Capsule-Shape	Roche Laboratories
NATAFORT	Natafort	12 mcg ; 60 mg ; 1000 IU ; 400 IU ; 11 IU ; 120 mg ; 1 mg ; 2 mg ; 3 mg ; 20 mg ; 10 mg	White	Coated Tablet		Warner Chilcott
ND; A	Janimine	10 mg	Orange	Coated Tablet		Abbott Laboratories
NE 2	Actonel with Calcium (Calcium Carbonate Tablets)	1250 mg	Light Blue	Tablet	Oval	Procter & Gamble
NE; 406	Didronel	400 mg	White	Tablet	Capsule-Shape, Scored	Procter & Gamble Pharmaceuticals
NE; A ;	Janimine	25 mg	Yellow	Coated Tablet		Abbott Laboratories
NEORAL 25 MG	Neoral	25 mg	Blue-Gray	Capsule, Liquid Filled	Oval	Novartis
NEORAL 100 MG	Neoral	100 mg	Blue-Gray	Capsule, Liquid Filled	Oblong	Novartis
NEXIUM 20 MG	Nexium	20 mg	Opaque, Amethyst with Two Yellow Bars	Capsule, Delayed Release		Astrazeneca
NEXIUM 40 MG	Nexium	40 mg	Opaque, Amethyst with 3 Yellow Bars	Capsule, Delayed Release		Astrazeneca
NICOTINE 14 MG/ DAY	Nicotine Transdermal System	14 mg/24 Hr	Opaque Tan	Patch, Extended Release	Square	Watson Laboratories
NICOTINE; 7 MG/ DAY	Nicotine Transdermal System	7 mg/24 Hours	Tan, Opaque	Patch	Square, Round Edges	Watson Laboratories
NICOTINE; 21 MG/ DAY	Nicotine Transdermal System	21 mg/24 Hours	Tan, Opaque	Patch	Square, Round Edges	Watson Laboratories
NIMOTOP	Nimotop	30 mg	Ivory	Capsule, Liquid Filled		Bayer Pharmaceutical
NL; A ;	Janimine	50 mg	Peach	Coated Tablet		Abbott Laboratories
NM	K-Tab	10 meq	Yellow	Extended-Release Tablet		Abbott Laboratories
NMI	Fe50	50 mg	Off White	Tablet		UCB Pharma
NO ; 4	Ondansetron Hydrochloride	4 mg	White	Tablet	Oval	Ranbaxy Pharmaceuticals
NO ; 8	Ondansetron Hydrochloride	8 mg	Yellow	Tablet	Oval	Ranbaxy Pharmaceuticals

IMPRINT	BRAND/GENERIC NAME	STRENGTH	COLOR	FORM	SHAPE	MANUFACTURER
NO DOZ	NO Doz	100 mg	White	Tablet	Circle	Bristol-Myers Squibb
NOLUDAR	Noludar	300 mg	Amethyst and White	Capsule		Roche Laboratories
NORCO; 539	Norco 10/325	10 mg ; 325 mg	Yellow	Tablet	Capsule-Shape, Scored	Watson Laboratories
NORCO; 729	Norco 7.5/325	325 mg ; 7.5 mg	Light Orange	Tablet	Capsule-Shape, Scored	Watson Laboratories
NORMOZIDE; 227	Normozide	200 mg ; 25 mg	White	Coated Tablet	Capsule-Shape, Scored	Schering
NORMOZIDE; 235	Normozide	100 mg ; 25 mg	Light Brown	Coated Tablet	Capsule-Shape, Scored	Schering
NORMOZIDE; 391 ;	Normozide	300 mg ; 25 mg	Blue	Coated Tablet	Capsule-Shape, Scored	Schering
NORPRAMIN; 25 ;	Norpramin	25 mg	Yellow	Tablet		Sanofi-Aventis U.S.
NORPRAMIN; 50 ;	Norpramin	50 mg	Green	Tablet		Sanofi-Aventis U.S.
NORPRAMIN; 75 ;	Norpramin	75 mg	Orange	Tablet		Sanofi-Aventis U.S.
NORPRAMIN; 100 ;	Norpramin	100 mg	Peach	Tablet		Sanofi-Aventis U.S.
NORPRAMIN; 150 ;	Norpramin	150 mg	White	Tablet		Sanofi-Aventis U.S.
NORTRIPTYLINE; DAN; 10 MG	Nortriptyline Hydrochloride	10 mg	Opaque Deep Green and Opaque White	Capsule		Watson Laboratories
NORTRIPTYLINE; DAN; 25 MG	Nortriptyline Hydrochloride	25 mg	Opaque Deep Green and Opaque White	Capsule		Watson Laboratories
NORTRIPTYLINE; DAN; 50 MG	Nortriptyline Hydrochloride	50 mg	Opaque White	Capsule		Watson Laboratories
NORTRIPTYLINE; DAN; 75 MG	Nortriptyline Hydrochloride	75 mg	Opaque Deep Green	Capsule		Watson Laboratories
NORVASC; 2.5 ;	Norvasc	2.5 mg	White	Tablet	Diamond-Shaped, Flat-Faced, Beveled Edge	Pfizer
NORVASC; 5 ;	Norvasc	5 mg	White	Tablet	Eight-Sided, Elongated, Flat-Aced, Beveled Edge	Pfizer
NORVASC; 10 ;	Norvasc	10 mg	White	Tablet	Flat-Faced, Beveled Edge, Circle	Pfizer
NOVAFED A ;	Novafed A	120 mg ; 8 mg	Red and Orange	Extended-Release Capsule	Capsule-Shape, Red Opaque with Orange Transparent Body	Aventis Pharmaceuticals
NOVAFED; 104	Novafed	120 mg	Orange and Brown	Controlled-Release Capsule	Capsule-Shape	Aventis Pharmaceuticals
NOVO NORDISK LOGO	Prandin	1 mg	Yellow	Tablet	Biconvex	Novo Nordisk
NOVO NORDISK LOGO (BULL)	Prandin	0.5 mg	White	Tablet	Biconvex	Novo Nordisk
NOVO NORDISK LOGO (BULL)	Prandin	2 mg	Peach	Tablet	Biconvex	Novo Nordisk
NPR LE 375	Prevacid Naprapac 375 - Naprosyn	375 mg	Pink	Tablet	Oval	Takeda Pharmaceuticals
NPR LE 500	Prevacid Naprapac 500 - Naprosyn	500 mg	Yellow	Tablet	Capsule-Shape	Takeda Pharmaceuticals
NPR; LE; 375	Naprosyn	375 mg	Pink	Tablet	Oval	Roche Laboratories
NRP104 20MG	Vyvanse	20 mg	Ivory	Capsule		Shire Us
NRP104 30MG	Vyvanse	30 mg	Orange, White	Capsule		Shire Us
NRP104 40MG	Vyvanse	40 mg	Blue-Green, White	Capsule		Shire Us
NRP104 50MG	Vyvanse	50 mg	Blue, White	Capsule		Shire Us
NRP104 60MG	Vyvanse	60 mg	Aqua Blue	Capsule		Shire Us
NRP104 70MG	Vyvanse	70 mg	Blue, Orange	Capsule		Shire Us
NT 26 ;	Neurontin	800 mg	White	Coated Tablet	Oval	Parke-Davis
NT; 0; RJS	Nature-Throid	32.4 mg	Tan	Tablet	Round, Compressed, Bisected Scored	Western Research Laboratories
NT; 1; RJS ;	Nature-Throid	64.8 mg	Tan	Tablet	Round, Compressed, Bisected Scored	Western Research Laboratories
NT; 2; RJS ;	Nature-Throid	129.6 mg	Tan	Tablet	Round, Compressed, Bisected Scored	Western Research Laboratories
NT; 3; RJS ;	Nature-Throid	194.4 mg	Tan	Tablet	Circle, Compressed	Western Research Laboratories
NT; 16 ;	Neurontin	600 mg	White	Coated Tablet	Circle	Parke-Davis
NVR R20	Ritalin LA	20 mg	White	Capsule, Extended Release		Novartis Pharmaceuticals
NVR ; J 125	Exjade	125 mg	Off-White	Tablet for Suspension	Circle	Novartis Pharmaceuticals
NVR ; J 250	Exjade	250 mg	Off-White	Tablet for Suspension	Circle	Novartis Pharmaceuticals
NVR ; J 500	Exjade	500 mg	Off-White	Tablet for Suspension	Circle	Novartis Pharmaceuticals
NVR D5	Focalin Xr	5 mg	Light Blue	Capsule, Extended Release		Novartis Pharmaceuticals
NVR D10	Focalin Xr	10 mg	Light Caramel	Capsule, Extended Release		Novartis Pharmaceuticals
NVR D15	Focalin Xr	15 mg	Green	Capsule, Extended Release		Novartis Pharmaceuticals
NVR D20	Focalin Xr	20 mg	White	Capsule, Extended Release		Novartis Pharmaceuticals
NVR R10	Ritalin LA	10 mg	Light Brown, White	Capsule, Extended Release		Novartis Pharmaceuticals
NVR R30	Ritalin LA	30 mg	Yellow	Capsule, Extended Release		Novartis Pharmaceuticals
NVR R40	Ritalin LA	40 mg	Light Brown	Capsule, Extended Release		Novartis Pharmaceuticals
NVR SI	Gleevec	100 mg	Orange with Red Ink	Capsule		Novartis
NVR/TKI ;	Tasigna	200 mg	Light Yellow Opaque	Capsule		Novartis
NVR; EH	Zelnorm	6 mg	White to Yellow Marbled	Tablet	Circle, Flat	Novartis Pharmaceuticals
NVR; SL	Gleevec	400 mg	Dark Yellow to Brownish Orange	Tablet	Oval	Novartis
NZ; 150; G	Nizatidine	150 mg	Light Yellow and Dark Yellow	Capsule		Par Pharmaceutical
NZ; 300; G	Nizatidine	300 mg	Light Brown	Capsule		Par Pharmaceutical
O-IR; PF5MG	Oxyir	5 mg	Beige and Orange	Capsule		Purdue Pharmaceutical Products
O-M; 180	Ortho Tri-Cyclen Lo White Tablet	0.025 mg ; 0.18 mg	White	28-Day Tablet Pack	Circle	Ortho-Mcneil Pharmaceutical
O-M; 215	Ortho Tri-Cyclen Lo Light Blue Tablet	0.215 mg ; 0.025 mg	Light Blue	28-Day Tablet Pack	Circle	Ortho-Mcneil Pharmaceutical

IMPRINT	BRAND/GENERIC NAME	STRENGTH	COLOR	FORM	SHAPE	MANUFACTURER
O-M; 250	Ortho Tri-Cyclen Lo Dark Blue Tablet	0.025 mg ; 0.25 mg	Dark Blue	28-Day Tablet Pack	Circle	Ortho-Mcneil Pharmaceutical
O-M; 650	Ultracet	325 mg ; 37.5 mg	Light Yellow	Coated Tablet	Capsule-Shape	Ortho-Mcneil Pharmaceutical
OGT; 918	Zavesca	100 mg ;	White	Capsule		Actelion Pharmaceuticals
OMNICEF	Omnicef	300 mg	Lavender and Turquoise	Capsule		Abbott Laboratories
ONE A DAY	One-A-Day Plus Extra C Adult Formula	5000 IU ; 1.5 mg ; 1.7 mg ; 20 mg ; 400 IU ; 15 IU ; 0.4 mg ; 500 mg ; 2 mg ; 6 mcg		Tablet		Bayer Consumer Care
OP 701	Vivactil	5 mg	Orange	Tablet	Oval	Odyssey Pharmaceuticals
OP 702	Vivactil	10 mg	Yellow	Tablet	Oval	Odyssey Pharmaceuticals
OP 704 ;	Urecholine	25 mg	Yellow	Tablet	Circle	Odyssey Pharmaceuticals
OP 706	Antabuse	250 mg	White	Tablet	Circle	Odyssey Pharmaceuticals
OP 707	Antabuse	500 mg	White	Tablet	Circle	Odyssey Pharmaceuticals
OP 718 ;	Surmontil	25 mg	Opaque Blue, Yellow	Capsule		Odyssey Pharmaceuticals
OP 719 ;	Surmontil	50 mg	Opaque Blue, Orange	Capsule	Capsule-Shape	Odyssey Pharmaceuticals
OP 720 ;	Surmontil	100 mg	Opaque Blue, White	Capsule		Odyssey Pharmaceuticals
OP; 706	Disulfiram	250 mg	White	Tablet	Circle	Odyssey Pharmaceuticals
ORAP 1	Orap	1 mg	White	Tablet	Oval	Gate Pharmaceuticals
ORAP 2 ; LEMMON	Orap	2 mg	White	Tablet	Oval	Gate Pharmaceuticals
ORETIC	Oretic	25 mg	White	Tablet	Circle	Abbott Laboratories
ORETIC	Oretic	50 mg	White	Tablet	Circle, Scored	Abbott Laboratories
ORG; 07	Jenest 28 White Tablet	35 mcg ; 0.5 mg	White	28-Day Tablet Pack	Circle	Organon Teknika
ORG; 14	Jenest 28 Peach Tablet	35 mcg ; 1 mg	Peach	28-Day Tablet Pack	Circle	Organon Teknika
ORGANON; 388	Cotazyme-S	5,000 USP units ; 20,000 USP units ; 20,000 USP units		Capsule		Organon
ORGANON; 393	Zymase	12,000 USP units ; 24,000 USP units ; 24,000 USP units	White and Green	Capsule		Organon
ORGANON; 542	Wigraine	1 mg ; 100 mg	White	Tablet	Circle	Organon
ORGANON; 790	Hexadrol	1.5 mg	Peach	Tablet		Organon
ORGANON; 791	Hexadrol	0.75 mg	White	Tablet		Organon
ORGANON; 792	Hexadrol	0.5 mg	Yellow	Tablet		Organon
ORGANON; 798	Hexadrol	4 mg	Green	Tablet		Organon
ORGANON; K2S	Mircette Yellow Tablet	0.01 mg	Yellow	Tablet	Circle	Organon
ORGANON; T4R ;	Mircette White Tablet	0.15 mg ; 0.02 mg	White	28-Day Tablet Pack	Circle	Organon
ORGANON; TR5	Desogen White Tablet	0.03 mg ; 0.15 mg	White	28-Day Tablet Pack	Circle	Organon
ORGANON; TZ3 ;	Remeron	15 mg	Yellow	Coated Tablet	Oval, Scored	Organon
ORGANON; TZ5 ;	Remeron	30 mg	Red-Brown	Coated Tablet	Scored, Oval	Organon
ORGANON; TZ7	Remeron	45 mg	White	Coated Tablet	Oval	Organon
ORINASE; 250	Orinase	250 mg	White	Tablet	Circle, Scored	Upjohn
ORINASE; 500	Orinase	500 mg	White	Tablet	Circle, Scored	Pharmacia & Upjohn
ORTHO; 0.35	Micronor	0.35 mg	Light Green	28-Day Tablet Pack	Circle	Ortho-Mcneil Pharmaceutical
ORTHO; 0214	Grifulvin V	500 mg	White	Tablet		Ortho-Mcneil Pharmaceutical
ORTHO; 75	Ortho-Novum 7/7/7-21 Light Peach Tablet	35 mcg ; 0.75 mg	Light Peach	21-Day Tablet Pack	Circle	Ortho-Mcneil Pharmaceutical
ORTHO; 75	Ortho-Novum 7/7/7-28 Light Peach Tablet	35 mcg ; 0.75 mg	Light Peach	28-Day Tablet Pack	Circle	Ortho-Mcneil Pharmaceutical
ORTHO; 135	Ortho-Novum 1/35-21	35 mcg ; 1 mg	Peach	21-Day Tablet Pack	Circle	Ortho-Mcneil Pharmaceutical
ORTHO; 135	Ortho-Novum 1/35-28 Peach Tablet	35 mcg ; 1 mg	Peach	28-Day Tablet Pack	Circle	Ortho-Mcneil Pharmaceutical
ORTHO; 135	Ortho-Novum 7/7/7-21 Peach Tablet	1 mg ; 35 mcg	Peach	21-Day Tablet Pack	Circle	Ortho-Mcneil Pharmaceutical
ORTHO; 135	Ortho-Novum 7/7/7-28 Peach Tablet	1 mg ; 35 mcg	Peach	28-Day Tablet Pack	Circle	Ortho-Mcneil Pharmaceutical
ORTHO; 135	Ortho-Novum 10/11-21 Peach Tablet	1 mg ; 35 mcg	Peach	21-Day Tablet Pack	Circle	Ortho-Mcneil Pharmaceutical
ORTHO; 150	Ortho-Novum 1/50-21	1 mg ; 50 mcg	Yellow	21-Day Tablet Pack	Circle	Ortho-Mcneil Pharmaceutical
ORTHO; 180	Ortho Tri-Cyclen 21 White Tablet	0.18 mg ; 0.035 mg	White	21-Day Tablet Pack	Circle	Ortho-Mcneil Pharmaceutical
ORTHO; 180	Ortho Tri-Cyclen 28 White Tablet	0.18 mg ; 0.035 mg	White	28-Day Tablet Pack	Circle	Ortho-Mcneil Pharmaceutical
ORTHO; 211	Grifulvin V	250 mg	White	Tablet		Ortho-Mcneil Pharmaceutical
ORTHO; 215	Ortho Tri-Cyclen 21 Light Blue Tablet	0.215 mg ; 0.035 mg	Light Blue	21-Day Tablet Pack	Circle	Ortho-Mcneil Pharmaceutical
ORTHO; 215	Ortho Tri-Cyclen 28 Light Blue Tablet	0.215 mg ; 0.035 mg	Light Blue	28-Day Tablet Pack	Circle	Ortho-Mcneil Pharmaceutical
ORTHO; 250	Ortho-Cyclen 21	0.25 mg ; 0.035 mg	Blue	21-Day Tablet Pack	Circle	Ortho-Mcneil Pharmaceutical
ORTHO; 250	Ortho-Cyclen 28 Blue Tablet	0.25 mg ; 0.035 mg	Blue	28-Day Tablet Pack	Circle	Ortho-Mcneil Pharmaceutical
ORTHO; 250	Ortho Tri-Cyclen 21 Blue Tablet	0.035 mg ; 0.25 mg	Blue	21-Day Tablet Pack	Circle	Ortho-Mcneil Pharmaceutical
ORTHO; 250	Ortho Tri-Cyclen 28 Blue Tablet	0.25 mg ; 0.035 mg	Blue	28-Day Tablet Pack	Circle	Ortho-Mcneil Pharmaceutical
ORTHO; 535	Modicon 21	0.5 mg ; 35 mcg	White	21-Day Tablet Pack	Circle	Ortho-Mcneil Pharmaceutical
ORTHO; 535	Modicon 28 White Tablet	0.5 mg ; 35 mcg	White	28-Day Tablet Pack	Circle	Ortho-Mcneil Pharmaceutical
ORTHO; 535	Ortho-Novum 7/7/7-21 White Tablet	0.5 mg ; 35 mcg	White	21-Day Tablet Pack	Circle	Ortho-Mcneil Pharmaceutical
ORTHO; 535	Ortho-Novum 7/7/7-28 White Tablet	0.5 mg ; 35 mcg	White	28-Day Tablet Pack	Circle	Ortho-Mcneil Pharmaceutical
ORTHO; 535	Ortho-Novum 10/11-21 White Tablet	35 mcg ; 0.5 mg	White	21-Day Tablet Pack	Circle	Ortho-Mcneil Pharmaceutical
ORTHO; 1570	Protostat	250 mg	White	Tablet	Capsule-Shape	Ortho-Mcneil Pharmaceutical
ORTHO; 1571	Protostat	500 mg	White	Tablet	Capsule-Shape	Ortho-Mcneil Pharmaceutical
ORTHO; D; 150	Ortho-Cept 21	0.15 mg ; 0.03 mg	Orange	21-Day Tablet Pack	Circle	Ortho-Mcneil Pharmaceutical
ORTHO; D; 150	Ortho-Cept 28 Orange Tablet	0.15 mg ; 0.03 mg	Orange	28-Day Tablet Pack	Circle	Ortho-Mcneil Pharmaceutical
ORUVAIL; 100	Oruvail	100 mg	Pink and Dark Green with Two Radial Bands	Capsule		Wyeth Pharmaceuticals
ORUVAIL; 150	Oruvail	150 mg	Pink and Light Green with Two Radial Bands	Capsule		Wyeth Pharmaceuticals

IMPRINT	BRAND/GENERIC NAME	STRENGTH	COLOR	FORM	SHAPE	MANUFACTURER
ORUVAIL; 200	Oruvail	200 mg	Pink and White with Two Radial Bands	Capsule		Wyeth Pharmaceuticals
OSTIVA	Ostiva	0.565 mg ; 0.25 mg ; 500 mg ; 50 mg ; 200 IU ; 1.2 mg		Tablet	Oval	Sciele Pharma
OV; 12	Desoxyn	5 mg	White	Tablet		Ovation Pharmaceuticals
OV; 31; T	Tranxene T-Tab	3.75 mg	Blue	Tablet	T-Shaped, Scored	Ovation Pharmaceuticals
OV; 32; T	Tranxene T-Tab	7.5 mg	Peach	Tablet	T-Shaped, Scored	Ovation Pharmaceuticals
OV; 33; T	Tranxene T-Tab	15 mg	Lavender	Tablet	T-Shaped, Scored	Ovation Pharmaceuticals
OV; 44	Tranxene-Sd Half Strength	11.25 mg	Blue	Tablet		Ovation Pharmaceuticals
OV; 45	Tranxene-Sd	22.5 mg	Tan	Extended-Release Tablet		Ovation Pharmaceuticals
OX ; 10	Oxandrolone	10 mg	White	Tablet	Capsule-Shape	Watson Laboratories
OXYROL; 3.9 MG/ DAY	Oxytrol	3.9 mg/24 Hours		Patch	Rectangle	Watson Laboratories
P	Panadol Junior	160 mg	White	Tablet	Oval	Bayer Consumer Care
P 067	Oxazepam	10 mg	Pink Opaque	Capsule		Actavis Elizabeth
P 069 ;	Oxazepam	15 mg	Red Opaque	Capsule		Actavis Elizabeth
P 073 ;	Oxazepam	30 mg	Maroon Opaque	Capsule		Actavis Elizabeth
P 741	Tizanidine Hydrochloride	4 mg	Yellow	Tablet	Circle	Actavis Elizabeth
P 742	Tizanidine Hydrochloride	2 mg	Yellow	Tablet	Capsule-Shape	Actavis Elizabeth
P 771	Diphenoxylate Hydrochloride and Atropine Sulfate	2.5 mg ; 0.025 mg	White	Tablet	Circle	Par Pharmaceutical
P&G; 402	Didronel	200 mg	White	Tablet	Rectangle	Procter & Gamble Pharmaceuticals
P; 02	Mercaptopurine	50 mg	Light Yellow	Tablet	Diamond	Par Pharmaceutical
P; 53; LEDERLE	Ext Phenytoin Sodium	100 mg	Clear	Capsule		Lederle Laboratories
P; 771	Atropine and Diphenoxylate Hydrochloride	0.025 mg ; 2.5 mg	White	Tablet	Circle	Par Pharmaceutical
P; 4600	Benzonatate	100 mg	Yellow	Capsule, Liquid Filled	Oval	Warner Chilcott
P; PRAVACOL 20; ;	Pravigard Pac	81 mg ; 20 mg	Yellow Tablet and White Tablet	Tablet		Bristol-Myers Squibb
P; PRAVACOL 20; ;	Pravigard Pac	325 mg ; 20 mg	Yellow Tablet and White Tablet	Tablet		Bristol-Myers Squibb
P; PRAVACOL 40; ;	Pravigard Pac	81 mg ; 40 mg	Green Tablet and White Tablet	Tablet		Bristol-Myers Squibb
P; PRAVACOL 40; ;	Pravigard Pac	325 mg ; 40 mg	Green Tablet and White Tablet	Tablet		Bristol-Myers Squibb
P; US; 144	Amiodarone Hydrochloride	100 mg	White	Tablet	Circle	Upsher-Smith Laboratories
P-D 270	Nardil	15 mg	Orange	Tablet	Biconvex	Parke-Davis
P-D 915 ;	Loestrin 24 Fe - White Tablet	1 mg ; 20 mcg	White	Tablet	Circle	Warner Chilcott
P-D ; CENTRAX; 553	Centrax	10 mg	Aqua	Capsule		Parke-Davis
P-D; 007	Dilantin Infatabs	50 mg	Yellow	Tablet, Chewable	Triangle, Scored	Parke-Davis
P-D; 141; 2	Diazepam	2 mg	White	Tablet	Oval	Parke-Davis
P-D; 142; 5	Diazepam	5 mg		Tablet	Triangle	Parke-Davis
P-D; 143; 10	Diazepam	10 mg	White	Tablet	Circle	Parke-Davis
P-D; 160	Pyridium Plus	0.3 mg ; 15 mg ; 150 mg		Tablet		Warner Chilcott
P-D; 200	Brondecon	200 mg ; 100 mg		Tablet		Parke-Davis
P-D; 201	Brondecon	200 mg ; 100 mg	Pink	Tablet		Parke-Davis
P-D; 202	Procan SR	250 mg	Green	Sustained-Release Tablet	Circle	Parke-Davis
P-D; 207	Procan SR	1000 mg	Red	Sustained-Release Tablet	Circle, Scored	Parke-Davis
P-D; 214	Choledyl SA	400 mg	Pink	Extended-Release Tablet		Parke-Davis
P-D; 221	Choledyl SA	600 mg	Tan	Extended-Release Tablet		Parke-Davis
P-D; 237	Zarontin	250 mg	Orange	Capsule		Parke-Davis
P-D; 260	Euthroid-1/2	30 mcg ; 7.5 mcg		Tablet		Parke-Davis
P-D; 261	Euthroid-1	60 mcg ; 15 mcg		Tablet		Parke-Davis
P-D; 262	Euthroid-2	120 mcg ; 30 mcg		Tablet		Parke-Davis
P-D; 263	Euthroid-3	180 mcg ; 45 mcg		Tablet		Parke-Davis
P-D; 271	Amitril	100 mg	Brown and Mustard	Coated Tablet		Parke-Davis
P-D; 272	Amitril	10 mg	Tan	Coated Tablet		Parke-Davis
P-D; 273	Amitril	25 mg	Coral	Coated Tablet		Parke-Davis
P-D; 274	Amitril	50 mg	Blue-Purple	Coated Tablet		Parke-Davis
P-D; 275	Amitril	75 mg	Green	Coated Tablet		Parke-Davis
P-D; 276	Centrax	10 mg	Blue	Tablet		Parke-Davis
P-D; 278	Amitril	150 mg	Orange	Coated Tablet		Parke-Davis
P-D; 365 ;	Dilantin Kapseals	30 mg	White with Pink Band	Extended-Release Capsule		Parke-Davis
P-D; 393	Milontin	500 mg		Capsule		Parke-Davis
P-D; 407	Cyclopar	250 mg	Scarlet and Flesh	Capsule		Parke-Davis
P-D; 471	Benadryl Capsule	25 mg	Pink and White	Capsule		Pfizer Consumer Health Care
P-D; 525	Celontin	300 mg	Yellow with Orange Band	Capsule		Parke-Davis
P-D; 529	Humatin	250 mg		Capsule		Monarch Pharmaceuticals
P-D; 531	Dilantin with Phenobarbital	100 mg ; 32 mg	White and Purple with Black Band	Capsule		Parke-Davis
P-D; 537	Celontin	150 mg	Yellow with Brown Band	Capsule		Parke-Davis
P-D; 540	Ponstel	250 mg	Ivory with a Blue Band	Capsule		First Horizon Pharmaceutical
P-D; 557	Verapamil Hydrochloride	80 mg		Tablet		Warner Chilcott
P-D; 573	Verapamil Hydrochloride	120 mg		Tablet		Warner Chilcott
P-D; 697	Cyclopar	500 mg	Orange and Flesh	Capsule		Warner Chilcott
P-D; 737; LOPID	Lopid	600 mg	White	Coated Tablet	Circle, Scored	Parke-Davis
P-D; 849	Quinidine Sulfate	200 mg		Tablet		Parke-Davis
P-D; CENTRAX; 552	Centrax	5 mg	Celery	Capsule		Parke-Davis
P-D; CENTRAX; 554	Centrax	20 mg	Yellow	Capsule		Parke-Davis
P2 ; G ;	Paroxetine Hydrochloride	20 mg	White	Tablet	Circle	Watson Pharma

IMPRINT	BRAND/GENERIC NAME	STRENGTH	COLOR	FORM	SHAPE	MANUFACTURER
P3 ; G ;	Paroxetine Hydrochloride	30 mg	White	Tablet	Circle	Watson Pharma
P4; LL	Pathilon	25 mg	Pink	Coated Tablet	Circle, Convex	Lederle Laboratories
P5; G	Pindolol	5 mg	White	Tablet	Circle	Par Pharmaceutical
P10; G	Pindolol	10 mg	White	Tablet	Circle	Par Pharmaceutical
P20	Pantoprazole Sodium	20 mg	Yellow	Tablet, Delayed Release	Oval	Wyeth Pharmaceuticals
P20	Protonix	20 mg	Yellow	Tablet, Delayed Release	Oval	Wyeth Pharmaceuticals
P46 ;	Amytal Sodium	250 mg/ampule		Solution for Injection		Eli Lilly
PA46 ;	Benzonatate	100 mg	Yellow	Capsule, Liquid Filled		Barr Laboratories
PA83	Benzonatate	200 mg	Yellow	Capsule, Liquid Filled		Barr Laboratories
PAD 0107	Clotrimazole	10 mg	White	Lozenge/troche	Circle	Paddock Laboratories
PAD 0116 ;	Benzphetamine Hydrochloride	50 mg		Tablet	Circle	Paddock Laboratories
PAD 112	Moexipril Hydrochloride	15 mg	Dark Beige	Tablet	Circle	Paddock Laboratories
PALI 3	Invega	3 mg	White	Tablet, Extended Release		Janssen
PALI 6	Invega	6 mg	Beige	Tablet, Extended Release		Janssen
PALI 9	Invega	9 mg	Pink	Tablet, Extended Release		Janssen
PANMYCIN; 250 MG	Panmycin	250 mg	Yellow and Gray	Capsule		Upjohn
PAR 282	Propranolol Hydrochloride	60 mg	Aqua Blue, White Opaque	Capsule, Extended Release		Par Pharmaceutical
PAR 328	Propranolol Hydrochloride	80 mg	Aqua Blue Opaque	Capsule, Extended Release		Par Pharmaceutical
PAR 329	Propranolol Hydrochloride	120 mg	Aqua Blue Opaque, Dark Blue Opaque	Capsule, Extended Release		Par Pharmaceutical
PAR 330	Propranolol Hydrochloride	160 mg	Dark Blue Opaque	Capsule, Extended Release		Par Pharmaceutical
PAR 845	Glimepiride	1 mg	Pink	Tablet	Rectangle	Par Pharmaceutical
PAR 846	Glimepiride	2 mg	Green	Tablet	Rectangle	Par Pharmaceutical
PAR 847	Glimepiride	4 mg	Blue	Tablet	Rectangle	Par Pharmaceutical
PAR 867	Dronabinol	2.5 mg	Cream	Capsule, Liquid Filled	Oblong	Par Pharmaceutical
PAR 868	Dronabinol	5 mg	Opaque Brown	Capsule, Liquid Filled	Oblong	Par Pharmaceutical
PAR 869	Dronabinol	10 mg	Orange	Capsule, Liquid Filled	Oblong	Par Pharmaceutical
PAR; 009	Isosorbide Dinitrate	30 mg	Blue	Tablet	Circle	Par Pharmaceutical
PAR; 015	Meclizine Hydrochloride	50 mg	Yellow and Blue	Tablet	Oval, Scored; Multiple Layered	Par Pharmaceutical
PAR; 016	Chlorzoxazone	250 mg	Orange	Tablet	Circle, Scored	Par Pharmaceutical
PAR; 020	Isosorbide Dinitrate	5 mg	White	Tablet	Circle, Scored	Par Pharmaceutical
PAR; 021	Isosorbide Dinitrate	10 mg	White	Tablet	Scored, Circle	Par Pharmaceutical
PAR; 022	Isosorbide Dinitrate	20 mg	Green	Tablet	Circle, Scored	Par Pharmaceutical
PAR; 027	Hydralazine Hydrochloride	25 mg	Peach	Tablet	Circle, Convex	Par Pharmaceutical
PAR; 028	Hydralazine Hydrochloride	50 mg	Peach or Blue	Tablet	Round or Oval	Par Pharmaceutical
PAR; 029	Hydralazine Hydrochloride	10 mg	Pink	Tablet	Circle	Par Pharmaceutical
PAR; 034	Meclizine Hydrochloride	12.5 mg	Blue	Tablet	Oval	Par Pharmaceutical
PAR; 035	Meclizine Hydrochloride	25 mg	Yellow	Tablet	Teardrop-Shape	Par Pharmaceutical
PAR; 043	Cyproheptadine Hydrochloride	4 mg	White	Tablet	Circle, Scored; Compressed	Par Pharmaceutical
PAR; 054	Imipramine Hydrochloride	10 mg	Yellow	Tablet	Triangle	Par Pharmaceutical
PAR; 055	Imipramine Hydrochloride	25 mg	Brown	Tablet	Circle	Par Pharmaceutical
PAR; 056	Imipramine Hydrochloride	50 mg	Green	Coated Tablet		Par Pharmaceutical
PAR; 056	Imipramine Hydrochloride	50 mg	Green	Tablet	Circle	Par Pharmaceutical
PAR; 061	Fluphenazine Hydrochloride	1 mg	White	Coated Tablet	Circle	Par Pharmaceutical
PAR; 062	Fluphenazine Hydrochloride	2.5 mg	Blue	Coated Tablet	Circle	Par Pharmaceutical
PAR; 064	Fluphenazine Hydrochloride	10 mg	Orange	Coated Tablet	Circle	Par Pharmaceutical
PAR; 067	Indomethacin	25 mg	Light Green or White and Blue	Capsule		Par Pharmaceutical
PAR; 068	Indomethacin	50 mg	Light Green or White and Blue	Capsule		Par Pharmaceutical
PAR; 076	Fluphenazine Hydrochloride	5 mg	Dark Pink	Coated Tablet	Circle	Par Pharmaceutical
PAR; 083	Dexamethasone	0.25 mg	Pale Orange	Tablet	Five-Sided, Scored	Par Pharmaceutical
PAR; 084	Dexamethasone	0.5 mg	Pale Yellow	Tablet	Five-Sided, Scored	Par Pharmaceutical
PAR; 085	Dexamethasone	0.75 mg	Pale Blue	Tablet	Five-Sided, Scored	Par Pharmaceutical
PAR; 086	Dexamethasone	1.5 mg	Pale Pink	Tablet	Five-Sided, Scored	Par Pharmaceutical
PAR; 087	Dexamethasone	4 mg	White	Tablet	Five-Sided, Scored	Par Pharmaceutical
PAR; 095	Metronidazole	250 mg	White	Coated Tablet	Circle	Par Pharmaceutical
PAR; 104	Allopurinol	100 mg	White	Tablet	Circle, Flat Bevel	Par Pharmaceutical
PAR; 105	Allopurinol	300 mg	Orange	Tablet	Circle	Par Pharmaceutical
PAR; 110	Clonidine Hydrochloride	0.1 mg	Green	Tablet	Round; Bisected Scored	Par Pharmaceutical
PAR; 111	Clonidine Hydrochloride	0.2 mg	Yellow	Tablet	Round; Bisected Scored	Par Pharmaceutical
PAR; 112	Clonidine Hydrochloride	0.3 mg	Blue	Tablet	Round; Bisected Scored	Par Pharmaceutical
PAR; 113	Clonidine Hydrochloride and Chlorthalidone	15 mg ; 0.1 mg	White	Tablet	Round; Flat-Faced; Beveled Edge; Bisected Scored	Par Pharmaceutical
PAR; 114	Metronidazole	500 mg	White	Tablet	Capsule-Shape	Par Pharmaceutical
PAR; 115	Clonidine Hydrochloride and Chlorthalidone	15 mg ; 0.2 mg	Blue	Tablet	Circle, Flat-Faced; Beveled Edge	Par Pharmaceutical
PAR; 116	Clonidine Hydrochloride and Chlorthalidone	15 mg ; 0.3 mg	White	Tablet	Round; Concave; Bisected Scored	Par Pharmaceutical
PAR; 117	Amiloride Hydrochloride	5 mg	Yellow	Tablet	Circle, Compressed	Par Pharmaceutical
PAR; 118	Propantheline Bromide	15 mg	Light Peach	Tablet	Circle	Par Pharmaceutical
PAR; 119	Nystatin	500,000 units	Brown	Coated Tablet	Circle	Par Pharmaceutical
PAR; 121	Hydralazine Hydrochloride	100 mg	Peach	Tablet	Circle	Par Pharmaceutical
PAR; 129	Dexamethasone	6 mg	Pale Green	Tablet	Five-Sided, Scored	Par Pharmaceutical
PAR; 133	Amitriptyline Hydrochloride	10 mg	Pink	Tablet	Circle	Par Pharmaceutical
PAR; 134	Amitriptyline Hydrochloride	25 mg	Green	Tablet	Circle	Par Pharmaceutical
PAR; 135	Amitriptyline Hydrochloride	50 mg	Brown	Tablet	Circle	Par Pharmaceutical
PAR; 136	Amitriptyline Hydrochloride	75 mg	Purple	Tablet	Circle	Par Pharmaceutical
PAR; 137	Amitriptyline Hydrochloride	100 mg	Orange	Tablet	Circle	Par Pharmaceutical
PAR; 138	Amitriptyline Hydrochloride	150 mg	Peach	Tablet	Circle	Par Pharmaceutical
PAR; 139	Sulfamethoxazole and Trimethoprim	400 mg ; 80 mg	White	Tablet		Par Pharmaceutical

IMPRINT	BRAND/GENERIC NAME	STRENGTH	COLOR	FORM	SHAPE	MANUFACTURER
PAR; 140	Sulfamethoxazole and Trimethoprim	800 mg ; 160 mg	White	Tablet		Par Pharmaceutical
PAR; 143	Hydralazine Hydrochloride and Hydrochlorothiazide	25 mg ; 25 mg	White	Capsule		Par Pharmaceutical
PAR; 144	Hydralazine Hydrocloride and Hydrochlorothiazide	50 mg ; 50 mg	White and Black	Capsule		Par Pharmaceutical
PAR; 145	Hydralazine Hydrochloride and Hydrochlorothiazide	100 mg ; 50 mg	Powder Blue and Light Blue	Capsule		Par Pharmaceutical
PAR; 162; 400	Ibuprofen	400 mg	White	Tablet	Circle	Par Pharmaceutical
PAR; 163; 600	Ibuprofen	600 mg	White	Tablet	Oval	Par Pharmaceutical
PAR; 164	Benztropine Mesylate	0.5 mg	White	Tablet	Circle, Scored	Par Pharmaceutical
PAR; 165	Benztropine Mesylate	1 mg	White	Tablet	Scored, Oval	Par Pharmaceutical
PAR; 166	Benztropine Mesylate	2 mg	White	Tablet	Circle, Scored	Par Pharmaceutical
PAR; 181	Perphenazine and Amitriptyline Hydrochloride	10 mg ; 2 mg	Blue	Coated Tablet	Circle	Par Pharmaceutical
PAR; 182	Perphenazine and Amitriptyline Hydrochloride	2 mg ; 25 mg	Orange	Coated Tablet	Circle	Par Pharmaceutical
PAR; 183	Perphenazine and Amitriptyline Hydrochloride	4 mg ; 10 mg	Salmon	Coated Tablet	Circle	Par Pharmaceutical
PAR; 184	Perphenazine and Amitriptyline Hydrochloride	4 mg ; 25 mg	Yellow	Coated Tablet	Circle	Par Pharmaceutical
PAR; 185	Perphenazine and Amitriptyline Hydrochloride	4 mg ; 50 mg	Orange	Coated Tablet	Circle	Par Pharmaceutical
PAR; 186	Methyldopa and Hydrochlorothiazide	250 mg ; 15 mg	Green	Coated Tablet	Circle	Par Pharmaceutical
PAR; 187	Methyldopa and Hydrochlorothiazide	250 mg ; 25 mg	White	Coated Tablet	Capsule-Shape	Par Pharmaceutical
PAR; 188	Methyldopa and Hydrochlorothiazide	30 mg ; 500 mg	Yellow	Coated Tablet	Oval	Par Pharmaceutical
PAR; 189	Methyldopa and Hydrochlorothiazide	500 mg ; 50 mg	Pink	Coated Tablet	Oval	Par Pharmaceutical
PAR; 193	Flurazepam Hydrochloride	15 mg	White and Powder Blue	Capsule		Par Pharmaceutical
PAR; 194	Flurazepam Hydrochloride	30 mg	Powder Blue	Capsule		Par Pharmaceutical
PAR; 200; 682	Ofloxacin	200 mg	White	Tablet	Capsule-Shape	Par Pharmaceutical
PAR; 202	Methyldopa and Chlorothiazide	150 mg ; 250 mg	Beige	Coated Tablet	Circle	Par Pharmaceutical
PAR; 203	Methyldopa and Chlorothiazide	250 mg ; 250 mg	Green	Coated Tablet	Circle	Par Pharmaceutical
PAR; 213	Orphengesic	25 mg ; 30 mg ; 385 mg	White and Green	Tablet	Circle, Flat; Double Layered	Par Pharmaceutical
PAR; 214	Orphengesic Forte	50 mg ; 60 mg ; 770 mg	White and Green	Tablet	Capsule-Shaped; Bisected; Double Layered Scored	Par Pharmaceutical
PAR; 216; 800	Ibuprofen	800 mg	White	Tablet	Capsule-Shape	Par Pharmaceutical
PAR; 217	Doxepin Hydrochloride	10 mg	Opaque Buff	Capsule		Par Pharmaceutical
PAR; 218	Doxepin Hydrochloride	25 mg	Opaque Ivory and White	Capsule		Par Pharmaceutical
PAR; 219	Doxepin Hydrochloride	50 mg	Opaque Ivory	Capsule		Par Pharmaceutical
PAR; 220	Doxepin Hydrochloride	75 mg	Bright Light Green	Capsule		Par Pharmaceutical
PAR; 221	Doxepin Hydrochloride	100 mg	White and Bright Light Green	Capsule		Par Pharmaceutical
PAR; 222	Doxepin Hydrochloride	150 mg	Opaque White and Blue	Capsule		Par Pharmaceutical
PAR; 223	Haloperidol	0.5 mg	White	Tablet	Circle, Scored; Flat; Compressed	Par Pharmaceutical
PAR; 224	Haloperidol	1 mg	Yellow	Tablet	Circle, Scored; Flat; Compressed	Par Pharmaceutical
PAR; 225	Haloperidol	2 mg	Pink	Tablet	Circle, Scored; Flat; Compressed	Par Pharmaceutical
PAR; 226	Haloperidol	5 mg	Green	Tablet	Circle, Scored; Flat; Compressed	Par Pharmaceutical
PAR; 227	Haloperidol	10 mg	Aqua	Tablet	Circle, Scored; Flat; Compressed	Par Pharmaceutical
PAR; 240	Temazepam	15 mg	Opaque White and Dark Green	Capsule		Par Pharmaceutical
PAR; 241	Temazepam	30 mg	Opaque White	Capsule		Par Pharmaceutical
PAR; 246	Carisoprodol and Aspirin	325 mg ; 200 mg	White and Light Lavender	Tablet	Circle, Double-Layered	Par Pharmaceutical
PAR; 249	Methocarbamol and Aspirin	325 mg ; 400 mg	White and Pink	Tablet	Circle, Double Layered; Compressed	Par Pharmaceutical
PAR; 258	Metaproterenol Sulfate	10 mg	White	Tablet	Circle, Scored; Compressed	Par Pharmaceutical
PAR; 259	Metaproterenol Sulfate	20 mg	White	Tablet	Circle, Scored; Compressed	Par Pharmaceutical
PAR; 289	Megestrol Acetate	20 mg	White	Tablet	Round, Bisected Scored	Par Pharmaceutical
PAR; 290	Megestrol Acetate	40 mg	White	Tablet	Round, Bisected Scored	Par Pharmaceutical
PAR; 300; 683	Ofloxacin	300 mg	White	Tablet	Capsule-Shape	Par Pharmaceutical
PAR; 400; 684	Ofloxacin	400 mg	White	Tablet	Capsule-Shape	Par Pharmaceutical
PAR; 412	Metoprolol Tartrate	50 mg	Light Pink	Coated Tablet	Circle	Par Pharmaceutical
PAR; 413	Metoprolol Tartrate	100 mg	Light Blue	Coated Tablet	Circle	Par Pharmaceutical
PAR; 444	Captopril	12.5 mg	White	Tablet	Oval	Par Pharmaceutical
PAR; 445	Captopril	25 mg	White	Tablet	Circle	Par Pharmaceutical
PAR; 446	Captopril	50 mg	White	Tablet	Circle	Par Pharmaceutical
PAR; 447	Captopril	100 mg	White	Tablet	Circle	Par Pharmaceutical
PAR; 448 ;	Alprazolam	0.25 mg	Light Yellow	Tablet	Oval, Scored	Par Pharmaceutical
PAR; 449	Alprazolam	0.5 mg	Dark Yellow	Tablet	Oval	Par Pharmaceutical
PAR; 467	Ibuprofen	400 mg	White	Coated Tablet	Capsule-Shape	Par Pharmaceutical
PAR; 468	Ibuprofen	600 mg	White	Coated Tablet	Capsule-Shape	Par Pharmaceutical
PAR; 473	Orphengesic Forte	100 mg ; 60 mg ; 770 mg	Blue and White	Tablet	Capsule-Shape, BI-Layered, Scored	Par Pharmaceutical
PAR; 544	Ranitidine Hydrochloride	150 mg		Tablet		Par Pharmaceutical
PAR; 545	Ranitidine Hydrochloride	300 mg		Tablet		Par Pharmaceutical
PAR; 556	Lisinopril	2.5 mg	White	Tablet	Oval	Par Pharmaceutical
PAR; 557	Lisinopril	5 mg	White	Tablet	Capsule-Shape	Par Pharmaceutical
PAR; 558	Lisinopril	10 mg	White	Tablet	Circle	Par Pharmaceutical
PAR; 559	Lisinopril	20 mg	White	Tablet	Circle	Par Pharmaceutical
PAR; 560	Lisinopril	40 mg	White	Tablet	Circle	Par Pharmaceutical
PAR; 635	Lisinopril	30 mg	White	Tablet	Circle	Par Pharmaceutical

IMPRINT	BRAND/GENERIC NAME	STRENGTH	COLOR	FORM	SHAPE	MANUFACTURER
PAR; 651; 5	Torsemide	5 mg	White	Tablet	Circle, Scored	Par Pharmaceutical
PAR; 652; 10	Torsemide	10 mg	White	Tablet	Circle, Scored	Par Pharmaceutical
PAR; 653; 20	Torsemide	20 mg	White	Tablet	Circle, Scored	Par Pharmaceutical
PAR; 654; 100	Torsemide	100 mg	White	Tablet	Circle, Scored	Par Pharmaceutical
PAR; 701	Clomiphene Citrate	50 mg	White	Tablet	Circle, Scored	Par Pharmaceutical
PAR; 707; 5	Buspirone Hydrochloride	5 mg	Peach	Tablet	Oval	Par Pharmaceutical
PAR; 708; 10	Buspirone Hydrochloride	10 mg	Peach	Tablet	Oval	Par Pharmaceutical
PAR; 721; 555	Buspirone Hydrochloride	15 mg	Peach	Tablet	Rectangle, Scored	Par Pharmaceutical
PAR; 724	Hydroxyurea	500 mg		Capsule		Par Pharmaceutical
PAR; 725; 7.5	Buspirone Hydrochloride	7.5 mg	Peach	Tablet	Oval	Par Pharmaceutical
PAR; 726	Doxycycline Hyclate	50 mg	Buff and White	Capsule		Par Pharmaceutical
PAR; 727	Doxycycline Hyclate	100 mg	Brown and Cream	Capsule		Par Pharmaceutical
PAR; 876	Paroxetine Hydrochloride	10 mg	White	Tablet		Par
PAR; 877	Paroxetine Hydrochloride	20 mg	White	Tablet		Par
PAR; 878	Paroxetine Hydrochloride	30 mg	White	Tablet		Par
PAR; 879	Paroxetine Hydrochloride	40 mg	White	Tablet		Par
PARAFLEX; MCNEIL	Paraflex	250 mg	Orange or Peach	Tablet		Ortho-Mcneil Pharmaceutical
PARAFON FORTE DSC; MCNEIL	Parafon Forte Dsc	500 mg	Light Green	Tablet		Mcneil Pharmaceutical
PARLODEL; 2 1/2 ;	Parlodel	2.5 mg	White	Tablet	Square, Scored	Novartis
PARLODEL; 5 MG; TRIANGLE(S)	Parlodel	5 mg	Caramel and White	Capsule, Liquid Filled		Novartis
PARNATE; SKF	Parnate	10 mg	Rose-Red	Tablet	Circle	Glaxosmithkline
PAXIL CR; 12.5	Paxil Cr	12.5 mg	Yellow	Controlled-Release Tablet	Circle	Glaxosmithkline
PAXIL CR; 25	Paxil Cr	25 mg	Pink	Controlled-Release Tablet	Circle	Glaxosmithkline
PAXIL CR; 37.5	Paxil Cr	37.5 mg	Blue	Controlled-Release Tablet	Circle	Glaxosmithkline
PAXIL; 10	Paxil	10 mg	Yellow	Film-Coated Tablet	Oval	Glaxosmithkline
PAXIL; 20	Paxil	20 mg	Pink	Film-Coated Tablet	Oval	Glaxosmithkline
PAXIL; 30	Paxil	30 mg	Blue	Film-Coated Tablet	Oval	Glaxosmithkline
PAXIL; 40	Paxil	40 mg	Green	Film-Coated Tablet	Oval	Glaxosmithkline
PBA ;	Proglycem	50 mg	Orange and Clear	Capsule		Schering
PCC 0843 VALEANT	Phrenilin with Caffeine and Codeine	40 mg ; 325 mg ; 30 mg ; 50 mg	Opaque Lavender, Opaque White	Capsule		Valeant Pharmaceuticals
PCE; ABBOTT LOGO	Pce Dispertab	333 mg	White with Pink Speckles	Tablet	Oval	Abbott Laboratories
PD 144	Femhrt	1 mg ; 5 mcg	White	Tablet	D-Shape	Warner Chilcott
PD 145	Femhrt	0.5 mg ; 2.5 mcg	White	Tablet	Oval	Warner Chilcott
PD 425	Tilia Fe - White Square Tablet	30 mcg ; 1 mg	White	Tablet	Square	Watson Pharma
PD 427	Tilia Fe - White Triangular Tablet	1 mg ; 20 mcg	White	Tablet	Triangle	Watson Pharma
PD 555	Tilia Fe - White Round Tablet	35 mcg ; 1 mg	White	Tablet	Circle	Watson Pharma
PD 622	Femcon Fe - Brown Tablet	75 mg	Brown	Tablet	Circle	Warner Chilcott
PD DILANTIN 100MG	Dilantin	100 mg	Opaque White, Orange	Capsule, Extended Release		Pfizer Us Pharmaceuticals Group
PD; 220	Accuretic	20 mg ; 12.5 mg	Pink	Coated Tablet	Triangle, Scored	Parke-Davis
PD; 222	Accuretic	10 mg ; 12.5 mg	Pink	Coated Tablet	Elliptical, Scored, Biconvex	Parke-Davis
PD; 223	Accuretic	20 mg ; 25 mg	Pink	Coated Tablet	Circle, Biconvex	Parke-Davis
PD; 352; 200	Rezulin	200 mg	Yellow	Coated Tablet	Oval	Parke-Davis
PD; 353; 400	Rezulin	400 mg	Tan	Coated Tablet	Oval	Parke-Davis
PD; 357; 300	Rezulin	300 mg	White	Coated Tablet	Oval	Parke-Davis
PD; 527; 5	Accupril	5 mg	Brown	Coated Tablet	Circle, Scored	Parke-Davis
PD; 530; 10	Accupril	10 mg	Brown	Coated Tablet	Triangle	Parke-Davis
PD; 532; 20	Accupril	20 mg	Brown	Coated Tablet	Circle	Parke-Davis
PD; 535; 40	Accupril	40 mg	Brown	Coated Tablet	Circle	Parke-Davis
PD; NEURONTIN 100 MG	Neurontin	100 mg	White	Capsule		Parke-Davis
PD; NEURONTIN 300 MG	Neurontin	300 mg	Yellow	Capsule		Parke-Davis
PD; NEURONTIN 400 MG	Neurontin	400 mg	Orange	Capsule		Parke-Davis
PE	Sudafed Pe	10 mg	Red	Tablet	Circle	Johnson & Johnson Consumer Products
PEDIACARE; CC	Pediacare for Ages 6-12 Cough-Cold	1 mg ; 5 mg ; 15 mg	Pink	Tablet, Chewable		Pharmacia & Upjohn
PERCODAN	Percodan	325 mg ; 4.8355 mg	Yellow	Tablet	Circle	Endo Pharmaceuticals
PF; 100 ;	Ms Contin	100 mg	Gray	Tablet, Extended Release	Circle	Purdue Pharmaceutical Products
PF; C275	Cardioquin	275 mg	White	Tablet		Purdue Pharmaceutical Products
PF; M15	Ms Contin	15 mg	Blue	Tablet, Extended Release	Circle	Purdue Pharmaceutical Products
PF; M30	Ms Contin	30 mg	Lavender	Tablet, Extended Release	Circle	Purdue Pharmaceutical Products
PF; M60	Ms Contin	60 mg	Orange	Tablet, Extended Release	Circle	Purdue Pharmaceutical Products
PF; M200	Ms Contin	200 mg	Green	Tablet, Extended Release	Capsule-Shape	Purdue Pharmaceutical Products
PF; MI; 15	Msir	15 mg	White	Tablet	Circle, Scored	Purdue Pharmaceutical Products
PF; MI; 30	Msir	30 mg	White	Tablet	Capsule-Shape, Scored	Purdue Pharmaceutical Products
PF; MSIR; 15; THIS END UP	Msir	15 mg	White and Blue	Capsule		Purdue Pharmaceutical Products
PF; MSIR; 30; THIS END UP	Msir	30 mg	Gray and Lavender	Capsule		Purdue Pharmaceutical Products
PF; T; 500	Trilisate 500 mg	293 mg ; 362 mg	Salmon	Coated Tablet		Purdue Pharmaceutical Products

IMPRINT	BRAND/GENERIC NAME	STRENGTH	COLOR	FORM	SHAPE	MANUFACTURER
PF; T; 750	Trilisate 750 mg	544 mg ; 440 mg	White	Coated Tablet		Purdue Pharmaceutical Products
PF; T; 1000	Trilisate 1000 mg	587 mg ; 725 mg	Red	Coated Tablet		Purdue Pharmaceutical Products
PF; U; 200	Uniphyl	200 mg	White	Controlled-Release Tablet	Circle	Purdue Pharmaceutical Products
PF; U; 400	Uniphyl	400 mg	White	Timed-Release Tablet		Purdue Pharmaceutical Products
PF; U; 600	Uniphyl	600 mg		Extended-Release Tablet		Purdue Pharmaceutical Products
PF; U200	T-Phyl	200 mg	White	Extended-Release Tablet		Purdue Pharmaceutical Products
PFEIFFER	Mycinettes	15 mg ; 2.5 mg	Yellow	Lozenge/troche	Circle	Pfeiffer Pharmaceuticals
PFIZER ; CDT 051	Caduet	5 mg ; 10 mg	White	Tablet		Pfizer
PFIZER ; CDT 052 ;	Caduet	5 mg ; 20 mg	White	Tablet		Pfizer
PFIZER ; CDT 054 ;	Caduet	40 mg ; 5 mg	White	Tablet		Pfizer
PFIZER ; CDT 058 ;	Caduet	5 mg ; 80 mg	White	Tablet		Pfizer
PFIZER ; CDT 101 ;	Caduet	10 mg ; 10 mg	Blue	Tablet		Pfizer
PFIZER ; CDT 102	Caduet	10 mg ; 20 mg	Blue	Tablet		Pfizer
PFIZER ; CDT 104	Caduet	10 mg ; 40 mg	Blue	Tablet		Pfizer
PFIZER ; CDT 108 ;	Caduet	10 mg ; 80 mg	Blue	Tablet		Pfizer
PFIZER ; CDT 251 ;	Caduet	2.5 mg ; 10 mg	White	Tablet		Pfizer
PFIZER ; CDT 252	Caduet	2.5 mg ; 20 mg	White	Tablet		Pfizer
PFIZER ; CDT 254 ;	Caduet	2.5 mg ; 40 mg	White	Tablet		Pfizer
PFIZER ; MVC 300 ;	Selzentry	300 mg	Blue	Tablet	Oval	Pfizer
PFIZER 306	Zithromax	250 mg	Pink	Tablet	Capsule-Shape	Pfizer
PFIZER 432; MINIZIDE	Minizide 2	2 mg ; 0.5 mg	Blue-Green, Pink	Capsule		Pfizer
PFIZER PGN 25	Lyrica	25 mg	White	Capsule		Pfizer
PFIZER PGN 50	Lyrica	50 mg	White	Capsule		Pfizer Us Pharmaceuticals Group
PFIZER PGN 75	Lyrica	75 mg	Orange, White	Capsule		Pfizer Us Pharmaceuticals Group
PFIZER PGN 100	Lyrica	100 mg	Orange	Capsule		Pfizer Us Pharmaceuticals Group
PFIZER PGN 150	Lyrica	150 mg	White	Capsule		Pfizer Us Pharmaceuticals Group
PFIZER PGN 200	Lyrica	200 mg	Light Orange	Capsule		Pfizer
PFIZER PGN 225	Lyrica	225 mg	Light Orange, White	Capsule		Pfizer
PFIZER PGN 300	Lyrica	300 mg	White, Orange	Capsule		Pfizer
PFIZER STN 12.5 MG	Sutent	12.5 mg	Orange	Capsule		Pfizer
PFIZER STN 25 MG	Sutent	25 mg	Caramel, Orange	Capsule		Pfizer
PFIZER STN 50 MG	Sutent	50 mg	Caramel	Capsule		Pfizer
PFIZER; 095; VIBRA ;	Vibramycin	100 mg	Blue	Capsule		Pfizer
PFIZER; 015	Tetracyn	250 mg	Black and White	Capsule		Pfizer
PFIZER; 016	Tetracyn	500 mg	Blue and White	Capsule		Pfizer
PFIZER; 072; TERRAMYCIN	Terramycin	125 mg		Capsule		Pfizer
PFIZER; 073	Terramycin	250 mg	Clear Yellow	Capsule		Pfizer
PFIZER; 073; TERRAMYCIN	Terramycin	250 mg	Yellow	Capsule		Pfizer
PFIZER; 084	Terramycin	250 mg	Yellow	Coated Tablet		Pfizer
PFIZER; 088	Terrastatin	250 mg ; 250000 U	Pink and Yellow	Capsule		Pfizer
PFIZER; 094	Vibramycin Hyclate	50 mg	Blue and White	Capsule		Pfizer
PFIZER; 094; VIBRA	Vibramycin	50 mg	Blue and White	Capsule		Pfizer Laboratories
PFIZER; 095	Vibramycin Hyclate	100 mg	Blue	Capsule		Pfizer
PFIZER; 099; VIBRA-TABS ;	Vibra-Tabs	100 mg		Coated Tablet	Circle	Pfizer
PFIZER; 105	Pfizerpen VK	250 mg	White	Tablet		Pfizer
PFIZER; 106	Pfizerpen VK	500 mg	White	Tablet		Pfizer
PFIZER; 180	Vistrax 5	5 mg ; 25 mg	White	Tablet		Pfizer
PFIZER; 181	Vistrax 10	10 mg ; 25 mg	Black and White	Tablet		Pfizer
PFIZER; 220; SUSTAIRE	Sustaire	100 mg	White	Delayed-Release Tablet		Pfizer
PFIZER; 221; SUSTAIRE ;	Sustaire	300 mg	White	Delayed-Release Tablet		Pfizer
PFIZER; 308	Zithromax	600 mg	White	Coated Tablet	Oval, Modified	Pfizer Laboratories
PFIZER; 335	Sterane	5 mg	White	Tablet	Oval	Pfizer Laboratories
PFIZER; 375	Renese	1 mg	White	Tablet	Circle, Scored	Pfizer
PFIZER; 376	Renese	2 mg	Yellow	Tablet	Circle, Scored	Pfizer
PFIZER; 377	Renese	4 mg	White	Tablet	Circle, Scored	Pfizer
PFIZER; 378	Trovan/zithromax Compliance Pak Trovafloxacin	100 mg	Blue	Coated Tablet	Circle	Pfizer Laboratories
PFIZER; 378	Trovan	100 mg	Blue	Coated Tablet	Circle	Pfizer
PFIZER; 379	Trovan	200 mg	Blue	Coated Tablet	Oval	Pfizer
PFIZER; 396	Geodon	20 mg	Blue and White	Capsule		Pfizer Laboratories
PFIZER; 397	Geodon	40 mg	Blue	Capsule		Pfizer Laboratories
PFIZER; 398	Geodon	60 mg	White	Capsule		Pfizer Laboratories
PFIZER; 399	Geodon	80 mg	Blue and White	Capsule		Pfizer Laboratories
PFIZER; 411	Glucotrol	5 mg	White	Tablet		Pfizer Us Pharmaceuticals Group
PFIZER; 412	Glucotrol	10 mg	White	Tablet	Diamond Shaped, Scored	Pfizer Us Pharmaceuticals Group
PFIZER; 430; MINIZIDE	Minizide 1	1 mg ; 0.5 mg	Blue-Green	Capsule		Pfizer
PFIZER; 431; MINIPRESS	Minipress	1 mg	White	Capsule		Pfizer

IMPRINT	BRAND/GENERIC NAME	STRENGTH	COLOR	FORM	SHAPE	MANUFACTURER
PFIZER; 437; MINIPRESS	Minipress	2 mg	Pink and White	Capsule		Pfizer
PFIZER; 438; MINIPRESS	Minipress	5 mg	Blue and White	Capsule		Pfizer
PFIZER; 441	Moderil	0.25 mg	Yellow	Tablet	Oval, Scored	Pfizer
PFIZER; 442	Moderil	0.5 mg	Salmon; Orange	Tablet	Oval, Scored	Pfizer
PFIZER; 446	Renese-R	2 mg ; 0.25 mg	White	Tablet		Pfizer
PFIZER; 541; VISTARIL ;	Vistaril	25 mg	Dark Green and Light Green	Capsule		Pfizer
PFIZER; 542; VISTARIL ;	Vistaril	50 mg	Dark Green and White	Capsule		Pfizer
PFIZER; 543; VISTARIL ;	Vistaril	50 mg	Dark Green and Pink	Capsule		Pfizer
PFIZER; 550	Zyrtec	5 mg	White	Tablet	Rectangle	Pfizer Us Pharmaceuticals Group
PFIZER; 551 ;	Zyrtec	10 mg	White	Tablet	Rectangle	Pfizer Us Pharmaceuticals Group
PFIZER; NSR; 25 ;	Inspra	25 mg	Yellow	Tablet	Diamond	Pfizer
PFIZER; NSR; 50 ;	Inspra	50 mg	Pink	Tablet	Diamond	Pfizer
PFIZER; TKN; 125	Tikosyn	125 mcg	Light Orange and White	Capsule		Pfizer Laboratories
PFIZER; TKN; 250	Tikosyn	250 mcg	Peach	Capsule		Pfizer Laboratories
PFIZER; TKN; 500	Tikosyn	500 mcg	Peach and White	Capsule		Pfizer Laboratories
PFIZER;VOR50	Vfend	50 mg	White	Coated Tablet	Circle	Pfizer Laboratories
PFIZER;VOR200	Vfend	200 mg	White	Coated Tablet	Capsule-Shape	Pfizer Laboratories
PG; 11	Helidac Therapy: Part I	262.4 mg	Pink	Tablet, Chewable	Circle	Procter & Gamble Pharmaceuticals
PG; 12	Helidac Therapy: Part III	500 mg	Pale Orange and White	Capsule		Procter & Gamble Pharmaceuticals
PHILLIPS	Phillips' Gelcaps	90 mg ; 83 mg	White	Capsule, Liquid Filled		Bayer Consumer Care
PIROXICAM; EGIS; 111	Piroxicam	10 mg	Blue and Red	Capsule		Ranbaxy Pharmaceuticals
PIROXICAM; EGIS; 112	Piroxicam	20 mg	Red	Capsule		Ranbaxy Pharmaceuticals
PK	Kaletra	133.3 mg ; 33.3 mg	Orange	Capsule		Abbott Laboratories
PL 500	Amoxicillin/clavulanate Potassium	500 mg ; 125 mg	White	Tablet	Oval	Par Pharmaceutical
PL 875	Amoxicillin/clavulanate Potassium	875 mg ; 125 mg	White	Tablet	Capsule-Shape	Par Pharmaceutical
PL AT8	Amoxicillin	875 mg	Pink	Tablet	Capsule-Shape	Par Pharmaceutical
PL C40	Amoxicillin/clavulanate Potassium	400 mg ; 57 mg	Mottled Pink	Tablet, Chewable	Circle	Par Pharmaceutical
PL CT4	Amoxicillin	400 mg	Pale Pink	Tablet, Chewable	Circle	Par Pharmaceutical
PL; AT8	Amoxicillin	875 mg	Pink	Tablet	Capsule-Shape	Ivax Pharmaceuticals
PLACIDYL; 500	Placidyl	500 mg	Red	Capsule, Liquid Filled		Abbott Laboratories
PLACIDYL; 750	Placidyl	750 mg	Green	Capsule, Liquid Filled		Abbott Laboratories
PLAQUENIL	Hydroxychloroquine Sulfate	200 mg	White with Black Ink	Tablet	Oval	Sanofi-Aventis U.S.
PLAQUENIL; P62	Plaquenil	200 mg	White	Tablet	Capsule-Shape	Sanofi-Aventis U.S.
PLEGINE; 35	Plegine	35 mg		Tablet		Wyeth Pharmaceuticals
PLENDIL; 450	Plendil	2.5 mg	Sage Green	Tablet, Extended Release	Circle	Astrazeneca
PLENDIL; 451	Plendil	5 mg	Red-Brown	Tablet, Extended Release	Circle	Astrazeneca
PLENDIL; 452	Plendil	10 mg	Red-Brown	Tablet, Extended Release	Circle	Astrazeneca
PLETAL; 50	Pletal	50 mg	White	Tablet	Triangle	Otsuka America Pharmaceutical
PLETAL; 100	Pletal	100 mg	White	Tablet	Circle	Otsuka America Pharmaceutical
PLIVA 563 ;	Cyclobenzaprine Hydrochloride	10 mg	Yellow	Tablet	Circle	Teva Pharmaceuticals
PLIVA 648 ;	Fluoxetine Hydrochloride	20 mg	Green Band, White Opaque	Capsule		Barr Laboratories
PN	Optinate - Prenatal Vitamin Tablet	10 IU ; 120 mg ; 3 mg ; 3.4 mg ; 20 mg ; 12 mcg ; 20 mg ; 30 mg ; 50 mg ; 90 mg ; 30 mcg ; 6 mg ; 200 mg ; 2 mg ; 15 mg ; 1 mg ; 400 IU	White	Tablet	Oval	First Horizon Pharmaceutical
PN; SANOFI	Prenatal Vitamin Ultra	400 IU ; 30 IU ; 20 mg ; 50 mg ; 120 mg ; 3 mg ; 3.4 mg ; 20 mg ; 12 mcg ; 90 mg ; 0.15 mg ; 250 mg ; 2 mg ; 25 mg ; 1 mg ; 4000 IU	Beige	Coated Tablet	Egg-Shape	Sanofi Pharmaceuticals
PP; 551	Metizol	250 mg	White	Tablet	Circle	Glenwood
PP; 1304	Pseudo-Chlor SR	120 mg ; 8 mg	Blue and Clear	Sustained-Release Capsule		Novartis Generics
PPP; 784; DURICEF; 500 MG	Duricef	500 mg	Maroon and Whtie	Capsule		Bristol-Myers Squibb
PPP; 785	Duricef	1 GM	White to Off White	Tablet	Oval	Bristol-Myers Squibb
PR 10 ; G	Pravastatin Sodium	10 mg	Whiteto Off-White	Tablet	Ovoid-Rectangular	Par Pharmaceutical
PR 20 ; G	Pravastatin Sodium	20 mg	Whiteto Off-White	Tablet	Ovoid-Rectangular	Par Pharmaceutical
PR 40 ; G	Pravastatin Sodium	40 mg	Whiteto Off-White	Tablet	Ovoid-Rectangular	Par Pharmaceutical
PR 80 ; G	Pravastatin Sodium	80 mg	White to Off-White	Tablet	Oval	Mylan Pharmaceuticals
PRAVACHOL 40 P ;	Pravachol	40 mg	Green	Tablet	Rectangle	Bristol-Myers Squibb
PRAVACHOL; 10; P ;	Pravachol	10 mg	Pale Pink or Peach	Tablet	Rectangle, Biconvex, Rounded	Bristol-Myers Squibb
PRAVACHOL; 20; P ;	Pravachol	20 mg	Yellow	Tablet	Rectangle, Rounded, Biconvex	Bristol-Myers Squibb
PRECOSE; 25	Precose	25 mg	White	Tablet	Circle	Bayer Pharmaceutical
PRECOSE; 50	Precose	50 mg	White to Yellow	Tablet		Bayer Pharmaceutical
PRECOSE; 100	Precose	100 mg	White to Yellow	Tablet		Bayer Pharmaceutical

IMPRINT	BRAND/GENERIC NAME	STRENGTH	COLOR	FORM	SHAPE	MANUFACTURER
PREMARIN 0.3	Premarin	0.3 mg	Green	Tablet	Oval	Wyeth Pharmaceuticals
PREMARIN 0.45	Premarin	0.45 mg	Blue	Tablet	Oval	Wyeth Pharmaceuticals
PREMARIN 0.625	Premarin	0.625 mg	Maroon	Tablet	Oval	Wyeth Pharmaceuticals
PREMARIN 0.9	Premarin	0.9 mg	White	Tablet	Oval	Wyeth Pharmaceuticals
PREMARIN 1.25	Premarin	1.25 mg	Yellow	Tablet	Oval	Wyeth Pharmaceuticals
PREMPRO	Premphase Conjugated Estrogens and Medroxyprogesterone	0.625 mg ; 5 mg	Light-Blue	Coated Tablet	Oval	Wyeth Pharmaceuticals
PREMPRO	Prempro Single Tablet	2.5 mg ; 0.625 mg	Peach	Tablet	Oval	Wyeth Pharmaceuticals
PRENATE DHA	Prenate Dha	27 mg ; 50 mg ; 300 mg ; Less Than or Equal TO 50 mg ; 85 mg ; 200 IU ; 10 IU ; 25 mg ; 1 mg ; 12 mcg ; 150 mg	Opaque Blue-Green	Capsule, Liquid Filled		Sciele Pharma
PRENATE; ADVANCE	Prenate Advance	50 mg ; 90 mg ; 200 mg ; 2 mg ; 25 mg ; 1 mg ; 400 IU ; 30 IU ; 120 mg ; 3 mg ; 3.4 mg ; 20 mg ; 2 mcg ; 20 mg ; 30 mg	White	Tablet	Oval	First Horizon Pharmaceutical
PRILOSEC; 10; 606	Prilosec	10 mg	Apricot and Amethyst	Enteric-Coated Tablet		Astrazeneca
PRILOSEC; 20; 742	Prilosec	20 mg	Amethyst	Timed-Release Capsule		Astrazeneca
PRINZIDE ; MSD 142	Prinzide	20 mg ; 25 mg	Peach	Tablet	Circle	Merck & Company
PRO DM	Protuss DM	600 mg ; 60 mg ; 30 mg	White	Sustained-Release Tablet	Film-Coated, Scored	First Horizon Pharmaceutical
PROCANBID; 500	Procanbid	500 mg	White	Tablet, Extended Release	Circle	Monarch Pharmaceuticals
PROCANBID; 1000	Procanbid	1000 mg	Gray	Tablet, Extended Release	Circle	Monarch Pharmaceuticals
PROCARDIA 20; PFIZER 261	Procardia	20 mg	Orange and Light Brown	Capsule, Liquid Filled		Pfizer Laboratories
PROCARDIA XL; 30	Procardia XL	30 mg	Rose Pink	Extended-Release Tablet	Circle, Biconvex	Pfizer Laboratories
PROCARDIA XL; 60	Procardia XL	60 mg	Rose Pink	Extended-Release Tablet	Circle, Biconvex	Pfizer Laboratories
PROCARDIA XL; 90	Procardia XL	90 mg	Rose Pink	Extended-Release Tablet	Circle, Biconvex	Pfizer Laboratories
PROCARDIA; PFIZER 260	Procardia	10 mg	Orange	Capsule, Liquid Filled		Pfizer Laboratories
PROLOPRIM 09A	Proloprim	100 mg	White	Tablet	Circle	Monarch Pharmaceuticals
PROPACET	Propacet 100	650 mg ; 100 mg	White	Coated Tablet	Oblong, Convex	Teva Pharmaceuticals
PROPACET; 100; LEMMON	Propacet	650 mg ; 100 mg	White	Coated Tablet	Oblong	Teva Pharmaceuticals
PROPECIA; P	Propecia	1 mg	Tan	Coated Tablet	Eight-Sided, Convex	Merck & Company
PROSED/DS	Prosed DS	81.6 mg ; 36.2 mg ; 10.8 mg ; 9 mg ; 0.12 mg	Dark Blue	Tablet	Circle	Ferring Pharmaceuticals
PROSTIGMIN; 15; ICN	Prostigmin	15 mg	White	Tablet	Flat, Bevel-Edged	Valeant Pharmaceuticals
PROTONIX	Pantoprazole Sodium	40 mg	Yellow	Tablet, Delayed Release	Oval	Wyeth Pharmaceuticals
PROTONIX	Protonix	40 mg	Yellow	Tablet, Delayed Release	Oval	Wyeth Pharmaceuticals
PROTOPAM; 500	Protopam	500 mg	White	Tablet	Circle	Wyeth Pharmaceuticals
PROVENTIL; 2; 252	Proventil	2 mg	White	Tablet	Circle	Schering
PROVENTIL; 4; 573	Proventil	4 mg	White	Tablet	Circle, Scored, Compressed	Schering
PROVERA 2.5	Provera	2.5 mg	Orange	Tablet	Circle	Pharmacia & Upjohn
PROVERA; 5	Provera	5 mg	White	Tablet	Six-Sided, Scored	Pharmacia & Upjohn
PROVERA; 10	Provera	10 mg	White	Tablet	Circle	Pharmacia & Upjohn
PROVIGIL; 100 MG	Provigil	100 mg	White	Tablet	Capsule-Shape	Cephalon
PROVIGIL; 200 MG	Provigil	200 mg	White	Tablet	Capsule-Shape, Scored	Cephalon
PROZAC; 10	Prozac	10 mg	Green	Tablet	Elliptical-Shaped, Scored	Eli Lilly
PS; 20	Periostat	20 mg	White	Tablet		Galderma
PU; 700	Dostinex	0.5 mg	White	Tablet	Capsule-Shape	Pharmacia & Upjohn
PURDUE	Dhc Plus	16 mg ; 256.4 mg ; 30 mg	Light Aqua and Bluish-Green	Capsule		Purdue Pharmaceutical Products
PURINETHOL 04A	Purinethol	50 mg	Pale Yellow to Buff	Tablet		Gate Pharmaceuticals
P-XL; 12 MG	Palladone	12 mg	Cinnamon	Extended-Release Capsule		Purdue Pharma
P-XL; 16 MG	Palladone	16 mg	Pink	Extended-Release Capsule		Purdue Pharma
P-XL; 24 MG	Palladone	24 mg	Blue	Extended-Release Capsule		Purdue Pharma
P-XL; 32 MG	Palladone	32 mg	White	Extended-Release Capsule		Purdue Pharma
QUARZAN; 2.5; ROCHE	Quarzan	2.5 mg	Green and Red Opaque	Capsule		Roche Products
QUARZAN; 5; ROCHE	Quarzan	5 mg	Green and Grey Opaque	Capsule		Roche Products
QUINIDEX; AHR	Quinidex Extentabs	300 mg	White	Extended-Release Tablet		Wyeth Consumer Healthcare
R ; 027 ;	Alprazolam	0.25 mg	White	Tablet	Circle	Actavis Elizabeth
R ; 029 ;	Alprazolam	0.5 mg	Peach	Tablet	Circle	Actavis Elizabeth
R ; 031 ;	Alprazolam	1 mg	Blue	Tablet	Circle	Actavis Elizabeth
R ; 83	Alprazolam	0.5 mg	White to Off-White	Tablet, Extended Release	Circle	Actavis Elizabeth
R ; 128 ;	Clonidine Hydrochloride	0.2 mg	Orange	Tablet	Circle	Actavis Elizabeth
R ; 129	Clonidine Hydrochloride	0.3 mg	Orange	Tablet	Circle	Actavis Elizabeth
R ; 538 ;	Carbidopa and Levodopa	10 mg ; 100 mg	Mottled Dark Blue	Tablet	Circle	Actavis Elizabeth
R ; 539 ;	Carbidopa and Levodopa	25 mg ; 100 mg	Mottled Yellow	Tablet	Circle	Actavis Elizabeth
R ; M	Risperidone	0.25 mg	White	Tablet	Circle	Mylan Pharmaceuticals
R 039 ;	Alprazolam	2 mg	Yellow	Tablet	Rectangle	Actavis Elizabeth
R 58 ; 4	Acetaminophen/codeine	300 mg ; 60 mg	White to Off White	Tablet	Circle	Actavis Elizabeth
R 127 ;	Clonidine Hydrochloride	0.1 mg	Orange	Tablet	Circle	Actavis Elizabeth
R 179	Tizanidine Hydrochloride	2 mg	White to Off White	Tablet	Oval	Par Pharmaceutical

IMPRINT	BRAND/GENERIC NAME	STRENGTH	COLOR	FORM	SHAPE	MANUFACTURER
R 180	Tizanidine Hydrochloride	4 mg	White to Off White	Tablet		Par Pharmaceutical
R 636 ;	Gabapentin	600 mg	Light Green	Tablet	Capsule-Shape	Actavis Elizabeth
R 637	Gabapentin	800 mg	Light Gray	Tablet	Capsule-Shape	Actavis Elizabeth
R 665 ;	Gabapentin	100 mg	Light Brown, White	Capsule		Actavis Elizabeth
R 666 ;	Gabapentin	300 mg	Light Brown, Yellow	Capsule		Actavis Elizabeth
R 667	Gabapentin	400 mg	Light Brown, Orange	Capsule		Actavis Elizabeth
R 728	Metformin Hydrochloride	750 mg	Light Orange	Tablet, Extended Release	Capsule-Shape	Actavis Elizabeth
R 751 ;	Glyburide/metformin Hydrochloride	1.25 mg ; 250 mg	White to Off-White	Tablet	Capsule-Shape	Actavis Elizabeth
R 752	Glyburide/metformin Hydrochloride	2.5 mg ; 500 mg	Yellow	Tablet	Capsule-Shape	Actavis Elizabeth
R 753	Glyburide/metformin Hydrochloride	5 mg ; 500 mg	Blue	Tablet	Capsule-Shape	Actavis Elizabeth
R 756	Citalopram Hydrobromide	20 mg	Pink	Tablet	Capsule-Shape	Actavis Elizabeth
R 757	Citalopram Hydrobromide	40 mg	White to Off-White	Tablet	Capsule-Shape	Actavis Elizabeth
R 2577	Diltiazem Hydrochloride - Once-A-Day Dosage	180 mg	Aqua Blue, Dark Green Opaque	Capsule, Extended Release		Actavis Elizabeth
R 2578	Diltiazem Hydrochloride - Once-A-Day Dosage	240 mg	Dark Green Opaque	Capsule, Extended Release		Actavis Elizabeth
R 2579	Diltiazem Hydrochloride - Once-A-Day Dosage	300 mg	Dark Green Opaque, Light Gray	Capsule, Extended Release		Actavis Elizabeth
R 2588	Diltiazem Hydrochloride - Once-A-Day Dosage	120 mg	Light Gray Opaque	Capsule, Extended Release		Actavis Elizabeth
R 2694	Ramipril	1.25 mg	White	Capsule		Actavis Elizabeth
R 2695	Ramipril	2.5 mg	Yellow Opaque	Capsule		Actavis Elizabeth
R 2696	Ramipril	5 mg	Light Brown	Capsule		Actavis Elizabeth
R 2697	Ramipril	10 mg	Gray	Capsule		Actavis Elizabeth
R 2778	Propranolol Hydrochloride	60 mg	White Opaque, Yellow Opaque	Capsule, Extended Release		Actavis Elizabeth
R 2779	Propranolol Hydrochloride	80 mg	Yellow Opaque	Capsule, Extended Release		Actavis Elizabeth
R 2781	Propranolol Hydrochloride	160 mg	Gray Opaque	Capsule, Extended Release		Actavis Elizabeth
R; 023	Aspirin/butalbital/caffeine	50 mg ; 325 mg ; 40 mg	White	Tablet	Circle	Actavis Elizabeth
R; 026	Phenobarbital	15 mg	White	Tablet	Circle	Actavis Elizabeth
R; 028	Phenobarbital	30 mg	White	Tablet	Circle	Actavis Elizabeth
R; 063	Lorazepam	2 mg	White	Tablet		Actavis Elizabeth
R; 076	Temazepam	15 mg	Green and White	Capsule		Actavis Elizabeth
R; 077	Temazepam	30 mg	White	Capsule		Actavis Elizabeth
R; 8	Lozol	2.5 mg	White	Coated Tablet	Eight-Sided	Aventis Pharmaceuticals
R; 33	Clonazepam	0.5 mg	Pink	Tablet	Circle	Actavis Elizabeth
R; 34	Clonazepam	1 mg	Yellow	Tablet	Circle	Actavis Elizabeth
R; 35	Clonazepam	2 mg	White	Tablet	Circle	Actavis Elizabeth
R; 57	Lorazepam	0.5 mg	White	Tablet	Circle	Actavis Elizabeth
R; 59	Lorazepam	1 mg	White	Tablet	Circle	Actavis Elizabeth
R; 121	Pramilet FA	0.15 mg ; 0.085 mg ; 60 mg ; 3 ; 2 mg ; 3 mg ; 3 mcg ; 40 mg ; 4000 IU ; 400 IU ; 1 mg ; 10 mg ; 1 mg ; 250 mg ; 100 mcg ; 10 mg		Coated Tablet		Ross Products
R; 143	Carbamazepine	200 mg	White	Tablet	Circle	Actavis Elizabeth
R; 221	Hydrochlorothiazide	25 mg	Peach	Tablet		Actavis Elizabeth
R; 222	Hydrochlorothiazide	50 mg	Peach	Tablet		Actavis Elizabeth
R; 224; 2.5	Minoxidil	2.5 mg	White	Tablet	Circle, Scored	Watson Laboratories
R; 225; 10	Minoxidal	10 mg	White	Tablet	Circle, Scored	Watson Laboratories
R; 229; 0.5	Haloperidol	0.5 mg	White	Tablet	Circle	Watson Laboratories
R; 230; 1	Haloperidol	1 mg	Yellow	Tablet	Circle	Watson Laboratories
R; 231; 2	Haloperidol	2 mg	Purple	Tablet	Circle	Watson Laboratories
R; 232; 5	Haloperidol	5 mg	Green	Tablet	Circle	Watson Laboratories
R; 233; 10	Haloperidol	10 mg	Green-Blue	Tablet	Circle	Watson Laboratories
R; 234; 20	Haloperidol	20 mg	Salmon	Tablet	Circle	Watson Laboratories
R; 269	Metoclopramide	10 mg	White	Tablet	Circle	Actavis Elizabeth
R; 316	Phentermine Hydrochloride	37.5 mg	White	Tablet	Capsule-Shape	Alpharma
R; 348	Propylthiouracil	50 mg	White	Tablet	Circle	Actavis Elizabeth
R; 439	Trazodone Hydrochloride	50 mg	White	Tablet	Circle	Actavis Elizabeth
R; 497	Nifedipine	10 mg	Yellow	Capsule, Liquid Filled		Actavis Elizabeth
R; 530	Nifedipine	20 mg	Red-Brown	Capsule, Liquid Filled		Actavis Elizabeth
R; 550	Diclofenac Sodium DR	50 mg	White	Tablet, Enteric Coated	Circle	Actavis Elizabeth
R; 551	Diclofenac Sodium DR	75 mg	White	Tablet, Enteric Coated	Circle	Actavis Elizabeth
R; 571	Indapamide	2.5 mg	White	Tablet	Circle	Actavis Elizabeth
R; 597	Indapamide	1.25 mg	Orange	Tablet	Circle	Actavis Elizabeth
R; 599	Etodolac	400 mg	Light Gray	Tablet	Egg-Shape	Actavis Elizabeth
R; 605	Acyclovir	200 mg	Green	Capsule		Actavis Elizabeth
R; 606	Acyclovir	400 mg	White	Tablet	Circle	Actavis Elizabeth
R; 607	Acyclovir	800 mg	Pastel Green	Tablet	Oval	Actavis Elizabeth
R; 611	Pentoxifylline	400 mg	Yellow	Tablet, Extended Release	Oblong	Actavis Elizabeth
R; 620	Isosorbide Mononitrate	20 mg	Blue	Tablet	Circle	Actavis Elizabeth
R; 631	Isosorbide Mononitrate	10 mg	Blue	Tablet	Circle	Actavis Elizabeth
R; 632	Etodolac	500 mg	White	Tablet	Egg-Shape	Actavis Elizabeth
R; 642	Doxazosin Mesylate	1 mg	White	Tablet	Circle	Actavis Elizabeth
R; 643	Doxazosin Mesylate	2 mg	White	Tablet	Capsule-Shape	Actavis Elizabeth
R; 644	Doxazosin Mesylate	4 mg	White	Tablet	Capsule-Shape	Actavis Elizabeth
R; 645	Doxazosin Mesylate	8 mg	White	Tablet	Circle	Actavis Elizabeth
R; 672	Spironolactone	50 mg	White	Tablet	Oval	Actavis Elizabeth

IMPRINT	BRAND/GENERIC NAME	STRENGTH	COLOR	FORM	SHAPE	MANUFACTURER
R; 673	Spironolactone	100 mg	White	Tablet	Circle	Actavis Elizabeth
R; 714	Tramadol Hydrochloride	50 mg	White	Tablet	Oval	Actavis Elizabeth
R; 717	Diclofenac Sodium	100 mg	Yellow	Tablet, Extended Release	Circle	Actavis Elizabeth
R; 747	Pentoxifylline	400 mg	Yellow	Tablet, Extended Release	Capsule-Shape	Actavis Elizabeth
R; 4374	Propoxyphene with Aspirin and Caffeine	32.4 mg ; 65 mg ; 389 mg		Capsule		Teva Pharmaceuticals
R; 4956	Triamterene and Hydrochlorothiazide	75 mg ; 50 mg	Yellow	Tablet		Watson Laboratories
R; 7621	VI-Daylin/f Multivitamin Plus Iron Chewable Tablet	60 mg ; 0.3 mg ; 1.05 mg ; 1.2 mg ; 1.05 mg ; 4.5 mcg ; 13.5 mg ; 12 mg ; 1 mg ; 2500 IU ; 400 IU ; 15 IU		Tablet, Chewable		Ross Products
R; 7626	VI-Daylin/f Multivitamin Chewable Tablet	1.05 mg ; 4.5 mg ; 1 mg ; 2500 IU ; 400 IU ; 15 IU ; 0.3 mg ; 1.05 mg ; 1.2 mg ; 13.5 mg ; 60 mg		Tablet, Chewable		Ross Products
R0.5 ;	Risperdal M-Tab	0.5 mg	Light Coral	Tablet, Disintegrating	Circle	Janssen Pharmaceutica Products
R1 ;	Risperdal M-Tab	1 mg	Light Coral	Tablet, Disintegrating	Square	Janssen Pharmaceutica Products
R2 ;	Risperdal M-Tab	2 mg	Coral	Tablet, Disintegrating	Square	Janssen Pharmaceutica Products
R3 ;	Risperdal M-Tab	3 mg	Coral	Tablet, Disintegrating	Circle	Janssen Pharmaceutica Products
R4 ;	Risperdal M-Tab	4 mg	Coral	Tablet, Disintegrating	Circle	Janssen Pharmaceutica Products
R5 ; M	Risperidone	0.5 mg	Beige	Tablet	Circle	Mylan Pharmaceuticals
R11 ; M	Risperidone	1 mg	White	Tablet	Circle	Mylan Pharmaceuticals
R12 ; M	Risperidone	2 mg	Beige	Tablet	Circle	Mylan Pharmaceuticals
R13 ; M	Risperidone	3 mg	White	Tablet	Circle	Mylan Pharmaceuticals
R14 ; M	Risperidone	4 mg	Beige	Tablet	Circle	Mylan Pharmaceuticals
R2780	Propranolol Hydrochloride	120 mg	Gray Opaque, Yellow Opaque	Capsule, Extended Release		Actavis Elizabeth
RAPAMUNE 1 MG	Rapamune	1 mg	White	Tablet	Triangle	Wyeth Pharmaceuticals
RAPAMUNE 2 MG	Rapamune	2 mg	Yellow to Beige	Tablet	Triangle	Wyeth Pharmaceuticals
RB 81 ;	Zolpidem Tartrate	5 mg	Pink	Tablet	Capsule-Shape	Ranbaxy Pharmaceuticals
RB 82 ;	Zolpidem Tartrate	10 mg	White to Off-White	Tablet	Capsule-Shape	Ranbaxy Pharmaceuticals
RB41	Cefprozil	250 mg	White to Off-White	Tablet	Oval	Ranbaxy Pharmaceuticals
RB42	Cefprozil	500 mg	White to Off-White	Tablet	Oval	Ranbaxy Pharmaceuticals
RC; 80	Panixine Disperdose	125 mg	Light Yellow	Tablet	Capsule-Shape, Scored	Ranbaxy Pharmaceuticals
RC; 81	Panixine Disperdose	250 mg	Light Yellow	Tablet	Capsule-Shape, Scored	Ranbaxy Pharmaceuticals
RC41 ;	Pravastatin Sodium	10 mg	Dark Yellow to Yellow	Tablet	Circle	Ranbaxy Pharmaceuticals
RC59 ;	Glimepiride	8 mg	Blue	Tablet	Capsule-Shape	Ranbaxy Pharmaceuticals
RD; 12	Nephro-Vite RX Vitamin B Complex and C Supplement	60 mcg ; 1.7 mg ; 60 mg ; 1 mg ; 300 mcg ; 20 mg ; 10 mg ; 10 mg ; 1.5 mg	Yellow	Tablet	Circle	Watson Laboratories
RE 72	Hydrochlorothiazide	12.5 mg	Light Orange	Tablet	Circle	Ranbaxy Pharmaceuticals
RE 73 ;	Hydrochlorothiazide	25 mg	Light Orange	Tablet	Circle	Ranbaxy Pharmaceuticals
RE 74 ;	Hydrochlorothiazide	50 mg	Light Orange	Tablet	Circle	Ranbaxy Pharmaceuticals
RE16	Sertraline Hydrochloride	25 mg	White	Tablet	Capsule-Shape	Ranbaxy Pharmaceuticals
RE20	Atenolol	50 mg	White to Off-White	Tablet	Circle	Ranbaxy Pharmaceuticals
RE21	Atenolol	100 mg	White to Off-White	Tablet	Circle	Ranbaxy Pharmaceuticals
REBETOL; 200 MG; SCHERING LOGO	Rebetol	200 mg	White	Capsule		Schering
REDUX	Redux	15 mg	Opaque White	Capsule		Wyeth-Ayerst Laboratories
REGLAN; 5; SP ;	Reglan	5 mg	Green	Tablet	Circle	UCB Pharma
REGLAN; SP; 10 ;	Reglan	10 mg	Pink	Tablet	Capsule-Shape	UCB Pharma
REL900 ;	Lovaza	1 GM	Light Yellow	Capsule, Liquid Filled		Reliant Pharmaceuticals
RELAFEN 500	Relafen	500 mg	White	Tablet	Oval	Glaxosmithkline
RELAFEN 750	Relafen	750 mg	Beige	Tablet	Oval	Glaxosmithkline
RENAGEL; 400	Renagel	400 mg	White	Coated Tablet	Oval	Genzyme
RENAGEL; 800	Renagel	800 mg	White	Coated Tablet	Oval	Genzyme
RENVELA 800	Renvela	800 mg	White	Tablet	Oval	Genzyme
REP; 20; PFIZER	Relpax	20 mg	Orange	Tablet	Circle	Pfizer Laboratories
REP; 40; PFIZER	Relpax	40 mg	Orange	Tablet	Circle	Pfizer Us Pharmaceuticals Group
RESCRIPTOR; 200 MG	Rescriptor	200 mg	White	Tablet	Capsule-Shape	Agouron Pharmaceuticals
REV 5 MG	Revlimid	5 mg	White Opaque	Capsule		Celgene
REV 10 MG	Revlimid	10 mg	Blue/green, Pale Yellow	Capsule		Celgene
REV 15 MG	Revlimid	15 mg	Powder Blue, White Opaque	Capsule		Celgene
REV 25 MG	Revlimid	25 mg	White Opaque	Capsule		Celgene
RG; F50	Fluconazole	50 mg	White or Almost White	Tablet	Rounded Rectangle	Barr Laboratories
RG; F100	Fluconazole	100 mg	White or Almost White	Tablet	Rounded Rectangle	Barr Laboratories
RG; F150	Fluconazole	150 mg	White or Almost White	Tablet	Oblong, Convex	Barr Laboratories
RG; F200	Fluconazole	200 mg	White or Almost White	Tablet	Rounded Rectangle	Barr Laboratories
RIB; 200; ROCHE	Copegus	200 mg	Light Pink	Tablet	Oval	Roche Laboratories

IMPRINT	BRAND/GENERIC NAME	STRENGTH	COLOR	FORM	SHAPE	MANUFACTURER
RIBA 200	Ribasphere	200 mg	White Opaque	Capsule		Par Pharmaceutical
RIFADIN; 150 ;	Rifadin	150 mg	Maroon and Scarlet	Capsule		Sanofi-Aventis U.S.
RIFADIN; 300 ;	Rifadin	300 mg	Maroon and Scarlet	Capsule		Sanofi-Aventis U.S.
RIFAMATE	Rifamate	300 mg ; 150 mg	Red	Capsule		Sanofi-Aventis U.S.
RIFATER	Rifater	50 mg ; 300 mg ; 120 mg	Light Beige	Tablet	Circle	Sanofi-Aventis U.S.
RIKER; 125; PLUS	Theolair-Plus	125 mg ; 100 mg		Tablet	Circle	3M Pharmaceuticals
RIKER; 161	Disipal	50 mg	Green	Tablet	Circle	3M Pharmaceuticals
RIKER; 193	Estomul-M	500 mg ; 45 mg	Pink	Tablet	Capsule-Shape	3M Pharmaceuticals
RIKER; 250; PLUS	Theolair-Plus	250 mg ; 200 mg		Tablet		3M Pharmaceuticals
RIKER; 265	Rauwiloid	2 mg	Brown	Tablet	Circle	3M Pharmaceuticals
RIKER; TEPANIL	Tepanil	25 mg	White	Tablet		3M Pharmaceuticals
RIKER; TEPANIL; TEN-TAB	Tepanil Ten-Tab	75 mg	White	Timed-Release Tablet		3M Pharmaceuticals
RL	Marinol	2.5 mg	White	Capsule, Liquid Filled	Circle	Roxane Laboratories
RL	Marinol	5 mg	Dark Brown	Capsule, Liquid Filled	Circle	Roxane Laboratories
RL	Marinol	10 mg	Orange	Capsule, Liquid Filled	Circle	Roxane Laboratories
RLI 54 698	Zonisamide	50 mg	Gray, White Opaque	Capsule		Roxane Laboratories
RLI 54 889	Zonisamide	100 mg	Gray Opaque, Red	Capsule		Roxane Laboratories
RLI 54 944	Zonisamide	25 mg	White, White Opaque	Capsule		Roxane Laboratories
RO; L3	Boniva	2.5 mg	White	Tablet	Oblong	Roche Laboratories
ROBAXIN; 500; SP	Robaxin	500 mg	Light Orange	Coated Tablet	Circle	Schwarz Pharma
ROBAXIN; 750; SP	Robaxin-750	750 mg	Orange	Coated Tablet	Capsule-Shape	Schwarz Pharma
ROBITAB; 8217	Robicillin VK	250 mg	White	Tablet	Circle, Scored	Wyeth Consumer Healthcare
ROBITAB; 8227	Robicillin VK	500 mg	White	Tablet	Circle, Scored	Wyeth Consumer Healthcare
ROBITAB; 8317	Robimycin	250 mg	Green	Enteric-Coated Tablet		Wyeth Consumer Healthcare
ROCHE 0245	Invirase	200 mg	Green Opaque, Light Brown	Capsule		Roche Laboratories
ROCHE 30 MG	Tamiflu	30 mg	Light Yellow	Capsule		Roche Laboratories
ROCHE 45 MG	Tamiflu	45 mg	Grey	Capsule		Roche Laboratories
ROCHE 75 MG	Tamiflu	75 mg	Grey, Light Yellow	Capsule		Roche Laboratories
ROCHE SQV 500	Invirase	500 mg	Light Orange to Greyish or Brownish Orange	Tablet	Oval	Roche Laboratories
ROCHE; 05; KLONOPIN	Klonopin	0.5 mg	Orange	Tablet	Circle, K-Shaped Perforation	Roche Pharmaceuticals
ROCHE; 0246	Fortovase	200 mg	Opaque Beige	Capsule, Liquid Filled		Roche Laboratories
ROCHE; 1; KLONOPIN	Klonopin	1 mg	Blue	Tablet	Circle, K-Shaped Perforation	Roche Pharmaceuticals
ROCHE; 2; KLONOPIN	Klonopin	2 mg	White	Tablet	Circle, K-Shaped Perforation	Roche Pharmaceuticals
ROCHE; 16	Noludar	50 mg	White	Tablet		Roche Laboratories
ROCHE; 17	Noludar	200 mg	White	Tablet		Roche Laboratories
ROCHE; 19	Noludar	50 mg	Purple and White	Capsule		Roche Laboratories
ROCHE; 136	Valcaps	2 mg	Blue and White	Capsule		Roche Pharmaceuticals
ROCHE; 137	Valcaps	5 mg	Blue and Yellow	Capsule		Roche Pharmaceuticals
ROCHE; 139	Valcaps	10 mg	Black and Blue	Capsule		Roche Pharmaceuticals
ROCHE; 274	Anaprox	275 mg	Blue	Tablet	Oval, Biconvex	Roche Laboratories
ROCHE; AZO; GANTANOL	Azo Gantanol	0.5 GM ; 100 mg	Red	Coated Tablet		Roche Pharmaceuticals
ROCHE; AZO; GANTRISIN	Azo Gantrisin	500 mg ; 50 mg	Red	Coated Tablet		Roche Pharmaceuticals
ROCHE; BUMEX 0.5	Bumex	0.5 mg	Light Green	Tablet	Oval	Roche Pharmaceuticals
ROCHE; BUMEX 1	Bumex	1 mg	Yellow	Tablet	Oval	Roche Pharmaceuticals
ROCHE; BUMEX 2	Bumex	2 mg	Peach	Tablet	Oval	Roche Pharmaceuticals
ROCHE; C; MOGADON; 5	Mogadon	5 mg	White	Tablet	Barrel, Biplane, Scored	Valeant Pharmaceuticals
ROCHE; C; MOGADON; 10	Mogadon	10 mg	White	Tablet	Biplane, Scored, Barrel	Valeant Pharmaceuticals
ROCHE; CYTOVENE; 250	Cytovene	250 mg	Opaque Green	Capsule		Roche Laboratories
ROCHE; GANTRISIN	Gantrisin	0.5 GM	White	Tablet	Circle, Scored	Roche Pharmaceuticals
ROCHE; POSICOR; 50	Posicor	50 mg	Pale Yellow	Tablet	Biconvex, Hexagon	Roche Laboratories
ROCHE; POSICOR; 100	Posicor	100 mg	Light Orange	Tablet	Biconvex, Hexagon	Roche Laboratories
ROCHE; PROSTIGMIN	Prostigmin	15 mg	White	Tablet		Roche Laboratories
ROCHE; XENICAL; 120	Xenical	120 mg	Dark Blue	Capsule		Roche Laboratories
RORER; 82	Lozol	2.5 mg	White	Tablet	Circle	Aventis Pharmaceuticals
RP; 51	Dextrostat	5 mg	Yellow	Tablet	Circle, Scored	Shire Pharmaceuticals
RP; 52	Dextrostat	10 mg	Yellow	Tablet	Circle, Double-Scored	Shire Pharmaceuticals
RPR; 0514	Combipatch	0.05 mg/day ; 0.14 mg/day		Patch	Square	Novartis
RPR; 0525	Combipatch	0.05 mg/day ; 0.25 mg/day		Patch	Square	Novartis
RPR; 202	Rilutek	50 mg	White	Tablet	Capsule-Shape	Sanofi-Aventis U.S.
RPR; 352	Slo-Phyllin	200 mg	White	Tablet	Circle	Aventis Pharmaceuticals
RPR; 5100	Penetrex	200 mg	Light Blue	Coated Tablet	Circle	Aventis Pharmaceuticals
RPR; 5140	Penetrex	400 mg	Dark Blue	Coated Tablet	Circle	Aventis Pharmaceuticals
RS; 117	Ergoloid Mesylate	0.5 mg	White	Tablet	Oval	3M Pharmaceuticals
RS; 119	Ergoloid Mesylate	1 mg	White	Tablet	Oval	3M Pharmaceuticals
RS; 142 ;	Diethylpropion Hydrochloride	75 mg	White	Tablet	Oval	3M Pharmaceuticals
RUSS; 702	Femcet	50 mg ; 325 mg ; 40 mg	Lavender	Capsule		UCB Pharma
RVT20	Revatio	20 mg	White	Tablet	Circle	Pfizer
RX 496 ;	Hydrocodone Bitartrate and Acetaminophen	7.5 mg ; 750 mg	White to Off-White	Tablet	Circle	Ranbaxy Pharmaceuticals

IMPRINT	BRAND/GENERIC NAME	STRENGTH	COLOR	FORM	SHAPE	MANUFACTURER
RX 497 ;	Hydrocodone Bitartrate and Acetaminophen	10 mg ; 325 mg	White to Off-White	Tablet	Circle	Ranbaxy Pharmaceuticals
RX 498 ;	Hydrocodone Bitartrate and Acetaminophen	10 mg ; 500 mg	White to Off-White	Tablet	Circle	Ranbaxy Pharmaceuticals
RX 532	Lisinopril	5 mg	Light Pink	Tablet	Circle	Ranbaxy Pharmaceuticals
RX 533	Lisinopril	10 mg	Light Pink	Tablet	Circle	Ranbaxy Pharmaceuticals
RX 534	Lisinopril	20 mg	Light Rust	Tablet	Circle	Ranbaxy Pharmaceuticals
RX 535	Lisinopril	40 mg	Light Yellow	Tablet	Circle	Ranbaxy Pharmaceuticals
RX 552	Clorazepate Dipotassium	3.75 mg	Blue	Tablet	Circle	Ranbaxy Pharmaceuticals
RX 553	Clorazepate Dipotassium	7.5 mg	Peach	Tablet	Circle	Ranbaxy Pharmaceuticals
RX 554	Clorazepate Dipotassium	15 mg	Red	Tablet	Circle	Ranbaxy Pharmaceuticals
RX 555	Raniclor	125 mg	Yellow	Tablet, Chewable	Circle	Ranbaxy Pharmaceuticals
RX 556	Raniclor	187 mg	Yellow	Tablet, Chewable	Circle	Ranbaxy Pharmaceuticals
RX 557	Raniclor	250 mg	Yellow	Tablet, Chewable	Circle	Ranbaxy Pharmaceuticals
RX 558	Raniclor	375 mg	Yellow	Tablet, Chewable	Circle	Ranbaxy Pharmaceuticals
RX 560 ;	Hydrocodone Bitartrate and Acetaminophen	5 mg ; 500 mg	White to Off-White	Tablet	Capsule-Shape	Ranbaxy Pharmaceuticals
RX 599	Lisinopril	30 mg	Rust	Tablet	Circle	Ranbaxy Pharmaceuticals
RX 627 ;	Gabapentin	100 mg	White Opaque	Capsule		Ranbaxy Pharmaceuticals
RX 628 ;	Gabapentin	300 mg	Ivory Opaque	Capsule		Ranbaxy Pharmaceuticals
RX 629 ;	Gabapentin	400 mg	Orange Opaque	Capsule		Ranbaxy Pharmaceuticals
RX 725	Clarithromycin	250 mg	Light Yellow	Tablet	Capsule-Shape	Ranbaxy Pharmaceuticals
RX 726	Clarithromycin	500 mg	Light Yellow	Tablet	Capsule-Shape	Ranbaxy Pharmaceuticals
RX; 7	Lorazepam	0.5 mg	White	Tablet	Circle	Ranbaxy Pharmaceuticals
RX; 504	Acyclovir	400 mg	White	Tablet	Oval	Ranbaxy Pharmaceuticals
RX; 505	Acyclovir	800 mg	White	Tablet	Oval	Ranbaxy Pharmaceuticals
RX; 514	Amoxicillin	125 mg	Pink	Tablet, Chewable	Oval	Ranbaxy Pharmaceuticals
RX; 514	Amoxicillin	125 mg	Pink Mottled	Tablet, Chewable	Oval, Biconvex	Ranbaxy Pharmaceuticals
RX; 514	Dispermox	125 mg	Pink	Tablet, Chewable	Circle	Ranbaxy Pharmaceuticals
RX; 515	Amoxicillin	250 mg	Pink	Tablet, Chewable	Circle	Ranbaxy Pharmaceuticals
RX; 515	Amoxicillin	250 mg	Pink Mottled	Tablet, Chewable	Circle, Flat-Faced, Bevel-Edged	Ranbaxy Pharmaceuticals
RX; 515	Dispermox	250 mg	Pink	Tablet, Chewable	Oval	Ranbaxy Pharmaceuticals
RX; 522	Enalapril Maleate	2.5 mg	Yellow	Tablet	Circle, Biconvex, Scored	Ranbaxy Pharmaceuticals
RX; 523	Enalapril Maleate	5 mg	White	Tablet	Biconvex, Scored, Circle	Ranbaxy Pharmaceuticals
RX; 524	Enalapril Maleate	10 mg	Red-Brown	Tablet	Circle, Biconvex	Ranbaxy Pharmaceuticals
RX; 525	Enalapril Maleate	20 mg	Orange	Tablet	Circle, Biconvex	Ranbaxy Pharmaceuticals
RX; 536	Hydrochlorothiazide and Lisinopril	12.5 mg ; 10 mg	Pale Blue	Tablet	Circle	Ranbaxy Pharmaceuticals
RX; 537	Hydrochlorothiazide and Lisinopril	12.5 mg ; 20 mg	Yellow	Tablet	Circle	Ranbaxy Pharmaceuticals
RX; 538	Hydrochlorothiazide and Lisinopril	25 mg ; 20 mg	Peach	Tablet	Circle	Ranbaxy Pharmaceuticals
RX; 565	Dispermox	200 mg	Light Pink	Tablet for Suspension	Circle	Ranbaxy Pharmaceuticals
RX; 567	Dispermox	400 mg	Light Pink	Tablet for Suspension	Circle	Ranbaxy Pharmaceuticals
RX; 652	Acyclovir	200 mg	White	Capsule		Ranbaxy Pharmaceuticals
RX; 654	Amoxicillin	250 mg	Yellow	Capsule		Ranbaxy Pharmaceuticals
RX; 654	Dispermox	250 mg	Yellow	Capsule		Ranbaxy Pharmaceuticals
RX; 655	Amoxicillin	500 mg	Maroon and Yellow	Capsule		Ranbaxy Pharmaceuticals
RX; 655	Dispermox	500 mg	Maroon	Capsule		Ranbaxy Pharmaceuticals
RX; 657	Cephalexin	500 mg	Dark Green and Light Green	Capsule		Ranbaxy Pharmaceuticals
RX; 658	Cefaclor	250 mg	Blue and Green	Capsule		Ranbaxy Pharmaceuticals
RX; 659	Cefaclor	500 mg	Blue and Green	Capsule		Ranbaxy Pharmaceuticals
RX; 675	Cephalexin	250 mg	Green and White	Capsule		Ranbaxy Pharmaceuticals
RX; 676	Cephalexin	500 mg	Dark Green and Light Green	Capsule		Ranbaxy Pharmaceuticals
RX; 677	Propoxyphene Hydrochloride	65 mg	Pink	Capsule		Ranbaxy Pharmaceuticals
RX; 678	Propoxyphene Hydrochloride Compound	389 mg ; 32.4 mg ; 65 mg	White and Red	Capsule		Ranbaxy Pharmaceuticals
RX; 679	Seconal Sodium	100 mg	Orange	Capsule		Ranbaxy Pharmaceuticals
RX; 680	Tuinal	50 mg ; 50 mg	Blue and Orange	Capsule		Ranbaxy Pharmaceuticals
RX; 681	Nalfon 200	200 mg	White and Ocher	Capsule		Ranbaxy Pharmaceuticals
RX; 682	Nalfon	300 mg	Yellow and Ocher	Capsule		Ranbaxy Pharmaceuticals
RX; 694	Minocycline Hydrochloride	50 mg	White Opaque	Capsule		Ranbaxy Pharmaceuticals
RX; 695	Minocycline Hydrochloride	75 mg	Gray Opaque	Capsule		Ranbaxy Pharmaceuticals
RX; 696	Minocycline Hydrochloride	100 mg	Opaque Gray and White	Capsule		Ranbaxy Pharmaceuticals
RX; 701	Etodolac	400 mg	Yellow	Coated Tablet	Oval	Ranbaxy Pharmaceuticals
RX; 713	Amoxicillin and Clavulanate Potassium	500 mg ; 125 mg	White	Tablet	Oval, Scored	Ranbaxy Pharmaceuticals
RX; 714	Etodolac	500 mg	Blue	Coated Tablet	Oval	Ranbaxy Pharmaceuticals
RX; 715	Ofloxacin	300 mg	White	Tablet	Oblong	Ranbaxy Pharmaceuticals
RX; 716	Ofloxacin	200 mg	White	Tablet	Oblong	Ranbaxy Pharmaceuticals
RX; 717	Ofloxacin	400 mg	White	Tablet	Oblong	Ranbaxy Pharmaceuticals
RX; 736	Benazepril Hydrochloride	5 mg	Light Yellow	Tablet	Circle	Ranbaxy Pharmaceuticals
RX; 737	Benazepril Hydrochloride	10 mg	Dark Yellow	Tablet	Circle	Ranbaxy Pharmaceuticals
RX; 738	Benazepril Hydrochloride	20 mg	Light Pink	Tablet	Circle	Ranbaxy Pharmaceuticals
RX; 739	Benazepril Hydrochloride	40 mg	Dark Pink	Tablet	Circle	Ranbaxy Pharmaceuticals
RX; 741	Phenobarbital	15 mg	White	Tablet		Ranbaxy Pharmaceuticals
RX; 742	Phenobarbital	30 mg	White	Tablet		Ranbaxy Pharmaceuticals
RX; 743	Phenobarbital	60 mg	White	Tablet		Ranbaxy Pharmaceuticals
RX; 744	Phenobarbital	100 mg	White	Tablet		Ranbaxy Pharmaceuticals
RX; 745	Morphine Sulfate	10 mg	White	Tablet		Ranbaxy Pharmaceuticals
RX; 746	Morphine Sulfate	15 mg	White	Tablet		Ranbaxy Pharmaceuticals
RX; 747	Morphine Sulfate	30 mg	White	Tablet		Ranbaxy Pharmaceuticals
RX; 748	Codeine Phosphate	30 mg	White	Tablet		Ranbaxy Pharmaceuticals
RX; 749	Codeine Phosphate	60 mg	White	Tablet		Ranbaxy Pharmaceuticals
RX; 751	Cefuroxime Axetil	250 mg	Blue	Tablet	Capsule-Shape	Ranbaxy Pharmaceuticals
RX; 752	Cefuroxime Axetil	500 mg	Blue	Tablet		Ranbaxy Pharmaceuticals
RX; 752	Cefuroxime	500 mg	Blue	Tablet	Oblong	Ranbaxy Pharmaceuticals
RX; 753	Amoxicillin and Clavulanate Potassium Chewable	200 mg ; 28.5 mg	Pink	Tablet	Circle	Ranbaxy Pharmaceuticals

IMPRINT	BRAND/GENERIC NAME	STRENGTH	COLOR	FORM	SHAPE	MANUFACTURER
RX; 754	Amoxicillin and Clavulanate Potassium Chewable	400 mg ; 57 mg	Pink	Tablet	Circle	Ranbaxy Pharmaceuticals
RX; 760	Amoxicillin	200 mg	Pink	Tablet, Chewable		Ranbaxy Pharmaceuticals
RX; 760	Dispermox	200 mg	Pink	Tablet, Chewable	Circle	Ranbaxy Pharmaceuticals
RX; 761	Amoxicillin	400 mg	Pink	Tablet, Chewable		Ranbaxy Pharmaceuticals
RX; 761	Dispermox	400 mg	Pink	Tablet, Chewable	Circle	Ranbaxy Pharmaceuticals
RX; 762	Amoxicillin	500 mg	Pink	Tablet	Capsule-Shape	Ranbaxy Pharmaceuticals
RX; 762	Dispermox	500 mg	Pink	Tablet	Capsule-Shape	Ranbaxy Pharmaceuticals
RX; 763	Amoxicillin	875 mg	Pink	Tablet	Capsule-Shape	Ranbaxy Pharmaceuticals
RX; 763	Dispermox	875 mg	Pink	Tablet	Capsule-Shape	Ranbaxy Pharmaceuticals
RX; 773	Lorazepam	1 mg		Tablet		Ranbaxy Pharmaceuticals
RX; 774	Lorazepam	2 mg	White	Tablet	Circle	Ranbaxy Pharmaceuticals
RX5	Lisinopril	2.5 mg	Light Pink	Tablet	Circle	Ranbaxy Pharmaceuticals
RX6	Simvastatin	5 mg	Peach	Tablet	Circle	Ranbaxy Pharmaceuticals
RX130	Doxycycline	50 mg	Light Blue	Tablet	Circle	Ranbaxy Pharmaceuticals
RX131	Doxycycline	75 mg	Green	Tablet	Circle	Ranbaxy Pharmaceuticals
RX132	Doxycycline	100 mg	Dark Blue	Tablet	Circle	Ranbaxy Pharmaceuticals
RX165	Sertraline Hydrochloride	50 mg	White	Tablet	Capsule-Shape	Ranbaxy Pharmaceuticals
RX166	Sertraline Hydrochloride	100 mg	White	Tablet	Capsule-Shape	Ranbaxy Pharmaceuticals
RX167	Sertraline Hydrochloride	150 mg	White	Tablet	Capsule-Shape	Ranbaxy Pharmaceuticals
RX168	Sertraline Hydrochloride	200 mg	White	Tablet	Capsule-Shape	Ranbaxy Pharmaceuticals
RX509	Amoxicillin and Clavulanate Potassium	875 mg ; 125 mg	White	Tablet	Capsule-Shape	Ranbaxy Pharmaceuticals
RX520	Cefpodoxime Proxetil	100 mg	White to Off White	Tablet	Capsule-Shape	Ranbaxy Pharmaceuticals
RX521	Cefpodoxime Proxetil	200 mg	White to Off White	Tablet	Capsule-Shape	Ranbaxy Pharmaceuticals
RX549	Quinapril	10 mg	White to Off-White	Tablet	Circle	Ranbaxy Pharmaceuticals
RX550	Quinapril	20 mg	White to Off-White	Tablet	Circle	Ranbaxy Pharmaceuticals
RX551	Quinapril	40 mg	White to Off-White	Tablet	Circle	Ranbaxy Pharmaceuticals
RX596 ;	Pravastatin Sodium	20 mg	Dark Yellow to Yellow	Tablet	Circle	Ranbaxy Pharmaceuticals
RX597 ;	Pravastatin Sodium	40 mg	Dark Yellow to Yellow	Tablet	Circle	Ranbaxy Pharmaceuticals
RX598	Pravastatin Sodium	80 mg	Dark Yellow to Yellow	Tablet	Capsule-Shape	Ranbaxy Pharmaceuticals
RX632	Fluoxetine	40 mg	Opaque Green, Opaque Orange	Capsule		Ranbaxy Pharmaceuticals
RX656	Cephalexin	250 mg	Dark Green and White	Capsule		Ranbaxy Pharmaceuticals
RX686	Fluoxetine	10 mg	Light Green, Opaque Light Green	Capsule		Ranbaxy Pharmaceuticals
RX687	Fluoxetine	20 mg	Opaque Green, Yellow	Capsule		Ranbaxy Pharmaceuticals
RX692	Clindamycin Hydrochloride	150 mg	Light Green, Opaque Turquoise Blue	Capsule		Ranbaxy Pharmaceuticals
RX693	Clindamycin Hydrochloride	300 mg	Opaque Turquoise Blue	Capsule		Ranbaxy Pharmaceuticals
RX709	Ciprofloxacin	250 mg	White to Off White	Tablet	Circle	Ranbaxy Pharmaceuticals
RX710	Ciprofloxacin	500 mg	White to Off White	Tablet	Oblong	Ranbaxy Pharmaceuticals
RX711	Ciprofloxacin	750 mg	White to Off White	Tablet	Oblong	Ranbaxy Pharmaceuticals
RX776	Fosinopril Sodium	20 mg	White to Off White	Tablet	Circle	Ranbaxy Pharmaceuticals
RX777	Fosinopril Sodium	40 mg	White to Off White	Tablet	Circle	Ranbaxy Pharmaceuticals
RX790	Simvastatin	10 mg	Peach	Tablet	Circle	Ranbaxy Pharmaceuticals
RX791	Simvastatin	20 mg	Tan	Tablet	Circle	Ranbaxy Pharmaceuticals
RX792	Simvastatin	40 mg	Brick Red	Tablet	Circle	Ranbaxy Pharmaceuticals
RX793	Simvastatin	80 mg	Brick Red	Tablet	Circle	Ranbaxy Pharmaceuticals
RX803	Fluconazole	50 mg	Pink	Tablet	Circle	Ranbaxy Pharmaceuticals
RX804	Fluconazole	100 mg	Pink	Tablet	Circle	Ranbaxy Pharmaceuticals
RX805	Fluconazole	150 mg	Pink	Tablet	Circle	Ranbaxy Pharmaceuticals
RX806	Fluconazole	200 mg	Pink	Tablet	Circle	Ranbaxy Pharmaceuticals
RX860	Metformin Hydrochloride	500 mg	Off White	Tablet, Extended Release	Capsule-Shape	Ranbaxy Pharmaceuticals
RYNA 1708	Ryna-12x	25 mg ; 60 mg ; 200 mg	Blue	Tablet	Oval	Medpointe
S 063	Agrylin	0.5 mg	White	Capsule		Shire Pharmaceuticals
S 064	Agrylin	1 mg	Gray	Capsule		Shire Pharmaceuticals
S CAFERGOT; P-B 78/35 SUPPOSITORY	Cafergot P-B	2 mg ; 100 mg ; 0.25 mg ; 60 mg		Suppository		Novartis Pharmaceuticals
S/T; DS; 911	Sulfamethoxazole and Trimethoprim	800 mg ; 160 mg	White	Tablet	Oval, Convex, Scored	Teva Pharmaceuticals
S; 5	Selegiline Hydrochloride	5 mg	White	Tablet	Shield-Shape	Mylan Pharmaceuticals
S; 15; WYETH; 317	Serax	15 mg	Yellow	Tablet	Five-Sided	Faulding Laboratories
S; 20; LESCOL	Lescol	20 mg	Brown and Light Brown	Capsule		Novartis Pharmaceuticals
S; 40; LESCOL	Lescol	40 mg	Brown and Gold	Capsule		Novartis Pharmaceuticals
S; 62	Seasonale	0.03 mg ; 0.15 mg	Pink	Tablet	Circle	Barr Laboratories
S; 78/22 ;	Bellergal	20 mg ; 0.3 mg ; 0.1 mg	Pink	Coated Tablet	Circle	Novartis Pharmaceuticals
S; 78; 240	Sandimmune	25 mg	Pink	Capsule	Oval	Novartis Pharmaceuticals
S; 78; 241	Sandimmune	100 mg	Dusty Rose	Capsule	Oblong	Novartis Pharmaceuticals
S; 78; 242	Sandimmune	50 mg	Yellow	Capsule	Oblong	Novartis Pharmaceuticals
S; 78-2	Mellaril	10 mg	Bright Chartreuse	Coated Tablet		Novartis
S; 78-8	Mellaril	15 mg	Pink	Coated Tablet		Novartis
S; 770	Sorbitrate	5 mg	Green	Tablet	Oval, Scored	Astrazeneca
S; 780	Sorbitrate	10 mg	Yellow	Tablet	Oval, Scored	Astrazeneca
S; 810	Sorbitrate	5 mg	Green	Tablet, Chewable	Circle, Scored	Astrazeneca
S; 820	Sorbitrate	20 mg	Blue	Tablet	Oval, Scored	Astrazeneca
S; AHG ;	Naqua	2 mg	Pink	Tablet	Character-Shape, Scored	Schering
S; AHH ;	Naqua	4 mg	Aqua	Tablet	Character-Shape, Scored	Schering
S; ANB ;	Etrafon-A	4 mg ; 10 mg	Orange	Coated Tablet		Schering
S; ANE	Etrafon-Forte	25 mg ; 4 mg	Red	Coated Tablet		Schering-Plough
S; HYDERGINE 1 ;	Hydergine	1 mg	White	Tablet	Circle	Novartis

IMPRINT	BRAND/GENERIC NAME	STRENGTH	COLOR	FORM	SHAPE	MANUFACTURER
S; HYDERGINE; LC; 1 MG	Hydergine Lc	1 mg	Off White	Capsule		Novartis
S; MELLARIL; 25	Mellaril	25 mg	Light Tan	Coated Tablet		Novartis
S; MELLARIL; 50	Mellaril	50 mg	White	Coated Tablet		Novartis
S; MELLARIL; 100	Mellaril	100 mg	Light Green	Coated Tablet		Novartis
S; MELLARIL; 150	Mellaril	150 mg	Yellow	Coated Tablet		Novartis
S; MELLARIL; 200	Mellaril	200 mg	Pink	Coated Tablet		Novartis
S10 ;	Sarafem	10 mg	Cream	Tablet	Circle	Warner Chilcott
S15 ;	Sarafem	15 mg	White	Tablet	Circle	Warner Chilcott
S20 ;	Sarafem	20 mg	Yellow	Tablet	Circle	Warner Chilcott
S190	Lunesta	1 mg	Light Blue	Tablet	Circle	Sepracor
S191	Lunesta	2 mg	White	Tablet	Circle	Sepracor
S193	Lunesta	3 mg	Dark Blue	Tablet	Circle	Sepracor
S405 250	Fosrenol	250 mg	White to Off-White	Tablet, Chewable	Circle	Shire Us
S405 500	Fosrenol	500 mg	White to Off- White	Tablet, Chewable	Circle	Shire Us
S405 750	Fosrenol	750 mg	White to Off- White	Tablet, Chewable	Circle	Shire Us
S405 1000	Fosrenol	1000 mg	White to Off-White	Tablet, Chewable	Circle	Shire Us
S476	Lialda	1.2 GM	Red-Brown	Tablet, Delayed Release	Oval	Shire Us
SA ; NVR	Gleevec	100 mg	Very Dark Yellow to Brownish Orange	Tablet	Circle	Novartis Pharmaceuticals
SAL 5	Pilocarpine Hydrochloride	5 mg	White	Tablet	Circle	Actavis Elizabeth
SAL 7.5	Pilocarpine Hydrochloride	7.5 mg	Blue	Tablet	Circle	Actavis Elizabeth
SAL; 5 ;	Salagen	5 mg	White	Tablet	Circle	Eisai
SAL; 7.5	Salagen	7.5 mg	Blue	Tablet	Circle	Eisai
SAN 60	Sanctura Xr	60 mg	Orange, White	Capsule, Extended Release		Allergan
SANDOZ; 78/71 ;	Sanorex	1 mg	White	Tablet	Elliptical; Scored	Novartis Pharmaceuticals
SANDOZ; 78; 36 ;	Cafergot P-B	100 mg ; 1 mg ; 30 mg ; 0.125 mg	Green	Coated Tablet		Novartis Pharmaceuticals
SANDOZ; 78; 38	Cedilanid	0.5 mg	Salmon	Coated Tablet		Novartis Pharmaceuticals
SANDOZ; 78; 48	Gynergen	1 mg	Ivory Gray	Coated Tablet		Novartis
SANDOZ; 78; 54	Methergine	0.2 mg	Purple	Tablet		Novartis Pharmaceuticals
SANDOZ; 78; 58	Sansert	2 mg	Yellow	Coated Tablet	Circle	Novartis Pharmaceuticals
SANDOZ; 78; 66	Sanorex	2 mg	White	Tablet	Circle, Scored	Novartis Pharmaceuticals
SANDOZ; S	Belladenal Spacetabs	0.25 mg ; 50 mg	Multi-Colored	Tablet		Novartis Pharmaceuticals
SANDOZ-S ;	Bellergal Spacetabs	0.2 mg ; 0.6 mg ; 40 mg	Multi-Colored	Tablet		Novartis
SANDOZ-S; 78; 33	Caffergot	100 mg ; 2 mg		Suppository		Novartis Pharmaceuticals
SANKYO; C; 12	Benicar	5 mg	Yellow	Tablet	Circle	Daiichi Sankyo
SANKYO; C; 14	Benicar	20 mg	White	Tablet	Circle	Daiichi Sankyo
SANKYO; C01	Welchol	625 mg	White	Tablet		Daiichi Sankyo
SANKYO; C22	Benicar HCT	20 mg ; 12.5 mg	Reddish-Yellow	Tablet	Circle	Daiichi Sankyo
SANKYO; C23	Benicar HCT	40 mg ; 12.5 mg	Reddish-Yellow	Tablet	Oval	Daiichi Sankyo
SANKYO; C25	Benicar HCT	40 mg ; 25 mg	Pink	Tablet	Oval	Daiichi Sankyo
SB 4890	Requip	0.25 mg	White	Tablet	Five-Sided	Glaxosmithkline
SB 4891	Requip	0.5 mg	Yellow	Tablet	Five-Sided	Glaxosmithkline
SB 4892	Requip	1 mg	Green	Tablet	Five-Sided	Glaxosmithkline
SB 4893	Requip	2 mg	Pale Yellowish-Pink	Tablet	Five-Sided	Glaxosmithkline
SB 4894	Requip	5 mg	Blue	Tablet	Five-Sided	Glaxosmithkline
SB 4895	Requip	3 mg	Pale to Moderate Reddish-Purple	Tablet	Five-Sided	Glaxosmithkline
SB 4896	Requip	4 mg	Pale Brown	Tablet	Five-Sided	Glaxosmithkline
SB; 39	Coreg	3.125 mg	White	Coated Tablet	Oval	Glaxosmithkline
SB; 4140	Coreg	6.25 mg	White	Coated Tablet	Oval	Glaxosmithkline
SB; 4141	Coreg	12.5 mg	White	Coated Tablet	Oval	Glaxosmithkline
SB; 4142	Coreg	25 mg	White	Coated Tablet	Oval	Glaxosmithkline
SB; 5500	Albenza	200 mg	White to Off-White	Coated Tablet	Circle, Biconvex, Bevel-Edged	Glaxosmithkline
SC ; P	Verapamil Hydrochloride	120 mg	Light Violet	Tablet, Extended Release	Oval	Ranbaxy Pharmaceuticals
SCHERING 402 ;	Theovent Long-Acting	125 mg	Dark Green and Yellow	Timed-Release Capsule		Schering
SCHERING; 011	Celestone	0.6 mg	Pink	Tablet	Circle, Compressed, Scored	Schering
SCHERING; 095 ;	Polaramine Repetabs	4 mg	Light Red	Timed-Release Tablet	Oval	Schering
SCHERING; 148 ;	Polaramine Repetabs	6 mg	Bright Red	Timed-Release Tablet	Oval	Schering
SCHERING; 228	Fulvicin P/g	125 mg	White	Tablet	Scored, Compressed	Schering
SCHERING; 251	Paxipam	20 mg	Orange	Tablet	Compressed, Scored	Schering
SCHERING; 311 ;	Oreton Methyl	10 mg	White	Tablet	Circle	Schering
SCHERING; 432 ;	Coriforte	130 mg ; 30 mg ; 500 G ; 4 mg ; 190 mg	Red and Yellow	Capsule		Schering
SCHERING; 507	Fulvicin P/g	250 mg	White	Tablet	Scored, Compressed	Schering
SCHERING; 525	Eulexin	125 mg	Opaque, Two-Toned Brown	Capsule		Schering
SCHERING; 538	Paxipam	40 mg	White	Tablet	Compressed, Scored	Schering
SCHERING; 753	Theovent Long-Acting	250 mg	Dark Green and Clear	Timed-Release Capsule		Schering
SCHERING; 820	Polaramine	2 mg	Red	Tablet	Oval, Compressed	Schering
SCHERING; 901	Chlor-Trimeton Decongestant	60 mg ; 4 mg	Blue	Tablet		Schering-Plough
SCHERING; 970 ;	Oreton Methyl	10 mg	Pink to Lavender	Tablet	Oval	Schering
SCHERING; AGT ;	Polaramine Repetabs	2 mg	Red	Tablet	Oval, Compressed	Schering
SCHERING; AUF ;	Fulvicin-U/f	250 mg	White	Tablet	Compressed, Scored	Schering
SCHERING; AUG ;	Fulvicin-U/f	500 mg	White	Tablet	Compressed, Scored	Schering
SCHERING; JE ;	Oreton Methyl	25 mg	Peach	Tablet	Circle	Schering
SCHERING; KEM ;	Meticorten	1 mg	White	Tablet	Compressed	Schering
SCHWARZ 620; 20	Monoket	20 mg	White	Tablet	Circle	UCB Pharma
SCHWARZ; 053 ;	Fedahist Gyrocaps	10 mg ; 65 mg	White and Yellow	Timed-Release Capsule		Schwarz Pharma
SCHWARZ; 055 ;	Fedahist Timecaps	8 mg ; 120 mg	Clear	Timed-Release Capsule		Schwarz Pharma
SCHWARZ; 0920	Dilatrate-SR	40 mg	Pink and Clear with White Beads	Capsule, Extended Release		UCB Pharma
SCHWARZ; 525	Ku-Zyme Hp	30000 U ; 30000 U ; 8000 U	White	Capsule		UCB Pharma

IMPRINT	BRAND/GENERIC NAME	STRENGTH	COLOR	FORM	SHAPE	MANUFACTURER
SCHWARZ; 532	Levsin/SL	0.125 mg	White	Tablet	Eight-Sided, Scored	Schwarz Pharma
SCHWARZ; 534 ;	Levsin-PB	0.125 mg ; 15 mg	Pink	Tablet	Circle, Scored	Schwarz Pharma
SCHWARZ; 610; 10	Monoket	10 mg	White	Tablet	Circle	UCB Pharma
SCHWARZ; 2489; VERELAN; 180 MG	Verelan	180 mg	Yellow and Gray	Capsule, Extended Release		UCB Pharma
SCHWARZ; 2490; VERELAN; 120 MG	Verelan	120 mg	Yellow	Capsule, Extended Release		UCB Pharma
SCHWARZ; 2491; VERELAN; 240 MG	Verelan	240 mg	Blue and Yellow	Capsule, Extended Release		UCB Pharma
SCHWARZ; 2495; VERELAN; 360 MG	Verelan	360 mg	Lavender and Yellow	Capsule, Extended Release		UCB Pharma
SCHWARZ; 4085; 100 MG	Verelan Pm	100 mg	White and Amethyst	Capsule, Extended Release		UCB Pharma
SCHWARZ; 4086; 200 MG	Verelan Pm	200 mg	Amethyst	Capsule, Extended Release		UCB Pharma
SCHWARZ; 4087; 300 MG	Verelan Pm	300 mg	Lavender and Amethyst	Capsule, Extended Release		UCB Pharma
SCHWARZ; 4122	Ku-Zyme	1200 U ; 15000 U ; 15000 U	Yellow and White	Capsule		UCB Pharma
SCHWARZ; 4175	Kutrase	2400 U ; 30000 U ; 30000 U	Green and White	Capsule		UCB Pharma
SCI 500	Sular	8.5 mg	Oyster	Tablet, Extended Release	Circle	Sciele Pharma
SCI 501	Sular	17 mg	Yellow Cream	Tablet, Extended Release	Circle	Sciele Pharma
SCI 502	Sular	25.5 mg	Mustard	Tablet, Extended Release	Oblong	Sciele Pharma
SCI 503	Sular	34 mg	Burnt Orange	Tablet, Extended Release	Oblong	Sciele Pharma
SCS; 3; 30	Low-Ogestrel White Tablet	0.3 mg ; 0.03 mg	White	28-Day Tablet Pack	Circle	Watson Laboratories
SCS; 5762	Piroxicam	20 mg	Orange Opaque	Capsule		Scs Pharmaceuticals
SEARLE; 6	Tri-Norinyl 21-Day	0.5 mg ; 35 mcg	Blue	21-Day Tablet Pack	Circle	Watson Laboratories
SEARLE; 7	Tri-Norinyl 21 Day Yellow-Green Tablet	1 mg ; 35 mcg	Yellow-Green	21-Day Tablet Pack	Circle	Watson Laboratories
SERAX; 10; 51; WYETH	Serax	10 mg	Pink and White	Capsule		Faulding Laboratories
SERAX; 15; 6; WYETH	Serax	15 mg	Red and White	Capsule		Faulding Laboratories
SERAX; 30; 52; WYETH	Serax	30 mg	Maroon and White	Capsule		Faulding Laboratories
SEROQUEL 25	Seroquel	25 mg	Peach	Tablet	Circle	Astrazeneca
SEROQUEL 50	Seroquel	50 mg	White	Tablet	Circle	Astrazeneca
SEROQUEL 100	Seroquel	100 mg	Yellow	Tablet	Circle	Astrazeneca
SEROQUEL 200	Seroquel	200 mg	White	Tablet	Circle	Astrazeneca
SINA 6301	Sina-12x	200 mg ; 25 mg	Purple	Tablet	Capsule-Shape	Medpointe
SINEQUAN; ROERIG; 534	Sinequan	10 mg	Pink and Red	Capsule		Pfizer Roerig
SINEQUAN; ROERIG; 535	Sinequan	25 mg	Pink and Blue	Capsule		Pfizer Roerig
SINEQUAN; ROERIG; 536	Sinequan	50 mg	Pink and White	Capsule		Pfizer Roerig
SINEQUAN; ROERIG; 537	Sinequan	150 mg	Blue	Capsule		Pfizer Roerig
SINEQUAN; ROERIG; 538	Sinequan	100 mg	Blue and White	Capsule		Pfizer Roerig
SINEQUAN; ROERIG; 539	Sinequan	75 mg	White	Capsule		Pfizer Roerig
SINGULAIR ; MRK 117	Singulair	10 mg	Beige	Tablet	Square	Merck & Company
SINGULAIR ; MRK 275	Singulair	5 mg	Pink	Tablet, Chewable	Circle	Merck & Company
SINGULAIR ; MRK 711	Singulair	4 mg	Pink	Tablet, Chewable	Oval	Merck & Company
SK ; PP	Verapamil Hydrochloride	180 mg	Light Pink	Tablet, Extended Release	Oval	Ranbaxy Pharmaceuticals
SKF; 25	Vontrol	25 mg	Orange	Tablet	Circle	Glaxosmithkline
SKF; 101	SK-Ampicillin	250 mg	Yellow and White	Capsule		Glaxosmithkline
SKF; 102	SK-Ampicillin	500 mg	Yellow and White	Capsule		Glaxosmithkline
SKF; 107	SK-Ampicillin	125 mg	White, Scored	Tablet, Chewable		Glaxosmithkline
SKF; 111	SK-Penicillin G	400,000 units	White	Tablet		Glaxosmithkline
SKF; 112	SK-Penicillin G	800000 U	White	Tablet	Capsule-Shape	Glaxosmithkline
SKF; 116	SK-Penicillin VK	250 mg	White	Tablet		Glaxosmithkline
SKF; 117	SK-Penicillin VK	500 mg		Tablet		Glaxosmithkline
SKF; 120	SK-Amitriptyline	10 mg	White	Tablet		Glaxosmithkline
SKF; 121	SK-Amitriptyline	25 mg	Green	Tablet		Glaxosmithkline
SKF; 122	SK-Digoxin	0.25 mg	White	Tablet		Glaxosmithkline
SKF; 123	SK-Amitriptyline	50 mg	Yellow	Tablet		Glaxosmithkline
SKF; 124	SK-Amitriptyline	75 mg	Green	Tablet		Glaxosmithkline
SKF; 126	SK-Tetracycline	250 mg	Pink and White	Capsule		Glaxosmithkline
SKF; 127	SK-Tetracycline	500 mg	Pink and White	Capsule		Glaxosmithkline
SKF; 129	SK-Niacin	50 mg	White	Tablet		Glaxosmithkline
SKF; 130	SK-Niacin	100 mg	White	Tablet		Glaxosmithkline
SKF; 131	SK-Amitriptyline	100 mg	Yellow	Tablet		Glaxosmithkline
SKF; 132	SK-Amitriptyline	150 mg	White	Tablet		Glaxosmithkline
SKF; 133	SK-Bamate	200 mg		Tablet		Glaxosmithkline

IMPRINT	BRAND/GENERIC NAME	STRENGTH	COLOR	FORM	SHAPE	MANUFACTURER
SKF; 134	SK-Bamate	400 mg	White	Tablet		Glaxosmithkline
SKF; 136	SK-Phenobarbital	15 mg	White	Tablet		Glaxosmithkline
SKF; 137	SK-Phenobarbital	30 mg	White	Tablet		Glaxosmithkline
SKF; 163	SK-Soxazole	500 mg	White	Tablet		Glaxosmithkline
SKF; 169	SK-Reserpine	0.25 mg	White	Tablet		Glaxosmithkline
SKF; 171	SK-Quinidine Sulfate	200 mg	White	Tablet		Glaxosmithkline
SKF; 173	SK-Apap	650 mg	White	Tablet	Capsule-Shape	Glaxosmithkline
SKF; 174	SK-Apap	325 mg	White	Tablet		Glaxosmithkline
SKF; 176	SK-Chloral Hydrate	500 mg	Green	Tablet		Glaxosmithkline
SKF; 303	SK-Diphenhydramine	25 mg	Green	Capsule		Glaxosmithkline
SKF; 304	SK-Diphenhydramine	50 mg	White and Green	Capsule		Glaxosmithkline
SKF; 310	SK-Propantheline	15 mg	White	Tablet	Circle	Glaxosmithkline
SKF; 316	SK-Petn	10 mg	White	Tablet		Glaxosmithkline
SKF; 317	SK-Petn	20 mg	White	Tablet		Glaxosmithkline
SKF; 319	SK-Oxycodone with Aspirin	325 mg ; 4.5 mg ; 0.38 mg	White	Tablet	Oval	Glaxosmithkline
SKF; 320	SK-Oxycodone with Acetaminophen	325 mg ; 5 mg	White	Tablet	Circle	Glaxosmithkline
SKF; 321	SK-Pramine	10 mg	Blue	Tablet		Glaxosmithkline
SKF; 322	SK-Pramine	25 mg	Blue	Tablet		Glaxosmithkline
SKF; 323	SK-Pramine	50 mg	Blue	Tablet		Glaxosmithkline
SKF; 324	SK-Apap	325 mg ; 15 mg	White	Tablet		Glaxosmithkline Consumer
SKF; 326	SK-Apap	30 mg ; 325 mg	White	Tablet		Glaxosmithkline
SKF; 327	SK-Apap	325 mg ; 60 mg	White	Tablet		Glaxosmithkline
SKF; 339	SK-Prednisone	5 mg	White	Tablet		Glaxosmithkline
SKF; 340	SK-Furosemide	20 mg		Tablet		Glaxosmithkline
SKF; 341	SK-Furosemide	40 mg		Tablet		Glaxosmithkline
SKF; 363	SK-Hydrochlorothiazide	25 mg		Tablet		Glaxosmithkline
SKF; 364	SK-Hydrochlorothiazide	50 mg		Tablet		Glaxosmithkline
SKF; 367	SK-Erythromycin	250 mg	Yellow	Tablet		Glaxosmithkline
SKF; 369	SK-Erythromycin	500 mg	Yellow	Coated Tablet	Capsule-Shape	Glaxosmithkline
SKF; 371	SK-Thioridazine Hydrochloride	10 mg		Tablet		Glaxosmithkline
SKF; 372	SK-Thioridazine	25 mg		Tablet		Glaxosmithkline
SKF; 373	SK-Thioridazine	50 mg		Tablet		Glaxosmithkline
SKF; 374	SK-Dexamethasone	0.5 mg	Light Yellow	Tablet		Glaxosmithkline
SKF; 375	SK-Thioridazine Hydrochloride	100 mg		Tablet		Glaxosmithkline
SKF; 376	SK-Dexamethasone	0.75 mg	Light Blue	Tablet		Glaxosmithkline
SKF; 377	SK-Dexamethasone	1.5 mg	Pink	Tablet		Glaxosmithkline
SKF; 379	SK-Dipyridamole	25 mg		Tablet		Glaxosmithkline
SKF; 380; 50MG	SK-Dipyridamole	50 mg		Tablet		Glaxosmithkline
SKF; 381; 75MG	SK-Dipyridamole	75 mg		Tablet		Glaxosmithkline
SKF; 403	SK-Triamcinolone	2 mg	Pink	Tablet		Glaxosmithkline
SKF; 404	SK-Triamcinolone	4 mg	White	Tablet		Glaxosmithkline
SKF; 406	SK-Triamcinolone	8 mg	Yellow	Tablet		Glaxosmithkline
SKF; 409	SK-Tolbutamide	500 mg	Peach-Orange	Tablet	Circle	Glaxosmithkline
SKF; 419	SK-Chlorothiazide	250 mg	White	Tablet	Circle	Glaxosmithkline
SKF; 420	SK-Chlorothiazide	500 mg	White	Tablet	Circle	Glaxosmithkline
SKF; 423	SK-Diphenoxylate	2.5 mg ; 0.025 mg	White	Tablet		Glaxosmithkline
SKF; 426	SK Metronidazole	250 mg	Off-White	Tablet		Glaxosmithkline
SKF; 441	SK-Lygen	5 mg	Pink	Capsule		Glaxosmithkline
SKF; 442	SK-Lygen	10 mg	Pink and Orange	Capsule		Glaxosmithkline
SKF; 443	SK-Lygen	25 mg	Orange	Capsule		Glaxosmithkline
SKF; 463	SK-65	65 mg	Gray and White	Capsule		Glaxosmithkline
SKF; 468	SK-65 Compound	32.4 mg ; 65 mg ; 389 mg	Orange and Gray	Capsule		Glaxosmithkline
SKF; 470	SK-Methocarbamol	500 mg	White	Tablet	Oval	Glaxosmithkline
SKF; 471	SK-Methocarbamol	750 mg	White	Tablet	Oval	Glaxosmithkline
SKF; 474	SK-65	650 mg ; 65 mg	Orange	Tablet	Capsule-Shape	Glaxosmithkline
SKF; 494	SK-Apap	300 mg ; 15 mg	White	Tablet	Circle	Glaxosmithkline
SKF; 499	SK-Probenecid	500 mg	White	Coated Tablet		Glaxosmithkline
SKF; 499	SK-Probenecid	500 mg	White	Tablet	Capsule-Shape, Scored	Glaxosmithkline
SKF; A70	Anspor	250 mg	Orange and White	Capsule		Glaxosmithkline Consumer
SKF; A71	Anspor	500 mg	Orange	Capsule		Glaxosmithkline
SKF; A90	Benzedrine	15 mg	Purple and Clear	Capsule		Glaxosmithkline
SKF; A91	Benzedrine	5 mg		Tablet		Glaxosmithkline
SKF; A92	Benzedrine	10 mg	Peach	Tablet		Glaxosmithkline
SKF; C26	Combid	10 mg ; 5 mg	Yellow & Clear	Capsule		Glaxosmithkline Consumer
SKF; C66	Compazine	5 mg	Yellow-Green	Coated Tablet	Circle	Glaxosmithkline
SKF; C67	Compazine	10 mg	Yellow-Green	Coated Tablet	Circle	Glaxosmithkline
SKF; D14	Cytomel	5 mcg	White	Tablet	Circle	Glaxosmithkline
SKF; D16	Cytomel	25 mcg	White	Tablet	Circle, Scored	Glaxosmithkline
SKF; D17	Cytomel	50 mcg	White	Tablet	Circle, Scored	Glaxosmithkline
SKF; D62	Darbid	5 mg	Pink	Tablet	Circle	Glaxosmithkline
SKF; E33	Dibenzyline	10 mg	Red, Coral	Capsule		Glaxosmithkline Consumer
SKF; H06	Dyrenium	50 mg		Capsule		Glaxosmithkline Consumer
SKF; H07	Dyrenium	100 mg	Red	Capsule		Glaxosmithkline Consumer
SKF; H74	Eskabarb	65 mg		Capsule		Glaxosmithkline Consumer
SKF; H76	Eskabarb	97 mg	Blue & Clear	Capsule		Glaxosmithkline Consumer
SKF; J10	Eskalith Cr	450 mg	Yellow	Controlled-Release Tablet	Circle	Glaxosmithkline
SKF; J20	Eskaphen B	0.25 Gr ; 5 mg	Peach	Tablet		Glaxosmithkline
SKF; J66	Eskatrol	15 mg ; 7.5 mg	White and Clear	Capsule		Glaxosmithkline
SKF; K60	Fortespan	150 mg ; 10,000 USP units ; 400 USP units ; 6 mg ; 6 mg ; 6 mg ; 15 mcg ; 60 mg	Red and Clear	Capsule		Glaxosmithkline
SKF; P36	Prydon	0.4 mg ; 0.305 mg ; 0.06 mg ; 0.035 mg ; 1 Gr	Blue and Clear	Capsule		Glaxosmithkline

IMPRINT	BRAND/GENERIC NAME	STRENGTH	COLOR	FORM	SHAPE	MANUFACTURER
SKF; RIDAURA	Ridaura	3 mg	Opaque Brown and Opaque Tan	Capsule		Connetics
SKF; S03	Stelazine	1 mg	Blue	Coated Tablet	Circle	Glaxosmithkline
SKF; S04	Stelazine	2 mg	Blue	Coated Tablet	Circle	Glaxosmithkline
SKF; S06	Stelazine	5 mg	Blue	Coated Tablet	Circle	Glaxosmithkline
SKF; S07	Stelazine	10 mg	Blue	Coated Tablet	Circle	Glaxosmithkline
SKF; T63	Thorazine	30 mg	Orange and Natural	Sustained-Release Capsule		Glaxosmithkline
SKF; T64	Thorazine	75 mg	Orange and Natural	Sustained-Release Capsule		Glaxosmithkline
SKF; T66	Thorazine	150 mg	Orange and Natural	Sustained-Release Capsule		Glaxosmithkline
SKF; T67	Thorazine	200 mg	Opaque Orange Cap and Natural Body	Sustained-Release Capsule		Glaxosmithkline
SKF; T69	Thorazine	300 mg	Opaque Orange Cap and Natural Body	Sustained-Release Capsule		Glaxosmithkline
SKF; T73	Thorazine	10 mg	Orange	Coated Tablet	Circle	Glaxosmithkline
SKF; T74	Thorazine	25 mg	Orange	Coated Tablet	Circle	Glaxosmithkline
SKF; T76	Thorazine	50 mg	Orange	Coated Tablet	Circle	Glaxosmithkline
SKF; T77	Thorazine	100 mg	Orange	Coated Tablet	Circle	Glaxosmithkline
SKF; T79	Thorazine	200 mg	Orange	Coated Tablet	Circle	Glaxosmithkline
SKF; V23	Trophite	10 mg ; 25 mcg	Pink	Tablet		Glaxosmithkline
SKF; V24	Troph-Iron	25 mcg ; 10 mg	Pink	Tablet		Glaxosmithkline
SL ; 400	Gleevec	400 mg	Very Dark Yellow to Brownish Orange	Tablet	Oval	Novartis Pharmaceuticals
SL; 433	Trazodone	50 mg	White	Tablet	Circle, Scored	Warner Chilcott
SL; 434	Trazodone	100 mg	White	Tablet	Circle, Scored	Warner Chilcott
SL; 459	Theophylline	300 mg	White	Sustained-Release Tablet	Capsule-Shaped, Bisected Scored	Novartis Generics
SLO-BID; 50 MG; RPR	Slo-Bid Gyrocaps	50 mg	White and Clear with White Pellets	Capsule	Oblong	Aventis Pharmaceuticals
SLO-BID; 75 MG; RPR	Slo-Bid Gyrocaps	75 mg	White and Clear with White Pellets	Extended-Release Capsule	Oblong	Aventis Pharmaceuticals
SLO-BID; 100 MG; RPR	Slo-Bid Gyrocaps	100 mg	White and Clear with White Pellets	Capsule	Oblong	Aventis Pharmaceuticals
SLO-BID; 125 MG; RPR	Slo-Bid Gyrocaps	125 mg	White and Clear with White Pellets	Extended-Release Capsule	Oblong	Aventis Pharmaceuticals
SLO-BID; 200 MG; RPR	Slo-Bid Gyrocaps	200 mg	White and Clear with White Pellets	Capsule	Oblong	Aventis Pharmaceuticals
SLO-BID; 300 MG; RPR	Slo-Bid Gyrocaps	300 mg	White and Clear with White Pellets	Extended-Release Capsule	Oblong	Aventis Pharmaceuticals
SOLATENE; ROCHE	Solatene	30 mg	Blue and Green	Capsule		Roche Pharmaceuticals
SOMA 250	Soma	250 mg	White	Tablet	Circle	Meda Pharmaceuticals
SOMA 350	Soma	350 mg	White	Tablet	Circle	Meda Pharmaceuticals
SORIATANE 10MG	Soriatane	10 mg	Brown, White	Capsule		Stiefel Laboratories
SORIATANE 25MG	Soriatane	25 mg	Yellow, Brown	Capsule		Stiefel Laboratories
SP 2309 1 0	Niferex-Pn Forte	250 mg ; 2 mg ; 1 mg ; 60 mg ; 20 mg ; 3 mg ; 30 IU ; 400 IU ; 25 mg ; 5000 IU ; 3.4 mg ; 10 mg ; 0.2 mg ; 12 mcg ; 80 mg ; 4 mg	White	Coated Tablet	Capsule-Shape	Ther-RX
SP; 111	Nulev	0.125 mg	White	Tablet, Disintegrating	Circle	UCB Pharma
SP; 351	Kemstro	10 mg	White	Disintegrating Tablet	Circle	Schwarz Pharma
SP; 352	Kemstro	20 mg	White	Disintegrating Tablet	Circle	Schwarz Pharma
SP; 431 ;	Proventil Repetabs	4 mg	White	Timed-Release Tablet	Circle	Schering
SP; 538	Levbid	0.375 mg	Light Orange	Tablet, Extended Release	Capsule-Shape	Schwarz Pharma
SP; 712	Uniretic	12.5 mg ; 7.5 mg	Yellow	Tablet	Oval	UCB Pharma
SP; 720	Uniretic	12.5 mg ; 15 mg	White	Tablet	Oval	UCB Pharma
SP; 725	Uniretic	25 mg ; 15 mg	Yellow	Tablet	Oval	UCB Pharma
SP; 2104; 500; 5	CO-Gesic	5 mg ; 500 mg	White	Tablet		UCB Pharma
SP; 2164; 750 MG	Mono-Gesic	750 mg	Pink	Coated Tablet	Oval, Scored	Schwarz Pharma
SP; 2209; 131/05	Niferex-Pn	312 mg ; 10 mg ; 4000 IU ; 400 IU ; 80 mg ; 60 mg ; 50 mg ; 3 mg ; 3 mcg ; 3 mg ; 2 mg	Blue	Coated Tablet	Oval	Ther-RX
SP; 4330	Niferex-150 Forte	1 mg ; 150 mg ; 25 mcg	Red and Clear with Brown Beads	Capsule		Ther-RX
SP; ADH ;	Trilafon	2 mg	Gray	Coated Tablet		Schering
SP; ADJ ;	Trilafon	8 mg	Gray	Coated Tablet		Schering
SP; ADK ;	Trilafon	4 mg	Gray	Coated Tablet		Schering
SP; ADM ;	Trilafon	16 mg	Gray	Coated Tablet		Schering
SP; ANA ;	Etrafon 2-10	10 mg ; 2 mg	Deep Yellow	Coated Tablet		Schering
SP; ANC ;	Etrafon	25 mg ; 2 mg	Pink	Coated Tablet		Schering
SP; WDR ;	Permitil	2.5 mg	Light Orange	Tablet	Oval, Compressed, Scored	Schering
SP; WEG ;	Permitil	10 mg	Light Red	Tablet	Oval, Compressed, Scored	Schering
SP; WFF ;	Permitil	5 mg	Purple-Pink	Tablet	Oval, Compressed, Scored	Schering
SP22 ;	Levatol	20 mg	Yellow	Tablet	Capsule-Shape	UCB Pharma
SP371; 20	Fluxid	20 mg	White	Disintegrating Tablet	Circle, Biconvex	Schwarz Pharma
SP372; 40	Fluxid	40 mg	White	Disintegrating Tablet	Circle, Biconvex	Schwarz Pharma
SPD417 SPD417 100 MG	Equetro	100 mg	Opaque Bluish Green, Opaque Yellow	Capsule, Extended Release		Validus Pharmaceuticals
SPD417 SPD417 200 MG	Equetro	200 mg	Opaque Blue, Opaque Yellow	Capsule, Extended Release		Validus Pharmaceuticals
SPD417 SPD417 300 MG	Equetro	300 mg	Blue, Opaque Yellow	Capsule, Extended Release		Validus Pharmaceuticals

IMPRINT	BRAND/GENERIC NAME	STRENGTH	COLOR	FORM	SHAPE	MANUFACTURER
SPI	Amitiza	8 mcg	Pink	Capsule, Liquid Filled	Oval	Takeda Pharmaceuticals
SPI	Amitiza	24 mcg	Orange	Capsule, Liquid Filled	Oval	Takeda Pharmaceuticals
SQUIBB; 28	Imipramine Hydrochloride	25 mg		Tablet		Bristol-Myers Squibb
SQUIBB; 39	Imipramine Hydrochloride	10 mg		Tablet		Bristol-Myers Squibb
SQUIBB; 40	Imipramine Hydrochloride	50 mg		Tablet		Bristol-Myers Squibb
SQUIBB; 45	Desipramine Hydrochloride	25 mg		Tablet		Bristol-Myers Squibb
SQUIBB; 63	Ergoloid Mesylates	1 mg		Tablet		Bristol-Myers Squibb
SQUIBB; 105	Sulindac	150 mg		Tablet		Bristol-Myers Squibb
SQUIBB; 107	Sulindac	200 mg		Tablet		Bristol-Myers Squibb
SQUIBB; 133	Clorazepate	3.75 mg		Tablet		Bristol-Myers Squibb
SQUIBB; 138	Smz-Tmp 400/80	400 mg ; 80 mg	White	Tablet	Circle, Scored	Bristol-Myers Squibb
SQUIBB; 139	Chlorpropamide	100 mg	Blue	Tablet	Circle	Bristol-Myers Squibb
SQUIBB; 152	Chlorpropamide	250 mg	Blue	Tablet	Circle	Bristol-Myers Squibb
SQUIBB; 157	Clorazepate Dipotassium	7.5 mg	Peach	Tablet	Circle, Scored	Bristol-Myers Squibb
SQUIBB; 159	Oxazepam	30 mg		Capsule		Bristol-Myers Squibb
SQUIBB; 160	Ethril	250 mg	Pink	Tablet		Bristol-Myers Squibb
SQUIBB; 161	Ethril	500 mg	Pink	Tablet		Bristol-Myers Squibb
SQUIBB; 162	Chlorthalidone	25 mg	Yellow	Tablet	Circle	Bristol-Myers Squibb
SQUIBB; 163	Clorazepate	15 mg	Pink	Tablet	Circle, Scored	Bristol-Myers Squibb
SQUIBB; 171	Smz-Tmp 800/160	800 mg ; 160 mg	White	Tablet	Oval, Scored	Bristol-Myers Squibb
SQUIBB; 180	Chlorthalidone	50 mg		Tablet		Bristol-Myers Squibb
SQUIBB; 187	Chlorthalidone	100 mg	White	Tablet	Circle	Bristol-Myers Squibb
SQUIBB; 192	Ascorbic Acid	50 mg		Tablet		Bristol-Myers Squibb
SQUIBB; 193	Perphenazine with Amitriptyline 2/10	2 mg ; 10 mg	Blue	Coated Tablet	Circle	Bristol-Myers Squibb
SQUIBB; 195	Tolazamide	100 mg	White	Tablet	Circle	Bristol-Myers Squibb
SQUIBB; 196	Ascorbic Acid	250 mg		Tablet		Bristol-Myers Squibb
SQUIBB; 202	Dicloxacillin Sodium	250 mg	Blue and White or Green and Light Green	Capsule		Bristol-Myers Squibb
SQUIBB; 203	Dicloxacillin Sodium	500 mg	Blue and White or Green and Light Green	Capsule		Bristol-Myers Squibb
SQUIBB; 211	Cloxacillin Sodium	250 mg		Capsule		Bristol-Myers Squibb
SQUIBB; 212	Cloxacillin Sodium	500 mg		Capsule		Bristol-Myers Squibb
SQUIBB; 230	Trimox	250 mg	Green	Capsule		Bristol-Myers Squibb
SQUIBB; 243	Corgard	100 mg		Tablet		Bristol-Myers Squibb
SQUIBB; 259	Perphenazine and Amitriptyline 2/25	2 mg ; 25 mg	Orange	Coated Tablet	Circle	Bristol-Myers Squibb
SQUIBB; 267	Perphenazine and Amitriptyline 4/10	10 mg ; 4 mg	Salmon	Coated Tablet	Circle	Bristol-Myers Squibb
SQUIBB; 271	Perphenazine and Amitriptyline 4/25	25 mg ; 4 mg	Yellow	Coated Tablet	Circle	Bristol-Myers Squibb
SQUIBB; 274	Trazodone	50 mg	White	Tablet	Circle	Bristol-Myers Squibb
SQUIBB; 275	Triamterene and Hydrochlorothiazide	25 mg ; 50 mg		Capsule		Bristol-Myers Squibb
SQUIBB; 277	Tolazamide	250 mg		Tablet		Bristol-Myers Squibb
SQUIBB; 279	Isosorbide Dinitrate	40 mg		Tablet		Bristol-Myers Squibb
SQUIBB; 280	Indomethacin	25 mg	Green	Capsule		Bristol-Myers Squibb
SQUIBB; 286	Quinidine Gluconate	324 mg	White	Sustained-Release Tablet	Circle	Bristol-Myers Squibb
SQUIBB; 289	Clonidine	0.1 mg		Tablet		Bristol-Myers Squibb
SQUIBB; 295	Indomethacin	50 mg	Green	Capsule		Bristol-Myers Squibb
SQUIBB; 297	Engran	1.5 mg ; 6000 U ; 400 U ; 3 mg ; 3 mg ; 2 mg ; 2 mcg ; 20 mg ; 5 mg ; 75 mg ; 100 mg ; 0.15 mg ; 45 mg ; 1 mg ; 1 mg	Blue	Tablet		Bristol-Myers Squibb
SQUIBB; 298	Lorazepam	0.5 mg	White	Tablet	Circle	Bristol-Myers Squibb
SQUIBB; 300	Prazosin Hydrochloride	1 mg		Capsule		Bristol-Myers Squibb
SQUIBB; 325	Trifluoperazine	10 mg	Lavender	Coated Tablet	Circle	Bristol-Myers Squibb
SQUIBB; 327	Triamterene and Hydrochlorothiazide	25 mg ; 50 mg		Tablet		Bristol-Myers Squibb
SQUIBB; 341	Theragran-Z	2 mg ; 22.5 mg ; 1 mg ; 0.6 mg ; 0.68 mg ; 200 mg ; 10 mg ; 10 mg ; 5 mg ; 5 mcg ; 12 mg ; 10000 IU ; 400 IU ; 15 mg ; 100 mg ; 20 mg ; 150 mcg	Brown	Tablet	Capsule-Shape	Bristol-Myers Squibb
SQUIBB; 348	Indomethacin SR	75 mg	Green and Clear	Capsule		Bristol-Myers Squibb
SQUIBB; 355	Valadol	325 mg	White	Tablet		Bristol-Myers Squibb
SQUIBB; 357	Valadol	120 mg	Yellow	Tablet, Chewable		Bristol-Myers Squibb
SQUIBB; 359	Furosemide	20 mg	White	Tablet	Oval	Bristol-Myers Squibb
SQUIBB; 360	Furosemide	40 mg	White	Tablet	Circle	Bristol-Myers Squibb
SQUIBB; 365	Trifluoperazine	1 mg	Lavender	Coated Tablet	Circle	Bristol-Myers Squibb
SQUIBB; 368	Trifluoperazine	2 mg	Lavender	Coated Tablet	Circle	Bristol-Myers Squibb
SQUIBB; 371	Digitoxin	0.1 mg		Tablet		Bristol-Myers Squibb
SQUIBB; 386	Carisoprodol	350 mg	White	Tablet	Circle	Bristol-Myers Squibb
SQUIBB; 399	Trifluoperazine	5 mg	Lavender	Coated Tablet	Circle	Bristol-Myers Squibb
SQUIBB; 400	Prazosin Hydrochloride	2 mg		Capsule		Bristol-Myers Squibb
SQUIBB; 408	Lorazepam	1 mg	White	Tablet	Circle	Bristol-Myers Squibb
SQUIBB; 433	Methyldopa	500 mg	White	Coated Tablet	Circle	Bristol-Myers Squibb
SQUIBB; 447	Methyldopa	250 mg	White	Coated Tablet	Circle	Bristol-Myers Squibb
SQUIBB; 457	Mycostatin	100000 U	Ivory	Tablet		Bristol-Myers Squibb

IMPRINT	BRAND/GENERIC NAME	STRENGTH	COLOR	FORM	SHAPE	MANUFACTURER
SQUIBB; 476 ;	Engram-Hp	30 mg ; 9 mg ; 4000 IU ; 200 IU ; 10 mg ; 0.4 mg ; 325 mg ; 75 mcg ; 50 mg ; 0.85 mg ; 1.25 mg ; 4 mcg		Tablet		Bristol-Myers Squibb
SQUIBB; 487	Lorazepam	2 mg	White	Tablet	Circle	Bristol-Myers Squibb
SQUIBB; 488	Metronidazole	250 mg	White	Tablet	Circle	Bristol-Myers Squibb
SQUIBB; 500	Prazosin Hydrochloride	5 mg		Capsule		Bristol-Myers Squibb
SQUIBB; 504	Kenacort	2 mg	White	Tablet		Bristol-Myers Squibb
SQUIBB; 511	Kenacort	1 mg	White	Tablet		Bristol-Myers Squibb
SQUIBB; 512	Kenacort	4 mg	White	Tablet		Bristol-Myers Squibb
SQUIBB; 518	Kenacort	8 mg	Yellow	Tablet		Bristol-Myers Squibb
SQUIBB; 520	B Complex with Vitamin C	10 mg ; 10 mg ; 2 mg ; 4 mcg ; 300 mg ; 100 mg		Tablet		Bristol-Myers Squibb
SQUIBB; 534	Clonidine	0.3 mg		Tablet		Bristol-Myers Squibb
SQUIBB; 538	Rautrax-N Modified	50 mg ; 2 mg ; 400 mg		Tablet		Bristol-Myers Squibb
SQUIBB; 539	Rautrax-N	400 mg ; 50 mg ; 4 mg		Tablet		Bristol-Myers Squibb
SQUIBB; 549	Iron with Vitamin C	50 mg ; 25 mg		Tablet		Bristol-Myers Squibb
SQUIBB; 560	Disopyramide	100 mg		Capsule		Bristol-Myers Squibb
SQUIBB; 567	Disopyramide	150 mg		Capsule		Bristol-Myers Squibb
SQUIBB; 572	Metronidazole	500 mg	White	Tablet	Oblong	Bristol-Myers Squibb
SQUIBB; 573	Ora-Testryl	5 mg		Tablet		Bristol-Myers Squibb
SQUIBB; 574	Oxazepam	10 mg		Capsule		Bristol-Myers Squibb
SQUIBB; 598	Neomycin Sulfate	350 mg		Tablet		Bristol-Myers Squibb
SQUIBB; 599	Oxazepam	15 mg		Capsule		Bristol-Myers Squibb
SQUIBB; 602	Naturetin with K	500 mg ; 2.5 mg		Tablet		Bristol-Myers Squibb
SQUIBB; 615	Propoxyphene Hydrochloride	65 mg	Green and Orange	Capsule		Bristol-Myers Squibb
SQUIBB; 619	Propoxyphene Hydrochloride and A.P.C.	227 mg ; 162 mg ; 32.4 mg ; 65 mg	Green and Gray	Capsule		Bristol-Myers Squibb
SQUIBB; 622	Meclofenamate	50 mg	Maroon and Pink	Capsule		Bristol-Myers Squibb
SQUIBB; 623	Noctec	250 mg	Red	Capsule		Bristol-Myers Squibb
SQUIBB; 626	Noctec	500 mg	Red	Capsule		Bristol-Myers Squibb
SQUIBB; 629	Meclofenamate	100 mg	Maroon and White	Capsule		Bristol-Myers Squibb
SQUIBB; 630	Methyldopa and Hydrochlorothiazide	250 mg ; 15 mg	Red	Coated Tablet	Circle	Bristol-Myers Squibb
SQUIBB; 637	Nydrazid	100 mg		Tablet		Bristol-Myers Squibb
SQUIBB; 645	Methyldopa and Hydrochlorothiazide	250 mg ; 25 mg	Pink	Coated Tablet	Circle	Bristol-Myers Squibb
SQUIBB; 649	Trigot	0.5 mg	White	Tablet		Bristol-Myers Squibb
SQUIBB; 652	Methyldopa and Hydrochlorothiazide	500 mg ; 30 mg	Red	Coated Tablet	Oval	Bristol-Myers Squibb
SQUIBB; 654	Trigot	1 mg	White	Tablet		Bristol-Myers Squibb
SQUIBB; 671	Methyldopa and Hydrochlorothiazide	50 mg ; 500 mg	Pink	Coated Tablet	Oval	Bristol-Myers Squibb
SQUIBB; 685	Rautrax	50 mg ; 400 mg ; 400 mg		Tablet		Bristol-Myers Squibb
SQUIBB; 692	Tolbutamide	500 mg	White	Tablet		Bristol-Myers Squibb
SQUIBB; 693 ;	Hydrochlorothiazide	25 mg	White	Tablet		Bristol-Myers Squibb
SQUIBB; 694 ;	Hydrochlorothiazide	50 mg	White	Tablet		Bristol-Myers Squibb
SQUIBB; 718	Chlordiazepoxide Hydrochloride	5 mg	Carmel and Yellow	Capsule		Bristol-Myers Squibb
SQUIBB; 723	Phenytoin Sodium	100 mg	White	Extended-Release Capsule		Bristol-Myers Squibb
SQUIBB; 727	Chlordiazepoxide Hydrochloride	10 mg	Carmel and Black	Capsule		Bristol-Myers Squibb
SQUIBB; 736	Chlordiazepoxide Hydrochloride	25 mg	Carmel and White	Capsule		Bristol-Myers Squibb
SQUIBB; 738	Temazepam	15 mg	Pink	Capsule		Bristol-Myers Squibb
SQUIBB; 749 ;	Cephalexin	250 mg	Swedish Orange and Gray	Capsule		Bristol-Myers Squibb
SQUIBB; 780	Rau-Sed	0.25 mg		Tablet		Bristol-Myers Squibb
SQUIBB; 788	Vitamin B-12	25 mcg		Capsule		Bristol-Myers Squibb
SQUIBB; 802	Clorazepate Dipotassium	3.75 mg	White	Capsule		Bristol-Myers Squibb
SQUIBB; 829	Chlorothiazide	500 mg	White	Tablet	Compressed	Bristol-Myers Squibb
SQUIBB; 831	Vitamin E	200 mg		Tablet		Bristol-Myers Squibb
SQUIBB; 838	Clorazepate	7.5 mg		Capsule		Bristol-Myers Squibb
SQUIBB; 845	Allopurinol	100 mg	White	Tablet	Circle	Bristol-Myers Squibb
SQUIBB; 849	Multiple Vitamins and Minerals	3 mg ; 22.5 mg ; 5000 IU ; 30 IU ; 500 mg ; 20 mg ; 20 mg ; 100 mg ; 25 mg ; 0.15 mg ; 25 mg ; 0.8 mg ; 50 mcg ; 27 mg ; 0.1 mg ; 50 mg ; 5 mg		Tablet		Bristol-Myers Squibb
SQUIBB; 851	Triamterene and Hydrochlorothiazide	75 mg ; 50 mg	Yellow	Tablet	Circle, Scored	Bristol-Myers Squibb
SQUIBB; 883	Doxycycline Hyclate	50 mg	White and Brown	Capsule, Liquid Filled		Bristol-Myers Squibb
SQUIBB; 884	Doxycycline Hyclate	100 mg	Brown	Capsule, Liquid Filled		Bristol-Myers Squibb
SQUIBB; 889	Vitamin E	74 mg		Capsule		Bristol-Myers Squibb
SQUIBB; 897	Doxycycline Hyclate	100 mg	Orange	Coated Tablet		Bristol-Myers Squibb
SQUIBB; 915	Vitamin B-1	50 mg		Tablet		Bristol-Myers Squibb
SQUIBB; 916	Vitamin B-1	100 mg		Tablet		Bristol-Myers Squibb
SQUIBB; 921	Vesprin	10 mg	Pink	Tablet		Bristol-Myers Squibb
SQUIBB; 922	Vesprin	25 mg	White and Orange	Tablet		Bristol-Myers Squibb
SQUIBB; 923	Vesprin	50 mg	Green	Tablet		Bristol-Myers Squibb
SQUIBB; 963	Trazodone	100 mg		Tablet		Bristol-Myers Squibb
SQUIBB; 1535	Loxapine Succinate	50 mg		Capsule		Bristol-Myers Squibb

IMPRINT	BRAND/GENERIC NAME	STRENGTH	COLOR	FORM	SHAPE	MANUFACTURER
SQUIBB; E.T.	E.T. the Extraterrestrial Children's Chewable Vitamins	60 mg ; 2 mg ; 6 mcg ; 5000 IU ; 400 IU ; 30 IU ; 0.4 mg ; 1.5 mg ; 1.7 mg ; 20 mg	Purple, Orange and Pink	Tablet, Chewable		Bristol-Myers Squibb
SQUIBB; E.T.	E.T. the Extraterrestrial Children's Chewable Vitamins with Iron	5000 IU ; 400 IU ; 30 IU ; 0.4 mg ; 1.5 mg ; 1.7 mg ; 20 mg ; 18 mg ; 60 mg ; 2 mg ; 6 mcg	Purple, Orange and Pink	Tablet, Chewable		Bristol-Myers Squibb
SQUIBB; W048	Dicloxacillin Sodium	250 mg		Capsule		Bristol-Myers Squibb
SQUIBB; W058	Dicloxacillin Sodium	500 mg		Capsule		Bristol-Myers Squibb
SQUIBB; W134	Lithium Carbonate	300 mg		Capsule		Bristol-Myers Squibb
SQUIBB; W460	Desipramine Hydrochloride	50 mg		Tablet		Bristol-Myers Squibb
SQUIBB; W470	Desipramine Hydrochloride	75 mg		Tablet		Bristol-Myers Squibb
ST ; PP	Verapamil Hydrochloride	240 mg	Light Green	Tablet, Extended Release	Capsule-Shape	Ranbaxy Pharmaceuticals
STARLIX; 60	Starlix	60 mg	Pink	Tablet	Circle, Bevel Edged	Novartis
STARLIX; 120	Starlix	120 mg	Yellow	Tablet	Oval	Novartis
STUART	Orexin Softab	10 mg ; 5 mg ; 25 mcg	Pink	Tablet	Circle, Biconvex	Johnson & Johnson Merck Consumer Pharmaceuticals
STUART; 380	Kasof	240 mg	Brown	Capsule		Johnson & Johnson Merck Consumer Pharmaceuticals
STUART; 450	Mylicon	40 mg	White	Tablet	Circle, Biconvex	Johnson & Johnson Merck Consumer Pharmaceuticals
STUART; 650	Ferancee	150 mg ; 3.1 Gr	Brown and Gold	Tablet, Chewable		Johnson & Johnson Merck Consumer Pharmaceuticals
STUART; 851	Mylanta II	40 mg ; 400 mg ; 400 mg	Green and White	Tablet, Chewable		Johnson & Johnson Merck Consumer Pharmaceuticals
STUART; 858	Mylicon 80	80 mg	Pink	Tablet, Chewable	Circle, Beveled	Johnson & Johnson Merck Consumer Pharmaceuticals
STUARTNATAL LOGO	Duet Dha - Dha Softgel Capsule	400 mg	Translucent Gold	Capsule, Liquid Filled	Oval	Xanodyne Pharmaceuticals
STUARTNATAL LOGO	Duet Dha Ec - Dha Softgel Capsule	400 mg	Frosted Gold	Capsule, Liquid Filled	Oval	Xanodyne Pharmaceuticals
SUPRAX; LL; 200	Suprax	200 mg	White	Coated Tablet	Rectangle, Scored, Convex	Lederle Laboratories
SUPRAX; LL; 400	Suprax	400 mg	White	Coated Tablet	Rectangle, Scored, Convex	Lederle Laboratories
SUSTIVA; 50 MG	Sustiva	50 mg	Gold and White	Capsule		Bristol-Myers Squibb
SUSTIVA; 200 MG	Sustiva	200 mg	Gold	Capsule		Bristol-Myers Squibb
SUSTIVA; SUSTIVA	Sustiva	600 mg	Yellow	Coated Tablet	Capsule-Shape	Bristol-Myers Squibb
SW; 200	Skelid	200 mg	White to Off-White	Tablet	Circle	Sanofi-Aventis U.S.
SX	Xifaxan	200 mg	Pink	Tablet	Circle	Salix Pharmaceuticals
SYNTEX	Norminest Fe-28 Blue Tablet	0.5 mg ; 0.035 mg	Blue	28-Day Tablet Pack		Roche Laboratories
SYNTEX; 2902	Anadrol	50 mg	White	Tablet		Roche Laboratories
SYNTEX; TORADOL; T	Toradol Oral	10 mg		Coated Tablet	Circle	Roche Laboratories
SYNTHROID; 25 ;	Synthroid	25 mcg	Orange	Tablet		Abbott Laboratories
SYNTHROID; 50 ;	Synthroid	50 mcg	White	Tablet		Abbott Laboratories
SYNTHROID; 75 ;	Synthroid	75 mcg	Violet	Tablet		Abbott Laboratories
SYNTHROID; 88 ;	Synthroid	88 mcg	Olive	Tablet	Circle, Scored	Abbott Laboratories
SYNTHROID; 100 ;	Synthroid	100 mcg	Yellow	Tablet		Abbott Laboratories
SYNTHROID; 112 ;	Synthroid	112 mcg	Rose	Tablet		Abbott Laboratories
SYNTHROID; 125 ;	Synthroid	125 mcg	Brown	Tablet		Abbott Laboratories
SYNTHROID; 137	Synthroid	137 mcg	Turquoise	Tablet		Abbott Laboratories
SYNTHROID; 150 ;	Synthroid	150 mcg	Blue	Tablet		Abbott Laboratories
SYNTHROID; 175	Synthroid	175 mcg	Lilac	Tablet		Abbott Laboratories
SYNTHROID; 200 ;	Synthroid	200 mcg	Pink	Tablet		Abbott Laboratories
SYNTHROID; 300 ;	Synthroid	300 mcg	Green	Tablet		Abbott Laboratories
SZ 183	Cafergot	1 mg ; 100 mg	Beige	Tablet	Circle	Novartis Pharmaceuticals
T	Potassium Bicarbonate	25 meq	Orange	Effervescent Tablet	Circle	Watson Laboratories
T	Tessalon Perles	100 mg	Yellow	Capsule		Forest Pharmaceuticals
T 25	Tarceva	25 mg	White	Tablet	Circle	Osi Pharmaceuticals
T 100	Tarceva	100 mg	White	Tablet	Circle	Genentech
T 150	Tarceva	150 mg	White	Tablet	Circle	Genentech
T; 93	Isoniazid	100 mg		Tablet		Eli Lilly
T; 107	Tenormin	25 mg	White	Tablet	Circle, Flat	Astrazeneca
T; 109	Carbamazepine	200 mg	White	Tablet	Circle	Teva Pharmaceuticals
T0R; ORGANON	Cyclessa Light Yellow Tablet	0.025 mg ; 0.1 mg	Light Yellow	Coated Tablet	Circle	Organon
T1R; ORGANON	Cyclessa Red Tablet	0.15 mg ; 0.025 mg	Red	Coated Tablet	Circle	Organon
T6R; ORGANON	Cyclessa Orange Tablet	0.125 mg ; 0.025 mg	Orange	Coated Tablet	Circle	Organon
T7 ; M	Tramadol Hydrochloride	50 mg	White	Tablet	Circle	Mylan Pharmaceuticals
T36	Calcium Gluconate	1 GM		Tablet		Eli Lilly
TAGAMET; 200; SKF	Tagamet	200 mg	Light-Green	Coated Tablet	Circle	Glaxosmithkline
TAGAMET; 800; SB	Tagamet	800 mg	Light-Green	Coated Tablet	Oval	Glaxosmithkline
TAK RAM-8	Rozerem	8 mg	Pale Orange-Yellow	Tablet	Circle	Takeda Pharmaceuticals
TAP LOGO PREVACID 30 ;	Prevacid	30 mg	Black, Opaquepink	Capsule, Delayed Release		Takeda Pharmaceuticals
TAP LOGO; PREVACID 15	Prevacid Naprapac 375 - Prevacid	15 mg	Green, Pink	Capsule, Delayed Release		Takeda Pharmaceuticals
TAP LOGO; PREVACID 15	Prevacid Naprapac 500 - Prevacid	15 mg	Green, Pink	Capsule, Delayed Release		Takeda Pharmaceuticals
TAP; 200 MG	Spectracef	200 mg	White with Blue Ink	Coated Tablet	Circle	Tap Pharmaceuticals
TAPLOGO PREVACID 15 ;	Prevacid	15 mg	Green, Pink	Capsule, Delayed Release		Takeda Pharmaceuticals
TARACTAN; ROCHE 10	Taractan	10 mg	Light Coral	Coated Tablet		Roche Pharmaceuticals
TARACTAN; ROCHE 25	Taractan	25 mg	Coral	Coated Tablet		Roche Pharmaceuticals
TARACTAN; ROCHE 50	Taractan	50 mg	Pinkish Orange	Coated Tablet		Roche Pharmaceuticals

IMPRINT	BRAND/GENERIC NAME	STRENGTH	COLOR	FORM	SHAPE	MANUFACTURER
TARACTAN; ROCHE 100	Taractan	100 mg	Reddish Brown	Coated Tablet		Roche Pharmaceuticals
TARGRETIN	Targretin	75 mg	Off-White	Capsule	Oblong	Eisai
TARKA; 182; KNOLL TRIANGLE ;	Tarka 2/180 mg	180 mg ; 2 mg	Pink	Sustained-Release Tablet	Oval	Abbott Laboratories
TARKA; 241; KNOLL TRIANGLE ;	Tarka 1/240 mg	1 mg ; 240 mg	White	Sustained-Release Tablet	Oval	Abbott Laboratories
TARKA; 242; KNOLL TRIANGLE ;	Tarka 2/240 mg	2 mg ; 240 mg	Gold	Sustained-Release Tablet	Oval	Abbott Laboratories
TARKA; 244; KNOLL TRIANGLE ;	Tarka 4/240 mg	4 mg ; 240 mg	Red-Brown	Sustained-Release Tablet	Oval	Abbott Laboratories
TAVIST; 78/72 ;	Tavist	2.68 mg	White	Tablet	Circle, Scored	Novartis Pharmaceuticals
TEGISON; 10; ROCHE	Tegison	10 mg	Brown and Green	Capsule	Oval	Roche Pharmaceuticals
TEGISON; 25; ROCHE	Tegison	25 mg	Brown and Caramel	Capsule	Oval	Roche Pharmaceuticals
TEGRETOL ; 27 27 ;	Tegretol	200 mg	Pink	Tablet	Capsule-Shape	Novartis
TEGRETOL ; 52 52 ;	Tegretol	100 mg	Pink, Red Speckled	Tablet, Chewable	Circle	Novartis
TEMOZOLOMIDE 5 MG SP	Temodar	5 mg	White	Capsule		Schering
TEMOZOLOMIDE; 20 MG; SP	Temodar	20 mg	Off-White with Brown Ink	Capsule		Schering
TEMOZOLOMIDE; 100 MG; SP	Temodar	100 mg	Off-White with Blue Ink	Capsule		Schering
TEMOZOLOMIDE; 250 MG; SP	Temodar	250 mg	Off-White with Black Ink	Capsule		Schering
TEN K	Ten-K	750 mg	White	Timed-Release Tablet	Capsule-Shape, Scored	Novartis
TENEX ; 1 RP	Tenex	1 mg	Light Pink	Tablet	Diamond	A.H. Robins
TENORETIC; 115	Tenoretic 50	25 mg ; 50 mg	White	Tablet	Round, Biconvex, Bisected Scored	Astrazeneca
TENORETIC; 117 ;	Tenoretic 100	25 mg ; 100 mg	White	Tablet	Circle, Biconvex	Astrazeneca
TENORMIN; 101	Tenormin	100 mg	White	Tablet	Circle, Flat	Astrazeneca
TENORMIN; 105	Tenormin	50 mg	White	Tablet	Round, Flat, Bisected Scored	Astrazeneca
TENUATE; 25	Tenuate	25 mg	White	Tablet	Circle	Sanofi-Aventis U.S.
TENUATE; 75	Tenuate Dospan	75 mg	White	Tablet, Extended Release	Capsule-Shape	Sanofi-Aventis U.S.
TH; 0; RJS ;	Westhroid	32.4 mg	Tan	Tablet	Round, Compressed, Bisected Scored	Western Research Laboratories
TH; 1; RJS ;	Westhroid	64.8 mg	Tan	Tablet	Round, Compressed, Bisected Scored	Western Research Laboratories
TH; 2; RJS ;	Westhroid	130 mg	Tan	Tablet	Circle, Compressed	Western Research Laboratories
TH; A	Cylert	18.75 mg	White	Tablet	Monogrammed, Grooved	Abbott Laboratories
THEO-24; 100 MG; UCB; 2832 ;	Theo-24	100 mg	Yellow-Orange and Clear	Extended-Release Capsule		UCB Pharma
THEO-24; 200 MG; UCB; 2842 ;	Theo-24	200 mg	Red-Orange and Clear	Extended-Release Capsule		UCB Pharma
THEO-24; 300 MG; UCB; 2852 ;	Theo-24	300 mg	Red and Clear	Extended-Release Capsule		UCB Pharma
THEO-24; 400 MG; UCB; 2902 ;	Theo-24	400 mg	Pink and Clear	Extended-Release Capsule		UCB Pharma
THEO-BID; 260	Theo-Bid Duracap	260 mg	Clear	Extended-Release Capsule		UCB Pharma
THEOBID; 130 ;	Theobid Duracap JR.	130 mg	Clear with White Beads	Capsule		UCB Pharma
THEOBID; 260 ;	Theobid Duracap	260 mg	Clear with White Beads	Capsule		UCB Pharma
THEOPHYL	Theophyl-SR	250 mg	Green and Clear	Timed-Release Capsule		Mcneil Pharmaceutical
THEOPHYL; 100	Theophyl Chewable	100 mg	White	Tablet, Chewable	Circle	Mcneil Pharmaceutical
THEOPHYL; 125	Theophyl-SR	125 mg	Yellow and Clear	Timed-Release Capsule		Mcneil Pharmaceutical
THEOPHYL; 225	Theophyl-225	225 mg	White	Tablet	Triangle, Scored	Mcneil Pharmaceutical
THER-RX ; 195	Precare Premier	15 mg ; 50 mg ; 6 mcg ; 3.5 IU ; 3 mg ; 3.4 mg ; 20 mg ; 50 mg ; 1 mg ; 12 mcg ; 250 mcg ; 30 mg ; 35 mg ; 25 mg ; 2 mg ; 50 mg	Peach	Tablet		Ther-RX
THER-RX 148	Encora - AM and Pm	100 mg ; 10 mg ; 50 IU ; 650 mg ; 550 mg	Pink	Capsule, Liquid Filled		Ther-RX
THER-RX 200	Primacare One	30 mg ; 30 mg ; 25 mg ; 170 IU ; 30 IU ; 1 mg ; 25 mg ; 150 mg ; 20 mg ; 7 mg ; 300 mg	Purple	Capsule, Liquid Filled		Ther-RX
THER-RX 218	Primacare One	7 mg ; 150 mcg ; 50 mg ; 5 mg ; 50 mg ; 500 mg ; 25 mg ; 800 IU ; 15 IU ; 1.5 mg ; 10 mg ; 50 mg ; 1 mg ; 300 mcg ; 100 mg ; 20 mg	Purple	Capsule, Liquid Filled		Ther-RX
THER-RX 220	Primacare Advantage - AM Dose	650 mg ; 10 mg ; 50 IU	Opaque Pink	Capsule, Liquid Filled	Oval	Ther-RX
THER-RX; 014	Precare Conceive	60 mg ; 200 mg ; 30 mg ; 30 IU ; 3 mg ; 3.4 mg ; 20 mg ; 50 mg ; 1 mg ; 100 mg ; 12 mcg ; 15 mg ; 2 mg	Yellow	Coated Tablet	Diamond	Ther-RX

IMPRINT	BRAND/GENERIC NAME	STRENGTH	COLOR	FORM	SHAPE	MANUFACTURER
THER-RX; 019	Premesis RX	75 mg ; 12 mcg ; 1 mg ; 200 mg	Blue	Tablet	Oval	Ther-RX
THER-RX; 025	Precare	250 mg ; 40 mg ; 3.5 mg ; 6 mcg ; 3 mg ; 3.4 mg ; 20 mg ; 20 mg ; 1 mg ; 12 mcg ; 50 mg ; 15 mg ; 2 mg ; 50 mg	Peach	Tablet	Coated, Partially Bisected Scored	Ther-RX
THER-RX; 128	Strongstart	225 mg ; 40 mg ; 30 IU ; 15 mg ; 7 mg ; 1 mg ; 12 mg ; 35 mg ; 2 mg ; 75 mcg ; 45 mcg ; 50 mcg ; 30 mg ; 25 mg ; 400 IU ; 3 mg ; 3.4 mg ; 400 IU ; 90 mcg ; 20 mg ; 50 mg	White	Tablet	Oval	Ther-RX
THER-RX; 137	Strongstart	250 mg ; 50 mg ; 35 mg ; 3.5 mg ; 15 mg ; 50 mg ; 1 mg ; 6 mcg ; 2 mg ; 10 mg	Orange	Tablet, Chewable		Ther-RX
THX 164	Niferex-150 Forte	1 mg ; 25 mcg ; 50 mg ; 100 mg ; 50 mg ; 60 mg ; 0.8 mg	Clear, Red	Capsule		Ther-RX
THX; 024	Precare	3.5 mg ; 1 mg ; 50 mg ; 15 mg ; 2 mg ; 50 mg ; 2 mg ; 250 mg ; 40 mg ; 6 mcg	Orange Speckled	Tablet, Chewable	Circle	Ther-RX
TI 01 LOGO	Spiriva	18 mcg	Light Green	Capsule		Pfizer
TI; A	Cylert	37.5 mg	Orange	Tablet	Monogrammed, Grooved	Abbott Laboratories
TIAZAC; 120	Tiazac	120 mg	Lavender	Extended-Release Capsule		Forest Pharmaceuticals
TIAZAC; 180	Tiazac	180 mg	White and Blue-Green	Extended-Release Capsule		Forest Pharmaceuticals
TIAZAC; 240	Tiazac	240 mg	Blue-Green and Lavender	Extended-Release Capsule		Forest Pharmaceuticals
TIAZAC; 300	Tiazac	300 mg	White and Lavender	Extended-Release Capsule		Forest Pharmaceuticals
TIAZAC; 360	Tiazac	360 mg	Blue-Green	Extended-Release Capsule		Forest Pharmaceuticals
TIAZAC; 420	Tiazac	420 mg	White	Extended-Release Capsule		Forest Pharmaceuticals
TIGAN; M079	Tigan	300 mg	Purple	Capsule		Monarch Pharmaceuticals
TJ; A	Cylert	75 mg	Tan	Tablet	Monogrammed, Grooved	Abbott Laboratories
TK; A	Cylert	37.5 mg	Orange	Tablet, Chewable	Monogrammed, Grooved	Abbott Laboratories
TL; 001	Methylprednisolone	4 mg	White	Tablet	Oval, Quadrisected Scored	Ranbaxy Pharmaceuticals
TL; 113	Prochlorperazine Maleate	5 mg	Yellow-Green	Tablet	Circle, Scored	Par Pharmaceutical
TL; 115	Prochlorperazine Maleate	10 mg	Light Green	Tablet	Circle, Scored	Par Pharmaceutical
TMC114 ; 300	Prezista	300 mg	Orange	Tablet	Oval	Tibotec Therapeutics
TO	Detrol	1 mg	White	Tablet	Circle	Pharmacia & Upjohn
TO 60	Fareston	60 mg	White to Off-White	Tablet	Circle	Schering
TOLECTIN DS; MCNEIL	Tolectin DS	400 mg	Orange	Capsule		Ortho-Mcneil Pharmaceutical
TOLECTIN; 200; MCNEIL	Tolectin	200 mg	White	Tablet		Ortho-Mcneil Pharmaceutical
TOLECTIN; 600; MCNEIL	Tolectin 600	600 mg	Orange	Tablet	Oval	Ortho-Mcneil Pharmaceutical
TOLINASE; 100	Tolinase	100 mg	White	Tablet	Circle, Scored	Pharmacia & Upjohn
TOLINASE; 250 ;	Tolinase	250 mg	White	Tablet	Circle, Scored	Pharmacia & Upjohn
TOLINASE; 500 ;	Tolinase	500 mg	White	Tablet	Circle, Scored	Pharmacia & Upjohn
TONOCARD; 707	Tonocard	400 mg	Yellow	Coated Tablet	Oval, Scored	Astrazeneca
TONOCARD; 709	Tonocard	600 mg	Yellow	Coated Tablet	Scored, Oblong	Astrazeneca
TOP; 15 MG	Topamax Sprinkle Capsule	15 mg	White and Clear with White Spheres	Capsule		Ortho-Mcneil Pharmaceutical
TOP; 25 MG	Topamax Sprinkle Capsule	25 mg	White and Clear with White Spheres	Capsule		Ortho-Mcneil Pharmaceutical
TORADOL; ROCHE	Toradol	10 mg	White	Tablet	Circle	Roche Laboratories
TPV 250	Aptivus	250 mg	Pink	Capsule, Liquid Filled	Oblong	Boehringer Ingelheim Pharmaceuticals
TR 50 ; G	Tambocor	50 mg	White	Tablet	Circle	Graceway Pharmaceuticals
TR 100 ; G	Tambocor	100 mg	White	Tablet	Circle	Graceway Pharmaceuticals
TR 125 G	Triazolam	0.125 mg	White	Tablet	Oblong	Mylan Pharmaceuticals
TR 150 ; G	Tambocor	150 mg	White	Tablet	Oval	Graceway Pharmaceuticals
TR 250 G	Triazolam	0.25 mg	Pale Yellow	Tablet	Oblong	Mylan Pharmaceuticals
TR; 125; G	Triazolam	0.125 mg	White	Tablet	Oval	Par Pharmaceutical
TR; 250; G	Triazolam	0.25 mg	Pale Yellow	Tablet	Oval, Scored	Par Pharmaceutical
TRANDATE; 100	Trandate	100 mg	Orange	Coated Tablet	Circle, Scored	Glaxosmithkline
TRANDATE; 200	Trandate	200 mg	White	Coated Tablet	Circle, Scored	Glaxosmithkline
TRANDATE; 300	Trandate	300 mg	Peach	Coated Tablet	Circle, Scored	Glaxosmithkline
TRANSDERM-NITRO; 0.1 MG/HR	Transderm-Nitro	0.1 mg/hr	Tan	Patch	Circle	Novartis Generics
TRANSDERM-NITRO; 0.2 MG/HR	Transderm-Nitro	0.2 mg/hr	Tan	Patch	Oblong	Novartis Generics
TRANSDERM-NITRO; 0.4 MG/HR	Transderm-Nitro	0.4 mg/hr	Tan	Patch	Oblong	Novartis Generics
TRANSDERM-NITRO; 0.6 MG/HR	Transderm-Nitro	0.6 mg/hr	Tan	Patch	Oblong	Novartis Generics
TRANSDERM-NITRO; 0.8 MG/HR	Transderm-Nitro	0.8 mg/hr	Tan	Patch	Circle	Novartis Generics

IMPRINT	BRAND/GENERIC NAME	STRENGTH	COLOR	FORM	SHAPE	MANUFACTURER
TRENTAL	Trental	400 mg	Pink	Tablet, Extended Release	Oblong	Sanofi-Aventis U.S.
TRIAD; UAD; 305	Triad	325 mg ; 50 mg ; 40 mg	White	Capsule		Uad Laboratories
TRIANGLE; 516	Benazepril Hydrochloride	5 mg	Light Orange	Tablet	Circle	Watson Pharma
TRIANGLE; 517	Benazepril Hydrochloride	10 mg	Orange	Tablet	Circle	Watson Pharma
TRIANGLE; 518	Benazepril Hydrochloride	20 mg	Peach	Tablet	Circle	Watson Pharma
TRIANGLE; 519	Benazepril Hydrochloride	40 mg	Orange-Red	Tablet	Circle	Watson Pharma
TRIANGLE; 521; 3	Acetaminophen and Codeine Phosphate	300 mg ; 15 mg	White	Tablet	Circle, Scored	Andrx Pharmaceuticals
TRIANGLE; 522; 3	Acetaminophen and Codeine Phosphate	300 mg ; 30 mg	White	Tablet	Circle	Watson Pharma
TRIANGLE; 523; 4	Acetaminophen and Codeine Phosphate	300 mg ; 60 mg	White	Tablet	Circle	Watson Pharma
TRIANGLE; 756	Benazepril Hydrochloride and Hydrochlorothiazide	5 mg ; 6.25 mg	White	Tablet		Andrx Pharmaceuticals
TRIANGLE; 757	Benazepril Hydrochloride and Hydrochlorothiazide	10 mg ; 12.5 mg	Purple	Tablet		Andrx Pharmaceuticals
TRIANGLE; 758	Benazepril Hydrochloride and Hydrochlorothiazide	12.5 mg ; 20 mg	Pink	Tablet		Andrx Pharmaceuticals
TRIANGLE; 759	Benazepril Hydrochloride and Hydrochlorothiazide	25 mg ; 20 mg	Red	Tablet		Andrx Pharmaceuticals
TRIANGLE; 791	Lovastatin	10 mg	White to Off-White	Tablet	Circle	Watson Pharma
TRIANGLE; 792	Lovastatin	20 mg	White to Off-White	Tablet	Circle	Watson Pharma
TRIANGLE; 793	Lovastatin	40 mg	White to Off-White	Tablet	Circle	Watson Pharma
TRIMPEX; 100; ROCHE	Trimpex	100 mg	White	Tablet	Circle, Scored	Roche Pharmaceuticals
TRIMPEX; 100; ROCHE	Trimpex	100 mg	White	Tablet	Oval, Scored	Roche Laboratories
TRINSICON-M; GLAXO	Trinsicon M	240 mg ; 15 mcg ; 75 mg ; 110 mg	Dark Pink and Dark Red	Capsule		Glaxosmithkline
TRITEC; STOMACH-SHAPED LOGO	Tritec	400 mg	Blue	Coated Tablet	Eight-Sided, Elongated	Glaxosmithkline
TTC; 091	Anaplex SR	8 mg ; 120 mg	Blue and Clear	Sustained-Release Capsule		Ecr Pharmaceuticals
TUMS	Tums Anti-Gas/antacid	500 mg ; 20 mg	Assorted	Tablet	Circle	Glaxosmithkline Consumer
TY; A	Tranxene-Sd	22.5 mg	Peach	Extended-Release Tablet	Circle	Abbott Laboratories
TYLENOL CODEINE 3 ; MCNEIL ;	Tylenol with Codeine No. 3	300 mg ; 30 mg	White	Tablet	Circle	Mcneil Pharmaceutical
TYLENOL; CODEINE; 2	Tylenol with Codeine No. 2	300 mg ; 15 mg	White	Tablet	Circle	Mcneil Pharmaceutical
TYLENOL; CODEINE; 4 ;	Tylenol with Codeine No. 4	300 mg ; 60 mg	White	Tablet	Circle	Mcneil Pharmaceutical
TYLENOL; COLD	Tylenol Cold Multi-Symptom	325 mg ; 2 mg ; 30 mg ; 15 mg	Light Yellow	Tablet		Mcneil Consumer Healthcare Division of Mcneil
TYLENOL; COLD	Tylenol Cold Multi-Symptom	325 mg ; 2 mg ; 30 mg ; 15 mg	Yellow	Tablet	Circle	Mcneil Consumer Healthcare Division of Mcneil
TYLENOL; COLD; DM; 80	Children's Tylenol Cold DM	0.5 mg ; 80 mg ; 3.75 mg ; 7.5 mg		Tablet, Chewable	Flat-Faced, Beveled	Mcneil Consumer Healthcare Division of Mcneil
TYLOX; MCNEIL	Tylox	5 mg ; 500 mg	Red	Capsule		Ortho-Mcneil Pharmaceutical
TZ; 1	Remeron Soltab	15 mg	White	Tablet, Disintegrating	Circle	Organon
TZ; 2	Remeron Soltab	30 mg	White	Tablet	Circle	Organon
TZ; 4	Remeron Soltab	45 mg	White	Tablet	Circle	Organon
TZ5 ; ORGANON	Remeron	30 mg	Red-Brown	Tablet	Oval	Organon
U	Colestid	1 GM	Yellow	Coated Tablet	Circle	Pharmacia & Upjohn
U	Unicap	1.7 mg ; 20 mg ; 2 mg ; 6 mcg ; 5000 IU ; 400 IU ; 15 IU ; 60 mg ; 0.4 mg ; 1.5 mg	Yellow	Capsule		Upjohn
U	Unicap M	15 mg ; 1 mg ; 5 mg ; 5000 IU ; 400 IU ; 15 IU ; 60 mg ; 0.4 mg ; 1.5 mg ; 1.7 mg ; 20 mg ; 2 mg ; 6 mcg ; 10 mg ; 150 mcg ; 18 mg ; 2 mg	Tan	Tablet		Johnson & Johnson Consumer Products
U	Unicap M Plus Iron	5 mg ; 35 mg ; 1.5 mg ; 10 mcg ; 2.5 mg ; 2.5 mg ; 50 mg ; 20 mg ; 0.5 mg ; 5 mg ; 2 mcg ; 10 IU ; 50 mg ; 0.15 mg ; 1 mg ; 1 mg ; 6 mg	Tan	Coated Tablet		Upjohn
U	Unicap Plus Iron	1.5 mg ; 1.7 mg ; 20 mg ; 10 mg ; 60 mg ; 2 mg ; 6 mcg ; 18 mg ; 5000 IU ; 400 IU ; 15 IU ; 0.4 mg	Red	Coated Tablet		Upjohn
U	Unicap Senior	15 mg ; 1 mg ; 5 mg ; 60 mg ; 2 mg ; 6 mcg ; 10 mg ; 5000 IU ; 15 IU ; 0.4 mg ; 1.2 mg ; 1.7 mg ; 14 mg ; 10 mg ; 150 mcg ; 2 mg	Blue	Tablet		Johnson & Johnson Consumer Products
U; 26 ;	Sandril	0.25 mg	Green	Tablet		Eli Lilly
U; 60	Keflex	1 GM	Green	Tablet		Eli Lilly
U; 94 ;	Xanax	2 mg	White	Tablet	Oblong	Pharmacia & Upjohn
U; 201 ;	Lorcet Plus	650 mg ; 7.5 mg	White	Tablet	Capsule-Shape, Scored	Uad Laboratories

IMPRINT	BRAND/GENERIC NAME	STRENGTH	COLOR	FORM	SHAPE	MANUFACTURER
U; 3617	Vantin	100 mg	Light Orange	Tablet	Circle	Pharmacia & Upjohn
U; 3618	Vantin	200 mg	Coral Red	Tablet	Circle	Pharmacia & Upjohn
U; 3761	Rescriptor	100 mg	White	Tablet	Capsule-Shape	Agouron Pharmaceuticals
U-S 147 ; P200	Pacerone	200 mg	Pink	Tablet	Circle	Upsher-Smith Laboratories
U-S 180 ;	Divalproex Sodium	125 mg	Rose	Tablet, Delayed Release	Capsule-Shape	Upsher-Smith Laboratories
U-S 181 ;	Divalproex Sodium	250 mg	Peach	Tablet, Delayed Release	Capsule-Shape	Upsher-Smith Laboratories
U-S 182 ;	Divalproex Sodium	500 mg	Light Pink	Tablet, Delayed Release	Capsule-Shape	Upsher-Smith Laboratories
U-S 144 ; P	Pacerone	100 mg	White	Tablet	Circle	Upsher-Smith Laboratories
UAD; 111	E-Lor	650 mg ; 65 mg	Orange	Tablet	Capsule-Shape, Film-Coated	Uad Laboratories
UAD; 400	Eudal-SR	120 mg ; 400 mg	White	Sustained-Release Tablet	Capsule-Shape, Scored	Uad Laboratories
UAD; 1120	Lorcet-HD	5 mg ; 500 mg	Maroon	Capsule		Uad Laboratories
UAD; 2304	Dital	105 mg	Lavender and Clear	Extended-Release Capsule		Uad Laboratories
UAD; 2404	Vertab	50 mg	Opaque Blue	Capsule		Uad Laboratories
UAD; 6350	Lorcet 10/650	10 mg ; 650 mg	Light Blue	Tablet	Capsule-Shape	Uad Laboratories
UAD; CEZIN S; 811	Cezin-S	50 IU ; 200 mg ; 50 mg ; 10 mg ; 10 mg ; 5 mg ; 4 mg ; 2 mg ; 80 mg ; 0.5 mg ; 70 mg ; 10000 IU ; 50 IU	Yellow	Capsule		Uad Laboratories
UAD; ENDAFED; 206	Endafed	120 mg ; 12 mg	Blue and Clear	Sustained-Release Capsule		Uad Laboratories
UC ABBOTT LOGO	Prosom	1 mg	White	Tablet		Abbott Laboratories
UCB 500XR	Keppra Xr	500 mg	White	Tablet, Extended Release	Oblong	UCB Pharma
UCB 579 10 MG	Metadate Cd	10 mg	Green, White	Capsule, Extended Release		UCB Pharma
UCB 580 20 MG	Metadate Cd	20 mg	Blue, White	Capsule, Extended Release		UCB Pharma
UCB 581 30 MG	Metadate Cd	30 mg	Reddish-Brown, White	Capsule, Extended Release		UCB Pharma
UCB 582 40 MG	Metadate Cd	40 mg	White, Yellow Ivory	Capsule, Extended Release		UCB Pharma
UCB 583 50 MG	Metadate Cd	50 mg	Purple, White	Capsule, Extended Release		UCB Pharma
UCB 584 60 MG	Metadate Cd	60 mg	White	Capsule, Extended Release		UCB Pharma
UCB; 250	Keppra	250 mg	Blue	Coated Tablet	Oblong, Scored	UCB Pharma
UCB; 250	Keppra	250 mg	Blue	Coated Tablet	Scored, Oblong	UCB Pharma
UCB; 364 ;	Trinsicon	110 mg ; 15 mcg ; 75 mg ; 0.5 mg ; 240 mg	Dark Pink and Dark Red	Capsule		UCB Pharma
UCB; 500	Keppra	500 mg	Yellow	Coated Tablet	Oblong, Scored	UCB Pharma
UCB; 500 ;	Lortab Asa	5 mg ; 500 mg	Dark Pink	Tablet	Capsule-Shape	UCB Pharma
UCB; 612 ;	Duratuss	120 mg ; 600 mg	White	Extended-Release Tablet	Oval, Scored	UCB Pharma
UCB; 620 ;	Duratuss G	1200 mg	White	Extended-Release Tablet	Capsule-Shape, Scored	UCB Pharma
UCB; 640	Duratuss Gp	1200 mg ; 120 mg	White	Extended-Release Tablet	Oval, Coated, Scored	UCB Pharma
UCB; 750	Keppra	750 mg	Orange	Coated Tablet	Oblong, Scored	UCB Pharma
UCB; 901 ;	Lortab 2.5/500	500 mg ; 2.5 mg	White with Pink Specks	Tablet	Capsule-Shaped, Bisected Scored	UCB Pharma
UCB; 902 ;	Lortab 5/500	500 mg ; 5 mg	White with Blue Specks	Tablet	Capsule-Shaped, Bisected Scored	UCB Pharma
UCB; 903 ;	Lortab 7.5/500	7.5 mg ; 500 mg	White with Green Specks	Tablet	Capsule-Shaped; Bisected Scored	UCB Pharma
UCB; 910 ;	Lortab 10/500	500 mg ; 10 mg	Pink	Tablet	Capsule-Shape	UCB Pharma
UCBB; 316 ;	Vicon Forte	80 mg ; 10 mcg ; 10 mg ; 2 mg ; 4 mg ; 1 mg ; 150 mg ; 10 mg ; 70 mg ; 25 mg ; 5 mg ; 8000 IU ; 50 IU	Orange and Black	Capsule		UCB Pharma
UD; ABBOTT LOGO	Prosom	2 mg	Pink	Tablet		Abbott Laboratories
UIC ; NVR	Exforge	10 mg ; 160 mg	Light Yellow	Tablet	Oval	Novartis
ULTRASE; MT6	Ultrase Mt6	19500 U ; 6000 U ; 19500 U	Yellow	Extended-Release Capsule		Axcan Scandipharm
ULTRASE; MT12	Ultrase Mt12	39,000 units ; 12,000 units ; 39,000 units	White and Yellow	Capsule		Axcan Scandipharm
ULTRASE; MT18	Ultrase Mt18	58,500 units ; 18,000 units ; 58,500 units	Gray and White	Capsule		Axcan Scandipharm
ULTRASE; MT20	Ultrase Mt20	20,000 units ; 65,000 units ; 65,000 units	Light Gray and Yellow	Capsule		Axcan Scandipharm
ULTRASE; MT24	Ultrase Mt24	78,000 units ; 24,000 units ; 78,000 units	Gray and Orange	Capsule		Axcan Scandipharm
ULTRASE; MT30	Ultrase Mt30	97500 U ; 97500 U ; 30000 U	Gray	Extended-Release Capsule		Axcan Scandipharm
UM	Dronabinol	2.5 mg	White	Capsule	Circle	Watson Pharma
UM	Dronabinol	5 mg	Dark Brown	Capsule	Circle	Watson Pharma
UM	Dronabinol	10 mg	Orange	Capsule	Circle	Watson Pharma
UPJOHN	Uticillin K	250 mg		Tablet		Upjohn
UPJOHN 949	Uracil Mustard	1 mg	Yellow and Dark Blue	Capsule		Upjohn
UPJOHN; 15	Cortisone Acetate	5 mg	White	Tablet	Circle, Scored	Pharmacia & Upjohn
UPJOHN; 23	Cortisone Acetate	10 mg	White	Tablet	Circle, Scored	Pharmacia & Upjohn
UPJOHN; 34	Cortisone Acetate	25 mg	White	Tablet	Circle, Scored	Pharmacia & Upjohn
UPJOHN; 243	Alkets	780 mg ; 130 mg ; 65 mg	Pink	Tablet, Chewable		Pharmacia & Upjohn
URS785 ;	Urso 250	250 mg	White	Tablet	Oval	Axcan Scandipharm
URS790 ;	Urso Forte	500 mg	White	Tablet	Oval	Axcan Scandipharm
US	Hemocyte	324 mg	Maroon	Tablet	Circle	U.S. Pharmaceutical

IMPRINT	BRAND/GENERIC NAME	STRENGTH	COLOR	FORM	SHAPE	MANUFACTURER
US	Hemocyte Plus	324 mg ; 10 mg ; 6 mg ; 5 mg ; 15 mcg ; 1 mg ; 30 mg ; 10 mg ; 80 mg ; 70 mg ; 4 mg ; 2 mg ; 200 mg	Maroon	Capsule		Us Pharmaceutical Corporation
US	Hemocyte-F	324 mg ; 1 mg	Maroon	Tablet	Circle	U.S. Pharmaceutical
US ; 2.5	Oxandrolone	2.5 mg	White	Tablet	Oval	Upsher-Smith Laboratories
US ; TANDEM F	Tandem F	162 mg ; 115.2 mg ; 1 mg	Light Brown, Red	Capsule	Capsule-Shape	U.S. Pharmaceutical
US ; TANDEM-OB	Tandem Ob	10 mg ; 6 mg ; 5 mg ; 15 mcg ; 1 mg ; 30 mg ; 10 mg ; 18.2 mg ; 6.9 mg ; 1.3 mg ; 0.8 mg ; 162 mg ; 115.2 mg ; 200 mg	Blue, Pink	Capsule	Capsule-Shape	U.S. Pharmaceutical
US ; TANDEM-PLUS	Tandem Plus	162 mg ; 115.2 mg ; 200 mg ; 10 mg ; 6 mg ; 5 mg ; 15 mcg ; 1 mg ; 30 mg ; 10 mg ; 18.2 mg ; 1.3 mg ; 0.8 mg	Pink	Capsule	Capsule-Shape	U.S. Pharmaceutical
US; 016	Folgard RX 2.2	0.5 mg ; 2.2 mg ; 25 mg	Yellow	Tablet	Oval	Upsher-Smith Laboratories
US; 017	Folgard	0.8 mg ; 10 mg ; 0.115 mg	Green	Tablet	Circle	Upsher-Smith Laboratories
US; 027	Pentoxil	400 mg	Light Pink	Extended-Release Tablet	Capsule-Shape	Upsher-Smith Laboratories
US; 12; 80	Sorine	80 mg	White	Tablet	Capsule-Shape	Upsher-Smith Laboratories
US; 13; 120	Sorine	120 mg	White	Tablet	Capsule-Shape	Upsher-Smith Laboratories
US; 14; 160	Sorine	160 mg	White	Tablet	Capsule-Shape	Upsher-Smith Laboratories
US; 15; 240	Sorine	240 mg	White	Tablet	Capsule-Shape	Upsher-Smith Laboratories
US; 67; 500	Niacor	500 mg	White	Tablet	Oval, Scored	Upsher-Smith Laboratories
US; 500	Salsitab	500 mg	Blue	Tablet	Circle	Upsher-Smith Laboratories
US; 750	Salsitab	750 mg	Blue	Tablet	Capsule-Shape	Upsher-Smith Laboratories
US; CENOGEN ULTRA; 140	Cenogen Ultra	10 mg ; 1.3 mg ; 0.8 mg ; 324 mg ; 200 mg ; 10 mg ; 6 mg ; 5 mg ; 15 mcg ; 1 mg ; 30 mg	Blue and Pink	Capsule		Us Pharmaceutical Corporation
USB; 001	Hexalen	50 mg	Clear	Capsule		Mgi Pharma
USL; 8	Potassium Chloride	600 mg	Blue	Sustained-Release Tablet	Circle	Upsher-Smith Laboratories
USL; 10	Potassium Chloride	750 mg	White	Sustained-Release Tablet	Circle	Upsher-Smith Laboratories
USL; 80	Zinc Sulfate	220 mg	Pink	Capsule		Upsher-Smith Laboratories
USV; 82	Lozol	2.5 mg	White	Tablet	Circle	Aventis Pharmaceuticals
V	Zelapar	1.25 mg	Pale Yellow	Tablet, Disintegrating		Valeant Pharmaceuticals
V ; TASMAR 100	Tasmar	100 mg	Beige	Tablet	Six-Sided	Valeant Pharmaceuticals
V ; TASMAR 200	Tasmar	200 mg	Reddish Brown	Tablet	Six-Sided	Valeant Pharmaceuticals
V; 4	Vospire ER	4 mg	Green	Coated Tablet	Circle	Odyssey Pharmaceuticals
V; 8	Vospire ER	8 mg	White	Extended-Release Tablet	Circle	Odyssey Pharmaceuticals
VALEANT 0247	Cesamet	1 mg	Purple, White	Capsule		Valeant Pharmaceuticals
VALEANT PF0844	Phrenilin Forte	50 mg ; 650 mg	Amethyst Opaque	Capsule		Valeant Pharmaceuticals
VALPROIC; 250; 0364	Valproic Acid	250 mg	Off-White	Capsule		Watson Laboratories
VALRELEASE 15; ROCHE	Valrelease	15 mg	Yellow and Blue	Sustained-Release Capsule		Roche Pharmaceuticals
VALTREX 1 GRAM	Valtrex	1 GM	Blue	Tablet	Capsule-Shape	Glaxosmithkline
VALTREX 500 MG	Valtrex	500 mg	Blue	Tablet	Capsule-Shape	Glaxosmithkline
VENTOLIN; 4; GLAXO	Ventolin	4 mg	White	Tablet	Circle, Compressed	Glaxosmithkline
VENTOLIN; 200; GLAXO	Ventolin Rotacaps	200 mcg	Light Blue and Clear	Capsule, Liquid Filled		Glaxosmithkline
VESANOID 10; ROCHE	Vesanoid	10 mg	Orange-Yellow and Red-Brown	Capsule		Roche Laboratories
VGC; 450	Valcyte	450 mg	Pink	Tablet	Oval, Convex	Roche Laboratories
VGR; 25; PFIZER	Viagra	25 mg	Blue	Coated Tablet	Diamond, Rounded	Pfizer Laboratories
VGR; 50; PFIZER	Viagra	50 mg	Blue	Coated Tablet	Diamond, Rounded	Pfizer Laboratories
VGR; 100; PFIZER	Viagra	100 mg	Blue	Coated Tablet	Diamond, Rounded	Pfizer Laboratories
VICODIN	Vicodin	5 mg ; 500 mg	White	Tablet		Abbott Laboratories
VICODIN HP	Vicodin Hp	10 mg ; 660 mg	White	Tablet	Oval	Abbott Laboratories
VICODIN; ES	Vicodin Es	7.5 mg ; 750 mg	White	Tablet	Oval, Scored	Abbott Laboratories
VIOKASE; 9111	Viokase 8	8000 U ; 30000 U ; 30000 U	Tan	Tablet	Circle, Compressed	Paddock Labs
VISKEN; 5; 78/111	Visken	5 mg	White	Tablet	Circle, Scored	Novartis Pharmaceuticals
VISKEN; 10; 78/73	Visken	10 mg	White	Tablet	Circle, Scored	Novartis Pharmaceuticals
VOLMAX; 4	Volmax	4 mg	Light Blue	Extended-Release Tablet	Six-Sided	Muro Pharmaceutical
VOLMAX; 4	Volmax	4 mg	Light Blue	Sustained-Release Tablet	Six-Sided	Muro Pharmaceutical
VOLMAX; 8	Volmax	8 mg	White	Extended-Release Tablet	Six-Sided	Muro Pharmaceutical
VOLMAX; 8	Volmax	8 mg	White	Sustained-Release Tablet	Six-Sided	Muro Pharmaceutical
VP; A ;	Vicoprofen	7.5 mg ; 200 mg	White	Coated Tablet	Circle, Convex	Abbott Laboratories
W 25 ; 701 ;	Effexor	25 mg	Peach	Tablet	Shield-Shape	Wyeth Pharmaceuticals
W 37.5 ; 781 ;	Effexor	37.5 mg	Peach	Tablet	Shield-Shape	Wyeth Pharmaceuticals
W 50	Pristiq	50 mg	Light Pink	Tablet, Extended Release	Triangle	Wyeth Pharmaceuticals
W 50 ; 703 ;	Effexor	50 mg	Peach	Tablet	Shield-Shape	Wyeth Pharmaceuticals
W 75 ; 704 ;	Effexor	75 mg	Peach	Tablet	Shield-Shape	Wyeth Pharmaceuticals

IMPRINT	BRAND/GENERIC NAME	STRENGTH	COLOR	FORM	SHAPE	MANUFACTURER
W 100	Pristiq	100 mg	Reddish-Orange	Tablet, Extended Release	Triangle	Wyeth Pharmaceuticals
W 100 ; 705	Effexor	100 mg	Peach	Tablet	Shield-Shape	Wyeth Pharmaceuticals
W 764	Nefazodone	100 mg	White to Off White	Tablet	Capsule-Shape	Watson Laboratories
W 765	Nefazodone	150 mg	Orange	Tablet	Capsule-Shape	Watson Laboratories
W 766	Nefazodone	200 mg	Yellow	Tablet	Capsule-Shape	Watson Laboratories
W 767	Nefazodone	250 mg	White to Off White	Tablet	Capsule-Shape	Watson Laboratories
W 923	Enalapril Maleate	2.5 mg	White	Tablet	Circle	Ranbaxy
W 1714 ;	Potassium Chloride	20 meq	White to Off-White	Tablet, Extended Release	Capsule-Shape	Schering
W 1715 ;	Potassium Chloride	10 meq	Mottled White to Off-White	Tablet, Extended Release	Capsule-Shape	Schering
W EFFEXOR XR 37.5	Effexor Xr	37.5 mg	Grey, Peach	Capsule, Extended Release		Wyeth Pharmaceuticals
W EFFEXOR XR 75	Effexor Xr	75 mg	Peach	Capsule, Extended Release		Wyeth Pharmaceuticals
W EFFEXOR XR 150	Effexor Xr	150 mg	Dark Orange	Capsule, Extended Release		Wyeth Pharmaceuticals
W; 0.45/1.5	Prempro Single Tablet	0.45 mg ; 1.5 mg	Gold	Tablet	Oval	Wyeth Pharmaceuticals
W; 0.625/5	Prempro Single Tablet	0.625 mg ; 5 mg	Light Blue	Tablet	Oval	Wyeth Pharmaceuticals
W; 2.5	Isordil	2.5 mg	Yellow	Tablet	Circle	Wyeth Pharmaceuticals
W; 5	Isordil	5 mg	Pink	Tablet	Circle	Wyeth Pharmaceuticals
W; 641	Triphasil-21 Brown Tablet	0.03 mg ; 0.05 mg	Brown	21-Day Tablet Pack	Circle	Wyeth Pharmaceuticals
W; 641	Triphasil-28 Brown Tablet	0.03 mg ; 0.05 mg	Brown	Tablet	Circle	Wyeth Pharmaceuticals
W; 642	Triphasil-21 White Tablet	0.04 mg ; 75 mcg	White	21-Day Tablet Pack	Circle	Wyeth Pharmaceuticals
W; 642	Triphasil-28 White Tablet	75 mcg ; 0.04 mg	White	Tablet	Circle	Wyeth Pharmaceuticals
W; 643	Triphasil-21 Light Yellow Tablet	0.03 mg ; 0.125 mg	Light Yellow	21-Day Tablet Pack	Circle	Wyeth Pharmaceuticals
W; 643	Triphasil-28 Light Yellow Tablet	0.125 mg ; 0.03 mg	Light Yellow	Tablet	Circle	Wyeth Pharmaceuticals
W; 718	Buspirone Hydrochloride	15 mg	White	Tablet	Oval, Scored	Watson Laboratories
W; 906 ;	Ranitidine Hydrochloride	150 mg	White	Tablet	Six-Sided	Ranbaxy Pharmaceuticals
W; 907 ;	Ranitidine Hydrochloride	300 mg	White	Tablet	Capsule-Shape	Ranbaxy Pharmaceuticals
W; 912	Alesse 21	0.1 mg ; 20 mcg	Pink	21-Day Tablet Pack	Circle	Wyeth Pharmaceuticals
W; 912	Alesse 28 Pink Tablet	20 mcg ; 0.1 mg	Pink	Tablet	Circle	Wyeth Pharmaceuticals
W; 965	Bethanechol Chloride	5 mg	White	Tablet	Oval	Ranbaxy Pharmaceuticals
W; 966	Bethanechol Chloride	10 mg	Pink	Tablet	Oval	Ranbaxy Pharmaceuticals
W; 967	Bethanechol Chloride	25 mg	Light Yellow	Tablet	Oval	Ranbaxy Pharmaceuticals
W; 968	Bethanechol Chloride	50 mg	Yellow	Tablet	Oval	Ranbaxy Pharmaceuticals
W; C; 270	Nardil	15 mg	Orange	Tablet		Pfizer
W; DILACOR XR; 120 MG ;	Dilacor Xr	120 mg	Pink and Flesh	Extended-Release Capsule		Watson Laboratories
W; DILACOR XR; 180 MG ;	Dilacor Xr	180 mg	Lavender and Flesh	Extended-Release Capsule		Watson Laboratories
W; DILACOR XR; 240 MG ;	Dilacor Xr	240 mg	Light Blue and Flesh	Extended-Release Capsule		Watson Laboratories
W; M; 31 ;	Mebaral	32 mg	White	Tablet		Ovation Pharmaceuticals
W; M; 32 ;	Mebaral	50 mg	White	Tablet		Ovation Pharmaceuticals
W; M; 33 ;	Mebaral	100 mg	White	Tablet		Ovation Pharmaceuticals
W; M; 87	Mytelase Chloride	10 mg	White	Tablet		Sanofi-Aventis U.S.
W; MERRELL; 547	Quinamm	260 mg	White	Tablet	Circle	Aventis Pharmaceuticals
W; T51	Talwin Nx	0.5 mg ; 50 mg	Yellow	Tablet	Oblong	Sanofi-Aventis U.S.
WALLACE 0692	Tussi-12 D	60 mg ; 10 mg ; 40 mg	Pink	Tablet	Capsule-Shape	Meda Pharmaceuticals
WALLACE; 431	Lufyllin-400	400 mg	White	Tablet	Capsule-Shape	Meda Pharmaceuticals
WALLACE; 521	Lufyllin	200 mg	White	Tablet		Meda Pharmaceuticals
WALLACE; 541	Lufyllin-GG	200 mg ; 200 mg	Yellow	Tablet	Circle	Meda Pharmaceuticals
WALLACE; 673	Ryna-12	25 mg ; 60 mg	Buff	Tablet	Oblong	Meda Pharmaceuticals
WALLACE; 717	Rynatuss	60 mg ; 5 mg ; 10 mg ; 10 mg	Brown	Tablet	Capsule-Shape	Meda Pharmaceuticals
WATSON 343 ;	Verapamil Hydrochloride	80 mg	White	Tablet	Circle	Watson Laboratories
WATSON 300	Furosemide	20 mg	White	Tablet	Circle	Watson Laboratories
WATSON 301	Furosemide	40 mg	White	Tablet	Circle	Watson Laboratories
WATSON 302	Furosemide	80 mg	White	Tablet	Circle	Watson Laboratories
WATSON 344 ;	Verapamil Hydrochloride	80 mg	Light Peach	Tablet	Circle	Watson Laboratories
WATSON 345 ;	Verapamil Hydrochloride	120 mg	White	Tablet	Circle	Watson Laboratories
WATSON 346 ;	Verapamil Hydrochloride	120 mg	Peach	Tablet	Circle	Watson Laboratories
WATSON 363	Clorazepate Dipotassium	3.75 mg	Light Blue	Tablet	Circle	Watson Laboratories
WATSON 364	Clorazepate Dipotassium	7.5 mg	Light Beige	Tablet	Circle	Watson Laboratories
WATSON 365	Clorazepate Dipotassium	15 mg	Pink	Tablet	Circle	Watson Laboratories
WATSON 369 ; 5 MG	Loxapine Succinate	5 mg	White	Capsule		Watson Laboratories
WATSON 370 ; 10 MG	Loxapine Succinate	10 mg	White and Yellow	Capsule		Watson Laboratories
WATSON 371 ; 25 MG	Loxapine Succinate	25 mg	White and Green	Capsule		Watson Laboratories
WATSON 372 ; 50 MG	Loxapine Succinate	50 mg	White and Blue	Capsule		Watson Laboratories
WATSON 403	Verapamil Hydrochloride	40 mg	White	Tablet	Circle	Watson Laboratories
WATSON 404	Verapamil Hydrochloride	40 mg	Light Peach	Tablet	Circle	Watson Laboratories
WATSON 685; 5-50 ;	Amiloride Hydrochloride and Hydrochlorothiazide	5 mg ; 50 mg	Peach	Tablet	Circle	Watson Laboratories
WATSON 706; 2-10 ;	Perphenazine and Amitriptyline Hydrochloride	10 mg ; 2.04 mg	Blue	Coated Tablet	Circle	Watson Laboratories
WATSON 707; 2-25 ;	Perphenazine and Amitriptyline Hydrochloride	25 mg ; 2 mg	Orange	Coated Tablet	Circle	Watson Laboratories
WATSON 708; 4-10 ;	Perphenazine and Amitriptyline Hydrochloride	10 mg ; 4 mg	Salmon	Coated Tablet	Circle	Watson Laboratories
WATSON 709; 4-25 ;	Perphenazine and Amitriptyline Hydrochloride	25 mg ; 4 mg	Yellow	Coated Tablet	Circle	Watson Laboratories

IMPRINT	BRAND/GENERIC NAME	STRENGTH	COLOR	FORM	SHAPE	MANUFACTURER
WATSON 714 65-650 ;	Acetaminophen and Propoxyphene Hydrochloride	650 mg ; 65 mg	Orange	Tablet	Oblong	Watson Laboratories
WATSON 749	Oxycodone and Acetaminophen	325 mg ; 5 mg	White	Tablet	Circle	Watson Laboratories
WATSON 824	Oxycodone and Acetaminophen	500 mg ; 7.5 mg	White	Tablet	Capsule-Shape	Watson Laboratories
WATSON 825	Oxycodone and Acetaminophen	650 mg ; 10 mg	White	Tablet	Capsule-Shape	Watson Laboratories
WATSON 932	Oxycodone and Acetaminophen	325 mg ; 10 mg	White	Tablet	Circle	Watson Laboratories
WATSON 933	Oxycodone and Acetaminophen	325 mg ; 7.5 mg	White	Tablet	Circle	Watson Laboratories
WATSON 3330 ;	Cyclobenzaprine Hydrochloride	7.5 mg	White	Tablet	Circle	Watson Laboratories
WATSON 3546	Butalbital, Aspirin, Caffeine and Codeine Phosphate	30 mg ; 50 mg ; 40 mg ; 325 mg	Blue and Yellow	Capsule		Watson Laboratories
WATSON 3256 ;	Cyclobenzaprine Hydrochloride	5 mg	White	Tablet	Circle	Watson Laboratories
WATSON; 15/30	Levora 0.15/30-28 White Tablet	0.15 mg ; 30 mcg	White	28-Day Tablet Pack	Circle	Watson Laboratories
WATSON; 15-30	Levora 0.15/30-21	0.15 mg ; 30 mcg	White	21-Day Tablet Pack	Circle	Watson Laboratories
WATSON; 50/30	Trivora-21 Blue Tablet	30 mcg ; 50 mcg	Blue	21-Day Tablet Pack	Circle	Watson Laboratories
WATSON; 50/30	Trivora-28 Blue Tablet	50 mcg ; 30 mcg	Blue	28-Day Tablet Pack	Circle	Watson Laboratories
WATSON; 75/40	Trivora-21 White Tablet	75 mcg ; 40 mcg	White	21-Day Tablet Pack	Circle	Watson Laboratories
WATSON; 75/40	Trivora-28 White Tablet	40 mcg ; 75 mcg	White	28-Day Tablet Pack	Circle	Watson Laboratories
WATSON; 125/30	Trivora-21 Pink Tablet	30 mcg ; 125 mcg	Pink	21-Day Tablet Pack	Circle	Watson Laboratories
WATSON; 125/30	Trivora-28 Pink Tablet	30 mcg ; 125 mcg	Pink	28-Day Tablet Pack	Circle	Watson Laboratories
WATSON; 235 ;	Nor-Qd	0.35 mg	Yellow	Tablet	Circle	Watson Pharma
WATSON; 240; 0.5 ;	Lorazepam	0.5 mg	White	Tablet	Circle	Watson Laboratories
WATSON; 241; 1 ;	Lorazepam	1 mg	White	Tablet	Circle	Watson Laboratories
WATSON; 242; 2 ;	Lorazepam	2 mg	White	Tablet	Circle, Scored	Watson Laboratories
WATSON; 254	Brevicon 28-Day Blue Tablet	0.5 mg ; 0.035 mg	Blue	28-Day Tablet Pack	Circle	Watson Laboratories
WATSON; 254 ;	Tri-Norinyl 28 Day Blue Tablet	35 mcg ; 0.5 mg	Blue	28-Day Tablet Pack	Circle	Watson Laboratories
WATSON; 259 ;	Tri-Norinyl 28 Day Yellow-Green Tablet	1 mg ; 35 mcg	Yellow-Green	28-Day Tablet Pack	Circle	Watson Laboratories
WATSON; 265	Norinyl 1/50 White Tablet	1 mg ; 50 mcg	White	28-Day Tablet Pack	Circle	Watson Laboratories
WATSON; 303	Indomethacin	25 mg	Green	Capsule		Watson Laboratories
WATSON; 304	Indomethacin	50 mg	Green	Capsule		Watson Laboratories
WATSON; 305 ;	Propranolol Hydrochloride	10 mg	Orange	Tablet	Circle	Watson Laboratories
WATSON; 306 ;	Propranolol Hydrochloride	20 mg	Blue	Tablet	Circle	Watson Laboratories
WATSON; 307 ;	Propranolol Hydrochloride	40 mg	Green	Tablet	Circle	Watson Laboratories
WATSON; 308 ;	Propranolol Hydrochloride	80 mg	Yellow	Tablet	Circle	Watson Laboratories
WATSON; 309; 50	Doxycycline	50 mg	Green and Yellow	Capsule		Watson Laboratories
WATSON; 310; 100	Doxycycline	100 mg	Green	Capsule		Watson Laboratories
WATSON; 312	Metoclopramide Hydrochloride	10 mg	White	Tablet	Round; Bisected Scored	Watson Laboratories
WATSON; 332	Lorazepam	0.5 mg	White	Tablet	Circle, Scored	Watson Laboratories
WATSON; 333	Lorazepam	1 mg	White	Tablet	Circle, Scored	Watson Laboratories
WATSON; 334	Lorazepam	2 mg	White	Tablet	Circle, Scored	Watson Laboratories
WATSON; 335	Acyclovir	400 mg	White to Off-White	Tablet	Oval	Watson Laboratories
WATSON; 336	Acyclovir	800 mg	White to Off-White	Tablet	Oval	Watson Laboratories
WATSON; 338	Diclofenac Sodium	50 mg	White to Off-White	Delayed-Release Tablet	Circle, Biconvex, Enteric-Coated	Watson Laboratories
WATSON; 347; 12.5 ;	Hydrochlorothiazide	12.5 mg	Teal and White	Capsule		Watson Laboratories
WATSON; 348 ;	Triamterene and Hydrochlorothiazide	75 mg ; 50 mg	Yellow	Tablet	Circle, Scored	Watson Laboratories
WATSON; 349 ;	Hydrocodone Bitartrate and Acetaminophen	500 mg ; 5 mg	White	Tablet	Capsule-Shape	Watson Laboratories
WATSON; 352 ;	Propranolol Hydrochloride	60 mg	Pink	Tablet	Circle	Watson Laboratories
WATSON; 353	Propranolol Hydrochloride	90 mg	Lavender	Tablet	Circle	Watson Laboratories
WATSON; 357	Methyldopa and Hydrochlorothiazide	250 mg ; 15 mg	Off-White	Coated Tablet	Circle	Watson Laboratories
WATSON; 358	Methyldopa and Hydrochlorothiazide	250 mg ; 25 mg	White	Coated Tablet	Circle	Watson Laboratories
WATSON; 359	Methyldopa and Hydrochlorothiazide	30 mg ; 500 mg	Off-White	Coated Tablet	Circle	Watson Laboratories
WATSON; 360	Methyldopa and Hydrochlorothiazide	500 mg ; 50 mg	White	Coated Tablet	Circle	Watson Laboratories
WATSON; 366	Fenoprofen Calcium	600 mg	Peach	Coated Tablet	Oblong, Scored	Watson Laboratories
WATSON; 367	Fenoprofen Calcium	200 mg	White and Yellow	Capsule		Watson Laboratories
WATSON; 368	Fenoprofen Calcium	300 mg	Yellow	Capsule		Watson Laboratories
WATSON; 373	Maprotiline Hydrochloride	25 mg	Peach	Coated Tablet	Oval	Watson Laboratories
WATSON; 374	Maprotiline Hydrochloride	50 mg	Peach	Coated Tablet	Circle	Watson Laboratories
WATSON; 375	Maprotiline Hydrochloride	75 mg	White	Coated Tablet	Oval	Watson Laboratories
WATSON; 379 ;	Amoxapine	25 mg	White	Tablet	Circle, Scored	Watson Laboratories
WATSON; 380 ;	Amoxapine	50 mg	Orange	Tablet	Circle, Scored	Watson Laboratories
WATSON; 381 ;	Amoxapine	100 mg	Blue	Tablet	Circle, Scored	Watson Laboratories
WATSON; 382 ;	Amoxapine	150 mg	Orange	Tablet	Circle, Scored	Watson Laboratories
WATSON; 383	Zovia 1/35e-21	35 mcg ; 1 mg	Light Pink	21-Day Tablet Pack	Circle	Watson Laboratories
WATSON; 383	Zovia 1/35e-28 Light Pink Tablet	1 mg ; 35 mcg	Light Pink	28-Day Tablet Pack	Circle	Watson Laboratories
WATSON; 384	Zovia 1/50e-21	1 mg ; 50 mcg	Pink	21-Day Tablet Pack	Circle	Watson Laboratories
WATSON; 384	Zovia 1/50e-28 Pink Tablet	1 mg ; 50 mcg	Pink	28-Day Tablet Pack	Circle	Watson Laboratories
WATSON; 385 ;	Hydrocodone Bitartrate and Acetaminophen	7.5 mg ; 500 mg	White	Tablet	Capsule-Shape	Watson Laboratories
WATSON; 387 ;	Hydrocodone Bitartrate and Acetaminophen	750 mg ; 7.5 mg	White	Tablet	Oblong	Watson Laboratories
WATSON; 388 ;	Hydrocodone Bitartrate and Acetaminophen	2.5 mg ; 500 mg	White	Tablet	Oblong	Watson Laboratories
WATSON; 395; 50; 0.5 ;	Pentazocine and Naloxone Hydrochloride	0.5 mg ; 50 mg	Green	Tablet	Capsule-Shape	Watson Laboratories
WATSON; 396; 25; 650	Pentazocine and Acetaminophen	25 mg ; 650 mg	Light Aqua	Tablet	Capsule-Shape	Watson Laboratories
WATSON; 401	Albuterol Sulfate	2 mg	White	Tablet	Circle	Watson Laboratories
WATSON; 402	Albuterol Sulfate	4 mg	White	Tablet	Circle	Watson Laboratories
WATSON; 405	Lisinopril	2.5 mg	White	Tablet	Circle	Watson Laboratories
WATSON; 406	Lisinopril	5 mg	White	Tablet	Capsule-Shape	Watson Laboratories
WATSON; 407	Lisinopril	10 mg	Light Blue	Tablet	Circle	Watson Laboratories
WATSON; 408	Lisinopril	20 mg	Yellow	Tablet	Circle	Watson Laboratories
WATSON; 409	Lisinopril	40 mg	Yellow	Tablet	Circle	Watson Laboratories

IMPRINT	BRAND/GENERIC NAME	STRENGTH	COLOR	FORM	SHAPE	MANUFACTURER
WATSON; 414	Estropipate	0.75 mg	Yellow	Tablet	Circle, Scored	Watson Laboratories
WATSON; 415	Estropipate	1.5 mg	Peach	Tablet	Circle, Scored	Watson Laboratories
WATSON; 416	Estropipate	3 mg	Blue	Tablet	Circle, Scored	Watson Laboratories
WATSON; 424	Triamterene and Hydrochlorothiazide	37.5 mg ; 25 mg	Light Green	Tablet	Circle, Scored	Watson Laboratories
WATSON; 425	Butalbital, Aspirin, Caffeine and Codeine Phosphate	50 mg ; 325 mg ; 40 mg ; 30 mg	Blue and Yellow	Capsule		Watson Laboratories
WATSON; 430	Carbidopa and Levodopa	10 mg ; 100 mg	Blue	Tablet	Circle, Scored	Watson Laboratories
WATSON; 431	Carbidopa and Levodopa	25 mg ; 100 mg	Tan	Tablet	Circle, Scored	Watson Laboratories
WATSON; 432	Carbidopa and Levodopa	25 mg ; 250 mg	Blue	Tablet	Scored, Circle	Watson Laboratories
WATSON; 437	Acebutolol Hydrochloride	200 mg	Red and Gray	Capsule		Watson Laboratories
WATSON; 438	Acebutolol Hydrochloride	400 mg	Maroon and Green	Capsule		Watson Laboratories
WATSON; 444	Guanfacine Hydrochloride	1 mg	Pink	Tablet	Circle	Watson Laboratories
WATSON; 451	Guanabenz Acetate	4 mg	Orange	Tablet	Circle	Watson Laboratories
WATSON; 452	Guanabenz Acetate	8 mg	Gray	Tablet	Circle	Watson Laboratories
WATSON; 453	Guanfacine Hydrochloride	2 mg	Peach	Tablet	Circle	Watson Laboratories
WATSON; 454	Gemfibrozil	600 mg	White	Coated Tablet	Scored, Oval	Watson Laboratories
WATSON; 460	Glipizide	5 mg	White	Tablet	Circle, Scored	Watson Laboratories
WATSON; 461	Glipizide	10 mg	White	Tablet	Circle, Scored	Watson Laboratories
WATSON; 462	Metoprolol Tartrate	50 mg	Pink	Tablet	Circle, Scored	Watson Laboratories
WATSON; 463	Metoprolol Tartrate	100 mg	Blue	Tablet	Circle, Scored	Watson Laboratories
WATSON; 466	Tramadol Hydrochloride	50 mg	White	Tablet	Circle	Watson Laboratories
WATSON; 485	Acetaminophen, Butalbital and Caffeine	325 mg ; 50 mg ; 40 mg	White	Tablet		Watson Laboratories
WATSON; 487	Estradiol	1 mg	Gray	Tablet	Scored, Circle	Watson Laboratories
WATSON; 488	Estradiol	2 mg	Light Green	Tablet	Circle, Scored	Watson Laboratories
WATSON; 491; 150MG	Mexiletine Hydrochloride	150 mg	Brown and Light Brown	Capsule		Watson Laboratories
WATSON; 492; 200MG ;	Mexiletine Hydrochloride	200 mg	Brown	Capsule		Watson Laboratories
WATSON; 493; 250MG ;	Mexiletine Hydrochloride	250 mg	Brown and Light Green	Capsule		Watson Laboratories
WATSON; 498	Doxycycline Hyclate	100 mg	Blue	Capsule		Watson Laboratories
WATSON; 499	Doxycycline Hyclate	100 mg	Beige	Coated Tablet	Circle	Watson Laboratories
WATSON; 500; 50MG ;	Doxycycline Hyclate	50 mg	Blue and White	Capsule		Watson Laboratories
WATSON; 502 ;	Hydrocodone Bitartrate and Acetaminophen	7.5 mg ; 650 mg	Pink	Tablet	Capsule-Shape	Watson Laboratories
WATSON; 503 ;	Hydrocodone Bitartrate and Acetaminophen	650 mg ; 10 mg	Light Green	Tablet	Capsule-Shape	Watson Laboratories
WATSON; 504	Indapamide	2.5 mg	White	Coated Tablet	Circle	Watson Laboratories
WATSON; 507	Necon 0.5/35-21	0.5 mg ; 35 mcg	Light Yellow	21-Day Tablet Pack	Circle	Watson Laboratories
WATSON; 507	Necon 0.5/35-28 Light Yellow Tablet	0.5 mg ; 35 mcg	Light Yellow	28-Day Tablet Pack	Circle	Watson Laboratories
WATSON; 507	Necon 10/11-21 Light Yellow Tablet	0.5 mg ; 35 mcg	Light Yellow	21-Day Tablet Pack	Circle	Watson Laboratories
WATSON; 507	Necon 10/11-28 Light Yellow Tablet	0.5 mg ; 35 mcg	Light Yellow	28-Day Tablet Pack	Circle	Watson Laboratories
WATSON; 508	Necon 1/35-21	1 mg ; 35 mcg	Yellow	21-Day Tablet Pack	Circle	Watson Laboratories
WATSON; 508	Necon 1/35-28 Yellow Tablet	1 mg ; 35 mcg	Yellow	28-Day Tablet Pack	Circle	Watson Laboratories
WATSON; 508	Necon 10/11-21 Yellow Tablet	1 mg ; 35 mcg	Yellow	21-Day Tablet Pack	Circle	Watson Laboratories
WATSON; 508	Necon 10/11-28 Yellow Tablet	1 mg ; 35 mcg	Yellow	28-Day Tablet Pack	Circle	Watson Laboratories
WATSON; 510	Necon 1/50-21	1 mg ; 50 mcg	Blue	21-Day Tablet Pack	Circle	Watson Laboratories
WATSON; 517	Hydrocodone Bitartrate and Acetaminophen	660 mg ; 10 mg	White	Tablet	Oval	Watson Laboratories
WATSON; 524	Trinessa White Tablet	0.18 mg ; 0.035 mg	White	28-Day Tablet Pack	Circle	Watson Laboratories
WATSON; 525	Trinessa Light Blue Tablet	0.215 mg ; 0.035 mg	Light Blue	28-Day Tablet Pack	Circle	Watson Laboratories
WATSON; 526	Mononessa	0.25 mg ; 0.035 mg	Blue	Tablet	Circle	Watson Laboratories
WATSON; 526	Trinessa Blue Tablet	0.25 mg ; 0.035 mg	Blue	28-Day Tablet Pack	Circle	Watson Laboratories
WATSON; 527	Indapamide	1.25 mg	Orange	Coated Tablet	Circle	Watson Laboratories
WATSON; 528	Estradiol	0.5 mg	White	Tablet	Circle, Scored	Watson Laboratories
WATSON; 540	Hydrocodone Bitartrate and Acetaminophen	10 mg ; 500 mg	Blue	Tablet	Capsule-Shape	Watson Laboratories
WATSON; 544 ;	Desipramine Hydrochloride	75 mg	Orange	Coated Tablet	Circle	Watson Laboratories
WATSON; 545 ;	Desipramine Hydrochloride	100 mg	Peach	Coated Tablet	Circle	Watson Laboratories
WATSON; 575	Trihexyphenidyl Hydrochloride	2 mg	White	Tablet	Circle, Scored	Watson Laboratories
WATSON; 576	Trihexyphenidyl Hydrochloride	5 mg	White	Tablet	Circle, Scored	Watson Laboratories
WATSON; 582	Propafenone Hydrochloride	150 mg	White	Coated Tablet	Circle, Scored	Watson Laboratories
WATSON; 583	Propafenone Hydrochloride	225 mg	White	Coated Tablet	Circle, Scored	Watson Laboratories
WATSON; 585	Diclofenac Potassium	50 mg	Brown	Coated Tablet	Circle	Watson Laboratories
WATSON; 594; 25 MG	Clomipramine Hydrochloride	25 mg	Blue	Capsule		Watson Laboratories
WATSON; 595; 50 MG	Clomipramine Hydrochloride	50 mg	Yellow	Capsule		Watson Laboratories
WATSON; 596; 75 MG	Clomipramine Hydrochloride	75 mg	Green	Capsule		Watson Laboratories
WATSON; 605 ;	Labetalol Hydrochloride	100 mg	Beige	Coated Tablet	Circle, Scored	Watson Laboratories
WATSON; 606 ;	Labetalol Hydrochloride	200 mg	White	Coated Tablet	Circle, Scored	Watson Laboratories
WATSON; 607 ;	Labetalol Hydrochloride	300 mg	Blue	Coated Tablet	Circle, Scored	Watson Laboratories
WATSON; 613	Butalbital, Acetaminophen and Caffeine	500 mg ; 40 mg ; 50 mg	Light Blue	Tablet	Capsule-Shape, Scored	Watson Laboratories
WATSON; 617	Morphine Sulfate	100 mg	Gray	Extended-Release Tablet	Circle	Watson Laboratories
WATSON; 629	Nora-Be	0.35 mg	White	Tablet	Circle	Watson Laboratories
WATSON; 630	Microgestin Fe 1/20 White Tablet	20 mcg ; 1 mg	White	28-Day Tablet Pack	Circle	Watson Laboratories
WATSON; 631	Microgestin Fe 1.5/30 Green Tablet	1.5 mg ; 30 mcg	Green	28-Day Tablet Pack	Circle	Watson Laboratories
WATSON; 632	Microgestin Fe 1/20 Brown Tablet	75 mg	Brown	28-Day Tablet Pack	Circle	Watson Laboratories

IMPRINT	BRAND/GENERIC NAME	STRENGTH	COLOR	FORM	SHAPE	MANUFACTURER
WATSON; 632	Microgestin Fe 1.5/30 Brown Tablet	75 mg	Brown	28-Day Tablet Pack	Circle	Watson Laboratories
WATSON; 632	Microgestin Fe Brown Tablet	75 mg	Brown	Tablet	Circle	Watson Laboratories
WATSON; 637	Pentoxifylline	400 mg	Red	Tablet, Extended Release	Oblong	Andrx Pharmaceuticals
WATSON; 639	Doxazosin Mesylate	1 mg	White	Tablet	Circle, Biconvex, Scored	Watson Laboratories
WATSON; 640	Doxazosin Mesylate	2 mg	Light Orange	Tablet	Circle, Biconvex, Scored	Watson Laboratories
WATSON; 641	Doxazosin Mesylate	4 mg	Light Orange	Tablet	Circle, Biconvex, Scored	Watson Laboratories
WATSON; 642	Doxazosin Mesylate	8 mg	Green	Tablet	Circle, Biconvex, Scored	Watson Laboratories
WATSON; 654	Sotalol Hydrochloride	80 mg	Light Blue	Tablet	Oval, Scored	Watson Laboratories
WATSON; 655	Sotalol Hydrochloride	160 mg	Light Blue	Tablet	Oval, Scored	Watson Laboratories
WATSON; 656	Sotalol Hydrochloride	240 mg	Light Blue	Tablet	Oval, Scored	Watson Laboratories
WATSON; 657	Buspirone Hydrochloride	5 mg	White	Tablet	Oval, Biconvex, Scored	Watson Laboratories
WATSON; 658	Buspirone Hydrochloride	10 mg	White	Tablet	Oval, Biconvex, Scored	Watson Laboratories
WATSON; 662; 120	Diltiazem Hydrochloride	120 mg	Pink and White	Extended-Release Capsule		Watson Laboratories
WATSON; 663; 180	Diltiazem Hydrochloride	180 mg	Pink and White	Extended-Release Capsule		Watson Laboratories
WATSON; 664; 240	Diltiazem Hydrochloride	240 mg	Red and White	Extended-Release Capsule		Watson Laboratories
WATSON; 665	Sotalol Hydrochloride	120 mg	Light Blue	Tablet	Oval, Scored	Watson Laboratories
WATSON; 667; 400 ;	Etodolac	400 mg	Yellow	Coated Tablet	Capsule-Shape	Watson Laboratories
WATSON; 668	Enalapril Maleate	2.5 mg	White to Off-White	Tablet	Circle, Biconvex, Scored	Watson Laboratories
WATSON; 669	Enalapril Maleate	5 mg	White to Off-White	Tablet	Circle	Watson Laboratories
WATSON; 670	Enalapril Maleate	10 mg	Pink with White Speckles	Tablet	Circle	Watson Laboratories
WATSON; 671	Enalapril Maleate	20 mg	Peach with White Speckles	Tablet	Circle, Biconvex	Watson Laboratories
WATSON; 682; 0.25 ;	Alprazolam	0.25 mg	White	Tablet	Oval, BI-Convex	Watson Laboratories
WATSON; 683; 0.5 ;	Alprazolam	0.5 mg	Peach	Tablet	Oval, BI-Convex	Watson Laboratories
WATSON; 684; 1 ;	Alprazolam	1 mg	Blue	Tablet	Oval, BI-Convex	Watson Laboratories
WATSON; 686; 10 ;	Baclofen	10 mg	White	Tablet	Oval	Watson Laboratories
WATSON; 687; 20 ;	Baclofen	20 mg	White	Tablet	Circle	Watson Laboratories
WATSON; 688; 12.5 ;	Captopril	12.5 mg	White	Tablet	Capsule-Shape, Scored	Watson Laboratories
WATSON; 689; 25 ;	Captopril	25 mg	White	Tablet	Circle, Quadrisect-Scored	Watson Laboratories
WATSON; 690; 50 ;	Captopril	50 mg	White	Tablet	Egg-Shape	Watson Laboratories
WATSON; 691; 100 ;	Captopril	100 mg	White	Tablet	Egg-Shape	Watson Laboratories
WATSON; 693; 500 ;	Chlorzoxazone	500 mg	Green	Tablet	Capsule-Shape, Partial-Scored	Watson Laboratories
WATSON; 695; 10 ;	Doxepin Hydrochloride	10 mg	Scarlet and Pink	Capsule		Watson Laboratories
WATSON; 696; 25 ;	Doxepin Hydrochloride	25 mg	Blue and Pink	Capsule		Watson Pharma
WATSON; 697; 50 ;	Doxepin Hydrochloride	50 mg	Pink and Flesh	Capsule		Watson Laboratories
WATSON; 698; 200 ;	Hydroxychloroquine Sulfate	200 mg	White	Coated Tablet	Oval	Watson Laboratories
WATSON; 700; 25 ;	Hydroxyzine Hydrochloride	25 mg	Green	Coated Tablet	Circle	Watson Laboratories
WATSON; 704; 50 ;	Hydroxyzine Hydrochloride	50 mg	Yellow	Coated Tablet	Circle	Watson Laboratories
WATSON; 710; 5 ;	Pindolol	5 mg	White	Tablet	Circle, Scored	Watson Laboratories
WATSON; 711; 10 ;	Pindolol	10 mg	White	Tablet	Circle, Scored	Watson Laboratories
WATSON; 712; 10 MG ;	Piroxicam	10 mg	Light Blue and White	Capsule		Watson Laboratories
WATSON; 713; 20 MG ;	Piroxicam	20 mg	Light Blue	Capsule		Watson Laboratories
WATSON; 726; 50	Meperidine Hydrochloride	50 mg	White	Tablet	Circle	Watson Laboratories
WATSON; 727; 100	Meperidine Hydrochloride	100 mg	White	Tablet	Circle	Watson Laboratories
WATSON; 728; 500	Etodolac	500 mg	Blue	Coated Tablet	Capsule-Shape	Watson Laboratories
WATSON; 735; 200	Etodolac	200 mg	Gray and Brown	Capsule		Watson Laboratories
WATSON; 736; 300	Etodolac	300 mg	Gray and Swedish Orange	Capsule		Watson Laboratories
WATSON; 737; 5; 500 MG	Oxycodone and Acetaminophen	5 mg ; 500 mg	White and Red	Capsule		Watson Laboratories
WATSON; 744; 1	Estazolam	1 mg	White	Tablet	Diamond, Scored	Watson Laboratories
WATSON; 745; 2	Estazolam	2 mg	Pink	Tablet	Diamond, Scored	Watson Laboratories
WATSON; 746	Clonazepam	0.5 mg	Yellow	Tablet	Circle	Watson Laboratories
WATSON; 747	Clonazepam	1 mg	Aqua	Tablet	Circle	Watson Laboratories
WATSON; 748	Clonazepam	2 mg	White	Tablet	Circle	Watson Laboratories
WATSON; 760 ;	Ranitidine	150 mg	Beige	Coated Tablet	Circle	Watson Laboratories
WATSON; 771; 18.75	Pemoline	75 mg	White	Tablet	Circle, Scored	Watson Laboratories
WATSON; 772; 37.5	Pemoline	37.5 mg	Peach	Tablet	Circle, Scored	Watson Laboratories
WATSON; 773; 18.75	Pemoline	75 mg	Yellow	Tablet	Circle, Scored	Watson Laboratories
WATSON; 774	Oxycodone Hydrochloride	5 mg	White	Tablet	Circle, Scored	Watson Laboratories
WATSON; 775 ;	Diltiazem Hydrochloride	30 mg	Blue	Tablet	Circle, Scored	Watson Laboratories
WATSON; 776 ;	Diltiazem Hydrochloride	60 mg	White	Tablet	Circle	Watson Laboratories
WATSON; 777 ;	Diltiazem Hydrochloride	90 mg	Blue	Tablet	Oblong	Watson Laboratories
WATSON; 778 ;	Diltiazem Hydrochloride	120 mg	White	Tablet	Oblong, Scored	Watson Laboratories
WATSON; 780 ;	Sucralfate	1 G	Light Blue	Tablet	Oblong	Watson Laboratories
WATSON; 781 ;	Clomiphene	50 mg	White	Tablet	Circle	Watson Laboratories
WATSON; 782 ;	Diethylpropion Hydrochloride	75 mg	White	Extended-Release Tablet	Capsule-Shape	Watson Laboratories
WATSON; 783 ;	Diethylpropion Hydrochloride	25 mg	White	Tablet	Circle	Watson Laboratories
WATSON; 784 ;	Carisoprodol	350 mg	White	Tablet	Circle	Watson Laboratories
WATSON; 785; 5MG ;	Chlordiazepoxide Hydrochloride	5 mg	Green and Yellow	Capsule		Watson Laboratories
WATSON; 787; 25MG ;	Chlordiazepoxide Hydrochloride	25 mg	Green and White	Capsule		Watson Laboratories
WATSON; 790 ;	Methylprednisolone	4 mg	White	Tablet		Watson Laboratories
WATSON; 791 ;	Naproxen	500 mg	White	Tablet	Capsule-Shape	Watson Laboratories
WATSON; 792 ;	Naproxen Sodium	275 mg	White	Tablet	Oval	Watson Laboratories
WATSON; 793 ;	Naproxen Sodium	550 mg	Green	Tablet	Oval	Watson Laboratories
WATSON; 794; 10MG	Dicyclomine	10 mg	Dark Blue	Capsule		Watson Laboratories
WATSON; 795 ;	Dicyclomine Hydrochloride	20 mg	Blue	Tablet	Circle	Watson Laboratories
WATSON; 796 ;	Sulfasalazine	500 mg	Mustard	Tablet	Round, Bisected Scored	Watson Laboratories

IMPRINT	BRAND/GENERIC NAME	STRENGTH	COLOR	FORM	SHAPE	MANUFACTURER
WATSON; 802 ;	Meclizine Hydrochloride	12.5 mg	Blue and White	Tablet	Oval	Watson Laboratories
WATSON; 804 ;	Meprobamate	200 mg	White	Tablet	Circle	Watson Laboratories
WATSON; 805 ;	Meprobamate	400 mg	White	Tablet	Convex, Circle	Watson Laboratories
WATSON; 806 ;	Methocarbamol	500 mg	White	Tablet	Circle	Watson Laboratories
WATSON; 807	Methocarbamol	750 mg	White	Tablet	Capsule-Shape	Watson Laboratories
WATSON; 808 ;	Desipramine Hydrochloride	25 mg	Yellow	Coated Tablet	Circle	Watson Laboratories
WATSON; 809 ;	Desipramine Hydrochloride	50 mg	Green	Coated Tablet	Circle	Watson Laboratories
WATSON; 820	Oxycodone and Aspirin	4.5 mg ; 0.38 mg ; 325 mg	Yellow	Tablet	Circle, Scored	Watson Laboratories
WATSON; 821 ;	Naproxen	250 mg	White	Tablet	Circle	Watson Laboratories
WATSON; 826; 20 MG	Fluoxetine Hydrochloride	10 mg	Light Green	Capsule		Watson Laboratories
WATSON; 827; 20 MG	Fluoxetine Hydrochloride	20 mg	Light Green and White	Capsule		Watson Laboratories
WATSON; 838	Ketorolac Tromethamine	10 mg	White	Coated Tablet	Circle, Convex	Watson Laboratories
WATSON; 841	Bisoprolol and Hydrochlorothiazide	6.25 mg ; 2.5 mg	Yellow	Tablet	Circle, Biconvex	Watson Laboratories
WATSON; 842	Bisoprolol and Hydrochlorothiazide	5 mg ; 6.25 mg	Pink	Tablet	Circle, Biconvex	Watson Laboratories
WATSON; 847	Ogestrel White Tablet	0.5 mg ; 0.5 mg	White	28-Day Tablet Pack	Circle	Watson Laboratories
WATSON; 848 ;	Ogestrel White Tablet	0.5 mg ; 0.05 mg	White	28-Day Tablet Pack	Circle	Watson Laboratories
WATSON; 850 ;	Acetaminophen and Codeine Phosphate	300 mg ; 15 mg	White	Tablet	Circle, Flat-Faced, Beveled Edge	Watson Laboratories
WATSON; 851 ;	Acetaminophen and Codeine Phosphate	300 mg ; 30 mg	White	Tablet	Circle, Scored	Watson Laboratories
WATSON; 852 ;	Acetaminophen and Codeine Phosphate	300 mg ; 60 mg	White	Tablet	Circle, Scored	Watson Laboratories
WATSON; 853	Acetaminophen and Hydrocodone Bitartrate	325 mg ; 10 mg	Yellow	Tablet	Capsule-Shape	Watson Laboratories
WATSON; 860	Lisinopril and Hydrochlorothiazide	10 mg ; 12.5 mg	Pink	Tablet	Circle	Watson Laboratories
WATSON; 861	Lisinopril and Hydrochlorothiazide	20 mg ; 12.5 mg	Light Blue	Tablet	Circle	Watson Laboratories
WATSON; 862	Lisinopril and Hydrochlorothiazide	20 mg ; 25 mg	Pink	Tablet	Circle	Watson Laboratories
WATSON; 885	Lisinopril	30 mg	Yellow	Tablet	Circle	Watson Laboratories
WATSON; 892	Jolivette	0.35 mg	Green	Tablet		Watson Laboratories
WATSON; 913	Norco 5/325	5 mg ; 325 mg	White with Orange Specks	Tablet	Capsule-Shape, Scored	Watson Laboratories
WATSON; 3159	Ursodiol	300 mg	White	Capsule		Watson Laboratories
WATSON; 3191	Pyridostigmine Bromide	60 mg	White	Tablet		Watson Laboratories
WATSON; 3202	Hydrocodone Bitartrate and Acetaminophen	5 mg ; 325 mg	White with Orange Specks	Tablet	Capsule-Shape	Watson Laboratories
WATSON; 3203	Hydrocodone Bitartrate and Acetaminophen	7.5 mg ; 325 mg	Light Orange	Tablet	Capsule; Bisected Scored	Watson Laboratories
WATSON; 3219	Aspirin, Caffeine and Butalbital	325 mg ; 50 mg ; 40 mg	Yellow and Green	Capsule		Watson Laboratories
WATSON; LOXITANE; 5 MG ;	Loxitane	5 mg	Opaque Green	Capsule		Watson Laboratories
WATSON; LOXITANE; 10 MG ;	Loxitane	10 mg	Dark Green and Yellow	Capsule		Watson Laboratories
WATSON; LOXITANE; 25 MG ;	Loxitane	25 mg	Dark Green and Light Green	Capsule		Watson Laboratories
WATSON; LOXITANE; 50 MG ;	Loxitane	50 mg	Dark Green and Blue	Capsule		Watson Laboratories
WATSON;259	Norinyl 1+35	1 mg ; 0.35 mg	Yellow-Green	Tablet	Circle	Watson Pharma
WBB	Mol-Iron	195 mg	Brown	Tablet		Schering-Plough Healthcare Products
WC	Tedral Expectorant	130 mg ; 24 mg ; 8 mg	White	Tablet		Parke-Davis
WC ; 720 / 1/2	Estrace	0.5 mg	White to Off-White	Tablet	Oval	Warner Chilcott
WC ; 721 / 1	Estrace	1 mg	Light Purple	Tablet	Oval	Warner Chilcott
WC ; 722 / 2	Estrace	2 mg	Green	Tablet	Oval	Warner Chilcott
WC 389	Femtrace	0.45 mg	Cream	Tablet	Circle	Warner Chilcott
WC 390	Femtrace	0.9 mg	White	Tablet	Circle	Warner Chilcott
WC 391	Femtrace	1.8 mg	Yellow	Tablet	Circle	Warner Chilcott
WC; 010	Chlorpromazine Hydrochloride	10 mg		Tablet		Warner Chilcott
WC; 025	Chlorpromazine Hydrochloride	25 mg		Tablet		Warner Chilcott
WC; 030	Methyldopa and Hydrochlorothiazide	15 mg ; 250 mg		Tablet		Warner Chilcott
WC; 031	Methyldopa and Hydrochlorothiazide	250 mg ; 25 mg		Tablet		Warner Chilcott
WC; 032	Methyldopa and Hydrochlorothiazide	500 mg ; 30 mg	Dark Red	Tablet	Circle	Warner Chilcott
WC; 033	Methyldopa and Hydrochlorothiazide	500 mg ; 50 mg	Grey	Tablet	Circle	Warner Chilcott
WC; 050	Chlorpromazine Hydrochloride	50 mg		Tablet		Warner Chilcott
WC; 070 ;	Propranolol Hydrochloride	10 mg		Tablet		Warner Chilcott
WC; 071 ;	Propranolol Hydrochloride	20 mg		Tablet		Warner Chilcott
WC; 072 ;	Propranolol Hydrochloride	40 mg		Tablet		Warner Chilcott
WC; 073 ;	Propranolol Hydrochloride	60 mg		Tablet		Warner Chilcott
WC; 074 ;	Propranolol Hydrochloride	80 mg		Tablet		Warner Chilcott
WC; 084	Gemfibrozil	600 mg	White	Coated Tablet	Circle, Scored	Warner Chilcott
WC; 100	Chlorpromazine Hydrochloride	100 mg		Tablet		Warner Chilcott
WC; 117	Diphenoxylate Hydrochloride and Atropine	2.5 mg ; 0.025 mg	White	Tablet	Circle	Warner Chilcott
WC; 121	Chlorthalidone	50 mg		Tablet		Warner Chilcott
WC; 123	Chlorthalidone	25 mg		Tablet		Warner Chilcott

IMPRINT	BRAND/GENERIC NAME	STRENGTH	COLOR	FORM	SHAPE	MANUFACTURER
WC; 141	Diazepam	2 mg		Tablet		Warner Chilcott
WC; 142	Diazepam	5 mg		Tablet		Warner Chilcott
WC; 201	Chlorpromazine Hydrochloride	200 mg		Tablet		Warner Chilcott
WC; 227	Natachew	1000 IU ; 400 IU ; 11 IU ; 120 mg ; 1 mg ; 2 mg ; 3 mg ; 20 mg ; 10 mg ; 12 mcg ; 29 mg	Tan Speckled	Tablet, Chewable	Circle, Scored	Warner Chilcott
WC; 230	Tedral	130 mg ; 24 mg ; 8 mg	White	Tablet		Parke-Davis
WC; 238	Tedral-25	24 mg ; 25 mg ; 130 mg	Salmon and Pink	Tablet		Parke-Davis
WC; 242	Carbamazepine	100 mg	Pink Speckled	Tablet, Chewable	Circle, Scored	Warner Chilcott
WC; 243	Carbamazepine	200 mg		Tablet		Warner Chilcott
WC; 271	Amitriptyline	100 mg		Tablet		Warner Chilcott
WC; 272	Amitriptyline	10 mg		Tablet		Warner Chilcott
WC; 273	Amitriptyline	25 mg		Tablet		Warner Chilcott
WC; 274	Amitriptyline	50 mg		Tablet		Warner Chilcott
WC; 275	Amitriptyline	75 mg		Tablet		Warner Chilcott
WC; 278	Amitriptyline	150 mg		Tablet		Warner Chilcott
WC; 402	Amcill	250 mg		Capsule		Warner Chilcott
WC; 404	Amcill	500 mg		Capsule		Warner Chilcott
WC; 420 ;	Quinine Sulfate	5 Gr		Capsule		Warner Chilcott
WC; 440	Furosemide	20 mg	White	Tablet	Oval	Warner Chilcott
WC; 441 ;	Furosemide	40 mg	White	Tablet	Circle	Warner Chilcott
WC; 442 ;	Furosemide	80 mg	White	Tablet	Circle	Warner Chilcott
WC; 443	Clonidine Hydrochloride	0.1 mg		Tablet		Warner Chilcott
WC; 444	Clonidine Hydrochloride	0.2 mg		Tablet		Warner Chilcott
WC; 445	Clonidine Hydrochloride	0.3 mg		Tablet		Warner Chilcott
WC; 451	Clorazepate Dipotassium	3.75 mg		Tablet		Warner Chilcott
WC; 452	Clorazepate Dipotassium	7.5 mg		Tablet		Warner Chilcott
WC; 453	Clorazepate Dipotassium	15 mg		Tablet		Warner Chilcott
WC; 551	Oxazepam	15 mg	Yellow	Tablet	Circle, Biconvex	Warner Chilcott
WC; 557	Verapamil Hydrochloride	80 mg	White	Tablet		Warner Chilcott
WC; 573	Verapamil Hydrochloride	120 mg	White	Tablet		Warner Chilcott
WC; 606	Aspirin	5 Gr	White	Tablet		Warner Chilcott
WC; 615	Minocycline Hcl	50 mg	Olive and Brown	Capsule		Warner Chilcott
WC; 616	Minocycline Hcl	100 mg	White and Olive	Capsule		Warner Chilcott
WC; 634 ;	Acetaminophen and Codeine No. 2	300 mg ; 15 mg		Tablet		Warner Chilcott
WC; 635 ;	Acetaminophen and Codeine No. 3	300 mg ; 30 mg	White	Tablet	Circle	Warner Chilcott
WC; 637 ;	Acetaminophen and Codeine No. 4	300 mg ; 60 mg	White	Tablet	Flat	Warner Chilcott
WC; 640	Acetaminophen	325 mg	White	Tablet	Circle	Warner Chilcott
WC; 648	Penapar VK	250 mg		Tablet		Warner Chilcott
WC; 672	Erythromycin Stearate	250 mg		Tablet		Warner Chilcott
WC; 673	Penapar VK	500 mg		Tablet		Warner Chilcott
WC; 702	Hydrochlorothiazide	25 mg		Tablet		Warner Chilcott
WC; 710	Hydrochlorothiazide	50 mg		Tablet		Warner Chilcott
WC; 712	Spironolactone with Hydrochlorothiazide	25 mg ; 25 mg		Tablet		Warner Chilcott
WC; 713	Spironolactone	25 mg		Tablet		Warner Chilcott
WC; 725	Aspirin with Codeine Phosphate No. 2	325 mg ; 15 mg		Tablet		Warner Chilcott
WC; 726	Aspirin with Codeine Phosphate No. 3	30 mg ; 325 mg		Tablet		Warner Chilcott
WC; 727	Aspirin with Codeine Phosphate No. 4	60 mg ; 325 mg		Tablet		Warner Chilcott
WC; 730	Amoxicillin	250 mg		Capsule		Warner Chilcott
WC; 731	Amoxicillin	500 mg	Red and Pink	Capsule		Warner Chilcott
WC; 784	Potassium Chloride	10 meq		Extended-Release Tablet		Warner Chilcott
WC; 800	Chlordiazepoxide Hydrochloride	5 mg		Capsule		Warner Chilcott
WC; 801	Chlordiazepoxide Hydrochloride	10 mg		Capsule		Warner Chilcott
WC; 802	Chlordiazepoxide Hydrochloride	25 mg		Capsule		Warner Chilcott
WC; 808	Cephradine	250 mg		Capsule		Warner Chilcott
WC; 809	Cephradine	500 mg		Capsule		Warner Chilcott
WC; 813 ;	Doxycycline Hyclate	100 mg		Tablet		Warner Chilcott
WC; 829 ;	Doxycycline Hyclate	50 mg		Capsule		Warner Chilcott
WC; 830 ;	Doxycycline Hyclate	100 mg		Capsule		Warner Chilcott
WC; 832	Amiloride Hydrochloride and Hydrochlorothiazide	5 mg ; 50 mg	Yellow	Tablet	Circle	Warner Chilcott
WC; 833	Triamterene and Hydrochlorothiazide	50 mg ; 75 mg	Yellow	Tablet	Round, Bisected Scored	Warner Chilcott
WC; 849	Quinidine Sulfate	200 mg		Tablet		Warner Chilcott
WC; 850	Duraquin	330 mg	White	Sustained-Release Tablet		Warner Chilcott
WC; 850	Quinidine Gluconate	330 mg		Tablet		Warner Chilcott
WC; 865 ;	Methyldopa	250 mg	Blue	Tablet	Circle	Warner Chilcott
WC; 866 ;	Methyldopa	500 mg	Blue	Tablet	Circle	Warner Chilcott
WC; 878	Metoclopramide Hydrochloride	10 mg		Tablet		Warner Chilcott
WC; 919	Erythromycin Stearate	500 mg		Tablet		Warner Chilcott
WC; 929	Nelova 0.5/35e-21	0.5 mg ; 35 mcg	Light Yellow	21-Day Tablet Pack	Circle	Warner Chilcott
WC; 929	Nelova 0.5/35e-28 Light Yellow Tablet	0.5 mg ; 35 mcg	Light Yellow	28-Day Tablet Pack	Circle	Warner Chilcott
WC; 929	Nelova 10/11-21 Light Yellow Tablet	35 mcg ; 0.5 mg	Light Yellow	21-Day Tablet Pack	Circle	Warner Chilcott
WC; 929	Nelova 10/11-28 Light Yellow Tablet	0.5 mg ; 35 mcg	Light Yellow	28-Day Tablet Pack	Circle	Warner Chilcott

IMPRINT	BRAND/GENERIC NAME	STRENGTH	COLOR	FORM	SHAPE	MANUFACTURER
WC; 930	Nelova 1/35e-21	1 mg ; 35 mcg	Dark Yellow	21-Day Tablet Pack	Circle	Warner Chilcott
WC; 930	Nelova 1/35e-28 Dark Yellow Tablet	1 mg ; 35 mcg	Dark Yellow	28-Day Tablet Pack	Circle	Warner Chilcott
WC; 930	Nelova 10/11-21 Dark Yellow Tablet	1 mg ; 35 mcg	Dark Yellow	21-Day Tablet Pack	Circle	Warner Chilcott
WC; 930	Nelova 10/11-28 Dark Yellow Tablet	1 mg ; 35 mcg	Dark Yellow	28-Day Tablet Pack	Circle	Warner Chilcott
WC; 940	R-Tannate	25 mg ; 8 mg ; 25 mg	Buff	Tablet	Capsule-Shape	Warner Chilcott
WC; 942	Nelova 1/50m-21	1 mg ; 50 mcg	Light Blue	21-Day Tablet Pack	Circle	Warner Chilcott
WC; 942	Nelova 1/50m-28 Light Blue Tablet	1 mg ; 50 mcg	Light Blue	28-Day Tablet Pack	Circle	Warner Chilcott
WC; 945	Dicloxacillin Sodium	250 mg		Capsule		Warner Chilcott
WC; 946	Dicloxacillin Sodium	500 mg		Capsule		Warner Chilcott
WC; 951	Potassium Chloride	8 meq		Extended-Release Capsule		Warner Chilcott
WC; 977	Temazepam	15 mg		Capsule		Warner Chilcott
WC; 978	Temazepam	30 mg		Capsule		Warner Chilcott
WC; 979	Acetaminophen and Propoxyphene Hydrochloride	65 mg ; 650 mg		Tablet		Warner Chilcott
WC; 980	Acetaminophen and Propoxyphene Napsylate	650 mg ; 100 mg		Tablet		Warner Chilcott
WC; 981	Haloperidol	0.5 mg		Tablet		Warner Chilcott
WC; 982	Haloperidol	1 mg		Tablet		Warner Chilcott
WC; 983	Haloperidol	2 mg		Tablet		Warner Chilcott
WC; 984	Haloperidol	5 mg		Tablet		Warner Chilcott
WC; 985	Clonidine Hydrochloride and Chlorthalidone	0.1 mg ; 15 mg		Tablet		Warner Chilcott
WC; 986	Clonidine Hydrochloride and Chlorthalidone	0.2 mg ; 15 mg		Tablet		Warner Chilcott
WC; 987	Clonidine Hydrochloride and Chlorthalidone	0.3 mg ; 15 mg		Tablet		Warner Chilcott
WC; 988	Flurazepam Hydrochloride	15 mg	Peach and Orange	Capsule		Warner Chilcott
WC; 989	Flurazepam Hydrochloride	30 mg	Peach and Strawberry	Capsule		Warner Chilcott
WELLBUTRIN SR; 100	Wellbutrin SR	100 mg	Blue	Sustained-Release Tablet	Circle, Biconvex	Glaxosmithkline
WELLBUTRIN SR; 150	Wellbutrin SR	150 mg	Purple	Sustained-Release Tablet	Circle, Biconvex	Glaxosmithkline
WELLBUTRIN XL; 150	Wellbutrin XL	150 mg	White to Yellow	Tablet	Circle	Glaxosmithkline
WELLBUTRIN XL; 300	Wellbutrin XL	300 mg	White to Yellow	Tablet	Circle	Glaxosmithkline
WELLBUTRIN; 75	Wellbutrin	75 mg	Yellow-Gold	Coated Tablet	Biconvex, Circle	Glaxosmithkline
WELLBUTRIN; 100	Wellbutrin	100 mg	Red	Coated Tablet	Circle, Biconvex	Glaxosmithkline
WELLBUTRIN; SR; 200	Wellbutrin SR	200 mg	Light Pink	Sustained-Release Tablet	Circle, Biconvex	Glaxosmithkline
WELLBUTRIN; XL; 150	Wellbutrin XL	150 mg	Creamy White to Pale Yellow	Extended-Release Tablet	Circle	Glaxosmithkline
WELLBUTRIN; XL; 300	Wellbutrin XL	300 mg	Creamy White to Pale Yellow	Extended-Release Tablet	Circle	Glaxosmithkline
WELLCOME; U3B	Tabloid	40 mg	Green-Yellow	Tablet	Circle, Scored	Glaxosmithkline
WELLCOME; ZOVIRAX; 200	Zovirax	200 mg	Blue	Capsule		Glaxosmithkline
WEST-WARD 475	Prednisone	5 mg	White	Tablet	Circle	Novartis Generics
WEST-WARD; 477	Prednisone	20 mg	Peach	Tablet	Circle, Scored	Novartis Generics
WESTWARD; FLURAZEPAM; 15	Flurazepam Hydrochloride	15 mg	Blue and White	Capsule		Novartis Generics
WESTWARD; FLURAZEPAM; 30	Flurazepam Hydrochloride	30 mg	Blue	Capsule	Oblong	Novartis Generics
WH-SCS; 5752	Piroxicam	10 mg	Opaque Orange and Opaque Light Blue	Capsule		Lederle Laboratories
WH-SCS; 5762	Piroxicam	20 mg	Opaque Orange	Capsule		Lederle Laboratories
WINTHROP; T; 37	Talacen	25 mg ; 650 mg	Pale Blue	Tablet		Sanofi-Aventis U.S.
WKJ ;	Permitil Chronotab	1 mg	Yellow	Tablet		Schering
WPI ; 11 17	Mirtazapine	15 mg	White to Off-White	Tablet	Oval	Watson Laboratories
WPI ; 3462	Sertraline Hydrochloride	200 mg	White	Tablet	Capsule-Shape	Watson Laboratories
WPI 339	Diclofenac Sodium	75 mg	White	Tablet, Delayed Release	Circle	Watson Laboratories
WPI 839	Bupropion Hydrochloride SR	150 mg	White	Tablet, Extended Release	Circle	Watson Laboratories
WPI 844	Glipizide	5 mg	Orange	Tablet, Extended Release	Circle	Watson Laboratories
WPI 845	Glipizide	10 mg	White to Off-White	Tablet, Extended Release	Circle	Watson Laboratories
WPI 858	Bupropion Hydrochloride SR	100 mg	White	Tablet, Extended Release	Circle	Watson Laboratories
WPI 867	Bupropion Hydrochloride	150 mg	White	Tablet, Extended Release	Circle	Watson Laboratories
WPI 900	Glipizide	2.5 mg	Light Orange	Tablet, Extended Release	Circle	Watson Laboratories
WPI 1118	Mirtazapine	30 mg	Yellow	Tablet	Oval	Watson Laboratories
WPI 1119	Mirtazapine	45 mg	White to Off-White	Tablet	Oval	Watson Laboratories
WPI 3177	Citalopram Hydrobromide	20 mg	White	Tablet	Circle	Watson Laboratories
WPI 3178	Citalopram Hydrobromide	40 mg	White	Tablet	Circle	Watson Laboratories
WPI 3332	Bupropion Hydrochloride XL	300 mg	White to Off-White	Tablet, Extended Release, 24 Hr	Circle	Watson Laboratories
WPI 3385	Bupropion Hydrochloride SR	200 mg	White	Tablet, Extended Release	Circle	Watson Laboratories
WPI 3416	Apap/butalbital/caffeine	325 mg ; 50 mg ; 40 mg	White	Tablet	Capsule-Shape	Watson Laboratories

IMPRINT	BRAND/GENERIC NAME	STRENGTH	COLOR	FORM	SHAPE	MANUFACTURER
WPI; 2455	Metformin Hydrochloride	1000 mg	Light Peach	Tablet		Watson Laboratories
WPI; 2713	Metformin Hydrochloride	500 mg	Light Peach	Tablet	Capsule-Shape	Watson Laboratories
WPI; 2775	Metformin Hydrochloride	850 mg	Light Peach	Tablet	Capsule-Shape	Watson Laboratories
WPI; 3111	Methylphenidate Hydrochloride	20 mg	White	Extended-Release Tablet	Oval	Watson Laboratories
WPI; 3137	Nizatidine	150 mg	Buff	Capsule		Watson Laboratories
WPI; 3138	Nizatidine	300 mg	Light Brown	Capsule		Watson Laboratories
WYETH; 1	Equanil	400 mg	White	Tablet		Wyeth Pharmaceuticals
WYETH; 2	Equanil	200 mg	White	Tablet		Wyeth Pharmaceuticals
WYETH; 10	Isordil	10 mg	White	Tablet	Circle	Wyeth Pharmaceuticals
WYETH; 13	Amphojel	600 mg	White	Tablet		Wyeth Pharmaceuticals
WYETH; 19	Phenergan	12.5 mg	Orange	Tablet		Wyeth Pharmaceuticals
WYETH; 22	Aludrox	233 mg ; 83 mg		Tablet, Chewable		Wyeth Pharmaceuticals
WYETH; 27	Phenergan	25 mg	White	Tablet		Wyeth Pharmaceuticals
WYETH; 28	Sparine	50 mg	Orange	Coated Tablet	Circle	Wyeth Pharmaceuticals
WYETH; 29	Sparine	25 mg	Yellow	Coated Tablet	Circle	Wyeth Pharmaceuticals
WYETH; 33	Equanil Wyseals	400 mg	Yellow	Coated Tablet	Circle	Wyeth Pharmaceuticals
WYETH; 33	Wyseals	400 mg	Yellow	Coated Tablet		Wyeth Pharmaceuticals
WYETH; 53	Omnipen	250 mg	Violet and Pink	Capsule		Wyeth Pharmaceuticals
WYETH; 56	Ovral	0.5 mg ; 50 mcg	White	21-Day Tablet Pack	Circle	Wyeth Pharmaceuticals
WYETH; 56	Ovral-28 White Tablet	0.5 mg ; 50 mcg	White	28-Day Tablet Pack	Circle	Wyeth Pharmaceuticals
WYETH; 57	Unipen	250 mg	Green and Yellow	Capsule		Wyeth Pharmaceuticals
WYETH; 59	Pen-Vee K	250 mg	White	Tablet		Wyeth Pharmaceuticals
WYETH; 62	Ovrette	75 mcg	Yellow	28-Day Tablet Pack	Circle	Wyeth Pharmaceuticals
WYETH; 71	Mazanor	1 mg	White	Tablet	Circle, Scored	Wyeth Pharmaceuticals
WYETH; 73, W; 4	Wytensin	4 mg	Orange	Tablet	Five-Sided	Wyeth Pharmaceuticals
WYETH; 74; W; 8	Wytensin	8 mg	Grey	Tablet	Five-Sided	Wyeth Pharmaceuticals
WYETH; 75	Nordette-21	30 mcg ; 0.15 mg	Light Orange	21-Day Tablet Pack	Circle	Wyeth Pharmaceuticals
WYETH; 75	Nordette-28 Light Orange Tablet	0.15 mg ; 30 mcg	Light Orange	28-Day Tablet Pack	Circle	Wyeth Pharmaceuticals
WYETH; 78	Lo/ovral	0.3 mg ; 30 mcg	White	21-Day Tablet Pack	Circle	Wyeth Pharmaceuticals
WYETH; 78	Lo/ovral-28 - White Tablet	0.3 mg ; 30 mcg	White	Tablet	Circle	Wyeth Pharmaceuticals
WYETH; 91	Equagesic	200 mg ; 325 mg	Orange and Pink	Tablet	Circle	Wyeth Pharmaceuticals
WYETH; 92; W; 16	Wytensin	16 mg	White	Tablet	Five-Sided	Wyeth Pharmaceuticals
WYETH; 119	Amphojel	300 mg	White	Tablet	Circle	Wyeth Pharmaceuticals
WYETH; 138	A-M-T	162 mg ; 250 mg		Tablet		Wyeth Pharmaceuticals
WYETH; 200	Sparine	100 mg	Pink	Coated Tablet	Circle	Wyeth Pharmaceuticals
WYETH; 227	Phenergan	50 mg	Pink	Tablet		Wyeth Pharmaceuticals
WYETH; 261	Mepergan Fortis	50 mg ; 25 mg	Maroon	Capsule		Wyeth Pharmaceuticals
WYETH; 308	Meperidine Hydrochloride	50 mg	Tablet	Tablet	Scored, Circle	Wyeth Pharmaceuticals
WYETH; 309	Omnipen	500 mg	Violet and Pink	Capsule		Wyeth Pharmaceuticals
WYETH; 313	Aspirin	300 mg		Tablet		Wyeth Pharmaceuticals
WYETH; 322	Chloral Hydrate	500 mg	Red	Capsule		Wyeth Pharmaceuticals
WYETH; 360	Pathocil	250 mg	Purple and White	Capsule		Wyeth Pharmaceuticals
WYETH; 389	Tetracycline Hydrochloride	250 mg	Blue and Yellow	Capsule		Wyeth Pharmaceuticals
WYETH; 390	Pen-Vee K	500 mg	White	Tablet		Wyeth Pharmaceuticals
WYETH; 434	Phenergan-D	60 mg ; 6.25 mg	Orange and White	Tablet		Wyeth Pharmaceuticals
WYETH; 464	Unipen	500 mg	White	Coated Tablet		Wyeth Pharmaceuticals
WYETH; 471	Tetracycline Hydrochloride	500 mg	Blue and Yellow	Capsule		Wyeth Pharmaceuticals
WYETH; 472	Basaljel	608 mg		Capsule		Wyeth Pharmaceuticals
WYETH; 473	Basaljel	608 mg		Tablet		Wyeth Pharmaceuticals
WYETH; 559	Wymox	250 mg	Gray and Green	Capsule		Wyeth Pharmaceuticals
WYETH; 560	Wymox	500 mg	Gray and Green	Capsule		Wyeth Pharmaceuticals
WYETH; 576	Wyamycin S	250 mg	Yellow	Coated Tablet		Wyeth Pharmaceuticals
WYETH; 578	Wyamycin S	500 mg	Pink	Coated Tablet		Wyeth Pharmaceuticals
WYETH; 593	Pathocil	500 mg	Purple and White	Capsule		Wyeth Pharmaceuticals
WYETH; 614	Cyclapen W	250 mg	Yellow	Tablet	Capsule-Shape, Scored	Wyeth Pharmaceuticals
WYETH; 615	Cyclapen W	500 mg	Yellow	Tablet		Wyeth Pharmaceuticals
WYETH; 4120	Cyclospasmol	100 mg	Orange	Coated Tablet		Wyeth Pharmaceuticals
WYETH; 4124	Cyclospasmol	200 mg	Blue	Capsule		Wyeth Pharmaceuticals
WYETH; 4140	Isordil Tembids	40 mg	Clear Blue and Transparent	Capsule		Wyeth Pharmaceuticals
WYETH; 4148	Cyclospasmol	400 mg	Red and Blue	Capsule		Wyeth Pharmaceuticals
WYETH; 4152	Isordil Titradose	5 mg	Pink	Tablet		Wyeth Pharmaceuticals
WYETH; 4153	Isordil Titradose	10 mg	White	Tablet		Wyeth Pharmaceuticals
WYETH; 4154	Isordil Titradose	20 mg	Green	Tablet		Wyeth Pharmaceuticals
WYETH; 4159	Isordil Titradose	30 mg	Blue	Tablet		Wyeth Pharmaceuticals
WYETH; 4169	Synalgos	6.25 mg ; 356.4 mg ; 30 mg	Maroon and Gray	Capsule		Wyeth Pharmaceuticals
WYETH; 4175	Synalgos-Dc-A	16 mg ; 356.4 mg ; 30 mg	Green and Gray	Capsule		Wyeth Pharmaceuticals
WYETH; 4177; SECTRAL; 200	Sectral	200 mg	Purple and Orange	Capsule		Wyeth Pharmaceuticals
WYETH; 4179; SECTRAL; 400	Sectral	400 mg	Brown and Orange	Capsule		Wyeth Pharmaceuticals
WYETH; 4181; ORUDIS 50	Orudis	50 mg	Dark Green and Light Green	Capsule		Wyeth Pharmaceuticals
WYETH; 4186; ORUDIS 25	Orudis	25 mg	Dark Green and Red	Capsule		Wyeth Pharmaceuticals
WYETH; 4187; ORUDIS 75	Orudis	75 mg	Dark Green and White	Capsule		Wyeth Pharmaceuticals
WYETH; 4188; C	Cordarone	200 mg	Pink	Tablet	Circle, Convex-Faced	Wyeth Pharmaceuticals
WYETH; 4191	Synalgos-Dc	16 mg ; 356.4 mg ; 30 mg	Blue and Gray	Capsule		Wyeth-Ayerst Laboratories
WYETH; 4192	Isordil Titradose	40 mg	Green	Tablet		Wyeth Pharmaceuticals
X; 0.5	Alprazolam	0.5 mg	White	Extended-Release Tablet	Five-Sided	Pharmacia & Upjohn
X; 0.5	Xanax Xr	0.5 mg	White	Tablet, Extended Release	Five-Sided	Pharmacia & Upjohn
X; 1	Xanax Xr	1 mg	Yellow	Extended-Release Tablet	Square	Pharmacia & Upjohn
X; 2	Xanax Xr	2 mg	Blue	Tablet, Extended Release	Circle	Pharmacia & Upjohn

IMPRINT	BRAND/GENERIC NAME	STRENGTH	COLOR	FORM	SHAPE	MANUFACTURER
X; 3	Xanax Xr	3 mg	Green	Extended-Release Tablet	Triangle	Pharmacia & Upjohn
X; 10	Uroxatral	10 mg	White and Yellow	Tablet, Extended Release	Circle	Sanofi-Aventis U.S.
X1 ; STUARTNATAL LOGO	Duet Dha - Dha Softgel Capsule	430 mg	Translucent Gold	Capsule, Liquid Filled	Oval	Xanodyne Pharmaceuticals
XANAX; 0.25	Xanax	0.25 mg	White	Tablet	Oval	Pharmacia & Upjohn
XANAX; 0.5	Xanax	0.5 mg	Peach	Tablet	Oval	Pharmacia & Upjohn
XANAX; 1.0	Xanax	1 mg	Blue	Tablet	Oval	Pharmacia & Upjohn
XELODA; 150	Xeloda	150 mg	Light Peach	Coated Tablet	Oblong	Roche Laboratories
XELODA; 500	Xeloda	500 mg	Peach	Coated Tablet	Oblong	Roche Laboratories
XP; A; 10	Amicar	500 mg	White	Tablet	Circle, Scored	Xanodyne Pharmaceuticals
XP; A; 20	Amicar	1000 mg	White	Tablet	Oblong, Scored	Xanodyne Pharmaceuticals
XR 200	Seroquel Xr	200 mg	Yellow	Tablet, Extended Release	Capsule-Shape	Astrazeneca LP
XR 300	Seroquel Xr	300 mg	Pale Yellow	Tablet, Extended Release	Capsule-Shape	Astrazeneca LP
XR 400	Seroquel Xr	400 mg	White	Tablet, Extended Release	Capsule-Shape	Astrazeneca LP
Y	Xyzal	5 mg	White	Tablet	Oval	Sanofi-Aventis U.S.
YSP 173	Zolpidem Tartrate	10 mg	White	Tablet	Circle	Actavis Elizabeth
YSP 174	Zolpidem Tartrate	5 mg	White	Tablet	Circle	Actavis Elizabeth
Z	Zomig-Zmt	2.5 mg	White	Disintegrating Tablet	Circle	Medpointe
Z 4	Zofran Odt	4 mg	White	Tablet, Disintegrating	Circle	Glaxosmithkline
Z 8	Zofran Odt	8 mg	White	Tablet, Disintegrating	Circle	Glaxosmithkline
Z 50 MG 2130	Nitrofurantoin Macrocrystals	50 mg	Pink Opaque, White Opaque	Capsule		Teva Pharmaceuticals
Z 100 MG 2131	Nitrofurantoin Macrocrystals	100 mg	Pink Opaque, White Opaque	Capsule		Teva Pharmaceuticals
Z; 5	Zomig-Zmt	5 mg	White	Disintegrating Tablet	Circle, Flat Faced, Bevelled	Medpointe
Z; 2083	Hydrochlorothiazide	25 mg	Peach	Tablet	Circle	Ivax Pharmaceuticals
Z; 2089	Hydrochlorothiazide	50 mg	Peach	Tablet	Circle	Ivax Pharmaceuticals
Z; 2186	Propoxyphene Hydrochloride	65 mg	Pale Pink	Capsule		Ivax Pharmaceuticals
Z; 2190	Probenecid	500 mg	Yellow	Coated Tablet	Capsule-Shape	Novartis Generics
Z; 2193	Probenecid with Colchicine	500 mg ; 0.5 mg	White	Tablet	Capsule-Shape	Novartis Generics
Z; 2218	Sulfisoxazole	500 mg	White	Tablet	Circle, Scored	Ivax Pharmaceuticals
Z; 2345	Procainamide Hydrochloride	250 mg	Yellow	Capsule		Ivax Pharmaceuticals
Z; 2347	Procainamide Hydrochloride	500 mg	Yellow and Orange	Capsule		Ivax Pharmaceuticals
Z; 2485	Hydrochlorothiazide	100 mg	Light Orange	Tablet	Circle	Ivax Pharmaceuticals
Z; 2662; 10	Famotidine	10 mg		Tablet		Ivax Pharmaceuticals
Z; 2907	Furosemide	40 mg	White	Tablet	Circle	Ivax Pharmaceuticals
Z; 2908	Furosemide	20 mg	White	Tablet	Oval	Ivax Pharmaceuticals
Z; 2909	Hydroxyzine Pamoate	50 mg	Green and White	Capsule		Ivax Pharmaceuticals
Z; 2911	Hydroxyzine Pamoate	25 mg	Dark Green and Light Green	Capsule		Ivax Pharmaceuticals
Z; 2929	Cyproheptadine Hydrochloride	4 mg	White	Tablet	Round-Flat, Bisected Scored	Ivax Pharmaceuticals
Z; 2931	Methyldopa	250 mg	White	Coated Tablet	Circle	Ivax Pharmaceuticals
Z; 2932	Methyldopa	500 mg	White	Coated Tablet	Circle	Ivax Pharmaceuticals
Z; 2959	Ergoloid Mesylates SL	1 mg	White	Tablet	Oval	Ivax Pharmaceuticals
Z; 2971	Metronidazole	250 mg	White	Tablet	Circle	Ivax Pharmaceuticals
Z; 2971 ;	Helidac Therapy: Part II	250 mg	White	Tablet	Circle	Procter & Gamble Pharmaceuticals
Z; 2984	Doxycycline Hyclate	50 mg	Blue and White	Capsule		Ivax Pharmaceuticals
Z; 3001	Quinine Sulfate	260 mg	White	Tablet	Circle	Teva Pharmaceuticals
Z; 3007	Metronidazole	500 mg	White	Tablet	Oblong	Ivax Pharmaceuticals
Z; 3626	Doxycycline Hyclate	100 mg	Orange	Coated Tablet	Circle	Ivax Pharmaceuticals
Z; 3690; 5	Prochlorperazine Maleate	5 mg	Gold	Tablet	Circle	Ivax Pharmaceuticals
Z; 3691; 10	Prochlorperazine Maleate	10 mg	Gold	Tablet	Circle	Ivax Pharmaceuticals
Z; 3925; 2	Diazepam	2 mg	White	Tablet	Circle	Ivax Pharmaceuticals
Z; 3926; 5	Diazepam	5 mg	Yellow	Tablet	Circle	Ivax Pharmaceuticals
Z; 3927; 10	Diazepam	10 mg	Light Blue	Tablet	Circle	Ivax Pharmaceuticals
Z; 4029	Indomethacin	25 mg	Green	Capsule		Ivax Pharmaceuticals
Z; 4030	Indomethacin	50 mg	Green	Capsule		Ivax Pharmaceuticals
Z; 4096; 10 ;	Baclofen	10 mg	White	Tablet	Circle, Flat, Scored	Ivax Pharmaceuticals
Z; 4097; 20 ;	Baclofen	20 mg	White	Tablet	Circle, Flat, Scored	Ivax Pharmaceuticals
Z; 4172	Quinine Sulfate	325 mg	White	Capsule		Ivax Pharmaceuticals
Z; 4226	Guanabenz Acetate	4 mg	Peach	Tablet	Circle, Compressed	Ivax Pharmaceuticals
Z; 4227	Guanabenz Acetate	8 mg	Grey	Tablet	Round, Compressed, Bisected Scored	Ivax Pharmaceuticals
Z; 4235; 20	Nadolol	20 mg	White	Tablet	Circle	Ivax Pharmaceuticals
Z; 4236; 40	Nadolol	40 mg	White	Tablet	Circle	Ivax Pharmaceuticals
Z; 4237; 80	Nadolol	80 mg	White	Tablet	Circle	Ivax Pharmaceuticals
Z; 4238; 120	Nadolol	120 mg	White	Tablet	Oblong	Ivax Pharmaceuticals
Z; 4239; 160	Nadolol	160 mg	White	Tablet	Oblong	Ivax Pharmaceuticals
Z; 4259	Indapamide	2.5 mg	White	Coated Tablet	Circle	Ivax Pharmaceuticals
Z; 4262; 1.25	Indapamide	1.25 mg	Orange	Tablet	Circle	Ivax Pharmaceuticals
Z; 4288; 20 MG	Nicardipine Hydrochloride	20 mg	Opaque White	Capsule		Ivax Pharmaceuticals
Z; 4289; 30 MG	Nicardipine Hydrochloride	30 mg	Light Blue Opaque	Capsule		Ivax Pharmaceuticals
Z; 4338; 5 MG	Terazosin Hydrochloride	5 mg	Red and White	Capsule		Ivax Pharmaceuticals
Z; 4804	Oxazepam	10 mg	Blue and White	Capsule		Ivax Pharmaceuticals
Z; 4805	Oxazepam	15 mg	Clear	Capsule		Ivax Pharmaceuticals
Z; 4806	Oxazepam	30 mg	Orange and White	Capsule		Ivax Pharmaceuticals
Z; 5624; 300 MG	Nizatidine	300 mg	Light Brown and White	Capsule		Ivax Pharmaceuticals
Z; LA; BOCK	Zephrex LA	120 mg ; 600 mg	Orange	Tablet, Extended Release	Oval	Sanofi-Synthelabo
ZANTAC 150 ; GLAXO ;	Zantac 150	150 mg	Peach	Tablet	Five-Sided	Glaxosmithkline
ZANTAC; 150; 427	Zantac 150 Efferdose	150 mg	White to Pale Yellow	Tablet, Effervescent	Circle	Glaxosmithkline

IMPRINT	BRAND/GENERIC NAME	STRENGTH	COLOR	FORM	SHAPE	MANUFACTURER
ZANTAC; 150; GLAXO	Zantac 150 Geldose	150 mg	Beige	Gel/jelly		Glaxosmithkline
ZANTAC; 300; GLAXO	Zantac 300 Geldose	300 mg	Beige	Gel/jelly		Glaxosmithkline
ZBN	Arava	10 mg	White	Tablet	Circle	Sanofi-Aventis U.S.
ZBO	Arava	20 mg	Yellow	Tablet	Triangle	Sanofi-Aventis U.S.
ZBP	Arava	100 mg	White	Coated Tablet	Circle	Aventis Pharmaceuticals
ZE; 74	Erythromycin Ethylsuccinate	400 mg	Mottled Pink	Tablet	Oval	Abbott Laboratories
ZENECA; ACCOLATE; 10	Accolate	10 mg	White	Coated Tablet	Circle, Biconvex, Mini	Astrazeneca
ZENECA; ACCOLATE; 20	Accolate	20 mg	White	Coated Tablet	Circle	Astrazeneca
ZENITH; 200 MG; 4171	Quinine Sulfate	200 mg	White	Capsule		Ivax Pharmaceuticals
ZENITH; 4266; 200	Acyclovir	200 mg	Opaque White	Capsule		Ivax Pharmaceuticals
ZESTORETIC; 141	Zestoretic	12.5 mg ; 10 mg	Peach	Tablet	Circle, Biconvex	Astrazeneca
ZESTORETIC; 142	Zestoretic	12.5 mg ; 20 mg	White	Tablet	Circle, Biconvex	Astrazeneca
ZESTORETIC; 145	Zestoretic	25 mg ; 20 mg	Peach	Tablet	Biconvex, Circle	Astrazeneca
ZESTRIL; 2 1/2; 135	Zestril	2.5 mg	White	Tablet	Circle, Biconvex	Astrazeneca
ZESTRIL; 10; 131	Zestril	10 mg	Pink	Tablet	Circle, Biconvex	Astrazeneca
ZESTRIL; 20; 132	Zestril	20 mg	Red	Tablet	Circle, Biconvex	Astrazeneca
ZESTRIL; 30; 133	Zestril	30 mg	Red	Tablet	Circle, Biconvex	Astrazeneca
ZESTRIL; 40; 134	Zestril	40 mg	Yellow	Tablet	Circle, Biconvex	Astrazeneca
ZESTRIL; 130	Zestril	5 mg	Pink	Tablet	Capsule-Shape, Biconvex, Scored	Astrazeneca
ZG ZENITH 30MG 4289	Nicardipine Hydrochloride	30 mg	Light Blue Opaque	Capsule		Barr Laboratories
ZG ZENITH 20MG 4288	Nicardipine Hydrochloride	20 mg	White Opaque	Capsule		Barr Laboratories
ZOFRAN 4	Zofran	4 mg	White	Tablet	Oval	Glaxosmithkline
ZOFRAN 8	Zofran	8 mg	Yellow	Tablet	Oval	Glaxosmithkline
ZOLOFT; 25 MG	Zoloft	25 mg	Light Green	Coated Tablet	Capsule-Shape, Scored	Pfizer
ZOLOFT; 50 MG	Zoloft	50 mg	Light Blue	Tablet	Capsule-Shape	Pfizer
ZOLOFT; 100 MG	Zoloft	100 mg	Light Yellow	Tablet	Capsule-Shape	Pfizer
ZOMIG; 2.5	Zomig	2.5 mg	Yellow	Coated Tablet	Circle, Biconvex, Scored	Medpointe
ZOMIG; 5	Zomig	5 mg	Pink	Tablet	Biconvex	Medpointe
ZOVIRAX; 800	Zovirax	800 mg	Light Blue	Tablet	Oval	Glaxosmithkline
ZOVIRAX; TRIANGLE	Zovirax	400 mg	White	Tablet	Shield-Shape	Glaxosmithkline
ZTM500 ; PFIZER	Zithromax	500 mg	Pink	Tablet	Capsule-Shape	Pfizer
ZYBAN; 150	Zyban	150 mg	Purple	Sustained-Release Tablet	Circle, Biconvex	Glaxosmithkline
ZYRTEC; C5	Zyrtec Chewable	5 mg	Purple	Tablet, Chewable	Circle	Pfizer Laboratories
ZYRTEC; C10	Zyrtec Chewable	10 mg	Purple	Tablet, Chewable	Circle	Pfizer Laboratories
ZYRTEC-D	Zyrtec-D 12 Hour	5 mg ; 120 mg	White	Tablet, Extended Release	Circle	UCB Pharma
ZYVOX; 400 MG	Zyvox	400 mg	White	Coated Tablet	Oblong, Compressed	Pharmacia & Upjohn
ZYVOX; 600 MG	Zyvox	600 mg	White	Coated Tablet	Capsule-Shape, Compressed	Pharmacia & Upjohn

Key to Controlled Substances Categories

Products listed with the symbols shown below are subject to the Controlled Substances Act of 1970. These drugs are categorized according to their potential for abuse. The greater the potential, the more severe the limitations on their prescription.

CATEGORY	INTERPRETATION
CII	**HIGH POTENTIAL FOR ABUSE.** Use may lead to severe physical or psychological dependence. Prescriptions must be written in ink, or typewritten and signed by the practitioner. Verbal prescriptions must be confirmed in writing within 72 hours, and may be given only in a genuine emergency. No renewals are permitted.
CIII	**SOME POTENTIAL FOR ABUSE.** Use may lead to low-to-moderate physical dependence or high psychological dependence. Prescriptions may be oral or written. Up to 5 renewals are permitted within 6 months.
CIV	**LOW POTENTIAL FOR ABUSE.** Use may lead to limited physical or psychological dependence. Prescriptions may be oral or written. Up to 5 renewals are permitted within 6 months.
CV	**SUBJECT TO STATE AND LOCAL REGULATION.** Abuse potential is low; a prescription may not be required.

Key to FDA Use-in-Pregnancy Ratings

The U.S. Food and Drug Administration's use-in-pregnancy rating system weighs the degree to which available information has ruled out risk to the fetus against the drug's potential benefit to the patient. The ratings, and their interpretation, are as follows:

CATEGORY	INTERPRETATION
A	**CONTROLLED STUDIES SHOW NO RISK.** Adequate, well-controlled studies in pregnant women have failed to demonstrate a risk to the fetus in any trimester of pregnancy.
B	**NO EVIDENCE OF RISK IN HUMANS.** Adequate, well-controlled studies in pregnant women have not shown increased risk of fetal abnormalities despite adverse findings in animals, or, in the absence of adequate human studies, animal studies show no fetal risk. The chance of fetal harm is remote, but remains a possibility.
C	**RISK CANNOT BE RULED OUT.** Adequate, well-controlled human studies are lacking, and animal studies have shown a risk to the fetus or are lacking as well. There is a chance of fetal harm if the drug is administered during pregnancy; but the potential benefits may outweigh the potential risk.
D	**POSITIVE EVIDENCE OF RISK.** Studies in humans, or investigational or post-marketing data, have demonstrated fetal risk. Nevertheless, potential benefits from the use of the drug may outweigh the potential risk. For example, the drug may be acceptable if needed in a life-threatening situation or serious disease for which safer drugs cannot be used or are ineffective.
X	**CONTRAINDICATED IN PREGNANCY.** Studies in animals or humans, or investigational or post-marketing reports, have demonstrated positive evidence of fetal abnormalities or risk which clearly outweighs any possible benefit to the patient.

U.S. FOOD AND DRUG ADMINISTRATION

Medical Product Reporting Programs

MedWatch (24-hour service) **800-332-1088**
Reporting of problems with drugs, devices, biologics (except vaccines), medical foods, and dietary supplements.

Vaccine Adverse Event Reporting System (24-hour service) **800-822-7967**
Reporting of vaccine-related problems.

Mandatory Medical Device Reporting **240-276-3000**
Reporting required from user facilities regarding device-related deaths and serious injuries.

Veterinary Adverse Drug Reaction Program **888-332-8387**
Reporting of adverse drug events in animals.

Division of Drug Marketing, Advertising, and Communication (DDMAC) **301-796-1200**
Inquiries from health professionals regarding product promotion.

USP Medication Errors **800-233-7767**
Reporting of medication errors or near-errors to help avoid future problems through improvement in product names and packaging.

Information for Health Professionals

Center for Drug Evaluation and Research Drug Information Hotline **301-827-4573**
Information on human drugs including hormones.

Center for Biologics Office of Communications **301-827-2000**
Information on biological products including vaccines and blood.

Center for Devices and Radiological Health **301-827-4573**
Automated request for information on medical devices and radiation-emitting products.

Emergency Operations **301-443-1240**
Emergencies involving FDA-regulated products, tampering reports, and emergency Investigational New Drug requests.

Office of Orphan Products Development **301-827-3666**
Information on products for rare diseases.

General Information

General Consumer Inquiries **888-463-6332**
Consumer information on regulated products/issues.

Freedom of Information **301-827-6500**
Requests for publicly available FDA documents.

Office of Public Affairs **301-827-6250**
Interviews/press inquiries on FDA activities.

Center for Food Safety and Applied Nutrition **888-723-3366**
Information on food safety, seafood, dietary supplements, women's nutrition, and cosmetics.

Consumer Information Service, Center for Devices and Radiological Health **800-638-2041**
Information on medical devices, mammography facilities, and radiation-emitting products.

POISON CONTROL CENTERS

The American Association of Poison Control Centers (AAPCC) uses a single, nationwide emergency number to automatically link callers with their regional poison center. This toll-free number, **800-222-1222**, also works for **teletype lines (TTY)** for the hearing-impaired and **telecommunication devices (TTD)** for individuals who are deaf. However, a few local poison centers and the ASPCA/Animal Poison Control Center are not part of this nationwide system and continue to use separate numbers.

Most of the centers listed below are certified by the AAPCC. **Certified centers are marked by an asterisk after the name**. Each has to meet certain criteria. It must, for example, serve a large geographic area; it must be open 24 hours a day and provide direct-dial or toll-free access; it must be supervised by a medical director; and it must have registered pharmacists or nurses available to answer questions from the public.

Within each state, centers are listed alphabetically by city. Some state poison centers also list their original emergency numbers (including TTY/TDD) that only work within that state. For these listings, callers may use either the state number or the nationwide 800 number.

ALABAMA

BIRMINGHAM

Regional Poison Control Center, The Children's Hospital of Alabama (*)

1600 7th Ave. South
Birmingham, AL 35233-1711
Business: 205-939-9201
Emergency: 800-222-1222
www.chsys.org

TUSCALOOSA

Alabama Poison Center (*)

2503 Phoenix Dr.
Tuscaloosa, AL 35405
Business: 205-345-0600
Emergency: 800-222-1222
800-462-0800 (AL)
www.alapoisoncenter.org

ALASKA

JUNEAU

Alaska Poison Control System

Section of Injury Prevention and EMS
410 Willoughby Ave., Room 103
Box 110616
Juneau, AK 99811-0616
Business: 907-465-3027
Emergency: 800-222-1222
www.chems.alaska.gov

(PORTLAND, OR)

Oregon Poison Center (*) Oregon Health and Science University

3181 SW Sam Jackson Park Rd.
Portland, OR 97239
Business: 503-494-8600
Emergency: 800-222-1222
www.oregonpoison.com

ARIZONA

PHOENIX

Banner Poison Control Center (*) Banner Good Samaritan Medical Center

901 E. Willetta St.
Suite 207-A
Phoenix, AZ 85006
Business: 602-253-3334
Emergency: 800-222-1222
www.bannerpoisoncontrol.com

TUCSON

Arizona Poison and Drug Information Center

1295 N. Martin Ave.
Tucson, AZ 85724
Business: 520-626-7899
Emergency: 800-222-1222
www.pharmacy.arizona.edu/outreach/poison/

ARKANSAS

LITTLE ROCK

Arkansas Poison and Drug Information Center College of Pharmacy - UAMS

4301 West Markham St.
Mail Slot 522-2
Little Rock, AR 72205-7122
Business: 501-686-6161
Emergency: 800-222-1222
800-376-4766 (AR)
TDD/TTY: 800-641-3805

ASPCA/ANIMAL POISON CONTROL CENTER

1717 South Philo Rd.
Suite 36
Urbana, IL 61802
Business: 217-337-5030
Emergency: 888-426-4435
800-548-2423
www.aspca.org/apcc

CALIFORNIA

FRESNO/MADERA

California Poison Control System-Fresno/Madera Div.(*) Valley Children's Hospital

9300 Valley Children's Place
MB15
Madera, CA 93638-8762
Business: 559-622-2300
Emergency: 800-222-1222
800-876-4766 (CA)
TDD/TTY: 800-972-3323
www.calpoison.org

SACRAMENTO

California Poison Control System-Sacramento Div.(*) UC Davis Medical Center

2315 Stockton Blvd.
Sacramento, CA 95817
Business: 916-227-1400
Emergency: 800-222-1222
800-876-4766 (CA)
TDD/TTY: 800-972-3323
www.calpoison.org

SAN DIEGO

California Poison Control System-San Diego Div. (*) UC San Diego Medical Center

200 West Arbor Dr.
San Diego, CA 92103-8925
Business: 858-715-6300
Emergency: 800-222-1222
800-876-4766 (CA)
TDD/TTY: 800-972-3323
www.calpoison.org

SAN FRANCISCO

California Poison Control System-San Francisco Div.(*) San Francisco General Hospital University of California San Francisco

Box 1369
San Francisco, CA 94143-1369
Business: 415-502-6000
Emergency: 800-222-1222
800-876-4766 (CA)
TDD/TTY: 800-972-3323
www.calpoison.org

COLORADO

DENVER

Rocky Mountain Poison and Drug Center (*)

777 Bannock St.
Mail Code 0180
Denver CO 80204-4028
Business: 303-739-1100
Emergency: 800-222-1222
TDD/TTY: 303-739-1127 (CO)
www.RMPDC.org

CONNECTICUT

FARMINGTON

Connecticut Regional Poison Control Center (*) University of Connecticut Health Center

263 Farmington Ave.
Farmington, CT 06030-5365
Business: 860-679-4540
Emergency: 800-222-1222
TDD/TTY: 866-218-5372
http://poisoncontrol.uchc.edu

DELAWARE

(PHILADELPHIA, PA)

The Poison Control Center (*) Children's Hospital of Philadelphia

34th St. & Civic Center Blvd.
Philadelphia, PA 19104-4399
Business: 215-590-2100
Emergency: 800-222-1222
TDD/TTY: 215-590-8789
www.poisoncontrol.chop.edu

DISTRICT OF COLUMBIA

WASHINGTON, DC

National Capital Poison Center (*)

3201 New Mexico Ave.
Suite 310
Washington, DC 20016
Business: 202-362-3867
Emergency: 800-222-1222
www.poison.org

FLORIDA

JACKSONVILLE

Florida Poison Information Center-Jacksonville (*)
Shands Jacksonville Medical Center

655 West 8th St.
Box C23
Jacksonville, FL 32209
Business: 904-244-4465
Emergency: 800-222-1222
http://fpicjax.org

MIAMI

Florida Poison Information Center-Miami (*)
University of Miami–Department of Pediatrics

P.O. Box 016960
Miami, FL 33101
Business: 305-585-5250
Emergency: 800-222-1222
www.miami.edu/poison-center

TAMPA

Florida Poison Information Center-Tampa (*)
Tampa General Hospital

P.O. Box 1289
Tampa, FL 33601-1289
Business: 813-844-7044
Emergency: 800-222-1222
www.poisoncentertampa.org

GEORGIA

ATLANTA

Georgia Poison Center (*)
Hughes Spalding Children's Hospital, Grady Health System

80 Jesse Hill Jr. Dr., SE
P.O. Box 26066
Atlanta, GA 30303-3050
Business: 404-616-9237
Emergency: 800-222-1222
404-616-9000 (Atlanta)
TDD: 404-616-9287
www.georgiapoisoncenter.org

HAWAII

(DENVER, CO)

Rocky Mountain Poison and Drug Center (*)

777 Bannock St.
Mail Code 0180
Denver CO 80204-4028
Business: 303-739-1100
Emergency: 800-222-1222
www.RMPDC.org

IDAHO

(DENVER, CO)

Rocky Mountain Poison and Drug Center (*)

777 Bannock St.
Mail Code 0180
Denver CO 80204-4028
Business: 303-739-1100
Emergency: 800-222-1222
www.RMPDC.org

ILLINOIS

CHICAGO

Illinois Poison Center (*)

222 South Riverside Plaza
Suite 1900
Chicago, IL 60606
Business: 312-906-6136
Emergency: 800-222-1222
TDD/TTY: 312-906-6185
www.illinoispoisoncenter.org

INDIANA

INDIANAPOLIS

Indiana Poison Control Center (*)
Clarian Health Partners
Methodist Hospital

I-65 at 21st St.
Indianapolis, IN 46206-1367
Business: 317-962-2335
Emergency: 800-222-1222
800-382-9097
317-962-2323 (Indianapolis)
TTY: 317-962-2336
www.clarian.org/poisoncontrol

IOWA

SIOUX CITY

Iowa Statewide Poison Control Center
Iowa Health System and the University of Iowa Hospitals and Clinics

401 Douglas St., Suite 402
Sioux City, IA 51101
Business: 712-279-3710
Emergency: 800-222-1222
712-277-2222 (IA)
www.iowapoison.org

KANSAS

KANSAS CITY

University of Kansas Poison Control Hospital Center

3901 Rainbow Blvd.
Room B400
Kansas City, KS 66160-7231
Business 913-588-6638
Emergency: 800-222-1222
800-332-6633 (KS)
TDD: 866-238-0677
www.kumed.com/poison

KENTUCKY

LOUISVILLE

Kentucky Regional Poison Center (*)
Kosair Children's Hospital

PO Box 35070
Louisville, KY 40232-5070
Business: 502-629-7264
Emergency: 800-222-1222
www.krpc.com

LOUISIANA

MONROE

Louisiana Drug and Poison Information Center (*)
University of Louisiana at Monroe

700 University Ave.
Monroe, LA 71209-6430
Emergency: 800-222-1222

MAINE

PORTLAND

Northern New England Poison Center

Maine Medical Center
22 Bramhall St.
Portland, ME 04102
Business: 207-662-0111
Emergency: 800-222-1222
207-871-2879 (ME)
TDD/TTY: 207-662-4900 (ME)
www.nnepc.org

MARYLAND

BALTIMORE

Maryland Poison Center (*)
University of Maryland at Baltimore
School of Pharmacy

220 Arch St.
Office Level 1
Baltimore, MD 21201
Business: 410-706-7604
Emergency: 800-222-1222
TDD: 410-706-1858
www.mdpoison.com

(WASHINGTON, DC)

National Capital Poison Center (*)

3201 New Mexico Ave.
Suite 310
Washington DC 20016
Business: 202-362-3867
Emergency: 800-222-1222
TDD/TTY: 202-362-8563 (MD)
www.poison.org

MASSACHUSETTS

BOSTON

Regional Center for Poison Control and Prevention (*)
(Serving Massachusetts and Rhode Island)
Children's Hospital Boston

300 Longwood Ave.
Boston, MA 02115
Business: 617-355-6609
Emergency: 800-222-1222
TDD/TTY: 888-244-5313
www.maripoisoncenter.com

MICHIGAN

DETROIT

Regional Poison Control Center (*)
Children's Hospital of Michigan

4160 John R. Harper
Professional Office Bldg.
Suite 616
Detroit, MI 48201
Business: 313-745-5335
Emergency: 800-222-1222
TDD/TTY: 800-356-3232
www.mitoxic.org/pcc

GRAND RAPIDS

DeVos Children's Hospital Regional Poison Center (*)

100 Michigan St., NE
Grand Rapids, MI 49503
Business: 616-391-3690
Emergency: 800-222-1222
http://poisoncenter.devoschildrens.org

MINNESOTA

MINNEAPOLIS

Minnesota Poison Control System (*) Hennepin County Medical Center

701 Park Ave.
Mail Code RL
Minneapolis, MN 55415
Business: 612-873-3144
Emergency: 800-222-1222
www.mnpoison.org

MISSISSIPPI

JACKSON

Mississippi Regional Poison Control Center, University of Mississippi Medical Center

2500 North State St.
Jackson, MS 39216
Business: 601-984-1680
Emergency: 800-222-1222
http://poisoncontrol.umc.edu

MISSOURI

ST. LOUIS

Missouri Regional Poison Center (*) Cardinal Glennon Children's Hospital

7980 Clayton Rd.
Suite 200
St. Louis, MO 63117
Business: 314-772-5200
Emergency: 800-222-1222
TDD/TTY: 314-612-5705
www.cardinalglennon.com

MONTANA

(DENVER, CO)

Rocky Mountain Poison and Drug Center (*)

777 Bannock St.
Mail Code 0180
Denver CO 80204-4028
Business: 303-739-1100
Emergency: 800-222-1222
TDD/TTY: 303-739-1127
www.RMPDC.org

NEBRASKA

OMAHA

The Poison Center (*) Children's Hospital

8401 W. Dodge St., Suite 115
Omaha, NE 68114
Business: 402-955-5555
Emergency: 800-222-1222
www.nebraskapoison.com

NEVADA

(DENVER, CO)

Rocky Mountain Poison and Drug Center (*)

777 Bannock St.
Mail Code 0180
Denver CO 80204-4028
Business: 303-739-1100
Emergency: 800-222-1222
www.RMPDC.org

(PORTLAND, OR)

Oregon Poison Center (*) Oregon Health and Science University

3181 SW Sam Jackson Park Rd.
Portland, OR 97239
Business: 503-494-8600
Emergency: 800-222-1222
www.oregonpoison.com

NEW HAMPSHIRE

(PORTLAND, ME)

Northern New England Poison Center

Maine Medical Center
22 Bramhall St.
Portland, ME 04102
Business: 207-662-0111
Emergency: 800-222-1222
www.nnepc.org

NEW JERSEY

NEWARK

New Jersey Poison Information and Education System (*) UMDNJ

140 Bergen St. Suite G1600
Newark, NJ 07101
Business: 973-972-9280
Emergency: 800-222-1222
TDD/TTY: 973-926-8008
www.njpies.org

NEW MEXICO

ALBUQUERQUE

New Mexico Poison and Drug Information Center (*)

MSC09/5080
1 University of New Mexico
Albuquerque, NM 87131-0001
Business: 505-272-4261
Emergency: 800-222-1222
http://HSC.UNM.edu/pharmacy/poison

NEW YORK

BUFFALO

Western New York Regional Poison Control Center (*) Women and Children's Hospital of Buffalo

219 Bryant St.
Buffalo, NY 14222
Business: 716-878-7654
Emergency: 800-222-1222
www.wnypoison.org

MINEOLA

Long Island Regional Poison and Drug Information Center (*) Winthrop University Hospital

259 First St.
Mineola, NY 11501
Business: 516-663-2650
Emergency: 800-222-1222
TDD: 516-747-3323 (Nassau)
631-924-8811 (Suffolk)
www.lirpdic.org

NEW YORK CITY

New York City Poison Control Center (*) NYC Dept. of Health

455 First Ave., Room 123
New York, NY 10016
Business: 212-447-8152
Emergency: (English) 800-222-1222
212-340-4494
212-POISONS (212-764-7667)

Emergency: (Spanish) 212-VENENOS (212-836-3667)
TDD: 212-689-9014
www.nyc.gov/html/doh/html/poison/poison.shtml

ROCHESTER

Finger Lakes Regional Poison and Drug Information Center (*) University of Rochester Medical Center

601 Elmwood Ave.
Box 321
Rochester, NY 14642
Business: 585-273-4155
Emergency: 800-222-1222
TTY: 585-273-3854
www.fingerlakespoison.org

SYRACUSE

Upstate New York Poison Center (*) SUNY Upstate Medical University

750 East Adams St.
Syracuse, NY 13210
Business: 315-464-7078
Emergency: 800-222-1222
TTY: 315-464-5424
www.upstatepoison.org

NORTH CAROLINA

CHARLOTTE

Carolinas Poison Center (*) Carolinas Medical Center

PO Box 32861
Charlotte, NC 28232-2861
Business: 704-512-3795
Emergency: 800-222-1222
www.ncpoisoncenter.org

NORTH DAKOTA

BISMARK

ND Department of Health Injury Prevention Program North Dakota Poison Center

600 E. Boulevard Ave.
Bismark, ND 58505
Business: 612-873-3144
Emergency: 800-222-1222
www.ndpoison.org

OHIO

CINCINNATI

Cincinnati Drug and Poison Information Center (*) Cincinatti Children's Hospital

3333 Burnet Ave.
Cincinnati, OH 45229
Business: 513-636-5063
Emergency: 800-222-1222
TDD/TTY: 800-253-7955
www.cincinnatichildrens.org/dpic

CLEVELAND

Greater Cleveland Poison Control Center Rainbow Babies and Children's Hospital

11100 Euclid Ave.
MP 6007
Cleveland, OH 44106-6007
Business: 216-844-1573
Emergency: 800-222-1222
www.uhhospitals.org/rainbowchildren/tabid/195/Default.aspx

COLUMBUS

Central Ohio Poison Center (*) Nationwide Children's Hospital

700 Children's Dr.
Columbus, OH 43205-2696
Business: 614-355-0435
Emergency: 800-222-1222
TTY: 614-228-2272
www.bepoisonsmart.com

OKLAHOMA

OKLAHOMA CITY

Oklahoma Poison Control Center (*) College of Pharmacy at OU Medical Center

940 Northeast 13th St.
Room 3N3510
Oklahoma City, OK 73104
Business: 405-271-5062
Emergency: 800-222-1222
www.oklahomapoison.org

OREGON

PORTLAND

**Oregon Poison Center (*)
Oregon Health and Science University**

3181 S.W. Sam Jackson Park Rd.
Portland, OR 97239
Business: 503-494-8600
Emergency: 800-222-1222
www.ohsu.edu/poison

PENNSYLVANIA

PHILADELPHIA

**The Poison Control Center (*)
Children's Hospital of Philadelphia**

34th Street & Civic Center Blvd.
Philadelphia, PA 19104-4399
Business: 215-590-2100
Emergency: 800-222-1222
215-386-2100 (PA)
TDD/TTY: 215-590-8789
www.poisoncontrol.chop.edu

PITTSBURGH

**Pittsburgh Poison Center (*)
Children's Hospital of Pittsburgh**

3705 Fifth Ave.
Pittsburgh, PA 15213
Business: 412-390-3300
Emergency: 800-222-1222
412-681-6669
www.chp.edu/clinical/03a_poison.php

RHODE ISLAND

(BOSTON, MA)

**Regional Center for Poison Control and Prevention (*)
Children's Hospital Boston**
(Serving Massachusetts and Rhode Island)

300 Longwood Ave., IC Smith Bldg
Boston, MA 02115
Business: 617-355-6609
Emergency: 800-222-1222
TDD/TTY: 888-244-5313
www.maripoisoncenter.com

SOUTH DAKOTA

(MINNEAPOLIS, MN)

Hennepin Regional Poison Center (*) Hennepin County Medical Center

701 Park Ave., Mail Code RL
Minneapolis, MN 55415
Business: 612-873-3144
Emergency: 800-222-1222
www.mnpoison.org

SIOUX FALLS

**Sanford Poison Center (*)
USD Medical Center**

1305 W. 18th St.
Box 5039
Sioux Falls, SD 57117-5039
Business: 605-328-6670
Emergency: 800-222-1222
www.sdpoison.org

TENNESSEE

NASHVILLE

Tennessee Poison Center (*)

1161 21st Ave. South
501 Oxford House
Nashville, TN 37232-4632
Business: 615-936-0760
Emergency: 800-222-1222
www.poisonlifeline.org

TEXAS

AMARILLO

**Texas Panhandle Poison Center (*)
Texas Tech University Health Sciences Center**

1501 S. Coulter Dr.
Amarillo, TX 79106
Business: 806-354-1630
Emergency: 800-222-1222
www.poisoncontrol.org

DALLAS

**North Texas Poison Center (*)
Texas Poison Center Network
Parkland Health and Hospital System**

5201 Harry Hines Blvd.
Dallas, TX 75235
Business: 214-589-0911
Emergency: 800-222-1222
www.poisoncontrol.org

EL PASO

**West Texas Regional Poison Center (*)
Thomason Hospital**

4815 Alameda Ave.
El Paso, TX 79905
Business 915-534-3800
Emergency: 800-222-1222
www.poisoncontrol.org

GALVESTON

**Southeast Texas Poison Center (*)
The University of Texas Medical Branch**

301 University Blvd.
Galveston, TX 77555-1175
Business: 409-772-9142
Emergency: 800-222-1222
www.poisoncontrol.org

SAN ANTONIO

**South Texas Poison Center (*)
The University of Texas Health Science Center–San Antonio**

7703 Floyd Curl Dr., MSC 7849
San Antonio, TX 78229-3900
Business: 210-567-5762
Emergency: 800-222-1222
www.poisoncontrol.org

TEMPLE

**Central Texas Poison Center (*)
Scott & White Memorial Hospital**

2401 South 31st St.
Temple, TX 76508
Business: 254-724-7401
Emergency: 800-222-1222
www.poisoncontrol.org

UTAH

SALT LAKE CITY

**Utah Poison Control Center (*)
University of Utah**

585 Komas Dr.
Salt Lake City, UT 84108
Business: 801-587-0600
Emergency: 800-222-1222
http://uuhsc.utah.edu/poison

VERMONT

(PORTLAND, ME)

Northern New England Poison Center

Maine Medical Center
22 Bramhall St.
Portland, ME 04102
Business: 207-662-0111
Emergency: 800-222-1222
www.nnepc.org

VIRGINIA

CHARLOTTESVILLE

**Blue Ridge Poison Center (*)
University of Virginia Health System**

PO Box 800774
Charlottesville, VA 22908-0774
Business: 434-924-0347
Emergency: 800-222-1222
www.healthsystem.virginia.edu/brpc

RICHMOND

**Virginia Poison Center (*)
Virginia Commonwealth University Medical Center**

600 E. Broad St. Suite 640
P.O. Box 980522
Richmond, VA 23298-0522
Business: 804-828-4780
Emergency: 800-222-1222
804-828-9123
www.poison.vcu.edu

WASHINGTON

SEATTLE

Washington Poison Center (*)

155 NE 100th St.
Seattle, WA 98125-8007
Business: 206-517-2359
Emergency: 800-222-1222
www.wapc.org

WEST VIRGINIA

CHARLESTON

**West Virginia Poison Center (*)
WVU Charleston Division**

3110 MacCorkle Ave. SE
Charleston, WV 25304
Business: 304-347-1212
Emergency: 800-222-1222
www.wvpoisoncenter.org

WISCONSIN

MILWAUKEE

Wisconsin Poison Center

Suite CC 660
P.O. Box 1997
Milwaukee, WI 53201
Business: 414-266-2952
Emergency: 800-222-1222
TDD/TTY: 414-266-2542
www.wisconsinpoison.org

WYOMING

(OMAHA, NE)

**The Poison Center (*)
Children's Hospital**

8401 W. Dodge St., Suite 115
Omaha, NE 68114
Business: 402-955-5555
Emergency: 800-222-1222
www.nebraskapoison.com

DRUG INFORMATION CENTERS

ALABAMA

BIRMINGHAM

Drug Information Service
University of Alabama
UAB Hospital Pharmacy
Drug Information-JT1720
619 S. 19th St.
Birmingham, AL 35249-6860
Mon.-Fri. 7 AM-4 PM
205-934-2162
www.health.uab.edu/pharmacy

Global Drug Information Service
Samford University
McWhorter School of Pharmacy
800 Lakeshore Dr.
Birmingham, AL 35229-7027
Mon. 8 AM-9 PM
Tues.-Fri. 8 AM-4:30 PM
205-726-2519 or 2891
www.samford.edu/schools/pharmacy/dic/index.html

HUNTSVILLE

Huntsville Hospital Drug Information Center
101 Sivley Rd.
Huntsville, AL 35801
Mon.-Fri. 8 AM-4:30 PM
256-265-8284

ARIZONA

TUCSON

Arizona Poison and Drug Information Center
1259 N. Martin Ave.
Drachman Hall B308
Tucson, AZ 85724
7 days/week, 24 hours
520-626-6016
800-222-1222 (**Emergency**)
www.pharmacy.arizona.edu

ARKANSAS

LITTLE ROCK

Arkansas Drug Information Center
4301 W. Markham St.
Slot 522-2
Little Rock, AR 72205
Mon.-Fri. 8:30 AM-5 PM
501-686-6161
(Little Rock area only - **for healthcare professionals only**)
888-228-1233
(AR only - **for healthcare professionals only**)

CALIFORNIA

LOS ANGELES

Los Angeles Regional Drug Information Center
LAC & USC Medical Center
1200 N. State St.
Trailer 25
Los Angeles, CA 90033
Mon.-Fri. 8 AM-4 PM
Closed 12 PM to 1 PM
323-226-7741

SAN DIEGO

Drug Information Service
University of California San Diego Medical Center
200 West Arbor Dr.
MC 8925
San Diego, CA 92103-8925
Mon.-Fri. 9 AM-5 PM
619-543-6971
(**for healthcare professionals only**)

STANFORD

Drug Information Center
University of California
Stanford Hospital and Clinics
300 Pasteur Dr.
Room H-0301
Stanford, CA 94305
Mon.-Fri. 8 AM-4 PM
650-723-6422

COLORADO

DENVER

Rocky Mountain Poison and Drug Center
990 Bannock St.
(Physical address)
777 Bannock St.
(Mailing address)
Denver, CO 80264
303-739-1100
800-222-1222 (**Emergency**)
www.rmpdc.org

CONNECTICUT

HARTFORD

Drug Information Center
Hartford Hospital
P.O. Box 5037
80 Seymour St.
Hartford, CT 06102
Mon.-Fri. 8:30 AM-5 PM
860-545-2221
860-545-2961(After 5 PM)
www.hartfordhospital.org

NEW HAVEN

Drug Information Center
Yale-New Haven Hospital
20 York St.
New Haven, CT 06540-3202
Mon.-Fri. 9 AM-5 PM
203-688-2248
www.ynhh.org/patients/pharmacy.html

DISTRICT OF COLUMBIA

Drug Information Service
Howard University Hospital
Room BB06
2041 Georgia Ave. NW
Washington, DC 20060
Mon.-Fri. 8:30 AM-4 PM
202-865-7413

FLORIDA

FT. LAUDERDALE

Nova Southeastern University College of Pharmacy
Drug Information Center
3200 S. University Dr.
Ft. Lauderdale, FL 33328
Mon.-Fri. 9 AM-5 PM
954-262-3103
http://pharmacy.nova.edu

GAINESVILLE

Drug Information & Pharmacy Resource Center
Shands Hospital at University of Florida
1600 SW Archer Rd.
Gainesville, FL 32610-0316
Mon.-Fri. 9 AM-5 PM
352-265-0408
(**for healthcare professionals only**)
http://shands.org/professional/druginfo

JACKSONVILLE

Drug Information Service
Shands Jacksonville
655 W. 8th St.
Jacksonville, FL 32209
Mon.-Fri. 8:30 AM-5 PM
904-244-4185
(**for healthcare professionals only**)
904-244-4700
(**for consumers, Mon.-Fri. 9:30 AM-4 PM**)
http://jax.shands.org/education/pharmacy/contact.asp

ORLANDO

Orlando Regional Drug Information Service
Orlando Regional Healthcare System
1414 Kuhl Ave., MP 192
Orlando, FL 32806
Mon.-Fri. 8 AM-4 PM
321-841-8715

TALLAHASSEE

Drug Information Education Center
Florida Agricultural and Mechanical University
College of Pharmacy and Pharmaceutical Sciences
Tallahassee, FL 32307
Mon.-Fri. 9 AM-5 PM
850-599-3064

WEST PALM BEACH

Drug Information Center
Nova Southeastern University, West Palm Beach
3970 RCA Blvd., Suite 7006A
Palm Beach Gardens, FL 33410
Mon.-Fri. 9 AM-5 PM
561-622-8682, ext 5655
(**for healthcare professionals only**)

GEORGIA

ATLANTA

Emory University Hospital
Dept. of Pharmaceutical Services-Drug Information
1364 Clifton Rd. NE
Atlanta, GA 30322
Mon.-Fri. 9 AM-4 PM
404-712-4644
(**for healthcare professionals only**)

Drug Information Service
Northside Hospital
1000 Johnson Ferry Rd. NE
Atlanta, GA 30342
Mon.-Fri. 9 AM-4 PM
404-851-8676 (GA only)

COLUMBUS

Columbus Regional Drug Information Center
710 Center St.
Columbus, GA 31902
Mon.-Fri. 8 AM-4:30 PM
706-571-1934
(**for healthcare professionals only**)

IDAHO

POCATELLO

Idaho Drug Information Service
Idaho State University
College of Pharmacy
970 S. 5th Ave.
Campus Box 8092
Pocatello, ID 83209
Mon.-Thur. 8:30 AM-5 PM
Fri. 8:30 AM-3 PM
208-282-4689
800-334-7139 (ID only)
http://pharmacy.isu.edu

ILLINOIS

CHICAGO

Drug Information Center
Northwestern Memorial Hospital
Feinberg Pavilion, LC 700
251 E. Huron St.
Chicago, IL 60611
Mon.-Fri. 8:30 AM-5 PM
312-926-7573

Drug Information Center
University of Illinois at Chicago
833 S. Wood St.
MC 886
Chicago, IL 60612-7231
Mon.-Fri. 8 AM-4 PM
312-996-3681
(for healthcare professionals only)
312-996-5332
(for consumers, Mon.-Fri. 9 AM-12 PM)
www.uic.edu/pharmacy

HARVEY

Drug Information Center
Ingalls Memorial Hospital
1 Ingalls Dr.
Harvey, IL 60426
Mon.-Fri. 8 AM-7 PM
Sat. 9 AM-3:30 PM
708-915-4300

HINES

Drug Information Service
Hines Veterans Administration Hospital
Pharmacy Services
MC119
P.O. Box 5000
Hines, IL 60141-5000
Mon.-Fri. 8 AM-4:30 PM
708-202-2573

PARK RIDGE

Drug Information Center
Advocate Lutheran General Hospital
1775 Dempster St.
Park Ridge, IL 60068
Mon.-Fri. 7:30 AM-4 PM
847-723-8128
(for healthcare professionals only)

INDIANA

INDIANAPOLIS

Drug Information Center
St. Vincent Hospital and Health Services
2001 W. 86th St.
Indianapolis, IN 46260
Mon.-Fri. 8 AM-4 PM
317-338-3200
(for healthcare professionals only)

Drug Information Service
Clarian Health Partners
Pharmacy Department I-65 at 21st St.
Room CG04
Indianapolis, IN 46202
Mon.-Fri. 8 AM-4:30 PM
317-962-1750

MUNCIE

Drug Information Center
Ball Memorial Hospital
2401 University Ave.
Muncie, IN 47303
Mon.-Fri. 8 AM-4:30 PM
765-747-3033

IOWA

DES MOINES

Regional Drug Information Center
Mercy Medical Center-Des Moines
1111 Sixth Ave.
Des Moines, IA 50314
Mon.-Fri. 8 AM-4:30 PM
(regional service; in-house service answered 7 days/ week, 24 hours)
515-247-3286

IOWA CITY

Drug Information Center
University of Iowa Hospitals and Clinics
200 Hawkins Dr.
Iowa City, IA 52242
Mon.-Fri. 8 AM-4:30 PM
319-356-2600

KANSAS

KANSAS CITY

Drug Information Center
University of Kansas Medical Center
3901 Rainbow Blvd.
Kansas City, KS 66160
Mon.-Fri. 8:30 AM-4:30 PM
913-588-2328

KENTUCKY

LEXINGTON

University of Kentucky
Central Pharmacy
Chandler Medical Center
800 Rose St., C-114
Lexington, KY 40536-0293
7 days/week, 24 hours
859-323-5642
859-323-6289

LOUISIANA

MONROE

Louisiana Drug and Poison Information Center
University of Louisiana at Monroe College of Pharmacy
Sugar Hall
Monroe, LA 71209-6430
Mon.-Thur. 8 AM-4:30 PM
Fri. 8 AM-11:30 AM
318-342-1710

NEW ORLEANS

Xavier University Drug Information Center
Tulane University Hospital and Clinic
1440 Canal St.
Suite 808
New Orleans, LA 70112
Mon.-Fri. 9 AM-5 PM
504-588-5670

MARYLAND

ANDREWS AFB

Drug Information Services
79 MDSS/SGQP
1050 W. Perimeter Rd.
Suite D1-119
Andrews AFB, MD 20762-6660
Mon.-Fri. 7:30 AM-5 PM
240-857-4565

BALTIMORE

Drug Information Service
Johns Hopkins Hospital
600 N. Wolfe St.
Carnegie 180
Baltimore, MD 21287-6180
Mon.-Fri. 8:30 AM-5 PM
410-955-6348
www.hopkinsmedicine.org/pharmacy

Drug Information Service
University of Maryland
School of Pharmacy Pharmacy Hall Room 760
20 North Pine St.
Baltimore, MD 21201
Mon.-Fri. 8:30 AM-5 PM
410-706-7568
(consumers only)
410-706-0898
(for healthcare professionals only)
www.pharmacy.umaryland.edu/umdi

EASTON

Drug Information
Pharmacy Dept.
Memorial Hospital
219 S. Washington St.
Easton, MD 21601
7 days/week, 7 AM-5:30 PM
410-822-1000, ext. 5645

MASSACHUSETTS

BOSTON

Drug Information Services
Brigham and Women's Hospital
75 Francis St.
Boston, MA 02115
Mon.-Fri. 7 AM-3 PM
617-732-5500, ext. 33696

WORCESTER

Drug Information Pharmacy
UMass Memorial Medical Center
Healthcare Hospital
55 Lake Ave. North
Worcester, MA 01655
Mon.-Fri. 8:30 AM-5 PM
508-856-3456
508-856-2775 (24-hour)

MICHIGAN

ANN ARBOR

Drug Information Service
Dept. of Pharmacy Services
University of Michigan Health System
1500 East Medical Center Dr.
UH B2D301
Box 0008
Ann Arbor, MI 48109-0008
Mon.-Fri. 8 AM-5 PM
734-936-8200

DETROIT

Drug Information Center
Department of Pharmacy Services
Detroit Receiving Hospital and University Health Center
4201 St. Antoine Blvd.
Detroit, MI 48201
Mon.-Fri. 9 AM-5 PM
313-745-4556
www.dmcpharmacy.org

LANSING

Drug Information Services
Sparrow Hospital
1215 East Michigan Ave.
Lansing, MI 48912
7 days/week, 24 hours
517-364-2444
www.sparrow.org

ROYAL OAK

Drug Information Services
William Beaumont Hospital
3601 West 13 Mile Rd.
Royal Oak, MI 48073-6769
Mon.-Fri. 8 AM-4:30 PM
248-898-4077

SOUTHFIELD

Drug Information Service
Providence Hospital
16001 West 9 Mile Rd.
Southfield, MI 48075
Mon.-Fri. 8 AM-4 PM
248-849-3125

MISSISSIPPI

JACKSON

Drug Information Center
University of Mississippi Medical Center
2500 N. State St.
Jackson, MS 39216
Mon.-Fri. 8 AM-4:30 PM
601-984-2060

MISSOURI

KANSAS CITY

University of Missouri-Kansas City
Drug Information Center
2464 Charlotte St., Suite 1220
Kansas City, MO 64108
Mon.-Fri. 9 AM-4 PM
816-235-5490

SPRINGFIELD

Drug Information Center
St. John's Hospital
1235 E. Cherokee St.
Springfield, MO 65804
Mon.-Fri. 8 AM-4:30 PM
417-820-3488

ST. JOSEPH

Regional Medical Center Pharmacy
5325 Faraon St.
St. Joseph, MO 64506
7 days/week, 24 hours
816-271-6141

MONTANA

MISSOULA

Drug Information Service
University of Montana School of Pharmacy and Allied Health Sciences
32 Campus Dr.
1522 Skaggs Bldg.
Missoula, MT 59812-1522
Mon.-Fri. 8 AM-5 PM
406-243-5254
800-501-5491
www.health.umt.edu/dis

NEBRASKA

OMAHA

Drug Informatics Service
School of Pharmacy
Creighton University
2500 California Plaza
Health Science Library
Room 204
Omaha, NE 68178
Mon.-Fri. 8:30 AM-4:30 PM
402-280-5101
http://druginfo.creighton.edu

NEW JERSEY

NEWARK

New Jersey Poison Information and Education System
140 Bergen St.
Newark, NJ 07107
Mon.-Fri. 8 AM- 5 PM
973-972-9280
800-222-1222 (**Emergency**)
www.njpies.org

NEW BRUNSWICK

Drug Information Service
Robert Wood Johnson University Hospital
Pharmacy Department
1 Robert Wood Johnson Pl.
New Brunswick, NJ 08901
Mon.-Fri. 8:30 AM-4:30 PM
732-937-8842

NEW MEXICO

ALBUQUERQUE

New Mexico Poison Center
University of New Mexico Health Sciences Center
MSC09 5080
1 University of New Mexico
Albuquerque, NM 87131
7 days/week, 24 hours
505-272-4261
800-222-1222 (**Emergency**)
http://hsc.unm.edu/pharmacy/poison

NEW YORK

BROOKLYN

International Drug Information Center
Long Island University
Arnold & Marie Schwartz College of Pharmacy & Health Sciences
75 DeKalb Ave.
RM-HS509
Brooklyn, NY 11201
Mon.-Fri. 9 AM-5 PM
718-488-1064
www.liu.edu

NEW HYDE PARK

Drug Information Center
St. John's University at Long Island Jewish Medical Center
270-05 76th Ave.
New Hyde Park, NY 11040
Mon.-Fri. 8 AM-3 PM
718-470-DRUG (3784)

NEW YORK CITY

Drug Information Center
Memorial Sloan-Kettering Cancer Center
1275 York Ave.
RM S-702
New York, NY 10021
Mon.-Fri. 9 AM-5 PM
212-639-7552

Drug Information Center
Mount Sinai Medical Center
1 Gustave Levy Pl.
New York, NY 10029
Mon.-Fri. 9 AM-5 PM
212-241-6619
(**for in-house healthcare professionals only**)

ROCHESTER

Finger Lakes Poison and Drug Information Center
University of Rochester
601 Elmwood Ave.
Rochester, NY 14642
Mon.-Fri. 8 AM-5 PM
585-275-3718
www.fingerlakespoison.org

NORTH CAROLINA

BUIES CREEK

Drug Information Center
School of Pharmacy
Campbell University
P.O. Box 1090
Buies Creek, NC 27506
Mon.-Fri. 8:30 AM-5:00 PM
910-893-1200, ext. 2701
800-760-9697, ext. 2701
800-327-5467 (NC only)
www.campbellpharmacy.net/resources/drug_info_center.html

CHAPEL HILL

University of North Carolina Hospitals
Drug Information Center
Dept. of Pharmacy
101 Manning Dr.
Chapel Hill, NC 27514
Mon.-Fri. 8 AM-4:30 PM
919-966-2373

DURHAM

Drug Information Center
Duke University Health Systems
DUMC Box 3089
Durham, NC 27710
Mon.-Fri. 8 AM-5 PM
919-684-5125

GREENVILLE

Eastern Carolina Drug Information Center
Pitt County Memorial Hospital
Dept. of Pharmacy Service
P.O. Box 6028
2100 Stantonsburg Rd.
Greenville, NC 27835
Mon.-Fri. 8 AM-5 PM
252-847-4257

WINSTON-SALEM

Drug Information Service Center
Wake-Forest University Baptist Medical Center
Medical Center Blvd.
Winston-Salem, NC 27157
Mon.-Fri. 8 AM-5 PM
336-716-2037
(**for healthcare professionals only**)

OHIO

ADA

Drug Information Center
Raabe College of Pharmacy
Ohio Northern University
Ada, OH 45810
Mon.-Thurs. 8:30 AM-5 PM
Fri. 8:30 AM-4 PM
419-772-2307
www.onu.edu/pharmacy/druginfo

CINCINNATI

Drug and Poison Information Center
Children's Hospital Medical Center
3333 Burnet Ave.
Cincinnati, OH 45229
Mon.-Fri. 9 AM-5 PM
513-636-5063 (Administration)
513-636-5111 (7 days/week, 24 hours)

CLEVELAND

Drug Information Service
Cleveland Clinic Foundation
9500 Euclid Ave.
Cleveland, OH 44195
Mon.-Fri. 8:30 AM-4:30 PM
216-444-6456
(for healthcare professionals only)

COLUMBUS

Drug Information Center
Ohio State University Hospital
Dept. of Pharmacy
Doan Hall 368
410 W. 10th Ave.
Columbus, OH 43210-1228
Mon.-Fri. 8 AM-4:30 PM
614-293-8679
(for in-house healthcare professionals only)

Drug Information Center
Riverside Methodist Hospital
3535 Olentangy River Road
Columbus, OH 43214
7 days/week, 24 hours
614-566-5425

TOLEDO

Drug Information Services
St. Vincent Mercy Medical Center
2213 Cherry St.
Toledo, Ohio 43608-2691
Mon.-Fri. 7 AM-5 PM
419-251-4227
www.rx.medctr.ohio-state.edu

OKLAHOMA

OKLAHOMA CITY

Drug Information Service
Integris Health
3300 Northwest Expressway
Oklahoma City, OK 73112
Mon.-Fri. 8 AM-4:30 PM
405-949-3660

Drug Information Center
OU Medical Center
1200 Everett Dr.
Oklahoma City, OK 73104
Mon.-Fri. 8 AM-4:30 PM
405-271-6226
Fax: 405-271-6281

TULSA

Drug Information Center
Saint Francis Hospital
6161 S. Yale Ave.
Tulsa, OK 74136
Mon.-Fri. 8 AM-4:30 PM
918-494-6339
(for healthcare professionals only)

PENNSYLVANIA

PHILADELPHIA

Drug Information Center
Temple University Hospital
Dept. of Pharmacy
3401 N. Broad St.
Philadelphia, PA 19140
Mon.-Fri. 8 AM-4:30 PM
215-707-4644

Drug Information Service
Dept. of Pharmacy
Thomas Jefferson University Hospital
111 S. 11th St.
Philadelphia, PA 19107-5089
Mon.-Fri. 8 AM-5 PM
215-955-8877

University of Pennsylvania Health System Drug Information Service
Hospital of the University of Pennsylvania
Department of Pharmacy
3400 Spruce St.
Philadelphia, PA 19104
Mon.-Fri. 8:30 AM-4 PM
215-662-2903

PITTSBURGH

Pharmaceutical Information Center
Mylan School of Pharmacy
Duquesne University
431 Mellon Hall
Pittsburgh, PA 15282
Mon.-Fri. 8 AM-4 PM
412-396-4600

UPLAND

Drug Information Center
Crozer-Chester Medical Center
Dept. of Pharmacy
1 Medical Center Blvd.
Upland, PA 19013
Mon.-Fri. 8 AM-4:30 PM
610-447-2851
(for in-house healthcare professionals only)

PUERTO RICO

SAN JUAN

Centro de Informacion de Medicamentos-CIM
Escuela de Farmacia-RCM
P.O. Box 365067
San Juan, PR 00936-5067
Mon.-Fri. 8 AM-4:30 PM
787-758-2525, ext. 1516

SOUTH CAROLINA

CHARLESTON

Drug Information Service
Medical University of South Carolina
150 Ashley Ave.
Rutledge Tower Annex
Room 604
P.O. Box 250584
Charleston, SC 29425-0810
Mon.-Fri. 9 AM-5:30 PM
843-792-3896
800-922-5250

SPARTANBURG

Drug Information Center
Spartanburg Regional Healthcare System
101 E. Wood St.
Spartanburg, SC 29303
Mon.-Fri. 8 AM-4:30 PM
864-560-6910

TENNESSEE

KNOXVILLE

Drug Information Center
University of Tennessee Medical Center at Knoxville
1924 Alcoa Highway
Knoxville, TN 37920-6999
Mon.-Fri. 8 AM-4:30 PM
865-544-9124

MEMPHIS

South East Regional Drug Information Center
VA Medical Center
1030 Jefferson Ave.
Memphis, TN 38104
Mon.-Fri. 6:30 AM-4 PM
901-523-8990, ext. 6720

Drug Information Center
University of Tennessee
875 Monroe Ave.
Suite 109
Memphis, TN 38163
Mon.-Fri. 8 AM-5 PM
901-448-5556

TEXAS

AMARILLO

Drug Information Center
Texas Tech Health Sciences Center
School of Pharmacy
1300 Coulter Rd.
Amarillo, TX 79106
Mon.-Fri. 8 AM-5 PM
806-356-4008

GALVESTON

Drug Information Center
University of Texas Medical Branch
301 University Blvd.
Galveston, TX 77555-0701
Mon.-Fri. 8 AM-5 PM
409-772-2734

HOUSTON

Drug Information Center
Ben Taub General Hospital
Texas Southern University/HCHD
1504 Taub Loop
Houston, TX 77030
Mon.-Fri. 8:30 AM-5 PM
713-873-3710

LACKLAND A.F.B.

Drug Information Center
Dept. of Pharmacy
Wilford Hall Medical Center
2200 Bergquist Dr.
Suite 1
Lackland A.F.B., TX 78236
7 days/week, 24 hours
210-292-5414

LUBBOCK

Drug Information and Consultation Service
Covenant Medical Center
3615 19th St.
Lubbock, TX 79410
7 days/week, 24 hours
806-725-0408

SAN ANTONIO

Drug Information Service
University of Texas Health Science Center at San Antonio
Department of Pharmacology
7703 Floyd Curl Drive
San Antonio, TX 78229-3900
Mon.-Fri. 8 AM-4 PM
210-567-4280

TEMPLE

Drug Information Center
Scott and White Memorial Hospital
2401 S. 31st St.
Temple, TX 76508
Mon.-Fri. 8 AM-5 PM
254-724-4636

UTAH

SALT LAKE CITY

Drug Information Service
University of Utah Hospital
421 Wakara Way
Suite 204
Salt Lake City, UT 84108
Mon.-Fri. 7:30 AM-5 PM
801-581-2073

VIRGINIA

HAMPTON

Drug Information Center
Hampton University School of Pharmacy
Hampton Harbors Annex
Hampton, VA 23668
Mon.-Fri. 9 AM-4 PM
757-728-6693

WEST VIRGINIA

MORGANTOWN

West Virginia Center for Drug and Health Information
West Virginia University
Robert C. Byrd Health Sciences Center
1124 HSN, P.O. Box 9520
Morgantown, WV 26506
Mon.-Fri. 8:30 AM-5 PM
304-293-6640
800-352-2501 (WV)
www.hsc.wvu.edu/SOP

WYOMING

LARAMIE

Drug Information Center
University of Wyoming
1000 East University Ave.
Dept 3375
Laramie, WY 82071
Mon.-Fri. 8:30 AM-4:30 PM
307-766-6988